GREENE'S
INFECTIOUS DISEASES OF THE DOG AND CAT

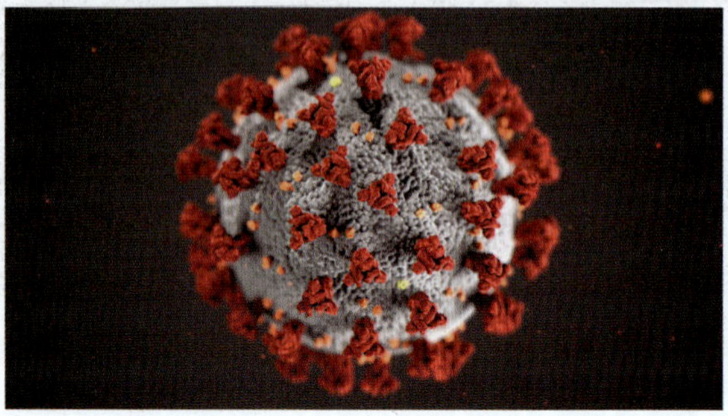

Photo credit: Alissa Eckert, MSMI; Dan Higgins, MAMS

GREENE'S INFECTIOUS DISEASES OF THE DOG AND CAT

Fifth Edition

Editor

Jane E. Sykes, BVSc (Hons) PhD MBA DACVIM
Professor,
Department of Medicine and Epidemiology,
University of California, Davis,
Davis, CA, USA

Section Editors

Shelley C. Rankin, BSc (Hons) PhD
Professor Emeritus of Microbiology,
University of Pennsylvania,
School of Veterinary Medicine,
Philadelphia, PA, USA;
Global Director of Microbiology and Molecular Diagnostics,
Zoetis Reference Laboratories, Zoetis,
Parsippany, NJ, USA

Mark G. Papich, DVM MS DACVCP
Professor of Clinical Pharmacology,
Burroughs Wellcome Fund Professor in Veterinary Pharmacology,
College of Veterinary Medicine,
North Carolina State University,
Raleigh, NC, USA

J. Scott Weese, DVM DVSc DACVIM FCAHS
Professor, Ontario Veterinary College,
Director, Centre for Public Health and Zoonoses,
University of Guelph,
Guelph, ON, Canada

Susan E. Little, DVM PhD DACVM
Regents Professor and
Krull-Ewing Professor of Veterinary Parasitology,
Center for Veterinary Health Sciences,
Oklahoma State University,
Stillwater, OK, USA

ELSEVIER

London New York Oxford Philadelphia St Louis Sydney 2023

Elsevier
3251 Riverport Lane
St. Louis, Missouri 63043

GREENE'S INFECTIOUS DISEASES OF THE DOG AND CAT, FIFTH EDITION ISBN: 978-0-323-50934-3

Previous editions copyrighted 2012, 2004, 2001, and 1996.

Library of Congress Control Number: 2021937118

Content Strategist: Jennifer Catando
Content Development Specialist: Joanne Scott/Meghan Andress
Project Manager: Julie Taylor
Design: Patrick C. Ferguson
Illustration Manager: Narayanan Ramakrishnan

Printed in India

Last digit is the print number: 9 8 7 6 5 4 3 2 1

CONTENTS

SECTION 3 Fungal Diseases

Jane E. Sykes

SECTION 4 Protozoal Diseases

Jane E. Sykes

SECTION 5 Metazoan Parasites and Parasitic Diseases

Susan E. Little

SECTION 6 Infectious Diseases of Body Systems and Clinical Problems

Jane E. Sykes

PREFACE

With a global zoonotic coronavirus pandemic which at the time of writing has infected over 480 million people and contributed to the death of over 6 million people worldwide, a knowledge of infectious diseases of companion animals has never been more important. To highlight this, the cover of this book features the iconic coronavirus virion as depicted by the Center for Disease Control and Prevention's medical illustrators, Dan Higgins and Alissa Eckhert.[1] In 2017-2018, the U.S. Pet Ownership & Demographics Sourcebook reported that there are 76.8 million owned dogs and 58.4 million owned cats in the United States, and that 38.4% of households own at least one dog and 25.4% own at least one cat,[2] so exposure of dogs and cats to a virus which is infecting up to 1 in 5 people tested in some parts of the United States[3] is significant. Many of the authors of this book have been called upon by governing bodies to consult on SARS-CoV-2 infections in dogs and cats, or by media outlets to inform the public about the risks of transmission of this virus to animals and back to their owners.

Every chapter in this fifth edition of *Greene's Infectious Diseases of the Dog and Cat* has received a major overhaul to ensure that the information provided is current, clinically relevant, and organized logically to help the reader find needed information. Illustrations and photographs have been updated, and the start of each chapter features a series of Key Points. Detailed information on the public health significance of each infection is provided, including information on related human conditions to inform not only those in the veterinary profession who are seeking to understand zoonotic potential, but also those in the human medical field who might be reading this book with interest in the veterinary perspective. Commenting on his coronavirus illustration, Higgins noted, "this virus, often referred to as invisible, suddenly has a face and is brought to life".[1] Thanks to the work of illustrators like Ted Huff and Kip Carter, I hope that the information and illustrations in this book do the same for all of the pathogens described.

In Part I, Section 1 focuses on diagnostic testing and epidemiological concepts. Information on antimicrobial pharmacology, including tables with drug doses, is located in Section 2. Principles of hospital infection control, now foremost in the operation of many veterinary clinics worldwide as a result of the pandemic, are detailed in Section 3, and specific pathogens and clinical syndromes are located in Part II. For the first time, the book contains a section on helminth and ectoparasite diseases. Inclusion of this section led to some angst over the book's title, as the definition of infection according to *Dorland's Medical Dictionary* is: "the invasion and multiplication of microorganisms in body tissues, which may be clinically inapparent or result in local cellular injury because of competitive metabolism, toxins, intracellular replication or antigen-antibody response."[4] As pointed out to me by one of the contributors to this book and a dear friend who seeks to ensure that my grammar and terminology are correct, non-protozoal parasites are not strictly microorganisms. In addition, some argue that while these parasites reproduce, they do not multiply in the host, so the term "infestation" is more appropriate. By another definition, infestation implies ectoparasitism, where the parasite is located externally to the host. Perhaps the title of this book should be "Infectious Diseases and Infestations of the Dog and Cat". Nevertheless, the term "infection" is widely used in both veterinary and human parasitology texts and so to avoid sounding awkward, that convention has been maintained.

I would like to acknowledge Dr. Craig Greene, Professor Emeritus at the University of Georgia, for his mentorship and inspiring me to pursue a career in clinical infectious diseases of dogs and cats. It was the early editions of this book which introduced me to the field, and I hope this edition will inspire more veterinarians who are beginning their careers. Much of the text in this edition builds upon Craig Greene's previous contributions, which are so significant they cannot even be quantified. Other mentors whose enthusiasm for infectious diseases, internal medicine and scientific writing has been a source of encouragement are Glenn Browning, Jane Armstrong, Peter Irwin, Robert Hardy, Richard Nelson, Edward Breitschwerdt, and Michael Lappin.

I would like to thank the Section Editors for their valuable input, all of the chapter contributors who made this book possible, and the team at Elsevier. Many friends and colleagues at the University of California-Davis, other veterinary academic and private practices, as well as those in industry have provided motivation and humor, even during challenging times (including bilateral broken wrists!). I would particularly like to acknowledge my family and pets here in the United States and in Australia, my running friends, the VMTH leadership team and colleagues in the medicine service, my MBA colleagues in Atlanta, and Missy Beall, Chandra Chandrashekar, Stuart Cohen, Jonathan "JD" Dear, Andrea Fascetti, Dennis Horter, Frédéric and Kristin Jacob, Christian Leutenegger, Richard Malik, Lindsay Merkel, Zach Mills, Nicole Nosek, Krystle Reagan, and George "GR" Thompson.

Jane E. Sykes BVSc (Hons) PhD MBA
DACVIM (Small Animal Internal Medicine)

1. De Zeen. https://www.dezeen.com/2020/05/14/covid-19-images-coronavirus-cdc-medical-illustrator-dan-higgins/.
2. American Veterinary Medical Association. U.S. Pet Ownership Statistics. 2020. https://www.avma.org/resources-tools/reports-statistics/us-pet-ownership-statistics.
3. Los Angeles Times. 1 in 5 coronavirus tests are positive in L.A. county, pointing to tough weeks ahead. 2021. https://www.latimes.com/california/story/2021-01-07/1-in-5-la-covid-tests-positive-surge.
4. Infection. *Dorland's Medical Dictionary*. 26th ed. Philadelphia: WB Saunders; 1985:664.

To the thousands of beloved dogs and cats of those who have lost their lives in the coronavirus pandemic.

ACKNOWLEDGMENTS

On behalf of all of the contributors to this text, the editor would like to acknowledge the significant contributions that the individuals below made to one or more chapters in the fourth edition of *Infectious Diseases of the Dog and Cat* (ed. Greene CE) and the first edition of *Canine and Feline Infectious Diseases* (ed. Sykes JE), which were used as the basis for many of the chapters in this edition by new authors. In particular, I would like to highlight the colossal editorial and authorship contributions of Craig E. Greene to all of the chapters in previous editions of this book.

Addie, Diane D.
Alvarez, Xavier
Baldwin, Claudia J.
Barr, Stephen C.
Barsanti, Jeanne A.
Bennett, D.
Bjöersdorff, Anneli
Boothe, Dawn M.
Bowen, Richard
Breitschwerdt, Edward B.
Bressler, Barrak M.
Brömel, Catharina
Calpin, Janet P.
Calvert, Clay A.
Carmichael, Leland E.
Center, Sharon A.
Clercx, Cecile
Cocayne, Christine G.
Cohn, Leah D.
Cramer, Sarah D.
Dawson, Susan
Day, Michael J.
DeBoer, Douglas J.
Decaro, Nicola
Didier, Elizabeth
Didier, Peter J.
Diniz, Pedro P.
Evermann, James F.
Favrot, Claude
Foil, Carol S.
Foley, Janet E.
Ford, Richard B.
Foreyt, William J.
Fox, James G.
Fyfe, Janet A.
Gaskell, Rosalind M.
Glaser, Carol A.
Goldstein, Richard E.
Gookin, Jody L.
Gorham, John
Greene, Craig E.
Greene, Russell T.
Hall, Gerryl G.
Harrus, Shimon
Hartmann, Katrin
Harvey, John W.
Ihrke, Peter J.
Jang, Spencer S.
Jones, Boyd R.
Jones, Robert L.
Kennedy, Frances A.
Kjos, Sonia A.
Koenig, Amie
Lappin, Michael E.
Legendre, Alfred M.
Levy, Julie K.
Levy, Steven A.
Lindsay, David S.
Löchelt, Martin
Love, Brenda C.
Lunn, Katherine F.
Macintire, Douglass K.
Malik, Richard
Mendez, Susana
Messick, Joanne B.
Moore, George E.
Nagle, Terry M.
Neer, Mark T.
Nelson, C. Thomas
Outerbridge, Catherine A.
Peeters, Dominique P.
Potter, Thomas M.
Powers, Edward L.
Reid, Hugh W.
Schatzberg, Scott J.
Schultz, Ronald D.
Sellon, Rance K.
Smith, Jo
Taboada, Joseph
Thomason, Justin D.
Waner, Trevor
Willoughby, Kim

LIST OF CONTRIBUTORS

Els Acke, MVM PhD DipECVIM-CA MANZCVS CertSAM
EBVS® European Veterinary Specialist in Small Animal Internal Medicine, IDEXX Vet Med Labor GmbH; University of Leipzig, Leipzig, Germany

Christopher B. Adolph, DVM MS DACVM (Parasitology)
Senior Veterinary Specialist, Veterinary Specialty Operations, Zoetis, USA, Companion Animal Division, Tulsa, OK, USA

Maria Afonso, DVM MSc Vet PhD MRCVS
Lecturer in Veterinary Anatomy, School of Veterinary Medicine, University of Glasgow, Glasgow, UK

Kelly E. Allen, MS PhD
Assistant Professor of Parasitology, Department of Veterinary Pathobiology, Center for Veterinary Health Sciences, Oklahoma State University, Stillwater, OK, USA

Boaz Arzi, DVM DAVDC DEVDC
Department of Surgical and Radiological Sciences, School of Veterinary Medicine, University of California, Davis Davis, CA, USA

Ingrid Balsa, MEd DVM DACVS (SA)
Department of Surgical and Radiological Sciences, School of Veterinary Medicine, University of California, Davis Davis, CA, USA

Gad Baneth, DVM PhD Dip ECVCP
Director, Koret School of Veterinary Medicine, Professor of Veterinary Medicine, The Rybak-Pearson Chair in Veterinary Medicine, Koret School of Veterinary Medicine, Hebrew University, Rehovot, Israel

Renee Barber, DVM PhD DACVIM (Neurology)
Assistant Professor, College of Veterinary Medicine, University of Georgia, Athens, GA, USA

Emi N. Barker, BSc BVSc PhD DipECVIM-CA MRCVS
Feline Centre, Langford Vets, Langford, UK; Bristol Veterinary School, University of Bristol, Langford, UK

Vanessa R. Barrs, BVSc (Hons) PhD MVetClinStud GradCertEd FANZCVS
Chair Professor of Companion Animal Health and Disease, Department of Veterinary Clinical Sciences, Jockey Club College of Veterinary Medicine and Life Sciences, City University of Hong Kong, Kowloon Tong, Hong Kong

Julia A. Beatty, BSc BVetMed PhD FANZCVS FRCVS
Chair Professor, and Head, Department of Veterinary Clinical Sciences, Jockey Club College of Veterinary Medicine and Life Sciences, City University of Hong Kong, Kowloon Tong, Hong Kong

Mikael Berg, MSc PhD
Swedish University of Agricultural Sciences, Department of Biomedical Sciences and Veterinary Public Health, Uppsala, Sweden

Adam J. Birkenheuer, DVM PhD DACVIM
Professor of Small Animal Internal Medicine, Andy Quattlebaum Distinguished Chair of Infectious Disease Research, College of Veterinary Medicine, North Carolina State University, Raleigh, NC, USA

Byron L. Blagburn, MS PhD DACVM (Hon) (Parasitology)
University Distinguished Professor, Department of Pathobiology, College of Veterinary Medicine, Auburn University, Auburn, AL, USA

Ross Bond, BVMS PhD DVD MRCVS DipECVD FHEA
Professor of Veterinary Dermatology, Department of Clinical Science and Services, Royal Veterinary College, Hatfield, UK

Dwight D. Bowman, MS PhD DACVM (Hon)
Professor of Parasitology, Department of Microbiology and Immunology, College of Veterinary Medicine, Cornell University, Ithaca, NY, USA

Edward B. Breitschwerdt, DVM DACVIM
Melanie S. Steele Professor of Medicine and Infectious Disease, Department of Clinical Sciences, College of Veterinary Medicine, North Carolina State University, Raleigh, NC, USA

Canio Buonavoglia, DVM
Professor of Infectious Diseases of Animals, Department of Veterinary Medicine, University of Bari, Valenzano, Italy

Brandy A. Burgess, DVM MSc PhD DACVIM DACVPM
Associate Professor of Epidemiology and Infection Control, Department of Population Health, College of Veterinary Medicine, University of Georgia, Athens, GA, USA

Jamie M. Burkitt Creedon, DVM DACVECC
Associate Professor of Clinical Small Animal Emergency and Critical Care, Department of Surgical and Radiological Sciences, School of Veterinary Medicine, University of California, Davis Davis, CA, USA

Barbara A. Byrne, DVM PhD DACVIM DACVM
Department of Pathology, Microbiology, and Immunology, University of California, Davis, Davis, CA, USA

Margret L. Casal, DVM MS PhD DipECAR
Professor of Medical Genetics, Reproduction, and Pediatrics, School of Veterinary Medicine, University of Pennsylvania, Philadelphia, PA, USA

Victoria J. Chalker, BSc PhD
Head, Science and Engineering Profession, United Kingdom Health Security Agency, London, UK

Bruno B. Chomel, DVM PhD
Professor Emeritus, Department of Population Health and Reproduction, University of California, Davis, Davis, CA, USA

Leah A. Cohn, DVM PhD DACVIM
Professor of Small Animal Medicine and Surgery, Department of Veterinary Medicine and Surgery, College of Veterinary Medicine, University of Missouri, Columbia, MO, USA

Lynette K. Cole, DVM DACVD
Department of Veterinary Clinical Sciences, The Ohio State University, College of Veterinary Medicine, Columbus, OH, USA

Stephen D. Cole, VMD MS DACVM
Assistant Professor of Microbiology (CE), Director of Clinical Microbiology, Department of Pathobiology, School of Veterinary Medicine, University of Pennsylvania, Philadelphia, PA, USA

Gary A. Conboy, DVM PhD DACVM
Professor Emeritus, Atlantic Veterinary College, University of Prince Edward Island, Charlottetown, Prince Edward Island, Canada

Roberto Cortinas, DVM PhD
Assistant Professor of Practice, School of Veterinary Medicine and Biomedical Sciences, University of Nebraska at Lincoln, Lincoln, NE, USA

Kimberly Coyner, DVM DACVD
Dermatology Clinic for Animals, Lacey, WA, USA

William T.N. Culp, VMD DACVS
Department of Surgical and Radiological Sciences, School of Veterinary Medicine, University of California, Davis Davis, CA, USA

Joshua B. Daniels, DVM PhD DACVM (Bacteriology)
Associate Professor, Department of Microbiology, Immunology, and Pathology, Colorado State University, Fort Collins, CO, USA

Autumn P. Davidson, DVM MS DACVIM
Staff Veterinarian, Veterinary Medical Teaching Hospital, University of California, Davis, Davis, CA, USA

Jonathan D. Dear, DVM MAS DACVIM
Associate Professor of Clinical Internal Medicine, Department of Medicine and Epidemiology, School of Veterinary Medicine, University of California, Davis Davis, CA, USA

Nicola Decaro, DVM PhD Dip ECVM
Professor of Infectious Diseases of Animals, Department of Veterinary Medicine, University of Bari, Valenzano, Italy

Amy E. DeClue, DVM MS DACVIM (SAIM)
Professor, Veterinary Internal Medicine, University of Missouri, College of Veterinary Medicine, Columbia, MO, USA

Dubraska Diaz-Campos, DVM PhD
Assistant Professor-Clinical Microbiology, Department of Clinical Sciences, The Ohio State University, Columbus, OH, USA

Pedro Paulo V.P. Diniz, DVM PhD
Director of Outcomes Assessment, Associate Professor in Small Animal Internal Medicine, College of Veterinary Medicine, Western University of Health Sciences, Pomona, CA, USA

Jitender P. Dubey, BVSc MVSc PhD FAAM DSc
United States Department of Agriculture, Agricultural Research Service, Beltsville Agricultural Research Center, Animal Parasitic Diseases Laboratory, Beltsville, MD, USA

Edward J. Dubovi, BA MA PhD
Professor of Virology, Animal Health Diagnostic Center, Department of Population Medicine and Diagnostic Sciences, College of Veterinary Medicine, Cornell University, Ithaca, NY, USA

Chrissy Eckstrand, DVM PhD DACVP
Assistant Professor, Washington State University, College of Veterinary Medicine, Washington Animal Disease Diagnostic Laboratory, Pullman, WA, USA

John A. Ellis, DVM PhD DACVP DACVM
Department of Veterinary Microbiology, Western College of Veterinary Medicine, University of Saskatchewan, Saskatoon, SK, Canada

David A. Elsemore, BA PhD
Associate Research Fellow, Assay Diagnostics, IDEXX Laboratories, Inc., Westbrook, ME, USA

Steven E. Epstein, DVM DACVECC
Professor of Clinical Small Animal Emergency and Critical Care, Department of Veterinary Surgical and Radiological Sciences, University of California, Davis, Davis, CA, USA

James F. Evermann, MS PhD
Professor of Clinical Virology, Department of Veterinary Clinical Sciences, College of Veterinary Medicine, Washington State University, Pullman, WA, USA

Janet E. Foley, DVM, PhD
Professor, Department of Medicine and Epidemiology, School of Veterinary Medicine, University of California, Davis, Davis, CA, USA

Urs Giger, Prof. Dr. med. vet. MS FVH Dipl. ACVIM-SA & ECVIM-CA (Internal Medicine) Dipl. ECVCP (Clinical Pathology)
Emeritus Charlotte Newton Sheppard Endowed Professor of Medicine, Chair, School of Veterinary Medicine, University of Pennsylvania, Philadelphia, PA, USA;
Emeritus Professor of Hematology, School of Medicine, University of Pennsylvania, Philadelphia, PA, USA;
Professor of Small Animal Internal Medicine, Vetsuisse, University of Zürich, Zürich, Switzerland

Ellie J.C. Goldstein, MD
Director, R. M. Alden Research Laboratory, Clinical Professor of Medicine, David Geffen School of Medicine at UCLA, Los Angeles, CA, USA

Jennifer Granick, DVM PhD DACVIM (SAIM)
Department of Veterinary Clinical Sciences, University of Minnesota, St. Paul, MN, USA

Isabella D.F. Gremião
Laboratory of Clinical Research on Dermatozoonoses in Domestic Animals, Evandro Chagas National Institute of Infectious Diseases, Oswaldo Cruz Foundation, Rio de Janeiro, Brazil

Amy M. Grooters, DVM DACVIM
Professor Emeritus, Companion Animal Medicine, Department of Veterinary Clinical Sciences, Louisiana State University, Baton Rouge, LA, USA

Danièlle A. Gunn-Moore, BSc(Hon) BVM&S PhD MANZCVS(Feline) FHEA FRSB FRCVS
Personal Chair of Feline Medicine, The Royal (Dick) School of Veterinary Studies and The Roslin Institute, The University of Edinburgh, Edinburgh, UK

Lynn Guptill, DVM PhD DACVIM
Department of Veterinary Clinical Sciences, Purdue University College of Veterinary Medicine, West Lafayette, IN, USA

Sarah A. Hamer, MS PhD DVM DACVPM (Epidemiology)
Department of Veterinary Integrative Biosciences, College of Veterinary Medicine and Biomedical Sciences, Texas A&M University, College Station, TX USA

Shimon Harrus, DVM PhD Dip ECVCP
Professor, Koret School of Veterinary Medicine, The Robert H. Smith Faculty of Agriculture, Food and Environment, The Hebrew University of Jerusalem, Rehovot, Israel

Katrin Hartmann, Dr. med. vet. Dr. habil. DipECVIM-CA
Clinic of Small Animal Medicine, Centre for Clinical Veterinary Medicine, Ludwig-Maximilians-University of Munich, Munich, Germany

Diana Henke, Dr. med. vet. Dip ECVN
Division of Neurological Sciences, Faculty of Veterinary Medicine, University of Bern, Bern, Switzerland

Emir Hodzic, DVM MSci PhD
Real-Time PCR Research and Diagnostic Core Facility, School of Veterinary Medicine, University of California, Davis Davis, CA, USA

Regina Hofmann-Lehmann, DVM FVH
Professor of Laboratory Medicine, Clinical Laboratory, Department of Clinical Diagnostics and Services, and Center for Clinical Studies, Vetsuisse Faculty, University of Zürich, Zürich, Switzerland

Elizabeth W. Howerth, DVM PhD ACVP
Department of Pathology, College of Veterinary Medicine, University of Georgia, Athens, GA, USA

Karin Hultin Jäderlund, DVM PhD DECVN
Professor of Veterinary Neurology, Norwegian University of Life Sciences, Department of Companion Animal Clinical Sciences, Ås, Norway

Kate F. Hurley, DVM MPVM DABVP
(Shelter Medicine Practice), Koret Shelter Medicine Program, University of California, Davis, Davis, CA, USA

Linda S. Jacobson, BVSc MMedVet PhD
Senior Manager, Shelter Medicine Advancement, Toronto Humane Society, Toronto, ON, Canada

Jonas Johansson Wensman, DVM PhD
Researcher, Associate Professor, Ruminant Medicine, Coordinator Global Development at VH Faculty, SLU Global, Swedish University of Agricultural Sciences, Department of Clinical Sciences, Uppsala, Sweden

Amy S. Kapatkin, DVM MAS DACVS
Professor, Department of Veterinary Surgical and Radiological Sciences, School of Veterinary Medicine, University of California, Davis, Davis, CA, USA

Marc Kent, DVM DACVIM (Internal Medicine and Neurology)
Department of Small Animal Medicine and Surgery, College of Veterinary Medicine, University of Georgia, Athens, GA, USA

Jennifer K. Ketzis, PhD Assoc Memb EVPC
Department of Biomedical Sciences, Ross University School of Veterinary Medicine, St. Kitts, West Indies

Linda Kidd, DVM PhD DACVIM
Professor, Small Animal Internal Medicine, Western University of Health Sciences, College of Veterinary Medicine, Pomona, CA, USA

Stacy Kraus, DVM
Koret Shelter Medicine Program, University of California, Davis Davis, CA, USA

Mark Krockenberger, BSc(Vet) BVSc PhD GradCertEdStud FANZVS (Veterinary Anatomical Pathology)
Professor of Veterinary Pathology, Associate Head of Veterinary Clinical Sciences, Registered Specialist Veterinary Pathologist, Sydney School of Veterinary Science, Marie Bashir Institute for Infectious Diseases and Biosecurity, The University of Sydney, Sydney, NSW, Australia

Michael R. Lappin, DVM PhD DACVIM
The Kenneth W. Smith Professor in Clinical Veterinary Medicine, Department of Clinical Sciences, College of Veterinary Medicine and Biomedical Sciences, Colorado State University, Fort Collins, CO, USA

Alice C.Y. Lee, DVM PhD DACVM (Parasitology)
Assistant Professor of Parasitology, Department of Comparative, Diagnostic, and Population Medicine, College of Veterinary Medicine, University of Florida, Gainesville, FL, USA

Tekla Lee-Fowler, DVM MS DACVIM (SAIM)
Associate Professor, College of Veterinary Medicine, Auburn University, Auburn, AL, USA

Susan E. Little, DVM PhD DACVM
Regents Professor and Krull-Ewing Professor of Veterinary Parasitology, Center for Veterinary Health Sciences, Oklahoma State University, Stillwater, OK, USA

Meryl P. Littman, VMD DACVIM
Professor Emerita of Medicine, University of Pennsylvania School of Veterinary Medicine, Philadelphia, PA, USA

Remo Lobetti, BVSc (Hons) MMedVet (Med) PhD Dip ECVIM (Internal Medicine)
Bryanston Veterinary Hospital, Bryanston, South Africa

Araceli Lucio-Forster, PhD
Lecturer, Department of Microbiology and Immunology, College of Veterinary Medicine, Cornell University, Ithaca, NY, USA

Jennifer A. Luff, VMD PhD DACVP
Associate Professor, Department of Population Health and Pathobiology, College of Veterinary Medicine, North Carolina State University, Raleigh, NC, USA

Hans Lutz, FVH FAMH
Professor Emeritus, Formerly: Clinical Laboratory, Vetsuisse Faculty, University of Zürich, Zürich, Switzerland

Mary Marcondes, DVM MSc PhD
Retired Professor, Small Animal Internal Medicine, School of Veterinary Medicine, São Paulo State University, Araçatuba, São Paulo, Brazil

Stanley L. Marks, BVSc PhD DACVIM (Internal Medicine, Oncology, Nutrition)
Professor of Small Animal Internal Medicine, Department of Medicine and Epidemiology, School of Veterinary Medicine, University of California, Davis, Davis, CA, USA

Sina Marsilio, Dr. med. vet. PhD DACVIM (SAIM) DECVIM-CA
Department of Medicine and Epidemiology, School of Veterinary Medicine, University of California, Davis Davis, CA, USA

Patrick L. McDonough, BS MS PhD
Professor Emeritus of Microbiology, Department of Population Medicine and Diagnostic Sciences, Cornell University College of Veterinary Medicine, Ithaca, NY, USA

Rodrigo C. Menezes, DVM PhD
Laboratory of Clinical Research on Dermatozoonoses in Domestic Animals, Evandro Chagas National Institute of Infectious Diseases, Oswaldo Cruz Foundation, Rio de Janeiro, Brazil

Lindsay Merkel, DVM DACVIM
Associate Professor, Small Animal Internal Medicine, Department of Veterinary Clinical Sciences, College of Veterinary Medicine, University of Minnesota, St Paul, MN, USA

W. Zach Mills, DVM MBA
Lieutenant Colonel (LTC), Veterinary Corp (VC), CACOM Preventive Medicine Veterinarian, 352d Civil Affairs Command, Fort Meade, MD; and Executive Director, Head of US Pet Veterinary Professional Services, Boehringer Ingelheim Animal Health USA, Inc., Duluth, GA, USA

Luisa H.M. Miranda, DVM MSc PhD
Lecturer of Veterinary Pathology, Sydney School of Veterinary Science, The University of Sydney, Sydney, NSW, Australia

George E. Moore, DVM PhD DACVIM DACVPM
Professor of Epidemiology, Department of Veterinary Administration, College of Veterinary Medicine, Purdue University, West Lafayette, IN, USA

Karen A. Moriello, DVM DACVD
Professor of Veterinary Dermatology and Allergy, University of Wisconsin, Madison, WI, USA

Alyssa C. Mourning, DVM DACVIM
Internal Medicine, BluePearl Veterinary Partners, Eden Prairie, MN, USA

John S. Munday, BVSc PhD DSc DACVP
Professor of Veterinary Pathology, School of Veterinary Science, Massey University, Palmerston North, New Zealand

Mathios E. Mylonakis, DVM Dr. med. vet.
Professor of Companion Animal Medicine, Companion Animal Clinic, School of Veterinary Medicine, Aristotle University of Thessaloniki, Thessaloniki, Greece

Yoko Nagamori, DVM MS DACVM
Zoetis PetCare, Veterinary Professional Services, Parsippany, NJ, USA

C. Thomas Nelson, DVM
Animal Medical Center of NE Alabama, Anniston, AL, USA

Anne B. Nordstoga, DVM PhD
Researcher, Norwegian Veterinary Institute, Oslo, Norway

Jacqueline M. Norris, BVSc MVS PhD MASM GradCertHigherEd
Professor of Veterinary Microbiology and Infectious Diseases, Associate Head of Research, Faculty of Science, Sydney School of Veterinary Science, Marie Bashir Institute for Infectious Diseases and Biosecurity, University of Sydney, Sydney, NSW, Australia

Carolyn R. O'Brien, BVSc MVetClinStud PhD FANZCVS
Registered Specialist in Feline Medicine, Melbourne Cat Vets, Fitzroy, Victoria, Australia

Conor O'Halloran, BVSc MSc PhD MRCVS
The Royal (Dick) School of Veterinary Studies and The Roslin Institute, The University of Edinburgh, Edinburgh, UK

Cynthia M. Otto, DVM PhD DACVECC DACVSMR
Professor of Working Dog Sciences and Sports Medicine, and Director, Penn Vet Working Dog Center, University of Pennsylvania School of Veterinary Medicine, Philadelphia, PA, USA

Mark G. Papich, DVM MS DACVCP
Professor of Clinical Pharmacology, Burroughs Wellcome Fund Professor in Veterinary Pharmacology, College of Veterinary Medicine, North Carolina State University, Raleigh, NC, USA

Colin R. Parrish, BSc PhD
John M. Olin Professor of Virology, Baker Institute for Animal Health, Department of Microbiology and Immunology, College of Veterinary Medicine, Cornell University, Ithaca, NY, USA

Niels C. Pedersen, BS DVM PhD
Professor Emeritus, Department of Medicine and Epidemiology, School of Veterinary Medicine, University of California, Davis, Davis, CA, USA

Andrew S. Peregrine, BVMS PhD DVM DEVPC DACVM
Associate Professor, Veterinary Parasitology, Department of Pathobiology, Ontario Veterinary College, University of Guelph, Guelph, ON, Canada

Sandro A. Pereira, DVM PhD
Laboratory of Clinical Research on Dermatozoonoses in Domestic Animals, Evandro Chagas National Institute of Infectious Diseases, Oswaldo Cruz Foundation, Rio de Janeiro, Brazil

Christine Petersen, DVM PhD
Director, Center for Emerging Infectious Diseases, Professor, Department of Epidemiology, College of Public Health, University of Iowa, Iowa City, IA, USA

John F. Prescott, MA VETMB PhD FCAHS
University Professor Emeritus, Department of Pathobiology, University of Guelph, Guelph, ON, Canada

Simon L. Priestnall, BSc Vet Path BVSc PhD DipACVP FRCPath
Professor of Veterinary Anatomic Pathology, Department of Pathobiology and Population Sciences, The Royal Veterinary College, Hatfield, UK

Barbara Qurollo, DVM MS
Associate Research Professor, Department of Clinical Sciences, College of Veterinary Medicine, North Carolina State University, Raleigh, NC, USA

Alan Radford, BSc BVSc PhD MRCVS
Institute of Infection, Veterinary and Ecological Sciences, University of Liverpool, Liverpool, UK

Shelley C. Rankin, BSc (Hons) PhD
Professor Emeritus of Microbiology, University of Pennsylvania, School of Veterinary Medicine, Philadelphia, PA, USA; Global Director of Microbiology and Molecular Diagnostics, Zoetis Reference Laboratories, Zoetis, Parsippany, NJ, USA

Krystle L. Reagan, DVM PhD DACVIM
Department of Medicine and Epidemiology, School of Veterinary Medicine, University of California, Davis, Davis, CA, USA

Mason V. Reichard, MS PhD
Professor, College of Veterinary Medicine, Oklahoma State University, Stillwater, OK, USA

Carol Reinero, DVM PhD DACVIM (SAIM)
Professor and Director of Comparative Internal Medicine Laboratory, University of Missouri, Columbia, Columbia, MO, USA

Meriam N. Saleh, PhD
Clinical Assistant Professor, Department of Veterinary Pathobiology, College of Veterinary Medicine and Biomedical Sciences, Texas A&M University, College Station, TX, USA

Sarah G.H. Sapp, PhD
Department of Population Health, College of Veterinary Medicine, University of Georgia, Athens, GA, USA

Ashley B. Saunders, DVM DACVIM (Cardiology)
Department of Small Animal Clinical Sciences, College of Veterinary Medicine and Biomedical Sciences, Texas A&M University, College Station, TX, USA

Tânia M.P. Schubach, DVM PhD
Laboratory of Clinical Research on Dermatozoonoses in Domestic Animals, Evandro Chagas National Institute of Infectious Diseases, Oswaldo Cruz Foundation, Rio de Janeiro, Brazil

Simone Schuller, Prof Dr. med. vet. DEA DECVIM-CA PhD
Department Clinical Veterinary Medicine, Division of Small Animal Internal Medicine, University of Bern, Bern, Switzerland

Valeria Scorza, MV PhD
Instructor, Department of Clinical Sciences, College of Veterinary Medicine and Biomedical Sciences, Colorado State University, Fort Collins, CO, USA

Rance K. Sellon, DVM PhD DACVIM
Associate Professor, Veterinary Clinical Sciences, Washington State University, College of Veterinary Medicine, Pullman, WA, USA

Claire R. Sharp, BSc BVMS(Hons) MS DACVECC
Senior Lecturer, School of Veterinary Medicine, College of Science, Health, Engineering and Education, Murdoch University, Murdoch, Western Australia, Australia

Deborah Silverstein, DVM DACVECC
Professor, Emergency and Critical Care, University of Pennsylvania School of Veterinary Medicine, Philadelphia, PA, USA

Ameet Singh, BSc DVM DVSc DACVS (SA)
Associate Professor, Department of Clinical Studies, Ontario Veterinary College, University of Guelph, Guelph, ON, Canada

Virginia Sinnott-Stutzman, DVM DACVECC
MSPCA Angell, Boston, MA, USA

Karen F. Snowden, DVM PhD DACVM (Parasitology)
Professor Emerita, Department of Veterinary Pathobiology, College of Veterinary Medicine and Biomedical Sciences, Texas A&M University, College Station, TX, USA

Laia Solano-Gallego, DVM PhD ECVCP
Professor, Dep. of Medicina i Cirurgia Animals, Facultat de Veterinària, Universitat Autònoma de Barcelona, Cerdanyola del Vallès, Barcelona, Spain

Miranda Spindel, DVM MS
Shelter Medicine Help, Fort Collins, CO, USA

Lindsay A. Starkey, DVM PhD DACVM (Parasitology)
Associate Professor of Parasitology, Department of Pathobiology, College of Veterinary Medicine, Auburn University, Auburn, AL, USA

Joshua A. Stern, DVM PhD DACVIM (Cardiology)
Professor of Cardiology, Department of Medicine and Epidemiology, School of Veterinary Medicine, University of California, Davis, Davis, CA, USA

Jean Stiles, DVM MS DACVO
Professor Emerita, Ophthalmology, Purdue University College of Veterinary Medicine, West Lafayette, IN, USA

Reinhard K. Straubinger, Dr. med. vet. PhD
LMU Institute for Infectious Diseases and Zoonoses, Ludwig-Maximilians-University of Munich, Munich, Germany

Jason W. Stull, VMD MPVM PhD DACVPM
Assistant Professor, The Ohio State University, College of Veterinary Medicine, Columbus, OH, USA; Assistant Professor, The University of Prince Edward Island, Atlantic Veterinary College, Charlottetown, Canada

Jane E. Sykes, BVSc (Hons) PhD MBA DACVIM
Professor, Department of Medicine and Epidemiology, University of California, Davis, CA, USA

Séverine Tasker, BSc BVSc PhD DSAM DipECVIM-CA FHEA FRCVS
Honorary Professor of Feline Medicine, Bristol Veterinary School, University of Bristol, Langford, UK; Chief Medical Officer, Linnaeus Veterinary Limited, Shirley, Solihull, UK

Jennifer E. Thomas, DVM DACVP
Clinical Assistant Professor, College of Veterinary Medicine, Oklahoma State University, Stillwater, OK, USA

Sara M. Thomasy, DVM PhD DACVO
Professor of Comparative Ophthalmology, Department of Surgical and Radiological Sciences, School of Veterinary Medicine, Department of Ophthalmology and Vision Science, School of Medicine, University of California, Davis Davis, CA, USA

Andrea Tipold, DVM Dip ECVN
Department of Small Animal Medicine and Surgery, University of Veterinary Medicine Hannover, Hannover, Germany

M. Katherine Tolbert, DVM PhD DACVIM (SAIM)
Clinical Associate Professor, Gastrointestinal Laboratory, Department of Small Animal Clinical Sciences, Texas A&M University, College Station, TX, USA

Thomas W. Vahlenkamp, DVM PhD
Professor, Institute of Virology, Center for Infectious Diseases, Faculty of Veterinary Medicine, University of Leipzig, Leipzig, Germany

Marc Vandevelde, Dr. med. vet. DipECVN
Professor Emeritus, Division of Neurological Sciences, Faculty of Veterinary Medicine, University of Bern, Bern, Switzerland

Nancy Vincent-Johnson, DVM MS DACVIM (SAIM) DACVPM
Veterinary Medical Officer, Chief Clinical Services, Fort Belvoir Veterinary Center, Fort Belvoir, VA, USA

Polina Vishkautsan, DVM DACVIM
Veterinary Specialty Center of Tucson, Tucson, AZ, USA

Trevor Waner, BVSc PhD Dip ECLAM
School of Veterinary Medicine, The Hebrew University of Jerusalem, Rehovot, Israel

J. Scott Weese, DVM DVSc DACVIM FCAHS
Professor, Ontario Veterinary College, Director, Centre for Public Health and Zoonoses, University of Guelph, Guelph, ON, Canada

Jodi L. Westropp, DVM PhD DACVIM
Professor, UC Davis School of Veterinary Medicine, Department of Veterinary Medicine and Epidemiology, Director, Veterinary Medical Continuing Education, Director, G.V. Ling Urinary Stone Analysis Lab, University of California, Davis Davis, CA, USA

Stephen D. White, DVM DACVD
Department of Medicine and Epidemiology, School of Veterinary Medicine, University of California, Davis, Davis, CA, USA

Jenessa A. Winston, DVM PhD DACVIM
Assistant Professor, Small Animal Internal Medicine, Department of Clinical Sciences, The Ohio State University, Columbus, OH, USA

Judit M. Wulcan, DVM MSc
School of Veterinary Medicine, Department of Pathology, Microbiology and Immunology, University of California, Davis Davis, CA, USA

Michael J. Yabsley, MS PhD
Professor, Daniel B. Warnell Professor in Forestry and Natural Resources, Department of Population Health, College of Veterinary Medicine and Warnell School of Forestry and Natural Resources, University of Georgia, Athens, GA, USA

PART I

Principles of Diagnosis, Treatment and Control of Infectious Diseases

Introduction to Part I

Part I of this book is divided into 3 sections: 1) Principles of Infectious Disease Diagnosis, 2) Anti-infective Drugs, and 3) Principles of Infection Control. The information presented is complementary to material provided in disease-specific chapters of this book (Part II). Drug doses for specific antiviral, antibacterial, antifungal, and antiparasitic drugs that are referred to in Part II are found in tables in the chapters on anti-infective therapy, together with key information on spectrum of activity, mechanism of action, and adverse effects. Vaccination strategies are discussed in Section 3, and the reader is referred to tables in the Appendix for guidance on vaccination intervals and adjustments based on animal lifestyle. A solid understanding of these principles facilitates a systematic and logical approach to diagnosis, treatment, and prevention of any infectious disease problem.

Section 1 Principles of Infectious Disease Diagnosis

Section 2 Anti-infective Drugs

Section 3 Principles of Infection Control

SECTION 1

Principles of Infectious Disease Diagnosis

Jane E. Sykes, Shelley C. Rankin

The accurate diagnosis of an infectious disease is critical to guide the effective treatment of an individual animal or outbreaks of disease in a population of animals. Making an accurate diagnosis requires an understanding of the principles of diagnostic testing and an understanding of the pathogenesis of the disease agent suspected. Some infectious diseases are distinctive enough to be identified clinically. However, many pathogens cause a wide spectrum of clinical signs, and a single clinical syndrome may result from infection with one of many pathogens. Diagnostic tests can generally be grouped into *organism detection tests* (culture, antigen tests, and nucleic acid tests) and *antibody detection tests.* In some situations (e.g., early in the course of illness, in immunosuppressed animals), organism detection tests are most appropriate. In others (e.g., chronic, persistent infectious diseases; identification of exposure in an animal population; acute diseases associated with an early rise in antibody titer that can be captured using acute and convalescent serology testing), antibody detection tests may be preferable. Increasingly, as new assays become available, the diagnosis and understanding of companion animal infectious diseases relies on the application of multiple diagnostic tests simultaneously.

This section, which focuses on diagnosis of companion animal infectious diseases, includes chapters on isolation of intracellular pathogens in cell culture, immunoassays, as well as clinically relevant information on specific diagnostic tests for bacteria, parasites, and fungi. Selection and collection of appropriate specimens for testing, how each test is performed, and how to best interpret the results are covered to inform and guide clinicians. A knowledge of the material presented in these chapters should provide the reader with a strong foundation in the appropriate selection and interpretation of diagnostic tests for all of the pathogens discussed in this book.

1

Isolation in Cell Culture

Edward J. Dubovi, Shelley C. Rankin

KEY POINTS

- With the increasing availability of nucleic acid–based testing and antigen capture ELISA tests, the use of cell culture for the diagnosis of infections caused by obligate intracellular pathogens in dogs and cats has decreased.
- Cell culture remains an important technique for: (1) nontargeted pathogen discovery, (2) amplification of viruses detected by molecular methods for genomic sequencing, (3) vaccine manufacture, and (4) virus neutralization assays. In certain instances, cell culture is the most sensitive and specific method for organism detection.
- Before collection of specimens, veterinary clinicians should communicate with the laboratory that is to perform the diagnostic testing to discuss the laboratory's capabilities with regard to pathogen detection and to discuss testing strategies within the context of the clinical event.
- Specimens are inoculated onto cell monolayers, and the presence of an infecting organism may be identified based on the detection of abnormal cell growth (cytopathic effects), or use of immunoassays or molecular assays for the specific agent of interest. Definitive identification of the infectious agent after growth in cell culture is by agent-specific fluorescent antibody staining or by nucleic acid–based tests.
- False-negative results may occur as a result of: (1) timing of specimen collection, (2) deterioration of organisms during transport, and (3) inability of the agent of interest to grow in the selected cell line used in the test system.
- As with all diagnostic tests, positive cell culture isolation results may not be the definitive link to the cause of an animal's signs because some organisms can be present without causing disease.

INTRODUCTION

Cell culture refers to the growth of eukaryotic cells under controlled conditions within the laboratory *(in vitro)*. Infectious agents that require living host cells for replication may be isolated in the natural host *(in vivo)*, in embryonated eggs *(in ovo)*, or in cell culture. The development of routine growth of eukaryotic cells under defined laboratory conditions in the late 1940s ushered in an era of rapid advancement in the characterization of viral pathogens as well as the development viral vaccines, e.g., poliovirus vaccine. Virus discovery was largely confined to research laboratories, but the expansion of commercial products and cell lines moved virus culture into diagnostic laboratories. By the 1980s, there was some thought that the discovery of most viral pathogens was complete. However, the start of a new era in pathogen discovery came with the identification of hepatitis C virus exclusively using molecular cloning techniques. It was recognized that more viral pathogens existed than could be grown in standard cell culture systems. The application of polymerase chain reaction (PCR) technology demonstrated the potential of molecular techniques (nucleic acid–based detection) in diagnostic testing. Use of next-generation sequencing (NGS) may result in identification of all viruses in existence within the next few years. The sensitivity and speed of molecular diagnostic assays has led to cell culture being used less often for routine clinical diagnostic purposes because of the longer turnaround times (days to weeks) and the cost to maintain a cell culture facility (Table 1.1). Nevertheless, isolation of viral and intracellular bacterial and protozoal pathogens in cell culture remains an important technique for the discovery of new pathogens, the propagation of isolates for research purposes, the generation of organisms for vaccination purposes, and the establishment of the efficacy of novel antimicrobial drugs. Vaccines for dogs and cats that are propagated in cell culture include those for canine distemper virus (CDV), canine adenovirus, parvovirus, rabies virus, and feline viral and chlamydial respiratory tract disease agents. Veterinary clinicians should remain aware of situations where cell culture may be the best technique to identify the presence of a novel infectious agent and the ideal methods for collection and submission of specimens. Knowledge of cell culture methods can help veterinary clinicians to submit the optimum specimens, to understand laboratory turnaround times, to be aware of potential complications, and to interpret results in the proper context.

SPECIMEN COLLECTION AND TRANSPORT

Although cell cultures can be used to propagate intracellular bacteria and protozoa, it is now most often used for the diagnosis of viral infections. Proactive communication between the clinician and the laboratory that performs viral isolation is recommended to improve the chances of a successful virus isolation. Many viruses have restricted host ranges and will only grow in cells from the affected species. Submitting specimens to a laboratory that does not have broad capabilities lowers the chances for a successful test outcome. Successful detection of viruses is also highly dependent on: (1) collecting the appropriate specimens, (2) the timing of specimen collection, and (3) rapid and proper specimen transport and processing. Thus, the actions of the veterinary clinician play a critical role in ensuring positive test results when a virus is present.

Information that should be discussed with the laboratory before specimen collection, and forwarded together with the specimen, includes the clinician's differential diagnosis, the patient signalment, history, clinical signs, immune status, travel history, and the number of animals affected (Box 1.1). This information is used to guide the selection of the best

TABLE 1.1 Alternatives to Cell Culture for Diagnosis of Obligate Intracellular Pathogens That Infect Dogs and Cats

System Affected and Most Common Agents	Other Diagnostic Tests Available
Respiratory Tract	
Canine respiratory coronavirus	RT-PCR
Canine adenovirus-2	PCR
Influenza viruses	RT-PCR, serum antibody detection
Canine parainfluenza virus	RT-PCR
Canine distemper virus	RT-PCR, antigen detection using FA
Canine herpesvirus	PCR, antigen detection using FA
Feline herpesvirus-1	PCR, IHC
Feline calicivirus	RT-PCR, IHC
Pneumovirus (both canine and feline)	RT-PCR
Eye	
Chlamydia felis	PCR
Feline herpesvirus	PCR
Canine herpesvirus	PCR
Central Nervous System	
Canine distemper virus	RT-PCR, antigen detection using FA, CSF antibody detection
West Nile virus	RT-PCR, IHC
Encephalitis viruses	RT-PCR, IHC
Gastrointestinal Tract	
Coronaviruses	RT- PCR
Canine distemper virus	RT- PCR, antigen detection using direct FA
Canine and feline parvovirus	PCR, antigen detection using direct FA
Reproductive System	
Canine herpesvirus	PCR
Congenital and Perinatal	
Canine herpesvirus	PCR
Feline herpesvirus-1	PCR
Blood	
Feline leukemia virus	PCR, antigen detection (ELISA)
Feline immunodeficiency virus	PCR, antibody detection
Anaplasma phagocytophilum	PCR, antibody detection
Rickettsia rickettsii	PCR, antibody detection
Ehrlichia canis	PCR, antibody detection

CSF, cerebrospinal fluid; *ELISA,* enzyme-linked immunosorbent assay; *FA,* fluorescent antibody; *IHC,* immunohistochemistry; *PCR,* polymerase chain reaction; *RT,* reverse transcriptase.

array of cell cultures to achieve a successful outcome. For example, there is very little value in attempting to isolate CDV from a fully immunized 6-year-old dog with neurological signs. In the absence of vaccination history, CDV would be on the top of the differential list. Some viruses, such as feline coronavirus (FCoV), are difficult to isolate in cell culture or grow slowly, whereas others, such as feline calicivirus (FCV), replicate readily and rapidly in cell culture, and the sensitivity of cell culture is high. Viruses differ with respect to the cell type in which they prefer to replicate. As a result, specimens should be sent to the laboratory with information on the specific viruses that are suspected, but the isolation procedure in the laboratory should be nontargeted in order to isolate all viruses in the specimen, even those unknown to the clinician.

BOX 1.1 Factors to be Discussed With Diagnostic Laboratories Before Collection of Specimens for Pathogen Isolation in Cell Culture

Patient species, breed, age, and environment
Number of animals affected
History and clinical signs
Immune status of the patient
Geographic location and travel history
Suspected infectious agents
Timing of specimen collection
Type and amount of specimen to be collected
Transport conditions, including timing and method of transportation

For acute viral infections, the timing of specimen collection is of paramount importance. Specimens should be collected as early as possible following the onset of clinical signs because viral shedding commences before the onset of signs and may continue for only a few days. The duration of viral shedding depends on the type of virus and the anatomic site sampled. For rotavirus infections, for example, fecal specimens may have undetectable agent as early as 48 hours after the onset of diarrhea. When multiple animals are affected, collection of specimens from more than one animal may increase the chance that an isolate will be obtained. If possible, antibody testing using acute and convalescent phase serology should be performed concurrently to help confirm the diagnosis (see Chapter 2).

Selection of the best specimen type and collection site for cell culture is optimized based on knowledge of the pathogenesis of the suspected infectious agent, because the optimum specimen collection site may not be the site where clinical signs are most severe. Submitting a blood sample for the isolation of canine influenza virus is largely without value as influenza virus replication in the dog is restricted to the respiratory tract. Specimen size should also be maximized (e.g., at least 5 mL of blood, body fluids, or lavage specimens) to increase the chance of a positive isolation with the use of multiple cell lines. Specimens from multiple collection sites, e.g., nasal and oropharyngeal swabs, can only enhance the chances for a successful agent detection. Swab specimens should be collected by placing a long-shafted swab in the area to be sampled, rotating the swab against the mucosa, and allowing the secretions to be absorbed for approximately 5 to 10 seconds. The type of swab used should be a plastic shaft with synthetic fiber as cotton/wood swabs may contain inhibitors that affect agent detection.

Swabs and small tissue specimens for virus isolation should be placed in buffered virus transport medium that contains antibiotics and protein stabilizer such as fetal bovine serum or bovine serum albumin. The transport medium can be obtained from the laboratory or purchased from other commercial sources.

Liquid specimens such as blood, CSF, and bronchoalveolar lavage fluid do not need to be placed in the transport medium prior to cell culture. Blood samples should be collected using sterile technique, with antiseptic preparation of the site of venipuncture, and can be submitted in EDTA anticoagulant tubes.

All specimens should be refrigerated on collection and transported as quickly as possible (preferably within 24 hours) to the laboratory because delayed transport can lead to a decrease in organism viability. If delays in excess of 2 to 3 days are anticipated, the specimen can be frozen, but whole blood should never be frozen as it becomes unusable for testing. Freezing should be avoided whenever possible, as it may lead to a loss of virus viability particularly in freezers available to clinicians. If freezing is unavoidable, freezing at −70°C is preferable to

TABLE 1.2 Specimen Collection Guide for Diagnosis of Viral and Intracellular Bacterial Infections of Companion Animals

System Affected	Possible Agents	Specimen Type
Respiratory tract	Dogs: respiratory coronaviruses, canine adenovirus, influenza viruses, parainfluenza virus, CDV, canine herpesvirus, canine pneumovirus Cats: FHV-1, FCV, influenza viruses, feline pneumovirus	Oropharyngeal swabs, nasal swabs,[1] transtracheal wash or bronchoalveolar lavage specimens: ideally 5–10 mL of fluid Lung tissue obtained at biopsy or necropsy, including an area adjacent to affected tissue
Eye	Dogs: canine herpesvirus, canine adenovirus Cats: FHV-1, *Chlamydia felis*	Conjunctival swab, scraping or biopsy
Central nervous system	Dogs: CDV, arboviruses	CSF: ideally at least 0.5–1 mL. Blood: at least 5 mL. Brain at necropsy
Gastrointestinal tract	Dogs: CDV, CPV, rotaviruses, canine coronavirus Cats: FCoV, FCV, noroviruses	Feces: ideally an olive-sized portion of formed feces or at least 5 mL of liquid stool Intestinal biopsies obtained using endoscopy or surgery, or intestinal tissue obtained at necropsy
Genital	Dogs: canine herpesvirus Cats: *Chlamydia felis*	Vesicle scrapings, vaginal swabs
Congenital and perinatal	Dogs: canine herpesvirus, CPV Cats: FHV-1, FeLV	Blood, tissues obtained at necropsy
Blood	Dogs: *Anaplasma phagocytophilum, Rickettsia rickettsii, Ehrlichia canis* Cats: FeLV, FIV, FCoV	Blood: ideally 8–10 mL

CDV, canine distemper virus; *CPV,* canine parvovirus; *FCoV,* feline coronavirus; *FCV,* feline calicivirus; *FeLV,* feline leukemia virus; *FHV-1,* feline herpesvirus-1; *FIV,* feline immunodeficiency virus.

freezing at –20°C, and shipping on dry ice is preferable. The laboratory should have a submission guide that should be checked for specimen handling recommendations.

Table 1.2 provides a guide to the recommended specimen types for isolation of viruses or obligate intracellular bacteria from companion animals. Specimens should be labeled with the patient data, the site(s) from which the specimen(s) was collected, and the date of specimen collection. Specimens should be placed inside leak-proof triple packaging and transported on wet ice or cold packs to the laboratory, especially if transport is expected to take longer than 1 hour. Sufficient absorbent materials should be placed within the secondary container in order to absorb all liquid in the sample in case of a spill. Specimens to be shipped must be labeled and handled according to governmental and International Air Transport Association (IATA) regulations for shipping materials known to contain "dangerous goods." This includes infectious substances classified as Category A or Category B substances, and dry ice. Category A infectious substances are those capable of causing permanent disability or life-threatening or fatal disease in otherwise healthy animals and humans.[2] Most specimens submitted by veterinarians belong to Category B, which are any infectious substances that do not fall under the criteria for inclusion in Category A. Updated documents providing guidance on regulations for the transport of infectious substances are provided online by the World Health Organization (WHO).[2] Permits may be required for the importation of international specimens.

DIAGNOSTIC METHODS

Maintenance of Cell Cultures in the Laboratory

In general, cells are grown as monolayers on specially coated plastic surfaces either in culture flasks or plates. The cells in the monolayer can be derived directly from an animal *(primary cell culture),* which tend to have a limited life span, or they may be immortalized *(continuous cell lines).* Primary cell cultures have two distinct advantages for the isolation of viruses. They are generally of a mixed cell population so that a virus that only grows in an endothelial cell, for example, could still be isolated, whereas a culture of only fibroblasts would fail to isolate that virus. Also, primary cultures may maintain differentiated characteristics that are essential for virus propagation. Early attempts to grow influenza virus in cell culture were met with sporadic success. Primary monkey kidney cultures showed modest success but passaged cells failed. This was because a key factor required for growth of influenza virus in cell culture is the presence of a cellular protease, which is lost upon primary cell passage. Further subculture of primary cell lines often reduces their sensitivity to viral infection. Primary cell cultures are produced by placing tissues in an enzymatic solution, such as trypsin or collagenase, in order to produce a single cell suspension. Primary cell cultures have been used widely for the isolation of intracellular pathogens of dogs and cats,[3–6] but are now infrequently used due to cost and availability of tissue samples.

Low-passage cell lines remain viable and useful for virus propagation for 20 to 30 population doublings. *Continuous cell lines* are the type of cell line used most commonly for diagnostic, research, and commercial purposes as they are easily obtainable and have predictable characteristics. These may have been derived from cancer cells (such as the widely used HeLa cell line derived from human cervical cancer cells of a patient named Henrietta Lacks),[7] or they may have spontaneously "immortalized" during culture of primary cells, or as is now common, they were developed by targeted genetic modifications. Two such immortalization modifications include expression of the large T antigen of SV 40 and the telomerase gene (hTERT). Immortalized cells may also be genetically modified so that they express virus receptor proteins. A prime example of this is the expression of the CDV lymphocyte receptor protein (SLAM) on Vero cells, which turns a tedious isolation procedure for CDV into one of the easiest virus isolation procedures. Continuous cell lines representing a wide variety of cell types are available from commercial suppliers (Table 1.3). Laboratories that perform virus isolation for disease diagnosis will generally inoculate multiple cell lines because different viruses from the same animal species may prefer to replicate in different cell types.

TABLE 1.3 Examples of Continuous Cell Lines Used for Isolation of Viruses and Intracellular Bacteria That Infect Dogs and Cats

Cell Line	Cell Origin	Pathogen(s)
Vero cells; recombinant Vero-SLAM cells	African Green monkey renal epithelial cells	CDV[11,12] *Rickettsia rickettsii*[13] *Toxoplasma gondii*[14]
Madin-Darby canine kidney cells (MDCK)	Kidney	CDV[8,15] Canine adenovirus[8,15] Canine herpesvirus[8,15] Parvoviruses[8,16] Canine parainfluenza virus[8] Canine calicivirus[4] Rotaviruses[17] Influenza viruses[18] FeLV[19] *Neospora caninum*[20]
Crandell-Rees feline kidney cells	Fetal kidney	FHV-1[21] FCV[21,22] FCoV[23] Parvoviruses[24] FIV[25]
HL-60	Human leukemia	*Anaplasma phagocytophilum*[26]
A-72	Canine fibroma	Canine adenovirus[27] Canine coronavirus[27] Canine parainfluenza virus[27] Canine herpesvirus[27] Canine parvovirus
McCoy	Mouse fibroblast	*Chlamydia felis*[28]
FCWF	*Felis catus* whole fetus, has characteristics of macrophages	FCoV[29] FHV-1[30]
DH-82	Monocyte/macrophage	*Ehrlichia canis*[31]

CDV, canine distemper virus; *FCoV*, feline coronavirus; *FCV*, feline calicivirus; *FeLV*, feline leukemia virus; *FHV-1*, feline herpesvirus-1; *FIV*, feline immunodeficiency virus.

Cells for culture are stored in the laboratory in liquid nitrogen tanks. The cells are thawed, dispersed in cell culture medium, and allowed to settle on the bottom of a plastic flask (Fig. 1.1). The cell culture medium keeps the cells moist and provides the cells with nutrients. *Minimum essential medium* (MEM), also known as *Eagle's MEM*, and *Dulbecco's medium* are examples of widely used synthetic cell culture media. The cell culture medium contains a balanced salt solution, essential amino acids, glucose, vitamins, and a bicarbonate buffering system. Variations of MEM are available, some of which contain nonessential amino acids, the pH indicator phenol red, and the pH buffering agent HEPES (4-(2-hydroxyethyl)-1-piperazineethanesulfonic acid), which helps to maintain a physiologic pH despite the increasing concentration of CO_2 that is produced as a result of cellular respiration. The medium often requires supplementation with animal serum, most commonly fetal bovine serum, which is essential for the establishment of primary cell cultures. Serum-free medium has been used successfully for culture of canine and feline viruses,[8] but it is impractical to use in a diagnostic laboratory if multiple cell lines are being used as each one would need to be adapted to serum-free conditions.

To prevent bacterial or fungal contamination when viral pathogens are cultured, careful attention to sterile technique is required. Cell propagation procedures are generally performed in a biosafety cabinet and the culture medium used for isolation procedures is always supplemented with broad-spectrum antibiotics (ciprofloxacin, gentamicin, ampicillin) with or without an antifungal agent (amphotericin B or nystatin). Even with these precautions, an occasional specimen will be unsuitable for the full isolation procedure due to overgrowth with bacteria or a fungus. Cell culture flasks are placed in a humidified incubator that maintains temperature usually at 37°C, and a gas mixture that typically contains 5% CO_2 if the cultures are open to the atmosphere.

The cell culture flasks are removed from the incubator and examined using an inverted, phase contrast binocular tissue culture microscope (see Fig. 1.1), which allows examination of unstained cells through the bottom of the flask. Cells grown for isolation procedures should be in a semiconfluent state so that they can continue to replicate in the early phases of the isolation procedure. Viruses such as canine parvovirus will not grow in nonreplicating cells. In order to passage the cells, the medium is removed, and a small volume of trypsin or EDTA solution is added to the monolayer. The monolayer is incubated with the solution for several minutes, after which the cells detach from the flask and are resuspended in medium. Depending on the cell type, one confluent monolayer may be "split" into 3 to 10 new cultures.

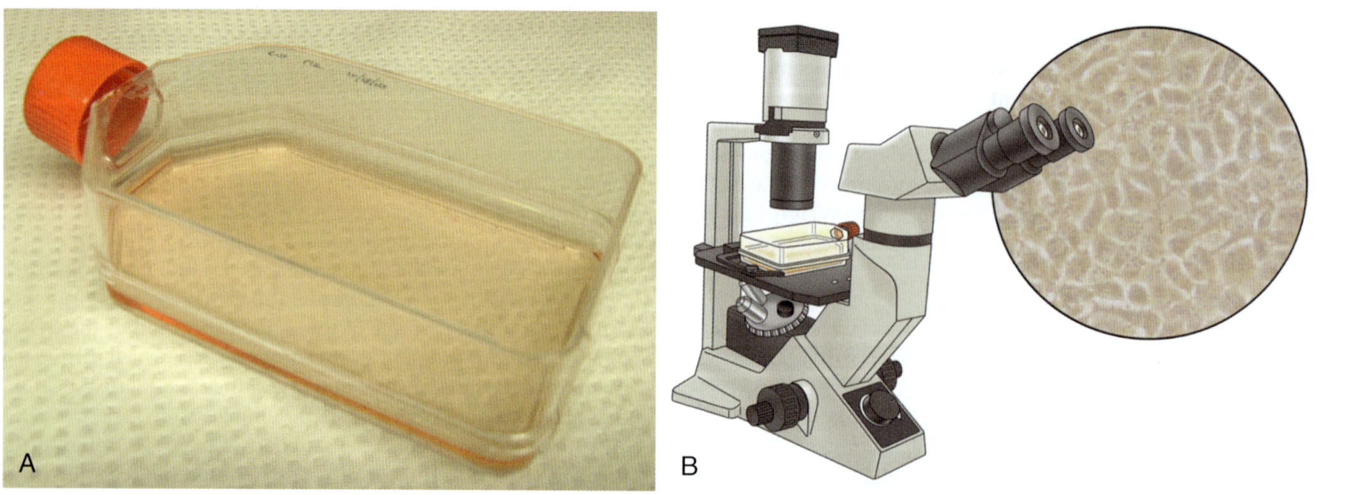

Fig. 1.1 (A) Plastic flask that contains cell culture medium. (B) A confluent cell monolayer is present at the bottom of the flask and can be visualized through the top of the flask using a binocular inverted microscope.

Occasionally, cell lines become cross-contaminated with other cell lines. The HeLa cell line is an example of a prolific and hardy cell line that commonly contaminates other cell cultures. Major cell line repositories such as the American Type Culture Collection (ATCC) use genetic typing methods to verify the identity of the cells in their collection. Receiving cell cultures from colleagues runs the risk that the culture may not be from the species claimed. Cell lines can also become easily contaminated with mycoplasmas, which pass through filters used to exclude other bacteria. The use of pipetting devices and biosafety cabinets has reduced the issue of mycoplasma contamination, but hundreds of lines are in use in research laboratories that are still contaminated. The presence of contaminating mycoplasmas can interfere with replication of other pathogens and cause alterations of cellular morphology. Mycoplasma contamination is detected using stains such as Hoechst stain (DNA stain), culture for *Mycoplasma* spp., and commercially available PCR assays that specifically detect mycoplasma DNA for the purpose of cell culture quality assurance.[9] Contamination of cell lines with noncytopathic viruses led to the spurious identification of animal viruses as human pathogens, particularly agents in the family *Paramyxoviridae*. Fetal bovine serum was certainly the source of bovine viral diarrhea virus that contaminated the Crandell-Rees feline kidney (CRFK) cell line frequently used for feline virus propagation.

Inoculation of Cell Cultures

Inoculation of a cell monolayer is accomplished by removal of overlying medium and adding a suspension of test material onto the cell monolayer. If tissue specimens are provided for culture, the specimens are disrupted in culture medium before they are inoculated onto the monolayer. Specimens may first be centrifuged to remove cell debris and bacteria. Passage through an appropriately sized filter can also be used before inoculation to remove bacteria. Organisms within the inoculum are then allowed to settle on the monolayer for approximately 1 to 3 hours before the residual inoculum is removed and fresh maintenance medium is added.

For detection of virus, the monolayer is then examined daily for evidence of cytopathic effect (CPE). CPE refers to the cellular changes induced by viral replication in the cell culture monolayer and includes cell lysis, cell rounding, or cell fusion (syncytium formation). The presence of CPE is determined by the comparison of inoculated cultures with uninoculated (control) cultures. The presence of a particular viral

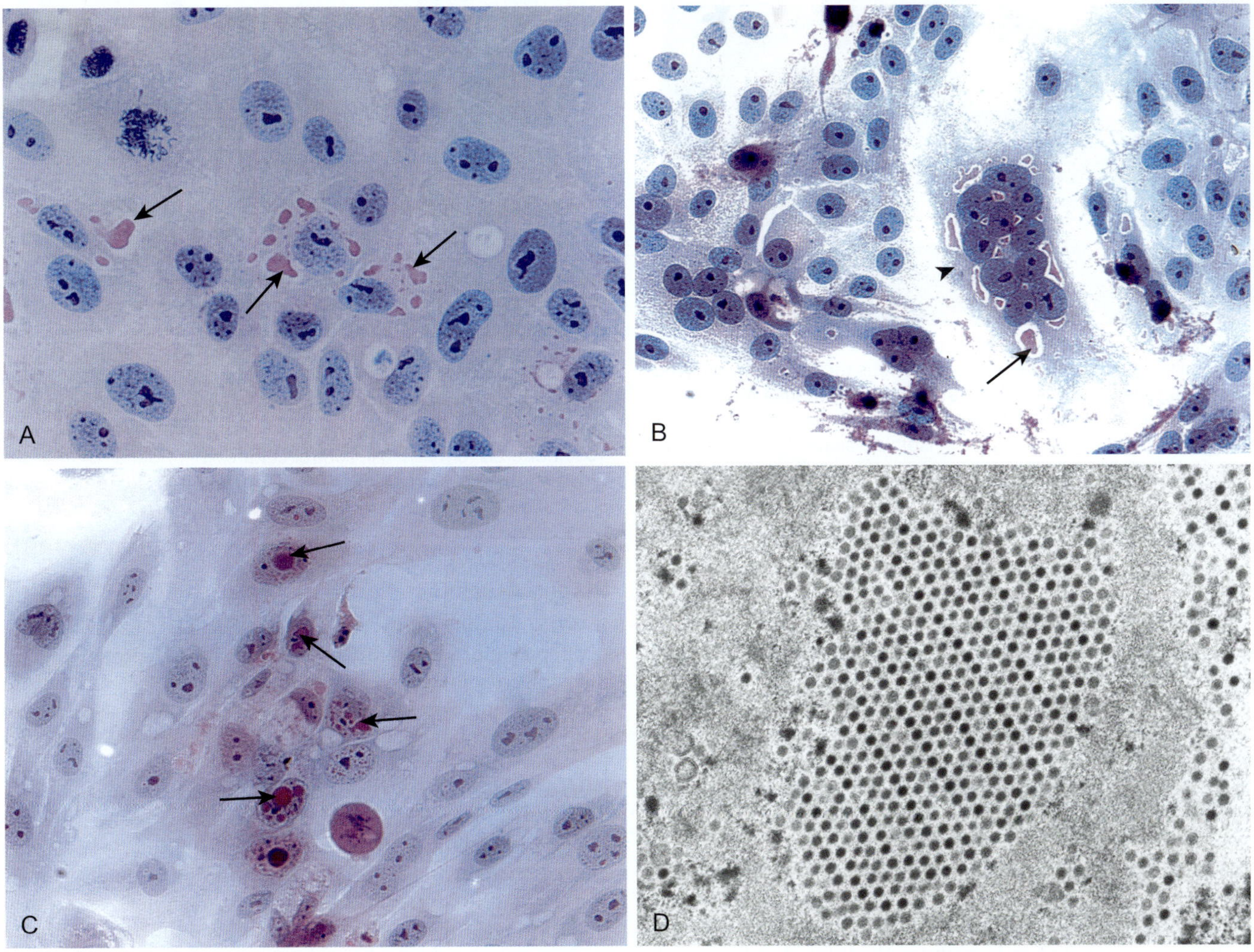

Fig. 1.2 Typical inclusions and abnormal cell morphology in virus-infected cells. (A) Reovirus inclusions *(arrows)* in infected Vero cells. (B) Canine distemper virus inclusions *(arrow)* and syncytium *(arrowhead)* in infected Vero cells. (C) Bovine adenovirus 5 intranuclear inclusions *(arrows)* in primary bovine kidney cells. (D) Transmission electron micrograph of an untyped adenovirus (gorilla) inclusion in A549 cells. (From Maclachlan NJ, Dubovi EJ. *Fenner's Veterinary Virology*. 4th ed. New York: Academic Press; 2011.)

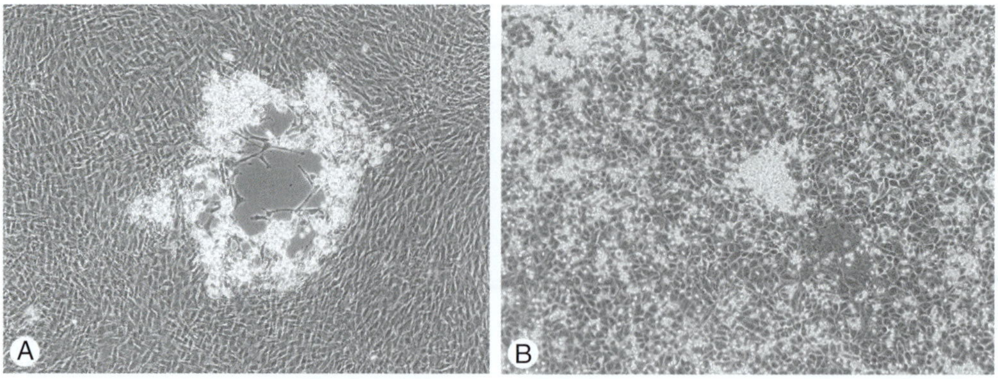

Fig. 1.3 (A) Cytopathic effect produced by a herpesvirus in feline lung cells. Note focal area of rounded and detached cells. (B) Hemadsorption: chicken erythrocytes adsorb to parainfluenza virus-infected cells that have incorporated hemagglutinin into the plasma membrane. (Courtesy of E. Dubovi, Cornell University.)

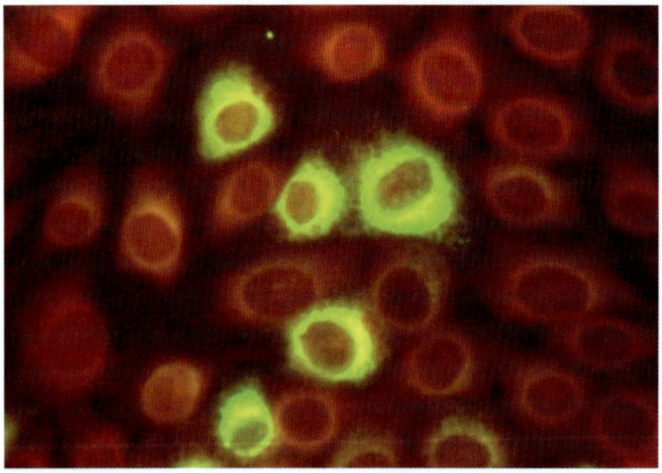

Fig. 1.4 Indirect fluorescent antibody detection of noncytopathic virus-infected cells. A cell monolayer exposed to virus for 72 hours was fixed with cold acetone. Fixed cells were stained with a mouse monoclonal antibody specific for bovine viral diarrhea virus, followed by a goat anti-mouse serum tagged with fluorescein isothiocyanate. (From Maclachlan NJ, Dubovi EJ. *Fenner's Veterinary Virology.* 4th ed. New York: Academic Press; 2011.)

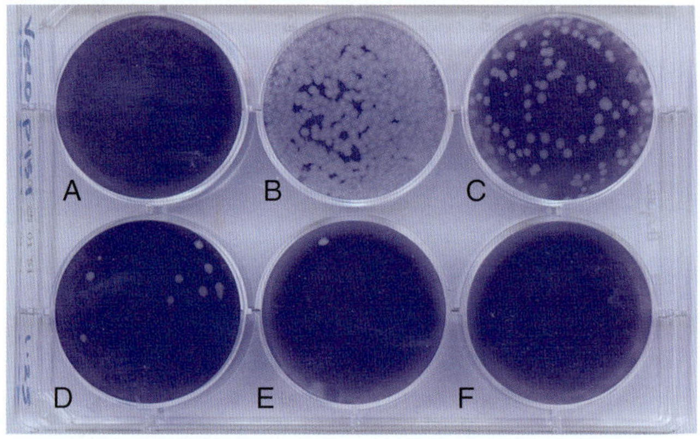

Fig. 1.5 Determination of the concentration of infectious virus using a plaque assay. Vero cell monolayers were inoculated with serial 10-fold dilutions of vesicular stomatitis virus. After a 1-hour adsorption period, cultures were overlaid with 0.75% agarose in cell culture medium containing 5% fetal bovine serum. Cultures were incubated for 3 days at 37°C in a 5% humidified CO_2 atmosphere. The agarose overlay was removed and cultures fixed and stained with 0.75% crystal violet in 10% buffered formalin. (A) Control culture. (B–F) Serial 10-fold dilution of virus: (B) 10^{-3}, (C) 10^{-4}, (D) 10^{-5}, (E) 10^{-6}, (F) 10^{-7}. (From Maclachlan NJ, Dubovi EJ. *Fenner's Veterinary Virology.* 4th ed. New York: Academic Press; 2011.)

pathogen is suspected by the appearance of characteristic CPE for that pathogen after a predicted incubation period (Fig. 1.2). For example, CPE induced by FCV is characterized by cell rounding and detachment that can occur within 24 hours, and within 16 hours for highly virulent strains.[10] Examination of the cell monolayer using light microscopy after fixation and staining can reveal additional diagnostic features, such as the presence of inclusion bodies and syncytium formation. Some viruses are relatively noncytopathogenic. The presence of some of these viruses can be demonstrated by adding washed erythrocytes to the monolayer and examination of the monolayer for evidence of hemadsorption (Fig. 1.3). Hemadsorption results from incorporation of viral surface hemagglutinin molecules into the plasma membranes of the cell culture monolayer. Parainfluenza viruses from many animal species are examples of hemadsorbing viruses that produce minimal CPE. Other, more sensitive and specific methods for identification of an organism that has infected a cell culture monolayer include fixation and staining of the monolayer with specific fluorescent antibodies (Fig. 1.4), use of molecular techniques such as PCR, or use of electron microscopy.

Plaque Assays

In 1915, with the discovery of viruses that infect bacteria, came the development of a laboratory procedure that had a profound effect on many aspects of virology. This procedure was the *plaque assay*, which permitted simple determination of the quantity of virus in a specimen. With the advent of cell culture, the same type of assay was developed for those viruses that are cytolytic for the host cells. Serial dilutions of virus are added to monolayers of susceptible cells. The monolayers are then overlaid with agar or methylcellulose, which restricts the spread of the virus to those cells adjacent to the initially infected cell. After an incubation time defined by the type of virus, "holes" in the monolayer, or *plaques*, can be visualized (Fig. 1.5). The monolayer can then be stained to make the plaques easier to see, and the number of plaques are counted in order to determine the amount of virus in the inoculum. Plaque assays are commonly used by researchers to assess the efficacy of antiviral treatments through reduction of plaque formation. This same principle of a reduction in plaque number is used to assess the amount of antibody in a serum sample. The plaque reduction

TABLE 1.4 Biosafety Levels (BSLs) Set for Diagnosis of Laboratory Practices

Level	Risk	Examples	Example Precautions
BSL 1	Minimal potential hazard to human health and the environment	CAdV-1, nonpathogenic *Escherichia coli*	Gloves, standard microbiologic practices using bench-top techniques. Routine decontamination practices (hand washing, routine bench disinfection, autoclaving of infectious waste)
BSL 2	Moderate potential hazard to human health and the environment. Organisms cause mild disease or are difficult to contract as laboratory aerosols. Agents for which effective vaccines or antibiotic treatment exist.	Most veterinary viruses, including influenza viruses	Access to the laboratory restricted when work is taking place; extreme precautions with sharp contaminated materials; use of appropriate biosafety cabinets when generation of aerosols possible. Eye protection. No requirement for directional airflow into the laboratory
BSL 3	Dangerous agents that can be transmitted by aerosol.	West Nile virus Equine encephalitis viruses, *Rickettsia rickettsii, Coxiella burnetii, Mycobacterium tuberculosis*	Laboratory is located away from high-traffic areas. Restricted laboratory access when work in progress; double door entry, ventilation providing airflow into the room, exhaust air not recirculated; special practices and protective clothing for BSL 3, including biosafety cabinet use; special floor and ceiling materials specified
BSL 4	Dangerous and exotic agents that pose a high risk of aerosol-transmitted laboratory infections, or which produce severe or fatal disease in humans	Ebola virus Marburg virus Smallpox virus Lassa fever virus	Hazmat suit and self-contained oxygen system, entrance containing multiple showers, a vacuum room, an ultraviolet light room, and multiple airlocked doors. Strict control of laboratory access to authorized personnel

neutralization test is widely used to test for antibodies to West Nile virus, Zika virus, and many other arboviruses where there is significant cross-reactivity among the neutralizing antibodies.

Laboratory Safety Concerns That Relate to Cell Culture

The processing of specimens in a biological safety cabinet not only serves to protect cultures from contamination but also acts to protect the laboratory worker from laboratory-acquired infections. Cell cultures alone are considered biohazards and disposal of the cultures and culture fluids must follow the guidelines for disposal of regulated medical waste. Most viruses grown in veterinary diagnostic laboratories are classified as pathogens that should be handled with biosafety level 2 (BSL 2) equipment and procedures. BSLs range from 1 through 4 (Table 1.4). In the United States, the Centers for Disease Control and Prevention (CDC) defines the biosafety procedures and classifies pathogens as to the BSLs needed to safely work with the pathogens. It is important that veterinary clinicians are aware that isolation of hazardous pathogens can only be conducted in specially designed and accredited laboratories.

INTERPRETATION OF RESULTS

Negative Results

Reasons for negative test results using virus isolation are numerous, so the clinician should not assume that a virus is not present when a negative test result is obtained (Box 1.2). Negative test results can occur due to: (1) a lack of viral shedding by the animal at the time of specimen collection, (2) the binding of antibodies to viruses within the specimen, (3) inadequate organism numbers at the anatomic site of specimen collection, or (4) loss of organism viability during transportation to the laboratory. Loss of viral viability is more likely to occur with enveloped viruses such as CDV than with nonenveloped, hardy viruses such as canine parvovirus or FCV. Negative test results can also occur when the cell line inoculated is not sensitive to the virus present in the specimen. This could be because the wrong cell line was used to test for a virus that could be cultured, or a viral pathogen existed in the sample for which no cell line was capable of growing *in vitro*, e.g., canine circovirus.

BOX 1.2 Reasons for Negative Test Results Following Isolation of Viruses in Cell Culture

- Virus not causing the disease
- No viral shedding at the time of sampling
- No viral shedding at the site of sampling
- Antibody interference with viral infectivity for cell culture
- Inadequate organism numbers at the anatomic site of specimen collection
- Loss of organism viability during transportation to the laboratory
- Overgrowth of one viral pathogen by another
- Overgrowth by bacterial or fungal agents
- Lack of cell sensitivity for the virus (wrong cell type inoculated)
- Laboratory inexperience with techniques required for virus isolation and identification

Inconclusive test results can also occur if the cultures are overgrown by bacteria or fungi before a virus test on the cells can be done. Although treatment of the viral transport and culture media with antimicrobials can help prevent this, resistant bacteria or fungi may still be present. Sometimes, multiple viruses are present within a specimen, and one virus overgrows another. For example, this can occur with mixed infections with FCV and FHV-1 in cats with upper respiratory tract disease. FCV rapidly infects CRFK cells and produces CPE, which obscures the concurrent presence of FHV-1.

Positive Results

It is imperative that veterinary clinicians be aware that the detection of a virus in a specimen does not always imply that the organism is the cause of the animal's clinical signs. This is especially true for specimens collected from the respiratory or gastrointestinal tracts, where multiple infectious agents may be present concurrently, and in many cases, viruses can replicate in these locations without causing clinical signs of illness. This is not as big an issue with virus isolation as it is with PCR panel tests where multiple potential pathogens are detected. In some animals, the development of severe clinical signs is more likely when there is simultaneous presence of multiple infectious agents. As noted previously for specimens that test negative, the presence of one agent may also obscure the presence of another, more significant organism (such as with FCV and FHV-1 co-infections), which could result in the incorrect assumption that only one organism is the cause of an animal's disease.

REFERENCES

1. Heikkinen T, Marttila J, Salmi AA, et al. Nasal swab versus nasopharyngeal aspirate for isolation of respiratory viruses. *J Clin Microbiol.* 2002;40(11):4337–4339.
2. World Health Organization guidance on regulations for the Transport of Infectious Substances 2019-2020. https://apps.who.int/iris/bitstream/handle/10665/325884/WHO-WHE-CPI-2019.20-eng.pdf?ua=1.
3. Schobesberger M, Zurbriggen A, Summerfield A, et al. Oligodendroglial degeneration in distemper: apoptosis or necrosis? *Acta Neuropathol.* 1999;97(3):279–287.
4. Maeda Y, Tohya Y, Matsuura Y, et al. Early interaction of canine calicivirus with cells is the major determinant for its cell tropism in vitro. *Vet Microbiol.* 2002;87(4):291–300.
5. Le LP, Rivera AA, Glasgow JN, et al. Infectivity enhancement for adenoviral transduction of canine osteosarcoma cells. *Gene Ther.* 2006;13(5):389–399.
6. Hemphill A, Vonlaufen N, Golaz JL, et al. Infection of primary canine duodenal epithelial cell cultures with *Neospora caninum*. *J Parasitol.* 2009;95(2):372–380.
7. Skloot R. The Immortal Life of Henrietta Lacks. Crown Publishers: New York.
8. Mochizuki M. Growth characteristics of canine pathogenic viruses in MDCK cells cultured in RPMI 1640 medium without animal protein. *Vaccine.* 2006;24(11):1744–1748.
9. Young L, Sung J, Stacey G, et al. Detection of Mycoplasma in cell cultures. *Nat Protoc.* 2010;5:929–934.
10. Ossiboff RJ, Sheh A, Shotton J, et al. Feline caliciviruses (FCVs) isolated from cats with virulent systemic disease possess in vitro phenotypes distinct from those of other FCV isolates. *J Gen Virol.* 2007;88(t 2):506–517.
11. Narang HK. Ultrastructural study of long-term canine distemper virus infection in tissue culture cells. *Infect Immun.* 1982;36(1):310–319.
12. Lan NT, Yamaguchi R, Uchida K, et al. Growth profiles of recent canine distemper isolates on Vero cells expressing canine signaling lymphocyte activation molecule (SLAM). *J Comp Pathol.* 2005;133(1):77–81.
13. Cory J, Yunker CE, Ormsbee RA, et al. Plaque assay of rickettsiae in a mammalian cell line. *Appl Microbiol.* 1974;27(6):1157–1161.
14. Buckley SM. Survival of *Toxoplasma gondii* in mosquito cell lines and establishment of continuous infection in Vero cell cultures. *Exp Parasitol.* 1973;33(1):23–26.
15. Cornwell HJ, Weir AR, Wright NG, et al. The susceptibility of a dog kidney cell-line (MDCK) to canine distemper, infectious canine hepatitis and canine herpesvirus. *Res Vet Sci.* 1970;11(6):580–582.
16. Basak S, Compans W. Polarized entry of canine parvovirus into an epithelial cell line. *J Virol.* 1989;63(7):3164–3167.
17. England JJ, Poston RP. Electron microscopic identification and subsequent isolation of a rotavirus from a dog with fatal neonatal diarrhea. *Am J Vet Res.* 1980;41(5):782–783.
18. Bao L, Xu L, Zhan L, et al. Challenge and polymorphism analysis of the novel (H1N1) influenza virus to normal animals. *Virus Res.* 2010;151(1):60–65.
19. Essex M, Kawakami TG, Kurata K. Continuous long-term replication of feline leukemia virus (FeLV) in an established canine cell culture (MDCK). *Proc Soc Exp Biol Med.* 1972;139(1):295–299.
20. Nishikawa Y, Iwata A, Nagasawa H, et al. Comparison of the growth inhibitory effects of canine IFN-alpha, -beta, and -gamma on canine cells infected with *Neospora caninum* tachyzoites. *J Vet Med Sci.* 2001;63(4): 445–458.
21. Crandell RA, Fabricant CG, Nelson-Rees WA. Development, characterization, and viral susceptibility of a feline (*Felis catus*) renal cell line (CRFK). *In Vitro.* 1973;9(3):176–185.
22. Kreutz LC, Seal BS, Mengeling WL. Early interaction of feline calicivirus with cells in culture. *Arch Virol.* 1994;136(1–2):19–34.
23. Van Hamme E, Dewerchin HL, Cornelissen E, et al. Attachment and internalization of feline infectious peritonitis virus in feline blood monocytes and Crandell feline kidney cells. *J Gen Virol.* 2007;88(Pt 9):2527–2532.
24. Hirasawa T, Tsujimura N, Konishi S. Multiplication of canine parvovirus in CRFK cells. *Nippon Juigaku Zasshi.* 1985;47(1):89–99.
25. Talbott RL, Sparger EE, Lovelace KM, et al. Nucleotide sequence and genomic organization of feline immunodeficiency virus. *Proc Natl Acad Sci USA.* 1989;86(15):5743–5747.
26. Goodman JL, Nelson C, Vitale B, et al. Direct cultivation of the causative agent of human granulocytic ehrlichiosis. *N Engl J Med.* 1996;334(4):209–215.
27. Binn LN, Marchwicki RH, Stephenson EH. Establishment of a canine cell line: derivation, characterization, and viral spectrum. *Am J Vet Res.* 1980;41(6):855–860.
28. Wills PJ, Johnson L, Thompson RG. Isolation of *Chlamydia* using McCoy cells and Buffalo green monkey cells. *J Clin Pathol.* 1984;37(2):120–121.
29. Mochizuki M, Mitsutake Y, Miyanohara Y, et al. Antigenic and plaque variations of serotype II feline infectious peritonitis coronaviruses. *J Vet Med Sci.* 1997;59(4):253–258.
30. Horimoto T, Kasaoka T, Tuchiya K, et al. An improved method for hemagglutinin extraction from feline herpesvirus type 1-infected cell line. *Nippon Juigaku Zasshi.* 1989;51(1):177–183.
31. Iqbal Z, Chaichanasiriwithaya W, Rikihisa Y. Comparison of PCR with other tests for early diagnosis of canine ehrlichiosis. *J Clin Microbiol.* 1994;32(7):1658–1662.

2

Immunoassays

Jane E. Sykes, Shelley C. Rankin, Rance K. Sellon, James F. Evermann

KEY POINTS

- Immunoassays are commonly used in practice to detect antigen or antibody in body fluids. Immunoassays are also used to assess the need for vaccination for certain pathogens, and the need to provide booster vaccinations for animals in high-risk (e.g., kennels, catteries) environments.
- The term *serology* is most often used to refer to assays that detect antibody in serum.
- Immunoassays that detect antigen or antibody in animals suspected to have an infectious disease include enzyme-linked immunosorbent assay (ELISA), enzyme immunoassay (EIA), colloidal gold-based immunochromatographic assay (GICA), immunofluorescence assay (IFA), immunohistochemistry (IHC), western immunoblotting, agglutination tests, agar gel immunodiffusion (AGID), complement fixation (CF), and serum neutralization assays.
- Positive immunoassay results do not always imply active infection, and negative results do not rule out infection (e.g., mucosal infection).
- When interpreting the results of immunoassays, veterinarians should know what is being measured (antigen or antibody), and consider the likelihood of antigen or antibody being present in relation to the onset of illness, whether the positive test result is consistent with clinical signs, the animal's vaccination history, and immune status. The possibility of false-positive results due to immunologic cross-reactivity, as well as the analytical sensitivity and specificity of the test used (i.e., the test's performance), must also be considered.
- Additional assays, such as nucleic acid amplification tests, may be required to support or confirm a diagnosis made by an immunoassay.

INTRODUCTION

Serology is the measurement of antigen-antibody interactions for diagnostic purposes, but is most often used to refer to the detection of antibodies in serum. Assays used to measure antigen-antibody interactions can also be used on body fluids other than serum such as plasma, urine, CSF, thoracic or abdominal fluids, and aqueous humor. Assays have been designed that detect specific classes of antibodies, most commonly IgG or IgM. Methods used to detect specific antibodies can also be applied to detect specific antigens.

Assays that measure antigen-antibody interactions for diagnostic purposes are broadly referred to as *immunoassays*. Some types of immunoassay include enzyme-linked immunosorbent assay (ELISA), immunofluorescence assay (IFA), colloidal gold-based immunochromatographic assay (GICA), complement fixation (CF), agglutination tests, agar gel immunodiffusion (AGID or gel ID tests), and western blotting.[1] Many of these assays involve the use of *polyclonal antibodies* or, more commonly, *monoclonal antibodies,* which are commercially available. Polyclonal antibodies are produced in animals (e.g., rabbits or horses) as a normal response to antigen exposure. Monoclonal antibodies are derived from murine antigen-primed B cells that are fused with tumor cells to create a hybridoma cell culture line. Once in culture, virtually unlimited amounts of antibody are produced with a high degree of antigenic specificity.

In general, a blood sample is *seroreactive* (or *seropositive*) if it contains antibodies to a particular organism. Some immunoassays, such as ELISA and IFA, provide quantitative results, expressed as optical density units (ODs) or titers (e.g., 1:800, or *reciprocal titer* = 800). Exposure of an immunocompetent individual to an infectious agent results in a rise in antibody titer over time (Fig. 2.1). The first antibody class to be produced by plasma cells is IgM, after which IgG synthesis by plasma cells occurs. When infection by a pathogen occurs for the first time, there is a lag phase of 5 to 7 days before IgM antibodies can be detected in the blood *(primary antibody response).* Over time, the antibody titer, composed predominantly of IgG antibodies, increases, and if the infectious agent is cleared by the host immune system, there is a progressive decline in the titer over weeks to months. The speed and magnitude by which the antibody titer rises depends on host factors and the infectious agent involved. For some diseases, such as leptospirosis, a significant rise occurs within 3 to 4 days of the onset of clinical signs. In secondary, or anamnestic, immune responses, the lag phase is shorter, the antibody titer increases more rapidly and to a greater magnitude, and antibodies may persist for longer periods of time (months to years).

Serologic diagnosis of infectious diseases relies on an understanding of the timing of the antibody response in relation to development of clinical signs. The results of serologic testing are interpreted differently for acute infections than they are for chronic, persistent, or mucosal infections. *For infections with a short incubation period,* such as leptospirosis or Rocky Mountain spotted fever, antibody is often undetectable (i.e., the patient is seronegative) in the first week of illness, although recently available assays offer potential for earlier diagnosis of leptospirosis because of IgM detection.[2] In general, an increase in antibody titers over a 2- to 4-week period then occurs. *Seroconversion* is consistent with recent infection, and at least a fourfold increase in titer is required for the change to be considered significant (e.g., 1:4 to 1:16; 1:128 to 1:512). Because serologic test results can differ between laboratories that perform the same assay, the same laboratory should be used to determine the acute and the convalescent titer. Rather than an increase in titer, a fourfold decline in the antibody titer also may

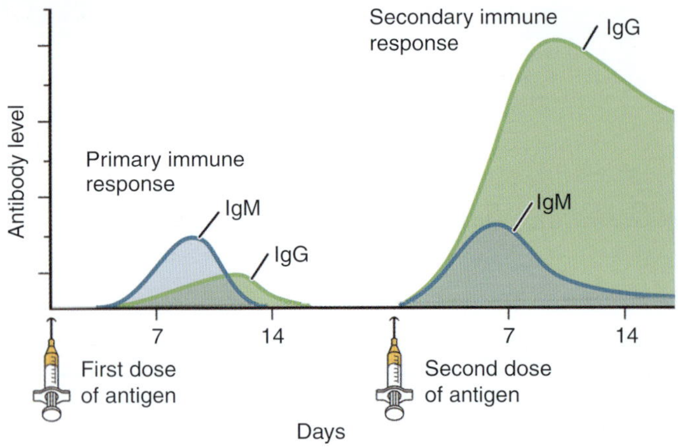

Fig. 2.1 Time course of primary and secondary immune responses, showing relative amounts of IgM and IgG produced at different times after antigen exposure. (Modified from Tizard IR. *Veterinary Immunology*. 8th ed. St Louis: Saunders; 2008.)

be consistent with recent infection, depending on the stage of illness at which serologic testing is performed. *For chronic, persistent infections,* such as those caused by FIV or *Ehrlichia canis*, a single, positive antibody titer can indicate active infection. Titer increases do not occur when infection persists beyond 1 to 2 months, and so acute- and convalescent-phase serology is not useful for diagnosis of chronic infections.

SPECIMEN COLLECTION AND TRANSPORT

Blood collected for antibody testing should be allowed to clot, or collected in a serum separator tube. Once the serum is separated, it can be removed and refrigerated or frozen. Serum can be refrigerated for up to a week before it is shipped to the laboratory. If testing is to be delayed for longer than a week, serum should be frozen at –20°C or –80°C. Serum can be stored frozen (frost-free freezers not recommended) for years without loss of antibody titer. For serum and other body fluid specimens collected for antigen testing, assay results may be more susceptible to variation with specimen storage. The laboratory should always be contacted in order to determine specimen storage and handling requirements.

DIAGNOSTIC METHODS

Immunofluorescence and Immunoperoxidase Antibody Assays

Direct IFA (also known as direct FA) detects *antigen* in clinical specimens. IFA involves the use of an antibody that has been tagged (*conjugated*) with a fluorescent label (such as fluorescein isothiocyanate) to detect the presence a specific antigen. IFA is performed directly on a glass slide, and fluorescence is detected by microscopy. The sensitivity of direct IFA is too low to detect individual virus particles or soluble antigen, so usually IFA detects accumulated antigen present in association with eukaryotic or bacterial cells in smears or tissues fixed on a glass slide. If the antigen is intracellular, pretreatment of the slide to permeabilize the cells may be necessary. The glass slide is then incubated with a solution that contains the fluorescent antibody, washed to remove unbound antibody, and the slide examined using a fluorescence microscope (Fig. 2.2). Examples of the use of direct IFA in veterinary medicine include detection of *Giardia* oocysts, FeLV within nucleated cells in peripheral blood or bone marrow, or CDV within epithelial cells from a conjunctival scraping, or lymphocytes

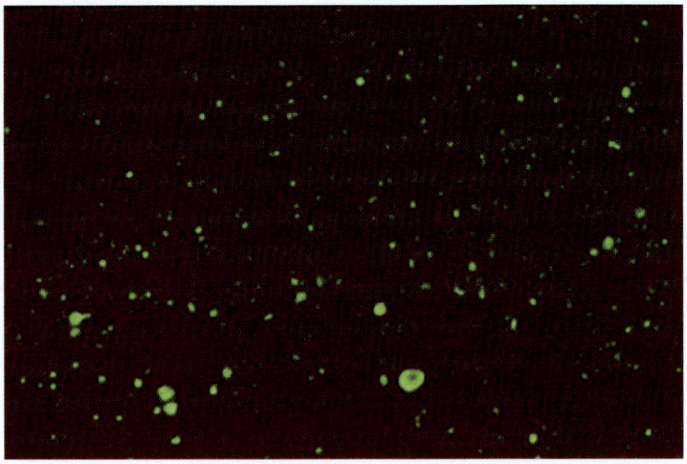

Fig. 2.2 Direct fluorescent antibody stain of brain tissue for rabies virus. Frozen tissue sections are stained with a commercial reagent that contains monoclonal antibodies specific for the rabies virus nucleocapsid. Antibodies are labeled with fluorescein. (From Centers for Disease Control and Prevention. Direct Fluorescent Antibody Test. https://www.cdc.gov/rabies/diagnosis/direct_fluorescent_antibody.html. Accessed April 28, 2022.)

from a peripheral blood smear. Nonspecific fluorescence can result in false positives using these methods, but this can be overcome with the inclusion of proper controls and technical expertise.

An alternative to the use of a fluorescein-conjugated antibody is the use of an antibody that has been conjugated to an enzyme such as horseradish peroxidase (immunoperoxidase). A substrate, most commonly 3,3′-diaminobenzidine (DAB), is then added to the slides. In the presence of hydrogen peroxide, DAB is converted to an insoluble brown precipitate which can be visualized using conventional light microscopy. This technique is known as *immunocytochemistry*. The same method, when applied to tissue sections, is known as *immunohistochemistry* (IHC; Fig. 2.3).

Indirect IFA (also known as IFA testing, or IFAT) is generally used to establish a serum *antibody* titer to an infectious agent, but it can also be used to detect antigen. When used to detect antigen, it is more sensitive than direct IFA. For measurement of antibody titer, patient serum is serially diluted in the laboratory and reacted with a known antigen that has been fixed to glass slides commercially manufactured for this purpose. Slides are then washed to remove unbound nonspecific antibody. A *secondary antibody*, conjugated to a fluorescent label and designed to react with the bound patient antibodies (e.g., dog IgG or dog IgM), is applied to the slides, which are washed again. The slides are then examined using a fluorescence microscope. The highest dilution of serum that results in specific fluorescence is reported as the antibody titer to the infectious agent of interest. Examples of the use of indirect IFA for serologic testing in dogs and cats include quantitative serology for some tick-borne infectious agents (e.g., *E. canis*, *Anaplasma* spp.), and antibody titer measurements to determine if an individual animal has adequate concentrations of specific IgG (e.g., to CDV).

Veterinary IFAs have been marketed that allow multiple antigen (or antibody) targets to be mounted on novel platforms, such as fluorescent beads or wells on the surface of a spinning silicon disc that resembles a compact disc. Automated silicon disc–based assays allow rapid and simultaneous analysis of hundreds of specimens, with dramatic reduction in labor associated with traditional IFAs or ELISAs, and reduced chance of false-positive or -negative assay results due to human error. A bead-based assay is currently available in the United States for detection of antibody to *Borrelia burgdorferi* (see Chapter

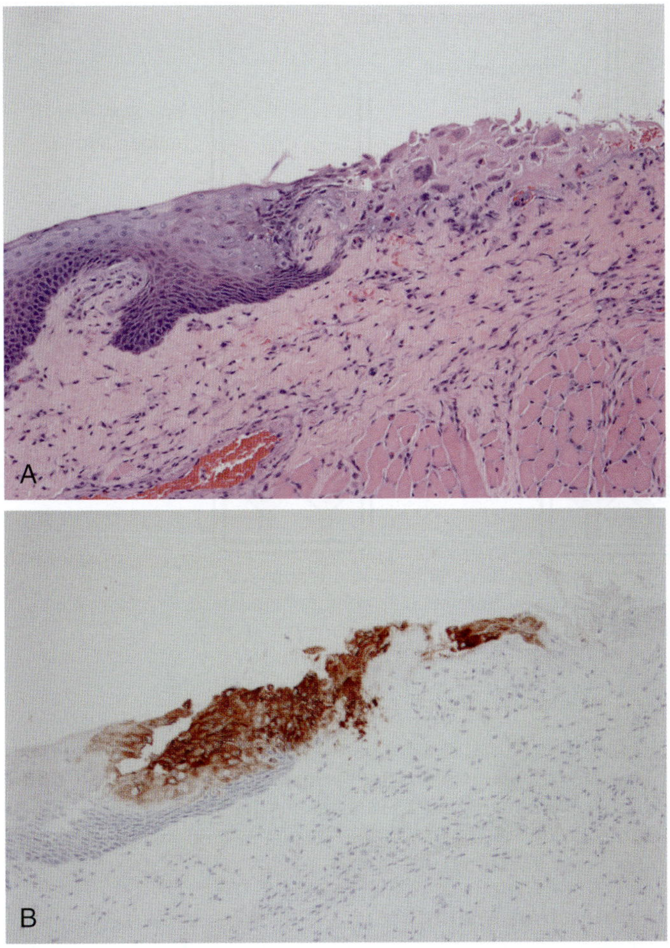

Fig. 2.3 Immunohistochemistry. (A) Hematoxylin and eosin–stained section of a lingual ulcer from a cat infected with feline herpesvirus-1. (B) The brown stained cells lining the ulcer are positive using an immunohistochemical stain for feline herpesvirus-1. (Courtesy of Dr. Patricia Pesavento, School of Veterinary Medicine, University of California, Davis.)

69) (Lyme Disease Multiplex Testing for Dogs, Animal Health Diagnostic Laboratory, Cornell University, NY, USA). A silicon disc–based assay is available in the United States for detection of antibodies to *B. burgdorferi, E. canis,* and *Anaplasma phagocytophilum* and antigen to *Dirofilaria immitis* (Accuplex 4, Antech Diagnostics, Irvine, CA, USA).

Enzyme-Linked Immunosorbent Assay (ELISA)

ELISA (also known as *enzyme immunoassay*)-based strategies can be used to detect antibody, whole antigen, or immunogenic peptides (those peptide sequences of a protein capable of inducing an immune response). In the laboratory, ELISA is usually performed in a polystyrene microtiter plate. However, modifications of the test, such as flow-through (as seen with SNAP tests by IDEXX Laboratories, ME, USA[3]), in which antigen or capture antibody is immobilized on a polyethylene matrix, are widely used as in-clinic assays in veterinary practices (e.g., for diagnosis of feline retrovirus, heartworm, *Giardia, Leishmania*, and tick-borne bacterial infections) (Fig. 2.4). For *antigen* detection, an unknown quantity of antigen in a clinical specimen is immobilized in the wells of the plate. The antigen is either bound directly to the surface of the plate, or is bound through the use of a *capture antibody*, an antibody adherent to the plate surface that specifically binds the antigen of interest *(sandwich ELISA)*. The antigen is then detected with an antibody, or for a sandwich ELISA, a second antibody, that is conjugated to an enzyme such as immunoperoxidase, and the substrate is added. This results in a color change, which can be read visually or using an ELISA plate reader (Fig. 2.5). The plate reader records optical density of the wells in comparison with that of the control wells, allowing assessment of the quantity of antigen present. The plates are washed with a detergent solution between steps, and this can be automated using an ELISA plate washer. Sandwich ELISAs have been used for detection of FeLV antigen in cat blood. In *competitive ELISA*, the test specimen (e.g., dog serum) that contains an unknown amount of antibody is mixed with a known amount of labeled antibody. The mixture is added to wells that contain known amounts of a capture antigen, and the labeled and unlabeled antibodies compete for antigen binding. The more

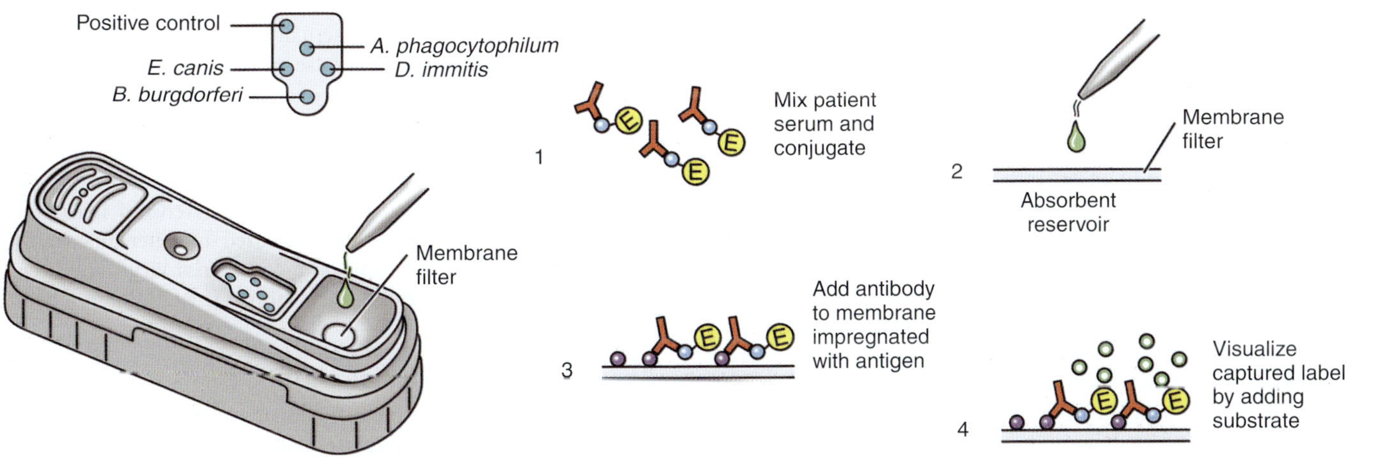

Fig. 2.4 Flow-through immunoassay device (IDEXX Laboratories, Inc.). Specific antigen (e.g., a recombinant protein) or antibody is immobilized on a membrane in the device in a spot or line. Patient serum that may or may not contain target antigen or antibody is mixed with a solution that contains conjugated antibody or antigen *(1)*. The solution is allowed to flow through the device, where it becomes captured on the membrane *(2 and 3)*. The device is activated (snapped), which releases wash and substrate reagents within the device. A positive reaction appears as a colored bar, or in this case, a dot *(4)*. Color development in designated spots on the membrane can indicate the presence of antibody to *Anaplasma* spp., *Ehrlichia* spp., and *Borrelia burgdorferi*, or the antigen of *Dirofilaria immitis*.

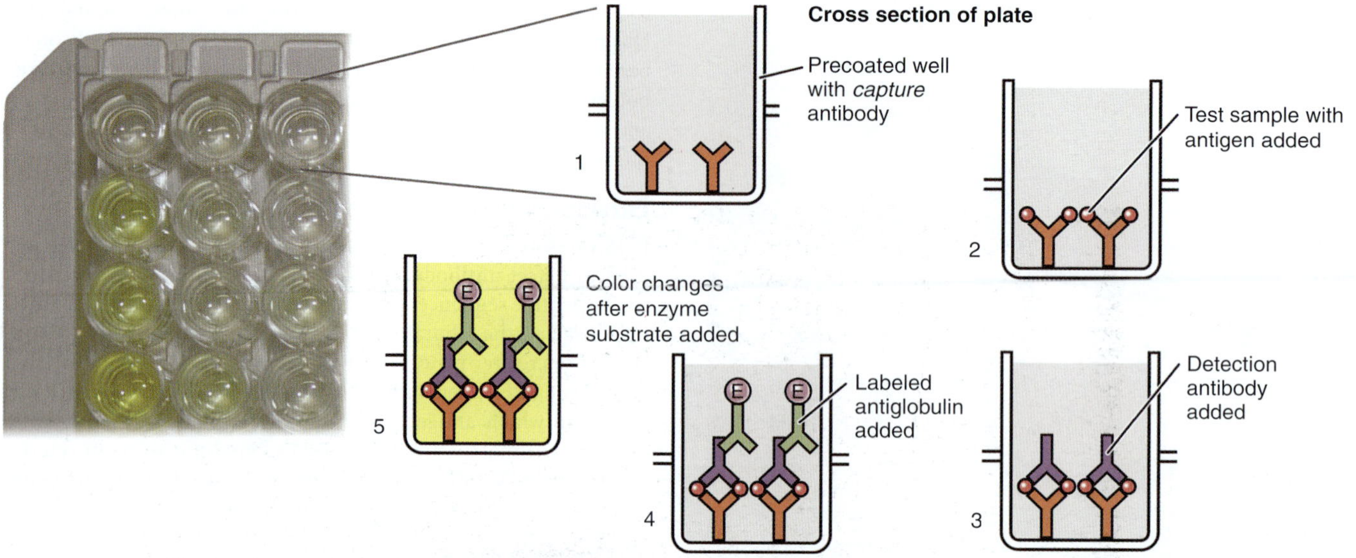

Fig. 2.5 Sandwich ELISA. An antibody is immobilized in the plate, which binds antigen in a test specimen. The antigen is then detected using an antibody that is conjugated to an enzyme such as immunoperoxidase, and the substrate is added, which results in a color change. (Modified from Tizard IR. *Veterinary Immunology.* 8th ed. St Louis: Saunders; 2008.)

labeled antibody that binds, the less antibody is present in the test specimen. Other variations of competitive ELISAs also exist.

For measurement of *antibody* titers, serial dilutions of serum can be added to a known amount of antigen fixed on a plate, and the antibodies detected using a secondary antibody.

Modifications of the ELISA test using the same principles of antibody or antigen binding to a substrate, and capture and detection strategies are also used in veterinary medicine. Examples include lateral-flow immunochromatographic tests whereby antigen or capture antibody is immobilized on a membrane filter, and detection of the antibody or antigen of interest is facilitated by gold nanoparticles (GICA), or colored nanobeads of other types, colored latex beads or fluorescent labels.[4] Because these assays do not use enzyme conjugates, they are not considered ELISAs. Paper-based platforms for immunochromatographic assays have also been explored to reduce cost and enhance ease of disposal.[5]

Western Immunoblotting

Western immunoblotting, also known as *western blotting,* is used to detect antibodies to an infectious agent in serum. After physical and/or chemical disruption of an organism, the organism's proteins are separated on the basis of molecular weight using vertical sodium dodecyl sulfate–polyacrylamide gel electrophoresis (SDS-PAGE). The protein bands are then transferred *(blotted)* to a nitrocellulose membrane using an electric current. The membrane is cut into vertical strips, and each strip is incubated with patient serum. If there are antibodies in the serum to antigens from the organism of interest, the antibodies bind to the specific antigens on the strip. The antigen-antibody complexes can then be visualized as discrete bands using secondary antibody-based immunoperoxidase detection methods. The pattern of band reactivity is specific for an immune response to that organism (Fig. 2.6). Western blotting has been offered commercially for the diagnosis of FIV infection and *B. burgdorferi* infection and has been used in research laboratories as the gold standard for the detection of antibody responses to vector-borne pathogens such as *E. canis.* In the case of FIV infection, western blotting has been used to confirm positive ELISA test results.[6] In the case of *B. burgdorferi* infection, western blotting has been evaluated for its ability to differentiate between the response to vaccination and natural exposure,[7] although some ELISA systems that incorporate a synthetic peptide identical to one expressed during natural infection offer this ability (see Chapter 69).

Agglutination Testing

Agglutination tests detect antibody or antigen and involve agglutination of bacteria, red cells, or antigen- or antibody-coated latex particles. Such tests rely on the bivalent nature of antibodies, which can cross-link particulate antigens. Serial dilutions of serum are tested for their ability to cause or inhibit agglutination, and the highest dilution that causes or inhibits agglutination is reported as the antibody or antigen titer. IgM causes agglutination more effectively than IgG. If excess antibody is present, particles may become so coated with antibody that agglutination is actually inhibited. This is called the *prozone effect* and can result in false-negative test results if serum is not adequately diluted. Examples of agglutination tests used to diagnose infectious diseases of dogs and cats include the microscopic agglutination test (MAT) for serologic diagnosis of leptospirosis (agglutination of live leptospires) and the cryptococcal antigen latex agglutination test (agglutination of antibody-coated latex beads). Hemagglutination inhibition (HI) is used to determine antibody titers to canine parvovirus and canine influenza virus, and it evaluates the ability of serum to inhibit erythrocyte agglutination by these viruses.

Agar Gel Immunodiffusion (AGID)

For AGID (gel ID or double diffusion) tests, round wells are cut in a layer of agar on a plastic plate using a punch. One well, usually the central well, is filled with a soluble antigen, and the other wells are filled with patient serum. A positive antibody control specimen is included in each assay. The reagents are allowed to diffuse into the agar, and when antibodies and antigen meet in optimal proportions (the *point of equivalence*), immune complexes form resulting in a visible line of precipitate between the antigen well and wells that contain positive serum (Fig. 2.7). Immunodiffusion

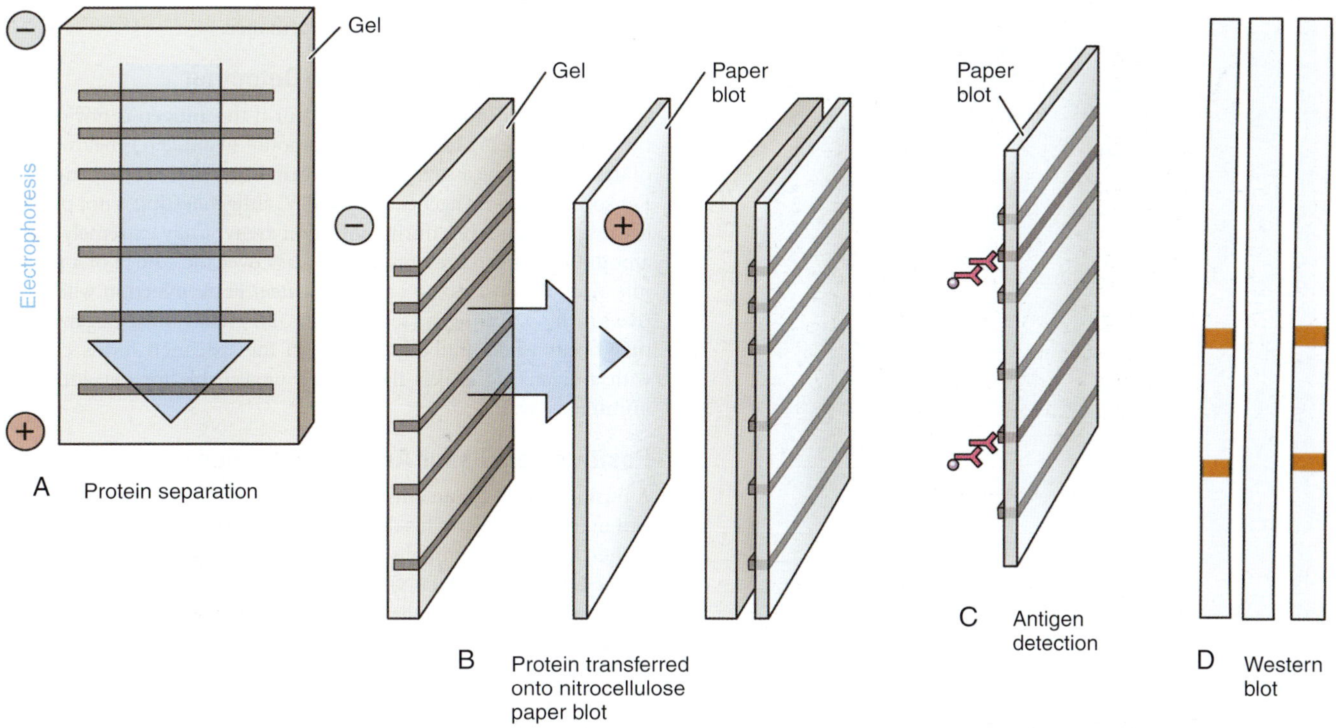

Fig. 2.6 Western blotting (immunoblotting). (A) Purified viruses or bacteria are disrupted and subjected to electrophoresis along the length of a polyacrylamide gel so that the proteins are separated according to their molecular weight. (B) The protein bands are transferred to a nitrocellulose paper membrane and (C) incubated with patient serum and then a labeled secondary antibody. (D) The outside strips represent a western blot that shows antibody reactivity to the antigens of feline immunodeficiency virus, while the middle strip reflects an absence of antibody reactivity.

tests are most often used to detect antibodies to fungal pathogens, such as *Aspergillus fumigatus*,[8] *Coccidioides* spp.,[9] and *Blastomyces* spp.,[10] and are also used to detect antibodies to *Brucella canis*.

Serum Neutralization

Serum neutralization is a technique used to determine the antibody titer to a virus. Serial dilutions of serum are mixed with a known quantity of virus particles. The mixture is incubated to allow the antibodies in the serum to bind to the virus particles, and the mixture is then added to a confluent cell monolayer. The highest dilution of serum that inhibits viral replication in the monolayer (as determined by examination for cytopathic effect or immunostaining) is the antibody titer reported by the laboratory. Serum neutralization can be used to detect antibodies to CDV and several respiratory viruses that infect dogs and cats.

Complement Fixation (CF) Testing

CF tests have largely been superseded by the use of ELISA-based tests. CF tests detect antibodies in serum. The test uses sheep red blood cells (RBCs), anti–sheep RBC antibody, and unheated guinea pig serum as a source of complement. Under normal circumstances, when these three reagents are mixed, the result is hemolysis which occurs when complement binds to antibody-coated RBC and triggers formation of the membrane attack complex, with resultant pore formation. In the CF test, a known antigen is added to patient serum heat-treated to inactivate complement in the test sample. When antigen-specific antibodies are present in the serum, addition of antigen leads to formation of antigen-antibody complexes. Guinea pig complement is then added to the mixture and is bound by the complexes. The resultant mixture is thus unable to lyse sensitized sheep RBCs. A lack of hemolysis indicates a positive CF test.

INTERPRETATION OF IMMUNOASSAY RESULTS

Interpretation of results of serology or immunoassay tests requires that the clinician knows whether the test detects antibody or antigen (Tables 2.1 and 2.2), and, if designed to detect antibody, whether the test is IgM-specific (detects early antibody responses), IgG-specific, or detects both immunoglobulin classes. Beyond diagnosis of infection, antigen detection assays can, when used serially during treatment for some infections (e.g., cryptococcosis; see Chapter 82), offer the additional advantage of predicting success (declining antigen concentrations) or failure (static or rising antigen concentrations) of therapy.

Immunoassay results should be interpreted in the context of the organism causing the infection, specifically the timing of antigen and antibody appearance in the body fluid being tested, and the prevalence of the infection in the population. Finally, the sensitivity and specificity of the test itself (i.e., the *analytical sensitivity and specificity*), which are determined during test validation should be available from the laboratory that performs the test (see also Chapter 7, Box 7.1). Some immunoassays that detect antigen will not generate a positive result unless a large amount of antigen is present in the specimen provided (low analytical sensitivity). Assays with low analytical specificity more commonly yield false-positive test results when testing animals from populations in which the prevalence of true positive test results is low, i.e., the prevalence of infection in the population is low. In this situation, a positive test has a *low positive predictive value*, and confirmatory testing may be required. A quality assurance program should be in effect in the diagnostic laboratory to ensure that specimens submitted are of adequate quality, that sufficient technical expertise is present to perform

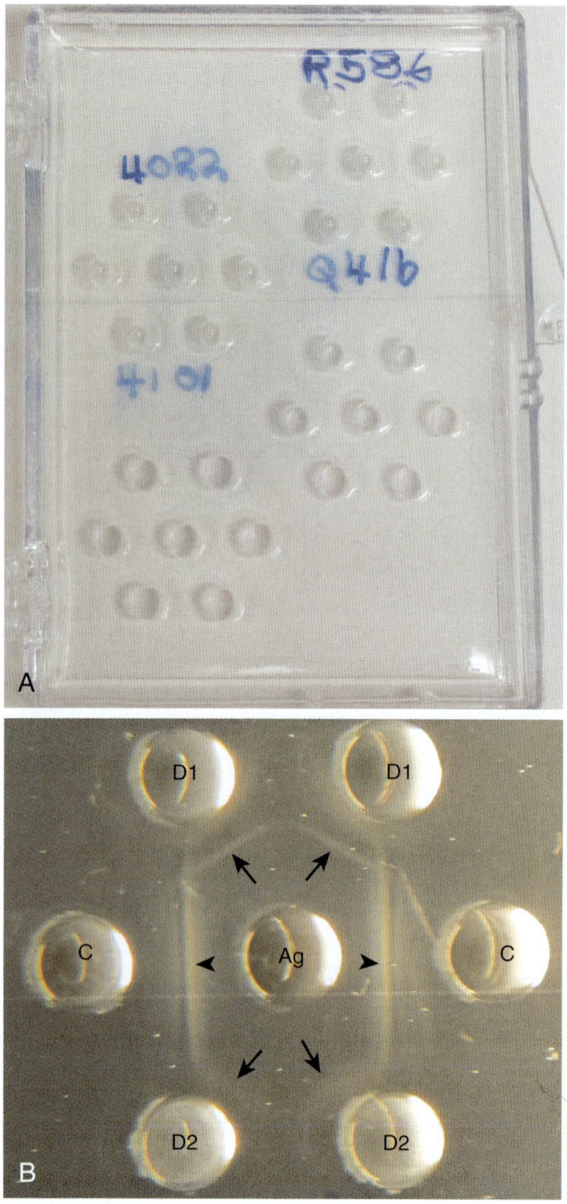

Fig. 2.7 (A) Gel immunodiffusion (or double diffusion) system used for detection of antibodies to *Aspergillus fumigatus, Histoplasma capsulatum, Blastomyces dermatitidis,* and *Coccidioides* spp. (Meridian Bioscience, Inc.). The kit consists of an agar diffusion medium in a small plastic tray that contains four arrays of six wells arranged around a central well. An antigen preparation for each of the fungal species is placed in the central well of each array. (B) Positive gel immunodiffusion for *Aspergillus fumigatus*. The central well *(Ag)* contains a purified carbohydrate preparation from mycelial phase cultures of *Aspergillus fumigatus, Aspergillus niger,* and *Aspergillus flavus*. The top two wells *(D1)* and the bottom two wells *(D2)* contain serum from two dogs (dog 1 and dog 2) with nasal aspergillosis (performed in duplicate for each dog). After the wells are loaded, the plate is incubated at room temperature for 24 hours. Precipitin lines form when the antigen and antibody diffuse out of each well and form immune complexes. A light box is used to illuminate the plate so the precipitin bands are visible. Both dogs are positive for antibody to the *Aspergillus* species tested *(small arrows)*, although the reaction is strongest for dog 1. The arrowheads point to the precipitin lines generated by the positive control antibodies *(C)*.

the tests, and that appropriate control assays are included with each test run to ensure proper assay performance.

Negative Results for Antigen Detection

A negative result for antigen will occur if the antigen is not present in the specimen being tested or if the amount of antigen is below the limit of detection of the assay (e.g., low worm burden in heartworm disease). For some infectious agents, such as FIV, antigen testing is not performed because antigen levels during infection are typically extremely low. The amount of antigen present can also vary over the course of a particular infection. For instance, a cat with a *latent* FeLV infection will be negative for the p27 antigen (see Chapter 32). Finally, false-negative results may occur when antibody present in the specimen forms complexes with antigen and makes the antigen unavailable for detection by the immunoassay.

Positive Results for Antigen Detection

A positive result for an antigen can indicate the presence of the organism in the specimen. This does not necessarily imply that the pathogen is the cause of an animal's clinical signs. Antigen can also be present in the absence of intact, viable organisms. Positive results can follow recent vaccination with the organism of interest. For example, positive parvovirus antigen test results have been suspected when tests have been performed on feces obtained several days after attenuated live parvovirus vaccination of kittens or puppies.[11,12] False positives can occur as a result of antigenic cross-reactivity with some other substance or organism in the specimen. An example is positive serum and urine antigen assays for *Aspergillus* spp. in dogs treated with Plasmalyte infusions or those infected with other molds such as *Paecilomyces* spp.[13]

Negative Results for Antibody Detection

A negative result for the presence of antibodies will occur if the patient has not been exposed to the infectious agent of interest, or if the patient has not had time to develop detectable antibody concentrations. For example, negative IgG antibody tests early in the course of illness are common with leptospirosis and canine granulocytic anaplasmosis. In this situation, a convalescent titer is required for diagnosis using serology. False-negative antibody test results can occur in severely immunosuppressed animals, such as in cats with advanced FIV infection that no longer can mount an immune response, or cats with advanced FIP (attributed to all patient antibody bound to viral particles and thus unable to bind to test substrate antigen). False-negative results may also occur because the test lacks sensitivity (i.e., low analytical sensitivity), or if the test detects the wrong class of immunoglobulin, e.g., IgG when infection is primarily mucosal and stimulating IgA production.[14]

Positive Results for Antibody Detection

A positive result for IgG antibody suggests *previous infection* with a pathogen but does not necessarily indicate active infection. Paired IgG titers spaced 1 to 4 weeks apart are required to document active infection. A single positive result for IgM-specific assays may indicate a recent infection or a chronic infection that continues to stimulate the immune system. Previous immunization may lead to positive results and is the basis for measurement of antibody titers to assess the need for additional vaccination[15] (see Chapter 20). If an infection is chronic and persistent, such as with FIV infection, positive results indicate active infection, provided there has been no history of previous FIV vaccination in a cat's lifetime. False-positive results for antibody may occur when antigenic cross-reactivity occurs. For example, dogs recovering from *Leptospira* infection have been shown to test positive on some immunoassays for the related spirochete *B. burgdorferi*.[16]

TABLE 2.1 Guidelines for Interpretation of Test Results Using Immunoassays That Detect Antigen

Antigen Test Result	Possible Explanation	Further Considerations
Negative	Pathogen of interest not present	Confirm with additional diagnostic test if necessary, (e.g., alternative antigen assay, antibody assay or NAAT)
	Antigen present, but quantity below limit of detection	Consider an antibody assay or NAAT
	Antigen present, but complexed by antibody and not available for detection	Consider an antibody assay or NAAT
	Technical error or reagent failure	Identified with inclusion of appropriate laboratory controls
	Poor assay analytical sensitivity (prone to give false-negative results)	Use an alternative assay
Positive	Pathogen of interest present	Confirm with additional diagnostic test if necessary, especially in regions with a low prevalence of infection. Antigen presence may not imply that the pathogen is the cause of disease
	Antigen present, but viable microbe absent	Confirm with additional diagnostic test
	Vaccine antigen present	Obtain vaccination history and consider a test that discriminates between vaccine and wild-type organisms, if available
	Cross-reactive antigen present from another substance or pathogen	Obtain history and consider the likelihood of infection with related agents
	Technical error	Identified with inclusion of appropriate controls by the laboratory
	Poor assay analytical specificity	Use alternative assay

NAAT, nucleic acid amplification test.

TABLE 2.2 Interpretation of Test Results Using Immunoassays That Detect Antibody

Antibody Test Result	Possible Explanation	Troubleshooting Suggestions
Negative	Exposure to pathogen of interest did not occur	Confirm with additional diagnostic test if necessary
	Too early in course of infection/illness	Obtain convalescent titer; consider an antigen test or NAAT for early diagnosis
	Severe immunosuppression	Consider an antigen test or NAAT
	Technical error	Identified with inclusion of appropriate controls by the laboratory
	Poor assay analytical sensitivity (prone to give false-negative results)	Use alternative assay
Positive	Previous natural exposure to the pathogen of interest	If infection is chronic and persistent, positive test results may equal active infection
	Previous immunization against the pathogen of interest	Obtain vaccination history; consider use of assays that discriminate between natural exposure and vaccine antibody, if available
	Immunologic cross-reactivity	Obtain history and consider the likelihood of previous exposure to related agents
	Technical error	Identified with inclusion of appropriate controls by the laboratory
	Poor assay specificity (prone to give false-positive results)	Use alternative assay. Consider the use of a confirmatory test, especially in regions with low disease prevalence

NAAT, nucleic acid amplification test.

REFERENCES

1. Day MJ. Introduction to antigen and antibody assays. *Topics Compan Anim Med.* 2015;30(4):128–131.
2. Lizer J, Grahlmann M, Hapke H, et al. Evaluation of a rapid IgM detection test for diagnosis of acute leptospirosis in dogs. *Vet Rec.* 2017;180:517.
3. O'Connor TP. SNAP assay technology. *Topics Compan Anim Med.* 2015;30(4):132–138.
4. O' Farrell B. Lateral flow technology for field-based applications—basics and advanced developments. *Topics Compan An Med.* 2015;30(4):139–147.
5. Costa MN, Veigas B, Jacob JM, et al. A low cost, safe, disposable, rapid and self-sustainable paper-based platform for diagnostic testing: lab on paper. *Nanotechnology.* 2014;25(094006).
6. Levy J, Crawford C, Hartmann K, et al. American Association of Feline Practitioners' feline retrovirus management guidelines. *J Feline Med Surg.* 2008;10(3):300–316.
7. Leschnik MW, Kirtz G, Khanakah G, et al. Humoral immune response in dogs naturally infected with *Borrelia burgdorferi* sensu lato and in dogs after immunization with a *Borrelia* vaccine. *Clin Vaccine Immunol.* 2010;17(5):828–835.
8. Pomrantz JS, Johnson LR, Nelson RW, et al. Comparison of serologic evaluation via agar gel immunodiffusion and fungal culture of tissue for diagnosis of nasal aspergillosis in dogs. *J Am Vet Med Assoc.* 2007;230(9):1319–1323.
9. Pappagianis D, Zimmer BL. Serology of coccidioidomycosis. *Clin Microbiol Rev.* 1990;3(3):247–268.

10. Spector D, Legendre AM, Wheat J, et al. Antigen and antibody testing for the diagnosis of blastomycosis in dogs. *J Vet Intern Med.* 2008;22(4):839–843.
11. Patterson EV, Reese MJ, Tucker SJ, et al. Effect of vaccination on parvovirus antigen testing in kittens. *J Am Vet Med Assoc.* 2007;230(3):359–363.
12. Greene CE Decaro N. Canine viral enteritis. In: Greene CE, ed. *Infectious Diseases of the Dog and Cat.* 4th ed. St. Louis: Elsevier; 2012:67–80.
13. Garcia RS, Wheat LJ, Cook AK, et al. Sensitivity and specificity of a blood and urine galactomannan antigen assay for diagnosis of systemic aspergillosis in dogs. *J Vet Intern Med.* 2012;26:911–919.
14. Wilson HL, Gerdts V, Babiuk LA. Mucosal vaccine development for veterinary and aquatic diseases. In: Kiyono H, Pascual DW, eds. *Mucosal Vaccines: Innovation for Preventing Infectious Diseases.* 2nd ed. London: Academic Press; 2020:811–829.
15. Roth JA, Spickler AR. Duration of immunity induced by companion animal vaccines. *Anim Health Res Review.* 2010;11(2):165–190.
16. Shin SJ, Chang YF, Jacobson RH, et al. Cross-reactivity between *B. burgdorferi* and other spirochetes affects specificity of serotests for detection of antibodies to the Lyme disease agent in dogs. *Vet Microbiol.* 1993;36(1–2):161–174.

3

Isolation and Identification of Aerobic and Anaerobic Bacteria

Stephen D. Cole, Shelley C. Rankin

KEY POINTS

- Aerobic Specimens: Specimens should be from appropriate anatomical sites and should be transported to the laboratory in transport medium as quickly as possible. Clinicians should never hesitate to contact their laboratory with questions.
- Anaerobic Specimens: Biopsies or aspirates are preferred for anaerobic culture. Specimens should be transported in oxygen-free containers.
- Microscopic Examination: A Gram stain can differentiate gram-positive and gram-negative organisms in clinical material. This can be important in the selection of antimicrobials before culture results are available. Acid-fast stains (such as Ziehl-Neelsen) are used to identify organisms such as *Mycobacterium* and *Nocardia.*
- Bacterial Culture: Aerobic culture of bacterial organisms typically requires 18 to 48 hours of incubation on a variety of media at 35°C to 37°C. Some organisms require other conditions (i.e., different temperature, longer incubation, etc.); therefore, communication of suspected fastidious pathogens to the laboratory is critical to help the laboratory select the most appropriate media and conditions.
- Blood Culture: Blood culture requires specialized medium or transport containers. A negative blood culture does not rule out bacteremia and should be interpreted in the context of clinical signs.
- Skin: Most commonly, the best skin specimens are from intact pustules. These are ruptured and contents collected. Alternatively, swabs from underneath crusts or over epidermal collarettes may be submitted to a laboratory. Punch biopsy of decontaminated skin should be considered for deep pyoderma.
- Body Fluids: Fluids should be collected aseptically and transported in a sterile container on ice. In general, 1–5 mL of fluid should be submitted.
- Tissues: Tissues should be submitted in a small amount of nonbacteriostatic sterile saline in a sterile container and shipped on ice. Tissues will be macerated with sterile technique in the laboratory prior to culture.
- Airway Specimens: Routine culture of upper airway specimens is not recommended due to high likelihood of contamination. Lower airway specimens should be collected by transtracheal wash, endotracheal wash, or bronchoalveolar lavage.
- Feces: Fecal culture is only performed routinely for the isolation of pathogens such as *Salmonella* and *Campylobacter.*
- Urine: Cystocentesis is the best method to obtain urine for culture. Urine specimens are plated with a quantitative loop and are incubated aerobically. Bladder biopsies or uroliths can also be considered for culture.
- Bacterial Identification: Most laboratories use phenotypic (biochemical) approaches to identify the species of bacteria isolated. Methods such as matrix-assisted laser desorption ionization time-of-flight (MALDI-TOF) mass spectroscopy or DNA sequencing are now being used more commonly.
- Susceptibility Testing: Susceptibility to antimicrobial drugs may be determined using a variety of methods. Methods are either dilution (i.e., broth microdilution) or diffusion based (i.e., Kirby-Bauer disc diffusion or ETEST strips). When possible, minimum inhibitory concentration (MIC) should be determined and considered during therapy. MIC values are interpreted by the laboratory using standardized "breakpoints" as susceptible (S), intermediate (I), or resistant (R).

INTRODUCTION

Factors that influence the detection of clinically relevant organisms in specimens collected from dogs and cats are:

1. An appropriate level of suspicion for the presence of a bacterial infection;
2. Development of a list of differential diagnoses that reflects the types of bacterial pathogens that might be the cause of clinical signs because of the requirement of some bacteria for special transport conditions, culture conditions, or prolonged incubation;
3. Collection of a sufficient amount of specimen;
4. Collection of the correct type of specimen;
5. Specimen collection from the correct anatomic location; and
6. Proper handling, storage, and transport of the specimen, which should be sent with a request for culture to the laboratory within acceptable time limits.

These factors cannot be overemphasized. Without them, time and money invested in collection of specimens and culture is wasted.

Given the increasing prevalence of multidrug resistance among bacteria that infect dogs and cats, veterinarians should attempt to confirm a bacterial infection at a normally sterile site by requesting microscopic evaluation of direct smears and culture by a laboratory, whenever possible, before the choice is made to administer an antimicrobial drug.

The purpose of this chapter is to provide information in regard to the correct way to collect and handle specimens for culture before

TABLE 3.1 Suggested Specimen Types for Bacterial Culture from Selected Anatomic Sites and Likely Pathogens Present

Specimen Type	Suggested Volume for Culture	Likely Pathogens Present
Blood	≥10 mL for patients weighing >10 kg, or 1% of patient blood volume	Gram-positive and gram-negative aerobes. Common contaminants are coagulase-negative staphylococci, *Corynebacterium* spp., *Bacillus* spp., and *Propionibacterium* spp.
Cerebrospinal fluid	≥0.5 mL	Gram-positive and gram-negative aerobes, anaerobes, *Brucella* spp. (dogs), *Nocardia* spp., *Actinomyces* spp.,[22] *Mycoplasma* spp. (cats)[23]
Middle ear	Aspirate of fluid or pus through tympanic membrane	Gram-positive and gram-negative aerobes, anaerobes, *Mycoplasma* spp., *Actinomyces* spp.[23,24]
Skin	Swab from epidermal collarette or ruptured pustule (superficial pyoderma); biopsy from which dermis has been removed (deep pyoderma)	Gram-positive aerobes (especially staphylococci), rarely *Pseudomonas aeruginosa*
External ear	Swab ear canal after removing debris and crusts from the canal	Gram-positive aerobes, *P. aeruginosa*
Cornea	Scrape or swab exposed corneal stroma and inoculate directly onto media. Referral to veterinary ophthalmologist recommended	Gram-positive aerobes, *Mycoplasma* spp., *P. aeruginosa*[25]
Abdominal fluid	1–5 mL	Gram-negative and gram-positive aerobes, anaerobes, *Actinomyces* spp.
Pleural fluid	1–5 mL	Gram-negative and gram-positive aerobes, anaerobes, *Actinomyces* spp., *Nocardia* spp., *Mycoplasma* spp.
Feces	Fresh whole stools preferred. Avoid swabs or fecal loops containing fecal matter due to low specimen size. Submit in clean, dry leak-proof container	*Escherichia coli*, *Salmonella* spp., *Clostridium perfringens*, *Clostridiodes difficile*, *Campylobacter* spp., *Anaerobiospirillum* spp.
Urine	1–5 mL urine collected using cystocentesis	Gram-negative and gram-positive aerobes, *Corynebacterium urealyticum*
Bronchoalveolar lavage specimens	1–5 mL	Gram-positive and gram-negative aerobes, anaerobes (aspiration pneumonia), *Mycoplasma* spp., rarely *Mycobacterium* spp.

they are sent to the laboratory, and to outline bacteriologic procedures performed in the microbiology laboratory that are of relevance to the small animal clinician.

SPECIMEN COLLECTION AND TRANSPORT

Specimens for Aerobic Bacterial Culture

Veterinary clinicians should collect specimens for culture using an *appropriate method* from the *correct anatomic site*. Collection of a sufficient *amount* of specimen is very important. Table 3.1 suggests optimal specimen types for detection of bacteria from specific anatomic sites. Attempts should always be made to prevent contamination with commensal bacteria during specimen collection. Clinicians should contact their laboratory before collecting specimens that are not routine to ensure optimal collection. Specimens should always be labeled with the patient's name, patient number, source of specimen, and the date and time of collection, and should be labeled, packaged, and transported according to regional and national regulations.

Specimens should be transported to the laboratory immediately where possible. If transport requires longer than 2 hours, appropriate transport medium should be used and specimens in transport medium should not be refrigerated. Fluid specimens or those that are not in transport medium should be refrigerated. Although specimens in transport medium can be held for up to 72 hours, culture of specimens older than 24 hours should be avoided if possible, even if they have been refrigerated or placed in transport media, because of increased likelihood of false-negative results with longer storage times. False-positive results can also occur with polymicrobial specimens if

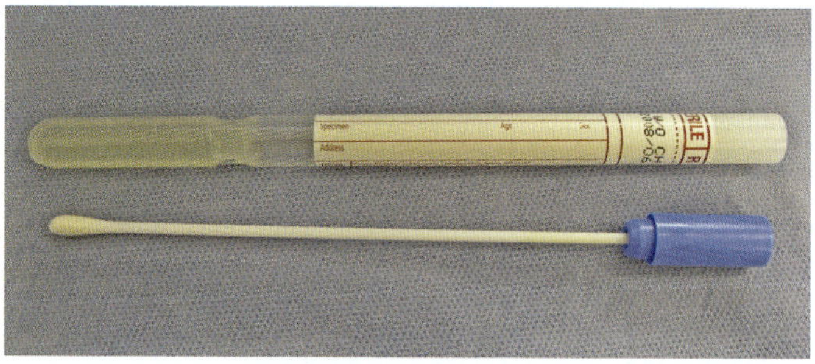

Fig. 3.1 Swab system containing transport medium for aerobic bacterial culture.

overgrowth occurs during transport. Transport medium for bacterial culture is usually supplied in a plastic tube with one or two swabs attached to the tube's cap (Fig. 3.1). The medium is designed to maintain bacterial viability without causing significant growth. It usually consists of a small amount of agar, reagents that maintain pH, a colorimetric pH indicator that indicates whether oxidation has occurred, and specific factors that maintain the viability of certain pathogens. Some organisms, such as chlamydiae and leptospires, have specific transport medium requirements.

Specimens for Anaerobic Bacterial Culture

When anaerobes are suspected, aspirates or biopsies should be obtained rather than swabs, and the specimen should be stored at room temperature and not refrigerated. This is because oxygen diffuses into cold specimens more rapidly than specimens held at room temperature. If this is not possible, separate specimens should be collected for aerobic and anaerobic culture. Specimens for anaerobic culture should preferably be transported in an oxygen-free container.

DIAGNOSTIC METHODS

Microscopic Examination of Direct Smears

A Gram stain prepared from the specimen can permit the rapid preliminary diagnosis of infection and determine whether the organism(s) present are gram positive or gram negative (Box 3.1; Fig. 3.2). This helps guide the clinician to select an appropriate empiric therapy, if necessary, while awaiting the results of culture and susceptibility testing. If sufficient material is available, examination of a direct smear also helps to determine whether a specimen is adequate for culture and aids interpretation of culture results. For swab or aspirate specimens, clinicians should consider providing a separate specimen for a direct smear in addition to a specimen for culture.

BOX 3.1 Procedure for Gram Staining

Heat-fix specimen on the slide by passing the slide two to three times over a gentle flame, or fix in 95% methanol for 2 minutes, and then air dry.
Flood with crystal violet solution for 15 to 60 seconds (10 g of 90% dye in 500 mL absolute methanol).
Wash with water.
Flood with iodine for 15 to 60 seconds (6 g of I_2 and 12 g of KI in 1800 mL of water).
Decolorize with acetone-alcohol (400 mL of acetone in 1200 mL of 95% ethanol)
Wash immediately.
Counterstain with safranin for 15 to 60 seconds (10 g of dye in 1 L of water).
Wash, blot dry, and examine using light microscopy.

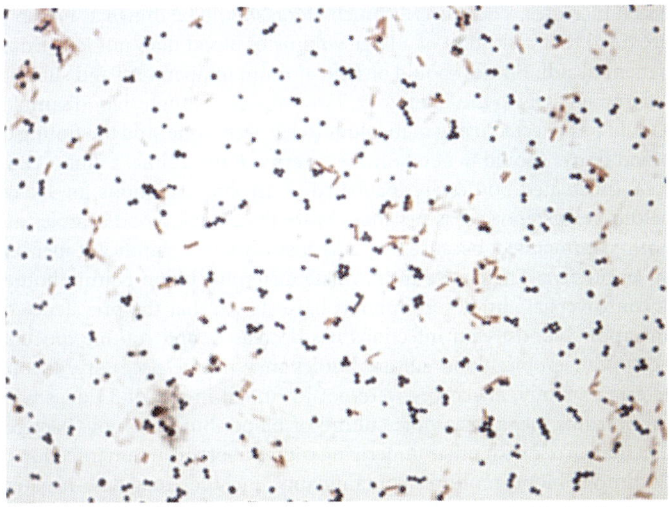

Fig. 3.2 Gram-stained smear of gram-positive cocci *(dark blue)* and gram-negative rods *(red)* (1600× oil magnification).

Acid-fast stains can be used on smears to assist in the identification of *Nocardia* and *Mycobacterium* spp., as well as on fecal smears to detect some parasitic oocysts, such as those of *Cryptosporidium*. These organisms stain magenta as a result of their high cell wall mycolic acid content, which in turn results in their resistance to decolorization after staining (which is often performed using an acid-alcohol solvent, hence the term *acid-fast*). Examples of acid-fast staining methods are the *Ziehl-Neelsen, Fite's,* and *Kinyoun* stains.

Bacterial Culture

Diagnostic bacterial culture requires appropriate laboratory facilities, proper BSL 2 containment, properly trained individuals, reference strains for quality control testing, and the use of standard protocols.[1] Media used for bacterial culture may be categorized as general-purpose, enriched, selective, differential, and specialized (Table 3.2). Some media belong to more than one of these categories. For example, MacConkey agar is both a selective and a differential medium (Fig. 3.3). Media for culture contains a nutrient source, most commonly peptones (hydrolyzed animal or vegetable substances), and is adjusted to a specific pH. Solid medium contains agar, which is derived from seaweed. Other nutrients may be added based on specific organism requirements. More than 100 different types of bacteriology media exist, most of which can be purchased as prepared plates or broth.

In the laboratory, media for bacterial culture should be warmed to room temperature before inoculation, and damaged media, such as dehydrated medium or medium that has changed color, should not be used. Medium is stored in the dark at 2°C to 8°C and discarded when it reaches its expiration date. After plating, incubation is most commonly performed at 35°C to 37°C in air for a minimum of 2 days. Conditions vary for specific bacteria, and growth in 3% to 5% CO_2 is preferred by some fastidious organisms. The laboratory should be informed, by providing an adequate clinical history, when pathogens with special culture requirements are suspected, such as *Campylobacter, Mycoplasma, Actinomyces, Nocardia,* and *Mycobacterium* spp. These organisms require special media or prolonged incubation times (e.g., weeks). Specimens for anaerobic culture should be plated onto appropriate media immediately and incubated in an anaerobic environment. Anaerobic containers, which create an anaerobic environment

TABLE 3.2 Types of Media Used in Bacteriology

Medium Type	Attributes	Example
Transport	Nonnutritive liquid or semisolid medium. Promotes organism viability without allowing significant growth	Amies transport medium
General-purpose	Allows growth of most aerobic and facultatively anaerobic organisms	Sheep blood agar
Enriched	Promotes growth of fastidious organisms that require specific nutrients, e.g., *Francisella*	Chocolate agar, which is enriched with heat-treated blood, which gives it a brown color
Selective	Selects for growth of certain organisms while inhibiting others	MacConkey agar, which is selective for gram-negative bacteria
Differential	Aids in preliminary identification of organisms based on colony appearance	MacConkey agar, which promotes pink colony formation by organisms that ferment lactose
Specialized	Selects for a specific pathogen through the addition of specific nutrients	Anaerobic medium, which contains hemin, vitamin K, and reducing agents

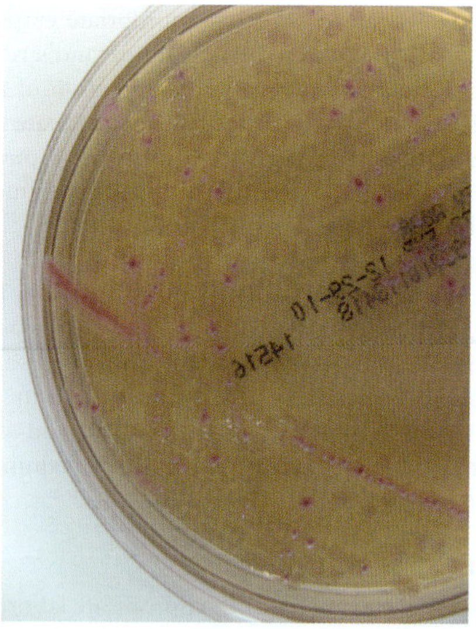

Fig. 3.3 Growth of bacteria on MacConkey medium that shows the selective and differential qualities of the medium. The medium contains substances that inhibit the growth of gram-positive bacteria. By using the lactose available in the medium, bacteria such as *Escherichia coli*, *Enterobacter* spp., and *Klebsiella* spp. produce acid when they grow on the medium, which lowers the pH of the agar and results in the formation of red to pink colonies.

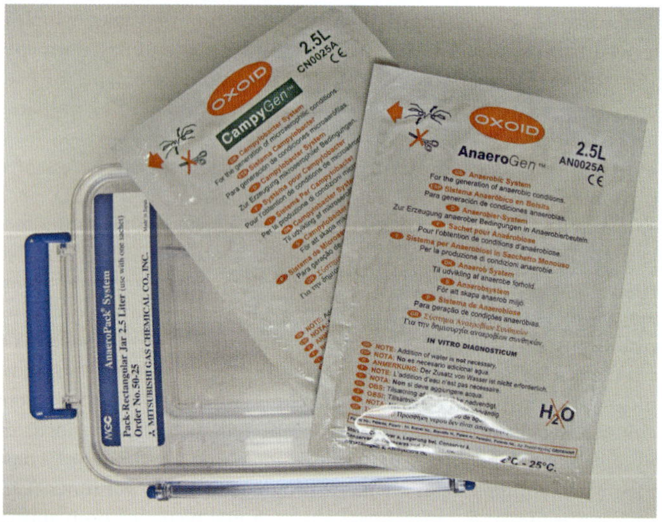

Fig. 3.4 System for isolation of anaerobic and microaerophilic bacteria. The packets are opened, and the sachets inside are placed into the container with the inoculated plates. The container is sealed immediately. The sachets contain ascorbic acid. Atmospheric oxygen in the container is rapidly absorbed and replaced with carbon dioxide in an exothermic reaction process. After an appropriate incubation period, the container is opened and the plates inspected for growth. An anaerobic indicator can be placed within the box to ensure that the proper conditions are maintained.

through the use of gas-generating reagents, can be used for incubation (Fig. 3.4). Because anaerobes grow more slowly than aerobes, anaerobic cultures should be held for 7 days before being reported as negative.

Blood and Intravascular Catheters

Bacteremic animals may be continuously or intermittently bacteremic. Because of intermittent bacteremia, multiple, separate specimens that each contain 10 mL or more of blood are recommended. Pediatric bottles are available that can be inoculated with as little as 1.5 mL of blood, although the chance of a positive isolation increases as the blood volume tested increases. Therefore, as much blood should be drawn as possible, provided that collection of a large volume of blood does not jeopardize patient health. Bottles should be held at room temperature and submitted immediately to the laboratory. Two, and ideally three, blood samples should be collected using meticulous sterile technique, and the timing of blood draws should depend on the severity of the animal's illness (Box 3.2). Inoculated bottles are incubated in aerobic conditions for 7 days before being reported as negative. More than three blood samples are not recommended, because they add cost without a significant increase in sensitivity.[2] The choice to inoculate anaerobic blood culture bottles is controversial. Studies in humans have shown that the prevalence of anaerobic bloodstream infections has decreased, and routine inoculation of anaerobic blood culture bottles may not be necessary. In one veterinary study, anaerobes were not identified in any of 33 dogs with endocarditis using anaerobic culture of blood, but anaerobic bacteremia may occur with other underlying causes of bloodstream infections.[2] Common blood culture contaminants include coagulase-negative staphylococci, and *Bacillus*, *Corynebacterium*, and *Propionibacterium* spp. When only one blood culture is positive for one of these organisms, contamination is likely, but the presence of multiple positive blood cultures from separate sites suggests true bacteremia.

Blood culture media contain the anticoagulant, sodium polyanethol sulfonate (SPS), which is less inhibitory to bacterial growth than other anticoagulants. Some blood culture media (e.g., BD BACTEC Plus) contain resin beads that bind antimicrobial drugs in the patient's blood specimen, so they do not inhibit bacterial growth (Fig. 3.5). The detection of bacterial growth in blood culture systems can be automated using instrumentation that measures emission of fluorescence or a colorimetric change in a sensor. The change occurs as CO_2 concentrations within the bottle increase, which indicates the presence of bacterial growth. Some instruments detect pressure changes in the head of the bottle. The culture is monitored at regular intervals by the instrument to optimize early detection of bacterial growth. Positive blood culture bottles are then evaluated by performing a Gram stain of the broth, and subculture to appropriate media.

BOX 3.2 Suggested Procedure for Obtaining Samples for Aerobic Bacterial Blood Culture

Shave site.

Clean skin with 10% povidone iodine or 1%–2% tincture of iodine, swabbing concentrically from the center; allow to dry (wait for 1 minute).

If a catheter must be used for specimen collection, clean access port with 70% alcohol and allow to dry. Avoid collection from a catheter if possible.

Clean stopper on top of the culture tube or bottle with 70% alcohol; allow to dry (wait for 1 minute).

Perform venipuncture using sterile gloves to palpate the vein.

Inoculate blood culture bottle without changing the needle.

Space cultures based on severity of illness before starting antimicrobial therapy.

- Acute febrile illness: antimicrobials need to be changed or started immediately; two sets from separate sites, all within 10 minutes. Consideration could be given to drawing a third set using a resin bottle just before administering the second dose of antimicrobials (i.e., when trough drug concentrations are present)
- Acute endocarditis: three sets from three separate sites, within 1–2 hours
- Nonacute disease: three sets from separate sites within 24 hours, spaced at intervals of at least 3 hours

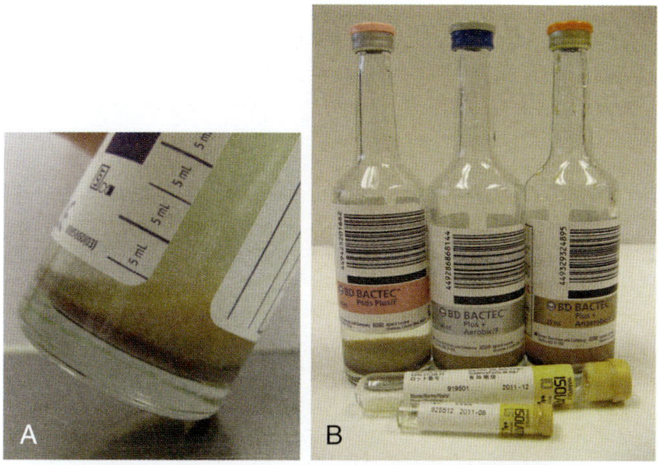

Fig. 3.5 Blood culture systems. (A) BACTEC system showing resin beads that bind antimicrobial drugs. (B) Pediatric, aerobic, and anaerobic BACTEC systems for blood culture together with adult and pediatric WAMPOLE Isolator tubes *(front)* for lysis-centrifugation culture of blood.

Another blood culture system is the Isolator lysis-centrifugation system (DuPont, Wilmington, DE, USA) (see Fig. 3.5B). In this system, blood is added to a tube that contains anticoagulant and a reagent that induces RBC lysis. The tube is centrifuged, and the pellet is plated onto agar media and incubated. This method allows colony counts to be obtained. The tubes allow isolation not only of aerobes but also some anaerobic bacteria.

Culture of intravascular catheter tips is performed to determine whether a catheter is a source of bacteremia and should only be performed simultaneously with blood culture. The catheter is removed after cleaning the skin around the catheter site with alcohol, and the distal 5 cm is aseptically removed into a sterile tube and submitted immediately.[3] In the laboratory, the catheter tip is rolled onto an agar plate and incubated overnight or placed in a thioglycollate enrichment broth, incubated overnight, and plated the following day. The result of catheter culture alone should not change treatment. Therefore, in most situations, blood culture may be all that is required.

Skin

For dogs with superficial pyoderma, specimens for culture should ideally be collected from a pustule. No surface disinfection should be performed. The hair should be clipped using sterile scissors; clippers should be avoided. A pustule is lanced with a sterile narrow-gauge needle, and pus on the needle or exuding from the pustule is applied to a sterile swab, which can then be placed in transport medium for transport to the laboratory. If a pustule cannot be found, cultures can also be obtained by lifting crusts and swabbing beneath the crust, or rolling the swab across an epidermal collarette two to three times. Papules can be cultured by biopsy after surface disinfection with 70% alcohol, allowing the surface to dry, and use of a 3- to 4-mm punch and sterile surgical instruments to collect the biopsy, which is then submitted in transport medium or a small amount of sterile saline. The biopsy site can then be sutured closed.

For deep pyoderma, a biopsy of the lesion should also be obtained after surface disinfection with 70% alcohol. The dermis should be excised with a sterile blade and the biopsy submitted as just described.

For dogs and cats with wounds, aspirates and deep tissue biopsies after surgical dissection are always preferable to swab specimens. Swab specimens are often contaminated by surface microorganisms, contain only a small amount of material, and are not amenable to optimal anaerobic transport. For this reason, collection of pus from fistulous tracts using a swab should also be avoided. If an abscess is present, an aspirate of the abscess fluid should be collected and submitted for aerobic and anaerobic culture. For dogs and cats with cellulitis, an aspirate can be attempted by injecting a small volume of sterile saline into the lesion and aspirating back into a syringe, although bacterial yields may be low and biopsy may be required in some cases.

Body Fluids

Usually, 1 to 5 mL of body fluid is required for culture. Fluid can be inoculated into blood culture bottles in the laboratory or alongside the patient. Body fluids that have the potential to clot should be submitted to the laboratory in a tube that contains an appropriate ratio of anticoagulant. In the laboratory, body fluids with volumes that exceed 1 mL may be concentrated using centrifugation and the pellet resuspended in a smaller volume (e.g., 0.5 mL) of the supernatant fluid before inoculation onto agar.

For CSF, the chance of organism isolation also increases when the volume submitted is maximized. If possible, at least 0.5 mL should be submitted for culture. CSF specimens should be immediately transported to the laboratory, preferably at room temperature.

Tissue Specimens

Attempts should be made to obtain as large a tissue specimen as possible for culture. The use of swabs to collect specimens for culture during surgical procedures is discouraged because of insufficient specimen size. Small pieces of tissue can be submitted in a small amount of sterile, nonbacteriostatic saline. In the laboratory, the tissue is minced using aseptic procedures to release organisms before smears are prepared and broth media inoculated. Because an anaerobic environment can be maintained within pieces of tissue greater than or equal to 1 cm^3 in volume, these are suitable for anaerobic culture without oxygen-free transport. Such tissue specimens may be stored at room temperature for up to 24 hours.

Airway Specimens

Specimens from the upper respiratory tract are generally contaminated with commensal bacteria. Isolation of organisms such as *Staphylococcus* and *Corynebacterium* spp., and *Escherichia coli* should be interpreted with caution. Aerobic bacterial culture of a nasal lavage specimen may be indicated in cats with chronic rhinosinusitis if an antimicrobial-resistant organism is suspected, in particular *Pseudomonas aeruginosa*. Isolation of *Bordetella bronchiseptica* may also have clinical significance in dogs and cats with signs of upper respiratory tract disease. Growth of *Mycoplasma* spp. from the nasal cavity has uncertain clinical significance, because *Mycoplasma* spp. can be isolated from the nasal cavities of both healthy cats and cats with rhinosinusitis.[4–7]

Specimens from the lower respiratory tract may be collected using transtracheal, endotracheal, or bronchoalveolar lavage. Bronchial brush specimens may also be submitted for culture after placing them in 1 mL of sterile nonbacteriostatic saline. The presence of intracellular bacteria on cytologic examination is consistent with a bacterial infection rather than contamination. Anaerobic culture could be considered for animals with aspiration pneumonia or migrating plant awn foreign body pneumonia.

Feces

Whole stools or swabs that contain fecal matter should be processed within 1 to 2 hours or refrigerated as soon as possible after specimen collection and submitted within 24 hours. The specimens should not be contaminated with barium or urine. Rectal swabs that contain fecal

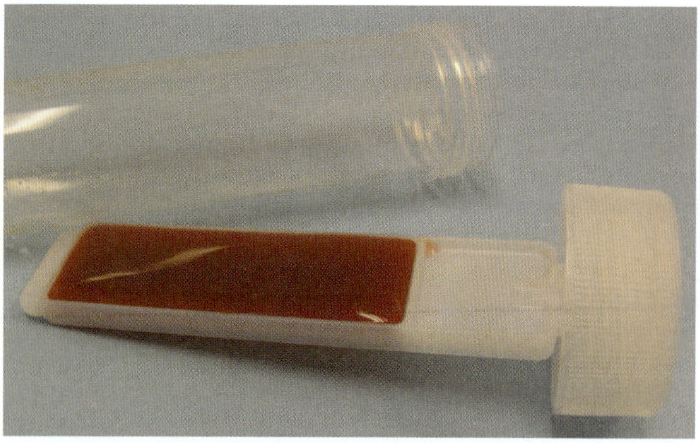

Fig. 3.6 Media paddle available for screening urine for the presence of an aerobic bacterial infection. The paddle is impregnated on each side with selective and nonselective media (in this case, eosin methylene blue medium, shown, and cysteine lactose electrolyte-deficient (CLED) media, on underside, respectively). The paddle is flooded with urine, incubated, and inspected for growth. Eosin methylene blue medium is red and selects for growth of gram-negative enteric organisms. CLED medium is initially green but turns yellow in the presence of lactose-fermenting organisms.

material can be immersed in transport medium until processing in accordance with the instructions of the swab manufacturer. Testing of more than one sequential specimen may improve detection of fecal pathogens due to the low sensitivity of fecal culture methods. Selective media are required for isolation of *Salmonella*. Because *Clostridium perfringens* and *Clostridioides difficile* are commonly detected in normal stool specimens, toxin antigen testing may be more appropriate than culture to determine the role these organisms may be playing in diarrhea (see Chapter 64). Special medium is also required for isolation of *Campylobacter* (see Chapter 65).

Urine

Urine should be collected using cystocentesis whenever possible. Collection of urine via sterile catheterization in male dogs is acceptable when cystocentesis is not possible. Quantitative cultures should always be performed. For specimens obtained by cystocentesis, any level of bacterial growth is significant, although most urinary tract infections contain greater than or equal to 10^3 CFU/mL of bacteria. For urine specimens obtained via catheter from male dogs, bacterial growth of greater than or equal to 10^5 CFU/mL has been considered significant.[8] Only aerobic bacterial culture is routinely indicated. Anaerobic urine culture may be indicated when there is radiologic evidence of emphysematous cystitis. Urine specimens should be submitted to the laboratory as soon as possible and may be refrigerated for up to 24 hours. Special urine transportation tubes can be used to preserve bacteria within the specimen, provided they are appropriate for the volume of urine collected (e.g., BD Vacutainer urine culture and sensitivity tube). Urine "paddles" are also available for in-house veterinary use. These allow inexpensive screening for the presence or absence of bacteria (Fig. 3.6). The paddles have media impregnated on them, are designed to be incubated in the clinic, and can provide some information on the infecting bacterial species present and the number of CFU/mL. Positive paddles can then be submitted to the laboratory for culture and susceptibility testing, although this does not always permit accurate identification of all bacteria present in mixed infections (see Chapter 127).

For animals with a urinary catheter in place and a suspected urinary tract infection, culture of the catheter tip is not recommended because it is generally contaminated with commensal organisms from the urethra. Instead, a urine specimen should be obtained by aspiration from a new urinary catheter, or, if feasible, using cystocentesis. If a catheter is used to collect the specimen, several milliliters of urine should be removed and discarded first to clear the catheter. Urine culture should never be performed from collection bag specimens. In the case of infection-induced urolithiasis (struvite urolithiasis), some clinicians choose to culture uroliths obtained at cystotomy.

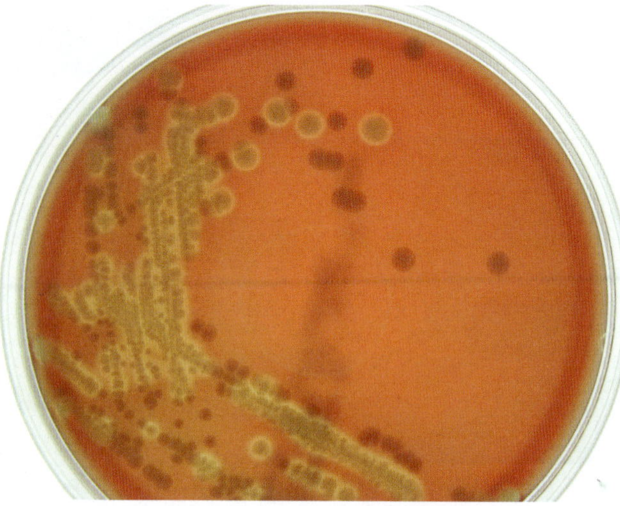

Fig. 3.7 Mixture of beta-hemolytic and nonhemolytic enteric bacteria growing on blood agar. Beta-hemolysis is characterized by complete clearing of the agar around each colony.

Fastidious and Unculturable Organisms

Some bacteria, such as *Bartonella* spp., *Borrelia/Borreliella (incertae sedis) burgdorferi*, and *Leptospira* spp., require special culture conditions (see Chapters 68–70). Others, such as hemotropic *Mycoplasma* species, are unculturable, and DNA amplification methods such as PCR are required for detection of these organisms. Cell culture is required to propagate certain bacteria. Examples include *Chlamydia felis* and tick-borne pathogens such as *Anaplasma phagocytophilum*.

Bacterial Identification

Following aerobic or anaerobic culture, presumptive bacterial identification can be made on the basis of colony morphology and microscopic morphology (e.g., Gram stain characteristics, rods or cocci). Further differentiation is generally based on a series of additional phenotypic tests, which are selected based on microscopic morphology and whether the organism is gram negative, gram positive, aerobic, or anaerobic. Microbiology laboratories use published methods to identify bacteria.[9] Preliminary tests used to identify gram-positive aerobic cocci include the presence or absence of hemolysis on a blood agar plate (for streptococci) (Fig. 3.7), a positive or negative catalase test, and the production of coagulase (for staphylococci). Identification of gram-negative aerobic bacilli relies on whether or not the organism ferments lactose, indole production, oxidase production, and the production of a variety of other enzymes. Assessment of motility and the ability to ferment carbohydrates are also used to differentiate bacteria. Biochemical test strips are available that allow multiple tests to be performed simultaneously (e.g., API strips, bioMérieux, Marcy L'Étoile, France) (Fig. 3.8) so that identification can be made within 24 to 48 hours. Automated identification systems that consist of a microtiter tray containing a variety of biochemical reagents (e.g., Sensititre, TREK Diagnostics, Cleveland, OH, USA and VITEK 2, bioMerieux, Marcy L'Etoile, France) are also in use in some veterinary diagnostic

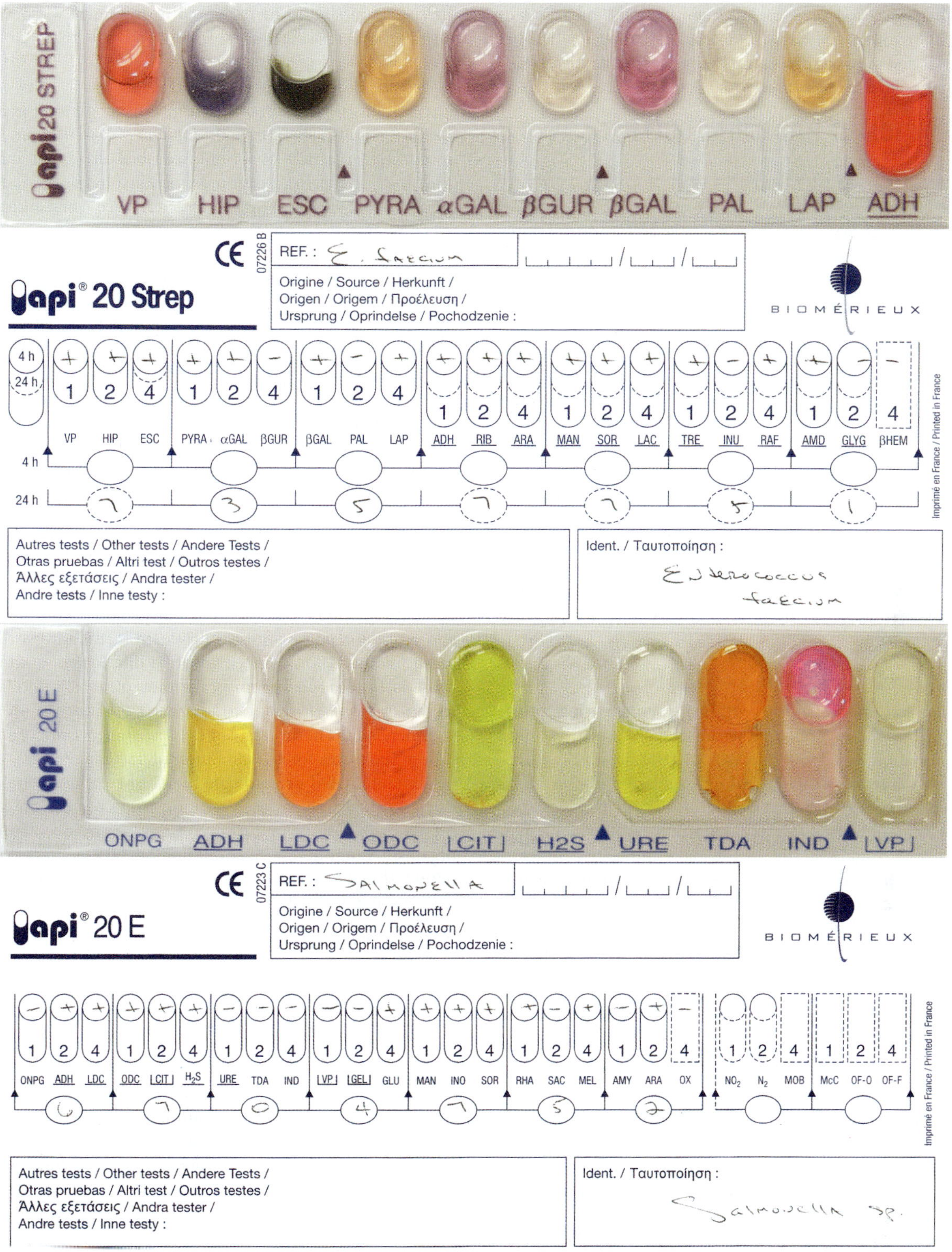

Fig. 3.8 API bacterial identification strips. Only the left half of the reaction strip is shown. Top (api20Strep): *Enterococcus faecium*. Bottom (api20E): *Salmonella* spp. Positive reactions are assigned a numerical code on the handwritten strip. The codes in each three-well group are added to generate a new (seven-number) code that can be used to identify the organism.

laboratories. Speciation of some *Mycobacterium* spp. requires analysis of mycolic acid content using high-performance liquid chromatography. Recently, the availability of MALDI-TOF mass spectrometry instrumentation (i.e., the Bruker Biotyper and VITEK MS systems) has revolutionized bacterial identification in the clinical microbiology laboratory. These systems use mass spectrometry to rapidly (on average in 6 minutes) and accurately (often >95%) identify organisms to the species level based on their chemical composition, provided a reference spectrum for the organism is available in the database used for comparison. Although the instrumentation is expensive, the ultimate cost is lower than with conventional biochemical methods because of reduction in labor and reagent costs.[10] Molecular methods such as 16S rRNA gene PCR and sequencing are also being used to identify organisms to the species level (see Chapter 6).

INTERPRETATION OF BACTERIAL CULTURE RESULTS

Specimens That Test Negative

Negative results (or lack of growth) using bacterial culture do not imply the absence of bacteria. Negative test results can occur as a result of inadequate specimen size (such as when swabs or aspirates are submitted), when there are inadequate organism numbers at the site of specimen collection, when overgrowth with commensal organisms occurs, or when there is loss of organism viability during transportation to the laboratory. The last is particularly problematic for anaerobic bacteria, and specimens for anaerobic culture ideally should reach the laboratory within 24 hours of collection. Antimicrobial therapy at the time of culture may affect culture results. Some postulate that neutrophils and their byproducts may also affect culture results (i.e., abscesses).

Negative test results can also occur when the organism is not inoculated onto the correct media or sufficient time is not allowed for growth. Clinicians must consider whether fastidious or slow-growing organisms might be present and inform the laboratory if they are suspected. Poor laboratory quality control procedures may also lead to false-negative test results. Use of an accredited laboratory can help minimize such problems.

Specimens That Test Positive

The detection of bacterial organisms within a specimen using culture does not imply that the organism is the cause of an animal's clinical signs. Contamination is a common cause of false-positive cultures. Isolation of only one or two colonies of coagulase-negative staphylococci, or *Bacillus*, *Corynebacterium*, or *Propionibacterium* spp., suggests contamination. Isolation of large numbers of a single type of bacteria from a normally sterile site is usually clinically significant, especially when supported by cytologic evidence of bacteria within phagocytes. A significant proportion of animals have positive urine cultures without clinical signs. Current guidelines suggest that in the absence of clinical signs or immunosuppression, animals with subclinical bacteriuria should not be treated.[11] A prospective study of adult cats with subclinical bacteriuria showed no difference in survival in the absence of treatment to healthy control cats.[12]

ANTIMICROBIAL SUSCEPTIBILITY TESTING

Importance of Antimicrobial Susceptibility Testing

Given the increasing recognition of antimicrobial resistance among bacteria that are isolated from small animal patients, determination of antimicrobial susceptibility can be as, or more, important to the clinician than the identity of the infecting organism. The result of antimicrobial susceptibility testing is generally available 2 to 3 days after submission of a specimen for culture. In animals that are critically ill, empiric antimicrobial therapy may already have been initiated by the time this result is available. The susceptibility results may show that the organism is resistant to a drug being used, in which case the drug should be changed to one that the organism tests susceptible to. The susceptibility pattern can also help to identify an alternate drug when the patient does not tolerate the initial drug prescribed. Susceptibility testing may indicate that the organism is susceptible to a more narrow-spectrum (and generally less expensive) antimicrobial drug than the drug initially prescribed, in which case the spectrum should be narrowed to minimize the development of antimicrobial resistance.

Methods of Susceptibility Testing

Susceptibility testing can be performed using dilution methods or diffusion methods. The *minimum inhibitory concentration* (MIC) is the lowest concentration of an antimicrobial drug that inhibits visible growth of an organism over a defined incubation period, most commonly 18 to 24 hours. The MIC is determined using dilution methods, which involve exposing the organism to twofold dilutions of an antimicrobial drug. The concentration range used varies with the drug and the organism being tested. *In vitro* factors that influence MIC include the composition of the medium, the size of the inoculum, incubation conditions, and the presence of resistant bacterial subpopulations within the inoculum. Standard protocols are published by the Clinical and Laboratory Standards Institute (CLSI) that specify medium composition and pH, inoculum size, inoculation procedures, agar depth, and incubation conditions, as well as quality control requirements.[9] Failure to comply with these protocols can lead to erroneous results, so laboratories that adhere to CLSI standards should be used whenever possible. MIC testing does not take into account *in vivo* factors such as postantibiotic effect and the effects of protein binding on antimicrobial drug activity (see Chapter 8).

Dilution Methods

Dilution methods include *broth macrodilution, broth microdilution,* and *agar dilution.* The most widely used method in North America is broth microdilution, whereby twofold dilutions of antimicrobials are made in a broth medium in a microtiter plate (Fig. 3.9). Pre-prepared frozen or freeze-dried microtiter plates for inoculation are available commercially. The results can be determined using visual examination of the plates for the inhibition of bacterial growth, or by the use of semiautomated or automated instrumentation. Dilutions can also be performed in agar, each dilution being poured onto a plate in a standardized fashion and allowed to set before inoculating it with the organism(s) of interest. Agar dilution can be used to perform susceptibility testing of fastidious bacteria with special medium requirements, such as *Campylobacter* spp.

Diffusion Methods

Diffusion methods include gradient diffusion (also known as ETEST) and disc diffusion. The ETEST involves use of a plastic strip coated with an antimicrobial gradient on one side and an MIC interpretive scale on the other side (Fig. 3.10A). An agar plate is inoculated with the organism of interest so that subsequent growth of the organism forms a "lawn" rather than individual colonies (i.e., *inoculation to confluence*). At the time of inoculation, the strips are applied to the surface of the plate. The antimicrobial drug diffuses into the medium, resulting in an elliptical zone of growth inhibition around the strip. The MIC is read at the point of intersection of the ellipse with the MIC scale on the strip. Although the strips are expensive, ETESTs have the advantage of being adaptable to use with fastidious organisms and anaerobes.

Disc diffusion, also known as Kirby-Bauer antibiotic testing, involves application of commercially available drug-impregnated filter paper discs to the surface of an agar plate that has been inoculated to confluence with the organism of interest. Commercially available, mechanical disc-dispensing devices can be used to apply several discs simultaneously to the surface of the agar. The drug diffuses radially through the agar, the concentration of the drug decreasing as the distance from the disc increases. This results in a circular zone of growth inhibition around the disc, the diameter of which correlates inversely to the MIC (Fig. 3.10B). The zone diameters are interpreted on the basis

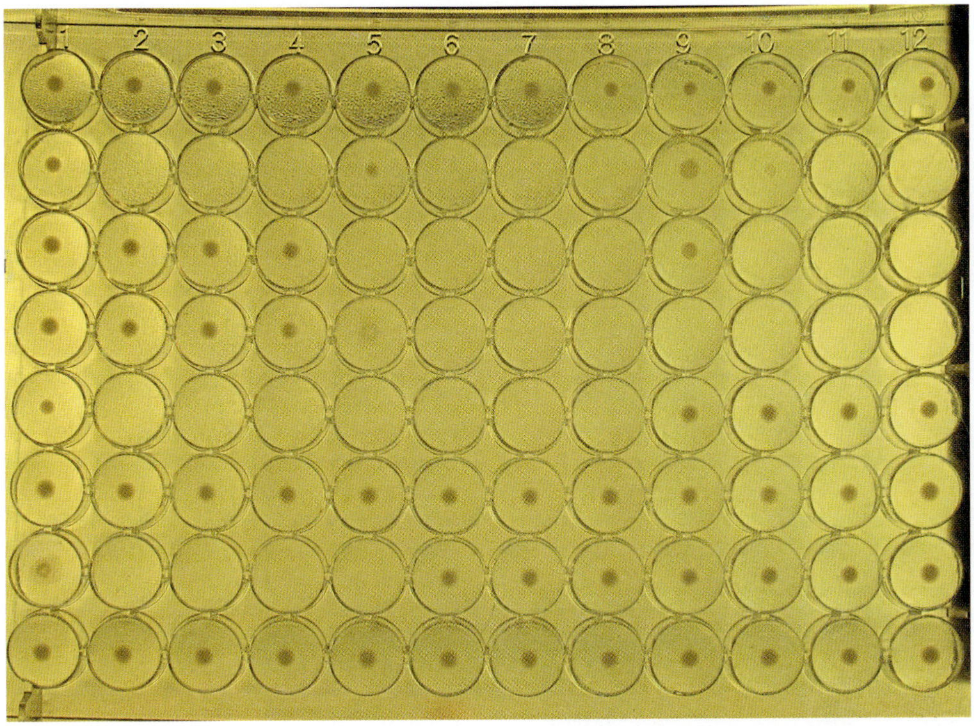

	1	2	3	4	5	6	7	8	9	10	11	12
A	AMP 0.25	AMP 0.5	AMP 1	AMP 2	AMP 4	AMP 8	AMP 16	OXA+ 0.25	OXA+ 0.5	OXA+ 1	OXA+ 2	OXA+ 4
B	AUG2 4/2	AUG2 8/4	AUG2 16/8	AUG2 32/16	AMI 4	AMI 8	AMI 16	AMI 32	FOX 2	FOX 4	FOX 8	FOX 16
C	TIC 8	TIC 16	TIC 32	TIC 64	POD 2	POD 4	POD 8	POD 16	TIM2 8/2	TIM2 16/2	TIM2 32/2	TIM2 64/2
D	SXT 0.5/9.5	SXT 1/19	SXT 2/38	FOV 0.25	FOV 0.5	FOV 1	FOV 2	FOV 4	FOV 8	FAZ 4	FAZ 8	FAZ 16
E	GEN 1	GEN 2	GEN 4	GEN 8	IMI 1	IMI 2	IMI 4	IMI 8	CLI 0.5	CLI 1	CLI 2	CLI 4
F	PEN 0.06	PEN 0.12	PEN 0.25	PEN 0.5	PEN 1	PEN 2	PEN 4	PEN 8	DOX 2	DOX 4	DOX 8	POS
G	XNL 0.25	XNL 0.5	XNL 1	XNL 2	XNL 4	MAR 0.25	MAR 0.5	MAR 1	MAR 2	RIF 1	RIF 2	POS
H	ENRO 0.25	ENRO 0.5	ENRO 1	ENRO 2	ERY 0.5	ERY 1	ERY 2	ERY 4	CHL 4	CHL 8	CHL 16	POS

AMP, ampicillin; AUG2, amoxicillin/clavulanic acid (2:1 ratio); TIC, ticarcillin; SXT, trimethoprim/sulfamethoxazole; GEN, gentamicin; PEN, penicillin; XNL, ceftiofur; ENRO, enrofloxacin; FOV, cefovecin; AMI, amikacin; POD, cefpodoxime; IMI, imipenem; ERY, erythromycin; MAR, marbofloxacin; OXA+, oxacillin + 2% NaCl; FOX, cefoxitin; TIM2, ticarcillin/clavulanic acid (constant 2); CLI, clindamycin; DOX, doxycycline; CHL, chloramphenicol; FAZ, cefazolin; RIF, rifampin; POS, positive control.

Fig. 3.9 Broth microdilution to determine the minimum inhibitory concentration (MIC). A series of wells contain an antimicrobial drug at twofold dilutions in a standard format. One custom plate format is shown (TREK Diagnostic Systems Sensititre Companion Animal MIC plate). A pellet of bacteria (in this case, *Escherichia coli* from an infected feline esophagostomy tube site) settles on the bottom of each well when growth fails to be inhibited by the antimicrobial drug concentration tested in that well. The cutoff MICs that define susceptibility versus resistance are published by the Clinical and Laboratory Standards Institute in the USA. This isolate was reported as resistant to ampicillin (AMP) (>16 mg/mL), resistant to amoxicillin-clavulanic acid (AUG2) (8/4 mg/mL), susceptible to amikacin (AMI) (8 mg/mL), susceptible to cefoxitin (FOX) (8 mg/mL), resistant to ticarcillin (TIC) (>64 mg/mL), susceptible to cefpodoxime (POD) (≤2 mg/mL), susceptible to ticarcillin-clavulanic acid (TIM2) (16 mg/mL), resistant to trimethoprim-sulfamethoxazole (SXT) (>2/38 mg/mL), susceptible to gentamicin (GEN) (2 mg/mL), susceptible to imipenem (IMI) (≤1 mg/mL), resistant to doxycycline (DOX) (>8 mg/mL), resistant to enrofloxacin (ENRO) and marbofloxacin (MAR) (both >2 mg/mL), and resistant to chloramphenicol (CHL) (>16 mg/mL). The MICs for ceftiofur (XNL), cefovecin, and cefazolin were ≤0.25, 1, and ≤4 mg/mL respectively, but because breakpoints for these drugs are not available for *E. coli* isolated from feline skin and soft tissue infections, only the MIC was reported and not the interpretation (whether the isolate was susceptible or resistant). Results for some drugs tested, such as oxacillin (OXA+), are not reported for gram-negative bacteria because these drugs are used to treat gram-positive bacterial infections. CLI, clindamycin; ERY, erythromycin; PEN, penicillin; RIF, rifampin; POS, positive control.

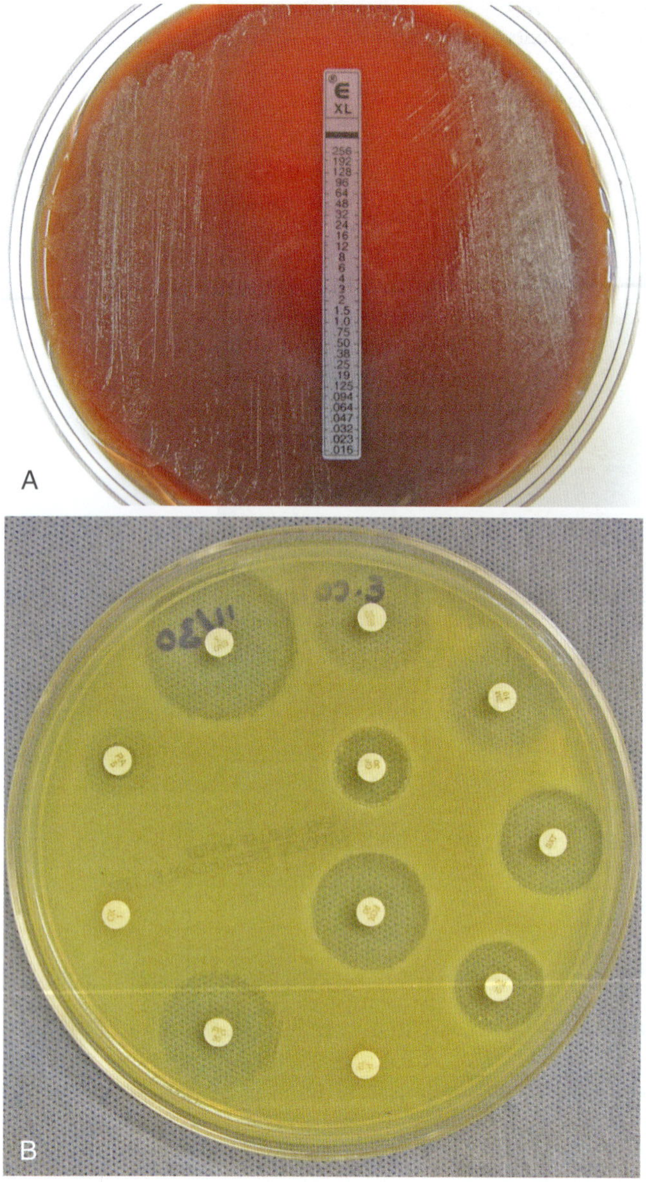

Fig. 3.10 Alternatives to broth microdilution for antimicrobial susceptibility testing. (A) ETEST that shows susceptibility of a *Bacteroides fragilis* isolate to amoxicillin-clavulanic acid. The strip in the center is impregnated with a gradient of antimicrobial drug (in this case, amoxicillin-clavulanic acid), with the highest concentration at the top of the strip. The MIC is read at the point (the ellipsis) where bacterial growth is no longer inhibited by the strip (0.19 μg/mL in this case). (B) Disc diffusion (also known as Kirby-Bauer testing) for *Escherichia coli* showing varying degrees of resistance to different antimicrobial drugs, reflected by zones of growth inhibition around discs containing each antimicrobial drug.

BOX 3.3 Factors Used by Standards Agencies to Establish Breakpoints for Antimicrobial Susceptibility Testing

Bacterial Factors

- Evaluation of MIC distributions for each bacterial species. These tend to be normally distributed (see Fig. 3.10; available for different antimicrobial drugs at www.eucast.org)[13]
- Knowledge of bacterial resistance mechanisms, as determined using phenotypic or genetic testing (e.g., testing for altered penicillin binding proteins in staphylococci)

Pharmacokinetics of the antimicrobial drug when used at a specific dosage regimen in the animal species of interest, including protein binding, taking into account variation among individuals

Pharmacodynamic indices (e.g., whether killing is concentration or time dependent) for the antimicrobial drug as they relate to organism killing (see Chapter 8)

Clinical response rates in humans and animal models, which are based on prospective, randomized controlled clinical studies with well-defined dosage regimens

of guidelines published by CLSI (see Definition of MIC Breakpoints, next), and the organisms are reported as susceptible, intermediate, or resistant. Zone diameters may not correlate precisely with MIC values, and regression line analysis should not be used to extrapolate MICs from zones of inhibition. Disc diffusion can only be used to test rapidly growing organisms that have consistent growth rates, for which criteria for interpretation of zone sizes are available.

Definition of MIC Breakpoints

In vitro susceptibility test results predict *in vivo* drug efficacy. Once susceptibility testing has been performed, organisms are classified on the susceptibility panel report as "susceptible" (S), "resistant" (R), and in some cases "intermediate" (I). The growth of a "susceptible" organism is predicted to be inhibited by antimicrobial drug concentrations that are usually achievable in blood and tissues using normal dosage regimens. "Intermediate" isolates have MICs that approach usually attainable blood and tissue levels and for which response rates may be lower than those of susceptible isolates. This category implies clinical efficacy in urine, where the drugs are normally concentrated (e.g., enrofloxacin and amoxicillin) or when a higher-than-normal dose of a drug can be used. "Resistant" isolates are predicted to grow in the usually achievable concentrations of drug in blood and tissues. So how does the laboratory predict *in vivo* susceptibility on the basis of an *in vitro* test? The laboratory uses MIC breakpoints (or, for disc diffusion testing, zone diameters) that are established, published, and revised regularly by committees affiliated with standards agencies such as the CLSI. If the MIC determined in the microbiology laboratory is lower than or equal to a published breakpoint for that organism-drug combination, the organism is defined as susceptible. Breakpoints are established on the basis of multiple factors (Box 3.3), which include: (1) a knowledge of MIC distributions and resistance mechanisms for each organism-drug combination (Fig. 3.11),[13] (2) clinical response rates in humans and animal models, (3) how the drug is distributed and metabolized in the body (pharmacokinetics), and (4) whether the drug is concentration dependent or time dependent as it relates to antibacterial effect (pharmacodynamics) (see Box 3.3).[14] For simplicity, MIC breakpoints are established for antimicrobial drug concentrations in the bloodstream and are based on a specific dosage regimen for the antimicrobial drug tested. This dosage regimen is selected by the standards agency involved. Because some antimicrobials are concentrated extensively in urine, some veterinary laboratories may offer urine MIC panels, which provide breakpoints for lower urinary tract infections. These breakpoints are higher than corresponding serum MIC breakpoints, so a greater proportion of organisms tested are classified as "susceptible." Urine MIC panels have been controversial because the possibility of concurrent pyelonephritis (tissue drug concentrations rather than urine concentrations) cannot always be ruled out. Breakpoints may be reevaluated when new mechanisms of resistance appear in bacteria or when new data are generated that improve understanding of the pharmacokinetics and pharmacodynamics of an antimicrobial drug.

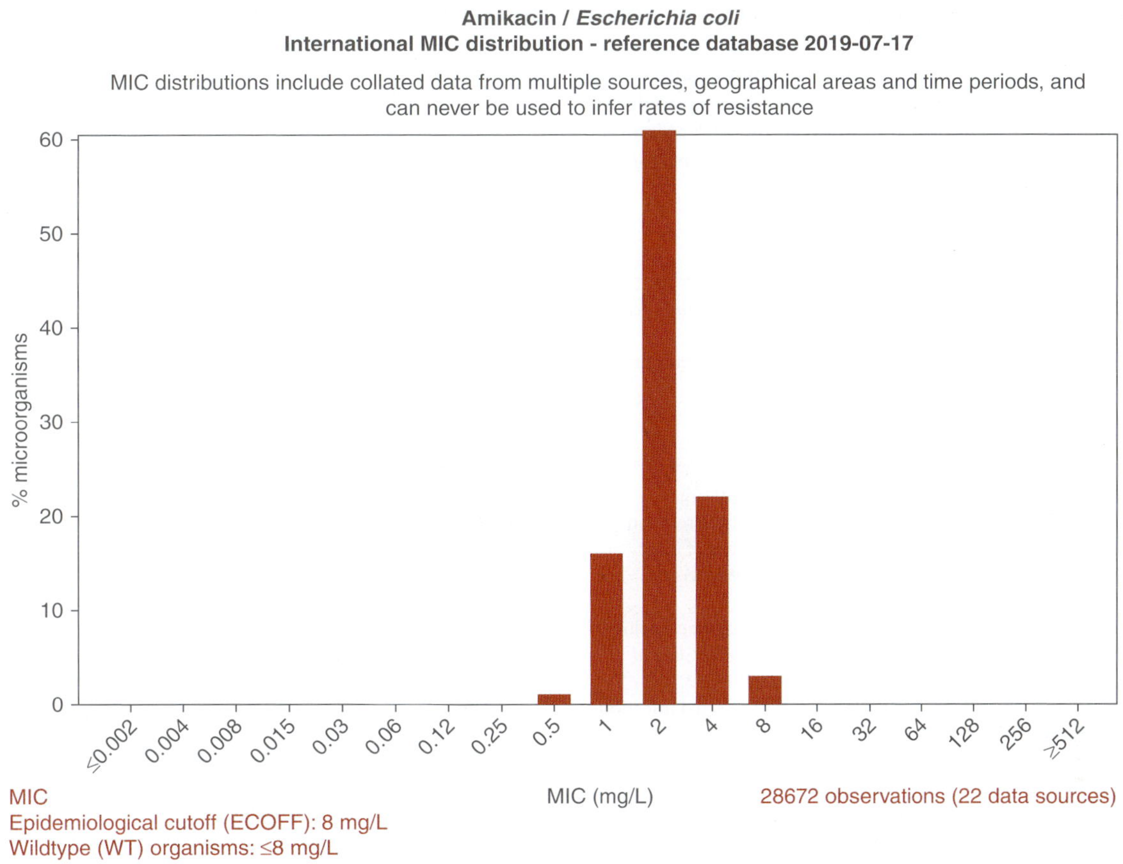

Fig. 3.11 Histogram that shows the distribution of amikacin minimum inhibitory concentrations (MICs) for isolates of *Escherichia coli*. The MICs are normally distributed. (From www.eucast.org.)

For infections in sites such as the CNS, the clinician needs to consider whether or not: (1) an antimicrobial will penetrate that site, (2) the drug is appropriate and safe, and (3) a higher dose is necessary to achieve adequate concentrations. The clinician must also consider factors such as immunosuppression and other concurrent illness or drug therapy when treating infections on the basis of antimicrobial susceptibility test results.

The bacterial species isolated determines which antimicrobials the laboratory selects for inclusion in susceptibility panels. For example, susceptibility to cephalosporins should not be reported for enterococci because of intrinsic resistance. Some antimicrobial drugs (e.g., vancomycin, linezolid, imipenem) should be reserved for treatment of multiple-drug resistant organisms that cause life-threatening infections. Consultation with a professional with expertise in infectious diseases or antimicrobial pharmacology is recommended before these drugs are selected.

Minimum and Serum Bactericidal Concentration

The *minimum bactericidal concentration* (MBC) is the minimum concentration of an antimicrobial drug that is bactericidal. It is determined by reculturing *(subculturing)* broth dilutions that inhibit growth of a bacterial organism (i.e., those at or above the MIC). The broth dilutions are streaked onto agar and incubated for 24 to 48 hours. The MBC is the lowest broth dilution of antimicrobial that prevents growth of the organism on the agar plate. Failure of the organism to grow on the plate implies that only nonviable organisms are present. The use of MBCs has been advocated by some for treatment of serious infections (such as endocarditis) or for treatment of immunosuppressed patients. Their value has been controversial, and they are not widely performed in human or veterinary medicine.

Serum bactericidal testing (SBT) is performed in the same manner as the MBC test, but uses the serum of a patient that has been treated with an antimicrobial. Serum is usually collected at expected peak and trough serum concentrations. SBT can be used to determine whether a patient has been adequately dosed, and to ensure that the antimicrobial is having the desired effect on the organism. Some data are available to support specific peak and trough SBT results required for the optimal treatment of human endocarditis, osteomyelitis, and cancer chemotherapy patients.[15–18] The SBT has not been widely used or evaluated for infections in dogs and cats and remains controversial in human medicine.

Mutant Prevention Concentration

The *mutant prevention concentration* (MPC) is the lowest antimicrobial drug concentration required to block the growth of the least susceptible bacterial cell in high-density bacterial populations.[19] Concentrations of antimicrobial in the zone between the MIC and the MPC (also known as the *mutant selection window*) allow selective amplification of resistant mutants.[20] This range is considered to be a "danger zone" for therapeutic drug concentrations. Minimizing the length of time that the antimicrobial drug concentration remains in the mutant selection window in vivo may reduce the likelihood for resistance selection during treatment.[21] The MPC cannot be extrapolated from the MIC. It is estimated using the standard agar dilution method used to estimate MIC, but with a larger inoculum (≥10^9 instead of 10^5 organisms), so as to include resistant subpopulations of bacteria. Administration of higher doses of antimicrobial drugs that exceed the MPC may increase the chance of toxicity to the patient, but offsets the chance of selection for resistant organisms, even though infection may be cured with lower doses.[20,21] Although first evaluated for the fluoroquinolones, data are accumulating regarding the usefulness of the MPC for other drug classes. MPC estimations are currently not routinely performed in veterinary diagnostic laboratories.

SUGGESTED READINGS

Drlica K, Zhao X. Mutant selection window hypothesis updated. *Clin Infect Dis*. 2007;44(5):681–688.

Turnidge JL, Paterson DL. Setting and revising antimicrobial susceptibility breakpoints. *Clin Microbiol Rev*. 2007;20(3):391–408.

REFERENCES

1. Clinical and Laboratory Standards Institute. http://www.clsi.org.
2. Sykes JE, Kittleson MD, Pesavento PA, et al. Evaluation of the relationship between causative organisms and clinical characteristics of infective endocarditis in dogs: 71 cases (1992-2005). *J Am Vet Med Assoc*. 2006;228(11):1723–1734.
3. Thomson RB. Specimen collection, transport, and processing: bacteriology. In: Murray PR, Barron EJ, Jorgensen JP, et al., eds. *Manual of Clinical Microbiology*. 9th ed. Washington, DC: ASM Press; 2007:291–333.
4. Veir JK, Ruch-Gallie R, Spindel ME, et al. Prevalence of selected infectious organisms and comparison of two anatomic sampling sites in shelter cats with upper respiratory tract disease. *J Feline Med Surg*. 2008;10(6):551–557.
5. Johnson LR, Drazenovich NL, Foley JE. A comparison of routine culture with polymerase chain reaction technology for the detection of *Mycoplasma* species in feline nasal samples. *J Vet Diagn Invest*. 2004;16(4):347–351.
6. Randolph JF, Moise NS, Scarlett JM, et al. Prevalence of mycoplasmal and ureaplasmal recovery from tracheobronchial lavages and of mycoplasmal recovery from pharyngeal specimens in cats with or without pulmonary disease. *Am J Vet Res*. 1993;54(6):897–900.
7. Tan RJS, Lim EW, Ishak B. Ecology of mycoplasmas in clinically healthy cats. *Aust Vet J*. 1977;53(11):515–518.
8. Ling GV. *Lower Urinary Tract Diseases of Dogs and Cats*. St Louis: Mosby; 1995:116.
9. Murray PR, Barron EJ, Jorgensen J, et al., eds. *Manual of Clinical Microbiology*. 9th ed. Washington, DC: ASM Press; 2007.
10. Bizzini A, Greub G. Matrix-assisted laser desorption ionization time-of-flight mass spectrometry, a revolution in clinical microbial identification. *Clin Microbiol Infect*. 2010;16(11):1614–1619.
11. Weese JD, Blondeau JM, Boothe D, et al. Antimicrobial use guidelines for treatment of urinary tract disease in dogs and cats: Antimicrobial Use Guidelines Working Group of the International Society for Companion Animal Infectious Diseases. *Vet Med Int*. 2011:263768.
12. White JD, Cave NJ, Grinberg A, et al. Subclinical bacteriuria in older cats and its association with survival. *J Vet Intern Med*. 2016;30(6):1824–1829.
13. European Committee on Antimicrobial Susceptibility Testing. http://www.eucast.org.
14. Turnidge JL, Paterson DL. Setting and revising antimicrobial susceptibility breakpoints. *Clin Microbiol Rev*. 2007;20(3):391–408.
15. Klastersky J, Daneau D, Swings G, et al. Antibacterial activity in serum and urine as a therapeutic guide in bacterial infections. *J Infect Dis*. 1974;129(2):187–193.
16. Reller LB. The serum bactericidal test. *Rev Infect Dis*. 1986;8(5):803–808.
17. Weinstein MP, Stratton CW, Ackley A, et al. Multicenter collaborative evaluation of a standardized serum bactericidal test as a prognostic indicator in infective endocarditis. *Am J Med*. 1985;78(2):262–269.
18. Weinstein MP, Stratton CE, Hawley HB, et al. Multicenter collaborative evaluation of a standardized serum bactericidal test as a predictor of therapeutic efficacy in acute and chronic osteomyelitis. *Am J Med*. 1987;83(2):218–222.
19. Blondeau JM, Hansen G, Metzler K, et al. The role of PK/PD parameters to avoid selection and increase of resistance: mutant prevention concentration. *J Chemother*. 2004;16(suppl 3):1–19.
20. Drlica K, Zhao X. Mutant selection window hypothesis updated. *Clin Infect Dis*. 2007;44(5):681–688.
21. Zhao X, Drlica K. A unified anti-mutant dosing strategy. *J Antimicrob Chemother*. 2008;62(3):434–436.
22. Radaelli ST, Platt SR. Bacterial meningoencephalomyelitis in dogs: a retrospective study of 23 cases (1990-1999). *J Vet Intern Med*. 2002;16(2):159–163.
23. Sturges BK, Dickinson PJ, Kortz GD, et al. Clinical signs, magnetic resonance imaging features, and outcome after surgical and medical treatment of otogenic intracranial infection in 11 cats and 4 dogs. *J Vet Intern Med*. 2006;20(3):648–656.
24. Cole LK, Kwochka KW, Kowalski JJ, et al. Microbial flora and antimicrobial susceptibility patterns of isolated pathogens from the horizontal ear canal and middle ear in dogs with otitis media. *J Am Vet Med Assoc*. 1998;212(4):534–538.
25. Tolar EL, Hendrix DV, Rohrback BW, et al. Evaluation of clinical characteristics and bacterial isolates in dogs with bacterial keratitis: 97 cases (1993-2003). *J Am Vet Med Assoc*. 2006;228(1):80–85.

4

Laboratory Diagnosis of Fungal Infections

Barbara A. Byrne, Shelley C. Rankin

KEY POINTS

- Fungi often grow more slowly than bacteria and can have specific culture media and incubation requirements. Many pathogenic fungi are dangerous to culture because they produce airborne conidia (spores) that may lead to laboratory-acquired infections.
- The clinician should notify the diagnostic laboratory if a fungal infection is suspected. Providing a list of suspected pathogens facilitates safe and successful culture of pathogenic fungi. The animal's signalment, clinical abnormalities, travel history, history of immunosuppressive drug therapy, and the results of cytologic or histopathologic examination should be considered.
- Specimens should be collected and transported as for bacterial culture. Refrigeration inhibits growth of some fungi, and freezing often prevents isolation of fungi from clinical specimens.
- Direct microscopic examination of specimens may provide presumptive identification of a fungal pathogen.
- Most pathogenic fungi remain predictably susceptible to antifungal drugs. Drug resistance among some pathogenic fungi has been documented, and the demand for antifungal susceptibility testing has increased. For some fungal pathogens, isolation, identification, and susceptibility testing before initiation of therapy may be advantageous.

INTRODUCTION AND DEFINITIONS

Fungi are eukaryotic microorganisms that secrete enzymes to digest organic material in the environment. The resultant nutrients are absorbed through a specialized fungal cell wall (known as *chemotrophic nutrition*). A basic understanding of fungal terminology facilitates communication between clinicians, microbiologists, and pathologists. Fungal organisms have two basic morphologic forms:

1. Molds—molds exist as filaments known as *hyphae,* which may be divided into cellular compartments *(septate hyphae).* Fungi with nonseptate or infrequently septate hyphae belong to the class Zygomycetes. A mass of filaments is known as a *mycelium.* A granule formed *in vivo* by a compacted mat of fungal filaments is a *eumycetoma* (as opposed to an *actinomycotic mycetoma*, which is a mycetoma formed by filamentous bacteria).
2. Yeasts—yeasts are single-celled organisms that reproduce by budding. In some cases, buds do not detach from the parent cell, but instead form a chain. Elongated chains of buds may resemble hyphae. These are termed *pseudohyphae* (Fig. 4.1).

Many pathogenic fungi exist as a mold in the environment, but convert to a yeast form in tissues. These fungi are called *dimorphic fungi.* Temperature can be a trigger for this conversion, and some dimorphic fungi convert from the yeast form in the animal to the infectious mold stage in the laboratory and pose a risk for laboratory personnel.

Molds can be further grouped using their asexual characteristics. Hyphomycetes (most pathogenic molds) can be categorized either as *moniliaceous* or *dematiaceous.* The hyphae and spores (conidia) of moniliaceous hyphomycetes lack visible melanin (*hyaline*) (e.g., *Aspergillus* spp.). The hyphae and spores of *dematiaceous* hyphomycetes have visible melanin (pigmented) (e.g., *Cladophialophora* spp.).

Molds reproduce by producing spores that can be produced following sexual reproduction. Sexual reproduction involves the fusion of haploid nuclei from two hyphal structures, which is followed by meiosis. Asexual reproduction (through mitosis) generates conidia that are identical to the parent cell. The asexual stage of a fungus is known as an *anamorph*, whereas the sexual stage is known as a *teleomorph*. Many fungi have two different species names to reflect these stages. For example, the teleomorph of *Cryptococcus neoformans* has been previously referred to as *Filobasidiella neoformans*. Formally, the teleomorph name has been designated to take precedence and can be used to describe both stages. Asexual reproduction predominates in most fungi, including in the laboratory during growth in culture. Thus, certain fungi, such as *C. neoformans*, have been more widely known by their anamorph name. Teleomorphs of some fungal organisms have not yet been described. Some organisms can exist in more than one asexual form, and therefore have had more than two names. Because of the confusion that has existed, with the recent Amsterdam Declaration of Fungal Nomenclature ("one fungus = one name"), there has been a move to use of only one name to describe fungal species.[1]

Diagnosis of fungal infections in animals requires laboratory procedures that include direct microscopic examination of a clinical specimen, isolation, and identification of a fungus. Diagnosis is often supported by immunologic tests to detect fungal antigen or host antibody to the fungus. Many direct specimen examinations and some antigen tests are now within the scope of POC diagnostic procedures for use in the primary veterinary practice. The development of improved methods for the rapid diagnosis of fungal infection has been directed at prepackaged identification kits, serologic kits, and molecular assays.[2] Confirmation of the identification of a specific fungus isolated from an infection frequently will be made by a specialty reference laboratory.

SPECIMEN COLLECTION AND TRANSPORT

Specimens collected for fungal isolation should be representative of the focus of infection and of adequate size or volume to permit direct examination and inoculation of media. Specimens should be obtained from an active site of infection as indicated by clinical and clinicopathologic examinations. In disseminated fungal infections,

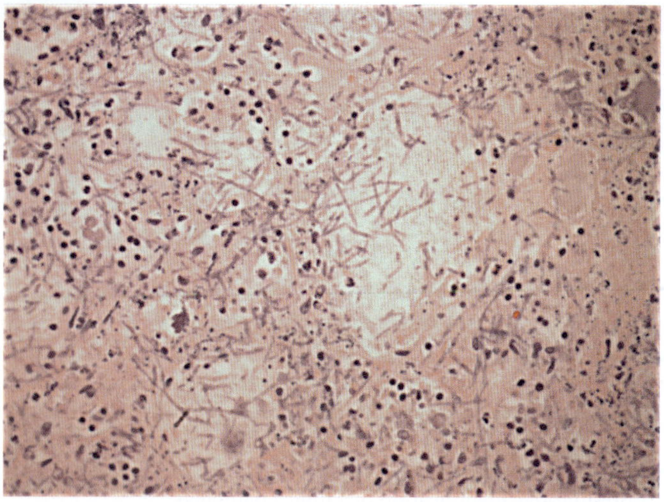

Fig. 4.1 Histopathology of the thyroid gland from a 13-year old female spayed poodle mix with disseminated *Candida albicans* infection. The dog had been treated with prednisone, cyclosporine, and azathioprine for refractory immune-mediated hematologic disease. Note intralesional pseudohyphae (hematoxylin and eosin stain, 400× magnification).

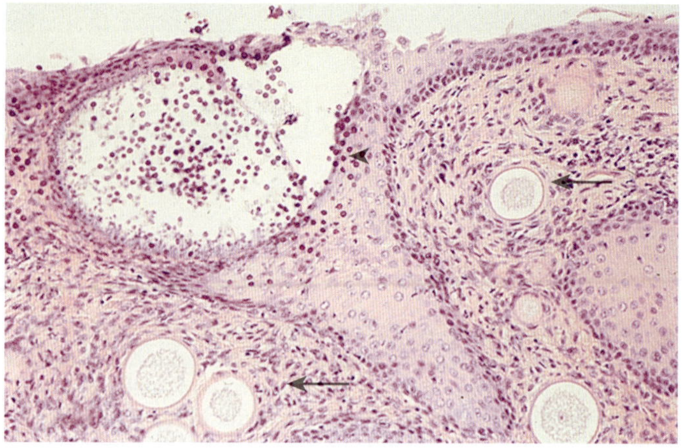

Fig. 4.2 Histopathology of a nasal polyp from a dog caused by *Rhinosporidium* spp. There are juvenile sporangia (arrows) and a mature sporangium that contains many endospores (arrowhead). (hematoxylin and eosin stain, 500× magnification). (Courtesy Spencer S. Jang, University of California, Davis, CA.)

blood culture for fungus may be indicated. Systemic mycoses are usually acquired via the respiratory tract and samples of lung tissue or airway exudate are often used. In certain disseminated mycotic infections, urine and lymph node tissue may also be appropriate specimens.[3]

For dermatophyte culture, lesions should be gently cleaned with 70% alcohol. The use of iodine should be avoided as it can inactivate dermatophytes. Surface antisepsis aids in minimizing the collection of environmental bacterial and fungal contaminants, thereby ensuring a meaningful result rather than contamination of cultures. Specimens for dermatophyte culture are best obtained by plucking hairs and crusts from the margin of the lesion. Use of a Wood's lamp may identify hairs infected with some dermatophyte species such as *Microsporum canis* (see Chapter 78). Skin scrapings can also be used for dermatophyte isolation. Brushings of affected lesions with a new, unused toothbrush can be useful for dermatophyte detection.[4] Nails are collected by clipping after treatment with 70% alcohol. Crumbled material from under the claw may be the best specimen, or an entire claw can be submitted. A biopsy may be required if fungi fail to grow from hair, scrapings, or swab specimens. Biopsy specimens should be divided and a portion placed in 10% buffered formalin for histopathologic examination to help confirm dermatophytosis. Skin scrapings, claw material, hair, and toothbrush specimens can be collected in a clean paper envelope or a sterile tube for transport to the laboratory. Envelopes are preferred to tubes because tubes retain moisture that can promote overgrowth of contaminants. Storage is best at room temperature because refrigeration can be harmful for some dermatophytes.

Swab specimens are of limited value for fungal isolation, and their use is discouraged. If no alternative collection method is available, specimens collected on swabs in a bacteriological transport medium should be inoculated onto suitable media without delay. Cotton swab specimens should not be used to make direct smears because recovery rates are poor.

Blood for fungal culture is collected directly after skin antisepsis into conventional or biphasic blood culture bottles, automated blood culture systems, or lysis-centrifugation systems.[5–7] Blood samples taken from indwelling intravenous catheters are not recommended because this may lead to growth of clinically insignificant fungi that grow and form a biofilm on the catheter.[5,7] Urine is best collected via cystocentesis. Urinary catheters may be colonized with yeast biofilms that can result in inaccurate diagnosis of funguria. Stool specimen cultures for diagnosis of fungal infections of the gastrointestinal tract are misleading since many fungi may be present in these specimens without associated disease; intestinal biopsy specimens for histologic examination are preferred. Body fluids and contents of masses suspected to contain fungi are collected through fine-needle aspiration or respiratory lavage/brushing. Large volumes that can be used for centrifugation are ideal. At least 3 mL of CSF is desirable if possible. Surgically collected material should be handled aseptically pending direct examination and culture. Corneal lesions are sampled by scraping with a sterile spatula, a surgical blade, or a nylon brush.

When rapid (<2 hours) transfer to the laboratory is not possible, storage and transport at room temperature is preferred. If transport requires longer periods, appropriate media should be used and the specimen should be refrigerated to prevent bacterial overgrowth.[6] Refrigeration may delay or inhibit proliferation of slow-growing fungi.

Urine specimens may be refrigerated for up to 24 hours before culture. Most bacteria and yeasts will multiply in urine held at room temperature. The laboratory should be informed if the patient is receiving antifungal drug treatment, which may interfere with fungal isolation.

Blood culture bottles can be held at room temperature for up to 24 hours. CSF and fluids from serous cavities and joints should be processed as soon as possible. CSF should be held at room temperature if not cultured immediately. Other sterile fluids should be held overnight under refrigeration.

Nasal biopsies and excised polyps may be divided between sterile containers for fungal isolation with 10% buffered formalin for histologic examination to assist with diagnosis of rhinosporidiosis or nasal aspergillosis (Fig. 4.2). Tissue may be moistened with a small amount of sterile saline.

Specimens should be labeled with the patient identification, source of specimen, and date and time of collection, and labeled, packaged, and transported according to regional and global regulations for shipping of infectious substances. Careful packaging and transport

TABLE 4.1 Microscopic Description of Some Common Fungal Pathogens of Dogs and Cats

Organism	Yeast or Hyphae	Diameter (μm)	Description	Geographic Distribution
Blastomyces spp.	Yeast	8–15	Round with thick, often refractile cell wall and broad-based budding	Southeastern and south central United States, upper Midwest region
Histoplasma spp.	Yeast	2–5	Oval to round, often found in clusters within macrophages	Ohio and Mississippi river valleys, and California, United States; Central America
Cryptococcus spp.	Yeast	2–15	Round to oval, narrow-based budding, sometimes forming chains of organisms. Large capsule (see Fig. 4.6). Poorly encapsulated variants are rarely encountered	Worldwide, common in Australia and western North America
Coccidioides spp.	Spherule	10–200	Spherules vary in size and may contain endospores ("pomegranate-like"). Using cytology, they appear as empty and collapsed, deeply basophilic structures.	Central California, Arizona, Nevada, Texas; Central and South America
Sporothrix schenckii	Yeast	2–6	Oval, round, or cigar-shaped, occasionally budding. May be found intracellularly and extracellularly. Difficult to find in dogs but may be abundant in cats	Temperate and tropical zones worldwide. Most common in South and Central America
Malassezia spp.	Yeasts and pseudohyphae	3–8 (yeast), 5–10 (pseudohyphae)	Round to oval; when budding, have a "footprint" appearance (see Fig. 4.7)	Worldwide
Candida spp.	Yeast and pseudohyphae	3–4 (yeast), 5–10 (pseudohyphae)	Usually yeasts with a single bud or pseudohyphae with multiple constrictions (see Fig. 4.1)	Worldwide
Dermatophytes	Hyphae	3–15	Septate hyaline hyphae, arthroconidia may be visible along hair shafts (see Fig 4.4)	Worldwide
Aspergillus spp.	Hyphae	4–6	Septate hyaline hyphae with uniform diameter that branch at 45-degree angles (see Fig. 4.3)	Worldwide
Scedosporium spp., *Paecilomyces* spp.	Hyphae	3–12	Septate hyaline hyphae that tend to branch at wider angles than *Aspergillus* spp. (45–90 degrees)	Worldwide
Basidiobolus and *Conidiobolus* (zygomycosis)	Hyphae	10–30	Wide, non- or poorly septate irregular hyaline hyphae, branching at right angles, may be twisted or folded. Poorly stained using hematoxylin and eosin stain	Tropical and subtropical regions of the Americas, Africa, southeast Asia, and Australia
Phialophora, Exophiala, Cladophialophora, Bipolaris (phaeohyphomycosis or dematiaceous molds)	Hyphae	1.5–6	Pigmented hyphae, budding cells with single septa and chains of swollen round cells. May form granules	Worldwide
Pythium insidiosum	Hyphae	4–9	Sparsely septate, hyaline hyphae with 90-degree branches, detectable using hematoxylin and eosin stain	Tropical, subtropical, and some temperate regions of the world

is particularly important for specimens suspected to contain fungal pathogens. If organisms such as *Coccidioides*, *Blastomyces*, or *Histoplasma* spp. might be present, the laboratory should be advised and specimens marked appropriately. This information will assist the laboratory in selecting appropriate media, incubation conditions, and safety precautions.

DIAGNOSTIC METHODS

Microscopic Examination of Direct Smears

Examination of a direct smear before inoculation of media allows presumptive identification of many fungi by the laboratory (Table 4.1; Fig. 4.3). This helps the clinician make initial treatment decisions and guides media selection by the laboratory.

The search for fungal structures may involve preparation of stained or unstained wet mounts, fixed stained smears, and histologic sections. Some of these techniques are simple and rapid and may provide the clinician with a presumptive or even definitive diagnosis and a time-saving guide to therapy (Table 4.2). Others require more specialized stains or laboratory procedures.

Wet Mounts

Specimens may be suspended on a slide in saline, water, or 10% potassium hydroxide (KOH). If tissue granules are present, they can be examined by the laboratory for hyphae and cultured. Examination of smears begins under low magnification (100×) and with subdued light, with the condenser lowered. When structures suggestive of fungal elements are seen, higher magnification (400×) is used for examination.

KOH preparations can be used to examine specimens for dermatophyte hyphae and arthroconidia. The KOH clears keratinaceous and cellular debris, but fungal elements are left intact. The hair or skin scraping to be examined is placed into a drop of 10% KOH on a slide (Fig. 4.4A). The material may require soaking in KOH before further processing. Crusty material is teased apart with forceps, covered with a coverslip, and passed over an open flame several times, with care taken not to boil the mixture. The slide is then examined for fungal elements (Fig. 4.4B and C). If no organisms are observed, the slide is reexamined in 30 minutes. A more sensitive modification of the KOH preparation uses chlorazol black E and dimethylsulfoxide (DMSO, Delasco, Council Bluffs, IA, USA) which stains hyphae and/or arthroconidia green against a gray background. A mixture of 20% KOH and 36% DMSO or 25% KOH or sodium hydroxide with 5% glycerol increases penetration and clarity of specimens. Clearing of claw material may require up to 2 hours.

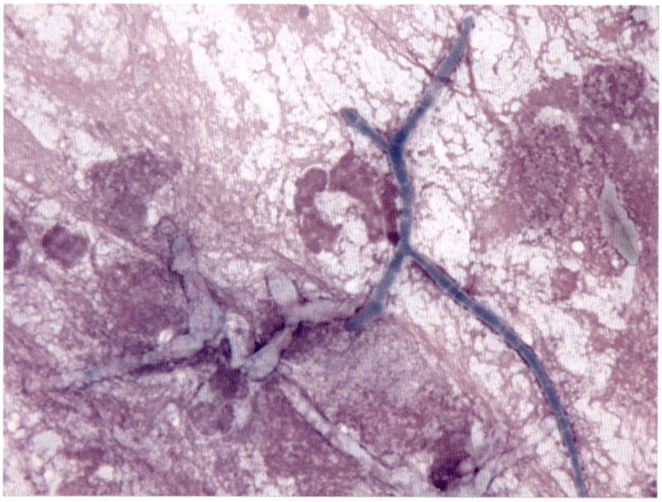

Fig. 4.3 Direct smear of an aspirate from a mediastinal mass of a 6-year-old female spayed labrador retriever with disseminated *Aspergillus deflectus* infection. Note hyphae with parallel walls that branch at 45-degree angles. Stain uptake by some hyphae is poor (Wright stain, 1000× magnification).

India ink or nigrosin (1% aqueous), when mixed on a slide with fluids or exudates, particularly CSF, containing *Cryptococcus* spp., provides a dark background that outlines the large capsules surrounding the yeast cells (see Chapter 82). Placing a drop of the specimen and a drop of India ink separately on a slide and then adding a coverslip allows for an optimal mixture gradient to form. However, less than 50% of culture-positive human CSF samples are detected by this method, so it is relatively insensitive.[5]

Less readily available methods of unstained wet mount visualization include phase microscopy, which improves visibility of fungal structures against a background of tissue debris, and fluorescence microscopy, in which specimens are prepared by mixing with an equal volume of 10% to 20% KOH and 0.5% calcofluor white (Difco, Detroit, MI, USA). Using a fluorescence microscope with a 365-nm exciter filter and a barrier filter that transmits light at 410 nm, fungal walls fluoresce (Fig. 4.5).

Fixed Smears

A Gram stain can be performed on most routine clinical specimens and can detect most fungi. Yeasts generally stain gram positive and molds tend to be gram negative or unstained. Yeasts are often detected because they retain the primary crystal violet stain (Fig. 4.6). The cell walls of molds often appear as unstained filaments. The usefulness of Gram stain for presumptive identification is generally limited to *Blastomyces, Candida, Cryptococcus, Malassezia* (Fig. 4.7), and *Geotrichum* spp., or the yeast form of *Sporothrix schenckii* spp. complex.

Romanowsky-type stains, such as Wright, Giemsa, and Diff-Quik, will stain fungi, especially yeasts, and are the stains of choice for *Histoplasma* spp. (see Chapter 81).

Histopathologic Findings

Routine hematoxylin and eosin stain of formalin-fixed paraffin-embedded tissue permits detection of fungi that cause systemic mycoses (coccidioidomycosis, histoplasmosis, blastomycosis, and cryptococcosis). Hyphae of filamentous fungi may also be detected; these can

TABLE 4.2 Stains and Reagents Used for Direct Examination of Fungi in Clinical Specimens

Stain or Reagent	Usage	Text Figures/Disadvantages
Gram	Stains bacteria, yeasts, and other fungi	*Cryptococcus* (Fig. 4.6); *Malassezia pachydermatis* (Fig. 4.7); some fungi stain variably or not at all
Potassium hydroxide	Clearing tissue and cellular debris from variety of specimens to provide greater visibility of fungal elements	Dermatophytes (Fig. 4.4); artifacts develop after preparation time; experience required
India ink	Observation for presence or absence of capsules of fungal cells against a dark background	*Cryptococcus* (see Chapter 82); problems of artifacts can occur in the stain, poor sensitivity
Calcofluor white	A fluorescent brightener binding to polysaccharide such as cellulose and chitin	Detects variety of fungal elements; requires a fluorescent microscope
Wright	Stain for cytologic examination of peripheral blood, bone marrow, body fluids, and organ impressions	*Histoplasma* (see Chapter 81); *Aspergillus* (see Chapter 86); *Candida* (see Chapter 85); *Prototheca* (see Chapter 90); limited use
Gomori's methenamine silver	Detection of fungal elements in histologic section	Fig. 4.8; not readily available to most clinical bacteriology laboratories
Periodic acid–Schiff reaction	Detection of fungal elements in histologic section	Fig. 4.8; not readily available to most clinical bacteriology laboratories
Hematoxylin and eosin	Routine histologic stain used for detection of some fungal elements	*Rhinosporidium* (Fig. 4.2); usually requires large numbers of organisms to be detected with this stain

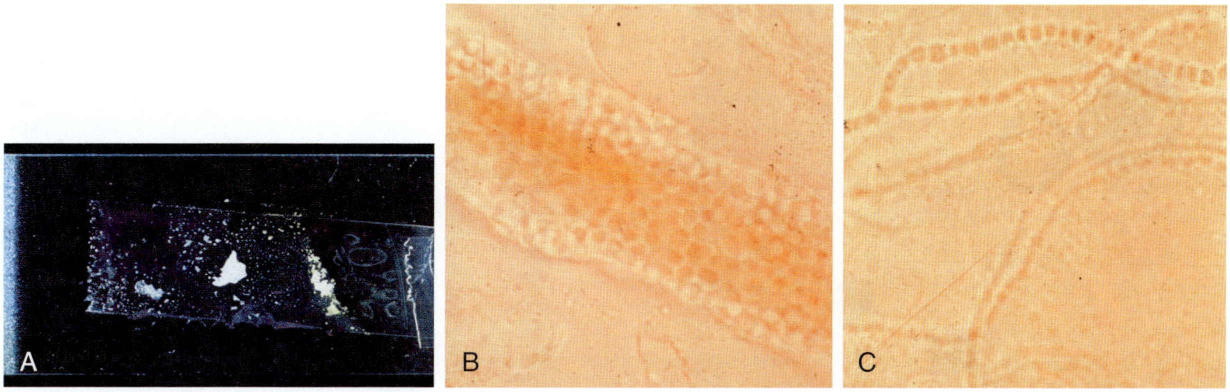

Fig. 4.4 (A) Hairs from a crusty skin lesion using a potassium hydroxide preparation (40× magnification) with (B) arthroconidia along or on the hair shaft or (C) chains of arthroconidia embedded in crusty material. (Courtesy Spencer S. Jang, University of California, Davis, CA.)

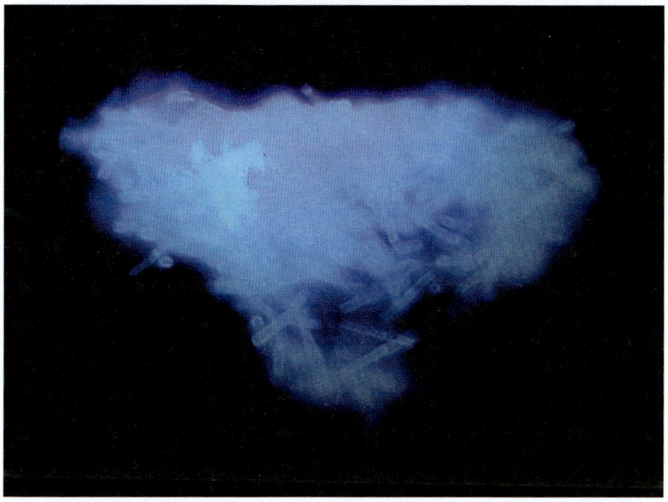

Fig. 4.5 Calcofluor white stain of a mat of *Aspergillus fumigatus* hyphae (1000× magnification).

be distinguished as septate or nonseptate and pigmented or nonpigmented, helping with their classification. A more fungal-specific stain is periodic acid–Schiff, which makes mycotic elements appear dark red against a contrasting background (Fig. 4.8A), or Gomori's methenamine silver (Fig. 4.8B), which stains fungal structures brownish-black against a pale green background. Many laboratories use hematoxylin with eosin as a counterstain or hematoxylin alone, which permits better pathologic characterization of the lesion than do other procedures. Mayer's mucicarmine stain colors the capsule of *Cryptococcus* spp. red.

Fungal Culture

Before culture, clinical specimens must be prepared for inoculation on fungal growth media. Body fluids are usually centrifuged by the laboratory to concentrate fungal organisms. The sediment is then resuspended in a smaller volume of supernatant and inoculated onto media. If biopsy specimens are submitted, the tissues are minced before they are inoculated onto media.[6] Tissue grinding should be avoided because it can be harmful to fragile hyphal structures. Scrapings, swab specimens, and hair may be inoculated directly onto fungal media. For dermatophyte culture, toothbrush bristles or hairs (using sterile forceps) may be pressed into the agar.

Many types of media are available for fungal isolation, and no single medium is optimal for all pathogens (Table 4.3). Special media are available for differentiation of fungal species (see Fungal Identification). Media that contain antibacterial agents (usually chloramphenicol or gentamicin) are used to culture specimens that are likely to contain bacteria. Cycloheximide is added to dermatophyte test medium (DTM) to inhibit the growth of contaminant saprophytic molds. All plates should be sealed with oxygen-permeable shrink seal or tape to prevent exposure of laboratory personnel to potentially dangerous conidia and to minimize contamination with saprophytic mold species.

Use of the Isolator system (Wampole Laboratories, Princeton, NJ, USA) improves the sensitivity of fungal isolation, including of *Histoplasma*, *Coccidioides*, and *Cryptococcus* spp. from blood.[7] This system involves lysis and centrifugation of 1 to 10 mL of blood. The supernatant is removed through the blood culture bottle stopper, and the concentrate is removed from the sediment and plated onto media. It can be difficult to detect molds with conventional broth-based blood culture systems, but yeast can be isolated, particularly *Candida* spp. Nevertheless, molds may be isolated from broth-based blood culture systems, provided incubation periods are long enough. Several commercial broth-based blood culture systems support growth of fungi.[8,9]

Inoculated media is incubated at temperatures lower than those used for bacterial isolation: ~25°C or 30°C. Cultures are examined daily during the first week of incubation and twice weekly thereafter for 4 weeks before being called negative. Plates or tubes that grow filamentous fungi should be opened only in a biologic safety cabinet.

Fungal Identification

Identification of cultured fungi is based on colony morphology (size, color, and consistency), fungal growth rate, appearance of hyphae or yeast, asexual or sexual reproductive structures, physiologic tests, antigenic characteristics, matrix-assisted laser desorption/ionization time-of-flight mass spectrometry (MALDI-TOF MS) analysis, and/or molecular analysis.

Yeast colonies resemble bacterial colonies and can be moist, dry, mucoid (Fig. 4.9A), or waxy. Mold colonies are generally dry, wrinkled, or heaped. Some molds such as zygomycetes (*Mucor, Rhizopus* spp.) grow rapidly, filling a Petri dish within 2 or 3 days. Others may not appear for a week or more and may remain as smaller colonies. Fruiting structures that produce conidia may appear as black specks in a colorless aerial mycelium (e.g., *Aspergillus niger*). Fruiting structures may be intensely pigmented, as seen by the green to blue-green colors of *Aspergillus fumigatus*. Some fungi produce soluble red or yellow pigment that diffuses through the medium (e.g., *Microsporum canis*). In others, pigment is confined to hyphae and

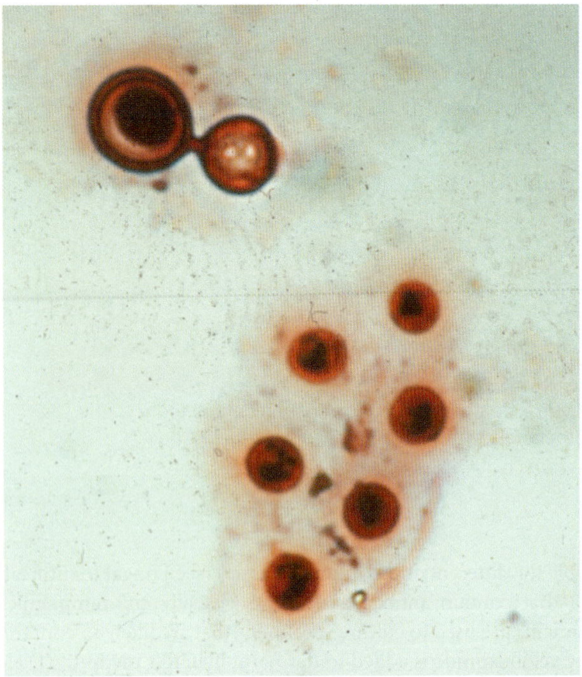

Fig. 4.6 *Cryptococcus spp.* Nasal granuloma of a cat. Budding forms, top; hazy zone around the six cells below represent capsules (Gram stain, 500× magnification). (Courtesy Spencer S. Jang, University of California, Davis, CA.)

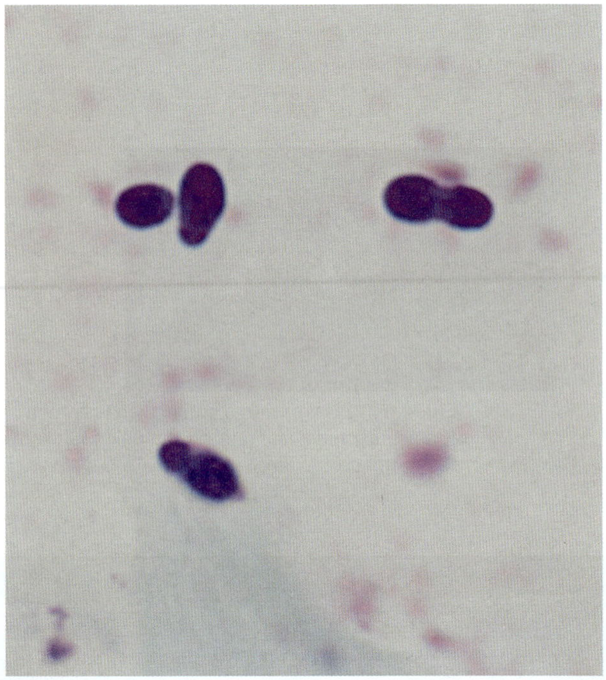

Fig. 4.7 *Malassezia* sp. ear exudate, dog. Broad-based budding yeast cells have "shoe print" appearance (Gram stain, 1000× magnification). (Courtesy Spencer S. Jang, University of California, Davis, CA.)

may be observed either on the surface or on the reverse side of the colony (Fig. 4.9B). The surface of the colony varies according to mycelial growth patterns from smooth ("glabrous") to powdery, velvety, and cottony. On DTM, dermatophytes rapidly utilize peptones in the medium, which leads to alkaline conditions and a red color change to the agar, often visible around the same time a mycelium appears. Molds that cause this color change should still be examined microscopically as some saprophytic molds may also cause the same color change; conversely, occasional dermatophytes fail to change or very slowly change the medium to red. As mentioned previously, agars with mold growth should not be opened outside of a biosafety cabinet.

Phenotypic identification of isolated molds is based on microscopic examination for hyphal characteristics: broad versus narrow, septate versus nonseptate, pigmented (dematiaceous) (Fig. 4.10) versus nonpigmented, conidia, and their supporting structures.

Microscopic examination of molds generally uses teased preparations or clear cellophane tape mounts from cultures prepared using appropriate precautions in a biosafety cabinet. Morphologic fungal structures are better preserved in their natural interrelationships in *lactophenol aniline blue (LPAB) tape mounts* (Figs. 4.11 and 4.12) or in a *slide culture.* To prepare a LPAB mount, tape is touched to the surface of a colony and placed sticky-side down in a drop of LPAB on a glass slide. Low-power microscopy aids early detection of mycelial growth, and macroconidia and microconidia of dermatophytes (Figs. 4.13 and 4.14). *Slide culture* permits LPAB examination of undisturbed fungal structures, and should not be performed for dangerous pathogens such as *Blastomyces* spp. or *Coccidioides* spp.

The *germ tube test* allows differentiation of *Candida albicans* from other *Candida* species. A standard serum, 0.5 to 1 mL, is inoculated with suspect *Candida* growth and incubated at 35°C for 2 to 3 hours. A drop of this suspension is then examined microscopically for germ tubes which can be seen sprouting from yeast cells (blastoconidia), which indicate the presence of *C. albicans* (Fig. 4.15).

A variety of broth or solid media are also used for fungal identification. For example, using chromogenic *Candida* agar can differentiate *Candida* spp., because each species has a specific colony morphology and color on this medium.[10] Commercially available test strips allow multiple biochemical identification tests for yeasts to be performed simultaneously (e.g., API 20C AUX Yeast Identification Kit, bioMérieux or RapID YEAST PLUS, Remel).[11] Other commonly used differential media include cornmeal agar for the demonstration of chlamydoconidia of *C. albicans, Trichophyton* agars for the identification of *Trichophyton* spp., and Christensen's urea agar for production of urease by *Cryptococcus, Rhodotorula, Trichophyton,* and *Trichosporon* spp.[12]

A recent innovation in identification of fungi is MALDI-TOF MS.[13–16] With this method, a yeast or mold isolate of unknown identification is spotted onto a stainless-steel slide target. A matrix is added that imparts a charge when the sample is struck with a laser and proteins fragment into peptides that pass through a vacuum tube at a rate determined by size and charge to hit a detector creating a peptide "spectrum." The spectrum of the test sample is compared to a database of spectra from known fungi, resulting in rapid (within minutes) identification. Yeast colonies can be directly transferred to the target slide, and identification is made within minutes. Molds generally require an extraction procedure before spotting the protein extract on the target for successful identification.

Fungal isolates can be identified to genus or species level by many other molecular-based methods. Both morphologic examination as well as molecular methods may be needed to identify some fungi definitively. Broad-spectrum 28S rRNA polymerase chain reaction (PCR) assays followed by testing with specific nucleic acid probes can be used.[17] A multiplex PCR approach for identification of a battery of commonly encountered yeasts and molds has also been described.[18] Commercially available DNA probes such as the AccuProbe (San Diego, CA, USA) are available for identification of fungal agents such as *Coccidioides, Blastomyces,* and *Histoplasma* spp. PCR-sequencing, especially of rRNA gene segments, can also be used for identification purposes. At present, the most commonly used regions are the D2

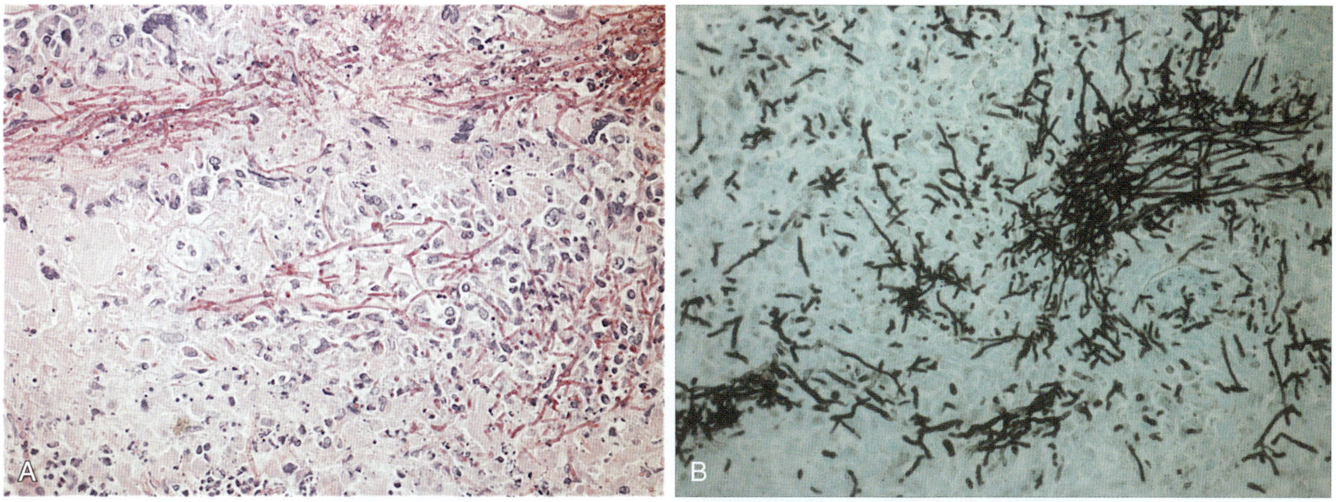

Fig. 4.8 Histopathology of the kidney from a 2-year-old female spayed German shepherd dog with disseminated paecilomycosis. (A) Periodic acid–Schiff stain. The fungal hyphae stain bright pink. (B) Gomori's methenamine silver stain. The fungal hyphae stain black (400× magnification).

TABLE 4.3 Isolation Media for Fungi

Type of Medium	Selective Features	Indications/Limitation in Mycologic Diagnosis
Sabouraud dextrose agar	Low pH; some formulations may have antibacterial agents	Cultivation of all fungi
Brain-heart infusion agar	None	Cultivation of all fungi
Potato flake/potato dextrose agar	Low pH, highly nutritious for most fungi	Cultivation of all fungi; induces sporulation of fungi
Inhibitory mold agar	Gentamicin, sometimes chloramphenicol	Cultivation of fungi when bacterial contamination is suspected; not for dermatophytes
Dermatophyte test media	Gentamicin, chloramphenicol, and cycloheximide; phenol red is color indicator	Dermatophyte isolation; media turns to red with dermatophyte growth; not for detection of conidia; may produce atypical colony growth; natural pigmentation obscured; nondermatophytes may turn yellow medium to red
Rapid sporulation medium	Cycloheximide and chloramphenicol; bromthymol blue is color indicator	For dermatophytes; media turns to blue-green to blue with dermatophyte growth; allows detection of conidia and pigment development for identification

variable region of the large-subunit rRNA gene and/or the internal transcribed spacer (ITS) regions (ITS-5.8S rRNA-ITS2).[19]

Direct Detection of Fungal DNA

Genus-specific, species-specific, or universal fungal primers can be used in PCR assays to detect fungal DNA in clinical specimens. Subsequent sequencing of PCR products also allows identification of fastidious or noncultivatable fungi. Real-time PCR can be used on peripheral blood for diagnosis of disseminated aspergillosis or *Candida* infections in people.[16,20–22] PCR assays have been used to identify *Pythium insidiosum* in specimens from dogs, and PCR-sequencing has been described for successful identification of *A. fumigatus* in formalin-fixed paraffin-embedded lung tissue from dogs.[23,24] Detection of dermatophyte DNA can aid in diagnosis of dermatophytosis.[25] Molecular-based test results should always be combined with clinical findings and, where possible, confirmed by morphologic features of the agent in tissues and/or in culture before making a final diagnosis.

Antigen and Serologic Testing

Assays designed to detect fungal antigens or antifungal antibodies in body fluids or blood are increasingly available. During cryptococcal infections, fungal capsule polysaccharide is produced abundantly, and its antigen can be detected in peripheral blood. Both latex agglutination and enzyme-linked immunoassays have been developed for cryptococcal antigen detection (see Chapters 2 and 82). Testing of body fluids, particularly urine, is available for diagnosis and treatment of histoplasmosis and blastomycosis (see Chapters 80 and 81).[26] An antigen-based test is also available for the detection of disseminated aspergillosis in dogs, and has shown high clinical sensitivity, although cross-reactivity with other fungi may occur (see Chapter 86).[27] Agar gel immunodiffusion for detection of anti-*Aspergillus* antibody has specificity for diagnosis of nasal aspergillosis, but negative results do not rule out infection.[28] An ELISA has been developed for diagnosis of pythiosis (see Chapter 88).[29]

INTERPRETATION OF FUNGAL CULTURE RESULTS

False-negative and false-positive results can occur with all types of diagnostic tests for fungal pathogens; therefore, results must be interpreted by taking into account the fungal species isolated, clinical signs, the results of cytology and histopathology, and the clinical picture.

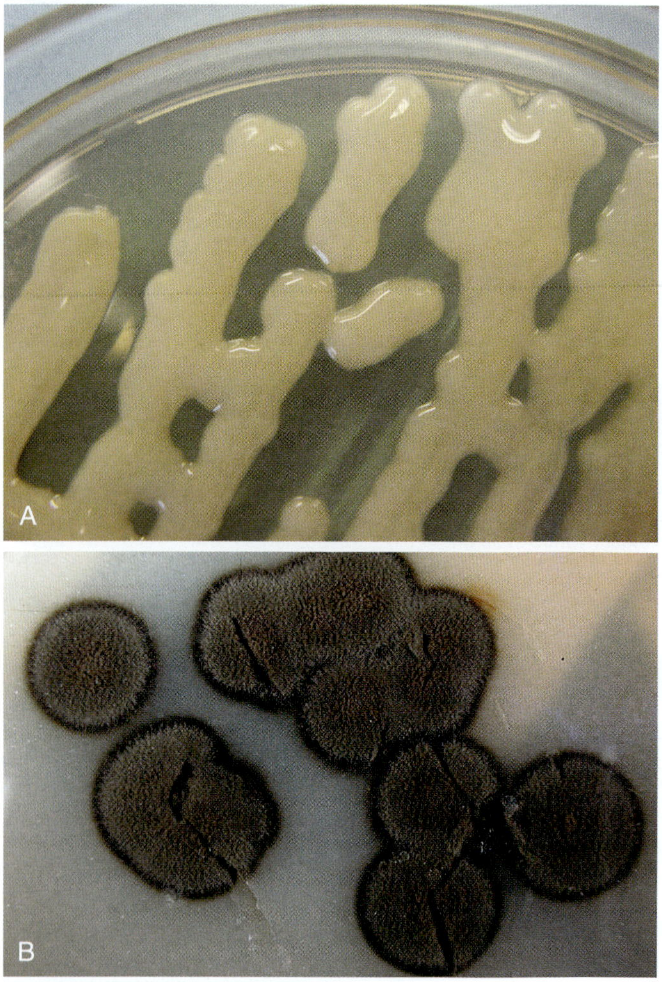

Fig. 4.9 Colony appearance. (A) Growth of *Cryptococcus gattii* yeast on potato flake agar. (B) Growth of *Cladophialophora bantiana*, a pigmented (dematiaceous) mold, isolated from canine brain tissue on potato flake agar.

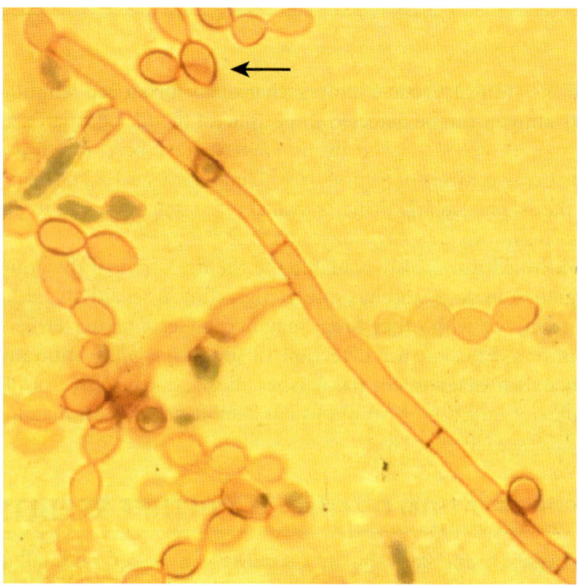

Fig. 4.10 *Cladophialophora bantiana* in culture. Oval conidia occurring in chains. Note dematiaceous (dark-pigmented) appearance of some conidia *(arrow)* and mycelium (lactophenol aniline blue, 200× magnification). (Courtesy Spencer S. Jang, University of California, Davis, CA.)

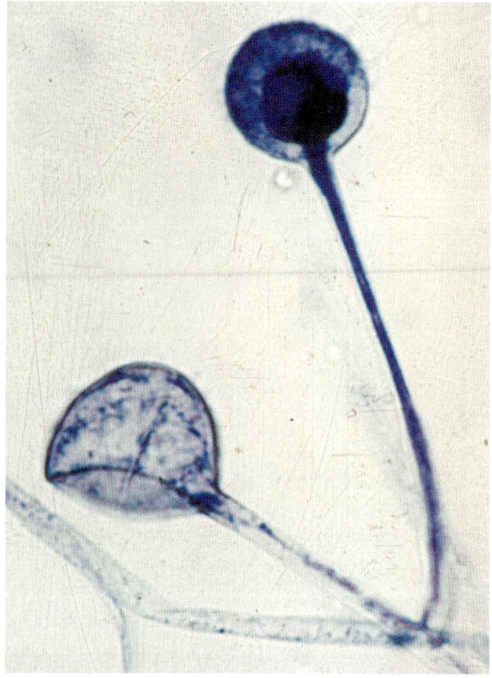

Fig. 4.11 *Mucor* in culture. Sporangia form on sporangiophores; note nonseptate, broad hyphae (lactophenol aniline blue, 200× magnification). (Courtesy Spencer S. Jang, University of California, Davis, CA.)

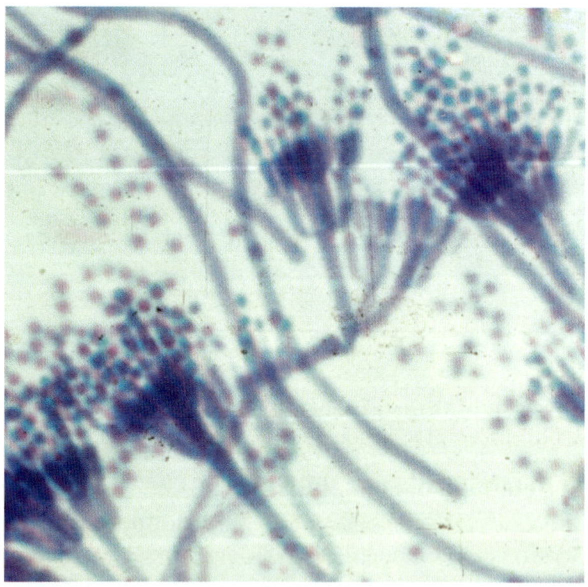

Fig. 4.12 *Penicillium* sp. fruiting structures (lactophenol aniline blue, 500× magnification). (Courtesy Spencer S. Jang, University of California, Davis, CA.)

Specimens That Test Negative

Negative test results can occur for many reasons, including, but not limited to, inadequate specimen size (such as when swabs or aspirates are submitted), inadequate organism numbers at the site of specimen collection, overgrowth with contaminating bacteria or saprophytic fungi, or loss of organism viability during specimen transportation. If a patient is receiving antifungal drugs but has not completely cleared the infection, culture may be negative.

False-negative test results can also occur when the specimen is not inoculated onto the correct media or insufficient time is allowed for

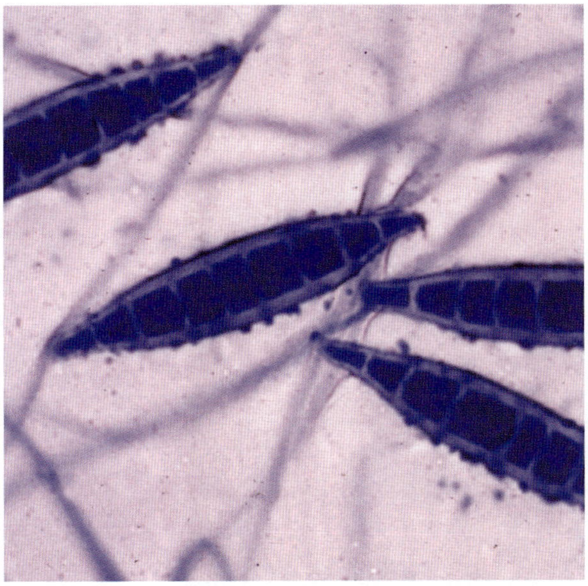

Fig. 4.13 *Microsporum canis* in culture. Rough and thick-walled multicellular spindle-shaped macroconidia. Note curved, pointed ends (lactophenol aniline blue, 200× magnification). (University of California, Davis, CA.)

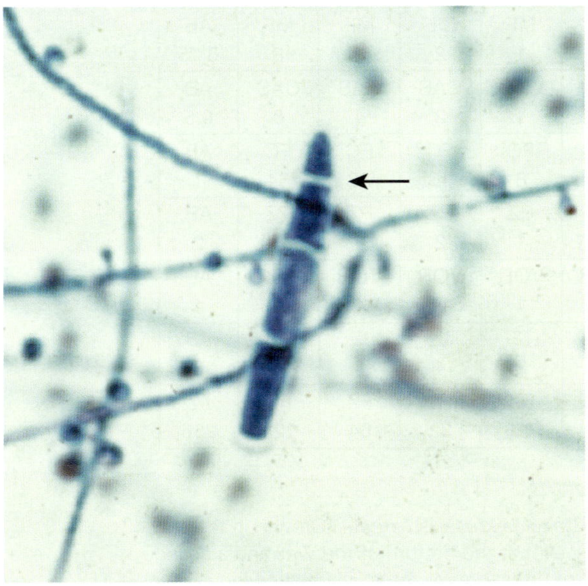

Fig. 4.14 *Trichophyton mentagrophytes* in culture. Spherical microconidia and one thin-walled, multicellular, cigar-shaped macroconidium *(arrow)* (lactophenol aniline blue, 200× magnification). (Courtesy Spencer S. Jang, University of California, Davis, CA.)

growth. It is critical that clinicians inform the laboratory if a specific fungal infection is suspected, and what organism might be involved. Poor laboratory quality control procedures may also lead to false-negative test results. Use of an accredited diagnostic laboratory can help minimize such problems.

Specimens That Test Positive

The detection of fungal organisms within a specimen does not always imply that they are the cause of clinical signs. Contamination by saprophytic fungi, especially *Aspergillus* or *Penicillium* spp., is the most common cause of false-positive fungal cultures. Organisms are more likely to be clinically significant when cytologic examination of a stained smear from the original specimen also demonstrates the presence of fungal organisms, especially in the presence of inflammation.

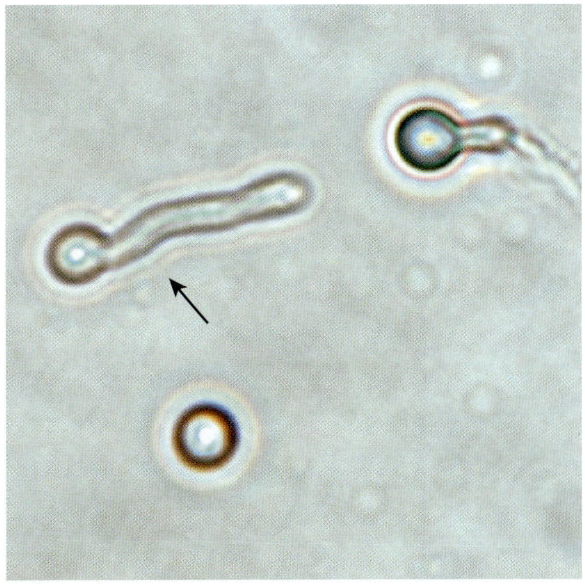

Fig. 4.15 Germ tube test. Formation of germ tube *(arrow)* characteristic of *Candida albicans*. Blastoconidia on left (wet mount, 200× magnification). (Courtesy Richard Walker, University of California, Davis, CA.)

ANTIFUNGAL SUSCEPTIBILITY TESTING

Resistance to antifungal agents has now been documented for a variety of fungal pathogens, and intrinsic resistance to certain antifungal antimicrobials has been recognized.[30] This has led to an increased demand for antifungal susceptibility testing by clinicians. Fortunately, the reproducibility of antifungal susceptibility testing has improved in recent years, and MIC breakpoints that define susceptibility and resistance (see Chapter 10) have been established for many fungal pathogens to aid in the treatment of fungal infections in humans. Although veterinary breakpoints are still lacking, antifungal susceptibility testing allows comparison of the activity of two or more antifungal drugs, and serial testing of isolates from a single patient allows the development of resistance to be monitored over time. Methods of susceptibility testing that have been adapted for yeast and mold infections include broth microdilution, antifungal impregnated strips (ETEST, bioMérieux, France), and disc diffusion test (see Chapter 10). Common antifungal agents tested include amphotericin B, itraconazole, fluconazole, voriconazole, posaconazole, caspofungin, and flucytosine (Fig. 4.16). Limitations of antifungal susceptibility testing include the slow growth of fungal pathogens (when compared to bacteria), and the fact that some fungi may grow as yeasts or molds depending on media and incubation conditions. Partial inhibition of growth over a wide range of antifungal drug dilutions may also occur (a phenomenon known as *trailing*). Criteria have been set for interpretation of MICs in the presence of trailing for different antifungal drugs.[31] MALDI-TOF MS has been used to determine antifungal drug susceptibility among *Candida* spp. and in the future may overcome some of the difficulties in testing that currently exist.[32]

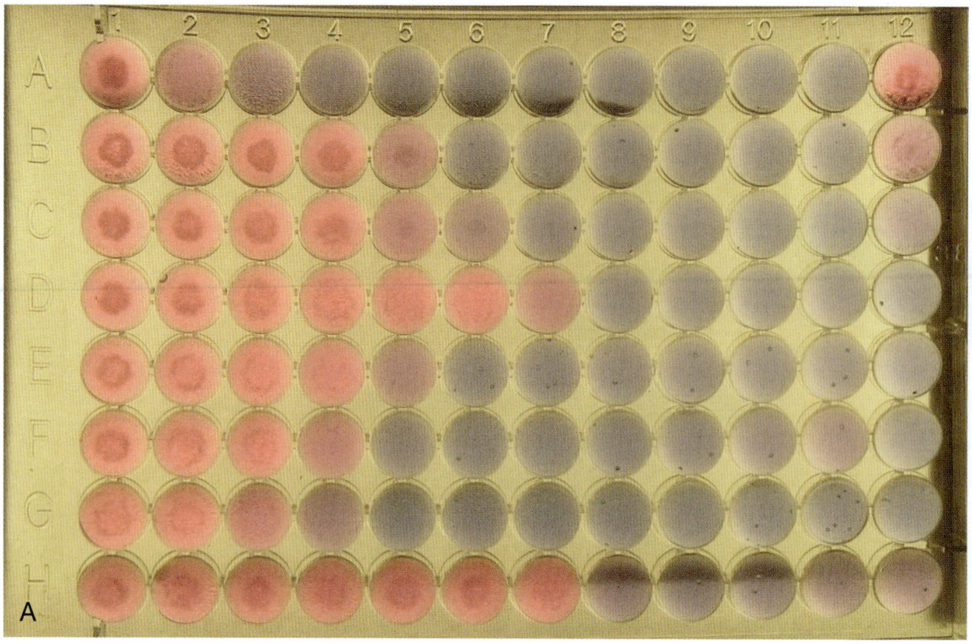

	1	2	3	4	5	6	7	8	9	10	11	12
A	POS	AND 0.015	AND 0.03	AND 0.06	AND 0.12	AND 0.25	AND 0.5	AND 1	AND 2	AND 4	AND 8	AB 0.12
B	MF 0.008	MF 0.015	MF 0.03	MF 0.06	MF 0.12	MF 0.25	MF 0.5	MF 1	MF 2	MF 4	MF 8	AB 0.25
C	CAS 0.008	CAS 0.015	CAS 0.03	CAS 0.06	CAS 0.12	CAS 0.25	CAS 0.5	CAS 1	CAS 2	CAS 4	CAS 8	AB 0.5
D	FC 0.06	FC 0.12	FC 0.25	FC 0.5	FC 1	FC 2	FC 4	FC 8	FC 16	FC 32	FC 64	AB 1
E	PZ 0.008	PZ 0.015	PZ 0.03	PZ 0.06	PZ 0.12	PZ 0.25	PZ 0.5	PZ 1	PZ 2	PZ 4	PZ 8	AB 2
F	VOR 0.008	VOR 0.015	VOR 0.03	VOR 0.06	VOR 0.12	VOR 0.25	VOR 0.5	VOR 1	VOR 2	VOR 4	VOR 8	AB 4
G	IZ 0.015	IZ 0.03	IZ 0.06	IZ 0.12	IZ 0.25	IZ 0.5	IZ 1	IZ 2	IZ 4	IZ 8	IZ 16	AB 8
H	FZ 0.12	FZ 0.25	FZ 0.5	FZ 1	FZ 2	FZ 4	FZ 8	FZ 16	FZ 32	FZ 64	FZ 128	FZ 256

B

Fig. 4.16 Minimum inhibitory concentration (MIC) assay for a *Candida krusei* isolate. (A) Growth in the presence of the antifungal drug is characterized by formation of a pellet at the bottom of the well and a change in the color of the medium from purple to pink. (B) Schematic of the same microtiter plate showing antifungal drug dilutions. Organisms are defined as susceptible, intermediate, or resistant based on MIC cutoffs (breakpoints or interpretive criteria) set by regulatory bodies such as the Clinical and Laboratory Standards Institute in the United States using human interpretive criteria. The report to the clinician would not/should not provide interpretations but would provide MIC values of anidulafungin (0.12 ug/mL), micafungin (0.25 ug/mL), caspofungin (1 ug/mL), flucytosine (8 ug/mL), voriconazole (0.12 ug/mL), itraconazole (0.25 ug/mL), fluconazole (128 ug/mL), posaconazole (0.25 ug/mL), and amphotericin B (≤0.12 ug/mL). AB, amphotericin B; AND, anidulafungin; CAS, caspofungin; FC, 5-flucytosine; FZ, fluconazole; IZ, itraconazole; MF, micafungin; POS, positive control; PZ, posaconazole; VOR, voriconazole.

SUGGESTED READINGS

Wickes BL, Romanelli AM. Diagnostic mycology: Xtreme challenges. *J Clin Microbiol*. 2020;58. e01245–19.

Berkow EL, Lockhart SR, Ostrosky-Zeichner L. Antifungal susceptibility testing: current approaches. *Clin Microbiol Rev*. 2020;33:e00069–19.

REFERENCES

1. Hawksworth DL, Crous PW, Redhead SA, et al. The Amsterdam Declaration on Fungal Nomenclature. *IMA Fungus*. 2011;2:105–112.
2. Yeo SF, Wong B. Current status of nonculture methods for diagnosis of invasive fungal infections. *Clin Microbiol Rev*. 2002;15:465–484.

3. Schultz RM, Johnson EG, Wisner ER, et al. Clinicopathologic and diagnostic imaging characteristics of systemic aspergillosis in 30 dogs. *J Vet Intern Med*. 2008;22:851–859.
4. Moriella KA. Management of dermatophyte infections in catteries and multiple-cat households. *Vet Clin North Am Small Anim Pract*. 1990;20:1457–1474.
5. Barenfanger J. Improving the clinical utility of microbiology data: an update. *Clin Microbiol Newslett*. 2003;25:1–8.
6. McGowan KL. Specimen collection, transport, and processing: mycology. In: Versalovic J, Carroll KC, Funke G, et al., eds. *Manual of Clinical Microbiology*. 10th ed. Washington, DC: American Society for Microbiology Press; 2011:1756–1766.
7. Reimer LG, Wilson ML, Weinstein MP. Update on detection of bacteremia and fungemia. *J Clin Microbiol*. 1997;10:444–465.
8. McDonald LC, Weinstein MP, Fune J, et al. Controlled comparison of BacT/ALERT FAN aerobic medium and BATEC fungal blood culture medium for detection of fungemia. *J Clin Microbiol*. 2001;39:662–664.
9. Taniguchi T, Ogawa Y, Kasai D, et al. Three cases of fungemia in HIV-infected patients diagnosed through the use of mycobacterial blood culture bottles. *Intern Med*. 2010;49:2179–2183.
10. Hospenthal DR, Murray CK, Beckius ML, et al. Persistence of pigment production by yeast isolates grown on CHROMagar *Candida* medium. *J Clin Microbiol*. 2002;40:4768–4770.
11. Wadlin JK, Hanko G, Stewart R, et al. Comparison of three commercial systems for identification of yeasts commonly isolated in the clinical microbiology laboratory. *J Clin Microbiol*. 1999;37:1967–1970.
12. St-Germain G, Summerbell R. *Identifying Fungi: A Clinical Laboratory Handbook*. 2nd ed. Belmont, CA: Star Publishing; 2011.
13. Angeletti S. Matrix assisted laser desorption time of flight mass spectrometry (MALDI-TOF MS) in clinical microbiology. *J Microbiol Methods*. 2017;138:20–29.
14. Cassagne C, Normand AC, Ollivier CL, et al. Performance of MALDI-TOF MS platforms for fungal identification. *Mycoses*. 2016;59:678–690.
15. Iriart X, Lavergne RA, Fillaux J, et al. Routine identification of medical fungi by MALDI-TOF: performance of the new VITEK MS using a new time-effective strategy. *J Clin Microbiol*. 2012;50:2107–2110.
16. Van Burik J, Myaerson D, Schreckhise RW, et al. Panfungal PCR assay for detection of fungal infection in human blood specimens. *J Clin Microbiol*. 1998;36:1169–1175.
17. Sandu GS, Kline BC, Sockman L, et al. Molecular probes for diagnosis of fungal infections. *J Clin Microbiol*. 1995;33:2913–2919.
18. Luo G, Mitchell TG. Rapid identification of pathogenic fungi directly from cultures by using multiplex PCR. *J Clin Microbiol*. 2002;40:2860–2865.
19. Hendolin PH, Paulin L, Koukila-Kahkola P, et al. Panfungal PCR and multiplex liquid hybridization for detection of fungi in tissue specimens. *J Clin Microbiol*. 2000;38:4186–4192.
20. Kami M, Fukui T, Ogawa S, et al. Use of real-time PCR on blood samples for diagnosis of invasive aspergillosis. *Clin Infect Dis*. 2001;33:1504–1512.
21. Mikulsk M, Furfaro E, Viscoli C. Non-cultural methods for the diagnosis of invasive fungal disease. *Expert Rev Anti Infect Ther*. 2015;13:104–117.
22. Phoompoung P, Chayakulkeeree M. Recent progress in the diagnosis of pathogenic *Candida* species in blood culture. *Mycopathologia*. 2016;181:363–369.
23. Adamama-Moraitou KK, Pardali D, Day MJ, et al. *Aspergillus fumigatus* bronchopneumonia in a Hellenic shepherd dog. *J Am Anim Hosp Assoc*. 2011;47:e13–e18.
24. Grooters AM, Gee MK. Development of a nested polymerase chain reaction assay for the detection and identification of *Pythium insidiosum*. *J Vet Intern Med*. 2002;16:147–152.
25. Cafarchia C, Gasser RB, Figueredo LA, et al. An improved molecular diagnostic assay for canine and feline dermatophytosis. *Med Mycol*. 2013;51:136–143.
26. Wheat LJ. Laboratory diagnosis of histoplasmosis: update. *Semin Respir Infect*. 2000;16:131–140.
27. Garcia RS, Wheat LJ, Cook AK, et al. Sensitivity and specificity of a blood and urine galactomannan antigen assay for the diagnosis of systemic aspergillosis in dogs. *J Vet Intern Med*. 2012;26:911–919.
28. Pomrantz JS, Johnson LR, Nelson RW, et al. Comparison of serologic evaluation via agar gel immunodiffusion and fungal culture of tissue for diagnosis of nasal aspergillosis in dogs. *J Am Vet Med Assoc*. 2007;230:1319–1323.
29. Grooters AM, Leise BS, Lopez MK, et al. Development and evaluation of an enzyme-linked immunosorbent assay for the serodiagnosis of pythiosis in dogs. *J Vet Intern Med*. 2002;16:142–146.
30. Fisher MC, Hawkins NJ, Sanglard D, et al. World emergence of resistance to antifungal drugs challenges human health and food security. *Science*. 2019;360:739–742.
31. Berkow EL, Lockhart SR, Ostrosky-Zeichner L. Antifungal susceptibility testing: current approaches. *Clin Microbiol Rev*. 2020;33:e00069–19.
32. Marinach C, Alanio A, Palous M, et al. MALDI-TOF MS-based drug susceptibility testing of pathogens: the example of *Candida albicans* and fluconazole. *Proteomics*. 2009;9:4627–4631.

5

Diagnostic Techniques for Identification of Parasites

Susan E. Little, Yoko Nagamori

KEY POINTS

- Parasites are responsible for some of the easiest, and also some of the most difficult, infections to diagnose in clinical practice.
- When organisms are present in large numbers, diagnosis can be quickly achieved by direct microscopic examination of appropriate specimens. However, in many cases, parasites responsible for an infection are not present in high numbers, are not shed or circulating at the time of specimen collection, or are difficult to identify because of their small size, subtle diagnostic features, or damage associated with handling or delay in specimen submission.
- Immunologic and molecular assays are increasingly available to circumvent these difficulties. Nonetheless, direct microscopic examination of feces, blood, or other clinical specimens is still the most common approach for diagnosis of most parasitic infections.
- Many assays described in this chapter can be readily performed in clinic by trained personnel. However, because confirmation and consultation are often desired when making a diagnosis of an unusual parasite, collection and preservation of specimens for submission to veterinary diagnostic laboratories are also discussed.
- The geographic distribution of parasites is constantly changing. Novel parasites are occasionally encountered by veterinarians who may not be familiar with relatively uncommon organisms that can infect patients in a given geographic area. Submission of appropriate specimens to a diagnostic laboratory with parasitology expertise is critically important to accurately identify organisms in cases of unusual parasites or apparent treatment failures.

MICROSCOPIC EXAMINATION

Microscopic Examination of Feces

Eggs, larvae, cysts, and oocysts of several helminth and protozoan parasites are commonly found in fecal specimens. To ensure fragile stages of some protozoa (such as trophozoites of *Giardia* or *Tritrichomonas*) remain intact, fecal specimens should be examined as quickly as possible after collection. When examination of feces is delayed and the specimen is held at room temperature, eggs of hookworms may hatch, which results in larvae in the feces. However, most helminth eggs and larvae, as well as the cysts and oocysts of protozoa, will still be evident and fully recoverable from refrigerated or fixed specimens.

Collection and Storage of Feces

To maximize sensitivity and specificity, at least 5 g of feces should be collected and placed in a clean, dry, air-tight container. Freshly shed feces is ideal as specimens collected from the ground often contain free-living nematode larvae that may confound diagnosis. The amount of material retrieved by use of a fecal wand is insufficient for diagnostic testing of most intestinal parasites. Although interpretation of a positive result on direct smear from a fecal wand specimen is possible, a negative result is meaningless because of the small amount of feces examined.[1]

When the presence of trophozoites is suspected, the fecal specimen should be held at room temperature and examined within 30 minutes after collection. If specimens cannot be examined immediately, feces should be refrigerated. Tightly sealed, refrigerated specimens may be examined for cysts, oocysts, eggs, or larvae, all of which are hardier than trophozoites and persist in the environment for several days after collection.[2]

When *Tritrichomonas blagburni* (syn. *foetus*) is suspected, the saline flush technique may be employed to collect a fecal specimen; specimens obtained from nondiarrheic or dry stools are unsuitable. Stopping treatment for several days before testing is also recommended.[2] The saline flush technique involves passage of a rubber catheter into the proximal colon followed by administration and gentle reaspiration of 10 mL of sterile saline. Water should not be used because this will lyse trophozoites. The fecal-saline solution is then examined directly under the microscope for trophozoites, or a drop is inoculated into a fecal culture pouch for parasite isolation (see Trichomoniasis, Chapter 102). Alternatively, the saline flush contents are centrifuged and the pellet submitted for molecular analysis.[2]

Examination of Feces

Recommended microscopic procedures for diagnosis of intestinal parasites are listed in Table 5.1. Because dogs and cats are predators and dogs are coprophagous, some parasite stages found in fecal specimens may be the result of material the animal has ingested rather than true parasitism. For example, oocysts of *Eimeria* spp. are often observed in canine fecal specimens following ingestion of herbivore feces, usually those of a rabbit, deer, horse, or cow. In these cases, treatment is not indicated.

Direct saline smear. The direct smear technique, which can be performed on diarrheic or formed fecal specimens, is most important when trophozoites are present. No concentration of the specimen is achieved, and this approach is a poor choice to diagnose infection with other intestinal parasites. To enhance detection, the substage condenser of the microscope should be adjusted to maximize contrast. When available, phase-contrast or dark-field microscopy may aid in the demonstration of motile trophozoites (Fig. 5.1), but these are not necessary for reliable identification of motile protozoa.

TABLE 5.1 **Recommended Microscopic Procedures for the Diagnosis of Common Gastrointestinal Parasites of the Dog and Cat**

Organism	Stage	Procedure[16]
Protozoa		
Cystoisospora Sarcocystis, Hammondia, Besnoitia, and *Cryptosporidium*	Oocysts	Sheather's sugar centrifugation flotation technique
Giardia	Trophozoites	Direct smear, occasionally seen on flotation
	Cysts	Direct smear, zinc sulfate centrifugation flotation technique
Tritrichomonas foetus	Trophozoites	Direct smear
Nematodes		
Ancylostoma spp., *Uncinaria* spp.	Eggs	Sheather's sugar or zinc sulfate centrifugation flotation technique
Physaloptera spp.	Eggs	Fecal sedimentation; occasionally found on direct smear
Strongyloides stercoralis	Larvae	Baermann examination; occasionally found on direct smear
Toxocara spp.	Eggs	Sheather's sugar or zinc sulfate centrifugation flotation technique
Trichuris spp.	Eggs	Sheather's sugar centrifugation flotation technique
Cestodes		
Dipylidium caninum	Eggs	Observation of proglottids; rarely found on Sheather's sugar centrifugation flotation technique
Echinococcus spp., *Taenia* spp.	Eggs	Occasionally found on Sheather's sugar centrifugation flotation technique
Mesocestoides spp.	Eggs	Occasionally found on Sheather's sugar centrifugation flotation technique
Spirometra spp., *Diphyllobothrium latum*	Eggs	Sheather's sugar centrifugation flotation technique
Trematodes		
Alaria spp.	Eggs	Fecal sedimentation
Nanophyetus salmincola	Eggs	Fecal sedimentation

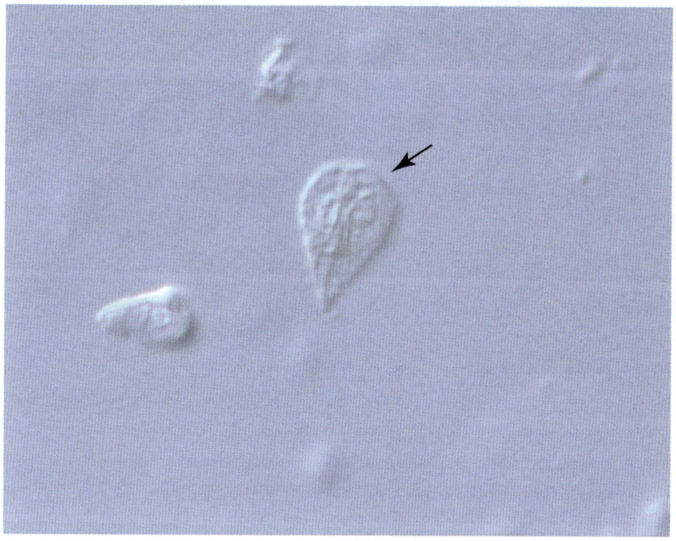

Fig 5.1 Unstained *Giardia* trophozoite *(arrow)* as viewed with phase-contrast microscopy showing morphologic details such as nuclei, median body, and flagella.

A direct smear is made by placing a drop of isotonic saline on a clean microscope slide and then mixing in a very small amount of fecal material (Fig. 5.2A). The amount that adheres to the tip of a wooden applicator stick is sufficient. A coverslip is then applied, and the slide is systematically scanned using the 10× objective but alternating with the 40× objective whenever structures morphologically resembling protozoan trophozoites or cysts are encountered. The fecal-saline mixture should be transparent enough that newsprint can be easily read through the material. A smear prepared with too much fecal material cannot be accurately interpreted. Motility and structural features of protozoa are best examined using the high-dry objective (40× to 43×). The oil immersion objective (100×) is not recommended for examination of fresh wet mounts because pressure on the coverslip from the oil objective displaces the fluid medium between the coverslip and the slide, making viewing difficult. If necessary, once motility has been observed, stain may be added to the smear to aid in identification of organisms.[1]

Stained smear. Although not required, adding stain to the wet mount through the edge of the coverslip may aid in visualizing internal structures of some protozoa. For example, although *Pentatrichomonas* spp. usually have five anterior flagella and *T. blagburni* usually has three anterior flagella, it is difficult to identify these organisms using living or unstained specimens. Special stains, such as silver staining, are needed to highlight flagella and other diagnostic features of trophozoites.[3]

Iodine is the most common stain used to reveal the internal structure of protozoans and is especially useful to confirm the identity of *Giardia* cysts and trophozoites. The iodine stains the cytoplasm of cysts dark gold, while the nuclei remain pale and refractile. Other stains used to identify protozoa in feces include methylene blue, acid methyl green, aqueous eosin, and crystal violet. Methylene blue is useful to identify trophozoites, especially those of *Entamoeba histolytica,* whereas acid methyl green stains the macronucleus of *Balantidium coli.* Aqueous eosin and crystal violet are both negative stains, which stain fecal debris but leave parasitic cysts and trophozoites unstained and highlighted by the stained background.[4]

Fecal flotation. Fecal concentration methods are often necessary to detect protozoal cysts or oocysts and common helminth eggs

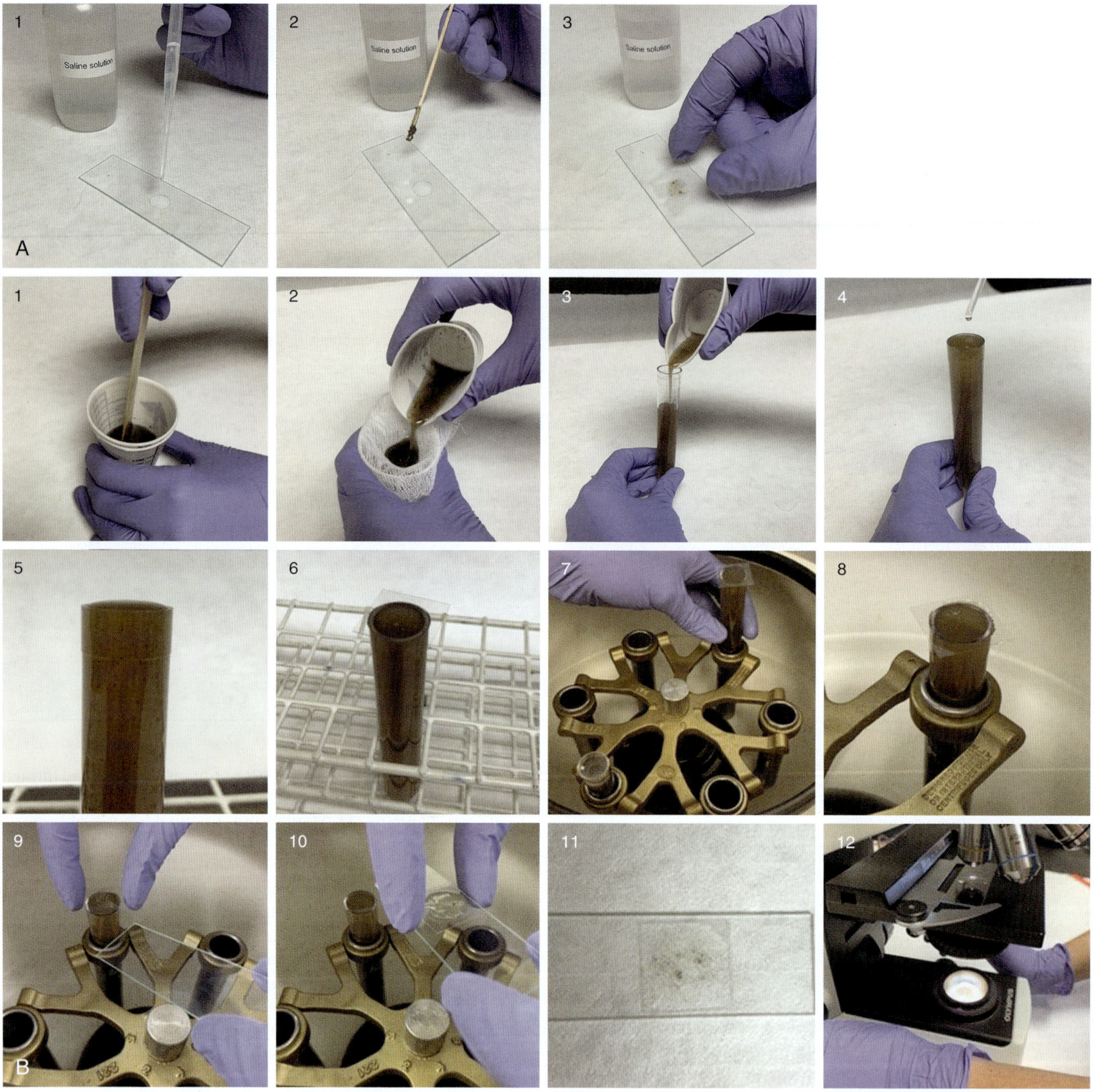

Fig. 5.2 (A) Procedure for direct fecal smear. 1. A drop of isotonic saline on a clean microscope slide. 2. An amount of fecal material is placed on the tip of a wooden applicator stick. 3. This material is stirred into the saline. A coverslip is applied and the slide is examined with the microscope. (B) Fecal procedure using swinging bucket rotor centrifuge. 1. About 5 to 10 g of feces are mixed with water to a liquid consistency. 2. The mixture is strained with gauze. 3. The strained feces-flotation solution mixture is poured into a 15-mL conical centrifuge tube. 4. Flotation solution is added. 5. A final amount is added to form a reverse meniscus at the top of the tube. 6. A coverslip is then placed on top of the meniscus. 7. The tube is placed in the centrifuge and a second tube filled with water is used to balance it. 8. A coverslip is added on the top and it is centrifuged with the coverslip in place. 9. After centrifugation, the coverslip is removed. 10. The coverslip is transferred, along with the adherent fluid, face down on a slide. 11. The unstained slide is transferred to a microscope. 12. The slide is examined as described in the text for this procedure. (Photographs provided by Kellee Sundstrom and Megan Lineberry, Oklahoma State University.)

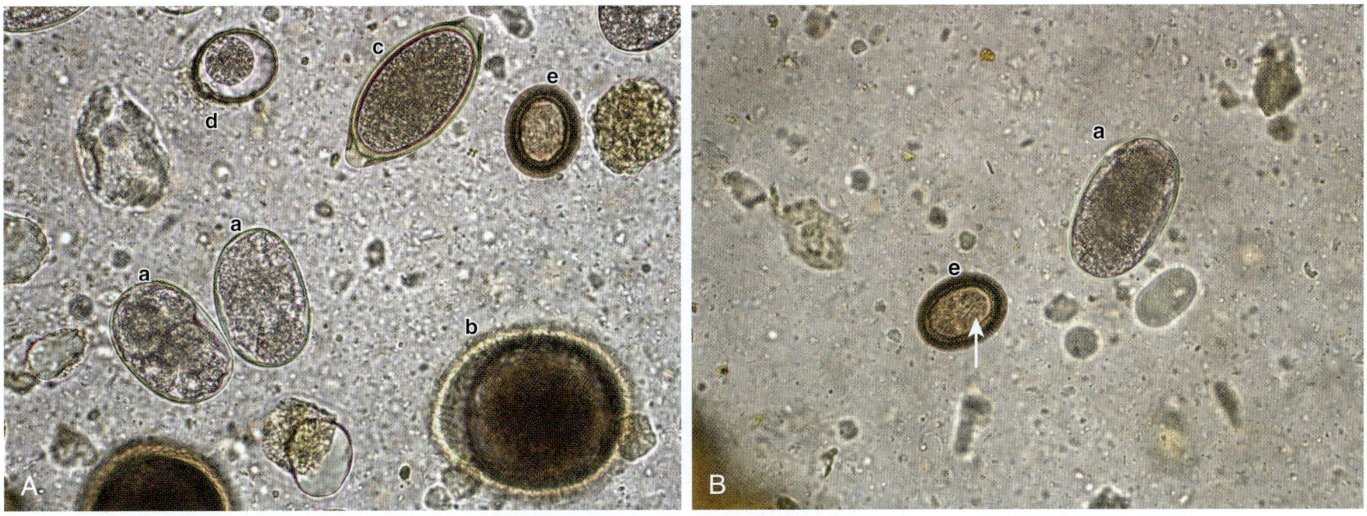

Fig. 5.3 (A) Eggs of *Ancylostoma caninum (a)*, *Toxocara canis (b)*, *Trichuris vulpis (c)*, *Cystoisospora canis (d)*, and *Taenia* sp. *(e)* in canine fecal flotation. (B) Closer view of eggs of *A. caninum (a)* and *Taenia* sp. *(e)* showing distinct hooks *(arrow)* within a *Taenia* sp. egg.

or larvae (see Table 5.1; Fig. 5.3). Sugar or salt solutions are used with centrifugation to concentrate parasites present in several grams of feces into a small volume of fluid that can be examined on a single slide. Alone, standard sodium nitrate tabletop flotation is not sensitive enough to identify infections with many intestinal parasites, although high-intensity infections consisting of numerous coccidial oocysts, ascarid eggs, or hookworm eggs may be detected. Although inactivated by the hypertonic solution and frequently lysed, trophozoites, especially those of *Giardia*, may also occasionally be seen on fecal flotation. Most platyhelminth eggs are considered too heavy to reliably float in common flotation solutions, and thus sedimentation is preferred. However, eggs of some cestodes and trematodes (e.g., *Taenia*, *Spirometra*, or *Alaria* spp.) may occasionally be recovered using flotation.

Solutions used in centrifugal fecal flotation methods include zinc sulfate and Sheather's sugar; a water wash may be included to assist in the examination of very mucoid or fatty fecal specimens. Feces are washed by combining 2 to 3 g of feces with 5 to 10 mL of water, straining the mixture through a double layer of cheesecloth, centrifuging for 5 to 10 minutes at approximately 650 × *g*, and then discarding the supernatant. The sediment is then mixed with 10 to 12 mL 33% zinc sulfate solution (specific gravity of 1.18) or Sheather's sugar solution (specific gravity of 1.25), strained through cheesecloth, and centrifuged for 5 to 10 minutes at approximately 650 × *g*.[1]

When available, a centrifuge with a swinging bucket rotor is ideal for the flotation step (Fig. 5.2B). The strained feces-flotation solution mixture is poured into a 15-mL conical centrifuge tube, and enough flotation solution is added to form a reverse meniscus at the top of the tube. A coverslip is then placed on top of the meniscus and the tube spun with the coverslip in place. A second tube of equal volume is needed to balance the centrifuge. Once completed, the coverslip is removed and transferred along with the adherent fluid face down on a slide, and the slide is examined (see Fig. 5.2B).

If only a fixed-angle bucket rotor is available, the feces-flotation solution mixture can be poured into a 15-mL centrifuge tube to the point at which it is almost full but does not spill when placed into the centrifuge bucket (approximately 13 mL). The tube is then spun without a coverslip. The top layer of the centrifuged material can be collected by carefully touching the base of a small test tube or a microbiologic loop to the surface and then transferring the adherent fluid to a slide. A coverslip is then applied and the preparation examined using a microscope.

Slides should be completely examined using the 10× and, when necessary, the 40× objective. Scanning a slide at low power (×4) is not sufficient to allow detection of many nematode eggs and most protozoan diagnostic stages.[1] Quantification methods such as the Wisconsin or modified McMaster egg counting techniques are not used for routine canine and feline fecal flotation. Some diagnostic laboratories add a comment on the report about the relative number of eggs, cysts, or oocysts detected. Nonetheless, it is critical to start with an adequate amount of feces to optimize sensitivity.

Fecal sedimentation. Sedimentation is used only for detection of helminths that shed heavier eggs (see Table 5.1). Eggs of several trematodes, cestodes, and even some nematodes (e.g., *Physaloptera* spp.) are not routinely recovered on fecal flotation. When these infections are suspected, either simple or centrifugal sedimentation, as described below, should be performed. Concentration is not as great with sedimentation as it is with flotation, but heavier eggs are more likely to be detected with these methods than by direct smear of feces alone.

For simple sedimentation, 100 mL of either tap water or saline is combined in a beaker with approximately 10 g of feces, strained through cheesecloth into a second beaker, and then allowed to settle for 1 hour. The supernatant is then decanted, more water added, and the settling step repeated. A small amount of sediment is then placed on a slide, a coverslip applied, and the slide scanned using the 10× objective. Some protocols recommend use of a smaller amount of feces and water combined in a test tube rather than in a beaker. Centrifugation accelerates the separation, but if mucus or fat are present, the fecal material should first be combined with Hemo-De (Scientific Safety Solvents, Keller, TX, USA) to facilitate separation of eggs. For centrifugal sedimentation, 1 g of feces is mixed with 10 mL of either 10% formalin or water and poured into a glass or polypropylene centrifuge tube and Hemo-De is added. The tube is capped and vigorously shaken, then centrifuged for 5 minutes at 650 × *g*. An applicator stick is used to break the top plug of debris so that both the debris plug and the supernatant can be decanted. The remaining sediment is placed on a slide, a coverslip applied, and the slide examined using the 10× objective.[1]

Baermann assay. The Baermann assay is used to recover motile nematode larvae, such as lungworm larvae (see Chapter 117) and

TABLE 5.2 Practical Techniques for the Diagnosis of Blood and Systemic Parasitic Infections

Organism	Blood Films	Aspirates	Tissue Impressions	Histologic Sections	Serologic Techniques
Babesia spp.	+	–	–	–	+
Cytauxzoon felis	+	–	+	+	–
Dirofilaria immitis	+	–	–	–	+
Hepatozoon americanum	+/–	–	+	+	–
Hepatozoon canis	+	–	+	+	–
Leishmania spp.	–	+	+	+	+
Neospora caninum	–	+	+	+	+
Platynosomum fastosum	–	–	–	+	–
Toxoplasma gondii	–	+	+	+	+
Trypanosoma cruzi	+	+	+	+	+

+, useful or indicated; –, not used or recommended.

Strongyloides stercoralis (see Chapter 116), from feces (see Table 5.1). The assay should only be performed with fresh feces. Results will be confounded by larvae from hatched hookworm eggs in specimens even just a few days old, as well as by the presence of free-living nematode larvae in feces collected from the ground. Approximately 10 g of feces is placed in a double layer of cheesecloth, secured by a rubber band, and suspended at the top of a disposable wine glass with a hollow stem. The apparatus is then filled with room temperature water to completely immerse the feces and held at room temperature for 8 to 16 hours. Any larvae present in the feces will migrate into the water and collect at the base of the hollow stem. After resting, the feces is removed and discarded and a small amount of fluid removed from the base of the stem with a pipette, placed on a slide, a coverslip applied, and examined for larvae using the 4× or 10× objective.[1]

Preservation of Feces

No specific preservation or addition of fixative is necessary before routine fecal flotation for common gastrointestinal parasites. If submission will be delayed a few days, refrigeration is recommended to prevent growth of mold and delay development of nematode eggs. If examination is delayed for several days and there is a desire to preserve protozoa, fresh feces can be mixed with a preservative before shipment. Enough fixative solution should be added to the feces to ensure adequate fixation. Some commonly used solutions include polyvinyl alcohol (PVA) and 10% formalin.[4] Ten percent formalin solution is an appropriate fixative for specimens suspected to contain *Cryptosporidium,* because formalin fixation, unlike fixation with PVA, does not interfere with immunodetection assays employed to detect *Cryptosporidium* (e.g., direct fluorescent antibody).

Potassium dichromate (1%) is the solution of choice for storing specimens that contain oocysts of coccidia because it allows the oocysts to sporulate, permitting the precise measurements of sporocysts and sporozoites and complete evaluation of oocyst structure that are needed for identification.[5] A 2% solution of sulfuric acid is an acceptable alternative to 1% potassium dichromate. Historically, PVA has been considered the best choice for fixing trophozoites because permanently stained slides can be prepared from PVA-fixed fecal material. However, both PVA, which contains mercuric chloride, and potassium dichromate are potent toxins and should be handled with great care. Less toxic, more environmentally safe commercial substitutes for PVA have become available, including Proto-Fix (AlphaTec Systems, Vancouver, WA, USA) and ECOFIX (Meridian Diagnostics, Cincinnati, OH, USA).[6]

Microscopic Examination of Whole Blood

Diagnostic stages of parasites may be detected both in fresh blood and in blood collected into anticoagulants. Microfilaria are often detected in EDTA-anticoagulated blood by direct examination of a saline wet mount of whole blood or by Knott test (see Chapter 111). In contrast, the most common method used to detect protozoa in blood is by microscopic examination of a stained blood smear. Bloodborne and systemic parasites that can be detected in stained blood smears or in fresh wet mounts are listed in Table 5.2.

Collection of Blood Specimens

Appropriate collection procedures for blood are dictated, in part, by the parasites suspected to be the cause of disease. If diagnosis requires blood smear examination, care should be taken during blood collection and handling to avoid hemolysis that may destroy parasites. Smears from fresh whole blood should be made immediately after collection; blood collected into EDTA anticoagulant can be submitted for smears to be made at a later time or for examining blood for microfilaria.[7] Some protozoa, especially *Babesia* spp., are more easily found in the peripheral circulation of microcapillary beds; detection of these parasites may be enhanced by collecting from an ear margin or clipped toenail.

Testing for Microfilaria

When present in high numbers, microfilaria may be found in saline wet mounts of whole blood. However, the modified Knott test, which concentrates any microfilaria present in 1 mL of blood, allows more sensitive detection. To prepare a wet mount, a small drop of anticoagulated whole blood is placed on a slide, a drop of saline added, the specimen briefly mixed, a coverslip applied, and the material directly examined using the 10× objective for any microfilaria present. Relative numbers and motility patterns of microfilaria present on a direct wet mount can support a diagnosis of *Dirofilaria immitis* infection. However, accurate measurement of microfilaria with an ocular micrometer is only readily achieved using a Knott test.

To perform the modified Knott test, 1 mL of EDTA-anticoagulated whole blood is placed in a centrifuge tube and 9 mL of 2% formalin added. The specimen is capped and mixed briefly to lyse the red blood cells, then centrifuged at 650 × *g* for 5 minutes. The supernatant is discarded and a drop of 0.1% methylene blue added to the sediment. Stained material is then transferred to a microscope slide using a pipette, a coverslip applied, and the specimen examined using the 10× objective for microfilaria. In the modified Knott test, microfilaria will be immobilized, fully extended, and readily measured and examined for key features that allow confirmation of their identity as either *D. immitis* or one of the other species that may be found in the blood. The stain highlights microfilarial nuclei, aiding identification (see Chapter 111 for additional tests for heartworm disease).

Preparation of Blood Films

Examination of dried blood films is often useful for diagnosis of protozoal infections. Thick films allow examination of a larger volume of blood, which increases sensitivity, but thin films are necessary for morphologic identification. If possible, multiple slides (at least two thick and two thin) should be prepared and submitted unstained.[3]

Thin films are prepared by placing a small drop of blood at one end of a clean microscope slide and then using a second slide to spread the blood. Blood should not be pushed across the slide because this may rupture parasites. To prepare thick films, two or three drops of blood are placed on a clean microscope slide and spread with the corner of another slide in a circular motion over a 2-cm area. Fresh blood should be stirred on the slide for an additional 30 seconds to prevent formation of fibrin strands. EDTA-anticoagulated blood does not need to be stirred after spreading.[3]

Both thick and thin films should be air dried at room temperature on a flat surface. The choice of stain will determine the need for additional preparation and fixation before staining. Some stains require thick films to be laked (immersed in distilled water to lyse erythrocytes) before staining. Thin films that are not stained within 48 hours should be fixed in 100% methanol. All films should be stored in a cool, dry, clean place in a sealed box.[3]

Staining Blood Films

Giemsa, Wright, and Wright-Giemsa are the most commonly used stains to detect and identify hemoprotozoa on blood smears. Diff-Quik can be used, but both detection of the presence of protozoa and subsequent morphologic identification to species may be more difficult.[7] Giemsa-stained blood smears have the added advantage of permanency; Wright-stained blood smears fade over time.

Examination of Blood Films

Stained blood films may be examined with or without a coverslip. When a coverslip is not used, a drop of immersion oil can be placed on the stained smear to reduce diffraction and facilitate microscopic examination at low power and with the high-dry objectives. Additional immersion oil should then be added and the feathered edge of the stained smear examined closely using the oil immersion objective. If preferred, a thin (#1) coverslip can be applied with neutral mounting medium before examination. The mounting medium prevents the coverslip from moving around on the stained smear and also reduces diffraction in a manner similar to immersion oil applied directly to the smear.[3] One advantage of using a coverslip is that it allows the slide to be thoroughly cleaned with lens cleaner and reexamined at a later date by another diagnostician; the surfaces of stained smears that do not have a coverslip cannot be cleaned.

Examination of Intact Parasites

Intact metazoan parasites are often recovered from vomit, feces, skin, or from other tissues collected at surgery or necropsy. Whenever possible, all available specimens should be submitted for morphologic identification to a diagnostic veterinary parasitology laboratory. Helminths may be submitted fresh in saline or, if submission will be delayed, fixed in dilute (5%) formalin; the 10% formalin used for preservation of tissues can destroy helminth structures needed for full identification. Arthropods should be submitted in 70% ethanol. All specimens from which nucleic acid will be collected for molecular identification or comparison should be placed in 70% ethanol. Formalin-fixed specimens are of limited value for molecular evaluation.

Microscopic Examination of Other Specimens

Parasites may sometimes be found on histologic examination of biopsy specimens, tissues collected at necropsy, or on cytology. Ideally, intact helminths or arthropods will be submitted directly for identification. Although intact stages of parasites may be detected and identified on microscopic examination of aspirates or impression smears and protozoa can be identified in histologic sections (see Table 5.2), thin sections of only one portion of a large metazoan parasite often precludes complete identification.

Histopathology

Parasites may be found on histologic examination of tissues with routine hematoxylin and eosin staining. Accurate identification of metazoan parasites in thin sections requires both advanced training in histoparasitology and sections made in a location that shows key features of the parasite. When tissue sections are limited or when stages are small (such as microfilaria in skin biopsies), definitive identification to genus and species by microscopy alone may not be possible. For protozoa, entire organisms are usually present on sections and identification is more readily achieved. Special stains may be used to improve detection or enhance morphologic characteristics of the stage of parasite seen, allowing more confident identification. Tissue specimens to be examined by histology for protozoan parasites should be collected and submitted quickly for frozen section evaluation when an immediate diagnosis is desired, or they should be placed in 10% formalin if processing will be delayed. Tissues on which electron microscopy will be performed should be placed in a glutaraldehyde-based fixative.[3]

Cytologic Examination of Other Body Fluids

Parasites are only rarely found on direct microscopic examination of aqueous humor, CSF, synovial fluid, urine, transtracheal wash, or bronchoalveolar lavage. *Giardia* trophozoites may occasionally be seen in duodenal aspirates collected at endoscopy. To determine if motile protozoa are present, all body fluids should be examined by direct smear immediately after collection; storage of specimens for even a short time may result in lysis of organisms and subsequent failure to detect infection. Specimens are processed for examination by centrifuging collected fluid at 2000 × *g* for 5 minutes and then making smears with the sediment and adding a small amount of associated fluid. After drying, smears should be stained as described for blood smears and examined for protozoa. Eggs of some nematodes (e.g., *Pearsonema plica*, *Dioctophyme renale*) may be found in urine sediment and directly identified (see Chapter 116). Similarly, larvae of some nematodes will be present in specimens collected by transtracheal wash or bronchoalveolar lavage; centrifugation of these specimens and direct microscopic examination of sediment enhances likelihood of detection.

Fine-Needle Aspirates

Parasites, especially protozoa, are occasionally found in fine-needle aspirates of lymph node, spleen, liver, or bone marrow. Dried smears of fine-needle aspirates are stained with Giemsa, Wright, or Wright-Giemsa and examined for protozoa as described for blood smears. Occasionally, some stages of metazoan parasites may also be found on lymph node aspirates including microfilaria and *Demodex* spp. mites.[8,9]

Impression Smears

Examination of stained impression smears of superficial lesions or of tissue collected at biopsy or necropsy may also reveal parasites, usually protozoa (e.g., *Leishmania* spp.). For this reason, impression smears should be made of all biopsy material when a parasitic infection is suspected.

Collection of Parasites from Skin

Large arthropods such as ticks, fleas, or lice should be placed in 70% ethanol and submitted intact for identification. A fine-toothed flea comb will often facilitate recovery of larger arthropods. However, mites are more readily recovered intact on skin scrapes, by swabbing ears (e.g., *Otodectes cynotis*), or by collecting dander and examining for superficial mites (e.g., *Cheyletiella yasguri*). Occasionally, larger arthropods (e.g., *Cuterebra*) or nematodes (e.g., *Dracunculus*) may be present in subcutaneous cysts or found emerging from dermal ulcers. Whenever possible, these organisms should be removed and submitted intact for identification.

To perform a skin scrape, a sterile scalpel blade is dipped in mineral oil and then used to abrade the affected area of skin; the material adherent to the blade is then transferred to a microscope slide. To enhance recovery of mites, collecting several scrapes from different areas of affected skin is recommended.[10] When ear mites are suspected, a swab with a small amount of mineral oil is used to transfer aural exudate to a slide. A drop of mineral oil is added if needed, a coverslip applied, and the material carefully examined for mites. Whenever skin mites are suspected, a fecal specimen should also be submitted for flotation. This is particularly important in cats, as mites may be removed during grooming and not detected on a skin scrape but will be found intact and can be readily identified by fecal flotation.[11]

CULTURE, ANIMAL INOCULATION, AND XENODIAGNOSIS

Culture and Animal Inoculation

Fecal Culture

Fecal culture for parasites is occasionally helpful in small animal practice. Specialized diagnostic laboratories that perform fecal culture for parasites should be identified before specimen submission. The specimen should be fresh and sent by the most rapid means available. Preservative should not be added. In addition, attempts should be made to identify parasites present in feces as specifically as possible based on their morphologic appearance before submitting specimens for culture.

Although fecal culture for diagnosis of parasites is not common, specific media have been developed that support the growth of *T. blagburni.* The InPouch TF test (BioMed Diagnostics, White City, OR, USA) is a useful in-clinic culture technique for identification of *T. blagburni* in cat feces. The test consists of a sterile pouch that contains liquid media. The media is inoculated with feces and held at room temperature with contents examined every 48 hours for evidence of motile trichomonads. Fecal specimens collected by clients for culture or microscopic examination for *T. blagburni* should be submitted fresh, not frozen or placed in fixative, kept warm and moist, free of cat litter, and unrefrigerated before testing in the clinic.[2] *Pentatrichomonas* spp., another flagellate occasionally found in diarrheic feces of dogs and cats, grows slowly in medium in which *T. blagburni* readily replicates.[12] Therefore, it is not likely that *Pentatrichomonas* spp. would be isolated in commercial pouch systems.

Blood Culture and Animal Inoculation

Although usually reserved for research projects, blood culture and animal inoculation are occasionally performed to detect and document the presence of protozoa. However, because these are rarely performed for clinical diagnosis, arrangement should be made with the laboratory before submission of specimens and specific instructions obtained on specimen collection and handling. In general, whole blood is collected aseptically into EDTA and then submitted to the laboratory as soon as possible.

Culture of Other Specimens

In some cases, culture of tissue aspirates, biopsy specimens, or body fluids other than blood may be desired. When indicated, an aliquot of the specimen collected for cytologic evaluation is placed in a sterile tube at the time of collection. Culture or animal inoculation can then be performed with this specimen as indicated. Rapid submission to an appropriate diagnostic laboratory will increase the likelihood of successfully culturing any protozoa present. To facilitate the process and receive exact instructions on specimen handling and submission, the diagnostic laboratory to be used should be contacted before collection of specimens.

Xenodiagnosis

Xenodiagnosis is a rarely performed procedure for clinical diagnosis. Laboratory-reared, parasite-free arthropods are allowed to feed on suspected infected hosts, and then, after appropriate time for development has elapsed, the arthropods are examined for the presence of parasites. Xenodiagnosis has historically been used for the diagnosis of trypanosomiasis but may also be useful to detect other protozoa.

ANTIGEN DETECTION

Parasite antigen present in clinical specimens may be detected by ELISA, by staining via direct FA, or by immunohistochemistry (see Chapter 2). Antigen may be excreted into blood or feces or, in the case of some protozoa detected by FA microscopy, be present on the surface of the parasite (Fig. 5.4). Although not a perfect substitute for direct

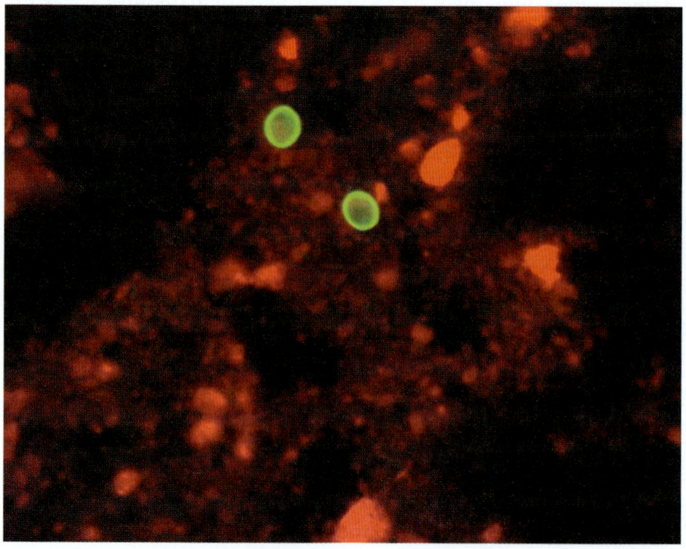

Fig. 5.4 Fluorescent antibody assay for detection of *Giardia* cysts in a fecal smear.

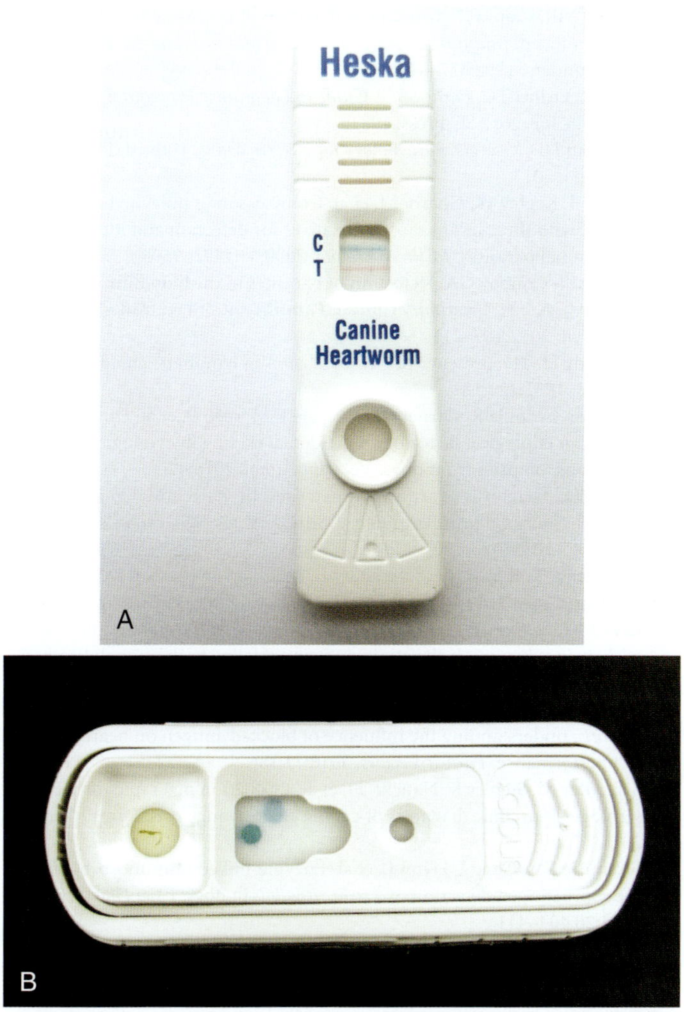

Fig. 5.5 (A) SoloStep CH Heartworm Test (Heska Laboratories, Loveland, CO, USA) positive for antigen of *Dirofilaria immitis.* (B) SNAP *Giardia* Test (IDEXX Laboratories, Westbrook, ME, USA) positive for soluble *Giardia* antigens.

microscopic examination, these assays enhance detection of parasites that are present in low numbers in clinical specimens or that are not yet patent and thus not shedding stages into blood or feces at all or in adequate numbers to allow microscopic detection.

Commercial immunodiagnostic assays are available for detection and identification of several helminths and protozoa. POC antigen tests are used on whole blood, serum, or plasma to diagnose infection with *D. immitis* in practice (Fig. 5.5A), and in diagnostic laboratories with microtiter plate assays. In some specimens, antigen may be present but trapped in immune complexes, which precludes detection. Treatment of the specimen to disrupt these immune complexes can increase sensitivity of detection.[13] Antigen tests are also available to detect *Angiostrongylus vasorum*, the French heartworm, in endemic areas.[14] Fecal antigen tests that detect ascarids, hookworms, and whipworms in the intestinal lumen are currently only available through a single commercial reference laboratory (IDEXX Laboratories, Inc., Westbrook, ME, USA).[15,16]

The stages of several common intestinal protozoa, including cysts of *Giardia* (Fig. 5.5B) and *E. histolytica* and oocysts of *Cryptosporidium* spp., can be detected in fecal specimens using antigen tests. Some of the assays used were originally developed for diagnosis of human infections. Care should be taken to optimize performance attributes of any assay not approved for use in veterinary specimens. At present, the Companion Animal Parasite Council (www.capcvet.org) only recommends *Giardia* antigen detection tests be used in clinically ill animals. Because other parasites may be present and because false-negative results can occur, these tests should always be performed along with microscopic examination of feces after centrifugal concentration. Parasite antigen can also sometimes be detected in fine-needle aspirates and biopsy specimens. Aliquots of specimens should be placed in a separate sterile tube at the time of collection and submitted to appropriate laboratories for direct FA or immunohistochemistry. Matching specimens should always be submitted for simultaneous cytologic or histologic examination whenever direct FA or immunohistochemical detection is pursued.

MOLECULAR DETECTION

Detection of parasite-specific nucleic acid sequences in patient specimens provides direct evidence of current or recent infection. In addition, larger metazoan parasites can often be identified by molecular methods when only damaged or partial specimens are available, precluding morphologic identification, provided the nucleic acid has not been damaged by fixation. A molecular approach to metazoan identification can prove particularly useful when attempting to distinguish between morphologically similar or identical organisms but should always be used as a complementary approach rather than the sole means of parasite identification. The most commonly used molecular techniques to detect or identify parasites in a diagnostic laboratory are PCR and in situ hybridization (see Chapter 6).

PCR has been used extensively for detection of *Giardia* spp. and *Cryptosporidium* spp. in feces from both dogs and cats, and for detection of *T. blagburni* in cats. Some PCR assays can distinguish between human-associated genotypes of *Giardia* spp. and those found only in dogs or cats.[17] Molecular diagnostic assays for intestinal protozoa are also available through diagnostic laboratories to screen animals with diarrhea. Some laboratories prefer fresh or frozen feces for PCR, whereas others suggest that a small amount (approximately 100 mg) of feces should be placed into a tube filled with 3 to 5 mL of 70% isopropyl alcohol and shipped at room temperature to the diagnostic laboratory.[2] PCR primers that amplify *T. blagburni* DNA can also amplify *Pentatrichomonas* spp. DNA, necessitating additional steps in identification, such as restriction enzyme digestion or sequencing of PCR products, to make a definitive diagnosis.[12]

PCR is also useful to evaluate blood specimens for the presence of hemoprotozoa; commercial diagnostic assays are available for *Babesia* spp., *Hepatozoon* spp., and *Cytauxzoon felis.* Whole blood specimens to be submitted for PCR should be collected into new blood tubes containing the anticoagulant specified by the laboratory; EDTA is the most common anticoagulant used. PCR can also be performed on specimens of other body fluids, fine-needle aspirates, and biopsy specimens. In situ hybridization is only performed at specialized research laboratories for a few protozoa.

SEROLOGIC TESTING

Feline heartworm antibody assays are widely used to determine if cats have been previously infected with *D. immitis* larvae (see Chapter 111). Serologic assays that detect antibodies to protozoa often are available through diagnostic laboratories. Indirect FA is the most commonly used platform, but ELISA, immunochromatographic strip (Fig. 5.6), and parasite agglutination tests are also available.

Individual laboratories should be consulted before submitting specimens. Care should be taken to prevent hemolysis during specimen collection or handling. Serum separated from the clot may be frozen before testing.

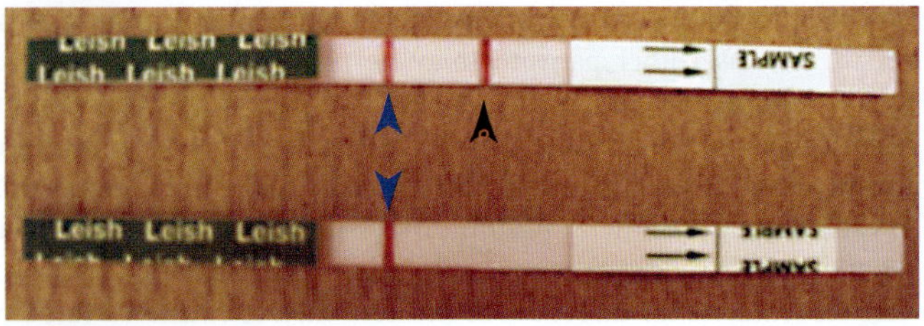

Fig. 5.6 Canine Kalazar *Detect* Rapid Test (InBios International, Seattle, WA, USA) for detection of antibody to *Leishmania* spp. Results shown include positive *(upper strip at black arrowhead)* and negative *(lower strip no black arrowhead)*. *Blue arrowheads* are reagent control-positive result.

Serologic testing for parasites has several advantages, including ease of specimen collection and low cost of most procedures. However, most of these assays are based on detection of IgG, which develops often after clinical disease has begun and remains elevated for months to years after initial infection, complicating interpretation of a single titer in a clinically ill animal. Diagnosis of active infection with an IgG-based test is supported by demonstrating a fourfold change in titer in two paired serum specimens collected 2 to 4 weeks apart. Some IgM-based tests are available. However, the presence of IgM antibodies in the serum does not correlate directly with clinical illness in all animals. Many healthy animals have detectable antibodies to protozoa, and immunosuppressed animals may not develop antibodies despite infection and clinical disease. Different assays vary in sensitivity and specificity, and there is potential for serologic cross-reactivity (e.g., among *Babesia* species). When necessary, the diagnostic laboratory performing the assay should be consulted for assistance in interpretation of results.

REFERENCES

1. Zajac AM, Conboy GA. Fecal examination for the diagnosis of parasitism. In: Zajac AM, Conboy GA, eds. *Veterinary Clinical Parasitology*. 8th ed. Ames: Wiley-Blackwell; 2012:3–169.
2. Tolbert MK, Gookin J. *Tritrichomonas foetus*: a new agent of feline diarrhea. *Compend Contin Educ Pract Vet*. 2009;31:374–381.
3. Lappin MR, Calpin JP. Laboratory diagnosis of protozoal infections. In: Greene CE, ed. *Infectious Diseases of the Dog and Cat*. 2nd ed. Philadelphia: WB Saunders; 1998:437–441.
4. Ash LR, Orihel TC. *Parasites: A Guide to Laboratory Procedures and Identification*. Chicago: ASC Press; 1987.
5. Bowman DD. *Georgis' Parasitology for Veterinarians*. 10th ed. Philadelphia: Saunders; 2013.
6. Jensen B, Kepley W, Guarner J, et al. Comparison of polyvinyl alcohol fixative with three less hazardous fixatives for detection and identification of intestinal parasites. *J Clin Microbiol*. 2000;38:1592–1598.
7. Zajac AM, Conboy GA. Detection of parasites in the blood. In: Zajac AM, Conboy GA, eds. *Veterinary Clinical Parasitology*. 8th ed. Ames: Wiley-Blackwell; 2012:185–211.
8. El-Gindy H. The presence of *Demodex canis* in lymphatic glands of dogs. *JAVMA*. 1952;121:181.
9. Paździor-Czapula K, Otrocka-Domagała I, Myrdek P, et al. *Dirofilaria repens*, an etiological factor or an incidental finding in cytologic and histopathologic biopsies from dogs. *Vet Clin Pathol*. 2018;47:307–311.
10. Greiner E. Diagnosis of arthropod parasites. In: Zajac AM, Conboy GA, eds. *Veterinary Clinical Parasitology*. 8th ed. Ames: Wiley-Blackwell; 2012:217–303.
11. Silbermayr K, Joachim A, Litschauer B, et al. The first case of *Demodex gatoi* in Austria, detected with fecal flotation. *Parasitol Res*. 2013;112:2805–2810.
12. Levy MG, Gookin JL, Poore M, et al. *Tritrichomonas foetus* and not *Pentatrichomonas hominis* is the etiologic agent of feline trichomonal diarrhea. *J Parasitol*. 2003;89:99–104.
13. Little S, Saleh M, Wohltjen M, Nagamori Y. Prime detection of *Dirofilaria immitis*: understanding the influence of blocked antigen on heartworm test performance. *Parasit Vectors*. 2018;11:186.
14. Schnyder M, Stebler K, Naucke TJ, et al. Evaluation of a rapid device for serological in-clinic diagnosis of canine angiostrongylosis. *Parasit Vectors*. 2014;7:72.
15. Elsemore DA, Geng J, Flynn L, et al. Enzyme-linked immunosorbent assay for coproantigen detection of *Trichuris vulpis* in dogs. *J Vet Diagn Invest*. 2014;26:404–411.
16. Elsemore DA, Geng J, Cote J, et al. Enzyme-linked immunosorbent assays for coproantigen detection of *Ancylostoma caninum* and *Toxocara canis* in dogs and *Toxocara cati* in cats. *J Vet Diagn Invest*. 2017;29:645–653.
17. McDowall RM, Peregrine AS, Leonard EK, et al. Evaluation of the zoonotic potential of *Giardia duodenalis* in fecal samples from dogs and cats in Ontario. *Can Vet J*. 2011;52:1329–1333.

6

Molecular Diagnostic Methods for Pathogen Detection

Emir Hodzic, Jane E. Sykes, Shelley C. Rankin

KEY POINTS

- Molecular diagnostic tests that detect nucleic acids, such as PCR assays, are now widely available for diagnosis of companion animal infectious diseases.
- Molecular diagnostic tests include tests that involve detection and amplification of nucleic acids (nucleic acid amplification tests [NAAT]), or probe-based assays that do not involve nucleic acid amplification.
- Specimens for these assays should be collected using aseptic technique in order to minimize contamination.
- Interpretation of molecular diagnostic test results requires knowledge of the problems and pitfalls of each type of assay. The results of testing at one laboratory may differ from those at another because of variations in assay design.
- With increased automation, laboratory proficiency testing, improved quality assurance, and standardization of reporting, the availability and utility of molecular diagnostic tests for companion animal infectious diseases continues to increase.

INTRODUCTION

One of Koch's postulates states that a microorganism must be isolated from a diseased organism and grown in pure culture in order to prove that it causes disease. This poses a problem, as many microorganisms are particular and fastidious in their growth requirements and cannot be cultivated on artificial media. Two major reasons have emerged to explain why most microbial agents cannot be cultured: (1) some only grow under specific nutritional conditions offered by the host, and (2) some microorganisms only grow in the presence of other microbial species.[1]

Commonly used methods of pathogen detection include microscopy, culture, biochemical methods, immunologic methods, and molecular methods.[2–8] As none of these methods are 100% sensitive and specific, it is recommended that multiple types of diagnostic assays be applied, depending on specimen type, clinical signs, and the suspected pathogen.[9] Traditional bacteriology can be time consuming because organisms have to be cultured, and usually a series of biochemical tests must be completed for identification.[10] Molecular diagnostic methods are suited to the detection of organisms that are not easily found using cytology or histopathology, are slow growing or difficult to culture, or when a rapid (<12 hours) diagnosis is required. Other applications are shown in Box 6.1.[11,12]

Although techniques for the amplification of pathogen-specific DNA sequences such as PCR are sensitive, there remain limits to this sensitivity when working with clinical specimens. Impurities within some specimens can inhibit PCR assays, and the use of small volumes for DNA extraction means that cells often have to be concentrated to increase sensitivity.[13]

ESSENTIAL PREREQUISITES FOR A POSITIVE OUTCOME WITH MOLECULAR DIAGNOSTIC TESTS

As for culture, the accuracy of molecular diagnostic tests depends on the appropriate specimen selection, collection, and transportation (Chapter 1).

Specimen Collection and Transport

When collecting specimens for molecular diagnostics, the timing of collection relative to the course of disease and the best specimen type must be considered. For acute diseases, molecular assays are most useful early in the course of disease. For chronic diseases, timing is less critical. Knowledge of organism shedding patterns can help to determine the most appropriate timing of specimen collection. For example, *Leptospira* organisms are primarily present in blood in the first week of acute illness, after which they may be shed in the urine.[14] Specimens should be collected before administration of antimicrobial drugs, although this is less critical than for specimens that are to be cultured.

Although specimen processing is usually well standardized in the diagnostic laboratory, *pre-analytical procedures* that occur before specimens arrive at the laboratory have considerable variability. For example, false-negative results may occur due to specimen degradation during transport. The main concerns during specimen transport and storage include specimen integrity, contamination, specimen identity, and the risk of environmental hazards due to infectious material. Because contamination can occur outside the PCR laboratory as well as within the laboratory, collection of specimens for nucleic acid testing should be performed aseptically to reduce the risk of false-positive results. Gloves should be worn, and disposable instruments should be used (e.g., disposable blades, punch biopsy instruments).[15–17] The recommendations for specimen collection and transport presented here are based on the guidelines published by the CLSI.[18] These guidelines are updated on a regular basis and ensure that detection of nucleic acids within clinical specimens is optimal.

For detection of pathogens that contain DNA (i.e., all bacteria, fungi, some viruses), either fresh or frozen specimens should be submitted. In general, DNA is stable in tissue for up to 24 hours at 2°C to 8°C, at least 2 weeks at –20°C, and at least 2 years at –70°C.[18] All specimens must be promptly transported to the diagnostic laboratory, preferably within 2 hours. In general, specimens for detection of bacterial agents should not be stored for more than 24 hours, and no more than 2 to 3 days at 4°C for viruses.[19] Specimens should not be stored

BOX 6.1 Applications of Nucleic Acid–Based Assays

Application	Example
Detection of microbes that are not easily detected using light microscopic examination of tissues or smears	*Bartonella* spp., viral pathogens
Detection of microbes that are difficult or impossible to culture	Hemotropic mycoplasmas, *Bartonella* spp., *Mycobacterium* spp., *Brucella* spp.
Rapid detection of microbes to allow early institution of infection control measures	Influenza virus, FCV, *Mycobacterium tuberculosis*
Detection of microbes that are hazardous to culture in the laboratory	H1N1 influenza virus, West Nile virus
Detection of microbes in the face of inactivating substances such as antimicrobials or formalin	Retrospective identification of an infecting microorganism in formalin-fixed, paraffin-embedded tissues after histopathology
Detection of antimicrobial resistance genes	*mecA*, the gene for methicillin resistance, in staphylococci
Detection of novel pathogens using broad-spectrum PCR and sequencing	*Bartonella henselae*,[11] hemotropic mycoplasmas[12]
Monitoring organism load as a measure of disease progression or response to treatment	FIV viral load
Identification of a cultured organism to the species level	*Nocardia* and *Actinomyces* spp., many fungi

FCV, feline calicivirus; *FIV*, feline immunodeficiency virus; *PCR*, polymerase chain reaction.

in frost-free freezers, as these undergo repeated freeze-thaw cycling, which can be associated with DNA degradation.[20] Box 6.2 outlines recommendations based on specimen type.[21]

RNA is highly susceptible to degradation during storage and transport. Swabs and body fluids should be immediately sent to the laboratory on wet ice. Tissue should ideally be snap-frozen at –70°C within half an hour of collection and shipped on dry ice without being thawed in the interim. RNA is stable for at least 2 years at or below –70°C. Naturally occurring ribonucleases can continue to degrade RNA at –20°C.

The optimal amount of tissue specimen for molecular testing is 1 to 2 g, although more or less may be required depending on the cellularity of the specimen.[18] Tissues stored in formalin, especially for prolonged periods, are suboptimal for PCR because the formalin cross-links the DNA in the specimen. Tissues fixed briefly in formalin (less than 18 hours) and then embedded in paraffin are preferable to tissues stored in formalin, because the formalin is removed during the embedding process. Paraffin-embedded specimens should only be used when no other specimens are available.[18]

Specimen Preparation in the Laboratory

Molecular detection methods depend more and more on proper *specimen preparation*. Clinical specimens are very heterogeneous (stool, plasma, CSF), so preparation must be a factor to consider in order to achieve results within a reasonable amount of time. The overall goals of specimen preparation are: (1) to concentrate the target, because pathogens may be present at low concentrations and molecular detection methods commonly use small volumes of specimen for nucleic acid extraction; (2) to remove or reduce the effects of inhibitory substances; and (3) to reduce

BOX 6.2 Guidelines for Collection and Transport of Specimens for NAAT

Specimen Type	Collection and Transport Recommendations
Whole blood and bone marrow	Use only EDTA or acid citrate dextrose (ACD) anticoagulant. Heparin may inhibit PCR.[21] The use of hemolyzed samples and frozen blood should be avoided if possible. DNA: Submit samples held at room temperature within 24 hours of collection. Samples can be stored at 2°C to 8°C for 72 hours, or at –20°C or ≤ –70°C for prolonged storage (removal of erythrocytes recommended). RNA: Use stabilization solution or send immediately to the laboratory on wet ice. For storage, freeze serum, plasma, or buffy coat specimens at ≤ –70°C.
Tissue specimens	Optimal specimen is 1 to 2 g of fresh tissue. Rinse blood from tissue using sterile saline. Wrap in saline-moistened gauze or paper. Avoid excessive dilution. Formalin-fixed, paraffin-embedded tissues can be used when no other specimen is available but are not optimal. DNA: Transport fresh tissue immediately to the laboratory on wet ice. Any storage should be at ≤ –70°C, preferably after snap-freezing in liquid nitrogen. RNA: Use stabilizing solution, process within 1 hour of collection, or snap-freeze in liquid nitrogen and store at ≤ –70°C.
Cerebrospinal fluid	DNA: Transport at 2°C to 8°C or freeze at –20°C or ≤ –70°C. RNA: Chill immediately on wet ice and deliver to the laboratory within 4 hours. Otherwise freeze immediately (removal of contaminating erythrocytes recommended) and ship on dry ice.
BAL fluid	Transport at room temperature within 24 hours of collection. If a delay is anticipated, store for up to 72 hours at 2°C to 8°C or freeze at ≤ –70°C.
Urine	Minimize storage at room temperature. Storage and transport should be according to the specific assay performed.
Feces	Use preserved specimen transport container or transport under refrigeration at 2°C to 8°C.

NAAT, nucleic acid amplification tests; *BAL*, bronchoalveolar lavage.

the heterogeneity of specimens in order to ensure negligible variations in serially collected specimens. If homogenized thoroughly, pooling of specimens facilitates high-throughput analysis in some cases.[8,13,22]

Quality assurance and *quality control* in the diagnostic laboratory must be taken into consideration. Components that are required for validation and verification of microbiologic diagnostic tests or test systems should include: (1) internal and external controls in each run; (2) participation in interlaboratory test results comparison; (3) validation of employee competence; (4) calibration and maintenance of instruments; and (5) correlation with clinical findings.[23,24]

MOLECULAR METHODS FOR PATHOGEN DETECTION

The ultimate goal of a molecular diagnostic test is rapid, sensitive, and accurate pathogen detection. Molecular diagnostics offer many

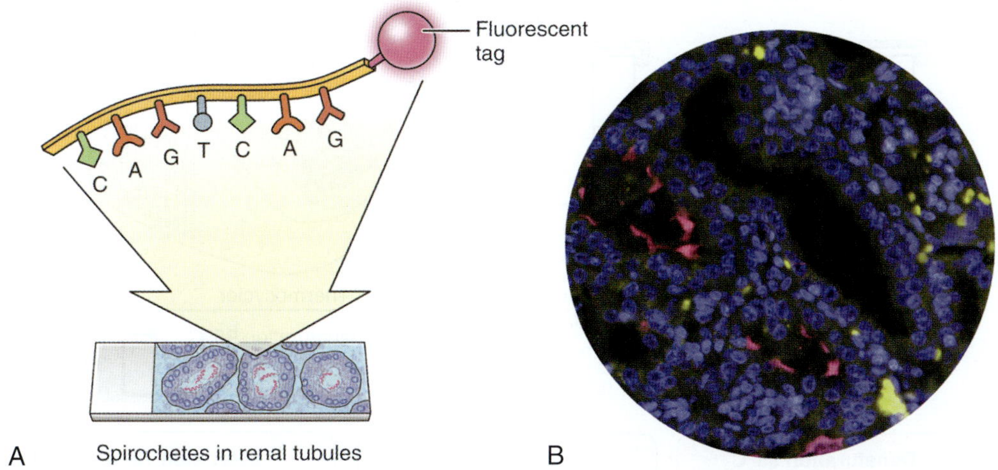

Fig. 6.1 (A) Fluorescence *in situ* hybridization (FISH). A nucleic acid probe that is complementary to a segment of leptospiral DNA that has been tagged with a fluorescent label is incubated with a tissue section on a slide. (B) Unbound probe is washed away and the section is examined using fluorescence microscopy. (*Leptospira* FISH image courtesy Dr. Richard Goldstein.)

advantages over traditional microbiologic and immunologic methods for pathogen detection. These include faster processing time as well as the potential for more accurate species identification and strain typing, which has resulted in a vastly improved understanding of infectious disease epidemiology. Molecular diagnostics has also revolutionized pathogen detection, evaluation of emerging novel infections, surveillance, early detection of bio-threat agents, and antimicrobial resistance profiling.[7,25]

Molecular assay types include endpoint (conventional) PCR, RT-PCR, real-time quantitative PCR (qPCR), isothermal amplification,[26,27] terminal restriction fragment length polymorphism (T-RFLP),[28] nucleic acid sequencing,[29] high-resolution melt analysis,[30] DNA microarrays,[31] tissue arrays,[32] and fluorescent-labelled in situ hybridization (FISH).[33,34] Despite the development of this broad range of amplification technologies, qPCR remains the most widely used method in both research and diagnostic laboratories for pathogen detection.[28,35]

Specimens vary considerably in physical properties, chemical composition, and microbial diversity, so molecular detection methods are typically developed for complex specimen types. For example, fecal matter is a complex mixture of undigested or partially digested food components as well as viable and nonviable microbial cells, with many inhibitors. The use of appropriate amplification controls by the laboratory facilitates detection of false negatives due to the presence of inhibitors. Other special requirements of molecular detection technology in order to ensure reliable results include proper establishment of quality-assured procedures, laboratory set-up, and proper training of staff in order to minimize the chance of contamination and false positives.

Direct Hybridization

Direct hybridization uses labeled oligonucleotide probes to detect bacteria, which are usually directed to 16S rRNA sequences specific to the species, genus, or other phylogenetic level of interest (Fig. 6.1). The oligonucleotide probes are small DNA or RNA segments that bind to complementary sequences within DNA or RNA molecules.[33] One end of the probe is designated the 5-prime (5′) end, and the other is the 3-prime (3′) end. A variety of oligonucleotide probes are available commercially as kits for detection of human pathogens. Some of these can also be used to detect the same pathogens in specimens from dogs or cats. Probes are widely used in human clinical microbiology laboratories to identify organisms that have been grown in culture (e.g., Gen-Probe Inc., San Diego, CA).

Probe hybridization can be performed on a nitrocellulose membrane *(solid-phase hybridization)*; on formalin-fixed, paraffin-embedded sections mounted on a microscope slide (*in situ hybridization*); or in solution *(liquid-phase hybridization)*. For solid-phase hybridization, the probe is reacted with microorganism DNA that has been immobilized on the membrane. Unbound probe is washed away, and the bound probe is detected using fluorescence, chemiluminescence, radioactivity, or color development (in the same way that bound antibody or antigen is detected in an ELISA or IFA assay). For *in situ* hybridization, formalin-fixed, paraffin-embedded specimens are sectioned and mounted on a special slide. The sections are deparaffinized, dried, and incubated with a solution that contains the probe, so both the presence and the location of the target pathogen within tissues can be identified. *In situ* hybridization assays that include a fluorescent-labeled probe are referred to as *fluorescence in situ hybridization* (FISH) assays (see Fig. 6.1).[33,36] The optimum specimen for FISH is a tissue that has been snap-frozen in liquid nitrogen after being embedded in optimal cutting temperature (OCT) medium.[18] FISH has been increasingly used to identify intralesional bacteria in companion animals, including: dogs with bacterial endocarditis,[37] histiocytic ulcerative colitis,[38] hepatitis,[39] and Lyme nephritis[40]; cats with small intestinal lymphoma;[41] and dogs and cats with gastric helicobacteriosis.[42]

Because liquid-phase hybridization occurs in solution, unbound probe cannot be washed away. To overcome this problem, a chemiluminescent acridinium ester label is attached to the probe. A subsequent chemical hydrolysis step selectively degrades only unbound probe. On addition of peroxides, the intact (hybridized) probe then emits light.[43]

Although not yet widely used for veterinary applications, *peptide nucleic acid (PNA) probes* are now increasingly available to detect target DNA. PNA probes are uncharged peptides that mimic DNA and bind to complementary DNA sequences just as a nucleic acid probe would.[44,45] PNA probes lack the net negative charge of nucleic acid probes; therefore, the electrostatic repulsion that normally occurs when two negatively charged DNA strands hybridize does not occur. The result is a more stable and specific binding of the probe to its target, which in turn can be associated with increased assay sensitivity and specificity.

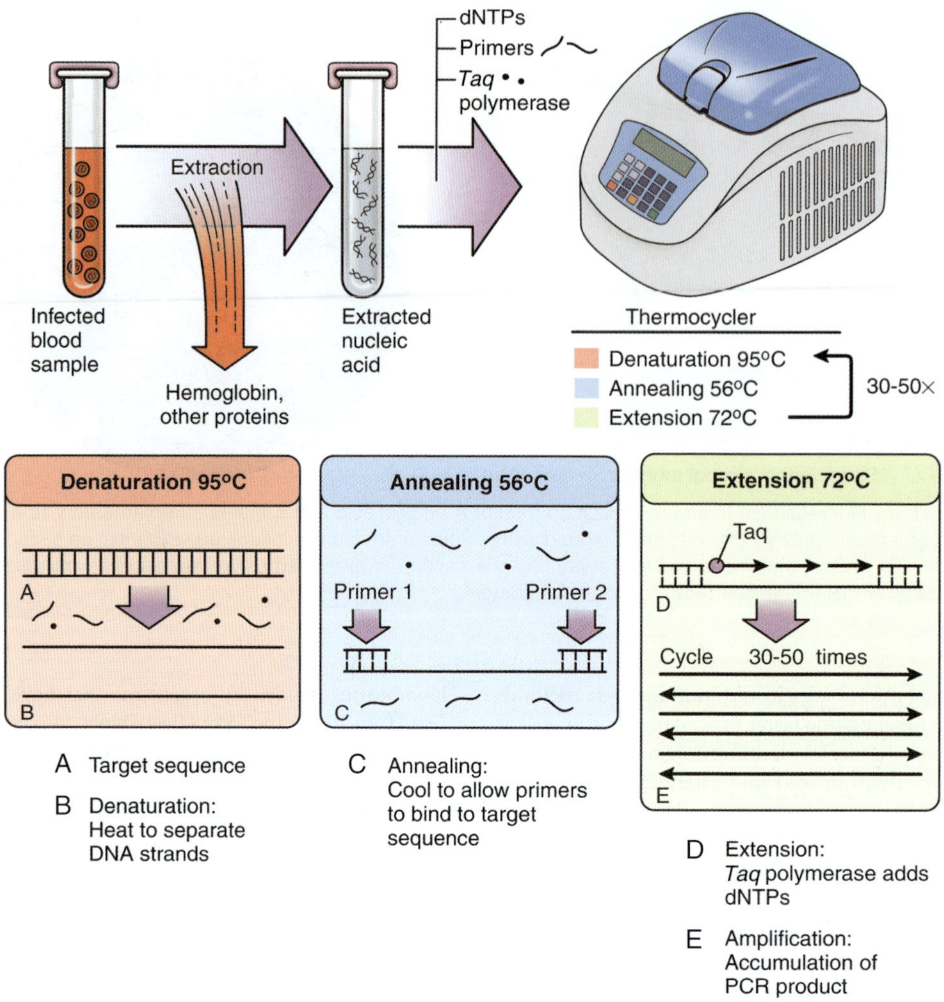

Fig. 6.2 Endpoint PCR assay. Two primers are hybridized on either side of a specific segment of a pathogen's DNA. Also present in the reaction mixture are the enzyme *Taq* polymerase, and free nucleotides for making new DNA. After addition of extracted DNA from a clinical specimen, a thermocycler is used to rapidly and repeatedly heat and cool the tubes through denaturation, annealing, and extension steps. The segment of pathogen DNA is repeatedly copied, with logarithmic accumulation of the PCR product.

Branched DNA assays and *hybrid capture assays* are highly sensitive hybridization methods that include steps to intensify the signal generated from probe hybridization.[46,47] They are not yet widely used in veterinary medicine.

Nucleic Acid Amplification

The general principles of all nucleic acid amplification technologies share common characteristics that fall into three categories: (1) target amplification systems, (2) probe amplification systems, and (3) signal amplification. These all use enzyme-mediated processes (a heat-stable DNA polymerase, such as that derived from *Thermophilus aquaticus,* a bacterium that is adapted to live in hot springs), two oligonucleotide primers, four deoxynucleotide triphosphates (dNTPs; G, T, A, and C), reaction buffer, and a target (a genomic or complementary DNA fragment). A solution (mastermix) is created in the laboratory that includes the polymerase, appropriate primers, dNTPs, and buffer, and this is then divided into aliquots for addition of DNA that has been extracted from the specimen. Once assembled, the reaction is placed in a thermal cycler, an instrument that subjects the reaction to a series of different temperatures for set amounts of time. Each round of temperature and time adjustments is referred to as one cycle of amplification. Each PCR cycle theoretically doubles the number of target DNA segments (amplicon) in the reaction. The end result is the production of millions to billions of copies of the targeted sequence in a matter of hours, and in each case, the amplification products (amplicons) can serve as templates for subsequent rounds of amplification.

Nucleic acid amplification methods include not only PCR methods (i.e., endpoint PCR, RT-PCR, nested PCR, multiplex PCR, qPCR, digital PCR [dPCR]), but also alternative technologies, such as such as strand-displacement amplification, loop-mediated isothermal amplification, ligase chain reaction, and nucleic acid sequence–based amplification.[36,48]

Types of PCR assays are broadly divided into three main groups: (1) *endpoint PCR*, (2) *qPCR*, and (3) *dPCR*.

Endpoint PCR

Endpoint PCR assays (previously referred to as *conventional* PCR assays) are the simplest PCR assays and although still widely for research purposes, their use for diagnostic purposes has decreased. In this method, nucleic acids (genomic DNA and/or total RNA) are extracted from biological specimens using a commercially available extraction kit. A pair of primers, roughly 20 nucleotides long, is then used to bracket a desired DNA sequence, which is subsequently copied using a DNA polymerase enzyme (Fig. 6.2). Initially the DNA is

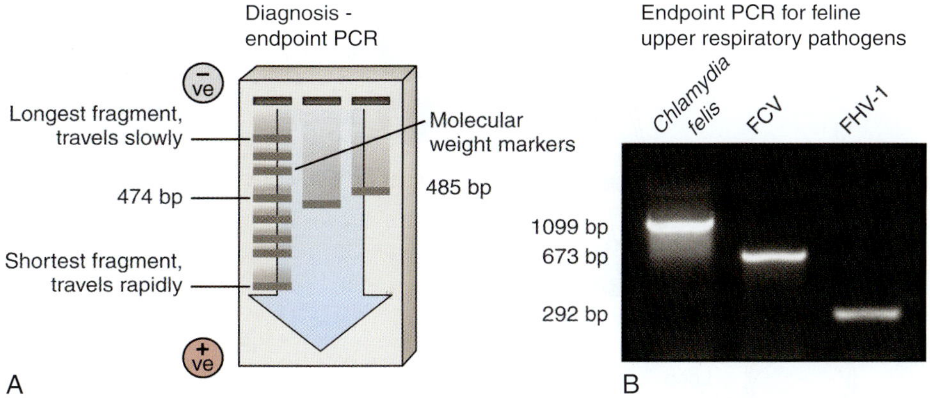

Fig. 6.3 Agarose gel electrophoresis showing detection of PCR products in an endpoint PCR assay. The longer the PCR product, the more slowly it moves through the gel. The size of the product can be estimated by running it alongside a molecular weight standard, which is available commercially. *FCV,* feline calicivirus; *FHV-1,* feline herpesvirus-1.

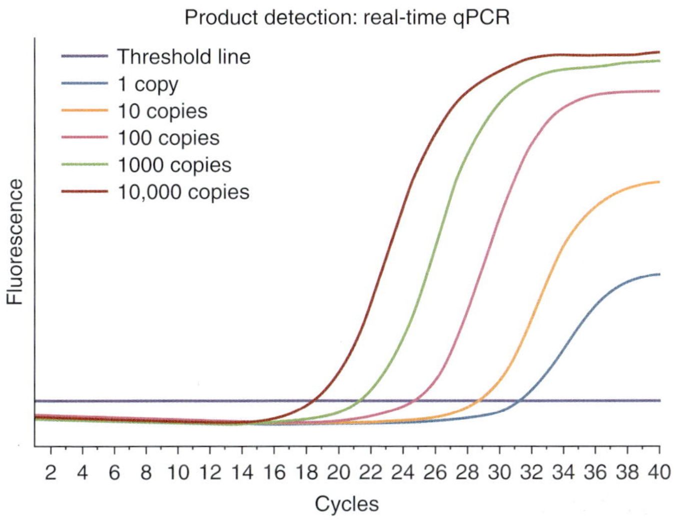

Fig. 6.4 Plot showing the emission of fluorescence during PCR product formation in real-time PCR as the number of cycles of denaturation, annealing, and extension increases. The C_T value is the number of PCR cycles required for the fluorescent signal to rise above a threshold value for fluorescence.

heated to 95°C, which causes the paired strands of DNA to separate (*denature*). Next, the tubes are cooled to a specific annealing temperature (usually 50°C to 65°C), which allows the primers to bind to their respective sequences. Finally, the tubes are heated to 72°C. This is the temperature at which the DNA polymerase adds dNTPs to the primers, extending the primers as it copies the sequence of the template DNA. The three-step cycle is repeated 30 to 50 times, which results in logarithmic accumulation of a PCR product that is an exact copy of the segment of DNA between the two primers.[7,8,36,17]

Products of PCR amplification are separated using agarose gel electrophoresis, stained with a dye that intercalates DNA (such as ethidium bromide), and the resulting fluorescent DNA bands are visualized using ultraviolet transillumination. The longer the PCR product, the more slowly it moves through the gel during electrophoresis. When a series of molecular weight markers are run alongside the end product of PCR, the size of the PCR product can be estimated (Fig. 6.3). The true identity of the product can then be confirmed using sequencing or by transferring it to a membrane and performing DNA hybridization with a specific probe. The process of loading the PCR product in agarose gels requires that the PCR tubes be opened, which can lead to aerosolization of PCR amplicons. These amplicons can then contaminate reagents, equipment, and tubes that are used for running subsequent PCR assays. Unless proper controls are included, false positives resulting from such contamination may go unidentified and lead to erroneous reporting of results.[49]

Real-Time Quantitative PCR (qPCR)

For diagnostic purposes, endpoint PCR assays have largely been superseded by qPCR, which monitors the accumulation of PCR product while the reaction takes place, usually through detection of fluorescence.[50] This provides quick, sensitive, quantitative detection of PCR products in a closed-tube format, thereby significantly reducing the risk of contamination and false-positive test results.[51,52] qPCR assays are amenable to automation, and reactions are generally loaded onto covered 96- or 384-well plates. Loading can be done robotically, further reducing the possibility of contamination and manual loading errors. qPCR instruments consist of a thermal cycler with an integrated excitation light source, a fluorescence detection system, and software. The software performs the quantitative analysis of detected fluorescence during the assay (Fig. 6.4). These instruments can simultaneously detect different wavelengths of light.[53,54] Special carousel thermocyclers are also available that rapidly heat and cool the reactions, which are placed in specially designed glass capillaries. As a result, some PCR assays can be completed in 45 minutes, instead of the 4 to 5 hours required for endpoint assays.[55]

Detection chemistries used in real-time quantitative PCR. The choice of probe chemistry used to detect PCR products in qPCR assays influences assay sensitivity and specificity, and so it can be helpful for clinicians to have an awareness of the approaches used. Fluorescent chemistries available that allow detection of target sequences during amplification can be categorized into two types: (1) double-stranded DNA (dsDNA) intercalating dyes (i.e., SYBR Green I, SYBR Gold, EvaGreen, LC Green, BOXTO, ResoLight, BEBO, SYTO, YO-PRO-1), and (2) fluorophore-labeled, sequence-specific oligonucleotide probes, which are designed to bind to the target sequence being amplified.[53,54,56]

When free in solution, dsDNA intercalating dyes exhibit little fluorescence, but when in contact with dsDNA, the dye intercalates between nucleic bases and assumes a conformation that emits fluorescence at a particular wavelength upon excitation. The fluorescent signal from a reaction is proportional to the amount of dsDNA present, and will increase as the target is amplified. Because there is no probe,

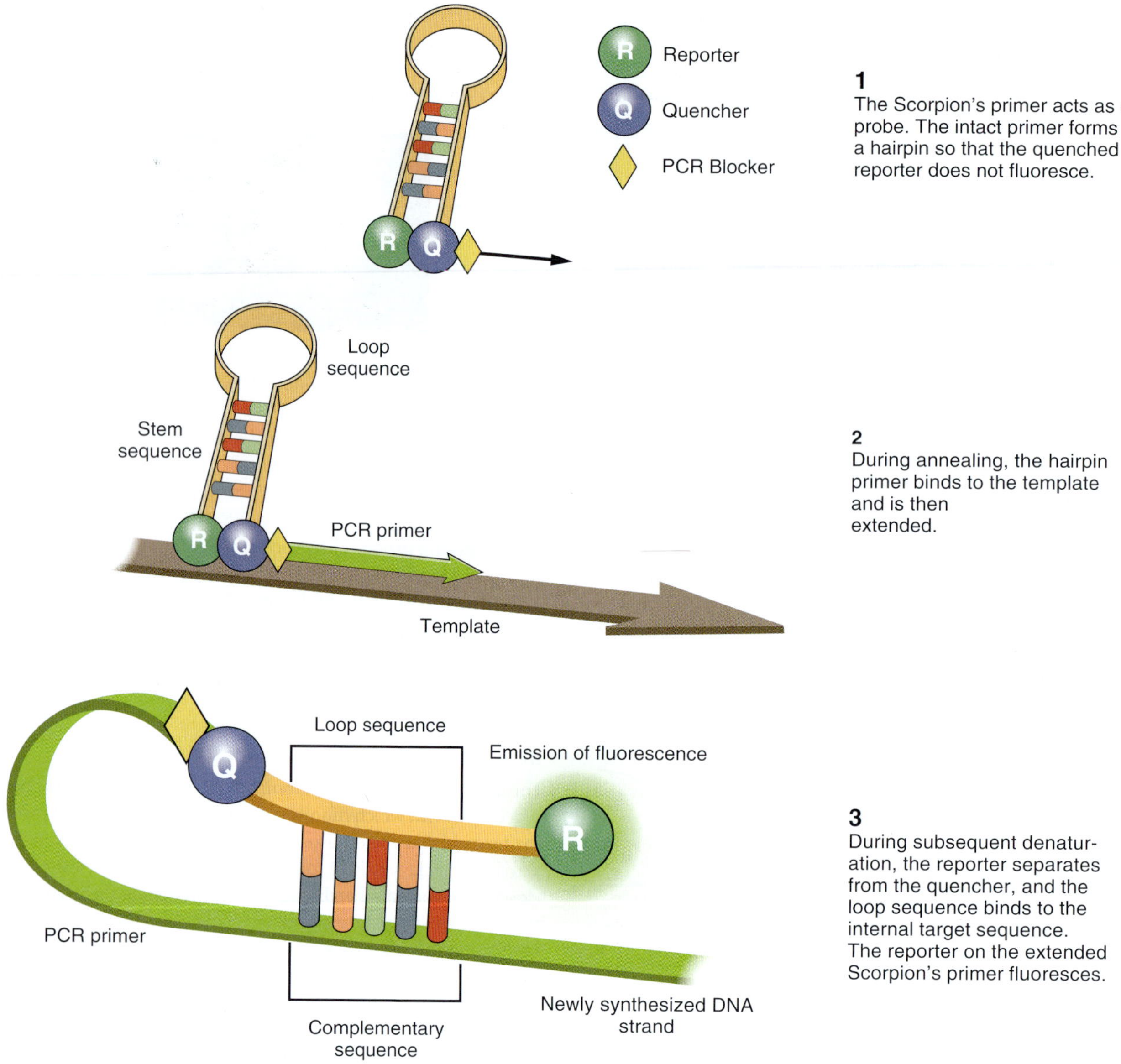

Fig. 6.5 Scorpions probe-primer assay.

carefully designed primers are required to ensure high specificity for the pathogen of interest. Intercalating dyes require melt-curve analysis to identify different reaction products. As a result, the presence of nonspecific products in a qPCR reaction may contribute to the overall fluorescence and affect the accuracy of quantification. Also, intercalating dyes cannot be used for multiplex reactions (reactions that target multiple pathogens in the same tube).[7,53]

Fluorophore primer- and probe-based chemistries can differ in their sequence geometry and binding mechanism, but nearly all share a fluorescent reporter dye partnered with a quencher dye, which are usually attached to an oligonucleotide probe. The quencher is a chromophore designed to absorb the fluorescent signal from the reporter dye when they are in close proximity, taking advantage of Förster Resonance Energy Transfer (FRET), to ensure specific fluorescence detection only in presence of amplified product. This can be accomplished by attaching a quencher molecule to the nucleic acid probe, and devising some mechanism by which the reporter and quencher become separated from one another when the probe binds to its specific target.[57] Fluorophore-labeled oligonucleotides used in the PCR reaction have been divided into three subgroups[54]:

(1) *Primer-probe* assays (e.g., Scorpions, Amplifluor, LUX, Cyclicons, Angler). In this case, one of the two PCR primers is connected to a probe by a quencher dye. The probe has a hairpin loop conformation that brings the quencher dye close to a fluorescent reporter dye attached to the 5′ end of the probe. Fluorescence emitted from primer-probe is detected and measured during the denaturation or extension phase of the qPCR. A commonly used *primer-probe* assay is Scorpions, which improves signals, has low background, and simple design.[58] During the course of PCR, the hairpin loop unfolds and the loop region of the probe hybridizes to the newly synthesized target sequence, causing the reporter dye to separate from the quencher dye and emit fluorescence (Fig. 6.5).

(2) *Probe assays* use a linear oligonucleotide that is complementary to the target nucleic acid sequence in addition to the primers, which is expected to anneal between the two primers. The oligonucleotide probe is labeled with a reporter dye on the 5′ end and quencher

dye on the 3′ end fluorophore, although the opposite orientation can also be used. The close proximity of the quencher dye to the reporter dye on the probe inhibits the reporter dye from emitting fluorescence. There are two types of probes used: (a) *hydrolysis probes* (e.g., TaqMan, Minor Groove Binding [MGB]-TaqMan, Snake assay), and (b) *hybridization probes* (e.g., Hybprobe or FRET, Molecular Beacons, HyBeacon, MGB-Pleiades, MGB-Eclipse, ResonSense, Yin-Yang or displacing). Hydrolysis probes rely on the 5′–3′ exonuclease activity of Taq polymerase. When the *Taq* DNA polymerase copies the section of DNA between the two primers, it encounters the probe and chops it into pieces, because it has inherent exonuclease activity. This causes the reporter dye to separate from the quencher dye. The reporter dye then emits fluorescence, which can be measured using a spectrophotometer.[53,54,59–61] The amount of fluorescent signal detected is directly proportional to the amount of the target amplified during the PCR reaction.[7,54] Many veterinary laboratories that offer probe-based PCR assays use TaqMan probes. MGB-TaqMan probes are designed to improve target DNA-binding specificity and sensitivity, and are becoming widely used for diagnosis of microbial pathogens. An example of a hybridization probe assay is the FRET probe assay. FRET probe assays use two probes that are predicted to lie adjacent to one another on the target sequence. The first probe is tagged at the 3′ end with one fluorophore, and the second probe contains a second fluorophore at the 5′ end, and a phosphate group attached to its 3′ end to prevent DNA amplification. When the two dyes come together during annealing, one fluorophore transfers its energy to the other, causing it to emit fluorescence, which can then be detected.[62] Currently there are only rare reports of the use of this technology for diagnosis in veterinary medicine.

(3) *Probes that are analogues of nucleic acids* (PNA, LNA, ZNA, non-natural bases: Plexor primer, Tiny-Molecular Beacon) are much shorter than nucleic acid probes due to the higher binding affinity of the analogue nucleic acid bases to standard DNA, and they are more stable in biological fluids. An analogue may have alterations in its phosphate backbone, pentose sugar (either ribose or deoxyribose) or nucleobases. Such probes only need to be 8–9 bases long.[53,54]

Primer and probe design. Primers are a critical component of PCR reactions. The primers are extended by the polymerase upon binding to the pathogen target DNA, and are designed to bind to the opposite strand to facilitate exponential amplification, which is the hallmark of PCR. The DNA polymerase synthesizes the new DNA copy by moving from the 5′ end toward the 3′ end. Both the sequence of the primers and that of the target sequence can affect the efficiency of PCR. A number of free and commercially available software programs are available for the purpose of designing primers. The following are important considerations when primers are designed:

- *Primer specificity*, as nonspecific amplification of nontarget DNA is one of the greatest challenges for successful target amplification. The specificity of primers and probes are verified using commercial software programs.
- *Primer length* (typically 16 to 28 nucleotides long).
- *Amplicon length* (usually 100 to 250 base pairs).
- *Primer G and C base pair content*, which is maintained between 35% and 65%.
- *Primer 3′ end stability*, which can contribute to nonspecific primer extension by Taq DNA polymerase, especially if the binding of the 3′ nucleotide bases is relatively tight to the nontarget template. Primers with very high 3′ terminal stability (as determined using a software program) are usually rejected.
- *Primer melting temperature (Tm).* Most primer design software programs can predict melting (annealing) temperature based on the nucleotide composition of the primers under evaluation.[7,54,63] The Tm of each primer used must be similar so that they anneal at the same temperature during PCR.

Validation and optimization of qPCR assays. In theory, the amount of fluorescence emitted during each PCR cycle doubles, and it is proportional to the number of copies of pathogen DNA in the clinical specimen. However, imperfections that result from variable pre-assay conditions, assay design, and improper data analysis can lead to inaccurate results and erroneous diagnostic conclusions. Before being used for diagnostic purposes, qPCR assays must be shown to be *sensitive, specific, reproducible,* and *efficient* through validation and verification. A number of factors can be altered to obtain optimum assay performance, which will lead to higher molecular sensitivity, specificity, and precision.

During validation of PCR assays, the laboratory uses the assay to test serial dilutions of a known amount of target DNA. For qPCR, *the limit of detection* is the lowest number of copies of the target DNA or RNA sequence that the assay can detect (also known as *analytical sensitivity*). The results are used to create a graph known as a *standard curve.* This consists of the logarithm of the initial starting quantity of DNA on the x-axis and the *quantification cycle (Cq; also known as cycle threshold* [C_T]) *values* obtained on the y-axis (see Fig. 6.4). Cq represents the number of cycles that elapse before fluorescence is detectable above a threshold value set by the thermocycler manufacturer. A standard curve is commonly generated using a 10-fold serial dilution series of at least five template concentrations. The standard curve can then be used to predict the amount of target DNA in a clinical specimen based on the Cq value.

The standard curve should result in a slope that demonstrates good efficiency, accuracy, and sensitivity. The efficiency of a qPCR reaction is the degree to which the polymerase converts reagents to produce target amplicons. Factors that affect the efficiency of a qPCR reaction include amplicon length and sequence, primer sequence, impurities and inhibitors in the sample, and cycling conditions. Once the standard curve is generated, the efficiency of the reaction is calculated from the slope of the log-linear portion of the standard curve (10-1/slope-1). A qPCR assay that has an *efficiency* of 100% doubles the number of copies of template in every PCR cycle. Efficiencies below 90% are unacceptable for quantitative assays, and ideally efficiency should be greater than 95%. Ideally, this is compared with a similar curve that uses dilutions of the standard DNA spiked into a clinical specimen, to show that inhibitors within the specimen do not affect efficiency.[64,65]

From a diagnostic standpoint, a qPCR assay may lack sensitivity (many false negatives) if the assay fails to detect all possible strains of a target organism. This can occur if the probe or primers are strain specific, rather than species specific, and many strains of the target organism exist with variable sequences (as is the case with RNA pathogens such as FCV). As part of the validation process, the assay should be shown to be *inclusive* and detect as many strains or variants as possible.

A qPCR assay has poor *analytical specificity* if false positives occur as a result of contamination or because of manual loading error. Specificity may also be poor if the primers bind to and initiate amplification of DNA from unrelated organisms or the host animal (i.e., cat, dog, human DNA). Specificity is tested during the validation process by showing that the qPCR assay fails to amplify DNA from clinical specimens that contain organisms that are genetically related to the target organism, as well as organisms that may be expected to be contaminating normal flora.[64]

BOX 6.3 Methods that may Be Used To Minimize Contamination in Diagnostic Laboratories that Perform Nucleic Acid Amplification Assays

Separation of rooms for DNA extraction, PCR and postamplification detection
Robotic DNA extraction
Automated detection of PCR products (real-time qPCR)
Opening one specimen tube at a time
Use of screw-top caps rather than snap-top tubes to prevent splashing
Use of filter-plugged pipette tips
Use of negative extraction controls and negative template controls in every run
Routine monitoring for contamination using wipes
Standard clean-up protocol that inactivates nucleic acids
Use of positive control samples of low concentration
Use of dUTP and uracil-*N*-glycosylase in the PCR mastermix

The results of qPCR assays must also be repeatable. *Repeatability* is determined for qPCR assays by determining whether the Cq value varies significantly for the same specimen when tested multiple times. Usually intra-assay (within the same run) and inter-assay (across different runs) variations are measured.[66]

Analysis of qPCR assay results. Data analysis includes an examination of the raw qPCR data, an evaluation of their quality and reliability, and the generation of reportable results. The output of a qPCR assay is an amplification curve, which is subject to background fluorescence (see Fig. 6.4). A range of factors affect the degree of background fluorescence, including choice of plasticware, unquenched probe fluorescence, and signal carryover into the neighboring sample wells. In well-designed assays, the background is low compared with the amplified signal. However, variation in the background signal may affect quantification comparisons between different specimens, so the laboratory must correct for baseline variations.

Most laboratories run approximately 40 cycles of amplification, and so specimens that generate Cq values less than 40 are considered to be positive. Said another way, if PCR proceeds to 40 cycles without emission of fluorescence (Cq = 40), then the target DNA is not detectable in the specimen, and the result is reported as negative. The lower the Cq value, the more target DNA (= organism load) is present in the specimen, because fewer cycles elapse before fluorescence is detected. Because specimen size varies, the Cq value may be normalized to the approximate number of host cells present in the specimen. Knowledge of organism load may have prognostic value for some infections, can allow infection to be monitored over time with treatment, and may be useful to differentiate low-level colonization from active infection causing clinical signs (see Interpretation of Results, later). At the time of writing, veterinary diagnostic laboratories performing PCR assays variably report organism loads to the clinician.[67]

Prevention of PCR Contamination and Quality Assurance

PCR contamination can be difficult to eradicate once it occurs, so prevention of contamination is critical (Box 6.3). Laboratories should include negative controls in every run, and a positive control should be included to ensure that the assay is working, preferably one that is also subjected to the nucleic acid extraction process. The positive control should contain a low concentration of DNA, because abundant DNA used as a positive control may serve as a source of contamination for other assays. Many laboratories run two separate negative controls. One of the negative controls contains mastermix and nuclease-free water in place of nucleic acid that has been extracted from a specimen. The other consists of water or a known negative specimen that is subjected to the extraction process to ensure that contamination does not occur during extraction (negative extraction control). When 96- or 384-well plate formats are used, negative control wells are interspersed among the test wells to monitor for plate contamination.[67]

In order to prevent contamination, some laboratories use deoxyuracil triphosphate (dUTP) instead of deoxythymidine triphosphate (dTTP) in the PCR mastermix. This substitution results in generation of PCR products that contain uracil (U) in place of thymidine (T). The enzyme uracil-*N*-glycosylase (UNG) is also added to the mix. This enzyme destroys DNA amplicons that contain deoxyuracil residues, and eliminates any contaminating DNA amplicons from previous reactions *before* PCR amplification begins. When the reaction mix is heated in the initial denaturation step, the UNG is destroyed.[68]

Many biological specimens contain components that inhibit PCR, such as hemoglobin, myoglobin, bile salts, humic acids, urea, and collagen,[13] and require extensive purification. However, extensive purification leads to losses and is expensive. Complete removal of inhibitors may not be possible. Various methods can be used to assess the presence of inhibitors within clinical specimens, as follows:

1. Determine the PCR efficiency in a test sample by subjecting serial dilutions of the sample to PCR.[69]
2. Use a *reference gene* (formerly known as a *housekeeping gene*). A reference gene is an endogenous amplification control gene that copurifies with the target nucleic acid and is amplified at the same time as the target pathogen DNA using a separate set of primers and probes. Amplification of a reference gene is usually performed on a separate aliquot of the extracted specimen at the same time as the assay for the target pathogen. Reference genes are typically host (dog or cat) genes that are expected to be present in the sample, such as canine or feline glyceraldehyde-3-phosphate dehydrogenase (GAPDH), histone, or 18S DNA. A negative reference gene PCR assay result (or a high Cq value for the assay, which is equivalent to a weak positive result) suggests that inhibitors may be present in the specimen, or that DNA in the submitted specimen may have degraded during storage or transport. Some qPCR assays use an *internal reference gene control*, in which a reference gene is amplified within the same reaction mix (known as multiplexing, see later in this chapter) with the qPCR assay for the target microorganism.
3. Use an *exogenous control, also known as a spike or SPUD gene.* The spikes typically consist of a chemically synthesized nucleic acid template (RNA or DNA, depending on the target) and two primers specific to the template and are run in the presence of SYBR Green I dye or a specific probe. The spike template is amplified in a separate control reaction, resulting in a characteristic Cq. Alongside this control reaction, the exogenous control is also spiked into specimens and the fluorescence emitted from the spike is compared with that emitted from the control. When inhibitors are not present, the Cq from the spiked clinical specimen will remain the same as the control, whereas in the presence of a contaminated specimen the Cq is higher.[70,71]

Variations of Polymerase Chain Reaction Assays

Variations of polymerase chain reaction include reverse-transcriptase qPCR, nested PCR, and multiplex PCR.

Reverse-Transcriptase qPCR

Reverse-transcriptase qPCR (RT-qPCR) is used for detection of pathogen RNA (such as RNA viruses) and gene expression studies. After extraction of total RNA from clinical specimens using a commercial kit or automated platform, the enzyme *reverse transcriptase* is used together with dNTPs to transcribe RNA into complementary DNA

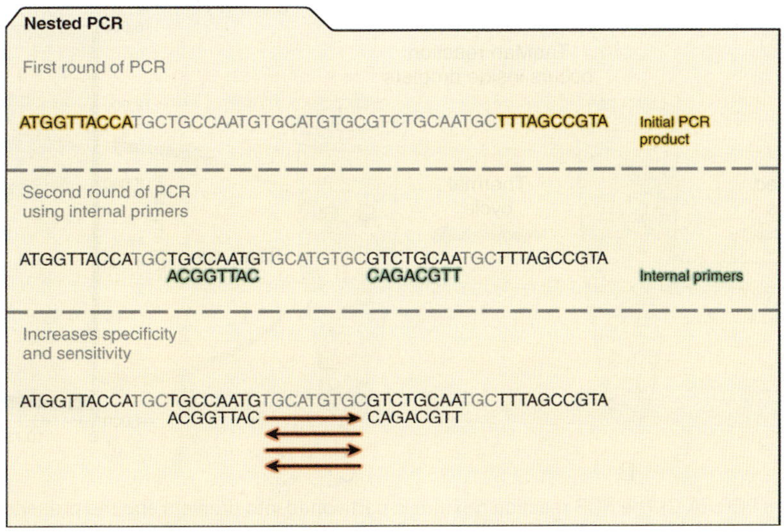

Fig. 6.6 Nested PCR. A second set of internal primers are used in a second round of PCR to increase the sensitivity and specificity of the assay.

(cDNA). The RT step can be initiated with *oligo(dT) primers* (primers that anneal to a poly-A tail), *random primers* (a mixture of primers with randomly assigned bases), a mixture of the two, or gene-specific primers. Subsequently, the cDNA is then used as the template for qPCR amplification.[72,73]

Nested PCR

In nested PCR, a small amount of amplified PCR product is subjected to a second round of PCR using another set of internal primers (Fig. 6.6). Having an additional set of primers increases the specificity of the PCR assay and also greatly increases its sensitivity.[74] Unfortunately, the increased sensitivity means that false positives due to contamination can be extremely problematic with this method, and it has lost popularity for diagnostic purposes.

Multiplex PCR

Multiplex PCR assays use multiple sets of primers *in the same reaction tube* to simultaneously detect multiple organisms (or multiple genes from the same organism). Duplex PCR assays can detect two organisms, and triplex PCR assays can detect three organisms. The potential downside of multiplex reactions is that if one organism is present in higher abundance, this may reduce the sensitivity of the assay for the other target organisms because amplification of the abundant pathogen DNA consumes reagents that are then unavailable for amplification of the other pathogen. Successful multiplexing results from careful experimental design and optimization of reaction conditions.[64,75,76]

Isothermal PCR

Isothermal PCR is a process that amplifies nucleic acids at a constant temperature, and has been the basis for in-clinic PCR assay development, because an expensive thermocycler is not required. Dozens of complex different isothermal amplification methods have been published, and some have reached the practice environment in human medicine (e.g., Loopamp MALARIA, Human Diagnostics Worldwide) and most recently in veterinary medicine (e.g., PCRun, Biogal). Examples include rolling-circle amplification and loop-mediated isothermal amplification (LAMP). In-clinic assays involve a DNA extraction step, followed by addition of reagents required for amplification, incubation in a heated block (e.g., 60°C for 1 hour), then detection of the PCR product. Detection of the products of PCR either involves the use of a lateral-flow disposable nucleic acid detection device (into which the tube containing the amplified DNA is inserted), or a small benchtop bioilluminator device that can semi-quantify the amount of DNA present in the reaction.[77] Isothermal in-clinic assays have been marketed for *Leptospira* spp., *Ehrlichia canis*, *Anaplasma platys*, *Leishmania* spp., *Babesia canis*, CPV, feline panleukopenia virus, and *Mycoplasma haemofelis*, which allow detection of a PCR product within 75 minutes. In one study, the clinical sensitivity and specificity of one assay for *M. haemofelis* (PCRun, Biogal) was compared with that of an endpoint PCR assay. Using one extraction method, the sensitivity and specificity was 94% and 96%, respectively; using a more crude extraction method recommended by the manufacturer, the sensitivity and specificity was 78% and 96%, respectively.[78] When compared with a qPCR assay, a *Leishmania* POC PCR assay offered in Europe by the same manufacturer also had high clinical specificity (100%) but low sensitivity (10% to 57%, depending on specimen type).[77] Sensitivity was also low (30%) and specificity high (100%) for an *E. canis* POC assay when compared with qPCR in experimentally infected dogs.[79] It was suggested that this may be because larger quantities of DNA must be present within a specimen for detection by the POC assays compared with detection by qPCR, based on the specimen types that tested positive for *Leishmania* and the stage of *E. canis* infection when positive results were obtained using the POC assays.[77] An insulated isothermal PCR (iiPCR) POC assay (POCKIT Nucleic Acid Analyzer, GeneReach USA, Lexington, MA) for *Babesia gibsoni* was shown to have high clinical sensitivity (90%) and specificity (99%) when compared with a qPCR assay (IDEXX Laboratories Inc., Westbrook, ME, USA), and generated results within 2 hours.[80]

DNA Microarrays

One of the limitations of culture is the inability to detect a target pathogen when it exists in a matrix that contains a large number of additional organisms. With microarray technology, the products of PCR amplification of a universal bacterial gene (such as bacterial 16S rRNA) can be hybridized onto a solid platform that contains thousands to more than a million oligonucleotide probes. These either hybridize to bacterial 16S rRNA genes; genus-, species-, or strain-specific genes; genes that specify resistance to antimicrobials; or toxin genes. The products of amplification are labeled with fluorescent dyes and the amplicon-probe interactions are measured using a laser scanner and analyzed by

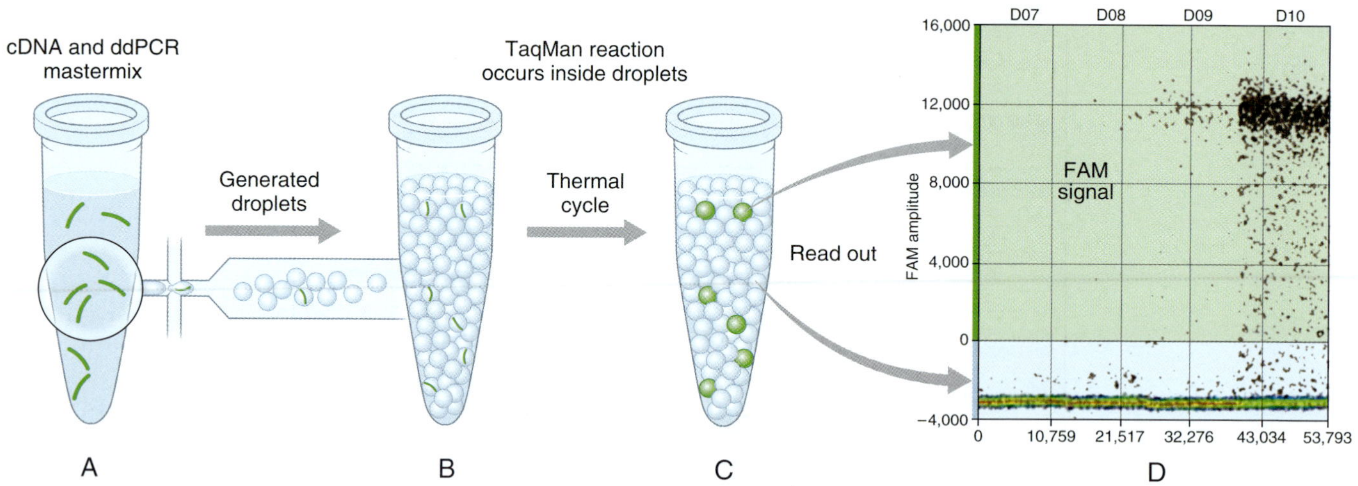

Fig. 6.7 Digital PCR. (A-C) The PCR reaction mixture is partitioned into droplets and the presence or absence of fluorescence from each droplet is measured. (D) The fraction of fluorescing droplets can be used to determine the number of target molecules present per droplet using Poisson distribution statistics.

a computer. Examples are PhyloChip (Second Generation Solutions), which has been widely used to analyze microbial communities using 16S bacterial rRNA probes, and Prove-It Sepsis (Mobidiag, Finland), which detects 60 species of bacteria and 13 fungi, as well as the *mecA* resistance gene, in blood specimens within a 3.5-hour time frame.

Digital PCR (dPCR)

First described in 1992,[81] dPCR is a refinement of PCR that can be used to more accurately quantify nucleic acids (including DNA, cDNA, methylated DNA, or RNA). In contrast to traditional PCR, the assembled reaction mixture is separated into a large number of individual portions (in microwell plates, capillaries, oil emulsions, or other chambers) and the reaction is carried out on each partition individually. After multiple cycles of PCR, the samples are checked as to whether they fluoresce or not. Poisson statistics are then used to measure the quantity of DNA present, and use of a calibration curve is not necessary; the fraction of fluorescing droplets predicts the number of target copies per droplet (Fig. 6.7). This separation allows a more reliable collection and sensitive measurement of nucleic acid amounts. It provides absolute quantification, because the number of droplets fluorescing due to proper amplification are determined, rather than DNA quantity being extrapolated using a calibration curve. The interest in dPCR has grown over the last 10 years because technologic progress makes it practical, with unparalleled precision, absolute quantification, flexibility, and increasingly affordable. dPCR may also be more reproducible and less susceptible to inhibition than qPCR. The method has been useful for viral/pathogen detection and quantification, gene expression studies, food testing, detection of point mutations, and clonal amplification for next-generation sequencing.[82,83]

INTERPRETATION OF PCR ASSAY RESULTS

A properly designed and highly efficient qPCR assay can detect very few copies (one or two) of a targeted gene, but both viable and nonviable organisms can be detected, which may be an obstacle for the clinician when trying to determine the significance of a positive qPCR result in light of an animal's disease. An understanding of the pathogenesis of infectious diseases and organism shedding patterns is crucial when interpreting positive qPCR results. Correct interpretation of the results relies on knowledge of the methods used by a laboratory and their advantage and disadvantages.

BOX 6.4 Factors that Should Be Considered When Interpreting NAAT Results

Test Result	Reason
Negative	Organism not present
	Too few organisms present
	Insufficient specimen size
	Wrong specimen type
	Improper timing of specimen collection
	Patient receiving antimicrobial therapy
	Specimen degradation during storage of transport
	Assay reagent failure
	Assay inhibitors present or extraction failure
	Reagents consumed in a multiplex assay
	Assay does not detect all strains
Positive	Viable or nonviable organisms present and causing disease
	Viable or nonviable organisms present but not causing disease
	Vaccine organisms present
	Contamination
	Loading errors
	Assay cross-reaction with other pathogens or host DNA in the specimen

NAAT, nucleic acid amplification test.

Factors that can lead to *negative test results* are shown in Box 6.4. An example of the use of the wrong specimen type would be submission of blood for a *Borrelia burgdorferi* qPCR test, when *B. burgdorferi* is found predominantly in connective tissue,[84] and only in blood for a short period of time during early infection. As discussed in this chapter, assay inhibition and specimen degradation can be identified by interpretation of reference gene control assay results, which should be performed by the laboratory; therefore, the clinician should use reliable laboratories and ensure that they use quality controls.

Factors that must be considered when interpreting *positive test results* are shown in Box 6.4. The most common reason for false-positive test results for assays that involve DNA amplification is contamination. Loading errors, in which specimen extracts are inadvertently loaded into the wrong wells on a microtiter plate, may also lead to false-positive results and are reduced with the use of automated methods. Because of the exquisite sensitivity of qPCR, the significance of a true positive result should be interpreted with a caution. The organism may be part of the normal flora or carried subclinically (e.g., latent FHV-1 in a nasal biopsy). Several US veterinary laboratories offer qPCR "panels" for diagnostic purposes, whereby qPCR assays for several different pathogens are performed in separate reaction wells (one per pathogen) on nucleic acid extracted from a single clinical specimen. This high-throughput panel format allows assays to be offered at a substantial discount over the cost of multiple individual assays. This type of testing can occasionally result in unexpected positive test results, such as a positive result for the *Clostridium perfringens* toxin gene in a cat with diarrhea that is suspected to have trichomoniasis. In this situation, the *C. perfringens* may be an incidental finding and unrelated to the clinical problem, because healthy cats can have such toxin genes in their feces (see Chapter 64). As with any laboratory test, positive results need to be interpreted in light of the clinical history, clinical signs, and the pathogenesis of the disease in question. A positive result can also occur if an attenuated live vaccine for the target organism was recently administered. Because qPCR detects both viable and nonviable organisms, qPCR can be positive for days after antimicrobials have been administered, when culture is negative.[85–87] The duration of qPCR positivity after treatment depends on the sample type tested and the target pathogen.

CHALLENGES OF CURRENT MOLECULAR DETECTION METHODS

The reliability of a molecular diagnostic test depends on its detection limit. Some methods have limited ability to detect low numbers of organisms without steps to amplify the population in advance of PCR. Culture-based enrichment has been used reliably to expand a pathogen's population, but this technique is a time-consuming step in the analysis.[88]

Molecular techniques have limitations, such as those that relate to inhibition of PCR, lack of sensitivity in chronic infections, and differentiation of vaccine organisms from true pathogens. Often, multiple different types of diagnostic tests (culture, PCR, serology) must be performed for successful pathogen detection, and a correct diagnosis relies on interpretation of these results in light of the total clinical picture.

Pathogens are most accurately identified by sequencing the entire chromosome, or one or more genes of the unknown organism, and comparing the sequences generated to others in an identification database such as Genbank. Sequences can be generated using PCR-based technology. This technology, known as *whole genome sequencing*, can be used to identify fungi, bacteria, and viruses. It can be used to identify slow-growing organisms, or even those that cannot be cultured. The major disadvantage of whole genome sequencing is the high costs associated with it in terms of dedicated facilities, personnel training, time, and consumables.

REFERENCES

1. Lamoth F, Greub G. Fastidious intracellular bacteria as causal agents of community-acquired pneumonia. *Expert Rev Anti Infect Ther.* 2010;8:775–790.
2. Murray PR, Baron EJ, Pfaller MA, et al. *Manual of Clinical Microbiology.* 6th ed. Washington, DC: American Society for Microbiology; 1995:1482.
3. Gracias KS, McKillip JL. A review of conventional detection and enumeration methods for pathogenic bacteria in food. *Can J Microbiol.* 2004;50:883–890.
4. Petti CA. Detection and identification of microorganisms by gene amplification and sequencing. *Clin Infect Dis.* 2007;44:1108–1114.
5. Lazcka O, Del Campo FJ, Munoz FX. Pathogen detection: a perspective of traditional methods and biosensors. *Biosens Bioelectron.* 2007;22:1205–1217.
6. Nayak M, Kotian A, Marathe S, et al. Detection of microorganisms using biosensors-a smarter way towards detection techniques. *Biosens Bioelectron.* 2009;25:661–667.
7. Pestana EA, Belak S, Diallo A, et al. *Early, Rapid and Sensitive Veterinary Molecular Diagnostics - Real Time PCR Applications.* Dordrecht, Netherlands: Springer; 2010:310.
8. Yousef AE. Detection of bacterial pathogens in different matrices: current practices and challenges. In: Zourob M, Elwary S, Turner A, eds. *Principles of Bacterial Detection: Biosensors, Recognition Receptors and Microsystems.* New York, NY: Springer; 2008:31–47.
9. Pickup RW. Development of molecular methods for the detection of specific bacteria in the environment. *J Gen Microbiol.* 1991;137:1009–1019.
10. Kaspar CW, Tartera C. Methods for detecting pathogens in food and water. *Methods Microbiol.* 1990;22:497–534.
11. Anderson B, Sims K, Regnery R, et al. Detection of *Rochalimaea henselae* DNA in specimens from cat scratch disease patients by PCR. *J Clin Microbiol.* 1994;32:942–948.
12. Willi B, Boretti FS, Cattori V, et al. Identification, molecular characterization, and experimental transmission of a new hemoplasma isolate from a cat with hemolytic anemia in Switzerland. *J Clin Microbiol.* 2005;43:2581–2585.
13. Radstrom P, Knutsson R, Wolffs P, et al. Pre–PCR processing: strategies to generate PCR-compatible samples. *Mol Biotechnol.* 2004;26:133–146.
14. Greenlee JJ, Bolin CA, Alt DP, et al. Clinical and pathologic comparison of acute leptospirosis in dogs caused by two strains of *Leptospira kirschneri* serovar grippotyphosa. *Am J Vet Res.* 2004;65:1100–1107.
15. Endler G, Slavka G. Stability of the specimen during preanalytic. In: Kessler HH, ed. *Molecular Diagnostics of Infectious Diseases.* Graz, Austria: Deutsche Nationalbibliothek; 2010:25–34.
16. Gimenez-Marin A, Rivas-Ruiz F, Perez-Hidalgo Mdel M, et al. Pre-analytical errors management in the clinical laboratory: a five-year study. *Biochem Med.* 2014;24:248–257.
17. Bustin SA. A history of MIQE guidelines. In: Nour AMA, Pfaffl MW, eds. *MIQE & qPCR iBook: How to Apply the MIQE Guidelines - a Visual, Interactive and Practical qPCR Guide.* 2nd ed. Freising, Germany: bioMCC; 2016:10–44.
18. Rainen L, Arbique JC, Asthana D, et al. Collection, transport, preparation, and storage of specimens for molecular methods; approved guideline. *Clinical and Laboratory Standards Institute, MM13-A.* 2005;25:1–45.
19. Miller JM, Holmes HT. Specimen collection, transport, and storage. In: Murray PR, ed. *Manual of Clinical Microbiology.* 6th ed. Washington, DC: ASM Press; 1995:19–33.
20. Lahiri DK, Schnabel B. DNA isolation by a rapid method from human blood samples: effects of MgCl2, EDTA, storage time, and temperature on DNA yield and quality. *Biochem Genet.* 1993;31:321–328.
21. Beutler E, Gelbart T, Kuhl W. Interference of heparin with the polymerase chain reaction. *Biotechniques.* 1990;9:166.
22. Rabenau HF, Raggam RB, Salzer HJF. Choice of adequate sample material. In: Kessler HH, ed. *Molecular Diagnostics of Infectious Diseases.* Graz, Austria: Deutsche Nationalbibliothek; 2010:1–24.
23. Raggam RB, Kessler HH, Rabenau HF. Quality assurance and quality control in the routine molecular diagnostic laboratory. In: Kessler HH, ed. *Molecular Diagnostics of Infectious Diseases.* Gratz, Austria: Bibliographic Nationalbibliothek; 2010:35–46.
24. Madej RM, Davis J, Holden MJ, et al. International standards and reference materials for quantitative molecular infectious disease testing. *J Mol Diagn.* 2010;12:133–143.
25. Yang S, Rothman RE. PCR-based diagnostics for infectious diseases: uses, limitations, and future applications in acute-care settings. *Lancet Infect Dis.* 2004;4:337–348.
26. Gill P, Ghaemi A. Nucleic acid isothermal amplification technologies: a review. *Nucleos Nucleot Nucleic Acids.* 2008;27:224–243.
27. Zanoli LM, Spoto G. Isothermal amplification methods for the detection of nucleic acids in microfluidic devices. *Biosensors.* 2013;3:18–43.
28. Sibley CD, Peirano G, Church DL. Molecular methods for pathogen and microbial community detection and characterization: current and poten-

tial application in diagnostic microbiology. *Infect Genet Evol.* 2012;12:505–521.

29. Su Z, Ning B, Fang H, et al. Next-generation sequencing and its applications in molecular diagnostics. *Expert Rev Mol Diagn.* 2011;11:333–343.
30. Heideman DA, Lurkin I, Doeleman M, et al. KRAS and BRAF mutation analysis in routine molecular diagnostics: comparison of three testing methods on formalin-fixed, paraffin-embedded tumor-derived DNA. *J Mol Diagn.* 2012;14:247–255.
31. Jordan BR. Is there a niche for DNA microarrays in molecular diagnostics? *Expert Rev Mol Diagn.* 2010;10:875–882.
32. Mohapatra G, Betensky RA, Miller ER, et al. Glioma test array for use with formalin-fixed, paraffin-embedded tissue: array comparative genomic hybridization correlates with loss of heterozygosity and fluorescence in situ hybridization. *J Mol Diagn.* 2006;8:268–276.
33. Vasavirama K. Molecular probes and their applications. *Int J LifeSc Bt & Pharm Res.* 2013;2:32–42.
34. Horbinski C, Miller CR, Perry A. Gone FISHing: clinical lessons learned in brain tumor molecular diagnostics over the last decade. *Brain Pathol.* 2011;21:57–73.
35. Marilynn R, Fairfax SH. Quantitative PCR: an introduction. In: Grody WW, Nakamura RM, Strom CM, Kiechle FL, eds. *Molecular Diagnostics: Techniques and Aplications for the Clinical Laboratory.* San Diego, CA: Elsevier; 2010:3–14.
36. Procop GW. Molecular diagnostics for the detection and characterization of microbial pathogens. *Clin Infect Dis.* 2007;45(suppl 2):S99–S111.
37. Kornreich BG, Craven M, McDonough SP, et al. Fluorescence in-situ hybridization for the identification of bacterial species in archival heart valve sections of canine bacterial endocarditis. *J Comp Pathol.* 2012;146:298–307.
38. Mansfield CS, James FE, Craven M, et al. Remission of histiocytic ulcerative colitis in Boxer dogs correlates with eradication of invasive intramucosal *Escherichia coli*. *J Vet Intern Med.* 2009;23:964–969.
39. Im J, Burney DP, McDonough SP, et al. Canine hepatitis associated with intrahepatic bacteria in three dogs. *J Am Anim Hosp Assoc.* 2018;54:65–70.
40. Hutton TA, Goldstein RE, Njaa BL, et al. Search for *Borrelia burgdorferi* in kidneys of dogs with suspected "Lyme nephritis". *J Vet Intern Med.* 2008;22:860–865.
41. Hoehne SN, McDonough SP, Rishniw M, et al. Identification of mucosa-invading and intravascular bacteria in feline small intestinal lymphoma. *Vet Pathol.* 2017;54:234–241.
42. Jergens AE, Pressel M, Crandell J, et al. Fluorescence in situ hybridization confirms clearance of visible *Helicobacter* spp. associated with gastritis in dogs and cats. *J Vet Intern Med.* 2009;23:16–23.
43. Arnold Jr LJ, Hammond PW, Wiese WA, et al. Assay formats involving acridinium-ester-labeled DNA probes. *Clin Chem.* 1989;35:1588–1594.
44. Padilla E, Manterola JM, Rasmussen OF, et al. Evaluation of a fluorescence hybridisation assay using peptide nucleic acid probes for identification and differentiation of tuberculous and non-tuberculous mycobacteria in liquid cultures. *Eur J Clin Microbiol Infect Dis.* 2000;19:140–145.
45. Zhang N, Appella DH. Advantages of peptide nucleic acids as diagnostic platforms for detection of nucleic acids in resource-limited settings. *J Infect Dis.* 2010;201(suppl 1):S42–S45.
46. Andras SC, Power JB, Cocking EC, et al. Strategies for signal amplification in nucleic acid detection. *Mol Biotechnol.* 2001;19:29–44.
47. Nolte FS, Caliendo AM. Molecular microbiology. In: Versalovic J, Carroll KC, Funke G, Jorgensen JH, Landry ML, Warnock DW, eds. *Manual of Clinical Microbiology.* 10th ed. Washington, DC: ASM Press; 2011:27–59.
48. Fakruddin M, Mannan KS, Chowdhury A, et al. Nucleic acid amplification: alternative methods of polymerase chain reaction. *J Pharm BioAllied Sci.* 2013;5:245–252.
49. Lee PY, Costumbrado J, Hsu CY, et al. Agarose gel electrophoresis for the separation of DNA fragments. *J vis exp: JoVE.* 2012.
50. Heid CA, Stevens J, Livak KJ, et al. Real time quantitative PCR. *Genome Res.* 1996;6:986–994.
51. Csordas AT, Barak JD, Delwiche MJ. Comparison of primers for the detection of *Salmonella enterica* serovars using real-time PCR. *Lett Appl Microbiol.* 2004;39:187–193.
52. Raoult D, Fournier PE, Drancourt M. What does the future hold for clinical microbiology? *Nat Rev Microbiol.* 2004;2:151–159.
53. Shipley GL. An introduction to real-time PCR. In: Dorak MT, ed. *Real-Time PCR.* London, UK: Taylor & Francis Group; 2007:1–38.
54. Navarro E, Serrano-Heras G, Castano MJ, et al. Real-time PCR detection chemistry. *Clin Chim Acta.* 2015;439:231–250.
55. Cockerill FR 3rd . Application of rapid-cycle real-time polymerase chain reaction for diagnostic testing in the clinical microbiology laboratory. *Arch Pathol Lab Med.* 2003;127:1112–1120.
56. Flynn JM, Sowers BA. qPCR oligonucleotide synthesis and design. In: Nour AMA, Pfaffl MW, eds. *The qPCR and dPCR MIQE Guidelines. A success story!.* 2nd ed. 2016:115–154. Online.
57. Didenko VV. DNA probes using fluorescence resonance energy transfer (FRET): designs and applications. *Biotechniques.* 2001;31:1106–1116, 1118, 1120–1121.
58. Whitcombe D, Theaker J, Guy SP, et al. Detection of PCR products using self-probing amplicons and fluorescence. *Nat Biotechnol.* 1999;17:804–807.
59. Bustin SA. Quantification of mRNA using real-time reverse transcription PCR (RT-PCR): trends and problems. *J Mol Endocrinol.* 2002;29:23–39.
60. McKillip JL, Drake M. Real-time nucleic acid-based detection methods for pathogenic bacteria in food. *J Food Prot.* 2004;67:823–832.
61. Keer JT. Quantitative real-time PCR analysis. In: Keer JT, Birch L, eds. *Essencials of Nucleic Acid Analysis. A Robust Approach.* Cambridge: The Royal Society of Chemistry; 2008:132–155.
62. Cardullo RA, Agrawal S, Flores C, et al. Detection of nucleic acid hybridization by nonradiative fluorescence resonance energy transfer. *Proc Natl Acad Sci U S A.* 1988;85:8790–8794.
63. Wang X, Seed B. High-throughput primer and probe design. In: Dorak MT, ed. *Real-time PCR.* London, UK: Taylor & Francis Group; 2007:93–106.
64. Bustin SA, Benes V, Garson JA, et al. The MIQE guidelines: minimum information for publication of quantitative real-time PCR experiments. *Clin Chem.* 2009;55:611–622.
65. Pfaffl MW. Relative quantification. In: Dorak MT, ed. *Real-Time PCR.* London, UK: Taylor & Francis Group; 2007:63–82.
66. Allen CA, Payne SL, Harville M, et al. Validation of quantitative polymerase chain reaction assays for measuring cytokine expression in equine macrophages. *J Immunol Methods.* 2007;328:59–69.
67. Adams PS. Data analysis and reporting. In: Dorak MT, ed. *Real-Time PCR.* London, UK: Taylor & Francis Group; 2007:39–62.
68. Longo MC, Berninger MS, Hartley JL. Use of uracil DNA glycosylase to control carry-over contamination in polymerase chain reactions. *Gene.* 1990;93:125–128.
69. Stahlberg A, Aman P, Ridell B, et al. Quantitative real-time PCR method for detection of B-lymphocyte monoclonality by comparison of kappa and lambda immunoglobulin light chain expression. *Clin Chem.* 2003;49:51–59.
70. Nolan T, Hands RE, Ogunkolade W, et al. SPUD: a quantitative PCR assay for the detection of inhibitors in nucleic acid preparations. *Anal Biochem.* 2006;351:308–310.
71. Kubista M, Svec D, Bjorkman J, et al. Quality control in qPCR. In: Nour AMA, Pfaffl MW, eds. *The qPCR and dPCR MIQE Guidelines. A success story!* 2016:191–209. Online.
72. Nolan T, Hands RE, Bustin SA. Quantification of mRNA using real-time RT-PCR. *Nat Protoc.* 2006;1:1559–1582.
73. Krishnan GB, Pennington RE. Reverse transcription. In: Nour AMA, Pfaffl MW, eds. *The qPCR and dPCR MIQE Guidelines. A success story!* 2016:100–114. Online.
74. Lu JJ, Chen CH, Bartlett MS, et al. Comparison of six different PCR methods for detection of *Pneumocystis carinii*. *J Clin Microbiol.* 1995;33:2785–2788.
75. Sun. Nucleic extraction and amplification. In: Grody WW, Nakamura RM, Strom CM, Kiechle FL, eds. *Molecular Diagnostics: Techniques and Applications for the Clinical Laboratory.* San Diego, CA: Elsevier; 2010:35–48.
76. Cai HY, Caswell JL, Prescott JF. Nonculture molecular techniques for diagnosis of bacterial disease in animals: a diagnostic laboratory perspective. *Vet Pathol.* 2014;51:341–350.
77. Selder R, Weber K, Bergmann M, et al. Sensitivity and specificity of an in-clinic point-of-care PCR test for the diagnosis of canine leishmaniasis. *Vet J.* 2018;232:46–51.

78. Hawley J, Yaaran T, Maurice S, et al. Amplification of *Mycoplasma haemofelis* DNA by a PCR for point-of-care use. *J Vet Diagn Invest.* 2018;30:140–143.
79. Waner T, Nachum-Biala Y, Harrus S. Evaluation of a commercial in-clinic point-of-care polymerase chain reaction test for *Ehrlichia canis* DNA in artificially infected dogs. *Vet J.* 2014;202:618–621.
80. Cooke KL, Frenzer P, Tucker SJ, et al. Rapid diagnosis of *Babesia gibsoni* by point-of-need testing by insulated isothermal PCR in dogs at high risk of infection. *J Vet Intern Med.* 2018;32:232–235.
81. Sykes PJ, Neoh SH, Brisco MJ, et al. Quantitation of targets for PCR by use of limiting dilution. *Biotechniques.* 1992;13:444–449.
82. Huggett JF, Foy CA, Benes V, et al. The digital MIQE guidelines: minimum information for publication of quantitative digital PCR experiments. *Clin Chem.* 2013;59:892–902.
83. Bizouarn F. Introduction to digital PCR. In: Biassoni R, Raso A, eds. *Quantitative Real-Time PCR.* New York, NY: Springer; 2014:27–42.
84. Aguero-Rosenfeld ME, Wang G, Schwartz I, et al. Diagnosis of Lyme borreliosis. *Clin Microbiol Rev.* 2005;18:484–509.
85. Bockenstedt LK, Mao J, Hodzic E, et al. Detection of attenuated, noninfectious spirochetes in *Borrelia burgdorferi*-infected mice after antibiotic treatment. *J Infect Dis.* 2002;186:1430–1437.
86. Braddock JA, Tasker S, Malik R. The use of real-time PCR in the diagnosis and monitoring of *Mycoplasma haemofelis* copy number in a naturally infected cat. *J Feline Med Surg.* 2004;6:161–165.
87. Sykes JE, Studdert VP, Browning GF. Comparison of the polymerase chain reaction and culture for the detection of feline *Chlamydia psittaci* in untreated and doxycycline-treated experimentally infected cats. *J Vet Intern Med.* 1999;13:146–152.
88. Pusterla N, Byrne BA, Hodzic E, et al. Use of quantitative real-time PCR for the detection of *Salmonella* spp. in fecal samples from horses at a veterinary teaching hospital. *Vet J.* 2010;186:252–255.

7

Clinical Epidemiology in Infectious Diseases and Interpretation of Diagnostic Tests

Janet E. Foley, Rance K. Sellon, W. Zach Mills, James F. Evermann, Jane E. Sykes, Shelley C. Rankin

KEY POINTS

Epidemiology

- Epidemiology is the study of the distribution and determinants of health-related states or events in populations and the application of these principles to control health outcomes.
- The epidemiologic triangle highlights how disease outcomes depend upon: (1) pathogen factors, (2) host factors, and (3) environment.
- *Endemic* or *enzootic disease* refers to a disease that is established in a population and occurs regularly in that population at a background level, whereas an *epidemic* or *outbreak* occurs whenever cases are widespread in the community and exceed this baseline level.
- Molecular typing methods that can be used to study the epidemiology of an infectious disease include multilocus sequence typing, pulsed-field gel electrophoresis, and whole genome sequencing.
- Spatial epidemiology involves use of modeling to determine factors that influence the geographic distribution of an infectious disease.
- Multiple logistic regression analysis is often used to identify factors that increase the risk of an infectious disease while controlling for confounding.

Diagnostic Test Interpretation

- Diagnostic tests can be divided into *organism detection tests* and *antibody detection tests.*
- Before requesting a diagnostic test, veterinarians need to have an understanding of the clinical sensitivity and specificity of that test, what the target of the test is (e.g., antigen, DNA, or antibody), and whether the test is appropriate for the purpose it is being applied for. An understanding of the pathogenesis of the infectious disease, including shedding patterns and sites, and whether a carrier state or latency occurs, is critical for interpretation of test results.

CLINICAL EPIDEMIOLOGY

Epidemiologic Concepts in Infectious Disease

Epidemiology is the study of the distribution and determinants of health-related states or events in specified populations and the application of these principles to control health outcomes.[1] Clinical epidemiology can be used in medical practice to evaluate diagnostic tests, determine causality, analyze risk factors associated with the likelihood of acquiring a disease, and compile prognostic factors that will determine the course of a particular disease.

The concept of the *epidemiologic triangle* is useful in clinical epidemiology of infectious disease. The epidemiologic triangle is a model that highlights how disease outcomes are interdependent of: (1) pathogen factors, (2) host factors, and (3) environment.[2–4] Pathogen factors include the ability to survive in the environment, the propensity of the microorganism to spread, virulence factors and the manner in which they are expressed, resistance to antimicrobial drugs, and the ability to evade host immune defenses. Numerous host factors have the potential to influence infection and disease, including sex, breed, age, and immune status.[5] Environmental factors include physical (e.g., local terrain or climate), biological (e.g., insect vectors), and social (e.g., households vs. catteries). The epidemiology of FIP is a good example of the concept of the epidemiologic triangle. The prevalence of the fatal disease, FIP, in catteries can be as high as 5%, whereas the prevalence in one-cat or two-cat households is 0.02% (see Chapter 31). This increased prevalence in catteries reflects higher levels of low-virulence strains of FCoV in the environment, increased viral replication from acquired immune suppression caused by concurrent infections, pregnancy, stress of crowding, and host cat genetic factors.[6,7] These factors are thought to accelerate the accumulation of virus mutations that allow the virus to infect macrophages and cause FIP.

The progression of an infectious disease is a continuum that begins in a particular environment and a unique, susceptible (or naïve) host. Once there is exposure to an infectious agent, the timing of clinical signs (if any), and shedding of pathogens, vary depending on the individual host and the type of pathogen involved. There may then be an incubation period before the onset of clinical signs, during which time an animal may shed infectious organisms. Death or complete recovery may follow, or the host may become a carrier in the absence of clinical signs. Carrier hosts may either shed organisms (e.g., FCV infections), or harbor persistent infections in the absence of shedding. Hosts that are carriers of vector-borne pathogens do not shed organisms but may act as reservoir hosts that transmit pathogens to vectors when they feed. For example, *Ehrlichia canis* establishes a chronic, subclinical infection in dogs that can last years, providing a reservoir for infection of uninfected ticks.[8–10] Other pathogens can establish regressive or latent infections (e.g., FeLV [as provirus] or FHV-1 [in the trigeminal ganglia]), and later reactivation and shedding of these pathogens can occur with immune suppression. Typically, infected animals that show clinical signs are thought to be the most highly infectious to other at-risk animals and humans because they shed larger quantities of organisms and/or have signs (such as sneezing) that facilitate transmission.

Analysis of contact patterns within and among populations can reveal targets for interventions that prevent spread of infectious diseases. In order to persist, some pathogens require frequent interhost transmission and constant exposure to susceptible hosts, others chronically persist in their hosts, and others succeed as a result of prolonged survival in the environment (e.g., CPV-2). It is also important to consider the potential for interspecies spread of infectious microorganisms, as for rabies, CPV-2, and influenza viruses.[8,11–14]

The potential for an infectious disease to occur in an "outbreak" or epidemic/epizootic is a concern for infectious disease epidemiologists. *Endemic* or *enzootic disease* refers to a disease that is established in a population and occurs regularly in that population at a background level. *Hyperendemic* refers to persistent, high levels of disease. An *epidemic* occurs whenever cases are widespread in the community and exceed this background level, and a *pandemic* is an epidemic that occurs over several countries or continents. An *outbreak* carries the same meaning as an epidemic but is generally used to refer to the occurrence of a greater-than-normal level of disease within a specific geographic region. Epidemics or outbreaks occur when there is an increase in the quantity or virulence of a pathogen, when a pathogen is introduced into new regions with naïve hosts, when the mode of transmission of a pathogen is enhanced, when there is a change in host susceptibility, and/or when factors increase host exposure or permit a change in the mode of transmission.[15] Outbreaks can be *common-source* (when hosts are all exposed to an infectious agent from the same source), *propagated* (when there is transmission from one host to another), *mixed* (comprising both common-source and propagated features), or *other* (where disease occurs neither as a result of common-source exposure or propagation; introduction of a vector-borne infectious disease is one example).[15]

To some extent, epidemics can be predicted using mathematical tools such as compartment models, which are sets of inter-related differential equations that model instantaneous changes in numbers of individuals who are either: (1) susceptible (S) to infection (not previously infected, or recovered but not immune); (2) currently infected (I); or (3) recovered and immune (R). This Susceptible-Infected-Recovered (SIR) model is the simplest version of a compartment model, but more elaborate models can allow for many additional factors such as no immunity, an exposed but not yet infectious state (E), arthropod vectors, and other complexities.

A crucially important value that derives from an SIR model is R_0 (R naught; also known as basic reproductive rate or basic reproduction number).[16] R_0 is meant to be a measure of the contagiousness of a disease that takes into account host behavior and pathogen characteristics; it is the number of cases that are expected to occur after the introduction of a single infectious individual into a fully susceptible population. A value of R_0 that exceeds 1 predicts continuation of an epidemic. When $R_0 < 1$, the epidemic is expected to die out. The magnitude of R_0 can correlate with the potential size of an epidemic and can be used to determine the proportion of the population that may need to be vaccinated to prevent ongoing transmission. However, it is not a measure of the severity of an infectious disease or the speed of a pathogen's spread through a population of hosts. The calculation of R_0 generally requires mathematical models that are developed using assumptions about the mechanisms of disease transmission in a population. It has been noted that R_0 is readily susceptible to misapplication and misinterpretation because many researchers that use R_0 lack sufficient training in the mathematical techniques required to accurately calculate R_0. For example, a simple R_0 may not be applicable to diseases where there is no recovered and immune state, or once the population comprises a mix of naïve and recovered individuals. Nevertheless, it remains a useful benchmark by which to compare magnitudes of predicted epidemics of different diseases or disease in different types of populations (Box 7.1, Figs. 7.1–7.3).

BOX 7.1 Terms Used in Clinical Epidemiology

Confounding: A spurious association between a risk factor and dependent outcome, caused by a variable that influences both the independent and dependent variable.

Etiologic (or Attributable) Fraction or Risk: The difference between the incidence of disease in a group of individuals exposed to a risk factor and in a group that are not exposed.

Etiologic Predictive Value: A value that informs how well a single test for a single pathogen predicts the true underlying cause of clinical signs in the circumstances where there is no single best test and when some individuals may be infected with an agent but not show signs (a carrier).

Fit-for-Purpose: An assay is "fit for purpose" if test methods and related procedures are appropriate for specific diagnostic applications in order for the test results to be of relevance.[17]

Sensitivity: The number of truly infected, test-positive individuals divided by the total number of infected individuals. This indicates how well the test detects all truly infected individuals (Fig. 7.1).

Specificity: The number of test-negative individuals who are truly uninfected, divided by the total number of uninfected individuals. This allows assessment of the likelihood of a false-positive test result.[18]

Positive Predictive Value: The positive predictive value (PPV) is the probability that an animal that has tested positive is infected with the pathogen of concern.[17]

Negative Predictive Value: The negative predictive value (NPV) is the probability that an animal that has tested negative is not infected with the pathogen of concern. The positive and negative predictive values depend on the prevalence of the disease in the regional animal population (Fig. 7.1).[17]

Risk Factor: Any characteristic or exposure that may modify the likelihood of developing a disease or being test positive. Risk factors may be positive (increasing probability of disease) or negative (protective).

Odds Ratio (OR): The relative odds of an outcome occurring (e.g., a positive test result) when there is a particular exposure or risk factor, compared with the odds of the outcome occurring in the absence of that exposure. An OR significantly greater than 1 implies that a risk factor increases likelihood of the outcome; an OR < 1 means the risk factor is protective; and an OR = 1 means that the risk factor has no effect on the outcome (Fig. 7.2).

Relative Risk: The ratio of the rate of infection or disease in animals exposed to a risk factor compared with those animals not exposed to the risk factor. As with OR, individuals with risk factors that impose a relative risk greater than 1 have increased risk of disease (Fig. 7.2).

Receiver Operating Characteristic (ROC) Curve: Plots of true-positive rates (sensitivity, y-axis) against false-positive rates (1-specificity, x-axis) for a test at different cutoff values used to define a positive test result. ROC analysis is often used to help determine the cutoff point that optimizes sensitivity and specificity. As cutoff values decrease, sensitivity increases while specificity decreases, and vice versa. The overall performance of a diagnostic test can be measured by determining the area under the ROC curve (AUC). The closer the AUC is to 1, the better the overall diagnostic performance of the test. The closer the AUC is to 0.5 (straight line, or "chance diagonal"), the closer the diagnostic test performance is to pure chance for distinguishing positive from negative results (Fig. 7.3).

Infection (disease)

Assay	Present	Absent	
Positive	a True positive (TP)	b False positive (FP)	a + b
Negative	c False negative (FN)	d True negative (TN)	c + d
	a + c	b + d	

$$\text{Sensitivity} = \frac{a}{a+c} = TP \qquad \text{Prevalence} = \frac{a+c}{a+b+c+d}$$

$$\text{Specificity} = \frac{d}{b+d} = TN \qquad \text{Accuracy} = \frac{a+d}{a+b+c+d}$$

$$\text{Positive predictive value} = \frac{a}{a+b} \qquad \text{Negative predictive value} = \frac{d}{c+d}$$

Fig. 7.1 Calculation of sensitivity, specificity, prevalence, accuracy, and positive and negative predictive value using a 2 × 2 table.

	Disease (case)	No Disease (control)	
Risk factor present	A	B	A + B
Risk factor absent	C	D	C + D
	A + C	B + D	

$$\text{Relative risk (RR)} = \frac{A}{A+B} \div \frac{C}{C+D}$$

$$\text{Odds ratio (OR)} = \frac{AD}{BC}$$

Attributable risk (AR) % = P(RR − 1) ÷ [1+ P(RR − 1)] × 100
(P = prevalence of exposure)

Fig. 7.2 Calculation of relative risk, odds ratio, and attributable risk using a 2 × 2 table.

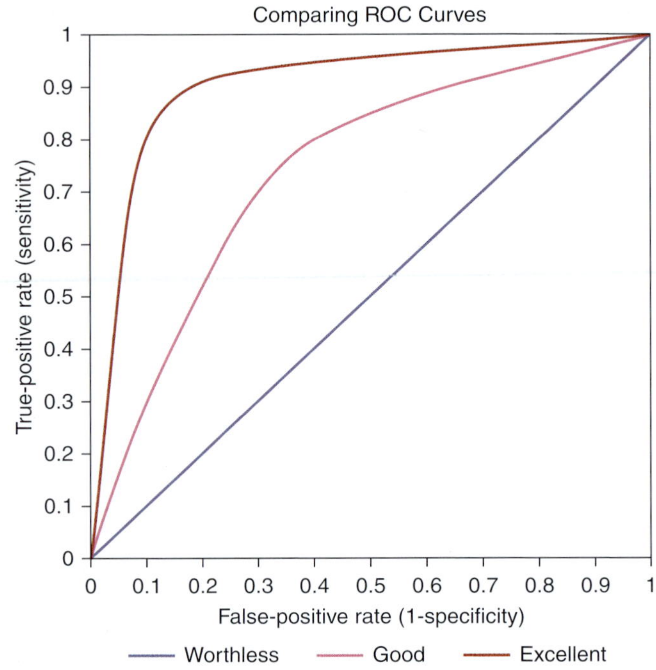

Fig. 7.3 Receiver operating characteristic (ROC) curves. Each curve represents excellent, good, and worthless assays that have been plotted on the same graph. Test accuracy depends on the degree to which the test separates those with and without the infectious disease of interest. Accuracy is represented by the area under the ROC curve (AUC). The test is perfect if the AUC is 1; an AUC of 0.5 represents a worthless test. An AUC above 0.8 is considered to be a good assay. (From Interpreting Diagnostic Tests. Thomas G. Tape, MD. University of Nebraska Medical Center; http://gim.unmc.edu/dxtests/roc3.htm)

Molecular Epidemiology

Molecular epidemiology focuses on how nucleic acid–based data can inform understanding of disease etiology, transmission, and distribution. Nucleic acid–based approaches can be used to understand pathogen transmission pathways, the evolution and spread of virulence genes, and host-microbe interactions and disease pathogenesis. Molecular epidemiology can reveal changes in evolving and emerging pathogens, their spread in space and emergence in new hosts, and their relationship with the environment.

Some molecular techniques used to study epidemiology target a small portion of a pathogen's genetic material, such as a single gene or intergenic region. Such assays can be used to document the presence of a pathogen in a host population, or to describe genetic relationships among multiple related strains and species of pathogens. Targets for single-gene studies must be chosen with care because DNA sequences that are relatively conserved among different strains are not as informative for epidemiologic studies as sequences that are moderately variable. In contrast, highly variable genes may not allow strains to be grouped at the level of resolution intended. The epidemiologic analysis of some microbes can be complicated by the diversity of evolutionary mechanisms by which microbes mutate (e.g., horizontal gene transmission by plasmids, transposons, viral vectors, homologous recombination, and other processes) that create downstream impacts on genetic lineages. *Multilocus sequence typing* (MLST) is a commonly used epidemiologic strain typing method that is referred to throughout this book. In classical MLST, a series of DNA segments (typically 7) from different parts of the genome (loci) are amplified using PCR and sequenced. The sequences of the collection of loci from different strains are compared. For example, MLST has been used to describe strains of *Leptospira interrogans* that might derive from different reservoir host species,[19] and an MLST protocol is a standard typing method for comparing *Cryptococcus* isolates.[20] Another frequently used strain typing method for comparing bacteria isolated from different sources is pulsed-field gel electrophoresis (PFGE). With PFGE, the entire genome of an organism is digested with one or more restriction enzymes which recognize specific short sequences of DNA and cut the DNA into fragments at these sequences (e.g., SmaI, which cuts in the center of the sequence "CCCGGG"). A pulsing electrical field is then used to move the DNA fragments through an agarose gel such that they are sorted by size. The sorted pattern of fragments is characteristic of each bacterial genotype and these "fingerprints" can be compared. Strains that have identical fingerprints are generally regarded to have originated from a common source. *Whole genome sequencing (WGS)* is now practical for the molecular epidemiology of most viruses and bacteria and in some cases has replaced techniques such as PFGE and classical MLST. A hybrid approach that is increasingly being applied is core genome MLST (cgMLST), whereby the sequences of hundreds of core genes are compared among isolates following WGS. For example, a cgMLST approach that uses 545 core genome sequences has been used to type leptospiral strains.[21] This method has high discrimination power and allows identification of species, sequence types, and most probable serogroups, allowing tracking of *Leptospira* strains in different hosts and over time.[22]

Molecular typing methods have been used to recognize genetic changes in pathogens that might correlate with increased or reduced virulence (as might occur when a virus adapts to a host), the emergence of viruses that have jumped a host-species barrier, and to detect antimicrobial-resistant bacterial strains.[7,12–14,23,24] An important cause for disease emergence is when a microbe gains the ability to cross a host-species barrier, as occurred with the emergence of CIV H3N8 (Fig. 7.4). Diagnosis requires suspicion that this has occurred so that a test can be applied in the new species. As pathogens spread, molecular tools help detect changing patterns of genetic relatedness and movement, a science called *phylogenetics*. Phylogenetic approaches have been used, for example, to monitor the northward spread of a particularly aggressive but cryptic lineage of the brown dog tick, *Rhipicephalus sanguineus*, in the United States.[25]

Spatial Epidemiology

Spatial epidemiology is the study of the geographic distributions of pathogens, vectors, diseases, and risk factors for these distributions. It incorporates *spatially implicit models*, whereby precise locations of geographic regions are not accounted for but implied by a model, and *spatially explicit work*, such as risk mapping of disease, whereby precise locations are known.[26] Spatially implicit models are often based on metapopulations, which are dynamic groups of small "patches" (areas in space), each with a small subpopulation, and each connected to other patches.[27] For infectious disease modeling, the subpopulation that resides in a patch would typically be a group of host individuals. Use of metapopulations in small animal medicine is uncommon, but interested readers are referred to the suggested readings list for further information.[28]

Spatial epidemiology uses maps and studies features of disease and underlying factors, such as clustering of disease in space and time, association of disease with spatially patterned risk factors (such as soil type, weather conditions, location of water sources), and changes in disease distributions. Mapping approaches commonly use geographic information system (GIS), a computer-based system that employs widely used software applications such as GRASS or ArcMap. These applications manage spatial data, produce maps, and allow for spatial modeling and analysis. Data are mapped and often color-coded to highlight degrees of risk. Once data are mapped, clusters of risk factors or disease can be assessed visually and analyzed using statistical approaches. Merging spatial information about a disease with data on risk can allow for hypothesis testing, such as whether disease

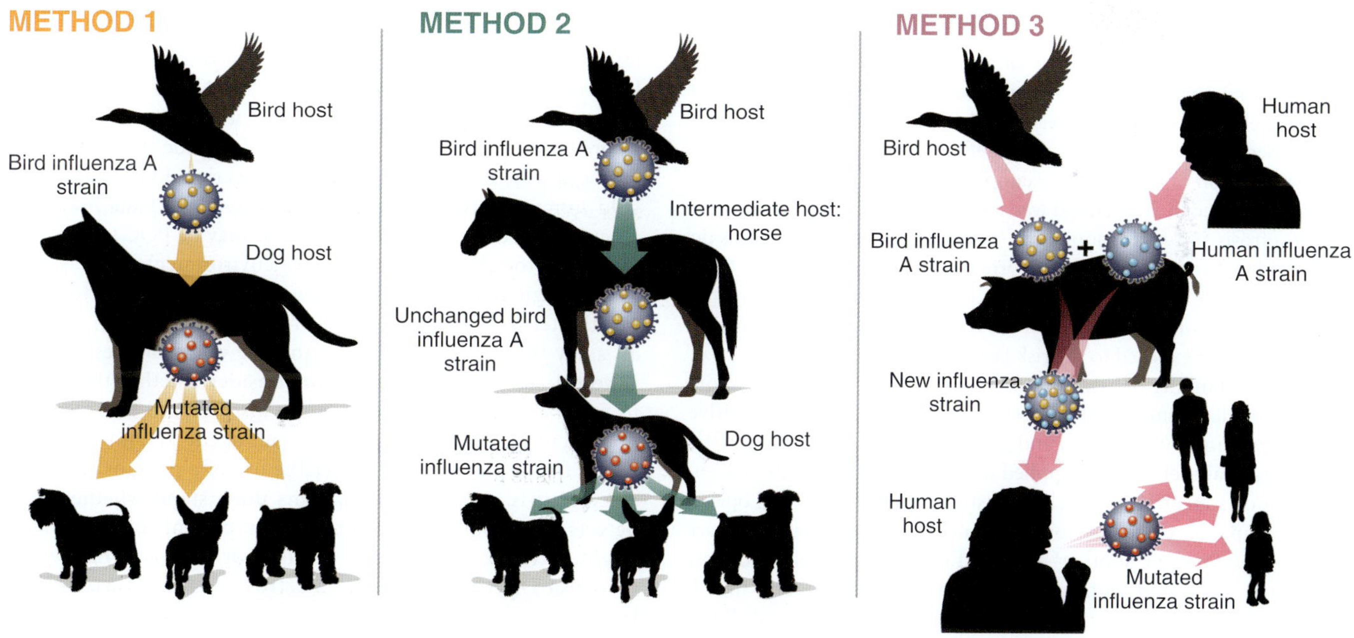

Fig. 7.4 Spread of viruses from one host species to another, with subsequent spread of infection to susceptible hosts. Influenza viruses are particularly good at crossing host-species barriers following recombination events and genetic drift. Method 1: Without further genetic change, a bird influenza A virus strain can move directly from an aquatic bird to another species, with subsequent evolution of the virus and spread within the new host species population. Method 2: The virus moves directly from an aquatic bird to an intermediate host, and then to a new host species, again with subsequent evolution and spread within the new host species population. Canine influenza virus H3N8 emerged as a result of mutation of equine influenza virus H3N8 (genetic drift), with subsequent spread to the general dog population and sustained spread within animal shelters. Equine influenza virus H3N8 was thought to have originated from birds. Recently, the overall prevalence of infection in the dog population has since declined, with some suggesting that extinction may have occurred at the time of writing. Method 3: Two different influenza virus strains from host species infect the same cells in an intermediate host, which results in generation of a recombinant virus that then spreads from the intermediate host to new hosts. There may be further mutations that allow the virus to then spread within the new host population.

is significantly associated with proximity of water sources or other predictors. GIS has also been used to examine theory of disease spread; this has been done for plague and rabies.[29,30]

Integrating Clinical Epidemiology into Practice

Primary data on infections, diseases, results of diagnostic testing, and risk factors are collected by veterinarians and diagnostic laboratories. These data are routinely used in practice to diagnose disease and inform medical management and preventative strategies for pets. They have also been used to provide information on human disease, such as when dogs act as sentinels for human disease. Clear recommendations for the expectations and limitations of diagnostic assays for diagnoses or screening are increasingly available via online technical bulletins and assay kit package inserts, and veterinarians interpreting these bulletins must have an understanding of concepts such as analytical sensitivity and specificity (how a test performs in the laboratory) and how they might relate to clinical sensitivity and specificity (how a test performs when applied to a population of animals with and without infection).[31]

Increased sensitivity and specificity of newer molecular and serologic diagnostic assays has resulted in more rapid turnaround and reduced costs. Commercial diagnostic laboratories, corporate veterinary practices, and medical scientific literature make valuable contributions to our knowledge of infectious disease epidemiology because the results of testing large numbers of specimens with the same assay are now available for analysis. These data provide evidence to inform decisions regarding vaccination frequency, which vaccines to use, what populations of animals are at elevated risk, and how likely animals are to serve as carriers and reservoirs of infection. Such data are needed for biosecurity and are particularly helpful if reported back to the clinicians and clients.

Risk Analysis

Through risk analysis, the relative importance of different risk factors associated with an animal's susceptibility to infection and disease can be assessed. Relative risk can be determined by studying groups of animals with defined risk factors (cohorts) over defined time periods for development of infection or disease. For example, introduction of a tetravalent leptospira vaccine in Switzerland was associated with a marked decrease in leptospirosis and AKI among dogs.[32] Relative risk and odds ratios do not provide information about the proportion of cases resulting from exposure to a risk factor. These values are determined by calculating the attributable risk, which accounts for the relative risk and the proportion of the population exposed to the risk factor (see Fig. 7.2).

An understanding of associations between disease and risk factors can inform decisions about targeted diagnostic testing, preventive management and intervention, and prognostication. Although a variety of statistical methods are applied depending on the study design, one common statistical approach is logistic regression analysis. Logistic regression analysis evaluates how a dependent binary variable (*binary* meaning one thing or another—diseased or not, test positive or test negative) is associated with independent variables (e.g., sex, breed, species, outdoor access) or risk factors. This highly flexible tool allows multiple risk factors to be assessed simultaneously, takes into account interactions among risk factors, controls for confounding effects, and can identify the strength of an association with each risk factor. In contrast, *univariate* analysis only allows the effect of one risk factor to be assessed at a time and does not take into account interactions or control for confounding. The ability of logistic regression analysis to control for confounding is particularly important. For example, univariate analysis might reveal that an increased frequency of leptospira vaccination increases the risk of adverse events such as anaphylaxis. However, young animals are vaccinated more frequently than older animals, and the increased rate of reactions might be due to age rather than frequency of vaccination. Logistic regression analysis controls for these effects and typically identifies a smaller number of significant risk factors when compared with univariate analysis of all of the individual risk factors included in the regression analysis.

DIAGNOSTIC TESTING FOR INFECTIOUS DISEASES

Diagnostic Versus Screening Assays

Veterinarians use diagnostic tests to diagnose acute or chronic infectious disease. The same assay may be used to assess the prevalence of disease, infection, or exposure in populations. A single assay may be validated for one or more intended purposes by optimizing its performance characteristics for each purpose. An assay that is used as a *screening assay* (to rule out an infectious disease agent) should have a high diagnostic sensitivity and a high negative predictive value. Screening an animal to show that it is free of a disease should be done with the assumption that the animal is truly free of the disease because the disease prevalence in the population represented by the animal is zero, or extremely low (e.g., *Brucella canis*). Screening tests are generally associated with a lower diagnostic specificity and positive results should be confirmed by a test with high specificity for the pathogen of interest. Clinicians need to be aware of problems associated with using tests that have been designed and validated as diagnostic tests for screening purposes in animals that are unlikely to have the disease of interest.

Types of Diagnostic Tests

Diagnostic tests for infectious diseases can be broadly divided into: (1) organism detection tests, and (2) antibody detection tests. *Organism detection tests* include culture/isolation, which detects viable pathogens; tests that detect antigen(s) of a pathogen (e.g., direct IFA, IHC, antigen detection ELISA); and tests that detect pathogen DNA or RNA such as PCR and isothermal amplification (collectively known as nucleic acid amplification tests [NAAT]), and fluorescent *in situ* hybridization (FISH). *Antibody detection tests* provide evidence of previous exposure to a pathogen and include indirect IFA assays, HI, serum neutralization, antibody detection ELISA, and colloidal gold immunochromatographic assays (GICA). Tests may be available through diagnostic laboratories or may be POC tests, which can be used in the clinic or low-resource environments such as shelters.

Serologic tests are often assumed to be antibody detection tests, but the term "serologic assay" (or immunoassay) can also refer to an assay that detects antigen if the use of antibodies is employed in test design. Clinicians need to consider whether they are trying to make a diagnosis of an *infectious disease* (and that also includes documenting *exposure* to an infectious agent) or show that the animal is free of disease. Whenever the use of a diagnostic test is considered, it is critical that clinicians understand whether the assay detects viable pathogens (culture), components of a pathogen that might be viable or nonviable (antigen or DNA), or not replicating (proviral DNA in the case of a retrovirus infection), or antibodies (exposure). The purpose of a particular test is important when syndromic panels, which are designed to detect multiple infectious agents and/or antibodies to those agents, are requested. For example, diarrhea panels are available that include culture for enteric pathogens, antigen ELISA assays for clostridial organisms, and PCR for bacteria, viruses and parasites that commonly cause diarrhea in particular animal hosts. There are also immunoassays such as the IDEXX SNAP 4Dx Plus test (IDEXX Laboratories Inc., USA) and the Antech AccuPlex 4 assay (Antech Diagnostics, USA) that detect vector-borne pathogens (Table 7.1). Use of such panels can occasionally produce unexpected positive results that may be difficult to interpret.[33] A positive PCR test result is not always a marker for active shedding or for disease status because pathogen nucleic acids

TABLE 7.1 Examples of Commercially Available Diagnostic Panels that May Be Selected for Diagnosis of Companion Animal Infectious Diseases

PCR Panel	Targets
Canine respiratory panel	Canine adenovirus-2 RNA Canine distemper virus RNA Canine parainfluenza virus RNA Canine influenza virus H3N8 RNA Canine influenza virus H3N2 RNA Canine herpesvirus DNA Canine respiratory coronavirus RNA *Bordetella bronchiseptica* DNA *Streptococcus equi* subsp *zooepidemicus* DNA
Feline respiratory panel	Feline herpesvirus-1 DNA Feline calicivirus RNA *Chlamydia felis* DNA *Mycoplasma felis* DNA *Bordetella bronchiseptica* DNA
Canine diarrhea panel	Canine parvovirus-2 DNA Canine enteric coronavirus RNA *Giardia duodenalis* DNA *Clostridium perfringens* enterotoxin A gene DNA *Cryptosporidium* spp. DNA *Salmonella* spp. DNA Canine distemper virus RNA
Feline diarrhea panel	Feline panleukopenia virus DNA Feline coronavirus RNA *Giardia duodenalis* DNA *Tritrichomonas foetus* DNA *Clostridium perfringens* enterotoxin A gene DNA *Cryptosporidium* spp. DNA *Salmonella* spp. DNA *Toxoplasma gondii* DNA
Vector-borne disease panel	*Anaplasma phagocytophilum* DNA *Anaplasma platys* DNA *Bartonella* spp. DNA *Ehrlichia canis* DNA *Rickettsia* spp. DNA *Borrelia burgdorferi* DNA *Babesia* spp. DNA *Mycoplasma haemocanis* DNA
Canine blood transfusion panel	*Anaplasma phagocytophilum* DNA *Anaplasma platys* DNA *Ehrlichia canis* DNA *Rickettsia* spp. DNA *Borrelia burgdorferi* DNA *Babesia* spp. DNA *Bartonella* spp. DNA *Leishmania* spp. DNA *Mycoplasma haemocanis* DNA "*Candidatus* Mycoplasma haematoparvum" DNA
Feline blood transfusion panel	Feline leukemia virus DNA Feline leukemia virus RNA Feline immunodeficiency virus DNA Feline coronavirus RNA *Bartonella* spp. DNA *Mycoplasma haemofelis* DNA "*Candidatus* Mycoplasma haemominutum" DNA "*Candidatus* Mycoplasma turicensis" DNA

It is particularly important to understand whether panels consist of organism detection tests, antibody detection tests, or both, and the significance of a positive result for each target in light of the pathogenesis of disease.

may be present in latent and subclinical infections; or when animals have recovered but retain nonviable pathogens or free nucleic acids, damaged cells, or debris. Positive PCR results can also occur when specimens become contaminated with environmental DNA.[33] Positive test results must be assessed in light of the patient's history, clinical signs, physical examination findings, the reason the test was performed, results of other diagnostic testing, and a knowledge of the extent to which these organisms can be detected in healthy animals as opposed to those that are diseased.[18]

Serology is the foundation for serodiagnosis, serosurveillance, and studies of vaccine-induced immunity. Serodiagnosis can assist in the diagnosis of current disease, such as the use of IgM assays to detect acute infection, or the use of antigen ELISA testing for detection of heartworm and FeLV infection. Serodiagnostic assays that detect IgG can imply previous infection, while a fourfold (two-step) rise in antibody titer over 1–4 weeks (e.g., 1:4 to 1:16, 1:16 to 1:64) suggests recent, active infection. For some diseases, determination of serum antibody titers can also aid in assessment of vaccine-induced protection (see Chapter 20). For example, dogs with specific CDV and CPV antibody titers are generally considered protected against CDV- and CPV-induced diseases. Antibody titers do not correlate with protection for other diseases, such as leptospirosis. In addition, factors such as degree of environmental exposure, and level of natural and pharmacologic-induced immune suppression need to be considered when antibody titers are used to determine the need for booster vaccinations.

The limits of test sensitivity and timing of positive test results over the course of infection are important considerations in diagnosis. Early after exposure, during the acute phase of an infection, the best options for diagnosis are tests which are sensitive, detect the pathogen directly (e.g., antigen ELISA, PCR, culture), and are performed on the appropriate target specimen. Serology tests that detect antibodies can be negative early in the course of illness if clinical signs appear after a short (< 10 days) incubation period. Subsequently, IgM antibodies circulate, the presence of which usually correlates with recent infection, followed by longer lasting IgG which indicates exposure to a given, or cross-reacting, pathogen. As the infection matures, direct tests for antigen or nucleic acids reveal animals with acute clinical infection as well as those with latent infection and those which are carriers. For chronic diseases or diseases that occur after a long incubation period (e.g., Lyme borreliosis, FIP), determination of acute and convalescent phase titers over a 1- to 4-week period is generally not appropriate because a significant

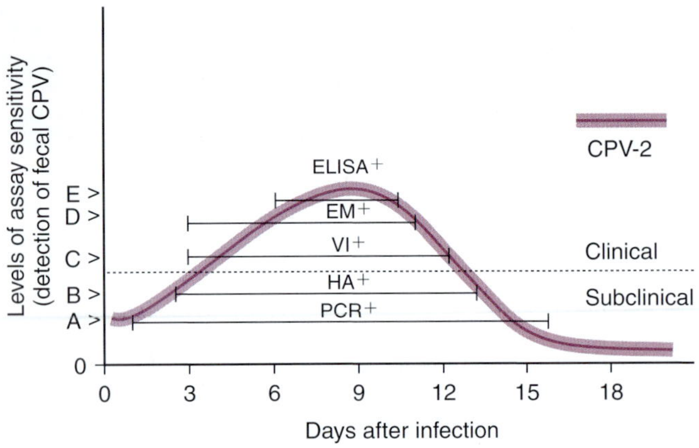

Fig. 7.5 Degrees of diagnostic assay sensitivity, with canine parvovirus (CPV) infection used as an example. There are five different types of assays *(A–E)*. Some assays are more appropriate for clinical diagnosis whereas others are more likely to detect low-level (subclinical) shedding. *ELISA,* enzyme-linked immunosorbent assay; *EM,* electron microscopy; *HA,* hemagglutination; *PCR,* polymerase chain reaction; *VI,* virus isolation.

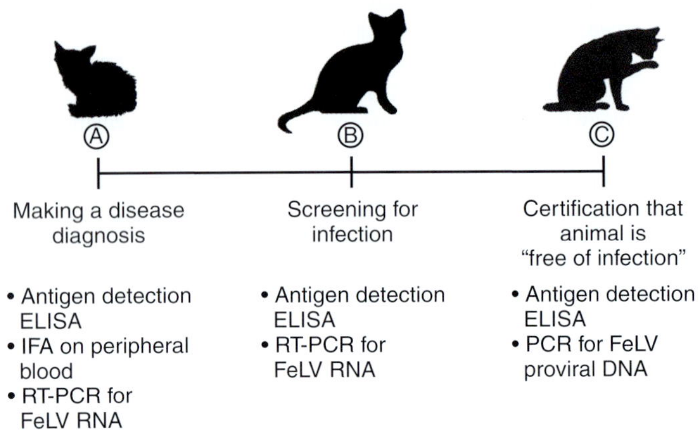

Fig. 7.6 Three reasons for using a diagnostic test. (A) Diagnosis of *disease* in a sick animal. In the case of FeLV infection, an antigen detection ELISA assay, IFA, or RT-PCR assay could be used to detect productive virus infection. However, detection of productive virus infection alone does not imply that the virus is responsible for clinical signs. (B) Screening for subclinical infection. For FeLV, this would involve use of a sensitive assay for productive virus infection, that is, an antigen detection ELISA assay or RT-PCR assay. (C) Certification that an animal is "free of infection" (e.g., for identification of blood donor cats). For FeLV, this might consist of an antigen detection ELISA assay *and* a provirus (DNA) PCR assay. *ELISA,* enzyme-linked immunosorbent assay; *FeLV,* feline leukemia virus; *IFA,* immunofluorescent antibody; *RT-PCR,* reverse transcriptase-polymerase chain reaction.

change in titer does not occur. When different test options are available, it is best to choose a test with appropriate sensitivity and specificity for the desired purpose, and to consider the prevalence of the disease in the patient population. As an example, dogs with clinical CPV-associated enteritis are likely to be CPV fecal antigen ELISA positive and PCR positive for CPV. Both tests are a good choice for the diagnosis of CPV enteritis; however, the latter can confirm active infection and also detect dogs that are subclinically infected or recently vaccinated with attenuated live vaccines (Fig. 7.5).[8] Some laboratories that perform real-time PCR results will report cycle threshold values, or an estimate of nucleic acid target copy number (see Chapter 6), with detection of nucleic acid in high copy number being more likely to relate to clinically significant infection than detection of nucleic acid in low copy number (e.g., some assays for CDV or FeLV infections). Depending on the pathogen, testing may lend itself to a diagnostic test hierarchy (Fig. 7.6). Multiple tests may need to be applied in parallel or in series to optimize diagnosis.

SUMMARY

The interface between disease diagnosis and clinical epidemiology has continued to be fortified by the ever-increasing knowledge of the importance of animal populations and their interactions with other animals and humans. With the development of molecular diagnostic assays, the finer details of how a pathogen sustains itself in a population by establishing short- and long-term carrier states have become more apparent. These assays have also shed light on how the potential for interspecies transmission impacts the nature of emerging infections. Although clinical epidemiology involves the understanding of health and disease in populations, it is fundamental in decision-making for the individual animal. An understanding of the epidemiologic features of a particular infectious disease facilitates the early identification of an outbreak, which in turn helps the clinician select the most appropriate diagnostic test and interpret the results of subsequent diagnostic testing. This early detection is essential for the development, implementation, and monitoring of prevention and control strategies.

SUGGESTED READINGS

Centers for Disease Control and Prevention. Principles of Epidemiology in Public Health Practice. 3rd ed. https://www.cdc.gov/csels/dsepd/ss1978/lesson1/section11.html.

Delamater PL, Street EJ, Leslie TF, et al. Complexity of the basic reproduction number (R_0). *Emerg Infect Dis.* 2019;25:1–4.

Foley J, Foley P, Pedersen N. The persistence of an SIS disease in a metapopulation. *J Appl Ecol.* 1999;36:555–563.

Obuchowski NA, Bullen JA. Receiver operating characteristic (ROC) curves: review of methods with applications in diagnostic medicine. *Physics Med Biol.* 2018;63. 07TR01.

REFERENCES

1. Last JM, Abramson JH, Freidman GD. *A Dictionary of Epidemiology.* New York: Oxford University Press; 2001.
2. Archie EA, Luikart G, Ezenwa VO. Infecting epidemiology with genetics: a new frontier in disease ecology. *Trends Ecol Evol.* 2009;24:21–30.
3. Case J, Chomel BB, Nicholson WL, et al. Serological survey of vector-borne zoonotic pathogens in pet cats from animal shelters and feral colonies. *J Feline Med Surg.* 2006;8:111–117.
4. Coyne KP, Dawson S, Radford AD, et al. Long-term analysis of feline calicivirus prevalence and viral shedding patterns in naturally infected colonies of domestic cats. *Vet Microbiol.* 2006;118:12–25.
5. Evermann JF, Kennedy M. Viral infections. In: Peterson M, Kutzler M, eds. *Small Animal Pediatrics.* Philadelphia: Elsevier; 2010:119–129.
6. Addie D, Belák S, Boucraut-Baralon C, et al. Feline infectious peritonitis. ABCD guidelines on prevention and management. *J Feline Med Surg.* 2009;11:594–604.
7. Brown MA, Troyer JL, Pecon-Slattery J, et al. Genetics and pathogenesis of feline infectious peritonitis virus. *Emerg Infect Dis.* 2009;15:1445–1452.
8. Evermann JF, Sellon R, Sykes J. Laboratory diagnosis of viral and rickettsial infections and epidemiology of infectious disease. In: Greene CE, ed. *Infectious Diseases of the Dog and Cat.* St. Louis: Elsevier; 2006:1–9.
9. Fritz CL. Emerging tick-borne diseases. *Vet Clin North America: Small Anim Prac.* 2009;39:265–278.

10. Mylonakis ME, Siarkou VI, Leontides L, et al. Evaluation of a serum-based PCR assay for the diagnosis of canine monocytic ehrlichiosis. *Vet Microbiol.* 2009;138:390–393.
11. Decaro N, Mari V, Campolo M, et al. Recombinant canine coronaviruses related to transmissible gastroenteritis virus of swine are circulating in dogs. *J Virol.* 2009;83:1532–1537.
12. Dubovi EJ, Njaa BL. Canine influenza. *Vet Clin North Am Small Anim Pract.* 2008;38:827–835.
13. Hoelzer K, Shackelton LA, Holmes EC, et al. Within-host genetic diversity of endemic and emerging parvoviruses of dogs and cats. *J Virol.* 2008;82: 11096–11105.
14. Kapil S, Allison RW, Johnston L, et al. Canine distemper virus strains circulating among North American dogs. *Clin Vaccine Immunol.* 2008;15:707–712.
15. Centers for Disease Control and Prevention. Principles of Epidemiology in Public Health Practice. 3rd ed. https://www.cdc.gov/csels/dsepd/ss1978/lesson1/section11.html.
16. Delamater PL, Street EJ, Leslie TF, et al. Complexity of the basic reproduction number (R_0). *Emerg Infect Dis.* 2019;25:1–4.
17. World Organisation for Animal Health. Principles and methods of validation of diagnostic assays for infectious diseases. In: *OIE Terrestrial Manual.* 2018:72–87.
18. Gordis L. *Epidemiology.* Philadelphia: Elsevier/Saunders; 2009:308.
19. Boonsilp S, Thaipadungpanit J, Amornchai P, et al. A single multilocus sequence typing (MLST) scheme for seven pathogenic *Leptospira* species. *PLoS Negl Trop Dis.* 2013;7. e1954.
20. Firacative C, Roe CC, Malik R, et al. MLST and whole-genome-based population analysis of *Cryptococcus gattii* VGIII links clinical, veterinary and environmental strains, and reveals divergent serotype specific subpopulations and distant ancestors. *PLoS Negl Trop Dis.* 2016;10. e0004861.
21. Guglielmini J, Bourhy P, Schiettekatte O, et al. Genus-wide *Leptospira* core genome multilocus sequence typing for strain taxonomy and global surveillance. *PLoS Negl Trop Dis.* 2019;13: e0007374.
22. |Grillova L, Picardeau M. Core genome multi-locus sequence typing analyses of *Leptospira* spp. using the bacterial isolate genome sequence database. *Methods Mol Biol.* 2020;2134:11–21.
23. Di Martino B, Di Rocco C, Ceci C, et al. Characterization of a strain of feline calicivirus isolated from a dog faecal sample. *Vet Microbiol.* 2009;139:52–57.
24. Morens DM, Folkers GK, Fauci AS. Emerging infections: a perpetual challenge. *Lancet Infect Dis.* 2008;8:710–719.
25. Villarreal Z, Stephenson N, Foley J. Possible northward introgression of a tropical lineage of *Rhipicephalus sanguineus* ticks at a site of emerging Rocky Mountain spotted fever. *J Parasitol.* 2018;104:240–245.
26. Ostfeld RS, Glass GE, Keesing F. Spatial epidemiology: an emerging (or re-emerging) discipline. *Trends Ecol Evol.* 2005;20:328–336.
27. Hess G, Randolph S, Arneberg P, et al. Spatial aspects of disease dynamics. In: Hudson P, et al. eds. *The Ecology of Wildlife Diseases.* Oxford: Oxford University Press; 2002:102–118.
28. Foley J, Foley P, Pedersen N. The persistence of an SIS disease in a metapopulation. *J Appl Ecol.* 1999;36:555–563.
29. Moore DA. Spatial diffusion of raccoon rabies in Pennsylvania, USA. *Prev Vet Med.* 1999;40:19–32.
30. Adjemian JZ, Foley P, Gage KL, et al. Initiation and spread of traveling waves of plague, *Yersinia pestis*, in the western United States. *Am J Trop Med Hygiene.* 2007;76:365–375.
31. Dunne G, Gurfield N. Local veterinary diagnostic laboratory, a model for the One Health initiative. *Vet Clin North Am Small Anim Pract.* 2009;39:373–384.
32. Francey T, Schweighauser A, Reber A, et al. Evaluation of changes in the epidemiology of leptospirosis in dogs after introduction of a quadrivalent antileptospiral vaccine in a highly endemic area. *J Vet Intern Med.* 2020;34:2405–2417.
33. Gunson R, Collins T, Carman W. Practical experience of high throughput real time PCR in the routine diagnostic virology setting. *J Clin Virol.* 2006;35:355–367.

SECTION 2

Anti-infective Drugs

Mark G. Papich

The majority of this book deals with diagnosis, pathology, and management of specific infectious diseases in dogs and cats. However, the book would not be complete without chapters on the agents used to treat and manage these infections. In this section, there are six chapters. The first chapter is a review of general principles of antimicrobial therapy. This chapter includes the importance of identifying the organism, pharmacokinetic properties of the agents, pharmacokinetic-pharmacodynamic (PK-PD) issues, and antimicrobial drug resistance. This introductory chapter sets the stage for the chapters that follow.

The remaining five chapters in Section 2 cover the major groups of drugs that are used to treat infections in dogs and cats: antiviral, antibacterial, antifungal, antiprotozoal, and antiparasitic agents. Included with the antiviral chapter is a section on immunomodulatory agents, which are often used to manage viral infections, but have also been used for other infectious diseases. Each of these chapters accompanies the specific sections on diseases that are contained in the majority of the book.

These chapters on specific antimicrobial agents include drugs that are approved by the US Food and Drug Administration (FDA), or regulatory authorities in other countries, for treating infections in dogs and cats. However, even with these approved agents available, there are still many unmet needs. The importance of these chapters lies in the realization that there are not always drugs approved by regulatory authorities to treat all of the infections encountered in dogs and cats. For example, there are no antiviral drugs approved in the United States for dogs and cats. Except for topical agents, there is only one antifungal agent approved. The available antibacterial agents do not cover many of the most important bacterial infections. Many antiprotozoal agents are used extralabel. Therefore, extralabel (off-label) human drugs or drugs approved for other animals are often used. Because the uses, dosing information, pharmacokinetics, and adverse effects are not available for these drugs on an approved drug label, these chapters are needed to provide veterinarians with a resource for the important characteristics of these agents. Each chapter includes state-of-the-art information available from published papers and experts who have studied these medications. The use of each drug listed is based on a consensus opinion of experts consistent with good clinical practice. Each chapter is referenced to original studies or the approved drug label to support the use. The recommendations, including dosages, listed in these chapters are based on the the best available evidence at the time this book was prepared. The authors cannot guarantee safety and efficacy of all the treatments discussed, and new information may emerge that was not known at the time the book was prepared.

8

Principles of Anti-infective Therapy

Jane E. Sykes, Mark G. Papich

KEY POINTS

- Use of antimicrobial drugs (AMDs) selects for resistant bacterial populations, both within the targeted bacterial population and also commensal bacterial populations.
- Bacterial mechanisms of drug resistance include production of enzymes that inactivate AMDs, drug exclusion through membrane alterations and efflux pumps, protection of target sites (e.g., ribosome), and modification of the site of action (or target) of the AMD.
- Strategies that minimize selection for drug resistance include: (1) confirmation of the presence of infection before AMD treatment is commenced, (2) proper identification of the infecting organism, (3) selection of agents with activity specific to the pathogen present, (4) administration of an adequate dose of AMD, and (5) administration of AMD for the proper duration of time (often as short as possible).
- Selection of an appropriate AMD should be based on the activity of the agent against the suspected pathogen; knowledge of drug pharmacokinetics, which includes bioavailability and tissue penetration; consideration of host factors such as concurrent illness, medications, or immunosuppression; and consideration of the agent's pharmacokinetic-pharmacodynamic (PK-PD) properties. The PK-PD properties include whether the drug exhibits concentration- or time-dependent antibacterial effects, which dictates the design of the dosage regimen.

INTRODUCTION

Antimicrobial drugs (AMDs; Box 8.1) have been considered one of the greatest inventions of the 20th century. The modern era of AMD treatment began with the discovery of sulfonamides in 1935.[1] In the 1940s, the therapeutic value of penicillin and streptomycin was discovered, and by 1950, the "golden age" of AMD therapy was underway. The increased use of AMDs in people, companion animals, and livestock has been accompanied by increased rates of antimicrobial resistance—in some instances, an alarming transition to multidrug resistance that has severely limited the available antimicrobial choices. Among 1,485 non-urinary *Escherichia coli* isolates from dogs in the United States from 2004 to 2011, there was a significant increase in the prevalence of resistance to cefazolin, cefoxitin, cephalothin, enrofloxacin, and tetracycline.[2] In the United Kingdom from 2003 to 2012, the prevalence of resistance among 14,555 clinical isolates of *Staphylococcus intermedius* group organisms (primarily *Staphylococcus pseudintermedius)* increased significantly.[3] Most of the veterinary isolates of *S. pseudintermedius* are MDR, which greatly limits the choices for treatment.[4] Clonal dissemination of methicillin-resistant *S. pseudintermedius*[5] and ESBL enzyme producing *E. coli* and *Klebsiella pneumoniae*[6,7] has been reported among companion animals worldwide. This has been compounded by a declining rate of development of new classes of AMDs for veterinary use, and increased scrutiny of the use of critically important human antimicrobial agents for administration to animals.

Antimicrobial resistance genes were present in microbes long before antimicrobial agents were used in therapy. Microbe populations generally consist of a mixture of genetically susceptible and resistant organisms. The use of AMDs exerts pressure that favors selection of the resistant microbes ("survival of the fittest") within both the targeted bacterial population and other commensal bacteria (which have the potential to become pathogenic when host defenses are impaired).

The risk of emergence of resistant bacterial strains depends on factors that include the size of the inoculum, ability of the bacteria to acquire mutations, the ability of host defenses to eliminate resistant bacteria, drug concentrations at the site of infection, and the duration of exposure to AMDs. Selection pressures are highest when bacteria are exposed to suboptimal dosage regimens (i.e., concentrations of drug below the level needed to kill or suppress the growth of the bacteria). In this scenario, the most susceptible strains are eliminated, but the more resistant strains flourish because of decreased competition. Resistant bacteria are not necessarily more virulent than susceptible bacteria, but they may require drugs not commonly used, or other measures not commonly used for treatment of the susceptible strains of bacteria.

According to the Infectious Disease Society of America, *antimicrobial stewardship* refers to coordinated interventions designed to improve and measure the appropriate use of antimicrobials by promoting the selection of the optimal AMD regimen, dose and duration of therapy, and route of administration.[7] Guidelines for prudent antimicrobial use have been published by several professional veterinary organizations and societies with the intention of reducing selection for resistant bacterial pathogens.[8–14] An AVMA taskforce on antimicrobial stewardship in companion animal practice has developed an antimicrobial stewardship program that includes client educational handouts and a series of antimicrobial use "dos and don'ts" for veterinary practitioners.[15]

BOX 8.1 Antimicrobial, Antibiotic, Antibacterial, Which Is Correct?

The terms "antibiotic," "antimicrobial," and "antibacterial" are often used interchangeably. They have different meanings that are often overlooked. An *antibiotic* is a natural chemical, produced by other organisms, that is designed to suppress the growth of other organisms (including bacteria, fungi, or protozoa). An *antimicrobial* is any compound, natural or synthetic, that suppresses microbial growth. An *antibacterial* is any compound that suppresses bacterial growth. The term "antimicrobial agent" is preferred by certain groups such as CLSI. Many times, even in this chapter, the terms are used interchangeably with the same meaning.

Specific guidelines regarding antimicrobial selection, dosing and duration of treatment for infections of the urinary tract, skin, and respiratory tract have been developed by consensus of the Antimicrobial Guidelines Working Group of the International Society for Companion Animal Infectious Diseases (www.iscaid.org). Veterinary hospitals are encouraged to adapt these guidelines or develop their own hospital-specific antimicrobial guidelines based on evaluation of the local prevalence (antibiograms) of AMD resistance and local prescribing practices. Strategies that may reduce the selection for antimicrobial resistance include documentation of the presence of infection; appropriate susceptibility testing; proper identification of the infecting organism; and the use of agents that are as specific for the pathogen as possible, at the proper dose and for the proper duration of time. There are older, outdated recommendations that recommended treatment for longer than necessary, which has led to a current trend to shorten the duration of antimicrobial therapy whenever possible for companion animals.

IDENTIFICATION OF THE INFECTING ORGANISM

The detection of fever or leukocytosis does not imply bacterial infection and the need for antibiotic treatment, especially given the relatively high prevalence of sterile inflammatory and immune-mediated diseases in dogs and viral infections in cats. Selection of the most appropriate AMD relies on knowledge of: (1) the presence of an infectious agent, (2) the type of infectious agent present, and (3) the likelihood of susceptibility of the agent to the AMD prescribed. In some cases, treatment with AMDs may not be necessary even though the cause of disease is bacterial. Some infections undergo spontaneous cures without the aid of an antibiotic. For example, a cat bite abscess can often be drained and resolved without the need to administer an antibiotic (see Chapter 75). Many transmissible respiratory infections, such as those belonging to the canine infectious respiratory disease complex, are self-limited and often spontaneously resolve without antibiotics.

In some situations, collection of a specimen for cytology or histopathology permits a diagnosis of infection to be established. Some difficult to grow or fastidious infectious agents, such as rickettsial and fungal pathogens, may be presumptively identified to the genus or species level based on their morphology. If skin cytology from a dog reveals cocci (a Gram stain is not necessary to confirm the presence of gram-positive cocci), then the presence of *S. pseudintermedius* is highly probable. If, on the other hand, cytology from an ear swab reveals rods, the possibility of *Pseudomonas aeruginosa* must be considered. In either case, this knowledge is valuable for selecting appropriate initial antibacterial therapy. The use of molecular diagnostic techniques, such as nucleic acid amplification tests (NAATs), can also allow rapid identification of an infecting organism, which can help to guide AMD selection. Many commercial laboratories now use MALDI-TOF MS for rapid identification and diagnosis of pathogens (see Chapter 3).

For example, identification of a vector-borne pathogen (e.g., *Rickettsia* spp., *Ehrlichia canis*) is helpful because doxycycline is usually the first drug of choice for the majority of these pathogens. Once the pathogen is identified, or presumptively identified, antibiotics can be administered that have a high probability of success based on typical susceptibility patterns for the wild-type strains. Unfortunately, there is now greater likelihood of encountering drug-resistant (non-wild-type) organisms. Therefore, in many instances, it has become important to collect specimens for culture and susceptibility testing before treatment with AMDs is commenced. Although there is an initial cost to the client for culture and susceptibility testing, long-term costs to the client may be reduced because prompt treatment with the most appropriate agent will decrease prescription of unnecessary or inappropriate AMDs, improved likelihood of rapid resolution of the underlying disorder with early diagnosis and appropriate treatment, and reduced need for more expensive, second- or third-line AMDs. Early attainment of therapeutic targets is important for rapid clinical resolution and decreased emergence of resistant bacteria.[16] Administration of AMDs without identification of the infectious agent can also decrease subsequent chances of successful culture and proper diagnosis if the problem does not resolve. Proper interpretation of culture and susceptibility panel results is also imperative. Practitioners should examine a culture report carefully and question whether a bacterial species isolated is truly the cause of infection as opposed to a contaminant or commensal. Among the agents listed as "susceptible" in a report, the clinician will have to decide on the best choice based on drug and patient characteristics. The reader is referred to Chapter 3 for more information on bacterial culture and susceptibility testing. The Clinical and Laboratory Standards Institute (CLSI) also provides an excellent resource for the interpretation of culture and susceptibility results for pathogens from animals.[17]

In animals with life-threatening infections, institution of AMD treatment is necessary before the results of culture and susceptibility become available. The choice of treatment at this stage can be based on cytology and knowledge of the type of infections that most commonly occur at the anatomic site involved (also known as *bacteriologic statistics*). Because of the life-threatening nature of these infections, the practice of "de-escalation" (as opposed to "escalation") is employed. This is the practice of initially selecting a highly active agent that has a high probability of successful elimination of the pathogen and initiating treatment quickly; then once the infectious agent has been identified, the drug spectrum should be changed or narrowed according to culture and susceptibility results. If the infection is life threatening, highly active agents such as an aminoglycoside or fluoroquinolone, or extended-spectrum β-lactam can be selected initially. Then, if culture and susceptibility show susceptibility to other β-lactam agents, treatment should be continued with these agents alone. Routine inclusion of an "antimicrobial time-out" 48 to 72 hours after initiating AMD therapy has been recommended when culture and susceptibility data or other clinical information becomes available. During this period, the clinician should reassess whether antimicrobial therapy should be continued, discontinued or modified.[15]

When available, use of regional or hospital-specific antibiograms can also help guide appropriate empirical antimicrobial therapy. A *regional antibiogram* lists commonly isolated species of bacteria and the likelihood of susceptibility to various AMDs based on cumulative culture and susceptibility data from a practice or region. The practitioner can then select the AMD based on the likelihood of a particular bacterial species being present at the site of an infection and its predicted resistance pattern. The term "antibiogram" has also been used incorrectly to describe an individual bacterial isolate's susceptibility pattern, so "regional antibiogram" is the recommended term to describe cumulative susceptibility data. Development of practice-specific antibiograms is recommended because antibiograms can differ considerably from one practice to another even within the same region, depending on factors such as clinician preference for AMD choices, the types of cases seen, and whether the patient population is primary or referral based.

CLASSIFICATION OF ANTIMICROBIAL DRUGS

AMDs may be classified based on their structure (e.g., β-lactams, fluoroquinolones), spectrum of activity (gram-positive versus gram-negative bacteria), mechanism of action (Table 8.1; Fig. 8.1), whether they are *bacteriostatic* (inhibit or slow growth) or *bactericidal* drugs, and their pharmacodynamic properties (see Pharmacodynamics of Antimicrobial Drugs, later).

The difference between bactericidal and bacteriostatic drugs has become more blurred in recent years. Some drugs are difficult to define because they may have different action on different bacterial species. The "static" versus "cidal" nature of many drugs depends on the concentration achieved. At low concentrations (e.g., 1 × MIC, 2 × MIC) they may be bacteriostatic, but at higher concentrations (e.g., 4 × MIC, 8 × MIC) they can be bactericidal. In reality, there are no examples where a bactericidal agent is preferred over a bacteriostatic agent based on available evidence and extensive evaluation from human clinical studies.[18] From a clinical perspective, it is more useful to describe drugs as time dependent versus concentration dependent rather than as bactericidal or bacteriostatic. This allows the clinician to consider the dosage regimen and dosing interval to optimize therapy.

Antibacterial drugs have also been classified for veterinary use as first-line, second-line, or third-line drugs[19] (in some guidelines, the authors use "first-choice," "second-choice," and so forth, and in the ISCAID guidelines the authors use first-tier, second-tier, third-tier, for the same meaning). First-line drugs are those that could be used for empirical selection in the absence of or pending the results of culture and susceptibility testing, and include amoxicillin, amoxicillin-clavulanate, cephalexin, doxycycline, minocycline, and trimethoprim-sulfonamides. Second-line drugs are those to be used

TABLE 8.1 Classification of Antimicrobial Drugs Based on Their Mechanism of Action

Mechanism Of Action	Antimicrobial Drug	Examples
Inhibition of cell wall synthesis	β-Lactams, glycopeptides, fosfomycin	Penicillin, cephalexin, meropenem, vancomycin
Cell membrane disruption	Polymyxins, daptomycin, aminoglycosides	Colistin, daptomycin, gentamicin, amikacin
Protein synthesis inhibition	Tetracyclines, aminoglycosides, chloramphenicol, lincosamides, macrolides, ketolides	Doxycycline, gentamicin, erythromycin, clindamycin, azithromycin, telithromycin
Inhibition of DNA replication	Fluoroquinolones	Enrofloxacin, marbofloxacin, pradofloxacin
Inhibition of folic acid metabolism	Trimethoprim-sulfonamides	Trimethoprim-sulfamethoxazole

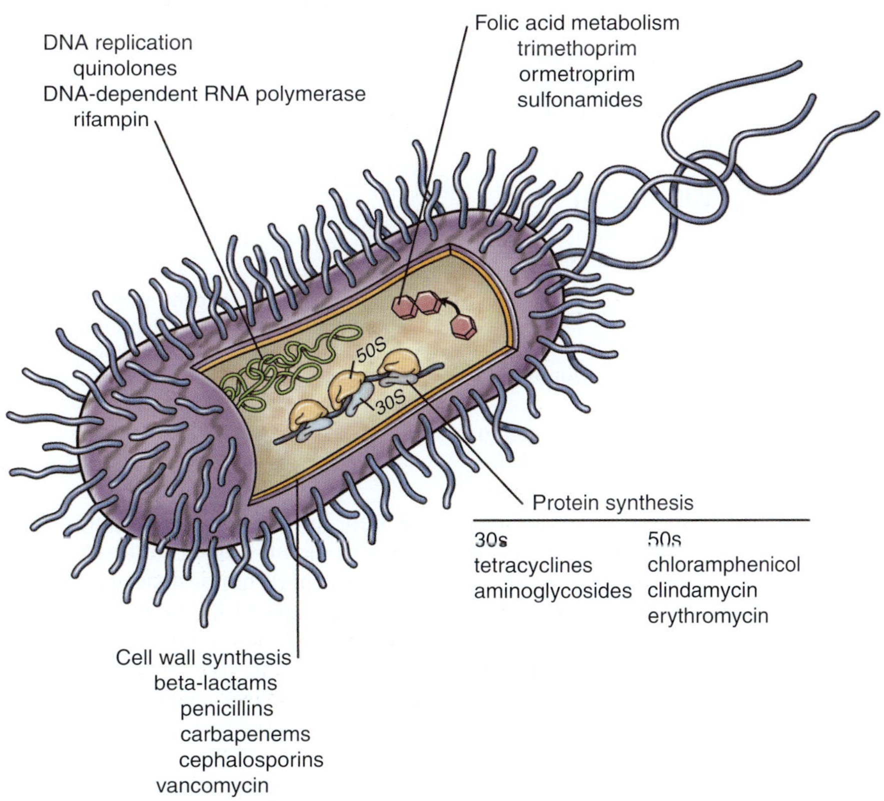

Fig. 8.1 Sites of action of antimicrobial drugs within the bacterial cell.

BOX 8.2 Criteria to Consider Before Administering a "Third-Line" Antibiotic

1. Infection must be documented based on clinical abnormalities and culture.
2. The infection is serious and has the potential to be life threatening if left untreated.
3. Resistance is documented to all other reasonable first- and second-line options.
4. The infection is potentially treatable.
5. The clinician may seek advice from an infectious disease clinician or a clinical microbiologist to discuss antimicrobial susceptibility test results, and to discuss the use of these agents if there is unfamiliarity with their use. In some instances, there may be other viable options (e.g., topical therapy).
6. The clinician should attempt for a duration of treatment that is as short as possible. (Prolonged treatment with these agents is usually unacceptable.)

on the basis of culture and susceptibility testing and because of the lack of any appropriate first-line options. These include piperacillin-tazobactam, amikacin, and third-generation cephalosporins. Some consensus documents (e.g., ISCAID guidelines, BSAVA guidelines) have considered some third-generation cephalosporins as appropriate first-line agents in special circumstances. Cefovecin may be considered when compliance may be a problem. Cefpodoxime proxetil has been considered by ISCAID to be either a "first- or second-tier" antibiotic because of its activity against staphylococci. Fluoroquinolones are usually considered second-tier antibiotics because fluoroquinolone exposure has been associated with emergence of antimicrobial resistance and treatment failures.[20] Fluoroquinolones could be considered as first-line drugs for dogs and cats suspected to have serious gram-negative bacterial infections that require treatment pending the results of culture and susceptibility testing.

The use of third-line drugs, including vancomycin, linezolid, rifampin, human-labeled third-generation cephalosporins (e.g., ceftazidime), and carbapenems such as imipenem and meropenem, is usually reserved for situations when certain criteria are met (Box 8.2).[19]

PHARMACODYNAMICS OF ANTIMICROBIAL DRUGS

Pharmacokinetic and pharmacodynamic parameters (PK-PD exposure relationships) are important determinants of the efficacy of AMDs and serve as the basis for determination of clinically effective dosage regimens and susceptibility breakpoints and for the development of guidelines for AMD use for specific types of infections.[21]

Antimicrobial activity is classified as *concentration dependent* or *time dependent*. AMDs that exhibit *concentration-dependent killing* are fluoroquinolones and aminoglycosides. These drugs work optimally when the peak concentration in the plasma (C_{max}) or the area under the curve (AUC) exceeds the MIC by a defined index factor (Fig. 8.2). These are typically bactericidal agents, and the ability to kill bacteria increases as the AMD concentrations are optimized. Target concentrations have been defined for laboratory animals and humans and have been extrapolated to veterinary patients. For example, the C_{max} to MIC ratio (C_{max}/MIC) should exceed 8 to 10 for optimum dosing of aminoglycosides. The AUC for a 24-hour interval to MIC ratio (AUC_{24}/MIC) should exceed approximately 100 for fluoroquinolones and exceed 90 for aminoglycosides. For some infections, a ratio of 125 for fluoroquinolones is better, and

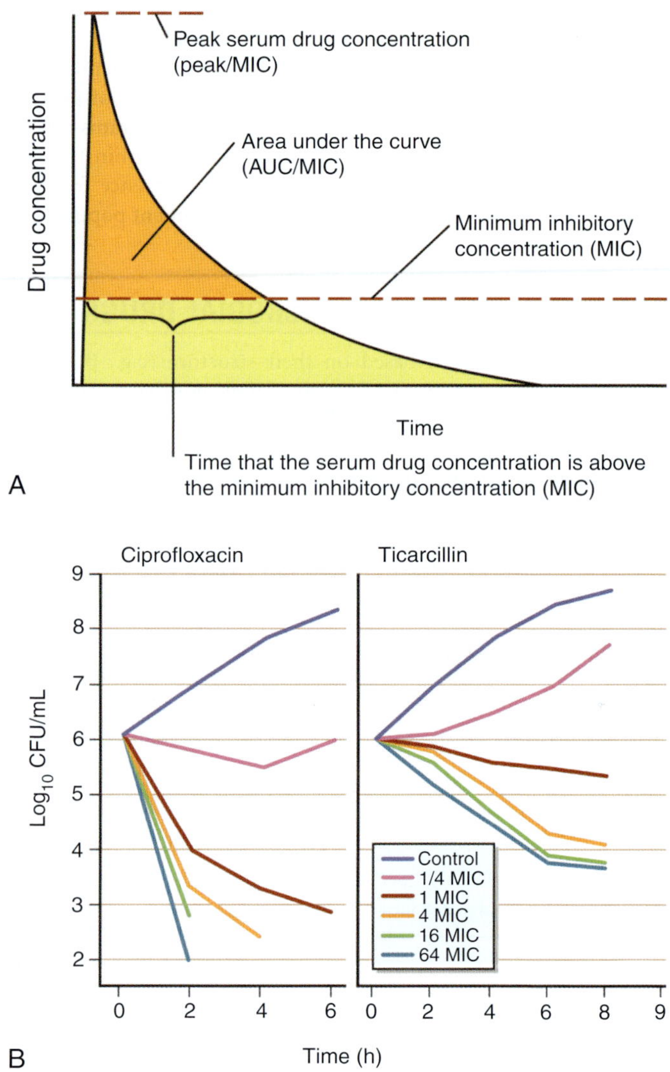

Fig. 8.2 Antimicrobial pharmacodynamics. (A) Antimicrobial drug (AMD) pharmacodynamics. Concentration-dependent drugs are most active when the peak concentration (C_{max}) or the area under the curve (AUC) in the plasma exceeds the MIC by a defined factor. For time-dependent drugs, outcome is correlated with the time that the AMD concentration at the site of infection spends above the MIC. This is usually expressed as the percent of time above the MIC during a 24-hour interval (T > MIC). (B) As AMD concentrations increase, the ability of concentration-dependent drugs such as fluoroquinolones (in this case, ciprofloxacin) to kill bacteria increases. As concentrations of time-dependent drugs such as β-lactam drugs (in this case, ticarcillin) increase, bacterial killing plateaus.

in some patients (e.g., immunocompromised patients with life-threatening infections), a ratio of 250 may be desirable. Drugs that exhibit concentration-dependent killing also have *postantibiotic effect* (PAE). The PAE is a persistent antimicrobial effect after drug concentrations at the site of infection fall below the MIC. The exact cause of the PAE varies with the drug, but it may result from irreversible binding of a drug to the target site. The duration of the PAE is influenced by the duration of antibiotic exposure, the drug concentration, the bacterial species present, and the class of antibiotic. For concentration-dependent antibiotics, administration of the total daily dose as a single dose every 24 hours is preferred to a smaller divided dose in order to maximize C_{max} or AUC. For aminoglycosides, this also reduces risk of kidney injury.

β-lactams (penicillins and cephalosporins) exhibit *time-dependent killing*. The activity of these drugs is maximized by the time above the MIC rather than the magnitude of the concentration. This is usually expressed as the percent of time above the MIC during a 24-hour interval (T > MIC). These drugs are most effective when administered multiple times a day or as continuous-rate infusions, in order to maintain drug concentrations at the site of infection. For some drugs (e.g., some cephalosporins), a long T > MIC is achieved by virtue of a long half-life. The required time above the MIC for an AMD varies with the pathogen present, the drug, and the site of infection. For a β-lactam antimicrobial (penicillin, cephalosporin), the desired target is a plasma concentration greater than the MIC maintained for at least 40% to 50% of the dosing interval.[21] Drug dosages that achieve these target concentrations in excess of an MIC for these periods can be calculated based on pharmacokinetic data. For time-dependent AMD with long half-lives (such as macrolides, clindamycin, vancomycin, and tetracyclines), efficacy is determined primarily by the extent to which the AUC exceeds the MIC. The magnitude of the target varies with each drug class, but in general an AUC/MIC ratio of the unbound drug > 25 is a desired target.

These parameters and indices constitute the PK-PD properties of the antimicrobial agent, also known as the PK-PD cutoff. As the MIC of an organism increases, it becomes more difficult to achieve these PK-PD targets (i.e., above the PK-PD cutoff), and organisms are regarded as resistant.

SITE OF INFECTION

In general, the concentration of an AMD at the site of infection should at least equal the MIC for the infecting organism, but the exact concentration and the duration of the concentration at the site varies with the class of antimicrobial. For some AMDs, the serum or plasma total (bound and unbound) drug concentrations may not reflect the drug concentration in tissues. Examples are the highly lipophilic macrolide antibiotics (e.g., azithromycin) for which the tissue drug concentration is much higher than plasma drug concentration because of sequestration inside cells. On the other hand, tissue concentrations greatly underestimate the plasma or serum drug concentration for poorly lipophilic agents such as aminoglycosides or β-lactams. Antimicrobial selection for different body sites are suggested in Box 8.3.

The concentration of an AMD at the site of infection is affected by factors such as lipid solubility, protein binding, pH at the site (or cell), and other factors reducing permeability, such as the presence of large amounts of pus, scar tissue, foreign material, devitalized tissue, and bone. Lipid-soluble drugs such as chloramphenicol, rifampin, fluoroquinolones, tetracyclines, and trimethoprim are most adept at crossing membranes, including the blood-brain, alveolar, and prostatic barriers. In contrast, poorly lipophilic, polar drugs such as penicillins and aminoglycosides do not cross lipid membranes and will not achieve adequate concentrations in tissues in which there is a barrier to penetration (e.g., prostate, brain, eye, or intracellular sites). In human patients, aminoglycosides and amphotericin B have been administered intrathecally to treat CNS infections,[22,23] but this is a rare treatment in veterinary medicine. In order to use β-lactam antibiotics to treat these infections, high doses are required because of a poorly penetrated blood-brain barrier. Even in the face of inflammation, the brain/blood concentration ratio of these drugs is low. Water-soluble AMDs are excreted in active form by the liver and concentrated in bile, such as tetracyclines, aminopenicillins, and cephalosporins; therefore, they are acceptable choices for susceptible hepatobiliary infections (see Chapter 126). Lower urinary tract infections can be successfully treated with drugs such as amoxicillin, amoxicillin-clavulanate, cephalosporins, and trimethoprim-sulfonamides, because these agents are highly concentrated in the urine of animals with healthy kidneys (see Chapter 127).

BOX 8.3 Examples Of Appropriate Initial Antimicrobial Drug Choices For Treatment Of Bacterial Infections In Different Anatomic Sites

Site	Appropriate Empiric Antimicrobial Drugs
Skin	Cephalexin Amoxicillin-clavulanate Clindamycin
Urinary tract	Amoxicillin Amoxicillin-clavulanate Cephalosporins Trimethoprim-sulfamethoxazole
Prostate	Trimethoprim-sulfamethoxazole Fluoroquinolones (enrofloxacin, marbofloxacin, orbifloxacin, levofloxacin)
Respiratory tract	Tetracyclines (doxycycline, minocycline) Fluoroquinolones
Intestinal tract (animals with hepatic encephalopathy)	Ampicillin Neomycin
Biliary tree	Amoxicillin-clavulanate Cephalosporins Fluoroquinolones
Brain	Metronidazole (anaerobes only) Fluoroquinolones Trimethoprim-sulfonamides
Bone	Clindamycin Cephalosporins Amoxicillin-clavulanate

OTHER HOST FACTORS

Other host factors that should be considered in AMD selection and route of administration include the following:

1. History of adverse drug reactions. These are most commonly gastrointestinal in dogs and cats, but may include hypersensitivity reactions. Examples include trimethoprim-sulfonamides and penicillins.
2. Age. The administration of systemic tetracyclines is contraindicated in young animals because of the potential for teeth discoloration (see Fig. 10.5). Doxycycline is less likely to produce this reaction if administered for a short course. Fluoroquinolones have the potential to cause cartilage and joint toxicity in dogs aged between 7 and 28 weeks.[24,25]
3. Species. Dogs and cats differ in their susceptibility to adverse drug reactions. For example, dogs can develop severe cutaneous reactions to 5-flucytosine. Dogs are the species most susceptible to adverse reactions to sulfonamides (see #4 below). Cats are susceptible to acute retinal degeneration following treatment with enrofloxacin doses above 5 mg/kg. Cats also are prone to esophageal ulceration from oral doxycycline hyclate or clindamycin hydrochloride. To avoid this effect, these drugs can be administered with a bolus of water or food to ensure passage of the medication into the stomach.

4. Sulfonamides. Dogs are the species most susceptible to reactions from sulfonamides (including trimethoprim-sulfonamides) because of an inability to acetylate the parent drug for elimination. Subsequently, some breeds of dog convert the drug to a cytotoxic metabolite that produces hypersensitivity-like reactions following trimethoprim-sulfonamide administration. Doberman pinschers may be at higher risk for this problem. Keratoconjunctivitis sicca (dry eye) is also a risk when administering sulfonamides to dogs.
5. Gastric acidity. The absorption of some AMDs, such as ketoconazole and itraconazole, is impaired by medications that suppress gastric acid production.
6. Concurrent medications. Drug interactions, such as concurrent use of drugs that require metabolism using cytochrome P450 enzymes, can affect the choice or dose of AMD used. For example, chloramphenicol and ketoconazole are well-known P450 enzyme inhibitors, whereas rifampin is an enzyme inducer. Fluoroquinolone and tetracycline antibiotics can chelate with divalent and trivalent cations, which inhibits oral absorption. Therefore, administration of these drugs with supplements containing aluminum, iron, magnesium, or calcium can diminish oral absorption.
7. Pregnancy. Penicillins, cephalosporins, aminoglycosides, and macrolides are generally considered safe during pregnancy. The volume of distribution in pregnancy is greater, and so higher doses may be required to achieve equivalent serum concentrations. On the other hand, azole antifungals, griseofulvin, and trimethoprim-sulfonamides carry risks during pregnancy.
8. Renal and hepatic function. The dose of AMDs that are dependent on renal elimination may require reduction in these animals with impaired renal function in order to minimize toxicity. For example, fluoroquinolones may be more likely to cause seizures or retinal toxicity in animals with kidney disease. The use of nephrotoxic drugs such as amphotericin B or aminoglycosides may be more likely to worsen kidney injury (and should be avoided) in animals with kidney disease.[26] Adverse effects may be more common when drugs that require hepatic metabolism, such as azole antifungals, metronidazole, rifampin, sulfonamides, or chloramphenicol, are administered to animals with impaired liver function.

ROUTE OF ADMINISTRATION

The most common routes of administration for AMDs in dogs and cats are topical, intravenous, intramuscular, subcutaneous, and oral. For localized infections of the skin, eye, or ear canal, topical administration has the advantage of delivering a high concentration of the AMD to the site, which may overcome bacterial resistance mechanisms and minimize systemic exposure to the drug. Parenteral administration, especially intravenous administration, provides maximum bioavailability when there may be questions regarding oral absorption or when oral medications must be avoided. This route is recommended for: (1) treatment of life-threatening infections, (2) systemic administration of antimicrobials with poor oral bioavailability (such as aminoglycosides and some injectable β-lactam antibiotics), and (3) when gastrointestinal signs or malabsorption preclude effective drug administration via the oral route. Because parenteral AMDs are generally administered in hospital, compliance with this mode of administration is also likely to be greater. Absorption may be delayed after subcutaneous or intramuscular administration when perfusion of these tissues is impaired; therefore, these routes are avoided unless the patient is well hydrated and tissues are well perfused. Peak plasma drug concentrations are achieved immediately after intravenous bolus administration. Therefore, bolus administration is an optimum approach for a concentration-dependent antimicrobial provided rapid injection does not produce toxicity (such as may occur with fluoroquinolones). For a time-dependent drug such as a β-lactam, a slow infusion, or a constant rate infusion (CRI) optimizes the time-dependent activity and can improve the outcomes in animals with severe infection.

Provided gastrointestinal function is healthy, administration of many oral AMDs results in acceptable bioavailability. For drugs that have oral absorption less than 100%, the low absorption is accounted for in the adjustment of the dosage regimen. However, it should be remembered that when oral absorption is low, more active drug remains in the intestine and may alter the intestinal bacterial population. Drugs with the highest oral bioavailability in dogs and cats are the fluoroquinolones; β-lactams have low and variable bioavailability depending on the drug. Nevertheless, once the animal can tolerate oral medications and its clinical condition becomes stable, a switch can be made from parenteral to oral antimicrobials. Peak plasma concentrations are always lower with oral administration than with intravenous administration, but for time-dependent drugs or for drugs that achieve efficacy on the basis of an AUC/MIC exposure relationship, this route is acceptable for a cure. Early switch from intravenous to oral therapy in human patients has gained increased favor in recent years because of reduced lengths of hospitalization, lowered costs, fewer intravascular catheter-related infections, and decreased selective pressure on nosocomial bacterial infections.[27–29] The oral bioavailability of some drugs can be maximized if they are administered with food (e.g., clavulanic acid-amoxicillin) or without food (e.g., azithromycin, tetracyclines). Some drugs are simply not absorbed orally and must be administered parenterally or by the topical route. These drugs include penicillin G, piperacillin, aminoglycosides, many cephalosporins (cefazolin, cefotaxime, cefoxitin), meropenem, imipenem, and vancomycin. Some drugs are not absorbed orally unless administered as a prodrug. An example is cefpodoxime proxetil. The proxetil portion of the molecule is cleaved off at the time of intestinal absorption to allow for adequate systemic concentrations.[30]

ANTIMICROBIAL RESISTANCE

Infectious agents may be intrinsically resistant to an AMD, or acquire resistance through genetic variations. *Intrinsic resistance* refers to the innate ability of an organism to resist the effects of an AMD owing to structural or functional characteristics of that organism. For example, enterococci are intrinsically resistant to cephalosporins because they lack the PBPs that bind these antibiotics.[31] Anaerobic bacteria are intrinsically resistant to aminoglycosides because oxygen is required for entry of the drug to the bacteria. Bacteria of the Enterobacterales (for example *E. coli* and *Enterobacter*) are intrinsically resistant to macrolide antibiotics. Mycoplasmas have intrinsic resistance to penicillins because they lack a cell wall. A list of *Intrinsic Resistance* is available in Appendix B of the CLSI VET01 document[32] and laboratories may use this information to avoid testing some drug-bacteria combinations.

Bacterial resistance should not be defined by whether they are *wild-type* or *non-wild-type bacteria.* Wild-type strains of bacteria are those that have an absence of acquired and mutational resistance mechanisms. Non-wild-type strains of bacteria are those that have the presence of an acquired or mutational resistance mechanism to the drug in question. Wild-type strains may include bacteria that have inherent resistance to antimicrobials as described above. However, clinical resistance, as defined below, is a measure of the bacteria to respond to clinically achievable drug concentrations. Wild-type bacteria can be clinically resistant (e.g., Enterobacterales are resistant to aminopenicillins), and non-wild-type bacteria can be susceptible to some antibacterial agents.

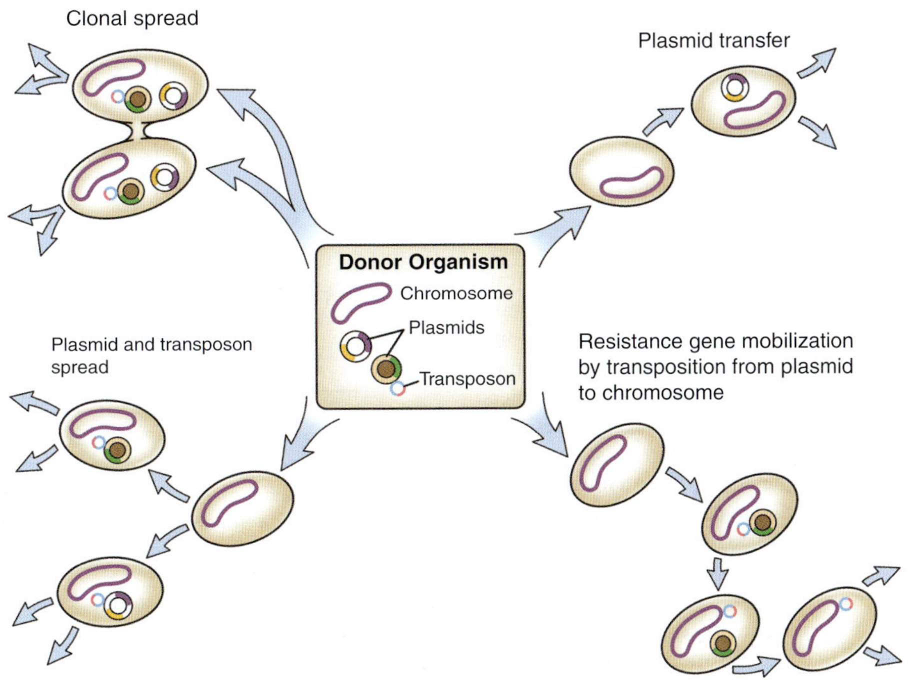

Fig. 8.3 Genetic mechanisms of resistance in bacteria.

The definition of *resistance* (or *clinical resistance*) used by CLSI relies on PK-PD cutoff targets, MIC distributions (wild-type cutoff), and clinical response (clinical cutoff). If sufficient drug concentrations can be achieved to attain a clinical cure—even in some cases when the bacteria are non-wild-type—the bacteria can be considered "susceptible." On the other hand, if drug concentrations after a standard dose cannot meet the PK-PD target defined for that drug-bug combination, the bacteria are reported as "resistant." In other words, the pathogen is considered resistant when standard dosage regimens cannot reach the PK-PD target of a particular C_{max}, AUC, or time above MIC.

Genetic resistance to an AMD may occur as a result of point mutations, DNA rearrangements, or acquisition of foreign DNA. Point mutations can result in alteration of the target site of an AMD, such as the susceptibility of bacterial DNA gyrase to fluoroquinolones.[33] DNA rearrangements may include inversions, deletions, duplications, insertions, or transpositions (including chromosome to plasmid) of large segments of DNA. The single most important mechanism of antibacterial resistance is acquisition of foreign DNA by horizontal transfer, especially that carried by plasmids and transposons.[34] Plasmids are circular, double-stranded DNA molecules that are capable of independent replication and can be transferred from one bacterial strain or species to another through the process of bacterial conjugation. Transposons are small, mobile segments of DNA that are flanked by inverted repeats and encode one or more resistance genes (Fig. 8.3). They depend on the chromosome or plasmids for replication. Plasmid-associated genes that confer AMD resistance are frequently on transposons and can move from the plasmid to the bacterial chromosome. A single plasmid may contain resistance genes for more than five different AMDs and represents an important mechanism for rapid spread of resistance genes among bacterial populations, including from one bacterial species to another.

Mechanisms of Antimicrobial Resistance

Antimicrobial Inactivation

Bacterial enzymes capable of inactivation of AMDs include β-lactamase enzymes, enzymes that modify aminoglycoside structure, chloramphenicol acetyltransferase, and macrolide (erythromycin) esterase. β-lactamase production is ubiquitous among *Staphylococcus* spp., and these enzymes hydrolyze penicillins and aminopenicillins, but not cephalosporins. β-lactamases are the most important mechanism of resistance to β-lactam antibiotics among gram-negative bacteria.[34] A vast array of β-lactamase enzymes have been discovered, which have been extensively classified into groups.[35,36] ESBLs can hydrolyze not only penicillins and first-generation cephalosporins, but also extended-spectrum cephalosporins such as cefotaxime and ceftazidime (which contain an oximino group). To date, ESBLs have only been described in gram-negative bacilli and are most commonly produced by *E. coli* and *K. pneumoniae*. Some, but not all, ESBLs can be inhibited by β-lactamase inhibitors such as clavulanic acid. The ESBL with the most importance at the present time for small animals are the CTX-M β-lactamases, which hydrolyze cefotaxime and other third-generation cephalosporins. Other types of β-lactamase enzymes include AmpC β-lactamases, which are encoded by chromosomal genes, and metallo-β-lactamases.[34,37] These types of β-lactamase enzymes are resistant to clavulanic acid. The most recent and alarming development has been the discovery of metallo-β-lactamases that can inactivate carbapenems such as meropenem and imipenem. These *carbapenemases* render the bacteria resistant to practically all available antibiotics.

Membrane Alteration

Protein channels called *porins* facilitate the passage of hydrophilic AMDs into gram-negative bacteria. Acquisition of porin mutations can result in conformational changes of or reduced expression of porins. The result is exclusion of AMDs such as β-lactams and fluoroquinolones.[38]

Efflux Pump Induction

Expression of efflux pumps by bacteria allows them to exclude certain AMDs. This is a major mechanism of resistance to tetracyclines in gram-negative bacteria. A variety of efflux pumps have been described.[39] Efflux pumps may not be specific for one particular class of antimicrobial; in other words, one MDR bacterial species can "pump" out different classes of drugs. Therefore, these have been termed "multidrug" efflux pumps and mediate multidrug resistance. The acquisition of MDR mechanisms greatly reduces the effective options for therapy. MDR organisms such as *P. aeruginosa* and *Acinetobacter baumannii* can utilize multidrug efflux pumps in concert with a variety of other resistance mechanisms, including β-lactamase enzyme production, drug target alterations, and AMD modification enzymes.

Target Modification

Methylation of ribosomal targets by bacterial methyltransferases can lead to resistance to tetracyclines, lincosamides, aminoglycosides, and especially macrolide antibiotics. Expression of altered PBPs is an important mechanism of resistance to β-lactam antimicrobials. Expression of PBP2a by staphylococci, which is encoded by the *mecA* gene, confers resistance to all β-lactam antimicrobials, including β-lactamase-resistant penicillins such as methicillin and oxacillin (methicillin-resistant staphylococci). Mutations of DNA gyrase can confer resistance to fluoroquinolones.[34] Resistance to trimethoprim-sulfonamides can result from altered dihydropteroate synthetase and dihydrofolate reductase enzymes.[40]

Target Protection

Target protection[41] is another mechanism of conferring resistance that serves a similar purpose as target modification. Target protection mechanisms are best known for tetracycline antibiotics; they can confer resistance to chloramphenicol and related drugs, oxazolidinones, fluoroquinolones, and others. In target protection, the target is not modified; instead, a target protection protein binds to the target to prevent the antibiotic from inhibiting the target mechanism.

Novel Approaches to Antimicrobial Drug Resistance

With rapid spread of MDR bacterial pathogens, alternatives to antibiotics have been investigated.[42] One approach is bacteriophage therapy. Bacteriophages are viruses that infect bacteria, and because of their specificity for certain bacterial species, they can deliver targets to one type of organism without harming others.[43,44] Bacteriophage infections may result in bacterial lysis, or delivery of a gene to the bacterial cell that increases its susceptibility to a given class of AMD.[42] Bacteriophage treatment may also be more successful than AMD treatment in the presence of biofilms, which impair antibiotic penetration. Barriers to implementation of phage therapy include the host immune response to the phage, bacterial resistance mechanisms, and uncertainties relating to dosing and the impact of other unidentified genes that might be present in bacteriophages. Other approaches that are under investigation include use of bacterial lysins, cationic antimicrobial peptides, antisense antibiotics, and antibacterial antibodies.[42] Bacterial lysins are derived from bacteriophages and are active only on gram-positive bacteria. Cationic antimicrobial peptides are derived from eukaryotic cells, have immunomodulatory properties, and rapidly kill a variety of bacteria.[45] Although it is difficult for bacteria to develop resistance to these peptides, multiple resistance mechanisms have been described. Antisense antibiotics are oligonucleotides that bind to the DNA of pathogenic microorganisms and inhibit gene expression.[46]

ANTIMICROBIAL DRUG COMBINATIONS

When an infectious agent is suspected but has not yet been identified, the use of AMD combinations is tempting because of the added broad spectrum of coverage that they provide. However, use of AMD combinations does not necessarily reduce the chance of selection for a resistant organism, adds expense, and may predispose to drug toxicity. Theoretically, drug combinations may have additive, synergistic, or antagonistic effects (Fig. 8.4). These properties are not as well established in clinical situations. For example, antagonism between

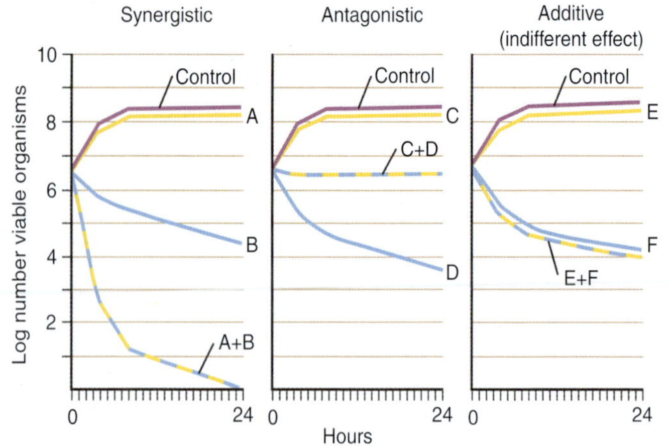

Fig. 8.4 Synergistic, antagonistic, and additive effects of antimicrobial drug combinations. Drugs used are referred to using letters of the alphabet. Control = no drug.

a bacteriostatic antibiotic (e.g., tetracycline) and a bactericidal antibiotic that requires bacterial growth for efficacy (e.g., a β-lactam) is also theoretically possible, but there is only one clinical example of this occurrence, published in the 1950s.[47] Such antagonism has not been replicated since that time.

The use of antibiotic combinations may be justified in some scenarios, such as:

1. Some drugs are administered in combination with other drugs to prevent rapid development of resistance compared with the use of a single agent. Examples are 5-flucytosine for antifungal treatment and rifampin in combination with macrolides for treatment of *Mycobacterium* spp. infections.
2. If a polymicrobial infection is present, combination drugs broaden the spectrum of activity.
3. If the nature of an infection is not known and infection is life threatening, it is reasonable to commence treatment with a broad-spectrum combination (e.g., a fluoroquinolone and a β-lactam), based on knowledge of the likely pathogen present and local prevalence of AMD resistance, pending the results of culture and susceptibility testing. Once the results of culture and susceptibility testing are available, de-escalation should be performed.
4. Certain combinations of AMD are synergistic for treatment of specific infections. For example, the combination of a β-lactam and an aminoglycoside may be synergistic for treatment of enterococcal infections, but not likely helpful for other infections. The relatively slow bactericidal activity of the β-lactam is enhanced by the addition of the aminoglycoside, such that shorter durations of treatment or extension of the dosing interval becomes possible without affecting outcome.[18] Combination therapy has been recommended for treatment of resistant *P. aeruginosa* infections, brucellosis, gastric helicobacteriosis, and some mycobacterial infections..
5. Some drugs are not effective against anaerobic bacteria (e.g., aminoglycosides and fluoroquinolones with the exception of pradofloxacin). They should be combined with an agent active against anaerobes (e.g., clindamycin or metronidazole) when a mixed infection with anaerobic and aerobic bacteria is suspected.
6. When a vector-borne pathogen is suspected, doxycycline may be administered until the results of further diagnostic tests confirm or eliminate this suspicion. In these cases, patients are frequently administered doxycycline in combination with another active agent to treat alternative bacterial infections that have not yet been ruled out.

MONITORING THE RESPONSE TO TREATMENT

The response to antimicrobial treatment is best monitored based on clinical assessment, which may include follow-up cytologic examination or cultures. However, in some situations such as bacterial cystitis, follow-up cultures are not recommended because the aim of AMD therapy is clinical cure rather than microbiological cure. Therapeutic drug monitoring can be used to ensure adequate serum drug concentrations when treating with aminoglycosides, vancomycin, and azole antifungal drugs, but these assays are rarely available in commercial veterinary diagnostic laboratories. Veterinary clinicians can check with local laboratories (e.g., human laboratories) to locate the availability of these assays in their area. It should be remembered that reference ranges for these laboratories are established from the human use of these drugs; veterinary therapeutic ranges are not established.

PROPHYLACTIC ANTIMICROBIALS

Prophylactic use of AMDs to prevent anticipated infections is controversial because of the increased risk of selecting for resistant microorganisms. In general, prophylactic AMD use is discouraged, with the exception of perioperative AMD therapy to prevent surgical infections when contamination is expected, treatment of deep bite wounds, and following chemotherapy when moderate to severe neutropenia develops (<1000 neutrophils/μL).[48] When used perioperatively to prevent surgical infections (e.g., orthopedic surgery) the administration should be as short as possible—rarely is there a need to extend the administration beyond the duration of the surgical procedure. For cancer chemotherapy prophylaxis, treatment for 3 to 7 days has been recommended if severe neutropenia is identified. Although more controversial, antimicrobial prophylaxis has also been suggested following chemotherapy in patients with a high risk of sepsis, including small breed dogs, those with hemic malignancy, and those treated with vincristine or doxorubicin.[48] In one prospective study, dogs administered trimethoprim-sulfadiazine following treatment of osteosarcoma or lymphoma with doxorubicin had significantly reduced hospitalization rate, nonhematologic toxicity, and gastrointestinal toxicity when compared with dogs that did not receive prophylactic antimicrobials.[49] Use of prophylactic antimicrobials for clean surgeries, routine elective surgery, dental procedures (in the absence of abscessation), and following placement of urinary catheters is strongly discouraged.

SUGGESTED READINGS

Weese JS, Giguere S, Guardabassi L, et al. ACVIM consensus statement on therapeutic antimicrobial use in animals and antimicrobial resistance. *J Vet Intern Med*. 2015;29(2):487–498.

Martinez MN, Papich MG, Drusano GL. Dosing regimen matters: the importance of early intervention and rapid attainment of the pharmacokinetic/pharmacodynamic target. *Antimicrob Agents Chemother*. 2012;56(6):2795–2805.

Papich MG. Pharmacokinetic-pharmacodynamic (PK-PD) modeling and the rational selection of dosage regimes for the prudent use of antimicrobial drugs. *Vet Microbiol*. 2014;171(3–4):480–486.

REFERENCES

1. Domagk G. Ein beitrag zur chemotherapie der bakteriellen infektionen. *Deut Med Wochenschr*. 1935;61(7):250–253.
2. Cummings KJ, Aprea VA, Altier C. Antimicrobial resistance trends among canine *Escherichia coli* isolates obtained from clinical samples in the northeastern USA, 2004-2011. *Can Vet J*. 2015;56(4):393–398.
3. Beever L, Bond R, Graham PA, et al. Increasing antimicrobial resistance in clinical isolates of *Staphylococcus intermedius* group bacteria and emergence of MRSP in the UK. *Vet Rec*. 2015;176(7):172.
4. Bemis DA, Jones RD, Frank LA, et al. Evaluation of susceptibility test breakpoints used to predict mecA-mediated resistance in *Staphylococcus pseudintermedius* isolated from dogs. *J Vet Diagn Invest*. 2009;21(1):53–58.
5. Perreten V, Kadlec K, Schwarz S, et al. Clonal spread of methicillin-resistant *Staphylococcus pseudintermedius* in Europe and North America: an international multicentre study. *J Antimicrob Chemother*. 2010;65(6):1145–1154.
6. Harada K, Shimizu T, Mukai Y, et al. Phenotypic and molecular characterization of antimicrobial resistance in *Klebsiella* spp. isolates from companion animals in Japan: clonal dissemination of multidrug-resistant extended-spectrum beta-lactamase-producing *Klebsiella pneumoniae*. *Front Microbiol*. 2016;7:1021.
7. Fishman N, Society for Healthcare Epidemiology of America, Infectious Diseases Society of America. Policy statement on antimicrobial stewardship by the Society for Healthcare Epidemiology of America (SHEA), the Infectious Diseases Society of America (IDSA), and the Pediatric Infectious Diseases Society (PIDS). *Infect Control Hosp Epidemiol*. 2012;33(4):322–327.
8. Weese JS, Giguere S, Guardabassi L, et al. ACVIM consensus statement on therapeutic antimicrobial use in animals and antimicrobial resistance. *J Vet Intern Med*. 2015;29(2):487–498.
9. Weese JS, Blondeau JM, Boothe D, et al. Antimicrobial use guidelines for treatment of urinary tract disease in dogs and cats: antimicrobial guidelines working group of the International Society for Companion Animal Infectious Diseases. *Vet Med Int*. 2011;2011:263768.
10. Hillier A, Lloyd DH, Weese JS, et al. Guidelines for the diagnosis and antimicrobial therapy of canine superficial bacterial folliculitis (antimicrobial guidelines working group of the International Society for Companion Animal Infectious Diseases). *Vet Dermatol*. 2014;25(163–175):e142–163.
11. Lappin MR, Blondeau J, Boothe D, et al. Antimicrobial use guidelines for treatment of respiratory tract disease in dogs and cats: antimicrobial guidelines working group of the International Society for Companion Animal Infectious Diseases. *J Vet Intern Med*. 2017;31(2):279–294.
12. American Animal Hospital Association. 2014 AAFP/AAHA Basic Guidelines for Judicious Therapeutic Use of Antimicrobials. www.aaha.org/aaha-guidelines/use-of-antimicrobials-configuration/use-of-antimicrobials/.
13. Morley PS, Apley MD, Besser TE, et al. Antimicrobial drug use in veterinary medicine. *J Vet Intern Med*. 2005;19(4):617–629.
14. Canadian Veterinary Medical Association. 2018 CVMA Guidelines for Veterinary Antimicrobial Use. www.canadianveterinarians.net/AMU-UAM. Accessed August 30, 2016.
15. American Veterinary Medical Association. Guidance for Antimicrobial Use in Companion Animal Practice. https://www.avma.org/KB/Resources/Reference/Pages/Guidance-for-Antimicrobial-Use-in-Companion-Animal-Practice.aspx.
16. Martinez MN, Papich MG, Drusano GL. Dosing regimen matters: the importance of early intervention and rapid attainment of the pharmacokinetic/pharmacodynamic target. *Antimicrob Agents Chemother*. 2012;56(6):2795–2805.
17. Clinical and Laboratory Standards Institute. Understanding susceptibility test data as a component of antimicrobial stewardship in veterinary settings. In: CLSI Report VET09. 1st ed. Wayne, PA: Clinical and Laboratory Standards Institute; 2019.
18. Wald-Dickler N, Holtom P, Spellberg B. Busting the myth of "static vs cidal": a systemic literature review. *Clin Infect Dis*. 2018;66(9): 1470–1474.
19. Weese JS. Investigation of antimicrobial use and the impact of antimicrobial use guidelines in a small animal veterinary teaching hospital: 1995-2004. *J Am Vet Med Assoc*. 2006;228(4):553–558.
20. Bakken JS. The fluoroquinolones: how long will their utility last? *Scand J Infect Dis*. 2004;36(2):85–92.
21. Papich MG. Pharmacokinetic-pharmacodynamic (PK-PD) modeling and the rational selection of dosage regimes for the prudent use of antimicrobial drugs. *Vet Microbiol*. 2014;171(3–4):480–486.
22. Johnson RH, Einstein HE. Amphotericin B and coccidioidomycosis. *Ann N Y Acad Sci*. 2007;1111(1):434–441.
23. Preston SL, Briceland LL. Intrathecal administration of amikacin for treatment of meningitis secondary to cephalosporin-resistant *Escherichia coli*. *Ann Pharmacother*. 1993;27(7–8):870–873.

24. Rosanova MT, Lede R, Capurro H, et al. Assessing fluoroquinolones as risk factor for musculoskeletal disorders in children: a systematic review and meta-analysis. *Arch Argent Pediatr.* 2010;108(6):524–531.
25. Sansone JM, Wilsman NJ, Leiferman EM, et al. The effect of fluoroquinolone antibiotics on growing cartilage in the lamb model. *J Pediatr Orthop.* 2009;29(2):189–195.
26. Munar MY, Singh H. Drug dosing adjustments in patients with chronic kidney disease. *Am Fam Physician.* 2007;75(10):1487–1496.
27. Broom J, Broom A, Adams K, et al. What prevents the intravenous to oral antibiotic switch? A qualitative study of hospital doctors' accounts of what influences their clinical practice. *J Antimicrob Chemother.* 2016;71(8):2295–2299.
28. Mertz D, Koller M, Haller P, et al. Outcomes of early switching from intravenous to oral antibiotics on medical wards. *J Antimicrob Chemother.* 2009;64(1):188–199.
29. Mazumder SA. Intravenous-to-Oral Switch Therapy; 2018. http://emedicine.medscape.com/article/237521-overview.
30. Papich MG, Davis JL, Floerchinger AM. Pharmacokinetics, protein binding, and tissue distribution of orally administered cefpodoxime proxetil and cephalexin in dogs. *Am J Vet Res.* 2010;71:1484–1491.
31. Williamson R, Calderwood SB, Moellering RC Jr, et al. Studies on the mechanism of intrinsic resistance to beta-lactam antibiotics in group D streptococci. *J Gen Microbiol.* 1983;129(3):813–822.
32. Clinical and Laboratory Standards Institute. VET01: Performance Standards for Antimicrobial Disk and Dilution Susceptibility Tests for Bacteria Isolated From Animals. 5th ed; 2019. https://clsi.org/standards/products/veterinary-medicine/documents/vet01/.
33. Arai K, Hirakata Y, Yano H, et al. Emergence of fluoroquinolone-resistant *Streptococcus pyogenes* in Japan by a point mutation leading to a new amino acid substitution. *J Antimicrob Chemother.* 2011;66(3):494–498.
34. Hawkey PM, Jones AM. The changing epidemiology of resistance. *J Antimicrob Chemother.* 2009;64(suppl 1). i3–10.
35. Bush K, Jacoby GA. Updated functional classification of beta-lactamases. *Antimicrob Agents Chemother.* 2010;54(3):969–976.
36. Jacoby GA, Munoz-Price LS. The new beta-lactamases. *N Engl J Med.* 2005;352(4):380–391.
37. Jacoby GA. AmpC beta-lactamases. *Clin Microbiol Rev.* 2009;22:161–182.
38. Pages JM, James CE, Winterhalter M. The porin and the permeating antibiotic: a selective diffusion barrier in Gram-negative bacteria. *Nat Rev Microbiol.* 2008;6(12):893–903.
39. Li XZ, Nikaido H. Efflux-mediated drug resistance in bacteria: an update. *Drugs.* 2009;69(12):1555–1623.
40. Skold O. Resistance to trimethoprim and sulfonamides. *Vet Res.* 2001;32(3–4):261–273.
41. Wilson DN, Hauryliuk V, Atkinson GC, et al. Target protection as a key antibiotic resistance mechanism. *Nat Rev Microbiol.* 2020;18(11):637–648.
42. Rios AC, Moutinho CG, Pinto FC, et al. Alternatives to overcoming bacterial resistances: State-of-the-art. *Microbiol Res.* 2016;191:51–80.
43. Gorski A, Miedzybrodzki R, Borysowski J, et al. Bacteriophage therapy for the treatment of infections. *Curr Opin Investig Drugs.* 2009;10(8):766–774.
44. O'Flaherty S, Ross RP, Coffey A. Bacteriophage and their lysins for elimination of infectious bacteria. *FEMS Microbiol Rev.* 2009;33(4):801–819.
45. Findlay B, Zhanel GG, Schweizer F. Cationic amphiphiles, a new generation of antimicrobials inspired by the natural antimicrobial peptide scaffold. *Antimicrob Agents Chemother.* 2010;54(10):4049–4058.
46. Bai H, Xue X, Hou Z, et al. Antisense antibiotics: a brief review of novel target discovery and delivery. *Curr Drug Discov Technol.* 2010;7(2):76–85.
47. Lepper MH, Dowling HF. Treatment of pneumococcic meningitis with penicillin compared with penicillin plus aureomycin; studies including observations on an apparent antagonism between penicillin and aureomycin. *AMA Arch Intern Med.* 1951;88(4):489–494.
48. Boudreaux B. Antimicrobial use in the veterinary cancer patient. *Vet Clin North Am Small Anim Pract.* 2014;44(5):883–891.
49. Chretin JD, Rassnick KM, Shaw NA, et al. Prophylactic trimethoprim-sulfadiazine during chemotherapy in dogs with lymphoma and osteosarcoma: a double-blind, placebo-controlled study. *J Vet Intern Med.* 2007;21(1):141–148.

9

Antiviral Chemotherapy and Immunomodulatory Drugs

Katrin Hartmann, Jane E. Sykes, Mark G. Papich

KEY POINTS

- Most antiviral drugs available for treatment of feline and canine viral infections are nucleoside analogues with greatest activity against retroviruses, herpesviruses, and coronaviruses.
- Antiviral drugs also affect the function of host cell machinery; therefore, they have considerable potential for toxicity.
- Antiviral drugs are widely used in human medicine for treatment of HIV, herpesvirus infection, and other viral infections. Much less is known about these medications in cats and dogs, and there are only few diseases of cats and dogs for which efficacy has been demonstrated.
- There are important differences between human and animal virus infections; therefore, it should not be assumed that the use of an antiviral agent in humans can be translated to a use in animals unless there is evidence of safety and efficacy.
- The most common indication for antiviral drugs in animals is treatment of FHV-1 infections with famciclovir and cidofovir. Zidovudine, an antiretroviral drug, has been used to treat FIV and FeLV infections. In addition, new antiviral drugs are now used to treat FIP.
- Antiviral drugs can act synergistically with immunomodulatory agents.
- Immunomodulators include microbial products, plant-derived immunomodulators, naturally occurring mammalian proteins, and synthetic drugs. The effect of many of these drugs on outcome in cats and dogs with infectious diseases has not been fully evaluated with well-designed studies.
- The parenteral use of natural or recombinant human cytokines in cats and dogs can produce neutralizing antibodies after 1 to 2 weeks of treatment, which can cross-react with endogenous proteins.
- Antiviral treatments are intended to suppress viral entry, multiplication, or transmission. Some of these antiviral agents can produce a remission or assist the patient's immune system to limit the course of the viral disease.

INTRODUCTION

This chapter describes the antiviral and immunomodulating agents used in cats and dogs. Unfortunately, there are limited approvals of drugs for these indications, and their use has relied on *in vitro* and *in vivo* studies, which have produced variable success. Only those drugs currently approved in the United States or Europe for use in animals or humans are discussed in this chapter with few exceptions of promising experimental drugs.

ANTIVIRAL DRUGS

Antiviral drug administration is still relatively uncommon in veterinary medicine, and the number of controlled studies of the efficacy of these drugs is limited. In contrast to antibacterial, antifungal, or antiprotozoal therapy, antiviral drugs are *virustatic*, that is, they do not inactivate viruses or achieve elimination of the virus. The benefit of these agents is to limit the spread of the virus, shorten duration of clinical signs, or improve patient well-being. Diagnosis of viral infections is often made after the viral replicative phase; thus, antiviral drugs are commonly used to treat chronic viral infections and to prevent reactivation of latent infections.

Antiviral drugs depend on host cell activity for their action. Subsequently, adverse effects in treated patients can be common, and many antiviral drugs active *in vitro* are not commercially available for this reason. Many others can only be given topically to avoid systemic toxicity. With the exception of feline interferon (IFN)-ω (not available in the United States), no antiviral drugs are specifically licensed for use in dogs and cats. Many human antiviral drugs were developed to treat HIV infection. Some of these compounds have activity against FIV, and sometimes FIV treatment studies were conducted to screen new compounds before their use in HIV-infected patients. Feline herpesvirus-1 (FHV-1) infection can be treated with several topical antiviral drugs (Table 9.1) and one promising oral compound.[1,2] New compounds for treatment of FIP are promising and undergoing evaluation (see Chapter 31).[3–5]

Some drugs used to treat FIP have been used investigationally or repurposed for investigations to treat humans with COVID-19 caused by SARS-CoV-2. A list of these agents are provided in Table 9.2. In dogs, treatment of viral infections is mainly supportive, and antiviral drugs are rarely used.

Antiviral drugs can be assigned to different drug classes based on the stage(s) of virus replication they interfere with (Table 9.3).[6,7] Potential targets in the retroviral replication process for antiviral drugs include binding of virus to specific cell surface receptors, entry into the cell and uncoating of the virus, reverse transcription of viral genome, integration of proviral DNA into host genome, viral protein processing, virion assembly and maturation, and virion release.[6,8,9] Combinations

TABLE 9.1 Antiviral Drugs in Use in Small Animals

Antiviral Drug	Mechanism Of Action	Human Applications	Small Animal Applications
Acyclovir/valacyclovir	Guanosine analogue. Interferes with viral DNA polymerase and DNA synthesis. Activity requires viral TK.	Treatment of herpesvirus infections, especially HSV and varicella-zoster virus	FHV-1 infections (poorly effective)
Penciclovir/famciclovir		Treatment of herpesvirus infections, especially HSV and varicella-zoster virus	FHV-1 infections
Cidofovir	Deoxycytidine monophosphate analogue. Activity independent of viral TK.	Systemic treatment of cytomegalovirus retinitis; topical treatment of papillomavirus infections	Topical treatment of FHV-1 ocular infections
Idoxuridine	Iodinated thymidine analogue. Interferes with viral DNA synthesis.	Topical treatment of HSV keratoconjunctivitis	Topical treatment of FHV-1 ocular infections
Trifluridine	Fluorinated thymidine analogue. Interferes with viral DNA synthesis.		
Vidarabine	Adenosine analogue. Interferes with viral DNA synthesis.		
Zidovudine	Thymidine analogue. Interferes with reverse transcription of virus RNA to DNA.	Systemic treatment of HIV infections	Systemic treatment of FIV and FeLV infections

FeLV, feline leukemia virus; *FHV-1,* feline herpesvirus-1; *FIV,* feline immunodeficiency virus; *HIV,* human immunodeficiency virus; *HSV,* herpes simplex virus; *TK,* thymidine kinase.

TABLE 9.2 Drugs of Clinical Interest in Veterinary Medicine Investigated for Treatment of Human Patients with COVID-19

Drug	Comment
Remdesivir	Although remdesivir has not been used in animals, it is chemically similar to the investigational antiviral drug GS-441524, which has been investigated for treating FIP.
Dexamethasone	Widely used corticosteroid anti-inflammatory medication in veterinary medicine. In human patients with COVID-19, it improves outcomes in severe cases by decreasing lung inflammation. It is commonly used as supportive treatment for FIP.
Hydroxychloroquine and chloroquine	Used on a limited basis in animals to treat some protozoal infections. Controversial results in patients with COVID-19.
Azithromycin	Often used in dogs and cats to treat bacterial infections (see Chapter 10). In human patients with COVID-19, the effects are controversial. NIH recommends against the use of hydroxychloroquine plus azithromycin, except in the context of a clinical trial, because of the potential for toxicities.
Ivermectin	Widely used antiparasitic agent in dogs and cats and a heartworm preventative. Theoretical potential for treatment of COVID-19 based on intracellular mechanisms, but concentrations achieved in patients with standard doses are not high enough to produce antiviral effects.
Famotidine	Widely used agent in dogs and cats to treat gastric problems exacerbated by high acidity. Investigated as a treatment for patients with COVID-19, but the mechanism of action is unknown.
Ascorbic acid (Vitamin C)	Antioxidant properties might protect host cells against infection-induced oxidative stress and can help host defenses against infection. NIH guidelines state there are insufficient data to recommend for or against use of vitamin C in noncritically ill patients or in critically ill patients.
Vitamin D	Used in some patients with COVID-19, but vitamin D supplements have not been shown to prevent or treat COVID-19.

FIP, feline infectious peritonitis; NIH, National Institute of Health.

of antiviral drugs with different mechanisms of action and combinations that include immunomodulatory drugs are increasingly used to treat human viral infections. For example, most HIV infection protocols consist of a combination of drugs that allows for a decrease in toxicity and reduction in selection for resistant mutants. Experience with combination treatment in cats and dogs is limited.

Nucleoside Reverse Transcriptase Inhibitors

The retroviral enzyme reverse transcriptase transcribes viral RNA into proviral DNA, which is subsequently integrated into the host cell's genome.[10] Compounds that inhibit this step have become the cornerstone of successful anti-HIV therapy. Reverse transcriptase inhibitors can be divided into three categories: nucleoside reverse transcriptase inhibitors (NRTIs), nucleotide reverse transcriptase inhibitors (NtRTIs), and non-nucleoside reverse transcriptase inhibitors (NNRTIs). Of these, NRTIs are the most commonly used drugs in human medicine.

NRTIs are analogues of mammalian 2′-deoxynucleosides and inhibit the polymerase function of the retroviral reverse transcriptase enzyme. Nucleosides are building blocks for the formation of DNA or RNA that are composed of a nitrogenous base and a five-carbon sugar (ribose or deoxyribose; Fig. 9.1). Like natural nucleosides, NRTIs must first be converted to a 5′-triphosphate form (nucleotide) through phosphorylation. In this form, they compete with host nucleotides and are incorporated into the elongating proviral DNA strand, thus functioning as competitive substrate inhibitors. However, NRTIs lack a 3′-hydroxyl group on the deoxyribose moiety, and this leads to strand termination as the subsequent nucleotide cannot form the next 5′-3′ phosphodiester bond necessary

TABLE 9.3 Classification of Antiviral Drugs

Category/Stage Of Replication Inhibited	Subcategory	Examples
Reverse transcriptase inhibitors	Nucleoside reverse transcriptase inhibitors	Zidovudine, fozivudine, didanosine, stavudine, zalcitabine, lamivudine, decitabine, gemcitabine
	Nucleotide reverse transcriptase inhibitors	Adefovir, tenofovir
	Non-nucleoside reverse transcriptase inhibitors	Suramin
DNA or RNA synthesis inhibitors	Nucleoside analogue DNA/RNA synthesis inhibitors	Acyclovir, valacyclovir, penciclovir, famciclovir, ganciclovir, cidofovir, idoxuridine, trifluridine, vidarabine, GS-441524, remdesivir
	Nucleotide synthesis inhibitors	Foscarnet, ribavirin
Protease inhibitors (maturation)		Nelfinavir, GC376
Entry inhibitors (virus attachment)	Receptor blockers Fusion inhibitors	Plerixafor
Integrase inhibitors (integration of proviral DNA)		Raltegravir
Nucleocapsid inhibitors (maturation)		Fused tetrathiocines, bis[1,2]dithiolo[1,4]thiazines and bis[1,2]dithiolopyrrole derivatives, 5-thieno-, 5-oxo-, 5-imino-1,2,3-dithiazole derivatives
Neuraminidase inhibitors (extrusion)		Oseltamivir, zanamivir, peramivir
Ion channel blockers (uncoating)		Amantadine
Antiviral amino acids		L-lysine

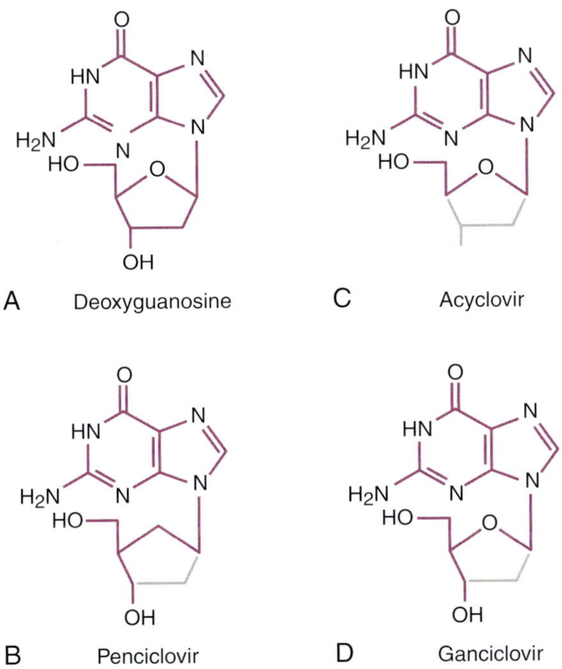

Fig. 9.1 Chemical structures of deoxyguanosine (a nucleoside) and anti-herpesviral nucleoside analogues. The grey portion is missing in the nucleoside analogues. (A) Deoxyguanosine. (B) Penciclovir. (C) Acyclovir. (D) Ganciclovir.

to extend the DNA strand. Latent viral infections are not affected because the replication of latent virus is suspended. However, reactivation of these infections can be prevented or reduced in frequency. Many NTRIs have documented *in vitro* activity not only against HIV but also against FIV, including zidovudine,[11,12] stavudine,[12–15] didanosine,[12,14] and zalcitabine.[14,16] To date, only zidovudine (AZT) has shown evidence of *in vivo* activity against feline retroviral infections with acceptable toxicity. Fozivudine, didanosine, stavudine, zalcitibine, lamivudine, decitabine, and gemcitabine might have *in vitro* activity against FIV and FeLV, but have not been evaluated in cats, have insufficient *in vivo* efficacy or are too toxic to administer to cats (Table 9.4). Therefore, discussion is limited to zidovudine.

Zidovudine (AZT)

Zidovudine (3′-azido-3′-deoxythymidine, AZT) is a thymidine analogue first synthesized in the 1960s as a potential anticancer agent.[11] In 1987, it was the first drug to be approved by the FDA for the treatment of HIV, and it remains an important component of HIV treatment protocols.[17,18] Inside host cells, it is converted to the active triphosphate form.

Zidovudine is available as a 10 mg/mL suspension and a 10 mg/mL injectable formulation. It has good oral bioavailability in cats and high distribution in tissues, including the CNS. It is metabolized to an inactive form by the liver and excreted by the kidneys. Dosage reduction has been recommended for cats with renal failure. Some cats treated with zidovudine develop dose-related hematologic adverse effects, most commonly nonregenerative anemia and neutropenia; therefore, the CBC should be monitored during treatment. Adverse effects can be confused with retrovirus-induced cytopenias.

Zidovudine inhibits FIV replication in infected cats. It reduces plasma viral load, improves the immunologic and clinical status of FIV-infected cats, increases quality of life, and prolongs life expectancy. In placebo-controlled trials, zidovudine improved stomatitis and increased the CD4:CD8 ratio in naturally FIV-infected cats.[19–23] Viral load was significantly lower in treated cats after 6 months of therapy compared with pre-treatment, while untreated cats showed a significant increase in viral load.[23] Neurologic abnormalities can improve with treatment, sometimes within days of therapy.[24] A decrease in viral load was even more significant when lamivudine was used in combination with zidovudine.[24] Zidovudine-resistant FIV mutants can arise after only 6 months' use as a result of a single-point mutation in the reverse transcriptase enzyme.[25–29]

Zidovudine is active against FeLV *in vitro*.[30–32]Activity against FeLV was also documented in experimentally infected cats when treatment was initiated less than 3 weeks after infection. When treated less than 1 week after experimental infection, cats were protected from bone marrow infection and persistent viremia.[32,33] In naturally infected cats,

TABLE 9.4 Nucleotide Reverse Transcriptase Inhibitors and Non-Nucleoside Reverse Transcriptase Inhibitors Evaluated for Treatment of Feline Retroviral Infections

Drug	Use In Humans	Use In Cats
Zidovudine	HIV	FIV and FeLV infection
Fozivudine	HIV	Insufficient *in vivo* activity against FIV
Didanosine	HIV	Activity *in vitro* against FeLV and *in vivo* against FIV, but causes toxic neuropathy
Stavudine	HIV	No *in vivo* data
Zalcitabine	HIV	No *in vivo* data for FIV; insufficient activity against FeLV; too toxic for use (thrombocytopenia, death)
Lamivudine	HIV	Insufficient activity in cats infected with FIV; too toxic for use (hematologic)
Decitabine	Myelodysplasia, HIV	*In vitro* activity against FeLV, *in vivo* activity unknown
Gemcitabine	Pancreatic neoplasia, HIV (in combination with decitabine)	*In vitro* activity against FeLV, *in vivo* activity unknown; might be too toxic for use (cytopenias)
Adefovir	Viral hepatitis	Insufficient *in vivo* activity against FeLV; active *in vivo* against FIV, but toxic (anemia)
Tenofovir	HIV	*In vitro* activity for FeLV and FIV, *in vivo* activity unknown; not available commercially
Suramin	Protozoal infections, neoplasia	FeLV *in vitro* activity; potentially very toxic; no long-term benefit in treated cats

FeLV, feline leukemia virus; *FIV,* feline immunodeficiency virus; *HIV,* human immunodeficiency virus.

however, treatment for 6 weeks did not lead to improvement of clinical, laboratory, immunologic, or virologic parameters.[34] Thus, the efficacy of zidovudine in FeLV-infected cats is less promising than in FIV-infected cats. Nevertheless, improvement in stomatitis, reduced antigenemia, and decreased incidence of lymphoma have been reported in naturally and experimentally infected cats treated with AZT.[22,35]

Nucleotide Reverse Transcriptase Inhibitors

NtRTIs also interact with the catalytic site of the viral reverse transcriptase and are incorporated into the elongating proviral DNA strand, causing strand termination.[36,37] They compete with the natural nucleotides and thus, also function as competitive substrate inhibitors. However, in contrast to NRTIs, NtRTIs contain a phosphate group and therefore need only two intracellular phosphorylation steps to be converted into their active forms.[36] This circumvents the first and often rate-limiting phosphorylation step.[37,38] Compounds in this group with *in vitro* activity against FIV are adefovir and tenofovir.

Non-Nucleoside Reverse Transcriptase Inhibitors

Unlike NRTIs and NtRTIs, which bind to the catalytic site of reverse transcriptase, NNRTIs interact with a single allosteric site of the enzyme[36] and are not incorporated into the proviral DNA strand.[37] They do not require intracellular activation.[9,37] The interaction with the allosteric site leads to conformational changes within reverse transcriptase.[39,40] This causes a decrease in the interaction between the DNA primer and the polymerase domain of the enzyme and inhibition of virus replication.[39,40] Most NNRTIs are highly specific for HIV. The only compound that has been used in veterinary medicine is suramin.

Nucleoside Analogue DNA/RNA Synthesis Inhibitors

The nucleoside analogue DNA/RNA synthesis inhibitors act similarly to the nucleotide analogues that inhibit reverse transcriptase, but mainly are used for treatment of herpesvirus infections. Nucleoside analogues used in human patients with herpesvirus infections are acyclovir and penciclovir, and their prodrugs valacyclovir and famciclovir, respectively. These drugs are activated by the herpesviral enzyme thymidine kinase (TK), which phosphorylates them to a monophosphate form. Host cell enzymes then phosphorylate the drugs further to triphosphate forms, which concentrate in virus-infected cells and interfere with viral DNA replication by inhibition of the viral DNA polymerase enzyme. The DNA polymerases of different herpesviruses are inhibited to varying degrees by each drug, and thus, not all herpesvirus infections are equally susceptible. Drug resistance results from reduced viral TK activity, altered TK, or altered viral DNA polymerase. The drugs cidofovir, idoxuridine, trifluridine, and vidarabine are not dependent on TK for phosphorylation. Therefore, they have greater host cell toxicity than other drugs that require phosphorylation such as acyclovir. One of those agents regularly used in cats is famciclovir. In small animal medicine, the drugs not depending on viral TK have been mainly used as topical treatments for ocular FHV-1 infections (Table 9.5).

New drugs have recently been developed that have strong efficacy against coronaviruses, including feline coronavirus (FCoV). The nucleoside analogue GS-441524 is the prodrug of remdesivir and thus closely related to remdesivir, the antiviral drug used to treat COVID-19. GS-441524 has recently been evaluated for treatment of FIP, and shows promise, but it is not yet commercially available.[3,5] Ultimately remdesivir may also prove to be an effective treatment for FIP, and more widely available than GS-441524.

Acyclovir

Acyclovir (acycloguanosine, 9-[2-hydroxyethoxymethyl]guanine) is a synthetic nucleoside analogue that is widely used to treat a variety of herpesvirus infections. It interferes with actively replicating herpesviruses, but not when in a latent stage. Acyclovir is given parenterally, orally, and topically in humans to treat mucocutaneous and genital herpesvirus infections caused by herpes simplex virus (HSV), varicella-zoster virus (e.g., shingles), and parenterally to treat herpesvirus encephalitis. Resistance of human herpesviruses to acyclovir occurs. Among the nucleoside analogues, acyclovir exhibits a particular selectivity for herpesvirus over host DNA polymerases because it is only activated in virus-infected cells, and the viral DNA polymerase is 10-fold more sensitive to the activated drug than the host enzyme.

In cats, acyclovir has been used systemically or topically to treat ocular FHV-1 infections. Oral administration of 50 mg/kg acyclovir to cats results in low peak plasma concentrations due to poor bioavailability.[41] Systemic administration can cause bone marrow toxicity.[41] When given in higher doses, the parent drug can precipitate in the renal tubules, causing obstructive nephropathy if diuresis is inadequate. In these cases, needle-shaped acyclovir crystals can be detected in the urine sediment.

TABLE 9.5 Antiviral Drugs Used for Treatment of Feline Herpesvirus Infections

Drug	Dose	Interval	Route	Comments
Famciclovir	90 mg/kg	q8h	PO	Reduce dose for cats with chronic kidney disease.
Cidofovir	0.5% solution	q12h	Topical ophthalmic	Monitor for ocular irritation. Solution prepared from commercial 7.5% intravenous solution by dilution in sterile saline. Diluted solution can be stored up to 6 months at 4°C, –20°C, and –80°C. Can also be obtained from compounding pharmacies.
Idoxuridine	0.1% solution or 0.5% ointment	q4h	Topical ophthalmic	Monitor for ocular irritation and ulceration. Compounding might be required.
Trifluridine	1% solution	q4h	Topical ophthalmic	Might be poorly tolerated.
Vidarabine	3% ointment	q4h	Topical ophthalmic	Well tolerated.
Lysine	250 mg (kittens) 500 mg (cats)	q12h	PO	Questionable efficacy. Bolus administration preferred over dietary supplementation.

CBC, complete blood (cell) count; *PO*, by mouth.

Urinalysis should be performed regularly in long-term acyclovir treatment. Renal failure is reversible with adequate rehydration.

Acyclovir is about 1000-fold less active against FHV-1 *in vitro* than against HSV, and is significantly less active against FHV-1 than other antiherpesviral drugs.[42–44] The main reason for poor efficacy against FHV-1 versus HSV is reduced phosphorylation by FHV-1 TK; the activity of this enzyme is markedly lower in FHV-1 than in HSV.[45] It has been suggested that acyclovir could be combined with human IFN-α or feline IFN-ω in cats because these drugs might have synergistic activity with acyclovir, as demonstrated *in vitro*.[46] Application of acyclovir as 0.5% ophthalmic ointment q5h in cats with ocular disease attributable to FHV-1 led to resolution of clinical signs after 10 days in a nonmasked, nonplacebo-controlled study.[47] However, in cats treated q8h, it took approximately twice as long. Therefore, frequent application (q4h) is necessary, and this, combined with its low activity against FHV-1, limits its use.

Valacyclovir

Valacyclovir (2-[(2-amino-1,6-dihydro-6-oxo-9*H*-purin-9-yl) methoxy] ethyl L-valinate hydrochloride) is a prodrug of acyclovir. It is the L-valine ester of acyclovir and has the same antiviral spectrum but a threefold to fivefold increase in oral bioavailability when compared with acyclovir. In humans, it is mainly used for treatment of herpes zoster, treatment of genital herpesvirus infection, and cytomegalovirus prophylaxis in kidney transplant recipients. In humans, it is rapidly absorbed orally and hydrolyzed to acyclovir and L-valine. Although plasma concentrations of acyclovir exceeding the IC_{50} for FHV-1 can be achieved after oral administration of this drug to cats, cats under treatment have developed renal tubular epithelial and hepatocellular necrosis, and severe bone marrow suppression.[48] Thus, valacyclovir should not be administered to cats.

Ganciclovir

Ganciclovir (2-amino-9-{[(1,3-dihydroxypropan-2-yl)oxy]methyl}-6,9-dihydro-3*H*-purin-6-one) is used to treat human herpesvirus infections.[49] Ganciclovir is a nucleoside analogue of 2′-deoxyguanosine and is phosphorylated to a deoxyguanosine triphosphate analogue, which is the active form. Ganciclovir resembles acyclovir except that it has an additional hydroxymethyl group on its acyclic side chain (see Fig. 9.1). In humans, ganciclovir is widely used to treat cytomegalovirus infections, which can be life threatening in immunocompromised individuals. Systemic administration of ganciclovir to humans is associated with a high incidence of adverse reactions, especially cytopenias and CNS signs; therefore, the use of ganciclovir is limited to humans with life-threatening or sight-threatening infections. It is available for oral or intravenous administration in humans, but is associated with more severe neurologic toxicity, neutropenia, and bacterial infections than is acyclovir.[50,51] Additionally, an intravitreal sustained-release ganciclovir implant has been developed for treatment of cytomegalovirus retinitis in humans,[52] and a 0.15% ophthalmic gel is commercially available for treatment of acute human herpetic keratitis.[53] A prodrug form with improved oral bioavailability (valganciclovir) also has been developed.[54] Ganciclovir is approximately 10-fold more active against FHV-1 *in vitro* than acyclovir.[42,43,55] Anecdotal reports of its topical administration to cats in Europe are very promising. However, safety, efficacy, and pharmacokinetics of ganciclovir or valganciclovir have not been reported in cats.

Penciclovir

Penciclovir (2-amino-9-[4-hydroxy-3-(hydroxymethyl)butyl]-6,9-dihydro-3H-purin-6-one) is a nucleoside deoxyguanosine analogue with a similar mechanism of action to acyclovir. Like acyclovir, it requires viral and cellular phosphorylation. However, it is present at much higher concentrations and for longer duration in cells than is acyclovir, which permits less frequent dosing. Penciclovir is absorbed poorly when given orally, and it is used mainly as a topical treatment (e.g., against HSV in herpes labialis). In a rabbit model of human HSV-1 keratitis, a 3% penciclovir ointment administered one, two, or four times daily decreased the severity of epithelial keratitis. Thus, a topical ophthalmic penciclovir ointment might be effective in cats with FHV-1 ocular disease, but there are no commercially available preparations available for ophthalmic use.[56] While 2-amino-9-(3-acetoxymethyl-4-isopropoxycarbonyloxybut-1-yl)- purine was not successful as an oral prodrug for penciclovir,[57] famciclovir is an effective prodrug of penciclovir with good oral bioavailability.

Whereas acyclovir showed very poor ability to inhibit FHV-1 replication *in vitro*, penciclovir and cidofovir were nearly equally highly effective. When the FHV-1 inoculation dose was raised, penciclovir was more active than cidofovir.[58,59] An implantable cylindrical device made from penciclovir-impregnated silicone for long-term, steady-state delivery of this drug suppressed primary infection of FHV-1 in a cell culture system.[60] Penciclovir-resistant mutants of FHV-1 with altered TK have been described.[59]

Famciclovir

Famciclovir is a prodrug of penciclovir with improved oral bioavailability. In humans with HSV infections and herpes zoster, famciclovir is as effective as acyclovir. In cats, penciclovir (and thus famciclovir) are much more potent inhibitors of FHV-1 replication than acyclovir.

In humans, famciclovir is well absorbed orally and rapidly metabolized to penciclovir.[61] This requires di-deacetylation to BRL42359 in blood, liver, or small intestine, with oxidation to penciclovir by hepatic aldehyde oxidase.[62–64] Most drug is eliminated unchanged in urine. In humans, concurrent food administration decreases peak plasma concentrations without affecting bioavailability. Neither famciclovir nor BRL42359 are active against FHV-1,[65] so metabolism to penciclovir is required. However, hepatic aldehyde oxidase activity in cats is minimal.[66] Famciclovir pharmacokinetics in the cat are complex and nonlinear (i.e., doubling of famciclovir dose does not lead to doubling of plasma penciclovir concentration), presumably due to saturation of the hepatic oxidase.[67,68] High plasma concentrations of BRL42359 accumulate,[67] but clinical responses occur in cats with both acute and chronic clinical signs of FHV-1 infection with negligible adverse effects.[69,70] Responses typically occur within a week of treatment. However, a single dose of famciclovir (125 or 500 mg) administered to cats at shelter intake was not efficacious in reducing clinical signs when 40% of the cats were already shedding FHV-1.[71]

There is controversy about the optimum famciclovir dose in cats. Doses used have ranged from 8 mg/kg q24h[70] to 140 mg/kg q8h.[72,73] In a masked, placebo-controlled trial, cats experimentally infected with FHV-1 and administered famciclovir at 90 mg/kg q8h PO achieved a peak plasma penciclovir concentration of 2100 ng/mL.[69] Compared with control cats, treated cats had reduced clinical signs, serum globulin concentrations, histologic evidence of conjunctivitis, viral shedding and serum FHV-1 titers, as well as increased conjunctival goblet cell density.[69] However, administration of one dose of 40 mg/kg PO to healthy cats achieved nearly identical plasma penciclovir concentrations to those achieved with a dose of 90 mg/kg.[74] Naturally infected client-owned cats with spontaneous disease administered famciclovir at 40 mg/kg q8h had tear penciclovir concentrations likely to be effective against FHV-1 for at least 3 hours after a dose of 40 mg/kg q8h.[73] Based on a study of healthy cats treated with famciclovir at 30, 40, or 90 mg/kg q12h or q8h, it was recommended that cats receive a dose of 90 mg/kg q12h because this regimen achieved comparable plasma and tear penciclovir concentrations to those achieved with 90 mg/kg q8h.[67] Furthermore, when famciclovir was administered to 59 client-owned cats, the median duration of therapy required for clinical improvement was significantly longer in cats administered 40 mg/kg (33 cats) than in cats treated with 90 mg/kg (26 cats).[72] Costs of care were estimated to be lower in the cats treated with the higher dose due to reduction in treatment duration, and potentially the number of recheck examinations required. Adverse events, which were mostly minor gastrointestinal signs, were reported in 17% of cats receiving 40 or 90 mg/kg q8h, with no difference between the two doses.[72] Although famciclovir is safer than acyclovir, cats administered famciclovir should be closely monitored, and assessment of the CBC and serum biochemistry panel should be considered in cats with known concurrent disease or cats expected to receive famciclovir for long periods. As in humans,[75] reduction in dose frequency should be considered in cats with renal disease.[67,72] Human famciclovir tablets are commonly too large for some cats and can be difficult to administer. Some veterinary compounding pharmacies have prepared oral formulations of compounded famciclovir for cats. However, testing of these formulations showed poor quality, inconsistency, and failure to show that the concentrations in these compounded forms were as stated on the label. These products made by veterinary compounding pharmacies failed to meet the United States Pharmacopeia (USP) (www.usp.org) compendial standards for compounded products and thus, cannot be recommended for cats. Instead, veterinarians are encouraged to use a pharmacy that adheres to the USP standard or modify the human-approved tablets.

Cidofovir

Cidofovir is a nucleotide analogue of deoxycytidine monophosphate. Thus, cidofovir already contains a monophosphate group,[76] and its metabolism to the active diphosphate form by host cellular enzymes is not dependent on viral TK. Therefore, it can be used to treat acyclovir- and famciclovir-resistant infections. Its safety arises from its relatively high affinity for viral DNA polymerase compared with human DNA polymerase.[77] In human patients, cidofovir is also used to treat cytomegalovirus retinitis. Cidofovir has extremely low (<5%) oral bioavailability, so it has to be administered intravenously, intravitreally, or topically. Cidofovir has a prolonged intracellular half-life, which enables infrequent parenteral dosing regimens in human patients (weekly, and then every other week for maintenance). Cidofovir applied q12h as a 0.5% or 1.0% ophthalmic solution in rabbit models of human herpetic keratoconjunctivitis was as effective as trifluridine q3–6h.[56,78] This makes it the topical treatment of choice for ocular FHV-1 infections. Local irritation and scarring of the nasolacrimal duct has been reported with topical administration in humans and rabbits with keratoconjunctivitis,[79,80] so treated cats should be monitored for nasolacrimal cicatrization. Cidofovir 0.5% retains efficacy when compounded with saline and refrigerated (4°C) or frozen (–20°C or –80°C) in plastic or glass for up to 6 months.[81] Cidofovir is highly active against FHV-1 *in vitro*.[42,43] It was also effective in a feline whole corneal explant model supporting FHV-1 replication.[82] In cats with experimental FHV-1 infection, cidofovir administration was associated with a significant improvement in clinical scores and ocular virus shedding when compared with placebo.[83]

Cidofovir also has *in vitro* activity against canine herpesvirus-1 (CHV-1).[84] Cidofovir was used to treat dendritic ulcerative keratitis in a 4-year-old dog associated with CHV-1 infection based on positive PCR results and rising serum antibody titers.[85] In dogs with experimentally induced ocular CHV-1 infection, application of topical 0.5% cidofovir ophthalmic solution q12h reduced duration of viral shedding, but caused ocular irritation leading to higher ocular disease scores and higher conjunctival and corneal leukocyte infiltration scores.[84]

Idoxuridine and Trifluridine

Idoxuridine and trifluridine are halogenated thymidine analogues that are phosphorylated by cellular enzymes to active triphosphate forms, which act as pyrimidine antagonists. Both drugs cause myelosuppression when given systemically, and so are only applied topically.[86,87] They are used in humans to treat HSV keratitis and dermatitis. When not commercially available, topical idoxuridine can be obtained from a compounding pharmacy as a 0.1% ophthalmic solution. Trifluridine is available as a 1% ophthalmic solution. Frequent application of both of these drugs is required (q4–6h). Local application is generally well tolerated, but prolonged use can cause corneal irritation or ulceration.[88] Trifluridine has better corneal penetration than idoxuridine,[89] but is more likely to cause ocular irritation in cats than idoxuridine.[90]

Idoxuridine and trifluridine are active against FHV-1 *in vitro*,[43,55] although both are more active against HSV.[43,55] In cats with ocular disease attributed to FHV-1, 0.1% idoxuridine solution was used q4–6h with improvement of clinical signs in three cats and no improvement or worsening in four cats.[87] Treatment with 1% trifluridine solution q4–8h was associated with improvement in one cat and no improvement or worsening in two cats.[87]

Corneal ulcerations associated with a naturally occurring CHV-1 infection appeared to respond to topical idoxuridine or trifluridine treatment.[91] Frequent topical ocular application of 1% trifluridine ophthalmic solution was well tolerated by dogs with experimentally induced recurrent ocular canine CHV-1 infection and reduced disease scores and viral shedding duration.[92]

Vidarabine

Vidarabine (9-β-D-arabinofuranosyladenine monohydrate, adenine arabinoside) is a purine nucleoside that is phosphorylated by host cellular enzymes to vidarabine triphosphate. It was originally developed as a cancer chemotherapeutic. Vidarabine triphosphate disrupts DNA synthesis by interfering with DNA polymerase. It has activity against herpesviruses, poxviruses, and retroviruses, as well as idoxuridine-resistant herpesvirus strains. In humans, it is used to treat smallpox and HSV keratitis, dermatitis, and encephalitis.[93] Systemic toxicity has restricted its use in veterinary practice to topical treatment as a 3% ophthalmic ointment. Local application in cats is well tolerated, but frequent application (q4–6h) is necessary.[90] Where not available commercially, it can be obtained from a compounding pharmacist.[2]

Vidarabine is active against FHV-1 *in vitro*[55] and has been used topically in ocular FHV-1 infections, although cidofovir has largely replaced its use because it can be applied less frequently. In a retrospective study of cats with ocular disease attributed to FHV-1, treatment with vidarabine was associated with improvement in one cat and no improvement or worsening in two cats.[87]

Vidarabine also has *in vitro* activity against FCoV,[94] but studies have not been performed to demonstrate efficacy in cats with FIP.

GS-441524

Treatment with the nucleoside analogue GS-441524, which is the prodrug of the COVID-19 antiviral drug remdesivir, reversed disease in 10 research cats when given subcutaneously once daily for 2 weeks.[3] Two of these cats required a second course of treatment, but were disease-free 8 months later. In a field study, 31 naturally infected cats without neurological or ocular FIP were treated with GS-441524 (2 mg/kg q24h SC, increasing to 4 mg/kg q24h SC).[5] Five of the cats died or were euthanized within 26 days of starting treatment. The remaining 26 cats received the full 12 weeks of treatment, and of these, 8 had relapses in 3 to 84 days, and the remaining 18 were healthy at the time of publication. In some of the cats that relapsed, remissions were obtained with another course of treatment, and ultimately, at the time of publication, 25 cats remained healthy. The time of diagnosis to the time of publication was 18 to 22 months. With increased availability of remdesivir following the COVID-19 pandemic, remdesivir might have the potential to be useful for treatment of FIP although it is less potent than GS-441524.

Nucleotide Synthesis Inhibitors

There are two types of nucleotide synthesis inhibitors: (1) pyrophosphate analogues that directly inhibit DNA and RNA polymerase (e.g., foscarnet) and (2) inhibitors of triphosphate synthesis that inhibit inosine monophosphate dehydrogenase, an essential enzyme for synthesis of nucleotides (e.g., ribavirin). Nucleotide synthesis inhibitors usually have a broad antiviral spectrum but also marked toxicity.

Foscarnet

Foscarnet (phosphonoformic acid, PFA) has *in vitro* activity against FIV, FeLV, and FHV-1.[95,96] However, its short half-life, poor oral absorption, and adverse effects have limited its use in cats. No *in vivo* studies in cats with virus infections have been published.

Ribavirin

Ribavirin (1-β-D-ribofuranosyl-1H-1,2,4-triazole-3-carboxamide, RTCA) is active against a significant number of feline and canine viruses *in vitro*, including FIV, FeLV, FHV-1, FCV, FCoV, Borna disease virus (BDV), as well as CDV and canine parainfluenza virus.[97–99] However, its clinical usefulness is limited because of its systemic toxicity, and it is not used in veterinary medicine. It is also no longer recommended for treatment in humans. Still, ribavirin might have the potential to be a promising drug for treating dogs with CDV. Further studies are required for understanding pharmacokinetics and toxicity of ribavirin in dogs.

Protease Inhibitors

Protease inhibitors are widely used to treat HIV infection and hepatitis C in humans. They prevent viral replication by selectively binding to viral proteases and blocking proteolytic cleavage of protein precursors needed for the production of infectious viral particles. Protease inhibitors currently on the market are highly selective for HIV and are not active against FIV. However, experimentally designed protease inhibitors had activity against FIV or FIV/HIV chimeras.[100–102] In addition, commercially available protease inhibitors, such as nelfinavir, have been evaluated for their activity against FCoV, and new protease inhibitors with potential activity against FCoV have been engineered.[103] The use of nelfinavir was also reported in a few cats with FIP in the field,[104,105] but toxicity and pharmacokinetics of nelfinavir in cats and its efficacy for treatment of FIP in controlled studies remains unknown.

GS376

Inhibitors that target 3C-like protease with broad-spectrum activity against important human and animal coronaviruses have recently been created.[106] One protease inhibitor (GS376) was shown to have activity against FCoV *in vitro*[107] and was effective to treat FIP in an experimental setting, but is not yet commercially available. Prolonged remissions were documented in some naturally infected cats. In one field study, 6 of 20 cats were in remission 18 months after 12 weeks of treatment, administered subcutaneously twice a day.[4] One of the challenges was treatment of neurologic FIP, likely because of failure of drug penetration of the CNS. Further field studies with this drug are required, and the compound is not yet commercially available.

Receptor Blockers

Receptor blockers belong to a group of antiviral drugs known as *entry inhibitors*, which also include fusion inhibitors. Receptor blockers are either homologs or antagonists of cellular viral receptors or co-receptors. If receptor blockers bind to the virus or to the cellular receptor, they inhibit attachment of the virus to the cell surface. Most receptor blockers on the market or under development are highly selective for HIV and not useful for veterinary medicine. One exception are bicyclams (e.g., plerixafor), because of the similarity between HIV and FIV in regards to chemokine receptor usage.[108–112] Plerixafor (1,1'-(1,4-phenylenbismethylene)-bis(1,4,8,11-tetraazacyclotetradecane)-octachlo-ride dehydrate, AMD3100) is the prototype bicyclam drug. It is used in humans for stem cell mobilization.[113] Plerixafor is active against FIV *in vitro*.[114] In naturally FIV-infected cats in a placebo-controlled double-blind clinical trial, treatment with plerixafor resulted in a significant decrease in provirus load, but also a decrease in serum magnesium levels, which however was not clinically relevant.[115] It has been administered to cats at a dose of 0.5 mg/kg q12h. Magnesium and calcium levels should be monitored during treatment.[115]

Integrase Inhibitors

The retroviral enzyme integrase catalyzes strand transfer (3′-end joining), which inserts both proviral DNA ends into a host cell chromosome. The high degree of conservation of integrase active sites for many retroviruses suggests that FIV and FeLV could be sensitive to integrase inhibitors.[116]

Raltegravir

In human patients, raltegravir is approved for treatment of HIV infections and is used in combination with other antiretroviral drugs.

Raltegravir is highly active *in vitro* against FeLV.[116,117] Concentrations in the effective range were not toxic to cell monolayers. However, raltegravir is partly eliminated as glucuronide. Some (but not all) glucuronide pathways are deficient in cats. This might increase the risk of toxicity in cats.[113] The efficacy and safety of raltegravir in a noncontrolled study of seven cats with experimentally induced progressive FeLV infection was investigated.[118] Raltegravir was administered at 40 mg q12h PO for 6.5 weeks and then 80 mg q12h PO for 2.5 weeks. The treatment reduced viremia in each cat, with up to 1 $\log_{10}$ reduction in viral RNA in four of seven cats, and the drug attained therapeutic plasma concentrations at both doses, with no adverse effects noted. However, viremia rebounded in all cats following drug removal. Raltegravir also had activity against FHV-1 in cell culture as well as in a feline whole corneal explant model.[82]

Nucleocapsid Inhibitors

Nucleocapsid inhibitors interact with viral assembly and disassembly through NCp7 zinc finger-targeted agents.[119] Such zinc finger inhibitors or zinc ejectors are compounds that interact adversely with zinc and cause them to release their zinc from its binding site, disrupting the conformation of the polypeptide chain and rendering the zinc fingers ineffective, thereby preventing them from performing their associated cellular functions. Zinc fingers are involved in mRNA regulation, reverse transcription, protection of synthesized viral DNA, transcription inhibition, and initial integration processes. Nucleocapsid inhibitors are used to treat HIV, but many other human viruses, such as Ebola virus, measles virus, and polio virus, have similar zinc finger motifs and could potentially benefit from zinc finger inhibitor technology. Several novel nucleocapsid inhibitors, such as fused tetrathiocines, bis[1,2]dithiolo[1,4]thiazines and bis[1,2]dithiolopyrrole derivatives, and 5-thieno-, 5-oxo-, and 5-imino-1,2,3-dithiazole derivatives, have been synthesized and evaluated for activity against FIV. These new compounds display potent nanomolar activity and low toxicity against FIV *in vitro*,[61,120,121] but they are not yet available.

Neuraminidase Inhibitors

Neuraminidase inhibitors prevent release of virus from the host cell. They inhibit virus replication by binding the viral enzyme neuraminidase, a viral surface glycoprotein. Oseltamivir is the only agent from this class that has been used in cats and dogs.

Oseltamivir

Oseltamivir, ethyl (3R,4R,5S)-5-amino-4-acetamido-3-(pentan-3-yloxy)-cyclohex-1-ene-1-carboxylate, is the prodrug of oseltamivir carboxylate, a potent inhibitor of influenza virus neuraminidase (Fig. 9.2). Oseltamivir is active against viruses that have neuraminidase in their envelope, including influenza viruses, parainfluenza viruses, and paramyxoviruses, and is used in the treatment and prophylaxis of influenza virus A and influenza virus B infections in humans. The viral neuraminidase cleaves sialic acid residues on the surface of infected cells, which allows new virus particles to be released from host cells. It also prevents aggregation of virus particles after they are released and facilitates spread of virus through the mucus of the respiratory tract by cleaving sialic acid residues in mucin.

Oseltamivir was the first orally active neuraminidase inhibitor to be commercially developed. It is a prodrug, which is hydrolyzed in the liver to an active metabolite, the free carboxylate of oseltamivir. A lipophilic side chain of the active drug binds to the viral neuraminidase, blocking its ability to cleave sialic acid residues, resulting in an inability of cells to release progeny virions. In humans and dogs, oseltamivir has high oral bioavailability.[122] Oseltamivir is used early in the course of human influenza to shorten the duration of illness by approximately 20 hours.

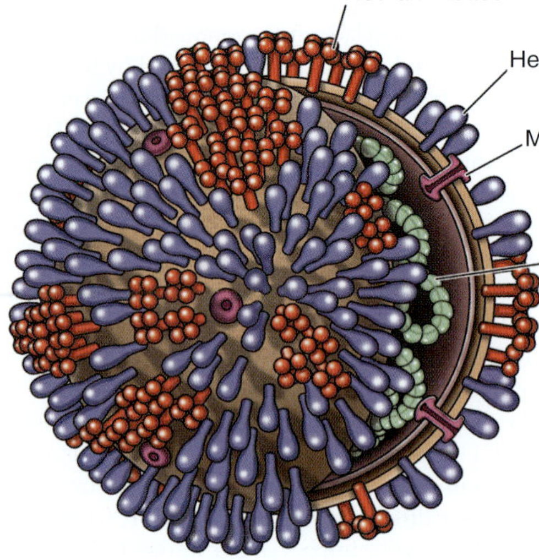

Fig. 9.2 Structure of an influenza virus. The M2 protein, which is only present in influenza A viruses, is inhibited by tricyclic amines such as amantadine. Oseltamivir inhibits the viral neuraminidase.

Oseltamivir has been used to treat canine parvovirus enteritis in puppies, with anecdotal reports of improved outcome. Although it does not have activity against CPV, and CPV does not possess a neuraminidase, it was used in a prospective, randomized, masked, placebo-controlled trial of 35 dogs with CPV-induced enteritis. Dogs treated with oseltamivir (2 mg/kg PO q12h) had no significant drop in their white blood cell count, whereas untreated dogs had white blood cell count decrease in the first 5 days of hospitalization.[123] Treated dogs also gained weight during hospitalization, whereas untreated dogs lost weight. However, there was no difference in hospitalization time, treatments needed, clinical scores, morbidity, or mortality between the two groups, and the number of dogs in each group was small. As CPV has no neuraminidase, it was hypothesized that oseltamivir instead might act on the neuraminidases of bacteria that are normally responsible for secondary bacterial infections in CPV enteritis, which are primarily those of the gastrointestinal tract. The role of bacterial neuraminidases in the pathogenesis of enteric bacterial infections and bacterial translocation is unknown. Bacterial neuraminidase enzymes might play a role in biofilm formation and help bacteria to invade mucin layers of the respiratory tract.[123,124] It has been suggested that gut bacteria might use neuraminidase to cleave sialic acid residues on gastrointestinal epithelial cells, which exposes receptor sites for bacterial adherence.

Ion Channel Blockers

The uncoating of viruses can be blocked by ion channel blockers that bind to viral proteins, such as influenza A virus M2 proteins, which normally function as ion channels for proton influx into the virus. Blocking the M2 protein leads to a pH change that inhibits viral fusion and internalization of the virus by endocytosis. Cycloalkylamine derivatives are used for this purpose in human medicine, mainly against influenza virus infections. Amantadine is the most important example of a cycloalkylamine derivative, and the only one that has been used in veterinary medicine. Related drugs include rimantadine, which has equal or greater efficacy to amantadine with reduced CNS adverse effects but more gastrointestinal irritation, and tromantadine, which is used topically to treat human herpesvirus infection. New experimental compounds that inhibit viroporins, viral proteins with ion channel activity that are possessed by several viruses, including FCoV, have been investigated *in vitro*,[125] but are not commercially available.

Amantadine

Amantadine (tricyclo[3,3,1,13,7]dec-l-ylamine hydrochloride, L-adamantanamine) is a stable cyclic amine with activity against enveloped RNA viruses. Amantadine was once applied as prophylaxis of human influenza, but it is rarely used for this indication currently because there are newer more potent agents available. As a dopaminergic drug, amantadine has been used to treat Parkinson's disease, cocaine dependence, and apathy in multiple sclerosis. It has also been also used in cats and dogs to treat neuropathic pain and osteoarthritis.[126] Data on the usefulness of amantadine in dogs and cats as an antiviral drug are limited. Amantadine was active against BDV *in vitro* in one study,[127] but in a different study, there was no *in vitro* activity in concentrations that were effective against influenza virus.[128] Anecdotal reports of successful outcomes following amantadine treatment exist in cats with BDV infection in northern Europe.

Antiviral Amino Acids

Amino acids and peptides can act as antivirals when they competitively inhibit translation and virus assembly.

L-Lysine

Initial interest in L-lysine arose from *in vitro* data and clinical trials in humans.[129]Arginine is essential for FHV-1[130] and HSV[131] replication, and it has been suggested that lysine antagonizes the availability or utilization of arginine by these viruses during protein synthesis. Protein fraction-I of the histone layer around the DNA of the eukaryotic or host cells is 28% L-lysine and 3% to 4% arginine. In contrast, the capsid protein composition of herpesviruses has approximately three times more arginine than lysine.[132] Thus, it was originally hypothesized to preferentially affect protein synthesis of the virus over that of the host because viral proteins had a higher arginine-to-lysine content than did human (and feline) proteins[132]; however, recent analyses suggested that the difference in feline and FHV-1 protein amino acid content is minimal.[133] Both an excess arginine and an absence of arginine interferes with the replication of HSV *in vitro*.[134,135] Excess L-lysine in the media has the same effect, likely by acting as an analogue of arginine, or by competing for cellular transport mechanisms, or both.[131,136] Markedly elevated L-lysine concentrations in combination with low arginine concentrations suppressed HSV-1[131,135] and FHV-1[130] replication *in vitro*. However, this did not occur with physiologic amino acid concentrations.[137] In a more recent study, various L-lysine concentrations did not inhibit *in vitro* replication of FHV-1 at arginine concentrations sufficient to maintain cell growth.[137] Thus, data on *in vitro* activity of L-lysine are controversial.

L-lysine is inexpensive and well tolerated in cats, with only mild and reversible gastrointestinal disturbances reported for some cats.[138] No adverse effects were seen in cats fed diets supplemented to up to 8.6% (dry matter) with L-lysine.[139] However, *in vivo* data regarding the efficacy of L-lysine in cats with FHV-1 infection are also contradictory. Although L-lysine is promoted by sponsors of dietary supplements for cats (which are not FDA regulated), the clinical results have not shown a benefit in naturally occurring infections. A recent meta-analysis, published by two biologists who owned cats with chronic FHV-1 infection presented multiple levels of evidence that L-lysine supplementation is not effective for the prevention or treatment of FHV-1 infection in cats.[133] Lysine does not antagonize arginine in cats, and evidence that low intracellular arginine concentrations would inhibit viral replication is lacking. Furthermore, lowering arginine levels is undesirable since cats cannot synthesize this amino acid themselves, and arginine deficiency might result in hyperammonemia, which could be fatal. Contradictory to this meta-analysis, administration of 500 mg L-lysine PO q12h beginning 6 hours before inoculation of cats with FHV-1 was associated with less severe conjunctivitis without a change in virus shedding when compared with placebo.[138] The effects of L-lysine administration on clinical signs and ocular shedding of FHV-1 were studied after reactivation of latent infection. Treated cats had fewer viral shedding episodes after stress of rehousing compared with the control group cats. Fewer cats and eyes had conjunctivitis, and onset of clinical signs of infection was delayed in cats receiving L-lysine.[140] In cats latently infected following experimental inoculation but without clinical signs at the time of the study, oral administration of 400 mg L-lysine q24h reduced viral shedding compared with placebo-treated cats.[140] However, in the only study to assess bolus administration of L-lysine in naturally infected cats, 144 shelter-housed cats received 250 mg (kittens) or 500 mg (adult cats) L-lysine q24h for their entire shelter stay. Outcomes were compared with an untreated control group. No significant treatment effect was detected for any parameter.[141] There was concern that the stress of tablet administration actually contributed to disease in these cats. Dietary supplementation with L-lysine also appears to have no beneficial impact on upper respiratory tract disease in shelters.[141–143] In fact, cats that received a supplemented diet had more severe disease and more frequent viral shedding than cats that received a nonsupplemented diet, despite a detectable increase in plasma lysine concentrations.[143] The supplemented diet did not affect plasma arginine concentration; therefore, altered arginine levels did not contribute to increased disease severity.[2] Thus, L-lysine has not demonstrated clear benefit in naturally occurring infections.

IMMUNOSTIMULANT DRUGS

"Immunomodulator" is a nonspecific term that has also been referred to as biologic response modifiers. These drugs include agents that suppress the immune system (e.g., glucocorticoids) and those that stimulate the immune system. In this chapter, only drugs that stimulate the immune system are discussed. Some of these compounds not only affect the immune system but also possess antiviral activity (e.g., IFNs). Probiotics also have immunomodulatory activity and have been used to treat viral infections (e.g., FHV-1).[83,144] These compounds are discussed in Chapter 125. Specific neutralizing antibodies (passive immunization), such as against FHV-1, FCV, FPV, CPV, CDV, and infectious canine hepatitis virus, have also been used for treatment of virus infections with variable results[145–147] but are not the subject of this chapter. Vaccines, such as intranasal vaccines, also have been used as therapeutic immunomodulators (see Chapter 20).

Categories of immunomodulators are shown in Table 9.6. Treatment of canine and feline viral infections with immunostimulating drugs has commonly produced disappointing results. Data from large, prospective, controlled clinical trials are lacking, and many are used infrequently or are not widely available (Table 9.7). Because of this, only those currently in use that appear to have some clinical benefit are discussed in detail. Doses of immunostimulants evaluated in dogs and cats are shown in Table 9.8.

Naturally Occurring Cytokines

Interferons

Interferons are polypeptide molecules that mediate antiviral and antigrowth responses and modulate the immune response.[148] A number of

TABLE 9.6 Immunostimulating Drugs Examined For Activity Against Canine and Feline Viral Infections

Category	Subcategory	Examples
Naturally occurring cytokines	Interferons	IFN-α, IFN-β, IFN-ω, IFN-γ
	Colony-stimulating factors	G-CSF, GM-CSF, erythropoietin
Naturally occurring biologic response modifiers	Mammalian- and insect-derived biologic response modifiers	Lactoferrin, melittin
	Microorganism-derived biologic response modifiers	Bacille Calmette-Guérin, staphylococcal protein A, staphylococcal phage lysate, *Serratia marcescens*, *Cutibacterium acnes*, parapoxvirus ovis (PIND-ORF)
	Plant-derived biologic response modifiers	Acemannan, polyprenyl immunostimulant, *Galanthus nivalis*-like compound, lambda-carrageenan, fucoidan, proanthocyanidin A2
Synthetic compounds	Antiparasitic and antibacterial compounds	Levamisole, diethylcarbamazine, mefloquine, ivermectin, doxycycline
	Other synthetic compounds	Pentoxifylline, propentofylline, leflunomide, indomethacin, suberoylanilide hydroxamine

G-CSF, granulocyte colony-stimulating factor; *GM-CSF,* granulocyte-macrophage colony-stimulating factor; *IFN,* interferon.

different interferons have been identified that are subdivided into type I, type II, and type III interferons.[149] IFN-α, IFN-β, IFN-ω, and IFN-γ have been used in veterinary medicine. The first three belong to type I IFNs, while IFN-γ is a type II IFN. Type I interferons (IFN-α, IFN-β, and IFN-ω) are produced by virus-infected cells,[88,150] whereas type II interferon (IFN-γ) is produced by activated T cells and natural killer cells in response to recognition of infected cells.[151]

Interferons bind to specific cell surface receptors and stimulate expression of proteins that interfere with various stages of viral replication.[152] Viral protein synthesis is not affected, so the antiviral activity of interferons is thought to be related to interference with later stages of viral replication, such as virion assembly and release.[150,153] Interferons also trigger virus-infected cells to undergo apoptosis.[151,153] Thus, interferons prevent the spread of virus from infected cells and aid in the clearance of viral infection.[151] Recombinant interferons that are commercially available, mostly used in cats and dogs, are human IFN-α and feline IFN-ω. IFN-γ plays a critical role in the clearance of intracellular pathogens by macrophages. Recombinant human IFN-γ has been used to treat chronic granulomatous disease caused by intracellular bacteria and fungi in humans, but few studies have been performed in cats and dogs. Low-dose feline IFN-γ and interleukin (IL)-12, experimentally prepared by a method known as *Sequential Kinetic Activated*, have been used in cats experimentally infected with FHV-1 with some success.[154] Recombinant adenoviruses engineered to contain IFN-γ genes had antiviral activity against CPV.[155]

Human Interferon-α. Naturally occurring IFN-α represents a group of more than 20 molecules that vary slightly in composition. They inhibit viral nucleic acid and protein synthesis. A variety of recombinant and natural human IFN-α preparations are available, including pegylated forms that have prolonged half-lives. IFN-α is active against many DNA and RNA viruses.[152] There are two common treatment regimens for use of IFN-α in cats, SC injection of high-dose (10^4 to 10^6 IU/kg q24h) IFN-α or oral application of low-dose (1 to 50 IU/kg q24h) IFN-α. When given parenterally to cats, human IFN-α becomes ineffective after 3 to 7 weeks because of development of neutralizing antibodies.[33] IFN-α can be given orally for a longer period, as no antibodies will develop during oral treatment. Given orally, IFN-α is inactivated by gastric acid and destroyed by trypsin and other proteolytic enzymes in the duodenum.[156] Therefore, immunomodulatory activity is thought to result from stimulation of oropharyngeal lymphoid tissue, which leads to cytokine release and a cascade of immunologic responses that ultimately act systemically.[157,158]

IFN-α is active against FIV *in vitro*.[159] Although it is sometimes used for treatment of FIV-infected cats, no controlled studies that evaluated the effect of high-dose parenteral human IFN-α in FIV-infected cats have been conducted. Use of low-dose oral human IFN-α in sick cats with natural FIV infections (50 IU/kg on the oral mucosa q24h for 7 days on alternating weeks for 6 months, followed by a 2-month break, and then repetition of the 6-month treatment) resulted in improvement of clinical signs in a placebo-controlled double-blind study.[160]

In vitro, FeLV replication is inhibited by human IFN-α.[161] Treatment of cats that had persistently high FeLV antigenemia with high-dose SC human IFN-α following experimental infection resulted in decreases in circulating FeLV antigen beginning 2 weeks after initiation of therapy.[33] However, because of anti-IFN-α antibody development, cats became refractory to therapy after several weeks.[33] In a placebo-controlled double-blind study in naturally FeLV-infected cats, a similar high-dose treatment regimen with human IFN-α (1×10^5 IU/kg SC q24h for 6 weeks) did not lead to improvement of clinical, laboratory, immunologic, or virologic parameters.[34] Low-dose oral IFN-α was used in a placebo-controlled study in experimentally induced FeLV infection.[157] Eight cats were treated with 0.5 IU/cat and five were treated with 5 IU/cat on 7 consecutive days on alternate weeks for a period of 1 month after challenge. There was no difference in development of viremia between groups, but treated cats had fewer clinical signs and longer survival times than the placebo group (with a better response in the cats given 0.5 IU). Uncontrolled field studies have reported apparent responses in a limited number of cats treated with low-dose oral IFN-α.[162,163] Significantly longer survival times were reported in 69 clinically affected cats treated with low-dose oral IFN-α (30 IU/kg for 7 consecutive days on a 1-week-on 1-week-off schedule) when compared with historical controls.[163] However, in a placebo-controlled study, treatment of sick client-owned FeLV-infected cats with the same protocol did not result in a significant difference in FeLV status, survival time, clinical or hematologic parameters, or subjective improvement in the owners' impression when compared with a placebo group.[164] Improvement in clinical signs and laboratory abnormalities in FeLV-infected cats were noted with low-dose oral IFN-α in other studies,[165,166] but concern was raised about evidence of a rebound effect after treatment was discontinued. These studies lacked a control group.

In vitro studies with dosages of 1×10^5 to 5×10^5 IU/mL of IFN-α showed reduced FHV-1 concentration and FHV-1-induced cytopathic effects without observable cytotoxicity to a feline corneal cell line[167] or Crandell-Rees feline kidney (CRFK) cells.[168] Administration of 108 IU/kg IFN-α SC q12h for 2 days (beginning a day before challenge) to 12 kittens experimentally infected with FHV-1 led to reduction of clinical signs over a 14-day period when compared with placebo.[169] FCV replication is also inhibited when cell cultures are treated with

TABLE 9.7 Immunostimulants with Unclear Benefit for Treatment of Canine and Feline Viral Infections

Name	Description	Proposed Mechanism	Activity
Melittin	26-amino acid peptide, component honey bee venom	Viral membrane lysis	*In vitro*, HIV, murine leukemia viruses, tobacco mosaic virus, HSV, FIV. Not effective in double-masked, placebo-controlled pilot study of 20 FIV-infected cats (500 μg/kg SC q12h for 6 weeks) or placebo.[226]
Staphylococcus aureus phage lysate and purified staphylococcal protein A (SPA)	Phage lysate: components of *Staphylococcus aureus* and a bacteriophage. Staphylococcal protein A (SPA): polypeptide purified from cell walls of *Staphylococcus aureus* Cowan I.	Combines with immune complexes at the Fc region of IgG. Activation of complement, T cells, natural killer cells, and IFN-γ production.	Available commercially for treatment of canine pyoderma (see Chapter 119). No clear benefit of SPA when used to treat cats with natural or experimental FeLV infections.[164,227]
Cutibacterium acnes (formerly *Propionibacterium acnes*)	Inactivated bacteria	Stimulates macrophage release of cytokines and IFNs, enhances T-cell and natural killer cell activity in mice	Used as adjunct treatment for chronic recurrent canine pyoderma (see Chapter 119). Moderately sized uncontrolled studies suggested clinical benefit in cats with FeLV infection in conjunction with supportive care, but no prospective or controlled studies have been performed.[228,229] In one study, 74 cats with experimentally induced FIP received *C. acnes*, SC IFN-α, a combination, or placebo. Administration of *C. acnes* in combination with IFN-α did not reduce mortality in treated *versus* untreated cats, but the mean survival time was prolonged for 3 weeks.[230]
Inactivated parapoxvirus avis (PIND-AVI) and parapoxvirus ovis (PIND-ORF) (Europe)	Inactivated poxviruses	"Paramunity inducers." Might induce IFNs and colony-stimulating factors and activate natural killer cells.	No benefit in placebo-controlled trials for treatment of FeLV infection,[231,232] feline upper respiratory tract disease,[233] or CPV infection.[234]
Acemannan	Mucopolysaccharide derived from aloe vera plant	Stimulates macrophages to secrete a variety of cytokines, including IFN-γ, TNF-α, prostaglandin E2, IL-1, and IL-6	Veterinary product available for intralesional injection of canine and feline tumors, including feline injection-site sarcomas.[235,236] Beneficial effects reported in uncontrolled trial of clinically affected FIV-infected cats for 12 weeks (IV or SC once weekly or PO q24h).[237] Immunostimulatory effects might promote viral replication. No clear benefit in a non-controlled trial of 50 cats with FeLV infection (2 mg/kg IP every 7 days for 6 weeks).[238]
Galanthus nivalis agglutinin	Mannose-binding plant lectin	Antineoplastic, antifungal, and antiviral activities. Blocks fusion of HIV with target cells and results in deletion of glycan in the HIV envelope protein, which triggers formation of neutralizing antibody against exposed epitopes.[239]	*In vitro* activity against feline coronavirus in combination with nelfinavir.[104]
Lambda-carrageenan	Seaweed extract that contains sulfated polysaccharides		*In vitro* activity against FHV-1. Ophthalmic application did not reduce clinical signs in small numbers of cats infected with FHV-1.[240]
Fucoidan	Sulfated polysaccharide in brown algae and brown seaweed	May inhibit viral infection by interfering with early steps of virus replication and inhibiting virus-mediated cell fusion.[241]	*In vitro* activity against CDV.[241]
Proanthocyanidin A2	Phenolic dimer, condensed tannin present in plants such as lychee	Antioxidant, anti-inflammatory, and antimicrobial properties.[242,243]	CDV.[244,245]
Mefloquine	4-quinolinemethanol derivative, antimalarial	Prevents viral replication	JC virus, FCV (additive with rfIFN-ω).[246]
Suberoylanilide hydroxamine	Synthetic compound	Binds to active site of histone deacetylases and chelates zinc ions. Antineoplastic, antifibrotic, and anti-inflammatory activity	Activates latent HIV infections for immune recognition and destruction.[247] When administered with food to 4 FIV latently infected research cats and 1 uninfected control cat, associated with an increase in FIV RNA and decrease in viral DNA burden.

CPV, canine parovirus; *FCV*, feline calicivirus; *FeLV*, feline leukemia virus; *FHV-1*, feline herpesvirus-1; *FIP*, feline infectious peritonitis; *FIV*, feline immunodeficiency virus; *HIV*, human immunodeficiency virus; *HSV*, herpes simplex virus; *IFN*, interferon; *IL*, interleukin; *JC virus*, John Cunningham virus; rfIFN-ω, recombinant feline interferon-ω; TNF, tumor necrosis factor.

TABLE 9.8 Doses of Commercially Available Immunomodulators Used to Treat Infectious Diseases of Dogs and Cats

Drug	Dose	Interval	Species	Route	Comments
Acemannan	2 mg/kg	Weekly	C	SC	For treatment of fibrosarcomas; efficacy unclear for FIV and FeLV infections
Feline recombinant interferon omega	1 million U/kg	q24h for 5 consecutive days on days 0, 14, and 60	C, D	SC	For FeLV infections
	0.1 million U/kg	q24	C	Oromucosal	For refractory caudal stomatitis associated with FCV infection
Filgrastim	5 μg/kg	q24h	C, D	SC	Monitor CBC weekly during treatment. Long-term use (>2 weeks) can lead to development of neutralizing antibodies.
Lactoferrin	200 mg powder or 40 mg/kg solution	q24h	C	Topical	For refractory gingivitis and stomatitis. Must be purchased from chemical suppliers
Lymphocyte T-cell immunomodulator	1 mL	Weekly	C	SC	For treatment of FeLV and FIV infections
Human recombinant interferon alpha	10^4 to 10^6 U/kg	q24h	C	SC	Monitor CBC weekly during parenteral treatment. Long-term parenteral use can lead to development of neutralizing antibodies
	1 to 50 U/cat	q24h		PO	
Pentoxifylline	15 mg/kg	q8h	D	PO	Benefits for treatment of FIP unclear. Co-administration of cytochrome P450 inhibitors may increase serum drug concentrations
	¼ of a 400 mg tablet	q8h	C		
Polyprenyl immunostimulant	3 mg/kg	Three times weekly	C	PO	Possible benefit for treatment of noneffusive FIP
Cutibacterium acnes, killed (formerly *Propionibacterium acnes*)	0.1 mg dogs < 7 kg 0.2 mg 7–20 kg 0.4 mg 20–34 kg 0.8 mg > 34 kg	Twice weekly. After 14 days, weekly until remission, and monthly thereafter to maintain remission	D	IV	For pyoderma. Available as a 0.4 mg/mL solution
Staphylococcus aureus phage lysate	0.5 mL	Once or twice weekly	D	SC	For pyoderma

CBC, complete blood count; *FCV*, feline calicivirus; *FeLV*, feline leukemia virus; *FIP*, feline infectious peritonitis; *FIV*, feline immunodeficiency virus.

IFN-α.[170] When IFN-α was given SC (10^5 IU/kg q24h for 14 days) to seven shelter cats with chronic upper respiratory tract disease that tested positive for FHV-1 or FCV by PCR, there was some improvement of clinical signs,[171] but further studies are needed to evaluate this approach in a larger cat population. IFN-α also has been administered orally to FHV-1 infected cats, but no controlled studies have been performed.[87] In cats with ocular disease, topical IFN-α q4-6h for 1 week beyond clinical resolution has been recommended. In cats with naturally occurring viral keratoconjunctivitis, ocular administration of high doses of IFN-α q12h for 14 days did not improve clinical disease or virus shedding when compared with saline.[172] With availability of famciclovir, topical IFN-α is used less frequently, or it is being used in combination with other drugs, based on observations of *in vitro* synergistic activity against FHV-1 or HSV-1 when combined with acyclovir.[46,173] Investigations of the efficacy of nucleoside analogues in combination with IFN-α in cats are warranted.

The antiviral activity of IFN-α against a FIP-causing FCoV strain was demonstrated *in vitro*.[174] A combination of IFN-α with ribavirin resulted in antiviral effects that were greater than the sum of the effects from either ribavirin or IFN-α alone,[174] but the combination was not effective *in vivo*. In one study, 74 cats (52 treated, 22 controls) with experimentally induced FIP received IFN-α, *Cutibacterium acnes*, a combination, or placebo. Prophylactic and therapeutic administration of high-dose (10^4 or 10^6 IU/kg) IFN-α did not reduce mortality in treated cats, but the mean survival time in cats treated with 10^6 IU/kg IFN-α with *C. acnes* was significantly prolonged for 3 weeks.[175]

IFN-α inhibits replication of CDV *in vitro*, with or without ribavirin,[176] but no *in vivo* studies have been published. IFN-α has been used to treat dogs with viral papillomatosis, but controlled studies are lacking.[177] In humans with papillomatosis, IFN-α has been used at 10^6 IU/person parenterally until regression occurred. A similar treatment regimen, intralesional injection or oral low-dose treatment, might be effective in dogs.

Feline Interferon-ω. Recombinant feline interferon-ω (IFN-ω) is licensed for use in cats and dogs in Europe, Asia, and Australia. It is not available in the United States. It has been used for treatment of viral infections in cats and dogs as well as for treatment of some tumors (e.g., feline mammary tumors)[178] and canine atopic dermatitis.[179] In healthy dogs, IFN-ω enhances the activities of whole blood cells, macrophages, and natural killer cells.[180] IFN-ω is produced in silkworms using a recombinant baculovirus. It can be used in cats for long periods without antibody development.[150] In FIV and FeLV infection, a dose of 10^6 IU/kg SC q24h on 5 consecutive days is suggested. No severe adverse effects have been reported in cats,[181] but transient lethargy, fever, vomiting, mild diarrhea, and anorexia have been documented in some treated cats, especially at higher doses (2.5×10^6 U/kg). Mild neutropenia, eosinophilia, and reversible increases of serum AST activity have also been described.[182] IFN-ω inhibits the replication of

FIV,[159] FeLV,[183] FCoV,[184] FHV-1 and FCV,[167,168,170] FPV and CPV,[184] and CDV[185] *in vitro*.

When used in a placebo-controlled multicenter trial to treat 62 naturally FIV-infected cats (10^6 IU/kg SC q24h on 5 consecutive days), there were no changes in survival in treated cats when compared with a placebo group, although some clinical improvement was noted.[181] In naturally FIV-infected cats housed in a shelter, clinical improvement was observed, but there was no control group included. Oral administration of a lower dose of IFN-ω (10^5 U/cat PO q24h for 90 days) to clinically affected, naturally FIV-infected cats was associated with improvement of clinical scores.[186] The improvement was not different from that observed in a historical control group treated with 10^6 IU/kg SC IFN-ω, which suggested that PO administration of the lower dose of IFN-ω could be used as an alternative to the licensed protocol at reduced cost. In a follow-up study of naturally FIV-infected cats treated either with PO or SC IFN-ω, there was no change in viremia and most cytokine concentrations measured,[187] which raised questions about the efficacy noted in the previous trials that lacked placebo-treated controls. It is possible that the clinical improvement observed resulted from an effect of IFN-ω on secondary infections rather than on the FIV infection itself.[150] Indeed, 16 naturally FIV- and/or FeLV-infected cats that were followed for 65 days during IFN-ω treatment had reduced excretion of co-infecting viruses (FCV, FHV-1, FCoV, and FPV).[88] Additional randomized, placebo-controlled, and double-blind studies are required to fully determine the efficacy of IFN-ω for treatment of FIV infections.

In one study, 48 cats with naturally occurring FeLV infection were treated with IFN-ω (10^6 IU/kg SC q24h SQ for 5 days). This treatment was applied three times, separated by several treatment-free weeks. There was a significant difference in the survival time of treated versus placebo-treated cats in a 9-month follow-up period, but not after 1 year.[181] Some clinical improvement was noted with IFN-ω treatment of FeLV-infected cats housed in a shelter, but no placebo group was included.[88] No studies have been published on the use of PO low-dose IFN-ω in FeLV-infected cats.

In an uncontrolled study, 12 cats that were suspected to have FIP were treated with IFN-ω in combination with glucocorticoids and supportive care.[188] Although most cats died, four cats with abdominal effusion survived 2 years, suggesting that treatment of cats with IFN-ω might increase survival time. In a randomized double-blind treatment trial, 34 cats with FIP were treated with glucocorticoids in conjunction with placebo or IFN-ω (10^6 IU/kg SC q48h until clinical improvement, then once weekly).[189] In all cats, FIP was confirmed by histology and/or immunohistochemical or immunofluorescent staining of FCoV antigen in effusion or tissue macrophages. Some cats in both groups survived for weeks to months (longest survival 200 days). There was, however, no significant difference in the mean survival time or quality of life of cats treated with IFN-ω when compared with placebo.[189]

At higher concentrations, the effect of IFN-ω on FHV-1 replication appears to be greater than that of IFN-α.[168] However, when used topically to treat experimentally infected cats with conjunctivitis, IFN-α had higher efficacy than IFN-ω, and cats treated with IFN-ω even had a worsened conjunctivitis score.[190] In cats with naturally occurring viral keratoconjunctivitis, ocular administration of IFN-ω q12h for 14 days did not improve clinical disease or virus shedding compared with treatment with saline solution.[172] In a noncontrolled field study, cats with suspected acute FCV infection showed improvement in clinical signs (e.g., upper respiratory tract disease or stomatitis) following treatment with IFN-ω (2.5×10^6 IU/kg IV q48h, 3 times).[191] However, in a placebo-controlled study, treatment with IFN-ω was not effective in ameliorating clinical signs.[192] In a prospective, randomized, placebo-controlled, double-blind clinical trial, 37 cats with acute FCV- and/or FHV-1-induced clinical signs were treated with IFN-ω (2.5×10^6/kg SC once, followed by 0.5×10^6 topically on the conjunctiva, intranasally, and orally q8h for 21 days). Treatment with IFN-ω was not effective in ameliorating clinical signs when compared with placebo, but accelerated a reduction in FCV load in infected cats.[192] Local injection of IFN-ω into oral lesions in cats with chronic gingivostomatitis, some of which were infected with FCV, was followed by some improvement, but the cats were also treated with other drugs and dental procedures, and a control group was not included.[193] In a controlled study, oromucosal administration of IFN-ω to cats with FCV-associated chronic gingivostomatitis had the same efficacy as glucocorticoid treatment, suggesting that IFN-ω might be an alternative to glucocorticoids.[194] In conclusion, data do not support the use of IFN-ω for treatment of FHV-1 infection, but there might be some efficacy for treatment of FCV infections, especially in cats with chronic gingivostomatitis.

In a case series that included five cats with cowpox virus pneumonia, two cats survived, both of which were treated with IFN-ω.[195] However, controlled studies are lacking.

When used to treat beagle puppies that were experimentally infected with CPV, the number of dogs that developed clinical signs did not differ significantly between the treated dogs and the placebo groups, but clinical signs were less severe in dogs treated with IFN-ω.[196] In one double-blind trial, 10 beagle puppies with experimentally induced CPV disease were randomized to two groups of five dogs each. Four days after challenge, one group was treated with saline and the other with IFN-ω (2.5×10^6 IU/kg IV q24h for 3 consecutive days). All five dogs in the placebo group died within 10 days. In the treated group, one animal died on day 2 after treatment was started, whereas the other four dogs recovered.[197] In a randomized, double-blind, multicenter field study in France, 92 dogs aged 1 to 28 months were treated with either IFN-ω (2.5×10^6 IU/kg IV q24h for 3 consecutive days) or placebo. Clinical signs in treated animals improved significantly in comparison with control animals, and in the IFN-ω group, 3 dogs died compared with 14 in the placebo group.[198] In a similar field study in Japan, mortality was also reduced in the dogs treated with IFN-ω (14/72) when compared with the control group (13/21).[199] These data suggest that IFN-ω improves clinical signs and reduces mortality due to CPV. There are no controlled studies of the use of IFN-ω to treat cats with panleukopenia. IFN-ω was not effective in preventing panleukopenia in cats after entering a cattery.[200]

Lymphocyte T-cell Immunomodulator

Lymphocyte T-cell immunomodulator (LTCI) is a protein derived from thymus epithelial cells. According to the product brochure, LTCI upregulates IL-2 production *in vitro* and regulates CD4 T-cell function. It was also reported to stimulate platelet production in mice with chemotherapy-induced thrombocytopenia. LTCI has been conditionally approved in the United States as an aid for treatment of FIV and FeLV infections, and for the associated signs of cytopenias and opportunistic infections, but controlled independent studies of the efficacy of LTCI in cats are required.

Naturally Occurring Biologic Response Modifiers

Lactoferrin

Commercial lactoferrin is a mammalian iron-binding glycoprotein of bovine origin with immunomodulatory properties. Lactoferrin is produced by the mucosal epithelial cells of all mammals and is present in secretions, especially in milk. It has been used for its local immunomodulatory effect in the oral cavity, and it has been shown to increase cellular phagocytic activity.[201] It binds iron, reducing its availability for bacteria, and thus has not only antibacterial but also antifungal, antiprotozoal, and antiviral activity, and its antitumor activity has also been investigated.[202] Lactoferrin inhibits influenza virus hemagglutination and cell infection.[203] A protective effect of lactoferrin during lethal bacteremia has been reported in mice.[204] Long-term oral administration of bovine lactoferrin to a dog with β_2-integrin-related neutrophil dysfunction was associated with increased neutrophil function and recovery from opportunistic infections.[205] Lactoferrin was also administered long term to two canine littermates with familial neutrophil dysfunction and improved their clinical signs.[206] Adverse effects have not been reported.

Topical application of lactoferrin (40 mg/kg q24h for 14 days) to the mouth of a small number of FIV-infected and noninfected cats with stomatitis was associated with improved appetite and reduced oral inflammation, salivation, and pain, and increased neutrophil phagocytic activity.[201] Treatment with lactoferrin might also have the potential to improve functions of overactivated lymphocytes by modulating the cell proliferation, cell cycle, and cytokine expression in cats in the terminal stage of FIV infection.[207] Lactoferrin has antiviral activity against FHV-1, CHV-1, and FCV *in vitro*.[208–210] No *in vivo* data are available so far in cats infected with FHV-1. Lactoferrin appeared to reduce the clinical signs in cats with chronic gingivostomatitis in one study, but it is unknown whether the cats were infected with FCV.[211] One cat with stomatitis and FCV infection was treated with lactoferrin powder (200 mg) that was applied directly to lesions for 22 months. Clinical signs began to resolve after 11 months, and resolution of clinical signs coincided with the cessation of FCV shedding.[212] However, the cat also received other medications, and because spontaneous resolution of this condition can occur, further studies are necessary.

Plant-Derived Biologic Response Modifiers

A few plant-derived biologic response modifiers are on the market, such as polyprenyl immunostimulant. Other plant extracts with antiviral activity have undergone preliminary *in vitro* assessment, but safety or clinical efficacy have not been reported.[213] Polyprenyl immunostimulant is a plant-derived veterinary biologic that is made of phosphorylated, linear polyisoprenols. *In vitro*, it upregulates synthesis of Th1 cytokines and has antiviral and antineoplastic properties.[214,215] Polyprenyl immunostimulant appeared to have a beneficial effect in two cats with histologically confirmed and one cat with suspected FIP without effusion.[216] One cat survived 14 months, and the other two cats were still in clinical remission after 24 and 28 months, respectively. In a field study, treatment with polyprenyl immunostimulant was evaluated in 60 cats that were suspected to have FIP by primary care and specialist veterinarians, but FIP was not confirmed. None of the cats had effusion. There was no control group. Of the 60 treated cats, 8/60 survived over 200 days and of those, 4/60 survived over 300 days. Veterinarians of treated cats that survived over 30 days reported improvements in clinical signs and behavior. The survival times were significantly longer in cats who were not treated with corticosteroids concurrently.[217] Use of polyprenyl immunostimulant might hold some promise for treatment of cats with FIP that have no effusion, while its use in cats with FIP with effusions has been disappointing. However, controlled studies in cats with confirmed FIP would be very important.

According to the manufacturer, cats with experimentally induced FHV-1 infection had a decreased severity and duration of upper respiratory tract signs when treated with polyprenyl immunostimulant in comparison with cats receiving placebo, but independent controlled studies are lacking.

Synthetic Compounds

Antiparasitic and Antibacterial Compounds

Some antiparasitic compounds nonspecifically stimulate cell-mediated or humoral immunity and thus have immunomodulatory activity. The antiparasitic agent ivermectin has been investigated for treating human patients with SARS-CoV-2 infection. Although ivermectin has theoretical potential for this use,[218] the concentrations achieved in patients with standard doses are not high enough to produce antiviral effects.[219] Some antibiotics also have immunomodulatory properties, including the macrolides, doxycycline, and metronidazole, but there are no prospective studies using these drugs in virus-infected cats and dogs.

Other Synthetic Compounds

Pentoxifylline and propentofylline are synthetic methylxanthines derived from theobromine. Propentofylline is marketed in Europe as a veterinary product. Both compounds are phosphodiesterase inhibitors with a variety of immunomodulatory properties. In rodents and humans, they inhibit tumor necrosis factor (TNF)-α, IL-1, IL-6, and IL-12 production, as well as activation of T and B cells, and increase neutrophil mobility and chemotaxis. They also increase erythrocyte cAMP levels, which results in increased erythrocyte deformability, lowered blood viscosity, and improved microcirculation and tissue perfusion. They decrease platelet aggregation and increase tissue plasminogen activator in patients with hyperaggregable platelets; thus, they can be useful for treatment of disorders that result in hypercoagulable states. Pentoxifylline has been evaluated as a treatment for equine endotoxemia. Despite decreases in TNF-α and IL-6 activity after incubation of equine monocytes with pentoxifylline *in vitro*, these effects did not occur in horses.[220] Beneficial effects of pentoxifylline are limited in horses when administered IV after challenge with endotoxin.[221] In dogs, pentoxifylline has been used to treat canine atopic dermatitis, dermatomyositis, and cutaneous vasculopathies,[222,223] as well as cognitive dysfunction in geriatric dogs.[224] In dogs, pentoxifylline has a low and unpredictable oral bioavailability and a short half-life, and q8h administration has been recommended. Adverse effects include vomiting and inappetence, which are more likely to occur when the tablets are crushed. Crushed tablets are also unpalatable to cats.

According to anecdotal reports, pentoxifylline has been used to treat some cats with FIP, with apparent improvement in clinical signs and survival time. However, when the closely related drug propentofylline was used in a double-blind trial of 23 cats with naturally occurring FIP, there was no difference in survival time, quality of life, amount of effusion, or TNF-α concentration in cats treated with propentofylline versus placebo.[225]

REFERENCES

1. Gould D. Feline herpesvirus-1: ocular manifestations, diagnosis and treatment options. *J Feline Med Surg*. 2011;13:333–346.
2. Thomasy SM, Maggs DJ. A review of antiviral drugs and other compounds with activity against feline herpesvirus type 1. *Vet Ophthalmol*. 2016;19(suppl 1):119–130.
3. Murphy BG, Perron M, Murakami E, et al. The nucleoside analog GS-441524 strongly inhibits feline infectious peritonitis (FIP) virus in tissue culture and experimental cat infection studies. *Vet Microbiol*. 2018;219:226–233.
4. Pedersen NC, Kim Y, Liu H, et al. Efficacy of a 3C-like protease inhibitor in treating various forms of acquired feline infectious peritonitis. *J Feline Med Surg*. 2018;20:378–392.
5. Pedersen NC, Perron M, Bannasch M, et al. Efficacy and safety of the nucleoside analog GS-441524 for treatment of cats with naturally occurring feline infectious peritonitis. *J Feline Med Surg*. 2019;21:271–281.
6. De Clercq E. Toward improved anti-HIV chemotherapy: therapeutic strategies for intervention with HIV infections. *J Med Chem*. 1995;38:2491–2517.
7. Palmisano L, Vella S. A brief history of antiretroviral therapy of HIV infection: success and challenges. *Annali Dell'istituto Superiore Di Sanita*. 2011;47:44–48.

8. Hartmann K. Antiviral and immunomodulatory chemotherapy. In: Greene CE, ed. *Infectious Diseases of the Dog and Cat*. 4th ed. St Louis, MO: Elsevier, Saunders; 2012:10–24.
9. Mohammadi H, Bienzle D. Pharmacological inhibition of feline immunodeficiency virus (FIV). *Viruses*. 2012;4:708–724.
10. Mitsuya H, Broder S. Strategies for antiviral therapy in AIDS. *Nature*. 1987;325:773–778.
11. Mitsuya H, Weinhold KJ, Furman PA, et al. 3'-Azido-3'-deoxythymidine (BW A509U): an antiviral agent that inhibits the infectivity and cytopathic effect of human T-lymphotropic virus type III/lymphadenopathy-associated virus in vitro. *Proc Natl Acad Sci U S A*. 1985;82:7096–7100.
12. Schwartz AM, McCrackin MA, Schinazi RF, et al. Antiviral efficacy of nine nucleoside reverse transcriptase inhibitors against feline immunodeficiency virus in feline peripheral blood mononuclear cells. *Am J Vet Res*. 2014;75:273–281.
13. Bisset LR, Lutz H, Boni J, et al. Combined effect of zidovudine (ZDV), lamivudine (3TC) and abacavir (ABC) antiretroviral therapy in suppressing in vitro FIV replication. *Antiviral Res*. 2002;53:35–45.
14. Smyth NR, McCracken C, Gaskell RM, et al. Susceptibility in cell culture of feline immunodeficiency virus to eighteen antiviral agents. *J Antimicrob Chemother*. 1994;34:589–594.
15. Balzarini J, Egberink H, Hartmann K, et al. Antiretrovirus specificity and intracellular metabolism of 2',3' -didehydro-2',3'-dideoxythymidine (stavudine) and its 5'-monophosphate triester prodrug So324. *Mol Pharmacol*. 1996;50:1207–1213.
16. North TW, North GL, Pedersen NC. Feline immunodeficiency virus, a model for reverse transcriptase-targeted chemotherapy for acquired immune deficiency syndrome. *Antimicrob Agents Chemother*. 1989;33:915–919.
17. Tressler R, Godfrey C. NRTI backbone in HIV treatment: will it remain relevant? *Drugs*. 2012;72:2051–2062.
18. Ezzell C. AZT given the green light for clinical treatment of AIDS. *Nature*. 1987;326:430.
19. Hartmann K, Donath A, Kraft W. AZT in the treatment of feline immunodeficiency virus infection: part 2. *Feline Pract*. 1995b;23:13–20.
20. Hartmann K, Donath A, Kraft W. AZT in the treatment of feline immunodeficiency virus infection: part 1. *Feline Pract*. 1995a;23:16–21.
21. Hartmann K. Feline immunodeficiency virus infection: an overview. *Vet J*. 1998;155:123–137.
22. Hartmann K, Donath A, Beer B, et al. Use of two virustatica (AZT, PMEA) in the treatment of FIV and of FeLV seropositive cats with clinical symptoms. *Vet Immunol Immunopathol*. 1992;35:167–175.
23. Gomez NV, Castillo VA, Gisbert MA, et al. Immune-endocrine interactions in treated and untreated cats naturally infected with FIV. *Vet Immunol Immunopathol*. 2011;143:332–337.
24. Gomez NV, Fontanals A, Castillo V, et al. Evaluation of different antiretroviral drug protocols on naturally infected feline immunodeficiency virus (FIV) cats in the late phase of the asymptomatic stage of infection. *Viruses*. 2012;4:924–939.
25. Smith RA, Remington KM, Preston BD, et al. A novel point mutation at position 156 of reverse transcriptase from feline immunodeficiency virus confers resistance to the combination of (-)-beta-2',3'-dideoxy-3'-thiacytidine and 3'-azido-3'-deoxythymidine. *J Virol*. 1998;72:2335–2340.
26. Medeiros Sde O, Abreu CM, Delvecchio R, et al. Follow-up on long-term antiretroviral therapy for cats infected with feline immunodeficiency virus. *J Feline Med Surg*. 2016;18:264–272.
27. McCrackin Stevenson MA, McBroom DG. In vitro characterization of FIV-pPPR, a pathogenic molecular clone of feline immunodeficiency virus, and two drug-resistant pol gene mutants. *Am J Vet Res*. 2001;62:588–594.
28. Remington KM, Chesebro B, Wehrly K, et al. Mutants of feline immunodeficiency virus resistant to 3'-azido-3'-deoxythymidine. *J Virol*. 1991;65:308–312.
29. Smith RA, Remington KM, Lloyd Jr RM, et al. A novel Met-to-Thr mutation in the YMDD motif of reverse transcriptase from feline immunodeficiency virus confers resistance to oxathiolane nucleosides. *J Virol*. 1997;71:2357–2362.
30. Hoover EA, Zeidner NS, Mullins JI. Therapy of presymptomatic FeLV-induced immunodeficiency syndrome with AZT in combination with alpha interferon. *Ann N Y Acad Sci*. 1990;616:258–269.
31. Tavares L, Roneker C, Postie L, et al. Testing of nucleoside analogues in cats infected with feline leukemia virus: a model. *Intervirology*. 1989;30(suppl 1):26–35.
32. Zeidner NS, Rose LM, Mathiason–DuBard CK, et al. Zidovudine in combination with alpha interferon and interleukin-2 as prophylactic therapy for FeLV-induced immunodeficiency syndrome (FeLV-FAIDS). *J Acquir Immune Defic Syndr*. 1990;3:787–796.
33. Zeidner NS, Myles MH, Mathiason-DuBard CK, et al. Alpha interferon (2b) in combination with zidovudine for the treatment of presymptomatic feline leukemia virus-induced immunodeficiency syndrome. *Antimicrob Agents Chemother*. 1990;34:1749–1756.
34. Stuetzer B, Brunner K, Lutz H, et al. A trial with 3'-azido-2',3'-dideoxythymidine and human interferon-alpha in cats naturally infected with feline leukaemia virus. *J Feline Med Surg*. 2013;15:667–671.
35. Nelson P, Sellon R, Novotney C, et al. Therapeutic effects of diethylcarbamazine and 3'-azido-3'-deoxythymidine on feline leukemia virus lymphoma formation. *Vet Immunol Immunopathol*. 1995;46:181–194.
36. De Clercq E. Anti-HIV drugs: 25 compounds approved within 25 years after the discovery of HIV. *Int J Antimicrob Agents*. 2009;33:307–320.
37. Ravichandran S, Veerasamy R, Raman S, et al. An overview on HIV-1 reverse transcriptase inhibitors. *Dig J Nanomater Biostruct*. 2008:171–187.
38. Cihlar T, Ray AS. Nucleoside and nucleotide HIV reverse transcriptase inhibitors: 25 years after zidovudine. *Antiviral Res*. 2010;85:39–58.
39. Xia Q, Radzio J, Anderson KS, et al. Probing nonnucleoside inhibitor-induced active-site distortion in HIV-1 reverse transcriptase by transient kinetic analyses. *Protein Sci*. 2007;16:1728–1737.
40. Das K, Martinez SE, Bauman JD, et al. HIV-1 reverse transcriptase complex with DNA and nevirapine reveals non-nucleoside inhibition mechanism. *Nat Stru Mol Biol*. 2012;19:253–259.
41. Owens JG, Nasisse MP, Tadepalli SM, et al. Pharmacokinetics of acyclovir in the cat. *J Vet Pharmacol Ther*. 1996;19:488–490.
42. van der Meulen K, Garre B, Croubels S, et al. In vitro comparison of antiviral drugs against feline herpesvirus 1. *BMC Vet Res*. 2006;2:13.
43. Maggs DJ, Clarke HE. In vitro efficacy of ganciclovir, cidofovir, penciclovir, foscarnet, idoxuridine, and acyclovir against feline herpesvirus type-1. *Am J Vet Res*. 2004;65:399–403.
44. Williams DL, Fitzmaurice T, Lay L, et al. Efficacy of antiviral agents in feline herpetic keratitis: results of an in vitro study. *Curr Eye Res*. 2004;29:215–218.
45. De Clercq E. Comparative efficacy of antiherpes drugs in different cell lines. *Antimicrob Agents Chemother*. 1982;21:661–663.
46. Weiss RC. Synergistic antiviral activities of acyclovir and recombinant human leukocyte (alpha) interferon on feline herpesvirus replication. *Am J Vet Res*. 1989;50:1672–1677.
47. Williams DL, Robinson JC, Lay E, et al. Efficacy of topical aciclovir for the treatment of feline herpetic keratitis: results of a prospective clinical trial and data from in vitro investigations. *Vet Rec*. 2005;157:254–257.
48. Nasisse MP, Dorman DC, Jamison KC, et al. Effects of valacyclovir in cats infected with feline herpesvirus 1. *Am J Vet Res*. 1997;58:1141–1144.
49. Smith KO, Galloway KS, Kennell WL, et al. A new nucleoside analog, 9-[[2-hydroxy-1-(hydroxymethyl)ethoxyl]methyl]guanine, highly active in vitro against herpes simplex virus types 1 and 2. *Antimicrob Agents Chemother*. 1982;22:55–61.
50. Ernst ME, Franey RJ. Acyclovir- and ganciclovir-induced neurotoxicity. *Ann Pharmacother*. 1998;32:111–113.
51. Burns LJ, Miller W, Kandaswamy C, et al. Randomized clinical trial of ganciclovir vs acyclovir for prevention of cytomegalovirus antigenemia after allogeneic transplantation. *Bone Marrow Transplant*. 2002;30:945–951.
52. Anand R, Nightingale SD, Fish RH, et al. Control of cytomegalovirus retinitis using sustained release of intraocular ganciclovir. *Archiv Ophthalmol*. 1993;111:223–227.
53. Chou TY, Hong BY. Ganciclovir ophthalmic gel 0.15% for the treatment of acute herpetic keratitis: background, effectiveness, tolerability, safety, and future applications. *Ther Clin Risk Manag*. 2014;10:665–681.
54. Jung D, Dorr A. Single-dose pharmacokinetics of valganciclovir in HIV- and CMV-seropositive subjects. *J Clin Pharmacol*. 1999;39:800–804.

55. Nasisse MP, Guy JS, Davidson MG, et al. In vitro susceptibility of feline herpesvirus-1 to vidarabine, idoxuridine, trifluridine, acyclovir, or bromovinyldeoxyuridine. *Am J Vet Res.* 1989;50:158–160.
56. Kaufman HE, Varnell ED, Thompson HW. Trifluridine, cidofovir, and penciclovir in the treatment of experimental herpetic keratitis. *Arch Ophthalmol.* 1998;116:777–780.
57. Choi WS, Im GJ, Kim DK, et al. Pharmacokinetic studies of 2-amino-9-(3-acetoxymethyl-4-isopropoxycarbonyl-oxybut-1-yl)purine, an oral prodrug for the antiviral agent penciclovir. *Drug Metabol Dispos.* 2001;29:945–949.
58. Hussein IT, Field HJ. Development of a quantitative real-time TaqMan PCR assay for testing the susceptibility of feline herpesvirus-1 to antiviral compounds. *J Virol Methods.* 2008;152:85–90.
59. Hussein IT, Menashy RV, Field HJ. Penciclovir is a potent inhibitor of feline herpesvirus-1 with susceptibility determined at the level of virus-encoded thymidine kinase. *Antiviral Res.* 2008;78:268–274.
60. Semenkow SL, Johnson NM, Maggs DJ, et al. Controlled release delivery of penciclovir via a silicone (MED-4750) polymer: kinetics of drug delivery and efficacy in preventing primary feline herpesvirus infection in culture. *Virol J.* 2014;11:34.
61. Asquith CR, Meli ML, Konstantinova LS, et al. Novel fused tetrathiocines as antivirals that target the nucleocapsid zinc finger containing protein of the feline immunodeficiency virus (FIV) as a model of HIV infection. *Bioorg Med Chem Let.* 2015;25:1352–1355.
62. Clarke SE, Harrell AW, Chenery RJ. Role of aldehyde oxidase in the in vitro conversion of famciclovir to penciclovir in human liver. *Drug Metab Dispos.* 1995;23:251–254.
63. Vere Hodge RA, Sutton D, Boyd MR, et al. Selection of an oral prodrug (BRL 42810; famciclovir) for the antiherpesvirus agent BRL 39123 [9-(4-hydroxy-3-hydroxymethylbut-l-yl)guanine; penciclovir]. *Antimicrob Agents Chemother.* 1989;33:1765–1773.
64. Filer CW, Allen GD, Brown TA, et al. Metabolic and pharmacokinetic studies following oral administration of 14C-famciclovir to healthy subjects. *Xenobiotica.* 1994;24:357–368.
65. Groth AD, Contreras MT, Kado-Fong HK, et al. In vitro cytotoxicity and antiviral efficacy against feline herpesvirus type 1 of famciclovir and its metabolites. *Vet Ophthalmol.* 2014;17:268–274.
66. Dick RA, Kanne DB, Casida JE. Identification of aldehyde oxidase as the neonicotinoid nitroreductase. *Chem Res Toxicol.* 2005;18:317–323.
67. Sebbag L, Thomasy SM, Woodward AP, et al. Pharmacokinetic modeling of penciclovir and BRL42359 in the plasma and tears of healthy cats to optimize dosage recommendations for oral administration of famciclovir. *Am J Vet Res.* 2016;77:833–845.
68. Thomasy SM, Maggs DJ, Moulin NK, et al. Pharmacokinetics and safety of penciclovir following oral administration of famciclovir to cats. *Am J Vet Res.* 2007;68:1252–1258.
69. Thomasy SM, Lim CC, Reilly CM, et al. Evaluation of orally administered famciclovir in cats experimentally infected with feline herpesvirus type-1. *Am J Vet Res.* 2011;72:85–95.
70. Malik R, Lessels NS, Webb S, et al. Treatment of feline herpesvirus-1 associated disease in cats with famciclovir and related drugs. *J Feline Med Surg.* 2009;11:40–48.
71. Litster AL, Lohr BR, Bukowy RA, et al. Clinical and antiviral effect of a single oral dose of famciclovir administered to cats at intake to a shelter. *Vet J.* 2015;203:199–204.
72. Thomasy SM, Shull O, Outerbridge CA, et al. Oral administration of famciclovir for treatment of spontaneous ocular, respiratory, or dermatologic disease attributed to feline herpesvirus type 1: 59 cases (2006-2013). *J Am Vet Med Assoc.* 2016;249:526–538.
73. Thomasy SM, Covert JC, Stanley SD, et al. Pharmacokinetics of famciclovir and penciclovir in tears following oral administration of famciclovir to cats: a pilot study. *Vet Ophthalmol.* 2012;15:299–306.
74. Thomasy SM, Whittem T, Bales JL, et al. Pharmacokinetics of penciclovir in healthy cats following oral administration of famciclovir or intravenous infusion of penciclovir. *Am J Vet Res.* 2012;73:1092–1099.
75. Boike SC, Pue MA, Freed MI, et al. Pharmacokinetics of famciclovir in subjects with varying degrees of renal impairment. *Clin Pharmacol Therap.* 1994;55:418–426.
76. Cihlar T, Chen MS. Identification of enzymes catalyzing two-step phosphorylation of cidofovir and the effect of cytomegalovirus infection on their activities in host cells. *Mol Pharmacol.* 1996;50:1502–1510.
77. Neyts J, Snoeck R, Schols D, et al. Selective inhibition of human cytomegalovirus DNA synthesis by (S)-1-(3-hydroxy-2-phosphonylmethoxypropyl)cytosine [(S)-HPMPC] and 9-(1,3-dihydroxy-2-propoxymethyl)guanine (DHPG). *Virology.* 1990;179:41–50.
78. Romanowski EG, Bartels SP, Gordon YJ. Comparative antiviral efficacies of cidofovir, trifluridine, and acyclovir in the HSV-1 rabbit keratitis model. *Invest Ophthalmol Visual Sci.* 1999;40:378–384.
79. Sherman MD, Feldman KA, Farahmand SM, et al. Treatment of conjunctival squamous cell carcinoma with topical cidofovir. *Am J Ophthalmol.* 2002;134:432–433.
80. Gordon YJ, Romanowski EG, Araullo-Cruz T. Topical HPMPC inhibits adenovirus type 5 in the New Zealand rabbit ocular replication model. *Invest Ophthalmol Visual Sci.* 1994;35:4135–4143.
81. Stiles J, Gwin W, Pogranichniy R. Stability of 0.5% cidofovir stored under various conditions for up to 6 months. *Vet Ophthalmol.* 2010;13:275–277.
82. Pennington MR, Fort MW, Ledbetter EC, et al. A novel corneal explant model system to evaluate antiviral drugs against feline herpesvirus type 1 (FHV-1). *J Gen Virol.* 2016;97:1414–1425.
83. Fontenelle JP, Powell CC, Veir JK, et al. Effect of topical ophthalmic application of cidofovir on experimentally induced primary ocular feline herpesvirus-1 infection in cats. *Am J Vet Res.* 2008;69:289–293.
84. Ledbetter EC, Spertus CB, Pennington MR, et al. In vitro and in vivo evaluation of cidofovir as a topical ophthalmic antiviral for ocular canine herpesvirus-1 infections in dogs. *J Ocul Pharmacol Therap.* 2015;31:642–649.
85. Gervais KJ, Pirie CG, Ledbetter EC, et al. Acute primary canine herpesvirus-1 dendritic ulcerative keratitis in an adult dog. *Vet Ophthalmol.* 2012;15:133–138.
86. Chin GN. Treatment of herpes simplex keratitis with idoxuridine and vidarabine: a double-blind study. *Ann Ophthalmol.* 1978;10:1171–1174.
87. Stiles J. Treatment of cats with ocular disease attributable to herpesvirus infection: 17 cases (1983-1993). *J Am Vet Med Assoc.* 1995;207:599–603.
88. Gil S, Leal RO, Duarte A, et al. Relevance of feline interferon omega for clinical improvement and reduction of concurrent viral excretion in retrovirus infected cats from a rescue shelter. *Res Vet Sci.* 2013;94:753–763.
89. O'Brien WJ, Edelhauser HF. The corneal penetration of trifluorothymidine, adenine arabinoside, and idoxuridine: a comparative study. *Invest Ophthalmol Visual Sci.* 1977;16:1093–1103.
90. Maggs DJ. Antiviral therapy for feline herpesvirus infections. *Vet Clin North Am Small Anim Pract.* 2010;40:1055–1062.
91. Ledbetter EC, Riis RC, Kern TJ, et al. Corneal ulceration associated with naturally occurring canine herpesvirus-1 infection in two adult dogs. *J Am Vet Med Assoc.* 2006;229:376–384.
92. Spertus CB, Mohammed HO, Ledbetter EC. Effects of topical ocular application of 1% trifluridine ophthalmic solution in dogs with experimentally induced recurrent ocular canine herpesvirus-1 infection. *Am J Vet Res.* 2016;77:1140–1147.
93. Schefold JC. Immunostimulation using granulocyte- and granulocyte-macrophage colony stimulating factor in patients with severe sepsis and septic shock. *Crit Care.* 2011;15:136.
94. Barlough JE, Scott FW. Effectiveness of three antiviral agents against FIP virus in vitro. *Vet Rec.* 1990;126:556–558.
95. Gobert JM, Remington KM, Zhu YQ, et al. Multiple-drug-resistant mutants of feline immunodeficiency virus selected with 2',3'-dideoxyinosine alone and in combination with 3'-azido-3'-deoxythymidine. *Antimicrob Agents Chemother.* 1994;38:861–864.
96. Swenson CL, Polas PJ, Cheney CM, et al. Prophylactic and therapeutic effects of phosphonoformate against feline leukemia virus in vitro. *Am J Vet Res.* 1991;52:2010–2015.
97. Povey RC. In vitro antiviral efficacy of ribavirin against feline calicivirus, feline viral rhinotracheitis virus, and canine parainfluenza virus. *Am J Vet Res.* 1978;39:175–178.
98. Mizutani T, Inagaki H, Araki K, et al. Inhibition of Borna disease virus replication by ribavirin in persistently infected cells. *Arch Virol.* 1998;143:2039–2044.

99. Elia G, Belloli C, Cirone F, et al. In vitro efficacy of ribavirin against canine distemper virus. *Antiviral Res.* 2008;77:108–113.
100. Lin YC, Happer M, Elder JH. Selection of drug-resistant feline immunodeficiency virus (FIV) encoding FIV/HIV chimeric protease in the presence of HIV-specific protease inhibitors. *J Virol.* 2013;87:8524–8534.
101. Lin YC, Perryman AL, Olson AJ, et al. Structural basis for drug and substrate specificity exhibited by FIV encoding a chimeric FIV/HIV protease. *Acta Crystallogr D.* 2011;67:540–548.
102. Lin YC, Torbett BE, Elder JH. Generation of infectious feline immunodeficiency virus (FIV) encoding FIV/human immunodeficiency virus chimeric protease. *J Virol.* 2010;84:6799–6809.
103. St John SE, Therkelsen MD, Nyalapatla PR, et al. X-ray structure and inhibition of the feline infectious peritonitis virus 3C-like protease: Structural implications for drug design. *Bioorg Med Chem Lett.* 2015;25:5072–5077.
104. Hsieh LE, Lin CN, Su BL, et al. Synergistic antiviral effect of *Galanthus nivalis* agglutinin and nelfinavir against feline coronavirus. *Antiviral Res.* 2010;88:25–30.
105. Tsai HY, Chueh LL, Lin CN, et al. Clinicopathological findings and disease staging of feline infectious peritonitis: 51 cases from 2003 to 2009 in Taiwan. *J Feline Med Surg.* 2011;13:74–80.
106. Kim Y, Mandadapu SR, Groutas WC, et al. Potent inhibition of feline coronaviruses with peptidyl compounds targeting coronavirus 3C-like protease. *Antiviral Res.* 2013;97:161–168.
107. Kim Y, Liu H, Galasiti Kankanamalage AC, et al. Reversal of the progression of fatal coronavirus infection in cats by a broad-spectrum coronavirus protease inhibitor. *PLoS Pathog.* 2016;12:e1005531.
108. Rucker J, Edinger AL, Sharron M, et al. Utilization of chemokine receptors, orphan receptors, and herpesvirus-encoded receptors by diverse human and simian immunodeficiency viruses. *J Virol.* 1997;71:8999–9007.
109. Willett BJ, Hosie MJ. The role of the chemokine receptor CXCR4 in infection with feline immunodeficiency virus. *Mol Membrane Biol.* 1999;16:67–72.
110. Wells TN, Proudfoot AE, Power CA, et al. Chemokine receptors - the new frontier for AIDS research. *Chem Biol.* 1996;3:603–609.
111. Willett BJ, Picard L, Hosie MJ, et al. Shared usage of the chemokine receptor CXCR4 by the feline and human immunodeficiency viruses. *J Virol.* 1997;71:6407–6415.
112. Donzella GA, Schols D, Lin SW, et al. AMD3100, a small molecule inhibitor of HIV-1 entry via the CXCR4 co-receptor. *Nat Med.* 1998;4:72–77.
113. Liles WC, Broxmeyer HE, Rodger E, et al. Mobilization of hematopoietic progenitor cells in healthy volunteers by AMD3100, a CXCR4 antagonist. *Blood.* 2003;102:2728–2730.
114. Egberink HF, De Clercq E, Van Vliet AL, et al. Bicyclams, selective antagonists of the human chemokine receptor CXCR4, potently inhibit feline immunodeficiency virus replication. *J Virol.* 1999;73:6346–6352.
115. Hartmann K, Stengel C, Klein D, et al. Efficacy and adverse effects of the antiviral compound plerixafor in feline immunodeficiency virus-infected cats. *J Vet Intern Med.* 2012;26:483–490.
116. Cattori V, Weibel B, Lutz H. Inhibition of feline leukemia virus replication by the integrase inhibitor raltegravir. *Vet Microbiol.* 2011;152:165–168.
117. Greggs WM 3rd, Clouser CL, Patterson SE, et al. Discovery of drugs that possess activity against feline leukemia virus. *J Gen Virol.* 2012;93:900–905.
118. Boesch A, Cattori V, Riond B, et al. Evaluation of the effect of short-term treatment with the integrase inhibitor raltegravir (Isentress) on the course of progressive feline leukemia virus infection. *Vet Microbiol.* 2015;175:167–178.
119. De Clercq E. New developments in anti-HIV chemotherapy. *Biochem Biophys Acta.* 2002;1587:258–275.
120. Asquith CR, Konstantinova LS, Laitinen T, et al. Evaluation of substituted 1,2,3-dithiazoles as inhibitors of the feline immunodeficiency virus (FIV) nucleocapsid protein via a proposed zinc ejection mechanism. *ChemMedChem.* 2016;11:2119–2126.
121. Asquith CR, Meli ML, Konstantinova LS, et al. Evaluation of the antiviral efficacy of bis[1,2]dithiolo[1,4]thiazines and bis[1,2]dithiolopyrrole derivatives against the nucelocapsid protein of the feline immunodeficiency virus (FIV) as a model for HIV infection. *Bioorg Med Chemis Let.* 2014;24:2640–2644.
122. Li W, Escarpe PA, Eisenberg EJ, et al. Identification of GS 4104 as an orally bioavailable prodrug of the influenza virus neuraminidase inhibitor GS 4071. *Antimicrob Agents Chemother.* 1998;42:647–653.
123. Savigny MR, Macintire DK. Use of oseltamivir in the treatment of canine parvoviral enteritis. *J Vet Emerg Critical Care.* 2010;20:132–142.
124. Soong G, Muir A, Gomez MI, et al. Bacterial neuraminidase facilitates mucosal infection by participating in biofilm production. *J Clin Invest.* 2006;116:2297–2305.
125. Takano T, Nakano K, Doki T, et al. Differential effects of viroporin inhibitors against feline infectious peritonitis virus serotypes I and II. *Arch Virol.* 2015;160:1163–1170.
126. Lascelles BDX, Gaynor JS, Smith ES, et al. Amantadine in a multimodal analgesia regimen for alleviation of refractory osteoarthritis pain in dogs. *J Vet Intern Med.* 2008;22:53–59.
127. Hallensleben W, Zocher M, Staeheli P. Borna disease virus is not sensitive to amantadine. *Arch Virol.* 1997;142:2043–2048.
128. Hurt AC, Selleck P, Komadina N, et al. Susceptibility of highly pathogenic A(H5N1) avian influenza viruses to the neuraminidase inhibitors and adamantanes. *Antiviral Res.* 2007;73:228–231.
129. Griffith RS, Norins AL, Kagan C. A multicentered study of lysine therapy in Herpes simplex infection. *Dermatol.* 1978;156:257–267.
130. Maggs DJ, Collins BK, Thorne JG, et al. Effects of L-lysine and L-arginine on in vitro replication of feline herpesvirus type-1. *Am J Vet Res.* 2000;61:1474–1478.
131. Griffith RS, DeLong DC, Nelson JD. Relation of arginine-lysine antagonism to herpes simplex growth in tissue culture. *Chemotherapy.* 1981;27:209–213.
132. Kaplan AS, Ben-Porat T. Synthesis of proteins in cells infected with herpesvirus, VI. Characterization of the proteins of the viral membrane. *Proc Natl Acad Sci U S A.* 1970;66:799–806.
133. Bol S, Bunnik EM. Lysine supplementation is not effective for the prevention or treatment of feline herpesvirus 1 infection in cats: a systematic review. *BMC Vet Res.* 2015;11:284.
134. Naito T, Irie H, Tsujimoto K, et al. Antiviral effect of arginine against herpes simplex virus type 1. *Int J Mol Med.* 2009;23:495–499.
135. Tankersley Jr RW. Amino acid requirements of herpes simplex virus in human cells. *J Bacteriol.* 1964;87:609–613.
136. Banos G, Daniel PM, Pratt OE. Saturation of a shared mechanism which transports L-arginine and L-lysine into the brain of the living rat. *J Physiol.* 1974;236:29–41.
137. Cave NJ, Dennis K, Gopakumar G, et al. Effects of physiologic concentrations of l-Lysine on in vitro replication of feline herpesvirus 1. *Am J Vet Res.* 2014;75:572–580.
138. Stiles J, Townsend WM, Rogers QR, et al. Effect of oral administration of L-lysine on conjunctivitis caused by feline herpesvirus in cats. *Am J Vet Res.* 2002;63:99–103.
139. Fascetti AJ, Maggs DJ, Kanchuk ML, et al. Excess dietary lysine does not cause lysine-arginine antagonism in adult cats. *J Nutri.* 2004;134:2042S–2045S.
140. Maggs DJ, Nasisse MP, Kass PH. Efficacy of oral supplementation with L-lysine in cats latently infected with feline herpesvirus. *Am J Vet Res.* 2003;64:37–42.
141. Rees TM, Lubinski JL. Oral supplementation with L-lysine did not prevent upper respiratory infection in a shelter population of cats. *J Feline Med Surg.* 2008;10:510–513.
142. Drazenovich TL, Fascetti AJ, Westermeyer HD, et al. Effects of dietary lysine supplementation on upper respiratory and ocular disease and detection of infectious organisms in cats within an animal shelter. *Am J Vet Res.* 2009;70:1391–1400.
143. Maggs DJ, Sykes JE, Clarke HE, et al. Effects of dietary lysine supplementation in cats with enzootic upper respiratory disease. *J Feline Med Surg.* 2007;9:97–108.
144. Lappin MR, Veir JK, Satyaraj E, et al. Pilot study to evaluate the effect of oral supplementation of *Enterococcus faecium* SF68 on cats with latent feline herpesvirus 1. *J Feline Med Surg.* 2009;11:650–654.

145. Bergmann M, Friedl Y, Hartmann K. Passive immunization in dogs and cats. *Tierarztl Prax Ausg K Kleintiere Heimtiere*. 2016;44:287–292.
146. Friedl Y, Schulz B, Knebl A, et al. Efficacy of passively transferred antibodies in cats with acute viral upper respiratory tract infection. *Vet J*. 2014;201:316–321.
147. Gerlach M, Proksch AL, Unterer S, et al. Efficacy of feline anti-parvovirus antibodies in the treatment of canine parvovirus infection. *J Small Animal Pract*. 2017;58:408–415.
148. Stark JJ, Dillman RO, Schulof R, et al. Interferon-alpha and chemohormonal therapy for patients with advanced melanoma: final results of a phase I-II study of the Cancer Biotherapy Research Group and the Mid-Atlantic Oncology Program. *Cancer*. 1998;82:1677–1681.
149. Klotz D, Baumgartner W, Gerhauser I. Type I interferons in the pathogenesis and treatment of canine diseases. *Vet Immunol Immunopathol*. 2017;191:80–93.
150. Domenech A, Miro G, Collado VM, et al. Use of recombinant interferon omega in feline retrovirosis: from theory to practice. *Vet Immunol Immunopathol*. 2011;143:301–306.
151. Goodbourn S, Didcock L, Randall RE. Interferons: cell signalling, immune modulation, antiviral response and virus countermeasures. *J Gen Virol*. 2000;81:2341–2364.
152. Gerlach N, Gibbert K, Alter C, et al. Anti-retroviral effects of type I IFN subtypes in vivo. *Euro J Immunol*. 2009;39:136–146.
153. Gomez-Lucia E, Collado VM, Miro G, et al. Effect of type-I interferon on retroviruses. *Viruses*. 2009;1:545–573.
154. Fiorito F, Cantiello A, Granato GE, et al. Clinical improvement in feline herpesvirus 1 infected cats by oral low dose of interleukin-12 plus interferon-gamma. *Comp Immunol Microbiol Infect Dis*. 2016;48:41–47.
155. Zhang K, Jin H, Zhong F, et al. Adenovirus-mediated canine interferon-gamma expression and its antiviral activity against canine parvovirus. *Acta Microbiol Sin*. 2012;52:1400–1407.
156. Cantell K, Pyhala L. Circulating interferon in rabbits after administration of human interferon by different routes. *J Gen Virol*. 1973;20:97–104.
157. Cummins JM, Beilharz MW, Krakowka S. Oral use of interferon. *J Interferon Cytokine Res*. 1999;19:853–857.
158. Koech DK, Obel AO. Efficacy of Kemron (low dose oral natural human interferon alpha) in the management of HIV-1 infection and acquired immune deficiency syndrome (AIDS). *East Afr Med J*. 1990;67:SS64–SS70.
159. Tanabe T, Yamamoto JK. Feline immunodeficiency virus lacks sensitivity to the antiviral activity of feline IFN-gamma. *J Interferon Cytokine Res*. 2001;21:1039–1046.
160. Pedretti E, Passeri B, Amadori M, et al. Low-dose interferon-alpha treatment for feline immunodeficiency virus infection. *Vet Immunol Immunopathol*. 2006;109:245–254.
161. Jameson P, Essex M. Inhibition of feline leukemia virus replication by human leukocyte interferon. *Antiviral Res*. 1983;3:115–120.
162. Tomkins DJ, Kwok SE, Douglas GR, et al. Sister chromatid exchange response of human diploid fibroblasts and Chinese hamster ovary cells to dimethylnitrosamine and benzo(a)pyrene. *Environ Mutagen*. 1982;4:203–214.
163. Weiss RC, Cummins JM, Richards AB. Low-dose orally administered alpha interferon treatment for feline leukemia virus infection. *J Am Vet Med Assoc*. 1991;199:1477–1481.
164. McCaw DL, Boon GD, Jergens AE, et al. Immunomodulation therapy for feline leukemia virus infection. *J Am Anim Hosp Assoc*. 2001;37:356–363.
165. Gomez-Lucia E, Collado VM, Miró G, et al. Follow-up of viral parameters in FeLV- or FIV-naturally infected cats treated orally with low doses of human interferon alpha viruses. *Viruses*. 11(9):845.
166. Gomez-Lucia E, Collado VM, Miró G, et al. Clinical and hematological follow-up of long-term oral therapy with type-I interferon in cats naturally infected with feline leukemia virus or feline immunodeficiency virus. *Animals (Basel)*. 2020;10(9):E1464.
167. Sandmeyer LS, Keller CB, Bienzle D. Effects of interferon-alpha on cytopathic changes and titers for feline herpesvirus-1 in primary cultures of feline corneal epithelial cells. *Am J Vet Res*. 2005;66:210–216.
168. Siebeck N, Hurley DJ, Garcia M, et al. Effects of human recombinant alpha-2b interferon and feline recombinant omega interferon on in vitro replication of feline herpesvirus-1. *Am J Vet Res*. 2006;67:1406–1411.
169. Cocker FM, Howard PE, Harbour DA. Effect of human alpha-hybrid interferon on the course of feline viral rhinotracheitis. *Vet Rec*. 1987;120:391–393.
170. Fulton RW, Burge LJ. Susceptibility of feline herpesvirus 1 and a feline calicivirus to feline interferon and recombinant human leukocyte interferons. *Antimicrob Agents Chemother*. 1985;28:698–699.
171. Fenimore A, Carter K, Fankhauser J, et al. Evaluation of intranasal vaccine administration and high-dose interferon- alpha2b therapy for treatment of chronic upper respiratory tract infections in shelter cats. *J Feline Med Surg*. 2016;18:603–611.
172. Slack JM, Stiles J, Leutenegger CM, et al. Effects of topical ocular administration of high doses of human recombinant interferon alpha-2b and feline recombinant interferon omega on naturally occurring viral keratoconjunctivitis in cats. *Am J Vet Res*. 2013;74:281–289.
173. Cerruti RL, Connell EV, Trown PW, et al. Synergistic interaction between interferon-alpha and acyclovir in the treatment of herpes simplex virus type 1 infection in mice. *Antiviral Res*. 1985;(Suppl 1):217–223.
174. Weiss RC, Oostrom-Ram T. Inhibitory effects of ribavirin alone or combined with human alpha interferon on feline infectious peritonitis virus replication in vitro. *Vet Microbiol*. 1989;20:255–265.
175. Weiss RC, Cox NR, Oostrom-Ram T. Effect of interferon or *Propionibacterium acnes* on the course of experimentally induced feline infectious peritonitis in specific-pathogen-free and random-source cats. *Am J Vet Res*. 1990;51:726–733.
176. Carvalho OV, Saraiva GL, Ferreira CG, et al. In-vitro antiviral efficacy of ribavirin and interferon-alpha against canine distemper virus. *Can J Vet Res*. 2014;78:283–289.
177. Calvert C. Canine viral papillomatosis. In: Greene CE, ed. *Infectious Diseases of the Dog and Cat*. 2nd ed. Philadelphia, PA: WB Saunders; 1998:49–51.
178. Penzo C, Ross M, Muirhead R, et al. Effect of recombinant feline interferon-omega alone and in combination with chemotherapeutic agents on putative tumour-initiating cells and daughter cells derived from canine and feline mammary tumours. *Vet Comp Oncol*. 2009;7:222–229.
179. Litzlbauer P, Weber K, Mueller RS. Oral and subcutaneous therapy of canine atopic dermatitis with recombinant feline interferon omega. *Cytokine*. 2014;66:54–59.
180. Kuwabara M, Nariai Y, Horiuchi Y, et al. Immunological effects of recombinant feline interferon-omega (KT-80) administration in the dog. *Microbiol Immunol*. 2006;50:637–641.
181. De Mari K, Maynard L, Sanquer A, et al. Therapeutic effects of recombinant feline interferon-omega on feline leukemia virus (FeLV)-infected and FeLV/feline immunodeficiency virus (FIV)-coinfected symptomatic cats. *J Vet Intern Med*. 2004;18:477–482.
182. Hampel V, Schwarz B, Kempf C, et al. Adjuvant immunotherapy of feline fibrosarcoma with recombinant feline interferon-omega. *J Vet Intern Med*. 2007;21:1340–1346.
183. Rogers R, Merigan TC, Hardy WD Jr, et al. Cat interferon inhibits feline leukaemia virus infection in cell culture. *Nat New Biol*. 1972;237:270–271.
184. Mochizuki M, Nakatani H, Yoshida M. Inhibitory effects of recombinant feline interferon on the replication of feline enteropathogenic viruses in vitro. *Vet Microbiol*. 1994;39:145–152.
185. Wang HJX, Yang L, Sun L, Wang H, Liu W. Comparison of antiviral activity between FeIFN-omega and FeIFN-alpha. *Sheng Wu Gong Cheng Xue Bao*. 2008;24:1556–1560.
186. Gil S, Leal RO, McGahie D, et al. Oral recombinant feline interferon-omega as an alternative immune modulation therapy in FIV positive cats: clinical and laboratory evaluation. *Res Vet Sci*. 2014;96:79–85.
187. Leal RO, Gil S, Duarte A, et al. Evaluation of viremia, proviral load and cytokine profile in naturally feline immunodeficiency virus infected cats treated with two different protocols of recombinant feline interferon omega. *Res Vet Sci*. 2015;99:87–95.
188. Ishida T, Shibanai A, Tanaka S, Uchida K, Mochizuki M. Recombinant feline interferon therapy of feline infectious peritonitis. In: Proceedings of the 2nd International FCoV/FIP Symposium; 2002:15. Glasgow, Scotland.
189. Ritz S, Egberink H, Hartmann K. Effect of feline interferon-omega on the survival time and quality of life of cats with feline infectious peritonitis. *J Vet Intern Med*. 2007;21:1193–1197.

190. Haid C, Kaps S, Gonczi E, et al. Pretreatment with feline interferon omega and the course of subsequent infection with feline herpesvirus in cats. *Vet Ophthalmol.* 2007;10:278–284.
191. Uchino TKR, Kouzuki S. Investigations of feline interferon and its therapeutic effects for field use: its therapeutics effects on feline calicivirus infection. *Jap J.* 1992;11:11.
192. Ballin AC, Schulz B, Helps C, et al. Limited efficacy of topical recombinant feline interferon-omega for treatment of cats with acute upper respiratory viral disease. *Vet J.* 2014;202:466–470.
193. Mihaljevic S. First clinical experiences with omega-interferon in the treatment of chronic gingivitis-stomatitis-oropharyngitis of cats. *Der Prakt Tierarzt.* 2003;84:350–361.
194. Hennet PR, Camy GA, McGahie DM, et al. Comparative efficacy of a recombinant feline interferon omega in refractory cases of calicivirus-positive cats with caudal stomatitis: a randomised, multi-centre, controlled, double-blind study in 39 cats. *J Feline Med Surg.* 2011;13: 577–587.
195. McInerney J, Papasouliotis K, Simpson K, et al. Pulmonary cowpox in cats: five cases. *J Feline Med Surg.* 2016;18:518–525.
196. Ishiwata K, Minagawa T, Kajimoto T. Clinical effects of the recombinant feline interferon-omega on experimental parvovirus infection in beagle dogs. *J Vet Med Sci.* 1998;60:911–917.
197. Martin V, Najbar W, Gueguen S, et al. Treatment of canine parvoviral enteritis with interferon-omega in a placebo-controlled challenge trial. *Vet Microbiol.* 2002;89:115–127.
198. de Mari K, Maynard L, Eun HM, et al. Treatment of canine parvoviral enteritis with interferon-omega in a placebo-controlled field trial. *Vet Rec.* 2003;152:105–108.
199. Minagawa T, Ishiwata K, Kajimoto T. Feline interferon-omega treatment on canine parvovirus infection. *Vet Microbiol.* 1999;69:51–53.
200. Paltrinieri S, Crippa A, Comerio T, et al. Evaluation of inflammation and immunity in cats with spontaneous parvovirus infection: consequences of recombinant feline interferon-omega administration. *Vet Immunol Immunopathol.* 2007;118:68–74.
201. Sato R, Inanami O, Tanaka Y, et al. Oral administration of bovine lactoferrin for treatment of intractable stomatitis in feline immunodeficiency virus (FIV)-positive and FIV-negative cats. *Am J Vet Res.* 1996;57:1443–1446.
202. Gibbons JA, Kanwar RK, Kanwar JR. Lactoferrin and cancer in different cancer models. *Front Biosci.* 2011;3:1080–1088.
203. Ammendolia MG, Agamennone M, Pietrantoni A, et al. Bovine lactoferrin-derived peptides as novel broad-spectrum inhibitors of influenza virus. *Pathog Glob Health.* 2012;106:12–19.
204. Zimecki M, Artym J, Chodaczek G, et al. Protective effects of lactoferrin in *Escherichia coli*-induced bacteremia in mice: relationship to reduced serum TNF alpha level and increased turnover of neutrophils. *Inflam Res.* 2004;53:292–296.
205. Kobayashi S, Abe Y, Inanami O, et al. Oral administration of bovine lactoferrin upregulates neutrophil functions in a dog with familial beta2-integrin-related neutrophil dysfunction. *Vet Immunol Immunopathol.* 2011;143:155–161.
206. Sato R, Kobayashi S, Abe Y, et al. Clinical effects of bovine lactoferrin on two canine cases with familial neutrophil dysfunction. *J Vet Med Sci.* 2012;74:1177–1183.
207. Kobayashi S, Sato R, Aoki T, et al. Effect of bovine lactoferrin on functions of activated feline peripheral blood mononuclear cells during chronic feline immunodeficiency virus infection. *J Vet Med Sci.* 2008;70:429–435.
208. Tanaka T, Nakatani S, Xuan X, et al. Antiviral activity of lactoferrin against canine herpesvirus. *Antiviral Res.* 2003;60:193–199.
209. Beaumont SL, Maggs DJ, Clarke HE. Effects of bovine lactoferrin on in vitro replication of feline herpesvirus. *Vet Ophthalmol.* 2003;6:245–250.
210. McCann KB, Lee A, Wan J, et al. The effect of bovine lactoferrin and lactoferricin B on the ability of feline calicivirus (a norovirus surrogate) and poliovirus to infect cell cultures. *J App Microbiol.* 2003;95: 1026–1033.
211. Hung YP, Yang YP, Wang HC, et al. Bovine lactoferrin and piroxicam as an adjunct treatment for lymphocytic-plasmacytic gingivitis stomatitis in cats. *Vet J.* 2014;202:76–82.
212. Addie DD, Radford A, Yam PS, et al. Cessation of feline calicivirus shedding coincident with resolution of chronic gingivostomatitis in a cat. *J Small Anim Pract.* 2003;44:172–176.
213. Bagla VP, McGaw LJ, Eloff JN. The antiviral activity of six South African plants traditionally used against infections in ethnoveterinary medicine. *Vet Microbiol.* 2012;155:198–206.
214. Danilov LL, Maltsev SD, Deyeva AV, et al. Phosprenyl: a novel drug with antiviral and immunomodulatory activity. *Arch Immunol Ther Exp.* 1996;44:395–400.
215. Vasil'ev AN, Ozherelkov SV, Kozlov V, et al. Antiviral and immunomodulating activity of polyprenyl phosphates in viral infections. *Antibiot Khimioter.* 2008;53:3–8.
216. Legendre AM, Bartges JW. Effect of polyprenyl immunostimulant on the survival times of three cats with the dry form of feline infectious peritonitis. *J Feline Med Surg.* 2009;11:624–626.
217. Legendre AM, Kuritz T, Galyon G, et al. Polyprenyl immunostimulant treatment of cats with presumptive non-effusive feline infectious peritonitis in a field study. *Front Vet Sci.* 2017;4:7.
218. Gonçalves K, Vasconcelos A, Barbirato D, et al. Therapeutic potential of ivermectin for COVID-19. *Authorea Preprints.* 2020 May 26.
219. Peña–Silva R, Duffull SB, Steer AC, et al. Pharmacokinetic considerations on the repurposing of ivermectin for treatment of COVID–19. *Br J Clin Pharmacol.* 2020 Jul 17.
220. Baskett A, Barton MH, Norton N, et al. Effect of pentoxifylline, flunixin meglumine, and their combination on a model of endotoxemia in horses. *Am J Vet Res.* 1997;58:1291–1299.
221. Barton MH, Moore JN, Norton N. Effects of pentoxifylline infusion on response of horses to in vivo challenge exposure with endotoxin. *Am J Vet Res.* 1997;58:1300–1307.
222. Nichols PR, Morris DO, Beale KM. A retrospective study of canine and feline cutaneous vasculitis. *Vet Dermatol.* 2001;12:255–264.
223. Marsella R, Olivry T. The ACVD task force on canine atopic dermatitis (XXII): nonsteroidal anti-inflammatory pharmacotherapy. *Vet Immunol Immunopathol.* 2001;81:331–345.
224. Siwak CT, Gruet P, Woehrle F, et al. Comparison of the effects of adrafinil, propentofylline, and nicergoline on behavior in aged dogs. *Am J Vet Res.* 2000;61:1410–1414.
225. Fischer Y, Ritz S, Weber K, et al. Randomized, placebo controlled study of the effect of propentofylline on survival time and quality of life of cats with feline infectious peritonitis. *J Vet Intern Med.* 2011;25:1270–1276.
226. Hartmann AD, Wilhelm N, Erfle V, et al. Clinical efficacy of melittin in the treatment of cats infected with the feline immunodeficiency virus. *Tierarztl Prax Ausg K Kleintiere Heimtiere.* 2016;44:417–423.
227. Lafrado LJ, Mathes LE, Zack PM, et al. Biological effects of staphylococcal protein A immunotherapy in cats with induced feline leukemia virus infection. *Am J Vet Res.* 1990;51:482–486.
228. Lies M. Volume of opinion warrants merit. *Vet Forum.* 1990;6:42.
229. Levy JK. FeLV and non-neoplastic felv-related disease. In: Ettinger SJ, Feldman EC, eds. Textbook of Veterinary Internal Medicine. Philadelphia: WB, Saunders; 2000:424–432.
230. Kelly EJ, Baldwin TJ, Chamberlain AP. Pathology in Practice. Dermatitis, cellulitis, and myositis caused by *S. marcescens* infection in a cat. *J Am Vet Med Assoc.* 2015;247:897–899.
231. Hartmann K, Block A, Ferk G, et al. Treatment of feline leukemia virus (FeLV) infection. *Vet Microbiol.* 1999;69:111–113.
232. Hartmann K, Block A, Ferk G, et al. Treatment of feline leukemia virus-infected cats with paramunity inducer. *Vet Immunol Immunopathol.* 1998;65:267–275.
233. Klimentowski S, Kolbl S, Fischer M. [The effectiveness of paramunization for the control of feline coryza]. *Berl Munch Tierarztl Wochenschr.* 1992;105:253–259.
234. Proksch AL, Unterer S, Truyen U, et al. Efficacy of the paramunity inducer PIND-ORF in the treatment of canine parvovirus infection. *Vet J.* 2014;202:340–347.
235. King GK, Yates KM, Greenlee PG, et al. The effect of acemannan immunostimulant in combination with surgery and radiation therapy on spontaneous canine and feline fibrosarcomas. *J Am Anim Hosp Assoc.* 1995;31: 439–447.

236. Harris C, Pierce K, King G, et al. Efficacy of acemannan in treatment of canine and feline spontaneous neoplasms. *Mol Biother.* 1991;3:207–213.
237. Yates KM, Rosenberg LJ, Harris CK, et al. Pilot study of the effect of acemannan in cats infected with feline immunodeficiency virus. *Vet Immunol Immunopathol.* 1992;35:177–189.
238. Sheets MA, Unger BA, Giggleman Jr GF, et al. Studies of the effect of acemannan on retrovirus infections: clinical stabilization of feline leukemia virus-infected cats. *Mol Biother.* 1991;3:41–45.
239. Wu L, Bao JK. Anti-tumor and anti-viral activities of *Galanthus nivalis* agglutinin (GNA)-related lectins. *Glycoconj J.* 2013;30:269–279.
240. Breitschwerdt EB, Davidson MG, Hegarty BC, et al. Prednisolone at anti-inflammatory or immunosuppressive dosages in conjunction with doxycycline does not potentiate the severity of *Rickettsia rickettsii* infection in dogs. *Antimicrob Agents Chemother.* 1997;41:141–147.
241. Trejo-Avila LM, Morales-Martinez ME, Ricque-Marie D, et al. In vitro anti-canine distemper virus activity of fucoidan extracted from the brown alga *Cladosiphon okamuranus. Virus Disease.* 2014;25:474–480.
242. Maldonado PD, Rivero-Cruz I, Mata R, et al. Antioxidant activity of A-type proanthocyanidins from *Geranium niveum* (Geraniaceae). *J Agric Food Chem.* 2005;53:1996–2001.
243. Shahat AA, Cos P, De Bruyne T, et al. Antiviral and antioxidant activity of flavonoids and proanthocyanidins from *Crataegus sinaica. Planta Medica.* 2002;68:539–541.
244. Galligioni V, Dal Pozzo F, Fontane G, et al. In vitro antiviral activity of proanthocyanidin A2 against canine distemper virus. *Afr J Tradit Complement Altern Med.* 2009;6:468–469.
245. Gallina L, Dal Pozzo F, Galligioni V, et al. Inhibition of viral RNA synthesis in canine distemper virus infection by proanthocyanidin A2. *Antiviral Res.* 2011;92:447–452.
246. McDonagh P, Sheehy PA, Fawcett A, et al. Antiviral effect of mefloquine on feline calicivirus in vitro. *Vet Microbiol.* 2015;176:370–377.
247. Shan L, Deng K, Shroff NS, et al. Stimulation of HIV-1-specific cytolytic T lymphocytes facilitates elimination of latent viral reservoir after virus reactivation. *Immunity.* 2012;36:491–501.

10

Antibacterial Drugs

Jane E. Sykes, Mark G. Papich

KEY POINTS

- An understanding of the mechanisms of action, spectrum of activity, pharmacokinetics, pharmacodynamics, and adverse effects of antibacterial drugs facilitates optimal treatment of bacterial infections while minimizing the chance for: (1) selection of resistant bacteria, (2) adverse reactions, and (3) drug interactions.
- The importance of appropriate administration of antibiotics, compliance issues, and potential adverse effects of the drug chosen should be discussed with the pet owner when antibiotics are prescribed.

INTRODUCTION

This chapter reviews the classification, mechanisms of action, spectrum of activity, resistance mechanisms, tissue penetration, clinical use, and adverse effects of the major classes of antibiotics used to treat dogs and cats. Antimicrobials have been grouped together in order according to their mechanism of action (cell wall synthesis, nucleic acid, and then protein synthesis inhibitors). Tables are dispersed throughout the text with drug dosages for each group of antibiotics. The reader is encouraged to review the accompanying text when using the tables. Not all antibiotics are reviewed here. Antibiotics that have specific uses, such as certain antimycobacterial drugs and nitrofurantoin, are reviewed in the relevant chapters of this book. Chapter 8 provides an overview of the basic principles of antimicrobial treatment and antimicrobial stewardship.

INHIBITORS OF CELL WALL SYNTHESIS

Inhibitors of cell wall synthesis include the beta-lactams (penicillins, cephalosporins, and carbapenems), fosfomycin, and glycopeptides.

Beta-Lactam Antibiotics

β-Lactam antibiotics have a β-lactam ring in their molecular structure (Fig. 10.1). They include penicillins, cephalosporins, monobactams, and carbapenems. They are bactericidal antibiotics (see Chapter 8) that bind covalently to and inhibit PBPs. These PBPs are needed to catalyze the cross-linking (or *transpeptidation*) of the peptidoglycan layer of bacterial cell walls, which is continuously remodeled by bacteria (Fig. 10.2). When PBPs are inactivated by β-lactam antibiotics, bacterial enzymes that hydrolyze the peptidoglycan cross-links during cell wall remodeling continue to function, which breaks down the cell wall further. The accumulation of peptidoglycan precursors also triggers activation of cell wall hydrolases, with further digestion of intact peptidoglycan. The end result is bacterial rupture.

The peptidoglycan layer of gram-positive bacteria is 50 to 100 times thicker than that of gram-negative bacteria and is highly cross-linked, which maintains the structural integrity of gram-positive bacteria.[1] Therefore, compared to gram-negative bacteria, gram-positive bacteria are more easily inactivated by β-lactam antibiotics and typically have lower MICs. Bacteria possess multiple PBPs, which are assigned numbers based on their molecular weight. PBPs vary in their affinities for different β-lactam antibiotics, which in part explains the difference in spectrum of activity and bactericidal action of β-lactam antibiotics. For example, inhibition of PBP1a and PBP1b leads to cell lysis, whereas inhibition of PBP2 results in rounded cells called spheroblasts. Drugs that produce rapid lysis (e.g., carbapenems) are the most bactericidal and have highest affinity for PBP1.

Resistance to β-lactam antibiotics was recognized soon after the discovery of penicillin in the 1930s. Resistance has increased gradually and is now common. Resistance results primarily from β-lactamase production.[2] It can also result from production of altered PBPs (such as PBP2a, which is encoded by the *mecA* gene and characterizes MRS) and, among gram-negative bacteria, exclusion of drugs that normally diffuse through porins to their site of action or removal by efflux transporters. Gram-negative β-lactamases are strategically located just beneath the outer LPS layer, which acts as the barrier to drug penetration. Gram-positive bacteria secrete β-lactamases into their immediate surroundings. There are hundreds of different β-lactamase enzymes that vary in their specificity for β-lactam drugs.

Most β-lactam antibiotics have a short half-life unless administered in slow-release formulations and exhibit time-dependent pharmacodynamics (see Chapter 8). Exceptions to this general description are described below. Drug concentrations should be maintained above the MIC (T > MIC) for approximately 50% of the dosing interval. For penicillins and carbapenems, T > MIC can be less than 50%, but aiming for a target of 50% ensures that most patients will have adequate exposure. Time of exposure (30% vs. 40%, vs. 50%, and so on) determines the extent of *in vitro* decline in CFUs in laboratory infection models, usually expressed as net bacterial stasis, 1-$\log_{10}$ reduction, 2-$\log_{10}$ reduction, or 3-$\log_{10}$- reduction in bacterial counts.[3] Immunosuppressed patients or severe life-threatening infection (e.g., pneumonia, sepsis) should have longer T > MIC than immunocompetent animals. To maintain this target, some β-lactam antibiotics with short half-lives require frequent administration or slow infusion. For other drugs, a long half-life prolongs the T > MIC to allow for infrequent administration. For example, cefpodoxime proxetil has a longer half-life than other oral cephalosporins, so it can be administered only once per day.

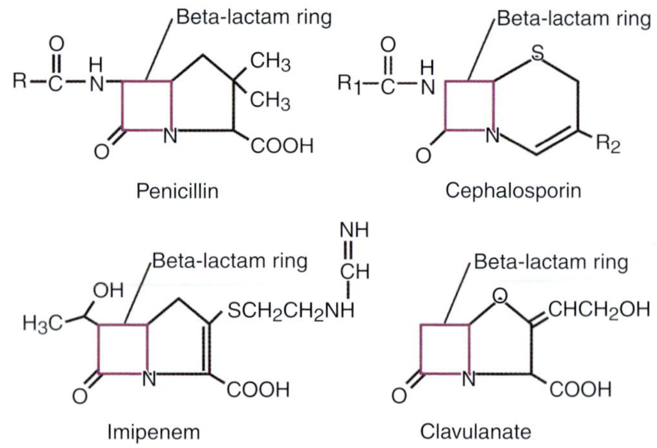

Fig. 10.1 Structure of β-lactam antibiotics.

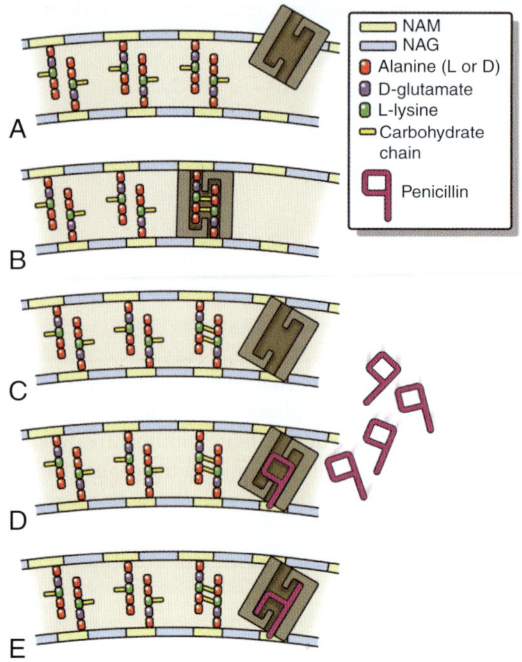

Fig. 10.2 Interference of peptidoglycan production by β-lactam antibiotics. The bacterial cell wall consists of *N*-acetylglucosamine *(NAG)* and *N*-acetylmuramic acid *(NAM)* subunits. (A) The penicillin-binding protein *(PBP, brown squares)* binds (B) peptide side chains and forms a cross-link. (C) The PBP dissociates from the wall once the cross-link has been formed. (D) Penicillins enter the active site of the PBP. (E) The β-lactam ring of the penicillin is irreversibly opened when it reacts with the PBP, which permanently blocks the active site.

Cefovecin has an extremely long half-life in dogs and cats and can be effective for some infections when administered at 14-day intervals. For other cephalosporins (e.g., injectable drugs with short half-lives such as ceftazidime), three- to four-times-daily dosing may be required for treatment of gram-negative bacterial infections.

Penicillins

Classification, Spectrum of Activity, and Resistance Mechanisms

Penicillins are derived from *Penicillium* molds. They are classified as naturally occurring penicillins such as penicillin G (benzyl penicillin), the semisynthetic aminopenicillins such as ampicillin and amoxicillin, penicillinase-resistant penicillins, and extended-spectrum penicillins. Table 10.1 shows the classification of the penicillins and their respective spectra of activity.

Penicillin G must be given parenterally because of poor oral absorption. Gram-positive bacteria that are susceptible to penicillin G are more susceptible to penicillin G than to aminopenicillins such as ampicillin. The aminopenicillins have some activity against gram-negative bacteria, but generally not bacteria of the Enterobacterales (e.g., *Escherichia coli*), or nonfermenters (e.g., *Pseudomonas aeruginosa*). Most of the gram-negative bacteria are resistant because they produce β-lactamases. Ampicillin and amoxicillin have an almost identical spectrum, but amoxicillin has approximately twice the oral absorption of ampicillin and is a better choice for oral administration.

Penicillinase-resistant penicillins (also known as β-lactamase-resistant penicillins or antistaphylococcal penicillins) such as methicillin have a structure that resists inactivation by staphylococcal β-lactamase enzymes. These drugs include methicillin, cloxacillin, and dicloxacillin. These drugs are rarely (if ever) used for small animal treatment today. Their oral absorption is poor, and many formulations are no longer available. Oxacillin is used by the laboratory to test for methicillin-resistant strains of *Staphylococcus* spp. This phenotypic test is highly reliable for detecting resistance caused by bacterial possession of the altered PBP2a, which leads to resistance to all β-lactam antibiotics.[4] It should be noted that that the cefoxitin test for this resistance mechanism in *Staphylococcus aureus* cannot be reliably used for *Staphylococcus pseudintermedius.*

Extended-spectrum penicillins (antipseudomonal penicillins) have enhanced activity against gram-negative bacteria, but must be given parenterally. Their short half-lives (less than 1 hour) frequently require administration or a CRI. These drugs include the carboxypenicillins, such as ticarcillin and carbenicillin, and piperacillin, an ureidopenicillin. The only agent in this group currently available is piperacillin, which is only available as the combination of piperacillin and tazobactam (discussed later in this chapter). Other drugs in this group have been withdrawn by the manufacturer.

Clavulanic acid, sulbactam, and tazobactam are β-lactamase inhibitors that are administered in conjunction with penicillins, which increase the spectrum of activity. β-Lactamase inhibitors possess weak intrinsic antibacterial activity. The combination of amoxicillin and clavulanate is a popular oral antibiotic for dogs, cats, and humans. The pharmacokinetics allow for oral absorption of both drugs (marketed for animals in a 1:4 ratio of clavulanate:amoxicillin) to maintain an effective plasma drug ratio throughout the dose interval. Sulbactam has been combined with ampicillin for IV injection. Sulbactam is not as active as clavulanic acid against some gram-negative β-lactamases. Tazobactam is combined with piperacillin. Piperacillin-tazobactam ("Pip-Taz") is a highly active combination against gram-positive and most gram-negative bacteria, including *P. aeruginosa* and many ESBL-producing Enterobacterales. Because of the short half-life in dogs (approximately 30 minutes), it must be administered IV frequently, or with a CRI. Ticarcillin-clavulanate, once a popular agent in veterinary hospitals, has been withdrawn from the manufacturer and is no longer available.

Clinical Use

Penicillin dosages for dogs and cats are listed in Table 10.2. The absorption and duration of activity of penicillins depends on the dose administered, the vehicle containing the drug, the solubility of the salt formulation, and the presence or absence of food. Penicillins are distributed to the extracellular fluid of most tissues. Because of low penetration across the blood-brain barrier and blood-ocular barrier, high doses are needed in order to attain effective levels in these tissues.

TABLE 10.1 Classification and Spectrum of Activity of Penicillin Antibiotics

Penicillin Group	Examples	Antibacterial Spectrum
Natural penicillins	Penicillin G	Gram-positive aerobic bacteria (especially streptococci) and anaerobes. *Pasteurella multocida* may also be susceptible
Aminopenicillins	Ampicillin Amoxicillin	Gram-positive aerobic bacteria (cocci and bacilli) and anaerobes; some susceptible gram-negative bacteria
Penicillinase-resistant penicillins	Methicillin Oxacillin Cloxacillin Dicloxacillin	Susceptible β-lactamase-producing gram-positive aerobic bacteria (*Staphylococcus* spp.). Less active against penicillinase-susceptible organisms than penicillin G
Extended-spectrum carboxypenicillins	Ticarcillin *(no longer available)* Carbenicillin *(no longer available)*	Increased activity against susceptible gram-negative aerobes, which includes *Pseudomonas aeruginosa*, *Proteus* spp., *Klebsiella*, and anaerobes. Some reduction in gram-positive spectrum. Destroyed by β-lactamases
Ureidopenicillins	Mezlocillin Piperacillin (always in combination with tazobactam)	Susceptible gram-positive and gram-negative aerobes, which include *Pseudomonas aeruginosa*. Some loss of anaerobic spectrum. Destroyed by β-lactamases
Penicillin–β-lactamase inhibitor combinations	β-Lactamase inhibitors: clavulanic acid, sulbactam, tazobactam. Examples: amoxicillin-clavulanate, piperacillin-tazobactam, ampicillin-sulbactam.	Susceptible β-lactamase-producing gram-positive and gram-negative aerobic bacteria and anaerobes

TABLE 10.2 Suggested Penicillin Dosages for Small Animals

Drug	Dose (mg/kg)	Interval (hours)	Species	Route	Comments	CLSI Breakpoints(µg/mL)
Penicillin G potassium or sodium	20,000–40,000 U/kg	6–8	D, C	IV, IM		≤8 for enterococci; ≤0.12 for staphylococci and streptococci
Ampicillin sodium	10–20	6–8	D, C	IV, IM, SC	Administer IV over 3 minutes. When reconstituted with sterile water to 250 mg/mL, vials should be used within 1 hour. When reconstituted with 0.9% NaCl to 45 mg/mL, stability is maintained for 48 hours if refrigerated	≤0.25 for staphylococci, streptococci, and gram-negative bacilli; ≤8 for canine urinary tract pathogens
Ampicillin-sulbactam	10–20	8	D, C	IV, IM	See ampicillin. Dose according to ampicillin component	≤8/4[a] for staphylococci and gram-negative bacteria
Amoxicillin	10–20	8–12	D, C	PO		See ampicillin.
Amoxicillin-clavulanate potassium	12.5–25	12	D, C	PO	More frequent or higher doses recommended for gram-negative infections	≤0.25/0.12[a] for staphylococci, streptococci, *Escherichia coli* and *Pasteurella multocida*
Ticarcillin disodium, ticarcillin-clavulanate[b] *(No longer available)*	33–50	4–6	D, C	IV	When reconstituted with 0.9% NaCl, stable for up to 14 days when refrigerated	≤64/2[a] for *Pseudomonas aeruginosa*, ≤16/2 for gram-negative enteric bacteria
Piperacillin sodium/ piperacillin-tazobactam[b]	40	6	D, C	IV	Reconstituted solution should be used within 7 days if refrigerated	See ticarcillin

[a]The "/" distinguishes the ticarcillin from clavulanic acid concentrations.
[b]It is recommended that the use of these drugs be reserved for life-threatening infections that are susceptible to these drugs but resistant to other drugs, on the basis of culture and susceptibility testing.
C, cats; *CLSI*, Clinical and Laboratory Standards Institute[41,42]; *D*, dogs; *IM*, intramuscular; *IV*, intravenous; *PO*, oral; *SC*, subcutaneous.

Penicillins undergo rapid renal elimination, and active drug is concentrated in the urine; therefore, they are useful for treatment of bacterial UTIs. Liver impairment has little effect on the pharmacokinetics of penicillins. In animals with kidney disease, increasing the length of the dose interval in proportion to the degree of kidney impairment should be considered to prevent accumulation from repeated doses. Potassium-containing penicillins should not be given IV to patients with oliguric acute kidney injury because of the risk of hyperkalemia.

Adverse Effects

Penicillins are generally well tolerated by dogs and cats. The most common adverse effects in dogs and cats are vomiting, diarrhea, and

TABLE 10.3 **Classification and Spectrum of Activity of Cephalosporin Antibiotics**

Cephalosporin Generation	Examples	Antibacterial Spectrum
First	Cephalexin Cefazolin Cefadroxil	Methicillin-susceptible staphylococci and streptococci and aerobes; some activity against gram-negative aerobes (especially cefazolin). Unpredictable activity against anaerobes
Second	Cefaclor Cefotetan *(no longer available)* Cefoxitin	Improved activity against gram-negative aerobes and anaerobes compared with first-generation drugs. Cefoxitin has greater stability against anaerobic β-lactamases (such as those produced by *Bacteroides* spp.) than other second-generation drugs
Third	Cefixime *(oral but no longer available)* Cefpodoxime *(only oral product in this group)* Ceftiofur Cefotaxime *(no longer available)* Ceftriaxone Cefovecin Ceftazidime	Activity primarily against gram-negative bacteria. Some drugs in this group have less activity against gram-positive bacteria and anaerobes
Fourth	Cefepime	Gram-positive cocci, gram-negative bacilli, many β-lactamase-producing gram-negative bacteria. Reserve for life-threatening infections where no other alternative is available

inappetence. These are more likely to occur with amoxicillin when clavulanic acid is administered concurrently. Hypersensitivity reactions that include fever, cutaneous reactions, immune-mediated cytopenias, and anaphylaxis are possible, especially in dogs, but are less common than in human patients (approximately 15% of people are allergic to penicillin). The use of penicillins should be avoided in animals with a history of such reactions. Rarely, rapid IV infusion or administration of high doses of penicillins to animals with co-existing renal failure is followed by development of neurologic signs, such as seizures. This effect is caused by inhibition of γ-aminobutyric acid (GABA) in the CNS. Pain or tissue reactions can occur when penicillins are administered IM or SC.

Cephalosporins

Classification and Spectrum of Activity

The cephalosporins were originally derived from *Acremonium* spp. (previously known as *Cephalosporium* spp.). They have been broadly grouped into first-, second-, third-, and fourth-generation cephalosporins based on their spectrum of activity. As the generation increases, there is an increase in gram-negative spectrum, and fourth-generation drugs have truly broad-spectrum activity (Table 10.3). An exception to this pattern is the newest addition to the group, ceftaroline. It has activity against MRS as a result of an affinity for PBP2a and has been considered a "fifth-generation" cephalosporin. Cephalosporins are resistant to staphylococcal β-lactamase, and the extended-spectrum cephalosporins (primarily third-generation drugs) are resistant to many gram-negative β-lactamases. However, bacterial plasmid-encoded ESBL enzymes and the chromosomally encoded AmpC β-lactamase can hydrolyze even third-generation cephalosporins and present an important therapeutic challenge. ESBLs are typically not detected using routine susceptibility testing but should be suspected when there is resistance among gram-negative bacteria to third-generation cephalosporins. A laboratory can confirm the presence of ESBL if an isolate is suspected.

Clinical Use

Cephalosporin dosages for cats and dogs are listed in Table 10.4. First-generation cephalosporins such as cephalexin are moderately absorbed orally and distributed into extracellular fluids. In general, they have poor penetration of the blood-brain barrier, even in the face of inflammation, but penetration into other extracellular fluids are sufficient. Most are excreted unchanged in the urine, and so are useful for treatment of UTIs. Cefazolin has greater activity against a wider range of bacterial isolates than the oral first-generation cephalosporins (e.g., cephalexin and cefadroxil).[5] Cefazolin has been a popular injectable antibiotic for perioperative use in small animals. This perioperative use of cefazolin is with the intention to prevent postsurgical infections, particularly in orthopedic surgery (see Chapter 121).

Use of second-, third-, and fourth-generation cephalosporins may be indicated when there is resistance to first-generation cephalosporins and there are no other reasonable alternatives available. Three third-generation cephalosporins are approved by the US FDA for use in small animals: ceftiofur, cefpodoxime proxetil, and cefovecin. These agents are approved for treatment of skin and soft tissue infections (cefpodoxime proxetil and cefovecin) and UTIs in dogs (ceftiofur). Although their use in small animal medicine has been controversial because of concerns that relate to selection for resistant bacteria,[6] there is no evidence at this time that these agents are more likely to select for resistance among isolates from dogs and cats than other agents. The injectable third-generation cephalosporins approved for humans have greater *in vitro* activity than cefpodoxime or cefovecin and occasionally have been used in dogs and cats (e.g., cefotaxime, ceftazidime, cefoperazone). Of these, ceftazidime is the most often used, and cefotaxime is no longer available in the United States. These drugs have a high degree of activity, but must be administered frequently by injection. Therefore, the use of these agents is limited to in-hospital use in which repeated IV injections or CRIs are possible.

Distribution and excretion into urine and bile is variable. Cefpodoxime proxetil is the most commonly used oral third-generation drug in small animals, approximately 50% of which is excreted in the urine in active form. Cefovecin is approved for use in dogs and cats in Europe and North America as a SC injection. The high protein binding and slow clearance result in a very long half-life in these species (approximately 7 days in cats and 5 days in dogs). Administration of cefovecin results in a duration of activity of at least 14 days in cats, and for at least 7 to 14 days in dogs (depending on the pathogen).

TABLE 10.4 Suggested Cephalosporin Dosages for Small Animals

Drug	Dose (mg/kg)	Interval (hours)	Route	Species	Comments	CLSI Breakpoints (µg/mL)
Cephalexin	25 15–20	12 12	PO	D C	Use 30 mg/kg q12h for pyoderma	≤2 for susceptible organisms.
Cefadroxil	22	12 24	PO	D C		See cephalexin
Cefazolin sodium	20–35	8	IV, IM	D, C	22 mg/kg q2h during surgery if indicated	See cephalexin
Cefaclor[b]	15–20	8	PO	D, C		≤8 for all susceptible organisms
Cefoxitin sodium[b]	30	6–8	IM, IV	D, C	Pain on injection IM	See cefaclor
Cefixime[b]	10	12	PO	D, C	Use 5 mg/kg q12–24h for urinary tract infections	≤1 for all susceptible organisms
Cefpodoxime proxetil[b]	5–10	24	PO	D[a]	Of all third-generation cephalosporins, most active against staphylococci. Less active against gram-negative and anaerobic infections	≤2 for all susceptible organisms
Ceftiofur sodium[b]	2.2–4.4	24	SC	D[a]	For treatment of otherwise resistant urinary tract infections	Not established for dogs and cats
Cefotaxime sodium[b] *(no longer available)*	50 20–80	126	IV, IM	D C	Partially metabolized by the liver to desacetyl cefotaxime which contributes to antibacterial activity. Good CNS penetration. Stable for 5 days in the refrigerator after reconstitution	See cefpodoxime
Ceftazidime[b]	30	6	IV	D, C	Potent antipseudomonal activity	≤4 for Enterobacterales, ≤8 for *Pseudomonas aeruginosa* and staphylococci
Cefovecin[b]	8	14 days	SC	D, C	Approved for use for skin and soft tissue infections and in some countries, urinary tract infections. Efficacy for treatment of infections in other sites not established	No approved breakpoint. ≤2 for all susceptible organisms is suggested
Cefepime[b]	40	6	IV, IM	D[a]	Reduce frequency in dogs with renal failure (q12–24h)	≤ 8 for all susceptible organisms

[a]Dose not established for cats.
[b]It is recommended that the use of most second-, third-, and fourth-generation cephalosporins be reserved for serious infections that are susceptible to those drugs but resistant to other reasonable alternatives on the basis of culture and susceptibility testing.
C, cats; *CLSI*, Clinical and Laboratory Standards Institute[41,42]; *CNS*, central nervous system; *D*, dogs; *IM*, intramuscular; *IV*, intravenous; *PO*, oral; *SC*, subcutaneous.

Adverse Effects

Adverse effects of cephalosporins in dogs and cats are similar to those of penicillins, with GI signs and hypersensitivity reactions being most frequent. Although the incidence is low, cross-sensitivity can occur between penicillins and cephalosporins, so cephalosporins should be used with caution in animals that have a history of reactions to penicillin. Injectable cephalosporins can cause phlebitis and pain on injection. Cephalosporins have the potential to cause false-positive results on test strips that use copper reduction for urine glucose detection. Certain cephalosporins, such as cefotetan (no longer available) and ceftriaxone, may exacerbate bleeding tendencies due to vitamin K antagonism.[7] Reversible bone marrow suppression has been reported in dogs given long-term high doses of ceftiofur, cefonicid, and cefazedone.[8]

Monobactams (Aztreonam)

Aztreonam is a synthetic β-lactam antibiotic that is resistant to some β-lactamases. It is effective against a wide range of gram-negative bacteria, including *P. aeruginosa,* but not gram-positive or anaerobic bacteria. In human medicine, aztreonam is used to treat patients with serious gram-negative infections who are allergic to penicillins and cannot tolerate aminoglycosides.[9] Dosages have not been established for dogs and it is rarely used.

Carbapenems

Spectrum of Activity and Clinical Use

Carbapenems are highly resistant to almost all bacterial β-lactamases and include imipenem, meropenem, ertapenem, and doripenem. Of these, meropenem is the most frequently used in small animals because it is easier to administer and has a favorable spectrum and few adverse effects. They penetrate the outer membrane of gram-negative bacteria more effectively than many other β-lactam antibiotics and bind to a variety of PBPs, which leads to rapid lysis of a broad spectrum of bacteria.[10] In contrast to other β-lactam antibiotics, carbapenems have a postantibiotic effect (see Chapter 8) similar to that of aminoglycosides and fluoroquinolones. Although effective against many gram-positive, gram-negative, and anaerobic bacterial infections, the use of carbapenems is reserved for treatment of serious, MDR gram-negative infections, especially caused by *E. coli, Klebsiella pneumoniae,* and

TABLE 10.5 **Suggested Carbapenem Dosages for Small Animals**

Drug	Dose (mg/kg)	Interval (hours)	Species	Route	Comments	CLSI Breakpoints (μg/mL)
Imipenem-cilastatin	5	6–8	D, C	IV, IM, SC	250–500 mg of reconstituted drug should be added to no less than 100 mL of fluids and administered IV over 30–60 minutes. Stable for 24 hours after reconstitution when refrigerated. For IM injections, reconstitute with 1% lidocaine	≤1 for Enterobacterales, ≤2 for *Pseudomonas aeruginosa*
Meropenem	10 (for *Escherichia coli*)	8	D	IV, IM, SC	SC injections may cause alopecia at the injection site.	Although an official breakpoint is not available at this time, use ≤1 μg/mL (S) for Enterobacterales (*E. coli*) and ≤2 μg/mL (S) for *P. aeruginosa*.
	30 (for *Pseudomonas aeruginosa*)	8	D	IV, IM, SC		
	10	12	C	IV, IM, SC		

Carbapenems should be used for serious infections resistant to other reasonable alternatives, on the basis of culture and susceptibility testing.
C, cats; *CLSI*, Clinical and Laboratory Standards Institute[41,42]; *D*, dogs; *IM*, intramuscular; *IV*, intravenous; *MIC*, minimum inhibitory concentration; *PO*, oral; *S*, susceptible; *SC*, subcutaneous.

P. aeruginosa, that are resistant to other antibiotics. MRS are resistant to carbapenems. Carbapenems must be administered parenterally because they are not absorbed after oral administration. Pharmacokinetics for meropenem have been reported for dogs.[11] Ertapenem has a narrower spectrum of activity and is less active against *P. aeruginosa* than the other agents. Dosages for dogs and cats are listed in Table 10.5.

The identification of carbapenemase production by some strains of gram-negative bacteria has raised great concern, because this confers resistance to a broad range of β-lactam antibiotics. Carbapenemase-producing *K. pneumoniae* (KPC), and carbapenem-resistent Enterobacterales (CRE), are resistant not only to all β-lactam antibiotics but also to fluoroquinolones and aminoglycosides.[12] *Klebsiella pneumoniae* that produce a plasmid-encoded metallo-β-lactamase enzyme (NDM-1) appeared in India in 2008 and have subsequently spread worldwide.[13] The only options left for treatment of these infections are tigecycline, polymyxins, and newly developed human drugs which have not been used in animals at this time.[14] The potential for spread of *K. pneumoniae* isolates that are resistant to all commercially available antibiotics now exists. Carapenemase (NDM-1) production has been detected in *E. coli* isolates from dogs and cats in the United States[15] and an *Acinetobacter lwoffii* isolate from a cat in China.[16]

Adverse Effects

Imipenem is degraded by dehydropeptidase-1, a brush border enzyme in the proximal renal tubules, which results in production of an inactive metabolite that is nephrotoxic. In order to prevent nephrotoxicity and maximize imipenem's antibacterial activity in the urine, imipenem is administered with cilastatin, which inhibits the dehydropeptidase-1 enzyme. Newer carbapenems such as meropenem are resistant to dehydropeptidase-1.

Adverse effects of carbapenems are otherwise rare and include vomiting, nausea, and pain on injection. Neurologic signs, including tremors, nystagmus, and seizures, can occur following rapid infusion of imipenem-cilastatin or in animals with renal insufficiency. Imipenem must be administered slowly in IV fluids (see Table 10.5). Slow administration is not required for meropenem, which is more soluble, and more stable after reconstitution. SC injections of meropenem have produced alopecia at the injection site,[17] but otherwise these injections have been very well tolerated and have eradicated infections associated with MDR gram-negative bacteria.

Glycopeptides

Mechanism of Action and Clinical Use

Glycopeptides are cyclic glycosylated peptide antimicrobials that inhibit the synthesis of peptidoglycan by binding to amino acids (D-alanyl-D-alanine) in the cell wall, preventing the addition of new units. Vancomycin, teicoplanin, and decaplanin are all glycopeptides. Only vancomycin has been used in small animals, but its use is rare.

Vancomycin was discovered in the 1950s, but has not been frequently used in small animals because it is not absorbed orally; therefore, IV infusion is required for treatment of systemic infections. When administered IV, it can be valuable for treatment of MDR gram-positive bacterial infections, such as MRS infections, resistant enterococcal infections, and encrusting cystitis caused by *Corynebacterium urealyticum*. The last is an emerging infection of dogs, cats, and immunocompromised human patients, treatment of which requires surgical debridement of the bladder in conjunction with glycopeptide administration.[18,19] Vancomycin is a valuable agent for treatment of MRS because resistance among these organisms is extremely rare and the bactericidal activity can be an advantage when treating immunocompromised patients. In human patients, oral vancomycin has been used to treat GI infections caused by resistant *Clostridioides difficile*.

Vancomycin-resistant methicillin-resistant *S. aureus* (MRSA) isolates are extremely rare in humans and have only been described in specific geographic locations. Vancomycin-resistant *S. pseudintermedius* isolates have not yet been described. Vancomycin-resistant enterococci (VRE) are well documented in human patients and can present a therapeutic challenge. Although currently rare, the existence of VRE has been reported in companion animals.[20,21] Resistance to vancomycin results from bacterial alteration of the terminal amino acid to which vancomycin binds. Because veterinary breakpoints for testing are not available, laboratories must use human interpretive categories for testing. In order to reduce inappropriate use of vancomycin, some laboratories do not report results for vancomycin susceptibility unless reporting is indicated on the basis of resistance in the remainder of the susceptibility panel.

There are new agents available for human medicine similar to vancomycin from the class of lipoglycopeptides. Dalbavancin (Dalvance) is a long-acting IV lipoglycopeptide, similar to telavancin (Vibativ). Oritavancin (Orbativ) is a long-acting IV lipoglycopeptide, similar to telavancin. The half-life of dalbavancin and oritavancin in humans is approximately 14 days, which allows for a single treatment. Telavancin (Vibativ) is a lipoglycopeptide for once-daily administration in humans. Because of the high cost of these drugs and reluctance to use valuable drugs for human use, the administration of these agents to animals for treatment of resistant infections has not been described.

Adverse Effects

Vancomycin is not commonly used to treat small animals, and so adverse reactions have not been well documented. The most common

TABLE 10.6 Suggested Vancomycin Dosages for Small Animals

Drug	Dose (mg/kg)	Interval (hours)	Species	Route	Comments	CLSI Breakpoints (µg/mL)
Vancomycin[a]	15	6–8	D	IV	Reconstituted drug is added to 0.9% NaCl or 5% dextrose and administered over 30 to 60 minutes. It can also be administered in 5% dextrose as a CRI, with a loading dose of 3.5 mg/kg, and then 1.5 mg/kg/hour IV. Therapeutic drug monitoring recommended to ensure that effective concentrations are achieved.	≤4 for *Enterococcus* and *Staphylococcus*
	12–15	8	C			

[a]The use of vancomycin should be reserved for gram-positive infections that are susceptible to vancomycin but resistant to all other reasonable alternatives, on the basis of culture and susceptibility testing.
C, cats; *CLSI*, Clinical and Laboratory Standards Institute[41,42]; *CRI*, constant-rate infusion; *D*, dogs; *IV*, intravenous.

reaction in human patients is the "red man syndrome" caused by histamine release after rapid infusion. This can be prevented through the use of antihistamines and slower infusion rates. Other adverse reactions are rare. Previously cited nephrotoxicity from vancomycin may be exaggerated because of its frequent co-administration with aminoglycosides, although a series of cases in dogs and cats with coexisting morbidities have been reported. Current formulations are of better quality and purity and less likely to produce kidney injury. Vancomycin is given by IV infusion over 30 to 60 minutes through a central or peripheral catheter (Table 10.6). Trough plasma concentrations can be monitored and should be greater than 10 µg/mL for skin and soft tissue infections, and 10 to 20 µg/mL for more complicated infections. Intramuscular administration should be avoided because it is painful and irritates tissues.

Fosfomycin

Mechanism of Action and Clinical Use

Fosfomycin is an antibiotic from *Streptomyces* spp. It is bactericidal and inactivates the bacterial enzyme UDP-*N*-acetylglucosamine-3-enolpyruvyltransferase (MurA), which catalyzes the first step in peptidoglycan synthesis. This is a unique mechanism of action that differs from that of β-lactam drugs and glycopeptides. Fosfomycin enters bacterial cells by the glucose-6-phosphate-inducible hexose monophosphate transport system and to a lesser extent, the L-alpha-glycerophosphate transport system. Bacteria with mutations of these transport systems can be resistant to fosfomycin. Other mechanisms of resistance include modification or overexpression of MurA or inactivation by plasmid-encoded bacterial enzymes such as *fosA, fosB, fosC,* and *fosX*.[22] Resistance in *E. coli* is currently rare, including among isolates from dogs and cats,[23] but fecal carriage of resistant isolates was detected in 2.4% and 0.8% of dogs and cats, respectively, from Hong Kong in 2008 to 2010.[24] Among 31 canine methicillin-resistant *S. pseudintermedius* isolates from North America, 84% were susceptible to fosfomycin.[25]

Clinical Use

Fosfomycin is available commercially as fosfomycin tromethamine. It has a broad-spectrum activity that includes aerobic and facultative gram-negative and gram positive bacteria. It is primarily indicated for treatment of MDR gram-positive and gram-negative bacterial UTIs, and in humans a single dose is recommended as a first-line treatment for acute uncomplicated cystitis. Fosfomycin exhibits concentration-dependent bacterial killing, with a long postantibiotic effect. The use of fosfomycin in veterinary medicine is currently limited by its high cost and relative unfamiliarity with the drug. Its use in dogs should be reserved for serious infections associated with clinical signs of lower urinary tract disease, where no other treatment option is available.

In humans, fosfomycin distributes widely into tissues after oral administration. It is not metabolized, and 54% to 65% of unaltered drug appears in the urine through glomerular filtration, attaining high concentrations in the urine.[22] Excellent tissue penetration and activity against biofilm is thought to be the result of the drug's low molecular weight and low plasma protein binding (< 0.5%).[26,27] This makes it appealing for treatment of bacterial prostatitis and pyelonephritis. Pharmacokinetic information for fosfomycin disodium when administered IM, SC, and PO (40 mg/kg and 80 mg/kg) has been described for dogs, but an oral dose that resulted in tissue concentrations necessary for effective bacterial killing was not established.[27] A combination of fosfomycin and clarithromycin was shown to have synergistic activity *in vitro* against *S. pseudintermedius* biofilm.[28]

Adverse Effects

In humans, fosfomycin administration is well tolerated, with the main adverse effect being diarrhea.[29] Administration of fosfomycin to dogs at a dose used to treat UTIs (40 mg/kg PO or IV q12h for 3 days) was not associated with hematologic or biochemical adverse effects, but young and adult cats developed acute kidney injury that was associated with tubular necrosis.[30] Therefore, until a safe dose has been established, fosfomycin should not be used to treat cats. More studies are also required to establish safe and effective doses of fosfomycin tromethamine for treatment of UTIs and systemic infections in dogs.

DRUGS THAT DISRUPT THE CELL MEMBRANE

Polymyxins

Mechanism of Action

The polymyxins are a group of closely related, cationic, cyclic peptides. Of the types A through E, polymyxin B and polymyxin E (colistin) are therapeutically most important. The most common use of this group in animals is from the formulations that contain polymyxins in a topical form, usually in combination with other agents (e.g., "triple antibiotic" that contains polymyxins B, neomycin, and bacitracin). Colistin is used as the last resort to treat serious gram-negative infections in humans. Polymyxins are cationic detergents that bind to LPS and increase the permeability of gram-negative bacteria. Most gram-negative organisms are susceptible. Increased use of polymyxins to treat infections in humans has been followed by appearance of resistant strains that most often have bacterial modifications of the lipid A component of LPS. Of major concern, plasmid-mediated resistance has been described in MDR *E. coli* from China that results from possession of the *mcr-1* gene, including among isolates from companion animals.[31] Other resistance mechanisms include complete loss of LPS and efflux pump mechanisms.[32]

Clinical Use and Adverse Effects

In dogs and cats, polymyxins are primarily used in combination with neomycin and bacitracin or tetracycline as topical preparations for treatment of localized ocular and otic infections. Colistin is given IV to humans to treat serious resistant infections. It has been the only agent active against some carbapenem-resistant Enterobacterales (CRE). Nephrotoxicity has limited the usefulness of these drugs for systemic therapy. Polymyxins are poorly absorbed when given orally and topically. They do not produce high plasma concentrations after parenteral administration, presumably because of high affinity for host cell membranes. Polymyxins diffuse poorly through biologic membranes and are excreted unchanged in urine.

Daptomycin

Daptomycin is a cyclic lipopeptide from *Streptomyces roseosporus* that is used parenterally in humans to treat serious infections caused by gram-positive bacteria (typically MRS and VRE). Daptomycin has a unique mechanism of action whereby it inserts into the bacterial cell membrane, which leads to permeabilization and depolarization of the membrane.[33] The extent to which this occurs depends on the amount of phosphatidylglycerol in the membrane, and resistant bacterial strains may have decreased synthesis of phosphatidylglycerol. Daptomycin has a bactericidal effect in a concentration-dependent manner. Adverse effects in human patients are uncommon but have included rhabdomyolysis and myalgia.[34] There are no reports of the use of daptomycin in dogs and cats.

NUCLEIC ACID INHIBITORS

Fluoroquinolones

Classification and Mechanism of Action

The fluoroquinolones bind to DNA gyrase (also known as topoisomerase II) and topoisomerase IV, enzymes that cleave DNA during DNA replication. The result is disruption of bacterial DNA and protein synthesis. For the veterinary fluoroquinolones enrofloxacin, orbifloxacin, and marbofloxacin, DNA gyrase is the primary target for gram-negative bacteria and topoisomerase IV is the primary target for gram-positive bacteria. Because topoisomerase IV has a lower affinity than DNA gyrase for this group of drugs, higher MICs are observed for gram-positive bacteria compared with the Enterobacterales.

Fluoroquinolones were created by addition of a fluorine group to nalidixic acid, which improves its spectrum of activity. Examples are enrofloxacin, ciprofloxacin, difloxacin, orbifloxacin, and marbofloxacin. Newer-generation fluoroquinolones inhibit *both* DNA gyrase and topoisomerase IV in gram-positive bacteria, leading to enhanced activity for treatment of gram-positive and anaerobic bacterial infections and reduced likelihood of selection for resistant mutants. Pradofloxacin, levofloxacin, moxifloxacin, and gatifloxacin are third-generation fluoroquinolones. The only antibiotic in this group approved for use in companion animals is pradofloxacin, which is approved for use in cats in the United States, and approved for both dogs and cats in European countries. Levofloxacin is a less expensive oral human generic drug in tablets that has become popular for oral use in dogs.

Resistance to fluoroquinolones results from DNA gyrase mutations, decreased bacterial permeability, and increased drug efflux.[35] Susceptibility to one fluoroquinolone generally predicts susceptibility to others, with the exceptions of third-generation fluoroquinolones (such as pradofloxacin) and ciprofloxacin, which has higher *in vitro* activity against *P. aeruginosa* than other fluoroquinolones.[36,37] There have been associations between fluoroquinolone use and increased emergence of resistance of some bacteria in human medicine. This has led to stewardship recommendations for limiting the use of fluoroquinolones to treat routine infections. The link between fluoroquinolone use and resistance in veterinary medicine has not been established in clinical patients, but has been demonstrated in research animals. Therefore, the consensus panel guidelines have recommended to reserve the administration of fluoroquinolones to small animals for cases where other antimicrobials may not be an option. Therefore, other “first-line” drugs are often available for most infections, and fluoroquinolones should be considered for cases that cannot tolerate other drugs, or when resistance to other drugs is more likely. Appropriate pharmacokinetic-pharmacodynamic (PK-PD) principles (discussed in Chapter 8) should be followed to reduce selection of resistant isolates.

Clinical Use

Fluoroquinolones are most valuable to treat gram-negative infections because there are often few oral medication alternatives for these infections. The fluoroquinolones are also effective for infections caused by staphylococci, but staphylococci tend to have higher MICs for fluoroquinolones than gram-negative bacteria. The activity of fluoroquinolones against anaerobes is variable. Pradofloxacin has the greatest activity, followed by marbofloxacin and enrofloxacin.[38] Fluoroquinolones are concentration-dependent antibiotics with a marked postantibiotic effect, so they are best administered as a single high daily dose. Doses for fluoroquinolones are listed in Table 10.7.

Fluoroquinolones are usually well absorbed after oral administration. Poor absorption occurs when they are complexed by divalent and trivalent cation-containing medications (e.g., antacids) and supplements (aluminum, calcium, iron, zinc). Use of these should be avoided if animals are receiving fluoroquinolones by the oral route, or separate the administration by at least 2 hours. Oral absorption of ciprofloxacin is lower and more variable in dogs than in humans, which necessitates administration of a higher dose. In one study, oral absorption of generic ciprofloxacin tablets in dogs was 58%, but the coefficient of variation was 45%.[39] In cats, only 22% to 33% of orally administered ciprofloxacin is absorbed. On the other hand, the human generic drug levofloxacin is absorbed almost completely in dogs and is preferred over ciprofloxacin, especially because canine-specific testing breakpoints have been established by CLSI.[40–42] Most fluoroquinolones are highly concentrated in the urine, so they are useful for treatment of UTIs. Enrofloxacin is metabolized to ciprofloxacin, which produces an additive effect because ciprofloxacin is active. Both drugs are subsequently excreted in the urine. Approximately half of the administered dose of marbofloxacin and orbifloxacin is excreted as unchanged drug in the urine.

Fluoroquinolones have variable protein binding, but this does not inhibit distribution to tissue fluids. Because of good lipophilicity, these drugs penetrate the prostate and respiratory secretions. They also penetrate the ear canal, but high doses may be required for treatment of bacteria with relatively high MIC values (e.g., *P. aeruginosa*).[43] Fluoroquinolones can attain high intracellular concentrations and can be used to treat infections caused by intracellular pathogens such as *Mycoplasma*, *Bartonella*, and some *Mycobacterium* spp.

Adverse Effects

Both oral and parenteral administration of fluoroquinolones can occasionally result in GI signs in dogs and cats, such as decreased appetite and vomiting. Rapid IV administration can cause systemic hypotension, tachycardia, and cutaneous erythema, possibly as a result of histamine release.[44] Neurologic signs, including tremors, ataxia, and seizures, can occur in dogs and cats treated with high doses of parenteral fluoroquinolones. Although not well understood, this is thought to result from fluoroquinolone interference with the binding of GABA to its receptors in the CNS.[45] In general, fluoroquinolones should be used cautiously in animals prone to seizures. Enrofloxacin causes

TABLE 10.7 Suggested Fluoroquinolone Dosages for Small Animals

Drug	Dose (mg/kg)	Interval (hours)	Species	Route	Comments	CLSI Breakpoints (μg/mL)
Enrofloxacin	5–20 5	24 24	D C[a]	IV, IM, PO IM, PO	Interactions can occur with certain oral medications (see text). Reduce dose or increase dosage interval with renal failure. Dilute in fluids (e.g., 1:10 dilution) and infuse IV over 30 minutes	≤0.5 μg/mL for susceptible infections. Use higher dosages (10–20 mg/kg) for organisms with MICs of 1 or 2 (except in cats). A dose of 5 mg/kg may be sufficient for UTIs
Ciprofloxacin hydrochloride	20–30 10	24 24	D, C D, C	PO IV	See enrofloxacin. Oral absorption may be limited (see text)	In humans, ≤0.25 μg/mL for susceptible infections (Enterobacterales) and ≤0.5 μg/mL for *Pseudomonas aeruginosa*, but for dogs, ≤ 0.03 μg/mL should be used.
Levofloxacin	23–25	24	D	PO	Human generic drug. Much better absorbed than ciprofloxacin in dogs	≤0.5 μg/mL for *E. coli*, ≤1 μg/mL for *Pseudomonas aeruginosa*
Marbofloxacin	2.75–5.5	24	D, C	PO	See enrofloxacin	≤1 μg/mL for susceptible infections. Use higher doses for bacteria with higher MICs
Orbifloxacin	2.5–7.5	24	D, C	PO	See enrofloxacin. Orbifloxacin suspension provides lower and more variable plasma levels than the tablets. A dose of 7.5 mg/kg should be used	See marbofloxacin
Difloxacin hydrochloride *(discontinued by manufacturer)*	5–10	24	D	PO	Urine concentrations may not be sufficient for treating UTIs	≤0.5 μg/mL for susceptible infections
Moxifloxacin	10	24	D, C	PO	Moxifloxacin has enhanced activity against gram-positive bacteria and anaerobes. In humans, urine concentrations are not sufficient for treatment of UTIs	No animal breakpoint is established.
Pradofloxacin	3[b] 5–7.5[c]	24	D, C C	PO	See moxifloxacin for spectrum of activity. Food reduces bioavailability. Appears effective for treatment of UTIs	≤0.25 μg/mL for susceptible infections

[a]The use of enrofloxacin to treat cats is controversial because of the potential for irreversible retinal toxicity and blindness. Do not exceed a dose of 5 mg/kg in cats. The use of alternative fluoroquinolones such as marbofloxacin, orbifloxacin, or pradofloxacin should be considered for cats.
[b]Tablet formulation. The use of pradofloxacin at high doses in dogs has been associated with myelosuppression and is off-label in the United States, but it is approved for both dogs and cats outside the United States at a dose of 3 mg/kg (tablets).
[c]Oral suspension for cats. The dose of the oral suspension for cats is higher (5–7.5 mg/kg) owing to reduced bioavailability.
C, cats; *CLSI,* Clinical and Laboratory Standards Institute[41,42]; *D,* dogs; *IM,* intramuscular; *IV,* intravenous; *MIC,* minimum inhibitory concentration; *PO,* oral; *UTI,* urinary tract infection.

hallucinations in humans, so it is not marketed or approved for treatment of humans.

Cats treated with high doses of enrofloxacin (generally > 5 mg/kg/day), especially parenteral enrofloxacin, have developed blindness resulting from acute retinal degeneration, manifested as bilateral mydriasis with tapetal hyperreflectivity.[46,47] This results from a functional defect in a fluoroquinolone transport protein in the cat, with subsequent accumulation of photoreactive drug in the retina.[48] In general, the blindness is irreversible, but if it is detected early and medication is discontinued, some resolution may occur. Orbifloxacin also can produce retinal injury in cats, but the dose needed for this reaction is much higher than doses used therapeutically. Studies of marbofloxacin (reported by the manufacturer) and pradofloxacin[49] showed no evidence of retinal toxicity in cats, even with high doses, although there are reports to the FDA of blindness in cats associated with the use of marbofloxacin. Cats with renal insufficiency or those treated with medications that increase plasma fluoroquinolone concentrations may be more likely to develop this adverse effect. Quinolones have limited solubility at alkaline pH and may crystallize in tissues. Dogs given high doses had subcapsular lenticular cataract formation and associated inflammation after treatment for 8 to 12 months.

Because they inhibit proteoglycan synthesis and chelate magnesium, fluoroquinolones can cause cartilage and joint toxicity in young animals, although the clinical importance of this has been questioned.[50,51] In general, prolonged (>7 days) use of fluoroquinolones during the period of rapid growth in dogs (from about 1 to 2 months of age to 28 weeks) should be avoided if possible. Cats are thought to be more resistant to development of cartilage toxicity. The US FDA has

TABLE 10.8 Suggested Metronidazole Dosages for Small Animals

Drug	Dose (mg/kg)	Interval (hours)	Species	Route	Comments
Metronidazole	15 10–15	12 24	D C	PO	Reduce dose by 50% in animals with hepatic dysfunction. An IV solution, metronidazole hydrochloride, is available but is highly acidic. It should be diluted in 100 mL of IV crystalloids and neutralized with 5 mEq sodium bicarbonate per 500 mg for a pH of 6–7. Diluted solutions are stable for 24 hours
Metronidazole benzoate	25	12	C	PO	More palatable formulation for cats may be available from some compounding pharmacies

C, cats; *D*, dogs; *IV*, intravenous; *PO*, oral.

recommended that fluoroquinolones be avoided in humans when other options exist because of the potential for neuromuscular (particularly tendon injury) adverse effects. Pradofloxacin has been associated with myelosuppression in dogs at doses greater than 10 mg/kg. All fluoroquinolones should be used cautiously in pregnant or lactating bitches.

Fluoroquinolones inhibit some cytochrome P450 enzymes, which decreases metabolism of other drugs. This occurs with theophylline in dogs; therefore, the dose of theophylline should be adjusted if administered concurrently. Like cephalosporins, fluoroquinolones can cause false-positive results on test strips for urine glucose detection. Cutaneous photosensitization occurs in human patients but is rare in animals. Other adverse effects reported in humans, but not in dogs and cats, include cardiac arrhythmias and QT interval prolongation, rupture of the aorta, pancreatitis, tendinitis and tendon rupture, altered glucose metabolism, and hepatic dysfunction.[52,53]

Metronidazole

Mechanism of Action and Spectrum of Activity

Metronidazole is a bactericidal nitroimidazole drug that is used primarily to treat anaerobic bacterial infections (both gram-negative and gram-positive), including those caused by *Bacteroides fragilis* and *Clostridium* spp., and infections with certain protozoa, such as *Giardia* spp. Metronidazole diffuses into bacterial cells as a prodrug and is activated in the cytoplasm. Once within the cell, the nitro group of metronidazole preferentially accepts electrons from electron transport proteins such as ferredoxin. A short-lived nitroso free radical is thus generated that damages DNA. The intermediate compounds then decompose into nontoxic, inactive end products.

Metronidazole has antioxidant properties that are believed to result from its ability to scavenge reactive oxygen species, and modulation of neutrophil activity.[54] It is often used at low doses to treat inflammatory bowel disease in dogs and cats,[55] but it is not known if the benefit is from the antibacterial activity or other effects on inflammatory cells. It has also been used to treat acute nonspecific diarrhea in dogs, but the value of this use has been questioned.[56,57]

Resistance to metronidazole is rare among anaerobes.[58] Mechanisms of resistance include reduced drug uptake and decreased reduction activity. Other proposed mechanisms include increased efflux, drug inactivation, and accelerated DNA repair.

Clinical Use

In dogs and cats, metronidazole is used to treat anaerobic bacterial and protozoal infections in a variety of tissues. Suggested doses are listed in Table 10.8. Metronidazole is rapidly and almost completely absorbed from the GI tract, diffuses across lipid membranes, and achieves therapeutic concentrations in tissue fluids. Metronidazole is metabolized by the liver. The metabolites, along with intact drug, are excreted in the urine.

Adverse Effects

The main adverse effect of metronidazole is neurotoxicity, which tends to occur with high doses (>30 mg/kg/day) or in animals with hepatic dysfunction. Clinical signs of neurotoxicity are reversible on discontinuation of the drug and include lethargy, truncal ataxia, hypermetria, intention tremors, head tilt, falling, vertical nystagmus, extensor rigidity, opisthotonos and seizures, and reflect injury to the vestibular system.[59,60] Although not fully understood, neurotoxicity is believed to result from antagonism of GABA in the cerebellar and vestibular systems. Neurologic signs resolve more quickly when treated with a low dose of diazepam (0.4 mg/kg PO q8h for 3 days), which confirms GABA antagonism as the potential mechanism.[59] Bilateral symmetrical cerebellar lesions, most commonly in the dentate nucleus, have been reported on MRI in human patients with metronidazole toxicity,[61] and multifocal necrotic foci were detected at necropsy in the brainstem of a cat.[60] Administration of metronidazole to animals with a history of metronidazole toxicosis is not recommended.[59]

Less commonly, metronidazole causes decreased appetite, vomiting, and diarrhea. Metronidazole suspension has a bitter taste that may be unpalatable to cats, which can be overcome by administration of the drug in gel capsules. Although not approved by the FDA, metronidazole benzoate is a more palatable formulation for cats and pharmacokinetic studies have demonstrated good absorption.[62] There have been concerns that relate to toxicity from the benzoic acid component of the formulation, which can cause CNS signs, blindness, and respiratory problems at high doses. However, this possibility is considered to be unlikely.[62] Because metronidazole benzoate is only 62% metronidazole (by weight), dosage adjustment is required when this formulation is used. Metronidazole inhibits hepatic microsomal enzymes and so may increase the concentration of drugs such as warfarin and cyclosporine. It also lowers serum lipid concentrations (including cholesterol concentrations) in human patients.[63] Metronidazole has been shown to be carcinogenic in mice and rats, and has been shown to cause reversible genotoxicity (DNA damage) in cats,[62] but there are no accounts of an increased rate of neoplasia in treated dogs or cats.

Rifamycins

Mechanism of Action and Spectrum of Activity

Named after the French crime movie *Rififi*, rifamycins are bactericidal antimicrobials that inhibit the β-subunit of DNA-dependent RNA polymerase in bacteria. This leads to impaired RNA synthesis. Only the semisynthetic drug rifampin (also known as rifampicin) has been used to any great extent in small animal medicine. Rifampin is active against staphylococci, streptococci, and only a few gram-negative organisms. When used as a component of antimycobacterial treatment regimens, it increases the chance of treatment success. Rifabutin is effective for treatment of some mycobacterial infections that are resistant to rifampicin.[64]

TABLE 10.9 **Suggested Rifampin Dose for Small Animals**

Drug	Dose (mg/kg)	Interval (hours)	Species	Route	Comments	CLSI Breakpoint (µg/mL)
Rifampin	5	12	D, C	PO	Preferably use in combination with other drugs. Avoid in animals with hepatic dysfunction. Do not administer with fatty meals. Drug interactions may occur (see text). Monitor liver enzymes with prolonged treatment. May impart a red-orange color to the urine and tears	≤1 for susceptible organisms (usually MICs of gram-positive bacteria fall below this breakpoint)

C, cats; *CLSI*, Clinical and Laboratory Standards Institute[41,42]; *D*, dogs; *MIC*, minimum inhibitory concentration; *PO*, oral.

It has been recommended that rifampin be used in combination with other antimicrobials to reduce the risk of emergence of rifampin resistance, which occurs quickly when rifampin is used alone. However, this applies primarily when it is used for long-term treatment, such as for mycobacterial infections. Monotherapy has been successful when rifampin has been used to treat MRS infections, which accounts for most of the current small animal use. Rifampin monotherapy has not been shown to be a risk factor for development of staphylococcal resistance. If combination treatment is pursued for treatment of MRS, there are often few effective alternatives with which to combine rifampin, because these infections are typically multidrug resistant. Resistance to rifampin results from a single mutation that leads to an altered RNA polymerase that does not effectively bind rifampin.

Clinical Use

One of the major advantages of rifampin is its high degree of lipid solubility, which provides the degree of intracellular penetration required for treatment of infections caused by intracellular bacteria such as *Mycobacterium* spp. and *Brucella canis*. Rifampin in combination with doxycycline has been used to treat bartonellosis.[65,66] Rifampin was not effective as monotherapy for treatment of *Ehrlichia canis* infections.[67] Because of its activity against staphylococci and the fact that it can be administered orally, it has been used for treatment of MRS infections in small animals. For other infections, rifampin is less attractive because of its adverse effect profile.

Rifampin dosing is shown in Table 10.9. Rifampin is rapidly absorbed from the GI tract and metabolized by the liver. Active metabolites are excreted in bile and, to a lesser extent, the urine. Approximately 75% to 90% of rifampin is bound to plasma proteins.

Adverse Effects

Vomiting, anorexia, and lethargy are common in dogs treated with rifampin, especially when it is administered together with other medications.[68] The drug can impart a red-orange color to the urine and, to a lesser extent, tears, saliva, the sclera, and mucous membranes. Rifampin can also be associated with increased serum liver enzyme activities and hepatopathy, especially with prolonged administration (> 36 days). Doses that exceed 10 mg/kg per day in dogs increase the risk of liver injury. When prescribing rifampin to dogs, it is advised to monitor serum liver enzyme activities and serum bilirubin concentration periodically. In humans, fever, cutaneous reactions, thrombocytopenia, acute intravascular hemolytic anemia, and acute tubulointerstitial nephritis have been reported, which appear to have an immune-mediated pathogenesis.[69] Rarely, pancreatitis has been reported in human patients receiving rifampin. Adverse effects have not been reported in cats, but some of these risks may apply to cats as well as dogs. Because of poor palatability, it is a challenge to administer to cats.

Rifampin is one of *the* most potent inducers of hepatic microsomal enzymes and efflux proteins, such as P-glycoprotein. Subsequently, it can increase the clearance of several co-administered drugs (thereby decreasing their efficacy), such as glucocorticoids, cyclosporine, itraconazole, isoniazid, barbiturates, theophylline, digoxin, and perhaps others. In human patients, recovery from the effect of rifampin on hepatic microsomal enzymes can take 4 weeks.[70]

Trimethoprim-Sulfonamides

Mechanism of Action

Trimethoprim and sulfonamides act synergistically to inhibit folic acid metabolism by bacteria. The combination interferes with purine and therefore DNA synthesis. Trimethoprim inhibits bacterial dihydrofolate reductase. Sulfonamides are chemical analogues of PABA and competitively inhibit the incorporation of PABA into dihydropteroic acid by the enzyme dihydropteroate synthetase, which also leads to decreased folic acid synthesis. Because folic acid is of dietary origin in animals, only bacterial purine synthesis is affected. When administered separately, each drug is bacteriostatic, but the combination is bactericidal and can broaden the spectrum. Preparations used to treat dogs and cats include a 1:5 ratio of trimethoprim to sulfonamide.

Resistance to trimethoprim-sulfonamide (TMS) antibiotics most commonly results from plasmid-mediated production of altered dihydrofolate reductase or dihydropteroate synthetase, with reduced binding affinities. Other mechanisms include overproduction of dihydrofolate reductase or PABA by bacteria, and reduced bacterial permeability to trimethoprim and sulfonamides. Multiple mechanisms may operate simultaneously.[71]

Clinical Use

TMS antibiotics have a broad spectrum of activity and can be used to treat gram-positive and many gram-negative bacterial infections, as well as some protozoal infections. Enterococci are intrinsically resistant to TMS antibiotics. Many anaerobic bacteria are not treated successfully because despite *in vitro* susceptibility, the drugs are less active in tissues where anaerobes proliferate. TMS antibiotics are the treatment of choice for nocardiosis. They have also been used successfully for prevention of bacterial infections in dogs being treated with myelosuppressive chemotherapeutics such as doxorubicin.[72] Prophylactic protocols have selected for resistant bacteria in humans,[73] but this has not been reported in animals. TMS combinations are available as either trimethoprim-sulfadiazine or trimethoprim-sulfamethoxazole (the latter is a human medical preparation), which are used interchangeably. However, the veterinary formulation of trimethoprim-sulfadiazine is rarely available commercially, and most veterinarians rely on trimethoprim-sulfamethoxazole. Equine formulations are usually trimethoprim-sulfadiazine. Although it is assumed that there is no difference in activity between the two formulations, this has not been sufficiently studied. The primary difference between the formulations is that sulfadiazine is more water soluble and is excreted in the urine in an unchanged form. A similar formulation to the TMS for use in veterinary medicine is ormetoprim-sulfadimethoxine, which has been

TABLE 10.10 Suggested Potentiated Sulfonamide Dosages for Small Animals

Drug	Dose (mg/kg)	Interval (hours)	Species	Route	Comments	CLSI Breakpoints (µg/mL)
Trimethoprim-sulfamethoxazole, trimethoprim-sulfadiazine	15–30[a]	12 (24 hour if using 30 mg/kg)	D, C	PO, IV	Avoid in animals with hepatic failure. Reduce dose in animals with renal insufficiency. Obtain baseline Schirmer tear test and monitor this and the CBC with prolonged treatment. Each 5-mL vial of the injectable preparation should be diluted in 75–125 mL of 5% dextrose and administered IV over 1 hour	≤2/38 for susceptible infections
Ormetoprim-sulfadimethoxine	55 on first day, and then 27.5[a]	24	D	PO	See trimethoprim-sulfamethoxazole	Use information for trimethoprim-sulfonamides

[a]Dose listed is for combined components (e.g., 5 mg of trimethoprim and 25 mg of sulfonamide).
C, cats; *CBC*, complete blood count; *CLSI*, Clinical and Laboratory Standards Institute[41,42]; *D*, dogs; *IV*, intravenous; *PO*, oral.

used for the same indications as TMS. Doses for TMS combinations are listed in Table 10.10.

Trimethoprim and sulfonamide combinations are well absorbed after oral administration. As a weak base, trimethoprim is able to penetrate the blood-prostate barrier and can be used to treat prostatic infections. Both trimethoprim and sulfonamides also penetrate the CNS. They are both metabolized to some extent by the liver. Both active drug and inactive metabolites appear in the urine. Reducing the dosage is unnecessary in renal failure unless it is severe. Active TMS is highly concentrated in urine and if tolerated, it is an appropriate first choice for treatment of UTIs in dogs and cats.[74]

Adverse Effects

TMS antimicrobials cause a wide range of adverse effects, which have somewhat limited their use. These reactions are primarily caused by the sulfonamide component. People who are "slow acetylators" of sulfonamides are more prone to adverse effects from sulfonamides and dogs can show similar effects because they cannot acetylate any medications.

GI signs such as vomiting can occur. Administration of trimethoprim-sulfamethoxazole suspension to cats often results in hypersalivation, anorexia, and vomiting. Other common adverse effects in dogs are hypersensitivity reactions and include keratoconjunctivitis sicca, fever, polyarthritis, cutaneous drug eruptions,[75,76] ITP, hemolytic anemia, hepatitis, pancreatitis, meningitis, interstitial nephritis, glomerulonephritis, and aplastic anemia (Fig. 10.3).[77–79] These events are relatively uncommon, but have been documented well enough in dogs that it has discouraged their routine use among some veterinary clinicians. Reversible hypothyroidism can occur after periods of treatment as short as 10 days.[80] Hepatic necrosis can occur as an idiosyncratic reaction.[81] Ormetoprim has been associated with neurologic signs in dogs, including tremors, anxiety, and seizures. Doberman pinschers may be more susceptible than other breeds to adverse effects of TMS because of their inability to detoxify certain sulfonamide metabolites; in another study, Samoyeds and miniature schnauzers also appeared to be more susceptible.[82,83]

Because of the risk of keratoconjunctivitis sicca in dogs, Schirmer tear tests should be performed before sulfonamides are administered and tear tests should be continued when prolonged treatment is required (e.g., greater than 1 week), and the drug should be avoided in dogs with keratoconjunctivitis sicca. The prognosis for return of lacrimation is poor, but topical cyclosporine appears to be effective in some

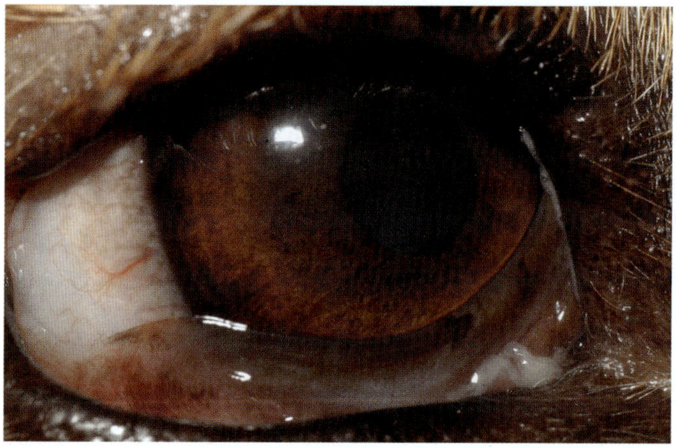

Fig. 10.3 Right eye of a 7-year-old intact male golden retriever that developed keratoconjunctivitis sicca after administration of trimethoprim-sulfamethoxazole for 3 weeks for septic peritonitis. The owner noticed the dog pawing at his eyes. Mucoid ocular discharge is present at the medial canthus. Schirmer tear test strip results were 0 mm for both eyes. (Image courtesy University of California, Davis Veterinary Ophthalmology service.)

cases. Sulfonamide cystolithiasis can occur in dogs treated with high doses of sulfonamides.[84] However, this effect is associated with the older, less soluble forms of sulfonamides. This adverse effect is rarely a concern with modern formulations.

PROTEIN SYNTHESIS INHIBITORS

Aminoglycosides

Mechanism of Action

All aminoglycosides contain an essential six-membered ring with amino-group substituents and are highly positively charged. Aminoglycosides with names that end in *-mycin* derive directly or indirectly from *Streptomyces* spp. (e.g., neomycin). Those with names ending in *-micin* are derived from *Micromonospora* (e.g., gentamicin).

Aminoglycoside mechanism of action is described by two processes. First, they bind electrostatically to the bacterial outer membrane and displace cell wall Mg^{2+} and Ca^{2+}, which normally link adjacent LPS molecules. This initial binding is greater in gram-negative bacteria than in gram-positive bacteria because of a greater presence of an outer

TABLE 10.11 **Suggested Aminoglycoside Dosages for Small Animals**

Drug	Dose (mg/kg)	Interval (hours)[a]	Species	Route	Comments	CLSI Breakpoints (µg/mL)
Gentamicin sulfate	9–14 5–8	24 24	D C	IV, IM, SC	Ensure adequate fluid and electrolyte balance during treatment. Avoid in animals with renal impairment. Monitor BUN and creatinine. Amikacin and tobramycin are more active against some gram-negative bacteria than gentamicin, but gentamicin is preferred for *Serratia* infections. Do not mix in vials with other drugs	≤2 for susceptible infections
Amikacin	15–30 10–14	24 24	D C	IV, IM, SC	See gentamicin	≤4 for susceptible infections (dogs)
Tobramycin sulfate	9–14 5–8	24 24	D C	IV, IM	See gentamicin. For nebulization, 160 mg of nebulization solution[b] q12h for 28 days. Preferred aminoglycoside for *Pseudomonas* infections	≤4 for susceptible infections
Kanamycin sulfate	20	24	D, C	IV or IM	See gentamicin. Less active than gentamicin and amikacin	≤16 for susceptible infections
Neomycin	10–20	6–12	D, C	PO	Not absorbed systemically; used to treat hepatic encephalopathy. Use cautiously in animals with renal disease and avoid use for > 14 days	Not applicable

[a]Once-daily administration is preferred except for enterococcal endocarditis, where the continuous presence of both an aminoglycoside and a penicillin is recommended (see Chapter 122).

[b]TOBI nebulization solution. Injectable tobramycin or gentamicin can be used but may be associated with bronchospasm. They should be diluted in 3 mL of sterile saline, and albuterol should be administered just before nebulization.

BUN, blood urea nitrogen; *C,* cats; *CLSI,* Clinical and Laboratory Standards Institute[41,42]; *D,* dogs; *IM,* intramuscular; *IV,* intravenous; *MIC,* minimum inhibitory concentration; *PO,* oral; *SC,* subcutaneous.

membrane in gram-negative organisms. The end result is disrupted cell permeability. The second mechanism of action is through protein synthesis inhibition. Aminoglycosides first enter the cell of susceptible bacteria. Because this is an oxygen-dependent process, anaerobes are intrinsically resistant to aminoglycosides. Once within the cell, aminoglycosides bind to the 30S subunit of the bacterial ribosome, which results in decreased protein synthesis.

Aminoglycosides, particularly gentamicin, amikacin, and tobramycin, are highly active compounds for which resistance is uncommon. The most common mechanism of aminoglycoside resistance is enzymatic modification of the drug by bacteria.[85] More than 50 modifying enzymes have been identified.[86] Reduced drug uptake by bacteria may also occur. Enterococci are intrinsically resistant to low levels (4 to 250 µg/mL) of aminoglycosides because of their anaerobic metabolism, and thus they require testing for high-level resistance. This is done in the microbiology laboratory using higher concentrations of aminoglycosides. Resistance to one aminoglycoside does not imply resistance to others. For example, tobramycin and amikacin are consistently more active than gentamicin against gram-negative bacteria. Kanamycin is one of the least active aminoglycosides. Because of these differences, a susceptibility panel should include gentamicin and either amikacin or tobramycin. Because of poor activity, aminoglycosides should not be used to treat infections caused by streptococci, regardless of the susceptibility test result. The activity against *Staphylococcus* spp. can vary, and may require a frequency of administration more than once per day to meet pharmacokinetic-pharmacodynamic (PK-PD) targets. Human guidelines state that aminoglycosides should always be used in combination with another antimicrobial agent (often a β-lactam antibiotic) for treating infections caused by *Staphylococcus* spp. Guidance on this use is not available in veterinary guidelines. Some susceptibility testing standards state that if a *Staphylococcus* spp. isolate is resistant to gentamicin, it should be reported resistant to all other aminoglycosides, regardless of the MIC. However, this recommendation does not exist in veterinary standards, and some *S. pseudintermedius* may test resistant to gentamicin, but susceptible to amikacin.[87]

Clinical Use

Aminoglycosides are primarily used to treat gram-negative bacterial infections and MDR staphylococcal infections. They also have activity against mycobacteria. They should not be used to treat anaerobic bacterial infections, and *Streptococcus* species, for which other more active agents are available (e.g., β-lactam antibiotics). Older recommendations suggest that aminoglycosides should be administered in combination with cell wall–active antimicrobial drugs (β-lactams and glycopeptides) for all infections, but this is no longer believed to be a therapeutic advantage. An exception may be for treating infections caused by *Staphylococcus* spp., but as noted above, this has not been studied in veterinary patients.

The aminoglycosides are water soluble, minimally bound to plasma proteins and poorly lipid soluble, so they penetrate tissue fluids well, but do not readily penetrate tissues that are dependent on lipid diffusion (prostate, brain, eye, or CSF). Penetration of bile is also poor. Oral absorption is negligible, and they should not be administered orally unless specifically intended to treat intestinal bacteria (e.g., oral neomycin for treatment of hepatic encephalopathy). Doses are shown in Table 10.11. Aminoglycosides also may be administered topically. Because they penetrate bronchial secretions poorly, nebulization has been used in order to overcome this problem in human patients as well as dogs with bronchopneumonia caused by MDR gram-negative bacteria (see Table 10.11).[88] Topical administration was also used successfully to treat *P. aeruginosa* bacteriuria in a dog with a cystostomy tube.[89] Gentamicin-impregnated beads and cement have been used successfully to treat MRS infections in orthopedic surgery. Aminoglycosides are excreted unchanged by the kidney and concentrate 25- to 100-fold in urine within an hour of drug administration, so they can be used to treat resistant gram-negative bacterial UTIs. They also accumulate in renal tissue and remain active for several days after dosing is discontinued. Because they are not well distributed into fat, dose reduction may be indicated for obese animals.

Despite their primary mechanism of action being protein synthesis inhibition, aminoglycosides are rapidly bactericidal with a prolonged, concentration-dependent postantibiotic effect. Transient high peak drug concentrations result in faster killing and greater bactericidal activity than lower concentrations over a prolonged period of time (i.e., they are concentration-dependent antimicrobial drugs). Once-daily dosing of a high dose of an aminoglycoside is therefore preferred because it achieves optimal bacterial killing but minimizes toxicity. In order to further minimize toxicity, aminoglycosides are generally infused slowly. In human patients, it is recommended they be administered over a 15- to 30-minute period; intramuscular or SC administration to dogs and cats achieves similar slow release into the circulation. Therefore, SC and intramuscular injections of water-soluble formulations of aminoglycosides are also acceptable routes of administration, although they may cause pain in some animals.

Adverse Effects

Aminoglycosides have the potential to cause nephrotoxicity, ototoxicity, and neuromuscular blockade. Their cationic structure and the high anionic phospholipid concentrations in the kidney and inner ear play an important role in toxicity. In the presence of GI ulceration or a compromised intestinal barrier, systemic absorption of orally administered aminoglycosides can occur, with associated nephrotoxicity or ototoxicity.[90] Nephrotoxicity has also followed local tissue administration of gentamicin in dogs and cats.[91,92]

Nephrotoxicity results from apoptosis and necrosis of renal tubular epithelial cells, and direct damage to the glomerulus as well. The mechanisms involved are complex.[93] Recovery can occur when the aminoglycoside is removed, but because aminoglycosides accumulate in renal tissue, the insult can persist for some time even after treatment is discontinued. Because of an understanding of the mechanisms of nephrotoxicity, preventative measures have been developed to mitigate kidney injury. Aminoglycosides bind to megalin-cubulin complexes on the surface of the cell and are endocytosed into the cytoplasm, where they accumulate in lysosomes. The lysosomes break down, with resultant drug leakage into the cytoplasm, where interference with mitochondrial function occurs. Aminoglycosides also bind membrane phospholipids and alter their turnover. Damaged renal tubular epithelial cells are shed into and obstruct the tubular lumen, which leads to a build-up of pressure within the glomerulus, leading to decreased glomerular filtration rate. Disrupted proximal tubular cell function leads to delivery of excessive water and electrolytes to the distal nephron, which in turn triggers tubuloglomerular feedback, with constriction of afferent arterioles and further decreases in the glomerular filtration rate.[93] Tubuloglomerular feedback is designed to protect the body from massive loss of water and electrolytes.

Risk factors for nephrotoxicity include older age, reduced renal function, concomitant liver disease, dehydration, electrolyte depletion, and concurrently administered nephrotoxic drugs, most commonly NSAIDs but also furosemide and cyclosporine. Although gentamicin nephrotoxicity can occur in young animals,[94] young age is not a contraindication to use of aminoglycosides, which are used widely to treat human neonatal sepsis.[95] In fact, one study indicates that neonatal puppies were more tolerant of kidney injury from gentamicin than older dogs.[94] This difference is attributed to the distribution of renal blood flow at birth. The chance of toxicity increases with more prolonged treatment periods (≥3 days). Gentamicin and amikacin are more toxic than tobramycin. Volume and salt loading do not decrease toxicity, but high levels of dietary calcium and protein have protective effects.[96] The best preventative measure is to avoid these drugs in any patients with preexisting kidney injury. If kidney injury develops after initiating treatment, the drug should be substituted with a safer drug. Urinary biomarkers such as neutrophil gelatinase-associated lipocalin (NGAL)[97] and urinary cystatin C[98] have been shown to be sensitive indicators of aminoglycoside-induced kidney injury in dogs and may be useful for monitoring treatment in the future.

Ototoxicity results from injury to the cochlear or the vestibular apparatus and is more likely to occur in animals with renal impairment or that are dehydrated. Cochlear toxicity results from damage to the hair cells of the organ of Corti, whereas vestibular toxicity results from damage to hair cells at the tip of the ampullae cristae. Auditory toxicity may be more common in dogs, whereas cats tend to develop vestibular toxicity.[99] Cochlear toxicity in dogs and cats may be underrecognized because it may be overlooked by pet owners. It may go unrecognized in animals because in humans it primarily affects the high frequencies.[100] In human patients, signs of vestibular toxicity can disappear with time because of compensatory mechanisms. Ototoxicity is generally irreversible, but in some human patients, gradual improvement in hearing can occur.[101]

Neuromuscular blockade is a rare but potentially life-threatening complication of aminoglycoside treatment. Severe neuromuscular blockade has not been reported in cats and dogs, but experimental studies show that it does occur when aminoglycosides are used in conjunction with some anesthetic agents.[102–104] Because of these concerns, aminoglycosides should be avoided in patients receiving anesthetic agents. Neuromuscular blockade results from decreased release of acetylcholine at neuromuscular junctions and decreased sensitivity of the postsynaptic neuron to acetylcholine. Autonomic blockade can also occur. The use of aminoglycosides should be avoided in animals with neuromuscular disease such as myasthenia gravis because aminoglycosides have the potential to exacerbate the clinical signs.[105]

Measurement of serum aminoglycoside concentrations can be used to ensure adequate plasma concentrations or to minimize toxicity.[106] Assays are offered by specialized veterinary pharmacology laboratories or through human hospitals. Aminoglycoside doses are designed to attain peak plasma concentrations approximately 8 to 10 times the MIC. If the MIC of the bacterial isolate is known, this, along with serum drug monitoring, may be used to derive individual specific therapy. Monitoring also may be useful to identify patients with disorders of drug elimination or distribution. Monitoring early in the course of therapy can identify patients with subclinical kidney disease. The effective volume of distribution for aminoglycosides is often higher in septic patients or animals that have a "third space" problem (such as pleural effusion), which may necessitate a higher dose. To perform therapeutic drug monitoring, the optimum time points are 1 hour after injection (C_{max}), followed by two additional time points in order to estimate the slope of the elimination curve. Trough levels could also be performed to minimize the chance of toxicity, with the recommendation that if high trough levels are detected, there is evidence of drug accumulation and the drug should be discontinued. In patients with normal renal function, trough levels with once-daily dosing should be in the "undetectable" range.

TABLE 10.12 Suggested Chloramphenicol Dosages for Small Animals

Drug	Dose (mg/kg)	Interval (hours)	Species	Route	Comments	CLSI Breakpoints (µg/mL)
Chloramphenicol	40–50 12.5–20	8 12	D C	PO	Avoid long-term use in cats. Monitor CBC with long-term use. Warn owners that human exposure to chloramphenicol may cause bone marrow disease. Drug interactions may occur (see text). Avoid in animals with hepatic failure	≤4 for streptococci, ≤8 for other susceptible bacteria
Florfenicol	20 22	6 8	D, C	PO, IM	Not approved for use in dogs and cats. Doses and adverse effects have not been well studied	See chloramphenicol

C, cats; *CBC*, complete blood count; *CLSI*, Clinical and Laboratory Standards Institute[41,42]; *D*, dogs; *IM*, intramuscular; *PO*, oral.

Chloramphenicol

Mechanism of Action and Spectrum of Activity

Chloramphenicol binds to the 50S subunit of the bacterial ribosome and inhibits bacterial protein synthesis. It is usually described as bacteriostatic, but there is some evidence that chloramphenicol may be more bactericidal than previously thought. Like other ribosomal inhibitors, chloramphenicol has a broad spectrum of activity, which includes gram-positive and gram-negative bacteria, anaerobes, and some rickettsial pathogens. Because chloramphenicol can cause aplastic anemia in humans, its use in humans has greatly diminished. The use in animals is limited to the treatment of MDR bacterial infections that are not susceptible to other veterinary-approved antimicrobial drugs. Thiamphenicol and florfenicol are related compounds, the availability of which varies from country to country. Although thiamphenicol was initially promoted as not inducing aplastic anemia in humans, cases of aplastic anemia have now been identified.[107] Florfenicol is more active than chloramphenicol and thiamphenicol, but has a shorter half-life in dogs and thus requires more frequent dosing (e.g., more often than every 8 hours) in this species. It was developed for food animal species where use of chloramphenicol is illegal. The only approved formulations of florfenicol for small animals are topical ear preparations for treating otitis (discussed below).

Resistance to chloramphenicols results from porin mutations, drug efflux, or production of chloramphenicol acetyltransferase enzymes, which inactivate the antibiotic.[108] Resistance to one chloramphenicol derivative predicts resistance to the others.

Clinical Use

Chloramphenicol and florfenicol may be useful for treatment of MRS infections, enterococcal infections, and ESBL-producing gram-negative bacterial infections. Chloramphenicol was approved in the United States for dogs many years ago (Chloromycetin 100-, 250-, and 500-mg tablets) for the labeled indication of "oral treatment of bacterial pulmonary infections, bacterial infections of the urinary tract, bacterial enteritis, and bacterial infections associated with canine distemper caused by susceptible organisms." Veterinary infectious disease experts believe that this old label indication is no longer valid. Moreover, the original approved dose of 55 mg/kg every 6 hours is probably too high. For the current use, there is a need to optimize dosage regimens and establish clinical breakpoints for dogs and cats.[109] Doses used today are shown in Table 10.12. Chloramphenicol is absorbed orally with or without food. Tablets and capsules have similar oral absorption, but the extent of oral absorption varies considerably among dogs. Chloramphenicol distributes well to extracellular fluids of most tissues. Less than 50% of the drug is bound to plasma protein. Because of its high degree of lipid solubility, it also diffuses to tissues with barriers, such as the CNS and the eye. Topical ophthalmic preparations achieve high concentration in the aqueous humor. In dogs, most absorbed chloramphenicol is metabolized by glucuronidation in the liver, with inactive metabolites excreted by the kidney. The use of chloramphenicol should therefore be avoided in animals with hepatic failure. Likewise, because of the requirement for elimination through glucuronidation, cats have longer elimination rates than dogs and are more susceptible to adverse effects. Provided renal failure is not present, sufficient active drug is excreted in the urine to enable treatment of UTIs that are resistant to other drugs, such as MRS and methicillin-resistant enterococci.

The most common use of florfenicol in dogs is the topical use for ear infections. There are two FDA-approved topical otic medications that contain florfenicol (in combination with corticosteroids and an antifungal agent) described below.

Adverse Effects

Exposure of humans to even small amounts of chloramphenicol has the potential to lead to irreversible aplastic anemia, an idiosyncratic reaction, weeks to months after discontinuing treatment. The reaction is rare (1 in 24,000 to 1 in 40,000 exposed humans) and most commonly occurs when human patients are treated with oral formulations.[110] Whether use of ophthalmic preparations in human patients poses a risk has been controversial.[111,112] Nevertheless, it is recommended that owners of pets being treated with chloramphenicol wear gloves when handling the drug and to avoid splitting or crushing tablets at home. Chloramphenicol commonly causes GI adverse effects in dogs and cats, including anorexia, hypersalivation, and vomiting.[113] Another adverse effect that has emerged since the more recent use in dogs is peripheral neuropathy. This manifests as pelvic limb ataxia, weakness, and neurologic defects.[113] It appears to be more common in large-breed dogs, with a mean body weight for dogs with pelvic limb weakness of 35.3 kg.[113] Because it may be confused with other neurologic diseases, veterinarians should review the drug history in affected patients. The problem resolves in most dogs after the drug is discontinued. High doses or prolonged treatment can result in *reversible* bone marrow suppression, which also usually resolves within days after discontinuation of treatment. High doses and prolonged treatment are needed to produce this effect in dogs, but cats are considerably more susceptible and can be at risk within 1 week of administration. Chloramphenicol is a potent inhibitor of P450 enzymes, and so the potential for significant drug interactions exists, including with NSAIDs, anticonvulsants, and analgesics. Dramatic increases in plasma methadone concentrations have been described in dogs treated concurrently with chloramphenicol.[114]

Florfenicol is available as an injectable antibiotic for livestock, a feed additive for pigs, and an oral agent for treating fish raised in aquaculture facilities. Florfenicol has not been widely used in dogs and cats because of inconvenient dose regimens and lack of an oral formulation. The safety of florfenicol in dogs and cats is undetermined. There are no safety studies reported from repeated doses, and caution should be exercised if it is used for treating drug-resistant infections in dogs and cats. Two exceptions are the topical forms approved for use in dogs by the FDA in 2014 and 2015. The product Osurnia contains 10 mg/mL florfenicol, 10 mg/mL terbinafine, and 1 mg/mL betamethasone acetate in a gel for topical administration. The product Claro contains florfenicol 15 mg/mL, terbinafine 13.3 mg/mL, and mometasone 2 mg/mL. The indication for each product is for the treatment of otitis externa in dogs associated with susceptible strains of bacteria (*S. pseudintermedius*) and yeast (*Malassezia pachydermatis*).

Macrolides, Lincosamides, and Ketolides

Classification and Mechanism of Action

The macrolides and lincosamides (clindamycin and lincomycin) are not chemically related but possess similar mechanisms of action, resistance, and antimicrobial activity. Macrolides, lincosamides, and the ketolide telithromycin inhibit protein synthesis by binding to the 50S subunit of bacterial ribosomes. Because they are weak bases, macrolides and lincosamides concentrate in the relatively acidic interior of leukocytes. The high concentrations in leukocytes may also produce immunomodulatory effects.[115–119] Macrolides, particularly the newer agents such as azithromycin, can impair leukocyte function, induce neutrophil apoptosis, interfere with superoxide production by mast cells, and suppress proinflammatory cytokine release.[115,116] These effects may suppress inflammatory reactions in some tissues, particularly the respiratory tract. These effects on immune cells and cytokine expression may be significant for treatment of respiratory infections in humans and cattle. However, the contribution of these properties to treatment of infections in dogs and cats is undetermined.

The first macrolide antibiotic discovered was erythromycin, a derivative of *Streptomyces erythreus*. Despite the common occurrence of GI adverse effects, poor GI absorption, and an extremely short half-life, erythromycin continues to have application in human medicine because of its safety in pregnancy and utility in human patients who are allergic to penicillin. Because these concerns are less important in dogs and cats, erythromycin is less commonly used in small animal patients. Adverse effects (primarily vomiting) and poor oral absorption are problems for the use in small animals and erythromycin has largely given way to the human oral drug, azithromycin, for treatment when a macrolide is indicated.

Since the discovery of erythromycin, several semisynthetic macrolides have become available. Azithromycin and other new macrolide antibiotics, such as clarithromycin and roxithromycin, have been referred to as "advanced-generation" macrolides. These have an extended spectrum of activity, with greater efficacy against atypical and some gram-negative bacteria, a longer duration of antimicrobial activity, longer half-life, improved GI absorption, greater intracellular concentrations, and a marked reduction in GI adverse effects. Clarithromycin has improved activity against streptococci and staphylococci compared with erythromycin and greater *in vitro* activity against mycobacteria. Telithromycin is an acid-stable, semisynthetic erythromycin derivative that has a 10-fold higher affinity for the 50S ribosomal subunit than erythromycin and achieves high intracellular concentrations in phagocytes. Its use is currently restricted for treatment of moderate to severe community-acquired pneumonia in human patients, based on concerns relating to adverse effects. There have been no reports of use of telithromycin to treat dogs or cats.

Azithromycin is the first drug in the group of *azalides*, which are semisynthetic derivatives of erythromycin. The structure of the newer agents includes basic nitrogen groups. They can have either two (di-basic) or three (tri-basic) nitrogen groups. The basic nitrogen groups on these newer agents produce a positive charge in an acidic environment below their pKa. The positive charge increases intracellular concentrations caused by ion trapping. It is this property that gives these agents such large intracellular distribution and a high volume of distribution. This property also renders these agents less active in acidic environments (e.g., some infected sites). Azithromycin is extensively concentrated within cells and is retained in tissues for prolonged periods, with a half-life of 30 hours in the dog and 35 hours in the cat. In human patients, a 5-day course provides therapeutic tissue concentrations for at least 10 days. Although azithromycin has an improved spectrum against some gram-negative bacteria (not Enterobacterales or *P. aeruginosa)*, it has less activity against gram-positive bacteria than erythromycin.[120,121]

Susceptibility to erythromycin often predicts susceptibility to other macrolide antimicrobial drugs. Susceptibility to erythromycin does not predict susceptibility to clindamycin in staphylococci due to the phenomenon of inducible clindamycin resistance (see Chapter 51). Resistance to macrolides and lincosamides results from decreased bacterial permeability (for gram-negative bacteria), alteration in the target site, increased drug efflux, and enzymatic inactivation of certain macrolides by bacterial esterases. Alteration in the target site involves production of a ribosomal methylase that adds a methyl group to the 50S subunit RNA, preventing the macrolide from binding to the ribosome. Expression of the methylase enzyme confers high-level resistance to azithromycin, clarithromycin, and also clindamycin.

Clinical Use

Macrolides and lincosamides are primarily used to treat gram-positive bacterial infections; they are ineffective against gram-negative bacteria of the Enterobacterales and nonfermenters such as *P. aeruginosa.* They are generally considered to be bacteriostatic. Doses are shown in Table 10.13. The use of erythromycin in small animals has declined tremendously since the availability of azithromycin and clindamycin, which are effective for similar indications. The main disadvantages of erythromycin are the adverse GI effects and poor oral absorption (described below). Erythromycin tablets have a protective coating to prevent degradation by gastric acid. After absorption, erythromycin is distributed well to most tissues and body fluids, with the exception of the CNS and urine. It is excreted in high concentrations in the bile, followed by enterohepatic circulation, and ultimately eliminated in the feces. Nonabsorbed drug is also present in the feces. It has activity against some anaerobes, spiral bacteria (particularly *Campylobacter*), and many intracellular bacteria. Tylosin has been used to treat chronic colitis in dogs[122] and is also active against *Campylobacter* and enteric *Clostridium* spp. Resolution of diarrhea in dogs treated with tylosin has been associated with increased fecal populations of *Enterococcus* spp. and lactic acid bacteria.[123]

Clarithromycin and azithromycin have considerably longer half-lives than erythromycin. The intracellular concentration of clarithromycin is about twofold to sixfold that in plasma. Clarithromycin is preferred over erythromycin or azithromycin for treatment of rapidly growing mycobacterial infections in dogs and cats (usually in combination with rifampin) (see Chapter 61). In humans, clarithromycin is extensively metabolized by the liver to a variety of specific active and

TABLE 10.13 Suggested Macrolide and Lincosamide Dosages for Small Animals

Drug	Dose (mg/kg)	Interval (hours)	Species	Route	Comments	CLSI Breakpoints (μg/mL)
Erythromycin	10–20	8	D, C	PO	Do not administer to rabbits or rodents, as this may cause fatal diarrhea. Drug interactions may occur (see text)	≤0.25 for streptococci and ≤0.5 for other susceptible organisms
Tylosin	5–15 8–11	12–24 12	D, C	PO IM	See erythromycin. For colitis in dogs, use 20 mg/kg q8h with food, and taper to as low as 5 mg/kg q24h if a response occurs[a]	
Clarithromycin	7.5	12	D, C	PO	Drug interactions may occur (see text). Consider dosage reduction in severe renal failure	≤2 for staphylococci. Respiratory cures may be possible for organisms with MICs up to 8, because drug concentrates within the lung
Azithromycin	5–10	24	D, C	PO	Extended intervals of q48h to q72h have been used for some indications (see text).	≤ 2 for susceptible bacteria. Serum MIC values may not predict tissue concentrations
Lincomycin hydrochloride	15–25	12	D, C	PO	See erythromycin. A dose of 10 mg/kg PO q12h has been suggested for pyoderma	0.25 for streptococci and ≤ 0.5 for other susceptible organisms
Clindamycin hydrochloride, clindamycin phosphate	11–33 11 10	12 24 12	D C D, C	PO PO IV, IM	See erythromycin. For IV administration, dilute 1:10 in 0.9% saline and administer over 30–60 minutes. The oral suspension may be unpalatable to cats. For toxoplasmosis, use 25 mg/kg q12h PO	See lincomycin

[a]20 mg/kg is equal to 1/8th teaspoon of tylosin phosphate (Tylan) for a 20-kg dog.

C, cats; *CLSI*, Clinical and Laboratory Standards Institute[41,42]; *D*, dogs; *IM*, intramuscular; *IV*, intravenous; *MIC*, minimum inhibitory concentration; *PO*, oral.

inactive metabolites, with some excretion of active drug and its metabolites into urine. Formation and excretion of these metabolites have not been well studied in dogs and cats.

Because of the prolonged concentrations of azithromycin in tissues and leukocytes, the plasma concentrations may fall below the MIC of pathogens, while still producing therapeutic benefit. Intracellular concentrations of azithromycin are 10- to 100-fold those in serum and can remain high within tissues several days after the drug has been discontinued. Despite the improved spectrum of activity of clarithromycin and azithromycin, with activity against some gram-negative bacteria and intracellular pathogens, many of these organisms are resistant. The primary indication for these antibiotics in small animals is in combination with other drugs such as rifampin for treatment of mycobacteriosis or bartonellosis, or atovaquone for treatment of certain systemic protozoal infections such as babesiosis and cytauxzoonosis. Azithromycin has been used to treat secondary bacterial infections in cats with URTD because its long half-life permits convenient dosing on an every-48- or every-72-hour basis. Despite its popularity for treating upper respiratory infections in cats, one study showed no benefit to this protocol over use of amoxicillin,[124] and the potential for overuse of azithromycin in this setting raises concerns in regard to selection for resistance to azithromycin. Despite the frequent administration of azithromycin for various infections (skin, soft tissue, respiratory), there are no well-controlled clinical studies that demonstrate effectiveness compared with placebo or other agents.

Lincomycin is active against gram-positive bacteria and has been used to treat staphylococcal pyoderma. However, the approved forms of lincomycin in many countries have largely been replaced by clindamycin. Clindamycin is nearly identical to lincomycin in structure. The only difference is the addition of chlorine replacing hydroxyl at one position, making clindamycin slightly more active against some bacteria than lincomycin, and better absorbed orally. An important difference is greater activity against anaerobic bacteria for clindamycin, which accounts for the common use to treat anaerobic infections in dogs and cats. Clindamycin has favorable pharmacokinetics in dogs and cats, and a variety of available formulations (tablets, capsules, oral liquid, and injection). Lincomycin and clindamycin are widely distributed in body tissues and fluids, including bile, peritoneal and pleural fluids, milk, placenta, prostatic fluid, and bone. Neither drug enters the CSF or ocular structures unless inflammation is present. Both drugs accumulate in neutrophils, macrophages, and abscesses. Clindamycin is also used to treat anaerobic bacterial infections, as well as toxoplasmosis and neosporosis (see Chapters 93 and 94).

Adverse Effects

Although otherwise very safe, erythromycin frequently causes vomiting, decreased appetite, and nausea because of stimulation of receptors of the GI hormone motilin, which increases GI smooth muscle activity.[125] In one of the pharmacokinetic studies conducted in dogs, IV and oral administration of various forms of erythromycin produced nausea and vomiting in *all* of the dogs in the study.[126] In the same study, administration of various oral formulations to dogs produced low, and likely ineffective, serum concentrations. Like other poorly absorbed oral antimicrobials, it can produce diarrhea due to changes in the GI flora. Although diarrhea and pseudomembranous colitis are serious complications of clindamycin treatment in humans, these problems are uncommon in small animals. Adverse effects are rarely reported for clarithromycin and azithromycin. Erythromycin and azithromycin inhibit P450 enzymes and so can increase the concentration of other drugs that are administered concurrently. Clarithromycin has been shown to decrease the metabolism of cyclosporine in dogs and cats.[127,128]

Clindamycin and lincomycin can cause vomiting and diarrhea, especially when clindamycin is used at high doses. Oral clindamycin

TABLE 10.14 Suggested Linezolid Dose for Small Animals

Drug	Dose (mg/kg)	Interval (hours)	Species	Route	Comments	CLSI Breakpoints (μg/mL)
Linezolid[a]	10	12	D, C	PO, IV	If administered with other drugs IV, the administration line should be flushed first	≤4 for staphylococci, ≤2 for *Enterococcus* spp.

[a]The use of linezolid should be reserved for gram-positive infections that are susceptible to linezolid but resistant to all other reasonable alternatives, on the basis of culture and susceptibility testing.
C, cats; *CLSI*, Clinical and Laboratory Standards Institute[41,42]; *D*, dogs; *IV*, intravenous; *PO*, oral.

can have an unpleasant taste in cats and the hydrochloride form can produce esophagitis.[129,130]

In human patients, telithromycin causes GI adverse effects, and there have also been rare reports of rashes, headache, visual disturbances, neuromuscular blockage, and acute liver failure. Use of telithromycin in dogs and cats has not been reported.

Oxazolidinones (Linezolid)

Mechanism of Action and Spectrum of Activity

Linezolid is a synthetic antibiotic used to treat infections caused by gram-positive bacteria that are resistant to other antimicrobial drugs, especially MRS and vancomycin-resistant staphylococci. It also can be used to treat MDR enterococci. Linezolid binds to the 50S ribosome and prevents formation of the initiation complex for protein synthesis.[131] This is a unique mechanism because other protein synthesis inhibitors interfere with polypeptide extension. Resistance to other protein synthesis inhibitors is not associated with resistance to linezolid. Rarely, resistance to linezolid is due to modification of the drug's target site, but this is extremely rare because several step mutations are necessary before resistance can occur. Previously, the high cost of oral linezolid limited its use in small animals. Brand name tablets (Zyvox) have been listed as US $120–$150 per tablet. However, the recent availability of generic tablets has reduced the cost to approximately 1/10 of the brand name tablet.

The use of linezolid has been limited to dogs and cats with resistant staphylococcal or enterococcal infections for which other antibiotics are not effective or have produced adverse effects.[132,133] Linezolid has favorable pharmacokinetics in dogs,[134] with nearly 100% oral absorption, which is not influenced by food (Table 10.14). The pharmacokinetics in cats has not been published. Because linezolid is bacteriostatic, plasma concentrations should be maintained above the MIC throughout the dosing interval.

In human patients, adverse effects include vomiting, diarrhea, and, rarely, thrombocytopenia or reversible pure red cell aplasia. In humans, the concern regarding bone marrow effects is increased after 2 weeks of treatment. There have been rare reports of bone marrow suppression in dogs from administration for more than 2 weeks, but it is undetermined if the changes were caused by other factors. Likewise, the authors are aware of cats that developed reversible PRCA after treatment with linezolid, but the cause was undetermined.

Linezolid is a type A monoamine oxidase inhibitor and so can interact with serotonin reuptake inhibitors.[135] It was originally considered for treatment of depression and anxiety in humans because of effects on the CNS. Although behavioral effects are unlikely to affect treatment in dogs and cats, there have been anecdotal accounts of minor behavior changes in dogs treated with linezolid.

From the limited experience in animals, linezolid appears to be well tolerated by dogs and cats, but more experience is needed to fully document efficacy and adverse effects. Despite the concern about monoamine oxidase inhibition and bone marrow suppression in human patients, these effects have not yet been documented in dogs or cats.

Tetracyclines

Mechanism of Action and Spectrum of Activity

Tetracyclines are bacteriostatic, time-dependent antibiotics with a broad spectrum of activity that includes gram-positive and gram-negative bacteria, some anaerobes, and atypical and intracellular pathogens such as spirochetes, *Mycoplasma* spp., and rickettsiae. Although the antibacterial spectrum is generally wide, one should not assume that bacteria are susceptible to these agents based on the human interpretive categories for susceptibility testing. Because of high protein binding of doxycycline to plasma proteins in animals, as well as lower and more variable oral absorption, the CLSI[41,42] breakpoint for antibacterial susceptibility testing is lower for dogs than for humans (cat breakpoints have not yet been established). For example, bacteria isolated from humans will be reported as "susceptible" to doxycycline if the MIC is ≤ 4 μg/mL, but the MIC must be ≤ 0.125 μg/mL for the isolate to be reported as susceptible for dogs. The corresponding breakpoints for minocycline are ≤ 4 μg/mL and ≤ 0.5 μg/mL, respectively. Clinical breakpoints are not established for cats, but a susceptible range is likely lower than that for dogs because of higher protein binding and lower oral absorption.

In contrast to the macrolides and clindamycin, which bind to the 50S ribosomal subunit, tetracyclines inhibit bacterial protein synthesis by binding to the 30S subunit. Thus, resistance to macrolides does not imply resistance to tetracyclines. The tetracyclines used most often to treat dogs and cats are doxycycline and minocycline. Clinical use of tetracycline and oxytetracycline is rare in the United States because of a lack of available formulations and lack of good quality data to guide dosing. In addition, doxycycline and minocycline have some distinct advantages. Doxycycline and minocycline are longer-acting drugs, more lipophilic, better absorbed orally, and have antibacterial activity that is better than other agents in this class. Doxycycline and minocycline also have antiinflammatory and immunomodulatory properties because of inhibition of inducible nitric oxide synthase and proinflammatory cytokines such as TNF-α.[136] These properties have led to the use of tetracyclines for treatment of immune-mediated dermatopathies in dogs[135] and plasmacytic pododermatitis in cats.[137] There is evidence for beneficial effects for treating osteoarthritis in dogs, but this use is uncommon. Delayed-release formulations that produce subantimicrobial doses have been developed for use in human patients with the inflammatory skin disease rosacea. Doxycycline and minocycline also are used to treat acne in humans. Although development of tetracycline resistance in bacterial flora has not been documented in association with the use of these preparations, the possibility has not been ruled out.[138]

Resistance to tetracyclines primarily results from porin mutations that exclude tetracyclines from the bacterial cell, and increased drug efflux, mediated by the *tetK* gene. Bacteria with *tetK* may still be susceptible to minocycline, but the presence of another gene, *tetM*,

TABLE 10.15 Suggested Tetracycline Dosages for Small Animals

Drug	Dose (mg/kg)	Interval (hours)	Species	Route	Comments	CLSI Breakpoints (µg/mL)
Tetracycline	15–20 4.4–11	8	D, C	PO IV, IM	Do not mix with food containing cations such as calcium, zinc, magnesium, iron, aluminum	≤2 for streptococci, ≤4 for other susceptible bacteria. Consider use of ≤1 for susceptible bacteria
Oxytetracycline	20 7.5–10	12	D, C	PO IV	See tetracycline. Administer on an empty stomach	See doxycycline
Doxycycline	5 10	12 24	D, C	PO, IV	For IV administration, dilute in 100 to 1000 mL of LRS or 5% dextrose and administer over 1 to 2 hours	≤0.125 µg/mL for *Staphylococcus pseudintermedius*, and gram-negative bacteria (*E. coli*, and other Enterobacterales)
Minocycline	5 8.8 (one 50-mg capsule)	12 24	D C	PO PO		≤0.5 µg/mL

C, cats; *CLSI*, Clinical and Laboratory Standards Institute[41,42]; *D*, dogs; *IM*, intramuscular; *IV*, intravenous; *LRS*, lactated Ringer solution; *PO*, oral.

confers resistance to all tetracyclines.[139] Therefore, resistance to doxycycline does not always imply resistance to minocycline.[140] The glycylcycline antibiotic tigecycline is a new parenteral antibiotic derived from minocycline that has greater activity than older agents, but is limited in use for treatment of MDR bacterial infections in humans.[141] For reasons that remain unclear, resistance to tetracyclines has not been a significant problem among intracellular pathogens such as *Chlamydia*, *Anaplasma*, and *Rickettsia* spp.[142]

Clinical Use

Doses are shown in Table 10.15. Doxycycline is the most commonly used tetracycline in dogs and cats and has fewer adverse effects than other tetracyclines. There is extensive experience with doxycycline in countries outside the United States because it is licensed for this use in Europe and other countries (e.g., Ronaxan tablets). It is the drug of choice for treatment of a variety of tick-borne infectious diseases, feline chlamydiosis, salmon poisoning disease, and leptospirosis. Many (approximately 50%) of *Staphylococcus* spp. are susceptible to doxycycline and minocycline using approved clinical breakpoints. However, because susceptibility is unpredictable, it is not a choice for empirical treatment. Doxycycline is commonly recommended for respiratory infections. In the ISCAID consensus guidelines for treatment of respiratory infections in dogs and cats,[143] doxycycline was recommended for many respiratory indications. Doxycycline was listed as the first-line drug option (i.e., first-choice) for five conditions: acute bacterial upper respiratory infection in cats, chronic bacterial upper respiratory infection in cats, CIRD complex (with a bacterial component), bacterial bronchitis in dogs and cats, and pneumonia in animals.

For treatment of vector-borne disease in dogs and cats caused by *E. canis* and other organisms, there is substantial clinical and experimental evidence for effectiveness from doxycycline at 10 mg/kg/day for 28 days, and perhaps lower doses. Two consensus statements[144,145] recommend doxycycline as the first drug of choice for these infections in dogs and cats. Another important use of doxycycline and minocycline is in the treatment of canine heartworm disease. This addition to heartworm treatment is based on the activity of these agents against *Wolbachia*, which is an obligate endosymbiont.[146] This use is considered a standard part of canine heartworm treatment and is discussed in the protocol available from the American Heartworm Society (see https://www.heartwormsociety.org/veterinary-resources/american-heartworm-society-guidelines).

Doxycycline can be administered once daily (usually 10 mg/kg), but twice-daily administration with a lower dose (5 mg/kg q12h) is frequently recommended. A lower dose given twice daily produces less GI problems (particularly vomiting) than a higher dose given once daily. Doxycycline is absorbed approximately 64% (average from all studies in dogs) from the GI tract and distributed to tissues at concentrations that often exceed the unbound plasma concentration, including the lung, bronchial secretions, liver, kidney, and, to some extent, the CNS. Minocycline can be administered as an adequate substitute for doxycycline if there are shortages in availability of doxycycline or high cost. Minocycline is more lipophilic than doxycycline, it is better absorbed orally, but oral absorption is inhibited by food.[147] (Feeding also may affect doxycycline oral absorption in dogs and cats, but this factor has not been studied.) Minocycline can produce a higher incidence of GI upset, particularly if the entire dose is administered once daily (as with doxycycline, twice-daily administration is most often recommended). Pharmacokinetic studies have shown that minocycline can be administered at similar doses as doxycycline (5 mg/kg PO q12h for dogs and 50 mg PO q24h for cats).[148,149] Higher doses have a tendency to cause vomiting in animals. Sucralfate can significantly decrease absorption of minocycline when administered concurrently because it can chelate to aluminum in this product.[150] Absorption of other tetracyclines from the GI tract is not as efficient as doxycycline and minocycline. Oral absorption is also inhibited by other di- and tri-valent cations (e.g., Fe^{+3}, Mg^{+2}). All tetracyclines are concentrated in bile. Urine concentrations of minocycline and doxycycline may not be as high as other agents that are strictly eliminated in the urine. However, the concentrations of minocycline and doxycycline may be high enough to bacteria shown to be susceptible according to the current CLSI minocycline and doxycycline breakpoints.[41,42]

Adverse Effects

The most common adverse effects of tetracyclines in dogs and cats are vomiting, decreased appetite, nausea, and diarrhea. These may be reduced when doxycycline hyclate tablets are administered intact (rather than being split or crushed) and by administering doxycycline with food, but the effect of feeding on oral absorption should be considered, as it has been shown to have a significant effect for minocycline.[147] The hyclate salt of doxycycline (containing hydrochloride) has been associated with esophagitis and esophageal strictures in cats (Fig. 10.4),[151] and life-threatening esophageal ulceration in a dog.[152] This is also a complication in humans.[153] A bolus of water or small meal should be administered immediately after dosing in order to prevent this complication, or a suspension rather than tablets should be used. Doxycycline monohydrate, another formulation available for humans, and available for

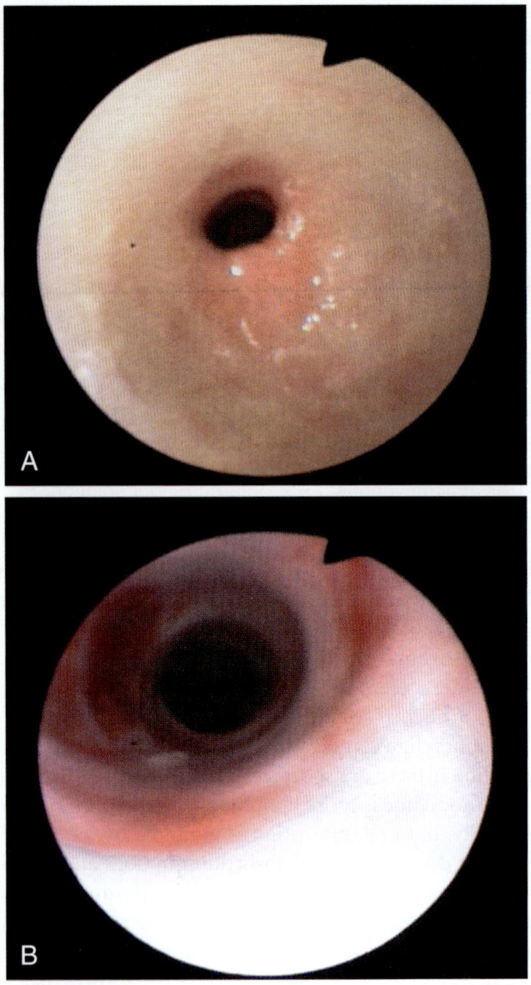

Fig. 10.4 (A) Esophageal stricture in a 9-year-old female spayed domestic shorthair cat that had been treated with doxycycline hyclate for possible hemoplasmosis. Regurgitation after eating commenced shortly after treatment was initiated. (B) The stricture was treated via repeated balloon dilatation; the image is taken immediately after the ballooning procedure was performed.

dogs and cats in some countries (e.g., Australia), has not been associated with esophageal erosions. To avoid problems with solid-dose oral forms or to decrease the cost of tablets, compounded formulations have been prepared for dogs and cats. Use of these formulations is discouraged unless the pharmacy can guarantee stability for the duration of treatment. Compounded, high-concentration (e.g., 33.3 mg/mL or 167 mg/mL) suspensions in aqueous vehicles have limited stability; suspensions in some vehicles do not retain their potency beyond 7 days.[154]

In dogs and cats with renal failure, tetracyclines other than doxycycline and minocycline should be avoided. Tetracyclines other than doxycycline can interfere with bone growth and cause significant and permanent gray-brown or yellow discoloration of the teeth (Fig. 10.5); therefore, their use is not recommended in puppies and kittens. Doxycycline is less likely to produce this effect because it binds calcium less avidly. As a result, the use of doxycycline in human pediatric medicine is now accepted for a short course.[155] All tetracyclines, including doxycycline, can cause hepatic failure and renal tubular necrosis. Cutaneous reactions (photosensitization) occur rarely in animals treated with tetracycline, but have been reported in humans.

IV preparations of doxycycline and minocycline are available but can be considerably more expensive than the oral formulations.

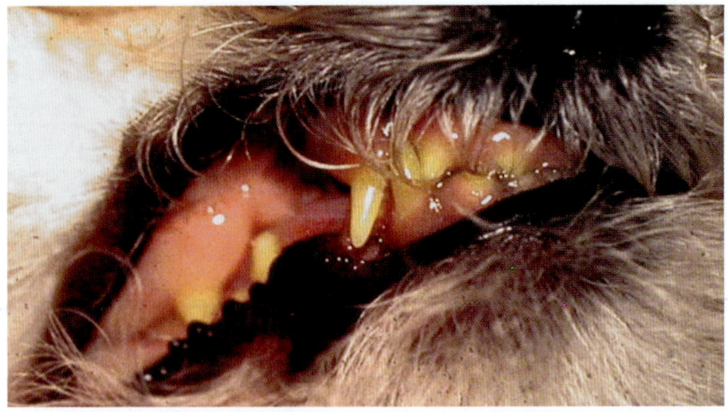

Fig. 10.5 Yellow discoloration of the teeth in a "puppy mill" puppy that was presumably treated with tetracycline antibiotics.

Doxycycline should be administered as a slow infusion (in humans, 1 to 2 hours is used). Thrombophlebitis can occur at the site of injection, and anaphylactic shock has been reported following parenteral administration of tetracycline to a dog.[156] On the other hand, although a slow IV infusion is also recommended for people with minocycline, the studies in dogs and cats used a short infusion of 5 minutes, without adverse events.[148,149]

Streptogramins

Quinupristin-dalfopristin is a combination of two streptogramin antibacterials in a 30:70 ratio. This combination is used for treatment of resistant gram-positive bacterial infections in humans. These agents act synergistically on the 50S ribosomal subunit to produce a bactericidal effect. This combination is approved to treat MRS and vancomycin-resistant *Staphylococcus* infections and *Enterococcus faecium* infections in humans. Quinupristin-dalfopristin is inactive against *Enterococcus faecalis.* Worldwide, a low rate of resistance exists among MDR gram-positive bacteria in humans and dogs; however, resistant strains have been identified that can methylate the ribosomal subunit, inactivate streptogramins, or that express efflux pumps.[157] Currently, there are no reports of use of quinupristin-dalfopristin in dogs and cats, which may relate to the drug's high cost, frequent adverse effects in humans, and the need to administer the drug intravenously through a central vein.[132]

SUGGESTED READINGS

Lappin MR, Blondeau J, Boothe D, et al. Antimicrobial use guidelines for treatment of respiratory tract disease in dogs and cats: antimicrobial guidelines working group of the International Society for Companion Animal Infectious Diseases. *J Vet Intern Med*. 2017;31:279–294.

Weese JS, Blondeau J, Boothe D, et al. International Society for Companion Animal Infectious Diseases (ISCAID) guidelines for the diagnosis and management of bacterial urinary tract infections in dogs and cats. *Vet J*. 2019;247:8–25.

Pennisi MG, Hofmann-Lehmann R, Radford AD, et al. *Anaplasma, Ehrlichia* and *Rickettsia* species infections in cats: European guidelines from the ABCD on prevention and management. *J Fel Med Surg*. 2017;19(5):542–548.

REFERENCES

1. Silhavy TJ, Kahne D, Walker S. The bacterial cell envelope. *Cold Spring Harb Perspect Biol*. 2010;2:a000414.
2. Gold HS, Moellering Jr RC. Antimicrobial-drug resistance. *N Engl J Med*. 1996;335:1445–1453.
3. Trang M, Dudley MN, Bhavnani SM. Use of Monte Carlo simulation and considerations for PK-PD targets to support antibacterial dose selection. *Curr Opin Pharmacol*. 2017;36:107–113.

4. Stapleton PD, Taylor PW. Methicillin resistance in *Staphylococcus aureus*: mechanisms and modulation. *Sci Prog.* 2002;85:57–72.
5. EUCAST. MIC and zone diameter distributions and ECOFFs. http://www.eucast.org/mic_distributions_and_ecoffs.
6. Lawrence M, Kukanich K, Kukanich B, et al. Effect of cefovecin on the fecal flora of healthy dogs. *Vet J.* 2013;198:259–266.
7. Williams KJ, Bax RP, Brown H, et al. Antibiotic treatment and associated prolonged prothrombin time. *J Clin Pathol.* 1991;44:738–741.
8. Deldar A, Lewis H, Bloom J, et al. Cephalosporin-induced changes in the ultrastructure of canine bone marrow. *Vet Pathol.* 1988;25:211–218.
9. Asbel LE, Levison ME. Cephalosporins, carbapenems, and monobactams. *Infect Dis Clin North Am.* 2000;14:435–447 (ix).
10. Zhanel GG, Wiebe R, Dilay L, et al. Comparative review of the carbapenems. *Drugs.* 2007;67:1027–1052.
11. Bidgood T, Papich MG. Plasma pharmacokinetics and tissue fluid concentrations of meropenem after intravenous and subcutaneous administration in dogs. *Am J Vet Res.* 2002;63:1622–1628.
12. Bratu S, Landman D, Alam M, et al. Detection of KPC carbapenem-hydrolyzing enzymes in *Enterobacter* spp. from Brooklyn, New York. *Antimicrob Agents Chemother.* 2005;49:776–778.
13. Marra A. NDM-1: a local clone emerges with worldwide aspirations. *Future Microbiol.* 2011;6:137–141.
14. Peleg AY, Hooper DC. Hospital-acquired infections due to gram-negative bacteria. *N Engl J Med.* 2010;362:1804–1813.
15. Shaheen BW, Nayak R, Boothe DM. Emergence of a New Delhi metallo-beta-lactamase (NDM-1)-encoding gene in clinical *Escherichia coli* isolates recovered from companion animals in the United States. *Antimicrob Agents Chemother.* 2013;57:2902–2903.
16. Sun Y, Ji X, Liu Y, et al. New Delhi metallo-beta-lactamase-1-producing acinetobacter lwoffii of companion animal origin in China. *Indian J Med Microbiol.* 2015;33:615–617.
17. Papich MG. *Saunders Handbook of Veterinary Drugs: Small and Large Animal.* 4th ed. St. Louis, MO: Elsevier Saunders; 2016.
18. Bailiff NL, Westropp JL, Jang SS, et al. *Corynebacterium urealyticum* urinary tract infection in dogs and cats: 7 cases (1996-2003). *J Am Vet Med Assoc.* 2005;226:1676–1680.
19. Briscoe KA, Barrs VR, Lindsay S, et al. Encrusting cystitis in a cat secondary to *Corynebacterium urealyticum* infection. *J Feline Med Surg.* 2010;12:972–977.
20. Lopez M, Tenorio C, Torres C. Study of vancomycin resistance in faecal enterococci from healthy humans and dogs in Spain a decade after the avoparcin ban in Europe. *Zoonoses Public Health.* 2013;60:160–167.
21. Abbott Y, Kirby BM, Karczmarczyk M, et al. High-level gentamicin-resistant and vancomycin-resistant *Enterococcus faecium* isolated from a wound in a dog. *J Small Anim Pract.* 2009;50:194–197.
22. Zhanel GG, Walkty AJ, Karlowsky JA. Fosfomycin: a first-line oral therapy for acute uncomplicated cystitis. *Can J Infect Dis Med Microbiol.* 2016;2016:2082693.
23. Hubka P, Boothe DM. In vitro susceptibility of canine and feline *Escherichia coli* to fosfomycin. *Vet Microbiol.* 2011;149:277–282.
24. Ho PL, Chan J, Lo WU, et al. Dissemination of plasmid-mediated fosfomycin resistance fosA3 among multidrug-resistant *Escherichia coli* from livestock and other animals. *J Appl Microbiol.* 2013;114:695–702.
25. DiCicco M, Weese S, Neethirajan S, et al. Fosfomycin susceptibility of canine methicillin-resistant *Staphylococcus pseudintermedius* isolates. *Res Vet Sci.* 2014;96:251–253.
26. Perez DS, Tapia MO, Soraci AL. Fosfomycin: uses and potentialities in veterinary medicine. *Open Vet J.* 2014;4:26–43.
27. Gutierrez OL, Ocampo CL, Aguilera JR, et al. Pharmacokinetics of disodium-fosfomycin in mongrel dogs. *Res Vet Sci.* 2008;85:156–161.
28. DiCicco M, Neethirajan S, Weese JS, et al. In vitro synergism of fosfomycin and clarithromycin antimicrobials against methicillin-resistant *Staphylococcus pseudintermedius. BMC Microbiol.* 2014;14:129.
29. Zhang CC, Weng TC, Su BA, et al. Salvage therapy with intravenous fosfomycin plus ceftriaxone for necrotizing fasciitis caused by penicillin-nonsusceptible *Streptococcus pneumoniae. J Microbiol Immunol Infect.* 2016;51:573–574.
30. Fukata T, Imai N, Shibata S. Acute renal insufficiency in cats after fosfomycin administration. *Vet Rec.* 2008;163:337–338.
31. Zhang XF, Doi Y, Huang X, et al. Possible transmission of mcr-1-harboring *Escherichia coli* between companion animals and human. *Emerg Infect Dis.* 2016;22:1679–1681.
32. Baron S, Hadjadj L, Rolain JM, et al. Molecular mechanisms of polymyxin resistance: knowns and unknowns. Int J Antimicrob Agents. 02016;48:583–591.
33. Taylor SD, Palmer M. The action mechanism of daptomycin. *Bioorg Med Chem.* 2016;24:6253–6268.
34. Seaton RA, Menichetti F, Dalekos G, et al. Evaluation of effectiveness and safety of high-dose daptomycin: results from patients included in the European Cubicin(®) Outcomes Registry and Experience. *Adv Ther.* 2015;32:1192–1205.
35. Robicsek A, Jacoby GA, Hooper DC. The worldwide emergence of plasmid-mediated quinolone resistance. *Lancet Infect Dis.* 2006;6:629–640.
36. Phillips I, King A. Comparative activity of the 4-quinolones. *Rev Infect Dis.* 1988;10(suppl 1):S70–S76.
37. Rubin J, Walker RD, Blickenstaff K, et al. Antimicrobial resistance and genetic characterization of fluoroquinolone resistance of *Pseudomonas aeruginosa* isolated from canine infections. *Vet Microbiol.* 2008;131:164–172.
38. Silley P, Stephan B, Greife HA, et al. Comparative activity of pradofloxacin against anaerobic bacteria isolated from dogs and cats. *J Antimicrob Chemother.* 2007;60:999–1003.
39. Papich MG. Ciprofloxacin pharmacokinetics and oral absorption of generic ciprofloxacin tablets in dogs. *Am J Vet Res.* 2012;73:1085–1091.
40. Madsen M, Messenger K, Papich MG. Pharmacokinetics of levofloxacin following oral administration of a generic levofloxacin tablet and intravenous administration to dogs. *Am J Vet Res.* 2019;80(10):957–962.
41. Clinical and Laboratory Standards Institute. Performance Standards for Antimicrobial Disk and Dilution Susceptibility Tests for Bacteria Isolated from Animals. In: *CLSI Standard VET01.* 6th ed. Wayne, PA: Clinical and Laboratory Standards Institute; 2021. Available from: www.CLSI.org.
42. Clinical and Laboratory Standards Institute. Performance Standards for Antimicrobial Disk and Dilution Susceptibility Tests for Bacteria Isolated from Animals. 5th ed. In: *CLSI supplement VET01S* Wayne, PA: Clinical and Laboratory Standards Institute; 2020. available from: www.CLSI.org.
43. Cole LK, Papich MG, Kwochka KW, et al. Plasma and ear tissue concentrations of enrofloxacin and its metabolite ciprofloxacin in dogs with chronic end-stage otitis externa after intravenous administration of enrofloxacin. *Vet Dermatol.* 2009;20:51–59.
44. Mori K, Maru C, Takasuna K. Characterization of histamine release induced by fluoroquinolone antibacterial agents in-vivo and in-vitro. *J Pharm Pharmacol.* 2000;52:577–584.
45. Christ W. Central nervous system toxicity of quinolones: human and animal findings. *J Antimicrob Chemother.* 1990;26(Suppl B):219–225.
46. Ford MM, Dubielzig RR, Giuliano EA, et al. Ocular and systemic manifestations after oral administration of a high dose of enrofloxacin in cats. *Am J Vet Res.* 2007;68:190–202.
47. Wiebe V, Hamilton P. Fluoroquinolone-induced retinal degeneration in cats. *J Am Vet Med Assoc.* 2002;221:1568–1571.
48. Ramirez CJ, Minch JD, Gay JM, et al. Molecular genetic basis for fluoroquinolone-induced retinal degeneration in cats. *Pharmacogenet Genomics.* 2011;21:66–75.
49. Messias A, Gekeler F, Wegener A, et al. Retinal safety of a new fluoroquinolone, pradofloxacin, in cats: assessment with electroretinography. *Doc Ophthalmol.* 2008;116:177–191.
50. Rosanova MT, Lede R, Capurro H, et al. Assessing fluoroquinolones as risk factor for musculoskeletal disorders in children: a systematic review and meta-analysis. *Arch Argent Pediatr.* 2010;108:524–531.
51. Sansone JM, Wilsman NJ, Leiferman EM, et al. The effect of fluoroquinolone antibiotics on growing cartilage in the lamb model. *J Pediatr Orthop.* 2009;29:189–195.
52. Heidelbaugh JJ, Holmstrom H. The perils of prescribing fluoroquinolones. *J Fam Pract.* 2013;62:191–197.

53. Committee on Infectious Diseases. The use of systemic fluoroquinolones. *Pediatrics.* 2006;118:1287–1292.
54. Narayanan S, Hunerbein A, Getie M, et al. Scavenging properties of metronidazole on free oxygen radicals in a skin lipid model system. *J Pharm Pharmacol.* 2007;59:1125–1130.
55. Jergens AE, Crandell J, Morrison JA, et al. Comparison of oral prednisone and prednisone combined with metronidazole for induction therapy of canine inflammatory bowel disease: a randomized-controlled trial. *J Vet Intern Med.* 2010;24:269–277.
56. Langlois DK, Koenigshof AM, Mani R. Metronidazole treatment of acute diarrhea in dogs: a randomized double blinded placebo–controlled clinical trial. *J Vet Intern Med.* 2020;34(1):98–104.
57. Shmalberg JW, Montalbano C, Morelli G, et al. A randomized double blinded placebo-controlled clinical trial of a probiotic or metronidazole for acute canine diarrhea. *Frontiers Vet Sci.* 2019;6:163.
58. Lofmark S, Edlund C, Nord CE. Metronidazole is still the drug of choice for treatment of anaerobic infections. *Clin Infect Dis.* 2010;50(suppl 1):S16–S23.
59. Evans J, Levesque D, Knowles K, et al. Diazepam as a treatment for metronidazole toxicosis in dogs: a retrospective study of 21 cases. *J Vet Intern Med.* 2003;17:304–310.
60. Olson EJ, Morales SC, McVey AS, et al. Putative metronidazole neurotoxicosis in a cat. *Vet Pathol.* 2005;42:665–669.
61. Moosa AN, Perkins D. Neurological picture. MRI of metronidazole induced cerebellar ataxia. *J Neurol Neurosurg Psychiatry.* 2010;81:754–755.
62. Sekis I, Ramstead K, Rishniw M, et al. Single-dose pharmacokinetics and genotoxicity of metronidazole in cats. *J Feline Med Surg.* 2009;11:60–68.
63. Jenkins DJ, Kendall CW, Hamidi M, et al. Effect of antibiotics as cholesterol-lowering agents. *Metabolism.* 2005;54:103–112.
64. Cavusoglu C, Karaca-Derici Y, Bilgic A. In-vitro activity of rifabutin against rifampicin-resistant *Mycobacterium tuberculosis* isolates with known rpoB mutations. *Clin Microbiol Infect.* 2004;10:662–665.
65. Dutta A, Schwarzwald HL, Edwards MS. Disseminated bartonellosis presenting as neuroretinitis in a young adult with human immunodeficiency virus infection. *Pediatr Infect Dis J.* 2010;29:675–677.
66. Liston TE, Koehler JE. Granulomatous hepatitis and necrotizing splenitis due to *Bartonella henselae* in a patient with cancer: case report and review of hepatosplenic manifestations of bartonella infection. *Clin Infect Dis.* 1996;22:951–957.
67. Theodorou K, Mylonakis ME, Siarkou VI, et al. Efficacy of rifampicin in the treatment of experimental acute canine monocytic ehrlichiosis. *J Antimicrob Chemother.* 2013;68:1619–1626.
68. Bajwa J, Charach M, Duclos D. Adverse effects of rifampicin in dogs and serum alanine aminotransferase monitoring recommendations based on a retrospective study of 344 dogs. *Vet Dermatol.* 2013;24(570–575):e135–576.
69. De Vriese AS, Robbrecht DL, Vanholder RC, et al. Rifampicin-associated acute renal failure: pathophysiologic, immunologic, and clinical features. *Am J Kidney Dis.* 1998;31:108–115.
70. Reitman ML, Chu X, Cai X, et al. Rifampin's acute inhibitory and chronic inductive drug interactions: experimental and model-based approaches to drug-drug interaction trial design. *Clin Pharmacol Ther.* 2011;89:234–242.
71. Then RL. Mechanisms of resistance to trimethoprim, the sulfonamides, and trimethoprim-sulfamethoxazole. *Rev Infect Dis.* 1982;4:261–269.
72. Chretin JD, Rassnick KM, Shaw NA, et al. Prophylactic trimethoprim-sulfadiazine during chemotherapy in dogs with lymphoma and osteosarcoma: a double-blind, placebo-controlled study. *J Vet Intern Med.* 2007;21:141–148.
73. Jacoby GA. Perils of prophylaxis. *N Engl J Med.* 1982;306:43–44.
74. Weese JS, Blondeau JM, Boothe D, et al. Antimicrobial use guidelines for treatment of urinary tract disease in dogs and cats: antimicrobial guidelines working group of the international society for companion animal infectious diseases. *Vet Med Int.* 2011;2011:263768.
75. Noli C, Koeman JP, Willemse T. A retrospective evaluation of adverse reactions to trimethoprim-sulphonamide combinations in dogs and cats. *Vet Q.* 1995;17:123–128.
76. Nuttall TJ, Malham T. Successful intravenous human immunoglobulin treatment of drug-induced Stevens-Johnson syndrome in a dog. *J Small Anim Pract.* 2004;45:357–361.
77. Trepanier LA. Idiosyncratic toxicity associated with potentiated sulfonamides in the dog. *J Vet Pharmacol Ther.* 2004;27:129–138.
78. Vasilopulos RJ, Mackin A, Lavergne SN, et al. Nephrotic syndrome associated with administration of sulfadimethoxine/ormetoprim in a dobermann. *J Small Anim Pract.* 2005;46:232–236.
79. Weiss DJ, Adams LG. Aplastic anemia associated with trimethoprim-sulfadiazine and fenbendazole administration in a dog. *J Am Vet Med Assoc.* 1987;191:1119–1120.
80. Brenner K, Harkin K, Schermerhorn T. Iatrogenic, sulfonamide-induced hypothyroid crisis in a Labrador Retriever. *Aust Vet J.* 2009;87:503–505.
81. Twedt DC, Diehl KJ, Lappin MR, et al. Association of hepatic necrosis with trimethoprim sulfonamide administration in 4 dogs. *J Vet Intern Med.* 1997;11:20–23.
82. Trepanier LA, Danhof R, Toll J, et al. Clinical findings in 40 dogs with hypersensitivity associated with administration of potentiated sulfonamides. *J Vet Intern Med.* 2003;17:647–652.
83. Cribb AE, Spielberg SP. An in vitro investigation of predisposition to sulphonamide idiosyncratic toxicity in dogs. *Vet Res Commun.* 1990;14:241–252.
84. Osborne CA, Lulich JP, Bartges JW, et al. Drug-induced urolithiasis. *Vet Clin North Am Small Anim Pract.* 1999;29:251–266 (xiv).
85. Garneau-Tsodikova S, Labby KJ. Mechanisms of resistance to aminoglycoside antibiotics: overview and perspectives. *Medchemcomm.* 2016;7:11–27.
86. Ramirez MS, Tolmasky ME. Aminoglycoside modifying enzymes. *Drug Resist Updat.* 2010;13:151–171.
87. Gold RM, Cohen ND, Lawhon SD. Amikacin resistance in *Staphylococcus pseudintermedius* isolated from dogs. *J Clin Microbiol.* 2014;52:3641–3646.
88. Sykes JE, Mapes S, Lindsay LL, et al. *Corynebacterium ulcerans* bronchopneumonia in a dog. *J Vet Intern Med.* 2010;24:973–976.
89. Torres AR, Cooke K. Intravesical instillation of amikacin for treatment of a lower urinary tract infection caused by *Pseudomonas aeruginosa* in a dog. *J Am Vet Med Assoc.* 2014;245:809–811.
90. Gookin JL, Riviere JE, Gilger BC, et al. Acute renal failure in four cats treated with paromomycin. *J Am Vet Med Assoc.* 1999;215:1821–1823, 1806.
91. Mealey KL, Boothe DM. Nephrotoxicosis associated with topical administration of gentamicin in a cat. *J Am Vet Med Assoc.* 1994;204:1919–1921.
92. Hayes G, Gibson T, Moens NM, et al. Intra-articular implantation of gentamicin impregnated collagen sponge causes joint inflammation and impaired renal function in dogs. *Vet Comp Orthop Traumatol.* 2016;29:159–163.
93. Lopez-Novoa JM, Quiros Y, Vicente L, et al. New insights into the mechanism of aminoglycoside nephrotoxicity: an integrative point of view. *Kidney Int.* 2011;79:33–45.
94. Cowan RH, Jukkola AF, Arant Jr BS. Pathophysiologic evidence of gentamicin nephrotoxicity in neonatal puppies. *Pediatr Res.* 1980;14:1204–1211.
95. Rao SC, Ahmed M, Hagan R. One dose per day compared to multiple doses per day of gentamicin for treatment of suspected or proven sepsis in neonates. *Cochrane Database Syst Rev.* 2006:CD005091.
96. Grauer GF, Greco DS, Behrend EN, et al. Effects of dietary protein conditioning on gentamicin-induced nephrotoxicosis in healthy male dogs. *Am J Vet Res.* 1994;55:90–97.
97. Kai K, Yamaguchi T, Yoshimatsu Y, et al. Neutrophil gelatinase-associated lipocalin, a sensitive urinary biomarker of acute kidney injury in dogs receiving gentamicin. *J Toxicol Sci.* 2013;38:269–277.
98. Sasaki A, Sasaki Y, Iwama R, et al. Comparison of renal biomarkers with glomerular filtration rate in susceptibility to the detection of gentamicin-induced acute kidney injury in dogs. *J Comp Pathol.* 2014;151:264–270.
99. Papich MG, Riviere JE. Aminoglycoside antibiotics. In: Riviere JE, Papich MG, eds. *Veterinary Pharmacology and Therapeutics.* 9th ed. Ames, IO: Wiley-Blackwell; 2009:915–935.

100. Lanvers-Kaminsky C, Zehnhoff-Dinnesen AA, Parfitt R, et al. Drug-induced ototoxicity: mechanisms, pharmacogenetics, and protective strategies. *Clin Pharmacol Ther*. 2017;101:491–500.
101. Gooi A, Hochman J, Wellman M, et al. Ototoxic effects of single-dose versus 19-day daily-dose gentamicin. *J Otolaryngol Head Neck Surg*. 2008;37:664–667.
102. Forsyth SF, Ilkiw JE, Hildebrand SV. Effect of gentamicin administration on the neuromuscular blockade induced by atracurium in cats. *Am J Vet Res*. 1990;51:1675–1678.
103. Martinez EA, Mealey KL, Wooldridge AA, et al. Pharmacokinetics, effects on renal function, and potentiation of atracurium-induced neuromuscular blockade after administration of a high dose of gentamicin in isoflurane-anesthetized dogs. *Am J Vet Res*. 1996;57:1623–1626.
104. Singh YN, Marshall IG, Harvey AL. Some effects of the aminoglycoside antibiotic amikacin on neuromuscular and autonomic transmission. *Br J Anaesth*. 1978;50:109–117.
105. Harnett MT, Chen W, Smith SM. Calcium-sensing receptor: a high-affinity presynaptic target for aminoglycoside-induced weakness. *Neuropharmacology*. 2009;57:502–505.
106. Papich MG. Therapeutic drug monitoring. In: Riviere JE, Papich MG, eds. *Veterinary Pharmacology and Therapeutics*. 9th ed. Ames, IO: Wiley-Blackwell; 2009:1328.
107. De Renzo A, Formisano S, Rotoli B. Bone marrow aplasia and thiamphenicol. *Haematologica*. 1981;66:98–104.
108. Schwarz S, Kehrenberg C, Doublet B, et al. Molecular basis of bacterial resistance to chloramphenicol and florfenicol. *FEMS Microbiol Rev*. 2004;28:519–542.
109. Maaland MG, Mo SS, Schwarz S, et al. In vitro assessment of chloramphenicol and florfenicol as second-line antimicrobial agents in dogs. *J Vet Pharmacol Ther*. 2015;38:443–450.
110. Wiholm BE, Kelly JP, Kaufman D, et al. Relation of aplastic anaemia to use of chloramphenicol eye drops in two international case-control studies. *BMJ*. 1998;316:666.
111. Fraunfelder FW, Fraunfelder FT. Restricting topical ocular chloramphenicol eye drop use in the United States. Did we overreact? *Am J Ophthalmol*. 2013;156:420–422.
112. Rayner SA, Buckley RJ. Ocular chloramphenicol and aplastic anaemia. Is there a link? *Drug Saf*. 1996;14:273–276.
113. Short J, Zabel S, Cook C, et al. Adverse events associated with chloramphenicol use in dogs: a retrospective study (2007-2013). *Vet Rec*. 2014;175:537.
114. KuKanich B, KuKanich K. Chloramphenicol significantly affects the pharmacokinetics of oral methadone in Greyhound dogs. *Vet Anaesth Analg*. 2015;42:597–607.
115. Giamarellos-Bourboulis EJ. Macrolides beyond the conventional antimicrobials: a class of potent immunomodulators. *Int J Antimicrob Agents*. 2008;31:12–20.
116. Schultz MJ. Macrolide activities beyond their antimicrobial effects: macrolides in diffuse panbronchiolitis and cystic fibrosis. *J Antimicrob Chemother*. 2004;54:21–28.
117. Parnham MJ, Erakovic Haber V, Giamarellos-Bourboulis EJ, et al. Azithromycin: mechanisms of action and their relevance for clinical applications. *Pharmacol Ther*. 2014;143:225–245.
118. Kovaleva A, Remmelts HH, Rijkers GT, et al. Immunomodulatory effects of macrolides during community-acquired pneumonia: a literature review. *J Antimicrob Chemother*. 2012;67:530–540.
119. Kanoh S, Rubin BK. Mechanisms of action and clinical application of macrolides as immunomodulatory medications. *Clin Microbiol Rev*. 2010;23:590–615.
120. Piscitelli SC, Danziger LH, Rodvold KA. Clarithromycin and azithromycin: new macrolide antibiotics. *Clin Pharm*. 1992;11:137–152.
121. Sivapalasingham S, Steigbigel N. Macrolides, clindamycin and ketolides. In: Mandell GL, Bennett JE, Dolin R, eds. *Mandell, Douglas and Bennett's Principles and Practice of Infectious Diseases*. 7th ed. Philadelphia, PA: Churchill Livingstone Elsevier; 2011:427–448.
122. Westermarck E, Skrzypczak T, Harmoinen J, et al. Tylosin-responsive chronic diarrhea in dogs. *J Vet Intern Med*. 2005;19:177–186.
123. Kilpinen S, Rantala M, Spillmann T, et al. Oral tylosin administration is associated with an increase of faecal enterococci and lactic acid bacteria in dogs with tylosin-responsive diarrhoea. *Vet J*. 2015;205:369–374.
124. Ruch-Gallie RA, Veir JK, Spindel ME, et al. Efficacy of amoxycillin and azithromycin for the empirical treatment of shelter cats with suspected bacterial upper respiratory infections. *J Feline Med Surg*. 2008;10:542–550.
125. Peeters TL. Erythromycin and other macrolides as prokinetic agents. *Gastroenterology*. 1993;105:1886–1899.
126. Albarellos GA, Kreil VE, Ambros LA, et al. Pharmacokinetics of erythromycin after the administration of intravenous and various oral dosage forms to dogs. *J Vet Pharmacol Ther*. 2008;31:496–500.
127. Katayama M, Kawakami Y, Katayama R, et al. Preliminary study of effects of multiple oral dosing of clarithromycin on the pharmacokinetics of cyclosporine in dogs. *J Vet Med Sci*. 2014;76:431–433.
128. Katayama M, Nishijima N, Okamura Y, et al. Interaction of clarithromycin with cyclosporine in cats: pharmacokinetic study and case report. *J Feline Med Surg*. 2012;14:257–261.
129. Beatty JA, Swift N, Foster DJ, et al. Suspected clindamycin-associated oesophageal injury in cats: five cases. *J Feline Med Surg*. 2006;8:412–419.
130. Glanemann B, Hildebrandt N, Schneider MA, et al. Recurrent single oesophageal stricture treated with a self-expanding stent in a cat. *J Feline Med Surg*. 2008;10:505–509.
131. Livermore DM. Linezolid in vitro: mechanism and antibacterial spectrum. *J Antimicrob Chemother*. 2003;51(suppl 2). ii9–16.
132. Papich MG. Selection of antibiotics for meticillin-resistant *Staphylococcus pseudintermedius*: time to revisit some old drugs?. *Vet Dermatol*. 2012;23:352–360. e364.
133. Foster JD, Trepanier LA, Ginn JA. Use of linezolid to treat MRSP bacteremia and discospondylitis in a dog. *J Am Anim Hosp Assoc*. 2014;50:53–58.
134. Beekmann SE, Gilbert DN, Polgreen PM. Toxicity of extended courses of linezolid: results of an Infectious Diseases Society of America Emerging Infections Network survey. *Diagn Microbiol Infect Dis*. 2008;62:407–410.
135. White SD, Rosychuk RA, Reinke SI, et al. Use of tetracycline and niacinamide for treatment of autoimmune skin disease in 31 dogs. *J Am Vet Med Assoc*. 1992;200:1497–1500.
136. Leite LM, Carvalho AG, Ferreira PL, et al. Anti-inflammatory properties of doxycycline and minocycline in experimental models: an in vivo and in vitro comparative study. *Inflammopharmacology*. 2011;19:99–110.
137. Bettenay SV, Mueller RS, Dow K, et al. Prospective study of the treatment of feline plasmacytic pododermatitis with doxycycline. *Vet Rec*. 2003;152:564–566.
138. McKeage K, Deeks ED. Doxycycline 40 mg capsules (30 mg immediate-release/10 mg delayed-release beads): anti-inflammatory dose in rosacea. *Am J Clin Dermatol*. 2010;11:217–222.
139. Thaker M, Spanogiannopoulos P, Wright GD. The tetracycline resistome. *Cell Mol Life Sci*. 2010;67:419–431.
140. Weese JS, Sweetman K, Edson H, et al. Evaluation of minocycline susceptibility of methicillin-resistant *Staphylococcus pseudintermedius*. *Vet Microbiol*. 2013;162:968–971.
141. Pankey GA. Tigecycline. *J Antimicrob Chemother*. 2005;56:470–480.
142. McOrist S. Obligate intracellular bacteria and antibiotic resistance. *Trends Microbiol*. 2000;8:483–486.
143. Lappin MR, Blondeau J, Boothe D, et al. Antimicrobial use guidelines for treatment of respiratory tract disease in dogs and cats: antimicrobial guidelines working group of the International Society for Companion Animal Infectious Diseases. *J Vet Intern Med*. 2017;31:279–294.
144. Pennisi MG, Hofmann-Lehmann R, Radford AD, et al. *Anaplasma, Ehrlichia* and *Rickettsia* species infections in cats: European guidelines from the ABCD on prevention and management. *J Fel Med Surg*. 2017;19(5):542–548.
145. Neer TM, Breitschwerdt EB, Greene RT, et al. Consensus statement on ehrlichial disease of small animals from the infectious disease study group of the ACVIM. *J Vet Intern Med*. 2002;16(3):309–315.
146. Savadelis MD, Day KM, Bradner JL, et al. Efficacy and side effects of doxycycline versus minocycline in the three-dose melarsomine canine adulticidal heartworm treatment protocol. *Parasites Vectors*. 2018;11(1):671.

147. Hnot ML, Cole LK, Lorch G, et al. Effect of feeding on the pharmacokinetics of oral minocycline in healthy research dogs. *Vet Dermatol.* 2015;26(399–405):e392–393.
148. Maaland MG, Guardabassi L, Papich MG. Minocycline pharmacokinetics and pharmacodynamics in dogs: dosage recommendations for treatment of meticillin-resistant *Staphylococcus pseudintermedius* infections. *Vet Dermatol.* 2014;25:182–190. e146–187.
149. Tynan BE, Papich MG, Kerl ME, et al. Pharmacokinetics of minocycline in domestic cats. *J Feline Med Surg.* 2016;18:257–263.
150. KuKanich K, KuKanich B, Harris A, et al. Effect of sucralfate on oral minocycline absorption in healthy dogs. *J Vet Pharmacol Ther.* 2014;37:451–456.
151. German AJ, Cannon MJ, Dye C, et al. Oesophageal strictures in cats associated with doxycycline therapy. *J Feline Med Surg.* 2005;7:33–41.
152. Sykes JE, Bailiff NL, Ball LM, et al. Identification of a novel hemotropic mycoplasma in a splenectomized dog with hemic neoplasia. *J Am Vet Med Assoc.* 2004;224:1946–1951. 1930–1941.
153. Morris TJ, Davis TP. Doxycycline-induced esophageal ulceration in the U.S. Military service. *Mil Med.* 2000;165:316–319.
154. Papich MG, Davidson G. Doxycycline potency after storage in a compounded formulation for animals. In: *American College of Veterinary Internal Medicine Forum.* Denver, CO, USA: 2011.
155. Volovitz B, Shkap R, Amir J, et al. Absence of tooth staining with doxycycline treatment in young children. *Clin Pediatr (Phila).* 2007;46:121–126.
156. Ward GS, Guiry CC, Alexander LL. Tetracycline-induced anaphylactic shock in a dog. *J Am Vet Med Assoc.* 1982;180:770–771.
157. Werner G, Cuny C, Schmitz FJ, et al. Methicillin-resistant, quinupristin-dalfopristin-resistant *Staphylococcus aureus* with reduced sensitivity to glycopeptides. *J Clin Microbiol.* 2001;39:3586–3590.

11

Antifungal Drugs

Polina Vishkautsan, Jane E. Sykes, Mark G. Papich

KEY POINTS

- Compared with antibacterial drugs, the range of antifungal drug classes available is limited. The azole class of antifungal agents is used for systemic treatment in most animal patients. The azoles have a similar mechanism of action, but can differ in their antifungal spectrum of activity, pharmacokinetics, and adverse effect profiles. Proper understanding of these factors is most likely to result in successful treatment with minimal adverse effects.
- Drug interactions occur with many antifungal drugs.
- Although therapeutic drug monitoring could improve treatment with the azole antifungals and 5-flucytosine, this is rarely done because of variable availability of clinical assays. If performed, the interpretation of the measured concentrations is based on guidelines for humans.
- Fungal infections often require prolonged treatment durations. This may be costly for some pet owners and can increase the risk of drug adverse effects.
- Fungal organisms that are resistant to certain antifungal drugs are increasingly recognized. Although antifungal susceptibility testing can identify resistant organisms, this is often not performed because there are no standards for interpreting susceptibility tests for veterinary pathogens and antifungal drugs used in veterinary medicine.

INTRODUCTION

In human medicine, an increase in the need for agents to treat fungal infections coincided with an increase in diseases that caused immunosuppression (e.g., HIV), or treatments with potent immunosuppressive drugs. In animals, immunosuppression can also underlie opportunistic fungal infections, and the importance of fungal infections in dogs and cats is increasingly recognized. It is anticipated that global climate changes also will increase fungal infections in mammals.[1]

With the exception of itraconazole, there are no antifungal drugs approved by regulatory authorities for use in dogs and cats. Therefore, veterinarians rely on extra-label use of human antifungal drugs, with indications and dosage regimens often extrapolated from human use. Because of differences in pharmacokinetics among species for these drugs, and differences in the susceptibility to adverse effects in dogs and cats compared with humans, this approach is not optimal, but because of experience with some of these agents, veterinarians are accumulating treatment guidelines to treat these infections. Fortunately, the clinical experience and pharmacokinetic data have expanded for these human drugs, which has allowed more precise antifungal treatment in animals. Efforts also have focused on the development of new, less toxic and more efficacious antifungal drugs and treatment regimens. This chapter reviews the classification, mechanisms of action, spectrum of activity, resistance mechanisms, pharmacokinetics, clinical use, and adverse effects of the major systemic antifungal drugs used to treat dogs and cats. Topical antifungal treatments are included in other chapters of this book relevant to specific infections.

Antifungal drug treatment is usually longer in duration then antibacterial drug treatment. One reason for this difference is that fungal organisms grow more slowly, and the drugs used (primarily azoles) are fungistatic, not fungicidal. The patient's immune system is also often compromised, which may be the underlying reason for the infection. Therefore, long-term treatment is needed to inhibit fungal growth and eradicate the infection. Antifungal drug treatment of animals that have deep mycoses often must be continued for months, and in some animals, it may be weeks before any clinical improvement is evident. Thus, a "trial-and-error" treatment approach with antifungal drugs is often not useful. In addition, disease often worsens within the first 1 to 2 weeks of treatment because of the host's inflammatory response to treatment effects. This may have severe consequences for the host when there is extensive involvement of the pulmonary parenchyma or the CNS. Concurrent treatment with an NSAID or, when CNS involvement is present, judicious use of a short course of anti-inflammatory glucocorticoids, may improve outcome in these situations.[2] The prognosis for animals with disseminated mold infections with reversible underlying immunosuppression (such as drug-induced immunosuppression) may be better than the prognosis for animals with no apparent underlying immunosuppressive disease.

AZOLE ANTIFUNGALS

Mechanism of Action, Classification, and Spectrum of Activity

Azole antifungal drugs inhibit sterol 14α-demethylase, a cytochrome P450-dependent fungal enzyme involved in synthesis of ergosterol, a key component of the fungal cell wall, from lanosterol. The result is the accumulation of 14α-methylsterols, which disrupt the fungal cell membrane (Fig. 11.1). The majority of the adverse effects and drug interactions observed with these drugs relate to the cross-inhibition of mammalian P450 enzymes (Table 11.1). Hence, adverse effects relating to reduced production of testosterone, cortisol, androgen, or cholesterol may be observed with some of the compounds. In addition, ketoconazole, itraconazole, and posaconazole inhibit the transport of several drugs (anticancer agents such as vincristine, macrocyclic lactones such as ivermectin) by the efflux transporter protein, P-glycoprotein, and can inhibit cytochrome P450 metabolizing enzymes, thus increasing the risk of toxicity of these drugs. All of the azole antifungals have the potential to be teratogenic and their use should be avoided in pregnancy.

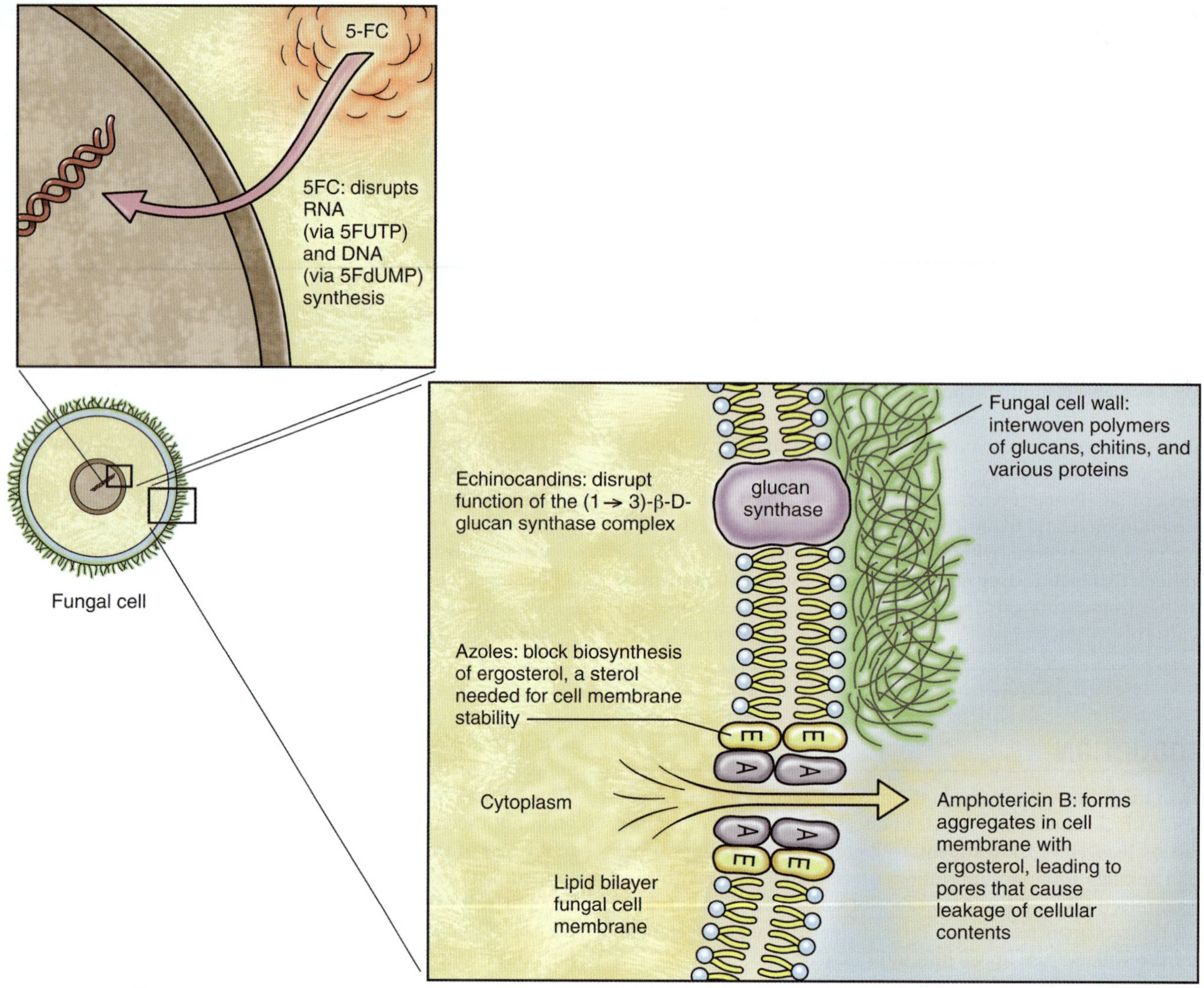

Fig. 11.1 Mechanism of action of antifungal drugs. *5FC,* 5-flucytosine; *5FdUMP,* 5-fluorodeoxyuridine monophosphate; *5FUTP,* 5-fluorouridine triphosphate; *A,* amphotericin B; *E,* ergosterol. (Modified from Rex JH, Stevens DA. Systemic antifungal agents. In: Mandell GL, Bennet JE, Dolin R, eds. *Mandell, Douglas and Bennett's Principles and Practice of Infectious Diseases.* 7th ed. Philadelphia, PA: Churchill Livingston Elsevier;2011:549–563.)

Azole antifungals are classified as imidazoles or triazoles based on whether they possess two or three nitrogen molecules in their azole ring. Ketoconazole, enilconazole, and clotrimazole are imidazoles. The latter two drugs have poor oral bioavailability and are used topically in veterinary medicine for the treatment of superficial mycoses (see Chapters 79 and 86). Triazole antifungal drugs, such as itraconazole and fluconazole, are more slowly metabolized and have less impact on mammalian sterol synthesis than do imidazoles. Imidazoles and triazoles have been widely used to treat a variety of mycoses, which include candidiasis, cryptococcosis, blastomycosis, histoplasmosis, coccidioidomycosis, dermatophytosis, sporotrichosis, and aspergillosis (Tables 11.2 and 11.3).

Unfortunately, resistance to azole antifungal drugs (intrinsic or acquired) has emerged among some fungi. Intrinsic resistance is reported for cryptic *Aspergillus* species, whereas acquired resistance is increasingly described for *Aspergillus fumigatus* isolates. Resistance results from mutations in the gene that encodes the C-14α demethylase enzyme (*cyp51A*), increased production of C-14α demethylase, and increased azole efflux by fungal cell membrane transporters. Resistant strains of *Aspergillus* have been identified in the environment and in human patients naïve to and previously exposed to azole therapy. Resistance was described in canine and feline isolates of *A. fumigatus,*[3] a feline isolate of *Aspergillus felis,*[4] a feline isolate of *Cryptococcus neoformans*[5] and *Cryptococcus gattii,* and a canine isolate of *Candida tropicalis.*[6] Methods for *in vitro* susceptibility testing have been standardized for human medicine,[7,8] with improved correlation between the results of *in vitro* susceptibility testing and clinical response. However, interpretive criteria for susceptibility testing are not available for veterinary uses and testing criteria are still needed for many drug-fungus combinations. Resistance to one azole does not always imply resistance to other azole antifungal drugs.

Ketoconazole

Spectrum of Activity and Clinical Use

Ketoconazole has largely been replaced by itraconazole for treatment of many mycoses, because of the high risk of adverse effects and drug interactions compared with triazole antifungal drugs. In some countries, ketoconazole has been abandoned for human use. Decreased human use has increased the cost of generic forms for veterinary use in recent years. Nevertheless, ketoconazole continues to be used in

TABLE 11.1 Substrates, Inhibitors, and Inducers of Cytochrome P-450

Function	CYP1A2	CYP2C19	CYP2C9	CYP2D6	CYP3A4
Substrates of isoenzyme	Caffeine Mexiletene Propranolol Theophylline Warfarin	Amitriptyline Clomipramine Cyclophosphamide Diazepam Omeprazole Voriconazole	Amitryptiline Losartan Piroxicam Sulfamethoxazole Warfarin	Amitryptiline Clomipramine Codeine Timolol Tramadol	Alprazolam Budesonide Calcium channel blockers Cisapride Colchicine Cyclosporine Doxorubicin Erythromycin Fentanyl Midazolam Sildenafil Vincristine
Inhibitors of isoenzyme	Acyclovir Allopurinol Cimetidine Ciprofloxacin Diltiazem Erythromycin Mexiletene Ofloxacin	Cimetidine Felbamate Fluconazole Fluoxetine Ketoconazole Omeprazole Voriconazole	Amiodarone Chlorpheniramine Isoniazid Metronidazole Phenylbutazone Sulfamethoxazole/ trimethoprim	Amiodarone Chlorpheniramine Fluoxetine Quinidine Ritonavir	Amiodarone Cimetidine Cyclosporine Danazol Diltiazem Fluconazole Itraconazole Ketoconazole Macrolides Omeprazole Posaconazole Quinidine Ritonavir Verapamil Voriconazole
Inducers of isoenzyme			Phenobarbital Rifampin		Griseofulvin Rifabutin Rifampin Ritonavir

TABLE 11.2 Spectrum of Activity and Tissue Distribution of Antifungal Drugs

Drug	Spectrum Of Activity	Tissue Distribution
Ketoconazole	Dimorphic fungi, *Malassezia* spp. Ineffective for aspergillosis.	Skin, bone, joint, lung. Poor CNS penetration.
Itraconazole	Dimorphic fungi and molds, *Malassezia* spp.	Skin, bone, lung. May enter the CNS and eye with inflammation.
Fluconazole	Some *Candida* spp., *Malassezia* spp., some dimorphic fungi. Poor efficacy against molds. *Aspergillus* spp. are intrinsically resistant.	Widely distributed including to the skin, lung, CNS, urine, and eye.
Voriconazole	Dimorphic fungi, yeasts, and molds with the exception of *Sporothrix schenckii* and zygomycetes.	CNS, eye, lung, bone. Does not penetrate the urinary tract.
Posaconazole	Dimorphic fungi, yeasts, and molds including zygomycetes and *Fusarium* spp.	Widely distributed.
Amphotericin B	Broad spectrum. Also active against *Leishmania* spp.	Limited penetration of the CNS and eye.
5-Flucytosine	*Cryptococcus* and *Candida* spp.	Widely distributed, which includes the CNS, eye, and urine.
Griseofulvin	Dermatophytes	Concentrates in skin.
Terbinafine	Activity highest for dermatophytes. To a lesser extent may have efficacy against other dimorphic and filamentous fungi in combination with another antifungal drug	Concentrates in skin and hair.
Caspofungin	*Candida* and *Aspergillus* spp. Not effective against *Cryptococcus* spp. or when given alone to treat *Coccidioides* spp.	Widely distributed. Poor penetration of the CNS and eye.

CNS, Central nervous system.

TABLE 11.3 Suggested Azole Antifungal Drug Doses for Dogs and Cats

Drug	Dose (mg/kg)	Interval (Hours)	Species	Route	Comments
Ketoconazole	10–15 5–10	12	D C	PO	Do not administer to pregnant animals. Monitor liver enzymes monthly during treatment. Drug interactions may occur (see text). Inhibits adrenal function. Antacids impair absorption.
Itraconazole	10 5 3–5 (dermatophytes)	24 12 24	D, C	PO	Do not administer to pregnant animals. Monitor liver enzymes monthly during treatment. Drug interactions may occur. Use of the oral suspension may warrant dose reduction to 3 mg/kg q24h. Monitor serum drug concentrations after 2 weeks if there is inadequate response to treatment (see text). Compounded formulations are unstable and should not be used. See Chapter 78 for treatment of dermatophytosis in cats.
Fluconazole	5–10 50 mg/cat	12 12–24	D C	PO	Do not administer to pregnant animals. Monitor liver enzymes during treatment. Drug interactions may occur.
Voriconazole	4–5 2.5	12 48–72	D C	PO	Use cautiously in animals with liver disease. In cats, a loading dose of 5 mg/kg should be given at the start of treatment, with the next dose 72 hours later. Therapeutic drug monitoring is strongly recommended in dogs and necessary in cats (see text).
Posaconazole	5 7.5 15	48 (oral tablet) 24 48	D C C	PO	Dose for dogs is for the delayed-release tablets. In cats, a loading dose of twice the daily maintenance dose is recommended. Longer intervals for dogs with oral tablets (e.g., q72h) may be considered. Utilize therapeutic drug monitoring for long-term treatment. Also see fluconazole. Antacids impair absorption.

C, cats; *D*, dogs; *PO*, by mouth.

veterinary medicine when the cost of other antifungal drugs is prohibitive. Clinical studies support the use for treatment of *Malassezia* dermatitis[9] and feline nasal and cutaneous cryptococcosis. The absorption of ketoconazole is improved when it is administered with food, and it is inhibited by concurrent use of antacids. Ketoconazole is highly protein bound, and is metabolized extensively by the liver. Nevertheless, moderate hepatic dysfunction does not alter blood concentrations of ketoconazole. Inactive products are excreted in bile, and to a lesser extent, the urine. Because of poor CNS penetration, it is ineffective for treatment of meningeal cryptococcosis and aspergillosis.[10] In one study, 38% of *A. fumigatus* isolates from dogs and cats had a ketoconazole MIC ≥ 8 µg/mL, which is higher than attainable plasma drug concentrations. Therefore, it may be an unsuitable choice for treatment of canine or feline sinonasal aspergillosis.[3]

Adverse Effects and Drug Interactions

The most common adverse effects of ketoconazole in dogs and cats are vomiting, anorexia, lethargy, and diarrhea.[11,12] These effects may be dose related. Administration of ketoconazole with food may reduce GI adverse effects. In addition, administration with food is important for optimum oral absorption because feeding stimulates acid secretion.[13] Mild increases in the activity of serum transaminases occur commonly during treatment, but do not warrant discontinuation of the drug. Less commonly, ketoconazole causes a clinically significant hepatitis, which may be accompanied by anorexia, vomiting, lethargy, increasing activities of serum ALT and ALP, and hyperbilirubinemia. The drug should be discontinued and liver enzymes monitored. After liver enzymes return to normal, consider an alternate antifungal agent for treatment. Hepatitis can occur at any time, and the onset may be extremely rapid. Pruritis and cutaneous erythema have been reported in fewer than 1% of dogs treated with ketoconazole.[11] Lightening of the haircoat color and cataract formation occur rarely.

Ketoconazole is a potent inhibitor of mammalian cytochrome P450 enzymes and efflux transporter proteins such as P-glycoprotein. Using *in vitro* assays to determine activity for dog cytochrome P450 enzymes, it was found that ketoconazole was a broad-spectrum inhibitor of all canine P450 enzymes tested.[14] Ketoconazole also can inhibit with P-glycoprotein transport. The consequence of this interaction is that oral absorption of some drugs may increase because of inhibition of the P-glycoprotein efflux transporter. This has been shown for cyclosporine, in which ketoconazole can greatly increase plasma drug concentrations of cyclosporine and reduce clearance by as much as 85%.[15] This property is used by some clinicians to increase blood levels of cyclosporine in dogs that are not responding to conventional doses of cyclosporine[16] or to reduce the cost of treatment.[17] There are concerns about whether use of ketoconazole in this way could contribute to antifungal drug resistance and increase the risk of adverse drug reactions. Ketoconazole can also produce adverse consequences by inhibiting P-glycoprotein at the blood-brain barrier. This effect increases CNS exposure to ivermectin in dogs, which results in toxicity.[11,18] It also inhibits testosterone and cortisol synthesis. As a result, it has been used to treat pituitary-dependent hyperadrenocorticism in dogs.[19] Transient infertility can occur during treatment of intact male animals. Ketoconazole should not be administered to pregnant animals.

Itraconazole

Spectrum of Activity and Clinical Use

Itraconazole is one of the most widely used azoles in veterinary medicine, and a veterinary formulation of itraconazole is available for treatment of feline dermatophytosis in North America and Europe

(Itrafungol, Elanco). Itraconazole has been used to treat blastomycosis, sporotrichosis, aspergillosis, coccidioidomycosis, dermatophytosis, histoplasmosis, phaeohyphomycosis, paecilomycosis, cryptococcosis, and *Malassezia* spp. infections. The use has included dogs and cats, but frequently extends to birds, and exotic animals. Itraconazole is highly lipophilic and practically insoluble in water. The capsule formulation of itraconazole contains sugar spheres coated with the drug, which increases surface area and solubility of the drug.[20] There are two oral solutions. The oral solution approved for use in cats is formulated as 10 mg/mL in a cherry and caramel flavor with hydroxypropyl-β-cyclodextrin, which maintains the solubility in solution. The approved human oral solution (Sporanox) contains exactly the same ingredients and solubilizing agent, in addition to other excipients such as sorbitol, propylene glycol, hydrochloric acid, and saccharin; therefore, it is expected that both formulations are bioequivalent. The formulation for cats is approved for treatment of dermatophytosis at a dose of 5 mg/kg/day on alternating weeks.[21] Itraconazole in capsules has variable absorption that is optimized when given with food because the acid secretion stimulated with feeding increases the drug solubility, which is necessary for dissolution and absorption. Because the oral solution is complexed with a solubilizing agent (beta cyclodextrin), it is dissolved in solution and administration of food does not influence absorption of this formulation. In humans and cats, oral solution is consistently better absorbed than the capsule formulation, regardless of feeding, and the capsule and oral solution are not bioequivalent and cannot be used interchangeably. Oral absorption of the solution in cats was 52%,[21] and oral absorption of the solution is 3–5 times higher than the capsules in cats.[21,22] Therefore, a dose reduction is indicated when switching from the oral capsule to the oral solution to reduce the chance of toxicity.[23] The difference between oral solution and oral capsule absorption is not as great in dogs compared with humans or cats.[24] Extent of oral absorption for the capsule was 85% that of the oral solution in dogs. The peak concentration (C_{MAX}) was 1.26 µg/mL and 1.54 µg/mL for the capsule and oral solution, respectively, when administered at the same dose.[24]

If the human formulation is used, administration of 3 mg/kg once daily to cats is usually adequate (see Table 11.3), but the approved label for cats lists 5 mg/kg daily on alternating weeks (1 week on; 1 week off). As with ketoconazole, concurrent administration of gastric acid suppressants (H_2-blockers, PPIs) may reduce absorption of the capsule. A generic capsule formulation of itraconazole (Patriot Pharmaceuticals) was slightly less bioequivalent in dogs when compared with the proprietary formulation, but pharmacokinetic data showed that therapeutic concentrations could still be achieved with its use.[20] Compounded formulations of itraconazole prepared by pharmacists from bulk powder have highly variable, poor, and even negligible oral absorption in animals,[20] in addition to being unstable formulations. As a result, compounded formulations should never be used in dogs and cats. In the authors' experience, treatment failures often occur when compounded itraconazole is used.

Like ketoconazole, itraconazole undergoes hepatic metabolism and inhibits metabolism of other P450-dependent drugs (e.g., cisapride, diazepam, cyclosporine; see Table 11.1). It is the only triazole antifungal drug that is converted to an active metabolite, hydroxyitraconazole.[25] Itraconazole is highly (99%) plasma protein bound and does not appear in the urine, CSF, or ocular tissues, although penetration of the CSF and eye may occur in the presence of inflammation. It accumulates in the skin and claws, which contributes to its long-lasting activity and allows for intermittent dosing for dermatophytes (e.g., 1 week on; 1 week off protocols).

As mentioned daily doses of 3–5 mg/kg are used in cats (see Table 11.3), and 10 mg/kg PO q24h in dogs. A loading dose of 20 mg/kg for the first dose has been used in dogs. However, in one study, the initial loading dose may have increased the risk of toxicity and did not appear to improve outcome.[26] Because of the variable absorption of oral itraconazole, monitoring of steady state plasma concentrations (e.g., 3 weeks after initiating treatment) may be helpful if clinical responses are suboptimal.[27] Trough plasma itraconazole concentrations between 0.5 and 1 µg/mL, as determined using high-performance liquid chromatography, were associated with therapeutic success in humans.[28,29] If the hydroxy metabolite is measured, combined itraconazole/hydroxyitraconazole concentrations of 2 to 4 µg/mL are preferred.

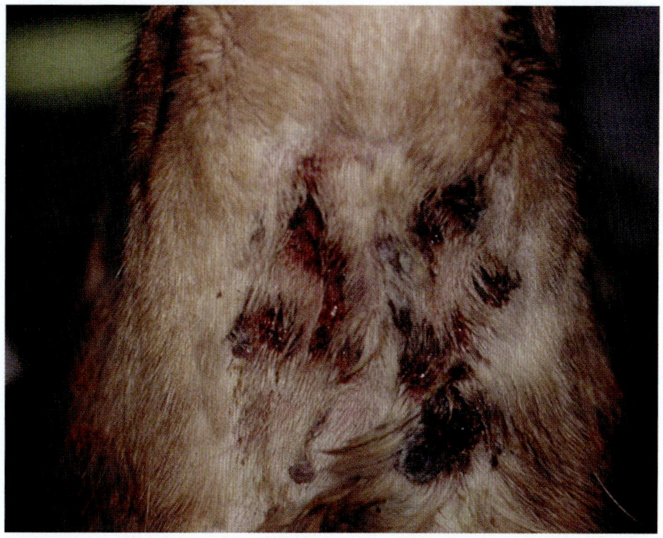

Fig. 11.2 Ulcerative skin lesions on the ventral aspect of the mandible of a golden retriever that had been treated with itraconazole for systemic blastomycosis.

Adverse Effects

The most common adverse effects of itraconazole in dogs and cats are vomiting and anorexia. Many effects are dose dependent. Dividing the total daily dose into twice-daily administration has been helpful in some animals to decrease GI adverse effects and improved absorption in human patients.[10] GI adverse effects may be more common with the oral solution. Mild to moderate increases in serum ALT activity commonly occur during treatment. If these elevations are not accompanied by inappetence or other liver enzyme elevations, treatment need not be discontinued. Significant hepatotoxicity, accompanied by anorexia, vomiting, and hyperbilirubinemia, is less likely to occur with itraconazole than with ketoconazole but has been reported in humans as well as in cats and dogs.[26,30–32] Hepatotoxicity more commonly occurs in dogs treated with 10 mg/kg/day,[26] but this dose may be necessary to attain the desired plasma drug concentration target.[24] Ulcerative or ulcerative-nodular skin lesions can occur in dogs, especially when doses of 10 mg/kg/day or higher are used (Fig. 11.2). Development of hepatitis or severe cutaneous ulceration should prompt discontinuation of the drug. It may be possible to reinstitute treatment at a lower dose once the adverse effects have resolved. Occasionally mild, focal cutaneous ulcerative lesions can resolve spontaneously, without discontinuation of treatment. Hepatic reactions also have been observed in cats. Although it is possible that this is a dose-related issue, a study in cats that administered 100 mg (total dose) q48h produced similar plasma drug concentrations in all cats, but hepatopathy occurred in 2 out of the 10 cats studied.[33] Evidence of hepatopathy was based on clinical laboratory tests during week 3 and week 5 of treatment (dose:

TABLE 11.4 Drugs that Are Substrates for the P-Glycoprotein Membrane Transporter Coded by ABCB1 (formerly known as MDR1)

Acepromazine	Ivermectin
Actinomycin D	Ketoconazole
Aldosterone	Levofloxacin
Amitriptyline	Loperamide
Butorphanol	Methylprednisolone
Cortisol	Milbemycin
Cyclosporine	Morphine
Dexamethasone	Moxidectin
Digoxin	Ondansetron
Diltiazem	Paclitaxel
Docetaxel	Phenothiazines
Doramectin	Selamectin
Docetaxel	Tacrolimus
Doxorubicin	Terfenadine
Doxycycline	Tetracycline
Eprinomectin	Verapamil
Erythromycin	Vinblastine
Itraconazole	Vincristine

P-glycoprotein is a membrane transporter responsible for transporting many drugs and other chemicals across membranes. A functional P-glycoprotein at the blood-brain barrier protects the brain from harmful effects of systemically administered drugs. P-glycoprotein may also be found at other important sites, such as the liver, placenta, kidney, and intestinal mucosa. Mutation of the gene that codes for P-glycoprotein (*ABCB1)* that produces a function deletion will expose some dogs (e.g., some herding breeds) to toxic concentrations of some drugs. Alternatively, if a drug is administered that is a P-glycoprotein inhibitor, it may decrease the effect of the membrane transporter and produce toxicity. Above are some of the P-glycoprotein substrates that may be effected by a mutation or drug inhibition.

12.3 and 26 mg/kg, respectively). Liver enzyme changes were accompanied by clinical signs (inappetence, icterus). After discontinuation of treatment, both cats recovered.

Itraconazole does not suppress adrenal and testicular function like ketoconazole, but can inhibit the metabolism of other P450 enzyme-dependent drugs, including cyclosporine, digoxin, cisapride, and vinca alkaloids (Tables 11.1 and 11.4). It can also interfere with P-glycoprotein transport of ivermectin, which results in increased plasma ivermectin concentrations.[34]

Fluconazole

Spectrum of Activity and Clinical Use

Fluconazole is the least active azole antifungal drug and has the narrowest spectrum of activity. The activity of fluconazole is limited to some *Candida*, *Cryptococcus*, and *Malassezia* spp., and some dimorphic fungi. Fluconazole has poor activity against molds, and *Aspergillus* spp. are intrinsically resistant to fluconazole. Some *Cryptococcus* spp. are resistant to fluconazole, and resistance can develop during treatment. Itraconazole is preferable to fluconazole for treatment of histoplasmosis, blastomycosis, sporotrichosis, and dermatophytosis, although fluconazole has been successfully used to treat coccidioidomycosis, blastomycosis, and *Malassezia* infections in dogs.[32]

Fluconazole is available as tablets, an oral suspension, and as an IV solution. The availability of generic fluconazole, and in turn, its cost, fluctuates. Approved generic fluconazole tablets are bioequivalent to the brand name formulation in humans. Similar bioequivalence is likely in animals. Fluconazole is more water soluble and stable than itraconazole, and the compounded oral suspensions can be used in animals with a 14-day beyond-use date. However, some compounded preparations of fluconazole for animals are unreliable, inconsistent, and of poor quality.[35] Veterinarians who prescribe the compounded formulation should use a reliable pharmacy that adheres to the compendial standards of the United States Pharmacopeia (www.usp.org).

Fluconazole is almost completely absorbed after oral administration, and bioavailability is not altered by food or gastric acidity. In contrast to itraconazole and ketoconazole, fluconazole is only weakly protein bound. Because it is more water soluble than other azoles, fluconazole diffuses into body fluids such as saliva, urine, joint fluid, and CSF. Therefore, it is the drug of choice for treating susceptible meningeal infection and UTIs caused by susceptible fungi. Renal excretion accounts for more than 90% of the elimination of fluconazole. The dosage should be decreased in animals with renal failure; this is especially important in patients receiving other P450-dependent drugs. Fluconazole will inhibit cytochrome P450 enzymes in dogs and alter the pharmacokinetics of some drugs metabolized by these enzymes.[36]

Adverse Effects

Adverse effects of fluconazole are uncommon to rare. When they occur, they are similar to those of itraconazole and include vomiting, anorexia, diarrhea, and increased liver enzymes. Dogs that fail to tolerate itraconazole may tolerate fluconazole without increases in liver enzymes.[32] Cutaneous rash, alopecia, cytopenias, and retinal edema with impaired vision have been reported in human patients.[37,38] In contrast to itraconazole, cutaneous ulceration has not been reported in dogs in association with fluconazole.

Voriconazole

Spectrum of Activity and Clinical Use

Voriconazole is a second-generation triazole that is derived from fluconazole. Voriconazole inhibits cytochrome P450-dependent 14-α lanosterol, an enzyme which catalyzes a key step in ergosterol synthesis, resulting in cell membrane disruption. This mechanism of action is fungicidal for *Aspergillus* spp. and fungistatic for other susceptible fungi. Therefore, in humans, it is the drug of choice for treatment of invasive aspergillosis.[39] It is also used to treat serious and refractory mold infections caused by *Scedosporium*, *Paecilomyces*, and *Fusarium* spp. Voriconazole is at least as active as itraconazole against veterinary isolates of *Cryptococcus* and *Candida* spp., and *A. fumigatus*.[40] It is not active against *Sporothrix* spp. or the zygomycetes.

Voriconazole is available as a tablet, oral suspension, and an IV solution in a sulfobutylether-β-cyclodextrin base. Like fluconazole, it has excellent oral bioavailability, but its absorption is reduced by food, and it should be administered prior to feeding. Voriconazole is poorly water soluble and moderately protein bound. It is extensively metabolized by hepatic cytochrome P450 enzymes and eliminated into bile. In humans, voriconazole has excellent tissue distribution and is considered the drug of choice for CNS and ocular infections. Maintenance of therapeutic concentrations in the CSF, aqueous humor, and synovial fluids in dogs appears to require twice-daily administration.[41] The cost of the human formulation has been very high; therefore, the use in dogs and cats has been uncommon. However, voriconazole has been used with some success to treat systemic mold infections in dogs.[42] Therapeutic drug monitoring is recommended because of individual variability in absorption and metabolism. The recommended trough concentration target in humans is between 1 and 5 mg/L.[28,29,39] Adverse effects can be seen above or at the high end of the concentration target.[43]

Adverse Effects

In humans, adverse effects of voriconazole include reversible visual effects such as photophobia and blurred vision, hallucinations, peripheral neuropathies, and photosensitization, as well as the same toxicities as other triazoles. Of all the triazoles, it is the most potent inhibitor of P450 enzymes. Voriconazole can induce its own metabolism over time in dogs and decrease plasma drug concentrations.[44] In a pharmacokinetic study in dogs, few of the dogs that were treated with voriconazole for 16 days exhibited mild to moderate loss of appetite and diarrhea. The authors have observed inappetence; increased serum liver enzyme activities; CNS signs, including ataxia and staring; and thinning of the haircoat and skin in dogs treated with voriconazole.

Pharmacokinetics in cats are much different than dogs. Whereas concentrations in dogs decrease with repeated doses, there is evidence that concentrations increase in cats with repeated doses.[43] Cats are very sensitive to adverse effects of voriconazole. When cats are treated with the same dose as dogs, they predictably develop inappetence as well as ocular and CNS signs including ataxia, pelvic limb paresis, mydriasis, apparent blindness, decreased pupillary light responses, and a decreased menace response.[45] Cardiac arrhythmias and hypokalemia can also occur. A pharmacokinetic study of voriconazole in cats suggested that the toxicity observed in cats results from a very long drug half-life.[43] Although additional studies are required, it may be possible to safely administer a low dose of voriconazole to cats every 2 to 3 days and still achieve therapeutic drug concentrations. It is recommended that this drug be avoided in cats or used at a low dose only if no other drug is available and therapeutic drug monitoring is used. Adverse effects in cats that were treated with a low dose of voriconazole every other day for 14 days included transient miosis when plasma drug concentrations were at the high end of the therapeutic range.[43] If voriconazole is used to treat cats, use of the tablet form is recommended, because administration of the oral suspension causes profuse salivation which in turn reduces drug availability.

Posaconazole

Spectrum of Activity and Clinical Use

Posaconazole (Noxafil) is a new azole antifungal drug, available as an oral suspension (40 mg/mL), a delayed-release tablet (100 mg), and an injectable solution. Topical otic preparations that contain posaconazole are approved for use in dogs. It is similar to itraconazole, but has a slightly different spectrum of activity and is more active (lower MIC values) than the other azole antifungal agents. In addition to other fungi in the spectrum of azoles, it is active against *Candida* and *Aspergillus* spp., Mucorales (formerly Zygomycetes) such as *Mucor* and *Rhizopus* spp., as well as *Fusarium* spp. It is used primarily in humans for *Aspergillus* and *Candida* spp. infections, but also is active against dermatophytes, *Histoplasma capsulatum, Blastomyces dermatitidis,* and *Coccidioides* and *Cryptococcus* spp. infections. The difference in activity compared with other azoles is the additional activity against *Mucorales* and *Fusarium* spp.[25,46] It has been efficacious for treatment of several refractory deep mycoses in animals, including aspergillosis and mucormycosis in cats and invasive aspergillosis in dogs.[38,47–49]

As with itraconazole, the absorption of posaconazole is improved by a meal, especially the presence of fatty food. Gastric acid suppression can reduce the bioavailability of posaconazole.[50] Delayed-release tablets were developed to overcome absorption limitations associated with the oral suspension.[51] The pharmacokinetics of posaconazole IV solution, oral suspension, and delayed-release tablets have been evaluated in dogs and cats.[46,52,53] The delayed-release tablet in dogs and the oral suspension in cats have a long half-life, which allows for once-daily or every other day administration.[46] The oral suspension has considerably lower bioavailability in dogs when compared with the delayed-release tablets; therefore, administration of the delayed-release tablets is preferred when possible. The human extended-release tablet (Noxafil) is very expensive; however, recently a much less expensive generic tablet has become available. The authors have several anecdotal accounts of successful use of this tablet as infrequently as every 3 days (dosing frequency confirmed with plasma concentration trough monitoring as described below).

Therapeutic drug monitoring is recommended in human patients due to variable plasma drug concentrations and risk of underexposure; in humans, the target plasma trough concentrations for treatment is > 1 µg/mL.[52] Posaconazole is highly protein bound (>95%) and undergoes hepatic metabolism, with some inhibition of P450 enzymes. Most administered posaconazole is eliminated in the feces. Data on CSF concentrations of posaconazole are not yet available, but it appears to be effective for treatment cryptococcosis in the CSF.

Adverse Effects

In humans, prolonged administration of oral posaconazole has been associated with GI adverse effects. Other treatment-related adverse events have been reported at a lower rate with posaconazole compared with other azole antifungal agents. Posaconazole appeared to be safe and well tolerated in long-term treatment of disseminated aspergillosis in dogs.[53] Increases in serum liver enzyme activities were not observed.[53] Adverse effects are less common in cats when compared with voriconazole, but information is limited at the time of writing.[47–49,52,54]

Other Azole Antifungals

Other azole drugs that are undergoing clinical trials in humans include ravuconazole, isavuconazole, albaconazole, and olorofim. Isavuconazole is a novel triazole agent that has recently been approved by the FDA for the treatment of aspergillosis and mucormycosis. It may have similar efficacy to voriconazole with fewer adverse effects. Isavuconazole has fungistatic activity against yeasts such as *Candida* and *Cryptococcus* spp., but appears to be fungicidal against *Aspergillus* spp.[55] Isavuconazole is available in oral and IV formulations. The IV formulation of isavuconazole is less nephrotoxic than that of voriconazole and posaconazole because it does not contain cyclodextrin. In humans, absorption of oral isavuconazole is excellent and unaffected by food or gastric pH. It is metabolized by P450 enzymes and does not achieve therapeutic concentrations in the urine. It appears to cross the blood-brain barrier and has been effective for treating CNS infections in humans.[56] The pharmacokinetics of isavuconazole in dogs and cats have not yet been reported.

Ravuconazole is structurally similar to fluconazole and voriconazole. In humans, it has a half-life of approximately 100 hours. It has activity against *Candida, Aspergillus, Cryptococcus, Histoplasma,* and *Coccidioides* spp. Its safety profile appears to be similar to that of fluconazole.[57]

Albaconazole is a triazole antifungal agent that has been developed for treatment of onychomycosis in human patients. There are currently no pharmacokinetic data for this drug in dogs and cats.

AMPHOTERICIN B

Mechanism of Action and Spectrum of Activity

AMB is a polyene macrolide antibiotic produced by *Streptomyces nodosus*. It is closely related to nystatin. AMB irreversibly binds sterols in fungal cell membranes, forming pores or channels with subsequent leakage of ions (see Fig. 11.1). Although generally considered to be fungistatic, at high doses it may be fungicidal. AMB also possesses immunomodulatory effects; it activates macrophages and enhances macrophage-killing capacity. This may help explain its efficacy against pathogens such as *Pythium insidiosum*, which lack cell wall ergosterol.

AMB has antifungal activity against all of the important small animal fungal pathogens. It is also active against *Leishmania* spp.[58–60] In human medicine, AMB is the preferred drug for treatment of rapidly progressive mycoses, immunosuppressed hosts, or fungal meningitis. Resistance to AMB is rare, although high MIC values have been observed for some molds including some isolates of *Aspergillus terreus*, *Paecilomyces* spp., and *Sporothrix schenckii*. The mechanism of resistance is not well understood, but it may relate to decreased cell wall ergosterol content.[61]

Clinical Use

AMB has poor aqueous solubility and is not absorbed from the GI tract. To administer IV, the conventional formulation is prepared as an emulsion in which it forms as a complex with the bile salt deoxycholate (Fungizone, AMB-D) (Box 11.1). The complex forms a colloid in water. Addition of electrolyte to the solution causes it to aggregate; therefore, it should be administered in 5% dextrose (D5W). It is not necessary to protect the infusion from light, as recommended in the past. In the bloodstream, AMB dissociates from deoxycholate and binds extensively to plasma proteins and cholesterol in membranes throughout tissues. Penetration of the vitreous humor and CSF is poor, but some animals with CNS infections may still respond to treatment. In human patients, AMB-D has been administered intrathecally to treat fungal meningitis and intraocularly following vitrectomy.[62]

A protocol for SC administration of AMB-D has been reported for treatment of cryptococcosis,[63] which may be less costly than IV administration. Sterile injection site abscesses occur in some animals treated using this protocol; therefore, IV administration is preferred whenever possible.

BOX 11.1 Suggested Amphotericin B Infusion Protocols for Dogs and Cats

Formulation	Protocol
All formulations	Obtain baseline CBC, kidney panel, and UA, and ensure adequate hydration before starting treatment. Recheck a kidney panel before each infusion. Administer three times weekly for 4 weeks or until azotemia is detected. For some infections, monthly administration of a single dose may be required to maintain remission.
Amphotericin B deoxycholate (IV route)	Reconstitute vial contents in sterile water to 5 mg/mL. Administer 0.9% NaCl IV at 1.5–2 times the calculated maintenance rate for 1 hour before and after AMB treatment. Ensure lines are flushed with D5W before infusing AMB.
	Dogs: Transfer 0.5 mg/kg to a 250- to 1000-mL bag of D5W (total fluid volume administered should be based on body weight and ability to tolerate a fluid load). Administer IV over 4–6 hours.
	Cats: Dilute 0.25 mg/kg in 30 mL of D5W and administer IV over 30 minutes to 1 hour.
Amphotericin B deoxycholate (SC route)	Transfer 0.5 mg/kg (cats) or 0.8 mg/kg (dogs) to bag containing 400 mL (cats) or 500 mL (dogs) of 0.45% NaCl in 2.5% dextrose. Administer SC. Fractious cats may need to be sedated or placed in a restraint bag. Sterile injection site abscess formation may occur with this protocol, especially with concentrations of amphotericin B > 20 mg/L.
Amphotericin B lipid complex (Abelcet)	Dilute to 1 mg/mL in D5W. Administer calculated dose IV over 1 to 2 hours.
	Dogs: 3 mg/kg
	Cats: 1 mg/kg

AMB, amphotericin B; *CBC*, complete blood count; *D5W*, 5% dextrose in water; *IV*, intravenous; *SC*, subcutaneous; *UA*, urinalysis.

Adverse Effects

The major adverse effect of AMB-D is kidney injury, which is dose dependent and transient if it is detected early and the drug is discontinued. Both an acute effect caused by renal vasoconstriction and a chronic cumulative effect from repeated administration occurs. Renal tubular acidosis, severe nephrogenic diabetes insipidus, hypokalemia, and hypomagnesemia can occur with treatment. Although performed rarely in dogs, aggressive IV fluid therapy and potassium supplementation has been needed in some severe cases in humans. Fluid-loading with sodium-containing fluids before the infusion may decrease nephrotoxicity.[64] Slow administration in a large volume of fluid also decreases nephrotoxicity. Concurrent use of other nephrotoxic drugs, such as aminoglycosides, should be avoided. In humans, AMB-D can also cause fever, chills, headache, nausea, vomiting, and, rarely, cytopenias and anaphylaxis.[64] Fever, inappetence, and vomiting also appear to occur in some dogs treated with AMB-D, and rarely nephrogenic diabetes insipidus. Phlebitis can occur at the IV infusion site. Other adverse effects noted in humans include infusion-related hypotension and hypochromic, normocytic anemia. NSAIDs can be administered to decrease pyrexia during treatment, but these should be used cautiously and with careful monitoring of renal parameters. Antiemetic agents are frequently administered at the time of infusion to decrease vomiting.

Lipid Formulations of AMB

Three lipid formulations of AMB are available (see Box 11.1). These are less nephrotoxic than AMB-D but are considerably more expensive. These formulations produce less injury to the kidneys because there is a lower rate of transfer of AMB to mammalian cell membranes and increased drug clearance from the blood by the mononuclear phagocyte system. This allows administration of a higher dose of the drug, sometimes with improved treatment efficacy. Nevertheless, kidney function should still be monitored. Selective uptake of lipid formulations by macrophages also facilitates treatment of pathogens that reside within macrophages, such as *Histoplasma* and *Leishmania* spp.

AMB colloidal dispersion (ABCD, Amphotec) contains AMB and cholesterol sulfate, which form disc-shaped particles. It is more likely to cause chills, fever, and hypotension in humans than AMB-D (80% vs. 12% for AMB-D), so it is given over 3–4 hours and with premedication.

Liposomal AMB (Ambisome) is a widely used formulation for treatment of human patients. It consists of AMB and a lipid mixture (phosphatidylcholine, cholesterol, and distearoyl phosphatidylglycerol). After reconstitution in D5W, it forms 80 nm vesicles. Nephrotoxicity and infusion-related reactions are much less common with liposomal AMB than with ABCD or AMB-D, and the drug appears to reach higher concentrations in the eye.[65] In human patients, it is used as salvage therapy for aspergillosis, cryptococcosis, and candidiasis.

AMB lipid complex (ABLC, Abelcet) is a mixture of AMB, dimyristoyl phosphatidylcholine, and dimyristoyl phosphatidylglycerol that forms ribbon-like sheets. ABLC is the most common formulation used

TABLE 11.5 Suggested 5-Flucytosine Drug Doses for Dogs and Cats

Drug	Dose (mg/kg)	Interval (Hours)	Species	Route	Comments
5-Flucytosine	25–50	6–8	C	PO	Monitor CBC. Use cautiously in animals with impaired renal function. Avoid use in dogs. Therapeutic drug monitoring is recommended in humans.

C, cats; *CBC,* complete blood count; *PO,* by mouth.

in veterinary medicine. Nephrotoxicity and infusion-related reactions are intermediate between AMB-D and liposomal AMB. It has been used in small animal patients to treat refractory cryptococcosis and cryptococcal meningitis and disseminated coccidioidomycosis, aspergillosis, blastomycosis, histoplasmosis, and pythiosis.

AMB cochleates are phosphatidylserine-calcium precipitates in the form of a continuous lipid bilayer sheet rolled up in a spiral. This formulation permits oral administration of AMB. Cochleates were effective when used to treat mouse models of candidiasis, aspergillosis, and most recently *S. schenckii.*[66] Cochleates remain under investigation on a research basis. Because of less experience for treating animals, significant toxicity has not been observed. Additional novel delivery systems that maintain the antimicrobial activity of AMB with reduced toxicity and improved tissue penetration are under development, such as nanoparticle formulations of AMB.[60]

5-FLUCYTOSINE

Mechanism of Action and Spectrum of Activity

Flucytosine is a fluorinated pyrimidine related to fluorouracil. It has activity only against *Cryptococcus* and *Candida* spp. These fungi deaminate flucytosine to 5-fluorouracil, which interferes with DNA replication and protein synthesis (see Fig. 11.1). Mammalian cells cannot convert flucytosine into 5-fluorouracil; therefore, injury to mammalian cells is limited. Flucytosine is synergistic with AMB and can be administered simultaneously to decrease emergence of resistance. Because marked drug resistance arises during treatment (secondary drug resistance), flucytosine must always be used in combination with other drugs, most commonly AMB. Resistance results from modifications in fungal enzymes that are required for drug uptake and metabolism.[61]

Clinical Use

The use of flucytosine in cats has been limited by its high cost, and toxicity means it cannot be used in dogs (see Adverse Effects). Flucytosine is absorbed well after oral administration and is minimally bound to plasma proteins. Penetration of the CSF and aqueous humor is excellent. In cats, flucytosine may be considered to treat severe or refractory cryptococcosis in combination with other agents. Because about 80% of the dose is excreted unchanged in the urine, high urinary concentrations can be achieved.

Adverse Effects

Administration of flucytosine should be avoided in dogs, which often develop a severe (but reversible) drug eruption within to 2 to 3 weeks of starting treatment. The combination of flucytosine and ketoconazole proved toxic to cats. The most common adverse effects of flucytosine therapy are myelosuppression and GI signs. The CBC should be monitored during treatment, and therapeutic drug monitoring should be considered. Myelosuppression is more likely to occur in patients receiving other myelosuppressive drugs. In humans, other adverse effects include rash and reversible increases in liver enzyme activities. Flucytosine toxicity may result from conversion of flucytosine to 5-fluorouracil by the intestinal microflora.

Kidney injury is another concern. The risk of flucytosine kidney injury is increased in animals with kidney disease; therefore, it should be avoided in animals with renal dysfunction unless they are monitored carefully (Table 11.5). In human patients, toxicity is correlated with 2-hour postpill concentrations greater than 100 mg/L, and concentrations of 30 to 80 mg/L are suggested for treatment of cryptococcosis.[28] Because AMB can cause impaired renal function, careful monitoring for toxicity is indicated when flucytosine is used in conjunction with AMB.

GRISEOFULVIN

Mechanism of Action and Spectrum of Activity

Griseofulvin is an oral antifungal drug derived from *Penicillium griseofulvum* that binds to fungal tubulin, leading to impaired microtubule function and mitotic arrest. It also has anti-inflammatory properties.[67] After administration, griseofulvin is rapidly deposited in keratin precursor cells in the skin and hair, but disappears from the stratum corneum within 48 to 72 hours of discontinuation of treatment. Griseofulvin is fungistatic and has a limited spectrum of activity. Because of narrow spectrum of activity, its use is limited to treatment of dermatophytosis. It is not effective against yeasts such as *Candida* and *Malassezia* spp. Resistance has been documented in some dermatophytes and may be due to altered tubulin.

Clinical Use

Because of the narrow spectrum of activity, need for prolonged duration of treatment, adverse effects, and availability of the azole antifungal agents, the use of griseofulvin has greatly diminished in small animal medicine.

The absorption of griseofulvin is increased when it is administered with a fatty meal or whole milk. The drug is available in microsized and ultramicrosized formulations, which improve absorption from the stomach and small intestine. Most veterinary preparations are microsized. The dose of the ultramicrosized formulation can be reduced by 50% because of improved absorption, but efficacy remains unchanged (Table 11.6). Prolonged treatment periods (months) are required for dermatophytosis (see Chapter 78).[68]

Adverse Effects

Griseofulvin is a potent inducer of cytochrome P450 enzymes and decreases the efficacy of other drugs metabolized by the same P450 enzymes (see Table 11.1) . Because it is extremely teratogenic, it should never be used to treat pregnant females, but can be used safely in male animals.[69] Other adverse effects of griseofulvin include inappetence, vomiting, and diarrhea. In cats, it can cause myelosuppression, which is generally reversible on discontinuation of treatment, but irreversible pancytopenia has been reported.[70] Myelosuppression may be more likely to occur in cats with FIV infection.[71] The CBC should be monitored every 2 weeks during treatment.

TABLE 11.6 Suggested Griseofulvin and Terbinafine Doses for Dogs and Cats

Drug	Dose (mg/kg)	Interval (Hours)	Species	Route	Comments
Griseofulvin (microsized)	25	12	D, C	PO	Administration with fatty food improves absorption. Dose may be increased to 50 mg/kg q12h for refractory infections. Avoid in cats with FIV infections. Do not use in pregnancy. Drug interactions possible. Monitor CBC.
Griseofulvin (ultramicrosized)	15	12	D, C	PO	Avoid in cats with FIV infections. Do not use in pregnancy. Drug interactions possible. Monitor CBC.
Terbinafine hydrochloride	30–40	24	D, C	PO	Administer with food.

C, cats; *CBC,* complete blood count; *D,* dogs; *FIV,* feline immunodeficiency virus; *PO,* by mouth.

TERBINAFINE

Mechanism of Action and Spectrum of Activity

Terbinafine is a synthetic allylamine that inhibits fungal squalene epoxidase, which blocks fungal lanosterol and ergosterol synthesis and leads to accumulation of toxic squalene, with resultant fungal cell lysis. A closely related drug of the same class is naftifine (Naftin), which is used as a topical cream for dermatophyte infections in humans. Terbinafine is most effective for treatment of dermatophytosis, but also has been used to treat *Malassezia* spp. dermatitis in dogs.[72] The efficacy of terbinafine for treatment of invasive fungal infections has not been well investigated.

Terbinafine efficacy for treating pythiosis has been inconsistent. It has been used both successfully[73] and unsuccessfully[74] in combination with other drugs to treat pythiosis in dogs. It also has *in vitro* activity against other dimorphic fungi and molds, although its activity is highest for dermatophytes.[75,76] Terbinafine may be synergistic when administered with other antifungal drugs, which may provide enhanced efficacy for treatment of refractory mycoses.[77] However, nondermatophyte molds including *Aspergillus* and *Fusarium* spp. have been detected in people with onychomycosis that failed to respond to terbinafine treatment.[78] Resistance has been reported in dermatophytes as a result of altered squalene epoxidase.[79]

Clinical Use

Terbinafine is available in 125 and 250 mg tablets (Lamisil, and generic forms) and a 1% topical cream (Lamisil available over the counter). Oral bioavailability in most species is moderate, ranging from 31% in cats to > 46% in dogs. It is better absorbed in dogs when given with food (see Table 11.6).[80]

In humans, it has the advantage of high lipophilicity and high concentrations attained in tissues such as stratum corneum, hair follicles, sebum-rich skin, and nails. In humans, after 12 days of therapy, the concentrations in stratum corneum exceed those in plasma by a factor of 75-fold. In cats after a daily dose of 30–40 mg/kg, the concentrations in hair may be 10-fold the serum concentrations and persist for weeks after discontinuation of treatment at 14 days.[81] However, these tissue concentrations have not been observed in dogs. A study in dogs showed that concentrations in canine skin, subcutaneous tissue, and sebum were not above the concentration needed to inhibit *Malassezia* spp.[82] Skin concentrations were only 1%–2% of serum concentrations.

Since terbinafine has become available as a less expensive generic product, the interest in its use in veterinary medicine has increased. Pharmacokinetic studies in which 30–35 mg/kg/day was administered to dogs[83,84] showed that sufficient concentrations can be maintained for most of the dose interval for susceptible fungi, but clinical studies are needed to confirm efficacy. By comparison, doses in humans are much lower at 125 mg twice daily (approximately 1.8 mg/kg q12h), with pediatric doses in the range of 4–8 mg/kg, once a day. The most common dose administered to dogs is 30–35 mg/kg once daily; and for cats, approximately 30 mg/kg/day, or ¼ tablet for small cats (62.5 mg), ½ tablet for medium size cats (125 mg), and one tablet for large cats (250 mg), all administered once daily. It should be administered for at least 14 days, but may be extended to 60 days.[85]

Results available to this point suggest that it is effective for the treatment of *Malassezia* dermatitis in dogs when given at 30 mg/kg PO, or 30 mg/kg twice weekly for at least 3 weeks.[86] However, the results also showed that this treatment produced insufficient resolution and only partial remission, even though there was clinical improvement in both groups.

There are two topical formulations approved for dogs, approved by the FDA in 2014 and 2015. The product Osurnia contains 10 mg florfenicol, 10 mg terbinafine, and 1 mg betamethasone acetate per mL in a gel for topical administration. The product Claro contains florfenicol 15 mg/mL, terbinafine 13.3 mg/mL, and mometasone 2 mg/mL. The indication for each product is for the treatment of otitis externa in dogs associated with susceptible strains of bacteria (*Staphylococcus pseudintermedius*) and yeast (*Malassezia pachydermatis*).

Adverse Effects

In dogs, reports of adverse effects of terbinafine are variable. One study reported effects in one-third of treated dogs, consisting of GI problems and increased hepatic enzymes. Another study[84] reported ocular problems in some dogs. Adverse effects can include GI signs, especially vomiting and increased liver enzyme activities, but these are uncommon. Facial pruritis has been reported in cats.[87]

ECHINOCANDINS

The echinocandins are lipopeptide antifungals that inhibit the formation of β-1,3-D-glucans in the fungal cell wall, a mechanism of action that is completely different from that for AMB and the azoles. The prototype drug is caspofungin acetate (Cancidas). Other drugs in this class are micafungin, anidulafungin, and most recently CD101 IV.[88] The use of these agents has been rare in dogs and cats.

Caspofungin is fungicidal against *Candida* spp., and fungistatic against *Aspergillus* spp. The echinocandins are ineffective against *Cryptococcus* spp., which possess little glucan synthase, and have been effective for treatment of *Coccidioides* spp. in a mouse model when used in conjunction with AMB,[89] as well as when used in combination with voriconazole for refractory human pediatric coccidioidomycosis.[90] Synergism has been reported when echinocandins are used in combination with other antifungal drugs.[91] In humans, the echinocandins are used primarily to treat invasive candidiasis and have some use in salvage therapy of aspergillosis.[56] They are used in a combination with a polyene in the treatment of mucormycosis.[56] Treatment with caspofungin induced remission in a dog with disseminated aspergillosis (1 mg/kg IV in 250 mL 0.9% NaCl over 1 hour, q24h).[43] Caspofungin is given once daily as a slow IV infusion. In human patients, it is extensively protein bound and metabolized slowly by the liver, with some renal excretion. It has limited ability to penetrate the CNS and eye.[92,93] The cost is similar to that of lipid formulations of AMB. Adverse effects noted in humans include fever, phlebitis, and increased activity of serum ALT (<20% of patients). The proper dose and extent to which adverse effects occur in dogs and cats is unknown, but administration of anidulafungin to a dog treated with caspofungin was associated with the development of a severe diffuse urticarial reaction.[43] CD101 is a novel echinocandin with a very long half-life in humans that is currently being developed as a once-weekly IV treatment for candidemia and invasive candidiasis.[88] It also has activity against a broad range of *Aspergillus* spp., including *A. terreus*.[94] Given the infrequent need for administration, it may represent a useful treatment in the future for disseminated aspergillosis in dogs, but the pharmacokinetics of echinocandins in dogs requires further investigation.

OROTOMIDES

Olorofim (F901318) belongs to a promising new class of antifungal agents known as the orotomides. It targets dihydroorotate dehydrogenase, which is involved in fungal pyrimidine synthesis; the mammalian enzyme is spared.[95] It is highly active against *Aspergillus* and also has activity against dimorphic fungi. There are currently no pharmacokinetic data for this drug in dogs and cats.

COMBINATION ANTIFUNGAL DRUG THERAPY

Azole antifungals are often administered in combination with other antifungal drugs for treatment of refractory or severe deep mycoses. In some patients, treatment is initiated with amphotericin-B for several days until the patient shows a favorable response, then treatment is switched to an oral azole antifungal agent for a longer period. However, few human observational studies and small-scale clinical trials have been published to support this practice.[96] There are no data as to whether the use of antifungal combinations in dogs and cats is more effective than monotherapy. Combined use of AMB and flucytosine is synergistic in treating cryptococcal infections in human patients; presumably, AMB facilitates penetration of flucytosine into the fungal cell. A combination of terbinafine or AMB and itraconazole is recommended for treatment of pythiosis in dogs. Because use of antifungal drug combinations is associated with an increased risk of drug adverse effects, this should be approached with careful consideration of available clinical information and individual patient factors.

OTHER ANTIFUNGAL TREATMENTS

In human patients, hyperbaric oxygen therapy has been used to treat some fungal infections in combination with antifungal drugs. Whether this is beneficial or harmful is controversial and requires further study.[97]

Other agents are administered topically and will not be discussed in detail here.

SUGGESTED READINGS

Mealey KL. Adverse drug reactions in veterinary patients associated with drug transporters. *Veterinary Clinics of North America: Small Animal Practice.* 2013;43:1067–1078.

Mealey KL, Fidel J. P-glycoprotein mediated drug interactions in animals and humans with cancer. *Journal of Veterinary Internal Medicine.* 2015;29:1–6.

Chang YL, Yu SJ, Heitman J, et al. New facets of antifungal therapy. *Virulence.* 2017;8:222–236.

Davis JL, and Maxwell L. Antifungal and antiviral drugs. In: Riviere JE, Papich MG, eds. *Veterinary Pharmacology and Therapeutics.* 10th ed. Hoboken, NJ: Wiley Blackwell; 2018:988–1032.

REFERENCES

1. Garcia-Solache MA, Casadevall A. Global warming will bring new fungal diseases for mammals. *MBio.* 2010;1.
2. Sykes JE, Sturges BK, Cannon MS, et al. Clinical signs, imaging features, neuropathology, and outcome in cats and dogs with central nervous system cryptococcosis from California. *J Vet Intern Med.* 2010;24:1427–1438.
3. Talbot JJ, Kidd SE, Martin P, et al. Azole resistance in canine and feline isolates of *Aspergillus fumigatus. Comp Immunol Microbiol Infect Dis.* 2015;42:37–41.
4. Barrs VR, van Doorn TM, Houbraken J, et al. *Aspergillus felis* sp. *nov.*, an emerging agent of invasive aspergillosis in humans, cats, and dogs. *PLoS One.* 2013;8:e64871.
5. Kano R, Okubo M, Yanai T, et al. First isolation of azole-resistant *Cryptococcus neoformans* from feline cryptococcosis. *Mycopathologia.* 2015;180:427–433.
6. Alvarez-Perez S, Garcia ME, Cutuli MT, et al. Acquired multi-azole resistance in *Candida tropicalis* during persistent urinary tract infection in a dog. *Med Mycol Case Rep.* 2016;11:9–12.
7. Clinical and Laboratory Standards Institute. M27-A3: Reference method for broth dilution antifungal susceptibility testing of yeasts. 2008:40.
8. Clinical and Laboratory Standards Institute. M38-A2: Reference method for broth dilution antifungal susceptibility testing of filamentous fungi; approved standard. 2008:52.
9. Negre A, Bensignor E, Guillot J. Evidence-based veterinary dermatology: a systematic review of interventions for *Malassezia* dermatitis in dogs. *Vet Dermatol.* 2009;20:1–12.
10. Rex JH, Stevens DA. Systemic antifungal agents. In: Mandell GL, Bennett JE, Dolin R, eds. *Mandell, Douglas and Bennett's Principles and Practice of Infectious Diseases.* 7th ed. Philadelphia, PA: Churchill Livingstone Elsevier; 2011:549–563.
11. Mayer UK, Glos K, Schmid M, et al. Adverse effects of ketoconazole in dogs: a retrospective study. *Vet Dermatol.* 2008;19:199–208.
12. Medleau L, Chalmers SA. Ketoconazole for treatment of dermatophytosis in cats. *J Am Vet Med Assoc.* 1992;200:77–78.
13. Zhou R, Moench P, Heran C, et al. pH-dependent dissolution in vitro and absorption in vivo of weakly basic drugs: development of a canine model. *Pharm Res.* 2005;22:188–192.
14. Aidasani D, Zaya MJ, Malpas PB, et al. In vitro drug-drug interaction screens for canine veterinary medicines: evaluation of cytochrome P450 reversible inhibition. *Drug Metab Dispos.* 2008;36:1512–1518.
15. Myre SA, Schoeder TJ, Grund VR, et al. Critical ketoconazole dosage range for ciclosporin clearance inhibition in the dog. *Pharmacology.* 1991;43:233–241.
16. Patricelli AJ, Hardie RJ, McAnulty JE. Cyclosporine and ketoconazole for the treatment of perianal fistulas in dogs. *J Am Vet Med Assoc.* 2002;220:1009–1016.
17. Mouatt JG. Cyclosporin and ketoconazole interaction for treatment of perianal fistulas in the dog. *Aust Vet J.* 2002;80:207–211.
18. Hugnet C, Lespine A, Alvinerie M. Multiple oral dosing of ketoconazole increases dog exposure to ivermectin. *J Pharm Sci.* 2007;10:311–318.
19. Lien YH, Huang HP. Use of ketoconazole to treat dogs with pituitary-dependent hyperadrenocorticism: 48 cases (1994-2007). *J Am Vet Med Assoc.* 2008;233:1896–1901.

20. Mawby DI, Whittemore JC, Genger S, et al. Bioequivalence of orally administered generic, compounded, and innovator-formulated itraconazole in healthy dogs. *J Vet Intern Med.* 2014;28:72–77.
21. Liang C, Shan Q, Zhong J, et al. Pharmacokinetics and bioavailability of itraconazole oral solution in cats. *J Feline Med Surg.* 2016;18:310–314.
22. Mawby D, Fowler L, Papich M, et al. Itraconazole absorption from proprietary and compounded formulations in healthy cats. *J Am Vet Med Assoc.* 2018;252:195–200.
23. Barone JA, Moskovitz BL, Guarnieri J, et al. Enhanced bioavailability of itraconazole in hydroxypropyl-beta-cyclodextrin solution versus capsules in healthy volunteers. *Antimicrob Agents Chemother.* 1998;42:1862–1865.
24. Hasbach AE, Langlois DK, Rosser EJ Jr, et al. Pharmacokinetics and relative bioavailability of orally administered innovator-formulated itraconazole capsules and solution in healthy dogs. *J Vet Intern Med.* 2017;31:1163–1169.
25. Pound MW, Townsend ML, Dimondi V, et al. Overview of treatment options for invasive fungal infections. *Med Mycol.* 2011;49:561–580.
26. Legendre AM, Rohrbach BW, Toal RL, et al. Treatment of blastomycosis with itraconazole in 112 dogs. *J Vet Intern Med.* 1996;10:365–371.
27. Pasqualotto AC, Denning DW. Generic substitution of itraconazole resulting in sub-therapeutic levels and resistance. *Int J Antimicrob Agents.* 2007;30:93–94.
28. Goodwin ML, Drew RH. Antifungal serum concentration monitoring: an update. *J Antimicrob Chemother.* 2008;61:17–25.
29. Hope WW, Billaud EM, Lestner J, et al. Therapeutic drug monitoring for triazoles. *Curr Opin Infect Dis.* 2008;21:580–586.
30. Gupta AK, Chwetzoff E, Del Rosso J, et al. Hepatic safety of itraconazole. *J Cutan Med Surg.* 2002;6:210–213.
31. McKay JS, Cox CL, Foster AP. Cutaneous alternariosis in a cat. *J Small Anim Pract.* 2001;42:75–78.
32. Foy DS, Trepanier LA. Antifungal treatment of small animal veterinary patients. *Vet Clin North Am Small Anim Pract.* 2010;40:1171–1188.
33. Middleton SM, Kubier A, Dirikolu L, et al. Alternate day dosing of itraconazole in healthy adult cats. *J Vet Pharmacol Ther.* 2016;39:27–31.
34. Ballent M, Lifschitz A, Virkel G, et al. Modulation of the P-glycoprotein-mediated intestinal secretion of ivermectin: in vitro and in vivo assessments. *Drug Metab Dispos.* 2006;34:457–463.
35. Laporte CM, Cruz-Espindola C, Thungrat K, et al. Quality assessment of fluconazole capsules and oral suspensions compounded by pharmacies located in the United States. *Am J Vet Res.* 2017;78:421–432.
36. KuKanich B, KuKanich K, Rankin D, et al. The effect of fluconazole on oral methadone in dogs. *Vet Anaesth Analg.* 2019;46:501–509.
37. Bradbury BD, Jick SS. Itraconazole and fluconazole and certain rare, serious adverse events. *Pharmacotherapy.* 2002;22:697–700.
38. Magrath GN, Pulido JS, Montero J, et al. Cystoid macular edema secondary to fluconazole toxicity. *Ocul Immunol Inflamm.* 2010;18:472–474.
39. Lat A, Thompson GR 3rd. Update on the optimal use of voriconazole for invasive fungal infections. *Infect Drug Resist.* 2011;4:43–53.
40. Okabayashi K, Imaji M, Osumi T, et al. Antifungal activity of itraconazole and voriconazole against clinical isolates obtained from animals with mycoses. *Nihon Ishinkin Gakkai Zasshi.* 2009;50:91–94.
41. Lemetayer JD, Dowling PM, Taylor SM, et al. Pharmacokinetics and distribution of voriconazole in body fluids of dogs after repeated oral dosing. *J Vet Pharmacol Ther.* 2015;38:451–456.
42. Schultz RM, Johnson EG, Wisner ER, et al. Clinicopathologic and diagnostic imaging characteristics of systemic aspergillosis in 30 dogs. *J Vet Intern Med.* 2008;22:851–859.
43. Vishkautsan P, Papich MG, Thompson GR 3rd, et al. Pharmacokinetics of voriconazole after intravenous and oral administration to healthy cats. *Am J Vet Res.* 2016;77:931–939.
44. Roffey SJ, Cole S, Comby P, et al. The disposition of voriconazole in mouse, rat, rabbit, guinea pig, dog, and human. *Drug Metab Dispos.* 2003;31:731–741.
45. Quimby JM, Hoffman SB, Duke J, et al. Adverse neurologic events associated with voriconazole use in 3 cats. *J Vet Intern Med.* 2010;24:647–649.
46. Kendall J, Papich MG. Posaconazole pharmacokinetics after administration of an intravenous solution, oral suspension, and delayed-release tablet to dogs. *Am J Vet Res.* 2015;76:454–459.
47. Evans N, Gunew M, Marshall R, et al. Focal pulmonary granuloma caused by *Cladophialophora bantiana* in a domestic short haired cat. *Med Mycol.* 2011;49:194–197.
48. Wray JD, Sparkes AH, Johnson EM. Infection of the subcutis of the nose in a cat caused by *Mucor* species: successful treatment using posaconazole. *J Feline Med Surg.* 2008;10:523–527.
49. McLellan GJ, Aquino SM, Mason DR, et al. Use of posaconazole in the management of invasive orbital aspergillosis in a cat. *J Am Anim Hosp Assoc.* 2006;42:302–307.
50. Krishna G, Moton A, Ma L, et al. Pharmacokinetics and absorption of posaconazole oral suspension under various gastric conditions in healthy volunteers. *Antimicrob Agents Chemother.* 2009;53:958–966.
51. Moore JN, Healy JR, Kraft WK. Pharmacologic and clinical evaluation of posaconazole. *Expert Rev Clin Pharmacol.* 2015;8:321–334.
52. Mawby DI, Whittemore JC, Fowler LE, et al. Posaconazole pharmacokinetics in healthy cats after oral and intravenous administration. *J Vet Intern Med.* 2016;30:1703–1707.
53. Corrigan VK, Legendre AM, Wheat LJ, et al. Treatment of disseminated aspergillosis with posaconazole in 10 dogs. *J Vet Intern Med.* 2016;30:167–173.
54. Krockenberger MB, Martin P, Halliday C, et al. Localised *Microsphaeropsis arundinis* infection of the subcutis of a cat. *J Feline Med Surg.* 2010;12:231–236.
55. Donnelley MA, Zhu ES, Thompson GR 3rd. Isavuconazole in the treatment of invasive aspergillosis and mucormycosis infections. *Infect Drug Resist.* 2016;9:79–86.
56. Schwartz S, Cornely OA, Hamed K, et al. Isavuconazole for the treatment of patients with invasive fungal diseases involving the central nervous system. *Med Mycol.* 2020;58:417–424.
57. Allen D, Wilson D, Drew R, et al. Azole antifungals: 35 years of invasive fungal infection management. *Expert Rev Anti Infect Ther.* 2015;13:787–798.
58. Oliva G, Roura X, Crotti A, et al. Guidelines for treatment of leishmaniasis in dogs. *J Am Vet Med Assoc.* 2010;236:1192–1198.
59. Sundar S, Chakravarty J, Agarwal D, et al. Single-dose liposomal amphotericin B for visceral leishmaniasis in India. *N Engl J Med.* 2010;362:504–512.
60. Chavez-Fumagalli MA, Ribeiro TG, Castilho RO, et al. New delivery systems for amphotericin B applied to the improvement of leishmaniasis treatment. *Rev Soc Bras Med Trop.* 2015;48:235–242.
61. Espinel-Ingroff A. Mechanisms of resistance to antifungal agents: yeasts and filamentous fungi. *Rev Iberoam Micol.* 2008;25:101–106.
62. Arthur RR, Drew RH, Perfect JR. Novel modes of antifungal drug administration. *Expert Opin Investig Drugs.* 2004;13:903–932.
63. Malik R, Craig AJ, Wigney DI, et al. Combination chemotherapy of canine and feline cryptococcosis using subcutaneously administered amphotericin B. *Aust Vet J.* 1996;73:124–128.
64. Laniado-Laborin R, Cabrales-Vargas MN. Amphotericin B: side effects and toxicity. *Rev Iberoam Micol.* 2009;26:223–227.
65. Goldblum D, Rohrer K, Frueh BE, et al. Ocular distribution of intravenously administered lipid formulations of amphotericin B in a rabbit model. *Antimicrob Agents Chemother.* 2002;46:3719–3723.
66. Batista-Duharte A, Lastre M, Romeu B, et al. Antifungal and immunomodulatory activity of a novel cochleate for amphotericin B delivery against *Sporothrix schenckii*. *Int Immunopharmacol.* 2016;40:277–287.
67. Moossavi M, Bagheri B, Scher RK. Systemic antifungal therapy. *Dermatol Clin.* 2001;19:35–52.
68. Moriello KA. Treatment of dermatophytosis in dogs and cats: review of published studies. *Vet Dermatol.* 2004;15:99–107.
69. von Heimendahl A, England GC, Sheldon IM. Influence of griseofulvin treatment on semen quality in the dog. *Anim Reprod Sci.* 2004;80:175–181.
70. Rottman JB, English RV, Breitschwerdt EB, et al. Bone marrow hypoplasia in a cat treated with griseofulvin. *J Am Vet Med Assoc.* 1991;198:429–431.
71. Shelton GH, Grant CK, Linenberger ML, et al. Severe neutropenia associated with griseofulvin therapy in cats with feline immunodeficiency virus infection. *J Vet Intern Med.* 1990;4:317–319.

72. Rosales MS, Marsella R, Kunkle G, et al. Comparison of the clinical efficacy of oral terbinafine and ketoconazole combined with cephalexin in the treatment of *Malassezia* dermatitis in dogs: a pilot study. *Vet Dermatol.* 2005;16:171–176.
73. Hummel J, Grooters A, Davidson G, et al. Successful management of gastrointestinal pythiosis in a dog using itraconazole, terbinafine, and mefenoxam. *Med Mycol.* 2011;49:539–542.
74. Pereira DI, Schild AL, Motta MA, et al. Cutaneous and gastrointestinal pythiosis in a dog in Brazil. *Vet Res Commun.* 2010;34:301–306.
75. Ryder NS. Activity of terbinafine against serious fungal pathogens. *Mycoses.* 1999;42(suppl 2):115–119.
76. Gupta AK, Kohli Y, Batra R. In vitro activities of posaconazole, ravuconazole, terbinafine, itraconazole and fluconazole against dermatophyte, yeast and non-dermatophyte species. *Med Mycol.* 2005;43:179–185.
77. Revankar SG, Nailor MD, Sobel JD. Use of terbinafine in rare and refractory mycoses. *Future Microbiol.* 2008;3:9–17.
78. Baudraz-Rosselet F, Ruffieux C, Lurati M, et al. Onychomycosis insensitive to systemic terbinafine and azole treatments reveals non-dermatophyte moulds as infectious agents. *Dermatology.* 2010;220:164–168.
79. Osborne CS, Leitner I, Hofbauer B, et al. Biological, biochemical, and molecular characterization of a new clinical *Trichophyton rubrum* isolate resistant to terbinafine. *Antimicrob Agents Chemother.* 2006;50:2234–2236.
80. Sakai MR, May ER, Imerman PM, et al. Terbinafine pharmacokinetics after single dose oral administration in the dog. *Vet Dermatol.* 2011;22:528–534.
81. Wang A, Ding H, Liu Y, et al. Single dose pharmacokinetics of terbinafine in cats. *J Feline Med Surg.* 2012;14:540–544.
82. Gimmler JR, White AG, Kennis RA, et al. Determining canine skin concentrations of terbinafine to guide the treatment of *Malassezia* dermatitis. *Vet Dermatol.* 2015;26:411–416. e495–416.
83. Williams MM, Davis EG, KuKanich B. Pharmacokinetics of oral terbinafine in horses and Greyhound dogs. *J Vet Pharmacol Ther.* 2011;34:232–237.
84. Sakai MR, May ER, Imerman PM, et al. Terbinafine pharmacokinetics after single dose oral administration in the dog. *Vet Dermatol.* 2011;22:528–534.
85. Moriello KA. Treatment of dermatophytosis in dogs and cats: review of published studies. *Vet Dermatol.* 2004;15:99–107.
86. Berger DJ, Lewis TP, Schick AE, et al. Comparison of once-daily versus twice-weekly terbinafine administration for the treatment of canine *Malassezia* dermatitis a pilot study. *Vet Dermatol.* 2012;23:418–e479.
87. Foust AL, Marsella R, Akucewich LH, et al. Evaluation of persistence of terbinafine in the hair of normal cats after 14 days of daily therapy. *Vet Dermatol.* 2007;18:246–251.
88. Sandison T, Ong V, Lee J, et al. Safety and pharmacokinetics of CD101 IV, a novel echinocandin, in healthy adults. *Antimicrob Agents Chemother.* 2017;61:e01627–16.
89. Gonzalez GM, Gonzalez G, Najvar LK, et al. Therapeutic efficacy of caspofungin alone and in combination with amphotericin B deoxycholate for coccidioidomycosis in a mouse model. *J Antimicrob Chemother.* 2007;60:1341–1346.
90. Levy ER, McCarty JM, Shane AL, et al. Treatment of pediatric refractory coccidioidomycosis with combination voriconazole and caspofungin: a retrospective case series. *Clin Infect Dis.* 2013;56:1573–1578.
91. Chen SC, Slavin MA, Sorrell TC. Echinocandin antifungal drugs in fungal infections: a comparison. *Drugs.* 2011;71:11–41.
92. Goldblum D, Fausch K, Frueh BE, et al. Ocular penetration of caspofungin in a rabbit uveitis model. *Graefes Arch Clin Exp Ophthalmol.* 2007;245:825–833.
93. Flattery AM, Hickey E, Gill CJ, et al. Efficacy of caspofungin in a juvenile mouse model of central nervous system candidiasis. *Antimicrob Agents Chemother.* 2011;55:3491–3497.
94. Pfaller MA, Messer SA, Rhomberg PR, et al. Activity of a long-acting echinocandin, CD101, determined using CLSI and EUCAST reference methods, against *Candida* and *Aspergillus* spp., including echinocandin- and azole-resistant isolates. *J Antimicrob Chemother.* 2016;71:2868–2873.
95. Oliver JD, Sibley GEM, Beckmann N, et al. F901318 represents a novel class of antifungal drug that inhibits dihydroorotate dehydrogenase. *PNAS.* 2016;113:12809–12814.
96. Panackal AA, Parisini E, Proschan M. Salvage combination antifungal therapy for acute invasive aspergillosis may improve outcomes: a systematic review and meta-analysis. *Int J Infect Dis.* 2014;28:80–94.
97. Grahl N, Shepardson KM, Chung D, et al. Hypoxia and fungal pathogenesis: to air or not to air? *Eukaryot Cell.* 2012;11:560–570.

12

Antiprotozoal Drugs

Jane E. Sykes, Mark G. Papich

KEY POINTS

- Antiprotozoal drugs often have a narrow spectrum of activity, although some are also active against bacteria and fungi. Many interfere with enzyme pathways specific to protozoal species that have little effect on the host.
- Many antiprotozoal agents are intended to inhibit growth, and treatment with antiprotozoal drugs may not consistently clear an infection.
- Resistance to antiprotozoal drugs is a growing problem among protozoal pathogens.
- Many antiprotozoal drugs with activity confined to the intestine have minimal to no adverse effects. However, some drugs have systemic effects that may limit their use.
- The availability of some antiprotozoal drugs is restricted in some countries.

INTRODUCTION

The use of antiprotozoal drugs in dogs and cats is frequently extrapolated from their use in human patients or food animal species. There are very few antiprotozoal agents approved for this use in veterinary medicine, and most are sulfonamides. The majority of these agents are used extralabel, and most antiprotozoal agents (coccidiostats mostly) in veterinary medicine are used in food producing animals (e.g., cattle, pigs, poultry) raised in close confinement. A review of the FDA list of approved animal drugs shows hundreds of products marketed for this purpose. Some antibacterial and antifungal drugs also have antiprotozoal activity, such as metronidazole, fluoroquinolones, trimethoprim-sulfonamides, clindamycin, and macrolides such as azithromycin, azoles, and amphotericin B (see Chapters 10 and 11 for a more detailed description of the use and adverse effects of these drugs). *In vitro* activity of antiprotozoal drugs, and monitoring of resistance, is more difficult for antiprotozoal drugs because standardized susceptibility testing is not routinely performed for these pathogens. Standards for testing do not exist for pathogens isolated from animals. In addition, many antiprotozoal drugs are designed to be active in the lumen of the intestine for treatment of intestinal protozoal infections, and the concentration of active drug in the intestinal lumen after oral administration is difficult to measure. Therefore, the concentration of drug to which these pathogens are exposed is often not known. The activity and dosage regimens of antiprotozoal drugs are often based on the results of clinical trials rather than pharmacokinetic-pharmacodynamic (PK-PD) concentration-exposure relationships between antiprotozoal drugs and the organism of interest.

Many antiprotozoal drugs are active only against a restricted range of protozoal species. To reflect this, drugs in this chapter are organized into antiprotozoal drugs primarily used for gastrointestinal infections; those with a broad spectrum of activity; those used to treat systemic protozoal infections (such as hepatozoonosis, toxoplasmosis, neosporosis, and sarcocystosis); those used to treat leishmaniosis; and those used to treat Chagas' disease. For many infections, treatment does not consistently result in parasitologic cure.

ANTIPROTOZOAL DRUGS USED PRIMARILY FOR GASTROINTESTINAL INFECTIONS

Amprolium

Amprolium is a thiamine analogue that is used to prevent and treat intestinal coccidiosis (Table 12.1). It is available as a feed additive for livestock and is sometimes administered in food or drinking water to puppies and kittens. To administer to dogs and cats, it is available as a 9.6% (9.6 g/100 mL) oral solution or a soluble powder in a 22.6 g packet, which then must be mixed with food. For treatment of coccidiosis, 1.25 g of 20% amprolium powder can be added to food or 30 mL of 9.6% amprolium solution to 3.8 L of drinking water for 7 days.

Adverse effects of anorexia or diarrhea are rare and primarily occur at high doses and with prolonged use. Central nervous system (CNS) signs can result from thiamine deficiency, which is reversible on addition of thiamine to the diet. However, thiamine supplementation may interfere with the drug's efficacy.

Benzimidazoles

Fenbendazole and Albendazole

Benzimidazoles bind to β-tubulin within a variety of helminths and protozoa. This leads to inhibition of tubulin polymerization and the formation of microtubules, with impaired cell division. Glucose uptake by parasites is also impaired. Resistance can result from production of altered β-tubulin by parasites, which reduces binding of benzimidazole drugs.

Fenbendazole is widely used to treat giardiasis in dogs and cats. It is safer than metronidazole, can be administered to young animals, and has higher efficacy, although treatment failure can still occur. A second course of treatment or administration of fenbendazole in combination with metronidazole can be effective in refractory cases. In one colony, elimination of infection was achieved when dogs were treated with fenbendazole for 10 days (instead of the typical use of 3 to 5 days), with bathing on day 5, separation into a clean facility, and disinfection of the original kennel. Dogs were returned to this kennel on day 7.[1] Administration with food may improve absorption, but the fat content of the food does not influence absorption.[2] Adverse effects

TABLE 12.1 Suggested Doses of Drugs Primarily Used to Treat Protozoal Infections of the Gastrointestinal Tract in Small Animals

Drug	Dose (mg/kg)	Interval (hours)	Species	Route	Duration (days)	Comments
Fenbendazole	50	24	C, D	PO	5–10	Giardiasis. May be administered with food. Safe in pregnancy.
Albendazole	25	12	C, D	PO	3	Giardiasis. May cause bone marrow suppression. Do not use in pregnancy.
Metronidazole	12–15	12	C, D	PO	5–7	Giardiasis. Use caution with hepatic insufficiency. Dose for metronidazole benzoate is 25 mg/kg, but with same interval.
Tinidazole	15	12–24	D, C	PO	5	Giardiasis. Administer with food or in capsules to reduce bitterness. Administered as a single dose in humans.
Ronidazole	30	24	C	PO	14	Tritrichomoniasis. Avoid doses ≥ 60 mg/kg/day. Compounded from powder.
Paromomycin	10	8	D	PO	5–10	Cryptosporidiosis. Caution in animals with diarrhea due to possible systemic absorption. Avoid in cats.
Nitazoxanide	100 mg/animal	12	D, C	PO	3	Cryptosporidiosis. Efficacy and safety unclear. Vomiting common in cats.
Amprolium	1.25 g of 20% powder or 30 mL of 9.6% solution to 3.8 L of water	24	D, C	PO	7	Cystoisosporiasis. Add to food. Do not administer for prolonged periods.
Sulfadimethoxine	55 on day 1, 27 thereafter	24	D, C	PO	3–23 or for 48 hours after signs resolve	Cystoisosporiasis with or without a dihydrofolate reductase inhibitor.

C, cats; *D*, dogs; *PO*, oral.

of fenbendazole are very rare but can include decreased appetite, vomiting, diarrhea, and rarely reversible pancytopenia.[3] At high doses used to treat *Mesocestoides* spp. peritonitis (100 mg/kg q12h), neurologic signs have been observed.[4] Febantel is metabolized to a benzimidazole compound and has been used in combination with praziquantel and pyrantel (Drontal Plus, Elanco, USA) to treat *Giardia* spp. infection in dogs, although efficacy at label dosages has been variable and some dogs can re-shed low numbers of cysts when treatment is discontinued.[5] Albendazole has an affinity for rapidly dividing cells, and although it is used extensively for treatment of parasitic infections in human patients, it been associated with anorexia and reversible bone marrow suppression in dogs and cats especially when high doses are administered for more than 5 days.[6] As a result, fenbendazole is used more commonly in small animals.

Nitroimidazoles

Protozoa reduce nitroimidazoles to nitro anion free radicals, which cause damage to parasite's DNA. Some nitroimidazoles are mutagens and carcinogens, but carcinogenesis has not been demonstrated in dogs and cats with long-term use. Because of this undocumented occurrence in animals or humans, some regulatory authorities have advocated for removal from the carcinogen list.

Metronidazole, ronidazole, and tinidazole have primarily been used to treat enteric protozoal infections. Benznidazole is specifically used to treat infections with *Trypanosoma cruzi*.

Metronidazole

Metronidazole is used to treat giardiasis in dogs and cats, although efficacy may be as low as 50%. It also has activity against amoebic infections. The clinical use and adverse effects of metronidazole are described in Chapter 10. In one study, addition of the probiotic SF68 to metronidazole treatment appeared to have clinical benefit when used to treat dogs with protozoal diarrhea in a shelter.[7] Doses of metronidazole used for treatment of giardiasis have the potential to be associated with neurotoxicity; therefore, fenbendazole is preferred because of greater safety and efficacy. Metronidazole can be combined with fenbendazole for refractory giardiasis.

In addition to neurotoxicity that is associated with high doses, metronidazole also has a very unpleasant taste, which is difficult to administer to dogs and cats. Subsequently some pharmacies will prepare a more palatable ester formulation (metronidazole benzoate) for oral administration. It is converted to the active form in the intestine, but on a weight-by-weight basis is only 62% metronidazole; therefore, dose adjustments must be performed when prescribing.

Tinidazole

Tinidazole is a 5-nitroimidazole that has amoebicidal, giardicidal, trichomonicidal, and anaerobic bactericidal activity. It is sometimes used as a single-dose treatment for giardiasis in human patients. The efficacy of tinidazole for treatment for giardiasis in dogs and cats has not been evaluated, and the half-life in dogs (4.4 hours) and cats (8.4 hours) is shorter than that in human patients (>12 hours).[8,9] Tinidazole is very well absorbed in dogs and cats, with a bioavailability of 100%. Adverse effects are similar to those of metronidazole. Like metronidazole, tinidazole has a bitter taste. It has not been effective for treatment of feline trichomoniasis.

Ronidazole

Ronidazole is the drug of choice for treatment of *Tritrichomonas foetus* infections, which are less responsive to metronidazole and tinidazole.[10–12] Ronidazole has not been approved by the US FDA for administration to dogs, cats or humans, and has been banned for use in food animals because of the potential for adverse effects in humans. Therefore, veterinarians have been cautioned about the use of the drug, and advised to prescribe it only when *T. foetus* infection has been confirmed.[13] Resistance to ronidazole has been identified in some isolates of *T. foetus* and is associated with treatment failure in infected cats.[14] Resistance is thought to result from increased oxygen-scavenging capacity by the parasite, whereby oxygen competes effectively with ronidazole and other nitroimidazoles for ferredoxin-bound electrons.

Ronidazole is absorbed rapidly and completely after oral administration to cats. Some compounded formulations may have decreased efficacy as a result of low ronidazole content or differences in drug release at the site of action (the large bowel). Because of rapid and complete absorption of immediate-release compounded oral forms, toxicity can occur if dosing recommendations are not followed. Decreased appetite, vomiting, and neurologic signs can occur in dogs and cats, especially at doses above 30 mg/kg q12h in cats and at doses as low as 10 mg/kg/day in dogs.[15] Once-daily dosing for 14 days is recommended because of the long half-life of the drug in cats.[13,16] Doses of 20 mg/kg or less may not effectively clear infection with *T. foetus*. Neurologic signs result from γ-aminobutyric acid (GABA) antagonism in the CNS and include ataxia, decreased mentation, agitation, tremors, and hyperesthesia, which occur up to 9 days after the start of treatment and resolve when the drug is discontinued.[15] Adverse effects may worsen for a few days after the drug is discontinued, after which time they slowly subside. A modified-release formulation that is delivered to the colon may have improved efficacy, but this was formulated in guar gum and is not available commercially, or readily prepared by compounding pharmacies.[16] When these capsules were administered to 10 cats at a dose of 30 mg/kg q24h, there were no adverse effects observed. Elimination of infection was achieved in 84% of treated cats, but because these cats were housed with placebo-treated cats, reinfections may have occurred.[17]

Owners should be advised to watch closely for adverse effects of drug therapy and discontinue treatment should signs of toxicity appear. The drug is contraindicated in pregnant or lactating queens.

Nitazoxanide

Nitazoxanide is a nitrothiazolyl-salicylamide derivative that has activity against *Giardia* and *Cryptosporidium* spp., *Sarcocystis neurona,* some anaerobic bacteria, *Helicobacter* spp., and *Campylobacter jejuni*. It inhibits the pyruvate-ferredoxin/flavodoxin oxidoreductase enzyme-dependent electron transfer reaction that is essential for anaerobic metabolism in these organisms. Resistance has been documented in *Giardia* spp.[18]

Reports of nitazoxanide use in dogs and cats have been rare. An equine formulation (Navigator, IDEXX Pharmaceuticals, USA) that was used to treat equine protozoal meningoencephalitis caused by *S. neurona* has been removed from the market due to concerns about adverse effects, primarily fatal enterocolitis. Doses have been extrapolated from those used for human patients. Nitazoxanide treatment of cats co-infected with *Cryptosporidium* spp. and *T. foetus* led to cessation of shedding during treatment, but infection was not eliminated.[19] Vomiting occurred frequently, especially at higher doses (75 mg/kg PO q12h). When used to treat dogs that were naturally infected with *Giardia* spp., nitazoxanide at doses of 75 mg/kg PO q12h and 150 mg/kg PO q12h on days 0 and 14 (7 dogs in each group) resulted in a dramatic reduction in the shedding of cysts when compared with an untreated control group.[20] Vomiting occurred in one dog treated with the high-dose protocol. In humans, nitazoxanide is rapidly absorbed from the gastrointestinal tract and metabolized to the active metabolite tizoxanide, which is highly protein bound. After hepatic glucuronidation, it is excreted in urine and bile.

ANTIBACTERIAL DRUGS WITH BROAD-SPECTRUM ANTIPROTOZOAL ACTIVITY

Folic Acid Antagonists

Trimethoprim, pyrimethamine, ormetoprim, and sulfonamides (sulfamethoxazole and sulfadiazine) inhibit parasite replication through folate antagonism. Synergistic combinations of sulfadiazine with trimethoprim or pyrimethamine are primarily used to treat toxoplasmosis, neosporosis, and intestinal coccidiosis (*Cystoisospora* spp. infections) in dogs and cats. A combination of pyrimethamine, trimethoprim-sulfadiazine, and clindamycin has also been used to treat *Hepatozoon americanum* infections.[21] Trimethoprim-sulfonamides are broadly used as antibacterial agents and the mechanisms of action, use, and adverse effects of trimethoprim and sulfonamides are discussed in Chapter 10.

Sulfadimethoxine

One of the most common oral anticoccidial agents administered to dogs and cats (especially animals in breeding facilities) is sulfadimethoxine, commonly known by its brand name Albon (Zoetis, USA). It is available as 125-, 250-, and 500-mg tablets and an oral suspension.

Pyrimethamine

Like trimethoprim, pyrimethamine inhibits dihydrofolate reductase, which is necessary for synthesis of thymidine. However, in contrast to trimethoprim, it has a greater affinity for the protozoal enzyme than the bacterial enzyme. Resistance to pyrimethamine can occur when parasites synthesize dihydrofolate reductase with an altered drug target site. Pyrimethamine is well absorbed after oral administration and penetrates a variety of tissues including the CNS. Hepatic metabolism and some renal excretion occur. Although clearance of pyrimethamine is not affected by renal disease, its use is cautioned in human patients with hepatic or renal insufficiency.

Pyrimethamine is well tolerated. Gastrointestinal signs such as vomiting, diarrhea, and decreased appetite occur in some treated animals. Bone marrow suppression can occur with prolonged treatment at higher doses as a result of folic acid deficiency. In human patients, concurrent administration of folinic acid is recommended when high doses are used for treatment of toxoplasmosis. Folinic acid, but not folic acid supplementation also reverses marrow suppression in dogs treated with pyrimethamine.[22] The CBC should be monitored weekly during treatment, and supplementation should be provided if leukopenia develops and continued treatment is necessary. Stomatitis, ulcerative glossitis, and exfoliative dermatitis have also been described in human patients as a result of folic acid deficiency. Other adverse effects of pyrimethamine-sulfadiazine combinations result from the sulfadiazine component (see Chapter 10).

Unlike trimethoprim-sulfadiazine, there are no approved formulations of pyrimethamine-sulfonamides for dogs and cats. Pyrimethamine is available as a single agent in tablets but should be administered with a sulfonamide for the best efficacy. Human formulation tablets of pyrimethamine have become extremely expensive in recent years. For example, in 2015, the price increased from $13.50 per pill to $750 per pill. Another alternative is a combination of pyrimethamine and sulfadiazine marketed as an oral formulation for horses (ReBalance, PRN Pharmaceutical, USA) to treat equine protozoal myeloencephalitis (EPM) in a formulation of 12.5 mg pyrimethamine and 250 mg sulfadiazine per mL. This product also has been administered to dogs and cats for treatment of some protozoal infections. Although off-label, it is a convenient formulation for small animal veterinarians. This formulation can be administered at a dose of 1 mg/kg pyrimethamine + 20 mg/kg sulfadiazine PO q24h. This is equivalent to 0.33 mL of the equine formulation per 4 kg of body weight for dogs and cats.

Macrolides and Lincosamides

Clindamycin, azithromycin, and clarithromycin are macrolide antibiotics with antiprotozoal activity. The use of these macrolides and lincosamides in dogs and cats as antibacterial agents and their adverse effects are discussed in Chapter 10. Clindamycin is the most widely used antiprotozoal for treatment of toxoplasmosis and neosporosis in dogs and cats, and has also been used in combination with diminazene aceturate and imidocarb dipropionate to treat canine babesiosis.[23] Although clindamycin inhibits shedding of *Toxoplasma gondii* oocysts by cats,[24] clinical efficacy of clindamycin for treatment of toxoplasmosis in dogs and cats has been questioned by experts and in published studies. An extended-release formulation of clindamycin achieved therapeutic serum concentrations for 60 hours in contrast to existing formulations, which achieved therapeutic concentrations for 12 hours.[25]

Trimethoprim-sulfonamides (discussed above) are a suitable alternative, or if clindamycin is used, pyrimethamine may be used in combination. In human patients, pyrimethamine and clindamycin are used as a substitute for pyrimethamine and sulfadiazine for treatment of toxoplasmosis in sulfadiazine-sensitive individuals. Azithromycin is used in combination with atovaquone for treatment of babesiosis and cytauxzoonosis.

Paromomycin (Aminosidine)

Paromomycin, also known as aminosidine, is the only aminoglycoside antibiotic that has efficacy against protozoa. It is poorly absorbed from the gastrointestinal tract and so has been used to treat enteric protozoal infections, particularly cryptosporidiosis. It is ineffective for treatment of tritrichomoniasis in cats.[12] Furthermore, when used to treat intestinal protozoal infections in cats, paromomycin has been absorbed systemically because of intestinal mucosal compromise, with resultant acute renal failure, deafness, and cataract formation.[26] As a result, its use has been limited. In human patients, paromomycin has been used topically to treat cutaneous leishmaniasis and parenterally to treat visceral leishmaniasis.[27] It had efficacy for treatment of nonazotemic leishmaniosis in dogs at 15 mg/kg SC q24h for 21 days, with no evidence of nephrotoxicity, although complete elimination of the parasite was not achieved.[28,29]

Tetracyclines and Ciprofloxacin

Doxycycline has primarily been used for malaria prophylaxis in humans. Ciprofloxacin is thought to inhibit DNA gyrase within a chloroplast organelle (the apicoplast) of apicomplexan parasites (see the triazines, later). It is an alternative to sulfadiazine for treatment of cystoisosporiasis in human patients. Tetracyclines and ciprofloxacin have not been widely used for prevention or treatment of protozoal infections in dogs and cats with the possible exception of doxycycline as part of combination treatment for babesiosis (see Chapter 97). Although ciprofloxacin was the fluoroquinolone of choice in the human studies, it has poor oral absorption in animals, especially in cats, and highly variable oral absorption in dogs. If indeed, ciprofloxacin is effective for some infections, it is anticipated that veterinary-labeled fluoroquinolones (enrofloxacin, marbofloxacin, orbifloxacin) would have similar effectiveness. When administered to animals, a portion of enrofloxacin is converted to ciprofloxacin. Another alternative for dogs is the human-labeled generic levofloxacin, which is available as an inexpensive tablet and has almost 100% bioavailability in dogs.[30]

ANTIPROTOZOAL DRUGS USED FOR SYSTEMIC PROTOZOAL INFECTIONS

Quinolone Derivatives

Atovaquone

Atovaquone is a hydroxynaphthoquinone that inhibits electron transport in protozoa by targeting the cytochrome bc_1 complex (Table 12.2). It has been used in combination with other antiprotozoal drugs as an alternative treatment for malaria, toxoplasmosis, and pneumocystosis in human patients.[18] In veterinary medicine, atovaquone is used in combination with azithromycin for treatment of *Babesia gibsoni*, *Babesia conradae*, *Babesia vulpes* (formerly *Babesia microti*-like or *Theileria annae*) infections and cytauxzoonosis (see Chapters 97 and 98). The drawback of using atovaquone is that it is expensive. Use of a compounded formulation in combination with azithromycin to treat 42 dogs with *B. gibsoni* infection resulted in pathogen clearance in 39 (93%) of dogs, and represents a more economical treatment protocol.[31] Resistance has been reported in *Plasmodium* spp., *T. gondii*, *Pneumocystis jirovecii*, *Cytauxzoon felis*, and canine *B. gibsoni* strains as a result of mutations in the cytochrome bc_1 complex.

Atovaquone is highly lipophilic and extensively protein bound. Little is known about atovaquone metabolism in dogs and cats. Its oral bioavailability increases significantly when food is administered concurrently. Atovaquone is available alone or in a formulation with proguanil for treatment and prevention of malaria in human patients. The combination formulation may cause vomiting and diarrhea in dogs, but otherwise atovaquone appears well tolerated by both dogs and cats.[32–34] In human patients, adverse effects have included gastrointestinal signs, headache, fever, and increased liver enzyme activities. Co-administration with metoclopramide, tetracycline, or rifampin significantly decreases plasma drug concentrations in humans and could possibly have similar effects in small animals.

A related drug, buparvaquone, which has been used to treat bovine theileriosis, was combined with azithromycin and used to treat dogs with *B. vulpes* infection. Two 5-mg/kg doses administered intramuscularly (IM) 48 hours apart were better tolerated than atovaquone, with similar outcomes as an atovaquone/azithromycin combination.[35] However, the pharmacokinetics and toxicity of buparvaquone in dogs have not been otherwise studied.

Decoquinate

Decoquinate is a 4-hydroxyquinolone coccidiostat that inhibits electron transport in protozoal mitochondria and interferes with sporozoite development. It likely has a similar mechanism of action to atovaquone, because resistance to atovaquone can result in cross-resistance to decoquinate.[36] Although developed as a feed additive coccidiostat for use in production animals, decoquinate can be used successfully and without adverse effects to prevent relapses in dogs that are chronically infected with *H. americanum*.[21] Decoquinate also appeared to be effective for treatment of *Sarcocystis* spp. myositis in a dog.[37] Its distribution and metabolism in dogs and cats have not been described.

Because there are no commercial formulations for small animals, the food animal feed additive is used. The decoquinate feed additive (27.2 g decoquinate per pound of premix) has been added to moist dog food at a rate of 0.5–1.0 tablespoons per 10 kg twice a day.

Aromatic Diamines

The aromatic diamines include imidocarb dipropionate, diminazene aceturate, pentamidine isethionate, and phenamidine isethionate. These drugs inhibit DNA synthesis in protozoa. In dogs, imidocarb and diminazene have been used most widely, primarily for treatment of *Babesia* spp. and *Hepatozoon canis* infections. In general, the use of imidocarb has been preferred over diminazene because of diminazene's narrow therapeutic index and concern about safety in animals. Pentamidine and phenamidine have also been used in dogs. Pentamidine isethionate is a second-line treatment for leishmaniasis in human patients and is used as an alternative to diminazene for treatment of African trypanosomiasis (see Chapter 100). Treatment of protozoal infections using aromatic diamines may not result in complete parasite elimination.

Imidocarb Dipropionate

Imidocarb dipropionate is primarily used to treat large *Babesia* spp. and *H. canis* infections in dogs. More effective agents have replaced imidocarb for treatment of canine monocytic ehrlichiosis and feline

TABLE 12.2 Suggested Doses of Drugs Primarily Used to Treat Systemic Protozoal Diseases Excluding Leishmaniosis and Trypanosomiasis in Small Animals

Drug	Dose (mg/kg)	Interval (hours)	Species	Route	Duration (days)	Comments
Pyrimethamine	0.5–1	24	D, C	PO	14–28	Primarily neosporosis, toxoplasmosis, and American hepatozoonosis. Use with a sulfonamide. Use caution with hepatic and renal insufficiency. Monitor CBC. Folinic acid supplementation (5 mg/day) may be required.
Pyrimethamine/ sulfadiazine	1 mg/kg pyrimethamine + 20 mg/kg sulfadiazine, in combination	24	D, C	PO	14–28	Available in an equine combination formulation with 250 mg sulfadiazine and 12.5 mg pyrimethamine per mL in a liquid suspension.
Clindamycin	22	12	D, C	PO		Toxoplasmosis, neosporosis, sarcocystosis, and American hepatozoonosis.
Azithromycin	10	24	D, C	PO	10	Babesiosis and cytauxzoonosis. Used with atovaquone.
Atovaquone	13.3–15	8	D,C	PO	10	Babesiosis and cytauxzoonosis with azithromycin. Administer with food.
Buparvaquone	5	Once, repeat in 48 hours	D	IM	N/A	Babesiosis. Pharmacokinetics has not been studied in dogs. Use with azithromycin.
Decoquinate	10–20	12	D	PO	≥365	American hepatozoonosis and sarcocystosis. Powder (6% decoquinate; 60 mg active ingredient per gram) is mixed with food. This equates to 0.5–1 tablespoon/10 kg body weight q12h.
Imidocarb dipropionate	6.6	Once, repeat in 14 days	D, C	Deep IM or SC	N/A	Large *Babesia* spp. infections. Caution with hepatic or renal insufficiency. Avoid use with other cholinesterase inhibitors.
Diminazene aceturate	3–5	Once	D	Deep IM	N/A	Babesiosis and African trypanosomiasis. Narrow therapeutic range.
Ponazuril	20–50	12–24	D	PO	3–28	Toxoplasmosis, neosporosis, cystoisosporiasis. Optimal dose, duration, efficacy, and adverse effects unknown.
Toltrazuril	10–30 5–10 30 15	24 24 Once Once, repeat in 10 days	D C (toxoplasmosis) C (coccidia) C (coccidia)	PO PO PO PO	3 2 N/A 3	Hepatozoonosis, cystoisosporiasis. One dose may be effective for cystoisosporiasis. Optimal dose and duration for hepatozoonosis unknown.

C, cats; *CBC*, complete blood count; *D*, dogs; *IM*, intramuscular; *N/A*, not applicable; *PO*, oral.

cytauxzoonosis, and its efficacy for treatment of *H. canis* infections does not appear to be high.[38]

Imidocarb is injected IM, twice, 2 weeks apart. It is generally well tolerated, except for acute effects shortly after injection. After injection, it can produce transient pain at the site of injection. Acute adverse effects result from its anticholinergic activity and include vomiting, shivering, hypersalivation, lacrimation, diarrhea, agitation, lethargy, pyrexia, and periorbital swelling. These generally resolve within a few hours. It appears to be eliminated in urine and feces.[39] A possible association between imidocarb treatment and acute renal tubular necrosis has been reported in dogs.[40] Massive hepatic necrosis was described after overdosage of dogs with 10 times the recommended dose.[41]

Diminazene Aceturate

Diminazene aceturate is administered parenterally, primarily to dogs, for treatment of babesiosis, trypanosomiasis, and infections with *Rangelia vitalii*, a protozoal pathogen of dogs from Brazil (see Chapter 105).[42] Diminazene aceturate is not readily available in the United States. Resistance to diminazene has been described in *B. gibsoni*.[43]

Although formulations for small animals are not available, a powdered commercial drug formulation (Veriben, Ceva Santé Animale, France) has been reconstituted with sterile water to a concentration of 7 mg/mL and administered IM at a dose of 3 mg/kg diminazene diaceturate for a pharmacokinetic study in cats.[44] The dose was well tolerated, but diminazene was eliminated quickly, with a half-life of only 1.7 hours and a peak concentration of only 0.5 μg/mL. The drug concentrations produced at this dose may not be consistently effective. Development of clinically effective doses from these data requires further studies. Diminazene was administered to seven cats experimentally infected with *Trypanosoma evansi* at a dose of 3.5 mg/kg IM on 5 consecutive days.[45] The treatment was 85.7% efficacious for elimination of the parasite, and no adverse effects were observed. The medication may be administered as a single treatment, or the dose can be repeated 72 to 96 hours after drug administration.

Although no adverse effects were observed in the study cited above, the doses of diminazene that are high enough to be consistently effective may produce concentrations that are toxic; therefore, caution is advised if it is used in clinical patients. Adverse effects include tachycardia and CNS signs such as ataxia, nystagmus, and opisthotonos. Death from diminazene toxicosis in association with neurologic signs and hemorrhagic necrosis within the CNS at necropsy has been described in dogs treated with consecutive daily doses.[46] In some protocols for *B. gibsoni* infections, diminazene administration has been followed a day later by treatment with imidocarb.

Triazine Antiprotozoals (Toltrazuril and Ponazuril)

Toltrazuril and its major metabolite ponazuril (toltrazuril sulfone, Marquis, Boehringer Ingelheim, USA) are triazine-based antiprotozoal drugs that have specific activity against apicomplexan coccidial infections. Toltrazuril is not available within the United States, but ponazuril and diclazuril are available in formulations used in other animals: ponazuril oral paste for horses, diclazuril oral pellets for horses, and diclazuril feed additive for poultry. In horses, these products are approved to treat EPM. Ponazuril and toltrazuril appear to act on a plastid-like chloroplast organelle (the *apicoplast*) in apicomplexan protozoa, which may have originally been acquired from a green alga.[47] This organelle contains a small circular genome and operates key biochemical pathways. Although their mechanism of action is unclear, triazines may inhibit metabolic enzymes or decrease pyrimidine synthesis within the apicoplast. The result of the action of these agents is to kill protozoa; therefore, their action is "cidal" rather than "static" against susceptible organisms.[48] Ponazuril and toltrazuril have been used in animals to treat cystoisosporiasis, toxoplasmosis, neosporosis, and EPM.[48] Triazine resistance has been described in coccidia from production animals.[49]

In dogs and cats, toltrazuril has been used to treat cystoisosporiasis and hepatozoonosis, although infection may persist in some animals.[21,50–55] In Europe, it is available in combination with the anthelmintic emodepside (Procox Oral Suspension for Dogs, Elanco Animal Health, Germany) for treatment of cystoisosporiasis and roundworm infections in puppies over 2 weeks of age. The suspension contains 18 mg/mL of toltrazuril, and a single 9-mg/kg dose is recommended. Toltrazuril appeared to be as effective as trimethoprim-sulfadiazine-clindamycin-pyrimethamine for treatment of canine American hepatozoonosis.[21] One dog with *H. canis* infection recovered after treatment with toltrazuril and trimethoprim-sulfamethoxazole,[55] but a toltrazuril and imidocarb combination did not offer benefit over treatment of *H. canis* infection with imidocarb alone.[56] A combination of toltrazuril/emodepside (15 mg/kg PO q24h for 6 days) and clindamycin (15 mg/kg PO q24h for 21 days) failed to eliminate infection in naturally infected dogs. When ponazuril paste was used to treat *Cystoisospora* spp. infections in dogs and cats in a shelter environment, a dose of 50 mg/kg PO q24h for 3 days appeared more effective in reducing shedding than a single dose of 50 mg/kg.[57] Doses of ponazuril used in other anecdotal reports of treatment of dogs and cats with cystoisosporiasis have ranged from 20 to 50 mg/kg for 2 to 5 days. In one dog, ocular toxoplasmosis that was refractory to clindamycin resolved after treatment with ponazuril for 28 days.[58]

The pharmacokinetics of the triazines in dogs has not been reported. In horses, ponazuril crosses the blood-brain barrier to some extent and achieves concentrations in CSF sufficient to inhibit protozoa. It has a long half-life in horses (>4 days) and in cattle (2 to 3 days). Because of its specific activity against apicomplexan parasites, significant toxicity in mammalian species has not been reported.

ANTILEISHMANIAL ANTIPROTOZOAL DRUGS

Antifungal Agents

Amphotericin B

Amphotericin B is a treatment of choice for human visceral leishmaniasis. The proposed mechanism of action is through binding to ergosterol in the protozoal membrane, which blocks the ability of *Leishmania* spp. to bind to and enter macrophages.[59] Lipid amphotericin B formulations have been used to treat leishmaniosis in dogs, although organism persistence and relapse have been reported in some dogs after twice-weekly treatment for up to 10 administrations (0.8 to 3.3 mg/kg IV).[60,61] In an effort to reduce selection for resistant parasites, the WHO recommends against the use of amphotericin B for treatment of canine leishmaniosis.[62] A full discussion of amphotericin B is provided in Chapter 11.

Azole Antifungals

Azole antifungals such as fluconazole have been used to treat cutaneous leishmaniasis in human patients. More effective antiprotozoal drugs are substituted for leishmaniosis. Posaconazole and ravuconazole also have activity against *T. cruzi* (see Chapter 100), and fluconazole has some activity against *Toxoplasma* spp. (see Chapter 93).

Antimony Compounds

Sodium stibogluconate (e.g., Pentostam, GlaxoSmithKline, UK) and *N*-methylglucamine antimoniate (meglumine antimoniate, Glucantime, Sanofi, France) are derived from the heavy metal antimony (Sb). They are called pentavalent antimony compounds (symbol Sb^{v}) because they contain Sb atoms that have five electrons in their outer shell. Pentavalent antimonials have been recommended as the first choice for treatment of *Leishmania* infections in humans and in dogs.[63] Their mechanism of action is still not completely clear, but it is thought that pentavalent antimony undergoes reduction to the more toxic trivalent version, possibly within macrophage phagolysosomes or within the parasite itself.[64] The trivalent compound inhibits protozoal enzymes and damages protozoal DNA.[65] Resistance to antimonials is an emerging problem in human *Leishmania* spp. isolates. This has led to the use of higher drug dosages, with an associated rise in the rate of drug toxicity. The availability of antimonial drugs is limited in the United States.

Both sodium stibogluconate and meglumine antimoniate are administered SC (Table 12.3). The treatment of choice for canine leishmaniosis

TABLE 12.3 Suggested Doses of Drugs Primarily Used to Treat Leishmaniosis or Chagas' Disease in Dogs

Drug	Dose (mg/kg)	Interval (hours)	Route	Duration (days)	Comments
Amiodarone	7.5	24	PO	—	Use with itraconazole, 5–10 mg/kg PO q24h
Meglumine antimoniate	75–100	24	SC	30–60	Leishmaniosis. Use with allopurinol. Available in ampules. Dose based on concentration of meglumine antimoniate. Caution in dogs with renal insufficiency.
Allopurinol	10	12	PO	At least 6–12 months	Leishmaniosis. Use with meglumine or miltefosine. Monitor CBC and serum chemistry in dogs with hepatic and renal insufficiency.
Miltefosine	2	24	PO	28	Leishmaniosis. Use with allopurinol.
Benznidazole	5–10	24	PO	60	Chagas' disease

CBC, complete blood count; *PO*, oral; *SC*, subcutaneous.

is a combination of meglumine antimoniate and allopurinol.[62,63,66] Complete clearance of the infection may not always occur.[67] After subcutaneous administration, more than 80% of meglumine antimoniate is eliminated by the kidneys. Pain at the site of injection is the most common adverse effect, and cutaneous abscesses or cellulitis may also occur.[68] Systemic adverse effects such as lethargy, vomiting, diarrhea, inappetence, and increased serum liver enzyme activities may be more likely to occur in the presence of renal failure, which can be a complication of leishmaniosis. Of concern, the administration of meglumine antimoniate to healthy dogs has led to renal tubular necrosis, in the absence of azotemia.[69] In human patients, other adverse effects include generalized arthralgias, abdominal pain, mild cytopenias, cardiotoxicity, and chemical pancreatitis.[27] Novel formulations of antimony compounds are under development for treatment of leishmaniosis, including lipid formulations and preparations that could be administered orally.[64]

Allopurinol

Allopurinol is a purine analogue. In parasites, allopurinol is metabolized to derivatives that are incorporated into RNA, which leads to impaired protein synthesis. Resistance can occur and appears to result from reduced activity of purine transporters and a reduced ability to accumulate purine.[70] In one study, resistance was associated with a decrease in copy number of the gene that encodes S-adenosylmethionine synthetase.[71] Although it has been used alone for treatment of canine leishmaniosis, allopurinol is most commonly used in combination with meglumine or miltefosine.

Allopurinol is rapidly absorbed from the gastrointestinal tracts of dogs. Peak drug concentrations occur 1 to 3 hours after administration.[72] Allopurinol is not bound to plasma proteins. Allopurinol rarely causes adverse effects in dogs. It inhibits mammalian xanthine oxidase, which results in decreased uric acid production from xanthine. As a result, long-term use can result in xanthine urolithiasis.[73] In human patients, allopurinol most commonly causes skin rashes. Gastrointestinal signs can also occur. Rarely administration of allopurinol to humans results in aplastic anemia or a hypersensitivity syndrome characterized by toxic epidermal necrolysis with hepatic and renal failure.[74,75] Serious adverse reactions are more likely to occur in human patients with renal insufficiency. At usual doses, allopurinol treatment leads to improvement in kidney lesions in dogs with leishmaniosis that have renal insufficiency.[76] Nevertheless, careful monitoring for adverse effects is indicated in these dogs (see Table 12.3). Serious drug interactions can occur when allopurinol is administered with azathioprine.

Miltefosine

Miltefosine is an effective alternative to pentavalent antimonials for treatment of leishmaniosis, although long-term outcomes were better in one study in dogs treated with meglumine.[66,77] It is a phospholipid analogue that activates cellular proteases in *Leishmania* spp., which results in apoptosis. It also appears to activate a Th1 cellular immune response, with production of IFN-γ and promotion of intracellular destruction of parasites by activated macrophages. Miltefosine is the first highly active oral drug for treatment of leishmaniosis. Nevertheless, despite clinical improvement in treated dogs, elimination of the parasite does not always occur.[66,78,79] Resistance to miltefosine can result from increased P-glycoprotein–mediated drug efflux and decreased drug uptake. Because miltefosine has a long half-life and must be administered for 28 days, selection for resistant isolates has been a concern, although resistant isolates from dogs have not yet been identified.

Over 90% of miltefosine is absorbed from the gastrointestinal tract of dogs after oral administration.[69] The half-life of miltefosine in the dog is approximately 6 days, so it accumulates until a steady-state plasma concentration is reached after 3 to 4 weeks of treatment. Clearance is believed to result from slow hepatic metabolism and excretion in bile. In dogs, adverse effects of treatment are mild and transient and consist of occasional vomiting and diarrhea.[80] In contrast to meglumine antimoniate, miltefosine does not appear to contribute to renal pathology in dogs.[66,69,81] It is teratogenic, so should be avoided in pregnancy.[82]

ANTIPROTOZOAL DRUGS FOR TREATMENT OF CHAGAS' DISEASE

Amiodarone

The combination of the antiarrhythmic amiodarone and an azole (itraconazole or posaconazole) has synergistic antiprotozoal activity against *T. cruzi*, and amiodarone has shown promise as an effective treatment for arrhythmias associated with chronic Chagas' disease in humans.[83] Amiodarone is a cationic lipophilic benzofuran. It is a class III antiarrhythmic that prolongs the action potential duration and the refractory period by inhibiting the repolarizing potassium channel. It also inhibits voltage-gated calcium channels. It is highly protein bound and lipophilic, with a high volume of distribution. Its antiprotozoal effects are the result of inhibition of calcium homeostasis, blockade of the action of the protozoal protease known as cruzipain, and inhibition of sterol production. It also has activity against *Leishmania* spp. and is an emerging treatment for human leishmaniasis, together with a related analogue, dronedarone. When used in a prospective, randomized trial in combination with itraconazole (10 mg/kg PO q24h) to treat dogs with naturally occurring Chagas' disease (7.5 mg/kg PO q24h), there was a significant reduction in mortality, clinical signs (such as lethargy and anorexia), electrocardiogram abnormalities, parasitemia, and overall survival time.[84] Adverse effects were primarily gastrointestinal and were associated with high plasma concentrations of itraconazole. Reduction of the itraconazole dose to attain plasma concentrations of 1 to 2 μg/mL was associated with resolution of adverse effects. Overall, the investigators reported that the combination was well tolerated.

Benznidazole

Benznidazole is a nitroimidazole that is used to treat acute Chagas' disease (see Chapter 100). It has been used alone and in combination with itraconazole, which may increase efficacy.[85] When used to treat chronic infections, although parasitemia is initially suppressed and systolic dysfunction controlled, the development of cardiomyopathy appears to be unaffected.[86] Benznidazole is activated by a parasite-specific nitroreductase to produce toxic metabolites.[87] Resistance can result from reduction in the level of activity of the nitroreductase and confers cross-resistance to nifurtimox.

Benznidazole is lipophilic, is readily absorbed from the gastrointestinal tract, and undergoes hepatic metabolism. In the United States, it is available from the CDC. The main adverse effect of treatment in dogs is vomiting. In human patients, it can cause skin rashes, peripheral neuropathy, and less commonly bone marrow suppression. It also has the potential to be carcinogenic.

Nifurtimox

Nifurtimox is a nitrofuran derivative used to treat Chagas' disease in humans. It has limited efficacy, with 70% parasitologic cure for acute disease and at best 20% for chronic disease. As with benznidazole, metabolic reduction of the nitro group by a trypanosome-specific nitroreductase leads to the formation of toxic metabolites. In human patients, it is well absorbed orally and undergoes hepatic metabolism. Gastrointestinal and neurologic signs are the primary adverse effects of nifurtimox, and like benznidazole, it has carcinogenic properties.[88] Severe adverse effects have precluded the use of nifurtimox in dogs.[89]

SUGGESTED READINGS

Reguera RM, Morán M, Perez-Pertejo Y, et al. Current status on prevention and treatment of canine leishmaniasis. *Vet Parasitol.* 2016;227:98–114.

Baneth G. Antiprotozoal treatment of canine babesiosis. *Vet Parasitol.* 2018;254:58–63.

Davis JL, Gookin JL. Antiprotozoan drugs. In: Riviere JE, Papich MG, eds. *Veterinary Pharmacology and Therapeutics.* 10th ed. Hoboken, NJ: Wiley Blackwell; 2018:1525.

REFERENCES

1. Saleh MN, Gilley AD, Byrnes MK, et al. Development and evaluation of a protocol for control of *Giardia duodenalis* in a colony of group-housed dogs at a veterinary medical college. *J Am Vet Med Assoc.* 2016;249:644–649.
2. McKellar QA, Galbraith EA, Baxter P. Oral absorption and bioavailability of fenbendazole in the dog and the effect of concurrent ingestion of food. *J Vet Pharmacol Ther.* 1993;16:189–198.
3. Gary AT, Kerl ME, Wiedmeyer CE, et al. Bone marrow hypoplasia associated with fenbendazole administration in a dog. *J Am Anim Hosp Assoc.* 2004;40:224–229.
4. Boyce W, Shender L, Schultz L, et al. Survival analysis of dogs diagnosed with canine peritoneal larval cestodiasis (*Mesocestoides* spp.). *Vet Parasitol.* 2011;180:256–261.
5. Bowman DD, Liotta JL, Ulrich M, et al. Treatment of naturally occurring, asymptomatic *Giardia* sp. in dogs with Drontal Plus flavour tablets. *Parasitol Res.* 2009;105(suppl 1):S125–S134.
6. Stokol T, Randolph JF, Nachbar S, et al. Development of bone marrow toxicosis after albendazole administration in a dog and cat. *J Am Vet Med Assoc.* 1997;210:1753–1756.
7. Fenimore A, Martin L, Lappin MR. Evaluation of metronidazole with and without *Enterococcus faecium* SF68 in shelter dogs with diarrhea. *Top Companion Anim Med.* 2017;32:100–103.
8. Lamp KC, Freeman CD, Klutman NE, et al. Pharmacokinetics and pharmacodynamics of the nitroimidazole antimicrobials. *Clin Pharmacokinet.* 1999;36:353–373.
9. Sarkiala E, Jarvinen A, Valttila S, et al. Pharmacokinetics of tinidazole in dogs and cats. *J Vet Pharmacol Ther.* 1991;14:257–262.
10. Gookin JL, Copple CN, Papich MG, et al. Efficacy of ronidazole for treatment of feline *Tritrichomonas foetus* infection. *J Vet Intern Med.* 2006;20:536–543.
11. Gookin JL, Stauffer SH, Coccaro MR, et al. Efficacy of tinidazole for treatment of cats experimentally infected with *Tritrichomonas foetus*. *Am J Vet Res.* 2007;68:1085–1088.
12. Kather EJ, Marks SL, Kass PH. Determination of the in vitro susceptibility of feline *Tritrichomonas foetus* to 5 antimicrobial agents. *J Vet Intern Med.* 2007;21:966–970.
13. Gookin JL, Hanrahan K, Levy MG. The conundrum of feline trichomonosis. *J Feline Med Surg.* 2017;19:261–274.
14. Gookin JL, Stauffer SH, Dybas D, et al. Documentation of in vivo and in vitro aerobic resistance of feline *Tritrichomonas foetus* isolates to ronidazole. *J Vet Intern Med.* 2010;24:1003–1007.
15. Rosado TW, Specht A, Marks SL. Neurotoxicosis in 4 cats receiving ronidazole. *J Vet Intern Med.* 2007;21:328–331.
16. LeVine DN, Papich MG, Gookin JL, et al. Ronidazole pharmacokinetics after intravenous and oral immediate-release capsule administration in healthy cats. *J Feline Med Surg.* 2011;13:244–250.
17. Grellet A, Makhlouf SE, Desquilbet L, et al. Efficacy of guar gum-based ronidazole capsules as a treatment for *Tritrichomonas foetus* infection in cats. *J Feline Med Surg.* 2017;19:177–184.
18. Muller J, Sterk M, Hemphill A, et al. Characterization of *Giardia lamblia* WB C6 clones resistant to nitazoxanide and to metronidazole. *J Antimicrob Chemother.* 2007;60:280–287.
19. Gookin JL, Levy MG, Law JM, et al. Experimental infection of cats with *Tritrichomonas foetus*. *Am J Vet Res.* 2001;62:1690–1697.
20. Moron-Soto M, Gutierrez L, Sumano H, et al. Efficacy of nitazoxanide to treat natural *Giardia* infections in dogs. *Parasit Vectors.* 2017;10:52.
21. Macintire DK, Vincent-Johnson NA, Kane CW, et al. Treatment of dogs infected with *Hepatozoon americanum*: 53 cases (1989-1998). *J Am Vet Med Assoc.* 2001;218:77–82.
22. Castles TR, Kintner LD, Lee CC. The effects of folic or folinic acid on the toxicity of pyrimethamine in dogs. *Toxicol Appl Pharmacol.* 1971;20:447–459.
23. Baneth G. Antiprotozoal treatment of canine babesiosis. *Vet Parasitol.* 2018;254:58–63.
24. Malmasi A, Mosallanejad B, Mohebali M, et al. Prevention of shedding and re-shedding of *Toxoplasma gondii* oocysts in experimentally infected cats treated with oral clindamycin: a preliminary study. *Zoonoses Public Health.* 2009;56:102–104.
25. Ortega E, Gutierrez L, Bernad MJ, et al. Evaluation of different oral formulations of clindamycin extended release in dogs. *Drug Res.* 2017;67:32–37.
26. Gookin JL, Riviere JE, Gilger BC, et al. Acute renal failure in four cats treated with paromomycin. *J Am Vet Med Assoc.* 1999;215:1821–1823. 1806.
27. Murray HW, Berman JD, Davies CR, et al. Advances in leishmaniasis. *Lancet.* 2005;366:1561–1577.
28. Athanasiou LV, Batzias GC, Saridomichelakis MN, et al. Pharmacokinetics and tolerability of aminosidine after repeated administrations using an optimal dose regimen in healthy dogs and in dogs with leishmaniosis. *Vet Parasitol.* 2014;205:365–370.
29. Athanasiou LV, Saridomichelakis MN, Kontos VI, et al. Treatment of canine leishmaniosis with aminosidine at an optimized dosage regimen: a pilot open clinical trial. *Vet Parasitol.* 2013;192:91–97.
30. Madsen M, Messenger K, Papich MG. Pharmacokinetics of levofloxacin following oral administration of a generic levofloxacin tablet and intravenous administration to dogs. *Am J Vet Res.* 2019;80:957–962.
31. Kirk SK, Levy JK, Crawford PC. Efficacy of azithromycin and compounded atovaquone for treatment of *Babesia gibsoni* in dogs. *J Vet Intern Med.* 2017;31:1108–1112.
32. Birkenheuer AJ, Levy MG, Breitschwerdt EB. Efficacy of combined atovaquone and azithromycin for therapy of chronic *Babesia gibsoni* (Asian genotype) infections in dogs. *J Vet Intern Med.* 2004;18:494–498.
33. Cohn LA, Birkenheuer AJ, Brunker JD, et al. Efficacy of atovaquone and azithromycin or imidocarb dipropionate in cats with acute cytauxzoonosis. *J Vet Intern Med.* 2011;25:55–60.
34. Matsuu A, Koshida Y, Kawahara M, et al. Efficacy of atovaquone against *Babesia gibsoni* in vivo and in vitro. *Vet Parasitol.* 2004;124:9–18.
35. Checa R, Montoya A, Ortega N, et al. Efficacy, safety and tolerance of imidocarb dipropionate versus atovaquone or buparvaquone plus azithromycin used to treat sick dogs naturally infected with the *Babesia microti*-like piroplasm. *Parasit Vectors.* 2017;10:145.
36. Pfefferkorn ER, Borotz SE, Nothnagel RF. Mutants of *Toxoplasma gondii* resistant to atovaquone (566C80) or decoquinate. *J Parasitol.* 1993;79:559–564.
37. Sykes JE, Dubey JP, Lindsay LL, et al. Severe myositis associated with *Sarcocystis* spp. infection in 2 dogs. *J Vet Intern Med.* 2011;25: 1277–1283.
38. De Tommasi AS, Giannelli A, de Caprariis D, et al. Failure of imidocarb dipropionate and toltrazuril/emodepside plus clindamycin in treating *Hepatozoon canis* infection. *Vet Parasitol.* 2014;200:242–245.
39. Vial HJ, Gorenflot A. Chemotherapy against babesiosis. *Vet Parasitol.* 2006;138:147–160.
40. Mathe A, Dobos-Kovacs M, Voros K. Histological and ultrastructural studies of renal lesions in *Babesia canis* infected dogs treated with imidocarb. *Acta Vet Hung.* 2007;55:511–523.
41. Kock N, Kelly P. Massive hepatic necrosis associated with accidental imidocarb dipropionate toxicosis in a dog. *J Comp Pathol.* 1991;104: 113–116.
42. Da Silva AS, Franca RT, Costa MM, et al. Experimental infection with *Rangelia vitalii* in dogs: acute phase, parasitemia, biological cycle, clinical-pathological aspects and treatment. *Exp Parasitol.* 2011;128:347–352.
43. Hwang SJ, Yamasaki M, Nakamura K, et al. Development and characterization of a strain of *Babesia gibsoni* resistant to diminazene aceturate in vitro. *J Vet Med Sci.* 2010;72:765–771.
44. Lewis KM, Cohn LA, Birkenheuer AJ, et al. Pharmacokinetics of diminazene diaceturate in healthy cats. *J Vet Pharmacol Ther.* 2012;35:608–610.

45. Silva ASD, Zanette RA, Wolkmer P, et al. Diminazene aceturate in the control of *Trypanosoma evansi* infection in cats. *Vet Parasitol.* 2009;165:47–50.
46. Echeverria JT, Soares RL, Crepaldi BA, et al. Clinical and therapeutic aspects of an outbreak of canine trypanosomiasis. *Rev Bras Parasitol Vet.* 2019;28:320–324.
47. Wiesner J, Reichenberg A, Heinrich S, et al. The plastid-like organelle of apicomplexan parasites as drug target. *Curr Pharm Des.* 2008;14:855–871.
48. Stock ML, Elazab ST, Hsu WH. Review of triazine antiprotozoal drugs used in veterinary medicine. *J Vet Pharmacol Ther.* 2018;41:184–194.
49. Stephen B, Rommel M, Daugschies A, et al. Studies of resistance to anticoccidials in *Eimeria* field isolates and pure *Eimeria* strains. *Vet Parasitol.* 1997;69:19–29.
50. Altreuther G, Gasda N, Schroeder I, et al. Efficacy of emodepside plus toltrazuril suspension (Procox® oral suspension for dogs) against prepatent and patent infection with *Isospora canis* and *Isospora ohioensis*-complex in dogs. *Parasitol Res.* 2011;109(suppl 1):S9–S20.
51. Altreuther G, Gasda N, Adler K, et al. Field evaluations of the efficacy and safety of Emodepside plus toltrazuril (Procox® oral suspension for dogs) against naturally acquired nematode and *Isospora* spp. infections in dogs. *Parasitol Res.* 2011;109(suppl 1):S21–S28.
52. Daugschies A, Mundt HC, Letkova V. Toltrazuril treatment of cystoisosporosis in dogs under experimental and field conditions. *Parasitol Res.* 2000;86:797–799.
53. Lloyd S, Smith J. Activity of toltrazuril and diclazuril against *Isospora* species in kittens and puppies. *Vet Rec.* 2001;148:509–511.
54. Petry G, Kruedewagen E, Bach T, et al. Efficacy of Procox® oral suspension for dogs (0.1% emodepside and 2% toltrazuril) against experimental nematode (*Toxocara cati* and *Ancylostoma tubaeforme*) infections in cats. *Parasitol Res.* 2011;109(suppl 1):S37–S43.
55. Voyvoda H, Pasa S, Uner A. Clinical *Hepatozoon canis* infection in a dog in Turkey. *J Small Anim Pract.* 2004;45:613–617.
56. Pasa S, Voyvoda H, Karagenc T, et al. Failure of combination therapy with imidocarb dipropionate and toltrazuril to clear *Hepatozoon canis* infection in dogs. *Parasitol Res.* 2011;109:919–926.
57. Litster AL, Nichols J, Hall K, et al. Use of ponazuril paste to treat coccidiosis in shelter-housed cats and dogs. *Vet Parasitol.* 2014;202:319–325.
58. Swinger RL, Schmidt Jr KA, Dubielzig RR. Keratoconjunctivitis associated with *Toxoplasma gondii* in a dog. *Vet Ophthalmol.* 2009;12:56–60.
59. Paila YD, Saha B, Chattopadhyay A. Amphotericin B inhibits entry of *Leishmania donovani* into primary macrophages. *Biochem Biophys Res Commun.* 2010;399:429–433.
60. Cortadellas O. Initial and long-term efficacy of a lipid emulsion of amphotericin B desoxycholate in the management of canine leishmaniasis. *J Vet Intern Med.* 2003;17:808–812.
61. Oliva G, Gradoni L, Ciaramella P, et al. Activity of liposomal amphotericin B (AmBisome) in dogs naturally infected with *Leishmania infantum*. *J Antimicrob Chemother.* 1995;36:1013–1019.
62. Solano-Gallego L, Koutinas A, Miro G, et al. Directions for the diagnosis, clinical staging, treatment and prevention of canine leishmaniosis. *Vet Parasitol.* 2009;165:1–18.
63. Oliva G, Roura X, Crotti A, et al. Guidelines for treatment of leishmaniasis in dogs. *J Am Vet Med Assoc.* 2010;236:1192–1198.
64. Frezard F, Demicheli C, Ribeiro RR. Pentavalent antimonials: new perspectives for old drugs. *Molecules.* 2009;14:2317–2336.
65. Lima MI, Arruda VO, Alves EV, et al. Genotoxic effects of the antileishmanial drug Glucantime. *Arch Toxicol.* 2010;84:227–232.
66. Manna L, Corso R, Galiero G, et al. Long-term follow-up of dogs with leishmaniosis treated with meglumine antimoniate plus allopurinol versus miltefosine plus allopurinol. *Parasit Vectors.* 2015;8:289.
67. Manna L, Reale S, Vitale F, et al. Real-time PCR assay in *Leishmania*-infected dogs treated with meglumine antimoniate and allopurinol. *Vet J.* 2008;177:279–282.
68. Ikeda-Garcia FA, Lopes RS, Ciarlini PC, et al. Evaluation of renal and hepatic functions in dogs naturally infected by visceral leishmaniasis submitted to treatment with meglumine antimoniate. *Res Vet Sci.* 2007;83:105–108.
69. Bianciardi P, Brovida C, Valente M, et al. Administration of miltefosine and meglumine antimoniate in healthy dogs: clinicopathological evaluation of the impact on the kidneys. *Toxicol Pathol.* 2009;37:770–775.
70. Kerby BR, Detke S. Reduced purine accumulation is encoded on an amplified DNA in *Leishmania mexicana amazonensis* resistant to toxic nucleosides. *Mol Biochem Parasitol.* 1993;60:171–185.
71. Yasur-Landau D, Jaffe CL, David L, et al. Resistance of *Leishmania infantum* to allopurinol is associated with chromosome and gene copy number variations including decrease in the S-adenosylmethionine synthetase (METK) gene copy number. *Int J Parasitol Drugs Drug Resist.* 2018;8:403–410.
72. Ling GV, Case LC, Nelson H, et al. Pharmacokinetics of allopurinol in Dalmatian dogs. *J Vet Pharmacol. Ther.* 1997;20:134–138.
73. Ling GV, Ruby AL, Harrold DR, et al. Xanthine-containing urinary calculi in dogs given allopurinol. *J Am Vet Med Assoc.* 1991;198:1935–1940.
74. Fagugli RM, Gentile G, Ferrara G, et al. Acute renal and hepatic failure associated with allopurinol treatment. *Clin Nephrol.* 2008;70:523–526.
75. Kim YW, Park BS, Ryu CH, et al. Allopurinol-induced aplastic anemia in a patient with chronic kidney disease. *Clin Nephrol.* 2009;71:203–206.
76. Plevraki K, Koutinas AF, Kaldrymidou H, et al. Effects of allopurinol treatment on the progression of chronic nephritis in canine leishmaniosis (*Leishmania infantum*). *J Vet Intern Med.* 2006;20:228–233.
77. Miro G, Oliva G, Cruz I, et al. Multicentric, controlled clinical study to evaluate effectiveness and safety of miltefosine and allopurinol for canine leishmaniosis. *Vet Dermatol.* 2009;20:397–404.
78. Manna L, Vitale F, Reale S, et al. Study of efficacy of miltefosine and allopurinol in dogs with leishmaniosis. *Vet J.* 2009;182:441–445.
79. Andrade HM, Toledo VP, Pinheiro MB, et al. Evaluation of miltefosine for the treatment of dogs naturally infected with *L. infantum* (=*L. chagasi*) in Brazil. *Vet Parasitol.* 2011;181:83–90.
80. Woerly V, Maynard L, Sanquer A, et al. Clinical efficacy and tolerance of miltefosine in the treatment of canine leishmaniosis. *Parasitol Res.* 2009;105:463–469.
81. Mateo M, Maynard L, Vischer C, et al. Comparative study on the short term efficacy and adverse effects of miltefosine and meglumine antimoniate in dogs with natural leishmaniosis. *Parasitol Res.* 2009;105:155–162.
82. Reguera RM, Moran M, Perez-Pertejo Y, et al. Current status on prevention and treatment of canine leishmaniasis. *Vet Parasitol.* 2016;227:98–114.
83. Stein C, Migliavaca CB, Colpani V, et al. Amiodarone for arrhythmia in patients with Chagas disease: a systematic review and individual patient data meta-analysis. *PLoS Negl Trop Dis.* 2018;12:e0006742.
84. Madigan R, Majoy S, Ritter K, et al. Investigation of a combination of amiodarone and itraconazole for treatment of American trypanosomiasis (Chagas' disease) in dogs. *J Am Vet Med Assoc.* 2019;255:317–329.
85. Cunha ELA, Torchelsen F, Cunha LM, et al. Benznidazole, itraconazole and their combination in the treatment of acute experimental Chagas' disease in dogs. *Exp Parasitol.* 2019;204:107711.
86. Santos FM, Lima WG, Gravel AS, et al. Cardiomyopathy prognosis after benznidazole treatment in chronic canine Chagas' disease. *J Antimicrob Chemother.* 2012;67:1987–1995.
87. Wilkinson SR, Taylor MC, Horn D, et al. A mechanism for cross-resistance to nifurtimox and benznidazole in trypanosomes. *Proc Natl Acad Sci U S A.* 2008;105:5022–5027.
88. Castro JA, de Mecca MM, Bartel LC. Toxic side effects of drugs used to treat Chagas' disease (American trypanosomiasis). *Hum Exp Toxicol.* 2006;25:471–479.
89. Barr SC. Canine Chagas' disease (American trypanosomiasis) in North America. *Vet Clin North Am Small Anim Pract.* 2009;39:1055–1064 (v–vi).

13

Antiparasitic Drugs

Lindsay A. Starkey, Byron L. Blagburn

KEY POINTS

- When considering choice of antiparasitic drugs, consultation of product labels, package inserts, regulatory documents, and current literature will provide the most up-to-date information regarding product availability and indications.
- Use of an approved product for the relevant host and parasite should be considered as the first-line treatment if available.
- Treatment for some parasitic infections, especially those caused by trematode and protozoan parasites, often requires the extra-label use of an approved drug or the use of a drug not approved for use in dogs and/or cats.
- Appropriate drug selection is only one component of treating parasitism. Use of a multimodal approach with multiple therapeutics that have unique mechanisms of action or alterations of the environment or host behavior is often necessary to appropriately break the life cycle and prevent a reinfection or reinfestation.
- Treatment failure is often due to one or many of a myriad of factors including but not limited to: inadequate dosage, improper storage, abbreviated duration, failure to control reinfection/reinfestation, lack of understanding of the life cycle, poor client compliance/adherence, or parasite resistance. Although resistance has been documented in the United States for a few parasites of dogs and/or cats, treatment failure secondary to any of the other listed reasons is still far more common.

INTRODUCTION

The antiparasitic market continues to grow with the advent of new pharmaceuticals and the combination of existing drugs; however, there still does not exist the single, perfect product to control all things parasite-related. Each patient is an individual, as are clients, therefore, several aspects must be considered in order to select the appropriate product for treatment of parasites or the prevention of common or potentially serious parasites. These include:

- Route of administration of the drug—some clients would prefer to administer a medication that resembles a treat rather than apply a topical product. Others may prefer something that remains on the outside of the animal rather than being administered orally. Topical treatment may be particularly important for animals undergoing a food trial or with specific food allergies. Some clients may like or dislike collars based on previous experience. Additionally, injectable options are available for some parasites and might be preferred by the clinician to control compliance.
- Duration of drug activity—some clients may opt for a longer-acting drug than a shorter-acting drug to reduce stressful interactions or to boost adherence.
- Host species—questions to be considered include: is the drug something that is metabolized differently by dogs versus cats? If using a drug not approved for use in dogs and cats, what are the potential adverse effects to be aware of? Have any adverse effects been reported that are breed-specific?
- Host life stage—is the animal young, geriatric, pregnant, lactating, to be used for breeding, or immunocompromised?
- Concurrent medications—some drugs potentiate the activity of others, while others are antagonistic and might reduce the efficacy of one another.
- Resistance profile—has resistance been reported for this parasite/drug combination; if so, how should efficacy be monitored, and what are other treatment options?
- Target parasites in the region—different parasites vary in their distribution and relative prevalence within the United States, so it is important to discuss local risks as well as the potential for travel-acquired parasites with the client.
- Transmission potential—are the parasites in question potential health hazards to other animals of the same species, different species, or even humans?

In this chapter, common antiparasitic drugs available for dogs and cats within the United States are organized in sections by the type of parasites targeted: helminths (nematodes, cestodes, and trematodes), insects, and acari. Extra-label uses of certain products are included provided there is supportive documentation in the literature. The product insert or label should be consulted, and veterinarians should strive to stay up-to-date on primary literature and regulatory changes regarding these commonly used products.

ANTHELMINTICS (TABLES 13.1–13.3)

Many products labeled for use in dogs and cats provide a broad spectrum of activity against common nematode and cestode parasites of pets, either as a treatment or preventive. However, there are a number of nematode parasites, a few cestodes, and most trematodes for which there is no label-approved treatment. Many anthelmintics can be safely used extra-label in dogs and cats. However, due to safety concerns, and because other treatment options are readily available, standard or elevated doses of large animal anthelmintics should not be used in dogs or cats. What follows is a summary of drug classes available in the United States with their labeled indications. Doses are also provided in Tables 13.1–13.3. Drugs are listed alphabetically by drug class (or drug if it is the only utilized drug within a drug class). Discussion is limited to the anthelmintic properties of these drugs; antiarthropod activity is addressed later in this chapter and antiprotozoal activity is discussed in Chapter 12.

TABLE 13.1 Recommended Treatments for Gastrointestinal and Systemic Nematode Parasites of Dogs and Cats[1–14]

Nemadote Parasites	Drugs	Species	Minimum Target Dose	Route	Frequency, Duration
Gastrointestinal Nematodes					
Ancylostoma spp.	Emodepside (+ praziquantel)	C	3 mg/kg	Transdermal	Once
	Fenbendazole	D, C[b]	50 mg/kg	PO	q24h for 3 days
	Febantel (+ pyrantel/praziquantel)	D	10–15 mg/kg	PO	Once
	Ivermectin	C	24 μg/kg	PO	Monthly
	Milbemycin oxime	D	0.5 mg/kg	PO	Monthly
		C	2 mg/kg	PO	Monthly
	Moxidectin	D	2.5 mg/kg	Transdermal	Monthly
		C	1 mg/kg	Transdermal	Monthly
		D	0.17 mg/kg	SC	q6 months
		D	0.5 mg/kg	SC	q12 months
	Moxidectin (+ fluralaner)	C	2 mg/kg	Transdermal	q2 months
	Pyrantel pamoate	D, C	5 mg/kg	PO	Once
	Selamectin	C	6 mg/kg	Transdermal	Monthly
Baylisascaris procyonis	Fenbendazole[a]	D	50 mg/kg	PO	q24h for 3 days
	Febantel (+ pyrantel/praziquantel)[a]	D	10–15 mg/kg	PO	Once
	Milbemycin oxime[a]	D	0.5 mg/kg	PO	Monthly
	Moxidectin[a]	D	2.5 mg/kg	Transdermal	Monthly
	Piperazine[a]	D, C	55–110 mg/kg	PO	Once, repeat 10 days later
	Pyrantel pamoate[a]	D	5 mg/kg	PO	Once
Physaloptera spp.	Pyrantel pamoate[a]	D, C	10–15 mg/kg	PO	q 2 weeks, for 3+ treatments
Spirocerca lupi	Doramectin[a]	D	400 μg/kg	PO or SC	q 1–2 weeks for 12 weeks
	Ivermectin[a]	D	400 μg/kg	PO or SC	q 1–2 weeks for 12 weeks
	Milbemycin oxime[a]	D	0.5 mg/kg	PO	Days 0, 7, 28, then monthly
Strongyloides spp.	Fenbendazole[a]	D, C[b]	50 mg/kg	PO	q24h for 5 days, repeat in 4 weeks
	Ivermectin[a]	D, C	200 μg/kg	SC	once and repeat in 2 weeks
	Ivermectin[a]	D, C	200–800 μg/kg	PO	q24h, twice
Toxocara spp.	Emodepside (+ praziquantel)	C	3 mg/kg	Transdermal	Once
	Fenbendazole	D, C[b]	50 mg/kg	PO	q24h for 3 days
	Febantel (+ pyrantel/praziquantel)	D	10–15 mg/kg	PO	Once
	Milbemycin oxime	D	0.5 mg/kg	PO	Monthly
		C	2 mg/kg	PO	Monthly
	Moxidectin	D	2.5 mg/kg	Transdermal	Monthly
		C	1 mg/kg	Transdermal	Monthly
	Moxidectin (+ fluralaner)	C	2 mg/kg	Transdermal	q2 months
	Piperazine	D, C	55–110 mg/kg	PO	Once, repeat 10 days later
	Pyrantel pamoate	D, C	5 mg/kg	PO	Once
	Selamectin	C	6 mg/kg	Transdermal	Monthly
Toxascaris leonina	Fenbendazole	D, C[b]	50 mg/kg	PO	q24h for 3 days
	Milbemycin oxime	D	0.5 mg/kg	PO	Monthly
		C	2 mg/kg	PO	Monthly
	Moxidectin	D	2.5 mg/kg	Transdermal	Monthly
	Piperazine	D, C	55–110 mg/kg	PO	Once, repeat 10 days later
Trichuris spp.	Fenbendazole	D	50 mg/kg	PO	q24h for 3 days
	Febantel (+ pyrantel/praziquantel)	D	10–15 mg/kg	PO	Once
	Milbemycin oxime	D	0.5 mg/kg	PO	Monthly
	Moxidectin	D	2.5 mg/kg	Transdermal	Monthly

TABLE 13.1 Recommended Treatments for Gastrointestinal and Systemic Nematode Parasites of Dogs and Cats[1–14]—cont'd

Nemadote Parasites	Drugs	Species	Minimum Target Dose	Route	Frequency, Duration
Uncinaria stenocephala	Fenbendazole	D, C[b]	50 mg/kg	PO	q24h for 3 days
	Febantel (+ pyrantel/praziquantel)	D	10–15 mg/kg	PO	Once
	Moxidectin	D	2.5 mg/kg	Transdermal	Monthly
		D	0.17 mg/kg	SC	q6 months
		D	0.5 mg/kg	SC	q12 months
	Pyrantel pamoate	D, C	5 mg/kg	PO	Once
Systemic Nematodes					
Aelurostrongylus abstrusus	Emodepside (+ praziquantel)[a]	C	3 mg/kg	Transdermal	Once
	Fenbendazole[a]	C[b]	20–50 mg/kg	PO	q24h for 5–15 days
	Ivermectin[a]	C	400 µg/kg	SC	Once and again in 2 weeks
	Moxidectin (+ imidacloprid)[a]	C	1 mg/kg	Transdermal	Monthly
	Selamectin[a]	C	6 mg/kg	Transdermal	Monthly
Crenosoma vulpis	Fenbendazole[a]	D	25–50 mg/kg	PO	q24h for 3–14 days
	Febantel (+ pyrantel/praziquantel)[a]	D	10–15 mg/kg	PO	q24h for 7 days
	Milbemycin oxime[a]	D	0.5 mg/kg	PO	Once
Dioctophyme renale	Surgical removal	D			
Dirofilaria immitis (preventative)	Eprinomectin (+ praziquantel)	C	0.5 mg/kg	Transdermal	Monthly
	Ivermectin	D	6 µg/kg	PO	Monthly
		C	24 µg/kg	PO	Monthly
	Milbemycin oxime	D	0.5 mg/kg	PO	Monthly
		C	2 mg/kg	PO	Monthly
	Moxidectin	D	2.5 mg/kg	Transdermal	Monthly
		C	1 mg/kg	Transdermal	Monthly
		D	0.17 mg/kg	SC	q6 months
		D	24 µg/kg	PO	Monthly
		D	0.5 mg/kg	SC	q12 months
	Selamectin	D, C	6 mg/kg	Transdermal	Monthly
Dirofilaria immitis (adulticide)	Melarsomine dihydrochloride	D	2.5 mg/kg	IM	3 injections total: once and then 2 injections 24 hours apart 1 month later
	Doxycycline[a]	D	10 mg/kg	PO	q12h for 4 weeks
	Minocycline[a]	D	5–10 mg/kg	PO	q12h for 4 weeks
Dirofilaria immitis (microfilaricidal)	Ivermectin[a]	D	6 µg/kg	PO	Monthly or more frequently
		D	50 µg/kg	PO	Once
	Levamisole[a]	D	10 mg/kg	PO	q12h for 14 days
	Milbemycin oxime[a]	D	0.5 mg/kg	PO	Monthly
	Moxidectin[c]	D	2.5 mg/kg	Transdermal	Monthly
		D	0.17 mg/kg	SC	q6 months
		D	0.5 mg/kg	SC	q12 months
		D	0.25 mg/kg	PO	Once
Eucoleus spp.	Fenbendazole[a]	D	50 mg/kg	PO	q24h for 14 days
	Milbemycin oxime[a]	D	2 mg/kg	PO	Once
	Moxidectin[a]	D	2.5 mg/kg	Transdermal	Monthly
Filaroides spp.	Fenbendazole[a]	D	50 mg/kg	PO	q24h for 7–21 days
Pearsonema spp.	Fenbendazole[a]	D,C[b]	50 mg/kg	PO	q24h; several doses may be required

[a]Use for these parasites or parasite stages is extra-label.
[b]Use in this host is extra-label.
[c]Only the transdermal formulation is approved for this use, the other 3 moxidectin formulations are extra-label.
NB: Always check package inserts for specific labeled indications and safety information. In some countries, use may be extra-label for some parasites/parasite stages or for some hosts, even if identified as on-label here.
C, cat; *D*, dog; *IM*, intramuscular injection; *PO*, oral; *SC*, subcutaneous injection.

TABLE 13.2 Available Heartworm Prevention Products for Dogs and Cats in the United States[1]

Macrocyclic Lactone Heartworm Preventives	Additional Actives	Species	Route/Duration
Eprinomectin	+ praziquantel	C	Transdermal, monthly[2]
Ivermectin	+ pyrantel	D	PO, monthly[2]
	+ pyrantel/praziquantel	D	PO, monthly
		D, C	PO, monthly
Milbemycin oxime	+ lufenuron	D	PO, monthly[2]
	+ lufenuron/praziquantel	D	PO, monthly
	+ praziquantel	D	PO, monthly
	+ spinosad	D	PO, monthly
		D, C	PO, monthly
Moxidectin	+ imidacloprid	D, C	Transdermal, monthly[2]
	+ pyrantel/sarolaner	D	PO, monthly
		D	Transdermal, monthly
		D	SC, q6 or q12 months
	+ fluralaner	C	Transdermal q2 months
Selamectin	+ sarolaner	C	Transdermal, monthly[2]
		D, C	Transdermal, monthly

NB: Always check package inserts for specific labeled indications and safety information.
C, cat; *D*, dog; *PO*, oral; *SC*, subcutaneous injection.

Benzimidazoles

Benzimidazoles have broad-spectrum label and extra-label indications. They bind to tubulin molecules within parasites, inhibiting microtubule formation and disrupting cell division. They may also block mitochondrial function by inhibiting fumarate reductase. Metabolism occurs within the liver if it occurs at all, elimination is via the bile.[15]

Fenbendazole

Fenbendazole is approved for use in dogs and is commonly used extra-label in cats. It is available as granules for dogs, and several suspension formulations are available for large animals. Bioavailability is increased when administered with food. Reported adverse effects include anorexia, vomiting, diarrhea, lethargy, and ataxia.[1,15]

Labeled indications for fenbendazole include the treatment of roundworms (*Toxocara canis, Toxascaris leonina*), hookworms (*Ancylostoma caninum, Uncinaria stenocephala*), whipworm (*Trichuris vulpis*), and tapeworm (*Taenia pisiformis*) in dogs when administered at the minimum target dose of 50 mg/kg PO q24h for 3 consecutive days.[1]

When fenbendazole is used in an extra-label manner, efficacy has been demonstrated against the nematodes *Aelurostrongylus abstrusus, Ancylostoma tubaeforme, Baylisascaris procyonis, Crenosoma vulpis, Eucoleus* spp., *Filaroides* spp., *Pearsonema* spp., *Strongyloides* spp., *T. leonina, Toxocara cati*, and *U. stenocephala* (see Table 13.1). For cestodes, efficacy has been demonstrated for *Mesocestoides* spp. tetrathyridial infection and other *Taenia* spp.; for trematodes, fenbendazole has efficacy against *Heterobilharzia americana, Nanophyetus salmincola*, and *Paragonimus kellicotti*[16–21] (see Table 13.3).

Fenbendazole has a wide margin of safety and is safe to use in pregnant and lactating animals, even for extended durations of time.[15] It is commonly used to mitigate the transmission of hookworm and roundworm infections in dogs from the pregnant bitch to puppies when dosed daily at a minimum target dose of 50 mg/kg, PO q24h, from day 40 of gestation through day 14 of lactation.[22]

Febantel

Febantel is a prodrug which is metabolized to both fenbendazole and oxfendazole within the host. It is not intended for use in pregnant animals, and use in cats is extra-label. Adverse effects include vomiting, diarrhea, transient salivation, and anorexia. Febantel is available as a tablet in combination with pyrantel pamoate and praziquantel.[1,15]

Labeled indications for febantel (in combination with pyrantel pamoate and praziquantel) include the treatment of roundworms (*T. canis, T. leonina*), hookworms (*A. caninum, U. stenocephala*), whipworms (*T. vulpis*), and tapeworms (*Dipylidium caninum, T. pisiformis*, and *Echinococcus* spp.) in dogs when administered at a minimum target dose of 10–15 mg/kg PO once.[1] This product has also been used extra-label for the treatment of *C. vulpis* infections (see Table 13.1).[2]

There is increasing evidence that the canine hookworm, *A. caninum* may be developing resistance to all approved canine anthelmintic classes (benzimidazoles, macrocyclic lactones, and pyrantel pamoate).[23,24] Research is currently focused on resistance biomarkers as well as development of an appropriate alternative treatment strategy. It is important to rule out opportunities for reinfection as a result of "larval leak", whereby parasite stages are released from the musculature or from a fecal-contaminated environment that contains infective hookworm larvae. Should ova be present on fecal flotation approximately 10 to 14 days following anthelmintic administration, adult parasites may not have died from anthelmintic treatment, which may be an indicator of a resistant population. Should ova be absent, the adult population was likely removed, therefore, resistance is unlikely.[23,24]

Emodepside

Emodepside is a cyclic depsipeptide. Cyclic depsipeptides bind to presynaptic latrophilin-like receptors in the pharynx and body wall muscle of nematodes resulting in flaccid paralysis and subsequent worm death.[1] Emodepside is only approved for use in cats in the United States as a transdermal (topical) product in combination with praziquantel.[1] Adverse effects include licking, excessive grooming, hypersalivation, lethargy, agitation, vomiting, diarrhea, eye irritation, respiratory irritation, tremors, ataxia, and erythema or alopecia at the application site. It also may interfere

TABLE 13.3 Recommended Treatments for Gastrointestinal and Systemic Platyhelminth Parasites of Dogs and Cats in the United States[2,16–21,25–27]

Platyhelminth Parasites	Drugs	Species	Minimum Target Dose (mg/kg)	Route	Frequency, Duration
Intestinal Cestodes					
Dipylidium caninum	Epsiprantel	D	5.5	PO	Once
		C	2.75	PO	Once
	Nitazoxanide[a]	D, C	100	PO	Once
	Praziquantel	D, C	5	PO or SC	Once
	Praziquantel (+ emodepside)	C	12	Transdermal	Once
	Praziquantel (+ eprinomectin)	C	10	Transdermal	Monthly
Dibothriocephalus (Diphyllobothrium) spp.	Praziquantel[a]	D, C	25	PO or SC	q24h for 2 days
Echinococcus spp.	Epsiprantel[a]	D	5.5	PO	Once
		C	2.75	PO	Once
	Praziquantel[a]	D, C	5	PO or SC	Once
	Praziquantel[a] (+ emodepside)	C	12	Transdermal	Once
	Praziquantel (+ eprinomectin)	C	10	Transdermal	Monthly
Mesocestoides spp.	Praziquantel[a]	D, C	5	PO or SC	Once
Spirometra spp.	Praziquantel[a]	D, C	25	PO or SC	q24h for 2 days
Taenia spp.	Epsiprantel	D	5.5	PO	Once
		C	2.75	PO	Once
	Fenbendazole	D, C[b]	50	PO	q24h for 3 days
	Nitazoxanide[a]	D, C	100	PO	Once
	Praziquantel[a]	D, C	5	PO or SC	Once
	Praziquantel (+ emodepside)	C	12	Transdermal	Once
	Praziquantel[a] (+ eprinomectin)	C	10	Transdermal	Monthly
Systemic Cestodes					
Dibothriocephalus (Diphyllobothrium) or *Spirometra* spp. (sparganosis)	Praziquantel[a]	D	25	PO or SC	q24h for 2+ days
Mesocestoides spp. (tetrathyridial infection)	Fenbendazole[a]	D	100	PO	q12h for 28 days
Intestinal Trematodes					
Alaria spp.	Praziquantel[a]	D, C	5	PO or SC	Once
Nanophyetus salmincola	Fenbendazole[a]	D	50	PO	q24h for 10–14 days
	Praziquantel[a]	D, C	20–30	PO or SC	Once
Platynosomum fastosum	Praziquantel[a]	C	20	IM	q24h for 3 days
Systemic Trematodes					
Heterobilharzia americana	Fenbendazole[a]	D	50	PO	q24h for 10+ days
	Praziquantel[a]	D	25	PO	q8h for 2+ days
Paragonimus kellicotti	Fenbendazole[a]	D	50	PO	q24h for 10+ days
	Praziquantel[a]	D	25	PO	q8h for 3 days

[a]Use may be extra-label.
[b]Use in this host is extra-label.
NB: Always check package inserts for specific labeled indications and safety information. In some countries, use may be extra label for some parasites/parasite stages or for some hosts, even if identified as on-label here.
C, cat; *D*, dog; *IM*, intramuscular injection; *PO*, oral; *SC*, subcutaneous injection.

with fetal development, therefore, should be used with caution in pregnant animals.[1,15]

Labeled indications (of the combination product with praziquantel) include the treatment of larval and adult stages of *A. tubaeforme* and *T. cati* when dosed at a minimum target dose of 3 mg/kg applied transdermally (topically) once. The combination with 12 mg/kg of praziquantel extends the labeled indications to include *D. caninum* and *Taenia taeniaeformis*.[2] When used extra-label, emodepside is effective for treatment of *A. abstrusus* infections in cats when dosed at the normal 3 mg/kg dose.[3]

Isoquinolones

Isoquinolones attack the parasite neuromuscular junction and the tegument resulting in increased cell membrane permeability to calcium, loss

TABLE 13.4 **Recommended Treatments for Insects of Dogs and Cats in the United States**[1,28,29]

Insects	Compounds	Species	Route	Frequency
Fleas	Adulticides:			
	Afoxolaner	D	PO	q 4 weeks
	Deltamethrin	D	CO	q 6 months
	Dinotefuran	D, C	TO, SP	q 4 weeks q 2+ weeks
	Fipronil	D, C	TO, SP	q 4 weeks
	Fluralaner	D, C	PO, TD	q 8 or 12 weeks
	Imidacloprid	D, C	TO, CO	q 4 weeks, q 8 months
	Indoxacarb	D, C	TO	q 4 weeks
	Lotilaner	D, C	PO	q 4 weeks
	Nitenpyram	D, C	PO	daily
	Sarolaner	D, C	PO, TD	q 4 weeks
	Selamectin	D, C	TD	q 4 weeks
	Spinetoram	C	TD	q 4 weeks
	Spinosad	D	PO	q 4 weeks
	Insect Growth Regulators:			
	Pyriproxyfen	D, C	TO	q 4 weeks
	S-methoprene	D, C	TO	q 4 weeks
	Insect Development Inhibitor:			
	Lufenuron	D, C	PO, SC	q 4 weeks, q 6 months
Flies	Deltamethrin	D	CO	q 6 months
	Permethrin	D	TO	q 4 weeks
Lice	Dinotefuran	D, C[b]	TO	q4 weeks
	Fipronil	D, C	TO, SP	q4 weeks
	Imidacloprid	D, C	TO	q4 weeks
	Selamectin[a]	D, C	TD	q4 weeks

[a]Use for these parasites is extra-label.
[b]Use in this host is extra-label.
Only compounds approved for use on animals by the EPA or FDA are included. NB: Always check package inserts for specific labeled indications and safety information. In some countries, use may be extra-label for some parasites/parasite stages or for some hosts, even if identified as on-label here.
C, cat; *CO,* collar; *D,* dog; *PO,* oral; *SC,* subcutaneous injection; *SP,* spray; *TD,* transdermal; *TO,* topical spot-on.

of intracellular calcium, and instantaneous contraction and paralysis. The tegument also experiences vacuolization and destruction. Adverse effects include vomiting, especially when given at high doses.[1,15]

Epsiprantel

Following oral administration, systemic absorption of epsiprantel is minimal. Subsequently, it is eliminated unchanged in the feces. Safety in pregnant animals has not been evaluated, but given the poor systemic absorption, safety in pregnant animals is likely.[15] Epsiprantel is available as a tablet with label indications for the treatment of *D. caninum* and *Taenia* spp. infections in dogs and cats (see Table 13.3).[1,16] Extra-label use against additional adult tapeworm species (such as *Echinococcus* spp. and *Mesocestoides* spp.) would be expected at labeled doses.[16]

Praziquantel

Praziquantel is completely absorbed following oral administration and is rapidly distributed, including across the blood-brain barrier. It is metabolized in the liver and predominantly excreted via the kidney. Praziquantel is safe in pregnant animals.[15] Oral, transdermal (topical), and injectable formulations are approved for treatment of common tapeworms, including *D. caninum, Taenia* spp., and/or *Echinococcus* spp. in dogs and/or cats in the United States.[1]

A variety of other praziquantel combination products are also available (in which the dose of praziquantel ranges 5–12 mg/kg as the minimum target dose). These are labeled for treatment of any or all of the following: *D. caninum, Taenia* spp., and/or *Echinococcus* spp. infections.[1] Praziquantel has been used extra-label in the treatment of the following infections: *Alaria* spp., *H. americana, Mesocestoides* spp. adults, *N. salmincola, P. kellicotti, Platynosomum fastosum,* and pseudophyllidean tapeworms (*Dibothriocephalus (Diphyllobothrium)* and *Spirometra* spp.)[2,16–21,25,26] (see Table 13.3). Resistance of *D. caninum* to standard doses of praziquantel has been reported; however, fleas must be completely under control before suspecting resistance is a problem.[30]

Macrocyclic Lactones

The macrocyclic lactones (avermectins and milbemycins) are widely used for prevention of *Dirofilaria immitis* infections (see Table 13.2), but this class of drugs has a broad spectrum of activity against a wide variety of nematodes (see Table 13.1) and arthropods (Table 13.4). Macrocyclic lactones are the by-products of *Streptomyces* spp. bacteria. They act on gamma-aminobutyric acid (GABA) and glutamate-gated chloride channels, which triggers an influx of chloride ions and the hyperpolarization of neurons, with subsequent paralysis and death. Metabolism does not occur and the drugs are excreted in the feces.[15] Adverse effects include vomiting, diarrhea, lethargy, hypersalivation, ataxia, brady/tachycardia, sinus arrhythmia, seizures, blindness, tremors, dehydration, depression, hyperthermia, coma, and death.[1,15] Signs of toxicity have been treated with supportive care and administration of physostigmine (to dogs) and neostigmine (to cats). Lipid emulsion infusion has also been used.[1]

All of the formulations approved for use in dogs are safe in dogs known to have the MDR1/ABCB1-1Δ mutation; however, higher doses should not be used in an extra-label manner, particularly in dog breeds in which this mutation has been more commonly described.[1,31]

Resistant biotypes of *D. immitis* are now circulating in naturally infected dogs, and all available macrocyclic lactone-based heartworm prevention products (with the exception of the feline product that contains eprinomectin) have failed in experimental studies when challenged with a known resistant *D. immitis* biotype. That being said, lack of compliance is still the primary consideration for apparent failure of efficacy of preventive products. Preventive products are still highly effective for prevention of adult heartworm infection and subsequent disease in dogs and cats.[32]

Eprinomectin

Eprinomectin is approved for use in cats in a transdermal (topical) formulation in combination with praziquantel. Eprinomectin is labeled for prevention of heartworm disease caused by *D. immitis*, adult and larval *T. cati* and *A. caninum*, and adult *Ancylostoma braziliense* infections when dosed at a minimum target dose of 0.5 mg/kg transdermally (topically) on a monthly basis in cats. The combination with praziquantel (minimum target dose of 10 mg/kg) extends the labeled indications to cover *D. caninum* and *E. multilocularis*.[1] This product should not be administered orally and has not been evaluated in pregnant animals.[1]

Ivermectin

Ivermectin is approved for use in dogs and cats at a minimum target dose of 6 μg/kg in dogs and 24 μg/kg in cats for the prevention of heartworm disease caused by *D. immitis* when administered PO on a monthly basis.[1] The higher dose in the cat product extends the labeled indications to include *A. tubaeforme*.[1] No teratogenesis was noted in pregnant animals when administered at four times the recommended dose.[15] Elevated doses of large animal formulations of ivermectin should not be used extra-label in dogs or cats. Adverse events consistent with ivermectin toxicity have been reported when the dose is increased above the label recommendation and combined with spinosad.[15,33,34]

Milbemycin Oxime

Milbemycin oxime is approved as a monthly oral tablet for dogs and cats. This drug is also available in combination with other active ingredients, lufenuron with or without praziquantel or spinosad, which can extend the labeled indications to include flea immature stages +/- tapeworms or adult fleas, respectively.[1,15] Milbemycin oxime at a minimum target dose of 0.5 mg/kg PO in dogs and 2 mg/kg PO in cats is indicated for the prevention of heartworm disease, treatment of *Ancylostoma* spp. and *Toxocara* spp. infections in dogs and cats, and *T. leonina* and *T. vulpis* infection in dogs.[1] Milbemycin oxime is safe for use in pregnant animals[1,15] and the oral formulation has been used extra-label for the treatment of *B. procyonis, C. vulpis, Demodex* spp., *D. immitis microfilaria, Eucoleus* spp., and *Spirocerca lupi*.[2,5,8,9] Outside the United States, milbemycin oxime has been combined with afoxolaner as a monthly broad spectrum parasite control product.[35]

Moxidectin

Moxidectin is available in three formulations: sustained-release injection, transdermal (topical), and oral.[1] All three formulations are approved for use as heartworm preventives. The sustained-release injection is also effective against existing hookworm infections.[1] Additional approved indications (please see product labels) for transdermal (topical) moxidectin in dogs include treatment of *D. immitis* circulating microfilariae in heartworm-positive dogs, sarcoptic mange mites, hookworms, ascarids, and whipworms. Imidacloprid has been added to extend the label claim to include fleas as well. There are two approved formulations of transdermal (topical) moxidectin available for cats. In addition to heartworm prevention, the product containing 1 mg/kg of moxidectin (+ imidacloprid) is labeled for ear mites, roundworms, hookworms, and fleas, while the product containing 2 mg/kg of moxidectin (+ fluralaner) is labeled for roundworms, hookworms, fleas, and ticks.[1] Extra-label uses of transdermal moxidectin products include *A. abstrusus* in cats, *B. procyonis* in dogs, several mites in dogs and cats, and *Eucoleus* spp. in dogs.[2,5,9,36–40] Oral moxidectin is available, in combination with pyrantel and sarolaner.[1]

Selamectin

Selamectin is approved as a monthly transdermal (topical) product for dogs and cats and is available alone or, for cats, in combination with sarolaner for added flea and tick control.[1,15] Labeled efficacy (please see product labels) includes prevention of heartworm disease, fleas, and ear mites. In cats, transdermal selamectin is also effective against hookworms and ascarids. In dogs, the label also includes treatment of *Sarcoptes scabiei* and *Dermacentor variabilis*.[1]

Melarsomine Dihydrochloride

Melarsomine dihydrochloride is an organoarsenical compound that inactivates parasite enzyme systems. It is only approved for use in dogs for the treatment of adult *D. immitis* as an IM injection.[2] It should not be given SC or IV. Following injection, it is rapidly absorbed and subsequently rapidly eliminated via the bile and kidneys.[15] Melarsomine dihydrochloride has a narrow therapeutic window and reported adverse effects include injection site reactions, increased liver enzyme activity, cough, gagging, lethargy, anorexia, fever, pulmonary congestion, and vomiting.[1,15] Dimercaprol can be used as an antidote in the case of an overdose. Safety has not been determined in pregnant animals.[15]

Melarsomine dihydrochloride is labeled to kill adult (> approximately 4-month-old) *D. immitis* when given as a series of IM injections. Both a two- and three-injection protocol are approved, however, both the American Heartworm Society and the CAPC recommend the three-injection protocol (2.5 mg/kg IM deep into the epaxial muscles, once on day 0 followed by two injections 24 hours apart 1 month later).[1,41,42] Heartworm treatment is often accompanied by adjunct therapies such as doxycycline or minocycline, glucocorticoids, exercise restriction, heartworm prevention, and a microfilaricidal treatment (if needed) (see Chapter 111).[11,41]

Nitazoxanide

Nitazoxanide is not approved for use in dogs and cats. It is available as tablets or a powder that can be mixed with water.[15] It is effective for treatment of refractory tapeworm infections (*D. caninum* or *Taenia* spp.) when used at a minimum target dose of 100 mg/kg PO once.[27] It is also used extra-label for the treatment of protozoal infections of dogs and cats (see Chapter 12 for more information on nitazoxanide).

Piperazine

Piperazine acts at the neuromuscular junction as a GABA agonist, resulting in worm paralysis. Its spectrum of activity is limited to roundworms. It is rapidly absorbed following oral administration and is excreted through the kidneys. Adverse effects include diarrhea, vomiting, and ataxia. No additional adverse effects have been noted when used in pregnant animals. Piperazine is available as a solution, soluble powder, and tablets.[15] Label indications for this parasiticide include the treatment for *Toxocara* spp. infections in dogs and cats with doses that range from 55 to 110 mg/kg PO.[1]

TABLE 13.5 Recommended Treatments for Ticks and Mites of Dogs and Cats in the United States[1,28,36–40,43,52]

Acari	Compounds	Species	Route	Frequency
Ticks (species)	Afoxolaner (Aa, Dv, Is, Rs)	D	PO	q 4 weeks
	Amitraz (NS)	D	CO	q 3 months
	Cyphenothrin (NS)	D	TO	q 4 weeks
	Deltamethrin (NS)	D	CO	q 6 months
	Etofenprox (NS)	C	TO	q 4 weeks
	Fipronil (NS)	D, C	TO, SP	q 4 weeks
	Flumethrin (NS)	D, C	CO	q 8 months
	Fluralaner (Aa, Dv, Is, Rs)	D	PO, TD	q 8 weeks (Aa), q 12 weeks (Dv, Is, Rs)
	Fluralaner (Dv, Is)	C	TD	q 8 weeks (Dv), q 8 or 12 weeks (Is)
	Isopropyl myristate (NS)	D, C	TO	as needed
	Lotilaner (Aa, Dv, Is, Rs)	D	PO	q 4 weeks
	Lotilaner (Is)	C	PO	q 4 weeks
	Permethrin (NS)	D	TO	q 4 weeks
	Sarolaner (Aa, Am, Dv, Is, Rs)	D	PO	q 4 weeks
	Sarolaner (Am, Dv, Is)	C	TD	q 4 weeks
	Selamectin (Dv)	D	TD	q 4 weeks
Mites (species)	Afoxolaner[a] (Ss, Oc, D)	D	PO	q 4 weeks
	Fipronil (Ss)	D	TO, SP	q 4 weeks
	Fluralaner[a] (Ss, Oc, D)	D, C	PO, TD	q 12 weeks
	Ivermectin (D)	D	PO	daily
	Ivermectin (Oc)	D, C	OT	once, repeat if needed
	Lotilaner[a] (Ss, D)	D	PO	q 4 weeks
	Milbemycin oxime	D	PO	daily
	Milbemycin oxime (Oc)	D, C	OT	once, repeat if needed
	Moxidectin (Ss, Oc, D[a])	D, C	TD	q 4 weeks (q 1–2 weeks for D)
	Sarolaner[a] (Ss, Oc, D)	D, C	PO, TD	q 4 weeks
	Selamectin (Ss, Oc)	D, C	TD	q 4 weeks (q 2 weeks for Ss)

[a]Use for these parasites is extra-label. Only compounds approved for use on animals by the EPA or FDA are included.
NB: Always check package inserts for specific labeled indications and safety information.
Aa, Amblyomma americanum; *C*, cat; *CO*, collar; *D*, dog; *D, Demodex* spp.; *Dv, Dermacentor variabilis*; *Is, Ixodes scapularis*; *NS*, not specified; *Oc, Otodectes cynotis*; *OT*, otic instillation; *PO*, oral; *Rs, Rhipicephalus sanguineus*; *SP*, spray; *Ss, Sarcoptes scabiei*; *TD*, transdermal; *TO*, topical spot-on.

Pyrantel pamoate

Pyrantel pamoate is a tetrahydropyrimidine that works as a nicotinic agonist at the neuromuscular junction, which results in muscle contraction followed by paralysis. It is poorly absorbed following oral administration, which accounts for its wide margin of safety. This product is safe to use in pregnant animals as well as very young animals. Excretion is mostly as unchanged drug in the feces. Tablets, chewables, and an oral suspension are available formulations for dogs and cats.[15] It is also available as a component of several combination products.[1]

Labeled indications in dogs and/or cats include treatment of *Ancylostoma* spp., *Toxocara* spp., *T. leonina*, and *Uncinaria* spp. infections when dosed at a minimum target dose of 5 mg/kg PO once.[1] An extra-label use includes the treatment of *B. procyonis* infections at the labeled dose of 5 mg/kg PO once in dogs.[5] Treatment for *Physaloptera* spp. in dogs and cats can be achieved using a minimum target dose of 10–15 mg/kg PO every 2 weeks for three or more treatments.[12]

ECTOPARASITICIDES

As for other parasiticides, the list of available products for the treatment of ectoparasites in dogs and cats continues to grow, although the market has recently seen the discontinuation or continued decline in use of some long-standing products used historically.[1,28] As new molecules are identified, the introduction of combination products with broader spectra of activity will likely follow. Documented resistance among fleas and/or ticks has been described for a number of currently approved compounds including carbamates, organophosphates, synthetic pyrethroids, and fipronil.[53–55] Decreased efficacy compared with historical data has also been shown in fleas with selamectin.[56] What follows is an alphabetical listing of drugs and/or drug classes used for the treatment of ectoparasites in dogs and/or cats. Doses are listed in Tables 13.4 and 13.5.

Amitraz

Amitraz is a formamidine which works by inhibition of mixed function oxidases and is an octopamine receptor agonist in arthropods. This results in hyperactivity and detachment of arthropods as well as reduced fecundity, oviposition, and egg hatchability. It functions mostly on acari (mites and ticks) and less so on insects. Adverse effects in dogs include transient sedation, lethargy, pruritus, gastrointestinal stasis and ileus, bradycardia, hypothermia, hypotension, hyperglycemia, hyperexcitability, respiratory depression, mydriasis, shock, disorientation, ataxia, tremors, coma, and seizures. Adverse effects can be offset by using yohimbine and atipamezole. Caution is recommended when using amitraz in diabetic animals as it can contribute to hyperglycemia. Caution is also recommended in pregnant animals. Amitraz is not for use in cats.[15]

Historically, a number of amitraz-based products such as dips and spot-ons were available for use in dogs; however, the only remaining amitraz product available for use in dogs in the United States is the amitraz 3-month collar for ticks (9%).[28]

Botanicals

Botanicals are molecules with insecticidal properties that are derived from plant materials and include rotenone, limonene, and the pyrethrins.[57–59] Various formulations for dogs and/or cats exist including shampoos, sprays, and dips. Rotenone, available as an ointment, is derived from plant roots and acts to inhibit mitochondrial respiratory enzymes. Limonene is a naturally occurring cyclic terpene derived from citrus fruit. Although reportedly noncarcinogenic with a low oral toxicity, in higher concentrations limonene causes dermal irritation. It is available as a medicated shampoo. Pyrethrin botanicals are derived from the plant *Chrysanthemum cinerariaefolium*. They interfere with neurotransmission by disrupting the transport of sodium and potassium ions, are rapidly biodegradable, and do not possess persistent activity. Pyrethrins are available as dips, shampoos, and sprays.[57–59]

Carbamates and Organophosphates

The carbamates and organophosphates (OPs) were historically used before the advent of newer, safer molecules with equivalent spectra of activity.[58,59] However, these compounds are still available, particularly as over-the-counter products, and therefore, they will be briefly covered here. They inhibit acetylcholinesterase, resulting in accumulation of acetylcholine at the nerve synapse, and overstimulation of the nerves. Carbamate binding to acetylcholinesterase is reversible, while OPs irreversibly bind the enzyme. Adverse effects include salivation, lacrimation, urination, diarrhea, dyspnea, vomiting, muscle fasciculations, weakness, and paralysis. Atropine can be used to reverse these clinical signs. Additionally, slow administration of pralidoxime (2PAM) can help reduce clinical signs associated with OP toxicity.[58,59] Idiosyncratic reactions have been reported in cats, young and thin animals, and sighthounds. These products may be available in spot-on, spray, powder, dip, and collar formulations for dogs and/or cats. Propoxur is a commonly used carbamate, whereas tetrachlorvinphos, coumaphos, diazinon, phosmet, pirimiphos, dichlorvos, and chlorpyrifos are OPs often included in products for pets.[58,59]

Fipronil

Fipronil is a phenylpyrazole insecticide/acaricide which can kill adult fleas, lice, and ticks. Some formulations are also labeled to control sarcoptic mange.[28,59] Fipronil acts on GABA and glutamate-gated chloride channels in the arthropod nervous system and is available in various formulations including sprays (0.29%) and monthly spot-ons (minimum target dose ranging from 6.01% to 9.8%). This drug is safe for use in dogs and cats and in pregnant animals. Adverse effects include irritation at the site of application and hypersensitivity reactions.[28]

Indoxocarb

Indoxocarb is an oxadiazine prodrug insecticide. Once in the mammalian host, it is metabolized and biotransformed into the decarbomethoxylated form which blocks voltage-gated sodium channels.[60] This drug has adulticidal as well as ovacidal and larvacidal properties against fleas.[61] Adverse effects include skin irritation at the site of application, redness, and pruritus. It should not be administered to pregnant animals. Indoxocarb is available as a spot-on formulation for target dogs and cats (minimum target dose of 15 mg/kg).[61,62]

Insect Development Inhibitors and Insect Growth Regulators

Insect development inhibitors (IDIs) and insect growth regulators (IGRs) exert their effects on the immature stages of fleas: eggs, larvae, and/or early pupae.[63] IDIs such as lufenuron interfere with the formation of chitin. IGRs mimic juvenile hormone, which subsequently interferes with the necessary signaling, thus halting proper development of the insect (e.g., methoprene and pyriproxifen).[63] Due to the unique mechanisms of action on insect-specific molecules, adverse effects are not reported in mammals. As many of these compounds are available in combination with other active ingredients, they should be used according to label recommendations when determining if safe in pregnant or young animals. Resistance to these molecules has not yet been reported. Lufenuron is available as a long-acting injectable preparation (minimum target dose of 10 mg/kg) or in combination with oral monthly heartworm prevention products (minimum target dose of 10 mg/kg).[1] It is excreted unchanged in bile. Methoprene is available as a spot-on, spray, collar, or shampoo formulation (minimum target doses ranging from 8.8% to 11.8%).[28] Its longevity is impacted by ultraviolet rays. Pyriproxyfen is available in combination with other insecticides and/or acaricides (minimum target doses ranging from 0.44% to 11.65%).[28]

Isopropyl Myristate

Isopropyl myristate is the ester of isopropyl alcohol and myristic acid. It acts by dissolving the outer wax layer of ticks, which results in uncontrolled desiccation and tick death. It is available as a spray (50%) for dogs and cats to kill ticks. It can be used as often as needed. Adverse effects include dermal and eye irritation[28]. The ester is also commonly found in a variety of human beauty products.

Isoxazolines

The isoxazolines work by selectively binding to and inhibiting the GABA-gated chloride channels. This results in hyperpolarization and generation of inhibitory postsynaptic potentials. Preferential binding to the GABA channels in insects and acari when compared with mammalian GABA channels results in a wide margin of safety. Reported adverse effects are often gastrointestinal or neurological (hypersalivation, weakness, tremor, ataxia, seizures).[43] The FDA has issued a class-wide statement regarding the potential for all of these drugs to elicit neurological adverse effects.[1] Safety in pregnant animals has not been evaluated for all of these products with the exception of fluralaner, which is reportedly safe to use in pregnant animals.[1] Metabolism of these molecules is minimal, and excretion is primarily through the bile.[43]

Isoxazolines have activity against fleas and ticks; however, the number of species of ticks and duration of activity against specific tick species present on the product label varies (see Table 13.5).[1] Isoxazolines also effectively kill (extra-label) several species of mites (see Table 13.5) as well as biting flies, lice, and mosquitoes (see Table 13.4) when administered according to the normal product regimen and dose.[38,40,44–52] Indeed, isoxazolines are becoming accepted as the treatment of choice for demodectic mange in dogs. Afoxolaner is available as a monthly chewable for dogs, dosed at a minimum target dose of 2.5 mg/kg.[1] Fluralaner is available in both chewable or transdermal formulations for dogs (minimum target dose of 25 mg/kg), and transdermal formulations for cats (minimum target dose of 40 mg/kg). Duration of activity is up to 12 weeks.[1] Lotilaner is available as a monthly chewable for dogs and cats, dosed at a minimum target dose of 20 mg/kg for dogs and 6 mg/kg for cats.[1] Sarolaner is available as a monthly chewable tablet for dogs (minimum target dose of 2 mg/kg) and a monthly transdermal formulation for cats (minimum target dose of 1 mg/kg).[1] Isoxazolines are available alone or, increasingly, in combination with macrocyclic lactones or other anthelmintics to provide broader-spectrum parasite control.

Macrocyclic Lactones

In addition to their efficacy as anthelmintics, macrocyclic lactones can be used to treat ectoparasites. Otic formulations of ivermectin (0.01%) and milbemycin (0.1%) oxime are available for the treatment of *Otodectes cynotis* infestations in cats.[28] Transdermal (topical) moxidectin is labeled for *O. cynotis* in cats and *Sarcoptes scabiei* in dogs,[1] and also is effective extra-label for treatment of *Demodex* spp. in dogs when used every 1–2 weeks.[38,64] Transdermal (topical) selamectin is labeled for treatment of flea adults, flea eggs, and *O. cynotis* infestations in dogs and cats; the dog formulation of selamectin is also labeled for treatment of *S. scabiei* and *Dermacentor variabilis* infestations. Selamectin is also effective extra-label against lice, including *Trichodectes canis* in dogs and *Felicola subrostratus* in cats.[29] Although necessary historically when other options were not available, high-dose, extra-label use of large animal macrocyclic lactone products for treatment of small animal ectoparasites (e.g., demodectic mange) may cause toxicity and is not recommended.[15]

Neonicotinoids

Neonicotinoids act on nicotinic acetylcholine receptors in insects.[65] Receptors in mammals and insects are structurally different; therefore, these compounds can be used safely in dogs and cats with little to no adverse effects. Excretion is primarily via the kidneys. Adverse effects include local erythema at the site of application and hyper salivation. These drugs should be used with caution in pregnant animals. Members of the class include dinotefuran, imidacloprid, and nitenpyram which have insecticidal activity against lice and adult fleas, as well as extra-label activity against additional insect species.[15,28,65] Dinotefuran is available as a spray (0.46%) or in combination with other active ingredients in a spot-on formulation (minimum target dose ranges from 4.95% to 22%). Imidacloprid is available as a daily oral medication (minimum target dose of 0.75 mg/kg) or in combination with other medications as a spot-on or collar (8.8%–10%). Nitenpyram is available as a daily oral product dosed at a minimum target dose of 1 mg/kg.

Spinosyns

Spinosyns are formed as a result of fermentation by the actinomycete *Saccharopolyspora spinosa.* They bind to nicotinic acetylcholine receptors in a location that differs from that of the neonicotinoids and to GABA-gated chloride channels. This activity results in hyperexcitation followed by paralysis in the insects.[66] Adverse effects in companion animals include inactivity, vomiting, inappetence, lethargy, and alopecia, erythema, and pruritis at the site of application. Spinosyns should be used with caution in pregnant animals and animals receiving extra-label (high) doses of ivermectin, because they can inhibit P-glycoprotein resulting in ivermectin toxicity. Spinosad is available as a monthly oral product either alone or with another drug in a broad-spectrum heartworm preventive and intestinal parasite control product (minimum target dose of 30 mg/kg). Spinetoram is available as a monthly 11.2% spot-on for use in cats.

Synthetic pyrethroids

In comparison with natural pyrethrins, synthetic pyrethroids are more potent, have a longer duration of action, and are more stable. These work to initially stimulate and then depress nerve cell function in insects and acari, with the end result being paralysis.[59,66] Adverse effects include skin or mucosal irritation, and for some compounds in cats (e.g., high-concentration permethrin), significant adverse effects include hyperexcitability, lethargy, ataxia, vomiting, tremors, seizures, hypersalivation, and death. Synthetic pyrethroids should be used with caution in pregnant animals and some products should be avoided in cats. A number of pyrethroids (most ending in the suffix –thrin) are available in over-the-counter formulations as spot-ons, collars, and shampoos. The most common ones utilized in dogs and/or cats are cyphenothrin, deltamethrin, etofenprox, flumethrin, and permethrin. Cyphenothrin and deltamethrin are fourth-generation synthetic pyrethroids that are available for use in dogs as a monthly spot-on (minimum target dose of 5.2%)[28] and a 6-month collar (minimum target dose of 4%), respectively. Etofenprox, while not a true synthetic pyrethroid, has the same mechanism of action. It is available as a spot-on (minimum target dose of 15%), spray, or shampoo for dogs and cats. Flumethrin is another fourth-generation synthetic pyrethroid that is available for use in dogs and cats as an 8-month collar (minimum target dose of 4.5%).[67,68] Permethrin is a third-generation synthetic pyrethroid that acts on sodium channels as well as chloride and calcium channels. It acts as a contact repellent as well as an insecticide and acaricide and is available in monthly spot-on formulations or sprays. The high concentration (minimum target dose ranges from 36.08% to 44.88%) in the monthly spot-on formulations is toxic to cats; however, the sprays have a lower concentration which can be tolerated by cats.

Synergists

Synergists inactivate mixed function oxidases such that insects are unable to detoxify insecticidal compounds. They are used to enhance the activity of other insecticidal compounds.[66] Commonly used compounds include piperonyl butoxide and N-octyl bicycloheptene dicarboximide (MGK 264) in a variety of formulations.

SUGGESTED READINGS

Papich MG. *Saunders Handbook of Veterinary Drugs: Small and Large Animal.* 4th ed. St. Louis: Elsevier; 2016.

CAPC. Companion Animal Parasite Council: Parasite Guidelines. https://capcvet.org/guidelines/.

REFERENCES

1. FDA. U.S. Food and Drug Administration: Freedom of Information Summaries; 2019. https://animaldrugsatfda.fda.gov/adafda/views/#/foiDrugSummaries.
2. Conboy G. Helminth parasites of the canine and feline respiratory tract. *Vet Clin North Am Small Anim Pract.* 2009;39:1109–1126.
3. Traversa D, Milillo P, Di Cesare A, et al. Efficacy and safety of emodepside 2.1%/praziquantel 8.6% spot-on formulation in the treatment of feline aelurostrongylosis. *Parasitol Res.* 2009;105(suppl 1):S83–S89.
4. Roberson EL, Burke TM. Evaluation of granulated fenbendazole (22.2%) against induced and naturally occurring helminth infections of cats. *Am J Vet Res.* 1980;41:1499–1502.
5. Bauer C. Baylisascariosis—infections of animals and humans with 'unusual' roundworms. *Vet Parasitol.* 2013;193:404–412.
6. Sivajothi S, Sudhakara RB. Cystitis due to *Capillaria* infection in a dog and its treatment. *J Parasit Dis.* 2017;41:627–628.
7. Paradies P, Iarussi F, Sasanelli M, et al. Occurrence of strongyloidiasis in privately owned and sheltered dogs: clinical presentation and treatment outcome. *Parasit Vectors.* 2017;10:345.
8. Bowman DD, Ulrich MA, Gregory DE, et al. Treatment of *Baylisascaris procyonis* infections in dogs with milbemycin oxime. *Vet Parasitol.* 2005;129:285–290.
9. Segev G, Rojas A, Lavy E, et al. Evaluation of a spot-on imidacloprid-moxidectin formulation (Advocate®) for the treatment of naturally occurring esophageal spirocercosis in dogs: a double-blinded, placebo-controlled study. *Parasit Vectors.* 2018;11:127.
10. Veronesi F, Morganti G, Di Cesare A, et al. A pilot trial evaluating the efficacy of a 10% imidacloprid/2.5% moxidectin spot-on formulation in the treatment of natural nasal capillariosis in dogs. *Vet Parasitol.* 2014;200:133–138.

11. Bowman DD, Atkins CE. Heartworm biology, treatment, and control. *Vet Clin North Am Small Anim Pract*. 2009;39:1127–1158.
12. Campbell KL, Graham JC. *Physaloptera* infection in dogs and cats. *Comp Cont Educat Pract Vet*. 1999;21:299.
13. Paradies P, Buonfrate D, Iatta R, et al. Efficacy of ivermectin to control *Strongyloides stercoralis* infection in sheltered dogs. *Acta Trop*. 2019;190:204–209.
14. Mesquita LR, Rahal SC, Faria LG, et al. Pre-and post-operative evaluations of eight dog following right nephrectomy due to *Dioctophyma renale*. *Vet Q*. 2014;34:167–171.
15. Papich MG. *Saunders Handbook of Veterinary Drugs: Small and Large Animal*. 4th ed. St. Louis: Elsevier; 2016.
16. Conboy G. Cestodes of dogs and cats in North America. *Vet Clin North Am Small Anim Pract*. 2009;39:1075–1090.
17. Peregrine AS. Flukes in Small Animals. Merck Veterinary Manual; 2014. https://www.msdvetmanual.com/digestive-system/gastrointestinal-parasites-of-small-animals/flukes-in-small-animals?query=flukes%20in%20small%20animals
18. Fabrick C, Bugbee A, Fosgate G. Clinical features and outcome of *Heterobilharzia americana* infection in dogs. *J Vet Intern Med*. 2010;24:140–144.
19. Headley SA, Scorpio DG, Vidotto O, Dumler JS. *Neorickettsia helminthoeca* and salmon poisoning disease: a review. *Vet J*. 2011;187:165–173.
20. Kuehn NF. Lung Flukes in Small Animals. Merck Veterinary Manual; 2013. https://www.merckvetmanual.com/respiratory-system/respiratory-diseases-of-small-animals/lung-flukes-in-small-animals.
21. Dubey JP, Miller TB, Sharma SP. Fenbendazole for treatment of *Paragonimus kellicotti* infection in dogs. *J Am Vet Med Assoc*. 1979;174: 835–837.
22. Burke TM, Roberson EL. Fenbendazole treatment of pregnant bitches to reduce prenatal and lactogenic infections of *Toxocara canis* and *Ancylostoma caninum* in pups. *J Am Vet Med Assoc*. 1983;183(9):987–990.
23. Kitchen S, Ratnappan R, Han S, et al. Isolation and characterization of a naturally occurring multidrug-resistant strain of the canine hookworm, *Ancylostoma caninum*. *Int J Parasitol*. 2019;49(5):397–406.
24. Castro PDJ, Kaplan RM. *Persistent Hookworm Infections in Dogs*; 2020. https://files.brief.vet/2020-07/Persistent%20Hookworm%20Infections%20in%20Dogs.pdf.
25. Bowman DD, Frongillo MK, Johnson RC, et al. Evaluation of praziquantel for treatment of experimentally induced paragonimiasis in dogs and cats. *Am J Vet Res*. 1991;52:68–71.
26. Lathroum CN, Shell L, Neuville K, et al. Efficacy of praziquantel in the treatment of *Platynosomum fastosum* in cats with natural infections. *Vet Sci*. 2018;5(2):35.
27. Euzeby J, Prom Tep S, Rossignol JF. Expérimentation des propriétés anthelminthiques de la nitazoxanide chez le chien, le chat et les ovins. *Revue Méd Vét*. 1980;10:687–696.
28. Environmental Protection Agency. Active Ingredient Dockets; 2019. https://www.regulations.gov.
29. Shanks DJ, Gautier P, McTier TL, et al. Efficacy of selamectin against biting lice on dogs and cats. *Vet Rec*. 2003;152:234–237.
30. Jesudoss Chelladurai J, Kifleyohannes T, Scott J, et al. Praziquantel resistance in the zoonotic cestode *Dipylidium caninum*. *Am J Trop Med Hyg*. 2018;99(5):1201–1205.
31. Geyer J, Janco C. Treatment of MDR1 mutant dogs with macrocyclic lactones. *Curr Pharm Biotechnol*. 2012;13(6):969–986.
32. Wolstenholme AJ, Evans CC, Jimenez PD, et al. The emergence of macrocyclic lactone resistance in the canine heartworm, *Dirofilaria immitis*. *Parasitology*. 2015;142(10):1249–1259.
33. Dunn ST, Hedges L, Sampson KE, et al. Pharmacokinetic interaction of the antiparasitic agents ivermectin and spinosad in dogs. *Drug Metab Dispos*. 2011;39(5):789–795.
34. Business Wire. Elanco Announces Comfortis® (Spinosad) for Cats and Small Dogs; 2012. https://www.businesswire.com/news/home/20120824005030/en/Elanco-Announces-Comfortis%C2%AE-spinosad-for-Cats-and-Small-Dogs.
35. EMA. European Medical Agency: Nexgard Spectra; 2019. https://www.ema.europa.eu/en/medicines/veterinary/EPAR/nexgard-spectra.
36. Heine J, Krieger K, Dumont P, et al. Evaluation of the efficacy and safety of imidacloprid 10% plus moxidectin 2.5% spot-on in the treatment of generalized demodicosis in dogs: results of a European field study. *Parasitol Res*. 2005;97(Suppl 1):S89–S96.
37. Mueller RS, Meyer D, Bensignor E, et al. Treatment of canine generalized demodicosis with a spot-on formulation containing 10% imidacloprid and 2.5% moxidectin (Advocate, Bayer Healthcare). *Vet Dermatol*. 2019;20(5–6):441–446.
38. Fourie JJ, Liebenberg JE, Horak IG, et al. Efficacy of orally administered fluralaner (Bravecto™) or topically applied imidacloprid/moxidectin (Advocate®) against generalized demodicosis in dogs. *Parasit Vectors*. 2015;8:187.
39. Short J, Gram D. Successful treatment of *Demodex gatoi* with 10% imidacloprid/1% moxidectin. *J Am Anim Hosp Assoc*. 2015;52(1):68–72.
40. Taenzler J, de Vos C, Roepke RKA, et al. Efficacy of fluralaner plus moxidectin (Bravecto®Plus spot-on solution for cats) against *Otodectes cynotis* infestations in cats. *Parasit Vectors*. 2018;11:595.
41. AHS. *American Heartworm Society: Canine Guidelines*. 2018. https://d3ft8sckhnqim2.cloudfront.net/images/pdf/2018_AHS_Canine_Guidelinesv3.pdf?1561995728.
42. CAPC. Companion Animal Parasite Council: Heartworm; 2016. https://capcvet.org/guidelines/heartworm/.
43. Weber T, Selzer PM. Isoxazolines: a novel chemotype highly effective on ectoparasites. *ChemMedChem*. 2016;11(3):270–276.
44. Beugnet F, Halos L, Larsen D, de Vos C. Efficacy of oral afoxolaner for the treatment of canine generalised demodicosis. *Parasite*. 2016;23:14.
45. Beugnet F, de Vos C, Liebenberg J, et al. Efficacy of afoxolaner in a clinical field study in dogs naturally infested with *Sarcoptes scabiei*. *Parasite*. 2016;23:26.
46. Carithers D, Crawford J, de Vos C, et al. Assessment of afoxolaner efficacy against *Otodectes cynotis* infestations of dogs. *Parasit Vectors*. 2016;9:635.
47. Taenzler J, de Vos C, Roepke RKA, et al. Efficacy of fluralaner against *Otodectes cynotis* infestations in dogs and cats. *Parasit Vectors*. 2017;10:30.
48. Taenzler J, Liebenberg J, Roepke RKA, et al. Efficacy of fluralaner administered either orally or topically for the treatment of naturally acquired *Sarcoptes scabiei* var. *canis* infestation in dogs. *Parasit Vectosr*. 2016;9:392.
49. Six RH, Becskei C, Mazaleski MM, et al. Efficacy of sarolaner, a novel oral isoxazoline, against two common mite infestations in dogs: *Demodex* spp. and *Otodectes cynotis*. *Vet Parasitol*. 2016;222:62–66.
50. Becskei C, De Bock F, Illambas J, et al. Efficacy and safety of a novel oral isoxazoline, sarolaner (Simparica™), for the treatment of sarcoptic mange in dogs. *Vet Parasitol*. 2016;222:56–61.
51. Snyder DE, Wiseman S, Liebenberg JE. Efficacy of lotilaner (Credelio™), a novel oral isoxazoline against naturally occurring mange mite infestation in dogs caused by *Demodex* spp. . *Parasit Vectors*. 2017;10:532.
52. Moog F, Brun J, Bourdeau P, et al. Clinical, parasitological, and serological follow-up of dogs with sarcoptic mange treated orally with lotilaner. *Case Rep Vet Med*. 2021:6639017.
53. Kunz SE, Kemp DH. Insecticides and acaricides: resistance and environmental impact. *Rev Sci Tech*. 1994;13(4):1249–1286.
54. Eiden AL, Kaufman PE, Oi FM, et al. Detection of permethrin resistance and fipronil tolerance in *Rhipicephalus sanguineus* (Acari: Ixodidae) in the United States. *J Med Entomol*. 2015;52(3):429–436.
55. Becker S, Webster A, Doyle RL, et al. Resistance to deltamethrin, fipronil and ivermectin in the brown dog tick, *Rhipicephalus sangineus sensu stricto*, Latreille (Acari: Ixodidae). *Ticks Tick Borne Dis*. 2019;10:1046–1050.
56. Dryden MW, Canfield MS, Bocon C, et al. In-home assessment of either topical fluralaner or topical selamectin for flea control in naturally infested cats in West Central Florida, USA. *Parasit Vectors*. 2018;11(1):422.
57. Coats JR. Risks from natural versus synthetic insecticides. *Annu Rev Entomol*. 1994;39:489–515.
58. Casida JE, Durkin KA. Neuroactive insecticides: targets, selectivity, resistance, and secondary effects. *Annu Rev Entomol*. 2013;58:99–117.
59. Lynn RC, Duquette RA. Antiparasitic Drugs. In: Bowman DD, ed. *Georgis' Parasitology for Veterinarians*. 11th ed. St. Louis, MO: Elsevier; 2021.
60. Wing KD, Andaloro JT, McCann SF, et al. Indoxacarb and the sodium channel blocker insecticides: chemistry, physiology and biology in

insects. In: Gilbert LI, ed. *Comprehensive Molecular Insect Science*. Elsevier; 2005:31–53.
61. Dryden MW, Payne PA, Smith V, et al. Efficacy of indoxacarb applied to cats against the adult cat flea, *Ctenocephalides felis*, flea eggs and adult flea emergence. *Parasit Vectors*. 2013;6:126.
62. Dryden MW, Payne PA, Smith V, et al. Evaluation of indoxacarb and fipronil (s)-methoprene topical spot-on formulations to control flea populations in naturally infested dogs and cats in private residences in Tampa FL. USA. *Parasit Vectors*. 2013;6:366.
63. Rust MK, Hemsarth WL. Intrinsic activity of IGRs against larval cat fleas. *J Med Entomol*. 2017;54:418–421.
64. Arther RG. Mites and lice: biology and control. *Vet Clin North Am Small Anim Pract*. 2009;39:1075–1090.
65. Matsuda K, Buckingham SD, Kleier D, et al. Neonicotinoids: insecticides acting on insect nicotinic acetylcholine receptors. *Trends Pharmacologic Sci*. 2001;22(11):573–580.
66. Beugnet FFranc M. Insecticide and acaricide molecules and/or combinations to prevent pet infestation by ectoparasites. *Trends Parasitol*. 2012;28(7):267–279.
67. Stanneck D, Rass J, Radeloff I, et al. Evaluation of the long-term efficacy and safety of an imidacloprid 10%/flumethrin 4.5% polymer matrix collar (Seresto®) in dogs and cats naturally infested with fleas and/or ticks in multicentre clinical field studies in Europe. *Parasit Vectors*. 2012;5:66.
68. Stanneck D, Kruedewagen EM, Fourie JJ, et al. Efficacy of an imidacloprid/flumethrin collar against fleas and ticks on cats. *Parasit Vectors*. 2012;5:82.

SECTION 3

Principles of Infection Control

Jane E. Sykes, J. Scott Weese

Infection control has typically been a slowly progressing and reactionary field, with incremental changes implemented based on new threats. While less ideal than a proactive approach, it has still led to major changes in routine infectious disease control measures and approaches in veterinary medicine, aimed at reducing disease risks in both patients and veterinary personnel. The emergence of the COVID-19 pandemic added a new dimension and led veterinary clinics across the globe to rethink their infection control practices in order to optimize safety for personnel, with the added focus of people as sources of veterinary occupational infections and reduction of intra-transmission of pathogens between personnel, not just from patients to personnel. The range of activities implemented or enhanced because of COVID-19, such as enhanced personal protective equipment use, distancing, attention to ventilation, better hand hygiene compliance, and enhanced environmental disinfection, undoubtedly also reduced the risk of hospital-associated infections among veterinary patients. This section addresses control of hospital-associated infections as well as control of infectious diseases in cat and dog populations; Chapter 19 addresses the epidemiology and transmission of zoonotic diseases and ways to reduce the risk of these diseases in immunocompromised people. Specific information on the public health risks of each disease is also provided in pathogen-specific chapters, including more information on equivalent human disorders.

Chapter 20 discusses immunization against infectious diseases. Types of vaccines, vaccine handling and administration, factors that influence the immune response to vaccines, serologic testing as a measure of vaccine efficacy, and adverse effects of vaccination are discussed. In addition, the appendix at the end of this book provides suggested immunization schedules for individual pets and shelter animals. The reader is also referred to chapters in Part II for more detailed information on prevention of specific infectious diseases.

14

Cleaning and Disinfection

J. Scott Weese

KEY POINTS

- Disinfection is a process that eliminates many or all microbes, but not bacterial spores, from inanimate objects. It is usually accomplished in hospital environments using liquid chemicals such as quaternary ammonium compounds or accelerated hydrogen peroxide. Proper cleaning is an essential step before disinfection to optimize disinfectant activity, and attention to contact time is also critical.
- *Antisepsis* reduces the number of microbes from living tissue and skin. Disinfectants are rarely used for skin antisepsis because they can cause injury to tissues and skin. Chlorhexidine is an example of a commonly used antiseptic.
- *Sanitation* is the reduction in the number of microorganisms on a surface to a safe level.
- *Sterilization* is the complete elimination of all microbes and can be accomplished in the hospital using techniques such as autoclaving.
- *Germicides* are agents that inactivate microorganisms, and include disinfectants, antiseptics, and sanitizers.
- Veterinarians must be aware of the advantages and disadvantages of different disinfectants, antiseptics, and sterilization processes in order to design and implement an optimal infection control program.
- Veterinarians should also be aware of items that represent environmental sources of pathogens and the optimal methods to disinfect those items.
- For detection of hospital bacterial contamination, routine culturing of the environment is not recommended. Fluorescent tagging methods may be useful for demonstration of efficacy of cleaning. In addition, direct observation may also be helpful to identify gaps in protocols and practices. ATP bioluminescence, which detects adenosine 5′-triphosphate (ATP) production by viable microbes in the environment, is a promising tracer to measure hospital contamination with bacteria.

INTRODUCTION

The hospital environment is not sterile, nor is it expected to be so. The environment, medical equipment, and virtually all other external surfaces are contaminated with a range of microbes, many being potential pathogens. The role of the environmental *microbiota*, the vast population of bacteria, viruses, fungi, Archaea, and parasites that exists in every facility, is hard to define; yet it is clear that the environment can be a source of infection of some situations. This risk varies greatly between different pathogens, with site and patient factors also greatly influencing the risk of disease.

Cleaning involves the removal of all visible organic and inorganic material from objects and surfaces through the use of manual or mechanical processes and detergent or enzymatic solutions (Box 14.1). *Sanitation* is the reduction in the number of microorganisms on a surface to a safe level. Sanitizers do not technically disinfect as they are weakly concentrated and have a limited contact time. These products are generally not used in healthcare settings, rather are used in food and water hygiene. *Disinfection* is the process that eliminates many or all microbes, but not bacterial spores, from inanimate objects. Factors that influence the efficacy of disinfection include the type of microorganism present, their number, the amount and type of organic matter present, the presence of biofilms, and the porosity of the surface to be disinfected. Some disinfectants kill spores with prolonged exposure times. These are known as *chemical sterilants*. When chemical sterilants are used at lower concentrations and for shorter contact times, they can inactivate all microbes except large numbers of bacterial spores, and are known as *high-level disinfectants*. *Low-level disinfectants* inactivate most vegetative bacteria, some fungi, and enveloped viruses, but not bacterial spores. *Intermediate-level disinfectants* inactivate mycobacteria, vegetative bacteria, most viruses, and most fungi.

Antisepsis is the process that reduces the number of microbes from living tissue and skin. Disinfectants are rarely used for skin antisepsis because they can cause injury to tissues and skin. *Germicides* are agents that inactivate microorganisms, and include disinfectants, antiseptics, and sanitizers.

Sterilization refers to complete elimination of all microbes, including bacterial spores, and is accomplished in hospital settings using processes such as pressurized steam, dry heat, ethylene oxide (ETO) gas, or liquid chemicals.

Cleaning, disinfection and sterilization are distinct practices with different goals and approaches. Understanding the differences between these practices is important for designing and implementing a proper environmental control program.

INDICATIONS FOR DISINFECTION AND STERILIZATION

Not all surfaces need to be treated similarly. According to the Spaulding method of classification for human healthcare, items to be sterilized or disinfected can be grouped into *critical*, *semicritical*, and *noncritical* items.[1] Critical items enter tissue or the vascular system, or are devices through which blood flows. These require sterilization before they can be used. Semicritical items are items that contact mucous membranes or nonintact skin, such as endoscopes. These generally require high-level disinfection. Noncritical items are items that contact intact skin, such as stethoscopes. Noncritical items generally require low-level or

BOX 14.1 Cleaning, Disinfection, and Sterilization Definitions

Sterilization	Complete elimination of all microbes, including bacterial spores. Accomplished in hospital settings using processes such as pressurized steam, dry heat, ethylene oxide gas, or liquid chemicals
Disinfection	Elimination of many or most microbes from an inanimate surface High-level disinfection: inactivation of all microbes except bacterial spores Intermediate-level disinfection: inactivation of mycobacteria, vegetative bacteria, most viruses, and most fungi, but not bacterial spores and many nonenveloped viruses Low-level disinfection: inactivation of most vegetative bacteria, some fungi, and enveloped viruses, but not bacterial spores, mycobacteria, or nonenveloped bacteria
Cleaning	Removal of gross debris through the use of manual or mechanical processes and detergent or enzymatic solutions. This results in removal of 90%–95% of the microbial burden

intermediate-level disinfection. However, it is clear that Spaulding's criteria are not absolute. For example, a fork contacts mucous membranes, yet human hospital cutlery does not undergo high-level disinfection. A food bowl would be a similar example in veterinary medicine. Therefore, these criteria should be used for general guidance, but consideration of the likelihood of contamination, the ability to properly clean and disinfect the item, body surfaces that will be exposed, and health status of patients who will be exposed is required to make final decisions on appropriate cleaning and disinfection practices.

CLEANING, SANITATION, DISINFECTION, AND STERILIZATION

Cleaning

Cleaning is the critical first step of disinfection or sterilization. It typically involves the use of water, combined with detergents or enzymatic agents. The physical aspects of cleaning remove the bulk of pathogens, as well as organic debris, leaving a surface that is more amenable to effective disinfection or sterilization, as these can be significantly impacted by the presence of organic debris. Cleaning also removes microorganisms that are resistant to many disinfectants, such as clostridial spores, nonenveloped viruses, and protozoa. Care should be taken when using high-pressure water sources (e.g., water hose or high-pressure washer) as these likely result in particle aerosolization and creates the potential for transmission and environmental contamination.

Cleaning and disinfection are typically two steps. While some products marketed as "cleaner-disinfectants" are available, efficacy data are sparse. A one-step approach is probably effective with a high-quality disinfectant and a relatively clean surface (e.g., a stainless steel examination table with minimal gross contamination), but it is optimistic to assume effective one-step cleaning and disinfection with moderate or high organic loads or with disinfectants that are readily inactivated by organic debris.

Disinfection

Typically, disinfection involves the use of liquid chemicals such as quaternary ammonium compounds or oxidizing agents. It is important to note that disinfection is a chemical process that can be impacted by the presence of organic debris, the type and level of microbial contamination, the concentration and contact time of the disinfectant, the nature of the item (e.g., porous, cracks, or crevices), and the temperature and pH during the disinfection process.

Disinfectants have variable properties that must be considered when selecting an appropriate product. There can be profound differences in spectrum, contact time, surface compatibility, impacts of organic debris, compatibility with cleaners, safety, environmental impacts, and cost (Table 14.1). These factors must be considered when designing a disinfection program for a facility. Ideally, a single disinfectant is used for most or all applications to reduce the likelihood of user error. However, in some situations, "regular" and "enhanced" disinfection practices may be reasonable. For example, a lower-level disinfectant such as a quaternary ammonium compound might be used routinely based on factors such as infection pressure and cost, with a more effective disinfectant (e.g., bleach, accelerated hydrogen peroxide [AHP]) reserved for pre-defined, higher-risk situations (e.g., puppy with diarrhea where parvovirus is a possibility). Clear documentation of cleaning and disinfection practices, including products, dilution, contact time, and lifespan, is required to reduce the risk of errors.

Glutaraldehyde

Glutaraldehyde is a saturated dialdehyde that is noncorrosive and can be used for high-level disinfection of materials that cannot undergo steam sterilization, such as rubber, plastics, and endoscopic equipment. It is not used as a general environment disinfectant.

Glutaraldehyde has broad-spectrum microbicidal activity. Aqueous solutions require activation by alkalinization to a pH of 7.5 to 8.5 for sporicidal activity to occur. When alkalinized, glutaraldehyde is used at a concentration of 2.4% for adequate periods of time, either chemical sterilization or high-level disinfection occurs, depending on the contact time. Contact times of at least 20 minutes (at or above 20°C) are required for high-level disinfection.

Once activated, 2.4% glutaraldehyde solution retains activity for 14 days, provided inadvertent dilution or excessive gross contamination does not occur. The solution is active in the presence of 2% organic matter. Inadvertent dilution can occur when endoscopes that contain fluid within their channels are immersed in the solution. Test strips are available from the manufacturer to monitor the activity of the solution (but not to attempt to extend the solution's expiration date).

Glutaraldehyde irritates mucous membranes of the respiratory and gastrointestinal tracts, so endoscopes must be rinsed properly after disinfection. It can also cause allergic contact dermatitis, but it is not mutagenic or carcinogenic. The wearing of nitrile rubber or butyl rubber gloves is recommended. Because of its relative expense and toxicity, it is not used to disinfect noncritical surfaces.

Ortho-phthalaldehyde (OPA)

OPA is a high-level disinfectant that contains 0.55% 1,2-benzenedicarboxaldehyde. It has excellent microbicidal, including sporicidal, activity, with a relatively short contact time. With a greater activity than glutaraldehyde, no need for activation, stability over a wide pH range, short contact time (12 minutes at or above 20°C, 5 minutes at 25°C), and lack of mucous membrane irritation, OPA is preferable to glutaraldehyde. While nonirritating, it will stain unprotected skin, and requires protective equipment during handling (gloves, eye and mouth protection, fluid-resistant gown) and adequate rinsing after disinfection. OPA is used for disinfection of equipment such as endoscopes. It is not used as an environmental disinfectant.

TABLE 14.1 **Characteristics of Selected Disinfectants**

Disinfectant Category	Activity In The Presence Of Organic Matter	Advantages	Disadvantages	Comments
Alcohols	Rapidly inactivated	Fast-acting No residue Relatively nontoxic	Rapid evaporation	Not appropriate for routine environmental disinfection Primarily used as antiseptics
Aldehydes	Good	Broad spectrum Relatively noncorrosive	Highly toxic	Used as an aqueous solution or as a gas (fumigation)
Chlorhexidine	Rapidly inactivated	Nontoxic	Incompatible with anionic detergents	Not appropriate for environmental disinfection Primarily used for antisepsis
Hypochlorites (bleach)	Rapidly inactivated	Broad spectrum, including spores Inexpensive Easy to access Low cost	Inactivated by cationic soaps/detergents and sunlight Frequent application required Corrosive	Commonly used for enhanced disinfection purposes. Corrosive and noxious properties typically preclude routine use.
Accelerated hydrogen peroxide	Good	Broad spectrum, including spores Shorter contact times Environmentally friendly	Cost	Excellent choice for environmental disinfection
Phenolics	Good	Broad spectrum Noncorrosive Stable in storage	Toxic to cats Unpleasant odor Incompatible with cationic or nonionic detergents	Some residual activity after drying. Little reason to use as an environmental disinfectant.
Quaternary ammonium compounds	Moderate	Stable in storage Nonirritating to skin Low toxicity Low cost Effective at high temperatures and pH	Incompatible with anionic detergents	Commonly used but provides relatively low-level disinfection Some residual activity after drying

Peracetic Acid

Peracetic acid belongs to the peroxygen family of compounds. When used at 50°C to 56°C in a specific peracetic acid reprocessing system, 0.2% solutions achieve sterilization in short time periods (30 to 45 minutes). Peracetic acid is active in the presence of organic matter. It is stable but can be corrosive and causes discoloration of endoscopes over time. Peracetic acid concentrates can cause irritation to mucous membranes and are corrosive to the eye and skin, but 0.2% solutions are generally nonirritating.

Potassium Peroxymonosulfate

Potassium peroxymonosulfate is an oxidizing agent that provides broad-spectrum disinfection, including activity against nonenveloped viruses and bacterial spores. Potassium peroxymonosulfate retains some activity in the presence of organic matter. It is corrosive and can cause serious skin and ocular burns at high concentrations, but ready-to-use solutions are nonirritating and less corrosive than bleach. The solution stains fabric and may damage surfaces, particularly metal, over time if rinsing is not performed. It is commonly used as an environmental disinfectant because of its many good properties; however, the potential for surface damage appears to be greater compared with many other disinfectants.

Hydrogen Peroxide

Hydrogen peroxide (H_2O_2) is a potent oxidizer, but standard H_2O_2 is not a good surface disinfectant because of its susceptibility to inactivation. AHP is an H_2O_2 solution that contains surfactants, an acid, and H_2O_2, providing broad-spectrum disinfection, including efficacy against bacterial spores, nonenveloped viruses, and dermatophytes.[2–4] With relatively short contact times and good activity in the presence of moderate organic loads, AHP has gained popularity as a disinfectant among healthcare institutions. Additionally, AHP has low toxicity, is environmentally friendly, and is compatible with most materials, giving it a combination of efficacy and practical use properties that is probably currently unsurpassed.

Sodium Hypochlorite (Bleach)

Hypochlorite is a potent oxidizing agent that provides broad-spectrum activity, including activity against nonenveloped viruses, bacterial spores, and dermatophytes. Household bleach, which contains 5.25% to 6.15% sodium hypochlorite, is readily available but must be diluted prior to use. The concentration of bleach that is used impacts both the required contact time and the level of disinfection. When used at a 1:10 dilution for a 10-minute contact time, household bleach is sporicidal but is irritating and can be highly corrosive to metal surfaces. For most clinical situations, 1:30 to 1:50 dilutions of household bleach provide more than 1000 ppm available chlorine and are effective for intermediate-level disinfection. Sodium hypochlorite is inactivated by organic matter, so cleaning is required before disinfection is performed. Hypochlorite is also light sensitive. Other disadvantages of bleach solutions are bleaching of colored fabric and the release of toxic chlorine gas when they are combined with other disinfectants such as quaternary ammonium compounds. Bleach is most often used for enhanced disinfection, targeting nonenveloped viruses, bacterial spores, or dermatophytes in response to specific cases or outbreaks. However, cost is probably the only benefit of using bleach rather than AHP.

Quaternary Ammonium Compounds

This class of disinfectants contains numerous different compounds, with generally similar activity. They are commonly used in veterinary clinics but provide relatively low-level disinfection in most situations. Although they are generally fungicidal, bactericidal, and virucidal for enveloped viruses, some bacteria are resistant, and there is little activity against nonenveloped viruses, bacterial spores, or dermatophytes. Some products have claims against nonenveloped viruses, but with higher concentrations and longer contact times. Contact times vary by product, so manufacturer recommendations should be followed; however, 10-minute contact times are often used. Advantages of this class include low cost, high stability, and low toxicity. If used as a primary disinfectant, having a protocol for enhanced disinfection with a more effective disinfectant (e.g., AHP) is needed for situations where resistant organisms are likely to be present (e.g., suspected parvovirus infection).

Phenolics

Phenolics are older disinfectants that are now uncommonly used in clinical environments. They are active against enveloped viruses and bacteria, but they are not sporicidal and have limited activity against fungi and nonenveloped viruses. Their main benefit is better activity in organic debris than some disinfectants, particularly quaternary ammoniums. They irritate skin and mucous membranes, and have the potential to be highly toxic if ingested by cats. Because of these limitations and the availability of other effective disinfectants, there is no indication for their use in veterinary facilities.

Alcohol

Ethyl alcohol and isopropyl alcohol are low-level disinfectants that will kill most bacteria, enveloped viruses, and some fungi. The optimum bactericidal concentration is 60% to 90% (volume/volume) in water. However, they do not destroy bacterial spores or penetrate proteinaceous material and are readily inactivated by organic debris. Therefore, they are not recommended for routine environmental disinfection. Alcohol is occasionally used for low-level disinfection of some patient contact items (e.g., thermometers); however, given the availability of other safe and more effective options, there is little indication to use alcohol for any disinfection procedures. Because alcohol is flammable and dries quickly, it can be difficult to achieve adequate contact times (≥ 1 minute).

Iodophors

Iodine solutions are primarily used as skin antiseptics. Formulations for disinfection are also available, which contain higher concentrations of free iodine than antiseptic preparations. An iodophor is a combination of iodine and a solubilizing agent (e.g., polyvinylpyrrolidone in povidone-iodine), which serves to provide a sustained-release form of iodine. Dilutions of iodophors are more active against microbes than concentrated povidone-iodine, so iodophors must be diluted correctly. Iodophors are bactericidal and virucidal. Their antibacterial activity does not persist for long periods on skin or in tissues, so frequent reapplication is required. Iodophors are relatively nontoxic and nonirritating. They are stable in solution but are inactivated by organic material, and they can stain plastics and, to some extent, tissues. There is no reason to use iodophors for environmental disinfection given the widespread availability of better disinfectants.

Chlorhexidine

Chlorhexidine is a cationic bisbiguanide that disrupts microbial cell membranes and precipitates cell contents. It is used widely for skin antisepsis in veterinary medicine but is a poor environmental disinfectant because of the low-level disinfection that it can achieve and the potential selection for chlorhexidine-resistant bacteria,[5,6] which could impact the efficacy of skin antisepsis and wound care. Anecdotally, outbreaks caused by pathogens with acquired chlorhexidine resistance (e.g., *Pseudomonas*) have been identified in facilities where chlorhexidine was used as a routine environmental disinfectant. As with iodophors, there is no reason to use chlorhexidine for environmental disinfection.

Sterilization

Steam Sterilization

Steam sterilization involves the use of saturated steam under pressure in an autoclave. This is the most effective form of sterilization, is nontoxic and inexpensive, and as a result is the most widely used in healthcare facilities. The use of steam under pressure allows lower temperatures to be used for shorter periods of time when compared with dry heat sterilization (Table 14.2). Cycle times vary depending on the autoclave used and whether items are wrapped or unwrapped, but are generally 30 minutes or less. There are two basic types of autoclaves; gravity displacement autoclaves and high-speed prevacuum sterilizers. Gravity displacement autoclaves admit steam at the top or sides of the autoclave, which displaces air through a drain vent at the bottom of the chamber (Fig. 14.1). High-speed prevacuum sterilizers rapidly pump air out of the sterilizer before steam is admitted. This leads to rapid penetration of steam into all surfaces. As a result, cycle and drying times can be reduced.

Before steam sterilization is performed, instruments should be cleaned thoroughly to remove organic and inorganic material, and then dried. All jointed items should be opened or unlocked, and items should not be crowded in the autoclave so that steam can circulate freely.

Assessment of autoclave efficacy is critical. Chemicals (e.g., indicator tape, indicator strips) are used to monitor temperature or both temperature and time and should be included outside and inside every autoclaved pack.[7] Both internal and external indicators should be used unless the internal indicator is visible through the packaging.[7] The external indicator should be evaluated by the individual removing packs from the autoclave, and the internal indicator should be evaluated by the individual opening the pack at the time of use. Biological indicators, most often consisting of *Geobacillus stearothermophilus* spores,[7] should be used on a regular basis. This is the only method that confirms actual sterilization, and the frequency of testing varies with the frequency of use and the types of items that are autoclaved. Weekly testing is probably appropriate for most veterinary hospitals, but more frequent use may be indicated in busy facilities and consideration should be given to including biological indicators with every load containing implantable devices.[7,8]

Failure of any of these methods to indicate effective sterilization must be immediately investigated. If internal or external indicators fail, the items must not be used and the event investigated. In the event of biological indicator failure (with or without external or internal indicator strip failure), any implantable items must be immediately recalled. Recall of other items is prudent but not considered necessary while the investigation ensues.[8] Three consecutive autoclave runs should be performed with biological indicators, and if any are positive, then all items processed since the last successful biological indicator run should be recalled and reprocessed.[7]

With any possible autoclave failure, an authorized individual should promptly service the autoclave. Biological indicator results should be recorded in an autoclave log to allow for proper tracking of autoclave function. Certified personnel should service autoclaves regularly as part of a preventive maintenance schedule.

Dry Heat Sterilization

Dry heat sterilization, using conditions such as 170°C for 60 minutes, 160°C for 120 minutes, or 150°C for 150 minutes,[9] is reserved for

TABLE 14.2 Recommended Conditions for Heat Sterilization

Sterilization Type	Conditions	Time
Gravity displacement steam	121°C (250°F), 106 kPa (15 lb/in²)[a]	30 minutes: wrapped items; 20 minutes: unwrapped items
	132°C (270°F), 30 lb/in²	15 minutes: wrapped items
High-speed prevacuum steam	132°C (270°F), 30 lb/in²	4 minutes
Dry heat	160°C (320°F)	2 hours at temperature, 3–3.5 hours with cooling
	170°C (340°F)	1 hour at temperature, 2–2.5 hours with cooling

[a]Pressure settings may vary. When possible, follow manufacturer's recommendations.

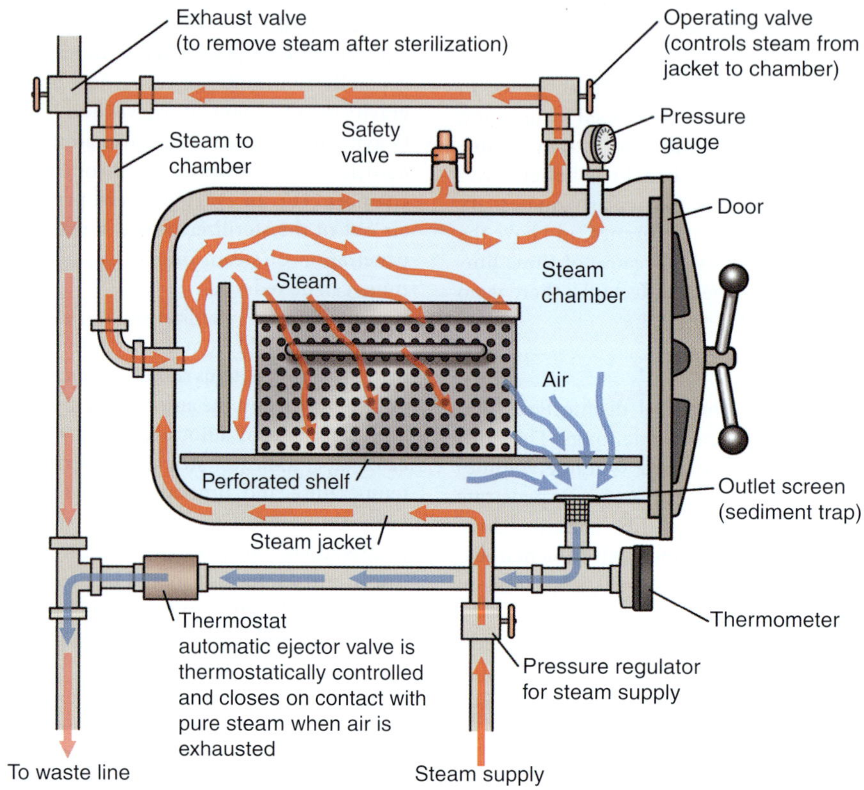

Fig. 14.1 Schematic illustration of gravity displacement sterilization. Steam is admitted at the top or sides of the autoclave, which displaces air through a drain vent at the bottom of the chamber.

materials that might be damaged by moisture or that are impenetrable to moist heat but can tolerate high temperatures. The advantages of lack of corrosive properties and good penetrating power are offset by the long cycle time. This method of sterilization is rarely performed in clinical situations.

Flash Sterilization

Flash sterilization refers to the rapid sterilization of unwrapped instruments and is usually performed as an emergency procedure in an operating room setting when time is insufficient to perform the preferred sterilization of wrapped items. This is most often indicated when an item is inadvertently contaminated during surgery and a sterile replacement is not available. In general, it is performed for 3 minutes at 132°C (270°F) and 27 to 28 lb/in². Each instrument must be carefully protected to ensure it does not become recontaminated during transport back to the operating room, usually in a "flash pan." Flash sterilization has occasionally been associated with an increased risk of intraoperative infections and patient injury in humans[10–12] and should not be used for routine purposes or in lieu of stocking an adequate number of surgical instruments or proper scheduling.

Gas Sterilization

ETO gas can be used to sterilize items that cannot withstand steam sterilization. ETO kills microorganisms through alkylation of protein, DNA, and RNA, providing broad-spectrum activity against even hardy organisms like mycobacteria, enveloped viruses, and bacterial spores. As with steam sterilization, a series of factors influence ETO efficacy including gas concentration, temperature, humidity, and time.[9] Typical recommended ranges for these factors are 450–1200 mg/mL, 29°C–65°C, 45%–85%, and 2–5 hours, respectively.[9] Cycle time (2–5 hours plus 8–12 hours of aeration at 50°C–60°C) and cost are disadvantages of this approach, as well as health and safety concerns with this flammable, explosive, and toxic chemical.[9]

Use of H_2O_2 vapor is a relatively new approach that takes advantage of the broad antimicrobial activity of H_2O_2, with the advantages of having no toxic byproducts (as H_2O_2 breaks down to water and oxygen)

TABLE 14.3 Recommended Concentration and Contact Times for Chemical Sterilants

Chemical/Combination	Concentration	Contact Time
Glutaraldehyde	2% or greater	10 hours
Glutaraldehyde + phenol	1.12% + 1.93%, respectively	12 hours
Accelerated hydrogen peroxide	7.5%	6 hours
Hydrogen peroxide + peracetic acid	7.35% + 0.23%, respectively	3 hours
Peracetic acid	0.2% or greater	50 minutes

and a shorter cycle time. H_2O_2 vapor is compatible with a wide range of materials and can effectively penetrate lumens with small internal diameters or long lengths (e.g., 1 mm of greater diameter and 125 mm or shorter length).[13]

As with steam sterilization, biological indicators should be used. *Bacillus* spores are used to assess ETO, while *G. stearothermophilus* spores are recommended for H_2O_2 vapor.[8] Biological indicators should be placed in the most challenging location in an autoclave load, typically in the center of the load.

Liquid Immersion Sterilization

Liquid immersion sterilization ("cold sterilization") involves the use of a variety of chemical sterilants. When used properly, true sterilization can be achieved; however, liquid immersion should be reserved for items that cannot be processed through other methods, as it is generally less effective and more prone to failure. Liquid immersion is likely more dependent on thorough cleaning than other sterilization methods, and is also presumably more prone to processing errors (e.g., improper dilution, inadequate contact time, improper pH, inadequate changing of solutions, and failure to ensure no air pockets are present), highlighting why this method should not be used for items that can be steam processed.

Examples of chemical sterilants with required concentrations and contact times are presented in Table 14.3. The time required to achieve sterilization is typically 3–12 hours,[7] although increasing the temperature can decrease the required time.[13] Manufacturer guidelines for concentration, temperature, and contact time must be followed.

After chemical processing, items typically need to be rinsed before being used on patients. This is a step that creates a risk of contamination if nonsterile water is used or if there is inadvertent contamination from hands, aerosols, or the environment. Care must be taken when handing and rinsing sterilized items. While items can be kept in the solution tray for a short period of time (e.g., for short transportation to the patient, with appropriate protocols to prevent spillage, or while awaiting a procedure), items should not be kept in chemical sterilants for prolonged storage.

"Cold sterile" solutions are often found in veterinary clinics and may contain critical items that come into contact with sterile patient sites. Often, these are used for relatively low-risk procedures such as minor laceration repairs, abscess drainage, or for items such as otoscope tips. Misuse of cold sterile solutions is widespread and bacterial contamination of cold sterile solutions has been identified in veterinary clinics,[14] likely as a result of inadequate pre-cleaning of instruments, inadequate contact time, adding dirty instruments to solutions containing "sterile" instruments, inadequate pH, inadequate changing of solutions, and inadequate dilution. Cold sterile solutions should not be used for surgical instruments or other items that come into contact with sterile sites, regardless of the minor nature of the procedure that will be performed.

Irradiation

Gamma irradiation is commonly used to sterilize disposable medical supplies such as catheters, gloves, syringes, and pharmaceuticals, but is not relevant for in-clinic sterilization.

SPECIFIC CONSIDERATIONS FOR EQUIPMENT CLEANING AND DISINFECTION

Thermometers

Rectal thermometers are at high risk of becoming contaminated with various pathogens. Outbreaks of disease caused by pathogens such as *Salmonella, Enterobacter cloacae,* and enterococci have been reported in humans in association with rectal thermometers, particularly in neonates and sometimes with fatal outcomes.[15–19] Similar reports are not available for veterinary medicine, but there is no reason to think the risk would be lower. The lack of veterinary data may simply reflect failure to identify or publish outbreaks rather than an inherently lower risk.

Human medicine has largely moved away from rectal thermometers, instead using oral or tympanic thermometers. Changes from rectal to tympanic thermometers have been associated with reduced incidence of vancomycin-resistant *Enterococcus* and *Clostridioides difficile* infections.[15] Moving away from rectal thermometers in animals would be ideal, yet practical alternatives are lacking. Tympanic thermometers may not be particularly accurate in animals,[20–22] and taking of oral temperatures is impractical, so rectal thermometers will likely continue to be widely used. Yet, measures can be taken to reduce the risk of pathogen transmission, including dedicating thermometers to individual patients and use of disposable thermometer covers,[23] as well as using proper disinfection practices.[18]

Any practice that involves cleaning and disinfection is accompanied by concerns about ineffective decontamination, either from inadequate protocols or inadequate compliance. Cleaning to remove gross contamination followed by wiping with a disinfectant such as AHP that is able to kill nonenveloped viruses and bacterial spores is the most practical approach, if disposable covers are not used. This is unlikely to completely eliminate pathogens but may be able to adequately reduce contamination to reduce disease risk.

Otoscope Cones

While manufactured as single-use items, otoscope cones are commonly reused in veterinary practices. Because of contact with the ear canal, contamination of otoscope cones is common.[24,25] When one considers the low cost of otoscope cones, it is hard to justify time-consuming disinfection methods. A practical approach would be to discard cones from patients with evidence of infectious disease and disinfect cones used on other patients. There has been limited study of disinfection methods, particularly when applied to naturally contaminated cones that are also contaminated with organic debris (e.g., exudates, ear wax) that might affect disinfection efficacy. Simply scrubbing or rinsing cones is minimally effective, and contamination can persist despite wiping with disinfectant-containing otoscope cone cleaning solutions.[26] Soaking in 2% chlorhexidine or a quaternary ammonium/EDTA product was shown to be effective with experimentally inoculated cones.[26] It is likely that cleaning to remove any visible debris followed by soaking in commonly used disinfectants would be effective, provided adequate disinfectant concentration and contact times are used, and that solutions are regularly changed. Regardless of the disinfectant used, cones should be rinsed with water prior to use.

Small Portable Medical Equipment

Patient-side medical equipment such as ultrasound machines can easily become contaminated with various pathogens[27] from direct contact with patients, other contaminated items, and hands of veterinary personnel. Specific recommendations are difficult to provide because of the variability in equipment surfaces. However, some basic concepts apply to all.

1. Prevention of contamination: While it is impossible to prevent all contamination, the incidence and degree of contamination can be limited by reducing direct patient contact with equipment as much as possible, using personal protective equipment (e.g., gloves) as indicated and using barriers (e.g., plastic sleeves) for high-risk (or all) cases. For patients that might be harboring a pathogen of particular concern, consideration should be given to whether the procedure is truly needed. Infection control concerns would rarely preclude performing a required diagnostic test, but if a test is not thought to be important, consideration should be given to cancelling or postponing the procedure, particularly if the item cannot be adequately disinfected.
2. Cleaning: Wiping to remove visible debris will greatly reduce any pathogen burden.
3. Disinfection: Specific disinfection approaches will vary with the surface material and characteristics, but wiping with a broadly efficacious environmental disinfect is usually practical and likely effective. Consideration must be given to sensitive equipment (e.g., ultrasound probe heads) and manufacturer guidelines should be consulted with respect to compatibility with different disinfectants.

Ophthalmoscopes and Other Handheld Instruments

Handheld equipment such as ophthalmoscopes and otoscopes are frequently touched and may be infrequently cleaned.[5] The role of these in pathogen transmission is completely unclear and probably limited; however, routine cleaning and disinfection of these (like any common hand contact surface) is indicated. There are no objective guidelines for frequency of cleaning and disinfection, but incorporating these items into a regular (e.g., weekly) schedule is logical, with additional cleaning and disinfection done on an as-needed basis after use on a potentially infectious patient. No disinfection efficacy studies are available, but removal of visible debris followed by wiping with disinfectant is practical. Some items may be more difficult to disinfect based on their design (e.g., many crevices) or surface materials, and those factors (and material compatibility) must be considered when choosing an approach to disinfection.

Clippers and Clipper Blades

As with any item used on multiple patients, clippers and clipper blades pose a potential but unquantified risk. Clippers and blades can be contaminated with the patient's skin microbiota, pathogens from other body sites, environmental bacteria, and opportunistic pathogens from human hands.[28] Risks increase when clippers are used on patients that are more likely to be shedding or contaminated with pathogens (e.g., infected wounds, pyoderma) and in patients or situations where there is an increased risk of disease (e.g., patients with wounds or those that are immunocompromised).

There has been no objective study of methods to disinfect clippers. In most situations, routine disinfection could involve cleaning to remove debris followed by spraying the clipper surface with a good quality environmental disinfectant. If there is concern about contamination with a highly transmissible or otherwise very concerning infectious agent, a more reliable method such as ETO gas or H_2O_2 vapor sterilization could be considered, although data about potential damage to clippers is lacking. Wiping or spraying clippers blades is not likely to be effective. Blades would have to be disassembled to provide adequate contact with disinfectant over the entire surface. Autoclaving blades is a more reliable approach, but requires an adequate supply of clipper blades to ensure that new blades are available whenever contamination may have occurred. Damage to blades from autoclaving is also a concern.

Computer Keyboard and Mouse

These items typically have abundant hand contact and can be contaminated with high microbial burdens.[29–33] With increasing use of electronic medical record systems, greater contact with computers during the course of patient care will increase contamination. Various approaches can be used to reduce the risk and implications of contamination. These include practices to prevent contamination (e.g., hand hygiene prior to using computers, use of keyboard covers) and those to reduce contamination (e.g., wiping with disinfectant wipes).

Phones

Personal or clinic-provided phones are almost ubiquitous in veterinary practice. Given frequent hand contact, contamination of phones and similar small electronic devices (e.g., pagers) is unsurprising and has been well described in both human and veterinary medicine.[34–39] Optimizing phone handling through ensuring hand hygiene is performed prior to phone contact is ideal, but good compliance is unlikely given the high incidence of phone use and the almost-reflexive answering of phones. Education to maximize hand hygiene prior to phone contact is still warranted. Routine disinfection of phones is indicated, although methods that are both effective and nondamaging are not well investigated. Using waterproof phone cases facilitates wiping and spraying with disinfectants, and should be encouraged.

MONITORING EFFICACY OF CLEANING AND DISINFECTION

Bacterial Culture

Routine bacterial culture of the general environment and routine nonsterile items is not recommended.[40] These types of items are not supposed to be sterile, and the relevance of "positive" bacterial cultures is questionable. Finding an opportunistic pathogen on an instrument might mean that it evaded cleaning and disinfection, no attempt was made to clean and disinfect, or that it was contaminated after successful cleaning and disinfection. If those cannot be differentiated, an effective response to the culture result is impossible to develop. Culture should be reserved for targeted situations where a clear action would result from positive versus negative cultures. This could be as part of an outbreak investigation, although environmental cultures are only useful in a small percentage of investigations. Culture could also be used as an educational tool to assess residual contamination after disinfection, but the information that is obtained is limited; there are better tools to assess routine cleaning (see fluorescent tagging below) and post-disinfection environmental cultures are best performed using

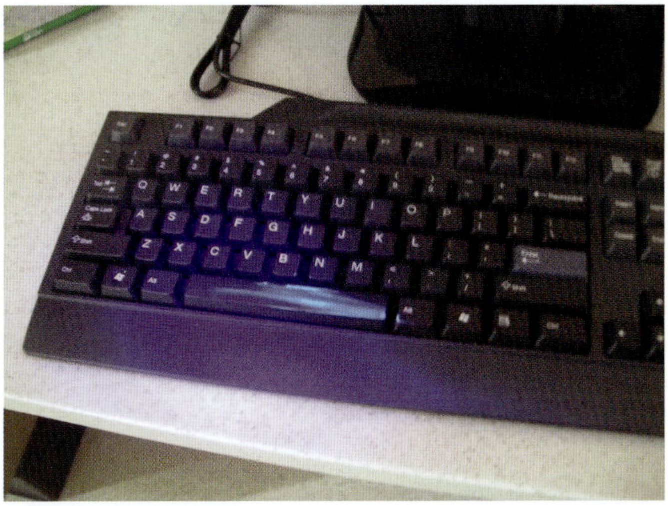

Fig. 14.2 Fluorescent tagging indicating lack of cleaning of the space bar of a computer keyboard.

specific laboratory methods that are not available from most diagnostic laboratories.

Fluorescent Tagging

Fluorescent tagging is a cost-effective and easy method for assessment of cleaning, but not disinfection. It involves application of a fluorescent dye that is not visible to the naked eye to various surfaces in a facility.[41] The dye is visible with ultraviolet light, and the "contaminated" sites can be assessed after a predetermined period of time to see if the dye has been removed, an indication of adequate cleaning (Fig. 14.2). When compared with culture, this can be done at very little cost and provide immediate information. Fluorescent tagging can be useful for periodic assessment as well as staff education.

Direct Observation

While typically unstructured and subjective, direct observation of cleaning and disinfection practices can be useful in a veterinary hospital. If done discretely, it allows for assessment of normal activities and potentially identification of gaps in protocols or practices. This can be done by clinicians with little effort, simply by paying attention to cleaning and disinfection practices that are regularly occurring during the course of a day. A more structured approach can be undertaken whereby specific practices or individuals are purposively monitored. However, this is more time consuming and if indiscrete, it can result in bias due to "the Hawthorne effect" (a change in behavior when the observer knows he/she is being observed). In situations where there are specific concerns about a practice or individual, this can be an effective approach. Remote observation can be performed using webcams[42,43] or closed circuit video, but data analysis can be very time consuming and associated with personnel and privacy concerns.

ATP Bioluminescence

More widely used in food production, ATP bioluminescence testing detects adenosine 5′-triphosphate (ATP), which is an excellent indicator of the presence of viable microbes. Various rapid, handheld systems are available to detect and quantify the bacterial burden on an environmental surface. While such testing has been used in healthcare situations,[44] the relevance of test results is currently unknown. As discussed above, general surfaces are not supposed to be sterile, and ATP bioluminescence does not differentiate between potential pathogens and harmless commensals. Readings can also be influenced by various chemicals,[45] some of which might be present on surfaces in a clinic. Currently, it is unclear how (or if) this technology could be applied in veterinary hospitals for infection control purposes.

SUGGESTED READINGS

Anderson MEC, Sargeant JM, Weese JS. Video observation of hand hygiene practices during routine companion animal appointments and the effect of a poster intervention on hand hygiene compliance. *BMC Vet Res.* 2014;10:106.

Weese JS, Lowe T, Walker M. Use of fluorescent tagging for assessment of environmental cleaning and disinfection in a veterinary hospital. *Vet Rec.* 2012;171:217.

REFERENCES

1. Spaulding EH. Chemical disinfection of medical and surgical materials. In: Lawrence C, Block SS, eds. *Disinfection, Sterilization and Preservation.* Philadelphia: Lea & Febiger; 1968:517–531.
2. Alfa MJ, Lo E, Wald A, et al. Improved eradication of *Clostridium difficile* spores from toilets of hospitalized patients using an accelerated hydrogen peroxide as the cleaning agent. *BMC Infect Dis.* 2010;10:268.
3. Perez J, Springthorpe VS, Sattar SA. Activity of selected oxidizing microbicides against the spores of *Clostridium difficile*: relevance to environmental control. *Am J Infect Control.* 2005;33:320–325.
4. Moriello KA. Kennel disinfectants for *Microsporum canis* and *Trichophyton* sp. *Vet Med Int.* 2015;2015:853–857.
5. Brooks SE, Walczak MA, Hameed R, et al. Chlorhexidine resistance in antibiotic-resistant bacteria isolated from the surfaces of dispensers of soap containing chlorhexidine. *Infect Control Hosp Epidemiol.* 2002;23:692–695.
6. Naparstek L, Carmeli Y, Chmelnitsky I, et al. Reduced susceptibility to chlorhexidine among extremely-drug-resistant strains of *Klebsiella pneumoniae. J Hosp Infect.* 2012;81:15–19.
7. Rutala WA, Weber DJ, Healthcare Infection Control Practices Advisory Committee. Guideline for Disinfection and Sterilization in Healthcare Facilities, 2008. https://www.cdc.gov/infectioncontrol/pdf/guidelines/disinfection-guidelines-H.pdf.
8. Jefferson JA. Central services. In: Association for Professionals in Infection Control. *APIC Text of Infection Control and Epidemiology.* Washington, DC: APIC; 2009.
9. Rutala W, Weber D. Infection control: the role of disinfection and sterilization. *J Hosp Infect.* 1999;43:S43–S55.
10. Babcock HM, Carroll C, Matava M, et al. Surgical site infections after arthroscopy: outbreak investigation and case control study. *Arthroscopy.* 2003;19:172–181.
11. Hood E, Stout N, Catto B. Flash sterilization and neurosurgical site infections: guilt by association. *Am J Infect Control.* 1997;25:156.
12. Rutala WA, Weber DJ, Chappell KJ. Patient injury from flash-sterilized instruments. *Infect Control Hosp Epidemiol.* 1999;20:458.
13. Rutala WA, Weber DJ. Cleaning, disinfection and sterilization. In: Association for Professionals in Infection Control. *APIC Text of Infection Control and Epidemiology.* Washington, DC: APIC; 2009.
14. Murphy CP, Weese JS, Reid-Smith RJ, et al. The prevalence of bacterial contamination of surgical cold sterile solutions from community companion animal veterinary practices in southern Ontario. *Can Vet J.* 2010;51:634–636.
15. Brooks S, Khan A, Stoica D, et al. Reduction in vancomycin-resistant *Enterococcus* and *Clostridium difficile* infections following change to tympanic thermometers. *Infect Control Hosp Epidemiol.* 1998;19:333–336.
16. Im SW, Chow K, Chau PY. Rectal thermometer mediated cross-infection with *Salmonella wandsworth* in a paediatric ward. *J Hosp Infect.* 1981;2:171–174.
17. Livornese LL, Dias S, Samel C, et al. Hospital-acquired infection with vancomycin-resistant *Enterococcus faecium* transmitted by electronic thermometers. *Ann Int Med.* 1992;117:112–116.
18. McAllister TA, Roud JA, Marshall A, et al. Outbreak of *Salmonella* Eimsbuettel in newborn infants spread by rectal thermometers. *Lancet.* 1986;1:1262–1264.

19. van den Berg RW, Claahsen HL, Niessen M, et al. *Enterobacter cloacae* outbreak in the NICU related to disinfected thermometers. *J Hosp Infect.* 2000;45:29–34.
20. Garner S. Ear versus rectal temperature in dogs and cats. *Vet Rec.* 2011;168:248.
21. Greer RJ, Cohn LA, Dodam JR, et al. Comparison of three methods of temperature measurement in hypothermic, euthermic, and hyperthermic dogs. *J Am Vet Med Assoc.* 2007;230:1841–1848.
22. Sousa MG, Carareto R, Pereira-Junior VA, et al. Comparison between auricular and standard rectal thermometers for the measurement of body temperature in dogs. *Can Vet J.* 2011;52:403–406.
23. Donkers LE, van Furth AM, van der Zwet WC, et al. *Enterobacter cloacae* epidemic on a neonatal intensive care unit due to the use of contaminated thermometers. *Ned Tijdschr Geneeskd.* 2001;145:643–647.
24. Korkmaz H, Cetinkol Y, Korkmaz M. Cross-contamination and cross-infection risk of otoscope heads. *Eur Arch Oto-Rhino-Laryngol.* 2013;270:3183–3186.
25. Kirby AL, Rosenkrantz WS, Ghubash RM, et al. Evaluation of otoscope cone disinfection techniques and contamination level in small animal private practice. *Vet Dermatol.* 2010;21:175–183.
26. Newton HM, Rosenkrantz WS, Muse R, et al. Evaluation of otoscope cone cleaning and disinfection procedures commonly used in veterinary medical practices: a pilot study. *Vet Dermatol.* 2006;17:147–150.
27. Weese JS, DaCosta T, Button L, et al. Isolation of methicillin-resistant *Staphylococcus aureus* from the environment in a veterinary teaching hospital. *J Vet Intern Med.* 2004;18:468–470.
28. Masterson TM, Rodeheaver GT, Morgan RF, et al. Bacteriologic evaluation of electric clippers for surgical hair removal. *Am J Surg.* 1984;148:301–302.
29. Bender JB, Schiffman E, Hiber L, et al. Recovery of staphylococci from computer keyboards in a veterinary medical centre and the effect of routine cleaning. *Vet Rec.* 2012;170:414.
30. Dumford DM, Nerandzic MM, Eckstein BC, et al. What is on that keyboard? Detecting hidden environmental reservoirs of *Clostridium difficile* during an outbreak associated with North American pulsed-field gel electrophoresis type 1 strains. *Am J Infect Control.* 2009;37:15–19.
31. Fraser MA, Girling SJ. Bacterial carriage of computer keyboards in veterinary practices in Scotland. *Vet Rec.* 2009;165:26–27.
32. Hartmann B, Benson M, Junger A, et al. Computer keyboard and mouse as a reservoir of pathogens in an intensive care unit. *J Clin Monit Comput.* 2004;18:7–12.
33. Wilson AP, Hayman S, Folan P, et al. Computer keyboards and the spread of MRSA. *J Hosp Infect.* 2006;62:390–392.
34. Brady RR, Fraser SF, Dunlop MG, et al. Bacterial contamination of mobile communication devices in the operative environment. *J Hosp Infect.* 2007;66:397–398.
35. Goldblatt JG, Krief I, Klonsky T, et al. Use of cellular telephones and transmission of pathogens by medical staff in New York and Israel. *Infect Control Hosp Epidemiol.* 2007;28:500–503.
36. Jeske H-C, Tiefenthaler W, Hohlrieder M, et al. Bacterial contamination of anaesthetists' hands by personal mobile phone and fixed phone use in the operating theatre. *Anaesthesia.* 2007;62:904–906.
37. Lee YJ, Yoo C-G, Lee C-T, et al. Contamination rates between smart cell phones and non-smart cell phones of healthcare workers. *J Hosp Med.* 2013;8:144–147.
38. Pal P, Roy A, Moore G, et al. Keypad mobile phones are associated with a significant increased risk of microbial contamination compared to touch screen phones. *J Infect.* 2013;4:65–68.
39. Julian T, Singh A, Rousseau J, et al. Methicillin-resistant staphylococcal contamination of cellular phones of personnel in a veterinary teaching hospital. *BMC Res Notes.* 2012;5:193.
40. Haley RW, Quade D, Freeman HE, et al. The SENIC Project. Study on the efficacy of nosocomial infection control (SENIC Project). Summary of study design. *Am J Epidemiol.* 1980;111:472–485.
41. Weese JS, Lowe T, Walker M. Use of fluorescent tagging for assessment of environmental cleaning and disinfection in a veterinary hospital. *Vet Rec.* 2012;171:217.
42. Anderson MEC, Sargeant JM, Weese JS. Video observation of hand hygiene practices during routine companion animal appointments and the effect of a poster intervention on hand hygiene compliance. *BMC Vet Res.* 2014;10:106.
43. Anderson MEC, Weese JS. Video observation of sharps handling and infection control practices during routine companion animal appointments. *BMC Vet Res.* 2015;11:185.
44. Moore G, Smyth D, Singleton J, et al. The use of adenosine triphosphate bioluminescence to assess the efficacy of a modified cleaning program implemented within an intensive care setting. *Am J Infect Control.* 2010;38:617–622.
45. Omidbakhsh N, Ahmadpour F, Kenny N. How reliable are ATP bioluminescence meters in assessing decontamination of environmental surfaces in healthcare settings?. *PloS One.* 2014;9. e99951.

15

Prevention of Infectious Diseases in Hospital Environments

Brandy A. Burgess, J. Scott Weese

KEY POINTS

- Healthcare-associated infections (HAIs) increase morbidity, mortality, duration of hospitalization, and cost of care.
- The aim of a hospital infection control program is to reduce the incidence of HAIs in patients, staff, and visitors to a veterinary hospital, and consists of infectious disease control personnel, a written protocol, training, and documentation.
- This chapter describes the key components of an infection control program, which describes practices that minimize transmission of infectious agents such as hand washing, use of protective clothing, cleaning and disinfection, antimicrobial stewardship, appropriate disposal of infectious agents, control of vectors and pests, and surveillance efforts. The protocol can also be used to educate staff about specific transmission precautions for infectious diseases seen within a practice.
- Details on sterilization, disinfection, and antisepsis are covered in Chapter 14.

INTRODUCTION

Optimal patient care cannot be realized without effectively managing risks related to healthcare-associated infections (HAIs).[1] It is well recognized in human healthcare that HAIs result in increased morbidity and mortality as well as increased hospitalization stays among affected patients, and can significantly increase the cost of care.[2] In 2002, there were approximately 4.5 HAIs per 100 human hospital admissions in the United States—accounting for an estimated 5.8% of deaths—representing one of the top 10 causes of deaths in the United States.[3] In human medicine, the Study on the Efficacy of Nosocomial Infection Control (SENIC), conducted in US healthcare facilities (1970–1976) demonstrated that HAI rates could be reduced by as much as 32% if hospitals employed trained infection control personnel, conducted some sort of surveillance, and had a system for reporting results back to stakeholders.[4] While we do not have equivalent data in support of our efforts in veterinary infection control, it is not unreasonable to assume a similar impact on infection rates when these practices are employed.

In veterinary medicine, we are just beginning to gain some perspective on the occurrence of HAIs among patients. Historically, much of the focus has been on epidemic disease as the majority of veterinary teaching hospitals (VTHs) regularly recognize outbreaks of HAIs among patients.[5] These disease epidemics tend to garner attention when they have significant impacts on patient morbidity and mortality.[6] Despite this, it is important to monitor endemic (i.e., baseline) rates of HAIs—the occurrence of which likely impacts a greater number of patients. That being said, data on endemic rates of HAIs among veterinary patients are limited. A single study, using syndromic surveillance, estimated that the endemic rate of HAIs in critical care units at small animal referral hospitals was 16.3% of dogs (95% confidence interval [CI] 14.3–18.5) and 12% of cats (95% CI 9.3–15.5).[7] This study focused on the occurrence of seven different syndromes in critical care patients including intravenous catheter site inflammation, urinary tract inflammation, acute respiratory disorders, gastrointestinal disorders, surgical site inflammation, fever of unknown origin, and bacteremia. It is important to keep in mind that critical care patients are likely to be more susceptible to the development of an HAI due to severe compromise and the invasive nature of their care, and so the rate would be expected to be lower in the general patient population.

Throughout this chapter, the term *infection control* will be used to encompass all practices intended to prevent the introduction and spread of infectious agents within a population. While traditionally, biosecurity (preventing the introduction of an agent into a population) and biocontainment (controlling the spread of an infectious agent after introduction into a population) are different, it is somewhat difficult to make this distinction in a veterinary hospital. By their very nature, clinics treat sick animals that are likely to introduce infectious agents into the hospital population. Therein lies the importance of incorporating infection control strategies into the daily practice of veterinary medicine.

Ethics of Infectious Disease Prevention

As veterinarians, we have ethical obligations laid before us by our oath to protect the individual patient (*relief of animal suffering*), protect the animal population of the present and the future (*protection of animal health and welfare*), and protect people (*promotion of public health*).[8] Incorporation of infection control strategies into the practice of medicine is critical if we are to address these interwoven responsibilities. Although veterinary infection control is in its infancy, there is an emerging minimum standard recognized in veterinary medicine—we must give due effort to infection control—no matter if we are practicing in a hospital, in a shelter, or caring for an individual or population of animals.[9]

Veterinarian's Role in Infectious Disease Prevention

Taking all reasonable precautions to reduce the foreseeable risks associated with infectious disease transmission among personnel and patients, i.e., infection control, is fundamental to provision of excellent patient care. While the majority of VTHs have formalized infection control programs, decidedly fewer small animal hospitals report having formalized programs.[5,10,11] Infection prevention and control recommendations have been developed by the Canadian Committee on Antibiotic Resistance (CCAR).[12] This guidance document provides specific recommendations for the development of a comprehensive program focusing on recognized best practices for small animal veterinary clinics. The National Association of State and Public Health Veterinarians (NASPHV) has also developed a "model infection control plan for veterinary practices." However, it provides few details and is very limited in scope, focusing mostly on zoonotic disease prevention, an important component of a comprehensive program.[13]

In the United States, veterinarians have both a legal obligation to "furnish to each of his employees employment and a place of employment which are free from recognized hazards that are causing or are likely to cause death or serious physical harm to his employees" [The General Duty Clause of the Occupational Safety and Health Act of 1970, 29 U.S.C. § 654 Sec.5,],[14] as well as a clear responsibility to recommend measures to reduce the risk of zoonotic pathogen transmission and counsel clients and personnel to seek medical attention in the event of zoonotic pathogen exposure.[15] Regulations may vary in other countries, but the essence remains the same. While this is a responsibility that is shared with human physicians, the reality is that neither rarely engages the other in such discussions[16] and understanding of zoonotic disease risks and animal-related infection control measures by physicians tends to be limited. Interestingly, research shows that while physicians believe it to be the responsibility of public health officials and veterinarians, veterinarians believe it to be the responsibility of physicians and public health officials.[17] This often leads to significant gaps, as both relevant groups assume the other is taking the responsibility.

Level of Infectious Disease Prevention

The minimum level of infectious disease prevention is unique to each facility, taking into account the patient population, level of disease risk, the risk aversion of facility stakeholders, and the standards set by the rules and regulations of the state's board of veterinary medicine. Thus, while there are core principles, specific practices within a program will vary.[9]

Disease risk and risk aversion may change over time. Thus, programs must be dynamic and rely upon organized surveillance efforts that provide data upon which to base decisions.[9] For example, during a regional outbreak of canine influenza, it may be prudent to implement additional precautions when caring for dogs with signs of upper respiratory tract disease or those with a travel history to affected regions. Rules and regulations of the region in which the practice is located establish, in part, the minimum standard of practice. For example, the State of Colorado veterinary medicine rules and regulations state that "all veterinarians must maintain a sanitary environment in which they care for patients…they are responsible for ensuring that their work is done in a clean environment and within the standard of care".[18] While this is somewhat vague, there is a clear implication that infection control is an important component in the practice of quality veterinary care. The NASPHV has developed the "compendium of veterinary standard precautions for zoonotic disease prevention in veterinary personnel" which can serve as a valuable resource when determining the level of infectious disease prevention practiced on a daily basis.[19]

Importance of Infectious Disease Prevention

HAIs are commonly linked with outbreaks of disease among hospitalized patients, and zoonotic infections are commonly identified as important occupational hazards among personnel.[5] While outbreaks receive the most attention, the occurrence of endemic disease likely has an impact on a greater number of patients. Infection control programs should be designed with the intention of protecting personnel, patients, and the hospital from foreseeable risks—preventing endemic disease from becoming epidemic disease. In so doing, we can create an environment for the delivery of optimal patient care. Infectious disease prevention in the hospital environment involves protection of: (1) personnel; (2) patients; and (3) the hospital.

1. *Protect personnel*: Veterinarians are occupationally at risk for development of zoonotic infections when compared with members of the general public (i.e., individuals not working with animals).[20] Approximately 61% of > 1,400 human pathogens are considered to be zoonotic, as are an estimated 75% of emerging infectious agents.[21] Veterinarians are exposed to zoonotic pathogens on a daily basis and may be among the first individuals exposed to emerging pathogens. A case example—the majority of zoonotic infections during the 2003 prairie dog-associated monkeypox virus outbreak in Wisconsin (the first reported outbreak outside of Africa) occurred in veterinary staff, who were found to be inconsistently using personal protective equipment (PPE).[22] With this in mind, it is critical to ensure that minimum preventive measures are being used in daily practice. The veterinary standard precautions as outlined by NASPHV is a good reference upon which to base a practice's minimum expectations and standards with respect to the prevention of disease transmission.[19]
2. *Protect patients:* Hospitalization comes with the inherent risk of HAI. Not all infections are preventable—even in hospitals that practice excellent infection control. By their very nature, hospitals congregate many patients from many different households and geographic locations, in various states of immune compromise, many of which may receive invasive treatments or immunosuppressive therapies. This creates a situation where not only are these patients at an increased risk from potential pathogens derived from their own resident flora, but are also at an increased risk for transmission of potential pathogens among patients and personnel. Despite the majority of VTHs accredited by the American Veterinary Medical Association (AVMA) reportedly having a formalized infection control program, 82% have still identified outbreaks of HAIs in a 5-year time span.[5] This undoubtedly represents the tip of the iceberg, as it is likely that endemic rates are higher and impact a greater number of patients. A formalized infection control program should not simply promote the use of recognized best practices, but should strive to educate personnel on the purpose of the program—in other words, the "why"—to encourage program compliance and preventing the endemic from becoming the epidemic.
3. *Protect the hospital:* Infectious disease prevention programs aim to mitigate the baseline transmission risk to prevent its escalation to epidemic levels. We can calculate the direct costs associated with these efforts, both in supplies and personnel time, but it is difficult to truly know the cost of an averted outbreak. Although hospital outbreaks are not uncommon, the costs associated with such an event typically go unreported. Many VTHs report restricting patient admissions (58% of those surveyed) or closing part of the facility (32% of those surveyed) to aid in mitigation efforts.[5] One VTH reported a financial loss of US$4.12 million associated with an outbreak of *Salmonella enterica* serovar Newport that resulted in a partial facility closure.[6] While it is relatively simple to quantify direct losses (i.e., hard costs), indirect losses related to client confidence, emotional stress, lost teaching opportunities, diminished morale of hospital personnel, and poor public relations are more difficult to enumerate. With this in mind, the upfront investment in education and prevention program development and maintenance are essential. While all infectious disease transmission cannot be prevented, strategies can be employed that reduce the baseline transmission risk to an acceptable endemic level.

ANTIMICROBIAL STEWARDSHIP

Antimicrobial stewardship is fundamental to the veterinarians' role in providing optimal patient care as well as safeguarding public health. As antimicrobial resistance (AMR) becomes an increasing animal health concern and use of antimicrobials in animals attracts escalating scrutiny, the need to effectively and logically use antimicrobials is paramount. While emergence of AMR is an inherent risk of antimicrobial use, an array of measures can be implemented to reduce and improve antimicrobial use, ideally with benefits to the patient and the population (both human and animal). The intent of an antimicrobial stewardship program is to improve patient outcomes while minimizing unintended consequences through coordinated efforts advocating the appropriate use (selection, dosing, route, and duration) of antimicrobials. Antimicrobial stewardship is in its infancy in veterinary medicine, with informal use of many strategies but few organized and comprehensive antimicrobial stewardship programs.

AMR can affect the ability to treat individual patients as well as control infectious diseases in animal populations. Many HAIs can be attributed to bacteria resistant to antimicrobials (e.g., *Escherichia coli, Enterococcus* spp.*, Acinetobacter baumannii, Staphylococcus pseudintermedius, and Staphylococcus aureus).*[23–25]

Controlling the emergence of AMR involves both the prevention of selection of resistant microorganisms (i.e., antimicrobial stewardship) and prevention of the spread of resistant organisms (i.e., infection control programs).[26,27] AMR can evolve through the accumulation of chromosomal mutations or the transfer of resistance genes between bacteria from different taxonomic and ecologic groups through mobile genetic elements (e.g., plasmids, transposons, or bacteriophages). Acquired resistance genes can confer resistance to a single antimicrobial, a single antimicrobial class, or a broad group of antimicrobials. Theoretically, all uses of antimicrobial drugs have the potential to select for resistant bacterial populations by providing a survival advantage for resistant bacteria. Genes associated with AMR to one antimicrobial can be linked to resistance genes against other antimicrobials as well as to disinfectants, thereby promoting the development of multidrug-resistant strains that may be more difficult to treat and eliminate from the hospital environment.[28–30]

Risk factors for the emergence of resistance in companion animals are poorly understood. In addition to volume of antimicrobial drug use, other factors likely play a role, including inappropriate dosing regimens (sub-therapeutic dosing, inadequate or excessive duration of therapy) and poor client compliance. There is increasing evidence that AMR in humans may affect pets, and as antimicrobial-resistant pathogens increase in the human population, exposure of pets may be inevitable. This is perhaps best demonstrated with methicillin-resistant *S. aureus* (MRSA)[31,32] but is also a concern with other pathogens such as enterococci and Enterobacterales.

Antimicrobials should be used judiciously.[33] Judicious use implies careful consideration before use and should incorporate the use of adequate doses at correct intervals for appropriate clinical indications, selection of narrow-spectrum antimicrobials specific for the isolated organisms (ideally based on antimicrobial susceptibility testing), selection of antimicrobials against which the isolated organisms are not prone to develop resistance, switching antimicrobials following failure of empiric therapy only after an effective treatment period, restriction of indiscriminate use of antimicrobial drugs (i.e., limit use to ill or at-risk animals and treat only as long as needed to achieve clinical response), and use of topical or local rather than systemic therapy whenever possible.[33]

Antimicrobial stewardship programs apply strategies based on local antimicrobial use and resistance patterns (i.e., facility and/or regionally specific) to reduce and improve use of antimicrobial drugs (Table 15.1). Antimicrobial drugs should be used when there is a reasonable expectation of favorably impacting patient outcomes,[34] and consideration should be given to controlling disease without their use. Not all infections are bacterial in nature, and not all bacterial infections require systemic antimicrobial therapy. Local therapy such as incision and drainage, and the use of local biocides or antimicrobials may be appropriate in some situations. The client's money should be invested in a proper work-up because: (1) early diagnostic intervention to detect diseases that can cause signs suggestive of bacterial infections (e.g., viral infections, immune-mediated or inflammatory conditions, or neoplasia) can eliminate the need for empirical use of antimicrobial drugs,[34] and (2) bacterial infection is almost always secondary to an underlying cause, and resolution of the underlying condition can result in the elimination of secondary bacterial infections without the use of antimicrobial drugs. In addition, failure to resolve the underlying cause only leads to recurrence of bacterial infection after antimicrobial drug therapy is discontinued. Voluntary restrictions on use can be an important component of a stewardship program; however, specific criteria must be provided to guide the "appropriate" use of antimicrobial drugs considered to be "critically important" to public health (e.g., carbapenems). The World Health Organization (WHO) has defined "critically important" antimicrobial drug classes to be classes that: (1) are the only, or are one of limited therapies, to treat serious bacterial infections in humans, and (2) are used to treat infections in people caused by bacteria transmitted from or that may acquire resistance genes from nonhuman sources.[35] For example, criteria that may need to be met prior to the use of restricted drugs may include: (1) that the infection must be documented based on clinical abnormalities and culture; (2) these drugs should be reserved for infections that are life threatening, not for subclinical infections; (3) resistance to all other reasonable options and susceptibility to the chosen antimicrobial must be documented; (4) infection must be potentially treatable; and (5) the clinician should contact the hospital expert (e.g., infectious disease control officer or a clinical microbiologist) to discuss antimicrobial susceptibility test results, determine whether there are any other viable options, and confirm that a restricted antimicrobial is necessary (see Table 15.1).

While antimicrobial stewardship programs can improve patient outcomes, they should not be relied upon as a primary prevention strategy. Inevitably, microorganisms will be exposed to antimicrobials in veterinary hospitals resulting in patient exposure to resistant bacteria in the hospital environment. Consequently, infection control precautions must be used to reduce the spread of resistant organisms from patient to patient and patients to personnel, and to reduce the likelihood of resistant bacteria becoming established in the hospital environment.

ROUTES OF TRANSMISSION

Transmission of microorganisms can occur via contact (direct or indirect), airborne transmission (aerosol or droplet formation), or be vector borne. Many preventive measures disrupt one or more of these routes of transmission. Transmission can occur among members of the same population (horizontal) or succeeding generations through genetic material (vertical). Spread of an agent to offspring by the placenta, during birth, or in milk is considered to be horizontal transmission. Not all infectious agents are transmissible. For example, systemic mycotic infections originate from soil rather than spreading between individuals.

Reservoirs and Carriers

The *reservoir* of an infectious microorganism is the natural habitat where the agent normally lives and multiplies. For example, *Leptospira*

TABLE 15.1 Key Aspects of an Antimicrobial Stewardship Program[129]

Program team members	Multidisciplinary team	• Infectious disease specialist • Clinical pharmacist with infectious disease training • Clinical microbiologist • Infection control expert • Hospital epidemiologist
Core strategies	Prospective surveillance, intervention, and feedback	• Audit and report use of specific drugs and patient outcomes to stakeholders (e.g., prescribers, administration)
	Antimicrobial restriction	• Restrict use of drugs considered to be "critically important" to public health[35] to approved indications by using: • Formulary restriction, and/or • Preauthorization with justification
	Education	• Provision of foundational knowledge can influence prescribing practices, increase compliance, and improve program buy-in • Combine in-service trainings and e-mail alerts with written guidelines and data from active surveillance (i.e., prospective surveillance and interventions)
Supplemental strategies	Guidelines and clinical pathways	• Evidence-based practice guidelines based on local microbiology and resistance patterns • Implementation should be incorporated with education and reporting use and patient outcomes
	Streamlining and de-escalation of therapy	• Discontinue empirical therapy based on clinical response or culture results, reconsider treatment after 48 hours • Eliminate redundant combination therapy
	Automatic stop orders	• Evidence-based discontinuation of therapy to limit therapy duration (e.g., perioperative prophylaxis automatically discontinued at 2 days unless justification provided for extended therapy)
	Dose optimization	• Base dosing on patient characteristics, causative organism, site of infection, and pharmacokinetics of the antimicrobial drug
	Clinical decision-making computerized support system	• Provide local epidemiological information and its potential impact on courses of therapy • Provide warnings regarding intended therapy based on guidelines and local patterns
Microbiology laboratory	Pathogen identification and susceptibility testing	• Timely and accurate microbial pathogen identification • Susceptibility testing based on Clinical and Laboratory Standards Institute (CLSI) Guidelines • Prioritization of tested antimicrobials • Selective reporting of susceptibility profiles
Determining program impact	Process measures	• Did intervention change antimicrobial use?
	Outcome measures	• Did intervention reduce adverse outcomes (e.g., antimicrobial resistance, adverse drug events)?

(Derived from Dellit TH, Owens RC, McGowan JE Jr, et al. Infectious Diseases Society of America and the Society for Healthcare Epidemiology of America guidelines for developing an institutional program to enhance antimicrobial stewardship. *Clin Infect Dis*. 2007;44:159–177.)

and systemic mycotic agents such as *Histoplasma* and *Cryptococcus* can survive in inanimate reservoirs such as soil and water. Alternatively, agents may exist in animate reservoirs known as *carriers*. Carriers can be clinically or subclinically infected, or they may be latently infected, shedding organisms intermittently in association with reactivation of an infection.

Contact Transmission

Contact transmission can be direct or indirect (vehicle). *Direct contact transmission* involves direct physical contact or close proximity between the reservoir host and the susceptible individual. Venereal transmission of *Brucella canis* between dogs and bite transmission of FIV between cats are examples of direct contact transmission. Direct transmission can be prevented through the use of separation or barrier nursing precautions. *Indirect contact transmission or vehicle transmission* involves the transfer of infectious organisms from the reservoir or carrier to a susceptible host (i.e., animal or person) indirectly by animate or inanimate intermediates known as vehicles or fomites. Indirect transmission depends on the ability of an agent to survive environmental conditions. Common animate fomites are human hands, while common inanimate fomites include stethoscopes, thermometers, doorknobs, keyboards, food dishes, or cages. Canine and feline parvoviruses are often spread via fomites due to the relatively long period of environmental persistence of these viruses. Prevention of indirect transmission may include adherence to rigorous hand hygiene protocols, barrier nursing precautions, or the use of dedicated equipment for infectious disease cases.

Common-source transmission involves simultaneous exposure of a significant number of individuals within a population to a vehicle contaminated by an infectious agent. The vehicles of common-source infections are usually blood products, drugs, food, and water. An example would be a food-source outbreak of *Salmonella* gastroenteritis.

TABLE 15.2 Microorganism Susceptibility to Common Chemical Disinfectants[130]

Susceptibility	Microorganism	Effective Disinfectant Classes
Highly susceptible	Mycoplasmas	Acids, alcohols, aldehydes, alkalis, biguanides, halogens, peroxygens, phenols, QACs
Susceptible	Gram-positive vegetative bacteria	Alcohol, aldehydes, alkalis, biguanides, halogens, peroxygens, some phenols, QACs
	Enveloped viruses	
	Gram-negative vegetative bacteria	
	Fungal spores	Some alcohols, aldehydes, biguanides, halogens, peroxygens, some phenols, some QACs
Resistant	Nonenveloped viruses	Aldehydes, halogens, peroxygens
	Mycobacteria	Alcohol, aldehydes, some alkalis, halogens, some peroxygens, some phenols
Highly resistant	Bacterial endospores	Some acids, aldehydes, halogens (high concentration), peroxygens
	Protozoal oocysts	Ammonium hydroxide, halogens (high concentration), some phenols
Extremely resistant	Prions	Generally resistant to chemical disinfection, sodium hypochlorite (high concentration)

Acids: hydrochloric acid, acetic acid, citric acid; alcohols: ethyl alcohol, isopropyl alcohol; aldehydes: formaldehyde, paraformaldehyde, glutaraldehyde; alkalis: sodium hydroxide, ammonium hydroxide, sodium carbonate; biguanides: chlorhexidine, novalsan, hibistat; halogens: hypochlorite, iodine; peroxygens: hydrogen peroxide, peroxyacetic acid, Virkon, Accel, Rescue; phenolics: TekTrol; quaternary ammonium compounds (QACs): Lysol, Roccal.

(Derived from Quinn PJ, Markey BK. Disinfection and Disease Prevention in Veterinary Medicine. In: Block SS, ed. *Disinfection, Sterilization, and Preservation.* 5th edn. Philadelphia: Lippincott Williams & Wilkins; 2001.)

Airborne Transmission

Airborne transmission may occur via aerosol transmission or droplet transmission. Respiratory pathogens such as canine influenza virus and *Histoplasma* spp. are commonly spread by this means. *Aerosol transmission* is the spread of very small airborne particles (generally < 100 μm in diameter). Freshly aerosolized particles rarely remain airborne for more than 1 minute unless they are smaller than 5 μm in diameter, at which point they can remain airborne for some time and even travel relatively long distances.[36] Droplet nuclei, which are desiccated aerosolized particles 1–10 μm in diameter, can also be carried alone or on dust particles by air currents for extended periods and distances.[37] Prevention of aerosol transmission often requires isolating the infected animal in its own air space, or at a minimum maintenance of significant separation between patients.

Droplet transmission occurs with larger particles generated during coughing and sneezing or during diagnostic procedures such as draining an abscess, wound irrigation, or performing endoscopy. Droplets generally do not remain airborne for long and typically only travel short distances from the source. Droplets from respiratory, fecal, or genitourinary secretions of dogs and cats generally do not travel farther than 4 or 5 feet unless there are wind currents or particularly forceful coughing, sneezing, or splashing. Separation of patients, use of barrier nursing precautions, and performance of procedures in low-traffic areas can prevent droplet transmission.

Vector-Borne Transmission

Vector-borne transmission involves transmission of infectious agents via invertebrate animals such as flies, fleas, ticks, and mosquitoes. Vectors can transmit through mechanical or biologic means, depending on the infectious agent's ability to multiply or propagate while being carried either externally or internally by the vector. *Mechanical vectors* carry the agent without agent multiplication or propagation. For example, vectors such as flies may transfer organisms externally on their feet or internally within their intestinal tracts. *Biologic vectors* carry an agent that multiplies within the vector before transmission. For example, transmission of the plague bacillus, *Yersinia pestis,* by fleas occurs in this manner. True biologic (developmental or cyclo-propagative) transmission by arthropod vectors involves an obligate developmental stage in the life cycle of the vector. Some protozoal pathogens (e.g., *Leishmania, Hepatozoon* and *Trypanosoma*) have a developmental life cycle in a vector.

Within a vector, agents can be transmitted transovarially (to successive generations of the vector, e.g., *Rickettsia rickettsii*) or transstadially (during molting from one vector stage to the next, e.g., *Anaplasma phagocytophilum*).

Implementation of vector control programs can reduce vector-borne transmission. Patients should be examined for external parasites and, if found, should be treated to reduce the risk of transmission. If other health concerns preclude treatment, these patients should be segregated from the general hospital population and provided with dedicated grooming equipment.

PREVENTATIVE MEASURES

Cleaning, Disinfection, and Sterilization

Cleaning, sanitation, disinfection, and sterilization are discussed in Chapter 14. Vegetative bacteria are relatively susceptible to most disinfectants; however, resistance to specific disinfectants can be present in certain microorganisms, either inherently or through acquisition of resistance genes. Enveloped viruses are quite susceptible to disinfectants; however, nonenveloped viruses tend to be resistant. Protozoal cysts, mycobacteria, and bacterial spores are highly resistant to disinfection and sanitation (Table 15.2). Prions, the proteinaceous agents that cause transmissible degenerative (spongiform) encephalopathies, are the most resistant infectious agents known.

Hospital Attire

Historically, the "white coat" has symbolized expertise and professionalism. However, white coats also serve to protect the clinician from contaminating their daily attire that may be worn from their homes to work and back again. White coats and neck ties are commonly identified as potential fomites with upwards of 60% of human hospital staff uniforms found to be colonized with potential pathogenic bacteria,[38] including MRSA, on up to 16% of white coats and 32% of neck ties tested.[39] Consequently, attire policies are commonly included in hospital infectious disease prevention programs.

TABLE 15.3 Indications for Hand Hygiene in Veterinary Practice

Hand Washing and Disinfection	Wearing of Latex Gloves
1. At times of arrival or leaving hospital	1. Before wound management
2. Before and after every patient contact	2. Before performing surgical or endoscopic procedures
3. After touching surfaces or objects likely to be contaminated	3. Before placing indwelling catheter
4. After handling patients likely to be colonized with resistant organisms	4. Before handling particularly susceptible patients (e.g., immune compromised, indwelling tubes/catheters)
5. Before preparing food or medications for patients	5. Before handling potential infectious patients
6. After removing gloves	6. Before handling disinfectants
7. After contact with body fluids	7. Handling of patients if you are immune compromised
8. After personal functions (e.g., smoking, sneezing, coughing, nose blowing, use of restroom)	

Hospital Attire in Nonsurgical Areas

Daily attire for hospital personnel in nonsurgical areas should strike a balance between professional appearance with the potential role clothing may play in pathogen transmission. Personnel should be encouraged to wear dedicated hospital attire (clothing and footwear) that is not worn outside of the clinic environment to prevent transportation of pathogens to and from locations outside the hospital. For all hospital personnel, footwear must be safe, protective (i.e., closed-toe), and cleanable (i.e., constructed of a nonporous material). Standard protective outerwear (e.g., white coat) should be neat and clean, with an adequate supply on hand to allow personnel to change at least daily and whenever outerwear becomes contaminated.

Hospital Attire in Surgical Areas

Dedicated attire for hospital personnel in surgical areas is intended to decrease patient exposure to potential pathogens and reduce the risk for surgical site infections. Typically, surgical attire includes scrubs, gowns, caps, masks, gloves, and dedicated footwear/footwear covers. While there are limited data to support these practices, dedicated surgical area footwear has been shown to significantly lower the level of contamination as compared with outdoor footwear,[40] and wearing a cover-gown when leaving the surgical area has been shown to greatly reduce bacterial contamination on surgical scrubs.[41] While the clinical implications of this finding are as yet unrealized, personnel should be encouraged to use either dedicated footwear or shoe covers when in surgical areas, and to wear a cover-gown upon leaving a surgical area or to don clean surgical scrubs prior to re-entry.

Healthcare Laundry

Healthcare laundry is a potential fomite and may include an assorted inventory of textiles such as scrubs and lab coats, surgical towels and drapes, and cage blankets and towels. The goal is to achieve hygienically clean laundry (i.e., laundered items pose a negligible transmission risk to patients and personnel).[42] Laundering reduces microbial contamination through mechanical, thermal, and chemical means. It begins by collecting point-of-use items and, with minimal handling, transportation to a central laundry area. Healthcare laundry may be laundered on-site or sent to a commercial laundry service. If managed on-site, visible debris should be removed before washing. Washing should begin with a rinse, a wash cycle with laundry chemicals and additives, followed by a clean water rinse. Washing with detergent and water temperature of 71.6°F (22°C) achieves a 3 log reduction of microorganisms per cm^2, whereas washing in water temperature of 160°F (71°C) achieves a 5 log reduction.[42] An additional 2 log reduction can be expected with a hot dryer or ironing.[42] Laundered items should be stored to ensure they are not contaminated before use.

Personnel should be encouraged to use dedicated hospital attire that is not worn outside of the hospital environment. Facilities are encouraged to provide a laundry service (on-site or a commercial laundry service) for hospital attire, in particular scrubs and lab coats, to reduce the risk this may pose to the household when taking these items home for laundering. Attire that is taken home for laundering should be transported in a sealed bag and laundered immediately. Personnel should take care to not contaminate themselves or the home environment and practice rigorous hand hygiene after handling contaminated laundry.

Hand Hygiene

One of the most important infection control measures is proper hand hygiene.[19,43–46] Hand contamination increases over time while attending to patients without gloving.[47,48] Use of soap and water or alcohol-based hand sanitizers is critically important to reduce the likelihood for transmission. Hand hygiene should be performed before and after each patient contact and before touching other surfaces or supplies (Table 15.3).

Hand Washing

The mechanical action of hand washing reduces the organic debris and transient microorganisms on the skin, and, with the addition of antimicrobial soap, may inactivate or inhibit the growth of microorganisms (Table 15.4).[19,49] Hand washing should be performed using a biocide-containing hand soap before and after every patient contact, after handling blood or other body fluids, and after the removal of PPE including gloves. Bar soaps should not be used in a healthcare setting and soap containers should be discarded when empty to reduce the potential for creating a reservoir for biocide-resistant bacteria. Wall dispensers should be cleaned and disinfected before refilling. Because frequent hand washing can compromise skin integrity, which increases the risk for bacterial colonization as well as decrease compliance with hand hygiene protocols,[49,50] lotions and moisturizers should also be provided to promote healthy skin. Detailed information on proper hand hygiene is available from the Centers for Disease Control and Prevention (CDC).[45]

Alcohol-Based Hand Sanitizers

Alcohol-based hand sanitizers are a widely available, effective and practical alternative to traditional hand washing.[48] These have rapid and broad-spectrum activity with little risk of emerging resistance. In healthcare settings, the CDC recommends the use of hand sanitizers that contain 60%–95% ethyl or isopropyl alcohol.[51] While hand size impacts total hand coverage, application of 2 mL or 3 mL of product achieves 90% palm or dorsum coverage, respectively.[52] The use of soap and water, rather than an alcohol-based hand sanitizer, is recommended when there is gross contamination with organic debris or when exposure to alcohol-resistant pathogens such as clostridial spores or parvovirus might have occurred.[51] Alcohol-based products can be especially useful when skin is likely to become compromised

TABLE 15.4 Recommended Methods for Hand Hygiene

Method		Description
Hand washing	Removes dirt and some transient bacteria	• Cleaning hands with conventional soap and water
Antiseptic hand washing	Removes and kills transient and some resident bacteria	• Cleaning and disinfecting hands with combination soap and antiseptic solution • Technique: 1) Completely wet hands and wrists in running stream of warm water—keep hands lower than elbows to avoid recontamination 2) Apply soap-antiseptic combination over front and back of hands 3) Rub all surfaces of hands and wrists, interlace fingers, and lather for manufacturers recommended time (15–30 seconds) 4) Thoroughly rinse hands in clear running water 5) Dry hands thoroughly with disposable towel 6) Turn off faucets with towel
Hand sanitizer	Removes and kills transient and some resident bacteria ***Note:*** *Use products containing 60%–95% ethyl or isopropyl alcohol*[51]	• Place hand sanitizer in readily available locations (e.g., kennel side) 1) Dispense 2–3 mL onto hands 2) Rub all hand surfaces for 15 seconds 3) Let disinfectant dry thoroughly before handling objects **Note:** Not effective in the presence of organic debris or for alcohol-resistant pathogens (e.g., clostridial spores, parvovirus)
Resources		
Hand hygiene in healthcare settings—Hand hygiene guidance[45]		https://www.cdc.gov/handhygiene/providers/guideline.html

due to frequent hand washing or when soap and water are unavailable. Although the cost of alcohol-based hand sanitation can be greater than cost of hand washing, it may bring improved compliance.[53]

Gloves

Glove use is intended to decrease pathogen transmission risk by providing a barrier to protect caregivers and patients. However, gloves are often misused in veterinary settings, potentially leading to greater contamination of people, patients, and the environment. In general, gloving should be considered an adjunct to, and not a replacement for, proper hand hygiene as glove failures are relatively common although typically unrecognized by the wearer.[54,55] Glove use is recommended when personnel expect to contact blood, body fluids, mucous membranes, or nonintact skin.[51] Gloves should be changed and not washed when moving from a contaminated to clean site on a single patient or moving between patients.[51] Additionally, gloves should be removed before touching other surfaces (e.g., countertops, keyboards, phones, or doorknobs) or accessing supplies (e.g., carts, bandage kits, cupboards, and supply rooms). Consideration should be given to double gloving when collecting samples from a patient in isolation or when glove contamination is expected. This will allow the removal of the outer, potentially contaminated, glove before labeling samples or removing PPE.

Hand Hygiene Compliance

While most veterinary personnel believe hand hygiene is important in the prevention of infectious disease transmission and zoonoses,[56,57] overall compliance can be low (14%–20% of hand hygiene opportunities) among small animal practitioners, with lower compliance before patient contacts (3% of opportunities) versus after patient contacts (26%) or between patient contacts (41%–48%).[56,58–60] Practitioner-reported obstacles to compliance include forgetfulness, damage to skin from frequent hand washing, being too busy, and a lack of available hand hygiene supplies.[57,60] There have been conflicting reports on the benefits of hand hygiene awareness campaigns. Signage may improve hand washing technique,[58] and incorporation of an educational component may improve compliance (see Table 15.3).[59]

Barrier Nursing Precautions

"Barrier nursing" precautions (i.e., the use of PPE) are widely used to minimize transmission and to reduce exposure of immunocompromised patients or personnel to potential pathogens. In veterinary settings, this usually includes the use of disposable gowns, gloves, facial protection, and implementation of footwear hygiene (i.e., footwear covers or use of footbaths or footmats). The intent is to create a barrier between "clean" and "dirty" to prevent the contamination of skin or underlying clothing with a potential pathogen from the patient or the environment.[61,62] Use of such precautions is not a panacea. A recent systematic review reported contamination rates from 25% to 100% irrespective of the type of PPE being used.[63] The effective implementation of barrier precautions not only requires a financial investment but an investment in time for proper donning and doffing of PPE and an investment in the education of personnel on the rationale for its use.

Barrier Gowns

Permeable gowns are typically used for general animal care, while impermeable gowns are recommended when splashes are expected (e.g., flushing wounds or draining abscesses). In general, disposable gowns should not be reused even on the same patient. If using washable (i.e., reusable) gowns, they should be appropriately laundered between uses. When donning and doffing gowns, the wearer must only touch the outside of the gown to limit cross-contamination.

Gloves

See the section in this chapter on hand hygiene.

Facial Protection

Face shields or glasses with a mask protect the mucous membranes of the eyes, nose, and mouth from potentially infectious materials. Consideration should be given to their use anytime there may be a splash or a spray hazard (e.g., when flushing wounds or draining abscesses).

Footwear Hygiene

Footwear hygiene includes the use of disposable footwear covers and/or disinfectant footbaths or footmats. Environmental contamination is commonly associated with outbreaks within veterinary hospitals.[64,65] Therefore, it is crucial that footwear be clean before moving to a new environment, either within the hospital or external to the hospital. Footwear should be easily cleaned and there may be additional requirements for safety (e.g., closed-toe shoes). When caring for patients in isolation or those who are immunocompromised, footwear should be able to be disinfected or dedicated to the care of an individual patient (see Footbaths/footmats).

Transmission-Based Precautions

Transmission-based precautions are instituted for patients with confirmed or suspected infections that are known to be transmitted via a particular route—airborne, droplet, or contact.[66]

Airborne precautions prevent the transmission of infectious agents by droplet nuclei. In human medicine, this typically involves isolation in a single-bed, negative-pressure room, barrier nursing precautions, and a high-density respirator (N95) mask. These masks resemble surgical masks but filter 1-µm particles with an efficiency of at least 95%, and must be properly fitted to the individual wearer by trained personnel. Airborne precautions are rarely necessary in hospitals that treat only dogs and cats, but should be considered for animals suspected to have pneumonic plague, tularemia, or a *Mycobacterium tuberculosis* infection.

Droplet precautions are used to prevent transmission by large-particle aerosols. This requires the use of barrier nursing precautions, but does not require a negative-pressure room. Droplet precautions apply to dogs and cats with transmissible respiratory disease. In human medicine, barrier precautions for droplet precautions include facial protection.

Contact precautions are indicated for animals with infections that can be transmitted by direct contact with the patient or through fomite contact (see Barrier Nursing Precautions).

Movement Restrictions, Separation, and Isolation

Managing the flow of traffic and restriction of movement (i.e., separation or isolation) of patients and personnel are important infection control strategies. Efforts should be made to minimize contact between infectious disease suspects and the general hospital population and to minimize their time spent in common areas (e.g., waiting areas or common service areas such as radiology). In general, the flow of patients and personnel should be from clean to dirty areas and from low to high pathogen risk areas. Separation and isolation strategies serve to limit environmental contamination and decrease the likelihood of contact between patients and personnel. The potential infectious disease status of all patients should be considered as early as possible—before arriving at the hospital, based on history, signalment or clinical signs, or during initial examination or hospitalization. The earlier that risks can be identified, the earlier the animal can be separated or isolated and the lower the risk to other patients and personnel. If it is known in advance that an animal with a suspected or known infectious disease is to be seen at the hospital, efforts should be made to admit the patient directly into an examination or isolation room, bypassing the waiting area. Special consideration should be given if a patient is from a shelter or breeding facility, as these are considered high-risk populations.

Separation

Separation is the establishment of hospital areas with differing levels of biosecurity. The degree of separation achieved is dictated by physical and operational limitations of the facility, and may be related to the species (e.g., dogs and cats), age (e.g., adult or neonate), severity of disease (e.g., critical care or elective surgery cases), or type of patient (i.e., inpatient vs. outpatient). Designated hospital areas may include critical care units and isolation units. Equipment and, possibly, personnel should ideally be dedicated to a particular hospital area for patient management. If movement of personnel or equipment is to occur, it should be governed by clearly defined infection control protocols (e.g., use of protective clothing, hand hygiene, and disinfection of equipment between areas).

Isolation

Isolation is a higher level of separation that not only limits contacts but also minimizes personnel and patient traffic in the area. Some facilities may incorporate video monitoring to ensure adequate observation while limiting high-risk contacts. Patients with suspected or confirmed transmissible infectious disease should be evaluated and managed in an area isolated from the main hospital population. In general, patients should be considered for separation and isolation if they have gastrointestinal disease (e.g., diarrhea or enteritis), acute respiratory disease (especially if febrile), abortion/fetal loss, neonatal death or disease, alopecic skin lesions that may represent dermatophytosis or sarcoptic mange, fever with or without other clinical signs, or acute onset neurologic disease. Whether a dedicated isolation facility or just contact precautions are used during hospitalization depends on the regional prevalence of transmissible infections in a specific practice area and the likelihood of one of those infections in the patient under evaluation.

At times, it may be necessary to use common hospital facilities or equipment (e.g., radiology, surgery, and endoscopy) for diagnostics or treatment of an infectious disease case or suspect. Proper communication in advance with veterinary team members located in these common areas about the risks is essential, and every effort should be made to use these areas at the end of the day, with thorough cleaning and disinfection immediately after use.

Footbaths and Footmats

The use of footbaths/footmats is a common strategy employed by VTHs, more so in large animal hospitals than in small animal hospitals.[67] Use of both footbaths and footmats can decrease bacterial counts on footwear.[67–69] However, efficacy depends on frequency of disinfectant replenishment, amount of organic debris on footwear and in the footbath/footmat, the type of disinfectant used, and compliance. Footmats and footbaths also serve as a visual indicator to personnel regarding the risk level of a particular area and may deter foot traffic. When footmats and footbaths are used, care should be taken to instruct personnel on proper use and to mitigate any slip hazard by providing a walk-off mat for surfaces that may become slippery when wet.

Environmental Infection Control

Environmental contamination is commonly associated with epidemic disease in large animal hospitals[6,64,65] and is increasingly recognized as a contributor to outbreaks in companion animal hospitals.[70,71] For some pathogens, the environment is a clear source of infection and a major contributor to disease (e.g., canine parvovirus), but for others, environmental transmission is mainly of concern in specific high-risk environments such as veterinary hospitals, kennels, or shelters (e.g., *Clostridioides difficile*).[70] With this in mind, environmental cleaning and disinfection is a cornerstone of an effective infection control program.

Cleaning and Disinfection

The simple act of scrubbing with a detergent can reduce bacterial load on a concrete surface by 90%.[73] When followed by the application of an appropriate disinfectant (i.e., class, concentration, and contact time), this can be reduced by an additional 6%.[72] Cleaning should remove all visible organic debris (e.g., feces, urine, nasal exudate, and blood) from surfaces because this can render disinfectants less effective. Many bacteria form biofilms in the environment. These organized bacterial communities produce protective extracellular polymer matrices that promote surface adhesion and protect them from environmental insult (e.g., disinfectants). Environmental biofilms are a source of potential pathogens as well as AMR genes.[73–75] Scrubbing with detergent is required to break up and remove biofilms from cleanable surfaces.

Chemical disinfection is a chemical reaction that is affected by the presence of organic debris as well as conditions such as temperature and UV light (i.e., sunlight). Many commercial products are available for environmental disinfection. When selecting a product, it is important to be cognizant of the major classes of disinfectants, their activity against different pathogens, and conditions that may limit their effectiveness (see Table 14.1). The products used should be registered by governmental agencies such as the US Environmental Protection Agency (EPA), used at label-indicated concentrations and contact times, and all safety precautions recommended by the manufacturer should be followed.

Routine Cleaning and Disinfection

Routine cleaning and disinfection attempts to minimize the burden of potential pathogens in the environment to a level that is inconsequential. Facility-specific protocols should be developed, written down, reviewed at least annually, and made readily accessible to all personnel. Routine cleaning and disinfection should occur regularly in areas used to house and manage all patients—not just areas reserved for suspected or confirmed infectious diseases—as well as personnel areas. While patient examination and treatment areas should be cleaned between each patient, all areas should also have a general daily cleaning with attention to corners, under cabinets, handles, and faucets. Cracks and crevices should be repaired, and dirt floors and porous surfaces (e.g., untreated wood or unsealed concrete) should be avoided as these cannot be effectively disinfected. If porous surfaces cannot be replaced, they can be rendered less porous by painting or sealing the surface.

Enhanced Cleaning

Enhanced cleaning should be completed immediately after use in areas known to have housed patients with suspected or confirmed infectious disease. This may include use of a higher-order disinfectant (e.g., accelerated peroxygen), with attention paid to surfaces that may be easily contaminated but overlooked in general cleaning (e.g., cabinet handles, keyboards, and faucets). Equipment used on such patients should be handled in a manner that minimizes contamination of hospital surfaces and cleaning and disinfection should occur prior to reuse. Aerosol application of disinfectants with appropriate safety measures (including respiratory protection for personnel) can be used as an adjunct to traditional cleaning to manage difficult-to-reach areas such as overhead areas.[76–78]

Common Use Equipment

Level of Disinfection for Patient Care Equipment (Table 15.5).[79]

Critical patient care equipment includes items that may enter a sterile field or the vascular system (e.g., surgical instruments, implants, intravenous catheters). If contaminated, these items carry a high risk for infection. Critical items should either be purchased as sterile or they should be sterilized before use. *Semi-critical patient care equipment* includes items that may contact mucous membranes or nonintact skin (e.g., anesthesia equipment, bronchoscope). These items should have high-level disinfection with chemical disinfectants performed before reuse, with the goal to eliminate all microorganisms except bacterial spores. *Noncritical patient care equipment* includes items that may contact intact skin, but not mucous membranes (e.g., blood pressure cuff). These items should have intermediate- or low-level disinfection with chemical disinfectants performed before reuse, with the goal to eliminate vegetative bacteria and most fungi and viruses. Intermediate-level disinfection is used in the presence of organic debris, while low-level disinfection is typically used in its absence.

Surgical Instruments, Equipment, and Power Tools

While historically cold sterilization has been used in medicine, it should not be used for instrument or implant sterilization when steam or ethylene oxide sterilization is available. With cold sterilization, there is likely greater potential for contamination and incomplete sterilization,[79] and HAIs have also been reported in human medicine associated with reprocessing of reusable medical and surgical instruments.[80] Surgical power tools may present a significant challenge in decontamination. Often having intricate, structurally complex designs, they can accumulate tissue and proteinaceous material which may harbor potential pathogens and disrupt the cleaning and disinfection process.[81,82] All manufacturer decontamination recommendations should be followed to ensure proper sterilization before reuse.

Anesthesia and Nebulizer Equipment

Small animal breathing systems have a tendency to harbor environmental microorganisms of low pathogenicity.[83] Contamination is typically greater in proximal tubing than in more distal tubing and the number of bacteria decreases over time.[83] As such, for routine uses, sterilization is not considered to be necessary. At a minimum, tubing

TABLE 15.5 Recommended Levels of Microbial Disinfection[79]

Level	Expected Effect	When to Use
High	• Elimination of all viruses and vegetative bacteria • Elimination of most bacterial spores and fungi	• Critical patient care equipment (may enter sterile field or vascular system; e.g., surgical instruments, implants, intravenous catheters) • Semi-critical patient care equipment (contact with mucous membranes or non-intact skin; e.g., anesthesia equipment, bronchoscope)
Intermediate	• Elimination of all vegetative bacteria • Elimination of most viruses and fungi	• In the presence of organic debris • Noncritical patient care equipment (contact with intact skin, but not mucous membranes; e.g., blood pressure cuff)
Low	• Elimination of most vegetative bacteria, fungi, enveloped viruses • Equivalent to sanitation	• Used in absence of organic debris • Noncritical patient care equipment (contact with intact skin, but not mucous membranes; e.g., blood pressure cuff)

(Derived from Rutala WA, Weber DJ. Disinfection and sterilization: an overview. *Am J Infect Control.* 2013;41:S2–5.)

should be scrubbed with a detergent to disrupt biofilm and high-level disinfection should be used, as this equipment is considered to be semi-critical. Routine disinfection of breathing systems can be achieved by soaking equipment in an antiseptic (selected due to the potential for contact with mucous membranes) such as chlorhexidine (2% solution) for 15 to 30 minutes, or accelerated hydrogen peroxide, following by thorough rinsing.[84] For nebulizers and humidifiers, flushing hydrogen peroxide (20% by volume in water) through the system with periodic sterilization is recommended. Special consideration should be given to equipment used on patients with suspected or confirmed contagious agents that may require additional measures (i.e., sterilization) before reuse or require disposal.

Endoscopic Equipment

Endoscopic equipment is very complex and intricate, with narrow channels for aspiration, flushing, and equipment passage. As such, endoscopic equipment cannot be sterilized. However, they are semi-critical, so should undergo high-level disinfection. While equipment should be cleaned and disinfected per manufacturers recommendations, a six-step process has been recommended for endoscope reprocessing: (1) pre-cleaning with function control, (2) manual brush cleaning and leak test, (3) rinse, (4) disinfection, (5) final rinse and drying, and (6) safe storage to avoid contamination.[85] Proper cleaning, including use of a brush to scrub channels before disinfection is critical as incomplete cleaning can result in HAIs (e.g., *Pseudomonas*).[86] After cleaning, disinfection can be achieved by soaking in alkaline glutaraldehyde for 10 minutes followed by a sterile water rinse. There are also automated endoscope reprocessing systems that use performic acid,[87] hydrogen peroxide vapor, or other disinfectants. Disinfectants can be corrosive to metal parts and should be thoroughly rinsed from any equipment after the proper contact time has been achieved.

Other Diagnostic Equipment (e.g., Ultrasound, ECG)

While ideally, diagnostic equipment would be dedicated to a particular service or hospital area, this may be impractical due to cost (e.g., ultrasound). Therefore, protocols should be developed to ensure proper cleaning and disinfection before equipment is moved from patient to patient and between hospital areas. Manufacturers' recommendations should be followed when cleaning and disinfecting specialty equipment.

Animal Holding and Housing Areas

General principles of environmental disinfection apply to cage and run cleaning, with removal of organic debris, scrubbing with detergent, rinsing, use of an adequate disinfectant, and provision of an appropriate concentration and contact time as key determinants of success. If high-pressure washing is used (i.e., PSI > 80–100), care should be taken as microorganisms can aerosolize and may result in small surface defects that preclude effective cleaning and disinfection.

Animal Feeding Dishes and Water Bowls

Pet food and water dishes are a recognized reservoir for potential pathogens in the home environment and presumably also in the hospital environment.[88] These items should be properly cleaned and disinfected before reuse. Generally, the use of a dishwasher is preferred to manual washing as higher water temperatures can be achieved that will eliminate many microorganisms, with the exception of bacterial spores.

Waste Management

An important part of effective infection prevention is proper management of medical and infectious waste. The AVMA has published general guidelines to aid veterinary practices in developing waste management programs,[89] which also must be in compliance with federal, state, and local laws.[90] Of particular interest in the United States is the Federal Medical Waste Tracking Act of 1988 (MWTA) which is regulated by the EPA. This act applies to veterinary medical waste that is considered to be a public health hazard. According to the MWTA, waste generators are liable for medical waste from its creation to final disposal, irrespective of the use of a waste management company.

Definitions for medical and infectious waste are provided by state laws and regulations. These definitions typically include information regarding waste infectivity, waste categories (e.g., sharps, tubing, fecal waste), and which facilities are required to comply with these regulations.[89] It is recommended that veterinary hospitals separate medical and infectious waste as it is generated.[89] Medical and infectious waste may include items such as needles, bandages, or bedding contaminated by bodily excretions, such as blood, nasal exudates, urine, or feces, or by tissue removed during medical or surgical treatment. Care should be taken to deter patient access to waste containers, and efforts should be made to reduce the likelihood for vector transmission by insects, rodents, or clinic cats and dogs. Appropriate disposal methods, such as autoclaving and incineration, will depend upon the suspected or confirmed infectious agent as well as local regulations.

Outdoor Elimination or Exercise Areas

Grass and/or dirt exercise and elimination areas are impossible to decontaminate. If possible, outside areas should be designated for use based on the risk for shedding a potential pathogen (e.g., *Salmonella*, *Leptospira*) by creating dedicated space for use by generally healthy patients, immunocompromised patients, and patients with suspected or confirmed transmissible infections. Consideration should be given to installing an outdoor surface such as a concrete pad (heated if it is to be used in a cold climate) that can be cleaned and disinfected after use by a potentially infectious case. If use of a grass/dirt area is unavoidable, "cleaning" should involve removal of all feces, cutting the grass to facilitate sunlight penetration, and "resting" the area (i.e., allowing sufficient time for infectious agent to become inactivated) before use by other patients. Alternatively, dirt can be removed and replaced after use by an infectious disease case.

Handling of Sharps

Sharps handling practices receive considerable attention in human medicine because of the risk of transmission of blood-borne pathogens. Significant injury or illness can follow sharps injuries including transmission of infectious agents and allergic or inflammatory reactions from exposure to medications.

Needle and Sharps Injuries

Needle and sharps injuries are most commonly associated with handling of syringes (64%), suture needles (51%), and scalpel blades (35%).[91] Career estimates for needle stick injury incidence rates range from 83% among veterinarians to 78%–93% among veterinary technicians,[92,93] and annual estimates for needle stick injury incidence rates range from 44% among veterinarians to 46% among veterinary technicians.[92,93] Needle recapping is common in veterinary medicine,[94] and approximately one-third of veterinary personnel report doing so due to a lack of an appropriate container for disposal.[92]

Needle and Sharps Handling Practices

The Compendium of Veterinary Standard Precautions, developed by the NASPHV, recommends that all hospital personnel receive specific training regarding safe sharps handling and risks associated with the handling of sharps. In general, only trained personnel should restrain patients and needles should not be bent prior to use. Needle caps should never be removed using your mouth and when uncapped, needles should not be passed to another individual nor carried throughout the clinic. If recapping a needle is necessary, the one-handed scoop method should be used—place the cap on a horizontal surface, and while holding a syringe with an attached needle in one hand, use the needle to scoop up the cap without using the other hand, securing the cap by pushing it on a hard surface.[19] To facilitate safe disposal of sharps, approved sharps containers should be placed in all areas used for patient management. To avoid sharps injuries (which can promote transmission of blood-borne zoonotic pathogens), forceps should be used to remove uncapped needles from syringes (or preferably dispose of as a unit) and also to remove scalpel blades from nondisposable scalpel handles (see Waste Management).

Control of Vectors and Rodents

Pest management should be an integrated program that utilizes pesticides, traps, and environmental controls to block access to buildings and create unfavorable environments for pest survival.[19] Environmental controls include sealing of access points, storage of food in sealed containers, elimination of rodent nesting sites, removal of standing water, installation of window screens, and the prompt disposal of waste. Both insects and rodents can serve as biologic or mechanical vectors for dissemination of pathogens. Flies have been shown to carry *Salmonella* as mechanical vectors.[95–97] Clinic cats or dogs can serve as biologic or mechanical vectors for infectious agents as well as be a source of antimicrobial-resistant bacteria.[98,99] Use of a pest control company is strongly encouraged to develop an integrated pest control program that is facility specific.

MONITORING INFECTION CONTROL PROGRAM EFFECTIVENESS

Assessment of an infection control program's efficacy is integral to program effectiveness and promotes compliance. Because infectious diseases emerge and re-emerge, it is imperative to ensure existing protocols are reviewed and updated. Additionally, identifying program limitations may lead to permanent policy change or temporary change to mitigate a transient risk. For example, during a regional outbreak of canine influenza, it may be prudent to implement additional precautions for dogs with upper respiratory signs or those with a travel history to impacted regions.

Surveillance activities can be used to assess program effectiveness and allow early detection of adverse events so that mitigation efforts can be rapidly instituted. Consideration should be given to the surveillance method (i.e., active, passive, syndromic) and type of surveillance (e.g., monitoring patients and/or the environment). Surveillance and monitoring for control of nosocomial infections in veterinary hospitals has been described in detail elsewhere.[100–102]

Surveillance Methods

Surveillance is the systematic collection, analysis, and interpretation of events in a population to enable tailored responses to adverse events or outcomes. A surveillance system has two components: (1) a monitoring system and (2) a critical limit at which a predetermined action will be taken to mitigate a perceived risk. Surveillance data allows for a facility to establish baseline or an expected level of a particular outcome, process, or event. Facility managers can then track this level to detect a deviation from what is normally expected and rapidly instigate corrective actions.

Active Surveillance

Active surveillance is conducted to identify an outcome or indicator of interest, e.g., performing fecal cultures on all dogs fed raw food diets in the home environment. This type of surveillance provides typically high-quality primary data, but is costly both financially and in personnel time. Active surveillance is most commonly used in large veterinary hospitals and may be used for targeted surveillance of high-risk patient groups.

Passive Surveillance

Passive surveillance is the use of information that has been collected for another purpose (e.g., diagnostic laboratory specimens). This type of surveillance is relatively inexpensive and simple to perform, but is considered a secondary data source. As such, there is limited control over the quality of the data. Many hospitals use passive surveillance data to monitor for resistant organisms and resistance patterns.

Syndromic Surveillance

Syndromic surveillance uses nonspecific indicators of disease (e.g., "diarrhea") that are identified before a definitive diagnosis can be determined. This type of surveillance is relatively easy to perform but relies upon formalized definitions to allow for monitoring. Syndromic surveillance can be a useful screening tool to implement enhanced infection control practices and mandatory testing protocols.

Patient Monitoring

Patient monitoring may be active (e.g., performing fecal cultures on all inpatients on admission for *Salmonella*), passive (e.g., summarizing laboratory tests to identify MRSA isolates), or involve observing for a particular syndrome (e.g., fevers in hospitalized patients).

While continuous surveillance can be performed, targeted surveillance of high-risk or high-cost problems is an efficient way to assess program efficacy.[103] It allows for a focused effort on a particular type of patient (e.g., all patients vs. inpatients vs. critical care patients), a specific pathogen (e.g., *Salmonella* or MRSA), or a specific syndrome (e.g., diarrheic or febrile patients). Incorporation of patient monitoring into an infection control program should be facility specific, and reflect the availability of resources and level of risk aversion of stakeholders, previous disease outbreak experiences, and disease prevalence in the area.

Environmental Monitoring

Environmental monitoring allows assessment of program effectiveness through the identification of residual contamination. It also can be instrumental in detecting reservoirs of potential pathogens.[101,104] Considerations are the type of specimens collected, the method of specimen collection, the detection method, laboratory selection, and available resources (both equipment and personnel time). Detection methods must be appropriately validated and optimized for that intended purpose. In general, if environmental testing is to be used, it should be performed regularly to establish a baseline level to which future findings can be compared. It should be remembered that the hospital environment is not expected to be sterile, and the presence of opportunistic pathogens is not unexpected. Environmental surveillance can provide important information during outbreaks, assist evaluation of endemic disease, act as an educational tool for personnel and evaluate the impact of interventions. However, results may be confusing, misleading, and counter-productive if testing is improperly implemented and interpreted.

Multiple methods have been described for environmental sampling including the use of electrostatic wipes or sterile sponges that are cultured for specific microorganisms[104,105] or contact plates (e.g., Rodac plates) to enumerate nonspecific bacterial growth.[106–108] In general, sampling a larger surface area will tend to provide a more representative sample and will likely be a more sensitive method for detection. Focusing sampling efforts on high-traffic areas (e.g., examination areas and common hallways) or on identifying environmentally persistent pathogens (e.g., *Salmonella*) can decrease costs associated with monitoring, but may provide limited information regarding the scope of the problem. As such, more inclusive follow-up sampling may need to be performed.

Program Compliance

Compliance with infection control protocols is critical to program success, yet it is one of the most challenging aspects of program implementation. Despite veterinarians expressing concern about risks associated with gastrointestinal parasites and bacteria, approximately one-half report "always" washing their hands between patient contacts or before eating, and only one-quarter report using appropriate PPE when evaluating a patient for gastrointestinal disease.[56]

Program compliance stems from creating a "safety culture." A strong safety culture should have norms and rules that explicitly define risks and provide guidelines, it should place safety as a priority and motivate personnel to act accordingly, and it should use reflexivity to understand risk and risk mitigation.[109] In practice, this might include leading by example, development of an education and training program, regular reporting of surveillance efforts, and creation of an infection control committee that will encourage and empower participation in program development and improvement. Personnel should be reminded that the program has been implemented to protect people, patients, and the practice, that it is necessary to provide optimal patient care, and that the program is only as good as those practicing the infection control measures agreed upon by the practice.

SPECIALIZED AREAS OF CONCERN

Healthcare-Associated Infections

HAIs are those that are acquired in a healthcare facility. These may be the result of indigenous microflora or exogenous microorganisms from other sources. Infections incubating at the time of admission to a facility are not classified as HAIs, although this distinction can be difficult to determine. In human healthcare, HAIs increase the duration of hospitalization, patient morbidity and mortality, and the overall cost of care.[2] They are one of the top 10 causes of human deaths in the United States, with an estimated 5.8% of deaths in 2002 being associated with HAIs.[3]

While we lack similar data in veterinary medicine, in 2006, 82% of accredited VTHs surveyed reported outbreaks of HAIs among patients in the previous 5 years and 32% reported zoonotic infections among personnel in the previous 2 years.[5] Among adult dogs and cats admitted to critical care units, approximately 16.3% and 12%, respectively, experienced HAI during hospitalization based on syndromic surveillance conducted at five participating VTHs over a 12-week period.[7] These estimates are derived from critical care patients that generally have systemic illness and thus greater immune compromise than the general patient population, and are more commonly subjected to invasive procedures and placement of indwelling catheters.

Peripheral Intravenous Catheterization

Peripheral intravenous catheterization is commonly associated with insertion site inflammation,[7] and places patients at risk for developing an HAI as it also creates a portal of entry for potential pathogens. Pathogens can gain venous access by migrating down the catheter itself or be introduced through a contaminated catheter tip, hub, or infusates. Catheter-tip culture-positive rates of 25% have been reported among dogs and cats admitted to a critical care unit[110] and 15% among noncritical patients.[111] Bacterial species commonly detected include *Enterobacter* and *Staphylococcus*.[110,111] While it is difficult to determine if catheter tips become contaminated during placement or seeding from another source, it is recommended that the catheter be placed after aseptic preparation of the insertion site—a 1-minute scrub with chlorhexidine followed by an alcohol application.[112,113] Catheter site preparation solutions and materials should be stored in closed containers and should not be refilled. They should be discarded when empty or cleaned and autoclaved before being refilled. Proper hand hygiene should be practiced before contacting the insertion site or placing a catheter. Catheter hub colonization accounts for approximately 70% of catheter-related sepsis in human patients receiving parenteral nutrition.[114] Thus, it has been recommended that the catheter hub be cleaned with alcohol or iodine before use of a sterile needle and syringe to administer medications.[113]

Catheter sites should be checked daily for evidence of thrombophlebitis (e.g., pain, swelling, redness, and discharge).[113] While inflammation itself may not necessitate catheter removal, it increases the risk of infection and can be difficult to distinguish from infection. Consequently, if these signs are observed, the catheter should be promptly removed and the catheter replaced at an alternative site. Aseptic catheter removal is recommended if catheter-tip culture is to follow (which should only be performed if there is evidence of infection at the catheter site): the site should be scrubbed as was done prior to catheter insertion, and the catheter then removed and the tip cut with sterile scissors and placed in a sterile red top tube with a drop of sterile saline to prevent desiccation for submission to the laboratory (avoiding excessive dilution). As a general guideline, a count > 15 CFU suggests a true infection as opposed to mere contamination.[115]

Catheter stabilization reduces the potential for thrombophlebitis. To restrict movement, a small amount of a broad-spectrum antimicrobial ointment should be applied at the point of catheter penetration through the skin and the site should be covered with a sterile occlusive dressing. The date and time of catheter insertion should be recorded. It is recommended that intravenous catheters be removed after 72 hours, although there is little objective data to support this practice. With modern catheter materials, proper placement, and close monitoring, longer-term catheterization is becoming more widely accepted. Catheters made of polytetrafluoroethylene, silicone elastomer, or polyurethane are more resistant to the adherence of microorganisms than are catheters made of polyvinyl chloride or polyethylene.[116] In addition, iodinated alcohol solutions within catheter hubs, chlorhexidine-silver-sulfadiazine or antibacterial-impregnated catheters, and antibacterial-impregnated sponges have been evaluated.[117]

Urinary Catheterization

Urinary catheterization can be associated with urinary tract inflammation[7] and disrupt normal urinary tract defense mechanisms, including normal flow of urine. Urinary catheters permit retrograde migration of commensal organisms that inhabit the prepuce, vagina, and distal urethra into the normally sterile portions of the urinary tract.[118] Prior to urinary catheter placement, external genitalia should be thoroughly cleansed and catheterization performed under aseptic conditions.

Many urinary tract infections (UTIs) occur within the first 3 days of catheterization,[118,119] with the risk for UTI increasing by 27% for every additional day of catheterization.[120] A complicating factor in most veterinary studies is a failure to differentiate subclinical bacteriuria from bacterial cystitis, particularly since treatment of subclinical bacteriuria is not generally recommended.[121] While closed systems are commonly used in human medicine, open systems are frequently used in veterinary medicine (but have been discouraged). Interestingly, the incidence of UTIs was found to be similar among dogs admitted to a critical care unit when using closed (8.3%) versus open (11.1%) urine collection systems for a median of 2-day duration.[122]

Antimicrobial therapy during catheterization can increase the risk for UTI if in place for more than a few days.[119,120] Therefore, it should be avoided unless there is clinical evidence of bacterial cystitis and/or the patient is deemed to be at high risk for upper UTI. In such cases, treatment should be initiated with the understanding that the goal of treatment is to ameliorate clinical signs, not eliminate infection, and the catheter should be removed as soon as possible.

Aquatic Equipment Used in Physical Therapy

With proper management, aquatic equipment (e.g., whirlpools, water treadmills) poses a low risk for pathogen transmission among patients and personnel. Equipment should be kept clean and free of hair and debris. Water chemistry levels should be checked daily and managed appropriately (chlorine:1–3 parts per million [ppm]; pH: 7.2–7.8; and alkalinity 80–120 ppm).[123]

Patients with a recent history of diarrhea or those with known or suspected resistant infections should be excluded, and patients with visibly soiled haircoats should be brushed and bathed prior to treatment. Facilities should develop protocols in the case of a fecal accident, which may include the use of a filtration system and/or complete removal of water and cleaning and disinfection appropriate for the equipment. The CDC provides recommendations for pool and hot tub owners that may be useful in protocol development.[124]

Immunocompromised Patients and Personnel

Patients and personnel can be immunocompromised as a result of disease (e.g., cancer, diabetes mellitus), medical treatment (e.g., chemotherapeutics), age (i.e., young and old), or pregnancy. While all general recommendations for the prevention of infectious diseases in this chapter are applicable to patients and personnel, particular consideration should be given to the use of barrier precautions to prevent exposure of immunocompromised animals and personnel.

Immunocompromised personnel should discuss any necessary work restrictions and precautions in light of their specific condition with their personal physician and/or an infectious disease doctor. Of particular concern for pregnant veterinary personnel are exposures to toxoplasmosis, lymphocytic choriomeningitis, brucellosis, listeriosis, psittacosis, and Q fever.[19] If possible, veterinary hospitals should establish a relationship with a doctor who is prepared to consult on zoonotic exposures with staff members.

Blood and Blood Component Transfusion Infectious Disease Prevention

Safe blood banking in veterinary medicine relies upon screening of healthy donors using the best available diagnostic tests. The American College of Veterinary Internal Medicine (ACVIM) has published a consensus statement providing guidelines for managing blood donor programs.[125] Blood donor selection should be based on a thorough history, physical examination, and initial clinicopathologic screening (e.g., CBC and biochemistry panel). Suitable donors should then be screened for pathogens that meet at least three of the following criteria: (1) pathogen causes clinical infection in blood recipients; (2) pathogen can be carried subclinically by otherwise healthy-appearing donors; (3) pathogen can be detected using culture or molecular methods in blood; and (4) infection in the recipient may be life threatening or difficult to treat.[125] At a minimum, blood donors should be tested yearly, with more frequent testing for geographically important agents and among animals with exposure to known risk factors (e.g., ticks) for development of infectious disease.[125] The ACVIM consensus statement provides detailed recommendations for specific agents of concern.[125]

Breeding, Boarding, and Shelter Facilities

Many of the general recommendations for the prevention of infectious diseases in this chapter are applicable to breeding, boarding, and shelter facilities. Additional recommendations unique to these facilities are presented in the next three chapters in this book. Many of these facilities have a significant transient population as well as resident animals. Protocols should be developed to reduce the risk to resident animals through separation of transient and resident animals, monitoring for signs of infectious disease, and determining required vaccinations and parasite prevention for all animals. Animals are often stressed on intake, which is exacerbated by high stocking densities, being grouped with unknown animals, and poor nutrition; immune compromise results. High-stocking densities also facilitate infectious disease transmission. Maintenance of separate animal groups, often by species and age, is critical to prevention of infectious disease transmission.

Facility managers need to be cognizant of the maximum capacity for care and strive to maintain populations below this level. The Farm Animal Welfare Council (FAWC) offers guiding principles when managing animal populations that equally apply to dog and cat populations in breeding, boarding, or shelter facilities. In 1979, the FAWC put forward the "Five Freedoms" for animals kept by man: (1) freedom from hunger and thirst; (2) freedom from discomfort; (3) freedom from pain, injury, or disease; (4) freedom to express normal behavior; and (5) freedom from fear and distress. By incorporating these principles into facility management protocols, facility managers are ensuring the health and welfare of the animals, including the prevention of infectious diseases. The Association of Shelter Veterinarians and the American Humane Association have each published detailed guidelines regarding shelter management, standard operating procedures, and standards of care.[126,127] The United States Department of Agriculture–Animal and Plant Health Inspection Service (USDA:APHIS) has published guidance documents for dog kennels and breeding facilities.[128]

Further useful online resources are shown in Table 15.6.

TABLE 15.6 Infection Control Web References

Entity	Website
American Veterinary Medical Association (AVMA) AVMA Policies: Regulation of Veterinary Medical Waste	https://www.avma.org/resources-tools/avma-policies/regulation-veterinary-medical-waste
Canadian Committee on Antibiotic Resistance (CCAR) Infection prevention and control best practices for small animal veterinary clinics	https://www.oahn.ca/resources/ipc-best-practices/
Centers for Disease Control and Prevention (CDC) Hand hygiene in healthcare settings: Guidelines Hand hygiene in healthcare settings: Hand hygiene basics Residential pool or hot tub owners: Cleaning and remediation Residential pool or hot tub owners: Disinfection and testing	www.cdc.gov/handhygiene/Guidelines.html www.cdc.gov/handhygiene/Basics.html; www.cdc.gov/healthywater/swimming/residential/cleaning-remediation.html; www.cdc.gov/healthywater/swimming/residential/disinfection-testing.html
National Association for State and Public Health Veterinarians	www.nasphv.org/documentsCompendia.html
World Health Organization (WHO) Critically important antimicrobials for human medicine. 5th revision	http://apps.who.int/iris/bitstream/10665/255027/1/9789241512220-eng.pdf?ua=1

REFERENCES

1. Morley PS. Evidence-based infection control in clinical practice: if you buy clothes for the emperor, will he wear them? *J Vet Intern Med.* 2013;27:430–438.
2. Calfee DP. Crisis in hospital-acquired, healthcare-associated infections. *Annu Rev Med.* 2012;63:359–371.
3. Klevens RM, Edwards JR, Richards Jr CL, et al. Estimating health care-associated infections and deaths in U.S. hospitals, 2002. *Public Health Rep.* 2007;122:160–166.
4. Haley RW, Culver DH, White JW, et al. The efficacy of infection surveillance and control programs in preventing nosocomial infections in US hospitals. *Am J Epidemiol.* 1985;121:182–205.
5. Benedict KM, Morley PS, Van Metre DC. Characteristics of biosecurity and infection control programs at veterinary teaching hospitals. *J Am Vet Med Assoc.* 2008;233:767–773.
6. Dallap Schaer BL, Aceto H, Rankin SC. Outbreak of salmonellosis caused by *Salmonella enterica* serovar Newport MDR-AmpC in a large animal veterinary teaching hospital. *J Vet Intern Med.* 2010;24:1138–1146.
7. Ruple-Czerniak A, Aceto HW, Bender JB, et al. Using syndromic surveillance to estimate baseline rates for healthcare-associated infections in critical care units of small animal referral hospitals. *J Vet Intern Med.* 2013;27:1392–1399.
8. American Veterinary Medical Association. Veterinarian's Oath. https://www.avma.org/resources-tools/avma-policies/veterinarians-oath.
9. Morley P, Anderson M, Burgess B. Report of the third Havemeyer workshop on infection control in equine populations. *Equine Vet J.* 2012.
10. Murphy CP, Reid-Smith RJ, Weese JS, et al. Evaluation of specific infection control practices used by companion animal veterinarians in community veterinary practices in southern Ontario. *Zoonoses Public Health.* 2010;57:429–438.
11. Lipton BA, Hopkins SG, Koehler JE, et al. A survey of veterinarian involvement in zoonotic disease prevention practices. *J Am Vet Med Assoc.* 2008;233:1242–1249.
12. Canadian Committee on Antibiotic Resistance. *Infection Prevention and Control Best Practices for Small Animal Veterinary Clinics.* 2020. https://www.oahn.ca/resources/ipc-best-practices/.
13. National Association of State and Public Health Veterinarians. Model infection control plan for veterinary practices. 2015. www.nasphv.org/Documents/ModelInfectionControlPlan.docx.
14. Morey RS. The general duty clause of the occupational safety and health act of 1970. *Harvard Law Rev.* 1973;86:988–1005.
15. Babcock S, Marsh AE, Lin J, et al. Legal implications of zoonoses for clinical veterinarians. *J Am Vet Med Assoc.* 2008;233:1556–1562.
16. Grant S, Olsen CW. Preventing zoonotic diseases in immunocompromised persons: the role of physicians and veterinarians. *Emerg Infect Dis.* 1999;5:159–163.
17. Gauthier JL, Richardson DJ. Knowledge and attitudes about zoonotic helminths: a survey of Connecticut pediatricians and veterinarians. *Compend Contin Educ Pract. Vet.* 2002;24:4–9.
18. Colorado State. Board of Veterinary Medicine. Rule 4 CCR 727-1: Veterinary medicine rules and regulations. 2011. https://casetext.com/regulation/colorado-administrative-code/department-700-department-of-regulatory-agencies/division-727-state-board-of-veterinary-medicine/rule-4-ccr-727-1-veterinary-medicine-rules-and-regulations.
19. Williams CJ, Scheftel JM, Elchos BL, et al. Compendium of veterinary standard precautions for zoonotic disease prevention in veterinary personnel: National Association of State Public Health Veterinarians: Veterinary Infection Control Committee 2015. *J Am Vet Med Assoc.* 2015;247:1252–1277.
20. Baker WS, Gray GC. A review of published reports regarding zoonotic pathogen infection in veterinarians. *J Am Vet Med Assoc.* 2009;234:1271–1278.
21. Taylor LH, Latham SM, Woolhouse ME. Risk factors for human disease emergence. *Philos Trans R Soc Lond B Biol Sci.* 2001;356:983–989.
22. Croft DR, Sotir MJ, Williams CJ, et al. Occupational risks during a monkeypox outbreak, Wisconsin, 2003. *Emerg Infect Dis.* 2007;13:1150–1157.
23. Boerlin P, Eugster S, Gaschen F, et al. Transmission of opportunistic pathogens in a veterinary teaching hospital. *Vet Microbiol.* 2001;82:347–359.
24. Sidhu MS, Oppegaard H, Devor TP, et al. Persistence of multidrug-resistant *Staphylococcus haemolyticus* in an animal veterinary teaching hospital clinic. *Microb Drug Resist.* 2007;13:271–280.
25. Francey T, Gaschen F, Nicolet J, et al. The role of *Acinetobacter baumannii* as a nosocomial pathogen for dogs and cats in an intensive care unit. *J Vet Intern Med.* 2000;14:177–183.
26. Besser TE, Hancock D, Davis MA. The veterinarian's role in controlling the emergence and dissemination of drug-resistant bacteria. *J Vet Med Educ.* 2003;30:136–139.
27. Warren DK, Fraser VJ. Infection control measures to limit antimicrobial resistance. *Critical Care Med.* 2001;29:N128–N134.
28. Levy SB, Marshall B. Antibacterial resistance worldwide: causes, challenges and responses. *Nat Med.* 2004;10:S122–S129.
29. Sidhu MS, Heir E, Leegaard T, et al. Frequency of disinfectant resistance genes and genetic linkage with beta-lactamase transposon Tn552 among clinical staphylococci. *Antimicrob Agents Chemother.* 2002;46:2797–2803.
30. Rajamohan G, Srinivasan VB, Gebreyes WA. Molecular and functional characterization of a novel efflux pump, AmvA, mediating antimicrobial and disinfectant resistance in *Acinetobacter baumannii. J Antimicrob Chemother.* 2010;65:1919–1925.
31. Soares Magalhães RJ, Loeffler A, Lindsay J, et al. Risk factors for methicillin-resistant *Staphylococcus aureus* (MRSA) infection in dogs and cats: a case-control study. *Vet Res.* 2010;41:55.
32. Weese JS, Dick H, Willey BM, et al. Suspected transmission of methicillin-resistant *Staphylococcus aureus* between domestic pets and humans in veterinary clinics and in the household. *Vet Microbiol.* 2006;115:148–155.
33. American Veterinary Medical Association. AVMA Policy: Judicious therapeutic use of antimicrobials. 2008. https://www.avma.org/KB/Policies/Pages/Judicious-Therapeutic-Use-of-Antimicrobials.aspx.
34. Weese JS, Giguere S, Guardabassi L, et al. ACVIM consensus statement on therapeutic antimicrobial use in animals and antimicrobial resistance. *J Vet Intern Med.* 2015;29:487–498.

35. World Health Organization. *Critically Important Antimicrobials for Human Medicine.* 6th Revision; 2019. https://www.who.int/publications/i/item/9789241515528.
36. Baskerville A. Mechanisms of infection in the respiratory tract. *N Z Vet J.* 1981;29:235–238.
37. Duguid JP. The size and the duration of air-carriage of respiratory droplets and droplet-nuclei. *J Hyg.* 1946;44:471–479.
38. Wiener-Well Y, Galuty M, Rudensky B, et al. Nursing and physician attire as possible source of nosocomial infections. *Am J Infect Control.* 2011;39:555–559.
39. Haun N, Hooper-Lane C, Safdar N. Healthcare personnel attire and devices as fomites: a systematic review. *Infect Contr Hosp Epidemiol.* 2016;37:1367–1373.
40. Amirfeyz R, Tasker A, Ali S, et al. Theatre shoes - a link in the common pathway of postoperative wound infection? *Ann R Coll Surg Engl.* 2007;89:605–608.
41. Copp G, Mailhot CB, Zalar M, et al. Covergowns and the control of operating room contamination. *Nurs Res.* 1986;35:263–268.
42. Sehulster LM. Healthcare laundry and textiles in the United States: review and commentary on contemporary infection prevention issues. *Infect Contr Hosp Epidemiol.* 2015;36:1073–1088.
43. Burke JP. Infection control - a problem for patient safety. *N Engl J Med.* 2003;348:651–656.
44. Healthcare Infection Control Practices Advisory Committee and Hand-Hygiene Task Force, et al. Guideline for hand hygiene in health-care settings. *J Am Coll Surg.* 2004;198:121–127.
45. Centers for Disease Control and Prevention. Hand Hygiene in Health-care Settings: Hand Hygiene Guidance; 2020. https://www.cdc.gov/handhygiene/providers/guideline.html.
46. Larson E. A causal link between handwashing and risk of infection? Examination of the evidence. *Infect Contr Hosp Epidemiol.* 1988;9:28–36.
47. Pittet D, Dharan S, Touveneau S, et al. Bacterial contamination of the hands of hospital staff during routine patient care. *Arch Intern Med.* 1999;159:821–826.
48. Traub-Dargatz JL, Weese JS, Rousseau JD, et al. Pilot study to evaluate 3 hygiene protocols on the reduction of bacterial load on the hands of veterinary staff performing routine equine physical examinations. *Can Vet J.* 2006;47:671–676.
49. Larson E. Hygiene of the skin: when is clean too clean? *Emerg Infect Dis.* 2001;7:225–230.
50. Larson E. Skin hygiene and infection prevention: more of the same or different approaches? *Clin Infect Dis.* 1999;29:1287–1294.
51. Boyce JM, Pittet D. Guideline for hand hygiene in health-care settings. Recommendations of the Healthcare Infection Control Practices Advisory Committee and the HICPAC/SHEA/APIC/IDSA Hand Hygiene Task Force. Society for Healthcare Epidemiology of America/Association for Professionals in Infection Control/Infectious Diseases Society of America. *MMWR Recomm Rep.* 2002;51:1–45.
52. Zingg W, Haidegger T, Pittet D. Hand coverage by alcohol-based handrub varies: volume and hand size matter. *Am J Infect Control.* 2016;44:1689–1691.
53. Boyce JM. Antiseptic technology: access, affordability, and acceptance. *Emerg Infect Dis.* 2001;7:231–233.
54. Korniewicz DM, Garzon L, Seltzer J, et al. Failure rates in nonlatex surgical gloves. *Am J. Infect Control.* 2004;32:268–273.
55. Burrow R, Pinchbeck G. Study of how frequently surgeons' gloves are perforated during operations. *Vet Rec.* 2006;158:558–561.
56. Wright JG, Jung S, Holman RC, et al. Infection control practices and zoonotic disease risks among veterinarians in the United States. *J Am Vet Med Assoc.* 2008;232:1863–1872.
57. Anderson ME, Weese JS. Self-reported hand hygiene perceptions and barriers among companion animal veterinary clinic personnel in Ontario, Canada. *Can Vet J.* 2016;57:282–288.
58. Anderson ME, Sargeant JM, Weese JS. Video observation of hand hygiene practices during routine companion animal appointments and the effect of a poster intervention on hand hygiene compliance. *BMC Vet Res.* 2014;10:106.
59. Shea A, Shaw S. Evaluation of an educational campaign to increase hand hygiene at a small animal veterinary teaching hospital. *J Am Vet Med Assoc.* 2012;240:61–64.
60. Nakamura RK, Tompkins E, Braasch EL, et al. Hand hygiene practices of veterinary support staff in small animal private practice. *J Small Anim Pract.* 2012;53:155–160.
61. Weese JS. Barrier precautions, isolation protocols, and personal hygiene in veterinary hospitals. *Vet Clin North Am Equine Pract.* 2004;20:543–559.
62. Goldmann DA. The role of barrier precautions in infection control. *J Hosp Infect.* 1991;18(Suppl A):515–523.
63. Verbeek JH, Ijaz S, Mischke C, et al. Personal protective equipment for preventing highly infectious diseases due to exposure to contaminated body fluids in healthcare staff. *Cochrane Database Syst Rev.* 2016;4:CD011621.
64. Dunowska M, Morley PS, Traub-Dargatz JL, et al. Comparison of *Salmonella enterica* serotype Infantis isolates from a veterinary teaching hospital. *J Appl Microbiol.* 2007;102:1527–1536.
65. Steneroden KK, Van Metre DC, Jackson C, et al. Detection and control of a nosocomial outbreak caused by *Salmonella* Newport at a large animal hospital. *J Vet Intern Med.* 2010;24:606–616.
66. Siegel JDRE, Jackson M, Chiarello L. *Guidelines for Isolation Precautions: Preventing Transmission Of Infectious Agents in Healthcare Settings*; 2007. https://www.cdc.gov/infectioncontrol/guidelines/isolation/index.html.
67. Morley PS, Morris SN, Hyatt DR, et al. Evaluation of the efficacy of disinfectant footbaths as used in veterinary hospitals. *J Am Vet Med Assoc.* 2005;226:2053–2058.
68. Dunowska M, Morley PS, Patterson G, et al. Evaluation of the efficacy of a peroxygen disinfectant-filled footmat for reduction of bacterial load on footwear in a large animal hospital setting. *J Am Vet Med Assoc.* 2006;228:1935–1939.
69. Hornig KJ, Burgess BA, Saklou NT, et al. Evaluation of the efficacy of disinfectant footmats for the reduction of bacterial contamination on footwear in a large animal veterinary hospital. *J Vet Intern Med.* 2016;30:1882–1886.
70. Weese JS, Armstrong J. Outbreak of *Clostridium difficile*-associated disease in a small animal veterinary teaching hospital. *J Vet Intern Med.* 2003;17:813–816.
71. Kuzi S, Blum SE, Kahane N, et al. Multi-drug-resistant *Acinetobacter calcoaceticus-Acinetobacter baumannii* complex infection outbreak in dogs and cats in a veterinary hospital. *J Small Anim Pract.* 2016;57:617–625.
72. Walters A. Hard surface disinfection and its evaluation. *J Appl Bacteriol.* 1967;30:56–65.
73. Hall-Stoodley L, Costerton JW, Stoodley P. Bacterial biofilms: from the natural environment to infectious diseases. *Nat Rev Microbiol.* 2004;2:95–108.
74. Stewart PS, Costerton JW. Antibiotic resistance of bacteria in biofilms. *Lancet.* 2001;358:135–138.
75. Joseph B, Otta SK, Karunasagar I. Biofilm formation by *Salmonella* spp. on food contact surfaces and their sensitivity to sanitizers. *Int J Food Microbiol.* 2001;64:367–372.
76. Saklou NT, Burgess BA, Van Metre DC, et al. Comparison of disinfectant efficacy when using high-volume directed mist application of accelerated hydrogen peroxide and peroxymonosulfate disinfectants in a large animal hospital. *Equine Vet J.* 2016;48:485–489.
77. Dunowska M, Morley PS, Hyatt DR. The effect of Virkon S fogging on survival of *Salmonella enterica* and *Staphylococcus aureus* on surfaces in a veterinary teaching hospital. *Vet Microbiol.* 2005;105:281–289.
78. Patterson G, Morley PS, Blehm KD, et al. Efficacy of directed misting application of a peroxygen disinfectant for environmental decontamination of a veterinary hospital. *J Am Vet Med Assoc.* 2005;227:597–602.
79. Rutala WA, Weber DJ. Disinfection and sterilization: an overview. *Am J Infect Control.* 2013;41:S2–S5.
80. Southworth PM. Infections and exposures: reported incidents associated with unsuccessful decontamination of reusable surgical instruments. *J Hosp Infect.* 2014;88:127–131.
81. Tosh PK, Disbot M, Duffy JM, et al. Outbreak of *Pseudomonas aeruginosa* surgical site infections after arthroscopic procedures: Texas, 2009. *Infect Control Hosp Epidemiol.* 2011;32:1179–1186.
82. Deshpande A, Smith GW, Smith AJ. Biofouling of surgical power tools during routine use. *J Hosp Infect.* 2015;90:179–185.
83. Pelligand L, Hammond R, Rycroft A. An investigation of the bacterial contamination of small animal breathing systems during routine use. *Vet Anaesth Analges.* 2007;34:190–199.

84. Crawford S, Weese JS. Efficacy of endotracheal tube disinfection strategies for elimination of *Streptococcus zooepidemicus* and *Bordetella bronchiseptica*. *J Am Vet Med Assoc*. 2015;247:1033–1036.
85. Jung M, Beilenhoff U. Hygiene: the looming Achilles heel in endoscopy. *Visceral Med*. 2016;32:21–28.
86. Srinivasan A, Wolfenden LL, Song X, et al. An outbreak of *Pseudomonas aeruginosa* infections associated with flexible bronchoscopes. *N Engl J Med*. 2003;348:221–227.
87. Rutala WA, Weber DJ. New disinfection and sterilization methods. *Emerg Infect Dis*. 2001;7:348–353.
88. Scott E, Duty S, Callahan M. A pilot study to isolate *Staphylococcus aureus* and methicillin-resistant *Staphylococcus aureus* from environmental surfaces in the home. *Am J Infect Control*. 2008;36:458–460.
89. Brody MD. AVMA guide for veterinary medical waste management. *J Am Vet Med Assoc*. 1989;195:440–452.
90. American Veterinary Medical Association. Waste disposal by veterinary practices: What goes where? 2008. https://www.avma.org/PracticeManagement/Administration/Pages/Waste-Disposal-by-Veterinary-Practices-What-Goes-Where.aspx.
91. Leggat PA, Smith DR, Speare R. Exposure rate of needlestick and sharps injuries among Australian veterinarians. *J Occup Med Toxicol*. 2009;4:25.
92. Fowler HN, Holzbauer SM, Smith KE, et al. Survey of occupational hazards in Minnesota veterinary practices in 2012. *J Am Vet Med Assoc*. 2016;248:207–218.
93. Weese JS, Faires M. A survey of needle handling practices and needlestick injuries in veterinary technicians. *Can Vet J*. 2009;50:1278–1282.
94. Anderson ME, Weese JS. Video observation of sharps handling and infection control practices during routine companion animal appointments. *BMC Vet Res*. 2015;11:185.
95. Morley PS, Strohmeyer RA, Tankson JD, et al. Evaluation of the association between feeding raw meat and *Salmonella enterica* infections at a Greyhound breeding facility. *J Am Vet Med Assoc*. 2006;228:1524–1532.
96. Wales AD, Carrique-Mas JJ, Rankin M, et al. Review of the carriage of zoonotic bacteria by arthropods, with special reference to *Salmonella* in mites, flies and litter beetles. Zoonoses Public Health. 2010; 57:299–314.
97. Mian LS, Maag H, Tacal JV. Isolation of *Salmonella* from muscoid flies at commercial animal establishments in San Bernardino County, California. *J Vector Ecol*. 2002;27:82–85.
98. Guardabassi L, Schwarz S, Lloyd DH. Pet animals as reservoirs of antimicrobial-resistant bacteria. *J Antimicrob Chemother*. 2004;54: 321–332.
99. Wall PG, Davis S, Threlfall EJ, et al. Chronic carriage of multidrug resistant *Salmonella typhimurium* in a cat. *J Small Anim Pract*. 1995;36:279–281.
100. Morley PS. Biosecurity of veterinary practices. *Vet Clin North Am Food Anim Pract*. 2002;18:133–155 (vii).
101. Morley PS. Surveillance for nosocomial infections in veterinary hospitals. *Vet Clin North Am Equine Pract*. 2004;20:561–576 (vi–vii).
102. Burgess BA, Morley PS. Veterinary hospital surveillance systems. *Vet Clin North Am: Small Animal Pract*. 2015;45:235–242.
103. Haley RW. The scientific basis for using surveillance and risk factor data to reduce nosocomial infection rates. *J Hosp Infect*. 1995;30(Suppl):3–14.
104. Burgess BA, Morley PS, Hyatt DR. Environmental surveillance for *Salmonella enterica* in a veterinary teaching hospital. *J Am Vet Med Assoc*. 2004;225:1344–1348.
105. Ruple-Czerniak A, Bolte DS, Burgess BA, et al. Comparison of two sampling and culture systems for detection of *Salmonella enterica* in the environment of a large animal hospital. *Equine Vet J*. 2013;46:499–502.
106. Hacek DM, Trick WE, Collins SM, et al. Comparison of the Rodac imprint method to selective enrichment broth for recovery of vancomycin-resistant enterococci and drug-resistant Enterobacteriaceae from environmental surfaces. *J Clin Microbiol*. 2000;38:4646–4648.
107. Lemmen SW, Hafner H, Zolldann D, et al. Comparison of two sampling methods for the detection of gram-positive and gram-negative bacteria in the environment: moistened swabs versus Rodac plates. *Int J Hyg Environ Health*. 2001;203:245–248.
108. Stockton KA, Morley PS, Hyatt DR, et al. Evaluation of the effects of footwear hygiene protocols on nonspecific bacterial contamination of floor surfaces in an equine hospital. *J Am Vet Med Assoc*. 2006;228:1068–1073.
109. Clarke S. Safety culture: under-specified and overrated? *Int J Management Rev*. 2000;2:65–90.
110. Marsh-Ng ML, Burney DP, Garcia J. Surveillance of infections associated with intravenous catheters in dogs and cats in an intensive care unit. *J Am Anim Hosp Assoc*. 2007;43:13–20.
111. Seguela J, Pages JP. Bacterial and fungal colonisation of peripheral intravenous catheters in dogs and cats. *J Small Anim Pract*. 2011;52:531–535.
112. Dorey-Phillips CL, Murison PJ. Comparison of two techniques for intravenous catheter site preparation in dogs. *Vet Rec*. 2008;162:280–281.
113. Tan RH, Dart AJ, Dowling BA. Catheters: a review of the selection, utilisation and complications of catheters for peripheral venous access. *Aust Vet J*. 2003;81:136–139.
114. Linares J, Sitges-Serra A, Garau J, et al. Pathogenesis of catheter sepsis: a prospective study with quantitative and semiquantitative cultures of catheter hub and segments. *J Clin Microbiol*. 1985;21:357–360.
115. Goldmann DA, Pier GB. Pathogenesis of infections related to intravascular catheterization. *Clin Microbiol Rev*. 1993;6:176–192.
116. Ashkenazi S, Weiss E, Drucker MM. Bacterial adherence to intravenous catheters and needles and its influence by cannula type and bacterial surface hydrophobicity. *J Lab Clin Med*. 1986;107:136–140.
117. Mermel LA. New technologies to prevent intravascular catheter-related bloodstream infections. *Emerg Infect Dis*. 2001;7:197–199.
118. Ogeer-Gyles J, Mathews K, Weese JS, et al. Evaluation of catheter-associated urinary tract infections and multi-drug-resistant *Escherichia coli* isolates from the urine of dogs with indwelling urinary catheters. *J Am Vet Med Assoc*. 2006;229:1584–1590.
119. Smarick SD, Haskins SC, Aldrich J, et al. Incidence of catheter-associated urinary tract infection among dogs in a small animal intensive care unit. *J Am Vet Med Assoc*. 2004;224:1936–1940.
120. Bubenik LJ, Hosgood GL, Waldron DR, et al. Frequency of urinary tract infection in catheterized dogs and comparison of bacterial culture and susceptibility testing results for catheterized and noncatheterized dogs with urinary tract infections. *J Am Vet Med Assoc*. 2007;231:893–899.
121. Weese JS, Blondeau JM, Boothe D, et al. International Society for Companion Animal Infectious Diseases (ISCAID) guidelines for the diagnosis and management of bacterial urinary tract infections in dogs and cats. *Vet J*. 2019;247:8–25.
122. Sullivan LA, Campbell VL, Onuma SC. Evaluation of open versus closed urine collection systems and development of nosocomial bacteriuria in dogs. *J Am Vet Med Assoc*. 2010;237:187–190.
123. Centers for Disease Control and Prevention. Residential Pool or Hot Tub Owners - Disinfection and Testing; 2017. https://www.cdc.gov/healthywater/swimming/residential/disinfection-testing.
124. Centers for Disease Control and Prevention. Residential pool or hot tub owners - cleaning and remediation; 2016. https://www.cdc.gov/healthywater/swimming/residential/cleaning-remediation.html.
125. Wardrop KJ, Birkenheuer A, Blais MC, et al. Update on canine and feline blood donor screening for blood-borne pathogens. *J Vet Intern Med*. 2016;30:15–35.
126. Smith M. *Operational Guide for Animal Care and Control Agencies: Sanitation and Disease Control in the Shelter Environment*; 2010. https://www.americanhumane.org/publication/animal-shelter-operational-guide-sanitation-and-disease-control-in-the-shelter-environment/.
127. Newbury S, Blinn MK, Bushby PH, et al. *Guidelines for Standard of Care in Animal Shelters*; 2010. https://www.sheltervet.org/assets/docs/shelter-standards-oct2011-wforward.pdf.
128. United States Department of Agriculture. Animal Welfare - Publications Forms and Guidance Documents. Last accessed July 14, 2019.
129. Dellit TH, Owens RC, McGowan JE Jr, et al. Infectious Diseases Society of America and the Society for Healthcare Epidemiology of America guidelines for developing an institutional program to enhance antimicrobial stewardship. *Clin Infect Dis*. 2007;44:159–177.
130. Quinn PJ, Markey BK. Disinfection and disease prevention in veterinary medicine. In: Block SS, ed. *Disinfection Sterilization Adn Preservation*. 15th ed. Philadelphia: Lippincott, Williams & Wilkins; 2001:1069–1103.

16

Prevention and Management of Infectious Diseases in Multiple-Cat Environments

Miranda Spindel, Jane E. Sykes

KEY POINTS

- Multiple-cat environments are those that contain at least five cats, and include multiple-cat homes, breeding catteries, pet stores, research catteries, shelters, foster or rescue homes, boarding facilities, and feral cat colonies.
- The risk of infectious disease in multiple-cat environments can be reduced by: (1) minimizing individual and population risk factors for infectious disease and (2) movement control.
- Minimizing individual and population risk factors involves attention to overall cat numbers and density, ensuring cats are in stable groups, provision of adequate cage space and hiding areas, use of disposable equipment, proper sanitation that involves use of disinfectants with activity against nonenveloped viruses, attention to air flow and quality, arthropod control, minimizing the ratio of juvenile to adult cats, and ensuring that cats are well nourished and receive preventative treatments for infectious diseases where available. Surveillance programs that allow early detection of increased morbidity and mortality can also reduce risk of infectious diseases.
- Movement control involves segregation of cats into healthy holding, public access, quarantine, and isolation areas. Order of attention to cats should be healthy, quarantined, and then isolated cats.
- Important infectious diseases in multiple-cat populations include infectious respiratory tract disease, GI disease, dermatophytosis, feline retrovirus infections, and FIP. Caregivers in multiple-cat environments should be able to recognize clinical signs associated with these conditions and have an understanding of the approach to their diagnosis, treatment, and prevention as outlined in this chapter. They should also understand the potential for zoonotic transmission of some of the pathogens involved.

INTRODUCTION

Multiple-cat environments are those that contain at least five cats. They include multiple-cat homes, breeding catteries, pet stores, research catteries, shelters, foster or rescue homes, veterinary hospitals, grooming and boarding facilities, and feral cat colonies. The prevalence of infectious disease in multiple-cat environments is often high because it is correlated with animal density and population size, and because resources for disease control may be limited. Many important feline infectious diseases that are common in multiple-cat environments are chronic, difficult to treat, or both. Thus, efficient management and disease prevention are paramount for success in multiple-cat husbandry.

Some degree of exposure to infectious agents is inevitable, given the ubiquitous nature of viruses such as FHV-1 and FCV and the environmental persistence of others such as FPV. Infectious diseases may be transmitted directly by immediate or close contact between reservoir and susceptible hosts, or indirectly through inanimate vehicles (fomites), air, or droplets, or various mechanical or biologic vectors (see Chapter 15). Whether infection becomes important in a multiple-cat setting depends on host, environment, and pathogen attributes.[1] Pathogen attributes include virulence, dose, and route of pathogen inoculation. Virulence is not under the control of the person who manages the feline population, but dose and route of infection can be. Environment and host contributors to infectious diseases also are important targets for minimizing spread of these diseases. This chapter reviews infectious disease management strategies in multiple-cat environments and provides an overview of several major infectious syndromes.

GENERAL MANAGEMENT STRATEGIES

Management of infectious diseases in multiple-cat environments should emphasize good husbandry and preventive medicine. Colony immunity—the resistance of a group of animals to invasion and spread of an infectious agent—should be maximized, as should the *colonization resistance* (CR) of each individual. CR is defined as the innate and acquired capability of an animal to resist infectious disease and includes behaviors (such as avoidance of filth), physical barriers (mucus, epithelium, fur), physical and chemical attributes of the host (low gastric pH, intestinal peristalsis, urine flow, mucociliary escalator), classical immunity, and resident microflora. Animals with impaired CR (e.g., cats infected with FIV, geriatric or immunosuppressed cats, cats receiving antimicrobials) not only are more susceptible to disease but also reduce the overall colony immunity.

Ideally, a preventive management program should be implemented by a team consisting of at least a veterinarian and staff member or volunteer who are familiar with the physical structure of the cats' environment, animal care staff and operations, and other details. Effective management of a multiple-cat environment to decrease risk of infection includes: (1) minimizing population and individual risk factors for infectious disease and (2) movement control, which is the regulation of access to other cats and fomites that could transmit infection.

Minimizing Population and Individual Risk Factors

Risk factors for disease should be systematically evaluated and corrected if possible. Risk factors include environmental factors and population characteristics. The two most important risk factors in multiple-cat environments are: (1) total cat numbers and (2) density, or the number of cats per unit space. Other intrinsic environmental risk factors include caging strategies, stresses (e.g., dogs, noise, unstable social structures), rate of new cat introduction, sanitation, air flow and quality, healthy cat programs, insect and vermin control, and season and climate. Population risk factors include population age composition, inbreeding status, breeds housed in the group, and presence of concurrent diseases.

Cat Numbers and Density

Cat numbers and density should be kept as low as possible, with an emphasis on minimizing (or properly segregating) the proportion of kittens and immunocompromised cats. If group housing strategies are employed, caging in stable cat groups should allow for some social interactions but not fighting. Cages should provide plenty of opportunities for cats to hide, vertical space, natural light and air, and windows through which cats can look. More detail on optimal group housing can be found elsewhere.[2,3]

Housing

Cages for individual cats should be more than sterile boxes because the increased susceptibility to disease caused by stress outweighs the reduction achievable by ease of cleaning. Environmental enrichment (hiding places, vertical spaces, and things for cats to look at and play with) is very important (Figs. 16.1 and 16.2).[3] Cages should not extend all the way to the ground (bottom cages at least 1 foot off the ground), and sick cats should never be housed above healthy cats. Sick cats with suspected infectious diseases should be in isolation. *All* components of the environment should be disposable or able to be completely cleaned and disinfected. Any potentially nondisposable items should be kept in closed rooms and decontaminated or disposed of when the group of cats has finished with them.

Sanitation

Sanitation is important and often improperly addressed. The main sources of infectious diseases are not cages, but rather the cats, and environmental components that become contaminated and cannot be or are not sanitized, such as carpets and human hands and clothing. Cleanliness is essential in any multiple-cat environment whether the cats are comingled in groups or individually housed. A disinfectant with activity against environmentally resistant microbes such as parvoviruses, calicivirus, and dermatophytes should be in routine use (see Chapter 14 and Table 15.2). For decontamination of *Toxoplasma gondii* and other coccidial oocysts, scalding water or ammonia solutions are required (see Public Health Considerations, Chapters 93 and 104). A protocol that outlines daily, weekly, and monthly routine sanitation procedures should be developed, updated regularly, and posted where it can be visually referenced. Protocols should also exist that cover sanitation procedures to be used during outbreaks of specific infectious diseases.

Air Flow and Quality

Air flow and quality are significant factors in the management of multiple-cat environments, but their importance is overrated. The advantages of increasing air turnover from 10 to 15 changes per minute are not enormous, but the increase in expense is. In general, the greater the population density, the greater the need for increased number of air changes per hour. By far the most efficient way to achieve quality air is to open windows or have indoor-outdoor catteries. Most cats do not need air conditioning as long as they have fresh water, protection from rain, and shade. However, in cold weather, cats need warmth. Optimally, temperature should be maintained at 50°F–80°F and humidity at 30%–70%.[4] Feline respiratory pathogens are not primarily transmitted via aerosol, but it is still important to ensure that air quality is healthy in order to minimize exposure risks and improve the respiratory defenses of the animals. Air ducts and ventilation areas should be cleaned regularly. If uncomfortable environmental conditions exist for humans (e.g., chemical fumes, dust), these should be corrected for the animals as well.

Population Risk Factors

Population risk factors for infectious disease include population age composition, degree of inbreeding, breeds housed, and presence of concurrent diseases. Many of the risk factors that increase the likelihood of endemic or epidemic disease in multiple-cat environments are also factors that increase risks for individual cats. Individual cats are more prone to infectious disease if they are very young, especially if they are colostrum-deprived, or very old; if they are stressed or malnourished; or if they are already incubating an infection. In cats, inbreeding per se is not a risk factor, but being a member of a more susceptible pedigree may be a risk.

Healthy Cat Programs and Vaccinations

Healthy cat programs and arthropod control minimize individual risk factors for infectious disease, maximize colony immunity, and provide a systematic opportunity for cats to be evaluated and either treated or removed from the population if they are not healthy. Routine screening of cats should be performed immediately on intake. Intake examinations should include a complete physical examination, core vaccination, and parasiticide treatment for hookworms and roundworms at minimum. Thereafter, according to the guidelines published by the Association of Shelter Veterinarians (Guidelines for Standards of Care in Animal Shelters),[3] apparently healthy animals that have been in care longer than a month should be weighed and have a body score recorded by trained individuals at least monthly. Veterinary examinations should be performed twice each year or more frequently if problems are identified. Geriatric, ill, or debilitated animals should be examined by a veterinarian for appropriate case management.

Vaccination on entry should be performed for healthy cats and kittens over 4 weeks of age. Because the use of vaccines must be tailored for individual situations, vaccine programs may differ for each multiple-cat environment. Vaccination has four potential disadvantages: (1) some vaccines cause mild disease or transient immunosuppression; (2) parenteral, adjuvanted vaccines have been associated with injection-site sarcoma formation; (3) vaccination can create false-positive serologic and molecular test results; and (4) use of vaccines may lead to a false sense of security that cats are adequately protected and other preventive management practices can be neglected. These disadvantages should be considered when selecting the type of vaccine(s), timing, and route of administration.

Minimally, initial vaccination should be directed at prevention of FPV, FHV-1, FCV and rabies virus infections. Choice of type of vaccine product and route of administration may vary depending on the population. Attenuated live vaccines for FHV-1, FCV, and FPV are preferred in many high-turnover environments such as rescues and shelters due to the rapid onset of immunity they provide. Inactivated virus vaccines must be administered at least twice at 2- to 4-week intervals before effective immunity is produced and thus are inappropriate in populations such as shelters where turnover rates can be rapid. Inactivated vaccines may be advantageous in facilities where vaccine-associated diseases are unacceptable (e.g., in research catteries) or in immunocompromised or pregnant animals. The reader is referred to Chapter 20 for advantages and disadvantages of different vaccine types.

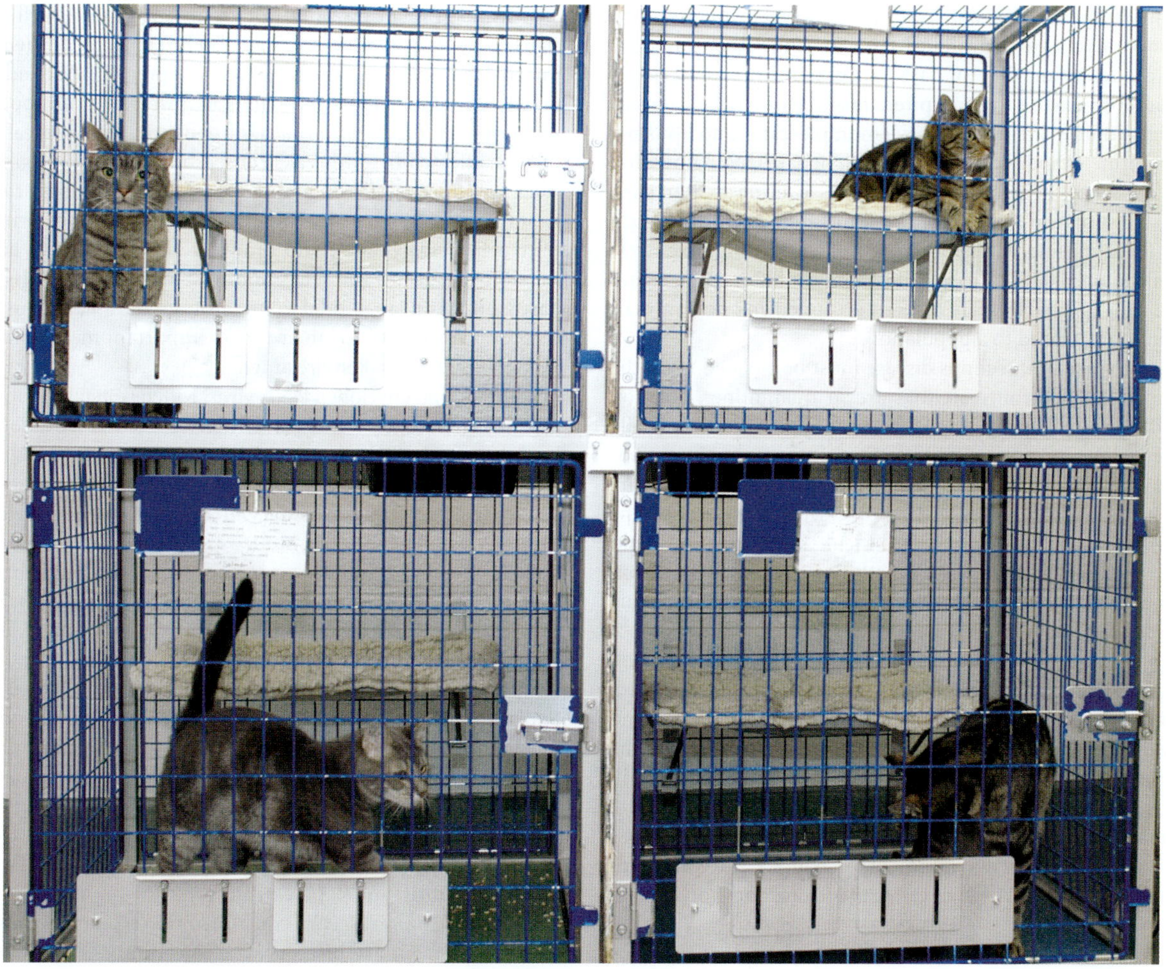

Fig. 16.1 Good husbandry is vital to an effective preventive medicine program.

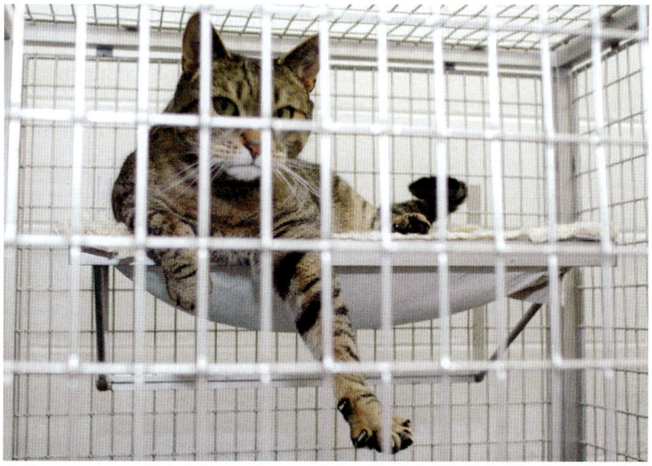

Fig. 16.2 Hammocks can reduce stress for cats in multiple-cat environments.

The panleukopenia fraction of the intranasal FVRCP vaccine has had questionable efficacy in field settings; therefore, it is not recommended as a sole vaccination for cats and kittens in high-risk environments.

The veterinarian and manager should inspect the animals and premises for arthropods regularly, for which there should be zero tolerance. Fleas and ticks transmit vector-borne diseases and have the potential to contribute to allergic dermatopathies. Cats can be infested with lice, ear mites, and mange mites. If any arthropods are seen during a routine inspection, the entire premises should be cleaned and treated with an approved pesticide, and every cat should receive treatment for ectoparasites. Monthly ectoparasite preventative treatments should be provided if needed to ensure that no cats are infested.

Surveillance for Morbidity and Mortality

It is important to track and to identify causes of mortality and morbidity in a population to better plan and implement infectious disease management programs. Necropsies should be performed after unexplained deaths, especially in shelters, breeding and research catteries, pet stores, and veterinary clinics. When infectious causes are suspected, laboratories should be advised of tentative diagnoses before the necropsy, if possible, and if possible multiple animals should be examined.

Movement Control

All animal facilities should minimally have the ability to separate animals into four physically separate defined areas: (1) healthy holding; (2) public (adoption, sales, etc.); (3) quarantine; and (4) isolation. Flow of human and animal movement and animal separation will depend to a degree on the type of facility and its design.

Healthy holding is typically an area where animals that are newly admitted and apparently healthy are housed. Upon admission, cats should receive healthy-cat care treatments and be observed daily by personnel qualified to perform physical examinations and detect clinical signs of infectious disease. *Quarantine* is a holding area for animals that may have been or are known to have been exposed to an infectious disease but are not yet showing clinical signs. In some situations, cats may require a quarantine time of days to weeks prior to entering a group to attempt to ensure the group remains free of clinical signs of disease. In high-volume shelters that have multiple-cat group housing, effective quarantine of individual animals can be challenging because new animals are always being admitted to the quarantine area. In such cases, the next best option may be cohort admission. There are different methods for admitting and structuring cohorts to minimize stress and risk of infectious disease. These include grouping by sex, age, and in an all-in/all-out approach where capacity is capped and new animals are not continuously added to a population.

Cats showing signs of infectious disease must be isolated from the general population and from cats that are in quarantine. Isolation spaces should be physically separated, low-traffic areas that are ideally located some distance from healthy cat areas. In some facilities, isolation may not be achievable on-site or may require closing an entire group area. In a small cattery or foster home setting, a cat could be isolated in a bathroom; however, it is difficult for owners to avoid transmitting infectious agents on their clothing, shoes, and skin from a sick cat to other cats. Cats with dermatophytosis, URTD, or diarrhea should ideally be moved to a true isolation ward and the presence of co-infections should be assumed when formulating management. Isolation should be a space that can easily be cleaned and disinfected, with easy entry and exit for staff, a separate air supply if possible, and low traffic. In some situations, isolation may be performed within the same building that general population housing occurs, whereas in others, a veterinary clinic or separate facility may need to be utilized. Population management becomes critical when incidence of infectious disease rises in multiple-cat environments. Facilities and programs must have an understanding of their capacity for care and work within it.

To reduce transmission of infectious agents, a specific order of care should be followed: (1) feed and clean healthy kittens and queens and then healthy cats, (2) feed and clean quarantined cats, and finally, (3) feed and clean isolated cats. In a large facility, isolated cats should be handled by personnel who are not handling the healthy cats. Only if absolutely necessary should a caregiver attend to healthy cats after attending to cats in isolation, and then only if the caregiver has changed clothes and shoes and washed all exposed skin.

IMPORTANT INFECTIOUS SYNDROMES IN MULTIPLE-CAT ENVIRONMENTS

The following section provides an overview of important infectious diseases in multiple-cat environments, with an emphasis on major clinical signs, diagnostic tests, and prevention measures that are relevant in this scenario. The reader is referred to pathogen-specific chapters in this book for more detail on each disease.

Respiratory Tract Disease

Etiologic Agents and Clinical Signs

Respiratory tract disease is the most prevalent and easily recognizable infectious problem in multiple-cat environments, and it is also the most difficult problem to manage.[5] The causative agents of URTD are common, easily transmitted, and cannot be completely prevented through vaccination. In general, minimizing severity and frequency of respiratory outbreaks in a population should be the goal, rather than eliminating disease, which is usually impossible.

FCV and FHV-1 are the most common causes of feline URTD.[6] Bacterial pathogens that contribute to disease include *Bordetella bronchiseptica, Chlamydia felis*, and *Mycoplasma* spp. (see Chapters 34, 35, 49, 55, and 57). The possibility of SARS-CoV2 infection in cats showing signs of respiratory illness should also be considered when exposure to infected humans has occurred (see Chapter 43). Secondary bacterial invaders include *Staphylococcus* spp., *Streptococcus* spp., *Pasteurella multocida*, and *Escherichia coli*. Infrequently, multiple-cat populations may be affected by outbreaks caused by unusual emerging pathogens such as influenza viruses and *Streptococcus equi* subsp. *zooepidemicus*. Respiratory pathogens are highly infectious and are primarily transmitted in ocular, nasal, and oral secretions. Although aerosol transmission can occur, the maximum distance for transmission is 4 feet, based on the average tidal volume of an adult cat. Thus, fomite and direct cat-cat transmission are more important means of transmission in most multiple-cat environments.[7]

FHV-1 is an enveloped DNA virus. Kittens often acquire the infection at a very young age because parturition results in reactivation of shedding by the queen. Later in life, transmission of FHV-1 requires intimate contact between cats. After infection, the virus persists in the trigeminal nerve. Intermittent reactivation results in upper respiratory signs, especially during stressful periods or immunosuppressive events. Disease signs may include conjunctivitis, anterior uveitis, serous ocular discharge with secondary bacterial infection and mucopurulent discharge, or keratitis with or without dendritic ulceration. Ulcerative and necrotizing facial dermatitis has been described in some cats with FHV-1 infection.[8]

FCV is a nonenveloped RNA virus with a high rate of mutation and is antigenically and genetically diverse.[9,10] Respiratory shedding of virus occurs for at least 10 to 14 days and commonly occurs for months in shelters and kittens. FCV infection can cause conjunctivitis and rhinitis with serous ocular discharge, caudal stomatitis, pneumonia, transient fever and limping, and immune-complex polyarthritis and gingivitis. Hypervirulent strains of FCV can cause facial and limb edema, hepatitis, and pancreatitis.[11]

Bordetella bronchiseptica contributes to respiratory tract signs, often in association with respiratory viral infection.[12,13] If it is protected and in a moist environment, *B. bronchiseptica* can survive for weeks. Cats may have mild primary bordetellosis with conjunctivitis and mild oculonasal discharge or develop pneumonia. Occasionally, signs of URTD in cats from multiple-cat environments are caused by *C. felis*, an obligate intracellular bacterial pathogen that survives poorly in the environment. The reservoir for this pathogen is feline conjunctival and genital mucosa. Chlamydiosis is often acquired shortly after weaning and is typically manifested as conjunctivitis. Feline disease attributed to mycoplasmas, which also survive poorly in the environment, include URTD, conjunctivitis, and arthritis. The role of mycoplasmas as primary URTD pathogens in cats has been controversial, given that they commonly are recovered from clinically healthy cats.

Although uncommonly documented in the literature, several agents associated with feline URTD have zoonotic potential. *Bordetella bronchiseptica* has rarely been associated with the disease in immunocompromised individuals.[14] *Chlamydia felis* infection has been documented in one immunocompromised individual with conjunctivitis.[15] Avian influenza H7N2 isolated in an outbreak of feline respiratory disease was also isolated from the veterinarian caring for the cats.[16]

Diagnosis

Although there are clinical signs that are more characteristic of some infections than others, clinical signs overlap and co-infections occur; therefore, specific diagnostic testing is required to identify the causal agents. Gingivostomatitis or extensive oral ulceration are suggestive of FCV infection. Lameness and joint pain suggest infection with *Mycoplasma* spp. or FCV. Cough may suggest *cattery cough (B. bronchiseptica* tracheitis). Keratitis and corneal ulceration suggest FHV-1 infection. Chronic sinusitis, often with turbinate destruction, may be from infection with either FHV-1 or FCV infection followed by secondary bacterial infection. Fever develops most commonly with FHV-1 or FCV infections.

In general, diagnostic testing should be performed when the results will change therapy or management, when there are increases in prevalence or severity of disease, or when there is a decrease in response to therapies that have previously been effective. In any population, testing a percentage of the population versus one or two representative animals will give a better representation of disease trends because virtually all of the pathogens can be found in clinically healthy cats. Both clinically ill and apparently healthy but exposed populations should ideally be tested. It can also be helpful to test animals who have entered a facility at different times. Before specimens are collected, the diagnostic laboratory should be consulted with for specimen collection and storage information. It is also important to contact the laboratory in advance and notify them if large numbers of specimens are to be submitted. No single test has perfect sensitivity and specificity, and combinations of tests may be required to optimize understanding. PCR is commonly performed for respiratory pathogen diagnosis, and because of its sensitivity, results must always be interpreted in relation to clinical information. Virus isolation and necropsy with histopathology may also be helpful.

Management and Prevention

URTD is best managed in a population by minimizing its severity and prevalence.[1] Infected and exposed cats may have recurring disease, and few multiple-cat populations (except specific pathogen-free research catteries) are free of URTD.

Vaccination. All cats in multiple-cat environments should receive vaccination for FHV-1 and FCV as part of a regular, routine core vaccination program. Because vaccination against panleukopenia is also considered core, these three components are often administered simultaneously. Attenuated live vaccines should be selected over inactivated products, unless there is a risk of pregnancy such as in a breeding facility. Intranasal vaccines can be used in young kittens to overcome maternal antibody, but parenteral vaccination is also required to protect cats from FPV infection. Vaccines for bordetellosis and chlamydiosis are noncore, and recommended for use when documented problems exist in a population. For additional information on vaccination selection and schedules in multiple-cat populations, see the Appendix.

Stress reduction. Every effort should be made to minimize stress as physical, emotional, and environmental stress strongly contributes to development of URTD. Changes in housing, nutrition, human interactions, and length of stay all play a role in optimizing cats' resistance to disease.

Population management. Increased animal density increases the chance of exposure to infectious agents. Additionally, when the number of animals requiring medical care increases, the resources per animal decrease. Sanitation is more difficult, treatment is more time consuming, and quality care is more difficult to provide. Multiple-cat environments with significant URTD may need help to establish clear-cut capacity guidelines in order to break a cycle of progressively worsening URTD.

Sanitation. It is critical that multiple-cat environments have a documented sanitation plan in place. Good sanitation limits pathogen accumulation and minimizes fomite spread. With the exception of FCV, most respiratory agents are very labile in the environment and are easy to inactivate with routine sanitation products and practices. Proper use of a routine disinfectant such as accelerated hydrogen peroxide or potassium peroxymonosulfate will inactivate FCV and all other respiratory pathogens in the environment. Attention must be paid to the role of humans in disease transmission. Animals should be handled, whenever possible, based on age and health status. This means that the youngest and most immunocompromised should be handled before the immunocompromised population. Supplies should be dedicated to specific areas of the facility. Although URTD pathogens are not primarily transmitted via aerosol, it is still important to pay attention to air quality in order to minimize exposure risks and improve respiratory defenses. Optimal temperature is 50°F–80°F, humidity 30%–70%, and air exchange rate 10–15/hour.[2,3] Because few facilities are ideal, it is generally best to focus on how to optimize ventilation. Air ducts and ventilation areas should be cleaned regularly.

Surveillance. Regular physical examinations and good electronic medical records that are maintained from the time of intake can help with early identification of disease. Caregivers need to have the knowledge and training to identify and document important clinical signs, and understand the steps to follow if significant changes are noted. Careful record keeping facilitates monitoring of trends or outbreaks of infectious disease developing in populations that might not be recognized in a large population on a day-to-day basis. Once identified, specific strategies can be implemented to improve animal health and welfare.

Segregation. Cats with URTD should ideally be isolated. Although cats can continue to shed URTD pathogens for weeks to months after clinical recovery, it is not practical in most multiple-cat environments to isolate for this length of time, and subclinical shedding is common in cat populations. Instead, once clinical signs have resolved (when shedding is likely to be greatest) and treatment is completed, cats typically are returned to the healthy areas. If virulent systemic calicivirus infections are suspected, isolation is particularly important. Some facilities may designate "URTD recovery" areas for these cats, but most recognize that respiratory pathogens are ubiquitous in group environments and it is virtually impossible to create a URTD-free zone. Reduction of stress is more critical.

Treatment

Individual cats with URTD should receive nursing care, humidification, and fluids if needed and should be encouraged to eat. Since the majority of infections are viral, antimicrobials should be reserved for inappetent cats that have mucopurulent discharges. Specific antiviral drugs may be valuable to treat severe FHV-1 infection (see Chapters 9 and 34). It is *not* appropriate to treat a whole population of affected cats with antimicrobials because most are infected with viruses, and widespread antimicrobial use adversely affects resident microflora, increases susceptibility to additional infections, and promotes antimicrobial resistance.

Prognosis

Most cats with acute URTD recover within 1 or 2 weeks with supportive care. However, mortality is possible in kittens or immunocompromised patients. Many cats that recover from acute URTD become chronic carriers of FHV-1 and FCV and may experience recurrent clinical signs in the future. Some cats will develop chronic rhinosinusitis.

Gastrointestinal Disease

Etiologic Agents and Clinical Signs

A multitude of bacterial, viral, protozoal, and parasitic agents can cause diarrhea and vomiting, and co-infections are common. Conditions common to multiple-cat environments such as stress, dietary change, intestinal parasitism, and immunocompromise can contribute to clinical signs. The major GI pathogens of concern in multiple-cat environments are FPV, *Salmonella*, *Campylobacter*, *Cystoisospora* and *Cryptosporidium* spp.,

Giardia duodenalis and, *Tritrichomonas blagburni* (see Chapters 30, 62, 65, 104, 103, 101, and 102 respectively). Infections with *T. blagburni* are especially prominent in purebred cats.[17,18] The primary mode of transmission for each of these pathogens is fecal-oral. Clinical signs include anorexia, variable appetite, weight loss or poor body condition, vomiting, large, small or mixed bowel diarrhea, flatulence, weakness, fever, or dehydration. *Salmonella* and *Campylobacter* spp., and some species of *Cryptosporidium* and *Giardia* have the potential to be zoonotic.

FPV is a small nonenveloped DNA virus that causes life-threatening diarrhea, vomiting, and immunosuppression. FPV has prolonged environmental persistence, is resistant to many chemical disinfectants, and is highly contagious.[19] FPV has a tropism for rapidly dividing cells such as epithelial cells of the GI tract, leukocyte precursors in bone marrow, and cerebellar Purkinje cells in neonatal or very young kittens. The incubation period is between 3 days and 2 weeks but is usually 5 to 7 days. Animals younger than 6 months are most likely to develop severe disease, whereas adult animals can have mild disease that is indistinguishable from diarrhea of any other cause. Infection with FPV typically manifests as vomiting and diarrhea that lead to dehydration. Sometimes illness progresses so rapidly that sudden death ensues within hours, and before vomiting and diarrhea develop. Infection is usually accompanied by immunocompromise, which can predispose the animal to bacteremia, shock, and death. Kittens infected in late gestation or in the first 1 to 2 weeks after birth experience damage to the Purkinje cells resulting in poor gross motor control from the cerebellum, although other peripheral nerves and the cerebrum remain intact.

Cats with salmonellosis may be subclinically infected, have diarrhea as the only sign, or be systemically ill. Clinical signs can include vomiting, small, large or mixed bowel diarrhea, and fever. Hematologic values in cats are sometimes suggestive of panleukopenia with neutropenia that has a severe left shift. *Salmonella* endotoxin creates a massive disruption of the host inflammatory mechanisms, resulting in release of acute-phase proteins with fever, vasodilation, increased vascular permeability, thrombosis, hypovolemia, disseminated intravascular coagulation, shock, and death.

Campylobacter spp. are zoonotic gram-negative, motile, curved, rod-shaped bacteria. Infection results in a range of clinical signs from no signs in carriers to severe diarrhea. *Campylobacter upsaliensis* has been associated with outbreaks of hemorrhagic gastroenteritis in populations of dogs and cats and in daycare centers for children.[20–22] Often, diarrhea associated with campylobacteriosis is self-limiting, but mortality can occur in debilitated, dehydrated, or very young animals should extensive nursing care not be feasible.

Diarrhea caused by *Giardia* and *Cryptosporidium* spp. is most severe in young and immunosuppressed animals. *Tritrichomonas blagburni* also tends to affect young adult purebred cats and causes large bowel diarrhea signs. *Cystoisospora* spp. are found very commonly in kittens in small numbers. The number of asexual reproductive cycles appears to be programmed; only two or three occur in any one host individual, and infection is self-limiting. When clinical signs of cystoisosporiasis occur, they typically manifest as profuse, watery diarrhea in kittens.

Diagnosis

As for respiratory pathogens, diagnosis of GI pathogens can be difficult because healthy animals can be infected, so it is difficult to determine the clinical relevance of a positive test result in an individual animal. Exhaustive testing is expensive and difficult, and often fails to identify a specific cause. Testing of multiple healthy and sick animals and comparing the results in each group may help to elucidate the cause.

Diagnostic testing should be performed whenever panleukopenia is suspected, as the consequences of this virus infecting a population can be devastating. Some of the commercially available fecal ELISA assays designed for the detection of parvovirus antigen in canine feces can be used for cats. A CBC may be also informative. False-positive ELISA antigen test results have the potential to occur as a result of recently administered vaccine virus; thus, cats should not be diagnosed with FPV enteritis unless they have appropriate clinical signs or very low blood leukocyte counts. Finally, if any cats die, a necropsy with histopathology should be performed.

While many bacterial and protozoal pathogens present in multiple-cat environments have zoonotic potential, healthy cats with normal stools are not considered human health risks, and testing beyond routine fecal flotation is generally not recommended for cats with normal stools. The AAFP Zoonoses Guidelines committee recommends that laboratory tests to evaluate diarrhea start with a fecal flotation, fecal wet mount examination, rectal cytology, and an acid-fast stain for *Cryptosporidium* spp.[23] Failure to find protozoal cysts on flotation or direct smear does not rule them out as contributing to the diarrhea because these assays have low sensitivity in early infection. *Cryptosporidium* and *Giardia* spp. in feces are more easily detected with ELISA or direct FA (available from commercial laboratories).

Enteropathogenic bacteria can be detected using aerobic, microaerophilic, and anaerobic culture, although it can be difficult to understand the clinical significance of the results. Routine microaerophilic culture on selective agar often is conducted at elevated temperatures (e.g., 42°C) and may fail to yield growth of less thermotolerant strains. Anaerobic culture can be performed on selective media, and immunologic assays can be used to detect *Clostridioides difficile* toxin A. Enteric PCR panels are also available that can detect DNA of a variety of enteric pathogens, which again are best interpreted when applied to multiple affected animals and in conjunction with the results of other diagnostic assays (see Chapters 63 and 64).

Management and Prevention

Surveillance should include regular quantification of the level of GI disease present, including the number of cases in which specific pathogens are identified. Animals can best resist GI infections when they are otherwise healthy and well nourished, not stressed, have intact resident bacterial microflora, and have been appropriately vaccinated. Problems arise in high-density catteries with high turnover of animals, highly susceptible animals, and changes in diet. It should be ensured that kittens receive colostrum. Less frequent but thorough disinfection is preferred to daily cursory disinfection, although spot cleaning should be performed every day. Because many enteropathogens are difficult to inactivate, the environment should be as dry as possible, exposed to UV light, and decontaminated with a disinfectant with activity against nonenveloped viruses. In some facilities, a 14-day intake quarantine is helpful. If the facility has an inadequate amount of space and holding time for a functional quarantine, the next best option is cohort admission.

Treatment

If necessary, empiric treatment of diarrhea may include use of antimicrobials, motility modulators, a bland diet, or anti-inflammatory agents. Antimicrobials can contribute to gut dysbiosis. Drugs to reduce gut motility and diarrhea increase retention time of all luminal contents, including pathogens that can exacerbate the disease. Bismuth subsalicylate should be used carefully in cats because they have very low tolerance for salicylic acid. Even use of bland diets can be counterproductive if cats reject them. Ensuring proper hydration and nutrition should be the focus whenever possible, which may require administration of subcutaneous or intravenous fluids, and tube feeding of inappetent cats.

Dermatophytosis

Etiologic Agents and Clinical Signs

Dermatophytosis (ringworm) is a fungal infection of the hair, nails, and superficial layers of the skin. Dermatophytes most commonly isolated from infected cats are *Microsporum canis*, *Microsporum gypseum*, and *Trichophyton mentagrophytes*. Dermatophytosis poses a significant management issue for multiple-cat environments because it is highly contagious, zoonotic, treatment can be lengthy, and environmental decontamination difficult. Dermatophyte infections tend to be most common in warm, humid environments, and in juvenile animals. Overcrowded conditions are a major risk factor for outbreaks. Early and accurate diagnosis of dermatophytosis in a multiple-cat environment is critical because environmental contamination can rapidly become difficult to contain.

Dermatophytes are divided into anthropophilic, zoophilic, and geophilic species. Anthropophilic species have evolved on humans and only rarely affect animals. Zoophilic species (e.g., *M. canis*) have adapted to animals, but may spread to humans. Geophilic species (e.g., *T. mentagrophytes*) are soil-adapted, and less commonly affect humans than animals. Although there are numerous species of dermatophytes that can affect cats, 90% of dermatophytosis in multiple-cat environments is thought to be due to *M. canis*.[24] For zoophilic species, infective arthrospores develop within the hair or skin, and the most important route of transmission is via direct animal-to-animal contact. For geophilic dermatophyte species, infective arthrospores can be present within the soil.

Dermatophytosis is acquired through contact with infective spores which can persist in the environment for weeks to months. The skin acts as a mechanical barrier, so any type of cutaneous trauma increases an animal's susceptibility to dermatophytosis. Grooming, clipping, or ectoparasites can all result in microabrasions to the skin. Dermatophyte spores can also be transmitted via fomites (e.g. towels, bowls, clippers, kennels) and potentially via airborne modes of transmission if fans or other air circulating devices are in use.

Dermatophyte conidia gain access to keratinized epithelium, then germinate, and mycelia enter cornified strata. As arthroconidia develop in tissue, clinical signs develop because of fungal products such as elastase, collagenase, and keratinase and as a result of allergic responses to the fungi. The incubation period for ringworm is between 4 days and 4 weeks. Infection finally may be resolved by cell-mediated immunity in weeks or months, although some carriers remain chronically infected. Severe or chronic disease prevalence is higher in geriatric cats, those younger than 1 year, Persian cats, cats infected with retroviruses, those that are pregnant or lactating, malnourished, or being given anti-inflammatory drugs, or those that have cancer or are stressed.

Cats with dermatophytosis classically exhibit circular areas of alopecia, broken hairs, crusting, and scaling. However, the clinical appearance is extremely variable. Lesions may be localized to the head or generalized and can vary in severity from minimal crusting and scaling to severely ulcerative, inflammatory lesions. The most common locations include the face, ears, feet, and tail. Subclinical carriage is also widespread. Pruritus may or may not be present. Some cats may present with a miliary dermatitis. Because the clinical signs are so variable, diagnosis should never be based on clinical signs alone. Major differential diagnoses include any disease that causes multifocal areas of alopecia, scale, and crusts, allergies such as atopic dermatitis, external parasites such as fleas and mites, cheyletiellosis, and demodicosis.

Dermatophytosis is also a zoonosis. Disease is most likely to affect very young, old, immunocompromised individuals, although healthy individuals can also become infected.

Diagnosis

Cats in multiple-cat environments can be screened for dermatophytosis using several complementary diagnostic tools: history, visual examination, Wood's lamp examination, PCR, direct examination of fluorescing hairs, and fungal culture. These tools can be used when cats enter a program, and/or when responding to a potential outbreak. It should be known if cats are littermates, from the same environment/home, and littermates or those living in contact with other animals should be treated as infected. A careful visual examination for dermatological issues should be a part of each cat's physical examination. Examination with a Wood's lamp can then be performed on any suspect lesions. In order for a Wood's lamp to be of use, proper technique must be followed with a lamp of sufficient quality (see Chapter 78). Wood's lamps emit long-wave, UVA light (320–400 nm). Infected hairs fluoresce because the fungus in the hair follicle deposits a metabolite on the growing hair shaft. Only *M. canis* produces this metabolite, and this bright apple-green fluorescence is thought to be seen in about 50% of *M. canis*-affected animals. Direct microscopic examination is performed on hairs plucked from the periphery of suspect and/or fluorescing lesions. Hair is cleared of keratin by suspending it in 10% to 20% potassium hydroxide. The slide is then gently heated for 15 to 20 seconds or allowed to stand for 30 minutes at room temperature before being examined. Infected hairs appear swollen and frayed, with loss of normal structure. Arthroconidia and hyphae occasionally can be seen.

Molecular assays are available for detection of dermatophyte DNA. PCR can be especially helpful early in the screening process and when monitoring treatment. However, because PCR is very sensitive, a positive result can be the result of active infection, fomites, or nonviable fungal organisms following successful treatment and fungal culture.[25]

Specimens for fungal culture are collected by plucking hair from the edge of the lesion or running a new toothbrush through the coat. If a toothbrush is used, the brush should be run over the cat's body until hairs are visible in the tines of the brush. If lesions are identified, they should be brushed last to minimize dispersal of spores. Hairs or toothbrush tines are placed onto an appropriate agar such as dermatophyte test medium (DTM) or rapid sporulation medium (RSM) that contain antibacterial and antifungal drugs to discourage growth of contaminants. DTM contains phenol red, which turns red in the presence of alkaline metabolites produced primarily by dermatophytes and a few saprophytes. Bromothymol blue in RSM turns blue-green in the presence of dermatophytes. Plates should be incubated between 27°C and 30°C for up to 3 weeks and should be observed daily for visible fungal mycelia and color change. When candidate dermatophytes are observed, hyphae should be examined under the microscope for the characteristic conidia (most easily seen on RSM) to confirm the diagnosis. This step, which is often skipped, is essential. The morphology and presence of macroconidia and microconidia are essential for confirmation and identification of dermatophytes.

Management and Prevention

Management of dermatophytosis in cat populations requires regular screening as described above in order to promote early recognition of disease and implement a plan for response if an outbreak occurs. Animals with positive culture results and possibly affected or exposed animals should be isolated. Staff members should wear gloves, smocks or coveralls, and boots or shoe covers while working with affected cats. After contact with dermatophyte-infected cats, staff members should not contact healthy cats until they have showered and changed clothes. Affected animals should not be allowed into the main facility until several weeks after clinical recovery and when weekly culture results have been negative for 2 consecutive weeks. Because dermatophyte spores are very hardy in the environment and resistant to many disinfectants, emphasis should be placed on thorough and repeated environmental decontamination. This is most effective in multiple-cat environments that are designed to be easily sanitized. Food bowls, litter pans, grooming instruments, bedding, and other potential fomites such as toys should be disposable or able to be decontaminated. A 1:10 bleach solution with at least a 10-minute contact time, or accelerated hydrogen peroxide are appropriate disinfectant choices. Washable items can be cleaned in a dishwasher if it has a water temperature of at least 43.3°C (110°F).

Treatment

Although many cats will spontaneously recover from dermatophytosis within months, when dermatophytosis is confirmed in a multiple-cat environment, the risk of outbreak generally leads to initiation of early treatment. Oral antifungal drug therapy in combination with topical treatments are recommended. Topical treatment reduces contamination of the environment and aids in elimination of infection.[25] Clipping, which should be performed *gently* with a number 10 blade, removes infected hairs and therefore reduces environmental contamination, and can be useful for long-haired or matted cats. However, clipping can also introduce infected spores into the environment if not done carefully, so it is not recommended as a routine treatment. Miconazole and lime-sulfur dip (4%) used twice weekly are the most efficacious topical treatments. Many other creams, ointments, and shampoos have disappointing results. Systemic therapy in combination with topical therapy helps to shorten the course of infection because of its activity on fungus within the hair follicles. Itraconazole, fluconazole, and terbinafine are appropriate choices. In multiple-cat environments, it is recommended that treatment continue until two fungal cultures or PCR tests taken 1 week apart are negative.

Retrovirus Infections

Etiologic Agent and Clinical Signs

FeLV and FIV are retroviruses that infect cats worldwide. The prevalence of infection varies greatly depending on age, health, environment, and lifestyle. Despite reduction in prevalence due to vaccination and screening, these viral infections remain a concern where groups of cats are in close contact. In a 2008 study of 18,000 cats, the prevalence of FeLV infection (antigenemia) was 2.3%, and FIV antibodies were detected in 2.5% of cats.[26] A 2017 study of 62,301 cats showed a prevalence of 3.1% for FeLV and 3.6% for FIV.[27] Sick cats and cats allowed outdoor access have a higher prevalence of infection compared with healthy cats. Although some characteristics can be used to predict likelihood of infection (age, sex, health status, and lifestyle), all cats are potentially at risk and it is recommended that each individual cat's status be known. Multiple cat programs should have procedures and policies in place to identify and segregate infected cats from the healthy population, as this is the most effective means of reducing transmission. Neither viruses are currently considered to be zoonotic.

Cats typically acquire FeLV through the oronasal route. Viremic cats shed infectious virus in multiple body fluids, including saliva, nasal secretions, feces and urine, and milk. Examples of activities that allow transmission include grooming, fighting, biting, or transfer during pregnancy or nursing. Transmission through use of shared litterboxes or feeding dishes is possible but less common. FeLV infection is sometimes referred to as "the friendly cat disease" because it can be transmitted by grooming and cohabitating without overt fighting.

In contrast, FIV infection most often affects fighting male cats. The virus is shed in high quantities in saliva, and the primary mode of transmission is through bite wounds. However, transmission has been documented in groups of cats where no fighting has been observed. Sexual transmission and transmission from queen to kitten are uncommon.

Acute FeLV infection is rarely associated with observable clinical signs. There may be transient leukopenia, fever and lethargy, but these signs are generally so mild that they are not noticed by caregivers or are attributed to other causes. Many cats recover from this phase and become regressively infected, without further impact (see Chapter 32). Cats with regressive infections are not viremic; however, FeLV provirus DNA is integrated into the cat's genome and can be detected with DNA-based PCR assays. In cats with progressive infection, the virus replicates in the lymphatic tissues and then the bone marrow. These cats become viremic, and generally develop FeLV-associated diseases. Common clinical signs in cats that develop progressive infection include anemia, opportunistic infections, lymphoma, and gingivitis, and progressively infected cats often succumb to such diseases after several years. When kittens are infected *in utero*, they often do not survive to birth or are stillborn.

FIV infection is often subclinical for years, eventually followed by overt clinical disease in some cats (see Chapter 33). After infection, the cat develops a high viremia followed by host immune-induced significant reductions in circulating virus load. As with FeLV, the acute phase of FIV is transient, nonspecific, and often mild, including fever, reduced appetite, and enlarged lymph nodes. Even though the cat's immune response suppresses viremia, the cat remains infected. Cats then enter the prolonged subclinical period that can last for years. Progressive immune dysfunction during this phase culminates in the chronic phase of illness, sometimes referred to as "feline AIDS" where opportunistic infections, chronic inflammatory disease, oral disease, and a host of secondary conditions occur. Severe URTD, hemotropic *Mycoplasma* infection, and neoplastic disease are common.

Diagnosis

Ideally, all cats should be tested for retrovirus infection because of the consequences of infection and because identification and segregation of infected cats is the most effective method to prevent spread. Testing one cat as a proxy for another or pooling samples from multiple cats for testing is inappropriate. Testing on admission to a program is recommended when group/colony housing is the case. When cats are not comingling, testing on admission is optional but still recommended. Testing is also optional for managed feral colonies in part because neutering reduces fighting which limits transmission. Proper test interpretation is critical. Most FeLV infections are identified by p27 antigen ELISA assays. Most cats and kittens test positive on soluble antigen tests within 28 days of exposure; however, this can vary. When antigen testing is negative and recent exposure is possible (such as on admission), a repeat test should be performed or recommended a minimum of 28 days from the last potential exposure. Kittens may be tested at any time, as there is not a risk of maternal antibody interfering with test results. Some kittens may take weeks to months to test positive if maternal transmission has occurred. A positive ELISA test suggests viremia and true infection for many cats; when prevalence of disease is low, the risk of a false positive increases significantly. This means it is important to confirm positive test results using a different manufacturer's test or an IFA test, which can be performed on blood or bone marrow at any time. A positive IFA indicates a cat that is likely to be persistently infected, whereas cats with positive antigen tests but negative IFA tests may ultimately become regressor cats. If a second antigen test in 30–60 days is still positive, regressive infection is unlikely. PCR assays are positive both in cats with regressive and progressive infections. Cats with discordant results may require repeated testing until the discordance resolves, and should be considered infectious until then.

Cats should be screened for FIV infection using an antibody ELISA. PCR assays are not sensitive enough for screening. Maternal antibodies can interfere with FIV testing in kittens, but false-positive test results rarely occur at 4 months of age and are very unlikely by 6 months.

Management and Prevention

The decision about how to manage retrovirus-infected cats in multiple-cat environments depends on many factors, including the mission and philosophy of the program, the physical facility, and other resources available. Infected cats can have an excellent quality of life for years; however, they have a contagious, potentially fatal infection and their condition requires appropriate housing and care to prevent transmission and maintain welfare and well-being. Cats that are housed individually pose no transmission risk and this may be an option in some programs. Because even moderately immunosuppressed cats are more susceptible to infection, cats with retrovirus infection can contribute disproportionately to the load of other pathogenic organisms in a multiple-cat environment, thereby increasing risks for other resident cats. In programs where isolation is unrealistic, grouping FeLV-positive cats together and grouping FIV-positive cats together could be considered. This is not ideal, as these cats are immunosuppressed and may transmit a variety of pathogens to each other. It is not recommended to comingle FeLV- or FIV-positive cats with a retrovirus-negative population. Cats must be well nourished, protected from stress and other infectious diseases, and treated for secondary conditions. If the program places cats in homes, either through sale or adoption, new owners should be informed of any positive FeLV/FIV status, the meaning of positive test results, advised to keep cats indoors, and provided with recommendations for care and treatment of these cats. In group environments, the FeLV vaccine can provide protection and is recommended. Because the vaccine requires two doses spaced apart by 2 to 4 weeks for efficacy, use in TNR programs is not advised. Cats should test negative before vaccination, the vaccine should never be considered a replacement for test and segregation as a control strategy, and there is no benefit to vaccinating an already infected cat. In locations where the FIV vaccine remains available, FIV vaccination makes screening difficult because vaccinated cats develop antibodies and therefore have positive ELISA assay results (see Chapter 33). For this reason, the FIV vaccine has not been generally recommended. If ever used, cats should be microchipped and vaccination documented in the medical record in association with the microchip number.

Treatment

Retrovirus-positive cats should receive biannual wellness examinations. A CBC is recommended annually for FIV-infected cats and semi-annually for FeLV-infected cats. Serum biochemistry testing should be performed annually. Spay or neuter is advised for these cats and vaccination decisions are based on individual cats' needs. Inactivated vaccines are generally recommended due to the potential for vaccine-associated disease in an immunocompromised animal. Retrovirus-positive cats should be housed indoors and treated regularly with parasiticides. Studies evaluating antiviral and immunomodulatory drug therapy in cats with retrovirus infections have met with somewhat disappointing results, although the use of oral IFN-α has shown some benefit for cats with stomatitis (see Chapter 33).

Prognosis

It is important to remember that healthy cats that test positive for FeLV may become regressor cats and never develop disease. Even cats that are persistently infected can remain healthy for several years with proper care. Similarly, lifespan may not be negatively impacted by FIV infection, and with supportive care for stomatitis and other secondary infections, even cats with advanced FIV infection can have a good quality of life for many months.

Feline Infectious Peritonitis

Etiology and Clinical Signs

FIP is the disease caused by FCoV, an enveloped RNA virus. Most strains of FCoV have low pathogenicity, and as such either do not cause disease, or just mild enteritis. Transmission of these strains is by the fecal-oral route. In multiple-cat groups, 40% to 60% of the cats shed virus in their feces at any given time, and virtually all cats have positive coronavirus serum antibody test results. Contaminated litter-boxes are a major source of infection. However, transmission can also occur indirectly through fecal particles on the fur, and fomites on caregivers' clothing, hands, and sanitation implements.[28]

Low-virulence FCoVs replicate primarily in enterocytes, but also can also be found in other tissues (as a result, the term "feline enteric coronavirus" has been used to describe these strains). Subsequently, most cats eliminate infection. Persistently infected carrier cats predominantly harbor FCoV in their colonic mucosa, facilitating prolonged fecal shedding of virus.[29,30]

A small percentage of cats go on to develop FIP as a result of an interplay between an aberrant immune response and mutation of the virus that allows it to enter macrophages and cause a systemic vasculitis. FIP most commonly develops in 1- to 3-year-old cats from multiple-cat environments and in cats over the age of 12 or in immunocompromised cats, including kittens and retrovirus-positive cats; however, cats of any age and health status can be affected.

Two clinical forms of FIP exist, the effusive ("wet") form and noneffusive ("dry") form, and some cats may initially develop noneffusive disease and progress to effusive disease, or have both forms concurrently. The time between initial exposure and development of FIP varies greatly. Effusive FIP typically progresses more rapidly, over several weeks, with accumulation of moderate- to high-protein effusions in the thorax or abdomen, which leads to dyspnea or abdominal distention. In noneffusive FIP, pyogranulomas develop within a variety of tissues, which can lead to formation of masses and organ failure. Noneffusive FIP may result from a partially successful cell-mediated immune response and signs may not be apparent for months to years. Clinical signs vary depending on the affected organ system and include fever, icterus, ascites, dyspnea, abdominal lymphadenopathy, thickened intestinal loops or abdominal masses, irregular renomegaly, uveitis, and neurologic signs.

Once it develops, FIP is progressive and fatal. Virulent FIP viruses are not shed from the intestinal tract, so FIP is not transmitted from one cat to another. In multiple-cat populations, apparent "outbreaks" of FIP can occur, which are thought to relate to the accumulation of factors that promote virus replication and mutation within individual cats (e.g., genetic susceptibility, concurrent infections, malnourishment, overcrowding, high juvenile to adult cat ratio; see Chapter 31). FCoVs do not infect humans, so there is no risk of zoonotic transmission.

Diagnosis

Obtaining a definitive diagnosis of FIP can be challenging. Clinical signs and laboratory abnormalities are nonspecific. The presence of marked hyperglobulinemia can add support to the diagnosis, and the likelihood of FIP is increased if the characteristic high-protein, low-cellularity effusion is identified. Unfortunately, many cats do not develop these abnormalities. Ultimately, diagnosis is based on a composite of history, signalment, clinical observations, physical examination, laboratory findings, and specific diagnostic testing.

Regardless of the magnitude of the antibody titer, diagnosis of FIP should never be made on the basis of serology alone. Generally, a positive titer result only indicates exposure to a coronavirus, which is more often a low-virulence FCoV strain. Very high (e.g., > 1:3200) titers may be suggestive of FIP in conjunction with consistent clinical signs.

Although some assays are more likely to detect strains with mutations associated with virulence, real-time RT-PCR assays cannot reliably differentiate between low-virulence FCoVs and FIP viruses. Ultimately, the only way to confirm a diagnosis of FIP is to identify coronavirus antigen with immunohistochemical stains in consistent lesions within biopsies or at necropsy. Immunocytochemistry can also be performed on aspirates or cytospins of effusion fluid, but the sensitivity of this method is lower and false-positive results are possible if the technician performing the assay is not adequately experienced.

Management and Prevention

FCoV infections can generally only be eradicated in very small groups of cats (≤ 4 per housing unit). An intranasal vaccine is available, but it has limited efficacy and must be given *before* FCoV exposure, which typically occurs before the age of administration (16 weeks). Prevention of FIP should focus on minimizing overcrowding, fecal contamination, concurrent infections, and the juvenile to adult cat ratio.[31] In breeding catteries, the use of male cats that generate offspring that develop FIP should be avoided for further breeding efforts.

Treatment and Prognosis

Supportive care and use of oral prednisolone at anti-inflammatory doses are currently the mainstay of treatment. In some cats, treatment with prednisolone can lead to complete remissions, but ultimately, weeks to over a year later, disease relapses. There have been encouraging advancements in antiviral drug therapy for FIP (see Chapters 9 and 31), but none of these drugs are commercially available at the time of writing.

SUGGESTED READINGS

Kessler M, Turner D. Socialization and stress in cats (*Felis silvestris catus*) housed singly and in groups and in groups in animal shelters. *Anim Welf.* 1999;8:15–26.

Rochlitz I. Recommendations for the housing of cats in the home, in catteries and animal shelters, in laboratories and in veterinary surgeries. *J Feline Med Surg.* 1999;1:181–191.

Newbury S, Blinn MK, Bushby PA, et al. CASV Guidelines for Standards of Care in Animal Shelters. https://www.sheltervet.org/assets/docs/shelter-standards-oct2011-wforward.pdf.

REFERENCES

1. Kessler M, Turner D. Socialization and stress in cats (*Felis silvestris catus*) housed singly and in groups and in groups in animal shelters. *Anim Welf.* 1999;8:15–26.
2. Rochlitz I. Recommendations for the housing of cats in the home, in catteries and animal shelters, in laboratories and in veterinary surgeries. *J Feline Med Surg.* 1999;1:181–191.
3. Newbury S, Blinn MK, Bushby PA, et al. ASV Guidelines for Standards of Care in Animal Shelters. https://www.sheltervet.org/assets/docs/shelter-standards-oct2011-wforward.pdf.
4. American Veterinary Medical Association. AVMA Companion Animal Care Guidelines; 2008. https://www.avma.org/KB/Policies/Pages/Companion-Animal-Care-Guidelines.aspx.
5. Gaskell R, Gaskell C. Respiratory disease. *Vet Q.* 1997;19:S48.
6. Ford RB. Role of infectious agents in respiratory disease. Feline infectious diseases. *Vet Clin N Am Small Anim Pract.* 1993;23:17–35.
7. Scarlett J. Feline upper respiratory disease. In: Miller L, Hurley K., eds. *Infectious Disease Management in Animal Shelters.* Ames, IA: Wiley-Blackwell; 2009: 125–146
8. Hargis AM, Ginn PE. Feline herpesvirus 1-associated facial and nasal dermatitis and stomatitis in domestic cats. *Vet Clin North Am Small Anim Pract.* 1999;29:1281–1290.
9. Kreutz LC, Johnson RP, Seal BS. Phenotypic and genotypic variation of feline calicivirus during persistent infection of cats. *Vet Microbiol.* 1998;l59:229–236.
10. Radford AD, Bennett M, McArdle F, et al. The use of sequence analysis of a feline calicivirus (FCV) hypervariable region in the epidemiological investigation of FCV related disease and vaccine failures. *Vaccine.* 1997;15:1451–1458.
11. Pedersen NC, Elliott JB, Glasgow A, et al. An isolated epizootic of hemorrhagic-like fever in cats caused by a novel and highly virulent strain of feline calicivirus. *Vet Microbiol.* 2000;73:281–300.
12. Binns SH, Dawson S, Speakman AJ, et al. Prevalence and risk factors for feline *Bordetella bronchiseptica* infection. *Vet Rec.* 1999;144:575–580.
13. Speakman AJ, Dawson S, Binns SH, et al. *Bordetella bronchiseptica* infection in the cat. *J Small Anim Pract.* 1999;40:252–256.
14. Datz C. *Bordetella* infections in dogs and cats: pathogenesis, clinical signs and diagnosis. *Compen Cont Edu Pract Vet.* 2003;25(12):896–900.
15. Browning GF. Is *Chlamydophila felis* a significant zoonotic pathogen? *Austral Vet J.* 2004;82:695–696.
16. Marinova-Petkova A, et al. Avian unfluenza A(H7N2) virus in humans exposed to sick cats, New York, USA, 2016. *Emerg Infect Dis.* 2017;23(12):2046–2049.
17. Gunn-Moore D, Tennant B. *Tritrichomonas foetus* diarrhoea in cats. Vet Rec 160:850-851.
18. Gookin J, et al. Efficacy of ronidazole for treatment of *Tritrichomonas foetus* infection. *J Vet Intern Med.* 2006;20(3):536–543. 2007.
19. Tuzio H. Feline panleukopenia In: Miller L, Hurley K, eds. *Infectious Disease Management in Animal Shelters.* Ames, IA: Wiley-Blackwell; 2009: 183–196.
20. Goossens H, Vlaes L, Butzler JP, et al. *Campylobacter upsaliensis* enteritis associated with canine infections. *Lancet.* 1991;337:1486.
21. Hald B, Madsen M. Healthy puppies and kittens as carriers of *Campylobacter* spp., with special reference to *Campylobacter upsaliensis. J Clin Microbiol.* 1997;35:3351–3352.
22. Patton CM, Shaffer N, Edmonds P, et al. Human disease associated with "*Campylobacter upsaliensis*" (catalase-negative or weakly positive *Campylobacter* species) in the United States. *J Clin Microbiol.* 1989;27:66–73.
23. Brown RR, Elston TH, et al. Feline zoonoses guidelines from the American Association of Feline Practitioners. *Comp Cont Ed Pract Vet.* 2003;25:936–965.
24. Moriello K. Diagnosis and treatment of dermatophytosis in dogs and cats. *Vet Dematol.* 2017;28:266–e268.
25. Moriello K. Management of dermatophyte infections in catteries and multiple cat households. *Vet Clin North Am Small Anim Pract.* 1990;20:1457–1474.
26. Levy JK, et al. Seroprevalence of feline leukemia virus and feline immunodeficiency virus infection among cats in North America and risk factors for positivity. *J Am Vet Med Assoc.* 2006;228:371–376.
27. Burling AN, Levy JK, Scott HM, et al. Seroprevalences of feline leukemia virus and feline immunodeficiency virus infection in cats in the United States and Canada and risk factors for seropositivity. *J Am Vet Med Assoc.* 2017;251:187–194.
28. Foley JE, Poland A, Carlson J, et al. Patterns of feline coronavirus infection and fecal shedding from cats in multiple-cat environments. *J Am Vet Med Assoc.* 1997;210:1307–1312.
29. Kipar A, Meli ML, Babtiste KE. Sites of feline coronavirus persistence in healthy cats. *J Gen Virol.* 2010;91:1698–1707.
30. Vogel L, Van der Lubben M, Te Lintelo EG, et al. Pathogenic characteristics of persistent feline enteric coronavirus infection in cats. *Vet Res.* 2010;41:71.
31. Pedersen NC. A review of feline infectious peritonitis virus infection: 1963–2008. *J Feline Med Surg.* 2009;11:225–258.

17

Prevention and Management of Infection in Canine Populations

Kate F. Hurley, Stacy Kraus, Jane E. Sykes

KEY POINTS

- Dog populations may be transient or stable. Transient populations have the greatest susceptibility to infectious diseases.
- The key for control of infectious disease in dog populations is ensuring capacity is appropriate and controlling dog movement to limit transmission of disease.
- Other important preventative measures are proper disinfection, reduction of stressors, use of parasite preventatives, vaccination, routine health surveillance, and in animal shelters, active management of length of stay.
- Many pathogens in dog populations have the potential to be transmitted to humans that are in contact with infected dogs. Attention to infection control protocols therefore promotes the health of humans as well as the dog population.

CHARACTERISTICS OF DOG POPULATIONS

Dog populations may be transient or stable. Transient populations are usually associated with veterinary hospitals; grooming and boarding facilities; community animal shelters; communal areas such as dog daycare facilities, dog parks, and dog shows; rescue organizations; retail outlets; suppliers that acquire and condition dogs for resale; and research kennels that do not maintain long-term residents. Relatively stable adult canine populations are found in kennels that support purebred interests (breeding or performance), in those that produce puppies for commercial pet channels, in research kennels that maintain long-term residents, and in multiple-pet households. Characteristics of both stable and transient populations can be noted in many settings including households, shelters, sanctuaries, and breeding and performance kennels.

Regardless of their purpose, all dog populations share general features, including close proximity of residents, some means of confinement, systems for sanitation and husbandry, and some means to deliver preventative and individual animal health care. The type and prevalence of infectious disease that occurs in a population depends on the regional prevalence of an infectious disease and the characteristics of both the facility and the dog population. For example, CPV can persist long-term in some environments if not effectively inactivated or removed. The disease is unlikely to be significant in a population of adult, vaccinated dogs, whereas populations that include naïve puppies are likely to experience a higher incidence of infection and disease. Disease caused by pathogens that survive poorly in the environment, such as those involved in canine infectious respiratory disease complex (CIRDC) (see Chapter 28), is more likely to occur when there are environmental stressors and crowding. Animal shelters offer unique challenges because transient dogs can subclinically be shedding pathogens common to the larger community.

Two extremely important management concepts in population medicine are defining capacity (management of population density) and control of movement of dogs within and among populations (e.g., segregation). Also of importance is proper environmental management of any facility in which a canine population is housed.

Regardless of the type of facility, strong preventative health care is necessary. A comprehensive population infection control program requires planning. Veterinary professionals are essential in the identification of risk factors for disease, to help direct the development of policies and procedures, and in the assessment of effectiveness of these measures.[1] Planned preventative care management is far more efficient and cost-effective compared with purely therapeutic or reactive management to infection outbreaks. In addition, thorough education and training of owners, managers, and staff is critical to successful implementation of a plan.

Zoonoses are of concern in all dog populations, particularly those with a high level of public interaction such as dogs in shelters and pet stores. Specific strategies, including training and availability of personal protective equipment (PPE), should be in place to ensure that staff and public health risks are minimized. Pathogens that have the potential to cause disease in humans in poorly managed environments are listed in Table 17.1.

DISEASE TRANSMISSION

Periodic introduction of disease into canine populations is inevitable, especially in transient populations. The likelihood that disease introduction will lead to transmission within a given population depends on the virulence of the organism introduced, the mechanism of transmission, the immunity of the dog population, and environmental factors that influence level of exposure. In populations where dogs are singly housed, direct transmission is of minimal importance. If dogs have direct contact with one another through open cage panels or are allowed to intermingle during cleaning, the direct route of transmission becomes more significant. The most common method of spread among singly housed dogs is likely to be transmission via contaminated fomites, such as hands, clothing and footwear, equipment, or surfaces. Droplet and aerosol transmission are concerns for canine respiratory pathogens such as CDV and CIVs. Pathogens such as CPV that are not normally airborne can nonetheless be spread by power sprayers or via dust spread by high-power fans. Vector-borne transmission can be an issue in populations where external parasites or biting insects are not controlled.[2]

TABLE 17.1 Examples of Pathogens with the Potential to Cause Disease in Humans in Contact with Dog Populations and Their Mode of Transmission

Pathogen Group	Pathogen Name	Route of Transmission
Viruses	Rabies virus	Bites
Bacteria	*Anaplasma phagocytophilum*	Ticks
	Bartonella spp.[a]	Fleas, needle-stick injuries, ticks?
	Bordetella bronchiseptica	Respiratory: droplets, fomites, close contact with infected dogs
	Brucella canis	Close contact with urinary, respiratory secretions from infected dogs, especially breeding kennels
	Campylobacter spp.	Fecal-oral
	Clostridioides difficile and *Clostridium perfringens* (toxigenic)	Fecal-oral
	Coxiella burnetii	Contact with placental materials
	Leptospira spp.	Contact with urine
	Multidrug-resistant bacteria (e.g., *Staphylococcus* spp., pathogenic *Escherichia coli*)	Contact with skin, urine, feces; infections of preexisting wounds; bites
	Hemotropic *Mycoplasma* spp. (e.g., "*Candidatus* Mycoplasma haematoparvum")[a]	Ticks?
	Pasteurella spp.[a]	Bites, preexisting wound infections
	Salmonella spp.[a]	Fecal-oral
	Streptococcus equi subsp. *zooepidemicus*	Respiratory droplets, other?
	Rickettsia rickettsii and other *Rickettsia* spp.	Ticks
Fungi	Dermatophytes[a]	Direct contact
	Malassezia spp.[a]	Direct contact
Protozoa	*Cryptosporidium* spp.[a]	Fecal-oral
	Giardia spp.	Fecal-oral (some assemblages)
Helminths	*Dipylidium caninum*	Fleas
	Toxocara canis	Fecal-oral
Arthropods	*Sarcoptes scabiei*	Direct contact
	Fleas	Direct contact, environmental
	Ticks (especially *Rhipicephalus sanguineus*)	Direct contact, environmental

[a] Most significant disease in the immunocompromised.

Environmental factors that influence transmission include population density; kennel design; the extent to which populations are segregated effectively; sanitation; and conditions such as ventilation, noise, and humidity.

MANAGEMENT OF POPULATION DENSITY

Maintaining population density within the capacity of the organization and facility is the foundation for a successful infectious disease management program. Crowding is a profound risk factor for transmission of infectious diseases in any population. For example, every day a dog spends in a shelter, they increase their risk of infectious respiratory disease by 3%. A greater burden is placed on air-handling systems, noise tends to increase with more barking dogs present, and the stress associated with crowded conditions will increase susceptibility to disease. If an increase in density is not accompanied by a commensurate increase in staffing, daily care for each animal may be compromised. This can lead to failures in key husbandry practices such as cleaning, monitoring for illness, and prompt isolation of potentially infectious dogs. A vicious cycle can easily ensue as the number of sick dogs increases. Daily treatment will require even more staff time, and individualized care is further jeopardized. The level of infectious pathogens increases in the environment, and spread of infection continues.

To avoid overcrowding, the appropriate capacity of the facility must first be determined. Maximum capacity should be calculated and not exceeded. Ideally, the population should be maintained at no more than 80% of capacity, to allow flexibility for management of dogs with special needs and to prepare for unexpected influxes. Capacity depends on the number of appropriate housing units and available staff time and can vary by subpopulations. For example, capacity for puppies cannot be the same as that for adult dogs, because special housing is required to prevent exposure of puppies to infectious disease. According to the National Animal Care and Control Association,[3] in a shelter situation, 15 minutes per dog is required for minimal daily care and cleaning (9 minutes for cleaning and 6 minutes for feeding). More time will be required to care for animals if the facility design prohibits efficient cleaning. It is more labor intensive if dogs must be removed from their kennels to a holding area that must be disinfected between uses. Optimally, dogs should be housed in a double-sided run where the dog can be moved to one side while the other side is being cleaned (Fig. 17.1). Additional time must also be allocated for medical care, socialization, and other special needs depending on the type of facility and the population in its care. In order to calculate staff capacity of an organization, available total staff time for care is divided by the number of minutes required per dog. For example, in a facility that has one staff member providing 8 hours of care/day for dogs requiring 30 minutes of care each, the staff capacity is 16 dogs. Documenting facility and staff capacities compared to actual average daily animal census on a monthly basis can be helpful for organizations experiencing a great deal of variation in daily population over the course of a year, such as shelters and some boarding facilities (Figs. 17.2 and 17.3).

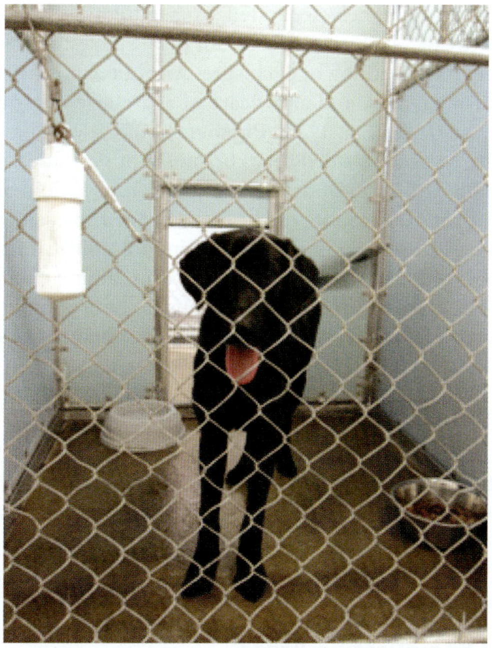

Fig. 17.1 Double-sided run with a sliding door that separates the two halves. This allows the dog some control over its environment and permits cleaning and care without removing the dog from the run. (From Greene, *Infectious Diseases of the Dog and Cat*, 4e. Figure 96-3, p. 1126.)

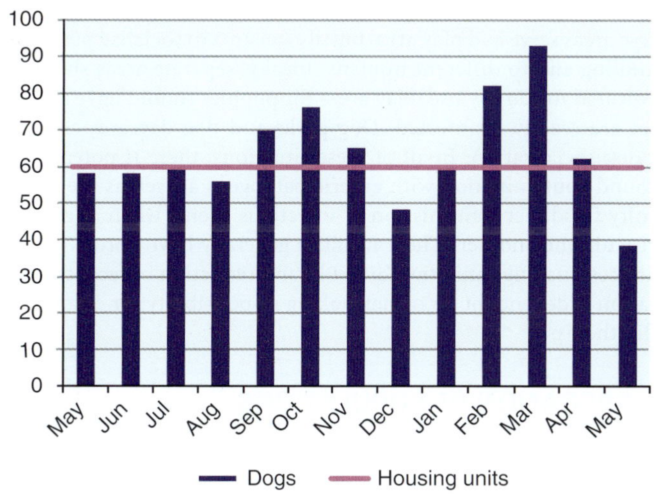

Fig. 17.2 Graph comparing facility capacity to average daily canine population by month over a 1-year period. In this facility, the number of housing units was inadequate for 6 of the 13 months recorded, resulting in chronic overcrowding. (Modified from Greene, *Infectious Diseases of the Dog and Cat*, 4e. Figure 96-1, p. 1125.)

The average daily population for the month is calculated by summing the daily population for each month and dividing by the number of days in that month.

Length of Stay and Pathway Planning

In contrast to some populations in which decreased transience is associated with decreased risk of infectious disease introduction and transmission, increased length of stay (LOS) has been identified as one of the most important risk factors for disease in animal shelters. This is likely due to the relationship between LOS and crowding and its associated risks: for a given number of dogs admitted to a shelter,

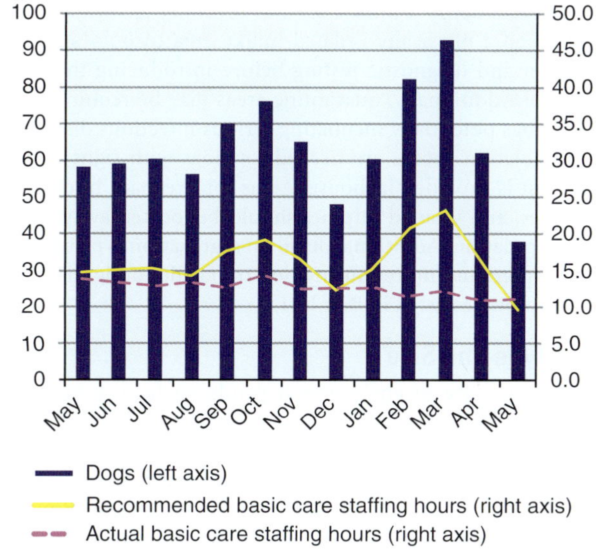

Fig. 17.3 Graph comparing staff capacity (total number of minutes available for care of dogs) with average daily canine population by month over a 1-year period. In this shelter, staffing at times was less than half the level required to provide the recommended minimum 15 minutes of daily care per dog. (Modified from Greene, *Infectious Diseases of the Dog and Cat*, 4e. Figure 96-2, p 1125.)

doubling of the LOS will double the population density on a daily basis. Active management of LOS is therefore a foundation of a successful disease control program in a shelter (or other setting with a fixed capacity and limited control over the rate of new admissions). Ideally, "pathway planning" should begin as soon as an animal is admitted in order to identify the shortest pathway to the best possible outcome for the animal. This can be facilitated by admitting animals that do not need admission on an emergency basis using an appointment system. Needed services such as spay/neuter surgery should be scheduled as soon as possible. Daily population rounds, in addition to identifying health concerns, should include an assessment of any needed actions to help move the dog safely through the system. These could include contacting possible owners or interested parties, marketing the dog for adoption, or evaluating rescue options. Prolonged stray holds often do not assist in increasing return to owner rates and the benefit of these should be carefully weighed against the risks of increased LOS. Ideally, long stray holds should be replaced by active programs to contact owners and reunite dogs with their families. Importantly, rushing to euthanasia or another suboptimal outcome is not a method to manage LOS. Rather, the overall average should be reduced by removing bottlenecks and rapidly identifying barriers, allowing adequate time to care for dogs with more complex needs or requiring a longer shelter stay.

KENNEL DESIGN AND LAYOUT AS IT RELATES TO POPULATION HEALTH

The building layout and defined activity zones will vary based on the mission and function of each facility. Specific zones should be separated and designated by signage to minimize transmission of disease. Some units have a public zone (e.g., veterinary hospitals, boarding and grooming facilities, shelters) that can include an entry area, housing areas, and activity areas. All units should have a restricted zone that includes rooms where animals are received, are held once entering the facility, and are examined for health assessment and treatment. Some facilities, such as breeding facilities and some shelters, need a physically isolated intake area to hold animals for observation and diagnostic testing before introducing them to the population. Additionally, quarantine areas may be required for isolation of dogs potentially incubating serious infectious diseases, and separate isolation rooms are needed for dogs with signs of disease if treatment is provided in-house. Areas for pregnant bitches, nursing puppies, and weaned puppies should be located away from the general population. Additional detail on segregation is provided later in this chapter, and more information on facility design is available from the resources listed in Box 17.1.[4]

Kennel Type and Size

The minimum size of enclosures depends on factors such as dog breeds housed and duration of housing. Recommendations have been published by the Association of Shelter Veterinarians,[5] the Animal and Plant Health Inspection Service, Department of Agriculture of the United States,[6] and the National Research Council (Box 17.1).[7] Barring medical conditions that require limited movement, enclosures must be of sufficient size to allow dogs to assume normal postures without touching the sides of the enclosure and to urinate and defecate away from feeding and sleeping areas; must accommodate bedding; and must allow for expression of a range of normal behaviors. Size and quality of housing will need to be greater for dogs housed for longer time periods (more than 2 weeks) and for whom no other avenue for exercise, play, and socialization is routinely provided. In production units or shelters, areas for pregnant bitches, nursing bitches, and litters are needed. Space should be adequate for the bitches to separate themselves from the litter. Enclosures should have solid barriers between adjacent enclosures to minimize transmission of pathogens.

BOX 17.1 Animal Welfare and Kennel Management Resources

Association of Shelter Veterinarians Guidelines for Standards of Care in Animal Shelters:
https://www.sheltervet.org/guidelines-for-standards-of-care-in-animal-shelters.

Animal and Plant Health Inspection Service, U.S. Department of Agriculture:
Animal Welfare Act and Animal Welfare Regulations. Specifications for the humane handling, care, treatment, and transportation of dogs and cats: https://www.aphis.usda.gov/animal_welfare/downloads/bluebook-ac-awa.pdf. 2019:111-134.

Center for Food Security and Public Health:
Infection control: https://www.cfsph.iastate.edu/zoonoses/zoonotic-disease-prevention/

Humane Society of the United States:
Animal welfare: https://humanepro.org/store

National Animal Control Association:
http://www.nacanet.org

National Research Council:
Guide for the Care and Use of Laboratory Animals, ed 8 (2011). National Academies Press. http://grants.nih.gov/grants/olaw/Guide-for-the-Care-and-Use-of-Laboratory-Animals.pdf

University of California, Davis, Koret Shelter Medicine Program:
https://www.sheltermedicine.com/

University of Wisconsin-Madison Shelter Medicine Program:
https://www.uwsheltermedicine.com/library/resources/developing-infectious-disease-policies-and-protocols-in-an-animal-shelter

Double-sided kennels separated by a guillotine door facilitate cleaning, provide separation of areas for eating or resting versus elimination, facilitate cleaning of enclosures without exposing animals to water or disinfectants, and allow care of aggressive dogs with minimal risk to staff (see Fig. 17.1). Puppies should always be housed in easily sanitized double-sided cages or runs that permit easy and efficient cleaning and care. Doors on kennels or runs should be secure.

Outdoor runs of concrete can be easily cleaned and sanitized. Runs built of gravel, dirt, or grass are challenging to sanitize and may harbor microbes and parasites, especially in warm, humid climates. Daily removal of feces from these areas is essential to limit contamination of the soil, and puppies or dogs with unknown vaccination history should not be exposed to these areas.

Surfaces and Flooring

Buildings should be constructed of materials that can be easily cleaned and disinfected. Concrete facilitates sanitation, provided it is sealed to make the surface impervious. Floor treatments should be coved up the wall of the kennel area and other areas where dogs may walk to facilitate cleaning. Floors should gradually slope to a drainage system to which dogs do not have access.

Play and Socialization Areas

Play and socialization areas can serve different functions in different units. In the shelter environment, these areas can serve to enrich the environment with fresh air and sunshine and to permit dog-human interaction. They can also serve as a place for supervised play between selected dogs. In a breeding establishment or shelter housing puppies, these areas serve as a play area, but also an area to socialize puppies to handling and to different humans. Ideally, separate areas should be dedicated for puppy use. Play areas for puppies should have surfaces that are readily disinfected. Dog parks and dog daycares are areas of dog socialization. In all of these situations, there is potential for ground contamination with enteric pathogens as well as the opportunity for direct transmission of infectious agents when dogs interact with one another. These facilities generally have porous ground surfaces, making sanitation difficult, and reduction of fecal contamination is dependent on owners taking responsibility for cleaning up after their pet.

SEGREGATION OF POPULATIONS

It is generally impractical, and often not desirable, to isolate healthy, compatible dogs from one another during confinement.[8] However, segregation of transient subpopulations is critical for infectious disease control. Less stringent precautions are required for healthy, adult dogs that are currently vaccinated, whereas greater care can be taken when handling vulnerable or infectious individuals.

Characteristics of Effective Segregation

Ideally, separate air supplies should be used for subpopulations, particularly for isolation of dogs with respiratory infections. At minimum, clear visual barriers should delineate physically separate areas stocked with separate equipment and supplies. Color coding of equipment can help ensure that it stays in the designated area. Appropriate PPE should be worn in areas housing puppies, sick dogs, or dogs with unknown or high-risk health histories. This includes long-sleeved tops and long pants or jump suits. Either hands should be thoroughly washed or sanitized before and after entering separate areas, or gloves should be worn and changed between areas. Sanitizer should be available outside each kennel and filled regularly. Gloves should be worn when handling sick dogs, because hand washing is not sufficient to reliably inactivate all pathogens. Shoe covers or dedicated boots should also be worn in areas housing sick dogs, because foot baths are not sufficient to reliably prevent transmission of disease.[9]

Categories for Segregation

Puppies

Because maternal antibodies may prevent effective immunization until approximately 16 to 20 weeks of age, puppies should always be housed and handled with special attention to infectious disease control. Puppies from different litters should not be cohoused unless both groups have been treated for parasites and there is a very low historical incidence of infectious disease.

Dogs with Unknown Health History

Some vaccines take a week or more to provide full protection, and the incubation period for many infectious diseases is a week or longer. Therefore animals with unknown vaccination or health history should initially be housed in easily sanitized areas and be attended to after the healthy resident dog population. True quarantine for newly admitted or acquired dogs is only viable when additional dogs are not admitted to the population during the quarantine period. This can be used for boarding and breeding facilities and some limited-intake shelters or sanctuaries. However, true quarantine is rarely feasible nor necessary in shelters, and the increased LOS associated with quarantine generally outweighs any benefit of this practice. Instead, newly admitted dogs should be vaccinated immediately upon intake, examined by trained staff, and observed for the first several days of care to monitor for any signs of ill health.

Dogs with Known Exposure to Contagious Pathogens

Dogs with a known history of exposure to CPV, CDV, or other serious contagious pathogens should be assessed for risk of infection based on history, degree of exposure, and antibody titers if appropriate.[10] At-risk dogs should be housed separately for the incubation period of the disease in question (see Dogs with Infectious Disease). If dogs develop illness during the quarantine period, risk assessment must be repeated for remaining dogs and the quarantine period restarted for dogs at risk of new exposure.

Dogs with Infectious Disease

Dogs with known or suspected infectious diseases should be housed in isolation. Ideally, separate isolation housing should be available for dogs with different conditions (e.g., suspected respiratory versus GI infections). At minimum, each dog in an isolation area should be handled with infectious disease precautions (Box 17.2).

Depending on the purpose of the facility, additional categories for segregation may be desirable, including maternity or nursing wards and areas for dogs that are to be rehomed or that require special care or monitoring.

BOX 17.2 Minimum Requirements When Husbanding Dogs in Isolation

1. Care for all healthy, resident animals before entering isolation facility.
2. Don personal protective equipment (PPE: gown or coveralls, gloves, shoe covers, or boots).
3. Avoid wetting animal during cleaning.
4. Examine animal and perform any required treatments.
5. Provide fresh food and clean water.
6. Remove PPE and put disposables in trash or put reusables in laundry.
7. Repeat steps 1 through 6 for each animal in the isolation ward.
8. Do not reenter resident facility.

DISINFECTION, SANITATION, AND PEST CONTROL

One of the cornerstones of prevention and control of disease in populations is a thorough cleaning and disinfection program. It is important that staff have a sound understanding of the major contagious pathogens of dogs, how they are transmitted, the degree to which they persist in the environment, and how they are best inactivated. Posted wall charts can facilitate access to this information. Decontamination of clothing, equipment, and hands as well as surfaces must be systematically addressed.

Effective cleaning and disinfection are dependent on knowing where to disinfect, choosing the right products, and following the essential steps in a disinfection protocol (see Chapter 14).[11] Proper cleaning procedures, including removal of organic material, rinsing before application of disinfectant, and attention to contact times are necessary. The order in which rooms and zones are cleaned and disinfected should proceed from areas housing healthy animals to those housing more vulnerable populations (e.g., puppies or newly admitted dogs) and finally to areas housing sick dogs. If this is not practical for logistical reasons, a change of PPE between areas can serve a similar purpose. Areas accessible to the general public should not be overlooked when developing a plan. Good management procedures, such as traffic patterns; holding, isolation, and quarantine protocols; vector control; washing and sanitation of feed and water bowls; and laundry procedures should be developed and modified when necessary. Education and regular training are key to success.

Pest control can be challenging in animal facilities, and the types of pests may vary with the region. Insects and rodents can contribute to disease outbreaks because they can be mechanical vectors of pathogens or reservoir hosts. All animal waste and spilled animal feed should be frequently removed from floors and feed bins and trash receptacles should be secured shut. Integrated pest management (prevention, nonchemical control when possible, and monitoring) can be effective, although commercial rodent/insect control programs, with careful assessment for safety of any chemical application, may be necessary.

OTHER ENVIRONMENTAL FACTORS

Attention to proper ventilation, humidity, temperature, sound and lighting levels is important to maintain the comfort of animals and caregivers and to reduce disease. Heating, ventilation, and air conditioning (HVAC) systems that share air through the system can serve as a vehicle to circulate pathogens throughout the facility, although other environmental factors such as population density and sanitation can outweigh this risk in most facilities. Separate HVAC systems are ideal and, if strategically placed (e.g., isolation facilities, nursery areas), can help minimize transmission of pathogens. In addition, good HVAC systems remove excessive moisture, dust, irritating gases, and chemical fumes. HVAC systems should not run only based on temperature adjustment, as this may lead to inadequate fresh air exchange during times of year when the temperature is mild. Humidity should be minimized by keeping the animal care areas and dogs as dry as possible. Physical drying of runs helps to keep dogs dry and comfortable and decreases odor and growth of mold and bacteria. Temperature should be maintained within a range that maintains animal comfort.[7] General guidelines are available (e.g., the AVMA recommends a range of 60 to 80°F); however, temperature requirements will vary depending on factors such as age, breed, and medical condition. Daily temperatures should be monitored using a high-low thermometer. Relative humidity should also be checked before husbanding the area. Barking dogs can increase the noise levels above those mandated by the Occupational Safety and Health Administration (see Guidelines for Standards of

Care in Animal Shelters, Box 17.1). Ear-protective devices should be worn to protect staff in these environments. Noise reduction is also advisable to reduce dog and human stress. Good lighting is essential in order to observe and inspect the behavior and physical condition of dogs, as well as for effective cleaning. Natural lighting can benefit both dogs and humans. Controlling the light-dark cycles (12 hours on, 12 hours off) maintains circadian rhythm.[7]

HOST FACTORS

Many pathogens commonly associated with respiratory or GI disease outbreaks can also be isolated from apparently healthy dogs. The likelihood of illness is influenced by the virulence of the pathogen, infective dose, and the host's innate and acquired immunity. Most pathogens also predispose to coinfections because they suppress normal host immune responses or damage host barriers. Immunity can be supported by controlling these coinfections, minimizing stress, and promoting normal behaviors such as self-grooming, eating, drinking, and developing a care routine.

Vaccination

Vaccination can largely prevent certain systemic infectious diseases in canine populations (e.g., parvovirus and canine distemper) and can reduce the frequency and severity of others, such as CIRDC. Vaccination programs should be tailored to the needs of the specific population. For transient kennel populations, such as shelters and boarding facilities, the focus of vaccination is on rapid protection from the limited subset of pathogens most likely to spread in this environment, including CDV, CPV, parainfluenza virus, adenovirus, and *Bordetella bronchiseptica.* Most dogs entering animal shelters may have insufficient titers for protection against CDV and CPV infection.[12] Although some attenuated live vaccines provide a degree of protection within hours to days, ideally vaccines should be given at least a week before entry into a kennel environment to optimize protection (see Chapter 20 and Appendix). If vaccination before entry is not possible, vaccines should be given immediately on admission for all dogs over 4 weeks of age. Inactivated vaccines may not provide protection until 10 to 14 days after a booster vaccine is administered, and for this reason will have limited benefit in highly transient dog populations such as many shelters. For stable kennel populations, infectious disease risk is likely to be lower and vaccination considerations are more similar to those in pet dogs, taking into account the exposure risks particular to the environment and the dog's lifestyle.

Parasite Control

External and internal parasite control is important to support animal health, to prevent contamination of the environment with resistant life cycle stages, to reduce transmission of vector-borne pathogens, and to protect public health. Animals and the environment should be treated as product information dictates to control fleas, ticks, and other external parasites. All animals should be treated with endoparasite preventatives (see Box 17.1)[13] and for heartworm depending on regional and environmental risk of exposure. Treatment for intestinal parasites should ideally be completed before entry into a kennel (e.g., for boarding kennels); otherwise, treatment should be initiated immediately on entry, and animals should be housed in easily cleaned environments until treatment has been completed. Diagnostic testing for internal parasites, when indicated, should ideally be performed at the time of entry to a facility and in the event of disease problems.

Nutrition

For dogs in transient populations such as shelters and boarding kennels, nutritional intake may be compromised by stress, unfamiliar or contaminated food, or competition with kennel mates when dogs are housed in groups. The goal of a feeding program for dogs housed for short periods is to support adequate nutritional intake, avoid anorexia, and prevent diarrhea. Unless the specific diet and amount of food the dog is normally fed are known, a high-quality diet appropriate to the life stage of the animal should be fed initially at the high end of the manufacturer's recommended amount.

Behavioral Wellness/Enrichment

In addition to being a welfare consideration in itself, behavioral wellness programs contribute to infectious disease control by reducing stress and supporting normal self-maintenance behaviors. For all dog populations, infectious disease control must be balanced with enrichment programs. However, LOS is a substantial risk factor for infectious disease in animal shelters, and enrichment can help maintain the behaviors and show dogs in natural settings that can lead to more rapid adoption or other positive outcomes. For dogs that have been vaccinated on intake and observed to be free of signs of infectious disease when monitored for several days, the benefits of out-of-cage enrichment and playgroups generally outweighs the small increased risk of infectious disease transmission. Even for dogs that cannot safely be removed from their runs, training and enrichment can be offered via clicker training, treats, and toys provided by facility staff members.

HEALTH MONITORING

Routine health monitoring of individuals ensures that health problems are promptly identified, treatment is implemented, and infectious disease spread prevented. Monitoring the population as a whole provides a means to evaluate success of husbandry procedures and detect emerging trends in population health. The larger and more transient the population, the more important a formal health monitoring system becomes. However, even for relatively small or stable populations, such as rescue homes, breeding kennels, and sanctuaries, a monitoring system should be established to prevent subtle health problems from being overlooked.

The first component of health monitoring is a thorough physical examination performed on entry to the population. This is important even for facilities admitting dogs in presumed good health. An entry examination documents preexisting conditions, and identifies problems that require treatment or special handling precautions. Results of the examination should be documented and accessible. Provided they remain apparently healthy, dogs in stable populations should be examined at least biannually; more frequent examinations should be performed in populations with higher turnover of animals and caregivers.

For transient populations, "daily rounds" should also be performed during which every animal is visually examined. This should occur before cleaning so that if potentially contagious conditions are identified, steps can be taken to prevent fomite transmission to other dogs in the course of care. Minimum daily observations include a visual assessment of the kennel and dog, including attitude; behavior; presence and character of urine and feces; whether food has been eaten; and any clinical signs such as respiratory, cutaneous, or GI signs. Daily observations should be recorded so patterns of illness can be monitored both for individual dogs and the population as a whole.[14] Example protocols and monitoring sheets can be found at academic shelter medicine sites online (see Box 17.1).[15,16]

In the event of an increase in frequency or severity of signs suggestive of infectious disease, diagnostics should be performed to identify the cause. Specimens should ideally be obtained from 10% to 30% of the population, or at least 5 to 10 acutely affected dogs. The frequency and timing of shedding should be considered when obtaining specimens for pathogen detection; for instance, the peak shedding period for canine influenza virus precedes clinical signs, so specimens from exposed as well as affected dogs should be tested. If any dog dies or is euthanized with clinical signs of an unidentified illness, necropsy should be considered if an infectious disease is suspected, and is strongly recommended if more than one animal dies with similar signs. At a minimum, specimens should be obtained and held for later testing if further cases are identified.[17] Tissues should be placed in formalin, refrigerated, and frozen so that histopathology, bacterial culture, and nucleic acid amplification assays can be performed if needed. Bacterial culture of specimens held at 4°C for longer than 24 hours is not recommended due to loss of bacterial viability or overgrowth by contaminating bacteria or fungi (see Chapter 3 for more information).

RECORD KEEPING

Thorough medical record keeping is a key component to proper management of dog populations. Each dog should have a record that includes its origin, signalment, history and physical examination including description, and any identification number (e.g., microchip number). Preventative medications should be documented (e.g., anthelmintic used, dose, and route). Details of diagnostic tests performed and their results should be recorded. Reproductive history and findings, including breeding dates, should be recorded for both male and female breeding dogs to assist with prediction of whelping dates and fertility assessments. Reproductive status (intact versus spayed or castrated) should be included. In production units, number of puppies, viability, congenital abnormalities, birth weight, and daily weights should be recorded. Any abnormalities or adverse events following treatment should also be recorded. In small facilities, written records may be kept, but electronic record-keeping systems are commercially available for some types of facilities (e.g., shelters) and can be critical for proper tracking of disease over time.

In addition to the individual record, records to assess the population are also beneficial for health assessment, incidence or prevalence of disease, LOS or animal care days, and other established performance measures based on the facility mission. Tracking current disease rates and comparing them to previous rates can provide incentives for beneficial changes to preventative health protocols. The ability to retrieve valuable information is based on accurate recording of information, and careful assessment.

COMMUNITY HEALTH

Because of the potential for transmission of zoonotic infectious diseases from dog populations to humans, maintaining dog population health is an important component of supporting community health. Although development of a comprehensive infection control plan represents a significant investment of resources, the ultimate return is healthier animals, more successful organizations, and safer communities.

SUGGESTED READINGS

Hurley KF, Baldwin CJ. Developing infectious disease policies and protocols in an animal shelter. In: Petersen CA, Dvorak G, Spickler SR, eds. *Maddie's Infection Control Manual for Animal Shelters*. Ames, IA: Center for Food Security and Public Health, Iowa State University, College of Veterinary Medicine; 2008:66–78.

REFERENCES

1. Hurley KF, Baldwin CJ. Developing infectious disease policies and protocols in an animal shelter. In: Petersen CA, Dvorak G, Spickler SR, eds. *Maddie's Infection Control Manual for Animal Shelters*. Ames, IA: Center for Food Security and Public Health, Iowa State University, College of Veterinary Medicine; 2008:66–78.
2. Tzipory N, Crawford PC, Levy JK. Prevalence of *Dirofilaria immitis, Ehrlichia canis*, and *Borrelia burgdorferi* in pet dogs, racing greyhounds, and shelter dogs in Florida. *Vet Parasitol*. 2010;171:136–139.
3. National Animal Care and Control Association. https://www.nacanet.org/.
4. University of California Davis Koret Shelter Medicine Program. Facility Design, Shelter Animal Housing and Shelter Population Management; 2019. https://www.sheltermedicine.com/library/resources/?r=daily-monitoring-summary-sheet.
5. Association of Shelter Veterinarians. Guidelines for Standards of Care in Animal Shelters; 2010. https://www.sheltervet.org/assets/docs/shelter-standards-oct2011-wforward.pdf.
6. Animal and Plant Health Inspection Service. *Department of Agriculture. Animal Welfare Act and Animal Welfare Regulations. Specifications for the Humane Handling, Care, Treatment and Transportation of Dogs and Cats*; 2019. https://www.aphis.usda.gov/animal_welfare/downloads/bluebook-ac-awa.pdf.
7. National Research Council of the National Academies. *Guide for the Care and Use of Laboratory Animals*. 8th ed. Washington, D. C: The National Academies Press; 2011. https://grants.nih.gov/grants/olaw/Guide-for-the-Care-and-Use-of-Laboratory-Animals.pdf.
8. Mertens PA, Unshelm J. Effects of group and individual housing on the behavior of kennelled dogs in animal shelters. *Anthrozoös*. 1996;9:40–41.
9. Stockton KA, Morley PS, Hyatt DR, et al. Evaluation of the effects of footwear hygiene protocols on nonspecific bacterial contamination of floor surfaces in an equine hospital. *J Am Vet Med Assoc*. 2006;228:1068–1073.
10. O'Quin J. Outbreak management. In: Miller L, Hurley KF, eds. *Infectious Disease Management in Animal Shelters*. 2nd ed. Ames, IA: Wiley-Blackwell; 2021:113–142.
11. The Center for Food Security and Public Health, Iowa State University College of Veterinary Medicine. Disinfection; 2021. https://www.cfsph.iastate.edu/infection-control/disinfection/.
12. Lechner ES, Crawford PC, Levy JK, et al. Prevalence of protective antibody titers for canine distemper virus and canine parvovirus in dogs entering a Florida animal shelter. *J Am Vet Med Assoc*. 2010;236:1317–1321.
13. Companion Animal Parasite Council. CAPC Guidelines; 2021. https://capcvet.org/guidelines/.
14. Hurley KF. Implementing a population health plan in an animal shelter: goal setting, data collection and monitoring, and policy development. In: Miller L, Zawistowski S, eds. *Shelter Medicine for Veterinarians and Staff*. Ames, IA: Blackwell; 2004:211–235.
15. University of Wisconsin-Madison Shelter Medicine. Instructions for Daily Monitoring of Animal Health and Behavior; 2015. https://www.uwsheltermedicine.com/library/resources/instructions-for-daily-monitoring-of-animal-health-and-behavior.
16. UC Davis Koret Shelter Medicine Program. Daily Monitoring Summary Sheet; 2021. https://www.sheltermedicine.com/library/resources/?r=daily-monitoring-summary-sheet.
17. Pesavento PA. Necropsy techniques. In: Miller L, Hurley KF, eds. *Infectious Disease Management in Animal Shelters*. Ames, IA: Wiley-Blackwell; 2009:107–122.

18

Considerations and Management of Infectious Diseases of Community (Unowned, Free-Roaming) Cats

Linda S. Jacobson

KEY POINTS

- During their lifetimes, community cats can move along the socialization spectrum and between owned and unowned status. They may interact with pet cats, humans, and wildlife. These factors impact infectious disease identification, risk assessment, and control.
- Community cats can carry zoonotic pathogens such as rabies, toxoplasmosis, bartonellosis, and zoonotic helminths.
- Pathogens of particular importance for the cats are retroviral infections, FPV, upper respiratory pathogens, and intestinal parasites.
- Disease prevalence is difficult to ascertain, as most surveys rely on convenience sampling of apparently healthy cats during TNR programs. The magnitude of disease risk to humans and pet cats is likely to be overstated based on pathogen surveys alone, particularly those using antibodies.
- Infectious disease management is focused on high priorities such as vaccination for rabies and other core pathogens. TNR programs offer opportunities for vaccination and parasite control.
- Individuals working with community cats should be vaccinated against rabies, avoid contact with cats that are not anesthetized, and use common-sense precautions such as wearing gloves and frequent hand washing.

INTRODUCTION

Unowned, free-roaming cats occupy a unique ethical, emotional, cultural and ecological niche from which they interface with pet cats, humans, and wildlife. Feral cats are essentially wild, yet are genetically identical to the companions that share our homes, and only a generation from domestication. This has significant implications for pathogen transmission and management.

Domestic cats are classified by ownership status; access to the outdoors; and degree of socialization to, and dependence on, humans.[1] *Feral cats* are unowned, unsocialized, and able to survive independently.[2,3] In urban areas, they often live in groups, or colonies, typically ranging from 2 to 12 members.[4,5] People frequently provide food and shelter for unowned urban cats.[6,7] *Managed colonies* are those whose populations are controlled through surgical sterilization programs, known as TNR.[8] The term *stray* typically refers to socialized cats that have been lost or abandoned. These cats may lose their socialization to humans over time.[2] *Pet cats* are owned and socialized to humans. A substantial proportion have access to the outdoors; this is the norm in many countries and varies according to personal and cultural preferences, rural or urban location, country and climate.[9–11]

Feline subpopulations are not static and cats can move among them during their lifetimes.[2,12] "Feral" cats can therefore be difficult to distinguish from "strays". Further, definitions vary and are used loosely and interchangeably. As a result, *community cat* is now used as an umbrella term for unowned, free-roaming cats, regardless of socialization status.[2,4] This terminology will be used in this chapter. The emphasis is on cats presumed to be feral/unsocialized—by designation or based on having been trapped and sterilized.

Cats are present on every continent except Antarctica, and are the most widespread terrestrial carnivores on earth.[13] Reliable estimates of community cat populations are important for effective management,[9] but are difficult to obtain. The range of published estimates can be so wide as to be almost meaningless—for example, 10 to 120 million for the United States and Canada[9]—and there are no estimates at all for most regions. The interchange among domestic cat subpopulations and the reclusive nature of free-living cats make community cats uniquely difficult to quantify.[9] Feline population dynamics have important implications for disease transmission. Variables include sex, home range, proximity to humans, movement among colonies, and population density.[1,12]

INFECTIOUS DISEASES IN COMMUNITY CATS: GENERAL CONSIDERATIONS

Areas of disagreement between community cat and wildlife advocates include public health concerns; transmission of pathogens to pet cats and other species; public nuisance; predation on wildlife, extinction of native species and disruption of ecosystems; and the welfare of the cats themselves.[8] These disagreements complicate attempts to understand and mitigate infectious disease risks.

The ease of sampling cats during TNR programs has generated a large number of recent pathogen surveys (Tables 18.1–18.6 and Figs. 18.1–18.3). It can be helpful to use a free-living population as a sentinel for emerging disease threats and zoonotic disease risks. However, the connections between pathogen prevalence and disease risk are frequently unclear. Serologic studies reflect previous exposure and may provide little information about clinical illness, reservoir status, or transmission risk. A salient example is *Toxoplasma gondii* infection, for

TABLE 18.1 Prevalence of Viral, Rickettsial, Chlamydial and Mycoplasma Pathogens in Community and Pet Cats: Selected Surveys 2009–2019

	Community Cats		Pet Cats			
Organism (Assay Target)	**No. Tested**	**Prevalence**	**No. Tested**	**Prevalence**	**Country**	**Reference**
FCV (Ab)	610	45.1%	974	32.9%	China	130
	205	86.6%	262	77.6%	France	20
	151	85.4%			Italy	69
	299	94.3%			Korea	7
FCoV (Ab)	105	13.3%	107	14.0%	Korea	131
FCoV (PCR)	105	4.8%	107	8.4%	Korea	131
	127	29.9%			United States	108
FHV-1 (Ab)	205	62.0%	264	24.0%	France	20
	151	37.1%			Italy	69
	299	97.9%			Korea	7
FIV (Ab)	130	10.0%			Belgium	132
	302	19.3%			Belgium	28
	96	5.2%			Canada	101
	174	33.9%			Egypt	133
	41	0.0%			Ethiopia	134
	219	22.0%	273	10.0%	France	20
	316	6.6%			Italy	25
	137	8.8%			Italy	16
	66	3.0%			Korea	67
	302	3.6%			Korea	7
	347	9.2%			Spain	112
	632	7.9%			Spain	24
	267	10.0%			United States	19
	1,128	1.1%			United States	26
	2,020	11.6%	44,812	3.2%	United States, Canada	62
	101	21.8%	75	8.0%	W. Indies	135
	115	16.5%	23	26.1%	W. Indies	136
FIV (Ab and PCR)	30	6.6%	200	6.0%	Brazil	66
FIV (PCR)	11	36.4%	24	0.0%	W. Indies	137
FeLV (Ag)	130	4.6%			Belgium	132
	302	0.7%			Belgium	28
	96	3.1%			Canada	101
	174	4.6%			Egypt	133
	41	0.0%			Ethiopia	134
	316	3.8%			Italy	25
	137	3.6%			Italy	16
	66	12.1%			Korea	67
	302	23.2%			Korea	7
	346	4.0%			Spain	112
	632	6.3%			Spain	24
	1,128	2.5%			United States	26
	2,020	5.6%	44,812	3.0%	United States, Canada	62
	101	0.0%	75	0.0%	W. Indies	135
FeLV (Ag and PCR)	30	0.0%	200	3.0%	Brazil	66
Mycoplasma haemofelis (PCR)	95	3.1%			Canada	99
	138	8.7%	456	2.2%	Spain	103
	260	10.8%			Spain	33
"*Candidatus* Mycoplasma haemominutum" (PCR)	95	8.4%			Canada	99
	138	8.7%	456	7.9%	Spain	103
	260	22.3%			Spain	33
Hemotropic *Mycoplasma* spp., (PCR)	117	47.9%			Korea	102
	70	54.3%			Korea	67
	302	32.5%			Korea	7
	138	15.9%	456	9.0%	Spain	103
	260	33.1%			Spain	33
FPV (Ab)	205	15.9%	264	36.6%	France	20
	151	45.7%			Italy	69
	298	79.2%			Korea	7

Ab, antibody; *Ag*, antigen; *FCV*, feline calicivirus; *FCoV*, feline coronavirus; *FeLV*, feline leukemia virus; *FHV-1*, feline herpesvirus-1; *FIV*, feline immunodeficiency virus; *FPV*, feline panleukopenia virus; *PCR*, polymerase chain reaction.

TABLE 18.2 Prevalence of Bacterial Pathogens in Community and Pet Cats: Selected Surveys 2009–2019

	Community Cats		Pet Cats			
Organism (Assay Target)	**No. Tested**	**Prevalence**	**No. Tested**	**Prevalence**	**Country**	**Reference**
Bartonella henselae (Ab)	112	35.7%			Korea	102
	302	34.8%			Korea	7
Bartonella spp. (Ab)	178	59.0%			Egypt	133
	46	10.9%			Ethiopia	134
	1,300	23.1%			Italy	138
	272	45.0%			United States	19
	101	52.5%	75	50.7%	W. Indies	135
Bartonella spp. (PCR)	116	2.6%			Australia	40
	65	45.6%	86	54.4%	Brazil	139
	95	2.1%			Canada	101
	179	30.7%	155	18.7%	Israel	14
	329	4.3%	320	1.6%	Portugal	98
Borrelia burgdorferi (PCR)	329	3.3%	320	0.9%	Portugal	98

Ab, antibody; *PCR*, polymerase chain reaction.

TABLE 18.3 Prevalence of Endoparasites in Community and Pet Cats: Selected Surveys 2009–2019

	Community Cats		Pet Cats			
Organism (Assay Target)	**No. Tested**	**Prevalence**	**No. Tested**	**Prevalence**	**Country**	**Reference**
Aelurostrongylus abstrusus (Obs)	125	16.8%	22	9.1%	Denmark	88
	125	8.0%			Greece	140
	48	10.4%			Spain	92
	287	0.3%			Spain	112
	168	6.5%	299	0.7%	Switzerland	86
Ancylostomatidae (Obs)	68	1.5%			Poland	82
Ancylostoma spp. (Obs)	48	18.8%			Spain	92
	846	11.2%			United States	83
Cestodes (Obs: feces)	127	14.2%			United States	108
Cestodes (Obs: necropsy)	50	80.0%			Iran	141
	48	75.0%			Gran Canaria I.	92
Dipylidium caninum (Obs: feces)	133	2.2%			Brazil	84
	68	4.4%			Poland	82
	287	1.4%			Spain	112
	459	4.6%			Spain	24
	168	2.4%	299	0.0%	Switzerland	86
Dipylidium caninum (Obs: necropsy)	50	58.0%			Iran	141
	51	29.4%			Iran	38
	48	64.6%			Gran Canaria I.	92
	162	53.1%			Spain	142
Dirofilaria immitis (Ab)	137	8.0%			W. Indies	143
Dirofilaria immitis (Ag)	287	8.4%	364	1.4%	China	90
	174	3.4%			Egypt	133
	137	5.1%			W. Indies	143
Dirofilaria immitis (Obs: microscopy)	103	1.0%			Iran	144
	64	0.0%	106	0.0%	Malaysia	91
Dirofilaria immitis (Obs: necropsy)	36	11.1%			Cayman Islands	89
	48	0.0%			Spain	92
Dirofilaria immitis (PCR)	235	6.0%			Korea	145
Hookworms (Obs)	133	87.9%			Brazil	84
	168	4.2%	299	0.0%	Switzerland	86
	127	70.1%			United States	108

Continued

TABLE 18.3 Prevalence of Endoparasites in Community and Pet Cats: Selected Surveys 2009–2019—cont'd

	Community Cats		Pet Cats			
Organism (Assay Target)	**No. Tested**	**Prevalence**	**No. Tested**	**Prevalence**	**Country**	**Reference**
Intestinal helminths (Obs: necropsy)	51	86.3%			Iran	38
	50	80.0%			Iran	141
	48	77.1%			Spain	92
Intestinal parasites (Obs: feces)	133	77.3%			Brazil	84
	100	76.0%			Canada	85
	590	51.3%	560	48.7%	Greece	45
	51	56.9%			Iran	38
	68	48.5%			Poland	82
	48	77.1%			Spain	92
	287	26.5%			Spain	112
	459	29.2%			Spain	24
	168	77.4%	299	11.7%	Switzerland	86
	846	63.9%			United States	83
Roundworms (Obs)	127	12.6%			United States	108
Taenia hydatigena (Obs: necropsy)	51	19.6%			Iran	38
Taenia taeniaeformis (Obs: necropsy)	50	60.0%			Iran	141
	51	86.3%			Iran	38
	48	31.3%			Spain	92
	162	3.1%			Spain	142
Taenia spp. (Obs: feces)	78	15.0%			Canada	101
	100	3.0%			Canada	85
	68	8.8%			Poland	82
	287	6.9%			Spain	112
	459	8.3%			Spain	24
	168	37.5%	299	1.7%	Switzerland	86
	846	7.7%			United States	83
Toxocara cati (Obs)	133	2.2%			Brazil	84
	78	34.0%			Canada	101
	100	70.0%			Canada	85
	51	86.3%			Iran	38
	68	27.9%			Poland	82
	48	20.8%			Spain	92
	287	7.7%			Spain	112
	459	11.7%			Spain	24
	168	54.8%	299	3.0%	Switzerland	86
	846	44.6%			United States	83
Trichuris vulpis (Ab)	65	38.5%			United States	146
	35	74.3%			W. Indies	146
Trichuris vulpis (Obs)	48	2.1%			Spain	92
	65	26.2%			United States	146
	35	68.6%			W. Indies	146

Ab, antibody; *Ag*, antigen; *Obs*, observation.

which antibodies in serum are common but oocysts in feces are rare (see Table 18.5). Surveys of zoonotic pathogens in community cats rarely refer to the prevalence of clinical disease in the human population, or the likelihood of human exposure, in the region. Claims about zoonotic disease risks posed by community cats therefore often remain theoretical and unsupported.

Evolving diagnostic methods and differing methods among studies further complicate interpretation. The increasing use of highly sensitive molecular assays has the potential to significantly increase the perception of disease threats without a true change in prevalence. For example, in one study PCR detected *Bartonella* in 94% of samples, but culture only 35.7%.[14] False-positive results or laboratory error may falsely elevate the apparent prevalence of a pathogen.[15,16] Necropsy studies demonstrate high prevalence of intestinal helminths, particularly cestodes, compared with fecal flotation (see Tables 18.3 and 18.6 and Figure 18.1).

The concept of disease ecology moves beyond detection of antibodies or pathogens in convenience samples, and takes into account co-infections, climate, habitat type, transmission biology, disease vectors, population dynamics, and density (Fig. 18.4).[17,18] Increasingly, anthropogenic climate change and habitat fragmentation are included in attempts to understand disease dynamics.[19] This type of approach

TABLE 18.4 Prevalence of Ectoparasites in Community and Pet Cats: Selected Surveys 2009–2019

	Community Cats		Pet Cats			
Organism (Assay)	**No. Tested**	**Prevalence**	**No. Tested**	**Prevalence**	**Country**	**Reference**
Cheyletiella spp. (Obs)	341	2.1%			Greece	147
	493	2.4%			United States	35
Ctenocephalides felis (Obs)	341	24.3%			Greece	147
	632	2.7%			Spain	24
Ectoparasites (Obs)	65	65.1%	147	23.9%	Spain	148
	637	13.6%			Spain	24
Felicola subrostratus (Obs)	341	0.6%			Greece	147
Fleas (Obs)	96	9.6%			Canada	101
	51	60.8%			Iran	38
	673	71.6%			United States	95
Notoedres cati (Obs)	341	2.4%			Greece	147
Otodectes cynotis (Obs)	130	2.3%			Belgium	132
	341	15.8%			Greece	147
	632	10.6%			Spain	24
	493	25.2%			United States	35
	673	19.4%			United States	95
Ticks (Obs)	673	18.7%			United States	95

Obs, observation.

TABLE 18.5 Prevalence of Protozoal Infections in Community and Pet Cats: Selected Surveys 2009–2019

	Community Cats		Pet Cats			
Organism (Assay Target)	**No. Tested**	**Prevalence**	**No. Tested**	**Prevalence**	**Country**	**Reference**
Babesia spp. (PCR)	329	4.6%	320	8.8%	Portugal	98
Coccidia (Obs)	127	12.6%			United States	108
Cryptosporidium spp. (Obs)	50	18.0%			Iran	149
Cryptosporidium spp. (PCR)	127	11.0%			United States	108
Giardia spp. (Obs)	68	2.9%			Poland	82
	287	2.4%			Spain	112
	459	5.0%			Spain	24
	168	0.6%	299	0.7%	Switzerland	86
	846	1.2%			United States	83
Giardia spp. (PCR)	127	7.9%			United States	108
Hepatozoon spp. (PCR)	329	9.7%	320	7.5%	Portugal	84
Isospora felis (Obs)	133	24.8%			Brazil	84
	78	14.0%			Canada	101
	287	6.3%			Spain	112
	846	9.7%			United States	83
Isospora rivolta (Obs)	133	16.5%			Brazil	84
Isospora spp. (Obs)	100	9.0%			Canada	85
	68	11.8%			Poland	82
	459	2.5%			Spain	24
	168	16.7%	299	3.0%	Switzerland	86
Leishmania spp. (PCR)	329	9.4%	320	10.3%	Portugal	98
Neospora caninum (Ab)	134	3.7%	138	2.2%	Brazil	150
Sarcocystis neurona (Ab)	134	6.0%	138	2.2%	Brazil	150
Sarcocystis spp. (Obs)	168	0.6%	299	0.0%	Switzerland	86

Continued

TABLE 18.5 Prevalence of Protozoal Infections in Community and Pet Cats: Selected Surveys 2009–2019—cont'd

	Community Cats		Pet Cats			
Organism (Assay Target)	**No. Tested**	**Prevalence**	**No. Tested**	**Prevalence**	**Country**	**Reference**
Toxoplasma gondii (Ab)	228	12.3%			Australia	17
	94	29.8%			Canada	101
	1,261	31.7%	5,284	18.1%	China	73
	180	95.6%			Egypt	133
	48	85.4%			Ethiopia	134
	203	30.5%			Italy	25
	79	32.9%			Italy	16
	107	64.5%			Iran	151
	1,363	9.0%	123	3.3%	Japan	152
	112	50.0%			Korea	102
	50	12.0%	100	0.0%	Korea	74
	298	7.7%			Korea	7
	194	24.2%			Portugal	153
	495	82.0%			Qatar	154
	59	84.7%			Spain	155
	346	53.5%			Spain	112
	356	24.2%			Spain	24
	101	27.7%	75	30.7%	W. Indies	135
	272	45.0%			United States	19
Toxoplasma gondii (Obs)	78	1.3%			Canada	101
	287	0.0%			Spain	112
	459	0.0%			Spain	24
	168	0.0%	299	1.3%	Switzerland	86
Toxoplasma gondii (PCR)	127	0.0%			Iran	72
	50	0.0%	100	0.0%	Korea	74
	300	4.7%			Korea	75
Tritrichomonas (PCR)	3	0.0%			W. Indies	136
	127	0.8%			United States	108
Trichomonads (Obs)	100	0.0%	5	20.0%	Canada	85
	115	0.0%	37	0.0%	W. Indies	136

Ab, antibody; *PCR*, polymerase chain reaction; *Obs*, observation.

TABLE 18.6 Summary of Prevalence of Intestinal Parasites and Ectoparasites in Community Cats

Pathogen	Fecal Flotation	Necropsy
Intestinal parasites	58.4	
Intestinal helminths		81.1
Roundworms (nematodes)		
Ancylostomatidae	10.5	
Hookworm species	54.1	
Aelurostrongylus abstrusus	8.4	
Toxocara cati	36.0	
Tapeworms (cestodes)		
Cestodes	14.2	77.5
Taenia spp	12.5	
Dipylidium caninum	3.0	51.3
Taenia taeniaeformis		45.2
Protozoa		
Isospora spp.	12.4	
Ectoparasites		
Ectoparasites	39.4	
Fleas	33.8	
Otodectes cynotis	14.7	

From Tables 18.3–18.5.
Data are shown as average percentage prevalence for available surveys.

is rare in the community cat literature, possibly because these populations are studied using techniques drawn from clinical veterinary medicine rather than wildlife biology.

Males and older cats often have higher pathogen prevalence in surveys, most likely because of their larger range and greater number of contacts with other animals, while kittens are at higher risk of clinical illness from GI and respiratory pathogens. Prevalence would be expected to vary locally based on expected transmission dynamics (e.g., direct versus vector-borne). However, prevalence patterns did not correlate with population density and caregiver activity in a Korean study.[7]

Altered risk of infection in community cats, compared with their fed and sheltered counterparts, is related to hunting and foraging behaviors; requirements for shelter; antagonistic interactions, particularly among males; and larger home ranges.[20] Malnutrition, parasites, and co-infections may predispose community cats to infection. Dozens of studies include data from both pets and community cats, allowing a cautious assessment of the risks posed by being outdoors and receiving little or no primary health care (see Tables 18.1–18.5).

The extent of morbidity and mortality from infectious diseases is also difficult to assess in free-living populations. Cats that become debilitated often seek hiding places, making it less likely that those dying of disease will be identified[21] or that ill cats will be present when population sampling is performed. Studies of community cat health are typically limited to observation from a distance or examination while anesthetized.[22–25] In the United States, community cats have been reported to be relatively healthy—0.5% were

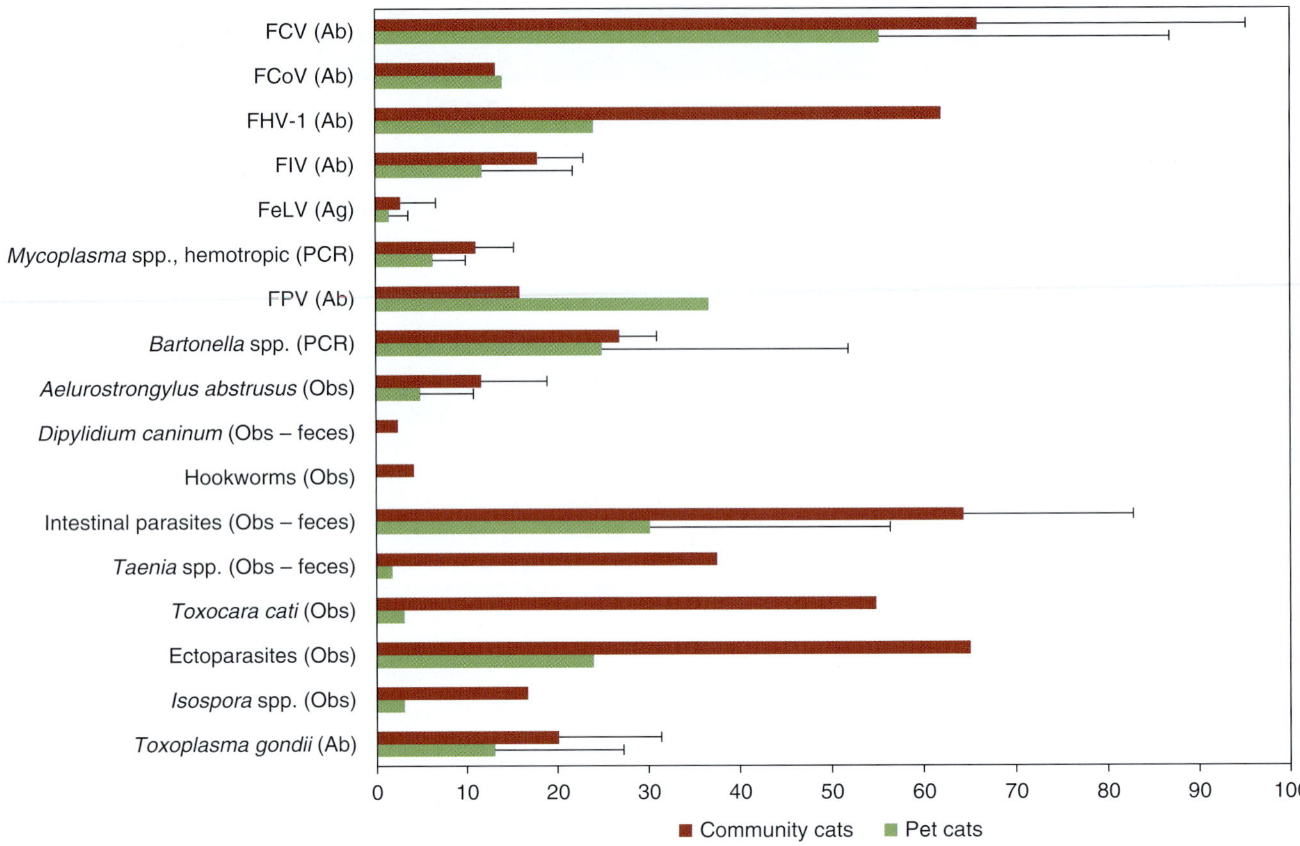

Fig. 18.1 Prevalence of selected pathogens in community cats and pet cats. Prevalence shown is the average percentage prevalence from surveys that included both community cats and pet cats. Standard deviation is shown if more than one study was included. *Ab,* antibody; *Ag,* antigen; *FCV,* feline calicivirus; *FCoV,* feline coronavirus; *FeLV,* feline leukemia virus; *FHV-1,* feline herpesvirus-1; *FIV,* feline immunodeficiency virus; *FPV,* feline panleukopenia virus; *Obs,* observed; *PCR,* polymerase chain reaction. (From Tables 18.1–18.5. References used: 14,20,45,62,66,73,74,86,88,98,103,130,131,135,136,139,148,152.)

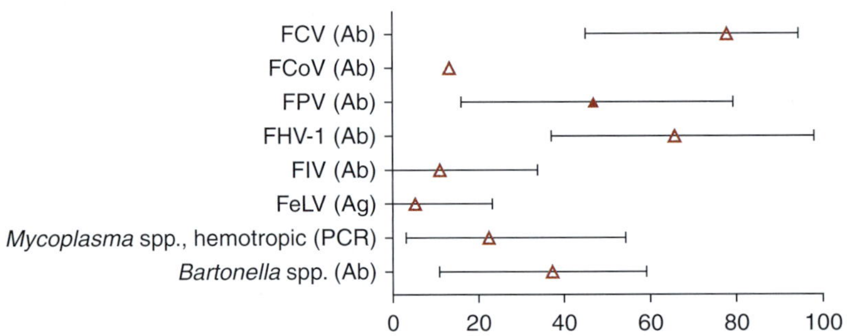

Fig. 18.2 Prevalence of selected viral, mycoplasmal, and bacterial pathogens in community cats. Percentage prevalence is shown as mean and range from surveys of community cats. *Ab,* antibody; *Ag,* antigen; *FCV,* feline calicivirus; *FCoV,* feline coronavirus; *FeLV,* feline leukemia virus; *FHV-1,* feline herpesvirus-1; *FIV,* feline immunodeficiency virus; *FPV,* feline panleukopenia virus; *PCR,* polymerase chain reaction. (From Tables 18.1–18.5. References used: 7,16,19,20,24-26,28,33,62,66,67,69,101–103,112,130–136,138.)

euthanized for serious health concerns and 0.2% to 0.3% died in care.[4,26,27] However, community kitten mortality is high, with 75% of kittens dying or disappearing before 6 months of age.[21] European studies showed variable proportions (<10% to 58.9%) of adult community cats in poor health, based on body condition score and other criteria.[24,25,28,29] Kittens were more likely to be emaciated than adults (72.7% vs. 45.8%).[22] Observations suggestive of infectious disease were emaciation, anemia, stomatitis, skin conditions, and URTD.[5,24,25,30–32]

Anemia was common in community cats in Italy[25,33] but uncommon elsewhere.[27] There was a significant association between being FIV-antibody positive and reduced red cell count (but not reduced hematocrit), with no significant associations found for FeLV-antigen positive status or seropositivity for *T. gondii*.[25] There was a significant association between testing positive for *Rickettsia* spp. by PCR and ocular disease, but no associations between being PCR positive for other vector-borne pathogens and other variables, including anemia and

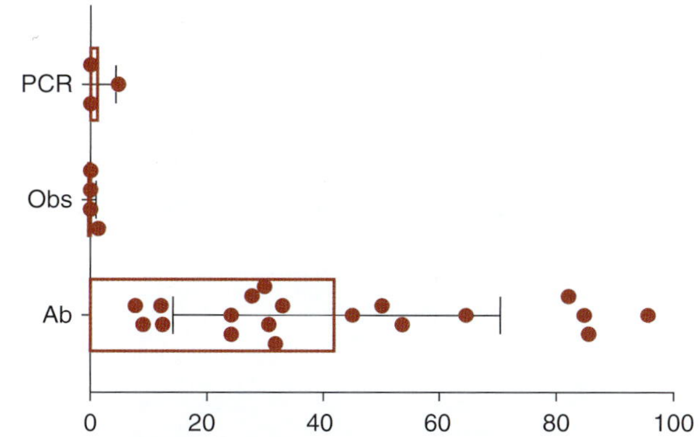

Fig. 18.3 Prevalence of *Toxoplasma* infection in surveys of community cats, showing the contrast among prevalence values for different diagnostic methods. Data are shown as percentage prevalence for individual surveys, with mean and standard deviation for multiple studies. *Ab,* antibody; *Obs,* observed; *PCR,* polymerase chain reaction. (From Tables 18.1–18.5). References used: 7,16,17,19,24,25,72–75,89,99,100,110,131–133,149–153

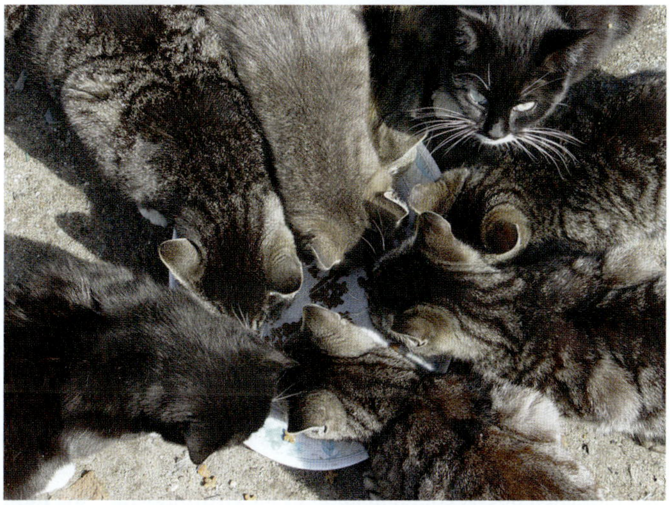

Fig. 18.4 Disease transmission in community cats is influenced by caregiver activity and population density. (Courtesy of Meredith Weiss, Neighborhood Cats, New York.)

thrombocytopenia.[34] The presence of *Cryptococcus*, ear mites, or fleas was not associated with overt clinical disease in most cats assessed.[32,35–37] Subclinical disease is to be expected in free-living populations where some susceptible individuals succumb to disease, directly or indirectly, and others live in equilibrium with infectious agents.[33]

Pathogen prevalence is highly variable among community cat populations (see Tables 18.1–18.5) and can differ markedly among geographic areas, rural and urban cat populations, or even different parts of the same city.[7,38–40] Some pathogens are restricted to certain parts of the world, where they can be very common. For example, high burdens of *Platynosoma* hepatic trematodes, which occur in tropical or subtropical regions, were found in community cats in Brazil[41] and zoonotic fish-borne trematodes are common in Kuwait and Korea.[39,42]

INFECTIOUS DISEASE RISKS TO HUMANS AND OTHER ANIMALS

Zoonotic diseases of concern in community cat populations include rabies, toxoplasmosis, bartonellosis, bite wound infections, toxocariasis, and ancylostomiasis.[43,44] Zoonotic disease risk from community cats should be examined "locally or at least with careful attention to environmental and ecologic conditions,"[27] as these affect cat density, pathogen presence and prevalence, contact with humans and the potential for pathogens to persist in the environment, as well as types and numbers of vectors and intermediate hosts.

There is no compelling evidence that the zoonotic disease risk presented by community cats is high or increasing. Risks may be different in developing countries, for which this type of information is less frequently reported and direct or indirect exposures may differ. However, it is striking that in the face of increasing numbers of TNR programs throughout the world, reports of TNR-related infectious disease outbreaks in humans are lacking. It remains the case, as pointed out more than a decade ago, that "there is concern about the possibility of cats transmitting diseases to humans, but in reviewing the literature there is little information on the actual frequency of zoonotic diseases in which cats can be implicated."[8]

Community cats may not pose a higher risk of zoonotic disease transmission than pet cats (particularly those with access to the outdoors).[1,3,27,45,46] In one study, infection prevalence did not differ between community and pet cats for FIV, FeLV, *Cryptosporidium* spp., *Giardia* spp., or *Toxocara cati*, while community cats had higher seroprevalence for *Bartonella henselae* and *T. gondii*.[27] The potential for direct transmission of pathogens by community cats is limited by their lack of intimate contact with humans and the short duration of contact when it occurs. Of greatest concern may be cats as sources of environmental contamination with pathogens such as *T. cati*, hookworm, and *T. gondii*.

Cat bites account for 5%–25% of reported animal bites.[47–49] The epidemiology differs from dog bites in almost every respect.[48] The majority of cat bites have been from community cats and most are self-reported as provoked.[48,49] In addition to the main concern of rabies transmission, there is a high risk of bacterial infection from cat bites because they tend to result in puncture wounds on the extremities and often transmit *Pasteurella multocida*, a fast-growing infection in humans (see Chapter 75).[47,50]

Cats may pose infectious disease risks to wildlife and vice versa. Some parasites, such as the cat flea (*Ctenocephalides felis*), occur on a large number of wildlife species.[51] Wild felids and domestic cats are susceptible to, or reservoirs for, a variety of shared pathogens.[19,52,53] Exposure of wild felids to domestic cat pathogens may be increasing through habitat fragmentation and compacted range.[52,53] Ingestion of cats may be a route of transmission of FeLV to large predatory felids.[52] In general, however, community cats are concentrated around human settlements and are unlikely to have much contact with nonurban wildlife.[54]

Pathogens can be transmitted among pet cats with access to the outdoors and community cats, among community cat colonies during TNR programs, among cats entering animal shelters, and among geographically separated populations in the case of shelter transport programs.

IMPORTANT INFECTIOUS DISEASES OF COMMUNITY CATS

Rabies

Community cats have been presented as a serious rabies threat in the United States based on the fact that more domestic cats now test positive than dogs.[55] The number of positive cats increased from 192 in 1988, when this shift was first reported,[56] to 270 in 2001,[57] but has remained within a similar range (with some fluctuations) since then.[58] More than 90% of rabies in the United States and Canada is found in wildlife, and > 99% of 50,000 annual rabies deaths in humans worldwide are estimated to be transmitted by dogs.[58–60] One presumptive and two confirmed human cases of feline-transmitted rabies have been reported in the United States since 1960.[61] Despite low numbers, the potential for rabies in free-roaming cats, low vaccination rates, and sporadic human exposure are continued cause for concern.

Feline Immunodeficiency Virus and Feline Leukemia Virus Infections

Retrovirus prevalence in community cats can be highly variable among studies and regions (see Table 18.1). A large study in the United States and Canada showed significantly higher prevalence among feral and stray cats than among owner-relinquished cats.[62] Adult age, male sex, and illness are associated with higher seroprevalence of FIV, but being an intact versus neutered male is less consistently significant.[28,62–64] In one study, the prevalence of FIV reached 100% in feral male cats older than 4 years.[20] Socially dominant males are most likely to be infected, since transmission is most often associated with fighting.[65] Females may be infected when males bite them on the neck during mating.[65]

Geography and population density affect retrovirus transmission patterns,[66] with a tendency toward higher prevalence in southern regions of Europe and North America, especially for FIV.[28] Urban strays have a promiscuous mating system associated with higher population density, compared with a polygynous system in rural areas.[7,65] This may result in fewer antagonistic interactions among urban cats and could explain why FIV is more prevalent in rural cats.[7,65] FeLV infection prevalence was higher in districts with high caregiver activity;[7] this may be due to higher population density. Most studies do not show a difference between males and females for FeLV antigenemia, and prevalence has not differed between urban and rural habitats.[67]

Feline Panleukopenia Virus and Respiratory Infections

Morbidity and mortality data for FPV, FHV, and FCV infections in community cats are lacking. Given the ubiquity and importance of these infections in domestic cats, they can be presumed to cause significant morbidity and mortality in free-roaming populations and could contribute to high kitten mortality (Fig. 18.5).

Variable proportions of community cats have evidence of exposure to and/or protective antibodies against FPV, FHV, and FCV (see Table 18.1).[7,20,68,69] This can be attributed to natural exposure, with some contribution from vaccination in managed colonies. FPV seroprevalence was higher in community cats than in unvaccinated owned cats, possibly reflecting concentration in areas where environmental virus load was higher.[20] Seroprevalence of this infection was higher in districts with low colony caregiver activity. This was suggested to be related to foraging behavior resulting from lower availability of food. There was an unexpected negative association between FCV seroprevalence and population density.[7]

Community cats with URTD were more likely to test PCR positive for FCV, *Chlamydia felis*, and *Mycoplasma felis* than cats without clinical signs.[70] *Chlamydia felis* was the most prevalent pathogen. A low prevalence of FHV infection was thought to be related to lower population density compared with other groups tested, as well as not having been subjected to the stress of shelter confinement.[70] Shedding of respiratory pathogens at intake to a shelter did not differ between stray and owner-surrendered cats, and in both groups it was ≤ 5% for all organisms other than *M. felis* (>20%).[71] The cumulative risk of developing URTD over time was higher for stray cats.

Toxoplasma gondii Infection

Cats and other felids are reservoirs of infection for *T. gondii* in humans, livestock, and wildlife.[10,27,72–74] Seroprevalence is highly variable in both unowned and owned cats. In studies where the status of the cats

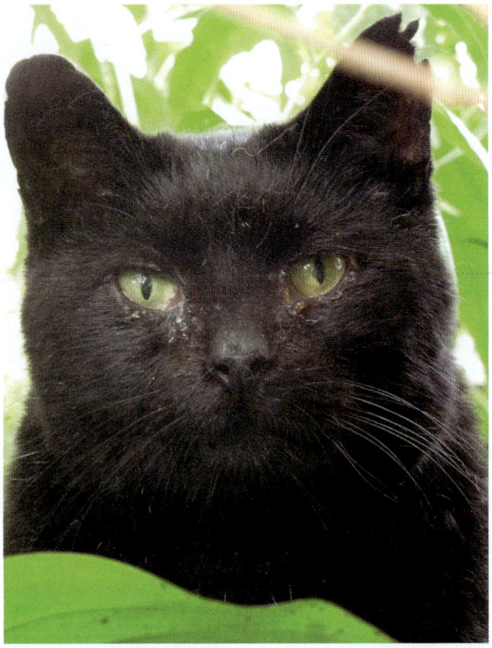

Fig. 18.5 Upper respiratory infections cause morbidity in community cats and are likely to contribute to kitten mortality. (Courtesy Sara Slater, Annex Cat Rescue, Toronto, Canada.)

was specified, the seroprevalence in feral cats was 9% to 84% (mean, 48.5%) compared with 18% to 85% (mean, 37.2%) for owned cats.[10]

The seroprevalence for *T. gondii* increases with age due to cumulative risk of exposure over time,[73] and may reflect increased lifespan rather than increased risk. Free-ranging kittens are typically exposed early in life, shed large numbers of oocysts for a short period, then become refractory to infection (see Chapter 93).[75] Oocyst shedding is brief, as reflected by low prevalence in studies using fecal flotation and fecal PCR (see Table 18.5 and Fig. 18.3), and seroprevalence may not correlate well with human infection or environmental contamination. Despite: (1) an increase in the population of cats; (2) increased contact with community cats through TNR and colony caregiving; and (3) high estimated oocyst contamination of the environment,[76] the number of cases of human toxoplasmosis decreased in the United States from 1999 to 2004.[77]

Toxoplasma gondii is more likely to be spread through environmental contamination in urban areas and through ingestion of infected paratenic hosts in rural regions.[7] The density of feral cats is not a reliable predictor of infection risk to native species, as transmission can occur at low cat densities.[17] Feeding commercial food to colonies might reduce infection rates by reducing predation on intermediate hosts.[7,78]

Endoparasite Infestations

Internal parasites, some of which have zoonotic potential, are common in community cats, which serve as an important reservoir through direct contact and environmental contamination.[45,79–82] As with other infections, a clear link between cat population, parasite prevalence, and clinical human infections rarely appears in the literature. Kittens are more likely to be infected, and more likely to carry high parasite burdens, than adults.[83] Co-infections are more common in community cats than in shelter or owned cats and are found in a substantial proportion, and sometimes the majority, of cats[83–86] (see Table 18.3).

Toxocara cati is the most important helminth in community cats (see Table 18.3).[81,83] Human toxocariasis is one of the most common zoonoses worldwide, but the role of cats is unclear. Interestingly, after pet dogs were banned from Iceland in 1924 (the ban was lifted in 1984), adult humans exposed to cats remained seronegative for *Toxocara*.[87]

Hookworms, which may have zoonotic potential, are found less consistently and the risk varies geographically (see Table 18.3).[81] Whipworms are infrequently reported, although the prevalence of infection is high in some populations. The risk of lungworm (*Aelurostrongylus abstrusus*) infection is higher in community cats due to ingestion of intermediate hosts.[45,88] With some exceptions, *Dirofilaria immitis* is rare or absent in community cat studies,[89–91] but should be considered in highly endemic areas (see Table 18.3).

Cestode infestations are underdiagnosed in fecal surveys due to intermittent shedding of proglottids,[83] and may be a greater source of morbidity in community cats than is appreciated. Prevalence can be very high in necropsy studies (see Table 18.3).[81,92] *Dipylidium caninum* and *Taenia taeniformis* are frequently found, with other cestodes being regionally common.[81] Cats are not currently implicated in transmission of zoonotic cestodes,[93] but surveillance is warranted. Community cats did not carry mature forms of *Echinococcus multilocularis* in a highly endemic area, but eggs have been reported in cat feces elsewhere.[93] *Taenia hydatigena* was common in cats in one study.[38]

Ectoparasite Infestations

Ctenocephalides felis is the most important ectoparasite of community cats, with reported prevalence ranging from 0% to 100% (mean, 32.3%).[51] Most infested cats have no clinical skin disease.[36] Flea infestations can be associated with zoonoses such as flea-borne rickettsiosis[94] and bartonellosis. *Otodectes cynotis* is the only mite of importance in community cats (see Table 18.4),[35,95] and infected cats are frequently clinically normal.[35–37] Tick infestations in cats may be underestimated due to grooming behavior and underdiagnosis of infection by immature stages.[95] However, tick-borne pathogens are rarely identified in community cats and were not associated with anemia or thrombocytopenia.[34,96–98]

Other Infections

The SARS-CoV-2 pandemic prompted initial fears that community cats could become a reservoir for infection for humans and other species. This now appears unlikely, but reasonable precautions should be observed at the community cat–human interface, particularly during TNR clinics.[99,100]

Bartonella, a potentially zoonotic pathogen that is primarily transmitted by fleas, is widespread in the community cat population. Seroprevalence is often higher than PCR-based prevalence (see Table 18.2). Prevalence was significantly higher in urban community cats, disproving a hypothesis that vector-borne disease would be more common in rural areas.[7] Hemotropic mycoplasma infections (see Table 18.1) are more common in male community cats,[101–103] supporting the role of fighting as an important means of transmission (see Chapter 58). Infections are often subclinical and may not be associated with anemia.[33,67] In studies from Europe, warm weather has been associated with increased prevalence.[33,103]

Despite predation on birds and the ability to contract Influenza under some circumstances, community cats have not played an important role in the transmission of avian influenza viruses (see Table 18.1).[104,105] However, a large feline outbreak of H7N2 virus infection in a New York shelter, which was associated with a single instance of cat-to-human transmission highlights the need for continued vigilance.[106]

Infections with *Leptospira*, *Toxascaris*, *Cryptosporidium*, *Giardia*, *Leishmania*, *Tritrichomonas*, and *Cryptococcus* spp., and dermatophytes appear to be uncommon in community cats, but for some of these pathogens, studies in different geographic regions are lacking.[24,32,81,107–114]

MANAGEMENT OF INFECTIOUS DISEASES IN COMMUNITY CATS

Rational infectious disease management in community cats requires strategic local decision-making based on clinical disease concerns (for both cats and humans), rather than on pathogen prevalence data alone. Public health records can assist in assessing local zoonotic disease risk.

Population Control

Regardless of attitudes toward community cats, interest groups share the goal of reducing free-roaming populations in order to decrease shelter intake and euthanasia, pathogen transmission, zoonotic disease risk, and predation on birds and wildlife. Community cats contribute disproportionately to feline population growth.[21,23] Reported sterilization rates now range from 0% to 68%, depending on colony management and the socioeconomic status of colony caregivers.[6,7,9,22,26,30,67,115] Sterilization rates for pet cats range from 12% in disadvantaged communities to 80%–98% in communities with access to more resources.[26,30,115–117] Sterilized cats are typically healthier, with improved welfare and increased longevity.[29,118,119] Sterilized cats are also less likely to transmit pathogens that are largely spread through mating and mating-related fighting (e.g., FIV).

The most devastating "disease" of domestic cats is shelter euthanasia. Euthanasia rates are highest for unsocialized cats. Nonlethal population control through TNR has been effective in decreasing shelter intake and reducing euthanasia.[1,4,26,119–121] As numbers decline, shelters can focus on other proactive programs that improve feline welfare. Community kittens can be rescued in greater numbers and socialized community cats can be adopted or transferred.[4,26,115] Colony caregivers play an increasingly important role in controlling disease and improving health and welfare for community cats.[5,22,29,30]

Despite its positive impact, TNR is resource intensive and not universally successful.[119,122] It is most effective in concert with other strategies—animal control policies not to pick up healthy community cats; community engagement and education, particularly around abandonment; targeted (rather than random) TNR; return-to-field; low-cost and pediatric spay/neuter programs for owned cats; universal sterilization before adoption; and supporting the changing culture around the way cats are viewed and valued.

TNR offers the opportunity to assess the health of community cats and provide vaccination, parasite control and additional health care, as practically feasible. It also allows sample collection for disease surveillance. This is likely to become increasingly important as transport programs grow to include more cats, and concerns over importation of infectious diseases grow. In order to mitigate risk, receiving organizations must be cognizant of infectious disease patterns at source locations.

Vaccination

The WHO recommends vaccination rather than population control for reducing transmission of canine rabies,[60] and the 2013 AAFP Advisory Panel recommended that cats in TNR programs receive FVRCP and 3- to 4-year rabies vaccines at the time of surgery.[123] Most community cat programs administer rabies vaccines at TNR.[124] This is an important contribution to public health efforts and helps create a transmission barrier between domestic cats and wildlife. More than 90% of rabid cats in the United States are found in southeastern states, where the raccoon rabies virus variant is endemic.[58] Rabies vaccination at TNR is imperative in such areas.

While rabies boosters should ideally be administered, a single vaccine is likely to provide long-term, or even lifelong, immunity.[60,125–127] A single vaccine at the time of TNR surgery resulted in protective titers against rabies in 98% of cats and protective titers against FPV, FHV, and FCV in the majority.[68]

Among cats with bite wounds and abscesses, 2% of those vaccinated against FeLV tested positive for the disease compared with 14% of unvaccinated cats.[128] The benefit of a single FeLV vaccination in feral cats undergoing TNR is unknown, but this could be considered in high-prevalence populations. Targeting kittens for FeLV vaccination would be most cost-effective, given the higher susceptibility of this age group to infection.

Parasite Control

Parasite control is high in the needs hierarchy, from both welfare and public health perspectives. Younger cats excrete more fecal eggs than adults[82] and are more severely affected clinically. This should be a target group for parasite control. Reducing parasite burdens, even transiently, is likely to be beneficial. Because unsocialized cats should only be handled after they are anesthetized, treatment is limited to topical and injectable products. The value of a single treatment for adults at TNR is questionable. Providing deworming treatment at colony feeding stations could lead to parasite resistance because of sporadic and potentially subtherapeutic treatment in a high-burden environment. Compared with untreated community cats, communally housed shelter cats with outdoor access and sporadic deworming had 49.5% prevalence of intestinal parasites compared with 77.3% in untreated community cats.[84] This suggests a limited benefit of sporadic deworming.

It must be accepted that some zoonotic parasites such as roundworms and hookworms cannot be controlled, similar to the case for wildlife species. Therefore, risk mitigation procedures to reduce human exposure should be in place in regions in which humans are at higher risk and for those working closely with community cats.

Control of Retrovirus Infections

Sterilization is expected to reduce retrovirus transmission through prevention of reproduction and decreased inter-cat aggression.[128] However, despite the growth in TNR, there was no overall decline in feline retrovirus prevalence in the United States in the decade to 2010.[62,63] This may be related to variable and often low sterilization rates. Subsequent large-scale surveys, reflecting TNR programs over the past decade, will be of great interest. Retrovirus infection prevalence decreased over time when strategies included sterilization, removal of positive cats, and vaccination against FeLV.[28,119] The effect of sterilization on prevalence was not examined separately.

The ethics of euthanasia of healthy cats that test positive for retroviruses are questionable.[28] False-positive test results are common when disease prevalence is low, and confirmatory tests are impractical in TNR settings. Testing healthy free-roaming cats for these diseases is not currently recommended, as removing them from the population is unlikely to significantly impact population prevalence, and resources are better directed to sterilization and vaccination.[2,154] Removal of positive cats from colonies might also affect colony social dynamics in ways that could influence pathogen transmission.

Education and Safety Precautions

Safe handling of community cats is essential to prevent injury, infection, and euthanasia for suspected rabies in the event of bite incidents. In their natural environment, unsocialized cats are wary of humans and will seek to hide or escape if approached. However, unsocialized cats are likely to bite defensively in fear when handled, such as when animal control personnel attempt to capture a cat by hand or place a cat in a carrier for transportation. Anyone who works with community cats should receive rabies vaccines. Gloves, and preferably gauntlets, should be worn when handling these cats. Many communities and shelters are now familiar with humane trapping methods, and information about safe and humane trapping and handling is readily available.[129]

Education initiatives must include those that relate to appropriate hand hygiene when community cats are handled or when exposed to their environment; avoidance of unessential handling of free-roaming cats; encouragement of pet owners to keep their pets indoors and provide adequate preventive care; and sterilization of pet cats.

SUGGESTED READINGS

Chalkowski K, Wilson AE, Lepczyk CA, et al. Who let the cats out? A global meta-analysis on risk of parasitic infection in indoor versus outdoor domestic cats (*Felis catus*). *Biol Lett.* 2019;15:20180840.

Fischer SM, Quest CM, Dubovi EJ, et al. Response of feral cats to vaccination at the time of neutering. *J Am Vet Med Assoc.* 2007;230:52–58.

Hellard E, Fouchet D, Santin-Janin H, et al. When cats' ways of life interact with their viruses: a study in 15 natural populations of owned and unowned cats (*Felis silvestris catus*). *Prev Vet Med.* 2011;101:250–264.

Levy JK, Wilford CL. Management of stray and feral community cats. In: Miller L, Zawistowski S, eds. *Shelter Medicine for Veterinarians and Staff.* Ames, IA: Wiley-Blackwell; 2013:669–688.

REFERENCES

1. Levy JK, Crawford PC. Humane strategies for controlling feral cat populations. *J Am Vet Med Assoc.* 2004;225:1354–1360.
2. Levy JK, Wilford CL. Management of stray and feral community cats. In: Miller L, Zawistowski S, eds. *Shelter Medicine for Veterinarians and Staff.* Ames, IA: Wiley-Blackwell; 2013:669–688.
3. Slater MR, Shain S. Feral cats: an overview. In: Salem DJ, Rowan AN, eds. *The State of the Animals.* 3rd ed. Washington, D.C.: Humane Society Press; 45–53.
4. Spehar DD, Wolf PJ. Integrated return-to-field and targeted trap-neuter-vaccinate-return programs result in reductions of feline intake and euthanasia at six municipal animal shelters. *Front Vet Sci.* 2019;6:1–13.
5. Tan K, Rand J, Morton J. Trap-neuter-return activities in urban stray cat colonies in Australia. *Animals.* 2017;7:46.
6. Finkler H, Hatna E, Terkel J. The impact of anthropogenic factors on the behavior, reproduction, management and welfare of urban, free-roaming cat populations. *Anthrozoös.* 2015;24:31–49.
7. Hwang J, Gottdenker NL, Oh D-H, et al. Disentangling the link between supplemental feeding, population density, and the prevalence of pathogens in urban stray cats. *Peer J.* 2018;6:e4988.
8. Robertson SA. A review of feral cat control. *J Feline Med Surg.* 2008;10:366–375.
9. Flockhart DTT, Coe JB. Multistate matrix population model to assess the contributions and impacts on population abundance of domestic cats in urban areas including owned cats, unowned cats, and cats in shelters. *PloS One.* 2018;13:1–34.
10. Dabritz HA, Conrad PA. Cats and *Toxoplasma*: implications for public health. *Zoonoses Public Health.* 2010;57:34–52.
11. Blancher P. Estimated number of birds killed by house cats (*Felis catus*) in Canada. *Avian Conserv Ecol.* 2013;8.
12. Slater MR. Behavioral ecology of free-roaming community cats. In: Weiss E, Mohan-Gibbons H, Zawistowski S, eds. *Animal Behaviour for Veterinarians and Staff.* Ames, IA: Wiley Blackwell; 2015:102–128.
13. Kitts-Morgan SE. Sustainable ecosystems: domestic cats and their effect on wildlife populations. *J Anim Sci.* 2015;93:848–859.
14. Gutiérrez R, Morick D, Gross I, et al. *Bartonellae* in domestic and stray cats from Israel: Comparison of bacterial cultures and high-resolution melt real-time PCR as diagnostic methods. *Vector Borne Zoonotic Dis.* 2013;13:857–864.
15. Lilly EL, Wortham CD. High prevalence of *Toxoplasma gondii* oocyst shedding in stray and pet cats (*Felis catus*) in Virginia, United States. *Parasites Vectors.* 2013;6:266.
16. Spada E, Proverbio D, Migliazzo A, et al. Serological and molecular evaluation of *Leishmania infantum* infection in stray cats in a nonendemic area in northern Italy. *ISRN Parasitol.* 2013:916376.
17. Hollings T, Jones M, Mooney N, et al. Wildlife disease ecology in changing landscapes: Mesopredator release and toxoplasmosis. *Int J Parasitol Parasites Wildl.* 2013;2:110–118.

18. Lewis JS, Logan KA, Alldredge MW, et al. The effects of demographic, social, and environmental characteristics on pathogen prevalence in wild felids across a gradient of urbanization. *PloS One.* 2017;12(11):e0187035.
19. Bevins SN, Carver S, Boydston EE, et al. Three pathogens in sympatric populations of pumas, bobcats, and domestic cats: implications for infectious disease transmission. *PloS One.* 2012;7(2):e31403.
20. Hellard E, Fouchet D, Santin-Janin H, et al. When cats' ways of life interact with their viruses: a study in 15 natural populations of owned and unowned cats (*Felis silvestris catus*). *Prev Vet Med.* 2011;101:250–264.
21. Nutter FB, Jay F, Stoskopf MK. Reproductive capacity of free roaming cats. *Am J Vet Med Assoc.* 2004;225:9–12.
22. Gunther I, Raz T, Klement E. Association of neutering with health and welfare of urban free-roaming cat population in Israel, during 2012-2014. *Prev Vet Med.* 2018;157:26–33.
23. Wallace JL, Levy JK. Population characteristics of feral cats admitted to seven trap-neuter-return programs in the United States. *J Feline Med Surg.* 2006;8:279–284.
24. Montoya A, García M, Gálvez R, et al. Implications of zoonotic and vector-borne parasites to free-roaming cats in central Spain. *Vet Parasitol.* 2018;251:125–130.
25. Spada E, Proverbio D, della Pepa A, et al. Seroprevalence of feline immunodeficiency virus, feline leukaemia virus and *Toxoplasma gondii* in stray cat colonies in northern Italy and correlation with clinical and laboratory data. *J Feline Med Surg.* 2012;14:369–377.
26. Levy JK, Isaza NM, Scott KC. Effect of high-impact targeted trap-neuter-return and adoption of community cats on cat intake to a shelter. *Vet J.* 2014;201:269–274.
27. Nutter FB, Dubey JP, Levine JF, et al. Seroprevalences of antibodies against *Bartonella henselae* and *Toxoplasma gondii* and fecal shedding of *Cryptosporidium* spp, *Giardia* spp, and *Toxocara cati* in feral and pet domestic cats. *J Am Vet Med Assoc.* 2004;225:1394–1398.
28. Garigliany M, Jolly S, Dive M, et al. Risk factors and effect of selective removal on retroviral infections prevalence in Belgian stray cats. *Vet Rec.* 2015;6. 45–45.
29. Gilhofer EM, Windschnurer I, Troxler J, et al. Welfare of feral cats and potential influencing factors. *J Vet Behav.* 2019;30:114–123.
30. Zito S, Walker J, Gates MC, et al. A preliminary description of companion cat, managed stray cat, and unmanaged stray cat welfare in Auckland, New Zealand using a 5-component assessment scale. *Front Vet Sci.* 2019;6:40.
31. Castro-Prieto J, Andrade-Núñez MJ. Health and ecological aspects of stray cats in old San Juan, Puerto Rico: Baseline information to develop an effective control program. *P R Health Sci J.* 2018;37:110–114.
32. Danesi P, Furnari C, Granato A, et al. Molecular identity and prevalence of *Cryptococcus* spp. nasal carriage in asymptomatic feral cats in Italy. *Med Mycol.* 2014;52:667–673.
33. Spada E, Proverbio D, Galluzzo P, et al. Prevalence of haemoplasma infections in stray cats in northern Italy. *ISRN Microbiol.* 2014;2014:1–8.
34. Spada E, Proverbio D, Galluzzo P, et al. Molecular study on selected vector-borne infections in urban stray colony cats in northern Italy. *J Feline Med Surg.* 2014;16:684–688.
35. Milley C, Dryden M, Rosenkrantz W, et al. Comparison of parasitic mite retrieval methods in a population of community cats. *J Feline Med Surg.* 2017;19:657–664.
36. Akucewich LH, Philman K, Clark A, et al. Prevalence of ectoparasites in a population of feral cats from north central Florida during the summer. *Vet Parasitol.* 2002;109:129–139.
37. Perego R, Proverbio D, De Giorgi GB, et al. Prevalence of otitis externa in stray cats in northern Italy. *J Feline Med Surg.* 2013;16:483–490.
38. Yakhchali M, Hajipour N, Malekzadeh-Viayeh R, et al. Gastrointestinal helminths and ectoparasites in the stray cats (Felidae: *Felis catus*) of Ahar municipality, northwestern Iran. *Iran J Parasitol.* 2017;12:298–304.
39. Shin S-S, Oh D-S, Ahn K-S, et al. Zoonotic intestinal trematodes in stray cats (*Felis catus*) from riverside areas of the Republic of Korea. *Korean J Parasitol.* 2015;53:209–213.
40. Dybing NA, Jacobson C, Irwin P, et al. *Bartonella* species identified in rodent and feline hosts from island and mainland Western Australia. *Vector Borne Zoonotic Dis.* 2016;16:238–244.
41. Ramos DG de S, Santos ARGLO, Da Costa Freitas L, et al. Feline platynosomiasis: analysis of the association of infection levels with pathological and biochemical findings. *Rev Bras Parasitol Veterinária.* 2017;26:54–59.
42. El-Azazy OME, Abdou N-EMI, Khalil AI, et al. Potential zoonotic trematodes recovered in stray cats from Kuwait municipality, Kuwait. *Korean J Parasitol.* 2015;53:279–287.
43. Nardoni S, Mugnaini L, Papini R, et al. AVMA policy: free-roaming abandoned and feral cats. *J Am Vet Med Assoc.* 2016;23:164–167.
44. Taetzsch SJ, Bertke AS, Gruszynski KR. Zoonotic disease transmission associated with feral cats in a metropolitan area: a geospatial analysis. *Zoonoses Public Health.* 2018;65:412–419.
45. Symeonidou I, Gelasakis AI, Arsenopoulos K, et al. Feline gastrointestinal parasitism in Greece: Emergent zoonotic species and associated risk factors. *Parasite Vectors.* 2018;11:227.
46. Luria BJ, Levy JK, Lappin MR, et al. Prevalence of infectious diseases in feral cats in Northern Florida. *J Fel Med Surg.* 2004;6:287–296.
47. Ellis R, Ellis C. Dog and cat bites (corrected version). *Am Fam Phys.* 2014;90:239–243.
48. Wright J. Reported cat bites in Dallas: characteristics of the cats, the victims, and the attack events. *Public Health Rep.* 1990;105:420–424.
49. Patrick GR, O'Rourke KM. Dog and cat bites: Epidemiologic analyses suggest different prevention strategies. *Public Health Rep.* 1998;113:252–257.
50. Abrahamian FM, Goldstein EJC. Microbiology of animal bite wound infections. *Clin Microbiol Rev.* 2011;24:231–246.
51. Clark NJ, Seddon JM, Šlapeta J, et al. Parasite spread at the domestic animal - wildlife interface: anthropogenic habitat use, phylogeny and body mass drive risk of cat and dog flea (*Ctenocephalides* spp.) infestation in wild mammals. *Parasit Vectors.* 2018;11:8.
52. Foley JE, Swift P, Fleer KA, et al. Risk factors for exposure to feline pathogens in California mountain lions (*Puma concolor*). *J Wildl Dis.* 2013;49:279–293.
53. Meli ML, Cattori V, Martínez F, et al. Feline leukemia virus and other pathogens as important threats to the survival of the critically endangered Iberian lynx (*Lynx pardinus*). *PloS One.* 2009;4:e4744.
54. Ferreira JP, Leitão I, Santos-Reis M, et al. Human-related factors regulate the spatial ecology of domestic cats in sensitive areas for conservation. *PloS One.* 2011;6:e25970.
55. Gerhold RW, Jessup DA. Zoonotic diseases associated with free-roaming cats. *Zoonoses Public Health.* 2013;60:189–195.
56. CDC. Rabies surveillance, United States; 1988. https://www.cdc.gov/mmwr/preview/mmwrhtml/00001458.htm.
57. Krebs JW, Noll HR, Rupprecht CE, et al. Rabies surveillance in the United States during 2001. *J Am Vet Med Assoc.* 2002;221:1690–1701.
58. Ma X, Monroe BP, Cleaton JM, et al. Rabies surveillance in the United States during 2017. *J Am Vet Med Assoc.* 2018;253:1555–1568.
59. Government of Canada. Rabies Cases in Canada 2018. http://www.inspection.gc.ca/animals/terrestrial-animals/diseases/reportable/rabies/2018-rabies-in-canada/eng/1550860268670/1550860329289.
60. World Health Organization. *WHO Expert Consultation on Rabies Third Report.* 2018.
61. CDC. Recovery of a patient from clinical rabies —, 2011; 2012 https://www.cdc.gov/mmwr/preview/mmwrhtml/mm6104a1.htm.
62. Burling AN, Levy JK, Scott HM, et al. Seroprevalences of feline leukemia virus and feline immunodeficiency virus infection in cats in the United States and Canada and risk factors for seropositivity. *J Am Vet Med Assoc.* 2017;251:187–194.
63. Levy JK, Scott HM, Lachtara JL, et al. Seroprevalence of feline leukemia virus and feline immunodeficiency virus infection among cats in North America and risk factors for seropositivity. *J Am Vet Med Assoc.* 2006;228:371–376.
64. Chhetri BK, Berke O, Pearl DL, et al. Comparison of risk factors for seropositivity to feline immunodeficiency virus and feline leukemia virus among cats: a case-case study. *BMC Vet Res.* 2015;11:1–7.
65. Courchamp F, Say L, Pontier D. Transmission of feline immunodeficiency virus in a population of cats (*Felis catus*). *Wildl Res.* 2000;27:603–611.
66. Lacerda LCC, Silva ANN, Freitas JSS, et al. Feline immunodeficiency virus and feline leukemia virus: frequency and associated factors in cats in northeastern Brazil. *Genet Mol Res.* 2017;16(2):gmr16029633.

67. Hwang J, Gottdenker N, Min M-S, et al. Evaluation of biochemical and haematological parameters and prevalence of selected pathogens in feral cats from urban and rural habitats in South Korea. *J Fel Med Surg*. 2016;18:443–451.
68. Fischer SM, Quest CM, Dubovi EJ, et al. Response of feral cats to vaccination at the time of neutering. *J Am Vet Med Assoc*. 2007;230:52–58.
69. Dall'Ara P, Labriola C, Sala E, et al. Prevalence of serum antibody titres against feline panleukopenia, herpesvirus and calicivirus infections in stray cats of Milan, Italy. *Prev Vet Med*. 2019;167:32–38.
70. McManus CM, Levy JK, Andersen LA, et al. Prevalence of upper respiratory pathogens in four management models for unowned cats in the Southeast United States. *Vet J*. 2014;201:196–201.
71. Gourkow N, Lawson JH, Hamon SC, et al. Descriptive epidemiology of upper respiratory disease and associated risk factors in cats in an animal shelter in coastal western Canada. *Can Vet J*. 2013;54:132–138.
72. Rahimi MT, Daryani A, Sarvi S, et al. Cats and *Toxoplasma gondii*: a systematic review and meta-analysis in Iran. *Onderstepoort J Vet Res*. 2015;82:1–10.
73. Ding H, Gao Y-M, Deng Y, et al. A systematic review and meta-analysis of the seroprevalence of *Toxoplasma gondii* in cats in mainland China. *Parasit Vectors*. 2017;10:27.
74. Kim SE, Choi R, Kang SW, et al. Prevalence of *Toxoplasma gondii* infection in household and feral cats in Korea. *J Parasit Dis*. 2017;41:823–825.
75. Jung BK, Lee SE, Lim H, et al. *Toxoplasma gondii* B1 gene detection in feces of stray cats around Seoul, Korea and genotype analysis of two laboratory-passaged isolates. *Korean J Parasitol*. 2015;53:259–263.
76. Torrey EF, Yolken RH. *Toxoplasma* oocysts as a public health problem. *Trends Parasitol*. 2013;29:380–384.
77. Jones JL, Kruszon-Moran D, Sanders-Lewis K, et al. *Toxoplasma gondii* infection in the United States, 1999–2004, decline from the prior decade. *Am J Trop Med Hyg*. 2018;77:405–410.
78. Edelhofer R, Prossinger H. Infection with *Toxoplasma gondii* during pregnancy: Seroepidemiological studies in Austria. *Zoonoses Public Health*. 2010;57:18–26.
79. Khademvatan S, Abdizadeh R, Rahim F, et al. Stray cats gastrointestinal parasites and its association with public health in Ahvaz City, south western of Iran. *Jundishapur J Microbiol*. 2014;7:e11079.
80. Chalkowski K, Wilson AE, Lepczyk CA, et al. Who let the cats out? A global meta-analysis on risk of parasitic infection in indoor versus outdoor domestic cats (*Felis catus*). *Biol Lett*. 2019;15:20180840.
81. Crawford HM, Calver MC, Fleming PA. A case of letting the cat out of the bag — why trap-neuter-return is not an ethical solution for stray cat (*Felis catus*) management. *Animals*. 2019;9:171.
82. Szwabe K, Blaszkowska J. Stray dogs and cats as potential sources of soil contamination with zoonotic parasites. *Ann Agric Environ Med*. 2017;24:39–43.
83. Nagamori Y, Payton ME, Duncan-Decocq R, et al. Fecal survey of parasites in free-roaming cats in northcentral Oklahoma, United States. *Vet Parasitol Reg Stud Reports*. 2018;14:50–53.
84. Pereira PF, Barbosa A da S, Moura APP de, et al. Gastrointestinal parasites in stray and shelter cats in the municipality of Rio de Janeiro, Brazil. *Rev Bras Parasitol Veterinária*. 2017;26:383–388.
85. Raab O, Greenwood S, Vanderstichel R, et al. A cross-sectional study of *Tritrichomonas foetus* infection in feral and shelter cats in Prince Edward Island, Canada. *Can Vet J*. 2016;57:265–270.
86. Zottler E-MM, Bieri M, Basso W, et al. Intestinal parasites and lungworms in stray, shelter and privately owned cats of Switzerland. *Parasitol Int*. 2019;69:75–81.
87. Woodruff AW, De Savigny DH, Hendy-Ibbs PM. Toxocaral and toxoplasmal antibodies in cat breeders and in Icelanders exposed to cats but not to dogs. *Br Med J*. 1982;284:309–310.
88. Olsen CS, Willesen JL, Pipper CB, et al. Occurrence of *Aelurostrongylus abstrusus* (Railliet, 1898) in Danish cats: a modified lung digestion method for isolating adult worms. *Vet Parasitol*. 2015;210:32–39.
89. Darby B, Dickinson C, Gaskins L, et al. Prevalence of heartworm infection in the feral cat population of Grand Cayman. *J Feline Med Surg Open Reports*. 2019;5:2055116919838083.
90. Hou H, Cao L, Ren W, et al. Seroprevalence of *Dirofilaria immitis* in cats from Liaoning province, northeastern China. *Korean J Parasitol*. 2017;55:673–677.
91. Al-Abd NM, Nor ZM, Kassim M, et al. Prevalence of filarial parasites in domestic and stray cats in Selangor State, Malaysia. *Asian Pac J Trop Med*. 2015;8:705–709.
92. Rodríguez-Ponce E, González JF, de Felipe MC, et al. Epidemiological survey of zoonotic helminths in feral cats in Gran Canaria island (Macaronesian archipelago-Spain). *Acta Parasitol*. 2016;61:443–450.
93. Umhang G, Forin-Wiart M-A, Hormaz V, et al. *Echinococcus multilocularis* detection in the intestines and feces of free-ranging domestic cats (*Felis s. catus*) and European wildcats (*Felis s. silvestris*) from northeastern France. *Vet Parasitol*. 2015;214:75–79.
94. Nelson K, Maina AN, Brisco A, et al. A 2015 outbreak of flea-borne rickettsiosis in san Gabriel valley, Los Angeles county, California. *PLoS Negl Trop Dis*. 2018;12:e0006385.
95. Thomas JE, Staubus L, Goolsby JL, et al. Ectoparasites of free-roaming domestic cats in the central United States. *Vet Parasitol*. 2016;228:17–22.
96. Kelly PJ, Köster L, Li J, et al. Survey of vector-borne agents in feral cats and first report of *Babesia gibsoni* in cats on St Kitts, West Indies. *BMC Vet Res*. 2017;13:331.
97. André MR, Herrera HM, de Jesus Fernandes S, et al. Tick-borne agents in domesticated and stray cats from the city of Campo Grande, state of Mato Grosso do Sul, midwestern Brazil. *Ticks Tic-borne Dis*. 2015;6:779–786.
98. Maia C, Ramos C, Coimbra M, et al. Bacterial and protozoal agents of feline vector-borne diseases in domestic and stray cats from southern Portugal. *Parasit Vectors*. 2014;7:115.
99. Sharun K, Dhama K, Pawde AM, et al. SARS-CoV-2 in animals: potential for unknown reservoir hosts and public health implications. *Vet Q*. 2021;41:181–201.
100. Weese JS. COVID-19 in animals review. Part 1: cats. *Worms & Germs Blog*. 2020. https://www.wormsandgermsblog.com/2020/10/articles/animals/cats/covid-in-animals-review-part-1-cats/
101. Stojanovic V, Foley P. Infectious disease prevalence in a feral cat population on Prince Edward Island, Canada. *Can Vet J*. 2011;52:979–982.
102. Hwang J, Gottdenker N, Oh D-H, et al. Infections by pathogens with different transmission modes in feral cats from urban and rural areas of Korea. *J Vet Sci*. 2017;18:541–545.
103. Díaz-Regañón D, Villaescusa A, Ayllón T, et al. Epidemiological study of hemotropic mycoplasmas (hemoplasmas) in cats from central Spain. *Parasit Vectors*. 2018;11:140.
104. Gordy JT, Jones CA, Rue J, et al. Surveillance of feral cats for influenza A virus in North Central Florida. *Influenza Other Respir Viruses*. 2012;6:341–347.
105. Zhao F-R, Zhou D-H, Zhang Y-G, et al. Detection prevalence of H5N1 avian influenza virus among stray cats in eastern China. *J Med Virol*. 2015;87:1436–1440.
106. Marinova-Petkova A, Jang Y, Lynch B, et al. Avian influenza A (H7N2) virus in human exposed to sick cats, New York, USA, 2016. *Emerg Infect Dis*. 2017;23:2046–2049.
107. Can H, Döşkaya M, Özdemir HG, et al. Seroprevalence of *Leishmania* infection and molecular detection of *Leishmania tropica* and *Leishmania infantum* in stray cats of İzmir, Turkey. *Exp Parasitol*. 2016;167:109–114.
108. Andersen LA, Levy JK, McManus CM, et al. Prevalence of enteropathogens in cats with and without diarrhea in four different management models for unowned cats in the southeast United States. *Vet J*. 2018;236:49–55.
109. Dybing NA, Jacobson C, Irwin P, et al. *Leptospira* species in feral cats and black rats from Western Australia and Christmas Island. *Vector Borne Zoonotic Dis*. 2017;17:319–324.
110. Zaidi S, Bouam A, Bessas A, et al. Urinary shedding of pathogenic *Leptospira* in stray dogs and cats, Algiers: a prospective study. PloS One. 13(5):e0197068.
111. Gomard Y, Lagadec E, Humeau L, et al. Feral cats do not play a major role in leptospirosis epidemiology on Reunion Island. *Epidemiol Infect*. 2019;147:e97.
112. Miró G, Rupérez C, Checa R, et al. Current status of *L. infantum* infection in stray cats in the Madrid region (Spain): implications for the recent outbreak of human leishmaniosis? *Parasit Vectors*. 2014;7:112.

113. Akhtardanesh B, Sharifi I, Mohammadi A, et al. Feline visceral leishmaniasis in Kerman, southeast of Iran: serological and molecular study. *J Vector Borne Dis.* 2017;54:96–102.
114. Proverbio D, Perego R, Spada E, et al. Survey of dermatophytes in stray cats with and without skin lesions in northern Italy. *Vet Med Int.* 2014;2014:565470.
115. Johnson KL, Cicirelli J. Study of the effect on shelter cat intakes and euthanasia from a shelter neuter return project of 10,080 cats from March 2010 to June 2014. *Peer J.* 2014;2:e646.
116. Humane Canada. *Cats in Canada 2017: A Five-Year Review of Cat Overpopulation*; 2017. https://humanecanada.ca/our-work/focus-areas/companion-animals/cats-in-canada-2017-a-five-year-review-of-cat-overpopulation/.
117. The Humane Society of the United States. Pets by the Numbers. https://www.humanesociety.org/resources/pets-numbers.
118. Scott KC, Levy JK, Gorman SP, et al. Body condition of feral cats and the effect of neutering. *J Appl Anim Welf Sci.* 2002;5:203–213.
119. Kreisler RE, Cornell HN, Levy JK. Decrease in population and increase in welfare of community cats in a twenty-three year trap-neuter-return program in Key Largo, FL: the ORCAT Program. *Front Vet Sci.* 2019;6:1–14.
120. Toronto Feral Cat Coalition & Animal Alliance. *Feral Cat Management in Canada: Lessons Learned in Toronto*; 2018. https://www.animalalliance.ca/wp-content/uploads/2019/01/7129_Feral-Report_2018_V2-SM-rev-FINAL.pdf.
121. Levy JK, Gale DW, Gale LA. Evaluation of the effect of a long-term trap-neuter-return and adoption program on a free-roaming cat population. *J Am Vet Med Assoc.* 2006;222:42–46.
122. Stoskopf MK, Nutter FB. Analyzing approaches to feral cat management - one size does not fit all. *J Am Vet Med Assoc.* 2005;225:1361–1964.
123. Scherk MA, Ford RB, Gaskell RM, et al. 2013 AAFP feline vaccination advisory panel report. *J Feline Med Surg.* 2014;16:66.
124. Alley Cat Rescue. Alley Cat Rescue's National Feral Cat Survey; 2012. https://www.prnewswire.com/news-releases/alley-cat-rescues-national-feral-cat-survey-157263395.html.
125. Moore MC, Davis RD, Kang Q, et al. Comparison of anamnestic responses to rabies vaccination in dogs and cats with current and out-of-date vaccination status. *J Am Vet Med Assoc.* 2015;246:205–211.
126. Soulebot JP, Brun A, Chappuis G, et al. Experimental rabies in cats: Immune response and persistence of immunity. *Cornell Vet.* 1981;71:311–325.
127. Frymus T. Feline Rabies: European Advisory Board on Cat Diseases. 2020 http://www.abcdcatsvets.org/rabies/.
128. Goldkamp CE, Levy JK, Edinboro CH, et al. Seroprevalences of feline leukemia virus and feline immunodeficiency virus in cats with abscesses or bite wounds and rate of veterinarian compliance with current guidelines for retrovirus testing. *J Am Vet Med Assoc.* 2008;232:1152–1158.
129. Kortis B, Weiss M, Frazier A, et al. Neighborhood Cats TNR Handbook. https://www.neighborhoodcats.org/resources/books-videos-more.
130. Wang K, Pei Z, Hu G. First report of feline calicivirus (FCV) infection in stray cats in northeast China. *Pol J Vet Sci.* 2017;20:595–598.
131. Dong-Jun A, Jeoung H-Y, Jeong W, et al. Prevalence of Korean cats with natural feline coronavirus infections. *Virol J.* 2011;8:455.
132. Bollez A, De Rooster H, Furcas A, et al. Prevalence of external ear disorders in Belgian stray cats. *J Feline Med Surg.* 2018;20:149–154.
133. Al-Kappany YM, Lappin MR, Kwok OCH, et al. Seroprevalence of *Toxoplasma gondii* and concurrent *Bartonella* spp., feline immunodeficiency virus, feline leukemia virus, and *Dirofilaria immitis* infections in Egyptian cats. *J Parasitol.* 2011;97:256–258.
134. Tiao N, Darrington C, Molla B, et al. An investigation into the seroprevalence of *Toxoplasma gondii, Bartonella* spp., feline immunodeficiency virus (FIV), and feline leukaemia virus (FeLV) in cats in Addis Ababa, Ethiopia. *Epidemiol Infect.* 2013;141:1029–1033.
135. Dubey JP, Lappin MR, Kwok OCH, et al. Seroprevalence of *Toxoplasma gondii* and concurrent *Bartonella* spp., feline immunodeficiency virus, and feline leukemia virus infections in cats from Grenada, West Indies. *J Parasitol.* 2009;95:1129–1133.
136. Yao C, Köster L, Halper B, et al. Failure to detect *Tritrichomonas foetus* in a cross-sectional survey in the populations of feral cats and owned outpatient cats on St Kitts, West Indies. *J Feline Med Surg Open Reports.* 2018;4:2055116918782584.
137. Kelly PJ, Stocking R, Gao D, et al. Identification of feline immunodeficiency virus subtype-B on St. Kitts, West Indies by quantitative PCR. *J Infect Dev Ctries.* 2011;5:480–483.
138. Brunetti E, Fabbi M, Ferraioli G, et al. Cat-scratch disease in northern Italy: Atypical clinical manifestations in humans and prevalence of *Bartonella* infection in cats. *Eur J Clin Microbiol Infect Dis.* 2013;32:531–534.
139. André MR, Dumler JS, Herrera HM, et al. Assessment of a quantitative 5' nuclease real-time polymerase chain reaction using the nicotinamide adenine dinucleotide dehydrogenase gamma subunit (nuoG) for *Bartonella* species in domiciled and stray cats in Brazil. *J Feline Med Surg.* 2016;18:783–790.
140. Diakou A, Di Cesare A, Barros LA, et al. Occurrence of *Aelurostrongylus abstrusus* and *Troglostrongylus brevior* in domestic cats in Greece. *Parasites Vectors.* 2015;8:4–9.
141. Hajipour N, Imani Baran A, Yakhchali M, et al. A survey study on gastrointestinal parasites of stray cats in Azarshahr (East Azerbaijan province, Iran). *J Parasit Dis.* 2016;40:1255–1260.
142. Waap H, Gomes J, Nunes T. Parasite communities in stray cat populations from Lisbon, Portugal. *J Helminthol.* 2014;88:389–395.
143. Fernandez C, Chikweto A, Mofya S, et al. A serological study of *Dirofilaria immitis* in feral cats in Grenada, West Indies. *J Helminthol.* 2010;84:390–393.
144. Khodabakhsh M, Malmasi A, Mohebali M, et al. Feline dirofilariosis due to *Dirofilaria immitis* in Meshkin Shahr district, northwestern Iran. *Iran J Parasitol.* 2016;11:269–273.
145. Park HJ, Lee SE, Lee WJ, et al. Prevalence of *Dirofilaria immitis* infection in stray cats by nested PCR in Korea. *Korean J Parasitol.* 2014;52:691–694.
146. Geng J, Elsemore DA, Oudin N, et al. Diagnosis of feline whipworm infection using a coproantigen ELISA and the prevalence in feral cats in southern Florida. *Vet Parasitol Reg Stud Reports.* 2018;14:181–186.
147. Lefkaditis MA, Sossidou AV, Panorias AH, et al. Urban stray cats infested by ectoparasites with zoonotic potential in Greece. *Parasitol Res.* 2015;114:3931–3934.
148. Segura F, Pons I, Miret J, et al. The role of cats in the eco-epidemiology of spotted fever group diseases. *Parasit Vectors.* 2014;7:1–13.
149. Mirzaghavami M, Sadraei J, Forouzandeh M. Detection of *Cryptosporidium* spp. in free ranging animals of Tehran, Iran. *J Parasit Dis.* 2016;40:1528–1531.
150. Meneses IDS de, Andrade MR, Uzêda RS, et al. Frequency of antibodies against *Sarcocystis neurona* and *Neospora caninum* in domestic cats in the state of Bahia, Brazil. *Rev Bras Parasitol Veterinária.* 2014;23:526–529.
151. Tehrani-sharif M, Jahan S, Alavi SM, et al. Seroprevalence of *Toxoplasma gondii* antibodies of stray cats in Garmsar, Iran. *J Parasit Dis.* 2015;39:306–308.
152. Matsuu A, Yokota S, Ito K, et al. Seroprevalence of *Toxoplasma gondii* in free-ranging and feral cats on Amami Oshima island, Japan. *J Vet Med Sci.* 2017;79:1853–1856.
153. Duarte A, Castro I, Pereira da Fonseca IM, et al. Survey of infectious and parasitic diseases in stray cats at the Lisbon Metropolitan Area, Portugal. *J Feline Med Surg.* 2010;12:441–446.
154. Boughattas S, Behnke J, Sharma A, et al. Seroprevalence of *Toxoplasma gondii* infection in feral cats in Qatar. *BMC Vet Res.* 2017;13:4–9.
155. Millán J, Cabezón O, Pabón M, et al. Seroprevalence of *Toxoplasma gondii* and *Neospora caninum* in feral cats (*Felis silvestris catus*) in Majorca, Balearic Islands, Spain. *Vet Parasitol.* 2009;165:323–326.
156. Little S, Levy J, Hartmann K, et al. 2020 AAFP Feline Retrovirus Testing and Management Guidelines. *J Feline Med Surg.* 2020;22:5–30.

19

Companion Animal Zoonoses in Immunocompromised and Other High-Risk Human Populations

Jason W. Stull

KEY POINTS

- Immunodeficiencies are common in people and may be congenital or acquired. It is estimated that up to 20% of the North American population and approximately 60% of North American households have some degree of immunosuppression.
- Up to 60% of households own pets, most commonly dogs or cats. Pet ownership may predispose high-risk people to zoonotic diseases. In addition, high-risk people often experience more severe disease, a longer duration of symptoms, or more severe or unexpected complications when compared with others. In general, the mental and physical benefits of pet ownership outweigh the risks, so education of pet owners to reduce the risks is important.
- Veterinarians play a key role in educating the public about ways to reduce the risk of zoonotic diseases, and should provide both written and verbal communications on this topic to pet owners. This should be documented in the medical record.
- Over 250 organisms are known to cause zoonotic infections, with over 70 of these involving companion animals. The most common zoonotic pathogens, their mode of transmission, clinical signs in humans, and prevention methods are reviewed in this chapter.

OVERVIEW OF HUMAN IMMUNODEFICIENCY SYNDROMES

Immunodeficiencies are frequently identified in people and result from numerous physiologic and pathologic processes (Box 19.1). Immune system defects generally increase the risk of infectious disease. Immunodeficiencies are categorized as congenital or acquired. Congenital immunodeficiencies, resulting from genetic disorders, increase susceptibility to infectious disease, depending on the type and penetrance of the defect.[1] One or more arms of the immune system (e.g., B cells, T cells) may be affected. Alternatively, immunodeficiencies are acquired, resulting from nongenetic factors, such as extremes of age (i.e., less than 5 years of age, greater than 65 years of age), pregnancy, or an immunocompromised state. Transplants (i.e., bone marrow and solid organ), infectious diseases (e.g., HIV infection), metabolic diseases (e.g., diabetes mellitus), splenectomy, cancers, and treatment with immunosuppressive drugs or chemotherapeutics most commonly contribute to an immunocompromised state.[2] The term "high-risk" is often used to denote individuals who have one or more congenital or acquired immunodeficiencies.

The mechanism of immunodeficiency varies with the cause of the immunodeficiency. Examples of mechanisms include incomplete immune development (children), waning immune response (elderly), temporary hormone-induced suppression (pregnancy), or specific abnormalities that result from congenital or acquired immunodeficiencies (e.g., metabolic derangements that result in inhibition of lymphocyte maturation and function).[3–5] Specific immune deficiency syndromes may increase risk for particular pathogens (e.g., neonates and invasive salmonellosis); however, this area is poorly understood.[6] Concurrent factors, such as other illnesses, burns, or indwelling tubes, catheters, or implants, increase the risk of infection by loss of natural barriers to infectious agents. Additionally, children and some individuals with developmental disabilities may have suboptimal hygiene practices or higher-risk contacts that further increase risk.[7]

It is estimated that 1 in 500 individuals in the United States is born with a defect in one or more components of the immune system.[5] More than 1.2 million people in the United States are infected with HIV, and approximately 10% do not know they are infected.[8] Each year approximately 50,000 people in the United States receive solid organ or bone marrow transplants.[9] There are approximately 25,000 splenectomies performed each year in the United States[10] in addition to the thousands of functionally hyposplenic patients, all of whom are considered at increased risk for infectious disease. In addition, there are many individuals with other underlying conditions that have less pronounced but still significant effects on the immune system, such as diabetes mellitus, renal disease, and cirrhosis. Pregnant women also have varying degrees of immunodeficiency; it is estimated that 2% of the population of the United States is pregnant at any given time.[11] Taken together, up to 20% of the North American population has some degree of immunosuppression (i.e., considered high-risk) with an even greater proportion of households having at least one high-risk individual (estimated as 59% of households in one study).[12,13]

PREVALENCE AND ADVANTAGES OF PET OWNERSHIP

Up to 60% of households with high-risk people in North America[12,14,15] and elsewhere[16] have pets. Dogs and cats are the most common pets residing in households with high-risk people, but other species (e.g., reptiles, birds, exotics, rodents) are also reported.[14,16] Additionally, pets are often acquired by high-risk individuals or households with a high-risk family member. In one study, 20% of households with

BOX 19.1 Factors Associated with Immunocompromise in Humans

Age	Fetuses, infants, preschoolers (less than 5 years of age), older adults (greater than 65 years of age)
Health Issues	Hospitalization, concurrent illness, autoimmune disease, organ transplantation, AIDS, diabetes mellitus, Cushing's syndrome, chronic renal failure, pregnancy, burns, leukopenia, cancer, congenital immunodeficiencies, hepatic cirrhosis, malnutrition, splenectomy, splenic dysfunction, myelosuppression, other reasons for immunocompromise
Therapeutic Agents	Cancer chemotherapy, immunosuppressive drug therapy, antimicrobial drugs
Medical Instrumentation and Procedures	Catheters, indwelling tubes, synthetic implants, splenectomy

children diagnosed with cancer acquired a new pet after their child was diagnosed.[14]

The mental and physical benefits that companion animals provide are great, and the risk for acquiring infections from pets is overall low. However, high-risk individuals are at greater risk for pet-associated infections than others, knowledge of disease risks is generally poor, and such individuals often engage in practices that put them or household members at increased risk for infections.[7,12,14] Helping the public and health professionals recognize both health benefits and risks associated with pets, as well as providing specific recommendations for precautions while handling and caring for pets can reduce risk of infection. The information in this chapter emphasizes zoonoses that are more commonly identified in high-risk individuals. However, because zoonoses can affect immunocompetent people, many of the principles pertain to anyone with pets.

RISKS OF COMPANION ANIMAL-ASSOCIATED ZOONOSES IN HUMANS

Zoonoses are infectious diseases that are naturally transmitted from living animals to humans.[17] High-risk people who own pets are at greater risk of contracting zoonotic diseases than those without pets (Box 19.2). In addition, high-risk people often experience more severe disease, a longer duration of symptoms, or more severe or unexpected complications than others.[18,19] For example, individuals infected with HIV are at 20–100 times greater risk of *Salmonella* bacteremia than those without HIV infection[18]; individuals with hematological malignancy are at 8 times the risk of *Salmonella* gastroenteritis and 2 times the risk of *Campylobacter* gastroenteritis than those without malignancy[19]; alcoholics, asplenic individuals, and immunocompromised individuals are at risk for severe (often fatal) *Capnocytophaga canimorsus* infection following dog/cat licks or bites[20]; and *Bordetella bronchiseptica* can cause severe illness in immunocompromised individuals,[21] while others rarely experience disease.

Despite the increased disease risk, to date, few studies have determined what proportion of human disease is attributable to contact with pets. For instance, it is estimated that 14% of all human illness caused by enteric pathogen groups is attributable to direct or indirect animal contact[22]; it is likely that pets are responsible for a relatively small component of this. In a separate study, cats or dogs were estimated to be responsible for 26% of all reported zoonotic human enteric infections for which contact with animals or their environment was the likely mode of transmission.[23] The true scope of pet-associated disease remains unknown partly due to a relative absence of reportable pet-associated pathogens (in people and animals) and complicating factors such as multiple non-pet exposure sources and subclinical shedding by pets.[24] This results in challenges relating to risk communication and decision-making, especially when attempting to weigh disease risks against benefits of pet ownership.

BOX 19.2 Mechanisms of Transmission of Zoonotic Infections

Zoonoses (dogs and cats to humans)	Bite, saliva, scratch, or close physical contact	Rabies, tularemia, pasteurellosis, *Capnocytophaga* infection, bartonellosis, dermatophytosis, *Malassezia pachydermatis* infection, sporotrichosis
	Droplet	Bordetellosis, plague, tularemia, coxiellosis, rhodococcosis
	Fecal-oral	Campylobacteriosis, yersiniosis, salmonellosis, toxoplasmosis, cryptosporidiosis, giardiasis, ancylostomiasis, toxocariasis
	Urine or genital secretions	*Escherichia coli* infections (pathogenic strains including ExPEC), canine brucellosis, leptospirosis, coxiellosis
Shared Vector-Acquired Zoonoses	Tick or flea vector	Ehrlichiosis, Rocky Mountain spotted fever, *Rickettsia felis* infection, borreliosis, plague, tularemia, bartonellosis, dipylidiasis
Sapronoses (environmentally acquired)	Inhalation or cutaneous inoculation	Anthrax, listeriosis, *Mycobacterium avium*–complex infection, blastomycosis, histoplasmosis, cryptococcosis, coccidioidomycosis, aspergillosis, pneumocystosis, microsporidiosis
Anthroponoses (humans to dogs and cats)		Group A streptococcal infections, *Streptococcus pneumoniae* infection, methicillin-resistant *Staphylococcus aureus* infections, *Clostridioides difficile* infection, *Mycobacterium tuberculosis* infection, *Entamoeba histolytica* infection, SARS-CoV-2 infection (COVID-19)

Given the high frequency of pet exposure and low reported pet-associated disease incidence, overall, pet-associated disease incidence is suspected to be low.[12,25–27] However, this should not negate awareness of important and severe disease in high-risk individuals.

People can acquire pet-associated zoonoses through numerous routes (see Box 19.2). Organisms can be acquired through contact with the skin and mucous membranes (e.g., bites, scratches, direct or indirect contact with animal saliva, urine and other body fluids), ingestion of animal fecal material, and inhalation of aerosols or droplets. Vector-borne pathogens can be transmitted from dogs and cats to humans when vectors feed on co-habitating humans. In some cases, dogs and cats bring vectors that are already infected with an organism closer to people. Many zoonoses have multiple routes of infection, so identification of a zoonotic pathogen in a pet-owning person does not necessarily indicate pet-related transmission.

Some pathogens are maintained in nature by replication of the organism in soil or water, on vegetation, or in decaying carcasses or animal excreta and can infect both humans and animals (*sapronoses*). For these pathogens, both humans and animals can acquire infections in a similar manner but independently of each other; in most cases, infected animals do not represent a direct infection risk for people (see Box 19.2). Instead, when animals get these infections, they act as sentinels for the risk of human infection in the region. Some zoonotic pathogens are maintained in humans (*anthroponoses*). Some of these infections can affect animals such as dogs and cats that may then transmit the infection to other animals or people, but this is not the most likely route of human infection.

Barriers to Prevention of Pet-Associated Zoonotic Diseases

One of the barriers to prevention of pet-associated zoonotic disease is low knowledge of these disease risks among the public and other healthcare professionals, which includes those at an increased risk for disease.[12,14] This may partly result from limited education of high-risk pet owners on the topic.[12,14,15] In one study, 94% of surveyed physicians in the United States stated they never or rarely initiated discussions about zoonoses with patients with HIV infection or AIDS.[28] Few veterinary (58%) and human medical (4%) practices make educational materials on zoonotic diseases available to clients or patients.[28,29] This is unfortunate, as several studies suggest that high-risk individuals are open to educational opportunities from healthcare providers and veterinary personnel.[12,14]

In order to provide targeted education and recommendations to clients with high-risk household members, veterinarians must be aware of the presence of high-risk household members or others that frequently contact household pets. As an additional barrier, veterinarians infrequently gather this information from clients.[14,28,30] Evidence suggests that many clients are comfortable providing veterinary personnel with human healthcare information to assist in determining the high-risk status of household members; yet if veterinary personnel do not ask, many clients will not provide this information.[14]

Perhaps one of the largest challenges is that the subject of pet-associated zoonoses falls at the intersection of veterinary and human medicine. In order to effectively address this area, multiple disciplines (e.g., human healthcare, veterinary healthcare) need to communicate. Unfortunately, evaluations of this area document poor interdisciplinary communication.[28,30,31] In one study, 100% of physicians and 97% of veterinarians in the United States claimed to never or rarely contact individuals of the other profession when looking for advice on zoonotic disease risks or cases.[28] Without a strong collaborative approach among healthcare disciplines, pet contact recommendations coming from a single healthcare group may be overly conservative or lacking due to limited knowledge of the area.

Although veterinarians generally are better prepared than human family practitioners to answer questions about animal diseases and human risks, patients, especially those who are immunocompromised, may not view them as the primary providers of this information.[14] Paradoxically, physicians seem to be uncomfortable discussing zoonotic diseases with their clients and view the veterinarian as playing a more important role in this service. In surveys of medical and veterinary professionals, physicians felt that public health officials and veterinarians should be responsible for this task.[32] When questioned about educating clients on the risk of zoonotic diseases, a much greater percentage of veterinarians felt comfortable with this task than did physicians.[30]

Veterinarians can be an important source of information about health risks of pet ownership and precautionary measures for high-risk people so that they can safely keep their pets. The latest guidelines from a number of public health and infectious disease organizations recommend that rather than give up their pets, immunocompromised people take simple precautions to prevent infection (see Recommendations).[3,13,25,33–38] A number of resources are available for clients or other healthcare professionals that provide a balanced view of health risks and benefits of pet ownership (Box 19.3).

Veterinarians can demonstrate their willingness and expertise to provide advice and guidance for zoonosis prevention by having signs or brochures in their waiting rooms, posting information on their website or similar social media channels, and actively engaging clients in the topic through client and patient intake questionnaires. Offering regional talks on pet care, zoonoses, and prevention may be particularly valued by the public. It is important to recognize that human health information may fall under country-specific privacy laws. In the United States, the Health Insurance Portability and Accountability Act (HIPAA) states that information about a person's health status is considered confidential and protected.[39] Therefore, veterinary staff need to ensure that any human health information obtained (e.g., client health status, immunocompromising conditions in household members or those frequently spending time with the client's pets) is adequately protected when recorded.[40] Often this is best achieved in veterinary medicine by keeping all written human health information general, including medical record notes and questions and responses contained in patient intake questionnaires. Additionally, a signed consent from clients is advisable when specific human health information is recorded or clients authorize veterinary team members to discuss their protected health information with a physician. Example disclosure forms are available.[40]

OCCUPATIONAL AND ENVIRONMENTAL FACTORS THAT INCREASE RISK OF ZOONOSES

Veterinarians, animal health workers, and those working or training in settings with high animal contact (e.g., pet shops, shelters) may be at greater risk for zoonoses.[41–43] During their careers, approximately two-thirds of veterinarians report a major animal-related injury that results in lost work or hospitalization.[44,45] In two studies, 28% and 47% of veterinarians in the United States reported development of a zoonotic infection during the course of their veterinary work.[29,46] Zoonoses most frequently reported included dermatophytosis, bartonellosis, and cat and dog bite infections. Similar risks exist for other veterinary personnel and students.[43,47] Within-clinic zoonotic transmission of pathogens such as methicillin-resistant *Staphylococcus aureus* (MRSA) and *Salmonella* has also been reported.[48–50] Suboptimal use of personal protective equipment may be partly responsible for the increased zoonotic disease risk in the veterinary profession.[51]

LEGAL IMPLICATIONS OF ZOONOSES FOR VETERINARIANS

Veterinarians have an inherent responsibility to advise pet owners on their risk of contracting zoonoses.[52,53] The use of both written (e.g., brochures, website materials) and verbal approaches are useful. It is important to clearly document all oral and written communications regarding these topics in the medical record, including whether a client declines veterinary advice. Veterinarians must advise clients to seek human healthcare advice when they suspect a zoonotic infection has occurred or is likely to occur. Veterinarians must also report zoonotic diseases where public health laws dictate, and must also protect their

BOX 19.3 Resources for High-Risk Pet Owners, Veterinary Personnel, and Healthcare Workers

Level	Resource	Comments On Audience/Content
International	World Organization for Animal Health (www.oie.int)	Association responsible for improving animal health worldwide
	World Health Organization (www.who.int)	Association responsible for improving human health worldwide
National and Regional	American Veterinary Medical Association (www.avma.org)	Provides updated information on zoonotic diseases in pets
	Centers for Disease Control and Prevention – Healthy Pets, Healthy People (www.cdc.gov/healthypets)	Resource highlighting zoonotic diseases in various animal species; risks and recommendations for organ transplant patients, infants and young children, and pregnant women; information on recent animal-associated disease outbreaks in people. Numerous brochures on pet-associated diseases in high-risk individuals
	Centers for Disease Control and Prevention – Handwashing: Clean Hands Save Lives (www.cdc.gov/handwashing)	Hand washing guidelines for veterinarians, healthcare workers, and pet owners
	Companion Animal Parasite Council (capcvet.org)	Information and recommendations for parasitic diseases; prevalence maps of select pathogens in dogs and cats for United States and Canada
	National Association of State Public Health Veterinarians (www.nasphv.org)	Information and guidelines for zoonotic disease prevention. Compendium of measures to prevent disease associated with animals in public settings
	Pet Partners (petpartners.org)	Information on service dogs; online educational module on infection control training for animal-assisted therapy handlers and healthcare members
	Pets are Loving Support (PALS) (www.palsatlanta.org), Pets are Wonderful Support (PAWS), PETS-DC (www.petsdc.org)	Aim to preserve the human-animal bond for vulnerable community members. Affiliates located in many major cities
	Medline Plus, Pets and the Immunocompromised Person (https://medlineplus.gov/ency/article/003967.htm)	Information for high-risk clients
	Centers for Disease Control and Prevention Foundation, Preventing Infections During Cancer Treatment – Caring for Your Pet (www.preventcancerinfections.org/health-tip-sheet/caring-your-pet)	Information for cancer patients
	Worms and Germs Blog (www.wormsandgermsblog.com)	Numerous factsheets on pet-associated diseases designed for pet owners, veterinarians, and human healthcare providers; additional resources on the topic
	Grace SF. Assessing client risk for zoonotic disease transmission – questions to ask. Clinician's Brief; 2008. http://www.cliniciansbrief.com/columns/39/assessing-client-risk-zoonotic-disease-questions-ask	Information for veterinarians
	Stull JW, Landers T. Bridging the veterinary–human healthcare communication divide. Veterinary Team Brief; 2017. https://www.cliniciansbrief.com/article/bridging-veterinary-human-healthcare-communication-divide	Information for veterinarians

employees through education on preventative measures. For information on prevention measures, consult the Recommendations section in this chapter and the *Compendium of Veterinary Standard Precautions for Zoonotic Disease Prevention in Veterinary Personnel*, published by the National Association of State Public Health Veterinarians online and in print.[54]

BENEFITS OF PET OWNERSHIP

Risks of zoonotic infection need to be balanced against the mental and physical health benefits of pet contact, especially for those who are ill or at increased risk of infections.[55,56] The emotional bond between owners and animals can be as important to the owner as human relationships and provides similar psychological benefits.[57] In many cases, pets are considered family members. Positive health outcomes including reduction in stress, depression, systemic blood pressure, and favorable lipid profiles have been associated with animal interaction.[56–59] Benefits have also been documented in the healthcare setting with reductions in pain and improved morale reported among those participating in animal-assisted therapy.[55]

Benefits from pet contact have been equally observed among individuals at high risk of pet-associated infections.[57–59] Children brought up with companion animals often have better social skills, self-esteem, and empathy than children without pets.[60] In adults and the elderly, studies have documented an association between pets and reduced risk of cardiovascular disease and improved psychological and physical well-being.[61] Health benefits are also well documented in individuals who are immunocompromised. Although illness and disability often alienate individuals from their family, friends, and acquaintances, pets provide continued and unconditional companionship and help their owners overcome the deleterious effects of loneliness.[62]

Given the many argued health benefits of pet ownership and contact, it may be more detrimental to the well-being of immunocompromised people to lose their pet companions than to risk acquiring a zoonotic infection. However, such people should understand the health risks and, perhaps most importantly, be aware of measures that can be taken to reduce infection risks while maintaining the strong bond with pets.

SPECIFIC DISEASE INFORMATION FOR HIGH-RISK INDIVIDUALS

More than 250 organisms are known to cause zoonotic infections, with over 70 of these involving companion animals (see Box 19.2). Given the growing molecular and epidemiologic evidence of the interspecies exchange of pathogens, such as MDR bacteria, this number is likely to increase.[63] Of these, only a subset is of greatest importance for high-risk people due to the severity of infection and overall frequency of infections (Table 19.1). Most of these zoonoses are more likely to be acquired from sources other than dogs and cats (e.g., the environment, other animal hosts, or people). Nevertheless, pet ownership does pose a risk to immunocompromised people and should be considered. Further, many are readily preventable, so client awareness and education is important. The reader is referred to respective chapters elsewhere in this book for additional information on each infection.

Bartonellosis

Bartonella spp. are small, fastidious, gram-negative, arthropod-borne, intracellular bacilli. The genus includes numerous species, 13 of which are believed or known to be associated with human disease.[64] Cats and dogs serve as reservoirs for infection of people.[64] Domestic cats serve as the primary reservoir for *Bartonella henselae* and *Bartonella clarridgeiae,* which cause cat scratch disease (CSD) and potentially life-threatening infections in humans.

CSD most commonly occurs from a cat scratch or cat bite, as claws and teeth can become contaminated with feces from infected fleas, or through direct flea bites.[64] Bartonellosis often manifests as subacute solitary or regional lymphadenomegaly and fever in immunocompetent people. More severe disease, such as bacteremia, endocarditis, neuroretinitis, and proliferative lesions on the skin, liver, or spleen can occur in high-risk patients (Fig. 19.1). Children (especially those aged 5–9 years) appear to be at greatest risk of CSD.[65]

Flea control is essential for reducing the spread of *Bartonella* spp. infection among cats, dogs, and humans. Additionally, attention to proper training and handling of cats and dogs to reduce bites and scratches is critical for households with high-risk people. Bite and scratch avoidance is particularly important for animals most likely to be infected (e.g., kittens, feral cats, outdoor cats, cats with fleas). Declawing is not a recommended strategy to reduce zoonotic infection; however, nails can be clipped to reduce the chance of their lacerating the skin. Keeping cats indoors can reduce risk of infection and is recommended in high-risk households. Guidelines aimed at reducing infections in HIV-infected persons recommend these individuals only acquire cats greater than 1 year of age that are in good health, reduce bites and scratches (in part by avoiding rough play), maintain flea control, promptly wash bites and scratches, and prevent cats from licking wounds.[66] It is reasonable to extend these recommendations beyond those with HIV infections to all high-risk households.

Bordetella bronchiseptica Infection

Bordetella bronchiseptica is a gram-negative coccobacillus commonly found in the respiratory tracts of many mammals, including cats and dogs, and is well known as a contributor to canine infectious respiratory disease complex. Humans are unusual hosts for this agent; exposure to infectious dogs or cats, or the attenuated live intranasal vaccine has been implicated in human infection, although proof that the vaccine causes human infection is lacking.[67,68] In immunocompetent people, *B. bronchiseptica* has been occasionally associated with mild upper respiratory tract infections.[67] In immunocompromised individuals, infection remains rare, however disease may be moderate to severe in affected individuals with sinusitis, tracheobronchitis, pneumonia, bacteremia, endocarditis, peritonitis, and meningitis. People with cystic fibrosis may be especially vulnerable to severe infection.[21,69–73]

Although bordetellosis is uncommon, it has been recommended that severely immunocompromised people, their pets, or both avoid contact with animals in animal shelters, dog kennels, catteries, or animal shows, where the infection is more prevalent or respiratory disease has been observed in animals. If necessary, vaccination of an immunocompromised person's pets can be considered to help control the spread of an outbreak of infection, preferably with the inactivated vaccine.[68]

Brucellosis

Humans most often become infected with *Brucella canis* through contact with the organism in canine genital secretions or from laboratory culture. Dogs may shed the organism in urine, saliva, and respiratory secretions; however, fluids from these routes generally have fewer organisms than genital secretions and are of lower risk for human infection. Infections in people are rarely reported; however, this may be a combination of low occurrence, unapparent clinical disease, and missed cases due to challenges in organism detection and limited testing.[74] Of the reported human cases, high-risk individuals are often involved. Immunocompromised patients (e.g., infected with HIV, cirrhosis) have been infected with *B. canis* as a result of contact with household dogs, resulting in bacteremia, fever, endocarditis, and peritonitis.[75–78] Several clinical *B. canis* infections in young children have been reported following contact with puppies.[79,80]

Individuals with infected dogs should be counseled on potential zoonotic disease risks; local public and agriculture health regulations may dictate the approach to *B. canis*-positive dogs.[81] In all circumstances, infected dogs should be neutered to help reduce the public health risk should they be kept as pets. Hygiene practices (e.g., hand washing, use of protective outerwear) should be carefully observed around aborting bitches. High-risk individuals should avoid contact with dogs with known or suspected brucellosis (such as dogs from breeding kennels that have had abortions or reproductive failure). The zoonotic risk of a neutered animal is low, but concerns about keeping an infected animal in the household with a high-risk person may be valid. Households with high-risk members should prevent unrestricted outdoor access of dogs, especially if contact with other dogs, notably strays, is likely.

Campylobacteriosis

Campylobacteriosis is caused by a microaerophilic group of gram-negative, curved, motile rods that are commensal flora of animals. Fecal-oral, foodborne, and waterborne modes of transmission are the principal avenues for human infection. *Campylobacter* spp. are frequently isolated from dogs and cats (especially younger than 1 year of age) recently acquired from pet stores, kennels, animal shelters, or pounds. Puppies and kittens with diarrhea have been most commonly associated with human infections.[82] Signs of infection in humans are intense abdominal discomfort, bloody diarrhea, fever, tenesmus, and fecal leukocytosis. Immunocompromised and young individuals are at the greatest risk for infection and severe disease. Immunosuppressed individuals with AIDS develop recurrent diarrhea, dehydration, and bacteremia. Dog-associated *Campylobacter* transmission to people has been well documented, including a large national (USA) outbreak of MDR *Campylobacter jejuni*, involving over 100 human cases (24% hospitalized) linked to puppy exposure.[83–87] Young children who live with a puppy are perhaps at greatest risk for infection.[83]

TABLE 19.1 Predominant Disease Manifestations of Dog and Cat Zoonoses of Importance for High-Risk People

Pathogen (Chapter)	Disease	Signs in Dogs and Cats	Signs in Immunocompetent Human Hosts	Predisposing Conditions	Signs in Immunocompromised Hosts
Viral					
Cowpox virus (38)	Cowpox	Usually in cats, rare in dogs: solitary crusted skin lesion on head, neck, or thoracic limbs to disseminated skin lesions with secondary bacterial infections, abscesses, fever, inappetence, lethargy, oculonasal discharge, diarrhea, and death	Usually mild, with a crusted skin lesion, sometimes with fever, headache, and nausea. Rarely more severe with large painful skin lesions with systemic illness requiring hospitalization and prolonged recovery	Atopic eczema, alcoholism, and drug abuse	Increased risk for severe form
Bacterial					
Bartonella spp. (70)	Cat scratch disease	Usually subclinical	Regional lymphadenopathy	HIV-AIDS, liver or kidney transplant, abnormal cardiac valve	Bacillary angiomatosis, peliosis hepatis, endocarditis
Bordetella bronchiseptica (55)	Bordetellosis	Cough	Pertussis-like syndrome	Malignancy, AIDS, malnutrition, chronic renal failure	Pneumonia, pleural effusion, sepsis, peritonitis
Campylobacter (65)	Campylobacteriosis	Diarrhea, especially in young animals	Abdominal discomfort, large-bowel diarrhea, fever	Young (<5 years old), HIV-AIDS	Recurrent diarrhea, dehydration, bacteremia
Capnocytophaga (75)	None	Subclinical	Wound infections	Asplenia/hyposplenia, alcoholism, elderly	Sepsis, pneumonia, soft tissue infection
Clostridioides difficile (64)	CDAD	Subclinical or diarrhea	Antibacterial-associated diarrhea, nosocomial diarrhea	Advanced age, long healthcare facility stays, gastrointestinal surgery, chemotherapy, organ transplantation	Similar to immunocompetent, but at increased risk for CDAD and have a poorer prognosis
Coxiella burnetii (48)	Q fever	Typically subclinical	Asymptomatic or mild flu-like illness, occasionally hepatitis, pneumonia, myocarditis, pericarditis, encephalitis	Previous cardiac valvulopathy, chronic steroid therapy, solid organ transplants, alcoholism, cirrhosis	Pneumonia, endocarditis, osteomyelitis, and chronic hepatitis; for pregnant women, spontaneous abortion, intrauterine growth retardation, premature delivery, fetal death
Escherichia coli (63)	Traveler's diarrhea	Enteric forms (especially neonatal kittens and puppies): vomiting, diarrhea, dehydration, anorexia, lethargy, weakness and death. Extraintestinal forms: UTI, emphysematous cystitis, severe acute hemorrhagic pneumonia	Enteric forms: severe acute diarrhea sometimes complicated by hemolytic uremic syndrome. Extraintestinal forms: UTI, sepsis, pneumonia, meningitis, and various multiorgan infections and abscesses	HIV-AIDS, cancer, leukemia, aplastic anemia, chemotherapy, glucocorticoids, diabetes mellitus, transplant patients, liver disease, autoimmune disease, malnutrition, alcoholism	Increased risk for both enteric and extraintestinal forms
Francisella tularensis (74)	Tularemia, rabbit fever, deer-fly fever	Subclinical to fever, lymphadenomegaly, draining wounds	Ulceroglandular or glandular illness	Older age, alcoholism, diabetes mellitus, transplantation, AIDS	Prolonged infection or death
Pasteurella spp. (75)	Pasteurellosis	Subclinical	Local cellulitis	Cirrhosis of liver and other chronic liver diseases, solid organ malignancies, glucocorticoid use, diabetes mellitus, prosthetic joints	Bacteremia or sepsis, endocarditis, osteomyelitis, pneumonia, endophthalmitis
Salmonella spp. (62)	Salmonellosis	Diarrhea or subclinical infections to bacteremia with osteomyelitis, meningitis, pneumonia, fever, and abortion	Usually self-limiting gastroenteritis with mucoid diarrhea and hematochezia	AIDS, age (<5 years old, elderly), diabetes mellitus, renal disease with dialysis, prosthetic heart valves, aplastic anemia, chemotherapy, malignancy	Refractory or life-threatening diarrhea; extraintestinal illness with absence of diarrhea including bacteremia, sepsis, meningitis, osteomyelitis, endocarditis

Continued

TABLE 19.1 Predominant Disease Manifestations of Dog and Cat Zoonoses of Importance for High-Risk People—cont'd

Fungal					
Dermatophytes; *Microsporum canis, Trichophyton* spp. (78)	Ringworm	Subclinical or lesions with circular alopecia, scaling, erythema, pruritis, hyperpigmentation, claw infections	Circular alopecia, scaling, crusting	Age (premature infants), HIV-AIDS, immunosuppressive medications with organ transplantation, autoimmune diseases	Same as immunocompetent, atypical signs, (e.g., disseminated cutaneous infections)
Malassezia pachydermatis (79)	*Malassezia* dermatitis	Normal skin flora in healthy animals. Can become pathogenic with skin inflammation, chronic glucocorticoid therapy, endocrine disorders, immunocompromise. Clinically presents as otitis externa, seborrheic skin with possible alopecia, lichenification, crusting, scaling, and pigmentation	Not normally found on human skin, asymptomatic	Age (infants in neonatal ICUs)	Bacteremia, UTIs, meningitis
Parasitic					
Cryptosporidium parvum, Cryptosporidium canis, Cryptosporidium felis (103)	Cryptosporidiosis	Subclinical in immunocompetent adult dogs and cats. Diarrhea, especially in young animals, kittens with FeLV or FIV infection, or immunocompromised dogs (e.g., CPV, CDV, intestinal lymphoma)	Diarrhea, abdominal cramps, nausea, vomiting	HIV-AIDS, malnutrition in children, organ transplantation, hyper IgM syndrome, cancers, chemotherapy	Prolonged intractable diarrhea, extraintestinal infection of the biliary and respiratory tracts
Giardia duodenalis (101)	Giardiasis	Subclinical or diarrhea, soft, light-colored, frothy, mucoid stools, flatulence, failure to thrive	Watery, foul-smelling diarrhea with flatus, abdominal distention	Malnutrition and chronic diarrhea in infants and children, nephrotic syndrome or lymphoma, age (older adults), AIDS and other immunodeficiencies; agammaglobulinemia, gastric surgeries, and reduced gastric acid	Prolonged diarrhea (more refractory to therapy)
Strongyloides stercoralis (116)	Strongyloidiasis	Subclinical; occasionally diarrhea, pneumonia, dermatitis in puppies	Subclinical, rash, diarrhea, abdominal pain	Immunosuppressive drugs, hematologic malignancy, human T-cell lymphotropic virus-1 (HTLV-1) infection	Abdominal pain, vomiting, diarrhea, intestinal obstruction, peritonitis, cough, hemoptysis, meningitis
Toxocara canis, Toxocara cati (112)	Toxocariasis	Subclinical; occasionally failure to gain weight, abdominal distension, respiratory signs in juveniles; enteritis in adults	Asymptomatic	Youth (less than 6 years of age for visceral larval migrans; mean age of 8–16 years for ocular larval migrans)	Visceral larval migrans (cough, fever, seizures), ocular larval migrans (unilateral vision loss, strabismus, chorioretinal granuloma, retinal detachment)
Toxoplasma gondii (93)	Toxoplasmosis	Subclinical, occasional diarrhea in kittens	Asymptomatic, self-limiting lymphadenopathy, chorioretinitis	Pregnancy (unborn fetus), HIV-AIDS, chemotherapy, cancer, especially bone marrow or organ transplantation, long-term glucocorticoid use	CNS complications (focal neurologic deficits, cognitive dysfunction, altered mental status); in pregnant women spontaneous abortion, prematurity or stillbirth; in neonates fever, microcephaly, hydrocephalus, hepatosplenomegaly, jaundice, seizures, chorioretinitis

AIDS, acquired immunodeficiency syndrome; *CDAD, Clostridioides difficile*–associated diarrhea; *CDV*, canine distemper virus; *CNS*, central nervous system; *CPV*, canine parvovirus; *CSD*, cat scratch disease; *FeLV*, feline leukemia virus; *FIV*, feline immunodeficiency virus; *GI*, gastrointestinal; *HIV*, human immunodeficiency virus; *ICU*, intensive care unit.

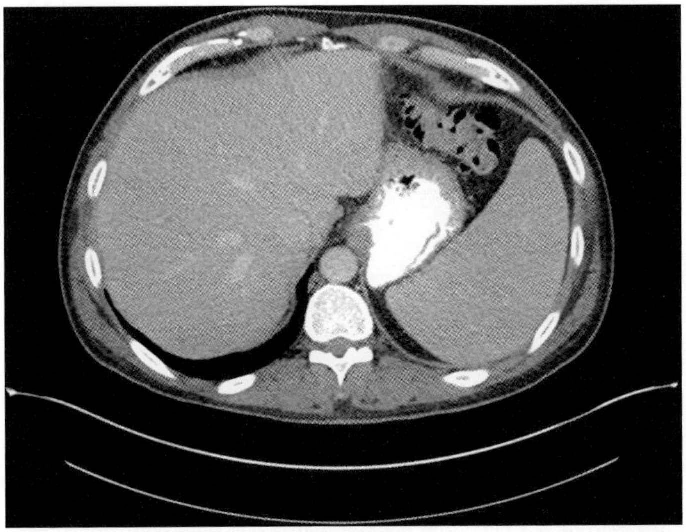

Fig. 19.1 Bartonellosis-associated hepatosplenomegaly (CT image) in a person with AIDS admitted for prolonged fever. The patient lived with many flea-infested cats and reported a recent cat scratch. (Photograph courtesy of Shandra Day and Shu-Hua Wang, Columbus, Ohio, USA.)

Preventative measures among high-risk people include avoidance of animals with diarrhea and adoption of pets younger than 1 year of age or from pet stores, kennels, or shelters. Washing hands after handling pets or their feces, and especially before eating is the most important precaution.

Capnocytophaga Infection

Capnocytophaga canimorsus is a gram-negative, rod-shaped organism that is found in the oral flora of dogs, cats, and other animals.[20] Transmission of *Capnocytophaga* is most commonly from a dog bite, although other types of contact with dogs or cats can also result in transmission.[88,89] Specific serovars of *C. canimorsus* appear to be linked with human infection.[90] In one review, a history of a cat or dog bite was present in 89% of 28 cases.[91] In the remaining cases, contact with salivary secretions on mucosal or broken skin surfaces may have been involved in transmission. Cats and dogs should not be allowed to lick a person's open cuts or wounds or have contact with medical devices, such as peritoneal dialysis equipment.[92] The clinical manifestations of *Capnocytophaga* infection in people range from cellulitis to fulminant sepsis. Although the condition is considered rare, it is likely that the infection is under-reported because the organism is difficult to culture by routine methods. Most cases in people are associated with an underlying immune disorder or a similar immunocompromising condition (e.g., alcoholism). Individuals with splenectomy are at increased risk, but other conditions can render a patient functionally asplenic or hyposplenic, such as sickle cell disease, alcoholism, and cirrhosis. Signs of infection are acute severe cellulitis and bacteremia, which may develop within 24 to 48 hours after the bite. The mortality associated with this organism is often at or greater than 20%. For those who survive, neurological sequelae are common.[89,93] Prevention involves bite and scratch avoidance and prompt treatment (e.g., washing with soap and water, antimicrobials as indicated). All individuals, especially high-risk people, should be advised to consult with a physician as soon as possible following an animal bite or severe scratch. Prophylactic antimicrobials are often administered to high-risk individuals in these situations. Pets should never be permitted to lick or otherwise have contact with wounds, ulcers, or skin lesions.

Clostridioides difficile Infection

Clostridioides difficile (previously *Clostridium difficile*) is a rod-shaped, gram-positive, anaerobic, spore-forming bacterium. Pathogenic strains can produce toxin A, an enterotoxin, and toxic B, a cytotoxin. *Clostridioides difficile* is an important cause of antimicrobial-associated diarrhea in humans, with an estimated 223,900 *C. difficile* infection (CDI)-related hospitalizations and at least 12,800 deaths each year in the United States.[94] Individuals at increased risk for CDI include those with recent antimicrobial use, hospitalized patients, the elderly, those receiving PPIs, and individuals with underlying immunosuppressive disease or chronic illnesses.[95]

The role of *C. difficile* as a pathogen in dogs and cats is controversial. Reports of animals as confirmed sources of infection for humans are lacking. However, dogs and cats can develop infection and shed the organism, with isolates often indistinguishable from those found in people.[96] Therapy dogs visiting human hospitals frequently (58/102; 58%) had positive culture results for *C. difficile* with 71% of the isolates being toxigenic strains.[97] Dogs became colonized with *C. difficile* (in addition to MRSA) during visits to the human hospital. The risk of acquisition is higher in dogs that lick patients or accept treats during visits.[98] In one study, residing with a pet was a risk factor for *C. difficile* colonization of immunocompromised individuals, and the organism was found to contaminate the environment of affected households.[99] In a study of dogs and cats owned by patients with CDI, probable transmission between the patient and pet was documented in 3/14 (21%) of the contacts.[100]

As with other potentially zoonotic enteric infections, avoidance of contact with feces or fecal-contaminated surfaces, use of gloves when cleaning up pet feces, frequent hand washing, and prompt diagnosis and treatment of animals that develop diarrhea are important precautions for high-risk individuals. Animal exposure to infected people and contaminated fomites, especially in healthcare facilities, should be avoided if possible.

Cowpox Virus Infection

Cowpox infection is a disease currently confined to Eurasia and is caused by a virus of the genus *Orthopoxvirus*. Cats acquire the pathogen from contact with infected rodents.[101] Cat-to-human transmission, often acquired through an abrasion in the skin, is the most common cause of human infection.[102] Cowpox infection in healthy individuals is often clinically mild, with the development of one to several pox lesions, nausea, pyrexia, and headaches.[102] In severe cases, often associated with immune suppression or preexisting skin disease, infection can cause large, painful skin lesions and systemic illness that can require hospitalization and even result in death (Fig. 19.2).[103] The use of simple hygiene practices, such as hand washing and use of gloves, reduction of cat-rodent contact in regions where the virus is present, and bite and scratch avoidance are recommended to avoid transmission.[101,103,104]

Coxiellosis

Q fever (coxiellosis) is caused by *Coxiella burnetii*, a small, gram-negative, obligately intracellular bacterial pathogen. Illness in humans due to Q fever can be acute or chronic. In the immunocompetent host, most acute infections are either asymptomatic or a self-limiting, febrile illness. Occasionally, granulomatous hepatitis, pneumonia, myocarditis, pericarditis, or encephalitis can occur, with an increased risk of these manifestations in high-risk individuals.[105–107] Endocarditis is the most frequent manifestation of chronic Q fever, with patients with existing valvulopathy at particularly increased risk.[108] Other features of chronic infections include infections of aneurysms and vascular grafts, osteomyelitis, and chronic hepatitis.[105] Individuals with solid organ transplants, alcoholic cirrhosis, or on chronic steroid therapy are also at increased risk for developing chronic Q fever.[105] Pregnant women deserve special mention because both the fetus and mother are at risk. Pregnant women can develop systemic disease or endocarditis,

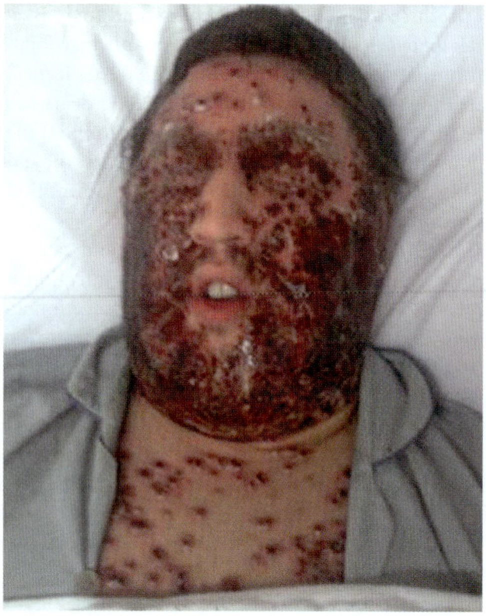

Fig. 19.2 Severe diffuse skin lesions of cowpox infection in a person with preexisting eczema. (Photograph courtesy Richard Lawn, Stafford, UK, letter to the editor of *Veterinary Record,* May 15, 2010, page 631, volume 166.)

while spontaneous abortion, intrauterine growth retardation, premature delivery, or fetal death can also occur.[109] Dormant *C. burnetii* can reactivate during subsequent pregnancies.

The primary reservoirs for human Q fever infection are cattle, goats, and sheep, but cats can be an important reservoir of Q fever in the urban setting.[110,111] Dogs are a less frequent source.[112] Infection in animals is usually not clinically apparent. Infected animals contaminate the environment by excretion of the organisms in placental tissues and in their milk. Parturient cats have been linked to human outbreaks of Q fever.[113] Raw meat has been implicated in the transmission of *C. burnetii* to cats and people.[114]

High-risk individuals described in this section should avoid contact with placental tissues of animals, periparturient animals, and newborn animals. Because coxiellosis has developed in humans exposed to parturient cats, protective gloves and outerwear, including masks and protective eyewear, should be worn by all individuals performing procedures in which there is contact with the genital tissues or secretions of parturient or aborting animals.

Cryptosporidiosis

Cryptosporidiosis is an intestinal infection caused by *Cryptosporidium* spp., ubiquitous, coccidian parasites of vertebrates. *Cryptosporidium parvum* is the least host-specific species, and infects people and many animal species including dogs and cats. *Cryptosporidium canis* and *Cryptosporidium felis* are predominant species in dogs and cats, respectively. Although these two species do not commonly infect humans,[115] they have been known to infect immunocompromised individuals, so are considered zoonotic.[116,117]

Cryptosporidium oocysts are infective as soon as they are shed in the feces, and the infective dose is very low, making direct transmission possible by any potential fecal-oral route, such as through contact with contaminated fur, soil, hands, clothing, or water. The oocysts are highly resistant to chemical and biological destruction, and remain infectious in cool, moist conditions for many months. They can survive in freshwater and saltwater and in chemically treated swimming pool water.

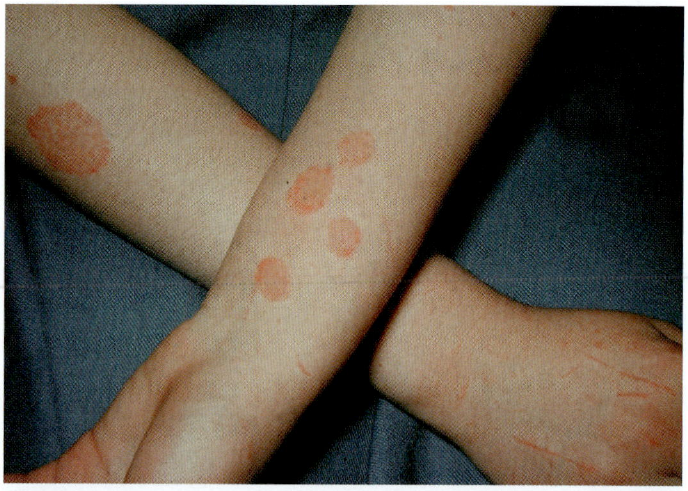

Fig. 19.3 Dermatophytosis (*Microsporum canis*) lesions on forearms of child with recent history of contact with a dog with dermatophytosis. (Photograph courtesy of Nordau Kanigsberg, Ottawa, Ontario, Canada.)

Immunocompetent human patients can be asymptomatic, but they may also experience a range of symptoms, including diarrhea, cramps, nausea, vomiting, and fever that typically lasts for 5 to 10 days. Cryptosporidiosis appears to be very common in individuals with certain immunocompromising conditions (e.g., estimated pooled global prevalence of 14% in HIV-infected people).[118] Immunocompromised individuals (e.g., HIV-AIDS, malnourished children, transplant recipients, hyper IgM syndrome, hematologic neoplasia, and cancer patients on chemotherapy) are at risk for severe, intractable disease that may be fatal.[119–121] Ownership of dogs and cats as pets has not been shown to increase the risk of cryptosporidiosis in immunocompetent persons.[122] In one study of people infected with HIV with and without cryptosporidiosis, pets were not a major risk factor for infection.[123]

Caution is advised when any *Cryptosporidium* species are found in a pet dog or cat. High-risk individuals should be particularly careful to avoid fecal contact, especially when the animal has diarrhea. Disposable gloves should be worn if contact with feces is unavoidable; hands should be immediately washed after glove removal. High-risk owners should seek veterinary advice promptly if their pets develop diarrhea. Stray animals or pets with diarrhea should not be adopted by high-risk individuals.

Dermatophytosis

Dermatophytosis in pets is most commonly caused by the zoophilic fungi *Microsporum canis, Microsporum gypseum,* and *Trichophyton* spp., and cats and dogs can serve as carriers. *Microsporum canis* is the most commonly implicated organism, especially in cats. Humans can acquire dermatophyte infections through contact with clinically affected or healthy animals or humans as well as contaminated fomites, such as household surfaces, bedding, and clothing. Classic skin lesions in humans consist of circular alopecia, scaling, crusting, and ulceration (Fig. 19.3).

Immunocompromised individuals can develop signs similar to those in immunocompetent patients or can have atypical signs such as adult tinea capitis (infection of the scalp involving the skin and hair), nail infections, or disseminated cutaneous infections.[124,125] Severe zoonotic dermatophytosis has been reported in humans with AIDS, systemic lupus erythematosus, and transplant patients on immunosuppressive medication.[126–129] One outbreak occurred in a neonatal intensive care unit (ICU) among premature infants with low birth weight and multiple medical problems.[130] A nurse who worked in the unit had acquired a cat and subsequently developed a recurrent clinical *M. canis* infection. The cat was taken to a veterinary dermatologist, who made the diagnosis of *M. canis* infection. The nurse was taken off duty and underwent treatment, and the unit instituted strict enhanced cleaning and disinfection procedures. This case underscores the importance of good communication among veterinarians, their clients, and their clients' physicians to help prevent or respond to infections, in this case dermatophytosis, where an animal might be involved.[131] Other outbreaks among neonates in hospitals have also been reported.[132,133]

Prevention of pet-associated zoonotic dermatophytosis involves avoidance of contact with infected animals, use of barriers (e.g., gloves) when handling infected animals, effective therapy of infected animals, and cleaning and disinfection of contaminated living spaces. Immunocompromised pet owners should seek veterinary care early should their pets develop skin lesions. Given the increased likelihood of infection, colonization, or contamination of shelter animals, such animals are not ideally suited for households with immunocompromised individuals. If such clients choose to acquire a pet from a shelter, temporary housing of the animal in a separate location for several weeks to ensure they are healthy and not incubating pathogens is recommended.

Escherichia coli Infections

Escherichia coli are gram-negative, rod-shaped bacteria that belong to the resident flora of the intestinal tract of humans and animals and are ubiquitous in the environment. The pathogenicity of individual strains varies depending on pathogen virulence factors and their interplay with host immunity.

In humans, diarrhea caused by virulent pathotypes can be acute, severe, watery, mucoid, bloody, or persistent and possibly complicated by hemolytic uremic syndrome. Extraintestinal pathogenic *E. coli* (ExPEC) is the most common cause of UTIs in people and can cause a variety of other infections, such as sepsis, pneumonia, and arthritis. High-risk individuals are at increased risk of infection and severe disease.[134]

Human-, dog- and cat-derived *E. coli* strains share similar resistance patterns, genotypes, and virulence factors, which suggests the possibility of zoonotic transmission.[135,136] Transmission of enterohemorrhagic *E. coli* (0157) from a dog to a sick child was implicated in one report. Two family dogs and cattle on a farm were colonized with the same strain as the child. No contact between the cattle and child was reported, but close contact between the dogs and child had occurred.[137]

Humans are most often infected as a result of consumption of contaminated food or exposure to other humans with diarrhea, and confirmed transmission from dogs and cats has not been reported. However, humans, dogs, and cats can share pathogenic types of *E. coli*. Because high-risk individuals are at increased risk for clinical illness and complications, these individuals should practice a high level of hygiene to reduce fecal-oral transmission. This includes frequent hand washing after animal fecal exposure, frequent removal and disposal of pets' feces, preferably by an immunocompetent individual, ensuring pets remain clean of urine and fecal material, and ensuring that sick pets are promptly seen by a veterinarian for early diagnosis and treatment. Raw or inadequately cooked diets, especially with meat or poultry ingredients, and unpasteurized dairy products are known potential sources of *E. coli* and should not be fed to pets who come into contact with high-risk people.

Giardiasis

The cause of giardiasis is *Giardia duodenalis*, a ubiquitous, extracellular protozoan found in the intestinal tracts of vertebrate animals and humans. *Giardia duodenalis* has been categorized into seven genetic assemblages (A–G), each adapted to a specific range of hosts. Humans can be infected with assemblages A1, A2, and B. Dogs can be infected with assemblages A1, B, C, and D. Cats can be infected with assemblages A1 and F. Rarely, dog- and cat-specific assemblages infect people.[138]

Giardiasis is reported most frequently in young children.[139] The primary sign in immunocompetent humans is watery, foul-smelling diarrhea with flatus and abdominal distention. Asymptomatic shedding can occur and is usually self-limiting. Patients with immunodeficiencies, such as common variable immunodeficiency and X-linked agammaglobulinemia, a history of gastric surgery, reduced gastric acid, and lymphoma have increased risk of infection and are often more difficult to treat.[140] AIDS patients are not at increased risk of infection, but can be refractory to treatment, with development of chronic diarrhea and malabsorption.[33]

Zoonotic transmission from dogs and cats is most likely to result from direct fecal contamination.[141] Because assemblage determination is not currently practical in a clinical setting, any infected dog or cat should be considered a potential source of infection for humans. Dogs and cats younger than 6 months of age and those with diarrhea are most commonly shedding *Giardia* and should be avoided as pets by high-risk people.[142] Off-leash park practices have been associated with an increased risk for *Giardia* shedding in dogs, therefore should also be avoided by such individuals.[143] Infected humans are of equal or greater concern as a potential source of infection to high-risk individuals and should generally be the first line of consideration when investigating illness in a person or instituting prevention measures. High-risk people should avoid contact with animal fecal material; if contact is required, gloves should be worm and hands washed immediately afterward.

Leptospirosis

Leptospirosis is caused by several serovars of the spirochete *Leptospira interrogans* that can infect dogs, cats, and a wide variety of other animals. Spirochetes are shed in the urine into water or moist environments. Humans become infected by contact of their mucous membranes, cuts, or skin abrasions with contaminated water or urine. The clinical signs of leptospirosis in people can vary widely from an inapparent influenza-like illness to a severe fatal disease with hepatic and renal failure as well as hemorrhagic pneumonia.

Infected dogs have been reported as the source of infection for people, although such reports are poorly documented in the literature.[144] Precautions for high-risk people include limiting exposure of pets by keeping cats indoors and dogs in a fenced yard or on a leash when outdoors, promptly seeking diagnosis and treatment for illness in pets, and vaccinating dogs against leptospirosis. Shortly after treatment with appropriate antimicrobial drugs (i.e., 48 hours), the urine of infected dogs is no longer likely to be infectious; therefore, prompt recognition and treatment is critical in reducing zoonotic risk.[144]

Malassezia pachydermatis Infection

Malassezia pachydermatis is a ubiquitous, lipophilic, commensal yeast found on the skin and mucocutaneous areas of animals, including dogs and cats. This yeast species most frequently colonizes dogs, whereas cats are colonized by this and other *Malassezia* species. *Malassezia* can be transmitted to humans through direct contact. One study[145] suggested that humans become contaminated with *M. pachydermatis* while contacting dogs with or without dermatitis. In this study, PCR detected *M. pachydermatis* on approximately 93% of the human participants. Although *M. pachydermatis* can colonize humans exposed to pets, clinical manifestations are most common in infants and immunocompromised adults.[146]

Malassezia pachydermatis is not a normal skin commensal in humans; however, humans can harbor it subclinically. *Malassezia pachydermatis* was identified as a cause of nosocomial infection in 15 infants in a hospital ICU.[147] It was isolated from the blood, urinary tract, CSF, tracheal aspirates, skin, and an intravenous catheter tip from affected infants. The source of infection was not certain, but it was considered likely that the infection was transmitted by healthcare workers infected by their pet dogs at home. All 15 isolates from the infants, the hands of one nurse, and skin of three of the healthcare workers' pet dogs that were sampled had matching genotypes of *M. pachydermatis* isolates. Improving hand washing stopped the spread of this infection cluster.[147]

Multidrug-Resistant Bacterial Infections

An estimated 2.8 million people annually in the United States develop MDR bacterial infections and at least 35,000 people die as a direct result of these infections.[94] The level of evidence for transmission between pets and people varies with the bacterial species. It is currently thought that many of these MDR bacteria are predominantly human pathogens, with people serving as the main reservoir, but that household pets can become colonized or infected, thus serving as a secondary source for human infection.

Methicillin-Resistant Staphylococcal Infections

Staphylococcus aureus is a human-adapted commensal that causes opportunistic infections. *Staphylococcus aureus* can also infect other animal species, including dogs and cats. MRSA has become an important public health concern due to its antimicrobial resistance to beta-lactam antimicrobials, and often to additional antimicrobial classes. MRSA is usually harbored by humans in their nasal passages, notably healthcare workers including veterinarians, who may develop infections or remain colonized for extended periods and inadvertently transmit the pathogen to others. Transfer of MRSA can also occur between humans and animals.[63] Although transfer can be bidirectional, humans are the most important source of MRSA for dogs or cats in human hospital, veterinary hospital, and community settings.[63,98,148,149] For example, dogs that visited human healthcare facilities were at five times the risk of acquiring MRSA than dogs involved in other interventions.[98]

In contrast, *Staphylococcus pseudintermedius* is the most common commensal of the skin of dogs. Reports of this organism causing infection and disease in humans are rare, but anecdotally increasing, and in some instances, isolates from diseased humans have been methicillin-resistant (MRSP), making therapy difficult.[150]

Judicious use of antimicrobials by veterinarians and physicians and strict infection control practices, especially hand hygiene, can help reduce the chance of MRSA and MRSP infections spreading among animal health workers in veterinary practices as well as to pet owners. High-risk individuals who live with dogs or cats that are known to be infected or colonized with MRSP or MRSA should perform hand hygiene immediately after pet contact and avoid contact with any infected sites on the animal.

Other Multidrug-Resistant Infections

Extended-spectrum beta-lactamases (ESBLs) are plasmid-mediated enzymes that hydrolyze beta-lactams and critical third-generation cephalosporins used to treat resistant bacterial infections in humans, thus inactivating a wide range of antimicrobials. ESBL-producing members of the order Enterobacterales (e.g., *E. coli*, *Klebsiella pneumoniae*, *Salmonella*) have become a focus of public health due to an increased frequency of human infections with these organisms, treatment challenges, and extension of infections into both hospital and community settings. Clinical manifestations are similar to those for nonresistant organisms, including UTI, bacteremia, splenic abscess, and sepsis. Although less widespread than in humans, ESBL-producing Enterobacterales have now been identified in dogs and cats.[151,152] Pet ownership has been documented as a risk factor for ESBL colonization in people.[153] Further, identical pulse field gel electrophoresis (PFGE) profiles of ESBL *E. coli* were detected in 9.5% (4/42) of isolate pairs from dogs and owners.[135] Resistance to other important antimicrobial classes (e.g., carbapenem, colistin) has recently been identified in companion animals.[154–157] Transmission of these organisms between people and their pets is possible and represents an important public health concern.[157]

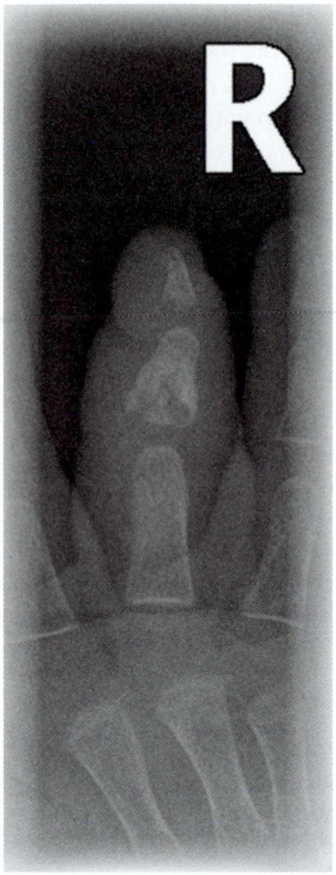

Fig. 19.4 Radiograph showing osteomyelitis (presumed *Pasteurella*) of the finger following a cat bite in a 4-month-old child. (Photograph courtesy of Jason Brophy, Ottawa, Ontario, Canada.)

Pasteurellosis

Pasteurella multocida is a gram-negative coccobacillus that colonizes the oral cavities of cats and dogs. *Pasteurella multocida* is a leading cause of animal bite wound infections in both immunocompetent and high-risk individuals. Like immunocompetent individuals, high-risk individuals also develop local soft tissue infections but are predisposed to develop more invasive, systemic infections, including sepsis, pneumonia, osteomyelitis, endocarditis, and meningitis (Fig. 19.4). Human infants less than 1 month of age who are exposed to dogs or cats appear to have a high risk for severe disease, with predisposition to meningitis.[158] In infants, most cases involve nontraumatic contact between the child and pet (e.g., licking or sniffing).[158] Nonbite exposures (e.g., scratches or lick contamination of mucous membranes, open wounds, or surgical sites) are also reported in adults, especially those at high risk for pet-associated infections.[159,160] Cirrhosis of the liver is one of the most common predisposing conditions associated with severe *Pasteurella* infections in adults,[161] but other predisposing conditions such as neoplasia, organ transplantation, recent joint implants, and polycystic kidney disease have been reported.[159,160] The elderly may also be predisposed to complications and death following *Pasteurella* infection, with an 8% fatality proportion in one study.[162] Severe *Pasteurella* peritonitis among individuals undergoing peritoneal dialysis who own pets (notably cats) has been reported, drawing attention to the need of educating patients on strict hygiene measures and avoiding pet contact with the dialysis equipment (especially in bag exchange areas).[163,164] The urgency of seeking treatment is illustrated by a case report of a 64-year-old man with cirrhosis who developed sepsis after a cat bite. Although he did seek medical care, it was 48 hours after the bite, and he died within 72 hours of the bite.[165]

Prevention measures focus on bite and scratch avoidance and prompt wound treatment. Pets should never be permitted to lick or otherwise have contact with wounds, surgery sites, dialysis or similar healthcare equipment, or skin lesions or be permitted to lick faces or ears of high-risk people.

Salmonellosis

Salmonella spp., a gram-negative, facultative anaerobic, rod-shaped bacterial species, infects mammals, birds, reptiles, amphibians, fish, and invertebrates. Exposure to contaminated food, such as meat and eggs, account for most human infections. The most well-known pet-related exposures have occurred with reptiles (notably turtles) and amphibians, in part due to their high frequency of subclinical carriage.[166,167] Healthy dogs and cats that live in low-stress environments are unlikely to be colonized with *Salmonella*; however, some factors increase colonization prevalence. Animals that are more likely to shed *Salmonella* include cats that have access to the outdoors and prey on wild birds,[131] young, debilitated, stressed, or immunocompromised dogs and cats[168] and those fed raw food diets containing meat or poultry, both commercial and homemade.[169,170] In one study, risk factors for *Salmonella* colonization in dogs were contact with livestock; treatment with a probiotic in the past 30 days; consumption of a commercial or homemade raw food diet, raw meat and eggs, or a homemade cooked diet; or the presence of more than one dog in a household.[171] Pets generally shed *Salmonella* in feces, although bacteriuria has been reported and potentially poses a human health risk.[172]

Salmonella-infected dogs and cats are usually subclinically infected or have acute diarrhea, but severe disease can occur. Symptoms in humans vary from a self-limiting gastroenteritis to bacteremia, fever, septic arthritis, abscesses, endocarditis, meningitis, or pneumonia. Immunocompromised people, young children, and older adults are predisposed to clinical illness. In addition to enteritis, high-risk individuals often suffer from extraintestinal infections (e.g., endocarditis, bacteremia, and sepsis).[173,174] People infected with HIV are at 20–100 times greater risk of *Salmonella* bacteremia than those without HIV infection.[18]

Animals that reside with high-risk individuals should only be fed canned or dry commercial food or well-cooked homemade food. Any dairy or animal-based (egg, meat) products or treats should be cooked or (high-pressure) pasteurized. If raw or undercooked products are fed, care should be taken to reduce cross-contamination during food preparation or feeding, and high-risk individuals should not have contact with animal feces. The use of stainless steel bowls for feeding, which are easier to disinfect, and gloves during feces clean-up are advised. Hands should be washed immediately after contact with animal feces, whether or not gloves are worn. Cats should be kept indoors.

Reptile-associated salmonellosis in high-risk individuals is often severe and can lead to bacteremia and meningitis, which can be fatal. High-risk people should avoid contact with reptiles, amphibians, exotic species (e.g., hedgehogs), rodents, young chicks, and ducklings and should exercise caution when visiting petting zoos or farms.[175–178]

Strongyloidiasis

Strongyloides stercoralis, sometimes referred to as the human threadworm, is a nematode found in the tropics, subtropics, and limited foci within the United States and Europe.[179] Humans are the principle hosts, although dogs (and rarely cats) can be infected and potentially serve as a source for human infection.[180] Young puppies, especially those housed in groups, are most likely to be infected.[181,182] Humans generally become infected with *S. stercoralis* from penetration of the skin by infective larvae in the soil.

In immunocompetent humans, most strongyloidiasis infections are asymptomatic. Occasionally, a localized, pruritic rash starting at the site of larval penetration occurs. Signs may progress to diarrhea and abdominal pain, with chronic infections leading to pruritis around the anus and perineum.[183] Immunocompromised individuals are at increased risk for severe, complicated strongyloidiasis, including hyperinfection and disseminated strongyloidiasis syndromes. The greatest risk factor for severe infection is high-dose glucocorticoid use, although other immunocompromising conditions including neoplasia and human T-cell lymphotropic virus-1 infection also increase disease risk.[179,184,185] In cases of severe strongyloidiasis, gastrointestinal symptoms are common, including abdominal pain, nausea, vomiting, diarrhea, and ileus, which can lead to intestinal obstruction. Ulceration of the intestinal mucosa can produce hemorrhage, peritonitis, and sepsis. Cough, hemoptysis, respiratory difficulties, and meningitis can result from migrating larvae.[183] High mortality (approaching 100%) is associated with untreated disseminated strongyloidiasis, and even with treatment mortality may exceed 25%.[179]

Dogs and cats likely have a minimal role in human strongyloidiasis. There is limited existing evidence of zoonotic transmission. In one study, an individual who worked in a dog colony was diagnosed with strongyloidiasis, and dogs in the facility were subsequently shown to be shedding *S. stercoralis* in their feces.[182] Individuals (especially those who are immunocompromised) who work closely with large groups of young dogs, such as breeding kennel and pet store workers, are likely those at any reasonable zoonotic risk for *S. stercoralis*. In these situations, measures to reduce individuals' exposure to dog feces will reduce any dog-associated *S. stercoralis* risk.

Toxocariasis

Toxocara canis and *Toxocara cati* are roundworms (ascarids) of the dog and cat, respectively. Nonembryonated eggs are passed in feces by dogs and cats into the environment where they become infective after several weeks. Humans become infected through consumption of infective eggs (e.g., contaminated soil, tissues of infected animals such as cattle and birds, contaminated fruits, and vegetables).[186] Human infections occur wherever there are dogs and cats. Given the time required for eggs to become infective, direct exposure with infected dogs and cats is of limited transmission potential, although there is some concern for contaminated dog/cat hair to serve as a source of human infection.[187] Contamination of the outdoor environment is common in many regions, and infective eggs are able to survive for extended periods under extreme climatic conditions leading to high levels of contamination and risk of human exposure.[188]

Although exposure to *Toxocara* spp. and subsequent antibody development is common, clinical disease is generally rare.[189] Adults do not typically develop clinical disease, while children, especially those with a history of pica or living in unsanitary conditions, appear to be at the greatest risk for toxocariasis.[189,190] VLM, where infective *Toxocara* spp. larvae migrate throughout the tissues of the infected person, may present as cough, fever, headache, wheezing, and seizures. Children under 6 years of age are most frequently diagnosed with VLM.[189] Ocular larval migrans (OLM), where infective larvae migrate into the eye, often presents as unilateral vision loss or strabismus with endophthalmitis, retinitis, chorioretinal granuloma, or retinal detachment. Children diagnosed with OLM are generally older than those diagnosed with VLM.[186,189]

Proper deworming of cats and dogs (especially of puppies, kittens, bitches, and nursing dams) is important to reduce environmental contamination and zoonotic risk.[191] Given the required time for eggs to become infective, prompt removal of feces further reduces zoonotic risks. As human infection relies on consumption of infective eggs, hand washing especially following contact with high-risk material (e.g., puppy/kitten environments, soil) and prohibiting pica are critical to human disease prevention.

Toxoplasmosis

Toxoplasma gondii is an obligate intracellular protozoan found worldwide. Although cats are the definitive hosts for the organism, humans can acquire infection through consumption of raw or undercooked meat, from vertical transmission to the fetus during pregnancy, and from soil contaminated with cat feces.[192] Although toxoplasmosis can be acquired by ingestion of oocysts shed by infected cats, infection in humans living in industrialized countries is usually caused by ingestion of undercooked meats, especially goat, mutton, or pork.[193]

In immunocompetent humans, *T. gondii* infection is often asymptomatic, whereas in others a self-limiting lymphadenopathy or mild influenza-like illness develops. In contrast, immunosuppressed individuals may develop serious illness with encephalitis, pneumonitis, or myocarditis. The unborn fetus, individuals with HIV-AIDS, or those on chemotherapy are at particular high risk for complications.

Congenital human toxoplasmosis is typically the result of an acute asymptomatic infection in the mother, and the risk of transmission to the fetus is dependent on the stage of pregnancy. The chance of transmission to the fetus is approximately 25% if the mother is exposed in the first trimester, 55% in the second trimester, and 65% in the third.[194] If the mother is infected early in pregnancy, spontaneous abortion, premature delivery, or stillbirth may result. Features seen in infants born to women infected later in pregnancy include fever, microcephaly, hydrocephalus, hepatosplenomegaly, jaundice, seizures, and chorioretinitis. Some infants are asymptomatic at birth and develop complications months, or even years, later. Results from a combination of serologic tests are needed to accurately determine whether a pregnant female or her fetus is infected.

Immunocompromised individuals, notably those with HIV-AIDS and cancer, are at approximately twice the risk of *T. gondii* infection compared with immunocompetent individuals.[195] Toxoplasmosis affects approximately 10% of AIDS patients and is thought to be responsible for at least 30% of CNS complications.[196] CNS involvement may result in focal neurologic deficits, cognitive dysfunction, and altered mental status in patients in late stages of HIV infection.[196] Individuals with cancer, particularly with bone marrow cancer, or those who receive organ transplantation or long-term glucocorticoid therapy are vulnerable to infection. Importantly, most cases of CNS toxoplasmosis are a result of reactivation of latent infections (often acquired through consumption of undercooked meat) rather than recent exposure.

The overall risk of becoming infected by cats in the urban household is low when compared with other modes of exposure (e.g., soil, food).[192,197] Oocysts must sporulate to be infectious, a process that takes 1 to 5 days. Because feces do not generally remain on the fur, direct contact with cats is an unlikely source of infection. Because of their environmental resistance, oocysts can enter the freshwater and marine water supplies and cause disease in humans or animals that ingest contaminated water or invertebrates harboring these organisms. Outbreaks have been associated with contamination of municipal water supplies by oocysts from feral or wild felids.[195–201]

Immunosuppressed people should wear gloves and wash their hands after contact with soil or raw meat. Cat litter boxes should be changed daily, preferably by an immunocompetent person. Hands should be washed after changing the litter box, gardening, or after other contact with the soil. All raw fruits and vegetables should be washed well before consumption, and raw meats should not contact foods that are to be eaten raw or cutting boards used to prepare them. Sandboxes should be covered when not in use.

In order to reduce exposure, cats of immunocompromised people should be kept inside and fed only commercial diets or well-cooked home-prepared diets. Patients do not have to part with their cats or have them tested for toxoplasmosis, either serologically or by fecal examination. However, cats that have serologic positive test results are likely protected from oocyst shedding because shedding is transient and generally occurs only after initial exposure. Despite the infrequency of cat-associated toxoplasmosis, many physicians, including obstetrician-gynecologists, still focus on cat litter disposal measures and overlook other potential sources of food ingestion or environmental exposure.[202] Veterinarians should be prepared to discuss this important topic with misinformed clients and healthcare professionals.

Tularemia

Francisella tularensis is an intracellular, highly pleomorphic, gram-negative coccobacillus, which is endemic in many regions of the world. The organism is typically found in lagomorphs (rabbits and hares), rodents, and arthropods. *Francisella tularensis* is transmissible to humans in infectious doses as low as 10 to 50 bacteria when inhaled. Both immunocompetent and immunocompromised people are affected; the clinical presentation ranges from cutaneous ulcers to pneumonia and rarely death. Individuals with advanced age, alcohol abuse, diabetes mellitus, organ transplantation, and AIDS are more likely to have severe infection.[203–205]

Although most human cases occur following arthropod bites and contaminated aerosols (e.g., aerosols generated by mowing over infected rabbit carcasses), more than 70 human cases of tularemia acquired from cats and dogs have been reported.[206–208] Both clinically healthy and sick cats and dogs can transmit tularemia; some cases involved a bite, but in others, casual contact was the only exposure.[207] Transmission to humans is likely due to the presence of organisms in an animal's mouth or claws.

Prevention of tularemia is primarily through reduction of the risk of tick and other arthropod bites to people and pets. Individuals such as hunters who handle potentially infected animals should wear gloves to prevent the introduction of the organism through cuts or abrasions, and game meat should be cooked. To prevent aerosol exposure, dead animals should be removed from grassy areas before mowing. Control of arthropod vectors, prevention of hunting by cats and dogs (e.g., by keeping cats indoors, control of dogs when outdoors), and prevention of cat bites and scratches in areas where tularemia is endemic are the primary means of reducing the infection risk from pets.

Vector-Borne Infections

Numerous arthropods transmit infections to people (e.g., RMSF, ehrlichiosis, Lyme borreliosis). The mammalian reservoirs of these infections are often wildlife species, and dogs and cats are not a direct source of infections for humans. Instead, they act as sentinels for infection, or they bring the shared vectors closer to humans. Sufficient duration of tick attachment is important in the successful transmission of many of these diseases. Therefore, good ectoparasite control for humans and pets can help to reduce the threat of infection.

Other Zoonoses

Numerous other pathogens have been identified as or suspected to be transmitted from cats or dogs to people (see Box 19.2). To date, these other pet-associated infections have not been documented with any greater frequency in high-risk individuals than in the general population; however, this area is currently under continued investigation. New zoonotic pathogens emerge and the epidemiology of existing zoonotic pathogens evolve, highlighting the importance of continued surveillance, research, and education in this rapidly changing and complex field. As an example, in 2020 the SARS-CoV-2 virus rapidly spread throughout the world resulting in the COVID-19 pandemic. While suspected to be of animal origin, COVID-19 spread predominately human-to-human. Yet, infection and illness in household pets was documented (transmitted from infectious people, anthroponoses) underscoring the close connection between human and pet infectious diseases. The references at the end of this chapter and the Public Health Considerations sections in other chapters in this book provide a more extensive review of all companion animal-associated zoonoses.

RECOMMENDATIONS ON ANIMAL OWNERSHIP AND CONTACT FOR HIGH-RISK INDIVIDUALS

Recommendations for animal ownership and contact have been established for patients in high-risk groups (see Box 19.3).[3,13,25,33–38] Guidelines are also available for animal-assisted interventions in healthcare facilities[209,210] and animals housed or visiting schools and other public settings.[176] Recommendations target common exposure routes and disease risk and severity. Human and veterinary healthcare providers should provide advice in a manner that is sensitive to the possible psychological benefits of pet ownership. It is rarely necessary for a high-risk individual to part with pets. In most cases, handling pets does not pose more risk for high-risk individuals than contact with other people or the environment. However, simple measures can further reduce the risk of pet-associated zoonoses. Many factors that increase the propensity of animals to carry pathogens (exposure to pathogens through food/water, other domestic animals, wildlife or the environment) are modifiable. Further, owners can often institute routines that reduce the chance of exposure to a pathogen from their companion animals.

Pet Selection

Because infectious diseases, including zoonoses, are more prevalent in puppies or kittens, when acquiring a new pet, households with high-risk individuals should seek mature, healthy dogs or cats with a known history from established vendors. Stray animals or animals being housed in areas of high population density, such as humane shelters, pet-breeding facilities, pounds, puppy or kitten mills, or crowded pet stores, are more likely to harbor pathogens. High-risk individuals should avoid contact with dogs and cats less than 6 months of age. Contact with, or purchase of reptiles, amphibians, rodents, exotic species (e.g., hedgehogs), and young poultry (e.g., chicks) should be avoided. Any newly acquired pet should be examined by a veterinarian before being introduced to a household, especially one with high-risk individuals. In some cases, individuals may wish to wait to acquire a new pet, such as if an individual's immunocompromised state is transient or variable until immune suppression is stable.

Personal Hygiene

High-risk people should perform hand hygiene (wash their hands with soap and water or use alcohol-based hand sanitizer) frequently, and always after handling pets or pet excretions. Hand hygiene is especially important before touching mucous membranes or other vulnerable sites—this includes before eating, smoking, performing dental hygiene, and having contact with medical devices and corrective lenses. Any bites or scratches from animals should be promptly washed. Given the increased risk for infections, high-risk individuals should promptly consult with their healthcare provider regarding the need for antimicrobial prophylaxis following bites or scratches. Pets should be strictly prohibited from licking open wounds, broken skin, mucous membranes (i.e., face licking), or medical devices such as intravascular catheters. Saliva should be washed from hands or open wounds. Rubber gloves should be worn by high-risk individuals when oral medication is given to pets, or someone else should assume these responsibilities. Bite wounds are probably the most common health risk faced by high-risk individuals. Pets that are aggressive in behavior or play should not be kept by households with high-risk people, and such households should take concerted efforts to reduce development of such behaviors through early training. Children should be taught not to startle feeding or sleeping animals.

Handling of Excrement

High-risk people should reduce contact with pet feces and animal-derived pet treats by use of gloves or a plastic bag, or another immunocompetent household member should perform these tasks. Hands should be washed after gloves are removed. Diarrheic stools are particularly challenging to remove without becoming exposed to enteropathogens. Animals with diarrhea should be bathed as needed. If contact cannot be avoided, high-risk individuals should wear rubber gloves during cleaning of diarrheic or other stools and use household bleach (5.25% sodium hypochlorite solution) at a dilution of 1 ounce per quart of water (1750 ppm) and 10 minutes of contact time for disinfection. Similar precautions can be recommended for handling other body fluids, including blood, urine, and saliva.

Daily cleaning of feline litter boxes can prevent *Toxoplasma* infection. Feline litter boxes should not be placed in food preparation areas and should be cleaned by a nonpregnant, immunocompetent adult. Creation of litter box dust can be avoided by using bag liners and dust-free litter. Although the litter box should be emptied outdoors or in well-ventilated areas to prevent inhalation, litter should be directed to a landfill and not placed directly into the environment. Cats should be prevented from jumping on kitchen counters or dining tables.

Dogs should be discouraged from coprophagia or drinking from the toilet. Within communities, animals should be restricted from defecating in child play areas, including playgrounds. Parks should have well-marked, designated areas for pets, playground sandboxes should be kept covered when not in use, and owners should promptly pick up and properly dispose of their pets' excrement. Children should be closely observed in certain environments to avoid pica, and should be taught (and observed) to effectively wash their hands, especially after playing in soil or having higher-risk contact with animals or the environment.

Care of Pets Owned by High-Risk Individuals

Pets in households with high-risk individuals should receive routine vaccinations and routine screening and prevention for endoparasites and ectoparasites based on history and lifestyle. Pets should be neutered to decrease roaming tendencies and behavioral problems. Serologic testing for FeLV and FIV is recommended for cats. Although FeLV and FIV pose no chance of infecting humans, infected cats are more susceptible to other infectious diseases, including zoonoses. Yearly physical examinations are important to maintain the health of the pet. Veterinary attention should be sought immediately for any pet that develops illness. Pets should be bathed regularly if needed, and the haircoat should be brushed regularly and matted fur removed. Claws should be trimmed on a regular basis to reduce the chance of scratch injuries, but declawing of cats is not indicated. Routine visual inspection for ticks and fleas is indicated based on the area and lifestyle of the pet. For ticks, pets should be checked daily or immediately after leaving tick-infested areas. Any attached ticks should be removed with gloves, a tick removal device, or tweezers, and hands should be washed after removal. Ticks should not be removed or crushed with bare, exposed hands.

Only canned or dry commercial food or well-cooked home-prepared food should be fed to pets in households with high-risk individuals. Dairy or animal-based (egg, meat) products or treats should be cooked or (high-pressure) pasteurized. Pets should be fed in a designated nonkitchen area to reduce opportunities for cross-contamination between pet food, human food, and common human-touch surfaces near eating locations. Pets should be prevented from coprophagia, scavenging, hunting, and feeding on carrion or garbage. They may need to be leashed or confined, or be supervised outdoors. Cats should be kept indoors or bells placed on their collars to scare prey and other wildlife. Access to outside surface water or toilet bowl water should be restricted.

Additional Recommendations for High-Risk Workers in Veterinary Clinics and Other High Animal-Contact Settings

High-risk workers in veterinary clinics and other animal-contact settings should discuss any necessary work restrictions and precautions with their physician. In general, high-risk individuals in these settings should avoid handling animals with suspected or known zoonotic diseases. Such individuals should strictly follow infection control principles, including hand hygiene and use of personal protective equipment (e.g., single use gloves, gowns). Based on the level of immunosuppression, routine glove use should be considered when handling all animals; however, strict hand hygiene after every patient contact and immediately after glove removal is most important. Gloves should always be worn when having contact with animal fluids, wounds, or feces (e.g., when performing a complete physical examination). Prevention of animal bites, scratches, and sharps injuries is important. Training for all staff on pet-associated zoonotic disease risks and prevention within and outside the veterinary clinic should be required and documented. Staff knowledge on this topic should be periodically assessed.

Animals in Human Healthcare Facilities

Dogs and cats are frequently permitted to enter human healthcare facilities and interact with human patients.[210–212] Zoonotic disease protocols at facilities are often lacking, or those responsible for the animals may have limited understanding of zoonotic diseases and prevention measures.[213] Zoonotic disease outbreaks associated with animals in healthcare have been described.[85,210] Guidelines are available to reduce the risk of zoonotic disease transmission in healthcare environments.[209,210,214] These recommendations incorporate recommendations for households with high-risk members, with a few important additions. In healthcare facilities, only dogs (not cats) should be used for animal-assisted activities. Dogs should be at least 1 year (ideally 2 years) of age, kept on leash at all times, have passed a temperament evaluation specific for the encountered conditions, should be healthy (i.e., without history of vomiting or diarrhea within the past week and no known or suspected communicable diseases), and not been fed in the past 90 days raw or dehydrated foods or treats of animal origin (excluding those high-pressure pasteurized or γ-irradiated). Hand hygiene should occur and be stressed before and after every animal contact. The reader is referred to specific guidelines for additional information such as required training for handlers, restricted areas within healthcare facilities, and recommendations for other animal groups, such as service animals, research animals, and personal pet visitation.[210]

SUGGESTED READINGS

Harpaz R, Dahl RM, Dooling KL. Prevalence of immunosuppression among US adults, 2013. *J Am Med Assoc*. 2016;316:2547–2548.

Babcock S, Marsh AE, Lin J, et al. Legal implications of zoonoses for clinical veterinarians. *J Am Vet Med Assoc*. 2008;233:1556–1562.

REFERENCES

1. McNicholl J. Host genes and infectious diseases. *Emerg Infect Dis*. 1998;4:423–426.
2. Harpaz R, Dahl RM, Dooling KL. Prevalence of immunosuppression among US adults, 2013. *J Am Med Assoc*. 2016;316:2547–2548.
3. Mani I, Maguire JH. Small animal zoonoses and immuncompromised pet owners. *Topic Comp Anim Med*. 2009;24:164–174.
4. Kourtis AP, Read JS, Jamieson DJ. Pregnancy and infection. *N Engl J Med*. 2014;371:1077.
5. Abbas AK, Lichtman AH, Pillai S. *Congenital and Acquired Immunodeficiencies. Cellular and Molecular Immunology*. Philadelphia: Saunders; 2007:463–488.
6. Sauteur PM, Relly C, Hug M, et al. Risk factors for invasive reptile associated salmonellosis in children. *Vector Borne Zoonotic Dis*. 2013;13:419–421.
7. Stull JW, Peregrine AS, Sargeant JM, et al. Pet husbandry and infection control practices related to zoonotic disease risks in Ontario, Canada. *BMC Publ Health*. 2013;13:520.
8. Centers for Disease Control and Prevention. HIV in the United States and Dependent Areas. https://www.cdc.gov/hiv/statistics/overview/ataglance.html.
9. US Department of Health and Human Services. Organ Procurement and Transplantation Network. https://optn.transplant.hrsa.gov/.
10. Sumaraju V, Smith LG, Smith SM. Infectious complications in asplenic hosts. *Infect Dis Clin North Am*. 2001;15:551–565.
11. Ventura SJ, Curtin SC, Abma JC, et al. Estimated pregnancy rates and rates of pregnancy outcomes for the United States, 1990-2008. *Natl Vital Stat Rep*. 2012;60:1–21.
12. Stull JW, Peregrine AS, Sargeant JM, et al. Household knowledge, attitudes and practices related to pet contact and associated zoonoses in Ontario, Canada. *BMC Publ Health*. 2012;12:553.
13. Trevejo RT, Barr MC, Robinson RA. Important emerging bacterial zoonotic infections affecting the immunocompromised. *Vet Res*. 2005;36:493–506.
14. Stull JW, Brophy J, Sargeant JM, et al. Knowledge, attitudes, and practices related to pet contact by immunocompromised children with cancer and immunocompetent children with diabetes. *J Pediatr*. 2014;165:348–355 e342.
15. Conti L, Lieb S, Liberti T, et al. Pet ownership among persons with AIDS in three Florida counties. *Am J Public Health*. 1995;85:1559–1561.
16. Abarca VK, Lopez Del PJ, Pena DA, et al. Pet ownership and health status of pets from immunocompromised children, with emphasis in zoonotic diseases. *Rev Chilena Infectol*. 2011;28:205–210.
17. Hubalek Z. Emerging human infectious diseases: anthroponoses, zoonoses, and sapronoses. *Emerg Infect Dis*. 2003;9:403–404.
18. Hung CC, Hung MN, Hsueh PR, et al. Risk of recurrent nontyphoid *Salmonella* bacteremia in HIV–infected patients in the era of highly active antiretroviral therapy and an increasing trend of fluoroquinolone resistance. *Clin Infect Dis*. 2007;45:e60–e67.
19. Gradel KO, Norgaard M, Dethlefsen C, et al. Increased risk of zoonotic *Salmonella* and *Campylobacter* gastroenteritis in patients with haematological malignancies: a population-based study. *Ann Hematol*. 2009;88:761–767.
20. Gaastra W, Lipman LJ. *Capnocytophaga canimorsus*. *Vet Microbiol*. 2010;140:339–346.

21. Ner Z, Ross LA, Horn MV, et al. *Bordetella bronchiseptica* infection in pediatric lung transplant recipients. *Pediatr Transplant.* 2003;7:413–417.
22. Hale CR, Scallan E, Cronquist AB, et al. Estimates of enteric illness attributable to contact with animals and their environments in the United States. *Clin Infect Dis.* 2012;54(suppl 5):S472–S479.
23. Whitfield Y, Johnson K, Hobbs L, et al. Descriptive study of enteric zoonoses in Ontario, Canada, from 2010 - 2012. *BMC Publ Health.* 2017;17(1):217.
24. Day MJ, Breitschwerdt E, Cleaveland S, et al. Surveillance of zoonotic infectious disease transmitted by small companion animals. *Emerg Infect Dis.* 2012;18:e1.
25. Angulo FJ, Glaser CA, Juranek DD, et al. Caring for pets of immunocompromised persons. *Can Vet J.* 1995;36:217–222.
26. Rijks JM, Cito F, Cunningham AA, et al. Disease risk assessments involving companion animals: an overview for 15 selected pathogens taking a European perspective. *J Comp Pathol.* 2016;155:S75–S97.
27. Lothstein K, Fisher B, Li Y, et al. Zoonotic infections in pediatric patients with acute leukemia. *Pediatr Blood Cancer.* 2013;60:E160–E162.
28. Hill WA, Petty GC, Erwin PC, et al. A survey of Tennessee veterinarian and physician attitudes, knowledge, and practices regarding zoonoses prevention among animal owners with HIV infection or AIDS. *J Am Vet Med Assoc.* 2012;240:1432–1440.
29. Lipton BA, Hopkins SG, Koehler JE, et al. A survey of veterinarian involvement in zoonotic disease prevention practices. *J Am Vet Med Assoc.* 2008;233:1242–1249.
30. Grant S, Olsen CW. Preventing zoonotic diseases in immunocompromised persons: the role of physicians and veterinarians. *Emerg Infect Dis.* 1999;5:159–163.
31. Root Kustritz MV, Molgaard LK, Tegzes JH. Frequency of interactions between veterinarians and other professionals to guide interprofessional education. *J Vet Med Educ.* 2013;40:370–377.
32. Gauthier JL, Richardson DJ. Knowledge and attitudes about zoonotic helminths: a survey of Connecticut pediatricians and veterinarians. *Compend Contin Educ Pract Vet.* 2002;24(Suppl):4–9.
33. Glaser CA, Angulo FJ, Rooney JA. Animal-associated opportunistic infections among persons infected with the human immunodeficiency virus. *Clin Infect Dis.* 1994;18:14–24.
34. Pickering LK, Marano N, Bocchini JA, et al. Exposure to nontraditional pets at home and to animals in public settings: risks to children. *Pediatrics.* 2008;122:876–886.
35. Hemsworth S, Pizer B. Pet ownership in immunocompromised children: a review of the literature and survey of existing guidelines. *Eur J Oncol Nurs.* 2006;10:117–127.
36. Yokoe D, Casper C, Dubberke E, et al. Safe living after hematopoietic cell transplantation. *Bone Marrow Transplant.* 2009;44:509–519.
37. Kaplan JE, Benson C, Holmes KH, et al. Guidelines for prevention and treatment of opportunistic infections in HIV-infected adults and adolescents: recommendations from CDC, the National Institutes of Health, and the HIV Medicine Association of the Infectious Diseases Society of America. *Morb Mortal Wkly Rep.* 2009;58:1–207.
38. Avery RK, Michaels MG. Strategies for safe living after solid organ transplantation. *Am J Transplant.* 2013;13:304–310.
39. US Department of Health and Human Services. Health Information Privacy; 2017. https://www.hhs.gov/hipaa/index.html.
40. Stull JW, Landers T. Bridging the veterinary–human healthcare communication divide. *Clinician's Brief.* 2017:50–53.
41. Haagsma JA, Tariq L, Heederik DJ, et al. Infectious disease risks associated with occupational exposure: a systematic review of the literature. *Occ Environ Med.* 2012;69:140–146.
42. Halsby KD, Walsh AL, Campbell C, et al. Healthy animals, healthy people: zoonosis risk from animal contact in pet shops, a systematic review of the literature. *PloS One.* 2014;9:e89309.
43. Sánchez A, Prats-van der Ham M, Tatay-Dualde J, et al. Zoonoses in veterinary students: a systematic review of the literature. *PloS One.* 2017;12:e0169534.
44. Scheftel JM, Elchos BL, Cherry B, et al. Compendium of veterinary standard precautions for zoonotic disease prevention in veterinary personnel: National Association of State Public Health Veterinarians Veterinary Infection Control Committee 2010. *J Am Vet Med Assoc.* 2010;237:1403–1422.
45. Baker WS, Gray GC. A review of published reports regarding zoonotic pathogen infection in veterinarians. *J Am Vet Med Assoc.* 2009;234:1271–1278.
46. Jackson J, Villarroel A. A survey of the risk of zoonoses for veterinarians. *Zoonoses Public Health.* 2012;59:193–201.
47. Fowler HN, Holzbauer SM, Smith KE, et al. Survey of occupational hazards in Minnesota veterinary practices in 2012. *J Am Vet Med Assoc.* 2016;248:207–218.
48. Wright JG, Tengelsen LA, Smith KE, et al. Multidrug-resistant *Salmonella* Typhimurium in four animal facilities. *Emerg Infect Dis.* 2005;11:1235–1241.
49. Cherry B, Burns A, Johnson GS, et al. *Salmonella* Typhimurium outbreak associated with veterinary clinic. *Emerg Infect Dis.* 2004;10:2249–2251.
50. Weese JS, Dick H, Willey BM, et al. Suspected transmission of methicillin-resistant *Staphylococcus aureus* between domestic pets and humans in veterinary clinics and in the household. *Vet Microbiol.* 2006;115:148–155.
51. Venkat H, Yaglom HD, Adams L. Knowledge, attitudes, and practices relevant to zoonotic disease reporting and infection prevention practices among veterinarians - Arizona, 2015. *Prev Vet Med.* 2019;169:104711.
52. Marsh AE, Babcock S. Legal implications of zoonotic disease transmission for veterinary practices. *Vet Clin North Am Small Anim Pract.* 2015;45:393–408 (vii).
53. Babcock S, Marsh AE, Lin J, et al. Legal implications of zoonoses for clinical veterinarians. *J Am Vet Med Assoc.* 2008;233:1556–1562.
54. Williams CJ, Scheftel JM, Elchos BL, et al. Compendium of veterinary standard precautions for zoonotic disease prevention in veterinary personnel: National Association of State Public Health Veterinarians: Veterinary Infection Control Committee 2015. *J Am Vet Med Assoc.* 2015;247:1252–1277.
55. Johnson R. Psychosocial and therapeutic aspects of human-animal interaction. In: Rabinowitz P, Conti L, eds. *Human-Animal Medicine: Clinical Approaches to Zoonoses Toxicants and Other Shared Health Risks.* St Louis, MO: Saunders; 2010:432.
56. Levine GN, Allen K, Braun LT, et al. Pet ownership and cardiovascular risk: a scientific statement from the American Heart Association. *Circulation.* 2013;127:2353–2363.
57. Siegel JM, Angulo FJ, Detels R, et al. AIDS diagnosis and depression in the Multicenter AIDS Cohort Study: the ameliorating impact of pet ownership. *AIDS Care.* 1999;11:157–170.
58. Melson GF. Child development and the human–companion animal bond. *Am Behav Sci.* 2003;47:31–39.
59. Raina P, Waltner-Toews D, Bonnett B, et al. Influence of companion animals on the physical and psychological health of older people: an analysis of a one-year longitudinal study. *J Am Geriatr Soc.* 1999;47:323–329.
60. Melson GF, Schwarz RL, Beck AM. Importance of companion animals in children's lives: implications for veterinary practice. *J Am Vet Med Assoc.* 1997;211:1512–1518.
61. Friedmann E, Thomas SA. Pet ownership, social support, and one-year survival after acute myocardial infarction in the Cardiac Arrhythmia Suppression Trial (CAST). *Am J Cardiol.* 1995;76:1213–1217.
62. Carmack BJ. The role of companion animals for persons with AIDS/HIV. *Holist Nurs Pract.* 1991;5:24–31.
63. Morris DO, Lautenbach E, Zaoutis T, et al. Potential for pet animals to harbour methicillin-resistant *Staphylococcus aureus* when residing with human MRSA patients. *Zoonoses Public Health.* 2012;59:286–293.
64. Breitschwerdt EB. Bartonellosis: one health perspectives for an emerging infectious disease. *ILAR J.* 2014;55:46–58.
65. Nelson CA, Saha S, Mead PS. Cat-scratch disease in the United States, 2005-2013. *Emerg Infect Dis.* 2016;22:1741–1746.
66. Mofenson LM, Brady MT, Danner SP, et al. Guidelines for the prevention and treatment of opportunistic infections among HIV-exposed and HIV-infected children: recommendations from CDC, the National Institutes of Health, the HIV Medicine Association of the Infectious Diseases Society of America, the Pediatric Infectious Diseases Society, and the American Academy of Pediatrics. *Morb Mortal Wkly Rep.* 2009;58:1–166.

67. Wernli D, Emonet S, Schrenzel J, et al. Evaluation of eight cases of confirmed *Bordetella bronchiseptica* infection and colonization over a 15-year period. *Clin Microbiol Infect.* 2011;17:201–203.
68. Gisel JJ, Brumble LM, Johnson MM. *Bordetella bronchiseptica* pneumonia in a kidney-pancreas transplant patient after exposure to recently vaccinated dogs. *Transpl Infect Dis.* 2010;12:73–76.
69. Woolfrey BF, Moody JA. Human infections associated with *Bordetella bronchiseptica. Clin Microbiol Rev.* 1991;4:243–255.
70. Register KB, Sukumar N, Palavecino EL, et al. *Bordetella bronchiseptica* in a paediatric cystic fibrosis patient: possible transmission from a household cat. *Zoonoses Public Health.* 2012;59:246–250.
71. Goldberg JD, Kamboj M, Ford R, et al. 'Kennel cough' in a patient following allogeneic hematopoietic stem cell transplant. *Bone Marrow Transplant.* 2009;44:381–382.
72. Powers HR, Shah K. *Bordetella bronchiseptica* bloodstream infection in a renal transplant patient. *Transpl Infect Dis.* 2017;19(6):e12774.
73. Szvalb AD, Rolston KV, Mori N, et al. Infections with the agent of 'kennel cough' in patients with cancer. *J Infect.* 2019;78(1):48–53.
74. Krueger WS, Lucero NE, Brower A, et al. Evidence for unapparent *Brucella canis* infections among adults with occupational exposure to dogs. *Zoonoses Public Health.* 2014;61:509–518.
75. Lucero NE, Maldonado PI, Kaufman S, et al. *Brucella canis* causing infection in an HIV-infected patient. *Vector Borne Zoonotic Dis.* 2010;10:527–529.
76. Javeri H, Jamieson S, Sehgal R, et al. *Brucella canis* peritonitis. *Infection.* 2014;42:195–197.
77. Lawaczeck E, Toporek J, Cwikla J, et al. *Brucella canis* in a HIV-infected patient. *Zoonoses Public Health.* 2011;58:150–152.
78. Marzetti S, Carranza C, Roncallo M, et al. Recent trends in human *Brucella canis* infection. *Comp Immunol Microbiol Infect Dis.* 2013;36:55–61.
79. Dentinger CM, Jacob K, Lee LV, et al. Human *Brucella canis* infection and subsequent laboratory exposures associated with a puppy, New York City, 2012. *Zoonoses Public Health.* 2015;62:407–414.
80. Lucero NE, Corazza R, Almuzara MN, et al. Human *Brucella canis* outbreak linked to infection in dogs. *Epidemiol Infect.* 2010;138:280–285.
81. National Association of State Public Health Veterinarians. Public Health Implications of *Brucella canis* Infections in Humans; 2012. http://www.nasphv.org/Documents/BrucellaCanisInHumans.pdf.
82. Fullerton KE, Ingram LA, Jones TF, et al. Sporadic *Campylobacter* infection in infants: a population-based surveillance case-control study. *Pediatr Infect Dis J.* 2007;26:19–24.
83. Tenkate TD, Stafford RJ. Risk factors for *Campylobacter* infection in infants and young children: a matched case-control study. *Epidemiol Infect.* 2001;127:399–404.
84. MacDonald E, White R, Mexia R, et al. Risk factors for sporadic domestically acquired *Campylobacter* infections in Norway 2010-2011: a national prospective case-control study. *PloS One.* 2015;10:e0139636.
85. Moffatt C, Appuhamy R, Andrew W, et al. An assessment of risk posed by a *Campylobacter*-positive puppy living in an Australian residential aged-care facility. *Western Pac Surveill Response J. Philippines.* 2014;1–6.
86. Mughini Gras L, Smid JH, Wagenaar JA, et al. Increased risk for *Campylobacter jejuni* and *C. coli* infection of pet origin in dog owners and evidence for genetic association between strains causing infection in humans and their pets. *Epidemiol Infect.* 2013;141:2526–2535.
87. Montgomery MP, Robertson S, Koski L, et al. Multidrug-resistant *Campylobacter jejuni* outbreak linked to puppy exposure - United States, 2016-2018. *Morb Mortal Wkly Rep.* 2018 21;67(37):1032–1035.
88. Wilson JP, Kafetz K, Fink D. Lick of death: *Capnocytophaga canimorsus* is an important cause of sepsis in the elderly. *BMJ Case Rep.* 2016;2016:bcr2016215450.
89. Hastbacka J, Hynninen M, Kolho E. *Capnocytophaga canimorsus* bacteremia: clinical features and outcomes from a Helsinki ICU cohort. *Acta Anaesthesiol Scand.* 2016;60:1437–1443.
90. Hess E, Renzi F, Karhunen P, et al. *Capnocytophaga canimorsus* capsular serovar and disease severity, Helsinki Hospital District, Finland, 2000-2017. *Emerg Infect Dis.* 2018;24(12):2195–2201.
91. de Boer MG, Lambregts PC, van Dam AP, et al. Meningitis caused by *Capnocytophaga canimorsus*: when to expect the unexpected. *Clin Neurol Neurosurg.* 2007;109:393–398.
92. Al-Fifi YS, Sathianathan C, Murray BL, et al. Pets are 'risky business' for patients undergoing continuous ambulatory peritoneal dialysis. *Can J Infect Dis Med Microbiol.* 2013;24:e96–e98.
93. van Samkar A, Brouwer MC, Schultsz C, et al. *Capnocytophaga canimorsus* meningitis: three cases and a review of the literature. *Zoonoses Public Health.* 2016;63:442–448.
94. Centers for Disease Control and Prevention. *Antibiotic Resistance Threats in the United States*; 2019. https://www.cdc.gov/drugresistance/pdf/threats-report/2019-ar-threats-report-508.pdf.
95. Martin JS, Monaghan TM, Wilcox MH. *Clostridium difficile* infection: epidemiology, diagnosis and understanding transmission. *Nat Rev Gastroenterol Hepatol.* 2016;13:206–216.
96. Arroyo LG, Kruth SA, Willey BM, et al. PCR ribotyping of *Clostridium difficile* isolates originating from human and animal sources. *J Med Microbiol.* 2005;54:163–166.
97. Lefebvre SL, Waltner-Toews D, Peregrine AS, et al. Prevalence of zoonotic agents in dogs visiting hospitalized people in Ontario: implications for infection control. *J Hosp Infect.* 2006;62:458–466.
98. Lefebvre SL, Reid-Smith RJ, Waltner-Toews D, et al. Incidence of acquisition of methicillin-resistant *Staphylococcus aureus, Clostridium difficile,* and other health-care-associated pathogens by dogs that participate in animal-assisted interventions. *J Am Vet Med Assoc.* 2009;234:1404–1417.
99. Weese JS, Finley R, Reid-Smith RR, et al. Evaluation of *Clostridium difficile* in dogs and the household environment. *Epidemiol Infect.* 2010;138:1100–1104.
100. Loo VG, Brassard P, Miller MA. Household transmission of *Clostridium difficile* to family members and domestic pets. *Infect Control Hosp Epidemiol.* 2016;37:1342–1348.
101. Mostl K, Addie D, Belak S, et al. Cowpox virus infection in cats: ABCD guidelines on prevention and management. *J Feline Med Surg.* 2013;15:557–559.
102. Baxby D, Bennett M, Getty B. Human cowpox 1969-93: a review based on 54 cases. *Br J Dermatol.* 1994;131:598–607.
103. Lawn R. Risk of cowpox to small animal practitioners. *Vet Rec.* 2010;166:631.
104. Switaj K, Kajfasz P, Kurth A, et al. Cowpox after a cat scratch - case report from Poland. *Ann Agric Environ Med.* 2015;22:456–458.
105. Raoult D, Tissot-Dupont H, Foucault C, et al. Q fever 19851998. Clinical and epidemiologic features of 1,383 infections. *Medicine (Baltim).* 2000;79:109–123.
106. Schoffelen T, Kampschreur LM, van Roeden SE, et al. *Coxiella burnetii* infection (Q fever) in rheumatoid arthritis patients with and without anti-TNFalpha therapy. *Ann Rheum Dis.* 2014;73:1436–1438.
107. Yilmaz G, Ozturk B, Memikoglu O, et al. An unusual manifestation of Q fever: peritonitis. *J Infect Public Health.* 2015;8:373–376.
108. Straily A, Dahlgren FS, Peterson A, et al. Surveillance for Q fever endocarditis in the United States, 1999-2015. *Clin Infect Dis.* 2017 13;65(11):1872–1877.
109. Carcopino X, Raoult D, Bretelle F, et al. Q Fever during pregnancy: a cause of poor fetal and maternal outcome. *Ann N Y Acad Sci.* 2009;1166:79–89.
110. Langley JM, Marrie TJ, Covert A, et al. Poker players' pneumonia. An urban outbreak of Q fever following exposure to a parturient cat. *N Engl J Med.* 1988;319:354–356.
111. Tozer SJ, Lambert SB, Strong CL, et al. Potential animal and environmental sources of Q fever infection for humans in Queensland. *Zoonoses Public Health.* 2014;61:105–112.
112. Buhariwalla F, Cann B, Marrie TJ. A dog-related outbreak of Q fever. *Clin Infect Dis.* 1996;23:753–755.
113. Malo JA, Colbran C, Young M, et al. An outbreak of Q fever associated with parturient cat exposure at an animal refuge and veterinary clinic in southeast Queensland. *Aust N Z J Public Health.* 2018;42(5):451–455.
114. Shapiro A, Bosward K, Mathews K, et al. Molecular detection of *Coxiella burnetii* in raw meat intended for pet consumption. *Zoonoses Public Health.* 2020;67(4):443–452.
115. Lucio-Forster A, Griffiths JK, Cama VA, et al. Minimal zoonotic risk of cryptosporidiosis from pet dogs and cats. *Trends Parasitol.* 2010;26:174–179.

116. Bowman DD, Lucio-Forster A. Cryptosporidiosis and giardiasis in dogs and cats: veterinary and public health importance. *Experimental Parasitol.* 2010;124:121–127.
117. Lucca P, De Gaspari EN, Bozzoli LM, et al. Molecular characterization of *Cryptosporidium* spp. from HIV infected patients from an urban area of Brazil. *Rev Inst Med Trop SP.* 2009;51:341–343.
118. Wang ZD, Liu Q, Liu HH, et al. Prevalence of *Cryptosporidium*, microsporidia and *Isospora* infection in HIV-infected people: a global systematic review and meta-analysis. *Parasit Vectors.* 2018 9;11(1):28.
119. Acikgoz Y, Ozkaya O, Bek K, et al. Cryptosporidiosis: a rare and severe infection in a pediatric renal transplant recipient. *Pediatr Transplant.* 2012;16:E115–E119.
120. Krause I, Amir J, Cleper R, et al. Cryptosporidiosis in children following solid organ transplantation. *Pediatr Infect Dis J.* 2012;31:1135–1138.
121. Hunter PR, Nichols G. Epidemiology and clinical features of *Cryptosporidium* infection in immunocompromised patients. *Clin Microbiol Rev.* 2002;15:145–154.
122. Roy SL, DeLong SM, Stenzel SA, et al. Risk factors for sporadic cryptosporidiosis among immunocompetent persons in the United States from 1999 to 2001. *J Clin Microbiol.* 2004;42:2944–2951.
123. Glaser CA, Safrin S, Reingold A, et al. Association between *Cryptosporidium* infection and animal exposure in HIV-infected individuals. *J Acquir Immune Defic Syndr.* 1998;17:79–82.
124. Bournerias I, De Chauvin MF, Datry A, et al. Unusual *Microsporum canis* infections in adult HIV patients. *J Am Acad Dermatol.* 1996;35:808–810.
125. Chen CH, Wen MC, Cheng CH, et al. Infectious alopecia in a dog breeder after renal transplantation. *J Chin Med Assoc.* 2008:477–480.
126. Berg JC, Hamacher KL, Roberts GD. Pseudomycetoma caused by *Microsporum canis* in an immunosuppressed patient: a case report and review of the literature. *J Cutan Pathol.* 2007;34:431–434.
127. King D, Cheever LW, Hood A, et al. Primary invasive cutaneous *Microsporum canis* infections in immunocompromised patients. *J Clin Microbiol.* 1996;34:460–462.
128. Tlacuilo-Parra A, Guevara-Gutierrez E, Mayorga J, et al. Onychomycosis in systemic lupus erythematosus: a case control study. *J Rheumatol.* 2003;30:1491–1494.
129. Voisard JJ, Weill FX, Beylot-Barry M, et al. Dermatophytic granuloma caused by *Microsporum canis* in a heart-lung recipient. *Dermatology.* 1999;198:317–319.
130. Drusin LM, Ross BG, Rhodes KH, et al. Nosocomial ringworm in a neonatal intensive care unit: a nurse and her cat. *Infect Control Hosp Epidemiol.* 2000;21:605–607.
131. Taylor DJ, Philbey AW. *Salmonella* infections in garden birds and cats in a domestic environment. *Vet Rec.* 2010;167:26–27.
132. Mossovitch M, Mossovitch B, Alkan M. Nosocomial dermatophytosis caused by *Microsporum canis* in a newborn department. *Infect Control (Thorofare).* 1986;7:593–595.
133. Snider R, Landers S, Levy ML. The ringworm riddle: an outbreak of *Microsporum canis* in the nursery. *Pediatr Infect Dis J.* 1993;12:145–148.
134. Safi M, Achour W, Baaboura R, et al. Distribution of virulence associated traits among urine *Escherichia coli* isolates from patients in onco-hematology. *J Infect Chemother.* 2016;22:221–224.
135. Carvalho AC, Barbosa AV, Arais LR, et al. Resistance patterns, ESBL genes, and genetic relatedness of *Escherichia coli* from dogs and owners. *Braz J Microbiol.* 2016;47:150–158.
136. Johnson JR, Johnston B, Clabots CR, et al. Virulence genotypes and phylogenetic background of *Escherichia coli* serogroup O6 isolates from humans, dogs, and cats. *J Clin Microbiol.* 2008;46:417–422.
137. Hogg RA, Holmes JP, Ghebrehewet S, et al. Probable zoonotic transmission of verocytotoxigenic *Escherichia coli* O 157 by dogs. *Vet Rec.* 2009;164:304–305.
138. Strkolcova G, Madar M, Hinney B, et al. Dog's genotype of *Giardia duodenalis* in human: first evidence in Europe. *Acta Parasitol.* 2015;60:796–799.
139. Painter JE, Gargano JW, Collier SA, et al. Giardiasis surveillance — United States, 2011-2012. *Morb Mortal Wkly Rep. Suppl.* 2015;64:15–25.
140. Doglioni C, De Boni M, Cielo R, et al. Gastric giardiasis. *J Clin Pathol.* 1992;45:964–967.
141. Thompson RCA. The zoonotic significance and molecular epidemiology of *Giardia* and giardiasis. *Vet Parasitol.* 2004;126:15–35.
142. Bouzid M, Halai K, Jeffreys D, et al. The prevalence of *Giardia* infection in dogs and cats, a systematic review and meta-analysis of prevalence studies from stool samples. *Vet Parasitol.* 2015;207:181–202.
143. Smith AF, Rock M, Neumann N, et al. Urban park-related risks for *Giardia* spp. infection in dogs. *Epidemiol Infect.* 2015;143:3277–3291.
144. Sykes JE, Hartmann K, Lunn KF, et al. 2010 ACVIM small animal Consensus statement on leptospirosis: diagnosis, epidemiology, treatment, and prevention. *J Vet Intern Med.* 2011;25:1–13.
145. Morris DO. *Malassezia pachydermatis* carriage in dog owners. *Emerg Infect Dis.* 2005;11:83–88.
146. Fan YM, Huang WM, Li SF, et al. Granulomatous skin infection caused by *Malassezia pachydermatis* in a dog owner. *Arch Dermatol.* 2006;142:1181–1184.
147. Welbel SF, McNeil MM, Pramanik A, et al. Nosocomial *Malassezia pachydermatis* bloodstream infections in a neonatal intensive care unit. *Pediatr Infect Dis J.* 1994;13:104–108.
148. Heller J, Kelly L, Reid SW, et al. Qualitative risk assessment of the acquisition of Meticillin-resistant *Staphylococcus aureus* in pet dogs. *Risk Anal.* 2010;30:458–472.
149. Hoet AE, van Balen J, Nava-Hoet RC, et al. Epidemiological profiling of methicillin-resistant *Staphylococcus aureus*-positive dogs arriving at a veterinary teaching hospital. *Vector Borne Zoonotic Dis.* 2013;13:385–393.
150. Starlander G, Borjesson S, Gronlund-Andersson U, et al. Cluster of infections caused by methicillin-resistant *Staphylococcus pseudintermedius* in humans in a tertiary hospital. *J Clin Microbiol.* 2014;52:3118–3120.
151. Abdel-Moein KA, Samir A. Occurrence of extended spectrum beta-lactamase-producing Enterobacteriaceae among pet dogs and cats: an emerging public health threat outside health care facilities. *Am J Infect Control.* 2014;42:796–798.
152. Dierikx CM, van Duijkeren E, Schoormans AH, et al. Occurrence and characteristics of extended-spectrum-beta-lactamase- and AmpC-producing clinical isolates derived from companion animals and horses. *J Antimicrob Chemother.* 2012;67:1368–1374.
153. Meyer E, Gastmeier P, Kola A, et al. Pet animals and foreign travel are risk factors for colonisation with extended-spectrum beta-lactamase-producing *Escherichia coli. Infection.* 2012;40:685–687.
154. Ewers C, Klotz P, Leidner U, et al. OXA-23 and ISAba1-OXA-66 class D beta-lactamases in *Acinetobacter baumannii* isolates from companion animals. *Int J Antimicrob Agents.* 2017;49:37–44.
155. Guerra B, Fischer J, Helmuth R. An emerging public health problem: acquired carbapenemase-producing microorganisms are present in food-producing animals, their environment, companion animals and wild birds. *Vet Microbiol.* 2014;171:290–297.
156. Shaheen BW, Nayak R, Boothe DM. Emergence of a New Delhi metallo-beta-lactamase (NDM-1)-encoding gene in clinical *Escherichia coli* isolates recovered from companion animals in the United States. *Antimicrob Agents Chemother.* 2013;57:2902–2903.
157. Zhang XF, Doi Y, Huang X, et al. Possible transmission of mcr-1-harboring *Escherichia coli* between companion animals and human. *Emerg Infect Dis.* 2016;22:1679–1681.
158. Guet-Revillet H, Levy C, Andriantahina I, et al. Paediatric epidemiology of *Pasteurella multocida* meningitis in France and review of the literature. *Eur J Clin Microbiol Infect Dis.* 2013;32:1111–1120.
159. Ferguson KB, Bharadwaj R, MacDonald A, et al. *Pasteurella multocida* infected total knee arthroplasty: a case report and review of the literature. *Ann R Coll Surg Engl.* 2014;96:e1–e4.
160. Christenson ES, Ahmed HM, Durand CM. *Pasteurella multocida* infection in solid organ transplantation. *Lancet Infect Dis.* 2015;15:235–240.
161. Koch CA, Mabee CL, Robyn JA, et al. Exposure to domestic cats: risk factor for *Pasteurella multocida* peritonitis in liver cirrhosis? *Am J Gastroenterol.* 1996;91:1447–1449.

162. Körmöndi S, Terhes G, Pál Z, et al. Human pasteurellosis health risk for elderly persons living with companion animals. *Emerg Infect Dis.* 2019;25(2):229–235.
163. Poliquin PG, Lagace-Wiens P, Verrelli M, et al. *Pasteurella* species peritoneal dialysis-associated peritonitis: household pets as a risk factor. *Can J Infect Dis Med Microbiol.* 2015;26:52–55.
164. Mirzai S, Rifai A, Tidrick A, et al. A case report on *Pasteurella multocida* peritoneal dialysis-associated peritonitis: when cats think medical equipment are toys. *Case Rep Nephrol.* 2019:5150695.
165. Drenjancevic IH, Ivic D, Drenjancevic D, et al. Fatal fulminant sepsis due to a cat bite in an immunocompromised patient. *Wien Klin Wochenschr.* 2008;120:504–506.
166. Walters MS, Simmons L, Anderson TC, et al. Outbreaks of salmonellosis from small turtles. *Pediatrics.* 2016;137.
167. Mettee Zarecki SL, Bennett SD, Hall J, et al. US outbreak of human *Salmonella* infections associated with aquatic frogs, 2008-2011. *Pediatrics.* 2013;131:724–731.
168. Van Immerseel F. Cats as a risk for transmission of antimicrobial drug–resistant *Salmonella. Emerg Infect Dis.* 2004;10:2169–2174.
169. Nemser SM, Doran T, Grabenstein M, et al. Investigation of *Listeria, Salmonella*, and toxigenic *Escherichia coli* in various pet foods. *Foodborne Pathog Dis.* 2014;11:706–709.
170. Lenz J, Joffe D, Kauffman M, et al. Perceptions, practices, and consequences associated with foodborne pathogens and the feeding of raw meat to dogs. *Can Vet J.* 2009;50:637–643.
171. Leonard EK, Pearl DL, Finley RL, et al. Evaluation of pet-related management factors and the risk of *Salmonella* spp. carriage in pet dogs from volunteer households in Ontario (2005-2006). *Zoonoses Public Health.* 2011;58:140–149.
172. Fauth E, Freeman LM, Cornjeo L, et al. *Salmonella* bacteriuria in a cat fed a *Salmonella*-contaminated diet. *J Am Vet Med Assoc.* 2015;247:525–530.
173. Ngwube A, Jackson S, Dixon T, et al. Disseminated *Salmonella* osteomyelitis in a 2-year-old with sickle cell disease. *Clin Pediatr (Phila).* 2012;51:594–601.
174. Clohessy P, Branley J. Nontyphoidal *Salmonella* prosthetic valve endocarditis. *Intern Med J.* 2012;42:1065.
175. Loharikar A, Vawter S, Warren K, et al. Outbreak of human *Salmonella* Typhimurium infections linked to contact with baby poultry from a single agricultural feed store chain and mail-order hatchery, 2009. *Pediatr Infect Dis J.* 2013;32:8–12.
176. National Association of State Public Health Veterinarians. Compendium of measures to prevent disease associated with animals in public settings. *J Am Vet Med Assoc.* 2013;243:1270–1288.
177. Stull JW, Stevenson KB. Zoonotic disease risks for immunocompromised and other high-risk clients and staff promoting safe pet ownership and contact. *Vet Clin North Am Small Anim Pract.* 2015;45:377–392.
178. Notes from the field: Multistate outbreak of human *Salmonella* Typhimurium infections linked to contact with pet hedgehogs - United States, 2011-2013. *Morb Mortal Wkly Rep.* 2013;62:73.
179. Mejia R, Nutman TB. Screening, prevention, and treatment for hyperinfection syndrome and disseminated infections caused by *Strongyloides stercoralis. Curr Opin Infect Dis.* 2012;25:458–463.
180. Thamsborg SM, Ketzis J, Horii Y, et al. *Strongyloides* spp. infections of veterinary importance. *Parasitology.* 2017;144:274–284.
181. Goncalves ALR, Machado GA, Goncalves-Pires MRF, et al. Evaluation of strongyloidiasis in kennel dogs and keepers by parasitological and serological assays. *Vet Parasitol.* 2007;147:132–139.
182. Georgi JR, Sprinkle CL. A case of human strongyloidosis apparently contracted from asymptomatic colony dogs. *Am J Trop Med Hyg.* 1974;23:899–901.
183. Puthiyakunnon S, Boddu S, Li Y, et al. Strongyloidiasis: an insight into its global prevalence and management. *PLoS Negl Trop Dis.* 2014;8:e3018.
184. Norsarwany M, Abdelrahman Z, Rahmah N, et al. Symptomatic chronic strongyloidiasis in children following treatment for solid organ malignancies: case reports and literature review. *Trop Biomed.* 2012;29:479–488.
185. Qu TT, Yang Q, Yu MH, et al. A fatal *Strongyloides Stercoralis* hyperinfection syndrome in a patient with chronic kidney disease: a case report and literature review. *Medicine (Baltim).* 2016;95:e3638.
186. Macpherson CNL. The epidemiology and public health importance of toxocariasis: a zoonosis of global importance. *Int J Parasitol.* 2013;43:999–1008.
187. Keegan JD, Holland CV. A comparison of *Toxocara canis* embryonation under controlled conditions in soil and hair. *J Helminthol.* 2013;87:78–84.
188. Traversa D, di Regalbono AF, Di Cesare A, et al. Environmental contamination by canine geohelminths. *Parasite Vector.* 2014;7:9.
189. Woodhall DM, Fiore AE. Toxocariasis: a review for pediatricians. *J Pediatric Infect Dis Soc.* 2014;3:154–159.
190. Lee RM, Moore LB, Bottazzi ME, et al. Toxocariasis in North America: a systematic review. *PLoS Negl Trop Dis.* 2014;8:e3116.
191. Overgaauw PA, van Knapen F. Veterinary and public health aspects of *Toxocara* spp. *Vet Parasitol.* 2013;193:398–403.
192. Dabritz HA, Conrad PA. Cats and *Toxoplasma:* implications for public health. *Zoonoses Public Health.* 2010;57:34–52.
193. Guo M, Buchanan RL, Dubey JP, et al. Qualitative assessment for *Toxoplasma gondii* exposure risk associated with meat products in the United States. *J Food Prot.* 2015;78:2207–2219.
194. Desmonts G, Couvreur J. Congenital toxoplasmosis. A prospective study of 378 pregnancies. *N Engl J Med.* 1974;290:1110–1116.
195. Wang ZD, Liu HH, Ma ZX, et al. *Toxoplasma gondii* infection in immunocompromised patients: a systematic review and meta-analysis. *Front Microbiol.* 2017 9;8:389.
196. Pereira-Chioccola VL, Vidal JE, Su C. *Toxoplasma gondii* infection and cerebral toxoplasmosis in HIV-infected patients. *Future Microbiol.* 2009;4:1363–1379.
197. Opsteegh M, Kortbeek TM, Havelaar AH, et al. Intervention strategies to reduce human *Toxoplasma gondii* disease burden. *Clin Infect Dis.* 2015;60:101–107.
198. Torrey EF, Yolken RH. *Toxoplasma* oocysts as a public health problem. *Trends Parasitol.* 2013;29:380–384.
199. Balasundaram MB, Andavar R, Palaniswamy M, et al. Outbreak of acquired ocular toxoplasmosis involving 248 patients. *Arch Ophthalmol.* 2010;128:28–32.
200. Aramini JJ, Stephen C, Dubey JP, et al. Potential contamination of drinking water with *Toxoplasma gondii* oocysts. *Epidemiol Infect.* 1999;122:305–315.
201. Bowie WR, King AS, Werker DH, et al. Outbreak of toxoplasmosis associated with municipal drinking water. The BC *Toxoplasma* Investigation Team. *Lancet.* 1997;350:173–177.
202. Jones JL, Krueger A, Schulkin J, et al. Toxoplasmosis prevention and testing in pregnancy, survey of obstetrician-gynaecologists. *Zoonoses Public Health.* 2010;57:27–33.
203. Khoury JA, Bohl DL, Hersh MJ, et al. Tularemia in a kidney transplant recipient: an unsuspected case and literature review. *Am J Kidney Dis.* 2005;45:926–929.
204. Sarria JC, Vidal AM, Kimbrough RC, et al. Fatal infection caused by *Francisella tularensis* in a neutropenic bone marrow transplant recipient. *Ann Hematol.* 2003;82:41–43.
205. Weile J, Seibold E, Knabbe C, et al. Treatment of tularemia in patient with chronic graft-versus-host disease. *Emerg Infect Dis.* 2013;19:771–773.
206. Capellan J, Fong IW. Tularemia from a cat bite: case report and review of feline-associated tularemia. *Clin Infect Dis.* 1993;16:472–475.
207. Larson MA, Fey PD, Hinrichs SH, et al. *Francisella tularensis* bacteria associated with feline tularemia in the United States. *Emerg Infect Dis.* 2014;20:2068–2071.
208. Kwit NA, Schwartz A, Kugeler KJ, et al. Human tularaemia associated with exposure to domestic dogs: United States, 2006-2016. *Zoonoses Public Health.* 2019;66(4):417–421.
209. Writing Panel of Working Group, Lefebvre SL, Golab GC, et al. Guidelines for animal-assisted interventions in health care facilities. *Am J Infect Control.* 2008;36:78–85.

210. Murthy R, Bearman G, Brown S, et al. Animals in healthcare facilities: recommendations to minimize potential risks. *Infect Control Hosp Epidemiol.* 2015;36:495–516.
211. Waltner-Toews D. Zoonotic disease concerns in animal-assisted therapy and animal visitation programs. *Can Vet J.* 1993;34:549–551.
212. Schuurmans L, Enders-Slegers MJ, Verheggen T, et al. Animal-assisted interventions in Dutch nursing homes: a survey. *J Am Med Dir Assoc.* 2016;17:647–653.
213. Lefebvre SL, Waltner-Toews D, Peregrine A, et al. Characteristics of programs involving canine visitation of hospitalized people in Ontario. *Infect Control Hosp Epidemiol.* 2006;27:754–758.
214. Hardin P, Brown J, Wright ME. Prevention of transmitted infections in a pet therapy program: an exemplar. *Am J Infect Control.* 2016;44:846–850.

20

Immunization

Jane E. Sykes

KEY POINTS

- Active immunization can partially or completely protect dogs and cats from severe consequences of infection with a variety of different pathogens, and in some cases it reduces shedding of these pathogens.
- Vaccines contain attenuated live microorganisms, inactivated microorganisms, or portions of these organisms. They also contain preservatives and may contain adjuvants.
- Failure of immunization can occur with improper storage or administration of vaccines, a large challenge dose, host factors such as concurrent infections or disease, and interference by maternal antibody.
- Other adverse effects of vaccine administration are uncommon to rare but include hypersensitivity reactions, disease induced by live attenuated vaccine organisms, and injection-site sarcomas in cats.
- The decision to administer a vaccine should be based on discussion of risks and benefits between the veterinarian and pet owner. This should be documented in the medical record.
- Guidelines for vaccine selection and administration have been published by a number of veterinary bodies, such as the AAFP, AAHA, AVMA, and WSAVA; suggestions can also be found in the Appendix.

INTRODUCTION

Immunization refers to artificial induction of immunity or protection from infectious disease and may be *active* or *passive*. In contrast, *vaccination* is the administration of an antigenic product. It follows that not all vaccinations are associated with successful immunization. *Active immunization* involves administration of vaccines that stimulate CMI or humoral immunity, or both, to a specific pathogen. Sometimes active immunization can also enhance nonspecific immunity, leading to reduction in disease caused by nontarget pathogens. *Passive immunization* refers to the administration of antibodies in order to provide temporary protection from disease and can occur through acquisition of MDA transplacentally in colostrum or milk; or treatment with preparations that contain specific or nonspecific immunoglobulins (see Chapter 9, Antiviral Chemotherapy and Immunomodulatory Drugs, and Chapter 21, for post-exposure prophylaxis for rabies.). Readers are referred to advanced immunology texts for detailed descriptions of the physiology of active and passive immunity.[1]

The goal of immunization is to generate a protective immune response of prolonged duration against a specific infectious disease, with minimal adverse effects. Because of the potential for adverse effects, vaccination should be performed only if there is a risk for significant morbidity or mortality from an infectious disease. Since the 1950s, a large number of vaccines for dogs and cats have been developed and marketed worldwide, and more are in development. Nevertheless, it is estimated that even in developed countries such as the United States, only 30% to 50% of dogs are properly immunized, and possibly an even smaller proportion of cats.[2,3] Appropriate vaccination of a larger proportion of the pet population may assist in reduction of the prevalence of infectious diseases through the induction of herd immunity (although the concept of herd immunity has been controversial following the COVID-19 pandemic). Protection of 70% of the population can be effective in reducing the prevalence of diseases when communicability is low, such as with rabies. However, with diseases such as CPV enteritis, where the virus is resistant and large quantities of virus are shed, the percentage of protection may need to be much higher to prevent outbreaks.

With the appearance of injection-site sarcomas (ISSs) in cats and increased recognition of leptospirosis in small-breed dogs, increased emphasis has been placed on vaccine safety. Three-yearly vaccination protocols for some vaccines have been recommended, with administration of other vaccines based on exposure risk. Manufacturers have also worked to purify vaccines and minimize adjuvant content without compromising vaccine efficacy. Vaccines have had a profound influence in the control of infectious disease, and for many vaccines the benefits of vaccination outweigh the risks. The massive injection of resources into vaccine research as a result of the COVID-19 pandemic has accelerated the design and production of safer yet highly efficacious vaccines for humans, and this will undoubtedly impact the nature of companion animal vaccines in the future.

VACCINE COMPOSITION AND TYPES OF VACCINES

A vaccine is a suspension of attenuated live or inactivated microorganisms, or parts thereof, that is administered to induce immunity. Currently available vaccines are primarily for bacterial or viral diseases, because the relatively small number of surface antigens on viruses and bacteria makes immunoprophylaxis more successful when compared with protozoal, fungal, or parasitic diseases. In addition to protective antigens, vaccines may contain preservatives and stabilizers as well as specific antimicrobials to preserve the antigen and inhibit bacterial and fungal growth within the vaccine. Some vaccines also contain an *adjuvant* to enhance the immune response to the antigen. Adjuvants increase the uptake of antigen by antigen-presenting cells, activate and mature antigen-presenting cells, induce production of immunoregulatory cytokines, activate inflammasomes, and induce local inflammation and cellular recruitment.[4,5] The most widely used adjuvants are particulate delivery system adjuvants, such as those that contain aluminum salt precipitates including aluminum hydroxide (Table 20.1).[4] Alum adjuvants are thought to activate the innate immune system after being detected by nucleotide-binding oligomerization domain (NOD)-like receptors (NLRs), and they preferentially stimulate Th2 responses.

TABLE 20.1 Types of Adjuvants

Category	Adjuvant Example
Delivery Systems	Aluminum salts
Mineral salts	Calcium phosphate
Lipid particles	Incomplete Freund's adjuvant
Microparticles	PLA (polylactic acid), PLG (poly[lactide-coglycolide])
Immune Potentiators	Muramyl dipeptide
	Lipopolysaccharide
	Imidazoquinolones (e.g., imiquimod)
	Saponins

Modified from Apostolico Jde S, Lunardelli VA, Coirada FC, et al. Adjuvants: classification, modus operandi, and licensing. *J Immunol Res.* 2016;2016:1459394.

Other adjuvants include immune potentiators such as saponin, which is present in a canine *Leishmania* vaccine. Immune potentiators activate innate immune responses by activating pattern recognition receptors (PRRs), including Toll-like receptors, NLRs, and the retinoic acid-inducible gene-I-like receptors (RLRs), which are expressed by immune cells. With an improved understanding of the mechanism of action of different adjuvants, it is possible to manipulate immune responses to vaccines by using different combinations of adjuvants.

Attenuated live vaccines (or modified live vaccines) contain microorganisms that are artificially manipulated so as to negate or greatly reduce their virulence, or are field strains of low virulence. Repeated passage through cell culture is the most common means of attenuation, but it can also be achieved through artificial manipulation of a pathogen's genome. Because they replicate in the host, organisms in attenuated live vaccines usually stimulate an immune response that most closely mimics the protection that results from natural infection. Vaccination with attenuated live CPV and CDV vaccines in the absence of MDA can result in protective immune responses within 3 days of a single injection, which may be followed by immunity that lasts many years, if not for life.[6–8] Partial immunity after vaccination with attenuated live CDV and FPV vaccines can occur within hours.[3,9,10] In addition, vaccine organisms that are shed can serve to immunize other animals in a population. However, the potential for reversion to virulence or vaccine-induced disease exists. Vaccine-induced disease is most likely to occur in highly immunosuppressed animals, including neonates less than 4 weeks of age. Attenuated live vaccines also have the potential to cause some immunosuppression in their own right,[11,12] or they may shift the balance from Th1 to Th2 immune responses.[13] Rarely, this can lead to clinical disease. For example, an outbreak of salmonellosis was reported in cats after use of a high-titer attenuated live FPV vaccine.[14] Very rarely, contamination of attenuated live vaccines has occurred with other potentially pathogenic microorganisms present within cell cultures used to propagate the vaccine. Bluetongue virus grew undetected in one commercial release of canine vaccine in the early 1990s, and caused abortions, cardiac failure, and respiratory distress in pregnant bitches vaccinated in the last trimester of gestation.[15] A more contemporary example is the detection of the feline endogenous retrovirus RD-114 in cell lines used to produce vaccines for dogs and cats in Japan and the United Kingdom.[16] This virus is capable of infecting canine cell lines and concern has been raised about its potential to cause immunosuppression or neoplastic disease, should it adapt to dogs.

Generally speaking, *inactivated vaccines* are less effective than attenuated vaccines, because replication in the host does not occur. They produce weaker immune responses of shorter duration, and more frequent booster immunizations may be required. With the exception of rabies, two initial doses of vaccine 3 to 4 weeks apart are essential to produce an effective immune response, and if more than 6 weeks elapses between these doses, it has been recommended that the series should be repeated.[2,17] Full protection may not develop until 2 to 3 weeks after the last dose. Beyond the initial vaccination series, it is not clear whether lapsed annual boosters require the series to be restarted. This is not always considered necessary for human immunization[18] but has been suggested for dogs when more than 2 or 3 years elapse between boosters.[17] Inactivated vaccines often (but not always) contain adjuvant as well as a large infectious dose to improve immunogenicity. The immune response to inactivated vaccines is often of shorter duration than the immune response to attenuated live vaccines. Inactivated vaccines are safer than attenuated live vaccines for use during pregnancy and in very young or debilitated animals, although it is possible that systemic allergic reactions could still jeopardize pregnancy. Although bacterins have traditionally been associated with a greater likelihood of allergic reactions than attenuated live vaccines, newer inactivated vaccines are safer and have reaction rates that more closely approach those of live attenuated vaccines.[19] The maximum duration of immunity (DOI) that is induced by commercially available bacterins for dogs and cats remains largely unknown, partly because challenge studies that evaluate long-term DOI are prohibitively expensive. Recent studies looking at the DOI for canine leptospirosis vaccines demonstrate protection that lasts at least 12 months,[20,21] with one study demonstrating reduction in leptospiremia and leptospiruria in dogs challenged 15 months after vaccination.[20] Some inactivated virus vaccines have been shown to have DOIs in excess of 7 years in cats.[22] Caution is required when extrapolation is made from the DOI for one product to that for a similar product from a different manufacturer, because it may not be equivalent. Although bacterins usually do not protect all animals from infection, they may prevent clinical illness. In some cases, natural infection of vaccinated animals serves to further boost the immune response, and this can influence DOI in the field. The advantages and disadvantages of attenuated live and inactivated vaccines are shown in Table 20.2.

Subunit vaccines contain specific structural components of a microbe that stimulate a protective immune response, together with adjuvant. They contain reduced amounts of foreign protein, which minimizes the potential for hypersensitivity reactions.

Recombinant DNA vaccines are created through manipulation of the DNA of a pathogen in the laboratory, with the negation of pathogen virulence. Sometimes this also can allow diagnostic tests to differentiate naturally infected from vaccinated animals (DIVA), because of differences in the antibody response evoked by the vaccine. There are several different types of recombinant DNA vaccines:

1. Recombinant subunit vaccines. These are produced by cloning one or more genes for a protective antigen into an expression vector, such as in *Escherichia coli*. The protein expressed by the bacteria is then purified and used in the vaccine (Fig. 20.1A). An example of a recombinant subunit vaccine is the Lyme recombinant OspA vaccine (Recombitek Lyme, Boehringer Ingelheim) and the Lyme recombinant OspA/chimeric OspC vaccine (Vanguard CrLyme, Zoetis) (see Chapter 69). Recombinant subunit protein vaccines have a DOI similar to that of inactivated whole-agent vaccines.
2. Deletion mutant vaccines. These are produced by deleting virulence genes from a pathogen while protective antigens are left in place. There are currently no such vaccines commercially available for dogs and cats, but their development has been described for FHV-1[23] and FCoV.[24]
3. Vectored vaccines. These are produced by inserting genes for one or more protective antigens into the genome of a virus. The virus replicates in the host and expresses the antigens but is nonpathogenic

TABLE 20.2 Comparison of Conventional Whole-Agent Attenuated Live and Inactivated Vaccines

	Attenuated Live	Noninfectious/Inactivated
Advantages	Rapid onset of immunity Sustained immunity after single dose May immunize others in populations Improved breakthrough of maternal antibody interference Improved stimulation of cell-mediated immunity Can administer via the mucosal route Lower risk of hypersensitivity reactions	Safe, even in immunocompromised and pregnant animals Do not interfere with development of immunity from other vaccines Stable in storage
Disadvantages	Potential for reversion to virulence Virulence in the immunocompromised Contraindicated in pregnancy May cause immune suppression Can interfere with development of immunity if administered within days to 2 weeks of another vaccine Less stable in storage Potential for vaccine contamination	Slow onset of immunity Multiple boosters required Often highly adjuvanted, with greater potential for adverse effects Reduced degree of protection compared with attenuated live vaccines Poor breakthrough of maternal antibody interference Restricted to parenteral use
Indications	Routine vaccination Outbreaks Production of mucosal immunity	Pregnancy (when needed) Immunocompromised animals Attenuated live options not available
Availability	Canine parvovirus enteritis (P) Canine adenovirus infection (P, IN, PO) Canine distemper (P) Canine parainfluenza (P, IN, PO) Feline panleukopenia (P, IN) Feline herpesvirus infection (P, IN) Feline calicivirus infection (P, IN) Feline infectious peritonitis (IN) *Bordetella bronchiseptica* (IN; D, C) (PO; D) *Chlamydia felis* (P)	Rabies (D, C) Canine influenza (H3N8, H3N2) Canine coronavirus enteritis *Babesia canis* Leptospirosis Lyme borreliosis *Bordetella bronchiseptica* (D) Feline panleukopenia virus Feline calicivirus Feline herpesvirus-1 Feline leukemia virus Feline immunodeficiency virus *Chlamydia felis*

C, cats; *D*, dogs; *IN*, intranasal; *P*, parenteral; *PO*, oral.

(Fig. 20.1B). Vaccines can be engineered to protein epitopes that are important for the agent's attachment, replication, development, or spread within the host. Multiple genes can be inserted, including those for cytokines such as IL-2, which can enhance the immune response to the simultaneously generated immunogenic proteins. One potential problem with genetically engineered vector vaccines is that the host can mount an immune response to the vector. For example, a recombinant vaccinia virus expressing FeLV gp70 envelope protein was not successful in producing antiviral antibodies in cats.[25] Instead, inoculated cats developed neutralizing antibody against the vaccinia virus. Currently available vectored vaccines for dogs and cats use canarypox virus as a vector, and include vaccines for rabies, CDV, and FeLV infection (Purevax FeLV, Boehringer Ingelheim; Recombitek Canine Distemper, Boehringer Ingelheim; Purevax Feline Rabies, Boehringer Ingelheim). Commercially available oral rabies vaccines with poxviruses as vectors have also been used to protect wildlife. Other vectors have also been used experimentally to create dog and cat vaccines, such as CAdV[26] and myxoma virus.[27]

4. DNA vaccines. These consist of naked DNA that encodes the antigens required for protective immunity. The DNA is injected directly to the animal intramuscularly using an inoculation system. The DNA is then taken up by host cells and translated into antigen. Both humoral and cell-mediated immune responses are produced, but inefficient uptake, concerns about modification of the host genome, and limited studies showing efficacy are disadvantages.[28] Formulations with nanoparticles, cationic lipids, protein polymers, or biodegradable microspheres allow for oral or intranasal delivery and result in significant production of secretory IgA production at mucosal sites. DNA vaccines are stable, resisting extremes in temperature, making their storage and preservation more practical and less expensive. Although they have been developed and tested experimentally, DNA vaccines are not available commercially for use in dogs and cats.
5. mRNA vaccines. mRNA vaccines are a relatively new type of vaccine that have entered widespread use following the COVID-19 pandemic (Moderna and Pfizer vaccines). mRNA vaccines are created in the laboratory from a linear DNA template using a phage RNA polymerase. They offer many advantages over other vaccine types; they are noninfectious and do not integrate into other nucleic acid molecules, so insertional mutagenesis is not of concern; they are degraded by normal host physiological processes; there is also no chance of an immune response to a vector virus; and they have inherent immunostimulatory activity, so can be nonadjuvanted. They elicit strong humoral and cellular immune responses. The instability of mRNA has been a limiting factor, however technological advancements have led to manipulations in mRNA composition and reagents that facilitate uptake of mRNA, protect it from being degraded, and prolong the immune response. The manufacture of mRNA vaccines also has the potential to be highly scalable, inexpensive and rapid. Based on

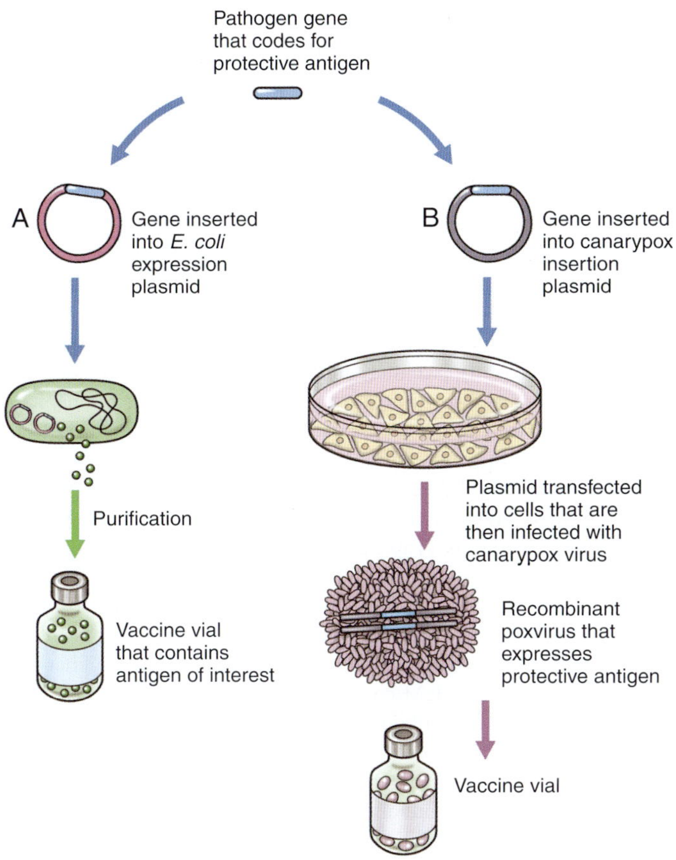

Fig. 20.1 Examples of recombinant DNA vaccines. (A) Recombinant subunit vaccine. The gene of interest is inserted into an expression vector such as a plasmid taken up by *Escherichia coli*, which subsequently produces large amounts of an immunogenic protein. This is purified and used in the vaccine. (B) Vectored vaccine. The gene or genes of interest are inserted into a canarypox or vaccinia vector, which is then inoculated into an animal. Replication of the vector within the host is followed by expression of the immunogenic protein. (From Sykes JE. *Canine and Feline Infectious Diseases*. 1st ed. Elsevier; 2014.)

the success of COVID-19 mRNA vaccines in terms of safety and efficacy, the appearance of mRNA vaccines for prevention of companion animal infectious diseases in the future is likely.

VACCINE STORAGE, HANDLING, AND ADMINISTRATION

Vaccines should be stored and administered according to label recommendations, which generally means refrigeration at 4°C (39.2°F). Inactivation of vaccines can occur if they are inadvertently frozen or heated to excessive temperatures, exposed to excessive amounts of light, or used beyond their expiration date. Hands should be washed before preparation and administration of the vaccine. Lyophilized products should be reconstituted with the proper diluent, and different vaccines should not be mixed in the same syringe or vial. Reconstituted products should be used immediately after reconstitution. Although it has been recommended that attenuated live vaccines be discarded if more than 1 hour has lapsed since reconstitution,[17] no published reports exist of the viability of vaccine organisms over time after reconstitution or of the ability of stored, reconstituted vaccine to elicit an immune response. In particular, the immunogenicity of distemper virus vaccines may be compromised if vaccines are improperly stored and handled, given the poor ability of this virus to survive in the environment. Vaccines should only be used in the animal species for which they are labeled, or serious adverse effects or failure of immunization can occur.

To reduce the likelihood of an adverse reaction, the number of vaccines administered should be minimized to core vaccines and those required based on risk assessment.[2] If vaccines for multiple different pathogens are to be administered simultaneously, they should be injected at distant sites, or, if possible, a combination vaccine should be used. Simultaneous vaccination for more than one pathogen does not appear to interfere with immune responses to each component of the vaccine,[29–31] and vaccine manufacturers must demonstrate that the protection that occurs for a specific pathogen after vaccination with a combination product equals the protection that occurs when a vaccine for only that pathogen is given (known as *interference testing*). The results of multiple studies have shown lack of interference with immunity in dogs and cats when antigens are used in combination.[32–35] In contrast, successive parenteral administration of different attenuated live vaccines at 3 to 14 day intervals has the potential to interfere with immune responses. An interval of 4 weeks is preferred for human patients.[18,36] Inactivated vaccines do not produce interference in this way.[18] Although anesthesia and surgery do not appear to interfere with immune responses to vaccination,[37] if possible, administration of vaccines to animals that are under anesthesia should be avoided because adverse reactions may be difficult or impossible to recognize in this situation. It is not necessary to re-administer an intranasal vaccine if the animal coughs or sneezes after administration.

The site and route of administration, product, serial number, expiry date, results of any serologic tests, and individual who administered the vaccine should be recorded for each vaccine administered. It has also been recommended that the date for the next vaccination be noted on the vaccination certificate, and that there be documentation that relevant information was provided to the client and that the client authorized vaccination. Veterinarians are expected to educate their clients about infectious disease risks for their pets, to inform clients of the risks and benefits of particular vaccines, and to handle and administer products in accordance with the manufacturer's guidelines and commonly accepted standards of practice.

COMPONENTS OF THE IMMUNE RESPONSE

The immune response is divided into innate and adaptive immune responses. The innate immune response is nonspecific and acts as an immediate line of defense against an infection. Components of the innate immune response consist of natural killer cells, which recognize host cells that are infected by viruses; complement, which is activated by bacterial cell wall components; and phagocytes, such as macrophages and dendritic cells. The adaptive immune response develops over several days and involves presentation of antigen by dendritic cells in association with the major histocompatibility complex and stimulation of B- and T-cell responses, together with the formation of memory B cells. The nature of the innate response influences the subsequent adaptive response. Cells of the innate immune system possess PRRs that can recognize patterns that are characteristic for various pathogens (PAMPs), including Toll-like receptors and NLRs. PAMPs are under investigation for use as adjuvants in human and animal vaccines in order to create improved T-cell immune responses.[38,39]

DETERMINANTS OF IMMUNOGENICITY

All vaccines that are available for dogs and cats induce CMI with induction of immunologic memory and a booster effect on repeat administration. Although the presence of antibody correlates with protection for some pathogens, such as CDV and CPV, a lack of antibody does not infer a lack of protection, because of the presence of CMI, which is more difficult to measure.

Vaccines rarely protect all vaccinated individuals from infection and disease. In particular, vaccines for canine and feline respiratory pathogens do not prevent disease but can reduce the prevalence and severity of disease as well as reduce the number of organisms shed. Limited immunity following vaccination is especially likely for infections for which immunity after natural infection is partial or short-lived.

The ability of a vaccine to induce an immune response depends not only on the target pathogen, vaccine composition, and route of administration but also on host factors such as age, nutrition, pregnancy status, stress, concurrent infections, and immune status, including the presence or absence of passively acquired antibody (Box 20.1). Some of these factors may also influence vaccine safety. Some animals may have an impaired ability to respond to vaccination. These dogs have been termed *nonresponders*.[2,40] This situation is probably rare if efficacious vaccines are used and booster vaccines are administered. Young dogs less than 1 year of age, have a significantly reduced response to vaccination with rabies virus vaccines when compared with adult dogs.[41] Small-breed dogs have a greater serologic response to rabies vaccines than large-breed dogs.[42] Administration of vaccines to febrile animals, animals with other infectious diseases, or animals with moderate to severe illness should be avoided if possible until 2 to 3 weeks after recovery has occurred, because the immune response to the vaccine may be suboptimal.

Failure of immunization can result from an inadequate dose of antigen. Thus, division of a single vaccine dose for administration to a larger number of dogs and cats, small-breed dogs as opposed to large-breed dogs, or young kittens as opposed to older kittens, may lead to failure of immunization. Veterinarians should not split vaccine doses because this shifts the liability from the vaccine manufacturer to the veterinarian if vaccine failure occurs. Immunization can also fail in the face of an overwhelming challenge dose.

BOX 20.1 Factors That Can Affect Immune Responses to Vaccines

Target pathogen (e.g., respiratory versus systemic pathogen)
Vaccine composition (e.g., inadequate adjuvant)
Route of administration
Young age
Breed/genetic factors
Nutrition
Pregnancy status
Concurrent moderate to severe illness
Fever
Immunosuppressive drugs
Presence of maternal antibody
Improper vaccine storage and administration
Vaccination with an attenuated live viral vaccine within last 3 days to 2 weeks
Inadequate time allowed for immunization before exposure to field organisms

The route of administration can influence the type of immune response generated. Subcutaneous administration is associated primarily with an IgG response, and rarely induces high levels of secretory IgA antibodies. In contrast, intranasal administration results in an IgA and, to a lesser extent, an IgG response. Immunogenicity and safety may be compromised when a vaccine is administered using the incorrect route.

In young animals, the presence of MDA inhibits endogenous IgG production through negative feedback mechanisms. The presence of MDA may also neutralize vaccine antigens and interfere with effective immunization. In dogs, a small proportion of MDA (approximately 10%) is acquired transplacentally and protects puppies that are deprived of colostrum for a short time after birth. In contrast, feline neonates appear to be born without transplacentally acquired antibodies.[43] IgM has been detected in some kittens at birth, likely as a result of perinatal production of IgM, because IgM is too large to cross the placental barrier.[43] Most MDA in dogs is acquired from colostrum, and to a lesser extent, from milk (Table 20.3). In dogs, colostral/milk IgG, IgA, and IgM concentrations are >120-fold, >110-fold, and >10-fold that of serum, respectively, and the IgG concentration in mammary secretions decreases to that of serum within the first 4 weeks of lactation. In contrast, in one study in cats, colostral IgG was only twofold higher than in serum, and IgA and IgM concentrations were actually lower.[43] The absorption of colostral antibodies occurs in the duodenum and jejunum via membrane Fc receptors on the intestinal epithelium that facilitate transport of IgG into the systemic circulation. The process is maximal within 24 hours of birth but also occurs to a limited degree throughout the remainder of the nursing period. The amount of antibody absorbed is also inversely proportional to the size of the litter. Once absorbed, the immunoglobulin from colostrum can give the neonate a titer that can equal or exceed that of the dam in some instances. Over time, the MDA declines at a characteristic half-life that is specific for each disease-producing agent (Table 20.4).[44–56] Antibody class is also important with respect to titer loss. Overall in kittens, the half-lives of maternally derived IgG and IgA in one study were 4.4 and 1.9 days, respectively, whereas in dogs, half-lives were 10 and 4–5 days, respectively. Maternally derived IgG in kittens was lowest at around 3 to 4 weeks of age, and serum IgG and IgA increased dramatically at 5 to 7 weeks of age. These results suggested that kittens may be susceptible to infectious diseases at about 1 month of age, perhaps as much as 2 weeks earlier than puppies.[43]

Despite these findings, it is important to recognize that there is considerable individual variation, with some animals maintaining high concentrations of maternal antibody for months. The persistent presence of MDA is one of the most common reasons for vaccine failure in dogs and cats. Any MDA titer against CPV has the potential to interfere with immunization. The amount of MDA in a puppy or

TABLE 20.3 Relative Proportions of Maternally Derived Antibody Obtained Transplacentally Versus from Colostrum for Selected Canine Infectious Diseases

	SERUM TITER OF NEONATE		
	% of Dam's Titer		% of Neonate's Titer
Disease	Presuckle	Postsuckle	Obtained in Utero/ Obtained from Colostrum
Canine distemper	3	77	4/96
Infectious canine hepatitis	NR	92	NR/NR
Canine parvoviral infection	5.7	60	10/90

NR, not reported.
Modified from Greene CE, Levy JK. Immunoprophylaxis. In: Greene CE, ed. *Infectious Diseases of the Dog and Cat.* 4th ed. Philadelphia: Elsevier; 2011.

TABLE 20.4 Half-Life of Maternally Derived Immunoglobulins in Neonatal Dogs and Cats

Pathogen	Half-Life (Days)	Usual Duration of Protection (Weeks)[a]
Canine distemper virus[47]	8.4	9–12
Canine parvovirus[49,50]	9.7	10–14
Canine adenovirus-1[44]	8.4	9–12
Feline panleukopenia virus[52]	9.5	8–14
Feline leukemia virus[53]	15.0	6–8
Feline herpesvirus-1[45,46,51]	18.5	6–8
Feline calicivirus[48,54]	15.0	10–14
Feline coronavirus[56]	7.0	4–6
Feline immunodeficiency virus[55]	12.5	12

[a]The duration of maternal antibody protection usually corresponds to the interval over which vaccines are ineffective.
Modified from Greene CE, Levy JK. Immunoprophylaxis. In: Greene CE, ed. *Infectious Diseases of the Dog and Cat*. 4th ed. Philadelphia: Elsevier; 2011.

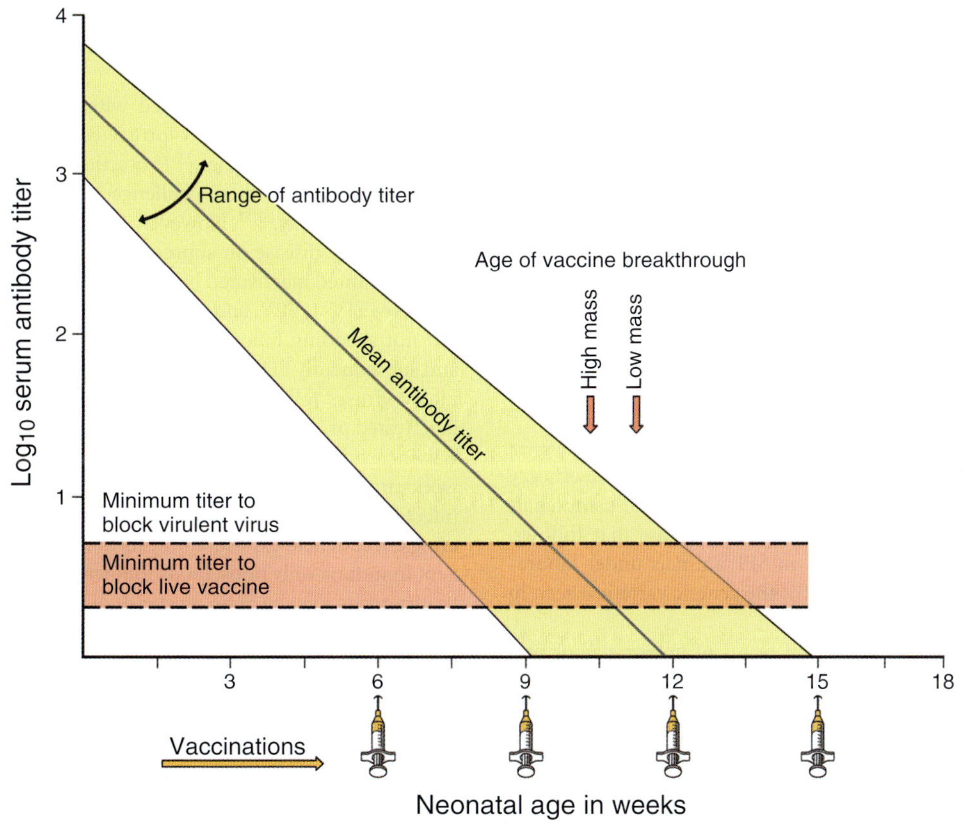

Fig. 20.2 Influence of maternally derived antibody (MDA) on immunization. Puppies and kittens acquire variable amounts of MDA transplacentally and through colostrum after birth. This binds to vaccine antigens and inhibits the immune response. A series of vaccines are administered to maximize the chance of inducing an immune response as MDA concentrations decline. The *window of susceptibility* is the period of time when MDA concentrations are high enough to interfere with immunization, but not sufficient to prevent natural infection. High antigen mass vaccines provide protection earlier than low mass vaccines. (From Greene CE, Schultz RD. Immunoprophylaxis. In: Greene CE, ed. *Infectious Diseases of the Dog and Cat.* 3rd ed. St Louis, MO: Saunders; 2006.)

kitten at any one point in time cannot be predicted because it varies depending on the titer of the dam and the amount of colostrum ingested after birth. As a result, a *series* of vaccinations, given every 2 to 4 weeks through 16 to 18 weeks of age, have been administered to puppies and kittens in order to increase the chance that successful immunization will occur soon after the decline of MDA titers to sufficiently low concentrations (Fig. 20.2). Nevertheless, a window always exists when MDA concentrations are high enough to interfere with immunization, but not sufficient to prevent natural infection. This window is known as the *window of susceptibility* or the *window of vulnerability*. The WSAVA has recommended that the vaccination typically given at 1 year of age instead be administered at 6 months of age, as the purpose of this booster was to ensure effective vaccination of animals that still had maternal antibody at the end of the vaccination series.

TABLE 20.5 Manufacturer's Claims for Vaccine Efficacy and Safety

Claim	Comment
Prevention of Infection	Products able to prevent all colonization or replication of the challenge organism in a vaccinated animal
Prevention of Disease	Products shown to be highly effective in preventing clinical disease in vaccinated animals. The 95% confidence interval estimate of efficacy must be at least 80%.
Aid in Disease Prevention	Products shown to prevent disease by a clinically significant amount which is usually less than that required to support a claim of disease prevention.
Aid in Disease Control	Products that alleviate disease severity, reduce disease duration, or delay disease onset.

The use of recombinant vector vaccines can overcome the interference by MDA, although the extent to which this applies in animals that have passive immunity to the vector virus (i.e., immunity transferred from a dam that was immunized with a recombinant vector vaccine) requires clarification. Because replication of the vector is aborted, the immune response to the vector itself may be reduced. As a result, passive transfer of neutralizing antibody titers to the vector may not occur. Mucosal vaccines can also provide greater protection in the face of MDA because the mucosal immune system matures shortly after birth.[57,58]

Whenever possible, animals should be isolated until sufficient time has elapsed for proper immunization. For most parenteral and mucosal vaccines, this is 1 week (and at the absolute minimum, 3 days) after inoculation. Vaccine failure can also occur in animals that are incubating the disease for which vaccination is performed at the time of vaccination.

VACCINE EFFICACY AND CHALLENGE STUDIES

The gold standard methodology for determination of vaccine efficacy is to expose vaccinated and unvaccinated animals to the same challenge dose and measure the severity of clinical disease that follows. These challenge studies are performed in SPF animals under laboratory conditions, which may not represent the genetic variation seen in some breed lines or field conditions.

Vaccine efficacy is often expressed in terms of *preventable or prevented fraction* (Table 20.5), which is the proportion of vaccinated animals that do not develop a disease after challenge compared with those unvaccinated animals that do develop the disease.

The formula is calculated as follows:

$$\text{Prevented fraction} = \frac{\text{Prevalence (\%) of disease in nonvaccinates} - \text{Prevalence (\%) in vaccinates}}{\text{Prevalence (\%) in nonvaccinates}}$$

It can also be expressed as mitigatable fraction (proportion with reduction in severity of clinical signs). Other claims include reduction of pathogen shedding, prevention of a specific clinical sign, or prevention of mortality. The level or degree of protection claim can therefore be limited.

After vaccine efficacy is determined in laboratory animals, a vaccine is subjected to field trials by a limited number of veterinarians before they are released for general use. Many products are initially marketed without complete knowledge of DOI or adverse effects. Manufacturers are receptive to reports of complications encountered by veterinarians and, in turn, keep the veterinary profession informed of continuing efficacy studies and potential complications.

Duration of Immunity

The DOI is important in determining the timing for booster vaccinations, and is determined by challenging animals with an infectious agent at variable periods of time after vaccination. With the exception of rabies vaccines, DOI of many marketed vaccines sold in the United States is not available because most challenges are performed several weeks after immunization. Vaccine manufacturers in the United States are not required to demonstrate longer DOI for already-licensed antigens. However, USDA guidelines do require DOI challenge studies for vaccines containing "newer" agents (i.e., those for which biologics were developed after ca. 2000), those likely to have shorter DOIs, and rabies virus vaccines.[59] The level of protection that must be demonstrated for long-term studies is generally less stringent than that for challenge studies obtained a few weeks after the primary vaccination series. Studies have shown DOIs of at least 3 years[60,61] and 4.75 years[6] for attenuated live CPV, CDV, and CAdV-2 vaccines. An inactivated canine rabies vaccine was shown to have a DOI of a minimum of 3 years, with clinical signs developing in 28 (88%) of 32 vaccinated dogs and 30 (97%) of 31 unvaccinated dogs.[62] Minimum DOIs of at least 1 year have been established for *Borrelia burgdorferi*,[63–65] *Leptospira*,[66–68] and intranasal *Bordetella bronchiseptica* vaccines in dogs,[69,70] although the latter two vaccines typically reduce infection and shedding but do not eliminate it altogether.

Laboratory kittens vaccinated with an inactivated vaccine against FHV-1, FCV, and FPV were protected against challenge with FPV 7 years after the initial series.[22] Protection against FHV-1 and FCV was only partial because these challenged cats developed respiratory signs of varying severity.[22,71] However, immunization lessened the severity of respiratory disease on subsequent challenge. Cats vaccinated with a nonadjuvanted inactivated bivalent FCV vaccine that contained attenuated live FHV-1, FPV, and *Chlamydia felis* had reduction in clinical signs but not shedding following challenge with a heterologous FCV strain and subsequently FHV-1.[72] The degree of protection against feline respiratory viruses following challenge 2 to 4 weeks after vaccination with inactivated or attenuated live vaccines has been similar,[73] although there is some evidence of slight waning of immunity in the period between 4 weeks and 1 year after vaccination, possibly to a greater extent for FHV-1 infection.[73–75] These studies do not take into account the natural boostering effect of field exposure for cats that contact other cats. Cats that are kept in indoor-only households following vaccination with no exposure to other cats may be at greatest risk of contracting severe disease when exposure ultimately occurs years later. This exposure could occur at a veterinary clinic if adequate precautions are not taken during examination (handwashing and proper disinfection of fomites in the examination room). Alternatively, the stress of visiting a veterinary clinic could lead to reactivation of latent FHV-1 infection in these cats.

A 2-year DOI study was conducted for an inactivated FeLV vaccine in which kittens were vaccinated at 8 and 11 weeks of age, then challenged 2 years after vaccination.[76] Persistent viremia developed in all of the 11 control cats but only 2 of 12 vaccinated cats. In another study, cats received one of four commercially available vaccines at 15 to 16 and 18 to 19 weeks of age, and a fifth group of cats served as unvaccinated control cats.[77] Four months following their final of two vaccinations, the cats were challenged with virulent FeLV, and the incidence of persistent viremia was determined. Two of the vaccines had a measured prevented fraction of 100%, whereas the other two had a fraction of 57% and 29%, respectively.

More information on vaccine efficacy and DOI can be found in chapters in this book relating to specific infectious diseases for which vaccines are available. Vaccines produced by different manufacturers, for the same antigen, may not necessarily have equal efficacy or DOI, because they may contain different adjuvants, strains, and organism titers.

MEASUREMENT OF THE IMMUNE RESPONSE

For some infections, such as rabies, CDV, CPV, and FPV, the presence of detectable circulating antibodies after MDA has waned (i.e., from age 20 weeks) correlates with protection. Thus, serologic assays such as hemagglutination-inhibition (for detection of CPV antibodies) and virus neutralization (for CDV, CAdV-1, CPV, and FPV) have been used in dogs and cats to decide whether vaccination is necessary, and also as a predictor of long-term DOI. Serologic testing has also been used to clear pets for travel; for example, immunity to rabies virus can be predicted using the rapid fluorescent focus inhibition test (a modified virus neutralization method) or fluorescent antibody virus neutralization (see Chapter 21), although protective serum antibody titers are generally not accepted as an alternative to vaccination where there is a legal requirement for vaccination against rabies.

Although positive antibody titers are associated with protection from some infections, an animal with no titer may still be resistant to challenge because of CMI, which is not measured. Conversely, an animal with a positive antibody titer has the potential to develop disease after challenge, possibly because of overwhelming exposure, immune suppression, or emergence of variant strains. Infections where the presence of detectable circulating antibodies does not correlate with protection include leptospirosis; respiratory and gastrointestinal viral and bacterial infections (where mucosal secretory IgA correlates better with protection); and chronic, persistent infections such as leishmaniosis, FIV infection, FIP virus infection, bartonellosis, and babesiosis. For *B. burgdorferi* infections, the presence of detectable antibodies to the conserved outer surface protein OspA present in vaccines can correlate with protection, because this neutralizes the pathogen within the tick during ingestion of a blood meal (see Chapter 69). However, the presence of other anti-*Borrelia* antibodies may not imply protection because reinfection with new strains can occur and the spirochete can persist in the face of the host immune response. Accurate and reliable rapid POC assays for measurement of antibody responses in dogs and cats are now available, although they still remain more expensive than vaccination. Assays are available for CDV, CPV, CAdV-1 and FPV (VacciCheck, Spectrum Labs, AZ/Biogal, Galed Labs, Kibbutz Galed, Israel; TiterCHEK CDV/CPV, Zoetis, NJ, USA). These have reduced the problems associated with variability of results among different laboratories, and insufficient validation of some assays. Measurement of antibody titers may be considered for animals that have had previous adverse responses to vaccination, particularly susceptible breeds (e.g., Rottweilers and CPV infection). The WSAVA has suggested that puppies could be tested at least 4 weeks after the final puppy vaccine to decide whether further vaccination for CDV or CPV is necessary; if the titer is positive, the next booster would not be required for 3 years.[2] Negative titers should prompt additional vaccination for these puppies.

Rapid POC serologic assays have also been used to make decisions regarding isolation or euthanasia in shelter situations, through identification of immune animals.[78] In the face of an outbreak, incoming seronegative animals can be vaccinated and fostered before returning them to the shelter. Unfortunately, it is not always possible to know if positive titers represent recent infection, and animals that test positive may still shed virus and pose a risk to other animals. In young puppies and kittens, positive results may represent persistent MDA or the presence of active immunity, and MDA does not have the same ability to protect against infection. POC serologic assays can also be used to decide whether pregnant animals are susceptible in a shelter environment and thus minimize adverse reactions to attenuated live vaccines in this group of animals (see Appendix). A study that evaluated the performance of one ELISA assay (TiterCHEK CPV/CDV) found that for CPV antibodies, the sensitivity and specificity of the assay was 92% and 94%, respectively, when compared with hemagglutination inhibition; and for CDV, it was 76% and 92%, respectively, when compared with serum neutralization.[79]

EFFECT OF AGE AND IMMUNOSUPPRESSION ON IMMUNE RESPONSES

Age-related declines in the immune response to vaccination can be a concern for the timing and frequency of booster vaccination for older dogs and cats.[80] However, geriatric dogs and cats rarely die of vaccine-preventable infectious diseases, even when not vaccinated for many years.[8] Compared with mice and humans, relatively little is known about the effect of age on the immune system of dogs and cats. No difference in the concentration of serum IgG was found between young and aged German shepherd dogs.[81] Compared with most Labrador retriever age groups, older members have decreased lymphocyte stimulation responsiveness to mitogens and increased percentages of their lymphocytes as total T cells, but a decreased percentage of CD4+ cells.[82,83] In dogs of various breeds, 32 young (3.15 ± 0.8 years) and 33 old dogs (12.1 ± 1.3 years) were vaccinated against CDV, CPV, and rabies.[84] No differences between old and young dogs were noted in postvaccination titers against any of the viruses. Results of one study were that senior cats had higher serum IgA and IgM but lower leukocyte counts and lower absolute values of T cells, B cells, and natural killer cells compared with young adult cats.[85]

Administration of glucocorticoids, even at immunosuppressive doses, has been shown to not interfere with the immune response to vaccination. In one study, unvaccinated 13-week-old puppies were treated with prednisolone at 1 or 10 mg/kg q12h for a week, q24h for a second week, then q48h for a third week, then vaccinated for CDV and challenged 3 days later. Although the prednisolone-treated puppies had decreased lymphocyte responsiveness, all vaccinated puppies were resistant to challenge. However, dogs treated with methotrexate and antithymocyte serum developed vaccine-induced distemper after CDV vaccination.[86] In another study, there was no difference in rabies antibody titers following vaccination in dogs treated with dexamethasone (0.25 mg/kg) and untreated dogs.[87]

ADVERSE REACTIONS TO VACCINES

A vaccine is needed if an infectious disease causes significant morbidity and mortality. Vaccines should prevent more disease than they cause. In order to produce protective immunity, a vaccine *must* stimulate a reaction in an animal, both at the site of injection and systemically. This may cause clinical signs. Ideally, the signs are mild and either unnoticeable or acceptable to the pet owner. In rare situations, adverse reactions are severe enough to threaten a pet's life. Sometimes, enhanced efficacy leads to a reduction in vaccine safety. Veterinarians are encouraged to report adverse reactions to vaccines to a technical service veterinarian employed for this purpose by the vaccine manufacturer. In some countries, the drug company then reports details of the adverse reaction to drug regulatory authorities. In the United Kingdom, the Veterinary Medicines Directorate has been evaluating adverse vaccine reactions since 1985, and the absolute number of adverse reactions to different vaccine types were published for dogs and cats until 2013.[88–96] The number of reports increased slightly over this period, but these broad numerator data represent a variety of factors, potentially affected by increased reporting, increased reports of perceived (rather than true) adverse reactions, more widespread vaccination, an increase in pet ownership, and so on, rather than a true increase in adverse events. An understanding of the true nature and

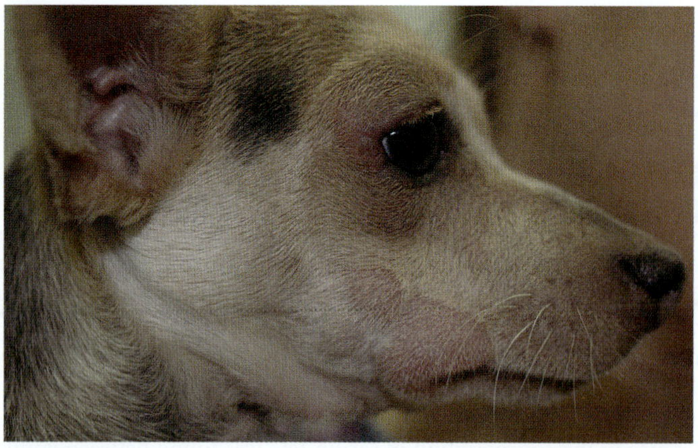

Fig. 20.3 Facial edema and hyperemia in a 4-month-old intact male Chihuahua mix after vaccination with a bacterin vaccine. (Courtesy Dr. Stephen D. White, University of California, Davis Veterinary Dermatology Service.)

incidence of adverse effects associated with vaccination requires much more detailed information, and has also been hampered by underreporting and variable delays between vaccination and the inconsistent appearance of potential, more chronic systemic adverse effects.[97] In addition, correlation of adverse reactions to vaccine administration in young animals may be difficult because of the uniform and frequent administration of vaccines to this group. For example, it has been difficult to prove a connection between vaccination for distemper and development of hypertrophic osteopathy in Weimaraner dogs. Nevertheless, it has been suggested that lines of Weimaraners that develop this problem following vaccination with attenuated live vaccines be vaccinated instead with recombinant canarypox CDV vaccines.[98] Despite claims of many antivaccination advocates, epidemiologic analysis has not revealed any correlation between vaccination within the last 3 months and ill health in dogs.[99] Of interest, analysis of survey responses from 2261 veterinarians from the United States and Canada in early 2020 identified a positive correlation between the existence of organized antivaccination movements against mandatory vaccination of children in the community and the number of clients resistant to pet vaccination.[100]

Immune-Mediated Vaccine Reactions

Type I Hypersensitivity Reactions

Type I hypersensitivity reactions occur when allergens cross-link IgE molecules that are bound to receptors on mast cells and basophils and trigger degranulation. Clinical signs of type I hypersensitivity responses that occur after vaccine administration include facial or periorbital edema, urticaria, cutaneous hyperemia, generalized pruritus, salivation, hypotensive shock, tachypnea, vomiting, diarrhea, collapse, and even death (Fig. 20.3). Vomiting and respiratory distress are common in cats. These signs generally occur within 24 hours of vaccine administration; anaphylaxis usually begins within minutes. The estimated incidence of anaphylaxis after vaccination of dogs and cats is 1 in 5,000 to 1 in 50,000 and depends on the vaccines used. One retrospective study evaluated 1.23 million dogs and nearly 0.5 million cats from more than 300 Banfield hospitals in the United States in 2002 through 2005. In this study, vaccine-associated adverse effects that were listed as vaccine reactions, allergic reactions, anaphylaxis, urticaria, and/or cardiac arrest were documented within 3 days of vaccine administration in 38.2 per 10,000 dogs and 47.4 per 10,000 cats.[30,101] Reactions coded as "allergic" or "anaphylaxis" were reported in approximately 1 in 785 dogs and 1 in 1,200 cats. Reactions coded as anaphylaxis constituted

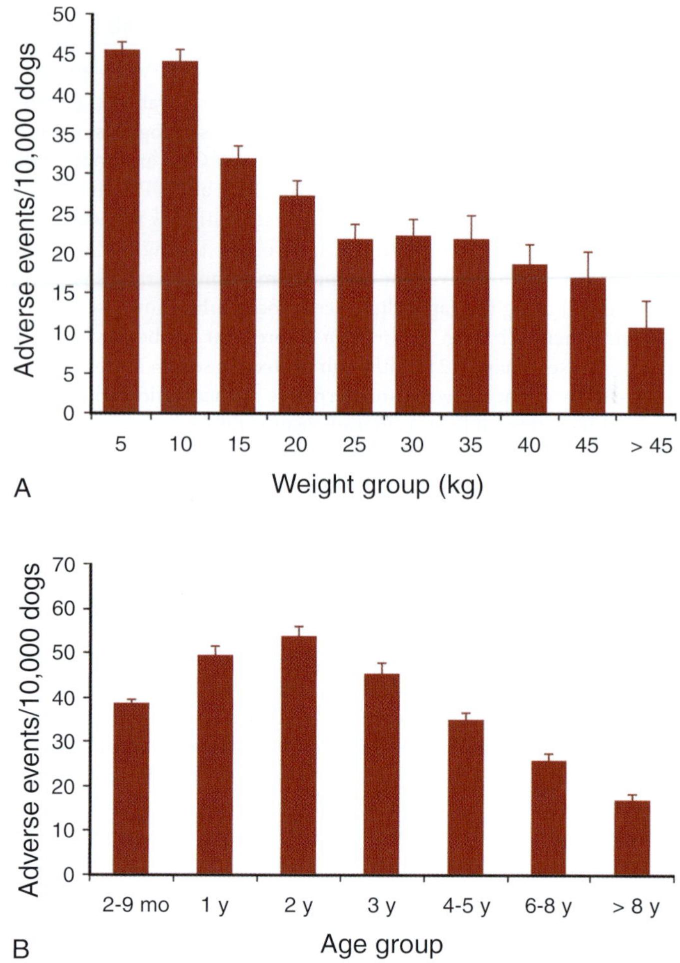

Fig. 20.4 Correlation between (A) body weight and (B) age and the occurrence of vaccine-associated adverse effects within 3 days of vaccination in dogs. (From Moore GE, Guptill LF, Ward MP, et al. Adverse events diagnosed within three days of vaccine administration in dogs. *J Am Vet Med Assoc.* 2005;227(7):1102–1108.)

only 5% of these reactions. Death occurred in 1 in 400,000 dogs and 1 in 125,000 cats that received vaccines, and all 3 dogs and 1 of the 4 cats that died received four or more doses of a vaccine (i.e., more than one vaccine product administered simultaneously). Most reactions in dogs (73%) occurred on the day the vaccine was administered (day 0), 19% occurred on day 1, 6% on day 2, and 3% on day 3. Data from the UK Veterinary Products Committee report indicated anaphylaxis in 1 in 385,000 vaccinated dogs and 1 in 555,000 cats.[40]

Vaccines that contain large amounts of adjuvant, certain preservatives, or inactivated bacteria with proinflammatory outer surface components are more likely to cause reactions. Proteins present in fetal calf serum and stabilizers such as gelatin within the vaccine may also be responsible for allergic reactions.[102] In the Banfield study, the risk of reactions increased with the number of vaccine doses (i.e., volume of vaccine in milliliters) administered per office visit.[30] Small-breed dogs, such as miniature dachshunds, pugs, Boston terriers, miniature pinschers, and Chihuahuas, were more susceptible to development of acute vaccine reactions, and the risk of a vaccine-related adverse event increased as body weight decreased. The risk of vaccine-related adverse events was four times greater in dogs that weighed 5 kg or less than in those that weighed more than 45 kg (Fig. 20.4). Adverse events increased in frequency with age up until 2 years in dogs and 1 year in cats, after which the frequency progressively declined to rates lower than that observed in animals less than 1 year of age (see Fig. 20.4). The decrease in frequency with older age may have occurred because of owners' unwillingness to have their pets vaccinated if a previous reaction occurred. Sexually intact dogs were less likely to develop adverse reactions than neutered dogs, but the opposite was true for cats.[22,34] Female cats were more likely to exhibit reactions than male cats. Because there is some evidence that vaccination can increase allergen-specific IgG and IgE in allergic dogs,[103] it has been suggested that atopic dogs receive booster vaccinations during nonallergenic seasons or disease-free intervals.[99]

The treatment of choice for anaphylaxis is epinephrine, together with other supportive treatments such as intravenous fluids and supplemental oxygen if necessary (Box 20.2). Antihistamines (e.g., diphenhydramine, IV or IM) and glucocorticoids (e.g., IV methylprednisolone sodium succinate) can be administered to dogs with less severe reactions. Vaccination should be avoided in animals with a history of severe reactions, although legal requirements for rabies vaccination may need to be considered in some geographic locations. Treatment with an antihistamine 20 to 30 minutes before vaccination could be considered in animals with a history of milder reactions. These animals should also be monitored closely in the hospital for several hours after vaccine administration. It has been suggested that in the future, commercial production of low-dose vaccines for small-breed dogs might be more appropriate, given their increased risk of reactions and more marked serologic responses to vaccination.[104] Preparations are currently available that are half the volume of previous preparations (0.5 mL instead of 1 mL), but the amount of vaccine antigen and adjuvant remains unchanged.

BOX 20.2 Considerations for Treatment of Anaphylaxis

- Place intravenous catheter
- Epinephrine (adrenaline): Initially, 0.01 mg/kg of a 1:1000 dilution IV; repeat every 5 to 15 minutes as needed to a maximum of 0.3 mg in patients < 40 kg and 0.5 mg in patients > 40 kg.
- Isotonic crystalloid 40–50 mL/kg (D) or 20–30 mL/kg (C) by IV infusion over 10 minutes; consider further resuscitation up to a total of 90 mL/kg (D) or 50 mL/kg (C).
- Supplemental oxygen
- Diphenhydramine 2 mg/kg IM or IV (D, C)[a]
- Methylprednisolone sodium succinate 2–6 mg/kg IV (D, C)[a]

[a] Not a substitute for epinephrine and intravenous fluids.
C, cats; *D*, dogs; *IM*, intramuscular; *IV*, intravenous.

Other Hypersensitivity Reactions, Including Autoimmune Disease

Type II hypersensitivity reactions occur when IgG and IgM bind to cell surface antigens and fix complement, with target cell lysis or removal of target cells by macrophages within reticuloendothelial tissues. Inactivated bacterial vaccines are most likely to serve as a nonspecific trigger because of the immune-enhancing effects of adjuvants and bacterial cell walls. Another potential mechanism is molecular mimicry, where vaccine antigens mimic host antigens, resulting in immunologic cross-reactivity against certain host tissues. Concerns have been raised that vaccination may predispose certain genetically susceptible individuals to immune-mediated cytopenias, although as in human medicine, studies of dogs and cats to date have failed to conclusively document vaccines as causes of these and other chronic diseases.[36,100] Immune-mediated hemolytic anemia was suspected to occur following parvovirus vaccination, possibly due to the hemagglutinating properties of the virus and the high antigen mass in some of these vaccines,[105] but a later retrospective case-control study found no association.[106] Transient thrombocytopenia can occur after vaccination in some dogs.[107] In one study, dogs developed antithyroglobulin antibodies after vaccination, although this was not associated with development of hypothyroidism.[108] Cats that are vaccinated with CRFK cell-derived vaccines develop antibodies against the CRFK proteins alpha-enolase and annexin A2.[109] Whether production of these antibodies has clinical significance remains to be determined.

Type III hypersensitivity reactions are characterized by immune-complex deposition in tissues and may be a consequence of immunization with certain vaccines. For example, anterior uveitis and subclinical

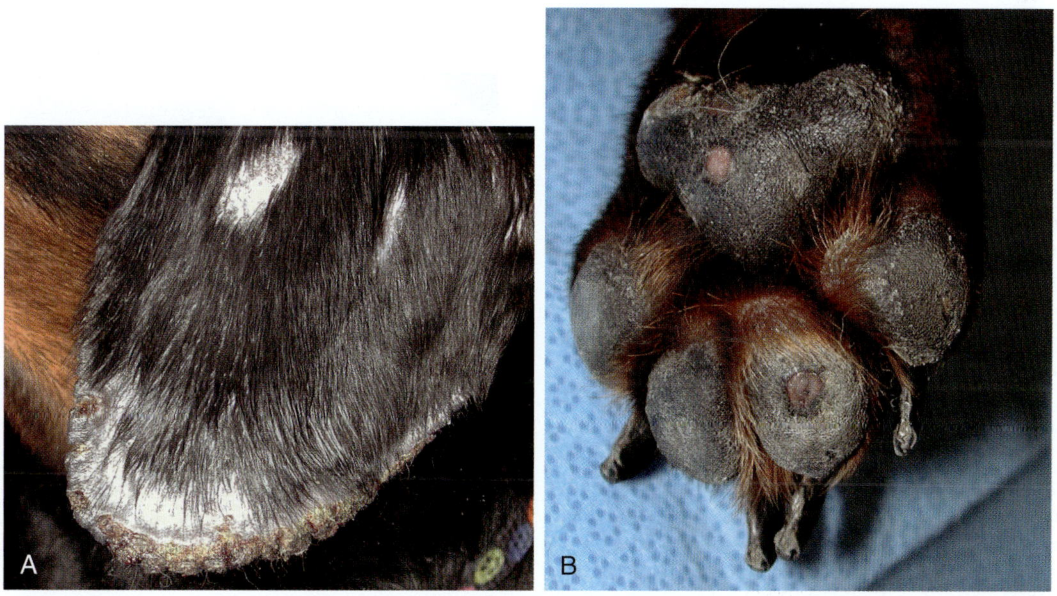

Fig. 20.5 Ischemic dermatopathy suspected to be associated with rabies virus vaccination that involved (A) the pinnae and (B) footpads of a 1-year-old male dachshund. The rabies vaccine was administered several months before the onset of signs. (Courtesy Dr. Stephen D. White, University of California, Davis Veterinary Dermatology Service.)

nephritis developed in 0.4% of dogs receiving CAdV-1 vaccine. This vaccine was replaced by CAdV-2 vaccines, which do not produce these lesions. A cutaneous vasculitis has been described after vaccination of dogs and cats with rabies virus vaccines ("rabies vaccine-induced vasculitis")[110–112] (Fig. 20.5). This can occur at the site of vaccine administration, and in some animals, a multifocal ischemic dermatopathy and myopathy that affects sites such as the pinnal margins, periocular areas, tail tip, and paw pads has been reported to occur 1 to 5 months after the appearance of the initial skin lesion.[112] The multifocal dermatopathy and myopathy has been reported to resolve after treatment with pentoxifylline and vitamin E. Additional evidence is required to strengthen the association between the multifocal condition and rabies vaccination. Similarly, concerns have been raised about a possible temporal association between vaccination and immune-mediated polyarthritis in some dogs,[113] but this association remains unproven. Immune-mediated polyradiculoneuritis, a type IV hypersensitivity reaction (delayed-type hypersensitivity), occurred after vaccination of dogs with suckling-mouse brain-derived inactivated rabies vaccines, which are no longer available.[114] Subsequent re-exposure resulted in more severe and prolonged paralysis. Granuloma formation at the site of vaccine administration also represents a type IV hypersensitivity reaction.

Despite the lack of conclusive evidence for an association between vaccination with currently available vaccines and autoimmune disease, it is possible that vaccination may be associated with dysregulation of the immune response in predisposed individuals. Therefore, vaccination is often withheld if not absolutely necessary in dogs and cats with a history of autoimmune disease. Serum titers could also be assessed to gauge the need for specific immunization in these animals.

Vaccine Organism-Induced Disease

Disease occasionally results from replication of microorganisms present in a vaccine, although severe disease is uncommon with currently available vaccines. Fever and lethargy are the most common adverse effects of vaccination and result from cytokine production in response to the vaccine. These are transient and usually resolve within 1 to 2 days.

In the past, the use of attenuated rabies virus vaccines resulted in ascending paralytic disease in a proportion of cats and dogs. This led to a change to inactivated, adjuvanted rabies vaccines. Administration of attenuated parvovirus vaccines (parenteral or intranasal) to pregnant cats and dogs can lead to cerebellar disease in the fetus, and these vaccines have the potential to cause severe disease if shed vaccine virus infects colostrum-deprived neonates that are less than 2 weeks of age.[2] A febrile lameness syndrome rarely can occur in young kittens vaccinated with certain FCV vaccines.[115,116] This usually develops 7 to 21 days after vaccination and resolves within 7 days with supportive care. Some CDV vaccines have been associated with postvaccinal distemper in young puppies.[117] As a result, vaccination with live attenuated CDV, CPV, and FPV (cats) vaccines should be avoided when possible in pregnant animals, puppies and kittens less than 6 weeks of age, and animals receiving potent anticancer chemotherapy drugs. Some CDV vaccine strains, such as Rockborn-like strains, are more virulent than others, and these may cause postvaccinal distemper in young puppies or severely immunocompromised dogs, and continue to circulate and contribute to distemper in the dog population.[118] The safest attenuated live CDV vaccines contain the Onderstepoort strain. Vaccination of certain exotic pet, zoo, and wildlife species, such as ferrets, with any attenuated live CDV vaccine for dogs can also lead to postvaccinal distemper.[119,120] For animals with chronic immunocompromise, the use of inactivated vaccines has been recommended if immunization is deemed necessary. However, inactivated vaccines may have reduced efficacy in immunocompromised animals compared with healthy animals.

The use of mucosal (e.g., intranasal) vaccines for respiratory pathogens in dogs and cats can be followed by development of mild to moderate, transient upper respiratory tract signs. There have been concerns that mucosal *B. bronchiseptica* vaccines may cause respiratory disease in immunosuppressed humans who inhale the vaccine directly during administration or who contact vaccine organisms that are subsequently shed by the vaccinated dog,[121,122] but definitive proof of this is still required (see Chapter 55). Inadvertent parenteral administration of the avirulent live intranasal *B. bronchiseptica* vaccine to dogs can lead to local injection-site reactions and, occasionally, fatal hepatic necrosis.[123] Inadvertent parenteral administration of mucosal *B. bronchiseptica* vaccines should be treated with subcutaneous fluids at the site of administration and an oral antibiotic likely to be effective against *B. bronchiseptica*, such as doxycycline. The ASPCA Poison Control Center also recommends injection of a gentamicin sulfate solution into the affected area (2 to 4 mg/kg gentamicin sulfate in 10 to 30 mL of saline).[3] Doxycycline treatment could be continued for 5 to 7 days. Dogs that develop hepatic necrosis may need more aggressive supportive care.

Local Cutaneous Reactions and Injection-Site Sarcomas

Local cutaneous reactions are common adverse effects of vaccination, especially in cats, and include pain, swelling, irritation, and abscess formation. In dogs, focal alopecia or discoloration of the haircoat at the vaccination site can also occur (Fig. 20.6). Inactivated vaccines that contain adjuvant have been most commonly incriminated. Focal cutaneous granulomas and sometimes permanent focal alopecia have been most commonly reported after inactivated rabies vaccine administration to breeds such as Maltese terriers and bichon frisé.

In the late 1980s, an increase in inflammatory injection-site reactions at the sites of rabies vaccine administration were noted in canine and feline biopsy specimens sent to the University of Pennsylvania. Shortly thereafter, sarcomas were observed at these sites in cats in the United States, with a 25% increase each year from 1987 to 1991 (Fig. 20.7).[124] This followed: (1) the change from attenuated live to inactivated rabies vaccines, (2) increased use of rabies vaccines in cats, and (3) the introduction of FeLV vaccines. The national incidence of sarcoma

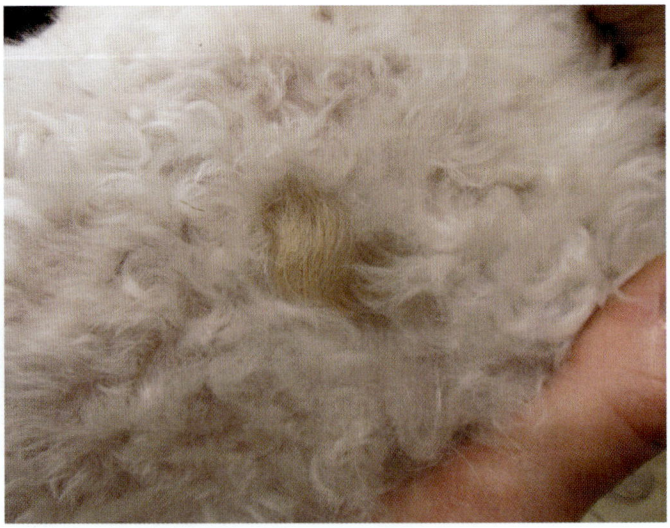

Fig. 20.6 A 2-year-old female toy poodle/Maltese terrier mix that developed focal alopecia at the site of vaccination followed by regrowth of hair with an altered color and texture. (Courtesy Nicole Pierce, University of California, Davis, Class of 2013.)

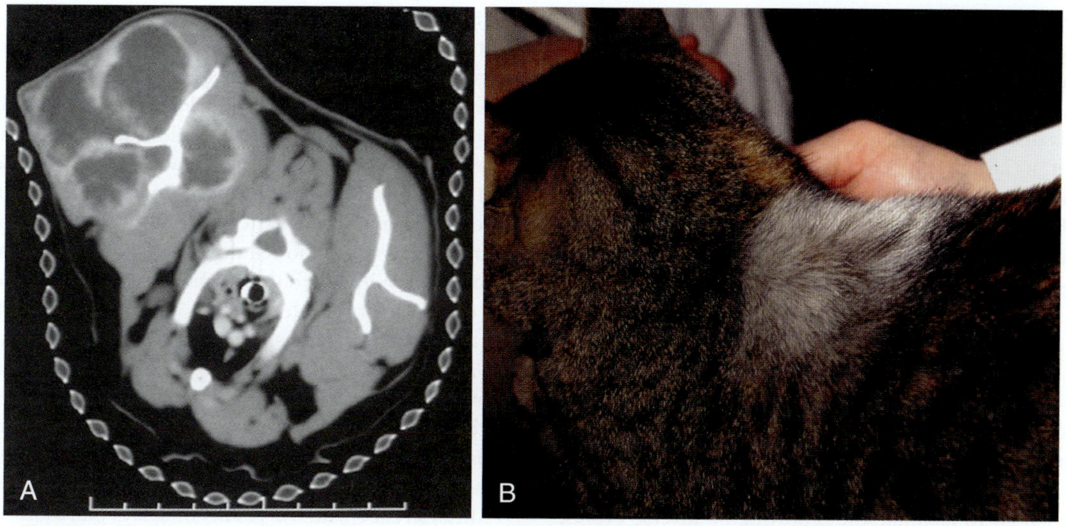

Fig. 20.7 (A) Computed tomographic image of an injection-site sarcoma over the scapula of a 12-year-old male neutered domestic shorthair cat. (B) Discoloration of the haircoat after radiation therapy.

formation is estimated to be 0.6 to 2 sarcomas per 10,000 cats that are vaccinated.[125,126] In contrast, in the United Kingdom, it was 0.21 per 10,000 vaccine doses sold between 1995 and 1999[126] and 1 per 5,000 to 12,500 vaccination visits in 2013.[127] The interval between tumor development and the last rabies vaccine typically ranges from 2 months to 10 years. Most tumors are fibrosarcomas, but other types of sarcomas can also occur. The term feline ISS is preferred to vaccine-associated sarcoma because the sarcomas have arisen at sites where other medications, including long-acting glucocorticoids, meloxicam, and intralesional cisplatin, have been injected.[128,129] The FDA also lists injection-site neoplasms as reported adverse effects following cefovecin injection. In addition, sarcomas have been identified at the site of a deep, nonabsorbable suture[130]; a retained abdominal surgical sponge[131]; microchip implantation[132,133]; and an indwelling port for subcutaneous fluids administration.[134] Feline ISSs differ histologically and are more aggressive in behavior than sarcomas at other sites. They are characterized by perivascular infiltration of lymphocytes and macrophages at the tumor periphery, a central area of necrosis and infiltration by tumor cells. The rate of metastasis has been estimated at 10%–28%,[135,136] with the most common site of metastasis being the lung.[137]

Although development of ISSs is clearly linked to administration of FeLV, rabies, and other vaccines, development of sarcomas is not related to the use of specific brands or types of vaccine within an antigen class (with the exception of recombinant vaccines, which have been associated with a decreased risk of ISS[138]), reuse of syringes, needle gauge, use and shaking of multidose vials, or concomitant viral infection.[139] There is also a lack of evidence that aluminum-containing vaccines are associated with a higher risk of sarcoma development than aluminum-free vaccines. There has been concern that adjuvant stimulates an intense inflammatory response that predisposes to sarcoma formation. One study showed that inactivated vaccines were approximately 10 times more likely to be associated with ISSs when administered at the pelvic limb site than nonadjuvanted recombinant vaccines.[138] An *in vitro* study that involved exposure of feline fibroblasts to aluminum chloride salts promoted cell cycle progression and cell growth, suggesting that aluminum alone may be capable of tumorigenesis in the absence of inflammation.[140] A study from Switzerland suggested that a decline in the incidence of feline ISSs may have followed introduction of a nonadjuvanted FeLV vaccine.[141]

Nevertheless, neither attenuated live, recombinant, nor inactivated vaccines are risk-free, and the connection between adjuvants and ISSs remains controversial.[142] There is some evidence that administration of cold vaccine may also be more likely to be associated with sarcoma formation, but this also requires verification.[139] To date, no oncogenic viruses have been identified in association with the sarcomas despite searches for FeLV, FIV, feline sarcoma virus, FFV, polyomavirus, and papillomaviruses.[143–147]

Treatment of ISSs involves aggressive surgical resection together with full-course radiation therapy because of the high incidence of recurrence. Radiation therapy may be delivered preoperatively, targeting the entire tumor plus a 3- to 5-cm margin, or postoperatively.[148] Median times to reported recurrence are 2 months to > 16 months, and recurrence may be manifested as multiple new tumors that develop along the surgical scar site. Advanced imaging using CT or MRI is necessary to determine the full extent of the tumor before surgery. In assessing tumor size, one study showed that CT is more accurate than physical examination, especially for larger tumors.[149] Possible adverse effects of radiation include mild to moderate cutaneous burns, hypopigmentation of the hair in the field (see Fig. 20.7B), and damage to the spinal cord, lungs, and kidneys within the field, although the last is rare. Use of computer-based radiation treatment plans and linear accelerators that incorporate imaging technology can help to reduce the size of the radiation field. In one study, the median survival time for cats treated with postsurgical curative radiation therapy was 43 months.[150] Most of these cats had clean margins after surgical resection of the tumor. In contrast, the median survival times for cats treated with coarse fractionated radiation therapy was 24 months. These cats generally had macroscopic disease or dirty margins. Postoperative brachytherapy using iridium-192 implants has also been used, with a median disease-specific survival time of 1242 days; local failure rate was still 55% and distant failure rate was 14% due to lung metastasis.[151] Adjuvant chemotherapy with carboplatin, single-agent doxorubicin, or epirubicin also has been associated with improved outcome in some studies.[150,152] *In vitro* sensitivity of ISS cells to carboplatin has been demonstrated.[153] Administration of toceranib to affected cats did not appear to result in clinical response in one study.[154] Administration of a recombinant canarypox vector expressing IL-2 at the tumor site commencing just before brachytherapy and continuing on day 7, 14, 21, 35 and 49 in 71 cats with ISSs resulted in a significantly longer time to relapse (> 730 days) when compared with surgery and radiation therapy alone (287 days).[155] This product was approved by the European Medicines Agency in 2013 (Oncept IL-2, Boehringer Ingelheim Vetmedica GmbH) and was conditionally licensed by the USDA in 2015 to delay postsurgical recurrence of feline fibrosarcoma in adult cats with stage I disease.

In order to prevent death from sarcoma formation in cats, a task force, the Vaccine-Associated Feline Sarcoma Task Force (VAFSTF) in North America recommended that rabies vaccines be administered as distally as possible on the right pelvic limb, and leukemia vaccines be administered as distally as possible on the left pelvic limb ("rabies right, leukemia left"). Care should be taken not to administer the vaccine too proximally or in the flank region, because tumors in these locations cannot be resected as effectively.[156] Vaccination of the cat in a crouched position may result in inadvertent administration into a more proximal location. The AAFP suggested that other core vaccines should be administered below the right elbow.[126] These recommendations were not adopted by the WSAVA, which suggested that vaccination sites be rotated from year to year.[2] The tail has also been used.[157] Both groups recommended that the interscapular region be avoided because vaccine constituents can pool in this region and contribute to a chronic inflammatory response. In addition, both groups recommended that the sites of administration and the product and batch number be documented to facilitate the reporting of adverse events. Excessive administration of vaccines to cats should be minimized. Owners should be advised to monitor injection sites for 3 months after vaccines are administered. The AAFP recommends performance of an incisional biopsy if a mass: (1) persists for 3 months or longer after injection; (2) becomes larger than 2 cm in diameter; or (3) continues to increase in size 1 month after injection (the "3-2-1 rule").[126]

In accordance with the VAFSTF recommendations, the anatomic location, shape, and size of masses that develop at injection sites should be documented, and an incisional or tru-cut biopsy performed. Fine-needle aspiration and excisional biopsy are not recommended because excisional biopsy is unlikely to be sufficient treatment should a sarcoma be present. If the mass is malignant, routine laboratory tests and thoracic radiography should be performed, together with CT or MRI of the mass if client finances allow. A veterinary oncologist should be consulted, and if possible, referral to a specialist surgeon or oncologist is recommended. Wide excision that includes at least a 3-cm margin (and preferably 5-cm margin) is necessary, together with one fascial plane beneath the mass,[158] and the entire piece of tissue excised should be submitted for histopathology and evaluation of surgical margins. Additional treatment, such as radiation therapy, chemotherapy, and immunotherapy (where available) can improve outcome. Cats should be reevaluated at 3-month intervals for at least 1 year after surgery.

Interference with Diagnostic Test Results

Vaccination has the potential to interfere with the results of assays that detect the antibody response to infection or assays that detect components of a pathogen itself.

Interference with antibody test results can be specific for the target pathogen or nonspecific. Nonspecific interference results from cross-reactivity between antibodies to vaccine components (such as albumin) and the reagents used in serodiagnostic tests, but it is rarely a problem. More commonly, specific interference occurs, resulting in false-positive test results for the infection targeted by the diagnostic test. This especially problematic if: (1) vaccination does not completely protect against infection, (2) the results of antibody tests are required for diagnosis, and (3) infection is chronic and persistent, and so identification of recent natural infection through seroconversion is usually not possible. For example, the inactivated FIV vaccine that is still available in some countries (Fel-O-Vax FIV, Boehringer Ingelheim) does not provide 100% protection, but vaccinated cats develop antibodies to the vaccine virus. These antibodies are detected by some ELISA and Western blot immunoassays used for diagnosis of FIV infection. In the absence of a history of vaccination, and in kittens older than 6 months of age, positive antibody test results for FIV indicate active infection.[159] PCR can be used to detect FIV infection in infected cats that have a history of vaccination with FIV vaccines, but PCR can occasionally be negative in cats with active infection, so a negative PCR result does not rule out natural infection with FIV. Vaccine interference with serodiagnosis can occur after vaccination of dogs for influenza or leptospirosis, but because both of these diseases are acute, seroconversion can be used for diagnosis of recent infection in vaccinated dogs. Some serologic assays differentiate between vaccinated and naturally infected animals (DIVA). Although not designed with that intent, the Antigen Rapid and Witness (Zoetis) generally only test positive for antibodies to FIV in truly infected cats, and are negative in uninfected cats that have been previously vaccinated. Serologic assays that detect the C6 antigen of *B. burgdorferi* do not detect antibodies that result from immunization with Lyme vaccines. The development of recombinant vaccines that stimulate a pattern of antibody responses that differ from those that result from natural infection can help to overcome issues related to differentiation of naturally infected and vaccinated animals.

Interference with the results of assays *that detect the pathogen itself (as opposed to the antibody response)* occurs after vaccination with attenuated live vaccine organisms that are shed by animals after vaccination. For example, cats may test positive using ELISA assays for FPV antigen after vaccination with attenuated live FPV vaccines, although for some assays, the rate at which this occurs is very low.[160] PCR tests can be positive for days to several weeks after vaccination with attenuated live vaccines.[161,162] In some cases, sequence analysis of the PCR product can sometimes allow differentiation between vaccine and field strains, but this is currently performed only on a research basis.[163] Rapid PCR assays have also been designed that differentiate between vaccine and field strains of some pathogens, such as CDV or *B. bronchiseptica.*[164,165] Quantification of organism numbers present in a specimen through the use of real-time PCR assays (e.g., for CDV) may shed light on whether natural infection (high organism load) or vaccination (low organism load) has occurred.

VACCINE SELECTION

The advantages and disadvantages of vaccines and vaccine combinations that are currently available on the market are provided in the relevant sections of this book for each infection entitled "Immunity and Vaccination." Suggested vaccination schedules for individual pets and shelter animals that are based on recommendations provided by the AAHA, the AAFP, the International Society of Feline Medicine (ISFM), and WSAVA are summarized in tables in the Appendix.[2,17,126,166–173]

To facilitate vaccine selection, vaccines for dogs and cats have been divided by various task forces into core vaccines, noncore vaccines, and those that are generally not recommended.

Core vaccines are recommended for all animals with an unknown vaccination history. The diseases involved have significant morbidity and mortality and are widely distributed, and in general, vaccination results in good protection from disease. All shelter animals should be vaccinated with core vaccines before entry to a shelter or at the time of entry if immunization ahead of time is not possible. Canine core vaccines include vaccines for CPV, CDV, CAdV, and rabies for countries where rabies is endemic. The leptospirosis vaccine also has been recommended as a core vaccine by the BSAVA[174] and some academic veterinary hospitals. The core feline vaccines are those for FHV-1, FCV, FPV, and rabies.

Noncore vaccines are optional vaccines that should be considered in light of exposure risk, that is, based on geographic distribution and the lifestyle of the pet. Vaccines considered as noncore vaccines for dogs are CPIV, CIV, *B. bronchiseptica, Leptospira* spp. (core in some statements), and *B. burgdorferi.* Optional or noncore vaccines for cats include FeLV, FIV, *C. felis,* and *B. bronchiseptica* vaccines.

Several other vaccines for infectious diseases are currently available on the market. For dogs, these are vaccines for CCoV, FIP, and rattlesnake envenomation. The reports of the AVMA and the AAHA canine vaccine task force, as well as the WSAVA guidelines, have listed the CoV vaccine as not generally recommended. Reasons for listing vaccines as not generally recommended are that "the diseases are either of little clinical significance or respond readily to treatment," evidence for efficacy of these vaccines is minimal, and they may "produce adverse events with limited benefit." Two studies examined outcomes following rattlesnake vaccination with the *Crotalus atrox* vaccine. One study used a mouse model and demonstrated improved survival following challenge with western diamondback venom, but not with northern Pacific or southern Pacific rattlesnake venom.[175] One retrospective study included 15 dogs that had received the rattlesnake vaccine and 256 dogs that had not received the vaccine. No significant difference was found between canine snakebite severity scores and a history of having received the vaccine.[176] Of concern, anaphylactic shock was reported in two dogs that had been previously vaccinated with the *C. atrox* vaccine following first-time envenomation, the authors hypothesizing that the vaccine was the initial inciting trigger.[177] For cats, the intranasal FIP vaccine is not generally recommended by the AAFP or the WSAVA because most cats are infected with FCoV before the age for initial vaccination (16 weeks), and the vaccine contains a CoV type that differs from the type that causes most infections (see Chapter 31).

VACCINATION OF EXOTIC CARNIVORES

Many nondomestic carnivores are vaccinated for diseases of dogs and cats with commercially available canine and feline vaccines. Unless absolutely necessary, attenuated live products should not be used in exotic species because they may cause clinical illness, and the potential always exists for reversion of the attenuated strain to virulence in a foreign host. Inactivated and recombinant vaccines should be used only after safety and efficacy have been demonstrated in the specific exotic species. Oral recombinant-vectored rabies vaccines have been used to control rabies in wildlife. The recombinant canarypox virus-vectored CDV vaccine has been proven safe and effective in ferrets and has been recommended to protect other captive wildlife species that are susceptible to distemper.[178,179] Recommendations for vaccination of captive wild canids and felids can be found elsewhere.[179]

Vaccination of wolf hybrids and Bengal cat hybrids has been controversial because they are considered wildlife, and efficacy of canine and feline vaccines in these species has not been proven. Vaccinating these animals creates legal and ethical issues for veterinarians and public health officials. In jurisdictions where these animals are not legal pets, they should not be vaccinated; however, veterinarians can decide to vaccinate in areas where ownership is allowed. The owner should be provided with written notice as part of informed consent that efficacy of vaccines is not proven in these animals.

VACCINATION REQUIREMENTS FOR TRANSPORT OF ANIMALS

Interstate shipment of animals with infectious diseases or those that have recently been exposed to infectious diseases is prohibited within the United States. Each state has established guidelines that generally include a physical examination and current rabies vaccination. Information about pet travel is available online in the current regulations of the USDA,[180] Department of Agriculture in Canada,[181] Department of Agriculture and Natural Resources in Australia,[182] Department of Environment, Food and Rural Affairs in the United Kingdom,[183] and similar bureaus in other countries. Worldwide travel regulations are also available at http://www.pettravel.com/passportnew.cfm.

In the European Economic Community, animals can move between member countries provided they show no signs of disease, are identified by tattoo or implanted microchip, are vaccinated using a WHO-approved vaccine certified by an official veterinarian, and are accompanied by an animal passport clearly identifying the individual.

For information regarding serologic testing and proof of rabies immunization for transport of animals, see Chapter 21.

SUGGESTED READINGS

Baker C, Pickering L, Chilton L, et al. General recommendations on immunization—recommendations of the advisory Committee on immunization practices (ACP). *MMWR Recomm Rep (Morb Mortal Wkly Rep)*. 2011;60(2):1–64.

Day MJ, Horzinek MC, Schultz RD. WSAVA guidelines for the vaccination of dogs and cats. *J Small Anim Pract*. 2016;57(1):E1–E45.

Larson LJ, Newbury S, Schultz R.D. Canine and feline vaccinations and immunology. In: Miller L, Hurley K eds. *Infectious Disease Management in Animal Shelters*. Ames, IO: Wiley-Blackwell; 2009:61–82.

Moore GE, HogenEsch H. Adverse vaccinal events in dogs and cats. *Vet Clin North Am Small Anim Pract*. 2010;40:393–407.

Welborn LV, DeVries JG, Ford R, et al. 2011 AAHA canine vaccination guidelines. *J Am Anim Hosp Assoc*. 2011;47:1–42.

Stone AE, Brummet GO, Carroza EM, et al. 2020 AAHA/AAFP Feline Vaccination Guidelines. *J Fel Med Surg*. 2020;22:813–830. https://www.aaha.org/aaha-guidelines/2020-aahaaafp-feline-vaccination-guidelines/feline-vaccination-home/

REFERENCES

1. Abbas AK, Lichtman AHH, Pillai S. *Cellular and Molecular Immunology*. 8th ed. Philadelphia, PA: Elsevier Saunders; 2015.
2. Day MJ, Horzinek MC, Schultz RD, et al. WSAVA Guidelines for the vaccination of dogs and cats. *J Small Anim Pract*. 2016;57:E1–E45.
3. Larson LJ, Newbury S, Schultz RD. Canine and feline vaccinations and immunology. In: Miller L, Hurley K, eds. *Infectious Disease Management in Animal Shelters*. Ames, IO: Wiley-Blackwell; 2009:61–82.
4. Apostolico Jde S, Lunardelli VA, Coirada FC, et al. Adjuvants: classification, modus operandi, and licensing. *J Immunol Res*. 2016;2016:1459394.
5. De Gregorio E, D'Oro U, Wack A. Immunology of TLR-independent vaccine adjuvants. *Curr Opin Immunol*. 2009;21:339–345.
6. Abdelmagid OY, Larson L, Payne L, et al. Evaluation of the efficacy and duration of immunity of a canine combination vaccine against virulent parvovirus, infectious canine hepatitis virus, and distemper virus experimental challenges. *Vet Ther*. 2004;5:173–186.
7. Schultz RD. Duration of immunity for canine and feline vaccines: a review. *Vet Microbiol*. 2006;117:75–79.
8. Schultz RD, Thiel B, Mukhtar E, et al. Age and long-term protective immunity in dogs and cats. *J Comp Pathol*. 2010;142(suppl 1):S102–108.
9. Brun A, Chappuis G, Precausta P, et al. Immunisation against panleukopenia: early development of immunity. *Comp Immunol Microbiol Infect Dis*. 1979;1:335–339.
10. Larson LJ, Schultz RD. Effect of vaccination with recombinant canine distemper virus vaccine immediately before exposure under shelter-like conditions. *Vet Ther*. 2006;7:113–118.
11. Mastro JM, Axthelm M, Mathes LE, et al. Repeated suppression of lymphocyte blastogenesis following vaccinations of CPV-immune dogs with modified live CPV vaccines. *Vet Microbiol*. 1986;12:201–211.
12. Phillips TR, Jensen JL, Rubino MJ, et al. Effects of vaccines on the canine immune system. *Can J Vet Res*. 1989;53:154–160.
13. Strasser A, May B, Teltscher A, et al. Immune modulation following immunization with polyvalent vaccines in dogs. *Vet Immunol Immunopathol*. 2003;94:113–121.
14. Foley JE, Orgad U, Hirsh DC, et al. Outbreak of fatal salmonellosis in cats following use of a high-titer modified-live panleukopenia virus vaccine. *J Am Vet Med Assoc*. 1999;214(67–70):43–64.
15. Wilbur LA, Evermann JF, Levings RL, et al. Abortion and death in pregnant bitches associated with a canine vaccine contaminated with bluetongue virus. *J Am Vet Med Assoc*. 1994;204:1762–1765.

16. Yoshikawa R, Shimode S, Sakaguchi S, et al. Contamination of live attenuated vaccines with an infectious feline endogenous retrovirus (RD-114 virus). *Arch Virol*. 2014;159:399–404.
17. Welborn LV, DeVries JG, Ford R, et al. 2011 AAHA canine vaccination guidelines. *J Am Anim Hosp Assoc*. 2011;47:1–42.
18. Baker C, Pickering L, Chilton L, et al. General recommendations on immunization – recommendations of the Advisory Committee on Immunization Practices (ACP). *MMWR Recomm Rep (Morb Mortal Wkly Rep)*. 2011;60:1–64.
19. Yao PJ, Stephenson N, Foley JE, et al. Incidence rates and risk factors for owner-reported adverse events following vaccination of dogs that did or did not receive a *Leptospira* vaccine. *J Am Vet Med Assoc*. 2015;247:1139–1145.
20. Grosenbaugh DA, Pardo MC. Fifteen-month duration of immunity for the serovar Grippotyphosa fraction of a tetravalent canine leptospirosis vaccine. *Vet Rec*. 2018;182:665.
21. Wilson S, Stirling C, Thomas A, et al. Duration of immunity of a multivalent (DHPPi/L4R) canine vaccine against four *Leptospira* serovars. *Vaccine*. 2013;31:3126–3130.
22. Scott FW, Geissinger CM. Long-term immunity in cats vaccinated with an inactivated trivalent vaccine. *Am J Vet Res*. 1999;60:652–658.
23. Kruger JM, Sussman MD, Maes RK. Glycoproteins gl and gE of feline herpesvirus-1 are virulence genes: safety and efficacy of a gl-gE deletion mutant in the natural host. *Virology*. 1996;220:299–308.
24. Balint A, Farsang A, Szeredi L, et al. Recombinant feline coronaviruses as vaccine candidates confer protection in SPF but not in conventional cats. *Vet Microbiol*. 2014;169:154–162.
25. Gilbert JH, Pedersen NC, Nunberg JH. Feline leukemia virus envelope protein expression encoded by a recombinant vaccinia virus: apparent lack of immunogenicity in vaccinated animals. *Virus Res*. 1987;7:49–67.
26. Hu RL, Liu Y, Zhang SF, et al. Experimental immunization of cats with a recombinant rabies-canine adenovirus vaccine elicits a long-lasting neutralizing antibody response against rabies. *Vaccine*. 2007;25:5301–5307.
27. McCabe VJ, Spibey N. Potential for broad-spectrum protection against feline calicivirus using an attenuated myxoma virus expressing a chimeric FCV capsid protein. *Vaccine*. 2005;23:5380–5388.
28. Jorritsma SH, Gowans EJ, Grubor-Bauk B, et al. Delivery methods to increase cellular uptake and immunogenicity of DNA vaccines. *Vaccine*. 2016;34:5488–5494.
29. King GE, Hadler SC. Simultaneous administration of childhood vaccines: an important public health policy that is safe and efficacious. *Pediatr Infect Dis J*. 1994;13:394–407.
30. Moore GE, Guptill LF, Ward MP, et al. Adverse events diagnosed within three days of vaccine administration in dogs. *J Am Vet Med Assoc*. 2005;227:1102–1108.
31. Offit PA, Quarles J, Gerber MA, et al. Addressing parents' concerns: do multiple vaccines overwhelm or weaken the infant's immune system? *Pediatrics*. 2002;109:124–129.
32. Bergman JG, Muniz M, Sutton D, et al. Comparative trial of the canine parvovirus, canine distemper virus and canine adenovirus type 2 fractions of two commercially available modified live vaccines. *Vet Rec*. 2006;159:733–736.
33. Guiot AL, Cariou C, Krogmann V, et al. Compatibility between a rabies vaccine and a combined vaccine against feline rhinotracheitis, FCV, FPLV and FeLV, and *Chlamydophila felis*. *Vet Rec*. 2008;162:690–692.
34. Jacobs AA, Bergman JG, Theelen RP, et al. Compatibility of a bivalent modified-live vaccine against *Bordetella bronchiseptica* and CPiV, and a trivalent modified-live vaccine against CPV, CDV and CAV-2. *Vet Rec*. 2007;160:41–45.
35. Kanellos T, Sutton DJ, Salisbury CF, et al. Combined administration in a single injection of a feline multivalent modified live vaccine against FHV, FCV, and FPLV together with a recombinant FeLV vaccine is both safe and efficacious for all four major feline viral pathogens. *J Feline Med Surg*. 2008;10:346–354.
36. Orenstein WA, Pickering LK, Mawle A, et al. Immunization. In: Mandell GL, Bennett GE, Dolin R, eds. *Principles and Practice of Infectious Diseases*. Philadelphia, PA: Churchill Livingstone, Elsevier; 2010:3917–3949.
37. Reese MJ, Patterson EV, Tucker SJ, et al. Effects of anesthesia and surgery on serologic responses to vaccination in kittens. *J Am Vet Med Assoc*. 2008;233:116–121.
38. Coffey TJ, Werling D. Therapeutic targeting of the innate immune system in domestic animals. *Cell Tissue Res*. 2011;343:251–261.
39. Li P, Wang F. Polysaccharides: candidates of promising vaccine adjuvants. *Drug Discov Ther*. 2015;9:88–93.
40. Day MJ. Vaccine side effects: fact and fiction. *Vet Microbiol*. 2006;117:51–58.
41. Kennedy LJ, Lunt M, Barnes A, et al. Factors influencing the antibody response of dogs vaccinated against rabies. *Vaccine*. 2007;25:8500–8507.
42. Berndtsson LT, Nyman AK, Rivera E, et al. Factors associated with the success of rabies vaccination of dogs in Sweden. *Acta Vet Scand*. 2011;53:22.
43. Casal ML, Jezyk PF, Giger U. Transfer of colostral antibodies from queens to their kittens. *Am J Vet Res*. 1996;57:1653–1658.
44. Carmichael LE, Robson DS, Barnes FD. Transfer and decline of maternal infectious canine hepatitis antibody in puppies. *Proc Soc Exp Biol Med*. 1962;109:677–681.
45. Edwards BG, Buell DJ, Acree WM. Evaluation of a new feline rhinotracheitis virus vaccine. *Vet Med Small Anim Clin*. 1977;72:205–209.
46. Gaskell RM. Studies on feline viral rhinotracheitis virus with particular reference to the carrier state. PhD thesis: University of Bristol, Bristol, UK; 1975.
47. Gillespie JH, Baker JA, Burgher J, et al. The immune response of dogs to distemper virus. *Cornell Vet*. 1958;48:103–126.
48. Johnson RP. Immunity to feline calicivirus in kittens. PhD thesis. University of Guelph, Guelph, Ontario, Canada; 1980.
49. Pollock RV, Carmichael LE. Maternally derived immunity to canine parvovirus infection: transfer, decline, and interference with vaccination. *J Am Vet Med Assoc*. 1982;180:37–42.
50. Pollock RV, Carmichael LE. Use of modified live feline panleukopenia virus vaccine to immunize dogs against canine parvovirus. *Am J Vet Res*. 1983;44:169–175.
51. Povey RC. A review of feline viral rhinotracheitis (feline herpesvirus I infection). *Comp Immunol Microbiol Infect Dis*. 1979;2:373–387.
52. Scott FW, Csiza CK, Gillespie JH. Maternally derived immunity to feline panleukopenia. *J Am Vet Med Assoc*. 1970;156:439–453.
53. Jarrett O, Russell PH, Stewart MF. Protection of kittens from feline leukaemia virus infection by maternally-derived antibody. *Vet Rec*. 1977;101:304–305.
54. Johnson RP, Povey RC. Transfer and decline of maternal antibody to feline calicivirus. *Can Vet J*. 1983;24:6–9.
55. MacDonald K, Levy JK, Tucker SJ, et al. Effects of passive transfer of immunity on results of diagnostic tests for antibodies against feline immunodeficiency virus in kittens born to vaccinated queens. *J Am Vet Med Assoc*. 2004;225:1554–1557.
56. Pedersen NC, Boyle JF, Floyd K, et al. An enteric coronavirus infection of cats and its relationship to feline infectious peritonitis. *Am J Vet Res*. 1981;42:368–377.
57. Jonsdottir I. Maturation of mucosal immune responses and influence of maternal antibodies. *J Comp Pathol*. 2007;137(suppl 1):S20–S26.
58. Siegrist CA. The challenges of vaccine responses in early life: selected examples. *J Comp Pathol*. 2007;137(suppl 1):S4–9.
59. United States Department of Agriculture Animal and Plant Health Inspection Service. Veterinary Services Memorandum. 800.202; 2016. https://www.aphis.usda.gov/animal_health/vet_biologics/publications/memo_800_202.pdf.
60. Gill M, Shrivas J, Morozov I, et al. Three-year duration of immunity for canine distemper, adenovirus, and parvovirus after vaccination with a multivalent canine vaccine. *Int J Appl Res*. 2004;2:227–235.
61. Gore TC, Lakshmanan N, Duncan KL, et al. Three-year duration of immunity in dogs following vaccination against canine adenovirus type-1, canine parvovirus, and canine distemper virus. *Vet Ther*. 2005;6:5–14.
62. Lakshmanan N, Gore TC, Duncan KL, et al. Three-year rabies duration of immunity in dogs following vaccination with a core combination vaccine against canine distemper virus, canine adenovirus type-1, canine parvovirus, and rabies virus. *Vet Ther*. 2006;7:223–231.

63. Chu HJ, Chavez Jr LG, Blumer BM, et al. Immunogenicity and efficacy study of a commercial *Borrelia burgdorferi* bacterin. *J Am Vet Med Assoc.* 1992;201:403–411.
64. LaFleur RL, Callister SM, Dant JC, et al. One-year duration of immunity induced by vaccination with a canine Lyme disease bacterin. *Clin Vaccine Immunol.* 2010;17:870–874.
65. Wikle RE, Fretwell B, Jarecki M, et al. Canine Lyme disease: one-year duration of immunity elicited with a canine OspA monovalent Lyme vaccine. *Int J Appl Res Vet Med.* 2006;4:23–28.
66. Klaasen HL, Molkenboer MJ, Vrijenhoek MP, et al. Duration of immunity in dogs vaccinated against leptospirosis with a bivalent inactivated vaccine. *Vet Microbiol.* 2003;95:121–132.
67. Klaasen HL, van der Veen M, Sutton D, et al. A new tetravalent canine leptospirosis vaccine provides at least 12 months immunity against infection. *Vet Immunol Immunopathol.* 2014;158:26–29.
68. Minke JM, Bey R, Tronel JP, et al. Onset and duration of protective immunity against clinical disease and renal carriage in dogs provided by a bi-valent inactivated leptospirosis vaccine. *Vet Microbiol.* 2009;137:137–145.
69. Jacobs AA, Theelen RP, Jaspers R, et al. Protection of dogs for 13 months against *Bordetella bronchiseptica* and canine parainfluenza virus with a modified live vaccine. *Vet Rec.* 2005;157:19–23.
70. Lehar C, Jayappa H, Erskine J, et al. Demonstration of 1-year duration of immunity for attenuated *Bordetella bronchiseptica* vaccines in dogs. *Vet Ther.* 2008;9:257–262.
71. Lappin MR, Andrews J, Simpson D, et al. Use of serologic tests to predict resistance to feline herpesvirus 1, feline calicivirus, and feline parvovirus infection in cats. *J Am Vet Med Assoc.* 2002;220:38–42.
72. Jas D, Frances-Duvert V, Vernes D, et al. Three-year duration of immunity for feline herpesvirus and calicivirus evaluated in a controlled vaccination-challenge laboratory trial. *Vet Microbiol.* 2015;177:123–131.
73. Scott FW. Evaluation of a feline viral rhinotracheitis-feline calicivirus disease vaccine. *Am J Vet Res.* 1977;38:229–234.
74. Poulet H. Alternative early life vaccination programs for companion animals. *J Comp Pathol.* 2007;137(suppl 1):S67–S71.
75. Povey RC, Koonse H, Hays MB. Immunogenicity and safety of an inactivated vaccine for the prevention of rhinotracheitis, caliciviral disease, and panleukopenia in cats. *J Am Vet Med Assoc.* 1980;177:347–350.
76. Jirjis FF, Davis T, Lane J, et al. Protection against feline leukemia virus challenge for at least 2 years after vaccination with an inactivated feline leukemia virus vaccine. *Vet Ther.* 2010;11:E1–E6.
77. Torres AN, O'Halloran KP, Larson LJ, et al. Feline leukemia virus immunity induced by whole inactivated virus vaccination. *Vet Immunol Immunopathol.* 2010;134:122–131.
78. Crawford PC, Levy JK, Leutenegger C. Use of antibody titers and quantitative PCR as risk assessment tools for management of an outbreak of canine distemper and parvovirus. In: *Proceedings of the American College of Veterinary Internal Medicine Forum, Denver, CO.*; 2011.
79. Litster AL, Pressler B, Volpe A, et al. Accuracy of a point-of-care ELISA test kit for predicting the presence of protective canine parvovirus and canine distemper virus antibody concentrations in dogs. *Vet J.* 2012;193:363–366.
80. HogenEsch H, Thompson S. Effect of ageing on the immune response of dogs to vaccines. *J Comp Pathol.* 2010;142(suppl 1):S74–S77.
81. Strasser A, Teltscher A, May B, et al. Age-associated changes in the immune system of German shepherd dogs. *J Vet Med A Physiol Pathol Clin Med.* 2000;47:181–192.
82. Greeley EH, Ballam JM, Harrison JM, et al. The influence of age and gender on the immune system: a longitudinal study in Labrador retriever dogs. *Vet Immunol Immunopathol.* 2001;82:57–71.
83. Heaton PR, Blount DG, Devlin P, et al. Assessing age-related changes in peripheral blood leukocyte phenotypes in Labrador retriever dogs using flow cytometry. *J Nutr.* 2002;132:1655S–1657S.
84. HogenEsch H, Thompson S, Dunham A, et al. Effect of age on immune parameters and the immune response of dogs to vaccines: a cross-sectional study. *Vet Immunol Immunopathol.* 2004;97:77–85.
85. Campbell DJ, Rawlings JM, Koelsch S, et al. Age-related differences in parameters of feline immune status. *Vet Immunol Immunopathol.* 2004;100:73–80.
86. Slater EA. The response to measles and distemper virus in immunosuppressed and normal dogs. *J Am Vet Med Assoc.* 1970;156:1762–1766.
87. Blancou J, Milward F, Toma B. Vaccination against rabies in carnivores treated with corticoids. *Rec Med Vet.* 1981;157:651–657.
88. National Office of Animal Health. NOAH Compendium of Data Sheets for Animal Medicines. https://www.noahcompendium.co.uk/home.
89. Davis G, Rooney A, Cooles S, et al. Suspected adverse events, 2012. *Vet Rec.* 2013;173:573–576.
90. Dyer F, Brown E, Cooles S, et al. Suspected adverse reactions, 2008. *Vet Rec.* 2009;165:162–164.
91. Dyer F, Diesel G, Cooles S, et al. Suspected adverse reactions, 2009. *Vet Rec.* 2010;167:118–121.
92. Dyer F, Mulugeta R, Spagnuolo-Weaver M, et al. Suspected adverse reactions, 2004. *Vet Rec.* 2005;156:561–563.
93. Dyer F, Spagnuolo-Weaver M, Cooles S, et al. Suspected adverse reactions, 2007. *Vet Rec.* 2008;163:69–72.
94. Dyer F, Spagnuolo-Weaver M, Cooles S, et al. Suspected adverse reactions, 2006. *Vet Rec.* 2007;160:748–750.
95. Dyer F, Diesel G, Cooles S, et al. Suspected adverse events, 2011. *Vet Rec.* 2012;170:640–643.
96. Davis G, Cooles S, Vasan N. Suspected adverse events, 2013. *Vet Rec.* 2015;176:11–14.
97. Moore GE, HogenEsch H. Adverse vaccinal events in dogs and cats. *Vet Clin North Am Small Anim Pract.* 2010;40:393–407.
98. Greene CE, Levy JK. Immunoprophylaxis. In: Greene CE, ed. *Infectious Diseases of the Dog and Cat.* 4th ed. Philadelphia, PA: Elsevier Saunders; 2011:1185–1188.
99. Edwards DS, Henley WE, Ely ER, et al. Vaccination and ill-health in dogs: a lack of temporal association and evidence of equivalence. *Vaccine.* 2004;22:3270–3273.
100. Kogan LR, Hellyer PW, Rishniw M. American and Canadian veterinarians' perceptions on dog and cat core vaccination rates and the impact of the human medicine anti-vaxx movement on veterinary medicine. *Can Vet J.* 2021;62:247–252.
101. Moore GE, DeSantis-Kerr AC, Guptill LF, et al. Adverse events after vaccine administration in cats: 2,560 cases (2002-2005). *J Am Vet Med Assoc.* 2007;231:94–100.
102. Ohmori K, Masuda K, Maeda S, et al. IgE reactivity to vaccine components in dogs that developed immediate-type allergic reactions after vaccination. *Vet Immunol Immunopathol.* 2005;104:249–256.
103. Tater KC, Jackson HA, Paps J, et al. Effects of routine prophylactic vaccination or administration of aluminum adjuvant alone on allergen-specific serum IgE and IgG responses in allergic dogs. *Am J Vet Res.* 2005;66:1572–1577.
104. Day MJ. Vaccine safety in the neonatal period. *J Comp Pathol.* 2007;137(suppl 1):S51–S56.
105. Duval D, Giger U. Vaccine-associated immune-mediated hemolytic anemia in the dog. *J Vet Intern Med.* 1996;10:290–295.
106. Carr AP, Panciera DL, Kidd L. Prognostic factors for mortality and thromboembolism in canine immune-mediated hemolytic anemia: a retrospective study of 72 dogs. *J Vet Intern Med.* 2002;16:504–509.
107. Straw B. Decrease in platelet count after vaccination with distemper-hepatitis (DH) vaccine. *Vet Med Small Anim Clin.* 1978;73:725–726.
108. Scott-Moncrieff JC, Azcona-Olivera J, Glickman NW, et al. Evaluation of antithyroglobulin antibodies after routine vaccination in pet and research dogs. *J Am Vet Med Assoc.* 2002;221:515–521.
109. Whittemore JC, Hawley JR, Jensen WA, et al. Antibodies against Crandell Rees feline kidney (CRFK) cell line antigens, alpha-enolase, and annexin A2 in vaccinated and CRFK hyperinoculated cats. *J Vet Intern Med.* 2010;24:306–313.
110. Nichols PR, Morris DO, Beale KM. A retrospective study of canine and feline cutaneous vasculitis. *Vet Dermatol.* 2001;12:255–264.
111. Wilcock BP, Yager JA. Focal cutaneous vasculitis and alopecia at sites of rabies vaccination in dogs. *J Am Vet Med Assoc.* 1986;188:1174–1177.

112. Vitale CB, Gross TL, Magro CM. Vaccine-induced ischemic dermatopathy in the dog. *Vet Dermatol.* 1999;10:131–142.
113. Kohn SL, Garner M, Bennett D, et al. Polyarthritis following vaccination in four dogs. *Vet Comp Orthoped Traumatol.* 2003;16:6–10.
114. Gehring R, Eggars B. Suspected post-vaccinal acute polyradiculoneuritis in a puppy. *J S Afr Vet Assoc.* 2001;72:96.
115. Dawson S, Gaskell RM. Problems with respiratory virus vaccination in cats. *Compend Contin Educ Pract Vet.* 1993;15:1347–1369.
116. Dawson S, McArdle F, Bennett D, et al. Investigation of vaccine reactions and breakdowns after feline calicivirus vaccination. *Vet Rec.* 1993;132:346–350.
117. Cornwell HJ, Thompson H, McCandlish IA, et al. Encephalitis in dogs associated with a batch of canine distemper (Rockborn) vaccine. *Vet Rec.* 1988;122:54–59.
118. Martella V, Blixenkrone-Moller M, Elia G, et al. Lights and shades on an historical vaccine canine distemper virus, the Rockborn strain. *Vaccine.* 2011;29:1222–1227.
119. Bush M, Montali RJ, Brownstein D, et al. Vaccine-induced canine distemper in a lesser panda. *J Am Vet Med Assoc.* 1976;169:959–960.
120. Carpenter JW, Appel MJ, Erickson RC, et al. Fatal vaccine-induced canine distemper virus infection in black-footed ferrets. *J Am Vet Med Assoc.* 1976;169:961–964.
121. Berkelman RL. Human illness associated with use of veterinary vaccines. *Clin Infect Dis.* 2003;37:407–414.
122. Gisel JJ, Brumble LM, Johnson MM. *Bordetella bronchiseptica* pneumonia in a kidney-pancreas transplant patient after exposure to recently vaccinated dogs. *Transpl Infect Dis.* 2010;12:73–76.
123. Toshach K, Jackson MW, Dubielzig RR. Hepatocellular necrosis associated with the subcutaneous injection of an intranasal *Bordetella bronchiseptica*-canine parainfluenza vaccine. *J Am Anim Hosp Assoc.* 1997;33:126–128.
124. Hendrick MJ, Shofer FS, Goldschmidt MH, et al. Comparison of fibrosarcomas that developed at vaccination sites and at nonvaccination sites in cats: 239 cases (1991-1992). *J Am Vet Med Assoc.* 1994;205:1425–1429.
125. Gobar GM, Kass PH. World Wide Web-based survey of vaccination practices, postvaccinal reactions, and vaccine site-associated sarcomas in cats. *J Am Vet Med Assoc.* 2002;220:1477–1482.
126. Scherk MA, Ford RB, Gaskell RM, et al. 2013 AAFP Feline Vaccination Advisory Panel report. *J Feline Med Surg.* 2013;15:785–808.
127. Dean RS, Pfeiffer DU, Adams VJ. The incidence of feline injection site sarcomas in the United Kingdom. *BMC Vet Res.* 2013;9:17.
128. Martano M, Morello E, Iussich S, et al. A case of feline injection-site sarcoma at the site of cisplatin injections. *J Feline Med Surg.* 2012;14:751–754.
129. Munday JS, Banyay K, Aberdein D, et al. Development of an injection site sarcoma shortly after meloxicam injection in an unvaccinated cat. *J Feline Med Surg.* 2011;13:988–991.
130. Buracco P, Martano M, Morello E, et al. Vaccine-associated-like fibrosarcoma at the site of a deep nonabsorbable suture in a cat. *Vet J.* 2002;163:105–107.
131. Haddad JL, Goldschmidt MH, Patel RT. Fibrosarcoma arising at the site of a retained surgical sponge in a cat. *Vet Clin Pathol.* 2010;39:241–246.
132. Carminato A, Vascellari M, Marchioro W, et al. Microchip-associated fibrosarcoma in a cat. *Vet Dermatol.* 2011;22:565–569.
133. Daly MK, Saba CF, Crochik SS, et al. Fibrosarcoma adjacent to the site of microchip implantation in a cat. *J Feline Med Surg.* 2008;10:202–205.
134. McLeland SM, Imhoff DJ, Thomas M, et al. Subcutaneous fluid port-associated soft tissue sarcoma in a cat. *J Feline Med Surg.* 2013;15:917–920.
135. Couto CG, Macy DW. Review of treatment options for vaccine-associated feline sarcoma. *J Am Vet Med Assoc.* 1998;213:1426–1427.
136. Hershey AE, Sorenmo KU, Hendrick MJ, et al. Prognosis for presumed feline vaccine-associated sarcoma after excision: 61 cases (1986-1996). *J Am Vet Med Assoc.* 2000;216:58–61.
137. Kobayashi T, Hauck ML, Dodge R, et al. Preoperative radiotherapy for vaccine associated sarcoma in 92 cats. *Vet Radiol Ultrasound.* 2002;43:473–479.
138. Srivastav A, Kass PH, McGill LD, et al. Comparative vaccine-specific and other injectable-specific risks of injection-site sarcomas in cats. *J Am Vet Med Assoc.* 2012;241:595–602.
139. Kass PH, Spangler WL, Hendrick MJ, et al. Multicenter case-control study of risk factors associated with development of vaccine-associated sarcomas in cats. *J Am Vet Med Assoc.* 2003;223:1283–1292.
140. AbdelMageed MA, Foltopoulou P, McNiel EA. Feline vaccine-associated sarcomagenesis: is there an inflammation-independent role for aluminium? *Vet Comp Oncol.* 2018;16:E130–E143.
141. Graf R, Guscetti F, Welle M, et al. Feline injection site sarcomas: data from Switzerland 2009-2014. *J Comp Pathol.* 2018;163:1–5.
142. Kass PH. Prevention of feline injection-site sarcomas: is there a scientific foundation for vaccine recommendations at this time? *Vet Clin North Am Small Anim Pract.* 2018;48:301–306.
143. Ellis JA, Jackson ML, Bartsch RC, et al. Use of immunohistochemistry and polymerase chain reaction for detection of oncornaviruses in formalin-fixed, paraffin-embedded fibrosarcomas from cats. *J Am Vet Med Assoc.* 1996;209:767–771.
144. Kidney BA, Ellis JA, Haines DM, et al. Evaluation of formalin-fixed paraffin-embedded tissues obtained from vaccine site-associated sarcomas of cats for DNA of feline immunodeficiency virus. *Am J Vet Res.* 2000;61:1037–1041.
145. Kidney BA, Ellis JA, Haines DM, et al. Comparison of endogenous feline leukemia virus RNA content in feline vaccine and nonvaccine site-associated sarcomas. *Am J Vet Res.* 2001;62:1990–1994.
146. Kidney BA, Haines DM, Ellis JA, et al. Evaluation of formalin-fixed paraffin-embedded tissues from vaccine site-associated sarcomas of cats for polyomavirus DNA and antigen. *Am J Vet Res.* 2001;62:828–832.
147. Kidney BA, Haines DM, Ellis JA, et al. Evaluation of formalin-fixed paraffin-embedded tissues from vaccine site-associated sarcomas of cats for papillomavirus DNA and antigen. *Am J Vet Res.* 2001;62:833–839.
148. Saba CF. Vaccine-associated feline sarcoma: current perspectives. *Vet Med. (Auckl).* 2017;8:13–20.
149. Ferrari R, Di Giancamillo M, Stefanello D, et al. Clinical and computed tomography tumour dimension assessments for planning wide excision of injection site sarcomas in cats: how strong is the agreement? *Vet Comp Oncol.* 2017;15:374–382.
150. Eckstein C, Guscetti F, Roos M, et al. A retrospective analysis of radiation therapy for the treatment of feline vaccine-associated sarcoma. *Vet Comp Oncol.* 2009;7:54–68.
151. Bloch J, Rogers K, Walker M, et al. Treatment of feline injection-site sarcoma with surgery and iridium-192 brachytherapy: retrospective evaluation of 22 cats. *J Feline Med Surg.* 2020;22:313–321.
152. Bray J, Polton G. Neoadjuvant and adjuvant chemotherapy combined with anatomical resection of feline injection–site sarcoma: results in 21 cats. *Vet Comp Oncol.* 2016;14:147–160.
153. Maxwell EA, Phillips H, Schaeffer DJ, et al. In vitro chemosensitivity of feline injection site-associated sarcoma cell lines to carboplatin. *Vet Surg.* 2018;47:219–226.
154. Holtermann N, Kiupel M, Hirschberger J. The tyrosine kinase inhibitor toceranib in feline injection site sarcoma: efficacy and side effects. *Vet Comp Oncol.* 2017;15:632–640.
155. Jas D, de Fornel-Thibaud P, Guigal PM, et al. A clinical trial to evaluate the efficacy of an adjuvant immunotherapy of feline injection-site sarcomas, in association with surgery and brachytherapy. In: *International Society of Feline Medicine Conference, Riga, Latvia*; 2014.
156. Shaw SC, Kent MS, Gordon IK, et al. Temporal changes in characteristics of injection-site sarcomas in cats: 392 cases (1990-2006). *J Am Vet Med Assoc.* 2009;234:376–380.
157. Carwardine D, Friend E, Toscano M, et al. UK owner preferences for treatment of feline injection site sarcomas. *J Small Anim Pract.* 2014;55:84–88.
158. Phelps HA, Kuntz CA, Milner RJ, et al. Radical excision with five-centimeter margins for treatment of feline injection-site sarcomas: 91 cases (1998-2002). *J Am Vet Med Assoc.* 2011;239:97–106.

159. Levy JK, Crawford PC, Slater MR. Effect of vaccination against feline immunodeficiency virus on results of serologic testing in cats. *J Am Vet Med Assoc.* 2004;225:1558–1561.
160. Patterson EV, Reese MJ, Tucker SJ, et al. Effect of vaccination on parvovirus antigen testing in kittens. *J Am Vet Med Assoc.* 2007;230:359–363.
161. Decaro N, Crescenzo G, Desario C, et al. Long-term viremia and fecal shedding in pups after modified-live canine parvovirus vaccination. *Vaccine.* 2014;32:3850–3853.
162. Ruch-Gallie R, Moroff S, Lappin MR. Adenovirus 2, *Bordetella bronchiseptica*, and parainfluenza molecular diagnostic assay results in puppies after vaccination with modified live vaccines. *J Vet Intern Med.* 2016;30:164–166.
163. Hirasawa T, Yono K, Mikazuki K. Differentiation of wild- and vaccine-type canine parvoviruses by PCR and restriction-enzyme analysis. *Zentralbl Veterinarmed B.* 1995;42:601–610.
164. Iemura R, Tsukatani R, Micallef MJ, et al. Simultaneous analysis of the nasal shedding kinetics of field and vaccine strains of *Bordetella bronchiseptica. Vet Rec.* 2009;165:747–751.
165. Si W, Zhou S, Wang Z, et al. A multiplex reverse transcription-nested polymerase chain reaction for detection and differentiation of wild-type and vaccine strains of canine distemper virus. *Virol J.* 2010;7:86.
166. Addie D, Belak S, Boucraut-Baralon C, et al. Feline infectious peritonitis. ABCD guidelines on prevention and management. *J Feline Med Surg.* 2009;11:594–604.
167. Egberink H, Addie D, Belak S, et al. *Bordetella bronchiseptica* infection in cats. ABCD guidelines on prevention and management. *J Feline Med Surg.* 2009;11:610–614.
168. Frymus T, Addie D, Belak S, et al. Feline rabies. ABCD guidelines on prevention and management. *J Feline Med Surg.* 2009;11:585–593.
169. Gruffydd-Jones T, Addie D, Belak S, et al. *Chlamydophila felis* infection. ABCD guidelines on prevention and management. *J Feline Med Surg.* 2009;11:605–609.
170. Klingborg DJ, Hustead DR, Carry-Galvin EA, et al. AVMA's principles of vaccination. *J Am Vet Med Assoc.* 2001;219:575–576.
171. Radford AD, Addie D, Belak S, et al. Feline calicivirus infection. ABCD guidelines on prevention and management. *J Feline Med Surg.* 2009;11:556–564.
172. Thiry E, Addie D, Belak S, et al. Feline herpesvirus infection. ABCD guidelines on prevention and management. *J Feline Med Surg.* 2009;11:547–555.
173. Truyen U, Addie D, Belak S, et al. Feline panleukopenia. ABCD guidelines on prevention and management. *J Feline Med Surg.* 2009;11:538–546.
174. Association BSAV. *Vaccination.* 2017.
175. Cates CC, Valore EV, Couto MA, et al. Comparison of the protective effect of a commercially available western diamondback rattlesnake toxoid vaccine for dogs against envenomation of mice with western diamondback rattlesnake (*Crotalus atrox*), northern Pacific rattlesnake (*Crotalus oreganus oreganus*), and southern Pacific rattlesnake (*Crotalus oreganus helleri*) venom. *Am J Vet Res.* 2015;76:272–279.
176. Witsil AJ, Wells RJ, Woods C, et al. 272 cases of rattlesnake envenomation in dogs: Demographics and treatment including safety of F(ab')2 antivenom use in 236 patients. *Toxicon.* 2015;105:19–26.
177. Petras KE, Wells RJ, Pronko J. Suspected anaphylaxis and lack of clinical protection associated with envenomation in two dogs previously vaccinated with *Crotalus atrox* toxoid. *Toxicon.* 2018;142:30–33.
178. Stephensen CB, Welter J, Thaker SR, et al. Canine distemper virus (CDV) infection of ferrets as a model for testing Morbillivirus vaccine strategies: NYVAC- and ALVAC-based CDV recombinants protect against symptomatic infection. *J Virol.* 1997;71:1506–1513.
179. Miller RE, Fowler M. *Fowler's Zoo and Wild Animal Medicine.* Vol. 8. St. Louis, MO: Elsevier Saunders; 2015.
180. US Department of Agriculture. Bring your pet into the United States from a foreign country (Import). 2017. https://www.aphis.usda.gov/aphis/pet-travel/bring-pet-into-the-united-states.
181. Canadian Department of Agriculture. Bringing animals to Canada: Importing and travelling with pets. 2018. http://www.inspection.gc.ca/animals/terrestrial-animals/imports/policies/live-animals/pets/eng/1326600389775/1326600500578.
182. Australian Department of Agriculture. Bringing cats and dogs to Australia. 2021. http://www.agriculture.gov.au/cats-dogs.
183. Department for Environment Food and Rural Affairs. Bringing your pet dog, cat or ferret to Great Britain. https://www.gov.uk/take-pet-abroad.

PART II

Specific Infectious Diseases and Their Etiologic Agents

Introduction to Part II

The remainder of this book is devoted to information on major infectious diseases of dogs and cats and the pathogens involved. The first 5 sections cover viral, bacterial, fungal, protozoal, and parasitic diseases, and the last section covers clinical problems associated with different body systems. For most infectious diseases, information on each disease is organized in a standard format: Etiologic Agent and Epidemiology, Clinical Features (including clinical signs and their pathogenesis, and physical examination findings), Diagnosis (laboratory findings, imaging findings, specific diagnostic assays, and pathologic findings), Treatment and Prognosis (including tables with drug doses), Immunity and Vaccination, Prevention, and Public Health Aspects. Whenever possible, a case example has been provided to illustrate how the principles discussed in the chapter can be applied to clinical cases. Since the last edition, in addition to the case examples, a key points section at the start of the chapter summarizes the most important information about each disease, illustrations have been updated, and a series of suggested readings has been added. Some pathogens that were previously described as part of a complex (e.g., canine infectious respiratory disease complex) now are described in separate chapters, because our understanding of these pathogens has increased. Multiple infections of public health importance are covered, such as SARS-CoV-2 infections in dogs and cats, leptospirosis, zoonotic vector-borne bacterial diseases such as Lyme disease and rickettsioses, bite and scratch wound infections; sporotrichosis, toxoplasmosis, leishmaniosis, toxocariasis, ticks, fleas, and multidrug resistant bacterial infections. That is just to name a few. Choose your favorite bug! However, I would recommend those who suffer from nightmares refrain from reading parasite chapters at bedtime…

SECTION 1

Viral Diseases

Jane E. Sykes

Our knowledge of viral diseases has expanded considerably in recent years with the advent of nucleic acid–based approaches to diagnosis, including application of rapid whole genome sequencing platforms. New viruses have been discovered, such as canine pneumovirus (Chapter 28), *Felis catus* gammaherpesvirus (Chapter 34), and several papillomaviruses (Chapter 40). The availability of sensitive, quantitative nucleic acid amplification tests has changed our understanding of the pathogenesis of diseases such as feline leukemia virus infection (Chapter 32), which has also led us to rethink our approach to diagnosis. Antiviral drugs such as famciclovir and remdesivir promise improved treatment outcomes for cats with feline infectious peritonitis (Chapter 31) and feline herpesvirus infections (Chapter 34). The appearance of new influenza virus variants (Chapter 25) and SARS-CoV-2 (Chapter 43) has highlighted the susceptibility of cats and dogs to emerging viral infections as well as the importance of the human-animal bond. However, diseases such as rabies (Chapter 21) also continue to be a threat to public health, and veterinary efforts to control these diseases in dogs and cats worldwide remain critical.

21

Rabies

Bruno B. Chomel, Jane E. Sykes

KEY POINTS

- First Described: Circa the second millennium BC, Mesopotamia.[1]
- Cause: Rabies virus (family *Rhabdoviridae*, genus *Lyssavirus*).
- Primary Mode of Transmission: Biting, with inoculation of saliva containing the virus.
- Affected Hosts: All warm-blooded animals. Main reservoir hosts include foxes, coyotes, jackals, dogs, wolves, raccoons, raccoon-dogs, skunks, mongooses, ferret-badgers, and a wide range of bat species. Accidental hosts (depending on the virus strains that infect them) include cats, cattle, sheep, goats, horses, ferrets, primates, and woodchucks.
- Geographic Distribution: Classic (genotype 1) rabies is found worldwide, except for Australia, New Zealand, Iceland, the United Kingdom, Japan, most of western Europe, Fiji, Hawaii, and Guam. However, bat-borne lyssaviruses are present in some of these countries (Australia, western Europe including the United Kingdom).
- Major Clinical Signs: Variable fever, lethargy, behavioral changes, pupillary dilation, ataxia, lower motor neuron paresis or paralysis (including of the muscles of mastication), vestibular signs (including a head tilt), dysphagia, dysphonia, tremors, seizures, ptyalism.
- Differential Diagnoses: Distemper virus infection; Aujeszky's disease (pseudorabies in dogs and cats), West Nile virus infection; equine encephalitis virus infection; bacterial, protozoal, or fungal meningoencephalitis; toxins such as strychnine; CNS trauma; spinal neoplasia; granulomatous meningoencephalitis.
- Public Health Significance: Rabies is a deadly zoonosis and domestic dogs remain the main source of human infection worldwide, accounting for more than 95% of human cases. In the United States, most human rabies is associated with bat contact.

ETIOLOGIC AGENT AND EPIDEMIOLOGY

Rabies is a deadly, zoonotic, neurologic disease caused by a bullet-shaped, enveloped, single-stranded RNA virus that belongs to the genus *Lyssavirus* (from Lyssa, the Greek goddess of madness, rage, and frenzy) (Fig. 21.1). The viral genome encodes five structural proteins: a nucleocapsid (N) protein, a phosphoprotein (P), a matrix (M) protein, a glycoprotein (G), and an RNA-dependent RNA polymerase (L). The virus is fragile in the environment, and readily inactivated by a variety of disinfectants, soaps, ultraviolet light, and heat. It can survive up to 3 to 4 days in carcasses at 20°C, and longer with refrigeration.[2,3] Freezing tissues at temperatures less than –20°C may prolong survival of the virus for years. However, freezing samples in a household-type freezer with subsequent defrosting cycles will destroy the virus for subsequent detection.

Currently, the lyssaviruses are classified into 16 species (Table 21.1).[4,5] The major rabies species are assigned to genotypes 1 through 7. Classic rabies virus belongs to genotype 1. The remaining lyssavirus genotypes primarily infect bats and less frequently cause fatal human encephalitis, which is clinically indistinguishable from classic rabies.[6] Thus, although Australia, New Zealand, Iceland, the United Kingdom, Japan, most of western Europe, Fiji, Hawaii, and Guam are designated terrestrial rabies-free, lyssaviruses that infect bats capable of causing fatal encephalitis in humans exist in some of these regions, such as Australia or western Europe including the United Kingdom (Fig. 21.2). Suspected spillover of European bat lyssavirus to domestic cats and sheep in Europe has been described. North, Central, and South America are unique because both terrestrial mammals and bats are only infected with genotype 1. The remaining information in this chapter pertains only to genotype 1 rabies virus infections.

Infection with rabies virus most commonly occurs as a result of inoculation of virus-containing saliva into a bite wound, in the large majority of the cases after a dog bite. Other routes of transmission reported in species other than dogs and cats are rare and include corneal or solid-organ transplantation in human patients[7]; aerosol transmission, such as that occurring within caves containing large numbers of bats[8,9]; transmission after ingestion of infected tissues[9,10]; and butchering of infected dogs.[11]

All warm-blooded animals are susceptible to rabies, although dogs, wild carnivores, and bats are considered the main natural reservoirs of rabies virus. Main reservoir hosts include foxes, coyotes, jackals, dogs, wolves, raccoons, raccoon-dogs, skunks, mongooses, ferret-badgers, and a wide range of bat species. Accidental hosts (depending on the rabies virus strains that infect them) include cats, cattle, sheep, goats, horses, ferrets, primates, and woodchucks. Marsupials, including opossums, have a lower degree of susceptibility. Some bird species can be experimentally infected but do not develop clinical signs and are unlikely hosts.[12] Rabies in a domestic fowl that had been bitten by a dog was described in India.[13]

Not every bite from a rabid animal leads to rabies virus infection, and infection may not always culminate in death, unless clinical signs develop. Factors influencing the outcome after a bite from a rabid animal include the proximity of the bite site to the CNS, the degree of innervation of the bite site, the age of the host (young animals are more susceptible), the amount of virus inoculated, and the neuroinvasiveness of the rabies virus variant involved. If left untreated, up to 60% of humans bitten by a rabid dog on the head or neck develop rabies compared with up to 40% of those bitten on the hand and 10% of those bitten on the trunk or leg.[14]

Rabies viruses that circulate within a certain geographic region are adapted to specific dominant reservoir hosts. Examples in the United States are bat rabies virus variants and raccoon or skunk rabies virus variants. All rabies virus variants can infect and cause disease in animals other than their reservoir hosts (spillover hosts). The possibility of a subclinical carrier state, especially in bats, has been suggested based on the detection of rabies virus antibody and, rarely, the virus itself in some reservoir host species that are not showing signs of illness.[6] The recognition of dogs that survived rabies in Ethiopia has raised concern about subclinical carriage in dogs.[15]

Owing to mandatory vaccination and control programs, domestic animal rabies in the United States has decreased in prevalence, whereas wildlife rabies has increased (Fig. 21.3). The dog rabies virus variant was considered eradicated from the United States at the beginning of the 21st century. Currently, cats are more commonly reported with rabies in the United States (about 300 cases/year) than dogs (fewer than 100 cases/year), most likely reflecting rabies vaccination practices and pet behavior, as pet cats are more likely to roam (Fig. 21.4A). No feline rabies virus variant has been described. In developed countries, the geographic distribution of feline and canine rabies follows that of regions where wildlife rabies is endemic. Most cats and dogs are infected with the rabies virus variant that is associated with the major wildlife reservoir host in their respective geographic location (Fig. 21.4B). In the United States, rabid cats are most often reported from the northeastern, mid-Atlantic, and south-Atlantic states, with lesser numbers from the north and south central states. The eastern distribution of feline rabies follows the distribution of raccoon rabies.[16,17] Rarely, cats are infected from bats. Rabies in dogs and cats is most commonly reported from the north central, south central, and Atlantic states (see Fig. 21.4A). In the four contiguous US states, dogs are mainly infected with rabies virus variants from raccoons or skunks. Because of the long incubation period, infected dogs have also been imported into the United States from other countries where canine rabies variants are endemic.[18,19] In Europe, the major wildlife reservoir species have been foxes and raccoon dogs, and in South Africa, jackals and mongooses predominate. In Western Europe, fox rabies has largely been eliminated as a result of mass vaccination campaigns. Spillover occurs from wildlife reservoir hosts to domestic animal species, which subsequently contact humans. Nevertheless, the vast majority of human cases in North America result from contact with infected bats, which are present in all states except Hawaii (see Public Health Aspects). Rabies in rodents and lagomorphs is rare, possibly because they are always killed by the bite of a rabid animal. In the United States, most reports have been from woodchucks in raccoon rabies endemic areas.[20] A few cases of rabies in pet ferrets, rabbits, and a pet guinea pig have been described.[21]

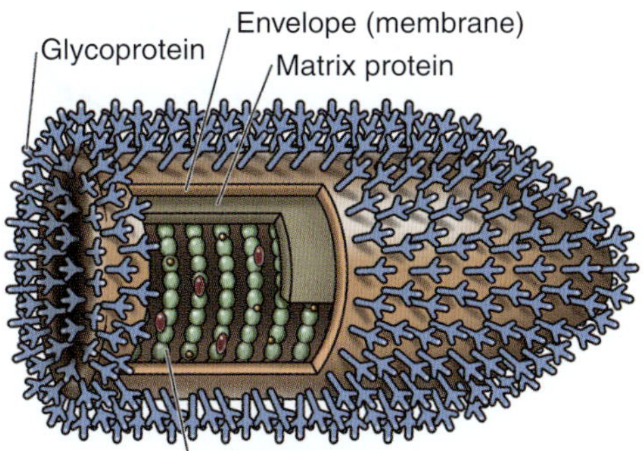

Fig. 21.1 Structure of a rabies virus virion.

Although rabies occurs in cats and dogs of any age, it is most frequently reported in young dogs and cats, with a median age of 1 year for both cats and dogs in one study; 75% of animals were 3 years of age or younger.[22] Rabies can occur in puppies and kittens that have not yet reached the age at which routine rabies vaccination is approved, which is an emerging issue as a result of illegal importation of pet dogs from countries where dog rabies is endemic. Male dogs may be slightly more predisposed, and most dogs and cats with rabies have not been neutered and live in rural environments, frequently being unrestrained

TABLE 21.1 Current Taxonomy of Lyssaviruses

Species (Genotype)	Potential Vector/Reservoir	Geographic Distribution
Rabies virus (1)	Carnivores (worldwide); bats (Americas)	Worldwide (with the exception of several islands)
Lagos bat virus (2)	Fruit (frugivorous) bats (*Megachiroptera*)	Africa
Mokola virus (3)	Unknown	Sub-Saharan Africa
Duvenhage virus (4)	Insectivorous bats	Southern Africa
European bat lyssavirus 1 (5)	Insectivorous bats (*Eptesicus serotinus*)	Europe
European bat lyssavirus 2 (6)	Insectivorous bats (*Myotis* spp.)	Europe
Australian bat lyssavirus (7)	Frugivorous and insectivorous bats (*Megachiroptera/Microchiroptera*)	Australia
Aravan virus	Insectivorous bats (*Myotis* spp.)	Central Asia
Khujand virus	Insectivorous bats (*Myotis* spp.)	Central Asia
Irkut virus	Insectivorous bats (*Myotis* spp.)	East Siberia
West Caucasian bat virus	Insectivorous bats (*Miniopterus* spp.)	Caucasian region
Shimoni bat virus	*Hipposideros commersoni*	East Africa
Bokeloh bat lyssavirus	Insectivorous bats (*Myotis* spp.)	Europe
Ikoma virus	Unknown	Africa
Gannoruwa bat lyssavirus	Unknown	Asia
Lleida bat lyssavirus	Insectivorous bats (*Miniopterus* spp.)	Europe (Spain)
Taiwan bat lyssavirus	Insectivorous bats	Taiwan

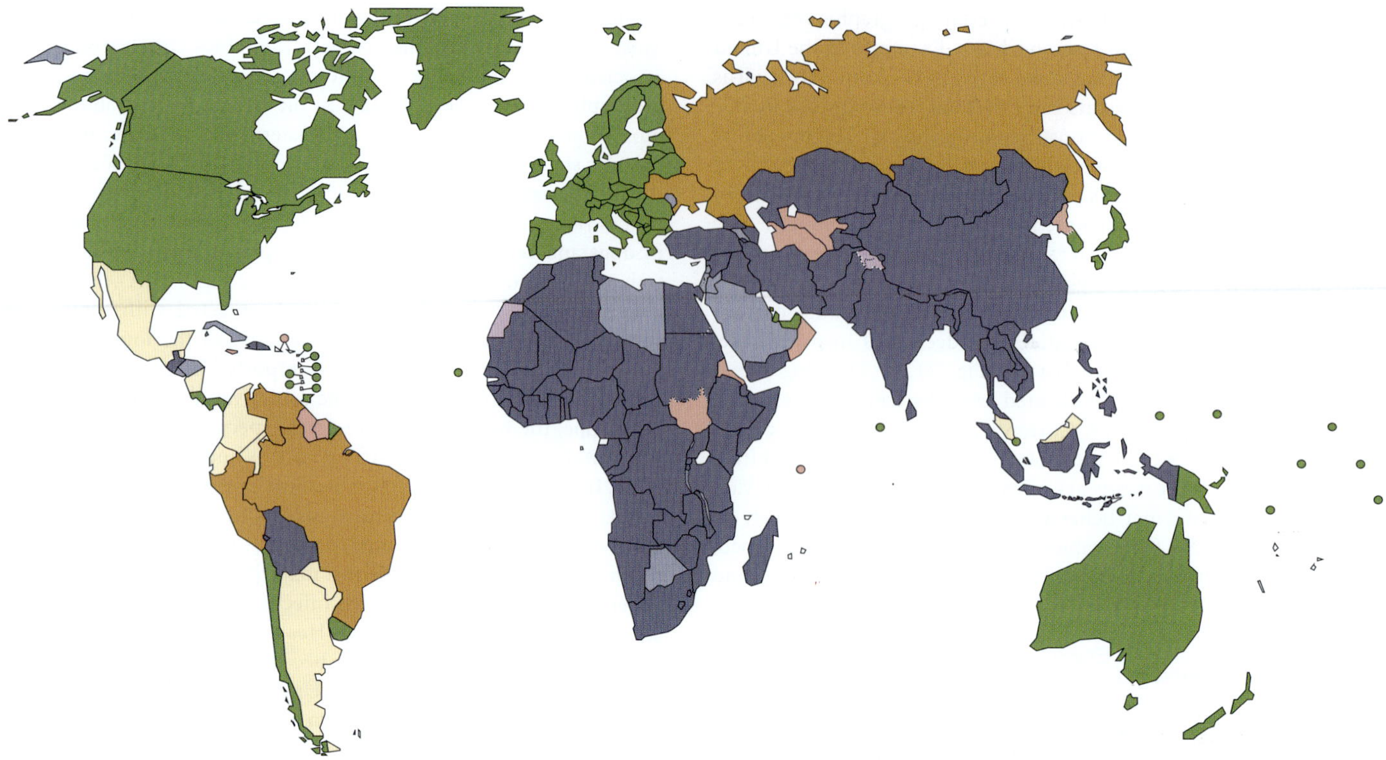

- Endemic dog-transmitted human rabies: dog rabies and dog-transmitted human rabies present in the country
- Endemic dog rabies: dog rabies in the majority of the country, but no dog-transmitted human rabies cases
- Sporadic dog-transmitted rabies: dog rabies in few areas of the country with sporadic human cases
- Controlled dog rabies: few cases of dog rabies in limited areas of the country but no dog-transmitted human rabies cases
- No dog rabies: zero dog rabies and zero dog-transmitted human rabies cases (except from imported)
- No information
- Not applicable

Fig. 21.2 Endemicity of dog rabies and dog-transmitted human rabies, 2016. (From the World Health Organization, Weekly Epidemiological Record No 7.© WHO 2017. All rights reserved © OMS 2017.)

at night.[16,22] In the United States, some degree of seasonality occurs for rabies in dogs and cats, which correlates with seasonal increases in rabid raccoons and skunks.[16,22] For the majority of cats and dogs with rabies, a history of known contact with wild animals or a wound is lacking.

CLINICAL FEATURES

Pathogenesis and Clinical Signs

After inoculation into the subcutaneous tissues and muscle, rabies virus replicates locally within muscle cells, with the nicotinic acetylcholine receptor on the postsynaptic muscle membrane being the main receptor for the virus.[23] It is thought to bud into the synaptic cleft, and then attach to peripheral nerve endings, in part using the neuronal cell adhesion molecule (NCAM) and p75NTR as receptors. Local replication around the bite site can continue for months before the virus exclusively enters peripheral motor nerve endings. It is no longer thought that sensory and autonomic nerves are involved.[23] The virus then travels in a retrograde fashion up nerve axons at a rate of 3 mm/hour, with virus replication and assembly occurring within the neuronal cell body, followed by transport to and budding from another synapse.[9] Once the virus is within the CNS, there is massive viral replication within neurons (Fig. 21.5), but without histopathologic evidence of damage to those neurons. The spinal cord, medulla oblongata, periaqueductal gray matter, limbic system, and cerebellum are particularly affected. The virus also moves outwards from the CNS in somatic and autonomic nerves and is deposited in a variety of tissues, including cardiac and skeletal muscle, the eye, the kidney, pancreas, nerves around hair follicles, and the salivary glands. Production of new virions through budding from the plasma membranes occurs primarily within the salivary glands, which results in the shedding of virus that can be transmitted to other hosts. Thus, the presence of virus in the saliva indicates that the CNS has been infected. In some animals, death occurs before the saliva becomes infected. Virus is shed by some dogs for up to 13 days before the onset of clinical signs, but more often the period of virus shedding before onset of clinical signs in dogs and cats is 1 to 5 days.[24]

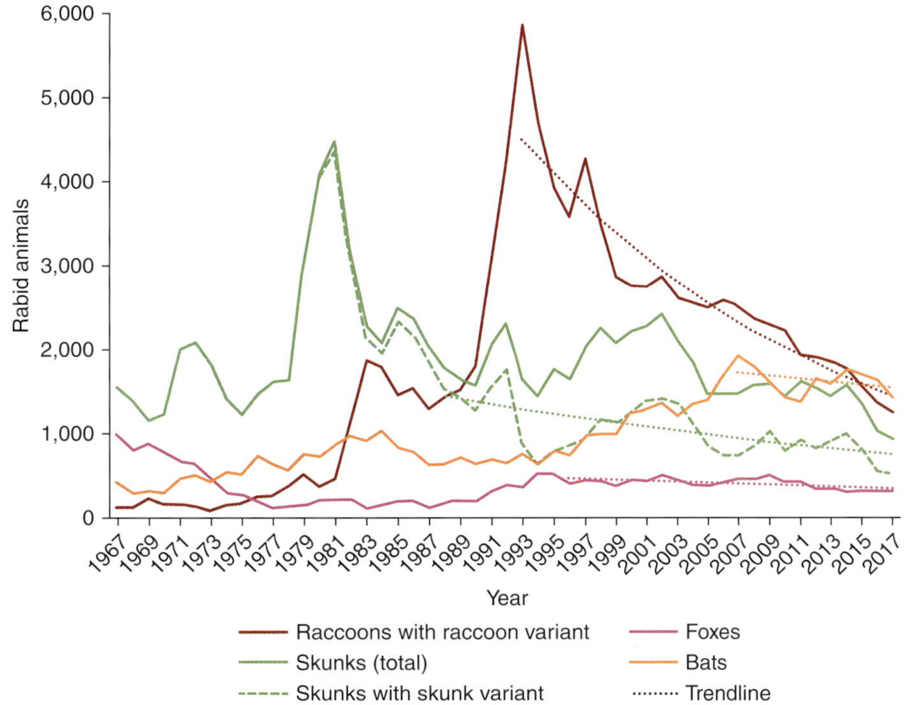

Fig. 21.3 Cases of rabies among wildlife in the United States, by year and species, 1966 to 2017. (From Ma X, Monroe BP, Cleaton JM, et al. Rabies surveillance in the United States during 2017. *J Am Vet Med Assoc.* 2018;253:1555–1568.)

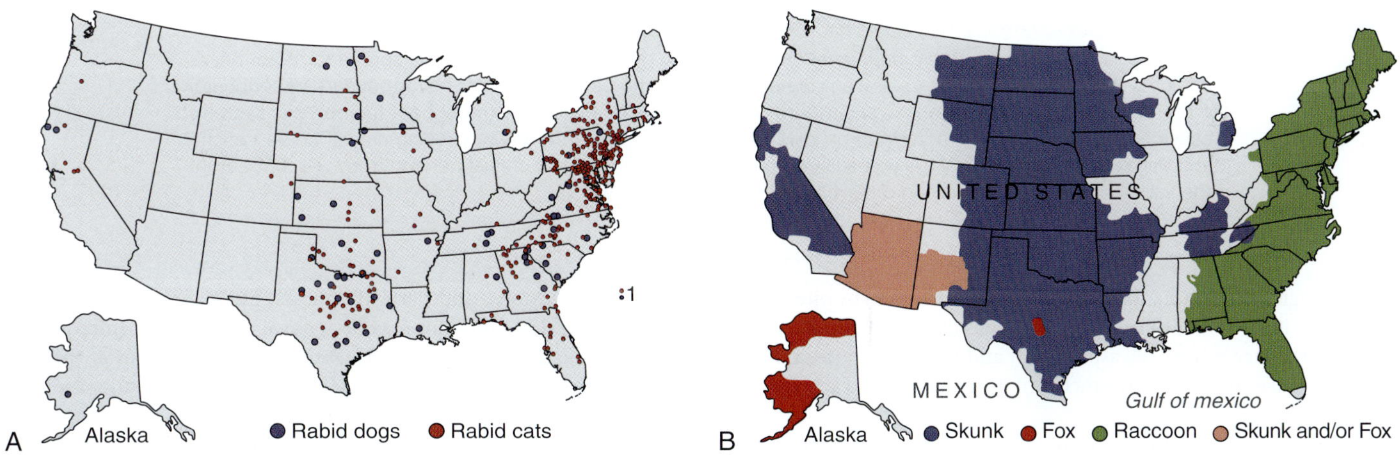

Fig. 21.4 (A) Reported cases of rabies that involve cats and dogs, by county, during 2017. Note the overlap with the distribution of wildlife reservoir hosts in B. (B) Approximate distribution of major rabies virus variants among mesocarnivores in the United States from 2013 through 2020. As a result of oral rabies vaccination programs, infection with the Texas gray fox rabies virus variant has not been reported from Texas since 2013 (central red region in Texas). Also, in California, skunk rabies virus variant infections between 2016 and 2020 have been limited to central California. (A and B modified from Ma X, Monroe BP, Cleaton JM, et al. Rabies surveillance in the United States during 2017. *J Am Vet Med Assoc.* 2018;253:1555–1568 and Ma X, Bonaparte S, Toro M, et al. Rabies surveillance in the United States during 2020. *J Am Vet Med Assoc.* 2022; May 5:1–9.)

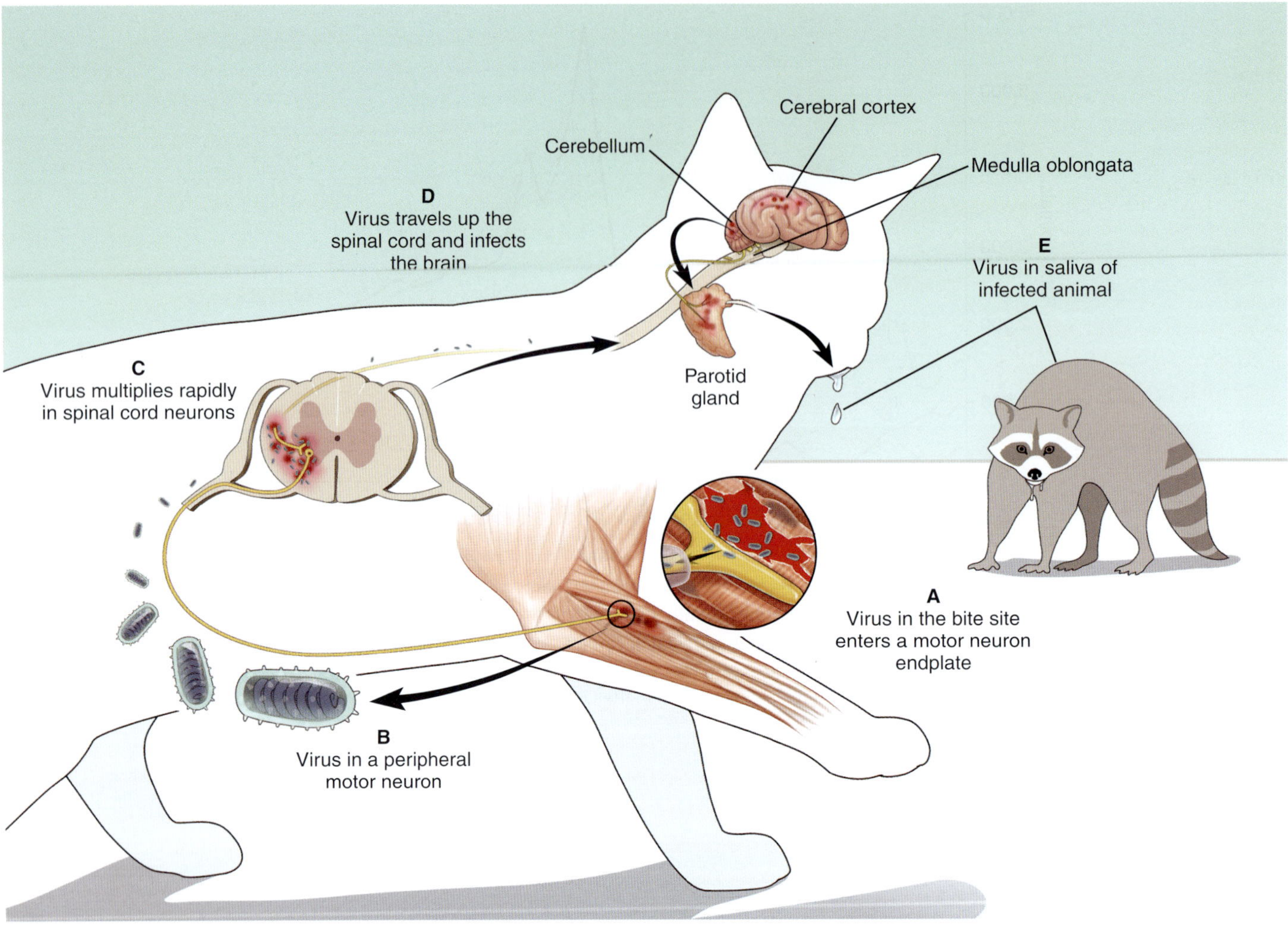

Fig. 21.5 A, Rabies virus enters peripheral nerves, or may replicate in myocytes and spread to motor nerve endings. B, Retrograde intra-axonal (centripetal) spread to the central nervous system occurs in peripheral motor nerves. C, Virus replicates in spinal cord neurons and spreads rapidly throughout the nervous system, causing progressive lower motor neuron paralysis. D, Virus enters the brain, causing cranial nerve deficits and behavioral changes. E, Virus spreads centrifugally in peripheral and cranial nerves, from which it enters the salivary glands and saliva and other tissues.

Although uncommon, infection by routes other than by bite is possible. After ingestion, the virus can infect cells of the oral mucosa, taste buds, pulmonary system (by aspiration), and intestinal mucosa. From these sites, virus migrates up branches of the cranial nerves and spreads to the brainstem.

The precise mechanism by which rabies virus causes fatal disease remains unknown. Clinical signs probably result from impaired neuronal function due to alteration of neuronal networks,[9,23] and occur after an incubation period that ranges from just over a week to 6 months or more. Most dogs and cats develop disease 1 to 2 months after exposure. In general, the closer the bite site is to the CNS, the shorter the incubation period. The incubation period is also influenced by the host species, age, degree of innervation of the bite site, neuroinvasiveness of the rabies virus variant, and the amount of virus inoculated. Although 90% of humans develop disease within 6 months of exposure, incubation periods of 6 years or more have been reported.[25–27]

The clinical presentations of rabies virus infection have been divided into excitatory ("furious") and paralytic ("dumb") forms. Three phases have been described in the progression of the disease, the prodromal, furious, and paralytic phases, but the stages are variable and may overlap, and signs may be atypical (Table 21.2). Infrequently, there is a history of a wound, or wounds are still present at the time neurologic signs occur. Unfortunately, rabies is infrequently suspected as the possible diagnosis at the time rabid animals are examined by veterinarians.[16,22]

When it occurs, the *prodromal phase* lasts 2 to 3 days in dogs and 1 to 2 days in cats, and is characterized by a variable fever, licking or chewing at the bite site, and behavioral changes. Dogs and cats may become lethargic, anorexic, apprehensive, restless, or reclusive, and vomiting may occur.[16] Some animals become more docile or affectionate. Pupillary dilation, sometimes with decreased pupillary light reflexes, may occur. The *furious phase* occurs in approximately two thirds of affected cats and dogs[28] and lasts 0 to 7 days. Clinical signs result from forebrain involvement and include irritability, anxiousness or excitability, hyperesthesia, hypersalivation, vocalization, roaming, and aggression (Fig. 21.6). Affected animals may try to eat foreign objects, which may become lodged within the GI tract, or they may attack their surroundings or moving objects. Some animals develop prolapse of the nictitans, ataxia, vestibular signs, abnormal sexual behaviors, and grand mal seizures. Tremors; staring, or a wild, spooky, or blank look in the eyes; increased vocalization; and compulsive running can occur in cats, which also often develop aggressive behavior.[16,22,29] The *paralytic phase* develops 1 to 10 days after the onset of clinical signs and is characterized by flaccid paralysis, which is ascending and often initially involves the bitten extremity. Neurologic examination reveals flaccid paralysis with absent segmental reflexes. Laryngeal paralysis may lead to a change in the sound or pitch of a dog's bark or cat's meow. Hypersalivation results from paralysis of the pharyngeal muscles, and a "dropped jaw" can occur as a result of masticatory muscle paralysis, especially in dogs, which may appear to owners as if they are choking.

If euthanasia is not performed, coma and death usually occurs within a week of the onset of signs, with a few animals dying as long as 10 days after the onset of illness. Death is associated with multiorgan failure, especially cardiac and respiratory failure. Recovery from rabies is extremely rare. Experimentally, some dogs have recovered from clinical rabies days to months after being infected with certain rabies virus strains.[30,31]

TABLE 21.2 Major Clinical Findings in 183 Cats and 119 Dogs with Rabies in the United States

Sign	Percentage of Cats	Percentage of Dogs
Aggression	55	31
Ataxia	30	49
Irritability	34	23
Anorexia	22	38
Lethargy	20	37
Hypersalivation	14	41
Dysphagia	10	30
Lameness	18	16
Limb paralysis	17	29
Jaw paralysis	3	29
Dysphonia	16	9
Hyperesthesia	10	17
Seizures	8	14
Fever	3	14

From Eng TR, Fishbein DB. Epidemiologic factors, clinical findings, and vaccination status of rabies in cats and dogs in the United States in 1988. National Study Group on Rabies. *J Am Vet Med Assoc.* 1990;197:201–209.

DIAGNOSIS

Rabies should be suspected in dogs and cats evaluated for sudden onset of behavioral changes and flaccid paralysis, especially in rabies-endemic regions, or in animals imported from rabies-endemic countries. Although a particularly high degree of suspicion is warranted for animals that lack a vaccination history for rabies, the disease has been reported in partially and completely vaccinated dogs and cats,[16,22,29] so a history of rabies vaccination should not be used to dismiss suspicion for rabies.

Laboratory Abnormalities

No specific or characteristic hematologic or biochemical changes have been reported in dogs and cats with rabies. Mild anemia was reported in one dog.[32] Analysis of the CSF may be unremarkable or show an increase in CSF protein concentration and mild to marked CSF pleocytosis. Small lymphocytes account for most of the differential cell count.[32]

Electromyography in one dog revealed abnormalities consistent with impaired neuromuscular transmission, including moderate fibrillations, positive sharp waves, and an absent M wave.[32] Changes suggestive of denervation have also been described in humans with rabies.[33]

Diagnostic Imaging

Magnetic Resonance Imaging Findings

Findings on MRI in dogs with rabies have included hyperintense lesions on T2-weighted images, especially in the midbrain, thalamus, and basal

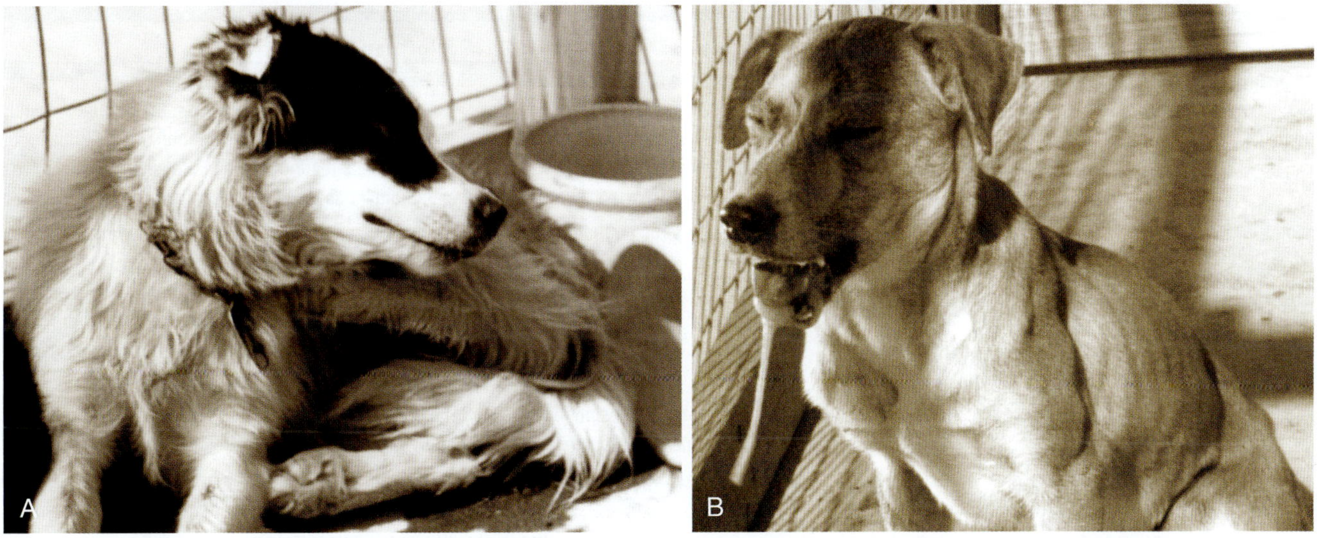

Fig. 21.6 (A) Dog with paralytic stage of rabies in sternal recumbency with torticollis. (B) Dog with rabies. Note open jaw and visible tongue with excessive salivary secretions resulting from the inability to swallow. (Courtesy CDC, Atlanta, USA.)

ganglia, that do not enhance with contrast.[34] In human patients with rabies, no significant abnormalities may be present on MRI, or MRI may show hyperintensities on T2-weighted images, especially in association with the gray matter. Lesions are frequently described in the medulla, pons, basal ganglia, and thalamus and reflect concentrations of rabies virus antigen.[35] Contrast enhancement can be present in comatose human patients but is usually not detected early in the course of illness. CT commonly does not reveal lesions in humans with rabies.

Microbiologic Testing

Diagnostic assays for rabies in dogs and cats are listed in Table 21.3.

Direct Fluorescent Antibody Testing and Immunohistochemistry

Rabies virus diagnosis is generally based on direct fluorescent antibody (DFA) staining for virus on impression smears of brain tissue obtained at necropsy. This is rapid, sensitive, and economic and is performed only in qualified laboratories that have been approved by local or state public health departments. In the United States, a national standardized protocol for rabies testing is published by the CDC.[36] False-negative results with DFA staining are rare when compared with mouse inoculation testing,[37] and all animals with virus in their saliva test positive. A direct rapid IHC test is also available, which has a similar sensitivity and specificity and does not require a fluorescence microscope.[38]

If rabies is suspected, the animal should be handled with extreme caution (see Prevention). Humane euthanasia should be performed, and the entire head should be submitted as soon as possible to public health authorities, so as not to delay postexposure prophylaxis measures for exposed individuals (see Public Health Aspects). Opening the skull using a saw generates aerosols and is not recommended. Although not optimal, if the head is not available, the spinal cord can be submitted. Tissues should be refrigerated and not frozen for optimal test sensitivity. Approved shipping containers should be used, which must be labeled with appropriate warnings.

Antemortem, DFA testing has been used to detect rabies virus in corneal touch impressions and frozen skin biopsy sections from the nuchal area in humans[39,40] or the region of the whiskers in dogs and cats. The sensitivity of this method is as low as 25%, and it should not be used for clinical diagnosis in dogs and cats suspected to have rabies. DFA staining has also been used for detection of rabies virus antigen in extracranial tissues at necropsy, including the tongue, salivary glands, adrenal glands, pancreas, GI tract, and myocardium.[41,42]

Serologic Diagnosis

Serologic tests for rabies virus antibodies are often negative in affected animals, as a result of immune evasion by the virus during the incubation period and possibly also virus-induced immunosuppression after the onset of clinical signs. If seroconversion occurs, it is typically late in the course of illness. Prior vaccination for rabies may result in confusing results. Determination of acute and convalescent titers on serum and determination of CSF antibody titers can aid in the diagnosis of human rabies.[40] In dogs and cats, serologic testing is most commonly used to document proof of prior vaccination, which is required for importation into rabies-free countries. It is not suitable for determining the need for booster vaccinations.[43]

Serologic methods include virus neutralization assays and ELISA assays.[44] The gold standard of rabies serology is the rapid fluorescent focus inhibition test (RFFIT), a virus neutralization assay, which assesses the ability of antibodies to prevent viral replication in cell culture. The fluorescent antibody virus neutralization (FAVN) test has been accepted as an alternative for determining titers in animals before importation. A minimum titer of 0.5 U/mL is required before importation to rabies-free countries is permitted.

Virus Isolation and Mouse Inoculation

Rabies virus can be isolated in a variety of cell culture lines, although isolation may be less sensitive than nucleic acid–based detection methods.[45] Virus isolation and inoculation of mice with tissue from affected patients can be used to confirm rabies virus infection by public health authorities when DFA testing of brain tissue is negative.

TABLE 21.3 Diagnostic Assays Available for Rabies in Dogs and Cats

Assay	Specimen Type	Target	Performance
Direct fluorescent antibody staining or immunohistochemistry	Brain, spinal cord, skin biopsies (latter not recommended in animals), other extracranial tissues	Rabies virus N (nucleocapsid) protein	High sensitivity and specificity on the brain tissue; because a single negative result does not rule out rabies, confirmatory tests such as mouse inoculation or RT-PCR is required for specimens testing negative. Sensitivity when used on extracranial tissues is relatively low.
Serology	Serum or CSF	Antirabies virus antibodies	Virus neutralization assays are the gold standard for serology, although ELISA assays are also available. Rarely useful for diagnosis of rabies, as the antibody response is delayed and so titers are often negative. Titers often determined before importation of animals into rabies-free countries.
Histopathology	Brain, spinal cord	Intracytoplasmic eosinophilic inclusions (Negri bodies)	Detection of Negri bodies has low sensitivity and is currently rarely used as a diagnostic test
RT-PCR	Brain, spinal cord, saliva, CSF, extracranial tissues	Rabies virus RNA	Rapid (within hours), has the potential to be very sensitive and specific; can be used to identify rabies genotypes and strains.

RT-PCR, real-time polymerase chain reaction; *CSF,* cerebrospinal fluid.

Molecular Diagnosis Using Nucleic Acid–Based Testing

Nucleic acid detection techniques are increasingly employed to detect rabies virus in tissues and may ultimately replace techniques such as isolation and histopathology.[46] RT-PCR assays have been used to rapidly detect the RNA of rabies virus and other lyssaviruses in dogs, cats, and humans and, when used on brain tissue, are sensitive and specific, the results correlating with those of DFA testing.[47–49] RT-PCR can be used to detect virus in a decomposing tissue, when the results of other assays might be negative.[50,51] Genetic analysis of resultant PCR products can also be used to identify lyssavirus genotypes and rabies virus variants (see Table 21.1).[52] For antemortem diagnosis in human patients, saliva is more likely to test positive than CSF. A nuchal biopsy specimen can also be tested.[53] The same appears to be true in dogs and cats, although again, attempts to make an antemortem diagnosis of rabies are not recommended in animals.[54] The sensitivity of RT-PCR for detection of rabies virus in the saliva of rabid dogs was 87%, so a negative result does not rule out a diagnosis of rabies.

Pathologic Findings

Gross Pathologic Findings

Gross lesions are generally absent in the CNS of dogs and cats with rabies. Lesions consistent with a previous wound or traumatic event may be present elsewhere on the body.

Histopathologic Findings

Rabies virus infection results in a remarkably mild, nonsuppurative polioencephalomyelitis. Changes include mild neuronal degeneration and neuronophagia, which may be followed by neuronal necrosis.[32] Lymphoplasmacytic perivascular cuffing and focal microglial hyperplasia are frequently described. The longer the duration of illness, the more pronounced the nonsuppurative inflammatory response. Sometimes, a spongiform encephalopathy with vacuolization in the gray matter is present.[21] In some animals, eosinophilic intracytoplasmic viral inclusion bodies (Negri bodies) are identified (Fig. 21.7). Negri bodies are considered a hallmark of rabies virus infection and are most commonly seen in tissues such as the pons, thalamus, hypothalamus, and hippocampus. They are generally only seen once neurologic signs have developed, and only in about 50% of animals that test positive using DFA testing. Inclusions that resemble Negri bodies have been described in the brain of cats and ruminants without rabies, and so the potential for confusion and a false-positive diagnosis of rabies exists.[55]

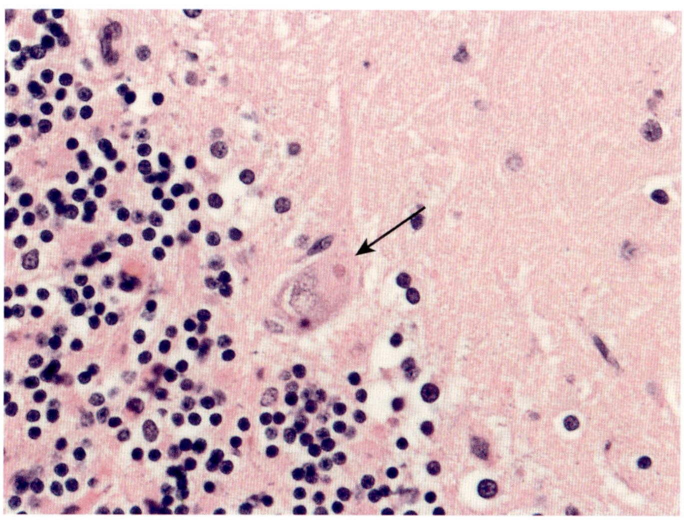

Fig. 21.7 Negri body *(arrow)* in a neuron within the central nervous system (hematoxylin and eosin stain, ×400). (From Kumar V, Abbas AK, Aster JC. *Robbins & Cotran Pathologic Basis of Disease.* 10th ed. Philadelphia, PA: Elsevier; 2021.)

TREATMENT AND PROGNOSIS

Immediate euthanasia and testing of dogs and cats suspected to have clinical signs of rabies is recommended. Once clinical signs have developed, rabies is almost always fatal and very few humans have survived. Most have been children, and several of those individuals had been vaccinated for rabies before the onset of illness. In all individuals, moderate to severe neurologic sequelae persisted. A 17-year-old girl in Texas survived clinical rabies without the need for intensive care.[56] Although a controversial treatment, after treatment with induced coma (the "Milwaukee protocol"), an 8-year old girl survived rabies that may have been acquired after a scratch from a stray cat.[57] Rarely, dogs inoculated experimentally with certain canine rabies virus variants have recovered from rabies encephalitis, sometimes with intermittent shedding of rabies virus in saliva after recovery.[31]

IMMUNITY AND VACCINATION

In most cases of human rabies, no immune response is detectable at 7 to 10 days after the onset of clinical signs. Rabies virus may evade immune recognition through rabies virus phosphoprotein-induced disruption of IFN signaling, as well as inhibition of apoptosis and destruction of invading T cells.[23,58] This may explain the relative lack of an inflammatory response within the CNS.

Currently available vaccines for cats and dogs contain inactivated virus or are canarypox-vectored recombinant rabies (cats) vaccines. Attenuated live rabies vaccines are no longer available in the United States because of their association with occasional postvaccinal rabies encephalitis in dogs and cats.[59] Vaccinia poxvirus-vectored glycoprotein recombinant vaccines are only used for wildlife vaccination.

In the United States, all dogs and cats should be vaccinated for rabies at 3 or 4 months of age (depending on local regulations), with a booster dose 1 year later, then every 3 years with approved inactivated vaccines, or annually with recombinant vaccines (see Chapter 20). It has been recommended that rabies vaccines be administered as distally as possible in the right pelvic limb, to allow better understanding of which vaccines are associated with sarcoma formation and to permit complete removal of sarcomas by amputation should they develop.[60,61] Canine rabies vaccination is required by law within most of the United States, and vaccines must be administered only by (or under the direct supervision of) a veterinarian.[62] Effective vaccination of at least 70% of the dog population is required to prevent rabies epizootics.[63] Owners who fail to comply with state or local requirements should be reported to the public health authorities.

Although rare, rabies has been reported in vaccinated animals, especially when vaccinations are not up to date.[29] Dogs and cats less than 1 year of age are not considered immunized until 28 days after the initial vaccination.[62] Because of a rapid anamnestic response, an animal is considered fully vaccinated immediately after booster vaccination.

The use of inactivated rabies virus vaccines in cats has been associated with formation of injection site sarcomas.[64,65] More commonly, rabies virus vaccination is associated with pain at the injection site, lameness, transient fever, and local cutaneous reactions, such as alopecia, focal cutaneous vasculitis, and focal granulomas.[66] A more generalized ischemic skin disease characterized by variable alopecia, crusting, erosions, and ulcers on the pinnal margins, periocular areas, tail tip, and paw pads has been described that occurs several months after rabies virus vaccination of dogs and begins with a lesion at the site of vaccination (see Chapter 20).[67]

Oral vaccinia-vectored recombinant rabies vaccines, which express the rabies virus glycoprotein, have been used in Europe and subsequently North America to control the spread of rabies in wild animals such as foxes, raccoons, and coyotes.[68] Canine and feline rabies vaccines are not approved for use in wild animals, which include wild animal hybrids such as wolf hybrids and Savannah cats. Wolf hybrids and Savannah cats are considered unvaccinated when decisions must be made regarding quarantine and euthanasia (Table 21.4).

PREVENTION

Prevention of rabies is dependent on widespread education of the public regarding the need to vaccinate dogs and cats for rabies, and the risks of wildlife contact. Control of stray dogs and cats and wild animal vaccination programs also help to prevent the disease. Ownership and importation of wild animals and hybrids is discouraged; in July 2021, the CDC issued a ban on the importation of dogs from rabies-endemic countries (113 countries in total). Puppies and kittens that have not yet reached the age for rabies vaccination should be kept away from wildlife.

According to US regulations, unvaccinated dogs and cats that have been exposed to a rabid animal should be euthanized immediately or vaccinated and placed in strict isolation, without direct contact with people or other animals, for 6 months.[62] If the biting animal is a wild animal that is unavailable for testing, the biting animal is presumed to be rabid.

For dogs and cats that are overdue for a booster vaccination, there are two possible outcomes: (1) if the animals have appropriate documentation of having received a USDA-licensed rabies vaccine at least once previously, they should immediately receive veterinary medical care for assessment, wound cleansing, and booster vaccination. The animal should be kept under the owner's control and observed for 45 days; and (2) if appropriate documentation is lacking, they should immediately receive veterinary medical care for assessment and wound cleansing, and local public health authorities should be consulted.[62]

Dogs and cats that are currently vaccinated should be revaccinated immediately (within 48 hours), kept under the owner's control, and observed for 45 days. Any illness in isolated or confined animals should be reported to local public health officials. If clinical signs suggestive of rabies develop, euthanasia and rabies testing should be performed. Ferrets that are overdue for a booster vaccination should be evaluated on a case-by-case basis.

Animals suspected to have rabies should be isolated from other animals and humans and handled with extreme caution, using heavy leather gloves, catch poles, and cages for restraint. Care should be taken not to allow people's skin to come into contact with salivary secretions. Signs that warn of the possibility of rabies should be placed on the cages of animals that are hospitalized for any period of time. If the risk of rabies is low, the animal should be confined and observed for 10 days. The clinician in charge should keep a list of all in-contact personnel during that period, and procedures should be minimized. High-risk rabies suspects should be confined in isolation using an established hospital protocol. Marked improvement in an animal's condition that occurs during a 10-day period is not consistent with a diagnosis of rabies. All specimens submitted to the laboratory should be labeled with warning labels.

TABLE 21.4 Procedures Required by Public Health Officials for Prevention of Rabies According to the Compendium of Animal Rabies Prevention and Control[42]

Situation	Rabies Vaccination History	Procedure	Rationale
Dog or cat exposed[a] to a rabid wild animal or wild animal that is unavailable for testing	Unvaccinated, dog or cat	Euthanize immediately or place in strict isolation for 6 months. Administer rabies vaccine on isolation or up to 28 days before release.	The quarantine period is based on the known incubation period for rabies. Animals that develop signs consistent with rabies during quarantine should be euthanized and tested for rabies.
	Not up to date with booster vaccinations (no proof of prior vaccination for dogs or cats). Not up to date for ferrets.	Contact public health authorities who decide procedures (revaccination or euthanasia) based on biting species, local prevalence of rabies, timing of previous vaccinations.	
	Vaccinated, dog or cat Or not up-to-date with booster vaccinations, but proof of prior vaccination.	Revaccinate, and keep under owner's control and observation for 45 days.	
Human bitten by a healthy dog or cat	Any	Confine animal and observe daily for 10 days; report illness that develops immediately to public health authorities. If signs of rabies develop, euthanize and test for rabies. Vaccination should not be performed until after the isolation period is complete.	Dogs and cats shedding rabies virus within the saliva will develop illness and die within the 10-day quarantine period.
Human bitten by a stray or unwanted dog or cat		Euthanize biting animal immediately and submit for rabies testing.	
Human bitten by a known rabid animal	Vaccinated, human	Vaccinate (1 mL) on day 0 and day 3 intramuscularly, in the upper deltoid muscle.	
	Unvaccinated, human	Postexposure prophylaxis: injection of human rabies immune globulin infiltrated at the bite site, followed by vaccination (1 mL) on days 0, 3, 7 and 14 (and 28 only for immunocompromised persons)	

[a]Exposure for rabies constitutes introduction of the virus into bite wounds, open cuts in skin, or onto mucous membranes from saliva or other potentially infectious material such as neural tissue.

Compendium updates are available online at http://www.nasphv.org/documentsCompendia.html.

Modified from Brown CM, Slavinski S, Ettestad P, Sidwa TJ, Sorhage FE. Compendium of Animal Rabies Prevention and Control, 2016. *J Am Vet Med Assoc.* 2016;248:505–517.

PUBLIC HEALTH ASPECTS

Each year, more than 50,000 people die from rabies worldwide. Approximately half of those numbers occur in India alone, and it has been estimated that 3 billion people continue to be at risk of rabies virus infection in more than 100 countries.[69] A large proportion of these people are children who have been attacked by rabid dogs. In the United States, human deaths due to rabies have decreased from more than 100 per year in the early 20th century to 2–3 per year.[70] Most humans in the United States are infected as a result of contact with insectivorous bats, which often appear injured or are behaving abnormally (including flying during the day), and, depending on the bat species, around 5% to 40% of dead or ill bats submitted for testing have rabies.[71,72] Seemingly insignificant contact with tiny bats, particularly the eastern pipistrelle and silver-haired bats, is reported in many human rabies cases (cryptic bat rabies). Despite the high prevalence of raccoon rabies in the eastern United States, only three human deaths (including one organ recipient) associated with a raccoon rabies variant have been reported.[71,72]

Prodromal signs of rabies in humans include malaise, fever, and pain, itching, or paresthesia at the site of the bite. People with furious rabies become nervous and hyperexcitable, after which signs of hydrophobia, aerophobia, confusion, and aggression develop. Autonomic signs such as hypersalivation, vomiting, miosis or mydriasis, excessive sweating, and priapism may occur. Paralytic rabies can be confused with Guillain-Barré syndrome.[40]

Sick domestic and wild animals that bite humans in regions where rabies is endemic and that subsequently die should be tested for rabies without delay. Prompt and aggressive treatment of wounds including irrigation under pressure with 20% aqueous soap solution, and application of a greater than 50% ethanol solution or povidone-iodine, can dramatically reduce the risk of contracting rabies after a bite.

The chain of events that must occur after a dog or cat bites a human are listed in Table 21.4 and depend on whether the animal is owned or stray, and on the animal's vaccination status.[62] Public health authorities must be notified when potential exposure occurs and make the final decision as to how these animals are handled.

Postexposure prophylaxis (PEP) is administered to humans after a bite from a known or suspected rabid animal. In the United States, it consists of an injection of human rabies immune globulin (H-RIG), ideally with at least half of the whole dose in the region of a bite site as soon as possible within the first 7 days of the bite, followed by a 4-dose vaccination regimen by the IM route on days 0, 3, 7 and 14 (and 28 in immunocompromised individuals) in the upper deltoid muscle with 1 mL of vaccine.[73] Fewer than 5 humans develop rabies each year in the United States, but PEP is given to 20,000 to 40,000 people each year, with on average 50 people receiving PEP for each rabies case investigated.

Depending on the risk, certain individuals may receive prophylactic vaccines against rabies. These individuals include veterinarians, veterinary students and staff, dog catchers, rabies researchers, rabies diagnosticians, wildlife workers, and travelers visiting rabies-enzootic regions. After exposure to a rabid animal, administration of immunoglobulin to these individuals is not necessary. Instead, rabies vaccine boosters are given immediately and 3 days later. The major vaccine in use in the United States is the human diploid cell vaccine (HDCV), although in developing countries, access to this vaccine is limited. Among animal workers, antibody titers are generally checked every 2 years, with administration of a booster dose if necessary.

SUGGESTED READINGS

Dietzschold B, Li J, Faber M, et al. Concepts in the pathogenesis of rabies. *Future Virol.* 2008;3:481–490.

Blanton JD, Wallace RM. The ancient curse: rabies. *Microbiol Spectr.* 2015;3(6).

Lackay SN, Kuang Y, Fu ZF. Rabies in small animals. *Vet Clin North Am Small Anim Pract.* 2008;38:851–861 (ix).

CDC. Public health response to a rabid kitten: four states, 2007. *MMWR Morb Mortal Wkly Rep.* 2008;56(51–52):1337–1340.

CDC. Recovery of a patient from clinical rabies: California, 2011. *MMWR Morb Mortal Wkly Rep.* 2012;61:61–65.

National Association of State Public Health Veterinarians, Compendium of Animal Rabies Prevention and Control Committee, Brown CM, et al. Compendium of animal rabies prevention and control. *J Am Vet Med Assoc.* 2016;248:505–517.

REFERENCES

1. Adamson PB. The spread of rabies into Europe and the probable origin of this disease in antiquity. *J R Asiat Soc GB Irel.* 1977;2:140–144.
2. Lewis VJ, Thacker WL. Limitations of deteriorated tissue for rabies diagnosis. *Health Lab Sci.* 1974;11:8–12.
3. Matouch O, Jaros J, Pohl P. Survival of rabies virus under external conditions. *Vet Med (Praha).* 1987;32:669–674.
4. World Health Organization. Rabies classification. https://www.who-rabies-bulletin.org/site-page/classification.
5. Troupin C, Dacheux L, Tanguy M, et al. Large-scale phylogenomic analysis reveals the complex evolutionary history of rabies virus in multiple carnivore hosts. *PLoS Pathog.* 2016;12:e1006041.
6. Warrell MJ, Warrell DA. Rabies and other lyssavirus diseases. *Lancet.* 2004;363:959–969.
7. Maier T, Schwarting A, Mauer D, et al. Management and outcomes after multiple corneal and solid organ transplantations from a donor infected with rabies virus. *Clin Infect Dis.* 2010;50:1112–1119.
8. Davis PL, Bourhy H, Holmes EC. The evolutionary history and dynamics of bat rabies virus. *Infect Genet Evol.* 2006;6:464–473.
9. Dietzschold B, Li J, Faber M, et al. Concepts in the pathogenesis of rabies. *Future Virol.* 2008;3:481–490.
10. Fischman HR, Ward 3rd FE. Oral transmission of rabies virus in experimental animals. *Am J Epidemiol.* 1968;88:132–138.
11. Wertheim HF, Nguyen TQ, Nguyen KA, et al. Furious rabies after an atypical exposure. *PLoS Med.* 2009;6:e44.
12. Jorgenson RD, Gough PM, Graham DL. Experimental rabies in a great horned owl. *J Wildl Dis.* 1976;12:444–447.
13. Baby J, Mani RS, Abraham SS, et al. Natural rabies infection in a domestic fowl (*Gallus domesticus*): a report from India. *PLoS Negl Trop Dis.* 2015;9:e0003942.
14. Cleaveland S, Fevre EM, Kaare M, et al. Estimating human rabies mortality in the United Republic of Tanzania from dog bite injuries. *Bull World Health Organ.* 2002;80:304–310.
15. Fekadu M. Asymptomatic non-fatal canine rabies. *Lancet.* 1975;1(7906):569.
16. Fogelman V, Fischman HR, Horman JT, et al. Epidemiologic and clinical characteristics of rabies in cats. *J Am Vet Med Assoc.* 1993;202:1829–1833.
17. McQuiston JH, Yager PA, Smith JS, et al. Epidemiologic characteristics of rabies virus variants in dogs and cats in the United States, 1999. *J Am Vet Med Assoc.* 2001;218:1939–1942.
18. Castrodale L, Walker V, Baldwin J, et al. Rabies in a puppy imported from India to the USA, March 2007. *Zoonoses Public Health.* 2008;55:427–430.
19. Monroe BP, Yager P, Blanton J, et al. Rabies surveillance in the United States during 2014. *J Am Vet Med Assoc.* 2016;248:777–788.
20. Childs JE, Colby L, Krebs JW, et al. Surveillance and spatiotemporal associations of rabies in rodents and lagomorphs in the United States, 1985-1994. *J Wildl Dis.* 1997;33:20–27.
21. Lackay SN, Kuang Y, Fu ZF. Rabies in small animals. *Vet Clin North Am Small Anim Pract.* 2008;38:851–861 (ix).

22. Eng TR, Fishbein DB. Epidemiologic factors, clinical findings, and vaccination status of rabies in cats and dogs in the United States in 1988. National Study Group on Rabies. *J Am Vet Med Assoc.* 1990;197:201–209.
23. Davis BM, Rall GF, Schnell MJ. Everything you always wanted to know about rabies virus (but were afraid to ask). *Annu Rev Virol.* 2015;2:451–471.
24. Fekadu M, Shaddock JH, Baer GM. Excretion of rabies virus in the saliva of dogs. *J Infect Dis.* 1982;145:715–719.
25. Dimaano EM, Scholand SJ, Alera MT, et al. Clinical and epidemiological features of human rabies cases in the Philippines: a review from 1987 to 2006. *Int J Infect Dis.* 2011;15:e495–e499.
26. Johnson N, Fooks A, McColl K. Human rabies case with long incubation, Australia. *Emerg Infect Dis.* 2008;14:1950–1951.
27. Shankar SK, Mahadevan A, Sapico SD, et al. Rabies viral encephalitis with probable 25 year incubation period! *Ann Indian Acad Neurol.* 2012;15:221–223.
28. Tepsumethanon V, Lumlertdacha B, Mitmoonpitak C, et al. Survival of naturally infected rabid dogs and cats. *Clin Infect Dis.* 2004;39:278–280.
29. Murray KO, Holmes KC, Hanlon CA. Rabies in vaccinated dogs and cats in the United States, 1997-2001. *J Am Vet Med Assoc.* 2009;235:691–695.
30. Fekadu M, Baer GM. Recovery from clinical rabies of 2 dogs inoculated with a rabies virus strain from Ethiopia. *Am J Vet Res.* 1980;41:1632–1634.
31. Fekadu M, Shaddock JH, Baer GM. Intermittent excretion of rabies virus in the saliva of a dog two and six months after it had recovered from experimental rabies. *Am J Trop Med Hyg.* 1981;30:1113–1115.
32. Barnes HL, Chrisman CL, Farina L, et al. Clinical evaluation of rabies virus meningoencephalomyelitis in a dog. *J Am Anim Hosp Assoc.* 2003;39:547–550.
33. Gadre G, Satishchandra P, Mahadevan A, et al. Rabies viral encephalitis: clinical determinants in diagnosis with special reference to paralytic form. *J Neurol Neurosurg Psychiatry.* 2010;81:812–820.
34. Laothamatas J, Wacharapluesadee S, Lumlertdacha B, et al. Furious and paralytic rabies of canine origin: neuroimaging with virological and cytokine studies. *J Neurovirol.* 2008;14:119–129.
35. Tirawatnpong S, Hemachudha T, Manutsathit S, et al. Regional distribution of rabies viral antigen in central nervous system of human encephalitic and paralytic rabies. *J Neurol Sci.* 1989;92:91–99.
36. CDC. Collection of Samples for Diagnosis of Rabies in Animals. http://www.cdc.gov/rabies/specific_groups/laboratories/index.html.
37. Beauregard M, Boulanger P, Webster WA. The use of fluorescent antibody staining in the diagnosis of rabies. *Can J Comp Med Vet Sci.* 1965;29:141–147.
38. Lembo T, Niezgoda M, Velasco-Villa A, et al. Evaluation of a direct, rapid immunohistochemical test for rabies diagnosis. *Emerg Infect Dis.* 2006;12:310–313.
39. Crepin P, Audry L, Rotivel Y, et al. Intravitam diagnosis of human rabies by PCR using saliva and cerebrospinal fluid. *J Clin Microbiol.* 1998;36:1117–1121.
40. Madhusudana SN, Sukumaran SM. Antemortem diagnosis and prevention of human rabies. *Ann Indian Acad Neurol.* 2008;11:3–12.
41. Jogai S, Radotra BD, Banerjee AK. Rabies viral antigen in extracranial organs: a post-mortem study. *Neuropathol Appl Neurobiol.* 2002;28:334–338.
42. Li Z, Feng Z, Ye H. Rabies viral antigen in human tongues and salivary glands. *J Trop Med Hyg.* 1995;98:330–332.
43. National Association of State Public Health Veterinarians, Compendium of Animal Rabies Prevention and Control Committee, Brown CM, et al. Compendium of animal rabies prevention and control, 2016. *J Am Vet Med Assoc.* 2016;248:505–517.
44. Moore SM, Hanlon CA. Rabies-specific antibodies: measuring surrogates of protection against a fatal disease. *PLoS Negl Trop Dis.* 2010;4:e595.
45. Panning M, Baumgarte S, Pfefferle S, et al. Comparative analysis of rabies virus reverse transcription-PCR and virus isolation using samples from a patient infected with rabies virus. *J Clin Microbiol.* 2010;48:2960–2962.
46. Fooks AR, Johnson N, Freuling CM, et al. Emerging technologies for the detection of rabies virus: challenges and hopes in the 21st century. *PLoS Negl Trop Dis.* 2009;3:e530.
47. Gupta PK, Singh RK, Sharma RN, et al. Preliminary report on a single-tube, non-interrupted reverse transcription-polymerase chain reaction for the detection of rabies virus in brain tissue. *Vet Res Commun.* 2001;25:239–247.
48. Kamolvarin N, Tirawatnpong T, Rattanasiwamoke R, et al. Diagnosis of rabies by polymerase chain reaction with nested primers. *J Infect Dis.* 1993;167:207–210.
49. Wadhwa A, Wilkins K, Gao J, et al. A pan-Lyssavirus Taqman real-time RT-PCR assay for the detection of highly variable rabies virus and other lyssaviruses. *PLoS Negl Trop Dis.* 2017;11:e0005258.
50. David D, Yakobson B, Rotenberg D, et al. Rabies virus detection by RT-PCR in decomposed naturally infected brains. *Vet Microbiol.* 2002;87:111–118.
51. Lopes MC, Venditti LL, Queiroz LH. Comparison between RT-PCR and the mouse inoculation test for detection of rabies virus in samples kept for long periods under different conditions. *J Virol Methods.* 2010;164:19–23.
52. Wacharapluesadee S, Hemachudha T. Ante- and post-mortem diagnosis of rabies using nucleic acid-amplification tests. *Expert Rev Mol Diagn.* 2010;10:207–218.
53. CDC. Human rabies: Virginia, 2009. *MMWR Morb Mortal Wkly Rep.* 2010;59:1236–1238.
54. Saengseesom W, Mitmoonpitak C, Kasempimolporn S, et al. Real-time PCR analysis of dog cerebrospinal fluid and saliva samples for ante-mortem diagnosis of rabies. *Southeast Asian J Trop Med Public Health.* 2007;38:53–57.
55. Szlachta HL, Habel RE. Inclusions resembling Negri bodies in the brains of nonrabid cats. *Cornell Vet.* 1953;43:207–212.
56. CDC. Presumptive abortive human rabies: Texas, 2009. *MMWR Morb Mortal Wkly Rep.* 2010;59:185–190.
57. CDC. Recovery of a patient from clinical rabies: California, 2011. *MMWR Morb Mortal Wkly Rep.* 2012;61:61–65.
58. Lafon M. Subversive neuroinvasive strategy of rabies virus. *Arch Virol Suppl.* 2004:149–159.
59. Pedersen NC, Emmons RW, Selcer R, et al. Rabies vaccine virus infection in three dogs. *J Am Vet Med Assoc.* 1978;172:1092–1096.
60. Morrison WB, Starr RM. Vaccine-associated feline sarcomas. *J Am Vet Med Assoc.* 2001;218:697–702.
61. Shaw SC, Kent MS, Gordon IK, et al. Temporal changes in characteristics of injection-site sarcomas in cats: 392 cases (1990-2006). *J Am Vet Med Assoc.* 2009;234:376–380.
62. Brown CM, Conti L, Ettestad P, et al. Compendium of animal rabies prevention and control, 2011. *J Am Vet Med Assoc.* 2011;239:609–617.
63. World Health Organization. Rabies. http://www.who.int/mediacentre/factsheets/fs099/en/.
64. Kass PH, Spangler WL, Hendrick MJ, et al. Multicenter case-control study of risk factors associated with development of vaccine-associated sarcomas in cats. *J Am Vet Med Assoc.* 2003;223:1283–1292.
65. Srivastav A, Kass PH, McGill LD, et al. Comparative vaccine-specific and other injectable-specific risks of injection-site sarcomas in cats. *J Am Vet Med Assoc.* 2012;241:595–602.
66. Wilcock BP, Yager JA. Focal cutaneous vasculitis and alopecia at sites of rabies vaccination in dogs. *J Am Vet Med Assoc.* 1986;188:1174–1177.
67. Vitale CB, Gross TL, Magro CM. Vaccine-induced ischemic dermatopathy in the dog. *Vet Dermatol.* 1999;10:131–142.
68. Sidwa TJ, Wilson PJ, Moore GM, et al. Evaluation of oral rabies vaccination programs for control of rabies epizootics in coyotes and gray foxes: 1995-2003. *J Am Vet Med Assoc.* 2005;227:785–792.
69. Wunner WH, Briggs DJ. Rabies in the 21 st century. *PLoS Negl Trop Dis.* 2010;4:e591.
70. Nigg AJ, Walker PL. Overview, prevention, and treatment of rabies. *Pharmacotherapy.* 2009;29:1182–1195.
71. Balsamo GA, Ratard RC. Epidemiology of animal rabies and its practical application to pre- and postexposure prophylaxis, Louisiana, 1988 to 2007. *Vector Borne Zoonotic Dis.* 2010;10:283–289.
72. Shankar V, Orciari LA, De Mattos C, et al. Genetic divergence of rabies viruses from bat species of Colorado, USA. *Vector Borne Zoonotic Dis.* 2005;5:330–341.
73. Minnesota Deparment of Health http://www.health.state.mn.us/diseases/rabies/risk/postexposure.html.

22

Canine Distemper Virus Infection

Jane E. Sykes, Marc Vandevelde

KEY POINTS

- First Described: 1905, Henri Carré, France.[1]
- Cause: CDV (family *Paramyxoviridae,* subfamily *Paramyxovirinae,* genus *Morbillivirus*).
- Affected Hosts: Dogs and other Canidae such as coyotes, foxes, and wolves; Procyonidae (raccoons, pandas); Mustelidae (ferrets, mink, skunks, otters); non-human primates. Large wild Felidae can also be affected.
- Geographic Distribution: Worldwide.
- Mode of Transmission: Oronasal contact with virus in secretions or excretions, droplet nuclei, and large-particle aerosol transmission.
- Major Clinical Signs: Fever, lethargy, inappetence, vomiting, diarrhea, dehydration, tachypnea, cough, conjunctivitis, neurologic signs, footpad and nasal planum hyperkeratosis.
- Differential Diagnoses: Canine parvovirus infection, other infectious causes of gastroenteritis, other causes of canine infectious respiratory disease, rabies, parasitic GI and respiratory disease, toxins such as lead and ethylene glycol, GI foreign body, dietary indiscretion, protozoal meningoencephalitis, systemic fungal infections such as cryptococcosis, portosystemic shunting with hepatic encephalopathy.
- Human Health Significance: CDV has been used as a model to study measles virus infection. The white matter lesions in the brain are considered to be a model for multiple sclerosis. There is some evidence that it may be involved in the pathogenesis of Paget's disease, a chronic, focal skeletal disorder of the elderly. Distemper outbreaks in primates raise concern about zoonotic potential of CDV.

ETIOLOGY AND EPIDEMIOLOGY

Canine distemper is an important disease of domestic dogs and wild animals worldwide. It is caused by CDV, an enveloped, pleomorphic negative-stranded RNA virus that belongs to the genus *Morbillivirus* (family *Paramyxoviridae*). CDV is closely related to the human measles virus and rinderpest virus and has been used as a model to study the pathogenesis of measles virus infections. The outer envelope of CDV contains hemagglutinin (H) and fusion (F) proteins, which are important in cellular attachment and entry (Fig. 22.1). Infection of dogs can lead to a severe, multisystemic disease that primarily affects the GI, respiratory, and neurologic systems (Fig. 22.2).

The host species spectrum of CDV is unusually wide. It includes terrestrial as well as aquatic mammals and affects the orders Carnivora (in 12 families that include Canidae, Mustelidae, Procyonidae, and Felidae), Rodentia (four families), Primates (two families), Artiodactyla (three families), and Proboscidea (one family).[2] Ferrets also are highly susceptible to distemper, but domestic cats are not affected. Virus shed by wildlife species such as raccoons can infect domestic dogs, but virus that is shed by dogs may also be a significant threat to wildlife populations, with catastrophic outbreaks of disease and high mortality rates.[3,4] A high prevalence of anti-CDV antibodies was detected in coyotes, red foxes, and gray foxes from Pennsylvania, USA, which raised concerns about the degree of spillover occurring between domestic dog and wild canid populations.[5] In domestic dogs with signs of infectious upper respiratory disease ("kennel cough"), distemper is an important differential diagnosis, and distemper can also mimic CPV enteritis. In fact, dual infections with CDV and CPV are probably underrecognized. Despite minor genetic variation, CDV isolates are serologically homogeneous. However, various strains differ in their pathogenicity, which may affect the severity and extent or type of clinical disease. Certain isolates, such as Snyder Hill, A75/17, and R252 strains, are highly virulent and neurotropic. The Snyder Hill strain causes polioencephalomyelitis, whereas the latter two strains cause demyelination. Other strains vary in their ability to cause CNS lesions. Properties of proteins coded by the N- and M-genes also affect viral persistence[6] and the ability to cause CNS disease.

Worldwide, a growing number of geographic lineages (also referred to as genotypes or clades) of CDV exist based on sequence analysis of the H-gene: Asia-1, Asia-2, Asia-4, India-1/Asia-5, America-1, America-2, Europe-1/South America-1, Europe-2 (Europe wildlife), South America-2, South America-3, Arctic, Rockborn-like, Africa-1, and Africa-2.[7] In the United States, vaccine strains belong to the America-1 lineage, whereas most field strains belong to the America-2 lineage. Strains that belong to the Europe-2 and Europe-3 lineages have also been detected in North American dogs.[1,8–10] In 2021, additional lineages were detected in wildlife in Ontario, Canada (Canada-1)[11] and red pandas in China.[12] Whether strains contained in CDV vaccines provide adequate protection against all wild-type viruses that currently circulate has been controversial. For example, one recent case series described CNS lesions associated with CDV infection in 4 vaccinated dogs, 2 of which were found to be infected with South American wild-type strains not included in the vaccine.[13] However, most disease in vaccinated dogs likely reflects failure of adequate vaccination, rather than lack of strain cross-reactivity.

Contact among recently infected (subclinical or diseased) animals maintains the virus in a population, and the birth of puppies helps provide a susceptible population for infection. Dogs that are not properly vaccinated can become infected after stress, immunosuppression, or contact with diseased individuals. Based on results of serosurveys, the infection rate is considered to be higher than the disease rate,[14] which reflects a certain degree of natural and vaccine-induced immunity in the general dog population. Many susceptible dogs can become subclinically infected but eliminate the virus without showing signs of illness. Although most recovered dogs clear the virus completely, some may harbor virus in their CNS.

The prevalence rate of spontaneous distemper in cosmopolitan dogs is greatest between 3 and 6 months of age, correlating with the loss of MDAs in puppies after weaning. In contrast, in susceptible, isolated populations of dogs, the disease is severe and widespread, affecting all ages. Increased susceptibility among breeds has been suspected but not proven.

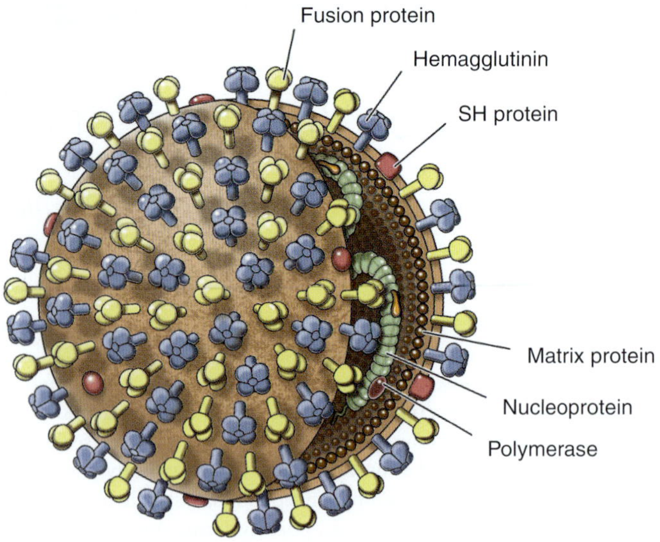

Fig. 22.1 Structure of CDV. The outer envelope contains hemagglutinin (H) and fusion (F) proteins, which are connected to the nucleocapsid by a matrix (M) protein, which is the most abundant protein in the virion. (From Sykes JE. *Canine and Feline Infectious Diseases*. Elsevier; 2014.)

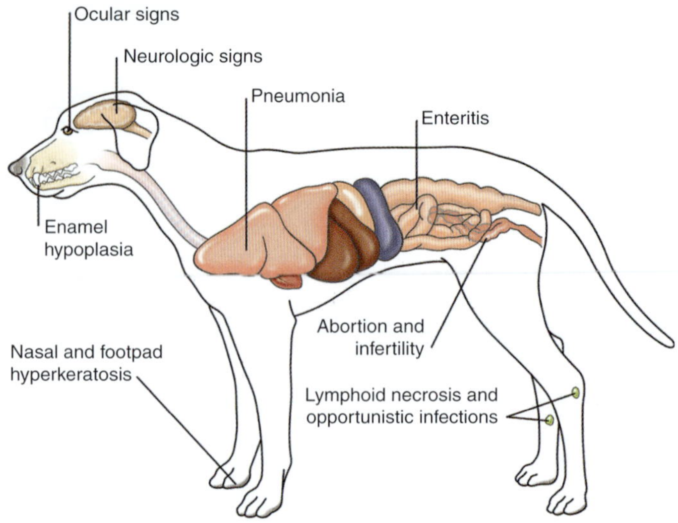

Fig. 22.2 Anatomic sites targeted by CDV infection. (From Sykes JE. *Canine and Feline Infectious Diseases*. Elsevier; 2014.)

Brachycephalic dogs have been reported to have a lower prevalence of disease, mortality, and sequelae compared with dolichocephalic breeds. Although vaccination has reduced the incidence of the disease, distemper still remains important where large numbers of young dogs with inadequate immunity are housed together, such as in kennels, large breeding facilities, and shelter environments. Puppies that have lost their maternal antibody are predisposed in regions where vaccination is performed, but occasionally disease occurs in older, vaccinated dogs.[15–17] Distemper also occurs in regions where vaccination of dogs is not performed or is poorly timed. As an enveloped virus, CDV is susceptible in the environment (surviving less than 1 day at room temperature) and is readily inactivated by heat, drying, and disinfectants; thus, contact between infected dogs is important to maintain transmission of the virus.

CLINICAL FEATURES

Pathogenesis and Clinical Signs

CDV is highly contagious and is spread through droplet nuclei and large-particle aerosol transmission. Dogs are generally exposed to CDV through contact with infected oronasal secretions, which may be shed by subclinically or clinically affected dogs. The virus initially infects monocytes within lymphoid tissue in the upper respiratory tract and tonsils and is subsequently disseminated via the lymphatics and blood to the entire reticuloendothelial system (Fig. 22.3). Within 24 hours PI, CDV multiplies in tissue macrophages and spreads in these cells via local lymphatics to tonsils and bronchial lymph nodes.[18] By days 4 to 6 PI, virus multiplication occurs within lymphoid follicles in the spleen, the gut-associated lymphatic tissue of the lamina propria of the stomach and small intestines, the mesenteric lymph nodes, and Kupffer cells in the liver. The viral hemagglutinin binds to a molecule on the surface of host cells known as the signaling lymphocytic activation molecule (SLAM, also known in humans as CD150). SLAM is a membrane glycoprotein of the immunoglobulin superfamily. It is important for cell entry by CDV as well as other morbilliviruses and is a key molecule in the pathogenesis of disease.[19] SLAM is expressed by immature thymocytes, activated lymphocytes, macrophages, and dendritic cells. Direct viral destruction of a significant proportion of the lymphocyte population, and especially CD4+ T cells, occurs within the blood, tonsils, thymus, spleen, lymph nodes, bone marrow, mucosa-associated lymphoid tissue, and hepatic Kupffer cells (Fig. 22.4).[20–22] Massive destruction of lymphocytes results in an initial lymphopenia and transient fever, which occurs a few days after infection. Acute CDV infection causes lymphocytic apoptosis, T-cell depletion, and long-lasting immunosuppression.[22–24] Prenatal and neonatal distemper infections can result in immunodeficiency in surviving puppies and can make concurrent infections with other viruses such as parvovirus, bacteria such as *Clostridium piliforme*, or protozoa such as *Neospora caninum* more severe.[25,26]

Further spread of CDV to epithelial and CNS tissues on days 8 to 9 PI probably occurs hematogenously as a cell-associated and plasma-phase viremia using the nectin 4 receptor[27] and its intensity depends on the dog's humoral and cell-mediated immune status. By day 14 PI, animals with adequate CDV antibody titers and cell-mediated cytotoxicity clear the virus from most tissues early on and show no clinical signs of illness. Recovery from CDV infection is associated with long-term immunity and cessation of viral shedding. Dogs with intermediate levels of cell-mediated immune responsiveness with delayed antibody titers by days 9 to 14 PI experience viral spread to their epithelial tissues. Clinical signs that develop may eventually resolve as antibody titer increases and virus is cleared from most body tissues.

By days 9 to 14 PI, in dogs with poor immune status, there is spread of virus to many tissues, including skin, exocrine and endocrine glands, and epithelium of the GI, respiratory, and genitourinary tracts. Clinical signs of disease in these dogs are usually dramatic and severe, and virus usually persists in their tissues until death. A frequent site of persistence is the skin, notably the foot pads ("hard pad disease") associated with hyperkeratosis and parakeratosis with vesicle, pustule, and inclusion body formation.[28] Virus entering the footpad epithelium during the viremic period causes proliferation of basal keratinocytes, resulting in the observed hyperkeratosis; however, neither the virus nor its nucleic acid appears to persist indefinitely.[29–31] Cytokine expression is upregulated in virus-infected footpad epidermal cells.[32,33] Alteration in the viral H protein gene sequence has been associated with this viral adaptation.[34]

Neuroinvasion occurs when viremia is of sufficient magnitude, which depends on the quality of the systemic immune response mounted by the host. In dogs, free or lymphocyte-associated virus can enter the brain by crossing the blood-brain barrier or the CSF via the choroid plexus, where it spreads to periventricular and subpial structures explaining the distribution of the ensuing lesions.[35] At least in

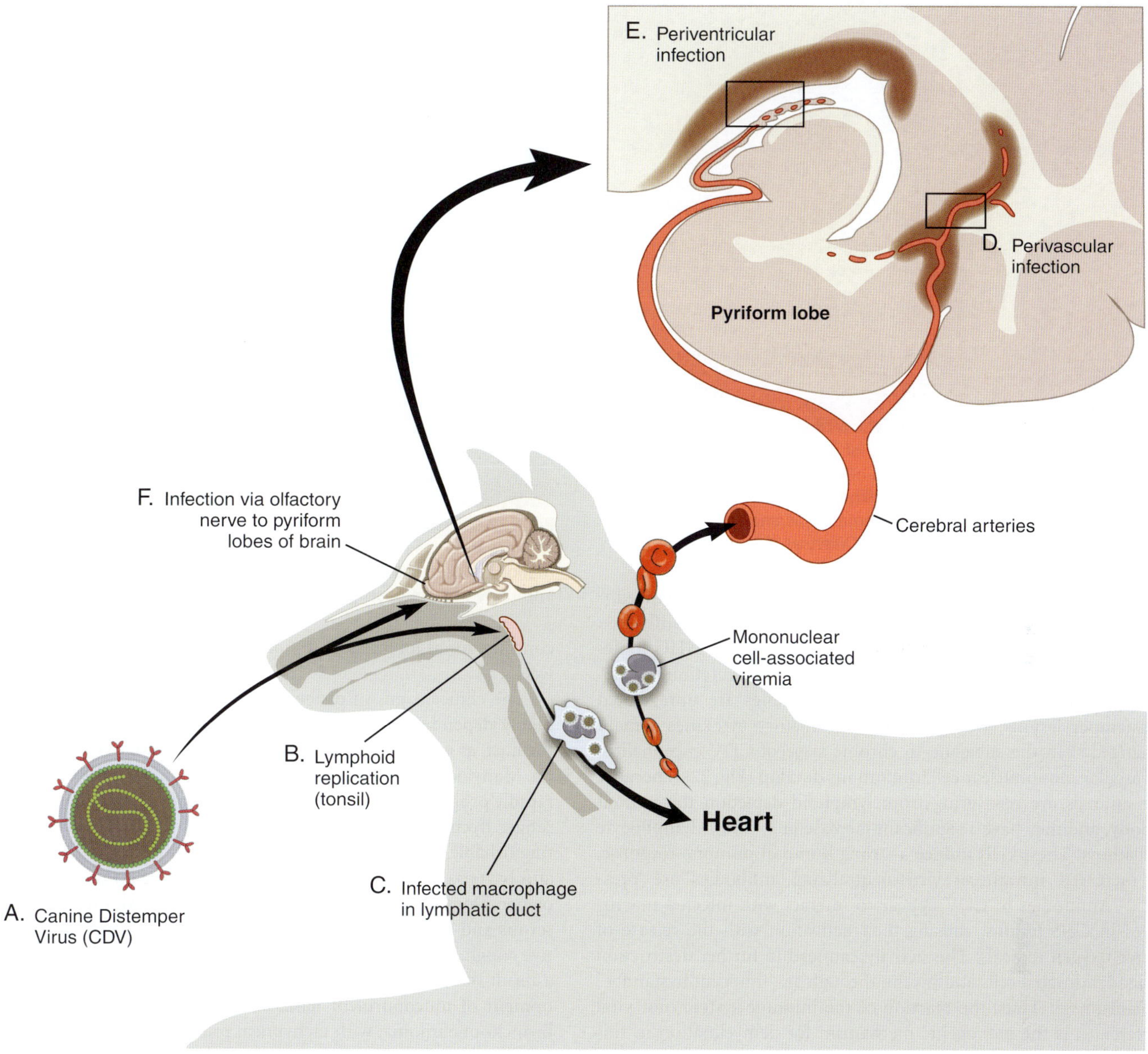

Fig. 22.3 Pathogenesis of distemper virus infection. *A,* CDV enters the respiratory tract via aerosols and colonizes the local lymphoid tissues such as the tonsils. *B,* Primary viral replication occurs in the tonsils, retropharyngeal nodes, bronchial lymph nodes, and GI lymphoid tissue. *C,* From these sites of primary replication, mononuclear cell-associated viremia occurs. *D,* Virus enters the CNS via the cerebral circulation and is deposited in the perivascular spaces of fine blood vessels. *E,* Alternatively, virus enters the vessels of the choroid plexus and eventually the CSF and ventricular system. *F,* As an uncommon phenomenon in dogs, CDV can travel from the nasal passage, through the cribiform plate and anterograde via the olfactory nerve to the olfactory bulb and CNS. There it localizes, predominantly in the pyriform lobes of the cerebral cortex.

ferrets, CDV can spread from the olfactory mucosa through the olfactory bulb and nerve to the brain. It is possible that selective polioencephalomalacia of rhinencephalic structures (including the pyriform and temporal lobes) in young puppies may result from olfactory invasion by CDV.[36]

The type of lesion produced and the course of infection within the CNS depend on numerous factors, including the age and immunocompetence of the host at the time of exposure, the neurotropic and immunosuppressive properties of the virus, and the time after infection at which lesions are examined. Gray matter lesions are the result of neuronal infection and necrosis and can lead to polioencephalomalacia. However, neuronal infection can also occur with minimal evidence of cytolysis and accumulation of viral inclusion bodies. Demyelination occurs in the white matter following productive viral replication in microglial and astroglial cells (Fig. 22.5). In oligodendrocytes, which produce myelin, infection is restricted to viral transcription without translation, which likely leads to metabolic dysfunction and degeneration of oligodendroglial cells. The end result is demyelination via a downregulation of myelin gene expression.[35] Other studies suggest that demyelination may be secondary to axonal damage.[37]

Because of immunosuppression, classical signs of inflammation are lacking in acute lesions, but there is a marked increase in CD8+ T cells throughout the CNS in dogs with acute distemper in response to the presence of the CDV nucleocapsid protein and increased Il-8

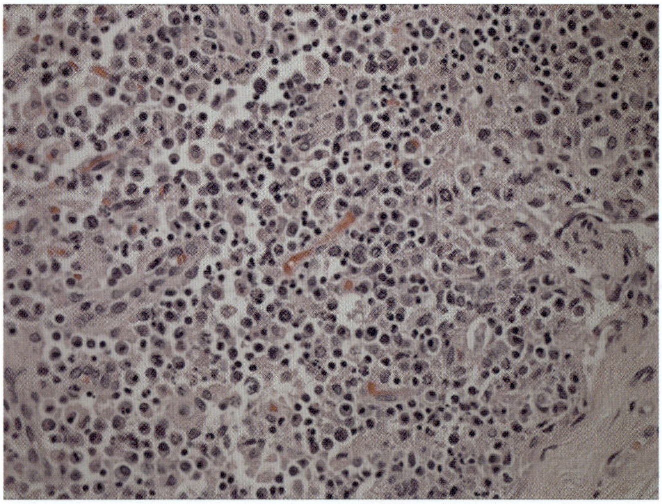

Fig. 22.4 Lymph node histopathology of a 5-month-old German shepherd mix with distemper. The dog had been adopted from a shelter and subsequently developed neurologic signs, diarrhea, and pneumonia. There is marked lymphoid necrosis. Hematoxylin and eosin stain. (From Sykes JE. *Canine and Feline Infectious Diseases.* Elsevier; 2014.)

activity.[38,39] Diffuse MHCII upregulation has also been recognized,[40] which may result from elevated levels of IFN-γ; this is frequently seen in viral infections in general.[41] Besides upregulation of MHC molecules, microglial cells in distemper exhibit enhanced secretion of reactive oxygen radicals.[42] Proinflammatory cytokines are upregulated in distemper lesions, whereas anti-inflammatory cytokines remain unchanged.[43] In the subacute to chronic stage of CDV encephalitis, perivascular mononuclear cell infiltrations develop (Fig. 22.6) because these animals are recovering from lymphoid depletion throughout the body, and they have a significant increase in T- and B-lymphocyte populations. These cells induce a strong humoral immune response, and increased intrathecal virus-neutralizing antibodies are present.[44,45] Antibodies to CDV appear to interact with infected macrophages in CNS lesions, causing their activation with the release of reactive oxygen radicals. This activity can lead to further destruction of oligodendroglial cells and myelin through an "innocent bystander" mechanism.[46,47] Thus, the reaction of the immune system, not viral interference, is the pathogenic mechanism for demyelination in this phase. If viral spread through the CNS has been extensive by the time the host immune system responds to the virus, widespread damage occurs with a fatal outcome. Some animals may recover because CDV is completely cleared from the inflammatory lesions. Frequently, CDV persists in the brain,[48] and keeps driving the inflammatory response and collateral white matter damage, which results in a chronic progressive or rarely a chronic relapsing disease. Persistence is related to noncytolytic cell-to-cell spread of viral nucleocapsids. By the time the infection is detected by the immune system, with an associated inflammatory response, CDV has already spread further to an area remote from the inflammatory focus. Thus, CDV "outruns" the immune system by rapidly spreading through the astroglial network using an as-yet unknown glial receptor. "Old dog encephalitis" is an exceedingly rare, poorly characterized form of distemper, manifested as a chronic progressive demyelinating panencephalitis similar to subacute sclerosing panencephalitis, a measles virus–induced disease in children. The term "old dog encephalitis" is a misnomer, because affected dogs are not necessarily old. Virus has been detected within the brains of these dogs with immunohistochemistry and RT-PCR assays.[25]

CDV is shed in all secretions and excretions from as early as day 5 after infection, before the onset of clinical signs. Shedding of virus can continue for as long as 3 to 4 months, but usually resolves after 1 to 2 weeks.

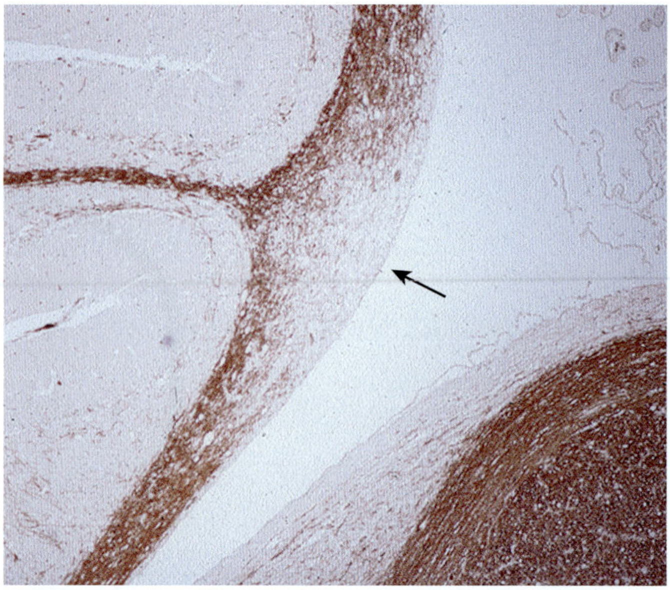

Fig. 22.5 Histopathology showing acute noninflammatory demyelination, with loss of myelin staining *(arrow)*. There is minimal inflammation in these lesions, which are typical for dogs with poor anti-CDV immunity (myelin-basic protein immunostain ×20).

The clinical signs of distemper in dogs vary dramatically and are highly dependent on virus strain and the age and immune status of the host, as well as concurrent infections with other viruses and bacteria. Many dogs experience subclinical infection, whereas others exhibit rapidly progressive infection followed by death. The incubation period ranges from 3 to 6 days. Respiratory or GI tract signs may be indistinguishable from those caused by other respiratory or enteric viruses and bacteria, or signs may be so mild that they go unnoticed by the owner. Dogs with respiratory involvement may exhibit fever, bilateral serous and nasal ocular discharges, conjunctivitis, and a nonproductive cough. Secondary bacterial infection, which occurs unhindered as a result of virus-induced immunosuppression, can lead to the development of mucopurulent nasal and ocular discharges and bacterial bronchopneumonia, with tachypnea, productive cough, lethargy, and decreased appetite. Viral destruction of the GI tract epithelium can result in inappetence, vomiting, diarrhea, electrolyte abnormalities, and dehydration. Dogs that mount an intermediate or delayed immune response may recover from acute illness but fail to eliminate the virus completely, which leads to a spectrum of more chronic disease manifestations, which often involve the uvea, lymphoid organs, footpads, and especially the CNS. Opportunistic infections can also develop in these dogs, whereas dogs developing nasal and digital hyperkeratosis usually have various neurologic complications.

Neurologic manifestations usually begin 1 to 3 weeks after recovery from systemic illness; however, no way is known to predict which dogs will develop neurologic disorders. Neurologic signs can also coincide with multisystemic illness, or less commonly, they can occur weeks to months later. Neurologic signs frequently develop in the presence of nonexistent or very mild extraneural signs.[49] Neurologic signs, whether acute or chronic, are typically progressive. Chronic relapsing neurologic deterioration with an intermittent recovery and a later, superimposed acute episode of neurologic dysfunction can occur. Neurologic complications of canine distemper are the most significant factors affecting prognosis and recovery from infection. Neurologic signs vary according to the area of the CNS involved. Hyperesthesia

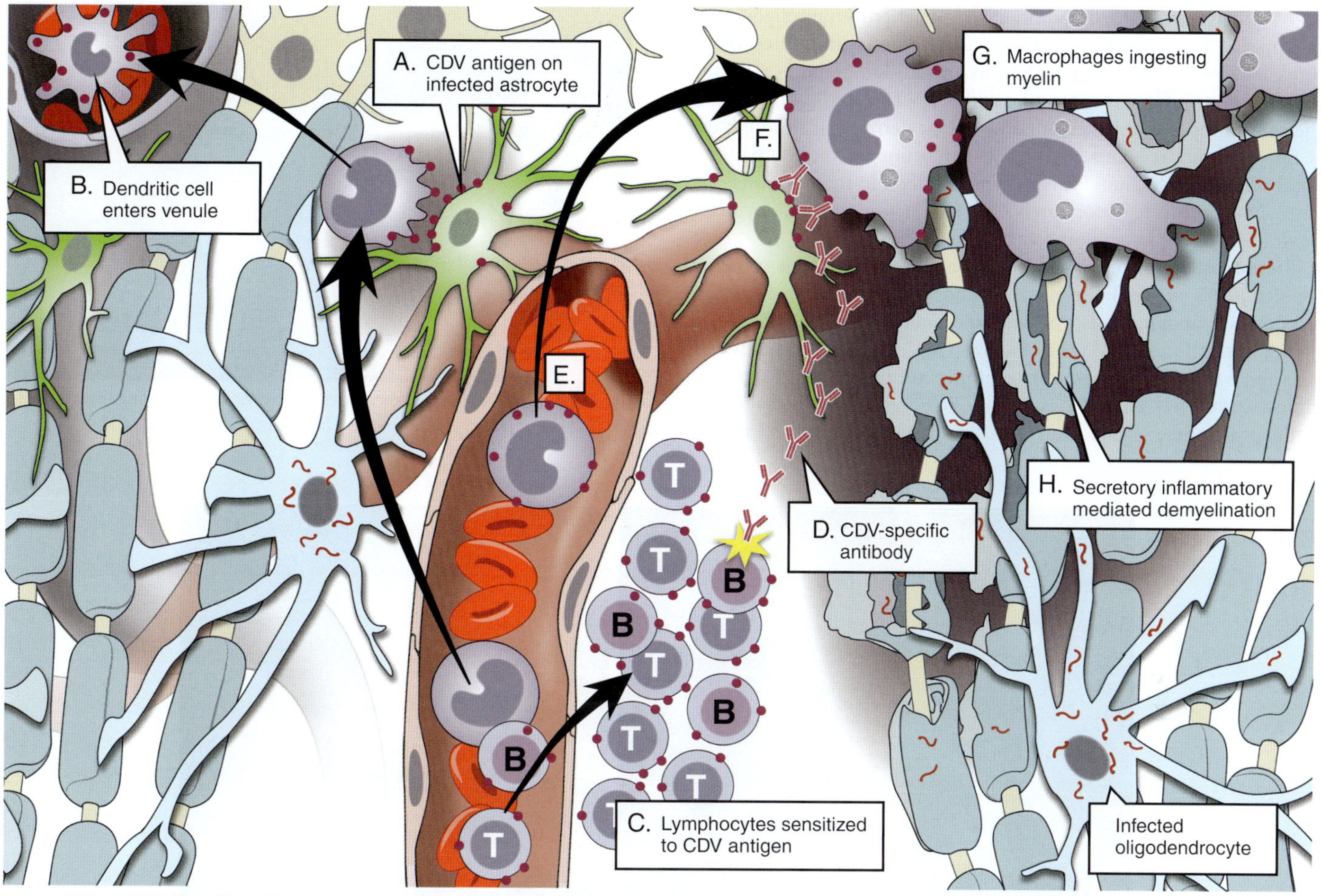

Fig. 22.6 Chronic perivascular cuffing with demyelination. For periods after viral infection, low quantities of unenveloped viral nucleocapsids remain in astrocytes with minimal cellular inflammatory response. Virus may also be found in oligodendrogliocytes and some neurons as untranslated viral RNA. *A,* CDV antigens are expressed on the surface of astrocytes. Signaling lymphocyte activation molecule (SLAM) on the surface of immune cells such as dendritic cells interacts with this viral antigen. *B,* Macrophages activated by the viral interaction transform to dendritic cells and emigrate from the CNS via venules and enter the systemic circulation, traveling to lymph nodes. There they present antigen to T cells and cause CDV-specific activation of other immunocytes. *C,* Lymphocytes, now sensitized to CDV antigens, enter the CNS via the blood vessel as a result of immune recruitment. Perivascular cuffing occurs with antigen-directed B cells and $CD8^+$ and $CD4^+$ T cells. *D,* B cells synthesize and release CDV-specific antibody. *E,* Similarly, sensitized mononuclear cells enter the perivascular space of the CNS with increased expression of cytokines (interleukin [IL]-6, IL-8, IL-12, and tumor necrosis factor-α) as a heightened immune response against the virus. *F,* CDV-specific antibody from the B cells that has become bound to surface antigen of infected astrocytes attracts activated monocyte/macrophages, displaying increased major histocompatibility complex class II and SLAM molecule expression. These bind to the Fc portion of this bound antibody, triggering antibody-dependent, cell-mediated cytotoxicity. In this process, activated macrophages secrete "highly active molecules" (e.g., matrix metalloproteinases, their associated inhibitors, and reactive oxygen radicals). These radiate into surrounding tissue, further damaging the blood-brain barrier, myelin, and other cellular elements in a "bystander" mechanism. *G,* Myelin unraveling and fragmentation occur as a result of the inflammation and necrosis. *H,* Macrophages ingest degenerating myelin and necrotic debris as a part of the clean-up process.

and cervical or paraspinal rigidity can be found in some dogs as a result of meningeal inflammation. Seizures, cerebellar and vestibular signs, paraparesis or tetraparesis with sensory ataxia, and myoclonus are common. Seizures can be of any type, depending on the region of the forebrain that is damaged by the virus. Myoclonus, the involuntary twitching of muscles in a forceful simultaneous contraction, can be present without other neurologic signs. The rhythmic flexor-extensor contractions of myoclonus can be present while a dog is awake, although they more commonly occur during sleep. Although considered specific for CDV infection, myoclonus can also be seen in other paramyxovirus infections of dogs and cats and, less commonly, in other inflammatory conditions of the CNS.[50] Ocular signs of persistent CDV infection include uveitis, chorioretinitis, keratoconjunctivitis sicca (KCS), keratitis, and optic neuritis, which may be associated with blindness. KCS is thought to result from damage to the lacrimal gland by CDV.[22] It may be transient or permanent, and can lead to keratitis and corneal ulceration. The virus itself can also infect the corneal epithelial and stromal cells. Young puppies infected with CDV before the eruption of permanent dentition can have severe damage to the enamel, dentin, or roots of their teeth. Enamel or dentin can show an irregular appearance in addition to partial eruption, oligodontia, or impaction of teeth. Enamel hypoplasia with or without neurologic signs may be an incidental finding in an older dog and is relatively pathognomonic for prior infection with CDV (Fig. 22.7). Infection of the skin can lead to a vesicular and pustular dermatitis, although this is uncommonly recognized. Persistent infection of the footpad and nasal planum epithelium leads to hyperkeratosis in these regions (Fig. 22.8). Myocarditis has been rarely described in puppies, with evidence of viral inclusions in cardiomyocytes at necropsy.[51]

Immunosuppression results from lymphopenia, necrosis of hematopoietic cells in the bone marrow, and dendritic cell malfunction. Lymphocyte apoptosis also occurs independent of viral infection of lymphocytes. The viral V protein allows CDV to replicate rapidly in T cells and is critical in CDV-mediated immunosuppression. This protein almost completely antagonizes IFN-α, TNF-α, IL-6, IFN-γ, and IL-2 in the acute phase of infection.[22] Finally, the nucleocapsid (N) protein

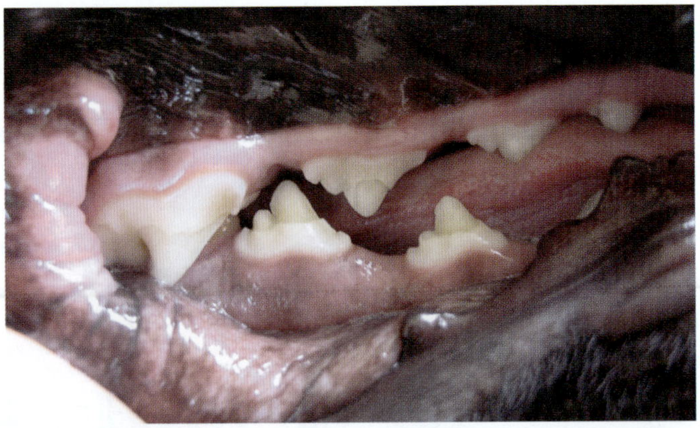

Fig. 22.7 Enamel hypoplasia induced by CDV infection. (From Sykes JE. *Canine and Feline Infectious Diseases*. Elsevier; 2014.)

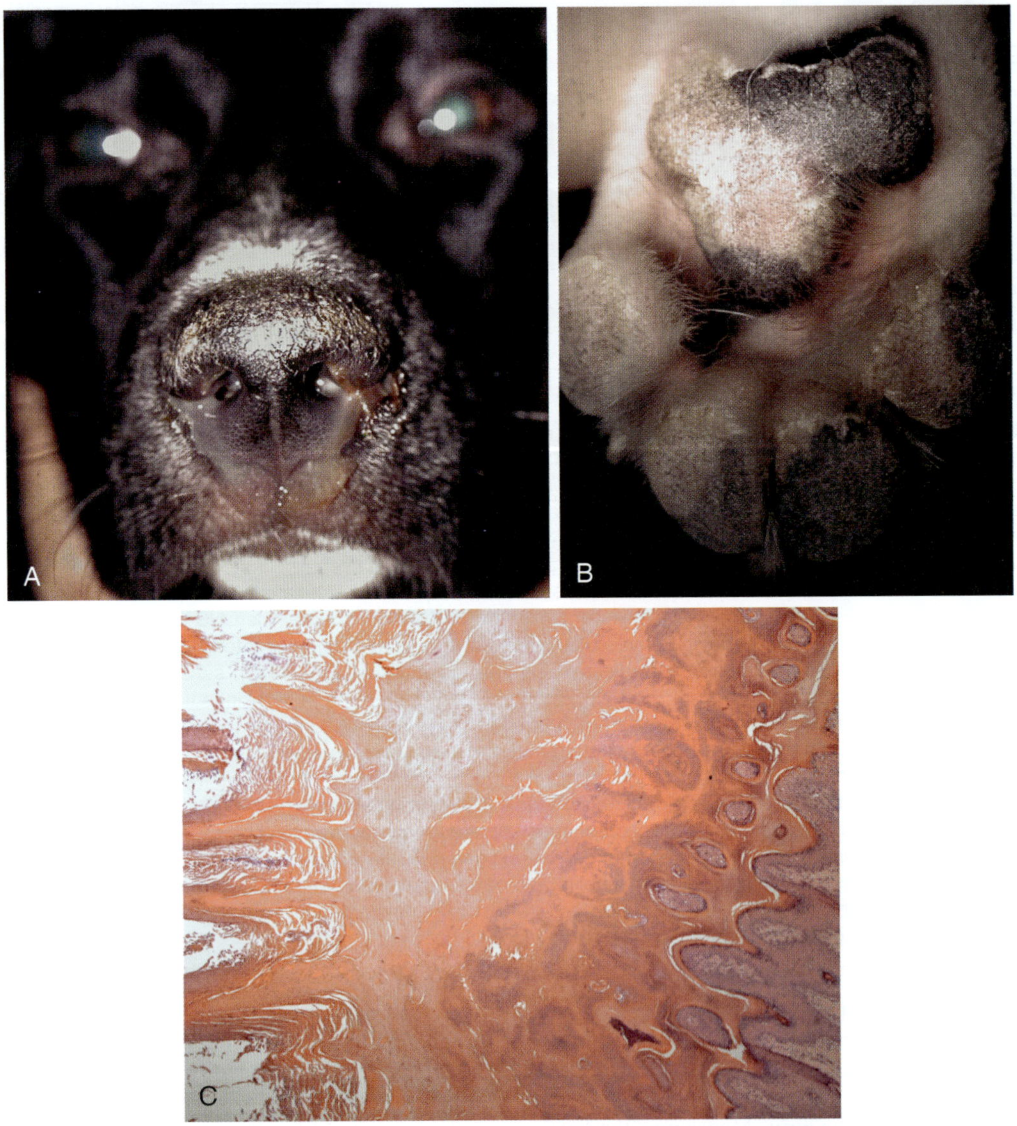

Fig. 22.8 Nasal planum (A) and footpad (B) hyperkeratosis induced by CDV infection in a 4-month-old border collie mix with conjunctivitis, mucopurulent nasal and ocular discharge, and myoclonus. Blepharospasm is also present. (C) Histopathology of the footpad of a 1-year-old German shepherd mix with distemper. Marked hyperkeratosis is evident. Hematoxylin and eosin stain, 40× magnification. (From Sykes JE. *Canine and Feline Infectious Diseases*. Elsevier; 2014.)

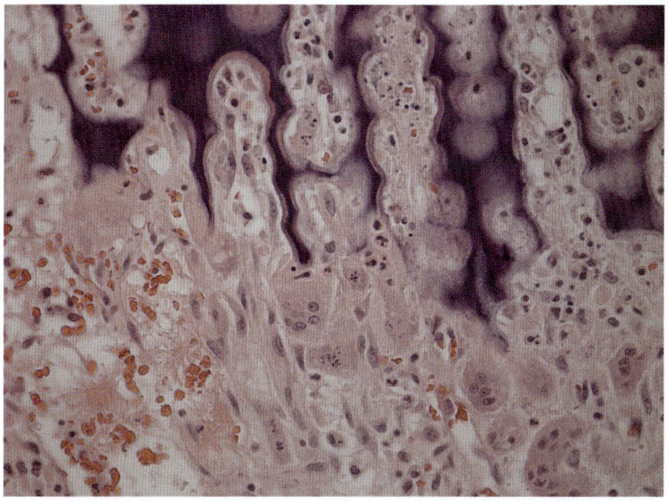

Fig. 22.9 Severe, neutrophilic osteomyelitis with submetaphyseal osteonecrosis and extensive bony resorption in a 4-month-old intact male Labrador retriever mix with distemper. The dog was seen for lethargy, mild diarrhea, fever, and reluctance to stand; joint pain was detected on physical examination. Direct IFA on urine sediment was positive for CDV, but a conjunctival scrape tested negative with direct IFA. Necropsy also revealed pneumonia with intracytoplasmic and intranuclear viral inclusions. Hematoxylin and eosin stain. (From Sykes JE. *Canine and Feline Infectious Diseases.* Elsevier; 2014.)

of morbilliviruses binds to the CD32 (Fc-γ) receptor on B cells, which results in impaired differentiation of B cells into plasma cells.[52] When the virus binds this receptor on dendritic cells, impaired antigen presentation by dendritic cells results, which disrupts T-cell function. The most common secondary infections in distemper are secondary bacterial infections that contribute to bronchopneumonia. *Bordetella bronchiseptica* is a common copathogen. Dogs may be diagnosed with bordetellosis in the early stages of distemper, and the underlying CDV infection may be overlooked. Other opportunistic infections that have been identified in dogs with distemper include toxoplasmosis,[53] salmonellosis,[54], nocardiosis,[55,56] and generalized demodecosis. Infection with *Pneumocystis carinii* was associated with CDV infection in a mink,[57] and concurrent neosporosis and canine distemper was reported in a raccoon.[58]

Uncommonly, CDV infection has been associated with metaphyseal bone lesions in young dogs as a result of infection of osteoclasts, osteoblasts, and osteocytes.[59] Infected cells undergo degeneration and necrosis, and metaphyseal osteosclerosis occurs (Fig. 22.9). This may lead to pain and lameness. CDV RNA has also been detected in bone cells of dogs with hypertrophic osteodystrophy, and CDV may play a role in this disease.[60] It has been shown that CDV surface proteins promote osteoclast formation.[61]

Finally, transplacental infections with CDV may be associated with infertility, stillbirth, or abortion and with neurologic signs in puppies that are less than 4 to 6 weeks of age.

Physical Examination Findings

Physical examination findings in dogs with distemper depend on the severity and chronicity of the disease, but include fever (occasionally up to 106°F or 41.1°C), conjunctivitis, serous to mucopurulent ocular and nasal discharges, blepharospasm and photophobia, tonsillar enlargement and hyperemia, tachypnea, and increased lung sounds (see Fig. 22.8). Cough may occur during the examination. Dehydration may also be present, especially in dogs with GI and severe neurologic signs. Rarely, a measles-like cutaneous rash or pustular dermatitis is evident.

Dogs with chronic disease can be thin or emaciated and show hyperkeratosis of the nasal planum and footpads. Puppies with hyperkeratosis, also known as "hardpad," have thickened, crusty footpads that resemble those of adult dogs (see Fig. 22.8). Myoclonus (involuntary twitching of isolated muscle groups) is common and, when mild, is most readily detected when affected puppies are at rest. Other neurologic signs include obtundation, seizures, tremors, opisthotonos, tetraparesis, paraparesis, delayed placing reactions, ataxia, and, less commonly, behavioral abnormalities, compulsive pacing, and vestibular signs such as a head tilt, nystagmus, strabismus, and circling.[15] Progressive lower motor neuron signs and hyperesthesia were described in one 4-month-old dog in association with a focal cervical spinal cord lesion on MRI.[62] Focal seizures may be localized to the head and jaw, with accompanying foamy hypersalivation ("chewing gum" seizures). Vocalization and apparent blindness can also occur. In addition to conjunctivitis and ocular discharge, an ophthalmologic examination may reveal corneal edema, corneal ulceration, aqueous flare, chorioretinitis, uveitis, or optic neuritis. Markedly decreased Schirmer tear test results and positive fluorescein tests may be present.[63] Optic neuritis appears as a large, pale, fluffy, optic disc with no physiologic depression. Rarely, lameness may be observed.

Dogs that have recovered from CDV infection may have evidence of dental abnormalities and enamel hypoplasia (see Fig. 22.7); healed chorioretinitis lesions, which appear as hyperreflective circular lesions ("gold medallion lesions"); keratoconjunctivitis sicca; or residual neurologic signs, especially myoclonus.

DIAGNOSIS

Practical diagnosis of canine distemper is primarily based on clinical suspicion. A characteristic history of a 3- to 6-month-old unvaccinated puppy with a compatible illness supports the diagnosis. Establishment of a diagnosis of distemper is most easily accomplished in dogs that have the full spectrum of clinical abnormalities, and especially when myoclonus is present, because there are few other diseases that cause this array of clinical signs. In dogs with isolated respiratory, GI, or neurologic signs, antemortem diagnosis is more challenging because these signs are less specific, laboratory diagnostic assays can be insensitive, and the presence of attenuated live vaccine virus can lead to false-positive results. A combination of laboratory tests may be required to establish the diagnosis, and the finding of a negative result for any assay does not rule out distemper. Sensitivity for detection of CDV using assays that detect virus may also be increased by testing of multiple specimens from different anatomic locations, such as various combinations of blood, urine, conjunctival smears, and CSF. In dogs with respiratory signs, the presence of conjunctivitis, blepharospasm, and ocular discharge should raise suspicion for distemper. Distemper should always be considered as a diagnosis in young dogs with neurologic signs, whether or not respiratory or GI signs are present. Finally, clinicians should maintain a high suspicion for the presence of concurrent infections such as parvoviral enteritis, concurrent respiratory viral infection, or bordetellosis.

Laboratory Abnormalities

Complete Blood Count

The CBC in dogs with acute distemper most commonly reveals mild anemia and an absolute lymphopenia caused by lymphoid depletion. This frequently persists in very young dogs with rapidly progressive systemic or neurologic signs. The lymphocyte count may also be normal, especially in more chronic distemper. Thrombocytopenia (as low as 30,000 cells/μL) and regenerative anemia have been found in experimentally infected neonates (aged less than 3 weeks) but have not been consistently recognized in older or spontaneously infected dogs

TABLE 22.1 Complete Blood Count Findings at Admission in 50 Dogs Diagnosed with Distemper at the UC Davis VMTH

Test	Reference Range	Percent Below the Reference Range	Percent Within the Reference Range	Percent Above the Reference Range	Range for Dogs with Distemper
Hematocrit (%)	40–55	80	20	0	17–53
MCV (fL)	65–75	26	72	2	58–80
MCHC (g/dL)	33–36	10	74	16	28–37
Neutrophils (cells/μL)	3000–10,500	12	32	56	16–27,765
Band neutrophils (cells/μL)	0–rare	0	72	28	0–4442
Monocytes (cells/μL)	150–1200	4	62	34	24–5202
Lymphocytes (cells/μL)	1000–4000	54	42	4	110–5575
Eosinophils (cells/μL)	0–1500	0	100	0	0–1114
Platelets (cells/μL)	150,000–400,000	14	66	20	17,000–594,000

Note: adult reference ranges were used.

TABLE 22.2 Findings on Serum Biochemistry Analysis in 27 Dogs with Distemper at the UC Davis VMTH

Test	Reference Range	Percent Below the Reference Range	Percent within the Reference Range	Percent Above the Reference Range	Range for Dogs with Distemper	Number of Dogs Tested
Sodium (mmol/L)	145–154	56	40	5	106–158	26
Potassium (mmol/L)	3.6–5.3	12	79	9	2.8–5.9	26
Chloride (mmol/L)	108–118	40	56	5	65–130	26
Bicarbonate (mmol/L)	16–26	0	86	14	16–34	26
Calcium (mg/dL)	9.7–11.5	25	68	7	5.1–12.7	27
Phosphorus (mg/dL)	3.0–6.2	7	50	43	2.6–10.0	27
Creatinine (mg/dL)	0.3–1.2	11	89	0	0–1.2	27
BUN (mg/dL)	5–21	7	91	2	0.6–25	27
Albumin (g/dL)	3.0–4.4	68	32	0	0.9–3.7	27
Globulin (g/dL)	1.8–3.9	7	82	11	1.5–5.3	27
Cholesterol (mg/dL)	135–361	9	86	5	88–385	26
Total bilirubin (mg/dL)	0–0.2	0	80	20	0–0.8	26
ALT (U/L)	19–67	7	75	18	8–389	26
ALP (U/L)	21–170	0	77	23	28–322	26

Note: adult reference ranges were used by the laboratory.

(Table 22.1). Neutropenia, monocytopenia, can occur, and occasionally these are severe. Neutrophilia with a left shift and toxic neutrophils may be present.

Serum Biochemical Tests

Abnormalities on the serum biochemistry panel in dogs with distemper are nonspecific and include electrolyte changes that occur with vomiting and diarrhea such as hyponatremia, hypokalemia, and hypochloridemia (Table 22.2). Hypoalbuminemia and associated hypocalcemia are also common. Mild increases in liver enzyme activities occur in some dogs, which may reflect hypoxia or secondary infections that occur as a result of translocation of intestinal bacteria.

Urinalysis

No specific urinalysis findings are reported in dogs with distemper.

CSF Analysis

Abnormalities of the CSF are detectable in dogs with neurologic signs of distemper; however, dogs with acute noninflammatory demyelinating encephalomyelitis may have normal CSF analysis results. Increases in protein (more than 25 mg/dL) and cell count (more than 10 cells/μL with a predominance of lymphocytes) are characteristic of subacute to more chronic, inflammatory forms of CDV encephalomyelitis.[15] Increased anti-CDV antibody (see section on serology) in CSF could be definitive evidence of distemper encephalitis because antibody is locally produced. An antibody ratio can help identify the effect of nonspecific leakage of distemper-specific IgG into the CSF from serum by dividing the concentration of distemper-specific IgG in CSF by that of IgG in serum and comparing the result with a corresponding CSF-serum antibody ratio for another infectious agent such as CAdV or CPV. If the ratio for CDV is higher than that for CAdV or CPV, then *de novo* local production of CSF antibody caused by CNS infection with distemper is expected. Alternatives are to compare the CDV-specific CSF-serum ratio with the ratio of IgG or albumin in CSF and serum.[64] In acute CNS infections, some mononuclear cells may contain large (15 to 10 μm), oval homogenous eosinophilic intracytoplasmic inclusions.[21] More effective is direct FA on cytospin preparations of CSF cells (see following text).

Diagnostic Imaging

Plain Radiography

When present, abnormalities on thoracic radiography in dogs with distemper include pulmonary interstitial to alveolar infiltrates and consolidation compatible with bronchopneumonia, especially in the cranial and ventral lung lobes.

Magnetic Resonance Imaging

Dogs with distemper encephalomyelitis can have normal MRI findings. Hyperintense lesions and loss of contrast between gray and white matter in the cerebellum and/or the brainstem have been described in T2-weighted images, which correspond to demyelination on histopathology.[65] Multifocal T2 and fluid-attenuated inversion recovery (FLAIR) hyperintensities can occur in other locations in the brain, and there may be mild meningeal contrast enhancement (Fig. 22.10).

Microbiologic Tests

Microbiologic tests for CDV infection are shown in Table 22.3.

Virus Isolation

Growth in pulmonary macrophages or lymphocytes was once considered an essential feature of virulent CDV isolates, whereas isolation of virulent CDV has been difficult in routine cell cultures. Currently, dog lymphocyte cultures,[66] marmoset lymphoid cell line (B95a),[66] and, probably most effective, SLAM transfected Vero cell lines[22] are routinely used. Cultures are monitored for giant cell (syncytia) formation, a characteristic cytopathic effect of CDV or by immunofluorescence. Because of defective viral replication, specimens from dogs with chronic or vaccine-induced encephalitis may not yield successful

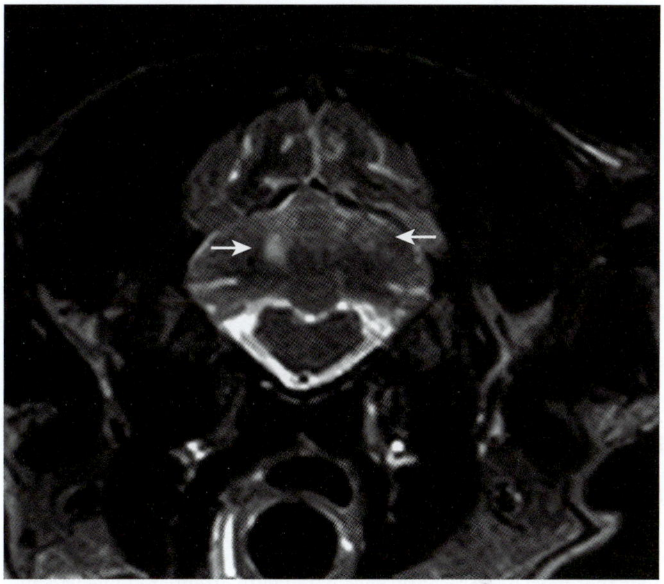

Fig. 22.10 Transverse section of the head at level of the cerebellum of a dog with demyelinating distemper encephalitis. T2 sequence. Multiple areas of hyperintensity of the white matter *(arrows)*.

TABLE 22.3 Diagnostic Assays Available for Distemper in Dogs

Assay	Specimen Type	Target	Performance
Virus isolation	Conjunctival and nasal swabs, blood, urine, transtracheal wash specimens, necropsy specimens	CDV	False negatives can occur in specimens that contain low numbers of virus particles. Attenuated live vaccine virus may also be isolated. Not widely offered for routine diagnostic purposes
Direct immunostaining (such as direct fluorescent antibody)	Smears made from conjunctival scrapings, urine sediment, respiratory lavage specimens, impression smears of tissue specimens	CDV antigen	False negatives can occur in specimens that contain low numbers of virus particles. False positives can occur if nonspecific fluorescence is incorrectly interpreted as a positive result. Possibility of false positives after recent vaccination with attenuated live CDV vaccines
Distemper ELISA antigen assay	See Virus isolation	CDV antigen	Inexpensive and rapid. Sensitivity and specificity in naturally infected dogs have not been well established. False positives can occur for weeks after vaccination with attenuated live CDV vaccines
RT-PCR	See Virus isolation	CDV RNA	Sensitivity and specificity can vary depending on assay design. Testing specimens from multiple anatomic sites or combining PCR assays with other diagnostic tests for CDV improves sensitivity. Attenuated live vaccine virus may be detected for days to weeks after vaccination. Because of the high sensitivity of some assays, the significance of a positive result in relation to disease may be difficult to interpret; quantitative assays may help distinguish between natural infection (high virus load) and vaccination (low virus load). False-negative results can occur when virus levels are low or as a result of degradation of viral nucleic acid during specimen transport
Serology (IgG and IgM ELISA; SN)	Serum and/or CSF	Antibodies against CDV antigens	Acute and convalescent sera are required for diagnosis of acute distemper, so diagnosis is retrospective. False positives can occur with recent CDV vaccination
Histopathology	Usually necropsy specimens, but also skin biopsies (such as footpad biopsies)	Eosinophilic intracytoplasmic and intranuclear inclusions; CDV antigen with immunostaining or CDV RNA with *in situ* hybridization	If available, *in situ* hybridization may be most sensitive for detection of virus in tissues

SN, serum neutralization.

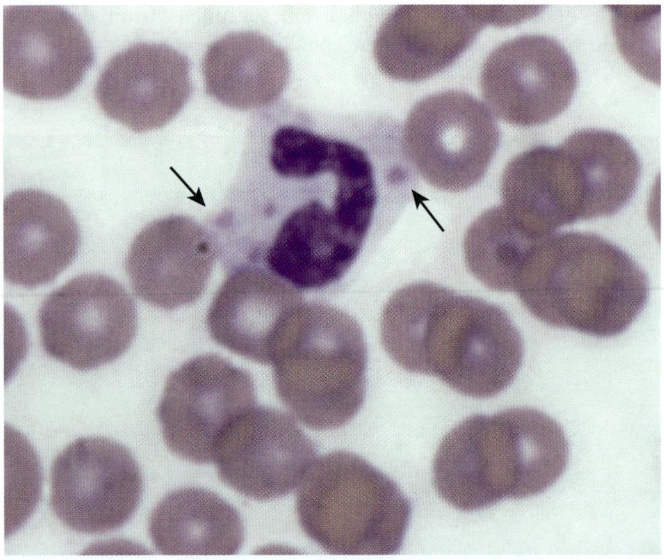

Fig. 22.11 Intracytoplasmic inclusions *(arrows)* in a circulating leukocyte of a 4-month-old border collie mix with distemper. (From Sykes JE. *Canine and Feline Infectious Diseases.* Elsevier; 2014.)

cultures. Wild-type virus must be distinguished from vaccine virus in dogs that have been recently vaccinated with attenuated live vaccines.

Cytologic Demonstration of CDV Inclusions

Intracytoplasmic viral inclusions can occasionally be seen in circulating blood cells of affected dogs, especially early in infection (although they also can be seen in chronic infections) (Fig. 22.11). Inclusions may also be visible in the cytoplasm of conjunctival epithelial cells. Epithelial cells can be scraped from the conjunctiva using a curette after application of a topical ophthalmic local anesthetic preparation. The cells are smeared onto a glass slide, stained with a Romanowsky or Wright-Leishman stain, and examined with light microscopy. Unfortunately, this has low sensitivity for diagnosis of distemper.[67] Intracytoplasmic distemper inclusions can be detected in the early phase of disease by examination of stained peripheral blood films, in low numbers in circulating lymphocytes, and with even less frequency in monocytes, neutrophils, and erythrocytes. Wright-Leishman-stained inclusions in lymphocytes are large (up to 3 μm), single, oval, gray structures, whereas erythrocytic inclusions (which are most numerous in polychromatophilic cells) are round and eccentrically placed and appear light blue. The sizes of erythrocytic inclusions are between those of metarubricyte nuclei and Howell-Jolly bodies. Buffy coat and bone marrow examination can improve the chances of detecting inclusions. Electron microscopy has confirmed that these inclusions consist of paramyxovirus-like nucleocapsids.

Immunostaining for CDV Antigen

Direct immunostaining of cells in conjunctival scrapings, CSF, or blood films is helpful in acute phases of illness. In chronic cases, it may be less rewarding because antibody coating or elimination of viral antigen may yield negative results. Immunostaining is more sensitive than identification of CDV inclusions with routine stains,[67] but false negatives still occur when low quantities of virus are present in the specimen.

Direct IFA techniques are often used in practice to detect CDV antigen in a variety of cell types, including conjunctival epithelial cells, leukocytes in a buffy coat smear, urine sediment, CSF cells (Fig. 22.12A), bone marrow, or tissues obtained at necropsy (Fig. 22.12B). Enzyme-antibody labelling can also be used (Fig. 22.12C).

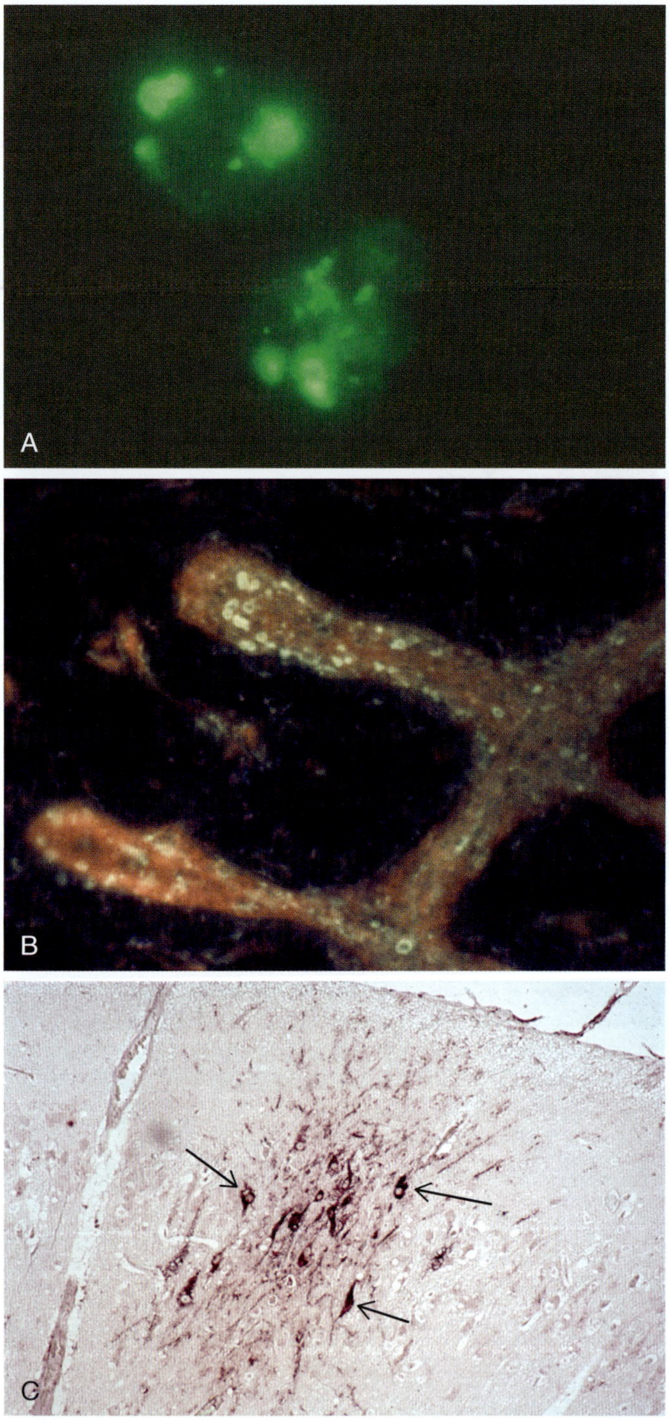

Fig. 22.12 (A) Immunofluorescent staining of CDV antigen in CSF cells (×1000). (B) Immunofluorescence highlighting CDV in a footpad biopsy. (C) Histopathology showing CDV RNA in neurons of cerebral cortex as detected using in situ hybridization *(arrows)*.

Transient false-positive results might occur after vaccination with attenuated live vaccines, so the results must be interpreted with caution in recently vaccinated dogs. False positives also have the potential to occur if nonspecific fluorescence is interpreted as a positive result by inexperienced laboratory technicians. Smears should be made on precleaned slides, air-dried thoroughly, and preferably fixed in acetone for 5 minutes before transport to the laboratory. At the laboratory, they are stained directly or indirectly with fluorescein or enzyme-conjugated CDV antibody.

Positive staining in conjunctival and genital epithelium is usually detected only within the first 3 weeks PI, when systemic illness is apparent. Virus also disappears in these tissues after the first 1 to 2 weeks of clinical illness (21 to 28 days PI) as antibody titers rise in association with clinical recovery. Virus can be detected for longer periods in epithelial cells and macrophages from the lower respiratory tract, and transtracheal washings can be obtained accordingly for diagnosis. Virus also persists for at least 60 days in the skin, uveal tissue, footpad, and CNS. In a series of clinically diagnosed cases of distemper, good correlation between direct FA and PCR was found.[67] Positive direct FA also correlated well with viral isolation.[8] Further research is required to understand the prevalence of and influence of vaccination on false-positive direct IFA results for diagnosis of distemper.

Antigen Detection ELISA Assays

ELISA assays that detect CDV antigen in serum (see Table 22.3) are available commercially as in-practice kits in some countries, but large well-controlled studies on their effectiveness are scant. Low sensitivity and false positives in dogs that were naturally infected with distemper were found in early assays.[68] Newer techniques such as lateral flow (immunochromatography) assay had improved sensitivity equivalent to that of an RT-PCR assay when applied to conjunctival swab specimens, but sensitivity was 90% and 86% when the assay was applied to blood lymphocytes and nasal swab specimens from dogs with distemper.[69] Sandwich-dot ELISA for the detection of CDV in clinically affected dogs showed an excellent correlation with direct electron microscopic demonstration of CDV.[70]

Molecular Diagnosis Using Nucleic Acid–Based Testing

The most sensitive laboratory technique for detection of CDV is the RT-PCR. A positive PCR result is indicative of infection, although not always associated with clinical illness. False-negative PCR results can occur if the virus is present in low concentrations at the site from which specimens are collected, or as a result of improper sample handling and extraction procedures or degradation of viral RNA during specimen collection and transport to the laboratory. In outbreak situations, collection of specimens from multiple dogs (at least 5 to 10) may increase the chance of positive test results.[71] Quantitative PCR is very sensitive and correlates well with viral isolation in experimentally infected dogs.[72] PCR also correlates very well with immunohistochemistry for CDV.[73]

RT-PCR assays are offered by a number of commercial veterinary diagnostic laboratories for diagnosis of distemper, sometimes as part of a panel that includes assays for other canine respiratory pathogens (see Chapter 124). Most assays detect a portion of the N protein gene. RT-PCR can be performed on whole blood, buffy coat, skin biopsies, conjunctival scrapings, urine, CSF, transtracheal washes, nasal and oropharyngeal swabs, and a variety of other tissues collected at necropsy (e.g., lung, small intestine, stomach, kidney, brain, bladder, lymphoid tissues). In one study of a limited number of experimentally infected dogs, conjunctival swabs were superior to whole blood, nasal flushes, and urine for PCR diagnosis of CDV infection,[74] whereas another study of naturally infected dogs showed highest viral loads in blood, followed by conjunctival swabs, and then urine.[75] At the time of writing, several POC PCR assays have been developed for detection of CDV. With further clinical validation and refinement, these assays have the potential to facilitate rapid and accurate diagnosis in veterinary clinics, shelters, and other poor-resource environments.[76,77]

RT-PCR is more sensitive than direct FA, but false positives may be more likely to occur after vaccination with attenuated live virus vaccines (not the recombinant vaccine), because most RT-PCR assays that are currently available for routine diagnostic purposes do not distinguish between vaccine and wild-type strains. Assays have been developed that differentiate between field and vaccine strains of CDV, but these are not commercially available.[78] Quantitation of RT-PCR results has been used to differentiate between shedding of attenuated vaccine virus (low viral load) from natural infection (high viral load) (e.g., Canine Distemper Quant RealPCR Test, IDEXX Laboratories, Portland, ME).[79] False-positive test results should not occur after use of *recombinant* CDV vaccines. A sensitive nested RT-PCR followed by an MspI restriction enzyme digestion step enabled to differentiate CDV field and vaccine strains using restriction fragment length polymorphism (RFLP) analysis.[80] More research is needed to clarify the influence of vaccination on the results of RT-PCR for distemper. The diagnosis is strengthened when positive PCR assay results are combined with positive results of other assays such as direct IFA.

Serologic Diagnosis

Neutralizing anti-CDV antibodies directed against the membrane proteins (H and F) of the virus appear 10 to 20 days PI, and can persist for the life of a recovered animal. They can be measured in the laboratory using serum neutralization (SN) assays (see Chapter 2), which is the gold standard against which other techniques are evaluated. Indirect FA testing has also been used to measure postvaccination titers, and results are comparable to those of SN.[81] ELISA assays are simpler and can be performed more rapidly, and these currently have similar sensitivity and specificity as SN.[82] Although sometimes less specific, whole-virus ELISA has been used to detect serum IgG and IgM antibodies to CDV. Increased specificity has been achieved using recombinant N protein–based ELISA in dogs.[83–86] Antibody to N and P proteins may appear 6 to 8 days PI when measured by ELISA. An ELISA based on CDV-H, which may be more relevant to assess protection, has also been developed.[87] Use of serology for diagnosis of distemper is complicated by the confounding effect of vaccination. This is especially true in shelter environments where all dogs are vaccinated on intake. High IgG titers are ambiguous and can indicate either past or present infection with CDV or past vaccination against CDV. Nevertheless, a fourfold rise in titer over a 2- to 4-week period supports recent infection. Acute and convalescent sera should be submitted to the same laboratory, because inter-laboratory variation in assay results occurs. Dogs with delayed-onset CDV encephalomyelitis have high levels of antibody in the CSF when compared with serum,[88] but should still be interpreted with caution. Increased titers of serum IgM-neutralizing antibody can be measured in dogs that survive the acute phase of infection and usually disappear by 3 months. Dogs that fail to develop significant titers of IgM or IgG post inoculation eventually die or have to be euthanized because of severe clinical illness.[89] High serum IgM titers have been more accurate in detecting acute clinical distemper cases (81%) compared with chronic progressive inflammatory encephalitis (60%). Transient IgM increases to CDV NP can also be seen for up to 3 weeks after first, but not after second, immunization with CDV vaccine.[84]

The results of serologic tests can be used to assess the need for vaccination, and also to determine which dogs are protected and therefore of low risk for development of disease and to some extent, virus shedding in outbreak situations. SN titers of at least 1:16 to 1:20 correlate with protection after vaccination. Titers of 1:100 or more correlate with protection in puppies that have received maternal antibodies.[90] One study showed a high (95%) prevalence of positive titers (≥ 10) using SN in 97 healthy client-owned adult dogs, and no appreciable increase in titers after vaccination.[91] Age less than 2 years was associated with lack of pre-vaccination antibodies. As a result, the authors suggested routine testing may be more appropriate than regular vaccination in adult dogs. Because of the presence of CMI, negative serologic results do not imply lack of protection. POC ELISA assays are also available for semiquantitative measurement of antibodies to CDV. One assay in this respect (Synbiotics TiterCHEK CDV/CPV, now offered by Zoetis) had a sensitivity of 76% and a specificity of 92% compared with SN when performed as a POC assay.[92] The low sensitivity would tend to overestimate the need for vaccination, which is preferable to an assay with low specificity, which might result in unnecessary exposure of a susceptible dog to infected dogs. In a 2021 study that evaluated the sensitivity and specificity of 4 POC tests available in Europe (ImmunoComb Canine VacciCheck, Biogal; TiterCHEK CDV-CPV, Zoetis; FASTest CDV-CPV Ab, Megacor; CanTi Check, Fassisi) using SN as the gold standard, specificity was high in 40 SPF dogs but poor for all assays in 176 dogs with acute or chronic illness. Sensitivity varied from 40 to 100%.[93]

Pathologic Findings

Gross Pathologic Findings

In addition to physical examination abnormalities described earlier, gross pathologic findings in canine distemper include thymic atrophy, pulmonary congestion and consolidation, liquid intestinal contents, and lymph node congestion and enlargement. Less common findings are mild pleural, pericardial, and/or peritoneal effusion and, uncommonly, visceral congestion and ecchymotic hemorrhages and meningeal congestion. In some dogs, gross necropsy abnormalities are minimal. Concurrent external and intestinal parasitic infections may also be identified.

Histopathologic Findings

Multifocal demyelinating lesions are pathognomonic for CDV infection (Fig. 22.13). Acute noninflammatory lesions include disseminated gray matter lesions with neuronal infection and degeneration and, characteristically, demyelination with spongy vacuolation of white matter and reactive gliosis. In surviving animals, patchy areas of demyelination are replaced by hypertrophic astrocytes and macrophages that are ingesting myelin. The most severe white matter changes in the CNS can be found in the lateral cerebellar peduncles, the dorsolateral medulla adjacent to the fourth ventricle, the deep cerebellar white matter, the optic nerves and tracts, and the spinal cord.[94] In one study of 17 dogs submitted for necropsy, the lumbosacral, thoracolumbar, cervical, and cervicothoracic regions were affected in 13, 11, 9, and 9 dogs, respectively.[95] Lesions in the lateral and dorsal funiculi were most common, and white matter lesions consisted of demyelination (17 dogs), astrocytosis (17), microgliosis (17), gemistocytes (11), and non-suppurative inflammation (10). Gray matter lesions included gliosis (8), non-suppurative inflammation (7), and malacia (5). Intracytoplasmic or intranuclear inclusions can be found

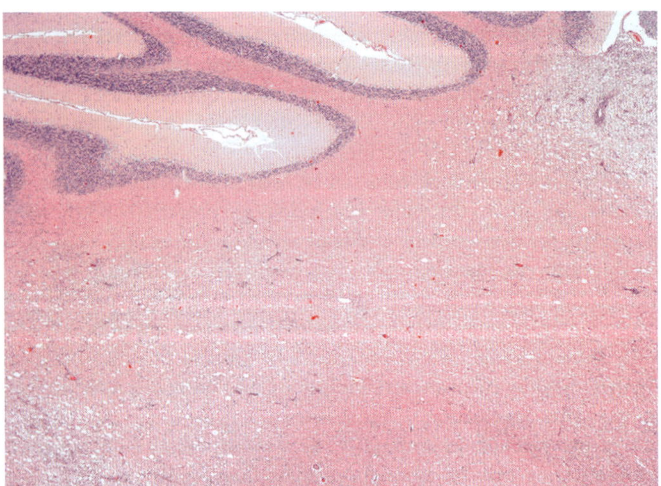

Fig. 22.13 Inflammatory demyelinating lesions (upper right and lower left corner) in cerebellar white matter. Hematoxylin and eosin stain.

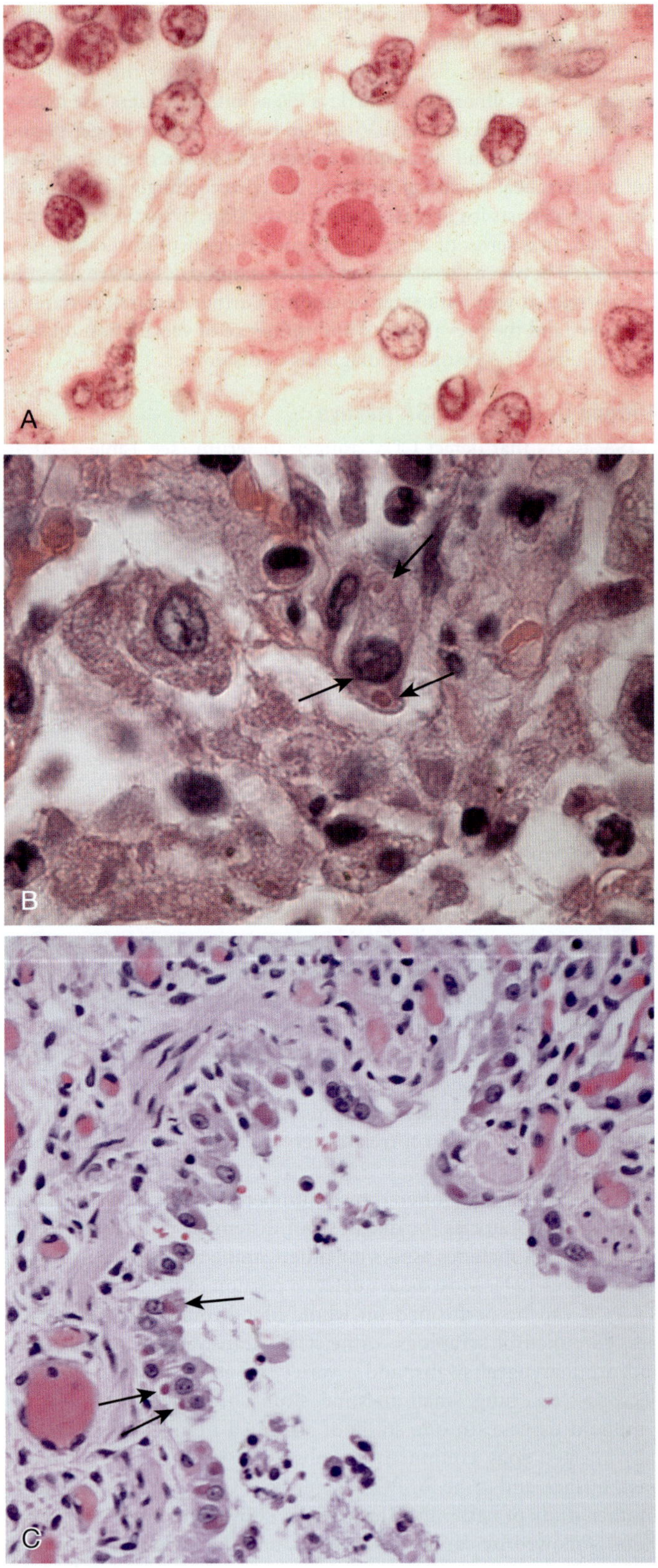

Fig. 22.14 (A) Neuron with multiple intracytoplasmic and intranuclear inclusion bodies in the cerebellum of a dog with distemper. Hematoxylin and eosin stain, 1000× oil magnification. (B) Eosinophilic intracytoplasmic and intranuclear viral inclusions *(arrows)* in the lung of the dog from Figure 22.4. Hematoxylin and eosin stain, 1000× oil magnification. (C) Bronchial epithelium from a dog infected with CDV. Intracytoplasmic inclusions are abundant *(arrows)*. Hematoxylin and eosin stain. (B, from Sykes JE. *Canine and Feline Infectious Diseases*. Elsevier; 2014. C, courtesy of Dr. Patricia Pesavento, University of California, Davis Veterinary Anatomic Pathology service.)

predominantly in astrocytes and neurons (Fig. 22.14). Chronic lesions are characterized by widespread perivascular lymphoplasmacytic infiltration, particularly in areas of demyelination. Demyelinating lesions can be more widespread and severe than lesions in dogs with acute encephalitis. Lesions of vaccine-induced distemper are typically those of a necrotizing polioencephalitis of the caudal brainstem with preference for the ventral pontine nuclei. Inclusions can be found in the nucleus or cytoplasm of astrocytes and neurons. Infection of the lungs leads to a lymphocytic and histiocytic interstitial pneumonia with proliferation of the alveolar epithelium; neutrophilic bronchopneumonia occurs as a result of secondary bacterial infection. There is often widespread lymphoid depletion and necrosis in all reticuloendothelial tissues (see Fig. 22.4), although lymphoid hyperplasia may be observed in dogs with chronic distemper. Epithelial cell necrosis may be present in the dental ameloblast layer, trachea, and bladder mucosa.

The diagnosis of CDV infection is supported by the presence of multifocal demyelination and eosinophilic intracytoplasmic or intranuclear inclusion bodies, which are 1 to 5 μm in diameter and occur in a variety of cell types, but especially in neurons, astrocytes, microglial cells, conjunctival epithelial cells, bladder epithelium, footpad epithelium, and sometimes lymphocytes (see Fig. 22.14). Less commonly, syncytia may be identified, such as in lymph nodes, lung, and brain. Confirmation of the presence of CDV in tissues can be established with the use of immunostaining, *in situ* hybridization, or RT-PCR (Fig. 22.15).

TREATMENT AND PROGNOSIS

When required, the mainstay of treatment for CDV infection is supportive care. No specific antiviral drug is available for treatment of CDV infection in living animals. R ribavirin,[96] 5-ethynyl-1-β-D-ribofuranosylimidazole-4-carboxamide (EICAR),[97] 6-methylmercaptopurine riboside,[98] caffeic acid,[99] various flavonoids,[98] and others all have anti-CDV activity but have only been tested *in vitro*. In view of the central role of membrane fusion in CDV pathogenesis,[100] fusion inhibitors would potentially be powerful antiviral drugs. High effectiveness of such drugs has been proven *in vitro* but they have not yet been tested *in vivo*.[101,102] Likewise, treatment of distemper with type 1 IFNs largely remains theoretical.[103,104] The old paradigm of treating distemper with hyperimmune sera was rekindled by an immunotherapy with porcine anti-CDV antibodies which decreased mortality in puppies with natural CDV infection.[105] The basic problem remains that CDV persists inside cells and immunoglobulins do not penetrate the blood-brain barrier.

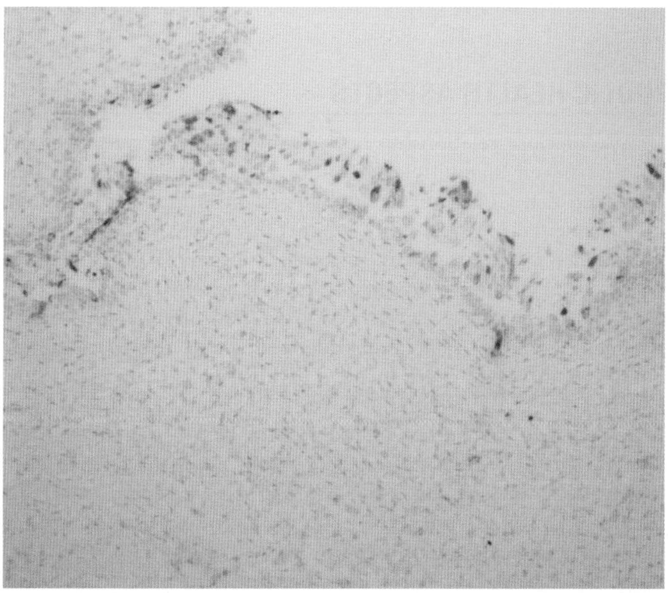

Fig. 22.15 Immunohistochemistry that shows CDV antigen (brown staining) in bladder transitional epithelial cells from a 2-year-old male neutered Australian cattle dog infected with CDV that had been recently adopted from a shelter and developed cough, ataxia, blindness, and seizures. (From Sykes JE. *Canine and Feline Infectious Diseases.* Elsevier; 2014.)

Dogs with mild respiratory or GI distemper may recover spontaneously without treatment. Dogs with severe respiratory and GI disease may require hospitalization and treatment with IV fluids, antimicrobial drugs for secondary bacterial pneumonia, oxygen supplementation, nebulization, and coupage. Ideally, these dogs should be housed in isolation, although in many veterinary hospitals, isolation may not permit treatment with oxygen and adequate monitoring. Under these circumstances, dogs could be housed under strict barrier precautions where oxygen and critical care can be provided. When possible, collection of a respiratory lavage specimen for culture and susceptibility is recommended for dogs with secondary bacterial pneumonia. When this is not possible, the use of antimicrobial drugs likely to be effective against *Bordetella bronchiseptica* (such as doxycycline) is recommended (see Chapter 55). Dogs with severe bronchopneumonia may require treatment with parenteral broad-spectrum antimicrobial drug combinations, such as ampicillin and a fluoroquinolone. Other supportive treatments include enteral nutrition, artificial tears for dogs with KCS, and antiemetics. Parenteral nutrition should be used only if absolutely necessary, because of the immunosuppression that occurs with CDV infection and possibility of nosocomial infections. Vitamin A supplementation before experimental infection reduced morbidity and mortality associated with CDV infection in ferrets,[106] but its usefulness as a treatment for canine distemper requires further investigation. Administration of daily oral vitamin A for 2 days to children younger than 2 years of age with measles reduces the risk of mortality and pneumonia-specific mortality, and because levels of serum retinol in children with severe measles are typically low, vitamin A treatment for these children is recommended by the American Association of Pediatrics.[107] Ascorbic acid has also been advocated as a treatment for distemper in dogs, but its efficacy remains unproven.[90]

Owners of dogs with respiratory and GI illness should be warned that CNS signs have the potential to develop weeks to even months after apparent recovery. Unfortunately, the development of CNS signs is unpredictable. When neurologic signs occur, they rarely resolve and may be progressive. Seizures, myoclonus, or optic neuritis are three neurologic manifestations in dogs that can be tolerated by many owners. As with myoclonus in humans, treatment can lessen the severity of the muscle contractions but rarely eliminates it.[108] Botulinum toxin appeared to have a beneficial effect on myoclonus in one clinical distemper case.[109] Recommendations have been made to administer anticonvulsants after the onset of systemic disease but before the development of seizures. No evidence shows that anticonvulsants prevent entry of the virus into the CNS; however, they can suppress irritable foci from causing seizures, which may prevent seizure circuits from becoming established. Information on seizure treatment in dogs can be found elsewhere.[110] Glucocorticoid therapy to reduce inflammation or CNS edema may have variable success for control of the blindness or papillary dilation from optic neuritis or other neurologic signs associated with vaccine-induced or chronic inflammatory forms of encephalitis. Any other oxygen radical scavenger could theoretically be beneficial in view of the neuropathogenesis of distemper.[35]

IMMUNITY AND VACCINATION

Immunity to CDV requires antibodies as well as cell-mediated immunity. Recovery from natural infection provides lifelong immunity. Distemper can be effectively prevented through immunization with attenuated live or recombinant vaccines. Inactivated vaccines do not provide sufficient protection and are not available in the United

States. In contrast, proper vaccination with attenuated live vaccines can provide long-lasting (at least 3 to 5 years), sterile immunity.[111] Attenuated live vaccines should be given to pet puppies every 3 to 4 weeks, commencing no earlier than 6 weeks of age. Maternal antibodies are usually absent by 12 to 14 weeks of age, and so the last vaccine should be given no sooner than 16 weeks of age (consider extension to 16 to 20 weeks in breeding kennels and shelters).[111] Ideally, pups should be isolated for at least 7 to 10 days after the last vaccine is administered (see Appendix). For dogs older than 16 weeks of age that are brought to the veterinarian for their first vaccination, two doses of vaccine should be given 3 to 4 weeks apart, although a single dose may provide protection. A booster is recommended by AAHA at 1 year and then no earlier than every 3 years thereafter.[111] The WSAVA recommends administration of the 1-year booster at 6 months.[112] For shelter dogs, vaccination should be performed as soon as possible before entry into the shelter. A single vaccine given even hours before entry can provide protection from severe disease.[113,114] Infection can still occur, but disease severity is lessened.

Although generally safe and effective when used according to label recommendations, attenuated live CDV vaccine virus can cause encephalitis when administered to immunocompromised dogs and puppies less than 6 weeks of age, and severe disease can occur in susceptible species such as ferrets and certain wildlife species. Administration of attenuated live CDV vaccines to dams immediately after whelping has been associated with the development of encephalitis in the puppies, and it was suggested that vaccine virus shed by the dam may cause disease in the pups.[115] Postvaccinal encephalitis usually occurs 3 to 20 days after vaccination and has been associated with certain batches of vaccines that contain the Rockborn strain.[116] Neurologic signs such as ataxia may be reversible in some dogs. Seizures may be progressive and irreversible. Some distemper vaccines available on the market still contain the Rockborn strain, and Rockborn-like viruses have been isolated from dogs with distemper, which may represent residual virulence of vaccine virus or circulation of vaccine-derived Rockborn-like viruses in the dog population.[117] Attenuated live CDV vaccines have been incriminated as a cause of hypertrophic osteodystrophy, especially in young Weimaraner dogs,[90,118] but there is a paucity of published evidence that supports the association.

A canarypox-vectored recombinant vaccine that expresses the H and F glycoproteins of CDV is also available for prevention of canine distemper (Boehringer Ingelheim). This vaccine induces a 3-year duration of immunity, protects dogs from severe disease when administered hours before shelter admission, can protect puppies from virulent CDV infection in the face of maternal antibody, and can be used in pregnant bitches and puppies as young as 4 weeks of age in the face of an outbreak or in heavily contaminated environments.[112,119] The recombinant vaccine has replaced the use of canine measles vaccines, which were previously used to overcome maternal antibody in the face of distemper outbreaks. Whether the recombinant vaccine overcomes maternal antibody that is directed against the canarypox-vectored vaccine virus as effectively as it overcomes maternal antibody against the attenuated CDV vaccine virus requires further evaluation. Further study of the relative efficacy of the recombinant and attenuated live vaccines in heavily contaminated environments such as shelters is also required. The canarypox-vectored recombinant vaccine is also the vaccine of choice for ferrets, and a specific ferret vaccine is available (Purevax Ferret Distemper, Boehringer Ingelheim).

Vaccine strains of CDV, such as Onderstepoort, Snyder Hill, and Lederle, belong to the America-1 lineage, but field strains that circulate in North America belong primarily to the America-2 lineage. Concern has been raised that these vaccines may not adequately protect against infection with field strains, but cross-neutralization studies suggest that antigenic differences are not sufficient to warrant changes in the current vaccines. The development of distemper in vaccinated dogs may reflect failure of vaccine efficacy as a result of the improper administration of vaccines, improperly timed vaccination series, or the use of vaccines that have been stored and handled inappropriately. The last is especially important for CDV vaccines because attenuated live vaccine virus is so labile. Vaccines should be stored in a refrigerator that maintains an internal temperature of 0°C to 4°C and reconstituted with the proper diluent immediately (within 1 hour) before administration. It has been recommended that vaccine held for longer than 1 hour after reconstitution be discarded.[111] A second dose should be given if some of the vaccine is found on the haircoat after administration.

PREVENTION

Properly timed vaccination is the key to prevention of CDV infection. Puppies with declining maternal antibody titers should be kept away from other dogs until the vaccination series is complete. In shelter situations, dogs with signs of respiratory or GI disease should be held well away from other dogs (at least 25 feet has been suggested[71]) and handled only after apparently healthy dogs have been cared for. Puppies should always be separated from adult dogs using equipment designated only for that area, and overcrowding should be prevented. Quarantine for CDV is difficult because the incubation period for development of neurologic signs may be as long as 6 weeks. Wildlife species such as raccoons can also shed CDV and were suspected as a source of infection in an outbreak that occurred in a Chicago shelter, when raccoons and dogs were co-transported in the back of a vehicle.[71] Routine cleaning and disinfection of contaminated surfaces readily eliminates virus in the environment. Proper nutrition may also help to prevent disease due to CDV. Isolated vitamin A deficiency is a major risk factor for severe measles and death in humans and distemper in ferrets. Retinoids interfere with replication of measles virus *in vitro* through a type I IFN-dependent mechanism.[120] The impact of nutritional status on disease due to CDV requires further investigation.

PUBLIC HEALTH ASPECTS

Because of close relationship between measles virus and CDV and the observation of multiple CD outbreaks in primates, it has been speculated that CDV could potentially adapt to humans. A number of experimental *in vitro* studies support this speculation, but there is no evidence *in vivo*; these are reviewed elsewhere.[121] It is likely that measles virus immunity would also protect against CDV. Both CDV and measles virus have played a controversial role in Paget's disease of bone, a common skeletal disorder characterized by focal abnormalities of increased bone turnover, which is associated with bone pain, deformity, and pathologic fractures.[122] Paget's disease most often occurs in the elderly, men are more likely to be affected than women, and the overall prevalence of the disease has decreased in many geographic locations.[123] Genetic factors clearly play a role in the disease, but in some studies, the RNA of paramyxoviruses that include CDV has been detected within lesions.[124] Other studies have failed to detect the nucleic acid of CDV in lesions, and contamination has been suggested as a reason for positive test results.[122] However, CDV has been shown to infect and replicate in human osteoclast precursors, further raising concern about the possibility of zoonotic transmission of CDV.[125]

CASE EXAMPLE

Signalment

"Molly", a 1.5-year-old female spayed golden retriever from Sacramento, CA.

History

Molly was evaluated for a 1-month-long history of abnormal behavior that included stumbling, failure to catch balls, and loss of interest in activity. She also had a 1-year history of seizures, which were thought to be due to idiopathic epilepsy and which were treated with phenobarbital (4 mg/kg PO q12h) and potassium bromide (17 mg/kg PO q12h). This was associated with a decrease in seizure frequency. Two weeks after the onset of abnormal behavior, Molly was taken to a local veterinary clinic. A serum phenobarbital concentration at that time was 50 μg/mL (therapeutic range, 10 to 40 μg/mL). The phenobarbital dose was decreased (1.4 mg/kg PO q24h), but Molly began circling to the left, head pressing, pacing, and vocalizing. She also stopped responding to the owners when they called her name, and two episodes of vomiting were noted. In the week before evaluation, Molly refused to eat dry food, but ate canned dog food. Her thirst had decreased and she was voluntarily urinating in the house. A serum phenobarbital concentration was repeated 2 days before she was evaluated and was 13 μg/mL. Molly had been vaccinated regularly (CDV, CPV, CAdV-2, and parainfluenza) and received monthly flea, tick, and heartworm prophylaxis.

Current Medications

Phenobarbital (1.4 mg/kg PO q24h); potassium bromide (17 mg/kg PO q12h).

Physical Examination

Body weight: 23.2 kg

General: Obtunded but hydrated. T = 101.7°F (38.7°C), HR = 60 beats/min, RR = 36 breaths/min, mucous membranes pink, CRT = 1 s.

Integument, eyes, ears, nose, and throat: No clinically significant abnormalities were identified. A full ophthalmologic examination was also unremarkable.

Musculoskeletal: Body condition score was 5/9. Molly was ambulatory on all four limbs.

Cardiovascular, respiratory, GI, and urogenital systems: No clinically significant findings were identified. All peripheral lymph nodes were normal sized. Average systolic blood pressure (10 measurements) was 120 mm Hg.

Neurologic Examination

Mentation: Obtunded and not responsive to verbal and most tactile stimuli; head pressing.

Gait/posture: Compulsive circling and leaning to the left was present.

Cranial nerves: No clinically significant abnormalities were identified.

Postural reactions: Placing reactions were absent in the left thoracic and left and right pelvic limbs.

Segmental reflexes: Diminished biceps and withdrawal reflexes were present, left thoracic limb only.

Panniculus: No abnormalities detected.

Spinal palpation: Pain was elicited in several regions along the spine. Resisted cervical ventroflexion.

Neuroanatomic localization: Diffuse cerebral or thalamic disease; C6 to T2 myelopathy

Laboratory Findings

CBC: HCT 37.9% (40–55%), MCV 68 fL (65–75 fL), MCHC 35.4 g/dL (33–36 g/dL), WBC 7510 cells/μL (6000–13,000 cells/μL), neutrophils 4859 cells/μL (3000–10,500 cells/μL), lymphocytes 2155 cells/μL (1000–4000 cells/μL), monocytes 338 cells/μL (150–1200 cells/μL), 427,000 platelets/μL (150,000–400,000 platelets/μL).

Serum chemistry profile: Sodium 141 mmol/L (145–154 mmol/L), potassium 4.4 mmol/L (4.1–5.3 mmol/L), chloride 109 mmol/L (105–116 mmol/L), bicarbonate 21 mmol/L (16–26 mmol/L), phosphorus 3.9 mg/dL (3.0–6.2 mg/dL), calcium 12.2 mg/dL (9.9–11.4 mg/dL), BUN 6 mg/dL (8–31 mg/dL), creatinine 0.6 mg/dL (0.5–1.6 mg/dL), glucose 109 mg/dL (70–118 mg/dL), total protein 6.1 g/dL (5.4–7.4 g/dL), albumin 2.7 g/dL (2.9–4.2 g/dL), globulin 3.4 g/dL (2.3–4.4 g/dL), ALT 132 U/L (19–67 U/L), AST 62 U/L (21–54 U/L), ALP 155 U/L (15–127 U/L), CK 399 U/L (46–320 U/L), GGT 10 U/L (0–6 U/L), cholesterol 291 mg/dL (135–345 mg/dL), total bilirubin 0.2 mg/dL (0–0.4 mg/dL).

Serum ionized calcium: 1.39 mmol/L.

Urinalysis: SpG 1.014; pH 7.0, few amorphous crystals. No other abnormalities detected.

Serum bromide concentration: 1.1 mg/mL (therapeutic range, 1.0–2.0 mg/mL).

Serum phenobarbital concentration: 1.4 μg/mL (result rechecked, therapeutic range, 15–40 μg/mL).

Serum bile acids: Pre-meal, 14 μmol/L (reference range, 0–12 μmol/L); post-meal, 16 μmol/L (reference range, 0–16 μmol/L).

Imaging Findings

Thoracic radiographs: No clinically significant abnormalities were present.

Spinal radiographs: Disc space narrowing was present between the sixth and seventh cervical vertebrae and to a greater extent between the seventh cervical and first thoracic vertebrae.

Abdominal ultrasound: No significant lesions were identified.

MRI: Precontrast: Multiple small regions of hyperintensity were noted on dual echo and FLAIR sequences, one of which was in the left thalamus along the third ventricle and another diffusely along the lateral aspect of the right thalamus. There was a linear region of hyperintensity along the right parietal and temporal lobes. On T1-weighted postcontrast images, a small focus of contrast enhancement was noted in the ventral aspect of the right thalamus in the region of hyperintensity on the precontrast fluid-weighted sequences. Impressions: Multifocal, relatively non–contrast-enhancing lesions in the cerebrum and thalamus suggestive of cerebral edema, encephalitis, or small infarcts.

Electroencephalography: No abnormalities were detected.

CSF Analysis

	Lumbar	Cisternal
Protein (mg/dL)	31	21
Total RBC (cells/μL)	111	2
Total nucleated cells (cells/μL)	1	3
Neutrophils (%)	0	0
Small mononuclear cells (%)	92	80
Large mononuclear cells (%)	8	20
Microscopic evaluation	Mild to moderate lymphocytic reactivity	Marginal mononuclear (lymphocytic) pleocytosis

Treatment and Outcome

Molly was hospitalized for a week during the diagnostic workup and treated with IV fluids and potassium bromide (35 mg/kg PO q12h). She became progressively more obtunded and showed additional neurologic signs of circling to the right and positional horizontal nystagmus with a fast phase to the right. The narrowed disc spaces were thought to represent intervertebral disc disease, and granulomatous meningoencephalitis was suspected. Potassium bromide was discontinued, and treatment with phenobarbital (5 mg/kg PO q12h), reinstituted. Dexamethasone was administered (0.2 mg/kg, IV q24h), but there was minimal improvement, and euthanasia was elected.

Continued

CASE EXAMPLE—cont'd

Necropsy Findings

Brain, cerebrum: Severe, generalized, chronic neuronal loss, axonal necrosis, and myelin degeneration with abundant eosinophilic inclusion bodies and canine distemper antigen (immunohistochemistry).

Brain and spinal cord (C1 to T7), corticospinal tracts: Severe, diffuse axonal necrosis and myelin degeneration.

Brain, cerebrum, and meninges: Generalized, lymphoplasmacytic, perivascular cuffing.

Tonsil, lymph nodes (mandibular, mesenteric, thoracic): Mild, multifocal lympholysis with intranuclear and intracytoplasmic eosinophilic inclusion bodies and canine distemper antigen.

Diagnosis

Chronic distemper encephalitis with demyelination ("old dog encephalitis").

Comments

Distemper was not suspected in this dog because of the dog's older age and history of vaccination. Initial infection may have occurred before vaccination was complete, vaccination may have been improperly performed, or the dog may have been a vaccine nonresponder, which is believed to occur rarely. The previous diagnosis of epilepsy further complicated the identification of distemper as an underlying cause. This case example highlights the importance of including distemper on the differential diagnosis list for young adult dogs with neurologic signs, because of the chronic course of disease that can occasionally occur. Additional laboratory tests that might or might not have been helpful for diagnosis of distemper in this dog include comparison of serum antibody titers to CDV in the CSF and serum, and RT-PCR for CDV on CSF. Neurologic signs were progressive in this dog and largely unresponsive to anticonvulsant drugs, and so the prognosis was extremely poor.

SUGGESTED READINGS

Beineke A, Puff C, Seehusen F, et al. Pathogenesis and immunopathology of systemic and nervous canine distemper. *Vet Immunol Immunopathol.* 2009;127:1–18.

Newbury S. Canine distemper virus. In: Miller L, Janeczko S, Hurley K, eds. *Infectious Disease Management in Animal Shelters.* 2nd ed. Ames, IA: Wiley-Blackwell;2021:256–273.

Strebel PM, Orenstein WA. Measles. *N Engl J Med.* 2019;381:349–357.

REFERENCES

1. Gamiz C, Martella V, Ulloa R, et al. Identification of a new genotype of canine distemper virus circulating in America. *Vet Res Commun.* 2011;35:381–390.
2. Martinez-Gutierrez M, Ruiz-Saenz J. Diversity of susceptible hosts in canine distemper virus infection: a systematic review and data synthesis. *BMC Vet Res.* 2016;12:78.
3. Craft ME, Volz E, Packer C, et al. Distinguishing epidemic waves from disease spillover in a wildlife population. *Proc Biol Sci.* 2009;276:1777–1785.
4. Sun Z, Li A, Ye H, et al. Natural infection with canine distemper virus in hand-feeding Rhesus monkeys in China. *Vet Microbiol.* 2010;141:374–378.
5. Kimpston, C. N., Hatke, A. L., Castelli, B., et al. High prevalence of antibodies against canine parvovirus and canine distemper virus among coyotes and foxes from Pennsylvania: implications for the intersection of companion animals and wildlife. *Microbiol Spectr.* 2022;Jan 26:e0253221.
6. Stettler M, Beck K, Wagner A, et al. Determinants of persistence in canine distemper viruses. *Vet Microbiol.* 1997;57:83–93.
7. Bhatt M, Rajak KK, Chakravarti S, et al. Phylogenetic analysis of haemagglutinin gene deciphering a new genetically distinct lineage of canine distemper virus circulating among domestic dogs in India. *Transbound Emerg Dis.* 2019;66:1252–1267.
8. Kapil S, Neel T. Canine distemper virus antigen detection in external epithelia of recently vaccinated, sick dogs by fluorescence microscopy is a valuable prognostic indicator. *J Clin Microbiol.* 2015;53:687–691.
9. Panzera Y, Calderon MG, Sarute N, et al. Evidence of two co-circulating genetic lineages of canine distemper virus in South America. *Virus Res.* 2012;163:401–404.
10. Ke GM, Ho CH, Chiang MJ, et al. Phylodynamic analysis of the canine distemper virus hemagglutinin gene. *BMC Vet Res.* 2015;11:164.
11. Giacinti, J. A., Pearl, D. L., Ojkic, D., et al. Genetic characterization of canine distemper virus from wild and domestic animal submissions to diagnostic facilities in Canada. *Prev Vet Med.* 2022;*198*:105535.
12. Wang, R., Wang, X., Zhai, J., et al. A new canine distemper virus lineage identified from red pandas in China. *Transbound Emerg Dis.* 2021; Nov 1:Online ahead of print.
13. Feijóo, G., Yamasaki, K., Delucchi, L., & Verdes, J. M. Central nervous system lesions caused by canine distemper virus in 4 vaccinated dogs. *J Vet Diagn Invest.* 2021;*33*:640–647.
14. Corrain R, Di Francesco A, Bolognini M, et al. Serosurvey for CPV-2, distemper virus, ehrlichiosis and leishmaniosis in free-ranging dogs in Italy. *Vet Rec.* 2007;160:91–92.
15. Amude AM, Alfieri AA, Alfieri AF. Clinicopathological findings in dogs with distemper encephalomyelitis presented without characteristic signs of the disease. *Res Vet Sci.* 2007;82:416–422.
16. Blixenkrone-Moller M, Svansson V, Have P, et al. Studies on manifestations of canine distemper virus infection in an urban dog population. *Vet Microbiol.* 1993;37:163–173.
17. Richards TR, Whelan NC, Pinard CL, et al. Optic neuritis caused by canine distemper virus in a Jack Russell terrier. *Can Vet J.* 2011;52:398–402.
18. Appel MJ. Pathogenesis of canine distemper. *Am J Vet Res.* 1969;30:1167–1182.
19. Yanagi Y, Takeda M, Ohno S. Measles virus: cellular receptors, tropism and pathogenesis. *J Gen Virol.* 2006;87:2767–2779.
20. Beineke A, Puff C, Seehusen F, et al. Pathogenesis and immunopathology of systemic and nervous canine distemper. *Vet Immunol Immunopathol.* 2009;127:1–18.
21. von Messling V, Milosevic D, Cattaneo R. Tropism illuminated: lymphocyte-based pathways blazed by lethal morbillivirus through the host immune system. *Proc Natl Acad Sci U S A.* 2004;101:14216–14221.
22. von Messling V, Svitek N, Cattaneo R. Receptor (SLAM [CD150]) recognition and the V protein sustain swift lymphocyte-based invasion of mucosal tissue and lymphatic organs by a morbillivirus. *J Virol.* 2006;80:6084–6092.
23. Krakowka S, Higgins RJ, Koestner A. Canine distemper virus: review of structural and functional modulations in lymphoid tissues. *Am J Vet Res.* 1980;41:284–292.
24. Kumagai K, Yamaguchi R, Uchida K, et al. Lymphoid apoptosis in acute canine distemper. *J Vet Med Sci.* 2004;66:175–181.
25. Headley SA, Amude AM, Alfieri AF, et al. Molecular detection of canine distemper virus and the immunohistochemical characterization of the neurologic lesions in naturally occurring old dog encephalitis. *J Vet Diagn Invest.* 2009;21:588–597.
26. Headley SA, Shirota K, Baba T, et al. Diagnostic exercise: Tyzzer's disease, distemper, and coccidiosis in a pup. *Vet Pathol.* 2009;46:151–154.
27. Alves L, Khosravi M, Avila M, et al. SLAM- and nectin-4-independent noncytolytic spread of canine distemper virus in astrocytes. *J Virol.* 2015;89:5724–5733.
28. Maeda H, Ozaki K, Takagi Y, et al. Distemper skin lesions in a dog. *Zentralbl Veterinarmed A.* 1994;41:247–250.
29. Engelhardt P, Wyder M, Zurbriggen A, et al. Canine distemper virus associated proliferation of canine footpad keratinocytes in vitro. *Vet Microbiol.* 2005;107:1–12.
30. Grone A, Engelhardt P, Zurbriggen A. Canine distemper virus infection: proliferation of canine footpad keratinocytes. *Vet Pathol.* 2003;40:574–578.

31. Grone A, Groeters S, Koutinas A, et al. Non-cytocidal infection of keratinocytes by canine distemper virus in the so-called hard pad disease of canine distemper. *Vet Microbiol.* 2003;96:157–163.
32. Grone A, Doherr MG, Zurbriggen A. Up-regulation of cytokeratin expression in canine distemper virus-infected canine footpad epidermis. *Vet Dermatol.* 2004;15:168–174.
33. Grone A, Doherr MG, Zurbriggen A. Canine distemper virus infection of canine footpad epidermis. *Vet Dermatol.* 2004;15:159–167.
34. Rivals JP, Plattet P, Currat-Zweifel C, et al. Adaptation of canine distemper virus to canine footpad keratinocytes modifies polymerase activity and fusogenicity through amino acid substitutions in the P/V/C and H proteins. *Virology.* 2007;359:6–18.
35. Vandevelde, M., & Zurbriggen, A. Demyelination in canine distemper virus infection: a review. *Acta Neuropathol.* 2005;*109*:56–68.
36. Lisiak JA, Vandevelde M. Polioencephalomalacia associated with canine distemper virus infection. *Vet Pathol.* 1979;16:650–660.
37. Ulrich R, Puff C, Wewetzer K, et al. Transcriptional changes in canine distemper virus-induced demyelinating leukoencephalitis favor a biphasic mode of demyelination. *PLoS One.* 2014;9:e95917.
38. Tipold A, Moore P, Zurbriggen A, et al. Early T cell response in the central nervous system in canine distemper virus infection. *Acta Neuropathol.* 1999;97:45–56.
39. Tipold A, Vandevelde M, Wittek R, et al. Partial protection and intrathecal invasion of CD8(+) T cells in acute canine distemper virus infection. *Vet Microbiol.* 2001;83:189–203.
40. Alldinger S, Wunschmann A, Baumgartner W, et al. Up-regulation of major histocompatibility complex class II antigen expression in the central nervous system of dogs with spontaneous canine distemper virus encephalitis. *Acta Neuropathol.* 1996;92:273–280.
41. Tsai SC, Summers BA, Appel MJ. Interferon in cerebrospinal fluid. A marker for viral persistence of canine distemper encephalomyelitis. *Arch Virol.* 1982;72:257–265.
42. Stein VM, Czub M, Schreiner N, et al. Microglial cell activation in demyelinating canine distemper lesions. *J Neuroimmunol.* 2004;153:122–131.
43. Spitzbarth, I., Baumgartner, W., & Beineke, A. The role of pro-and anti-inflammatory cytokines in the pathogenesis of spontaneous canine CNS diseases. *Vet Immunol Immunopathol.* 2012;*147*:6–24.
44. Mitchell WJ, Summers BA, Appel MJ. Viral expression in experimental canine distemper demyelinating encephalitis. *J Comp Pathol.* 1991;104:77–87.
45. Wunschmann A, Alldinger S, Kremmer E, et al. Identification of CD4+ and CD8+ T cell subsets and B cells in the brain of dogs with spontaneous acute, subacute-, and chronic-demyelinating distemper encephalitis. *Vet Immunol Immunopathol.* 1999;67:101–116.
46. Botteron C, Zurbriggen A, Griot C, et al. Canine distemper virus-immune complexes induce bystander degeneration of oligodendrocytes. *Acta Neuropathol.* 1992;83:402–407.
47. Burge T, Griot C, Vandevelde M, et al. Antiviral antibodies stimulate production of reactive oxygen species in cultured canine brain cells infected with canine distemper virus. *J Virol.* 1989;63:2790–2797.
48. Muller CF, Fatzer RS, Beck K, et al. Studies on canine distemper virus persistence in the central nervous system. *Acta Neuropathol.* 1995;89:438–445.
49. Tipold A, Vandevelde M, Jaggy A. Neurological manifestations of canine distemper virus infection. *J Small Anim Pract.* 1992;33:466–470.
50. Tipold A. Diagnosis of inflammatory and infectious diseases of the central nervous system in dogs: a retrospective study. *J Vet Intern Med.* 1995;9:304–314.
51. Kim, D. Y., Zinn, M. M., Odemuyiwa, S. O., et al. Myocarditis caused by naturally acquired canine distemper virus infection in 4 dogs. *J Vet Diagn Invest.* 2021;*33*:167–169.
52. Kerdiles YM, Cherif B, Marie JC, et al. Immunomodulatory properties of morbillivirus nucleoproteins. *Viral Immunol.* 2006;19:324–334.
53. Ehrensperger F, Pospischil A. Spontaneous mixed infections with distemper virus and *Toxoplasma* in dogs. *Dtsch Tierarztl Wochenschr.* 1989;96:184–186.
54. Smith HW, Buxton A. Incidence of Salmonellae in faces of dogs suffering from distemper. *Nature.* 1950;166:824.
55. Fawi MT, Tag el Din MH, el-Sanousi SM. Canine distemper as a predisposing factor for *Nocardia asteroides* infection in the dog. *Vet Rec.* 1971;88:326–328.
56. Ribeiro MG, Salerno T, Mattos-Guaraldi AL, et al. Nocardiosis: an overview and additional report of 28 cases in cattle and dogs. *Rev Inst Med Trop Sao Paulo.* 2008;50:177–185.
57. Dyer NW, Schamber GJ. Pneumocystosis associated with canine distemper virus infection in a mink. *Can Vet J.* 1999;40:577–578.
58. Lemberger KY, Gondim LF, Pessier AP, et al. *Neospora caninum* infection in a free-ranging raccoon (*Procyon lotor*) with concurrent canine distemper virus infection. *J Parasitol.* 2005;91:960–961.
59. Baumgartner W, Boyce RW, Alldinger S, et al. Metaphyseal bone lesions in young dogs with systemic canine distemper virus infection. *Vet Microbiol.* 1995;44:201–209.
60. Mee AP, Gordon MT, May C, et al. Canine distemper virus transcripts detected in the bone cells of dogs with metaphyseal osteopathy. *Bone.* 1993;14:59–67.
61. Wang W, Feng W, Li D, et al. Fusion and hemagglutinin proteins of canine distemper virus promote osteoclast formation through NF-kappaB dependent and independent mechanisms. *Exp Cell Res.* 2019;378:171–181.
62. Green, L., Cook, L., Martinez, M., & Green, E. Distemper encephalomyelitis presenting with lower motor neuron signs in a young dog. *J Am Anim Hosp Assoc.* 2020;*56*:127–132.
63. de Almeida DE, Roveratti C, Brito FL, et al. Conjunctival effects of canine distemper virus-induced keratoconjunctivitis sicca. *Vet Ophthalmol.* 2009;12:211–215.
64. Tipold A, Pfister H, Vandevelde M. Determination of the IgG index for the detection of intrathecal immunoglobulin synthesis in dogs using an ELISA. *Res Vet Sci.* 1993;54:40–44.
65. Bathen-Noethen A, Stein VM, Puff C, et al. Magnetic resonance imaging findings in acute canine distemper virus infection. *J Small Anim Pract.* 2008;49:460–467.
66. Appel MJ, Pearce-Kelling S, Summers BA. Dog lymphocyte cultures facilitate the isolation and growth of virulent canine distemper virus. *J Vet Diagn Invest.* 1992;4:258–263.
67. Athanasiou LV, Kantere MC, Kyriakis CS, et al. Evaluation of a direct immunofluorescent assay and/or conjunctival cytology for detection of canine distemper virus antigen. *Viral Immunol.* 2018;31:272–275.
68. Soma T, Ishii H, Hara M, et al. Detection of canine distemper virus antigen in canine serum and its application to diagnosis. *Vet Rec.* 2003;153:499–501.
69. An DJ, Kim TY, Song DS, et al. An immunochromatography assay for rapid antemortem diagnosis of dogs suspected to have canine distemper. *J Virol Methods.* 2008;147:244–249.
70. Li Z, Zhang Y, Wang H, et al. Sandwich-dot enzyme-linked immunosorbent assay for the detection of canine distemper virus. *Can J Vet Res.* 2013;77:303–308.
71. Newbury S. Canine distemper virus. In: Miller L, Janeczko S, Hurley K, eds. *Infectious Disease Management in Animal Shelters.* 2nd ed. Ames, IA: Wiley-Blackwell; 2021:256–273.
72. Sehata G, Sato H, Ito T, et al. Use of quantitative real-time RT-PCR to investigate the correlation between viremia and viral shedding of canine distemper virus, and infection outcomes in experimentally infected dogs. *J Vet Med Sci.* 2015;77:851–855.
73. Nemeth NM, Oesterle PT, Campbell GD, et al. Comparison of reverse-transcription real time PCR and immunohistochemistry for the detection of canine distemper virus infection in raccoons in Ontario, Canada. *J Vet Diagn Invest.* 2018;30:319–323.
74. Kim D, Jeoung SY, Ahn SJ, et al. Comparison of tissue and fluid samples for the early detection of canine distemper virus in experimentally infected dogs. *J Vet Med Sci.* 2006;68:877–879.
75. Elia G, Decaro N, Martella V, et al. Detection of canine distemper virus in dogs by real-time RT-PCR. *J Virol Methods.* 2006;136:171–176.
76. Brown AT, McAloose D, Calle P, et al. Development and validation of a portable, point-of-care canine distemper virus qPCR test. *PLoS One.* 2020;15:e0232044.

77. Wang J, Wang J, Li R, et al. Evaluation of an incubation instrument-free reverse transcription recombinase polymerase amplification assay for rapid and point-of-need detection of canine distemper virus. *J Virol Methods*. 2018;260:56–61.
78. Si W, Zhou S, Wang Z, et al. A multiplex reverse transcription-nested polymerase chain reaction for detection and differentiation of wild-type and vaccine strains of canine distemper virus. *Virol J*. 2010;7:86.
79. IDEXX Laboratories. IDEXX Reference Laboratories offers the Canine Distemper Virus (CDV) Quant RealPCR™ Test. 2017. Available at: https://www.idexx.com/files/idexx-introduces-cdv-quant-realpcr.pdf.
80. Fischer CD, Ikuta N, Canal CW, et al. Detection and differentiation of field and vaccine strains of canine distemper virus using reverse transcription followed by nested real time PCR (RT-nqPCR) and RFLP analysis. *J Virol Methods*. 2013;194:39–45.
81. Twark L, Dodds WJ. Clinical use of serum parvovirus and distemper virus antibody titers for determining revaccination strategies in healthy dogs. *J Am Vet Med Assoc*. 2000;217:1021–1024.
82. Gray LK, Crawford PC, Levy JK, et al. Comparison of two assays for detection of antibodies against canine parvovirus and canine distemper virus in dogs admitted to a Florida animal shelter. *J Am Vet Med Assoc*. 2012;240:1084–1087.
83. von Messling V, Harder TC, Moennig V, et al. Rapid and sensitive detection of immunoglobulin M (IgM) and IgG antibodies against canine distemper virus by a new recombinant nucleocapsid protein-based enzyme-linked immunosorbent assay. *J Clin Microbiol*. 1999;37:1049–1056.
84. Barben G, Stettler M, Jaggy A, et al. Detection of IgM antibodies against a recombinant nucleocapsid protein of canine distemper virus in dog sera using a dot-blot assay. *Zentralbl Veterinarmed A*. 1999;46:115–121.
85. Latha D, Geetha M, Ramadass P, et al. Development of recombinant nucleocapsid protein based IgM-ELISA for the early detection of distemper infection in dogs. *Vet Immunol Immunopathol*. 2007;119:278–286.
86. Latha D, Geetha M, Ramadass P, et al. Evaluation of ELISA based on the conserved and functional middle region of nucleocapsid protein to detect distemper infection in dogs. *Vet Microbiol*. 2007;120:251–260.
87. Cho KH, Kim J, Yoo HA, et al. Use of hydrophilic extra-viral domain of canine distemper virus H protein for enzyme-linked immunosorbent assay development. *J Vet Sci*. 2014;15:503–509.
88. Johnson GC, Fenner WR, Krakowka S. Production of immunoglobulin G and increased antiviral antibody in cerebrospinal fluid of dogs with delayed-onset canine distemper viral encephalitis. *J Neuroimmunol*. 1988;17:237–251.
89. Kubo T, Kagawa Y, Taniyama H, et al. Retrospective serological analysis of spontaneous CDV infection in 192 dogs. *J Vet Med Sci*. 2008;70:475–477.
90. Greene CE, Appel MJ. Canine distemper. In: Greene CE, ed. *Infectious Diseases of the Dog and Cat*. 3rd ed. Philadelphia, PA: WB Saunders; 2006:9–21.
91. Bergmann, M., Freisi, M., Zablotski, Y., et al. Prevalence of neutralizing antibodies to canine distemper virus and response to vaccination in client-owned adult healthy dogs. *Viruses*. 2021;*13*:945.
92. Litster AL, Pressler B, Volpe A, et al. Accuracy of a point-of-care ELISA test kit for predicting the presence of protective canine parvovirus and canine distemper virus antibody concentrations in dogs. *Vet J*. 2012;193:363–366.
93. Bergmann, M., Zablotski, Y., Rieger, A., et al. Comparison of four commercially available point-of-care tests to detect antibodies against canine distemper virus in dogs. *Vet J*. 2021;*273*:105693.
94. Thomas WB, Sorjonen DC, Steiss JE. A retrospective evaluation of 38 cases of canine distemper encephalomyelitis. *J Am Anim Hosp Assoc*. 1993;29:129–133.
95. Areco, W. V. C., Todo, L. A. S., de Avila, N. C., et al. Histopathological features of spinal cord lesions in dogs with distemper-associated demyelinating leucoencephalomyelitis. *J Comp Pathol*. 2021;*189*:110–119.
96. Dal Pozzo F, Galligioni V, Vaccari F, et al. Antiviral efficacy of EICAR against canine distemper virus (CDV) in vitro. *Res Vet Sci*. 2010;88:339–344.
97. Wyde PR, Moore-Poveda DK, De Clercq E, et al. Use of cotton rats to evaluate the efficacy of antivirals in treatment of measles virus infections. *Antimicrob Agents Chemother*. 2000;44:1146–1152.
98. Carvalho OV, Botelho CV, Ferreira CG, et al. In vitro inhibition of canine distemper virus by flavonoids and phenolic acids: implications of structural differences for antiviral design. *Res Vet Sci*. 2013;95:717–724.
99. Wu ZM, Yu ZJ, Cui ZQ, et al. In vitro antiviral efficacy of caffeic acid against canine distemper virus. *Microb Pathog*. 2017;110:240–244.
100. Plattet P, Alves L, Herren M, et al. Measles virus fusion protein: structure, function and inhibition. *Viruses*. 2016;8:112.
101. Hardes K, Becker GL, Lu Y, et al. Novel furin inhibitors with potent anti-infectious activity. *Chem Med Chem*. 2015;10:1218–1231.
102. Kalbermatter D, Shrestha N, Ader-Ebert N, et al. Primary resistance mechanism of the canine distemper virus fusion protein against a small-molecule membrane fusion inhibitor. *Virus Res*. 2019;259:28–37.
103. Klotz D, Baumgartner W, Gerhauser I. Type I interferons in the pathogenesis and treatment of canine diseases. *Vet Immunol Immunopathol*. 2017;191:80–93.
104. Klotz D, Gerhauser I. Interferon-stimulated genes—mediators of the innate immune response during canine distemper virus infection. *Int J Mol Sci*. 2019;20:1620.
105. Liu PC, Chen CA, Chen CM, et al. Application of xenogeneic anti-canine distemper virus antibodies in treatment of canine distemper puppies. *J Small Anim Pract*. 2016;57:626–630.
106. Rodeheffer C, von Messling V, Milot S, et al. Disease manifestations of canine distemper virus infection in ferrets are modulated by vitamin A status. *J Nutr*. 2007;137:1916–1922.
107. Strebel PM, Orenstein WA. Measles. *N Engl J Med*. 2019;381:349–357.
108. Caviness JN, Brown P. Myoclonus: current concepts and recent advances. *Lancet Neurol*. 2004;3:598–607.
109. Schubert T, Clemmons R, Miles S, et al. The use of botulinum toxin for the treatment of generalized myoclonus in a dog. *J Am Anim Hosp Assoc*. 2013;49:122–127.
110. Charalambous M, Shivapour SK, Brodbelt DC, et al. Antiepileptic drugs' tolerability and safety—a systematic review and meta-analysis of adverse effects in dogs. *BMC Vet Res*. 2016;12:79.
111. American Animal Hospital Association Canine Vaccination Task Force. 2011 AAHA canine vaccination guidelines. *J Am Anim Hosp Assoc*. 2011;47:1–42.
112. Day MJ, Horzinek MC, Schultz RD, et al. WSAVA guidelines for the vaccination of dogs and cats. *J Small Anim Pract*. 2016;57:E1–E45.
113. Larson LJ, Schultz RD. Effect of vaccination with recombinant canine distemper virus vaccine immediately before exposure under shelter-like conditions. *Vet Ther*. 2006;7:113–118.
114. Andrukonis, A., Brown, K. M., Hall, N. J., & Protopopova, A. Intake vaccinations reduced signs of canine respiratory disease during an outbreak at an animal shelter. *Front Vet Sci*. 2021;*8*:627580.
115. McCandlish IA, Cornwell HJ, Thompson H, et al. Distemper encephalitis in pups after vaccination of the dam. *Vet Rec*. 1992;130:27–30.
116. Cornwell HJ, Thompson H, McCandlish IA, et al. Encephalitis in dogs associated with a batch of canine distemper (Rockborn) vaccine. *Vet Rec*. 1988;122:54–59.
117. Martella V, Blixenkrone-Moller M, Elia G, et al. Lights and shades on an historical vaccine canine distemper virus, the Rockborn strain. *Vaccine*. 2011;29:1222–1227.
118. Harrus S, Waner T, Aizenberg, et al. Development of hypertrophic osteodystrophy and antibody response in a litter of vaccinated Weimaraner puppies. *J Small Anim Pract*. 2002;43:27–31.
119. Larson LJ, Schultz RD. Three-year duration of immunity in dogs vaccinated with a canarypox-vectored recombinant canine distemper virus vaccine. *Vet Ther*. 2007;8:101–106.
120. Trottier C, Colombo M, Mann KK, et al. Retinoids inhibit measles virus through a type I IFN-dependent bystander effect. *FASEB J*. 2009;23:3203–3212.
121. Duque-Valencia J, Sarute N, Olarte-Castillo X, et al. Evolution and interspecies transmission of canine distemper virus—an outlook of the diverse evolutionary landscapes of a multi-host virus. *Viruses*. 2019;11:582.
122. Ralston SH, Afzal MA, Helfrich MH, et al. Multicenter blinded analysis of RT-PCR detection methods for paramyxoviruses in relation to Paget's disease of bone. *J Bone Miner Res*. 2007;22:569–577.
123. Cooper C, Harvey NC, Dennison EM, et al. Update on the epidemiology of Paget's disease of bone. *J Bone Miner Res*. 2006;21(suppl 2):P3–P8.
124. Mee AP, Dixon JA, Hoyland JA, et al. Detection of canine distemper virus in 100% of Paget's disease samples by in situ-reverse transcriptase-polymerase chain reaction. *Bone*. 1998;23:171–175.
125. Selby PL, Davies M, Mee AP. Canine distemper virus induces human osteoclastogenesis through NF-kappaB and sequestosome 1/P62 activation. *J Bone Miner Res*. 2006;21:1750–1756.

23

Infectious Canine Hepatitis and Feline Adenovirus Infection

Nicola Decaro

KEY POINTS

- First Described: Infectious canine hepatitis (ICH) was first described in 1947 in Sweden (Rubarth)[1]; CAdV-1 was first isolated in chick embryos in 1951.[2] An adenovirus was first isolated from a cat in 1999 and was further characterized in 2019.[3]
- Cause: Canine adenovirus-1 and feline adenovirus 1 (family *Adenoviridae,* genus *Mastadenovirus*, species *Canine mastadenovirus A*).
- Affected Hosts: Dogs, coyotes, foxes, wolves, bears, skunks (CAdV-1); domestic cats (FAdV-1).
- Geographic Distribution: Worldwide (CAdV-1); the distribution of FAdV-1 is unclear, but antibodies have been detected in cats in Europe and North America.
- Mode of Transmission: Direct contact with infected saliva, feces and urine, and contaminated fomites.
- Major Clinical Signs in Dogs: Fever, lethargy, inappetence, vomiting, hemorrhagic diarrhea, abdominal pain, dehydration, conjunctivitis, petechial hemorrhages, tachypnea, cough, corneal edema ("blue eye"), icterus or neurologic signs. The spectrum of clinical signs in cats requires further study, but disseminated infection has been described.
- Differential Diagnoses (ICH): Other systemic viral diseases such as parvoviral enteritis and canine distemper, enteric viral and bacterial infections, hepatotoxicosis (e.g., mushrooms), dicumarol poisoning, Rocky Mountain spotted fever, GI foreign body, dietary indiscretion, leptospirosis, portosystemic shunting with hepatic encephalopathy, disseminated fungal infections (especially systemic candidiasis), systemic protozoal infections (especially sarcocystosis, toxoplasmosis, or African trypanosomiasis), hemic neoplasia (especially lymphoma).
- Human Health Significance: CAdV-1 does not infect humans. FAdV-1 is related to human adenovirus-1 but the zoonotic significance of this virus is unknown.

CANINE ADENOVIRUS INFECTION

ETIOLOGY AND EPIDEMIOLOGY

Infectious canine hepatitis (ICH) is an uncommonly recognized disease of dogs that is caused by CAdV-1, a nonenveloped, icosahedral double-stranded DNA virus that is antigenically related to CAdV-2 (see Chapter 28) (Fig. 23.1). As with other adenoviruses, CAdV-1 is highly resistant to environmental inactivation, surviving disinfection with various chemicals such as chloroform, ether, acid, and formalin, and is stable when exposed to certain frequencies of ultraviolet radiation. The virus survives for days at room temperature on soiled fomites and remains viable for months at temperatures below 4°C. Inactivation of CAdV-1 occurs after 5 minutes at 50°C to 60°C, which makes steam cleaning a plausible means of disinfection. Chemical disinfection has also been successful when iodine, phenol, and sodium hydroxide are used; however, all are potentially caustic.[4]

There are 50 different species within the genus *Mastadenovirus*, and within these species, there are many different adenovirus types; for example, 7 human adenovirus species (designated *Human mastadenovirus A* though *G*) including 85 different types have been described.[3] Disease caused by CAdV-1 (now referred to as *Canine mastadenovirus A* by the International Committee on Taxonomy of Viruses) was first observed in farmed red foxes (*Vulpes vulpes*) and consequently named epizootic fox encephalitis due to the neurological disorders observed in the affected animals.[5] ICH was reported in dogs a few years later and based on the similar clinical course and pathology, Carl Sven Rubarth suggested a common etiology for the two diseases,[1] which were subsequently known as Rubarth's disease. The etiological agent, CAdV-1, was isolated a decade later[2] and attenuated through passages on canine and swine cell lines to produce vaccines. In 1961, another adenovirus of dogs, CAdV-2, was isolated from dogs with laryngotracheitis or tracheobronchitis.[6] ICH has been reported in free-ranging foxes and other wild carnivores belonging to the families *Canidae*, *Ursidae*, *Procyonidae*, and *Mustelidae*. A fatal infection was reported in an otter (*Lutra lutra*).[7] In addition to these carnivores, serum antibodies have also been detected in marine mammals including walruses (*Odobenus rosmarus*) and sea lions (*Eumetopias jubatus*).[8-10] The high prevalence of naturally occurring serum neutralizing antibodies in the unvaccinated feral and wildlife dog population suggests that subclinical infection is widespread.[11-14]

ICH has been described worldwide and most commonly occurs in dogs that are less than 1 year of age, but it was frequently reported in adult dogs before widespread vaccination for ICH was introduced. CAdV-1 has been isolated from all body tissues and secretions of dogs during the acute stages of the disease. By 10 to 14 days post inoculation (PI), using traditional methods the virus can be found only in the kidneys and is excreted in the urine for at least 6 to 9 months. However, molecular tools have proved that CAdV-1 viremia and shedding can last for several weeks. Aerosol transmission of the virus via the urine is unlikely, given that susceptible dogs housed 6 inches apart from virus shedders do not become infected. Viral spread can occur by contact with fomites, including feeding utensils and hands.[4]

The strong antigenic relationship between CAdV-1 and CAdV-2 is clinically important, because parenteral vaccines that contain CAdV-2 protect against infection with CAdV-1 and vice versa. After the introduction of CAdV vaccines, ICH largely disappeared, but over the past decade it has reemerged in dogs and wildlife, with published reports of disease from Italy, France, Switzerland, UK, Brazil, Australia, and the United States.[14-27] Disease in Europe has been associated with puppy trading from kennels in eastern European countries and possibly spillover of virus circulating

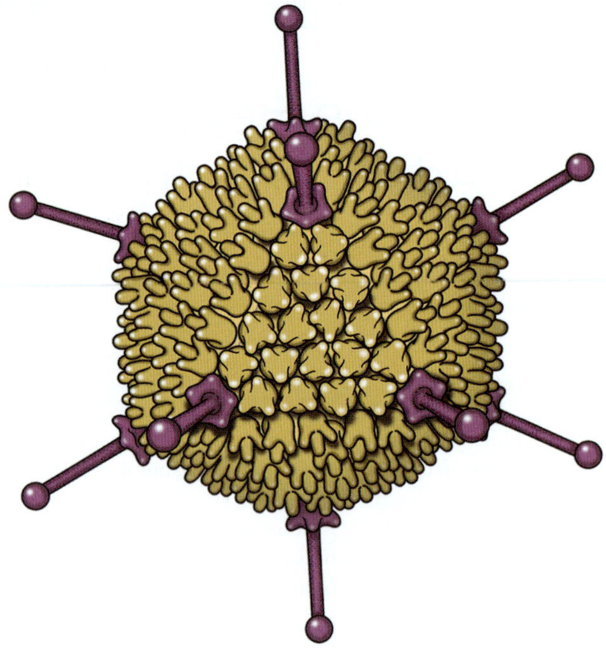

Fig. 23.1 Structure of canine adenovirus. The virus is a non-enveloped, icosahedral virus with fibers *(purple)* that radiate outwards from the virion.

in wildlife.[28] In Italy, three outbreaks occurred in shelters and the others involved purebred puppies imported from Hungary a few days before the onset of clinical signs. Several of the dogs were coinfected with other viruses, such as CDV, CPV, or CCoV.[18] Encephalopathy due to CAdV-1 infection was described in nine 5-week-old Labrador retriever puppies from Arkansas in the United States, all of which belonged to the same litter.[17] The litter was from an unvaccinated bitch. Mixed infections with CAdV-1, CAdV-2, CDV, CPV, and *Neospora caninum* were reported in puppies in Brazil,[29] and a coinfection with CAdV-1 and *Pasteurella pneumotropica* was documented in Italy in a 2-month-old male German shepherd with fever, lethargy, and cachexia.[21] These case descriptions confirm that CAdV-1 continues to circulate in the dog population and can result in severe disease in young dogs when vaccination does not occur, is improperly timed, and stress, coinfections and overcrowded conditions prevail. In addition, it is possible that emergence of new strains, such as through viral recombination, may be associated with reduced efficacy of vaccination. A recombinant CAdV-1 strain that has some genetic characteristics of CAdV-2 was reported to cause acute and fatal disease in a 6-month-old rottweiler and an 11-week-old poodle mix from South Australia in 2013.[26] Both dogs had received vaccines for CAdV-2, although the age of these dogs when the last vaccine in the series was given was not reported, so it is possible they were vaccinated in the face of persistent MDA. Rarely, CAdV-2 infection has been associated with neurologic signs in dogs.[30]

CLINICAL FEATURES

Pathogenesis and Clinical Signs

CAdV-1 is shed in saliva, feces, and urine, and transmission occurs through direct dog-to-dog contact or contact with contaminated fomites such as hands, utensils, and clothing. Ectoparasites such as fleas and ticks are also potential mechanical vectors.[28,31]. Airborne transmission does not appear to be important. After natural oronasal exposure, the virus initially localizes in the tonsils (Fig. 23.2), where it spreads to regional lymph nodes and lymphatics before reaching the blood through the thoracic duct. Using virus isolation to detect the virus, viremia lasts 4 to 8 days PI, whereas using molecular assays, CAdV-1 can be detected for several weeks in the blood.[32] Viremia results in rapid dissemination of the virus to other tissues and body secretions, including saliva, urine, and feces. The duration of viral shedding is variable, but urinary shedding has the potential to last 6 to 9 months. Hepatic parenchymal cells and vascular endothelial cells of many tissues, including the CNS, are prime targets of viral localization and injury. Initial cellular injury of the liver, kidney, and eye is associated with cytotoxic effects of the virus. A sufficient antibody response by day 7 PI clears the virus from the blood and liver and restricts the extent of hepatic damage. Widespread centrilobular to panlobular hepatic necrosis is often fatal in experimentally infected dogs, which may be accompanied by a persistently low virus neutralization antibody titer (less than 1:4). Acute hepatic necrosis can be self-limiting and centrilobularly restricted such that hepatic regeneration occurs in dogs that survive this phase of the disease. Dogs that demonstrate a partial neutralizing antibody titer (> 1:16, but < 1:500) by day 4 or 5 PI may develop chronic active hepatitis and hepatic fibrosis. Persistent hepatic inflammation continues, possibly as a result of chronic latent hepatic infection. Dogs immune to parenteral challenge with CAdV-1 are still susceptible to respiratory disease via aerosolized viral particles.[4]

Both virulent and attenuated live strains of CAdV-1 produce renal lesions. As detected by immunofluorescence and ultrastructural evaluation, virus initially localizes in the glomerular endothelium in the viremic phase of disease and produces glomerular injury. An increase in neutralizing antibody at approximately 7 days PI is associated with the glomerular deposition of circulating immune complexes (CICs) and transient proteinuria. Glomerular lesions contain deposits of viral antigen, immunoglobulin (Ig)G, IgM, and C3.[4,33,34] CAdV-1 is not detected in the glomerulus after 14 days PI; however, it persists in renal tubular epithelium. Tubular localization of the virus is primarily associated with viruria, and only a transient proteinuria occurs. A mild focal interstitial nephritis is found in recovered dogs. However, in contrast to liver disease, there is a lack of evidence that chronic progressive renal disease results from infection by CAdV-1.[4]

Clinical complications of ocular localization of CAdV-1 occur in approximately 20% of naturally infected dogs and in less than 1% of dogs after vaccination with attenuated live CAdV-1 vaccines. The development of ocular lesions begins during viremia, which develops 4 to 6 days PI. The virus enters the aqueous humor from the blood and replicates in corneal endothelial cells. Severe anterior uveitis and corneal edema develop 7 to 14 days PI, a period corresponding to an increase in neutralizing antibody titer (Fig. 23.3). Deposition of CICs with complement fixation results in chemotaxis of inflammatory cells into the anterior chamber and extensive corneal endothelial damage. Disruption of the intact corneal endothelium, which serves to pump fluid from the cornea into the anterior chamber, results in corneal stromal edema. Uveitis and edema are usually self-limiting unless additional complications or massive endothelial destruction occurs. Clearing of corneal edema coincides with endothelial regeneration and restoration of the hydrostatic gradient between the corneal stroma and aqueous humor. Recovery of the eye is usually apparent by 21 days PI. If the inflammatory changes are severe enough to block the filtration angle, increased intraocular pressure can result in glaucoma and hydrophthalmos.[4]

Complications are often associated with the pathogenesis of ICH. DIC, a frequent complication, begins in the early viremic phase of the disease and can be triggered by endothelial cell damage, with widespread activation of coagulation, or hepatic malfunction, with decreased clearance of activated clotting factors. Decreased hepatic synthesis of clotting factors in the face of excessive consumption compounds the bleeding defect. Although the cause of death in ICH is uncertain, the liver is a primary site of viral injury. Hepatic insufficiency and hepatic encephalopathy can result in a semicomatose state and death. Some dogs die so suddenly that liver damage with clinical evidence of hepatic failure does not have time to occur. Death in these

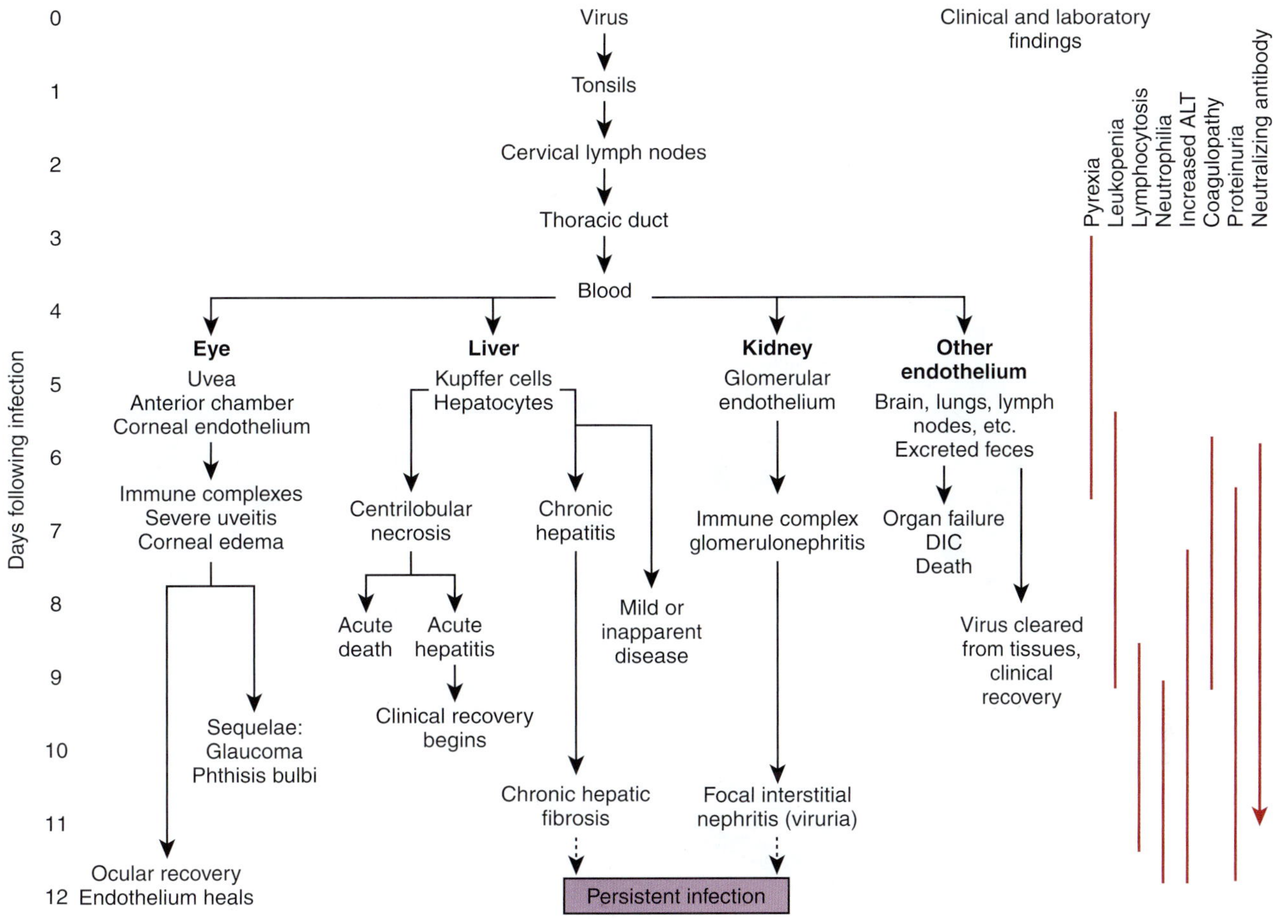

Fig 23.2 Pathogenesis of CAdV-1 infection.

dogs can result from damage to the brain, lungs, and other vital parenchymal organs or from the development of DIC.[4]

The incubation period in dogs is of 4 to 6 days after ingestion of infectious material and 6 to 9 days after direct contact with infected dogs.[23,24] Coinfections with CCoV, CDV, or CPV can exacerbate the disease, increasing mortality.[22,35-38]

ICH is most frequently recognized in dogs younger than 1 year, although unvaccinated dogs of all ages can be affected. Many infected dogs probably show no signs of illness.[4,28,31] Three overlapping disease syndromes have been described. The first is peracute disease with circulatory collapse, coma, and death after a brief illness that lasts less than 24 to 48 hours. The second, more commonly described syndrome is acute disease, which is associated with high morbidity and reported mortality rates of around 10% to 30%.[4] Dogs with acute disease either recover or die within a 2-week period. The third is a more chronic form that occurs in dogs with partial immunity, with death due to hepatic failure weeks (subacute disease) or months (chronic infection) after initial infection.[39]

Clinical signs in dogs that survive the acute viremic period include vomiting, abdominal pain, and diarrhea with or without evidence of hemorrhage. In the early phase of infection, fever (103° F to 106°F [39.4°C to 41.1°C]), tachycardia, and tachypnea may occur. Fever may be transient or biphasic. Tonsillitis, usually associated with pharyngitis and laryngitis, is common. Cough and increased breath sounds may be present in dogs with pneumonia. Cervical lymphadenomegaly can occur with subcutaneous edema of the head, neck, and dependent portions of the trunk. Abdominal pain and hepatomegaly are usually apparent. There may be widespread petechial and ecchymotic hemorrhages, epistaxis, and bleeding from venipuncture sites. Icterus is uncommon in acute ICH, but it is found in some dogs that survive the acute fulminant phase of the disease. Abdominal distention is caused by accumulation of serosanguineous fluid or hemorrhage. CNS signs, including lethargy, disorientation, seizures, or coma, can develop at any time after infection. In foxes and rarely in domestic dog pups, CNS signs can be seen in the absence of other systemic manifestations.[17] The development of neurologic signs may also represent hepatic encephalopathy, intracranial thrombosis or hemorrhage, or, as occurred in one outbreak, concurrent infection with CDV.[18]

Mildly affected dogs may recover after the initial febrile phase. Clinical signs of these uncomplicated cases of ICH frequently last 5 to 7 days before improvement. Persistent signs may be found in dogs with a concurrent viral infection such as canine distemper or in dogs that develop chronic hepatitis. More severe or additional clinical signs occur in dogs that are coinfected with other pathogens.[18,19,21,22,36-38]

Glomerulonephritis usually occurs about 1 to 2 weeks after the acute signs resolve. Infection of the glomerular endothelium is followed by a persistent tubular infection, interstitial nephritis, and viruria, but chronic renal failure has not been described.[33,34] Corneal edema and anterior uveitis usually occur when clinical recovery begins and may be the only clinical abnormalities seen in some dogs. Dogs with corneal edema show blepharospasm, photophobia, and serous ocular discharge. Corneal edema usually begins at the limbus and spreads centrally (Fig. 23.4). Ocular pain, present during the early stages of infection, usually subsides once edema is diffuse. However, pain may return with the development of glaucoma or corneal ulceration and

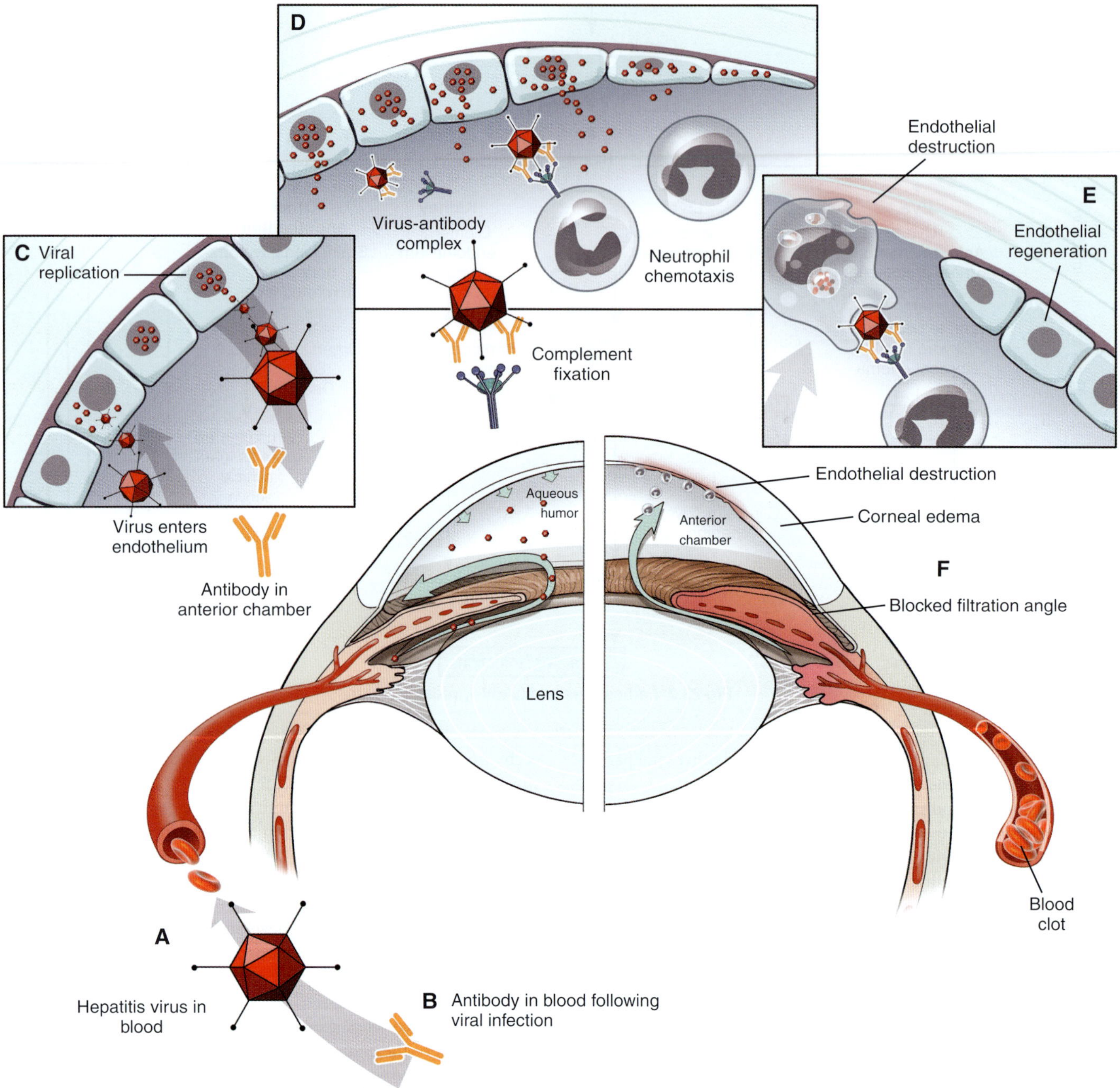

Fig. 23.3 Sequential pathogenesis of CAdV-1 infection in the eye. A, During the viremic period, CAdV-1 enters the eye via the uveal tract, localizing in vascular endothelial cells of the choroid and causing mild uveitis. Virus also enters the aqueous humor and localizes in the corneal endothelial cells. B, A CAdV-1-specific antibody response reaches the eye via the uveal tract and enters the aqueous humor in the presence of virus. C, Virus is free in the aqueous and endothelial cells and there is viral-antibody complex formation and intranuclear inclusion body formation. D, There is complement fixation on virus-immune complexes free and in endothelial cells to chemotaxis of neutrophils. More severe uveitis and corneal endothelial injury occurs. E, Corneal endothelial cell loss allows aqueous to enter the cornea causing corneal edema (blue eye). After mononuclear phagocytes remove virus-immune complexes, and inflammation subsides, corneal endothelium regenerates. F, Uveal inflammation may lead to blockage of the filtration angle and subsequent glaucoma.

perforation. Occasionally, corneal edema fails to resolve for months and may be associated with complications such as glaucoma.[40] In older literature, the Afghan hound was reportedly susceptible to this complication.[41]

In experimental infections with CAdV-1, chronic hepatitis with extensive fibrosis was observed in some dogs that recovered from acute illness, with survival for up to 8 months.[39] The virus could not be found in hepatic lesions from these dogs. Attempts to detect CAdV-1 in the liver of other dogs with chronic active hepatitis using PCR assays have to date been unrewarding.[42-44]

Physical Examination Findings

Physical examination findings in dogs with acute ICH vary, but can include lethargy, dehydration, fever (up to 106°F or 41°C), mild to severe congestion and enlargement of the tonsils, pallor, conjunctivitis, peripheral lymphadenopathy, tachypnea, increased breath sounds, and tachycardia. In some reports, serous to mucopurulent ocular and nasal discharge have been observed, but these may have resulted from coinfections with other respiratory viruses.[28] Abdominal palpation may reveal hepatomegaly, splenomegaly, or abdominal pain. Icterus is uncommon but can occur in dogs with a more prolonged course of disease. Peripheral edema that involves the head, neck, and ventral abdomen has been described.[44] Puppies with CAdV-1 encephalitis may show circling, vocalization, head pressing, ataxia, and blindness.[17] Coagulopathies may be manifested as cutaneous or mucosal petechial hemorrhages, epistaxis, or prolonged bleeding from venipuncture sites.

Ocular complications occur in at least 20% of affected dogs. Unilateral or, less commonly, bilateral corneal edema may be observed, which initially develops at the limbus and is occasionally associated with blepharospasm, photophobia, and a serous ocular discharge.[40] Unilateral involvement may progress to bilateral involvement over several days. Using a slit lamp, the cornea is markedly thickened, and there is episcleral and ciliary injection. Uveitis may also be apparent. Corneal ulceration and increased intraocular pressure has also been described in dogs with corneal edema, the latter of which may result in blindness.[40]

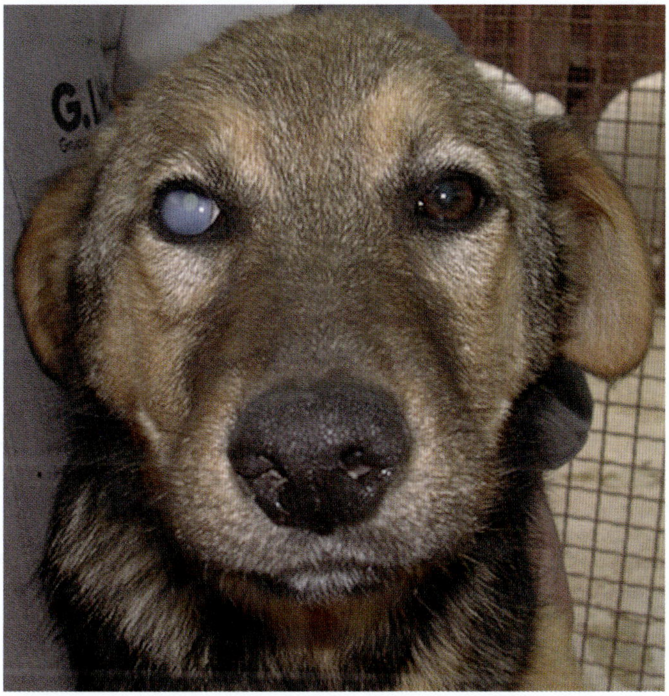

Fig. 23.4 Young adult dog with corneal edema from an Italian shelter outbreak of CAdV-1 infection. (Dr. Nicola Decaro, Department of Veterinary Medicine, University of Bari, Italy.)

DIAGNOSIS

ICH should be suspected in any dog less than 1 year of age that has a questionable vaccination history and signs of fever, respiratory, GI, and hepatic disease, and certainly in any young dog that develops corneal edema. Diagnosis is easily achieved at necropsy when characteristic intranuclear inclusion bodies are seen in tissues, but the sensitivity and specificity of this finding is unknown. Inclusion bodies may be seen on impression smears of liver biopsies or tissue obtained at necropsy. Antemortem diagnosis is challenging owing to the lack of commercially available assays and the disease may be underdiagnosed (Table 23.1). Serologic (antibody) assays are available, but they provide only a retrospective diagnosis, and interpretation of these assays may be a challenge when there is a history of vaccination or active circulation of CAdV-2.[31]

Laboratory Abnormalities

Complete Blood Count

Findings reported on the CBC in dogs with ICH are variable and include leukopenia, anemia, normoblastosis, and moderate to severe thrombocytopenia. Leukopenia (< 2000 cells/μL) occurs early in the course of infection and may be profound. Initially there is lymphopenia, then progressive neutropenia until death.[45] Bandemia and toxic changes may also be present. Occasionally leukocytosis is observed.[37] Leukocytosis and lymphocytosis may occur as part of the recovery process.

TABLE 23.1 Diagnostic Assays Available for Infectious Canine Hepatitis

Assay	Specimen Type	Target	Performance
Histopathology	Usually necropsy specimens, but also liver biopsy	Hepatic necrosis with intranuclear inclusions; CAdV-1 antigen with immunohistochemistry	True sensitivity and specificity of inclusion visualization unknown. Liver biopsy may not be feasible because of coagulopathies
PCR and real-time PCR	EDTA-blood; rectal, conjunctival, and nasal swabs; urine; tissues collected at necropsy	CAdV-1 DNA	Sensitivity and specificity may vary depending on assay design. Assays discriminating between CAdV-1 and CAdV-2 are available. The significance of a positive result from urine may be difficult to interpret due to subclinical shedding. False-negative results may occur as a result of PCR assay inhibition by components of feces
Virus isolation	All body secretions, tissues	CAdV-1	Sensitive, but generally only available as a research tool. No discrimination between CAdV-1 and CAdV-2

Serum Biochemical Tests

Changes on the serum biochemistry profile include increased activity of serum ALT (sometimes >1000 U/L), AST, and ALP; hyperbilirubinemia; hypoglycemia; and hypoalbuminemia.[46] The degree of increased activities of serum transaminases and ALP depends on the time of sampling and the magnitude of hepatic necrosis. These enzyme increases continue until day 14 PI, after which they decline, although they may persist or recur in dogs that develop chronic hepatitis. Of diagnostic importance, the increase in ALT activity, a measure of hepatocellular necrosis, is often disproportionately higher than the increase in serum bilirubin. This disparity, which is typical for ICH and differentiates it from most other causes of widespread hepatic necrosis, results from the predominant centrilobular nature of the necrosis. In contrast, the periportal, peripheral lobular regions are spared. Serum protein alterations, detectable only on serum electrophoresis, are a transient increase in α2-globulin by 7 days PI and by a delayed increase in γ-globulin, which peaks 21 days PI.[4]

Measures of hepatic function, such as serum ammonia or bile acid concentrations, can be increased during the acute course of ICH or later in dogs that develop hepatic fibrosis. Similarly, hypoglycemia may be found in dogs in the terminal phases of the disease. Determination of serum ammonia concentration may facilitate diagnosis of hepatic encephalopathy in dogs with neurologic signs.

Urinalysis

The urinalysis of dogs with ICH may reveal proteinuria, hyaline and granular cylindruria, hematuria, and bilirubinuria. Proteinuria (primarily albuminuria) is a reflection of the renal damage caused by the virus and can usually be detected on random urinalysis because the concentration is greater than 50 mg/dL. The increase in glomerular permeability can result from localization of the virus in the glomerulus in the initial stages of infection. Alternatively, as the disease progresses, glomeruli become damaged by CICs or as an effect of DIC.[4]

Coagulation Profile

In addition to thrombocytopenia, coagulation abnormalities reported in ICH reflect the presence of DIC and hepatic failure and include prolonged PT, markedly prolonged APTT (to 6 to 7 times control values), decreased factor VIII activity, hypofibrinogenemia, and increased fibrinogen degradation product concentrations. Platelet function assays have shown reduced platelet adhesion.[45]

Diagnostic Imaging

Findings on plain radiography and abdominal sonography in dogs with ICH have not been reported. Possible findings on plain radiography are a normal to slightly enlarged liver, and poor detail as a result of abdominal effusion or young age.

Microbiologic Tests

Virus Isolation

CAdV-1 can be readily isolated in a variety of cell types, such as Madin-Darby canine kidney (MDCK) cells.[8,9] In dogs with acute illness, any body fluid or tissue is likely to contain sufficient virus for isolation. The optimal necropsy specimens are kidney, lung, and lymphoid tissues; liver is rich in arginase, which inhibits virus isolation in cell culture.[46] Viral growth in cells is manifested as cell rounding, cluster formation, and detachment. Immunofluorescence (IF) can detect viral antigens in infected cell cultures and in acetone-fixed tissue sections or smears. As a consequence of viral replication, intranuclear inclusion bodies may be evident within cells after staining with H&E.[17,18,31] However, virus isolation, even if followed by detection of viral antigens, is not able to distinguish between infection with CAdV-1 and CAdV-2. This is important since CAdV-2 can be sporadically isolated from organs and feces of either vaccinated or acutely infected dogs, while CAdV-1 can be often detected in the respiratory secretions, trachea, and lungs.[31] In addition, virus isolation is not widely offered by commercial veterinary diagnostic laboratories.

Serologic Diagnosis

Serologic tests are available for detection of IgG and IgM against CAdV-1, which include ELISA assays, hemagglutination inhibition, and serum neutralization. However, due to cross-reactivity with CAdV-2, diagnosis of ICH cannot rely only on serological testing. In addition, dogs with acute disease may die before they develop antibodies to the virus.[39] For dogs that recover from illness, a recent history of vaccination may complicate interpretation of acute and convalescent phase serology. In the absence of a vaccination history, a fourfold rise in titer over a 2- to 3-week period together with compatible clinical signs is supportive of the diagnosis of ICH. Titers that follow natural infection may be higher than those that follow vaccination. Rapid serological tests, based on the ELISA technology, are available for determination of postvaccination antibodies.

Molecular Diagnosis

Due to the antigenic relatedness of the two CAdV types, distinction between CAdV-1 and CAdV-2 requires molecular testing. PCR amplification followed by restriction fragment length polymorphism analysis (see Chapters 6 and 7) using the endonucleases *Pst*I and *Hpa*II generates differential patterns.[48] Endpoint (conventional) PCR assays for rapid detection of CAdV-1 in clinical specimens such as nasal, rectal, and ocular swabs and blood, as well as tissue obtained at necropsy, have been described. These include assays that differentiate between CAdV-1 and CAdV-2 (Fig. 23.5).[23] Because of the rarity of the disease, the clinical sensitivity and specificity of these assays are not well understood. A SYBR® Green real-time PCR assay has been introduced for CAdV detection and differentiation.[49] A duplex real-time PCR assay based on the TaqMan technology for simultaneous detection and characterization of CAdV-1 and CAdV-2 was developed by using a single primer pair and virus-specific probes.[45,50] This assay was highly sensitive (at least 1 to 2 logs more than endpoint PCR) and showed a good linearity over a range of nine orders of magnitude, which allows a precise calculation of DNA load in samples that contain widely varying amounts of virus.

The results of PCR assays on urine may be more difficult to interpret than those for other specimens, because of the potential for chronic shedding from this site in the absence of clinical signs. Assays that specifically detect CAdV-1 differentiate between virulent CAdV-1 virus and vaccine virus, because vaccines for ICH all contain only CAdV-2.

Pathologic Findings

Gross Pathologic Findings

Findings on necropsy or biopsy examination of tissues from dogs can usually confirm a diagnosis of ICH. Dogs that die during the acute phase of the disease are often in good body condition, with edema and hemorrhage of superficial lymph nodes and cervical subcutaneous tissue. Icterus is mild or not usually apparent. The abdominal cavity may contain fluid that varies from clear to bright red in color. Petechial and ecchymotic hemorrhages are often present on serosal surfaces. The liver is enlarged, dark, and mottled in appearance, and a prominent fibrinous exudate is usually found on the liver surface and in the interlobar fissures (Fig. 23.6). Typically, the gallbladder is thickened and edematous and has a bluish-white opaque appearance. Fibrin can be deposited on other abdominal serosal surfaces, giving them a ground-glass appearance. Intraluminal GI hemorrhage is a frequent finding. The spleen is enlarged and bulges on the cut surface.

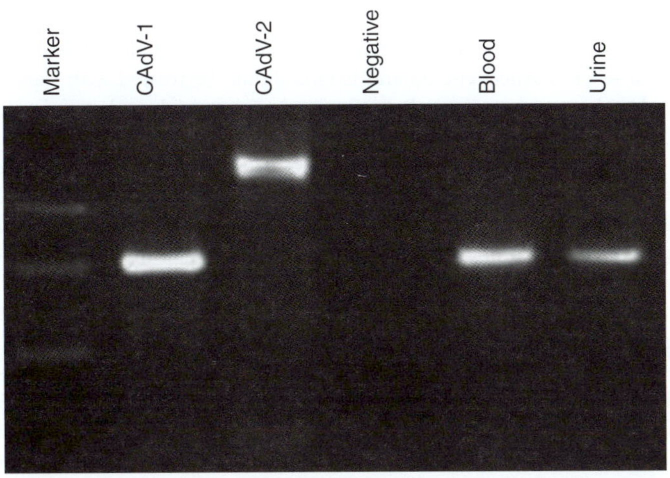

Fig. 23.5 PCR assay for detection of CAdV-1 and CAdV-2. Lane 1, molecular weight marker. Lane 2, positive control for CAdV-1 (508 base pair [bp] product). Lane 3, positive control for CAdV-2 (1030 bp). Lane 4, negative control (rectal swab from a dog negative for CAdV-1/CAdV-2). Lanes 5 and 6, clinical specimens positive for CAdV-1 (EDTA-blood and urine collected from the case example 2 weeks after initial examination).

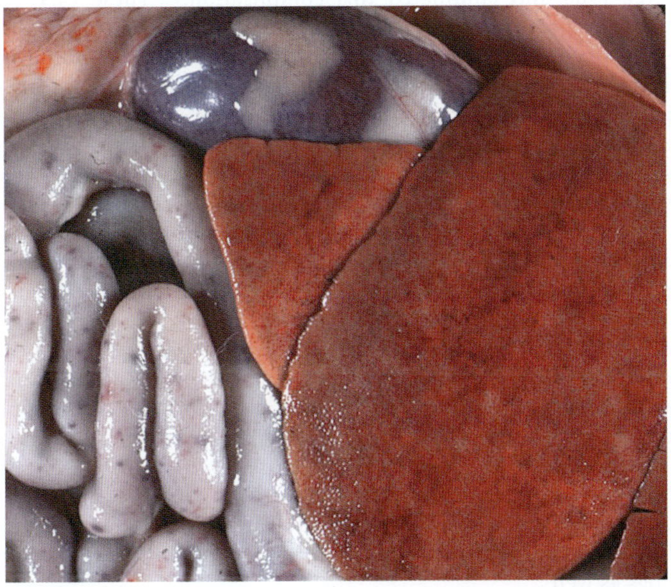

Fig. 23.6 Infectious canine hepatitis, hepatic necrosis, liver, dog. The liver from dogs with infectious canine hepatitis can be slightly enlarged and friable with a blotchy yellow discoloration. Sometimes fibrin is evident on the capsular surface. Note the petechiae on the serosal surface of the intestines caused by vascular damage. (Courtesy Dr. M.D. McGavin, College of Veterinary Medicine, University of Tennessee. In Zachary JF, McGavin MD. *Pathologic Basis of Veterinary Disease*, 5th ed. St. Louis, MO: Mosby; 2012.)

Variable gross lesions in other organs include multifocal hemorrhagic renal cortical infarcts. The lungs have multiple, patchy, gray-to-red areas of consolidation. Hemorrhagic and edematous bronchial lymph nodes are found. Scattered hemorrhages, present on coronal section of the brain, are primarily located in the midbrain and caudal brainstem. Ocular lesions, when present, are characterized by corneal opacification and clouding of the aqueous humor.

In dogs with chronic disease, the liver may be small, firm, and nodular. The kidneys may be studded with multiple white foci (0.5 cm diameter) that extend from the renal pelvis to the outer cortex. Ocular sequelae from the acute disease can include either glaucoma or phthisis bulbi.[4]

Histopathologic Findings

Histopathologic examination of the liver of dogs that die of acute hepatitis usually reveals widespread centrilobular to panlobular necrosis. In dogs with mild hepatocellular necrosis, the margin between necrotic and viable hepatocytes is sharply defined within the liver lobule. Preservation of the underlying support stroma allows for eventual hepatic regeneration. Only in severe cases does coagulation necrosis of entire hepatic lobules prevent regeneration. Neutrophilic and mononuclear cell infiltrates are associated with the removal of underlying necrotic tissue. Bile pigment rarely accumulates in most cases because of the transient nature of hepatocellular necrosis and the frequent lack of peripheral lobular involvement of portal regions. Intranuclear inclusions are initially found in Kupffer's cells and later in viable hepatic parenchymal cells. Subacute to chronic hepatic disease is marked by sporadic foci of necrosis with neutrophilic, mononuclear, and plasma cell infiltration and is found in dogs with partial immunity that survive initial stages of infection.

Historically, CAdV-1 has been observed with direct fluorescent antibody in hepatocytes of recovered dogs with chronic hepatic inflammation. PCR and histochemical staining of tissues have been used to examine for CAdV-1 in the livers of dogs with naturally occurring ICH, chronic hepatitis, and hepatic fibrosis.[44] Although the dogs with known ICH have had positive test results, CAdV-1 has not been detected in studies that used PCR on liver specimens from dogs with idiopathic acute or chronic hepatitis.[43]

Widespread histologic alterations occur in other organs as a result of endothelial injury caused by the virus. The gallbladder has marked subserosal edema, but the epithelium remains intact. Viral inclusions are initially found in the renal glomeruli but are later found in renal tubular vascular endothelium. Focal interstitial accumulations of neutrophils and mononuclear cells are found in the renal cortex and medulla. These mild changes often progress to focal interstitial fibrosis.[51] Lymphoid organs, including the lymph nodes, tonsils, and spleen, are congested with neutrophilic and mononuclear cell infiltrates. Lymphoid follicles are dispersed with central areas of necrotic foci. Intranuclear inclusions can be found in vascular endothelial cells and histiocytes. The lungs have thickened alveoli with septal cell and peribronchial lymphoid accumulations. Alveoli in consolidated areas are filled with an exudate consisting of erythrocytes, fibrin, and fluid. Mucosal and submucosal edema with focal subserosal hemorrhage is found in the intestinal tract. Widespread vascular degeneration and tissue hemorrhage and necrosis are associated with the presence of intravascular fibrin thrombi.

Swollen, desquamated endothelial cells in meningeal vessels often contain intranuclear inclusions. Mononuclear cuffing is present around small vessels throughout the parenchyma of the CNS.[17] Mild endothelial proliferation and mononuclear perivascular infiltration persist for at least 3 weeks after clinical recovery.

Ocular changes are characterized by granulomatous iridocyclitis with corneal endothelial disruption and corneal edema. Iridial and ciliary vessels are congested with inflammatory cells that are also present in the iris and filtration angle.

The inclusion bodies seen in ICH have been classified as Cowdry type A or B. They are often multiple basophilic inclusions and are present in both ectodermal and mesodermal tissues. Their relative abundance in the liver makes this the optimal tissue for impression smears obtained by biopsy or at necropsy (Fig. 23.7). Initial hypertrophy of the cell nucleus is followed by peripheral margination of the chromatin network and nucleolus, which forms a central, dark-staining nuclear remnant surrounded by a halo of chromatin. The initial inclusions are acidophilic but become basophilic as the chromatin marginates. Care must be taken to distinguish inclusions from faintly staining hepatocyte nucleoli.[4,31]

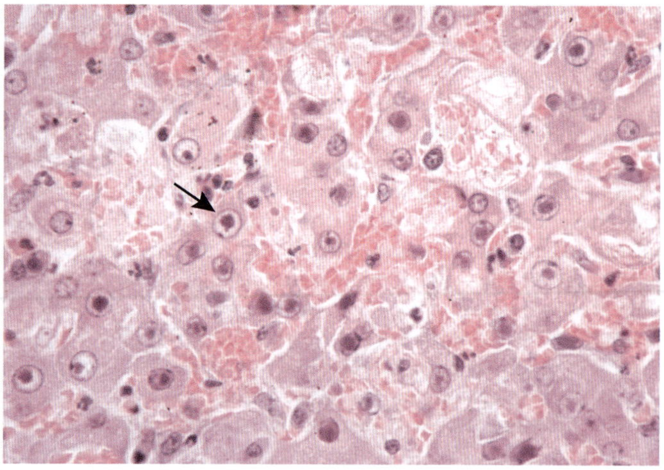

Fig. 23.7 Infection of hepatocytes and endothelial cells with CAdV-1 produces characteristic basophilic intranuclear inclusions surrounded by a clear zone that separates them from the marginated chromatin *(arrow)*. H&E stain. (Courtesy Dr. W. Crowell, College of Veterinary Medicine, The University of Georgia and Noah's Archive, College of Veterinary Medicine, The University of Georgia. In Zachary JF, McGavin M. *Pathologic Basis of Veterinary Disease*, 5th ed. St. Louis, MO: Mosby; 2012.)

TREATMENT AND PROGNOSIS

Supportive Care

Clinical management of dogs that develop ICH is primarily supportive. In the absence of complicating factors, clinical recovery and hepatocellular regeneration can occur with centrilobular necrosis. It may be difficult to determine whether neurologic signs are related to hepatic encephalopathy or viral encephalitis. Measurement of blood glucose or ammonia concentrations may be helpful.

Immediate placement of an indwelling intravenous catheter is required for severely affected dogs; however, because of coagulopathy, care must be taken to minimize hemorrhage. Fluid therapy with a polyionic isotonic fluid such as Ringer's solution can correct losses from vomiting and diarrhea. Replacement of clotting factors and platelets through administration of fresh plasma or whole blood may be necessary in conjunction with anticoagulant therapy in dogs with coagulopathies.

In comatose dogs, possible hypoglycemia should be addressed by administration of 50% glucose (0.5 mL/kg, IV, over 5 minutes). Hypoglycemia is likely to recur if continuous infusion of hypertonic glucose is not maintained. Hypertonic glucose infusion should be continued at a rate not greater than 0.5 to 0.9 g/kg per hour. Treatment of hepatic encephalopathy is directed at reducing protein catabolism by colonic bacteria and ammonia resorption in the renal tubules. Ammonia production can be reduced by administering restricted protein diets and management of GI hemorrhage. Evacuation of the colon by administration of warm water enemas may also retard ammonia absorption. Nonabsorbable oral antibacterials such as neomycin have been advocated to reduce ammonia-producing bacteria in the intestine, but their effectiveness is questionable. Acidification of the colonic contents can also be achieved by feeding oral lactulose to nonvomiting animals. Renal resorption of ammonia can be reduced by administration of parenteral or oral potassium and correction of metabolic alkalosis.

Other medications that may be indicated include antiemetics, antacids, sucralfate, whole blood or plasma transfusions, and colloids such as hetastarch. The use of parenteral broad-spectrum antimicrobial drugs should be considered for dogs with hemorrhagic gastroenteritis that may develop bacteremia as a result of bacterial translocation. After fluorescein staining has shown no evidence of corneal ulceration, dogs with severe corneal edema and uveitis should be treated with topical ophthalmic preparations that contain glucocorticoids and atropine to prevent development of glaucoma.

Prognosis depends on the severity of disease, which reflects the immune status of the affected dog and possibly the virus strain. There is a possibility that recovered dogs may develop chronic hepatitis or chronic glomerulonephritis, but the extent to which this truly occurs is unknown.

IMMUNITY AND VACCINATION

Immunity to natural infection with CAdV-1 is probably lifelong. Effective vaccines have been available and widely used as part of core vaccine programs for dogs for many years. Immunity after immunization with attenuated live vaccines lasts at least 3 years and probably longer, up to 9 years according to challenge and serological studies.[52] Early vaccines, which contained CAdV-1, were associated with the development of corneal edema and glomerulonephritis in a small percentage (<1%) of immunized dogs. Replacement of attenuated live CAdV-1 with CAdV-2 occurred after 1980 and eliminated this complication.[53] These vaccines have the potential to cause transient respiratory signs and tonsillitis in dogs if accidental inhalation occurs, so care should be taken not to aerosolize the vaccine during administration. MDA persists until puppies are 12 to 16 weeks of age and interferes with immunization when virus neutralization titers are high. Vaccines should be administered every 3 to 4 weeks from 6 weeks of age, with the last vaccine given no earlier than 16 weeks of age (see Appendix). After completing the puppy series at 16 weeks or older and vaccinating again at 26 or 52 weeks of age, revaccination need not be done more often than every 3 years. In the absence of MDA, attenuated live vaccines protect against ICH as early as 5 days after vaccination. Revaccination can be avoided, especially in immunocompromised dogs or dogs with a history of postvaccination reactions in the presence of specific antibodies, which can be easily determined by commercially available serological assays.[54] The presence of serum antibody, regardless of titer, in an actively immunized dog over the age of 20 weeks is correlated with protection.[55] Vaccine virus may be shed from the respiratory tract by dogs after vaccination, which has the potential to immunize other dogs as well.

Although extensive vaccination has greatly reduced the incidence of CAdV-1 infection, reemergence of ICH in western Europe has been associated to parallel trading of pups with uncertain sanitary status from the eastern European countries. Currently, there are few data on the molecular epidemiology of CAdV-1, but it is commonly accepted that vaccine breaks occur very rarely with CAdV-2 vaccines, since the viruses are genetically stable. Accordingly, CAdV-1 infection in vaccinated dogs has been associated with MDA interference in the early life of the pups rather than the emergence of variants genetically distant from the prototype strains contained in commercially available vaccines.[18]

PREVENTION

The best means of prevention of ICH is proper vaccination. Additional control measures that could be considered in locations where outbreaks occur, such as in shelters, include proper disinfection, isolation, and prevention of overcrowding and other coinfections, which may worsen disease. Because contact with wild animal species such as coyotes, wolves, and foxes that might be shedding the virus may also be a source of infection for dogs, exclusion of these species from interactions with domestic dogs may also serve to prevent the disease.

PUBLIC HEALTH ASPECTS

In humans, species C adenoviruses are considered to be the most clinically significant adenovirus species, as they can become latent in an episomal form in immune cells and reactivate in immunocompromised patients.[3] There is currently no evidence that CAdV-1 infects humans. However, there is some evidence that adenoviruses that infect cats may have the capability of infecting humans (see Feline Adenovirus Infection).

FELINE ADENOVIRUS INFECTION

In cats, clinical disease caused by adenovirus infection is most likely to occur in immunocompromised animals.[56,57] In studies of cats in Hungary, Scotland, the Netherlands, the Czech Republic, and the United States, serologic findings indicated adenovirus exposure in 15%, 10%, 20%, 25%, and 26% of cats, respectively.[3,58,59] However, the clinical findings of disseminated adenovirus infection have only been described in detail in one cat.[60,61] Inclusion body hepatitis in a black panther was suggestive of adenovirus infection; however, the causative agent could not be confirmed by electron microscopy or through virus isolation.[62]

The cat with disseminated adenovirus infection was an 8-year-old, spayed female, domestic shorthair cat. Physical examination findings included mental obtundation and oral mucosal petechiae. Abnormal hematologic findings included leukopenia (2100 cells/μL) and thrombocytopenia (73,000/μL). There was no apparent response to treatment with IV lactated Ringer's solution, dexamethasone, and vitamin K, and the cat died 4 hours after initial examination. At necropsy, the abdominal cavity and pericardial sac were filled with serous fluid. Serosal and mucosal surfaces of the small and large intestines were diffusely dark red with scattered serosal petechiae, and there was dark red fluid intestinal contents. The liver and kidneys were enlarged, and the liver had an accentuated lobular pattern. Abdominal fluid tested positive for FeLV p27 antigen and was negative for FIV antibody. An adenovirus particle was identified by electron micrography of intestinal contents. Histologically, there was moderate lymphoid depletion and peripheral hemorrhage in lymphoid tissue. Endothelial cells were detached from intramyocardial arteries (Fig. 23.8). Nuclei of these sloughed cells were large and pleomorphic, and many contained intranuclear inclusion bodies. Multiple round eosinophilic inclusions were present in some nuclei, with amphophilic granular inclusions filling other nuclei. Some nuclei were almost filled with well-delineated basophilic inclusions, with margination of the small amount of surrounding chromatin (Fig. 23.8, *inset*). Some nuclei had indistinct borders, resulting in a "smudge cell" appearance. The cytoplasm of sloughed endothelial cells was eosinophilic.

Throughout the GI tract, there was diffuse submucosal edema. Diffuse superficial necrotizing and hemorrhagic enteritis was present in the small intestine. Necrosis was more severe in the ileum, with full-thickness mucosal necrosis over Peyer's patches. Sections of colon were comparably affected, with particularly severe mucosal necrosis overlying areas of submucosal lymphoid tissue. Submucosal and mesenteric blood vessels at all levels of the GI tract had endothelial lesions as described in the heart. Similar vascular lesions were seen in small hepatic arteries, pulmonary arteries, trachea, thymic remnant, urinary bladder, thyroid gland, adrenal gland, bone marrow, spleen, lymph node, and kidney.

Electron microscopic examination of detached endothelial cells revealed intranuclear viral particles measuring approximately 65 nm in diameter (Fig. 23.9). Some of these particles were icosahedral, with dense central cores. In some areas, viral particles formed loose crystalline arrays.

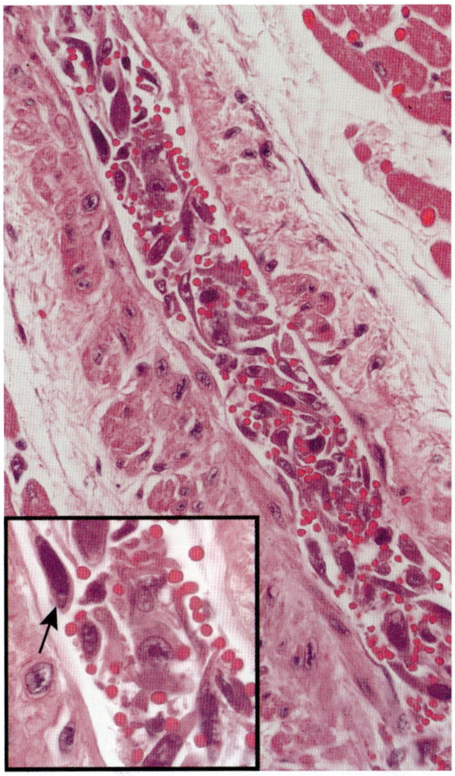

Fig. 23.8 Photomicrograph of an intramyocardial artery from a cat with disseminated adenovirus infection. Endothelial cells are sloughing. Spindle-shaped cells within the arterial lumen have large, pleomorphic nuclei, some with inclusion bodies (H&E stain, ×400). **Inset,** Nucleus containing an inclusion body (*arrow*; H&E stain, ×1000). (Courtesy Frances A. Kennedy, Michigan State University, East Lansing, MI.)

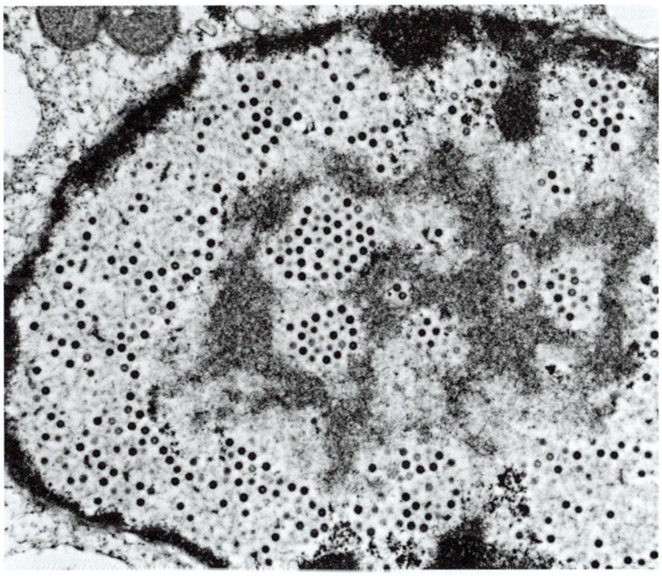

Fig. 23.9 Electron micrograph of an endothelial cell from a cat with disseminated adenovirus infection. There are intranuclear viral particles. Moderate autolytic change is responsible for disruption of adenoviral arrays (×17,900). (From Kennedy FA, Mullaney TP. Disseminated adenovirus infection in a cat. *J Vet Diagn Invest.* 1993;5:273-276.)

Because adenoviruses are generally considered to be relatively host-specific,[1] healthy horses, dogs, and one goat on the property were unlikely sources of infection for this cat. Other cats on the property were also apparently healthy. It is possible that FeLV-associated immunocompromise predisposed this cat to disseminated adenovirus infection. Leukopenia may have been a consequence of FeLV infection, terminal endotoxemia, or both. Thrombocytopenia was most likely consequent to consumption secondary to vascular lesions.

Results of serologic studies in cats, measuring serum antibody to feline adenovirus, have indicated that persistent subclinical adenovirus infection exists in the feline population. Risk factors for seroreactivity are age and the presence of respiratory or GI signs.[63] However, to date, only one case of adenovirus infection in a cat has been confirmed using molecular methods.[3,59] The affected cat had transient hepatic failure, and the results of serologic testing supported the possibility of adenovirus infection. Adenovirus hexon capsid nucleic acid was detected in two rectal swabs taken 1 year apart and a pharyngeal swab taken at the second time point. This finding suggests that, in addition to persistent subclinical infections, chronic shedding of adenovirus may be possible in cats.

Feline adenovirus is not considered to cause disease in humans, although there are few reports that describe the possibility of interspecies transmission. In one report of a 1-year-old girl with gastroenteritis, a fecal specimen from the child was positive for an adenovirus strain that exhibited a high degree of homology to a feline adenovirus.[12] No cats were kept in the household. A feline adenovirus isolate was also described that could replicate in both monkey Vero cells and human HeLa cells.[11] In a large epidemiological survey for adenoviruses in humans in Brazil, a nasopharyngeal aspirate of a child contained a strain that had a hexon gene sequence with 100% nucleotide identity to feline isolates.[13] Most recently, the adenovirus isolated from a rectal swab from the cat with hepatitis in the late 1990s was shown to replicate in human and feline cell lines, exhibited serologic cross-reactivity with human adenoviruses, and had high sequence homology to species C human adenoviruses.[3,59] It was proposed that the virus be named FeAdV-1.[3] In contrast, the cat with disseminated disease and FeLV infection was infected with an adenovirus that was distinct from human adenoviruses,[64] which currently remains unnamed.

CASE EXAMPLE

Signalment

"Pablo," 2-year-old male American pit bull terrier from Bari, Italy.

History

Pablo lived indoors but contacted other dogs at a building site, to which he was occasionally brought. Pablo was unvaccinated, and was fed commercial dry food. The owner reported a 2-day history of inappetence, lethargy, and respiratory distress before taking Pablo to a veterinary clinic. As a puppy, Pablo had severe gastroenteritis of unknown etiology.

Physical Examination

Body weight: 23.3 kg.

General: Lethargic, not fully responsive, with evidence of respiratory distress. Temperature = 103.1°F (39.4°C), HR = 70 beats/min, RR = 48 breaths/min, mucous membranes slightly pale, CRT = 2 s.

Integument, eyes, ears, nose, and throat: Mild tonsillitis.

Musculoskeletal: Ambulatory on all four limbs. No clinically significant abnormalities.

Cardiovascular, respiratory, gastrointestinal, and urogenital systems: Increased breath sounds diffusely. Tense abdomen, with severe cranial abdominal pain. Moderate peripheral lymphadenopathy, mainly involving the retropharyngeal lymph nodes. Prepucial edema and hemorrhages were observed.

Laboratory Findings

CBC: HCT 36.3% (37–55%)MCV 73.2 fL (60–77 fL), MCHC 38.2 g/dL (30–37.5 g/dL), WBC 13,510 cells/μL (5500–16,900 cells/μL), neutrophils 11,440 cells/μL (2000–12,000 cells/μL), lymphocytes 1112 cells/μL (500–4900 cells/μL), monocytes 65 cells/μL (30–2000 cells/μL), platelets 27,000/μL (175,000–500,000 platelets/μL)

Serum chemistry profile: BUN 13 mg/dL (7–27 mg/dL), creatinine 1.0 mg/dL (0.5–1.8 mg/dL), glucose 89 mg/dL (74–143 mg/dL), total protein 4.6 g/dL (5.5–7.5 g/dL), albumin 2.01 g/dL (2.5–4.0 g/dL), globulin 2.6 g/dL (1.8–3.9 g/dL), ALT 698 U/L (10–100 U/L), AST 700 U/L (0–50 U/L), ALP 155 U/L (23–212 U/L), creatine kinase 458 U/L (10–200 U/L), GGT 0 U/L (0–7 U/L), cholesterol 201 mg/dL (110–320 mg/dL), total bilirubin 0.1 mg/dL (0–0.9 mg/dL)

Serum protein electrophoresis: There was a slight reduction of the albumin fraction (43.6%, reference range 45.0–55.0%) and an increase in the α2-globulin fraction (18.2%, normal range 8.0–14.0%). The albumin/globulin ratio was 0.77.

Urinalysis: SpG 1.033; pH 6.5, 1+ protein, 1+ bilirubin, 1+ hemoprotein, no glucose, no WBC, rare RBC, 2+ epithelial cells, few granular casts.

Imaging Findings

Thoracic radiographs: The cardiovascular and pulmonary structures appeared within normal limits. Pulmonary interstitial and alveolar infiltration were evident along with a moderate pleural effusion.

Abdominal ultrasound: A moderate abdominal effusion was present. Spleen, liver, and gallbladder walls were enlarged and hypoechoic. Multiple enlarged, hypoechoic mesenteric, and splenic lymph nodes were observed.

Fecal Examination

Fecal flotation and sedimentation: Negative for parasites.

Molecular Assays

EDTA-blood, fecal, and nasal swab specimens were submitted for molecular detection of canine parvovirus, coronavirus, adenoviruses, and distemper virus using PCR-based assays. All specimens tested positive for CAdV-1.

Diagnosis

Infectious canine hepatitis.

Treatment

Supportive care was provided with IV fluids, oxygen supplementation, and anti-inflammatory drugs; S-adenosylmethionine (20 mg/kg PO q24h) was also administered.

Follow-up

At a recheck 2 weeks later, there was marked clinical improvement. The dog was fully responsive, energetic, with slight pallor of the mucus membranes and a temperature of 100.9°F (38.3°C). Thoracic auscultation and abdominal palpation were unremarkable, and preputial hemorrhages had resolved. There was persistent generalized lymphadenopathy. Liver enzyme activities were normal. A CBC showed anemia (HCT 27.3%), leukocytosis (WBC 29120 cells/μL), neutrophilia (23,160 cells/μL), monocytosis (4280 cells/μL), and thrombocytosis (660,000 platelets/μL). Urinalysis findings were unremarkable. Blood-EDTA and urine samples tested still positive for CAdV-1 by endpoint PCR see (Fig. 23.5).

Comments

The clinical course of ICH in this dog was atypical since there was no overt gastroenteric involvement. This was likely due to the age of the affected animal since it is well known that the pathogenic potential of CAdV-1 is higher in young pups than in adult dogs. The detection of the viral DNA 2 weeks after the dog was first examined is in agreement with the long-term viremia and shedding observed for CAdV-1. (Case example courtesy of Dr. Vito Manfredi, Ambulatorio Veterinario Stella Alpina, Triggiano, Italy.)

SUGGESTED READINGS

Decaro N, Campolo M, Elia G, et al. Infectious canine hepatitis: an "old" disease reemerging in Italy. *Res Vet Sci*. 2007;83:269–273.

Wong M, Woolford L, Hasan NH, et al. A novel recombinant canine adenovirus type 1 detected from acute lethal cases of infectious canine hepatitis. *Viral Immunol*. 2017;30:258–263.

Ongradi J, Chatlynne LG, Tarcsai KR, et al. Adenovirus isolated from a cat is related to human adenovirus 1. *Front Microbiol*. 2019;10:1430.

REFERENCES

1. Rubarth S. An acute virus disease with liver lesion in dogs (hepatitis contagiosa canis): a pathologico-anatomical and etiological investigation. *Acta Path Microbiol Scand*. 1947. suppl 69.
2. Miles JA, Parry HB, Larin NM, et al. Cultivation of canine hepatitis virus in embryonated hen's eggs and its subsequent transmission to dogs. *Nature*. 1951;168:699–700.
3. Ongradi J, Chatlynne LG, Tarcsai KR, et al. Adenovirus isolated from a cat is related to human adenovirus 1. *Front Microbiol*. 2019;10:1430.
4. Greene CE. Infectious canine hepatitis and canine acidophil cell hepatitis. In: Greene CE, ed. *Infectious Diseases of the Dog and Cat*. 1st ed. Philadelphia: WB Saunders; 1998:22–28.
5. Green RG, Ziegler NR, Green BB, et al. Epizootic fox encephalitis. I. General description. *Am J Hyg*. 1930;12:109–129.
6. Ditchfield J, Macpherson LW, Zbitnew A. Association of canine adenovirus (Toronto a 26/61) with an outbreak of laryngotracheitis ("kennel cough"): a preliminary report. *Can Vet J*. 1962;3:238–247.
7. Park NY, Lee MC, Kurkure NV, et al. Canine adenovirus type 1 infection of a Eurasian river otter (*Lutra lutra*). *Vet Pathol*. 2007;44:536–539.
8. Burek KA, Gulland FM, Sheffield G, et al. Infectious disease and the decline of Steller sea lions (*Eumetopias jubatus*) in Alaska, USA: insights from serologic data. *J Wildl Dis*. 2005;41:512–524.
9. Philippa JD, Leighton FA, Daoust PY, et al. Antibodies to selected pathogens in free-ranging terrestrial carnivores and marine mammals in Canada. *Vet Rec*. 2004;155:135–140.
10. Robinson AJ, Crerar SK, Waight Sharma N, et al. Prevalence of serum antibodies to canine adenovirus and canine herpesvirus in the European red fox (*Vulpes vulpes*) in Australia. *Aust Vet J*. 2005;83:356–361.
11. Almberg ES, Mech LD, Smith DW, et al. A serological survey of infectious disease in Yellowstone National Park's canid community. *PloS One*. 2009;4:e7042.
12. Grinder M, Krausman PR. Morbidity-mortality factors and survival of an urban coyote population in Arizona. *J Wildl Dis*. 2001;37:312–317.
13. Gur S, Acar A. A retrospective investigation of canine adenovirus (CAV) infection in adult dogs in Turkey. *J S Afr Vet Assoc*. 2009;80:84–86.
14. Thompson H, O'Keeffe AM, Lewis JC, et al. Infectious canine hepatitis in red foxes (*Vulpes vulpes*) in the United Kingdom. *Vet Rec*. 2010;166:111–114.
15. Balboni A, Mollace C, Giunti M, et al. Investigation of the presence of canine adenovirus (CAdV) in owned dogs in Northern Italy. *Res Vet Sci*. 2014;97:631–636.
16. Balboni A, Verin R, Morandi F, et al. Molecular epidemiology of canine adenovirus type 1 and type 2 in free-ranging red foxes (*Vulpes vulpes*) in Italy. *Vet Microbiol*. 2013;162:551–557.
17. Caudell D, Confer AW, Fulton RW, et al. Diagnosis of infectious canine hepatitis virus (CAV-1) infection in puppies with encephalopathy. *J Vet Diagn Invest*. 2005;17:58–61.
18. Decaro N, Campolo M, Elia G, et al. Infectious canine hepatitis: an "old" disease reemerging in Italy. *Res Vet Sci*. 2007;83:269–273.
19. Headley SA, Alfieri AA, Fritzen JT, et al. Concomitant canine distemper, infectious canine hepatitis, canine parvoviral enteritis, canine infectious tracheobronchitis, and toxoplasmosis in a puppy. *J Vet Diagn Invest*. 2013;25:129–135.
20. Muller C, Sieber-Ruckstuhl N, Decaro N, et al. Infectious canine hepatitis in 4 dogs in Switzerland. *Schweiz Arch Tierheilkd*. 2010;152:63–68.
21. Pintore MD, Corbellini D, Chieppa MN, et al. Canine adenovirus type 1 and *Pasteurella pneumotropica* coinfection in a puppy. *Vet Ital*. 2016;52:57–62.
22. Pratelli A, Martella V, Elia G, et al. Severe enteric disease in an animal shelter associated with dual infections by canine adenovirus type 1 and canine coronavirus. *J Vet Med B Infect Dis Vet Public Health*. 2001;48:385–392.
23. Walker D, Abbondati E, Cox AL, et al. Infectious canine hepatitis in red foxes (*Vulpes vulpes*) in wildlife rescue centres in the UK. *Vet Rec*. 2016;178:421.
24. Knowles S, Bodenstein BL, Hamon T, et al. Infectious canine hepatitis in a brown bear (*Ursus arctos horribilis*) from Alaska, USA. *J Wildl Dis*. 2018;54:642–645.
25. Balboni A, Dondi F, Agnoli C, et al. Novel sequence variants of viral hexon and fibre genes in two dogs with canine adenovirus type 1-associated disease. *Vet J*. 2017;223:73–75.
26. Wong M, Woolford L, Hasan NH, et al. A novel recombinant canine adenovirus type 1 detected from acute lethal cases of infectious canine hepatitis. *Viral Immunol*. 2017;30:258–263.
27. Dowgier G, Lahoreau J, Lanave G, et al. Sequential circulation of canine adenoviruses 1 and 2 in captive wild carnivores, France. *Vet Microbiol*. 2018;221:67–73.
28. Cabasso VJ. Infectious canine hepatitis virus. *Ann N Y Acad Sci*. 1962;101:498–514.
29. Headley SA, Oliveira TES, Pereira AHT, et al. Canine morbillivirus (canine distemper virus) with concomitant canine adenovirus, canine parvovirus-2, and *Neospora caninum* in puppies: a retrospective immunohistochemical study. *Sci Rep*. 2018;8:13477.
30. Chander V, Sharma GK, Bhatt M, et al. Isolation and genetic characterization of canine adenovirus 2 from a domestic dog showing neurological symptoms. *Braz J Microbiol*. 2021:1–8.
31. Decaro N, Martella V, Buonavoglia C. Canine adenoviruses and herpesvirus. *Vet Clin North Am Small Anim Pract*. 2008;38:799–814 (viii).
32. Decaro N. Unpublished observations.
33. Hervas J, Gomez-Villamandos JC, Perez J, et al. Focal mesangial-sclerosing glomerulonephritis and acute-spontaneous infectious canine hepatitis: structural, immunohistochemical and subcellular studies. *Vet Immunol Immunopathol*. 1997;57:25–32.
34. Morrison WI, Nash AS, Wright NG. Glomerular deposition of immune complexes in dogs following natural infection with canine adenovirus. *Vet Rec*. 1975;96:522–524.
35. Baker JA, Richards MG, Brown AL, et al. Infectious Hepatitis in Dogs. In: *Proceedings of the 87th Annual Meeting of the American Veterinary Medical Association*; 1950:242–248.
36. Ducatelle R, Maenhout D, Coussement W, et al. Dual adenovirus and distemper virus pneumonia in a dog. *Vet Q*. 1982;4:84–88.
37. Kobayashi Y, Ochiai K, Itakura C. Dual infection with canine distemper virus and infectious canine hepatitis virus (canine adenovirus type 1) in a dog. *J Vet Med Sci*. 1993;55:699–701.
38. Stookey JL, VanZwieten MJ, Whitney GD. Dual viral infections in two dogs. *J Am Vet Med Assoc*. 1972;161:1117–1121.
39. Gocke DJ, Preisig R, Morris TQ, et al. Experimental viral hepatitis in the dog: production of persistent disease in partially immune animals. *J Clin Invest*. 1967;46:1506–1517.
40. Curtis R, Barnett KC. The ocular lesions of infectious canine hepatitis. 1. Clinical features. *J Small Anim Pract*. 1973;14:375–389.
41. Curtis R, Barnett KC. Canine adenovirus-induced ocular lesions in the Afghan hound. *Cornell Vet*. 1981;71:85–95.
42. Bexfield NH, Andres-Abdo C, Scase TJ, et al. Chronic hepatitis in the English springer spaniel: clinical presentation, histological description and outcome. *Vet Rec*. 2011;169:415.
43. Boomkens SY, Slump E, Egberink HF, et al. PCR screening for candidate etiological agents of canine hepatitis. *Vet Microbiol*. 2005;108:49–55.
44. Chouinard L, Martineau D, Forget C, et al. Use of polymerase chain reaction and immunohistochemistry for detection of canine adenovirus type 1 in formalin-fixed, paraffin-embedded liver of dogs with chronic hepatitis or cirrhosis. *J Vet Diagn Invest*. 1998;10:320–325.
45. Wigton DH, Kociba GJ, Hoover EA. Infectious canine hepatitis: animal model for viral-induced disseminated intravascular coagulation. *Blood*. 1976;47:287–296.
46. Beckett SD, Burns MJ, Clark CH. A study of the blood glucose, serum transaminase, and electrophoretic patterns of dogs with infectious canine hepatitis. *Am J Vet Res*. 1964;25:1186–1190.

47. Carmichael LE. Identification of a canine adenovirus (infectious canine hepatitis virus) inhibitor in dog liver extracts as arginase. *Infect Immun.* 1972;6:348–354.
48. Assaf R, Marsolais G, Yelle J, et al. Unambiguous typing of canine adenovirus isolates by deoxyribonucleic acid restriction-endonuclease analysis. *Can J Comp Med.* 1983;47:460–463.
49. Balboni A, Dondi F, Prosperi S, et al. Development of a SYBR Green real-time PCR assay with melting curve analysis for simultaneous detection and differentiation of canine adenovirus type 1 and type 2. *J Virol Methods.* 2015;222:34–40.
50. Dowgier G, Mari V, Losurdo M, et al. A duplex real-time PCR assay based on TaqMan technology for simultaneous detection and differentiation of canine adenovirus types 1 and 2. *J Virol Methods.* 2016;234:1–6.
51. Wright NG. Interstitial nephritis in a dog associated with infectious canine hepatitis virus. *Vet Rec.* 1970;86:92–93.
52. Schultz RD, Thiel B, Mukhtar E, et al. Age and long-term protective immunity in dogs and cats. *J Comp Pathol.* 2010;142(suppl 1):S102–S108.
53. Bass EP, Gill MA, Beckenhauer WH. Evaluation of a canine adenovirus type 2 strain as a replacement for infectious canine hepatitis vaccine. *J Am Vet Med Assoc.* 1980;177:234–242.
54. Decaro N, Buonavoglia C, Barrs VR. Canine parvovirus vaccination and immunisation failures: are we far from disease eradication? *Vet Microbiol.* 2020;247:108760.
55. Day MJ, Horzinek MC, Schultz RD, et al. WSAVA Guidelines for the vaccination of dogs and cats. *J Small Anim Pract.* 2016;57:E1–E45.
56. Brown CC, Baker DC, Barker IK. Alimentary system. In: Maxie JG, ed. *Jubb, Kennedy and Palmer's Pathology of Domestic Animals.* 5th ed. Philadelphia, PA: Saunders Elsevier; 2007:1–296.
57. Caswell JL, Williams KJ. Respiratory system. In: Maxie JG, ed. *Jubb, Kennedy and Palmer's Pathology of Domestic Animals.* 5th ed. Philadelphia, PA: Saunders Elsevier; 2007:523–653.
58. Lakatos B, Farkas J, Adam E, et al. Serological evidence of adenovirus infection in cats. *Arch Virol.* 2000;145:1029–1033.
59. Lakatos B, Farkas J, Egberink HF, et al. Detection of adenovirus hexon sequence in a cat by polymerase chain reaction (short communication). *Acta Vet Hung.* 1999;47:493–497.
60. Kennedy FA. Feline adenovirus infection. In: Greene CE, ed. *Infectious Diseases of the Dog and Cat.* 2nd ed. Philadelphia, PA: WB Saunders; 1998.
61. Kennedy FA, Mullaney TP. Disseminated adenovirus infection in a cat. *J Vet Diagn Invest.* 1993;5:273–276.
62. Gupta PP. Inclusion body hepatitis in a black panther (*Panthera pardus pardus*). *Zentralbl Veterinarmed B.* 1978;25:858–860.
63. Lakatos B, Knotek Z, Farkas J, et al. Adenovirus infection in cats. An epidemiological survey in the Czech Republic. *Acta Vet Brno.* 1999;68:275–280.
64. Lakatos B, Hornyak A, Forgach P, et al. Detection of a putative novel adenovirus by PCR amplification, sequencing and phylogenetic characterisation of two gene fragments from formalin-fixed paraffin-embedded tissues of a cat diagnosed with disseminated adenovirus disease. *Acta Vet Hung.* 2017;65:574–584.

24

Canine Herpesvirus Infection

Autumn P. Davidson, Jane E. Sykes, Margret L. Casal

KEY POINTS

- Cause: CHV-1 (*Canid alphaherpesvirus 1*), genus *Varicellovirus,* subfamily *Alphaherpesvirinae,* family *Herpesviridae*, a cytocidal species-specific alphaherpesvirus. An Epstein-Barr (EBV)-like gamma herpesvirus has been described in dogs with unclear clinical significance (described separately below).
- First Described: New York, United States, 1965.[1]
- Affected Hosts: CHV-1 only infects domestic and wild Canidae. Specific receptors on the canine cell surface have been identified that contribute to this specificity.
- Geographic Distribution: The distribution of CHV-1 is worldwide. Serosurveys of wild canid populations indicate a ubiquitous exposure. The seroprevalence in domestic dogs ranges from 15% to as high as 100% in some kennels. A higher seroprevalence exists in kenneled dogs or colony dogs than in household pets.
- Route of Transmission: Direct contact with mucosal secretions from the respiratory or genital tracts of infected canids.
- Major Clinical Signs: Abortion is the main sign of CHV-1 infection in bitches. Adult dogs may show URTD and keratitis. Neonates infected with CHV-1 may develop inappetence, failure to thrive, vocalization, tachypnea, diarrhea, neurologic signs, abdominal pain, nasal discharge, weight loss, mucosal petechiation, and death.
- Differential Diagnoses: For CHV-1, major differential diagnoses are bacterial sepsis and infections with other viruses such as CDV and CPV-2.
- Human Health Significance: CHV-1 does not infect humans.

CANINE HERPESVIRUS-1

ETIOLOGIC AGENT AND EPIDEMIOLOGY

CHV-1 is a double-stranded DNA enveloped virus that belongs to the family *Herpesviridae* (Fig. 24.1). Infections with the virus have been reported from the United States, Canada, Australia, Japan, England, and Germany. The virus has a genome that is approximately 125 kb long, and to date, whole genome sequence information suggests that isolates worldwide may be genetically very similar.[2,3] CHV-1 was first recognized in the mid-1960s in association with a fatal disease in puppies.[1] It is commonly blamed for acute neonatal puppy death or failure to thrive, sometimes termed the "fading puppy syndrome." When confirmed as a cause of disease, untreated CHV-1 infection in neonates can cause high (up to 100%) mortality among littermates. There is serologic evidence of widespread exposure of domestic dogs to CHV-1 worldwide, with seroprevalences ranging from 15% to as high as 100% in some kennels. A higher seroprevalence exists in kenneled dogs or dogs from colonies than in household pets. Serosurveys of wild canid populations indicate a ubiquitous exposure.[2,4–9]

Alphaherpesviruses are cytocidal, causing tissue necrosis and localized mucosal or generalized systemic infection, most often in young or immunosuppressed animals. The replication of CHV-1 is similar to that of other alphaherpesviruses. Synthesis of viral DNA and nucleocapsids occurs within the host cell nucleus, with the viral envelope being acquired at the nuclear membrane. The virus is transported through the endoplasmic reticulum and Golgi apparatus to the cell surface and released, although most of the virus remains intracellular. CHV-1 is temperature sensitive and prefers to replicate at temperatures less than 37°C. As an enveloped virus, CHV-1 is not stable in the environment and is readily inactivated by standard disinfectants and by heat above 40°C.[10] It is maintained in nature by persistence in its canine host and direct spread from infected animals.

CHV-1 persists in the ganglionic and lymphoid tissues of the oronasal and genital mucosae. Replication and shedding occurs at mucosal surfaces where temperatures are cooler. Recovery from CHV-1 disease is believed to be associated with lifelong latent infection of the neural ganglia. Periodic reactivation of shedding can occur following immunosuppression, such as that induced by pregnancy, transportation, overcrowding, or immunosuppressive drug therapy. Factors that predispose neonatal pups to generalized infection are hypothermia during the first 2–3 weeks of life and a lack of natural immunity if the dam is unexposed.[7,10] CHV-1 infection has not been reported in cats; CHV-1 shares only 51% genetic homology with FHV-1.[11]

CLINICAL FEATURES

Pathogenesis and Clinical Signs in Adult Dogs

Respiratory infection

Transmission of CHV-1 occurs through direct contact with mucosal secretions from the respiratory or genital tracts of infected animals. The incubation period is 6 to 10 days. The virus replicates in the epithelial cells of the oronasal and pharyngeal mucosa, the genital tract, and the regional lymphatics. CHV-1 is one of the viral etiologies of CIRD complex. In a temporal study in shelter dogs, CHV-1 was found in 9.6% of BAL and 12.8% of transtracheal wash specimens from necropsied dogs with endemic respiratory illness.[12] Compared with other incriminated pathogens for which the dogs had received vaccination, CHV-1–associated illness in this report was usually more severe, and its isolation rate was usually highest 3 to 4 weeks after the dog's introduction into the kennel. Signs associated with upper respiratory infection with CHV-1 can also be mild and transient. Healthy adult dogs

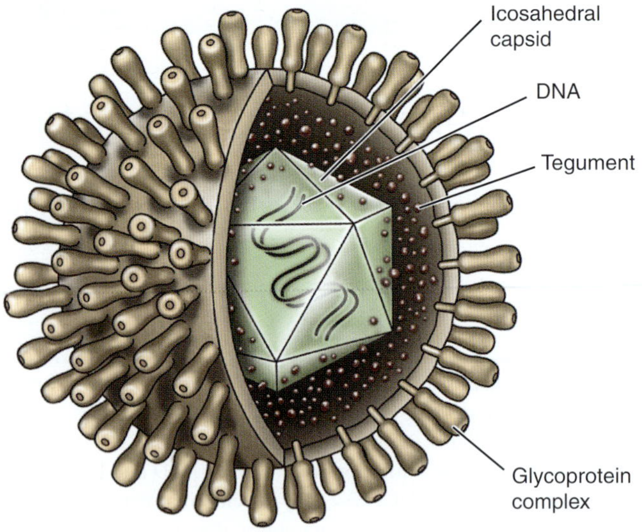

Fig. 24.1 Schematic structure of a herpesvirus. Herpesviruses are large, enveloped DNA viruses. The DNA is contained within an icosahedral capsid.

of either gender can develop mild upper respiratory signs (sneezing, serous oculonasal discharge, keratitis) for a few days but are otherwise usually clinically unaffected. The inherent immunity in a given breed of dog or in an individual dog likely plays an important role in protection against herpesvirus infections.

Genital infection

Infection with CHV-1 can cause genital infections and visible lesions in adult dogs. Primary genital infections in older bitches are characterized by lymphofollicular lesions, variable degrees of vaginal hyperemia, and occasionally petechial or ecchymotic submucosal hemorrhage (Fig. 24.2). No discomfort or vaginal discharge is noted in affected pregnant bitches, even in those that had abortions or stillbirths. Vesicular lesions have been noted during the onset of proestrus and regress during anestrus. Male dogs, with similar lesions over the base of the penis and preputial reflection, may have a preputial discharge. However, these lesions are nonspecific and not pathognomonic for CHV-1 infection. Occasionally herpesviruses have been isolated from papulovesicular lesions of the canine genital tract; such lesions may be recurrent episodes in previously infected bitches. Genital localization of the virus in bitches may be a means of venereal transmission of the virus, but it is most important as a source of infection for pups at birth. Spread of CHV-1 from seropositive males to susceptible females at the time of breeding does not appear to be a significant mode of transmission, although such a mechanism is believed to occur. Application of PCR assays has shown persistence of the virus in the lumbosacral ganglion, with presumed recrudescence and mucosal replication with subsequent shedding by the genital mucosae. Localized genital or respiratory infections and viral shedding can occur in the presence of circulating antibodies.[10]

Ocular infection

CHV-1 can be detected in conjunctival or corneal swab specimens from adult dogs. Because the prevalence of infection in apparently healthy dogs is high, associating positive test results with disease is difficult. However, CHV-1 is more prevalent in conjunctival swab specimens from dogs with conjunctivitis versus those without. Furthermore, CHV-1 has been found in dogs with naturally occurring dendritic corneal ulcerations that are considered pathognomonic lesions in other species. The development of dendritic keratitis was described in a dog with keratoconjunctivitis sicca that was treated with topical immunosuppressive drugs (cyclosporine and tacrolimus).[13] Conjunctivitis

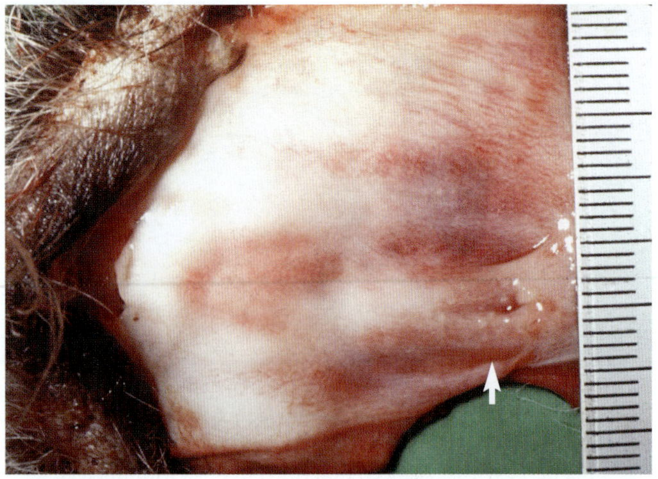

Fig. 24.2 Vaginitis associated with CHV-1 infection. *Arrow* points to a vesicular lesion. (Courtesy Akira Hashimoto, Hokkaido University, Sapporo, Japan.)

and ulcerative and nonulcerative keratitis were identified in an outbreak of ocular disease in a closed domestic dog colony; CHV-1 was incriminated as the cause by PCR and viral culture. Furthermore, experimental topical ocular inoculation of dogs produced a self-limiting ocular infection manifested by conjunctivitis and followed by latency. Infection, characterized by conjunctivitis, keratitis, and viral reshedding, was reactivated 8 months later by systemic administration of immunosuppressive doses of glucocorticoids. Topical ocular application of glucocorticoids was not associated with recrudescence of infection.[14–17]

Systemic disease

A fatal multisystemic infection by CHV-1 was reported in a 9-year-old spayed female bichon frisé with no evidence of underlying immunosuppression.[18] The dog was evaluated with clinical signs of vomiting and diarrhea, which were rapidly followed by death. At necropsy, there was multifocal necrosis with intranuclear inclusion bodies in the liver, adrenal glands, and small intestinal tract.

Pathogenesis and Clinical Signs in Fetuses and Neonates

In utero infection

Although neonatal infection usually is acquired at or soon after birth, transplacental transmission can also occur. Death of neonatal puppies younger than 1 week as a result of infection probably indicates *in utero* infection. The recently infected brood bitch generally shows no clinical signs. The effects of transplacental infection with CHV-1 depend on the stage of gestation at which infection occurs (Fig. 24.3). Resorption (apparent infertility) and abortion of stillborn or weak pups with no clinical signs in the dam have been reported. Although some puppies can survive such *in utero* infections and appear normal after delivery by cesarean section, others harbor the virus inapparently in their tissues. However, most pups develop systemic herpesvirus infection within 9 days of birth.[10]

Systemic neonatal infection

Transmission of CHV-1 can occur subsequent to close contact with infectious vaginal fluids during whelping or with vulvar or oronasal secretions in the postpartum period. Exposure of a naïve bitch to CHV-1 during the last 3 weeks of gestation results either in late-term abortion of a litter, or neonatal disease or death within the first few weeks of life, because inadequate periparturient maternal antibodies exist to allow passive immunity to be acquired by the neonates.

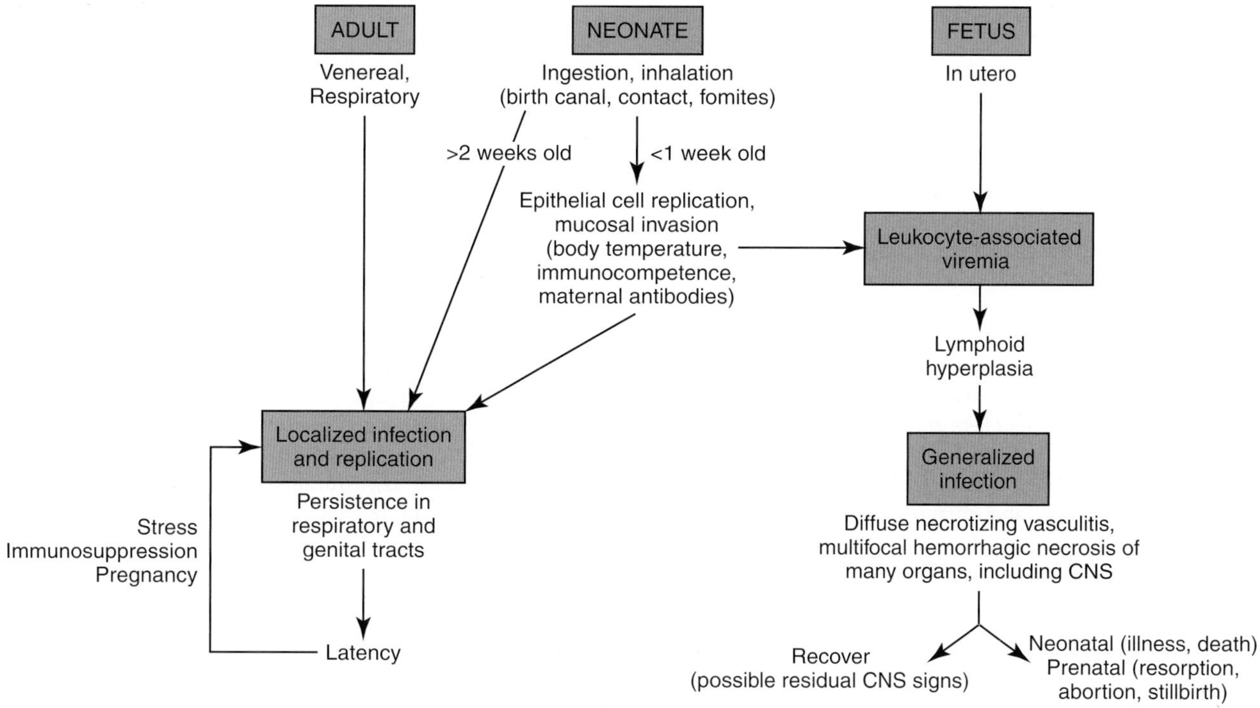

Fig. 24.3 Pathogenesis of canine herpesvirus-1 infection.

Puppies born to a naïve bitch may also become infected as a result of contact with other dogs in the home or kennel that shed virus. Neonatal CHV-1 infection is usually associated with an acute and fatal illness, primarily between 1 and 3 weeks of age. Immunity acquired from the dam appears to be important in the survival of infected neonates, as those suckling seropositive bitches can become subclinically infected while shedding virus from the oropharynx. The existence of maternal antibodies or immune lymphocytes acquired from milk may explain why naturally infected pregnant bitches that give birth to diseased puppies subsequently give birth to healthy litters. Serum antibody titers in previously infected pregnant bitches may also suppress viremia and spread of infection to the fetus.

CHV-1 replicates in the epithelial cells of the neonatal oronasal and pharyngeal mucosa, the genital tract, and the regional lymphatics. Replication and spread of the virus are facilitated by the presence of a low body temperature (33°C–35°C), which is present in oral and genital mucous membranes and in canine neonates. Temperature regulation of the newborn pup is not developed until 2 to 3 weeks of age, and neonatal rectal temperature is usually 1°C to 1.5°C (2°F to 3°F) lower than that of the adult dog. In addition to having a reduced capacity for temperature regulation, neonatal pups are incapable of an adequate febrile response. Cell-mediated immune functions are also suppressed at temperatures lower than 39°C, rendering hypothermic pups more susceptible to CHV-1 infection. The virus then enters the bloodstream by way of macrophages. Cell-associated viremia develops within 3 to 4 days of inoculation. Virus localization in the mononuclear phagocytic cells of the lymph nodes and spleen results in lymphoid hyperplasia and necrosis. Progressive multifocal hemorrhagic necrosis occurs in several organs; the highest concentrations of virus are found in the adrenal glands, kidneys, lungs, spleen, and liver. Lesions may be related to the vasculitis and marked thrombocytopenia that occurs during infection. Thrombocytopenia can result from DIC associated with widespread vascular endothelial damage and tissue necrosis. Ganglioneuritis of the trigeminal nerve is a frequent lesion in puppies infected by oronasal exposure. Meningoencephalitis can also occur in neonatal puppies,[19] but CNS signs are not always apparent. Puppies usually die from systemic illness before neurologic signs appear.

Clinical signs in the neonate are not specific and include incessant vocalization, poor nursing effort (with weight loss), diarrhea, and serous to hemorrhagic nasal discharge. Despite the muscular activity associated with crying, restlessness, and shivering, no increase in body temperature typically occurs. Neonates lose consciousness and may have opisthotonos and seizures just before death. Rectal temperatures become subnormal terminally, typically within 24 to 48 hours after the onset of clinical illness.

Some neonates develop mild clinical disease and subsequently recover. Ocular involvement was described in one recovering puppy.[20] Animals that survive systemic infection may develop persistent neurologic signs; normal survivors have also been reported.[21] Persistent shedding of CHV-1 for several weeks after recovery has been documented in recovering puppies.[20] Older (> 3 to 5 weeks of age) puppies exposed to CHV-1 may develop subclinical infection, or the course of disease may be less severe as a result of their ability to mount a febrile response. Latent infection also may develop.

Physical Examination Findings

Physical examination findings in dogs with URTD associated with CHV-1 infection may include cough and/or serous to mucopurulent ocular and nasal discharge. Genital infections in bitches may be manifested as lymphofollicular or papulovesicular lesions, vaginal hyperemia, and occasionally petechial or ecchymotic submucosal hemorrhage (see Fig. 24.2). Vesicular lesions have been noted during the onset of proestrus and regress during anestrus. Male dogs can also develop vesicular lesions over the base of the penis and preputial reflection, which are sometimes accompanied by preputial discharge. Dogs with ocular infections due to CHV-1 can show signs of blepharitis, conjunctivitis, ulcerative and nonulcerative keratitis, dendritic ulceration, and serous to mucopurulent ocular discharge.

CHV-1–infected neonates may have petechiation of the mucous membranes and an erythematous rash with papules or vesicles and subcutaneous edema of the ventral abdominal and inguinal region. Vesicles may be present in the vulva and vagina of female puppies, the prepuce of males, and the buccal cavity. An increased respiratory effort with tachypnea and vocalization is common. Abdominal distension and pain upon abdominal palpation occurs. Normal orientation and localization toward the dam is lacking, and the suckle reflex can be diminished.

DIAGNOSIS

Diagnosis of ocular, respiratory, and reproductive infection by CHV-1 in adult dogs usually involves application of NAATs to clinical specimens, but again there may be challenges distinguishing between positive tests due to latency or subclinical exposure and those associated with disease.

Antemortem diagnosis of CHV-1 infection in neonates can be challenging. Necropsy of at least one deceased littermate for diagnostic testing is usually required. A timely diagnosis facilitates correct therapeutic decisions and directs proper kennel management.

Laboratory Abnormalities

Hematologic and biochemical abnormalities in dogs with herpesvirus infections are nonspecific, but marked thrombocytopenia can be observed in neonatal puppies. A marked increase in the activity of serum ALT can be found in infected neonates.

Microbiologic Tests

Virus Isolation

CHV-1 can be isolated from several parenchymal organs of puppies that have died of acute systemic infection but is most commonly isolated from the adrenal glands, kidneys, lungs, spleen, lymph nodes, and liver. In animals that have recovered or are older, growth of CHV-1 is usually restricted to the oral mucosa, upper respiratory tract, and external genitalia. As noted, recrudescence of virus shedding may be provoked by administration of immunosuppressive doses of glucocorticoids and may also be precipitated by stressful situations, such as the introduction of unfamiliar dogs into a kennel. CHV-1 grows only in cultured cells of canine origin, primarily in dog kidney cells at an optimal temperature range of 35°C to 37°C. CHV-1 produces Cowdry type A intranuclear inclusions, which can be difficult to demonstrate and are most readily identified in tissues that have been fixed in Bouin's solution. FA techniques, electron microscopy, and PCR can be used to detect CHV in cell cultures. Diagnosis by virus isolation takes several days.[10]

Serologic Diagnosis

Antibody titers to CHV-1 are usually determined using virus neutralization assays. Neutralizing antibodies increase after infection and remain high for only 1 to 2 months; low titers may be detected for at least 2 years. Seropositivity indicates exposure, not necessarily active infection, although viral persistence and latent infection might be presumed. Serologic tests are not standardized, resulting in variation in results among laboratories. The main application of serologic diagnostic assays is in outbreak investigations, and acute and convalescent serologic testing may be required to document recent infections.

Molecular Diagnosis Using Nucleic Acid–Based Testing

Tissues obtained at necropsy, ocular or genital swabs, or respiratory lavage specimens (for dogs with respiratory disease) can be submitted for rapid molecular diagnosis using CHV-1–specific PCR assays. Nucleic acid detection has been evaluated in suspected cases of spontaneous CHV-1 infection and is the most reliable means of detecting latent infection in older animals. Nested PCR and *in situ* hybridization have been used to detect virus in formalin-fixed, paraffin-embedded tissues from naturally infected puppies.[22,23] In one study, real-time PCR was used to detect the shedding of CHV-1 in nasal and ocular secretions of puppies that recovered from systemic CHV-1 infection; other puppies in the litter died and CHV-1 was detected in the kidney, liver, lung and brain tissue.[20] Viral nucleic acid has been found within nuclei adjacent to and within hemorrhagic lesions in pups. Many epithelial cells, neurons, fibrocytes, cardiac myocytes, and hepatocytes contain virus. Nucleic acid testing for CHV-1 is offered by some university and commercial laboratories; clinicians should be aware of availability and turnaround time. Unfortunately, false-negative results have been observed from different laboratories or with different sampling methodologies and reduced viral load during latency; false-positive results can occur because of the high prevalence of clinically healthy dogs that are carriers of the virus.

Pathologic Findings

Gross Pathologic Findings

Gross changes in the kidneys at necropsy of pups infected with CHV-1 include multifocal petechial to ecchymotic subcapsular hemorrhages. The pleural surfaces may be mottled pink and red due to coagulation necrosis (Fig. 24.4A–D). Multifocal random acute necrosis of other organs, including the liver, pancreas, intestine, and adrenal glands, may also be apparent. Lesions may resemble those of bacterial sepsis.

Histopathologic Findings

Histopathology can be used to confirm CHV-1 infection in neonates but may be unrewarding if the timing of specimen collection is not optimal. Characteristic viral intranuclear inclusion bodies can be difficult to find. Histopathologic evaluation commonly reveals severe nephrosis (proximal renal tubular epithelial necrosis and renal pelvic epithelial apoptosis with swollen vesicular nuclei); diffuse severe hepatic congestion and inflammation with vacuolar hepatopathy (neutrophilic, histiocytic, and lymphocytic infiltration with apoptosis); acute severe necrotizing bronchointerstitial pneumonia with pulmonary edema and hemorrhage (terminal bronchiolar hemorrhage and edema with fibrin accumulation, macrophage infiltration, necrosis, and alveolar disruption); and thymic, lymph node, and splenic lympholysis (severe diffuse cortical lympholysis with sinus congestion). Findings on examination of the CNS include multifocal glial nodules, cerebellar cortical necrosis, and meningeal inflammation, although the inflammatory reaction may be minimal. Depending on the stage of cellular infection and method of fixation, basophilic or acidophilic inclusions may be noted, but they are less commonly identified than those found in other herpesvirus infections. Inclusions are more readily seen in the nasal epithelium or kidney than in areas of widespread necrosis, such as the lung or liver.[10] *In situ* hybridization has been used to document the location of CHV-1 DNA in the brain of affected neonates and showed nucleic acid in the granule neurons of the cerebellum, meningeal, and parenchymal endothelial cells, and randomly distributed neurons.[19]

TREATMENT AND PROGNOSIS

Respiratory and Ocular Infections

Treatment of respiratory infections typically requires only supportive care. Ocular disease caused by CHV-1 has been treated with topical idoxuridine, trifluridine, and cidofovir(see Chapter 9). Treatment with 0.5% cidofovir twice daily for 14 days decreased shedding but was associated with worsening of ocular signs, so it is not recommended.[24] Treatment of experimentally infected dogs with topical trifluridine six times daily for 2 days and then four times daily for 12 days led to reduction in clinical signs and viral shedding when compared with a placebo group, without evidence of toxicity.[25] In dogs that were experimentally infected with CHV-1, the application of topical ophthalmic 0.15% ganciclovir gel (one drop five times daily for 7 days, then one drop three times daily for 7 days) was effective in reducing clinical disease scores when compared with an untreated control group and was well tolerated.[13]

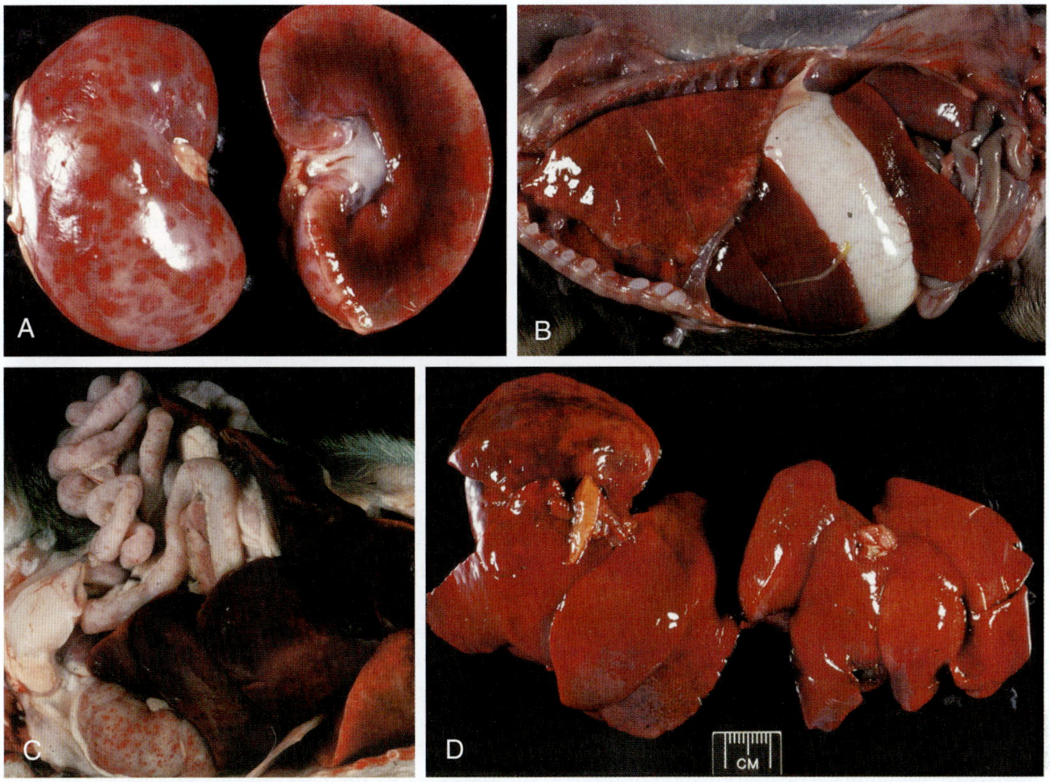

Fig. 24.4 (A) Kidneys from 12-day-old mastiff puppy from a litter of 17 puppies, 14 of which died. CHV-1 was isolated from the puppy. Gross changes include subcapsular hemorrhagic foci typical of (but not pathognomonic for) herpetic nephritis. On cut section, white and red cortical streaks are evident; a hemorrhagic medulla is evident. (B) Multifocal pink and red pleural mottling in the puppy described in A. Serosanguinous pleural fluid was present. Histopathology identified multiple areas of pulmonary necrosis and bronchopneumonia. (C) Small-intestinal serosal petechiation in the same puppy. Histopathology identified enterocyte necrosis consistent with CHV-1 infection. (D) Liver of the same puppy showing uniform firmness and diffuse mottle with rounded edges. Histopathology identified scattered multiple foci of acute hepatic coagulation necrosis; eosinophilic intranuclear inclusions typical of herpesviral inclusions were seen within viable hepatocytes. (Images courtesy JR Peauroi.)

Neonatal Infections

Treatment of puppies with CHV-1 infection is often unrewarding and rarely effective due the rapid progression of fulminant clinical signs. Residual cardiac and neurologic damage may occur in recovered animals. This possibility must be discussed with owners before considering antiviral treatment of an infected litter. Treatment of affected puppies with immune serum from seroconverted dams has been described but is typically ineffective. In some cases, mortality can be reduced during an outbreak by treating puppies with 1 to 2 mL of immune sera given intraperitoneally. Immune sera can be obtained by pooling sera from bitches that had recently given birth to litters of puppies that died of CHV-1 infection. Only one dose is required because of the short susceptibility period. This seems to reduce mortality, but its success depends on the presence of adequate levels of serum antibodies and administration of the sera *before* full development of systemic disease. If neurologic signs have already developed, they will likely persist.[10] Under experimental conditions in which body temperatures were elevated artificially *before* exposure to virus, puppies had reduced mortality, less severe clinical signs, and minimal pathologic changes. At elevated temperatures, viral growth in tissues was restricted compared with growth in conventionally reared pups. Pretreatment by raising ambient temperature could be considered for exposed but as yet unaffected puppies in a litter.[10]

An incompletely developed immune system and inadequate thermoregulation during the first days of life means neonates are vulnerable to systemic infection (by both bacterial and viral pathogens). The umbilicus of neonates should be treated with tincture of iodine immediately after birth to reduce contamination and prevent bacterial ascent into the peritoneal cavity (omphalitis-peritonitis). Neonatal bacterial peritonitis with bacteremia can cause rapid neonatal death if not recognized and treated promptly. Factors that predispose puppies to bacteremia and sepsis include endometritis in the bitch, a prolonged delivery/dystocia, feeding of replacement formulas, the use of ampicillin, stress, low birth weight (<350 g), and hypothermia with body temperatures less than 35.5°C (95°F). Bacterial organisms most frequently associated with bacteremia are *Escherichia coli*, streptococci, staphylococci, and *Klebsiella* spp. Commonly, a decrease in weight gain, failure to suckle, hematuria, persistent diarrhea, unusual vocalization, abdominal distention and pain, and sloughing of the extremities indicate sepsis. These signs are similar to those encountered with CHV-1 infection. Prompt therapy with broad-spectrum, bactericidal antibiotics; optimal nutrition via supported nursing, tube feeding, or bottle feeding; maintenance of body temperature; and appropriate fluid replacement are indicated. The third-generation cephalosporin ceftiofur sodium is an appropriate choice for treatment of neonatal sepsis.

Failure of a pup with the tentative diagnosis of neonatal sepsis to respond to antibacterial drug treatment should prompt consideration of CHV-1 infection. Specific antiviral therapy, if instituted in a timely manner, may reduce mortality from CHV-1 (see Chapter 9). Treatment of systemic CHV-1 infection with antiviral drugs such as 5-iodo-2-deoxyuridine has been unsuccessful, and few studies have been performed on newer antiviral agents that are effective for treatment of localized and CNS herpes simplex virus (HSV) infections in humans and laboratory animals. In one study, two 15-day-old pups died of CHV-1 infection. Five littermates were given a course of vidarabine as soon as the cause of the deaths was identified, and they all survived. The surviving pups had high (>1:64) neutralizing antibody titers 2 months later, indicating that they had been infected.[26] Vidarabine (cidofovir) is only available as a compounded ophthalmic solution. Acyclovir has activity against HSV (Table 24.1). Its use in dogs has not been well studied; one case report exists describing survival of 4 litter mates following confirmation of CHV-1 in 2 deceased 25-day-old puppies.[21] Valacyclovir, an acyclovir prodrug, increases bioavailability in humans to 50%. The efficacy of famciclovir, a prodrug for penciclovir, for treatment of CHV-1 infection requires further study, but the pharmacokinetics of famciclovir in dogs resembles that in humans; much lower doses may be required when compared with cats. Bovine lactoferrin, an iron-binding antimicrobial component of milk, has been reported to inhibit CHV in vitro experimentally. Lactoferrin is commercially available as a component of a topical product (Zymox) for dermatological application; its use on neonatal oronasal mucosa has been suggested if CHV exposure is suspected.[27]

IMMUNITY AND VACCINATION

Minimal transplacental transfer of immunity occurs in the dog. Adequate ingestion of colostrum must occur immediately postpartum for puppies to acquire passive immunity. The transmission of protective passive immunity (placental or colostral antibodies) to puppies depends on the prior existence of adequate serum maternal antibodies. Therefore, breeding bitches with exposure to CHV-1 earlier in life have the best opportunity to seroconvert and develop protective antibodies. This commonly occurs in kennels or at crowded canine events such as dog shows and trials. Documentation of an antibody titer to CHV-1 generally indicates the presence of adequate maternal antibodies.

Unexposed bitches must be strictly isolated from potential exposure during gestation and for at least 6 weeks postpartum to prevent acquisition and transmission of the virus to the fetus or neonates. Subsequent litters of the infected pregnant or postpartum bitch are usually normal because of acquisition of maternal antibodies; however, reactivation of maternal viral infection with stress, pregnancy, and immunosuppressive drugs has been reported.[28,29]

Because CHV-1 infects pups *in utero* or as neonates, active immunization can be considered only in the dam. Development of vaccines for CHV-1 has been hampered by the poor immunogenicity characteristic of the herpesviral vaccines developed for other species, such as FHV-1 vaccines. Immunization with a commercially inactivated vaccine in Europe resulted in fourfold increases in virus neutralization titers in most vaccinated dogs, but did not appear to provide long-term protection.[10] A lyophilized, inactivated, purified CHV-1 strain F205 vaccine prepared with enriched glycoproteins was used to vaccinate SPF bitches 10 days postcoitus and 6 weeks later near the end of gestation. The near-term booster was used to enhance the short-lived humoral response. As analyzed by PCR, 100% of pups born to these bitches were protected against clinical illness when challenged oronasally with CHV-1 at 3 days of age; in most instances (93.5% of 31 pups) they were also protected against viral infection. In contrast, a majority of challenged control pups (81% of 31 pups) died of generalized CHV disease between 6 and 14 days after challenge.[30] The vaccinated bitches and litters were kenneled with the control bitches and litters. A subunit vaccine using this inactivated strain is licensed for use in some European countries (Eurican Herpes 205, Boehringer Ingelheim, Germany). Revaccination with two doses of the vaccine is recommended at each pregnancy. In one study, adult dogs with experimentally induced latent CHV-1 infection were vaccinated and then treated with glucocorticoids in order to reactivate infection and disease. Vaccination did not prevent disease or viral shedding, but was associated with reduced clinical scores within a 2-week period after vaccination, and improved long-term (34 weeks) immune responses to the virus.[31] The vaccine is not currently available in the United States. Vaccination of naïve bitches before whelping makes sense; the effect of this vaccination on litters from previously seroconverted bitches needs to be demonstrated in a controlled study.

PREVENTION

On a practical basis, eradication of CHV-1 from a kennel is impossible. Screening for infected animals also is impractical, and owners should be advised that subsequent litters from an affected bitch have a very low risk of developing clinical illness. Accordingly, cesarean delivery or artificial insemination is not justified to reduce spread of infection. Artificial insemination could be used when a male that is known or suspected to be infected is bred to a primiparous naïve bitch, but the benefit of such a practice has not been studied.

As a preventive practice, care should be taken to ensure that the environmental temperature of newborn puppies is kept warm with heated whelping boxes, heat lamps, or other warming devices that do not cause excessive dehydration. Mild to absent clinical signs are

TABLE 24.1 Treatment for Canine Herpesvirus Infections

Drug	Dose	Route	Interval	Duration	Indication
Acyclovir[a]	10 mg/kg (0.01 mg/g)	Oral	q6h	5–7 days	Neonatal infections[b]
Famciclovir (feline)	90 mg/kg	Oral	q12h		Ocular infections
Lactoferrin (oral solution in spray form)		Swab oral mucosa	q12h		Suggested preventative approach in exposed puppies, evidence unclear
Trifluridine solution (1%)	One drop	Topical ophthalmic	Six times daily for 2 days, then four times daily for 12 days	14 days	Ocular infections
Ganciclovir gel (0.15%)	One drop	Topical ophthalmic	Five times daily for 7 days, then three times daily for 7 days	14 days	Ocular infections

[a]Available as 200-mg capsules. Contents of capsule are added to 10 mL of warm water. The powder does not dissolve; however, each pup receives 0.5 mL (10 mg) of the suspension orally every 6 hours. Famciclovir may be a safer and more efficacious choice for systemic treatment (see Chapter 9).
[b]Because of the small size of neonates, fluids or plasma therapy may have to be given intraperitoneally, intraosseously, or subcutaneously rather than the preferred intravenous route. Additional warming of the animals is essential.

common in dogs that have recovered from CHV-1 infection, with occasional rhinitis, vaginitis, or balanoposthitis. Viral shedding for 1 week generally ensues with introduction of new dogs in a kennel (stress), during concurrent illnesses, or in a dog with drug-induced immunosuppression. Such dogs can act as reservoirs of infection for neonates and should be separated from new litters. Clinically affected puppies shed large quantities of virus in their secretions for 2 to 3 weeks after recovery. Virus persists for only short periods in respiratory or vaginal secretions, so its spread is most common through immediate direct contact with infected animals or through fomites. CHV-1 outbreaks causing reproductive problems are most likely in large, open commercial breeding operations. Private breeders have the best success in avoiding exposure of naïve bitches and their offspring by operating a closed kennel during breeding.

PUBLIC HEALTH ASPECTS

In general, herpesviruses are very host specific, and CHV-1 is not known to infect humans.

CANINE GAMMAHERPESVIRUS

ETIOLOGIC AGENT AND EPIDEMIOLOGY

Gammaherpesviruses belong to the subfamily *Gammaherpesvirinae*. In humans, the primary gammaherpesviruses of disease significance are Epstein-Barr virus (EBV) (human gammaherpesvirus 4) and Kaposi's sarcoma-associated herpesvirus (human gammaherpesvirus 8). EBV is the cause of infectious mononucleosis and has been associated with a variety of lymphoproliferative disorders, nonlymphoid malignancies, and autoimmune conditions. Kaposi's sarcoma-associated herpesvirus causes nodular mass lesions in the skin, lymph nodes, and sometimes other organs.

Gammaherpesviruses can latently infect lymphocytes and cause lytic infections of epithelial cells and fibroblasts. Only a few studies have examined the prevalence and importance of gammaherpesvirus infections in dogs by examining blood and tissues for either gammaherpesviral, EBV or EBV-like particles, DNA, RNA, or antibodies.[32–40] Serologic evidence exists that dogs are exposed to gammaherpesviruses, and there is preliminary evidence of an EBV-like herpesvirus within B cells in dogs with malignancies.[34] Other studies suggest that gammaherpesviruses do not cause malignancies in dogs.[37,39]

In Taiwanese dogs, antibodies against EBV-specific polymerase, EBV-encoded DNA binding protein and EBV-specific thymidine kinase proteins were present in 10, 15, and 32 of 36 dogs tested, respectively.[32] When the presence of EBV-like DNA was investigated in both serum and WBC of 21 of these dogs, all serum samples were negative, but 15 WBC samples were positive for a partial EBV sequence using molecular testing. Serum antibodies were not present in all dogs with positive EBV-like viral DNA in their WBCs suggesting that latent infections may be possible in dogs.[32] Gammaherpesviruses have been detected in other carnivores, namely the lion (*Panthera leo*) and the spotted hyena (*Crocuta crocuta*) (the latter being more closely related to the dog) using PCR detection of both gammaherpesvirus-specific polymerase and glycoprotein B genes.[33] Another study aimed to determine the prevalence of EBV infection in dogs in the United Kingdom ($n = 112$) and the United States ($n = 104$) using serology and PCR to detect EBV in various tissue specimens.[36] An IFA demonstrated serum antibodies against EBV or EBV-like viruses in about a third of the British dogs and two thirds of the American dogs. All blood samples, lymphoma specimens, and all but one tonsil specimens were negative by PCR for EBV DNA. A study from Italy examined the prevalence of gammaherpesvirus infection in blood donor dogs. All nested PCRs performed to detect viral DNA in 54 dogs were negative.[35] However, as in other studies, the number of animals sampled was relatively small.

EBV is implicated as a contributor to idiopathic pulmonary fibrosis in humans, multinodular pulmonary fibrosis in horses, and pulmonary fibrosis in an experimental mouse model by causing epithelial injury.[40] There has been interest in a possible association between gammaherpesvirus infection and canine idiopathic pulmonary fibrosis (CIPF) in the West Highland white terrier.[38] Blood and lung specimens were obtained from affected and control dogs and tested for the presence of alpha-, beta-, and gamma-herpesviral DNA encoding a highly conserved region of a polymerase gene (*DOPL*) by PCR. None of the samples were positive.[38] However, the DNA was extracted from paraffin-embedded lung tissue, which often yields low-quality DNA.

More importantly, EBV in humans is associated with epithelial and hematological malignancies. This raises the question whether EBV or EBV-like gammaherpesvirus could be associated with malignancies in dogs. Two studies were unable to detect gammaherpesviral particles using a specific and degenerate PCRs in tissues and blood of dogs with lymphoma despite the presence of serum antibodies against EBV.[36,39] In another study, DNA was extracted from paraffin-embedded canine mammary tumors to study the relationship between EBV infections and malignancies.[37] Only one of 47 specimens examined was positive by nested PCR for the presence of viral DNA. EBV-like viral DNA and RNA as well as latent membrane protein-1 were detected in malignant lymph nodes from dogs with lymphoma.[34] Adding weight to evidence for a possible association between this infection and malignancy was the finding that the highest serum antibody titers were found in those dogs with B-cell lymphoma.[34]

Further studies will be needed to determine the pathogenicity of EBV, EBV-like, or other gammaherpesviruses in dogs and their association with canine malignancies. Currently, antibody titers and molecular assays for the detection of gammaherpesvirus infections are only performed in specialized laboratories.[35] Should a gammaherpesvirus be established as a cause or contributor to some types of lymphoma in dogs, treatment of lymphoma in dogs using chemotherapy alone may need to be reevaluated. In human patients with EBV infections, treatments such as adoptive immunotherapy (with EBV-specific cytotoxic T cells) have been used with some success, but use of antiviral drugs has been met with limited success.[41]

CASE EXAMPLE

Signalment

Two, 25-day-old female Labrador retriever puppies from a litter of eight whelped at a guide dog kennel in San Rafael, California.

History

Whelping was directly observed and occurred without incident; the pups showed normal weight gain (checked twice daily) and behavior until the last 24 hours. The litter nursed from birth, and the dam was normal. The dam was housed in a private home until a week prepartum, then was kenneled in the whelping facility with five other bitches in separate runs. Four days previously, the litter was vaccinated with an intranasal *Bordetella bronchiseptica* vaccine and dewormed with pyrantel pamoate according to routine preventative healthcare practice.

Current Medications

None.

Continued

CASE EXAMPLE—cont'd

Physical Examination

Physical examination of both puppies revealed hypothermia (rectal temperature 36.3°C [97°F] and 36.0°C [97°F], respectively), tachypnea, a markedly tense abdomen, and continuous vocalization.

Differential Diagnosis

Bacterial sepsis (*Escherichia coli, Streptococcus, Staphylococcus,* and *Klebsiella* most commonly), infections with CHV-1, *Bordetella bronchiseptica*, CAdV-2, CPIV, *Brucella canis*, CDV, *Neospora caninum, Toxoplasma gondii*.

Laboratory Findings

Fecal Examination: Negative for parasites or ova.

Necropsy Findings

Despite supportive care (exogenous warming, supplemental feeding with artificial bitch's milk [Esbilac Pet Ag, Inc.], subcutaneous lactated Ringer's solution, and ceftiofur sodium [2.5 mg/kg SC q12h]), the puppies died within 12 hours and then underwent necropsy examination. Tissues collected for histopathologic evaluation included kidney, liver, lung, thymus, mesenteric lymph node, and spleen.

Because of gross findings of hemorrhagic foci in the lungs and kidneys, renal tissue was submitted for a CHV-1–specific PCR assay. The PCR assay confirmed the presence of CHV-1 DNA in the renal tissue. Gross (foci of hemorrhage in the lungs and kidneys) and histopathologic evaluations of the deceased puppies were typical of CHV-1 but were not confirmatory because of the similarity of findings to those of neonatal bacterial sepsis. The presence of intranuclear inclusion bodies were suspected in macrophages from the lung of one puppy. Aerobic bacterial culture of the peritoneal cavity was negative for bacterial growth.

Diagnosis

Neonatal CHV-1 infection.

Treatment

Poor weight gain and vocalization were reported in two additional puppies. The primary differential diagnoses included neonatal bacteremia and CHV-1 infection. Because of the lack of response to therapy for bacterial infection in the two deceased puppies, the remaining six puppies were treated with acyclovir suspension (20 mg/kg PO q6h) for 7 days, and exogenous warming adequate to raise the rectal temperature to just above 37.7°C (100°F). Therapy was initiated the day before the PCR assay confirmed infection with CHV-1.

All six treated puppies survived and were successfully weaned between 5 and 6 weeks of age. All were placed in private homes and had uneventful subsequent health histories and normal behavior. Physical examinations including complete fundic evaluations were performed at 12 to 14 months of age and were normal in all. Two of the dogs have become active guide dogs for the blind, and one is an assistance dog for the hearing impaired. All remain physically normal at more than 26 months of age.

Comments

The epizootiology of this outbreak suggests that the puppies were born from a naïve bitch and exposed to CHV-1 from another carrier dog at days 14 to 17 after birth. Two of eight (25%) succumbed to the disease; two of the remaining six showed early clinical signs, after which antiviral therapy was initiated for all dogs.

SUGGESTED READINGS

England GCW. Clinical approach to the infertile bitch. In: England G, von Heimendahl A, eds. *BSAVA Manual of Canine and Feline Reproduction and Neonatology*. 2nd ed. England: BSAVA; 2010:51–63.

Casal M. Management and critical care of the neonate. In: England G, von Heimendahl A, eds. *BSAVA Manual of Canine and Feline Reproduction and Neonatology*. 2nd ed. England: BSAVA; 2010:135–165.

Kauffman LK, Baldwin CJ. Pregnancy loss in the bitch and queen. In: Bonagura JD, Twedt DC, eds. *Kirk's Current Veterinary Therapy XV*. St, Louis, MO: Elsevier; 2014:1003–1015.

Andrei G, Trompet E, Snoeck R. Novel therapeutics for Epstein-Barr virus. *Molecules*. 2019;24.

REFERENCES

1. Carmichael LE, Squire RA, Krook L. Clinical and pathologic features of a fatal viral disease of newborn pups. *Am J Vet Res*. 1965;26:803–814.
2. Papageorgiou KV, Suarez NM, Wilkie GS, et al. Genome sequence of canine herpesvirus. *PloS One*. 2016;11:e0156015.
3. Sarker S, Das S, Helbig K, et al. Genome sequence of an Australian strain of canid alphaherpesvirus 1. *Aust Vet J*. 2018;96:24–27.
4. Almberg ES, Mech LD, Smith DW, et al. A serological survey of infectious disease in Yellowstone National Park's canid community. *PloS One*. 2009;4:e7042.
5. Robinson AJ, Crerar SK, Waight Sharma N, et al. Prevalence of serum antibodies to canine adenovirus and canine herpesvirus in the European red fox (*Vulpes vulpes*) in Australia. *Aust Vet J*. 2005;83:356–361.
6. Nothling JO, Hussy D, Steckler D, et al. Seroprevalence of canine herpesvirus in breeding kennels in the Gauteng Province of South Africa. *Theriogenology*. 2008;69:276–282.
7. Ronsse V, Verstegen J, Onclin K, et al. Risk factors and reproductive disorders associated with canine herpesvirus-1 (CHV-1). *Theriogenology*. 2004;61:619–636.
8. Yesilbag K, Yalcin E, Tuncer P, et al. Seroprevalence of canine herpesvirus-1 in Turkish dog population. *Res Vet Sci*. 2012;92:36–39.
9. Ronsse V, Verstegen J, Onclin K, et al. Seroprevalence of canine herpesvirus-1 in the Belgian dog population in 2000. *Reprod Domest Anim*. 2002;37:299–304.
10. Greene CE. Canine herpesvirus infection. In: Greene CE, ed. *Infectious Diseases of the Dog and Cat*. 4 ed. Philadelphia, PA: WB Saunders; 2011:48–54.
11. Rota PA, Maes RK. Homology between feline herpesvirus-1 and canine herpesvirus. *Arch Virol*. 1990;115:139–145.
12. Erles K, Dubovi EJ, Brooks HW, et al. Longitudinal study of viruses associated with canine infectious respiratory disease. *J Clin Microbiol*. 2004;42:4524–4529.
13. Ledbetter EC, Nicklin AM, Spertus CB, et al. Evaluation of topical ophthalmic ganciclovir gel for the treatment of dogs with experimentally induced ocular canine herpesvirus-1 infection. *Am J Vet Res*. 2018;79:762–769.
14. Ledbetter EC, Dubovi EJ, Kim SG, et al. Experimental primary ocular canine herpesvirus-1 infection in adult dogs. *Am J Vet Res*. 2009;70:513–521.
15. Ledbetter EC, Hornbuckle WE, Dubovi EJ. Virologic survey of dogs with naturally acquired idiopathic conjunctivitis. *J Am Vet Med Assoc*. 2009;235:954–959.
16. Ledbetter EC, Kice NC, Matusow RB, et al. The effect of topical ocular corticosteroid administration in dogs with experimentally induced latent canine herpesvirus-1 infection. *Exp Eye Res*. 2010;90:711–717.
17. Ledbetter EC, Kim SG, Dubovi EJ. Outbreak of ocular disease associated with naturally-acquired canine herpesvirus-1 infection in a closed domestic dog colony. *Vet Ophthalmol*. 2009;12:242–247.
18. Gadsden BJ, Maes RK, Wise AG, et al. Fatal Canid herpesvirus 1 infection in an adult dog. *J Vet Diagn Invest*. 2012;24:604–607.
19. Jager MC, Sloma EA, Shelton M, et al. Naturally acquired canine herpesvirus-associated meningoencephalitis. *Vet Pathol*. 2017;54:820–827.
20. Losurdo M, Dowgier G, Lucente MS, et al. Long-term shedding of Canine alphaherpesvirus 1 in naturally infected newborn pups. *Res Vet Sci*. 2018;119:244–246.
21. Davidson AP, Grundy SA, Foley JE. Successful medical management of neonatal canine herpes: a case report. *Comm Therio*. 2003;3.

22. Decaro N, Amorisco F, Desario C, et al. Development and validation of a real-time PCR assay for specific and sensitive detection of canid herpesvirus 1. *J Virol Methods*. 2010;169:176–180.
23. Kim O. Optimization of in situ hybridization assay using non-radioactive DNA probes for the detection of canine herpesvirus (CHV) in paraffin-embedded sections. *J Vet Sci*. 2004;5:71–73.
24. Ledbetter EC, Spertus CB, Pennington MR, et al. In vitro and in vivo evaluation of cidofovir as a topical ophthalmic antiviral for ocular canine herpesvirus-1 infections in dogs. *J Ocul Pharmacol Ther*. 2015;31:642–649.
25. Spertus CB, Mohammed HO, Ledbetter EC. Effects of topical ocular application of 1% trifluridine ophthalmic solution in dogs with experimentally induced recurrent ocular canine herpesvirus-1 infection. *Am J Vet Res*. 2016;77:1140–1147.
26. Carmichael LE, Greene CE. Canine herpesvirus infection. In: Greene CE, ed. *Infectious Diseases of the Dog and Cat*. Philadelphia, PA: WB Saunders; 1990:252–258.
27. Tanaka T, Nakatani S, Xuan X, et al. Antiviral activity of lactoferrin against canine herpesvirus. *Antiviral Res*. 2003;60:193–199.
28. Malone EK, Ledbetter EC, Rassnick KM, et al. Disseminated canine herpesvirus-1 infection in an immunocompromised adult dog. *J Vet Intern Med*. 2010;24:965–968.
29. Okuda Y, Hashimoto A, Yamaguchi T, et al. Repeated canine herpesvirus (CHV) reactivation in dogs by an immunosuppressive drug. *Cornell Vet*. 1993;83:291–302.
30. Poulet H, Guigal PM, Soulier M, et al. Protection of puppies against canine herpesvirus by vaccination of the dams. *Vet Rec*. 2001;148:691–695.
31. Ledbetter EC, Kim K, Dubovi EJ, et al. Clinical and immunological assessment of therapeutic immunization with a subunit vaccine for recurrent ocular canine herpesvirus-1 infection in dogs. *Vet Microbiol*. 2016;197:102–110.
32. Chiou SH, Chow KC, Yang CH, et al. Discovery of Epstein-Barr virus (EBV)-encoded RNA signal and EBV nuclear antigen leader protein DNA sequence in pet dogs. *J Gen Virol*. 2005;86:899–905.
33. Ehlers B, Dural G, Yasmum N, et al. Novel mammalian herpesviruses and lineages within the Gammaherpesvirinae: cospeciation and interspecies transfer. *J Virol*. 2008;82:3509–3516.
34. Huang SH, Kozak PJ, Kim J, et al. Evidence of an oncogenic gammaherpesvirus in domestic dogs. *Virology*. 2012;427:107–117.
35. Marenzoni ML, Antognoni MT, Baldelli F, et al. Detection of parvovirus and herpesvirus DNA in the blood of feline and canine blood donors. *Vet Microbiol*. 2018;224:66–69.
36. Milman G, Smith KC, Erles K. Serological detection of Epstein-Barr virus infection in dogs and cats. *Vet Microbiol*. 2011;150:15–20.
37. Roa Lopez GA, Suarez JJ, Barato P, et al. Lack of association between Epstein-Barr virus and mammary tumours in dogs. *J Vet Res*. 2018;62:309–315.
38. Roels E, Dourcy M, Holopainen S, et al. No evidence of herpesvirus infection in West Highland white terriers with canine idiopathic pulmonary fibrosis. *Vet Pathol*. 2016;53:1210–1212.
39. Waugh EM, Gallagher A, McAulay KA, et al. Gammaherpesviruses and canine lymphoma: no evidence for direct involvement in commonly occurring lymphomas. *J Gen Virol*. 2015;96:1863–1872.
40. Williams KJ. Gammaherpesviruses and pulmonary fibrosis: evidence from humans, horses, and rodents. *Vet Pathol*. 2014;51:372–384.
41. Andrei G, Trompet E, Snoeck R. Novel therapeutics for Epstein-Barr virus. *Molecules*. 2019;24.

25

Influenza Virus Infections

Thomas W. Vahlenkamp, Jane E. Sykes

KEY POINTS

- Cause: In recent years, several influenza viruses have been transmitted from human (H1N1, H3N2), avian (H3N2, H7N2, H5N1, H5N6), or equine (H3N8) origin to dogs and cats. The transmitted avian influenza viruses (H5N1, H5N6) also included highly pathogenic viruses causing severe disease. Only CIVs H3N8 and H3N2 have exhibited sustained transmission within dog populations. The distinct differences in receptor preference among influenza viruses of different species cause a rather inefficient transmission of influenza viruses among different hosts.
- First Description: CIV H3N8 was first described in 2004 (Florida, USA) in the racing greyhound population.[1] CIV H3N2 emerged in 2006 in South Korea and China and spread to the USA in 2015.[2]
- Geographic Distribution: Worldwide with regional accumulation of cases.
- Mode of Transmission: Aerosol transmission or close contact, sometimes fomites.
- Major Clinical Signs: Mild respiratory disease, including frequent cough and fever, although infection of the lungs and more severe disease and death occur on occasion and are probably associated with mixed infections by other viruses or bacteria.
- Differential Diagnoses: Other viruses that cause similar signs are CAdV, parainfluenza virus, CRCoV, CHV, canine pneumovirus, and possibly reoviruses. In cats, FCV, FHV-1, and SARS-CoV-2 are other viruses that should be on the differential diagnosis list. Bacterial causes of upper respiratory tract disease such as *Bordetella bronchiseptica* and in cats, *Chlamydia felis,* must also be considered.
- Human Health Significance: The infections of dogs and cats with influenza viruses of different origins, including human, avian, and equine, along with the history of close contact of the companion animals with infected humans, birds, or horses in most of the reported cases have raised the concern that companion animals may act as host species contributing to the adaptation of avian viruses in mammals as well as a potential reservoir of mammalian influenza viruses to humans.

ETIOLOGY AND EPIDEMIOLOGY

Influenza viruses are in the family *Orthomyxoviridae*, and are negative-sense, single-stranded, RNA viruses that infect a variety of mammals and birds. Aquatic birds are generally subclinically infected reservoirs. Mammals, both domestic (swine, horses, dogs, ferrets) and nondomestic (mink, aquatic), poultry, and humans inadvertently can become infected with individual viral strains that spread among the various hosts.[3] Almost every winter, two genera of influenza viruses—influenza A and B—produce episodic outbreaks of an acute self-limiting febrile illness in susceptible humans. Influenza B and C are mainly human pathogens and are only rarely seen in animals. Influenza A viruses have the widest host species range and greatest mutability, and can rapidly evolve into new genetic subtypes.

Subtypes of influenza A viruses are specified by the antigenic nature of two surface glycoproteins (hemagglutinin [H1-H18] and neuraminidase [N1-N11]) (Table 25.1). Influenza viruses continuously evolve through point mutations in their nucleic acid that lead to a gradual "drift" in their genome, which encodes surface proteins. The immune response selects for new virus strains by allowing those strains that can escape the antibody-mediated response to replicate. This process results in continuous emergence of new strains every influenza season. In avian species, waterfowl are often the subclinical reservoir for influenza A viruses, whereas chickens and turkeys may develop disease after infection. The viruses are shed in the feces of aquatic birds and contaminate the environment where other hosts may become exposed. Influenza viruses in mammals primarily spread through the transfer of virus-containing respiratory secretions via aerosolized particles (smaller than 10 μm) from an infected to a susceptible individual. Fomite transmission through contact with contaminated surfaces or common usage items can also occur. Influenza A viruses cause generally mild respiratory disease or reduced egg production in avian hosts; however, mutations in strains with hemagglutinins of subtype H5 or H7 can sometimes result in highly pathogenic avian influenza virus (HPAIV) strains that can cause significant mortality in birds.

TABLE 25.1 Influenza A Virus Subtypes Identified in Dogs and Cats with Naturally Occurring Respiratory Disease

Species	Host Origin	Subtype	Location
Dog	Human	Pandemic H1N1/09	China, USA (NY), Mexico
	Avian	H3N2 CIV	South Korea, China, USA
		H3N1 CIV	South Korea
		H5N1	Thailand
		H5N2	China
	Equine	H3N8 CIV	USA
Cat	Human	Pandemic H1N1/09	USA, Italy, Canada
	Avian	H7N2 (LPAIV)	USA (NY)
		H5N1 (HPAIV)	Thailand, Europe
		H5N6 (HPAIV)	Asia, Europe, Africa

HPAIV, highly pathogenic avian influenza virus; *LPAIV,* low pathogenic avian influenza virus.

The genome of influenza viruses consists of eight different segments which allow for extensive reassortment of individual or multiple genome segments during coinfection of a single host species with two different influenza viruses (see Fig. 7.6). This drives evolution of influenza viruses in avian species and in mammals. For example, pigs can become simultaneously infected with both human and avian strains because the different sialic acid receptors in the respiratory epithelium allow simultaneous entry of swine, human, and avian influenza virus strains. Within the porcine host, novel influenza virus A strains can originate in a sudden and dramatic fashion, through antigenic "shift" from genetic reassortment. The genome segments of the progeny viruses may be derived from different species. Pigs are, therefore, believed to serve as a "mixing vessel" with regard to this genetic reassortment. If genetic recombination occurs, a new human influenza virus strain may arise with the ability to spread readily from swine back to people, but with a markedly different antigenic composition from the original infecting human strain. An antigenically distinct new strain may evolve to which the human population has no immunity.[4] Viruses that are naturally circulating in pig populations can occasionally also cause influenza in people who are occupationally exposed. Historically, these viruses are not transmitted efficiently among humans.[5] This also applies to virulent avian influenza virus strains that can occasionally spread directly to people, but causing only limited spread. Meat from poultry or swine does not pose a risk for human infections when it is properly cooked.

Most contemporary human infections have been associated with either influenza B viruses or the H1N1 and H3N2 subtypes of influenza A. Fever, myalgia, and signs of upper or lower respiratory tract infections are the most common manifestations in people. Mortality is the result of pulmonary complications. Dogs and cats, living in close proximity to their owners, may occasionally become infected during human influenza A outbreaks. Furthermore, dogs or cats coming in close proximity to birds, swine, or horses or eating uncooked meat by-products from these animals may contract these infections. Several influenza A subtypes have been detected in dogs and cats, with sustained transmission only documented for H3N8 and H3N2 viruses in dogs (Fig. 25.1).[6] Currently only H3N2 appears to be circulating in the dog population, with an active outbreak in Los Angeles, California, at the time of writing.

As enveloped viruses, influenza viruses are relatively susceptible to environmental influences. Their survival is prolonged by colder temperatures and moist conditions. Common disinfectants and warm environmental temperatures with low humidity are most effective in their inactivation. In the absence of organic material, most common disinfectants (1% sodium hypochlorite, quaternary ammonium compounds and 70% ethanol, aldehydes, and lipid solvents) inactivate the virus after 10 minutes' contact time. At pH 7.0, chlorine concentrations typically used in drinking water are sufficient to inactivate the avian virus after times of exposure as brief as 1 minute.[7] Ionizing radiation and acid (pH 2.0) are also virucidal. In the absence of disinfection, survival in moist conditions is not greater than 30 minutes at 56°C (133° F), a few hours at 55°C (132°F), several days at room temperature of 22°C (71°F), and at least a month when frozen. At room temperatures canine virus isolates survive on surfaces, clothing, or hands for 48, 24, or 12 hours, respectively.

INFLUENZA VIRUS INFECTIONS OF HUMAN ORIGIN

Experimental intranasal or intravenous infections of dogs with human influenza virus A,[8-11] B,[10,11] and C[12-15] types have provided convincing evidence that these viruses can replicate in dogs. However, clinical signs in infected animals have either been absent or consisted of a mild conjunctivitis, serous nasal discharge, and variable fever. With respect to natural infections, serologic responses to influenza A virus have been observed in dogs during human disease outbreaks.[16-19] Limited data, based on virus isolation from respiratory secretions, document sporadic natural transmission and subclinical infection of dogs with *human* H3N2 influenza A viruses[18,20-23] and type C viruses.[12,13] There is, however, no evidence for sustained transmissions of human influenza viruses in dogs. Species barriers may be too tight for natural transmission to occur[24] despite the fact that human influenza viruses readily replicate in Madin-Darby canine kidney (MDCK) cells.

Antibodies have been detected in the blood of healthy cats using HI against H3N2 influenza viruses.[10,16,18,25,26] No antibodies against subtypes H1, H2, and H4 through H8 were detected.[26] As human epidemics with influenza H3N2 viruses occurred in the countries of investigation, it might be that the cats had been exposed to this particular virus. Cats have also been experimentally infected with human (H3N2), avian (H7N3), and seal (H7N7) influenza viruses.[10,18,25,27] After infection, cats developed antibodies, sometimes even shed virus, but never showed clinical signs. In some studies, human influenza virus H3N2, H2N2, and influenza B virus infections could also be transmitted among experimental cats that were housed together. These earlier studies suggested that cats and dogs might represent yet another host for various influenza viruses in nature.[27]

Pandemic Influenza H1N1 Virus Infections

Before its spread to dogs and cats, the pandemic influenza A/H1N1/09 virus was only known to infect humans, pigs, horses, and birds. In dogs, the first detection of influenza A/H1N1/09 was reported from China. Two of 52 samples from sick dogs tested positive for the virus.

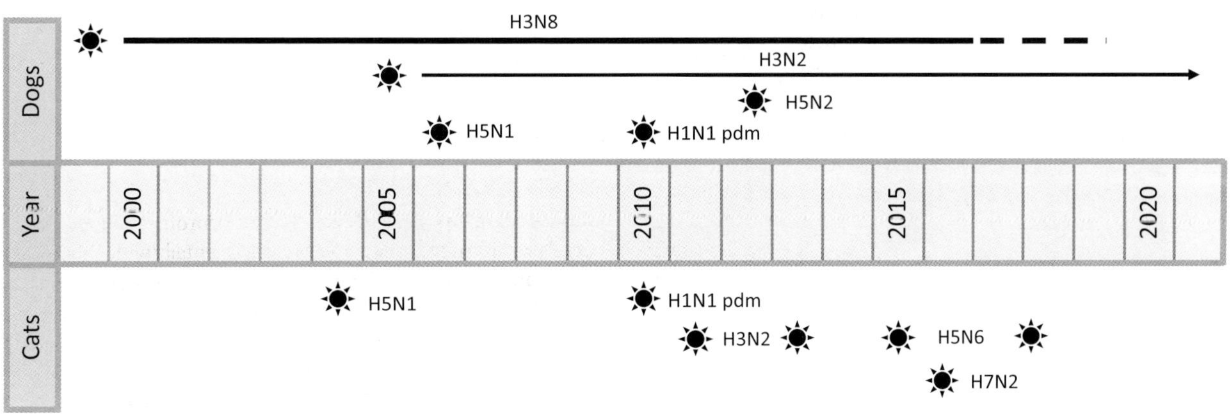

Fig. 25.1 Timeline of influenza virus infections from 1999–2021 in dogs and cats. H3N8 and H3N2 virus infections have been sustained in dog populations over several years with a recent case decline and possible disappearance of H3N8.

The viruses in the dogs had genomes that were 99% homologous to those of viruses from human H1N1 flu cases, confirming that the dogs were infected. In New York, a 13-year-old dog with respiratory illness associated with lethargy, cough, anorexia, and fever had radiographic evidence of pneumonia. The dog improved after therapy with fluids, antibacterials, and nebulization and was discharged from the hospital after 48 hours. Molecular testing confirmed that the dog was infected with the pandemic H1N1 virus.

In separate incidents, two cats from Iowa and Utah, one cat from California, and two cats from Oregon[28] developed respiratory signs after family members in the household suffered from influenza illness. One of the Iowa cats developed respiratory illness within 6 days after onset of respiratory disease in human family members.[29] The cat was afebrile and dehydrated on physical examination. Bilateral multifocal caudodorsal alveolar densities were observed on thoracic radiography (Fig. 25.2). Cytologic examination of bronchoalveolar wash specimens revealed foamy macrophages, nondegenerate neutrophils, and small lymphocytes. All of the cats had had serum antibody reactive to the pandemic influenza virus A/H1N1/09. The cats and their owners recovered, and there was no evidence that the cats transmitted the virus to humans. RT-PCR results targeting the influenza H1N1 virus were positive in one cat.[29] However, results are often negative, perhaps relating to the low rate and transient nature of viral shedding in heterologous hosts. In cats that died of H1N1 infections, severe necrotizing bronchointerstitial pneumonia has been found with virus present throughout tissues in the lower respiratory tract.[28]

Serological screening of domestic dogs and cats between 2011 and 2014 from animal shelters in 19 provinces of Thailand revealed only few exposed animals.[30] In total 932 sera from dogs and 79 cat sera were investigated. Six canine and one feline serum specimens were seroreactive to the pandemic H1N1 virus. At the same time, serosurveys conducted in Europe and Asia using ELISA revealed influenza-specific antibodies in the sera of domestic cats at low prevalence (1.5–2.5%).[31,32] In contrast, serosurveys conducted in Japan and the United States using HI assays for pandemic H1N1 virus revealed a prevalence exceeding 30% in domestic cats.[33] Antibody prevalences to human seasonal influenza H1N1 and H3N2 viruses in the cat sera investigated were 10.9 and 17.6%, respectively. It is also possible that variation in the sensitivity of different assays has contributed to the observed differences.

Because the degree of shedding of influenza A H1N1 virus by dogs and cats is low, there appears to be low risk of infecting more susceptible human hosts. Even swine infected with the A/H1N1/09 strain harbor it in tissues for no longer than 3 days after exposure.[34] Influenza H1N1 virus RT-PCR tests can be used for diagnosis.

Public Health Aspects

Because of the close association of pets with humans, concern has been raised that dogs and cats may be important in the spread or maintenance of influenza infection in people. Many reports exist of the presence in dogs and cats of antibodies against human influenza virus strains. Influenza infection that jumps between different species is often a self-limiting spread and is not efficiently transmitted between in-contact animals. No evidence suggests that the virus replicates sufficiently to spread from infected pets to humans. Because of their potential infection on a clinical or subclinical basis, dogs and cats may be useful as sentinel hosts for surveillance of influenza virus infections.[35]

INFLUENZA VIRUS INFECTIONS OF AVIAN ORIGIN

All influenza H and N subtypes can be found in varying combinations in different aquatic birds, which represent the natural reservoir of all influenza viruses. In aquatic birds, influenza virus infections are usually of low pathogenicity and not associated with clinical signs. Viral replication is mainly restricted to the GI tract and transmission of the infection

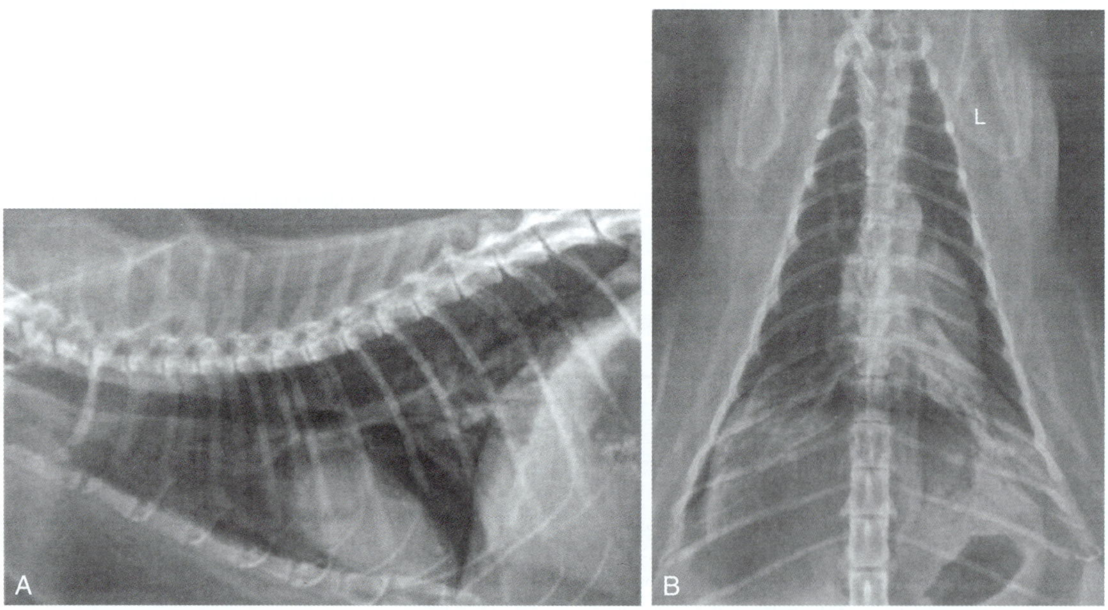

Fig. 25.2 Radiographs of the thorax of a cat with confirmed influenza A pandemic (H1N1) 2009 virus infection. (A) Right lateral view; (B) Dorsoventral view. Asymmetric soft-tissue opacities are evident in the right and left caudal lung lobes. An alveolar pattern, composed of air bronchograms with border-effaced (indistinct) adjacent pulmonary vessels, is most pronounced in the left caudal lobe *(L)*. A small gas lucency in the pleural space appears in the right caudal and dorsal thoracic cavity. An endotracheal tube is visible at the thoracic inlet on the lateral view in this moderately obese cat. (From Sponseller BA, Strait E, Jergens A, et al. Influenza A pandemic (H1N1) 2009 virus infection in domestic cat. *Emerg Infect Dis.* 2010;16:534-537.)

is facilitated by the cloacal-oral route. Avian influenza viruses subtype H5 and H7 are exceptional in that they can mutate at the hemagglutinin cleavage site, which leads to systemic spread and replication of the virus in the infected avian host. Therefore, avian influenza viruses subtype H5 and H7 are divided into low-pathogenic avian influenza viruses (LPAIVs) and HPAIVs based on their biological nature. In contrast to LPAIV infections, infections with HPAIVs are associated with diverse clinical signs in waterbirds and severe clinical signs in domestic poultry. Some of these viruses also acquire a broadened host spectrum.[3,36]

Avian influenza viruses preferentially infect cells that harbor a 2′-3′ sialic acid receptor linkage, whereas human influenza viruses infect cells that harbor a 2′-6′ sialic acid receptor linkage. This difference in receptor preference among these viruses is the reason for inefficient transmission of avian influenza viruses to mammalian hosts. Nevertheless, occasional virus transmissions to dogs and cats can occur.

Influenza H3N2 Virus Infections

CIV H3N2 was first recognized in South Korea and China in 2006, and likely arose from transfer of an avian influenza virus in 2005. The virus caused an outbreak of respiratory disease in South Korea in dogs at three veterinary clinics and one kennel.[2] All but one of the dogs at the clinics died. Infection with a closely related strain was found in southern China.[37] The virus then circulated throughout Korea and both northern and southern China, which was associated with some genetic drift. Clinical signs in affected dogs included fever, sneezing with nasal discharge, cough, and anorexia. The dogs had signs of severe pulmonary lesions at necropsy. In experimentally infected dogs, H3N2 is shed for up to 6 days after the onset of illness. Unlike the highly pathogenic avian-origin H5N1 strains, which produce respiratory and systemic illness, the avian-lineage H3N2 isolate, which adapted to spread among dogs, produced mild upper respiratory tract disease, including frequent cough and fever. However, infection of the lungs and more severe disease and death occur on occasion and are probably associated with mixed infections by other viruses or bacteria.[38]

In Asia, the virus has been most widespread among dogs in kennels and meat dog farms and markets. Given that live poultry markets in Asia have been identified as a major source of influenza viruses that spill over to infect new hosts, close physical contact between birds and dogs in these host-dense environments might have facilitated the emergence of the virus in dogs.[39] H3N2 influenza virus was introduced into the Chicago area in the United States from Asia in 2015, and has since caused widespread outbreaks of disease in dogs.[40] Despite local control measures, the virus continued circulating among dogs in and around Chicago and then appeared in southeastern states, for example, Georgia and North Carolina, although secondary outbreaks appear to have ended within a few months.[39] Continued infections in the Chicago area occurred, this time without evidence of secondary outbreaks. Multiple introductions of H3N2 influenza virus from Asia have re-seeded disease within the United States in different locations, with an active shelter outbreak in southern California at the time of writing (August 2021). Influenza H3N2 virus appears to have a relatively broad host range, infecting ferrets, guinea pigs, and cats after experimental challenge. Natural spillover of the virus from dogs to cats has been documented in South Korea and the United States, but those outbreaks were largely confined to the shelter populations where they emerged, and the viruses do not appear to undergo prolonged transmission in household cats, despite high level of viral shedding. Experimental inoculation of Korean or USA H3N2 strains into pigs resulted in poor replication, so infection of pigs from dogs appears to be unlikely, even though pigs are a common host of other H3N2 influenza viruses.

Dogs vaccinated with two doses of an inactivated adjuvanted H3N2 virus vaccine were protected against challenge infection with the avian-lineage canine influenza isolate.[41] In the USA, both monovalent and bivalent inactivated vaccines are available for prevention of CIV H3N8 and H3N2 infections. Two doses (2 to 4 weeks apart) are required to achieve protection, which limits their efficacy when used at entry in shelter and boarding environments.

Public Health Aspects

Human influenza H1N1 (pandemic and seasonal) and H3N2 viruses appear to be able to occasionally infect dogs. Although none of these infections is known to have resulted in major onward transmission among dogs, this might provide the opportunity for human influenza viruses to reassort with CIVs through natural coinfections in dogs. In the last decade, novel reassorted CIVs (H3N1, H3N2) have emerged in South Korea.[42,43] No transfers of either CIV subtype to humans have been documented. Nevertheless, the potential of dogs to act as virus mixing vessels or as sources of zoonotic infections exists.

Influenza H7N2 Virus Infections

In 2016 an outbreak of influenza H7N2 virus occurred in cats at several animal care shelters in the United States (New York, Pennsylvania). The first outbreak was detected in three facilities of the municipal animal shelter system in New York City. Transmission of the virus to an attending veterinary staff member warranted the use of additional precautions measures. By the end of the outbreak approximately 500 cats had been tested positive for this virus and retrospective serological analyses supported the existence of two human infections during this outbreak.[44] Sequence analysis revealed that the virus was phylogenetically related to a North American lineage low-pathogenic avian influenza H7N2 virus circulating in live poultry markets during 1996 and 2005.[45] While it is unknown how the index cat was exposed to the influenza H7N2 virus, the high rate of transmission among cats and concern about a possible zoonotic transmission mandated quarantine precautions. Person-to-person transmission was not observed, although the influenza H7N2 virus obviously is capable of eliciting mild illness in humans. Airborne transmission and/or direct contact with fomites of infected cats most probably contribute to the efficient transmission of the virus between cats and also to the transmission from cats to humans.[46] Therefore continued surveillance and transmission-based precautions are necessary during the treatment and care of influenza H7N2 virus–infected cats.

Highly Pathogenic Influenza H5N1 Virus Infections

HPAIV of subtype H5N1 originated in China in 1996 and spread to other countries in Southeast Asia until 2003. The viruses, continuously shaped by several reassortment events and by antigenic drift, established endemic infections, driven by subclinically infected duck populations in this area. An incursion of HPAIV H5N1 of the phylogenetic cluster 2.2 ("Qinghai lineage") into the wild bird population of northwestern China in 2005 marked the beginning of an unprecedented virus spread to other Asian regions, Europe, and Africa within a single year. Apart from causing severe clinical signs in gallinaceous bird populations, HPAIV H5N1 also exhibited a potential to infect mammals including humans. Next to humans, naturally infected mammal species were members of the order Carnivora (Canidae, Felidae, Mustelidae, and Viverridae).[47-50]

In dogs and cats, a fatal infection of a dog that ingested HPAIV H5N1–infected chicken carcasses was reported in Thailand in 2006.[51] Several outbreaks of HPAIV H5N1 infection have been reported in felids under natural conditions. The first outbreak was in 2003, when two tigers and two leopards died in a zoo in Suphanburi, Thailand after developing high fever and respiratory distress.[52] Shortly after, a clouded leopard died in a zoo in Chonburi, Thailand, from infection with influenza

H5N1. One month later, a tiger at the same zoo was found to be infected but recovered.[53] During an outbreak in a tiger zoo in Sriracha, Thailand, a total of 147 tigers died or were euthanized.[54] The first evidence that domestic cats were at risk of infection with HPAIV H5N1 was in 2004, when 3 domestic cats from a household in Thailand, in which 14 cats had died, testing positive for influenza H5N1.[53] The virus was also detected in a domestic cat in Thailand that had died following development of fever, dyspnea, seizures, and ataxia.[55]

Experimental inoculation of dogs with HPAIV H5N1 results in severe clinical illness.[56] Experimental infections using HPAIV H5N1 confirmed that cats can develop severe clinical signs after infection[24,57] or after ingestion of infected chicken.[24] The first cases of HPAIV H5N1 infection in domestic cats in Europe were detected during the outbreak of avian influenza on the German Isle of Rügen in February 2006, during which three free-roaming cats found dead were harboring the virus.[48] At approximately the same time, three cats that did not show clinical signs tested positive by RT-PCR for influenza virus H5N1 in an animal shelter in Graz, Austria, after an infected swan had been brought to the shelter.[58]

Phylogenetic analysis of the HPAIV H5N1 viruses from the dog and a cat from Thailand revealed that the virus was highly similar to the avian influenza virus circulating in poultry at the same time.[59] No genetic reassortment event was necessary for the transmission of the virus to the dog. In central Thailand, about 25% of 629 village dogs had positive test results for H5-specific antibodies.[60] It remains to be verified whether increased numbers of dogs with antibody-positive test results can be found in areas with a high prevalence of HPAIV infections in poultry or wild birds. In order to evaluate the potential of dogs to spread H5N1 influenza virus to humans, inoculation studies were performed with two different HPAIV H5N1 strains.[8,9] Short-term virus shedding from the nasal cavity was observed inconsistently and only with low titers. All of the inoculated dogs developed antibodies. Transmission of infection to in-contact dogs and cats was not observed.[8] Therefore, although dogs are susceptible to HPAIV H5N1, no evidence has been obtained for a major role of dogs in the spread of this virus.

As in dogs, infections of felids with HPAIV H5N1 have been documented in areas with HPAIV H5N1 infections in poultry or wild birds in the surrounding area.[29,52,58] Phylogenetic analyses have shown that viral isolates from cats and tigers are highly similar to the avian virus circulating in poultry at the same time, indicating that no genetic reassortment events with mammalian influenza viruses had occurred. Several point mutations have been identified that are associated with higher virulence in mammals; however, none of them seem to be essential for the infection in felids.[52,59,61,62] Sporadic fatal disease due to HPAIV H5N1 infection in domestic cats, leopards, and tigers received considerable public attention.[63] Infections in felids were reported in Asia (China, Thailand, Vietnam, Indonesia, Iraq) and Europe (Austria, Germany). The presence of antibodies and clinical evidence of HPAIV H5N1 infections in different species of wildcats (e.g., Asiatic golden cat, clouded leopard) have been reported from Cambodia.[64]

Despite the described sporadic HPAIV H5N1 cases in felids, the prevalence of infection among pet cats in European countries seems to be low. A study conducted in Germany included 171 cats having outdoor access in areas in which infected birds had been found at the time of investigation. Neither virus excretion nor antibodies were detected among the cats.[65] In Milan, Italy, there was no evidence of antibodies to HPAIV H5N1 in cats.[66] Because no outbreaks of avian influenza had occurred in the sampling area at that time, the likelihood of finding antibody-positive cats was most probably low. Because the tests performed in these studies are able to detect antibodies against all influenza A viruses, the investigations also confirmed that cats are not prone to infections with the seasonal influenza viruses circulating in humans. In contrast to these investigations, 8 (7%) of 111 feral cats tested in an unpublished study of the National Institute of Animal Health in Bangkok and 20% of 500 cats tested in Indonesia[67] had antibodies to influenza A H5N1. It is possible that cats are more susceptible to virus strains circulating in Asia compared with European virus strains, and thus, more cats become infected in Asia. Within HPAIV H5N1, at least two genetically and antigenically distinct lineages (clades 1 and 2) exist with different geographic distributions in Asia. Clade 1 was isolated mainly in Vietnam and Thailand, whereas clade 2 was found mainly in China and Indonesia. From there, the "Qinghai-like" sublineage spread to the Middle East, Europe, and Africa and separated into three different subclusters.[61,68] All Asian cases reported in felids were caused by infections with clade 1 viruses. The outbreak in domestic cats in Iraq and the fatal cases in Germany were caused by Qinghai-like clade 2 viruses. Therefore, cats seem to be susceptible to different circulating H5N1 virus strains.[61] It seems likely that the difference in prevalence among cats is caused by higher risk of exposure to the virus in Asia. Compared with the situation in Asia, only a relatively small number of wild birds and poultry farms were affected in Europe. Additionally, cats included in the European studies were pet cats, which were fed by their owners and thus would probably have been exposed to the virus only during bird hunting.

Pathogenesis

Infection of felids occurs mostly through direct contact with infected birds, particularly through ingestion of infected poultry.[24,52,54,55] Both inhalation and ingestion seem to be potential routes of virus entry.[24,69,70] The virus spreads to the lower respiratory tract, where it can cause severe pneumonia.[48,52,55] In the lungs, influenza H5N1 viruses in cats attach predominantly to type II pneumocytes and alveolar macrophages.[71] The predominant involvement of the lower respiratory tract and the inability of the virus to attach to cells of the upper respiratory tract may be a reason why cats excrete virus at relatively low concentrations.[24,71] Experimentally infected cats develop a significant rise in body temperature from day 1 PI, lethargy, protrusion of the nictitating membrane, conjunctivitis, and respiratory distress by day 2 PI. Unlike other influenza viruses, which usually have restricted replication in the mammalian respiratory tract, HPAIV H5N1 infection in cats leads to viremia and systemic infection. Severe necrosis and inflammation in many organs occur, with a fatal disease outcome. This has also been shown after experimental intratracheal and oculonasopharyngeal infection.[24,57,70] Virus can be detected in pharyngeal, nasal, and rectal swabs as well as urine specimens. Viral shedding starts between days 1 and 3 PI and lasts up to 7 days PI.[24,70] Ingestion of infected birds can be a route of transmission to cats under natural conditions.[24] Horizontal transmission through both the respiratory and gastrointestinal routes has been demonstrated in experimental infections[24] and was also assumed under natural conditions in the Sriracha tiger zoo outbreak in Thailand.[54]

Clinical Features

The incubation period appears to vary depending on the route of infection and is shorter after direct experimental infection through respiratory and oral routes (1 to 2 days) than after cat-to-cat transmission (5 days).[70,72] Clinical signs described in affected felids include fever, lethargy, dyspnea, conjunctivitis, and protrusion of the third eyelid.[24,52,54,55] Neurologic signs result from cerebral and cerebellar congestion and nonsuppurative meningoencephalitis accompanied by vasculitis.[54,55] Diarrhea, as described in affected poultry and also in humans infected with HPAIV H5N1,[73,74] has not been observed in affected cats. Sudden death may occur in cats as soon as 2 days after the onset of clinical signs.[54,55]

Infection of cats with HPAIV H5N1 also can result in subclinical infection. Three cats housed in an animal shelter in Austria shed virus after contact with an infected swan, and two cats developed antibodies to influenza H5N1 virus, but none developed clinical signs.[58]

Experimentally, the development of clinical signs is dose-dependent. Infection with a high viral dose results in virus shedding and fatal disease. When cats are exposed to a moderate dose, they do not develop clinical signs but seroconvert and shed only small amounts of virus. Cats exposed to a low dose of virus do not become infected.[57]

Laboratory abnormalities described in tigers include severe leukopenia and thrombocytopenia and increased activities of serum ALT and AST.[54] Markedly increased liver enzyme activities also have been found in diseased domestic cats.[48]

Diagnosis

Influenza should be considered as a diagnosis in cats that develop respiratory disease with outdoor access in regions with sporadic or endemic outbreaks of influenza virus H5N1 in birds. Because of the systemic replication of the virus in diseased dogs and cats, detection is possible not only in pharyngeal, nasal, and rectal swabs but also in fecal and urine specimens, organ tissues, and pleural fluid.[69,70,75] Pharyngeal swabs are convenient to obtain and will also detect subclinically infected cats.[57,58] Swabs should be placed in a sterile tube with a few drops of saline. Bacterial transport medium should not be used. Influenza virus RNA can be identified by RT-PCR with primers specific for the matrix (M) gene. A subtype-specific RT-PCR can then be used to identify involved hemagglutinin and neuraminidase genes.[48,52] Viral isolation can be performed by inoculation of swab suspensions into embryonated hen eggs or in cell cultures (e.g., MDCK) and be identified subsequently by RT-PCR or HI assays.[51,55,70] Immunohistochemistry can be used to detect influenza virus antigen in affected organs.[55,70] In-clinic tests designed to screen cats for infection are not commercially available. All tests that have been studied lacked the sensitivity to produce reliable results in specimens derived from experimentally infected cats.[65]

Antibodies to influenza viruses in serum specimens can be detected using viral neutralization assays within 3 weeks after infection.[57] HI assays and a commercially available, species-independent competitive ELISA assay based on the nucleoprotein are more sensitive for the detection of antibodies against influenza viruses. Both tests are able to detect antibodies within 2 weeks PI and may be used for serosurveillance studies.[57,58,76]

Treatment

Not much is known about the efficacy of antiviral treatment in cats infected with HPAIV H5N1. The neuraminidase inhibitor oseltamivir (Tamiflu, Roche, Nutley, NJ) has good antiviral activity against HPAIV H5N1 *in vitro*[77] and in experimentally infected mice and ferrets,[78,79] and is recommended for treatment and prophylaxis of HPAIV H5N1 infection in humans.[80] However, treatment with oseltamivir (75 mg/60 kg q12h) failed to protect tigers from infection and disease during the outbreak in the Sriracha zoo in 2004. This might be due to differences between humans and felids in drug pharmacokinetics and host metabolism.[54,62] Sequence analysis of the virus obtained from the treated tigers excluded the possibility that drug-resistant mutants had emerged.[62]

The prognosis for infected cats in the field is unclear. Subclinical infections are possible, but all domestic cats that developed clinical signs to date have died or had to be euthanized.

Prevention

Although sustained transmission of HPAIV H5N1 in cats in Asia and Europe has not occurred, the number of countries reporting these infections demonstrate that the transmissions are not exceptional single events but rather expected if the exposure or the infection pressure in the environment is high enough. The role of cats in the adaptation of HPAIV H5N1 to mammals remains to be elucidated and, therefore, vaccination regimens have been discussed. So far, however, no licensed influenza vaccine for cats is available.

An inactivated, adjuvanted heterologous whole-virus vaccine based on an LPAIV of subtype H5N6 protected cats even against a lethal high-dose challenge HPAIV H5N1 infection.[57] Vaccination induced high HPAIV H5N1 cross-reacting HI antibody titers before challenge. Vaccinated cats did not develop any clinical signs and showed a significant reduction in viral excretion.[57] Other experimental studies have used fowlpox virus expressing avian influenza virus H5 derived from an H5N8 influenza virus,[42] H5 from a H5N1 influenza virus,[81] or a canine adenovirus expressing H5 of a recent tiger isolate as a vaccine vector.[82] These vector-based vaccines have never been tested in challenge experiments. However, a recombinant vaccine with a canarypox vector producing the hemagglutinin protein protected cats against challenge with two HPAIV H5N1 isolates from humans.[29]

Public Health Aspects

Although dogs and cats are susceptible to infection with HPAIV H5N1, there is no evidence they play a major role in spread of this virus. There have been no reports of humans contracting the infection from diseased dogs or cats. However, preventative measures must be taken to minimize the risk of virus transmission to humans when cats or dogs are suspected to be infected with HPAIV H5N1. All natural infections in cats and dogs have been connected directly to the occurrence of HPAIV H5N1 in birds. Therefore, contact of dogs and cats with infected birds must be avoided. It has been advised to keep cats indoors in areas where HPAIV outbreaks occur. Cats should also not be fed uncooked poultry meat. If animals are suspected to be infected or infection is confirmed, they should be isolated and the number of contacts with them should be minimized. Personnel handling infected animals should wear protective clothing (gloves, face masks, etc.). Fractious cats should be sedated for handling. Proper quarantine, hygiene, and disinfection are important.

Transmission of infection from infected cats to dogs and from infected dogs to cats has been investigated experimentally with contact conditions similar to those common in pet households.[8] Cats and dogs had close contact and shared water and food bowls. At least under these conditions, no transmission occurred. Therefore, the risk of trans-species transmission of HPAIV H5N1 infections between dogs and cats seems to be low.

Highly Pathogenic Influenza H5N6 Virus Infections

The avian influenza H5N1 virus was the first influenza virus identified with a polybasic cleavage site in its haemagglutinin (therefore displaying a highly pathogenic phenotype) and that could infect cats. In recent years, another HPAIV (subtype H5N6) spread among poultry across Asia, Europe, and Africa. In China, HPAIV H5N6 emerged in 2013 and spread to Southeast Asia. In 2014, the first human H5N6 infection was reported in China. Analysis of fecal specimens from wild birds and one lung specimen from a dead domestic cat collected in areas with close proximity to the residence of the infected human revealed that some of the wild birds and also the cat died due to a H5N6 infection.[83] This was the first case of fatal H5N6 avian influenza virus infection in a domestic cat. Subsequent analyses during HPAIV H5N6 outbreaks in poultry and wild birds in South Korea in 2016 revealed three additional infected cats.[84] The cats displayed acute salivation, lethargy, and seizures, and died within 4 days of illness onset despite antimicrobial drug treatment. Virus isolated at necropsy from the three cats were similar to HPAIV H5N6 isolated in chicken farms nearby. Necropsy findings included bloody nasal discharge, severe pulmonary congestion and edema, splenomegaly, and necrotic lesions and influenza virus antigens in multiple visceral organs. It seems likely that the neurotropism of the virus was a key factor contributing to the sudden death of the animals.[84] Epidemiological investigations showed that the cats might have been infected by ingestion of (or contact with) infected wild birds, although the virus was not isolated from wild birds around the area at this time. Sequence analyses of H5N6 viruses isolated from cats in China in 2016 showed continued antigenic drift and antigenic shift. Analyzed influenza H5N6 viruses harbored individual genome segments from three different (H5N6, H9N2, H7N9) viruses.[85] This confirmed a continued evolution of the co-circulating avian influenza viruses in China. Due to the large distribution of H5N6 virus infections in birds and the few documented infections in cats, the probability of H5N6 virus transmission to cats can be assumed to be low. Nevertheless, avian influenza virus surveillance will be needed for mammals, including cats, during regional H5N6 outbreaks. Irrespective of and before the occurrence of HPAIV H5N1 and H5N6 infections in dogs, canine infection with LPAIV H5N2 was reported in China.[86]

INFLUENZA VIRUS INFECTIONS OF EQUINE ORIGIN

Clinically apparent influenza virus infection associated with sustained transmission in dogs occurred in the United States in Florida as early as 1999, when a strain of H3N8 equine influenza virus circulating in horses adaptively evolved via genetic mutation–induced alterations in the hemagglutinin protein and infected racing greyhounds.[1,87] The virus was first isolated during an outbreak of respiratory disease in dogs in 2004, and homologous isolates were found in greyhounds and other breeds in Florida and other states thereafter.[88] The spread of infection appeared to be sporadic and involve the integration of infected dogs into populations of susceptible dogs.

Canine Influenza H3N8 Virus Infections

The influenza H3N8 virus isolate from the Florida outbreak was determined to be a host-adapted CIV; it readily replicated in dogs and spread in a sporadic fashion throughout the United States. The virus has the entire genome of the equine virus with minor modifications in the hemagglutinin portion of the genome[88-90] resulting in five amino acid substitutions. Sequential examination of the canine isolates has revealed minor genetic alterations with the continuing trend of mutations typical of influenza viruses.[91] This modified H3N8 virus readily replicates and spreads between dogs[92] but does not establish a productive infection in horses.[75,93,94] The adapted CIV also does not replicate in avian species such as domestic chickens, turkeys, or ducks.[95]

Epidemiology

Retrospective antibody detection studies with genetic documentation in the United Kingdom and Australia between 2002 and 2007 have substantiated independent novel infections of dogs with equine H3N8 strains that were in direct or indirect contact with horses.[88,96-100] These represent individual episodes of exposure of dogs to infected horses, with limited replication and spread in dogs, rather than independent mutational adaptations to infect dogs. Horizontal spread among affected dogs in these outbreaks has not been demonstrated. In the United States, the virus that emerged in Florida spread widely for several years. Interconnected networks of dense susceptible host populations found in dog shelters and kennels probably enabled the long-term maintenance of the virus. The virus has subsequently become increasingly confined to areas in the northeastern United States.[39] Since 2016, influenza H3N8 virus has only been rarely identified in the USA,[40] and at the time of writing, the virus appears to be extinct.

In one experimental study, dogs cohoused with horses that were infected with an equine H3N8 isolate also became infected. However, although virus was found in the nasal passages of affected dogs, horizontal spread of the virus among dogs was not confirmed.[101] Similar findings were made in one natural outbreak where affected dogs were in direct contact with, or in the immediate vicinity of, infected horses.[99] However, dogs in that study did not become infected if their only exposure was to owners having contact with infected horses. Furthermore, infected dogs from that study were transported and kept with other dogs in urban locations, and no further spread of infection to contact dogs was found. Cross-species transmission of influenza virus from horses to dogs increases the concern for future respiratory infection outbreaks in dogs exposed to horses or possible new adaptations of the equine virus to preferentially infect dogs.

Pathogenesis

Experimental inoculation of the canine-adapted Florida virus isolate back into horses produced a milder illness in horses than that caused by the parental equine strain.[102] Mice can also be experimentally infected and develop respiratory tract inflammation.[103] Experimental intratracheal and intranasal inoculation of the laboratory-isolated virus into dogs produced fever (above 39° C [102.2° F]) for 2 days without signs of respiratory illness.[1] In other studies, intranasally infected 14- to 15-week-old antibody-negative pups developed respiratory signs and lung lesions with demonstrated viral replication and seroconversion.[104] These lesions were also found in further studies where adult dogs were infected by intranasal and intratracheal virus inoculation.[103] Although respiratory airway and lymph node inflammation is prominent, pulmonary involvement to the point of consolidation is uncommon in experimentally infected dogs.[88,103] Viral replication and shedding was greatest during the early incubation period, which lasted 2 to 4 days, and rapidly declined thereafter; lower-level shedding lasted up to 7 to 10 days. Shedding of CIV is of lower magnitude and shorter duration than that observed for influenza virus infections of other species. However, even subclinically infected dogs still shed virus, although at lower levels than more severely affected dogs.

Clinical Features

Subclinical infections can be documented by seroconversion without illness in dogs. However, after introduction of the virus into facilities with susceptible dogs, the severity of infection and prevalence of infection may be suddenly noticeably greater than with other causes of CIRD. The longer naïve dogs entering an endemic shelter reside, the more likely they are to become infected.[105] Clinical signs of affected dogs in the first identified outbreaks ranged from fever, tachypnea, and mucopurulent nasal discharge to self-limiting cough (10 to 14 days). As the infection has spread and vaccination has been implemented, the severity of signs and proportion of severely ill dogs has been reduced in those kennels. The most severe and persistent respiratory manifestations are associated with the development of pneumonia, which can be confirmed by thoracic radiography. Leukocytosis with a left shift may be found with evaluation of the hematologic parameters in dogs with pneumonia. Recovery occurs in a majority of infected dogs; a minority dies peracutely, and death is associated at necropsy with pulmonary, mediastinal, and pleural hemorrhages.[1,87,103] Infections in greyhound kennels have had the greatest severity of respiratory complications including pneumonia, which may relate to concurrent infection with group C streptococci and other bacteria.[87,103] Histologic changes included tracheitis, bronchitis, and suppurative bronchopneumonia (Fig. 25.3). Subsequent to these outbreaks, dogs that have had no history of respiratory illness may have high antibody titers against these viruses, indicating rapid spread of infection with subclinical illness in many dogs and to many other kennels, shelter facilities, and individual pets.

Diagnosis

Signs of CIV infection are similar to those caused by other agents of CIRD. Specific testing, although not always indicated in the clinical situation, should be performed to confirm the cause of illness. This is sometimes important in large outbreaks when causes must be confirmed to aid in control measures. A variety of tests can confirm the viral cause. For serum antibody determination, which is often the most reliable method, acute and convalescent samples should be taken within the first 7 days of illness

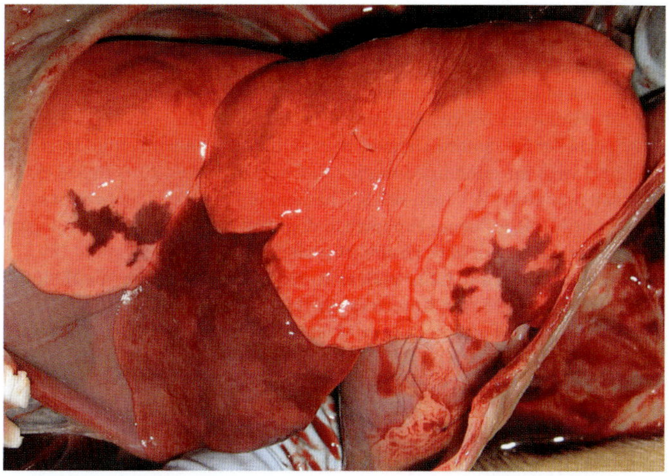

Fig. 25.3 Canine influenza virus–induced lung lesions in a young dog, 3 days after experimental exposure. Pulmonary congestion and consolidation and petechial hemorrhages are visible. (Courtesy Merck (MSD) Animal Health.)

and again 14 days later. Fourfold change in the antibody titer is indicative of active infection. Single positive titer determinations or lack of demonstration of a significant change in the titer only confirms exposure. Virus-specific antibody titers can be measured using HI and microneutralization assays.[1,88,106] The second method is the detection of virus, isolated from nasal (best) or pharyngeal (lower yield) swabs during the first 4 days of infection. Although tracheal or pulmonary washings may be superior, they involve additional cost and risk for collection from clinical patients. Virus can be cultivated in MDCK cells or embryonated eggs.[88] Specific antisera and RT-PCR can be used to identify the influenza virus subtype. RT-PCR can also be used directly from clinical specimens, preferably nasal swabs; however, as with viral isolation, results are usually only positive in the first 4 days of illness. Using immunohistochemical staining or in situ hybridization, virus can be detected throughout the respiratory tract in association with the inflammatory lesions. Pulmonary tissue should be submitted for culture, RT-PCR, or pathologic evaluation from dogs that die.

Clinical signs of this infection are similar to that caused by group C streptococci (*Streptococcus equi* subsp. *zooepidemicus*), which can cause outbreaks of acute, often fatal respiratory illness in many host species including kenneled dogs.

Treatment

Therapy with broad-spectrum antibacterials can reduce the severity of illness related to secondary bacterial infection and pneumonic complications; however, it does not offer a practical means of preventing virus spread and will not shorten the disease course in animals without significant secondary bacterial infections. Use of specific anti-influenza virus drugs, such as oseltamivir, is not recommended because their efficacy has not been investigated. Hospitalization, which is often required for severely affected animals, requires isolation and symptomatic therapy with parenteral fluids to maintain hydration. Recovery is generally within 2 to 3 weeks, although it can be longer in dogs that develop pneumonia.

Prevention

In experimental studies, recombinant-vectored H3 vaccines have increased virus-specific serum antibody concentrations in dogs and protected them against experimental challenge.[76,107] Vaccines against the infection in horses are commercially available. In dogs, vaccines are licensed in individual countries. An inactivated equine influenza virus vaccine was evaluated before availability of a canine influenza vaccine but did not provide protection.[88] A commercially available subcutaneous, adjuvanted, inactivated CIV H3N8 vaccine protected pups challenged 13 days after the second vaccination.[108] The severity of clinical signs, pathologic lesions, and magnitude of viral shedding were lower in vaccinated pups than in animals of the control group. HI antibody titers increased more dramatically after exposure to virulent challenge virus in vaccinated as compared to control pups. The vaccine is given as two 1-mL doses 2 to 4 weeks apart. It is recommended for dogs that have a lifestyle conducive to exposure to this virus and other respiratory tract infections. Dogs that are group-housed, in facilities with a high turnover of animals (e.g., animal shelters), or in densely populated communities with high viral prevalence are at greatest risk. Dogs in contact with horses might also be vaccinated; however, the cross-protection provided by the canine vaccine against the equine virus strains requires additional study. Those in individual households are least likely to contract infection. Pups should be at least 6 weeks old for the first injection. Annual vaccination is recommended. Because of the limited level and duration of shedding of influenza virus by infected dogs, the geographic spread of infection has been gradual and sporadic. Implementation of vaccination programs for dogs will help to control further spread of this virus.

Preventative measures should be exercised to prevent cross-species infection of influenza viruses where they are known to exist.[109] As influenza in horses is restricted to the respiratory tract and does not cause a systemic infection, viral transmission from horses to dogs through feeding raw horse meat is rather unlikely, although this feeding practice is common in management of certain sporting or working breeds such as greyhounds.

BOX 25.1 Online Resources for Influenza Infection of Dogs and Cats[a]

- Cornell University Veterinary Diagnostic Laboratory. Canine Influenza Information and Statistics in the United States. http://ahdc.vet.cornell.edu/news/civ.cfm.
- American Veterinary Medical Association. Canine Influenza. https://www.avma.org/resources-tools/animal-health-and-welfare/canine-influenza
- Centers for Disease Control and Prevention. Influenza in Animals. https://www.cdc.gov/flu/other/index.html
- Center for Food Security and Public Health. Iowa State University. Canine Influenza. http://www.cfsph.iastate.edu/Factsheets/pdfs/canine_influenza.pdf
- University of California-Davis Koret Shelter Medicine Program. Canine Influenza. https://www.sheltermedicine.com/library/resources/?r=canine-influenza

[a]Last accessed March 3, 2021.

Public Health Aspects

Although human influenza virus strains occasionally infect dogs and cats, there is no evidence that the canine influenza H3N8 virus can be spread from dogs to people.[110] Nevertheless, immunocompromised humans should generally avoid direct contact with animals having respiratory illness. Veterinarians should report concurrent human and animal respiratory outbreaks because of the rare chance that the human- or canine-adapted viruses may have changed species affinity with the risk of subsequent spread. There is no evidence that CIV infects other animals such as cats. Therapeutic and preventative measures should be used in management of ill dogs to minimize the spread of infection.

SUGGESTED READINGS (SEE ALSO BOX 25.1)

Borland S, Gracieux P, Jones M, et al. Influenza A virus infection in cats and dogs: a literature review in the light of the "One Health" concept. *Front Public Health*. 2020;8:83.

Parrish CR, Voorhees IEH. H3N8 and H3N2 canine influenza viruses: understanding these new viruses in dogs. *Vet Clin North Am Small Anim Pract*. 2019;49:643–649.

REFERENCES

1. Crawford PC, Dubovi EJ, Castleman WL, et al. Transmission of equine influenza virus to dogs. *Science*. 2005;310:482–485.
2. Song D, Kang B, Lee C, et al. Transmission of avian influenza virus (H3N2) to dogs. *Emerg Infect Dis*. 2008;14:741–746.
3. Vahlenkamp TW, Harder TC. Influenza virus infections in mammals. *Berl Munch Tierarztl Wochenschr*. 2006;119:123–131.
4. Wentworth DE, McGregor MW, Macklin MD, et al. Transmission of swine influenza virus to humans after exposure to experimentally infected pigs. *J Infect Dis*. 1997;175:7–15.
5. Van Reeth K. Avian and swine influenza viruses: our current understanding of the zoonotic risk. *Vet Res*. 2007;38:243–260.
6. Wasik BR, Voorhees IEH, Parrish CR: Canine and feline influenza, *Cold Spring Harb Perspec Med* 11, 2021. a038562.
7. Rice EW, Adcock NJ, Sivaganesan M, et al. Chlorine inactivation of highly pathogenic avian influenza virus (H5N1). *Emerg Infect Dis*. 2007;13:1568–1570.
8. Giese M, Harder TC, Teifke JP, et al. Experimental infection and natural contact exposure of dogs with avian influenza virus (H5N1). *Emerg Infect Dis*. 2008;14:308–310.
9. Maas R, Tacken M, Ruuls L, et al. Avian influenza (H5N1) susceptibility and receptors in dogs. *Emerg Infect Dis*. 2007;13:1219–1221.
10. Paniker CK, Nair CM. Experimental infection of animals with influenza-virus types A and B. *Bull World Health Organ*. 1972;47:461–463.
11. Todd JD, Cohen D. Studies of influenza in dogs. I. Susceptibility of dogs to natural and experimental infection with human A2 and B strains of influenza virus. *Am J Epidemiol*. 1968;87:426–439.
12. Manuguerra JC, Hannoun C. Natural infection of dogs by influenza C virus. *Res Virol*. 1992;143:199–204.
13. Manuguerra JC, Hannoun C, Simon F, et al. Natural infection of dogs by influenza C virus: a serological survey in Spain. *New Microbiol*. 1993;16:367–371.
14. Ohwada K, Kitame F, Homma M. Experimental infections of dogs with type C influenza virus. *Microbiol Immunol*. 1986;30:451–460.
15. Ohwada K, Kitame F, Sugawara K, et al. Distribution of the antibody to influenza C virus in dogs and pigs in Yamagata Prefecture, Japan. *Microbiol Immunol*. 1987;31:1173–1180.
16. Fyson RE, Westwood JC, Brunner AH. An immunoprecipitin study of the incidence of influenza A antibodies in animal sera in the Ottawa area. *Can J Microbiol*. 1975;21:1089–1101.
17. Madhavan HN, Agarwal SC. Sero-epidemiology of human and canine influenza in Pondicherry, South India, during 1971-1974. *Indian J Med Res*. 1976;64:835–840.
18. Romvary J, Rozsa J, Farkas E. Infection of dogs and cats with the Hong Kong influenza A (H3N2) virus during an epidemic period in Hungary. *Acta Vet Acad Sci Hung*. 1975;25:255–259.
19. Van Heerden J, Mills MG, Van Vuuren MJ, et al. An investigation into the health status and diseases of wild dogs (Lycaon pictus) in the Kruger National Park. *J S Afr Vet Assoc*. 1995;66:18–27.
20. Nikitin A, Cohen D, Todd JD, et al. Epidemiological studies of A-Hong Kong-68 virus infection in dogs. *Bull World Health Organ*. 1972;47:471–479.
21. Chang CP, New AE, Taylor JF, et al. Influenza virus isolations from dogs during a human epidemic in Taiwan. *Int J Zoonoses*. 1976;3:61–64.
22. Houser RE, Heuschele WP. Evidence of prior infection with influenza A/Texas/77 (H3N2) virus in dogs with clinical parainfluenza. *Can J Comp Med*. 1980;44:396–402.
23. Kilbourne ED, Kehoe JM. Demonstration of antibodies to both hemagglutinin and neuraminidase antigens of H3N2 influenza A virus in domestic dogs. *Intervirology*. 1975;6:315–318.
24. Kuiken T, Fouchier R, Rimmelzwaan G, et al. Feline friend or potential foe? *Nature*. 2006;440:741–742.
25. Paniker CK, Nair CM. Infection with A2 Hong Kong influenza virus in domestic cats. *Bull World Health Organ*. 1970;43:859–862.
26. Onta T, Kida H, Kawano J, et al. Distribution of antibodies against various influenza A viruses in animals. *Nihon Juigaku Zasshi*. 1978;40:451–454.
27. Hinshaw VS, Webster RG, Easterday BC, et al. Replication of avian influenza A viruses in mammals. *Infect Immun*. 1981;34:354–361.
28. Lohr CV, DeBess EE, Baker RJ, et al. Pathology and viral antigen distribution of lethal pneumonia in domestic cats due to pandemic (H1N1) 2009 influenza A virus. *Vet Pathol*. 2010;47:378–386.
29. Sponseller BA, Strait E, Jergens A, et al. Influenza A pandemic (H1N1) 2009 virus infection in domestic cat. *Emerg Infect Dis*. 2010;16:534–537.
30. Tangwangvivat R, Chanvatik S, Charoenkul K, et al. Evidence of pandemic H1N1 influenza exposure in dogs and cats, Thailand: a serological survey. *Zoonoses Public Health*. 2019;66:349–353.
31. Jeoung HY, Shin BH, Lee WH, et al. Seroprevalence of subtype H3 influenza A virus in South Korean cats. *J Feline Med Surg*. 2012;14:746–750.
32. Damiani AM, Kalthoff D, Beer M, et al. Serological survey in dogs and cats for influenza A (H1N1) pdm09 in Germany. *Zoonoses Public Health*. 2012;59:549–552.
33. Ibrahim M, Ali A, Daniels JB, et al. Post-pandemic seroprevalence of human influenza viruses in domestic cats. *J Vet Sci*. 2016;17:515–521.
34. Vincent AL, Lager KM, Harland M, et al. Absence of 2009 pandemic H1N1 influenza A virus in fresh pork. *PLoS One*. 2009;4:e8367.
35. Cleaveland S, Meslin FX, Breiman R. Dogs can play useful role as sentinel hosts for disease. *Nature*. 2006;440:605.
36. Alexander DJ, Brown IH. History of highly pathogenic avian influenza. *Rev Sci Tech*. 2009;28:19–38.
37. Li S, Shi Z, Jiao P, et al. Avian-origin H3N2 canine influenza A viruses in Southern China. *Infect Genet Evol*. 2010;10:1286–1288.
38. Jung K, Lee CS, Kang BK, et al. Pathology in dogs with experimental canine H3N2 influenza virus infection. *Res Vet Sci*. 2010;88:523–527.
39. Voorhees IEH, Glaser AL, Toohey-Kurth K, et al. Spread of canine influenza A(H3N2) Virus, United States. *Emerg Infect Dis*. 2017;23:1950–1957.
40. Parrish CR, Voorhees IEH. H3N8 and H3N2 canine influenza viruses: understanding these new viruses in dogs. *Vet Clin North Am Small Anim Pract*. 2019;49:643–649.
41. Lee C, Jung K, Oh J, et al.: Protective efficacy and immunogenicity of an inactivated avian-origin H3N2 canine influenza vaccine in dogs challenged with the virulent virus, *Vet Microbiol* 2010;143:184–188.
42. Song D, Moon HJ, An DJ, et al. A novel reassortant canine H3N1 influenza virus between pandemic H1N1 and canine H3N2 influenza viruses in Korea. *J Gen Virol*. 2012;93:551–554.
43. Na W, Lyoo KS, Song EJ, et al. Viral dominance of reassortants between canine influenza H3N2 and pandemic (2009) H1N1 viruses from a naturally co-infected dog. *Virol J*. 2015;12:134.
44. Poirot E, Levine MZ, Russell K, et al. Detection of avian influenza A(H7N2) virus infection among animal shelter workers using a novel serological approach-New York City, 2016-2017. *J Infect Dis*. 2019;219:1688–1696.
45. Marinova-Petkova A, Laplante J, Jang Y, et al. Avian influenza A(H7N2) virus in human exposed to sick cats, New York, USA, 2016. *Emerg Infect Dis*. 2017;23:2046–2049.
46. Blachere FM, Lindsley WG, Weber AM, et al. Detection of an avian lineage influenza A(H7N2) virus in air and surface samples at a New York City feline quarantine facility. *Influenza Other Respir Viruses*. 2018;12:613–622.
47. Beeler E. Influenza in dogs and cats. *Vet Clin North Am Small Anim Pract*. 2009;39:251–264.
48. Klopfleisch R, Wolf PU, Uhl W, et al. Distribution of lesions and antigen of highly pathogenic avian influenza virus A/Swan/Germany/R65/06 (H5N1) in domestic cats after presumptive infection by wild birds. *Vet Pathol*. 2007;44:261–268.
49. Roberton SI, Bell DJ, Smith GJ, et al. Avian influenza H5N1 in viverrids: implications for wildlife health and conservation. *Proc Biol Sci*. 2006;273:1729–1732.
50. Thiry E, Zicola A, Addie D, et al. Highly pathogenic avian influenza H5N1 virus in cats and other carnivores. *Vet Microbiol*. 2007;122:25–31.
51. Songserm T, Amonsin A, Jam-on R, et al. Fatal avian influenza A H5N1 in a dog. *Emerg Infect Dis*. 2006;12:1744–1747.
52. Keawcharoen J, Oraveerakul K, Kuiken T, et al. Avian influenza H5N1 in tigers and leopards. *Emerg Infect Dis*. 2004;10:2189–2191.

53. Enserink M, Kaiser J. Virology. Avian flu finds new mammal hosts. *Science*. 2004;305:1385.
54. Thanawongnuwech R, Amonsin A, Tantilertcharoen R, et al. Probable tiger-to-tiger transmission of avian influenza H5N1. *Emerg Infect Dis*. 2005;11:699–701.
55. Songserm T, Amonsin A, Jam-on R, et al. Avian influenza H5N1 in naturally infected domestic cat. *Emerg Infect Dis*. 2006;12:681–683.
56. Chen Y, Zhong G, Wang G, et al. Dogs are highly susceptible to H5N1 avian influenza virus. *Virology*. 2010;405:15–19.
57. Vahlenkamp TW, Harder TC, Giese M, et al. Protection of cats against lethal influenza H5N1 challenge infection. *J Gen Virol*. 2008;89: 968–974.
58. Leschnik M, Weikel J, Mostl K, et al. Subclinical infection with avian influenza A (H5N1) virus in cats. *Emerg Infect Dis*. 2007;13:243–247.
59. Amonsin A, Songserm T, Chutinimitkul S, et al. Genetic analysis of influenza A virus (H5N1) derived from domestic cat and dog in Thailand. *Arch Virol*. 2007;152:1925–1933.
60. Butler D. Thai dogs carry bird-flu virus, but will they spread it? *Nature*. 2006;439:773.
61. Weber S, Harder T, Starick E, et al. Molecular analysis of highly pathogenic avian influenza virus of subtype H5N1 isolated from wild birds and mammals in northern Germany. *J Gen Virol*. 2007;88:554–558.
62. Amonsin A, Payungporn S, Theamboonlers A, et al. Genetic characterization of H5N1 influenza A viruses isolated from zoo tigers in Thailand. *Virology*. 2006;344:480–491.
63. Harder TC, Vahlenkamp TW. Influenza virus infections in dogs and cats. *Vet Immunol Immunopathol*. 2010;134:54–60.
64. Desvaux S, Marx N, Ong S, et al. Highly pathogenic avian influenza virus (H5N1) outbreak in captive wild birds and cats, Cambodia. *Emerg Infect Dis*. 2009;15:475–478.
65. Marschall J, Schulz B, Harder Priv-Doz TC, et al. Prevalence of influenza A H5N1 virus in cats from areas with occurrence of highly pathogenic avian influenza in birds. *J Feline Med Surg*. 2008;10:355–358.
66. Paltrinieri S, Spagnolo V, Giordano A, et al. Influenza virus type A serosurvey in cats. *Emerg Infect Dis*. 2007;13:662–664.
67. MacKenzie D. Deadly H5N1 may be brewing in cats. *New Scientist*. 2007;193:6–7.
68. Salzberg SL, Kingsford C, Cattoli G, et al. Genome analysis linking recent European and African influenza (H5N1) viruses. *Emerg Infect Dis*. 2007;13:713–718.
69. Yingst SL, Saad MD, Felt SA. Qinghai-like H5N1 from domestic cats, northern Iraq. *Emerg Infect Dis*. 2006;12:1295–1297.
70. Rimmelzwaan GF, van Riel D, Baars M, et al. Influenza A virus (H5N1) infection in cats causes systemic disease with potential novel routes of virus spread within and between hosts. *Am J Pathol*. 2006;168:176–183. quiz 364.
71. van Riel D, Munster VJ, de Wit E, et al. H5N1 virus attachment to lower respiratory tract. *Science*. 2006;312:399.
72. Kuiken T, Holmes EC, McCauley J, et al. Host species barriers to influenza virus infections. *Science*. 2006;312:394–397.
73. Tran TH, Nguyen TL, Nguyen TD, et al. Avian influenza A (H5N1) in 10 patients in Vietnam. *N Engl J Med*. 2004;350:1179–1188.
74. Apisarnthanarak A, Kitphati R, Thongphubeth K, et al. Atypical avian influenza (H5N1). *Emerg Infect Dis*. 2004;10:1321–1324.
75. Rivailler P, Perry IA, Jang Y, et al. Evolution of canine and equine influenza (H3N8) viruses co-circulating between 2005 and 2008. *Virology*. 2010;408:71–79.
76. Karaca K, Dubovi EJ, Siger L, et al. Evaluation of the ability of canarypox-vectored equine influenza virus vaccines to induce humoral immune responses against canine influenza viruses in dogs. *Am J Vet Res*. 2007;68:208–212.
77. Hurt AC, Selleck P, Komadina N, et al. Susceptibility of highly pathogenic A(H5N1) avian influenza viruses to the neuraminidase inhibitors and adamantanes. *Antiviral Res*. 2007;73:228–231.
78. Leneva IA, Roberts N, Govorkova EA, et al. The neuraminidase inhibitor GS4104 (oseltamivir phosphate) is efficacious against A/Hong Kong/156/97 (H5N1) and A/Hong Kong/1074/99 (H9N2) influenza viruses. *Antiviral Res*. 2000;48:101–115.
79. Govorkova EA, Ilyushina NA, Boltz DA, et al. Efficacy of oseltamivir therapy in ferrets inoculated with different clades of H5N1 influenza virus. *Antimicrob Agents Chemother*. 2007;51:1414–1424.
80. Schunemann HJ, Hill SR, Kakad M, et al. WHO Rapid Advice Guidelines for pharmacological management of sporadic human infection with avian influenza A (H5N1) virus. *Lancet Infect Dis*. 2007;7:21–31.
81. Uhl EW, Harvey SB, Michel F, et al. Immunogenicity of avian H5N1 influenza virus recombinant vaccines in cats. *Viral Immunol*. 2010;23:221–226.
82. Gao YW, Xia XZ, Wang LG, et al. [Construction and experimental immunity of recombinant replication-competent canine adenovirus type 2 expressing hemagglutinin gene of H5N1 subtype tiger influenza virus]. *Wei Sheng Wu Xue Bao*. 2006;46:297–300.
83. Yu Z, Gao X, Wang T, et al. Fatal H5N6 avian influenza virus infection in a domestic cat and wild birds in China. *Sci Rep*. 2015;5:10704.
84. Lee K, Lee EK, Lee H, et al. Highly pathogenic avian influenza A(H5N6) in domestic cats, South Korea. *Emerg Infect Dis*. 2018;24:2343–2347.
85. Cao X, Yang F, Wu H, et al. Genetic characterization of novel reassortant H5N6-subtype influenza viruses isolated from cats in eastern China. *Arch Virol*. 2017;162:3501–3505.
86. Zhan GJ, Ling ZS, Zhu YL, et al. Genetic characterization of a novel influenza A virus H5N2 isolated from a dog in China. *Vet Microbiol*. 2012;155:409–416.
87. Yoon KJ, Cooper VL, Schwartz KJ, et al. Influenza virus infection in racing greyhounds. *Emerg Infect Dis*. 2005;11:1974–1976.
88. Dubovi EJ, Njaa BL. Canine influenza. *Vet Clin North Am Small Anim Pract*. 2008;38:827–835. viii.
89. von Grotthuss M, Rychlewski L. Influenza mutation from equine to canine. *Science*. 2006;311:1241–1242. Author reply 1241–1242.
90. Payungporn S, Crawford PC, Kouo TS, et al. Influenza A virus (H3N8) in dogs with respiratory disease, Florida. *Emerg Infect Dis*. 2008;14: 902–908.
91. Hoelzer K, Murcia PR, Baillie GJ, et al. Intrahost evolutionary dynamics of canine influenza virus in naive and partially immune dogs. *J Virol*. 2010;84:5329–5335.
92. Jirjis FF, Deshpande MS, Tubbs AL, et al. Transmission of canine influenza virus (H3N8) among susceptible dogs. *Vet Microbiol*. 2010;144:303–309.
93. Yamanaka T, Tsujimura K, Kondo T, et al. Infectivity and pathogenicity of canine H3N8 influenza A virus in horses. *Influenza Other Respir Viruses*. 2010;4:345–351.
94. Gibbs EP, Anderson TC. Equine and canine influenza: a review of current events. *Anim Health Res Rev*. 2010;11:43–51.
95. McKinley ET Spackman E, Pantin-Jackwood MJ. The pathogenesis of H3N8 canine influenza virus in chickens, turkeys and ducks. *Influenza Other Respir Viruses*. 2010;4:353–356.
96. Smith KC, Daly JM, Blunden AS, et al. Canine influenza virus. *Vet Rec*. 2005;157:599.
97. Newton R, Cooke A, Elton D, et al. Canine influenza virus: cross-species transmission from horses. *Vet Rec*. 2007;161:142–143.
98. Murcia PR, Baillie GJ, Daly J, et al. Intra- and interhost evolutionary dynamics of equine influenza virus. *J Virol*. 2010;84:6943–6954.
99. Kirkland PD, Finlaison DS, Crispe E, et al. Influenza virus transmission from horses to dogs, Australia. *Emerg Infect Dis*. 2010;16:699–702.
100. Daly JM, Blunden AS, Macrae S, et al. Transmission of equine influenza virus to English foxhounds. *Emerg Infect Dis*. 2008;14:461–464.
101. Yamanaka T, Nemoto M, Tsujimura K, et al. Interspecies transmission of equine influenza virus (H3N8) to dogs by close contact with experimentally infected horses. *Vet Microbiol*. 2009;139:351–355.
102. Long MT, Gibbs EP, Crawford PC, et al. Comparison of virus replication and clinical disease in horses inoculated with equine or canine influenza viruses. In: *Immunobiology of Influenza Virus Infection: Approaches for an Emerging Zoonotic Disease*. Athens, GA: 2007.
103. Castleman WL, Powe JR, Crawford PC, et al. Canine H3N8 influenza virus infection in dogs and mice. *Vet Pathol*. 2010;47:507–517.
104. Deshpande M, Abdelmagid O, Tubbs A, et al. Experimental reproduction of canine influenza virus H3N8 infection in young puppies. *Vet Ther*. 2009;10:29–39.

105. Holt DE, Mover MR, Brown DC. Serologic prevalence of antibodies against canine influenza virus (H3N8) in dogs in a metropolitan animal shelter. *J Am Vet Med Assoc*. 2010;237:71–73.
106. Kruth SA, Carman S, Weese JS. Seroprevalence of antibodies to canine influenza virus in dogs in Ontario. *Can Vet J*. 2008;49:800–802.
107. Rosas C, Van de Walle GR, Metzger SM, et al. Evaluation of a vectored equine herpesvirus type 1 (EHV-1) vaccine expressing H3 haemagglutinin in the protection of dogs against canine influenza. *Vaccine*. 2008;26:2335–2343.
108. Deshpande MS, Jirjis FF, Tubbs AL, et al. Evaluation of the efficacy of a canine influenza virus (H3N8) vaccine in dogs following experimental challenge. *Vet Ther*. 2009;10:103–112.
109. Crawford C, Spindel M. Canine influenza. In: Miller L, Hurley K, eds. *Infectious Disease Management in Animal Shelters*. Ames, IA: Wiley-Blackwell; 2009:173–180.
110. Krueger WS, Heil GL, Yoon KJ, et al. No evidence for zoonotic transmission of H3N8 canine influenza virus among US adults occupationally exposed to dogs. *Influenza Other Respir Viruses*. 2014;4:99–106.

26

Canine Parainfluenza Virus Infection

John A. Ellis

KEY POINTS

- Cause: CPIV is a paramyxovirus that is related to parainfluenza viruses and mumps virus in humans (family *Paramyxoviridae*, genus *Rubulavirus*).
- First Described: CPIV was first isolated from dogs with acute URTD in 1967.
- Affected Hosts: Canids. Experimental infections in rodents, cats, and ferrets have been reported, but are a questionable clinical significance.
- Geographic Distribution: Worldwide.
- Route of Transmission: Aerosol, direct contact, fomites.
- Major Clinical Signs: Nonspecific signs of URTD comprising harsh or honking cough, serous nasal discharge, conjunctivitis, and fever (uncomplicated disease). May predispose to lower respiratory tract disease (bronchitis, pneumonia) that is usually associated with secondary bacterial infections, such as *Bordetella bronchiseptica* infections. CPIV has also been rarely associated with neurologic and enteric diseases in dogs.
- Differential Diagnoses: Other causes of acute infectious URTD including, CAdV, CIV, CRCoV, CHV, *B. bronchiseptica*, and possibly reoviruses and canine pneumovirus. Less frequently, other causes of upper and lower respiratory diseases such as airway collapse, fungal or protozoal pneumonia, respiratory tract neoplasia, airway foreign bodies, chronic bronchitis, parasitic infections (such as *Filaroides, Oslerus, Capillaria, Paragonimus, Dirofilaria*), aspiration bronchopneumonia, left-sided congestive heart failure.
- Human Health Significance: None documented; clinical CPIV infections are limited to canids.

ETIOLOGIC AGENT AND EPIDEMIOLOGY

CPIV has a long, complicated history. It has been called Simian virus 5 (SV5), parainfluenza virus 5, canine parainfluenza 2, or, simply, CPIV.[1] It was first found in cultures of rhesus and cynomolgus monkey kidney cells in 1956[2] which led to a still somewhat unresolved controversy concerning its infectivity and pathogenicity in laboratory rodents and in humans.[1] CPIV was first isolated from dogs with respiratory disease in 1967.[3]

CPIV is in the genus *Rubulavirus* of the subfamily *Paramyxovirinae*, order *Mononegavirales,* of the family *Paramyxoviridae*.[4] Other important rubulaviruses that are distantly genetically and antigenically related to CPIV are human parainfluenza virus types 2 and 4 (HPIV-2 and HPIV-4, respectively) and mumps virus.[1,4] Parainfluenza viruses are spherical to pleomorphic and consist of a nucleocapsid that is surrounded by a lipid envelope.[1,4] CPIV has a single-stranded, nonsegmented, negative-sense RNA genome made up of approximately 15,000 nucleotides comprising seven genes that encode for eight proteins. The nucleocapsid or ribonucleoprotein (RNP) core of the virus includes the N or nucleoprotein, the phosphoprotein (P), and large (L) proteins. The matrix or M protein is the most abundant viral protein in an infected cell. It is located on the inner face of the forming envelope, and is essential in the assembly, budding, and release of progeny virions.[1,4] Hemagglutinin-neuraminidase (HN) and fusion (F) glycoproteins are found on spikes in the envelope; they mediate attachment to, and penetration of, the host cell, respectively, and are targets for protective antibody responses.[4] There are two other small nonstructural proteins: the small hydrophobic or SH protein that modulates apoptosis or "programmed cell death" in infected cells; and the V protein that affects interferon biology, the cell cycle, and apoptosis.[4] The RNA-dependent RNA polymerase is a nonstructural protein that is essential for the transcription of viral mRNA and replication of genomic RNA.

Like other single-stranded RNA viruses, CPIV exists as a diverse population of related viruses, or "quasispecies", rather than a single "species." Currently, there is little known about genomic and antigenic differences among CPIVs isolated from dogs, mostly because only a small number of field isolates have been examined.[1,5] Such differences could be related to virulence, and, potentially, to vaccine efficacy. Direct sequencing of CPIV isolates from one outbreak of respiratory disease in kennelled dogs revealed 100% sequence identity in PCR products amplified from two tracheal specimens, and these did not differ from the CPIV vaccine isolate.[6] Unfortunately, these products were from the N protein gene, which is highly conserved and probably unlikely to reveal differences among isolates.[4] Application of panels of monoclonal antibodies has revealed only minor differences in the HN, F, and P proteins among CPIV isolates.[1]

Infection and disease associated with CPIV are most prevalent in situations where dogs are commingled and crowded, such as during boarding, thereby enhancing the potential of droplet transmission (aerosol) of the virus.[1,7–13] CPIV spreads rapidly under these conditions and a large percentage of dogs can rapidly become infected. Certainly, based on what is known about human parainfluenza virus infections in environments such as hospitals and nurseries, fomites are likely important in transmission of CPIV.[4] In addition, the physiological sequelae of stress that accompany commingling situations are likely an important co-factor in CPIV infection, but are unexamined. Climate and seasonal weather variation in transmission and prevalence of infection are also likely to be important unexplored variables in CPIV in dogs.

Numerous historical and recent serological surveys and identification of CPIV in CIRD cases from many countries on several continents indicate a worldwide and widespread prevalence of CPIV infection.[1,7–13] The incidence of CPIV infection in outbreaks varies, as does the incidence of co-infections. Respiratory disease is generally more severe when co-infections are present.[1] There is less known about the prevalence of CPIV in household dogs, but it is probably much lower. A 2015 study documented CPIV in 3.2% of dogs without clinical signs of respiratory disease that were examined at animal shelters, providing an insight into the prevalence of subclinical infections.[14]

An area of controversy in the epidemiology of CPIV infections has been the host range of CPIV. Summarizing numerous studies, available data indicate that canids are the primary or only target species for clinical CPIV infections.[1] This includes wild canids, notably coyotes and foxes. Among other canids, CPIV-associated clinical disease has only been documented in ferrets, and that was only by experimental infection. CPIV seropositivity has been detected in some wild mustelids. Domestic cats have been experimentally infected with CPIV, but no disease resulted. Their possible role as reservoirs for dogs has not been completely excluded. Beyond carnivores, notably in laboratory rodents, the preponderance of evidence indicates that CPIV infections are restricted or abortive. Mice and hamsters can be infected, that is, CPIV can be recovered after "infection", but no disease or lesions result. The ability of CPIV to infect primates is more complicated and somewhat unresolved. Taken together, data indicate that CPIV is unlikely to be of clinical concern in immunocompetent humans. However, its zoonotic potential should probably not be completely discounted in immunosuppressed individuals, approximately 40% of whom own pets in the United States.[15]

CLINICAL SIGNS AND THEIR PATHOGENESIS

CPIV can cause a variety of clinical signs of variable severity including a dry, harsh, hacking cough for 2 to 6 days, several days of pyrexia, nasal discharge, pharyngitis, and tonsillitis.[1] Importantly, these signs are not specific for CPIV infection, and there are often co-infecting pathogens. This makes a clinical etiologic diagnosis difficult.

Since most dogs with uncomplicated CPIV infections recover, there is little documentation of lesions associated with CPIV infection in natural outbreaks. Available data indicate that the main CPIV-associated lesion is histologic tracheobronchitis that is similar to parainfluenza virus infections in other species.[1,4] There is necrosis of tracheal and bronchiolar epithelial cells and sometimes hyperplasia of mucosal epithelium (Fig. 26.1). This is accompanied by infiltration of the epithelium and lamina propria by a mixed population and inflammatory cells. Purulent exudate may be visible in the airways. These changes can lead to disruption of mucociliary function of ciliated epithelia, which can predispose infected animals to secondary bacterial pneumonia. Local inflammation and congestion in the olfactory mucosa can also result in a loss of sense of smell.[16]

Studies in children and puppies suggest that parainfluenza virus infections, especially when combined with other common respiratory pathogens, can have a lifelong impact on hyper-responsiveness in airways. Although there has been no recent work on this phenomenon in dogs, available data suggest that CPIV infection can have pulmonary physiologic and chronic inflammatory effects beyond those normally attributed to acute viral infection.[1,4]

Naturally occurring, uncomplicated, CPIV infections in dogs are usually self-limiting and restricted to the respiratory tract, primarily the upper respiratory tract. However, there have been a few reports of systemic infection, which have included involvement of the CNS and the GI tract. CPIV was isolated from an ataxic paretic puppy with encephalitis with hydrocephalus, and from a puppy with acute hemorrhagic enteritis.[1] Certainly, other paramyxoviruses with broader target cell tropisms, notably CDV, cause systemic disease in dogs, but involvement of CPIV in disease outside the respiratory tract is a rare event that may be attributable to viral strain differences.

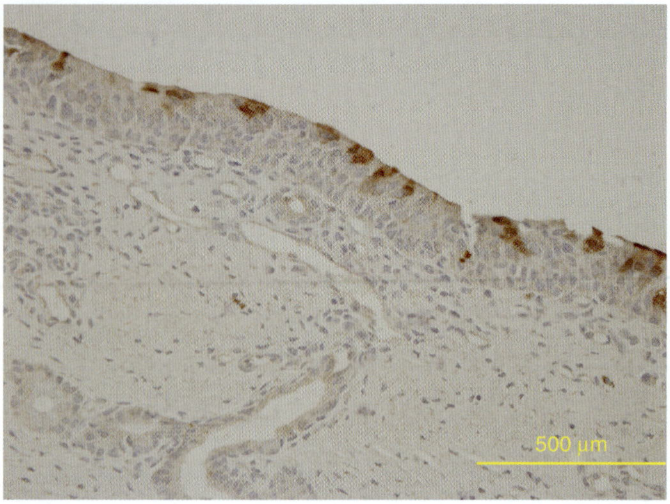

Fig. 26.1 Tracheitis in a calf with bovine parainfluenza virus-3 (BPIV-3) infection. Note numerous ciliated epithelial cells containing brown-staining viral antigens and associated mixed population of inflammatory cells in the epithelial layer and lamina propria.

DIAGNOSIS

As with CIRD pathogens in general, the most definitive antemortem diagnosis of CPIV infection involves detection of the virus in nasal secretions (Table 26.1).[1,4] Historically, this was done with cell culture. From a practical standpoint, use of polyester-tipped swabs are preferred for isolation.[1] CPIV readily grows in a variety of cell types from different host species origins.[1] The use of primary canine cells may improve the sensitivity of detection of field isolates. CPEs in inoculated cell cultures include intracytoplasmic inclusion bodies and syncytium formation, which varies among isolates, and hemadsorption with guinea pig erythrocytes.[1,4] Immunofluorescence (IF) staining is usually used to confirm CPIV infection. CPIV is relatively labile in storage and transport. Failure to account for this can result in false-negative results in isolation. Rapid diagnosis of CPIV can also be attempted by direct IFA staining of cells in smears of nasal swabs. Traditional culture methods have mostly been replaced by PCR detection. Usually these are multiplex PCR assays in the form of a "respiratory panel" that has the capability to detect multiple pathogens simultaneously.[8–13,17] These highly sensitive and specific tests are now in common usage and are available from commercial diagnostic laboratories in many countries. Two important caveats in their use are the timing of specimen collection (> 6–7 days after infection) and recent intranasal (IN) vaccination. Collection of specimens more than 6–7 days after infection risks a high likelihood of negative test results (due to the brief period of virus shedding). Collection of specimens within 3 weeks of IN vaccination is likely to lead to false-positive test results.

In an outbreak situation, serology can be a useful diagnostic approach, especially if dogs have been affected for more than a week. Acute and convalescent serum samples, optimally collected 10–14 days apart, should be used. Hemagglutination-inhibition, virus neutralization tests, or now, more frequently, ELISA tests can be used to measure CPIV-specific antibodies.[1] Factors to consider when using serological testing include the overall endemicity of infection, persistence of maternal antibodies, and routine vaccination, all of which can result in dogs having antibodies to CPIV in the absence of recent exposure. Such dogs may not have anamnestic antibody responses following infection.[1] Despite some limitations, serology using stored paired

TABLE 26.1 Diagnostic Assays Available for Parainfluenza Virus Infections in Dogs

Assay	Specimen Type	Target	Performance
Virus isolation	Conjunctival, nasal and caudal pharyngeal swabs, transtracheal and bronchoalveolar wash specimens, airway and lung specimens collected at necropsy	Virus	False negatives can occur in specimens that contain no or low numbers of virus particles. Attenuated live virus may also be isolated. May take several days and requires specialized techniques and expertise.
RT-PCR	See above	Parainfluenza virus RNA	Sensitivity and specificity may vary depending on assay design. Sensitivity may be low because of brief shedding. Attenuated live vaccine virus may be detected after mucosal vaccination. Because of subclinical shedding, the significance of a positive result may be difficult to interpret. False-negative results may occur as a result of degradation of viral nucleic acid during specimen transport.
Serology	Serum	Antibodies against parainfluenza virus (hemagglutination-inhibition, virus neutralization tests, ELISA)	Interpretation complicated by previous vaccination and exposure. May be useful when the exposed population is naïve and unvaccinated. Acute and convalescent sera required for diagnosis.
Histopathology	Necropsy specimens	Immunostaining	Can be used for diagnosis at necropsy. Immunostaining and/or PCR is required to definitively identify the presence of parainfluenza virus

serum samples may be the only approach to document CPIV infection in outbreak situations when virus detection attempts are not undertaken or fail to yield positive results. The presence of tracheobronchitis or bronchiolytic lesions in dogs that die of respiratory disease is suggestive of CPIV infection. CPIV infection in these cases can be documented using immunohistochemical staining[18]; however, if an affected dog has been sick for more than a week and has secondary bacterial pneumonia, CPIV may no longer be detectable in the lesions.

TREATMENT AND PROGNOSIS

As with most other acute respiratory virus infections, there is no specific therapy for CPIV infections other than supportive care. For most infections, disease is self-limiting. At the population level, control of CIRD including CPIV infection by vaccination alone is often inadequate, especially in high-density dog populations; therefore, attention to environmental co-factors is important. In a kennel or boarding facility, routine cleaning with one of the various commercially available disinfectants is recommended; because CPIV is an enveloped virus, it is susceptible to most disinfectants as well as desiccation. It is also important to clean or remove sources of fomites, which are probably an underappreciated means of transmission.[1,4] Adequate ventilation is also critical in reducing the airborne transmission of CPIV and other CIRD pathogens. Furthermore, 12 to 20 air exchanges per hour and maintenance of facilities at a relative humidity between 50% and 65% with ambient temperature between can 21°C and 23.8°C has been recommended. At the first signs of respiratory disease, infected animals should be isolated if possible. Once an outbreak has occurred, depopulation of the entire facility for up to 2 weeks may be necessary. Minimally, this should preclude exposure via shedding of CPIV by subclinically infected and recovering animals.

IMMUNITY AND VACCINATION

Vaccines for CPIV have been available since the late 1970s, when both IN and parenteral vaccines were developed.[1] Current CPIV vaccines are combination vaccines containing one or more respiratory or systemic pathogens, available for either parenteral or IN administration. Vaccine efficacy has been tested primarily in experimental infections. A limitation of experimental infection models is the usually mild or no disease that results from infection with attenuated CPIV strains that have been propagated in culture in the laboratory, often resulting in a less than robust test of vaccine-stimulated immunity. Nevertheless, both mucosal and parenteral vaccines, when administered properly, optimally at least 10 to 14 days before exposure, can confer clinical immunity as defined by reduced clinical disease and reduced viral shedding.[1] Although CPIV can be a component of core vaccines that are administered every 3 years, vaccination for CPIV and *Bordetella bronchiseptica* should be performed annually for dogs at risk. Therefore, different products must be used for vaccination in the second and third years of each cycle. The ability of IN CPIV-containing vaccines to stimulate rapidly induced local innate immunity and their potential use prior to commingling, or in outbreak situations has not been examined. Although somewhat controversial, both mucosal and systemic antibody responses are correlates of immunity; however, currently, the antibody response to CPIV in vaccinated dogs remains poorly characterized. Moreover, there is virtually nothing known about CMI in CPIV infections, although it is likely to be important, as in other respiratory paramyxoviral infections. Although not formally tested, it is likely that maternal antibodies interfere with priming of CPIV immunity by parenteral vaccination of puppies, as is the case with CDV, which may favor the use of an IN vaccine as a first dose. The comparative utility of IN and injectable CPIV vaccines in boosting of primed immune responses has not been examined. Beyond measuring antibody titers over time, there is very little known about the duration of clinical immunity conferred by vaccination or recovery from infection; it is probably shorter than the persistence of any detectable antibody. Despite gaps in the knowledge, priming through mucosal vaccination early in puppyhood, followed by boosting parenterally when maternal antibodies have decayed at 2–3 months of age, may be the most efficacious approach to immunoprophylaxis.[19]

SUGGESTED READINGS

Ellis JA, Krakowka GS. A review of canine parainfluenza virus infection in dogs. *J Am Vet Med Assoc.* 2012;240:273–284.

Weese JS, Stull J. Respiratory disease outbreak in a veterinary hospital associated with canine parainfluenza virus infection. *Can Vet J.* 2013;54:79–82.

REFERENCES

1. Ellis JA, Krakowka GS. A review of canine parainfluenza virus infection in dogs. *J Am Vet Med Assoc.* 2012;240:273–284.
2. Hull RN, Minner JR, Smith JW. New viral agents recovered from tissue cultures of monkey kidney cells. I. Origin and properties of cytopathogenic agents SV1, SV2, SV4, SV5, SV6, SV11, SV12, and SV15. *Am J Hyg.* 1956;63:204–215.
3. Binn LN, Eddy GA, Lazar EC, et al. Viruses recovered from laboratory dogs with respiratory disease. *Proc Soc Exp Biol Med.* 1967;126:140–145.
4. Karron RA, Collins PL. Parainfluenza viruses. In: Knipe DM, Howley PM, eds. *Fields Virology*. 6th ed. Philadelphia: Lippincott, Williams & Wilkins; 2013:1497–1526.
5. Lui C, Li X, Zhang J, et al. Isolation and genomic characterization of canine parainfluenza virus type 5 strain in China. *Arch Virol.* 2017;162:2337–2344.
6. Erles K, Dubovi EJ, Brooks JW, et al. Longitudinal study of viruses associated with canine infectious respiratory disease. *J Clin Microbiol.* 2004;42:4524–4529.
7. Ellis J, Anseeuw E, Gow S, et al. Seroepidemiology of respiratory (group 2) canine coronavirus, canine parainfluenza virus and *Bordetella bronchiseptica* infections in urban dogs in a humane shelter and in rural dogs in small communities. *Can Vet J.* 2011;52:861–868.
8. Weese JS, Stull J. Respiratory disease outbreak in a veterinary hospital associated with canine parainfluenza virus infection. *Can Vet J.* 2013;54:79–82.
9. Schulz BS, Kurz S, Weber K, et al. Detection of respiratory viruses and *Bordetella bronchiseptica* in dogs with acute respiratory tract infections. *Vet J.* 2014;201:365–369.
10. Viitanen S, Lappalainen A, Rajamaki MM. Co-infections with respiratory viruses in dogs with bacterial pneumonia. *J Vet Int Med.* 2015;29:544–551.
11. Joffe DJ, Lelewski R, Weese S, et al. Factors associated with development of canine infectious respiratory disease complex (CIRDC) in dogs in 5 Canadian small animal clinics. *Can Vet J.* 2016;57:46–51.
12. Monteiro FL, Cargnelutti JF, Martins M, et al. Detection of respiratory viruses in shelter dogs maintained under varying environmental conditions. *Braz J Microbiol.* 2016;47:876–881.
13. Decaro N, Mari V, Larocca V, et al. Molecular surveillance of traditional and emerging pathogens associated with canine infectious respiratory disease. *Vet Microbiol.* 2016;192:21–25.
14. Lavan R, Knesl O. Prevalence of canine infectious respiratory pathogens in asymptomatic dogs presented at US animal shelters. *J Small Anim Pract.* 2015;56:572–576.
15. Angulo FJ, Glaser CA, Juranek DD, et al. Caring for pets of immunocompromised owners. *J Am Vet Med Assoc.* 1994;205:1711–1718.
16. Myers LJ, Nusbaum KE, Swango LJ, et al. Dysfunction of sense of smell caused by canine parainfluenza virus infection of dogs. *Am J Vet Res.* 1988;49:188–190.
17. Altan E, Seguin MA, Leutenegger CM, et al. Nasal virome of dogs with respiratory infection signs include novel taupapillomviruses. *Virus Gene.* 2019;55:191–197.
18. Damian M, Morales E, Salas G, Trigo FJ. Immunohistochemical detection of antigens of distemper, adenovirus and parainfluenza viruses in domestic dogs with pneumonia. *J Comp Path.* 2005;133:289–293.
19. Lu S. Heterologous prime-boost vaccination. *Curr Opin Immunol.* 2009;21:346–351.

27

Canine Respiratory Coronavirus Infection

Canio Buonavoglia, Jane E. Sykes

KEY POINTS

- Causes: CRCoV belongs to the genus *Betacoronavirus* of the *Coronaviridae* family. It was thought to arise from bovine coronavirus (BoCoV) through a cross-species transmission event, as suspected for the closely related human coronavirus OC43 (HCoV-OC43).[1] Viruses of the *Betacoronavirus* genus are typically responsible for either respiratory or enteric disease. Enteric CCoV is a different coronavirus that belongs to the genus *Alphacoronavirus*.
- First Described: CRCoV was first reported in 2003 in a group of dogs newly introduced in a rehoming facility in the United Kingdom where enzootic respiratory disease was reported despite regular vaccination. The earliest report has been ascribed to an old sample collected in Canada in 1996 based on a retrospective study,[2] but earlier circulation cannot be ruled out.
- Affected Hosts: Natural infection with CRCoV has been reported only in dogs, supported by Koch's postulates by experimental infection.[3] Similarly, CCoV only causes disease in canids. However, in 2021 a recombinant CCoV was identified in humans with respiratory illness in Malaysia.
- Geographic Distribution: Both CRCoV and CCoV have been found worldwide. Serologic studies and molecular surveys have detected CRCoV in Europe, the United States and Canada, Japan, Korea, China and New Zealand, demonstrating a global distribution of CRCoV with various prevalence rates.
- Route of Transmission: CRCoV is a highly infectious pathogen with respiratory tropism. Oronasal transmission due to shedding of viral particles through respiratory secretions is considered preferential. In addition, CRCoV has been detected in the feces from naturally infected dogs,[4–6] thus suggesting a possible fecal-oral transmission, although this was not confirmed experimentally.[3]
- Major Clinical Signs: Like CCoV, CRCoV often causes subclinical infections. When disease occurs, CRCoV infection is associated with mild respiratory signs including nasal discharge, sneezing, and cough, which have been documented in natural and experimental infections. CRCoV is a significant contributor to the CIRD complex, predisposing dogs to secondary infections and more severe clinical signs. Occasionally, CRCoV has been detected in dogs with nonrespiratory disease, although whether this virus was responsible for the observed signs was unclear since other pathogens were also detected.[4] A hypervirulent strain of CCoV, known as pantropic CoV, can also infect the respiratory tract, but most affected dogs have shown GI and neurologic signs, in association with leukopenia.
- Differential Diagnoses: Differential diagnosis for CRCoV infection includes infection by other CIRD-associated pathogens, such as CAdV-2, CPIV, CHV-1, *Bordetella bronchiseptica*, *Mycoplasma cynos*, and *Streptococcus equi* subsp. *zooepidemicus*, together with influenza viruses, canine pneumovirus (CPnV), pantropic CCoV, and mammalian reovirus (MRV).
- Treatment and Prevention: For CRCoV, no specific treatment has been tested yet and, to date, vaccines are not available. Vaccines available for prevention of CCoV infection do not protect against CRCoV infection.
- Human Health Significance: There are no reports of disease caused by CRCoV in humans or animals other than dogs.[7] Nonetheless, animal CoVs are regarded as a potential threat by the scientific community, chiefly after the emergence of SARS CoVs and Middle East Respiratory Syndrome (MERS), since potential cross-species transmission may occur from animals to humans.

ETIOLOGIC AGENT AND EPIDEMIOLOGY

CRCoV belongs to the family *Coronaviridae* (order *Nidovirales,* subfamily *Coronavirinae*) that consists of pleomorphic virions of 80 to 120 nm in diameter, containing a positive-sense single-stranded RNA genome of the largest size among all RNA viruses. Due to the envelope, coronaviruses are susceptible in the environment and easily inactivated by commercial disinfectants and detergents. They are more likely to survive in the environment at cooler temperatures. Comparative analysis of coronavirus genomes shows an exceptional plasticity and a marked ability to evolve, generating new strains, genotypes, and serotypes, as a result of a high mutation rate, recombination events, and occasionally of interspecies transmission.[8] Phylogenetically, coronaviruses are classified into four genera, *Alpha-*, *Beta-*, *Gamma-*, and *Deltacoronavirus,* and several species. CRCoV is grouped with bovine coronavirus (BoCoV) and human coronavirus (HCoV) OC43 within the *Betacoronavirus-1* group, which is also defined as bovine-like compared with SARS-CoV-1 and SARS-CoV-2 that are referred to as *Betacoronavirus-2*.[9,10] With a few exceptions, CCoV mainly includes strains with enteric tropism and that belong to the genus *Alphacoronavirus-1,* closely related to FCoV, porcine transmissible gastroenteritis virus (TGEV), HCoV-229E, and HCoV-NL63.[11] All coronaviruses display a similar genome organization with five genes arranged in a conserved order. Two thirds of the genome comprises the replicase gene, which encodes for two overlapping open reading frames, ORF1a and ORF1b, which work as replication/transcription complex.[12] Downstream of the ORF1 gene there are four genes encoding for the structural proteins S, E, M, and N. The spike (S) glycoprotein mediates viral attachment to specific cell receptors driving host cell type binding and is the main inducer of virus-neutralizing antibodies. The E protein drives the assembly of the viral envelope, but is not essential for virus propagation. The membrane (M) protein constitutes the most abundant structural component. Finally, the nucleocapsid (N) protein is complexed with viral RNA, which shapes the core structure of the viral particles.[12] In addition, each coronavirus possesses group-specific accessory genes that are dispensable for viral replication *in vitro* but, as a rule, are maintained in field strains driving virus-host interactions and increasing virulence in natural hosts.[13] CRCoV possesses the canonic genome organization of the genus *Betacoronavirus*, with an additional accessory gene encoding for a surface hemagglutinin-esterase protein (HE)[14] and three accessory genes encoding for nonstructural proteins (*nsp*) that are scattered in the genome, namely ORF 2a, 4a, and 4b.[15] Since its first detection in 2003 in dogs from a rehoming center in the United Kingdom where enzootic respiratory disease was identified, CRCoV was clearly distinguished from CCoV by its molecular and pathologic features.[15,16] Serologic investigations have demonstrated that CRCoV is widespread. The highest seroprevalences to CRCoV have been found in Canada (59.1%) and the United States (54.7%), with lower prevalences from the United Kingdom (36.2%), Ireland (30.3%),[17] Italy (32.1%),[4] and New Zealand (29%).[18] Furthermore, circulation of CRCoV in Asia also has been reported, although with lower seroprevalences in Japan (17.8%)[19] and Korea (12.8%).[20] Due to the antigenic similarities between CRCoV and BoCoV, the bovine virus has often been used as antigen for CRCoV serologic surveys. Importantly, it has been shown experimentally that BoCoV can infect dogs, causing subclinical infection and seroconversion.[19] It is possible that dogs, chiefly in rural areas, have antibodies due to exposure to bovine viruses rather than CRCoV, which should be taken into account when interpreting the results of serologic investigations. Worldwide, at the time of writing, more than 25 dogs have been reported with evidence of natural infection by SARS-CoV-2 (the cause of COVID-19 in humans),[21,22] but most dogs have had no clinical signs and the extent to which this virus can cause disease in dogs remains unclear. Clinical signs and viral shedding did not occur in dogs that seroconverted following experimental infection.[23] Infection of pet dogs has followed exposure to infected humans, and there is currently no evidence of dog-to-human transmission (see Chapter 43 for detailed information on COVID-19 and animals).

Almost all the dogs tested on entry to the shelter in the United Kingdom where CRCoV was first detected seroconverted after 3 weeks, drastically increasing the seroprevalence from 30% to 99%.[16] Similarly, a high incidence of seroconversion has been described in Canada.[24] This indicates that the virus is highly contagious, spreading rapidly in groups of susceptible dogs. Increased prevalence is reported in high-density environments and dogs housed in shelters or kennels, especially after 2–3 weeks of residence in those environments. Dogs older than 6 months are also at increased risk for exposure.[17]

Molecular surveys using PCR have confirmed the circulation of CRCoV in dogs from several countries, with prevalences of 17.5% in the United Kingdom,[16] 7.2% in Italy,[25] 5% in Finland,[26] 9.8% in Germany,[27] and 2.1% in Japan.[5] Interestingly, CRCoV is uncommonly detected in healthy dogs, with 1.8% positive animals in the United States,[28] 0% in Germany,[27] and 4% in Austria.[29] Molecular characterization has identified several CRCoV strains, which suggests genetic diversification, possibly related to geographic patterns of evolution. Whether the observed genetic diversity also implies changes in the biologic features and/or virulence of the various strains requires further investigation.[15,30]

CLINICAL FEATURES

Pathogenesis and Clinical Signs

CRCoV has been primarily associated with respiratory disease. The multifactorial etiology of CIRD hinders a clear understanding of the pathogenesis of CRCoV infection, as synergic mechanisms with other respiratory pathogens impact the clinical course of the infection. Viral transmission mainly occurs via the oronasal route, through respiratory droplets propagated either directly or indirectly. In experimentally infected dogs, viral shedding from the oropharynx was detected at 4 and 6 days PI and lasted for 8–10 days. Sentinel dogs in close contact with inoculated dogs displayed the same shedding pattern.[3] Early shedding of viral particles from day 2 PI may be responsible for the rapid spread observed under natural conditions.[16] Histopathologic evaluation with IHC reveals CRCoV antigen in respiratory columnar epithelial cells within the trachea, bronchi, and major bronchioles.[2,31] Viral antigen has also been detected in ciliated epithelial and goblet cells within the trachea during experimental infections, with visible accumulations in cytoplasmatic vacuoles and on the luminal surface.[31] Replication of CRCoV in these locations negatively impacts ciliary function, interferes with antiviral defense provided by activation of the IFN-JAK/STAT signal transduction pathway within infected cells, and downregulates the expression of proinflammatory cytokines, such as IL-1β, IL-6, TNF-α, and chemokines, such as IL-8.[31] This predisposes to invasion and colonization by other viral and bacterial pathogens (Fig. 27.1).

CRCoV RNA also has been identified in the stools of infected dogs, suggesting a possible additional route of transmission. Attempts to re-isolate CRCoV from enteric samples of dogs actively shedding the virus at the oropharyngeal level were not successful, so it is possible that CRCoV may pass through the canine enteric tract mechanically without intestinal replication.[3] Further investigation is required to determine conclusively whether enteric shedding of the virus can play a role in transmission of CRCoV among dogs. Although CRCoV tropism seems to be restricted mainly to respiratory tissues, the virus has been occasionally detected in dogs with nonrespiratory signs, although co-infection with other pathogens may have been responsible for the observed clinical signs.[4,5] Therefore, a dual enteric-respiratory tropism is possible, as observed for BoCoV,[32] although the ability of the virus to replicate in the GI tract has not yet been demonstrated.

Mild respiratory signs such as nasal discharge, sneezing, and dry cough are the main clinical signs in dogs infected by CRCoV. Loss of appetite, lethargy, or weight loss and other nonspecific signs of illness could be observed when other CIRD-associated pathogens are also involved. This could explain the prolonged duration or the increased severity of the disease observed in some cases. CRCoV seems to be associated primarily with early-stage signs of CIRD, operating as a "quick-hit" respiratory pathogen, and creates conditions that promote more severe secondary infections when other environmental and medical-related factors are favorable. Whilst it is not clear if CRCoV should be considered a primary pathogen of CIRD, a role in the development of this disease complex has been confirmed repeatedly. Accordingly, CRCoV should be always included in the diagnostic algorithms when acute respiratory disease is reported.

Physical Examination Findings

CRCoV infection can result in nonspecific respiratory signs that include serous to mucopurulent ocular and nasal discharge, sneezing, and a dry cough. In dogs with tracheitis, cough may be easily elicited on manipulation of the trachea. To date, there is no evidence of severe disease associated with CRCoV infection. Fever, loss of appetite, and lethargy are rarely reported, and are mostly related to co-infections with other pathogens.[4] Lower respiratory tract signs may appear when secondary bacterial infections complicate the clinical course.

DIAGNOSIS

Laboratory Abnormalities

Information on CBC and serum chemistry profile findings during CRCoV infection is limited. Dogs infected experimentally with CRCoV show some CBC abnormalities.[3] Significant lymphocytosis was observed between days 6 and 14 PI. In addition, transient neutropenia was observed in a significant number of dogs. Some dogs have developed a mild bandemia and toxic changes within leukocytes. Usually, coronavirus infections trigger abnormalities in lymphocyte subsets, interfering with the immune function of the host in a manner that is specifically related with the viral tropism.[33] For betacoronaviruses, transient neutropenia has been reported for SARS CoVs[34,35] and BoCoV.[36] Whether CRCoV is able to modulate the immune system is unknown.

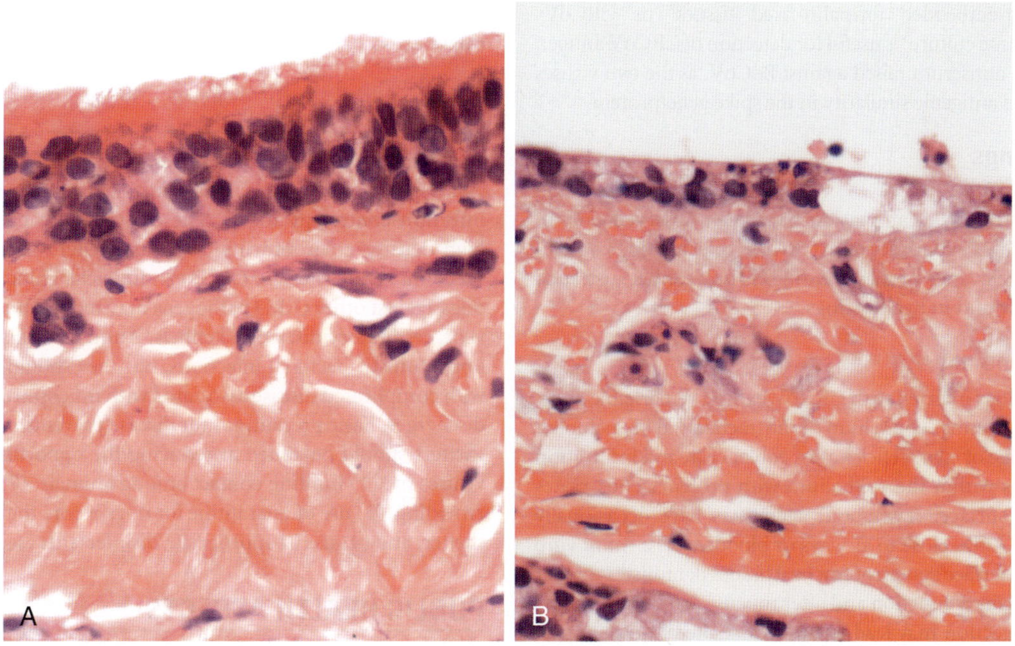

Fig. 27.1 Effect of canine respiratory coronavirus (CRCoV) infection on ciliated respiratory epithelial cells. (A) Respiratory epithelium immediately before inoculation with CRCoV. (B) The same cells 48 hours after inoculation with CRCoV. There is marked loss of cilia, thinning of the epithelium with individual cell necrosis, and sloughed necrotic cells on the surface. There are also occasional large vacuoles within the epithelium, which likely represent foci of cell loss secondary to viral replication. (Courtesy Dr. Simon Priestnall and Professor Joe Brownlie, Royal Veterinary College, UK.)

Microbiologic Tests

As observed for all the etiologic agents suspected to play a role in CIRD, clinical signs are generic and if sought, a definitive diagnosis of CRCoV infection must rely on specific microbiologic tests (Table 27.1). History of recent exposure to other dogs, rapid spread of the disease in a high population density environment, and short clinical course of the disease may support a diagnosis of CIRD, but these do not provide clues to the cause(s) of disease.

Virus Isolation and Molecular Diagnosis

Virus isolation for CRCoV can be difficult because some CRCoV strains are not adapted to grow *in vitro*. Virus propagation on human rectal tumor cell line HRT-18[37] can be successful. The supernatant of infected cell cultures agglutinates chicken erythrocytes at 4°C and mouse erythrocytes at room temperature, although this technique is not sensitive and is difficult to standardize.

In contrast, molecular-based methods are sensitive and specific tools for diagnosis of CRCoV infection. A quantitative real-time RT-PCR assay specific for detection of CRCoV has been developed,[6] and some commercial veterinary diagnostic laboratories offer respiratory PCR panels that include detection of CRCoV.

Specimens suitable for analysis can be collected from the nasal and oral cavities, the oropharynx and nasopharynx. Nasal and tracheal washes and lung lavage fluids from infected animals are expected to yield positive results.[3,6,38] At necropsy, nasal and palatine tonsils, trachea, bronchial lymph nodes, and lung tissues can be collected. Due to the limited period of viral shedding, negative results can occur when specimen collection occurs late after the onset of the clinical signs.

Serologic Testing

Serologic tests may provide information on the prevalence of exposure to CRCoV in dogs but are not recommended for diagnosis. Rapid seroconversion occurs in high density populations. Commercial kits are not available on the market, and either ELISA tests based on BoCoV antigen[4,16] or serum neutralization assays are used.[5] Because the HE protein of betacoronaviruses can agglutinate chicken and mouse erythrocytes, HI has been investigated for detection of antibodies to CRCoV. However, it appears to be poorly specific and sensitive, and not recommended for diagnosis.[4] An ELISA based on CRCoV antigen yielded results comparable to BoCoV-based ELISA assays.[17] IFA has been proposed as the gold standard for serologic testing based on comparative evaluation of sensitivity and specificity.

TABLE 27.1 Diagnostic Assays for Canine Respiratory Coronavirus Infections

Assay	Specimen Type	Target	Significance
Virus isolation (HRT-18 cells)	Nasal or oral swabs, respiratory lavage specimens	CRCoV	Poorly sensitive, difficult to perform.
RT-PCR	Nasal or oral swabs, respiratory lavage specimens	CRCoV RNA	Rapid, sensitive, and specific. Positive results do not imply disease causation because the virus can be found in healthy dogs.
Serology (ELISA, HI, or IFA)	Serum	Antibodies	Positive results reflect exposure. Acute and convalescent titers are required to document recent infection in association with respiratory signs. Assays based on HI have poor sensitivity and specificity and are not recommended.

CRCoV, canine respiratory coronavirus; *ELISA,* enzyme-linked immunosorbent assay; *HI,* hemagglutination-inhibition; *IFA,* immunofluorescent antibody; *RT-PCR,* reverse transcriptase-polymerase chain reaction.

IHC on paraffin-embedded formalin-fixed tissues[2] or CRCoV-inoculated tracheal tissue culture[3] is useful for detection of CRCoV antigen using a cross-reactive antiserum raised against BoCoV, as the two viruses share high genetic and antigenic similarity in the spike gene/protein.

Pathologic Findings

Gross Pathologic Findings

Gross lesions suggestive of inflammation have been observed only in the nares and trachea of experimentally CRCoV-infected dogs at necropsy.[3] The clinical relevance of these findings is unclear because such changes can also be found in healthy dogs.

Histopathologic Findings

On histopathology, dogs infected with CRCoV exhibit remarkable alteration of the ciliated columnar epithelium of the trachea and bronchioles. There is loss or damage of cilia, deficiency of goblet cells, and infiltration of inflammatory cells within the epithelium with proteinaceous material on the luminal surface.[3] Lymphoid aggregates have occasionally been observed in the lungs close to airways or blood vessels. An *in vitro* model using an air-interface system of tracheal tissues demonstrated that CRCoV may impair ciliary function and alter mucus secretion by goblet cells.[6] In addition, infection may lead to functional alteration of antiviral mechanisms, with significant reduction in the expression of proinflammatory cytokines and chemokines. CRCoV antigen can be found in columnar epithelial cells, goblet cells, and in multifocal aggregates dispersed on the luminal surface.[3,6] The same pattern was observed in specimens from two naturally infected dogs with bronchitis and suppurative bronchiolitis collected during an outbreak of distemper in a shelter.[2]

TREATMENT AND PROGNOSIS

There are no specific antiviral drugs available for treatment of dogs for CRCoV infection. However, CRCoV rarely causes complicated or severe disease. Treatment consists of supportive care for respiratory disease (see Chapter 28).

IMMUNITY AND VACCINATION

Vaccines are not available for prevention of CRCoV infection. Vaccines for CCoV are not expected to protect against CRCoV infection (or SARS-CoV-2 infection) because of the low antigenic relationships among the viruses.[17,36,39] Current guidelines for vaccination of dogs do not recommend vaccination because they have not been shown to protect effectively against pathogenic strains of CCoV.[40] CRCoV elicits a humoral immune response with seroconversion within 14 to 21 days PI in both natural and experimental infections.[3,37] The duration of CRCoV-induced immunity has not been evaluated yet, and it is not clear whether dogs with specific immunity are protected against reinfection or disease. In a serologic study of kennelled dogs, seropositivity was statistically associated with protection from respiratory signs, although 50% of seropositive dogs still developed signs. Serum neutralization tests have demonstrated a high degree of antigenic similarity among strains circulating in geographically distinct locations, which increases the likelihood that any vaccine developed in the future might cross-protect against strains that circulate worldwide.[3]

PREVENTION

Prevention involves reducing stress, control of co-infections with vaccination where available, and limiting transmission through proper infection control protocols. These aspects are particularly relevant in high-density environments, such as shelters, rehoming centers, and breeding kennels, where CIRD can impact significantly. Vaccination of dogs against other CIRD pathogens may reduce, but not completely prevent, respiratory disease in kennels. Antimicrobials can be used to treat opportunistic bacterial infections, but they should be reserved for dogs with complicated disease associated with mucopurulent ocular and nasal discharges. Basic precautions for disease prevention and management in shelters should be aimed at reducing the opportunities of exposure to viruses by: (1) limiting contact among animals, (2) prevention of overcrowding, (3) use of quarantine for dogs before their introduction in the shelter, and (4) use of appropriate disinfectants (see Chapter 17).

PUBLIC HEALTH ASPECTS

CRCoV appears to be a variant of BoCoV.[41] Whether the virus originated directly from BoCoV or from a common ancestor is not clear, although the two viruses are highly similar genetically and antigenically.[9] Dogs can be experimentally infected with an enteric BoCoV and SARS-CoV-2, with subclinical seroconversion.[19,23] Unlike other coronaviruses, BoCoV and SARS-CoV-2 seem to easily cross host species barriers.[42] Coronaviruses genetically and/or antigenically similar to BoCoV have been detected in water buffalo,[43] several deer species,[44] alpacas,[45] waterbuck,[46] and giraffe.[47] Furthermore, the virulent BoCoV enteric strain DB2 can cause mild diarrhea in avian hosts under experimental conditions.[48] BoCoV-like viruses have also been identified from humans.[49] The human enteric CoV strain 4408, which is genetically and antigenically closely related to BoCoV, was identified from a child with acute diarrhea. At the time of writing, natural infections with SARS-CoV-2 have been reported in a variety of host species, including domestic cats, dogs, hamsters, ferrets, mink, otters, white-tailed deer, and multiple captive wild felids (see Chapter 43).[21,22] Hamsters, rhesus macaques, rabbits, white-tailed deer, and ferrets have been infected experimentally.[50] Interspecies transmission and recombination are common events for coronaviruses, and several novel human coronaviruses, including SARS-CoV-2, have emerged in recent years from animal coronaviruses.[8] In a serologic survey of immunocompetent adult humans conducted in the United States before the 2019 pandemic, CRCoV-specific antibodies were not identified.[7] However, in 2021, a cluster of infections with CCoV-HuPn-2018, a coronavirus related to CCoV and a FCoV was recognized in children with respiratory illness in 2017–2018 from Malaysia.[51] The clinical significance and epidemiology of this coronavirus requires further investigation. Monitoring the circulation and diversity of animal coronaviruses is pivotal for readily identifying potential zoonotic risks and developing adequate strategies of prevention and control.

CASE EXAMPLE

Signalment

"Bruce," a 6-month-old intact male English bulldog puppy.

History

Bruce was acquired at 10 weeks of age from a breeder, and at that time the owner noticed stertorous breathing. Approximately 1 month later, Bruce developed signs of nasal discharge and cough. Bruce was examined at a local veterinary clinic at that time. Radiographic findings were suggestive of localized pneumonia. Treatment with clavulanic acid-amoxicillin for 10 days was associated with clinical improvement, but 3 days after the antimicrobials were discontinued, the signs returned. Reinstitution of antimicrobial treatment for 1 week again led to resolution of clinical signs. When the signs returned for a third time, they were more severe. Radiographs showed evidence of a hypoplastic trachea and a diffuse alveolar pattern, with the left lung fields more severely affected than the right. A CBC showed leukocytosis (21,430 cells/μL) due to neutrophilia (17,940 cells/μL). Serum chemistry profile was unremarkable. Bruce was hospitalized and treated with IV fluids, clavulanic acid-amoxicillin, enrofloxacin, and nebulization. This led to rapid clinical improvement, and after discharge from the hospital, antimicrobials were continued. The owner was also instructed to hand-feed meatballs to reduce the risk of aspiration of food. Approximately 5 weeks before evaluation at the UC Davis VMTH, Bruce played with another puppy that was diagnosed the following day with "kennel cough." A day later, Bruce began making retching sounds with increased respiratory effort, although these improved after 24 hours. Mucopurulent nasal discharge appeared 7 days after contacting the puppy. Since that time, the owner reported that Bruce had exhibited a deep nonproductive cough that was most apparent throughout the night, and cough was often worse after eating and drinking.

Current Medications

None

Other Medical History

Bruce had been properly vaccinated with an attenuated live CDV, CPV2, CAdV-2, and CPIV-3 vaccine. There are no other dogs in the household, only three adult cats, but Bruce frequently plays with other puppies. Bruce always had a good appetite and was fed canned commercial dog food. There has been no increased thirst or urination. Intermittent vomiting has been noticed since Bruce was acquired.

Physical Examination

Body weight: 11.0 kg

General: Bright, alert, responsive, hydrated. Temperature = 101.3°F, HR = 150 beats/minute, normal RR, mucous membranes pink, CRT = 2 seconds.

Integument: Clean haircoat. No evidence of ectoparasites. Moist dermatitis between skin folds.

Eyes, ears, nose, and throat: Severe epiphora, conjunctivitis, and mild scleral injection OU. Bilateral mucopurulent nasal discharge with normal airflow. Severe prognathism.

Musculoskeletal: BCS 4/9. Ambulatory, well-muscled.

Cardiovascular: Strong and bilaterally synchronous femoral pulses. No murmurs or arrhythmias on auscultation.

Respiratory: Increased upper airway sounds. Multiple episodes of nonproductive, deep, "honking" coughs (5–10 per episode) during examination. No abnormal findings on lung auscultation.

GI: No evidence of abdominal pain or other abnormalities on palpation. Small bladder noted.

Genitourinary: Single descended testicle. No other abnormalities detected.

Rectal examination: Unremarkable.

Lymph nodes: All within normal limits.

Laboratory Findings

CBC: HCT 37.5% (40%–55%), MCV 69.3 fL (65–75 fL), MCHC 33.1 g/dL (33–36 g/dL), WBC 15,690 cells/μL (6,000–13,000 cells/μL), neutrophils 11,265 cells/μL (3,000–10,500 cells/μL), lymphocytes 2,918 cells/μL (1,000–4,000 cells/μL), monocytes 1,098 cells/μL (150–1,200 cells/μL), platelets 430,000/μL (150,000–400,000 /μL).

Imaging Findings

Thoracic radiographs: There is a moderate bronchial pattern excessive for the patient's age. The cardiac silhouette and pulmonary vasculature appear within normal limits. There is a small amount of gas and fluid within the esophagus on the lateral projections. Within the viewable abdomen, abdominal serosal detail is adequate for the patient's age. The stomach has a small amount of gas. The gastric rugae are mildly prominent. There is a hemivertebra in the mid-thoracic vertebral column.

Neck: The soft palate is moderately to markedly thickened. There is increased opacity over the region of the larynx. The trachea is narrowed and appears to have a thick wall. The trachea-to-thoracic inlet ratio is 8.5%. The tympanic bullae are small and have thick walls.

Impressions: Brachycephalic syndrome. Hypoplastic trachea with suspected tracheitis. Hypoplastic bullae and vertebral anomaly consistent with the breed.

Microbiologic Testing

Respiratory real-time PCR panel: PCR positive for CRCoV and *Streptococcus equi* subsp. *zooepidemicus* on pooled nasal and ocular swabs. PCR negative for influenza virus (H3N8), CDV, CPIV, CAdV-2, CHV-1, and *Bordetella bronchiseptica*.

Diagnosis

Brachycephalic airway syndrome (BAS). Infection with CRCoV and *Streptococcus equi* subsp. *zooepidemicus*. Cryptorchidism.

Treatment

Treatment with enrofloxacin and amoxicillin-clavulanic acid was reinstituted, together with 0.1% dexamethasone ophthalmic drops for the conjunctivitis (OU q12h). The owner was also instructed to feed Bruce in an upright position to reduce the likelihood of aspiration. Clinical improvement occurred, with the cough limited to the night time, but signs again worsened when the antibiotics were discontinued. Three weeks after the initial examination, an esophagram was performed which identified a sliding hiatal hernia. Bronchoscopy and bronchoalveolar lavage (BAL) were performed. Airway examination revealed an elongated soft palate and everted laryngeal saccules. Bronchoscopy showed a markedly hypoplastic trachea with moderate mucus accumulation. All airways were mildly edematous with mild mucus and mild stenosis. The BAL showed moderate neutrophilic inflammation (40% neutrophils, 53% macrophages, 400 cells//μL) with some intracellular bacterial rods and occasional diplococci. Aerobic bacterial culture yielded moderate numbers of *B. bronchiseptica* and very small numbers of *Mycoplasma* spp. The *Bordetella* isolate was susceptible to amoxicillin-clavulanic acid, enrofloxacin, and doxycycline. A respiratory real-time PCR panel on BAL solution was negative for all pathogens. Two days after bronchoscopy, Bruce was anesthetized again. The soft palate and everted laryngeal saccules were resected, and a routine prescrotal closed castration was performed on the left testicle and the right retained testicle was removed via the same incision. Bruce recovered uneventfully and was discharged the following day with instructions to administer omeprazole and sucralfate, and to continue elevated feeding. Doxycycline (5 mg/kg PO q12h for 4 weeks) was prescribed for treatment of bordetellosis. Subsequently, his clinical signs improved markedly and there was no recurrence of clinical signs after antimicrobials were discontinued.

Comments

Bruce was infected with multiple respiratory pathogens including CRCoV, likely as a result of contact with other dogs. Some of his respiratory signs and conjunctivitis may have been caused by these organisms, and some may have resulted from aspiration pneumonia secondary to a hiatal hernia and BAS. It is possible that BAS predisposed Bruce to persistent infections with these organisms due to impaired host defenses. Interestingly, bacterial pneumonia was associated with a *Bordetella* and *Mycoplasma* infection, as confirmed by cytology and culture of BAL fluid. Although *Bordetella* was detected using culture, real-time PCR for *Bordetella* was negative, demonstrating the need for application of multiple types of microbiologic tests in some cases. Because resolution of BAS can reduce intrathoracic pressure and decrease herniation, surgical correction of the hiatal hernia was not performed. After 4 months, a repeat esophagram showed some evidence of persistent hiatal herniation and gastroesophageal reflux. However, because clinical signs were controlled, the owner was instructed just to monitor for any worsening of clinical signs that might trigger the need for surgery.

SUGGESTED READINGS

Erles K, Brownlie J. Canine respiratory coronavirus: an emerging pathogen in the canine infectious respiratory disease complex. *Vet Clin North Am Small Anim Pract*. 2008;38:815–825.

Mitchell JA, Brooks HW, Szladovits B, et al. Tropism and pathological findings associated with canine respiratory coronavirus (CRCoV). *Vet Microbiol*. 2013;162:582–594.

Priestnall SL. Canine respiratory coronavirus: a naturally occurring model of COVID-19? *Vet Pathol*. 2020;57:467–471.

REFERENCES

1. Vijgen L, Keyaerts E, Moës E, et al. Complete genomic sequence of human coronavirus OC43: molecular clock analysis suggests a relatively recent zoonotic coronavirus transmission event. *J Virol*. 2005;79:1595–1604.
2. Ellis JA, McLean N, Hupaelo R, et al. Detection of coronavirus in cases of tracheobronchitis in dogs: a retrospective study from 1971 to 2003. *Can Vet J*. 2005;46:447–448.
3. Mitchell JA, Brooks HW, Szladovits B, et al. Tropism and pathological findings associated with canine respiratory coronavirus (CRCoV). *Vet Microbiol*. 2013;162:582–594.
4. Decaro N, Desario C, Elia G, et al. Serological and molecular evidence that canine respiratory coronavirus is circulating in Italy. *Vet Microbiol*. 2007;121:225–230.
5. Yachi A, Mochizuki M. Survey of dogs in Japan for group 2 canine coronavirus infection. *J Clin Microbiol*. 2006;44:2615–2618.
6. Mitchell JA, Brooks H, Shiu KB, et al. Development of a quantitative real-time PCR for the detection of canine respiratory coronavirus. *J Virol Methods*. 2009;155:136–142.
7. Krueger WS, Heil GL, Gray GC. No serologic evidence for zoonotic canine respiratory coronavirus infections among immunocompetent adults. *Zoonoses Public Health*. 2013;60:349–354.
8. Coleman CM, Matthew B. Coronaviruses: important emerging human pathogens. *J Virol*. 2014;88:5209–5212.
9. Vijgen L, Keyaerts E, Lemey P, et al. Evolutionary history of the closely related group 2 coronaviruses: porcine hemagglutinating encephalomyelitis virus, bovine coronavirus, and human coronavirus OC43. *J Virol*. 2006;80:7270–7274.
10. Stout AE, Andre NM, Jaimes JA, et al. Coronaviruses in cats and other companion animals: where does SARS-CoV-2/COVID-19 fit? *Vet Microbiol*. 2020;247:108777.
11. Gorbalenya AE, Enjuanes L, Ziebuhr J, et al. Nidovirales: evolving the largest RNA virus genome. *Virus Res*. 2006;117:17–37.
12. Gorbalenya AE. Genomics and evolution of the Nidovirales. In: Perlman S, Gallagher T, Snijder EJ, eds. *Nidoviruses*. Washington, DC: ASM Press; 2008:15–28.
13. Enjuanes L, Brian D, Cavanagh D, et al. Family Coronaviridae. In: van Regenmortel MHV, Fauquet CM, Bishop DHL, et al., eds. *Virus Taxonomy, 7th Report of the International Committee on Taxonomy of Viruses*. San Diego: Academic Press; 2000:835–849.
14. de Groot RJ. Structure, function and evolution of the hemagglutinin-esterase proteins of corona and toroviruses. *Glycoconj J*. 2006;23:59–72.
15. Lorusso A, Desario C, Mari V, et al. Molecular characterization of a canine respiratory coronavirus strain detected in Italy. *Virus Res*. 2009;141:96–100.
16. Erles K, Toomey C, Brooks HW, et al. Detection of a group 2 coronavirus in dogs with canine infectious respiratory disease. *Virology*. 2003;310:216–223.
17. Priestnall SL, Brownlie J, Dubovi EJ, et al. Serological prevalence of canine respiratory coronavirus. *Vet Microbiol*. 2006;115:43–53.
18. Knesl O, Allan FJ, Shields S. The seroprevalence of canine respiratory coronavirus and canine influenza virus in dogs in New Zealand. *N Z Vet J*. 2009;57:295–298.
19. Kaneshima T, Hohdatsu T, Satoh K, et al. The prevalence of a group 2 coronavirus in dogs in Japan. *J Vet Med Sci*. 2006;68:21–25.
20. An DJ, Jeoung HY, Jeong W, et al. A serological survey of canine respiratory coronavirus and canine influenza virus in Korean dogs. *J Vet Med Sci*. 2010;72:1217–1219.
21. United States Department of Agriculture Animal and Plant Health Inspection Service. Confirmed Cases of SARS-CoV-2 in Animals in the United States; 2020.
22. World Organisation for Animal Health. *COVID-19 Portal: Events in Animals*; 2020. https://www.oie.int/en/scientific-expertise/specific-information-and-recommendations/questions-and-answers-on-2019novel-coronavirus/events-in-animals/.
23. Bosco-Lauth AM, Hartwig AE, Porter SM, et al. Experimental infection of domestic dogs and cats with SARS-CoV-2: pathogenesis, transmission, and response to reexposure in cats. *Proc Natl Acad Sci USA*. 2020;117:26382–26388.
24. Ellis J, Anseeuw E, Gow S, et al. Seroepidemiology of respiratory (group 2) canine coronavirus, canine parainfluenza virus, and *Bordetella bronchiseptica* infections in urban dogs in a humane shelter and in rural dogs in small communities. *Can Vet J*. 2011;52:861–868.
25. Decaro N, Mari V, Larocca V, et al. Molecular surveillance of traditional and emerging pathogens associated with canine infectious respiratory disease. *Vet Microbiol*. 2016;192:21–25.
26. Viitanen SJ, Lappalainen A, Rajamaki MM. Co–infections with respiratory viruses in dogs with bacterial pneumonia. *J Vet Intern Med*. 2015;29:544–551.
27. Schulz BS, Kurz S, Weber K, et al. Detection of respiratory viruses and *Bordetella bronchiseptica* in dogs with acute respiratory tract infections. *Vet J*. 2014;201:365–369.
28. Lavan R, Knesl O. Prevalence of canine infectious respiratory pathogens in asymptomatic dogs presented at US animal shelters. *J Small Anim Pract*. 2015;56:572–576.
29. Hiebl A, Auer A, Bagrinovschi G, et al. Detection of selected viral pathogens in dogs with canine infectious respiratory disease in Austria. *J Small Anim Pract*. 2019;60:594–600.
30. An DJ, Jeong W, Yoon SH, et al. Genetic analysis of canine group 2 coronavirus in Korean dogs. *Vet Microbiol*. 2010;141:4–52.
31. Priestnall SL, Mitchell JA, Brooks HW, et al. Quantification of mRNA encoding cytokines and chemokines and assessment of ciliary function in canine tracheal epithelium during infection with canine respiratory coronavirus (CRCoV). *Vet Immunol Immunopathol*. 2009;127:38–46.
32. Park SJ, Kim GY, Choy HE, et al. Dual enteric and respiratory tropisms of winter dysentery bovine coronavirus in calves. *Arch Virol*. 2007;152:1885–1900.
33. Gralinski LE, Baric RS. Molecular pathology of emerging coronavirus infections. *J Pathol*. 2015;235:185–195.
34. Wong RS, Wu A, To KF, et al. Haematological manifestations in patients with severe acute respiratory syndrome: retrospective analysis. *BMJ*. 2003;326:1358–1362.
35. Pereira MAM, de Almeida Barros IC, Verissimo AL, et al. Laboratory findings in SARS-CoV-2 infections: state of the art. *Rev Assoc Med Bras*. 2020;66:1152–1156.
36. Tråvén M, Näslund K, Linde N, et al. Experimental reproduction of winter dysentery in lactating cows using BCV-comparison with BCV infection in milk-fed calves. *Vet Microbiol*. 2001;81:127–151.
37. Erles K, Shiu KB, Brownlie J. Isolation and sequence analysis of canine respiratory coronavirus. *Virus Res*. 2007;124:78–87.
38. Erles K, Brownlie J. Canine respiratory coronavirus: an emerging pathogen in the canine infectious respiratory disease complex. *Vet Clin North Am Small Anim Pract*. 2008;38:815–825.
39. Priestnall SL, Pratelli A, Brownlie J, et al. Serological prevalence of canine respiratory coronavirus in southern Italy and epidemiological relationship with canine enteric coronavirus. *J Vet Diagn Invest*. 2007;19:176–180.
40. Day MJ, Horzinek MC, Schultz RD, et al. Vaccination Guidelines Group (VGG) of the World Small Animal Veterinary Association (WSAVA). WSAVA guidelines for the vaccination of dogs and cats. *J Small Anim Pract*. 2016;57:E1–E45.
41. Saif LJ. Bovine respiratory coronavirus. *Vet Clin North Am Food Anim Pract*. 2010;26:349–364.
42. Decaro N, Elia G, Campolo M, et al. Detection of bovine coronavirus using a TaqMan-based real-time RT-PCR assay. *J Virol Methods*. 2008;151:167–171.

43. Majhdi F, Minocha HC, Kapil S. Isolation and characterization of a coronavirus from elk calves with diarrhea. *J Clin Microbiol.* 1997;35:2937–2942.
44. Tsunemitsu H, el-Kanawati ZR, Smith DR, et al. Isolation of coronaviruses antigenically indistinguishable from bovine coronavirus from wild ruminants with diarrhea. *J Clin Microbiol.* 1995;33:3264–3269.
45. Jin L, Cebra CK, Baker RJ, et al. Analysis of the genome sequence of an alpaca coronavirus. *Virology.* 2007;365:198–203.
46. Alekseev KP, Vlasova AN, Jung K, et al. Bovine-like coronaviruses isolated from four species of captive wild ruminants are homologous to bovine coronaviruses, based on complete genomic sequences. *J Virol.* 2008;82:12422–12431.
47. Hasoksuz M, Alekseev K, Vlasova A, et al. Biologic, antigenic, and full-length genomic characterization of a bovine-like coronavirus isolated from a giraffe. *J Virol.* 2007;81:4981–4990.
48. Ismail MM, Cho KO, Ward LA, et al. Experimental bovine coronavirus in Turkey poults and young chickens. *Avian Dis.* 2001;45:157–163.
49. Zhang XM, Herbst W, Kousoulas KG, et al. Biological and genetic characterization of a hemagglutinating coronavirus isolated from a diarrhoeic child. *J Med Virol.* 1994;44:152–161.
50. Kumar A, Pandey SN, Pareek V, et al. Predicting susceptibility for SARS-CoV-2 infection in domestic and wildlife animals using ACE2 protein sequence homology. *Zoo Biol.* 2021;40:79–85.
51. Vlasova AN, Diaz A, Damtie D, et al. Novel canine coronavirus isolated from a hospitalized pneumonia patient, East Malaysia. *Clin Infect Dis.* 2021;ciab456.

28

Miscellaneous and Emerging Canine Respiratory Viral Infections

Simon L. Priestnall, Jane E. Sykes

KEY POINTS

- First Described: Respiratory disease in dogs was first described in 1961 in Canada (due to CAdV-2).[1] With the exception of SARS-CoV-2, the most newly recognized virus, canine hepacivirus, was described in the United States in 2011.[2]
- Proposed Causes: CAdV, CIV (and other influenza viruses), CPIV, CRCoV, CHV, canine pneumovirus, possibly reoviruses, bocaviruses, and canine hepacivirus.
- Geographic Distribution: Worldwide.
- Mode of Transmission: Aerosol transmission or close contact, sometimes fomites.
- Major Clinical Signs: Harsh or honking cough, serous nasal discharge, conjunctivitis, fever (uncomplicated disease). Fever, lethargy, inappetence, tachypnea, productive cough, mucopurulent nasal and ocular discharge, rarely death (complicated disease).
- Differential Diagnoses: Upper and lower respiratory diseases such as airway collapse, bordetellosis, *Streptococcus equi* subsp. *zooepidemicus* infection or other bacterial pneumonia, fungal or protozoal pneumonia, respiratory tract neoplasia, airway foreign bodies, chronic bronchitis, eosinophilic bronchopneumopathy or granulomatosis, parasitic infections (such as *Filaroides, Oslerus, Capillaria, Paragonimus, Dirofilaria*), aspiration bronchopneumonia, left-sided congestive heart failure.
- Human Health Significance: Viruses that cause CIRD generally are not considered zoonotic. However, the emergence of human influenza virus infections in dogs, particularly in eastern Asia, is a growing concern. At the time of writing, it remains unclear whether dogs can be a source of human infection with SARS-CoV-2.

ETIOLOGIC AGENTS AND EPIDEMIOLOGY

Canine viral respiratory disease is a widespread problem where large numbers of dogs are housed indoors together, such as in shelters, commercial dog colonies, and breeding facilities. The longer dogs are housed in a shelter situation, the greater the risk that respiratory illness will occur.[3] In shelter environments, CIRD, previously referred to as "kennel cough" or canine infectious tracheobronchitis, delays the placement of dogs in homes and can result in unmanageable costs related to treatment, quarantine, and isolation. CIRD occasionally occurs in owned dogs after a period of contact with large numbers of other dogs at dog parks, dog sporting events, or dog behavior classes. It can also occur after dogs (or dog owners) visit veterinary hospitals, boarding facilities, or pet daycare centers.

With the widespread clinical application of molecular diagnostic assays, it is increasingly apparent that the number of viruses that can infect the canine respiratory tract is much larger than previously thought. This has led to exciting new discoveries in the field of CIRD, and our knowledge of the pathogens involved continues to expand. Co-infections with multiple viruses and bacteria such as *Mycoplasma* spp., *Bordetella bronchiseptica*, and *Streptococcus equi* subspecies *zooepidemicus* are common and contribute to an increased severity of disease.[4–8] Younger age has also been associated with increased severity of disease.[5]

Viruses confirmed as causing or contributing to CIRD include CHV-1 (see Chapter 24), CAdV-2 (see Chapter 23), CDV (see Chapter 22), CPIV (see Chapter 26), CRCoV (see Chapter 27), and CIV (see Chapter 25). There is evidence that infection with canine pneumovirus (CPnV) may also be associated with respiratory disease.[4] CAdV-1 may also play a role when vaccination is not performed or when it is performed improperly.[7] CAdV-1 is discussed in more detail in Chapter 23 and will not be discussed further here. The extent to which SARS-CoV-2 causes respiratory disease in dogs is not clear; most infected dogs have shown no signs. Infections of dogs and cats with SARS-CoV-2 are covered in Chapter 43. The major bacterial causes of CIRD are covered in Chapters 50, 55 and 57.

Although most of the canine respiratory viruses have a worldwide distribution, their relative prevalence varies from year to year and between geographic locations. Even within a state or city, predominant pathogens may differ from one shelter and boarding kennel to another.

CDV, CHV-1, CPIV, CRCoV, CPnV, and CIV are enveloped viruses, so they survive poorly in the environment and are susceptible to a variety of disinfectants. Despite this, contact with virus that persists in the environment may be important for transmission in densely housed populations of dogs. CAdV-2 is a nonenveloped virus and has the potential to survive several weeks on fomites. Shedding times vary depending on the pathogen (Table 28.1). Diagnostic tests for respiratory viral pathogens are summarized in Table 28.2.

CANINE RESPIRATORY VIRUSES WITH ESTABLISHED PATHOGENICITY

Canine Herpesvirus-1

The extent to which CHV-1 plays a role in respiratory disease in dogs has been debated.[9] Experimental infections of dogs can result in rhinitis or signs of tracheobronchitis, and intraocular infection results in conjunctivitis and keratitis (Case Example and Fig. 28.1).[10–13] There is

TABLE 28.1 Major Viral Causes of Transmissible Respiratory Disease in Dogs

Organism	Incubation Period (Days)[a]	Shedding Period[a]	Environmental Survival
Canine adenovirus-1	4 to 9	6 to 9 months	Weeks to months
Canine adenovirus-2	3 to 6	1 to 2 weeks	Weeks to months
Canine distemper virus	3 to 6, longer for neurological signs	Weeks to months	Hours
Canine herpesvirus-1	6 to 10; may be longer with stress-induced reactivation	Unknown	Hours
Canine influenza virus	2 to 4	7 to 10 days (H3N8); H3N2 up to 21 days	Hours
Canine parainfluenza virus	3 to 10	8 to 10 days	Hours
Canine respiratory coronavirus	Probably days	6 to 8 days	Hours
Canine pneumovirus	Unknown	Unknown	Hours

[a]Incubation and shedding periods are approximate and may differ when co-infections or immunosuppression operate.

TABLE 28.2 Diagnostic Assays Available for Respiratory Viruses in Dogs

Assay	Specimen Type	Target	Performance
Virus isolation	Conjunctival, nasal and caudal pharyngeal swabs, transtracheal and bronchoalveolar lavage specimens, airway and lung specimens collected at necropsy	Virus	False negatives can occur in specimens that contain no or low numbers of virus particles. Attenuated live virus may also be isolated. May take several days and requires specialized techniques and expertise.
RT-PCR	See above	Viral RNA	Sensitivity and specificity may vary depending on assay design. Sensitivity may be low because of brief shedding for some viruses. Assays may not be available for all viruses or may not detect all virus strains. Testing specimens from multiple different anatomic sites, or combining PCR with other diagnostic tests can increase sensitivity. Attenuated live vaccine virus may be detected after vaccination. Because of subclinical shedding, the significance of a positive result may be difficult to interpret. False-negative results may occur as a result of degradation of viral nucleic acid during specimen transport.
Serology	Serum	Antibodies against respiratory viral antigens	Interpretation complicated by previous vaccination and exposure. May be useful when the exposed population is naïve and unvaccinated for the virus of interest. Acute and convalescent sera required for diagnosis.
Histopathology	Necropsy specimens	Viral inclusions; immunostaining	Can be used for diagnosis at necropsy. Detection of inclusions has low sensitivity and immunostaining and/or PCR is required to definitively identify the infecting virus

RT-PCR, reverse transcriptase-polymerase chain reaction.

evidence of widespread exposure to CHV-1 in dogs worldwide,[9] and a substantial proportion of the dog population may be latently infected. Like other herpesviruses, CHV-1 becomes latent in neurologic tissues, with precipitation of virus shedding by stress. Consistent with the time delay required for reactivation after stress, CHV-1 was most frequently detected 3 to 4 weeks after dogs were introduced to a rehoming center, whereas CRCoV and CPIV were most frequently detected in the first and second week. Dogs infected with CHV-1 were more likely to have severe respiratory disease, although severe respiratory disease itself might predispose dogs to the shedding of CHV-1.[9] Infection with CHV-1 was reported in association with fatal hepatic necrosis in an adult dog that lacked any evidence of immunosuppression.[14] More recently, CHV-1 has been associated with fatal pneumonia in four previously clinically healthy (nonimmunosuppressed) dogs in the United States[15] (Fig. 28.2); thus, the role of this virus as a primary respiratory pathogen in adult dogs may need to be further investigated. For more information on CHV-1 infections, the reader is referred to Chapter 24.

Canine Adenovirus-2

Adenoviruses are icosahedral DNA viruses that infect a variety of animal species. CAdV-2 is found worldwide and primarily infects the respiratory tract of dogs. Rarely, it has been implicated as a cause of enteritis in dogs, and it was found in the brains of puppies with neurologic signs.[16] The virus replicates in nonciliated bronchiolar epithelial cells; epithelial cells of the nasal mucosa, pharynx, and tonsillar crypts; mucous cells in the trachea and bronchi; and type 2 alveolar epithelial cells. CAdV-2 can also be isolated from retropharyngeal and bronchial lymph nodes as well as epithelial cells of the intestinal tract. Shedding typically ceases 1 to 2 weeks after initial infection. For more information on CAdV infections, the reader is referred to Chapter 23.

Canine Influenza Viruses

Influenza viruses are enveloped viruses with segmented single-stranded RNA genomes that belong to the family *Orthomyxoviridae* (see Chapter 25). Influenza viruses that cause disease in domestic animals belong to the genus *Influenzavirus A,* whereas influenza B and influenza C viruses primarily circulate among humans. Influenza A viruses are classified based on the genetic composition of their hemagglutinin (H) and neuraminidase (N) genes. To date, 16 H types and 9 N types have been identified, each of which are antigenically distinct.[17] The names of influenza viruses are specified as follows: influenza genus (A, B, or C)/host/geographic origin/strain number/year of

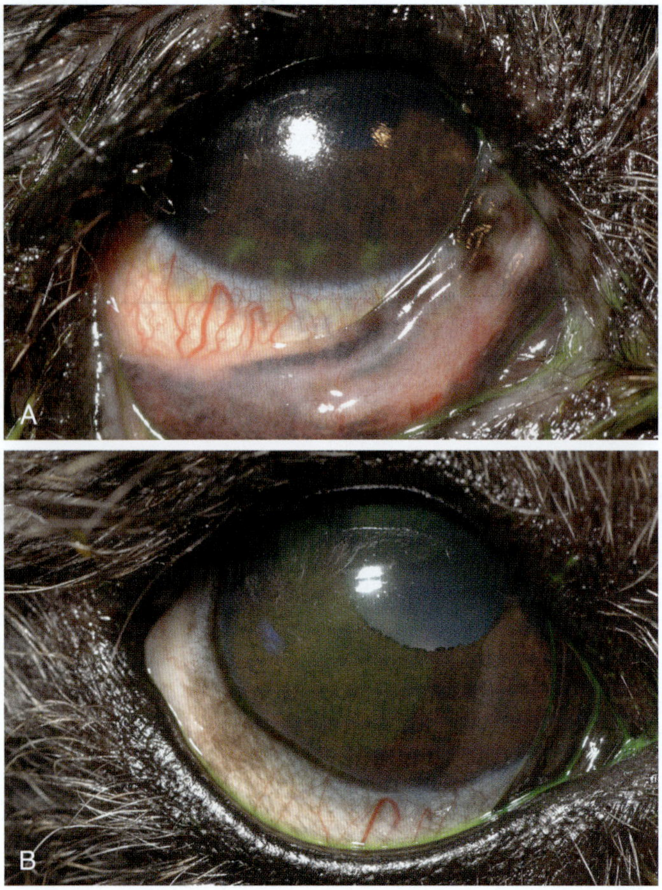

Fig. 28.1 (A) Right eye of a 10-year-old male neutered miniature schnauzer infected with bilateral conjunctivitis and dendritic ulceration associated with canine herpesvirus infection. Fluorescein uptake can be seen in a branching pattern at the limbus of the right eye. (B) The same dog 1 month later. Note diffuse stain uptake over at least 25% of the corneal surface. (Courtesy University of California, Davis Veterinary Ophthalmology Service.)

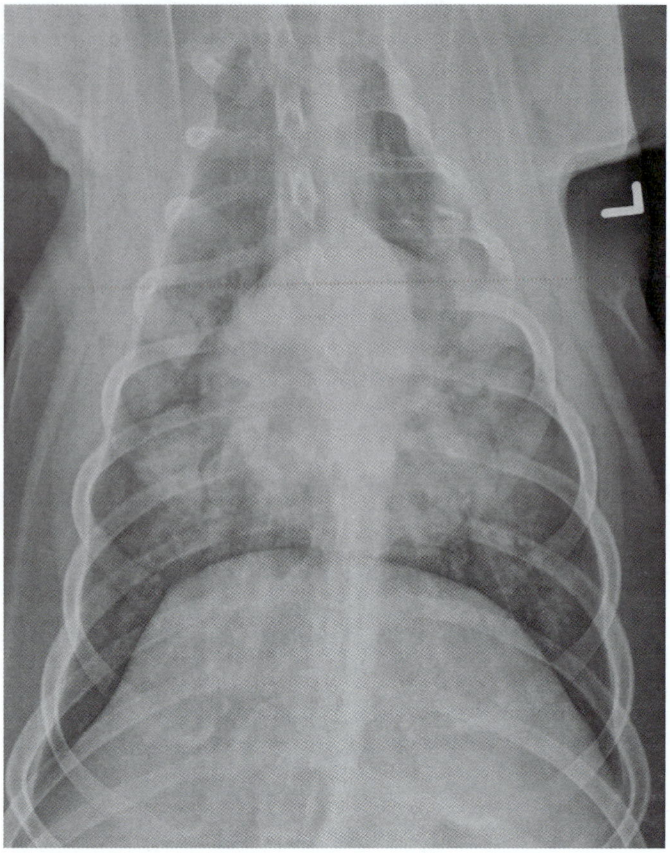

Fig. 28.2 Dorsoventral thoracic radiograph from a 2-year-old male neutered coonhound that had left a boarding facility 6 days previously with a moist, productive cough that subsequently progressed and was complicated by the development of fever and a mucopurulent nasal discharge. A complete blood count showed neutrophilia (17,840 cells/μL), increased numbers of band neutrophils (223 cells/μL), and monocytosis (3,345 cells/μL). Bronchopneumonia is present that involves the right cranial, right middle, and left cranial lung lobes. Interestingly, canine herpesvirus DNA was detected in a pooled extract from nasal, conjunctival, and oral swab specimens, as well as a whole blood sample using a PCR assay.

isolation and, in parentheses, H and N type—for example, A/canine/Florida/43/2004 (H3N8).[18] Extensive genomic rearrangements that occur within influenza A viruses allow for occasional cross-species transmission among birds and mammals. These rearrangements occur when two different viruses simultaneously infect a host, with subsequent genetic reassortment. Occasionally, cross-species transmission occurs without alteration of the viral genome.

In the United States, CIV emerged in racing greyhounds in Florida in 2003 and 2004,[18] where it caused hemorrhagic pneumonia and a high mortality. However, serologic evidence of infection in the greyhound dog population dates back to 1999.[19] Infections spread slowly and were subsequently reported in racing greyhounds and non-greyhounds in at least 38 American states. Outbreaks continued to occur in shelter situations for nearly a decade after the virus was discovered. The virus was an H3N8 virus that closely resembled an equine influenza virus, which suggested that an interspecies jump occurred without genetic reassortment.[18] Instead, accumulation of point mutations with minor amino acid changes occurred, with sustained transmission among dogs. The most significant outbreaks of disease due to CIV occurred in Florida, New England, Colorado, Wyoming, and Texas. In many other states, sustained transmission of the virus from one dog to another did not occur. The most significant risk factor for infection was indoor housing.[20] Virtually all cases to date involved dogs in kennels, animal shelters, or dog daycare facilities. Dogs of all ages and breeds are susceptible, but to date severe hemorrhagic pneumonia has occurred only in greyhounds.[21] The virus is shed for up to 7 to 10 days. CIV has retained the ability to infect horses, but horses develop only mild disease or no clinical signs.[21] The prevalence of infection as determined by real-time PCR has been gradually decreasing within the dog population. By the year 2020, some experts believed this virus was extinct or near extinction within the United States.

Avian-lineage H3N2 CIV emerged in South Korean dogs in 2007, and a similar virus was subsequently isolated from dogs in China.[22,23] Korean isolates were associated with epidemics of respiratory disease in kennels within veterinary clinics.[23] In February/March of 2015, an H3N2 virus was introduced into the Chicago area, likely as a result of importation of a dog from Korea, after which it spread to several other states within the United States, especially North Carolina and Georgia. Additional importation events may have contributed to an outbreak of infection in late 2017 in California. This virus caused more severe upper respiratory signs in dogs, and spread to a greater extent within the owned pet dog population when compared with the H3N8 virus. A novel H5N2 influenza virus was detected in a dog with respiratory disease in China.[24] Dogs are susceptible to infection with human influenza virus H1N1[25,26] and avian H5N1[27]; however, sustained transmission of these viruses in the dog population has not been reported. Limited infection of dogs with equine H3N8 viruses was detected in hounds in England[28] and during an equine influenza outbreak in Australia.[29] In England, disease was so severe that several hounds had to be euthanized, and subacute broncho-interstitial pneumonia was detected at necropsy.[28] The Australian dogs developed inappetence, lethargy, nasal discharge, and a cough that persisted for several weeks, but dog-to-dog transmission was not identified. Experimental transmission of H3N8 influenza virus from horses to dogs was documented in Japan, but infected dogs did not show signs of illness.[30]

Dogs are susceptible to both mammalian and avian-lineage influenza viruses, and as such reassortment of viruses following co-infection poses a potentially significant zoonotic risk to humans, particularly in the western world, who have more frequent and close contact with dogs than either poultry or pigs.

Canine Parainfluenza Viruses

CDV, CPIV, and CPnV belong to the family *Paramyxoviridae*, which are enveloped RNA viruses. CPIV belongs to the genus *Rubulavirus*. The virus infects dogs worldwide, replicates in epithelial cells of the upper respiratory tract, and often causes no signs or mild respiratory illness. CPIV was the most prevalent respiratory pathogen in a large study of dogs from the United States with respiratory disease,[5] as well as 138 dogs from Italy.[31] Respiratory disease may be more severe when co-infections with other pathogens such as *B. bronchiseptica* are present.[32] Viremia seems to be uncommon, but occasionally CPIV has been isolated from the liver, spleen, and kidneys. A strain of CPIV was also isolated from a dog with neurologic signs.[33] Virus is shed for up to 10 days after infection. CPIV is discussed further in Chapter 26. CDV is now rarely associated with typical CIRD, but should be considered in the differential diagnosis, especially if respiratory signs are severe or complicated by secondary bacterial pneumonia. The concurrent presence of GI or neurologic signs are also suggestive of distemper, but sometimes these may be overlooked or absent. The immunosuppressive effects of CDV infection may also predispose an animal to infection with other respiratory pathogens, and is discussed further in Chapter 22.

Canine Respiratory Coronavirus (CRCoV)

CRCoV belongs to the *Betacoronavirus* genus of the *Coronaviridae* family, most closely related to bovine coronavirus (BoCoV) and human coronavirus OC43 (see Chapter 27).[34] The betacoronavirus SARS-CoV-2 is less closely related (see Chapter 43),[35] but similarities in the pathogenesis of, epidemiology of, and immune response to CRCoV and SARS-CoV-2 have been noted.[36] CRCoV is serologically and genetically distinct from CCoV, an alphacoronavirus, which is typically an etiologic agent of enteric disease, although pantropic CCoV have recently been identified and are discussed later in this chapter.

CRCoV was first described in 2003 during an investigation into the pathogenesis of CIRD in a large UK rehoming center.[37] This study showed a strong association between exposure to CRCoV and the development of CIRD in dogs entering the kennel. Since the initial report, the global presence of CRCoV has been demonstrated.[4,38–49] Collective findings from outbreaks and clinical cases indicate that CRCoV is associated with mild respiratory disease during the early stages of CIRD, with typical clinical signs including a dry cough and nasal discharge.[8,37,50] CRCoV has been isolated from a wide range of respiratory and respiratory-associated lymphoid tissues (trachea, palatine tonsil, nasal cavity, nasal tonsil, bronchial lymph node, apical and diaphragmatic lung lobes, and lung lavage fluids). The trachea and nasal tonsil are the most common sites of infection and are also reported to have the highest viral loads.[51,52] Indisputably, CRCoV displays a clear preferential tropism for canine respiratory tissues, particularly those of the upper airways including ciliated epithelial and goblet cells of the trachea and bronchioles.

Histologic examination of the respiratory tissues from experimentally challenged dogs showed a clear and consistent association between exposure to CRCoV and inflammation in the nares and trachea, with significant injury, such as shortening and clumping, or loss of tracheal cilia.[52] These findings support the hypothesis that CRCoV causes damage to the mucociliary clearance mechanisms of the upper airways, which may predispose dogs to secondary infections (see Fig. 27.1). Further evidence in support of this was seen in an *in vitro* CRCoV-infected canine tracheal organ culture system, in which a moderate reduction in mucociliary clearance was observed.[53]

The discovery of CRCoV and the subsequent research into its pathogenesis has highlighted the importance of viruses in CIRD, not only through direct cellular damage but also through the less obvious effects on the host immune system. Combined, these effects can result in significant morbidity whilst predisposing to other more serious secondary infections.

NOVEL CANINE RESPIRATORY VIRUSES

Viruses believed to play a role in CIRD include CPnV, pantropic CCoVs, canine hepacivirus, canine bocaviruses (CBoV), and reoviruses. A study of 138 dogs either with clinical signs of CIRD or that had been exposed to dogs recently recovered from CIRD found that CPIV was still the most commonly detected viral pathogen.[31] These results mirror similar recent studies from several European countries and Canada.[4,54–56] Interestingly some of the established viral causes of CIRD, namely CHV-1, CAdV-2, and CDV are now infrequently or rarely isolated from clinical cases with more recently discovered viruses such as CRCoV, or novel agents such as CPnV, appearing to fill this niche. In the case of CDV and CAdV-2, this is likely associated with widespread use of effective vaccines, but CPIV is also included in most primary vaccine courses and yet still appears to be a persistent problem. The picture is far from clear though, with other studies appearing to show a relatively high prevalence of CIRD pathogens such as CAdV-2 (and even CDV) in subclinically infected shelter dogs.[57] For the novel agents discussed in the following sections, no vaccines are currently available. However, for at least some of the agents, this is the subject of a great deal of active research.

Canine Pneumovirus

CPnV was first described in 2010 following a retrospective study of respiratory disease in dogs from two animal shelters in the United States.[58] It was reported that after three passages in A72 cells, a CPE uncharacteristic of viruses commonly isolated from dogs was observed. After failing to identify other common agents, a pool of monoclonal antibodies against a human respiratory pathogen (human respiratory syncytial virus) was used, and fluorescent staining was observed in infected cell cultures. Degenerate primers were used to amplify three regions of the viral genome, and sequence analysis revealed that the unknown virus was closely related to murine pneumovirus (MPV), a common pathogen of research and commercial rodent colonies.[59]

In 2011 the full genome sequence of CPnV was completed and its place within the pneumovirus genus of the subfamily *Pneumovirinae* and family *Paramyxoviridae* was confirmed.[60] CPnV is closely related to a number of important human and veterinary respiratory pathogens, including human and bovine respiratory syncytial virus, human metapneumovirus, avian pneumovirus, and most closely, MPV.

Since its initial discovery, CPnV has been detected in kenneled and pet dogs in the United States, the United Kingdom, Asia, and continental Europe.[4,31,60–62] Whilst CPnV is readily detected in dogs with respiratory disease,[58,60] its role as a causative agent of disease has been unclear. Extensive serologic surveys and surveillance studies will be required to determine the presence of CPnV globally and to establish an association with clinical disease. A large multicenter European study of kenneled and pet dogs identified CPnV in 23.4% of 572 dogs using PCR, and there was a clear association between positive test results and clinical signs of respiratory disease.[4] CPnV was the most frequent virus detected in dogs with CIRD and a similar proportion of healthy dogs from New Zealand, highlighting perhaps an inconsistent role in disease causality, and the need to ensure diagnostic assays include the more novel viruses.

The pathogenesis of CPnV infection in dogs remains to be investigated. For other pneumovirus species, transmission occurs via contact with respiratory secretions and the apical airway epithelial cells are the principal targets for infection. Indeed, following an experimental inoculation of BALB/c mice, CPnV was shown to replicate effectively in the lungs, with viral antigen detected predominantly in the epithelial cells lining the bronchioles.[63]

The host immune response, in particular neutrophil activity, has been associated with tissue damage during pneumovirus infection.[17,34,41] In the mouse model, CPnV infection was associated with the induction of a local proinflammatory cytokine response and the presence of mild multifocal perivascular neutrophilic inflammation in the lung.[18,28] Compared with MPV infections, however, there were minimal histopathological changes, reduced neutrophil infiltration of the parenchyma, and no apparent hemorrhage or edema.[64] Similar reductions in neutrophil infiltration have been observed in MPV-challenged mice deficient in type 1 IFN receptors, or in the absence of IFN-γ signaling.[65,66] Pneumoviruses have developed many immune modulation strategies, particularly mechanisms for circumventing host type 1 IFN responses. It will be interesting to establish whether these reported findings are consistent in dogs, and if so, whether they are linked to IFN signaling and immunomodulatory mechanisms of the virus.

The glycoprotein (G) of related pneumovirus species mediates attachment to host cells, and as such contains the major neutralizing epitopes. Considered an important virulence factor, a high degree of genetic and antigenic variation is shown to exist within the G protein of RSV species, which frequently gives rise to escape mutants.[67] The G protein sequences of several isolates have been reported, and this led to the designation of A and B subtypes, both of which were identified in multiple locations across the United States, and included two strains isolated from cats.[64] The study compared group A and B viruses in the BALB/c mouse model, in which virus replication was detected as early as three days post intranasal inoculation, with peak levels at day 6 PI. Local cytokine production and inflammatory responses were examined and some differential responses between A and B strains were observed.[64] Whether a clinical outcome can be linked to subtype warrants further investigation, but for human RSV infections, the findings are conflicting. In addition to *in vivo* studies, it will be important to undertake clinical surveillance and to establish the degree of variation across the CPnV genome and in particular the G protein to determine whether variation is associated with pathogenicity in the dog.

Quantitative RT-PCR assay is becoming increasingly available commercially for CPnV. The recommended diagnostic specimens include nasal and pharyngeal swabs or respiratory lavage specimens. Necropsy specimens from the lung and upper airways are also suitable for testing with this assay.

Canine Reoviruses

Reoviruses (family *Reoviridae*, genus *Orthoreovirus*) are nonenveloped viruses with a segmented, double-stranded RNA genome. Mammalian reoviruses infect a variety of host species and have a worldwide distribution. The prefix *reo-* stands for *r*espiratory *e*nteric *o*rphan virus, which highlights the tropism of reoviruses for cells of the respiratory and GI tract, and their uncommon association with disease. Despite serologic evidence of widespread exposure to reoviruses in dogs,[68] they have been found only rarely in dogs with respiratory disease[69,70] and dogs with enteritis.[71] There are three mammalian reovirus serotypes, and all three have been detected in dogs. The role of reoviruses in disease causation in dogs is unclear because disease has not been reproducible experimentally; however, they may act synergistically with other respiratory pathogens to cause disease.

Pantropic Canine Coronavirus

CCoV has traditionally been considered an enteric pathogen of low virulence which is not only frequently isolated from dogs with diarrhea but is also detected in feces of dogs displaying no clinical signs.[20,72] In 2005, an outbreak of fatal systemic disease occurred in Italy; CCoV was detected in affected dogs in a range of tissues, including the lungs, where pulmonary lesions were observed. Although the clinical signs associated with the infection have been predominantly GI and neurologic, its presence in the lungs of infected dogs may suggest a role of this tissue in the pathogenesis of CIRD. To distinguish these infections from cases with a purely enteric tropism, the term *pantropic CCoV* has been applied.

CCoV isolates are grouped into CCoV type I isolates, which are closely related to feline coronavirus (FCoV) type I, and CCoV type II isolates, which comprise types IIa and IIb.[73] CCoV type IIb is closely related to transmissible gastroenteritis virus of swine (TGEV).[74,75] CCoV type IIa is the most prevalent of the types within the canine population; however, co-infections with CCoV types I and II are also common.[76]

The pantropic variant of CCoV was first isolated from an outbreak of systemic and fatal disease in dogs in a pet shop in Bari, Italy. Dogs exhibited lethargy, vomiting, hemorrhagic diarrhea, and neurologic signs.[77] All seven affected dogs were between 45 and 56 days of age and died within a few days of onset of clinical signs. At necropsy, gross findings were hemorrhagic enteritis and serosanguinous abdominal effusion, multifocal consolidation of the lungs, superficial hemorrhages within liver and spleen, petechial hemorrhages on lymph node surfaces, and multifocal hemorrhagic renal infarcts. Histopathologic examination showed a fibrinopurulent exudate within the bronchi, bronchioles, and alveoli, degeneration of bronchial and bronchiolar epithelia, fibrinoid vascular necrosis, alveolar hemorrhage, and edema.[78] Further extraintestinal lesions included lymphoid depletion within the spleen and acute renal infarcts. In the lungs, viral antigen was detected within bronchial and bronchiolar epithelial cells and alveolar septa as well as occasional arterial walls. The authors suggested that the vascular lesions observed may have led to the renal infarcts and abdominal effusion.

CCoV type IIa was isolated from the affected tissues and was detected by RT-PCR, whereas other canine viral or bacterial pathogens were not identified. The viral isolate CB/05 had a high sequence identity with FCoV type II strain 79-1683 within the spike gene.[77] Subsequent experimental infections produced similar clinical signs to those observed during the original outbreak, with a more severe clinical course in 2.5-month-old dogs than in 6-month-old dogs.[79] Infected dogs also exhibited lymphopenia with cell counts below 60% of the initial count. Further experimental studies showed depletion of CD4+ T cells for up to 30 days PI.[80]

Since the original report, additional outbreaks have occurred in Italy,[81] France, Belgium,[82] and Greece.[83] Clinical signs exhibited by pups during five outbreaks in Belgium and France included vomiting, diarrhea, and convulsions. CCoV was detected by RT-PCR in the lungs of affected dogs in all outbreaks. Pulmonary lesions were described as subacute interstitial pneumonia and alveolar edema. In four of the five outbreaks, CPV type 2c was detected in fecal specimens of affected dogs. Spleen and liver were tested by PCR for CPV-2c but were found to be negative. The authors suggest that infection with CPV-2c might facilitate systemic spread of CCoV. While the original pantropic isolate CB/05 is a CCoV type IIa, one outbreak in France was associated with CCoV type I.[82]

A large European surveillance study of 354 cases of fatal disease associated with clinical signs, including leukopenia, enteritis, respiratory distress, and/or neurologic signs, identified CCoV in extraintestinal tissues in 33 cases.[84] Of these, 24 were CCoV type IIa and 9 were CCoV type IIb, confirming that strains other than CCoV type IIa can cause systemic infection. In addition, similar to previous studies in France and Belgium, dogs with systemic CCoV infection were commonly co-infected with CPV-2.

Currently available inactivated vaccines against CCoV have been shown to be ineffective against challenge with pantropic CCoV type IIa[85]; the clinical signs, however, were milder in vaccinated dogs. To date, no consistent genetic marker has been identified for discrimination of enteric and pantropic CCoV strains. Of concern, a virus related to CCoV was recently detected in humans with respiratory illness in Malaysia.[86]

Canine Bocavirus

Bocaviruses contain a single-stranded DNA genome and are distinct from other members of the *Parvoviridae* family in that they possess an additional open reading frame (ORF) named NP1, between the nonstructural and structural coding regions. Most of the attention to date has focused on human bocavirus (HBoV), which is found ubiquitously worldwide, and, in particular, HBoV-1, which has been associated with respiratory disease. Initially, the frequent detection of HBoV-1 in asymptomatic individuals and the high viral co-infection rates detected in symptomatic cases indicated that HBoV-1 may exist only as a bystander. However, the application of improved diagnostics have demonstrated a high seroprevalence and a positive correlation between disease and high copy numbers of HBoV, providing increasing evidence that HBoV-1 is an important respiratory pathogen in humans.[72]

Before 2012, minute virus of canines (MVC) was the only known member of the *Bocavirus* genus to infect dogs. MVC typically causes only subclinical infection in adult dogs, but can also cause abortions in bitches and severe respiratory infections in newborn puppies.[87,88] In 2012, several novel species of CBoV were identified using novel primer walking molecular techniques.[89] Analysis of 35 CBoV variants indicated that these CBoVs represent a highly diverse group of viruses, which can be divided into three groups. Group A variants were significantly more prevalent in healthy dogs raised in controlled conditions than in diseased animals, and Group B (especially B1) and C variants were substantially more prevalent in dogs with respiratory disease.[89] The association between respiratory infections and CBoV positivity was most notable for shelter-housed dogs.

A clear relationship between CBoV and respiratory disease in dogs is yet to be established. Furthermore, it not known whether other viral pathogens were also present in the infected dogs (as is the case for HBoV-1). However, the higher prevalence of CBoV B and C variants in dogs with respiratory disease suggests that these viruses may infect diseased animals as opportunistic pathogens or enhance the severity of lesions in co-infections.[89] Evidence for the latter is provided by a study from China in which CBoV was detected in a number of fecal specimens from diarrheic dogs and often in mixed infections with other novel viruses.[90] Although bocaviruses remain only a putative cause of respiratory disease in dogs, there is currently much interest in their wider role as canine and feline pathogens.

Canine Hepacivirus

In 2011, a novel nonprimate hepacivirus (NPHV), tentatively named canine hepacivirus (CnNPHV), was identified in respiratory swab specimens collected from 9 of 33 dogs housed in rehoming shelters in the United States.[2] The dogs represented cases from five different outbreaks of respiratory disease. Six CnNHPV-positive dogs were identified in one outbreak, and three in a second outbreak in the same rehoming shelter 2 weeks later. The virus was also detected in liver specimens from five unrelated dogs which died from GI illness. A subsequent study from the United Kingdom identified the virus in the upper respiratory tract of shelter dogs with respiratory disease by RT-PCR and *in situ* hybridization, and found that it was associated with increased severity of histopathologic changes in the respiratory mucosa.[91]

Canine hepacivirus is the first NPHV to be described; subsequently, a closely related virus has also been detected in the serum samples of horses in the United Kingdom and United States.[92,93] Analysis of the NPHV sequences from dogs in the United Kingdom and United States has shown that they share a common ancestor, which existed in the 1980s, and that a cross-species transmission event may have occurred from horses to dogs around 1970.[94] Comparative phylogenetic analysis has confirmed that canine hepacivirus is the closest genetic relative of hepatitis C virus (HCV) to date.[2] HCV is associated with chronic hepatitis in humans, and the discovery of NPHVs may provide new insights into its origins. The discovery of a hepacivirus in dogs with respiratory disease is intriguing; however, a role for this novel virus in the pathogenesis of disease remains to be determined.

CASE EXAMPLE

Signalment

"Winnie," a 10-year-old male neutered miniature Schnauzer from Sacramento, CA

History

Winnie was brought to his local veterinarian because of a 1-day history of serous ocular and nasal discharge, and sneezing. Fever (103.5°F) was documented on physical examination, and enrofloxacin (2 mg/kg, PO q24h), bacitracin-neomycin-polymixin ophthalmic ointment (OU q8h) and diphenhydramine (2.2 mg/kg, PO q12h) were prescribed, which did not appear to reduce the severity of signs. A day later, he became lethargic, inappetent, polydipsic, and the owners described wheezing, continuous nasal discharge, and a moist cough, so he was brought to the UC Davis William R. Pritchard VMTH for a second opinion. Winnie had been vaccinated regularly for CDV, CAdV-2, CPV, rabies, *B. bronchiseptica*, and CPIV. He was recently cared for in a boarding facility for a week and had been home for the last 11 days. He also visited dog parks regularly and was exposed to grass awns. There were two other miniature Schnauzers at home, and both were currently well.

Current Medications

Enrofloxacin, 2 mg/kg PO q24h

Other Medical History

Increased activity of ALP was noted at a senior care visit 2 months before the onset of respiratory signs.

CASE EXAMPLE—cont'd

Physical Examination

Body weight: 9.4 kg

General: Lethargic but hydrated. Temperature = 100.8°F, HR = 104 beats/minute, RR = 12 breaths/minute, mucous membranes pink, CRT = 1–2 seconds.

Integument: No clinically significant abnormalities.

Eyes, ears, nose, and throat: Severe chemosis, hyperemia, and mucoid ocular discharge OU, profuse bilateral serous nasal discharge and decreased nasal airflow, hypersalivation, right tonsillar enlargement.

Musculoskeletal: BCS 5/9. Ambulatory on all four limbs.

Cardiovascular: No clinically significant abnormalities.

Respiratory: Stertorous respiratory noises. Increased respiratory effort with a normal RR. Referred wheezing noises in all lung fields on auscultation.

GI: Tense abdomen, hepatomegaly detected on palpation.

Rectal examination: No abnormalities detected.

Lymph nodes: All peripheral lymph nodes normal sized.

Ophthalmologic Examination

Both eyes were open. There was mucoid ocular discharge OU. PLRs (direct and consensual) were brisk and complete OU. No evidence of anisocoria. Menace response, dazzle and palpebral reflexes all complete OU. Globe position and movements normal OU. Periorbital palpation and globe retropulsion were normal. The dog behaved as if sighted.

OS: Lids normal, third eyelid hyperemic and edematous, moderate conjunctival hyperemia and chemosis, cornea clear, anterior chamber clear, no flare, vitreous normal, dilated fundic examination normal. There was iris atrophy, lens nuclear sclerosis, and a pinpoint incipient anterior cortical cataract just ventral to the center of the lens.

OD: Lids normal, prominent secretions at meibomian gland openings, third eyelid hyperemic and edematous, moderate conjunctival hyperemia and chemosis, cornea clear, anterior chamber clear, no flare, vitreous normal, dilated fundic examination normal. There was iris atrophy, lens nuclear sclerosis, and linear pigment deposition on the anterior lens capsule at the 5 o'clock position.

Schirmer tear test: 8 mm/minute OU

Introcular pressure: 16 mmHg OS, 17 mmHg OD

Fluorescein stain: multiple dendritic ulcers at the ventral peripheral cornea OD (see Fig. 28.1).

Laboratory Findings

CBC: HCT 53.5% (40%–55%), MCV 67.7 fL (65–75 fL), MCHC 35.3 g/dL (33–36 g/dL), 1 nucleated red cell/100 WBC, WBC 14,780 cells/μL, corrected WBC 14,600 cells/μL (6,000–13,000 cells/μL), neutrophils 10,804 cells/μL (3,000–10,500 cells/μL), band neutrophils 438 cells/μL (rare), lymphocytes 1,752 cells/μL (1,000–4,000 cells/μL), monocytes 1,460 cells/μL (150–1,200 cells/μL), eosinophils 0 cells/μL (0–1,500 cells/μL), platelets 216,000 platelets/μL (150,000–400,000 platelets/μL). A few highly reactive lymphocytes were noted.

Serum chemistry profile: sodium 142 mmol/L (145–154 mmol/L), potassium 6.1 mmol/L (3.6–5.3 mmol/L), chloride 102 mmol/L (105–116 mmol/L), bicarbonate 25 mmol/L (16–26 mmol/L), phosphorus 6.7 mg/dL (3.0–6.2 mg/dL), calcium 9.5 mg/dL (9.9–11.4 mg/dl), BUN 20 mg/dL (8–31 mg/dL), creatinine 0.7 mg/dL (0.5–1.6 mg/dL), glucose 80 mg/dL (60–104 mg/dL), total protein 5.7 g/dL (5.4–7.4 g/dL), albumin 2.2 g/dL (2.9–4.2 g/dL), globulin 3.5 g/dL (2.3–4.4 g/dL), ALT 564 U/L (19–67 U/L), AST 116 U/L (21–54 U/L), ALP 1024 U/L (15–127 U/L), GGT 10 U/L (0–6 U/L), cholesterol 195 mg/dL (135–345 mg/dL), total bilirubin 0.4 mg/dL (0–0.4 mg/dL).

Urinalysis: SpG 1.009; pH 8.5, negative for protein, bilirubin, hemoprotein, glucose; rare WBC/HPF, 0 RBC/HPF, 0–3 hyaline casts/HPF, few amorphous crystals, moderate degenerated cells, and amorphous debris in the sediment.

Imaging Findings

Thoracic and cervical radiographs: A mild to moderate bronchial and interstitial pattern was identified, and was most prominent in the caudal lung fields. A prominent fissure line was identified in the left lateral thorax. Cervical radiographs were unremarkable. Impressions: Pulmonary changes more significant than those related to age, but nonspecific.

Abdominal ultrasound: The cranial pole of the right adrenal was mild to moderately enlarged. A focal area of the cranial pole of the right kidney was mineralized and there was a mild increase in renal cortical echogenicity. The liver appeared sonographically normal. A small stone that measured approximately 3 mm was identified in the urinary bladder.

Microbiologic Testing

A nasal swab was collected and submitted for real-time PCR panel for canine respiratory pathogens, which included CHV-1, CIV, CDV, CPIV, CAdV-2, and *B. bronchiseptica.* The results were available 3 days later, and the swab was positive for CHV-1 DNA.

Diagnosis

Upper respiratory disease and keratitis associated with CHV-1 infection.

Treatment

Winnie was hospitalized in isolation and treated with 0.9% NaCl (30 mL/hour, IV), nebulization for 15 minutes q8h, clavulanic acid-amoxicillin (13.5 mg/kg PO q12h) and lubricating eye ointment (1 inch OU q4h). Clinical improvement occurred a day later and electrolyte abnormalities normalized. When the dendritic ulcers were detected, idoxuridine (0.1% ophthalmic solution, 2 drops OU q4–6h) was prescribed. Unfortunately, the owner was away for the next month, and the idoxuridine was not regularly administered by the dog's caregiver. At a recheck 5 weeks after the dog was first seen, the owner reported 80% improvement in Winnie's respiratory signs although he continued to sneeze approximately six times a day and was still pawing at his eyes. There was persistent conjunctival hyperemia and a fluorescein stain showed large, superficial areas of uptake over the central cornea OU (see Fig. 28.1). STT was 13 mm/minute OS and 8 mm/minute OD. A CBC was normal and the serum biochemistry profile showed persistently increased ALP (835 U/L) and GGT activities (12 U/L) and improvement in the serum ALT activity (124 U/L). The owner was instructed to administer idoxuridine as directed for an additional 2 weeks, as well as lubricating ointment, bacitracin-neomycin ophthalmic ointment (q8h OU), and L-lysine gel (2 mL [400 mg] q12h PO), separating the ophthalmic medications with administration of the idoxuridine first. At a recheck 2 weeks later, all signs had resolved. STT results were 14 mm/minute OS and 10 mm/minute OD, and there was no uptake of fluorescein. The idoxuridine was discontinued. Winnie had another episode of respiratory signs 4 months later, at which time the STT results were 15 mm/minute OU. Treatment with lubricating eye ointment and L-lysine was continued.

Comments

This is an unusual case of ocular and respiratory herpesviral infection. The early detection of dendritic ulcers allowed a definitive connection to be made between the clinical signs and positive PCR assay result. The negative PCR assay results for other respiratory pathogens do not rule out the possibility of co-infections with these organisms, because shedding of these organisms may have ceased or be at undetectable levels. Approximately 2 years later, mild serous nasal discharge returned which progressed to depigmentation of the planum nasale. A biopsy of the nasal planum showed epitheliotropic lymphoma. He was treated with multiagent chemotherapy for over a year without recurrence of the ocular signs.

SUGGESTED READINGS

Priestnall SL, Mitchell JA, Walker CA, et al. New and emerging pathogens in canine infectious respiratory disease. *Vet Pathol.* 2014;51:492–504.

Mitchell JA, Cardwell JM, Leach H, et al. European surveillance of emerging pathogens associated with canine infectious respiratory disease. *Vet Microbiol.* 2017;212:31–38.

Day MJ, Carey S, Clercx C, et al. Aetiology of canine infectious respiratory disease complex and prevalence of its pathogens in Europe. *J Comp Pathol.* 2020;176:86–108.

REFERENCES

1. Ditchfield J, Macpherson LW, Zbitnew A. Association of canine adenovirus (Toronto A 26/61) with an outbreak of laryngotracheitis ("kennel cough"): a preliminary report. *Can Vet J.* 1962;3:238–247.
2. Kapoor A, Simmonds P, Gerold G, et al. Characterization of a canine homolog of hepatitis C virus. *Proc Nat Acad Sci USA.* 2011;108:11608–11613.
3. Edinboro CH, Ward MP, Glickman LT. A placebo-controlled trial of two intranasal vaccines to prevent tracheobronchitis (kennel cough) in dogs entering a humane shelter. *Prev Vet Med.* 2004;62:89–99.
4. Mitchell JA, Cardwell JM, Leach H, et al. European surveillance of emerging pathogens associated with canine infectious respiratory disease. *Vet Microbiol.* 2017;212:31–38.
5. Maboni G, Seguel M, Lorton A, et al. Canine infectious respiratory disease: new insights into the etiology and epidemiology of associated pathogens. *PloS One.* 2019;14. e0215817.
6. Damian M, Morales E, Salas G, et al. Immunohistochemical detection of antigens of distemper, adenovirus and parainfluenza viruses in domestic dogs with pneumonia. *J Comp Pathol.* 2005;133:289–293.
7. Larson LJ, Henningson J, Sharp P, et al. Efficacy of the canine influenza virus H3N8 vaccine to decrease severity of clinical disease after cochallenge with canine influenza virus and *Streptococcus equi* subsp. *zooepidemicus. Clin Vacc Immunol.* 2011;18:559–564.
8. Erles K, Dubovi EJ, Brooks HW, et al. Longitudinal study of viruses associated with canine infectious respiratory disease. *J Clin Microbiol.* 2004;42:4524–4529.
9. Buonavoglia C, Martella V. Canine respiratory viruses. *Vet Res.* 2007;38:355–373.
10. Appel MJ, Menegus M, Parsonson IM, et al. Pathogenesis of canine herpesvirus in specific-pathogen-free dogs: 5- to 12-week-old pups. *Am J Vet Res.* 1969;30:2067–2073.
11. Ledbetter EC, Kim SG, Dubovi EJ, et al. Experimental reactivation of latent canine herpesvirus-1 and induction of recurrent ocular disease in adult dogs. *Vet Microbiol.* 2009;138:98–105.
12. Ledbetter EC, Dubovi EJ, Kim SG, et al. Experimental primary ocular canine herpesvirus-1 infection in adult dogs. *Am J Vet Res.* 2009;70:513–521.
13. Karpas A, Garcia FG, Calvo F, et al. Experimental production of canine tracheobronchitis (kennel cough) with canine herpesvirus isolated from naturally infected dogs. *Am J Vet Res.* 1968;29:1251–1257.
14. Gadsden BJ, Maes RK, Wise AG, et al. Fatal Canid herpesvirus 1 infection in an adult dog. *J Vet Diagn Invest.* 2012;24:604–607.
15. Kumar S, Driskell EA, Cooley AJ, et al. Fatal canid herpesvirus 1 respiratory infections in 4 clinically healthy adult dogs. *Vet Pathol.* 2015;52:681–687.
16. Benetka V, Weissenbock H, Kudielka I, et al. Canine adenovirus type 2 infection in four puppies with neurological signs. *Vet Rec.* 2006;158:91–94.
17. Webster RG, Bean WJ, Gorman OT, et al. Evolution and ecology of influenza A viruses. *Microbiol Rev.* 1992;56:152–179.
18. Crawford PC, Dubovi EJ, Castleman WL, et al. Transmission of equine influenza virus to dogs. *Science.* 2005;310:482–485.
19. Anderson TC, Bromfield CR, Crawford PC, et al. Serological evidence of H3N8 canine influenza-like virus circulation in USA dogs prior to 2004. *Vet J.* 2012;191:312–316.
20. Barrell EA, Pecoraro HL, Torres-Henderson C, et al. Seroprevalence and risk factors for canine H3N8 influenza virus exposure in household dogs in Colorado. *J Vet Intern Med.* 2010;24:1524–1527.
21. Crawford C, Spindel M. Canine influenza. In: Miller L, Hurley K, eds. *Infectious Disease Management in Animal Shelters.* Ames, IA: Wiley-Blackwell; 2009:173–180.
22. Lin Y, Zhao Y, Zeng X, et al. Genetic and pathobiologic characterization of H3N2 canine influenza viruses isolated in the Jiangsu Province of China in 2009-2010. *Vet Microbiol.* 2012;158:247–258.
23. Song D, Kang B, Lee C, et al. Transmission of avian influenza virus (H3N2) to dogs. *Emerg Infect Dis.* 2008;14:741–746.
24. Zhan GJ, Ling ZS, Zhu YL, et al. Genetic characterization of a novel influenza A virus H5N2 isolated from a dog in China. *Vet Microbiol.* 2012;155:409–416.
25. Lin D, Sun S, Du L, et al. Natural and experimental infection of dogs with pandemic H1N1/2009 influenza virus. *J Gen Virol.* 2012;93:119–123.
26. Dundon WG, De Benedictis P, Viale E, et al. Serologic evidence of pandemic (H1N1) 2009 infection in dogs. *Italy. Emerg Infect Dis.* 2010;16:2019–2021.
27. Chen Y, Zhong G, Wang G, et al. Dogs are highly susceptible to H5N1 avian influenza virus. *Virology.* 2010;405:15–19.
28. Daly JM, Blunden AS, Macrae S, et al. Transmission of equine influenza virus to English foxhounds. *Emerg Infect Dis.* 2008;14:461–464.
29. Kirkland PD, Finlaison DS, Crispe E, et al. Influenza virus transmission from horses to dogs, Australia. *Emerg Infect Dis.* 2010;16:699–702.
30. Yamanaka T, Nemoto M, Tsujimura K, et al. Interspecies transmission of equine influenza virus (H3N8) to dogs by close contact with experimentally infected horses. *Vet Microbiol.* 2009;139:351–355.
31. Decaro N, Mari V, Larocca V, et al. Molecular surveillance of traditional and emerging pathogens associated with canine infectious respiratory disease. *Vet Microbiol.* 2016;192:21–25.
32. Ellis JA, Krakowka GS. A review of canine parainfluenza virus infection in dogs. *J Am Vet Med Assoc.* 2012;240:273–284.
33. Evermann JF, Lincoln JD, McKiernan AJ. Isolation of a paramyxovirus from the cerebrospinal fluid of a dog with posterior paresis. *J Am Vet Med Assoc.* 1980;177:1132–1134.
34. Erles K, Shiu KB, Brownlie J. Isolation and sequence analysis of canine respiratory coronavirus. *Virus Res.* 2020;124:78–87.
35. Stout AE, Andre NM, Jaimes JA, et al. Coronaviruses in cats and other companion animals: where does SARS-CoV-2/COVID-19 fit? *Vet Microbiol.* 2003;247:108777.
36. Priestnall SL. Canine respiratory coronavirus: a naturally occurring model of COVID-19? *Vet Pathol.* 2020;57:467–471.
37. Erles K, Toomey C, Brooks HW, et al. Detection of a group 2 coronavirus in dogs with canine infectious respiratory disease. *Virology.* 2003;310:216–223.
38. More GD, Cave NJ, Biggs PJ, et al. A molecular survey of canine respiratory viruses in New Zealand. *N Z Vet J.* 2021;69:224–233.
39. Priestnall SL, Brownlie J, Dubovi EJ, et al. Serological prevalence of canine respiratory coronavirus. *Vet Microbiol.* 2006;115:43–53.
40. Decaro N, Desario C, Elia G, et al. Serological and molecular evidence that canine respiratory coronavirus is circulating in Italy. *Vet Microbiol.* 2007;121:225–230.
41. Priestnall SL, Pratelli A, Brownlie J, et al. Serological prevalence of canine respiratory coronavirus in southern Italy and epidemiological relationship with canine enteric coronavirus. *J Vet Diagn Invest.* 2007;19:176–180.
42. Ellis J, Anseeuw E, Gow S, et al. Seroepidemiology of respiratory (group 2) canine coronavirus, canine parainfluenza virus, and *Bordetella bronchiseptica* infections in urban dogs in a humane shelter and in rural dogs in small communities. *Can Vet J.* 2011;52:861–868.
43. Kaneshima T, Hohdatsu T, Satoh K, et al. The prevalence of a group 2 coronavirus in dogs in Japan. *J Vet Med Sci.* 2006;68:21–25.
44. Yachi A, Mochizuki M. Survey of dogs in Japan for group 2 canine coronavirus infection. *J Clin Microbiol.* 2006;44:2615–2618.
45. Mochizuki M, Yachi A, Ohshima T, et al. Etiologic study of upper respiratory infections of household dogs. *J Vet Med Sci.* 2008;70:563–569.
46. Soma T, Ishii H, Miyata K, et al. Prevalence of antibodies to canine respiratory coronavirus in some dog populations in Japan. *Vet Rec.* 2008;163:368–369.

47. An DJ, Jeong W, Yoon SH, et al. Genetic analysis of canine group 2 coronavirus in Korean dogs. *Vet Microbiol.* 2010;141:46–52.
48. An DJ, Jeoung HY, Jeong W, et al. A serological survey of canine respiratory coronavirus and canine influenza virus in Korean dogs. *J Vet Med Sci.* 2010;72:1217–1219.
49. Knesl O, Allan FJ, Shields S. The seroprevalence of canine respiratory coronavirus and canine influenza virus in dogs in New Zealand. *N Z Vet J.* 2009;57:295–298.
50. Erles K, Brownlie J. Investigation into the causes of canine infectious respiratory disease: antibody responses to canine respiratory coronavirus and canine herpesvirus in two kennelled dog populations. *Arch Virol.* 2005;150:1493–1504.
51. Mitchell JA, Brooks H, Shiu KB, et al. Development of a quantitative real-time PCR for the detection of canine respiratory coronavirus. *J Virol Methods.* 2009;155:136–142.
52. Mitchell JA, Brooks HW, Szladovits B, et al. Tropism and pathological findings associated with canine respiratory coronavirus (CRCoV). *Vet Microbiol.* 2013;162:582–594.
53. Priestnall SL, Mitchell JA, Brooks HW, et al. Quantification of mRNA encoding cytokines and chemokines and assessment of ciliary function in canine tracheal epithelium during infection with canine respiratory coronavirus (CRCoV). *Vet Immunol Immunopathol.* 2009;127:38–46.
54. Joffe DJ, Lelewski R, Weese JS, et al. Factors associated with development of Canine Infectious Respiratory Disease Complex (CIRDC) in dogs in 5 Canadian small animal clinics. *Can Vet J.* 2016;57:46–51.
55. Viitanen SJ, Lappalainen A, Rajamaki MM. Co-infections with respiratory viruses in dogs with bacterial pneumonia. *J Vet Intern Med.* 2015;29:544–551.
56. Schulz BS, Kurz S, Weber K, et al. Detection of respiratory viruses and *Bordetella bronchiseptica* in dogs with acute respiratory tract infections. *Vet J.* 2014;201:365–369.
57. Lavan R, Knesl O. Prevalence of canine infectious respiratory pathogens in asymptomatic dogs presented at US animal shelters. *J Small Anim Pract.* 2015;56:572–576.
58. Renshaw RW, Zylich NC, Laverack MA, et al. Pneumovirus in dogs with acute respiratory disease. *Emerg Infect Dis.* 2010;16:993–995.
59. Kraft V, Meyer B. Seromonitoring in small laboratory animal colonies. A five year survey: 1984-1988. *Zeitschrift fur Versuchstierkunde.* 1990;33:29–35.
60. Renshaw R, Laverack M, Zylich N, et al. Genomic analysis of a pneumovirus isolated from dogs with acute respiratory disease. *Vet Microbiol.* 2011;150:88–95.
61. Mitchell JA, Cardwell JM, Renshaw RW, et al. Detection of canine pneumovirus in dogs with canine infectious respiratory disease. *J Clin Microbiol.* 2013;51:4112–4119.
62. Piewbang C, Techangamsuwan S. Phylogenetic evidence of a novel lineage of canine pneumovirus and a naturally recombinant strain isolated from dogs with respiratory illness in Thailand. *BMC Vet Res.* 2019;15:300.
63. Percopo CM, Dubovi EJ, Renshaw RW, et al. Canine pneumovirus replicates in mouse lung tissue and elicits inflammatory pathology. *Virology.* 2011;416:26–31.
64. Glineur SF, Renshaw RW, Percopo CM, et al. Novel pneumoviruses (PnVs): evolution and inflammatory pathology. *Virology.* 2013;443:257–264.
65. Garvey TL, Dyer KD, Ellis JA, et al. Inflammatory responses to pneumovirus infection in IFN-alpha beta R gene-deleted mice. *J Immunol.* 2005;175:4735–4744.
66. Bonville CA, Percopo CM, Dyer KD, et al. Interferon-gamma coordinates CCL3-mediated neutrophil recruitment in vivo. *BMC Immunol.* 2009;10:14.
67. Sullender WM. Respiratory syncytial virus genetic and antigenic diversity. *Clin Microbiol Rev.* 2000;13:1–15.
68. Hwang CC, Mochizuki M, Maeda K, et al. Seroepidemiology of reovirus in healthy dogs in six prefectures in Japan. *J Vet Med Sci.* 2014;76:471–475.
69. Binn LN, Marchwicki RH, Keenan KP, et al. Recovery of reovirus type 2 from an immature dog with respiratory tract disease. *Am J Vet Res.* 1977;38:927–929.
70. Lou TY, Wenner HA. Natural and experimental infection of dogs with reovirus type 1: pathogenicity of the strain for other animals. *Am J Hygeine.* 1963;77:293–304.
71. Decaro N, Campolo M, Desario C, et al. Virological and molecular characterization of a mammalian orthoreovirus type 3 strain isolated from a dog in Italy. *Vet Microbiol.* 2005;109:19–27.
72. Jartti T, Hedman K, Jartti L, et al. Human bocavirus-the first 5 years. *Rev Med Virol.* 2012;22:46–64.
73. Decaro N, Buonavoglia C. An update on canine coronaviruses: viral evolution and pathobiology. *Vet Microbiol.* 2008;132:221–234.
74. Decaro N, Mari V, Campolo M, et al. Recombinant canine coronaviruses related to transmissible gastroenteritis virus of swine are circulating in dogs. *J Virol.* 2009;83:1532–1537.
75. Erles K, Brownlie J. Sequence analysis of divergent canine coronavirus strains present in a UK dog population. *Virus Res.* 2009;141:21–25.
76. Decaro N, Mari V, Elia G, et al. Recombinant canine coronaviruses in dogs, Europe. *Emerg Infect Dis.* 2010;16:41–47.
77. Buonavoglia C, Decaro N, Martella V, et al. Canine coronavirus highly pathogenic for dogs. *Emerg Infect Dis.* 2006;12:492–494.
78. Zappulli V, Caliari D, Cavicchioli L, et al. Systemic fatal type II coronavirus infection in a dog: pathological findings and immunohistochemistry. *Res Vet Sci.* 2008;84:278–282.
79. Decaro N, Campolo M, Lorusso A, et al. Experimental infection of dogs with a novel strain of canine coronavirus causing systemic disease and lymphopenia. *Vet Microbiol.* 2008;128:253–260.
80. Marinaro M, Mari V, Bellacicco AL, et al. Prolonged depletion of circulating CD4+ T lymphocytes and acute monocytosis after pantropic canine coronavirus infection in dogs. *Virus Res.* 2010;152:73–78.
81. Decaro N, Mari V, von Reitzenstein M, et al. A pantropic canine coronavirus genetically related to the prototype isolate CB/05. *Vet Microbiol.* 2012;159:239–244.
82. Zicola A, Jolly S, Mathijs E, et al. Fatal outbreaks in dogs associated with pantropic canine coronavirus in France and Belgium. *J Small Anim Pract.* 2012;53:297–300.
83. Ntafis V, Xylouri E, Mari V, et al. Molecular characterization of a canine coronavirus NA/09 strain detected in a dog's organs. *Arch Virol.* 2012;157:171–175.
84. Decaro N, Cordonnier N, Demeter Z, et al. European surveillance for pantropic canine coronavirus. *J Clin Microbiol.* 2013;51:83–88.
85. Decaro N, Elia G, Martella V, et al. Immunity after natural exposure to enteric canine coronavirus does not provide complete protection against infection with the new pantropic CB/05 strain. *Vaccine.* 2010;28:724–729.
86. Vlasova AN, Diaz A, Damtie D, et al. Novel canine coronavirus isolated from a hospitalized pneumonia patient, East Malaysia. *Clin Infect Dis.* 2021;ciab456.
87. Binn LN, Lazar EC, Eddy GA, et al. Recovery and characterization of a minute virus of canines. *Infect Immun.* 1970;1:503–508.
88. Carmichael LE, Schlafer DH, Hashimoto A. Pathogenicity of minute virus of canines (MVC) for the canine fetus. *Cornell Vet.* 1991;81:151–171.
89. Kapoor A, Mehta N, Dubovi EJ, et al. Characterization of novel canine bocaviruses and their association with respiratory disease. *J Gen Virol.* 2012;93:341–346.
90. Guo D, Wang Z, Yao S, et al. Epidemiological investigation reveals genetic diversity and high co-infection rate of canine bocavirus strains circulating in Heilongjiang province, Northeast China. *Res Vet Sci.* 2016;106:7–13.
91. El-Attar LM, Mitchell JA, Brooks Brownlie H, et al. Detection of non-primate hepaciviruses in UK dogs. *Virology.* 2015;484:93–102.
92. Burbelo PD, Dubovi EJ, Simmonds P, et al. Serology-enabled discovery of genetically diverse hepaciviruses in a new host. *J Virol.* 2012;86:6171–6178.
93. Lyons S, Kapoor A, Sharp C, et al. Nonprimate hepaciviruses in domestic horses, United Kingdom. *Emerg Infect Dis.* 2012;18:1976–1982.
94. Pybus OG, Theze J. Hepacivirus cross-species transmission and the origins of the hepatitis C virus. *Curr Op Virol.* 2016;16:1–7.

Canine Parvovirus Infections and Other Viral Enteritides

Colin R. Parrish, Jane E. Sykes

KEY POINTS

- First Described: 1978, worldwide, Appel and others.[1]
- Cause: CPV-2 variants (family *Parvoviridae,* subfamily *Parvovirinae,* genus *Protoparvovirus*)
- Affected Hosts: Dogs and other members of the order Carnivora, including coyotes, foxes, wolves, raccoons, otters, coatis, as well as occasional infections of large and small cats.
- Geographic Distribution: Worldwide.
- Route of Transmission: Direct contact with virus in feces and vomitus as well as contact with contaminated fomites.
- Major Clinical Signs: Fever, lethargy, inappetence, vomiting, diarrhea, dehydration. Sudden death or tachypnea due to myocarditis occurs rarely and only after infection of neonatal animals.
- Differential Diagnoses: CDV infection, other canine viral enteritides, dietary indiscretion, toxins, GI foreign body, enteric parasitic infections such as giardiasis and helminth infections, enteric bacterial infections such as salmonellosis, salmon poisoning disease, pancreatitis, hypoadrenocorticism, inflammatory bowel disease.
- Human Health Significance: CPV-2 variants do not infect humans.

ETIOLOGIC AGENT AND EPIDEMIOLOGY

CPV is the most widely recognized cause of transmissible viral diarrhea in dogs and one of the most common infectious diseases of dogs worldwide. It is caused by variants of CPV-2, which are members of the genus *Protoparvovirus.* CPV-2 emerged in the early to mid-1970s and caused a worldwide pandemic of illness in dogs in 1978.[2] The spread of the virus worldwide occurred over a remarkable period of about 6 months. CPV-2 may have been derived from virus related to feline panleukopenia virus (FPV); the first strain recognized was replaced by a mutant that was called CPV-2a during 1979 and 1980, and there have been a number of additional mutations in the viruses, although those are of unknown significance.[3,4] The more recent strains derived from CPV-2a may occasionally cause feline viral enteritis.[5–7] Feline parvoviral enteritis is further discussed in Chapter 30. CPV-2 variants are distinct from another parvovirus—canine bocavirus (previously, canine minute virus). That virus appears to have minimal pathogenic potential, although in the past it has been suggested to be associated with abortion in pregnant dogs or occasional disease in neonatal or adult dogs.[1,8–10]

Parvoviruses are small, nonenveloped, single-stranded DNA viruses (Fig. 29.1A) that can survive for long periods (months) in the environment under cool moist conditions. As a result, environmental and fomite transmission are important, likely including mechanical transfer by insects or rodents. CPV requires the presence of mitotically active cells in order to replicate so that there is a relationship between the ages of animals and the severity of clinical disease. Young animals (6 weeks to 6 months, but especially those less than 12 weeks of age) are more likely to develop severe illness; however, disease may also occur in unvaccinated or improperly vaccinated adult dogs. In North America, certain breeds (including Rottweilers, American pit bull terriers, Doberman pinschers, English springer spaniels, and German shepherd dogs) appear to be at increased risk for development of severe parvoviral enteritis,[11,12] but this appears not to be the case in other geographic locations. A seasonal distribution of disease has been reported in some geographic locations, which may reflect times when more puppies are present, or when dogs access the outdoors and contact virus in the environment. For example, in Saskatoon, Canada, dogs were three times more likely to be admitted with parvoviral enteritis in July, August, and September, compared with the rest of the year.[12] In Australia, increased case numbers were associated with warmer weather and lower rainfall.[13] In other studies, the seasonal pattern of disease differed or was nonexistent.[14,15] For dogs older than 6 months of age, intact males were twice as likely as females to develop parvoviral enteritis.[12] Surveillance studies from Australia also found a correlation between clusters of parvoviral enteritis and regions of relative socioeconomic disadvantage, which may be associated with use of vaccines and number of vaccinations given, while the treatment given varied with the socioeconomic status of the owners.[13,14,16]

A variety of viral pathogens have been shown or suggested to be associated with enteritis and diarrhea in dogs, including CDV (see Chapter 22), canine enteric coronavirus (Fig. 29.1B), rotavirus, astrovirus, adenovirus, calicivirus, and novel viruses that include noroviruses, sapovirus, kobuvirus, and possibly also a circovirus.[17–23] While some of these viruses appear to be common infections, they vary in their ability to cause clinical disease on their own. A variety of strains of canine norovirus have been detected in young dogs with diarrhea worldwide, as well as healthy dogs, with a prevalence of infection in dogs with gastroenteritis that has ranged from 2% to 40%.[18,23] Canine enteric coronavirus primarily causes mild diarrhea in puppies that are less than 6 weeks of age and may also be found in co-infections with other viral causes of gastroenteritis, including CPV-2 variants. Rarely, it has been associated with more significant diarrhea in young dogs or neonates.[24–26] This chapter focuses on canine parvoviral enteritis, which is the most widely recognized and pathogenic viral enteritis of dogs.

CLINICAL FEATURES

Pathogenesis and Clinical Signs

Transmission of parvovirus and other viral causes of gastroenteritis occurs by the fecal-oral or oronasal routes, after exposure to virus in

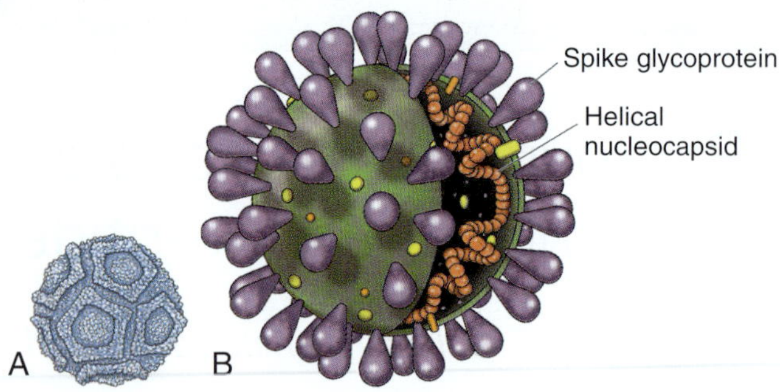

Fig. 29.1 (A) General structure of canine parvovirus. The virus is nonenveloped, 26 nm in diameter, and has icosahedral symmetry. (B) Structure of a coronavirus, which is an enveloped virus. Canine parvovirus is about one quarter the size of a coronavirus.

feces or vomit, or to virus persisting on fomites. Virus is shed for a few days before the onset of clinical signs, and shedding declines considerably after immune responses develop around 7 days.[27,28] The severity of clinical signs likely depends on stressors such as weaning and overcrowding, maternal antibody, and the presence of concurrent infections such as other enteric viral and parasitic infections. Mild or subclinical infections are probably widespread.

The incubation period for canine parvoviral enteritis is likely between 4 and 7 days. The virus initially replicates in the oropharyngeal lymphoid tissues, then free virus spreads widely in the plasma. Virus-infected lymphoid cells also may carry the virus around the body.[28] In older animals the virus will infect, replicate in, and kill rapidly dividing cells, which in puppies are found in higher proportions in the GI tract, thymus, lymph nodes, and bone marrow. Affected GI tissues include the epithelium of the tongue, oral cavity, esophagus, and intestinal tract, and especially the germinal epithelial cells of the small intestinal crypts. The destruction of the intestinal epithelium results in shortened crypts and incomplete epithelial coverage, resulting in loss of fluid regulation and diarrhea. Malabsorption and increased intestinal permeability result. Neutropenia results from not only infection of the marrow but also sequestration of neutrophils in the damaged GI tissue. Secondary bacterial infections of the GI tract, which may be followed by bacterial translocation, bacteremia, and endotoxemia play a key role in the pathogenesis of the disease. Mucosal candidiasis has also been described in puppies with parvoviral enteritis (see Chapter 85).

The outcome is clinical signs of fever, lethargy, inappetence, vomiting, diarrhea, rapid dehydration, and abdominal pain. Diarrhea is often liquid, foul-smelling, and may contain streaks of blood or frank blood. Dogs with canine parvoviral enteritis have evidence of disordered coagulation, with decreased antithrombin activities, prolonged APTT, increased thromboelastography maximum amplitude, and increased fibrinogen concentrations. Catheter and organ thrombosis may occur.[29] Secondary bacteremia may be associated with multiple organ failure and death.

Infection of the dam by CPV-2 variants early in gestation can lead to fetal infection that results in fetal death, resorption, or abortion, although these infections are rare due to the immunity that is found in most bitches by the time they are bred, which would prevent infection. Puppies infected *in utero* late in gestation or which lack maternal immunity and infected up to 2 weeks after birth may develop viral myocarditis due to viral infection of the dividing myocardial cells, which can result in sudden death or congestive heart failure.[30–32] Damage to the developing myocardium usually occurs up to the first 2 weeks of life, but clinical signs of myocardial damage may be delayed until up to 2 months of age. Cerebellar hypoplasia has been rarely reported in dogs after *in utero* infection,[33] but is more common in kittens infected

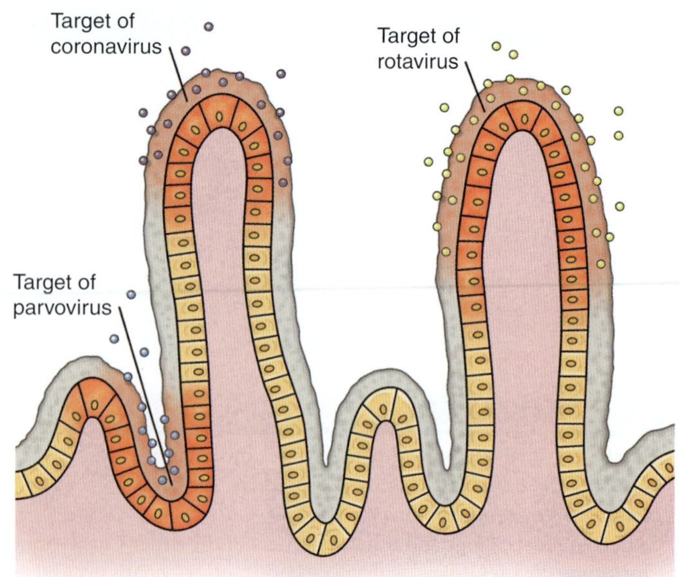

Fig. 29.2 Target sites of replication of selected enteric viral pathogens. The most pathogenic enteric viruses, such as canine parvovirus, replicate and destroy crypt epithelial cells.

with FPV (see Chapter 30). Generalized infection in neonatal puppies is rare, but when present may result in hemorrhaging and necrosis within the brain, liver, lungs, kidneys, lymphoid tissues, and GI tract.[34]

Neurologic signs in puppies with parvoviral enteritis may result from hypoxia secondary to myocarditis, hypoglycemia, or intracranial thrombosis or hemorrhage. The possibility of co-infection with CDV should also be considered.

In contrast to CPV-2 variants, the replication of less pathogenic enteric viruses is restricted to the intestinal tract, and the crypt epithelial cells are generally spared (Fig. 29.2). Canine enteric coronavirus, for example, infects the mature enterocytes at the tips of the villi. Crypt cell hyperplasia occurs to replace the damaged cells. The villi become shortened or distorted, which leads to malabsorption and diarrhea.

Physical Examination Findings

Physical examination of puppies with parvoviral enteritis often reveals fever (up to 41°C or 105°F), lethargy, weakness, dehydration, and abdominal tenderness and a fluid-filled intestinal tract on palpation (Fig. 29.3). Vomiting or diarrhea may occur during the examination, or there may be evidence of diarrhea or frank blood on the perineum or the rectal thermometer. Abdominal palpation may reveal a tubular mass as a result of intestinal intussusception. Ulcerative glossitis can occur in some puppies. Mucosal pallor, prolonged capillary refill time, or rarely hypothermia may be observed in some dogs.[35] Septic shock may be associated with tachycardia or bradycardia, mental obtundation, and poor pulse quality. Uncommonly, neurologic signs such as tremors and seizures are observed. Puppies with myocarditis may be tachypneic and have increased lung sounds as a result of congestive heart failure. Erythema multiforme has been reported in dogs with canine parvoviral enteritis; these dogs had generalized cutaneous and mucosal ulceration as well as swelling of the pinnae and paws.[36,37]

DIAGNOSIS

Laboratory Abnormalities

Complete Blood Count

The most common abnormalities found on the CBC are leukopenia, neutropenia, and lymphopenia (Table 29.1). Toxic neutrophils and monocytopenia may also be present. Only around one third of dogs had leukopenia in one study.[15,35] Leukopenia can develop after the onset of GI signs when puppies are first brought for examination. Some dogs have leukocytosis due to neutrophilia and monocytosis. Although the presence of leukopenia supports a diagnosis of parvoviral enteritis, other severe GI infections such as salmonellosis can also cause leukopenia and diarrhea, so it is not specific for parvoviral enteritis. Thrombocytosis or, less commonly, thrombocytopenia may also occur.[15,35] Some puppies develop anemia as a result of GI blood loss, which may be nonregenerative or become regenerative.

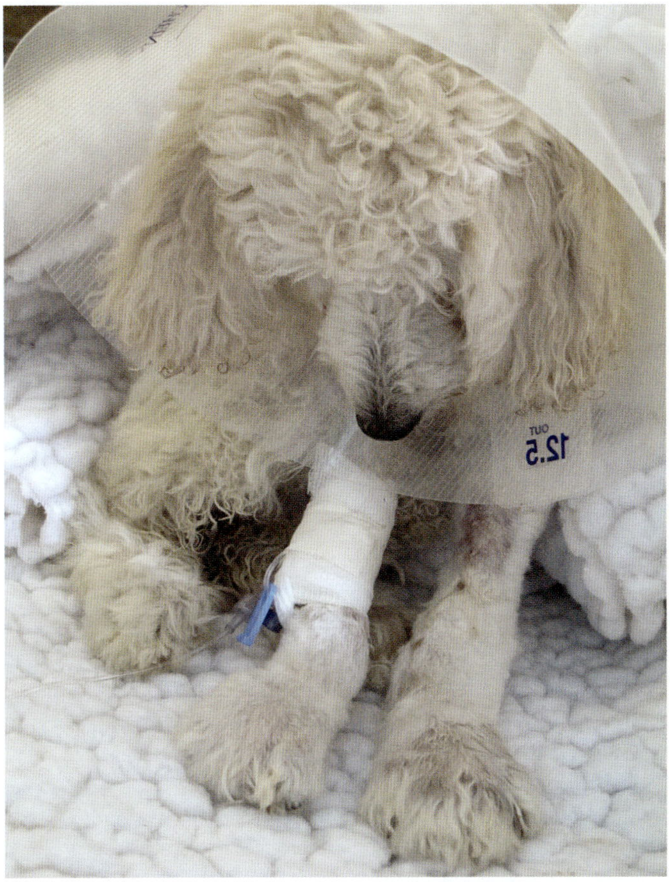

Fig. 29.3 Obtundation in a 3-month-old intact male standard poodle puppy with canine parvovirus enteritis. The dog had been vaccinated for canine parvovirus at 8 and 10 weeks of age.

Serum Biochemical Tests

The serum biochemistry panel in dogs with parvoviral enteritis often shows hypoproteinemia, hypoalbuminemia, and hypoglycemia. Mild hyperglycemia has also been reported. Electrolyte abnormalities such as hyponatremia, hypochloremia, and hypokalemia may occur (Table 29.2). Occasionally severe dehydration results in prerenal azotemia. Puppies with bacterial sepsis may develop increased liver enzyme activities and hyperbilirubinemia.

Coagulation Profile

Coagulation abnormalities have been reported in a small number of dogs with parvoviral enteritis. When abnormalities occur, findings include prolonged APTT, decreased antithrombin activity, increased fibrinogen concentrations, and increased thromboelastography maximum amplitude.[29] An increase in D-dimers or fibrin degradation products has not been reported. More research is warranted to understand the range of coagulation abnormalities that can occur in parvoviral enteritis.

Diagnostic Imaging

Plain Radiography

Plain abdominal radiography in dogs with parvoviral enteritis may show poor serosal detail (often due to lack of intra-abdominal fat in puppies) and a fluid- and gas-filled GI tract. Abdominal radiography is usually performed to assess for the presence of a GI foreign body.

Sonographic Findings

Findings on abdominal ultrasonography in canine parvoviral enteritis are nonspecific but can include a thickened GI mucosa, mild peritoneal effusion, fluid distention of the GI tract, and decreased GI motility. Mild mesenteric lymphadenomegaly may be present. Abdominal

TABLE 29.1 Complete Blood Count Findings at Admission in 45 Dogs Diagnosed with Canine Parvoviral Enteritis at the University of California Davis VMTH

Test	Reference Range	Percent Below The Reference Range (%)	Percent Within The Reference Range (%)	Percent Above The Reference Range (%)	Range For Dogs With CPV Enteritis	Number Tested
Hematocrit (%)	40–55	71	29	0	21–53	45
MCV (fL)	65–75	29	71	0	54–74	45
MCHC (g/dL)	33–36	24	69	7	30–37	45
Neutrophils (cells/μL)	3,000–10,500	56	31	13	8–22,453	45
Band neutrophils (cells/μL)	0-rare	0	31	69	0–1,582	45
Monocytes (cells/μL)	150 1200	20	60	20	11–2,475	45
Lymphocytes (cells/μL)	1,000–4,000	49	22	0	165–3,698	45
Eosinophils (cells/μL)	0–1,500	0	100	0	0–1,236	45
Platelets (cells/μL)	150,000–400,000	5	60	35	103,000–639,000	43

Note: Adult reference ranges were used by the laboratory.

CPV, canine parvovirus; *MCHC,* mean corpuscular hemoglobin concentration; *MCV,* mean corpuscular volume; VMTH, veterinary medical teaching hospital.

TABLE 29.2 Findings on Serum Biochemistry Analysis in 27 Dogs with Canine Parvoviral Enteritis at the University of California Davis VMTH

Test	Reference Range	Percent Below The Reference Range (%)	Percent Within The Reference Range (%)	Percent Above The Reference Range (%)	Range For Dogs With Parvoviral Enteritis	Number Of Dogs Tested
Sodium (mmol/L)	145–154	85	15	0	132–147	26
Potassium (mmol/L)	3.6–5.3	4	92	4	3.4–5.9	26
Chloride (mmol/L)	108–118	65	31	4	94–120	26
Bicarbonate (mmol/L)	16–26	8	92	0	14–25	26
Calcium (mg/dL)	9.7–11.5	30	70	0	7.4–11.5	27
Phosphorus (mg/dL)	3.0–6.2	0	52	48	3.1–12.3	27
Creatinine (mg/dL)	0.3–1.2	37	59	4	<0.2–1.6	27
BUN (mg/dL)	5–21	0	85	15	5–48	27
Albumin (g/dL)	3.0–4.4	70	30	0	0.9–3.8	27
Globulin (g/dL)	1.8–3.9	26	67	7	1.4–4.5	27
Cholesterol (mg/dL)	135–361	4	89	8	108–460	26
Total bilirubin (mg/dL)	0–0.2	0	89	12	0–1.7	26
ALT (U/L)	19–67	15	62	23	10–165	26
ALP (U/L)	21–170	0	42	58	56–397	26

Note: Adult reference ranges were used by the laboratory.
ALP, alkaline phosphatase; *ALT,* alanine aminotransferase; *BUN,* blood urea nitrogen; VMTH, veterinary medical teaching hospital.

TABLE 29.3 Diagnostic Assays Available for Canine Parvoviral Enteritis in Dogs

Assay	Specimen Type	Target	Performance
Fecal antigen ELISA	Feces	CPV antigen	Specificity for detection of virus nears 100%, but weak positives based on detection of vaccine virus may occur after immunization with attenuated live vaccines. False negatives are common (low sensitivity).
Hemagglutination assay	Feces	CPV antigen	Inexpensive and rapid. Sensitivity and specificity in naturally infected dogs unknown, but high titers are diagnostic if confirmed by hemagglutination inhibition with a specific antibody.
Histopathology	Usually necropsy specimens, especially gastrointestinal tissues	Crypt necrosis (sometimes with rare intranuclear inclusions); parvovirus antigen with IHC or parvovirus DNA with *in situ* hybridization	Can be used for diagnosis at necropsy.
PCR	Feces, tissue species	CPV DNA	Sensitivity and specificity vary depending on assay design. Attenuated live vaccine virus may be detected in feces for days to weeks after vaccination. Because of the high sensitivity of some assays, the significance of a positive result may be difficult to interpret. False-negative results may occur as a result of inhibition of PCR by components of feces.
Fecal electron microscopy	Feces	Virus particles	Not widely available, turnaround time can be slow, and may be expensive. Requires the presence of large amounts of virus.
Virus isolation	Feces, tissues	CPV	Difficult, not widely available. Used as a research tool.

CPV, canine parvovirus (refers to CPV-2 variants); *ELISA,* enzyme-linked immunosorbent assay; *IHC,* immunohistochemistry.

ultrasound is useful to confirm a diagnosis of secondary intestinal intussusception.

Microbiologic Tests

Diagnostic assays for canine parvoviral enteritis in dogs are listed in Table 29.3.

Fecal Parvovirus Antigen ELISA

The most widely used assay for diagnosis of canine parvoviral enteritis is a POC fecal antigen assay, which is performed on a rectal swab specimen. Several assays are available, and those are often based on specific antibodies to capture and detect the viruses in the feces. Although the details are proprietary, tests are generally updated regularly to ensure that all currently circulating strains that vary in antigenicity are detected.[38] Sensitivities of the different tests may vary, and false negatives are common due to viral shedding being transient, and also later after infection antibodies may bind to the viral antigen in the feces and block their reaction with the antibodies in the assay.[39,40] The sensitivities of three commercially available fecal antigen assays (SNAP Parvo test, IDEXX Laboratories GmbH, Germany; FASTest Parvo Strip, Scil Animal Care Company GmbH, Germany; Witness Parvo Card, Selectavet GmbH, Germany) were 50%, 40%, and 60%, respectively, when compared to immunoelectron microscopy, and 18%, 16%, and 26%, respectively, when compared with results of a fecal PCR assay.[38] Fecal PCR using quantitative PCR is generally more reliable, where high levels of viral DNA indicate infection (see below). A fecal antigen test for detection of CPV in specimens that contained high CPV DNA loads (>10^5 copies/mg of feces as determined with real-time PCR) showed 80%, 78%, and 77% positives, respectively.[38]

Comparison with PCR and immunoelectron microscopy of stool showed the specificities of the three commercially available antigen assays above were 98%, 98%, and 92%, respectively,[41] so false positives were uncommon. False-positive antigen tests can occur 4 to 8 days after vaccination with attenuated live CPV-2 vaccines, when virus is shed in feces in low amounts, but those are uncommon.[42,43]

Hemagglutination Testing

CPV agglutinates erythrocytes, and so the presence of the virus in stool can be detected with a simple hemagglutination test that involves mixing a suspension of feces with porcine or feline erythrocytes. Agglutination of erythrocytes in a microwell plate or on a slide may indicate the presence of parvovirus in the feces.[44,45] The presence of CPV as the hemagglutinating virus should be confirmed using a hemagglutination inhibition test with specific antibodies against the virus.

Molecular Diagnosis Using Nucleic Acid–Based Testing

Real-time PCR assays for detection of CPV-2 variants and other enteric viral pathogens (such as CCoV) are now the test of choice and may detect as few as 1,000 copies of viral DNA per milligram of stool, with fast turnaround times. PCR assays will detect virus when fecal antigen tests are negative or when canine enteric coronavirus infection is a potential cause of illness. However, true-positive PCR assay results for CPV can occur in dogs without signs of gastroenteritis or in dogs with chronic diarrhea, so that confirming the role of any specific virus will depend on the quantity of viral DNA detected and other diagnostic criteria. Attenuated live vaccine virus can also be detected in the feces with PCR assays after vaccination, although assays have been designed that can differentiate between vaccine and wild-type virus.[46] False-positive PCR results occur on occasions after vaccination,[43,45] although in some of the studies conducted many of the post-vaccination viral DNA were of natural infections and not the vaccine. Quantitation of virus loads in feces using real-time PCR is helpful for interpretation of the significance of a positive PCR assay result.

Fecal Electron Microscopy

Fecal electron microscopy is still offered by some institutions for diagnosis of viral enteritis, and may also facilitate diagnosis of other viral infections such as rotavirus, norovirus, and coronavirus infections. Large amounts of virus must generally be present for results to be positive, and skilled operators are required to accurately identify viruses present.

Virus Isolation

CPV variants can be isolated in canine and feline cells, but is relatively slow and expensive compared with other methods of virus detection.

Serology

Antibodies to CPV-2 can be measured in the laboratory using HI (see Chapter 2). In addition, POC ELISA assays are available for semiquantitative measurement of antibodies to CPV-2. These assays are generally used to assess the need for vaccination, rather than for diagnosis of CPV-2 enteritis.

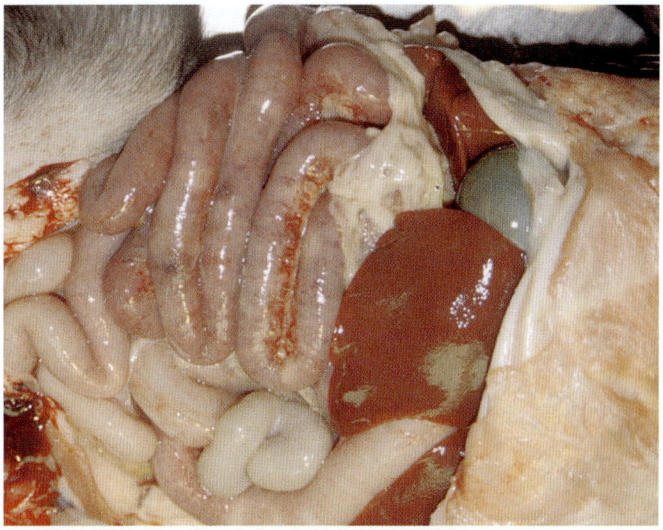

Fig. 29.4 Discoloration of the small intestinal wall and serosal hemorrhage in a puppy that died of canine parvoviral enteritis. (Courtesy University of California, Davis Veterinary Anatomic Pathology Service.)

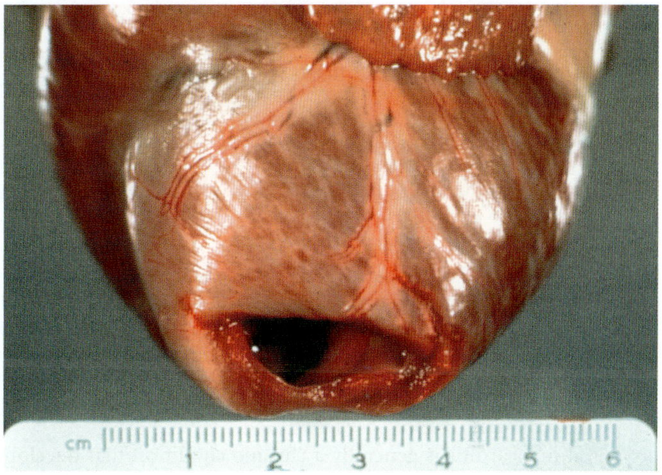

Fig. 29.5 Heart from a dog that died with canine parvovirus-2 myocarditis. Pale streaking of the myocardium is present. (Courtesy Pfizer Animal Health, Lincoln, NE.)

Pathologic Findings

Gross Pathologic Findings

Gross pathologic findings in dogs with CPV enteritis include thickening and discoloration of the intestinal wall with serosal hemorrhage (Fig. 29.4) and enlarged, edematous abdominal lymph nodes. The intestine may contain bloody liquid contents, and mucosal hemorrhage may be identified. Pale areas may be seen within the myocardium of dogs with parvoviral myocarditis (Fig. 29.5).

Histopathologic Findings

The major histopathologic finding in severely affected dogs is necrosis of the crypt epithelium in the small intestine, with widespread systemic lymphoid depletion and necrosis. The crypts of the small intestine are often dilated and distended with cellular debris and mucus (Fig. 29.6), along with signs of proliferation of crypt enterocytes. Intestinal villi are collapsed, shortened, and fused, with attenuation of the epithelial lining, and there may be mild to severe fibrinous inflammation and hemorrhage. Myeloid depletion may be found in the bone marrow.

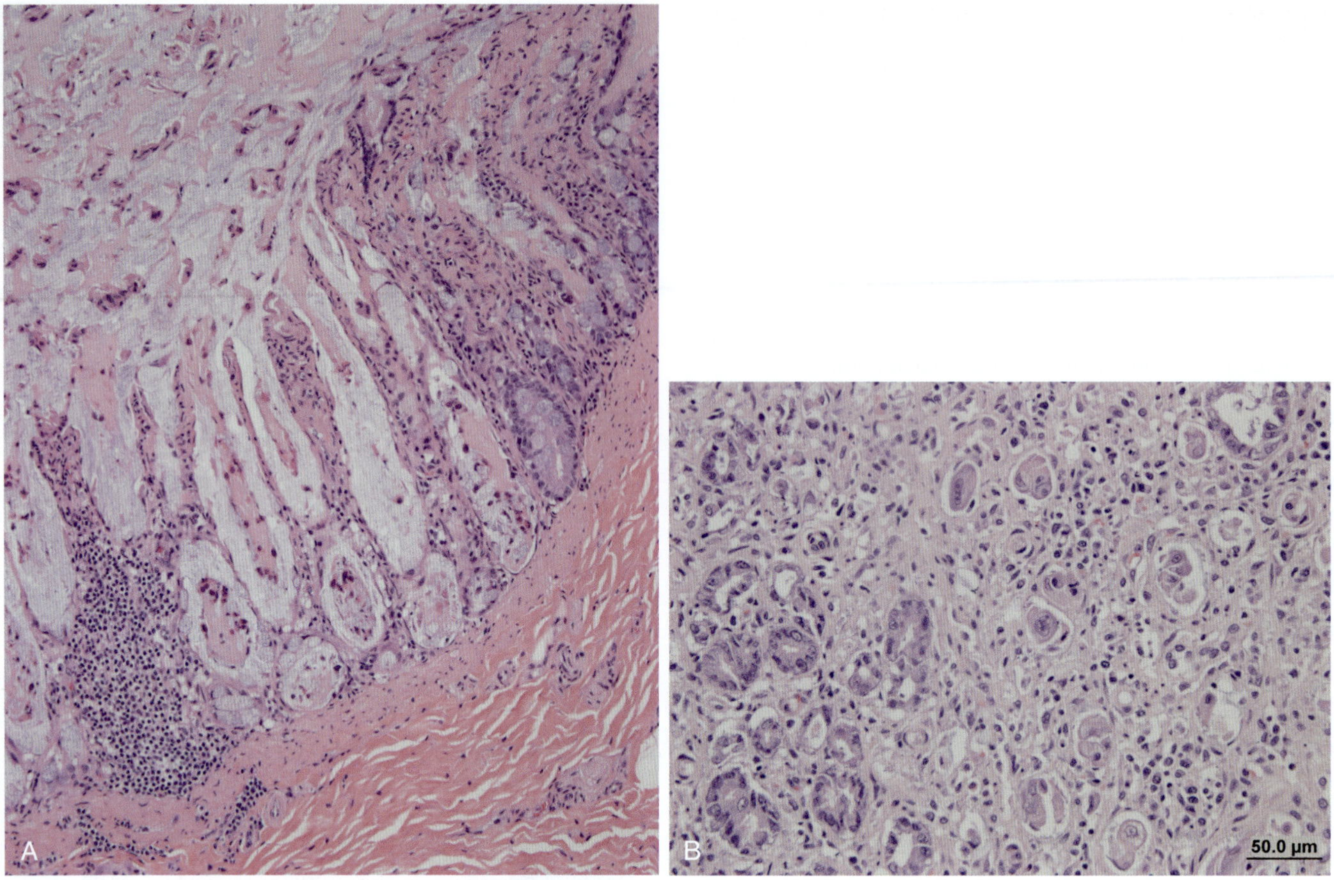

Fig. 29.6 (A) Segmental crypt necrosis in the ileum of a dog infected with a CPV-2 variant. There is severe loss of crypt epithelial cells. Hematoxylin and eosin (H&E) stain. (B) Jejunum of a dog after infection by a CPV-2 variant. Regenerating epithelial cells, which here are nested in an inflamed jejunal lamina, have a large and bizarre appearance and resemble adenoma cells. As a result, the disease has been termed *adenomatosis*. Parvovirus antigen was no longer detectable by immunohistochemistry at this stage. The crypts in the bottom left corner have a more normal appearance. H&E stain. (Courtesy Dr. Patricia Pesavento, University of California, Davis Veterinary Anatomic Pathology Service.)

Parvoviral myocarditis is generally a chronic condition that develops over a few weeks and is characterized by myocardial degeneration and necrosis, with a lymphocytic inflammatory infiltrate. Myocardial fibrosis can also be present. Rarely, CNS lesions consisting of leukoencephalomalacia have been described.[47] Viral intranuclear inclusions may be visible in some cells, especially the intestinal crypt epithelium. IHC and immunofluorescence can be used to detect viral antigen in the GI tract, marrow, lymphoid tissues, and rarely in the myocardium.[28] *In situ* hybridization (see Chapter 6) can also be used to detect virus in histopathology specimens and may have greater sensitivity than IHC.[48,49]

TREATMENT AND PROGNOSIS

Antimicrobial Treatment and Supportive Care

Treatment of CPV enteritis involves supportive care and treatment of secondary bacterial infections with antimicrobial drugs (Table 29.4). Whenever possible, the patient should be hospitalized in isolation as they may be shedding high levels of virus. Appropriate fluid therapy and maintenance of adequate blood glucose concentrations are the most critical aspects of treatment. Whenever possible, fluids should be given intravenously and supplemented as needed with potassium chloride and dextrose. Blood glucose concentrations should be monitored at least twice daily, and more frequent monitoring may be indicated if hypoglycemia is present. Although not generally recommended for puppies that are vomiting or dehydrated, administration of subcutaneous fluids and antimicrobial drugs in the home can result in recovery when client finances do not permit treatment in hospital.[50] Fluids administered subcutaneously should never be supplemented with dextrose, because dextrose is hyperosmotic and can cause further dehydration, as well as injection-site reactions. In one study of an outpatient protocol, 50% of 20 puppies required dextrose supplementation and 60% required potassium supplementation.[50]

An antimicrobial drug or drug combination with activity against gram-negative and anaerobic bacteria should be administered parenterally. Injectable ampicillin or cefazolin alone may be sufficient for many dogs, but puppies that have hemorrhagic diarrhea or evidence of sepsis should probably be treated with a combination of a penicillin and a fluoroquinolone, or a combination of a penicillin and an aminoglycoside. Use of fluoroquinolones in young, rapidly growing animals has been associated with cartilage damage (see Chapter 10), but when used for the short periods of time required to treat parvoviral enteritis, this may not be of significant concern. Proper hydration is critical before aminoglycosides are used because of their potential for nephrotoxicity.

Treatment with antiemetics (such as a metoclopramide constant-rate infusion, maropitant or parenteral ondansetron), H2 blockers such as famotidine, whole blood or plasma transfusions, colloids such as hetastarch, or partial or total parenteral nutrition may be indicated

TABLE 29.4 Medications that May Be Used in Conjunction with Fluid Therapy to Treat Canine Parvoviral Enteritis

Drug	Dose (mg/kg)	Route	Interval (Hours)
Ampicillin sodium	20	IV	6
Cefazolin sodium	20	IV	8
Enrofloxacin[a]	5	IV	24
Ondansetron	0.5 to 1	IV	12
Maropitant citrate	1	SC	24
Metoclopramide	1–2 mg/kg/day	IV	CRI
Famotidine	0.5	IV	12–24

[a]Has been associated with cartilage injury in growing animals. Prolonged use (>7 days) is not recommended. See Chapter 10.
CRI, constant-rate infusion; *IV*, intravenous; *SC*, subcutaneous.

in some dogs. Maropitant (1 mg/kg IV q24h) and ondansetron (0.5 mg/kg IV q8h) were shown to have similar efficacy in parvoviral enteritis.[51] Placement of a central line or multilumen catheter may be necessary in severely ill puppies, but strict sterile technique must be adhered to because of the potential for hospital-associated infection. In general, unless absolutely necessary, invasive surgical procedures and the use of parenteral nutrition solutions should be avoided in puppies with severe neutropenia. Whether plasma or hetastarch is the treatment of choice for dogs with low colloid oncotic pressure requires further study. Plasma may offer benefit over hetastarch in that it contains antibodies from immune dogs, but titers may not be sufficient to be beneficial, and most puppies show evidence of an antibody response within 3 days after onset of clinical signs. Hetastarch has anticoagulant properties that could be beneficial in light of the hypercoagulable state that has been documented in canine parvoviral enteritis, but these effects also have the potential to increase mortality, and hetastarch has been associated with acute kidney injury in critically ill human patients.[52] Early enteral nutrition with a nasogastric feeding tube was associated with reduced hospitalization times in one study, as compared to withholding food until vomiting had ceased (Fig. 29.7).[53] Gastric suction should be performed through the tube before food is administered. One study of 28 dogs with parvoviral enteritis suggested that use of an oral recuperation fluid might be associated with a more rapid return to oral food intake and greater caloric intake when compared with use of water.[54]

Other treatments that have been investigated include anti-endotoxin sera, recombinant bactericidal permeability-increasing (BPI) protein, recombinant granulocyte colony-stimulating factor (G-CSF), recombinant feline interferon-omega (rfIFN-ω, Virbagen omega), serum from immune animals, fecal microbiota transplantation, and oseltamivir. Anti-endotoxin sera, recombinant BPI protein, and human recombinant G-CSF were not found to be beneficial. Although neutrophil counts were higher and hospital times were shorter in dogs treated with recombinant canine G-CSF, survival times in these dogs were decreased.[55] There has been concern that treatment of parvovirus infections with G-CSF might cause harm because the increased cell turnover induced by the drug might promote parvovirus replication. However, in another nonrandomized, prospective, placebo-controlled clinical trial of 62 puppies with parvoviral enteritis, administration of recombinant G-CSF (5 μg/kg daily) was associated with improvement in hematological parameters; all dogs treated with recombinant G-CSF survived, whereas 5 of 31 dogs in the placebo group died.[56] Treatment

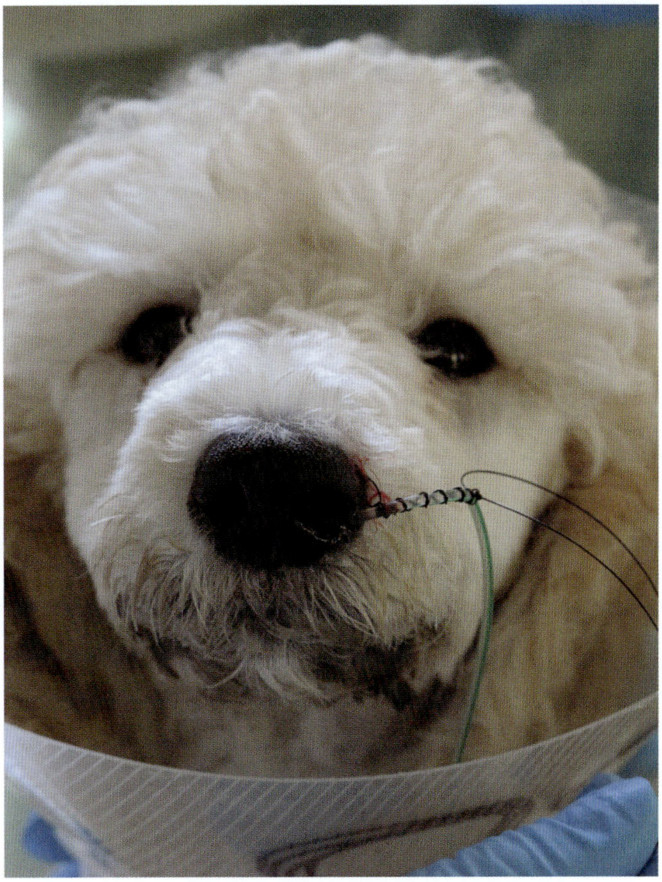

Fig. 29.7 Puppy in Fig. 29.3 after placement of a nasogastric feeding tube.

of puppies with parvoviral enteritis with rfIFN-ω in a number of placebo-controlled trials has been associated with reduced disease severity and, in some studies, significantly reduced mortality,[57] but it has not been beneficial for treatment of FPV infections (see Chapter 30 vaccine and wild-type virus). Administration of serum from cats with antibodies to FPV to puppies with parvoviral enteritis did not appear to be beneficial.[58] In a randomized prospective clinical trial of 66 puppies with hemorrhagic diarrhea that were fecal PCR positive for CPV, fecal microbiota transplantation (10 g of feces from a healthy dog diluted in 10 mL of saline per rectum, 6 to 12 hours after admission) was associated with faster resolution of diarrhea and shorter hospitalization times when compared with standard treatment.[59]

Oseltamivir inhibits the neuraminidase of influenza viruses and does not have specific antiparvoviral activity, but it has been suggested for treatment of CPV enteritis. As CPV does not possess a neuraminidase, it has been hypothesized that oseltamivir instead may act on the neuraminidases of bacteria that are normally responsible for secondary bacterial infections in parvovirus enteritis, primarily those of the GI tract. A single prospective, randomized, masked, placebo-controlled trial of 35 dogs with parvoviral enteritis showed that dogs treated with oseltamivir (2 mg/kg PO q12h) had no significant drop in their leukocyte count, whereas untreated dogs had a significant drop in their leukocyte count in the first 5 days of hospitalization.[60] Treated dogs also gained weight during hospitalization, whereas untreated dogs lost weight. However, there was no difference in hospitalization time, clinical scores, morbidity, or mortality between the two groups, and the number of dogs in each group was small. The authors acknowledged the potential concerns that relate to administration of an oral medication to dogs with enteritis, with possible variability in drug absorption.

Given the lack of proof of efficacy of this drug, and restrictions on its use for treatment of human influenza virus infections, its use in dogs is not encouraged. More information on canine G-CSF, rfIFN-ω, and oseltamivir can be found in Chapter 9 of this book.

Prognosis

The prognosis for viral enteritis in puppies varies with the severity of illness and the owners' ability to afford appropriate treatment. Many cases of CPV-2 infection are likely mild or subclinical and not recognized. However, for those that do develop enteritis the survival rates have ranged from 9% in untreated puppies to greater than 90% with aggressive treatment in tertiary referral hospitals.[11,35,61,62] Factors that have been related to mortality include the presence of initial leukopenia or lymphopenia, monocytopenia, neutropenia, and evidence of SIRS.[15,61,63] SIRS was defined as the presence of at least three of the following four criteria: HR greater than 140 beats/minute, temperature above 102.5°F or below 100°F, and WBC counts greater than 17,000 or less than 6,000 cells/μL (see Chapter 123). A 2020 study identified a model that could predict survival based on a combination of plasma antithrombin concentration, serum AST activity, serum lipase concentration, monocyte count, and lymohocyte count.[64] Survival may also be lower in Rottweilers than in other breeds and in young puppies (less than 7 to 12 weeks of age).[60] In Australia, euthanasia was more likely to occur in summer; among pedigree dogs, in hounds, gundogs, and non-sporting breed dogs; and in puppies less than 6 months of age, and if owners were socioeconomically disadvantaged.[16,61] Vomiting and lethargy at admission as well as lymphopenia and hypoalbuminemia have been associated with prolongation of hospitalization times by approximately 2 days.[15] Positive changes in leukocyte counts (and especially lymphocyte counts) as early as 24 hours after admission have been associated with survival.[63] In general, puppies that survive the first 3 to 4 days of treatment make complete recoveries. Complications of infection include bacteremia and septic shock, intestinal intussusception, aspiration pneumonia, and esophageal strictures. Some longer-term association with chronic gastroenteritis has been reported, possibly resulting from the damage to the intestine or from the antibody treatment that is often given.[65]

IMMUNITY AND VACCINATION

Immunity that follows natural infection by CPV-2 variants appears to provide lifelong protection against reinfection, as likely does immunization with attenuated live viral vaccines. Both attenuated live and inactivated CPV vaccines are available. With the possible exception of shelter environments, attenuated live vaccines should never be administered to pregnant bitches because they may cause disease in the developing fetus. If possible, pregnant bitches introduced into shelter environments should be tested for antibody to CPV before vaccination with attenuated live vaccines, and these dogs should only be vaccinated if they test negative. The use of inactivated vaccines is not recommended because of their short duration and low levels of protection, and for breeding bitches, they provide only very low levels of maternal immunity. There is a *window of vulnerability* for CPV-2 infection in puppies, which is the period when maternal antibody interferes with the vaccine virus's ability to replicate and stimulate an effective immune response, but is unable to prevent infection with virulent field virus (see Chapter 20 for a discussion of this concept). Small quantities of attenuated live vaccine virus are shed from the intestinal tract after immunization, but this should not be relied on to immunize other in-contact animals. Protection against challenge with field virus occurs for at least 3 years and likely for life after the initial puppy series is administered (see Chapter 20). Although not documented, exposure of dogs to virus in the environment may serve to boost immunity after vaccination.

The initial immunization series should be given every 3 to 4 weeks from 6 to 8 weeks of age, until no sooner than 14 to 16 weeks (16 to 20 weeks in breeding kennels or contaminated environments) because of persistence of sufficient titers of maternal antibody in some puppies until 16 to 20 weeks of age. After that, a vaccine should be administered at 6 months or 1 year of age, and every 3 years thereafter (see Appendix). Previously, the vaccination at 6 months was recommended at 1 year of age, but as the purpose of this vaccination was to immunize dogs that still retained maternal antibody at 16 to 20 weeks of age, the WSAVA has recommended shifting this to ensure those dogs were not vulnerable for several months (see Chapter 20).[66] Puppies should be isolated in the home environment until 7 to 10 days after the last booster. Attendance at organized puppy classes has been advocated as a way to promote socialization in this period, and currently there is no evidence that such activities increase risk for parvoviral enteritis. Serum antibody titers of at least 1:80 as determined with HI correlate well with protection.

There is some minor antigenic variation among strains of CPV-2 that are circulating among dogs, which have been given various names that include CPV-2a, CPV-2b, CPV-2c, and concern has been raised that currently available CPV vaccines may not provide adequate protection against infection by all CPV strains. However, failure of protection in a successfully vaccinated dog (where the vaccine virus infected and antibodies developed) is rare, and experimental challenge studies have demonstrated strong protection between the different viruses when dogs are immunized, suggesting adequate cross-protection.[67] Whether there are differences in maternal antibody protection of dogs to the different strains is not known.

Both inactivated and attenuated live vaccines are available for prevention or reduction of canine enteric coronavirus infection, but because the disease is generally mild or inapparent and primarily occurs in puppies younger than 6 weeks of age, their use has not been generally recommended.[68]

PREVENTION

Prevention of CPV-2 enteritis requires immunization and appropriate quarantine, isolation, cleaning, and disinfection procedures. Proper immunization provides complete protection against both infection and disease, and should be a central component of any strategy for managing this virus and its infection. Puppies that have not yet been successfully vaccinated should not be introduced into environments where there has been a history of parvoviral enteritis and where adequate environmental disinfection cannot be guaranteed. Environmental decontamination is challenging, and the virus is extremely resistant to many disinfectants, but parvoviruses can be inactivated with a freshly prepared 1 in 30 dilution of household bleach; potassium peroxymonosulfate (Trifectant, Virkon S); accelerated hydrogen peroxide; or high-level chemical disinfectants such as glutaraldehyde and *ortho*-phthalaldehyde, when contact times of at least 10 minutes are used (see Chapter 14 for more information on disinfection). These disinfectants will also inactivate other enteric viruses. Steam cleaning should be used on surfaces that cannot be otherwise disinfected, and dishwashers that attain temperatures of at least 75°C should be used to wash dishes. Even if steam cleaning is not available, thorough cleaning with detergents will reduce viral loads and likelihood of exposure.

For shelters, quarantine periods of 2 weeks have been recommended before introduction of puppies that might be shedding virus because shedding rarely continues for longer than 10 days.[68] The bathing of recovered puppies can help to remove virus that persists on the haircoat. Rodent and insect vector control can also be used to prevent spread of the virus in the environment. Outdoor grassy areas and dirt are difficult or impossible to adequately disinfect, and so only immunized animals should be allowed on these areas. However, virus levels will fall as virus likely becomes bound to soil and inactivated by sunlight. The use of bleach on these areas is not recommended because of adverse environmental effects from runoff.

The prevalence and impact of enteric viral infections can also be reduced through regular removal of fecal contamination, prolonged exposure of contaminated surfaces to sunlight and drying, and elimination of stressors such as overcrowding, transport, poor nutrition, and concurrent infections such as intestinal parasites.

PUBLIC HEALTH ASPECTS

In general, enteric viral pathogens of dogs, including CPV-2 variants, do not infect humans. However, recent detection of human norovirus genogroups in dogs have suggested the possibility of zoonotic transmission. In central Thailand, an outbreak of diarrhea in kenneled dogs and children that were in contact with the dogs was described; norovirus was detected using PCR in the dogs and children, and whole genome sequencing confirmed that virus isolated from the dogs was the same as that isolated from the children (genotype GII.4).[69] Other infectious causes of gastroenteritis in puppies have the potential to be zoonotic, and co-infections with these pathogens can occur, so caution should be maintained when handling puppies with diarrhea. Precautions used in isolation should be sufficient to prevent enteric zoonoses (see Chapter 15).

CASE EXAMPLE

Signalment

"Sam," an 8-week-old intact male Hungarian vizsla puppy from northern California.

History

Sam was acquired 6 days ago from a breeder, and was eating and active at that time. The next day Sam was examined at a local veterinary clinic, and a routine fecal examination revealed infection with *Giardia* and *Isospora* spp. Treatment with sulfamethoxazole was initiated, but 1 day later the puppy developed diarrhea. The next day, lethargy and vomiting were noted. Vomiting and diarrhea occurred every few hours. The diarrhea contained fresh blood and the vomitus consisted of clear, frothy fluid. Inappetence and intermittent vomiting continued for the next 2 days.

Current Medications

None

Other Medical History

Vaccination with an attenuated live CDV, CPV-2, and CPIV vaccine was performed when Sam was 6 weeks of age. There were no other dogs in the household, only one adult cat.

Physical Examination

Body weight: 4.2 kg.

General: Quiet, alert, responsive. Estimated to be 7% to 8% dehydrated, T = 103.4°F (39.7°C), HR = 240 beats/minute, RR = 36 breaths/minute, mucous membranes pale pink and tacky, CRT = 2 seconds.

Integument: Full, shiny haircoat. No ectoparasites were seen.

Eyes, ears, nose, and throat: Enophthalmos and a dry nasal planum were present.

Musculoskeletal: BCS 2/9. The dog was ambulatory, but emaciated and weak.

Cardiovascular: Weak but synchronous femoral pulses. No murmurs or arrhythmias on auscultation.

Respiratory: No clinically significant findings.

GI: No evidence of abdominal pain on palpation. Fluid-filled intestinal tract. Full urinary bladder noted.

Rectal examination: Bloody diarrhea was present on the thermometer. Rectal examination was not performed.

Lymph nodes: All lymph nodes were within normal limits.

Laboratory Findings

CDC: HCT 31.5% (40%–55%), MCV 62.6 fL (65–75 fL), MCHC 35.6 g/dl (33–36 g/dL), WBC 530 cells/μL (6,000–13,000 cells/μL), neutrophils 16 cells/μL (3,000–10,500 cells/μL), lymphocytes 504 cells/μL (1,000–4,000 cells/μL), monocytes 11 cells/μL (150–1,200 cells/μL), platelets clumped but appeared adequate.

Serum chemistry profile: sodium 143 mmol/L (145–154 mmol/L), potassium 3.8 mmol/L (3.6–5.3 mmol/L), chloride 106 mmol/L (108–118 mmol/L), bicarbonate 23 mmol/L (16–26 mmol/L), phosphorus 4.8 mg/dL (3.0–6.2 mg/dL), calcium 10.3 mg/dL (9.7–11.5 mg/dl), BUN 6 mg/dL (5–21 mg/dL), creatinine < 0.2 mg/dL (0.3–1.2 mg/dL), glucose 133 mg/dL (64–123 mg/dL), total protein 4.3 g/dL (5.4–7.6 g/dL), albumin 2.4 g/dL (3.0–4.4 g/dL), globulin 1.9 g/dL (1.8–3.9 g/dL), ALT 22 U/L (19–67 U/L), AST 15 U/L (19–42 U/L), ALP 179 U/L (21–170 U/L), creatine kinase 274 U/L (51–399 U/L), GGT < 3 U/L (0-6 U/L), cholesterol 278 mg/dL (135–361 mg/dL), total bilirubin 0.1 mg/dL (0–0.2 mg/dL), magnesium 2.0 mg/dL (1.5–2.6 mg/dL).

Imaging Findings

Abdominal radiographs: The stomach wall appeared thickened. Numerous round gas opacities were present in a loop of intestine in the right cranial abdomen, which were believed to represent gas in the ascending colon or duodenum. Multiple additional gas opacities were present in a loop of intestine in the mid-right abdomen at the level of the fourth lumbar vertebra. There was reduced serosal detail compatible with the age of the animal. Changes were considered consistent with the presence of gastroenterocolitis.

Microbiologic Testing

Fecal parvovirus antigen ELISA: Negative

Fecal enteric real-time PCR panel: PCR positive for CPV in fecal specimen. PCR negative for *Clostridium difficile* toxin A and toxin B genes, *Cryptosporidium* spp., *Salmonella* spp., and *Giardia* spp. DNA.

Fecal zinc sulfate centrifugal flotation: Negative for parasite ova.

Diagnosis

Enteritis and leukopenia secondary to CPV infection.

Treatment

Sam was admitted to isolation and treated aggressively with IV lactated Ringer's solution that was supplemented with 20 mEq KCl/L, famotidine (0.5 mg/kg IV q12h), ondansetron (0.5 mg/kg IV q12h), ampicillin (22 mg/kg IV q6h), and enrofloxacin (5 mg/kg IV q24h). Because of persistent vomiting, maropitant citrate (1 mg/kg IV q24h) was added as a second antiemetic. Blood glucose concentration was monitored three times daily, but supplementation with dextrose was not required. Bloody diarrhea that contained sloughed intestinal mucosa occurred every few hours for the first 24 hours. The neutrophil count was 9 cells/μL the following day, but by day 4 of hospitalization was 261 cells/μL, with 241 moderately toxic bands/μL and a lymphocyte count of 1,226 cells/μL. There was gradual clinical improvement during this time, and Sam began to ingest small quantities of cottage cheese and rice on day 4. He was discharged from the hospital on day 5.

Comments

Despite the negative fecal antigen ELISA assay, CPV enteritis was suspected in this dog based on the history, clinical signs, and severe leukopenia. The finding of leukopenia and diarrhea is not diagnostic for parvoviral enteritis, because it can also be caused by other severe enteritides such as salmonellosis. The positive fecal real-time PCR assay for CPV supported the diagnosis, but because positive fecal PCR results can occur in healthy dogs with some assays, and also after vaccination, the fecal PCR result alone did not confirm the diagnosis of CPV enteritis. The diagnosis was therefore made on the basis of the combination of findings. The neutropenia in this dog was profound. Infection likely occurred before the owner acquired the puppy because the diarrhea began only 2 days after the puppy was purchased.

SUGGESTED READINGS

Carmichael LE. An annotated historical account of canine parvovirus. *J Vet Med Ser B*. 2005;52(7–8):303–311.

Iris K, Leontides LS, Mylonakis ME, et al. Factors affecting the occurrence, duration of hospitalization and final outcome in canine parvovirus infection. *Res Vet Sci*. 2010;89:174–178.

Mylonakis ME, Kalli I, Rallis TS. Canine parvoviral enteritis: an update on the clinical diagnosis, treatment, and prevention. *Vet Med (Auckl)*. 2016;7:91–100.

REFERENCES

1. Carmichael LE. An annotated historical account of canine parvovirus. *J Vet Med Ser B*. 2005;52:303–311.
2. Hoelzer K, Parrish CR. The emergence of parvoviruses of carnivores. *Vet Res*. 2010;41:39.
3. Clegg SR, Coyne KP, Parker J, et al. Molecular epidemiology and phylogeny reveal complex spatial dynamics in areas where canine parvovirus is endemic. *J Virol*. 2011;85:7892–7899.
4. Voorhees IEH, Lee H, Allison AB, et al. Limited intrahost diversity and background evolution accompany 40 years of canine parvovirus host adaptation and spread. *J Virol*. 2019;94.
5. Battilani M, Balboni A, Ustulin M, et al. Genetic complexity and multiple infections with more Parvovirus species in naturally infected cats. *Vet Res*. 2011;42:43.
6. Ikeda Y, Nakamura K, Miyazawa T, et al. Feline host range of canine parvovirus: recent emergence of new antigenic types in cats. *Emerg Infect Dis*. 2002;8:341–346.
7. Truyen U, Evermann JF, Vieler E, et al. Evolution of canine parvovirus involved loss and gain of feline host range. *Virology*. 1996;215:186–189.
8. Eminaga S, Palus V, Cherubini GB. Minute virus as a possible cause of neurological problems in dogs. *Vet Rec*. 2011;168:111–112.
9. Ohshima T, Kawakami K, Abe T, et al. A minute virus of canines (MVC: canine bocavirus) isolated from an elderly dog with severe gastroenteritis, and phylogenetic analysis of MVC strains. *Vet Microbiol*. 2010;145:334–338.
10. Pratelli A, Buonavoglia D, Tempesta M, et al. Fatal canine parvovirus type-1 infection in pups from Italy. *J Vet Diagn Invest*. 1999;11:365–367.
11. Glickman LT, Domanski LM, Patronek GJ, et al. Breed-related risk factors for canine parvovirus enteritis. *J Am Vet Med Assoc*. 1985;187:589–594.
12. Houston DM, Ribble CS, Head LL. Risk factors associated with parvovirus enteritis in dogs: 283 cases (1982-1991). *J Am Vet Med Assoc*. 1996;208:542–546.
13. Kelman M, Barrs VR, Norris JM, et al. Socioeconomic, geographic and climatic risk factors for canine parvovirus infection and euthanasia in Australia. *Prev Vet Med*. 2020;174:104816.
14. Brady S, Norris JM, Kelman M, et al. Canine parvovirus in Australia: the role of socio-economic factors in disease clusters. *Vet J*. 2012;193:522–528.
15. Iris K, Leontides LS, Mylonakis ME, et al. Factors affecting the occurrence, duration of hospitalization and final outcome in canine parvovirus infection. *Res Vet Sci*. 2010;89:174–178.
16. Kelman M, Ward MP, Barrs VR, et al. The geographic distribution and financial impact of canine parvovirus in Australia. *Transbound Emerg Dis*. 2019;66:299–311.
17. Duijvestijn M, Mughini-Gras L, Schuurman N, et al. Enteropathogen infections in canine puppies: (Co-)occurrence, clinical relevance and risk factors. *Vet Microbiol*. 2016;195:115–122.
18. Martella V, Pinto P, Buonavoglia C. Canine noroviruses. *Vet Clin North Am Small Anim Pract*. 2011;41:1171–1181.
19. Li L, Pesavento PA, Shan T, et al. Viruses in diarrhoeic dogs include novel kobuviruses and sapoviruses. *J Gen Virol*. 2011;92:2534–2541.
20. Grellet A, Chastant-Maillard S, Robin C, et al. Risk factors of weaning diarrhea in puppies housed in breeding kennels. *Prev Vet Med*. 2014;117:260–265.
21. Melegari I, Marsilio F, Di Profio F, et al. Seroprevalence of sapovirus in dogs using baculovirus-expressed virus-like particles. *Virus Res*. 2018;251:1–5.
22. Soma T, Nakagomi O, Nakagomi T, et al. Detection of norovirus and sapovirus from diarrheic dogs and cats in Japan. *Microbiol Immunol*. 2015;59:123–128.
23. Bodnar L, Lorusso E, Di Martino B, et al. Identification of a novel canine norovirus. *Infect Genet Evol*. 2017;52:75–81.
24. Licitra BN, Whittaker GR, Dubovi EJ, et al. Genotypic characterization of canine coronaviruses associated with fatal canine neonatal enteritis in the United States. *J Clin Microbiol*. 2014;52:4230–4238.
25. Evermann JF, Abbott JR, Han S. Canine coronavirus-associated puppy mortality without evidence of concurrent canine parvovirus infection. *J Vet Diagn Invest*. 2005;17:610–614.
26. Ntafis V, Xylouri E, Radogna A, et al. Outbreak of canine norovirus infection in young dogs. *J Clin Microbiol*. 2010;48:2605–2608.
27. Macartney L, McCandlish IA, Thompson H, et al. Canine parvovirus enteritis 2: Pathogenesis. *Vet Rec*. 1984;115:453–460.
28. Meunier PC, Cooper BJ, Appel MJ, et al. Pathogenesis of canine parvovirus enteritis: sequential virus distribution and passive immunization studies. *Vet Pathol*. 1985;22:617–624.
29. Otto CM, Rieser TM, Brooks MB, et al. Evidence of hypercoagulability in dogs with parvoviral enteritis. *J Am Vet Med Assoc*. 2000;217:1500–1504.
30. Hayes MA, Russell RG, Babiuk LA. Sudden death in young dogs with myocarditis caused by parvovirus. *J Am Vet Med Assoc*. 1979;174:1197–1203.
31. Lenghaus C, Studdert MJ, Finnie JW. Acute and chronic canine parvovirus myocarditis following intrauterine inoculation. *Aust Vet J*. 1980;56:465–468.
32. Meunier PC, Cooper BJ, Appel MJ, et al. Experimental viral myocarditis: parvoviral infection of neonatal pups. *Vet Pathol*. 1984;21:509–515.
33. Schatzberg SJ, Haley NJ, Barr SC, et al. Polymerase chain reaction (PCR) amplification of parvoviral DNA from the brains of dogs and cats with cerebellar hypoplasia. *J Vet Intern Med*. 2003;17:538–544.
34. Lenghaus C, Studdert MJ. Generalized parvovirus disease in neonatal pups. *J Am Vet Med Assoc*. 1982;181:41–45.
35. Mylonakis ME, Kalli I, Rallis TS. Canine parvoviral enteritis: an update on the clinical diagnosis, treatment, and prevention. *Vet Med (Auckl)*. 2016;7:91–100.
36. Favrot C, Olivry T, Dunston SM, et al. Parvovirus infection of keratinocytes as a cause of canine erythema multiforme. *Vet Pathol*. 2000;37:647–649.
37. Woldemeskel M, Liggett A, Ilha M, et al. Canine parvovirus-2b-associated erythema multiforme in a litter of English Setter dogs. *J Vet Diagn Invest*. 2011;23:576–580.
38. Decaro N, Desario C, Beall MJ, et al. Detection of canine parvovirus type 2c by a commercially available in-house rapid test. *Vet J*. 2010;184:373–375.
39. Kantere MC, Athanasiou LV, Spyrou V, et al. Diagnostic performance of a rapid in-clinic test for the detection of canine parvovirus under different storage conditions and vaccination status. *J Virol Methods*. 2015;215–216:52–55.
40. Proksch AL, Unterer S, Speck S, et al. Influence of clinical and laboratory variables on faecal antigen ELISA results in dogs with canine parvovirus infection. *Vet J*. 2015;204:304–308.
41. Schmitz S, Coenen C, Konig M, et al. Comparison of three rapid commercial canine parvovirus antigen detection tests with electron microscopy and polymerase chain reaction. *J Vet Diagn Invest*. 2009;21:344–345.
42. Decaro N, Crescenzo G, Desario C, et al. Long-term viremia and fecal shedding in pups after modified-live canine parvovirus vaccination. *Vaccine*. 2014;32:3850–3853.
43. Freisl M, Speck S, Truyen U, et al. Faecal shedding of canine parvovirus after modified-live vaccination in healthy adult dogs. *Vet J*. 2017;219:15–21.
44. Carmichael LE, Joubert JC, Pollock RV. Hemagglutination by canine parvovirus: serologic studies and diagnostic applications. *Am J Vet Res*. 1980;41:784–791.
45. Marulappa SY, Kapil S. Simple tests for rapid detection of canine parvovirus antigen and canine parvovirus-specific antibodies. *Clin Vaccine Immunol*. 2009;16:127–131.

46. Decaro N, Elia G, Desario C, et al. A minor groove binder probe real-time PCR assay for discrimination between type 2-based vaccines and field strains of canine parvovirus. *J Virol Methods*. 2006;136:65–70.
47. Schaudien D, Polizopoulou Z, Koutinas A, et al. Leukoencephalopathy associated with parvovirus infection in Cretan hound puppies. *J Clin Microbiol*. 2010;48:3169–3175.
48. Nho WG, Sur JH, Doster AR, et al. Detection of canine parvovirus in naturally infected dogs with enteritis and myocarditis by in situ hybridization. *J Vet Diagn Invest*. 1997;9:255–260.
49. Waldvogel AS, Hassam S, Stoerckle N, et al. Specific diagnosis of parvovirus enteritis in dogs and cats by in situ hybridization. *J Comp Pathol*. 1992;107:141–146.
50. Perley K, Burns CC, Maguire C, et al. Retrospective evaluation of outpatient canine parvovirus treatment in a shelter-based low-cost urban clinic. *J Vet Emerg Crit Care*. 2020;30:202–208.
51. Sullivan LA, Lenberg JP, Boscan P, et al. Assessing the efficacy of maropitant versus ondansetron in the treatment of dogs with parvoviral enteritis. *J Am Anim Hosp Assoc*. 2018;54:338–343.
52. Groeneveld AB, Navickis RJ, Wilkes MM. Update on the comparative safety of colloids: a systematic review of clinical studies. *Ann Surg*. 2011;253:470–483.
53. Mohr AJ, Leisewitz AL, Jacobson LS, et al. Effect of early enteral nutrition on intestinal permeability, intestinal protein loss, and outcome in dogs with severe parvoviral enteritis. *J Vet Intern Med*. 2003;17:791–798.
54. Tenne R, Sullivan LA, Contreras ET, et al. Palatability and clinical effects of an oral recuperation fluid during the recovery of dogs with suspected parvoviral enteritis. *Top Companion Anim Med*. 2016;31:68–72.
55. Duffy A, Dow S, Ogilvie G, et al. Hematologic improvement in dogs with parvovirus infection treated with recombinant canine granulocyte-colony stimulating factor. *J Vet Pharmacol Ther*. 2010;33:352–356.
56. Armenise A, Trerotoli P, Cirone F, et al. Use of recombinant canine granulocyte-colony stimulating factor to increase leukocyte count in dogs naturally infected by canine parvovirus. *Vet Microbiol*. 2019;231:177–182.
57. de Mari K, Maynard L, Eun HM, et al. Treatment of canine parvoviral enteritis with interferon-omega in a placebo-controlled field trial. *Vet Rec*. 2003;152:105–108.
58. Gerlach M, Proksch AL, Unterer S, et al. Efficacy of feline anti-parvovirus antibodies in the treatment of canine parvovirus infection. *J Small Anim Pract*. 2017;58:408–415.
59. Pereira GQ, Gomes LA, Santos IS, et al. Fecal microbiota transplantation in puppies with canine parvovirus infection. *J Vet Intern Med*. 2018;32:707–711.
60. Savigny MR, Macintire DK. Use of oseltamivir in the treatment of canine parvoviral enteritis. *J Vet Emerg Crit Care*. 2010;20:132–142.
61. Ling M, Norris JM, Kelman M, et al. Risk factors for death from canine parvoviral-related disease in Australia. *Vet Microbiol*. 2012;158:280–290.
62. Otto CM, Jackson CB, Rogell EJ, et al. Recombinant bactericidal/permeability-increasing protein (rBPI21) for treatment of parvovirus enteritis: a randomized, double-blinded, placebo-controlled trial. *J Vet Intern Med*. 2001;15:355–360.
63. Goddard A, Leisewitz AL, Christopher MM, et al. Prognostic usefulness of blood leukocyte changes in canine parvoviral enteritis. *J Vet Intern Med*. 2008;22:309–316.
64. Franzo G, Corso B, Tucciarone CM, et al. Comparison and validation of different models and variable selection methods for predicting survival after canine parvovirus infection. *Vet Rec*. 2020;187–e76.
65. Kilian E, Suchodolski JS, Hartmann K, et al. Long-term effects of canine parvovirus infection in dogs. *PloS One*. 2018;13:e0192198.
66. WSAVA Vaccination Guidelines. https://wsava.org/global-guidelines/vaccination-guidelines/.
67. Hernandez-Blanco B, Catala-Lopez F. Are licensed canine parvovirus (CPV2 and CPV2b) vaccines able to elicit protection against CPV2c subtype in puppies?: a systematic review of controlled clinical trials. *Vet Microbiol*. 2015;180:1–9.
68. Ford RB, Larson LJ, McClure KD, et al. AAHA canine vaccination guidelines. *J Am Anim Hosp Assoc*. 2017;53:243–251. 2017.
69. Charoenkul K, Nasamran C, Janetanakit T, et al. Human norovirus infection in dogs, Thailand. *Emerg Infect Dis*. 2020;26:350–353.

30

Feline Panleukopenia Virus Infection and Other Feline Viral Enteritides

Jane E. Sykes, Colin R. Parrish

KEY POINTS

- First Described: In 1928, Verge and Christoforoni, France.[1]
- Cause: Feline panleukopenia virus (synonym of feline parvovirus; FPV); also canine parvovirus (CPV); (family *Parvoviridae*, subfamily *Parvovirinae*, genus *Protoparvovirus*, species *Carnivore protoparvovirus 1*).
- Affected Hosts: Domestic and wild cats; foxes, mink, and raccoons.
- Geographic Distribution: Worldwide.
- Mode of Transmission: Direct contact with virus in feces, vomitus, and contaminated fomites.
- Major Clinical Signs: Fever, lethargy, inappetence, vomiting, diarrhea, dehydration, sudden death. Neurologic signs (primarily due to cerebellar damage) may occur after infection of neonatal kittens.
- Differential Diagnoses: Other feline viral enteritides, toxins, GI foreign body, enteric parasitic infections such as giardiasis and nematode infections, enteric bacterial infections such as salmonellosis, pancreatitis, or inflammatory bowel disease. Congenital CNS defects should be considered in cats with neurologic signs.
- Human Health Significance: FPV is not known to infect humans, but was isolated from monkeys in one outbreak.

ETIOLOGY AND EPIDEMIOLOGY

Feline panleukopenia virus (FPV) is a parvovirus that causes enteritis and panleukopenia in domestic and wild cat species worldwide.[2–4] It has also been associated with disease in raccoons, mink, foxes, and African green monkeys (one outbreak). The virus can also replicate in ferrets without causing disease. Feline panleukopenia is sometimes confusingly referred to as "cat plague" and "feline distemper"; use of these terms is discouraged due to confusion with other diseases. In raccoons and mink, FPV has sometimes been named raccoon parvovirus or mink enteritis virus. FPV is a small, single-stranded nonenveloped DNA virus that is closely related to CPV-2. In contrast to CPV-2, which emerged in the late 1970s, the disease caused by FPV has been known since at least the 1920s.[1] FPV survives for long periods in the environment and resists disinfection, and generally only replicates in dividing cells (see Chapter 29).

Feline panleukopenia most often occurs in cats younger than 1 year of age, but the virus infects unvaccinated or inadequately vaccinated cats of all ages. The ages of affected cats vary from very young (in cases of cerebellar hypoplasia), up to over a year, but average ages of affected cats tend to be lower; in one study the mean was 4 months.[5,6] However, kitten deaths have been reported despite vaccination of kittens, possibly because successful vaccination is prevented by maternal antibodies, and kittens are exposed to large amounts of virus in the environment.[7,8] Outbreaks of panleukopenia in cats correlate seasonally with increases in susceptible newborn kitten numbers. Panleukopenia occurs most commonly in multicat households, and especially in animal shelter environments which contain higher numbers of kittens, and where new kittens are introduced frequently. It can also occur in cats with outdoor exposure, such as for barn, feral, and stray cats, which are most often not vaccinated. In various studies, the prevalence of protective antibody titers to FPV in feral or owned cats has been seen to vary widely, ranging from about 25% to 80%, suggesting both low rates of exposure to the virus and vaccination in some cases.[2,9] In some animal shelters, devastating outbreaks of panleukopenia have led to high mortalities (including euthanasia) of large numbers of cats.[6,10] Contact with other cats may not be present in the history because fomite transmission is so effective.[5] FPV replicates to a limited extent in dogs, but without disease or virus shedding. Some feline panleukopenia results from infection of cats by the related mink enteritis virus or, rarely (in less than 10% of cases), by CPV.[11–13]

Other viral pathogens that have been associated with gastroenteritis in cats include feline enteric coronavirus (see Chapter 31), FeLV, rotavirus, calicivirus, reovirus, and astrovirus. A torovirus-like agent has been associated with a syndrome of diarrhea and protrusion of the nictating membranes in cats.[14] Togavirus-like and picornavirus-like particles have been identified in the feces of Australian cats. Analysis of the feline fecal virome has also revealed the presence of circoviruses, picobirnaviruses, kobuvirus, polyomaviruses, and feline norovirus.[15–17] The clinical significance of many of these viruses as they relate to diarrhea in cats remains uncertain. Feline norovirus (family *Caliciviridae*) was detected in an outbreak of gastroenteritis in a shelter in New York state, where 6/14 8- to 12-week-old cats tested positive using PCR[18]; the virus has also been detected in an apparently healthy cat from Japan[19] and diarrheic cats from South Italy.[20] In the South Italy study, 3/48 (6.2%) of diarrheic cats from shelters tested positive using PCR, whereas 0/57 healthy shelter cats tested positive.[20] In addition, experimental infection of SPF cats was followed by vomiting, weight loss, and diarrhea, with virus shedding in stool for 8 days.[19,21] Molecular characterization of this virus has shown it belongs to genogroup GVI, a genotype that does not normally infect humans. Some feline norovirus and canine norovirus isolates have had high sequence homology, raising the possibility that interspecies transmission might be possible.[22] However, considerable diversity exists among norovirus strains from dogs and cats.[22]

CLINICAL FEATURES

Pathogenesis and Clinical Signs

The pathogenesis of FPV infection is similar to that of CPV infection (see Chapter 29). Transmission is by the fecal-oral route, and indirect transmission through contaminated fomites represents the most important means of infection. Like CPV, FPV enters cells using transferrin receptor type-1[23] and replicates in cells that are in the S-phase of the mitotic cycle. Initially, the virus replicates in oropharyngeal lymphoid tissue, after which it disseminates in blood to all tissues as a free virus viremia, as well as through infected lymphocytes. Infection of lymphoid tissues leads to lymphoid tissue necrosis. Infection of the marrow is associated with leukopenia, which is compounded by neutrophil sequestration in damaged GI tissue. The virus also replicates in and kills the small intestinal crypt epithelial cells, resulting in shortening of villi, increased intestinal permeability, and malabsorption.

Subclinical infection is probably widespread, especially in young adult or adult cats. Disease severity depends on combinations of factors such as age, immune status, and concurrent infections with other bacterial, parasitic, or viral pathogens, which increase the turnover rate of intestinal epithelial cells enhancing viral replication and cellular destruction. Co-infections can occur with feline enteric coronavirus, *Clostridium piliforme, Salmonella* spp., FeLV, or astroviruses.[24–27] Disease generally occurs after an incubation period of 2 to 7 days. Infection of kittens or adult cats results in clinical signs of fever, lethargy, vocalization, weakness, and inappetence, which may progress to profound dehydration, vomiting, sometimes watery to hemorrhagic diarrhea, and rapid loss of weight. Some cats develop only anorexia and lethargy, in the absence of vomiting, diarrhea, or leukopenia.[5,10,13] Secondary bacterial infections are associated with more severe signs of disease. Death usually results from complications relating to dehydration, electrolyte imbalances, hypoglycemia, hemorrhage, or bacteremia and endotoxemia.

In the developing fetus or neonate in a nonimmune queen, FPV may replicate in a variety of tissues that are not affected in older animals. Abortion, congenital abnormalities, or infertility can result from infection early in pregnancy, although the queen is generally otherwise unaffected. Later in pregnancy or in neonates up to approximately 1 week of age, viral destruction of Purkinje cells and granule precursor cells located in the cerebellar external granular layer leads to cerebellar hypoplasia (Fig. 30.1). The severity of infection can vary between kittens in a litter. Sometimes a portion of the litter fails to survive and the remainder develop neurologic signs.[28] Signs of cerebellar ataxia are nonprogressive and are most apparent when kittens begin to walk at about 2 to 3 weeks of age, although mentation and appetite are otherwise normal, and these kittens can sometimes make acceptable pets. Other developmental CNS abnormalities have been reported less commonly, and include hydrocephalus, porencephaly (cystic lesions within the cerebral hemispheres), or hydranencephaly (complete replacement of the cerebral hemispheres with cystic lesions). These abnormalities may be accompanied by signs of forebrain damage, such as seizures and behavioral changes. Unlike CPV, FPV appears to be able to infect neurons other than the cerebellar Purkinje cells, which are terminally differentiated cells.[29,30] Ocular lesions can also develop and include retinal folding, dysplasia and degeneration, and optic nerve hypoplasia.

The DNA of FPV has been detected in the myocardium of cats with hypertrophic, dilated, and restrictive cardiomyopathy, but was not detected in a subset of healthy control cats.[31] A study of cats with endomyocardial restrictive cardiomyopathy and myocarditis revealed no evidence of parvoviral DNA in archived heart tissue.[32] Additional studies to assess the role of FPV in feline myocarditis and cardiomyopathy are needed.

Fecal shedding of virus usually lasts for several days, and in some cats, it may persist for up to 6 weeks. However, a longitudinal study of clinically affected shelter kittens showed that shedding as determined using PCR ceased after day 14, suggesting isolation for at least 2 weeks after diagnosis may be needed to control spread.[33] Viral DNA may be detected in tissues by PCR for months or years after infection, but that is likely to be residual from the earlier infection and to be noninfectious.[34]

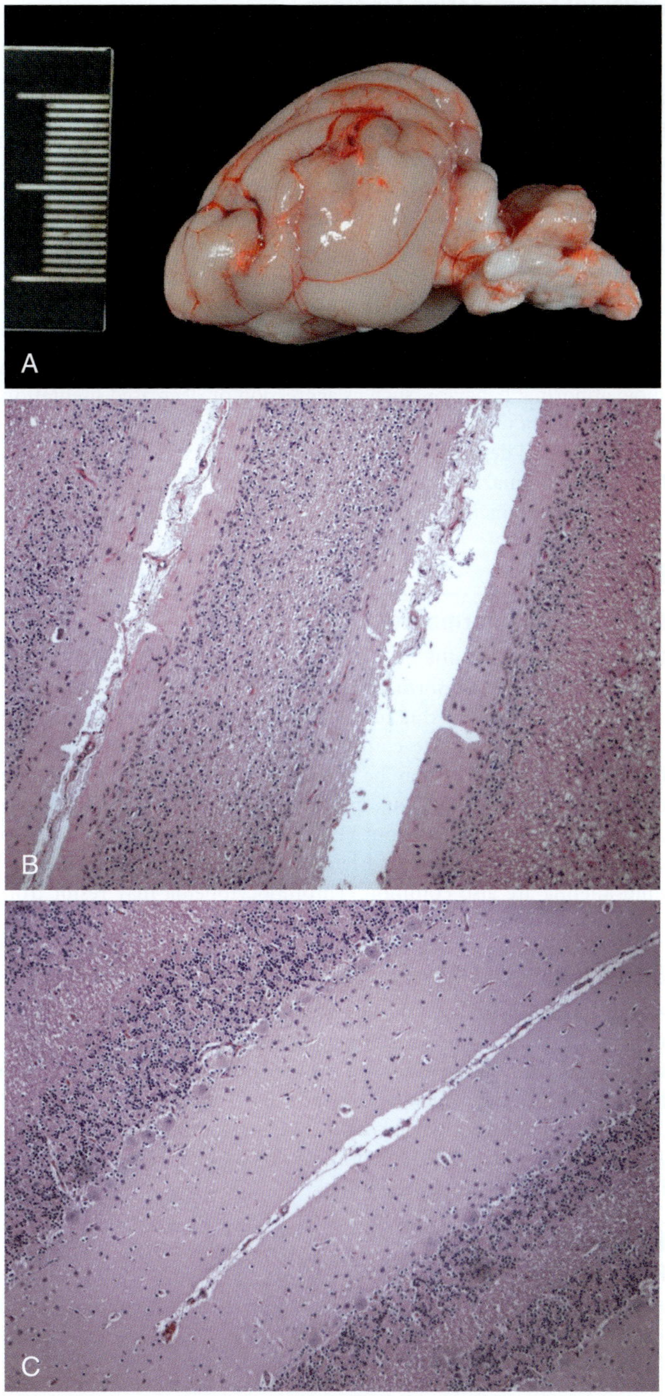

Fig. 30.1 (A) Hypoplasia of the cerebellum in an approximately 10-month-old cat that died of neurologic disease related to feline panleukopenia virus infection. (B) Severe cerebellar hypoplasia in a 1-year-old male neutered domestic short-hair cat that was euthanized for cerebellar signs and seizures. The neurologic signs had been present since the cat was found at approximately 4 months of age. There is a paucity of neurons and glial cells in all layers. (C) Normal feline cerebellum. Note the dramatically increased width of the molecular layer when compared with B. (A, Courtesy University of California, Davis Veterinary Pathology Service.)

Physical Examination Findings

The most common physical examination findings in cats with FPV infection are weakness, lethargy, and dehydration. Fever (103°F to 107°F; 39.5°C to 42.5°C) may be present early in the course of illness. Pain may be noted on palpation of the abdomen, or a hunched posture may be present. The perianal region may be contaminated with feces. Oral ulceration and mucosal pallor may be present in severely affected cats, and rarely, bacteremia may be accompanied by icterus. Terminally, affected cats may be hypothermic, bradycardic, and comatose.

Kittens with cerebellar damage are generally bright and alert but exhibit intention tremors, incoordination, ataxia, hypermetria, a broad-based stance, decreased postural reactions, a truncal sway, and absence of a menace response. Cats with forebrain disease may show abnormal behavior, such as aggression or decreased mentation. Examination of the ocular fundus may reveal folding of the retina, evidence of retinal degeneration with discrete gray spots, and optic nerve hypoplasia. Retinal lesions may be an incidental finding in older, recovered cats, which includes surviving cats with cerebellar hypoplasia.

DIAGNOSIS

Laboratory Abnormalities

Complete Blood Count

The most common abnormality on the CBC in feline panleukopenia is leukopenia, which is due to a neutropenia and lymphopenia (Box 30.1).[5,6,10] Total leukocyte counts may be as low as 50 cells/μL, and toxic band neutrophils may be present. However, in one study only 65% of 187 cats with panleukopenia were leukopenic, so an absence of leukopenia does not rule out FPV infection. Recovery may be associated with lymphocytosis and leukocytosis. Thrombocytopenia and mild anemia are also common. Thrombocytopenia may result from damage to the marrow or, possibly, DIC.

Serum Biochemical Tests

Serum biochemistry analysis may show hypoalbuminemia, hypoglobulinemia, and/or hypocholesterolemia; electrolyte abnormalities such as hyponatremia or hypernatremia, hypochloremia, hyperkalemia, or less commonly hypokalemia; and acid-base abnormalities (see Box 30.1). In severely affected cats, azotemia, increased serum activities of AST or ALT, or hyperbilirubinemia may be present. Hyperglycemia or hypoglycemia may also be identified.

Diagnostic Imaging

Plain Radiography

As in dogs with parvoviral enteritis, abdominal radiography in cats with panleukopenia may show evidence of poor serosal detail and a fluid- and gas-filled GI tract.

Magnetic Resonance Imaging Findings

MRI of cats with neurologic signs due to FPV may reveal evidence of cerebellar agenesis or hypoplasia. Rarely, hydrocephalus, porencephaly, or hydranencephaly can be detected.[28]

Microbiologic Tests

Diagnostic assays available for feline panleukopenia are listed in Table 30.1.

Serologic Diagnosis

Many kittens have maternal antibodies, while varying numbers of older animals have antibodies due to past infection or vaccination, so serology detecting IgG is of limited use for diagnosis of FPV-related disease. However, serologic assays that detect antibody against FPV may be used to assess the need for vaccination, in order to determine which cats are at risk for infection. The gold standard method for FPV serology is hemagglutination inhibition (HI), which measures the ability of serum to prevent agglutination of erythrocytes by the virus (see Chapter 2). Serum neutralization assays may also be used, and there is a relationship between neutralization and hemagglutination titers, with the neutralization assay being more sensitive at lower levels.[35] POC assays designed to detect antibody titers to CPV have a low sensitivity (28%) for detection of antibodies to FPV in cats.[36] A POC assay designed to detect feline antibodies (ImmunoComb Feline VacciCheck Test Kit, Biogal, Galed Labs, Israel) also had a low sensitivity (49%), although specificity was high.[36] The use of this test for risk analysis in shelter situations may therefore lead to inappropriate removal or isolation of cats with results indicating that they lack protective antibody titers (false negative), which might waste resources.[36] However, positive results should reliably indicate protection. The test can be performed quickly (30 minutes) and requires as little as 5 μL of serum or plasma, so provided it is understood that a negative result could mean either a protected or susceptible status, and a positive result equates to protection, the test still has the potential to provide useful information.

BOX 30.1 Prevalence of Laboratory Abnormalities in Cats with Panleukopenia

Leukopenia: 122/187 (65%)
Thrombocytopenia: 83/153 (54%)
Anemia: 91/187 (48%)
Neutropenia: 64/137 (47%)
Lymphopenia: 53/137 (39%)
Hypoalbuminemia: 45/101 (45%)
Hypochloremia: 40/112 (36%)
Hyponatremia: 41/127 (32%)
Hypoproteinemia: 46/153 (30%)
Hyperglycemia: 48/168 (29%)
Increased AST activity: 26/98 (27%)
Hyperkalemia: 30/132 (23%)
Increased BUN: 36/168 (21%)
Hyperbilirubinemia: 19/134 (14%)
Increased ALT activity: 18/135 (13%)
Increased creatinine: 12/155 (8%)
Hypokalemia: 9/132 (7%)
Hypernatremia: 8/127 (6%)
Hypoglycemia: 10/168 (6%)

Modified from Kruse BD, Unterer S, Horlacher K, et al. Prognostic factors in cats with feline panleukopenia. J Vet Intern Med. 2010;24:1271–1276.

Antigen Detection Enzyme-Linked Immunosorbent Assay

FPV can be detected in feces or rectal swabs using antigen assays designed to detect CPV.[37–39] The sensitivity and specificity of these assays varies from one assay to another and with the stage of infection because virus shedding may be transient. In general, false-negative results are common with these assays, but false positives are uncommon, so a positive test result in a cat with consistent clinical signs suggests a diagnosis of feline panleukopenia. The specificity of one POC device (SNAP Parvo, IDEXX Laboratories, Westbrook, ME, USA) was high; 54 of 55 positive assay results were confirmed with a PCR assay. However, in another study, the sensitivity of this assay was low compared with fecal PCR and it was not recommended for monitoring virus shedding.[33] Another study of 52 cats with diarrhea and 148 healthy cats showed variability in the sensitivity and specificity of five different test kits when compared with fecal electron microscopy.[39] Sensitivity ranged from 50% to 80%, and specificity ranged from 94% to 100%. This study included only 10 cats with FPV as determined

TABLE 30.1 Diagnostic Assays Available for Feline Panleukopenia

Assay	Specimen Type	Target	Performance
Canine parvovirus fecal antigen ELISA	Feces	Parvoviral antigen	Sensitivity varies with the assay used and the timing of specimen collection. False negatives are common, but a positive result generally indicates infection.
Histopathology	Usually necropsy specimens, especially GI tissues	Crypt necrosis with intranuclear inclusions; FPV antigen with IHC or IFA	Can be used for necropsy diagnosis
Polymerase chain reaction (PCR)	Feces, tissue samples	FPV DNA	Sensitivity and specificity varies depending on assay design. The extent to which attenuated live vaccine virus can be detected after vaccination is not well understood. Because of the high sensitivity of some assays, the significance of a positive result may be difficult to interpret. False-negative results may occur as a result of inhibition of PCR by components of feces.
Fecal electron microscopy	Feces	Virus particles	Not widely available, turnaround time can be slow, and may be expensive. Requires the presence of large amounts of virus.
Virus isolation	Feces, tissues	FPV	Difficult, not widely available. Used primarily as a research tool.

ELISA, Enzyme-linked immunosorbent assay; *FPV*, feline panleukopenia virus; *IFA*, immunofluorescent antibody; *IHC*, immunohistochemistry.

with electron microscopy. Real-time PCR is now more commonly used for laboratory diagnosis of FPV infections. Attenuated live viral vaccines may result in low levels of virus in the feces a few days after vaccination, but positive fecal antigen assay results after vaccination appear to be uncommon, but again vary with the test used.[40,41] There are a number of tests available in different regions of the world, including SNAP Parvo (IDEXX Laboratories) and the Witness Parvo (Zoetis, NJ, USA).

Fecal Electron Microscopy

Fecal electron microscopy is still offered by some institutions for diagnosis of viral enteritis. It may also facilitate diagnosis of other infections such as rotavirus, astrovirus, torovirus, calicivirus, norovirus, and coronavirus infections. Turnaround time may be slow, large amounts of virus must be present for results to be positive, and technical expertise is required to accurately identify virus in the stool. Due to its poor sensitivity and general lack of availability, it is not used for routine diagnosis.

Virus Isolation

FPV can be isolated in feline cells, but is a specialized procedure that takes several days to complete, so it is not commonly used for routine diagnosis.

Molecular Diagnosis Using Nucleic Acid–Based Testing

Specific real-time PCR assays for detection of FPV and differentiation of FPV from CPV-2 variants are now offered by most veterinary diagnostic laboratories as the most sensitive as well as the fastest and cheapest assay. They are generally offered as part of panels that screen for several potential enteric viral pathogens. These assays may be used on whole blood or feces. The extent to which these assays detect attenuated live vaccine virus after vaccination, or residual viral DNA in recovered animals requires further study.

Pathologic Findings

Gross Pathologic Findings

Gross pathologic findings in cats with feline panleukopenia include thymic involution; thickening, distention, and discoloration of the intestinal wall with serosal hemorrhage (Fig. 30.2); and enlarged, edematous mesenteric lymph nodes. The intestine may contain bloody liquid contents, and mucosal hemorrhage may be identified. Hemorrhages may be visible on the surface of other organs as well. In some cats, mild pleural or peritoneal effusion is present. Cats infected

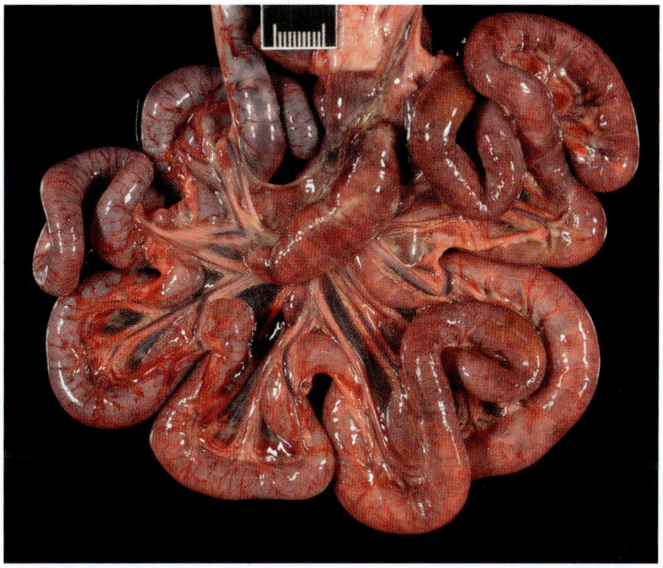

Fig. 30.2 Intestinal tract of a 2-year-old intact female domestic long-hair cat with severe feline panleukopenia. The intestinal loops are dilated and flaccid and discolored red to purple. Ruler = 1 cm.

prenatally may have cerebellar aplasia, or more commonly a small cerebellum (often half to three-quarters normal size).[42,43] Rarely other developmental CNS abnormalities such as hydrocephalus, hydranencephaly, or porencephaly are observed.

Histopathologic Findings

Histopathologic findings in the intestinal tract are similar to those described for CPV-2 infection, with crypt dilation and necrosis of crypt epithelial cells, accumulation of cellular debris, neutrophil infiltration, loss of villi, and submucosal edema throughout the small and large intestines; the jejunum and ileum are usually most severely affected (Fig. 30.3A). Acutely affected cats show widespread lymphoid depletion and there may be hyperplasia of mononuclear phagocytes. Intranuclear inclusions are found in some cats (Fig. 30.3B). Examination of the bone marrow may reveal bone marrow hypoplasia. Examination of the cerebellum shows cellular depletion; reactive astrocytosis may be present. Lymphocytic meningoencephalitis and neuronal necrosis,[44] as well as neuronal vacuolization[45] have been described in some cats. IHC or IFA may be used to document the presence of the virus within tissues (Fig. 30.3C).[46]

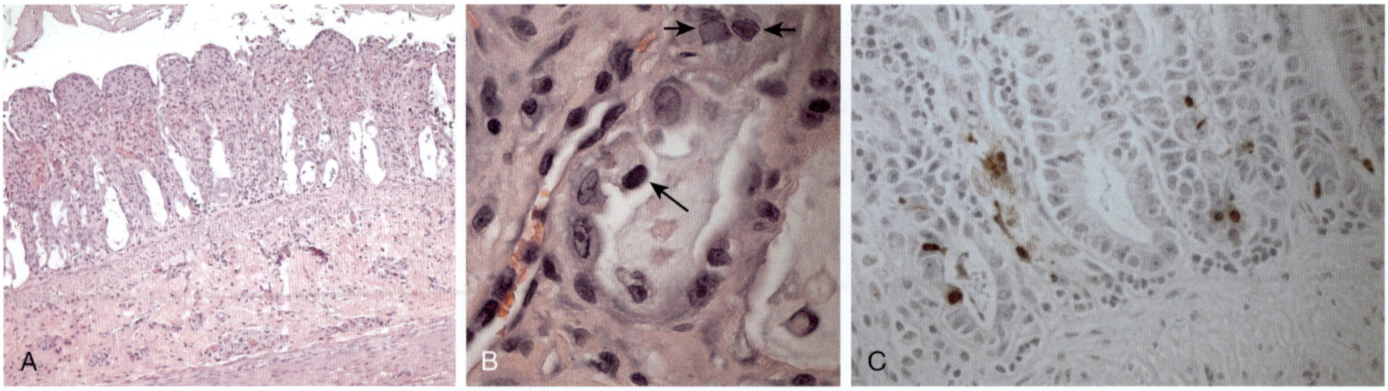

Fig. 30.3 (A) Histopathology of the jejunum from a kitten with panleukopenia. Villi are rounded and blunted with nearly complete epithelial loss and crypt dilation. Hematoxylin and eosin (H&E) stain. (B) Histopathology of the jejunum from a young barn cat that died after several days of profound weakness and neurologic signs. Six other cats in the barn died with the same signs. Mucosal crypts are dilated and contain debris, and intranuclear inclusions are present *(small arrows)*. Another cell *(large arrow)* is foamy and degenerate and has a hyperchromatic nucleus. H&E stain. (C) Same cat as in B. The presence of feline panleukopenia virus in the intestinal tract is confirmed with immunohistochemistry (brown stain). (Courtesy Dr. Patricia Pesavento, University of California, Davis Veterinary Anatomic Pathology Service.)

TREATMENT AND PROGNOSIS

Antimicrobial Treatment and Supportive Care

Treatment of cats with feline panleukopenia is with supportive care, especially IV crystalloids and parenteral antimicrobial drug treatment as for CPV-2 infections (see Chapter 29). Dextrose supplementation of fluids may be required, and blood glucose concentration should be monitored. Oral intake of food and water should be withheld until vomiting has ceased. Experience with early enteral nutrition has not been reported in cats, and extreme care is warranted to prevent aspiration pneumonia. Antiemetics such as metoclopramide or ondansetron may be effective. In contrast to canine parvoviral enteritis, treatment with rfIFN-ω has not been beneficial for treatment of feline panleukopenia, although increased antibody production and a reduced acute inflammatory response was observed.[47]

Prognosis

While there are an unknown number of mild or subclinical infections, when cats present with clinical disease the prognosis varies. Cats with panleukopenia that survive the first 5 days of treatment usually recover, although recovery is often more prolonged than it is for dogs with parvoviral enteritis. In cats with feline panleukopenia, survival rates vary between around 20% and 50%.[5,6,10] In one study, nonsurvivors had lower leukocyte and platelet counts than survivors, and cats with white cell counts below 1000/μL were almost twice as likely to die than those with white cell counts above 2500/μL. Only total leukopenia, and not lymphopenia, was correlated with mortality. Hypoalbuminemia and hypokalemia were also associated with an increased risk of mortality. Total T4 concentration was the only variable associated with survival in one study, and a cutoff value of 0.82 μg/mL was proposed for distinguishing survivors from nonsurvivors.[48] In contrast to dogs with parvoviral enteritis, mortality in cats with clinical disease does not appear to be correlated with age.

Cerebellar signs in kittens with cerebellar hypoplasia typically do not progress and may improve slightly as a result of compensatory responses from other senses such as vision.[49]

IMMUNITY AND VACCINATION

Recovery from feline panleukopenia is thought to confer lifelong immunity. Effective vaccines are widely available. An intranasal FPV, FHV-1, and FCV vaccine is available; its use has been controversial, because panleukopenia is a systemic disease. An outbreak of salmonellosis and panleukopenia occurred in one cattery that used an intranasal FPV vaccine.[7] No difference was noted in seroconversion rates between five cats vaccinated with the intranasal vaccine and five cats vaccinated with a parenteral attenuated live vaccine, but the number of cats in this study was small. In other studies of larger numbers of cats that were vaccinated with the parenteral vaccines, most seroconverted with protective antibody titers on day 7 and/or 28.[8,50]

Both inactivated and attenuated live vaccine types can induce protective antibody titers after vaccination in a high proportion of cats, although the attenuated live vaccine results in higher and more prolonged protective titers than the inactivated vaccine.[9,41] Provided maternally-derived antibody (MDA) is absent, immunity is present within 1 week after a single vaccination with an attenuated live viral vaccine[8,51] and most likely lasts for life.[52] Nevertheless, two doses, 3 to 4 weeks apart, have been recommended for initial vaccination with attenuated live vaccines in the absence of information about MDA. Two injections are always required for inactivated vaccines, and maximal immunity does not occur until 1 week after the second dose. However, even with an inactivated vaccine, challenge 7.5 years after vaccination was associated with protection.[53] The routine use of inactivated vaccines is discouraged, and those should be reserved for immunosuppressed cats or colostrum-deprived neonates that are less than 4 weeks of age, or when there is a need to vaccinate pregnant cats that are expected to carry the kittens to term. In general, and particularly in shelter situations, the use of attenuated live vaccines is recommended because of the slow onset of immunity and relatively low antibody titers associated with inactivated vaccines.[54] FPV vaccines protect cats against challenge with CPV-2 strains.[55,56] However, cross-reactivity of antibodies induced by FPV vaccination to CPV-2 was lower than that to FPV as determined using HI.[57]

The most common reason for vaccine failure is interference by MDA. Maternal antibody persists from 8 until 12 weeks, and possibly longer in some cats. Virus neutralization titers above 1:10 are likely to interfere with vaccination, and kittens with titers below 1:40 are generally considered to be susceptible to infection by FPV. Kittens should be vaccinated every 3 to 4 weeks from 6 to 8 weeks of age, and it is recommended that the last vaccine in the kitten series be given no earlier than 16 to 20 weeks of age. When there is a history of an outbreak situation, the final booster could be given at 16 to 20 weeks of age.[58,59] A booster should be administered at 6 months to 1 year, and every 3 years thereafter.

Vaccination of pregnant queens with attenuated live viral vaccines can cause cerebellar hypoplasia or fetal losses. The frequency with which this occurs is unknown, as many queens are immune by the time they are bred. As a result, it has been suggested that pregnant queens only be vaccinated with attenuated live FPV vaccines if they are being introduced into a shelter, where most are spayed upon arrival. Otherwise quarantine while immunization with inactivated vaccines should be performed. Alternatively, assessment for protective antibody titers with an in-house test kit (where available) could be performed.

PREVENTION

New kittens should not be introduced into households that previously contained cats infected with FPV unless they are fully vaccinated, or until a period of at least 2 weeks has elapsed along with thorough cleanup of the facilities. In the face of an outbreak, exposed and susceptible kittens may be effectively protected for 2 to 4 weeks through SC or intraperitoneal administration of 2 mL of type-matched serum from cats with a high antibody titer.[60] However, this is only effective when administered before the onset of clinical signs, and it can interfere with subsequent vaccination. For these kittens, it has been recommended that vaccination be withheld for 3 weeks after the serum has been administered. Passive immunization may be useful when cats are introduced into a shelter situation where a known problem exists. Repeated treatment with serum should be avoided because hypersensitivity reactions may occur. Prevention of feline panleukopenia should also include proper disinfection with disinfectants that are effective against parvoviruses, such as bleach, accelerated hydrogen peroxide, or potassium peroxymonosulfate (see Chapter 14) and, in shelter situations, isolation or removal of cats that develop GI illness, and separate housing for healthy kittens (see Chapter 16).

PUBLIC HEALTH ASPECTS

Although FPV is not known to infect humans, a unique strain of FPV was recently isolated from a diarrheic monkey in China that was associated with a large outbreak among monkeys in a colony.[61] This strain was shown to cause panleukopenia in inoculated cats. Whether other enteric viruses, such as some norovirus strains, can be transmitted between companion animals and people, remains unclear. One study that looked at a diverse array of animal noroviruses concluded that there was more evidence of human noroviruses in animals than animal noroviruses in humans, suggesting the possibility of reverse zoonoses.[62]

CASE EXAMPLE

Signalment

"Callie," a 2-year-old female intact domestic long-hair cat from Woodland, CA.

History

Callie was brought to an emergency clinic for acute onset of collapse and severe illness. The current owner had fostered the cat for 1 week after she was found as a stray. The cat had been nursing a litter of kittens. The kittens were 4 weeks old, being weaned and apparently healthy. Since being fostered, the cat had exhibited a progressive decrease in appetite and thirst, and her feces had become soft and pasty. The night before she was brought to the emergency clinic, she had been bathed, and afterwards she vomited bile-stained fluid twice and was placed on a heating pad. The following morning she was found laterally recumbent and minimally responsive.

Physical Examination

Body weight: 2.3 kg.

General: Stuporous mentation, estimated to be 8% to 10% dehydrated, T < 92°F (<33°C), HR = 132 beats/minute, RR = 32 breaths/minute, mucous membranes pale and tacky, unable to assess CRT. Fecal and urinary stains were present around the perineum and on the caudal aspect of the pelvic limbs.

Musculoskeletal: BCS 2/9. Diffuse muscle wasting was present. The cat was laterally recumbent and nonambulatory.

Cardiovascular: Weak femoral pulses. No murmurs or arrhythmias were detected.

GI and urogenital: The abdomen was soft and nonpainful on palpation. Fluid-filled intestinal loops were palpated, and the urinary bladder was small (<5 cm) and soft.

All other systems: No abnormalities were detected.

Laboratory Findings

CBC: HCT 46% (30%–50%), MCV 49.8 fL (42–53 fL), MCHC 30.4 g/dL (30–33.5 g/dL), WBC 150 cells/μL (4,500–14,000 cells/μL), neutrophils 0 cells/μL (2,000–9,000 cells/μL), lymphocytes 141 cells/μL (1,000–7,000 cells/μL), highly reactive lymphocytes 6 cells/μL, monocytes 3 cells/μL (50–600 cells/μL), platelets 32,000 platelets/μL (180,000–500,000 platelets/μL).

Serum chemistry profile: Sodium 141 mmol/L (151–158 mmol/L), potassium 4.0 mmol/L (3.6–4.9 mmol/L), chloride 111 mmol/L (117–126 mmol/L), bicarbonate 23 mmol/L (15–21 mmol/L), phosphorus 6.0 mg/dL (3.2–6.3 mg/dL), calcium 7.4 mg/dL (9.0–10.9 mg/dL), BUN 24 mg/dL (18–33 mg/dL), creatinine 0.5 mg/dL (1.1–2.2 mg/dL), glucose 68 mg/dL (63–118 mg/dL), total protein 3.2 g/dL (6.6–8.4 g/dL), albumin 1.6 g/dL (2.2–4.6 g/dL), globulin 1.6 g/dL (2.8–5.4 g/dL), ALT 125 U/L (27–101 U/L), AST 143 U/L (17–58 U/L), ALP 4 U/L (14–71 U/L), creatine kinase 2,409 U/L (73–260 U/L), GGT < 3 U/L (0–4 U/L), cholesterol 68 mg/dL (89–258 mg/dL), total bilirubin 0.2 mg/dL (0–0.2 mg/dL), magnesium 2.5 mg/dL (1.5–2.5 mg/dL).

Imaging

An abdominal ultrasound showed marked fluid distention of the small intestines.

Microbiologic Testing

In-clinic ELISA serology for FeLV antigen and FIV antibody: negative.

Treatment and Outcome

Callie was treated with active warming, and a central venous access line was placed. IV crystalloids (four warmed 60-mL boluses of lactated Ringer's solution [LRS], each given over 20 minutes) were administered, after which a venous acid-base panel showed a pH of 7.267 (7.31–7.46), bicarbonate of 17.5 mmol/L (14–22 mmol/L), base excess of −8.1 mmol/L (−4 to +2 mmol/L), pCO_2 of 39.7 mmHg (25–37 mmHg), lactate of 4.5 mEq/L (<2 mEq/L), glucose of 52 mg/dL, potassium of 3.1 mEq/L, sodium of 141 mEq/L, and ionized calcium of 1.17 (1.1–1.4 mmol/L). A dextrose bolus and ticarcillin-clavulanic acid (22 mg/kg, q6h, IV) were administered. The cat repeatedly vomited blood-tinged fluid, and so treatment with metoclopramide (0.02 mg/kg/hour) and famotidine (0.5 mg/kg, IV, q12h) was initiated. Aggressive crystalloid fluid therapy was continued (LRS supplemented with 30 mEq/L KCl and 2.5% dextrose), and treatment with hetastarch was also initiated. Systolic blood pressure (Doppler) was 60 to 90 mmHg, HR increased to 170 beats/minute, and rectal temperature increased to 100°F. When the CDC results were available, the cat was placed in the isolation ward.

Pasty diarrhea that contained sloughed mucosa occurred every 1 to 2 hours, which transitioned to liquid red feces over 24 hours. A CBC again showed absolute neutropenia and 15,000 platelets/μL. After another 24 hours, the cat's condition deteriorated despite aggressive treatment and monitoring. Partial parenteral nutrition was initiated. That evening, pyrexia developed (104.6°F) as well as tachypnea and increased respiratory effort. The owner elected euthanasia. The cat regurgitated approximately 200 mL of dark brown fluid at the time of euthanasia.

CASE EXAMPLE—cont'd

Gross Necropsy Findings

In the peritoneal cavity, 10 mL of semiopaque red fluid was present. Streaks of hemorrhage were noted throughout the skeletal muscle. Between the pylorus and the ileocecocolic junction, the serosa of the small intestinal tract was dark red to purple to black (see Fig. 30.2). The entire small and large intestinal tract was dilated and flaccid. The small intestinal mucosa was dark red to purple and contained a small amount of dark red mucoid material. The mesenteric lymph nodes were prominent, and their cut surface was discolored red to dark pink. The liver was pale yellow and extended beyond the costal arches. Numerous petechial hemorrhages were present on the serosal surface of the urinary bladder.

Histopathologic Findings

Within the duodenum, jejunum, and ileum, there was severe, subacute, diffuse necrotizing and fibrinohemorrhagic enteritis. The villi were necrotic, fused, and markedly blunted with a minimal inflammatory response. Necrosis extended into the crypts, and there was some evidence of a regenerative response that included enterocyte hypertrophy, karyomegaly, and rare mitotic figures. Mixed bacteria, which included small gram-negative rods and large numbers of gram-positive cocci, lined and effaced the denuded villi. There was diffuse lymphoid depletion in lymph nodes, as well as the mucosa-associated lymphoid tissue in the cecum and colon. Marked depletion of erythroid and myeloid precursors was present in the bone marrow. There were multifocal areas of hemorrhage in the skeletal and cardiac muscle, intestinal tract, and lungs, as well as fibrin thrombi in the lungs. FPV antigen was identified in intestinal epithelial cells using IHC. Culture of the jejunum for *Salmonella* spp. was negative.

Diagnosis

Feline panleukopenia.

Comments

The cat in this report was a stray with an unknown vaccination history, which demonstrates that severe disease can occur even in adult cats. Antemortem diagnostic testing for FPV with a fecal antigen ELISA assay or PCR assay was discussed with the owner, but was declined because of the high degree of suspicion for the disease and the lack of impact that a positive or negative result would have had on the treatment plan. Secondary bacterial sepsis was suspected. Additional co-infections with other viruses, such as FCoV, or enteropathogenic bacteria could not be ruled out. During the cat's treatment, one of the kittens in the litter died suddenly and the other developed signs of illness.

SUGGESTED READINGS

Barrs VR. Feline panleukopenia: a re-emergent disease. *Vet Clin North Am Small Anim Pract*. 2019;49:651–670.

Di Martino B, Di Profio F, Melegari I, et al. Feline virome-a review of novel enteric viruses detected in cats. *Viruses*. 2019;11.

Hosie MJ, Addie DD, Boucraut-Baralon C, et al. Matrix vaccination guidelines: 2015 ABCD recommendations for indoor/outdoor cats, rescue shelter cats and breeding catteries. *J Feline Med Surg*. 2015;17:583–587.

REFERENCES

1. Verge J, Christoforoni N. La gastroenterite infectieuse des chats; est-elle due a un virus filtrable. *C R Seances Soc Biol Fil*. 1928;99:312.
2. Barrs VR. Feline panleukopenia: a re-emergent disease. *Vet Clin North Am Small Anim Pract*. 2019;49:651–670.
3. Steinel A, Parrish CR, Bloom ME, et al. Parvovirus infections in wild carnivores. *J Wildl Dis*. 2001;37:594–607.
4. Stuetzer B, Hartmann K. Feline parvovirus infection and associated diseases. *Vet J*. 2014;201:150–155.
5. Kruse BD, Unterer S, Horlacher K, et al. Prognostic factors in cats with feline panleukopenia. *J Vet Intern Med*. 2010;24:1271–1276.
6. Litster A, Benjanirut C. Case series of feline panleukopenia virus in an animal shelter. *J Feline Med Surg*. 2014;16:346–353.
7. Addie DD, Toth S, Thompson H, et al. Detection of feline parvovirus in dying pedigree kittens. *Vet Rec*. 1998;142:353–356.
8. Bergmann M, Schwertler S, Reese S, et al. Antibody response to feline panleukopenia virus vaccination in healthy adult cats. *J Feline Med Surg*. 2018;20:1087–1093.
9. Fischer SM, Quest CM, Dubovi EJ, et al. Response of feral cats to vaccination at the time of neutering. *J Am Vet Med Assoc*. 2007;230:52–58.
10. Porporato F, Horzinek MC, Hofmann-Lehmann R, et al. Survival estimates and outcome predictors for shelter cats with feline panleukopenia virus infection. *J Am Vet Med Assoc*. 2018;253:188–195.
11. Battilani M, Balboni A, Ustulin M, et al. Genetic complexity and multiple infections with more parvovirus species in naturally infected cats. *Vet Res*. 2011;42:43.
12. Decaro N, Desario C, Miccolupo A, et al. Genetic analysis of feline panleukopenia viruses from cats with gastroenteritis. *J Gen Virol*. 2008;89:2290–2298.
13. Nakamura K, Sakamoto M, Ikeda Y, et al. Pathogenic potential of canine parvovirus types 2a and 2c in domestic cats. *Clin Diagn Lab Immunol*. 2001;8:663–668.
14. Muir P, Harbour DA, Gruffydd-Jones TJ, et al. A clinical and microbiological study of cats with protruding nictitating membranes and diarrhoea: isolation of a novel virus. *Vet Rec*. 1990;127:324–330.
15. Ng TF, Mesquita JR, Nascimento MS, et al. Feline fecal virome reveals novel and prevalent enteric viruses. *Vet Microbiol*. 2014;171:102–111.
16. Zhang W, Li L, Deng X, et al. Faecal virome of cats in an animal shelter. *J Gen Virol*. 2014;95:2553–2564.
17. Di Martino B, Di Profio F, Melegari I, et al. Feline virome: a review of novel enteric viruses detected in cats. *Viruses*. 2019;11.
18. Pinto P, Wang Q, Chen N, et al. Discovery and genomic characterization of noroviruses from a gastroenteritis outbreak in domestic cats in the US. *PloS One*. 2012;7:e32739.
19. Takano T, Kusuhara H, Kuroishi A, et al. Molecular characterization and pathogenicity of a genogroup GVI feline norovirus. *Vet Microbiol*. 2015;178:201–207.
20. Di Martino B, Di Profio F, Melegari I, et al. A novel feline norovirus in diarrheic cats. *Infect Genet Evol*. 2016;38:132–137.
21. Takano T, Hiramatsu K, Matsuyama M, et al. Viral shedding and clinical status of feline-norovirus-infected cats after reinfection with the same strain. *Arch Virol*. 2018;163:1503–1510.
22. Bodnar L, Lorusso E, Di Martino B, et al. Identification of a novel canine norovirus. *Infect Genet Evol*. 2017;52:75–81.
23. Hueffer K, Parker JS, Weichert WS, et al. The natural host range shift and subsequent evolution of canine parvovirus resulted from virus-specific binding to the canine transferrin receptor. *J Virol*. 2003;77:1718–1726.
24. Ikegami T, Shirota K, Goto K, et al. Enterocolitis associated with dual infection by *Clostridium piliforme* and feline panleukopenia virus in three kittens. *Vet Pathol*. 1999;36:613–615.
25. Lutz H, Castelli I, Ehrensperger F, et al. Panleukopenia-like syndrome of FeLV caused by co-infection with FeLV and feline panleukopenia virus. *Vet Immunol Immunopathol*. 1995;46:21–33.
26. Mochizuki M, Osawa N, Ishida T. Feline coronavirus participation in diarrhea of cats. *J Vet Med Sci*. 1999;61:1071–1073.
27. Moschidou P, Martella V, Lorusso E, et al. Mixed infection by feline astrovirus and feline panleukopenia virus in a domestic cat with gastroenteritis and panleukopenia. *J Vet Diagn Invest*. 2011;23:581–584.
28. Sharp NJ, Davis BJ, Guy JS, et al. Hydranencephaly and cerebellar hypoplasia in two kittens attributed to intrauterine parvovirus infection. *J Comp Pathol*. 1999;121:39–53.

29. Poncelet L, Garigliany M, Ando K, et al. Cell cycle S phase markers are expressed in cerebral neuron nuclei of cats infected by the feline panleukopenia virus. *Cell Cycle*. 2016;15:3482–3489.
30. Url A, Truyen U, Rebel-Bauder B, et al. Evidence of parvovirus replication in cerebral neurons of cats. *J Clin Microbiol*. 2003;41:3801–3805.
31. Meurs KM, Fox PR, Magnon AL, et al. Molecular screening by polymerase chain reaction detects panleukopenia virus DNA in formalin-fixed hearts from cats with idiopathic cardiomyopathy and myocarditis. *Cardiovasc Pathol*. 2000;9:119–126.
32. McEndaffer L, Molesan A, Erb H, et al. Feline panleukopenia virus is not associated with myocarditis or endomyocardial restrictive cardiomyopathy in cats. *Vet Pathol*. 2017;54:669–675.
33. Janke KJ, Jacobsen LS, Giacinti JA, et al. Fecal viral DNA shedding following clinical panleukopenia virus infection in shelter kittens: a prospective, observational study. *J Feline Med Surg*. 2022;24:337–343.
34. Allison AB, Kohler DJ, Fox KA, et al. Frequent cross-species transmission of parvoviruses among diverse carnivore hosts. *J Virol*. 2013;87:2342–2347.
35. Soma T, Ohta K, Yamashita R, et al. Anti-feline panleukopenia virus serum neutralizing antibody titer in domestic cats with the negative or low hemagglutination inhibition antibody titer. *J Vet Med Sci*. 2019;81:252–255.
36. Digangi BA, Gray LK, Levy JK, et al. Detection of protective antibody titers against feline panleukopenia virus, feline herpesvirus-1, and feline calicivirus in shelter cats using a point-of-care ELISA. *J Feline Med Surg*. 2011;13:912–918.
37. Abd-Eldaim M, Beall M, Kennedy M. Detection of feline panleukopenia virus using a commercial ELISA for canine parvovirus. *Vet Ther*. 2009;10:E1–E6.
38. Awad RA, Khalil WKB, Attallah AG. Epidemiology and diagnosis of feline panleukopenia virus in Egypt: clinical and molecular diagnosis in cats. *Vet World*. 2018;11:578–584.
39. Neuerer FF, Horlacher K, Truyen U, et al. Comparison of different in-house test systems to detect parvovirus in faeces of cats. *J Feline Med Surg*. 2008;10:247–251.
40. Bergmann M, Schwertler S, Speck S, et al. Faecal shedding of parvovirus deoxyribonucleic acid following modified live feline panleucopenia virus vaccination in healthy cats. *Vet Rec*. 2019;185:83.
41. Patterson EV, Reese MJ, Tucker SJ, et al. Effect of vaccination on parvovirus antigen testing in kittens. *J Am Vet Med Assoc*. 2007;230:359–363.
42. Csiza CK, De Lahunta A, Scott FW, et al. Pathogenesis of feline panleukopenia virus in susceptible newborn kittens II. Pathology and immunofluorescence. *Infect Immun*. 1971;3:838–846.
43. Resibois A, Coppens A, Poncelet L. Naturally occurring parvovirus-associated feline hypogranular cerebellar hypoplasia: A comparison to experimentally-induced lesions using immunohistology. *Vet Pathol*. 2007;44:831–841.
44. Kokosinska A, Maboni G, Kelly KM, et al. Lymphoplasmacytic meningoencephalitis and neuronal necrosis associated with parvoviral infection in cats. *Vet Pathol*. 2019;56:604–608.
45. Pfankuche VM, Jo WK, van der Vries E, et al. Neuronal vacuolization in feline panleukopenia virus infection. *Vet Pathol*. 2018;55:294–297.
46. Garigliany M, Gilliaux G, Jolly S, et al. Feline panleukopenia virus in cerebral neurons of young and adult cats. *BMC Vet Res*. 2016;12:28.
47. Paltrinieri S, Crippa A, Comerio T, et al. Evaluation of inflammation and immunity in cats with spontaneous parvovirus infection: consequences of recombinant feline interferon-omega administration. *Vet Immunol Immunopathol*. 2007;118:68–74.
48. Petini M, Drigo M, Zoia A. Prognostic value of systemic inflammatory response syndrome and serum concentrations of acute phase proteins, cholesterol, and total thyroxine in cats with panleukopenia. *J Vet Intern Med*. 2020;34:719–724.
49. Penderis J. The wobbly cat. Diagnostic and therapeutic approach to generalised ataxia. *J Feline Med Surg*. 2009;11:349–359.
50. Lappin MR, Veir J, Hawley J. Feline panleukopenia virus, feline herpesvirus-1, and feline calicivirus antibody responses in seronegative specific pathogen-free cats after a single administration of two different modified live FVRCP vaccines. *J Feline Med Surg*. 2009;11:159–162.
51. Jas D, Aeberle C, Lacombe V, et al. Onset of immunity in kittens after vaccination with a non-adjuvanted vaccine against feline panleucopenia, feline calicivirus and feline herpesvirus. *Vet J*. 2009;182:86–93.
52. Gore TC, Lakshmanan N, Williams JR, et al. Three-year duration of immunity in cats following vaccination against feline rhinotracheitis virus, feline calicivirus, and feline panleukopenia virus. *Vet Ther*. 2006;7:213–222.
53. Scott FW, Geissinger CM. Long-term immunity in cats vaccinated with an inactivated trivalent vaccine. *Am J Vet Res*. 1999;60:652–658.
54. Day MJ, Horzinek MC, Schultz RD, et al. WSAVA guidelines for the vaccination of dogs and cats. *J Small Anim Pract*. 2016;57:E1–E45.
55. Chalmers WS, Truyen U, Greenwood NM, et al. Efficacy of feline panleucopenia vaccine to prevent infection with an isolate of CPV2b obtained from a cat. *Vet Microbiol*. 1999;69:41–45.
56. Jack SC, Sutton D, Bhogle A, et al. FPL-vaccinated cats are protected from CPV2c and CPV2b challenge. *Vet Rec*. 2014;174:146.
57. Nakamura K, Ikeda Y, Miyazawa T, et al. Characterisation of cross-reactivity of virus neutralising antibodies induced by feline panleukopenia virus and canine parvoviruses. *Res Vet Sci*. 2001;71:219–222.
58. Hosie MJ, Addie DD, Boucraut-Baralon C, et al. Matrix vaccination guidelines: 2015 ABCD recommendations for indoor/outdoor cats, rescue shelter cats and breeding catteries. *J Feline Med Surg*. 2015;17:583–587.
59. Mostl K, Egberink H, Addie D, et al. Prevention of infectious diseases in cat shelters: ABCD guidelines. *J Feline Med Surg*. 2013;15:546–554.
60. Levy JK, Crawford PC, Collante WR, et al. Use of adult cat serum to correct failure of passive transfer in kittens. *J Am Vet Med Assoc*. 2001;219:1401–1405.
61. Yang S, Wang S, Feng H, et al. Isolation and characterization of feline panleukopenia virus from a diarrheic monkey. *Vet Microbiol*. 2010;143:155–159.
62. Villabruna N, Koopmans MPG, de Graaf M. Animals as reservoir for human norovirus. *Viruses*. 2019;11.

31

Feline Coronavirus Infections

Niels C. Pedersen, Jane E. Sykes

KEY POINTS

- First Described: 1963 (Holzworth, 1963)[1]; a viral etiology was not identified until the 1970s.
- Cause: Feline coronavirus (family Coronaviridae, genus Coronavirus).
- Affected Hosts: Cats and wild felids, especially cheetahs.
- Mode of Transmission: Fecal-oral (FECV), internal mutation (FIPV).
- Geographic Distribution: Worldwide.
- Major Clinical Signs: Fever, lethargy, inappetence, vomiting, diarrhea, dehydration, icterus, tachypnea, uveitis, neurologic signs, abdominal distention due to ascites.
- Differential Diagnoses: Toxoplasmosis, congestive heart failure, carcinomatosis, lymphoma, pancreatitis, rabies, cryptococcosis, bacterial peritonitis, pyothorax, bacterial meningitis, chronic stomatitis, multiple myeloma, FeLV or FIV infection.
- Human Health Significance: Feline coronaviruses do not infect humans.

ETIOLOGIC AGENT

Coronavirus Nomenclature

Coronaviruses have adapted themselves to many species of mammals and birds over the last 10,000 years, a brief period in the evolution of their hosts.[2] The myriad of resultant species, subspecies, clades (strains), and biotypes of coronaviruses are classified in the order *Nidovirales,* family *Coronaviridae,* and subfamily *Coronavirinae.* Members of the *Coronavirinae* are currently divided into four genera: *alpha-, beta-, gamma-,* and *delta-coronavirus.* The species *alphacoronavirus 1* contains the subspecies FCoV, the closely related CCoV, and porcine transmissible gastroenteritis virus (TGEV). SARS-CoV-2 viruses are distinct from feline coronaviruses; they belong to the *betacoronavirus* genus (see Chapter 43).

Feline coronaviruses occur in two distinct serotypes, I and II, based on virus neutralization using antisera to feline coronaviruses and canine coronaviruses.[3] It has been proposed that these be re-classified as clade A and B based on spike (*S*) gene sequencing.[4] Serotype I feline coronaviruses are distinctly of cat origin and are neutralized by antibodies to the predominant field isolates of FCoV, while type II feline coronaviruses are recombinants between type I FCoV and CCoV and are neutralized by CCoV antibodies.[5] Genetic variability in the degree of FCoV/CCoV recombination among modern isolates suggests that they are continuously occurring and evolving.[6] Seroype I feline coronaviruses predominate in Europe and the Americas, while up to 25% of feline coronaviruses from Asian countries are serotype II.[7–9] The recombination that leads to the serotype conversion involves the antibody binding site on the *S* gene that is responsible for virus neutralization and variable parts of the adjacent 3abc, E genes.

Like most RNA viruses, feline coronaviruses are undergoing constant genetic drift due to mutation and recombination, resulting in numerous closely related clades (strains) that genetically differ 10% or more from each other. These clades segregate along environmental and geographic lines.[10–12] One clade will usually predominate in environments where there is little movement of cats, such as shelters,[13] laboratory cat breeding facilities,[14] catteries, or geographic regions.[11]

The definitive classification of feline coronaviruses is the biotype (pathotype). Two biotypes exist in nature: feline enteric coronavirus (FECV) and feline infectious peritonitis virus (FIPV). The biotype names FECV and FIPV were originally assigned to these agents decades ago based on the diseases they caused. The name FECV should be used when referring to the virus found in feces of healthy cats, while the name FIPV refers to the putative virus found in tissues and effusions of cats with FIP.[15] The subspecies name FCoV should be used to describe features shared at the subspecies level. Therefore, the names FECV and FIPV will be primarily used for the rest of this discussion when describing the two vastly different diseases they cause.

Feline Coronavirus Structure and Replication

Coronaviruses acquired their name from the surface projections that resemble a corona or crown (see Fig. 29.1B). The FCoV genome contains a single positive strand of RNA containing 29,000 nucleotides, the longest among RNA viruses. The genome is made up of a single gene (1ab) that encodes for 16 nonstructural proteins involved in genome replication, four genes coding for structural proteins (S, M, N, E), and five accessory genes (3abc, 7ab). Proteins encoded by the accessory genes are not part of the virion structure and are involved in largely unknown host/virus interactions.[16] Coronaviruses employ a highly efficient replication strategy involving the creation of six nested overlapping capped RNAs that mimic cellular messenger RNA, thus enabling subversion of cellular pathways to aid in their replication.[16] Coronaviruses must convert their viral RNA to messenger RNA by an RNA-dependent RNA polymerase (replicase). Virion assembly begins in a replication-transcription complex made up of components of the endoplasmic reticulum and Golgi apparatus. Assembling virions then make their way to the cell surface through membrane structures and are released from the cell surface by exocytosis. This replication strategy is error prone and leads to mutations in single nucleotides, deletions, insertions, and recombination. Such mutations have been the source of genetically distinguishable strains, serotypes, biotypes, and even new subspecies and species.[17–19]

Coronaviruses make initial contact with their host cell membrane through a fusion peptide on the S protein followed by firm attachment between a second ligand on the S protein and a more distantly situated cellular receptor.[20] All group I coronaviruses including TGEV, HCV-229E, and serotype II feline coronaviruses use aminopeptidase N as a cellular receptor, while angiotensin-converting enzyme 2 (ACE2) is the attachment receptor for SARS-CoVs and the related human respiratory CoV NL63.[21–23] Bat and MERS coronaviruses use dipeptidyl peptidase 4 (DPP4) as a functional receptor. The actual *in vivo* cellular receptors for non-tissue culture–adapted strains of serotype I and II FECVs for intestinal epithelium and corresponding serotype I FIPVs for peritoneal macrophages are unknown.[16] Although it is likely that FECV utilizes conventional coronavirus type receptors to infect mature intestinal epithelial cells, the inability to culture FECV has stifled the search. There is increasing evidence that FIPVs may utilize Fc type receptors to enter host macrophages as immune complexes.[24]

Host Range

FCoV seropositivity, FECV fecal shedding, and/or occasional cases of FIP have been reported in the African lion, mountain lion, leopard, cheetah, jaguar, lynx, serval, caracal, European wild cat, Sand cat, and Pallas cat.[25–32] Although not extensively studied, it is assumed that wild and domestic Felidae are infected with the same FECVs.[33] There is no evidence that either FECV or FIPV is a pathogen of humans. Coronaviruses infecting humans have evolved from animal species other than cats (e.g., HCoV-229E, -MERS, -SARS-I (and likely SARS-CoV-2) from bats and HCoV-OC43 from cattle).[18,34]

EPIDEMIOLOGY

Feline Enteric Coronavirus

FECV was first identified during studies on why healthy cats in multicat environments were seropositive to FIPV but did not develop FIP.[35] The logical assumption was that FIP was an uncommon clinical manifestation of a ubiquitous and largely nonpathogenic coronavirus. Although fecal extracts from healthy cats in such environments caused seroconversion, no cases of FIP occurred. In contrast, a pure tissue culture FIPV caused fatal FIP in 80% or more of experimental exposures.[35] This was the first evidence that FIPV and FECV were distinctly different in their disease potential. Two strains of FECV were ultimately propagated by cat-to-cat passage using fecal extracts. The original FECV strain was designated FECV-UCD[35] and a second isolate FECV-RM.[14] Both strains belong to serotype I and have been used in experimental FECV infection studies.[10,36,37] FECV has proven extremely difficult to propagate in tissue culture because of its strict tropism for mature intestinal epithelial cells.[38,39]

FECV is ubiquitous in cats throughout the world and is enzootic in virtually all larger multicat environments, especially dense urban environment, shelters, sanctuaries, and foster homes with large numbers of kittens.[40] The only place found to be free of FECV has been the Falkland Islands, and attempts are being made to quarantine these cats from outside infection.[41] Over one half of healthy cats and 80% of cats with diarrhea from high-risk environments are fecal shedders over any given time and the shared use of litter pans greatly enhances direct fecal-oral spread. Indirect transmission can occur via fomites that contaminate the fur and are then ingested during grooming. The virus is also readily transmitted via litter dust and on the clothing and person of caregivers.[14,35] Survival in the environment is likely limited to 1 to 2 days, and the virus is susceptible to destruction by routine disinfectants and detergents, as well as prolonged exposure to UV light or drying. The infection rate among strictly outdoor cat populations is unknown, but likely decreases in proportion to population density and increasing age.

Kittens born in nature do not usually shed FECV until after 9–10 weeks of age,[12,42] an age period confirmed by experimental infection studies of kittens born to infected queens.[37,43] Therefore, kittens appear to be protected by some sort of natural immunity for the first months of life, although the exact nature of this immunity is unknown. However, it is most likely to be maternal in origin as it follows the kinetics of maternal protection for other common kittenhood pathogens. Immunity to FECV infection disappears after several months and coincides with the cessation of fecal shedding.[10,37] Secondary and tertiary infections are common in denser multicat environments where kittens are both an important primary target for infection as well as a major source for recurrent infections in older cats.

Feline Infectious Peritonitis Virus

FIP was first described as an "important disorder of cats" in 1963 at the Angell Memorial Animal Hospital, Boston.[1] Cases of FIP were subsequently reported in countries throughout the world.[44] In 1966, it was first proposed that FIP was caused by a virus,[45] and subsequently, virus particles were observed in the tissues of experimentally infected cats.[15] In the early 1970s, the similarities of the virus to members of the family *Coronaviridae*,[46] the recognition of non-effusive and effusive forms of disease,[47] and the neurologic and ocular forms of FIP were described.[48] Virulent FIPV was first propagated in autochthonous macrophage cultures[49] and later in tissue culture.[35,50] FECV was first reported in 1981 in a population of cats with periodic FIP.[35] The theory that FIPV arises within an individual cat as a result of mutation of FECV ("internal mutation") was first entertained in 1987.[51] Sequence-based evidence that FIPVs arose by internal mutation in cats infected with FECV was first published in 1998.[52]

The origin of the virus that causes FIP is unclear, but, like other coronaviruses, it may have originated from a coronavirus from another host species. FIP appeared about a decade after the initial descriptions of transmissible gastroenteritis (TGE) of pigs in North America.[53] Canine respiratory coronavirus (CRCoV) also underwent a similar change in organ predisposition due to recombination with bovine coronavirus (BoCV).[54] Another scenario is that FECV existed for a long time before FIP was first documented, but evolved to a strain that was much more likely to mutate to FIPV. It is noteworthy that TGEV in pigs was replaced worldwide by a much less pathogenic pneumotropic strain within 30 years[19] through simple mutations.[55] Yet another explanation may involve changes in the popularity of cats and feline husbandry in the post-WWII era. The numbers of pet cats have greatly increased during this period, pure breeding and cattery rearing became increasingly popular, the urban and suburban cat populations increased in density, and more cats, and kittens, were present in shelters. The large indoor multicat environments created by pure breeding and sheltering of free-roaming cats are known to favor FECV infection and FIP.[37,56,57] A final explanation involves FeLV infection, which also became rampant among indoor multicat households during this same period because of the increased movement of cats from the outdoors to the indoors and resultant close cat-to-cat contact. FeLV infection was a significant cofactor for FIP, being found in up to one half of cats with FIP during the 1970s.[58,59] Although the incidence of FIP dropped after FeLV infection was controlled, it quickly rebounded and is now higher than at any time. This rebound coincides with the increased demand for pedigreed cats and larger proportion of adoptions through kitten foster/rescue.

FIP currently causes the death of 0.3% to 1.4% of all cats seen at veterinary institutions worldwide.[60–62] The incidence among kittens from foster/rescue organizations, conventional shelters, and catteries is higher. In a study that examined mortality in 274 kittens from homes, shelters, or catteries from 1986 to 2000, FIP accounted for 6.2% of overall mortality, 3.6% of deaths in shelters, and 7.8% in catteries.[63] When it occurs, FIP is a highly fatal disease that occurs mainly in cats aged 3–18 months with few cases after 7 years of age. A second peak occurs among aged cats.[64]

Risk factors for FIP fall into two general categories: 1) factors that increase severity of FECV exposure, and 2) factors that negatively affect a cat's immune system during the first weeks or months before or after initial FECV exposure and following subsequent secondary infections. In one study, the most significant risk factors for FIP in catteries were younger age, proportion of cats with high coronavirus antibody titers, and the proportion of cats shedding coronaviruses.[65] Deficiencies in passive systemic and passive local (lactogenic) immunity caused by premature separation from queens may also play a role in increased FIP morbidity, and further studies are needed to determine the effect of early neutering, intense vaccination, over- or under-feeding, and concurrent infectious diseases. Ultimately, increased FECV replication leads to a greater number of FIPVs. Typical FECV infections generate thousands of progenies carrying at least one of the critical mutations. Innate immune responses can prevent tissue invasion and disease in situations where pathogen exposure is low. However, when exposure is high and innate immune defenses are weakened by environmental stresses, only strong adaptive immune responses will prevent disease.

The risk of FIP in kittens from different environments is closely related to the density of kittens. The highest kitten density and risk for FECV infection appears to be among foster/rescue groups, which concentrate on saving, socializing, neutering, and re-homing kittens.[40] Conventional mixed-species shelters may have a lower incidence of FIP, likely due to the increasingly common practice of intentionally or non-intentionally diverting younger kittens to foster/rescue facilities. FIP losses in high-risk environments such as dense urban environments, foster/rescue facilities, and catteries tend to occur unpredictably in clusters several weeks after spring and fall kitten seasons and can range from less than 1% to greater than 10% of kittens under 6–7 months of age.[65]

Every cattery with enzootic FECV infection is at risk of losing cats from FIP if they breed enough kittens over a long enough time. The risk of FIP appears to decrease over periods of 3 years in stable groups of cats, indicating an increase in population resistance.[66] This is most likely age related[67] and argues against the rapid turnover of breeding cats in catteries.

Pedigree cats have a higher incidence of FIP than random-bred cats.[62,68] The incidence of FIP has been followed in four typical catteries over a 5-year period.[65] Even though disease incidence was often less than 1%, spikes in mortality > 10% occurred in young cats and kittens at least once in 5 years.[65] In a study of 11,535 cats examined over a 16-year period, 1.3% of pedigreed cats developed FIP compared with 0.35% of random-bred cats.[60] Some studies show certain breeds to be more prone to FIP than others, although the exact breeds vary from one survey to another.[68,69] In a large survey of over 11,000 hospital patients, FIP was significantly higher in modern "designer"-type breeds such as Bengal, Birman, Himalayan, ragdoll, and rex than in older established breeds such as Burmese, Manx, Persian, Russian blue, and Siamese.[60] In contrast, a high incidence of FIP was reported in Burmese in Australia[69] and a low incidence in Burmese in Italy,[60] whereas Himalayan were found less susceptible in Australia[68] and more susceptible in Italy.[60] Male cats are at somewhat greater risk than females across several, but not all studies.[61]

The genetic basis for FIP susceptibility/resistance has been elusive. In one study comparing FIP deaths and pedigrees, a heritable risk for FIP accounted for up to 50% of risk.[70] Attempts to identify specific heritable genetic polymorphisms responsible for FIP susceptibility among Birman catteries naturally exposed to FIP failed to identify significant polymorphism linked to the disease phenotype.[71] Breeding for resistance by mating related resistant cats to each other increased susceptibility to experimental FIP, and it was concluded that inbreeding is the most significant genetic risk factor.[72]

CLINICAL FEATURES

Pathogenesis

Feline Enteric Coronavirus (Coronavirus Enteritis)

The pathogenesis of FIP usually begins when FECV infects kittens and presumably in older cats that have lost their immunity and become susceptible to repeat exposures. Primary FECV infection occurs in kittens at around 9 weeks of age when maternal protection is waning. Infections may also occur before 9 weeks where environmental exposures are high, and kittens are either bottle-fed or exposed to levels of virus that overcome any maternal immunity. A second group of cats over 10 years of age may also be at increased risk in association with other chronic diseases and weakening immunity (Fig. 31.1).[64]

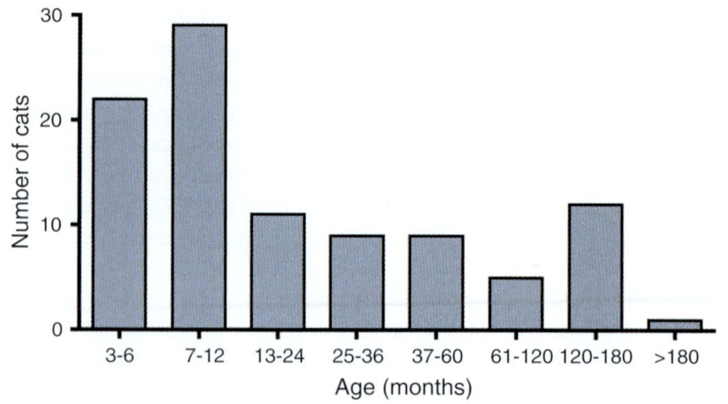

Fig. 31.1 Age distribution of 99 cats with necropsy-confirmed feline infectious peritonitis at the William R. Pritchard Veterinary Medical Teaching Hospital at UC Davis. An additional six cats were reported to be "juvenile" or kittens. There were 38 females (17 intact) and 66 males (22 intact).

Transmission of FECV is by the fecal-oral route. Infectious virions pass through the stomach intact, and there is evidence from cell cultures suggesting that trypsin and possibly other proteolytic enzymes may alter the surface spikes and play an important role in subsequent enteric coronavirus infectivity and cytopathicity.[73] FECV ultimately targets the mature apical epithelium at the tips of intestinal epithelium (see Fig. 29.2). Unlike TGEV of swine and BoCV infection of calves, which can cause severe and often fatal enteritis, FECV infection of cats is only a minimal pathogen and there is a weak statistical association with diarrhea. Its clinical importance is related to its propensity to mutate to the FIPV biotype. The comparative importance of FECV in diarrhea has been studied in shelter cats.[74] Twelve enteric pathogens were identified, including coronavirus, *Clostridium perfringens* enterotoxin A, *Cryptosporidium* spp., *Giardia* spp., *Cystoisospora* spp., hookworms, ascarids, *Salmonella* spp., astrovirus, FPV, FCV, and *Spirometra* spp. Of fecal specimens testing positive for one or more of these agents, FECV was the most common. Only FCoV was significantly (P = .03) more prevalent in cats with diarrhea (58%) than cats with normal feces (36%).

Virus is released when the apical epithelial cells undergo natural- or virus-induced apoptosis, with spread to adjacent and distant villi. FECV infection in 275 purebred cats from six catteries was studied by collection of fecal specimens for FECV RT-PCR every 1–3 months.[65] A large proportion of these cattery cats shed virus at any given time, but most manifested cycles of shedding and non-shedding. Similarly, all adult cats in an Abyssinian cattery shed virus in their feces at least once during the year and 4/15 cats were shedding greater than 75% of the time.[75] In a study of the persistence and evolution of endemic FECV infection in a closed cat-breeding facility, viral RNA was detected by RT-PCR in the feces of 36/42 cats (86%) tested and 4/5 cats were still shedding when tested 111 days later.[76] Two cats were then placed in strict isolation and virus shedding lasted up to 7 months in one animal. A viremic stage has not been confirmed. In a study of 50 healthy kittens and cats from a shelter that had feces tested, 28 were found to be FCoV shedders, but only two had detectable FCoV RNA in buffy coat cells.[77]

Experimental FECV infection studies were first conducted on SPF cats.[10,37,42] Clinical signs were frequently inapparent or consisted of transient diarrhea, occasionally preceded by vomiting. Fecal shedding, as determined by RT-PCR on rectal swabs, appeared within as little as 2 days[10,12] and was significantly higher in kittens than in older cats.[42] FECV was identified throughout the intestine through day 28, at which time occasional virus-positive macrophages were seen in the sinuses of reactive mesenteric lymph nodes.[12] The viral load was 10–100,000 times higher in the colon than in other sites in the intestine. FECV shedding remained at high levels for 2–10 months before eventually evolving into one of three excretion patterns: 1) persistent virus shedding at varying levels over 9–24 months; 2) periods of virus shedding interlaced with periods of non-shedding; and 3) cessation of virus shedding after 5–19 months.[37] The colon appears to be the main site of FECV persistence.[12] Active infection is associated with the appearance and rise in FCoV antibody titers and cessation of shedding with a marked drop in titers.[37] Pregnancy, parturition, and lactation have no influence on fecal shedding by queens, and methylprednisolone acetate treatment does not appear to induce non-shedders to shed and shedders to increase shedding.[37]

Feline Infectious Peritonitis Virus (Feline Infectious Peritonitis)

FIP is caused by specific mutants that occur during FECV infection.[52] These mutant FECVs lose tropism for the intestinal epithelium and gain tropism for monocyte/macrophages. This drastic switch in tropism leads to an entirely different disease, which closely resembles other macrophage-associated diseases such as tuberculosis, leprosy, the deep mycoses, and leishmaniosis. The anatomic sites where mutations occur are not clear, but one likely site is in the lymphoid tissues regional to the primary persistent infection site in the cecum and colon.[36] In a study of the effect of FECV coinfection in FIV immunocompromised laboratory cats, mutations capable of causing FIP occurred in 11% of primary FECV infections.[78] Given an incidence of around 1%, it is apparent that only about 1 in 100 FIPV mutations actually lead to FIP. FIPVs generated by internal mutation are genetically unique to each cat and are contained solely within infected macrophages in diseased tissues and effusions and have limited access to the outside. Therefore, cat-to-cat transmission is an infrequent occurrence and when it occurs, it presents as a self-limiting epizootic caused by the same virus.

Mutations in FECVs that lead to the switch in cell tropism occur in at least three identical regions of the viral genome. The most universal mutation site involves the putative fusion peptide on the spike (*S*) gene and consists of a single nucleotide change at either nucleotide 1058 or 1060. The M1058L mutation (methionine to leucine) occurs in 91.6% of all FIPVs. The S1060A mutation (serine to methionine) occurs in 4.3% of isolates.[79] Neither mutation is found in FECVs. Unfortunately, 4% or more of FIPV isolates do not have either mutation, which makes it difficult to identify their role in FIP pathogenesis. This site is most likely involved in how FIPV and FECV enter their respective host cells. One possibility is that subtle changes in the fusion domain inhibits infection of intestinal epithelium through its normal receptor and favors internalization of FIPV by peritoneal macrophages through alternative Fc receptors.

The second most consistent mutation to be associated with the FIPV biotype is in the accessory *3c* gene.[52] Most FIPV isolates have numerous mutations leading to significant amino acid changes in the 3′ region of the gene.[11] These mutations frequently lead to truncation of the gene and a totally nonfunctional 3c gene product, and are unique for each isolate.[11,52,79–82] The function of the 3c protein is unknown. The loss of a functional 3c protein in FIPVs appears to enhance viral replication in macrophage-like cells.[83]

A third site for FIPV mutations is in the S1/S2 cleavage region, which is involved in two thirds of FIPV isolates.[84] The S1 protein is cleaved from S2 in the Golgi network by the host protease furin. Mutations at this site are again unique to each FIPV and alter the efficiency of cleavage of the S protein by furin. Because the efficiency of furin cleavage is increased in many FIPV isolates, whereas in others it is decreased or unchanged, it is also difficult to ascribe a functional significance to mutations at this region of the FECV genome.

Bone marrow–derived monocytes are recruited into the sites of peritoneal macrophage infection, most likely by the effect of macrophage-derived cytokines on nearby endothelial cell adhesion proteins. The incoming monocytes evolve into M1 macrophages, again by the action of cytokines, evoking either a protective innate and adaptive T-cell immunity and no disease, or to a persistent infection, a flamboyant cytokine storm, immune-mediated inflammation, and disease.[24] The incubation period in naïve cats is 14 to 21 days, which corresponds with the appearance of first antibodies. The epitope responsible for both antibody-dependent enhancement (ADE) and *in vitro* virus neutralization is on the S protein of FIPV.[85] Complement is also bound to virus and antibody,[86] which facilitates the uptake of FIPV by macrophages[87,88] through Fc receptor binding. Immune complex formation contributes to venulitis by evoking Arthus- or immediate-type hypersensitivity reactions. Both neutrophils and macrophages are involved in this reaction.[89] The resultant vasculitis is manifested grossly by edema, hyperemia, micro-hemorrhage, thrombosis, and fibrosis. The vasculitis associated with effusive FIP often leads to coagulation abnormalities indicative of DIC.[90] However, clinical signs of DIC are uncommon.

It has been postulated that FIP is a balance between Th1- and Th2-mediated immunity.[24] In this scenario, non-effusive FIP is associated with a strong delayed-type hypersensitivity (DTH) and weak immediate-type hypersensitivity reactions, whereas effusive FIP is a result of strong immediate hypersensitivity and weak DTH reactions. This is reminiscent of cellular immune responses in lepromatous compared with tuberculoid leprosy of humans. Evidence for the role of T-cell immunity in FIP comes from research with a coronavirus that infects mice, mouse hepatitis virus (MHV). MHV, like FIPV, exists as two biotypes, enterotropic and polytropic. Certain polytropic laboratory strains of MHV cause a disease syndrome analogous to FIP of cats when they infect IFN-γ–deficient mice.[91] Infection with enterotropic MHV in immunocompetent mice is limited to the small intestine for the first week and then to the cecum and colon for the next 2 weeks. B-cell–deficient mice exposed to enterotropic MHV develop chronic subclinical infection restricted to the GI tract that lasts for 7–8 weeks. In contrast, T-cell–deficient mice infected with the same enterotropic MHV develop a multi-systemic, lethal, FIP-like disease. These mouse studies indicate that the FIPV mutations are preventing the T-cell immune responses normally associated with FECVs.

Clinical Signs

FIP tends to occur in two distinct forms with transitions often occurring between them. The classic wet, effusive, or non-parenchymatous form of FIP is a diffuse peritonitis associated with a large outpouring of inflammatory fluid from diseased venules on serosal surfaces, mesenteries, and omentum. Similar disease may also involve the thorax. Non-effusive ("dry") FIP is manifested by more focal and organized granulomatous lesions in organs such as the mesentericlymph nodes, cecum, colon, kidney, lungs, pericardium, eyes, brain, and spinal cord, and miscellaneous sites. Disease signs may evolve over weeks, months, and rarely a year or more. Wet FIP has been likened to the lepromatous form of human leprosy.

The dry, non-effusive, or parenchymatous form of FIP has been compared to the tuberculoid form of human leprosy. Dry FIP frequently begins as a brief episode of apparent or inapparent effusive disease, whereas non-effusive FIP can morph into effusive disease. A mixture of the two forms can also be seen at necropsy. There is ample evidence that infection may incubate for days, weeks, months, and rarely years before either resolving or clinically manifesting itself. This initial infection is most likely contained to foci of infection in organs such as the cecum, ileum, and colon, and associated lymph nodes. Clinical signs in this latent period may be inapparent or associated with retardation of growth, increased susceptibility to other common pathogens, or other vague signs of ill health. Once disease becomes apparent, it is usually progressive and fatal. However, there are reports of cats that make an apparent recovery, only to have clinical signs recur months and even years later.[56,92]

Both the non-effusive and effusive forms of FIP share many of the same initial clinical signs. The earliest overt signs include a progressively worsening lethargy, inappetence, and weight loss. Kittens and adolescent cats may be smaller than normal, have poor quality coats, may be less active, and suffer recurrent bouts of vague illnesses compared with siblings or cats of the same age. A fluctuating antibiotic-unresponsive fever

TABLE 31.1 Variability in Clinical Signs of Non-Effusive Feline Infectious Peritonitis

Anatomic Site	% of Cats with Associated Signs
Peritoneal cavity	58.0
Peritoneal and pleural cavities	22.0
Pleural cavity	11.0
Peritoneal cavity and eyes	2.8
Peritoneal cavity and CNS	1.9
Peritoneal and pleural cavities, CNS	0.9
Peritoneal and pleural cavities, eyes	0.9
Pleural cavity, CNS, eyes	0.9
Peritoneal cavity, CNS, eyes	0.9

CNS, central nervous system.
From Pedersen NC. Serologic studies of naturally occurring feline infectious peritonitis. *Am J Vet Res.* 1976;37:1449–1453.

TABLE 31.2 Variability in Clinical Signs of Non-Effusive Feline Infectious Peritonitis

Anatomic Site	% of Cats with Associated Signs
Peritoneal cavity	30
CNS	22
Eyes	14
CNS, eyes	8
Peritoneal cavity, eyes	7
Peritoneal and pleural cavities	4
Peritoneal and pleural cavities, CNS	3
Peritoneal and pleural cavities, eyes	2
Peritoneal cavity, CNS, eyes	2
Pleural cavity	1

CNS, central nervous system.
From Pedersen NC. Serologic studies of naturally occurring feline infectious peritonitis. *Am J Vet Res.* 1976;37:1449–1453.

is common with FIP and in one study, 22% of all cats presenting with a fever were ultimately found to have FIP.[93] Additional clinical manifestations vary greatly depending on the form and organ distribution of the inflammation. The timing of the subsequent disease course is also variable and ultimately fatal if untreated in almost all cases. Although the disease course for FIP is generally assumed to be a few days or weeks, some cats with either wet or dry FIP can survive for many weeks, months, and occasionally a year or more with just supportive care.

The effusive form of FIP is more common in kittens but also observed in adolescent, adult, and aged cats (Table 31.1). Effusions are observed solely in the abdomen in about 75% of cats, solely thoracic effusions in 10%–15%, and a mixture of thoracic and abdominal effusions in less than 10% of cases (see Table 31.1).[61] Abdominal effusions are manifested by abdominal distention and may be one of the first signs of FIP noted by the owners. Intact male cats may manifest scrotal enlargement due to inflammation of testicular tunics, whereas female cats with ascites may be considered pregnant and the disease discovered on spaying. Tachypnea may accompany thoracic effusion. Involvement of the CNS and eyes is seen in only about 10% of kittens with abdominal and/or thoracic effusions (see Table 31.1). Pericardial effusions are uncommon, either as a primary clinical manifestation or in combination with fluid accumulation in other body cavities.

About one fourth of cats with FIP have non-effusive or predominantly non-effusive FIP.[61] However, this proportion appears to be rising, either because of improved diagnosis or to an actual increase in incidence. The dry form also predominates in certain popular breeds such as the Birman[71] and Burmese.[69] The non-effusive form is also more apt to be subclinical[56,92,94] and may go unnoticed until host resistance is eventually overcome, and the disease becomes either effusive or involves the CNS and eyes. Clinical signs vary according to the organs that are involved. For instance, a disproportionate number of cats with non-effusive FIP develop neurologic and/or ocular disease (Table 31.2). A colonic form of the disease was first described in 1983 (Fig. 31.2).[95] FIP colitis is manifested by chronic diarrhea associated with mucus, fresh blood, and straining to defecate. The thickened colon, cecum, and ileocecocolic lymph nodes are readily palpated or visualized on abdominal ultrasound. FIP colitis has also been diagnosed at surgery for abdominal emergencies when a colonic pyogranuloma causes intestinal obstruction.

Neurologic disease is the sole presenting sign in about 22% of cats with non-effusive FIP, while an additional 7% is accompanied by detectable lesions in the peritoneal cavity (see Table 31.2). Ocular disease occurs as the sole manifestation in 14% of non-effusive FIP cases (see Table 31.2), while ocular disease plus CNS or other organ involvement occurs in 10% of cases. CNS involvement in cats with non-effusive FIP is varied in its clinical expression. Meningitis, ependymitis, and choroiditis with extension into adjacent tissues are common lesions in cats with brain involvement (Fig. 31.3). CNS involvement can manifest in early stages by spontaneous muscle twitches, atypical limb extension and swallowing motions, and brief episodes of staring. Signs will then progress slowly or rapidly to ataxia, usually worse in the pelvic limbs. Cerebellar-vestibular signs including nystagmus, head tilt or circling may be present. Hydrocephalus, secondary to disease of the choroid and ependyma, has also been documented[96–98] and can lead to dementia, personality changes (aggression, rage, hiding/withdrawal, etc.), or seizures.

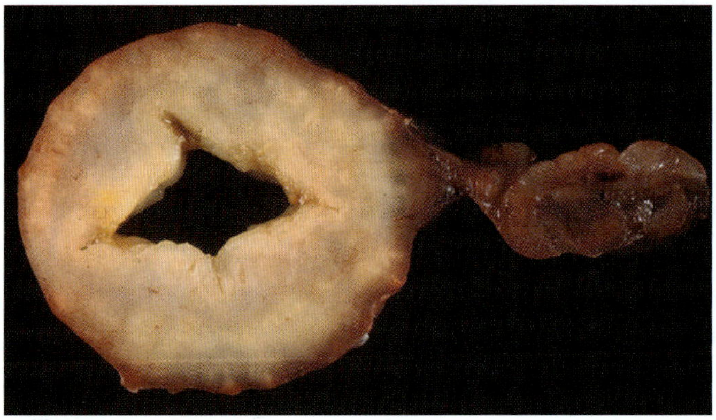

Fig. 31.2 Section of diseased colon removed at surgery from a 7-month-old female spayed domestic shorthair with anorexia and hematochezia. Histopathology showed severe, multifocal coalescing pyogranulomatous colitis and lymphadenitis typical of the colonic form of dry feline infectious peritonitis.

FIP is a major contributor to inflammatory/infectious disease of the spine.[99] Spinal involvement with FIP often leads to severe posterior paresis and urinary or fecal incontinence.

Once the virus enters the CNS or eyes, it is sheltered from the normal bloodborne immune responses. However, the infection is still capable of stimulating a systemic immune response as a result of lymphatic connections between the brain and cervical lymph nodes.[100] Such stimulation may explain why serum and CSF/aqueous antibody titers are so high in this form of FIP. This compartmentalization of infection and immune responses can lead to a scenario where virus-infected macrophages outside protected sites are eliminated, whereas infection in sites such as the brain and eye persist. This may also explain why many cats with CNS disease do not have noticeable extra-abdominal lesions (see Table 31.2).

Ocular FIP is usually manifested by a varying degree of uveitis and/or retinitis[101] that often starts in one and then progresses to involve both eyes (Fig. 31.4A–C). The earliest signs of anterior uveitis may be a discoloration of the iris, aqueous flare, and keratic precipitates. Although FIP is the major cause of uveitis in young cats, it can be confused with idiopathic uveitis. In one study, the duration of disease tended to be shorter in cats with FIP than in cats with idiopathic uveitis.[102] In another study of 92 cats with uveitis from the UK, cats with FIP uveitis had the youngest age (median 1.4 years) whereas those with neoplasia (such as lymphoma) had the oldest age (median 12.8 years), and cats with FIP or lymphoma were more likely to be purebred than cats with idiopathic uveitis.[103] Microbial nucleic acids, antigens, or antibodies against a causative agent were seldom found in the blood/serum of cats with idiopathic uveitis, whereas serum FCoV titers ≥ 1:6400 were detected only in cats with FIP. Aqueous humor contained predominantly neutrophils in cats with FIP and large reactive lymphocytes and plasma cells more frequently in cats with idiopathic uveitis. However, neither clinical nor cytologic assessment of anterior chamber contents reliably differentiated idiopathic uveitis from FIP.

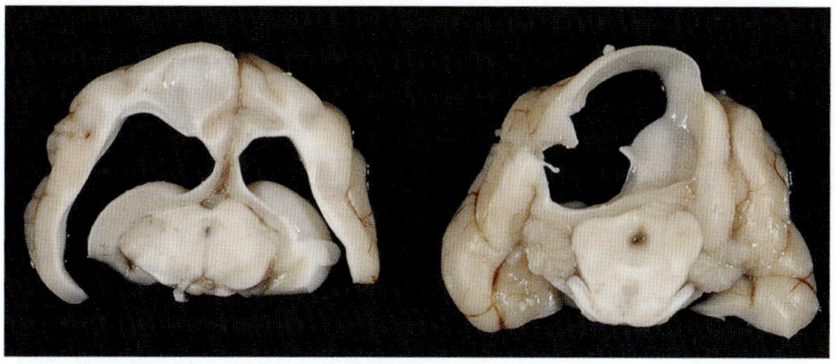

Fig. 31.3 Obstructive hydrocephalus in an 8-month-old male neutered exotic shorthair cat that developed ataxia and head tremors. Hydrocephalus and secondary cerebellar herniation were found at necropsy. Histopathology revealed severe, multifocal pyogranulomatous meningoencephalitis, choroiditis, and ventriculitis, and pyogranulomatous inflammatory lesions were also found throughout the thoracic and abdominal viscera. (Courtesy of the University of California, Davis Veterinary Pathology service.)

Retinitis is manifested by congestion of retinal blood vessels and hemorrhage that may be associated with retinal detachment and degeneration of the tapetum and optic disc. It can be unilateral or bilateral. Retinitis is often a sign of brain involvement and associated neurologic signs. Uncommon sites for extraperitoneal and extrapleural lesions, other than the CNS and eyes, include the oral cavity, nasal passages, testicles, and skin.

DIAGNOSIS

The diagnosis of FIP is based first and foremost on consideration of signalment (age, sex, and breed), environmental origin, disease history, abnormalities on physical examination (including effusions if present), and routine CBC and serum chemistry findings. There is sometimes enough evidence at this point to make a presumptive diagnosis of FIP, and whether more invasive diagnostic tests are warranted can be discussed with the owner.[104] The next step, if needed, is to choose tests that will either further increase the odds that the disease signs are due to FIP using "indirect tests" or attempt to provide a definitive diagnosis using "direct tests." It must be remembered that

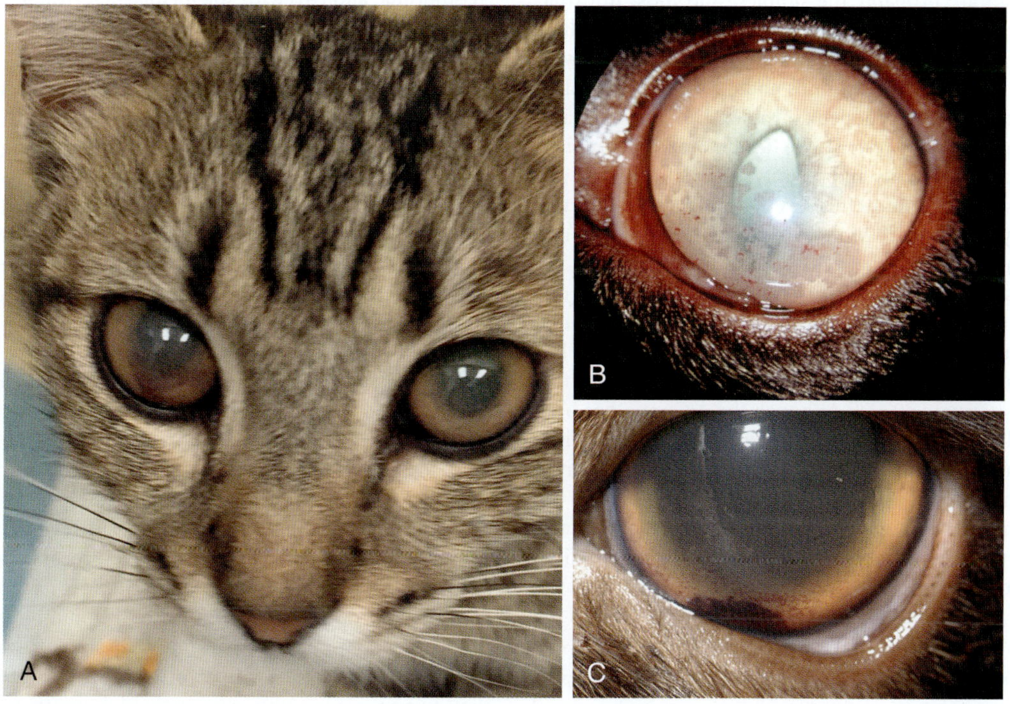

Fig. 31.4 Ocular signs associated with feline infectious peritonitis (FIP). (A) A 3-month-old male neutered domestic shorthair cat with acute bilateral uveitis associated with FIP. The anterior chamber of the left eye contains a large fibrinous clot. (B) Perivascular retinal lesions in a 7-month-old intact female domestic shorthair cat with FIP. (C) Keratic precipitates in a 5-year old intact male Burmese cat with FIP. (Courtesy of the University of California, Davis Veterinary Ophthalmology service.)

TABLE 31.3 Complete Blood Count Findings at Admission in 38 Cats with Necropsy-Confirmed Feline Infectious Peritonitis[a]

Test	Reference Range	Percent Below the Reference Range	Percent Within the Reference Range	Percent Above the Reference Range	Range For Cats With FIP	Number Tested
Hematocrit (%)	30–50	68	32	0	17–53	38
MCV (fL)	65–75	18	82	0	36–52	38
MCHC (g/dL)	33–36	5	58	37	28–36	38
RDW (%)	14–18	0	30	70	14–33	27
Neutrophils[b] (cells/μL)	2,000–9,000	3	26	71	416–49,313	38
Band neutrophils[b] (cells/μL)	0–rare	0	50	50	0–3,251	38
Metamyelocytes (cells/μL)	0	0	95	5	0–276	38
Monocytes (cells/μL)	50–600	5	71	24	0–820	38
Lymphocytes (cells/μL)	1,000–7,000	58	42	0	89–6,886	38
Eosinophils (cells/μL)	150–1,100	71	29	0	0–770	38
Platelets (cells/μL)	180,000–500,000	37	44	19	30,000–874,000	27[c]

[a]Cats seen at the William R. Pritchard Veterinary Medical Teaching Hospital at the University of California, Davis.
[b]22 (58%) had evidence of neutrophil toxic changes.
[c]A smear was evaluated manually for 37 cats. The presence of macroplatelets was reported for 18 (49%) of cats.
MCHC, mean corpuscular hemoglobin concentration; *MCV*, mean corpuscular volume; *RDW*, red cell distribution width.

no test is 100% sensitive and specific and that diagnostic sensitivity and specificity is strengthened by the inclusion of other supportive clinical findings.

Laboratory Abnormalities

Complete Blood Count and Serum Chemistry Profile

A CBC and serum chemistry panel that includes bilirubin, total protein, globulin, and albumin are probably the simplest and most informative indirect tests for FIP.[56,61,105] Common CBC abnormalities include nonregenerative anemia (anemia of inflammatory disease), leukocytosis with an absolute increase in neutrophils and a relative or absolute decrease in lymphocytes, and eosinopenia (Table 31.3). Occasionally, mild to moderate bandemia is present. The degree of lymphopenia is a good indicator of disease activity and severity, especially in cats with effusive FIP, whereas cats with non-effusive FIP often have low normal to normal lymphocyte counts.[106] Monocyte counts are variable and usually in the normal range.

An increased plasma total protein concentration is frequent in cats with FIP, especially in cats with non-effusive disease. Serum globulin concentration is frequently high and albumin concentration may be low (Table 31.4). This results in albumin-to-globulin ratios (A:G) ratios that are frequently below normal (<0.6).[61] Although the A:G ratio has been advocated as a useful test for FIP, the predictive value of the A:G ratio is very much dependent on the presence of other historical, clinical/physical, or laboratory abnormalities associated with the disease.[107]

FIP is perhaps the most common cause of hyperbilirubinemia in young cats, especially those with effusive FIP.[61] Hyperbilirubinemia is usually not associated with increased liver enzyme activity,[108] as the liver parenchyma is often spared in cats with FIP. Rather, bilirubin is a by-product of intravascular and extravascular destruction of RBCs by macrophages and a species deficiency in glucuronidation.[109]

Serum Protein Electrophoresis

Analysis of 155 serum specimens from cats with increased serum total protein or globulin concentration found that 136 (87.7%) had abnormal serum electrophoresis profiles, most commonly from a polyclonal increase in gamma globulins (Fig. 31.5).[110] Alpha and beta globulins are also increased in many FIP sera due to increased production of acute-phase reactants and complement proteins. The most common disease classification associated with serum protein abnormalities in the 155 feline sera was infectious/inflammatory disease (80/136; 58.8%), including 39 cats with a diagnosis of FIP. Monoclonal gammopathy was observed in four cats, including one with FIP, one with lymphoma, and two with splenic plasmacytoma.

Analysis of Effusions

The presence of a characteristic type of fluid in the peritoneal cavity and/or pleural cavity is one of the most diagnostic clinical features of FIP. Classic FIP effusions are usually yellow tinged (sometimes blue green), cloudy, high in protein (near or equal to plasma levels), and have white cell counts of 3,000 cells/μL or greater (Table 31.5). Red cells are often present but seldom in numbers that grossly tinge the fluid. The fluid color is due to the presence of bilirubin (yellow) or biliverdin (blue green). The deeper colored the fluid, the more red cell destruction is occurring and the more severe the inflammatory process. Classic FIP effusions are often viscous with an egg-white consistency, contain fibrin tags, and frequently form partial clots when placed in a serum tube.

Effusions from cats with more chronic and fibrotic disease may be clear or pale yellow, have protein content as low as 2.0 g/L, and cell counts nearer to 200 cells/μL. Such effusions are frequently and incorrectly called "modified transudates." However, they have their origin in inflammatory and not transudative processes and do not meet the established physical or physiologic criteria for a modified transudate.[111] A more appropriate term, if it existed, would be "modified exudate."

The exudate of FIP is unlike that seen in rare cases of bacterial peritonitis or in cats with pyothorax. These are much more purulent in appearance, with extremely high neutrophil counts and not as viscous or yellow tinged. The neutrophils in bacterial peritonitis are often toxic, whereas those in FIP fluid are typically mature. However, secondary bacterial infections have also been identified on occasion in cats with effusive FIP. Effusions associated with liver and heart

TABLE 31.4 Findings on Serum Biochemistry Analysis in 36 Cats with Necropsy-Confirmed Feline Infectious Peritonitis[a]

Test	Reference Range	Percent Below the Reference Range	Percent Within the Reference Range	Percent Above the Reference Range	Range For Cats With FIP	Number of Cats Tested
Sodium (mmol/L)	151–158	94	6	0	129–152	35
Potassium (mmol/L)	3.6–4.9	26	74	0	2.2–5.4	35
Chloride (mmol/L)	117–126	91	9	0	94–121	35
Bicarbonate (mmol/L)	15–21	8	75	17	12–25	36
Calcium (mg/dL)	9.0–10.9	56	44	0	6.6–10.6	36
Phosphorus (mg/dL)	3.2–6.3	8	69	22	1.9–8.4	36
Creatinine (mg/dL)	1.1–2.2	69	28	3	0.4–2.8	36
BUN (mg/dL)	18–33	56	31	14	10–58	36
Glucose (mg/dL)	63–118	0	47	53	63–381	36
Total protein (g/dL)	6.6–8.4	31	28	42	4.1–11.9	36
Albumin (g/dL)	2.2–4.6	50	50	0	0.9–3.6	36
Globulin (g/dL)	2.8–5.4	3	42	56	2.5–9.4	36
Cholesterol (mg/dL)	89–258	17	83	0	56–247	36
Total bilirubin (mg/dL)	0–0.2	0	40	60	0–5.3	36
ALT (U/L)	27–101	50	25	25	18–648	36
AST (U/L)	17–58	6	43	51	0–1554	36
ALP (U/L)	14–71	28	61	11	0–161	36
GGT (U/L)	0–4	0	96	4	0–5	23

[a]Cats seen at the William R. Pritchard Veterinary Medical Teaching Hospital at the University of California, Davis.

ALP, alkaline phosphatase; *ALT,* alanine aminotransferase; *AST,* aspartate aminotransferase; *BUN,* blood urea nitrogen; *GGT,* gamma-glutamyl transferase.

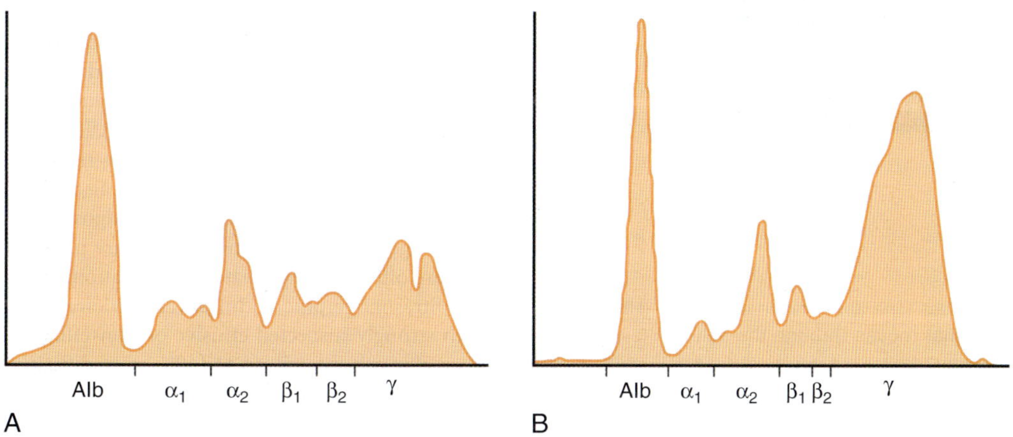

Fig. 31.5 (A) Densitometric scan of serum protein electrophoresis of normal feline serum. (B) Scan from a 9-month-old male neutered domestic shorthair cat with feline infectious peritonitis. There is a polyclonal gammopathy, represented by a broad peak in the γ-globulin region, with a mild decrease in the albumin and mild increases in the α_2 and β_1 fractions. (Redrawn from Baker RJ, Valli VE. Electrophoretic and immunoelectrophoretic analysis of feline serum proteins. *Am J Vet Res.* 1988;52:308–304.)

disease, lymphatic duct rupture (chylous effusions), and neoplasia seldom have the same overall physical and cellular characteristics as FIP effusions.

Rivalta test. The Rivalta test has been long used for diagnosing FIP-associated exudates.[105] The test involves placing a few drops of effusion into a weak acetic acid solution. The appearance of a ball ("jellyfish") of white flocculent material that moves through the solution indicates a positive test (Fig. 31.6). In a study of 497 cats with effusions, 35% of which had confirmed FIP, the Rivalta test had a sensitivity of 91% and a specificity of 66%, with a positive predictive value of 58% and a negative predictive value of 93%.[112] The diagnostic performance of the test increased when cats with lymphoma or bacterial infections were excluded, or when only cats of ≥ 2 years of age were considered. Therefore, the value of the Rivalta test for diagnosis of FIP increases as more diagnostic features of FIP are included and signs of other disorders excluded. Effusions that have low protein and cell counts, and are less inflammatory in origin, are unlikely to test positive and the interface between positive and negative is not always clear.

TABLE 31.5 Composition of Body Cavity Effusions from 21 Cats with Necropsy-Confirmed Feline Infectious Peritonitis[a]

Test	Range	Mean ± S.D.	Number of Cats Tested
Total protein (g/dL)	2.9–8.1	5.1 ± 1.8	21
RBC (cells/μL)	<100–38,600	ND	18
TNC (cells/μL)	200–13,200	3,683 ± 3,474	19
Neutrophils (%)	3–97	61 ± 28	21
Lymphocytes (%)	0–22	6 ± 6	21
Monocytes (%)	1–96	33 ± 26	21

[a]Cats seen at the William R. Pritchard Veterinary Medical Teaching Hospital at the University of California, Davis. Specimens included abdominal (n = 19) and pleural (n = 2) effusions.
RBC, red blood cells; *TNC,* total nucleated cell count.

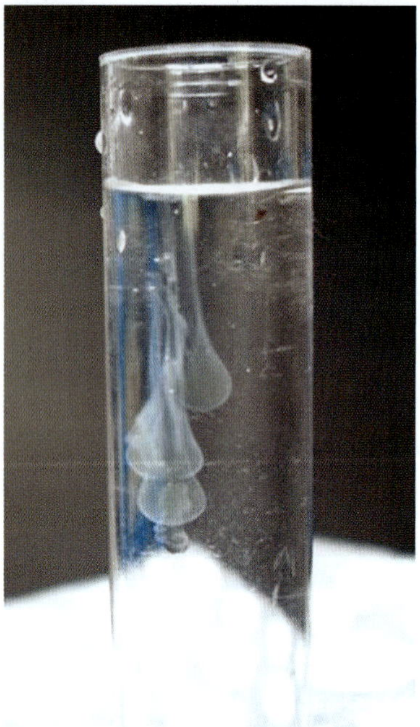

Fig. 31.6 Positive Rivalta test. The appearance of a ball ("jellyfish") of white flocculent material that moves through the solution (similar to a lava lamp) indicates a positive test.

Analysis of Cerebrospinal Fluid and Aqueous Humor

The results of CSF analysis were reported on cats with necropsy-confirmed FIP from five veterinary institutions from the United Kingdom, Australia, and United States.[113] Total protein concentration was increased (mean, 9.4 g/L; median, 3.6 g/L; range, 0.85–28.8 g/L) as was total nucleated cell count (mean, 196/μL; median, 171/μL; range, 15–479/μL). Neutrophils were the dominant cell in most cats, whereas lymphocytes and a mixture of neutrophils and lymphocytes were observed in a smaller proportion (Table 31.6).

α1-Acid Glycoprotein

α1-Acid glycoprotein (AGP) has been used extensively, particularly in parts of Europe, as an indicator test for FIP. AGP is hyposialylated in cats with FIP, but not in healthy cats or in cats with other diseases.[114] One study concluded that serum AGP could be used as a discriminating marker for FIP, but only when coupled with other risk factors or test results supportive of a diagnosis of FIP.[115] AGP serum concentrations of 1.5–2 μg/mL add further support to the diagnosis when the index of suspicion is high.

Diagnostic Imaging

Plain Radiography

Plain thoracic radiography may reveal pleural effusion, enlargement of the cardiac silhouette in cats with pericardial effusion, and pulmonary nodular or peribronchial infiltrates in cats with pyogranulomatous pneumonia (Fig. 31.7). Abdominal radiographs may show loss of peritoneal or retroperitoneal detail due to peritoneal effusion, hepatomegaly, splenomegaly, renomegaly, or mass lesions associated with the GI tract or abdominal lymph nodes.

Sonographic Findings

The diagnosis of FIP often depends on the ability to identify abdominal or thoracic effusions and to obtain a fluid specimen for analysis. Ultrasound can be helpful for identification and collection of small volumes of fluid (Fig. 31.8). Ultrasound can also locate lesions such as enlarged abdominal lymph nodes, kidney masses, or infiltrative lesions of the colon or other organs. Ultrasound-guided biopsies of such lesions may be required to obtain tissues for microscopic, IHC, or PCR testing. Ultrasonography may also be helpful for diagnosis of FIP in cats with neurologic or ocular signs, as abdominal lesions such as enlarged mesenteric lymph nodes are present in most of these cats and are often not appreciated on palpation.

Ultrasonographic findings were reviewed retrospectively in 16 cats with strongly suspected effusive or non-effusive FIP.[116] The liver was normal in echogenicity in 11 (69%) cats, diffusely hypoechoic in 3 cats,

TABLE 31.6 Composition of Cerebrospinal Fluid from 10 Cats with Necropsy-Confirmed Feline Infectious Peritonitis[a]

Test	Range	Median	Reference Range	Number of Cats Tested
Total protein (mg/dL)	44–4,079	639	<25 mg/dL	4[b]
RBC (cells/μL)	3–850	340	0	9
TNC (cells/μL)	26–2,637	303	0–2	10
Neutrophils (%)	4–90	73	NA	10
Lymphocytes (%)	5–89	19	NA	10
Monocytes (%)	0–20	7	NA	10

[a]Cats seen at the William R. Pritchard Veterinary Medical Teaching Hospital at the University of California, Davis.
[b]Insufficient quantity was available for protein determination.
RBC, red blood cells; *TNC,* total nucleated cell count, NA, not applicable.

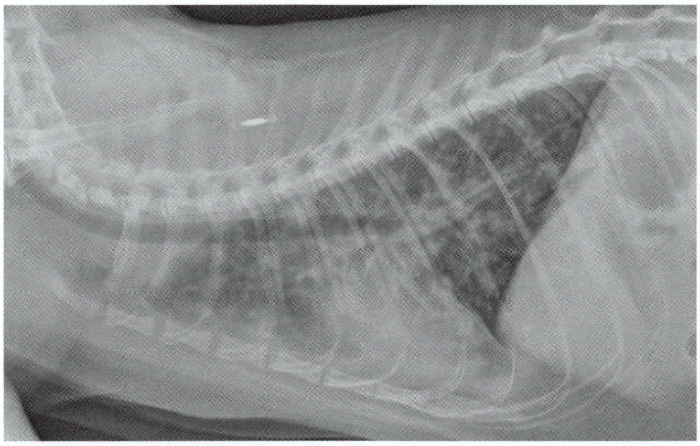

Fig. 31.7 Thoracic radiographs from a 9-month-old male neutered domestic shorthair cat with feline infectious peritonitis and pyogranulomatous pneumonia. There is a severe, diffuse, patchy alveolar and nodular interstitial pattern with thickening of the bronchial walls and mild pleural effusion.

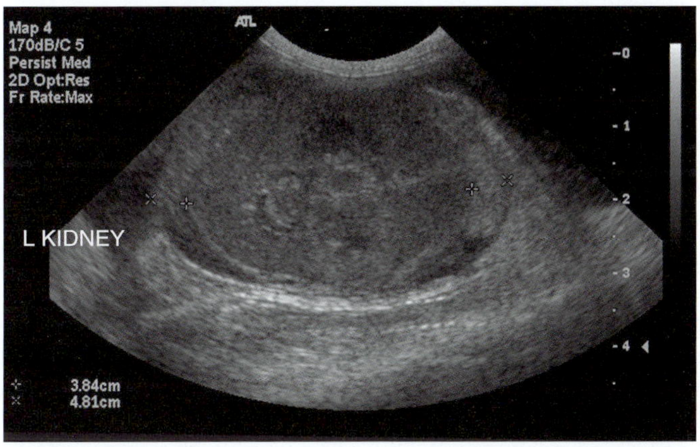

Fig. 31.8 Abdominal ultrasound of a 1-year-old male intact Scottish fold with feline infectious peritonitis. There is renal irregularity and subcapsular fluid, as well as moderate peritoneal effusion.

focally hyperechoic in 1 cat and focally hypoechoic in another. Five cats had a hypoechoic subcapsular rim in one or both kidneys. Free fluid was present in the peritoneal cavity in seven cats and in the retroperitoneal space in one cat. Abdominal lymphadenopathy was noted in nine cats. The spleen had normal echogenicity in 14 cats and was hypoechoic in 2 cats. One cat had bilateral orchitis, with loss of normal testicular architecture. The authors concluded that, while none of these ultrasonographic findings were specific for FIP, their significance was greatly increased when included with other suggestive findings.

Magnetic Resonance Imaging

MRI is a useful tool for diagnosis of neurologic FIP, particularly in combination with a compatible signalment, clinical presentation, and CSF analysis. MRI findings were described in 24 cats with necropsy-confirmed neurologic FIP.[113] Three distinct clinical syndromes were identified: T3-L3 myelopathy, central vestibular syndrome, and multifocal CNS disease. MRI abnormalities were detected in all cases and included meningeal contrast enhancement, ependymal contrast enhancement, ventriculomegaly, syringomyelia, and foramen magnum herniation (Fig. 31.9) All 24 cats were euthanized, with a median survival time of 14 days (range, 2–115) from onset of clinical signs. Histopathologic analysis identified perivascular pyogranulomatous

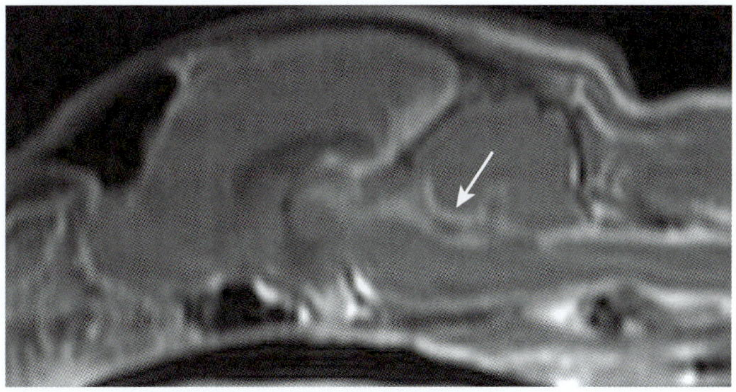

Fig. 31.9 T1-weighted post-contrast magnetic resonance imaging scan of an 8-month-old female domestic shorthair cat with neurologic feline infectious peritonitis. There was marked enhancement of the ependymal lining of the fourth ventricle *(arrow)* as well as the central canal, and moderate meningeal enhancement of the brainstem and cervical spinal cord. The feline coronavirus antibody titer was ≥ 1:20,480. A cerebrospinal fluid analysis showed marked, mixed, predominantly neutrophilic inflammation. (Courtesy University of California-Davis Veterinary Diagnostic Imaging Service.)

infiltrates, lymphoplasmacytic infiltrates, or both affecting the leptomeninges, choroid plexus, and periventricular parenchyma.

Microbiologic Tests (Table 31.7)

Serologic Diagnosis

The accepted gold standard method for detection of antibodies to FCoV is an IFA using cat cell lines with tissue culture–adapted FIPV-79-1146 as the antigen.[59,64] TGEV grown on pig cells or CCoV grown on dog cells can also be used. IFA serology is accurate if properly done, but controversy still exists over its diagnostic value as FECV and FIPV evoke identical type antibodies. Although antibody titers tend to be higher in cats with FIP, they also trend high among healthy cats in the same environments that produce FIP.[43,59] Nonetheless, there is some value in determination of FCoV antibody titers. Antibodies to FCoV appear within 2 weeks of FECV infection, typically to titers of around 1:100 to 1:400 and then drop to levels of 1:25 or lower in cats that develop immunity and cease shedding.[37] Cats with antibody titers ≥ 1:400 are almost always FECV shedders, and cats with titers of ≤ 1:25 are usually non-shedders.

Rising FCoV antibody titers can also indicate progression of subclinical FIP, but the opportunity or rationale for such sequential testing is limited. FCoV antibody titers were found to rise above their baseline among a colony of cats with enzootic FECV infection that were subsequently infected with FeLV that appeared to reactivate FIP (Fig. 31.10).[59] Most healthy FECV exposed cats have titers of 1:400 or less. Only a few healthy cats have FCoV titers of 1:1600, while titers ≥ 1:3200 (provided the assay is performed correctly) are highly suggestive of FIP[105] and can be considered definitive if coupled with other signs of FIP. However, there are some cats with FIP that have low or even negative FCoV titers.[117] This means that very high titers from a reliable laboratory support a diagnosis of FIP in combination with suggestive clinical signs, but low or negative titers cannot be used to rule out FIP. A progressive rise in titer over a period of several months may also indicate that FIP is changing from a subclinical to clinical form (see Fig. 31.10).

A 7b serum ELISA antibody test was developed on a faulty premise that FECVs lack the *7b* gene and hence do not produce the 7b protein, whereas FIPVs have the *7b* gene, produce the protein, and therefore evoke a 7b antibody response. However, virtually all field isolates of FIPVs and FECVs possess an intact *7b* gene and therefore both evoke anti-7b antibodies.[118] The 7b antibody test is essentially the same as

TABLE 31.7 Assays Available for Diagnosis of Feline Infectious Peritonitis

Assay	Specimen Type	Target	Performance
Fluorescent or immunoperoxidase antibody staining	Wash or effusion specimens, tissue aspirates, tissues obtained at biopsy or necropsy	FCoV	Gold standard for diagnosis. False negatives can occur in specimens that contain low numbers of macrophages or virus particles, or when virus is complexed by antibody. Immunofluorescence is more sensitive than immunoperoxidase methods. Nonspecific staining may be interpreted as positive results by untrained personnel.
Serology	Blood, CSF, aqueous humor, effusion fluid	FCoV antibody	Positive antibody titers reflect only antibodies to a coronavirus and are not specific for a diagnosis of FIP. Most cats in multicat households test positive. Negative titers can occur in cats with advanced FIP. High titers in cats that do not reside in multicat households and that have signs suggestive of FIP support the diagnosis. Interlaboratory variation in methodology and titer reporting occurs.
RT-PCR	Blood, wash or effusion specimens, tissue aspirates, tissues obtained at biopsy or necropsy	FCoV RNA	Does not differentiate between virulent and avirulent FCoV strains, and avirulent strains may be found in tissues and blood. However, cats with high copy numbers of FCoV RNA in extraintestinal tissues are more likely to have FIP than those with low copy numbers. Sensitivity and specificity may vary depending on assay design. False-negative results may occur when virus levels are low or as a result of degradation of viral nucleic acid during specimen transport.
Histopathology	Usually necropsy specimens, but also biopsies	Inflammatory lesions induced by FCoV (pyogranulomatous vasculitis)	Biopsy is often not feasible antemortem as a result of critical illness and coagulopathies.

CSF, cerebrospinal fluid; *FCoV,* feline coronavirus; *FIP,* feline infectious peritonitis; *RT-PCR,* reverse transcriptase-polymerase chain reaction.

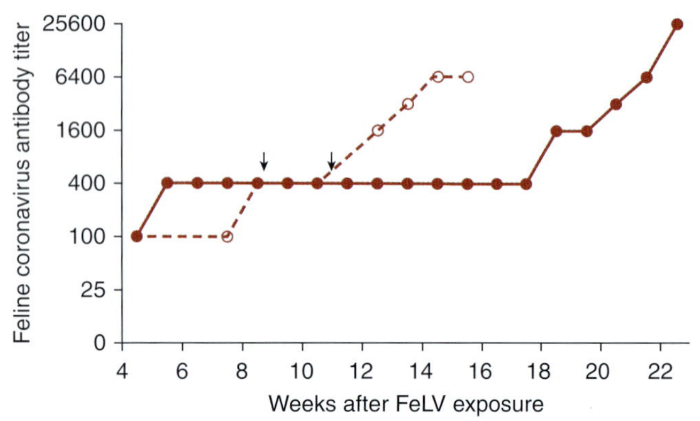

Fig. 31.10 Feline coronavirus (FCoV) antibody titers in two cats that were naturally infected with feline enteric coronavirus before being exposed to feline leukemia virus (FeLV) carriers. The FCoV titers began to rise 2 to 10 weeks after the cats became persistently FeLV viremic *(arrows)* and reached levels of 1:6400 to 1:25,600 just before death from feline infectious peritonitis (FIP). This figure demonstrates three features of FIP: (1) feline infectious peritonitis virus (FIPV) can remain dormant or subclinical for some time following FECV infection, (2) persistent FeLV infection has the potential to activate dormant or subclinical FIPV infection, and (3) rising FCoV antibody titers can be associated with disease progression.

other FCoV antibody tests. However, there are no good studies on how to interpret 7b antibody titers in context to disease status.

FCoV antibody tests have also been adapted to ELISA and rapid immunochromatographic test formats.[119,120] All are 96% to 100% sensitive in detecting antibody in blood or effusions. Serology on CSF has also been applied for diagnosis of neurologic FIP. In one study, the most useful antemortem indicators of neurologic FIP were positive IgG anti-CoV antibody titer in the CSF, increased serum total protein concentration, and MRI findings suggesting periventricular contrast enhancement, ventricular dilatation, and hydrocephalus.[96] However, in another study, CSF antibody was detected only in cats with serum titers of 1:4,096 to 1:16,384 and the investigators concluded that CSF antibodies were passively acquired.[121] In another attempt to measure local CNS antibody production in cats with FIP, an albumin quotient and IgG index were measured to determine whether proteins in the CSF were of blood or local origin. Neither the albumin quotient nor IgG index identified a pattern consistent with intrathecal IgG synthesis in cats with the CNS form of FIP.[122] In conclusion, it seems that coronavirus antibodies enter the CSF at high levels when they are also at very high levels in the serum.[123]

Molecular Diagnosis Using Nucleic Acid–Based Testing

PCR testing of feces for FCoV shedding is of limited value. The fecal virus is of the FECV biotype, even in cats with FIP. Furthermore, cats with FIP often shed FECV at low or negligible levels compared with healthy cats.[11,80,124] Routine testing of healthy cats by breeders to predict FIP problems should also be discouraged because the odds of healthy FECV shedders developing FIP are very low.[14,77] There is evidence, however, that the higher the proportion of cats in a cattery that shed coronavirus at a given time, and the higher the level of shedding, the more likely FIP will occur in the population.[65] This is an expensive and not a very accurate way of predicting future FIP risk. Testing of feces for FECV shedding can be theoretically used to eliminate FECV from a cat population such as was done in conjunction with FCoV serology in an experimental cat breeding facility.[14] However, such a use of RT-PCR must be coupled with sequential testing and proper quarantine facilities and procedures, as was done in this facility. Attempts to isolate FECV-negative kittens and cats in conventional housing with inadequate quarantine procedures are doomed to fail.

RT-PCR assays for replicating (mRNA) and non-replicating forms of FCoV were also used to screen the blood buffy coat cells and feces of 205 healthy shelter cats to predict whether they would develop FIP later.[77] Of 205 buffy coats, 1 (0.5%) tested positive for replicating forms of viral RNA (mRNA) and 9/205 (4.4%) for non-replicating RNA, whereas 28/50 (56%) fecal specimens tested positive for mRNA. None of the 10 cats with replicating or non-replicating forms of FCoV in their blood developed FIP over the subsequent 6 months.

The *7b* gene is often used as a target for FCoV PCR because it is the most abundant viral transcript and most likely to be detected. The *M* gene has also been targeted in some PCR assays, as it is highly conserved across all isolates.[125] The use of the *7b* RT-PCR for diagnostic purposes is based on the premise that FECVs will be only found in feces of healthy cats and FIPVs only in diseased tissues and effusions of cats with FIP. Although this test has excellent sensitivity and specificity when used to detect FECV in fecal specimens of healthy cats, test results for FIP tissues and effusions have been variable. In one study of 854 cats with ascites that were suspected to have FIP based on clinical signs, 95% of ascites specimens from purebred and 79% from random-bred cats tested positive by RT-PCR. This decreased with each increasing year of age, with 70% of effusions from purebred and 42% from random-bred cats of 12–24 months of age testing positive.[123] This variation with breed or age can best be explained by the filtering effect of known risk—pedigreed cats are more likely to develop FIP than random-bred cats and younger cats are more likely to have FIP than older cats. Therefore, the specificity and sensitivity of PCR tests for FIP should always be considered along with other risk factors.[126]

The specimen type also influences the results of molecular testing. PCR was performed on peripheral blood mononuclear cells (PBMCs) of 21 cats with FIP, serum from 26 cats with FIP, and cell-free abdominal or thoracic effusions of 36 cats with FIP, and results were compared to those from a control group with other diseases.[127] PCR had a sensitivity of 29% and specificity of 100% in PBMCs, 15% sensitivity and 86%–100% specificity in serum, and 89% sensitivity and 89%–100% specificity in cell-free body cavity effusions. When fluid and cellular fractions of ascites and blood were tested from cats with experimentally induced effusive abdominal FIP, most FCoV *7b* RNA was found in the cellular pellet of ascites fluid rather than in supernatant, and viremia was not reliably detected in serum or PBMCs.[128] Similar observations were made in cats with naturally occurring FIP.[129] Viral RNA levels are too low in whole blood, plasma, or blood cells to be reliably detected. When testing effusions, a fresh cell pellet is the preferred specimen to test. Tissues to be tested should be only from lesions, and lesions from cats with non-effusive FIP would be expected to have lower viral RNA loads than lesions from cats with effusive FIP.

In one study, FCoV PCR on CSF from cats with neurologic signs and other risk factors for FIP was highly sensitive and specific.[113,127] CSF was also a useful specimen when tested for both FCoV *7b* RNA and FCoV antibody by indirect IFA.[123] CSF antibody titers of 1:640 or greater were found only in cats with FIP and were always positive by RT-PCR.

There is now a more accurate understanding of the genetic make-up of FECV and FIPV isolates and the mutations leading to the FIPV biotype. Mutations in the ORF 3c and at the S1/S2 gene cleavage site are unique to each FIPV and are therefore not good candidates for a test that differentiates FECVs from FIPVs.[84,124] However, two SNP mutations in the fusion peptide of the S protein occur in around 96% of FIPVs detected in diseased tissues but never in true FECVs.[80] An RT-PCR test has been commercialized that detects FIPV-specific mutations in the *S* gene.

In theory, the *7b* RT-PCR assay should identify any FCoV RNA in a specimen, whereas the FIPV-specific test would determine whether the RNA belonged to the FECV or FIPV biotype. However, the FIPV-specific assay has much lower sensitivity than the FCoV-specific test. In specimens with high loads of FIPV-specific RNA, both tests will be positive and the presence of an FIPV can be confirmed. However, when the starting amount of FIPV RNA is low, the more sensitive *7b* FCoV test will be positive, but the less sensitive FIPV *S* gene test may be negative. In a study of 57 cats with proven FIP and 45 control cats

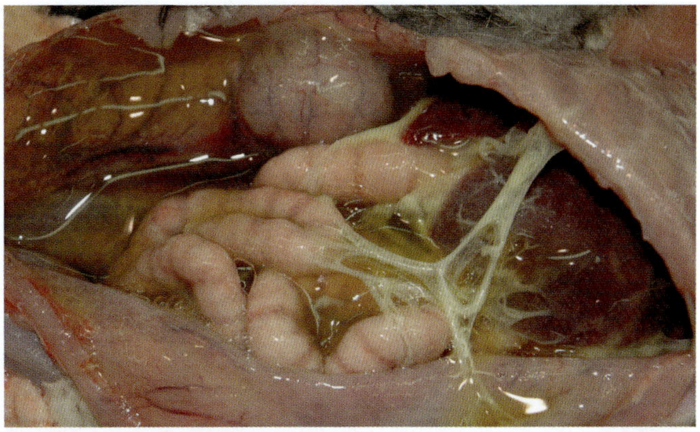

Fig. 31.11 Gross appearance of the abdominal cavity of a 10-month-old male intact domestic shorthair cat with acute effusive abdominal feline infectious peritonitis. Over 1.2 L of a mildly yellow-tinged effusion was removed from the abdominal cavity. (Courtesy Dr. Brian Murphy, University of California-Davis Veterinary Anatomic Pathology Service.)

without FIP, identification of *S* gene- mutated FCoVs as an additional step to the detection of FCoV alone only moderately increased specificity for tissue specimens (from 92.6% to 94.6%) and specificity was unchanged for fluid specimens (97.9%).[82] However, sensitivity was significantly decreased for the FIPV-specific tests for tissue (from 89.8% to 80.9%) and fluid specimens (from 78.4% to 60%). A further complication of the *S* gene mutation test for FIPVs is that these mutations are not found in all FIPV strains from the field.[80,130]

Pathologic Findings

Gross Pathologic Findings

Abdominal and/or thoracic effusions in cats with FIP range from a few milliliters to over a liter, and the color from nearly clear to a deep yellow (Fig. 31.11) The principal lesion is the pyogranuloma, which appears grossly as focal whitish plaques ranging from microscopic to several millimeters in diameter and most obvious on serosal surfaces of abdominal or thoracic organs and mesenteries (Fig. 31.12). The omentum and splenic mesentery are usually thickened by varying degrees of edema and fibrosis, the intestinal mesenteries cloudy, and the visceral and parietal serosal surfaces thickened with a ground-glass appearance. Focal hemorrhages are often seen in the omentum and splenic mesentery and the affected tissues stained yellow from bilirubin. Similar, but less defined, gross lesions can occur on the parietal and visceral surfaces of the chest, mediastinum, diaphragm, pericardium, heart, and lungs.

Lesions of non-effusive FIP can be classified as intra-peritoneal/pleural, extra-peritoneal/pleural, or both. They are less diffuse and more solitary than those of wet FIP, much larger, and more typical of classic, sometimes tumor-like, granulomas. The lesions are also more likely to extend down from the surface of organs into the underlying parenchyma, hence the alternative name of parenchymatous FIP. Almost 50% of cats with non-effusive FIP have disease localized to the peritoneal cavity and in 30% of cases solely abdominal lesions are present. Pleural cavity lesions occur in only 10% of cats with non-effusive FIP, usually in association with peritoneal disease. Abdominal lymph node involvement is often a primary manifestation of non-effusive FIP, especially in the subclinical form (Fig. 31.13).[56,92,94] The kidneys are also a major target (Fig. 31.14).[47] Although effusive and non-effusive FIP are considered distinct forms, they are in reality creations of opposing immediate-type hypersensitivity and DTH reactions to virus-infected macrophages and elements, and one or both reactions may be observed in individual cats.

Histopathologic Findings

The microscopic lesions of effusive FIP are characteristic, with the hallmark lesion being a vasculitis targeted at venules in the omentum,

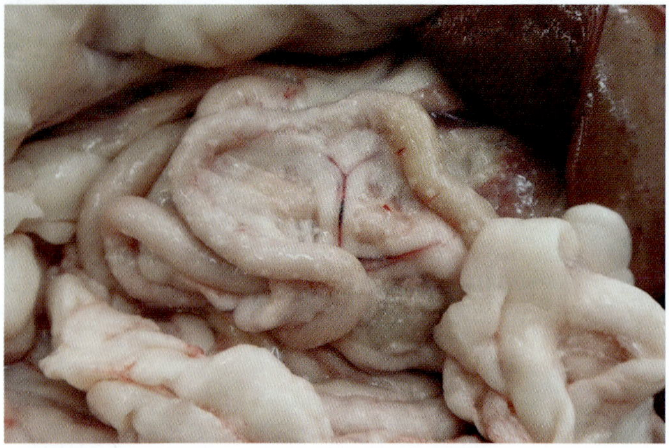

Fig. 31.12 Gross appearance of abdominal cavity of a cat with a more chronic form of effusive abdominal feline infectious peritonitis than shown in Fig. 31.11. The omentum is contracted and thickened and whitish plaques are seen on the surface of the gastrointestinal tract. (Courtesy Dr. Brian Murphy, University of California-Davis Veterinary Anatomic Pathology Service.)

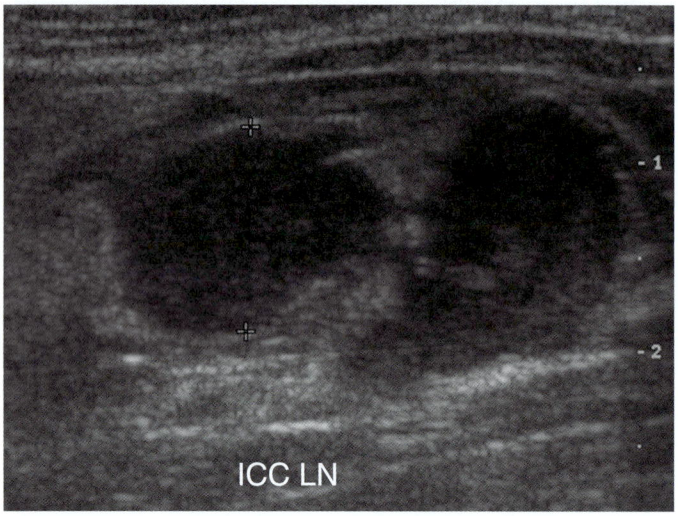

Fig. 31.13 Abdominal ultrasound image showing enlarged ileocolic lymph nodes in a 9-month-old domestic shorthair cat with non-effusive feline infectious peritonitis (FIP). Ileocolic lymph node enlargement is common to both forms of FIP and is the primary site of disease.

mesenteries and serosal surfaces of the abdomen, and pleural surfaces, mediastinum, and pericardium of the heart (Fig. 31.15A). A second characteristic lesion is the pyogranuloma, which consists of focal accumulations of macrophages and neutrophils adjacent to blood vessels. FIPV can be detected by IHC or immunofluorescence within these macrophages (Fig. 31.15B). Pyogranulomas tend to be more diffuse in acute cases and more defined with chronicity. Hyperemia and edema associated with more acute inflammation and loss of small vessel integrity is also more pronounced in severe cases, while this tends to be replaced by serous atrophy and fibrosis in more chronic cases.

Lesions of non-effusive FIP are centered around small aggregates of macrophages resembling the pyogranuloma of effusive FIP, but with a large rim of lymphocytic/plasmocytic infiltrate. Lesions tend to occur in the subcapsular parenchyma of abdominal organs such as the kidney, liver, colon, cecum, spleen, mesenteric lymph nodes, diaphragm, lungs, or pericardium rather than on the peritoneal or parietal serosa. Lesions appear to be remnants of an earlier serositis extending from the surface and into the underlying parenchyma along blood vessels. The ependyma and meninges are target tissues in the CNS and

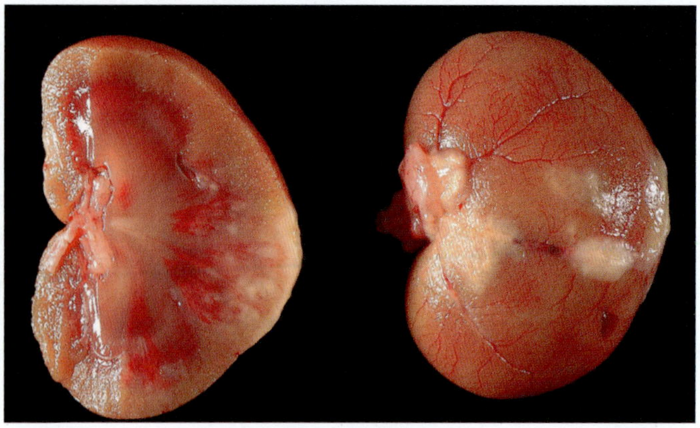

Fig. 31.14 Kidneys of the cat in Fig. 31.8. Multiple pale, tan, firm nodules expand the renal cortices and protrude from the cortical surfaces. (Courtesy D. Gasper and M. Jones, University of California-Davis Veterinary Anatomic Pathology Service.)

the uveal tract and retina in the eyes. Lesions in the skin, testicles, and nasal passages have also been described. The central pyogranulomas in non-effusive FIP are surrounded by dense infiltrates of lymphocytes and plasma cells that invade the surrounding parenchyma. The pyogranulomas contain fewer infected macrophages than those in cats with effusive FIP, which suggests that the host is better able to contain the infection in this form of FIP. Intermediate forms of effusive and non-effusive FIP may also be observed at necropsy. Intestinal[131] and renal lesions[47] of non-effusive FIP may be mistaken for neoplasia.[132] In the colonic form of the disease, foci of pyogranulomatous inflammation in the submucosa and muscularis mucosa surround pale pink-staining areas made up of collagen and sparse cells. These foci are encapsulated in turn by dense layers of fibrous tissue. FIPV antigen is found in large macrophages within the regions of active inflammation.

Immunohistochemistry. A definitive diagnosis of FIP cannot be made based solely on gross and microscopic pathologic features and requires proof of the presence of FIPV in tissues and in particular, macrophages within lesions. IHC on tissues collected at biopsy or necropsy can be as reliable as PCR, but accuracy is subject to many variables and requires excellent quality controls.[133,134] The greatest causes of false negatives and false positives include inadequate specimens, poor reagents, and reading errors. Immunofluorescence is more sensitive than immunoperoxidase staining but requires fresh frozen tissue sections with or without glycerol/resin protection medium. Immunoperoxidase staining can be performed on formalin-fixed tissues or cell pellets.

IHC of effusions from cats suspected to have FIP is strongly recommended, as effusions contain numerous virus-positive macrophages that can be concentrated onto slides. When the results of direct immunofluorescence on feline effusions were compared with histopathologic examination of tissues collected at necropsy in 17 cats, histopathology supported a diagnosis of FIP in 10/17 cases and ruled out FIP in 7/17 cases.[135] Antemortem immunofluorescence testing was positive in all 10 cases confirmed as FIP at necropsy. In the seven cats where FIP was ruled out at necropsy, IHC was negative in five cases and falsely positive in two cases. In another study, immunocytochemistry was 85% sensitive and 72% specific for the diagnosis of FIP from effusions.[136]

IHC can also be used to detect FIPV-infected macrophages within other specimens, such as CSF[137] or biopsy specimens.

TREATMENT

There is currently no approved, readily available, simple, or inexpensive treatment for FIP and the default treatment consists of drainage of fluid when necessary, anti-inflammatory doses of prednisolone, and reduction

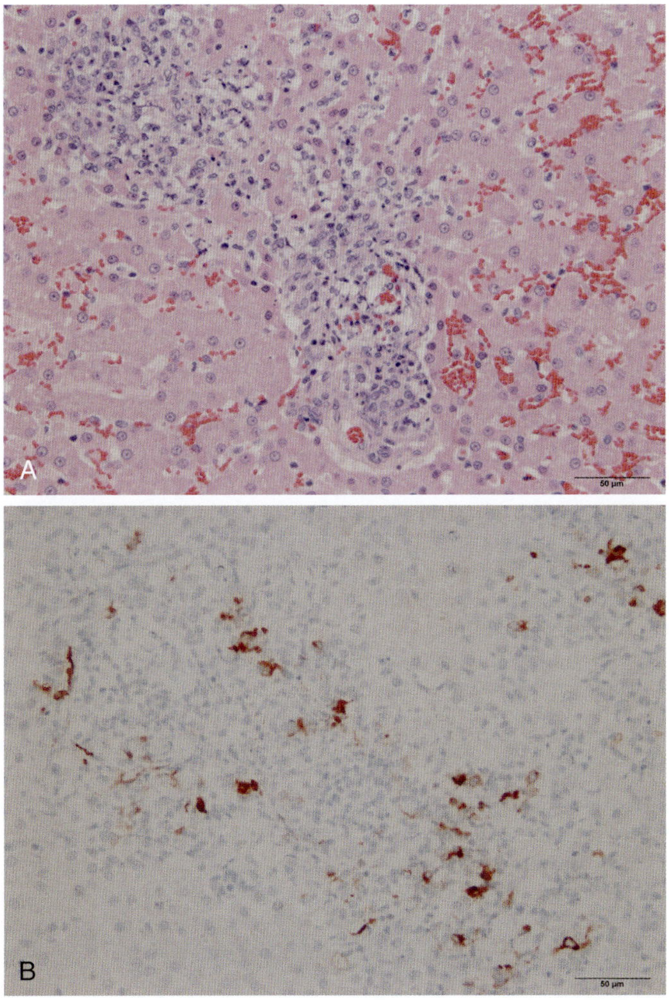

Fig. 31.15 (A) Histopathology of the liver of a cat with feline infectious peritonitis demonstrating pyogranulomatous hepatitis (hematoxylin and eosin stain). (B) Macrophages stain strongly positive for feline coronavirus antigen with immunohistochemistry. (Courtesy Dr. Patricia Pesavento, University of California-Davis Veterinary Anatomic Pathology Service)

of stress. Numerous available drugs, biologics, and nutritional supplements have been tried.[106] Antimicrobial drugs are seldom justified, as secondary bacterial infections are usually absent. Claims of cures have been made following many treatments, but these cures are uncommon and anecdotal. The problem is that there are no accurate mortality figures for FIP to evaluate any of these treatments. The only certainties are that older cats tend to live longer than younger cats and cats with non-effusive disease tend to live longer than cats with effusive FIP. Cats that are severely ill are also more likely to be euthanized upon diagnosis or shortly thereafter, whereas cats with milder disease are often treated supportively and kept alive longer, adding additional bias to mortality curves. Because of these factors, it is essential that a control population be included in studies of treatment effects on the disease. Survival time for cats with FIP also appear to be increasing over the last decade, which may relate to owner persistence with different treatments, or a true change in disease expression (either as a result of host genetics or virus factors).

Removal of abdominal effusion, except in cases where it interferes with breathing, is not recommended as it is rapidly replaced from body stores. Unnecessary removal of effusions can lead to hypoproteinemia and electrolyte disorders. Removal of thoracic effusions is frequently required to relieve dyspnea and can result in clinical improvement for several days or weeks. Removal of enlarged abdominal lymph nodes, intestinal masses, or single diseased kidney, is only indicated if life-threatening complications

TABLE 31.8 Suggested Drug Dosages for Treatment of Feline Infectious Peritonitis

Drug	Dose	Route	Interval (Hours)
Prednisolone	1–2 mg/kg	PO	12–24
Chlorambucil[a]	2 mg/cat	PO	48–72

[a]Monitor the complete blood count during treatment.

exist (e.g., intestinal blockage), as infection is almost always more widespread than clinically apparent. Other supportive care measures such as fluid therapy or placement of feeding tubes also may be required.

Anti-Inflammatory and Immunomodulating Drugs

Prednisolone and alkylating drugs such as chlorambucil have been used to reduce clinical signs in cats with FIP (Table 31.8), but there is no evidence that they significantly alter lifespan. Rather than using this less specific therapeutic approach, attempts have been made to inhibit the cytokine response. TNF inhibitors have been used to alleviate some of the signs of FIP and may decrease mortality when given in the initial stages of experimental FIPV infection.[138] Pentoxifylline has been shown to inhibit TNF-α production by macrophages and has been used to control vasculitis in humans. However, a study of 23 cats with proven FIP failed to detect an effect of a related drug, propentoxifylline, on the survival time, the quality of life, or any FIP-associated clinical or laboratory parameters.[139]

Nonspecific Immunostimulants

Anecdotal reports exist of cats presumed to be infected with FIP being cured or having their lives prolonged with a variety of non-specific immunomodulators (see Chapter 9). Polyprenyl immunostimulant (PI) is a plant extract claimed to prolong the lives, and possibly cure, some cats with mild forms of non-effusive FIP.[92,140] None of these biologics have been demonstrated to stimulate normal immune processes in healthy cats, and sufficiently powered randomized, placebo-controlled, double-masked studies of cats with confirmed FIP are lacking. A major problem is a lack of reliable survival statistics for cats treated with supportive care alone.[140]

Feline IFN-ω (Virbagen omega, Virbac) is a veterinary product widely marketed in Europe and Asia for treatment of many conditions of dogs and cats. It was proposed as a cure for cats with FIP in a study from Japan.[141] Twelve clinically ill cats were treated with a combination of a glucocorticoid and feline IFN-ω. Complete remission was observed in four cats and temporary remission in four cats. This study prompted widespread use of feline IFN-ω for treatment of FIP, except in countries where it was not approved for any veterinary use (including the United States). A subsequent double-blind, placebo-controlled study of 37 client-owned cats with predominately effusive FIP showed feline IFN-ω to lack efficacy.[142] Nonetheless, it continues to be used by some veterinarians to treat FIP and there have been anecdotal reports of occasional cats that have been cured. Human IFN-α given by injection or orally has also been used to treat cats with FIP, but it is immunogenic and is rendered ineffective after several weeks of use (see Chapter 9).

Nonspecific Viral Inhibitors

No virus disease of animals has commanded as much attention as FIP, and many drugs and biologics with inhibitory activity against FIPV in tissue culture have been studied. Many of the biologics studied inhibit FIPV by suppressing normal cellular processes that are usurped by the virus for its own replication, raising their toxicity for the cat. Others work by reacting with surface proteins and block infection in tissue culture but not in natural disease. These include cyclosporine and related immunophilins, vioporin inhibitors, pyridine N-oxide derivatives, chloroquine, plant lectins (*Hippeastrum* hybrid agglutinin, *Galanthus nivalis* agglutinin), ubiquitin inhibitors, and semisynthetic derivatives of glycopeptide antibiotics (vancomycin, teicoplanin).[83,120,143–150] Only chloroquine has been tested for efficacy in naturally occurring disease in cats. The clinical scores of cats in groups treated with chloroquine were only slightly better than those of cats in groups not treated with chloroquine and there was evidence of hepatotoxicity.[120]

Viral inhibitory peptides and silencing RNA molecules also have been used to inhibit FIPV replication in tissue culture. In one study, five overlapping peptides that span the heptad repeat (HR) region of the S protein of a type II FIPV strain (NTU-156) were used to inhibit virus replication by blocking the intercalation of the HR1 and HR2 regions necessary for S protein-mediated fusion.[151] One of the five peptides inhibited FIPV replication by 97%, and had a synergistic effect with human IFN-α. In another study, eight small synthetic interfering RNA (siRNA) that targeted four regions of the genome were used to inhibit replication of the serotype II FIPV strain 79-1146.[152] Two of the siRNAs (targeting the 5' leader sequence and the nucleocapsid gene) resulted in a > 95% reduction in virus replication *in vitro*. Similar results were obtained by other investigators using five siRNAs that targeted the 3′ leader sequence and nucleocapsid genes.[153] These investigators then incorporated their siRNAs into infectious HIV-derived replication competent plasmids, which were then used to infect cultured feline hematopoietic stem cells.[154] The stem cells then produced anti-CoV miRNA with a reduction in FCoV replication, thus taking the application of siRNAs one step closer, but still distant, from clinical application.

Targeted Antiviral Drug Therapy

The most successful antiviral therapies have involved drugs that target viral genes that regulate key processes in virus attachment, integration, or replication. Drugs used for related and unrelated RNA virus infection of humans can target at least two FCoV genes. One is the 3C-like protease[155,156] and the second is the replicase gene responsible for RNA-dependent RNA transcription of subgenomic RNA transcripts.[157]

Viral Protease Inhibitors

GC376, a 3C-like protease inhibitor, was the first specific antiviral drug tested against both experimental[156] and naturally occurring FIP.[155] GC376 is a prodrug which is broken down to the active moiety, GC373. GC373 is virtually identical to nirmatrelvir, the active component of Paxlovid (Pfizer) for treatment of COVID-19.[158] GC373 inhibits the 3C-like protease. Structural proteins of CoV are first transcribed from mRNAs as polyproteins, which are then cleaved by 3C-like proteases into individual proteins used in virion production. Preliminary *in vitro* tests showed that GC376 was effective in inhibiting FIPV replication at levels not toxic to cells.[156] Use of GC376 to treat cats with experimental FIPV infection resulted in cures when treatment was started at the onset of disease and continued for 2 to 4 weeks.[157] A field trial using 20 cats with naturally occurring FIP and twice-daily SC injections yielded mixed results.[155] There was dramatic clinical improvement in cats without neurologic signs within a few days of starting treatment, and 6 of 20 cats developed sustained remissions after 12 weeks of continuous treatment. However, relapses that occurred during treatment or after treatment led to euthanasia of 14 of the 20 cats. Development of neurologic disease during or after treatment was the major cause of failure. Adverse drug effects were manageable and consisted of injection site reactions and impaired development of permanent teeth.[155] At the time of writing, GC376 is under development for treatment of FIP and simultaneously being evaluated as a treatment for COVID-19 by Anivive Life Sciences.[159]

Nucleoside Analogues (RNA Transcription Inhibitors)

Ribavarin is a guanosine nucleoside analogue used once in combination with IFN for the treatment of hepatitis C. It is an *in vitro* inhibitor of FIPV[160] but had no effect on experimental FIPV infection.[161]

The adenosine nucleoside analogue GS-441524, the active form of the prodrug remdesivir (Gilead Sciences) is the most promising treatment for FIP tested to date. GS-441524 and related compounds have been developed as a result of research into possible treatments for human RNA viral diseases such as Ebola, Marburg, SARS-CoV-1 and SARS-CoV-2, and MERS. GS-441524 is the parent nucleoside of remdesivir (i.e., the active metabolite of remdesivir, a prodrug). Remdesivir was originally developed to treat hepatitis C in humans and has now been used extensively worldwide to treat COVID-19. GS-441524 is taken up by cells, phosphorylated stepwise to mono-, di-, and tri-phosphate forms, which then compete with cellular adenosine nucleotide for incorporation into replicating FIPV RNA (see also Chapter 9).[162] GS-441524 given SC demonstrated favorable pharmacokinetics in laboratory cats and was effective against experimental disease.[162] A field trial of 31 cats was conducted with various non-neurologic forms of FIP and drug given SC q24h for a minimum of 12 weeks.[163] Five of the 31 cats recruited to the trial had to be euthanized during the first few days of treatment due to the severity of their disease and complications, but 26 went on to be treated for 12 weeks or longer. Of the 26 cats, 25 achieved sustained disease remission following one or two cycles of treatment with no systemic signs of toxicity. Apparent cures were described by owners in over 50% of 393 cats treated at home with GS-441524, with a mean cost of treatment of $4920 (USD).[164]

There are several limitations of drugs like GC376 and GS-441524. The passage of both drugs into the CSF and aqueous humor is impeded by the blood/brain and blood/eye barriers, respectively.[157,162] Attempts to overcome this by increasing the drug dosage have not been successful for GC376, although clinical signs were greatly decreased.[155] Higher dosages of GS-441524 can overcome the blood/brain barrier in cats with neurologic FIP.[165] A second limitation has been cost. Treatment currently costs several thousand dollars for drug alone, but this cost is expected to decrease with time.[164] A final, and more important limitation, involves legal approval for veterinary use of closely related drugs that have been developed for humans against COVID-19. These drugs currently include the nucleoside analogues remdesivir[166] and molnupiravir,[167] and the viral protease inhibitor paxlovid.[158] These drugs have only conditional approval for in-hospital use against COVID-19 at the time of writing. There is a concern among large pharmaceutical companies that concurrent use of these or closely related drugs in animals would complicate the full approval process of drugs for human use. Without FDA approval, veterinarians were initially unwilling to use drugs that were not legally produced and sold. This led initially to a situation where a cure was available for the first time for FIP but no inclination to apply it in the field. However, the desperate need of cat owners for a treatment for FIP and willingness of companies in China to provide them the drugs quickly rendered these concerns moot. People concerned about FIP, particularly those involved in foster/rescue, were quick to embrace the treatment.[164] Their efforts resulted in tens of thousands of cats from around the world being successfully cured of FIP from 2017 onward. This success convinced some academic veterinarians to become involved.[164,168] The legality of using unapproved antivirals for treatment of diseases has also been overcome in some countries by allowing veterinarians to use conditionally approved drugs like remdesivir.[169] Hopefully, such arrangements will be short-lived as drugs like remdesivir, molnupiravir and paxlovid are given full approval for coronavirus disease in people. Full approval by national entities like the FDA will allow veterinarians to use them per label or extra label fashion when no approved animal equivalent is available, provided that they are compounded from federally approved drugs. (AVMA)

PROGNOSIS

The 1-year mortality for FIP is around 95% for cats treated with various non-virus–specific medications. Younger cats, which tend to have more acute and severe forms of FIP, have the shortest survival times, whereas older cats with less severe and more chronic forms of FIP tend to live longer. Marked pyrexia, lethargy, inappetence, weight loss, and icterus are indications of a poor prognosis. Lymphopenia is often associated with more fulminant disease, whereas higher counts are associated with more localized and less intense inflammation. Cats with pronounced abdominal effusions that are still active, eating, and maintaining weight are more likely to manifest lower-grade fever, clearer fluid, and less likely to be icteric. Apparent long-term cures have now been described for many cats treated with nucleoside analogues such as GS-441524 and remdesivir.

IMMUNITY

FECV immunity is mediated by humoral mucosal and systemic responses.[170] Secretory antibody responses in the gut most likely mirror IgG antibody levels in the blood. Antibodies measured by indirect IFA appear in the blood within 10 to 14 days of infection and rise to titers around 1:400 at the peak of shedding.[10,37] Serum antibody titers then fall to levels of 1:25 or less as virus shedding becomes intermittent and finally ceases.[37] Reinfections are common and resemble primary infections in the pattern of fecal shedding and antibody responses. Reinfection has also been observed in natural disease.[66] This pattern of infection is typical, as immunity to mucosal pathogens often requires a long period of exposure or persistence to develop and does not evoke strong memory.[171] Immunity to animal coronavirus vaccines is also notoriously poor.[172]

As noted earlier in this chapter, cellular immunity appears to be important in determining the outcome of FIPV infection. Humoral immunity is not thought to be nonprotective in FIP and contributes to disease pathogenesis. In a study of experimentally infected cats, investigators were unable to identify T-cell responses that might predict disease outcome during early infection with FIPV. However, on re-exposure to FIPV, antiviral T-cell responses appeared to be important in preventing disease.[173]

PREVENTION

Minimizing Exposure

Attempts have been made to eliminate FECV from cat populations. One approach used has been to isolate pregnant queens from all other cats and wean and isolate kittens at 4–6 weeks of age.[174] Even if the queen is shedding FECV, most kittens have sufficient maternal-derived immunity to resist infection until 9–10 weeks of age. After early weaning, kittens are strictly quarantined and tested for fecal FECV shedding at monthly intervals for several months to assure that they are free of the virus. Once free from FECV, prevention of infection requires a specific facility for noninfected cats and strict control of the movement of people to avoid introduction of the virus on fomites. It also precludes acquisition of new cats without strict testing and quarantine and limits introduction of cats, all of which defeat the purposes of pedigreed cat breeding.

FECV infection can also be allowed to burn itself out. In one study of naturally infected cats, FECV shedding dramatically decreased over 3 years, suggesting a type of herd immunity.[66] If a cattery or other multicat facility is closed to new susceptible cats, either from outside or from within (i.e., kittens bred in the facility), the proportion of fecal shedders will slowly decline. This can be facilitated through the testing of all the cats used to produce a FCoV-free population by fecal PCR or serology.[14] Cats that are negative by PCR and have low FCoV titers (≤1:25 by indirect IFA) are segregated to one facility and quarantined. Cats with strong positive PCR values and antibody titers ≥ 1:400 are eliminated, and cats with intermediate values are segregated to a second facility. This testing is repeated every month and within a year or less the result will be two separate groups of cats that should be free of infection with a minimum of loss of breeding stock. These procedures have been used to eliminate FECV infection from SPF experimental cat breeding colonies.[14]

A direct relationship exists between the extent of fecal shedding of FECV and FIP.[36,65] Cats over 3 years of age are also less apt to be FECV carriers. Therefore, the severity of FECV exposure and incidence of FIP can be diminished by reducing the numbers of breeding cats to a minimum and by decreasing the proportion of younger cats in a cat population. Breeding cats should be kept for longer periods of time to reduce the numbers of young cats introduced into the cattery. Adult cats are also less likely to shed other common pathogens, and when coupled with decreased kitten density, this can also reduce the incidence of upper respiratory and enteric infectious diseases. Catteries that remain free of FIP are often those that maintain six or less breeding queens with one or two toms. Unnecessary cats should be removed from the cattery whenever possible. Kitten production should be also minimized by more careful mate selection and breeding for quality rather than quantity.

Vaccination

Several potential FIP vaccines have been described over the last three decades.[56,57] These vaccines have had preventable fractions that range from 0% to 75%, and results from the field have been mixed.[108] Only one vaccine, Primucell FIP (Zoetis, Parsippany, NJ), has been successfully licensed and marketed in the United States and several other countries. This is an intranasal vaccine that contains a temperature-sensitive mutant of serotype II FIPV-DF2, and initial vaccination consists of two doses of the vaccine given 3 weeks apart.[175] Vaccination has not been shown to be effective when administered to cats less than 16 weeks of age, suggesting that the immune system must reach a more mature state of development than for other routinely used vaccines. The vaccine has been shown to be safe with no signs of ADE.[176] There are several aspects of the vaccine that limit its use in the field. It contains a serotype II strain of FIPV, while serotype I strains predominate in the field. Serotype I and II strains contain different virus-neutralizing epitopes. The vaccine is also without efficacy when administered to kittens less than 16 weeks of age, which is at least 6 weeks after kittens from multi-cat environments have been exposed to FECV. The vaccine may also lack efficacy in cats that have been previously exposed to FCoV.[108] In a placebo-controlled study of two high FIP–risk populations,[177] the vaccine was safe and efficacious in one population of cats that had low antibody titers to FCoV at the time of vaccination. It was concluded that vaccination could protect cats with no or low FCoV antibody titer. However, catteries with low CoV titers are at low risk for FIP, and titers are generally high among cattery, rescue, and shelter cats. Therefore, the target group for this vaccine would be cats exposed to uncommon serotype II strains of FECV, with less than a 1% risk of developing FIP after such exposure, and that are over 16 weeks of age and seronegative for FCoV exposure when vaccinated. Furthermore, vaccination of FCoV-naïve laboratory cats ≥ 16 weeks of age, was less than 70% effective against challenge exposure with a serotype II FIPV when adjusted for the survival rate of nonvaccinates.[175] As a result of these concerns, the AAFP has stated that, "at this time, there is insufficient evidence that the vaccine induces clinically relevant protection, and use of the vaccine is not recommended."[178]

Genetic Selection

Susceptibility to FIP in pedigreed cats appears to be 50% heritable in breeds studied.[70] Attempts to use positive selection in a laboratory setting to enhance resistance among random-bred cats failed, and the resultant inbreeding increased rather than decreased FIP susceptibility.[72] Genetic susceptibility appears to involve inheritance of numerous risk factors, some positive and others negative.[71,72] Because inbreeding is a much greater problem among pedigreed than random-bred cats, genetic factors play a proportionately greater role in catteries than in kitten rescues or shelters. Other host and environmental co-factors are of greater importance in random-bred populations. The fact that some breeds and lines of pedigreed cats are at greater genetic risk for FIP is a two-edged sword. Although inbreeding and artificial genetic bottlenecks may increase FIP risk in pedigreed cats, catteries can control which toms and queens are bred and may be able to associate certain breeding combinations with development of FIP. The practice of not using cats that have produced kittens that have died of FIP or that are in closely related lines known to have problems with FIP is widely accepted. Both toms and queens contribute genetic risk factors, but because toms produce many more kittens, the culling of problem toms rather than queens can be more effective.[70] Tom cats from lines with no history of FIP can overcome genetic deficiencies in queens, while breeding genetically deficient toms with deficient queens can rapidly bring FIP problems to the forefront.

PUBLIC HEALTH ASPECTS

There is no evidence that humans can become infected with FCoV. Most human coronaviruses, including SARS-CoV-2 (the cause of COVID-19), are beta- and not alpha-CoVs. SARS-CoV-2 can infect and cause disease in cats (see Chapter 43).[179] Other coronaviruses have been shown to cause FIP-like disease in ferrets and mice. If a coronavirus emerged that could cause similar clinical manifestations and outcomes in humans as FIPV can in cats, it would clearly represent a major threat to humans, and would without doubt be the subject of intense research.

CASE EXAMPLE

Signalment

"Ricky", a 9-month-old male castrated domestic shorthair from Sacramento, CA.

History

Ricky was obtained as a stray at 8 weeks of age by a local kitten rescue group and adopted by the owner at 3 months of age. He had experienced multiple upper respiratory tract infections before being adopted but was healthy when placed in a new home with one other cat. He was an indoor cat that was sometimes walked briefly outdoors.

Ricky was brought to a local veterinary clinic at 9 months of age because of an acute onset of increased thirst and urination. A serum chemistry panel showed hyperglobulinemia (7.7 mg/dL). The urine SpG was 1.025 with inactive sediment and culture negative for aerobic bacteria. Ricky stopped eating over the next 3 days and was returned to the clinic. Laboratory abnormalities at that time included a mature neutrophilia (11,904 cells/μL), lymphocytosis (5,104 cells/μL), eosinophilia (1,536 cells/μL), hyperglobulinemia (6.9 mg/dL), and hypoalbuminemia (2.4 mg/dL) with A:G ratio of 0.35. A FCoV antibody titer was positive at 1:400. Serology for *Toxoplasma gondii* was negative. Plain thoracic radiographs showed a mild interstitial pattern. Abdominal ultrasound showed a moderately enlarged mesenteric lymph that was reactive on aspiration. Ricky's appetite recovered when cyproheptadine was initiated for several weeks, after which treatment was discontinued. Ricky remained outwardly normal over the next 3 weeks, although occasional soft feces were noticed in the litter box. The owners were concerned about the possibility of FIP. The owner suspected FIP and wanted a second opinion.

Physical Examination

Ricky was bright, alert, and active on presentation with a weight of 4.2 kg, T = 103°F, HR = 200 beats/minute, and eupneic. His eyes, ears, nose, and throat were normal, and his BCS was 5/9. Thoracic auscultation did not reveal any abnormalities, and abdominal palpation was normal.

Laboratory Findings

A CBC demonstrated a slightly low HCT at 27.3%, a normal MCV and MCHC, and a leukocytosis of 24,950 cells/μL with neutrophilia (17,141 cells/μL), high normal lymphocytes (6,886 cells/μL), a monocyte count of 724 cells/μL, eosinophils of 200 cells/μL, and a slightly elevated platelet count (518,000/μL).

A serum chemistry profile demonstrated a normal sodium, potassium, chloride, bicarbonate, phosphorous, calcium, BUN, creatinine, and glucose. However, total protein concentration was greatly elevated at 10.7 g/dL with a low normal albumin (2.6 g/dL) and high globulin (8.1 g/dL) and A:G ratio of 0.32. Serum liver enzyme activities (ALT, AST, ALP, and GGT) were normal, as were the cholesterol and bilirubin concentrations. A serum protein electrophoresis showed a polyclonal gammopathy with a mild decrease in albumin and mild increases in the α_2 and β_1 fractions consistent with the acute-phase inflammatory response.

Imaging Findings

Ultrasound of the abdomen demonstrated moderate splenomegaly and a diffuse mesenteric lymphadenopathy. An aspirate of a mesenteric lymph node showed a heterogenous population of lymphocytes, predominated by small, mature lymphocytes and low numbers of intermediate and large reactive lymphocytes with scattered plasma cells and histiocytes. Immunocytochemistry using two different monoclonal antibodies to FCoV was negative.

Microbiologic Testing

FeLV antigen and FIV antibody serology were negative, as were blood cultures for *Bartonella clarridgeiae* and *Bartonella henselae*. Ricky was also seronegative for antibodies to *Ehrlichia canis*, *Anaplasma phagocytophilum*, *Rickettsia* spp., and whole blood PCR-negative for *A. phagocytophilum*, *Anaplasma platys*, *Bartonella* spp., *E. canis*, and *Mycoplasma haemofelis*. Aerobic and anaerobic bacterial cultures of mesenteric lymph node aspirates were negative; an FCoV 7b PCR on whole blood was also negative. Serology for FCoV antibodies was positive at 1:102,400.

Diagnosis

A tentative diagnosis of FIP was made based on Ricky's background, the marked polyclonal gammopathy, and extremely high CoV titer.

Treatment and Outcome

Ricky was treated with prednisolone (5 mg, PO, q12h for 7 days, followed by 5 mg, PO, q24h thereafter), and chlorambucil (2 mg, PO, every 3 days). After 6 weeks of treatment, Ricky appeared normal and CBC variables were within normal reference ranges. However, his total protein was 8.5 g/dL with a globulin of 4.5 g/dL and an abdominal ultrasound showed persistent, but mild mesenteric lymphadenomegaly. A repeat FCoV titer was 1:25,600 and treatment with feline IFN-ω was commenced at 4.5 million units, SC, once weekly.

Ricky was next seen 3 months later, at which time he appeared playful, his appetite was normal, and his body weight had remained stable at 4.5 kg. A CBC showed mild anemia (HCT 28.5%), with low normal WBC with neutrophils at 4,439 cells/μL and lymphopenia (468 cells/μL). A serum chemistry panel and abdominal ultrasound showed no abnormalities, which prompted discontinuation of the chlorambucil and IFN-ω and continuation of prednisolone.

Ricky was next seen 12 months after his illness, at which time he was apparently healthy. CBC findings were unchanged from the previous visit and his serum globulin concentration was 4.7 g/dL. The prednisolone dose was decreased to

Continued

CASE EXAMPLE—cont'd

5 mg q48h. One month later, albumin and globulin concentrations were 3.3 and 5.1 g/dL, respectively, and the prednisolone dose was reduced to 2.5 mg q48h. Two months later, a CBC was unremarkable, but the globulin had increased to 5.7 g/dL, abdominal ultrasound showed a mild enlargement of the mesenteric lymph nodes, and the serum CoV antibody titer was 1:409,600. The prednisolone dose was returned to 5 mg, PO, q24h, and 1 month later, the serum globulin concentration was 4.9 g/dL.

Ricky was still doing well clinically 1.5 months later, but a mid-abdominal mass was palpated on physical examination and the serum globulin concentration had increased again (5.6 g/dL). Abdominal ultrasound showed several moderately enlarged and hypoechoic lymph nodes in the ileocolic region, the largest of which measured 0.9 cm in diameter. The surrounding mesentery was focally hyperechoic. There was also focal hyperechoic retroperitoneal tissue surrounding the right kidney with scant retroperitoneal fluid. Attempts to obtain aspirates from the lymph nodes were unsuccessful. The prednisolone dose was increased to 5 mg, PO, q12h, and treatment with chlorambucil was reinstituted. Ricky became lethargic and anorectic over the next week. A CBC showed worsening anemia (HCT 24.3%) and persistent lymphopenia (782 cells/μL). His globulin concentration was increased (5.8 g/dL) and albumin normal (3.3 g/dL). A fourth FCoV antibody titer was 1:25,600. Treatment with cyproheptadine was initiated and the chlorambucil and pentoxifylline discontinued. The inappetence continued, he became persistently pyrexic (103.4°F to 104°F), and hematochezia and tachypnea developed over the next few days. HCT dropped to 16.5%, and hypokalemia, hyponatremia, and hypochloremia developed. Ricky was hospitalized and treated with 1 unit of packed RBCs, IV crystalloids, and parenteral antimicrobial drugs. Thoracic radiographs showed a severe, diffuse, patchy alveolar and nodular interstitial pattern with thickening of the bronchial walls and mild pleural effusion. A tracheobronchial lavage showed marked mixed, predominantly pyogranulomatous inflammation with moderate epithelial hyperplasia and some degenerate neutrophils. Immunocytochemistry with an anti-FCoV antibody was strongly positive (Fig. 31.16). Shortly thereafter he began to seize and was euthanized.

Necropsy Findings

A necropsy showed moderate to severe, multifocal to coalescing pyogranulomatous inflammation involving the parietal and visceral serosa of the spleen, liver, kidney, intestines, diaphragm, thoracic and abdominal walls, and pericardium. There was also multifocal pyogranulomatous splenitis, hepatitis, nephritis, meningoencephalitis, and pneumonia with pulmonary necrosis. Straw-colored effusion was present in the abdominal cavity, thoracic cavity, and pleural space. IHC was strongly positive for FCoV antigen.

Comments

This case was typical of several cats that start out with dry FIP localized primarily to the mesenteric lymph nodes. This has been previously described as the mildest clinical form of FIP. In this presentation, the host immune system can contain most of the infection to the primary target organ (i.e., the mesenteric lymph node), but the immune response is insufficient to bring about a complete cure and the disease becomes clinically apparent. In other such cases, the disease has been known to completely resolve or remain subclinical for many months and possibly years.[56,92] Although Ricky appeared to respond on several occasions to medications such as prednisolone and IFN-ω, there is reasonable evidence that none of these drugs are effective in altering the disease course,[160,163] and the ups and downs in clinical condition during these earlier stages would be as expected for this form of FIP. Ultimately, disease progressed and a diagnosis of FIP was confirmed with immunocytochemistry on a tracheobronchial lavage specimen. The terminal development of effusions is also more commonly recognized and has been referred to as 'dry-to-wet' FIP. It is often only when the disease becomes conspicuously effusive that the correct diagnosis is made. The PCR and immunocytochemistry results early during illness were false negatives, indicating that the level of virus in the samples at these early stages was below the sensitivity of the assay procedures or that sampling was inadequate. Drugs such as GC376, GS-441524, and remdesivir have shown promise for complete cure of disease in cases such as this, but were not available at the time this cat was alive.

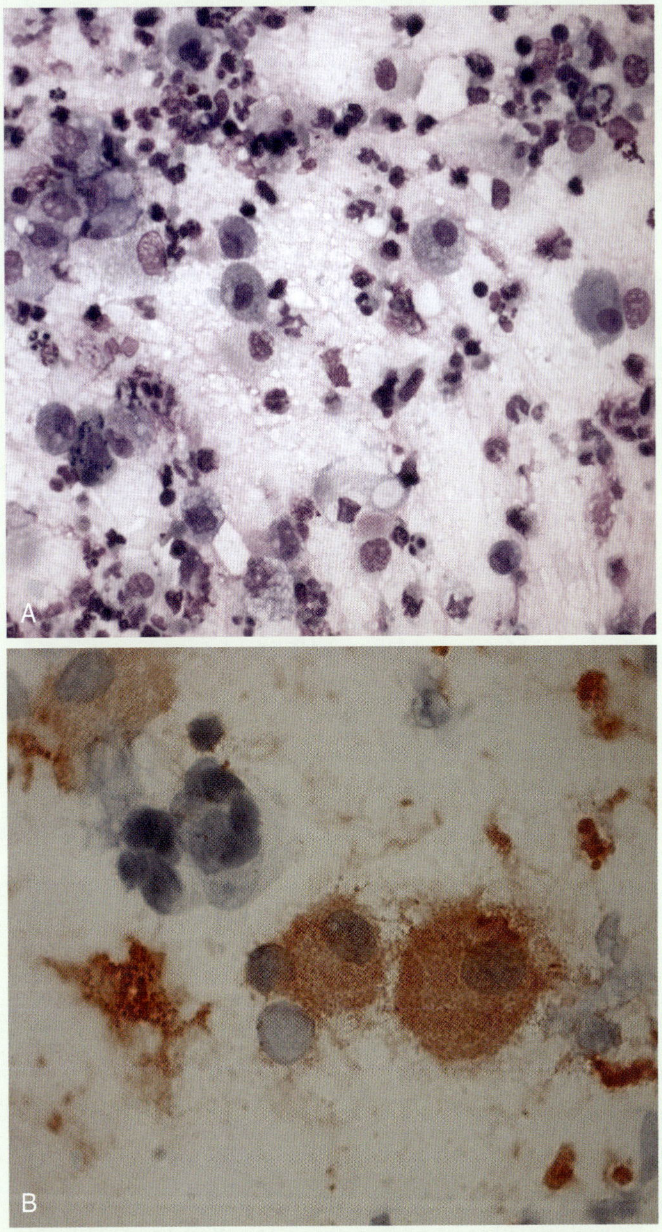

Fig. 31.16 (A) Cytospin preparation of a tracheobronchial lavage specimen from the cat in Fig. 31.7. The specimen was highly cellular (4,400 cells/μL) and the cells consisted of 42% degenerate neutrophils and nondegenerate neutrophils, 5% lymphocytes, and 53% macrophages. (B) Immunocytochemistry stain on the same specimen for coronavirus antigen showing positive staining in association with macrophages.

SUGGESTED READINGS

American Veterinary Medical Association. Compounding FAQ for veterinarians. https://www.avma.org/resources-tools/animal-health-and-welfare/animal-health/compounding/compounding-faq-veterinarians. Last accessed April 7, 2022.

Nadeau J, Evans S. Unlicensed GS-441524-like antiviral therapy can be effective for at-home treatment of feline infectious peritonitis. *Animals (Basel)*. 2021;11:2257.

Pedersen NC, Perron M, Bannasch M, et al. Efficacy and safety of the nucleoside analog GS-441524 for treatment of cats with naturally occurring feline infectious peritonitis. *J Feline Med Surg*. 2019;21:271–281.

Tasker S. Diagnosis of feline infectious peritonitis: Update on evidence supporting available tests. *J Feline Med Surg*. 2018;20:228–243.

REFERENCES

1. Holzworth J. Some important disorders of cats. *Cornell Vet*. 1963;53:157–160.
2. Wertheim JO, Chu DK, Peiris JS, et al. A case for the ancient origin of coronaviruses. *J Virol*. 2013;87:7039–7045.
3. Pedersen NC, Black JW, Boyle JF, et al. Pathogenic differences between various feline coronavirus isolates. *Adv Exp Med Biol*. 1984;173:365–380.
4. Whittaker GR, Andre NM, Millet JK. Improving virus taxonomy by recontextualizing sequence-based classification with biologically relevant data: the case of the alphacoronavirus 1 species. *mSphere*. 2018;3.
5. Herrewegh AA, Smeenk I, Horzinek MC, et al. Feline coronavirus type II strains 79-1683 and 79-1146 originate from a double recombination between feline coronavirus type I and canine coronavirus. *J Virol*. 1998;72:4508–4514.
6. Terada Y, Matsui N, Noguchi K, et al. Emergence of pathogenic coronaviruses in cats by homologous recombination between feline and canine coronaviruses. *PLoS One*. 2014;9:e106534.
7. Sharif S, Arshad SS, Hair-Bejo M, et al. Diagnostic methods for feline coronavirus: a review. *Vet Med Int*. 2010;2010.
8. An DJ, Jeoung HY, Jeong W, et al. Prevalence of Korean cats with natural feline coronavirus infections. *Virol J*. 2011;8:455.
9. Amer A, Siti Suri A, Abdul Rahman O, et al. Isolation and molecular characterization of type I and type II feline coronavirus in Malaysia. *Virol J*. 2012;9:278.
10. Vogel L, Van der Lubben M, te Lintelo EG, et al. Pathogenic characteristics of persistent feline enteric coronavirus infection in cats. *Vet Res*. 2010;41:71.
11. Pedersen NC, Liu H, Scarlett J, et al. Feline infectious peritonitis: role of the feline coronavirus 3c gene in intestinal tropism and pathogenicity based upon isolates from resident and adopted shelter cats. *Virus Res*. 2012;165:17–28.
12. Kipar A, Meli ML, Baptiste KE, et al. Sites of feline coronavirus persistence in healthy cats. *J Gen Virol*. 2010;91:1698–1707.
13. Addie DD, Schaap IA, Nicolson L, et al. Persistence and transmission of natural type I feline coronavirus infection. *J Gen Virol*. 2003;84:2735–2744.
14. Hickman MA, Morris JG, Rogers QR, et al. Elimination of feline coronavirus infection from a large experimental specific pathogen-free cat breeding colony by serologic testing and isolation. *Feline Pract*. 1995;23:96–102.
15. Zook BC, King NW, Robison RL, et al. Ultrastructural evidence for the viral etiology of feline infectious peritonitis. *Pathol Vet*. 1968;5:91–95.
16. Tekes G, Thiel HJ. Feline coronaviruses: pathogenesis of feline infectious peritonitis. *Adv Virus Res*. 2016;96:193–218.
17. Huang YW, Dickerman AW, Pineyro P, et al. Origin, evolution, and genotyping of emergent porcine epidemic diarrhea virus strains in the United States. *mBio*. 2013;4:e00737. e00713.
18. Chan JF, Lau SK, To KK, et al. Middle East respiratory syndrome coronavirus: another zoonotic betacoronavirus causing SARS-like disease. *Clin Microbiol Rev*. 2015;28:465–522.
19. Rasschaert D, Duarte M, Laude H. Porcine respiratory coronavirus differs from transmissible gastroenteritis virus by a few genomic deletions. *J Gen Virol*. 1990;71(Pt 11):2599–2607.
20. Jaimes JA, Whittaker GR. Feline coronavirus: insights into viral pathogenesis based on the spike protein structure and function. *Virology*. 2018;517:108–121.
21. Tresnan DB, Holmes KV. Feline aminopeptidase N is a receptor for all group I coronaviruses. *Adv Exp Med Biol*. 1998;440:69–75.
22. Tresnan DB, Levis R, Holmes KV. Feline aminopeptidase N serves as a receptor for feline, canine, porcine, and human coronaviruses in serogroup I. *J Virol*. 1996;70:8669–8674.
23. Tusell SM, Schittone SA, Holmes KV. Mutational analysis of aminopeptidase N, a receptor for several group 1 coronaviruses, identifies key determinants of viral host range. *J Virol*. 2007;81:1261–1273.
24. Watanabe R, Eckstrand C, Liu H, et al. Characterization of peritoneal cells from cats with experimentally-induced feline infectious peritonitis (FIP) using RNA-seq. *Vet Res*. 2018;49:81.
25. Colby ED, Low RJ. Feline infectious peritonitis. *Vet Med Small Anim Clin*. 1970;65:783–786.
26. Colly LP. Feline infectious peritonitis. *Vet Clin North Am Small Anim Pract*. 1973;3:34.
27. Gaffney PM, Kennedy M, Terio K, et al. Detection of feline coronavirus in cheetah (*Acinonyx jubatus*) feces by reverse transcription-nested polymerase chain reaction in cheetahs with variable frequency of viral shedding. *J Zoo Wildl Med*. 2012;43:776–786.
28. Juan-Salles C, Domingo M, Herraez P, et al. Feline infectious peritonitis in servals (*Felis serval*). *Vet Rec*. 1998;143:535–536.
29. Mwase M, Shimada K, Mumba C, et al. Positive immunolabelling for feline infectious peritonitis in an African lion (*Panthera leo*) with bilateral panuveitis. *J Comp Pathol*. 2015;152:265–268.
30. Pfeifer ML, Evermann JF, Roelke ME, et al. Feline infectious peritonitis in a captive cheetah. *J Am Vet Med Assoc*. 1983;183:1317–1319.
31. Tuch K, Witte KH, Wuller H. Feststellung deer feline infecktiösen Peritonitis (FIP) bei Hauskatzen und Leoparden in Deutschland. *Zentralblatt fur Veterinarmedizin Reihe B*. 1974;21:426–441.
32. Watt NJ, MacIntyre NJ, McOrist S. An extended outbreak of infectious peritonitis in a closed colony of European wildcats (*Felis silvestris*). *J Comp Pathol*. 1993;108:73–79.
33. Kennedy M, Kania S, Stylianides E, et al. Detection of feline coronavirus infection in southern African nondomestic felids. *J Wildl Dis*. 2003;39:529–535.
34. Holmes EC, Goldstein SA, Rasmussen AL, et al. The origins of SARS-CoV-2: a critical review. *Cell*. 2021;184(19):4848–4856.
35. Pedersen NC, Boyle JF, Floyd K. Infection studies in kittens, using feline infectious peritonitis virus propagated in cell culture. *Am J Vet Res*. 1981;42:363–367.
36. Kipar A, Baptiste K, Barth A, et al. Natural FCoV infection: cats with FIP exhibit significantly higher viral loads than healthy infected cats. *J Feline Med Surg*. 2006;8:69–72.
37. Pedersen NC, Allen CE, Lyons LA. Pathogenesis of feline enteric coronavirus infection. *J Feline Med Surg*. 2008;10:529–541.
38. Desmarets LM, Theuns S, Olyslaegers DA, et al. Establishment of feline intestinal epithelial cell cultures for the propagation and study of feline enteric coronaviruses. *Vet Res*. 2013;44:71.
39. Desmarets LM, Vermeulen BL, Theuns S, et al. Experimental feline enteric coronavirus infection reveals an aberrant infection pattern and shedding of mutants with impaired infectivity in enterocyte cultures. *Sci Rep*. 2016;6:20022.
40. Andersen LA, Levy JK, McManus CM, et al. Prevalence of enteropathogens in cats with and without diarrhea in four different management models for unowned cats in the southeast United States. *Vet J*. 2018;236:49–55.
41. Addie DD, McDonald M, Audhuy S, et al. Quarantine protects Falkland Islands (Malvinas) cats from feline coronavirus infection. *J Feline Med Surg*. 2012;14:171–176.
42. Pedersen NC, Sato R, Foley JE, et al. Common virus infections in cats, before and after being placed in shelters, with emphasis on feline enteric coronavirus. *J Feline Med Surg*. 2004;6:83–88.
43. Foley JE, Poland A, Carlson J, et al. Patterns of feline coronavirus infection and fecal shedding from cats in multiple-cat environments. *J Am Vet Med Assoc*. 1997;210:1307–1312.
44. Horzinek MC, Osterhaus AD. Feline infectious peritonitis: a coronavirus disease of cats. *J Small Anim Pract*. 1978;19:623–630.

45. Wolfe LG, Griesemer RA. Feline infectious peritonitis. *Pathol Vet.* 1966;3:255–270.
46. Ward JM. Morphogenesis of a virus in cats with experimental feline infectious peritonitis. *Virology.* 1970;41:191–194.
47. Montali RJ, Strandberg JD. Extraperitoneal lesions in feline infectious peritonitis. *Vet Pathol.* 1972;9:109–121.
48. Slauson DO, Finn JP. Meningoencephalitis and panophthalmitis in feline infectious peritonitis. *J Am Vet Med Assoc.* 1972;160:729–734.
49. Pedersen NC. Morphologic and physical characteristics of feline infectious peritonitis virus and its growth in autochthonous peritoneal cell cultures. *Am J Vet Res.* 1976;37:567–572.
50. Hitchcock LM, O'Reilly KJ, Beesley JE. In vitro culture of feline infectious peritonitis virus. *Vet Rec.* 1981;108:535–537.
51. Pedersen NC. Virologic and immunologic aspects of feline infectious peritonitis virus infection. *Adv Exp Med Biol.* 1987;218:529–550.
52. Vennema H, Poland A, Foley J, et al. Feline infectious peritonitis viruses arise by mutation from endemic feline enteric coronaviruses. *Virology.* 1998;243:150–157.
53. Doyle LP, Hutchings LM. A transmissible gastroenteritis in pigs. *J Am Vet Med Assoc.* 1946;108:257–259.
54. Lu S, Wang Y, Chen Y, et al. Discovery of a novel canine respiratory coronavirus support genetic recombination among betacoronavirus1. *Virus Res.* 2017;237:7–13.
55. Pensaert M, Callebaut P, Vergote J. Isolation of a porcine respiratory, non-enteric coronavirus related to transmissible gastroenteritis. *Vet Q.* 1986;8:257–261.
56. Pedersen NC. A review of feline infectious peritonitis virus infection: 1963-2008. *J Feline Med Surg.* 2009;11:225–258.
57. Pedersen NC. An update on feline infectious peritonitis: diagnostics and therapeutics. *Vet J.* 2014;201:133–141.
58. Cotter SM, Gilmore CE, Rollins C. Multiple cases of feline leukemia and feline infectious peritonitis in a household. *J Am Vet Med Assoc.* 1973;162:1054–1058.
59. Pedersen NC, Theilen G, Keane MA, et al. Studies of naturally transmitted feline leukemia virus infection. *Am J Vet Res.* 1977;38:1523–1531.
60. Pesteanu-Somogyi LD, Radzai C, Pressler BM. Prevalence of feline infectious peritonitis in specific cat breeds. *J Feline Med Surg.* 2006;8:1–5.
61. Riemer F, Kuehner KA, Ritz S, et al. Clinical and laboratory features of cats with feline infectious peritonitis: a retrospective study of 231 confirmed cases (2000-2010). *J Feline Med Surg.* 2016;18:348–356.
62. Rohrbach BW, Legendre AM, Baldwin CA, et al. Epidemiology of feline infectious peritonitis among cats examined at veterinary medical teaching hospitals. *J Am Vet Med Assoc.* 2001;218:1111–1115.
63. Cave TA, Thompson H, Reid SW, et al. Kitten mortality in the United Kingdom: a retrospective analysis of 274 histopathological examinations (1986 to 2000). *Vet Rec.* 2002;151:497–501.
64. Pedersen NC. Serologic studies of naturally occurring feline infectious peritonitis. *Am J Vet Res.* 1976;37:1449–1453.
65. Foley JE, Poland A, Carlson J, et al. Risk factors for feline infectious peritonitis among cats in multiple-cat environments with endemic feline enteric coronavirus. *J Am Vet Med Assoc.* 1997;210:1313–1318.
66. Addie DD, Toth S, Murray GD, et al. Risk of feline infectious peritonitis in cats naturally infected with feline coronavirus. *Am J Vet Res.* 1995;56:429–434.
67. Pedersen NC, Liu H, Gandolfi B, et al. The influence of age and genetics on natural resistance to experimentally induced feline infectious peritonitis. *Vet Immunol Immunopathol.* 2014;162:33–40.
68. Worthing KA, Wigney DI, Dhand NK, et al. Risk factors for feline infectious peritonitis in Australian cats. *J Feline Med Surg.* 2012;14:405–412.
69. Norris JM, Bosward KL, White JD, et al. Clinicopathological findings associated with feline infectious peritonitis in Sydney, Australia: 42 cases (1990-2002). *Aust Vet J.* 2005;83:666–673.
70. Foley JE, Pedersen NC. The inheritance of susceptibility to feline infectious peritonitis in purebred catteries. *Feline Pract.* 1996;24:14–22.
71. Golovko L, Lyons LA, Liu H, et al. Genetic susceptibility to feline infectious peritonitis in Birman cats. *Virus Res.* 2013;175:58–63.
72. Pedersen NC, Liu H, Durden M, et al. Natural resistance to experimental feline infectious peritonitis virus infection is decreased rather than increased by positive genetic selection. *Vet Immunol Immunopathol.* 2016;171:17–20.
73. Storz J, Rott R, Kaluza G. Enhancement of plaque formation and cell fusion of an enteropathogenic coronavirus by trypsin treatment. *Infect Immun.* 1981;31:1214–1222.
74. Sabshin SJ, Levy JK, Tupler T, et al. Enteropathogens identified in cats entering a Florida animal shelter with normal feces or diarrhea. *J Am Vet Med Assoc.* 2012;241:331–337.
75. Harpold LM, Legendre AM, Kennedy MA, et al. Fecal shedding of feline coronavirus in adult cats and kittens in an Abyssinian cattery. *J Am Vet Med Assoc.* 1999;215:948–951.
76. Herrewegh AA, Mahler M, Hedrich HJ, et al. Persistence and evolution of feline coronavirus in a closed cat-breeding colony. *Virology.* 1997;234:349–363.
77. Fish EJ, Diniz PPV, Juan YC, et al. Cross-sectional quantitative RT-PCR study of feline coronavirus viremia and replication in peripheral blood of healthy shelter cats in Southern California. *J Feline Med Surg.* 2018;20:295–301.
78. Poland AM, Vennema H, Foley JE, et al. Two related strains of feline infectious peritonitis virus isolated from immunocompromised cats infected with a feline enteric coronavirus. *J Clin Microbiol.* 1996;34:3180–3184.
79. Chang HW, Egberink HF, Halpin R, et al. Spike protein fusion peptide and feline coronavirus virulence. *Emerg Infect Dis.* 2012;18:1089–1095.
80. Chang HW, de Groot RJ, Egberink HF, et al. Feline infectious peritonitis: insights into feline coronavirus pathobiogenesis and epidemiology based on genetic analysis of the viral 3c gene. *J Gen Virol.* 2010;91:415–420.
81. Hora AS, Tonietti PO, Taniwaki SA, et al. Feline coronavirus 3c protein: a candidate for a virulence marker? *BioMed Res Int.* 2016;2016:8560691.
82. Barker EN, Tasker S, Gruffydd-Jones TJ, et al. Phylogenetic analysis of feline coronavirus strains in an epizootic outbreak of feline infectious peritonitis. *J Vet Intern Med.* 2013;27:445–450.
83. Hsieh LE, Huang WP, Tang DJ, et al. 3C protein of feline coronavirus inhibits viral replication independently of the autophagy pathway. *Res Vet Sci.* 2013;95:1241–1247.
84. Licitra BN, Millet JK, Regan AD, et al. Mutation in spike protein cleavage site and pathogenesis of feline coronavirus. *Emerg Infect Dis.* 2013;19:1066–1073.
85. Takano T, Tomiyama Y, Katoh Y, et al. Mutation of neutralizing/antibody-dependent enhancing epitope on spike protein and 7b gene of feline infectious peritonitis virus: influences of viral replication in monocytes/macrophages and virulence in cats. *Virus Res.* 2011;156:72–80.
86. Jacobse-Geels HE, Daha MR, Horzinek MC. Isolation and characterization of feline C3 and evidence for the immune complex pathogenesis of feline infectious peritonitis. *J Immunol.* 1980;125:1606–1610.
87. Dewerchin HL, Cornelissen E, Van Hamme E, et al. Surface-expressed viral proteins in feline infectious peritonitis virus-infected monocytes are internalized through a clathrin- and caveolae-independent pathway. *J Gen Virol.* 2008;89:2731–2740.
88. Dewerchin HL, Desmarets LM, Noppe Y, et al. Myosins 1 and 6, myosin light chain kinase, actin and microtubules cooperate during antibody-mediated internalisation and trafficking of membrane-expressed viral antigens in feline infectious peritonitis virus infected monocytes. *Vet Res.* 2014;45:17.
89. Kipar A, May H, Menger S, et al. Morphologic features and development of granulomatous vasculitis in feline infectious peritonitis. *Vet Pathol.* 2005;42:321–330.
90. Weiss RC, Dodds WJ, Scott FW. Disseminated intravascular coagulation in experimentally induced feline infectious peritonitis. *Am J Vet Res.* 1980;41:663–671.
91. Kyuwa S, Tagawa Y, Machii K, et al. MHV-induced fatal peritonitis in mice lacking IFN-gamma. *Adv Exp Med Biol.* 1998;440:445–450.
92. Legendre AM, Bartges JW. Effect of Polyprenyl Immunostimulant on the survival times of three cats with the dry form of feline infectious peritonitis. *J Feline Med Surg.* 2009;11:624–626.
93. Spencer SE, Knowles T, Ramsey IK, et al. Pyrexia in cats: retrospective analysis of signalment, clinical investigations, diagnosis and influence of

prior treatment in 106 referred cases. *J Feline Med Surg*. 2017;19:1123–1130.
94. Hugo TB, Heading KL. Prolonged survival of a cat diagnosed with feline infectious peritonitis by immunohistochemistry. *Can Vet J*. 2015;56:53–58.
95. Van Kruiningen HJ, Ryan MJ, Shindel NM. The classification of feline colitis. *J Comp Pathol*. 1983;93:275–294.
96. Foley JE, Lapointe JM, Koblik P, et al. Diagnostic features of clinical neurologic feline infectious peritonitis. *J Vet Intern Med*. 1998;12:415–423.
97. Fankauser R, Fatzer R. Meningitis and chorioependymitis granulomatosa der Katze. Mögliche beziehungen zur felinen infectiösen peritonitis (FIP). *Kleintier-Praxis*. 1977;22:19–22.
98. Krum S, Johnson K, Wilson J. Hydrocephalus associated with the noneffusive form of feline infectious peritonitis. *J Am Vet Med Assoc*. 1975;167:746–748.
99. Marioni-Henry K. Feline spinal cord diseases. *Vet Clin North Am Small Anim Pract*. 2010;40:1011–1028.
100. Louveau A, Smirnov I, Keyes TJ, et al. Structural and functional features of central nervous system lymphatic vessels. *Nature*. 2015;523:337–341.
101. Peiffer Jr RL, Wilcock BP. Histopathologic study of uveitis in cats: 139 cases (1978-1988). *J Am Vet Med Assoc*. 1991;198:135–138.
102. Wiggans KT, Vernau W, Lappin MR, et al. Diagnostic utility of aqueocentesis and aqueous humor analysis in dogs and cats with anterior uveitis. *Vet Ophthalmol*. 2014;17:212–220.
103. Wegg ML, Jeanes EC, Pollard D, et al. A multicenter retrospective study into endogenous causes of uveitis in cats in the United Kingdom. Ninety two cases. *Vet Ophthalmol*. 2021;24:591-598..
104. Tasker S. Diagnosis of feline infectious peritonitis: update on evidence supporting available tests. *J Feline Med Surg*. 2018;20:228–243.
105. Hartmann K, Binder C, Hirschberger J, et al. Comparison of different tests to diagnose feline infectious peritonitis. *J Vet Intern Med*. 2003;17:781–790.
106. Hartmann K, Ritz S. Treatment of cats with feline infectious peritonitis. *Vet Immunol Immunopathol*. 2008;123:172–175.
107. Jeffery U, Deitz K, Hostetter S. Positive predictive value of albumin: globulin ratio for feline infectious peritonitis in a mid-western referral hospital population. *J Feline Med Surg*. 2012;14:903–905.
108. Addie D, Belak S, Boucraut-Baralon C, et al. Feline infectious peritonitis. ABCD guidelines on prevention and management. *J Feline Med Surg*. 2009;11:594–604.
109. Court MH, Greenblatt DJ. Molecular genetic basis for deficient acetaminophen glucuronidation by cats: UGT1A6 is a pseudogene, and evidence for reduced diversity of expressed hepatic UGT1A isoforms. *Pharmacogenetics*. 2000;10:355–369.
110. Taylor SS, Tappin SW, Dodkin SJ, et al. Serum protein electrophoresis in 155 cats. *J Feline Med Surg*. 2010;12:643–653.
111. Zoia A, Slater LA, Heller J, et al. A new approach to pleural effusion in cats: markers for distinguishing transudates from exudates. *J Feline Med Surg*. 2009;11:847–855.
112. Fischer Y, Sauter-Louis C, Hartmann K. Diagnostic accuracy of the Rivalta test for feline infectious peritonitis. *Vet Clin Pathol*. 2012;41:558–567.
113. Crawford AH, Stoll AL, Sanchez-Masian D, et al. Clinicopathologic features and magnetic resonance imaging findings in 24 cats with histopathologically confirmed neurologic feline infectious peritonitis. *J Vet Intern Med*. 2017;31:1477–1486.
114. Ceciliani F, Grossi C, Giordano A, et al. Decreased sialylation of the acute phase protein alpha1-acid glycoprotein in feline infectious peritonitis (FIP). *Vet Immunol Immunopathol*. 2004;99:229–236.
115. Paltrinieri S, Giordano A, Tranquillo V, et al. Critical assessment of the diagnostic value of feline alpha1-acid glycoprotein for feline infectious peritonitis using the likelihood ratios approach. *J Vet Diagn Invest*. 2007;19:266–272.
116. Lewis KM, O'Brien RT. Abdominal ultrasonographic findings associated with feline infectious peritonitis: a retrospective review of 16 cases. *J Am Anim Hosp Assoc*. 2010;46:152–160.
117. Meli ML, Burr P, Decaro N, et al. Samples with high virus load cause a trend toward lower signal in feline coronavirus antibody tests. *J Feline Med Surg*. 2013;15:295–299.
118. Kennedy MA, Abd-Eldaim M, Zika SE, et al. Evaluation of antibodies against feline coronavirus 7b protein for diagnosis of feline infectious peritonitis in cats. *Am J Vet Res*. 2008;69:1179–1182.
119. Addie DD, le Poder S, Burr P, et al. Utility of feline coronavirus antibody tests. *J Feline Med Surg*. 2015;17:152–162.
120. Takano T, Katoh Y, Doki T, et al. Effect of chloroquine on feline infectious peritonitis virus infection in vitro and in vivo. *Antiviral Res*. 2013;99:100–107.
121. Boettcher IC, Steinberg T, Matiasek K, et al. Use of anti-coronavirus antibody testing of cerebrospinal fluid for diagnosis of feline infectious peritonitis involving the central nervous system in cats. *J Am Vet Med Assoc*. 2007;230:199–205.
122. Steinberg TA, Boettcher IC, Matiasek K, et al. Use of albumin quotient and IgG index to differentiate blood- vs brain-derived proteins in the cerebrospinal fluid of cats with feline infectious peritonitis. *Vet Clin Pathol*. 2008;37:207–216.
123. Soma T, Saito N, Kawaguchi M, et al. Feline coronavirus antibody titer in cerebrospinal fluid from cats with neurological signs. *J Vet Med Sci*. 2018;80:59–62.
124. Pedersen NC, Liu H, Dodd KA, et al. Significance of coronavirus mutants in feces and diseased tissues of cats suffering from feline infectious peritonitis. *Viruses*. 2009;1:166–184.
125. Hornyak A, Balint A, Farsang A, et al. Detection of subgenomic mRNA of feline coronavirus by real-time polymerase chain reaction based on primer-probe energy transfer (P-sg-QPCR). *J Virol Methods*. 2012;181:155–163.
126. Stranieri A, Giordano A, Paltrinieri S, et al. Comparison of the performance of laboratory tests in the diagnosis of feline infectious peritonitis. *J Vet Diagn Invest*. 2018;30:459–463.
127. Doenges SJ, Weber K, Dorsch R, et al. Detection of feline coronavirus in cerebrospinal fluid for diagnosis of feline infectious peritonitis in cats with and without neurological signs. *J Feline Med Surg*. 2016;18:104–109.
128. Pedersen NC, Eckstrand C, Liu H, et al. Levels of feline infectious peritonitis virus in blood, effusions, and various tissues and the role of lymphopenia in disease outcome following experimental infection. *Vet Microbiol*. 2015;175:157–166.
129. Felten S, Weider K, Doenges S, et al. Detection of feline coronavirus spike gene mutations as a tool to diagnose feline infectious peritonitis. *J Feline Med Surg*. 2017;19:321–335.
130. Longstaff L, Porter E, Crossley VJ, et al. Feline coronavirus quantitative reverse transcriptase polymerase chain reaction on effusion samples in cats with and without feline infectious peritonitis. *J Feline Med Surg*. 2017;19:240–245.
131. Harvey CJ, Lopez JW, Hendrick MJ. An uncommon intestinal manifestation of feline infectious peritonitis: 26 cases (1986-1993). *J Am Vet Med Assoc*. 1996;209:1117–1120.
132. Kipar A, Koehler K, Bellmann S, et al. Feline infectious peritonitis presenting as a tumour in the abdominal cavity. *Vet Rec*. 1999;144:118–122.
133. True LD. Quality control in molecular immunohistochemistry. *Histochem Cell Biol*. 2008;130:473–480.
134. Giori L, Giordano A, Giudice C, et al. Performances of different diagnostic tests for feline infectious peritonitis in challenging clinical cases. *J Small Anim Pract*. 2011;52:152–157.
135. Litster AL, Pogranichniy R, Lin TL. Diagnostic utility of a direct immunofluorescence test to detect feline coronavirus antigen in macrophages in effusive feline infectious peritonitis. *Vet J*. 2013;198:362–366.
136. Felten S, Matiasek K, Gruendl S, et al. Investigation into the utility of an immunocytochemical assay in body cavity effusions for diagnosis of feline infectious peritonitis. *J Feline Med Surg*. 2017;19:410–418.
137. Ives EJ, Vanhaesebrouck AE, Cian F. Immunocytochemical demonstration of feline infectious peritonitis virus within cerebrospinal fluid macrophages. *J Feline Med Surg*. 2013;15:1149–1153.
138. Doki T, Takano T, Kawagoe K, et al. Therapeutic effect of anti-feline TNF-alpha monoclonal antibody for feline infectious peritonitis. *Res Vet Sci*. 2016;104:17–23.
139. Fischer Y, Ritz S, Weber K, et al. Randomized, placebo controlled study of the effect of propentofylline on survival time and quality of life of

cats with feline infectious peritonitis. *J Vet Intern Med.* 2011;25:1270–1276.
140. Legendre AM, Kuritz T, Galyon G, et al. Polyprenyl immunostimulant treatment of cats with presumptive non-effusive feline infectious peritonitis in a field study. *Front Vet Sci.* 2017;4:7.
141. Ishida T, Shibanai A, Tanaka S, et al. Use of recombinant feline interferon and glucocorticoid in the treatment of feline infectious peritonitis. *J Feline Med Surg.* 2004;6:107–109.
142. Ritz S, Egberink H, Hartmann K. Effect of feline interferon-omega on the survival time and quality of life of cats with feline infectious peritonitis. *J Vet Intern Med.* 2007;21:1193–1197.
143. van der Meer FJ, de Haan CA, Schuurman NM, et al. Antiviral activity of carbohydrate-binding agents against Nidovirales in cell culture. *Antiviral Res.* 2007;76:21–29.
144. van der Meer FJ, de Haan CA, Schuurman NM, et al. The carbohydrate-binding plant lectins and the non-peptidic antibiotic pradimicin A target the glycans of the coronavirus envelope glycoproteins. *J Antimicrob Chemother.* 2007;60:741–749.
145. Pfefferle S, Schopf J, Kogl M, et al. The SARS-coronavirus-host interactome: identification of cyclophilins as target for pan-coronavirus inhibitors. *PLoS Pathog.* 2011;7:e1002331.
146. Tanaka Y, Sato Y, Sasaki T. Suppression of coronavirus replication by cyclophilin inhibitors. *Viruses.* 2013;5:1250–1260.
147. Balzarini J, Keyaerts E, Vijgen L, et al. Inhibition of feline (FIPV) and human (SARS) coronavirus by semisynthetic derivatives of glycopeptide antibiotics. *Antiviral Res.* 2006;72:20–33.
148. Balzarini J, Keyaerts E, Vijgen L, et al. Pyridine N-oxide derivatives are inhibitory to the human SARS and feline infectious peritonitis coronavirus in cell culture. *J Antimicrob Chemother.* 2006;57:472–481.
149. Keyaerts E, Vijgen L, Pannecouque C, et al. Plant lectins are potent inhibitors of coronaviruses by interfering with two targets in the viral replication cycle. *Antiviral Res.* 2007;75:179–187.
150. Takano T, Nakano K, Doki T, et al. Differential effects of viroporin inhibitors against feline infectious peritonitis virus serotypes I and II. *Arch Virol.* 2015;160:1163–1170.
151. Liu IJ, Tsai WT, Hsieh LE, et al. Peptides corresponding to the predicted heptad repeat 2 domain of the feline coronavirus spike protein are potent inhibitors of viral infection. *PLoS One.* 2013;8:e82081.
152. McDonagh P, Sheehy PA, Norris JM. In vitro inhibition of feline coronavirus replication by small interfering RNAs. *Vet Microbiol.* 2011;150:220–229.
153. Anis EA, Wilkes RP, Kania SA, et al. Effect of small interfering RNAs on in vitro replication and gene expression of feline coronavirus. *Am J Vet Res.* 2014;75:828–834.
154. Anis EA, Dhar M, Legendre AM, et al. Transduction of hematopoietic stem cells to stimulate RNA interference against feline infectious peritonitis. *J Feline Med Surg.* 2017;19:680–686.
155. Pedersen NC, Kim Y, Liu H, et al. Efficacy of a 3C-like protease inhibitor in treating various forms of acquired feline infectious peritonitis. *J Feline Med Surg.* 2018;20:378–392.
156. Kim Y, Mandadapu SR, Groutas WC, et al. Potent inhibition of feline coronaviruses with peptidyl compounds targeting coronavirus 3C-like protease. *Antiviral Res.* 2013;97:161–168.
157. Kim Y, Liu H, Galasiti Kankanamalage AC, et al. Reversal of the progression of fatal coronavirus infection in cats by a broad-spectrum coronavirus protease inhibitor. *PLoS Pathog.* 2016;12:e1005531.
158. Carr F. *Pfizer's new COVID 19 drug: paxlovid.* Dartmouth Undergraduate Journal of Science; 2021. Available at: https://sites.dartmouth.edu/dujs/2021/12/08/pfizers-new-covid-19-drug-paxlovid/.
159. Anivive. *Thanks to cats, one promising coronavirus treatment is already in development: the GC376 story*; 2022. Available at: https://anivive.com/coronavirus.
160. Barlough JE, Scott FW. Effectiveness of three antiviral agents against FIP virus in vitro. *Vet Rec.* 1990;126:556–558.
161. Weiss RC, Cox NR, Martinez ML. Evaluation of free or liposome-encapsulated ribavirin for antiviral therapy of experimentally induced feline infectious peritonitis. *Res Vet Sci.* 1993;55:162–172.
162. Murphy BG, Perron M, Murakami E, et al. The nucleoside analog GS-441524 strongly inhibits feline infectious peritonitis (FIP) virus in tissue culture and experimental cat infection studies. *Vet Microbiol.* 2018;219:226–233.
163. Pedersen NC, Perron M, Bannasch M, et al. Efficacy and safety of the nucleoside analog GS-441524 for treatment of cats with naturally occurring feline infectious peritonitis. *J Feline Med Surg.* 2019;21:271–281.
164. Jones S, Novicoff W, Nadeau J, et al. Unlicensed GS-441524-like antiviral therapy can be effective for at-home treatment of feline infectious peritonitis. *Animals (Basel).* 2021;11:2257.
165. Dickinson PJ, Bannasch M, Thomasy SM, et al. Antiviral treatment using the adenosine nucleoside analogue GS-441524 in cats with clinically diagnosed neurological feline infectious peritonitis. *J Vet Intern Med.* 2020;34:1587–1593.
166. Zhang S. *A much-hyped COVID-19 drug is almost identical to a black-market cat cure. The Atlantic*; 2020. Available at: https://www.theatlantic.com/science/archive/2020/05/remdesivir-cats/611341/.
167. Pedersen NC. The long history of Beta-d-N4-hydroxycytidine and its modern application to treatment of Covid-19 in people and FIP in cats. Available at: https://ccah.vetmed.ucdavis.edu/sites/g/files/dgvnsk4586/files/inline-files/Molnuparivir%20as%20a%20third%20antiviral%20drug%20for%20treatment%20of%20FIP%20v13_1.pdf; 2021.
168. Krentz D, Zenger K, Alberer M, et al. Curing cats with feline infectious peritonitis with an oral multi-component drug containing GS-441524. *Viruses.* 2021;13:2228.
169. Hughes D, Howard G, Malik R. *Treatment of FIP in cats with remdesivir. Clinical review.* The Veterinarian; 2021. Available at: https://www.turramurravet.com.au/wp-content/uploads/2021/07/FIP-Article_The-Veterinarian.pdf.
170. Pearson M, LaVoy A, Evans S, et al. Mucosal immune response to feline enteric coronavirus infection. *Viruses.* 2019;11:906.
171. Brandtzaeg P. Induction of secretory immunity and memory at mucosal surfaces. *Vaccine.* 2007;25:5467–5484.
172. Saif LJ. Animal coronavirus vaccines: lessons for SARS. *Dev Biol.* 2004;119:129–140.
173. Mustaffa-Kamal F, Liu H, Pedersen NC, et al. Characterization of antiviral T cell responses during primary and secondary challenge of laboratory cats with feline infectious peritonitis virus (FIPV). *BMC Vet Res.* 2019;15:165.
174. Addie DD, Jarrett O. Control of feline coronavirus infection in kittens. *Vet Rec.* 1990;126:164.
175. Gerber JD, Ingersoll JD, Gast AM, et al. Protection against feline infectious peritonitis by intranasal inoculation of a temperature-sensitive FIPV vaccine. *Vaccine.* 1990;8:536–542.
176. Reeves NC, Pollock RV, Thurber ET. Long-term follow-up study of cats vaccinated with a temperature-sensitive feline infectious peritonitis vaccine. *Cornell Vet.* 1992;82:117–123.
177. Fehr D, Holznagel E, Bolla S, et al. Placebo-controlled evaluation of a modified life virus vaccine against feline infectious peritonitis: safety and efficacy under field conditions. *Vaccine.* 1997;15:1101–1109.
178. Scherk MA, Ford RB, Gaskell RM, et al. 2013 AAFP feline vaccination advisory panel report. *J Feline Med Surg.* 2013;15:785–808.
179. Shi J, Wen Z, Zhong G, et al. Susceptibility of ferrets, cats, dogs, and other domesticated animals to SARS-coronavirus 2. *Science.* 2020;368:1016–1020.

32

Feline Leukemia Virus Infection

Katrin Hartmann, Regina Hofmann-Lehmann, Jane E. Sykes

KEY POINTS

- Cause: FeLV, a gammaretrovirus of domestic cats, is a member of the *Oncornavirus* subfamily of retroviruses. It contains a protein core with single-stranded RNA protected by an envelope.
- First Described: FeLV was first described in 1964 by William Jarrett and coworkers, when virus particles were seen budding from the membrane of malignant lymphoblasts from a cat with naturally occurring lymphoma. Although clusters of lymphoma cases occurring in households had always been observed, it was not until the discovery of FeLV that an infectious etiology was finally proven.
- Affected Hosts: In nature, FeLV mainly infects domestic cats. Some wild felids are also susceptible.
- Geographic Distribution: FeLV infection occurs worldwide. For many years after its discovery, FeLV was considered to account for most disease-related deaths in pet cats, and was responsible for more clinical syndromes than any other single agent.
- Route of Transmission: Prolonged close contact with salivary secretions is the most common mode of transmission, and less frequently FeLV is transmitted through biting, transplacental transmission, transmission through milk, and through blood transfusion.
- Major Clinical Signs: Most common clinical signs include lethargy, pallor, signs of stomatitis, signs of underlying lymphoma or leukemia, signs of immune-mediated disorders, or signs of opportunistic infections.
- Differential Diagnoses: For cats with immunosuppression, FIV infection is the primary differential diagnosis; for cats with stomatitis, FCV infection or FIV infection are the differential diagnoses; for cats with immune-mediated diseases and cytopenias, primary immune-mediated disease and other bone marrow diseases are the differential diagnoses.
- Human Health Significance: FeLV does not infect humans.

ETIOLOGIC AGENT AND EPIDEMIOLOGY

FeLV is a gammaretrovirus of domestic cats that belongs to the *Oncornavirus* subfamily of retroviruses. It was first described in 1964 by William Jarrett and coworkers, when virus particles were seen budding from the membrane of malignant lymphoblasts from a cat with naturally occurring lymphoma.[1-4] FeLV contains a protein core with single-stranded RNA protected by an envelope. FeLV is an exogenous agent that replicates within many tissues, including bone marrow, salivary glands, and respiratory epithelium. If the immune response does not intervene after initial infection, FeLV spreads to the bone marrow and infects hematopoietic precursor cells. All retroviruses, including FeLV, rely on a DNA intermediate for replication. The single-stranded RNA genome is reversely transcribed into DNA, which is integrated into the host's cell genome as *provirus* with the help of an integrase enzyme. After reverse transcription, synthesis of viral proteins occurs with assembly of the virions near the cell membrane and budding from the cell. Once the provirus is integrated, cell division results in daughter cells that also contain viral DNA. The ability of the virus to become part of the host's own DNA is crucial for the lifelong persistence of the virus after bone marrow infection.

Both exogenous (foreign, "pathogenic") and endogenous (inherited, mostly "nonpathogenic") retroviruses occur in cats.[5] Pathogenic exogenous viruses that can be transmitted horizontally from cat to cat include FeLV, FIV, and FFV (previously known as syncytium-forming virus, see Chapter 36), which is widespread but has a low pathogenicity.

On the basis of similarities in nucleotide sequences, it is likely that FeLV evolved from a virus in an ancestor of the rat. It is assumed that this event took place in the late Pleistocene up to 10 million years ago in the North African desert. Ancestral rats and cats roamed freely, and the virus was transmitted to cats through ingestion or a rat bite. The initial spread of FeLV among cats might have been inhibited by the aridity of the North African desert.[6]

FeLV is divided into several subgroups, but only subgroup FeLV-A is infectious and transmitted from cat to cat. The other subgroups (e.g., FeLV-B and FeLV-C) are not transmitted from cat to cat under natural circumstances but can be generated *de novo* in a FeLV-A-infected cat by mutation or recombination of the FeLV-A genome with cellular genes or genes from endogenous retroviruses in the cat's genome. The feline sarcoma virus (FeSV) also is a recombination of the FeLV-A genome with tumor-associated cellular genes (proto-oncogenes) and likewise is generated *de novo* in a FeLV-A-infected cat.

The endogenous counterparts of exogenous FeLV, termed enFeLVs, are integrated into the genome of domestic cats and closely related wild felids. EnFeLV is thought to have originated hundreds of thousands of years ago from cats that had eaten mice viremic with a murine leukemia virus (MuLV) that was able to incorporate its genome into the germline cells of the predator. This MuLV was then inherited by the feline offspring in a Mendelian manner. EnFeLVs are present in every cat and every feline cell. In contrast, more recently integrated endogenous elements can display polymorphisms among cats. As enFeLV elements are generally mutated and nonfunctional, they do not form infectious virions, although expression of short transcripts has been observed.[7] Recombination can occur between enFeLV and exogenous FeLV-A following infection, which can give rise to pathogenic viruses. Transduction of enFeLV *env* sequences encoding for the viral envelope can lead to development of FeLV-B or FeLV-D.[8-10] In addition, parts of, or the entire, *gag* genes of enFeLV have been identified in FeLV isolates from naturally infected cats.[11] Moreover, truncated envelope proteins encoded by enFeLV (FeLIX) can facilitate infection with fusion-defective exogenous FeLV by binding to the cellular receptor.[12] FeLIX activity was detected at a functional level in sera from domestic cats.[13] EnFeLV loads can vary among different cat populations and are influenced by the breed and gender of the cat.[14] An association between enFeLV loads and FeLV-A replication but not with outcome of FeLV infection was demonstrated.[15] Full-length enFeLV elements with putative functional open reading frames have been characterized.[16] These are present in only 9% to 15% of domestic cats suggesting that they are relatively recent additions to the feline genome.[17]

Other endogenous retroviral elements are also found in cats, such as RD-114, which is most closely related to an endogenous baboon retrovirus. RD-114 elements and RD-114-related sequences (RDRSs) likely entered the cat genome hundreds of thousands of years ago as a result of predation of early primates by ancestor cats, both before and after domestication.[18,19] No loci that encode infectious RD-114 could be found in the feline genome, but a virus nearly identical to RD-114 can be produced by recombination between two defective RD-114 virus-related proviruses.[20,21] Although there is no evidence of pathogenicity of RD-114 in cats, or an immune response to the virus, it could play a role in normal fetal differentiation.[22-24] Assays to screen for RD-114 infection in cell culture, and a method to establish cell lines with reduced risk of endogenous retroviruses have been developed.[25,26]

Various recombinations of RD-114, FeLV-related sequences, and the baboon endogenous virus have been characterized, now known as endogenous retroviruses of domestic cats (ERV-DCs). Several proviral clones have been identified and numbered according to their genomic insertions, for example, ERV-DC1, and classified into genotypes I, II, and III by phylogenetic analysis. Most contain deletions and mutations that render them noninfectious, but there are several ERV-DCs that are infectious in the domestic cat and can even infect human cell lines. Some of these are fixed in the cat genome, whereas others are mobile and have the potential to eventually disappear. Approximately one-third of cats tested in Japan carried ERV-DC10 loci.[8] It is unclear whether ERV-DCs are harmful or beneficial to the host. Hosts tend to tightly control their ERVs, particularly those with high transcriptional activity, for example by promotor methylation.[27]

FeLV Subgroups

FeLV subgroups are immunologically closely related but use different cellular receptors.[28-32] The three most established FeLV subgroups are FeLV-A, FeLV-B, and FeLV-C (Table 32.1). The cell surface entry receptor for FeLV-A is a putative thiamine transporter (THTR1) which is widely expressed in cat tissues. Therefore it was speculated that FeLV-A infection could disrupt thiamine uptake with pathological consequences.[33] Thiamine uptake was indeed blocked by FeLV-A; in feline fibroblasts that naturally express feline THTR1, this blockade resulted in a growth arrest at physiological concentrations of extracellular thiamine. THTR1 is highly conserved among different feline species (Iberian lynx, Asiatic and Indian lion, European wildcat, jaguarundi, domestic cat) and thus variations in the THTR1 sequence do not explain host species susceptibility differences.[34] FeLV-B uses Pit1 and Pit2 as receptors for virus entry; Pit1 and Pit2 normally function as sodium-dependent phosphate transporters.[28,32] The FeLV-C receptor (FLVCR) is a 12-transmembrane domain surface protein that exports heme from cells. FLVCR is required for erythroid maturation.[35-37] FLVCR is also important for development and maturation of CD4+ and CD8+ T cells.[38]

Only FeLV-A is transmitted horizontally from cat to cat in nature. The other subgroups evolve in FeLV-A-infected cats by mutation and recombination between FeLV-A and cellular or endogenous retroviral sequences contained in normal feline DNA. Subgroup B originates from recombination of FeLV-A with enFeLV. In one study of a closed colony of cats, multiple FeLV-B variants were generated in more than half of the cats infected with FeLV-A; horizontal transmission was also considered possible because of a high degree of genetic similarity of the variants among cats.[39] Subgroup C is less common and is the result of mutations in the *env* gene.[2]

Replication of FeLV-B and FeLV-C is usually only possible with the help of FeLV-A, because important genomic sequences are replaced in these recombinant viruses. Proposed FeLV-A helper functions include enhanced replication efficiency, immune evasion, and replication rescue for defective FeLV-B and FeLV-C virions. However, in newborn SPF kittens, experimental FeLV-B or FeLV-C infection was established without the presence of FeLV-A.[40,41] Moreover, by screening 300 field isolates using interference assays, two isolates, FeLV-2518 and FeLV-4314, displayed the FeLV-B phenotype alone in the absence of a fully functional helper FeLV-A virus.[42] Nevertheless, naturally infected cats usually carry FeLV-A either alone or in combination with FeLV-B, FeLV-C, or both. In consequence, if immunity to FeLV subgroup A is present, the cat has immunity to infection by any FeLV subtype.

In general, the pathogenicity of FeLV-B and FeLV-C, in combination with FeLV-A, is higher than that of FeLV-A alone.[43] Envelope protein differences among subtypes have been shown to be the major determinants of pathogenicity, but the mechanisms by which these differences influence pathogenesis are not well understood. FeLV-B infection is commonly associated with malignancies, especially thymic lymphoma. FeLV-C is mainly associated with nonregenerative anemia.[44]

Other FeLV subgroups have been described more recently. FeLV-D arises from recombination of FeLV-A and the *env* gene of a feline endogenous gammaretrovirus (ERV-DC), genotype I.[8,45] FeLV-D was detected in the blood or tumor tissues of three of 283 FeLV-infected cats, but its infectivity and pathogenicity remain unclear. Receptors for FeLV-D have not yet been identified. FeLV-T is highly cytolytic for T lymphocytes and causes severe immunosuppression[46-48] but is likely not important in the field. FeLV-T also uses Pit-1 as a receptor, like FeLV-B, but for reasons that remain unclear, the host ranges of FeLV-B and FeLV-T are not exactly the same.[32] FeLV-T is fusion-defective and requires the cofactor FeLIX to infect cells. As described earlier, FeLIX is a truncated envelope protein encoded by an endogenous FeLV, which can function as either a transmembrane protein or a soluble component to facilitate infection.[12,13,49] Another subgroup that can be found experimentally, "FeLV feline-acquired immunodeficiency syndrome" (FeLV-FAIDS) virus, is composed of FeLV-A and

TABLE 32.1 Host Cellular Receptors for Major FeLV Subtypes

FeLV Subtype	Receptor	Receptor Function	Comments
FeLV-A	FeTHTR1[29]	Thiamine transporter protein	Present in all cats with FeLV infection; transmitted exogenously
FeLV-B	FePit1 or FePit2[404]	Inorganic phosphate transporter protein	Results from recombination between FeLV-A and feline endogenous FeLV-related retrovirus sequences; can facilitate development of lymphoma or enhance neuropathogenicity
FeLV-C	FLVCR[405]	Heme transporter protein	Arises from point mutations in FeLV-A *env* gene; associated with nonregenerative anemia

FePit, feline Pit; *FeTHTR1,* feline thiamine transporter 1; *FLVCR,* FeLV-C receptor.

a highly immunopathogenic variant that infects CD4+ and CD8+ T lymphocytes and B lymphocytes in blood, lymph nodes, and myeloid cells.[50] Widespread proliferation of this virus greatly impairs the host immune response. In 2016, the subgroup FeLV-TG35-2 was described, which originated from a FeLV-infected cat, TG35, in Japan;[51] a folate transporter has been identified as a possible receptor.[52]

Virus Genome and Proteins

FeLV is a typical retrovirus (Fig. 32.1). It contains a single-stranded RNA molecule that is transcribed into proviral DNA by the enzyme reverse transcriptase (RT) and subsequently integrated into the host cellular genome. The gene sequence contains long terminal repeats (LTRs), which are repeated sequences that have regulatory function and control expression of the other viral genes but generally do not code for a protein product. From the 5′ to the 3′ end, the gene order is LTR-*gag-pol-env*-LTR (Table 32.2). LTR regions play a critical role in viral tissue tropism and pathogenicity. Within the LTRs, recurrent enhancer sequences (or upstream region enhancers [UREs]) are frequently found in cats with myeloid leukemias and could play a role in oncogenesis.[53,54] For example, the U3-LTR region has the ability to upregulate the NFκB signaling pathway via activation of Ras-Raf-IκB kinase and degradation of IκB.[55] The *gag* (group-associated antigen) gene encodes internal structural proteins, including p15, p12, p27, and p10. The p27 protein is produced in amounts that exceed that necessary for assembly of new virus particles. Thus, p27 is abundant in the cytoplasm of individual infected cells and also in the blood of infected cats, which is why most available immunochromatographic tests, such as ELISA and IFA assays, are designed to detect this protein, either free in plasma or within neutrophils and platelets, respectively. Free p27 is also detectable in tears and saliva. The *pol* (polymerase) gene encodes the viral enzymes RT, polymerase, and integrase. The *env* (envelope) gene encodes the envelope components gp70 and p15E. The envelope protein gp70 defines the virus subgroup and appears to be important for inducing immunity. Antibodies to gp70 result in neutralization of the virus and immunity to reinfection. Thus, gp70 is important in natural resistance and therefore as a target for vaccine production. The transmembrane protein p15E is thought to interfere with host cell immune responses, which facilitates viral persistence.[56]

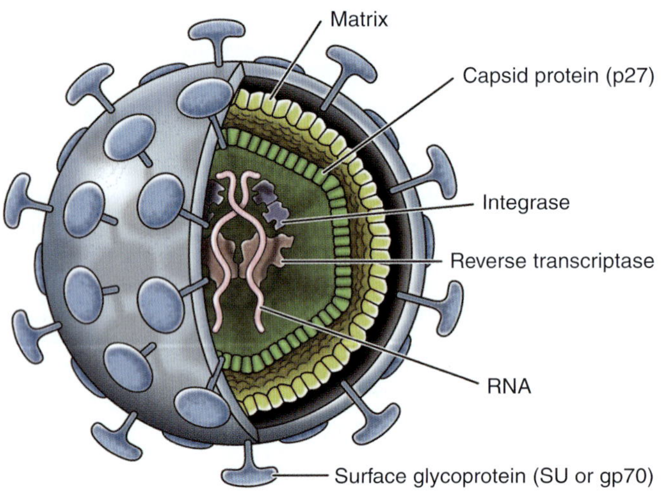

Fig. 32.1 Structure of feline leukemia virus. Gammaretroviruses contain two identical strands of RNA and associated enzymes, which include reverse transcriptase, integrase, and protease, packaged into a core composed of the capsid protein (p27) with a surrounding matrix, all enclosed by a phospholipid membrane envelope derived from the host cell. The envelope contains a gp70 glycoprotein and the transmembrane protein p15E.

Host Range

In nature, FeLV mainly infects domestic cats. Some wild felids are also susceptible. *In vitro*, FeLV also can replicate in nonfelid cell lines. FeLV-B replicates in cells derived from cats, dogs, cows, pigs, hamsters, monkeys, and humans; and FeLV-C replicates in cells of cats, dogs, guinea pigs, and humans.[1,57,58] Although certain human cell lines can be infected by FeLV-A, FeLV is not thought to pose a risk for humans; FeLV-A shed by cats carries carbohydrates on the virus envelope (α-Gal epitope) that are readily recognized by naturally occurring anti-αGal antibodies in humans, and the virus is neutralized by complement.[59] However, experimental FeLV infection with development of lymphoma could be induced in young dogs and marmosets.[60] In experimental infections with FeSV, fibrosarcomas also could be produced in nonfelids.[61] However, no reports exist on natural transmission of FeLV to nonfelids.

FeLV infection is enzootic in some wild felid populations, such as European wildcat populations. Introduction of FeLV into free-living and captive wild felid populations such as Florida panthers or the Iberian lynx has serious consequences for their health and survival. In several instances of FeLV infection in wild felids, contact with domestic cats was the source of infection. Within felids from lineage 8 (to which the domestic cat belongs), FeLV was isolated from the European wildcat (*Felis silvestris silvestris*).[62] FeLV-infected free-ranging European wildcats were reported in Great Britain, Switzerland, France, Germany, Portugal, and Spain.[63-69] Up to 49% of wildcats tested FeLV antigen–positive, but no evidence of FeLV-associated disease was found,

TABLE 32.2 Summary of the Genetic Map and Function of Feline Leukemia Virus Proteins

Gene	Location	Proteins	Function
gag	Core	p15	Matrix protein
		p12	Probably involved in the integration process
		p27	Capsid protein; used for antigen testing
		p10	Nucleocapsid protein
pol	Core	p14/PR	Protease
		p80/RT	Reverse transcriptase; enzyme copying viral RNA into complementary DNA strand
		p46/IN	Integrase
env	Envelope	gp70/SU	External surface unit; primary target for protective humoral immune response; FeLV subtype-specific antigens FeLV-A, FeLV-B, FeLV-C
		p15E/TM	Transmembrane protein; role in immunosuppression

although in one study the FeLV antigen–positive wildcats had poorer body condition than FeLV antigen–negative wildcats.[66] European wildcats that tested provirus-positive using PCR were significantly more often coinfected with feline hemoplasmas than FeLV provirus-negative wildcats.[70]

In the phylogenetic felid lineage 7 (the leopard cat lineage [genus *Otocolobus*]), FeLV antigen was detected in wild Pallas' cats (*Otocolobus* [*Felis*] *manul*) of the Daurian Steppe in Russia.[71]

FeLV has also been detected in lineage 6 felids (the puma lineage [genera *Puma* and *Acinonyx*]). Between 2002 and 2005, five Florida panthers died as a result of FeLV infection, with clinical signs of lymphadenopathy, anemia, and weight loss.[72,73] The outbreak likely originated from one cross-species transmission because the FeLV strain involved, FeLV-Pco, closely resembled a highly virulent FeLV strain of domestic cats. Due to the severity of the outbreak, a FeLV vaccination program for the Florida panthers was initiated. Evidence of FeLV infection was also detected in free-ranging Brazilian pumas,[74] free-ranging Brazilian jaguarundis (*Puma yagouaroundi*),[75] captive cheetahs (*Acinonyx jubats*),[76,77] and 5.4% of 490 California mountain lions sampled between 1990 and 2008.[78]

In the lynx lineage 5 (genus *Lynx*), FeLV was detected in an 11-month-old captive-bred bobcat (*Lynx rufus*) that had signs of lethargy, anorexia, neutropenia, lymphopenia, and nonregenerative anemia.[79] The bobcat had been in contact with a domestic cat (surrogate mother), which was suspected to be the source of the infection. Based on sequencing analysis, FeLV-A from domestic cats was also assumed to be the source of FeLV infection in critically endangered Iberian lynxes (*Lynx pardinus*) in Southern Spain.[80] FeLV provirus in the absence of detectable circulating antigen was detected in 6 of 21 lynxes between 1993 and 2003. A subsequent study on 77 of the approximately 200 remaining free-ranging Iberian lynxes in the same area between 2003 and 2007 revealed 14 FeLV provirus-positive animals, but at that time most of the animals were also antigen-positive.[81] During a 6-month period in 2007, about two-thirds of the FeLV-infected lynxes died.[82] High-throughput sequencing of the virus suggested that the virus most likely originated from domestic cats.[83] Many domestic cats and European wildcats were FeLV antigen–positive in the same area.[68,84] Preventative measures, including surveillance and vaccination programs for the Iberian lynx have therefore been introduced. Moreover, domestic cat populations should be controlled and vaccinated in order to reduce the infectious pressure on wildlife.

FeLV infection was also confirmed in several species of the ocelot lineage 4 (genus *Leopardus*), including free-ranging kodkods (*Leopardus guigna*) on a Chilean island, a captive ocelot (*Leopardus pardalis*) and a captive oncilla (*Leopardus tigrinus*) in Brazil,[85,86] and a margay (*Leopardus wiedii*) and pampas cats (*Leopardus pajeros*) in US zoological parks.[87] The pathogenic potential of FeLV in these felid species is unknown.

No studies are available on FeLV in felids of the lineages 3 and 2 (caracal and bay cat lineages), but multiple studies suggest that FeLV infection is absent in wild felids of the panthera lineage 1 (genus *Panthera*), a lineage that is not closely related to the domestic cat. FeLV infection was not detected in many studies of African lions (*Panthera leo*), Asian lions (*Panthera leo persica*), jaguars (*Panthera onca*), and Amur tigers (*Panthera tigris altaica*).[88-95] When a recombinant subunit FeLV vaccine was used in lions and tigers (*Panthera tigris*), no antibody response was observed.[96]

Prevalence

FeLV infection exists in domestic cats worldwide. Studies report a prevalence of 2.3% to 3.3% in the United States, 0% to 8.8% in Europe, 0% to 24.5% in Asia, and 0.5% to 21% in Australia.[97-116] Only cats on some islands such as Grenada, the West Indies, Isabela Island, and the Galapagos, have been found free of FeLV infection.[117-119]

The prevalence of FeLV infection varies depending on the health status of the cat population sampled.[120] In healthy free-roaming cats, the prevalence typically ranges from 1% to 8%.[98,101,103,120,121] In sick cats, the prevalence can be as high as 38%.[97,122,123]

The overall prevalence of FeLV infection used to be decreasing in many geographic areas.[97-99,101,103-105,123,124] The Tufts Veterinary Diagnostic Laboratory, where approximately 2000 serum samples are tested yearly for FeLV antigen, reported a decrease from 8% in 1989 to 4% in 1995.[125] In Germany, a steady decrease in FeLV prevalence from 6% to 1% was observed when investigating the FeLV infection rate from 1993 to 2002.[101] A study from Switzerland found a decrease from 9% to 3% in FeLV prevalence between 1990 and 2003.[126] The decrease in prevalence is most likely the result of test and removal programs at breeding facilities, the practice of testing cats at animal shelters before adoption, and the widespread use of vaccination. However, in more recent years, the prevalence of infection has plateaued.[101,126,127]

Models have been constructed to predict the dynamics of FeLV infection in cat populations. These predicted that FeLV dynamics depend on: (1) the size of the host population, and (2) the relationship between host density and the pattern of contacts of individual cats. They found no threshold population size for virus persistence in large populations but the possibility of FeLV extinction in small populations.[128] A study that included a large number of cats from the United States revealed a higher prevalence of FIV infections in the southern and eastern United States when compared to FeLV infection. In contrast, FeLV infections were more prevalent in the western United States when compared to FIV infections.[129] In a study of FeLV prevalence in 32 European countries, seven risk factors and three protective factors were found.[110] Among the risk factors was the geographic origin of the cat: FeLV prevalence was higher in southern countries compared to northern and western parts of Europe. Other risk factors included male intact sex, indoor and outdoor or outdoor-only residence, living in large groups of five or more animals, and being an ill cat.[110] Risk factors for FeLV and FIV infections are only slightly different. The prevalence of both infections is higher in cats that roam outside[101,103] because direct contact is required for transmission. Although fighting, free-roaming, intact male cats are still considered mainly at risk for acquiring FIV infection, the same factors can facilitate FeLV infection.[101,110,130] However, being male (neutered or not) and having access to the outdoors has a stronger impact on FIV prevalence than on FeLV prevalence, while presence of clinical illness is a stronger predictor for FeLV infection.[129]

Although FeLV transmission commonly occurs among infected queens and kittens and among cats living in prolonged close contact, aggressive behavior plays a greater role than previously reported.[131] Cats that exhibit aggressive behavior have a higher risk of FeLV infection,[101] and more than 8% of cats examined by veterinarians for fighting injuries were FeLV antigen–positive in one study, a prevalence considerably higher than in the clinically healthy cat population.[131]

Although no breeds are predisposed to being infected with FeLV, infection is less commonly found in purebred cats,[110] possibly because they are more commonly kept indoors. In addition, awareness in the cat-breeder community leads to frequent testing. In older studies, young age was considered a risk factor for FeLV infection. However, a study in the United States of 18,038 cats at 345 veterinary clinics and 145 animal shelters revealed that adult cats were more likely to be FeLV-infected than young cats.[103] In a study from Europe that included 6005 cats, cats aged 1 to 6 years were at greatest risk.[110] In another study, the median age of FeLV-infected cats was not lower than that of uninfected cats.[101]

This was unexpected because of the phenomenon of age-related resistance to FeLV infection.[132,133] However, because of increased awareness, more cats are tested for FeLV, FeLV infection is being recognized earlier, and medical care is provided during the initial stage of the disease. In addition, awareness among cat breeders and animal shelters has led to routine testing of new pets entering the household or shelter.

A genetic predisposition might contribute to a susceptibility of cats to FeLV infection. Analysis of single-nucleotide polymorphisms (SNPs) in the *APOBEC3H* gene of domestic cats showed that one of the SNPs was significantly correlated with the susceptibility to FIV and/or FeLV infections.[134]

With few exceptions, FeLV prevalence studies are based on detection of FeLV p27 antigen in blood. However, free antigen can usually only be detected in the blood of viremic cats (in progressively infected cats or in the early stage of regressive infection, see Pathogenesis), because those with regressive infections only harbor provirus, with no associated antigen production.[135] In a study from Switzerland, 7% of cats had both viral p27 antigen and provirus in blood, and 10% of cats had negative results for p27 antigen and positive results for proviral DNA in blood.[136] Comparable results were also found in a study from Germany where the number of antigen-positive, provirus-positive cats was similar to the number of antigen-negative, provirus-positive cats.[100]

Transmission

FeLV spreads through close contact between virus-shedding cats and susceptible cats. The transmission of FeLV occurs primarily via saliva. Viremic cats constantly shed millions of virus particles in saliva.[137,138] The concentration of virus in saliva and blood of healthy viremic cats is as high as it is in sick cats. Fighting and biting behavior,[101,131] as well as social behavior, such as sharing food and water dishes, mutual grooming, and using common litter areas, are the most effective means of transmission of FeLV. Although the virus can enter many tissues, body fluids, and secretions, urine and feces are less likely to be a source of infection for other cats. However, FeLV is shed in small amounts in feces and urine,[139,140] so fecal shedding of FeLV cannot fully be excluded as a mode of transmission.[140] FeLV RNA has been detected in fleas and their feces,[141,142] but flea transmission does not seem to play a major role in nature. Iatrogenic transmission can occur via contaminated needles, instruments, fomites, or blood transfusions.[143,144]

The viral envelope is lipid-soluble, and FeLV is readily inactivated in the environment (usually within minutes, but sometimes up to 48 hours). Therefore close contact among cats is usually required for spread of infection. Single cats kept strictly indoors are not at risk for acquiring infection. It is only because of latency (in regressively infected cats) and reactivation that viremia is occasionally detected in middle-aged to old cats that have lived alone indoors since they were adopted as kittens. A waiting period is not needed before introducing a new cat into a household after removal of an infected cat. FeLV transmission is not a risk in a veterinary hospital or boarding kennel scenario as long as cats are housed in separate cages, and routine cage disinfection and hand washing are performed between handling cats.[145]

Vertical transmission from mother to kittens occurs commonly. Neonatal kittens can be infected transplacentally or when the queen has close contact with them. Transmission also can occur in queens with regressive infection; FeLV transmission via milk to offspring from queens with FeLV antigen–negative test results has been described.[146] If *in utero* infection occurs, fetal resorption, abortion, and neonatal death can occur, although up to 20% of vertically infected kittens can survive the neonatal period to become progressively infected adults.[123] Newborn kittens from infected queens can have negative FeLV antigen test results at birth, but can test positive over subsequent weeks to months when viral replication accelerates. Thus, if the queen or any kitten in her litter is infected, the entire litter should be treated as if infected and isolated from uninfected cats.

Susceptibility to progressive infection, which is associated with persistent viremia and culminates in FeLV-associated disease, is highest in young kittens. It is more difficult in adult cats to achieve progressive infection after experimental infection, and depending on the FeLV strain used, experimental infection does not lead to progressive infection already in kittens older than 16 weeks of age.[132] Age-related resistance to FeLV also exists in nature. It has been suggested that age-related resistance might be related to a decline in the number of cellular receptors (THTR1) available for FeLV-A to enter target cells. Maturation of macrophage function might also play a role.[147] Thus, the risk of an adult cat becoming progressively infected after a brief interaction with a FeLV-shedding cat is very low.

CLINICAL FEATURES

Pathogenesis

Although outcome of infection mainly depends on immune status and age of the cat, it is also affected by pathogenicity of the virus. The outcome of FeLV infection thus also reflects genetic variation both in the virus and the host population. Certain viral mutations can increase the speed of disease onset, whereas others change disease outcome entirely, and it has been suggested that LTR and surface unit (SU) genes mediate a rapid pathogenesis with distinctive clinical features and oncogenic mechanisms.[123]

FeLV infection can have different courses. Once integrated into the cat genome, FeLV provirus can persist for years, and recurrence of viremia and disease can occur in some cats.[148,149] However, integrated viral DNA can also elicit solid protection and long-lasting maintenance of protective immunity.[150] The currently accepted stages of FeLV infection are: (1) abortive infection, (2) regressive infection, (3) progressive infection, and (4) focal or atypical infection.[150-152]

Although cats with only integrated proviral DNA without virus replication do not shed infectious virus in saliva, proviral DNA can be infectious via blood transfusion.[144] FeLV provirus and plasma viral RNA are usually detectable by PCR within 1 week of FeLV exposure, even if FeLV antigen is not. All cats with progressive and regressive infection can undergo this phase and develop similar proviral and plasma viral RNA loads in the peripheral blood during early infection.[150] However, later in the infection, proviral loads remain high in progressively infected cats but decrease in regressively infected cats.[136]

Abortive Infection

After initial infection, which most commonly occurs via oronasal routes, virus replicates in the local lymphoid tissue in the oropharyngeal area. In some immunocompetent cats, viral replication is halted by an effective humoral and cell-mediated immune response, and viremia does not occur.[135,151,153-156] Abortive infection has been observed infrequently after experimental FeLV inoculation with low inocula and is characterized by negative test results for culturable virus, antigen, viral RNA, and proviral DNA.[152,157] Thus, cats with abortive infection have high levels of neutralizing antibody, but neither FeLV antigen nor viral RNA or proviral DNA can be detected in the blood. In these cats, virus never spreads systemically, and infection usually remains undetected. Abortively infected cats have the same life expectancy as cats that have never been exposed to FeLV.[143] They have strong immunity and are protected against new viral challenges, probably for several years if not lifelong. Protective immunity is partly humoral and partly cellular, and antibody production is not necessarily required for protection; about 2% are protected without detectable antibodies.

Regressive Infection

Regressive infection follows an effective immune response, with containment of viremia before (or shortly after) the time of bone marrow infection. After initial infection, FeLV spreads systemically within lymphocytes and monocytes.[158] During this period, cats have positive results on ELISA antigen tests and shed virus. Cats can show lethargy, fever, or lymphadenomegaly resulting from lymphocytic hyperplasia during this phase. The virus spreads to target tissue, including thymus, spleen, lymph nodes, and salivary glands. In most cats, viremia lasts only a few weeks, but in some rare cases cats can overcome viremia even after many months.[159] On the other hand, some regressively infected cats are never antigen-positive.

In some cats, hematopoietic precursor cells in the bone marrow then become infected and produce infected neutrophils and platelets that circulate in the body.[158,160] A high level of viremia develops, and lymphoid organs and salivary glands become infected with up to 1×10^6 virus particles/mL of saliva. From this time point on, viral antigen is also detectable intracellularly in platelets and granulocytes by tests that detect large quantities of intracellular antigen, such as IFA. Even if bone marrow becomes infected, some cats can clear viremia (and develop regressive infection); however, the longer the viremia lasts, the less likely it will be contained. Once bone marrow cells are infected, cats will remain provirus-positive because proviral DNA persists in bone marrow stem cells. This has previously been referred to as "latent infection" of the marrow, but is now considered a stage of regressive infection. Once virus replication is contained, no intact virus is actively produced, so cats with regressive infection have negative results from routine tests (ELISA and IFA) that detect FeLV antigen. Regressive infection can only be detected using proviral PCR or culture of bone marrow samples in the presence of high doses of glucocorticoids. Productive infection can be reactivated spontaneously or with immune suppression with viremia and therefore positive results on antigen tests. Regressive infections can also reactivate in pregnancy, with reemergence of FeLV infection in kittens. Mammary glands of regressively infected queens can produce infectious viral particles with onset of lactation.[146]

Reactivation is more likely the earlier the stress factor occurs after the viremic phase. As time passes, regressive infections become more difficult to reactivate, even with high doses of glucocorticoids. Nevertheless, regressively infected cats stay provirus-positive and reactivation can take place many years after infection.[148,154] In one SPF cat that had been experimentally infected with FIV and FeLV, regressive FeLV infection occurred and the cat remained aviremic for over 8 years. Subsequently, a genetically altered FeLV virus reappeared with reactivation of viremia. This coincided with the development of multicentric lymphoma, likely because the immune system was by then, severely depleted due to the FIV infection.[148]

It is unclear how often regressive FeLV infection can result in FeLV-related disease. One study found a high prevalence of regressive infection in older cats at necropsy and suggested an association with hematologic changes and inflammatory processes.[161] In another study, two of 37 cats (5%) with nonregenerative cytopenias and negative FeLV antigen test had positive results with bone marrow provirus PCR.[162] FeLV provirus can be detected occasionally in lymphomas of some FeLV antigen–negative cats,[163-165] but a causative association has not been made. Cats from FeLV cluster households had a 40-fold higher incidence of FeLV antigen–negative lymphoma compared to cats from the general population. Two studies reported that regressive FeLV infections occurred in 50% to 52% of antigen-negative lymphomas in older cats (> 7 years),[164,166] while other groups found evidence of provirus in only 1 of 22,[167] in 1 of 10,[166] and in 0 of 50 FeLV antigen–negative lymphomas[169] suggesting that regressive infection is only rarely involved in tumor development.

Integrated FeLV provirus has the potential to interrupt or inactivate cellular genes in infected cells, or regulatory properties of viral DNA can alter expression of neighboring genes. In addition, because bone marrow microenvironment cells (e.g., myelomonocytic progenitor cells and stromal fibroblasts) provide a reservoir for regressive FeLV infections, provirus has the potential to alter cellular functions and contribute to the pathogenesis of myelosuppressive disorders. Finally, FeLV not only contributes its genes to the host, but also has been shown to appropriate (or "steal") cellular genes, which could have the potential to contribute to viral oncogenesis.[167,170,171] Replication-defective enFeLV can recombine with FeLV and thus produce infectious oncogenic particles. However, using next-generation RNA-sequencing, no expression of FeLV has yet been detected in feline tumor samples; in fact, there was even a decreased expression of endogenous retrovirus genes in lymphoma versus control specimens.[172]

Progressive Infection

In cats with progressive FeLV infection, extensive virus replication occurs, first in the lymphoid tissues and then in the bone marrow and in mucosal and glandular epithelial tissues in most infected cats.[56] Mucosal and glandular infection is associated with viral shedding, which persists for the life of the cat. Progressive infection is characterized by insufficient FeLV-specific immunity. Progressively infected cats have low levels of detectable neutralizing antibodies.[100,168] These cats usually develop FeLV-associated diseases that can be fatal.

Young and immunosuppressed cats are at higher risk for developing progressive infection. In a cat with a first-time single contact with a FeLV-shedding cat, the risk of developing progressive infection is less than 5%. However, if a shedding cat is introduced into a naïve group of cats, and the cats are housed together for an extended period, the risk increases to about 30%.[147]

Regressive and progressive infections can be distinguished by repeated testing for viral antigen in peripheral blood.[152] Many infected cats initially have positive antigen test results within 2 to 3 weeks after virus exposure. In case of regressive infection, cats will become negative in viral antigen tests 2 to 8 weeks later or, in rare cases, months later. Both progressive and regressive infections are almost always accompanied by persistent FeLV proviral DNA in blood. However, FeLV proviral and viral RNA loads in leukocytes, as analyzed by quantitative PCR, indicate that FeLV progressive infection is associated with secondary viremia of bone marrow origin, whereas regressive cats sustain only a nonproductive viral infection in low numbers of lymphocytes.[173] During acute infection, blood proviral and viral RNA loads of cats with progressive and regressive infections are not significantly different, which, however, changes after weeks.[136,151,152] Subsequently, cats with progressive infections have higher virus loads than cats with regressive infections, and virus loads within specific leukocyte subsets differ depending on the infection outcome.[160]

Focal or Atypical Infection

Focal infections or atypical infections have been reported as a rare form of infection in both experimental and natural infections. They are characterized by persistent atypical local viral replication in certain tissues, such as the spleen, lymph nodes, small intestine, or mammary glands.[146,174] This can lead to intermittent or low-grade production of p27 antigen. Therefore these cats can have weakly positive or discordant results in antigen tests, or positive and negative results can alternate. Queens with atypical infection of their mammary glands can transmit the virus to their kittens via milk in the face of negative antigen test results.[146]

Clinical Signs

Progressive infection with FeLV can result in tumors, hematologic disorders, immunosuppression, immune-mediated diseases, and other syndromes (including reproductive disorders, fading kitten syndrome, and neuropathy). The death rate of progressively infected cats in multicat households has been described as approximately 50% in 2 years and 80% in 3 years.[23,123] However, survival time of progressively infected cats kept indoors in single-cat households with good veterinary care can be much higher. Still, FeLV infection has the greatest impact on mortality in closed households with mixed endemic viral infections.[100,175] A large study in the United States compared the survival of more than 1000 FeLV-infected cats to more than 8000 age- and sex-matched uninfected control cats[103] and found that in FeLV-infected cats, median survival was 2.4 years compared to 6.0 years for control cats.

Most cats with FeLV-associated disease are evaluated not for tumors but for anemia or immunosuppression. Of 8642 FeLV-infected cats examined at US veterinary teaching hospitals, coinfections (including FIP, FIV infection, upper respiratory infection, hemotropic mycoplasmosis, and stomatitis) were the most frequent findings (15%), followed by anemia (11%), lymphoma (6%), leukopenia or thrombocytopenia (5%), and leukemia or myeloproliferative disease (4%).[176]

Disease expression can relate to virus factors, such as the FeLV subgroup (e.g., FeLV-B is primarily associated with tumors, FeLV-C is primarily associated with nonregenerative anemia), but clinical outcome is also strongly influenced by the age of the cat at the time of infection.[132] Neonatal kittens can develop marked thymic atrophy after infection ("fading kitten syndrome"), resulting in severe immunosuppression, wasting, and early death. As cats mature, they acquire resistance to infection. When older cats become infected, they tend to have abortive or regressive infections or, if they develop progressive infection, signs are milder and they usually have a more protracted period of apparent good health.[123]

Tumors

FeLV infection is most commonly associated with lymphoma and leukemia, and less commonly with other hematopoietic tumors. In addition, unusual forms of lymphoma, such as feline neurolymphomatosis[177] or other tumors, including osteochondromas, olfactory neuroblastoma, uterine adenocarcinoma, and cutaneous horns, have been described.

Feline oncornavirus cell membrane antigen (FOCMA) is an antigen present on the surface of transformed cells. FOCMA can be found on the surface of feline lymphoma and FeSV-induced fibrosarcoma cells but not on the surface of normal feline lymphocytes.[178,179] Many cats with FeLV in cluster households have antibodies against FOCMA. Those with the highest titers are most likely to remain free of malignancies. However, some cats that are viremic with a high FOCMA antibody titer can develop lymphoma or leukemia months or years later after the titer declined.[23] Currently, FOCMA is considered a nonhomogenous group of viral antigens that can, although not always, be present on the surface of FeLV-infected cells. At the least, FOCMA antibodies indicate exposure to FeLV but since tests for the detection of FOCMA are difficult to establish and to standardize, FOCMA is not considered to be of clinical value.

Lymphoma. Lymphomas and leukemias account for about 30% of all feline tumors, the highest proportion recorded in any animal species.[180-184] Progressively FeLV-infected cats have a 60-fold increased risk of lymphoma.[185] Lymphoma can affect up to 25% of cats with progressive FeLV infection, usually within 2 years after diagnosis of the infection. FeLV-induced lymphomas are mainly T-cell lymphomas.[186] Mediastinal lymphoma is the most common form (Fig. 32.2), followed

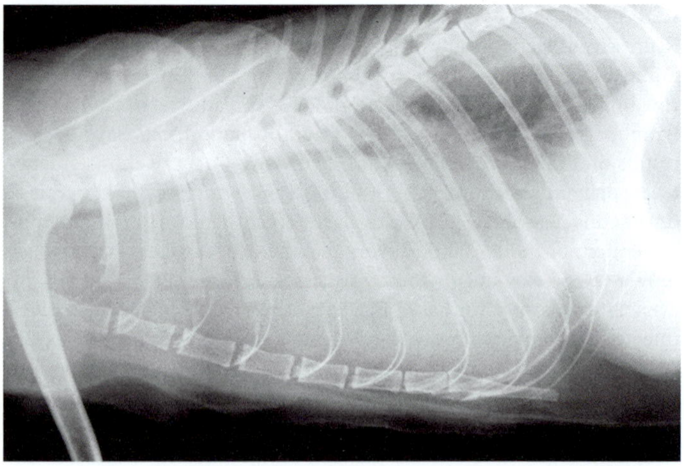

Fig. 32.2 Lateral thoracic radiograph of a cat with severe pleural effusion and mediastinal mass. The trachea is displaced dorsally, and the cardiac shadow is barely visible.

by multicentric lymphoma, although spinal, renal, ocular, and other forms of lymphoma are occasionally reported in progressively FeLV-infected cats.[187] In the past, young to middle-aged cats (median 7 years) were commonly diagnosed with lymphoma, but lymphoma is now a disease of mostly older cats with a median age of 11 years.[188] This also is likely a result of the decreasing prevalence of progressive FeLV infection as a contributing factor for development of lymphoma, as cats with FeLV-associated lymphoma are usually younger than cats with lymphoma without FeLV infection.[100] In addition, the incidence of FeLV antigen–negative lymphomas increased from approximately 18 cases per year before 1994 to approximately 32 cases per year from 1994 to 2003.[189]

In support of the association between FeLV infection and lymphoma, lymphoma can be induced in kittens by experimental FeLV infection;[190-192] cats naturally infected with FeLV have a higher risk of lymphoma than uninfected cats;[190,193] and in the past, when the prevalence of FeLV infection was higher, most cats with lymphoma had progressive FeLV infection. Previous studies showed that up to 80% of feline lymphomas and leukemias were FeLV-related.[194-197] A study conducted at a veterinary teaching hospital in Germany showed that from 1980 to 1995, 59% of cats with lymphoma were FeLV antigen–positive, but from 1996 to 1999, only 20% were positive.[188] In a study from the Netherlands, only 4 of 71 cats with lymphoma were FeLV antigen–positive, and 22 of these cats had mediastinal lymphoma, which previously was reported to be strongly associated with FeLV infection.[198]

The most important mechanism for the development of malignancy is insertion of the FeLV genome into the cellular genome near a cellular oncogene (most commonly *myc*). This results in activation and overexpression of that gene and uncontrolled proliferation of these cells. FeLV can also incorporate the oncogene to form a recombinant virus (e.g., FeLV-B, FeSV) which contains cellular oncogene sequences that are then rearranged and activated. When they enter a new cell, these recombinant viruses are oncogenic. Thus, FeLV-induced neoplasms are caused, at least in part, by somatically acquired insertional mutagenesis in which the integrated provirus activates a proto-oncogene or disrupts a tumor suppressor gene. In a study of 119 cats with lymphoma, transduction (insertion into) the *myc* locus had occurred in 38 cats (32%).[199] Transduction of the NOTCH2 gene by FeLV was described in a naturally infected cat with multicentric lymphoma.[200] Another study suggested that the U3-LTR region of FeLV could transactivate cancer-related signaling pathways through production of a noncoding 104-base RNA transcript that activates NF-κ B.[201] Twelve common integration sites for FeLV associated with lymphoma development have been identified in six loci: *c-myc, flvi-1, flvi-2* (contains *bmi-1*), *fit-1, pim-1,* and *flit-1*.[202] *C-myc* is a proto-oncogene, *bmi-1* and *pim-1* are myc-collaborators, *fit-1* appears to be closely linked to *myb*, and *flit-1* insertion was associated with overexpression of cellular genes, for example, activin-A receptor type II-like 1 (ACVRL1).[202] *Flit-1* was identified as an important proviral integration site. Of 35 FeLV-related tumors, 5 of 25 thymic lymphomas had proviral insertion within the *flit-1* locus, whereas none of four alimentary lymphomas, five of five multicentric lymphomas, and one T-lymphoid leukemia had rearrangements in this region. Some studies also show that variations in the FeLV surface glycoprotein can determine the development of tumors.[203] In one study, oncogene-containing retroviruses were experimentally generated by recombination events between viral and cellular sequences, a phenomenon called "oncogene capture," and a novel FeLV virus "FeLV-AKT" was designed that captured feline c-AKT1 in feline lymphoma. FeLV-AKT contains a *gag*-AKT fusion gene that encodes a myristoylated Gag matrix protein and the kinase domain of feline c-AKT1. It was therefore hypothesized that AKT might be involved in FeLV-associated oncogenesis.[204]

The predominant anatomical locations of lymphoma in cats in general are alimentary (approximately 50%) and extranodal (approximately 25%).[188,189,198,205,206] The majority of cats with alimentary and extranodal lymphoma (mainly kidney and nasopharyngeal) are now FeLV antigen–negative (96% and 89%, respectively),[188] suggesting most cats have other underlying etiologies, such as chronic inflammation or environmental and genetic factors. Several decades ago, 25% to 31% of renal lymphoma cases were associated with FeLV infection[195,206,207] compared with 0% to 6% in more recent studies.[163,188,198,208] A similar situation is seen in multicentric lymphoma; in the 1980s and 1990s, up to 69% of all lymphomas were multicentric, and 31% to 65% of these cats had progressive FeLV infection[164,195,206] compared with 0% to 13% of cats in more recent studies.[163,188,198,205] Mediastinal lymphoma is uncommon today (10%),[188] but many affected cats still have progressive FeLV infection with a prevalence ranging from 19% to 73%.[164,181,188,206,209] In a study from the Netherlands, where the general prevalence of FeLV was only 0.3%, 19% of cats with mediastinal lymphoma were progressively FeLV-infected, but of cats with lymphoma, all progressively infected cats had mediastinal lymphoma.[198] In a UK study, 9% of cats with mediastinal lymphoma were progressively FeLV-infected, which is higher than the general prevalence.[210]

The role of FeLV as a negative prognostic factor for lymphoma patients with regard to remission and survival times is discussed controversially, although more recent studies indicate a negative impact of FeLV infection in cats with lymphoma.[198,206,207,211] FeLV antigen–negative cats with lymphoma had significantly longer remission times (472 days) than FeLV antigen–positive cats (25 days) following treatment.[188] Median remission and survival times for FeLV antigen–positive cats were 27 and 37 days, respectively, and for FeLV antigen–negative cats, 146 and 170 days.[206] FeLV-associated lymphomas have a higher rate of mitoses than those that are FeLV-negative,[212] possibly indicating a more aggressive biological behavior that negatively affects outcome.

Leukemia. Leukemia in cats with FeLV infection most often involves lymphocytes, but all other hematopoietic cell lines can be affected, including granulocytic, erythroid, and megakaryocytic lines, resulting in myeloproliferative disease or MDS. The prognosis for cats with myeloproliferative diseases in general is poor.

Diagnosis of acute leukemia is made by CBC and bone marrow examination. Cytologic abnormalities of bone marrow include increased cellularity, megaloblastic maturation, increased myelofibrosis, and immature blast cells. FeLV variants that bear URE tandem repeats in their LTR can be associated with induction of both MDS and acute myeloid leukemia (AML) in cats. In one study, experimental infection of cats with FeLV clone33 (originating from a cat with AML) resulted in MDS in 41% of the cats, characterized by peripheral blood cytopenias and dysplastic changes in the bone marrow. Some of the cats with MDS eventually developed AML.[213]

Chronic leukemias are rare in cats and sometimes associated with FeLV.[214,215] They include well-differentiated chronic lymphocytic leukemia, chronic myelogenous leukemia, polycythemia vera, erythemic myelosis, and essential thrombocythemia. Cats with erythemic myelosis have nonregenerative or poorly regenerative anemia (12% to 15%) with normal neutrophil counts and variable thrombocytopenia. Abnormal erythrocyte stages are found in bone marrow and often in peripheral blood.[216]

Eosinophilic leukemia, polycythemia vera and essential thrombocythemia in cats have also been reported in association with FeLV infection.[217,218] Eosinophilic leukemia is difficult to distinguish from hypereosinophilic syndrome.

Fibrosarcoma. Fibrosarcomas that are associated with FeLV are caused by FeSV, a recombinant virus that develops in FeLV-A-infected cats by recombination of the FeLV-A genome with cellular oncogenes. Through a process of genetic recombination, FeSV acquires one of several oncogenes, such as *fes, fms,* or *fgr*. As a result, FeSV is an acutely transforming virus, causing a polyclonal malignancy with multifocal tumors arising simultaneously after a short incubation period. With the decrease in FeLV prevalence, FeSV has become very uncommon. FeSV-induced fibrosarcomas usually occur in young cats. Several strains of FeSV that have been identified from naturally occurring tumors are defective. They are unable to replicate without the presence of FeLV-A as a helper virus that supplies proteins (such as those coded by the *env* gene) to FeSV. The host range for FeSV depends on the helper FeLV-A. Fibrosarcoma cells express FOCMA just as lymphoma cells do. Experimental infection with FeSV causes tumors that progress in some cats and regress in others. Those in which the tumors regress have high FOCMA antibody titers.[219]

Fibrosarcomas caused by various strains of FeSV tend to grow rapidly, often with multiple cutaneous or subcutaneous nodules that are locally invasive and metastasize to the lung and other sites. Solitary fibrosarcomas in old cats are typically injection-site sarcomas and are not associated with FeSV or FeLV infection. These tumors are slower growing, locally invasive, slower to metastasize, and are occasionally curable by excision combined with radiation and/or gene therapy.

Experimentally, FeSV has also been associated with melanoma formation, showing that FeSV can transform cells of ectodermal and of mesodermal origin.[22] Intradermal or intraocular inoculation of FeSV into kittens produced melanomas in the skin or anterior chamber of the eye.[23] However, FeSV has not been associated with naturally occurring melanomas of cats.

Other Tumors. A number of other tumors have been found in FeLV-infected cats, but a link between FeLV infection and formation of these tumors has not been clearly established. Iris melanomas, for example, are not associated with FeLV infection as once was believed, as a result of one study in which 3 of 18 eyes had positive test results for FeLV-FeSV proviral DNA.[220] In a later study, however, immunohistochemical staining and PCR did not reveal FeLV or FeSV in the ocular tissues of any cats with iris melanomas.[221]

One case report described a metastatic uterine adenocarcinoma in a 2-year-old female Persian cat with progressive FeLV infection.[222] Osteochondromas (cartilaginous exostoses on flat bones) have also been described in FeLV-infected cats. Although histologically benign, they can cause significant morbidity if they put pressure on adjacent tissues such as the spinal cord or nerve roots.[223-225] The pathogenesis of these osteochondromas is unknown. Spontaneous feline olfactory neuroblastomas are aggressive, histologically inhomogenous tumors of the nose and pharynx and have high metastatic rates. Budding FeLV particles were found in the primary tumors and lymph node metastases, and FeLV DNA was found in tumor tissue.[226] Two of three cats described had positive FeLV antigen test results. The exact role of FeLV in the genesis of these tumors is uncertain. Cutaneous horns associated with benign hyperplasia of keratinocytes have also been described in FeLV-infected cats.[227]

Hematologic Disorders

Hematologic disorders described in association with FeLV include anemia (nonregenerative or regenerative); persistent, transient, or cyclic neutropenia; panleukopenia-like syndrome; platelet abnormalities (thrombocytopenia and platelet function abnormalities); and aplastic anemia (pancytopenia) (Fig. 32.3).

Anemia. In older literature, it was estimated that more than two-thirds of all nonregenerative anemias in cats were the result of FeLV infection. This is no longer the case because of the decrease in overall FeLV prevalence. In a 2009 study of 79 anemic cats, FeLV was found in only two cats, both of which had hemolytic anemia.[228] Approximately 10% of FeLV-associated anemias are regenerative.[229] Regardless of the cause, regenerative FeLV-associated anemias usually have a favorable response to treatment. Most FeLV-associated anemias, however, are nonregenerative and result from infection of hematopoietic stem cells and supporting stroma cells. In addition to the direct effect of the virus on erythropoiesis, secondary disorders can cause nonregenerative anemia in FeLV-infected cats.

Several mechanisms contribute to anemia in FeLV-infected cats (Table 32.3). Hemolytic anemia caused by secondary infection with hemotropic mycoplasmas can occur in FeLV-infected immunosuppressed cats. FeLV-induced IMHA also has been described. Affected cats can have positive Coombs' tests, autoagglutination, and spherocytosis. In a study on IMHA in cats, 2 of 19 cats had positive FeLV antigen test results.[230] However, in another study, Coombs' positive results in cats with anemia were not significantly associated with retrovirus or hemoplasma infection.[231] Regenerative anemia secondary to blood loss can occasionally occur as a result of FeLV-associated thrombocytopenia or platelet functional defects.

Pure red cell aplasia (PRCA) is a severe, nonregenerative anemia (hematocrit [HCT] < 15%). It can be caused by infection with FeLV-C through interactions of FeLV-C with cell surface receptors in the bone marrow.[232,233] Bone marrow examination shows an almost complete lack of erythroid precursors with normal myeloid and megakaryocytic precursors and an increased myeloid-erythroid ratio.[23,123] These cats typically have macrocytosis (rarely normocytosis) but no or few reticulocytes. Whenever macrocytic anemia occurs in a cat in the absence of reticulocytosis, FeLV infection should be suspected. The macrocytosis results from skipped mitoses during erythropoiesis. These cats do not have folate or vitamin B_{12} deficiencies. Iron is present in macrophages but not erythrocyte precursors. Serum erythropoietin (EPO) levels are markedly increased, indicating that anemia is not caused by an EPO deficiency.[123] Treatment with immunosuppressive drugs can result in resolution of anemia within 3 to 5 weeks; however, relapse occurs when treatment is discontinued.[234] An atypical presentation of PRCA in a 9-month-old, female, domestic longhair kitten with progressive FeLV infection was reported. Histological examination of the bone marrow revealed an almost complete absence of erythroid precursor cells and mild to moderate myelofibrosis. The cat also had very unusual CNS defects.[235]

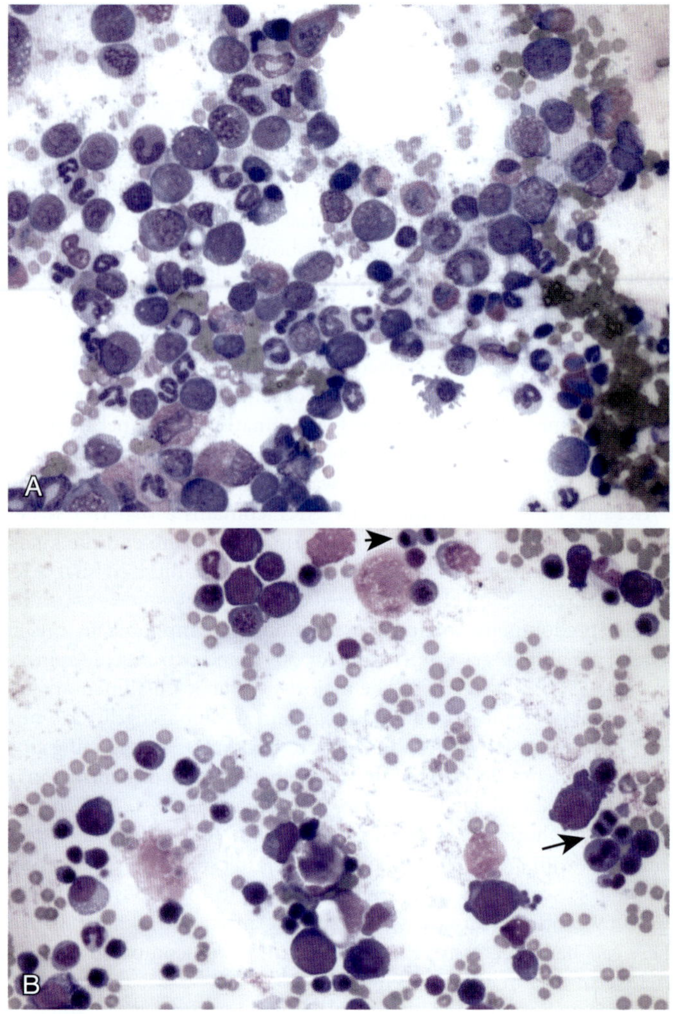

Fig. 32.3 Bone marrow abnormalities in cats with progressive FeLV infection. (A) Bone marrow aspirate cytology from a 6-month-old male neutered domestic shorthair cat that was evaluated for lethargy and fever. Acute leukemia, marked erythroid aplasia, marked granulocytic dysplasia, and increased eosinophilopoiesis are present. Megakaryocytic dysplasia was also identified. The G:E ratio was approximately 2950:1 with marked erythroid aplasia. Wright stain. (B) Bone marrow aspirate cytology from a 1-year-old male neutered domestic shorthair with progressive FeLV infection. Severe megaloblastic erythrodysplasia and mild megakaryocytic dysplasia were identified. The myeloid series was present but markedly decreased in all stages; the myeloid-to-erythroid ratio was estimated at 1:6.5 (compare with A). Nuclear to cytoplasmic asynchrony (megaloblastic change) is present, with immature nuclei in cytoplasm with hemoglobinization. Mitotic figures were present in moderate numbers and were seen in the late stages of the erythroid series *(arrows).*

Anemia of inflammatory disease can also contribute to anemia in FeLV-infected cats, specifically in association with secondary diseases. The HCT often increases spontaneously if the secondary disease or comorbidity is treated successfully.

Hematopoietic tumors, including lymphoma or leukemia, as well as opportunistic infectious agents, such as mycobacteria, can cause anemia as a result of myelophthisis. Bone marrow suppression with anemia can also result from MDS or myelofibrosis. Diagnosis of myelofibrosis requires a bone marrow core biopsy because aspiration is typically nondiagnostic.

Aplastic anemia can be present in FeLV-infected cats and is characterized by aplasia of all cell lines with severe pancytopenia. Bone

TABLE 32.3 Mechanisms of Anemia in Cats Infected with FeLV

Category	Underlying Mechanism
Decreased RBC production	Pure red cell aplasia (FeLV-C) Aplastic anemia Leukemia (myelophthisis) Myelofibrosis Anemia of inflammatory disease
RBC loss	Thrombocytopenia secondary to immune-mediated or bone marrow disease
Increased RBC destruction	FeLV-associated IMHA Coinfection with hemoplasmas

marrow is usually hypocellular or can show necrosis cytologically.[236] Cats with pancytopenia often had positive test results for FeLV antigen in earlier times, but in a study of 13 cats with aplastic anemia from 1996 to 2004, only two were FeLV antigen–positive.[237] In FeLV-infected cats, cyclic hematopoiesis with periodic fluctuation in reticulocytes, granulocytes, and platelets can be seen. FeLV can affect bone marrow accessory cell viability, growth, production, or all of these of hematopoietic progenitor growth-regulating substances by altering cytokine mRNA levels.[238-240] Cytologic examination of bone marrow aspirates reveals few precursors, and core biopsy specimens might be needed to obtain a diagnosis. Bone marrow transplantation has not been successful in these cats, but some respond to immunosuppressive drug therapy.

Platelet abnormalities. Thrombocytopenia can occur as a result of FeLV-induced bone marrow suppression or hematopoietic tumors. Immune-mediated thrombocytopenia can accompany IMHA in cats with underlying FeLV infection. The life span of platelets is shortened in some FeLV-infected cats. Giant platelets and thrombocytosis have been observed in some progressively infected cats.[229]

White blood cell abnormalities. FeLV can reduce leukocyte numbers and function.[241-243] Lymphopenia is seen in many cats with progressive FeLV infection. Affected cats can develop thymic atrophy and depletion of lymph node paracortical zones. In some cats, lymphopenia is characterized by preferential loss of CD4+ helper T cells, resulting in an inverted CD4/CD8 ratio.[244] More commonly, substantial losses of helper cells and cytotoxic suppressor cells (CD8+ cells) occur,[245] and in long-term FeLV infection, a significant decrease in both CD4+ and, to a lesser degree, CD8+ lymphocytes was demonstrated.[246]

Neutropenia is common in FeLV-infected cats[247] and generally occurs alone or in conjunction with other cytopenias. In some cases, myeloid hypoplasia of all granulocytic stages is observed, suggesting direct cytopathic infection of neutrophil precursors. In some neutropenic FeLV-infected cats, bone marrow maturation arrest can occur at the myelocyte and metamyelocyte stages. It has been hypothesized that an immune-mediated mechanism might be responsible in cases in which neutrophil counts recover with glucocorticoid treatment ("glucocorticoid-responsive neutropenia"). Glucocorticoid-responsive cyclic neutropenia also has been reported. The cycles are usually regular, ranging from 8 to 14 days. Bone marrow cytology during the neutropenic phase can indicate either granulocytic hyperplasia or hypoplasia, with a disproportionate number of cells in the promyelocytic stage. Cats with neutropenia commonly have recurrent fever or persistent bacterial infections, and some cats have persistent gingivitis. Neutrophils of progressively infected cats can also have decreased chemotactic and phagocytic function.[241]

Feline panleukopenia-like syndrome (FPLS) or FeLV-associated enteritis (FAE) consists of severe leukopenia (fewer than 3000 cells/μL) and enteritis and destruction of intestinal crypt epithelium that mimics feline panleukopenia caused by FPV. This syndrome might actually not be caused by FeLV alone, as initially thought, but by coinfection with FPV.[248] FAE is the preferred term because clinical signs are usually enteric, and include hemorrhagic diarrhea, vomiting, oral ulceration or gingivitis, anorexia, and weight loss.[249,250]

Immunosuppression and Secondary Infections

Diseases secondary to immunosuppression account for a large portion of the morbidity and mortality of FeLV-infected cats.[251-254] Progressively FeLV-infected cats are predisposed to secondary infections primarily because of immunosuppression similar to that in HIV infection, but immunosuppression is more severe than that associated with FIV infection.

The exact mechanisms by which FeLV damages the immune system are poorly understood. Specific pathogenic immunosuppressive variants, such as FeLV-T, have been described that require a membrane-spanning receptor molecule (Pit1) and a second co-receptor protein (FeLIX) to infect T lymphocytes.[48] The latter protein is expressed from an endogenous provirus arising from FeLV-A, which is similar to the FeLV receptor-binding protein of FeLV-B.[46] Affected cats can develop thymic atrophy and depletion of lymph node paracortical zones after infection.

Reduced leukocyte numbers and function associated with infection also contribute to immunosuppression. Many immune function tests of naturally FeLV-infected cats have been reported to be abnormal, including poor response to T-cell mitogens, prolonged allograft reaction, reduced immunoglobulin production, depressed neutrophil function, and complement depletion. Interleukin (IL)-2 and IL-4 are decreased in some cats,[123,239] but FeLV does not appear to suppress IL-1 production from infected macrophages. Increased TNF-α levels have been observed in serum of FeLV-infected cats as well as in FeLV-infected cells in culture. T cells of FeLV-infected cats produce lower levels of B-cell stimulatory factors than do those of noninfected cats, which becomes progressively more severe over time.[251]

Primary and secondary humoral antibody responses to specific antigens are delayed and decreased in FeLV-infected cats. Progressively FeLV-infected cats do not consistently mount an adequate immune response to vaccines, such as rabies.[255] Therefore a need for more frequent vaccinations (e.g., yearly) has been suggested for these cats.

There are many reports of FeLV-infected cats with concurrent bacterial, viral, protozoal, and fungal infections (Fig. 32.4), but there is little evidence to demonstrate that FeLV-infected cats have a higher prevalence of infections than cats without FeLV infection, or that response to anti-infective therapies are less effective in FeLV-infected cats. Thus, although FeLV is capable of causing immunosuppression, it should not be assumed that all concurrent infections in FeLV-infected cats result from the underlying FeLV infection. Secondary diseases that can be associated with FeLV include FIP, coccidiosis, and feline upper respiratory tract disease.[256,257] A few studies have focused on the role and the influence of FeLV infection on hemoplasma infection with controversial results, because in some studies, FeLV infection was a risk factor for hemoplasma infection,[258-261] whereas in other studies it was not.[262-265] Cats that were naturally infected with FeLV were more likely to develop and not eliminate *Bartonella henselae* infection; however, the course and clinical outcome of *Bartonella* infection was the same as in cats not coinfected with FeLV.[261,263,266,267] No association is generally found between FeLV infection and feline leishmaniosis[268-270] with the exception of one study, where the presence of *Leishmania*

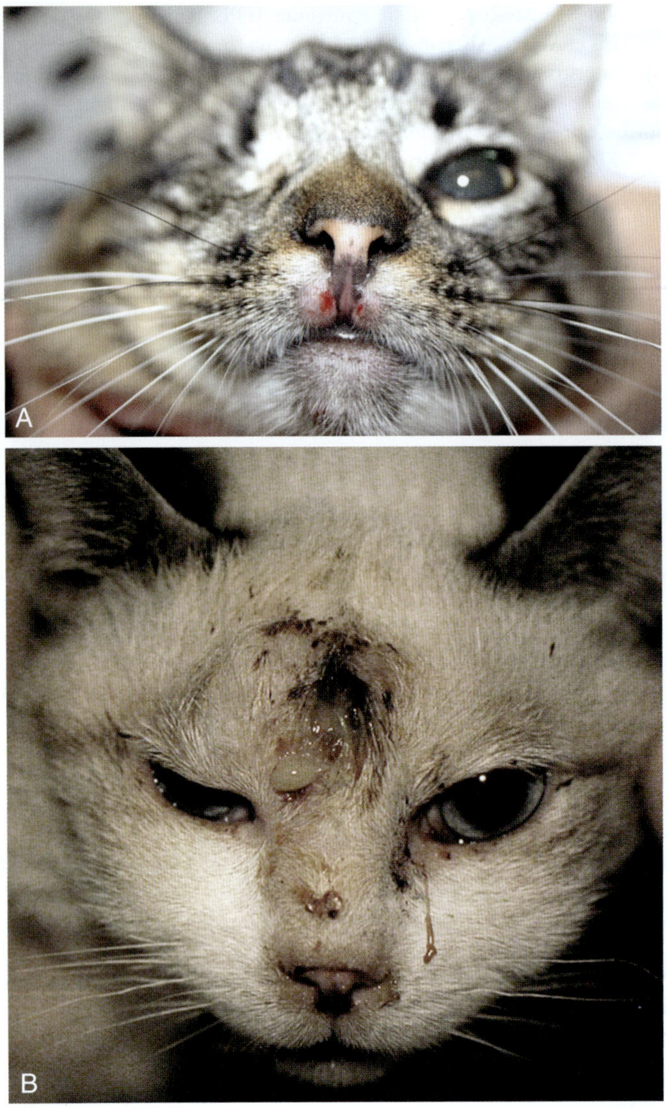

Fig. 32.4 Opportunistic infections in cats with progressive FeLV infection. (A) Ulceration of the nasal planum in a 6-month-old male neutered domestic medium hair cat with progressive FeLV infection as defined by positive ELISA antigen and IFA assays on peripheral blood. Chronic gingivostomatitis was also present, and FCV infection was suspected. (B) Severe nasal cryptococcosis in a Siamese cat from a cattery with endemic FeLV infection.

spp. antibodies and DNA was significantly associated with FeLV infection.[271] No association was found with rickettsial infections[272] or sporotrichosis in cats in Brazil.[273]

Skin infections occur in some FeLV-infected cats. Progressively FeLV-infected cats have a greater diversity of cutaneous and mucosal microflora compared with uninfected cats,[274] and infections associated with dermatologic conditions are usually caused by immunosuppression.[275] Traumatic injuries can be complicated by secondary bacterial infections or abscesses. Otitis externa and miliary dermatitis can be initiated by ectoparasites or allergies but persist because of secondary bacterial infections.

Most studies have not found an association between chronic gingivostomatitis and progressive FeLV infection,[276,277] although one study showed that cats with any oral inflammatory disease were more likely to be infected with FeLV than cats with healthy oral cavities.[278] One study investigated biopsy samples of oral mucosal biopsies of 27 cats with chronic gingivostomatitis and detected FeLV antigens by immunohistochemistry in the epithelium and inflammatory infiltrate of 29.6% of cats. FIV antigens were identified only in one, and FCV antigens in none of the cats using immunohistochemistry.[279]

Immune-Mediated Diseases

FeLV-infected cats can have immune-mediated diseases caused by an overactive or dysregulated immune response to the virus. Although humoral immunity to specific stimulation decreases in FeLV-infected cats, nonspecific increases of IgG and IgM have been noted. The loss of T-cell activity and the formation of antigen-antibody complexes contribute to immune dysregulation.[280] Antigens that can form antigen-antibody complexes include those associated with whole virus particles as well as free gp70, p27, or p15E proteins.[281,282] Immune-mediated diseases described in FeLV-infected cats include IMHA,[230] glomerulonephritis,[283] uveitis,[284,285] and polyarthritis.[227] A chronic polyarthritis syndrome can also be caused by FFV, and concurrent FIV infection can occur in either instance.[286] Although hyperglobulinemia is often associated with immune-mediated disorders, it does not appear to be more prevalent in progressively infected cats when compared with FIV-infected cats.[287] Hyperproteinemia is not significantly more prevalent in progressively infected cats than in uninfected cats, whereas FIV-infected cats are more likely than uninfected cats to display hyperglobulinemia.[280-282,287,288]

Other Syndromes

Other syndromes directly associated with FeLV infection include FeLV-associated neuropathy, reproductive disorders, and fading kitten syndrome.

Neuropathies. Neurologic dysfunction has been described in FeLV-infected cats. Most neurologic signs are associated with lymphoma and lymphocytic infiltrations of the brain or spinal cord, or secondary infectious diseases such as cryptococcosis, toxoplasmosis, FIP, or unusual diseases such as encephalitozoonosis or listeriosis.[289] However, in some cases an underlying cause is not apparent, even after necropsy. Anisocoria, mydriasis, central blindness, Horner's syndrome, or urinary incontinence caused by myelopathy[290] have been described in progressively FeLV-infected cats without morphologic changes. It is possible that FeLV has direct neurotoxic properties. Envelope glycoproteins of retroviruses can stimulate increased intracellular free calcium leading to neuronal death, as described in HIV-infected humans. A polypeptide of the FeLV envelope was found to cause dose-dependent neurotoxicity associated with alterations in intracellular calcium ion concentration, neuronal survival, and neurite outgrowth. The polypeptide of a FeLV-C strain was significantly more neurotoxic than the same peptide derived from a FeLV-A strain.[291,292]

Clinical signs in 16 cats with progressive FeLV infection and neurologic signs consisted of abnormal vocalization, hyperesthesia, and paresis progressing to paralysis. Some cats develop anisocoria or urinary incontinence during the course of their illness. Others have concurrent FeLV-related problems, such as myelodysplastic disease. Microscopically, white-matter degeneration with dilation of myelin sheaths and swollen axons has been identified in the spinal cord and brainstem of affected animals.[290] Immunohistochemical staining of affected tissues revealed consistent expression of FeLV p27 antigens in neurons, endothelial cells, and glial cells, and proviral DNA was amplified from multiple sections of the spinal cord.[290]

Reproductive disorders. FeLV-infected queens can transmit the virus transplacentally. Fetal resorption, abortion, and neonatal death can occur if *in utero* FeLV infection occurs. Apparent infertility is likely caused by early resorption of fetuses. Abortions usually occur late in gestation, with expulsion of normal-appearing fetuses. Bacterial endometritis can accompany abortions, particularly in cats with neutropenia.[23]

Fading kitten syndrome. Kittens born to infected queens can become exposed to FeLV transplacentally, but exposure also occurs at birth and throughout the nursing period. Some kittens become immune, but most become progressively infected and die at an early age with fading kitten syndrome, characterized by failure to nurse, dehydration, hypothermia, thymic atrophy, and death usually within the first 2 weeks of life.[123]

Physical Examination Findings

Physical examination findings in cats with progressive FeLV infection vary dramatically depending on the stage of infection and the secondary disease process present.[293,294] There might be no abnormalities, or cats can show signs of lethargy, fever, mucosal pallor, petechial hemorrhages, dehydration, peripheral lymphadenomegaly, thin body condition, stomatitis, subcutaneous abscesses, or upper respiratory tract disease. Anemic cats can have a hemodynamic heart murmur, tachypnea, or tachycardia, or can be icteric. Cats with severe anemia can be laterally recumbent or comatose and hypothermic. Cats with thymic lymphoma can be tachypneic and have decreased lung and cardiac sounds on thoracic auscultation as a result of pleural effusion, or heart sounds can be displaced caudally. Decreased compressibility of the cranial thorax can also be detected. Splenomegaly, hepatomegaly, renomegaly, intestinal masses, and/or abdominal lymph node enlargement can be detected on abdominal palpation of cats with multicentric lymphoma. Neurologic signs are detected infrequently when compared with signs of anemia or thoracic or abdominal lymphoma and include ataxia, anisocoria, and mydriasis. Although also relatively uncommon, uveitis can be identified, or there might be other ocular abnormalities as a result of intraocular lymphoma or coinfections with other pathogens.[293-295]

DIAGNOSIS

General Statement about Diagnostic Tests

Testing for FeLV and consequently preventing exposure of healthy cats to FeLV-infected cats is the most effective way to prevent the spread of infection.[296,297] FeLV vaccination should not be considered a substitute for testing. The European Advisory Board on Cat Diseases (ABCD) and AAFP have established guidelines for testing cats for FeLV.[297] According to these guidelines, the FeLV status of all cats should be known, because the infection has serious health consequences that influence patient management, both in illness and for wellness care. Failure to identify infected cats can lead to inadvertent exposure and transmission to uninfected cats. Misdiagnosis of infection in uninfected cats can lead to unnecessary changes in lifestyle or even euthanasia.[297] When bringing a new cat into an established household, a follow-up antigen test should be performed at least 90 days after the initial test or after a possible exposure to FeLV because cats could be in the early stage of infection at the time of the first test; and this test should be performed before bringing the cat into the home.[298]

Cats can be tested at any age (Fig. 32.5), because screening tests detect antigen and not antibodies, so neither maternal antibodies nor

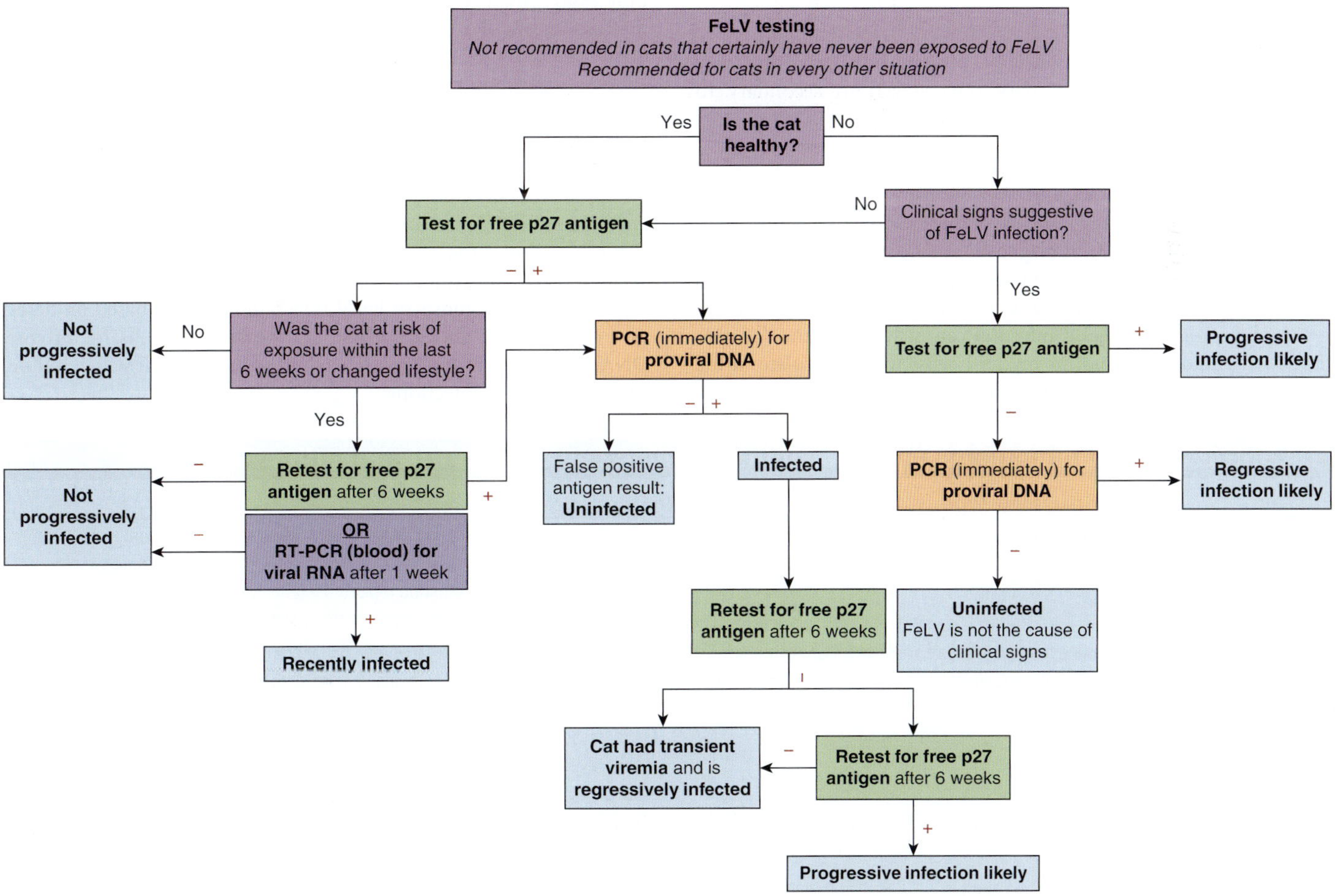

Fig. 32.5 Diagnostic algorithm for FeLV infection. (Redrawn from European Advisory Board on Cat Diseases (ABCD). www.abcdcatsvets.org.)

antibodies from vaccination interfere with testing. However, kittens that are infected as a result of maternal transmission might not test positive for weeks to months after birth.[299] It has been suggested that blood collected immediately after vaccination could contain detectable FeLV antigens from the vaccine itself, so diagnostic samples should be collected before FeLV vaccine administration.[300] It is not known how long this test interference persists. Cats can require retrovirus testing at different times in their lives.[297]

Laboratory Abnormalities

Complete Blood Count

The CBC in progressively FeLV-infected cats can be normal or show regenerative or nonregenerative anemia, neutropenia, lymphopenia, monocytopenia, and/or thrombocytopenia. Evidence of agglutination can be present in cats with IMHA. Moderate to marked leukocytosis due to neutrophilia and bandemia can also be present. Large numbers of circulating blasts, megakaryocytes, or dysplastic cells (such as erythrocytes with giant Howell-Jolly bodies) can be found in cats with leukemia or MDS. When compared to uninfected cats, progressively FeLV-infected cats were nearly fourfold more likely to be anemic, fivefold more likely to be thrombocytopenic, fourfold more likely to be neutropenic, and threefold more likely to have lymphocytosis.[288]

Serum Chemistry Profile

Findings on serum biochemistry analysis and urinalysis are nonspecific and reflect underlying secondary disease processes. Hyperbilirubinemia and bilirubinuria can be present in cats with immune-mediated hemolytic anemia or hemoplasma infection.[288]

Urinalysis

Cats with glomerulonephritis can be proteinuric. Bacteriuria may be identified in cats with urinary tract infections secondary to immunosuppression.

Bone Marrow Cytology and Histopathology

Both bone marrow aspirate and core biopsy specimens should be obtained in cats with pancytopenia or severe nonregenerative anemia. If aspirate results are not diagnostic, a core biopsy should be collected, because bone marrow aspirates from cats with aplastic anemia or myelofibrosis are typically of low cellularity. Bone marrow findings in cats with progressive FeLV infection can include evidence of neoplastic lymphoid, erythroid, or myeloid cells (which circulate in the peripheral blood of cats with leukemia); myelodysplasia; hypoplasia or aplasia of erythroid, myeloid, or megakaryocyte cell lines; erythroid, myeloid, and megakaryocyte hyperplasia despite peripheral cytopenias; and megakaryocyte hypoplasia. Cytochemical stains that identify cells of the myeloid lineage (such as alkaline phosphatase, peroxidase, Sudan black B, and nonspecific esterase), immunocytochemistry, or flow cytometry using antibodies that target cell surface cluster of differentiation (CD) molecules might be needed to definitively identify the cell type involved in some acute undifferentiated leukemias.[295]

Diagnostic Imaging

Plain Radiographs

Imaging findings in cats with FeLV infection can reflect a secondary disease process and are extremely variable. Cats with FeLV-associated thymic lymphoma have a mediastinal mass on thoracic radiography that can be accompanied by mild to severe pleural effusion.

Sonographic Findings

Abdominal sonography in cats with multicentric lymphoma can reveal hypoechoic and enlarged abdominal lymph nodes and enlargement; or hypoechogenicity, or mottling of the spleen, liver, or kidneys. Increased hepatic echogenicity can occur with liver lymphoma. Intestinal masses with loss of normal bowel wall layering can be detected in cases of intestinal lymphoma. Splenomegaly can sometimes be found in cats with immune-mediated cytopenias.

Microbiologic Tests

For diagnosis of FeLV infection, usually direct organism detection assays are preferred (Table 32.4). Routine tests are available that detect free FeLV p27 antigen in blood. Free FeLV antigen can be detected by ELISA or other immunochromatographic assays (ICGAs). Cell-bound antigen can be detected by IFA. Nucleic acid amplification assays can be used to detect FeLV DNA (provirus) or viral RNA, and virus isolation to demonstrate viable virus particles can also be performed in specialized laboratories. Detection of antibodies is necessary for demonstration of abortive infection. The presence of antibodies also can indicate protection against new infection. Table 32.5 shows the results of different diagnostic tests at different stages of FeLV infection.

In practice, diagnosis of FeLV infection is usually based on detection of FeLV p27 antigen. When also obtaining results for proviral DNA, progressively and regressively infected cats are detected, but not cats with abortive infections.

TABLE 32.4 Diagnostic Assays Available for Feline Leukemia Virus Infection

Assay	Specimen Type	Target	Performance
ELISA or immune-chromatographic tests for soluble FeLV antigen	Serum, plasma (whole blood)	Free FeLV p27 antigen	Confirmation is recommended in healthy cats with a second test from a different manufacturer or PCR. Positive antigen test results do not signify progressive infection, and the assay must be repeated 6 (and 12) weeks later or an IFA performed. Negative tests can occur in the first month of infection.
Proviral DNA PCR	Bone marrow, tissue, lymph node aspirates	Proviral DNA	Sensitivity and specificity may vary between laboratories. Assays that have demonstrated sensitivity and specificity may be useful to detect cats with regressive infection for elimination from blood donor programs, or to resolve the results of ELISA assays. Quantitative provirus PCR assays can be helpful for prediction of status (regressive vs. progressive) and outcome, although in some cats, repeated testing may be required over time to establish the status of infection.
RT-PCR	Blood, bone marrow	Viral RNA	Sensitivity and specificity may vary between laboratories. Never use in the absence of antigen testing
Virus isolation	Blood, bone marrow	Replication-competent FeLV virus	Difficult, not widely available. Used primarily as a research tool

TABLE 32.5 Characterization of Possible Outcomes of FeLV Infection

Parameter	Progressive Infection	Regressive Infection	Focal Infection (Rare)	Abortive Infection	No Infection
Viremia	Persistently positive	Undetectable or transiently positive	Absent	Absent	Absent
Replicating virus in blood (virus isolation from blood)	Positive	Negative (only positive during transient viremia or after reactivation)	Negative	Negative	Negative
Viral RNA in blood (RT-PCR of blood)	Positive	Blood: positive or negative	Negative	Negative	Negative
Free FeLV p27 antigen in blood (p27 ELISA or immunomigration on blood)	Positive ~ 3–6 weeks after infection	Negative (only positive during transient viremia or after reactivation)	Alternating or low positive	Negative	Negative
Intracellular FeLV p27 antigen in blood (IFA on blood smear)	Positive (~ 3 weeks after free p27 antigen tests)	Negative (only positive during transient viremia or after reactivation)	Negative or alternating	Negative	Negative
Provirus integration into host's genome	Yes	Yes	Yes (localized)	No	No
Proviral FeLV DNA in blood (PCR on whole blood)	Positive	Positive	Negative or low positive	Negative	Negative
Immune response	Poor	Good	Good	Very good	No
Anti-FeLV antibodies serum (different tests on serum/plasma)	Negative (or low titers)	Positive (high titers)	Positive (high titers)	Positive (variable titers)	Negative
Viral shedding	Yes (continuously); major source of FeLV infection	No (only during transient viremia or after reactivation)	Usually no (one report on shedding in milk)	No	No
Viral RNA saliva (RT-PCR on saliva)	Yes	No (only during transient viremia or after reactivation)	No	No	No
Transmission of infection via blood transfusion	Yes	Yes	Potentially	No	No
Reactivation of FeLV infection	No (infection already continuously active)	Possible (seldom; decreasing probability with increasing duration after exposure)	No (infection sequestered continuously active)	No	No
Consequences	FeLV-associated disease common	FeLV-associated disease uncommon (rarely lymphoma or bone marrow suppression), but common after reactivation	Unlikely	None	None
Prognosis	Poor	Good; poor after reactivation	Variable	Good	Good

Former terminology: progressive infection = persistent viremia; regressive infection = latent infection with or without previous transient viremia; abortive infection = regressor cat.
(Adapted from Hofmann-Lehmann R, Hartmann K. Feline leukaemia virus infection: a practical approach to diagnosis. *J Fel Med Surg.* 2020;22:831–846.)

Detection of FeLV Antigen

The mainstay of clinical testing for FeLV are ELISAs and other immunochromatography or rapid immunomigration assays, which are available for use as plate-based ELISAs or rapid POC tests. Plate-based ELISAs are offered by commercial veterinary diagnostic laboratories. IFA testing for viral antigen is still in use in some countries.[301] All of these assays detect free FeLV core protein p27, but POC assays and plate-based ELISAs are more sensitive than IFAs (the latter detects only intracellular antigen, so becomes positive later than ELISA, once the bone marrow has become infected). Cats with a positive POC test or plate-based ELISA and a negative IFA result are more likely to later develop a regressive infection than are cats with positive results on both assays. In general, to distinguish between regressive and progressive infection, cats should be retested for free p27 antigen 6 weeks after the first positive test result. If the result is still positive, the test should be repeated after another 6 weeks. If at this time the cat remains positive, it is most likely progressively infected and will develop FeLV-associated disease. To avoid the need for serial retesting, cats positive for FeLV free p27 antigen can be immediately retested using IFA. More than 90% of cats with positive IFA results have progressive infection.[181,301-304] A small number of cats with persistently positive ELISA and negative IFA results can have focal or atypical infections that are contained by the immune system.[303] A negative ELISA but positive IFA always represents either a false-negative ELISA result (which is rare) or a false-positive IFA result.

Plate-based ELISAs and POC assays. POC tests are the recommended screening tests for FeLV infection. A positive whole blood, serum, or plasma POC test or plate-based ELISA usually indicates that the cat is viremic. These assays usually become positive within 28 days after exposure, in the first phase of viremia, before the bone marrow is affected. Thus, positive results can reflect transient viremia (in cats becoming regressively infected) or persistent viremia (in progressively infected cats). However, false-positive results are possible, especially when whole blood is used on plate-based ELISAs and some POC tests (that are based on an ELISA principle, such as the SNAP [IDEXX Laboratories]), and particularly when samples are hemolyzed. Thus, plasma or serum should be used with plate-based ELISAs and the SNAP (IDEXX Laboratories). Immunochromatography-based POC tests contain a filtering membrane, so whole blood and serum/plasma do not produce different results.[305] Membrane-based tests eliminate separate washing steps and include positive and negative controls for each test sample. Several comparisons of different POC tests have been performed.[305-310] It is difficult to compare these studies because gold standards differ and tests with similar names can differ among countries or from one time period to the next. However, in general, sensitivities and specificities of different tests have been similar. Positive predictive values of most tests in those comparison studies were between 50% and 80%, whereas negative predictive values were close to 100%.[308] False-positive results are becoming more common because the decreasing prevalence of FeLV infection is leading to lower positive predictive values. Thus, in cat populations with a high prevalence of infection, for example, cats with thymic lymphoma, a positive test result is likely to be accurate, whereas in a lower-risk population, such as a population of indoor cats from single-cat households, a positive test should be viewed with more suspicion, and confirmatory tests should be performed, for example using a POC test from a different manufacturer or a provirus PCR assay.[123] Therefore in general, negative test results are reliable because of the low prevalence of infection in most populations, but positive results have to be interpreted carefully. If a second confirmatory test is positive, this significantly increases the predictive value.[305] POC tests or plate-based ELISAs have been also used on tear and saliva specimens;[311] however, this is not recommended because antigen shedding with saliva and tears is intermittent.

IFA. IFA on smears from blood or bone marrow detect cell-associated p27 antigen within infected blood cells, primarily neutrophils, and platelets. The earliest the test becomes positive after infection of the bone marrow is at about 3 weeks of viremia. IFA is not recommended as a screening test because cats in the first weeks of viremia that are already shedding virus and capable of transmitting infection are not detected. IFA can be used for prognostic reasons or to confirm positive and suspicious ELISA results. IFA requires special processing and fluorescent microscopy and must be performed by a qualified reference laboratory. Generally, two or more blood smears of good quality should be air-dried and mailed, unfixed, to the laboratory. As antigen is present at highest concentrations in neutrophils and platelets, false-negative results can occur when these two cell lines are deficient. False-positive results occur when smears are too thick, background fluorescence is high, or the test is prepared and interpreted by inexperienced personnel. Use of anticoagulated blood rather than fresh blood for preparing smears can also cause errors.[312,313] Variations in quality control among facilities have been reported, and careful attention should be paid to the selection of the reference laboratory.[123]

Molecular Diagnosis Using Nucleic Acid–Based Testing

PCR detects proviral DNA (integrated into the cellular genome of the cat), while RT-PCR detects viral RNA (of free replicating virus). PCR and RT-PCR can be performed on blood, saliva, bone marrow, and tissues. When performed under optimal conditions, PCR methods are the most sensitive tests for FeLV diagnosis and can help resolve cases with discordant antigen test results. However, they must be performed by experienced laboratories and should be well validated. Minor alterations in sample handling by laboratory personnel can destroy nucleic acid or introduce contamination, leading to either false-negative or false-positive results, respectively. There are no comparative studies of the diagnostic accuracy of various commercial laboratories offering FeLV PCR. Assays usually target conserved regions of the FeLV genome, but different PCR assays can vary in their analytical sensitivity and specificity. Minor strain variations can prevent binding of the primers, a step necessary to amplify the viral genome. Moreover, primers and probe must be designed to distinguish endogenous FeLV-like sequences from exogenous FeLV infection.

Quantitative real-time PCR and RT-PCR assays can be used to quantify provirus and viral RNA loads, respectively.[15,136,158,314-318] A clinically validated quantitative PCR assay is now available commercially (IDEXX Laboratories) that can help to ascertain whether a cat is progressively or regressively infected.[318]

PCR for detection of FeLV DNA. An important indication for performing proviral PCR on whole blood is to confirm a positive ELISA result, especially in low-prevalence populations. True-positive ELISA results are accompanied by high proviral loads.[136,319] In early infection, provirus PCR is positive earlier than antigen detection. Moreover, provirus PCR is useful to detect regressively infected cats, and prove absence of FeLV in a multicat environment, such as breeding colonies and catteries. Approximately 2% to 10% of cats with negative antigen tests have been positive for FeLV provirus by PCR.[100,136,137] Most of these cats remain antigen-negative, do not shed virus, and are unlikely to ever develop FeLV-associated diseases, but some can reactivate and then shed FeLV and develop FeLV-associated disease.[149] In addition, these cats can transmit infection if they act as blood donors.[144]

RT-PCR for detection of FeLV RNA. Most commercially available PCR assays for FeLV are based on detection of proviral DNA rather than viral RNA. If performed on blood (or serum or plasma), RT-PCR should always be positive when ELISAs are positive, thus indicating progressive infection. Cats with regressive infection are provirus-positive but most do not possess detectable viral RNA in the blood. If performed on blood (or serum or plasma), RT-PCR should always be positive when ELISA tests are positive. However, in some cats, plasma viral RNA can be found in the absence of FeLV antigen. In contrast, detection of viral RNA in saliva generally indicates viremia.[137,138] RT-PCR results from plasma and saliva can also be helpful in the very early phase of infection. Viral RNA can be detected in plasma or saliva by RT-PCR as early as 1 week after FeLV exposure—earlier than antigen testing by ELISA and even earlier than provirus PCR from blood.[139,319] RT-PCR in saliva has also been used to screen multicat households for FeLV shedders. Active salivary shedding as detected using RT-PCR was consistent in antigenemic cats, whereas non-antigenemic cats with a low proviral load did not shed viral nucleic acid in saliva. FeLV RNA is stable for more than 60 days in saliva specimens stored at room temperature, and in naturally infected cats, RT-PCR on saliva had a high sensitivity and specificity when compared to tests for antigen in blood.[100,137,138] If the cost of testing is a limitation in a multicat environment, pooled saliva specimens could be used for RT-PCR, as the assay can be sufficiently sensitive to detect a single infected cat in a pool of up to 30 specimens.[138]

Virus Isolation

Virus isolation is not practical for routine diagnosis because it is difficult and time-consuming to perform and requires special facilities. Where available, it can be used to confirm positive test results or to better understand a cat's infection status if other assays generate conflicting results.

Indirect Detection of Infection

FeLV-infected cats develop antibodies against several viral proteins. Recently, antibodies against the p15E protein have been demonstrated to be valuable predictors of FeLV exposure,[313] and now a new POC test detecting p15E antibodies is available in several European countries, but its usefulness under field conditions still has to be determined. In a study assessing the status of FeLV infection in the cat population of southern Germany, many cats that had never received FeLV vaccines had FeLV antibodies despite negative antigen and PCR test results, and thus were thought to be abortively infected.[100] FeLV low-dose exposure can result in antibody production during an abortive infection, with cats having anti-FeLV antibodies but no detectable FeLV antigen or DNA.[140,157]

Detection of antibodies is the only way to diagnose abortive FeLV infection. Cats with abortive FeLV infection do not get sick and will not shed the virus, and infection will not be reactivated. However, these cats are considered immune against new infection, and thus vaccination might not be necessary. Therefore to avoid overvaccination and injection-site sarcoma formation, tests for FeLV antibodies ultimately might be useful as prevaccination screening tests. The connection between the presence of antibodies and immunity, however, is not absolute, because some vaccinated cats will not develop antibodies,[100] and there will be cats that are protected against FeLV infection despite the absence of detectable antibodies.[319-323]

Pathologic Findings

Most of the pathologic findings in FeLV-infected cats reflect secondary infections or tumors. FeLV itself can sometimes lead to lymph node, CNS, or bone marrow changes.

Gross Pathologic Findings

Gross and histopathologic findings in cats with progressive FeLV infection usually reflect secondary disease processes. Lymphoma and evidence of myelodysplasia or leukemias are the most common findings, but secondary infections also can be detected.

Histopathologic Findings

Reactive lymphoid hyperplasia is a common finding in cats with progressive FeLV infection. Histology of the bone marrow can reveal lymphoma, leukemias, or myelodysplasia. The intestinal tracts of cats with FAE can show crypt cell necrosis and regeneration, lymphoplasmacytic infiltrates, and blunting and fusion of villi.[324] CNS lesions can include loss of axons and dilated myelin sheaths within the spinal cord.[290] Immunohistochemical stains can be applied to tissues, such as bone marrow or tumor tissue, to confirm the presence of FeLV antigen.[161,162,169,325]

TREATMENT

General Management of FeLV-Infected Cats

Disease in cats that test positive for FeLV antigen can be related or unrelated to FeLV infection. Management protocols for FeLV antigen–positive cats must include the housemates of the FeLV-infected cat (Box 32.1).[297,326,327]

BOX 32.1 Management of FeLV Infection in Multicat vs Individual Cat Households*

Multicat households

- FeLV is mainly transmitted through social contact, but also through biting and fighting.
- If a FeLV-infected cat lives in an otherwise negative household, it is likely that the other cats have already been infected and are immune to new infection.
- The risk of progressive infection in adult FeLV-negative cats is approximately 10 to 15% if they have lived together with a viremic cat.
- If owners refuse to separate housemates, uninfected cats should receive FeLV vaccination to enhance immunity. Owners should be informed that vaccination does not provide complete protection in these high-exposure environments.

Individual cat households

- FeLV-infected cats should be kept indoors to avoid transmission of FeLV to other cats and to reduce their risk of acquiring other infectious diseases.
- Vaccinations should be administered to FeLV-infected cats according to guidelines for immunocompromised cats. Progressively FeLV-infected cats might not be able to mount an adequate immune response to vaccines. Therefore more frequent vaccination (e.g., yearly) could be considered.
- FeLV-infected cats should have veterinary wellness visits at least semiannually to promptly detect changes in health status. A CBC, biochemistry profile, and urinalysis should be performed at least annually.
- Intact male and female cats should be neutered.
- Surgery is well tolerated, but perioperative antibiotic administration should be considered, especially if bacterial contamination of normally sterile anatomic sites is likely to occur.
- FeLV-infected cats can be housed in the same ward as other hospitalized patients, but in individual cages. They should not be placed in isolation.
- If FeLV-infected cats become sick, prompt identification of the secondary illness is essential to allow early therapeutic intervention. Most cats with FeLV infection respond as well as uninfected cats to appropriate medications, although a longer and more aggressive course of therapy might be needed.
- In general, the use of glucocorticoids or other immunosuppressive drugs should be avoided unless specifically indicated, e.g., for neoplastic or immune-mediated disease.

*See references[143,297,300]

FeLV-Infected Households

In households with one or more progressively FeLV-infected cats, all cats should be tested for FeLV antigen and provirus so that their status is known. It is likely that all cats in that household have been exposed and are progressively, regressively, or abortively infected. Cats with regressive or abortive infection are likely protected against new FeLV infection. Naïve cats should not be introduced, even if vaccinated. Shedding of virus generally occurs through salivary glands, and cat-to-cat transmission can occur by allogrooming, sharing of food and water bowls and litter boxes, and fighting and biting behavior. Cats within the household that have negative FeLV antigen test results will tend to outlive progressively infected cats. Therefore after months or years, all remaining cats will be antigen-negative and immune to new infection.

Individual FeLV-Infected Cats

FeLV-infected cats should be confined indoors to reduce the likelihood of secondary infections, but also to prevent spread of FeLV to other cats in the neighborhood. Good nutrition and husbandry are essential to maintain good health. Raw meat, eggs, and unpasteurized milk should be avoided because of the risk of acquiring foodborne bacterial or parasitic infections.[298]

In progressively infected cats, wellness visits to the veterinarian should occur at least semiannually. Visits should include a detailed history, a thorough physical examination including accurate body weight determination, and an ophthalmic examination. In addition, a CBC, biochemistry profile, urinalysis, and centrifugal fecal flotation should be performed at least yearly. Intact males and females should be neutered to reduce stress associated with estrus and mating behavior and to decrease the desire to roam outside. Surgery is generally well tolerated by subclinically infected cats. Perioperative antibiotic administration should be considered during surgeries and dental procedures.[297,298]

Vaccination with core vaccines (against FPV, FHV, and FCV) should be performed regularly and considered even more frequently than in non–FeLV-infected cats due to immunosuppression, even if the cat is kept strictly indoors. One field study could not find a difference in response to vaccination between progressively FeLV-infected and noninfected cats.[328] Ideally, FPV antibodies should be evaluated to confirm protection and to determine necessity to revaccinate in adult cats. If an owner cannot be convinced to keep a FeLV-infected cat inside, rabies vaccinations should be given (in accordance with state and local regulations). FeLV vaccines are not recommended in cats with known progressive or regressive FeLV infections because these vaccines have no effect on viremia, carrier state or elimination, or on development of FeLV-associated disease in an already infected cat and do not prevent reactivation of regressive infection.[329]

BOX 32.2 Suggested Management Recommendations for FeLV-infected Cats

If no clinical signs are present

- No treatment
- Cats should be kept strictly indoors

If clinical signs are present

- First assess for and treat underlying diseases, which may or may not be FeLV-related

Treatment of FeLV-infected cats with lymphoma

- Consider chemotherapeutic drug protocols (e.g., COP)
- Prognosis might be more guarded

Treatment of FeLV-infected cats with idiopathic anemia

- Consider transfusion
- Try erythropoietin or darbepoetin if nonregenerative
- If no effect, consider glucocorticoids for possible IMHA

Treatment of FeLV-infected cats with idiopathic neurological signs

- Consider zidovudine (5 mg/kg PO q12h)

Treatment of FeLV-infected cats with recurring bacterial infections

- Treat recurring bacterial infections promptly and using cidal antimicrobial drugs at appropriate doses
- Consider feline interferon omega if available (10^6 IU/kg SC q24h)

COP, cyclophosphamide, vincristine, prednisolone; *IMHA*, immune-mediated hemolytic anemia.

Treatment of FeLV-Associated Diseases

In most cases, secondary diseases in progressively FeLV-infected cats are treated as is for uninfected cats, and respond in a similar manner.[330] Prompt and accurate identification of FeLV-associated disease aids early intervention and a more successful outcome (Box 32.2). Nevertheless, the owner should be forewarned that response to treatment can sometimes take longer than expected. FeLV itself does not cause fever, so a search for a concurrent infection must be made in persistently febrile cats.

Glucocorticoids and other immunosuppressive drugs should be avoided whenever possible in FeLV-infected cats, unless clearly indicated. These drugs might compound the risk of secondary infections. Also, cats with regressive FeLV infection should not receive glucocorticoid treatment because it increases the risk of reactivation. Myelosuppressive drugs should also be avoided because they can potentiate the myelosuppressive syndromes caused by FeLV.

Tumors

Although the prognosis is worse for FeLV-associated tumors when compared with the same tumors in cats testing negative for FeLV,[198,206,331,332] some patients greatly benefit from antitumor therapy. Antitumor therapy should be applied with identical protocols used in non–FeLV-infected cats. In an older report of 38 cats with lymphoma treated with a COP (cyclophosphamide, vincristine, and prednisolone) protocol, 75% achieved complete remission with a median remission duration of 150 days and a 1-year remission rate of 20%.[333] The most frequent tumor in these cats was mediastinal lymphoma, and most cats were progressively infected with FeLV. In a later report, cats from the same geographic area were treated with the same protocol and had a complete remission rate of only 47%, with a median remission duration of 86 days.[334] In this group, few cats were progressively FeLV-infected, and the alimentary form of lymphoma was the most frequent.[334] Cats with acute leukemia are difficult to treat because the bone marrow becomes filled with neoplastic blast cells, which must be destroyed before the normal hematopoietic precursors can repopulate. This process can take 3 to 4 weeks. The remission rate in cats with acute lymphocytic leukemia treated initially with vincristine and prednisone is approximately 25%, whereas the rate in cats with AML treated with doxorubicin or cytosine arabinoside is close to zero.[23] A cat with suspected FeLV-associated chronic lymphocytic leukemia was successfully treated with a combination of prednisone, chlorambucil, cyclophosphamide, doxorubicin, and lomustine.[214] Secondary infections are common and must be treated quickly and aggressively, especially if they occur at the time of the granulocyte nadir. Although prophylactic antibiotics are not given routinely in the treatment of leukemia or lymphoma, broad-spectrum bactericidal antibiotics should be given to progressively FeLV-infected cats receiving tumor therapy, especially if fever or other signs of secondary infection occur.

FeSV-induced feline sarcomas should be treated early, with wide and deep surgical excision. If no metastases are present, but microscopic tumors remain after surgery, radiation can be successful in delaying recurrence.

Hematologic Disorders

Although hematologic disorders are sometimes irreversible in progressively FeLV-infected cats, the course can be cyclic and there can be some improvement with time. Treatment with blood transfusions or bone marrow–stimulating cytokines should be considered. Of 29 anemic (HCT < 20%) FeLV-infected cats treated with blood transfusions (over 2 weeks), the HCT returned to the reference range in eight cats. Glucocorticoid treatment can increase the lifespan of erythrocytes if the anemia is immune-mediated, and antibodies are present against erythrocytes or precursors, and some cats with FeLV-associated nonregenerative anemia respond well to high-dose prednisolone. Occasionally, secondary infections (e.g., hemoplasma infections) are responsible for the anemia, and these can be treatable. Even though EPO concentrations are often elevated in cats with FeLV-related anemia, treatment with recombinant human erythropoietin (rHuEPO) or darbepoetin can be helpful. RHuEPO treatment not only increases erythrocyte counts but also can increase platelet and megakaryocyte numbers.[335] In a study in FIV-infected cats, all rHuEPO-treated cats had a gradual increase in erythrocyte counts, hemoglobin concentrations, and HCT and increased white blood cell counts.[336] The recommended dose is 100 IU/kg SC q48 hours until the desired HCT (usually 30%) is reached and then as needed to maintain the HCT at 30%. A response might not be seen for 3 to 4 weeks, and if it does not occur, iron supplementation might be required. Iron should not be given to cats that have received transfusions because whole blood contains 0.5 mg/mL of iron, which increases risk of hepatic hemosiderosis. Anti-EPO antibodies can develop in 25% to 30% of rHuEPO-treated animals after 6 to 12 months. Binding of these antibodies to native EPO can result in bone marrow failure and refractory anemia. However, anti-EPO antibodies dissipate after discontinuation of treatment. Darbepoetin alpha is a synthetic EPO that possesses an additional two N-linked oligosaccharide chains, and seems to be less likely to induce production of anti-EPO antibodies in cats than EPO.

Neutropenia can lead to severe immunosuppression, and antibiotics can be necessary in some neutropenic cats to prevent secondary bacterial translocation and development of sepsis. Treatment with filgrastim (5 μg/kg SC q24h for up to 21 days) has caused transient responses. Potential adverse effects include bone discomfort, splenomegaly, allergic reactions, and fever.[336,337] Short-term increases in neutrophil counts can be followed by neutropenia with continued use of filgrastim because of development of dose-dependent neutralizing antibodies to this heterologous product after 10 days to 7 weeks. Thus, treatment should not be used for more than 3 weeks.[336,337] Another risk is development of persistent antibodies against endogenous feline granulocyte colony-stimulating factor (at higher dosages), with rebound neutropenia. One study suggested that filgrastim is contraindicated in FIV-infected cats because it led to increased viral load.[336] In a pilot study, a small number of naturally FeLV-infected cats were treated with filgrastim; however, treatment did not result in significant changes in neutrophil counts.[338] Other authors reported that filgrastim has been used in FeLV-infected cats with cyclic neutropenia with some success.[123] In some FeLV-infected cats, neutropenia is immune-mediated, and responds to immunosuppressive doses of glucocorticoids. In animals with myeloid hypoplasia and in the absence of myeloid precursors, direct effects of FeLV are suspected, and glucocorticoids should not be used. Thus, bone marrow aspiration and cytology should be performed before glucocorticoids are considered.

Antiviral Chemotherapy and Immunomodulators

Antiviral drugs and immunomodulators are sometimes used to treat FeLV-infected cats (Tables 32.6 to 32.8). Unfortunately, few large controlled studies have been conducted in naturally infected cats, and most of them have shown unclear or no benefit.[339-342] This section will focus on drugs that are currently commercially available. The reader is referred to Chapter 9 for more detailed information on mechanism of action, other uses, study outcomes, and adverse effects.

TABLE 32.6 Antiviral Drug Studies for Treatment of FeLV Infection

Drug Class	Drug	Efficacy *In Vitro*	Controlled Study *In Vivo*	Efficacy *In Vivo*	Comments	EBM Level (I–IV)
Nucleoside Reverse Transcriptase Inhibitors						
	Zidovudine	Yes[406–411]	Yes	No[342,411,412]	Not very effective	I
	Didanosine	Yes[410,411]	No	ND	Possibly effective, but no *in vivo* data available	IV
	Zalcitabine	Yes[411]	Yes	No[413–415]	Not very effective, but relatively toxic	II
	Decitabine	Yes[346]	No	ND	Possibly effective, but no *in vivo* data available	IV
	Gemcitabine	Yes[346]	No	ND	Possibly effective, but no *in vivo* data available	IV
Nucleotide Reverse Transcriptase Inhibitors						
	Adefovir	Yes[416]	Yes	Yes[340,416]	Poorly effective, but relatively toxic	I
	Tenofovir	Yes[346]	No	ND	Possibly effective, but likely also relatively toxic	IV
Non-Nucleoside Reverse Transcriptase Inhibitors						
	Suramin	No	No	ND	Weak efficacy in uncontrolled experimental studies	III
Nucleotide Synthesis Inhibitors						
	Foscarnet	Yes[417]	No	ND	Effective *in vitro*, but too toxic	IV
	Ribavirin	Yes[418]	No	ND	Effective *in vitro*, but too toxic	IV
Integrase Inhibitor						
	Raltegravir	Yes[345,346,419]	Yes	Yes[347]	Mildly effective with reduction of viremia in one experimental study, but viremia relapsed after drug removal	II

ND, Not determined; *EBM,* evidence-based medicine[420]

EBM grade I = This is the best evidence, comprising data obtained from properly designed, randomized controlled clinical trials in the target species (in this context cats).

EBM grade II = Data obtained from properly designed, randomized controlled studies in the target species with spontaneous disease in an experimental setting.

EBM grade III = Data based on nonrandomized clinical trials, multiple case series, other experimental studies, and dramatic results from uncontrolled studies.

EBM grade IV = Expert opinion, case reports, studies in other species, pathophysiological justification.

(Including EBM grades for judgment of the available efficacy data including expert opinion of the authors.)

TABLE 32.7 Immunomodulatory Drug Studies for Treatment of FeLV Infection

Drub Class	Drug	Efficacy *In Vitro*	Controlled Study *In Vivo*	Efficacy *In Vivo*	Comments	EBM Level (I–IV)
Interferons						
	Human interferon-α	Yes[421]	Yes (SC high dose)	No[342]	Ineffective in a placebo-controlled blinded field study	I
			Yes (PO low dose)	No[341]	Ineffective in a placebo-controlled blinded field study, contrary to some effect reported in case series	I
	Feline interferon-ω	Yes[422]	Yes (SC high dose)	Yes[423,424]	Some effect (most likely more on secondary infections)	I
Microorganism-Derived Biologic Response Modifiers						
	Mycobacterium spp.	ND	Yes	No[425]	Not effective in an experimental setting	II
	Staphylococcus spp.	ND	Yes	Yes[341]	Some effect on owners' subjective impression on the health of their cats in a placebo-controlled field study	I
	Cutibacterium acnes	ND	No	ND	Some effect based on anecdotal reports and case series	III
	Serratia marcescens	ND	No	ND	Likely ineffective based on an uncontrolled study	III
	Poxviruses	ND	Yes	No[339]	Ineffective in large placebo-controlled blinded field studies	I
Plant-Derived Biologic Response Modifiers						
	Acemannan	ND	No	ND	Ineffective based on uncontrolled studies	III
Antiparasitics						
	Levamisole	ND	No	ND	Likely not indicated, but controlled studies missing	IV
	Diethylcarbamazine	ND	Yes	No[426]	Ineffective in one experimental study	II

ND, Not determined; *EBM,* evidence-based medicine.[420]
EBM grade I = This is the best evidence, comprising data obtained from properly designed, randomized controlled clinical trials in the target species (in this context cats).
EBM grade II = Data obtained from properly designed, randomized controlled studies in the target species with spontaneous disease in an experimental setting.
EBM grade III = Data based on nonrandomized clinical trials, multiple case series, other experimental studies, and dramatic results from uncontrolled studies.
EBM grade IV = Expert opinion, case reports, studies in other species, pathophysiological justification.
(Including EBM grades for judgment of the available efficacy data including expert opinion of the authors.)

TABLE 32.8 Suggested Medications for Treatment of FeLV Infection

Drug	Dose	Route	Interval (Hours)	Comments
Zidovudine (AZT)	5 mg/kg	PO	12	Monitor CBC weekly during treatment for the first month, then monthly
Feline recombinant interferon-ω	1 million U/kg	SC	q24h for 5 consecutive days starting on days 0, 14, and 60	
Human recombinant interferon-α	1 to 50 U/cat	PO	24	

In general, human antiviral drugs used to treat cats have been less active against FeLV when compared to FIV. Most human antiviral drugs were developed for treatment of HIV infection, which is more closely related to FIV infection. Many drugs developed for humans, such as ribavirin,[343,344] have caused unacceptable toxicity in cats. Drugs that have been used in cats that were experimentally or naturally infected with FeLV include zidovudine (AZT), zalcitabine, adefovir, and suramin. Zidovudine has been administered to FeLV-infected cats with acceptable toxicity, but there has been no clear benefit on clinical outcomes. The same was true for adefovir. Some drugs, such as gemcitabine and tenofovir, have activity against FeLV *in vitro*, but their efficacy *in vivo* and toxicity in cats are so far unknown. The integrase inhibitor raltegravir was highly active against FeLV *in vitro*.[344,345] Raltegravir was administered at 40 mg q12h PO for 6.5 weeks, and then 80 mg q12h PO for 2.5 weeks. The treatment reduced viremia in each cat, with up to 1 $\log_{10}$ reduction in viral RNA in four of seven cats, and the drug attained therapeutic plasma concentrations at both doses, with no adverse effects noted. However, viremia rebounded in all cats following drug removal.[347]

Immunomodulators used to treat FeLV-infected cats have included human IFN-α, feline IFN-ω, staphylococcal protein A, *Cutibacterium acnes* (formerly *Propionibacterium acnes*), *Serratia marcescens* extract, poxvirus preparations, acemannan, levamisole, and diethylcarbamazine. Benefits of most of these drugs have not been clearly demonstrated (see Chapter 9), and some, such as levamisole, are too toxic for routine use.

Prognosis

Survival times for cats with FeLV infection vary considerably depending on the stage of infection, host immunity, and the strain of FeLV involved. Some older studies suggested that FeLV-infected cats live a maximum of 3 years after diagnosis, but these studies involved group-housed cats in multiple-cat FeLV-endemic environments. With proper care, FeLV-infected cats can live much longer than 3 years and, in fact, die at an older age from causes unrelated to their retroviral infection.[348] Most cats that are progressively infected with FeLV go on to develop FeLV-associated disease within 5 years of diagnosis.[175] A comparison of more than 800 progressively FeLV-infected cats and 8000 controls revealed a median survival time of 2.4 years for progressively FeLV-infected cats versus 6.3 years for controls.[300] Still, many progressively infected cats, especially adult cats, can live for several years with a good quality of life, and so euthanasia is not recommended solely on the basis of a persistently positive FeLV antigen test. Some cats with FeLV-associated lymphoma can have long-term remissions when treated with standard chemotherapy protocols. Proviral DNA load and p27 antigen concentration correlated with survival in one longitudinal study, with cats having both proviral DNA load and p27 antigen concentration above cutoff values of 4 $\times 10^5$ copies/mL and 37.5 ng/mL, respectively ("high positive" cats) having a median survival time of 1.37 years from time of enrollment; in contrast, over 90% of "low positive" cats were still alive at the end of the 4-year study.[318] In another study, cats with regressive infections also had evidence of a stronger immune response to the FeLV SU glycoprotein compared with cats in other outcome groups, as well as having evidence of virus-neutralizing antibodies.[349] These assays have the potential to be increasingly used in the future to predict outcome in cats that test positive for FeLV.

IMMUNITY

The majority of cats naturally exposed to FeLV will become immune to reinfection. This differs for other retrovirus infections, such as in FIV or HIV infection. As a result, although the mechanism of protection against FeLV and the role of neutralizing antibodies and cell-mediated immunity are still not completely understood, efficacious FeLV vaccines are commercially available.

Antibodies are at least partially protective. Experimentally, susceptible kittens can be protected from FeLV infection after passive immunization with sera containing high antibody concentrations against FeLV.[350] However, once persistent viremia is established, treatment with virus-neutralizing monoclonal antibodies is ineffective.[351] Most cats that overcome viremia exhibit high antibody titers to the virus,[352-354] and cats with regressive infection have higher antibody titers than cats with progressive infection.[136] Antibodies are directed against different components of the virus.[352]

Not all immune cats develop high antibody levels, and thus, cytotoxic T lymphocytes (CTLs) are also important.[352] Use of the recombinant FeLV canarypox vaccine did not induce antibodies to FeLV but cats were nonetheless protected from progressive infection.[319,322] CTLs specific for FeLV appear before virus-neutralizing antibodies, and the virus load in progressively FeLV-infected cats can be lowered after passive transfer of FeLV-specific CTLs stimulated *in vitro*, which suggests an important role of CTLs in FeLV immunity.[353,355]

VACCINATION

Vaccine Development and Efficacy

Cats with abortive and regressive FeLV infection mount an effective immune response and prevent or contain virus replication. This is a unique feature of FeLV infection and supports the idea that immune protection can be achieved through vaccination. Live attenuated vaccines produce a strong humoral immune response[356] but have the potential to establish infection or integrate into the host genome and later result in FeLV antigen–negative lymphomas. Most early inactivated FeLV vaccines were either poor immunogens, ineffective in preventing progressive FeLV infection, or enhanced tumor development. With refinement in cell culture conditions, large amounts of soluble FeLV antigens could be harvested in cell culture supernatants.[357] FeLV envelope antigen preparations alone were shown to provide protection if used in conjunction with potent adjuvants.[358] With such preparations, no viral genes could be introduced into host cells, circumventing the oncogenic potential of FeLV. The first vaccine based on soluble FeLV antigens was licensed in 1985, and then underwent further modifications to improve efficacy.

Although most FeLV vaccines effectively protect cats from progressive infection, there is controversy surrounding the degree of efficacy and which type of vaccine is most efficacious.[323] Few independent studies exist that compare the efficacy of vaccines. Testing protocols vary widely among studies, with differences in time periods assessed between vaccination and challenge, challenge strains, challenge doses, cats, and different methods of virus detection following challenge. Therefore meaningful comparison of studies is difficult if not impossible. To overcome age-related resistance, some studies used glucocorticoids for immunosuppression before intranasal challenge or performed parenteral FeLV exposure. These challenges produce a much higher proportion of infected control cats, reducing the overall number of cats needed for efficacy studies. The comparability of these challenges to natural exposure has been questioned.[147,359-362] However, some FeLV vaccines proved efficacious even under these severe challenge conditions, suggesting that the vaccines could also protect cats against FeLV infection under natural conditions. Some studies involved natural challenge, in which vaccinated and control cats were housed together with FeLV-shedding cats.[362,363] Although more comparable to a field situation, such natural challenge situations often fail to result in a high rate of progressive infection in unvaccinated control cats, leading to a low calculated efficacy of the vaccine and unsuitable data for vaccine approval. For example, for inactivated FeLV vaccines, European licensing authorities require that less than 20% of the vaccinated cats and more than 80% of the unvaccinated controls develop progressive infection.

There are three types of FeLV vaccines licensed: (1) classical inactivated whole virus vaccines; (2) genetically engineered recombinant subunit vaccines based on the FeLV envelope protein p45 (a nonglycosylated form of gp70 produced in bacteria);[364] and (3) infectious recombinant canarypox virus engineered to express the *env* and *gag*/part of *pol* genes of FeLV.[365] The recombinant FeLV p45 subunit vaccine was the first commercial recombinant vaccine for small animals and was demonstrated to be highly efficacious in protecting cats from progressive FeLV infection. Later, a recombinant canarypox vaccine became available in Europe, which is a different product than that licensed for use in the United States. An independent comparison of FeLV whole virus vaccines available in the United States revealed a very high efficacy for two of four vaccines tested.[366] There was absence of provirus integration and viral RNA in most cats vaccinated with the two whole virus vaccines, thus indicating sterile immunity (complete absence of viral RNA, proviral DNA, antigen, and culturable virus after challenge). These results contradicted with those from an earlier study that showed that neither one of the two whole virus vaccines nor the recombinant canarypox vaccine led to sterilizing immunity.[319] FeLV provirus was found to persist for years even after challenge in vaccinated cats, and recurrence of viremia and disease development was observed in some cats.[150] Thus, vaccination does not appear to consistently protect against development of regressive infection.

While inactivated whole virus and recombinant protein vaccines require adjuvants, the recombinant canarypox vaccine is a replication-defective live virus vaccine that does not require an adjuvant to induce protective immunity.[319,322] Cats protected by the recombinant canarypox vaccine have a higher ratio of FeLV-specific IFN-γ- to IL-10-producing cells than susceptible cats, in accordance with the known importance of CMI induced by this vaccine.[367] An improved version of the recombinant canarypox vaccine was produced by a target mutation within the FeLV envelope protein to delete the immunosuppressive domain p15E; this led to induction of a more pronounced cell-mediated immune response and to slightly increased vaccine efficacy.[367] Two studies that compared the recombinant vaccine to an inactivated vaccine have been the subject of controversial discussion. The first study claimed that an inactivated whole virus vaccine was superior in protecting cats from FeLV challenge (90% protection from progressive infection) compared to the recombinant canarypox vaccine (20% protection from progressive infection).[368] The validity of this study was debated, in part because an intercurrent parvovirus infection was probably introduced by a contaminated challenge virus preparation, which likely created immunosuppression. The challenge and parvovirus infection occurred within 3 weeks after the second vaccination, so likely impacted immunity to vaccination.[369] In the second study, immunosuppression was created using high doses of glucocorticoids during challenge, which occurred 3 months after the second vaccination.[370] Under these circumstances, the whole virus vaccine performed better (preventable fraction 100%) than the recombinant canarypox vaccine (preventable fraction 45%). Concerns were raised in response to this study because the severe immunosuppression during challenge likely specifically impacted CMI, which is critical for responses to recombinant canarypox vaccines.[371] In reaction to this, it was suggested that cats at risk for FeLV infection in the field might also be immunosuppressed.[372]

These debates aside, the administration of FeLV vaccines prolongs the life expectancy of FeLV-exposed cats.[151] FeLV vaccines are considered noncore vaccines, so are recommended for all cats with a potential FeLV exposure risk, such as cats permitted to roam outdoors or cats brought to or living in multicat environments with other cats of uncertain FeLV status. Cats kept strictly indoors are at risk if kept in multicat households in which some cats have outdoor access. In areas with high FeLV prevalence, vaccination of all kittens and juvenile cats up to 1 year of age should be considered, since the environment into which a kitten enters can rarely be predicted with certainty.[373,374] Additionally, kittens also have a particularly high risk of developing progressive infection after FeLV exposure. Recommendations for most vaccines are for two subcutaneous doses 3 to 4 weeks apart for initial protection followed by a vaccination 1 year later. FeLV vaccines should be given in the left pelvic limb as distally as possible.[374] Results of several studies indicate that FeLV vaccine-induced immunity persists for at least 12 months following vaccination, but likely much longer. Some vaccines are licensed for yearly boosters, some for up to 3-year boosters. Recommendations by different expert panels vary concerning the booster intervals of adult cats. In adult cats that have received appropriate initial two-dose immunization and a booster after 1 year, the need for subsequent vaccination and the booster interval is best determined by analysis of risk.[374] At-risk adult cats should continue to be vaccinated for FeLV annually, but cats at low risk of FeLV exposure can be vaccinated every 3 years.[374] In a study that addressed the duration of immunity in cats vaccinated with an adjuvanted inactivated whole virus vaccine, 10 of 12 cats vaccinated 2 years before FeLV exposure were protected from progressive infection, while all 11 controls were unprotected (preventable fraction 83%).[375] In another study using an inactivated whole virus vaccine, cats were exposed 8, 20, and 36 months after vaccination to FeLV. The outcome of the study was hampered by the age-related resistance, which meant that only 10 of the 32 control cats demonstrated progressive infection.[376] Nonetheless, only one of 44 vaccinated cats became progressively infected.

It is not necessary to administer vaccines from the same manufacturer for boosters.[377] Not all cats respond equally to FeLV vaccination, and immunosuppressed cats can fail to develop immunity.[378] In a 5-year field study of a colony of 30 domestic adult cats naturally exposed to FeLV infection, FeLV vaccination was effective in cats not infected with FIV, but failed to protect FIV-infected cats.[98] In contrast, in an experimental study using a recombinant FeLV p45 subunit vaccine, FIV-infected cats were successfully immunized and protected from FeLV challenge exposure in the early phase of infection.[379] No benefit of FeLV vaccination was observed in cats with progressive but subclinical FeLV infection on virus load or life expectancy.[329] Therefore FeLV vaccination is not recommended in progressively FeLV-infected cats. Vaccination of cats with a history of regressive or abortive infections should also not be necessary, since these cats most likely have protective immune response against FeLV. As described in the Diagnosis section, new antibody tests might be useful to detect immune cats, but their validity still has to be evaluated in the field.

FeLV Vaccination and Injection-Site Sarcomas

In early studies, a statistical association was demonstrated between FeLV and rabies vaccinations and later development of feline injection-site sarcomas (FISS) (see Chapter 20). However, in a subsequent multicenter case-control study in the United States and Canada, no single vaccine brand or manufacturer within antigen class could be identified as a risk factor for FISS development.[380] One study compared the subcutaneous tissue response to different FeLV vaccines. Three groups of 15 cats were injected with one of three FeLV multicomponent vaccines, a recombinant canarypox vaccine, a vaccine with a lipid-based adjuvant, and a vaccine adjuvanted with an alum-Quil A mixture. On days 7, 21, and 62 post vaccination, significantly less inflammation was associated with administration of the recombinant canarypox multicomponent vaccine. The inflammation was most severe in cats receiving the multicomponent vaccine containing FeLV p45 and an aluminum-based adjuvant.[381] Not only adjuvanted FeLV and rabies vaccines, but also other vaccines and injections of long-acting drugs, such as glucocorticoids, or injuries, such as through foreign bodies, and microchip implants were associated with the development of FISS in some case reports (see Chapter 20).

Some studies examined a possible role of FeLV and FeSV in the development of FISS, but could not detect either FeLV or FeSV in the tumors.[186] Furthermore, no other viruses, including FIV, FFV, polyomaviruses, or papillomaviruses were detected in tumor tissues.[382-385]

No evidence was found for the replication or expression of endogenous retroviruses in FISS.[383,385] In addition, feline primary cutaneous lymphomas were described in association with vaccination. A total of 17 cutaneous lymphomas with a history of vaccine injection at the site of tumor development were evaluated. Postinjection time of development ranged from 15 days to approximately 9 years in five cats. FeLV gp70 and/or p27 proteins were expressed in 10 of the 17 tumors. It was suggested that persistent inflammation induced by the injection and reactivation of FeLV expression might have contributed to the development of these tumors.[386] Chapter 20 describes recommendations to minimize the risk of FISS. Along these lines, no FeLV vaccinations should be administered to indoor-only cats or already immune cats,[387] and, thus, FeLV prevaccination testing is recommended.

PREVENTION

Preventative methods, including general precautions, testing and removal strategies, and vaccination, have been successful in significantly decreasing the prevalence of FeLV infection.[110]

FeLV is very fragile, surviving only minutes at most outside the host animal. Thus, direct contact among cats and immediate fomite transfer are the major risk factors, but transmission requires prolonged, close contact. Progressively infected cats should be physically separated from other cats in the environment. In a veterinary hospital, FeLV-shedding cats can be housed in the same ward with other hospitalized patients as long as they are housed in separate cages and certain precautionary measures are taken. Simple precautions (e.g., hand washing) and routine cleaning procedures prevent transmission in the hospital setting.

Cats with progressive FeLV infection should be housed in individual cages and confined to them throughout their hospitalization. They should never be placed in isolation with cats that have other infections, such as viral respiratory infections, because FeLV-infected cats may be immunosuppressed. Routine hospital infection-control precautions will prevent transmission of FeLV.

FeLV can be transmitted hematogenously; therefore all feline blood donors should be screened and confirmed to be free of infection before donating blood.[297,298,388] Pre–blood transfusion screening should include not only ELISA to detect FeLV antigen, but also provirus PCR testing because regressively infected cats (antigen-negative, provirus-positive) also transmit the virus, and blood product recipients can become regressively or even progressively FeLV-infected.[144] FeLV was also detected in the corneal tissues of cats by PCR and immunohistochemistry;[389] therefore screening potential corneal donors for FeLV infection is also generally warranted.

In the mid-1970s, test and removal programs were extremely effective for eliminating the virus from catteries. When testing was first implemented, the prevalence of FeLV in purebred catteries was 11%. Within 4 years, the rate was reduced to less than 2%. Today, FeLV infection should be considered an abnormality in a well-run cattery. Many stray-cat shelters also implement testing in their conditioning protocols, thus further reducing the rate of FeLV infection.[123,390]

PUBLIC HEALTH ASPECTS

Although FeLV can replicate in human cell lines,[391] no conclusive evidence of natural human infection with FeLV has been detected. Concerns that relate to the possibility of zoonotic transmission of FeLV infection have arisen from several observations. Firstly, some FeLV strains grow in human cell cultures.[392] Secondly, lymphoma has been induced by injection of large doses of virus into neonates of nonfeline species, such as pups and marmosets.[60] Thirdly, contact of humans with sick cats was linked to development of childhood leukemia, and the degree of contact between FeLV-infected cats and children with leukemia was double that of contact between healthy children and healthy cats.[393,394] Fourth, veterinarians were shown to have a higher death rate from leukemia than a control population of physicians and dentists.[22,359,395-397]

Despite these facts, FeLV does not appear to be a risk to humans. Some investigators have detected antibodies to FeLV in humans with leukemia and owners of progressively FeLV-infected cats.[398-401] On the other hand, studies using more specific radioimmunoassays obtained negative results. No human has ever been found to be viremic with FeLV. PCR was used without success to find FeLV sequences in blood and bone marrow of young and adult humans with leukemia.[402]

One study found that human blood cells are uniquely resistant to infection with FeLV due to the activity of cellular enzymes that mutate the viral genome. A second blockade to infection was identified that appears to suppress viral gene expression after the viral genome has integrated into the host cell genome. As cells derived from other normal human cell types are fully supportive of FeLV replication, innate resistance of blood cells could be critical in protecting against cross-species infection.[403] In conclusion, there is no evidence that FeLV is transmitted from cats to humans. Still, if immunosuppressed people live in close contact with FeLV-infected cats, there is a certain risk, not for FeLV infection but for infection by secondary pathogens that have the potential to be zoonotic.

CASE EXAMPLE

Signalment

"Mausi," a 6-year-old female spayed domestic shorthair from Munich, Germany.

History

Mausi was presented to the Ludwig-Maximilians-Universitaet Munich, Germany, Veterinary Medical Teaching Hospital, for lethargy and anorexia of 3 days' duration. Mausi had not eaten and not defecated during this time. There had been no change in urination.

At a local veterinary clinic on the first day of illness, a physical examination revealed fever (105.1°F or 40.6°C). Treatment with amoxicillin/clavulanic acid did not lead to clinical improvement. Mausi tested positive for FeLV antigen 2 years previously, after which time the cat had been housed exclusively indoors. There were three other cats in the household that were also indoor-only since Mausi was found to be infected with FeLV. A FeLV test had revealed that one other cat was FeLV antigen–positive, the other two cats were FeLV antigen–negative. None of the other three cats were ill. Mausi had not had any known toxin exposure, there were no recent changes in the environment, and the cat was fed a commercial dry cat food.

Current Medications

Amoxicillin/clavulanic acid PO.

Other Medical History

None.

CASE EXAMPLE—cont'd

Physical Examination

Body weight: 6.9 kg

General: Quiet, alert, responsive, well hydrated, T = 104.4°F (40.2°C), HR = 220 beats/min, RR = 36 breaths/min, mucous membranes pink, CRT = 1 s, haircoat unkempt.

Eyes, ears, nose, and throat (including dilated fundoscopic examination): Mild gingivitis.

Musculoskeletal: Body condition score 7/9. Normal ambulation.

Cardiovascular, respiratory, gastrointestinal, genitourinary, and lymph nodes: Mausi resented palpation of her cranial abdomen. No other clinically significant abnormalities were detected.

Laboratory Findings

CBC: HCT 24.6% (30%–50%), MCV 48.4 fL (42–53 fL), reticulocytes 7800 cells/μL, WBC 12,470 cells/μL (4500–14,000 cells/μL), neutrophils 10,438 cells/μL (2000–9000 cells/μL), band neutrophils 1,459 cells/μL (0–1000 cells/μL), lymphocytes 344 cells/μL (1000–7000 cells/μL), monocytes 229 cells/μL (0–1000 cells/μL), platelets 192,000 platelets/μL (180,000–500,000 platelets/μL).

On blood smear, the neutrophils showed mild toxicity.

Serum Chemistry Profile: Sodium 148 mmol/L (151–158 mmol/L), potassium 3.8 mmol/L (3.6–4.9 mmol/L), chloride 119 mmol/L (117–126 mmol/L), bicarbonate 18 mmol/L (15–21 mmol/L), phosphorus 3.9 mg/dL (3.2–6.3 mg/dL), calcium 9.5 mg/dL (9.0–10.9 mg/dL), BUN 19 mg/dL (18–33 mg/dL), creatinine 1.2 mg/dL (1.1–2.2 mg/dL), glucose 169 mg/dL (63–118 mg/dL), total protein 7.0 g/dL (6.6–8.4 g/dL), albumin 2.6 g/dL (2.2–4.6 g/dL), globulin 4.4 g/dL (2.8–5.4 g/dL), ALT 72 U/L (0–101 U/L), ALP 12 U/L (0–71 U/L), cholesterol 104 mg/dL (89–258 mg/dL), total bilirubin 0.2 mg/dL (0–0.2 mg/dL).

Urinalysis (cystocentesis): SpG 1.020; pH 7.0, 1+ protein, 2+ hemoprotein, 0–1 WBC/HPF, 0–2 RBC/HPF, some rods

Imaging Findings

Plain abdominal radiographs: The intestines were relatively empty. No masses were identified. Abdominal serosal detail appeared normal.

Abdominal sonography: The left kidney measured 4.2 cm in length and showed a mildly enlarged renal pelvis. The remainder of the abdomen was unremarkable.

Microbiologic and Virologic Testing

Aerobic bacterial urine culture: growth of *Escherichia coli* (sensitivity testing revealed that the *E. coli* was sensitive to pradofloxacin, but resistant to amoxicillin/clavulanic acid)

POC ELISA for FeLV antigen and FIV antibodies: positive for FeLV antigen, negative for FIV antibodies

Diagnosis

Progressive FeLV infection and acute pyelonephritis (characterized by fever, bacteriuria, and mild neutrophilia with left shift). Right renal agenesis (likely congenital).

Treatment

Mausi was hospitalized and treated with intravenous fluids, and initially, while awaiting the culture and susceptibility results, treated with amoxicillin/clavulanic acid (20 mg/kg, IV, q12h) and pradofloxacin (oral suspension 5 mg/kg, PO q24h). Rectal temperature normalized within 24 hours, and the cat started eating again. After 48 hours, hematocrit was 27.6%, neutrophil count was 5759 cells/μL with no bands or toxicity, and lymphocyte count was 917 cells/μL. As culture and susceptibility testing revealed an *E. coli* that was resistant to amoxicillin/clavulanic acid, but susceptible to pradofloxacin, amoxicillin/clavulanic acid treatment was discontinued, and Mausi was discharged from the hospital with instructions to continue pradofloxacin treatment for 1 month. Two weeks after the antibiotics had been discontinued, Mausi appeared healthy. A physical examination, CBC, kidney panel, urinalysis, and aerobic bacterial urine culture showed no abnormalities. Her hematocrit was 38.9%, and white blood cell count was 4620 cells/μL. One year later, Mausi remained clinically healthy, and a CBC showed a hematocrit of 38.2%, white blood cell count of 4500 cells/μL, neutrophil count of 3362 cells/μL, and a lymphocyte count of 905 cells/μL. Mausi remained alive and well with a normal CBC 4 years after she was initially seen for the pyelonephritis. Mausi died 2 years later, 7.5 years after first testing positive for progressive FeLV infection.

Comments

Even though this cat was initially seen for moderately severe illness in association with progressive FeLV infection, there was full clinical recovery with treatment and the cat remained alive and well for 6 additional years. Fever, bacteriuria, and neutrophilia with left shift were likely associated with pyelonephritis. The nonregenerative anemia likely represented an anemia of inflammatory disease, and the lymphopenia and the hyperglycemia were likely stress-induced.

The two FeLV antigen–negative cats most likely had been exposed to FeLV and had regressive or abortive FeLV infection, in which case they would be protected against new FeLV infection.

This case clearly demonstrates that other treatable diseases can be present in progressively FeLV-infected cats, long-term survival is possible, and that a search for the underlying cause of clinical signs and adequate treatment is always recommended.

SUGGESTED READINGS

Beall MJ, Buch J, Clark G, et al. Feline leukemia virus p27 antigen concentration and proviral DNA load are associated with survival in naturally infected cats. *Viruses*. 2021;13:302.

Little S, Levy J, Hartmann K, et al. AAFP feline retrovirus testing and management guidelines. *J Feline Med Surg*. 2020;22:5–30.

REFERENCES

1. Jarrett O, PH R. Differential growth and transmission in cats of feline leukemia viruses of subgroups A and B. *Int J Cancer*. 1978;21:466–472.
2. Jarrett O, Hardy Jr WD, Golder MC, et al. The frequency of occurrence of feline leukaemia virus subgroups in cats. *Int J Cancer*. 1978;21:334–337.
3. Jarrett WF, Martin WB, Crighton GW, et al. Transmission experiments with leukemia (lymphosarcoma). *Nature*. 1964; 202:566–567.
4. Willett BJ, Hosie MJ. Feline leukaemia virus: half a century since its discovery. *Vet J*. 2013;195:16–23.
5. Polani S, Roca AL, Rosensteel BB, et al. Evolutionary dynamics of endogenous feline leukemia virus proliferation among species of the domestic cat lineage. *Virology*. 2010;405:397–407.
6. Benveniste RE, Sherr CJ, Todaro GJ. Evolution of type C viral genes: origin of feline leukemia virus. *Science*. 1975;190:886–888.
7. Soe LH, Devi BG, Mullins JI, et al. Molecular cloning and characterization of endogenous feline leukemia virus sequences from a cat genomic library. *J Virol*. 1983;46:829–840.
8. Anai Y, Ochi H, Watanabe S, et al. Infectious endogenous retroviruses in cats and emergence of recombinant viruses. *J Virol*. 2012;86:8634–8644.

9. Overbaugh J, Riedel N, Hoover EA, et al. Transduction of endogenous envelope genes by feline leukaemia virus in vitro. *Nature.* 1988;332:731–734.
10. Stewart MA, Warnock M, Wheeler A, et al. Nucleotide sequences of a feline leukemia virus subgroup A envelope gene and long terminal repeat and evidence for the recombinational origin of subgroup B viruses. *J Virol.* 1986;58:825–834.
11. Kawamura M, Watanabe S, Odahara Y, et al. Genetic diversity in the feline leukemia virus gag gene. *Virus Res.* 2015;204:74–81.
12. Anderson MM, Lauring AS, Burns CC, et al. Identification of a cellular cofactor required for infection by feline leukemia virus. *Science.* 2000;287:1828–1830.
13. Sakaguchi S, Shojima T, Fukui D, et al. A soluble envelope protein of endogenous retrovirus (FeLIX) present in serum of domestic cats mediates infection of a pathogenic variant of feline leukemia virus. *J Gen Virol.* 2015;96:681–687.
14. Tandon R, Cattori V, Willi B, et al. Copy number polymorphism of endogenous feline leukemia virus-like sequences. *Mol Cell Probes.* 2007;21:257–266.
15. Tandon R, Cattori V, Gomes-Keller MA, et al. Quantitation of feline leukaemia virus viral and proviral loads by TaqMan real-time polymerase chain reaction. *J Virol Methods.* 2005;130:124–132.
16. Roca AL, Pecon-Slattery J, O'Brien SJ. Genomically intact endogenous feline leukemia viruses of recent origin. *J Virol.* 2004;78:4370–4375.
17. Roca AL, Nash WG, Menninger JC, et al. Insertional polymorphisms of endogenous feline leukemia viruses. *J Virol.* 2005;79:3979–3986.
18. Barbacid M, Stephenson JR, Aaronson SA. Evolutionary relationships between gag gene-coded proteins of murine and primate endogenous type C RNA viruses. *Cell.* 1977;10:641–648.
19. Miyazawa T, Shimode S, Nakagawa S. RD-114 virus story: from RNA rumor virus to a useful viral tool for elucidating the world cats' journey. *Uirusu.* 2016;66:21–30.
20. Beyer W, Mohring R, Drescher B, et al. Molecular cloning of an endogenous cat retroviral element (ECE 1): a recombinant between RD-114 and FeLV-related sequences. Brief report. *Arch Virol.* 1987;96:297–301.
21. Shimode S, Nakagawa S, Miyazawa T. Multiple invasions of an infectious retrovirus in cat genomes. *Sci Rep.* 2015;5:8164.
22. Cotter SM. Feline viral neoplasia. In: Greene CE, ed. *Infectious Diseases of the Dog and Cat.* 1st ed. Philadelphia: WB, Saunders; 1990:316–334.
23. Cotter SM. Feline viral neoplasia. In: Greene CE, ed. *Infectious Diseases of the Dog and Cat.* 2nd ed. Philadelphia: WB, Saunders; 1998:71–84.
24. Todaro GJ, Tevethia SS, Melnick JL. Isolation of an RD-114 related type-C virus from feline sarcoma virus-transformed baboon cells. *Intervirology.* 1973;1:399–404.
25. Fukuma A, Yoshikawa R, Miyazawa T, et al. A new approach to establish a cell line with reduced risk of endogenous retroviruses. *PLoS One.* 2013;8. e61530.
26. Narushima R, Tamura N, Iida M, et al. Detection of RD-114 virus by a reverse transcriptase assay based on product enhancement. *Biologicals.* 2012;40:421–425.
27. Kuse K, Ito J, Miyake A, et al. Existence of two distinct infectious endogenous retroviruses in domestic cats and their different strategies for adaptation to transcriptional regulation. *J Virol.* 2016;90:9029–9045.
28. Bupp K, Sarangi A, Roth MJ. Selection of feline leukemia virus envelope proteins from a library by functional association with a murine leukemia virus envelope. *Virology.* 2006;351:340–348.
29. Mendoza R, Anderson MM, Overbaugh J. A putative thiamine transport protein is a receptor for feline leukemia virus subgroup A. *J Virol.* 2006;80:3378–3385.
30. Rey MA, Prasad R, Tailor CS. The C domain in the surface envelope glycoprotein of subgroup C feline leukemia virus is a second receptor-binding domain. *Virology.* 2008;370:273–284.
31. Miyazawa T. Receptors for animal retroviruses. *Uirusu.* 2009;59:223–242.
32. Shojima T, Nakata R, Miyazawa T. Host cell range of T-lymphotropic feline leukemia virus in vitro. *Biochem Biophys Res Comm.* 2006;345:1466–1470.
33. Mendoza R, Miller AD, Overbaugh J. Disruption of thiamine uptake and growth of cells by feline leukemia virus subgroup A. *J Virol.* 2013;87:2412–2419.
34. Katrin Helfer-Hungerbuehler A, Cattori V, Bachler B, et al. Quantification and molecular characterization of the feline leukemia virus A receptor. *J Mol Epidemiol Evol Genetics Infect Dis.* 2011;11:1940–1950.
35. Khan AA, Quigley JG. Heme and FLVCR-related transporter families SLC48 and SLC49. *Mol Aspects Med.* 2013;34:669–682.
36. Fleming MD, Hamza I. Mitochondrial heme: an exit strategy at last. *J Clin Invest.* 2012;122:4328–4330.
37. Chiabrando D, Marro S, Mercurio S, et al. The mitochondrial heme exporter FLVCR1b mediates erythroid differentiation. *J Clin Invest.* 2012;122:4569–4579.
38. Philip M, Funkhouser SA, Chiu EY, et al. Heme exporter FLVCR is required for T cell development and peripheral survival. *J Immunol.* 2015;194:1677–1685.
39. Erbeck K, Gagne RB, Kraberger S, et al. Feline leukemia virus (FeLV) endogenous and exogenous recombination events result in multiple FeLV-B subtypes during natural infection. *J Virol.* 2021;95.e0035321.
40. Bechtel MK, Hayes KA, Mathes LE, et al. Recombinant feline leukemia virus (FeLV) variants establish a limited infection with altered cell tropism in specific-pathogen-free cats in the absence of FeLV subgroup A helper virus. *Vet Pathol.* 1999;36:91–99.
41. Sarma PS, Log T, Skuntz S, et al. Experimental horizontal transmission of feline leukemia viruses of subgroups A, B, and C. *J Natl Cancer Inst.* 1978;60:871–874.
42. Stewart H, Jarrett O, Hosie MJ, et al. Are endogenous feline leukemia viruses really endogenous? *Vet Immunol Immunopathol.* 2011;143:325–331.
43. Rojko J, Essex M, Trainin Z. Feline leukemia/sarcoma viruses and immunodeficiency. *Adv Vet Sci Comp Med.* 1988;32:57–96.
44. Jarrett O, Golder MC, Toth S, et al. Interaction between feline leukaemia virus subgroups in the pathogenesis of erythroid hypoplasia. *Int J Cancer.* 1984;34:283–288.
45. Ito J, Watanabe S, Hiratsuka T, et al. Refrex-1, a soluble restriction factor against feline endogenous and exogenous retroviruses. *J Virol.* 2013;87:12029–12040.
46. Barnett AL, Wensel DL, Li W, et al. Structure and mechanism of a coreceptor for infection by a pathogenic feline retrovirus. *J Virol.* 2003;77:2717–2729.
47. Lauring AS, Anderson MM, Overbaugh J. Specificity in receptor usage by T-cell-tropic feline leukemia viruses: implications for the in vivo tropism of immunodeficiency-inducing variants. *J Virol.* 2001;75:8888–8898.
48. Lauring AS, Cheng HH, Eiden MV, et al. Genetic and biochemical analyses of receptor and cofactor determinants for T-cell-tropic feline leukemia virus infection. *J Virol.* 2002;76:8069–8078.
49. Nakaya Y, Shojima T, Hoshino S, et al. Focus assay on FeLIX-dependent feline leukemia virus. *J Vet Med Sci.* 2010;72:117–121.
50. Quackenbush SL, Dean GA, Mullins JI, et al. Analysis of FeLV-FAIDS provirus burden and productive infection in lymphocyte subsets in vivo. *Virology.* 1996;223:1–9.
51. Miyake A, Watanabe S, Hiratsuka T, et al. Novel feline leukemia virus interference group based on the env gene. *J Virol.* 2016;90:4832–4837.
52. Miyake A, Kawasaki J, Ngo H, et al. Reduced folate carrier: an entry receptor for a novel feline leukemia virus variant. *J Virol.* 2019;93. e00269–19.
53. Matsumoto Y, Momoi Y, Watari T, et al. Detection of enhancer repeats in the long terminal repeats of feline leukemia viruses from cats with spontaneous neoplastic and nonneoplastic diseases. *Virology.* 1992,189.745–749.
54. Nishigaki K, Okuda M, Endo Y, et al. Structure and function of the long terminal repeats of feline leukemia viruses derived from naturally occurring acute myeloid leukemias in cats. *J Virol.* 1997;71:9823–9827.
55. Abujamra AL, Spanjaard RA, Akinsheye I, et al. Leukemia virus long terminal repeat activates NFkappaB pathway by a TLR3-dependent mechanism. *Virology.* 2006;345:390–403.
56. Rojko JL, Hoover EA, Mathes LE, et al. Pathogenesis of experimental feline leukemia virus infection. *J Natl Cancer Inst.* 1979;63:759–768.
57. Jarrett O, Laird HM, Hay D. Growth of feline leukaemia virus in human cells. *Nature.* 1969;224:1208–1209.

58. Sarma PS, Log T, Jain D, et al. Differential host range of viruses of feline leukemia-sarcoma complex. *Virology*. 1975;64:438–446.
59. Takeuchi Y, Porter CD, Strahan KM, et al. Sensitization of cells and retroviruses to human serum by (alpha 1-3) galactosyltransferase. *Nature*. 1996;379:85–88.
60. Rickard CG, Post JE, Noronha F, et al. Interspecies infection by feline leukemia virus: serial cell-free transmission in dogs of malignant lymphomas induced by feline leukemia virus. *Bibl Haematol*. 1973;39:102–112.
61. Anderson BC, Theilen GH. Continuing studies of feline sarcoma virus induced tumors in newborn lambs and in kittens: a model to study comparative neoplasia. *Eur J Cancer*. 1980;16:925–935.
62. Boid R, McOrist S, Jones TW, et al. Isolation of FeLV from a wild felid (*Felis silvestris*). *Vet Rec*. 1991;128:256.
63. McOrist S, Boid R, Jones TW, et al. Some viral and protozool diseases in the European wildcat (*Felis silvestris*). *J Wildl Dis*. 1991;27:693–696.
64. McOrist S. Diseases of the European wildcat (*Felis silvestris* Schreber, 1777) in Great Britain. *Rev Sci Technique*. 1992;11:1143–1149.
65. Leutenegger CM, Hofmann-Lehmann R, Riols C, et al. Viral infections in free-living populations of the European wildcat. *J Wildl Dis*. 1999;35:678–686.
66. Fromont E, Sager A, Leger F, et al. Prevalence and pathogenicity of retroviruses in wildcats in France. *Vet Rec*. 2000;146:317–319.
67. Duarte A, Fernandes M, Santos N, et al. Virological survey in free-ranging wildcats (*Felis silvestris*) and feral domestic cats in Portugal. *Vet Microbiol*. 2012;158:400–404.
68. Leon CI, Garcia-Bocanegra I, McCain E, et al. Prevalence of selected pathogens in small carnivores in reintroduction areas of the Iberian lynx (*Lynx pardinus*). *Vet Rec*. 2017.
69. Daniels MJ, Golder MC, Jarrett O, et al. Feline viruses in wildcats from Scotland. *J Wildl Dis*. 1999;35:121–124.
70. Willi B, Filoni C, Catao-Dias JL, et al. Worldwide occurrence of feline hemoplasma infections in wild felid species. *J Clin Microbiol*. 2007;45:1159–1166.
71. Naidenko SV, Pavlova EV, Kirilyuk VE. Detection of seasonal weight loss and a serologic survey of potential pathogens in wild Pallas' cats (*Felis [Otocolobus] manul*) of the Daurian Steppe, Russia. *J Wildl Dis*. 2014;50:188–194.
72. Brown MA, Cunningham MW, Roca AL, et al. Genetic characterization of feline leukemia virus from Florida panthers. *Emerg Infect Dis*. 2008;14:252–259.
73. Cunningham MW, Brown MA, Shindle DB, et al. Epizootiology and management of feline leukemia virus in the Florida puma. *J Wildl Dis*. 2008;44:537–552.
74. Filoni C, Catao-Dias JL, Bay G, et al. First evidence of feline herpesvirus, calicivirus, parvovirus, and *Ehrlichia* exposure in Brazilian free-ranging felids. *J Wildl Dis*. 2006;42:470–477.
75. Filoni C, Catao-Dias JL, Cattori V, et al. Surveillance using serological and molecular methods for the detection of infectious agents in captive Brazilian neotropic and exotic felids. *J Vet Diagn Invest*. 2012;24:166–173.
76. Briggs MB, Ott RL. Feline leukemia virus infection in a captive cheetah and the clinical and antibody response of six captive cheetahs to vaccination with a subunit feline leukemia virus vaccine. *J Am Vet Med Assoc*. 1986;189:1197–1199.
77. Marker L, Munson L, Basson PA, et al. Multicentric T-cell lymphoma associated with feline leukemia virus infection in a captive Namibian cheetah (*Acinonyx jubatus*). *J Wildl Dis*. 2003;39:690–695.
78. Foley JE, Swift P, Fleer KA, et al. Risk factors for exposure to feline pathogens in California mountain lions (*Puma concolor*). *J Wildl Dis*. 2013;49:279–293.
79. Sleeman JM, Keane JM, Johnson JS, et al. Feline leukemia virus in a captive bobcat. *J Wildl Dis*. 2001;37:194–200.
80. Luaces I, Domenech A, Garcia-Montijano M, et al. Detection of feline leukemia virus in the endangered Iberian lynx (*Lynx pardinus*). *J Vet Diagn Invest*. 2008;20:381–385.
81. Meli ML, Cattori V, Martinez F, et al. Feline leukemia virus and other pathogens as important threats to the survival of the critically endangered Iberian lynx (*Lynx pardinus*). *PLoS One*. 2009;4:e4744.
82. Meli ML, Cattori V, Martinez F, et al. Feline leukemia virus infection: a threat for the survival of the critically endangered Iberian lynx (*Lynx pardinus*). *Vet Immunol Immunopathol*. 2010;134:61–67.
83. Geret CP, Cattori V, Meli ML, et al. Feline leukemia virus outbreak in the critically endangered Iberian lynx (*Lynx pardinus*): high-throughput sequencing of envelope variable region A and experimental transmission. *Arch Virol*. 2011;156:839–854.
84. Millan J, Candela MG, Palomares F, et al. Disease threats to the endangered Iberian lynx (*Lynx pardinus*). *Vet J*. 2009;182:114–124.
85. Mora M, Napolitano C, Ortega R, et al. Feline immunodeficiency virus and feline leukemia virus infection in free-ranging guignas (*Leopardus guigna*) and sympatric domestic cats in human perturbed landscapes on Chiloe Island, Chile. *J Wildl Dis*. 2015;51:199–208.
86. Guimaraes AM, Brandao PE, de Moraes W, et al. Survey of feline leukemia virus and feline coronaviruses in captive neotropical wild felids from Southern Brazil. *J Zoo Wildl Med*. 2009;40:360–364.
87. Kennedy-Stoskopf S. Emerging Viral Infections in Large Cats. In: Fowler ME, Miller RE, eds. *Zoo and Wild Animal Medicine: Current Therapy*. 4th ed. Philadelphia, Pennsylvania: W. B. Saunders; 1999.
88. Harrison TM, McKnight CA, Sikarskie JG, et al. Malignant lymphoma in african lions (*Panthera leo*). *Vet Pathol*. 2010;47:952–957.
89. Driciru M, Siefert L, Prager KC, et al. A serosurvey of viral infections in lions (*Panthera leo*), from Queen Elizabeth National Park, Uganda. *J Wildl Dis*. 2006;42:667–671.
90. Ramanathan A, Malik PK, Prasad G. Seroepizootiological survey for selected viral infections in captive Asiatic lions (*Panthera leo persica*) from western India. *J Zoo Wildl Med*. 2007;38:400–408.
91. Ramsauer S, Bay G, Meli M, et al. Seroprevalence of selected infectious agents in a free-ranging, low-density lion population in the Central Kalahari Game Reserves in Botswana. *Clin Vaccine Immunol*. 2007;14:808–810.
92. Furtado MM, de Ramos Filho JD, Scheffer KC, et al. Serosurvey for selected viral infections in free-ranging jaguars (*Panthera onca*) and domestic carnivores in Brazilian Cerrado, Pantanal, and Amazon. *J Wildl Dis*. 2013;49:510–521.
93. Hofmann-Lehmann R, Fehr D, Grob M, et al. Prevalence of antibodies to feline parvovirus, calicivirus, herpesvirus, coronavirus, and immunodeficiency virus and of feline leukemia virus antigen and the interrelationship of these viral infections in free-ranging lions in east Africa. *Clin Diagn Lab Immunol*. 1996;3:554–562.
94. Endo Y, Uema M, Miura R, et al. Prevalence of canine distemper virus, feline immunodeficiency virus and feline leukemia virus in captive African lions (*Panthera leo*) in Japan. *J Vet Med Sci*. 2004;66:1587–1589.
95. Goodrich JM, Quigley KS, Lewis JC, et al. Serosurvey of free-ranging Amur tigers in the Russian far east. *J Wildl Dis*. 2012;48:186–189.
96. Risi E, Agoulon A, Allaire F, et al. Antibody response to vaccines for rhinotracheitis, caliciviral disease, panleukopenia, feline leukemia, and rabies in tigers (*Panthera tigris*) and lions (*Panthera leo*). *J Zoo Wildl Med*. 2012;43:248–255.
97. Arjona A, Escolar E, Soto I, et al. Seroepidemiological survey of infection by feline leukemia virus and immunodeficiency virus in Madrid and correlation with some clinical aspects. *J Clin Microbiol*. 2000;38:3448–3449.
98. Bandecchi P, Dell'Omodarme M, Magi M, et al. Feline leukaemia virus (FeLV) and feline immunodeficiency virus infections in cats in the Pisa district of Tuscany, and attempts to control FeLV infection in a colony of domestic cats by vaccination. *Vet Rec*. 2006;158:555–557.
99. Dorny P, Speybroeck N, Verstraete S, et al. Serological survey of *Toxoplasma gondii*, feline immunodeficiency virus and feline leukaemia virus in urban stray cats in Belgium. *Vet Rec*. 2002;151:626–629.
100. Englert T, Lutz H, Sauter-Louis C, et al. Survey of the feline leukemia virus infection status of cats in Southern Germany. *J Feline Med Surg*. 2012;14:392–398.
101. Gleich SE, Krieger S, Hartmann K. Prevalence of feline immunodeficiency virus and feline leukaemia virus among client-owned cats and risk factors for infection in Germany. *J Feline Med Surg*. 2009;11:985–992.
102. Hellard E, Fouchet D, Santin-Janin H, et al. When cats' ways of life interact with their viruses: a study in 15 natural populations of owned and unowned cats (*Felis silvestris catus*). *Prev Vet Med*. 2011;101:250–264.

103. Levy JK, Scott HM, Lachtara JL, et al. Seroprevalence of feline leukemia virus and feline immunodeficiency virus infection among cats in North America and risk factors for seropositivity. *J Am Vet Med Assoc*. 2006;228:371–376.
104. Muirden A. Prevalence of feline leukaemia virus and antibodies to feline immunodeficiency virus and feline coronavirus in stray cats sent to an RSPCA hospital. *Vet Rec*. 2002;150:621–625.
105. Yilmaz H, Ilgaz A, Harbour DA. Prevalence of FIV and FeLV infections in cats in Istanbul. *J Feline Med Surg*. 2000;2:69–70.
106. Bande F, Arshad SS, Hassan L, et al. Molecular detection, phylogenetic analysis, and identification of transcription motifs in feline leukemia virus from naturally infected cats in Malaysia. *Vet Med Int*. 2014;2014:760961.
107. Bande F, Arshad SS, Hassan L, et al. Prevalence and risk factors of feline leukaemia virus and feline immunodeficiency virus in peninsular Malaysia. *BMC Vet Res*. 2012;8:33.
108. Rypula K, Ploneczka-Janeczko K, Bierowiec K, et al. Prevalence of viral infections in cats in southwestern Poland in the years 2006 to 2010. *Berl Munch Tierarztl Wochenschr*. 2014;127:163–165.
109. Spada E, Proverbio D, della Pepa A, et al. Seroprevalence of feline immunodeficiency virus, feline leukaemia virus and *Toxoplasma gondii* in stray cat colonies in northern Italy and correlation with clinical and laboratory data. *J Feline Med Surg*. 2012;14:369–377.
110. Studer N, Lutz H, Saegerman C, et al. Pan-European study on the prevalence of the feline leukaemia virus infection - reported by the European Advisory Board on Cat Diseases (ABCD Europe). *Viruses*. 2019:11.
111. Sukhumavasi W, Bellosa ML, Lucio-Forster A, et al. Serological survey of *Toxoplasma gondii, Dirofilaria immitis*, feline immunodeficiency virus (FIV) and feline leukemia virus (FeLV) infections in pet cats in Bangkok and vicinities, Thailand. *Vet Parasitol*. 2012;188:25–30.
112. Westman M, Norris J, Malik R, et al. The diagnosis of feline leukaemia virus (FeLV) infection in owned and group-housed rescue cats in Australia. *Viruses*. 2019;11.
113. Cong W, Meng QF, Blaga R, et al. *Toxoplasma gondii, Dirofilaria immitis*, feline immunodeficiency virus (FIV), and feline leukemia virus (FeLV) infections in stray and pet cats (*Felis catus*) in northwest China: co-infections and risk factors. *Parasitol Res*. 2016;115:217–223.
114. Garigliany M, Jolly S, Dive M, et al. Risk factors and effect of selective removal on retroviral infections prevalence in Belgian stray cats. *Vet Rec*. 2016;178:45.
115. Hwang J, Gottdenker N, Min MS, et al. Evaluation of biochemical and haematological parameters and prevalence of selected pathogens in feral cats from urban and rural habitats in South Korea. *J Feline Med Surg*. 2016;18:443–451.
116. Najafi H, Madadgar O, Jamshidi S, et al. Molecular and clinical study on prevalence of feline herpesvirus type 1 and calicivirus in correlation with feline leukemia and immunodeficiency viruses. *Vet Res Forum*. 2014;5:255–261.
117. Dubey JP, Lappin MR, Kwok OC, et al. Seroprevalence of *Toxoplasma gondii* and concurrent *Bartonella* spp., feline immunodeficiency virus, and feline leukemia virus infections in cats from Grenada, West Indies. *J Parasitol*. 2009;95:1129–1133.
118. Kelly PJ, Moura L, Miller T, et al. Feline immunodeficiency virus, feline leukemia virus and *Bartonella* species in stray cats on St Kitts, West Indies. *J Feline Med Surg*. 2010;12:447–450.
119. Levy JK, Crawford PC, Lappin MR, et al. Infectious diseases of dogs and cats on Isabela island, Galapagos. *J Vet Intern Med*. 2008;22:60–65.
120. Little S, Sears W, Lachtara J, et al. Seroprevalence of feline leukemia virus and feline immunodeficiency virus infection among cats in Canada. *Can Vet J*. 2009;50:644–648.
121. Solano-Gallego L, Hegarty B, Espada Y, et al. Serological and molecular evidence of exposure to arthropod-borne organisms in cats from northeastern Spain. *Vet Microbiol*. 2006;118:274–277.
122. Harrus S, Klement E, Aroch I, et al. Retrospective study of 46 cases of feline haemobartonellosis in Israel and their relationships with FeLV and FIV infections. *Vet Rec*. 2002;151:82–85.
123. Levy JK. FeLV and non-neoplastic FeLV-related disease. In: Ettinger SJ, Feldman EC, eds. *Textbook of Veterinary Internal Medicine*. Philadelphia: WB, Saunders; 2000:424–432.
124. Englert T, Lutz H, Hartmann K. Untersuchung des FeLV-Status der süddeutschen Katzenpopulation. *Tierarztl Prax*. 2009;37:9.
125. Cotter SM. Changing epidemiology of FeLV. Florida: USA *Proceedings of the 15th Annual ACVIM Forum*. 1997:22–25.
126. Hofmann-Lehmann R, Gonczi E, Riond B, et al. Feline leukemia virus infection: importance and current situation in Switzerland. *Schweiz Arch Tierheilkd*. 2018;160:95–105.
127. Burling AN, Levy JK, Scott HM, et al. Seroprevalences of feline leukemia virus and feline immunodeficiency virus infection in cats in the United States and Canada and risk factors for seropositivity. *J Am Vet Med Assoc*. 2017;251:187–194.
128. Fromont E, Pontier D, Langlais M. Dynamics of a feline retrovirus (FeLV) in host populations with variable spatial structure. *Proc Biol Sci*. 1998;265:1097–1104.
129. Chhetri BK, Berke O, Pearl DL, et al. Comparison of risk factors for seropositivity to feline immunodeficiency virus and feline leukemia virus among cats: a case-case study. *BMC Vet Res*. 2015;11:30.
130. Galdo Novo S, Bucafusco D, Diaz LM, et al. Viral diagnostic criteria for feline immunodeficiency virus and feline leukemia virus infections in domestic cats from Buenos Aires, Argentina. *Rech Appl Market*. 2016;48:293–297.
131. Goldkamp CE, Levy JK, Edinboro CH, et al. Seroprevalences of feline leukemia virus and feline immunodeficiency virus in cats with abscesses or bite wounds and rate of veterinarian compliance with current guidelines for retrovirus testing. *J Am Vet Med Assoc*. 2008;232:1152–1158.
132. Hoover EA, Olsen RG, Hardy Jr WD, et al. Feline leukemia virus infection: age-related variation in response of cats to experimental infection. *J Natl Cancer Inst*. 1976;57:365–369.
133. Hosie MJ, Robertson C, Jarrett O. Prevalence of feline leukaemia virus and antibodies to feline immunodeficiency virus in cats in the United Kingdom. *Vet Rec*. 1989;125:293–297.
134. de Castro FL, Junqueira DM, de Medeiros RM, et al. Analysis of single-nucleotide polymorphisms in the APOBEC3H gene of domestic cats (*Felis catus*) and their association with the susceptibility to feline immunodeficiency virus and feline leukemia virus infections. *J Mol Epidemiol Evol Genetics Infect Dis*. 2014;27:389–394.
135. Rojko JL, Hoover EA, Quackenbush SL, et al. Reactivation of latent feline leukaemia virus infection. *Nature*. 1982;298:385–388.
136. Hofmann-Lehmann R, Huder JB, Gruber S, et al. Feline leukaemia provirus load during the course of experimental infection and in naturally infected cats. *J Gen Virol*. 2001;82:1589–1596.
137. Gomes-Keller MA, Gonczi E, Tandon R, et al. Detection of feline leukemia virus RNA in saliva from naturally infected cats and correlation of PCR results with those of current diagnostic methods. *J Clin Microbiol*. 2006;44:916–922.
138. Gomes-Keller MA, Tandon R, Gonczi E, et al. Shedding of feline leukemia virus RNA in saliva is a consistent feature in viremic cats. *Vet Microbiol*. 2006;112:11–21.
139. Cattori V, Tandon R, Riond B, et al. The kinetics of feline leukaemia virus shedding in experimentally infected cats are associated with infection outcome. *Vet Microbiol*. 2009;133:292–296.
140. Gomes-Keller MA, Gonczi E, Grenacher B, et al. Fecal shedding of infectious feline leukemia virus and its nucleic acids: a transmission potential. *Vet Microbiol*. 2009;134:208–217.
141. Vobis M, D'Haese J, Mehlhorn H, et al. The feline leukemia virus (FeLV) and the cat flea (*Ctenocephalides felis*). *Parasitol Res*. 2003;90 (suppl 3):S132–S134.
142. Vobis M, D'Haese J, Mehlhorn H, et al. Evidence of horizontal transmission of feline leukemia virus by the cat flea (*Ctenocephalides felis*). *Parasitol Res*. 2003;91:467–470.
143. Lutz H, Addie D, Belak S, et al. Feline leukaemia. ABCD guidelines on prevention and management. *J Feline Med Surg*. 2009;11:565–574.
144. Nesina S, Katrin Helfer-Hungerbuehler A, Riond B, et al. Retroviral DNA–the silent winner: blood transfusion containing latent feline leukemia provirus causes infection and disease in naive recipient cats. *Retrovirology*. 2015;12:105.

145. Addie DD, Boucraut-Baralon C, Egberink H, et al. Disinfectant choices in veterinary practices, shelters and households: ABCD guidelines on safe and effective disinfection for feline environments. *J Feline Med Surg.* 2015;17:594–605.
146. Pacitti AM, Jarrett O, Hay D. Transmission of feline leukaemia virus in the milk of a non-viraemic cat. *Vet Rec.* 1986;118:381–384.
147. Hoover EA, Mullins JI. Feline leukemia virus infection and diseases. *J Am Vet Med Assoc.* 1991;199:1287–1297.
148. Helfer-Hungerbuehler AK, Cattori V, Boretti FS, et al. Dominance of highly divergent feline leukemia virus A progeny variants in a cat with recurrent viremia and fatal lymphoma. *Retrovirology.* 2010;7:14.
149. Helfer-Hungerbuehler AK, Widmer S, Kessler Y, et al. Long-term follow up of feline leukemia virus infection and characterization of viral RNA loads using molecular methods in tissues of cats with different infection outcomes. *Virus Res.* 2015;197:137–150.
150. Hofmann-Lehmann R, Cattori V, Tandon R, et al. How molecular methods change our views of FeLV infection and vaccination. *Vet Immunol Immunopathol.* 2008;123:119–123.
151. Hofmann-Lehmann R, Cattori V, Tandon R, et al. Vaccination against the feline leukaemia virus: outcome and response categories and long-term follow-up. *Vaccine.* 2007;25:5531–5539.
152. Torres AN, Mathiason CK, Hoover EA. Re-examination of feline leukemia virus: host relationships using real-time PCR. *Virology.* 2005;332:272–283.
153. Madewell BR, Jarrett O. Recovery of feline leukaemia virus from non-viraemic cats. *Vet Rec.* 1983;112:339–342.
154. Pacitti AM, Jarrett O. Duration of the latent state in feline leukaemia virus infections. *Vet Rec.* 1985;117:472–474.
155. Pedersen NC, Meric SM, Ho E. The clinical significance of latent feline leukemia virus infection in cats. *Feline Pract.* 1984;14:32–48.
156. Post JE, Warren L. Reactivation of latent feline leukemia virus. In: Hardy WD, Essex M, McClelland AJ, eds. *Feline Leukemia Virus.* North Holland, New York: Elsevier; 1980:424–432.
157. Major A, Cattori V, Boenzli E, et al. Exposure of cats to low doses of FeLV: seroconversion as the sole parameter of infection. *Vet Res.* 2010;41:17.
158. Cattori V, Pepin AC, Tandon R, et al. Real-time PCR investigation of feline leukemia virus proviral and viral RNA loads in leukocyte subsets. *Vet Immunol Immunopathol.* 2008;123:124–128.
159. Hofmann-Lehmann R, Holznagel E, Aubert A, et al. Recombinant FeLV vaccine: long-term protection and effect on course and outcome of FIV infection. *Vet Immunol Immunopathol.* 1995;46:127–137.
160. Pepin AC, Tandon R, Cattori V, et al. Cellular segregation of feline leukemia provirus and viral RNA in leukocyte subsets of long-term experimentally infected cats. *Virus Res.* 2007;127:9–16.
161. Suntz M, Failing K, Hecht W, et al. High prevalence of non-productive FeLV infection in necropsied cats and significant association with pathological findings. *Vet Immunol Immunopathol.* 2010;136:71–80.
162. Stützer B, Muller F, Majzoub M, et al. Role of latent feline leukemia virus infection in nonregenerative cytopenias of cats. *J Vet Intern Med.* 2010;24:192–197.
163. Gabor LJ, Love DN, Malik R, et al. Feline immunodeficiency virus status of Australian cats with lymphosarcoma. *Aust Vet J.* 2001;79:540–545.
164. Jackson ML, Haines DM, Meric SM, et al. Feline leukemia virus detection by immunohistochemistry and polymerase chain reaction in formalin-fixed, paraffin-embedded tumor tissue from cats with lymphosarcoma. *Can Vet J.* 1993;57:269–276.
165. Wang J, Kyaw-Tanner M, Lee C, et al. Characterisation of lymphosarcomas in Australian cats using polymerase chain reaction and immunohistochemical examination. *Aust Vet J.* 2001;79:41–46.
166. Weiss AT, Klopfleisch R, Gruber AD. Prevalence of feline leukaemia provirus DNA in feline lymphomas. *J Feline Med Surg.* 2010;12:929–935.
167. Sheets RL, Pandey R, Jen WC, et al. Recombinant feline leukemia virus genes detected in naturally occurring feline lymphosarcomas. *J Virol.* 1993;67:3118–3125.
168. Beatty JA, Tasker S, Jarrett O, et al. Markers of feline leukaemia virus infection or exposure in cats from a region of low seroprevalence. *J Feline Med Surg.* 2011;13:927–933.
169. Stützer B, Simon K, Lutz H, et al. Incidence of persistent viraemia and latent feline leukaemia virus infection in cats with lymphoma. *J Feline Med Surg.* 2011;13:81–87.
170. Rezanka LJ, Rojko JL, Neil JC. Feline leukemia virus: pathogenesis of neoplastic disease. *Cancer Invest.* 1992;10:371–389.
171. Rohn JL, Linenberger ML, Hoover EA, et al. Evolution of feline leukemia virus variant genomes with insertions, deletions, and defective envelope genes in infected cats with tumors. *J Virol.* 1994;68:2458–2467.
172. Krunic M, Ertl R, Hagen B, et al. Decreased expression of endogenous feline leukemia virus in cat lymphomas: a case control study. *BMC Vet Res.* 2015;11:90.
173. Cattori V, Hofmann-Lehmann R. Absolute quantitation of feline leukemia virus proviral DNA and viral RNA loads by TaqMan real-time PCR and RT-PCR. *Methods Mol Biol.* 2008;429:73–87.
174. Hayes KA, Rojko JL, Tarr MJ, et al. Atypical localised viral expression in a cat with feline leukaemia. *Vet Rec.* 1989;124:344–346.
175. Addie DD, Dennis JM, Toth S, et al. Long-term impact on a closed household of pet cats of natural infection with feline coronavirus, feline leukaemia virus and feline immunodeficiency virus. *Vet Rec.* 2000;146:419–424.
176. Cotter SM. Management of healthy feline leukemia virus-positive cats. *J Am Vet Med Assoc.* 1991;199:1470–1473.
177. Mandrioli L, Morini M, Biserni R, et al. A case of feline neurolymphomatosis: pathological and molecular investigations. *J Vet Diagn Invest.* 2012;24:1083–1086.
178. Hardy Jr WD, Zuckerman EE, MacEwen EG, et al. A feline leukaemia virus- and sarcoma virus-induced tumour-specific antigen. *Nature.* 1977;270:249–251.
179. Vedbrat SS, Rasheed S, Lutz H, et al. Feline oncornavirus-associated cell membrane antigen: a viral and not a cellularly coded transformation-specific antigen of cat lymphomas. *Virology.* 1983;124:445–461.
180. Hardy WD Jr. Epidemiology of primary neoplasms of lymphoid tissues in animals. In: Twomey JJGR, ed. *Comprehensive Immunology of Lymphoreticular Neoplasms.* New York: Plenum Medical Book Company; 1978:129–180.
181. Hardy WD. Hematopoietic tumors of cats. *J Am Anim Hosp Assoc.* 1981;17:921–940.
182. Crighton GW. Lymphosarcoma in the cat. *Vet Rec.* 1969;84:329–331.
183. Dorn CR, Taylor DO, Hibbard HH. Epizootiologic characteristics of canine and feline leukemia and lymphoma. *Am J Vet Res.* 1967;28:993–1001.
184. Dorn CR, Taylor DO, Schneider R, et al. Survey of animal neoplasms in Alameda and Contra Costa Counties, California. II. Cancer morbidity in dogs and cats from Alameda county. *J Natl Cancer Inst.* 1968;40:307–318.
185. Shelton GH, Grant CK, Cotter SM, et al. Feline immunodeficiency virus and feline leukemia virus infections and their relationships to lymphoid malignancies in cats: a retrospective study (1968-1988). *J Acquir Immune Defic Syndr.* 1990;3:623–630.
186. Ellis JA, Jackson ML, Bartsch RC, et al. Use of immunohistochemistry and polymerase chain reaction for detection of oncornaviruses in formalin-fixed, paraffin-embedded fibrosarcomas from cats. *J Am Vet Med Assoc.* 1996;209:767–771.
187. Hartmann K. Role of retroviruses in feline lymphoma. *Viruses.* 2015;25:4–15.
188. Meichner K, Kruse DB, Hirschberger J, et al. Changes in prevalence of progressive feline leukaemia virus infection in cats with lymphoma in Germany. *Vet Rec.* 2012;171:348.
189. Louwerens M, London CA, Pedersen NC, et al. Feline lymphoma in the post-feline leukemia virus era. *J Vet Intern Med.* 2005;19:329–335.
190. Hardy Jr WD, Hirshaut Y, Hess P. Detection of the feline leukemia virus and other mammalian oncornaviruses by immunofluorescence. *Bibl Haematol.* 1973;39:778–799.
191. Jarrett O, Laird HM, Hay D. Determinants of the host range of feline leukaemia viruses. *J Gen Virol.* 1973;20:169–175.
192. Rickard CG, Post JE, Noronha F, et al. A transmissible virus-induced lymphocytic leukemia of the cat. *J Natl Cancer Inst.* 1969;42:987–1014.

193. Essex M, Cotter SM, Carpenter JL, et al. Feline oncornavirus-associated cell membrane antigen. II. Antibody titers in healthy cats from household and laboratory colony environments. *J Natl Cancer Inst.* 1975;54:631–635.
194. Cotter SM, Hardy Jr WD, Essex M. Association of feline leukemia virus with lymphosarcoma and other disorders in the cat. *J Am Vet Med Assoc.* 1975;166:449–454.
195. Francis DP, Cotter SM, Hardy Jr WD, et al. Comparison of virus-positive and virus-negative cases of feline leukemia and lymphoma. *Canc Res.* 1979;39:3866–3870.
196. Hardy Jr WD, McClelland AJ, Zuckerman EE, et al. Development of virus non-producer lymphosarcomas in pet cats exposed to FeLV. *Nature.* 1980;288:90–92.
197. Francis DP, Essex M, Hardy Jr WD. Excretion of feline leukaemia virus by naturally infected pet cats. *Nature.* 1977;269:252–254.
198. Teske E, van Straten G, van Noort R, et al. Chemotherapy with cyclophosphamide, vincristine, and prednisolone (COP) in cats with malignant lymphoma: new results with an old protocol. *J Vet Intern Med.* 2002;16:179–186.
199. Tsatsanis C, Fulton R, Nishigaki K, et al. Genetic determinants of feline leukemia virus-induced lymphoid tumors: patterns of proviral insertion and gene rearrangement. *J Virol.* 1994;68:8296–8303.
200. Watanabe S, Ito J, Baba T, et al. Notch2 transduction by feline leukemia virus in a naturally infected cat. *J Vet Med Sci.* 2014;76:553–557.
201. Forman LW, Pal-Ghosh R, Spanjaard RA, et al. Identification of LTR-specific small non-coding RNA in FeLV infected cells. *FEBS Lett.* 2009;583:1386–1390.
202. Fujino Y, Ohno K, Tsujimoto H. Molecular pathogenesis of feline leukemia virus-induced malignancies: insertional mutagenesis. *Vet Immunol Immunopathol.* 2008;123:138–143.
203. Bolin LL, Ahmad S, Levy LS. The surface glycoprotein of a natural feline leukemia virus subgroup A variant, FeLV-945, as a determinant of disease outcome. *Vet Immunol Immunopathol.* 2011;143:221–226.
204. Kawamura M, Umehara D, Odahara Y, et al. AKT capture by feline leukemia virus. *Arch Virol.* 2016;162:1031–1036.
205. Simon D, Eberle N, Laacke-Singer L, et al. Combination chemotherapy in feline lymphoma: treatment outcome, tolerability, and duration in 23 cats. *J Vet Intern Med.* 2008;22:394–400.
206. Vail DM, Moore AS, Ogilvie GK, et al. Feline lymphoma (145 cases): proliferation indices, cluster of differentiation 3 immunoreactivity, and their association with prognosis in 90 cats. *J Vet Intern Med.* 1998;12:349–354.
207. Mooney SC, Hayes AA, Matus RE, et al. Renal lymphoma in cats: 28 cases (1977-1984). *J Am Vet Med Assoc.* 1987;191:1473–1477.
208. Taylor SS, Goodfellow MR, Browne WJ, et al. Feline extranodal lymphoma: response to chemotherapy and survival in 110 cats. *J Small Anim Pract.* 2009;50:584–592.
209. Day MJ. Review of thymic pathology in 30 cats and 36 dogs. *J Small Anim Pract.* 1997;38:393–403.
210. Fabrizio F, Calam AE, Dobson JM, et al. Feline mediastinal lymphoma: a retrospective study of signalment, retroviral status, response to chemotherapy and prognostic indicators. *J Feline Med Surg.* 2014;16:637–644.
211. Brenn SH, Couto SS, Craft DM, et al. Evaluation of P-glycoprotein expression in feline lymphoma and correlation with clinical outcome. *Vet Comp Oncol.* 2008;6:201–211.
212. Valli VE, Jacobs RM, Norris A, et al. The histologic classification of 602 cases of feline lymphoproliferative disease using the National Cancer Institute working formulation. *J Vet Diagn Invest.* 2000;12:295–306.
213. Hisasue M, Nagashima N, Nishigaki K, et al. Myelodysplastic syndromes and acute myeloid leukemia in cats infected with feline leukemia virus clone33 containing a unique long terminal repeat. *Int J Cancer.* 2009;124:1133–1141.
214. Kyle KN, Wright Z. Apparent feline leukemia virus-induced chronic lymphocytic leukemia and response to treatment. *J Feline Med Surg.* 2010;12:341–344.
215. Weiss A. FeLV-associated chronic lymphocytic leukemia. *J Feline Med Surg.* 2010;12:995. author reply 996.
216. Comazzi S, Paltrinieri S, Caniatti M, et al. Erythremic myelosis (AML6er) in a cat. *J Feline Med Surg.* 2000;2:213–215.
217. Gelain ME, Antoniazzi E, Bertazzolo W, et al. Chronic eosinophilic leukemia in a cat: cytochemical and immunophenotypical features. *Vet Clin Pathol.* 2006;35:454–459.
218. De Bosschere H, Vander Stichele V. Essential thrombocythemia in a cat, associated with feline leukemia virus. *Tijdschr Diergeneeskd.* 2014;139:24–28.
219. Schaller JP, Essex M, Yohn DS, et al. Feline oncornavirus-associated cell membrane antigen. V. Humoral immune response to virus and cell membrane antigens in cats inoculated with Gardner-Arnstein feline sarcoma virus. *J Natl Cancer Inst.* 1975;55:1373–1378.
220. Stiles J, Bienzle D, Render JA, et al. Use of nested polymerase chain reaction (PCR) for detection of retroviruses from formalin-fixed, paraffin-embedded uveal melanomas in cats. *Vet Ophthalmol.* 1999;2:113–116.
221. Cullen CL, Haines DM, Jackson ML, et al. Lack of detection of feline leukemia and feline sarcoma viruses in diffuse iris melanomas of cats by immunohistochemistry and polymerase chain reaction. *J Vet Diagn Invest.* 2002;14:340–343.
222. Cho SJ, Lee HA, Hong S, et al. Uterine adenocarcinoma with feline leukemia virus infection. *Lab Anim Res.* 2011;27:347–351.
223. Lott-Stolz G. Short original report. Osteochondromatosis in the cat. *Schweiz Arch Tierheilkd.* 1988;130:635–638.
224. Pool RR, Carrig CB. Multiple cartilagenous exostoses in a cat. *Vet Pathol.* 1972;9:350–359.
225. Rosa C, Kirberger RM. Extraskeletal osteochondroma on a cat's elbow. *J South Afr Vet Assoc.* 2012;83:104.
226. Schrenzel MD, Higgins RJ, Hinrichs SH, et al. Type C retroviral expression in spontaneous feline olfactory neuroblastomas. *Acta Neuropathol.* 1990;80:547–553.
227. Pedersen NC. Feline leukemia virus infection. In: Ettinger SJ, Feldman EC, eds. *Feline Husbandry, Diseases and Management in the Multiple Cat Environment.* Goleta, CA: American Veterinary Publications; 1991:210–220.
228. Laberke S, Hartmann K. Differenzialdiagnostische Aspekte und Charakterisierung der Anämie bei 79 Katzen unter besonderer Berücksichtigung der Rolle von Infektionen mit felinen Hämoplasmen. *Tierarztl Prax.* 2009;37:33.
229. Shelton GH, Linenberger ML. Hematologic abnormalities associated with retroviral infections in the cat. *Sem Vet Med Surg.* 1995;10:220–233.
230. Kohn B, Weingart C, Eckmann V, et al. Primary immune-mediated hemolytic anemia in 19 cats: diagnosis, therapy, and outcome (1998-2004). *J Vet Intern Med.* 2006;20:159–166.
231. Tasker S, Murray JK, Knowles TG, et al. Coombs', haemoplasma and retrovirus testing in feline anaemia. *J Small Anim Pract.* 2010;51:192–199.
232. Quigley JG, Burns CC, Anderson MM, et al. Cloning of the cellular receptor for feline leukemia virus subgroup C (FeLV-C), a retrovirus that induces red cell aplasia. *Blood.* 2000;95:1093–1099.
233. Tailor CS, Willett BJ, Kabat D. A putative cell surface receptor for anemia-inducing feline leukemia virus subgroup C is a member of a transporter superfamily. *J Virol.* 1999;73:6500–6505.
234. Stokol T, B JT. Pure red cell aplasia in cats: 9 cases (1989-1997). *J Am Vet Med Assoc.* 1999;214:75–79.
235. Southard TL, Rodriguez-Ramos Fernandez J, Priest H, et al. Holoprosencephaly and pure red cell aplasia in a feline leukaemia virus-positive kitten. *J Comp Pathol.* 2016;154:239–242.
236. Shimoda T, Shiranaga N, Mashita T, et al. A hematological study on thirteen cats with myelodysplastic syndrome. *J Vet Med Sci.* 2000;62:59–64.
237. Weiss DJ. Aplastic anemia in cats - clinicopathological features and associated disease conditions 1996-2004. *J Feline Med Surg.* 2006;8:203–206.
238. Linenberger ML, Abkowitz JL. In vivo infection of marrow stromal fibroblasts by feline leukemia virus. *Exp Hematol.* 1992;20:1022–1027.
239. Linenberger ML, Deng T. The effects of feline retroviruses on cytokine expression. *Vet Immunol Immunopathol.* 1999;72:343–368.
240. Linenberger ML, Dow SW, Abkowitz JL. Feline leukemia virus infection downmodulates the production of growth-inhibitory activity by marrow stromal cells. *Exp Hematol.* 1995;23:1069–1079.

241. Hoffmann-Jagielska M, Winnicka A, Jagielski D, et al. Influence of naturally acquired feline leukemia virus (FeLV) infection on the phagocytic and respiratory burst activity of neutrophils and monocytes of peripheral blood. *Polish J Vet Sci.* 2005;8:93–97.
242. Lafrado LJ, Olsen RG. Demonstration of depressed polymorphonuclear leukocyte function in nonviremic FeLV-infected cats. *Cancer Invest.* 1986;4:297–300.
243. Wardini AB, Guimaraes-Costa AB, Nascimento MT, et al. Characterization of neutrophil extracellular traps in cats naturally infected with feline leukemia virus. *J Gen Virol.* 2010;91:259–264.
244. Quackenbush SL, Donahue PR, Dean GA, et al. Lymphocyte subset alterations and viral determinants of immunodeficiency disease induction by the feline leukemia virus FeLV-FAIDS. *J Virol.* 1990;64:5465–5474.
245. Hoffmann-Fezer G, Mortelbauer W, Hartmann K, et al. Comparison of T-cell subpopulations in cats naturally infected with feline leukaemia virus or feline immunodeficiency virus. *Res Vet Sci.* 1996;61:222–226.
246. Hofmann-Lehmann R, Holznagel E, Ossent P, et al. Parameters of disease progression in long-term experimental feline retrovirus (feline immunodeficiency virus and feline leukemia virus) infections: hematology, clinical chemistry, and lymphocyte subsets. *Clin Diagn Lab Immunol.* 1997;4:33–42.
247. Brown MR, Rogers KS. Neutropenia in dogs and cats: a retrospective study of 261 cases. *J Am Anim Hosp Assoc.* 2001;37:131–139.
248. Lutz H, Castelli I, Ehrensperger F, et al. Panleukopenia-like syndrome of FeLV caused by co-infection with FeLV and feline panleukopenia virus. *Vet Immunol Immunopathol.* 1995;46:21–33.
249. Kipar A, Kremendahl J, Grant CK, et al. Expression of viral proteins in feline leukemia virus-associated enteritis. *Vet Pathol.* 2000;37:129–136.
250. Kipar A, Kremendahl J, Jackson ML, et al. Comparative examination of cats with feline leukemia virus-associated enteritis and other relevant forms of feline enteritis. *Vet Pathol.* 2001;38:359–371.
251. Diehl LJ, Hoover EA. Early and progressive helper T-cell dysfunction in feline leukemia virus-induced immunodeficiency. *J Acquir Immune Defic Syndr.* 1992;5:1188–1194.
252. Ogilvie GK, Tompkins MB, Tompkins WA. Clinical and immunologic aspects of FeLV-induced immunosuppression. *Vet Microbiol.* 1988;17:287–296.
253. Pardi D, Hoover EA, Quackenbush SL, et al. Selective impairment of humoral immunity in feline leukemia virus-induced immunodeficiency. *Vet Immunol Immunopathol.* 1991;28:183–200.
254. Sykes JE. Immunodeficiencies caused by infectious diseases. *Vet Clin North Am Small Anim Pract.* 2010;40:409–423.
255. Franchini M. *Die Tollwutimpfung von mit FeLV infizierten Katzen (Thesis).* University of Zurich; 1990.
256. Reinacher M. Diseases associated with spontaneous feline leukemia virus (FeLV) infection in cats. *Vet Immunol Immunopathol.* 1989;21:85–95.
257. Reinacher M, Wittmer G, Koberstein H, et al. The significance of FeLV infection for diseases in necropsied cats. *Berl Munch Tierarztl Wochenschr.* 1995;108:58–60.
258. Bauer N, Balzer HJ, Thure S, et al. Prevalence of feline haemotropic mycoplasmas in convenience samples of cats in Germany. *J Feline Med Surg.* 2008;10:252–258.
259. Bergmann M, Englert T, Stuetzer B, et al. Risk factors of different hemoplasma species infections in cats. *BMC Vet Res.* 2017;13:52.
260. Sykes JE, Terry JC, Lindsay LL, et al. Prevalences of various hemoplasma species among cats in the United States with possible hemoplasmosis. *J Am Vet Med Assoc.* 2008;232:372–379.
261. de Bortoli CP, Andre MR, Seki MC, et al. Detection of hemoplasma and *Bartonella* species and co-infection with retroviruses in cats subjected to a spaying/neutering program in Jaboticabal, SP, Brazil. *Rev Bras Parasitol Vet.* 2012;21:219–223.
262. Jenkins KS, Dittmer KE, Marshall JC, et al. Prevalence and risk factor analysis of feline haemoplasma infection in New Zealand domestic cats using a real-time PCR assay. *J Feline Med Surg.* 2013;15:1063–1069.
263. Laberke S, Just F, Pfister K, et al. Prevalence of feline haemoplasma infection in cats in Southern Bavaria, Germany, and infection risk factor analysis. *Berl Munch Tierarztl Wochenschr.* 2010;123:42–48.
264. Macieira DB, de Menezes Rde C, Damico CB, et al. Prevalence and risk factors for hemoplasmas in domestic cats naturally infected with feline immunodeficiency virus and/or feline leukemia virus in Rio de Janeiro, Brazil. *J Feline Med Surg.* 2008;10:120–129.
265. Willi B, Boretti FS, Baumgartner C, et al. Prevalence, risk factor analysis, and follow-up of infections caused by three feline hemoplasma species in cats in Switzerland. *J Clin Microbiol.* 2006;44:961–969.
266. Bergmann M, Englert T, Stuetzer B, et al. Prevalence of *Bartonella* species infections in cats in Southern Germany. *Vet Rec.* 2017;180:325.
267. Buchmann AU, Kershaw O, Kempf VA, et al. Does a feline leukemia virus infection pave the way for *Bartonella henselae* infection in cats? *J Clin Microbiol.* 2010;48:3295–3300.
268. Martin-Sanchez J, Acedo C, Munoz-Perez M, et al. Infection by *Leishmania infantum* in cats: epidemiological study in Spain. *Vet Parasitol.* 2007;145:267–273.
269. Sobrinho LS, Rossi CN, Vides JP, et al. Coinfection of *Leishmania chagasi* with *Toxoplasma gondii*, feline immunodeficiency virus (FIV) and feline leukemia virus (FeLV) in cats from an endemic area of zoonotic visceral leishmaniasis. *Vet Parasitol.* 2012;187:302–306.
270. Spada E, Canzi I, Baggiani L, et al. Prevalence of *Leishmania infantum* and co-infections in stray cats in northern Italy. *Comp Immunol Microbiol Infect.* 2016;45:53–58.
271. Sherry K, Miro G, Trotta M, et al. A serological and molecular study of *Leishmania infantum* infection in cats from the Island of Ibiza (Spain). *Vector Borne and Zoonotic Diseases.* 2011;11:239–245.
272. Bergmann M, Englert T, Stuetzer B, et al. Prevalence of selected rickettsial infections in cats in Southern Germany. *Comp Immunol Microbiol Infect.* 2015;42:33–36.
273. Kitada AA, Favacho AR, Oliveira RV, et al. Detection of serum antibodies against *Bartonella* species in cats with sporotrichosis from Rio de Janeiro, Brazil. *J Feline Med Surg.* 2014;16:308–311.
274. Sierra P, Guillot J, Jacob H, et al. Fungal flora on cutaneous and mucosal surfaces of cats infected with feline immunodeficiency virus or feline leukemia virus. *Am J Vet Res.* 2000;61:158–161.
275. Piscopo SE. Feline retroviruses and the skin. *Vet Forum.* 2000:32–40.
276. Belgard S, Truyen U, Thibault JC, et al. Associations between infectious agents and chronic stomatitis in cats. *Berl Munch Tierarztl Wochenschr.* 2010;123:369–376.
277. Quimby JM, Elston T, Hawley J, et al. Evaluation of the association of *Bartonella* species, feline herpesvirus 1, feline calicivirus, feline leukemia virus and feline immunodeficiency virus with chronic feline gingivostomatitis. *J Feline Med Surg.* 2008;10:66–72.
278. Kornya MR, Little SE, Scherk MA, et al. Association between oral health status and retrovirus test results in cats. *J Am Vet Med Assoc.* 2014;245:916–922.
279. Rolim VM, Pavarini SP, Campos FS, et al. Clinical, pathological, immunohistochemical and molecular characterization of feline chronic gingivostomatitis. *J Feline Med Surg.* 2017;19:403–409.
280. Pedersen NC. Feline leukemia virus infection. In: Pedersen NC, ed. *Feline Infectious Diseases.* Santa Barbara, CA: American Veterinary Publications; 1988:83.
281. Day NK, O'Reilly-Felice C, Hardy Jr WD, et al. Circulating immune complexes associated with naturally occurring lymphosarcoma in pet cats. *J Immunol.* 1980;125:2363–2366.
282. Tuomari DL, Olsen RG, Singh VK, et al. Detection of circulating immune complexes by a Clq/protein A-ELISA during the preneoplastic stages of feline leukemia virus infection. *Vet Immunol Immunopathol.* 1984;7:227–238.
283. Anderson LJ, Jarrett WF. Membranous glomerulonephritis associated with leukaemia in cats. *Res Vet Sci.* 1971;12:179–180.
284. Brightman 2nd AH, Ogilvie GK, Tompkins M. Ocular disease in FeLV-positive cats: 11 cases (1981-1986). *J Am Vet Med Assoc.* 1991;198:1049–1051.
285. Jinks MR, English RV, Gilger BC. Causes of endogenous uveitis in cats presented to referral clinics in North Carolina. *Vet Ophthalmol.* 2016;19(suppl 1):30–37.
286. Oohashi E, Yamada K, Oohashi M, et al. Chronic progressive polyarthritis in a female cat. *J Vet Med Sci.* 2010;72:511–514.

287. Miro G, Domenech A, Escolar E, et al. Plasma electrophoretogram in feline immunodeficiency virus (FIV) and/or feline leukaemia virus (FeLV) infections. *J Vet Med.* 2007;54:203–209.
288. Gleich S, Hartmann K. Hematology and serum biochemistry of feline immunodeficiency virus-infected and feline leukemia virus-infected cats. *J Vet Intern Med.* 2009;23:552–558.
289. Raith K, Muntener T, Vandevelde M, et al. Encephalomyelitis resembling human and ruminant rhombencephalitis caused by *Listeria monocytogenes* in a feline leukemia virus-infected cat. *J Vet Intern Med.* 2010;24:983–985.
290. Carmichael KP, Bienzle D, McDonnell JJ. Feline leukemia virus-associated myelopathy in cats. *Vet Pathol.* 2002;39:536–545.
291. Fails AD, Mitchell TW, Rojko JL, et al. An oligopeptide of the feline leukemia virus envelope glycoprotein is associated with morphological changes and calcium dysregulation in neuronal growth cones. *J Neurovirol.* 1997;3:179–191.
292. Mitchell TW, Rojko JL, Hartke JR, et al. FeLV envelope protein (gp70) variable region 5 causes alterations in calcium homeostasis and toxicity of neurons. *J Acquir Immun Defic Syndr.* 1997;14:307–320.
293. Hartmann K. Clinical aspects of feline immunodeficiency and feline leukemia virus infection. *Vet Immunol Immunopathol.* 2011;143:190–201.
294. Hartmann K. Clinical aspects of feline retroviruses: a review. *Viruses.* 2012;4:2684–2710.
295. Sykes JE, Hartmann K. Feine leukemia virus infection. In: Sykes JE, ed. *Canine and Feline Infectious Diseases.* Philadelphia: WB, Saunders; 2013:224–238.
296. Little S, Bienzle D, Carioto L, et al. Feline leukemia virus and feline immunodeficiency virus in Canada: recommendations for testing and management. *Can Vet J.* 2011;52:849–855.
297. Little S, Levy J, Hartmann K, et al. AAFP feline retrovirus testing and management guidelines. *J Feline Med Surg.* 2020;22:5–30.
298. Levy JK, Richards J, Edwards D, et al. Feline retrovirus testing and management. *Compend Cont Educ Pract Vet.* 2001;22:652–657.
299. Levy JK, Crawford PC. Feline leukemia virus. In: Ettinger SJ, Feldman EC, eds. *Textbook of Veterinary Internal Medicine.* Philadelphia: WB, Saunders; 2005:653.
300. Levy J, Crawford C, Hartmann K, et al. American Association of Feline Practitioners' feline retrovirus management guidelines. 2008 *J Feline Med Surg.* 2008;10:300–316.
301. Hardy Jr WD, Zuckerman EE. Ten-year study comparing enzyme-linked immunosorbent assay with the immunofluorescent antibody test for detection of feline leukemia virus infection in cats. *J Am Vet Med Assoc.* 1991;199:1365–1373.
302. Jarrett O, Golder MC, Stewart MF. Detection of transient and persistent feline leukaemia virus infections. *Vet Rec.* 1982;110:225–228.
303. Jarrett O, Pacitti AM, Hosie MJ, et al. Comparison of diagnostic methods for feline leukemia virus and feline immunodeficiency virus. *J Am Vet Med Assoc.* 1991;199:1362–1364.
304. Lutz H, Pedersen NC, Durbin R, et al. Monoclonal antibodies to three epitopic regions of feline leukemia virus p27 and their use in enzyme-linked immunosorbent assay of p27. *J Immunol Methods.* 1983;56:209–220.
305. Hartmann K, Werner RM, Egberink H, et al. Comparison of six in-house tests for the rapid diagnosis of feline immunodeficiency and feline leukaemia virus infections. *Vet Rec.* 2001;149:317–320.
306. Hartmann K, Griessmayr P, Schulz B, et al. Quality of different in-clinic test systems for feline immunodeficiency virus and feline leukaemia virus infection. *J Feline Med Surg.* 2007;9:439–445.
307. Kim WS, Chong CK, Kim HY, et al. Development and clinical evaluation of a rapid diagnostic kit for feline leukemia virus infection. *J Vet Sci.* 2014;15:91–97.
308. Levy J. Performance of point-of-care Assays for FeLV and FIV. *Proceedings of the ACVIM Forum.* Denver, CO; 2016:772.
309. Pinches MD, Diesel G, Helps CR, et al. An update on FIV and FeLV test performance using a Bayesian statistical approach. *Vet Clin Pathol.* 2007;36:141–147.
310. Sand C, Englert T, Egberink H, et al. Evaluation of a new in-clinic test system to detect feline immunodeficiency virus and feline leukemia virus infection. *Vet Clin Pathol.* 2010;39:210–214.
311. Hawkins EC. Saliva and tear tests for feline leukemia virus. *J Am Vet Med Assoc.* 1991;199:1382–1385.
312. Weijer K, van Herwijnen R. Detection of FeLV antigen. *Vet Rec.* 1995;137:127.
313. Jarrett O. Detection of FeLV antigen. *Vet Rec.* 1995;137:127.
314. Arjona A, Barquero N, Domenech A, et al. Evaluation of a novel nested PCR for the routine diagnosis of feline leukemia virus (FeLV) and feline immunodeficiency virus (FIV). *J Feline Med Surg.* 2007;9:14–22.
315. Cattori V, Tandon R, Pepin A, et al. Rapid detection of feline leukemia virus provirus integration into feline genomic DNA. *Mol Cell Probes.* 2006;20:172–181.
316. Pinches MD, Helps CR, Gruffydd-Jones TJ, et al. Diagnosis of feline leukaemia virus infection by semi-quantitative real-time polymerase chain reaction. *J Feline Med Surg.* 2007;9:8–13.
317. Torres AN, O'Halloran KP, Larson LJ, et al. Development and application of a quantitative real-time PCR assay to detect feline leukemia virus RNA. *Vet Immunol Immunopathol.* 2008;123:81–89.
318. Beall MJ, Buch J, Clark G, et al. Feline leukemia virus p27 antigen concentration and proviral DNA load are associated with survival in naturally infected cats. *Viruses.* 2021;13:302.
319. Hofmann-Lehmann R, Tandon R, Boretti FS, et al. Reassessment of feline leukaemia virus (FeLV) vaccines with novel sensitive molecular assays. *Vaccine.* 2006;24:1087–1094.
320. Boenzli E, Hadorn M, Hartnack S, et al. Detection of antibodies to the feline leukemia virus (FeLV) transmembrane protein p15E: an alternative approach for serological FeLV detection based on antibodies to p15E. *J Clin Microbiol.* 2014;52:2046–2052.
321. Langhammer S, Hubner J, Kurth R, et al. Antibodies neutralizing feline leukaemia virus (FeLV) in cats immunized with the transmembrane envelope protein p15E. *Immunology.* 2006;117:229–237.
322. Poulet H, Brunet S, Boularand C, et al. Efficacy of a canarypox virus-vectored vaccine against feline leukaemia. *Vet Rec.* 2003;153:141–145.
323. Sparkes AH. Feline leukaemia virus and vaccination. *J Feline Med Surg.* 2003;5:97–100.
324. Reinacher M. Infektionen mit dem felinen Leukämie-Virus (FeLV) bei sezierten Katzen. *Kleintierpraxis.* 1987:56–72.
325. Santagostino SF, Mortellaro CM, Boracchi P, et al. Feline upper respiratory tract lymphoma: site, cyto-histology, phenotype, FeLV expression, and prognosis. *Vet Pathol.* 2015;52:250–259.
326. Hartmann K. Feline leukemia virus and feline immunodeficiency virus. In: Bonagura JD, Twedt DC, eds. *Kirk's Current Veterinary Therapy XIV.* St. Louis: Saunders Elsevier; 2009:1278–1283.
327. Hartmann K. Antiviral and immunomodulatory chemotherapy. In: Greene CE, ed. *Infectious Diseases of the Dog and Cat.* 4th ed. St Louis, Missouri: Elsevier, Saunders; 2012:10–24.
328. Bergmann M, Schwertler S, Speck S, et al. Antibody response to feline panleukopenia virus vaccination in cats with asymptomatic retrovirus infections: a pilot study. *J Feline Med Surg.* 2019;21:1094–1101.
329. Helfer-Hungerbuehler AK, Spiri AM, Riond B, et al. No benefit of therapeutic vaccination in clinically healthy cats persistently infected with feline leukemia virus. *Vaccine.* 2015;33:1578–1585.
330. Hartmann K. How I treat feline retrovirus infections. *NAVC Clinician's Brief.* 2012;5:79–84.
331. Ettinger SJ. Principles of treatment for feline lymphoma. *Clin Tech Small Anim Pract.* 2003:98–102.
332. Kristal O, Lana SE, Ogilvie GK, et al. Single agent chemotherapy with doxorubicin for feline lymphoma: a retrospective study of 19 cases (1994-1997). *J Vet Intern Med.* 2001;15:125–130.
333. Cotter SM. Treatment of lymphoma and leukaemia with cyclophosphamide, vincristine and prednisolone: II. Treatment of cats. *J Am Anim Hosp Assoc.* 1983;19:166–172.
334. Moore AS, Cotter SM, Frimberger AE, et al. A comparison of doxorubicin and COP for maintenance of remission in cats with lymphoma. *J Vet Intern Med.* 1996;10:372–375.
335. Ogilvie GK. Hematopoietic growth factors: frontiers for cure. *Vet Clin North Am Small Anim Pract.* 1995;25:1441–1456.
336. Arai MDJ, Lewis A, Yamamoto JK. The use of human hematopoietic growth factors (rhGM-CSF and rhEPO) as a supportive therapy for FIV-infected cats. *Vet Immunol Immunopathol.* 2000;77:71–92.

337. Greene CE, Watson ADJ. Immunoprophylaxis and immunotherapy. In: Greene CE, ed. *Infectious Diseases of the Dog and Cat*. 2nd ed. St Louis, Missouri: Elsevier Saunders; 1998:717–750.
338. Kraft W, Kuffer M. Treatment of severe neutropenias in dogs and cats with filgrastim. *Tierarztl Prax*. 1995;23:609–613.
339. Hartmann K, Block A, Ferk G, et al. Treatment of feline leukemia virus (FeLV) infection. *Vet Microbiol*. 1999;69:111–113.
340. Hartmann K, Donath A, Beer B, et al. Use of two virustatica (AZT, PMEA) in the treatment of FIV and of FeLV seropositive cats with clinical symptoms. *Vet Immunol Immunopathol*. 1992;35:167–175.
341. McCaw DL, Boon GD, Jergens AE, et al. Immunomodulation therapy for feline leukemia virus infection. *J Am Anim Hosp Assoc*. 2001;37:356–363.
342. Stuetzer B, Brunner K, Lutz H, et al. A trial with 3'-azido-2',3'-dideoxythymidine and human interferon-alpha in cats naturally infected with feline leukaemia virus. *J Feline Med Surg*. 2013;15:667–671.
343. Povey RC. Effect of orally administered ribavirin on experimental feline calicivirus infection in cats. *Am J Vet Res*. 1978;39:1337–1341.
344. Weiss RC, Cox NR, Boudreaux MK. Toxicologic effects of ribavirin in cats. *J Vet Pharmacol Ther*. 1993;16:301–316.
345. Cattori V, Weibel B, Lutz H. Inhibition of feline leukemia virus replication by the integrase inhibitor raltegravir. *Vet Microbiol*. 2011;152:165–168.
346. Greggs WM 3rd, Clouser CL, Patterson SE, et al. Discovery of drugs that possess activity against feline leukemia virus. *J Gen Virol*. 2012;93:900–905.
347. Boesch A, Cattori V, Riond B, et al. Evaluation of the effect of short-term treatment with the integrase inhibitor raltegravir (Isentress) on the course of progressive feline leukemia virus infection. *Vet Microbiol*. 2015;175:167–178.
348. Hartmann K. FeLV treatment strategies and prognosis. *Suppl Compend Cont Educ Pract Vet*. 2005;27:14.
349. Parr YA, Beall MJ, Levy JK, et al. Measuring the humoral immune response in cats exposed to feline leukaemia virus. *Viruses*. 2021;13:428.
350. Hoover EA, Schaller JP, Mathes LE, et al. Passive immunity to feline leukemia: evaluation of immunity from dams naturally infected and experimentally vaccinated. *Infect Immun*. 1977;16:54–59.
351. Weijer K, UytdeHaag FG, Jarrett O, et al. Post-exposure treatment with monoclonal antibodies in a retrovirus system: failure to protect cats against feline leukemia virus infection with virus neutralizing monoclonal antibodies. *Int J Cancer*. 1986;38:81–87.
352. Lutz H, Pedersen N, Higgins J, et al. Humoral immune reactivity to feline leukemia virus and associated antigens in cats naturally infected with feline leukemia virus. *Cancer Res*. 1980;40:3642–3651.
353. Flynn JN, Dunham SP, Watson V, et al. Longitudinal analysis of feline leukemia virus-specific cytotoxic T lymphocytes: correlation with recovery from infection. *J Virol*. 2002;76:2306–2315.
354. Russell PH, Jarrett O. The specificity of neutralizing antibodies to feline leukaemia viruses. *Int J Cancer*. 1978;21:768–778.
355. Flynn JN, Hanlon L, Jarrett O. Feline leukaemia virus: protective immunity is mediated by virus-specific cytotoxic T lymphocytes. *Immunology*. 2000;101:120–125.
356. Jarrett W, Mackey L, Jarrett O, et al. Antibody response and virus survival in cats vaccinated against feline leukaemia. *Nature*. 1974;248:230–232.
357. Wolff LH, Mathes LE, Olsen RG. Recovery of soluble feline oncornavirus-associated cell membrane antigen from large volumes of tissue culture fluids. *J Immunol Methods*. 1979;26:151–156.
358. Lewis MG, Mathes LE, Olsen RG. Protection against feline leukemia by vaccination with a subunit vaccine. *Infect Immun*. 1981;34:888–894.
359. Clark N, Kushner NN, Barrett CB, et al. Efficacy and safety field trials of a recombinant DNA vaccine against feline leukemia virus infection. *J Am Vet Med Assoc*. 1991;199:1433–1443.
360. Hines DL, Cutting JA, Dietrich DL, et al. Evaluation of efficacy and safety of an inactivated virus vaccine against feline leukemia virus infection. *J Am Vet Med Assoc*. 1991;199:1428–1430.
361. Legendre AM, Hawks DM, Sebring R, et al. Comparison of the efficacy of three commercial feline leukemia virus vaccines in a natural challenge exposure. *J Am Vet Med Assoc*. 1991;199:1456–1462.
362. Legendre AM, Mitchener KL, Potgieter LN. Efficacy of a feline leukemia virus vaccine in a natural exposure challenge. *J Vet Intern Med*. 1990;4:92–98.
363. Gruffydd-Jones TJ. A comparative study on the effects of a canarypox based recombinant leukaemia vaccine (Eurifel FeLV), against a natural FeLV challenge in cats. In: *Proceedings of the 24th World Small Animal Veterinary Association (WSAVA) Congress*. 2nd ed. Lyon, France; 1999.
364. Marciani DJ, Kensil CR, Beltz GA, et al. Genetically-engineered subunit vaccine against feline leukaemia virus: protective immune response in cats. *Vaccine*. 1991;9:89–96.
365. Tartaglia J, Jarrett O, Neil JC, et al. Protection of cats against feline leukemia virus by vaccination with a canarypox virus recombinant, ALVAC-FL. *J Virol*. 1993;67:2370–2375.
366. Torres AN, O'Halloran KP, Larson LJ, et al. Feline leukemia virus immunity induced by whole inactivated virus vaccination. *Vet Immunol Immunopathol*. 2010;134:122–131.
367. Schlecht-Louf G, Mangeney M, El-Garch H, et al. A targeted mutation within the feline leukemia virus (FeLV) envelope protein immunosuppressive domain to improve a canarypox virus-vectored FeLV vaccine. *J Virol*. 2014;88:992–1001.
368. Stuke K, King V, Southwick K, et al. Efficacy of an inactivated FeLV vaccine compared to a recombinant FeLV vaccine in minimum age cats following virulent FeLV challenge. *Vaccine*. 2014;32:2599–2603.
369. Hofmann-Lehmann R, Levy LS, Willett BJ. Comparing the efficacy of FeLV vaccines: comment on: Stuke, K. et al. Efficacy of an inactivated FeLV vaccine compared to a recombinant FeLV vaccine in minimum age cats following virulent FeLV challenge. Vaccine 2014;32(22):2599-2603. *Vaccine*. 2015;33:2737-2738.
370. Patel M, Carritt K, Lane J, et al. Comparative efficacy of feline leukemia virus (FeLV) inactivated whole-virus vaccine and canarypox virus-vectored vaccine during virulent FeLV challenge and immunosuppression. *Clin Vaccine Immunol*. 2015;22:798–805.
371. Poulet H, Thibault JC, Masias A. Immunosuppression in a comparative study of feline leukemia virus vaccines. *Clin Vaccine Immunol*. 2015;22:1294–1295.
372. Patel M, Carritt K, Lane J, et al. Reply to "Immunosuppression in a comparative study of feline leukemia virus vaccines". *Clin Vaccine Immunol*. 2015;22:1296–1297.
373. Richards JR, Elston TH, Ford RB, et al. The 2006 American Association of Feline Practitioners Feline Vaccine Advisory Panel report. *J Am Vet Med Assoc*. 2006;229:1405–1441.
374. Stone AE, Brummet GO, Carozza EM, et al. AAHA/AAFP feline vaccination guidelines. *J Feline Med Surg*. 2020;22:813–830. 2020.
375. Jirjis FF, Davis T, Lane J, et al. Protection against feline leukemia virus challenge for at least 2 years after vaccination with an inactivated feline leukemia virus vaccine. *Vet Ther*. 2010;11:E1–E6.
376. Wilson S, Greenslade J, Saunders G, et al. Difficulties in demonstrating long term immunity in FeLV vaccinated cats due to increasing age-related resistance to infection. *BMC Vet Res*. 2012;8:125.
377. Kanellos T, Sutton DJ, Salisbury CF, et al. Combined administration in a single injection of a feline multivalent modified live vaccine against FHV, FCV, and FPLV together with a recombinant FeLV vaccine is both safe and efficacious for all four major feline viral pathogens. *J Feline Med Surg*. 2008;10:346–354.
378. Hartmann K. ABCD Guidelines: Vaccination of Immunocompromised Cats. 2017. Available at: http://www.abcdcatsvets.org/vaccination-of-immunocompromised-cats/.
379. Lehmann R, Franchini M, Aubert A, et al. Vaccination of cats experimentally infected with feline immunodeficiency virus, using a recombinant feline leukemia virus vaccine. *J Am Vet Med Assoc*. 1991;199:1446–1452.
380. Kass PH, Spangler WL, Hendrick MJ, et al. Multicenter case-control study of risk factors associated with development of vaccine-associated sarcomas in cats. *J Am Vet Med Assoc*. 2003;223:1283–1292.
381. Day MJ, Schoon HA, Magnol JP, et al. A kinetic study of histopathological changes in the subcutis of cats injected with non-adjuvanted and adjuvanted multi-component vaccines. *Vaccine*. 2007;25:4073–4084.
382. Kidney BA, Ellis JA, Haines DM, et al. Evaluation of formalin-fixed paraffin-embedded tissues obtained from vaccine site-associated sarcomas of cats for DNA of feline immunodeficiency virus. *Am J Vet Res*. 2000;61:1037–1041.

383. Kidney BA, Haines DM, Ellis JA, et al. Evaluation of formalin-fixed paraffin-embedded tissues from vaccine site-associated sarcomas of cats for polyomavirus DNA and antigen. *Am J Vet Res.* 2001;62:828–832.
384. Kidney BA, Haines DM, Ellis JA, et al. Evaluation of formalin-fixed paraffin-embedded tissues from feline vaccine site-associated sarcomas for feline foamy virus DNA. *Am J Vet Res.* 2002;63:60–63.
385. Kidney BA, Haines DM, Ellis JA, et al. Evaluation of formalin-fixed paraffin-embedded tissues from vaccine site-associated sarcomas of cats for papillomavirus DNA and antigen. *Am J Vet Res.* 2001;62:833–839.
386. Roccabianca P, Avallone G, Rodriguez A, et al. Cutaneous lymphoma at injection sites: pathological, immunophenotypical, and molecular characterization in 17 cats. *Vet Pathol.* 2016;53:823–832.
387. Hartmann K, Day MJ, Thiry E, et al. Feline injection-site sarcoma: ABCD guidelines on prevention and management. *J Feline Med Surg.* 2015;17:606–613.
388. Pennisi MG, Hartmann K, Addie DD, et al. Blood transfusion in cats: ABCD guidelines for minimising risks of infectious iatrogenic complications. *J Feline Med Surg.* 2015;17:588–593.
389. Herring IP, Troy GC, Toth TE, et al. Feline leukemia virus detection in corneal tissues of cats by polymerase chain reaction and immunohistochemistry. *Vet Ophthalmol.* 2001;4:119–126.
390. Hosie MJ, Addie DD, Boucraut-Baralon C, et al. Matrix vaccination guidelines: 2015 ABCD recommendations for indoor/outdoor cats, rescue shelter cats and breeding catteries. *J Feline Med Surg.* 2015;17:583–587.
391. Nakata R, Miyazawa T, Shin YS, et al. Reevaluation of host ranges of feline leukemia virus subgroups. *Microbes Infect.* 2003;5:947–950.
392. Morgan RA, Dornsife RE, Anderson WF, et al. In vitro infection of human bone marrow by feline leukemia viruses. *Virology.* 1993;193:439–442.
393. Bross ID, Gibson R. Cats and childhood leukemia. *Journal of Medicine.* 1970;1:180–187.
394. Penrose M. Cat leukemia. *Br Med J.* 1970;1:775.
395. Blair A, Hayes Jr HM. Cancer and other causes of death among U.S. veterinarians, 1966-1977. *Int J Cancer.* 1980;25:181–185.
396. Fasal E, Jackson EW, Klauber MR. Mortality in California veterinarians. *J Chronic Dis.* 1966;19:293–306.
397. Gutenson NEM, Francis DP. Risk to humans from exposure to feline leukemia virus: epidemiological considerations. Viruses in naturally occurring cancers. *J Egypt Soc Parasitol.* 1980;7.
398. Caldwell GG, Baumgartener L, Carter C, et al. Seroepidemiologic testing in man for evidence of antibodies to feline leukemia virus and bovine leukemia virus. *Bibl Haematol.* 1975:238–241.
399. Jacquemin PC, Saxinger C, Gallo RC. Surface antibodies of human myelogenous leukaemia leukocytes reactive with specific type-C viral reverse transcriptases. *Nature.* 1978;276:230–236.
400. Olsen RG, Mathes LE, Yohn DS. Complement-fixation-inhibition as a test for antibodies in cats and humans to C-type RNA tumor virus antigen. *Bibl Haematol.* 1975:419–429.
401. Fink MA, Sibal LR, Plata EJ. Serologic detection of feline leukemia virus antigens or antibodies. *J Am Vet Med Assoc.* 1971;158(suppl 2):1070+.
402. Nowotny N, Uthman A, Haas OA, et al. Is it possible to catch leukemia from a cat? *J Egypt Soc Parasitol.* 1995;346:252–253.
403. Terry A, Kilbey A, Naseer A, et al. Barriers to infection of human cells by feline leukemia virus: insights into resistance to zoonosis. *J Virol.* 2017;91.
404. Anderson MM, Lauring AS, Robertson S, et al. Feline Pit2 functions as a receptor for subgroup B feline leukemia viruses. *J Virol.* 2001;75:10563–10572.
405. Keel SB, Doty RT, Yang Z, et al. A heme export protein is required for red blood cell differentiation and iron homeostasis. *Science.* 2008;319:825–828.
406. Hoover EA, Zeidner NS, Mullins JI. Therapy of presymptomatic FeLV-induced immunodeficiency syndrome with AZT in combination with alpha interferon. *Ann NY Acad Sci.* 1990;616:258–269.
407. Mathes LE, Polas PJ, Hayes KA, et al. Pre- and postexposure chemoprophylaxis: evidence that 3'-azido-3'-dideoxythymidine inhibits feline leukemia virus disease by a drug-induced vaccine response. *Antimicrobial Agents Chemother.* 1992;36:2715–2721.
408. Mukherji E, Au JL, Mathes LE. Differential antiviral activities and intracellular metabolism of 3'-azido-3'-deoxythymidine and 2',3'-dideoxyinosine in human cells. *Antimicrobial Agents Chemother.* 1994;38:1573–1579.
409. Tavares L, Roneker C, Johnston K, et al. 3'-Azido-3'-deoxythymidine in feline leukemia virus-infected cats: a model for therapy and prophylaxis of AIDS. *Cancer Res.* 1987;47:3190–3194.
410. Tavares L, Roneker C, Postie L, et al. Testing of nucleoside analogues in cats infected with feline leukemia virus: a model. *Intervirology.* 1989;30(suppl 1):26–35.
411. Zeidner NS, Rose LM, Mathiason-DuBard CK, et al. Zidovudine in combination with alpha interferon and interleukin-2 as prophylactic therapy for FeLV-induced immunodeficiency syndrome (FeLV-FAIDS). *J Acquir Immune Defic Syndr.* 1990;3:787–796.
412. Zeidner NS, Myles MH, Mathiason-DuBard CK, et al. Alpha interferon (2b) in combination with zidovudine for the treatment of presymptomatic feline leukemia virus-induced immunodeficiency syndrome. *Antimicrobial Agents Chemother.* 1990;34:1749–1756.
413. Hoover EA, Zeidner NS, Perigo NA, et al. Feline leukemia virus-induced immunodeficiency syndrome in cats as a model for evaluation of antiretroviral therapy. *Intervirology.* 1989;30(suppl 1):12–25.
414. Polas PJ, Swenson CL, Sams R, et al. In vitro and in vivo evidence that the antiviral activity of 2',3'-dideoxycytidine is target cell dependent in a feline retrovirus animal model. *Antimicrobial Agents Chemother.* 1990;34:1414–1421.
415. Zeidner NS, Strobel JD, Perigo NA, et al. Treatment of FeLV-induced immunodeficiency syndrome (FeLV-FAIDS) with controlled release capsular implantation of 2',3'-dideoxycytidine. *Antiviral Res.* 1989;11:147–160.
416. Hoover EA, Ebner JP, Zeidner NS, et al. Early therapy of feline leukemia virus infection (FeLV-FAIDS) with 9-(2-phosphonylmethoxyethyl) adenine (PMEA). *Antiviral Res.* 1991;16:77–92.
417. Swenson CL, Polas PJ, Cheney CM, et al. Prophylactic and therapeutic effects of phosphonoformate against feline leukemia virus in vitro. *Am J Vet Res.* 1991;52:2010–2015.
418. Greene CE, Watson ADJ. Antiviral drugs. In: Greene CE, ed. *Infectious Diseases of the Dog and Cat.* 2nd ed. St Louis, Missouri: Elsevier Saunders; 1998a:6–9.
419. Zhu Y, Antony JM, Martinez JA, et al. Didanosine causes sensory neuropathy in an HIV/AIDS animal model: impaired mitochondrial and neurotrophic factor gene expression. *Brain.* 2007;130:2011–2023.
420. Lloret A. The process of evidence-based medicine. *J Feline Med Surg.* 2009;11:529.
421. Jameson P, Essex M. Inhibition of feline leukemia virus replication by human leukocyte interferon. *Antiviral Res.* 1983;3:115–120.
422. Rogers R, Merigan TC, Hardy Jr WD, et al. Cat interferon inhibits feline leukaemia virus infection in cell culture. *Nature: New Biol.* 1972;237:270–271.
423. Gil S, Leal RO, Duarte A, et al. Relevance of feline interferon omega for clinical improvement and reduction of concurrent viral excretion in retrovirus infected cats from a rescue shelter. *Res Vet Sci.* 2013;94:753–763.
424. De Mari K, Maynard L, Sanquer A, et al. Therapeutic effects of recombinant feline interferon-omega on feline leukemia virus (FeLV)-infected and FeLV/feline immunodeficiency virus (FIV)-coinfected symptomatic cats. *J Vet Intern Med.* 2004;18:477–482.
425. Bachman D, Cockerell GL, de Noronha F, et al. Effect of bacille Calmette-Guerin immunotherapy on feline sarcoma virus-induced neoplasms in the cat. *Am J Vet Res.* 1982;43:475–480.
426. Nelson P, Sellon R, Novotney C, et al. Therapeutic effects of diethylcarbamazine and 3'-azido-3'-deoxythymidine on feline leukemia virus lymphoma formation. *Vet Immunol Immunopathol.* 1995;46:181–194.

33

Feline Immunodeficiency Virus Infection

Julia A. Beatty, Jane E. Sykes

KEY POINTS

- Cause: FIV (family *Retroviridae*, subfamily *Orthoretrovirinae*, genus *Lentivirus*).
- First Described: California, 1986;[1] serologic evidence of infection dates back to the 1960s.[2,3]
- Affected Hosts: Domestic and wild cats; hyenas.
- Geographic Distribution: Endemic worldwide.
- Mode of Transmission: Primarily biting. Queen-to-kitten transmission uncommon. Horizontal between housemates rare. Iatrogenic via blood transfusion possible.
- Major Clinical Signs: Most FIV-infected cats are subclinically infected for most or all of their lifetime. Signs include lethargy and fever, stomatitis, chronic GI signs, wasting, neurologic signs, high-grade lymphoma, immune-mediated diseases, and opportunistic infections.
- Differential Diagnoses: Variable depending on clinical signs.
- Human Health Significance: FIV does not infect humans. Immunosuppressed owners should be counseled regarding the risk of opportunistic pathogen exposure from any immunosuppressed pet.

ETIOLOGIC AGENT AND EPIDEMIOLOGY

FIV is an enveloped, RNA virus that belongs to the *Lentivirus* genus of the *Retroviridae*. It infects domestic and wild cats worldwide, as well as hyenas.[4] FIV strains are highly host-specific. Cross-species transmission, even among carnivore hosts, is rare.[5] Like HIV, FIV establishes a chronic, persistent infection that, in some cats, ultimately culminates in immunodeficiency. Because of its similarities to HIV, FIV infection in cats has been used as a research model for HIV infection in the past.[6] Thus, relative to other viral infections of companion animals, much is known about FIV pathogenesis.

Familiarity with retroviral structure and replication assists in understanding diagnostic, treatment, and prevention strategies for these infections. Like other retroviruses, FIV has a three-layered structure that is composed of an innermost genome-nucleocapsid complex with helical symmetry, an icosahedral capsid, and an envelope with glycoprotein spikes (Fig. 33.1). Each virion contains a duplicate, single-stranded RNA genome. The FIV genome contains three major genes: *gag*, which encodes the virion core proteins (capsid [p24], nucleocapsid [p10], and matrix [p15]); *pol,* which encodes the reverse transcriptase, protease, and integrase enzymes; and *env*, which encodes surface (gp120) and transmembrane (gp40) envelope glycoproteins.[7] Several accessory and regulatory genes are also encoded. FIV Env binds to CD134, the primary cell surface receptor, to initiate infection.[8] CD134 is expressed on feline CD4+ T cells, B cells, and activated macrophages. A conformational change in Env exposes the binding site for the co-receptor CXCR4, a chemokine receptor, triggering cell entry.[8] The viral envelope fuses with the cell membrane, and the capsid is released into the cytoplasm where reverse transcription occurs and a double-stranded DNA (dsDNA) copy of the retroviral genome is made. Additional sequences, known as *long terminal repeats* (LTRs), are added to either end of the viral genome. The virus then passes into the nucleus where the dsDNA copy integrates into the host genome; at this point, the integrated dsDNA becomes a *provirus.* Transcription of this proviral DNA, which is controlled by the LTRs, leads to synthesis of new virion components, and virus assembly and budding occur at the cell surface (Fig. 33.2). Depending on the cellular environment, proviral DNA may either be *latent,* whereby transcription does not occur, or be transcriptionally active. Latency is one mechanism by which retroviruses can evade the host immune system. Within an infected cat, FIV mutates frequently to create a pool of variant viruses. Point mutations introduced during reverse transcription and recombination between viruses that co-infect a single cell are the major mechanisms involved. Variable regions in *env* form the basis for the phylogenetic classification of FIV into major subtypes or clades, A to F. Regional variation in the prevalence of subtypes exists with subtypes A, B, and C being most common.[9,10] Classification of FIV subtypes has become complex because sequences used for subtyping do not detect all *env* recombinants. Additionally, recombinant subtypes, such as A/B, B/E, and A/B/C, are now recognized,[11,12] and the existence of additional subtypes likely. The heterogeneity of the virus complicates the design of molecular diagnostic tests and vaccines for FIV. The clinical relevance of subtype classification is not yet clear since subtype does not consistently predict clinical manifestations or vaccine protection.[13,14]

FIV is transmitted by direct inoculation of saliva or blood during fighting.[15,16] Other routes of transmission are of minor epidemiologic significance. Horizontal transmission of FIV between cats in stable households is rare.[17] Queen-to-kitten (prenatal, natal, and postnatal) transmission of FIV is documented infrequently, although primary infection of the queen during pregnancy may increase the risk of transmission.[18] Diagnosis of FIV infection in one kitten does not imply that the whole litter is infected.[19] Natural sexual transmission of FIV is not reported, although experimentally, FIV can be recovered from semen, and intravaginal exposure results in transmission.[20]

Detection of circulating antibodies has been used as a marker of infection in epidemiologic studies because FIV infection is lifelong. Seroprevalence varies from <5% to >20% depending on the region and the population tested (Table 33.1). FIV infection rates are particularly high in Australia and Japan. Two studies in Australia found that 14.6% and 15% of client-owned cats tested at veterinary clinics were seropositive.[21,22] In Japan, the overall seroprevalence was 23.2%, with up to one third of male cats testing positive.[23] Risk factors for FIV

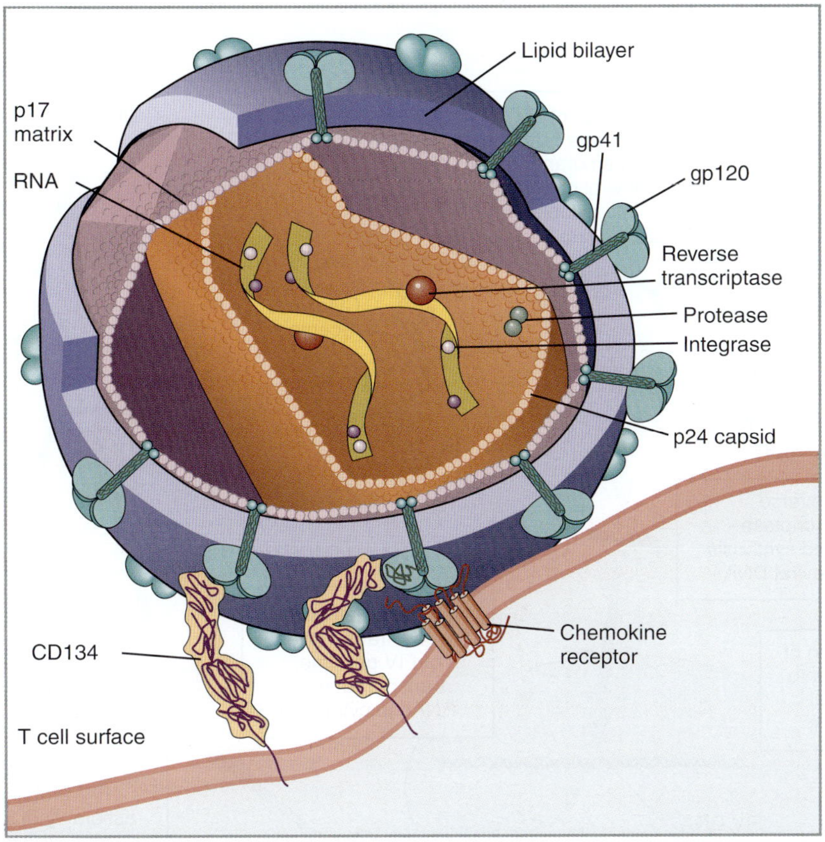

Fig. 33.1 An FIV virion is shown adjacent to the surface of a CD4+ T cell. Lentiviruses contain two identical strands of RNA (the viral genome) and associated enzymes, which include reverse transcriptase, integrase, and protease, packaged into a core composed of the p24 capsid protein with a surrounding p15 protein matrix, all enclosed by a phospholipid membrane envelope that is derived from the host cell. Viral encoded membrane proteins (gp40 and gp120) are bound to the envelope. CD134 (OX40), a member of the tumor necrosis factor receptor superfamily, and CXCR4, a chemokine receptor, on the host cell surface function as primary and co-receptor, respectively, for FIV.

infection are shown in Table 33.2. The mean age at diagnosis is 6 to 8 years, and 80% to 90% of cats are more than 2 years of age.[24] Male cats are up to 4.7 times more likely to be seropositive than female cats.[25] In a North American study, the prevalence of FIV infection in sick, feral cats was 18.2%, whereas that in healthy indoor cats was only 0.7%.[25] Occasionally, co-infections with FeLV occur, and results of some studies suggest that infection with one retrovirus is a risk factor for infection with the other.[26,27]

CLINICAL FEATURES

Pathogenesis and Clinical Signs

FIV infection is characterized by a progressive immune dysfunction which, in some infected cats, results in clinical signs suggestive of immune deficiency or inflammatory, immune-mediated or neoplastic disease.[1,28,29] The immunopathogenesis of FIV infection has been studied extensively in experimental infections of young cats housed in minimal disease environments. The immunologic changes documented in experimentally infected cats are rarely accompanied by clinical signs.[30] An improved understanding of the clinical course of FIV infection in naturally infected cats, which are typically infected in adulthood and exposed to infectious and environmental cofactors, awaits longitudinal field studies of FIV-infected cats and controls.

FIV infection can be broadly considered to progress in three stages: a transient primary stage, a chronic subclinical stage, and an advanced, clinical stage that is eventually terminal (Fig. 33.3). During the primary stage, which lasts for several weeks, the virus replicates rapidly and viremia is detectable by virus isolation and PCR.[31] Immune dysfunction begins soon after FIV infection. CD4+ T-cell numbers decline rapidly during the first weeks of infection. An early rise in an activated subpopulation of lymphocytes that expresses low levels of the CD8 molecule, CD8^{low}, exacerbates a reduced CD4:CD8 ratio.[32] Lymphocyte function is negatively impacted, for example, T-cell priming to novel antigens is disrupted within 5 weeks of experimental infection.[33] Dissemination of virus to lymphoid tissues occurs and virus can be detected in saliva within 3 weeks of experimental infection.[34] A strong immune response comprising CD8+, cytotoxic T cells, and antibodies to viral proteins is detectable from 2 to 6 weeks after experimental infection.[35] Virus replication is contained but, crucially, not cleared by the host immune system. Transient clinical signs sometimes accompany the primary stage. These include lethargy, anorexia, waxing and waning fever, neutropenia, and a lymphadenopathy due to reactive lymphoid hyperplasia (Fig. 33.4), which can persist for months.

The subclinical stage lasts for years and, often, for a cat's lifetime. Virus replication proceeds in peripheral lymph nodes,[36] but viremia is almost or completely absent. Hence, antigen testing is not used for FIV diagnosis. CD4+-cell numbers in the periphery rebound initially, then decline progressively.[37,38] Dysregulation of cytokine production contributes to impaired immunity to opportunistic pathogens. For example, primary challenge of clinically normal FIV-infected cats with

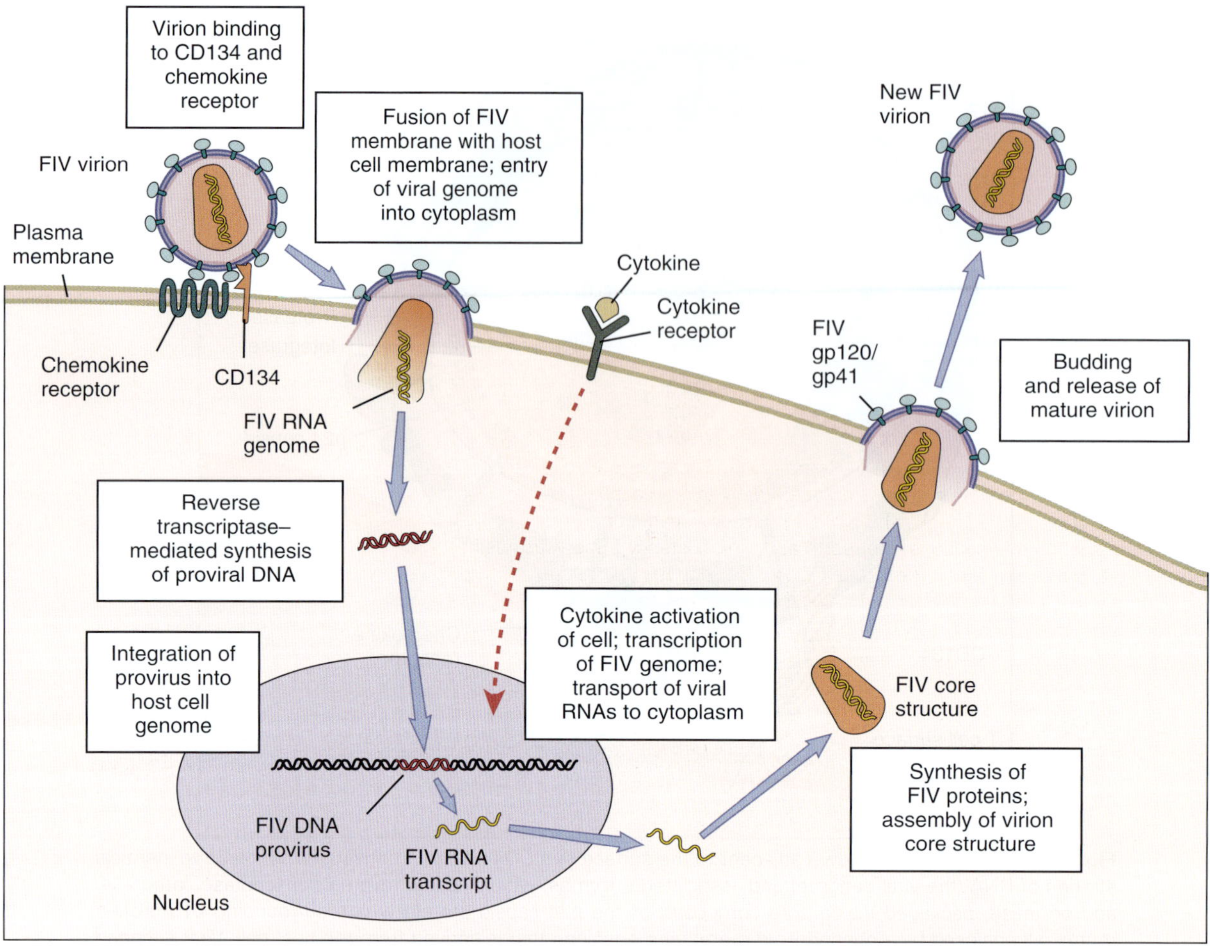

Fig. 33.2 The life cycle of feline immunodeficiency virus (FIV). The sequential steps from initial infection of a host cell to release of a new virus particle are shown. An infected cell produces many virions, each capable of infecting nearby cells, with subsequent spread of the infection.

TABLE 33.1 FIV Seroprevalence Estimates from Selected Regions (2009-)

Country Region	Population	Seroprevalence
United States and Canada	Client-owned and shelter cats	3.6%[124]
Germany	Client-owned cats	3.6%[27]
NW China	Client-owned and shelter cats	9.12%[125]
United Kingdom	Shelter cats	3% and 11.4%[126]
Malaysia	Client-owned cats	10%[127]
Australia	Client-owned cats	14-15%[21,22]
Singapore	Client-owned and shelter cats	16%[128]
Japan	Client-owned cats	23.2%[23]

TABLE 33.2 Risk Factors for FIV Infection

Variable	High Risk	Low Risk
Sex	Male	Female
Neuter Status	Unneutered	Neutered
Breed	Mixed Breed	Pure Breed
Environment	Free Roaming	Confined
Health Status	Sick	Healthy
Age	Adult	Juvenile

Toxoplasma gondii can result in severe, systemic toxoplasmosis compared with only mild, transient signs in FIV-uninfected cats.[39] Cats chronically infected with FIV produce less IL-2 and IL-12, and more IL-10 in response to *T. gondii* infection than control cats.[40] Innate as well as adaptive immunity is affected; defective natural killer (NK)-cell function delayed clearance of *Listeria monocytogenes* in experimental FIV infection.[41] Immune hyperactivation as well as suppression contributes to immune dysfunction in FIV infection. Polyclonal B-cell stimulation results in hypergammaglobulinemia.[42] Chronic antigenemia activates T-cell subpopulations which function as immune suppressors. These include CD4+ and CD8+ cells that express B7 and CTLA4, which contribute to immune anergy and apoptosis in lymph nodes, as well as CD4+CD25+ T-regulatory cells which function as nonspecific suppressors, thereby impacting immunity to FIV and to opportunistic pathogens.[43,44]

In some cats, clinical signs of advanced FIV infection eventually ensue. The advanced stage of FIV infection is characterized by profound lymphoid depletion, escape of virus from immunologic control, and clinical signs including opportunistic infections, neoplastic disease, myelosuppression, and neurologic disease (Table 33.3).[45–48] Immune dysfunction can manifest clinically as atypical and refractory

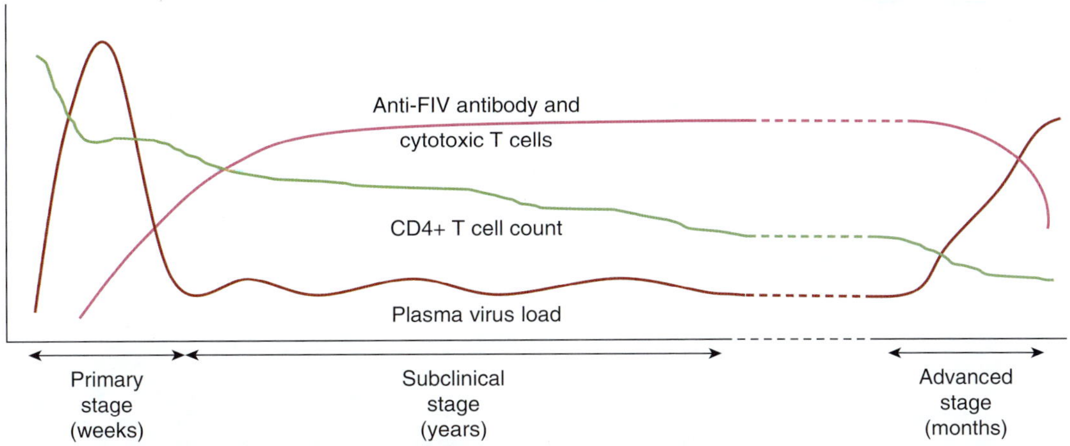

Fig. 33.3 Changes in virus load and CD4+ T-cell numbers over the course of infection with feline immunodeficiency virus (FIV). Viremia is detected early after infection and may be accompanied by systemic signs (primary stage). Plasma viremia then falls to very low levels and remains this way for many years (subclinical stage). Although this period is referred to as "clinical latency," the virus itself is not latent; there is ongoing production of virus and a steady decline in CD4+ T-cell counts. The rate of progression of the subclinical stage depends on factors such as the virus strain, co-infections with other agents that activate virus transcription, and host immunity. Some cats progress to the advanced stage of infection where signs of immunodeficiency develop, and plasma viremia increases. Advanced FIV infection is eventually terminal. Antibody production declines, and antibody tests may be negative in cats with advanced-stage disease, but polymerase chain reaction assays are usually positive.

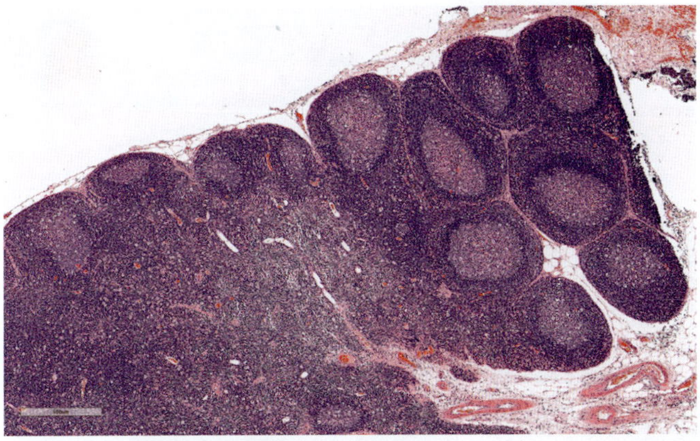

Fig. 33.4 Submandibular lymph node from a young cat in the primary stage of FIV infection with generalized lymphadenomegaly, showing prominent, irregular follicular hyperplasia (H&E staining). (Courtesy of Dr Laura Setyo.)

bacterial, viral, or parasitic infections (Fig. 33.5). Respiratory infections, bacterial pyoderma, generalized demodicosis, mycobacterial infection, disseminated cowpox, pulmonary cryptococcosis, sporotrichosis, and lungworm infections are reported.[28,49–51] Persistent cytopenias, particularly neutropenia or lymphopenia, are described in advanced FIV infection.[21,52] These infections are often more severe and less responsive to treatment than the same infections in immunocompetent cats. FIV infection has been linked to feline chronic gingivostomatitis (FCGS), a painful and debilitating condition that can greatly impact quality of life (Fig. 33.6).[53] The etiology of FCGS is ill-defined, and it is likely to be multifactorial. Epidemiologic evidence identifies FIV as a risk factor in some studies and, while FIV is clearly not causal, a role for the virus in disease manifestation and severity in infected cats seems likely.[54] Immune stimulation triggered by FIV may contribute to chronic oral inflammation, while immune suppression may delay clearance of other pathogens, such as FCV or secondary bacterial invaders. Significant differences in the oral microbiota of FIV-infected cats compared with uninfected cats, including higher relative abundance of fusobacteria and actinobacteria in FIV infection, have been demonstrated. The clinical significance of these findings awaits clarification.[55]

TABLE 33.3 Disease Diagnoses in 127 Cats with FIV Infection[a,b]

Disease	Cats Infected With FIV (n = 127)[c]	Controls (n = 210)[d]	P Value[e]
Intraocular inflammation	16	17	0.18
Stomatitis	21	11	< 0.001
Cardiomyopathy	21	17	0.02
Upper respiratory tract disease	13	9	0.03
Neurologic signs	16	24	0.75
Chronic kidney disease	23	40	0.83
Diabetes mellitus	9	18	0.63
Hyperthyroidism	11	14	0.49
Lymphoma	23	20	0.02
Squamous cell carcinoma (SCC)	12	9	0.057
Fibrosarcoma	2	9	0.17
Carcinomas other than SCC	4	12	0.28

[a]All cats were seen over the same time period at the UC Davis VMTH.
[b]Results should be interpreted with caution because the data were retrospectively collected. Some cats may have had undiagnosed disease, such as subclinical chronic kidney or cardiac disease. The pathogenesis of a disease process in FIV-positive cats might also differ from that found in FIV-negative cats.
[c]All cats were > 6 months of age and none had a history of FIV vaccination.
[d]All control cats were negative for FIV antibody at their visit to UC Davis.
[e]As determined by chi-square (univariate) analysis. The p values < 0.05 were significant.
Modified from Trott KA, Kass PH, Sparger EE, et al. A clinical case control study: clinical presentation of FIV-positive cats. University of California, Davis, STARS in Science Day. 2007; abstr.

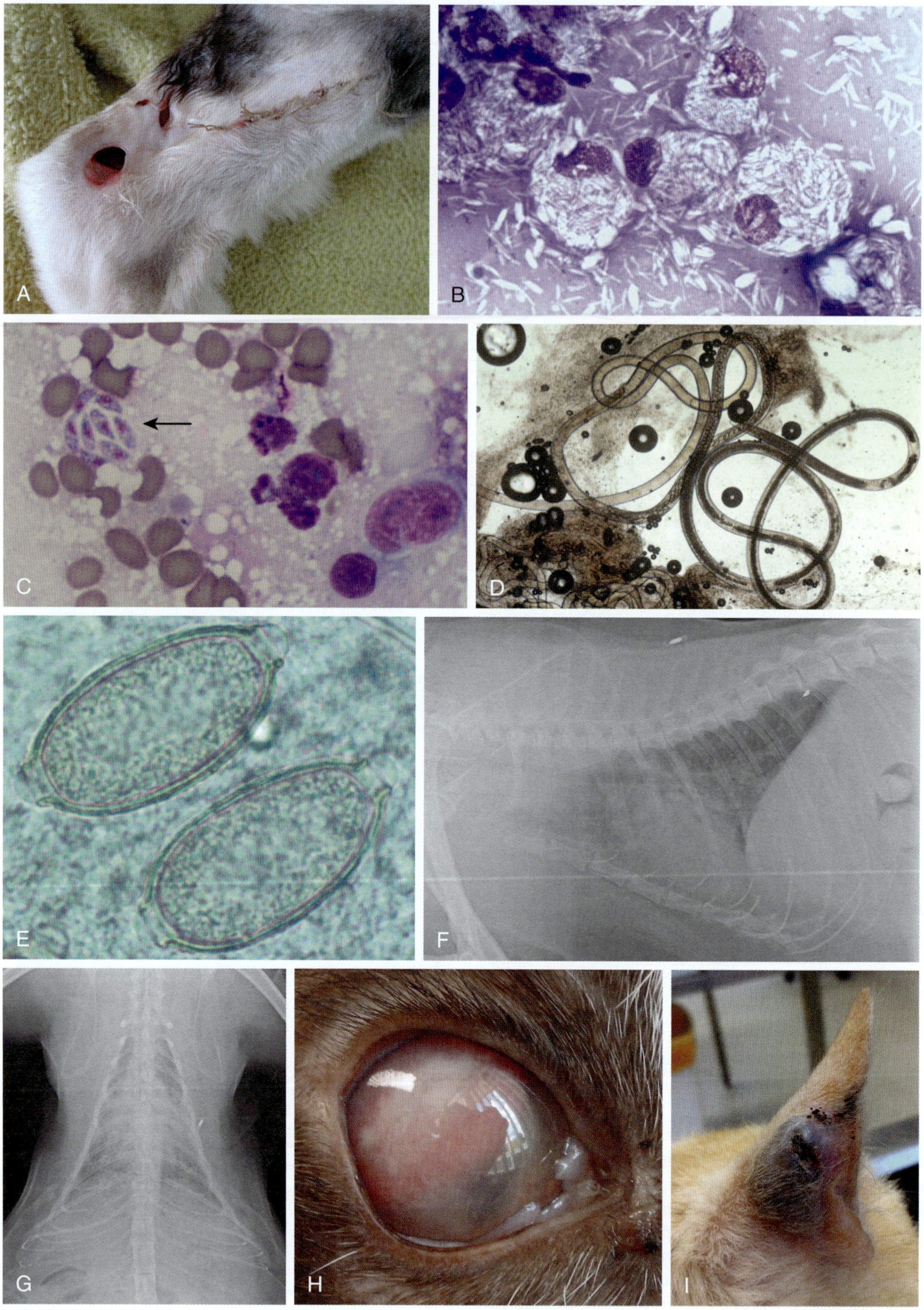

Fig. 33.5 (A) *Mycobacterium lepraemurium* infection causing a nonhealing hock wound in a 12-year-old cat with advanced-stage feline immunodeficiency virus (FIV) infection. (B) Fine-needle aspiration cytology of the lesion shown in A shows numerous negatively staining intracellular bacilli. Modified Wright-Giemsa. (C) Impression cytology of liver biopsy from a 9 year-old male, neutered FIV-infected cat investigated for a hepatopathy. *Toxoplasma gondii* tachyzoites *(arrow)* are surrounded by red blood cells. Modified Wright-Giemsa. (D) Bronchoalveolar lavage (BAL) fluid from an adult cat with advanced FIV infection shows a heavy burden of adult *Eucoleus aerophilus* and (E) characteristic ova. (F) Lateral and (G) ventrodorsal thoracic radiographs from a 9-year-old male, neutered domestic shorthair cat diagnosed with pulmonary cryptococcosis. The cat was investigated for a chronic cough. A generalized mixed, predominantly bronchointerstitial pulmonary pattern is seen on radiographs. *Cryptococcus* was cultured from BAL fluids. No yeasts had been identified on cytology of the BAL. (H) Extranodal (intraocular), high grade, B-cell lymphoma in advanced FIV infection. (I) Focal infection of the pinna of an adult cat with advanced FIV infection. *Cladophialophora carrionii*, a filamentous dematiaceous fungus, was cultured from the lesion and identified on polymerase chain reaction. The cat was on multiagent chemotherapy for nasal lymphoma that had been diagnosed 4 months prior. The phaeohyphomycosis was treated successfully with pinnectomy and oral posaconazole. The cat remained healthy for another 2 years until upper respiratory tract signs recurred and euthanasia was requested. Nasal cryptococcosis was diagnosed at necropsy.

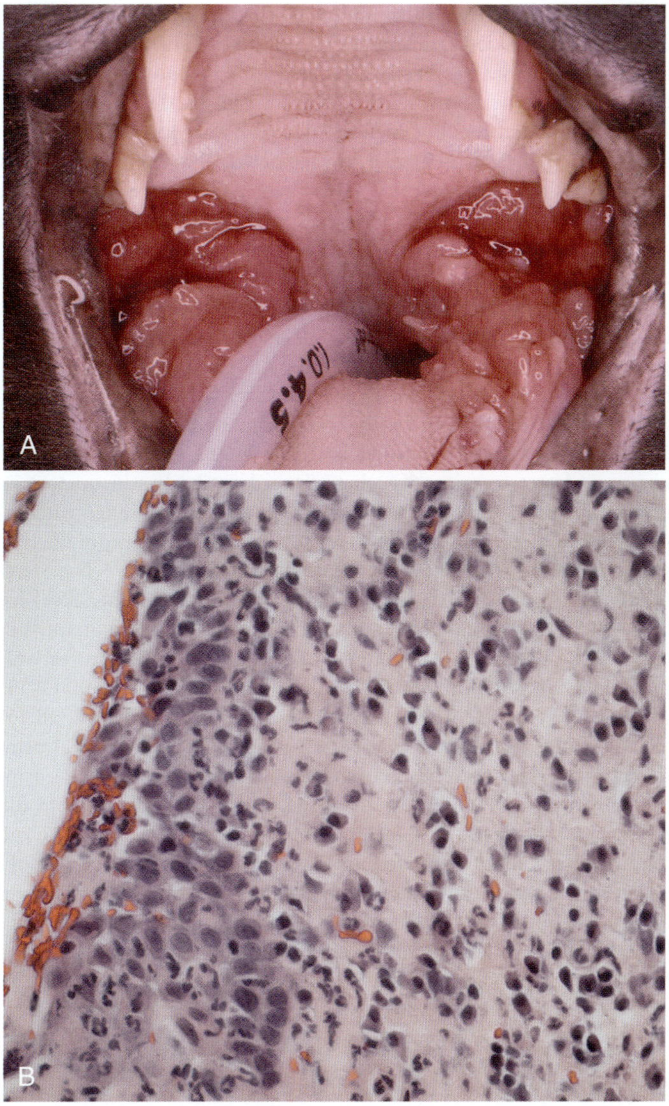

Fig. 33.6 Severe lymphoplasmacytic stomatitis in a cat infected with FIV. (A) There is marked hyperemia, ulceration, and proliferative lesions in the palatoglossal folds. (B) Histopathology of a biopsy from a cat with severe stomatitis associated with FIV infection. (A, From Bonello D, Roy CG, Verstraete FJM. Non-neoplastic proliferative oral lesions. In: Verstraete FJM, Lommer MJ, eds. *Oral and Maxillofacial Surgery in Dogs and Cats*. Philadelphia, PA: Saunders; 2011.)

The risk of lymphoma is increased in FIV-infected cats by fivefold to sixfold.[56] FIV-associated lymphomas are typically high-grade, extranodal, B-cell tumors, similar to HIV-associated diffuse large B-cell lymphoma.[57] Direct oncogenesis by FIV is rare. Integration site mapping demonstrated truncation of a gene on chromosome B3 and downregulation of the unaffected allele, consistent with a loss-of-function mutation, in a single case.[58] FIV-induced immune dysfunction may play a role in lymphomagenesis. Reduced CD4-cell counts, a known risk factor for HIV-associated lymphoma, have been demonstrated in cats developing FIV-associated lymphoma.[59] In HIV-associated lymphomas, co-infecting gammaherpesviruses are causal in 20%–100% of cases depending on the lymphoma subtype.[60] Whether *Felis catus gammaherpesvirus 1*, the lymphotropic gammaherpesvirus of domestic cats, is an infectious co-factor in FIV-associated lymphoma is under investigation.[61] Hyperstimulation of the B-cell compartment in FIV infection might also contribute to oncogenesis, with amplification of normal somatic mutations predisposing to B-cell tumors. Increased numbers of circulating B cells, plasma immunoglobulin, and IL-1 and IL-6, which stimulate B-cell proliferation and differentiation, have been documented in FIV-infected cats that develop lymphoma.[62] Many other neoplasms are described in FIV-infected cats, but the role of FIV, if any, in these cancers is unknown.

Severe unexplained weight loss can occur in advanced FIV infection. This resembles wasting syndrome, an AIDS-defining condition in HIV infection, described as weight loss of 10% or more over 30 days with no identifiable cause other than HIV infection. Wasting syndrome is multifactorial with changes in protein and lipid metabolism, altered energy requirements, anorexia, cytokine derangements, malabsorption, endocrinopathies, and myopathies all contributing. An increased risk for renal diseases in FIV infection is suspected, but a causal association has been difficult to prove. Renal proteinuria but not renal azotemia has been associated with natural FIV infection.[63]

FIV-associated neuropathology has been studied extensively as an experimental model for neurodegenerative diseases in HIV infection. The incidence of neurologic signs that accompany natural FIV infection is unknown. Following experimental infection, FIV provirus can be detected in the CNS from 2 to 4 weeks. The virus targets non-neuronal cells, primarily macrophages and microglia, resulting in a progressive encephalitis.[64] Histopathologic lesions are generally less severe in FIV infection than in HIV infection. This may, in part, be explained by the reduced macrophage tropism exhibited by FIV in comparison with HIV, since macrophages carry virus across the blood-brain and blood-CSF barriers. However, some FIV isolates induce severe neuropathology. Lesions may be clinically silent or induce progressive neurologic deficits including behavioral changes, stereotypic motor behaviors, increased aggression, delayed placing reactions, and reduced pupillary light reflexes.[65] In natural FIV infection, compulsive roaming, changes in sleeping patterns, aggression, seizures, ataxia, tremors, movement disorders, and paraparesis have been reported, but the extent to which other etiologies were excluded is unclear. Some deficits that accompany HIV-associated neurodegeneration (such as reduced concentration, memory or learning, and psychological problems)[66] cannot be routinely assessed in cats.

Perinatal FIV infection, although rare, has been associated with an accelerated disease course, abortion, stillbirth, low birth weights, reduced survival, and T-cell–deficient kittens.[67]

Physical Examination Findings

Cats infected with FIV are often clinically normal or display clinical signs that are unrelated to FIV infection. In the primary stage of FIV infection, cats may be febrile or show generalized peripheral lymphadenopathy. Common physical examination findings in cats with advanced disease include FCGS, chronic upper respiratory tract signs, otitis externa, pyoderma, and abscesses as well as a diverse spectrum of disease manifestations that relate to underlying opportunistic infections or neoplasia. Behavioral abnormalities such as obtundation, aggression, and cognitive impairment have been reported. Other neurologic abnormalities include ataxia, anisocoria, and abnormal segmental reflexes. Ocular abnormalities may result from the FIV infection itself, opportunistic infections, or lymphoma, and include anterior uveitis, hyphema, pars planitis, chorioretinitis, and/or glaucoma.

DIAGNOSIS

FIV-infected cats should be identified to optimize individual healthcare and to prevent infection of other cats. Indications for testing, modified from recommendations by the AAFP, are shown in Box 33.1.[68] Assessment of the clinical significance of FIV infection in a

BOX 33.1 Indications for Serologic Testing for FIV and FeLV

- Sick cats, even if they tested negative in the past
- All newly acquired cats or kittens (2 tests, at least 60 days apart)
- After exposure to a retrovirus-infected cat or a cat with unknown status, and especially after a bite wound (2 tests, at least 60 days apart)
- Cats that live in a household with other retrovirus-infected cats (annual retesting unless isolated)
- Before initial vaccination with FeLV or FIV vaccines
- Before any booster vaccination
- Before use as a blood donor (2 tests, at least 60 days apart)
- On entry to a shelter or before adoption (2 tests, at least 60 days apart); if financial resources are not available for this, cats should be held singly and postadoption testing (2 tests, at least 60 days apart) recommended before mingling with other cats occurs. The status of the other cats in the household should be known before new cats are introduced.
- For group-housed cats, before introduction (2 tests, at least 60 days apart if possible) and on an annual basis
- Testing is considered optional for feral cat trap-neuter-return programs

sick cat is challenging because the virus may, or may not, be contributing to the current clinical signs. Surrogate markers used to stage HIV infection in people, such as CD4+ T-cell counts and viral load, have not been extensively validated for use in cats.[48] It is reasonable to assume that FIV may be playing a role in infected cats with refractory or recurrent infections, infections with intracellular pathogens such as mycobacteria, opportunistic pathogens, and cases of high-grade B-cell lymphoma.

Laboratory Abnormalities

Laboratory abnormalities are not helpful for the diagnosis of FIV infection. If abnormalities are identified, they may be associated with intercurrent disease or may be a consequence of FIV infection itself. Abnormalities that are commonly reported in FIV infection are mild anemia, lymphopenia, neutropenia, and hyperglobulinemia.[52] Such changes should be interpreted cautiously in older sick cats where they are common regardless of FIV status.[21] Mild prolongations in APTT, thrombin time, and fibrinogen concentrations compared with controls have been reported in FIV-infected cats, although PT and platelet function are generally normal.

Microbiologic Tests

Commercial FIV tests detect either anti-FIV antibodies using immunoassays, or viral nucleic acid using PCR. Virus isolation from PBMCs is not commercially available.

Serologic Diagnosis

Serology is the first line for FIV testing. POC tests utilizing lateral-flow ELISA or immunochromatography technologies and diagnostic laboratory-based ELISA assays are in widespread use, have rapid turnaround times, and high sensitivities and specificities for antibody detection.[25,69,70] In cats over 6 months of age that have not been vaccinated against FIV, anti-FIV antibodies are a marker for FIV infection because the virus establishes a persistent infection.

In countries where commercial FIV vaccines are available, or in cats with a history of having been vaccinated for FIV, POC test selection is important. This is because vaccination with inactivated whole virus vaccines induce antibodies to a broad range of FIV proteins, and POC kits vary in their ability to distinguish vaccine-induced from infection-associated anti-FIV antibodies. This means that an uninfected cat that has been vaccinated for FIV can test positive on POC tests in some circumstances. The antigens used in POC kits vary among manufacturers but include p15, p24, and gp40. In a study of FIV-vaccinated ($n = 119$) and unvaccinated ($n = 239$) owned cats, two POC assays, Witness FeLV/FIV (Zoetis Animal Health, USA) and Anigen Rapid FIV/FeLV (BioNote, Korea), performed well in their ability to detect antibodies induced by natural FIV infection regardless of the cat's FIV vaccination status (PPV 70% and 100% and NPV 100% and 100%, respectively).[71] The high specificity of these kits for identifying FIV infection (98.1%) was confirmed in an independent study of 104 FIV-uninfected specific pathogen free (SPF) cats that had been vaccinated against FIV.[72] However, prospective studies of FIV-uninfected kittens and young cats vaccinated with the inactivated FIV vaccine have reported that both the Witness and Anigen POC kits may detect transient, vaccine-induced antibodies in up to 66% of vaccinates.[73,74] Some evidence suggests that interference with the results of Witness and Anigen assays by vaccination is more likely in young cats, and within several months of vaccination.[73,74] The SNAP FIV/FeLV Combo POC assay (IDEXX Corporation, Maine, USA) has high (94%–100%) sensitivity and specificity for detection of anti-FIV antibodies but does not distinguish between the antibody response induced by vaccination and that induced by natural infection. Of 119 FIV-vaccinated cats, of which only 5 were infected with FIV, all 119 tested positive using SNAP FIV/FeLV Combo compared with 11 using the Witness assay and 5 (all confirmed as infected using PCR) using the Anigen assay.[71] Clarification of the utility of POC kits from different manufacturers for determination of FIV infection status in cats that may have been vaccinated for FIV is expected. The reliability of a negative serologic test result is unchanged by a history of vaccination.

Other serologic assays, including IFA assays and Western blotting, have limited availability. Both are technically demanding, subject to interoperator variability in interpretation, and Western blotting may be less sensitive than ELISA assays when performed by some laboratories.[75]

Molecular Diagnosis Using Nucleic Acid–Based Testing

Molecular tests target integrated DNA provirus and some also detect viral RNA by qPCR. Variability in performance among laboratories has been demonstrated.[76] Commercial PCR assays have diagnostic sensitivity that is 5%–15% lower than that of serology, and diagnostic specificity that is similar to serology.[77–79] Sequence variability among isolates, low provirus or virus load, poor sample quality, and technical issues may all impact the sensitivity of PCR (see Chapter 6). FIV PCR should not be used to screen for FIV infection. Rather, FIV PCR can be used as an adjunct to serology to determine the true infection status of cats in certain circumstances, including seropositive cats that may have been vaccinated for FIV, seropositive cats less than 6 months of age, seronegative cats that may have been recently exposed to FIV, and seronegative cats where advanced-stage FIV is suspected. After experimental FIV challenge, PCR can detect viral RNA within 1 to 2 weeks and DNA within 3 weeks, but differences in virus strain, dose, and assay sensitivities mean that it is hard to predict how long after natural exposure PCR can be used to detect FIV infection.[31] Positive PCR test results indicate that the cat is almost certainly infected, whereas negative PCR results are inconclusive.

Interpretation and Confirmation of Serologic Test Results

Interpretation of the results of serologic screening requires the integration of clinical findings from the individual cat to guide whether repeat serology or PCR is indicated and what the timing of any repeat testing

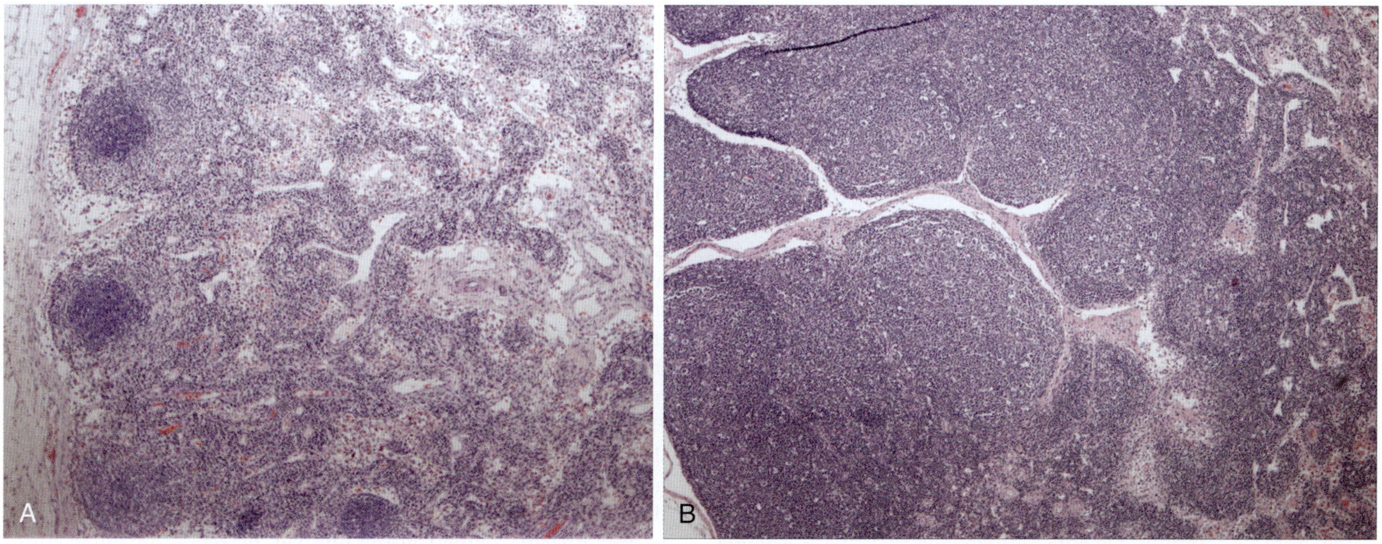

Fig. 33.7 (A) Depletion of paracortical areas in the mesenteric lymph node of an 8-year-old female spayed domestic shorthair with feline immunodeficiency virus infection that was euthanized as a result of the development of progressive neurologic signs. (B) Normal feline lymph node for comparison.

should be.[68] The time to seroconversion following natural infection is variable and can be prolonged.[68] If possible, a seronegative cat that may have been recently exposed should be isolated from FIV-infected cats or cats of unknown FIV status and retested after 60 days. Some cats in the terminal stage of FIV infection have impaired antibody production. These cats often have high plasma viral loads but are seronegative.[80] Thus, if advanced FIV infection is suspected, negative test results should be followed by PCR.

Confirmation of positive serologic test results is recommended. The testing methodology used for confirmation will depend on assessment of the cat's FIV infection risk, test availability, whether previous FIV vaccination can be ruled out, and financial considerations.

The following considerations apply regarding positive serologic test results:

Cats at low risk of infection. Confirmation of a positive serologic test result in cats with a low risk of infection, including healthy cats and indoor cats, is essential because the PPV of serology is low in low-risk groups. The reason for this is that the *prevalence of FIV* in a low-risk population approaches the *expected frequency of false positives*. So for each positive test result obtained in cats at low risk, there is a higher chance that the result is a false positive.

Maternally derived FIV antibodies can result in positive serologic test results in uninfected kittens. Positive serology results in cats under 6 months of age can be confirmed with PCR. Alternatively, serology can be repeated after 6 months of age.[68] Negative serologic test results in kittens are generally reliable.

Cats vaccinated with the inactivated FIV vaccine. As discussed above, where a history of vaccination for FIV is confirmed or cannot be ruled out, the Anigen Rapid FIV/FeLV or Witness FeLV/FIV is currently the preferred POC screening test. A positive result using one of these POC kits can be confirmed using the other kit, or a PCR test.

Pathologic Findings

Cats in the primary stage of FIV infection may have generalized lymphadenomegaly on gross necropsy. Histopathologic changes in lymph nodes, spleen, tonsils, and mucosa-associated lymphoid tissue include hyperplasia, follicular dysplasia, and expansion of B- and T-cell areas (see Fig. 33.4). These changes can persist for months or years. In advanced FIV infection, gross findings may include emaciation, stomatitis, and evidence of lymphoma or opportunistic infections. Advanced FIV infection is associated with lymphoid depletion (Fig. 33.7). Bone marrow pathologies include mild dysplasia, erythroid hypoplasia, and/or myeloid hyperplasia. Inflammatory changes may be seen within skeletal muscle and/or the GI tract. Histopathology of the CNS in cats infected with neurovirulent FIV strains may reveal mild lymphoplasmacytic meningitis, perivascular lymphocytic infiltrates, diffuse gliosis, microglial nodules, and mild neuronal degeneration and apoptosis.[65,81]

TREATMENT AND PROGNOSIS

Many sick FIV-infected cats have treatable diseases. The diagnosis of FIV infection in a sick cat can influence the differential diagnoses to include, for example, unusual opportunistic and parasitic infections. FIV status also guides treatment selection. Where antimicrobial drugs are indicated, selection should ideally be based on the results of susceptibility testing. Clinicians should be vigilant for drug reactions, as these may be more prevalent in FIV-infected cats. For example, severe drug-induced neutropenia following griseofulvin administration has been reported in FIV-infected cats.[82] Glucocorticoids may be indicated to treat intercurrent inflammatory or immune-mediated problems arising in FIV-infected cats. Glucocorticoids should be used judiciously, only where specifically indicated, and with close patient monitoring.

Investigation of chronic gingivostomatitis includes consideration of a range of contributing etiologies including FCV, inflammation associated with dental disease, immune-mediated and neoplastic causes, and eosinophilic granuloma complex.[53] The degree and duration of response to treatments such as dental cleaning, antimicrobial drugs, IFNs, and anti-inflammatory doses of glucocorticoids is variable. Extraction of premolars and molars is reported to improve signs in 60%–80% of cats with severe gingivostomatitis.[83]

In cats with intermediate- or high-grade lymphoma, there is no evidence that FIV infection *per se* is a negative prognostic indicator for response to multiagent chemotherapy, although data are limited. Close monitoring of the neutrophil count during chemotherapy is warranted. Where neurologic impairment is identified and localized in FIV-infected cats, investigation for potentially treatable causes is indicated. Management of FIV-associated wasting involves investigation for treatable underlying diseases (such as enteropathies and exocrine pancreatic insufficiency), supportive care, nutritional support, and appetite stimulation.

Severe or persistent cytopenias in FIV-infected cats should be investigated for treatable underlying causes since cytopenias are common in sick cats regardless of their FIV status.[21,52] There is currently no suitable supportive treatment for FIV-associated neutropenia. Recombinant human granulocyte colony-stimulating factor (rHuG-CSF) increased neutrophil counts in young cats that were experimentally infected with FIV in the short term, until antibodies to rHuG-CSF developed.[84] Cross-reactivity of induced antibodies to endogenous feline G-CSF risks refractory agranulocytosis. Pegylated feline G-CSF showed promising results with less frequent dosing, but this compound is not commercially available.[85] Anemia occurs with FIV infection, although less commonly than neutropenia. Recombinant human erythropoietin (rhEPO) was effective at increasing PCV in FIV-infected cats without inducing anti-rhEPO antibodies in one small study.[86] Darbepoetin, which is longer acting and less antigenic than rhEPO, is effective in cats,[87] although studies in FIV-infected cats are not reported.

Immune Modulation and Antiviral Therapies

Owners' expectations should be managed before embarking on a treatment trial with immunomodulators or antiviral drugs. FIV infection cannot be cured. The small chance of improving clinical signs should be balanced against the potential risks and costs involved, including monitoring costs. Data to support the use of immunomodulators in FIV infection are very limited (see Chapter 9).[88,89] Nonspecific immune stimulation risks unintended outcomes including increased virus replication and the activation of immune suppressor cells. In a placebo-controlled study using human recombinant interferon-alpha (rHuIFN-α) (50 IU/cat, oral transmucosal, q24h, 7 days on, 7 days off for 6 months) in natural FIV infection, no effect on plasma virus or provirus load was detected although improved clinical signs were reported.[90] Improvements in clinical parameters were also reported using recombinant feline interferon-omega (rFeIFN-ω, Virbagen Omega, Virbac) at 1 MU/kg, SC, q24h for 5 days, repeated on day 14 and 60, or a lower-dose oral protocol (0.1 MU/cat rFeIFN-ω, PO, q24h for 90 days).[91,92]

Antiretroviral therapies have dramatically improved the prognosis for HIV-infected humans. Combinations of drugs that inhibit HIV reverse transcriptase, protease, or integrase avoid the rapid emergence of drug-resistant mutants. Virus load and CD4 count are used to guide the timing of initiation of treatment, and to assess response in asymptomatic HIV-infected patients. In contrast, there are limited data to evaluate antiretrovirals in FIV infection and there are no licensed products. Combination therapy for FIV to avoid the emergence of resistant mutants is hampered by the limited choice of drugs; most inhibitors of HIV protease are not active against FIV, and data on potential inhibitors of FIV integrase are limited to their *in vitro* activity.[93] Several nucleoside analogues inhibit FIV reverse transcriptase, including zidovudine (3'-azido-3'-deoxythymidine), lamivudine (3TC, 2′,3′-dideoxy-3′-thiacytidine) and adefovir (PMEA, 9-(2-phosphonomethoxyethyl)adenine). Improvements in clinical scores, virus load, and CD4 counts are reported in some studies, but adverse effects, including anemia, neutropenia, and GI signs are common and can be severe. The pharmacokinetics of zidovudine has been studied in cats, and this drug was associated with improvement in stomatitis in a blinded, placebo-controlled study.[94,95] Monitoring of the CBC weekly for the first month and then monthly is advised. Treatment is not recommended for cats with myelosuppressive diseases. If HCT drops below 20%, zidovudine should be discontinued, after which anemia usually resolves in a few days.[68] Zidovudine-resistant FIV mutants can develop as early as 6 months from initiation of treatment.[96] Monotherapy with fozivudine (45 mg/kg PO q12h) reduced the viremia in cats with acute FIV infection but had no effect on viral load or immune function in chronic infection.[97] Plerixafor (AMD3100), a selective CXCR4 antagonist, has been evaluated in client-owned, FIV-infected cats.[98] A prospective, placebo-controlled, double-blind trial showed a mild reduction in proviral load, minimal adverse effects, and no emergence of resistance over a 6-week period, but there was no improvement in clinical or immunologic variables. As novel antivirals for potential clinical use in cats become available, their evaluation should include studies of *in vitro* efficacy, safety *in vivo*, pharmacokinetics, and blinded, placebo-controlled clinical trials.

Management of Healthy FIV-Infected Cats

Comprehensive international guidelines for the management of FIV-infected cats are available from the AAFP and the European Advisory Board on Cat Diseases (ABCD), with updates published periodically.[99,100] FIV-infected cats might benefit from small over multicat households because of reduced stress and reduced exposure to infectious agents. Over a 22-month period, clinical immunodeficiency was not detected in FIV-infected cats rehomed from a shelter into households of one or two cats.[101] By comparison, survival of FIV-infected cats in a multicat household of over 60 cats was significantly reduced, with lymphoma reported as the most common cause of death. FIV-infected cats should be prevented from roaming to prevent FIV transmission. The feeding of raw foods and hunting behavior should be avoided to reduce exposure to *T. gondii* and other foodborne pathogens. Cats should be neutered to reduce roaming and aggressive interactions with other cats.

A veterinary examination every 6 to 12 months will facilitate early detection of emerging health problems. Even apparently minor problems in FIV-infected cats should be fully investigated. A CBC, serum biochemistry panel, and urinalysis are recommended annually.[68] Optimal control of ectoparasites, endoparasites, dental prophylaxis, and diet should be discussed with owners. Perioperative antimicrobial drug treatment (i.e., during the procedure) could be considered for cats that undergo invasive surgery or dental treatments, but antimicrobial treatment need not be continued beyond this period.

The use of FHV, FCV, and FPV core vaccines raises several issues for FIV-infected cats: the potential for vaccine failure in the face of immune dysfunction, failure to contain modified live vaccine virus, and enhancement of FIV replication and immune dysfunction from vaccine-induced immunostimulation. Following a review of available evidence by the European ABCD, recommendations for vaccination of FIV-infected and other immunosuppressed cats with core vaccines have been published.[102] In summary, booster vaccinations are *not* recommended for adult FIV-infected cats kept indoors, unless indicated by anti-FPV antibody levels. If exposure to FPV, FHV, or FCV cannot be excluded, then vaccination using an inactivated product is recommended.

Hospitalized cats should not be housed in isolation facilities on the basis of their FIV status alone, since this places potentially immunosuppressed cats at risk of exposure to transmissible infectious diseases.

Prognosis

Controlled studies demonstrate comparable survival time between FIV-infected and uninfected cats.[21,27,103,104] In a study of almost 10,000 retrovirus tested pet cats, including 1,100 seropositive for FIV, the survival rate at 6 years was 65% compared with 90% for uninfected cats.[103] In the same study, if deaths during the first 100 days were excluded, survival of FIV-infected cats was 94% and 80% at 3 and 6 years, respectively, compared with controls. Even though a negative effect of FIV infection on survival is minor or nonexistent when groups of cats are studied, the effect of FIV infection on morbidity may be underestimated. Clinicians should maintain an index of suspicion for subtle consequences of immune dysfunction, even in cats reported as healthy by their owners.

In experimental studies, infection of neonatal cats is associated with more rapid progression and severity of disease than infection of young adult cats.[105,106] Progression to advanced-stage FIV can occur within 2 months in kittens, after which life spans are typically less than 1 year.[107] In the absence of surrogate markers that reliably predict disease progression, the prognosis for an individual FIV-infected cat should be determined regardless of its FIV status.

There is no clinical justification for the euthanasia of healthy cats on the basis of their FIV status. Rehoming of healthy FIV-infected cats to stable households of one or two cats and prevention from roaming is encouraged wherever possible over euthanasia.

IMMUNITY AND VACCINATION

A commercial, inactivated, adjuvanted, whole-virus FIV vaccine is currently marketed in Australia and New Zealand (Fel-O-Vax FIV, Boehringer Ingelheim) and Japan (Ferrovacs FIV, Zoetis JP) having been discontinued in the United States and Canada. The vaccine is licensed for use in healthy cats of at least 8 weeks of age as an aid in the prevention of infection. There has been longstanding controversy regarding the use of the FIV vaccine. One reason for this has been conflicting data from vaccine efficacy studies and the absence, until recently, of data on efficacy in the field. The FIV vaccine, which contains subtypes A (Petaluma) and D (Shizuoka), performs well in most published studies, inducing sterilizing immunity against homologous and heterologous strains such as subtype B viruses.[108,109] In studies performed by the vaccine developers, preventable fractions between 80% and 100% are reported as well as protection from contact challenge and a duration of immunity of 12 months or more.[110–117] In contrast, in an early independent experimental study, Fel-O-Vax FIV provided no protection against challenge with a subtype A isolate (Glasgow-8).[13] A study of 89 FIV-vaccinated cats and 212 unvaccinated cats in the field in Australia reported a protective rate of only 56%.[112] Five vaccine breakthroughs were identified, and all were subtype A, the most common subtype in circulation in Australia.[113,114] A New Zealand study of 185 cats with outdoor access found no protective effect from Fel-O-Vax FIV vaccination.[115] A second area of concern has been that FIV-uninfected cats vaccinated against FIV can test positive on serologic tests for FIV. Commercial PCR testing for FIV was introduced to assist in determining the true infection status of FIV-seropositive cats where prior vaccination was confirmed or could not be excluded. However, FIV POC serology assays from some manufacturers can identify FIV infection regardless of vaccination history in many circumstances (see Diagnosis).[71] FIV vaccination has been reclassified by the Vaccination Guideline Group (VGG) of the WSAVA from "not recommended" to "non-core."[116] The FIV vaccine should only be used for cats at high risk of infection, such as outdoor cats that fight with other cats. The initial vaccination should only be given to cats that test seronegative for FIV. Cat owners should be informed that protection is incomplete and that identification of subsequent infection may not be straightforward. There is also a risk of injection-site sarcoma. The initial vaccine dose is followed by two booster doses at 3- to 4-week intervals, followed by annual boosters so long as the risk persists.

PREVENTION

The most effective way to prevent FIV infection is to confine uninfected cats. Free-roaming cats are at high risk of FIV infection and they represent an important source of new infections. FIV-infected cats should also be confined to prevent new infections. Prevention of roaming reduces infectious disease risk, and also prevents trauma, straying, and hunting. Environmental enrichment is essential for confined cats. Where a cat from a multicat household is diagnosed with FIV infection, all cats in the household should be tested and no new cats introduced, as this may lead to conflict and increased fighting behavior. Isolation of FIV-infected cats in a household should be considered although the spread of FIV among cats in stable, closed households is uncommon.[17,117] In breeding catteries, infection can be prevented by screening all new introductions, preferably with a 2-month quarantine period followed by retesting and removal of all infected cats from the cattery. Transmission in shelters can be reduced by testing on intake, or housing cats singly and testing at, or shortly after, adoption, together with education of adopters regarding the need to retest.

FIV shed in secretions is rapidly inactivated in dry conditions. In veterinary hospitals, routine cleaning and disinfection procedures to prevent the spread of FHV-1, FCV, and FPV effectively eliminate any residual risk of environmental contamination. Standard practices to prevent nosocomial infections transferred in body fluids should be observed. Cats used as blood donors should be free from FIV infection since iatrogenic transmission by this route is almost certain.[118] Ideally, initial FIV serology should be repeated after 60 days and PCR testing is also advised before enrolling a potential blood donor.

PUBLIC HEALTH ASPECTS

Despite its similarities to HIV, FIV does not infect humans. Experimentally, productive infection of human cells *in vitro* and infection of nonhuman primates with FIV can be achieved.[119,120] A serosurvey of veterinary workers with occupational exposure found no evidence of FIV infection, and the human CD134 molecule does not support cellular entry by the virus.[121,122] However, immunosuppressed human patients, such as transplant recipients, should avoid handling any potentially immunosuppressed animal, or observe meticulous hygiene practices to avoid the possibility of exposure to shared, potentially fatal, opportunistic pathogens.[123]

CASE EXAMPLE

Signalment

"Arthur," an 11-year-old male neutered domestic shorthair from northern California.

History

Arthur was initially brought to his veterinarian for a 2-day history of lethargy and decreased appetite. Physical examination was unremarkable. Blood work showed HCT of 28% (reference range, 29%–38%), WBC count of 6,400 cells/μL with a normal differential, clumped platelets, mild hyperbilirubinemia (0.5 mg/dL), mild hypoalbuminemia (2.4 g/dL), and hyperglobulinemia (5.5 g/dL). He was treated with amoxicillin and mirtazapine, but lethargy and inappetence persisted. Serial hemograms performed over the subsequent 3 months showed progressive leukopenia due to a neutropenia and lymphopenia (Table 33.4), during which time Arthur was treated with orbifloxacin, with some improvement in his appetite and attitude. A bone marrow aspirate performed 5 weeks after the onset of illness showed myeloid hyperplasia with a left shift. Serology for FIV and FeLV was performed 11 weeks after onset of illness, and the cat was negative for FeLV antigen and had an equivocal test result for FIV antibody. Serum thyroxine concentration was low (0.7 μg/dL, reference range 1.1–3.3 μg/dL). The cat was referred for further evaluation.

Arthur was an indoor and outdoor cat and had a history of predation (mice and birds) and fighting with other cats in the neighborhood. His diet otherwise consisted of a commercial wet cat food. He was vaccinated regularly for rabies, FeLV, FHV-1, FCV, and FPV infections.

Current Medications

Orbifloxacin, 7 mg/kg PO q12h.

Other Medical History

Routine blood work had been performed 3 years previously, which showed a normal CBC, a globulin of 5 g/dL, a urine SpG of 1.069, and a T4 of 1.3. At that time, Arthur tested negative for FeLV antigen and positive for FIV antibody.

Physical Examination

Body weight: 3.1 kg

General: Quiet, alert, responsive, estimated to be 5% to 7% dehydrated, T = 103.9°F (39.9° C), HR = 144 beats/minute, RR = 50 breaths/minute, mucous membranes pale pink, CRT < 2 seconds. A dry haircoat with moderate amounts of scale was present. There was no evidence of ectoparasites.

Eyes, ears, nose, and throat (with dilated fundoscopic examination): Moderate gingivitis and absent mandibular canine teeth. No other clinically significant abnormalities were detected.

Musculoskeletal: BCS 2/9. Generalized muscle atrophy was noted. Ambulatory in all four limbs.

Cardiovascular: Aside from an intermittent gallop rhythm, no abnormalities were noted.

Respiratory: No abnormalities were detected.

GI and urogenital: Abdomen soft and nonpainful on palpation, mild hepatomegaly. Urinary bladder was small and soft.

Lymph nodes: All lymph nodes less than 1 cm in diameter.

Laboratory Findings

CBC: HCT 22.5% (30%–50%), MCV 47.5 fL (42–53 fL), MCHC 32.9 g/dL (30–33.5 g/dL), reticulocytes 7,400 cells/μL, WBCs 1,100 cells/μL (4,500–14,000 cells/μL), neutrophils 704 cells/μL (2,000–9,000 cells/μL), band neutrophils 99 cells/μL, lymphocytes 220 cells/μL (1,000–7,000 cells/μL), monocytes 77 cells/μL (50–600 cells/μL), platelets 32,000/μL (180,000–500,000/μL). Neutrophils showed moderate toxicity with many Döhle bodies, and there were many macroplatelets.

Serum chemistry profile: Sodium 149 mmol/L (151–158 mmol/L), potassium 3.1 mmol/L (3.6–4.9 mmol/L), chloride 115 mmol/L (117–126 mmol/L), bicarbonate 17 mmol/L (15–21 mmol/L), phosphorus 4.3 mg/dL (3.2–6.3 mg/dL), calcium 8.8 mg/dL (9.0–10.9 mg/dL), BUN 17 mg/dL (18–33 mg/dL), creatinine 1.1 mg/dL (1.1–2.2 mg/dL), glucose 158 mg/dL (63–118 mg/dL), total protein 8.1 g/dL (6.6–8.4 g/dL), albumin 3.0 g/dL (2.2–4.6 g/dL), globulin 5.1 g/dL (2.8–5.4 g/dL), ALT 121 U/L (27–101 U/L), AST 113 U/L (17–58 U/L), ALP 10 U/L (14–71 U/L), creatine kinase 278 U/L (73–260 U/L), GGT <3 U/L (0–4 U/L), cholesterol 204 mg/dL (89–258 mg/dL), total bilirubin 0.8 mg/dL (0–0.2 mg/dL), magnesium 2.4 mg/dL (1.5–2.5 mg/dL).

Antinuclear Antibody Serology

Positive at 1:32

Microbiologic and Virologic Testing

POC ELISA serology for FeLV antigen and FIV antibody: negative

FCoV antibody serology: negative at 1:25

Aerobic and anaerobic blood cultures (three specimens): negative

PCR for FIV proviral DNA: positive (cycle threshold value = 30, values < 40 are positive)

Imaging Findings

Abdominal ultrasound: Hepatomegaly was identified, and the spleen had a mottled echotexture. There was mild enlargement of the ileocecal lymph nodes and mild diffuse thickening of the small intestinal submucosal layer.

Thoracic radiographs: Cardiopulmonary structures were within normal limits.

Cytologic Findings

Liver aspiration cytology: A moderately bloody background contained scattered, variably sized clusters of uniform hepatocytes and low numbers of nucleated cells. The nucleated cells consisted of a mixture of nondegenerate neutrophils, lymphocytes, macrophages, and rare myeloid precursors. Several macrophages were erythrophagic. Interpretation: Possible mild myeloid extramedullary hematopoiesis.

Spleen aspiration cytology: The specimen was highly cellular with a pink background that contained a moderate amount of blood and scattered clumps of hemosiderin. A mixed population of lymphocytes was admixed with variable numbers of hematopoietic precursor cells. Hematopoietic precursors were primarily granulocytic precursors, with many progranulocytes. A few erythroid precursors, including erythroblasts, were noted. Plasma cells were moderately increased in number, and both immature and mature forms were seen. Several binucleated and rare trinucleated plasma cells and scattered immature lymphocytes were noted. Vacuolated macrophages were increased in number and often contained phagocytized erythrocytes or blue-green pigment consistent with hemosiderin. Scattered mitotic figures were noted. Interpretation: Moderate plasmacytosis, extramedullary hematopoiesis, and histiocytic hyperplasia with erythrophagocytosis and increased iron. The large number of immature plasma cells raised the possibility of plasma cell neoplasia; however, reactive plasmacytosis could not be ruled out.

Bone marrow aspiration cytology: Numerous hypercellular unit particles were present. A few mature megakaryocytes were noted. Hematopoietic cells consisted largely of myeloid precursors, with an estimated myeloid-to-erythroid ratio greater than 10. Myeloid cells showed orderly maturation to the band neutrophil stage, with few segmented neutrophils. Few erythroid precursors were noted, which included rare prorubricytes, rubricytes, and metarubricytes. Scattered well-differentiated plasma cells and a small amount of hemosiderin were noted. Interpretation: Marked myeloid hyperplasia, marked erythroid hypoplasia, and moderate megakaryocytic hypoplasia. The myeloid hyperplasia together with persistent neutropenia suggested myelodysplasia.

Continued

CASE EXAMPLE—cont'd

Serum protein electrophoresis: A mild increase in α2 globulins was present (1.34 g/dL, reference range, 0.4–0.9 g/dL) together with a broad-based gamma region. This was consistent with an acute-phase inflammatory response.

Diagnosis

Advanced stage of FIV infection, characterized by pancytopenia secondary to myelodysplasia; hepatopathy (open diagnosis).

Comments

The progression of FIV infection was apparent in this cat, which transitioned from a seropositive to a seronegative, PCR-positive state as a result of progressive decline in immune function and, ultimately, failure to produce antibodies. The cause of the hepatopathy was not identified. Blood cultures were negative, and spleen and liver aspiration cytology failed to reveal evidence of underlying neoplasia. Because of the plasmacytosis in the spleen, serum protein electrophoresis was performed to assist diagnosis of a plasma cell tumor (as supported by a monoclonal gammopathy), but this was not apparent. The cat was treated with clavulanic acid–amoxicillin without clinical improvement. Treatment with glucocorticoids was also offered because of the possibility of undiagnosed round cell neoplasia or immune-mediated neutropenia (in light of the myeloid hyperplasia combined with a positive antinuclear antibody test). The cat died at home 1 month later, and necropsy was not performed.

TABLE 33.4 Laboratory Abnormalities in a Cat with FIV Infection

	DAYS AFTER ONSET OF ILLNESS					
	39	**47**	**56**	**74**	**83**	**Reference Range**
Hematocrit (%)	29	29	33	27	22	30–50
White blood cells/μL	2,000	2,100	1,000	1,100	1,100	4,500–14,000
Neutrophils/μL	1,180	1,407	610	572	704	2,000–9,000
Lymphocytes/μL	700	588	340	462	220	1,000–7,000
Platelets/μL	191,000	196,000	Clumped	Clumped	32,000	180,000–500,000
FIV/FeLV serology[a]				Equivocal/negative	Negative/negative	

The cat was an 11-year-old male, neutered domestic shorthair that tested positive for antibodies to FIV 3 years earlier, at which time the CBC was normal.

[a]SNAP FIV/FeLV Combo Test, IDEXX Laboratories.

CBC, complete blood count; *FeLV*, feline leukemia virus; *FIV*, feline immunodeficiency virus.

SUGGESTED READINGS

Hartmann K. Clinical aspects of feline immunodeficiency and feline leukemia virus infection. *Vet Immunol Immunopathol.* 2011;143:190–201 (for a review of molecular pathogenetic mechanisms of disease).

Hosie MJ. Feline Immunodeficiency Virus. ABCD Guidelines; 2017. http://www.abcdcatsvets.org/feline-immunodeficiency/.

European Advisory Board on Cat Diseases. ABCD Guidelines on Vaccination in Immunosuppressed Cats. https://www.vaccicheck.nl/sites/default/files/documents/vaccination-guidelines/abcd-vaccination-guidelines/abcd_guidelines_on_vaccination_in_immunosuppressed_cats.pdf.

REFERENCES

1. Pedersen NC, Ho EW, Brown ML, et al. Isolation of a T-lymphotropic virus from domestic cats with an immunodeficiency-like syndrome. *Science.* 1987;235:790–793.
2. Gruffydd-Jones TJ, Hopper CD, Harbour DA, et al. Serological evidence of feline immunodeficiency virus infection in UK cats from 1975-76. *Vet Rec.* 1988;123:569–570.
3. Reid RW, Barr MC, Scott FW. Retrospective serologic survey for the presence of feline immunodeficiency virus-antibody. A comparison of ELISA and IFA techniques. *Cornell Vet.* 1992;82:359–369.
4. Troyer JL, Pecon-Slattery J, Roelke ME, et al. Seroprevalence and genomic divergence of circulating strains of feline immunodeficiency virus among Felidae and Hyaenidae species. *J Virol.* 2005;79:8282–8294.
5. Troyer JL, VandeWoude S, Pecon-Slattery J, et al. FIV cross-species transmission: an evolutionary prospective. *Vet Immunol Immunopathol.* 2008;123:159–166.
6. Elder JH, Lin Y, Fink E, et al. Feline immunodeficiency virus (FIV) as a model for study of lentivirus infections: parallels with HIV. *Current HIV Res.* 2010;8:73–80.
7. Talbott RL, Sparger EE, Lovelace KM, et al. Nucleotide sequence and genomic organisation of feline immunodeficiency virus. *Proc Natl Acad Sci U S A.* 1989;86:5743–5747.
8. Willett BJ, Hosie MJ. The virus–receptor interaction in the replication of feline immunodeficiency virus (FIV). *Curr Opin Virol.* 2013;3:670–675.
9. Sodora DL, Shpaer EG, Kitchell BE, et al. Identification of 3 feline immunodeficiency virus (FIV) env gene subtypes and comparison of the FIV and human immunodfeiciency virus Type1 evolutionary patterns. *J Virol.* 1994;68:2230–2238.
10. Bachmann MH, Mathiason-Dubard C, Learn GH, et al. Genetic diversity of feline immunodeficiency virus: dual infection, recombination, and distinct evolutionary rates among envelope sequence clades. *J Virol.* 1997;71:4241–4253.
11. Hayward JJ, Rodrigo AG. Molecular epidemiology of feline immunodeficiency virus in the domestic cat (*Felis catus*). *Vet Immunol Immunopathol.* 2010;134:68–74.
12. Beczkowski PM, Hughes J, Biek R, et al. Feline immunodeficiency virus (FIV) env recombinants are common in natural infections. *Retrovirology.* 2014;11:80.
13. Dunham SP, Bruce J, MacKay S, et al. Limited efficacy of an inactivated feline immunodeficiency virus vaccine. *Vet Rec.* 2006;158:561–562.
14. Nichols J, Litster A, Leutenegger CM. Relationship between viral subgroup, viral load and health status in a population of cats naturally infected with feline immunodeficiency virus. In: *Proceedings of the 2nd Symposium of the International Society for Companion Animal Infectious Diseases.* ; 2012. San Francisco, CA.

15. Yamamoto J, Hansen H, Ho E, et al. Epidemiologic and clinical aspects of feline immunodeficiency virus infection in cats from the continental United States and Canada and possible mode of transmission. *J Am Vet Med Assoc.* 1989;194:213.
16. Matteucci D, Baldinotti F, Mazzetti P, et al. Detection of feline immunodeficiency virus in saliva and plasma by cultivation and polymerase chain reaction. *J Clin Microbiol.* 1993;31:494–501.
17. Litster AL. Transmission of feline immunodeficiency virus (FIV) among cohabiting cats in two cat rescue shelters. *Vet J.* 2014;201:184–188.
18. Medeiros SO, Martins AN, Almeida Dias CG, et al. Natural transmission of feline immunodeficiency virus from infected queen to kitten. *Virol J.* 2012;9:99.
19. O'Neil LL, Burkhard MJ, Diehl LJ, et al. Vertical transmission of feline immunodeficiency virus. *AIDS Res Hum Retroviruses.* 1995;11:171–182.
20. Jordan HL, Howard J, Barr MC, et al. Feline immunodeficiency virus is shed in semen from experimentally and naturally infected cats. *AIDS Res Hum Retroviruses.* 1998;14:1087–1092.
21. Liem B, Dhand N, Pepper A, et al. Clinical findings and survival in cats naturally infected with feline immunodeficiency virus. *J Vet Intern Med.* 2013;27:798–805.
22. Westman ME, Paul A, Malik R, et al. Seroprevalence of feline immunodeficiency virus and feline leukaemia virus in Australia: risk factors for infection and geographical influences (2011–2013). *J Fel Med Surg Open Reports.* 2016;2:1–11.
23. Nakamura Y, Ura A, Hirata M, et al. An updated nation-wide epidemiological survey of feline immunodeficiency virus (FIV) infection in Japan. *J Vet Med Sci.* 2010;72:1051.
24. Sparger EE, Luciw PA, Elder JH, et al. Feline immunodeficiency virus is a lentvirus associated with an AIDS-like disease in cats. *AIDS.* 1989;3:S43–S49.
25. Levy JK, Scott HM, Lachtara JL, et al. Seroprevalence of feline leukemia virus and feline immunodeficiency virus infection among cats in North America and risk factors for seropositivity. *J Am Vet Med Assoc.* 2006;228:371–376.
26. Little S, Sears W, Lachtara J, et al. Seroprevalence of feline leukemia virus and feline immunodeficiency virus infection among cats in Canada. *Can Vet J.* 2009;50:644–648.
27. Gleich SE, Krieger S, Hartmann K. Prevalence of feline immunodeficiency virus and feline leukaemia virus among client-owned cats and risk factors for infection in Germany. *J Fel Med Surg.* 2009;11:985–992.
28. Yamamoto JK, Sparger E, Ho EW, et al. Pathogenesis of experimentally indiced feline immunodeficiency virus infection in cats. *Am J Vet Res.* 1988;49:1246–1258.
29. Torten M, Franchini M, Barlough J, et al. Progressive immune dysfunction in cats experimentally infected with feline immunodeficiency virus. *J Virol.* 1991;65:2225–2230.
30. English R, Nelson P, Johnson CM, et al. Development of clinical disease in cats experimentally infected with feline immunodeficiency virus. *J Infect Dis.* 1994;170:543.
31. Diehl LJ, Mathiasondubard CK, Onell LL, et al. Longitudinal assessment of feline immunodeficiency virus kinetics in plasma by use of a quantitative competitive reverse-transcriptase PCR. *J Virol.* 1995;69:2328–2332.
32. Willett BJ, Hosie MJ, Callanan JJ, et al. Infection with feline immunodeficiency virus is followed by the rapid expansion of a CD8+ lymphocyte subset. *Immunology.* 1993;78:1–6.
33. Bishop SA, Williams NA, Gruffydd-Jones TJ, et al. An early defect in primary and secondary T cell responses in asymptomatic cats during acute feline immunodeficiency virus (FIV) infection. *Clin Exp Immunol.* 1992;90:491–496.
34. Dean GA, Reubel GH, Moore PF, et al. Proviral burden and infection kinetics of feline immunodeficiency virus in lymphocyte subsets of blood and lymph node. *J Virol.* 1996;70:5165–5169.
35. Beatty JA, Willett BJ, Gault EA, et al. A longitudinal study of feline immunodeficiency virus-specific cytotoxic T lymphocytes in experimentally infected cats, using antigen-specific induction. *J Virol.* 1996;70:6199–6206.
36. Eckstrand CD, Hillman C, Smith AL, et al. Viral reservoirs in lymph nodes of FIV-infected progressor and long-term non-progressor cats during the asymptomatic phase. *PloS One.* 2016;1:e0146285.
37. Hoffmann-Fezer G, Thum J, Ackley C, et al. Decline in CD4+ cell numbers in cats with naturally acquired feline immunodeficiency virus infection. *J Virol.* 1992;66:1484–1488.
38. Ackley CD, Yamamoto J, Levy N, et al. Immunologic abnormalities in pathogen-free cats experimentally infected with feline immunodeficiency virus. *J Virol.* 1990;64:5652–5655.
39. Davidson MG, Rottman JB, English RV, et al. Feline immunodeficiency virus predisposes cats to acute generalized toxoplasmosis. *Am J Pathol.* 1993;143:1486–1497.
40. Levy JK, Ritchey JW, Rottman JB, et al. Elevated interleukin-10-to-interleukin-12 ratio in feline immunodeficiency virus-infected cats predicts loss of type 1 immunity to *Toxoplasma gondii*. *J Infect Dis.* 1998;178:503–511.
41. Simoes RD, Howard KE, Dean GA. In vivo assessment of natural killer cell responses during chronic feline immunodeficiency virus infection. *PloS One.* 2012;7:e37606.
42. Flynn JN, Cannon CA, Lawrence CE, et al. Polyclonal B-cell activation in cats infected with feline immunodeficiency virus. *Immunology.* 1994;81:626–630.
43. Tompkins MB, Bull ME, Dow JL, et al. Feline immunodeficiency virus infection is characterized by B7(+)CTLA4(+) T cell apoptosis. *J Infect Dis.* 2002;185:1077–1093.
44. Tompkins MB, Tompkins WA. Lentivirus-induced immune dysregulation. *Vet Immunol Immunopathol.* 2008;123:45–55.
45. Brown P, Hopper CD, Harbour D. Pathological features of lymphoid tissues in cats with natural feline immunodeficiency virus infection. *J Comp Pathol.* 1991;104:345–355.
46. Ishida T, Tomoda I. Clinical staging of feline immunodeficiency virus infection. *Jpn J Vet Sci.* 1990;52:645–648.
47. Diehl LJ, Mathiason-Dubard CK, O'Neil LL, et al. Induction of accelerated feline immunodeficiency virus disease by acute-phase virus passage. *J Virol.* 1995;69:6149–6157.
48. Goto Y, Nishimura Y, Mizuno T, et al. Quantification of viral ribonucleic acid in plasma of cats naturally infected with feline immunodeficiency virus. *Am J Vet Res.* 2000;61:1609–1613.
49. Taffin ERL, Casaert S, Claerebout E, et al. Morphological variability of *Demodex cati* in a feline immunodeficiency virus-positive cat. *J Am Vet Med Assoc.* 2016;249:1308–1312.
50. Ishida T, Washizu T, Toriyabe K, et al. Feline immunodfeiciency virus-infection in cats of Japan. *J Am Vet Med Assoc.* 1989;194:221–225.
51. Barrs VR, Martin P, Nicoll RG, et al. Pulmonary cryptococcosis and *Capillaria aerophila* infection in an FIV-positive cat. *Aust Vet J.* 2000;78:154–158.
52. Gleich S, Hartmann K. Hematology and serum biochemistry of feline immunodeficiency virus-infected and feline leukemia virus-infected cats. *J Vet Intern Med.* 2009;23:552–558.
53. Lommer MJ. Oral inflammation in small animals. *Vet Clin North Am Small Anim Pract.* 2013;43:555–571.
54. Kornya MR, Little SE, Scherk MA, et al. Association between oral health status and retrovirus test results in cats. *J Am Vet Med Assoc.* 2014;245:916–922.
55. Weese SJ, Nichols J, Jalali M, et al. The oral and conjunctival microbiotas in cats with and without feline immunodeficiency virus infection. *Vet Res.* 2015;46:21.
56. Shelton GH, Grant CK, Cotter SM, et al. Feline immunodeficiency virus and feline leukemia virus infections and their relationships to lymphoid malignancies in cats: a retrospective study (1968-1988). *J Acquir Immune Defic Syndr.* 1990;3:623–630.
57. Callanan JJ, Jones BA, Irvine J, et al. Histologic classification and immunophenotype of lymphosarcomas in cats with naturally and experimentally acquired feline immunodeficiency virus infections. *Vet Pathol.* 1996;33:264–272.
58. Beatty J, Terry A, MacDonald J, et al. Feline immunodeficiency virus integration in B-cell lymphoma identifies a candidate tumor suppressor gene on human chromosome 15q15. *Cancer Res.* 2002;62:7175–7180.
59. Poli A, Abramo F, Baldinotti F, et al. Malignant lymphoma associated with experimentally induced feline immunodeficiency virus infection. *J Comp Pathol.* 1994;110:319–328.

60. Carbone A, Cesarman E, Spina M, et al. HIV-associated lymphomas and gamma-herpesviruses. *Blood*. 2009;113:1213–1224.
61. McLuckie A, Barrs V, Lindsay S, et al. Molecular diagnosis of *Felis catus* gammaherpesvirus 1 (FcaGHV1) infection in cats of known retrovirus status with and without lymphoma. *Viruses*. 2018;10:128.
62. Beatty JA, Lawrence CE, Callanan JJ, et al. Feline immunodeficiency virus (FIV)-associated lymphoma: a potential role for immune dysfunction in tumourigenesis. *Vet Immunol Immunopathol*. 1998;65:309–322.
63. Baxter K, Levy J, Edinboro C, et al. Renal disease in cats infected with feline immunodeficiency virus. *J Vet Intern Med*. 2012;26:238–243.
64. Dow SW, Poss ML, Hoover EA. Feline immunodeficiency virus: a neurotropic lentivirus. *J Acquir Immune Defic Syndr*. 1990;3:65–668.
65. Meeker RB. Feline immunodeficiency virus neuropathogenesis: from cats to calcium. *J Neuroimmune Pharmacol*. 2007;2:154–170.
66. Shapshak P, Kangueane P, Fujimura RK, et al. Editorial NeuroAIDS review. *AIDS*. 2011;25:123–141.
67. Rogers AB, Hoover EA. Fetal feline immunodeficiency virus is prevalent and occult. *J Infect Dis*. 2002;186:895–904.
68. Levy J, Crawford C, Hartmann K, et al. 2008 American Association of Feline Practitioners' feline retrovirus management guidelines. *J Fel Med Surg*. 2008;10:300–316.
69. Hartmann K, Griessmayr P, Schulz B, et al. Quality of different in-clinic test systems for feline immunodeficiency virus and feline leukaemia virus infection. *J Fel Med Surg*. 2007;9:439–445.
70. Sand C, Englert T, Egberink H, et al. Evaluation of a new in-clinic test system to detect feline immunodeficiency virus and feline leukemia virus infection. *Vet Clin Pathol*. 2010;39:210–214.
71. Westman ME, Malik R, Hall E, et al. Determining the feline immunodeficiency virus (FIV) status of FIV-vaccinated cats using point-of-care antibody kits. *Comp Immunol Microbiol Infect Dis*. 2015;42:43–52.
72. Crawford C. Does a DIVA test exist for differentiating FIV infection from FIV vaccination? *J Vet Intern Med*. 2016;30:1475–1476.
73. Lappin M. Detection of feline immunodeficiency virus antibodies in serum of vaccinated cats using a commercially available kit. *ID20 J Vet Intern Med*. 2015;29:1257–1283.
74. Westman ME, Malik R, Hall E, et al. Duration of antibody response following vaccination against feline immunodeficiency virus. *J Fel Med Surg*. 2017;19:1055–1064.
75. Levy JK, Crawford PC, Slater MR. Effect of vaccination against feline immunodeficiency virus on results of serologic testing in cats. *J Am Vet Med Assoc*. 2004;225:1558–1561.
76. Crawford PC, Slater MR, Levy JK. Accuracy of polymerase chain reaction assays for diagnosis of feline immunodeficiency virus infection in cats. *J Am Vet Med Assoc*. 2005;226:1503–1507.
77. Morton JM, McCoy RJ, Kann RKC, et al. Validation of real-time polymerase chain reaction tests for diagnosing feline immunodeficiency virus infection in domestic cats using Bayesian latent class models. *Prev Vet Med*. 2012;104:136–148.
78. Pinches MDG, Diesel G, Helps CR, et al. An update on FIV and FeLV test performance using a Bayesian statistical approach. *Vet Clin Pathol*. 2007;36:141–147.
79. Litster A, Leutenegger C, Estrada M, et al. Diagnostic accuracy of a commercially available PCR test to detect feline immunodeficiency virus antigen. In: *Proceedings of the 2nd Symposium of the International Society for Companion Animal Infectious Diseases*; 2012. San Francisco, CA.
80. Dandekar S, Beebe AM, Barlough J, et al. Detection of feline immunodeficiency virus (FIV) nucleic acids in FIV-seronegative cats. *J Virol*. 1992;66:4040–4049.
81. Maingat F, Vivithanaporn P, Zhu Y, et al. Neurobehavioral performance in feline immunodeficiency virus infection: integrated analysis of viral burden, neuroinflammation, and neuronal injury in cortex. *J Neurosci*. 2009;29:8429–8437.
82. Shelton GH, Grant CK, Linenberger ML, et al. Severe neutropenia associated with griseofulvin therapy in cats with feline immunodeficiency virus infection. *J Vet Intern Med*. 1990;4:317–319.
83. Hennet P. Chronic gingivo-stomatitis in cats: long-term follow-up of 30 cases treated by dental extractions. *J Vet Dent*. 1997;14:15–21.
84. Phillips K, Arai M, Tanabe T, et al. FIV-infected cats respond to short-term rHuG-CSF treatment which results in anti-G-CSF neutralizing antibody production that inactivates drug activity. *Vet Immunol Immunopathol*. 2005;108:357–371.
85. Coleman JK, Sakagawa Y, Tanabe T, et al. Pegylated feline granulocyte colony-stimulating factor increases neutrophil levels in cats. *Vet J*. 2014;200:44–50.
86. Arai M, Darman J, Lewis A, et al. The use of human hematopoietic growth factors (rhGM-CSF and rhEPO) as a supportive therapy for FIV-infected cats. *Vet Immunol Immunopathol*. 2000;77:71–92.
87. Chalhoub S, Langston CE, Farrelly J. The use of darbepoetin to stimulate erythropoiesis in anemia of chronic kidney disease in cats: 25 cases. *J Vet Intern Med*. 2012;26:363–369.
88. Gingerich DA. Lymphocyte T-cell immunomodulator (LTCI): review of the immunopharmacology of a new veterinary biologic. *Int J Appl Res Vet Med*. 2008;6:61–68.
89. Pontzer CH, Yamamoto JK, Bazer FW, et al. Potent anti-feline immunodeficiency virus and anti-human immunodeficiency virus effect of IFN-tau. *J Immunol*. 1997;158:4351–4357.
90. Pedretti E, Passeri B, Amadori M, et al. Low-dose interferon-alpha treatment for feline immunodeficiency virus infection. *Vet Immunol Immunopathol*. 2006;109:245–254.
91. Domenech A, Miro G, Collado VM, et al. Use of recombinant interferon omega in feline retrovirosis: from theory to practice. *Vet Immunol Immunopathol*. 2011;143:301–306.
92. Gil S, Leal RO, McGahie D, et al. Oral recombinant feline interferon-omega as an alternative immune modulation therapy in FIV positive cats: clinical and laboratory evaluation. *Res Vet Sci*. 2014;96:79–85.
93. Savarino A, Pistello M, D'Ostilio D, et al. Human immunodeficiency virus integrase inhibitors efficiently suppress feline immunodeficiency virus replication in vitro and provide a rationale to redesign antiretroviral treatment for feline AIDS. *Retrovirology*. 2007;4:79.
94. Hartmann K, Donath A, Kraft W. AZT in the treatment of feline immunodeficiency virus infection, 1. *Feline Pract*. 1995;23:16–21.
95. Hartmann K, Donath A, Kraft W. AZT in the treatment of feline immunodeficiency virus infection, 2. *Feline Pract*. 1995;23:13–20.
96. Smith RA, Remington KM, Preston BD, et al. A novel point mutation at position 156 of reverse transcriptase from feline immunodeficiency virus confers resistance to the combination of (-)-beta-2 ',3 '-dideoxy-3 '-thiacytidine and 3 '-azido-3 '-deoxythymidine. *J Virol*. 1998;72:2335–2340.
97. Miller MM, Fogle JE. Administration of fozivudine tidoxil as a single-agent therapeutic during acute feline immunodeficiency virus infection does not alter chronic infection. *Viruses*. 2012;4:954.
98. Hartmann K, Stengel C, Klein D, et al. Efficacy and adverse effects of the antiviral compound plerixafor in feline immunodeficiency virus-infected cats. *J Vet Intern Med*. 2012;26:483–490.
99. Hosie MJ. Feline Immunodeficiency Virus. ABCD Guidelines; 2017. http://www.abcdcatsvets.org/feline-immunodeficiency/.
100. Little S, Levy J, Hartmann K, et al. 2020 AAFP feline retrovirus testing and management guidelines. *J Fel Med Surg*. 2020;22:5–30.
101. Bęczkowski PM, Litster A, Lin TL, et al. Contrasting clinical outcomes in two cohorts of cats naturally infected with feline immunodeficiency virus (FIV). *Vet Microbiol*. 2015;176:50–60.
102. European Advisory Board on Cat Diseases. ABCD Guidelines on Vaccination in Immunosuppressed Cats; 2017. https://www.vaccicheck.nl/sites/default/files/documents/vaccination-guidelines/abcd-vaccination-guidelines/abcd_guidelines_on_vaccination_in_immunosuppressed_cats.pdf.
103. Levy J, Lorentzen L, Shields J, et al. Long-term outcome of cats with natural FeLV and FIV infection. In: *Proceedings of the 8th International Feline Retrovirus Research Symposium*; 2006. Washington, DC.
104. Ravi M, Wobeser GA, Taylor SM, et al. Naturally acquired feline immunodeficiency virus (FIV) infection in cats from western Canada: prevalence, disease associations, and survival analysis. *Can Vet J*. 2010;51:271–276.
105. Pedersen NC, Leutenegger CM, Woo J, et al. Virulence differences between two field isolates of feline immunodeficiency virus (FIV-

APetaluma and FIV-CPGammar) in young adult specific pathogen free cats. *Vet Immunol Immunopathol.* 2001;79:53–67.

106. George JW, Pedersen NC, Higgins J. The effect of age on the course of experimental feline immunodeficiency virus infection in cats. *AIDS Res Hum Retroviruses.* 1993;9:897–905.
107. ONeil LL, Burkhard MJ, Obert LA, et al. Regression of feline immunodeficiency virus infection. *AIDS Res Hum Retroviruses.* 1997;13:713–718.
108. Pu R, Coleman J, Coisman J, et al. Dual-subtype FIV vaccine (Fel-O-Vax® FIV) protection against a heterologous subtype B FIV isolate. *J Fel Med Surg.* 2005;7:65–70.
109. Huang C, Conlee D, Loop J, et al. Efficacy and safety of a feline immunodeficiency virus vaccine. *Anim Health Res Rev.* 2004;5:295–300.
110. Huang C, Conlee D, Gill M, et al. Dual-subtype feline immunodeficiency virus vaccine provides 12 months of protective immunity against heterologous challenge. *J Fel Med Surg.* 2010;12:451–457.
111. Kusuhara H, Hohdatsu T, Okumura M, et al. Dual-subtype vaccine (Fel-O-Vax FIV) protects cats against contact challenge with heterologous subtype B FIV infected cats. *Vet Microbiol.* 2005;108:155–165.
112. Westman ME, Malik R, Hall E, et al. The protective rate of the feline immunodeficiency virus vaccine: an Australian field study. *Vaccine.* 2016;34:4752–4758.
113. Kann R, Kyaw–Tanner M, Seddon J, et al. Molecular subtyping of feline immunodeficiency virus from domestic cats in Australia. *Aust Vet J.* 2006;84:112–116.
114. Iwata D, Holloway SA. Molecular subtyping of feline immunodeficiency virus from cats in Melbourne. *Aust Vet J.* 2008;86:385–389.
115. Stickney A, Ghosh S, Cave NJ, et al. Lack of protection against feline immunodeficiency virus infection among domestic cats in New Zealand vaccinated with the Fel-O-Vax® FIV vaccine. *Vet Microbiol.* 2020;250:108865.
116. Day MJ, Horzinek MC, Schultz RD, et al. Guidelines for the vaccination of dogs and cats compiled by the vaccination guidelines group (VGG) of the World Small Animal Veterinary Association (WSAVA). *J Small Anim Pract.* 2016;57:E1–E45.
117. Addie DD, Dennis JM, Toth S, et al. Long-term impact on a closed household of pet cats of natural infection with feline coronavirus, feline leukaemia virus and feline immunodeficiency virus. *Vet Rec.* 2000;146:419–424.
118. Pennisi MG, Hartmann K, Addie DD, et al. Blood transfusion in cats. ABCD guidelines for minimising risks of infectious iatrogenic complications. *J Fel Med Surg.* 2015;17:588–593.
119. Johnston J, Power C. Productive infection of human peripheral blood mononuclear cells by feline immunodeficiency virus: Implications for vector development. *J Virol.* 1999;73:2491–2498.
120. Johnston JB, Olson ME, Rud EW, et al. Xenoinfection of nonhuman primates by feline immunodeficiency virus. *Curr Biol.* 2001;11:1109–1113.
121. Butera ST, Brown J, Callahan ME, et al. Survey of veterinary conference attendees for evidence of zoonotic infection by feline retroviruses. *J Am Vet Med Assoc.* 2000;217:1475–1479.
122. de Parseval A, Chatterji U, Morris G, et al. Structural mapping of CD134 residues critical for interaction with feline immunodeficiency virus. *Nat Struc Mol Biol.* 2005;12:60–66.
123. Fassbender P, Zange S, Ibrahim S, et al. Generalized cowpox virus infection in a patient with HIV, Germany, 2012. *Emerg Infect Dis.* 2016;22:553–555.
124. Burling AN, Levy JK, Scott HM, et al. Seroprevalences of feline leukemia virus and feline immunodeficiency virus infection in cats in the United States and Canada and risk factors for seropositivity. *J Am Vet Med Assoc.* 2017;251:187–194.
125. Cong W, Meng QF, Blaga R, et al. *Toxoplasma gondii, Dirofilaria immitis,* feline immunodeficiency virus (FIV), and feline leukemia virus (FeLV) infections in stray and pet cats (*Felis catus*) in northwest China: co-infections and risk factors. *Parasitol Res.* 2016;115:217–223.
126. Stavisky J, Dean RS, Molloy MH. Prevalence of and risk factors for FIV and FeLV infection in two shelters in the United Kingdom (2011-2012). *Vet Rec.* 2017;181:451.
127. Sivagurunathan A, Atwa AM, Lobetti R. Prevalence of feline immunodeficiency virus and feline leukaemia virus infection in Malaysia: a retrospective study. *JFMS Open Reports.* 2018;4. 2055116917752587.
128. Chan C, Beatty JA, Barrs VR, et al. Evidence for feline innumodeficiency virus, feline leukaemia virus, *Bartonella* spp., haemoplasmas and *Toxoplasma gondii* exposure in Singaporean cats. *J Vet Intern Med.* 2013;27:729.

34

Feline Herpesvirus Infections

Jane E. Sykes, Michael R. Lappin, Sara M. Thomasy, Julia A. Beatty

KEY POINTS

- First Described in Cats: FHV-1, 1958 (United States)[1]; *Felis catus* gammaherpesvirus 1 (FcaGHV1), 2014 (United States).[2]
- Causes: FHV-1, family *Herpesviridae,* an alphaherpesvirus; FcaGHV1, family *Herpesviridae,* genus *Percavirus,* a gammaherpesvirus. Molecular evidence of feline bovine herpesvirus 4 (genus *Rhadinovirus*) infections requires verification.
- Geographic Distribution: FHV-1, worldwide; FcaGHV1, worldwide.
- Mode of Transmission: FHV-1, close contact, fomite spread, to a lesser extent aerosols; FcaGHV1, under investigation, epidemiology supports biting as a plausible route.
- Major Clinical Signs: FHV-1, serous to mucopurulent nasal and ocular discharge, sneezing, stertor, conjunctivitis, keratitis, lingual or facial ulceration, fever, inappetence, tachypnea, cough, rarely death; FcaGHV1, most infections expected to be subclinical.
- Differential Diagnoses: Differential diagnoses for FHV-1 infection are other respiratory viral infections (FCV, influenza viruses), infections with bacteria such as *Bordetella bronchiseptica, Mycoplasma* spp., *Streptococcus* spp., or *Chlamydia felis*; other causes of rhinitis such as cryptococcosis, aspergillosis, neoplasia, foreign bodies, chronic idiopathic feline rhinosinusitis, nasopharyngeal stenosis, or nasopharyngeal polyps; feline chronic airway disease.
- Human Health Significance: Neither FHV-1 nor FcaGHV1 infects humans.

FELINE HERPESVIRUS-1 INFECTION

ETIOLOGY AND EPIDEMIOLOGY

FHV-1 causes ocular disease, URTD, and reproductive failure in domestic cats and wild Felidae. Feline URTD is a widespread and important contributor to morbidity and mortality where large numbers of cats are housed together, especially in overcrowded or stressful conditions.[3] Co-infections with other respiratory viral (especially FCV) and bacterial pathogens (including *Mycoplasma* spp., *Chlamydia felis,* and *Bordetella bronchiseptica*) are common. More information on other viral and bacterial causes of feline URTD can be found in Chapters 25, 35, 49, 50, 55, 57, and 124.

FHV-1 is a large, double-stranded DNA virus with a glycoprotein-lipid envelope that has a worldwide distribution. Most cats are exposed to FHV-1 during their lifetime. FHV-1 is an alphaherpesvirus that is closely related to canine herpesvirus-1, and to a lesser extent, herpes simplex virus (HSV). There is only a single serotype of FHV-1. Isolates are also genetically similar, yet some variation in strain virulence exists.[4] The complete genome sequences of more than 25 FHV-1 strains collected over a 40-year time period have been determined, revealing extremely low genetic diversity (0% to 0.01%).[5,6] In another study of 26 FHV-1 strains from multiple shelters in the United States, the overall interstrain genetic distance was 0.093%.[7]

Using culture, FHV-1 has been detected in 0% to 39% of cats with URTD, although in some catteries and shelters with endemic FHV-1 infection, the prevalence may be higher. When sensitive PCR assays are used to detect FHV-1, the prevalence of infection approaches 100% in some groups of cats with acute URTD.[8,9] The prevalence of shedding by apparently healthy cats has ranged from 0% to 10% but most often is less than 2%.[3,10–17] Virtually all infected cats develop latent infection, which occurs in the trigeminal ganglion, cranial cervical ganglion, and pterygopalatine ganglion.[18] FHV-1 DNA can also be detected in other tissues of the head, such as the cornea and nasal cavity, but this is thought to reflect chronic persistent infection rather than latency. Reactivation of shedding, with or without concurrent clinical signs of URTD, occurs in less than half of latently infected cats 4 to 12 days after stress (Fig. 34.1).[19] Examples of stressors include transportation (such as to a veterinary clinic, boarding or breeding facility, shelter, or cat show), lactation, housing changes, exposure to new cats, concurrent illness, or treatment with immunosuppressive drugs such as glucocorticoids or cyclosporine.[20] The duration of shedding after reactivation ranges from 1 to 13 days (mean, 7 days).[21,22] A refractory period of several months is thought to follow recovery from reactivation whereby cats are less likely to reactivate. Some cats reactivate more frequently than others, and therefore are of greater epidemiologic importance. Shedding that coincides with lactation results in infection of susceptible kittens, but whether or not they develop disease depends on their amount of MDA. On some occasions, kittens with low concentrations of MDA may become subclinically infected and become latent carriers without showing clinical signs.[19] Such a mechanism is obviously ideal for the virus because it can spread to the next generation without harming its host.

FHV-1 survives a maximum of 18 hours at room temperature and is readily inactivated by drying and most disinfectants. Because of this, transmission occurs primarily through close contact, although fomites remain a very important mode of transmission in crowded environments. Aerosol transmission is of lesser importance.[19,23] Aerosols generated by sneezing cats typically travel no further than a distance of 4 to 5 feet, and are not thought to be a major source of infection.

In one study, cats shedding FHV-1 at intake to shelters were at a greater risk of subsequently developing URTD following intake than cats that were not shedding pathogens,[24] whereas this was not the case for cats shedding FCV. Poor hygiene and overcrowding has been associated with an increased risk of URTD due to FHV-1 in shelters. Other risk factors include recent contact with cats outside a household, being of mixed breed, lack of vaccination, and young age.[25,26]

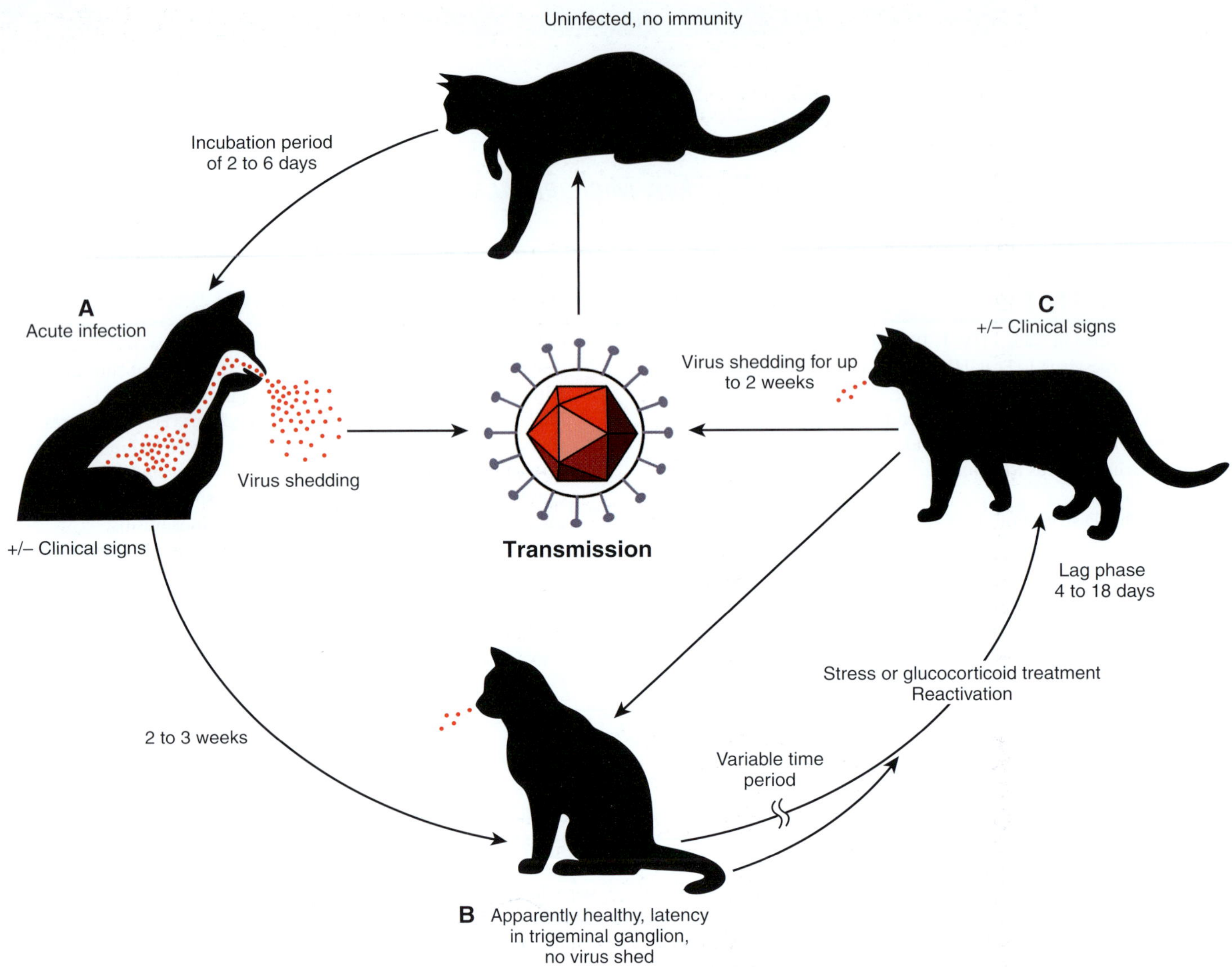

Fig. 34.1 Transmission of feline herpesvirus-1 infection and the carrier state. (A) After initial infection, clinical signs of upper respiratory tract disease (URTD) with virus shedding may occur after an incubation period of 2 to 6 days. Some cats may show no signs of illness. (B) Virtually all cats become latent carriers with persistence of virus latency-associated transcripts (LATs) within neurons of the trigeminal ganglia (see Fig. 34.2). (C) Reactivation of shedding occurs 4 to 18 days after stress, and may or may not be accompanied by clinical signs of URTD. These cats represent a source of infection for other cats.

CLINICAL FEATURES

Pathogenesis and Clinical Signs

Following direct or indirect contact with virus in respiratory secretions from the conjunctiva, nasal cavity, and oropharynx, FHV-1 replicates within the lymphoid and epithelial cells in the upper respiratory tract and causes cytolysis. FHV-1 also replicates in corneal epithelial cells.[27] During acute infection, the virus has been isolated from the conjunctiva, cornea, uveal tract, retina, optic nerve, ciliary ganglion, pterygopalatine ganglion, trigeminal ganglion, brainstem, visual cortex, cerebellum, and olfactory bulb.[18] Primary lung involvement may occur but is rare. Systemic infection with viremia occurs in some cats acutely infected with FHV-1 and may be more likely to occur in neonates and debilitated cats. During acute infection, the virus invades sensory nerve endings and is transported to the trigeminal ganglion and cranial cervical ganglion, where it becomes latent. Infection of the trigeminal ganglion can lead to ganglion cell death, increased numbers of glial cells, and lymphoplasmacytic inflammation.[18] In the latent state, the viral genome persists as a circular, histone-associated episome within neuronal cell nuclei, with no production of infectious virus (Fig. 34.2). In this state, production of virus proteins is greatly reduced in order to reduce host immune recognition. However, production of noncoding viral latency-associated transcripts (LATs) and microRNAs occurs at a higher rate. The LATs are thought to be important for maintenance of the latent state, possibly in part through inhibition of cellular apoptosis or other mechanisms of cell death or reduction of expression of lytic genes.[28] There is also evidence in HSV infections that a viral lytic protein, *infected cell polypeptide 0* (ICP0), is functional during latent infection, and important for production of LATs.[28]

Clinical signs of URTD can occur after an incubation period of 2 to 6 days, although longer incubation periods are also possible with lower challenge doses. Viral shedding occurs predominantly in ocular, nasal, and oral secretions as early as 24 hours after infection, and often before the onset of clinical signs. Clinical signs and shedding may also occur following reactivation of latent virus in the ganglia, whereby lytic genes are activated, viral transcription occurs, and there is anterograde

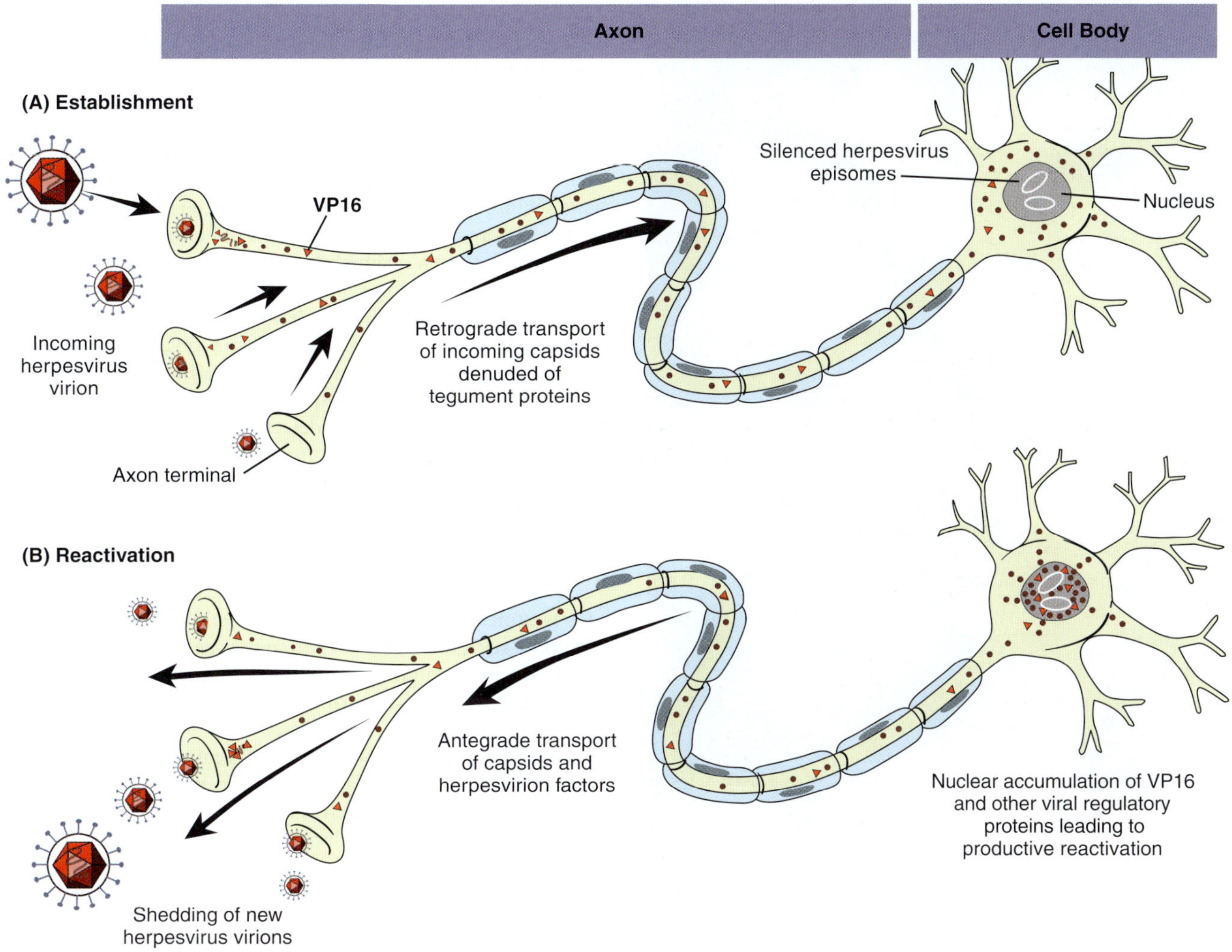

Fig. 34.2 Latency of herpes simplex virus-1 within neurons of the trigeminal ganglia. (A) Virus enters the nervous system via axon terminals of peripheral neurons that innervate the upper respiratory tract. There is retrograde transport of virus capsids to the cell body where the viral genome is delivered to the neuronal cell nucleus. Loss of the viral tegument protein VP16, which is required for virus replication, promotes latency in neurons as a circular (episomal) form. (B) Reactivation, with anterograde transport of new capsids and virions, is associated with accumulation of VP16 and other viral regulatory proteins as a result of increased virus replication secondary to immunosuppression. (Adapted from Wilson AC, Mohr I. A cultured affair: HSV latency and reactivation in neurons. *Trends Microbiol.* 2012;12:604–611.)

transport of virus to initial sites of infection or any region innervated by the ganglia, such as the cornea. Clinical signs range considerably in severity and chronicity, from no signs or mild serous ocular discharge to pneumonia and death. Mild signs of respiratory disease resolve spontaneously within 10 to 20 days. The most severe signs tend to occur in very young or elderly debilitated cats. Concurrent immunosuppressive illness or infection with other respiratory pathogens and opportunistic bacteria also profoundly influences disease severity.

Respiratory Tract Disease

Acute (<10 days' duration) clinical signs of URTD in cats infected with FHV-1 include fever, lethargy, conjunctivitis, blepharitis, and sneezing, which may be followed by development of mucopurulent ocular and nasal discharge, and, less commonly, cough or tachypnea (Fig. 34.3A). Severe sneezing has particularly been associated with FHV-1 infection when compared with infection with other respiratory pathogens. Mucopurulent discharges result from secondary bacterial infections with opportunistic pathogens such as *Streptococcus* spp., *Staphylococcus* spp., *Pasteurella multocida*, and *Escherichia coli*. Ocular and nasal discharges may become crusted, and kittens' eyelids may not open as a result of tenacious exudates. Closed eyelids may bulge as exudate accumulates behind adhered lids, a condition termed *ophthalmia neonatorum*. When severe, this can be followed by extensive corneal damage and rupture of the globe usually due to secondary bacterial keratitis. In neonatal infections caused by FHV-1, damage to upper respiratory epithelium may lead to osteolysis of the nasal turbinates and persistent or recurrent sinusitis and rhinitis. In kittens, concurrent corneal and conjunctival ulceration can result in formation of a symblepharon (adherence between the cornea and conjunctiva or two regions of ulcerated conjunctiva). When severe, symblephara can result in vision compromise or even blindness. FHV-1 infections may also lead to pharyngitis and laryngitis, which can be accompanied by clinical signs of gagging or obstructive respiratory patterns. Pneumomediastinum and subcutaneous emphysema were described in one cat with necrotizing bronchopneumonia and fibrinonecrotic tracheitis due to FHV-1 infection.[29] Although ulcerative glossitis, hypersalivation, and ulceration of the nasal planum, conjunctiva, and skin is more common and severe with FCV infection, it can also be

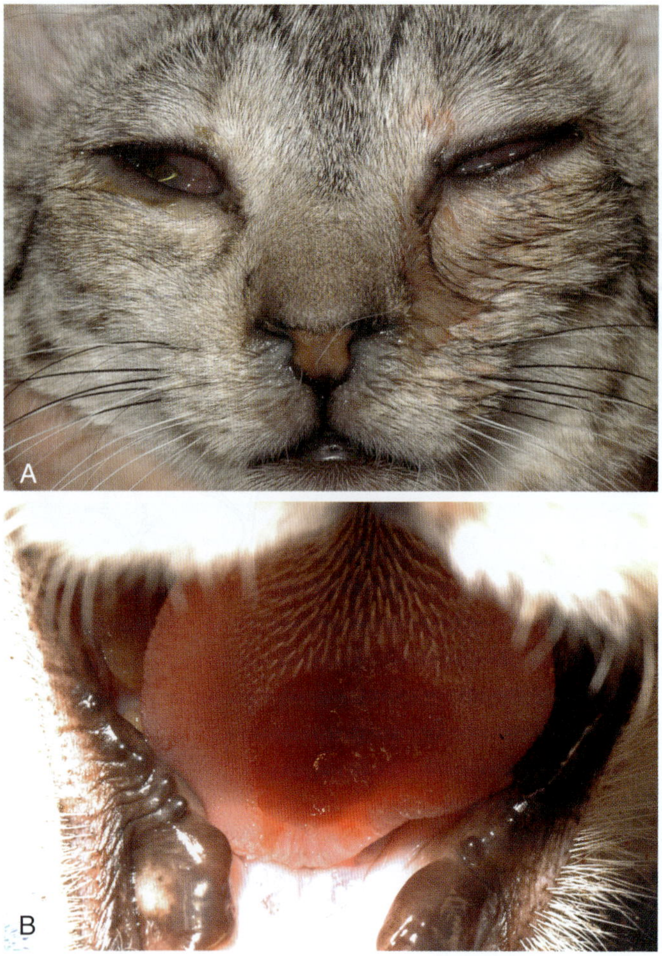

Fig. 34.3 Chemosis, mucopurulent ocular, and nasal discharge (A) and lingual ulceration (B) in a 6-month-old intact male domestic medium-hair cat with chronic nasal discharge and conjunctivitis. A conjunctival swab specimen tested positive with a PCR assay for feline calicivirus RNA and negative for feline herpesvirus-1, *Chlamydia felis*, and *Mycoplasma* spp. DNA. (Courtesy of the University of California, Davis Veterinary Ophthalmology Service.)

associated with FHV-1 infection (Fig. 34.3B). The role of FHV-1 in chronic rhinosinusitis in adult cats is unclear, but it is possible that repeated viral reactivation and progressive damage to the mucosa may play a role in this syndrome.

Ocular Disease

FHV-1 is an important cause of conjunctivitis, blepharitis, and corneal disease in cats, and has been implicated as a cause of acute and chronic ulcerative (epithelial) keratitis, stromal keratitis, eosinophilic keratitis, corneal sequestra, and uveitis.[30,31] Infection of cats with FHV-1 often results in conjunctivitis and ulcerative keratitis due to viral replication and thus direct cytotoxicity to the conjunctival and corneal epithelium, respectively.[27] While the presence of dendritic corneal ulcers in cats is pathognomonic for FHV-1 infection, these ulcers are less commonly identified as they rapidly enlarge to form superficial geographic ulcers. Cats with FHV-1 infection also exhibit decreases in conjunctival goblet cell density and tear film breakup time, and this resultant tear film instability likely contributes to the ongoing pathology of the conjunctiva and/or cornea.[32,33] Though infrequent, keratoconjunctivitis sicca can occur from damage to the ductules secondary to chronic herpetic blepharoconjunctivitis and/or neurogenic origin.[34] Stromal keratitis consisting of corneal cellular infiltrate and/or vascularization is a relatively uncommon manifestation of FHV-1 infection and occurs presumably as a result of the immune response to viral antigen in the corneal stroma.[30]

While the function that FHV-1 plays in the aforementioned syndromes is relatively clear, its role in the pathogenesis in eosinophilic keratitis, corneal sequestra, and uveitis remains nebulous and requires further study.[35] For example, FHV-1 DNA was detected using PCR in 55% of cats with corneal sequestra and 76% of scrapings from cats with eosinophilic keratitis in comparison with 5.9% of cats with normal corneas.[36] However, for corneal sequestra, brachycephalic cats were significantly less likely to have FHV-1 DNA in the specimens versus domestic shorthair and longhair breeds suggesting that nonviral factors such as corneal sensitivity and exposure likely play a role in its pathogenesis.[37] For eosinophilic keratitis, FHV-1 DNA was more likely to be detected in cats with a history and/or presence of a corneal ulcer at initial presentation.[38] However, it was not possible to discern if the cats with FHV-1 DNA and concurrent eosinophilic keratitis were experiencing primary herpetic disease or reactivation of latent virus in the trigeminal ganglion. Nevertheless, eosinophilic keratitis typically does not respond to antiviral medications, and immunosuppressive medications are often required for treatment. This suggests that this condition may result from an immune response to FHV-1 or another antigenic stimulus.[39] While reflex uveitis secondary to ulcerative herpetic keratitis is common, the role of FHV-1 in the pathogenesis of idiopathic anterior uveitis remains unclear.[38,40]

Studies of chronic HSV infections in rabbits suggest that this may relate to a significant decrease in corneal nerve density that occurs after 4 months of infection, which is associated with severe epithelial and stromal nerve damage with decreased corneal sensitivity, as well as formation of scar tissue in the central cornea.[41] A case report suggests a similar phenomenon exists in cats infected with FHV-1.[34]

Other Clinical Manifestations

FHV-1 can cause severe ulcerative and eosinophilic facial dermatitis, which is most likely to occur on the rostral muzzle and nasal planum, possibly reflecting viral spread to these sites following reactivation from the trigeminal ganglia (Fig. 34.4). A similar syndrome has also been described in cheetahs. Lesions have also been described elsewhere on the body in the absence of facial lesions.[42]

Multifocal necrotizing gastritis was described in one cat with concurrent necrotizing bronchopneumonia and laryngotracheitis in a cat with systemic FHV-1 infection.[43] Rarely, neurologic signs due to meningoencephalitis[44] and reproductive complications such as abortion and fetal resorption have been observed in infected cats, although it is unclear what role FHV-1 itself plays in the pathogenesis of reproductive failure. Abortion may be due to the severe systemic effects of the illness, rather than a direct effect of the virus itself.[19]

Physical Examination Findings

Acute Feline Herpesvirus-1 Infections

Physical examination findings in cats with acute viral URTD vary from mild serous ocular discharge and conjunctivitis to fever, severe mucopurulent ocular and nasal discharges, chemosis, dehydration, thin body condition, stertorous or stridorous respiration, tachypnea, increased breath sounds on thoracic auscultation, hypersalivation, and ulceration of the nasal planum, tongue, and lips. Because ulcerative lesions can occur at the base of the tongue near the larynx, examination of the entire tongue should be performed in cats that are febrile and inappetent, which may require sedation. Punctate or dendritic ulcerative keratitis may be seen in cats with acute FHV-1 infection.

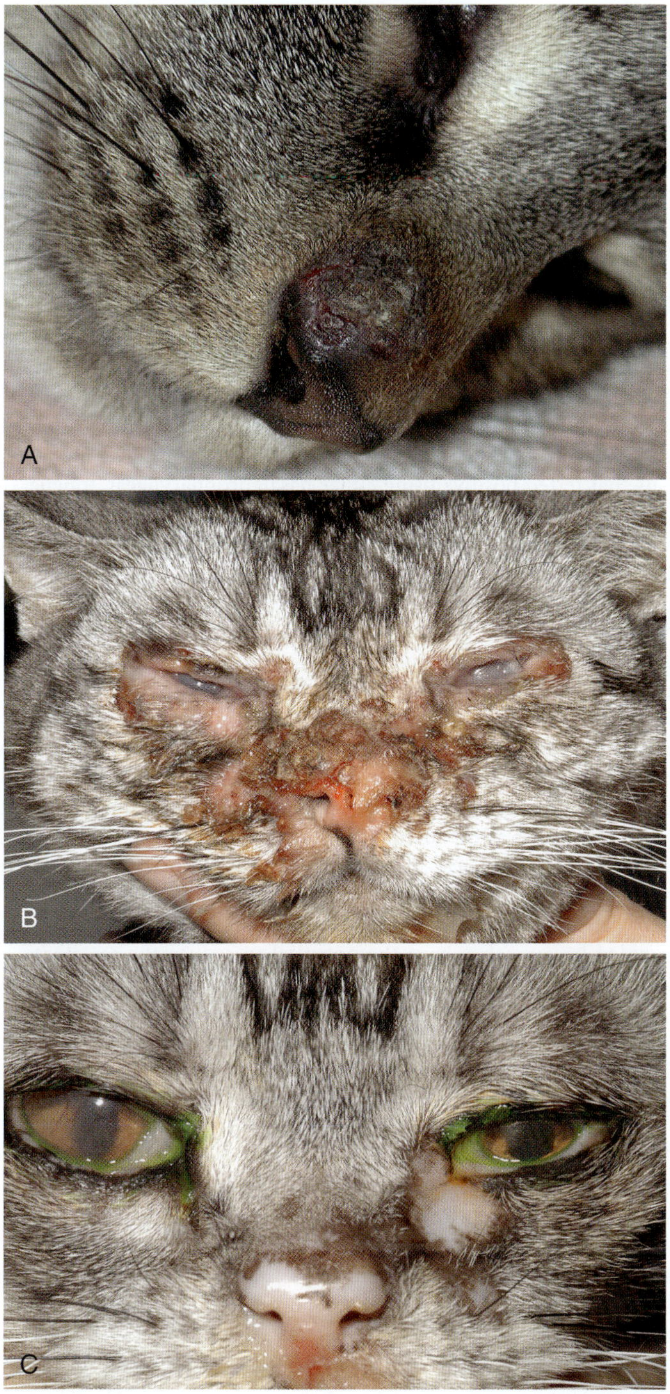

Fig. 34.4 Ulcerative and eosinophilic facial dermatitis secondary to feline herpesvirs-1 (FHV-1) infection. (A) A 3-year-old female spayed domestic shorthair with a 2-month history of a crusted lesion on the right dorsal muzzle. (B) A 14-year-old female spayed domestic shorthair with blepharokeratoconjunctivitis and severe ulcerative facial dermatitis. (C) Same cat as in B after 4 months of treatment with famciclovir. Fluorescein stain is present. Biopsy in both cats showed severe, diffuse, necrotizing, and eosinophilic dermatitis with a few intranuclear inclusions bodies. A PCR assay for FHV-1 DNA on a biopsy from the cat in B was positive. (Courtesy of the University of California, Davis Veterinary Dermatology and Ophthalmology Service.)

Chronic Feline Herpesvirus-1 Infections

Ophthalmic examination findings associated with chronic FHV-1 infection can vary widely and include serous to mucoid ocular discharge, blepharedema, conjunctival hyperemia and/or chemosis, corneal ulceration with edema, corneal vascularization, pigmentation, mineralization, and/or fibrosis, keratoconjunctivitis sicca, and brown or black discoloration to the stroma consistent with corneal sequestra (Fig. 34.5).[27,31,45] Eosinophilic keratitis manifests as superficial, pink to white vascularized proliferative lesions on the cornea and/or conjunctiva; the superotemporal quadrant is the most affected position in the cornea.[38] Herpetic facial dermatitis is manifested as cutaneous ulceration, erythema, exudation, and adherent crusts, most commonly around the nose and eyes but occasionally on the trunk and limbs.[46]

DIAGNOSIS

It is generally not possible to diagnose FHV-1 infection based on clinical signs alone, because other respiratory pathogens can cause similar clinical signs. The presence of corneal ulceration should raise suspicion for FHV-1 infection, but mixed infections occur and complicate diagnosis. A history of exposure to other cats provides support for a diagnosis of viral respiratory disease, but because FHV-1 infections can recrudesce with stress, potential or known exposure to other cats is not essential to implicate respiratory viruses as a cause of disease. Previous vaccination for FHV-1 does not rule out the possibility of FHV-1 infection. All cats with signs of URTD should have known retrovirus infection status because viral URTD is common in retrovirus-infected cats. When signs such as chronic nasal discharge are present, other etiologies should also be considered, such as fungal infections, neoplasia, and foreign bodies. Diagnosis of eosinophilic keratitis and ulcerative facial dermatitis may require corneal scrapings or skin biopsy, respectively.

Laboratory Abnormalities

There are no specific CBC, serum biochemical, or urinalysis abnormalities that aid in a diagnosis of FHV-1 infection. The CBC can be normal or show a mild to moderate neutrophilia, sometimes with band neutrophils or neutrophil toxicity. Lymphopenia may be present in severely affected cats. Serum biochemistry findings are usually unremarkable unless disease is severe or chronic.

Endotracheal lavage specimens from cats with pneumonia may show a suppurative or mixed exudate, sometimes with evidence of secondary bacterial infection. Aerobic bacterial culture and susceptibility testing, and culture for *Mycoplasma* spp. are indicated on wash specimens. Organisms such as *Pasteurella* spp., *Staphylococcus pseudintermedius*, *Streptococcus* spp., *E. coli*, *Klebsiella pneumoniae*, and some *Mycoplasma* spp. may infect the airways as opportunists. Bacterial culture of nasal swabs is generally not recommended because it often leads to growth of normal flora, which has no clinical relevance. However, resistant *Pseudomonas aeruginosa* infections can develop in some cats with chronic URTD that have been treated repeatedly with antimicrobial drugs.

Herpetic ulcerative keratitis may lead to secondary bacterial and/or fungal infection. Therefore, aerobic bacterial and/or fungal cultures should be considered in cases of feline ulcerative keratitis with stromal loss, malacia, and/or cellular infiltrate. If eosinophilic keratitis is suspected, a corneal scraping should be performed after administration of a topical anesthetic; abundant eosinophils with neutrophils and/or mast cells will typically be present.

Diagnostic Imaging

In uncomplicated FHV-1 infections, plain thoracic radiographs may be unremarkable or show a mild diffuse interstitial to bronchointerstitial pattern. Alveolar patterns or lung lobe consolidation can occur with secondary bacterial pneumonia.

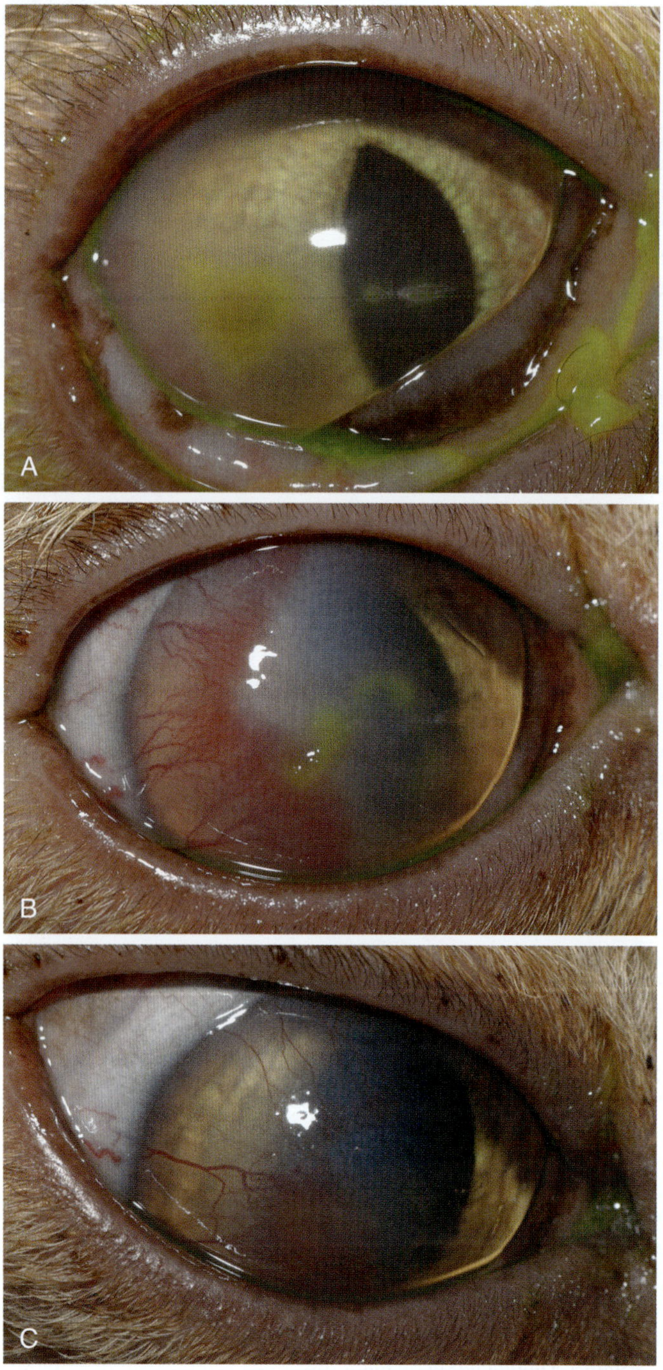

Fig. 34.5 (A) Ulcerative and stromal keratitis in a 2-year-old male neutered Rex cat. Feline herepesvirus-1 infection was suspected. Treatment with famciclovir (375 mg, PO, q8h), L-lysine (500 mg, PO, q12h), and cidofovir (0.5%; one drop, OD, q12h) was associated with clinical improvement over a 1-month period (B and C). The cat had a history of a corneal sequestrum and subsequently developed eosinophilic keratitis. (Courtesy of the University of California, Davis Veterinary Ophthalmology Service.)

Microbiologic Tests

Because many cats experience self-limiting disease, attempts to obtain an etiologic diagnosis of URTD should be made when disease persists for longer than 7 to 10 days or is complicated by pneumonia, with lethargy and inappetence. When outbreaks of respiratory disease occur in shelters or the pattern of endemic respiratory disease changes, attempts to make an etiologic diagnosis are also indicated and strongly encouraged. Because FHV-1 can be detected in apparently healthy cats, it may be difficult to know the significance of a positive test result in a single cat with signs of respiratory disease. In an outbreak situation, collection of multiple specimen types from several cats with and without clinical signs can facilitate diagnosis and allow interpretation of the significance of test results. In shelter situations or outbreaks of severe disease, necropsies can provide valuable information and should be performed by a veterinary pathologist as soon as possible after death or euthanasia. Tissues should be submitted for histopathology (in formalin), bacterial and virus isolation (fresh tissue), and PCR for respiratory viruses and bacteria (fresh or frozen tissue; see Chapter 6).

Assays available to detect FHV-1 include virus isolation, direct immunofluorescence, and PCR assays (Table 34.1). The use of both PCR and culture together offers the greatest sensitivity when it is important to obtain a diagnosis. One study suggested that use of nasal swab specimens results in detection of FHV-1 using PCR in 95% of cats that tested positive using either nasal, oropharyngeal, tongue, or conjunctival swab specimens,[47] but submitting swabs from multiple sites increases the chance of a positive test result, and FCV is more likely to be detected in oropharyngeal swabs.

Virus Isolation

Although not commonly performed for routine diagnosis, FHV-1 is readily isolated in cell culture. Virus isolation is offered to veterinarians by some commercial veterinary diagnostic laboratories that specialize in virology. Suitable specimens for isolation of FHV-1 include conjunctival, nasal, and oropharyngeal swabs, endotracheal or bronchoalveolar lavage specimens, or upper airway tissue or lung obtained at necropsy. If swabs are used for specimen collection, polyester-tipped swabs and specific virus transport media should be used, which are available from commercial testing laboratories. When conjunctival swabs are collected, the use of topical anesthetics should also be avoided because they have the potential to reduce the sensitivity of virus isolation.[48] Isolation may take several days. Sensitivity can be very low in cats with chronic manifestations of infection (more than 10 days after the onset of clinical signs). In cats with mixed FCV and FHV-1 infections, FCV may obscure the presence of FHV-1 because it produces cytopathic effects more rapidly.

Fluorescent Antibody Testing

FA that specifically detects FHV-1 can be applied to conjunctival smears or impression smears from lung tissue collected at necropsy. The effect of vaccination with attenuated live vaccines on direct FA test results has not been reported. The sensitivity of direct FA testing is lower than that of PCR or virus isolation,[49] and inexperienced laboratory personnel may misinterpret nonspecific fluorescence as a positive result.

Molecular Diagnosis Using Nucleic Acid–Based Testing

Panels of real-time PCR assays that detect feline respiratory pathogens are offered by some commercial veterinary diagnostic laboratories and are rapid and relatively inexpensive. These can include assays for FHV-1 and FCV, as well as bacteria such as *Mycoplasma* spp., *B. bronchiseptica*, and *C. felis*. The sensitivity and specificity of PCR assays for FHV-1 vary considerably among laboratories. Swabs of the nasal cavity, conjunctival sac, or caudal pharynx; respiratory lavage specimens; skin biopsies; or upper respiratory tract and lung tissue collected at necropsy are suitable specimens for testing. Topical anesthetics and fluorescein can reduce the sensitivity of PCR assays for human herpesviral infections,[50] and thus should be avoided, although one study showed no inhibitory effect of topical fluorescein or proxymetacaine in cats on FHV-1 PCR results.[51] False-negative PCR results can occur in cats with chronic infections that shed low amounts of virus. An

TABLE 34.1 Diagnostic Assays Available for FHV-1 Infections in Cats

Assay	Specimen Type	Target	Performance
Virus isolation	Conjunctival, nasal, and caudal pharyngeal swabs, transtracheal and bronchoalveolar lavage specimens, airway and lung specimens collected at necropsy	Virus	Negative results can occur if specimens contain no or low numbers of virus particles. May take several days and requires specialized techniques and expertise.
PCR	See Virus isolation	Viral nucleic acid	Sensitivity and specificity may vary depending on assay design. Sensitivity may be low because of brief shedding or low-level shedding in chronic infections. Testing specimens from multiple different anatomic sites or combining PCR with other diagnostic tests can increase sensitivity. Attenuated live vaccine virus may be detected after vaccination. Because of subclinical shedding, the significance of a positive result may be difficult to interpret.
Serology	Serum	Antibodies against FHV-1 antigens	Interpretation complicated by previous vaccination and exposure.
Histopathology	Necropsy or biopsy specimens	FHV-1 inclusions; immunostaining	Detection of FHV-1 inclusions has low sensitivity, and immunostaining and/or PCR is required to definitively identify the infecting virus.

FHV-1, feline herpesvirus-1.

isothermal PCR assay has been described that permits detection of FHV-1 within 20 minutes.[52]

Positive PCR assay results for FHV-1 should be interpreted with caution because cats with no clinical signs can shed FHV-1. In one shelter, a correlation between the quantity of FHV-1 present in pooled oropharyngeal and conjunctival swabs as determined using quantitative real-time PCR and the severity of histologic lesions within the nasal cavity was detected, with cycle threshold values less than 29 correlating with the most severe histologic lesions.[53] In the future, quantitation of viral nucleic acid within swabs may assist interpretation of the clinical significance of positive PCR results. Also, PCR can detect attenuated live vaccine virus that is shed after routine vaccination. However, this appeared to be an uncommon phenomenon in one study that used PCR to detect FHV-1 in 12 cats previously exposed to the virus over a 3-week period after vaccination with intranasal or parenteral attenuated live FHV-1 vaccines.[12] Additional studies are required to determine the prevalence of positive assay results after vaccination and their relationship to vaccine virus. In outbreak situations, false-positive PCR results have the potential to occur if swabs become contaminated with virus from the environment or the hands of personnel. Clean examination gloves should be worn for each cat, and the swab should touch only the anatomic site to be tested. In one randomized study of shelter cats, results of FHV-1 or *Mycoplasma* spp. PCR assays did not accurately predict response to cidofovir or topical tetracycline ointment, respectively.[54]

Serologic Diagnosis

Serologic assays (such as ELISA or serum neutralization assays) that detect antibodies to FHV-1 are offered on a commercial basis to veterinarians. Unfortunately, serology is not useful for diagnosis because of vaccine titer interference and the high prevalence of subclinical exposure to these viruses in the cat population. Serology has also been used to predict protection from infection, although cats with negative titers can still have some degree of immunity, and cats with positive titers may develop illness after challenge.

Pathologic Findings

Gross lesions in cats with FHV-1 infections include cutaneous and lingual ulcerations, evidence of conjunctivitis and keratitis, and mucopurulent exudate within the nasal cavity and trachea. In cats with pneumonia, the lungs may be edematous with diffuse or multifocal consolidated areas. Histopathology may show rhinitis, tracheitis, and/or alveolitis. Intranuclear viral inclusions may be found within epithelial cells of the upper respiratory tract (Fig. 34.6). Osteolytic changes within the nasal turbinates may also be identified. Virus can be detected in epithelial cells using IHC or FA staining. Skin biopsies from cats with ulcerative herpesviral dermatitis show epidermal hyperplasia, ulceration, and necrosis that extends into the superficial dermis, and infiltration with degenerated neutrophils, eosinophils, and fewer numbers of histiocytes, plasma cells, and lymphocytes. In some skin biopsies, intranuclear viral inclusions are identified.[45,55]

TREATMENT AND PROGNOSIS

Supportive care is the mainstay of treatment for acute FHV-1 infections and includes subcutaneous fluid therapy, antimicrobial drugs for secondary bacterial infections, and enteral nutrition. Antimicrobial therapy should be withheld for cats with acute (<10 days) illness that are otherwise appetent according to ISCAID Antimicrobial Use Guidelines[56] (Table 34.2). When inappetence and mucopurulent discharges are present, empiric treatment with a short course of doxycycline or amoxicillin is recommended for primary or secondary bacterial infections. Use of topical or systemic antiviral drugs is indicated for cats with severe or chronic clinical signs. Appetite stimulants may be useful in some cats, but if inappetence persists for longer than 3 days, feeding tube placement is indicated. Severely affected cats may require hospitalization in isolation and treatment with parenteral fluids, antimicrobial drugs, nebulization, and supplemental oxygen. Acute signs generally resolve within 2 to 3 weeks with supportive care, but some cats experience frequent disease relapses and chronic complications such as keratitis.

The use of antiviral drugs should be considered for cats with severe and recurrent or persistent manifestations of FHV-1 infection such as keratitis, severe conjunctivitis, and ulcerative dermatitis. Antiviral drugs are discussed in more depth in Chapter 9 (see Table 9.5 for dosages). A comprehensive review of antiviral drugs and other compounds with established or purported activity against FHV-1 can be found elsewhere (see Suggested Readings). Acyclovir and its prodrug, valacyclovir, cause unacceptable renal, bone marrow, and hepatic toxicity when administered systemically to cats, and so their

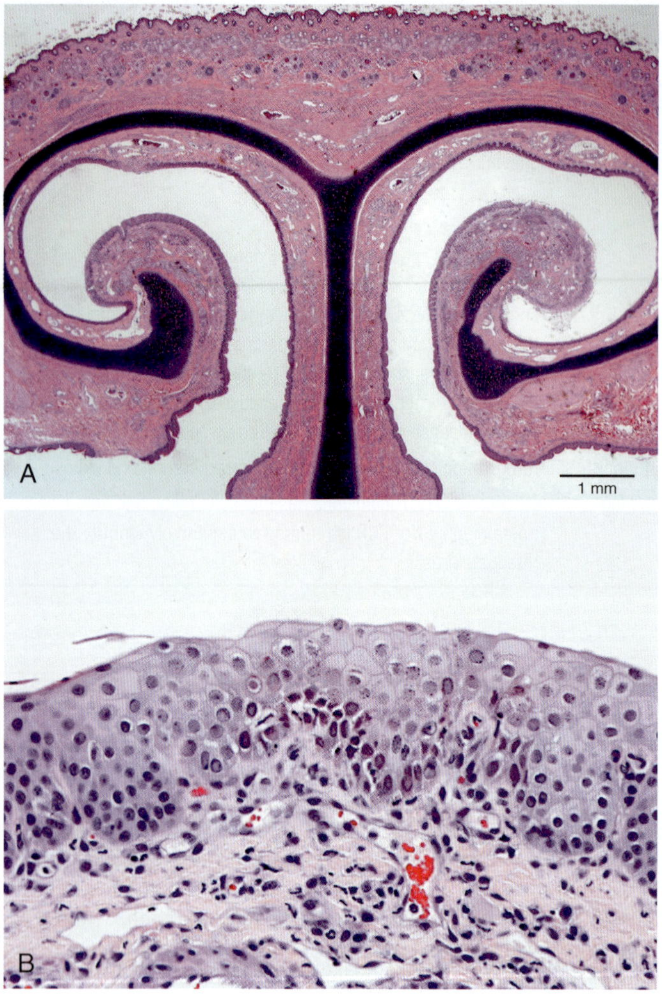

Fig. 34.6 (A) Cross-section of the nares of a shelter cat with rhinitis due to infection by feline herpesvirus-1. Ulceration is most severe on the right side. Hematoxylin and eosin stain. (B) Higher magnification of the nasal epithelium that shows rhinitis and the presence of intraepithelial, intranuclear inclusion bodies. (From Burns RE, Wagner DC, Leutenegger CM, et al. Histologic and molecular correlation in shelter cats with acute upper respiratory infection. *J Clin Microbiol.* 2011;49:2454–2460. Images courtesy Dr. Patricia Pesavento, University of California, Davis Veterinary Anatomic Pathology Service.)

use is not recommended.[57,58] By contrast, oral famciclovir is generally well tolerated by adult cats and kittens and results in significant clinical improvement and decreased viral shedding in cats with acute and chronic herpetic disease (see Fig. 34.5B and C).[59–61] When administered with other topical and systemic antibacterial drugs, owner-reported clinical response rates in a population of cats seen at a tertiary referral hospital were greater than 80%, with approximately 50% of cats showing marked improvement as assessed by clinicians.[59] Another study of 24 kittens with acute URTD showed no difference in clinical response when famciclovir was compared with doxycycline; however, FHV-1 was only detected using PCR in seven of these cats.[62] No difference in clinical outcome was also reported in a placebo-controlled study of shelter-housed cats with evidence of herpetic disease, although shedding of FHV-1 was reduced in famciclovir-treated cats.[63] Cats in this study were treated for 7 days, and famciclovir was evaluated both for prophylaxis and treatment. The recommended dose based on pharmacokinetic studies of famciclovir and its active metabolite, penciclovir, in plasma and tears is 90 mg/kg q12h.[64] Use of a single dose of famciclovir at intake of cats to shelters was ineffective at reducing shedding and disease.[65] Because viral strains that are resistant to famciclovir have been described,[66] the use of famciclovir should be reserved for severe or refractory infections to minimize further selection for resistance.

The active metabolite of famciclovir, penciclovir, also has potential to be a useful drug for local treatment of feline herpesviral infections since it has poor oral bioavailability.[67] Based on *in vitro* studies using corneal explants as well as a study of experimentally infected cats, the integrase inhibitor raltegravir also shows promise as a treatment for FHV-1 infections.[68,69]

Cidofovir and ganciclovir have shown the greatest promise as topical treatments due to their potency against FHV-1 *in vitro*. Furthermore, topical cidofovir decreases disease severity and viral shedding in experimentally infected cats[70], and has the advantage of requiring only twice-daily administration. Topical ganciclovir (0.15%) had excellent *in vitro* activity and was well tolerated when administered to 4 healthy cats q8h for 7 days.[71] Topical ophthalmic preparations that contain idoxuridine, trifluridine, vidarabine, or acyclovir can be used to treat herpetic keratitis, although the true efficacy of these drugs has not been well studied. Frequent topical application is required (4–6 times daily), and prolonged use may cause corneal and/or conjunctival irritation. Idoxuridine and vidarabine may be better tolerated by cats than trifluridine. In addition to topical and/or systemic antiviral drugs, topical administration of a mucinomimetic such as sodium hyaluronate is beneficial to address the decrease in conjunctival goblet density and concomitant tear film instability caused by FHV-1.[60]

Human recombinant IFN-α and recombinant feline IFN-ω inhibit FHV-1 replication *in vitro* and have been administered parenterally, topically (for keratitis), and orally to cats with FHV-1 infection.[72] Obvious clinical responses to treatment have not been uniformly observed, but controlled clinical trials that involve large numbers of cats are lacking. Topical administration of human recombinant IFN-α or recombinant feline IFN-ω had no benefit over saline in cats with naturally occurring viral keratoconjunctivitis.[73] Clinical improvement was noted when IFN-α was given subcutaneously 2 days before inoculation of cats with FHV-1,[74] and in 8 of 13 naturally infected cats treated with 10,000 U/kg SC for 14 days.[75] Parenteral administration may be followed by the development of neutralizing antibodies beyond 3 weeks of treatment. Use of a combination of low-dose, sequential kinetic activated (SKA) IL-12 and IFN-γ in a randomized, prospective, placebo-controlled study for 6 months was associated with clearance of infection as determined using endpoint (conventional) PCR in 12 of 15 treated cats.[76] Preliminary data suggest that administration of an intranasal FHV-1 and FCV vaccine may result in clinical improvement in cats with chronic URTD that have failed other therapies.[75]

Lysine has shown efficacy for treatment of herpesviral conjunctivitis in cats when administered as tablets[77] and may reduce reactivated shedding by latently infected cats.[78] However, when administered to shelter cats, there was no reduction in URTD, possibly because of the stress of tablet administration.[79] Dietary formulation with lysine has also been ineffective for management of URTD in shelters and in fact may contribute to a worsened outcome.[80] Various concentrations of lysine were not able to inhibit replication of FHV-1 *in vitro*.[81] On the basis of the lack of clear evidence supporting the use of lysine for prevention and treatment of FHV-1 infections in cats and concerns about adverse outcomes, it has been recommended by some that its use be discontinued.[82]

The use of glucocorticoids to treat refractory herpetic keratitis is controversial, because it may reactivate virus and worsen disease. The exception is eosinophilic keratitis which often requires treatment with

TABLE 34.2 Antimicrobials Used To Treat Feline Herpesvirus-1 Infections in Cats

Drug	Dose	Route	Interval	Duration (days)	Comments
Cidofovir	0.5% solution	Topical ophthalmic	q12h	Until resolution	Monitor for ocular irritation. Compounding may be required or a solution can be prepared from commercial 7.5% intravenous solution by dilution in sterile saline. Store diluted solution up to 6 months at 4°C, –20°C, and –80°C.
Idoxuridine	0.1% solution or 0.5% ointment	Topical ophthalmic	4–6 times daily	Until resolution	Monitor for ocular irritation. Compounding is required.
Vidarabine	3% ointment	Topical ophthalmic	4–6 times daily	Until resolution	Monitor for ocular irritation. Compounding is required.
Trifluridine	1% solution	Topical ophthalmic	4–6 times daily	Until resolution	May be poorly tolerated. Monitor for ocular irritation.
Famciclovir	90 mg/kg	PO	q12h	Until resolution	Monitor for inappetence and diarrhea.
Ganciclovir	0.15% gel	Topical ophthalmic	q8h	Until resolution	Monitor for ocular irritation.
Raltegravir	80 mg	PO	q12h	Until resolution	Monitor for adverse events given that safety testing was limited to a 2 week study in healthy cats experimentally infected with FHV-1.
Doxycycline	5 mg/kg q12h OR 10 mg/kg q24h	PO	24	7–10	For secondary bacterial infection. Hyclate suspension should be followed by administration of a bolus of water; compounded suspensions are not stable beyond 7 days.
Amoxicillin	22	PO	12	7–10	For secondary bacterial infection. Not active against mycoplasmas or *Chlamydia*.

topical glucocorticoids. Because the role of FHV-1 in this condition is unclear, topical antiviral medications such as cidofovir are often given concurrently. Topical glucocorticoids are contraindicated when corneal ulceration is present, so it is critical to apply fluorescein stain and carefully examine the corneas for retention of the dye. Cats with ulcerative eosinophilic keratitis may require systemic glucocorticoid treatment until the ulcers heal.

Superficial lamellar keratectomy may be required for chronic corneal ulceration and/or corneal sequestra that are nonresponsive to medical therapy.[83] Other surgical treatments for corneal sequestra include corneoconjunctival transposition, lamellar keratoplasty followed by corneal transplantation, amniotic membrane transplantation, conjunctival graft placement, or placement of acellular matrix.[84–86] For surgical interventions, referral to a veterinary ophthalmologist is recommended.

IMMUNITY AND VACCINATION

Immunity to FHV-1 depends on cell-mediated and systemic and local (mucosal IgA) humoral immune responses. Maternal antibody can persist until 14 weeks of age,[19] although other kittens may be susceptible to infection at 6 weeks of age.

Vaccines for FHV-1 have been available for decades, but these do not provide complete protection, and disease continues to be widespread in the cat population. Infection of kittens before completion of the primary vaccine series contributes to this problem. Both inactivated and attenuated live FHV-1 vaccines are available, and attenuated live vaccines are available for parenteral or intranasal administration. Inactivated vaccines contain adjuvant, and their use should be reserved for immunosuppressed cats (such as retrovirus-infected cats) or pregnant cats, if deemed necessary. A recent study showed that although total clinical score was not significantly different between the groups, clinical signs of respiratory disease in cats vaccinated with a single dose of an inactivated vaccine were significantly reduced when compared with cats vaccinated with an attenuated live vaccine following challenge 7 days later.[87] When infections are a problem in kittens in breeding catteries, vaccination of the queen before mating is preferable to vaccination during pregnancy and may prolong the duration of maternal antibody persistence.[88] Vaccination as early as 4 weeks of age (but not before) could be considered in catteries with high rates of viral URTD. The primary series should consist of vaccines administered every 3 to 4 weeks of age until no earlier than 16 weeks of age.

No FHV-1 vaccine prevents infection, the carrier state, or reactivation, but FHV-1 vaccines can reduce disease severity. Whether a cat contracts feline viral URTD after vaccination depends on factors such as virus strain virulence, the challenge dose, environmental temperature and humidity, and the presence of underlying immunosuppressive disease or other concurrent disease.

Vaccination with FHV-1 vaccines can reduce the duration of shedding, viral infectivity (presumably as a result of complexing of virus by antibody), and the load of latent virus in the trigeminal ganglia.[19,89,90] It is unclear if the frequency of reactivation is reduced, although this is the case for herpesviral vaccines in other species (such as the shingles vaccine for humans). The intranasal FHV-1 vaccine virus can itself become latent, but whether parenteral FHV-1 vaccine virus becomes latent is unknown.

Because FHV-1 strains are antigenically similar, the immune response to one FHV-1 strain cross protects against other FHV-1 strains.

Parenteral vaccines that contain FHV-1 are generally safe. Intranasal vaccines are less well tolerated by cats and can be occasionally followed by mild to moderate postvaccinal signs of URTD. This may be problematic in shelter environments where clinical signs of URTD warrant the need for separate housing. On the other hand, intranasal vaccines are advantageous in this situation because of rapid onset of immunity, with partial protection after 2 days and significant protection after 4 days.[19] They can also overcome maternal antibody at a young age, although some injectable vaccines may also still be effective at an early age. Concurrent administration of a parenteral and intranasal vaccine to naïve kittens was superior to parenteral vaccination alone in one challenge study.[91] Because vaccine virus is propagated in feline kidney cells, there has been concern that parenteral administration of feline vaccines might lead to chronic renal inflammation when immune responses to vaccine components cross-react with endogenous renal antigens.[92] Further studies are required to determine whether this is clinically important.

Vaccine boosters are recommended by the AAHA/AAFP 6 months after completion of the primary series, and at 3-yearly intervals thereafter in cats with low levels of exposure to respiratory viruses.[93] Titers tend to be low following vaccination and do not predict protection from infection, so they should not be used to decide whether to administer boosters. For cats in contaminated environments such as catteries, cats housed periodically in boarding facilities, or large multicat households with frequent introductions, annual vaccination may be more appropriate. The duration of immunity after vaccination remains incompletely understood. Although partial protection persists for several years after vaccination,[94] the degree of protection does wane with time, at least for cats that receive no natural boostering in the interim (i.e., from exposure to field virus). In one report, relative FHV-1 vaccine efficacy was 95%, when challenge occurred a few weeks after primary vaccination with an inactivated vaccine.[95] This compared with 52% when challenge occurred after 7.5 years.[96] In another study, a 50% reduction in clinical scores occurred after challenge 1 year after administration of an attenuated live FHV-1 vaccine, compared with around 75% after challenge 4 weeks after vaccination.[97] In the field, natural boostering as a result of contact with virus shed by other cats or subclinical reactivation may maintain immunity for longer periods of time.

PREVENTION

In addition to vaccination, reduction of stress and overcrowding is critical for prevention of disease caused by FHV-1. Proper hand washing and disinfection in shelters, boarding facilities, and veterinary hospitals to prevent fomite transmission is also very important, and dedicated food and water bowls should be used. Care of household cats by friends or neighbors should be recommended whenever possible rather than boarding to reduce the chance of infection or reactivation. Veterinarians should remember that all cats, whether apparently healthy or sick, can be a source of FHV-1 infection. Cats should be housed individually (unless they are from the same household and tolerate close proximity to one another). Barriers between cats should be impermeable, and cats with URTD should be separated by at least 4 to 5 feet to prevent aerosol transmission. If possible, cats that enter large multicat environments and shelters should be quarantined for 3 weeks to identify cats that are incubating disease. Use of tactics to reduce stress in shelter environments, such as creating spaces for cats to hide and "gentling" (gentle stroking and vocalizations) multiple times a day[24] can have a tremendous impact on reduction of disease caused by FHV-1 and viral shedding. Fostering in temporary homes can also reduce the prevalence of disease in shelter cats. When all other control measures fail in breeding catteries, early weaning and isolation of kittens from 4 weeks could be considered.

In one randomized trial of experimentally infected cats with chronic, subclinical FHV-1 infection, cats fed a probiotic with immune-modulating effects had less recurrent conjunctivitis than cats fed the control supplement, suggesting a prevention effect.[98]

In a different trial involving a similar model using housing change to induce mild stress, experimentally infected cats with chronic, subclinical FHV-1 infection that were housed in a room with a pheromone diffuser had decreased total stress scores and less sneezing when compared with cats housed is a room with a placebo diffuser.[99]

PUBLIC HEALTH ASPECTS

FHV-1 does not infect humans.

FELINE GAMMAHERPESVIRUS INFECTIONS

FELIS CATUS GAMMAHERPESVIRUS 1

FcaGHV1 infection is believed to be endemic worldwide. Blood samples from 1%–23.6% of cats from the Americas, Australasia, and Europe are positive for DNA using a FcaGHV1-specific qPCR.[2,100–104] Molecular studies do not detect all FcaGHV1 infections. Serology suggests that the true infection rate is at least double that indicated by molecular studies.[105] Age, sex, neuter status, health status, and co-infections have been identified as risk factors for FcaGHV1 infection with some regional variations.[2,100,101,106] Male sex and age over 2 years are important risk factors for FcaGHV1 DNA detection. FIV-infected cats are 5–10 times more likely to be positive for FcaGHV1 DNA than non-FIV–infected controls matched for age and sex,[2,100,103,104,106] and a UK study found that almost all FcaGHV1-infected cats were co-infected with at least one hemoplasma species.[101] Based on epidemiologic data, biting has been suggested as one potential route of FcaGHV1 transmission.[107]

Although generally host specific, some gammaherpesviruses can infect closely related hosts. If the alternate host is nonimmune, rapidly fatal disease can ensue, with malignant catarrhal fever of ruminants being a good example. FcaGHV1 infection of at least one nondomestic felid, the critically endangered Tsushima leopard cat, has been identified in Japan.[108]

Fortunately for a virus that is highly prevalent, it is likely that most FcaGHV1 infections are subclinical. Gammaherpesvirus infections in other species cause persistent infections that are typically clinically latent except in certain circumstances such as when CMI is compromised, when they can cause lymphoproliferative and neoplastic disorders.[109] The existence of a gammaherpesvirus in the domestic cat was first suggested by observations from the FIV cat model of HIV infection in humans. Both FIV and HIV infections increase the patient's risk of developing high-grade B-cell lymphomas.[110,111] Of HIV-associated lymphomas, 30% to 95%, depending on subtype, are causally linked to one or both of the gammaherpesviruses that infect humans, Epstein-Barr virus and Kaposi's sarcoma–associated herpesvirus. Whether FcaGHV1 plays a role in FIV-associated lymphomas is under investigation. Neither a molecular diagnosis of FcaGHV1 nor whole-blood FcaGHV1 load was related to outcome in 122 lymphoma cases compared with 71 controls matched for age and sex.[107] Interestingly, the same study identified shorter survival in FcaGHV1-positive lymphoma cases suggesting that prospective investigation of FcaGHV1 DNA detection as a prognostic marker for lymphoma may be warranted.

Diagnostic tests for FcaGHV1 are only available in a research setting. A qPCR targeting the glycoprotein B gene and serologic assays that detect antibodies recognizing ORF52 and ORF38 proteins have been described.[2,105]

OTHER GAMMAHERPESVIRUSES

Gammaherpesviruses infecting nondomestic Felidae have been identified in the puma (*Puma concolor*, PcoGHV1), African lion (*Panthera leo*, PleoGHV1), bobcat (*Lynx rufus*, LruGHV1 & 2), and ocelot (*Leopardus pardalis*, LpaGHV1).[2,112,113] To date, cross-species infectivity has been identified only for LruGHV1 which was detected in 13% of pumas in a US study.[2]

The bovine gammaherpesvirus, BHV4, has a wide host range and feline infections have been reported, but their prevalence and pathogenic potential remain controversial. Early experimental infections and disease association studies supporting a role for BHV4 in URTD and lower urinary tract disease have not been replicated. Molecular epidemiologic studies using nested or hemi-nested PCR to detect BHV4 DNA in free-ranging domestic cats reported divergent results; 26.9% of 104 blood samples from Michigan were BHV4 positive in one study,[114] whereas none of 101 cats from California, Colorado, and Florida tested PCR positive[115] suggesting that geographic variation in prevalence is likely.

CASE EXAMPLE

Signalment

"Boris," a 7-year-old male neutered Burmese cat from northern California.

History

Boris was brought to the University of California, Davis, VMTH for a 3-day history of inappetence, head shaking, gagging, hypersalivation, coughing, and sneezing. The gagging occurred throughout the day and occasionally was followed by vomiting. The vomit consisted of bile-stained fluid. Boris had not been drinking. He was taken to a local emergency clinic where bilateral serous nasal discharge was noted, and he was treated for 24 hours with IV crystalloid fluids and amoxicillin. Blood work showed hypokalemia (4.0 mEq/L, reference range 4.5–5.3 mEq/L), hyperglycemia (292 mg/dL, reference range 70–150 mg/dL), neutrophilia (12,920 cells/μL, reference range 2,500–12,500) and lymphopenia (136, reference range 1,500–7,000). FeLV and FIV serology was negative. A urinalysis showed a SpG of 1.050, pH of 7, and 1+ proteinuria and glucosuria. Lateral and dorsoventral radiographs of the thorax and abdomen showed moderate to severe gas distention of the proximal esophagus and stomach. Profuse salivation and gagging continued, and he was referred to a specialty clinic because of concerns for a possible GI foreign body. There had been no diarrhea, no history of travel or trauma, and no recent surgical procedures. A new indoor plant was brought into the house 2 days before the onset of clinical signs. He was last immunized for FHV-1, FCV, FPV, and rabies 1 year previously. Boris was housed completely indoors and was exposed to one other cat that only occasionally had access to the outdoors. His diet consisted of a commercial dry cat food.

Physical Examination

Body weight: 4.8 kg.

General: Lethargic, but responsive, 5% to 7% dehydrated. Held head extended and gagged and hypersalivated throughout the examination; seemed unable to swallow. Vomited bile-stained fluid once during the examination. T = 100.8°F (38.2°C), HR > 240 beats/minute, RR = 24 breaths/minute, mucous membranes pink, CRT = 1 second. The cat's haircoat was unkempt.

Eyes, ears, nose, and throat: Bilateral serous nasal discharge was present. A linear ulcer was identified on the right lateral aspect of the tongue.

Musculoskeletal: BCS was 4/9. Ambulatory.

Cardiovascular and respiratory: Other than tachycardia, no other abnormalities were detected.

GI and genitourinary: Mild abdominal distention was present.

Lymph nodes: All lymph nodes were < 1 cm in diameter.

Laboratory Findings

CBC: HCT 34.2% (30%–50%), MCV 51.0 fL (42–53 fL), MCHC 32.5 g/dL (30–33.5 g/dL), WBC 12,600 cells/μL (4,500–14,000 cells/μL), neutrophils 11,844 cells/μL (2,000–9,000 cells/μL), band neutrophils 126 cells/μL, lymphocytes 126 cells/μL (1,000–7,000 cells/μL), monocytes 252 cells/μL (50–600 cells/μL), eosinophils 126 cells/μL (150–1,100 cells/μL), platelets 989,000 platelets/μL (180,000–500,000 platelets/μL). The neutrophils showed slight toxicity, and there were a few Heinz bodies.

Serum chemistry profile: Sodium 141 mmol/L (151–158 mmol/L), potassium 4.0 mmol/L (3.6–4.9 mmol/L), chloride 108 mmol/L (117–126 mmol/L), bicarbonate 27 mmol/L (15–21 mmol/L), phosphorus 4.5 mg/dL (3.2–6.3 mg/dL), calcium 8.1 mg/dL (9.0–10.9 mg/dL), BUN 21 mg/dL (18–33 mg/dL), creatinine 1.1 mg/dL (1.1–2.2 mg/dL), glucose 212 mg/dL (63–118 mg/dL), total protein 5.1 g/dL (6.6–8.4 g/dL), albumin 2.2 g/dL (2.2–4.6 g/dL), globulin 2.9 g/dL (2.8–5.4 g/dL), ALT 83 U/L (27–101 U/L), AST 50 U/L (17–58 U/L), ALP 16 U/L (14–71 U/L), cholesterol 147 mg/dL (89–258 mg/dL), total bilirubin 0 mg/dL (0–0.2 mg/dL).

Imaging Findings

Endoscopy: Boris was anesthetized and an oral examination performed, which showed only mild dorsal pharyngeal lymphoid hyperplasia. Rhinoscopy showed a moderate amount of mucus and mild diffuse erythema of the nasal mucosa. Gastroduodenoscopy revealed focal areas of gastric erosion with hemorrhage.

Treatment

Boris was treated with IV crystalloid fluids (LRS with 20 mEq/L KCl at 20 mL/hour), ampicillin (23 mg/kg, IV, q8h), enrofloxacin (2.6 mg/kg, IV, q24h), sucralfate (0.25 g, PO, q8h), and famotidine (0.25 mg/kg, IV, q12h). He continued to hypersalivate, and he vomited approximately 100 mL of fluid twice daily. After the first day of hospitalization, the owners reported that their other cat had developed signs of URTD, with sneezing and nasal discharge. Enteral or parenteral nutrition was discussed with the owner, but on the evening of the second day of hospitalization, Boris was found gagging and cyanotic. He was taken to the intensive care unit but developed cardiorespiratory arrest. CPR was instituted and tracheal suction revealed yellow fluid consistent with possible aspiration. Although CPR was initially successful, Boris arrested again and died shortly afterward.

Necropsy Examination

Gross necropsy examination showed numerous lingual ulcerations, mostly pinpoint but some coalescing into larger ulcers up to 1 cm long and 0.5 cm wide. Both lungs were diffusely dark red, poorly collapsed, and oozed large amounts of clear fluid on cut surface. There was a small amount of yellow ascites fluid. Histopathology revealed marked, multifocal, acute to subacute necrotizing stomatitis, rhinitis, tracheitis, bronchiolitis, and alveolitis with intranuclear herpesviral inclusions in the bronchiolar epithelium. IFA testing on lung tissue was positive for FHV-1. Virus isolation was negative. Histopathology of GI biopsies collected at endoscopy and tissues collected at necropsy was unremarkable.

Comments

This cat died of a severe and overwhelming FHV-1 infection despite the fact that he was an adult cat that had been vaccinated regularly. Clinical signs of anorexia, gagging, and hypersalivation likely resulted from stomatitis, pharyngitis, and tracheitis. Histopathology with IFA staining confirmed the involvement of FHV-1. The negative virus isolation result may have been because of an insufficient sample size, inactivation of virus by antibody, or lack of viable virus in the specimen. Because FHV-1 survives poorly in the environment, it may deteriorate in clinical specimens during transport to the laboratory.

SUGGESTED READINGS

Thomasy SM, Shull O, Outerbridge CA, et al. Oral administration of famciclovir for treatment of spontaneous ocular, respiratory, or dermatologic disease attributed to feline herpesvirus type 1: 59 cases (2006-2013). *J Am Vet Med Assoc.* 2016;249:526–538.

Lappin MR, Blondeau J, Boothe D, et al. Antimicrobial Use Guidelines for Treatment of Respiratory Tract Disease in Dogs and Cats: Antimicrobial Guidelines Working Group of the International Society for Companion Animal Infectious Diseases. *J Vet Intern Med.* 2017;31:279–294.

Bol S, Bunnik EM. Lysine supplementation is not effective for the prevention or treatment of feline herpesvirus 1 infection in cats: a systematic review. *BMC Vet Res.* 2015;11:284.

Beatty JA, Troyer RM, Carver S, et al. *Felis catus* gammaherpesvirus 1; a widely endemic potential pathogen of domestic cats. *Virology.* 2014;460-461:100–107.

REFERENCES

1. Crandell RA, Maurer FD. Isolation of a feline virus associated with intranuclear inclusion bodies. *Proc Soc Exp Biol Med.* 1958;97:487–490.
2. Beatty JA, Troyer RM, Carver S, et al. *Felis catus* gammaherpesvirus 1; a widely endemic potential pathogen of domestic cats. *Virology.* 2014;460–461:100–107.
3. Helps CR, Lait P, Damhuis A, et al. Factors associated with upper respiratory tract disease caused by feline herpesvirus, feline calicivirus, *Chlamydophila felis* and *Bordetella bronchiseptica* in cats: experience from 218 European catteries. *Vet Rec.* 2005;156:669–673.
4. Hamano M, Maeda K, Mizukoshi F, et al. Experimental infection of recent field isolates of feline herpesvirus type 1. *J Vet Med Sci.* 2003;65:939–943.
5. Vaz PK, Job N, Horsington J, et al. Low genetic diversity among historical and contemporary clinical isolates of felid herpesvirus 1. *BMC Genom.* 2016;17:704.
6. Tai SH, Niikura M, Cheng HH, et al. Complete genomic sequence and an infectious BAC clone of feline herpesvirus-1 (FHV-1). *Virology.* 2010;401:215–227.
7. Lewin AC, Kolb AW, McLellan GJ, et al. Genomic, recombinational and phylogenetic characterization of global feline herpesvirus 1 isolates. *Virology.* 2018;518:385–397.
8. Veir JK, Ruch-Gallie R, Spindel ME, et al. Prevalence of selected infectious organisms and comparison of two anatomic sampling sites in shelter cats with upper respiratory tract disease. *J Feline Med Surg.* 2008;10:551–557.
9. Litster A, Wu CC, Leutenegger CM. Detection of feline upper respiratory tract disease pathogens using a commercially available real-time PCR test. *Vet J.* 2015;206:149–153.
10. Berger A, Willi B, Meli ML, et al. Feline calicivirus and other respiratory pathogens in cats with feline calicivirus-related symptoms and in clinically healthy cats in Switzerland. *BMC Vet Res.* 2015;11:282.
11. Fernandez M, Manzanilla EG, Lloret A, et al. Prevalence of feline herpesvirus-1, feline calicivirus, *Chlamydophila felis* and *Mycoplasma felis* DNA and associated risk factors in cats in Spain with upper respiratory tract disease, conjunctivitis and/or gingivostomatitis. *J Feline Med Surg.* 2017;19:461–469.
12. Ruch-Gallie RA, Veir JK, Hawley JR, et al. Results of molecular diagnostic assays targeting feline herpesvirus-1 and feline calicivirus in adult cats administered modified live vaccines. *J Feline Med Surg.* 2011;13:541–545.
13. Coutts AJ, Dawson S, Willoughby K, et al. Isolation of feline respiratory viruses from clinically healthy cats at UK cat shows. *Vet Rec.* 1994;135:555–556.
14. Shewen PE, Povey RC, Wilson MR. A survey of the conjunctival flora of clinically normal cats and cats with conjunctivitis. *Can Vet J.* 1980;21:231–233.
15. Wardley RC, Gaskell RM, Povey RC. Feline respiratory viruses: their prevalence in clinically healthy cats. *J Small Anim Pract.* 1974;15:579–586.
16. Bech-Nielsen S, Fulton RW, Cox HU, et al. Feline respiratory tract disease in Louisiana. *Am J Vet Res.* 1980;41:1293–1298.
17. Ellis TM. Feline respiratory virus carriers in clinically healthy cats. *Aust Vet J.* 1981;57:115–118.
18. Townsend WM, Jacobi S, Tai SH, et al. Ocular and neural distribution of feline herpesvirus-1 during active and latent experimental infection in cats. *BMC Vet Res.* 2013;9:185.
19. Gaskell R, Dawson S, Radford A, et al. Feline herpesvirus. *Vet Res.* 2007;38:337–354.
20. Lappin MR, Roycroft LM. Effect of ciclosporin and methylprednisolone acetate on cats previously infected with feline herpesvirus 1. *J Feline Med Surg.* 2015;17:353–358.
21. Gaskell RM, Povey RC. Re excretion of feline viral rhinotracheitis virus following corticosteroid treatment. *Vet Rec.* 1973;93:204–205.
22. Gaskell RM, Povey RC. Experimental induction of feline viral rhinotracheitis virus re-excretion in FVR-recovered cats. *Vet Rec.* 1977;100:128–133.
23. Gaskell RM, Povey RC. Transmission of feline viral rhinotracheitis. *Vet Rec.* 1982;111:359–362.
24. Gourkow N, Lawson JH, Hamon SC, et al. Descriptive epidemiology of upper respiratory disease and associated risk factors in cats in an animal shelter in coastal western Canada. *Can Vet J.* 2013;54:132–138.
25. Binns SH, Dawson S, Speakman AJ, et al. A study of feline upper respiratory tract disease with reference to prevalence and risk factors for infection with feline calicivirus and feline herpesvirus. *J Feline Med Surg.* 2000;2:123–133.
26. Sykes JE, Anderson GA, Studdert VP, et al. Prevalence of feline *Chlamydia psittaci* and feline herpesvirus 1 in cats with upper respiratory tract disease. *J Vet Intern Med.* 1999;13:153–162.
27. Nasisse MP, Guy JS, Davidson MG, et al. Experimental ocular herpesvirus infection in the cat. Sites of virus replication, clinical features and effects of corticosteroid administration. *Invest Ophthalmol Vis Sci.* 1989;30:1758–1768.
28. Raja P, Lee JS, Pan D, et al. A herpesviral lytic protein regulates the structure of latent viral chromatin. *mBio.* 2016;7.
29. Maes S, Van Goethem B, Saunders J, et al. Pneumomediastinum and subcutaneous emphysema in a cat associated with necrotizing bronchopneumonia caused by feline herpesvirus-1. *Can Vet J.* 2011;52:1119–1122.
30. Nasisse MP, English RV, Tompkins MB, et al. Immunologic, histologic, and virologic features of herpesvirus-induced stromal keratitis in cats. *Am J Vet Res.* 1995;56:51–55.
31. Nasisse MP, Guy JS, Stevens JB, et al. Clinical and laboratory findings in chronic conjunctivitis in cats: 91 cases (1983-1991). *J Am Vet Med Assoc.* 1993;203:834–837.
32. Lim CC, Cullen CL. Schirmer tear test values and tear film break-up times in cats with conjunctivitis. *Vet Ophthalmol.* 2005;8:305–310.
33. Lim CC, Reilly CM, Thomasy SM, et al. Effects of feline herpesvirus type 1 on tear film break-up time, Schirmer tear test results, and conjunctival goblet cell density in experimentally infected cats. *Am J Vet Res.* 2009;70:394–403.
34. Sebbag L, Pesavento PA, Carrasco SE, et al. Feline dry eye syndrome of presumed neurogenic origin: a case report. *JFMS Open Rep.* 2018;4. 2055116917746786.
35. Volopich S, Benetka V, Schwendenwein I, et al. Cytologic findings, and feline herpesvirus DNA and *Chlamydophila felis* antigen detection rates in normal cats and cats with conjunctival and corneal lesions. *Vet Ophthalmol.* 2005;8:25–32.
36. Nasisse MP, Glover TL, Moore CP, et al. Detection of feline herpesvirus 1 DNA in corneas of cats with eosinophilic keratitis or corneal sequestration. *Am J Vet Res.* 1998;59:856–858.
37. Kafarnik C, Fritsche J, Reese S. Corneal innervation in mesocephalic and brachycephalic dogs and cats: assessment using in vivo confocal microscopy. *Vet Ophthalmol.* 2008;11:363–367.
38. Dean E, Meunier V. Feline eosinophilic keratoconjunctivitis: a retrospective study of 45 cases (56 eyes). *J Feline Med Surg.* 2013;15:661–666.
39. Spiess AK, Sapienza JS, Mayordomo A. Treatment of proliferative feline eosinophilic keratitis with topical 1.5% cyclosporine: 35 cases. *Vet Ophthalmol.* 2009;12:132–137.
40. Powell CC, McInnis CL, Fontenelle JP, et al. *Bartonella* species, feline herpesvirus-1, and *Toxoplasma gondii* PCR assay results from blood and

aqueous humor samples from 104 cats with naturally occurring endogenous uveitis. *J Feline Med Surg.* 2010;12:923–928.
41. He J, Cosby R, Hill JM, et al. Changes in corneal innervation after HSV-1 latency established with different reactivation phenotypes. *Curr Eye Res.* 2017;42:181–186.
42. Sanchez MD, Goldschmidt MH, Mauldin EA. Herpesvirus dermatitis in two cats without facial lesions. *Vet Dermatol.* 2012;23:171–173. e135.
43. McGregor GF, Sheehan K, Simko E. Pneumonia and gastritis in a cat caused by feline herpesvirus-1. *Can Vet J.* 2016;57:147–150.
44. Hora AS, Tonietti PO, Guerra JM, et al. Felid herpesvirus 1 as a causative agent of severe nonsuppurative meningoencephalitis in a domestic cat. *J Clin Microbiol.* 2013;51:676–679.
45. Andrew SE. Ocular manifestations of feline herpesvirus. *J Feline Med Surg.* 2001;3:9–16.
46. Lee M, Bosward KL, Norris JM. Immunohistological evaluation of feline herpesvirus-1 infection in feline eosinophilic dermatoses or stomatitis. *J Feline Med Surg.* 2010;12:72–79.
47. Schulz C, Hartmann K, Mueller RS, et al. Sampling sites for detection of feline herpesvirus-1, feline calicivirus and *Chlamydia felis* in cats with feline upper respiratory tract disease. *J Feline Med Surg.* 2015;17:1012–1019.
48. Storey ES, Gerding PA, Scherba G, et al. Survival of equine herpesvirus-4, feline herpesvirus-1, and feline calicivirus in multidose ophthalmic solutions. *Vet Ophthalmol.* 2002;5:263–267.
49. Burgesser KM, Hotaling S, Schiebel A, et al. Comparison of PCR, virus isolation, and indirect fluorescent antibody staining in the detection of naturally occurring feline herpesvirus infections. *J Vet Diagn Invest.* 1999;11:122–126.
50. Goldschmidt P, Rostane H, Saint-Jean C, et al. Effects of topical anaesthetics and fluorescein on the real-time PCR used for the diagnosis of Herpesviruses and *Acanthamoeba* keratitis. *Br J Ophthalmol.* 2006;90:1354–1356.
51. Segarra S, Papasouliotis K, Helps C. The in vitro effects of proxymetacaine, fluorescein, and fusidic acid on real-time PCR assays used for the diagnosis of feline herpesvirus 1 and *Chlamydophila felis* infections. *Vet Ophthalmol.* 2011;14(suppl 1):5–8.
52. Wang J, Liu L, Wang J, et al. Recombinase polymerase amplification assay: a simple, fast and cost-effective alternative to real time PCR for specific detection of feline herpesvirus-1. *PLoS One.* 2017;12:e0166903.
53. Burns RE, Wagner DC, Leutenegger CM, et al. Histologic and molecular correlation in shelter cats with acute upper respiratory infection. *J Clin Microbiol.* 2011;49:2454–2460.
54. Zirofsky D, Rekers W, Powell C, et al. Feline herpesvirus 1 and *Mycoplasma* spp. conventional PCR assay results from conjunctival samples from cats in shelters with suspected acute ocular infections. *Top Companion Anim Med.* 2018;33:45–48.
55. Lamm CG, Dean SL, Estrada MM, et al. Pathology in practice. Herpesviral dermatitis. *J Am Vet Med Assoc.* 2015;247:159–161.
56. Lappin MR, Blondeau J, Boothe D, et al. Antimicrobial Use Guidelines for Treatment of Respiratory Tract Disease in Dogs and Cats: Antimicrobial Guidelines Working Group of the International Society for Companion Animal Infectious Diseases. *J Vet Intern Med.* 2017;31:279–294.
57. Owens JG, Nasisse MP, Tadepalli SM, et al. Pharmacokinetics of acyclovir in the cat. *J Vet Pharmacol Ther.* 1996;19:488–490.
58. Nasisse MP, Dorman DC, Jamison KC, et al. Effects of valacyclovir in cats infected with feline herpesvirus 1. *Am J Vet Res.* 1997;58:1141–1144.
59. Thomasy SM, Shull O, Outerbridge CA, et al. Oral administration of famciclovir for treatment of spontaneous ocular, respiratory, or dermatologic disease attributed to feline herpesvirus type 1: 59 cases (2006-2013). *J Am Vet Med Assoc.* 2016;249:526–538.
60. Thomasy SM, Lim CC, Reilly CM, et al. Evaluation of orally administered famciclovir in cats experimentally infected with feline herpesvirus type-1. *Am J Vet Res.* 2011;72:85–95.
61. Malik R, Lessels NS, Webb S, et al. Treatment of feline herpesvirus-1 associated disease in cats with famciclovir and related drugs. *J Feline Med Surg.* 2009;11:40–48.
62. Kopecny L, Maggs DJ, Leutenegger CM, et al. Effects of famciclovir in cats with spontaneous acute upper respiratory tract disease. *J Feline Med Surg.* 2019. 1098612X19857587.
63. Cooper AE, Thomasy SM, Drazenovich TL, et al. Prophylactic and therapeutic effects of twice-daily famciclovir administration on infectious upper respiratory disease in shelter-housed cats. *J Feline Med Surg.* 2019;21:544–552.
64. Sebbag L, Thomasy SM, Woodward AP, et al. Pharmacokinetic modeling of penciclovir and BRL42359 in the plasma and tears of healthy cats to optimize dosage recommendations for oral administration of famciclovir. *Am J Vet Res.* 2016;77:833–845.
65. Litster AL, Lohr BR, Bukowy RA, et al. Clinical and antiviral effect of a single oral dose of famciclovir administered to cats at intake to a shelter. *Vet J.* 2015;203:199–204.
66. Piret J, Boivin G. Resistance of herpes simplex viruses to nucleoside analogues: mechanisms, prevalence, and management. *Antimicrob Agents Chemother.* 2011;55:459–472.
67. Semenkow SL, Johnson NM, Maggs DJ, et al. Controlled release delivery of penciclovir via a silicone (MED-4750) polymer: kinetics of drug delivery and efficacy in preventing primary feline herpesvirus infection in culture. *Virol J.* 2014;11:34.
68. Pennington MR, Fort MW, Ledbetter EC, et al. A novel corneal explant model system to evaluate antiviral drugs against feline herpesvirus type 1 (FHV-1). *J Gen Virol.* 2016;97:1414–1425.
69. Spertus CB, Pennington MR, Van de Walle GR, et al. Effects of orally administered raltegravir in cats with experimentally induced ocular and respiratory feline herpesvirus-1 infection. *Am J Vet Res.* 2019;80:490–497.
70. Fontenelle JP, Powell CC, Veir JK, et al. Effect of topical ophthalmic application of cidofovir on experimentally induced primary ocular feline herpesvirus-1 infection in cats. *Am J Vet Res.* 2008;69:289–293.
71. Lewin AC, Liu C-C, Alling C, et al. *In vitro* efficacy of ganciclovir against feline herpesvirus-1 and assessment of ocular tolerability in healthy cats. *J Fel Med Surg.* 2021;23:400–404.
72. Thomasy SM, Maggs DJ. A review of antiviral drugs and other compounds with activity against feline herpesvirus type 1. *Vet Ophthalmol.* 2016;19(suppl 1):119–130.
73. Slack JM, Stiles J, Leutenegger CM, et al. Effects of topical ocular administration of high doses of human recombinant interferon alpha-2b and feline recombinant interferon omega on naturally occurring viral keratoconjunctivitis in cats. *Am J Vet Res.* 2013;74:281–289.
74. Cocker FM, Howard PE, Harbour DA. Effect of human alpha-hybrid interferon on the course of feline viral rhinotracheitis. *Vet Rec.* 1987;120:391–393.
75. Fenimore A, Carter K, Fankhauser J, et al. Evaluation of intranasal vaccine administration and high-dose interferon- alpha2b therapy for treatment of chronic upper respiratory tract infections in shelter cats. *J Feline Med Surg.* 2016;18:603–611.
76. Fiorito F, Cantiello A, Granato GE, et al. Clinical improvement in feline herpesvirus 1 infected cats by oral low dose of interleukin-12 plus interferon-gamma. *Comp Immunol Microbiol Infect Dis.* 2016;48:41–47.
77. Stiles J, Townsend WM, Rogers QR, et al. Effect of oral administration of L-lysine on conjunctivitis caused by feline herpesvirus in cats. *Am J Vet Res.* 2002;63:99–103.
78. Maggs DJ, Nasisse MP, Kass PH. Efficacy of oral supplementation with L-lysine in cats latently infected with feline herpesvirus. *Am J Vet Res.* 2003;64:37–42.
79. Rees TM, Lubinski JL. Oral supplementation with L-lysine did not prevent upper respiratory infection in a shelter population of cats. *J Feline Med Surg.* 2008;10:510–513.
80. Drazenovich TL, Fascetti AJ, Westermeyer HD, et al. Effects of dietary lysine supplementation on upper respiratory and ocular disease and detection of infectious organisms in cats within an animal shelter. *Am J Vet Res.* 2009;70:1391–1400.
81. Cave NJ, Dennis K, Gopakumar G, et al. Effects of physiologic concentrations of L-lysine on in vitro replication of feline herpesvirus 1. *Am J Vet Res.* 2014;75:572–580.
82. Bol S, Bunnik EM. Lysine supplementation is not effective for the prevention or treatment of feline herpesvirus 1 infection in cats: a systematic review. *BMC Vet Res.* 2015;11:284.
83. Jegou JP, Tromeur F. Superficial keratectomy for chronic corneal ulcers refractory to medical treatment in 36 cats. *Vet Ophthalmol.* 2015;18:335–340.

84. Laguna F, Leiva M, Costa D, et al. Corneal grafting for the treatment of feline corneal sequestrum: a retrospective study of 18 eyes (13 cats). *Vet Ophthalmol.* 2015;18:291–296.
85. Barachetti L, Giudice C, Mortellaro CM. Amniotic membrane transplantation for the treatment of feline corneal sequestrum: pilot study. *Vet Ophthalmol.* 2010;13:326–330.
86. Balland O, Poinsard AS, Famose F, et al. Use of a porcine urinary bladder acellular matrix for corneal reconstruction in dogs and cats. *Vet Ophthalmol.* 2016;19:454–463.
87. Summers SC, Ruch-Gallie R, Hawley JR, et al. Effect of modified live or inactivated feline herpesvirus-1 parenteral vaccines on clinical and laboratory findings following viral challenge. *J Feline Med Surg.* 2017;19:824–830.
88. Radford AD, Addie D, Belak S, et al. Feline calicivirus infection. ABCD guidelines on prevention and management. *J Feline Med Surg.* 2009;11:556–564.
89. Sussman MD, Maes RK, Kruger JM. Vaccination of cats for feline rhinotracheitis results in a quantitative reduction of virulent feline herpesvirus-1 latency load after challenge. *Virology.* 1997;228:379–382.
90. Sykes JE, Browning GF, Anderson G, et al. Differential sensitivity of culture and the polymerase chain reaction for detection of feline herpesvirus 1 in vaccinated and unvaccinated cats. *Arch Virol.* 1997;142:65–74.
91. Reagan KL, Hawley JR, Lappin MR. Concurrent administration of an intranasal vaccine containing feline herpesvirus-1 (FHV-1) with a parenteral vaccine containing FHV-1 is superior to parenteral vaccination alone in an acute FHV-1 challenge model. *Vet J.* 2014;201:202–206.
92. Whittemore JC, Hawley JR, Jensen WA, et al. Antibodies against Crandell Rees feline kidney (CRFK) cell line antigens, alpha-enolase, and annexin A2 in vaccinated and CRFK hyperinoculated cats. *J Vet Intern Med.* 2010;24:306–313.
93. Stone AE, Brummet GO, Carozza EM, et al. 2020 AAHA/AAFP feline vaccination guidelines. *J Feline Med Surg.* 2020;22:813–830.
94. Gore TC, Lakshmanan N, Williams JR, et al. Three-year duration of immunity in cats following vaccination against feline rhinotracheitis virus, feline calicivirus, and feline panleukopenia virus. *Vet Ther.* 2006;7:213–222.
95. Povey RC, Koonse H, Hays MB. Immunogenicity and safety of an inactivated vaccine for the prevention of rhinotracheitis, caliciviral disease, and panleukopenia in cats. *J Am Vet Med Assoc.* 1980;177:347–350.
96. Scott FW, Geissinger CM. Long-term immunity in cats vaccinated with an inactivated trivalent vaccine. *Am J Vet Res.* 1999;60:652–658.
97. Poulet H. Alternative early life vaccination programs for companion animals. *J Comp Pathol.* 2007;137(suppl 1):S67–S71.
98. Lappin MR, Veir JK, Satyaraj E, Czarnecki-Maulden G. Pilot study to evaluate the effect of oral supplementation of *Enterococcus faecium* SF68 on cats with latent feline herpesvirus 1. *J Feline Med Surg.* 2009;11(8):650–654.
99. Contreras ET, Hodgkins E, Tynes V, et al. Effect of a pheromone on stress-associated reactivation of feline herpesvirus-1 in experimentally inoculated kittens. *J Vet Intern Med.* 2018;32(1):406–417.
100. Ertl R, Korb M, Langbein-Detsch I, et al. Prevalence and risk factors of gammaherpesvirus infection in domestic cats in Central Europe. *Virol J.* 2015;12:146.
101. McLuckie A, Tasker S, Dhand NK, et al. High prevalence of *Felis catus* gammaherpesvirus 1 infection in haemoplasma-infected cats supports co-transmission. *Vet J.* 2016;214:117–121.
102. Caringella F, Desario C, Lorusso E, et al. Prevalence and risk factors for *Felis catus* gammaherpesvirus 1 detection in domestic cats in Italy. *Vet Microbiol.* 2019;238:108426.
103. Novacco M, Kohan NR, Stirn M, et al. Prevalence, geographic distribution, risk factors and co-infections of feline gammaherpesvirus infections in domestic cats in Switzerland. *Viruses.* 2019;11:721.
104. Kurissio JK, Rodrigues MV, Taniwaki SA, et al. *Felis catus* gammaherpesvirus 1 (FcaGHV1) and coinfections with feline viral pathogens in domestic cats in Brazil. *Ciência Rural.* 2018;48.
105. Stutzman-Rodriguez K, Rovnak J, VandeWoude S, et al. Domestic cats seropositive for *Felis catus* gammaherpesvirus 1 are often qPCR negative. *Virology.* 2016;498:23–30.
106. Tateno M, Takahashi M, Miyake E, et al. Molecular epidemiological study of gammaherpesvirus in domestic cats in Japan. *J Vet Med Sci.* 2017;79:1735–1740.
107. McLuckie A, Barrs VR, Lindsay S, et al. Molecular diagnosis of *Felis catus* gammaherpesvirus 1 (FcaGHV1) infection in cats of known retrovirus status with and without lymphoma. *Viruses.* 2018;10:128.
108. Makundi I, Koshida Y, Endo Y, et al. Identification of *Felis catus* gammaherpesvirus 1 in Tsushima leopard cats (*Prionailurus bengalensis euptilurus*) on Tsushima Island, Japan. *Viruses.* 2018;10:378.
109. Ackermann M. Pathogenesis of gammaherpesvirus infections. *Vet Microbiol.* 2006;113:211–222.
110. Shelton GH, Linenberger ML, Grant CK, et al. Hematologic manifestations of feline immunodeficiency virus infection. *Blood.* 1990;76:1104–1109.
111. Raphael BG, Knowles DM. Acquired immunodeficiency syndrome-associated non-Hodgkin's lymphoma. *Semin Oncol.* 1990;17:361–366.
112. Ehlers B, Dural G, Yasmum N, et al. Novel mammalian herpesviruses and lineages within the Gammaherpesvirinae: cospeciation and interspecies transfer. *J Virol.* 2008;82:3509–3516.
113. Lozano CC, Sweanor LL, Wilson-Henjum G, et al. Identification of novel gammaherpesviruses in ocelots (*Leopardus pardalis*) and bobcats (*Lynx rufus*) in Panama and Colorado, USA. *J Wildl Dis.* 2015;51:911–915.
114. Kruger JM, Venta PJ, Swenson CL, et al. Prevalence of bovine herpesvirus-4 infection in cats in Central Michigan. *J Vet Intern Med.* 2000;14:593–597.
115. Chiu E, Troyer RM, Lappin MR, et al. Bovine herpesvirus 4 DNA is not detected in free-ranging domestic cats from California, Colorado or Florida. *J Feline Med Surg.* 2017;19:235–239.

35

Feline Calicivirus Infections

Alan Radford, Maria Afonso, Jane E. Sykes

KEY POINTS

- First Described: 1957 (New Zealand, Fastier).[1]
- Causes: FCV, family *Caliciviridae,* genus *Vesivirus.*
- Affected Hosts: Domestic cat and many other Felidae. Similar viruses also isolated occasionally from dogs.
- Geographic Distribution: Worldwide.
- Primary Mode of Transmission: Oronasal, fomite spread.
- Major Clinical Signs: Oral ulceration, oculonasal discharges, lethargy. Less commonly lameness, lower respiratory tract infection, and signs of enteritis. Rare virulent forms may also cause edema, icterus, skin necrosis, and death.
- Differential Diagnosis: Differential diagnoses for FCV infection are other respiratory viral infections (FCV, influenza viruses), infections with bacteria such as *Bordetella bronchiseptica, Mycoplasma* spp., *Streptococcus* spp., or *Chlamydia felis;* other causes of rhinitis such as cryptococcosis, aspergillosis, neoplasia, foreign bodies, chronic idiopathic feline rhinosinusitis, nasopharyngeal stenosis, or nasopharyngeal polyps; feline chronic airway disease. For cats with oral ulcerations, exposure to caustic substances may be suspected.
- Human Health Significance: None known.

ETIOLOGY AND EPIDEMIOLOGY

FCV is a small, unenveloped, single-stranded RNA virus, a member of the *Vesivirus* genus of the *Calicivirus* family (Fig. 35.1 and Table 35.1). Both domestic cats and other members of the Felidae family can be infected.[2–5] Although dogs have their own genetically distinct calicivirus,[6,7] viruses antigenically and genetically related to FCV have also been detected in dogs with diarrhea (see Chapter 29),[8–10] and some epidemiologic evidence suggests a link between the two.[11] The role of FCV strains in canine disease and the significance of dogs as a reservoir of feline infection are not known. Other caliciviruses have been identified in cats, notably feline norovirus, but the role of this virus in disease is unknown.[12]

A large number of different strains of FCV exist, which vary slightly in antigenicity and pathogenicity, although they are all sufficiently cross-reactive to be classified as one serotype.[13] Although in general antigenicity is not associated with pathogenicity, some evidence suggests that FCV isolates collected from chronic stomatitis cases may show minor antigenic differences.[14,15] Genetically, FCV strains appear to represent one large diverse group, with little evidence of within-group clusters.[16–19] However, several studies have identified potential separate genotypes in Asia and Europe using longer genomic sequences which may provide for greater resolution.[20–24] Enteric strains appear to differ genetically from strains that cause respiratory disease, and appear more likely to resist trypsin, and bile treatment.[25,26] Considerable variability may be seen between individual isolates, particularly in immunogenic regions of the viral capsid gene.[22–28] This genetic diversity is useful epidemiologically in that it allows differentiation among FCV strains.[17,29–31]

Most strains of FCV are sufficiently related antigenically to induce some degree of cross-protective immunity, but cats can still be sequentially infected with different strains of virus and show varying degrees of clinical illness. Some isolates appear to be more immunogenic and cross-reactive than others. The most commonly used strains in vaccine products have been F9 and 255, but other strains have also been used, some in bivalent or trivalent FCV vaccines.[32–34] There is continued discussion over the degree of cross-protection afforded by such vaccines, particularly the original monovalent FCV vaccines. Some evidence indicates that they are still cross-reactive against the majority of field isolates, whereas other studies suggest that the percentage of isolates[17,35] neutralized by such vaccine strains may be decreasing, possibly as a result of immune selection pressures from widespread vaccine use.[17,36–38] Direct comparison between studies, however, can be difficult because results may vary according to factors such as the population tested (including perhaps whether sick or healthy cats are sampled), and the methodology used for testing. Nevertheless, structured, routine monitoring of vaccine efficacy against current field isolates would be useful.[17]

The ability to readily grow FCV in cell culture has led to its frequent use as a surrogate for calicivirus inactivation in disinfection studies, as well as more general studies of calicivirus structure and biology. FCV is moderately resistant in the external environment for days to several weeks on dried surfaces at room temperature, and longer in colder wetter conditions.[13] The virus is not as susceptible to the effects of disinfectants as other respiratory viruses such as FHV-1,[39] but useful disinfectants for both viruses are accelerated hydrogen peroxide or household bleach (5.25% sodium hypochlorite) diluted 1 part in 30 in water (1750 ppm) with added detergent.[40] The use of 5% sodium bicarbonate has also been shown to be effective and has been recommended by the ABCD.[41]

FCV infections are fairly widespread in the general cat population, with a generally higher prevalence in multicat households, shelters, and also in younger animals.[11,17,42–44] The virus is mainly shed in ocular, nasal, and oral secretions, and spread is largely by direct contact with an infected cat. Acutely infected animals are clearly one of the most important sources of virus, but infection also commonly occurs from clinically recovered carrier cats.[13] In some situations, particularly within a cattery, indirect transmission may occur. Contaminated secretions may be present on cages, on feeding and cleaning utensils, and on personnel. Some evidence suggests that feces from fleas fed on artificially FCV-infected blood may infect kittens oronasally,[45] but this is unlikely to be a significant source of infection. Aerosols are not thought to be of major importance for the spread of FCV; cats do not appear to be able to produce an infectious aerosol for this virus during normal respiration, although sneezed macrodroplets may transmit infection over a distance of 1 to 2 m (3 to 6 ft).

Despite vaccination, carriers are widespread in the population and are probably the main reason why FCV is so successful. An understanding of the FCV carrier state is important to help determine strategies for control. The carrier state is widespread in the cat population, with approximately 10% of household pets and 25% to 75% of shelter or colony cats testing positive for FCV shedding (Fig. 35.2).[17,43,46–48] As with other pathogens, FCV is likely to be common in situations of cat hoarding.[49] The virus persists in carriers in tonsillar and other oropharyngeal tissues. Although the precise mechanism of persistence is unclear, it is likely to include immune selection pressure driving antigenic variation in the viral capsid protein, which then allows the virus to evade the host immune response.[22,24,28] However other host, viral, and environmental factors also undoubtedly play a role.

In situations such as boarding and rescue facilities, many different FCV strains tend to be present, probably reflecting the relatively rapid turnover of carrier cats bringing in their own strains from different sources.[28,30] In contrast, in colonies of cats where FCV is endemic, in general only one or two distinct strains circulate.[28,30,50] Longitudinal studies of these endemically infected colonies have shown that although many cats appear to be long-term carriers, only a small minority (approximately 10%) are persistently infected, the remainder undergoing cycles of reinfection from within the colony.[50] Those with true persistent infection continuously evolve their own viral strain over time. Unlike FHV-1, there appears to be no latent phase for FCV carriers; FCV carriers shed virus more or less continuously.[51] The remainder of long-term carriers appear to undergo cycles of reinfection, either with a variant of the same strain, or in some cases, a different strain circulating within the colony. Interestingly, some cats within these endemic situations appeared to be resistant to infection, suggesting either age-related or genetically determined resistance.[51] These findings help explain: (1) the lower carriage rate of approximately 10% in household pets, where opportunity for reinfection is less likely to occur; and (2) the inability in some previous experimental studies to induce a carrier state in small groups of cats.

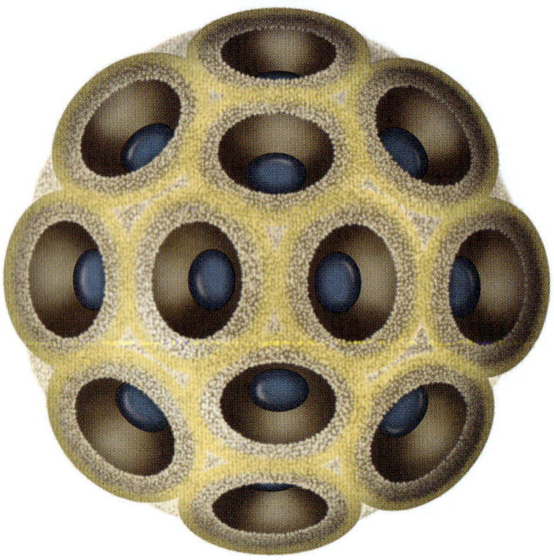

Fig. 35.1 Calicivirus structure.

CLINICAL FEATURES

Pathogenesis and Clinical Signs

The natural routes of infection for FCV are nasal, oral, and conjunctival. Viral replication mainly occurs in the oral and respiratory tissues, although some differences between strains can be found. Some strains have a predilection for the lung, and others have been found in synovial fluid macrophages.[52,53] Virus may also be found in visceral tissues, feces, and occasionally in the urine. Oral ulcers are the most prominent pathologic feature of FCV infection.[13] These ulcers begin as vesicles, which subsequently rupture, with necrosis of the overlying epithelium and infiltration of neutrophils at the periphery and the base. Healing takes place over 2 to 3 weeks.

Lower respiratory complications are dominated by multifocal desquamation of activated alveolar macrophages and less frequently occasional type II pneumocytes with fibrin exudation, consistent with diffuse alveolar damage. FCV has also been shown to infect and replicate in alveolar macrophages and, to a lesser extent, type II pneumocytes.[54] Although primary interstitial pneumonia can occur in FCV infection, particularly with more virulent strains, it has probably been overemphasized in the past as a result of experimental studies using aerosol challenge rather than the more natural oronasal routes. More recently it has been suggested that FHV-1 infection may facilitate secondary FCV infection of type II pneumocytes and alveolar macrophages.[54]

Lesions seen in FCV-infected joints consist of an acute synovitis with thickening of the synovial membrane and an increased amount of synovial fluid within the joint. In cases of FCV-associated virulent

TABLE 35.1 Clinically Relevant Caliciviruses

Virus	Host	Reservoirs	Geographic Distribution	Clinical Signs	Human Health Significance	Other
Rabbit hemorrhagic disease virus	Rabbit	May be transmitted by fleas, flies, and mosquitoes	Global	Often acute-onset fever, depression, and death	None	Used as a biological agent to control rabbit populations in Australia
Vesicular exanthema of swine virus	Pig	Sea mammals	West coast USA	Vesicular lesions similar to foot and mouth disease virus	None	Generally considered eradicated in pigs
Norovirus	Mainly human although some affect a range of species including mice, cattle, pigs, cats, and dogs	None known	Global	Human norovirus is generally considered the most common cause of acute gastroenteritis in people	Those noroviruses affecting non-human species are not considered zoonotic	FCV has been used to study calicivirus biology as, unlike most noroviruses, it grows readily in cell culture

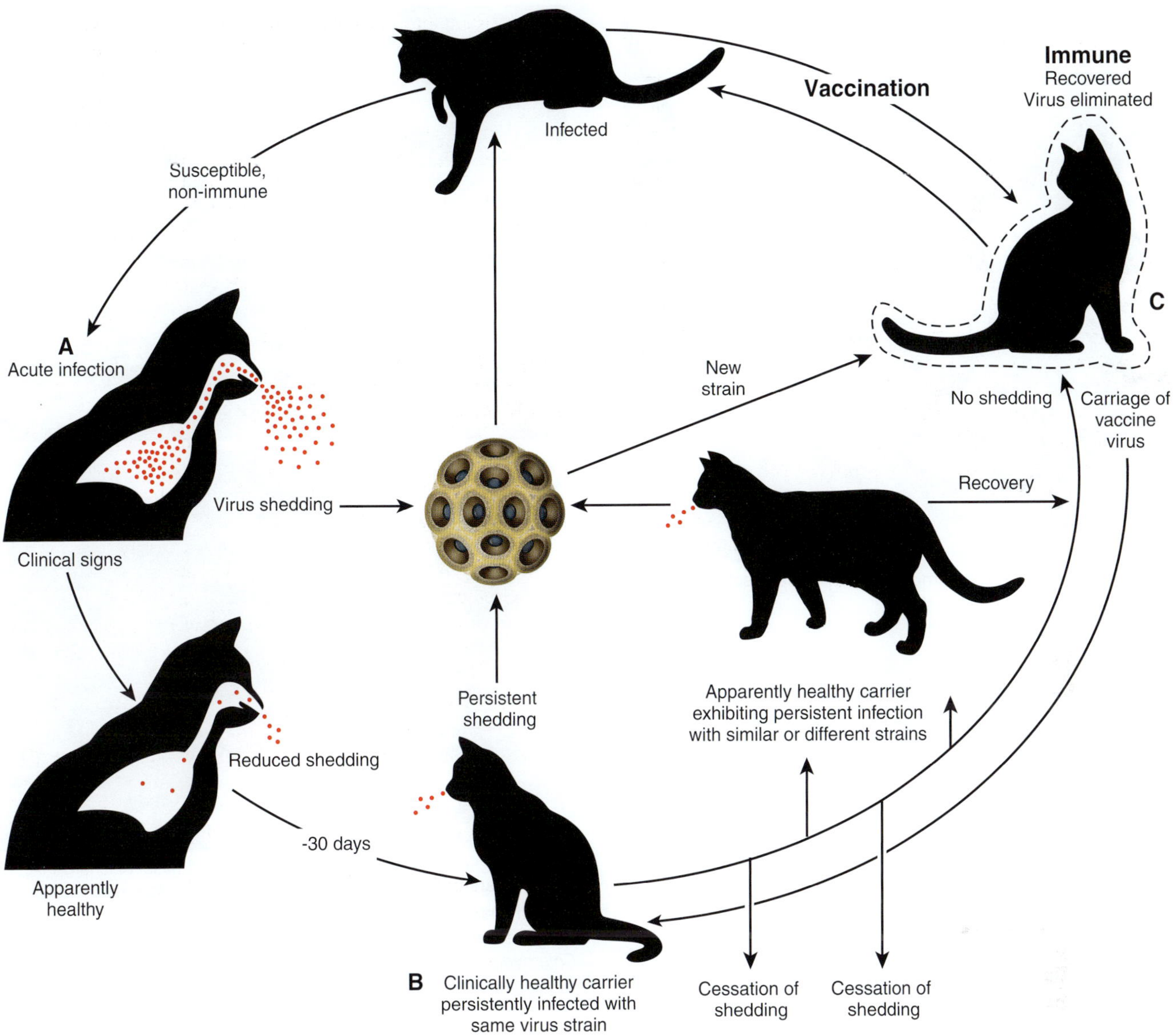

Fig. 35.2 Epidemiology of the FCV carrier state.

systemic disease (VSD), virus gains access to cellular compartments not normally associated with FCV infection.[55] Lesions are widespread and include subcutaneous edema, oral ulceration, and variable levels of cutaneous ulceration, particularly on the pinnae, paw pads, and nares.[51,56–58] Other lesions are more variable and include bronchointerstitial pneumonia and necrosis in the liver, spleen, and pancreas. Viral antigens have been detected in the skin, nasal mucosa, lung, pancreas, liver, and endothelial cells of the dermis associated with necrosis.[51,59]

Strains of FCV can differ in tropism and virulence. Therefore, a wide range of clinical signs may be seen. Most strains induce a fairly characteristic, mild syndrome characterized by pyrexia, oral ulceration, and mild respiratory and conjunctival signs. Signs of enteritis have been associated with some strains.[25,26] Some strains of FCV, however, are nonpathogenic; others are more virulent and may induce more severe systemic disease. Rarely, kittens may develop a fatal pneumonia.[54] Several outbreaks of a severe acute systemic febrile disease with high mortality have been described worldwide caused by particularly virulent strains of FCV (FCV-associated VSD [FCV-VSD]).[57,60,61]

In a typical case of FCV infection, early signs include lethargy and pyrexia. Oral ulceration is the most characteristic feature and may be the only clinical sign present, and it is possible that many cases go unreported (Fig. 35.3). Ulceration is usually on the tongue but can occur elsewhere in the mouth, on the lips, and on the nose. Skin ulceration on other parts of the body occurs rarely. Sneezing, conjunctivitis, and ocular and nasal discharges typically occur but are generally relatively mild.[62,63] Cats with oral ulcers may show hypersalivation. Some strains can cause pneumonia with associated dyspnea, and others have been associated with diarrhea.[25,26]

Other FCV isolates produce a febrile disease with lameness and pyrexia.[64] The lameness may or may not be associated with oral and respiratory signs, and it is likely that considerable overlap exists between the conditions. Affected cats are often dull and anorexic. In most cases, full recovery occurs within 24 to 48 hours. Acute lameness has also been observed after vaccination, and in some of these cases, viruses originating from live vaccines may be involved; this was particularly associated with one vaccine no longer licensed, and lameness following vaccination is now rare.[60]

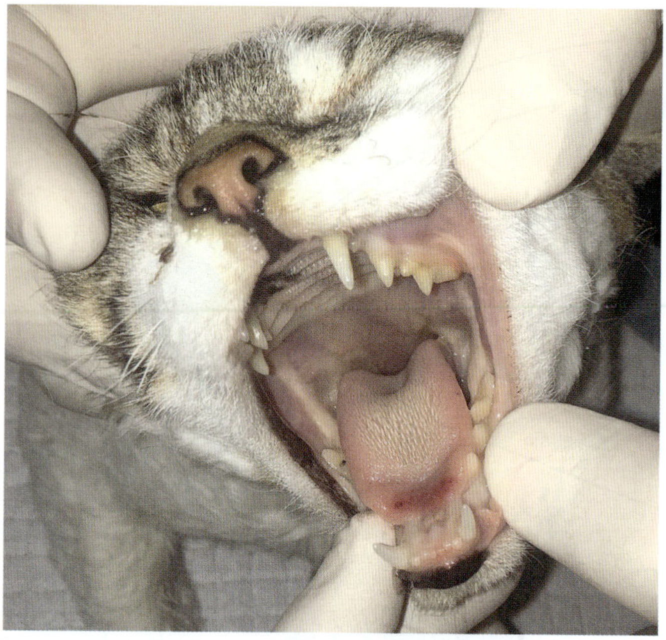

Fig. 35.3 Lingual ulceration and mucopurulent nasal discharge in a cat infected with FCV.

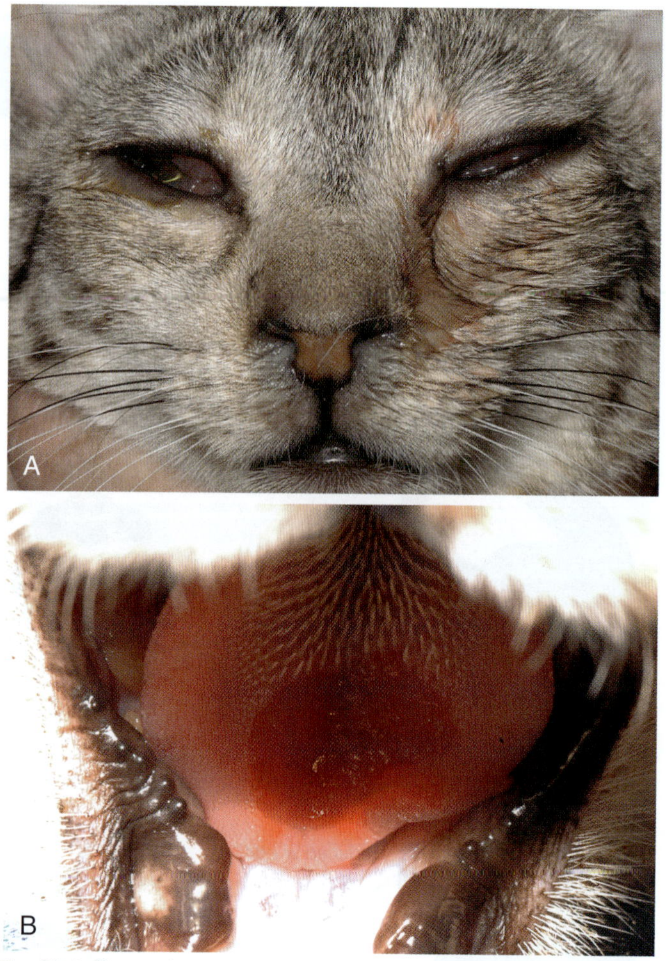

Fig. 35.4 Chemosis, mucopurulent ocular and nasal discharge (A); and lingual ulceration (B) in a 6-month-old intact male domestic medium-hair cat with chronic nasal discharge and conjunctivitis. A conjunctival swab specimen tested positive with PCR for FCV RNA and negative for FHV-1, *Chlamydia felis*, and *Mycoplasma* spp. (Courtesy of the University of California, Davis Veterinary Ophthalmology Service.)

Many of the described outbreaks of FCV-VSD are nosocomial infections, and each outbreak appears to have been caused by a different FCV strain.[55,57,58,65] Although highly contagious within a group of cats, all outbreaks have been contained, and the disease has not spread into the general population. Possible reasons for the appearance of such strains and for their subsequent disappearance are not understood but have been discussed elsewhere.[13,66] High mortality among affected cats and disease containment may be two important factors that limit spread of these outbreaks, though other factors may play a role.[66]

Cats with FCV-VSD variably show facial and paw edema, pyrexia, classic signs of oral ulceration and upper respiratory infection, icterus, epistaxis and hematochezia, and high mortality. Necropsy findings are again somewhat variable in individual cases but include pneumonia, hepatomegaly, pancreatitis, and pericarditis.[56,57,59,65,67,68] Many affected cats are fully vaccinated, suggesting that, as can occur with more typical strains of FCV, vaccines may not completely protect against these VSD-producing isolates. Although the outbreaks have been relatively well controlled with strict quarantine and isolation, given that FCV is an inherently variable pathogen, clinicians must remain vigilant for further outbreaks of this disease.

The chronic oral disease feline chronic gingivostomatitis complex has also been associated with FCV infection (see also Chapter 125).[69] The prevalence of this condition has been estimated at 0.7% of consultations in first opinion practice in the United Kingdom[70] and can be a particular problem because of the difficulty in treating this condition. In a number of studies, more than 80% of cats with chronic oral disease have been found to shed FCV compared with approximately 20% of controls,[66] but these figures may vary depending on the criteria used to select clinical cases and the diagnostic assays used.[71] Recent work has shown no correlation between FCV load and disease severity or outcome.[72] FCV infection has been associated with acute faucitis,[73] and in one colony of cats, chronic stomatitis developed after the accidental introduction of FCV.[74] However, other agents, in particular FIV, and various host factors are likely to be involved in the condition, and the pathogenesis is not yet fully understood.

Physical Examination Findings

Physical examination findings in cats with FCV infections vary from mild serous ocular discharge and conjunctivitis through to fever, severe mucopurulent ocular and nasal discharges, dehydration, stertorous respiration, tachypnea and/or respiratory difficulty, increased breath sounds on thoracic auscultation, hypersalivation, and ulceration of the nasal planum, tongue, and lips (Fig. 35.4). Because ulcerative lesions can occur at the base of the tongue near the larynx, examination of the entire tongue should be performed in cats that are febrile and inappetent, which may require sedation. Cats with VSD can have edema of the face and lips, icterus, cutaneous ulceration, evidence of petechial hemorrhages, and abdominal pain. Cats with feline chronic gingivostomatitis complex frequently test FCV positive. These animals may have ulceroproliferative caudal stomatitis or buccal/alveolar mucositis and exhibit pain on examination of the oral cavity (Fig. 35.5).

DIAGNOSIS

A range of pathogens other than FCV are associated with upper respiratory tract disease in the cat, notably FHV-1, but also *Bordetella bronchiseptica* and to a lesser extent *Chlamydia felis* (primarily ocular). Generally, FCV remains the most commonly detected pathogen in

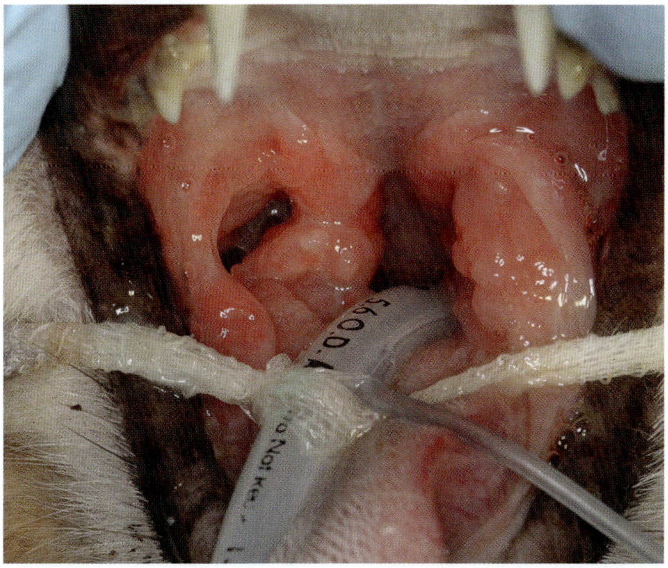

Fig. 35.5 Severe lymphoplasmacytic caudal stomatitis in a cat infected with FCV.

diseased cats, either alone or less frequently in mixed infections.[75] While clinical signs can be suggestive of one pathogen over another, they are rarely pathognomonic. Specific diagnostic testing for FCV is not always necessary, particularly in individual cases of relatively mild upper respiratory tract disease. However, identifying a causative agent may be helpful when disease is severe, warranting specific therapy, where multiple cats are involved, and where disease occurs in vaccinated cats.

Laboratory Abnormalities

There are no specific CBC, biochemistry profile, or urinalysis abnormalities that aid in a diagnosis of FCV infection. The CBC may be normal or show a mild to moderate neutrophilia, sometimes with band neutrophils or neutrophil toxicity, and lymphopenia in severely affected cats with secondary bacterial pneumonia. Hematological abnormalities in cats with VSD have included mild to severe anemia, thrombocytopenia, neutrophilia, and lymphopenia. Serum biochemistry findings in cats with viral respiratory disease are usually unremarkable unless disease is severe or chronic. Cats with VSD may have hypoalbuminemia, hyperbilirubinemia, mildly increased serum activities of ALT and AST, and mild to moderately increased serum CK activities. Serum CK activities up to 11,000 U/L can occur.[56] Cats with chronic stomatitis may have hyperglobulinemia due to a polyclonal gammopathy.

Tracheobronchial lavage specimens from cats with pneumonia may show a suppurative or mixed exudate, sometimes with evidence of sepsis. Aerobic bacterial culture with mycoplasma culture if possible is indicated on wash specimens, and antimicrobial susceptibilities should be obtained for any aerobic bacteria isolated. Organisms such as *Pasteurella* spp., *Staphylococcus pseudintermedius*, *Streptococcus* spp., *Escherichia coli*, *Klebsiella pneumoniae*, and some *Mycoplasma* spp. infect the airways as opportunists and are not considered to be primary pathogens. Bacterial culture of nasal swabs is generally not recommended because it often leads to growth of normal flora, which has no clinical relevance.

Diagnostic Imaging

In uncomplicated infections, plain thoracic radiographs may be unremarkable or show a mild diffuse interstitial to bronchointerstitial pattern. Alveolar patterns or lung lobe consolidation may occur with secondary bacterial pneumonia.

TABLE 35.2 Essential Features of Clinical Respiratory Disease Related to the Pathogen Involved

Feature	FHV-1	FCV[a]	Bb	ChF
Lethargy	+++	+	+	+
Sneezing	+++	+	++	+
Conjunctivitis	++	+	–	+++[b]
Hypersalivation	++	–[c]	–	–
Ocular discharge	+++	+	(+)	+++
Nasal discharge	+++	+	++	+
Oral ulceration	(+)	+++	–	–
Keratitis	+	–	–	–
Cough	(+)	–	++	–
Pneumonia	(+)	(+)	+	+/–
Lameness	–	+	–	–

[a]Strain variation exists. For FCV-associated VSD signs, see text.
[b]Often persistent.
[c]Evidence of ptyalism may be present in cats with lingual ulcerations.
+++, marked; ++, moderate; +, mild; (+), less common; +/–, subclinical; –, absent.
Bb, Bordetella bronchiseptica; ChF, Chlamydia felis.
Adapted from Monne Rodriguez JM, Soare T, Malbon A, et al. Alveolar macrophages are the main target cells in feline calicivirus-associated pneumonia. *Vet J.* 2014;201:156-165. Used with permission.

Microbiologic Tests

A presumptive diagnosis may be attempted based on clinical signs alone. For example, predominantly oral ulceration might indicate FCV infection, whereas marked sneezing with more severe respiratory and conjunctival signs might suggest infection by FHV-1 (Table 35.2). With *Chlamydia* infection, the main clinical sign is marked persistent conjunctivitis (see Chapter 49).

Confirmatory diagnosis of FCV is typically made by collection of oropharyngeal swabs for testing, and is generally sufficient (Table 35.3). However, addition of conjunctival or other specimens may modestly increase sensitivity of respiratory pathogen diagnosis.[76] Traditionally, viral isolation in feline cell cultures has been used to detect FCV.[77] Several RT-PCR assays have now been described, using various approaches including targeting different regions of the genome[78–80] and such molecular testing for FCV is now being widely used commercially. PCR and sequencing, particularly of the hypervariable region of the capsid gene, are useful for distinguishing between FCV isolates and have been extensively used to better understand the epidemiology of the disease.[17,66] Serology is generally not helpful in the diagnosis of FCV infection because of the high prevalence of seroreactivity from vaccination.

When an organism is detected in an animal with respiratory disease, it is reasonable to assume that the agent is involved in the disease process. However, especially for FCV and *Bordetella*, a relatively large number of clinically healthy cats will also be shedding the organisms. Therefore interpretation of a positive result may be problematic unless taken in conjunction with other factors, such as the characteristic clinical signs. Similarly for FHV-1, latently infected cats may also shed reactivated virus, and thus a positive result may also be unrelated to the observed clinical signs. In an epidemiologic context, however, a positive result indicates the cat has been infected with FHV-1 and thus has the potential to infect other cats. For FHV-1, quantitative PCR can

TABLE 35.3 Diagnostic Assays Available for FCV in Cats

Assay	Specimen Type	Target	Performance
Virus isolation	Oropharyngeal swabs, transtracheal and bronchoalveolar wash specimens, airway and lung specimens collected at necropsy	Whole virus (viable)	False negatives can occur in specimens that contain no or low numbers of virus particles. May take several days to weeks and requires specialized techniques and expertise
RT-PCR	See above	Conserved regions of the FCV genome	Sensitivity and specificity may vary depending on assay design. Sensitivity may be low because of brief shedding for some viruses or low-level shedding in chronic infections. Assays may not detect all virus strains. Testing specimens from multiple different anatomic sites, or combining PCR with other diagnostic tests can increase sensitivity. Attenuated live vaccine virus may be detected after vaccination. Because of subclinical shedding, the significance of a positive result may be difficult to interpret. False-negative results may occur as a result of degradation of viral nucleic acid during specimen transport. Results rapid (1–2 days)
Serology	Serum	Antibodies against FCV capsid antigens	Interpretation complicated by previous vaccination and exposure. May be useful in outbreak situations that involve a novel strain of FCV. May be useful to quantify immune responses and experimentally for estimates of cross-protection
Histopathology	Tissue specimens	Immunostaining for viral capsid antigens	Antigen load can be low even in positive samples. Strain variation again means false negatives may occur depending on the precise antibody used in the test. Particularly useful as an adjunct to the diagnosis of VSD.

VSD, virulent systemic disease.

provide additional information with respect to viral load and stage of infection, especially if consecutive samples are taken. In countries where intranasal vaccines are available, a positive result may be indicative of FHV-1 or FCV vaccine virus rather than wild-type viruses. FCV can be also detected in fecal specimens, although the significance of this is unknown.[2,81]

Pathologic Findings

Gross lesions in cats with FCV infections include cutaneous and lingual ulcerations, submandibular or retropharyngeal lymph node enlargement, mucosal hyperemia, and mucopurulent exudate within the nasal cavity and trachea. The oral ulcers most typical of FCV infection begin as vesicles, which subsequently rupture, with necrosis of the overlying epithelium and infiltration of neutrophils at the periphery and the base. Healing takes place over 2 to 3 weeks. Rarer lower respiratory complications are dominated by multifocal desquamation of activated alveolar macrophages and occasional type II pneumocytes with fibrin exudation, consistent with diffuse alveolar damage; FCV has been shown to infect and replicate in these cell types. Lesions seen in FCV-infected joints consist of an acute synovitis with thickening of the synovial membrane and an increased amount of synovial fluid within the joint; viral antigen in synovial macrophages suggests these cells may be permissive as seen in the lung.

Necropsy findings in cats with VSD have been variable. Gross lesions are widespread and include subcutaneous edema, ulceration of the mouth, and variable levels of ulceration of the skin particularly on the pinnae, pawpads, and nares. Frequently reported findings include individual hepatocellular necrosis and dissociation with minimal inflammation, acute interstitial pneumonia, and free pleural and abdominal fluid.[56,57,65,67] Acute necrotizing vasculitis of subcutaneous and oral submucosal vessels has been reported.[82] Intestinal crypt necrosis and pancreatitis have been reported in experimentally infected cats. Viral antigens have been detected in the skin, nasal mucosa, lung, pancreas, liver, and endothelial cells of the dermis associated with necrosis.

TREATMENT AND PROGNOSIS

Good nursing care is essential in cases of feline respiratory disease, and in milder cases is generally best given at home by the owner. Many cats will not eat because of an impaired sense of smell or oral ulceration, and thus they should be encouraged to eat by offering highly palatable, aromatic foods. Warm, freshly prepared food may have more appealing flavor and odor. Appetite stimulants may be effective in some cats. If eating is painful, baby foods or specialized proprietary or blended food may be helpful. Cats with severe illness may require hospitalization and fluid therapy, and when anorexia is prolonged, placement of a feeding tube may be indicated. Nasal discharges should be wiped away with saline. Mucolytic drugs (e.g., bromhexine hydrochloride) have been suggested to help clear airways in the more chronic phase, but conventional steam inhalation (e.g., placing the cat in a steamy room) or nebulizing saline also may be useful. Administration of pain medications and chlorhexidine mouthwashes may improve appetite for cats with painful oral ulcerations.

In most cases of viral respiratory disease, antibacterial treatment may not be required. Current guidelines suggest that antibacterials are only indicated when clinical signs persist for over 10 days and/or when the cat is systemically unwell; in such cases, doxycycline or amoxicillin/clavulanate are preferred.[83] Because swallowing solid tablets may be painful for cats, antibiotics may need to be given as syrups or long-acting injections, or through a feeding tube.

No specific antiviral drugs are available for treatment of FCV infections. Ribavirin is active in cell culture but was too toxic for *in vivo* use.[84,85] FCV strains show varying susceptibility to IFN *in vitro*.[86] Some authors advocate the use of IFN to treat feline chronic gingivostomatitis complex.[13,87] A synthetic antisense nucleotide sequence, phosphorodiaminate morpholino oligomer, which specifically binds to FCV, was trialed in kittens during natural outbreaks of FCV-VSD. The results suggested an increased survival in treated cats compared to untreated animals.[88] However, this was a small-scale study and such therapies are not commercially available.

IMMUNITY AND VACCINATION

For FCV, immunity has generally been measured by serum virus-neutralizing (VN) antibody levels. Systemic antibodies measured by VN have always been considered the hallmark of immunity for FCV and are certainly important in protection, as studies using mouse-cat chimeric antibodies have also shown.[89,90] However, some cats with no detectable FCV-VN antibody have demonstrated immunity to re-challenge with a heterologous strain, and several types of cell-mediated immune responses have been reported.[91] In a 2021 study, attenuated live vaccination of research cats induced cellular but not humoral cross-protective immune responses, highlighting the importance of non-humoral mechanisms of immunity against FCV.[92] For both FCV and FHV-1, local immune responses are also likely to be important. Nevertheless, for both viruses, a reasonable correlation has been shown with serologic (VN and ELISA) tests to predict resistance or susceptibility to disease after challenge.[32,93] The ultimate test of immunity is, of course, response to challenge.

With FCV infection, homologous VN antibody titers are generally higher than those in FHV-1 and are better correlated to protection,[32] and immunity is also longer lived. However, some variation exists, depending on the viral strain involved and whether homologous or heterologous protection is being considered. Reinfection with a second strain will generally boost responses to both strains. After vaccination against FCV, reasonable protection has been reported to last for at least 3 years, and moderate levels of antibody for at least 4 years.[93–96] However, this will likely depend on vaccine and challenge strain combinations evaluated.

For FCV, in most kittens, MDAs persist for 10 to 14 weeks.[13] However, there is considerable variation for both viruses. In one study, 20% to 26% of kittens had no detectable antibodies at 6 weeks of age.[97] In contrast, in some animals, levels of MDA that interfere with vaccination may persist until 12 to 14 weeks of age.[97–99] Low levels of MDA do not necessarily protect against subclinical infection.

Vaccines for FCV have been available for many years and vaccination has been relatively successful in controlling disease. However, disease can still be a problem, especially when cats are kept grouped together and when kittens lose their MDA before vaccination. FCV is very widespread in the cat population and carriers are common, ensuring plenty of exposure for naïve cats. Prevention and control, therefore, often require a combined approach of vaccination and management.

Three types of FCV vaccines are commercially available: attenuated live virus vaccines administered parenterally or IN, and inactivated virus vaccines given parenterally. The latter are generally adjuvanted, but products are available in some parts of the world where the inactivated FCV component is without adjuvant.

In previously unexposed cats, all vaccines induce reasonable protection against disease. There is increasing evidence that vaccinated animals shed less virus following subsequent challenge.[47,95] However, vaccination does not completely protect against infection or the development of the carrier state, and as a result, vaccinated animals can still act as an important reservoir of FCV infection in the population.

Several FCV strains are used in commercial vaccines, including strains F9 and 255. In addition, bivalent (G1/431) and trivalent vaccines have been developed and in some cases marketed, containing additional strains of FCV including those associated with VSD.[32,34,95,100,101] Most of these strains seem to protect against the majority of FCV isolates.[17,102] A 2021 study showed reduction in viral RNA loads, duration of RNAemia, and severity of clinical signs in cats vaccinated with a single attenuated live FCV strain (F9) and challenged at 46 and 99 weeks with heterologous strains.[103] However, for all vaccines, the antigenic diversity of FCV means that strains will probably vary in the degree of protection offered by different vaccines. Multivalent vaccines may increase the proportion of strains against which the vaccines are effective when compared to the individual antigens that they contain,[32,34,100,101,104,105] but more studies are needed to validate this.

FCV vaccines are only licensed to control acute upper respiratory tract disease. There is no evidence that vaccines affect the onset, development, or course of chronic stomatitis. For VSD, many outbreaks have been reported in vaccinated animals. Evidence for protection against VSD is perhaps conflicting. It is clear that several outbreaks have been reported in vaccinated animals. However, experimental challenge studies for some FCV vaccines have shown protection against individual VSD strains.[32,100] Taken together, it is likely that other potentially virulent strains exist in the field but remain undetected because they happen to be sufficiently neutralized by vaccination. However, all VSD outbreaks have so far been caused by distinct strains, and there is no evidence to suggest the virulent viruses have a unique antigenic profile, distinct from more typical strains.[55,66] Therefore it is likely that no vaccine will protect against all VSD strains. The priority for vaccine efficacy should be to demonstrate broad general cross reactivity against a wide range of strains of varying pathogenicity that remains stable over time.

Parenteral attenuated live vaccines should be administered carefully because clinical signs can be induced if the vaccine virus reaches the oral-respiratory mucosa (i.e., if the cat licks the injection site or if an aerosol is made with the syringe). Vaccine virus should not become systemic; however, replication of FCV vaccine virus after parenteral inoculation may sometimes occur, with the potential for disease in the vaccinated cat and spread to other cats.[13,106] However, genetic typing of FCV isolates from vaccine reactions has shown that the majority are associated with coincidental field virus infection, with vaccine-like viruses only being isolated rarely from either vaccine reactions or the general cat population.[28,29,50,60,107]

Intranasal vaccines induce strong protection, but mild to moderate adverse effects may develop, such as sneezing and oculonasal discharges. Intranasal vaccines, however, are useful for rapid (2 to 4 days) onset of protection.[108–110] Intranasal vaccines used in conjunction with parenteral vaccine on entry have reduced the severity of upper respiratory disease in cats introduced or maintained at contaminated shelters for 3 or more days.[111]

Inactivated adjuvanted FCV vaccines are also effective, and modern adjuvants have led to improvements in immunogenicity. Concerns about an association between adjuvanted vaccines and injection site sarcomas have led to marketing of a nonadjuvanted vaccine containing inactivated FCV antigens in some parts of the world, although the FHV-1 and feline panleukopenia fractions remain attenuated. Vaccination with an inactivated vaccine during pregnancy can help protect kittens by prolonging the duration of MDA. However, product information supplied by the manufacturer should be consulted to determine whether this is approved.

There is a general agreement that FCV vaccination is a core requirement for all cats, such that all cats should benefit from vaccine protection. However, the timing of such vaccines are complicated as local and national guideline groups—including the AAFP, the ABCD, and the WSAVA—seek to balance the desire to reduce injections (and hence sarcoma risk) with the need to ensure high levels of protection in the face of uncertain MDA levels and duration of immunity. In most cases, product data sheets advocate a primary kitten course with parenteral vaccines at approximately 9 and 12 weeks of age. A third vaccination may be considered 3 to 4 weeks later when MDA levels are believed to be high enough to interfere with the first two vaccines.[97–99,112] For example, a third kitten vaccine may be rationally introduced in populations of cats where MDA levels are unknown but where disease has occurred previously in young cats before the first booster (at 6 months or 1 year of age). Similarly, annual booster vaccines would be reserved for those adult cats perceived to be exposed to high-risk situations (e.g., boarding catteries and rescue shelters), with triennial vaccination being sufficient for cats at low risk (e.g., indoor cats; those living in areas of low cat densities where cat populations are generally stable). Such a tailored approach clearly requires an individual risk-benefit assessment to determine the most appropriate vaccination strategy for a particular cat. The different approaches to vaccination are reflected in practice where it seems a variable approach to vaccination is taken. The reader is referred to Chapter 20 for more information on immunization and the appendix for vaccination interval recommendations.

PREVENTION

Household Cats

After the first booster, pets should be vaccinated regularly against FCV and FHV-1 (1 to 3 years), the frequency depending on the individual cat's perceived risk, and also the specific vaccine being used and its duration of immunity claim. In general, however, for cats at low risk (e.g., indoor cats; those living in areas of low cat densities where cat populations are generally stable), triennial vaccination is likely to be sufficient, whereas cats exposed to high-risk situations (e.g., boarding catteries and rescue shelters) should be vaccinated annually. Ideally, to minimize the possibility of infectious disease, a friend or neighbor should feed the cat while the owner is on vacation, rather than boarding the cat in a cattery. Individual cats should be protected from stress and high-risk social contact as much as possible to avoid exposure.

Boarding Catteries

All cats entering a cattery should have an up-to-date vaccination record for FHV-1 and FCV.[46] In boarding catteries, where animals may be stressed and exposure to carriers is likely, annual boosters may be advisable. When rapid protection is required, the intranasal vaccine may be advisable. Clients should be aware that such vaccines themselves may induce mild clinical signs.

Cattery owners should not rely on vaccination alone for disease control because pathogens will inevitably be present either from the occasional cat incubating disease or from carriers. Thus, measures should be taken to prevent spread of infection and reduce the concentration of infectious agents in the environment (Box 35.1).

Shelter Facilities

In general, the same management measures apply as those with boarding catteries. Although this practice may be more difficult to achieve, molecular typing studies have demonstrated that limiting the spread of individual FCV isolates within a shelter is possible if good hygiene measures are used.[30,50] Because the immune status of cats in a rescue shelter is often unknown, incoming animals should ideally be quarantined from existing residents. Unless animals can be isolated on arrival for 3 to 4 weeks, parenteral vaccines may not have time to become effective.[95] Those with clinical signs should also be isolated. In these circumstances, use of intranasal vaccines may be advisable if available. Stress plays an important role in predisposing to infection and disease for a range of feline pathogens, and it is good practice to reduce stress levels where possible.[113] The reader is referred to Chapter 16 for more information on prevention of infectious diseases in shelter environments.

Breeding Catteries

If any cattery has contact, whether direct or indirect, with other cats, it is safest to assume that most will have some level of FCV infection unless proven otherwise by repeat diagnostic testing. In closed colonies trying to stay virus free, use of inactivated vaccines is preferable. Care should be taken to avoid bringing virus into the colony; any cat with a history of, or contact with, oral or respiratory disease may be a carrier. Vaccinated cats can also be carriers, and kittens can be infected subclinically because of MDA. This, in part, explains the risk of infection from cat shows, where many cats are FCV positive. However, the greatest risk of infection to disease-free households is likely to be from stud cats and new breeding stock when exposure is prolonged; introduction of such animals should ideally be from respiratory disease-free colonies.

Cats entering a disease-free colony should be quarantined for 3 weeks to identify animals incubating the disease. Cats should be tested for virus shedding at least twice a week during this time. This practice increases the probability of detecting FHV-1 (as virus may reactivate after a change of housing) and some FCV carriers that may be shedding only low levels of virus. Even so, the risk still exists of importing a latent FHV-1 carrier or a low-level FCV carrier that may be a source of infection. For most situations, the only reasonable course is to attempt disease control (Box 35.2).

PUBLIC HEALTH ASPECTS

Feline calicivirus is generally considered species-specific and poses no known human health risk. However, FCV has been used as a surrogate virus for the study of human norovirus because of shared biochemical and genomic properties between the two viruses. It was also used to develop a mask decontamination method to assess the ability to reuse N95 masks in the COVID-19 pandemic.[114]

BOX 35.1 Recommendations to Prevent the Spread of the FCV and Other Respiratory Viruses in Boarding Catteries

Admit only fully vaccinated cats, preferably revaccinated within a year before admission.

House cats individually with solid partitions between pens, unless cats are from same household.

Ensure that cage fronts are at least 1 m apart.

Put known carriers or cats with history of respiratory disease in a separate section, or at least at one end of the cattery, and clean, feed, and provide water to them last.

Ensure that surfaces of pen can be easily disinfected and that food and litter bowls can be easily removed without entering the pen (i.e., do not handle cats more than necessary).

Feed cats in same order each day and attend to each pen completely before moving on to the next.

Either disinfect hands between each pen or have individual rubber gloves for each pen, for use only with that pen.

Disinfect gloves thoroughly before use with a new boarder. Alternatively, use disposable gloves.

Wear rubber boots and step into a disinfectant bath if it is necessary to enter a pen.

Either use disposable food trays or have two sets of food bowls used on alternate days. Soak used set in a 1:30 household bleach (5.25% sodium hypochlorite) solution with detergent for several hours and then rinse and allow to dry until reuse 24 hours later.

Prepare food in a central area.

Use similar system to food bowls for litter trays.

When a cat goes home, thoroughly disinfect cage, allow to dry, and preferably leave empty for 2 days before reusing.

Reduce concentration of virus in the environment by providing adequate ventilation, low relative humidity, and optimal environmental temperatures.

Adapted from Monne Rodriguez JM, Soare T, Malbon A, et al. Alveolar macrophages are the main target cells in feline calicivirus-associated pneumonia. *Vet J.* 2014;201:156-165. Used with permission.

BOX 35.2 Feline Respiratory Disease Control Program in a Breeding Cattery with Endemic Disease

Provide regular vaccination.

Give booster vaccinations to queens either before mating or during pregnancy (inactivated vaccine only, if licensed for this use).

Keep cats as stress-free as possible, and use good management practices to reduce spread of viruses within the colony.

Avoid breeding queens with a history of oral or respiratory disease in their kittens.

Move queens into isolation at least 3 weeks before term so that the kittens are not exposed to carriers in the colony and that any shedding episode from the queen, as a result of the move, will end before parturition.

Wean kittens into isolation away from the queen as soon as feasible (ideally at 4 to 5 weeks before MDAs wane).

Vaccinate all kittens as soon as MDAs are at a noninterfering level (normally 9 or more weeks), and keep them in strict isolation until a week after the second dose (normally at 12 weeks, but in some cases after a third vaccination 3 to 4 weeks later).

Earlier FHV-1 and FCV vaccination schedules with intranasal (if available) or parenteral vaccines may be used, although these are not always licensed for early use and should be used with care. Parenteral vaccines can be given from 6 weeks of age, at 3-week intervals until 12 weeks, and if indicated, up to 15 to 16 weeks of age. Intranasal vaccination should be carried out 7 to 10 days or so before disease has been occurring and then again at 12 weeks. Some evidence indicates that multiple doses are not necessary, although they were originally advocated.

CASE EXAMPLE 1

Signalment

"Sam," a 1-year-old male neutered domestic shorthair cat from Orangevale, CA.

History

Sam's owner, a veterinary technician, reported a 4-day history of illness that began with ptyalism and progressed to inappetence and difficulty prehending both canned and dry food. The owner also noted that Sam's mouth had a foul odor. There had been no diarrhea, vomiting, coughing, or sneezing. He was an indoor-outdoor cat and was obtained as a kitten, with no previous health problems. There was one other 2-year-old cat in the household that was apparently healthy. Sam was up to date on vaccinations, which included vaccines for FCV, FHV-1, FPV, FeLV, and rabies.

Current Medications

None.

Physical Examination

Body weight: 5.6 kg

General: Quiet, alert, responsive, hydrated. Ambulatory on all four limbs. Temperature = 102.9°F (39.4°C), heart rate = 180 beats/min, respiratory rate = 48 breaths/min, mucous membranes pink, CRT = 1 s.

Integument: A normal haircoat was present and there was no evidence of ectoparasites.

Eyes, ears, nose, and throat: No significant abnormalities of the eyes, nose, or ears were noted. There was moderate ptyalism, and examination of the oral cavity revealed multiple ulcerations along the right lip and a 1-cm ulcer on the rostral aspect of the tongue.

Musculoskeletal: A body condition score of 6/9 was noted. No visible lameness or musculoskeletal abnormalities were noted.

Cardiovascular: Strong femoral pulses were noted. No murmurs or arrhythmias were detected on thoracic auscultation.

Respiratory, gastrointestinal, and genitourinary: No abnormalities detected.

Lymph nodes: There was mild enlargement of the right mandibular lymph node.

Laboratory Findings

Sam was anesthetized and a swab specimen was collected from the oropharynx. The specimen tested strongly positive for FCV using real-time PCR.

Diagnosis

FCV infection.

Treatment

While under anesthesia, an esophagostomy tube for administration of food and water was placed without complication. In addition, Sam was prescribed buprenorphine (1.5 mg PO q12h) for pain and oral sucralfate suspension in an attempt to coat the lingual ulcerations (1 mL PO q8h, at least 1 hour before buprenorphine). The feeding tube was removed 2 weeks later.

Comments

This case was interesting because of the sole finding of lingual ulcerations, without any other evidence of respiratory disease, which was so dramatic that a caustic cause of oral ulceration was suspected by the clinician on the case. The positive PCR test result does not prove that the cause of the oral ulcerations was FCV, because of the carrier state, but the strong positive test result in association with typical clinical signs in a young cat owned by a veterinary technician was strongly suggestive. The cat may have acquired infection from contact with other outdoor cats, or it is possible that the owner introduced the virus on her clothing or other fomites because she was unwittingly in contact with a carrier cat at her workplace. Although she was instructed to do her best to separate this cat from her other cat and disinfect her household with disinfectants that have activity against FCV, it is likely that her other cat had already been exposed. Fortunately, no clinical signs appeared in this cat. This case also illustrates the occurrence of disease in the face of proper vaccination, possibly because of lack of strain cross-protection.

CASE EXAMPLE 2

You provide veterinary care to a breeding colony of some five queens. On the 15th February, four 12-week-old kittens received their second attenuated live core FVRCP vaccine. One week later (22nd February), the four kittens developed lingual ulcers and fever.

The owners were extremely disappointed as they were not aware of previous infections in their colony. Because of the history of recent vaccination, the similarity of the signs to FCV infection, and the fact that an attenuated live vaccine was used, you submit plain oropharyngeal swabs in virus transport medium for diagnostic testing. Four days later, the results confirm that three of the kittens are infected with FCV. Oropharyngeal swabs were also submitted for *Bordetella bronchiseptica* isolation but were negative.

As a result of the positive tests for FCV, you discuss this case with the vaccine manufacturer as a potential adverse event. It is agreed that one of the kitten FCV isolates be typed and compared to the sequence of the virus in the vaccine. This sequence strongly suggested that the FCV infection in the breeding household did not originate from the vaccine, rather that the cats were infected with a distinct field strain of virus.

Several questions should be considered in regard to why the kittens were infected with FCV field viruses so soon after vaccination.

1. *Is FCV causing the disease?* It is possible the disease in the kittens was not caused by FCV. The prevalence of FCV carriers is high and therefore the FCV infection of these cats may have been incidental. However, the clinical signs were quite suggestive of FCV infection, so it seems reasonable to assume that the virus caused the disease.
2. *Why did these kittens develop clinical disease if they have already received vaccines?* The incubation period for FCV is generally approximately 2 to 7 days, although it may be longer in some cases. Therefore it seems likely that the kittens were infected approximately between the 15th and 20th February, 0 to 5 days after their second vaccination on the 13th February. At this stage, the kittens were not completely protected by the anamnestic response of vaccination. Therefore this case cannot be considered a failure of the vaccine to protect. This only becomes a concern when fully vaccinated animals develop clinical disease.
3. *Where did the virus isolated from the kittens come from?* The most likely origin of this field virus is other cats within the breeding household. The prevalence of FCV in households can be very high (up to 90%), unless there is strict isolation of the cats in the colony. Infection can remain clinically silent in fully vaccinated adult cats in such households. Clinical disease may only occur when kittens become infected in the immunity gap between the decline of MDA and onset of vaccine immunity. It can be useful to determine the extent of FCV (and FHV-1) infection in such colonies by testing some of the other cats, especially if clinical disease in kittens is a regular occurrence. Owners are sometimes surprised to learn that their adult cats have FCV (or FHV-1) infection when they have no clinical disease and have been regularly vaccinated. This is because FCV (and FHV-1) vaccines do not protect against the establishment of the carrier state.

From Pedersen NC, Elliott JB, Glasgow A, Poland A, Keel K. An isolated epizootic of hemorrhagic-like fever in cats caused by a novel and highly virulent strain of feline calicivirus. *Vet Microbiol* [Internet]. 2000 May 11;73:281-300.

SUGGESTED READINGS

Radford AD, Addie D, Belák S, et al. Feline calicivirus infection: ABCD Guidelines on Prevention and Management. *J Feline Med Surg*. 2009 Jul;11(7):556–564. Last updated November 2020. Available at: http://www.abcdcatsvets.org/feline-calicivirus-infection-2012-edition/.

Bordicchia M, Fumian TM, Van Brussel K, et al. Feline calicivirus virulent systemic disease: clinical epidemiology, analysis of viral isolates and in vitro efficacy of novel antivirals in Australian outbreaks. *Viruses*. 2021;13:2040.

REFERENCES

1. Fastier LB. A new feline virus isolated in tissue culture. *Am J Vet Res*. 1957;18:382–389.
2. Tian J, Liu D, Liu Y, et al. Molecular characterization of a feline calicivirus isolated from tiger and its pathogenesis in cats. *Vet Microbiol*. 2016;192:110–117.
3. Kadoi K, Kiryu M, Iwabuchi M, et al. A strain of calicivirus isolated from lions with vesicular lesions on tongue and snout. *New Microbiol*. 1997;20:141–148.
4. Driciru M, Siefert L, Prager KC, et al. A serosurvey of viral infections in lions (*Panthera leo*), from Queen Elizabeth National Park, Uganda. *J Wildl Dis*. 2006;42:667–671.
5. Harrison TM, Sikarskie J, Kruger J, et al. Systemic calicivirus epidemic in captive exotic felids. *J Zoo Wildl Med*. 2007;38:292–299.
6. Matsuura Y, Tohya Y, Nakamura K, et al. Complete nucleotide sequence, genome organization and phylogenic analysis of the canine calicivirus. *Virus Gene*. 2002;25:67–73.
7. Roerink F, Hashimoto M, Tohya Y, et al. Genetic analysis of a canine calicivirus: evidence for a new clade of animal caliciviruses. *Vet Microbiol*. 1999;69:69–72.
8. Di Martino B, Di Rocco C, Ceci C, et al. Characterization of a strain of feline calicivirus isolated from a dog faecal sample. *Vet Microbiol*. 2009;139:52–57.
9. Hashimoto M, Roerink F, Tohya Y, et al. Genetic analysis of the RNA polymerase gene of caliciviruses from dogs and cats. *J Vet Med Sci*. 1999;61:603–608.
10. Martella V, Pratelli A, Gentile M, et al. Analysis of the capsid protein gene of a feline-like calicivirus isolated from a dog. *Vet Microbiol*. 2002;85:315–322.
11. Binns SH, Dawson S, Speakman AJ, et al. A study of feline upper respiratory tract disease with reference to prevalence and risk factors for infection with feline calicivirus and feline herpesvirus. *J Feline Med Surg*. 2000;2:123–133.
12. Pinto P, Wang Q, Chen N, et al. Discovery and genomic characterization of noroviruses from a gastroenteritis outbreak in domestic cats in the US. *PLoS One*. 2012;7:e32739.
13. Radford AD, Addie D, Belak S, et al. Feline calicivirus infection. ABCD guidelines on prevention and management. *J Feline Med Surg*. 2009;11:556–564 Last updated November 2020. Available at: http://www.abcdcatsvets.org/feline-calicivirus-infection-2012-edition/.
14. Dawson S, McArdle F, Bennett M, et al. Typing of feline calicivirus isolates from different clinical groups by virus neutralisation tests. *Vet Rec*. 1993;133:13–17.
15. Poulet H, Brunet S, Soulier M, et al. Comparison between acute oral/respiratory and chronic stomatitis/gingivitis isolates of feline calicivirus: pathogenicity, antigenic profile and cross-neutralisation studies. *Arch Virol*. 2000;145:243–261.
16. Geissler K, Schneider K, Platzer G, et al. Genetic and antigenic heterogeneity among feline calicivirus isolates from distinct disease manifestations. *Virus Res*. 1997;48:193–206.
17. Afonso MM, Pinchbeck GL, Smith SL, et al. A multi-national European cross-sectional study of feline calicivirus epidemiology, diversity and vaccine cross-reactivity. *Vaccine*. 2017;35:2753–2760.
18. Coyne KP, Christley RM, Pybus OG, et al. Large-scale spatial and temporal genetic diversity of feline calicivirus. *J Virol*. 2012;86:11356–11367.
19. Hou J, Sanchez-Vizcaino F, McGahie D, et al. European molecular epidemiology and strain diversity of feline calicivirus. *Vet Rec*. 2016;178:114–115.
20. Sato Y, Ohe K, Murakami M, et al. Phylogenetic analysis of field isolates of feline calcivirus (FCV) in Japan by sequencing part of its capsid gene. *Vet Res Commun*. 2002;26:205–219.
21. Spiri AM, Theze J, Meli ML, et al. Genetic diversity and phenotypic associations of feline caliciviruses from cats in Switzerland. *J Gen Virol*. 2016;97:3253–3266.

22. Kreutz LC, Johnson RP, Seal BS. Phenotypic and genotypic variation of feline calicivirus during persistent infection of cats. *Vet Microbiol.* 1998;59:229–236.
23. Baulch-Brown C, Love D, Meanger J. Sequence variation within the capsid protein of Australian isolates of feline calicivirus. *Vet Microbiol.* 1999;68:107–117.
24. Radford AD, Bennett M, McArdle F, et al. Quasispecies evolution of a hypervariable region of the feline calicivirus capsid gene in cell culture and persistently infected cats. *Vet Microbiol.* 1999;69:67–68.
25. Di Martino B, Lanave G, Di Profio F, et al. Identification of feline calicivirus in cats with enteritis. *Transbound Emerg Dis.* 2020;67:2579–2588.
26. Guo J, Ding Y, Sun F, et al. Co-circulation and evolution of genogroups I and II of respiratory and enteric feline calicivirus isolates in cats. *Transbound Emerg Dis.* 2022; Jan 4. Online ahead of print.
27. Horimoto T, Takeda Y, Iwatsuki-Horimoto K, et al. Capsid protein gene variation among feline calicivirus isolates. *Virus Gene.* 2001;23:171–174.
28. Coyne KP, Gaskell RM, Dawson S, et al. Evolutionary mechanisms of persistence and diversification of a calicivirus within endemically infected natural host populations. *J Virol.* 2007;81:1961–1971.
29. Radford AD, Bennett M, McArdle F, et al. The use of sequence analysis of a feline calicivirus (FCV) hypervariable region in the epidemiological investigation of FCV related disease and vaccine failures. *Vaccine.* 1997;15:1451–1458.
30. Radford AD, Sommerville LM, Dawson S, et al. Molecular analysis of isolates of feline calicivirus from a population of cats in a rescue shelter. *Vet Rec.* 2001;149:477–481.
31. Sykes JE, Studdert VP, Browning GF. Detection and strain differentiation of feline calicivirus in conjunctival swabs by RT-PCR of the hypervariable region of the capsid protein gene. *Arch Virol.* 1998;143:1321–1334.
32. Poulet H, Jas D, Lemeter C, et al. Efficacy of a bivalent inactivated non-adjuvanted feline calicivirus vaccine: relation between in vitro cross-neutralization and heterologous protection in vivo. *Vaccine.* 2008;26:3647–3654.
33. Huang C, Hess J, Gill M, et al. A dual-strain feline calicivirus vaccine stimulates broader cross-neutralization antibodies than a single-strain vaccine and lessens clinical signs in vaccinated cats when challenged with a homologous feline calicivirus strain associated with virulent systemic disease. *J Feline Med Surg.* 2010;12:129–137.
34. Masubuchi K, Wakatsuki A, Iwamoto K, et al. Immunological and genetic characterization of feline caliciviruses used in the development of a new trivalent inactivated vaccine in Japan. *J Vet Med Sci.* 2010;72:1189–1194.
35. Smith SL, Afonso MM, Pinchbeck GL, et al. Temporally separated feline calicivirus isolates do not cluster phylogenetically and are similarly neutralised by high-titre vaccine strain FCV-F9 antisera in vitro. *J Feline Med Surg.* 2020;22:602–607.
36. Lauritzen A, Jarrett O, Sabara M. Serological analysis of feline calicivirus isolates from the United States and United Kingdom. *Vet Microbiol.* 1997;56:55–63.
37. Addie D, Poulet H, Golder MC, et al. Ability of antibodies to two new caliciviral vaccine strains to neutralise feline calicivirus isolates from the UK. *Vet Rec.* 2008;163:355–357.
38. Mochizuki M, Kawakami K, Hashimoto M, et al. Recent epidemiological status of feline upper respiratory infections in Japan. *J Vet Med Sci.* 2000;62:801–803.
39. Eleraky NZ, Potgieter LN, Kennedy MA. Virucidal efficacy of four new disinfectants. *J Am Anim Hosp Assoc.* 2002;38:231–234.
40. Addie DD, Boucraut-Baralon C, Egberink H, et al. Disinfectant choices in veterinary practices, shelters and households: ABCD guidelines on safe and effective disinfection for feline environments. *J Feline Med Surg.* 2015;17:594–605.
41. Spiri AM, Meil ML, Riond B, et al. Environmental contamination and hygienic measures after feline calicivirus field strain infections of cats in a research facility. *Viruses.* 2019;11:958.
42. Bannasch MJ, Foley JE. Epidemiologic evaluation of multiple respiratory pathogens in cats in animal shelters. *J Feline Med Surg.* 2005;7:109–119.
43. Helps CR, Lait P, Damhuis A, et al. Factors associated with upper respiratory tract disease caused by feline herpesvirus, feline calicivirus, *Chlamydophila felis* and *Bordetella bronchiseptica* in cats: experience from 218 European catteries. *Vet Rec.* 2005;156:669–673.
44. Pedersen NC, Sato R, Foley JE, et al. Common virus infections in cats, before and after being placed in shelters, with emphasis on feline enteric coronavirus. *J Feline Med Surg.* 2004;6:83–88.
45. Mencke N, Vobis M, Mehlhorn H, et al. Transmission of feline calicivirus via the cat flea (*Ctenocephalides felis*). *Parasitol Res.* 2009;105:185–189.
46. McManus CM, Levy JK, Andersen LA, et al. Prevalence of upper respiratory pathogens in four management models for unowned cats in the Southeast United States. *Vet J.* 2014;201:196–201.
47. Porter CJ, Radford AD, Gaskell RM, et al. Comparison of the ability of feline calicivirus (FCV) vaccines to neutralise a panel of current UK FCV isolates. *J Feline Med Surg.* 2008;10:32–40.
48. Zicola A, Saegerman C, Quatpers D, et al. Feline herpesvirus 1 and feline calicivirus infections in a heterogeneous cat population of a rescue shelter. *J Feline Med Surg.* 2009;11:1023–1027.
49. Polak KC, Levy JK, Crawford PC, et al. Infectious diseases in large-scale cat hoarding investigations. *Vet J.* 2014;201:189–195.
50. Coyne KP, Edwards D, Radford AD, et al. Longitudinal molecular epidemiological analysis of feline calicivirus infection in an animal shelter: a model for investigating calicivirus transmission within high-density, high-turnover populations. *J Clin Microbiol.* 2007;45:3239–3244.
51. Coyne KP, Dawson S, Radford AD, et al. Long-term analysis of feline calicivirus prevalence and viral shedding patterns in naturally infected colonies of domestic cats. *Vet Microbiol.* 2006;118:12–25.
52. Dawson S, Bennett D, Carter SD, et al. Acute arthritis of cats associated with feline calicivirus infection. *Res Vet Sci.* 1994;56:133–143.
53. Truyen U, Geissler K, Hirschberger J. Tissue distribution of virus replication in cats experimentally infected with distinct feline calicivirus isolates. *Berl Munch Tierarztl Wochenschr.* 1999;112:355–358.
54. Monne Rodriguez JM, Soare T, Malbon A, et al. Alveolar macrophages are the main target cells in feline calicivirus-associated pneumonia. *Vet J.* 2014;201:156–165.
55. Pesavento PA, Chang KO, Parker JS. Molecular virology of feline calicivirus. *Vet Clin North Am Small Anim Pract.* 2008;38:775–786 (vii).
56. Hurley KE, Pesavento PA, Pedersen NC, et al. An outbreak of virulent systemic feline calicivirus disease. *J Am Vet Med Assoc.* 2004;224:241–249.
57. Pedersen NC, Elliott JB, Glasgow A, et al. An isolated epizootic of hemorrhagic-like fever in cats caused by a novel and highly virulent strain of feline calicivirus. *Vet Microbiol.* 2000;73:281–300.
58. Deschamps JY, Topie E, Roux F. Nosocomial feline calicivirus-associated virulent systemic disease in a veterinary emergency and critical care unit in France. *JFMS Open Rep.* 2015;1:2055116915621581.
59. Pesavento PA, MacLachlan NJ, Dillard-Telm L, et al. Pathologic, immunohistochemical, and electron microscopic findings in naturally occurring virulent systemic feline calicivirus infection in cats. *Vet Pathol.* 2004;41:257–263.
60. Radford AD, Dawson S, Wharmby C, et al. Comparison of serological and sequence-based methods for typing feline calcivirus isolates from vaccine failures. *Vet Rec.* 2000;146:117–123.
61. Bordicchia M, Fumian TM, Van Brussel K, et al. Feline calicivirus virulent systemic disease: clinical epidemiology, analysis of viral isolates and in vitro efficacy of novel antivirals in Australian outbreaks. *Viruses.* 2021;13:2040.
62. Gerriets W, Joy N, Huebner-Guthardt J, et al. Feline calicivirus: a neglected cause of feline ocular surface infections? *Vet Ophthalmol.* 2012;15:172–179.
63. Stiles J. Ocular manifestations of feline viral diseases. *Vet J.* 2014;201:166–173.
64. TerWee J, Lauritzen AY, Sabara M, et al. Comparison of the primary signs induced by experimental exposure to either a pneumotrophic or a 'limping' strain of feline calicivirus. *Vet Microbiol.* 1997;56:33–45.
65. Reynolds BS, Poulet H, Pingret JL, et al. A nosocomial outbreak of feline calicivirus associated virulent systemic disease in France. *J Feline Med Surg.* 2009;11:633–644.
66. Radford AD, Coyne KP, Dawson S, et al. Feline calicivirus. *Vet Res.* 2007;38:319–335.
67. Coyne KP, Jones BR, Kipar A, et al. Lethal outbreak of disease associated with feline calicivirus infection in cats. *Vet Rec.* 2006;158:544–550.
68. Schorr-Evans EM, Poland A, Johnson WE, et al. An epizootic of highly virulent feline calicivirus disease in a hospital setting in New England. *J Feline Med Surg.* 2003;5:217–226.

69. Fried WA, Soltero-Rivera M, Ramesh A, et al. Use of unbiased metagenomic and transcriptomic analyses to investigate the association between feline calicivirus and feline chronic gingivostomatitis in domestic cats. *Am J Vet Res*. 2021;82:381–394.
70. Healey KA, Dawson S, Burrow R, et al. Prevalence of feline chronic gingivo-stomatitis in first opinion veterinary practice. *J Feline Med Surg*. 2007;9:373–381.
71. Tenorio AP, Franti CE, Madewell BR, et al. Chronic oral infections of cats and their relationship to persistent oral carriage of feline calici-, immunodeficiency, or leukemia viruses. *Vet Immunol Immunopathol*. 1991;29:1–14.
72. Druet I, Hennet P. Relationship between feline calicivirus load, oral lesions, and outcome in feline chronic gingivostomatitis (caudal stomatitis): retrospective study in 104 cats. *Front Vet Sci*. 2017;4:209.
73. Reubel GH, Hoffmann DE, Pedersen NC. Acute and chronic faucitis of domestic cats. A feline calicivirus-induced disease. *Vet Clin North Am Small Anim Pract*. 1992;22:1347–1360.
74. Waters L, Hopper CD, Gruffydd-Jones TJ, et al. Chronic gingivitis in a colony of cats infected with feline immunodeficiency virus and feline calicivirus. *Vet Rec*. 1993;132:340–342.
75. Nguyen D, Barrs VR, Kelman M, et al. Feline upper respiratory tract infection and disease in Australia. *J Feline Med Surg*. 2019;21:973–978.
76. Schulz C, Hartmann K, Mueller RS, et al. Sampling sites for detection of feline herpesvirus-1, feline calicivirus and *Chlamydia felis* in cats with feline upper respiratory tract disease. *J Feline Med Surg*. 2015;17:1012–1019.
77. Guo H, Miao Q, Zhu J, et al. Isolation and molecular characterization of a virulent systemic feline calicivirus isolated in China. *Infect Genet Evol*. 2018;65:425–429.
78. Meli ML, Berger A, Willi B, et al. Molecular detection of feline calicivirus in clinical samples: a study comparing its detection by RT-qPCR directly from swabs and after virus isolation. *J Virol Methods*. 2018;251:54–60.
79. Litster A, Wu CC, Leutenegger CM. Detection of feline upper respiratory tract disease pathogens using a commercially available real-time PCR test. *Vet J*. 2015;206:149–153.
80. Wilhelm B, Leblanc D, Leger D, et al. Farm-level prevalence and risk factors for detection of hepatitis E virus, porcine enteric calicivirus, and rotavirus in Canadian finisher pigs. *Can J Vet Res*. 2016;80:95–105.
81. Zhang W, Li L, Deng X, et al. Faecal virome of cats in an animal shelter. *J Gen Virol*. 2014;95:2553–2564.
82. Meyer A, Kershaw O, Klopfleisch R. Feline calicivirus-associated virulent systemic disease: not necessarily a local epizootic problem. *Vet Rec*. 2011;168:589.
83. Lappin MR, Blondeau J, Boothe D, et al. Antimicrobial use guidelines for treatment of respiratory tract disease in dogs and cats: antimicrobial guidelines working group of the International Society for Companion Animal Infectious Diseases. *J Vet Intern Med*. 2017;31:279–294.
84. Povey RC. Effect of orally administered ribavirin on experimental feline calicivirus infection in cats. *Am J Vet Res*. 1978;39:1337–1341.
85. Povey RC. In vitro antiviral efficacy of ribavirin against feline calicivirus, feline viral rhinotracheitis virus, and canine parainfluenza virus. *Am J Vet Res*. 1978;39:175–178.
86. Ohe K, Takahashi T, Hara D, et al. Sensitivity of FCV to recombinant feline interferon (rFeIFN). *Vet Res Commun*. 2008;32:167–174.
87. Matsumoto H, Teshima T, Iizuka Y, et al. Evaluation of the efficacy of the subcutaneous low recombinant feline interferon-omega administration protocol for feline chronic gingivitis-stomatitis in feline calicivirus-positive cats. *Res Vet Sci*. 2018;121:53–58.
88. Smith AW, Iversen PL, O'Hanley PD, et al. Virus-specific antiviral treatment for controlling severe and fatal outbreaks of feline calicivirus infection. *Am J Vet Res*. 2008;69:23–32.
89. Umehashi M, Imamura T, Akiyama S, et al. Post-exposure treatment of cats with mouse-cat chimeric antibodies against feline herpesvirus type 1 and feline calicivirus. *J Vet Med Sci*. 2002;64:1017–1021.
90. Umehashi M, Imamura T, Akiyama S, et al. Pre-exposure treatment of cats with anti-FHV-1 and anti-FCV mouse-cat chimeric antibodies. *J Vet Med Sci*. 2003;65:563–566.
91. Knowles JO, McArdle F, Dawson S, et al. Studies on the role of feline calicivirus in chronic stomatitis in cats. *Vet Microbiol*. 1991;27:205–219.
92. Spiri AM, Novacco M, Meli ML, et al. Modified-live feline calicivirus vaccination elicits cellular immunity against a current feline calicivirus field strain in an experimental challenge study. *Viruses*. 2021;13:1736.
93. Lappin MR, Andrews J, Simpson D, et al. Use of serologic tests to predict resistance to feline herpesvirus 1, feline calicivirus, and feline parvovirus infection in cats. *J Am Vet Med Assoc*. 2002;220:38–42.
94. Gore TC, Lakshmanan N, Williams JR, et al. Three-year duration of immunity in cats following vaccination against feline rhinotracheitis virus, feline calicivirus, and feline panleukopenia virus. *Vet Ther*. 2006;7:213–222.
95. Jas D, Aeberle C, Lacombe V, et al. Onset of immunity in kittens after vaccination with a non-adjuvanted vaccine against feline panleucopenia, feline calicivirus and feline herpesvirus. *Vet J*. 2009;182:86–93.
96. Scott FW, Geissinger CM. Long-term immunity in cats vaccinated with an inactivated trivalent vaccine. *Am J Vet Res*. 1999;60:652–658.
97. Dawson S, Willoughby K, Gaskell RM, et al. A field trial to assess the effect of vaccination against feline herpesvirus, feline calicivirus and feline panleucopenia virus in 6-week-old kittens. *J Feline Med Surg*. 2001;3:17–22.
98. Poulet H. Alternative early life vaccination programs for companion animals. *J Comp Pathol*. 2007;137(suppl 1):S67–S71.
99. Reese MJ, Patterson EV, Tucker SJ, et al. Effects of anesthesia and surgery on serologic responses to vaccination in kittens. *J Am Vet Med Assoc*. 2008;233:116–121.
100. Huang L, Krieg AM, Eller N, et al. Induction and regulation of Th1-inducing cytokines by bacterial DNA, lipopolysaccharide, and heat-inactivated bacteria. *Infect Immun*. 1999;67:6257–6263.
101. Poulet H, Brunet S, Leroy V, et al. Immunisation with a combination of two complementary feline calicivirus strains induces a broad cross-protection against heterologous challenges. *Vet Microbiol*. 2005;106:17–31.
102. Almeras T, Schreiber P, Fournel S, et al. Comparative efficacy of the Leucofeligen FeLV/RCP and Purevax RCP FeLV vaccines against infection with circulating feline calicivirus. *BMC Vet Res*. 2017;13:300.
103. Spiri AM, Riond B, Stirn M, et al. Modified live feline calicivirus vaccination reduces viral RNA loads, duration of RNAemia, and the severity of clinical signs after heterologous feline calicivirus challenge. *Viruses*. 2021;13:1505.
104. Hohdatsu T, Sato K, Tajima T, et al. Neutralizing feature of commercially available feline calicivirus (FCV) vaccine immune sera against FCV field isolates. *J Vet Med Sci*. 1999;61:299–301.
105. Wensman JJ, Samman A, Lindhe A, et al. Ability of vaccine strain induced antibodies to neutralize field isolates of caliciviruses from Swedish cats. *Acta Vet Scand*. 2015;57:86.
106. Pedersen NC, Hawkins KF. Mechanisms for persistence of acute and chronic feline calicivirus infections in the face of vaccination. *Vet Microbiol*. 1995;47:141–156.
107. Radford AD, Sommerville L, Ryvar R, et al. Endemic infection of a cat colony with a feline calicivirus closely related to an isolate used in live attenuated vaccines. *Vaccine*. 2001;19:4358–4362.
108. Gaskell R, Dawson S, Radford A, et al. Feline herpesvirus. *Vet Res*. 2007;38:337–354.
109. Lappin MR, Sebring RW, Porter M, et al. Effects of a single dose of an intranasal feline herpesvirus 1, calicivirus, and panleukopenia vaccine on clinical signs and virus shedding after challenge with virulent feline herpesvirus 1. *J Feline Med Surg*. 2006;8:158–163.
110. Lappin MR, Veir J, Hawley J. Feline panleukopenia virus, feline herpesvirus-1, and feline calicivirus antibody responses in seronegative specific pathogen-free cats after a single administration of two different modified live FVRCP vaccines. *J Feline Med Surg*. 2009;11:159–162.
111. Edinboro CH, Janowitz LK, Guptill-Yoran L, et al. A clinical trial of intranasal and subcutaneous vaccines to prevent upper respiratory infection in cats at animal shelter. *Feline Pract*. 1999;27:7–13.
112. Digangi BA, Levy JK, Griffin B, et al. Effects of maternally-derived antibodies on serologic responses to vaccination in kittens. *J Feline Med Surg*. 2012;14:118–123.
113. Mostl K, Egberink H, Addie D, et al. Prevention of infectious diseases in cat shelters: ABCD guidelines. *J Feline Med Surg*. 2013;15:546–554.
114. Alt J, Eveland R, Fiorello A, et al. Development and validation of technologies suitable for the decontamination and re-use of contaminated N95 filtering facepiece respirators in response to the COVID-19 pandemic. *J Hosp Infect*. 2022;19:141–148.

36

Feline Foamy (Syncytium-Forming) Virus Infection

Chrissy Eckstrand

KEY POINTS

- Cause: FFV, family *Retroviridae*, subfamily *Spumaretrovirinae.*
- First Described: 1969, United States.[1]
- Affected Hosts: Domestic cat and many other Felidae.
- Geographic Distribution: Worldwide.
- Route of Transmission: Unknown, but vertical transmission (*in utero* and/or mammary) and salivary transmission through close contact are hypothesized.
- Major Clinical Signs: An association between FFV infection and clinical disease remains unproven, but the virus has been detected in cats with idiopathic polyarthritis.
- Differential Diagnosis: Primary immune-mediated polyarthritis, polyarthritis secondary to other infections such as FeLV, FCV, *Chlamydia felis*, *Mycoplasma* spp. infection.
- Human Health Significance: Although foamy viruses can infect multiple cell lines, no known transmission from cats to humans has been documented.

ETIOLOGIC AGENT AND EPIDEMIOLOGY

FFV, previously known as "feline syncytium-forming virus," is a retrovirus in the family *Retroviridae*, subfamily *Spumaretrovirinae.*[2] Host-specific viruses of this genus have also been isolated from various mammalian species including cattle and nonhuman primates and often have no, or low, pathogenic potential.[3,4] Foamy viruses are atypical retroviruses in that viral particles bud from the endoplasmic reticulum, can contain DNA or RNA, and are highly cell-associated. Additionally, reverse transcription can occur late in the cell infection cycle.[2,5] Proviral DNA is integrated into the host cell chromosome, and persistent infection, with or without viral production, can result. The prevalence of FFV infection is high in both clinically healthy and diseased cats. At least two genotypes and serotypes have been identified, which share broad serologic cross-reactivity even to the serotype-specific ectodomain of the FFV Env-SU glycoprotein.[6–8] Virus has been isolated from primary cultures of tissue and body secretions in up to 90% of a population of cats.[9] More typically, the prevalence of infection in a cat population varies between 25% and 50%, depending on the age, geographic location, and local environment of the cats.[10–16] Furthermore, 50% or more of kittens born to FFV-infected queens are infected at birth,[15] and 15% of cultures from fetal cats are positive for the virus, suggesting that it can be transmitted vertically.[17] *In utero* infection probably occurs by the transfer of infected maternal leukocytes across the placenta, but infection may also be transmitted through milk of lactating animals.[15]

The highest prevalence of FFV infection is in roaming or outdoor cats, suggesting possible transmission through bite wounds (like FIV); however, epidemiologic evidence suggests that FFV is more likely transmitted by intimate social contact (like FeLV).[18] This is also supported by serologic evidence that male and female cats, with or without neutering, have an equal rate of seroreactivity.[14] Some wild cat species (*Felis silvestris, Felis iriomotensis,* and *Felis bengalensis*) also have a relatively high prevalence rate of seroreactivity to FFV; however, extensive surveys are not available.[13,19,20]

FFV is a nuisance to virologists and manufacturers of feline therapeutics like vaccines and mesenchymal stem cells because it often only becomes apparent in feline tissues and cell cultures after multiple passages.[21–23] *In vitro*, FFV is not highly host specific; in addition to cat cells, it infects cells of dogs, chickens, humans, and bats.[20] This is supported by evidence that foamy viruses utilize heparan sulfate, a ubiquitous cellular polysaccharide, as an attachment factor.[24] When FFV is produced, it is enveloped and has long glycoprotein spikes (Fig. 36.1A). Viral particles may accumulate in the host cell cytoplasm within membrane-bound vesicles, giving the cell a foamy appearance. In cell culture, it produces multinucleated syncytia within 1 to 2 weeks of growth in certain rapidly multiplying tissue cultures (Fig. 36.1B). Cell lysis is a late event because large syncytia are not viable. Syncytium formation in cell culture is not unique to FFV; it also has been associated with a variant of FeLV where an insertion into the FeLV envelope glycoprotein gene is responsible for this CPE.[25] FFV can be distinguished from FeLV, which is visualized only as it buds from the cell, whereas FFV often forms recognizable intracytoplasmic inclusions and preassembled nucleocapsids within the cytoplasm before budding (see Fig. 36.1A).

FFV has been considered an attractive retroviral vector for the delivery of feline vaccine antigens and heterologous genes because of its lack of apparent pathogenicity, and its suitability as such has been demonstrated.[26–30] The complete genome of FFV proviral DNA has been cloned, manipulated to be replication-competent or replication-deficient depending on the therapeutic purpose,[31,32] and explored for use in cats.[31–34]

CLINICAL FEATURES

Pathogenesis and Clinical Signs

FFV has never been unambiguously associated with disease. Many cats have been infected naturally and experimentally and had no

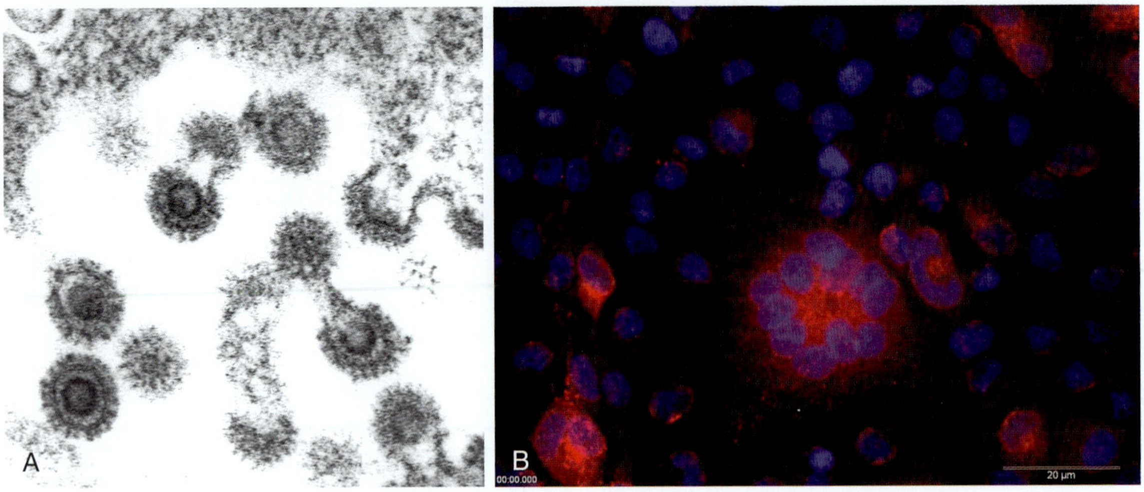

Fig. 36.1 Feline foamy virus (FFV) particles and proteins in productively FFV-infected Crandell-Rees Feline Kidney (CRFK) cells. (A) Thin-section electron microscopy of budding and released FFV particles displaying the regular Env glycoprotein spikes in the membrane surrounding the FFV core. CRFK cells were processed for electron microscopy 5 days after infection (Magnification: ×160,000). (B) Detection of FFV proteins in infected CRFK cells 2 days after infection. Protein antigens staining red are visible in a multinucleated cell. FFV-specific antigens were detected using FFV cat reference serum and a goat anticat IgG *(red)*. Nuclei were counterstained with Hoechst dye *(blue)*. A multinucleated FFV-induced syncytium (cell fusion, center) and cells displaying no cytopathic effects are positive for FFV antigens. (A, Courtesy Birgit Hub, Hanswalter Zentgraf, and Dragana Slavkovic, German Cancer Research Centre, Heidelberg. B, Courtesy Anne Bleiholder, German Cancer Research Centre, Heidelberg.)

clinical illness, a scenario that may reflect a very close virus-host co-adaptation.[35,36] Virus replication in the cat is a complex interplay between host immunity, host antiviral restriction factors such as APOBEC3 proteins, and virus accessory proteins, such as Bet, which counteracts APOBEC3.[37–40]

Reports about FFV pathogenicity are controversial and conflicting. Investigations into the presence of the virus in cats with chronic polyarthritis are quite variable with 100% of cats affected with chronic progressive polyarthritis in one study and 15% in another.[41,42] Concurrent FeLV infection was found in 70% of cats in the former study mentioned. The prevalence of infection with both viruses was 2 to 10 times greater than that in age-matched cats not having chronic progressive polyarthritis. By altering the host immune system, FeLV may potentiate the ability of FFV to produce disease. Combined infections with FFV and FIV are also frequently found.[42,43] However, co-infection with FFV and FIV did not increase the severity of FIV-induced illness in the early stages of the disease.[32] A combined infection is most likely a result of a common mode of transmission rather than a mutual pathogenic mechanism. FFV strains infect lymphoblastoid cells *in vitro*, producing altered replication, syncytia formation, and fragmentation of cellular DNA.[44] These features of apoptosis may be responsible for independent immune alterations in infected cats.

Immune-mediated polyarthritis is hypothesized to result from chronic antigenic stimulation and immune complex deposition. Arthritis that occurs in conjunction with FFV infection is characterized histologically in the acute stage as fibrinopurulent synovitis, and chronically as lymphoplasmacytic synovitis with synovial hyperplasia, loss of articular cartilage, pannus, and periosteal and subchondral bone remodeling.[45] An inherent genetic tendency may explain why certain male cats are more prone to developing disease despite the high prevalence of these viral infections in the general population. It is currently not clear whether FFV or any persisting feline virus contributes to arthritis or related immunopathologic disease of cats. Using PCR, FFV DNA was not detected in tissue from vaccine site-associated sarcomas from cats.[28]

Most FFV-infected cats show no clinical signs. Chronic progressive polyarthritis of cats generally affects naturally infected males between 1½ and 6 years of age.[41,46–49] Two forms of the disease have been described: one with osteoporosis and periarticular periosteal proliferation, the other with periarticular erosions, collapse of the joint space, and joint deformities. Lymphadenomegaly and arthralgias are caused by both types. In experimentally FFV-infected cats that were monitored for a 6-month period PI, histopathologic changes of mild glomerulonephritis and moderate interstitial pneumonia were observed[50]; however, no corresponding co-housed uninfected control cats were evaluated to substantiate the association of the virus infection with these mild lesions.

DIAGNOSIS

Microbiologic Tests

Serologic Diagnosis

FFV infections are associated with the production of virus-specific antibodies by the infected hosts. Therefore, assays based on immunodiffusion methods, IFA, immunoblotting, and ELISA are used to test for virus-specific antibodies.[16,41,42,51,52] Infected kittens can be detected at birth by culturing buffy coat cells from their peripheral blood. Animals are infected for life and develop persistent, nonprotective antibody titers to the virus.[53] For this reason, cats showing a serologic response toward FFV are presumed to be infected. Neonatal kittens born to infected queens lose their maternal antibody by 6 to 8 weeks of age if they are not infected. Serum antibody titers increase after this time if they become infected.[17]

Virus Isolation

In addition to serology, virus cultures to screen cats for infection by the detection of FFV-specific antigens and CPEs (syncytia) can be performed. Virus can be isolated from most tissues but requires one to four passages *in vitro*. IHC has been developed to detect the FFV Bet protein, and is predominantly present in cells of lymphoid organs such as the lymph nodes, tonsils, thymus, and spleen.[54] Additionally, FFV has been demonstrated in saliva.[53] It appears that FFV replication in peripheral blood leukocytes is suppressed by the host. This latent virus can be reactivated by co-cultivating buffy-coat leukocytes with permissive feline cells.[53]

Molecular Diagnosis Using Nucleic Acid–Based Testing

PCR can also be used directly to detect virus in blood leukocytes or cells of body fluids or tissues. There is a 100% correlation between seropositive results in cats and detection of proviral DNA in leukocytes.[52]

TREATMENT AND PREVENTION

FFV infection is lifelong and eradication therapies do not currently exist. Additionally, specific antiviral therapies have not been thoroughly investigated for use as infection is generally considered nonpathogenic. The antiviral drug tenofovir can salvage FFV-infected mesenchymal stem cells from CPEs when cultured *in vitro* for autologous mesenchymal stem cell therapy.[21]

Chronic progressive polyarthritis has no known cure, and the clinical and pathologic changes it causes usually are temporarily responsive for weeks to months to immunosuppressive therapy such as prednisolone (10–15 mg/day per cat) and cyclophosphamide (2.5 mg/day per cat, PO, for 4 days each week). Cats identified as having polyarthritis should be eliminated from research projects and removed from donating stem cells, vaccine production, and SPF colonies because an infectious or contagious etiology cannot be excluded.

PUBLIC HEALTH ASPECTS

All nonhuman primate species harbor distinct host-species specific strains of simian foamy viruses that are genetically different from FFV.[52] No data are available to document the existence of an authentic human foamy virus; however, people who are occupationally exposed to nonhuman primates have the highest rate of exposure and zoonotic infection to the different simian foamy viruses.[55] Other foamy viruses of domestic animals, including FFV, can infect a variety of cell types from different species *in vitro*. No transmission of these other viruses to people has been documented.[3,52] Furthermore, data from studies of seroreactivity among veterinarians and other people occupationally exposed to cats did not support an increased risk of infection.[56]

SUGGESTED READINGS

Pinto-Santini DM, Stenbak CR, Linial ML. Foamy virus zoonotic infections. *Retrovirology*. 2017;14:55.

Meiering CD, Linial ML. Historical perspective of foamy virus epidemiology and infection. *Clin Microbiol Rev*. 2001;14:165–176.

Inkpen H. Chronic progressive polyarthritis in a domestic shorthair cat. *Can Vet J*. 2015;56:621–623.

REFERENCES

1. Riggs JL, Oshirls, Taylor DO, et al. Syncytium forming agent isolated from domestic cats. *Nature*. 1969;222:1190–1191.
2. Linial ML. Foamy viruses are unconventional retroviruses. *J Virol*. 1999;73:1747–1755.
3. Bastone P, Truyen U, Lochelt M. Potential of zoonotic transmission of non-primate foamy viruses to humans. *J Vet Med B Infect Dis Vet Public Health*. 2003;50:417–423.
4. Materniak M, Hechler T, Lochelt M, et al. Similar patterns of infection with bovine foamy virus in experimentally inoculated calves and sheep. *J Virol*. 2013;87:3516–3525.
5. Roy J, Rudolph W, Juretzek T, et al. Feline foamy virus genome and replication strategy. *J Virol*. 2003;77:11324–11331.
6. Winkler IG, Flugel RM, Lochelt M, et al. Detection and molecular characterisation of feline foamy virus serotypes in naturally infected cats. *Virology*. 1998;247:144–151.
7. Phung HT, Ikeda Y, Miyazawa T, et al. Genetic analyses of feline foamy virus isolates from domestic and wild feline species in geographically distinct areas. *Virus Res*. 2001;76:171–181.
8. Bleiholder A, Löchelt M. Unpublished obervations; 2010. German Cancer Research Centre, Heidelberg, Germany.
9. Hackett AJ, Pfiester A, Arnstein P. Biological properties of a syncytia-forming agent isolated from domestic cats (feline syncytia-forming virus). *Proc Soc Exp Biol Med*. 1970;135:899–904.
10. Bleiholder A, Muhle M, Hechler T, et al. Pattern of seroreactivity against feline foamy virus proteins in domestic cats from Germany. *Vet Immunol Immunopathol*. 2011;143:292–300.
11. Jarrett O. Strategies of retrovirus survival in the cat. *Vet Microbiol*. 1999;69:99–107.
12. Lin JA, Cheng MC, Inoshima Y, et al. Seroepidemiological survey of feline retrovirus infections in cats in Taiwan in 1993 and 1994. *J Vet Med Sci*. 1995;57:161–163.
13. Miyazawa T, Ikeda Y, Maeda K, et al. Seroepidemiological survey of feline retrovirus infections in domestic and leopard cats in northern Vietnam in 1997. *J Vet Med Sci*. 1998;60:1273–1275.
14. Nakamura K, Miyazawa T, Ikeda Y, et al. Contrastive prevalence of feline retrovirus infections between northern and southern Vietnam. *J Vet Med Sci*. 2000;62:921–923.
15. Pedersen NC. Feline syncytium-forming virus. In: Appel MJ, ed. *Virus Infections of Carnivores*. New York: Elsevier; 1987:329–335.
16. Romen F, Pawlita M, Sehr P, et al. Antibodies against Gag are diagnostic markers for feline foamy virus infections while Env and Bet reactivity is undetectable in a substantial fraction of infected cats. *Virology*. 2006;345:502–508.
17. Hackett AJ, Manning JS. Comments on feline syncytia-forming virus. *J Am Vet Med Assoc*. 1971;158(suppl 2):948+.
18. Winkler IG, Lochelt M, Flower RL. Epidemiology of feline foamy virus and feline immunodeficiency virus infections in domestic and feral cats: a seroepidemiological study. *J Clin Microbiol*. 1999;37:2848–2851.
19. Daniels MJ, Golder MC, Jarrett O, et al. Feline viruses in wildcats from Scotland. *J Wildl Dis*. 1999;35:121–124.
20. Phung HT, Tohya Y, Shimojima M, et al. Establishment of a GFP-based indicator cell line to quantitate feline foamy virus. *J Virol Methods*. 2003;109:125–131.
21. Arzi B, Kol A, Murphy B, et al. Feline foamy virus adversely affects feline mesenchymal stem cell culture and expansion: implications for animal model development. *Stem Cells Dev*. 2015;24:814–823.
22. Hatama S, Otake K, Ohta M, et al. Reactivation of feline foamy virus from a chronically infected feline renal cell line by trichostatin A. *Virology*. 2001;283:315–323.
23. Kukedi A, Bartha A, Nagy B. Latent infection with feline syncytial virus of cell cultures prepared from the kidneys of new-born kittens. *Vet Microbiol*. 1988;16:9–14.
24. Plochmann K, Horn A, Gschmack E, et al. Heparan sulfate is an attachment factor for foamy virus entry. *J Virol*. 2012;86:10028–10035.
25. Rohn JL, Moser MS, Gwynn SR, et al. Vivo evolution of a novel, syncytium-inducing and cytopathic feline leukemia virus variant. *J Virol*. 1998;72:2686–2696.
26. Bastone P, Lochelt M. Kinetics and characteristics of replication-competent revertants derived from self-inactivating foamy virus vectors. *Gene Ther*. 2004;11:465–473.
27. German AC, Helps CR, Harbour DA. FIP: a novel approach to vaccination. Proceedings from the 2nd International FCoV/FIP Symposium, Glasgow, 4–7 August 2002. *J Feline Med Surg*. 2004;6:119–124.
28. Kidney BA, Haines DM, Ellis JA, et al. Evaluation of formalin-fixed paraffin-embedded tissues from feline vaccine site-associated sarcomas for feline foamy virus DNA. *Am J Vet Res*. 2002;63:60–63.
29. Kruger JM, Osborne CA. The role of uropathogens in feline lower urinary tract disease. Clinical implications. *Vet Clin North Am Small Anim Pract*. 1993;23:101–123.

30. Schwantes A, Ortlepp I, Lochelt M. Construction and functional characterization of feline foamy virus-based retroviral vectors. *Virology*. 2002;301:53–63.
31. Wirtz R, Lochelt M. Construction and analysis of genomic, full-length infectious foamy virus DNA clones. *Methods Mol Biol*. 2005;304:423–434.
32. Zenger E, Brown WC, Song W, et al. Evaluation of cofactor effect of feline syncytium-forming virus on feline immunodeficiency virus infection. *Am J Vet Res*. 1993;54:713–718.
33. Liu W, Lei J, Liu Y, et al. Feline foamy virus-based vectors: advantages of an authentic animal model. *Viruses*. 2013;5:1702–1718.
34. Schwantes A, Truyen U, Weikel J, et al. Application of chimeric feline foamy virus-based retroviral vectors for the induction of antiviral immunity in cats. *J Virol*. 2003;77:7830–7842.
35. Saib A. Non-primate foamy viruses. *Curr Top Microbiol Immunol*. 2003;277:197–211.
36. Switzer WM, Salemi M, Shanmugam V, et al. Ancient co-speciation of simian foamy viruses and primates. *Nature*. 2005;434:376–380.
37. Chareza S, Slavkovic Lukic D, Liu Y, et al. Molecular and functional interactions of cat APOBEC3 and feline foamy and immunodeficiency virus proteins: different ways to counteract host-encoded restriction. *Virology*. 2012;424:138–146.
38. Lochelt M, Romen F, Bastone P, et al. The antiretroviral activity of APOBEC3 is inhibited by the foamy virus accessory Bet protein. *Proc Natl Acad Sci U S A*. 2005;102:7982–7987.
39. Lukic DS, Hotz-Wagenblatt A, Lei J, et al. Identification of the feline foamy virus Bet domain essential for APOBEC3 counteraction. *Retrovirology*. 2013;10:76.
40. Munk C, Hechler T, Chareza S, et al. Restriction of feline retroviruses: lessons from cat APOBEC3 cytidine deaminases and TRIM5alpha proteins. *Vet Immunol Immunopathol*. 2010;134:14–24.
41. Pedersen NC, Pool RR, O'Brien T. Feline chronic progressive polyarthritis. *Am J Vet Res*. 1980;41:522–535.
42. Weissl K, Benetka V, Schachner E, et al. Osteoarthritis in cats and the possible involvement of feline calicivirus and feline retroviruses. *Wien Tierarztl Monatsschr*. 2012;99:123–133.
43. Bandecchi P, Matteucci D, Baldinotti F, et al. Prevalence of feline immunodeficiency virus and other retroviral infections in sick cats in Italy. *Vet Immunol Immunopathol*. 1992;31:337–345.
44. Ikeda Y, Itagaki S, Tsutsui S, et al. Replication of feline syncytial virus in feline T-lymphoblastoid cells and induction of apoptosis in the cells. *Microbiol Immunol*. 1997;41:431–435.
45. Craig L, Dittmer K, Thompson K. Bones and joints. In: Maxie MG, ed. *Jubb, Kennedy, and Palmer's Pathology of Domestic Animals*. 6th ed. St. Louis: Elsevier; 2016:158.
46. Moise NS, Crissman JW. Chronic progressive polyarthritis in a cat. *J Am Anim Hosp Assoc*. 1982;18:965–969.
47. Pedersen NC, Pool R, O'Brien T. Chronic progressive polyarthritis of the cat. *Feline Pract*. 1975;5:42–51.
48. Wilkinson GT, Robins GM. Polyarthritis in a young cat. *J Small Anim Pract*. 1979;20:293–297.
49. Inkpen H. Chronic progressive polyarthritis in a domestic shorthair cat. *Can Vet J*. 2015;56:621–623.
50. German AC, Harbour DA, Helps CR, et al. Is feline foamy virus really apathogenic? *Vet Immunol Immunopathol*. 2008;123:114–118.
51. Gaskin JM, Gillespie JH. Detection of feline syncytia-forming carrier state with a microimmunodiffusion test. *Am J Vet Res*. 1973;34:245–247.
52. Winkler IG, Lochelt M, Levesque JP, et al. A rapid streptavidin-capture ELISA specific for the detection of antibodies to feline foamy virus. *J Immunol Methods*. 1997;207:69–77.
53. Alke A, Schwantes A, Zemba M, et al. Characterization of the humoral immune response and virus replication in cats experimentally infected with feline foamy virus. *Virology*. 2000;275:170–176.
54. Weikel J, Lochelt M, Truyen U. Demonstration of feline foamy virus in experimentally infected cats by immunohistochemistry. *J Vet Med A Physiol Pathol Clin Med*. 2003;50:415–417.
55. Heneine W, Schweizer M, Sandstrom P, et al. Human infection with foamy viruses. *Curr Top Microbiol Immunol*. 2003;277:181–196.
56. Butera ST, Brown J, Callahan ME, et al. Survey of veterinary conference attendees for evidence of zoonotic infection by feline retroviruses. *J Am Vet Med Assoc*. 2000;217:1475–1479.

37

Paramyxovirus Infections

Hans Lutz, Claire R. Sharp, Jane E. Sykes

KEY POINTS

- Cause: Viruses of the family *Paramyxoviridae*; genera *Morbillivirus* (feline morbillivirus [FeMV], canine distemper virus [CDV]), *Henipavirus* (including Hendra virus [HeV] and Nipah virus], and the newly named *Rubulavirus* (previously paramyxovirus; mumps virus [MuV]).
- First Described: FeMV was first described in China in 2012.[1] CDV was first described in France in 1905.[2] HeV was first isolated in Queensland, Australia in 1994.[3] Nipah virus was first identified in humans in Malaysia in 1999. MuV was first described in 410 BC (Hippocrates).
- Affected Hosts: Domestic cats (FeMV); large wild Felidae, dogs and other Canidae, Procyonidae (raccoons, pandas), Mustelidae (ferrets, mink, skunks, otters), nonhuman primates (CDV); horses, humans, flying foxes (reservoirs), domestic cats (experimental infection only), guinea pigs (experimental), dogs (HeV); pigs, humans, fruit bats (reservoirs), domestic cats, dogs (Nipah virus); humans, dogs, cats (MuV).
- Geographic Distribution: Asia, Europe, North and South America (FeMV); northeastern Australia (HeV); Malaysia, Singapore, Bangladesh, India (Nipah virus); worldwide (MuV).
- Route of Transmission: Oronasal contact with virus in secretions or excretions, droplet nuclei, and large particle aerosol transmission.
- Major Clinical Signs: Paramyxoviruses cause infections of the CNS, and respiratory and urinary tracts. FeMV has been implicated in chronic kidney disease in cats, but its clinical significance remains unclear. Natural infections of dogs with HeV have been rare and subclinical. Natural infections of dogs and cats with Nipah virus are also rare, but death and severe respiratory signs have been described. MuV can cause parotitis with salivary gland enlargement.
- Differential Diagnoses: These include other causes of infectious respiratory disease; parasitic respiratory disease; toxins such as lead and ethylene glycol; other causes of infectious meningoencephalitis. Differential diagnosis for mumps include other causes of parotitis such as immune-mediated disease.
- Human Health Significance: FeMV is not known to infect humans. HeV and Nipah viruses cause serious infections of humans with high mortality. Mumps is a serious infection of humans but largely controlled by vaccination; periodic outbreaks still occur. Dogs and cats do not appear to be important in transmission of these viruses to humans.

INTRODUCTION

The *Paramyxoviridae* family includes, among others, feline morbillivirus (FeMV), canine distemper virus (CDV), *Henipavirus* (including Hendra virus [HeV] and Nipah virus), and *Rubulavirus* (including mumps virus [MuV]). These viruses affect domestic and wild felids, canids, procyonids, mustelids, and many more mammalian species. Transmission is by close contact, droplets, and aerosols. These infections, of which many occur around the world, can cause mild to serious diseases of the CNS, and respiratory and urinary tracts, but many infections are associated with no symptoms. Henipavirus infections in Asia and Australia are zoonotic diseases and can be very serious in humans, but are hardly transmitted to humans by cats and dogs.

Paramyxoviruses have been associated with emerging infectious diseases in a variety of species in recent decades, and as such are important viruses to both human and veterinary medicine.[4] This chapter focuses on paramyxovirus infections in cats, although infections of both dogs and cats with HeV, Nipah virus, and MuV are also described. Diagnostic testing for these latter three virus infections requires coordination with local public health authorities given their significance for human health.

FELINE MORBILLIVIRUS INFECTION

Until recently, the genus *Morbillivirus* was recognized to contain six species: CDV, measles virus, rinderpest virus (now eradicated), peste des petits ruminants virus, phocine distemper virus, and cetacean morbillivirus. Of these, only CDV had been known to affect felids, causing clinical signs in some large exotic felids, but not in domestic cats. In 2012 however, a novel FeMV was isolated from cats in Hong Kong and mainland China.[1]

This virus was officially recognized as the seventh species of the genus *Morbillivirus* in 2016. Early reports of FeMV infection were only in domestic cats, however in 2020 the virus was identified by RT-PCR in urine and homogenized kidney tissue from two black leopards (*Panthera pardus*) in Thailand.[5]

In 2012, FeMV RNA was identified by RT-PCR in 56 of 457 (12.3%) stray cats from Hong Kong.[1] Of the specimen types collected, urine was most commonly PCR positive for FeMV (53/56 cat specimens). Subsequently, many of these cats were shown to have antibodies to the FeMV N protein (54/56 RT-PCR positive cats were antibody positive). Additionally, 78/401 (19.5%) RT-PCR-negative cats were antibody positive, suggesting previous exposure. Concurrently, 1/16 diseased cats from mainland China was RT-PCR positive to FeMV in oral and rectal swabs.[1] To identify possible disease associations, necropsies were performed in two stray cats that were RT-PCR positive for FeMV.[1] Histology revealed renal tubular degeneration and necrosis in both cats, consistent with tubulointerstitial nephritis (TIN), the histologic correlate of CKD in cats. In a small case-control study of a further 27 stray cats, TIN was documented in 7/12 cats that were positive for FeMV using RT-PCR, but only 2/15 FeMV-negative cats ($P < .05$), suggesting an association between FeMV and TIN.[1] This first report suggesting an association between FeMV and TIN generated significant interest in the field, given the large disease burden of CKD in cats.[6]

Since its discovery, epidemiologic studies have now documented FeMV in domestic cats in Japan,[7–9] Europe,[10–14] the United States,[15] Brazil,[16] Malaysia,[17] and additional cases in China.[18]

To identify infected cats, most investigators have tested urine or kidney tissue specimens, reporting a prevalence of FeMV infection using RT-PCR that has ranged from 3%, in the northeastern United States,[15] to 52.9% (9/17 cats) in a multicat house that had close contact with a stray cat colony in Brazil.[16] While the mode of FeMV transmission is unknown, its higher prevalence in the aforementioned multicat household, as well as in colony cats,[19] suggests that close cat contact may be involved. Male predominance has also been reported in some molecular epidemiologic studies.[17,20]

The seroprevalence of FeMV has also varied widely, although fewer studies report the results of antibody testing. Seroprevalence of anti-FeMV antibodies has ranged from 21.2% in Japan[9,20] to 66.7% in the United Kingdom.[13] However, none of the FeMV serosurveys have employed virus neutralization (VN), the gold standard for diagnostic serology, and thus methodologic limitations may have resulted in inaccuracies in serologic data. Development of VN assays is needed to better understand the epidemiology of, and immune response to, FeMV.

Studies that have reported concurrent molecular and serological data identify four populations of cats: (1) those that have never been exposed to the virus (both RT-PCR and seronegative), (2) those that have been exposed, developed antibodies, and likely cleared the virus from their urine (RT-PCR negative, and seropositive), (3) those likely to be in the early stage of infection but without antibodies (RT-PCR positive but seronegative), and (4) those both RT-PCR and seropositive, suggesting both the presence of active viral shedding and circulating antibodies. At least some cats in the fourth group appear to be chronically infected.[14,15,19]

Several studies have attempted to investigate the role of FeMV infection in CKD in cats. Some have suggested an association,[10,20,21] while others have found no association.[9,13,16,17,19] Undoubtedly FeMV can be identified in cat urine, both by RT-PCR and virus isolation, and will grow after inoculation of CRFK cells. Additionally, some authors have identified FeMV in renal tubular epithelial cells by IHC.[1,13,22] Nonetheless, associations documented in some of these studies do not prove causation, and pathogenesis studies are needed. Of note, other morbilliviruses are not known to cause kidney disease, despite infecting epithelial cells of the urogenital tract.

Given that morbilliviruses are significant pathogens in a variety of host species, it is tempting to hypothesize that FeMV may cause pathology in cats. Morbilliviruses are classically lymphotropic and epitheliotropic, resulting in clinical signs affecting the skin, respiratory tract, GI tract, and CNS. Additionally, morbilliviruses classically result in immunosuppression. Whether or not FeMV results in a similar spectrum of disease in cats remains to be determined. Only two studies specifically evaluating *in vitro* FeMV cell tropism have been published, documenting FeMV replication in cat fibroblasts, lymphoid cells, and glial cells as well as in renal, pulmonary epithelial and primary brain cells. Feline morbillivirus genotype 2 (FeMV-GT2) also replicates readily in several types of lymphocytes.[23,24]

Evidence that FeMV can infect glial cells *in vitro*, in addition to occasional clinical reports of FeMV RT-PCR positivity of cat brain tissue,[19] suggest the potential for the virus to be neurotrophic, as is seen with other morbilliviruses. It remains unknown to what degree FeMV infection may explain historic evidence of a paramyxovirus-like agent in the CNS of stray and pet cats with subclinical focal demyelinating encephalitis.[25,26] Unfortunately at the time, while paramyxovirus-like nucleocapsids were observed using electron microscopy in fixed cat brain and optic nerve tissues, as well as explant cultures of CNS tissue co-cultivated with CRFK cells, the virus could not be definitively identified.[26]

Future FeMV research should focus on acute and chronic pathogenesis studies using experimental infections to understand the route of infection, transmission, viral receptor usage, and cell tropism of FeMV, in addition to the immune response to the virus, and the pathology it causes. Ultimately, if FeMV is identified as a pathogen, there will be a need for commercially available diagnostic tests, the development of effective vaccines, and even investigation of the role of antivirals for the treatment of active infection. Currently, testing for FeMV is being done on a research basis and not offered on a commercial basis, given the unclear role of FeMV in disease.

CANINE DISTEMPER VIRUS INFECTION IN CATS

CDV, which also belongs to the genus *Morbillivirus*, infects a wide variety of terrestrial carnivores. Information on CDV infection in dogs is covered in depth in Chapter 22. Domestic cats can be infected through experimental inoculation, but clinical signs do not develop. Virus-neutralizing antibodies to CDV have been detected in domestic cats housed in close proximity to dogs, but again, clinical illness has not been documented.[27,28] In contrast to domestic cats, large exotic Felidae are more susceptible to infection with CDV. CDV isolates from exotic felids are similar to virulent isolates from other carnivores, and infection likely originates from wildlife and/or domestic dogs in close proximity to exotic cats (Fig. 37.1).[29–39] Noncanid carnivores, such as raccoons and skunks, may also act as vectors of CDV for exotic cats in zoological gardens.[40]

There are several case reports implicating CDV in progressive neurologic disease, with or without respiratory signs, in exotic cats around the world, including an African lioness (*Panthera leo*),[41] Bengal tiger (*Panthera tigris tigris*),[42] both captive and free-ranging adult Siberian tigers (*Panthera tigris altaica*),[38,43] and two snow leopards (*Uncia uncia*).[44] Although isolation of CDV was not performed in many of these cases, the presence of consistent histologic lesions (non-suppurative encephalitis or meningoencephalitis), characteristic intranuclear inclusions, IHC, and serologic documentation of CDV antibodies provide strong support for CDV as the etiologic agent. The aforementioned snow leopards were co-infected with feline panleukopenia virus (FPV),[44] suggesting the possibility of FPV-induced immunosuppression. CDV was also implicated as the cause of death in an Iberian lynx (*Lynx pardinus*) in the Donana National Park in South-Western Andalusia, Spain.[45] The Iberian lynx is at present the most critically endangered felid, and the virus was closely related to that isolated from a stone marten (*Martes foina*) found close by. Thus, CDV represents a constant threat to free-ranging wild felids.

CDV has caused large outbreaks of disease in free-ranging wild felid populations.[46–48] The first such outbreak occurred in 1994, resulting in the death of a considerable proportion of lions in the Serengeti in Tanzania.[46,49–51] Clinical signs were primarily neurologic. Pathologic findings were encephalitis and pneumonia. Inclusion bodies immunologically cross-reacting with CDV proteins were identified in 14/19 lion specimens that were available for examination. A total of 71/83 serum samples were found to be positive for anti-CDV antibodies.[46]

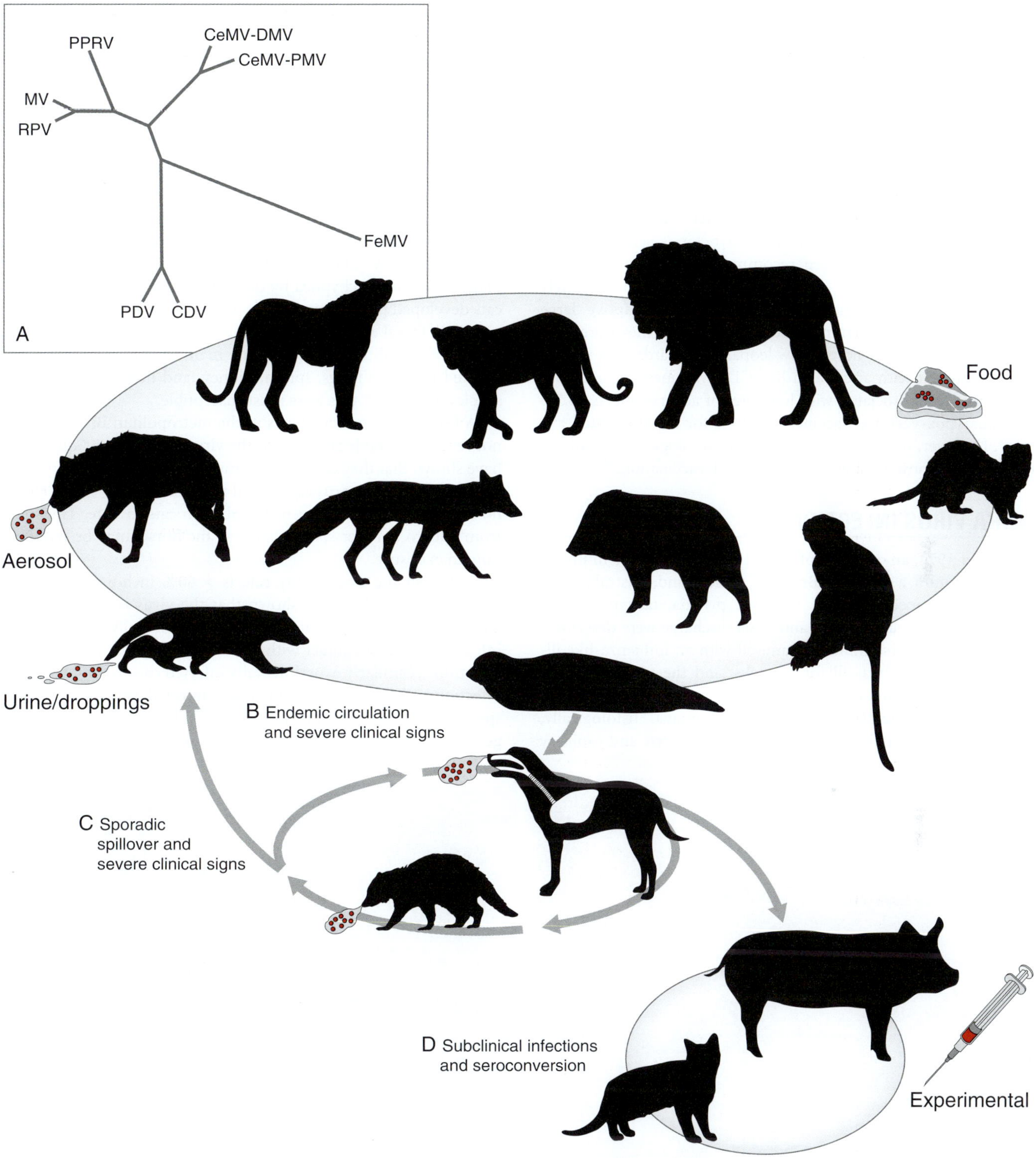

Fig. 37.1 Canine distemper virus (CDV) phylogeny and cross species transmission. A, Phylogenetic tree based on alignment of morbillivirus H glycoproteins. B–D, Illustration of cross-species transmission of CDV between multiple domestic and wildlife reservoir hosts. B, CDV infection circulates in dogs and raccoons due to population sizes large enough to maintain endemic transmission. C, Spillover and/or limited chains of transmission in a large number of wildlife species including various cat species, e.g., tiger, lynx, leopard, lion, and other Serengeti wildlife; North American wildlife, e.g., gray wolf, coyote, skunk, black-footed ferret, mink; European wildlife, e.g., European badger, fox; seals, and rhesus and cynomolgus macaques. D, Subclinical, self-limiting infection has been reported in experimentally infected cats and pigs. *CeMV-DMV,* cetacean morbillivirus/dolphin morbillivirus, *CeMV-PMV,* cetacean morbillivirus/porpoise morbillivirus, *FeMV,* feline morbillivirus; *MV,* measles virus, *PDV,* phocine distemper virus; *PPRV,* peste des petits ruminants virus; *RPV,* rinderpest virus.

Phylogenetic analysis suggested that the lion CDV isolate was closely related to the Onderstepoort strain of CDV, and may have originated from domestic dogs living around the Serengeti parks.[46] Purported contributors to the epizootic included hyenas transmitting the disease to local domestic dogs and lions, and loss of cross-immunization of lions by consumption of rinderpest-infected buffaloes when the closely related rinderpest virus was eradicated in the 1980s. To reduce the probability of further outbreaks of CDV in lions, a program to vaccinate the domestic dogs living around the parks was initiated.

CDV outbreaks have also occurred in captive lions, tigers, and leopards.[41,52,53] Affected cats developed anorexia, GI and/or respiratory signs, followed by CNS signs of ataxia, myoclonus, seizures, coma, and death. Vaccination has been recommended to protect captive large exotic Felidae, however vaccine efficacy remains incompletely documented.[54,55] A multi-institutional study of 812 captive large felids documented that canarypox-vectored CDV vaccines were used most commonly in tigers, lions, snow leopards, leopards, and jaguars (96.3%) compared with attenuated live CDV vaccines (3.7%). Both vaccine types were associated with low rates of adverse effects (0.5% for the canarypox-vectored vaccine, and 2.9% for the attenuated live vaccine). However, only 66% of animals with serologic data available experienced seroconversion at some point post-vaccination.[54]

HENDRA VIRUS INFECTION

In September 1994, an outbreak of acute respiratory disease in horses occurred in Hendra, a suburb of Brisbane, Queensland, Australia.[3,56,57] The horses developed anorexia, lethargy, pyrexia, tachypnea, and ataxia. Terminally, head pressing and nasal discharge were described. A stable hand and horse trainer became ill with an influenza-like illness. The stable hand was ill for 6 weeks, and the trainer died. A novel virus, HeV (genus *Henipavirus*), that was closely related to a *Morbillivirus* was isolated from the horses and humans. Histologically, the horses had interstitial pneumonia with pneumocyte and capillary degeneration.[58] Virus was detected in endothelial cells using immunofluorescence, as well as in CSF, brain tissue, and serum using PCR.[59] Necrotizing lymphadenitis is also common, and syncytial cells can be found in a variety of different organs. Anti-Nipah virus antibody can be used for IHC due to cross-reactivity (Fig. 37.2).

Since its first isolation, over 90 HeV-associated fatalities in horses and 4 human fatalities have been documented.[60] HeV is transmitted by excretions (saliva, feces, nasal discharge) of pteropid bats (flying foxes)[61] of which some species are now known to be reservoirs. A large number of laboratory animal species, including dogs and cats, were experimentally inoculated subcutaneously with the virus.[3,58] The dogs and cats had been vaccinated for common viral diseases but notably the dogs for CDV. The dogs did not become ill, but the cats developed inappetence and tachypnea by day 5 PI and died 1–2 days later. The cats developed pulmonary edema, hilar lymphadenomegaly, pneumonia, and pleural effusion, but neurologic signs were absent. Histologic lesions of vasculitis resembled those in affected horses. The virus was isolated from the lungs, spleen, kidney, and brain. Of all laboratory species inoculated, cats were most susceptible.

A limited serosurvey of cats in the metropolitan Brisbane area did not reveal detectable antibody to the virus.[3] Subsequent studies in cats have shown that they can be experimentally infected by nonparenteral routes and that the virus can spread naturally among cats.[62] However, no field infections have been described in cats to date. Transmission from bats to another species, such as the horse, may be required for human exposure.

Although the case fatality rate is > 60% in horses and humans, transmission studies have shown that the virus is not highly contagious. Horses in direct contact with experimentally infected cats and infected horses in contact with other horses or cats did not transmit infection.[63] Similarly experimentally infected cats did not transmit the infection to horses. In experimentally infected animals, regardless of species, virus was most prevalent in the kidney and urine, which suggests urinary transmission as the means of spread. Additionally, HeV

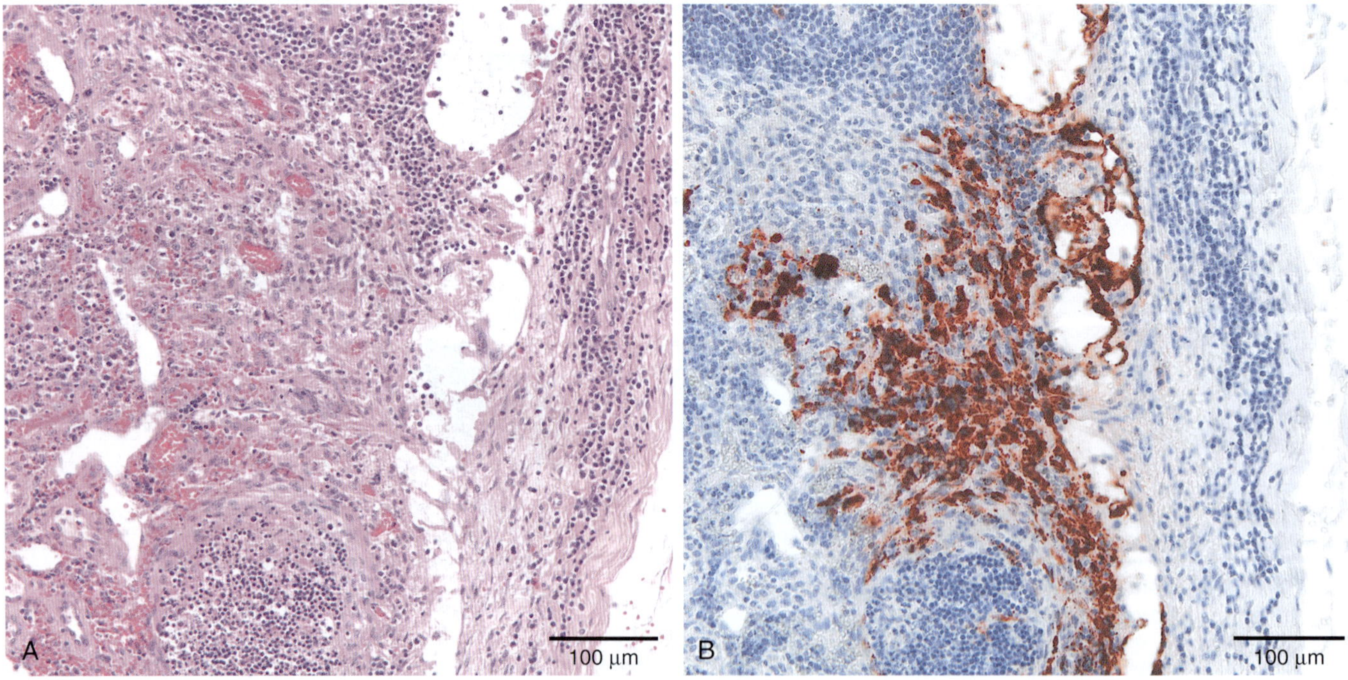

Fig. 37.2 (A) Histologic section of the lymph node from a horse with acute Hendra virus infection showing lymphadenitis with syncytial cell formation (hematoxylin and eosin stain). (B) Hendra virus antigen in a section adjacent to (A). Anti-Nipah N antibody. (From Middleton D. Hendra Virus. *Vet Clin North Am Equine Pract.* 2014;30:579–589.)

was isolated for up to 3 weeks after infection of a horse and 14 months in a human developing infection, suggesting viral persistence and a carrier state.

Natural infections with HeV have been reported in at least two dogs, and additional subclinical infections that were undetected may also have occurred. In 2013, HeV was detected by RT-PCR in the serum of a dog on the same farm as an infected horse in New South Wales, Australia.[64] This dog had been in close contact with the affected horse and was apparently exposed to the horse's blood after the horse was euthanized 14 days prior. The dog was apparently healthy and testing had been done as a surveillance effort. The dog also had virus neutralizing antibodies at a titer of 1:8. Because of concerns surrounding transmission risk, the dog was euthanized 2 days later. At necropsy, necrotizing vasculitis was detected in the dog's kidney, brain, lymph nodes, spleen, liver, intestine, and lungs. Small amounts of viral antigen were detected in the kidney, and many tissues were positive for HeV using RT-PCR; serum collected at necropsy had an antibody titer of 1:128.

The risk of transmission of HeV from dogs to horses or humans remains unknown, but it has been recommended that dogs be kept away from infected horses.[64] Experimentally infected dogs were shown to shed virus in nasal secretions at levels similar to those detected in horses.[65]

NIPAH VIRUS INFECTION

An outbreak of fatal human encephalitis during 1998 and 1999 in Malaysia was attributed to Nipah virus (genus *Henipavirus*), at that time a novel paramyxovirus acquired from swine.[66,67] Pigs, humans (primarily pig farmers), dogs, and cats were infected. As with HeV, fruit bats are reservoirs, which have a worldwide distribution, with spillover to other mammalian hosts. Although illness was reported in the other species, the disease in pigs was self-limiting and, in some cases, subclinical. Human infection was attributed to close contact with pigs. The role of dogs or cats as secondary sources of infection could not be excluded.

Since its emergence, over 700 cases of Nipah virus infection have occurred in humans in South and Southeast Asia, with a mortality rate of 40% to 70%.[66] Only one naturally infected cat has been described.[58] Results of serosurveys of feral cats in endemic areas suggest that transmission among bats and cats may be uncommon.[68] In experimentally infected cats, Nipah virus was similar in its behavior to that of the closely related HeV. Two cats were experimentally infected by the oronasal route with Nipah virus from an outbreak associated with respiratory and neurologic signs in pigs.[69] Respiratory and neurologic disease was observed in the cats, and virus was found in secretions of the oropharynx and excreted in urine. The virus causes widespread systemic vasculitis, especially the respiratory tract and CNS. Pulmonary lesions are giant cell pneumonia, and the secretions and tissues contain large amounts of virus. Transplacental infection also occurs in experimentally infected pregnant cats with resultant infection of kittens.[70,71] Experimental subunit vaccines containing soluble glycoprotein G of either HeV or Nipah virus protected cats against subsequent challenge with virulent Nipah virus.[72,73]

Dogs were suspected of being reservoirs of infection during the initial epidemic in humans.[74] Virus was identified by immunohistochemical staining of tissues in two dogs that died.[58] One of the dogs was found dead, and the other had fever, respiratory distress, conjunctivitis, and mucopurulent ocular and nasal discharge. Interstitial pneumonia, renal tubular necrosis, and nonsuppurative meningitis were described at necropsy.[58] Pigs were readily infected from fruit bats. Dogs were examined because they lived communally with pigs and humans and could have served as secondary reservoir hosts. Despite the high prevalence of seroreactivity among dogs at the time of the initial outbreak,[75] it was very low in dogs outside the immediate disease-endemic area.[76] Thus, infected dogs acted as dead-end hosts; infection did not spread in the absence of the infected pigs that had been depopulated.

MUMPS VIRUS INFECTION

MuV is a paramyxovirus causing parotitis and less frequently deafness, orchitis, and other clinical signs, with a high incidence in children aged between 5 and 9 years.[77] There are rare reports of the transmission of MuV to dogs with signs of lethargy and parotitis[78] and serologic evidence of exposure of cats.[79] After the introduction of vaccines in 1965, and routine vaccination of children, the incidence of disease in humans has decreased by 99%, but periodic outbreaks of disease still occur as a result of lack of vaccination or vaccine failure.[80,81] Dogs and cats do not play a significant role in transmission of MuV to humans.

AVIAN NEWCASTLE DISEASE VIRUS INFECTION

Avian Newcastle disease virus (genus *Paramyxovirus*) has not been reported to naturally infect cats, but has been experimentally inoculated into the CNS of domestic adult cats and kittens, producing disseminated encephalomyelitis.[82,83] Neonatal kittens can also be infected by intraocular or intranasal exposure to large quantities of virus. The incubation period following oculonasal administration of virus was relatively long (11 to 17 days) when compared with that after direct CNS inoculation (3 to 4 days). Clinical signs were seizures, head tilt, myoclonus, and progressive lower motor neuron paralysis. In some affected animals, behavioral alterations were present. A disseminated nonsuppurative meningoencephalitis was found histologically; virus appeared to spread throughout the nervous system along the descending and ascending neuronal pathways.

SUGGESTED READINGS

Choi EJ, Ortega V, Aguilar HC. Feline morbillivirus, a new paramyxovirus possibly asspciated with feline kidney disease. *Viruses*. 2020;12:E501.

Middleton D. Hendra virus. *Vet Clin North Am Equine Pract*. 2014;30:579–589.

Aditi SM. Nipah virus infection: a review. *Epidemiol Infect*. 2019;147:e95.

Rubin S, Eckhaus M, Rennick LJ, et al. Molecular biology, pathogenesis and pathology of mumps virus. *J Pathol*. 2015;235:242–252.

REFERENCES

1. Woo PCY, Lau SKP, Wong BHL, et al. Feline morbillivirus, a previously undescribed paramyxovirus associated with tubulointerstitial nephritis in domestic cats. *P Natl Acad Sci USA*. 2012;109:5435–5440.
2. Gamiz C, Martella V, Ulloa R, et al. Identification of a new genotype of canine distemper virus circulating in America. *Vet Res Commun*. 2011;35:381–390.
3. Murray K, Selleck P, Hooper P, et al. A morbillivirus that caused fatal disease in horses and humans. *Science*. 1995;268:94–97.
4. Thibault PA, Watkinson RE, Moreira-Soto A, et al. Zoonotic potential of emerging paramyxoviruses: knowns and unknowns. *Adv Virus Res*. 2017;98:1–55.
5. Piewbang C, Chaiyasak S, Kongmakee P, et al. Feline morbillivirus infection associated with tubulointerstitial nephritis in black leopards (*Panthera pardus*). *Vet Pathol*. 2020.
6. Beatty JA, Sharp CR, Duprex WP, et al. Novel feline viruses: emerging significance of gammaherpesvirus and morbillivirus infections. *J Feline Med Surg*. 2019;21:5–11.

7. Park ES, Suzuki M, Kimura M, et al. Identification of a natural recombination in the F and H genes of feline morbillivirus. *Virology.* 2014;468:524–531.
8. Furuya T, Sassa Y, Omatsu T, et al. Existence of feline morbillivirus infection in Japanese cat populations. *Arch Virol.* 2014;159:371–373.
9. Sakaguchi S, Nakagawa S, Yoshikawa R, et al. Genetic diversity of feline morbilliviruses isolated in Japan. *J Gen Virol.* 2014;95:1464–1468.
10. Lorusso A, Di Tommaso M, Di Felice E, et al. First report of feline morbillivirus in Europe. *Vet Ital.* 2015;51:235–237.
11. Marcacci M, De Luca E, Zaccaria G, et al. Genome characterization of feline morbillivirus from Italy. *J Virol Methods.* 2016;234:160–163.
12. Yilmaz H, Tekelioglu BK, Gurel A, et al. Frequency, clinicopathological features and phylogenetic analysis of feline morbillivirus in cats in Istanbul, Turkey. *J Feline Med Surg.* 2017;19:1206–1214.
13. McCallum KE, Stubbs S, Hope N, et al. Detection and seroprevalence of morbillivirus and other paramyxoviruses in geriatric cats with and without evidence of azotemic chronic kidney disease. *J Vet Intern Med.* 2018;32:1100–1108.
14. De Luca E, Crisi PE, Di Domenico M, et al. A real-time RT-PCR assay for molecular identification and quantitation of feline morbillivirus RNA from biological specimens. *J Virol Methods.* 2018;258:24–28.
15. Sharp CR, Nambulli S, Acciardo AS, et al. Chronic infection of domestic cats with feline morbillivirus, United States. *Emerg Infect Dis.* 2016;22:760–762.
16. Darold GM, Alfieri AA, Muraro LS, et al. First report of feline morbillivirus in South America. *Arch Virol.* 2017;162:469–475.
17. Mohd Isa NH, Selvarajah GT, Khor KH, et al. Molecular detection and characterisation of feline morbillivirus in domestic cats in Malaysia. *Vet Microbiol.* 2019;236:108382.
18. Ou JJ, Ye ST, Xu HB, et al. First report of feline morbillivirus in mainland China. *Arch Virol.* 2020;165:1837–1841.
19. De Luca E, Crisi PE, Marcacci M, et al. Epidemiology, pathological aspects and genome heterogeneity of feline morbillivirus in Italy. *Vet Microbiol.* 2020;240:108484.
20. Park ES, Suzuki M, Kimura M, et al. Epidemiological and pathological study of feline morbillivirus infection in domestic cats in Japan. *BMC Vet Res.* 2016;12.
21. Sieg M, Heenemann K, Rückner A, et al. Discovery of new feline paramyxoviruses in domestic cats with chronic kidney disease. *Virus Gene.* 2015;51:294–297.
22. Sutummaporn K, Suzuki K, Machida N, et al. Association of feline morbillivirus infection with defined pathological changes in cat kidney tissues. *Vet Microbiol.* 2019;228:12–19.
23. Sieg M, Busch J, Eschke M, et al. A new genotype of feline morbillivirus infects primary cells of the lung, kidney, brain and peripheral blood. *Viruses.* 2019;11:146.
24. Sakaguchi S, Koide R, Miyazawa T. In vitro host range of feline morbillivirus. *J Vet Med Sci.* 2015;77:1485–1487.
25. Cook RD, Wilcox GE. Primary demyelination in the central nervous system of cats. *Neuropathol Applied Neurobiol.* 1985;11:361–367.
26. Wilcox GE, Flower RL, Cook RD. Recovery of viral agents from the central nervous system of cats. *Vet Microbiol.* 1984;9:355–366.
27. Ikeda Y, Nakamura K, Miyazawa T, et al. Seroprevalence of canine distemper virus in cats. *Clin Diagn Lab Immunol.* 2001;8:641–644.
28. Lickey AL, Kennedy M, Patton S, et al. Serologic survey of domestic felids in the Peten region of Guatemala. *J Zoo Wildl Med.* 2005;36:121–123.
29. Biek R, Ruth TK, Murphy KM, et al. Factors associated with pathogen seroprevalence and infection in Rocky Mountain cougars. *J Wildl Dis.* 2006;42:606–615.
30. Cleaveland S, Appel MG, Chalmers WS, et al. Serological and demographic evidence for domestic dogs as a source of canine distemper virus infection for Serengeti wildlife. *Vet Microbiol.* 2000;72:217–227.
31. Driciru M, Siefert L, Prager KC, et al. A serosurvey of viral infections in lions (*Panthera leo*), from Queen Elizabeth National Park, Uganda. *J Wildl Dis.* 2006;42:667–671.
32. Fiorello CV, Noss AJ, Deem SL, et al. Serosurvey of small carnivores in the Bolivian Chaco. *J Wildl Dis.* 2007;43:551–557.
33. Franklin SP, Kays RW, Moreno R, et al. Ocelots on Barro Colorado Island are infected with feline immunodeficiency virus but not other common feline and canine viruses. *J Wildl Dis.* 2008;44:760–765.
34. Harrison TM, Mazet JK, Holekamp KE, et al. Antibodies to canine and feline viruses in spotted hyenas (*Crocuta crocuta*) in the Masai Mara National Reserve. *J Wildl Dis.* 2004;40:1–10.
35. Munson L, Marker L, Dubovi E, et al. Serosurvey of viral infections in free-ranging Namibian cheetahs (*Acinonyx jubatus*). *J Wildl Dis.* 2004;40:23–31.
36. Philippa JD, Leighton FA, Daoust PY, et al. Antibodies to selected pathogens in free-ranging terrestrial carnivores and marine mammals in Canada. *Vet Rec.* 2004;155:135–140.
37. Quigley KS, Evermann JF, Leathers CW, et al. Morbillivirus infection in a wild siberian tiger in the Russian Far East. *J Wildl Dis.* 2010;46:1252–1256.
38. Ramanathan A, Malik PK, Prasad G. Seroepizootiological survey for selected viral infections in captive Asiatic lions (*Panthera leo persica*) from western India. *J Zoo Wildl Med.* 2007;38:400–408.
39. Ramsauer S, Bay G, Meli M, et al. Seroprevalence of selected infectious agents in a free-ranging, low-density lion population in the Central Kalahari Game Reserves in Botswana. *Clin Vaccine Immunol.* 2007;14:808–810.
40. Junge RE, Bauman K, King M, et al. A serologic assessment of exposure to viral pathogens and *Leptospira* in an urban raccoon (*Procyon lotor*) population inhabiting a large zoological park. *J Zoo Wildl Med.* 2007;38:18–26.
41. Wood SL, Thomson GW, Haines DM. Canine distemper virus-like infection in a captive African lioness. *Can Vet J.* 1995;36:34–35.
42. Appel MJ. Canine distemper virus. In: Appel MJ, ed. *Virus Infections of Carnivores.* New York: Elsevier; 1987:133–159.
43. Gould DH, Fenner WR. Paramyxovirus-like nucleocapsids associated with encephalitis in a captive Siberian tiger. *J Am Vet Med Assoc.* 1983;183:1319–1322.
44. Fix ASRD, Hill HT. Feline panleukopenia virus and subsequent canine distemper virus infection in two snow leopards. *J Zoo Wildl Med.* 1989;20:273–281.
45. Meli ML, Simmler P, Cattori V, et al. Importance of canine distemper virus (CDV) infection in free-ranging Iberian lynxes (*Lynx pardinus*). *Vet Microbiol.* 2010;146:132–137.
46. Roelke-Parker ME, Munson L, Packer C, et al. A canine distemper virus epidemic in Serengeti lions (*Panthera leo*). *Nature.* 1996;379:441–445.
47. Gilbert M, Miquelle DG, Goodrich JM, et al. Estimating the potential impact of canine distemper virus on the Amur tiger population (*Panthera tigris altaica*) in Russia. *PloS One.* 2014;9:e110811.
48. Mourya DT, Yadav PD, Mohandas S, et al. Canine distemper virus in Asiatic lions of Gujarat State, India. *Emerg Infect Dis.* 2019;25:2128–2130.
49. Guiserix M, Bahi-Jaber N, Fouchet D, et al. The canine distemper epidemic in Serengeti: are lions victims of a new highly virulent canine distemper virus strain, or is pathogen circulation stochasticity to blame? *J Royal Soc, Interface.* 2007;4:1127–1134.
50. Morell V. Canine distemper virus. Serengeti's big cats going to the dogs. *Science.* 1994;264:1664.
51. Spencer JA, Bingham J, Heath R, et al. Presence of antibodies to canine distemper virus, canine parvovirus and canine adenovirus type 1 in free-ranging jackals (*Canis adustus* and *Canis mesomelas*) in Zimbabwe. *Onderstepoort J Vet Res.* 1999;66:251–253.
52. Appel MJ, Yates RA, Foley GL, et al. Canine distemper epizootic in lions, tigers, and leopards in North America. *J Vet Diagn Invest.* 1994;6:277–288.
53. Endo Y, Uema M, Miura R, et al. Prevalence of canine distemper virus, feline immunodeficiency virus and feline leukemia virus in captive African lions (*Panthera leo*) in Japan. *J Vet Med Sci.* 2004;66:1587–1589.
54. Georoff TA, Ramsay EC, Gyimesi ZS, et al. Review of canine distemper vaccination use and safety in North American captive large felids (*Panthera* spp.) from 2000 to 2017. *J Zoo Wildl Med.* 2020;50:778–789.
55. Appel MJ, Summers BA. Pathogenicity of morbilliviruses for terrestrial carnivores. *Vet Microbiol.* 1995;44:187–191.
56. Field HE, Breed AC, Shield J, et al. Epidemiological perspectives on Hendra virus infection in horses and flying foxes. *Aust Vet J.* 2007;85:268–270.
57. Middleton D. Hendra virus. *Vet Clin North Am Equine Pract.* 2014;30:579–589.

58. Hooper P, Zaki S, Daniels P, et al. Comparative pathology of the diseases caused by Hendra and Nipah viruses. *Microbes Infect.* 2001;3:315–322.
59. O'Sullivan JD, Allworth AM, Paterson DL, et al. Fatal encephalitis due to novel paramyxovirus transmitted from horses. *Lancet.* 1997;349:93–95.
60. Field HE. Hendra virus ecology and transmission. *Curr Opin Virol.* 2016;16:120–125.
61. Edson D, Field H, McMichael L, et al. Routes of Hendra virus excretion in naturally-infected flying-foxes: implications for viral transmission and spillover risk. *PLoS One.* 2015;10:e0140670.
62. Westbury HA, Hooper PT, Brouwer SL, et al. Susceptibility of cats to equine morbillivirus. *Aust Vet J.* 1996;74:132–134.
63. Williamson MM, Hooper PT, Selleck PW, et al. Transmission studies of Hendra virus (equine morbillivirus) in fruit bats, horses and cats. *Aust Vet J.* 1998;76:813–818.
64. Kirkland PD, Gabor M, Poe I, et al. Hendra virus infection in dog, Australia, 2013. *Emerg Infect Dis.* 2015;21:2182–2185.
65. Middleton DJ, Riddell S, Klein R, et al. Experimental Hendra virus infection of dogs: virus replication, shedding and potential for transmission. *Aust Vet J.* 2017;95:10–18.
66. Aditi SM. Nipah virus infection: a review. *Epidemiol Infect.* 2019;147:e95.
67. Amal NM, Lye MS, Ksiazek TG, et al. Risk factors for Nipah virus transmission, Port Dickson, Negeri Sembilan, Malaysia: results from a hospital-based case-control study. *Southeast Asian J Trop Med Public Health.* 2000;31:301–306.
68. Epstein JH, Abdul Rahman S, Zambriski JA, et al. Feral cats and risk for Nipah virus transmission. *Emerg Infect Dis.* 2006;12:1178–1179.
69. Middleton DJ, Westbury HA, Morrissy CJ, et al. Experimental Nipah virus infection in pigs and cats. *J Comp Pathol.* 2002;126:124–136.
70. Dimitrov DS, Wang LF. In utero transmission of Nipah virus: role played by pregnancy and vertical transmission in Henipavirus epidemiology. *J Infect Dis.* 2007;196:807–809.
71. Mungall BA, Middleton D, Crameri G, et al. Vertical transmission and fetal replication of Nipah virus in an experimentally infected cat. *J Infect Dis.* 2007;196:812–816.
72. McEachern JA, Bingham J, Crameri G, et al. A recombinant subunit vaccine formulation protects against lethal Nipah virus challenge in cats. *Vaccine.* 2008;26:3842–3852.
73. Mungall BA, Middleton D, Crameri G, et al. Feline model of acute Nipah virus infection and protection with a soluble glycoprotein-based subunit vaccine. *J Virol.* 2006;80:12293–12302.
74. Parashar UD, Sunn LM, Ong F, et al. Case-control study of risk factors for human infection with a new zoonotic paramyxovirus, Nipah virus, during a 1998-1999 outbreak of severe encephalitis in Malaysia. *J Infect Dis.* 2000;181:1755–1759.
75. Field H, Young P, Yob JM, et al. The natural history of Hendra and Nipah viruses. *Microbes Infect.* 2001;3:307–314.
76. Mills JN, Alim AN, Bunning ML, et al. Nipah virus infection in dogs, Malaysia, 1999. *Emerg Infect Dis.* 2009;15:950–952.
77. Latner DR, Hickman CJ. Remembering mumps. *PLoS Pathog.* 2015;11:e1004791.
78. Mitten RW, Fleming C, Gooey PD. Concurrent parotiditis (mumps) in a child and a dog. *Aust Vet J.* 1982;58:39.
79. Cuadrado RR. An epidemiological study on parainfluenza, DA and mumps virus infections in domestic animals in New England. *Bull World Health Organ.* 1965;33:803–808.
80. Choi KM. Reemergence of mumps. *Korean J Pediatr.* 2010;53:623–628.
81. Rubin S, Eckhaus M, Rennick LJ, et al. Molecular biology, pathogenesis and pathology of mumps virus. *J Pathol.* 2015;235:242–252.
82. Greene CE. Feline paramyxovirus encephalomyelitis. In: Greene CE, ed. *Infectious Diseases of the Dog and Cat.* 2nd ed. Philadelphia: WB Saunders; 1990:360–362.
83. Greene CE, Lutz H. Feline paramyxovirus infections. In: Greene CE, ed. *Infectious Diseases of the Dog and Cat.* 2nd ed. Philadelphia: WB Saunders; 1998:107–109.

38

Feline Poxvirus Infections

Conor O'Halloran

KEY POINTS

- First Described: Feline poxvirus infection was first described in the United Kingdom in 1978.[1–3]
- Causes: Poxviruses (family *Poxviridae*, genus *Orthopoxvirus*). Cowpox virus infection is by far the most frequently reported poxviral infection of both cats and dogs. Other poxvirus infections have also rarely been described in pets.[4,5]
- Affected Hosts: Cats, less often dogs, and a variety of other mammalian host species.
- Geographic Distribution: Cowpox virus is limited to Europe and Asia; infections with other poxviruses have been described in North America.
- Mode of Transmission: Entry through a break in the skin.
- Major Clinical Signs: Single or multiple, papular, and crusted skin lesions with fever, lethargy, hyporexia, and signs of pneumonia can also occur in affected cats.
- Differential Diagnoses: Allergic dermatitis, facial dermatitis caused by FHV-1, nocardiosis, mycobacteriosis, cutaneous lymphoma, autoimmune dermatoses such as pemphigus foliaceus, cutaneous drug reactions.
- Human Health Significance: Many poxviruses, including cowpox and orf viruses, are zoonotic, and owners of affected animals need to be advised of the threat to their health.

ETIOLOGIC AGENT AND EPIDEMIOLOGY

Cowpox virus is a member of the *Orthopoxvirus* genus within the family *Poxviridae*, which are large, enveloped, double-stranded DNA viruses. Other orthopoxviruses include smallpox virus (now eradicated), vaccinia virus (the smallpox vaccine virus), monkeypox virus (which is endemic to central Africa but was recently introduced to, and has since been eradicated from, North America), and a range of other mammalian orthopoxviruses.[1,2,4–9] All orthopoxviruses are closely related genetically and antigenically; therefore, vaccinia virus can be used to immunize against all orthopoxvirus infections. Cowpox virus has the largest genome of all the orthopoxviruses. Different strains of cowpox virus exist, as determined by both biologic characteristics and nucleotide sequence.[8,10–12] Whether these relate to geographic variation in the virus (and therefore its main hosts and pathogenicity) or a range of independent virus species is still to be determined. For the purpose of this chapter, they are regarded as a single viral species.

Despite its name and its original isolation from cows, cowpox is rarely described in cattle; rather, cowpox virus circulates primarily in wild rodents.[13,14] Cowpox virus has a wide incidental host range that includes not only rodents, cats, dogs, cattle, and humans but also a variety of captive wildlife mammals.[1,2,4,13,14] The main route of transmission among rodents is not known, although, as for many orthopoxviruses, the respiratory route is probably important.[1,2,4,6,8] In most incidental hosts, which include domestic animals and humans, the most frequent route of infection is through a break in the skin which gives rise to the "primary" lesion. The main reservoirs of cowpox virus are believed to be bank voles (*Myodes glareolus*), field voles (*Microtus agrestis*) and, to a slightly lesser extent, wood mice (*Apodemus sylvaticus*).[1,14] As these rodent species undergo annual population cycles, breeding mainly in the summer and fall months, viral transmission and prevalence has strong seasonality. Therefore, transmission to accidental hosts such as cats, dogs, people, and zoo animals also occurs mainly (but not exclusively) in the late summer, fall, and early winter.[4]

Cats probably become infected directly from rodent hunting, whereas infection in other species is often acquired from an amplifying intermediate host.[1,2] These are incidental hosts in which the virus replicates to higher titers than in the reservoir rodent hosts; thus, they bridge the epidemiologic gap between the reservoir and the host of interest. The main amplifying hosts for human cases of cowpox virus infection are the domestic cat (and, in the past, possibly cattle), followed by peri-domestic rodent species such as rats.[1,2,4,7] Rats can also be a source of infection for captive wildlife species. The virus is very hardy and survives in scabs for weeks or months, including in the environment, where it may be a source of human infection.

Reports of natural orthopoxvirus infection in wild or domestic dogs are rare. A natural orthopoxvirus infection, characterized by ulcerative dermatitis at the site of a suspected rat bite, was identified in a domestic dog in the United Kingdom.[15] This infection was likely caused by cowpox, because this has been the only orthopoxvirus in the United Kingdom since smallpox was eradicated.[8] Specific antibodies were found in 6% to 20% of foxes in Germany.[16,17] Intradermal inoculation of 2×10^5 plaque-forming units of cowpox virus into red foxes (*Vulpes vulpes*) produced mild skin lesions with minimal viral replication, and no lesions were found after oral dose administration of virus.[16,17] Another orthopoxvirus, murine ectromelia, has caused congenital disease in farm-raised silver foxes (*Vulpes* winter coat), blue foxes (*Alopex lagopus* winter coat), and mink (*Mustela vison*) in the Czech Republic.[18] A novel orthopoxvirus was described in 2018 in a 6-month-old cat from Italy with severe and rapidly progressing cutaneous disease that appeared to be more closely related to this virus than to cowpox virus.[5]

CLINICAL FEATURES

Pathogenesis and Clinical Signs

The outcome of feline infection is likely to depend on the viral strain, route and site of infection, dose of inoculated virus, and the concurrent presence of systemic immunosuppression, such as infection with exogenous retrovirus infections (FIV or FeLV) or, critically, the administration of systemic glucocorticoids.[1,2,4,8,19] In many hosts, such as humans, dogs, and cattle, the primary lesion of cowpox virus infection, plus perhaps some limited virus replication in draining lymph nodes, may be as far as disease progresses. In cats and many captive wild mammalian species, however, the virus replicates in monocytes and macrophages and spreads to multiple organs, particularly the lungs and the spleen. Here, the virus replicates further, giving rise to a secondary viremia, which is often associated with pyrexia and mild or occasionally severe systemic signs. In all species, infection most commonly presents externally as focal cutaneous lesions, which heal spontaneously, with no systemic signs. During the viremic period, virus can be isolated from the respiratory tract. Fatal necrotizing pneumonia has been described.[10]

The strain of the virus may also influence the clinical severity of disease.[20] For example, some cats within the United Kingdom were seen with large areas of focal dermal necrosis (eschars) with extensive erythema and edema, which may represent infection with a particularly virulent strain.

In many captive wild Felidae, pneumonia is more common than in domestic cats, and mortality is high.[21–23] Similarly, elephants and rhinoceroses in central European zoos develop severe systemic disease and often die—this can be such a severe disease that elephants are vaccinated in many European zoological parks. Reports of fatal cowpox in captive primates are rare, but high rates of subclinical seroconversion in other primate populations have been reported.[21–23] In wild rodent reservoir hosts, clinical signs are absent or, at least, subtle.[13,14] Population-level studies of naturally infected voles and mice show that infection may be associated with decreased fecundity and decreased survival. When lesions are seen in rodents, they are often in incidental rodent hosts such as rats.

Physical Examination Findings

The skin lesions first develop as papules, which become ulcers up to 1 cm in diameter that crust over and heal over 4 to 6 weeks (Fig. 38.1A and B). This leaves small patches of alopecia until the hair regrows. Lesions are most often found on the head, neck, or forelimbs. In cats such as Siamese breeds, the haircoat may grow back a darker color, and scars are often visible for years in cats if they are clipped. Although unproven, it has been suggested that some strains of cowpox virus may have increased pathogenicity, with infection culminating in large areas of cellulitis, cutaneous ulceration, and/or necrosis (Fig. 38.1C).[10,20]

DIAGNOSIS

Definitive diagnosis of poxvirus infections requires laboratory identification of the causative virus.[13,20,24,25] In Europe, where cowpox virus is endemic, clinical signs combined with identification of an orthopoxvirus frequently suffice to make a diagnosis. Elsewhere, however, more extensive laboratory tests, including sequence analysis, may be required to specifically identify the causative virus. Histopathology of biopsy specimens also yields characteristic findings that can raise strong suspicion for poxvirus infection.[10] Diagnostic test options are summarized in Table 38.1.

Microbiologic Tests

Cell Culture

The best specimens to collect for virus isolation are fresh skin lesions, although virus can be found in crusts from healing lesions for several weeks. No special transport media are required and specimens can be transported in any sterile container at room temperature.[24] The virus replicates in a variety of both feline and non-feline cell lines generating an obvious CPE, usually within 24 to 76 hours. Identification of the virus can then be performed using immunostaining or PCR assay and sequencing.

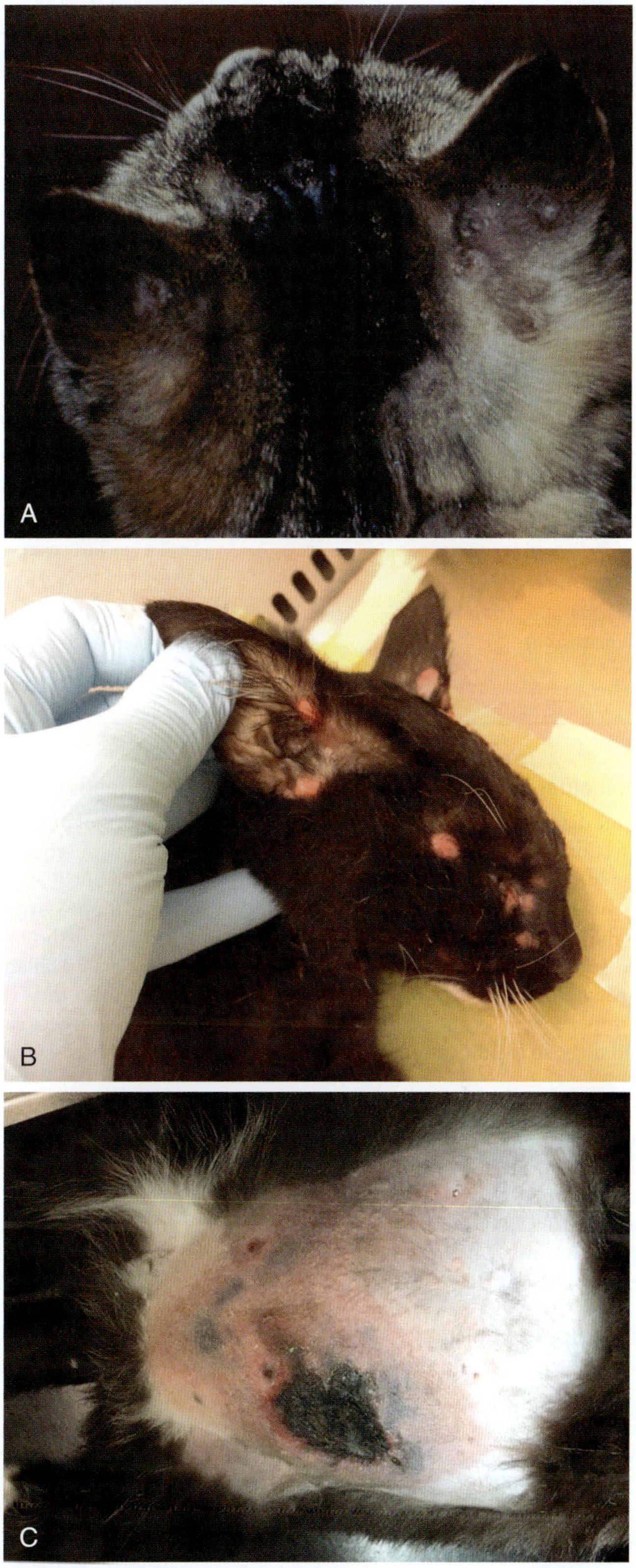

Fig. 38.1 (A and B) Secondary papules and crusted skin lesions in cats with cowpox virus infection. (C) Cat with more severe manifestation of cowpox virus infection, with a large area of cutaneous necrosis.

Electron microscopy can identify virus particles within skin lesions, is a more rapid approach to diagnosis than cell culture and is fairly sensitive (Fig. 38.2).[24] Negative-stained suspensions of skin lesion material allow typical orthopoxvirus particles to be seen in most cases.

TABLE 38.1 Diagnostic Assays Available for Poxvirus Infections

Assay	Specimen Type	Target	Performance
Virus isolation	Skin biopsies, crusts	Poxviruses	May not be widely available in some regions. Sensitive for diagnosis of orthopoxviruses
Polymerase chain reaction (PCR)	Skin biopsies, crusts	Poxvirus DNA	Sensitivity and specificity may vary depending on assay design; may not differentiate between orthopoxviruses. Availability on a commercial basis may be limited in some regions
Histopathology	Skin biopsies, necropsy specimens	Poxvirus inclusions	Confirmation of poxvirus infection requires immunohistochemistry or PCR
Electron microscopy	Skin crusts	Virus particles	May not be widely available, turnaround time can be slow, and may be expensive

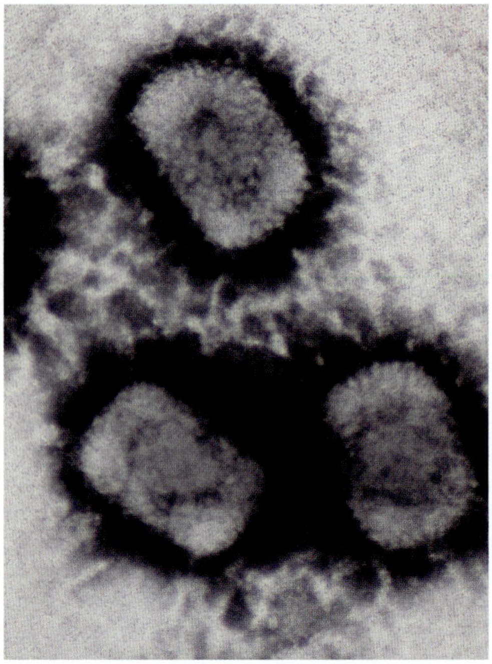

Fig. 38.2 Electron micrograph of a cowpox virus particle. In contrast, parapoxviruses have the appearance of a new ball of yarn, with thread-like surface tubules arranged in a criss-cross fashion.

Molecular Diagnosis Using Nucleic Acid–Based Testing

Some diagnostic laboratories offer PCR assays for diagnosis of poxvirus infection, which can be both sensitive and, if combined with sequencing, specific. Orthopoxviruses are so similar genetically that PCR assays targeted at many orthopoxvirus genes only identify orthopoxviruses to the genus level.[24] PCR assays that differentiate between orthopoxvirus species have been described, but such assays tend to be available through research or other specialist laboratories. Of course, in much of Europe, cowpox virus is the only orthopoxvirus known to infect cats and dogs, so identification to the species level is often not necessary.

Serologic Diagnosis

Serum assays including virus neutralization, HI, complement fixation, and ELISA can detect antibody to orthopoxvirus, but a rising titer is required to prove active infection.[24] However, the prevalence of orthopoxvirus antibodies in domestic cats in Europe is usually only 1% to 2%, so a consistent clinical history combined with an antibody titer is reasonably specific.[8]

Pathologic Findings

Histopathologic Findings

Characteristic histopathologic findings include suppurative dermatitis with evidence of necrosis and ulceration.[10] Epithelial hyperplasia, ballooning degeneration of keratinocytes and large, cytoplasmic eosinophilic viral inclusion bodies within keratinocytes are present (Fig. 38.3). IHC has been used to identify intracellular orthopoxvirus antigen in epidermal and follicular cells.[10]

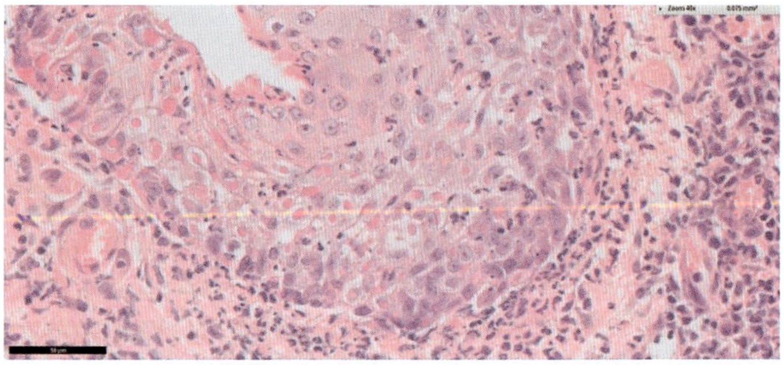

Fig. 38.3 Histopathology of a feline poxvirus lesion that shows epithelial hyperplasia and large numbers of eosinophilic intracytoplasmic inclusion bodies.

TREATMENT

Treatment is generally supportive as there are no antiviral drugs licensed to treat cowpox infections. Broad-spectrum antibacterials are recommended to treat secondary bacterial infections, if identified, and additional nonspecific therapy, including fluids, may be necessary. Glucocorticoids are considered contraindicated because they may exacerbate the condition. There appears to be an association between administration of glucocorticoids and progression of disease from limited skin lesions to pulmonary disease, which may be severe and even fatal.

Historically, most cats with cowpox-induced pneumonia died despite supportive treatment. In a recent case series, recombinant feline interferon-omega (rfIFN–ω, Virbagen Omega, Virbac, France) was used in four cats at a dose of 1 million international units (IU) given either IV or SC for 3 to 5 days (see Chapter 9).[26,27] Two of the cats with severe pneumonia survived. As this drug has been shown to be safe to use in cats, it could be considered for treatment of more severe cases. Other antiviral drugs could also be considered. The most promising antiviral in cats is famciclovir for the treatment of FHV-1 infections, but its efficacy against cowpox virus is unknown.[28] Vidarabine has activity against poxviruses *in vitro*, and cidofovir has broad-spectrum activity against poxviruses in humans, and cowpoxvirus in particular *in vitro* (see Chapter 9).[29,30] Cidofovir was also shown to protect mice from a lethal cowpox challenge. However, more research in cats is needed as this drug has been shown to be nephrotoxic in humans.

PUBLIC HEALTH ASPECTS

Human cowpox is rare (with one or two cases occurring each year in the United Kingdom), but cats are thought to be the source of more than 50% of these cases.[7,9] The risk of cat-to-human transmission is small if basic hygiene precautions are taken, and so this illness does not warrant euthanasia of the cat on public health grounds.

CASE EXAMPLE

Signalment

"Yogi," a 9-year-old entire male domestic shorthaired cat from Lancaster, Lancashire, United Kingdom.

History

Yogi was examined in September following the development of a swollen lateral digit of the left thoracic limb noted by owner over the last 3 days. The cat was in good general health, up to date with all routine parasite prevention and core vaccinations, and was an avid rodent hunter.

Physical Examination

The digit was swollen and erythematous but was not associated with lameness. The associated superficial cervical lymph node was mildly enlarged. Multiple, non-painful, haired crusts were present over the dorsum, but no other clinical abnormalities were detected. The patient was discharged with oral meloxicam for 7 days.

At the week recheck appointment, a number of crusts had fallen away and the alopecic areas oozed a serous to purulent discharge. Histopathology of punch biopsies revealed severe multifocal follicular dermatitis. The inflammatory cells present mainly consisted of neutrophils, macrophages, and fewer lymphocytes and plasma cells. There was multifocal ulceration of the overlying epidermis adjacent to moderately hyperplastic areas. Large eosinophilic intracytoplasmic inclusion bodies were seen in the epidermal and follicular epithelial cells characteristic of poxvirus infection.

Diagnosis

Poxvirus infection.

Treatment

Amoxicillin-clavulanic acid was initially prescribed to treat secondary bacterial pyoderma, but this was switched to cefovecin because the cat could not be medicated orally. IFN-ω (1 million U/kg IV q24h for 3 days) was also administered. The cat was monitored as an outpatient over 6 weeks, during which time there was complete resolution of the clinical signs.

SUGGESTED READINGS

Lanave G, Dowgier G, Decaro N, et al. Novel orthopoxvirus and lethal disease in cat, Italy. *Emerg Infect Dis.* 2018;24:1665–1673.

Jungwirth N, Puff C, Koster K, et al. Atypical cowpox virus infection in a series of cats. *J Comp Pathol.* 2018;158:71–76.

O'Halloran C, Del-Pozo J, Breheny C, et al. Unusual presentations of feline cowpox. *Vet Rec.* 2016;179:442–443.

REFERENCES

1. Bennett M, Gaskell CJ, Baxby D, et al. Feline cowpox virus infection. *J Small Anim Pract.* 1990;31:167–173.
2. Thomsett LR. Cowpox in cats. *J Small Anim Pract.* 1989;30:236–241.
3. Thomsett LR, Baxby D, Denham EM. Cowpox in the domestic cat. *Vet Rec.* 1978;103:567.
4. Chomel BB. Emerging and re-emerging zoonoses of dogs and cats. *Animals (Basel).* 2014;4:434–445.
5. Lanave G, Dowgier G, Decaro N, et al. Novel orthopoxvirus and lethal disease in cat, Italy. *Emerg Infect Dis.* 2018;24:1665–1673.
6. Backel K, Cain C. Skin as a marker of general feline health: cutaneous manifestations of infectious disease. *J Fel Med Surg.* 2017;19:1149–1165.
7. Baxby D, Bennett M. Low risk from feline cowpox. *Lancet.* 1990;336:1070–1071.
8. Naidoo J, Baxby D, Bennett M, et al. Characterization of orthopoxviruses isolated from feline infections in Britain. *Arch Virol.* 1992;125:261–272.
9. Schulze C, Alex M, Schirrmeier H, et al. Generalized fatal cowpox virus infection in a cat with transmission to a human contact case. *Zoonoses Public Health.* 2007;54:31–37.
10. Jungwirth N, Puff C, Koster K, et al. Atypical cowpox virus infection in a series of cats. *J Comp Pathol.* 2018;158:71–76.
11. Kaysser P, von Bomhard W, Dobrzykowski L, et al. Genetic diversity of feline cowpox virus, Germany 2000-2008. *Vet Microbiol.* 2010;141:282–288.
12. Tryland M, Sandvik T, Holtet L, et al. Antibodies to orthopoxvirus in domestic cats in Norway. *Vet Rec.* 1998;143:105–109.
13. Bennett M, Smith GL, Baxby D. Cowpox virus. In: Mahy BWJ, Regenmortel MHVV, eds. *Encyclopedia of Virology.* 3rd ed. Oxford: Academic Press; 2008.
14. Crouch AC, Baxby D, McCracken CM, et al. Serological evidence for the reservoir hosts of cowpox virus in British wildlife. *Epidemiol Infect.* 1995;115:185–191.
15. von Bomhard W, Mauldin EA, Breuer W, et al. Localized cowpox infection in a 5-month-old Rottweiler. *Vet Dermatol.* 2011;22:111–114.
16. Henning K, Czerny CP, Meyer H, et al. A seroepidemiological survey for orthopox virus in the red fox (*Vulpes vulpes*). *Vet Microbiol.* 1995;43:251–259.
17. Muller T, Henning K, Kramer M, et al. Seroprevalence of orthopox virus specific antibodies in red foxes (*Vulpes vulpes*) in the Federal State Brandenburg, Germany. *J Wildl Dis.* 1996;32:348–353.
18. Mahnel H, Holejsovsky J, Bartak P, et al. Congenital "ectromelia" in fur-bearing animals caused by Orthopoxvirus muris. *Tierarztl Prax.* 1993;21:469–472.
19. Bennett M, Gaskell CJ, Gaskell RM, et al. Poxvirus infection in the domestic cat: some clinical and epidemiological observations. *Vet Rec.* 1986;118:387–390.
20. O'Halloran C, Del-Pozo J, Breheny C, et al. Unusual presentations of feline cowpox. *Vet Rec.* 2016;179:442–443.
21. Baxby D, Ashton DG, Jones D, et al. Cowpox virus infection in unusual hosts. *Vet Rec.* 1979;104:175.
22. Bennett M, Baxby D. Cowpox. *J Med Microbiol.* 1996;45:157–158.
23. Kurth A, Nitsche A. Cowpox in zoo animals. In: Miller RE, Fowler ME, eds. *Fowler's Zoo and Wild Animal Medicine: Current Therapy.* St Louis: Elsevier Saunders; 2011:32–37.
24. Bennett M, Baxby D, Gaskell RM. The laboratory diagnosis of Orthopoxvirus infection in the domestic cat. *J Small Anim Pract.* 1985;26:653–661.
25. Ouschan C, Rest J, Peters S. Cowpox virus infection in a cat in Southwest Germany? A case presentation. *Wiener Tierarztliche Monatsschrift.* 2013;100:326–330.
26. McInerney J, Papasouliotis K, Simpson K, et al. Pulmonary cowpox in cats: five cases. *J Feline Med Surg.* 2016;18:518–525.
27. Li SF, Zhao FR, Shao JJ, et al. Interferon-omega: Current status in clinical applications. *Int Immunopharmacol.* 2017;52:253–260.
28. De Clercq E. Highlights in the discovery of antiviral drugs: a personal retrospective. *J Med Chem.* 2010;53:1438–1450.
29. De Clercq E. Potential of acyclic nucleoside phosphonates in the treatment of DNA virus and retrovirus infections. *Expert Rev Anti Infect Ther.* 2003;1:21–43.
30. De Clercq E. Clinical potential of the acyclic nucleoside phosphonates cidofovir, adefovir, and tenofovir in treatment of DNA virus and retrovirus infections. *Clin Microbiol Rev.* 2003;16:569–596.

39

Pseudorabies

Diana Henke, Marc Vandevelde

KEY POINTS

- First Described: 1902 (Hungary, Aujeszky).[1]
- Cause: Suid (porcine) herpesvirus-1 (family *Herpesviridae*, subfamily *Alphaherpesvirinae*, genus *Varicellovirus*).
- Affected Hosts: Domestic and feral swine, cattle, horses, sheep, goats, dogs, cats, bears, raccoons, foxes, hedgehogs, opossums, deer, Florida panther, jackals, coyotes, some nonhuman primates (macaques, marmosets), chickens, pigeons, geese, ducks, buzzards, sparrow hawks, rabbits, guinea pigs, rats and mice.
- Geographic Distribution: Worldwide.
- Major Clinical Signs: Fever, lethargy, hypersalivation, muscle stiffness, variable facial pruritis, ataxia, behavioral changes, vomiting, diarrhea, respiratory distress.
- Differential Diagnoses: Rabies, canine distemper, toxicoses (e.g., organophosphates, heavy metals, ethylene glycol, strychnine).
- Human Health Significance: Some cases of pseudorabies virus-induced encephalitis have been reported in humans.

ETIOLOGIC AGENT AND EPIDEMIOLOGY

Pseudorabies virus (PRV), also known as Aujeszky's disease virus or suid (porcine) herpesvirus-1 (SuHV-1), is an enveloped DNA virus, which belongs to the family *Herpesviridae*, subfamily *Alphaherpesviridae*, and genus *Varicellovirus*.[2] As with other herpesviruses, PRV can cause latent infection, with viral DNA being incorporated into the host cell genome. The virus is relatively resistant to environmental factors and can survive outside the host for several months under favorable climatic conditions. Survival of PRV depends on temperature (10 days at 37°C, 40 days at 25°C) and pH (optimum, 7), and it is quickly inactivated by drying and exposure to ultraviolet light.[3] The molecular biology of PRV has been extensively studied because PRV is probably one of the most used viruses in experimental neuroscience.[4]

Pseudorabies, the disease caused by PRV (also known as *Aujeszky's disease*, *mad itch*, and *infectious bulbar paralysis*) occurs in most countries of the world, except Australia, and has been responsible for massive economic losses to the swine industry.[5,6] The name pseudorabies was applied because the clinical signs caused by the virus in rabbits resembled those of rabies. In swine, clinical signs depend on the age at exposure and virus strain. Subclinical infections and shedding occur commonly. When they do develop signs, older pigs typically develop respiratory disease. Encephalitis occurs in adult pigs infected with virulent strains or in piglets; reproductive disease and fetal loss occurs in pregnant sows. Recovered pigs develop latent infection of neuronal tissues with reactivation and shedding of virus in nasal secretions following stress. In the past, clinical disease outbreaks have been reported in several European, South American, and Asian countries. Restricted endemic areas are in the United States, Mexico, Brazil, and China. However, a PRV surveillance scheme is lacking in many countries. Continuous large-scale vaccination, removal of wild-type infected animals, followed by elimination of all PRV antibody-positive animals resulted in the eradication of the disease from domestic pigs in large parts of continental Europe (including Finland, Sweden, Norway, the Netherlands, Denmark, Austria, Switzerland, Germany, Hungary, Slovakia), the United Kingdom, Mexico, Canada, the United States, and New Zealand.[7–10]

Although many mammalian species are susceptible to infection with PRV, it is predominantly a problem in pigs, the main reservoir of the virus.[5,6] However, cattle, goats, sheep, dogs, and cats are sporadically affected.[11–18] It does not appear to affect humans; most reports of possible human infection have been circumstantial and not documented. Infection frequently is subclinical in pigs because they have become well adapted to the virus. The disease is spread by commercial movement of infected pigs or contaminated pork products. Venereal transmission occurs when infected boars shed PRV in semen. Although wild animals such as Iberian lynx, raccoons, panthers,[19–21] and rodents may act as transient reservoirs, they are not important in maintaining the disease in nature. Their role is limited to temporary local spread of virus within enzootic areas. However, in many European countries, the United States, Brazil, and Japan, PRV infection is endemic in wild boars with strongly varying seroprevalences ranging from 0 to 100%, creating a reservoir for the virus.[22–26]

PRV infection in dogs and cats is thought to occur only in areas where the disease is enzootic in pigs. Such interaction has been documented by molecular biologic studies on viral isolates.[27,28] In fact, the occurrence of typical pseudorabies signs in companion animals can be the first indication that the disease is enzootic in the local pig population. Companion animals almost invariably are infected as a result of consuming contaminated raw pork.[12,29] Dogs also have developed pseudorabies after having bitten infected pigs.[30] Direct dog-to-dog spread has not been shown to occur.[31] However, one report described an outbreak in animals without direct contact with swine. Isolated strains of PRV showed considerable differences in DNA patterns to vaccine and isolated strains obtained from pigs in the same region.[11] Feline and canine cases have been reported in Poland, Italy, Austria, Argentina, Germany, Northern Ireland, China, Japan, and the southern United States (Florida, Oklahoma, Arkansas, Alabama).[11,12,14,15,28,30,32–34] These are primarily hunting dogs that contact wild swine,[35–39] which has followed global expansion in wild swine populations; disease in dogs may be more likely to occur in regions that have dense populations of wild swine, such as southern parts of the United States (Fig. 39.1) and regions of Europe such as Germany, France, Spain, Poland, and the Czech Republic.[37] Dogs that reside on swine farms may

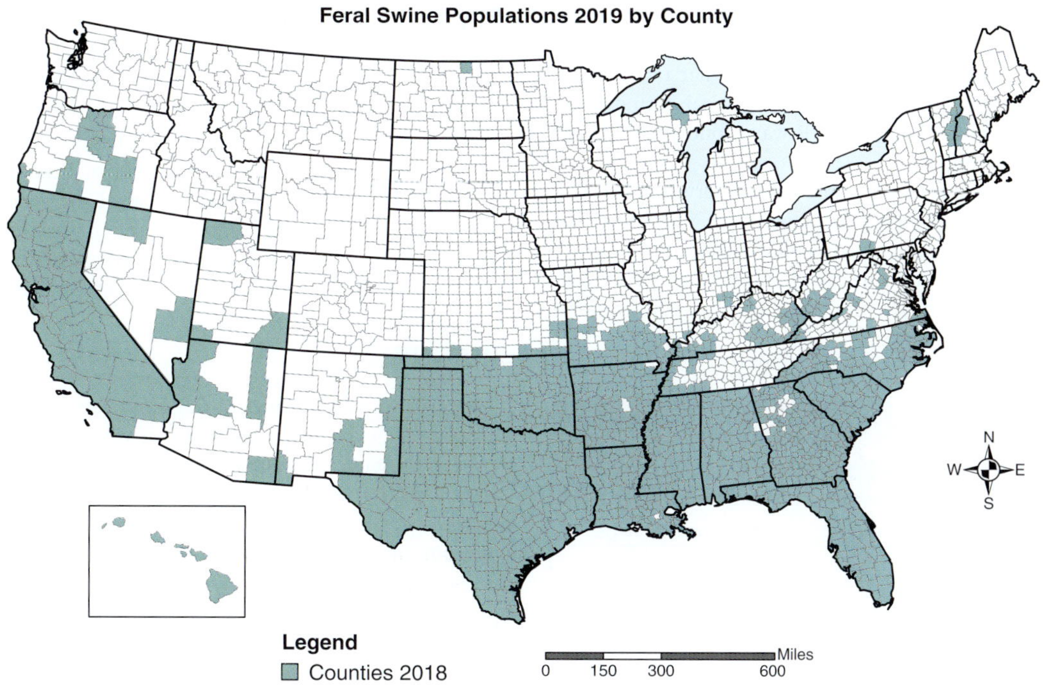

Fig. 39.1 Geographic distribution of wild swine in the United States. (From United States Department of Agriculture Animal and Plant Health Inspection Service; https://www.aphis.usda.gov.)

also become infected.[40] In some reports, packs of dogs have become infected after consumption of uncooked offal from infected pigs or pig carcasses.[41,42] Dogs of any age, sex, and breed can be affected, and dog-to-dog transmission does not occur, presumably because dogs do not shed sufficient virus to infect other hosts. Cats have the potential to be infected after ingestion of pork waste or infected rodents, but reports of naturally occurring Aujeszky's disease are extremely rare.[43] Because subclinical infections and nonspecific signs of disease are common in swine, identification of pseudorabies in dogs may be the first indication that disease is present in a swine herd or wild swine populations.

CLINICAL FEATURES

Pathogenesis and Clinical Signs

SuHV-1 is shed in the saliva and nasal discharges of swine, and transmission can occur by direct contact with these discharges, contact with aerosols from swine, and ingestion of infected swine carcasses or other infected animals, especially wild animals. The virus can survive on fomites and in carcasses for several weeks. Naturally acquired infection in dogs and cats occurs after ingestion of the virus, although a similar sequence of events occurs after parenteral inoculation of virus. PRV enters the nerve endings at the inoculation site and travels in retrograde fashion via the axoplasm of the nerve fibers to the brain, which results in ganglioneuritis and encephalitis. Infection can also lead to ganglioneuritis of the cardiac autonomic plexuses with associated myocardial degeneration[44] and degeneration of intestinal myenteric ganglia.[42] Clinical signs appear rapidly after a short incubation period that typically ranges from 1 to 6 days, but incubation periods up to 10 days have been reported.[41] Experimental studies in orally infected cats have shown that PRV replicates in the tonsils and travels from the oral mucosa via the sensory branches of the 9th and 10th cranial nerves to the nucleus tractus solitarius and area postrema in the medulla oblongata.[45] The 5th cranial nerve has been less frequently involved. Experimental infections in rats have shown that PRV spreads in a highly specific manner through synaptic connections.[46,47] Viral–cellular interactions have been studied in great detail in experimental models.[4]

The majority of dogs and cats that become infected develop severe clinical signs. The onset of clinical illness is hyperacute, and signs progress rapidly until death occurs (possibly as a result of acute myocarditis); the total course rarely lasts longer than 48 hours. With very few exceptions, pseudorabies is always fatal in dogs. Cats may be somewhat more resistant but have rarely recovered from the disease. The initial sign often noted by the owner is a change in behavior, such as inactivity, lethargy, and indifference, although some animals become aggressive or restless. Dyspnea; diarrhea, which may be hemorrhagic (e.g., hematemesis or melena); and vomiting are occasionally seen (Table 39.1). The dyspnea is often caused by severe pulmonary edema. Body temperature may be normal or abnormal, and hypersalivation is common. However, the most characteristic sign is intense pruritus, which usually occurs in the head region and rarely occurs in other areas such as the neck and shoulders. Affected dogs violently scratch their faces and ears and rub their heads against the floor or walls. One side of the head and neck may become swollen. Self-mutilation results in erythema, excoriation, and ulceration of the skin and underlying tissues (Fig. 39.2A and B). The scratching becomes increasingly frantic and may end in generalized seizures. Most of the other neurologic signs observed in PRV infection refer to lesions in the lower brainstem and consist of one or several deficits in cranial nerve function. These deficits are usually unilateral and include anisocoria, mydriasis, lack of direct or consensual pupillary light reflexes, trismus, paresis and paralysis of the facial muscles, head tilt, inability to swallow, and vocal changes.[28] Anisocoria and a hoarse voice are considered to be highly consistent signs in the cat. Less commonly observed neurologic signs include behavioral abnormalities such as aggression, generalized hyperesthesia, head pressing, and generalized seizures. The latter often occur as sequelae to frantic scratching. Paresis and paralysis of the limbs are sometimes noted shortly before death. Although less common, in some cats, death has been preceded predominantly by acute GI signs. Arrhythmias may occur as a result of myocarditis.[14,48,49] A variety of cardiac arrhythmias have been reported in experimentally infected dogs, which have included ventricular premature complexes, ventricular tachycardia, sinus arrest, atrial tachycardia, atrial fibrillation, wandering pacemaker, second-degree heart block, T- and P-wave abnormalities, and atrioventricular dissociation.

An atypical course of the disease has also been observed in cats that died suddenly without developing neurologic signs.[50] Pruritus has been absent in some cases of spontaneous PRV infection in dogs[15,51] and in experimental oral infection in cats.[45] In one case series, only 18% of dogs exhibited facial pruritis.[52] GI signs have been the predominant feature of some infected dogs.

TABLE 39.1 Clinical Signs Reported in a Retrospective Study of 25 Dogs with Pseudorabies from the United States[53]

Clinical Sign	Percentage Of Affected Dogs
Ptyalism	100
Anorexia	84
Ataxia	76
Wandering	64
Tachypnea	64
Dyspnea	60
Vocalization	56
Pruritis	52
Neck stiffness	48
Vomiting	36
Muscle spasms	36
Aggression	36
Trismus	28
Dysphagia	24
Abnormal pupillary light responses	20
Seizures	16
Mydriasis	12

Physical Examination Findings

Physical examination findings include lethargy, hypersalivation, dehydration, muscle stiffness, tachypnea or respiratory difficulty, and facial pruritis, excoriations, and edema due to self-trauma (see Fig. 39.2). Other neurologic signs that may be detected include ataxia, head tilt, circling, hyperesthesia, behavioral abnormalities, anisocoria, mydriasis, nystagmus, slow or absent pupillary light responses, recumbency, and coma. Fever may be identified early in the course of infection (up to 108°F),[53] but terminally, hypothermia may occur. A variety of cardiac arrhythmias may also be identified on physical examination.

DIAGNOSIS

Diagnosis of pseudorabies in dogs and cats is based on a compatible history (i.e., exposure to domestic or wild swine in regions where the virus is present), suggestive clinical signs, and histopathology and/or virus detection methods such as IFA staining, virus isolation, or PCR on tissues collected at necropsy (Table 39.2). Antemortem diagnosis of pseudorabies in dogs and cats using virus detection methods has not yet been described.

Laboratory Abnormalities

Hematologic or biochemical abnormalities are not found in pseudorabies. Electrocardiographic findings may include cardiac arrhythmias.[54] CSF may show increased protein concentration and mononuclear pleocytosis. This finding is strongly indicative of viral encephalitis but is not specific for pseudorabies.

Microbiologic Tests

Serologic Diagnosis

Virus neutralization, immunodiffusion, latex agglutination test, and ELISA methods commonly are used to detect serum antibody to PRV in pigs. Serologic studies have been valuable in determining the prevalence of disease in pig populations.[22] Serology has not been useful for antemortem diagnosis in dogs and cats. This likely reflects the rapid course of disease and insufficient time for antibody responses to develop.

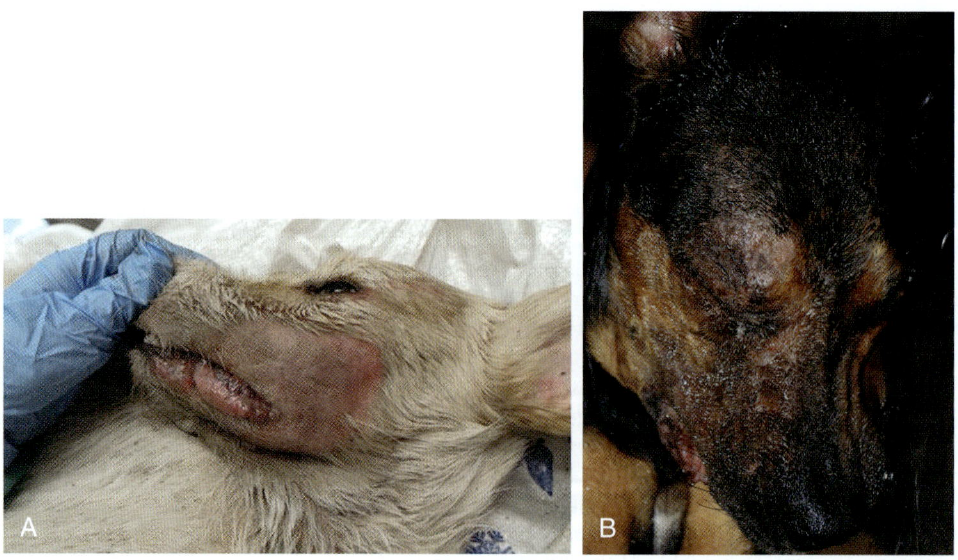

Fig. 39.2 (A and B) Dogs with pseudorabies and self-mutilation injuries. (A, From Ciarello FP, Moreno A, Miragliotta N, et al. Aujeszky's disease in hunting dogs after the ingestion of wild boar raw meat in Sicily (Italy): clinical, diagnostic and phylogenetic features. *BMC Vet Res* 18, 27 (2022). https://doi.org/10.1186/s12917-022-03138-2; B, From Cramer SD, Campbell GA, Njaa BL, et al. Pseudorabies virus infection in Oklahoma hunting dogs. *J Vet Diagn Invest.* 2011;23:915–923.)

TABLE 39.2 Diagnostic Assays Available for Pseudorabies in Dogs and Cats

Assay	Specimen Type	Target	Performance
Histopathology	Usually necropsy specimens, especially brainstem	Nonsuppurative meningoencephalitis with weakly eosinophilic intranuclear inclusions; SuHV-1 antigen with IHC, IFA, or DNA with *in situ* hybridization	Used for postmortem diagnosis.
Polymerase chain reaction (PCR)	CNS, tonsils, possibly self-traumatized skin biopsies or tonsillar swabs	SuHV-1 DNA	Unknown whether PCR could be used for antemortem diagnosis. Not widely available.
Virus isolation	CNS, tonsils, occasionally other tissues such as skin biopsies or the lung	SuHV-1	Specialized procedure. False negatives occur commonly.

CNS, central nervous system; *IFA,* immunofluorescent antibody; *IHC,* immunohistochemistry; *SuHV-1,* suid herpesvirus-1.

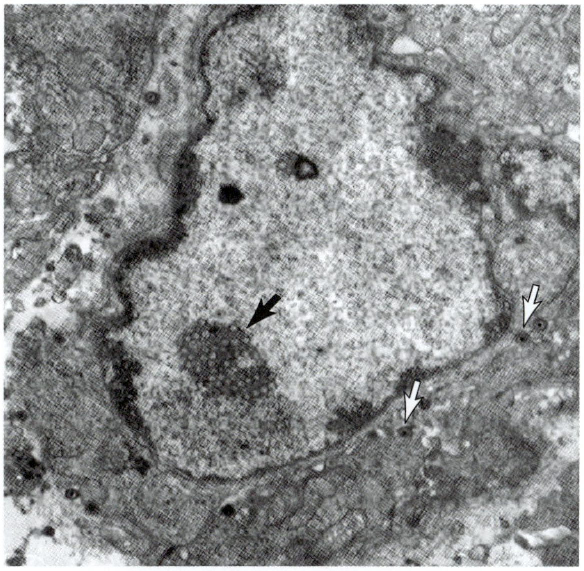

Fig. 39.3 Electron micrograph of pseudorabies virus (PRV)-infected cell culture. Intranuclear *(black arrow)* and cytoplasmic *(white arrows)* PRV viral particles. (Courtesy Dr. R. Maes, Michigan State University, East Lansing, MI.)

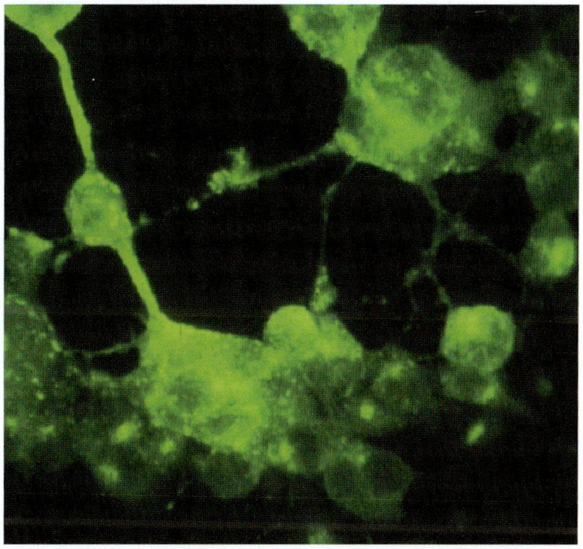

Fig. 39.4 Immunofluorescent antibody staining of cell culture infected with PRV. Note cytopathologic effect as multinucleated syncytia. (Courtesy Dr. R. Maes, Michigan State University, East Lansing, MI.)

Virus Isolation

Virus can be isolated in tissue culture from the lung and spleen and especially from brain and tonsils of animals with pseudorabies (Fig. 39.3). Although many cell lines have been used, most laboratories use pig kidney epithelial cells. A definite CPE consisting of syncytial formation is visible after 12 to 24 hours (Fig. 39.4). Virus isolation is not always easy in dogs, even in well-substantiated cases.[55] Pharyngeal washings, tonsillar swabs, and saliva are unsuitable for viral isolation in dogs.[56] Haired skin from regions of pruritis could be considered for testing.

Molecular Diagnosis Using Nucleic Acid–Based Testing

PCR for different viral genes is the method of choice to detect the presence of PRV in the porcine population.[57–59] In dogs and cats, besides IHC, rabbit inoculation test, and virus isolation, PCR has been used successfully to detect the virus at necropsy.[14,28] Whether these assays are useful for antemortem diagnosis is not known, but PCR could be attempted on specimens such as biopsies of pruritic regions or tonsillar swabs.

Pathologic Findings

No gross lesions are diagnostic of pseudorabies, with the exception of the skin lesions that result from intense pruritus. Gross pathologic abnormalities include evidence of facial dermatitis, tonsillar enlargement, and GI mucosal hyperemia and ulceration. In some cases, abnormal stomach contents have been noted because of pica. Pulmonary edema and congestion have been consistent findings. Focal myocarditis and ecchymosis have been found in dogs and cats. Histopathology of the tonsils reveals suppurative tonsillar inflammation, sometimes with necrosis. Lesions in the CNS are almost exclusively located in the brainstem and primarily involve cranial nerve nuclei.[14,60] They may be unilateral and consist of perivascular cuffing with mononuclear cells and pronounced proliferation of astrocytes and microglial cells (Fig. 39.5A and B). The areas of focal gliosis often show degeneration (karyorrhexis) in the center and may progress to the formation of microabscesses. Severe changes occur in neurons, with chromatolysis and disintegration of the nucleus (Fig. 39.5C). The most definitive finding is the presence of weak eosinophilic viral inclusion bodies in the nuclei of astrocytes and neurons. Viral-specific antigen or nucleic acid can be demonstrated in formalin-fixed, paraffin-embedded tissues with immunocytochemical methods[14,61] or *in situ* hybridization, respectively.[62,63] Inflammatory changes can also be found in the nerves and ganglia associated with the site of viral entry. Severe inflammation of the myenteric plexus in the alimentary canal of dogs naturally infected with PRV has also been reported.[64] Experimentally infected dogs had ganglioneuritis of autonomic nerves of the heart.[64]

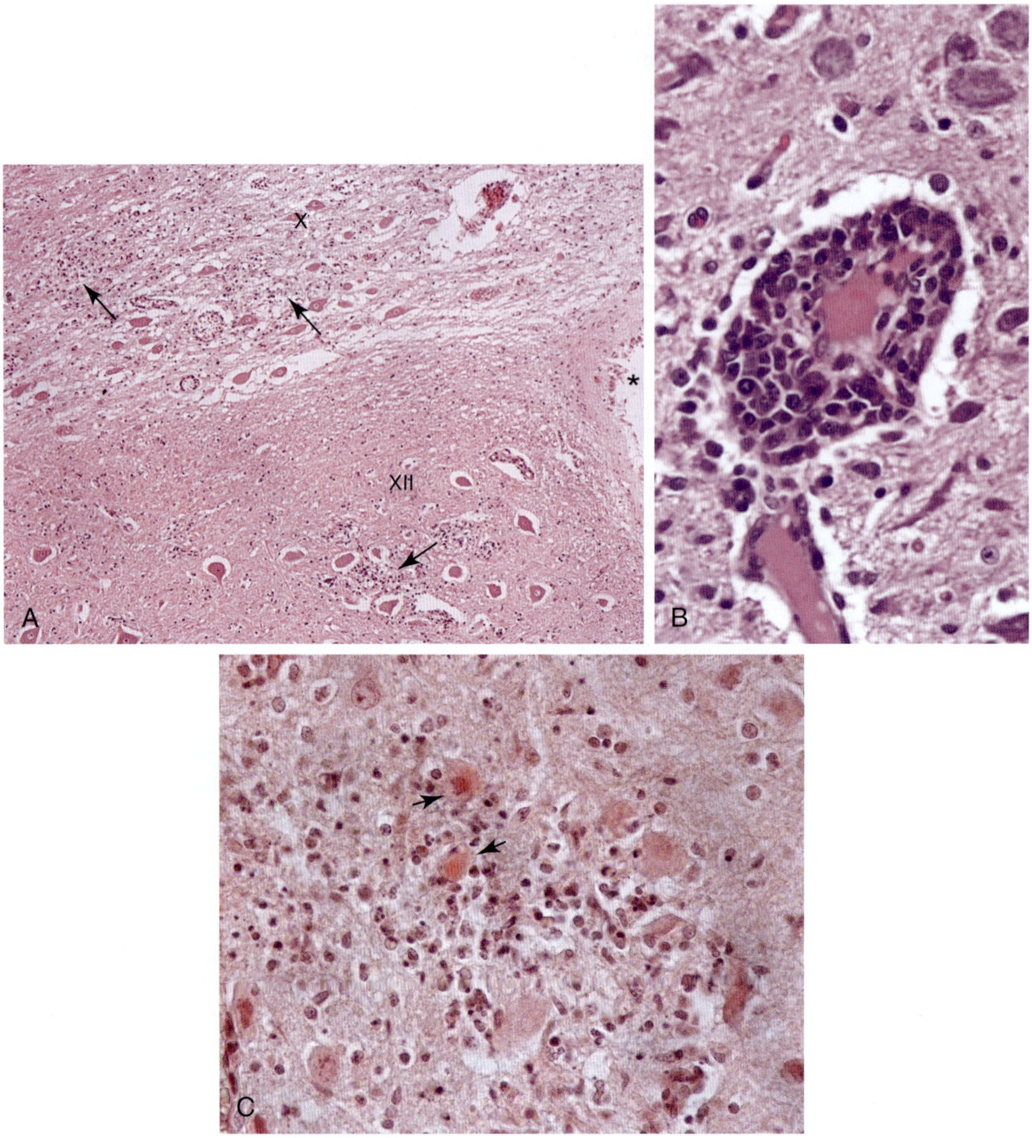

Fig. 39.5 Histologic findings of pseudorabies encephalitis in a dog. (A) Medulla oblongata (*asterisk*, fourth ventricle). Disseminated, inflammatory, mononuclear infiltration *(arrows)* in the nuclei of vagal (*X*) and hypoglossal (*XII*) nerves (H&E stain, ×40). (B) Mononuclear perivascular cuffing and gliosis in the brainstem (H&E stain, ×250). (C) Medulla oblongata, sensory nucleus of the trigeminal nerve. Widespread neuronal degeneration with chromatolysis and some eosinophilic shrunken neurons *(arrows)* associated with severe invasion of inflammatory cells (H&E stain, ×250). *H&E,* hematoxylin and eosin.

Diagnostic methods include IHC, immunofluorescence, or *in situ* hybridization on smears or frozen sections of various tissues. The brain and tonsils are the tissues of choice in such studies.

TREATMENT AND PROGNOSIS

Treatment of pseudorabies is generally futile because the disease is almost always fatal. Heavy sedation and anesthesia may lessen or relieve the itching and convulsions; however, nothing can alter the outcome of the disease. Treatment with anti-PRV serum did not improve the condition of a dog with Aujeszky's disease[51] and is considered to be ineffective in the prevention of infection.[31]

IMMUNITY AND VACCINATION

Although vaccines are used in swine to reduce losses in geographic locations where the disease is enzootic, vaccines are not available for dogs and cats because of the sporadic incidence of the disease. It is possible to vaccinate small animals against PRV, although this would be indicated only in endemic areas where exposure to infected domestic pigs and wild boars may occur. Natural infection with PRV has not been observed in vaccinated dogs and cats.[65] However, experimental vaccination challenge studies showed that it may be difficult to protect dogs with an inactivated vaccine, although most animals develop serum neutralizing antibodies to PRV.[31] Attenuated PRV vaccines may cause postvaccinal reactions that may be as lethal as the natural infection. PRV deletion mutants have been developed for vaccination of pigs.[10] Such "deletion" vaccines are safe and useful for controlling the disease because serologic surveys can distinguish between vaccine-induced and natural anti-PRV antibodies. Deletion vaccines have been tested in raccoons, albeit with limited success.[66] DNA vaccines have also been developed.[45] Human adenoviruses have been used as vectors for experimental immunization of cats against PRV antigens.[67] To the authors' knowledge, none of these modern vaccines have been systematically tested or applied in dogs and cats. Considerable progress has been made in the eradication of PRV infection in swine in many areas of the world.[10] As a result, Aujeszky's disease has become a very rare condition in dogs and cats, and the development and application of PRV vaccines in small animals have remained insignificant. In view of the extremely low frequency of the disease in dogs and cats, further developments are unlikely.

PREVENTION

Prevention is the most important means of control of PRV infection in dogs and cats. Pseudorabies can be effectively prevented by feeding only cooked food to dogs and cats, control of rodents, and prevention of contact between domestic swine (in regions where the disease is enzootic) and wild swine and dogs.

PUBLIC HEALTH ASPECTS

In general, humans appear to be refractory to infection with SuHV-1. However, cases of PRV-induced encephalitis, as determined by PCR in CSF samples have been discovered in humans working with pigs in China.[68]

SUGGESTED READINGS

Cramer SD, Campbell GA, Njaa BL, et al. Pseudorabies virus infection in Oklahoma hunting dogs. *J Vet Diagn Invest*. 2011;23:915–923.

Serena MS, Metz GE, Lozada MI, et al. First isolation and molecular characterization of Suid herpesvirus type 1 from a domestic dog in Argentina. *Open Vet J*. 2018;8:131–139.

REFERENCES

1. Aujeszky A. Uber eine neue infektienkrankheir bei haustieren. *Zentralbl Bakteriol I Orig*. 1902;32:353–357.
2. Mettenleiter TC. Aujeszky's disease (pseudorabies) virus: the virus and molecular pathogenesis–state of the art, June 1999. *Vet Res*. 2000;31:99–115.
3. Davies EB, Beran GW. Influence of environmental factors upon the survival of Aujeszky's disease virus. *Res Vet Sci*. 1981;31:32–36.
4. Pomeranz LE, Reynolds AE, Hengartner CJ. Molecular biology of pseudorabies virus: impact on neurovirology and veterinary medicine. *Microbiol Mol Biol Rev*. 2005;69:462–500.
5. Hoblet KH, Miller GY, Bartter NG. Economic assessment of a pseudorabies epizootic, breeding herd removal/repopulation, and downtime in a commercial swine herd. *J Am Vet Med Assoc*. 1987;190:405–409.
6. Yamane I, Ishizeki S, Yamazaki H. Aujeszky's disease and the effects of infection on Japanese swine herd productivity: a cross-sectional study. *J Vet Med Sci*. 2015;77:579–582.
7. Muller T, Batza HJ, Schluter H, et al. Eradication of Aujeszky's disease in Germany. *J Vet Med B Infect Dis Vet Public Health*. 2003;50:207–213.
8. Hahn EC, Fadl-Alla B, Lichtensteiger CA. Variation of Aujeszky's disease viruses in wild swine in USA. *Vet Microbiol*. 2010;143:45–51.
9. MacDiarmid SC. Aujeszky's disease eradication in New Zealand. *Aust Vet J*. 2000;78:470–471.
10. Freuling CM, Muller TF, Mettenleiter TC. Vaccines against pseudorabies virus (PrV). *Vet Microbiol*. 2016.
11. Salwa A. A natural outbreak of Aujeszky's disease in farm animals. *Pol J Vet Sci*. 2004;7:261–266.
12. Henderson JP, Graham DA, Stewart D. An outbreak of Aujeszky's disease in sheep in Northern Ireland. *Vet Rec*. 1995;136:555–557.
13. Liu H, Li XT, Hu B, et al. Outbreak of severe pseudorabies virus infection in pig-offal-fed farmed mink in Liaoning Province, China. *Arch Virol*. 2016.
14. Zhang L, Zhong C, Wang J, et al. Pathogenesis of natural and experimental Pseudorabies virus infections in dogs. *Virol J*. 2015;12:44.
15. Schoniger S, Klose K, Werner H, et al. Nonsuppurative encephalitis in a dog. *Vet Pathol*. 2012;49:731–734.
16. Hara M, Shimizu T, Fukuyama M, et al. Natural case of Aujeszky's disease in the dog in Japan. *Nihon Juigaku Zasshi*. 1987;49:645–649.
17. Matsuoka T, Iijima Y, Sakurai K, et al. Aujeszky's disease in a dog. *Nihon Juigaku Zasshi*. 1988;50:277–278.
18. Jin HL, Gao SM, Liu Y, et al. Pseudorabies in farmed foxes fed pig offal in Shandong province, China. *Arch Virol*. 2016;161:445–448.
19. Glass CM, McLean RG, Katz JB, et al. Isolation of pseudorabies (Aujeszky's disease) virus from a Florida panther. *J Wildl Dis*. 1994;30:180–184.
20. Masot AJ, Gil M, Risco D, et al. Pseudorabies virus infection (Aujeszky's disease) in an Iberian lynx (*Lynx pardinus*) in Spain: a case report. *BMC Vet Res*. 2017;13:6.
21. Wright JC, Thawley DG. Role of the raccoon in the transmission of pseudorabies: a field and laboratory investigation. *Am J Vet Res*. 1980;41:581–583.
22. Meier RK, Ruiz-Fons F, Ryser-Degiorgis MP. A picture of trends in Aujeszky's disease virus exposure in wild boar in the Swiss and European contexts. *BMC Vet Res*. 2015;11:277.
23. Sandfoss MR, DePerno CS, Betsill CW, et al. A serosurvey for *Brucella suis*, classical swine fever virus, porcine circovirus type 2, and pseudorabies virus in feral swine (*Sus scrofa*) of eastern North Carolina. *J Wildl Dis*. 2012;48:462–466.
24. Gaskamp JA, Gee KL, Campbell TA, et al. Pseudorabies virus and *Brucella abortus* from an expanding wild pig (*Sus scrofa*) population in southern Oklahoma, USA. *J Wildl Dis*. 2016;52:383–386.
25. Paes Rde C, Fonseca Jr AA, Monteiro LA, et al. Serological and molecular investigation of the prevalence of Aujeszky's disease in feral swine (*Sus scrofa*) in the subregions of the Pantanal wetland, Brazil. *Vet Microbiol*. 2013;165:448–454.
26. Mahmoud HY, Suzuki K, Tsuji T, et al. Pseudorabies virus infection in wild boars in Japan. *J Vet Med Sci*. 2011;73:1535–1537.
27. Goldberg TL, Weigel RM, Hahn EC, et al. Comparative utility of restriction fragment length polymorphism analysis and gene sequencing to the molecular epidemiological investigation of a viral outbreak. *Epidemiol Infect*. 2001;126:415–424.
28. Moreno A, Sozzi E, Grilli G, et al. Detection and molecular analysis of Pseudorabies virus strains isolated from dogs and a wild boar in Italy. *Vet Microbiol*. 2015;177:359–365.
29. Hara M, Shimizu T, Nemoto S, et al. The genome type of Aujeszky's disease virus isolated from a cat in Japan. *J Vet Med Sci*. 1991;53:1087–1089.
30. Cramer SD, Campbell GA, Njaa BL, et al. Pseudorabies virus infection in Oklahoma hunting dogs. *J Vet Diagn Invest*. 2011;23:915–923.
31. Pensaert MB, Commeyne S, Andries K. Vaccination of dogs against pseudorabies (Aujeszky's disease), using an inactivated-virus vaccine. *Am J Vet Res*. 1980;41:2016–2019.
32. Steinrigl A, Revilla-Fernandez S, Kolodziejek J, et al. Detection and molecular characterization of Suid herpesvirus type 1 in Austrian wild boar and hunting dogs. *Vet Microbiol*. 2012;157:276–284.
33. Pedersen K, Turnage CT, Gaston WD, et al. Pseudorabies detected in hunting dogs in Alabama and Arkansas after close contact with feral swine (*Sus scrofa*). *BMC Vet Res*. 2018;14:388.
34. Serena MS, Metz GE, Lozada MI, et al. First isolation and molecular characterization of Suid herpesvirus type 1 from a domestic dog in Argentina. *Open Vet J*. 2018;8:131–139.
35. Thaller D, Bilek A, Revilla-Fernandez S, et al. Diagnosis of Aujeszky's disease in a dog in Austria. *Wien Tierarztl Monatsschr*. 2006;93:62–67.
36. Cay AB, Letellier C. Isolation of Aujeszky's disease virus from two hunting dogs in Belgium after hunting wild boars. *Vlaam Diergeneeskd Tijdschr*. 2009;78:194–195.
37. Muller T, Hahn EC, Tottewitz F, et al. Pseudorabies virus in wild swine: a global perspective. *Arch Virol*. 2011;156:1691–1705.
38. Toma B, Dufour B. Transmission de la maladie d'Aujeszky des sangliers aux suides domestiques. *Epidemiol et Sante Anim*. 2004;45:115–119.
39. Buergelt CD, Romero CH, Chrisman CL. Pseudorabies in two dogs. *Vet Med*. 2000;95:439–442.
40. Quiroga MI, Nieto JM, Sur J, et al. Diagnosis of Aujeszky's disease virus infection in dogs by use of immunohistochemistry and in-situ hybridization. *Zentralbl Veterinarmed A*. 1998;45:75–81.

41. Hugoson G, Rockborn G. On the occurrence of pseudorabies in Sweden. II. An outbreak in dogs caused by feeding abattoir offal. *Zentralbl Veterinarmed B.* 1972;19:641–645.
42. Gore R, Osborne AD, Darke PG, et al. Aujeszky's disease in a pack of hounds. *Vet Rec.* 1977;101:93–95.
43. Hara M, Shimizu T, Nemoto S, et al. A natural case of Aujeszky's disease in the cat in Japan. *J Vet Med Sci.* 1991;53:947–949.
44. Olson GR, Miller LD. Studies on the pathogenesis of heart lesions in dogs infected with pseudorabies virus. *Can J Vet Res.* 1986;50:245–250.
45. Hagemoser WA, Kluge JP, Hill HT. Studies on the pathogenesis of pseudorabies in domestic cats following oral inoculation. *Can J Comp Med.* 1980;44:192–202.
46. Card JP, Rinaman L, Lynn RB, et al. Pseudorabies virus infection of the rat central nervous system: ultrastructural characterization of viral replication, transport, and pathogenesis. *J Neurosci.* 1993;13:2515–2539.
47. Enquist LW. Exploiting circuit-specific spread of pseudorabies virus in the central nervous system: insights to pathogenesis and circuit tracers. *J Infect Dis.* 2002;186(suppl. 2):S209–S214.
48. Apelt HJ. Aujeszky's disease in the dog and cat. *Tierarztl Prax.* 1983;11:223–228.
49. Egberink HF. Aujeszky's disease in dogs and cats. *Tijdschr Diergeneeskd.* 1990;115:349–353.
50. Howard DR. Pseudorabies in dogs and cats. In: Kirk RW, ed. *Current Veterinary Therapy*. Philadelphia: WB Saunders; 1986:1071–1072.
51. Richter JH, van der Vijver JW, Fischer RF, et al. An atypical case of Aujeszky's disease in a dog. *Tijdschr Diergeneeskd.* 1975;100:330–334.
52. Hawkins BA, Olson GR. Clinical signs of pseudorabies in the dog and cat: a review of 40 cases. *Iowa State Univ Vet.* 1985;47:116–119.
53. Monroe WE. Clinical signs associated with pseudorabies in dogs. *J Am Vet Med Assoc.* 1989;195:599–602.
54. Laval K, Enquist LW. The neuropathic itch caused by pseudorabies virus. *Pathogens.* 2020;9:254–282.
55. Akkermans JP. Aujeszky's disease and its problems. *Tijdschr Diergeneeskd.* 1981;106:332–337.
56. Tu L, Lian J, Pan Y, et al. Retrospective detection and phylogenetic analysis of pseudorabies virus in dogs in China. *Arch Virol.* 2021;166:91–100.
57. Ruiz-Fons F, Vidal D, Hofle U, et al. Aujeszky's disease virus infection patterns in European wild boar. *Vet Microbiol.* 2007;120:241–250.
58. Miao LF, Zhang CF, Chen CM, et al. Real-time PCR to detect and analyze virulent PPV loads in artificially challenged sows and their fetuses. *Vet Microbiol.* 2009;138:145–149.
59. Ma W, Lager KM, Richt JA, et al. Development of real-time polymerase chain reaction assays for rapid detection and differentiation of wild-type pseudorabies and gene-deleted vaccine viruses. *J Vet Diagn Invest.* 2008;20:440–447.
60. Fankhauser R, Fatzer R, Steck F, et al. Aujeszky's disease in dog and cat in Switzerland. *Schweiz Arch Tierheilkd.* 1975;117:623–629.
61. Ducatelle R, Coussement W, Hoorens J. Demonstration of pseudorabies viral antigen in thick and ultrathin tissue sections of young pigs using an immunogold method. *Am J Vet Res.* 1984;45:1913–1917.
62. Sehl J, Teifke JP. Comparative pathology of pseudorabies in different naturally and experimentally infected species: a review. *Pathogens.* 2020;9:633–656.
63. Vandevelde M. Pseudorabies. In: Green CE, ed. *Infectious Diseases of the Dog and Cat.* 1st ed. Philadelphia: WB Saunders; 1998:384–388.
64. Zhang L, Zhong C, Wang J, et al. Pathogenesis of natural and experimental pseudorabies virus infections in dogs. *Virology J.* 2015;12:44–54.
65. Akkermans JP. Vaccination of 'non-swine' against Aujeszky's disease. *Tijdschr Diergeneeskd.* 1980;105:1084–1085.
66. Weigel RM, Hahn EC, Scherba G. Survival and immunization of raccoons after exposure to pseudorabies (Aujeszky's disease) virus gene-deleted vaccines. *Vet Microbiol.* 2003;92:19–24.
67. Gonin P, Fournier A, Oualikene W, et al. Immunization trial of cats with a replication-defective adenovirus type 5 expressing the ENV gene of feline immunodeficiency virus. *Vet Microbiol.* 1995;45:393–401.
68. Xue Y, Hongzhi G, Chen L, et al. Characteristics of human encephalitis caused by pseudorabies virus: a case series study. *Int J Infect Dis.* 2019;87:92–99.

40

Papillomavirus Infections

Jennifer A. Luff, John S. Munday

KEY POINTS

- First Described: The transmissibility of canine papillomaviruses was described in the late 1800s; electron microscopic descriptions occurred in the late 1960s.[1,2] Papillomavirus infections of cats were not recognized until 1990.[3]
- Cause: Papillomaviruses (family *Papillomaviridae*).
- Affected Hosts: With the notable exception of bovine deltapapillomaviruses, papillomaviruses appear to have high species specificity.
- Geographic Distribution: Worldwide.
- Mode of Transmission: Cutaneous or mucosal inoculation, probably through microtrauma.
- Major Clinical Signs: Dogs: oral or cutaneous exophytic or endophytic papillomas, cutaneous pigmented plaques, possibly cutaneous and oral SCCs. Cats: cutaneous viral plaques, cutaneous Bowenoid *in situ* carcinomas, possibly cutaneous SCCs, oral papillomas, and feline sarcoids.
- Human Health Significance: Canine and feline papillomavirus do not infect humans.

ETIOLOGIC AGENTS AND EPIDEMIOLOGY

Papillomaviruses are small (30 to 60 nm), nonenveloped, icosahedral viruses with a circular double-stranded DNA genome (Fig. 40.1). They lack a lipid envelope, are resistant in the environment, and survive detergents and high temperatures. With rare exceptions, papillomaviruses are strictly host specific and have been identified in most mammalian species.[4]

Papillomaviruses infect keratinocytes at mucosal and cutaneous sites, most likely through microabrasions. Most papillomavirus infections are subclinical.[5] However, due to the ability of papillomaviruses to influence cell growth and regulation, infection by some papillomavirus types can result in marked proliferation of epithelial cells. This proliferation results in thickening and folding of the epidermis and the development of a hyperplastic, self-resolving papilloma (also referred to as a wart).[5] Less commonly, infection by papillomaviruses can influence the development of neoplasia (Box 40.1). In humans, whether infection remains asymptomatic, results in a papilloma, or promotes neoplasia is largely determined by the papillomavirus type[5] and the immune status of the host.[6] It is likely that the same is true for papillomavirus infections of dogs and cats, with both viral and host factors important in determining the manifestation of disease.

Due to the routine use of molecular testing, the number of different papillomavirus types identified in dogs and cats has expanded dramatically in recent years.[4] Papillomaviruses are classified on the basis of the L1 capsid gene nucleotide sequence.[7] At least 23 different types have been identified in dogs so far, with several additional novel types that have not been fully sequenced (Table 40.1).[8–24] These viruses have been classified into three distinct genera: *Lambdapapillomavirus, Taupapillomavirus, and Chipapillomavirus*.[10,25,26] In cats, six *Felis catus* papillomavirus (FcaPV) types have been fully sequenced with FcaPV1 classified within the *Lambdapapillomavirus* genus, FcaPV2 classified within the *Dyothetapapillomavirus* genus, and FcaPV3, 4, 5, and 6 likely to be classified within the *Taupapillomavirus* genus.[27–32] As with dogs, it appears likely that additional FcaPV types will be identified in the future.

The canine lambdapapillomaviruses include *Canis familiaris* papillomavirus (canine papillomavirus, CPV[†]) types 1 and 6.[8,10] CPV1 was the first CPV identified. This virus commonly infects young dogs, often resulting in numerous oral papillomas that spontaneously regress. This CPV has also rarely been associated with cutaneous endophytic (inverted) papillomas and invasive cutaneous SCCs.[33–37] CPV6 was identified from a single cutaneous papilloma that regressed spontaneously.[10] CPV19 was identified from a single oral papilloma.[22]

Taupapillomaviruses that have been identified in dogs include CPV types 2, 7, 13, 17, 21, 22, and 23. CPV2 has been identified within cutaneous papillomas and is only rarely associated with SCC.[18] However, in a research colony of dogs with X-linked severe combined immunodeficiency, CPV2 caused cutaneous papillomas that progressed to invasive and metastatic SCC.[38] CPV7 has thus far only been reported from a single cutaneous papilloma/*in situ* SCC.[10] CPV13 was identified from oral cytobrush specimens from a dog with oral papillomatosis.[9] CPV17 was identified as the likely cause of multiple oral SCCs in a dog.[39,40] CPV21, CPV22, and CPV23 were identified using viral metagenomics from nasal swabs and the association with clinical disease is currently unknown.[24]

Chipapillomaviruses include CPV types 3, 4, 5, 8, 9, 10, 11, 12, 14, 15, and 16. All of these chipapillomaviruses are associated with cutaneous pigmented plaques. CPV3 has been reported in multiple dogs, including a dog that developed numerous pigmented plaques and *in situ* SCC,[16] one dog with pigmented plaques,[41] one dog with pigmented plaques, basal cell carcinomas, SCCs, and trichoblastomas,[42] and one dog with a pigmented viral plaque that progressed to SCC.[36] CPV4 has been most commonly associated with pigmented plaques in pug dogs,[17,43–45] but other dog breeds can be affected.[41] CPV9 has been identified in several dogs with pigmented plaques,[12,19,41,46] including one dog that developed multicentric invasive SCC in association with its persistent pigmented plaques.[47] CPV12 has been identified in two dogs with pigmented plaques[20,41] and two additional related Basenji

[†] For the purposes of this chapter, CPV refers to canine papillomavirus, not canine parvovirus.

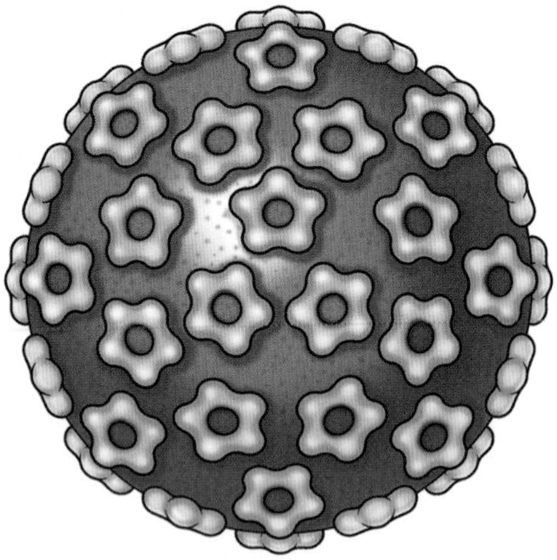

Fig. 40.1 Structure of a papillomavirus. The virus is nonenveloped and has an icosahedral capsid composed of two different capsid proteins (L1 and L2).

BOX 40.1 Spectrum of Clinical Manifestations Associated with Papillomavirus Infections in Dogs and Cats

Dogs
Oral papillomatosis
Cutaneous exophytic papillomas (warts)
Cutaneous endophytic papillomas (inverted warts)
Pigmented cutaneous plaques
Cutaneous *in situ* squamous cell carcinomas (SCCs)
Invasive cutaneous SCCs
Oral SCCs

Cats
Feline viral plaques
Bowenoid *in situ* carcinomas
Invasive cutaneous SCCs
Basal cell carcinomas
Oral papillomas
Feline sarcoids

dogs.[15] In one Basenji dog, the lesions progressed to invasive and metastatic SCC. The other Basenji dog developed metastatic SCC associated with pigmented plaques due to CPV16.[13,15] CPV16 has also been identified in two additional dogs with pigmented plaques that progressed to SCC.[36,48] CPV5 and CPV15 have been identified in small numbers of dogs with pigmented plaques,[10,41] while CPV types 8, 10, 11, and 14 have thus far only been identified from single cases of pigmented plaques.[11,12,14,21] CPV18 was originally identified within a pigmented plaque from a pug dog,[23] and has been identified in one additional pug dog with a pigmented plaque and basal cell tumor.[45] CPV20 is most likely a *Chipapillomavirus* based upon its sequence, but there is currently no reported information for this virus.

There have been several reports of pigmented plaques progressing to SCC. The associated CPV type, however, has only rarely been identified; therefore, it remains unknown whether pigmented plaques caused by a particular CPV type are at greater risk of progressing to SCC. Thus far, only CPV3, CPV9, CPV12, and CPV16 have been associated with malignant progression of pigmented plaques to invasive and metastatic SCC.[13,15,47] Overall, these are rare cases and there is

TABLE 40.1 Spectrum of Papillomavirus Types and Disease Associations in Dogs

Genus	CPV Type	Clinical Manifestation
Lambda	1	Oral papillomas, oral SCC[a], cutaneous papillomas
	6	Cutaneous papillomas (warts)
	19	Oral papilloma
Tau	2	Cutaneous papillomas
	7	Cutaneous papillomas, *in situ* SCC
	13	Oral papillomas
	17	Oral SCC[a]
Chi	3	Cutaneous pigmented plaques, *in situ* SCC
	4, 5, 8, 10, 11, 14, 15, 18	Cutaneous pigmented plaques
	9, 12, 16	Cutaneous pigmented plaques, *in situ* SCC, invasive SCC[a]

CPV, canine papillomavirus; *SCC,* squamous cell carcinoma.
[a]The majority of SCCs in dogs are not associated with papillomavirus infections.

currently no evidence to suggest that CPVs are a significant cause of either cutaneous or oral SCCs.[49–51]

Many of these CPV types have been identified in small numbers of dogs, and often from a single lesion or a single animal. Therefore, it is difficult to determine their prevalence, geographic distribution, biologic characteristics, or clinical behavior.

In general, lesions due to papillomavirus infection are more frequently recognized in dogs than in cats. In cats, infections by papillomaviruses are believed to cause feline viral plaques and Bowenoid *in situ* carcinomas (BISCs). As viral plaques can progress into BISCs,[52] these two lesions probably represent a continuum of papillomavirus-induced hyperplasia and dysplasia of the epidermis. BISCs have been previously referred to as multicentric SCCs *in situ*. However, as BISCs can develop as single lesions, and as BISCs contain histologic features not observed in sun-induced *in situ* SCCs, this term is not favored. In cats, papillomaviruses are also recognized to cause feline sarcoids (previously known as fibropapillomas) and oral papillomas. In cats, there is increasing evidence that papillomaviruses may influence the development of a proportion of cutaneous SCCs. While papillomaviral DNA has been occasionally detected in feline oral SCCs,[53–56] there is currently no evidence that feline oral SCCs are caused by papillomaviruses.[57]

Felis catus papillomavirus type 1. This *Lambdapapillomavirus* was initially identified in a feline viral plaque from a cat that was suspected to be immunosuppressed.[30] Subsequent research suggests that FcaPV1 is a rare cause of feline viral plaques. However, this papillomavirus was identified in two feline oral papillomas[58] and, as FcaPV1 is closely related to the papillomaviruses that cause oral papillomas in lions and snow leopards, this virus is the likely cause of oral papillomas in domestic cats.

Felis catus papillomavirus type 2. This *Dyothetapapillomavirus* currently appears to be the most common cause of papillomavirus-induced disease in cats. The majority of feline viral plaques and BISCs appear to be caused by infection with this papillomavirus type.[59] However, as FcaPV2 can be detected on the skin of most cats[60] and yet only a small proportion develop disease, host factors appear to be important for disease development. The importance of host factors is demonstrated by the observation that Devon Rex, and the closely related Sphinx, cats develop an unusually severe manifestation of FcaPV2-induced disease

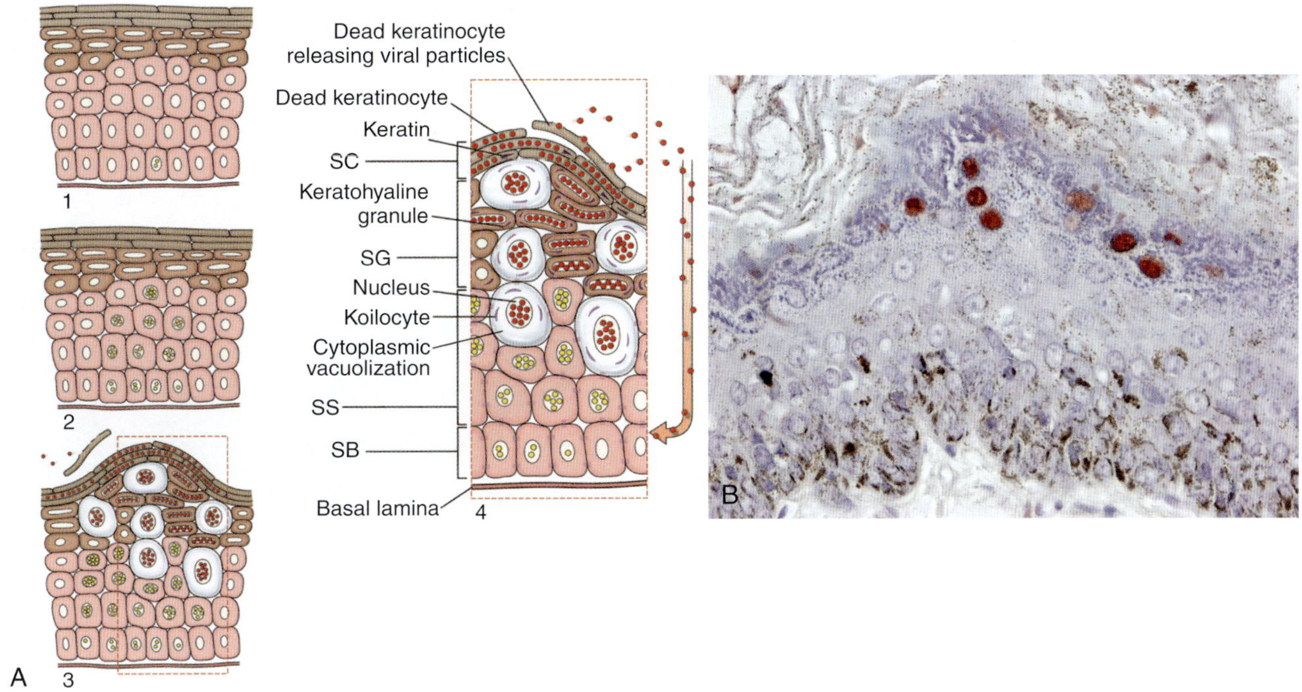

Fig. 40.2 Schematic representation of the events of papillomavirus infection in the epidermis. (A) 1, The primary infection occurs in a cell of the stratum basale *(SB)* after the virus gains entry via a microabrasion. The virus replicates and expresses the early proteins, which leads to increased cellular proliferation. 2, Progeny of the initial infected cells migrate laterally and move upward, where they accumulate in the stratum spinosum *(SS)* and stratum granulosum *(SG)*. 3, Cellular differentiation ultimately occurs, and large numbers of virions are produced in association with papilloma development. Virions are shed with exfoliating keratinocytes of the stratum corneum *(SC)*. 4, Detail from 3. (B) Immunoperoxidase staining of papillomavirus antigen in a cutaneous plaque from a dog. (B, Courtesy of Luff J, University of California, Davis. In: MacLachlan NJ, Dubovi EJ, eds. *Fenner's Veterinary Virology*. 4th ed. Burlington, MA: Academic Press [Elsevier]; 2011.)

early in life.[61,62] The host factors that are important in disease development are currently uncertain. Initial studies suggested immunosuppression predisposed to disease; however, both viral plaques and BISCs can develop without any detectible loss of immune function. This suggests that immunosuppression is not essential for disease development.

In addition to viral plaques and BISCs, there is increasing evidence that FcaPV2 is a significant cause of feline cutaneous SCCs. FcaPV2 DNA has been detected more frequently in SCCs than in non-SCC skin specimens,[59] papillomavirus-induced changes in cell regulatory proteins have been detected in SCCs that contain FcaPV2 DNA,[63] differences in biological behavior have been observed between SCCs with evidence of papillomavirus infection and those without,[64] and FcaPV2 oncogene RNA has been detected within a proportion of feline cutaneous SCCs.[65–67] Overall, FcaPV2 could influence the development of 30%–50% of feline cutaneous SCCs. SCCs from haired skin are most likely to contain evidence of a papillomaviral etiology. However, some evidence also suggests that FcaPV2 can act as a co-factor with sun exposure to promote SCC development.[68]

Felis catus papillomavirus types 3, 4, 5, and 6. These papillomaviruses will probably all be classified within the *Taupapillomavirus* genus. These types have been detected in association with pre-neoplastic or neoplastic skin lesions in cats. However, these seem to be less common causes of feline viral plaques, BISCs, and SCCs than FcaPV2.[27,31,32,69] Currently, it is uncertain whether lesions caused by these four papillomavirus types have a different clinical behavior to lesions caused by FcaPV2. However, these types may be more likely to result in the development of basal cell carcinomas.[70]

Feline sarcoids. Evidence suggests that these mesenchymal neoplasms are caused by cross-species infection with bovine papillomavirus (BPV) type 14.[71] BPV14 is a *Deltapapillomavirus* like BPV1 and BPV2, which are thought to cause equine sarcoids. It is interesting to note that BPV14 has not been detected in an equine sarcoid, and neither BPV1 nor BPV2 has been detected in a feline sarcoid. Evidence of viral replication is not present within feline sarcoids, and these are considered to be dead-end infections.[72] How the papillomavirus is transferred from cow to cat is currently unknown.

CLINICAL FEATURES

Pathogenesis, Clinical Signs, and Physical Examination Findings

Infection with papillomaviruses follows inoculation of the virus through microabrasions in the skin and mucous membranes caused by physical trauma. Initial infection and viral amplification occurs within keratinocytes of the stratum basale.[73] As basal keratinocytes undergo differentiation, early viral proteins (E proteins) are expressed and associate with regulators of the cell cycle to stimulate cell cycle progression.[73] This can lead to enhanced proliferation of cells in the stratum spinosum and stratum granulosum, with accumulation of infected cells and papilloma formation (Fig. 40.2). With the exception of feline sarcoids, which remain as latent (or nonproductive) infections, late viral products, including the virus capsid proteins (L1 and L2), are first expressed in cells of the stratum spinosum. Papillomaviruses are nonlytic viruses, and mature virions are shed with cells that exfoliate from the stratum corneum or the nonkeratinized cells of the mucous membranes. Infected cells develop a characteristic CPE, which consists of cytoplasmic vacuolization. Tens of thousands of virus particles are produced by each infected cell. Papillomaviruses can predispose to the neoplastic transformation of infected cells because their viral E6 and E7 proteins (also known as oncoproteins) alter normal cell cycle regulation and/or apoptosis.[74] For example, human "high-risk" papillomavirus types produce proteins that degrade p53 and retinoblastoma protein (pRb), which are important tumor suppressors.[75] Accidental integration of the DNA of human "high-risk" papillomavirus types into host cell DNA can result in a marked increase in papillomavirus oncogene expression. The resultant population of rapidly dividing and genetically unstable cells is greatly predisposed to neoplastic transformation.[74]

Canine Oral Papillomatosis

Canine oral papillomas most commonly occur in young dogs and often regress spontaneously over a 4- to 8-week period.[26] They can also occur as a result of immunosuppression, such as after treatment with cyclosporine, less commonly chronic glucocorticoid treatment, or chronic infection with *Ehrlichia canis*. Rarely, papillomas in the caudal oropharynx obstruct respiration. Oral papillomas can occur on the lips, mucocutaneous junctions, tongue, pharynx, eyelids, and infrequently haired skin[26] (Fig. 40.3). They may cause halitosis, ptyalism, and oral discomfort. Early lesions are smooth and raised, but as they enlarge they may become cauliflower-like. They may be pigmented or nonpigmented.

Canine Cutaneous Papillomas

Cutaneous exophytic and endophytic papillomas usually occur as solitary masses.[26] Exophytic papillomas are proliferative nodules, whereas endophytic papillomas are cup-shaped cutaneous nodules that range in size from 2 mm to 2 cm in diameter with a central keratin-filled depression. Cutaneous exophytic papillomas are wart-like projections that appear anywhere on the body, but especially the lower limbs and footpads. Single or multiple lesions can occur anywhere on the body (Fig. 40.4). They have also been described in the interdigital space.[38] Rarely, papillomas can form along sites of previous surgery.[76]

Canine Pigmented Plaques

Pigmented plaques can develop as single or multiple lesions on the skin and have variable degrees of pigmentation. The lesions usually range in size from 1 mm to 1 cm, but can become larger. They appear as dark (although this can be variable), hyperkeratotic flat lesions that are typically present on the ventrum or medial aspects of the limbs[48] (Fig. 40.5). Pugs and miniature schnauzers are considered to be predisposed, but many other breeds can be affected. The lesions can regress spontaneously over the course of a few months, but may persist in some dogs. These are generally not of clinical significance, although rarely they can progress to SCCs.[15,48,77]

Canine Squamous Cell Carcinomas

These neoplasms are often ulcerated, nodular masses that may be found alongside pigmented plaques or cutaneous papillomas when malignant transformation occurs. However, transformation of oral and cutaneous papillomas is rare, and most cases of canine SCCs are not associated with papillomavirus infection.[49–51]

Feline Viral Plaques

Plaques typically develop on older cats and often present as multiple, less than 1 cm in diameter, sessile, hairless, pigmented lesions. They tend to develop most frequently around the face, although they can develop anywhere on the body.

Bowenoid In Situ Carcinoma (BISC)

BISCs also typically develop on older animals, although have been reported in Devon Rex cats as young as 3 years of age.[61] Most cats with

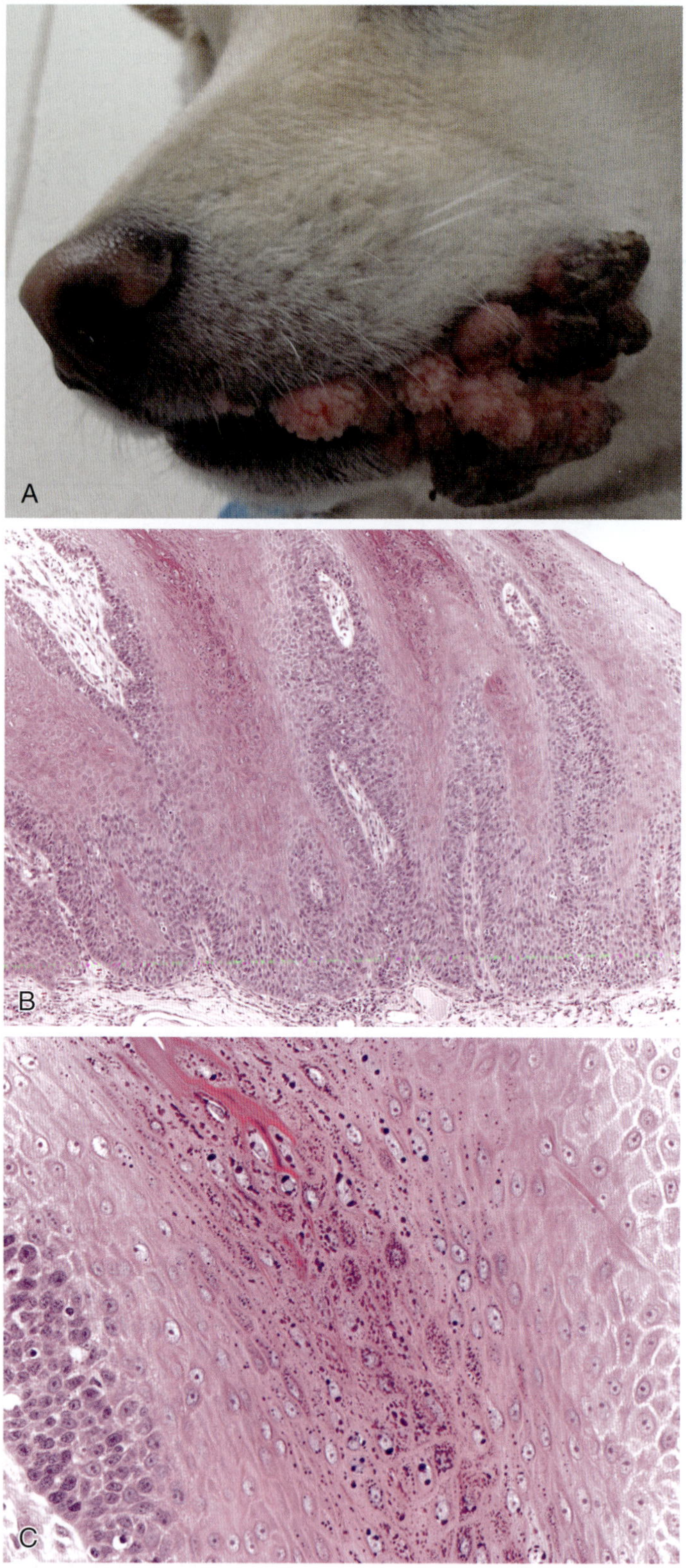

Fig. 40.3 (A) Oral papillomatosis in a 1.5-year-old male Shiba Inu. (B and C) Histology of an oral papilloma with characteristic exophytic projections of epidermal hyperplasia and increased keratohyalin granules. (A, Courtesy of Steven White, University of California at Davis, School of Veterinary Medicine, Dermatology Service.)

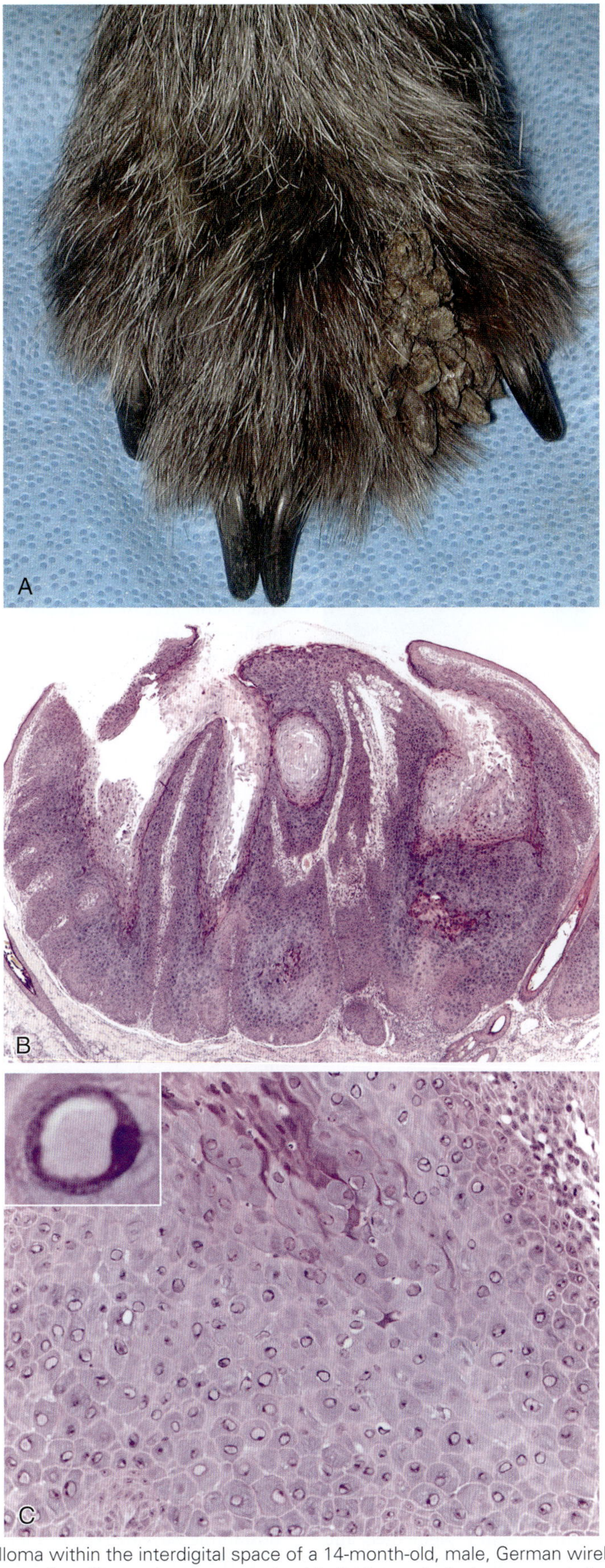

Fig. 40.4 (A) Papilloma within the interdigital space of a 14-month-old, male, German wirehaired pointer. (B) Histology of an inverted papilloma showing typical epithelial hyperplasia that occurs below the level of the surrounding normal skin. (C) Higher magnification of keratinocytes with characteristic blue-gray cytoplasm and prominent intranuclear inclusions *(inset)*. (A, Courtesy of Steven White, University of California at Davis, School of Veterinary Medicine, Dermatology Service.)

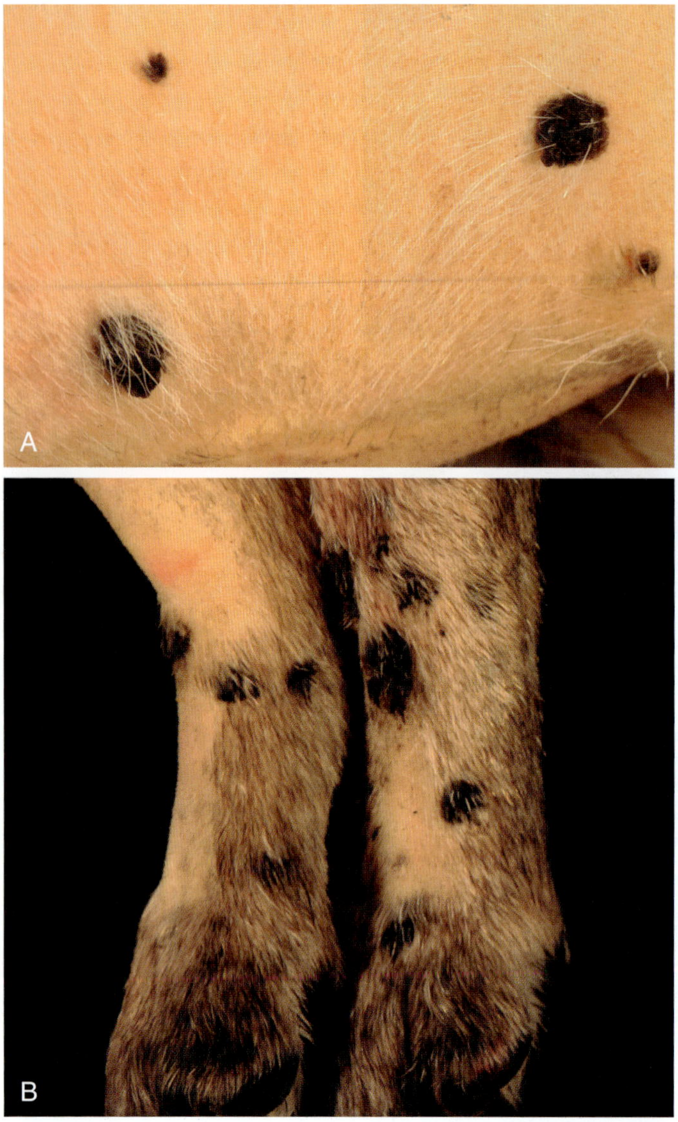

Fig. 40.5 (A and B) Multiple pigmented plaques on the ventral abdomen and limbs of a 10-year-old female, spayed pug dog. (Courtesy of Ashley Talley, North Carolina State University, College of Veterinary Medicine, Anatomic Pathology Service.)

BISCs will develop multiple lesions, although the development of a single lesion does not exclude BISC as a diagnosis.[78] BISCs most commonly involve the head and dorsum of cats (Fig. 40.6). They typically appear as roughly spherical hairless masses that can either be ulcerated or covered by orthokeratosis. They can be pigmented. Differentiation between a feline viral plaque and a BISC may not be possible clinically, but as a general rule, the larger the lesion is, the greater the likelihood of a BISC.

Feline Cutaneous Squamous Cell Carcinomas

These appear as ulcerated masses. Feline cutaneous SCCs can be subdivided into those that are caused by sun exposure and develop as a progression from actinic keratosis and those that are caused by papillomavirus infection and develop as a progression from a BISC. As sunlight appears to be the most common cause of feline cutaneous SCCs, these neoplasms most often occur in lightly pigmented and lightly haired areas of the body. SCCs that develop on the pinnae are the least likely to contain evidence of papillomavirus infection, while SCCs from haired, pigmented skin are most likely to have a putative papillomaviral etiology.

Feline Oral Papillomas

These lesions are rarely reported in middle-aged to older cats. However, as the papillomas do not cause clinical signs and are only discovered as an incidental finding, the true prevalence of oral papillomas in cats is unknown. Oral papillomas appear as multiple < 5-mm diameter pale raised lesions on the ventral surface of the tongue.[58]

Feline Sarcoids

Feline sarcoids have been described in cats from North America, New Zealand, the United Kingdom, Sweden, and Australia. They are thought to be caused by BPV14, and contact with cattle appears necessary for disease development. Affected cats are often young (<5 years), male, outdoor cats from rural environments.[79] Sarcoids typically appear as hairless, solitary, firm, exophytic masses. Although they most commonly develop around the mouth and nose, especially the nasal philtrum (Fig. 40.7), they have also been reported at other locations such as in digits, tail tip, eyelids, and pinnae.[79,80]

DIAGNOSIS

The history and gross appearance of oral papillomas in dogs is generally sufficient for diagnosis. For other papillomas and plaques, the diagnosis can be confirmed with biopsy and histopathology. A full-thickness biopsy that includes adjacent normal skin should be collected. The presence of papillomaviruses can be investigated using PCR, IHC, *in situ* hybridization, or electron microscopy, although these techniques are primarily used on a research basis. Caution should be used when interpreting the results of PCR assays because papillomaviruses can be detected on normal skin,[60,81] so results should be interpreted in association with clinical signs. While DNA *in situ* hybridization is considered less sensitive than PCR, this technique can confirm the location of papillomavirus DNA within the lesion. However, the presence of DNA within a lesion does not necessarily prove causality. Assays to detect papillomaviral oncogene RNA in a lesion have been used to further investigate whether the papillomavirus is likely to be influencing cell behavior or simply present within the lesion as an "innocent bystander."[15,65]

IHC and electron microscopy can be used to detect viral antigen and viral particles, respectively. These techniques can only detect papillomaviruses in lesions that contain viral replication. Typically, little or no viral replication is present in SCCs and sarcoids, which makes these techniques of reduced value to investigate a papillomavirus etiology of these lesions. In the authors' experience, few papillomavirus-induced lesions contain antipapillomavirus immunostaining in the absence of histologically detectible papillomavirus-induced cell changes. Canine and feline papillomavirus-specific reagents are not widely available, and care has to be taken to ensure cross-reactivity between the available antipapillomavirus antibodies and canine and feline papillomaviruses.

IHC to detect $p16^{CDKN2A}$ protein (p16) can also be used to investigate a possible papillomaviral etiology of a lesion. Papillomaviruses consistently alter normal cell regulation by degrading pRb. Loss of normal pRb function in a cell increases p16. Therefore, the detection of intense nuclear and cytoplasmic p16 immunostaining in a human oral SCC is considered consistent with a papillomaviral etiology.[82] Similarly, intense p16 immunostaining has been observed in association with loss of pRb in feline viral plaques, BISCs, and papillomavirus-associated SCCs.[75] Additionally, increased p16 immunostaining was observed in a feline oral papilloma and in a canine oral SCC that was associated with CPV17 infection.[40,58] The advantage of p16 immunostaining over papillomavirus immunostaining is that p16

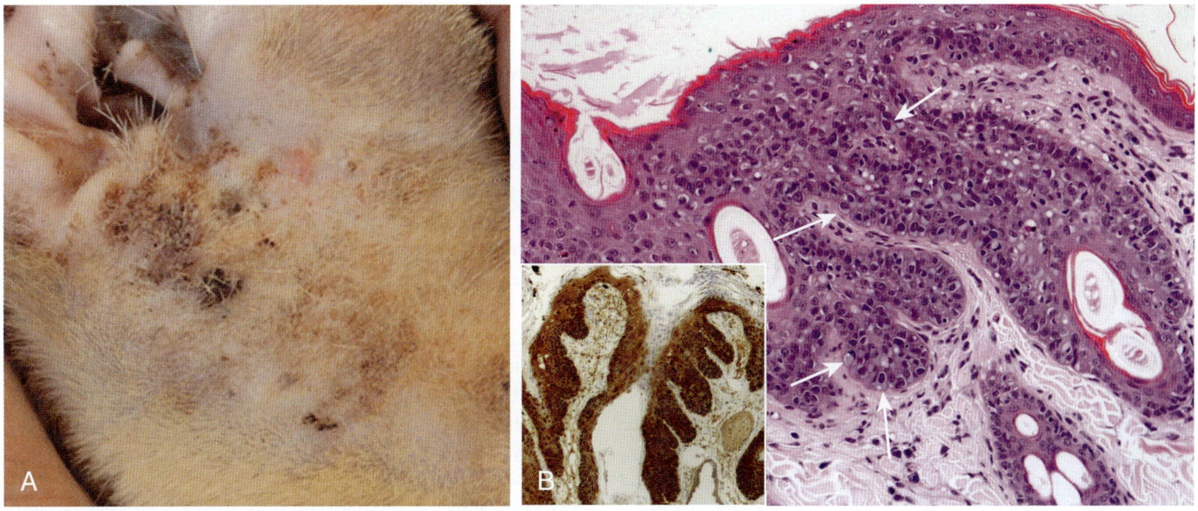

Fig. 40.6 (A) Bowenoid *in situ* carcinoma (BISC). These masses appear as single or multiple scaly or ulcerated plaques that are most common on the head and dorsum. (B) Histopathology of a BISC reveals hyperplasia and dysplasia involving the full thickness of the epidermis and extending into follicular infundibula. While this lesion contains prominent papillomavirus-induced cell changes *(arrows)*, such changes tend to be rare in advanced BISC lesions. The dysplastic cells contain a marked increase in p16CDKN2A *(inset)* suggesting that the papillomavirus has influenced cell cycle regulation by interfering with normal retinoblastoma protein function.

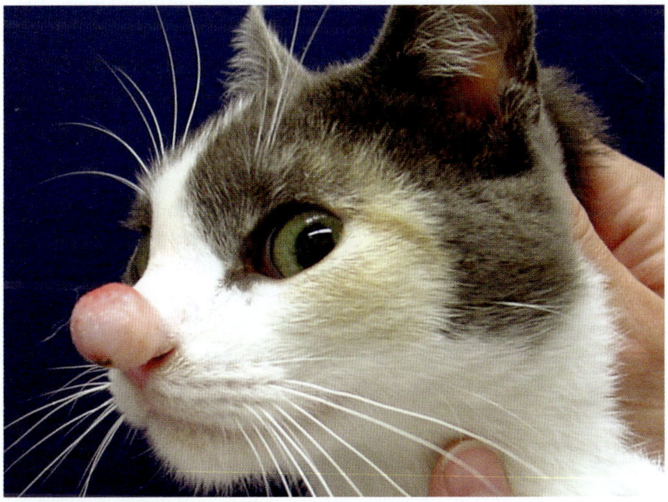

Fig. 40.7 Sarcoid of the nasal philtrum of a cat. The sarcoid recurred after repeated attempts at surgical excision. The sarcoid eventually began to interfere with eating and the cat was euthanized. (Courtesy of Dr. William Miller, Cornell University College of Veterinary Medicine and Dr Cameron Knight, University of Calgary.)

immunostaining is not dependent on active viral replication. In addition, the presence of increased p16 within a lesion that contains papillomavirus DNA provides evidence that the papillomavirus was altering cell regulation rather than being present as an incidental infection. However, a disadvantage of p16 immunostaining is that any cause of reduced pRb function will increase cell p16 and the specificity of this test for the detection of a papillomavirus etiology in dogs and cats has not been determined.

Microbiologic Tests

Molecular Diagnosis Using Nucleic Acid–Based Testing

PCR assays can be used to detect papillomaviruses within biopsy or cytobrush specimens from dogs and cats. Consensus primers are available to detect multiple different papillomavirus types. If unfixed tissue is available, either rolling circle amplification or next generation sequencing can be used to amplify whole circular genomic DNA.[26,29]

Pathologic Findings

Productive infection of an epithelial cell by a papillomavirus can result in papillomavirus-induced cell changes. Recognition of these changes is good evidence that the lesion was caused by papillomavirus infection. Furthermore, each papillomavirus genus appears to result in subtly different cell changes and so detection of these changes can be valuable to suggest the likely etiologic agent.[69] Papillomavirus infection can result in *koilocytosis*—cells with a dark shrunken nucleus surrounded by a clear cytoplasmic halo. Papillomavirus infection can also result in the development of large cells that have increased quantities of blue-gray fibrillar cytoplasm (see Fig. 40.4C). Less frequently, papillomaviruses can result in the development of prominent intracytoplasmic bodies, likely due to aggregates of keratin. Papillomaviruses can also be visible as amphophilic to basophilic intranuclear inclusions in the upper layers of the epidermis, although these inclusions tend to be transient and can sometimes be hard to differentiate from nucleoli (see Fig. 40.4C).

Histopathology of canine exophytic papillomas generally reveals exophytic projections of epidermal hyperplasia (acanthosis) with extensive hyperkeratosis and clumped keratohyalin granules in the stratum spinosum (see Fig. 40.3C). Endophytic papillomas are cup-shaped masses of epithelial hyperplasia that occur below the level of the surrounding normal skin (see Fig. 40.4B). Koilocytosis and intranuclear inclusions are often prominent (see Fig. 40.4C).

Histopathology of canine pigmented plaques reveals locally extensive epidermal hyperplasia, hyperkeratosis, hyperpigmentation, and clumped keratohyalin granules; koilocytes and viral inclusions are generally not observed.[26]

Feline viral plaques appear as focal well-demarcated areas of epidermal thickening. They frequently contain koilocytes and often contain cells that have increased quantities of blue-gray fibrillar cytoplasm.

BISCs also appear as well-demarcated foci of epidermal thickening; however, in contrast to a viral plaque, the thickened epidermis contains evidence of dysplasia (see Fig. 40.6). The cells within the basal cell layers typically become crowded and groups of cells can develop dorsoventrally aligned nuclei resulting in a "windblown" appearance. Papillomavirus-induced cell changes can be present within BISCs; however, they tend to be less frequent in advanced lesions. The presence of invasion of cells through the basement membrane prompts a classification of SCC.

SCCs that are associated with papillomavirus infection rarely have evidence of papillomavirus infection and histology cannot be used to predict which SCCs contain papillomaviral DNA.

Feline oral papillomas appear as a focus of thickened epithelium that is arranged as exophytic folds supported by a fibrovascular stalk. Papillomavirus-induced cell changes are present including the presence of prominent eosinophilic cytoplasmic bodies.[58]

Feline sarcoids appear as dermal fibroplastic proliferations. The overlying epidermis is mildly hyperplastic and includes long, thin rete ridges that extend into the tumor.[79] The characteristic epidermal changes allow differentiation from a fibrosarcoma. Papillomaviral replication does not occur in feline sarcoids, and these lesions do not contain papillomavirus-induced cell changes.

TREATMENT AND PROGNOSIS

The outcome of a papillomavirus infection depends on the papillomavirus type and as more information becomes available, certain papillomavirus types may be found to be more likely to result in neoplastic transformation, which may aid prognostication. The prognosis also appears to be influenced by host factors. The overwhelming majority of oral and cutaneous papillomas in young dogs regress spontaneously 4 to 16 weeks after onset of clinical signs. However, they may persist in older dogs, or when there is underlying immune compromise, and occasionally progress to malignancy.[36,37] If possible, underlying immunosuppression should be treated (for example, through removal or tapering of immunosuppressive drug treatment).

Lesions can be removed surgically if they cause physical obstruction or for cosmetic reasons, but surgical treatment may be followed by recurrence. As in human medicine, cryotherapy appears to be a useful technique to treat canine papillomas that persist. As seen in humans with warts, repeated treatments may be required for some canine papillomas.[83] Numerous other treatments have been proposed to accelerate resolution of a papilloma. However, because a high proportion of papillomas eventually spontaneously regress, definitively proving that a treatment influences resolution is difficult. Treatment with azithromycin (10 mg/kg PO q24h for 10 days) appeared to be effective in a prospective, randomized, double-blinded placebo-controlled clinical trial that included 12 dogs with oral papillomatosis and 5 dogs with cutaneous papillomatosis.[84] However, azithromycin has been subsequently reported to have been used without showing beneficial clinical effects. The use of topical or intralesional immunomodulators (such as imiquimod cream) and antiviral drugs (such as cidofovir) has shown promise for treatment of persistent papillomas in humans, but these treatments have not been evaluated for papillomas in dogs. Papilloma regression is dependent on CMI and there is no evidence that stimulating a humoral antibody response by autogenous vaccination influences resolution of a papilloma.

Canine pigmented plaques can persist, but transformation to invasive SCC is rare.[15,47] There are single case reports demonstrating successful treatment of extensive cutaneous pigmented plaques with carbon dioxide laser treatments[85] and the antineoplastic agent tigilanol tiglate.[86]

The behavior of feline viral plaques and BISCs is poorly understood. It appears that spontaneous regression is possible, although some lesions remain stable over a long period of time, and others progress to SCC.[87] Progression to SCC appears to be especially frequent and rapid in Devon Rex and Sphinx cats with subsequent metastases reported.[61,62] In a study of 12 cats with BISCs that were treated using topical imiquimod cream, partial resolution of a treated lesion was noted in all cats with 5 cats reported to have complete remission of at least one BISC lesion.[78] However, five cats developed erythema at the site of treatment and two cats showed signs of systemic toxicity. While this study showed some promise, no untreated cats with BISCs were included and whether or not imiquimod significantly alters the disease course in cats with BISCs remains unknown. It should also be noted that imiquimod does not have any specific action against papillomaviruses. Due to the surface location of BISCs, it appears likely that cryotherapy may be a potential treatment option, although there are no published studies using this as a treatment for BISCs in cats. As in humans, papillomavirus-associated feline cutaneous SCCs appear to have a more favorable prognosis than nonpapillomavirus-associated SCCs.[64]

Most feline oral papillomas probably spontaneously resolve and there is no evidence that they progress to oral SCCs in cats.[50,58]

Feline sarcoids often recur locally after surgical removal, but metastasis does not occur. Topical imiquimod cream did not appear to slow the disease progression in a cat with a feline sarcoid.[71]

IMMUNITY AND VACCINATION

Regression of a papilloma is associated with papillomavirus type-specific resistance to reinfection. Immunity to papillomaviruses comprises: (1) the host immune response to the virus and (2) a cell-mediated immune response to the tumor, which is ultimately responsible for tumor regression. This explains why new tumors may not occur, but old tumors persist and continue to grow in the face of an immune response to the virus, and immunization with the virus does not induce tumor regression. Papillomaviruses can evade the host immune response because infection is limited to the skin, and the immunogenic capsid protein is not expressed until the virus reaches the terminally differentiated outer layer. A variety of other mechanisms of immune evasion have been identified in human papillomavirus infections, including downregulation of the antiviral interferon response by papillomavirus proteins.[88]

PREVENTION

No vaccines are available for prevention of papillomavirus-induced disease in dogs and cats. While vaccination against CPV1 would be expected to prevent oral papillomas and a proportion of cutaneous papillomas, it appears unlikely that clients would pay for a vaccine to prevent a benign disease that almost always spontaneously resolves. An experimental vaccine against FcaPV2 was recently developed and shown to induce antibodies against this virus. However, the vaccine did not decrease the viral load on the skin of cats.[89] This suggests that any vaccine has to be given prior to first infection by the virus. As cats seem to be infected immediately after birth,[90] it appears to be hard to use vaccines to prevent FcaPV2-induced BISCs or SCCs in cats. Prevention of immunosuppressive conditions, such as retrovirus infections in cats, and cautious use of potent immunosuppressive drugs, such as cyclosporine, may reduce the chance of papillomavirus-induced disease.

PUBLIC HEALTH ASPECTS

More than 250 papillomavirus types infect humans. Papillomaviruses are relatively species specific, and there is no evidence that either CPV or feline papillomavirus infect humans.

CASE EXAMPLE

Signalment

"Oscar," an adult male neutered Rottweiler mix (Fig. 40.8).

History

Oscar was brought to the University of California-Davis, Veterinary Medical Teaching Hospital for examination after adoption by a veterinary student as a stray from an American Indian reservation in Arizona. The student was concerned about the possibility of malnourishment, a painful mouth, and pruritic skin disease. Since his rescue 5 days previously, the student had been feeding him four times daily with maintenance commercial wet and dry dog foods. His appetite had been ravenous and tapeworm segments had been observed in his feces. He had been isolated from other pets in the household.

Physical Examination

Body weight: 25.5 kg.

General: Bright and alert with normal mentation, nervous. T = 100.8°F (38.2°C), HR = 90 beats/minute, RR = 18 breaths/minute, mucous membranes pink, CRT = 1 second.

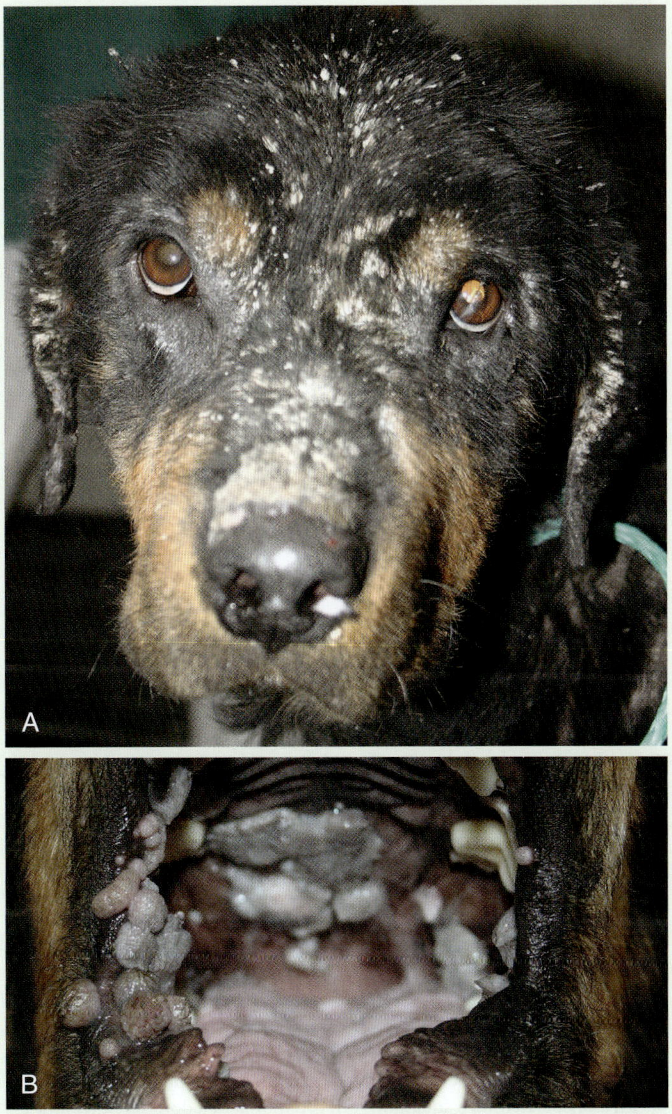

Fig. 40.8 (A) Adult male neutered Rottweiler with a high antibody titer to *Ehrlichia canis*, malnutrition, gastrointestinal parasitism, and sarcoptic mange. (B) Oral papillomatosis was present on oral examination and involved the hard and soft palates, buccal mucosa, and lips.

Integument: A dull haircoat was present. Patchy generalized alopecia with severe scaling, crusting, hyperpigmentation, ulceration, and lichenification was present on the face, pinnae and pinnal margins, shoulders, trunk, and extremities.

Eyes, ears, nose, and throat: Moderate mucoid discharge was present from both eyes. The incisor teeth were severely worn. Oral examination also revealed pain on opening the mouth and multiple pink to gray pedunculated masses that ranged from a few millimeters to over 1 cm in diameter on the buccal mucosa and gingiva, lateral aspect of the tongue, and on the hard and soft palates (see Fig. 40.8B). These were consistent with oral papillomatosis.

Musculoskeletal: BCS 1/9. Normal gait. No other musculoskeletal abnormalities were noted.

Cardiovascular and respiratory: No clinically significant abnormalities were detected.

GI and genitourinary: Abdominal palpation was within normal limits. Intact male with soft, symmetrical testes. Soft feces were noted on rectal examination.

Lymph nodes: Mandibular and superficial cervical nodes were enlarged (approximately 3 cm); the popliteal nodes were sized within normal limits.

Laboratory Findings

CBC: HCT 32.3% (40%–55%), MCV 64.3 fL (65–75 fL), MCHC 36.2 g/dL (33–36 g/dL), WBC 10,390 cells/μL (6,000–13,000 cells/μL), neutrophils 5,995 cells/μL (3,000–10,500 cells/μL), lymphocytes 1,891 cells/μL (1,000–4,000 cells/μL), monocytes 758 cells/μL (150–1,200 cells/μL), eosinophils 1,704 cells/μL (0–1,500 cells/μL), platelets 322,000 platelets/μL (150,000–400,000 platelets/μL), rare macroplatelets observed.

Serum chemistry profile: Sodium 144 mmol/L (145–154 mmol/L), potassium 4.8 mmol/L (3.6–5.3 mmol/L), chloride 108 mmol/L (108–118 mmol/L), bicarbonate 26 mmol/L (16–26 mmol/L), phosphorus 5.1 mg/dL (3.0–6.2 mg/dL), calcium 10.1 mg/dL (9.7–11.5 mg/dL), BUN 26 mg/dL (5–21 mg/dL), creatinine 0.7 mg/dL (0.3–1.2 mg/dL), glucose 108 mg/dL (64–123 mg/dL), total protein 7.7 g/dL (5.4–7.6 g/dL), albumin 2.9 g/dL (3.0–4.4 g/dL), globulin 4.8 g/dL (1.8–3.9 g/dL), ALT 48 U/L (19–67 U/L), AST 30 U/L (19–42 U/L), ALP 117 U/L (21–170 U/L), GGT < 3 U/L (0–6 U/L), cholesterol 210 mg/dL (135–361 mg/dL), total bilirubin 0.1 mg/dL (0–0.2 mg/dL).

Urinalysis: SpG 1.048; pH 5.0, negative protein (SSA), 1+ bilirubin; no hemoprotein, ketones or glucose; 1–2 WBC/HPF, rare RBC/HPF, rare bilirubin crystals, moderate sperm.

Cytology of superficial and deep skin scrapings: *Sarcoptes* mites were seen.

Imaging Findings

Lateral and dorsoventral thoracic radiographs were unremarkable. Abdominal ultrasonography revealed a small, 1-cm hypoechoic nodule in the body of the spleen. The remainder of the abdominal structures was within normal limits.

Microbiologic Testing

Lateral flow ELISA assay for antibodies to *E. canis, Anaplasma phagocytophilum,* and *Borrelia burgdorferi* and *Dirofilaria immitis* antigen (SNAP 4Dx Plus, IDEXX Laboratories, ME, USA): Positive for antibodies to *Ehrlichia* spp.

Vector-borne disease serology panel (*Babesia canis, A. phagocytophilum, E. canis, Rickettsia* spp. IFA): Positive for antibodies to *E. canis* (1:655,360) and *Rickettsia* spp. (1:40,960).

Fecal flotation: *Giardia* spp. cysts (<1 per 40× field), *Sarcoptes* mites (1 to 10 per 10× field).

Diagnosis

Canine oral papillomatosis; malnutrition; sarcoptic mange; suspected chronic canine monocytic ehrlichiosis; previous exposure to SFG rickettsias; giardiasis; cestodiasis.

CASE EXAMPLE—cont'd

Treatment

Oscar was treated with doxycycline (5 mg/kg PO q12h for 6 weeks) for ehrlichiosis, topical selamectin (every 2 weeks for a total of 6 weeks) for sarcoptic mange, praziquantel (5 mg/kg, once) for cestodiasis, cephalexin (22 mg/kg q12h for 4 weeks) for secondary bacterial pyoderma, and fenbendazole (50 mg/kg PO q24h for 3 days) for giardiasis. The owner was instructed to bathe him with an oatmeal shampoo twice weekly. At a recheck appointment 4 weeks later, Oscar weighed 31.5 kg. The skin lesions had improved, and new hair growth was noted. Pruritus was still present. More oral papillomas were present, and the owner described worsened halitosis. Mandibular lymph nodes remained enlarged. Treatment with cephalexin and doxycycline was continued for an additional 3 weeks. After 3 weeks, Oscar's bodyweight was 33.4 kg, the oral papillomas and mandibular lymphadenomegaly had resolved, and Oscar was vaccinated with CDV, canine parvovirus, CAdV, CPIV, and rabies virus vaccines and neutered.

Comments

The gross appearance of the oral lesions in this dog was sufficient to make a diagnosis of oral papillomatosis. Papillomatosis has been reported in other dogs with chronic *E. canis* infection, but the extent to which ehrlichiosis contributed to papillomatosis in this dog is unknown. The immunosuppression associated with malnutrition may also have played a role. Resolution of lesions occurred within 7 weeks after treatment of the immunosuppressive disorders, but papillomatosis can also resolve spontaneously over the same time period.

SUGGESTED READINGS

Lange CE, Favrot C. Canine papillomaviruses. *Vet Clin Small Anim Pract.* 2011;41:1183–1195.

Munday JS, Sharp CR, Beatty JA. Novel viruses: update on the significance of papillomavirus infections in cats. *J Fel Med Surg.* 2019;21:409–418.

Munday JS, Thomson NA, Luff JA. Papillomaviruses in dogs and cats. *Vet J.* 2017;225:23–31.

REFERENCES

1. Watrach AM. The ultrastructure of canine cutaneous papilloma. *Cancer Res.* 1969;29:2079–2084.
2. Watrach AM, Hanson LE, Meyer RC. Canine papilloma: the structural characterization of oral papilloma virus. *J Natl Cancer Inst.* 1969;43:453–458.
3. Carney HC, England JJ, Hodgin EC, et al. Papillomavirus infection of aged Persian cats. *J Vet Diagn Invest.* 1990;2:294–299.
4. Rector A, Van Ranst M. Animal papillomaviruses. *Virology.* 2013;445:213–223.
5. Munday JS. Bovine and human papillomaviruses: a comparative review. *Vet Pathol.* 2014;51:1063–1075.
6. Connolly K, Manders P, Earls P, et al. Papillomavirus-associated squamous skin cancers following transplant immunosuppression: one Notch closer to control. *Cancer Treat Rev.* 2014;40:205–214.
7. Bernard HU, Burk RD, Chen Z, et al. Classification of papillomaviruses (PVs) based on 189 PV types and proposal of taxonomic amendments. *Virology.* 2010;401:70–79.
8. Delius H, Van Ranst MA, Jenson AB, et al. Canine oral papillomavirus genomic sequence: a unique 1.5-kb intervening sequence between the E2 and L2 open reading frames. *Virology.* 1994;204:447–452.
9. Lange CE, Ackermann M, Favrot C, et al. Entire genomic sequence of novel canine papillomavirus type 13. *J Virol.* 2012;86:10226–10227.
10. Lange CE, Tobler K, Ackermann M, et al. Three novel canine papillomaviruses support taxonomic clade formation. *J Gen Virol.* 2009;90:2615–2621.
11. Lange CE, Tobler K, Lehner A, et al. A case of a canine pigmented plaque associated with the presence of a Chi-papillomavirus. *Vet Dermatol.* 2012;23. 76–e19.
12. Lange CE, Tobler K, Schraner EM, et al. Complete canine papillomavirus life cycle in pigmented lesions. *Vet Microbiol.* 2013;162:388–395.
13. Luff J, Mader M, Britton M, et al. Complete genome sequence of canine papillomavirus type 16. *Genome Announc.* 2015;3.
14. Luff J, Moore P, Zhou D, et al. Complete genome sequence of canine papillomavirus type 10. *J Virol.* 2012;86:11407.
15. Luff J, Rowland P, Mader M, et al. Two canine papillomaviruses associated with metastatic squamous cell carcinoma in two related Basenji dogs. *Vet Pathol.* 2016;53:1160–1163.
16. Tobler K, Favrot C, Nespeca G, et al. Detection of the prototype of a potential novel genus in the family Papillomaviridae in association with canine epidermodysplasia verruciformis. *J Gen Virol.* 2006;87:3551–3557.
17. Tobler K, Lange C, Carlotti DN, et al. Detection of a novel papillomavirus in pigmented plaques of four pugs. *Vet Dermatol.* 2008;19:21–25.
18. Yuan H, Ghim S, Newsome J, et al. An epidermotropic canine papillomavirus with malignant potential contains an E5 gene and establishes a unique genus. *Virology.* 2007;359:28–36.
19. Yuan H, Luff J, Zhou D, et al. Complete genome sequence of canine papillomavirus type 9. *J Virol.* 2012;86:5966.
20. Zhou D, Luff J, Paul S, et al. Complete genome sequence of canine papillomavirus virus type 12. *Genome Announc.* 2015;3.
21. Zhou D, Luff J, Usuda Y, et al. Complete genome sequence of canine papillomavirus type 11. *Genome Announc.* 2014;2.
22. Tisza MJ, Yuan H, Schlegel R, et al. Genomic sequence of canine papillomavirus 19. *Genome Announc.* 2016;4. e01380–16.
23. Lange CE, Diallo A, Zewe C, et al. Novel canine papillomavirus type 18 found in pigmented plaques. *Papillomavirus Res.* 2016;2:159–163.
24. Altan E, Seguin MA, Leutenegger CM, et al. Nasal virome of dogs with respiratory infection signs include novel taupapillomaviruses. *Virus Gene.* 2019;55:191–197.
25. Gil da Costa RM, Peleteiro MC, Pires MA, et al. An update on canine, feline and bovine papillomaviruses. *Transbound Emerg Dis.* 2017;64:1371–1379.
26. Lange CE, Favrot C. Canine papillomaviruses. *Vet Clin North Am Small Anim Pract.* 2011;41:1183–1195.
27. Dunowska M, Munday JS, Laurie RE, et al. Genomic characterisation of *Felis catus* papillomavirus 4, a novel papillomavirus detected in the oral cavity of a domestic cat. *Virus Gene.* 2014;48:111–119.
28. Lange CE, Tobler K, Markau T, et al. Sequence and classification of FdPV2, a papillomavirus isolated from feline Bowenoid in situ carcinomas. *Vet Microbiol.* 2009;137:60–65.
29. Munday JS, Dunowska M, Hills SF, et al. Genomic characterization of *Felis catus* papillomavirus-3: a novel papillomavirus detected in a feline Bowenoid in situ carcinoma. *Vet Microbiol.* 2013;165:319–325.
30. Tachezy R, Duson G, Rector A, et al. Cloning and genomic characterization of *Felis domesticus* papillomavirus type 1. *Virology.* 2002;301:313–321.
31. Munday JS, Dittmer KE, Thomson NA, et al. Genomic characterisation of *Felis catus* papillomavirus type 5 with proposed classification within a new papillomavirus genus. *Vet Microbiol.* 2017;207:50–55.
32. Carrai M, Van Brussel K, Shi M, et al. Identification of a novel papillomavirus associated with squamous cell carcinoma in a domestic cat. *Viruses.* 2020;12:124.
33. Bregman CL, Hirth RS, Sundberg JP, et al. Cutaneous neoplasms in dogs associated with canine oral papillomavirus vaccine. *Vet Pathol.* 1987;24:477–487.

34. Sundberg JP, Smith EK, Herron AJ, et al. Involvement of canine oral papillomavirus in generalized oral and cutaneous verrucosis in a Chinese Shar Pei dog. *Vet Pathol.* 1994;31:183–187.
35. Teifke JP, Lohr CV, Shirasawa H. Detection of canine oral papillomavirus-DNA in canine oral squamous cell carcinomas and p53 overexpressing skin papillomas of the dog using the polymerase chain reaction and non-radioactive in situ hybridization. *Vet Microbiol.* 1998;60:119–130.
36. Thaiwong T, Sledge DG, Wise AG, et al. Malignant transformation of canine oral papillomavirus (CPV1)-associated papillomas in dogs: an emerging concern? *Papillomavirus Res.* 2018;6:83–89.
37. Regalado Ibarra AM, Legendre L, Munday JS. Malignant transformation of a canine papillomavirus type 1-induced persistent oral papilloma in a 3-year-old dog. *J Vet Dent.* 2018;35:79–95.
38. Goldschmidt MH, Kennedy JS, Kennedy DR, et al. Severe papillomavirus infection progressing to metastatic squamous cell carcinoma in bone marrow-transplanted X-linked SCID dogs. *J Virol.* 2006;80:6621–6628.
39. Munday JS, Dunowska M, Laurie RE, et al. Genomic characterisation of canine papillomavirus type 17, a possible rare cause of canine oral squamous cell carcinoma. *Vet Microbiol.* 2016;182:135–140.
40. Munday JS, Tucker RS, Kiupel M, et al. Multiple oral carcinomas associated with a novel papillomavirus in a dog. *J Vet Diagn Invest.* 2015;27:221–225.
41. Luff JA, Affolter VK, Yeargan B, et al. Detection of six novel papillomavirus sequences within canine pigmented plaques. *J Vet Diagn Invest.* 2012;24:576–580.
42. Orbell HL, Munday JS, Orbell GMB, et al. Development of multiple cutaneous and follicular neoplasms associated with canine papillomavirus type 3 in a dog. *Vet Dermatol.* 2020;31:401–403.
43. Narama I, Kobayashi Y, Yamagami T, et al. Pigmented cutaneous papillomatosis (pigmented epidermal nevus) in three pug dogs; histopathology, electron microscopy and analysis of viral DNA by the polymerase chain reaction. *J Comp Pathol.* 2005;132:132–138.
44. Tanabe C, Kano R, Nagata M, et al. Molecular characteristics of cutaneous papillomavirus from the canine pigmented epidermal nevus. *J Vet Med Sci.* 2000;62:1189–1192.
45. Yu M, Chambers JK, Tsuzuki M, et al. Pigmented viral plaque and basal cell tumor associated with canine papillomavirus infection in Pug dogs. *J Vet Med Sci.* 2019;81:1643–1648.
46. Cavana P, Hubert B, Cordonnier N, et al. Generalized verrucosis associated with canine papillomavirus 9 infection in a dog. *Vet Dermatol.* 2015;26:209–210.
47. Munday JS, O'Connor KI, Smits B. Development of multiple pigmented viral plaques and squamous cell carcinomas in a dog infected by a novel papillomavirus. *Vet Dermatol.* 2011;22:104–110.
48. Alves CDBT, Weber MN, Guimarães LLB, et al. Canine papillomavirus type 16 associated to squamous cell carcinoma in a dog: virological and pathological findings. *Braz J Microbiol.* 2020;51:2087–2094.
49. Munday JS, Waropastrakul S, Gibson I, et al. Papillomaviral DNA sequences are not amplifiable from canine subungual squamous cell carcinomas. *N Z Vet J.* 2013;61:234–236.
50. Munday JS, French A, Harvey CJ. Molecular and immunohistochemical studies do not support a role for papillomaviruses in canine oral squamous cell carcinoma development. *Vet J.* 2015;204:223–225.
51. Porcellato I, Brachelente C, Guelfi G, et al. A retrospective investigation on canine papillomavirus 1 (CPV1) in oral oncogenesis reveals dogs are not a suitable animal model for high-risk HPV-induced oral cancer. *PloS One.* 2014;9:e112833.
52. Wilhelm S, Degorce-Rubiales F, Godson D, et al. Clinical, histological and immunohistochemical study of feline viral plaques and bowenoid in situ carcinomas. *Vet Dermatol.* 2006;17:424–431.
53. Munday JS, Knight CG, French AF. Evaluation of feline oral squamous cell carcinomas for p16CDKN2A protein immunoreactivity and the presence of papillomaviral DNA. *Res Vet Sci.* 2011;90:280–283.
54. Munday JS, French AF. *Felis catus* papillomavirus types 1 and 4 are rarely present in neoplastic and inflammatory oral lesions of cats. *Res Vet Sci.* 2015;100:220–222.
55. O'Neill SH, Newkirk KM, Anis EA, et al. Detection of human papillomavirus DNA in feline premalignant and invasive squamous cell carcinoma. *Vet Dermatol.* 2011;22:68–74.
56. Altamura G, Cardeti G, Cersini A, et al. Detection of *Felis catus* papillomavirus type-2 DNA and viral gene expression suggest active infection in feline oral squamous cell carcinoma. *Vet Comp Oncol.* 2020;18:494–501.
57. Chu S, Wylie TN, Wylie KM, et al. A virome sequencing approach to feline oral squamous cell carcinoma to evaluate viral causative factors. *Vet Microbiol.* 2020;240:108491.
58. Munday JS, Fairley RA, Mills H, et al. Oral papillomas associated with *Felis catus* papillomavirus type 1 in 2 domestic cats. *Vet Pathol.* 2015;52:1187–1190.
59. Munday JS, Kiupel M, French AF, et al. Amplification of papillomaviral DNA sequences from a high proportion of feline cutaneous in situ and invasive squamous cell carcinomas using a nested polymerase chain reaction. *Vet Dermatol.* 2008;19:259–263.
60. Thomson NA, Dunowska M, Munday JS. The use of quantitative PCR to detect Felis catus papillomavirus type 2 DNA from a high proportion of queens and their kittens. *Vet Microbiol.* 2015;175:211–217.
61. Ravens PA, Vogelnest LJ, Tong LJ, et al. Papillomavirus-associated multicentric squamous cell carcinoma in situ in a cat: an unusually extensive and progressive case with subsequent metastasis. *Vet Dermatol.* 2013;24:642–645. e161–162.
62. Munday JS, Benfell MW, French A, et al. Bowenoid in situ carcinomas in two Devon Rex cats: evidence of unusually aggressive neoplasm behaviour in this breed and detection of papillomaviral gene expression in primary and metastatic lesions. *Vet Dermatol.* 2016;27:215–e255.
63. Munday JS, Gibson I, French AF. Papillomaviral DNA and increased p16CDKN2A protein are frequently present within feline cutaneous squamous cell carcinomas in ultraviolet-protected skin. *Vet Dermatol.* 2011;22:360–366.
64. Munday JS, French AF, Gibson IR, et al. The presence of p16 CDKN2A protein immunostaining within feline nasal planum squamous cell carcinomas is associated with an increased survival time and the presence of papillomaviral DNA. *Vet Pathol.* 2013;50:269–273.
65. Thomson NA, Munday JS, Dittmer KE. Frequent detection of transcriptionally active *Felis catus* papillomavirus 2 in feline cutaneous squamous cell carcinomas. *J Gen Virol.* 2016;97:1189–1197.
66. Altamura G, Corteggio A, Pacini L, et al. Transforming properties of *Felis catus* papillomavirus type 2 E6 and E7 putative oncogenes in vitro and their transcriptional activity in feline squamous cell carcinoma in vivo. *Virology.* 2016;496:1–8.
67. Hoggard N, Munday JS, Luff J. Localization of *Felis catus* papillomavirus type 2 e6 and e7 RNA in feline cutaneous squamous cell carcinoma. *Vet Pathol.* 2018;55:409–416.
68. Munday JS, Kiupel M. Papillomavirus-associated cutaneous neoplasia in mammals. *Vet Pathol.* 2010;47:254–264.
69. Munday JS, Fairley R, Atkinson K. The detection of *Felis catus* papillomavirus 3 DNA in a feline bowenoid in situ carcinoma with novel histologic features and benign clinical behavior. *J Vet Diagn Invest.* 2016;28:612–615.
70. Munday JS, Thomson NA, Henderson G, et al. Identification of *Felis catus* papillomavirus 3 in skin neoplasms from four cats. *J Vet Diagn Invest.* 2018;30:324–328.
71. Munday JS, Thomson N, Dunowska M, et al. Genomic characterisation of the feline sarcoid-associated papillomavirus and proposed classification as Bos taurus papillomavirus type 14. *Vet Microbiol.* 2015;177:289–295.
72. Teifke JP, Kidney BA, Lohr CV, et al. Detection of papillomavirus-DNA in mesenchymal tumour cells and not in the hyperplastic epithelium of feline sarcoids. *Vet Dermatol.* 2003;14:47–56.
73. Doorbar J. The papillomavirus life cycle. *J Clin Virol.* 2005;32(suppl 1):S7–S15.
74. Moody CA, Laimins LA. Human papillomavirus oncoproteins: pathways to transformation. *Nat Rev Cancer.* 2010;10:550–560.
75. Munday JS, Aberdein D. Loss of retinoblastoma protein, but not p53, is associated with the presence of papillomaviral DNA in feline viral plaques, Bowenoid in situ carcinomas, and squamous cell carcinomas. *Vet Pathol.* 2012;49:538–545.
76. Munday JS, French AF, MacNamara AR. The development of multiple cutaneous inverted papilloma following ovariohysterectomy in a dog. *N Z Vet J.* 2010;58:168–171.
77. Stokking LB, Ehrhart EJ, Lichtensteiger CA, et al. Pigmented epidermal plaques in three dogs. *J Am Anim Hosp Assoc.* 2004;40:411–417.

78. Gill VL, Bergman PJ, Baer KE, et al. Use of imiquimod 5% cream (Aldara) in cats with multicentric squamous cell carcinoma in situ: 12 cases (2002-2005). *Vet Comp Oncol*. 2008;6:55–64.
79. Schulman FY, Krafft AE, Janczewski T. Feline cutaneous fibropapillomas: clinicopathologic findings and association with papillomavirus infection. *Vet Pathol*. 2001;38:291–296.
80. Munday JS, Knight CG. Amplification of feline sarcoid-associated papillomavirus DNA sequences from bovine skin. *Vet Dermatol*. 2010;21:341–344.
81. Lange CE, Zollinger S, Tobler K, et al. Clinically healthy skin of dogs is a potential reservoir for canine papillomaviruses. *J Clin Microbiol*. 2011;49:707–709.
82. Smeets SJ, Hesselink AT, Speel EJ, et al. A novel algorithm for reliable detection of human papillomavirus in paraffin embedded head and neck cancer specimen. *Int J Cancer*. 2007;121:2465–2472.
83. Richman AW, Kirby AL, Rosenkrantz W, et al. Persistent papilloma treated with cryotherapy in three dogs. *Vet Dermatol*. 2017;28. 625–e154.
84. Yagci BB, Ural K, Ocal N, et al. Azithromycin therapy of papillomatosis in dogs: a prospective, randomized, double-blinded, placebo-controlled clinical trial. *Vet Dermatol*. 2008;19:194–198.
85. Knight EC, Munday JS, Stone BM, et al. Carbon dioxide laser treatment of extensive pigmented viral plaque lesions in a golden retriever dog. *Vet Dermatol*. 2016;27. 442–e117.
86. Hansen N, Nicholas N, Pack G, et al. Progressive cutaneous viral pigmented plaques in three Hungarian Vizslas and the response of lesions to topical tigilanol tiglate gel. *Vet Med Sci*. 2017;4:53–62.
87. Munday JS, Peters-Kennedy J. Consistent detection of *Felis domesticus* papillomavirus 2 DNA sequences within feline viral plaques. *J Vet Diagn Invest*. 2010;22:946–949.
88. Stanley MA. Epithelial cell responses to infection with human papillomavirus. *Clin Microbiol Rev*. 2012;25:215–222.
89. Thomson NA, Howe L, Weidgraaf K, et al. *Felis catus* papillomavirus type 2 virus-like particle vaccine is safe and immunogenic but does not reduce FcaPV-2 viral loads in adult cats. *Vet Immunol Immunopathol*. 2019;213:109888.
90. Thomson NA, Thomas DG, Weidgraaf K, et al. *Felis catus* papillomavirus type 2 DNA loads on kittens are transient and do not reflect their susceptibility to infection. *J Feline Med Surg*. 2018;20:332–338.

41

Arthropod-Borne Viral Infections

Jane E. Sykes, Andrea Tipold

KEY POINTS

- First Described: Eastern equine encephalitis, 1831 (horses, Massachusetts)[1]; West Nile virus infection, 1937 (human, Uganda)[2]; tick-borne encephalitis virus, 1931 (humans, Austria);[3] African horse sickness virus, 1569 (horses, Africa).[4]
- Causes: RNA viruses that belong to the families *Togaviridae* (genus *Alphavirus*), such as eastern equine encephalitis virus; *Bunyaviridae,* such as La Crosse virus; *Reoviridae,* such as African horse sickness virus, and *Flaviviridae,* such as West Nile virus and tick-borne encephalitis virus.
- Affected Hosts: A variety of animal species including horses, humans, and dogs.
- Geographic Distribution: Follows that of the vector host. Eastern equine encephalitis virus is found in the eastern and southeastern United States, as well as Central and South America; West Nile virus is found in Africa, Asia, Middle East, Europe, and the United States; African horse sickness virus is found in Africa and the Middle East; tick-borne encephalitis virus is found in continental Europe and Asia.
- Mode of Transmission: Primarily mosquitoes, and for tick-borne encephalitis virus, *Ixodes* ticks. Dogs can be infected with African horse sickness virus by ingestion of horse meat, but *Culicoides* midges in addition to mosquitoes may also be involved in transmission of the virus to dogs.
- Major Clinical Signs: Fever (sometimes >105°F [40.6°C]), lethargy, neurologic signs, and sometimes systemic signs such as anorexia and diarrhea. African horse sickness virus also causes respiratory signs due to pulmonary edema.
- Differential Diagnoses: Rabies, distemper, pseudorabies; bacterial, protozoal, or fungal meningitis; meningoencephalitis of unknown origin (MUO); hemic neoplasia with CNS involvement. Differential diagnosis for African horse sickness virus infection also includes severe viral or bacterial respiratory tract diseases (e.g., influenza virus infection or *Streptococcus equi* subsp. *zooepidemicus* infection).
- Human Health Significance: Humans are susceptible to disease caused by many arboviruses. Dogs and cats are dead-end hosts and do not serve as reservoirs for human infection. Blood and tissues of affected dogs and cats should be handled with caution.

ETIOLOGY, EPIDEMIOLOGY, AND CLINICAL FEATURES

A large number of viruses that are spread by arthropod vectors (sometimes referred to as *arboviruses*, for *ar*thropod-*bo*rne *viruses*) can infect dogs and cats, often causing encephalitis (Box 41.1 and Table 41.1). These viruses are enveloped RNA viruses that are unstable in the environment and readily inactivated with routine disinfectants. Disease is sporadic, and for many arboviruses, only subclinical infections have been documented in dogs and cats. Arboviruses are maintained in vectors and often small rodent and/or avian reservoir hosts, and some of these reservoir hosts can develop illness in association with infection. The geographic distribution is dependent on that of the vectors and reservoir hosts. Dogs and cats, as well as other domestic animal and human hosts, are generally considered "dead-end" hosts that do not maintain sufficient viremia to infect arthropods (Fig. 41.1). Arboviruses replicate within the arthropod vector and are transmitted to vertebrate hosts when the vector feeds; this is followed by viremia and, in some cases, viral spread to the CNS and neuroinvasion, with subsequent neuronal necrosis and inflammation. When neurologic disease occurs, it has important public health significance, because the clinical signs can mimic those of rabies. Because humans have the potential to be infected with these viruses, serologic evidence of infection of dogs and cats in a region where disease in humans is not widely recognized can also have public health significance.

BOX 41.1 General Features of Arbovirus Infections as They Relate to Dogs and Cats

- Vector-borne RNA viruses
- Often mosquito borne
- Maintained among small wild vertebrate reservoir hosts, especially birds and/or rodents
- Geographic distribution follows that of vector host
- Seasonal distribution that reflects activity of the vector host
- May cause disease in humans and other domestic animals, especially horses
- Infection of dogs and cats is most often subclinical
- Dogs and cats are "dead-end" hosts
- Infection more prevalent in dogs than in cats
- Sporadic reports of disease, especially in young animals (<6 months)
- Neurologic signs accompanied by fever and sometimes other systemic signs (e.g., diarrhea)
- Histopathology shows neuronal necrosis, gliosis, and perivascular cuffing within the brain, which is predominantly nonsuppurative. Occasionally hepatitis and myocarditis are described

Alphavirus Infections (Family *Togaviridae*)

Alphaviruses are enveloped, single-stranded RNA mosquito-borne viruses that belong to the family *Togaviridae*. Members of this group that are of importance to human and animal health include Eastern,

TABLE 41.1 Arthropod-Borne Viral Infections of Dogs and Cats

Classification	Virus	Vector	Reservoir Hosts	Affected Hosts	Geographic Distribution
Family *Togaviridae*, genus *Alphavirus*	Eastern equine encephalitis virus (EEEV)	Mosquitoes (*Culiseta melanura, Coquillettidia* spp., *Aedes* spp., *Culex* spp.)	Birds	Humans (North American strains), horses, dogs, other domestic farm animal species and farmed and captive birds	Primarily southeastern (especially Georgia and Florida), eastern, and Great Lakes regions of the United States and the Caribbean Islands (North American EEEV strains); also Central America, Brazil, Guyana, Argentina (South American EEEV strains).
	Venezuelan equine encephalitis virus	Mosquitoes (*Psorophora confinnis, Aedes spp.*, *Culex* spp.)	Rodents	Horses, humans, possibly dogs	Southern United States (Florida), Central and South America (especially Colombia, Venezuela, Trinidad, Peru, Ecuador, Mexico)
	Ross River and Barmah Forest virus	Mosquitoes (*Ochlerotatus vigilax*)	Wallabies, kangaroos	Humans, dogs, cats	Australia, from Tasmania to Queensland
Family *Bunyaviridae*, genus *Orthobunyavirus*	La Crosse virus	Mosquitoes	Small mammals (chipmunks)	Humans, dogs	Eastern and Midwestern United States
Family *Bunyaviridae*, genus *Orthobunyavirus*	Tensaw virus	Mosquitoes (*Anopheles* spp.)	Rodents	Dogs, cattle	Southeastern United States
Family *Bunyaviridae*, genus *Phlebovirus*	Rift Valley fever virus	Mosquitoes (*Culex theileri, Aedes caballus*)	Ungulates (sheep)	Humans, dogs, cats	East Africa
Family *Flaviviridae*	West Nile virus	Mosquitoes	Birds	Horses, humans, birds, dogs	North, Central, and South America; Africa, the Middle East, Europe, Asia, Australia
	Tick-borne encephalitis virus	*Ixodes* ticks	Rodents, birds	Humans, horses, dogs; domestic animals are frequently infected subclinically	Europe, Asia
	St. Louis encephalitis virus	Mosquitoes (*Culex* spp.)	Birds	Humans, dogs, cats	United States, Canada, Central America, Caribbean Islands, Colombia, Brazil, Argentina
	Japanese encephalitis virus	Mosquitoes (*Culex* spp.)	Birds	Humans, dogs, cats, pigs, horses	Siberia, Japan, China, many far-east countries
	Powassan virus	Ticks (*Ixodes cookei, Ixodes marxi*)	Rodents	Sheep, humans, dogs	United States, Canada
	Louping-ill virus	Ticks (*Ixodes ricinus*)	Red grouse	Sheep, cattle, humans, dogs	Scotland, Ireland
	Wesselsbron virus	Mosquitoes (*Aedes* spp.)	Ungulates, sheep	Sheep, dogs	South Africa
	Yellow fever virus	Mosquitoes (*Aedes* spp.)	Nonhuman primates, humans	Humans, cats	South America, Africa
Family *Reoviridae*	African horse sickness virus	Midges (*Culicoides* spp.), mosquitoes	Zebra	Horses, dogs	Africa, Middle East, Mediterranean
	Bluetongue virus	Midges (*Culicoides* spp.)	Sheep	Sheep, dogs	Worldwide

Western, and Venezuelan encephalitis viruses, which cause disease in humans and horses in the Americas; and Ross River virus, which causes disease in humans in Australia and the Pacific islands. Venezuelan equine encephalitis virus (VEEV) primarily causes outbreaks of disease in horses and humans in Central and the northern parts of South America, although an outbreak occurred in Texas in 1971, and there is the potential for additional outbreaks in the United States.[5] Experimental infection of dogs with VEEV resulted in fever, leukopenia, and neurologic signs.[6] Although there is one possible report of encephalitis in a puppy due to a VEEV,[7] only eastern equine encephalitis virus (EEEV) is a significant cause of naturally occurring disease in dogs. Dogs have been used as sentinels for the presence of VEEV variants (such as Everglades virus) in epidemiologic serosurveys.[8] Western equine encephalitis virus causes encephalitis in dogs after experimental parenteral or intracerebral inoculation, but naturally occurring disease has not been described.[9]

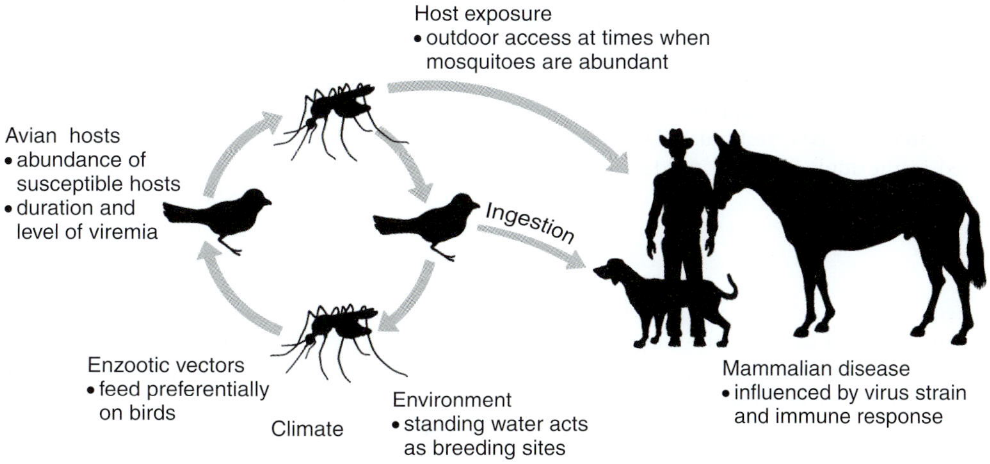

Fig. 41.1 West Nile virus transmission cycle and factors that influence arbovirus epidemiology. (From Sykes JE. *Canine and Feline Infectious Diseases*. Elsevier; 2014.)

Other alphaviruses cause subclinical seroconversion when they infect dogs under natural conditions. Ross River and Barmah Forest viruses are endemic in Australia, affecting kangaroos and wallabies as major mammalian reservoirs. Serum neutralizing antibodies are widespread in human and mammalian populations, and have been detected in dogs and cats. Dogs and cats that were experimentally fed infected mosquitoes were relatively resistant to both viral infections.[10] A few animals seroconverted, but none developed viremia or clinical signs. Therefore they are unlikely to be important reservoirs of these viruses.

EEEV is endemic in swampy areas of the southeastern United States,[11] where it is maintained in a variety of avian reservoir hosts. It causes disease in humans, horses, dogs, and other domestic animal species. Different viral lineages vary in pathogenicity for humans and horses. Human cases occur in the southeastern, eastern, and Great Lakes regions of the United States, but especially Florida, Georgia, Massachusetts, and New Jersey; there has been most recent expansion of the virus' geographic range in the New England region (Fig. 41.2A).[12–15] Most affected dogs have been reported from Georgia; dogs from New York state and Michigan have also been affected, as well as captive wolf pups in Michigan in 2019.[13,16,17] Dogs with signs of encephalitis have always been young (<7 months of age). Disease usually occurs in late spring or summer. Clinical signs include fever, lethargy, inappetence, and diarrhea, with rapid progression (within 1 to 2 days) to recumbency, tachypnea, miosis, nystagmus, tremors, seizures, and death.[11,16]

Bunyavirus Infections

Like togaviruses, bunyaviruses are enveloped, single-stranded RNA viruses. Clinically important bunyaviruses for animal and human health are the mosquito-borne viruses Rift Valley fever (genus *Phlebovirus*) and La Crosse (genus *Bunyavirus*) viruses; the tick-borne virus Crimean-Congo hemorrhagic fever virus (genus *Nairovirus*); and members of the genus *Hantavirus*, which are not transmitted by vectors and cause hemorrhagic febrile and respiratory illness in humans (see Chapter 43, Emerging and Miscellaneous Viral Infections). Serologic evidence of infection with some vector-borne bunyaviruses has been documented in dogs and cats.

Tensaw Virus

Tensaw virus is a bunyavirus found in the southeastern United States. It infects a variety of mammalian species, and although not considered a significant disease threat to humans, there is widespread human exposure to the virus, and it has rarely caused human encephalitis.[18] When inoculated into dogs and cats, it produced subclinical viremia, and mosquito-mediated transmission from infected dogs was demonstrated.[19]

Rift Valley Fever Virus

Rift Valley fever virus (genus *Phlebovirus*, family *Bunyaviridae*) causes widespread outbreaks of abortion and death in livestock in parts of Africa and the Arabian peninsula, often after heavy rainfall, which facilitates emergence of infected mosquitoes. Humans can also be infected, either as a result of mosquito-borne transmission, or contact with infected livestock tissues, fluids, or aborted material.[20] Disease in humans tends to be self-limiting, but 1% to 2% of infected humans can develop clinically significant hepatitis, retinitis, delayed-onset encephalitis, or hemorrhagic disease, the latter with high mortality. Because it threatens both livestock and human health, Rift Valley fever virus is of significant public health concern.

When experimentally inoculated subcutaneously into newborn puppies and kittens, Rift Valley fever virus can cause viremia with fever then neurologic signs (ataxia and seizures), terminal hypothermia, and death.[21–24] In contrast, older puppies and adult dogs show no clinical signs, but the virus can cause abortions and stillbirths in experimentally infected pregnant bitches.[21] Puppies were shown to transmit the virus to their mother and to other puppies, raising concern for the possible role of dogs in transmission of the virus to livestock or humans. Under natural conditions, it has been suggested that dogs might become infected through inhalation or ingestion of the virus from infected carcasses. Given that only neonatal puppies and kittens are capable of transmitting infection following experimental infection, the role of dogs and cats in the epidemiology of this disease seems to be of limited significance.

La Crosse Virus

La Crosse virus rarely causes naturally occurring disease in dogs.[25,26] La Crosse virus was named after La Crosse in Wisconsin, where it was first identified as a human pathogen, and is mostly found in the eastern and midwestern United States (Fig. 41.2B). The virus is maintained in rodents, especially Eastern gray squirrels and chipmunks. Vector infection can be lifelong, with transovarial transmission to subsequent generations of mosquitoes. La Crosse virus is a major cause of human pediatric encephalitis in North America, although mortality is low. Affected dogs have included an adult dog from Florida and three puppies from southern Georgia.[25,26] Mild fever, lethargy, ataxia, vestibular signs, and ultimately seizures occurred in the adult dog, and sudden death was reported in the puppies.

Reovirus Infections

Reoviruses are icosahedral, nonenveloped viruses. The major reovirus of significance to dogs and cats is African horse sickness virus (genus *Orbivirus*). As its name implies, African horse sickness virus causes outbreaks of disease in horses in Africa with high (90%) mortality. Infection occurs throughout sub-Saharan Africa, extending from Senegal to Somalia and South Africa. The disease also occurs sporadically in the Middle East, India, and Pakistan, and spread to Spain in 1966 and again in 1987, which resulted in significant equine mortality.[27] It is spread by biting *Culicoides imicola* midges; other biting insects may play a lesser role in transmission.[27] In horses, disease results from damage to the respiratory and cardiovascular systems, and has been divided into a mild febrile form; a peracute pulmonary form, with rapid death due to pulmonary edema; a subacute cardiac form characterized by fever and subcutaneous edema; and a mixed cardiopulmonary form.[4] Dogs are the only other animals capable of developing the severe form of disease. Dogs can be naturally infected, most commonly when they ingest infected horse meat, but there have also been reports of infection of dogs from South Africa without this history, suggesting the possibility of vector-borne transmission.[27,28] In further support of vector-borne transmission, most of these cases were seen during peak seasonal *Culicoides* midge activity (late summer). Many dogs show no clinical signs, but severe disease can occur. The incubation period is 1 to 2 weeks, followed by variable fever, lethargy, inappetence, and signs of pulmonary edema, including tachypnea, cough, and foamy nasal discharge. This can be followed by diarrhea and seizures, with high mortality.[27–29]

A reovirus with historical significance for dogs is bluetongue virus, which causes disease in sheep and to a lesser extent in cattle in Australia, the United States, Africa, the Middle East, Asia, and Europe. Natural disease caused by this virus in dogs is unlikely based on the observed low prevalence of seropositivity in dogs in endemic areas.[30] Abortion in pregnant bitches and their subsequent death occurred 7 to 9 days after vaccination with a bluetongue virus-contaminated, attenuated live virus combination canine vaccine in the early 1990s.[31,32] Lesions in

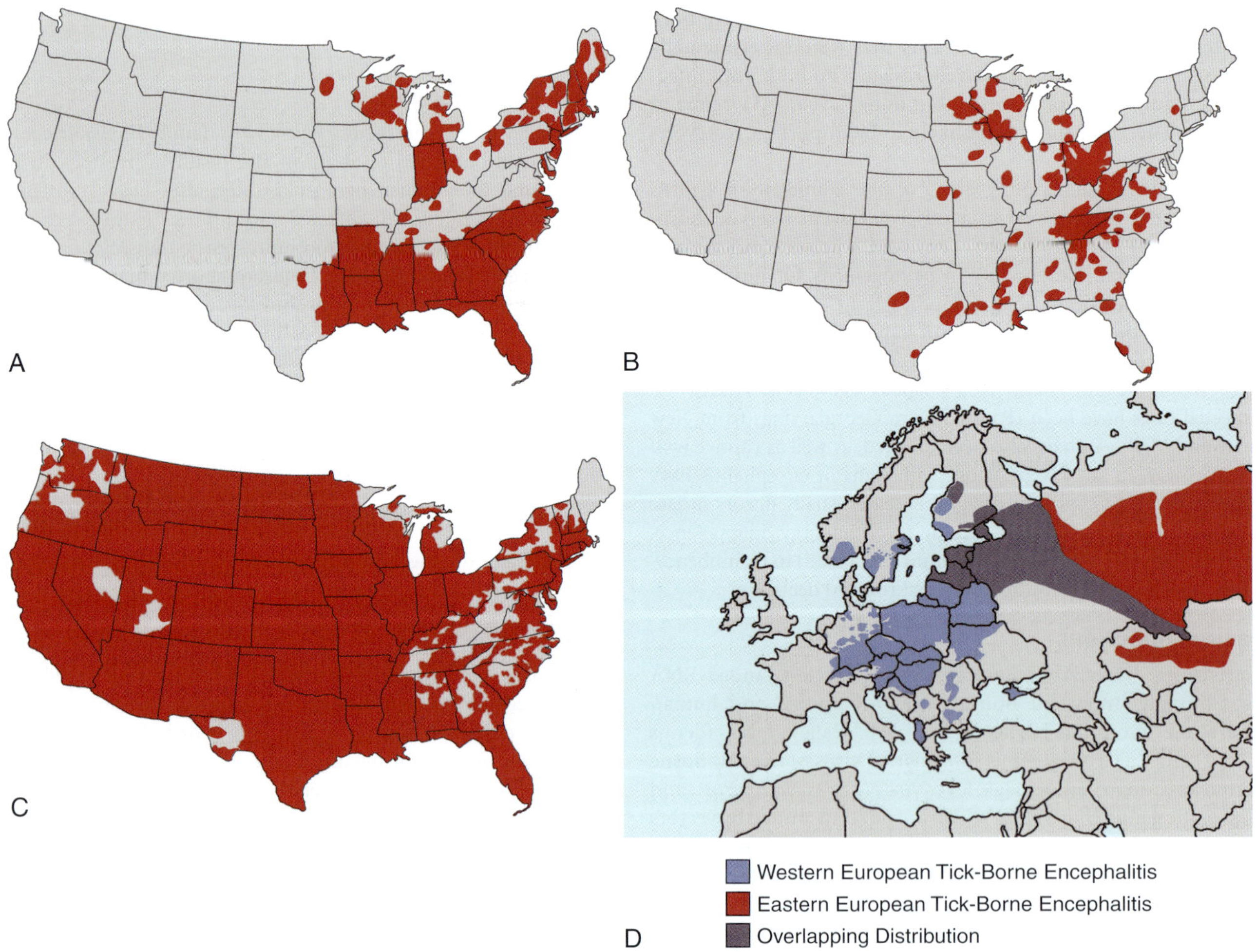

Fig. 41.2 Geographic distribution of some arboviruses that can cause disease in dogs and cats. (A) Regions in the USA with eastern equine encephalitis virus transmission. (B) Regions in the USA with La Crosse virus transmission. (C) Regions in the USA Regions with West Nile virus transmission. (D) Regions with tick-borne encephalitis virus transmission. (A–D, Modified from Sykes JE. *Canine and Feline Infectious Diseases*. Elsevier; 2014.)

the dam consisted of interstitial pneumonia, myocardial degeneration, hepatic vasculitis, and renal glomerulitis.[32]

Flavivirus Infections

Flaviviruses are small, icosahedral, enveloped viruses with a single-stranded RNA genome. Vector-borne flaviviruses (*flavi* = "yellow," Latin) of importance to human and animal health are the mosquito-borne viruses Japanese encephalitis virus, yellow fever virus, Murray Valley encephalitis virus, St. Louis encephalitis virus, Wesselsbron virus, Dengue viruses, and West Nile virus (WNV), as well as the tick-borne viruses inducing tick-borne encephalitis (TBE) virus, Louping-ill virus, and Powassan virus. Japanese encephalitis virus, Murray Valley encephalitis virus, and St. Louis encephalitis virus all belong to the *Japanese encephalitis complex*. Antibodies to some of these viruses have been detected in dogs and to a lesser extent, cats in serosurveys,[33–37] but serologic cross-reactivity among flaviviruses can occur. Although uncommon, WNV in the United States and TBE virus in Europe have been reported to cause disease in dogs on more than one occasion. One dog from Africa with fatal encephalitis was initially thought to be infected with Wesselsbron disease virus,[38] but the isolate was later confirmed to be WNV.[39]

West Nile Virus Infection

WNV was first isolated in 1937 from a woman in the West Nile region of Uganda.[2] In the 1950s, the virus was recognized in Israel as a cause of human neurologic disease in the elderly,[40] and subsequently was identified in other parts of Europe and South Africa. In 1999, it appeared in New York state, possibly by transport of infected humans, birds, or mosquitoes.[41] WNV then spread explosively westward across the United States, and by 2003, disease was detected across the United States to California (Fig. 41.2C). WNV also spread into Canada, Mexico, the Caribbean, and Central and South America, and is now one of the most broadly distributed arboviruses.[41,42] Several different variants of the virus exist, which differ in virulence. Strains circulating within the Western hemisphere, Europe, the Middle East, India, Africa, and Australia belong to WNV lineage 1; lineage 2 strains circulate in South Africa, Madagascar, and, now also Europe. Other lineages have also been reported, but these are not associated with outbreaks of human disease.

Although most of the natural transmission of WNV in the United States has been associated with three *Culex* subspecies (*pipiens*, *quinquefasciatus*, and *tarsalis*), WNV has been isolated from at least 65 mosquito species.[43–72] Transmission of WNV by mosquitoes increases in the warmer months, with peak activity in the northern hemisphere between July and October. Birds (especially passerines such as crows, jays, brown sparrows, and the American robin; shorebirds; owls; and hawks) are important reservoir hosts (see Fig. 41.1). Some avian species, such as brown sparrows, maintain high viremia in the absence of clinical signs, whereas crows develop high viremias and near-uniform mortality. Other modes of transmission include ingestion through predation of infected birds or rodents, blood transfusion, needle-stick injuries, and transplacental transmission. Increased ambient temperature is associated with increased efficiency of transmission from mosquitoes to birds. Disease primarily occurs in birds, humans, and horses, but disease has been reported in several other vertebrate species, including farmed alligators.[44] Most mammalian species develop a viremia of insufficient magnitude to infect feeding mosquitoes, but some exceptions occur, including among some rodent and lagomorph species.[45] Dogs develop low-titer viremia and are considered incompetent as amplifying hosts, but treatment of dogs with glucocorticoids before infection resulted in levels of viremia roughly 50 times that in untreated dogs.[46]

After inoculation, the virus replicates in keratinocytes, dendritic cells, and Langerhans cells. This is followed by spread to draining lymph nodes, further replication in lymph node macrophages, cell-associated viremia, and dissemination to peripheral organs.[43] The vast majority of infected humans experience no clinical signs. When signs occur in humans they follow an incubation period of 2 to as long as 21 days (usually 2 to 6 days). They are often mild and self-limiting and include fever, headache, myalgia, fatigue, GI symptoms, and a transient rash.[43,47] Rarely, hepatitis, pancreatitis, myocarditis, rhabdomyolysis, orchitis, uveitis, and chorioretinitis can occur. Severe neuroinvasive disease occurs in fewer than 1% of cases, is most common in the elderly, those with advanced immunosuppression, or people with chronic medical conditions. Severe disease is characterized by high fever, cervical rigidity, muscle weakness, seizures, and flaccid paralysis, and neurological signs may persist for over a year in those that recover. Fatality rates in humans with encephalitis are reported to be 3% to 19%.[45] Neurologic signs result from viral invasion of neurons in the brainstem, deep nuclei, and anterior horns within the spinal cord. Neuroinvasion appears to occur by both anterograde and retrograde axonal transport.[43,48] The innate immune system plays a critical role in control of WNV replication. Cellular immunity, mediated by CD4+ and CD8+ T cells, is essential for clearance of virus from the CNS, but in some cases, cellular immune responses appear to contribute to immunopathogenetic lesions in the CNS.[49]

Clinical signs in horses result from polioencephalomyelitis and include fever and neurologic signs such as ataxia, weakness, and muscle tremors.[50] Approximately two-thirds of horses recover. Infected wild birds can exhibit neurologic disease but are usually found dead. Myocarditis and meningoencephalitis are common necropsy findings in these birds.[51]

In dogs, there is widespread serologic evidence of infection, but disease is rare. Dogs have been widely used as sentinels for evidence of WNV in different geographic locations. Serologic surveys have revealed prevalences of 27% in Senegal in 2014, 62% in working dogs in Morocco in 2012,[52] 28% in Saskatchewan, Canada in 2008–2010,[53] 5% in New York City in 1999, 4.6% in China in 2011,[54] 18% in Harris County, Texas in 2005,[55] and 56% in Louisiana after Hurricane Katrina.[56] Cats also can become infected and seroconvert, but illness has not been described. Dogs that were experimentally infected with WNV using mosquitoes developed viremia of low magnitude and short duration, and failed to show clinical manifestations of illness, except for transient pyrexia in one dog.[57] Cats infected experimentally by feeding them infected mice remained healthy, and cats infected using mosquitoes developed transient fever, inappetence, and lethargy, with viremia that was more sustained than that in dogs.

Five clinically affected dogs have been described following natural infection. All, apart from a dog from Africa, resided in various parts of the United States (Missouri, Mississippi, California, and Illinois).[58–61] All of the dogs showed signs of fever and progressive neurologic disease. Neurologic signs included generalized tremors, ataxia, a head tilt, bobbing movements, altered mentation, cervical pain, abnormal placing reactions, and tetraparesis. Diarrhea, serous oculonasal discharge, conjunctivitis, abdominal pain, cardiac arrhythmias due to myocarditis, tachypnea, tachycardia, and a stiff gait associated with mild neutrophilic polyarthritis have been reported (Fig. 41.3). For all dogs, diagnosis was made at necropsy. In Europe, WNV infection was suspected at necropsy of dogs with encephalitis of unknown origin after detection of immunohistological precipitates using virus-specific antibodies; however, the infection was not confirmed using other techniques.[62]

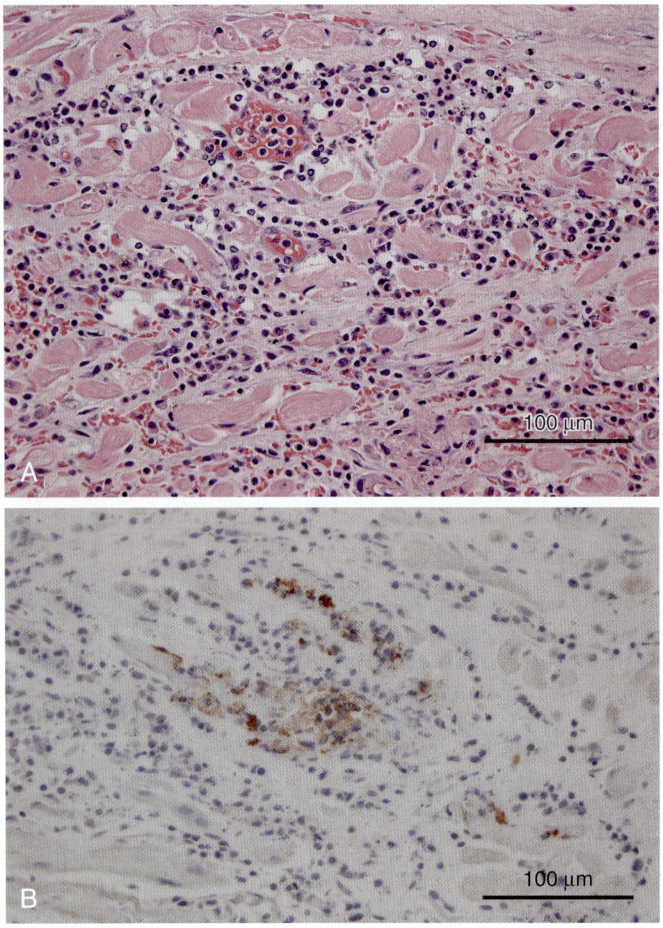

Fig. 41.3 Severe lymphocytic and neutrophilic myocarditis and vasculitis due to West Nile virus (WNV) infection with focally extensive hemorrhage and myonecrosis. (A) Hematoxylin and eosin stain. (B) Immunohistochemical stain showing WNV immunoreactivity within neutrophils and histiocytes *(brown)*. (From Cannon AB, Luff J, Brault C, et al. Acute encephalitis, polyarthritis and myocarditis associated with West Nile virus infection in a dog. *J Vet Intern Med.* 2006;20:1219–1223.)

Tick-Borne Encephalitis Virus

TBE virus is a notifiable disease that causes potentially fatal neurologic disease in humans in Europe and Asia, where it is the most important tick-borne viral disease of humans.[63] The virus is transmitted transstadially and to a lesser extent transovarially within infected ticks, and ticks can transmit the disease to each other while co-feeding, independent of systemic viremia in vertebrate hosts.[64] The primary reservoirs for the virus are small rodents such as mice and voles. Consumption of raw milk from infected ruminants (especially goats) is a lesser mode of transmission to humans (Fig. 41.4). TBE has been reported not only in humans, but also in dogs, horses, monkeys, and wild ruminants, but not in cats.

At least three subtypes of TBE virus exist, which vary in virulence and geographic distribution. The three predominant subtypes are designated the European, Siberian, and far-eastern subtypes,[65,66] although as of 2019 two additional subtypes have been proposed—the Baikalian and Himalayan subtypes.[66] The far-eastern subtype occurs in far-eastern Russia, Japan, Korea, and China and is the most virulent subtype, with mortality rates in humans that may exceed 20%. In much of Europe, *Ixodes ricinus* ticks spread the European subtype (Western and Central European TBE). *Ixodes persulcatus* ticks transmit the other viral subtypes in northeastern Europe, Russia, and far-east Asia (Eastern European TBE) (Fig. 41.2D).[67] Both Siberian and European subtypes may be found in eastern Europe. The disease was originally detected in 1937 in Austria (Central European TBE), but its geographic distribution has expanded rapidly so that the European subtype now occurs throughout Europe as far west as France and now possibly Belgium, the Netherlands, Northern Germany, and the United Kingdom.[37,66,68,69] Until very recently, TBE had not been reported in the United Kingdom and Ireland, but a related tick-borne flavivirus, Louping-ill virus, was known to be present. However, a recent surveillance effort in the United Kingdom detected TBE virus in ticks from the Norfolk/Suffolk (Thetford Forest) area, where the seroprevalence of flavivirus infection was highest.[66] No human or canine cases of TBE have yet been reported in the United Kingdom. An astonishing finding suggests that a specific adaptation of the tick populations to their respective TBE virus isolates occurs.[70]

In Europe, some of the highest incidence rates have occurred in central European countries, especially the Czech Republic.[71] Disease seasonality correlates with the activity of the tick in various parts of Europe.

In humans, signs of TBE occur in approximately one-third of infected individuals 4 to 28 days (and usually 7 to 14 days) after a tick bite and are usually biphasic.[66] In the first, viremic phase, fever, malaise, headache, myalgia, and vomiting occur, which resolve within 1 week. In some individuals, after an asymptomatic period that lasts 2 to 10 days, clinical signs return and are accompanied by signs of meningitis, meningoencephalitis, meningoencephalomyelitis, or meningoencephaloradiculitis. About 4 to 14% of cases are fatal, most often in the elderly,[72] but neurologic signs can persist for months or longer than a year. Co-infections with *Borrelia* (*Borreliella*) *burgdorferi* can occur. Vaccines are currently recommended for prevention of TBE in humans, and national vaccination programs have greatly reduced the incidence of disease.[73]

Subclinical infection of dogs with TBE virus is widespread, and so dogs have been important sentinels for the presence of the virus in new regions of Europe. Rarely, illness that resembles that in humans can occur in dogs. Affected dogs have been described from Sweden, Norway, Greece, Switzerland, Austria, Germany, the Czech Republic, and Italy.[63,74–77] Several reports have described disease in rottweilers, but it is not clear whether this represents a true breed predisposition. Signs in dogs include high fever (over 39°C [102.5°F]), lethargy, anorexia, and neurologic signs such as decreased mentation, behavioral changes such as aggression, delayed placing reactions, ataxia, flaccid paralysis, reduced segmental reflexes, neck pain, vestibular signs, tremors, tetraparesis, miosis, anisocoria, and generalized seizures.[63,67] These signs progress rapidly over several days to a week, sometimes culminating in death or euthanasia. In a 2021 long-term follow-up study of 54 dogs with TBE, the disease was clinically biphasic, with initial non-specific clinical signs followed by onset of neurologic deficits. The case fatality rate in that study was 33%.[77] Of the dogs that died, all died within 4 months, and of those that survived, 17% had residual neurologic signs. Neurologic sequelae were more often detected in older dogs and dogs with seizures at the time of initial evaluation. Because of the rapid progression of neurologic signs, the disease is sometimes mistaken for rabies. Recovery has been described rarely.

Louping-Ill Virus

Louping-ill virus is transmitted by *I. ricinus* ticks, which are the most abundant ticks in the United Kingdom, and mainly causes neurologic disease in sheep (especially weaned lambs) and red grouse, an economically important gamebird. This is in contrast to TBE virus,

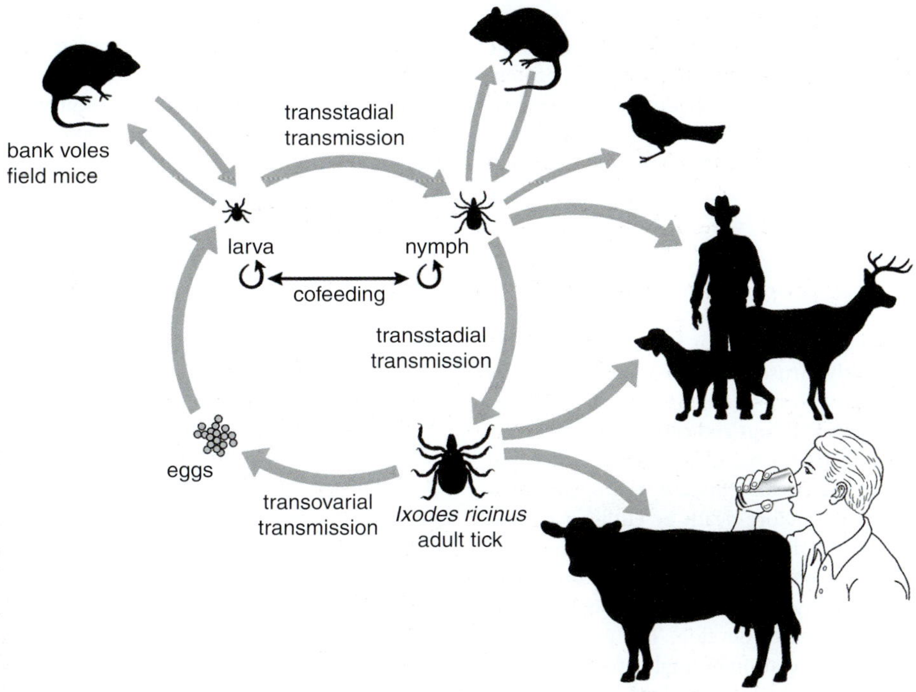

Fig. 41.4 Transmission cycle for tick-borne encephalitis virus. (From Sykes JE. *Canine and Feline Infectious Diseases*. Elsevier; 2014.)

which does not cause disease in sheep. Several different molecular types of the virus have been described that circulate in distinct geographic regions, and although the virus has been detected in Europe, disease predominantly occurs in rough pastures and upland heather moorland of Scotland, Cumbria, Wales, Devon, North Yorkshire, and Ireland (Fig. 41.5).[78,79] Red grouse and sheep, together with mountain hares, are considered to be important reservoir hosts, another important difference from TBE virus, which is maintained in small rodents. Red grouse are most often infected as a result of ingestion of infected ticks. The virus rarely causes encephalitis in other species, such as cattle, humans, horses, pigs, goats, farm-raised deer, and dogs.[79–82] Fewer than 50 cases have been reported in humans, but when disease caused by Louping-ill virus occurs in people it is typically a febrile illness that may be followed by neurological signs, and most often occurs in abattoir workers, farm workers, and laboratory staff.[79] Disease in cats has not been described. In sheep, mixed infections with *Anaplasma phagocytophilum* and Louping-ill virus can be associated with high mortality. Much of the efforts to prevent the disease have been to protect red grouse for hunting.[78]

Working sheepdogs and gun dogs are at increased risk of exposure. A virus that was genetically very similar to sheep-derived Louping-ill virus strains was identified in one infected dog.[82] The risk of infection is also highest in the spring and fall, when tick activity is greatest. Most dogs are probably subclinically infected. When clinical signs develop, initial signs are primarily caused by cerebellar dysfunction and include mild paresis, ataxia, and tremors. Within 24 hours, severe incoordination, tetraplegia, and opisthotonos may develop. In surviving dogs, recovery has been slow, and neurological signs may persist for months to years.

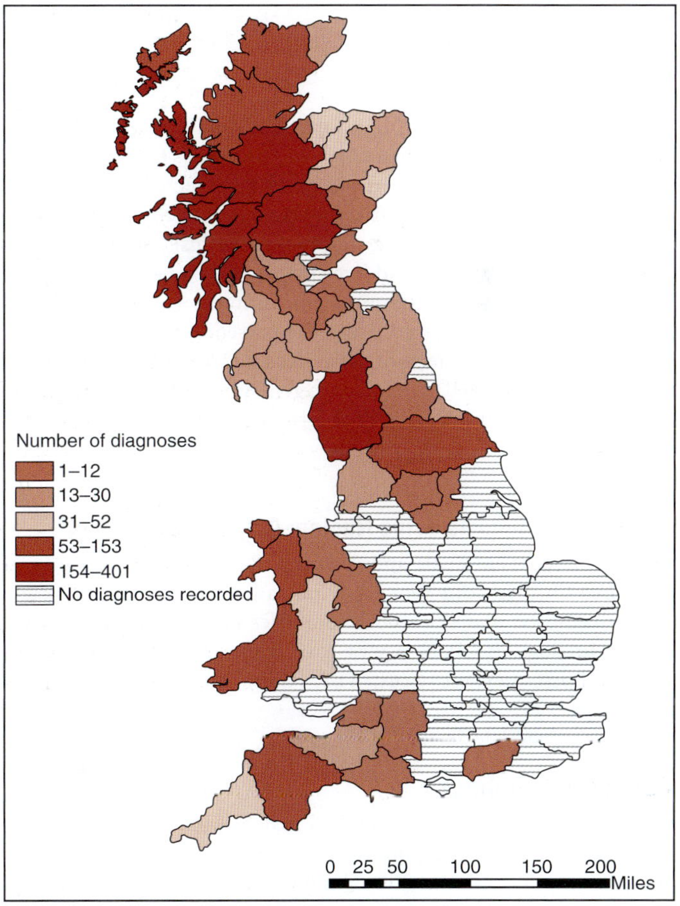

Fig. 41.5 Regions of the United Kingdom with Louping-ill virus transmission. (Modified from Jeffries CL, Mansfield KL, Phipps LP, et al. Louping ill virus: an endemic tick-borne disease of Great Britain. *J Gen Virol*. 2014;95:1005–1014.)

DIAGNOSIS

Laboratory Abnormalities and Diagnostic Imaging

Laboratory abnormalities in dogs with vector-borne viral encephalitis are nonspecific. No or minimal abnormalities may be detected in some dogs. Mild anemia, leukopenia, lymphopenia, or leukocytosis due to a neutrophilia (sometimes with a left shift) may occur. The CSF may also be unremarkable, or there may be increased protein concentration and mononuclear pleocytosis. MRI findings described in a puppy with EEEV infection consisted of changes consistent with multifocal meningoencephalitis with transtentorial and foramen magnum herniation.[83]

Microbiologic Tests

Serologic Diagnosis

Serologic assays such as serum neutralization or ELISAs are available for detection of antibodies to arboviruses through specialized veterinary diagnostic or research laboratories, and have primarily been used for epidemiologic serosurveys of dogs and cats. Serologic assays have, in general, not been very useful for diagnosis of acute viral encephalitis in dogs and cats. First, because disease is rare, arbovirus infections are often not suspected before death or euthanasia, and euthanasia is often performed early because of suspicion for rabies. Second, incubation periods are often short and disease in dogs progresses rapidly with a high mortality rate, so there is usually insufficient time for an antibody response to develop. The possibility of previous exposure confounds interpretation of single titers. Serologic assays have mainly been used to detect IgG and IgM in serum and CSF of dogs with TBE from Europe.[34] Demonstration of serum antiviral IgM is the standard diagnostic test for equine WNV disease, and in any species, a fourfold or greater rise in neutralization titer is evidence of an infection.

Virus Isolation

Arboviruses can be isolated in a variety of cell lines, and virus isolation has been used to detect WNV, TBE virus, La Crosse virus, and African horse sickness virus in naturally infected dogs.[25,59,84,85] Fresh or fresh-frozen brain or spinal cord homogenates from dogs with encephalitis are suitable specimens. Because viremia occurs, blood, CSF, lung, spleen, and liver might also be useful specimens for isolation.[59,63] Immunofluorescent antibody staining and RT-PCR assays can be used to confirm the presence of the virus in cell cultures.[11,59] Because many of these viruses can infect humans, specialized biosafety level 3 facilities are generally required. This limits the availability and practicality of virus isolation for routine diagnostic purposes.

Molecular Diagnosis Using Nucleic Acid–Based Testing

End point (conventional) and real-time RT-PCR assays have been described for many different arboviral pathogens. Specialized veterinary diagnostic and research laboratories generally perform these assays. In dogs, RT-PCR assays have been used to detect EEEV, African horse sickness virus, TBE (CSF), and WNV in clinical specimens.[11,27,28,59,83]

Pathologic Findings

In general, histopathology of the CNS in dogs with vector-borne viral infections reveals nonsuppurative meningoencephalitis or meningoencephalomyelitis, with multifocal mild to moderate gliosis, neuronal necrosis, and perivascular cuffing with lymphocytes, histiocytes, and plasma cells within Virchow-Robin spaces.[25,59,63] Neutrophils predominate within the meninges of dogs infected with EEEV.[11] Within brain tissue, inflammatory infiltrates in dogs infected with EEEV have been most prominent in the gray matter of the cerebral cortices and midbrains. Gray matter has also been preferentially infected in dogs with WNV encephalitis.[59] Pathologic changes in dogs with TBE are most severe in the gray matter of the brainstem and the cerebellum;[86–88] meningitis and spinal cord involvement have also been described.[63] In animals with Louping-ill virus infection, lesions have been concentrated in the spinal cord and cerebellum. Immunohistochemical reagents are available for detection of most arboviruses that can infect dogs, and have been used to detect antigen of WNV, La Crosse virus, African horse sickness virus, and TBE virus in CNS and other tissues of dogs.[26,27,59,73,88] In dogs with advanced TBE virus infection, viral antigen is not easily found, suggesting rapid clearance of the virus occurs early in the course of infection.

Extraneural lesions have mainly been reported in dogs infected with WNV and young puppies that were experimentally infected with Rift Valley fever virus, although foci of myocardial degeneration have been noted in dogs with naturally occurring EEEV. Dogs with African horse sickness virus infection had acute interstitial pneumonia and pleuritis (Fig. 41.6).[27] Multifocal to diffuse hepatocellular necrosis has been the most consistent finding in neonatal puppies and kittens infected with Rift Valley fever virus. Lesions in experimentally infected puppies and kittens showed poorly defined intrahepatic eosinophilic intranuclear

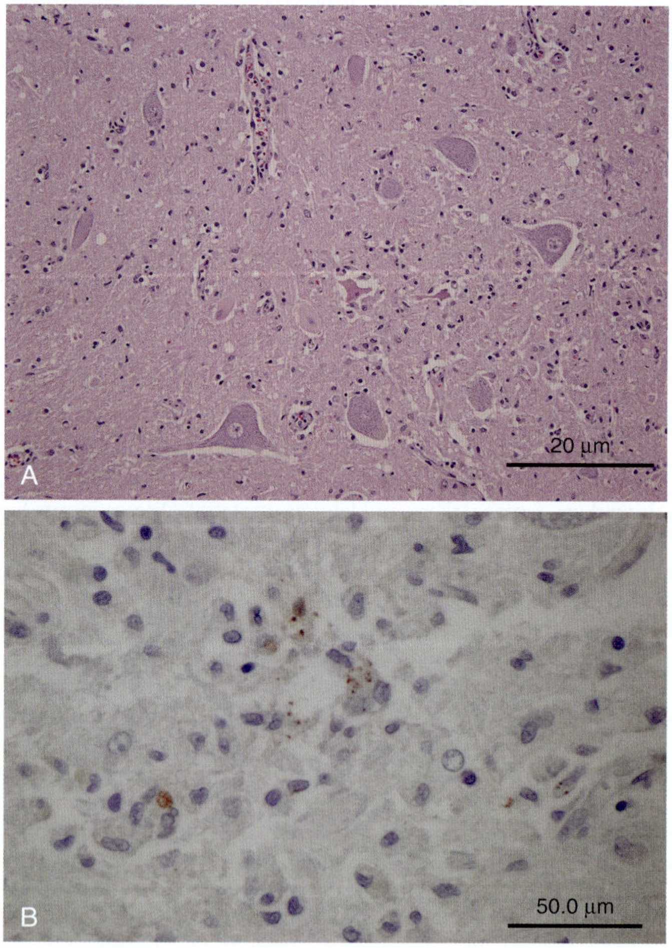

Fig. 41.6 Spinal cord segment of a dog with West Nile virus (WNV) encephalitis that shows gliosis and multiple degenerate neurons. (A) Hematoxylin and eosin stain. (B) Immunohistochemical stain showing WNV immunoreactivity *(brown)*. (From Cannon AB, Luff J, Brault C, et al. Acute encephalitis, polyarthritis and myocarditis associated with West Nile virus infection in a dog. *J Vet Intern Med*. 2006;20:1219–1223.)

inclusions and Councilmanlike bodies, which are more prominent in other hosts.[24] Lymphocytic and necrotizing myocarditis was present in some puppies and a kitten experimentally infected with Rift Valley fever virus, and several dogs naturally infected with WNV (Fig. 41.7). Other findings in dogs with WNV infection have included evidence of hepatic and renal tubular epithelial cell necrosis, adrenal gland cortical necrosis and lymphoid aggregates, neutrophilic pancreatitis, and mild plasmacytic synovitis.[58–61]

TREATMENT AND PROGNOSIS

Treatment of dogs with vector-borne viral encephalitis is supportive only. The prognosis appears to be poor, but because only a handful of infected dogs have been reported, the true prognosis is poorly understood. In virtually all dogs with neurologic signs, diagnosis has been made at necropsy. Some dogs with TBE recover with supportive care.[34] In the 2021 study of 54 dogs from Switzerland, the case fatality rate was 33%, and long-term neurological deficits occurred in 17% of the dogs.[77] Glucocorticoids have been used to treat some dogs and cats with viral encephalitides, but their use is controversial because of immunosuppression, and controlled studies are not available.

IMMUNITY AND VACCINATION

Exposure to vector-borne viruses appears to confer immunity to future infections with the same virus. Vaccines are not available for dogs because disease is uncommon to rare. However, vaccines are available and used widely in endemic areas to prevent flavivirus infections in humans (such as TBE, yellow fever, and Japanese encephalitis); WNV encephalitis in horses; and Louping-ill virus infection in sheep, cattle, and goats. Human vaccines have been used to prevent TBE in dogs, but there is limited evidence of the efficacy of these vaccines in dogs. Use of inactivated Louping-ill virus vaccines for sheep in dogs has resulted in fluid-filled swellings at the site of injection that may require surgical drainage, and dogs appear to require at least two injections to elicit a detectable serum antibody response.[89]

PREVENTION

The risk of arboviral infections in dogs and cats can be reduced through control of mosquito and tick vectors. Keeping pets indoors, especially at dawn and dusk when mosquitoes are most active, can also reduce exposure, provided mosquitoes are excluded through the use of proper screens and windows. For WNV, prevention of predation on dead birds or rodents may also reduce the risk of infection, and for African horse sickness, dogs should be prevented from consuming carcasses from dead horses in endemic areas. Drainage of standing water and removal of containers (tin cans, old tires, flower pots, clogged gutters, bunched tarpaulins) that act as breeding sites are important for mosquito control. Water in birdbaths should be changed at least weekly. Weeds and brush should be reduced. Human mosquito repellents that contain DEET (N,N-Diethyl-meta-toluamide) are not recommended for pets, because they can be toxic.[53] Some products labeled for tick prevention in dogs and cats may help to repel mosquitoes but are not likely to completely protect against mosquito bites. More information on tick prevention can be found in Chapter 13. Only products specifically labeled for cats should be used on cats or on dogs that are in contact with cats, because of the sensitivity of cats to permethrin toxicosis.[54]

PUBLIC HEALTH ASPECTS

Many arboviruses that cause disease in humans also infect dogs and cats. Dogs and cats are generally not considered reservoirs for transmission of virus to humans because they do not develop high-level or sustained viremia. As noted previously, dogs have been used as sentinels for the presence of these viruses in epidemiologic studies.

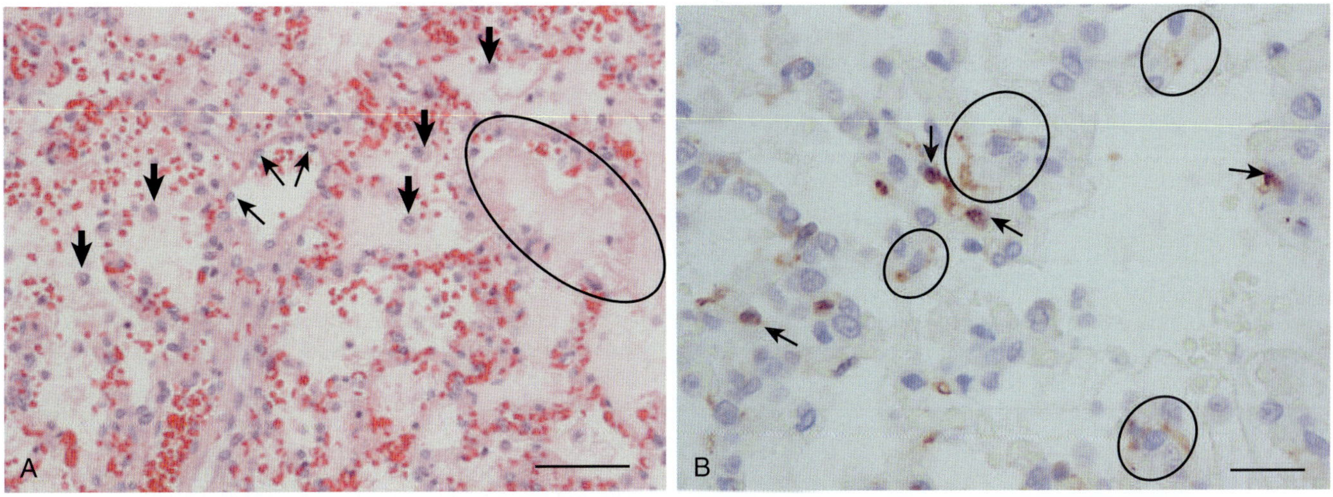

Fig. 41.7 Interstitial pneumonia with alveolar macrophage proliferation in a dog infected with African horse sickness virus. (A) Hematoxylin and eosin, 200× magnification. There is proteinaceous alveolar fluid and fibrin exudation *(oval)*, alveolar macrophage activation and proliferation *(large arrows)*, and marked vascular endothelial nuclear hyperactivation *(small arrows)*. (B) Immunohistochemical staining using African horse sickness-specific NS4 antibody, 400× magnification. There is positive solid staining of nuclear antigen *(arrows)*, and granular cytoplasmic staining of endothelial cells *(circles)*. (From O'Dell N, Arnot L, Janisch CE, et al. Clinical presentation and pathology of suspected vector transmitted African horse sickness in South African domestic dogs from 2006 to 2017. *Vet Rec*. 2018;182:715.)

CASE EXAMPLE

Signalment

"Paloma," a 13-year-old female spayed golden retriever–Irish setter mix from Vacaville in northern California.

History

Paloma was evaluated at the University of California, Davis, VMTH in September for a 3-day history of inappetence and lethargy. Two days before, physical examination by the referring veterinarian had revealed tachycardia (96 beats/min) and pyrexia (103.1°F or 39.5°C). Results of routine CBC, biochemistry tests, and a urinalysis did not reveal clinically significant abnormalities. The dog was treated with amoxicillin (20 mg/kg PO q12h) and enrofloxacin (10 mg/kg PO q12h), without improvement.

Physical Examination

Body weight: 28.6 kg.

General: Obtunded, 5% dehydrated. T = 106°F (41.1°C), HR = 140 beats/min, RR = 92 breaths/min, mucous membranes pink, CRT = 1 s.

Integument: No clinically significant abnormalities.

Eyes, ears, nose, and throat: Bilateral enophthalmos, mild serous ocular discharge, conjunctivitis, and nuclear sclerosis were present. Moderate to severe dental disease was present. Examination of the ocular fundus showed no abnormalities.

Musculoskeletal: Body condition score 4/9. Ambulatory on all four limbs, but generalized weakness was noted. Moderate atrophy of the temporalis, quadriceps, and gastrocnemius muscles was present.

Cardiovascular, respiratory, GI, urogenital, and lymphoid systems: Tachypnea and tachycardia were identified. There was mild cranial abdominal discomfort on palpation. All peripheral lymph nodes were normal sized.

Neurologic examination: Decreased placing reactions were noted in all four limbs, and there was pain on manipulation of the neck.

Laboratory Findings

CBC: HCT 37.5% (40%–55%), MCV 67.3 fL (65–75 fL), MCHC 34.4 g/dL (33–36 g/dL), WBC 6050 cells/µL (6000–13,000 cells/µL), neutrophils 5627 cells/µL (3000–10,500 cells/µL), lymphocytes 363 cells/µL (1000–4000 cells/µL), monocytes 61 cells/µL (150–1200 cells/µL), adequate platelet numbers (clumped on smear).

Serum chemistry profile: Sodium 144 mmol/L (145–154 mmol/L), potassium 4.0 mmol/L (3.6–5.3 mmol/L), chloride 110 mmol/L (108–118 mmol/L), bicarbonate 16 mmol/L (16–26 mmol/L), phosphorus 3.1 mg/dL (3.0–6.2 mg/dL), calcium 9.1 mg/dL (9.7–11.5 mg/dL), BUN 8 mg/dL (5–21 mg/dL), creatinine 0.6 mg/dL (0.3–1.2 mg/dL), glucose 86 mg/dL (64–123 mg/dL), total protein 5.7 g/dL (5.4–7.6 g/dL), albumin 2.3 g/dL (3.0–4.4 g/dL), globulin 3.4 g/dL (1.8–3.9 g/dL), ALT 25 U/L (19–67 U/L), AST 34 U/L (19–42 U/L), ALP 53 U/L (21–170 U/L), GGT 3 U/L (0–6 U/L), cholesterol 236 mg/dL (135–361 mg/dL), total bilirubin 0.3 mg/dL (0–0.2 mg/dL).

Imaging Findings

Thoracic, abdominal, spinal, and joint radiographs: No significant abnormalities were noted.

Abdominal ultrasound: Mild mesenteric and moderate sublumbar lymphadenomegaly was identified. The dog exhibited pain on ultrasound of the right cranial abdomen, but no abnormalities in this region were identified. Impressions: mesenteric and sublumbar lymphadenomegaly.

Microbiologic Testing

Aerobic and anaerobic blood cultures (five sequentially collected specimens): negative.

Serology for *Ehrlichia canis, Anaplasma phagocytophilum*, and *Borrelia burgdorferi* antibodies (POC assay, IDEXX Laboratories, ME, USA): negative.

Treatment

Paloma was treated with lactated Ringer's solution (3 mL/kg/h IV) with potassium chloride supplementation (20 mEq/L), amoxicillin (22 mg/kg PO q8h), enrofloxacin (10 mg/kg PO q24h), and doxycycline (5 mg/kg PO q12h). Physical examination on day 2 revealed persistent pyrexia (105.6°F), tachycardia (108 beats/min), and a stiff gait, but there was no evidence of joint pain or swelling on palpation. Cytologic analysis of synovial fluid collected from both carpal and tibiotarsal joints using arthrocentesis revealed mild suppurative and mononuclear inflammation.

On day 3, the dog became tetraparetic and was unable to stand for longer than a few seconds. Pyrexia (104.5°F) persisted, and treatment with dexamethasone sodium phosphate (0.2 mg/kg IV once) and hydromorphone (0.05 mg/kg IV once) was initiated. Neurologic examination disclosed mental dullness, decreased placing reactions in all four limbs, and normal segmental reflexes. Further evaluation for neurologic disease, such as imaging of the brain, CSF analysis, or both, was offered, but declined by the owner because of financial limitations. On day 4, the dog was normothermic, and sternally recumbent. Prednisone (1 mg/kg PO q12h) and metronidazole (10 mg/kg PO q8h) were added to the treatment regimen. Despite this treatment, by day 5, Paloma was laterally recumbent and obtunded. The owner elected euthanasia.

Necropsy Findings

Histopathologic findings at necropsy consisted of severe acute multifocal necrotizing perivascular and random neutrophilic pancreatitis; severe lymphocytic and neutrophilic myocarditis and vasculitis with myonecrosis; and mild, multifocal gliosis and perivascular to random lymphoplasmacytic and neutrophilic polioencephalomyelitis. The cervical spinal cord was the most severely affected. Mild perivascular plasmacytic synovitis was also present. Aerobic and anaerobic cultures of the liver, spleen, lung, and synovial fluid were negative. West Nile virus (WNV) antigen was detected with immunohistochemical stains within foci of encephalomyelitis and myocarditis. The virus was isolated from fresh-frozen lung tissue, and WNV RNA was detected using RT-PCR in the synovium, synovial fluid, spinal cord, heart, and kidney tissue.[59]

Diagnosis

Encephalitis, myocarditis, and polyarthritis associated with WNV infection.

Comments

This was a rare case of encephalitis and myocarditis associated with WNV infection in a dog. Disease occurred in September, the time of peak activity for virus transmission by mosquitoes (July to October).

SUGGESTED READINGS

Andrews C, Gerdin J, Patterson J, et al. Eastern equine encephalitis in puppies in Michigan and New York states. *J Vet Diagn Invest*. 2018;30:633–636.

O'Dell N, Arnot L, Janisch CE, et al. Clinical presentation and pathology of suspected vector transmitted African horse sickness in South African domestic dogs from 2006 to 2017. *Vet Rec*. 2018;182:715.

Holding M, Dowall SD, Medlock JM, et al. Tick-borne encephalitis virus, United Kingdom. *Emerg Infect Dis*. 2020;26:90–96.

Salat J, Ruzek D. Tick-borne encephalitis in domestic animals. *Acta Virol*. 2020;64:226–232.

Salat J, Hunady M, Schanilec P, et al. Experimental and natural infections of tick-borne encephalitis virus in dogs. *Viruses*. 2021;13:2039.

REFERENCES

1. Hanson RP. An epizootic of equine encephalomyelitis that occurred in Massachusetts in 1831. *Am J Trop Med Hyg*. 1957;6:858–862.
2. Smithburn KC, Hughs TP, Burke AW, et al. A neurotropic virus isolated from the blood of a native of Uganda. *Am J Trop Med Hyg*. 1940;20:471–492.
3. Schneider H. Über epidemische Meningitis serosa. *Wien Klin Wochenschr*. 1931;44:350.
4. Mellor PS, Hamblin C. African horse sickness. *Vet Res*. 2004;35:445–466.
5. Zehmer RB, Dean PB, Sudia WD, et al. Venezuelan equine encephalitis epidemic in Texas, 1971. *Health Serv Rep*. 1974;89:278–282.
6. Davis MH, Hogge Jr AL, Ferrell JF, et al. Mosquito transmission of Venezuelan equine encephalomyelitis virus from experimentally infected frogs. *Am J Trop Med Hyg*. 1966;15:227–230.
7. Habluetzel JE, Grimes JE, Pigott MB Jr. Serologic evidence of naturally occurring Venezuelan equine encephalomyelitis virus infection in a dog. *J Am Vet Med Assoc*. 1973;162:461–462.
8. Coffey LL, Crawford C, Dee J, et al. Serologic evidence of widespread everglades virus activity in dogs, Florida. *Emerg Infect Dis*. 2006;12:1873–1879.
9. Schlotthauer CF. The susceptibility of dogs to viruses of equine encephalomyelitis (western). *J Am Vet Med Assoc*. 1941;99:388–390.
10. Boyd AM, Kay BH. Assessment of the potential of dogs and cats as urban reservoirs of Ross River and Barmah Forest viruses. *Aust Vet J*. 2002;80:83–86.
11. Farrar MD, Miller DL, Baldwin CA, et al. Eastern equine encephalitis in dogs. *J Vet Diagn Invest*. 2005;17:614–617.
12. Centers for Disease Control and Prevention. *Eastern. Equine Encephalitis*; 2020. Available at: http://www.cdc.gov/easternequineencephalitis/tech/epi.html.
13. Oliver J, Lukacik G, Kramer LD, et al. Geography and timing of cases of eastern equine encephalitis in New York state from 1992 to 2012. *Vector Borne Zoonotic Dis*. 2016;16:283–289.
14. Molaei G, Armstrong PM, Graham AC, et al. Insights into the recent emergence and expansion of eastern equine encephalitis virus in a new focus in the Northern New England USA. *Parasit Vectors*. 2015;8:516.
15. Sun JA, Hallowell TC. Magnetic resonance imaging, clinicopathologic findings, and clinical progression of a puppy with confirmed Eastern equine encephalitis virus. *Can Vet J*. 2021;62:1298–1303.
16. Andrews C, Gerdin J, Patterson J, et al. Eastern equine encephalitis in puppies in Michigan and New York states. *J Vet Diagn Invest*. 2018;30:633–636.
17. Thompson KA, Henderson E, Fitzgerald SD, et al. Eastern equine encephalitis virus in Mexican wolf pups at zoo, Michigan, USA. *Emerg Infect Dis*. 2021;27:1173–1176.
18. McGowan JE, Jr Bryan JA, Gregg MB. Surveillance of arboviral encephalitis in the United States, 1955-1971. *Am J Epidemiol*. 1973;97:199–207.
19. Sudia WD, Coleman PH, Chamberlain RW. Experimental vector-host studies with Tensaw virus, a newly recognized member of the Bunyamwera arbovirus group. *Am J Trop Med Hyg*. 1969; 18:98–102.
20. Bird BH, McElroy AK. Rift Valley fever virus: Unanswered questions. *Antiviral Res*. 2016;132:274–280.
21. Walker JS, Remmele NS, Carter RC, et al. The clinical aspects of Rift Valley Fever virus in household pets. I. Susceptibility of the dog. *J Infect Dis*. 1970;121:9–18.
22. Walker JS, Stephen EL, Remmele NS, et al. The clinical aspects of Rift Valley Fever virus in household pets. II. Susceptibility of the cat. *J Infect Dis*. 1970;121:19–24.
23. Keefer GV, Zebarth GL, Allen WP. Susceptibility of dogs and cats to Rift Valley fever by inhalation or ingestion of virus. *J Infect Dis*. 1972;125: 307–309.
24. Mitten JQ, Remmele NS, Walker JS, et al. The clinical aspects of Rift Valley Fever virus in household pets. 3. Pathologic changes in the dog and cat. *J Infect Dis*. 1970;121:25–31.
25. Black SS, Harrison LR, Pursell AR, et al. Necrotizing panencephalitis in puppies infected with La Crosse virus. *J Vet Diagn Invest*. 1994;6:250–254.
26. Tatum LM, Pacy JM, Frazier KS, et al. Canine La Crosse viral meningoencephalomyelitis with possible public health implications. *J Vet Diagn Invest*. 1999;11:184–188.
27. O'Dell N, Arnot L, Janisch CE, et al. Clinical presentation and pathology of suspected vector transmitted African horse sickness in South African domestic dogs from 2006 to 2017. *Vet Rec*. 2018;182:715.
28. Van Sittert SJ, Drew TM, Kotze JL, et al. Occurrence of African horse sickness in a domestic dog without apparent ingestion of horse meat. *J S Afr Vet Assoc*. 2013;84:e1–5.
29. Van Rensberg IB, De Clerk J, Groenewald HB, et al. An outbreak of African horsesickness in dogs. *J S Afr Vet Assoc*. 1981;52:323–325.
30. Howerth EW, Dorminy M, Dreesen DW, et al. Low prevalence of antibodies to bluetongue and epizootic hemorrhagic disease viruses in dogs from southern Georgia. *J Vet Diagn Invest*. 1995;7:393–394.
31. Akita GY, Ianconescu M, MacLachlan NJ, et al. Bluetongue disease in dogs associated with contaminated vaccine. *Vet Rec*. 1994;134:283–284.
32. Evermann JF, McKeirnan AJ, Wilbur LA, et al. Canine fatalities associated with the use of a modified live vaccine administered during late stages of pregnancy. *J Vet Diagn Invest*. 1994;6:353–357.
33. Chang HC, Takashima I, Arikawa J, et al. Biotin-labeled protein-A enzyme-linked immunosorbent assay for the detection of Japanese encephalitis antibody in sera from humans, swine and several animal species. *J Virol Methods*. 1984;9:143–151.
34. Kokernot RH, Hayes J, Will RL, et al. Arbovirus studies in the Ohio-Mississippi Basin, 1964-1967. II. St. Louis encephalitis virus. *Am J Trop Med Hyg*. 1969;18:750–761.
35. Lindhe KE, Meldgaard DS, Jensen PM, et al. Prevalence of tick-borne encephalitis virus antibodies in dogs from Denmark. *Acta Vet Scand*. 2009;51:56.
36. Resnick MP, Grunenwald P, Blackmar D, et al. Juvenile dogs as potential sentinels for West Nile virus surveillance. *Zoonoses Public Health*. 2008;55:443–447.
37. Roelandt S, Heyman P, De Filette M, et al. Tick-borne encephalitis virus seropositive dog detected in Belgium: screening of the canine population as sentinels for public health. *Vector Borne Zoonotic Dis*. 2011;11:1371–1376.
38. Simpson VR, Kuebart G, Barnard B. A fatal case of Wesselsbron disease in a dog. *Vet Rec*. 1979;105:329.
39. Burt FJ, Grobbelaar AA, Leman PA, et al. Phylogenetic relationships of southern African West Nile virus isolates. *Emerg Infect Dis*. 2002;8:820–826.
40. Bernkopf H, Levine S, Nerson R. Isolation of West Nile virus in Israel. *J Infect Dis*. 1953;93:207–218.
41. Murray KO, Mertens E, Despres P. West Nile virus and its emergence in the United States of America. *Vet Res*. 2010;41:67.
42. Morshed M, Tang P, Petric M, et al. West Nile virus finally debuts in British Columbia 10 years after its introduction to North America. *Vector Borne Zoonotic Dis*. 2011;11:1221–1224.
43. Petersen LR, Brault AC, Nasci RS. West Nile virus: review of the literature. *J Am Med Assoc*. 2013;310:308–315.
44. Jacobson ER, Ginn PE, Troutman JM, et al. West Nile virus infection in farmed American alligators (*Alligator mississippiensis*) in Florida. *J Wildl Dis*. 2005;41:96–106.
45. Chancey C, Grinev A, Volkova E, et al. The global ecology and epidemiology of West Nile virus. *BioMed Res Int*. 2015;2015:376230.
46. Bowen RA, Rouge MM, Siger L, et al. Pathogenesis of West Nile virus infection in dogs treated with glucocorticoids. *Am J Trop Med Hyg*. 2006;74:670–673.
47. Hayes EB, Gubler DJ. West Nile virus: epidemiology and clinical features of an emerging epidemic in the United States. *Annu Rev Med*. 2006;57:181–194.
48. Maximova OA, Bernbaum JG, Pletnev AG. West Nile Virus spreads transsynaptically within the pathways of motor control: anatomical and ultrastructural mapping of neuronal virus infection in the primate central nervous system. *PLoS Negl Trop Dis*. 2016;10:e0004980.
49. Rossini G, Landini MP, Gelsomino F, et al. Innate host responses to West Nile virus: implications for central nervous system immunopathology. *World J Virol*. 2013;2:49–56.

50. Schuler LA, Khaitsa ML, Dyer NW, et al. Evaluation of an outbreak of West Nile virus infection in horses: 569 cases (2002). *J Am Vet Med Assoc.* 2004;225:1084–1089.
51. Steele KE, Linn MJ, Schoepp RJ, et al. Pathology of fatal West Nile virus infections in native and exotic birds during the 1999 outbreak in New York City, New York. *Vet Pathol.* 2000;37:208–224.
52. Durand B, Haskouri H, Lowenski S, et al. Seroprevalence of West Nile and Usutu viruses in military working horses and dogs, Morocco, 2012: dog as an alternative WNV sentinel species? *Epidemiol Infect.* 2016;144:1857–1864.
53. Gaunt MC, Waldner C, Taylor SM. Serological survey of West Nile virus in pet dogs from Saskatchewan, Canada. *Vector Borne Zoonotic Dis.* 2015;15:755–758.
54. Lan D, Ji W, Yu D, et al. Serological evidence of West Nile virus in dogs and cats in China. *Arch Virol.* 2011;156:893–895.
55. Resnick MP, Grunenwald P, Blackmar D, et al. Juvenile dogs as potential sentinels for West Nile virus surveillance. *Zoonoses Public Health.* 2008;55:443–447.
56. Levy JK, Lappin MR, Glaser AL, et al. Prevalence of infectious diseases in cats and dogs rescued following Hurricane Katrina. *J Am Vet Med Assoc.* 2011;238:311–317.
57. Austgen LE, Bowen RA, Bunning ML, et al. Experimental infection of cats and dogs with West Nile virus. *Emerg Infect Dis.* 2004;10:82–86.
58. Buckweitz S, Kleiboeker S, Marioni K, et al. Serological, reverse transcriptase-polymerase chain reaction, and immunohistochemical detection of West Nile virus in a clinically affected dog. *J Vet Diagn Invest.* 2003;15:324–329.
59. Cannon AB, Luff JA, Brault AC, et al. Acute encephalitis, polyarthritis, and myocarditis associated with West Nile virus infection in a dog. *J Vet Intern Med.* 2006;20:1219–1223.
60. Lichtensteiger CA, Heinz-Taheny K, Osborne TS, et al. West Nile virus encephalitis and myocarditis in wolf and dog. *Emerg Infect Dis.* 2003;9:1303–1306.
61. Read RW, Rodriguez DB, Summers BA. West Nile virus encephalitis in a dog. *Vet Pathol.* 2005;42:219–222.
62. Schaudien D, Schwab S, Linke S, et al. Lack of detectable West Nile virus RNA in brains and kidneys of dogs and cats with immunohistological precipitates using virus-specific antibodies. *Vet Microbiol.* 2008;132:171–176.
63. Pfeffer M, Dobler G. Tick-borne encephalitis virus in dogs: is this an issue? *Parasit Vectors.* 2011;4:59.
64. Randolph SE. Transmission of tick-borne pathogens between co-feeding ticks: Milan Labuda's enduring paradigm. *Ticks Tick Borne Dis.* 2011;2:179–182.
65. Ecker M, Allison SL, Meixner T, et al. Sequence analysis and genetic classification of tick-borne encephalitis viruses from Europe and Asia. *J Gen Virol.* 1999;80(Pt 1):179–185.
66. Holding M, Dowall SD, Medlock JM, et al. Tick-borne encephalitis virus, United Kingdom. *Emerg Infect Dis.* 2020;26:90–96.
67. Leschnik MW, Kirtz GC, Thalhammer JG. Tick-borne encephalitis (TBE) in dogs. *Int J Med Microbiol.* 2002;291(suppl 33):66–69.
68. Hira V, de Graaf JA, Rockx B, et al. Author's reply: the first tick-borne encephalitis case in The Netherlands: reflections and a note of caution. *Euro Surveill.* 2016;21:30356.
69. Völker I, Hoffmann B, Nessler J, et al. First tick borne encephalitis in a dog resident in Northern Germany. *Berl Muenchner Tieraerztl Wschr.* 2017:114–160.
70. Liebig K, Boelke M, Grund D, et al. Tick populations from endemic and non-endemic areas in Germany show differential susceptibility to TBEV. *Sci Rep.* 2020;10:15478.
71. Mansfield KL, Johnson N, Phipps LP, et al. Tick-borne encephalitis virus - a review of an emerging zoonosis. *J Gen Virol.* 2009;90:1781–1794.
72. Thomas SJ, Endy TP, Rothman AL, et al. Flaviviruses. In: Mandell GL, Bennett JE, Dolin R, eds. *Principles and Practice of Infectious Diseases.* 9th ed. Philadephia, PA: Churchill Livingstone, Elsevier; 2020 2019:2013–2039.
73. Kunz C, Heinz FX. Tick-borne encephalitis. *Vaccine.* 2003;21(suppl 1):S1–S2.
74. Weissenbock H, Suchy A, Holzmann H. Tick-borne encephalitis in dogs: neuropathological findings and distribution of antigen. *Acta Neuropathol.* 1998;95:361–366.
75. Hekrlova A, Kubicek O, Lany P, et al. Tick-borne encephalitis in dogs: application of "nested real-time RT-PCR" for intravital virus detection. *Berl Munch Tierarztl Wochenschr.* 2015;128:397–401.
76. Sievert C, Richter H, Beckmann K, et al. Comparison between proton magnetic resonance spectroscopy findings in dogs with tick-borne encephalitis and clinically normal dogs. *Vet Radiol Ultrasound.* 2017;58:53–61.
77. Kleeb C, Golini L, Beckmann K, et al. Canine tick-borne encephalitis: clinical features, survival rate and neurological sequelae: a retrospective study of 54 cases (1999-2016). *Front Vet Sci.* 2021;8:782044.
78. Gilbert L. Louping ill virus in the UK: a review of the hosts, transmission and ecological consequences of control. *Exp Appl Acarol.* 2016;68:363–374.
79. Jeffries CL, Mansfield KL, Phipps LP, et al. Louping ill virus: an endemic tick-borne disease of Great Britain. *J Gen Virol.* 2014;95:1005–1014.
80. MacKenzie CP. Recovery of a dog from louping-ill. *J Small Anim Pract.* 1982;23:233–236.
81. MacKenzie CP, Lewis ND, Smith ST, et al. Louping-ill in a working collie. *Vet Rec.* 1973;92:354–356.
82. Dagleish MP, Clark JJ, Robson C, et al. A fatal case of Louping-ill in a dog: immunolocalization and full genome sequencing of the virus. *J Comp Pathol.* 2018;165:23–32.
83. Sun JA, Hallowell TC. Magnetic resonance imaging, clinicopathologic findings, and clinical progression of a puppy with confirmed Eastern equine encephalitis virus. *Can Vet J.* 2021;62:1298–1303.
84. Gresikova M, Sekeyova M, Weidnerova K, et al. Isolation of tick-borne encephalitis virus from the brain of a sick dog in Switzerland. *Acta Virol.* 1972;16:88.
85. Salama SA, Dardiri AH, Awad FI, et al. Isolation and identification of African horsesickness virus from naturally infected dogs in Upper Egypt. *Can J Comp Med.* 1981;45:392–396.
86. Tipold A, Fatzer R, Holzmann H. Central European tick-borne encephalitis in dogs. *Kleintierpraxis.* 1993;38:619–628.
87. Weissenbock H, Holzmann H. Tick-borne encephalitis in Austrian dogs. *Vet Rec.* 1996;139:575–576.
88. Weissenbock H, Holzmann H. Immunohistochemical diagnosis of tick-borne encephalitis in Austrian dogs. *Wien Tierarztl Mnsch.* 1997;84:34–38.
89. Thomson JR, Reid HW. Louping ill virus vaccination of dogs. *Vet Rec.* 1987;120:94.

42

Bornavirus Infection

Jonas Johansson Wensman, Mikael Berg, Karin Hultin Jäderlund

KEY POINTS

- First Described: Staggering disease was first described in the 1970s in Sweden (Kronevi et al., 1974). It was linked to BoDV infection in 1995 in Sweden (Lundgren et al., 1995).
- Causes: Borna disease virus (BoDV) (species *Mammalian 1 orthobornavirus*), family *Bornaviridae.*
- Affected Hosts: *Mammalian 1 orthobornavirus* mainly affects horses and sheep, but also cats, dogs, other equids, and ungulates.
- Geographic Distribution: Europe (endemic in horses and sheep in Central Europe; in cats mainly reported in Sweden), worldwide serologic evidence of exposure in various species.
- Primary Mode of Transmission: Not entirely known. Reservoirs (small mammals) have been suggested.
- Major Clinical Signs: Gait disturbances and behavioral changes.
- Differential Diagnoses: Other feline encephalitides and neoplastic diseases affecting the CNS.
- Human Health Significance: A variant bornavirus has been associated with three cases of fatal encephalitis in breeders of variegated squirrels. Also, at least eight cases of BoDV-1 in humans have been described further emphasizing the zoonotic potential for BoDV-1, especially in endemic regions. The suggested association of BoDV and neuropsychiatric disorders in humans is however still highly controversial.

ETIOLOGIC AGENT AND EPIDEMIOLOGY

Naturally occurring clinical feline bornavirus infection, characterized by behavioral and motor dysfunction ("staggering disease"), was first described in Sweden.[1] Although BoDV infection has been reported in cats with ataxia and other neurologic signs in the United Kingdom, Japan, and Belgium,[2] a direct etiologic role of BoDV has not been established in these cases. One case of feline Borna disease (BD), verified by IHC, was reported from Switzerland.[3] Two dogs have been reported with BD, one from Austria[4] and the other from Japan.[5] BoDV has been detected in dogs in China, associated with importation of infected sheep from Germany.[6] A wild cat (*Lynx lynx*) in Sweden was also diagnosed with classic BD.[7] Feline BoDV isolates have however only been rarely reported.

BoDV is an enveloped, nonsegmented, negative-stranded RNA virus of the family *Bornaviridae* in the order *Mononegavirales.*[8] The genus *Orthobornavirus* consists of a number of new species such as *Mammalian 1 orthobornavirus*, *Elapid 1 orthobornavirus*, *Passeriform 1* and *2 orthobornavirus*, *Psittaciform 1* and *2 orthobornavirus*, and *Waterbird 1 orthobornavirus.* This chapter will only deal with *Mammalian 1 orthobornavirus* viruses. These viruses seem to be rather stable genetically, whereas the genetic variation within other virus species is considerably greater.

BoDV persistently resides within the CNS after natural and experimental infection of various animal species, ranging from birds to primates.[9] Historically, BoDV infected military horses in the endemic area around the city of Borna in Germany.[10] Cases of "classic BoDV encephalomyelitis", or "BD," in horses, sheep, and cattle seem to be restricted to endemic regions in Germany, Switzerland, and Austria. However, numerous other species may also be infected naturally, possibly including humans. Special concern was raised after fatal transmission of a bornavirus variant to three humans who were breeding variegated squirrels (*Sciurus variegatoides*),[11] indicating that some bornaviruses may be zoonotic.

Specific BoDV antibodies have been detected in horses and cats in various regions of the world. The disease in horses may be largely subclinical because the prevalence of antibodies in sera is much greater than the prevalence of clinical illness.[12] Based on serologic and nucleic acid screening, many feline infections are also subclinical. Serologic studies indicate that in addition to Europe, cats have been subclinically exposed in the Philippines, Indonesia, Turkey, Japan, and Australia.[13] BoDV antibodies have also been detected in cats with a wide variety of clinical signs. Although the clinical manifestations may not be directly caused by BoDV, it is possible that the virus is an opportunistic pathogen. Serologic results from two studies suggest that cats infected with FIV are more prone to BoDV infection.[14,15]

Disease associated with BoDV occurs most frequently in spring and summer,[13] and thus arthropod transmission has been suspected. A definitive reservoir host has not been documented, but rodents, insectivores, and birds are suspected. There are a number of recent reports of BoDV in various small mammals such as white-toothed shrews[16] and bank voles,[17] which indicate that different hosts exist in various geographical regions.

Viral RNA has been detected in feces and urine of naturally infected cats,[18] and in salivary, nasal, and conjunctival secretions of horses and sheep[12,19]; animals may become infected by direct contact with these secretions or with fomites, such as contaminated food or water. Infection does not appear to spread readily among cats. Epidemiologic studies suggest that risk factors for infection in cats are highest for intact males that hunt mice in rural woodland environments.[20]

CLINICAL FEATURES

Pathogenesis

BoDV is highly neurotropic and probably gains access to the CNS by transmucosal entry into nerve endings terminating in the olfactory, oropharyngeal, or GI mucosae.[21] Similar to the spread of rabies virus,

BoDV spreads into and throughout the CNS by intra-axonal transport and from there spreads centrifugally into the peripheral nerves.[22] Unlike rabies virus, the replication rate of BoDV is slow. The immune response to viral antigens is not protective but incites an immunopathologic response.[23] Neutralizing antibodies appear in the serum and CSF. This response fails to clear the infection; the inflammation subsides, and BoDV persists at low levels in the CNS of the host. In the CNS, BoDV infects neurons, astrocytes, oligodendrocytes, and ependymal cells. Experimental infection of feline astrocytes has been shown to impair their glutamate uptake function, a proposed mechanism for additional neuronal injury.[24] Interactions between BoDV and host proteins likely contribute to the development of clinical signs.[21,25,26]

In experimentally infected rats, acute-phase immunity is cellular, with T cells as the predominant cell infiltrate. With chronic infection, plasma cell infiltrates and antibody titers increase and may magnify the inflammatory reaction.[27] These findings are similar to those found with naturally infected cats with staggering disease, in which T cells predominate in the CNS and peripheral circulation,[28] with an intense IFN-γ gene expression in the CNS.[29] Cytotoxic CD8+ T cells are thought to induce this immune response against the virus. Antibody titers increase with persistent infection of the CNS.

Experimentally and naturally infected cats develop humoral immune responses to the BoDV proteins p24 and p40.[30] Serum antibodies to another BoDV protein, p10, have also been found in cats with ataxia.[31] In addition to the systemic humoral response, BoDV-specific antibodies are produced intracerebrally in naturally and experimentally infected cats.[30] Intracerebral inoculation of BoDV produces high antibody titers against the immunodominant proteins in CSF; however, natural infections induce a weak humoral immune response in cats, primarily directed against BoDV p24.[30]

Clinical signs

Affected cats are typically presented with a history of gait disturbances mixed with behavioral changes.[18,32] The gait is most often described as unsteady, predominantly in the pelvic limbs, with stiff and slow movements, as well as falling. At the same time, affected cats often become more social and affectionate, vocalize more frequently, with absent-minded behavior. Besides these overt neurological signs, > 40% of the cats are inappetent and approximately every fourth case exhibits constipation.[18,32] Otherwise, affected cats are apparently healthy.

Physical Examination Findings

On physical examination, almost half of affected cats are febrile (≥39.3°C).[18,32] About as many have an inability to retract the claws, predominantly of the pelvic limbs, and show signs of lumbosacral pain on palpation.[18,32] On neurologic examination, affected cats display varying degrees of proprioceptive ataxia with a stiff, stilted gait, sometimes with an abnormally stiff tail. As a rule, postural reactions and menace responses are absent or decreased. A majority of the affected cats is mildly obtunded and a similar proportion of cats exhibit increased vocalization throughout the whole examination.[18,32] In one study, 86% of affected cats behaved abnormally during a nociception test; their pupils dilated and their muscles flexed in response to a perceived painful stimulus, but they showed a reduced inclination to physically retreat from the painful stimulus.[18] Spinal reflexes are normal to exaggerated. Neurological deficits are bilateral and mainly symmetrical. Some clinical signs previously associated with other feline neurologic diseases, such as epileptic seizures, compulsive walking, lateralized vestibular syndrome, or facial paresis, are seldom included in the plethora of neurologic signs in cats with staggering disease.[18]

DIAGNOSIS

Laboratory abnormalities

Complete Blood Count and Serum Chemistry Profiles

Leukopenia, or a WBC count in the low-normal range, has been the only hematologic abnormality present in affected cats. Approximately 50% of the affected cats have had WBC counts below the reference range. Both neutrophil and lymphocyte counts have been at the lower end of the reference range. A few affected cats have had a slight increase in the activity of serum ALT.[18,32]

Cerebrospinal Fluid Analysis

On CSF analysis, a mononuclear pleocytosis is found in about one third of cats with staggering disease. The CSF protein content is increased (> 0.36 g/L) in approximately 50% of affected cats.[18,32] In a few cases, there has been evidence of previous intrathecal hemorrhage in the form of xanthochromia.

Microbiologic Tests

Because BoDV causes a persistent infection of the CNS, associating infection with clinical disease can be challenging. Therefore, positive test results using serologic and molecular methods support staggering disease as a tentative diagnosis when other explanations for clinical signs have been ruled out. Antibodies are most often detected using indirect IFA testing.[17] This method is considered to be specific, but insensitive. In one study, antibodies were found in 81% of cats with staggering disease compared with 16% in a control group.[18] Nested RT-PCR has been frequently used in research settings to detect BoDV RNA in peripheral blood monocytes or brain tissue.[33,34] This method is highly sensitive, but because of its inherent high risk of laboratory contamination, the results have been questioned.[35] To overcome this drawback, real-time RT-PCR assays have been developed and used to detect BoDV RNA in brain tissue, though its use as an antemortem clinical diagnostic tool has not yet been demonstrated.[36,37] Virus RNA has been detected mainly in blood in a few clinical cases in cats.[18]

Detection in the CNS of BoDV antigen by IHC, of BoDV RNA by *in situ* hybridization, or both in combination with neurohistopathologic alterations is considered the most reliable method of confirming active CNS disease. BoDV can be isolated from CNS tissue by inoculation of cell cultures or rats.[38]

Although lesions of feline BD resemble those of feline poliomyelitis, no evidence suggests that these disorders are related. The histologic and clinical features of BD should be contrasted with feline poliomyelitis, which predominantly affects the spinal cord, causing progressive lower motor neuron dysfunction with milder brainstem involvement (see Chapter 129).

Pathologic Findings

The inflammatory reaction in the CNS is characterized by a lymphohistiocytic or lymphoplasmacytic meningoencephalitis in the gray matter of the olfactory bulb, cerebral cortex, hippocampus, basal ganglia, and brainstem.[18,32] The spinal cord is affected to a lesser degree. Perivascular mononuclear cell infiltrates mainly consist of lymphocytes. The surrounding brain parenchyma is also affected, sometimes with neuronophagia and neuronal degeneration (Fig. 42.1). Inflammation of intra-abdominal ganglions may also be observed.

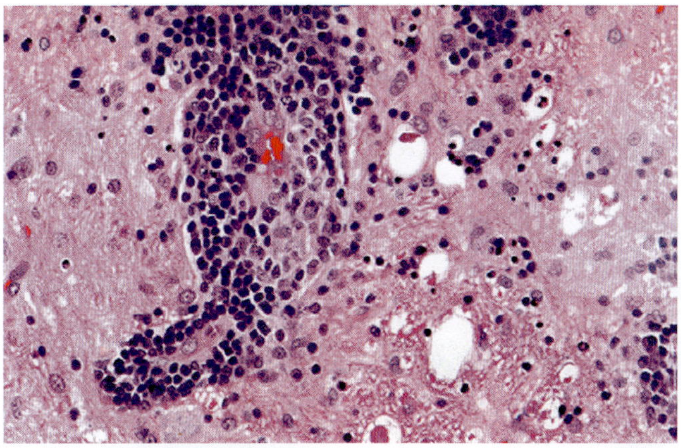

Fig. 42.1 Histopathologic findings showing characteristic nonsuppurative perivascular cuffs in gray matter of the CNS (Hematoxylin and eosin stain, ×200). (Courtesy Anna-Lena Berg, Medical Products Agency, Uppsala, Sweden.)

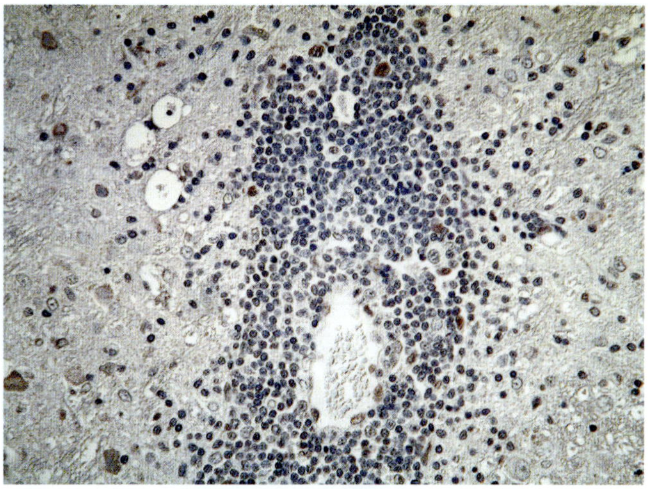

Fig. 42.2 Immunohistochemistry with Borna disease virus (BoDV) antigen (*brown staining*) within astrocytes. Anti-BoDV p24 antibody staining. (Courtesy Anna-Lena Berg, Medical Products Agency, Uppsala, Sweden.)

BoDV antigen and nucleic acid persist in brain tissue of cats, particularly within astrocytes, causing chronic inflammatory lesions (Fig. 42.2). In one cat, large amounts of virus but no inflammation were found within neurons, presumably from viral persistence by infection at an early age.[39]

BD in dogs has been characterized by a rapid onset of progressive intracranial CNS deficits that are similar to those in canine distemper.[4,5] Histopathologic lesions, which predominated in the forebrain and midbrain, have been characterized by a nonsuppurative meningoencephalitis with perivascular cuffing and diffuse mononuclear cell infiltrates of adjacent neuropil. Inflammatory cells in the cuffs largely comprise CD3+ T cells. Viral antigen and RNA can be detected in neurons using IHC and *in situ* hybridization.

TREATMENT AND PROGNOSIS

In the initial stage of staggering disease, supportive care such as IV fluids should be considered. In addition, antibacterial drugs, glucocorticoids, and/or the antiviral drug amantadine hydrochloride have been used in many cats. In a retrospective study of 54 affected cats, broad-spectrum antimicrobial drugs and glucocorticoids, as well as combinations of such medications, had a beneficial effect on survival time. Treatment with amantadine hydrochloride did not significantly increase survival time.[40] Treatment with glucocorticoids, especially at an early stage of disease, also has shown promise.[41] However, in the absence of controlled treatment trials, the effect of any therapy is anecdotal. Clinical signs progress within 1 to 4 weeks until the clinical condition either deteriorates, resulting in euthanasia,[18] or stabilizes and might improve slightly with time, still leaving most cats permanently afflicted with motor dysfunction, personality changes, or both (Fig. 42.3). In surviving cats, neurologic signs often eventually relapse. However, survival times for up to 7 years have been described.[40]

IMMUNITY AND VACCINATION

There is currently no available vaccine for BoDV infection.

PREVENTION

Because the mechanism of BoDV transmission is currently not completely understood, it is difficult to provide adequate advice on preventive measures. BoDV is inactivated by common decontamination methods, such as heat, detergents, and chlorine.

PUBLIC HEALTH ASPECTS

BoDV has been studied as a cause of human neuropsychiatric illnesses.[42,43] Antibodies to the virus have been detected in sera of patients with psychiatric disorders in various countries. The prevalence of BoDV-specific antibodies is fourfold higher in patients with HIV infection than in control patients.[44]

As in animals, controversy surrounds the significance of BoDV infection in humans.[45–47] The most definitive evidence of a link between infection and disease has been the detection of BDV-specific antigen and RNA in the brains of humans with hippocampal sclerosis and schizophrenia.[48–50] Also, a number of human fatal cases of encephalitis were described in association to BoDV-1 infection.[51] Thus, BoDV shall be considered to be a potential lethal zoonotic virus for both immunocompromised as well as fully healthy individuals. However, it is unclear how these patients were infected in the first place.

A variant bornavirus was associated with fatal encephalitis in breeders of variegated squirrels. In one squirrel, the same virus as detected in affected humans was found, suggesting direct transmission from apparently healthy squirrels to humans.[11]

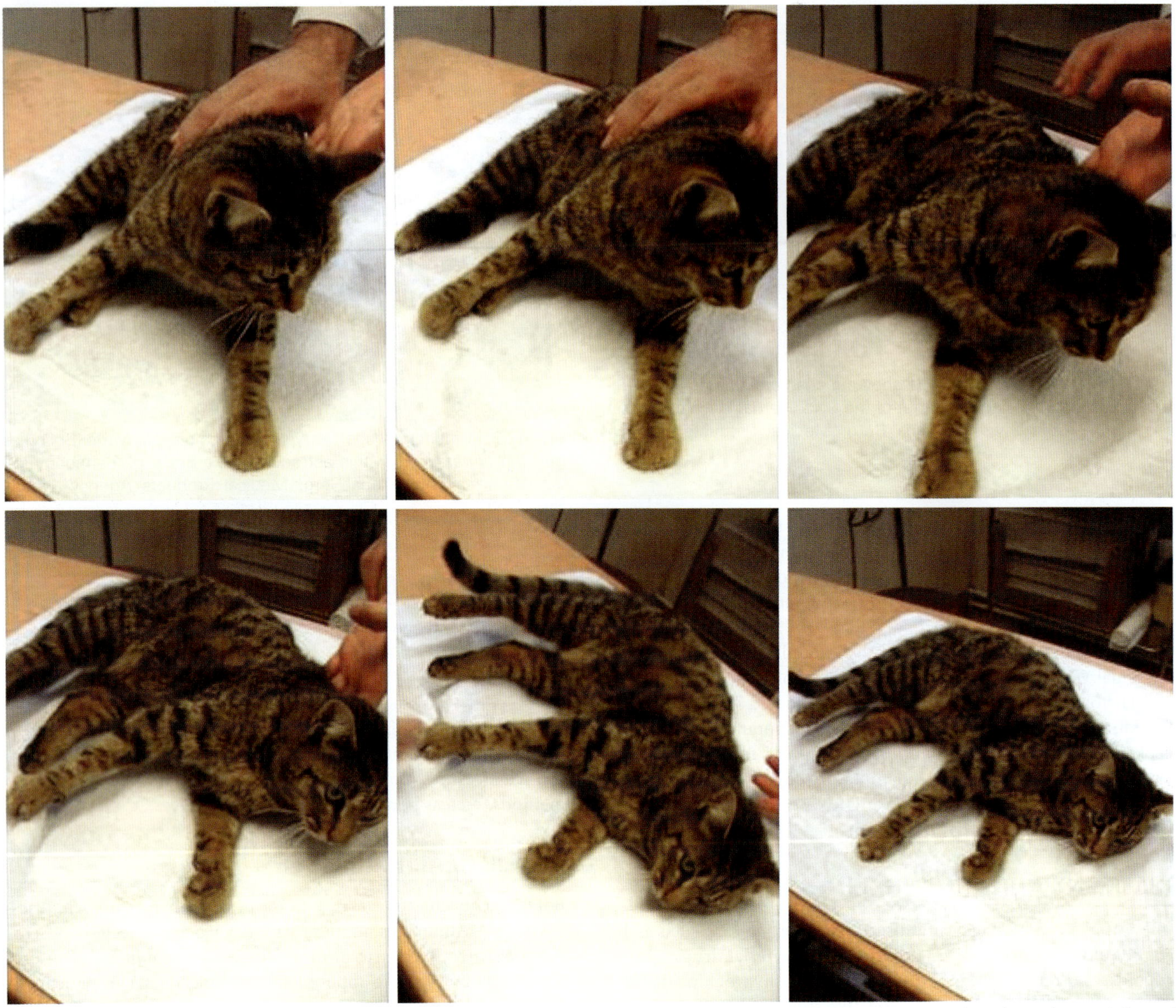

Fig. 42.3 A 2.5-year-old pregnant female cat with clinical signs of Borna disease virus infection. The series of photos show how the cat falls to the left (from upper left to lower right). The cat displayed a severe general proprioceptive ataxia with an absent menace response and decreased postural reactions in the thoracic and pelvic limbs.

CASE EXAMPLE

Signalment

"Teddy," a 4-year-old male, neutered, European shorthair cat from Alunda in the Uppsala area, Sweden.

History

Teddy was described to be ataxic 4 weeks before initial examination. Treatment with oral prednisolone and amoxicillin was initiated for a tentative diagnosis of staggering disease. Teddy improved somewhat initially, but ataxia then worsened. Over the 2 weeks leading up to initial examination, pelvic limb ataxia, "knuckling" of the thoracic limbs, and changes in behavior (abnormal degree of affection and increased vocalization) were noted. Although his appetite was unaffected, a 1-kg weight loss over the last month had occurred. He was up to date on vaccinations. Teddy was an outdoor cat from rural surroundings. There were three other cats in the household, and all were healthy.

Current Medications

Prednisolone 2.5 mg q24h PO.

Physical Examination

Body temperature = 38.5°C; body weight = 3.5 kg; BCS = 3/9; HR = 130 beats/minute; mucous membranes moist and pink. No significant abnormalities were noted during examination of lymph nodes, integument, eyes, ears, nose and throat, cardiovascular, respiratory, GI, or genitourinary organs.

Neurologic Examination

Mental status: Slightly obtunded. Behavior: Affectionate and meowing. Posture: Stiff limbs. Extension of the claws were noted in both thoracic and pelvic limbs. Gait: Teddy was ambulatory, with paraparesis and a severe ataxia, more pronounced in the pelvic limbs. The gait was stiff and stilted. Cranial nerves: Menace reactions were reduced, otherwise no abnormalities were noted. Postural reactions: The postural reactions in all four limbs were reduced. Spinal reflexes: A crossed extensor reflex was present in all four limbs, the other spinal reflexes were normal. Nociception: Teddy showed an abnormal response to toe stimulation, in that he vocalized but did not attempt to escape the nociceptive stimulus.

CASE EXAMPLE—cont'd

Laboratory Findings

CBC: Hemoglobin 162 g/L (80–150 g/L), WBC 4,200 cells/μL (5,500–9,500 cells/μL), neutrophils 2,900 cells/μL (2,500–12,500 cells/μL), eosinophils 0 cells/μL (0–1,500 cells/μL), lymphocytes 1,100 cells/μL (1,500–7,000 cells/μL), monocytes 100 cells/μL (100–1,000 cells/μL).

Serum chemistry profile: ALT <72 U/L (<60–120 U/L), ALP 24 U/L (<300 U/L), creatinine 1.1 mg/dL (0.7–1.9 mg/dL), albumin 4.6 g/dL (3.2–4.6 g/dL)

Serum protein electrophoresis: globulin 2.5 g/dL, α1-globulins 2 g/L (2–3 g/L), α2-globulins 9 g/L (11–17 g/L), β1-globulins 3 g/L (3–6 g/L), β2-globulins 2 g/L (1–3 g/L), γ-globulins 9 g/L (8–18 g/L).

Total T4: 26 mmol/L (7–35 mmol/L).

CSF analysis from the cerebellomedullary cistern: Clear and colorless. Mononuclear pleocytosis; erythrocytes 105/μL, leucocytes 58/μL, 100% mononuclear cells. Protein 0.75 g/L.

Serology: BoDV IFA in serum ≥ 1:160, BoDV IFA in CSF 1:5. Serology for *Toxoplasma* antibodies, CoV antibodies, FeLV antigen, and FIV antibodies negative in serum.

Real-time PCR for BoDV RNA in blood, urine, and CSF: Negative.

Diagnosis

Staggering disease. Teddy was euthanized a few days later due to further progression of signs.

Necropsy findings: Meningoencephalomyelitis, especially in the grey matter.

Comments

In this case, a diagnosis of staggering disease was strongly suspected based on the typical clinical signs and the positive serology, as well as ruling out other possible causes of disease.

SUGGESTED READINGS

Lutz H, Addie DD, Boucraut-Baralon C, et al. European Advisory Board on Cat Diseases. Borna disease virus infection in cats: ABCD guidelines on prevention and management. *J Feline Med Surg.* 2015;17(7):614–616.

Wensman JJ, Jäderlund KH, Holst BS, et al. Borna disease virus infection in cats. *Vet J.* 2014;201(2):142–149.

Wensman JJ, Jäderlund KH, Gustavsson MH, et al. Markers of Borna disease virus infection in cats with staggering disease. *J Feline Med Surg.* 2012;14(8):573–582.

REFERENCES

1. Kronevi T, Nordström M, Moreno W, et al. Feline ataxia due to nonsuppurative meningoencephalomyelitis of unknown aetiology. *Nord Vet Med.* 1974;26:720–725.
2. Kamhieh S, Flower RL. Borna disease virus (BDV) infection in cats. A concise review based on current knowledge. *Vet Q.* 2006;28:66–73.
3. Caplazi P, Melzer K, Goetzmann R, et al. Borna disease in Switzerland and in the principality of Liechtenstein. *Schweiz Arch Tierheilkd.* 1999;141:521–527.
4. Weissenböck H, Nowotny N, Caplazi P, et al. Borna disease in a dog with lethal meningoencephalitis. *J Clin Microbiol.* 1998;36:2127–2130.
5. Okamoto M, Kagawa Y, Kamitani W, et al. Borna disease in a dog in Japan. *J Comp Pathol.* 2002;126:312–317.
6. Zhang L, Wang X, Zhan Q, et al. Evidence for natural Borna disease virus infection in healthy domestic animals in three areas of western China. *Arch Virol.* 2014;159:1941–1949.
7. Degiorgis MP, Berg AL, Hård Af Segerstad C, et al. Borna disease in a free-ranging lynx (*Lynx lynx*). *J Clin Microbiol.* 2000;38:3087–3091.
8. Amarasinghe GK, Ayllón MA, Bao Y, et al. Taxonomy of the order *Mononegavirales*: update 2019. *Arch Virol.* 2019;164(7):1967–1980.
9. Kinnunen PM, Palva A, Vaheri A, et al. Epidemiology and host spectrum of Borna disease virus infections. *J Gen Virol.* 2013;94:247–262.
10. Dürrwald R, Ludwig H. Borna disease virus (BDV), a (zoonotic?) worldwide pathogen. A review of the history of the disease and the virus infection with comprehensive bibliography. *Zentralbl Veterinarmed B.* 1997;44:147–184.
11. Hoffmann B, Tappe D, Hoper D, et al. A variegated squirrel bornavirus associated with fatal human encephalitis. *N Engl J Med.* 2015;373:154–162.
12. Richt JA, Grabner A, Herzog S. Borna disease in horses. *Vet Clin North Am Equine Pract.* 2000;16:579–595 (xi).
13. Wensman JJ, Jaderlund KH, Holst BS, et al. Borna disease virus infection in cats. *Vet J.* 2014;201:142–149.
14. Huebner J, Bode L, Ludwig H. Borna disease virus infection in FIV-positive cats in Germany. *Vet Rec.* 2001;149:152.
15. Helps CR, Turan N, Bilal T, et al. Detection of antibodies to Borna disease virus in Turkish cats by using recombinant p40. *Vet Rec.* 2001;149:647–650.
16. Hilbe M, Herrsche R, Kolodziejek J, et al. Shrews as reservoir hosts of Borna disease virus. *Emerg Infect Dis.* 2006;12:675–677.
17. Kinnunen PM, Billich C, Ek-Kommonen C, et al. Serological evidence for Borna disease virus infection in humans, wild rodents and other vertebrates in Finland. *J Clin Virol.* 2007;38:64–69.
18. Wensman JJ, Jaderlund KH, Gustavsson MH, et al. Markers of Borna disease virus infection in cats with staggering disease. *J Feline Med Surg.* 2012;14:573–582.
19. Vahlenkamp TW, Konrath A, Weber M, et al. Persistence of Borna disease virus in naturally infected sheep. *J Virol.* 2002;76:9735–9743.
20. Berg AL, Reid-Smith R, Larsson M, et al. Case control study of feline Borna disease in Sweden. *Vet Rec.* 1998;142:715–717.
21. Wensman JJ. Bornaviruses. In: Munir M, ed. *Mononegaviruses of Veterinary Importance: Pathobiology and Molecular Diagnosis.* Wallingford, UK: CAB International; 2013.
22. Morales JA, Herzog S, Kompter C, et al. Axonal transport of Borna disease virus along olfactory pathways in spontaneously and experimentally infected rats. *Med Microbiol Immunol.* 1988;177:51–68.
23. Tizard I, Ball J, Stoica G, et al. The pathogenesis of bornaviral diseases in mammals. *Anim Health Res Rev.* 2016;1–18.
24. Billaud JN, Ly C, Phillips TR, et al. Borna disease virus persistence causes inhibition of glutamate uptake by feline primary cortical astrocytes. *J Virol.* 2000;74:10438–10446.
25. Wensman JJ, Leuchowius KJ, Yan J, et al. Visualization of Borna disease virus protein interactions with host proteins using in situ proximity ligation assay. *Br J Virol.* 2016;3:11–23.
26. Kamitani W, Ono E, Yoshino S, et al. Glial expression of Borna disease virus phosphoprotein induces behavioral and neurological abnormalities in transgenic mice. *Proc Natl Acad Sci U S A.* 2003;100:8969–8974.
27. Stitz L, Dietzschold B, Carbone KM. Immunopathogenesis of Borna disease. *Curr Top Microbiol Immunol.* 1995;190:75–92.
28. Berg AL, Johannisson A, Johansson M, et al. Peripheral and intracerebral T cell immune response in cats naturally infected with Borna disease virus. *Vet Immunol Immunopathol.* 1999;68:241–253.
29. Wensman JJ, Ilback C, Hjertstrom E, et al. Expression of interferon gamma in the brain of cats with natural Borna disease virus infection. *Vet Immunol Immunopathol.* 2011;141:162–167.
30. Johansson M, Berg M, Berg AL. Humoral immune response against Borna disease virus (BDV) in experimentally and naturally infected cats. *Vet Immunol Immunopathol.* 2002;90:23 33.
31. Ouchi A, Kishi M, Kobayashi T, et al. Prevalence of circulating antibodies to p10, a non-structural protein of the Borna disease virus in cats with ataxia. *J Vet Med Sci.* 2001;63:1279–1285.
32. Lundgren AL. Feline non-suppurative meningoencephalomyelitis. A clinical and pathological study. *J Comp Pathol.* 1992;107:411–425.
33. Sauder C, de la Torre JC. Sensitivity and reproducibility of RT-PCR to detect Borna disease virus (BDV) RNA in blood: implications for BDV epidemiology. *J Virol Methods.* 1998;71:229–245.

34. Zimmermann W, Dürrwald R, Ludwig H. Detection of Borna disease virus RNA in naturally infected animals by a nested polymerase chain reaction. *J Virol Methods.* 1994;46:133–143.
35. Staeheli P, Sauder C, Hausmann J, et al. Epidemiology of Borna disease virus. *J Gen Virol.* 2000;81:2123–2135.
36. Schindler AR, Vögtlin A, Hilbe M, et al. Reverse transcription real-time PCR assays for detection and quantification of Borna disease virus in diseased hosts. *Mol Cell Probes.* 2007;21:47–55.
37. Wensman JJ, Thoren P, Hakhverdyan M, et al. Development of a real-time RT-PCR assay for improved detection of Borna disease virus. *J Virol Methods.* 2007;143:1–10.
38. Lundgren AL, Zimmermann W, Bode L, et al. Staggering disease in cats: isolation and characterization of the feline Borna disease virus. *J Gen Virol.* 1995;76(Pt 9):2215–2222.
39. Berg AL, Berg M. A variant form of feline Borna disease. *J Comp Pathol.* 1998;119:323–331.
40. Sjödén L. Survival, quality of life and medical treatment of cats showing clinical signs of staggering disease. MSc Thesis. Department of Clinical Sciences. Uppsala: Swedish University of Agricultural Sciences; 2013.
41. Berg AL. Borna disease in cats. In: Bonagura JD, ed. *Kirk's Current Veterinary Therapy.* Philadelphia: Saunders; 1999:976–978.
42. Carbone KM. Borna disease virus and human disease. *Clin Microbiol Rev.* 2001;14:513–527.
43. Thakur R, Sarma S, Sharma B. Role of Borna disease virus in neuropsychiatric illnesses: are we inching closer? *Indian J Med Microbiol.* 2009;27:191–201.
44. Bode L, Riegel S, Ludwig H, et al. Borna disease virus-specific antibodies in patients with HIV infection and with mental disorders. *Lancet.* 1988;2:689.
45. Dürrwald R, Kolodziejek J, Herzog S, et al. Meta-analysis of putative human bornavirus sequences fails to provide evidence implicating Borna disease virus in mental illness. *Rev Med Virol.* 2007;17:181–203.
46. Schwemmle M, Jehle C, Formella S, et al. Sequence similarities between human bornavirus isolates and laboratory strains question human origin. *Lancet.* 1999;354:1973–1974.
47. Lipkin WI, Briese T, Hornig M. Borna disease virus - fact and fantasy. *Virus Res.* 2011;162:162–172.
48. Czygan M, Hallensleben W, Hofer M, et al. Borna disease virus in human brains with a rare form of hippocampal degeneration but not in brains of patients with common neuropsychiatric disorders. *J Infect Dis.* 1999;180:1695–1699.
49. De La Torre JC, Gonzalez-Dunia D, Cubitt B, et al. Detection of Borna disease virus antigen and RNA in human autopsy brain samples from neuropsychiatric patients. *Virology.* 1996;223:272–282.
50. Nakamura Y, Takahashi H, Shoya Y, et al. Isolation of Borna disease virus from human brain tissue. *J Virol.* 2000;74:4601–4611.
51. Niller HH, Angstwurm K, Rubbenstroth D, et al. Zoonotic spillover infection with Borna disease virus 1 leading to fatal human encephalitis, 1999-2019: an epidemiological investigation. *Lancet Infect Dis.* 2020;20(4):467–477.

43

Emerging and Miscellaneous Viral Infections

Jane E. Sykes

KEY POINTS

- The infectious diseases described in this chapter are either: (1) diseases of humans or other animals generally transmitted through contact with the secretions or excretions of rodents (hantaviruses, arenaviruses, and encephalomyocarditis virus), swine (hepatitis E virus), monkeys (Ebola virus), or bats (systemic coronaviruses); (2) common diseases of humans where the role of companion animals in transmission has been investigated (enteroviruses, SARS-CoV-2); (3) diseases of significant importance to the agricultural industry (foot-and-mouth disease virus, vesicular exanthema, encephalomyocarditis virus); or (4) significant diseases of potential prey of dogs and cats (rabbit hemorrhagic disease virus).
- Clinical illness has not always been confirmed in dogs and cats with these infections, but evidence of seroconversion to these viruses exists.
- In some cases, concern has been raised in the possible role of dogs and cats in zoonotic transmission; this has been heightened by the COVID-19 pandemic.
- In general, research suggests that dogs and cats do not play a major role in transmission of these viruses, but the potential exists should new viral variants emerge.

HANTAVIRUS INFECTION

ETIOLOGIC AGENTS AND EPIDEMIOLOGY

Hantaviruses are enveloped RNA viruses that belong to the family *Bunyaviridae*, which contains four other genera (*Nairovirus, Orthobunyavirus, Phlebovirus,* and *Tospovirus*), and are named after the Hantan River area in South Korea where the disease was first observed. Hantaviruses are the only members of the *Bunyaviridae* that are not transmitted by arthropod vectors (for comparison, see *Bunyaviridae* in Chapter 41, Arthropod-Borne Viral Infections). Each hantavirus strain of is uniquely adapted to a subclinically infected rodent, shrew, or bat reservoir, and humans usually become infected through contact with rodent feces, urine, or saliva. Direct physical contact with the rodents is not required, so aerosolized virus is the likely means of spread of infection between rodents and humans. Rodent bites have also been documented as a means of transmission.[1] Although humans are generally considered dead-end hosts, some strains (Andes virus in South America) can be directly transmitted between humans. Species differences exist among rodents as to the length of salivary excretion, with times ranging up to 1 year. Infected rodents are thought to harbor the virus in their lungs and kidneys for life.

Over 50 different hantavirus strains have been identified worldwide. Those that are pathogenic for humans cause two clinically distinct syndromes. *Hantavirus hemorrhagic fever with renal syndrome (HFRS)* is the vastly more common syndrome, and is caused by Hantan River, Seoul, Dobrava-Belgrade, and Saaremaa viruses in Europe, Asia, and Africa. *Hantavirus pulmonary syndrome* (*HPS*; also known as hantavirus cardiopulmonary syndrome), a pulmonary disease with 40%–50% mortality, occurs in North, Central, and South America. It is primarily caused by Sin Nombre virus in North America, which is carried by deer mice. In the United States, most human infections have occurred in the Four Corners states (Arizona, Colorado, New Mexico, and Utah), although only a few dozen cases are reported in North America annually (Fig. 43.1).[2] Monongahela, New York, Bayou, and Black Creek Canal viruses also cause HPS in North America and are found in eastern Canada and the eastern and southeastern regions of the United States. In South and Central America, a number of other viruses can cause HPS, including Andes virus in Argentina, Brazil, and Chile; Laguna Negra virus in Bolivia and Paraguay; and Choclo virus in Panama.[3]

The disease is more prevalent during seasons and years when population densities of rodents are highest. The greatest incidence of infection in humans occurs when their work or recreational activities expose them to rodents. Infections occur on farms, in suburbs, and in residential areas. In laboratory rats in the United States, infection by the Seoul virus has been controlled by serologic testing and by producing rodents from cesarean-derived stock maintained under strict barrier conditions.

Although human infections receive the most attention, dogs and cats have the potential to become infected following contact with rodents and rodent excreta. The possibility of hantavirus infection in cats was initially raised in a study from China that indicated that cat ownership was a risk factor for hantavirus infection in humans.[4] Several studies conducted worldwide have identified hantavirus antibodies in domestic cats, with seroprevalences of 5% in Austria,[5] 9.6% in Great Britain,[6] 16.9% in Belgium,[7] 2.9% in rural cats from the southwestern Canadian prairie,[8] and 2.8% in New Mexico and northeastern Arizona.[9] Cats that are allowed to roam or hunt outdoors have the highest seroprevalence, and in the Belgian study, cats and dogs living in forested areas had higher seroprevalence.[7] Hantavirus antigen was detected in the lungs of 2 of 100 cats that had a history of rodent hunting at necropsy.[10] The seroprevalence in dogs has been low, 4.9% in Belgium,[7] 0% in the Canadian prairie,[8] and 3.5% in New Mexico and Arizona.[9] At this time, it seems that neither coyotes nor dogs or cats appear to play a major role in the maintenance and transmission of Sin Nombre virus.

CLINICAL FEATURES

Pathogenesis and Clinical Signs

In cats and dogs, clinical hantavirus infection has never been documented, and so most or all infections are probably subclinical. Both

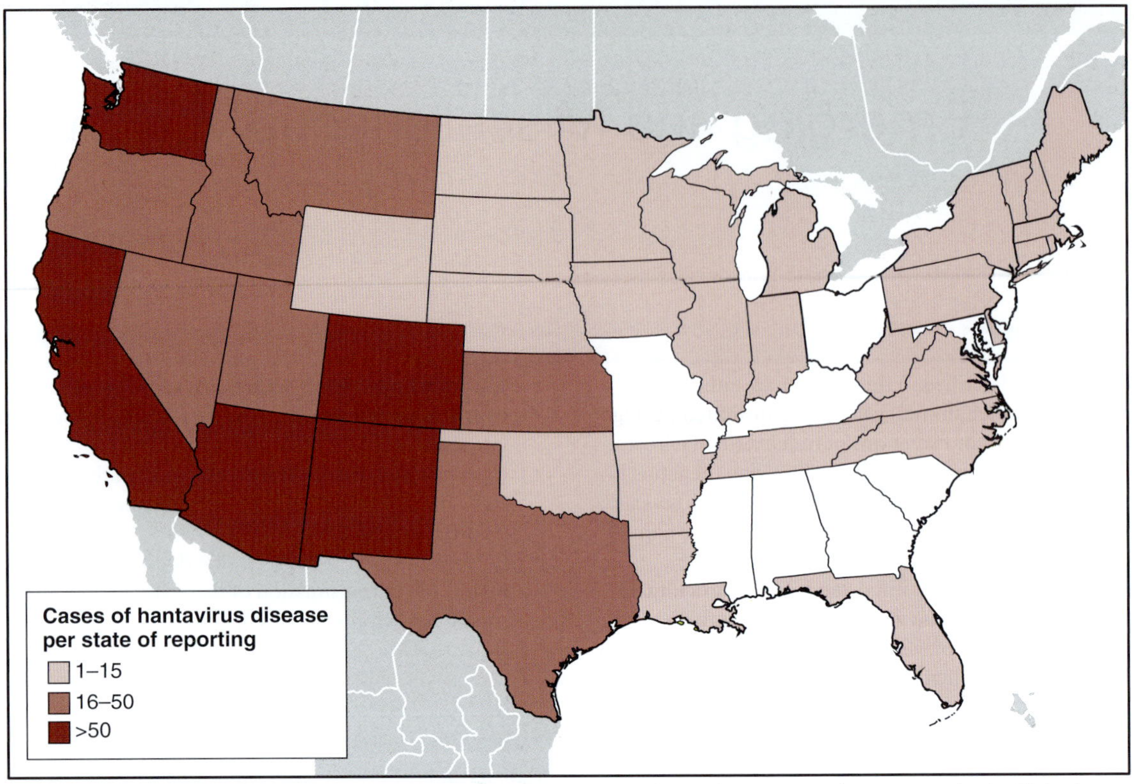

Fig. 43.1 Geographic distribution of cumulative reported hantavirus pulmonary syndrome cases in the United States. States that are not shaded had no cases reported. (Modified from the CDC; http://www.cdc.gov/hantavirus/surveillance/reporting-state.html. 2019.)

hantaviral syndromes result from vascular leakage, although the pathogenesis of this remains unclear.[1] In humans, hantavirus infection resembles leptospirosis, which is an important differential diagnosis.[11] The clinical manifestations depend on viral strain, but in general, HFRS is associated with fever, headache, abdominal pain, signs of renal dysfunction, thrombocytopenia, hemorrhagic diathesis, and sometimes neurologic signs. HPS is characterized by fever, myalgia, vomiting, abdominal pain, respiratory signs resulting from acute pulmonary edema, and circulatory collapse.[12] Some humans also develop renal insufficiency, although this is less common when compared with HFRS. Radiographs reveal acute bilateral pulmonary interstitial infiltrates. Most deaths associated with HPS are related to cardiogenic shock rather than pulmonary failure; therefore, the term "hantavirus cardiopulmonary syndrome" is more appropriate than "hantaviral pulmonary syndrome."[3]

DIAGNOSIS

The diagnosis of hantavirus infection in humans is made using serologic and molecular methods. Early in the course of illness, virus can be detected using RT-PCR in whole blood.[12] A serologic diagnosis can be made using a variety of serologic methods (most commonly ELISA) through detection of serum IgM, a fourfold increase in serum IgG, or detection of IgG or IgM against the N protein.

TREATMENT

In human patients, treatment includes cautious IV crystalloid fluid administration, colloids, electrolyte replacement, oxygen supplementation, blood pressure support, and dialysis.[12] Intravenous ribavirin has also been effective in the treatment of HFRS when used early in the course of illness. Excessive fluid administration must be avoided because it may increase the severity of pulmonary edema.

PUBLIC HEALTH ASPECTS

Avoidance of contact with rodents and their excreta is the most effective way to reduce the prevalence of disease. Masks, and in some cases respirators, should always be worn by people cleaning rodent-infested buildings. Areas to be cleaned should be thoroughly soaked with disinfectants such as dilute sodium hypochlorite before they are mopped. Vacuuming and sweeping should be avoided to minimize aerosolization.

ARENAVIRUS INFECTION

The arenaviruses are enveloped, single-stranded RNA viruses that generally infect rodents (genus *Mammarenavirus*, family *Arenaviridae*). At least eight different arenaviruses cause disease in humans, which range in severity. Each arenavirus species is usually associated with a particular rodent reservoir host. One of the most significant arenaviruses is lymphocytic choriomeningitis virus (LCV), an arenavirus of house mice (*Mus musculus*) that is found worldwide. Hamsters are also competent reservoirs. LCV is transmitted *in utero* or at birth and persists for the life of the rodent in high concentrations in tissues. Humans can become infected as a result of contact of mucous membranes or abraded skin with aerosols from infected rodents. Immunocompromised people are most susceptible; postnatal infections cause acute aseptic meningoencephalitis, whereas congenital infections produce CNS and ocular malformations.[13] Outbreaks in humans resulted from contact with pet or laboratory hamsters, including accidental transmission of the infection in organ recipients.[14–16] Other arenaviruses have more restricted geographic distributions (e.g., Lassa virus in West Africa and Whitewater Arroyo virus in the southwestern United States) and cause febrile or febrile hemorrhagic diseases in humans.

Outbreaks of rodent lymphocytic choriomeningitis infections have raised concern that domestic dogs or cats might serve as reservoirs or vectors of the virus for human exposure. Although puppies did not develop clinical illness after parenteral or cerebral inoculation,[17] they developed neutralizing antibody titers to the virus, and infection was transmitted from infected to noninfected puppies. Except for intranuclear inclusions in the adrenal cortex, pathologic changes were not observed. It is unlikely that dogs or cats become infected or spread the virus by natural exposure, because most human infections result from direct contact with rodents.

ENCEPHALOMYOCARDITIS VIRUS INFECTION

Encephalomyocarditis virus (also known as Cardiovirus A) is a small, nonenveloped RNA virus that belongs to the genus *Cardiovirus* in the family *Picornaviridae.* It infects a variety of domestic and wild animals worldwide, with rodents as subclinically infected reservoir hosts. Humans may also be infected. Most human infections are thought to be subclinical.[18] Rodents shed virus for up to 29 days after infection. Transmission is by the fecal-oral route, and infections typically occur through ingestion of contaminated food, water, or carcasses. Pigs are most susceptible and can develop myocarditis or transplacental infection with fetal death at various time periods of gestation. Disease in humans is rarely described, and can range from a mild febrile illness to meningoencephalitis.[18]

The extent to which encephalomyocarditis virus can cause disease in dogs and cats is unclear. In Austria, 0.5% of 200 cats were seropositive to encephalomyocarditis virus.[19] Encephalomyocarditis virus antigen was found in the brains of four dogs and four cats with nonsuppurative meningoencephalitis.[20] In China, an encephalomyocarditis virus (EMCV-C15) was detected in 4 of 69 serum specimens from dogs with fever and variable GI and respiratory signs using real-time PCR.[21] These four dogs were co-infected with canine parvovirus. The virus was subsequently propagated in cell culture, and experimental infection of 4-week-old puppies with the isolate was followed by development of pulmonary edema, myocarditis, pelvic limb paralysis and encephalitis. The virus was then detected in a variety of tissues, but especially the heart and brain, using RT-PCR. However, whether the experimentally infected dogs were tested for CPV infection was not reported.

ENTEROVIRUS INFECTIONS

Enteroviruses are tiny, nonenveloped, single-stranded RNA viruses that belong to the genus *Enterovirus* (family *Picornaviridae*). Viruses in this genus commonly infect humans worldwide and were previously separated into polioviruses, coxsackieviruses (types A and B), echoviruses, and as yet unclassified enteric viruses. However, because of recognized overlap in these viral groups, newer members of the genus are called enteroviruses (EVs), which are designated by a sequential numbering system (e.g., EV70). The genus also includes the human rhinoviruses (which cause the common cold) and poliovirus. EVs are environmentally resistant and infect humans primarily via the fecal-oral route, but are also shed in respiratory secretions and can contaminate fomites. After replication in submucosal lymphoid tissues, the viruses can spread systemically to various other tissues.

Dogs have been tested to determine whether they harbor a variety of human EVs because of the possible zoonotic potential (Table 43.1).[22–27] Similar information is not available for cats. Dogs are exposed to and can shed human EVs. Although dogs appear to become infected with these viruses, clinical signs have not been apparent. The viruses

TABLE 43.1 Human Enteroviruses Recovered From Apparently Healthy Dogs

Virus	Specimen	Geographic Location
Poliovirus 1	Feces	West Bengal[22]
	Feces	Costa Rica[23]
Echovirus 6	Feces	California[24]
	Nasopharynx, feces	New Mexico[24–26]
Echovirus 7	Feces	West Bengal[22]
Coxsackievirus A9, A20	Feces	Costa Rica[23]
Coxsackievirus B1	Nasopharynx, feces	Texas, New Mexico[24,25]
Coxsackievirus B3	Nasopharynx, feces	New Mexico[25]
Coxsackievirus B5	Nasopharynx, feces	New Mexico[25]
Unclassified enteroviruses	Feces	Philippines[27]

can be found in canine feces for a period of months, but whether the extended shedding results from persistence or reinfection is uncertain. EVs recovered from nasopharyngeal or fecal cultures of dogs have been grown in tissue culture and cause cytopathogenic effects, primarily in monkey kidney but not canine cell lines, supporting the fact that they are human viruses. Neutralization tests have shown them to be closely related to human isolates.[28,29] In some instances, EVs in canine feces were believed to be simply passing through the GI tract of dogs, rather than causing infection. Alternatively, they may be canine EVs antigenically related to human EVs, such as the recently discovered canine picornavirus.[30] Newer techniques to determine viral homogeneity by genetic analysis should shed light on this in the future.

Oral inoculation of dogs with echovirus 6 or coxsackievirus B1 produced minimal signs of enteric disease. Although virus could be isolated from the feces, seroconversion did not occur.[31,32] Although dogs shed these viruses in low amounts, viral spread to susceptible dogs has resulted in infection.[32] Whether infected dogs can be a source of human infection is uncertain. In one study, dog and cat ownership had a protective effect on EV infection in infants.[33]

EBOLA VIRUS INFECTION

Ebola virus is a filamentous, enveloped, single-stranded RNA virus that belongs to the genus *Ebolavirus* and family *Filoviridae* (Fig. 43.2). The virus causes vascular injury, leading to a fulminant hemorrhagic fever in human and nonhuman primates with a 40% to 80% mortality rate. Clinical signs in humans include fever, fatigue, abdominal pain, severe headache, vomiting, diarrhea, myalgia, arthralgia, weakness, and hemorrhages.[34] Death generally results from hypovolemic shock and multiorgan dysfunction. The first recorded description of the disease was in 1976 in Zaire (now the Democratic Republic of Congo), and the virus is named after the Ebola River where the first outbreak occurred. Various species of fruit bats act as reservoir hosts.[35] Humans become infected by contact with body fluids of other infected humans, or contact with other infected animals, especially bats. Infections have occurred as a result of handling meat of bats, nonhuman primates, or duikers (a species of antelope) (Fig. 43.3).[35] Healthcare workers have also been infected. Transmission is more likely later in the course of infection than in the first few days of clinical signs, and the incubation period is 2 to 21 days (average 8 to 10 days). Diagnosis of infection in humans is based on cell culture, serologic detection of antibodies or antigen, and/or detection of viral RNA with real-time RT-PCR assays.[36] Treatment is with aggressive supportive care, as no antiviral

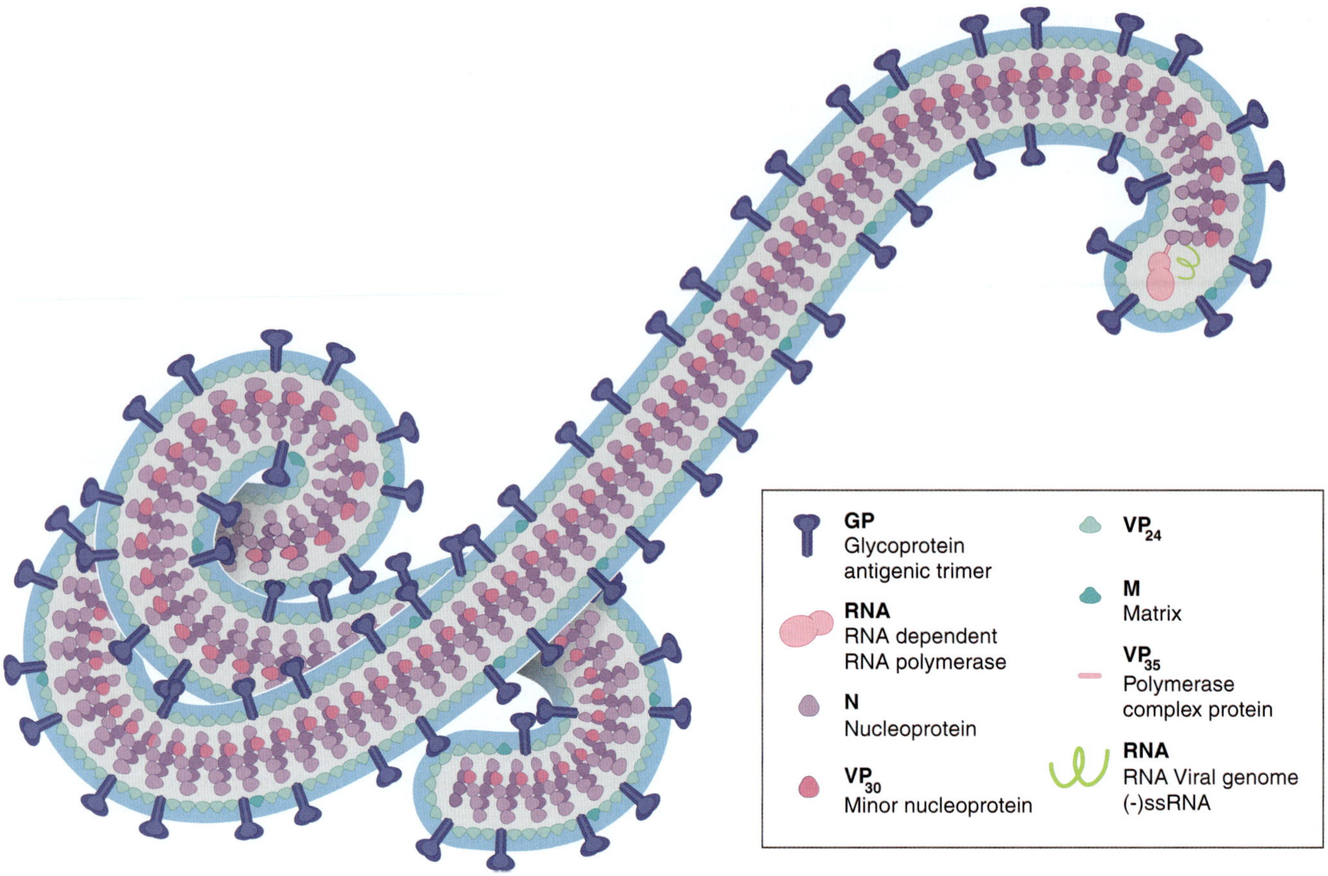

Fig. 43.2 Structure of the Ebola virus virion.

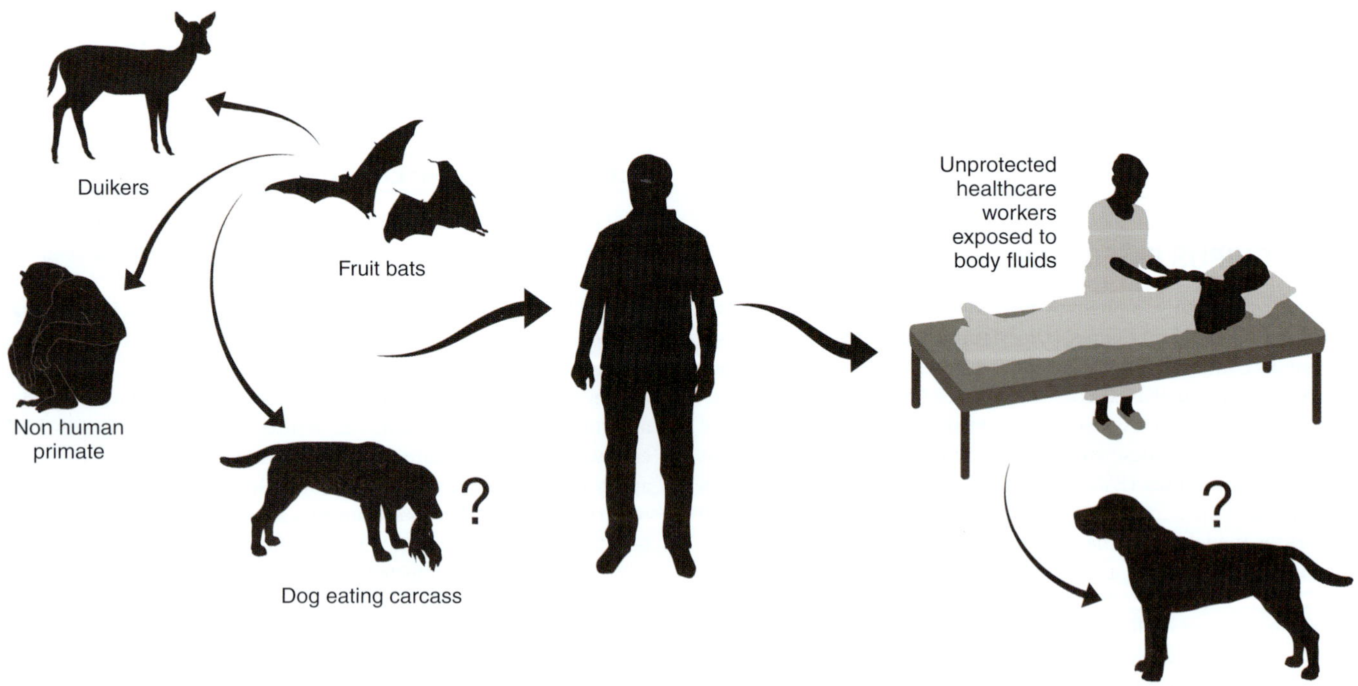

Fig. 43.3 Epidemiology of Ebola virus infection. (Adapted from CDC; https://www.cdc.gov/vhf/ebola/)

TABLE 43.2 Comparison of Features of the Four Major Hepatitis E Virus Genotypes of Significance to Human Health

Characteristics	Genotype 1	Genotype 2	Genotype 3	Genotype 4
Geographic location	Africa and Asia	Mexico, West Africa	Developed countries	China, Taiwan, Japan
Risk groups	Young adults	Young adults	Older adults (>40 years), males, and immunocompromised individuals	Young adults
Zoonotic transmission	No	No	Yes	Yes
Chronic infection	No	No	Yes	No
Outbreak occurrence	Common	Smaller scale	Uncommon	Uncommon

(Modified from the Centers for Disease Control and Prevention; https://www.cdc.gov/hepatitis/hev/hevfaq.htm. 2020.)

drugs have yet proven to be effective.[34] The virus can persist weeks to months in some recovered humans, and chronic infection of semen has led to sexual transmission. The possibility of development of an effective vaccine holds promise.[37]

The most significant outbreak began in Guinea in December 2013 and spread rapidly throughout West Africa. The outbreak continued to early 2016, affecting approximately 30,000 people and resulting in over 11,000 deaths.[34,38] During the outbreak, the virus underwent mutation that increased its tropism for human cells, and decreased its tropism for bat cells, which was thought to contribute to the size of the outbreak.[39] In August 2014, the WHO declared the outbreak was an international public health emergency. Human-to-human transmission occurred outside Africa in Madrid, Spain, and Dallas, Texas. In Spain, a nurse was infected when she cared for a patient with Ebola virus infection that was transferred from West Africa to Spain. She subsequently recovered. In Texas, a man contracted the disease after flying from Liberia to Dallas. Subsequently, two nurses that cared for him became infected. The man died, but the nurses recovered with supportive care.

Antibodies to Ebola virus have been detected in the serum of dogs,[38,40] raising concerns about the role of feral and domestic dogs in the transmission of Ebola virus. During the 2001-2002 outbreak of Ebola virus in Gabon, Africa, dogs were observed feeding on animal carcasses. The seroprevalence in dogs in the virus-epidemic area (25.2%) was higher than the seroprevalence in nonepidemic areas of Gabon (15.2%) or France (2%).[40] In another study that aimed to investigate the role of dogs as sentinels for human exposure to filoviruses, 47 (73%) of 64 dog serum specimens had evidence of exposure to filoviruses, and up to 100% of dog serum specimens from some regions where Ebola had occurred in humans had evidence of possible exposure to Ebola virus.[38] Neither Ebola virus antigens nor nucleotide sequences or cultivated virus were detected in any seropositive or seronegative dog blood specimens. Clinical signs have not been observed in exposed dogs, and whether they can serve as a source of infection for people remains uncertain. In 2014, the Spanish government ordered the pet dog of the nurse in Spain, "Excalibur," to be euthanized, and "Bentley," a Cavalier King Charles spaniel owned by one of the nurses in Dallas was quarantined under BSL-4 precautions for 3 weeks. Such precautions require considerable resources, including people trained in how to use and remove appropriate personal protective equipment (PPE). Suitable quarantine facilities were not available in Spain.[41] Although Excalibur was not tested for Ebola virus infection, no evidence of Ebola virus infection was detected in Bentley despite repeated testing over the course of the quarantine period. As a result of concerns about the role of companion animals in transmission of Ebola virus infection, the AVMA and CDC issued guidance statements for public health officials on pets of Ebola virus disease contacts and on quarantine of dogs and cats after exposure to a human with confirmed Ebola virus disease.[42] Quarantine is required for a minimum of 3 weeks after the pet was last exposed to a person with Ebola. In order to avoid quarantine, it is recommended that animals in contact with a person being monitored for development of symptoms be moved to another household, so that in the event symptoms do occur, those animals are not exposed.

HEPATITIS E VIRUS INFECTION

Hepatitis E virus (HEV) generally causes an acute self-limiting hepatitis in humans. Although previously considered a disease primarily occurring in developing tropical and subtropical countries, it has recently emerged as the most common cause of acute hepatitis in the United Kingdom.[43] Chronic infections that can culminate in cirrhosis can occur in immunosuppressed individuals such as transplant recipients.[44] The virus is icosahedral and nonenveloped, with a single-stranded positive-sense RNA genome, and belongs to the family *Hepeviridae*, genus *Orthohepevirus*. Strains that infect humans are classified into four genotypes; genotypes 1 and 2 exclusively infect humans, but genotypes 3 and 4 infect humans and other animal species, with pigs considered the predominant reservoir (Table 43.2).[44–46] Additional strains of HEV have been detected in other animal species, including chickens, rats, ferrets, and moose, but these are genetically distinct from those that infect humans.[45] All genotypes are shed in feces with fecal-oral contact as the means of transmission. Genotype 1 infection is the most common form of acute hepatitis in people in Asia, with most infections resulting from ingestion of water that has been contaminated with feces. Outbreaks of genotype 1 infection occur in developing countries in southeast and central Asia, the Middle East, and North Africa, especially after heavy rainfall and monsoons. Sporadic outbreaks caused by genotype 2 occur in Mexico and West Africa. Genotype 3 causes disease in developed countries and genotype 4 in China, Taiwan, and Japan. Foodborne transmission through consumption of undercooked pork, deer, and boar meat predominates for genotypes 3 and 4, and outbreaks are uncommon. Genotype 3 strains have also been detected in wild and farmed rabbits.[45] Contamination of water with pig feces can result in contamination of other foodstuffs, including shellfish and fruit.

Antibodies to HEV have been detected in cats and dogs worldwide, and an epidemiologic connection between pet ownership and human HEV infection has been implied because of the number of infected humans that have reported dog or cat contact.[47–49] Seroprevalences have been reported of approximately 20% in dogs and 6% in cats from China,[50,51] 0% in dogs and 8% in cats from Korea,[52] 28% of 287 dogs from South Korea,[38] 0.9% of 212 dogs in the United States,[53] 0.8% in dogs from the United Kingdom,[54] less than 1% in dogs and 2% in cats from Japan,[55,56] 7% in dogs from Brazil,[57] and 23% of 44 dogs from

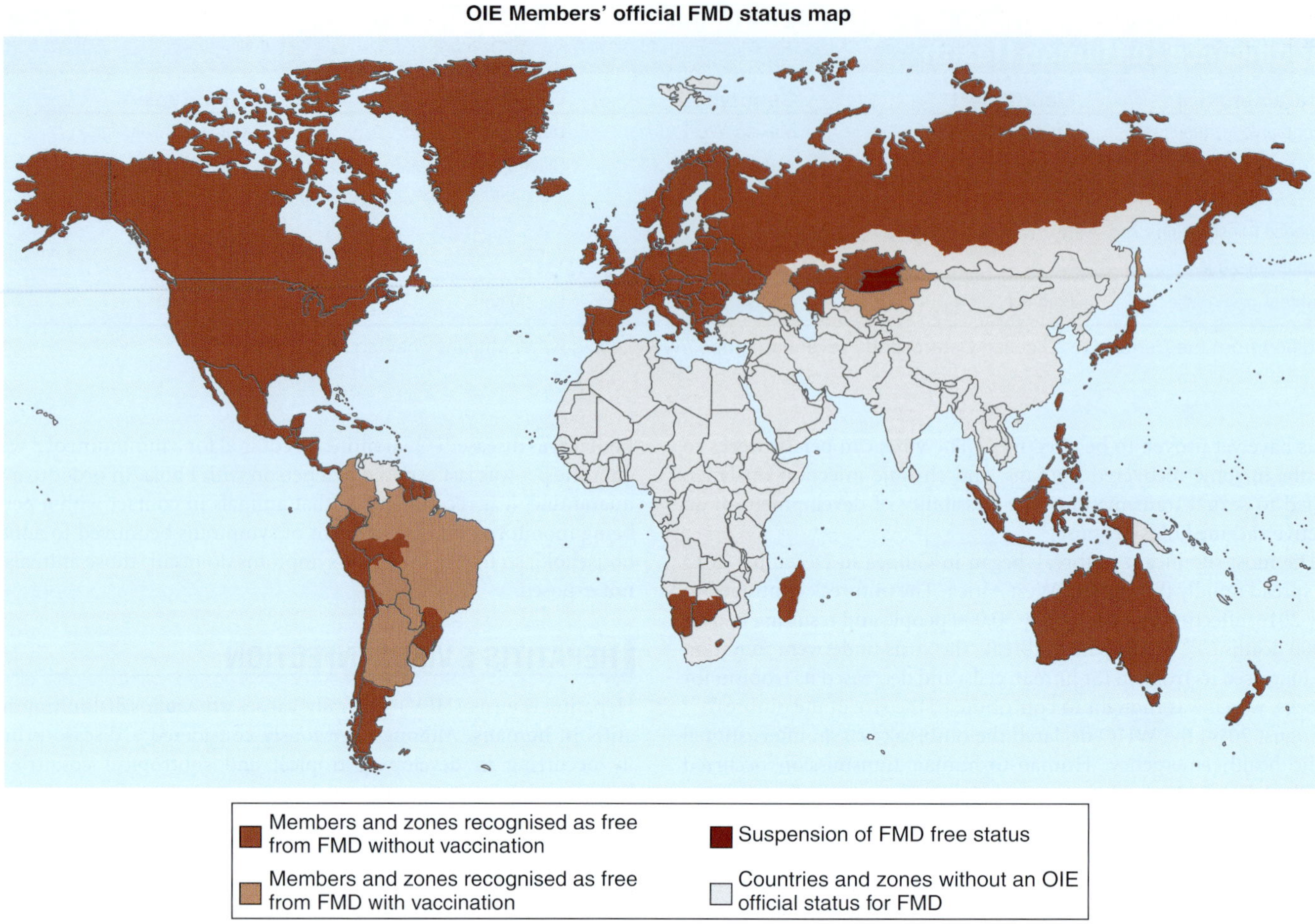

Fig. 43.4 World Health Organization Member Countries' foot-and-mouth disease (FMD) status. (From World Organization for Animal Health. Foot and Mouth Disease [FMD]. http://www.oie.int/en/disease/foot-and-mouth-disease/#ui-id-2. 2022. ©OIE 2022.)

India.[58] In China, dogs and cats were more likely to be seropositive if they shared kitchen scraps with humans, as opposed to being fed a commercial pet food.[51] However, attempts to detect HEV RNA in serum, liver, and feces from dogs and cats have consistently yielded negative results.[54,55,59,60] This included one attempt that used broadly reactive primers expected to detect strains divergent from those that infect humans.[54] Furthermore, pet veterinarians attending a conference in Portugal were not found to have an increased risk of seropositivity when compared with the general population,[61] whereas in the United States, swine veterinarians were much more likely to be seropositive than those who did not have contact with swine.[62] Currently, the evidence suggests that dogs and cats do not play an important role in transmission of HEVs to humans. Prevention of HEV infection involves general sanitation.

FOOT-AND-MOUTH DISEASE

Foot-and-mouth disease (FMD) is a highly contagious febrile vesicular disease of wild and domestic cloven-hoofed animals. It is caused by various strains of FMD virus, a nonenveloped RNA virus (genus *Aphthovirus*, family *Picornaviridae*). It occurs worldwide and has significant economic impact on the agricultural industry. Seven serotypes are recognized, named following their recognition in France, Germany, South Africa, and Pakistan (O, A, C, SAT1, SAT2, SAT3, Asia-1). Eradication has been variably successful in Australia, New Zealand, Japan, Europe, and North America, with the last outbreak in the United States occurring in 1929.[63] Many countries in South America are considered disease-free (Fig. 43.4).[64] The disease continues to be a problem in the Middle East, Africa, and parts of Asia, and reappearance of the disease in places it has been eradicated, usually as a result of accidental importation of contaminated meat (or pigs fed contaminated meat products) from countries where FMD persists, results in major economic losses. For example, the 2001 outbreak in the United Kingdom was estimated to cost US $12.3 to 13.8 billion.[63] Culling, restriction of movement, disinfection, monitoring, and vaccination are used to control the disease. Vaccines do not cross-protect among different strains, so they must be designed to target a particular outbreak strain.

Dogs and cats are resistant to infection and do not play a major role in spreading or harboring the disease under conditions of natural exposure. Dogs and cats can be experimentally infected,[65] but naturally occurring disease has not been recognized. Carnivores have the potential to become incidentally infected during outbreaks in herbivores by contacting these animals or their offal, but are only considered to play a role in transmission by acting as fomites. Dogs can also contribute to the spread of FMD by carrying remains of animals from one location to another.

Guidelines have been established for dog owners in areas known to have infected animals. Dogs in areas with infected animals must be leashed or enclosed to a confined space at all times. Dogs must not be walked across farmland and contact with livestock and wild animals should be prevented. Certain sporting activities involving dogs should not be allowed in quarantined areas. In the United Kingdom, concerns about the spread of FMD during the 2001 outbreak resulted in postponement of the Crufts Dog Show. Similarly, cats should be kept indoors as much as possible. Disinfectants suitable for inactivating the virus are 4% sodium carbonate, 0.5% citric acid, 4%–5% acetic acid, 1% potassium peroxymonosulfate, 3% sodium hypochlorite (2:3 ratio of gallons of household bleach to 3 gallons of water), or 2% sodium hydroxide.[66] Phenolic disinfectants, quaternary ammonium compounds, and biguanides are not effective. Halogens such as sodium hypochlorite or iodine are less effective because of inactivation by organic matter.

VESICULAR EXANTHEMA AND OTHER CALICIVIRUSES

Vesicular exanthema of swine is caused by a calicivirus that causes lesions on the mouth, lips, snout, and feet of pigs. It has only been reported in the United States, and not since 1959, but is of historic importance because it can be confused with FMD. Dogs have developed clinical signs of illness characterized by vesicular eruptions when outbreaks of vesicular exanthema virus infection have occurred in swine.[67] Virus was not definitely isolated in these cases. Experimentally infected dogs developed fever within 24 hours after inoculation and vesicular eruptions on their tongues and in their oral cavities.[67] These lesions healed within a few days. Virus was isolated from the spleen of a dog that became febrile after inoculation.

In 2018, several additional caliciviruses were isolated from military working dogs in the United States.[68] These were closely related to canine calicivirus. Further work will be required to determine their pathogenicity. A calicivirus (canine vesivirus) was isolated from dogs that died in 2015 during a focal outbreak of hemorrhagic gastroenteritis in a pet housing facility in Virginia, USA. Virus nucleic acid was found in association with areas of necrosis and hemorrhage in the intestinal tract, but also in the brain of a dog that had nonsuppurative meningoencephalitis.[69]

RABBIT HEMORRHAGIC DISEASE

Rabbit hemorrhagic disease (RHD), also known as *rabbit calicivirus disease*, is an acute, highly contagious, and often fatal disease of rabbits caused by rabbit hemorrhagic disease virus (RHDV, genus *Lagovirus*, family *Caliciviridae*). Transmission of the virus is by direct contact with secretions from infected rabbits or with infected fomites. The disease was first identified in China in 1984, spread rapidly to Europe, where it killed millions of domesticated rabbits in less than a year, and has now also been reported in other parts of Asia, Africa, Australia, New Zealand, and the Americas. In 2010, a new variant of the virus, RHDV2, emerged in France. The virus was introduced into Australia and held under quarantine to investigate its utility to control rabbit overpopulation, but escaped quarantine in 1995 and killed over 10 million rabbits within a 2-month period. Subsequently, it was deliberately and illegally introduced into New Zealand. In 2019 and 2020, it appeared in wild and domestic lagamorphs in the northwestern and southwestern United States, respectively.[70,71] By March of 2022, the virus had been identified in lagomorphs from 19 different US states.[72] Affected rabbits develop a febrile hemorrhagic disease, sometimes accompanied by icterus, neurologic signs, and cutaneous ulceration.

Only rabbits are susceptible to disease caused by RHDV. Feral cats in New Zealand have antibodies to RHDV, and the virus was detected using nested RT-PCR in the liver of one seropositive cat.[73] Cats fed rabbit livers infected with RHDV developed serologic titers to the virus, and RHDV RNA was detected in the tonsils, mesenteric lymph nodes, spleen, and liver. Even though large amounts of virus were found, clinical disease was not observed. Active replication of RHDV was not demonstrated.

SEVERE ACUTE RESPIRATORY CORONAVIRUS INFECTIONS

Severe acute respiratory syndrome coronaviruses are betacoronaviruses most closely related to betacoronaviruses isolated from bats. Other betacoronaviruses include OC43 and HKU1, the cause of common colds in humans; Middle Eastern Respiratory Syndrome (MERS) virus; canine respiratory coronavirus (CRCoV); and bovine coronavirus (BoCV) (Table 43.3). While also a betacoronavirus, CRCoV is more closely related to BoCV and OC43 than SARS-CoVs (Fig. 43.5).[74] The original SARS-CoV, which caused disease in humans from 2002 to 2004, was thought to be transmitted to farmed civets after recombination in bats.[75] When Himalayan palm civets were transported to Guangdong market in China, the virus spread among market civets; spillover to humans likely occurred in 2002, with spread of the virus that extended over the course of 2003. Civet cats are not true cats but small mammals that resemble weasels; they are more closely related to mongoose. The virus was also found in raccoon dogs at street markets. However, civets seemed like a more likely conduit than raccoon dogs because the virus was able to persist in infected animals for up to 2 weeks, and many infections were associated with restaurants where civet meat was prepared and served. Extensive culling of palm civets followed. SARS-CoV-1 causes respiratory illness in humans with pneumonia and lymphopenia after an incubation period of 2 to 10 days, with a case fatality rate of 9.6%.[76] The SARS outbreak ended by 2004, with no more cases resulting from person-to-person transmission since then. In total, there were about 8,000 cases in 30 countries,

TABLE 43.3 Major Coronaviruses of Humans and Animals That Belong to the Alpha- and Betacoronavirus Genera

Alphacoronavirus	Betacoronavirus
Human 229E (common cold)	Human OC43 (common cold)
Human NL63 (common cold)	Human HKU1 (common cold)
Feline coronavirus (FECV and FIPV) (serotypes I and II)	MERS-CoV (Middle Eastern respiratory syndrome) (systemic)
Canine coronavirus (serotypes I and II [a, b, c])	SARS-CoV (severe acute respiratory syndrome) coronavirus (systemic)
Transmissible gastroenteric virus of swine (TGEV)	SARS-CoV-2
Porcine epidemic diarrhea virus (PEDV)	Bovine coronavirus
	Canine respiratory coronavirus Equine coronavirus Murine hepatitis virus Porcine hemagglutinating encephalomyelitis virus

Deltacoronaviruses (such as wild avian coronaviruses, porcine deltacoronavirus) and gammacoronaviruses (such as avian infectious bronchitis virus) primarily infect birds.

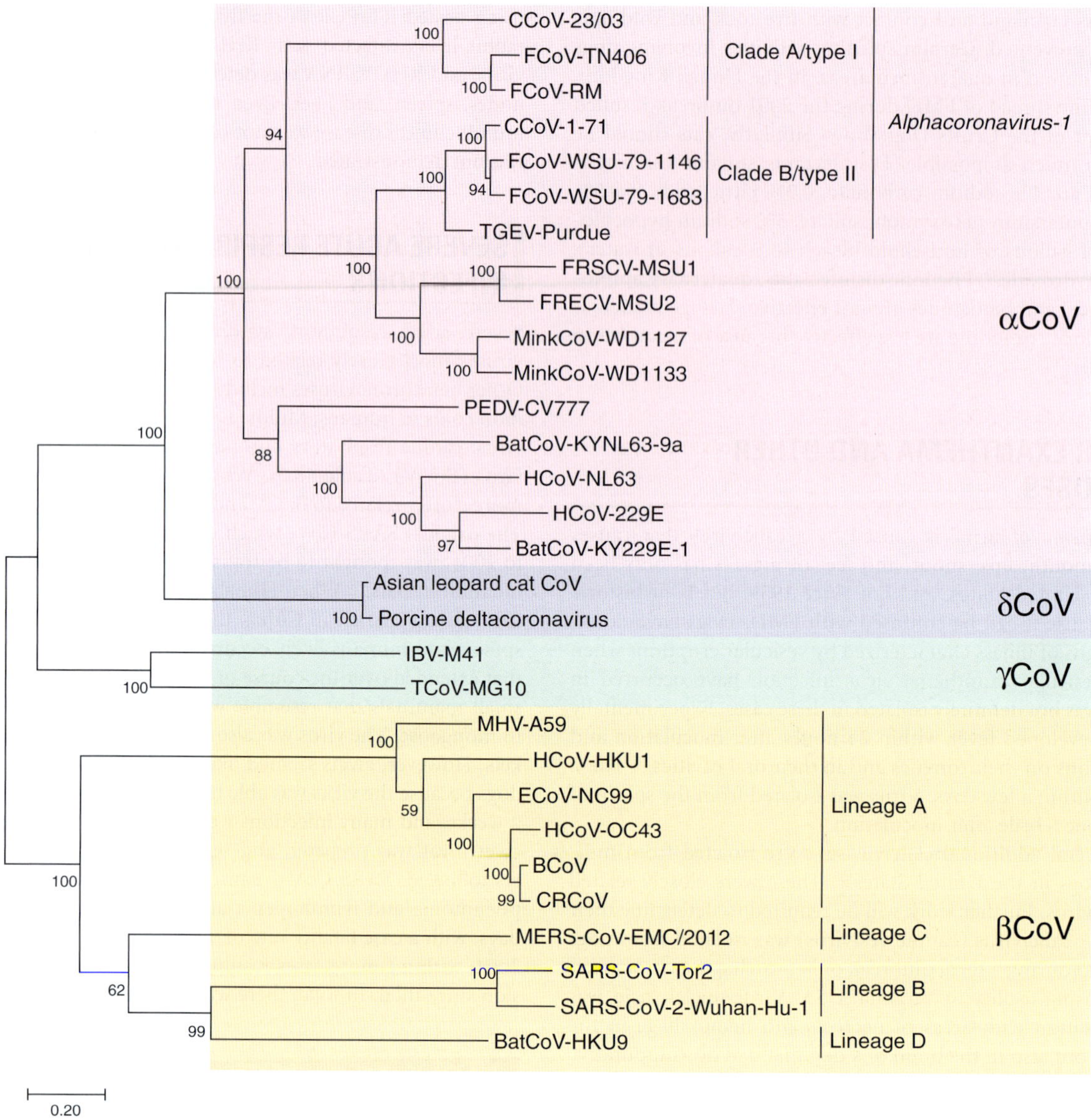

Fig. 43.5 Phylogenetic tree of selected coronaviruses based on spike protein sequences. The tree is drawn to scale, with branch lengths measured in the number of nucleotide substitutions per site. *BatCoV,* bat coronavirus; *BCoV,* bovine coronavirus; *CCoV,* canine coronavirus; *CRCoV,* canine respiratory coronavirus; *ECoV,* equine coronavirus; *FCoV,* feline coronavirus; *FRECV,* ferret enteric coronavirus; *FRSCV,* ferret systemic coronavirus; *HCoV,* human coronavirus; *IBV,* infectious bronchitis virus; *MERS-CoV,* Middle East respiratory syndrome coronavirus; *MHV,* murine hepatitis virus; *PEDV,* porcine epidemic coronavirus; *SARS-CoV,* severe acute respiratory syndrome coronavirus; *TCoV,* turkey coronavirus; *TGEV,* transmissible gastroenteritis virus. (Reprinted from Stout AE, Andre NM, Jaimes JA, et al. Coronaviruses in cats and other companion animals: Where does SARS-CoV-2/COVID-19 fit? *Vet Microbiol.* 2020;247:108777.)

including North America, South America, Europe, and Asia.[77] It was the search for other human coronaviruses at this time that led to the discovery of the common cold coronaviruses NL63 and HKU1.[78] It is generally believed that civets and raccoon dogs do not represent ongoing reservoirs of SARS-CoV-1. A small number of pet cats tested positive and seroconverted in a large outbreak of SARS that occurred in an apartment complex in Hong Kong.[79] In that outbreak, which involved over 300 people, there was evidence that airborne transmission of the virus was occurring as a result of hydraulic action of sewerage drainage pipes, so the situation was unusual.[80] Experimental infection of six ferrets and six cats was also accomplished.[79] None of the cats in that study had clinical signs, whereas several ferrets developed lethargy and one died. Infection was transmitted to a limited number of in-contact animals, and only ferrets developed clinical illness. However, pulmonary pathology was detected in the cats that was similar to that in humans.

MERS-CoV was first isolated from the lungs of a 60-year-old person who died from severe respiratory illness in Saudi Arabia in 2012.[81] Clinical manifestations range from none to severe pneumonia, acute renal failure, and septic shock. Since then, 2,984 confirmed cases have been reported with 858 deaths in 27 countries.[82] Three-quarters of patients had co-morbidities. All human cases have been associated with travel to the Arabian Peninsula. Only two infected humans have been reported in the United States.[83] Dromedary camels have been implicated as amplifying hosts based on the detection of antibodies in these camels as well as sequences resembling MERS-CoV in camels

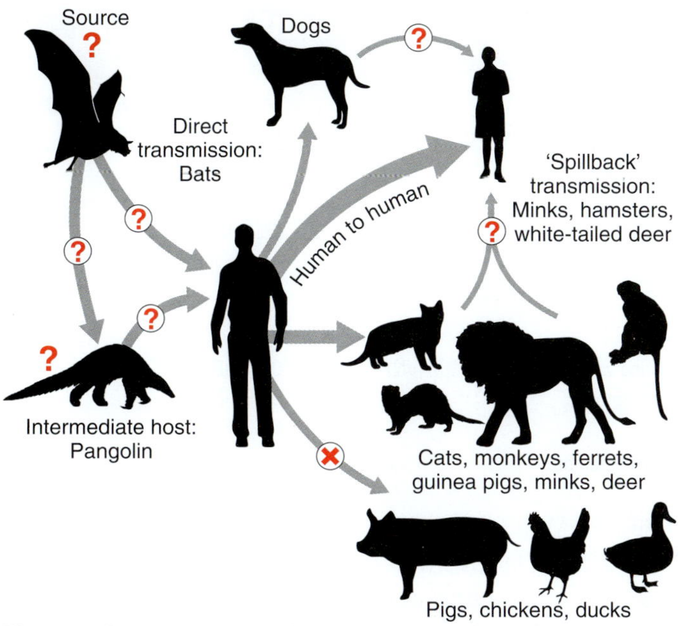

Fig. 43.6 Diagram representing our understanding of zoonotic and reverse zoonotic transmission of SARS-CoV-2 at the time of writing.

from the Arabian Peninsula. In addition, most people with the disease have a history of interactions with dromedary camels. However, the precise role that dromedaries play in the transmission of MERS remains unknown.[84] No sustained human-to-human transmission has been documented anywhere in the world.

SARS-CoV-2 infection emerged in late 2019 in Wuhan, China, as the cause of COVID-19, a highly contagious systemic viral disease that at the time of writing has infected nearly 500 million people worldwide and contributed to the death of over 6.1 million people.[85] COVID-19 occurs after an incubation period of 2 to 14 days, and consists of fever, myalgia and fatigue, respiratory signs (primarily cough and shortness of breath), GI signs, and anosmia and ageusia (loss of taste). Less frequently, stroke-like neurologic signs, cardiac arrhythmias due to myocarditis, and acute kidney injury have been described. Severe outcomes and death are more likely in older people and those with chronic conditions such as diabetes mellitus, chronic lung disease, and cardiovascular disease. Early in the pandemic, a case fatality rate of 10%–27% was reported in people over 85 years of age, 3% to 11% in those aged 65–84 years, 1% to 3% in those aged 55–64 years, <1% in those aged 20–54 years, and 0% in those aged less than 19 years.[86]

The precise origin of SARS-CoV-2 is not known (Fig. 43.6). The overwhelming majority of CoVs have been identified only in bats, and so bats are considered the major natural CoV reservoirs. However, two of the human common cold CoVs likely originated in rodents. Importantly, domestic animals are important intermediate hosts for transmission of CoVs to humans, and camelids, cattle, civet cats, dromedary camels, and pigs have all been implicated in this role.[87] Pangolins have been most closely studied as a possible amplifying host for SARS-CoV-2, because they have been shown to harbor genetically very similar CoV strains (albeit more different than those found in bats), coronavirus strains capable of infecting human cells, and are sold in Chinese food markets.[88] Considered the world's most trafficked mammal, pangolins have been trafficked for their scales, which are used in traditional Chinese medicine, and they are also a luxury food item. It has been suggested that the African swine fever outbreak in China may have contributed to emergence of SARS-CoV-2 because shortage of pork products drove an increased trade of farmed susceptible animals and wildlife as a source of food.[89] Accidental or deliberate release of an engineered virus from a laboratory (the "lab-leak theory") has also been suggested as a possible origin of the virus, but has been disputed on the basis of epidemiological studies or studies of the composition of the virus.[90,91]

The host receptor for SARS-CoV and SARS-CoV-2 is the angiotensin-converting enzyme 2 (ACE2) receptor, whereas MERS binds to the dipeptidyl peptidase 4 receptor. A receptor-binding domain (RBD) on the viral spike (S) protein interacts with the ACE2 receptor, which is followed by viral entry into host cells. The S protein must be activated before the virus can enter cells. This requires the synergistic action of host furin enzymes, which cleave the S protein into S1 and S2 components, and a cell surface serine protease enzyme known as serine 2 (TMPRSS2).[92] Although the amino acid sequence of the ACE2 receptor can influence whether a host species can be infected, other factors, such as the distribution and density of ACE2 receptor expression in tissues, host and virus factors influencing spike protein cleavage, the use of co-receptors (such as neuropilin 1), and the host immune response to infection, also influence species susceptibility and expression of clinical disease.[93]

Experimental infection studies have shown that cats and ferrets are capable of transmitting SARS-CoV-2 infection to other cats and ferrets, whereas dogs did not transmit infection to a small number of in-contact dogs.[94–97] Hamsters, rabbits, deer, American minks, raccoon dogs, deer mice, fruit bats, otters, and nonhuman primates are also susceptible to experimental infection.[98] At the time of writing, more than 200 pet dogs and cats worldwide have tested positive for SARS-CoV-2, with reports documented by the OIE and the USDA.[99,100] Most dogs and cats have been subclinically infected, or if signs are present, it has not been possible to determine whether they are associated with infection or due to an unrelated comorbidity.[100,101,102,103] A small number of animals died shortly after they tested positive, but co-morbidities explained the reason for death. However, one 4-month-old kitten from the United Kingdom was euthanized and viral pneumonia was confirmed at necropsy, with FA showing intralesional SARS-CoV-2 antigen.[104] Of 10 dogs and cats that tested positive for SARS-CoV-2 and then died or were euthanized in the United States, it was concluded that infection was an incidental finding in 8 animals, but was the cause of disease in one dog and one cat.[105] In a necropsy surveillance study of 5 animals in contact with infected humans, infection was confirmed in 3 cats and a tiger, but infection was not thought to be the cause of death in any of the cases. The remaining animal was a dog that died of bronchopneumonia, but this dog tested negative for SARS-CoV-2.[106]

A small number of infected dogs and cats have been reported to have cardiac disease at the time of death,[103,105] including the first dog reported to be infected with SARS-CoV-2. Suspected myocarditis was described in association with natural infection in 8 cats and 3 dogs in the United Kingdom.[107] However, cardiac disease and exposure to SARS-CoV-2 in pet dogs and cats is likely widespread, and no convincing evidence for an association between these and disease exists at the time of writing. The possibility remains that new variants of SARS-CoV-2 could arise that are more virulent in dogs and cats or more transmissible, so ongoing monitoring is critical.

Animals with positive test results have typically been in contact with infected owners. Evidence of transmission of infection from dogs or cats back to owners has not been documented, but remains theoretically possible. Mink on mink farms appear to be the most susceptible to infection and disease, with fatal infections reported. There has been evidence of mink-to-mink, mink-to-human, and mink-to-dog and cat transmission on mink farms worldwide. In addition, an outbreak of the delta variant of SARS-CoV-2 in Syrian hamsters in a pet shop in Hong Kong was followed by zoonotic transmission and then human-to-human transmission.[98] Extensive culling efforts associated

TABLE 43.4 Selected Studies Reporting the Prevalence of Antibodies to SARS-CoV-2 and Shedding of SARS-CoV-2 in Dogs

Location (Number of Dogs)	Dates	Population	Seroprevalence (%)	Virus Detection By PCR (Specimen Type)
France (12)[127]	Feb–Mar 2020	In close contact with veterinary students, some of which tested positive for SARS-CoV-2	0/12 (LIPS)[128]	
Hong Kong (15)[129]	Feb–Mar 2020	In contact with humans with COVID-19		2/15 (N, O)[a,b]
United States, Asia, Europe (2150)[116]	Feb–Apr 2020	Dogs with respiratory disease		0/2150 (PR)
Wuhan, China (9)[130]	Mar 2020	In contact with humans with COVID-19	1/9 (ELISA, VN)	0/9 (O, R)
Northern Italy (603)[131]	Mar–May 2020	High-prevalence regions, some living with infected humans, some with respiratory signs	15/451 (3.3) (VN)	0/303 (OP) 0/183 (N) 0/66 (R)
France (11)[101]	April 2020	In contact with humans with or suspected to have COVID-19		0/11 (NP, R)
Spain (12)[132]	Apr–May 2020	In contact with humans with COVID-19		0/12 (OP, R)
Texas, USA (59)[117]	Jun–Jul 2020	In contact with humans with COVID-19	7/59 (11.9) (VN)	1/59 (PR, R, B)[b]
Wuhan (910)[133]	Jan–Sep 2020	Random source, including shelters	16/910 (1.8) (ELISA)	
Chile (1)[118]	May–Sep 2020	In contact with humans with COVID-19	0/10 (ELISA)	
United States (WA and ID) (100)[120]	Apr 2020-Sep 2021	In contact with humans with COVID-19	33/81 (ELISA)	5/94 (N/OP)
Brazil (Rio de Janeiro) (29)[121]	May 2020-Oct 2020	In contact with humans with COVID-19	1/29 (VN)	8/29 (N/OP)

[a]Virus isolated.
[b]Virus sequence obtained.
B, body; *ELISA*, enzyme-linked immunosorbent assay; *F*, feces; *LIPS*, luciferase immunoprecipitation system; *N*, nasal; *NP*, nasopharyngeal; *O*, oral; *OP*, oropharyngeal; *PR*, pooled respiratory; *R*, rectal; *VN*, virus neutralization.

with these zoonotic transmission events have drawn considerable media attention. Recently, likely transmission from white-tailed deer to humans was described.[108] Concern has been raised that evolution of the virus in wildlife with subsequent "spillback" to humans could lead to additional pandemic waves, potentially with higher mortality. One study provided evidence that the highly transmissible Omicron variant may have evolved in mice, with subsequent spillback to humans,[109,110] although the true origin of the Omicron variant at the time of writing remains unknown.

In early April of 2020, a report was released of an infected tiger at the Bronx zoo in New York.[111] The tiger was tested because it developed a cough and inappetence and was in contact with a caregiver that was subclinically shedding SARS-CoV-2. In addition, the tiger's sister, two Siberian tigers, and three lions at the zoo were reported to also have clinical signs of respiratory illness. It was later published that there were two separate transmission events that involved the tigers and the lions, with the lions being infected with a slightly different variant than the tigers. Infected animals shed infectious virus in their respiratory secretions and feces.[112] Since then, there have been reports of other clinical infections in captive wild felids worldwide (puma, snow leopards, lions, and tigers)[113,114] Widespread vaccination of captive wildlife species and mink has been introduced to reduce morbidity and mortality in these species. The vaccine being used for this purpose in the United States at the time of writing is an experimental recombinant subunit vaccine (Zoetis, NJ, USA).[115]

Since the start of the pandemic, evidence has been accumulating in regard to the extent of infection of pet dogs and cats. One commercial veterinary diagnostic laboratory (IDEXX Laboratories, ME, USA) reported no positive PCR tests in 4,617 dogs and cats from Asia, Europe, and North America for which specimens were submitted for respiratory viral PCR testing from mid-February 2020 to mid-April 2020.[116] Instead, assays were positive for common respiratory pathogens such as FCV, *Bordetella bronchiseptica*, and *Mycoplasma cynos*. The seroprevalence has ranged from 0% to 40% in dogs and 0% to 44% in cats (Tables 43.4 and 43.5). The prevalence of positive PCR results has ranged from 0% to 13% in dogs and 0% to 25% in cats. Virus has been more often detected in respiratory swab specimens than in rectal swabs or feces, and shedding in cats has been documented in respiratory secretions for up to 25 days.[117] In many cases, full-length SARS-CoV-2 genome sequence has been obtained using next-generation sequencing platforms, and shown to match that of the animal's owner.[117–119] In a Texas study, SARS-CoV-2 infection was identified using PCR and sequencing in 3 of 17 (17.6%) cats and 1 of 59 (10.3%) dogs from 4 of 39 separate households. All PCR-positive animals were subclinically infected. In a study from Idaho and Washington, USA, signs of illness that could be consistent with COVID-19 were reported in 20% of dogs and 39% of cats that had been in contact with people with COVID-19.[120] Differences in prevalence may reflect variations in assay performance, the time of year, as well as the degree of contact between positive owners and sampled animals. Behaviors that promote close contact between humans and pets, such as sharing of food dishes and beds may increase risk of transmission.[120,121]

In general, the results of studies to date suggest that subclinical infection of dogs and cats with SARS-CoV-2 occurs commonly, although shedding of virus is relatively uncommon. Cats appear to be more susceptible to infection than dogs and may be able to show signs of respiratory illness and shed virus for over a week. Although domestic cats can transmit infection to other cats following experimental infection, the extent to which this occurs in the field remains unknown. However, veterinarians working in small animal practice have not been identified as at increased risk of infection and contact

TABLE 43.5 Selected Studies Reporting the Prevalence of Antibodies to SARS-CoV-2 and Shedding of SARS-CoV-2 in Cats

Location (Number of Cats)	Dates	Population	Seroprevalence (%)	Virus Detection By PCR (Specimen Type)
Wuhan, China (102)[134]	Jan–Mar 2020	Random source, some shelter cats	15/102 (14.7) (ELISA) 11/102 (10.7) (VN)	0/102 (NP, R)
United States, Asia, Europe (2466)[116]	Feb–Apr 2020	Cats with respiratory disease (being tested for other respiratory pathogens)		0/2466 (PR)
France (9)[127]	Feb–Mar 2020	In close contact with veterinary students, some of which tested positive for SARS-CoV-2	0/9 (LIPS)[128]	
Hong Kong (50)[119]	Feb–Aug 2020	In contact with humans with COVID-19		6/50 (12) (N, O, R)[a]
Wuhan, China (10)[130]	Mar 2020	In contact with humans with COVID-19	2/10 (ELISA, VN)	0/10 (O, R)
Northern Italy (316)[131]	Mar–May 2020	High-prevalence regions, some living with infected humans, some with respiratory signs	11/191 (5.8) (VN)	0/173 (OP) 0/78 (N) 0/30 (R)
United Kingdom (387)[104]	Mar–Jul 2020	Cats with respiratory disease (being tested for other respiratory pathogens)		1/387 (0.3) (OP)[a]
France (22)[101]	April 2020	In contact with humans with or suspected to have COVID-19		1/22 (4.5) (NP, R)[a]
Spain (8)[132]	Apr–May 2020	In contact with humans with COVID-19		1/8 (OP, R)
Germany (920)[135]	Apr–Sep 2020	Visiting veterinary hospitals with hematology testing	6/920 (0.7%) (ELISA, IFA)	
Chile[118]	May–Sep 2020	In contact with humans with COVID-19	1/12 (ELISA)	3/12 (25) (N, F)[a]
Texas, USA (17)[117]	Jun–Jul 2020	In contact with humans with COVID-19	7/16 (43.8) (VN)	3/17 (17.6)[a] (PR, R, B)
United States (WA and ID) (47)[120]	Apr 2020-Sep 2021	In contact with humans with COVID-19	13/32 (ELISA)	3/39 (N/OP)
Brazil (Rio de Janeiro) (29)[121]	May 2020-Oct 2020	In contact with humans with COVID-19	2/10 (VN)	4/10 (N/OP)

[a]Virus sequence obtained.

B, body; *ELISA*, enzyme-linked immunosorbent assay; *F*, feces; *LIPS*, luciferase immunoprecipitation system; *N*, nasal; *NP*, nasopharyngeal; *O*, oral; *OP*, oropharyngeal; *PR*, pooled respiratory; *R*, rectal; *VN*, virus neutralization.

with other humans continues to represent the main risk factor for human infection. Over time, it is possible that the virus could develop a greater propensity to cause illness in, or be shed by dogs and cats through further mutation, a situation that requires close monitoring. If this should occur, SARS-CoV-2 vaccines for companion animals may be needed. According to CDC recommendations, humans that test positive for SARS-CoV-2 should quarantine themselves with their pets, and limit contact with their pets in the household until the quarantine period is over (including distancing, wearing a mask in the house, hand washing, and if possible separating the pets and having others perform activities that require contact).[3] If their pet becomes sick, someone else in the household should take the pet to the veterinarian, and if possible, an initial telemedicine consultation should be organized. Veterinary clinics should question people that plan to bring animals in for care about potential infection by, or exposure to, SARS-CoV-2, as is done in human healthcare institutions. Updated guidance for veterinarians on appropriate prevention practices for different exposure situations is provided by the CDC, together with a variety of other resources.[122] Testing for SARS-CoV-2 may need to be done in conjunction with local public health authorities.[123]

Should a pet test positive for the virus, owners should interact with them as if there were a positive human in the household (although the pet should not be made to wear a mask). Owners can be referred to guidance from the CDC[3] and the AVMA[124] on SARS-CoV-2 and animals. The virus is readily susceptible to disinfectants, and temperatures that exceed 55°F can inactivate the virus in well under an hour.[125] At the time of writing, the risk of fomite transmission is considered low, generally less than 1 in 10,000 (see Suggested Readings), so the primary mode by which people are infected with SARS-CoV-2 is through respiratory droplet exposure.[126]

SUGGESTED READINGS

Sargianou M, Watson DC, Chra P, et al. Hantavirus infections for the clinician: from case presentation to diagnosis and treatment. *Crit Rev Microbiol.* 2012;38:317–329.

Biggar RJ, Woodall JP, Walter PD, et al. Lymphocytic choriomeningitis outbreak associated with pet hamsters. Fifty-seven cases from New York State. *JAMA.* 1975;232:494–500.

Leligdowicz A, Fischer WA 2nd, Uyeki TM, et al. Ebola virus disease and critical illness. *Crit Care.* 2016;20:217.

American Veterinary Medical Association. *Ebola virus.* 2019. Available at: https://www.avma.org/ebola-virus.

McElroy A, Hiraide R, Bexfield N, et al. Detection of hepatitis E virus antibodies in dogs in the United Kingdom. *PLoS One.* 2015;10. e0128703.

Hosie MJ, Epifano I, Herder V, et al. Detection of SARS-CoV-2 in respiratory samples from cats in the UK associated with human-to-cat transmission. *Vet Rec.* 2021;188:e247.

Hosie MJ, Hofmann-Lehmann R, Hartmann K, et al. Anthropogenic infection of cats during the 2020 COVID-19 pandemic. *Viruses.* 2021;13:185.

Centers for Disease Control and Prevention. Science Brief: SARS-CoV-2 and surface (fomite) transmission for indoor community environments. 2021. Available at: https://www.cdc.gov/coronavirus/2019-ncov/more/science-and-research/surface-transmission.html#ref7.

REFERENCES

1. Papa A, Vaheri A, LeDuc JW, et al. Meeting report: Tenth International Conference on Hantaviruses. *Antiviral Res.* 2016;133:234–241.
2. Centers for Disease Control and Prevention. Reported Cases of Hantavirus Disease. 2019. Available at: http://www.cdc.gov/hantavirus/surveillance/reporting-state.html.
3. Centers for Disease Control and Prevention. If You Have Pets. 2021. Available at: https://www.cdc.gov/coronavirus/2019-ncov/daily-life-coping/pets.html.
4. Xu ZY, Tang YW, Kan LY, et al. Cats: source of protection or infection? A case-control study of hemorrhagic fever with renal syndrome. *Am J Epidemiol.* 1987;126:942–948.
5. Nowotny N. The domestic cat: a possible transmitter of viruses from rodents to man. *Lancet.* 1994;343:921.
6. Bennett M, Lloyd G, Jones N, et al. Prevalence of antibody to hantavirus in some cat populations in Britain. *Vet Rec.* 1990;127:548–549.
7. Dobly A, Yzoard C, Cochez C, et al. Spatiotemporal dynamics of Puumala hantavirus in suburban reservoir rodent populations. *J Vector Ecol.* 2012;37:276–283.
8. Leighton FA, Artsob HA, Chu MC, et al. A serological survey of rural dogs and cats on the southwestern Canadian prairie for zoonotic pathogens. *Can J Public Health.* 2001;92:67–71.
9. Malecki TM, Jillson GP, Thilsted JP, et al. Serologic survey for hantavirus infection in domestic animals and coyotes from New Mexico and northeastern Arizona. *J Am Vet Med Assoc.* 1998;212:970–973.
10. Nowotny N, Weissenboeck H, Aberle S, et al. Hantavirus infection in the domestic cat. *JAMA.* 1994;272:1100–1101.
11. Goeijenbier M, Hartskeerl RA, Reimerink J, et al. The hanta hunting study: underdiagnosis of Puumala hantavirus infections in symptomatic non-travelling leptospirosis-suspected patients in the Netherlands, in 2010 and April to November 2011. *Euro Surveill.* 2014;19.
12. Sargianou M, Watson DC, Chra P, et al. Hantavirus infections for the clinician: from case presentation to diagnosis and treatment. *Crit Rev Microbiol.* 2012;38:317–329.
13. Bonthius DJ. Lymphocytic choriomeningitis virus: an underrecognized cause of neurologic disease in the fetus, child, and adult. *Semin Pediatr Neurol.* 2012;19:89–95.
14. Biggar RJ, Woodall JP, Walter PD, et al. Lymphocytic choriomeningitis outbreak associated with pet hamsters. Fifty-seven cases from New York State. *JAMA.* 1975;232:494–500.
15. Rousseau MC, Saron MF, Brouqui P, et al. Lymphocytic choriomeningitis virus in southern France: four case reports and a review of the literature. *Eur J Epidemiol.* 1997;13:817–823.
16. Bowen GS, Calisher CH, Winkler WG, et al. Laboratory studies of a lymphocytic choriomeningitis virus outbreak in man and laboratory animals. *Am J Epidemiol.* 1975;102:233–240.
17. Dalldorf G. Lymphocytic choriomeningitis of dogs. *Cornell Vet.* 1943;33:347–350.
18. Carocci M, Bakkali-Kassimi L. The encephalomyocarditis virus. *Virulence.* 2012;3:351–367.
19. Nowotny N. Serologic studies of domestic cats for potential human pathogenic virus infections from wild rodents. *Zentralbl Hyg Umweltmed.* 1996;198:452–461.
20. Schwab S, Herden C, Seeliger F, et al. Non-suppurative meningoencephalitis of unknown origin in cats and dogs: an immunohistochemical study. *J Comp Pathol.* 2007;136:96–110.
21. Luo YK, Liang L, Tang QH, et al. Isolation and characterization of encephalomyocarditis virus from dogs in China. *Sci Rep.* 2017;7:438.
22. Graves IL, Oppenheimer JR. Human viruses in animals in West Bengal: an ecological analysis. *Hum Ecol.* 1975;3:105–130.
23. Grew N, Gohd RS, Arguedas J, et al. Enteroviruses in rural families and their domestic animals. *Am J Epidemiol.* 1970;91:518–526.
24. Clapper WE. Comments on viruses recovered from dogs. *J Am Vet Med Assoc.* 1970;156:1678–1680.
25. Lundgren DL, Clapper WE, Sanchez A. Isolation of human enteroviruses from beagle dogs. *Proc Soc Exp Biol Med.* 1968;128:463–467.
26. Pindak FF, Clapper WE. Isolation of enteric cytopathogenic Human Orphan Virus Type 6 from dogs. *Am J Vet Res.* 1964;25:52–54.
27. Waldman EA, Moreira RC, Saez SG, et al. Human enterovirus infection in stray dogs. Some aspects of interest to public health. *Rev Inst Med Trop Sao Paulo.* 1996;38:157–161.
28. Lundgren DL, Meade GH, Clapper WE. Cross neutralization and gel double diffusion studies of enteroviruses isolated from beagle dogs. *Tex Rep Biol Med.* 1970;28:49–58.
29. Lundgren DL, Sanchez A, Magnuson MG, et al. A survey for human enteroviruses in dogs and man. Enterovirus survey. *Arch Gesamte Virusforsch.* 1970;32:229–235.
30. Woo PC, Lau SK, Choi GK, et al. Molecular epidemiology of canine picornavirus in Hong Kong and Dubai and proposal of a novel genus in Picornaviridae. *Infect Genet Evol.* 2016;41:191–200.
31. Lundgren DL, Hobbs CH, Clapper WE. Experimental infection of beagle dogs with Coxsackievirus type B1. *Am J Vet Res.* 1971;32:609–613.
32. Pindak FF, Clapper WE. Experimental infection of beagles with ECHO virus type 6. *Tex Rep Biol Med.* 1966;24:466–472.
33. Witso E, Cinek O, Aldrin M, et al. Predictors of sub-clinical enterovirus infections in infants: a prospective cohort study. *Int J Epidemiol.* 2010;39:459–468.
34. Leligdowicz A, Fischer WA 2nd, Uyeki TM, et al. Ebola virus disease and critical illness. *Crit Care.* 2016;20:217.
35. Kaner J, Schaack S. Understanding Ebola: the 2014 epidemic. *Global Health.* 2016;12:53.
36. Broadhurst MJ, Brooks TJ, Pollock NR. Diagnosis of ebola virus disease: past, present, and future. *Clin Microbiol Rev.* 2016;29:773–793.
37. Sridhar S. Clinical development of Ebola vaccines. *Ther Adv Vaccines.* 2015;3:125–138.
38. Haun BK, Kamara V, Dweh AS, et al. Serological evidence of Ebola virus exposure in dogs from affected communities in Liberia: A preliminary report. *PLoS Negl Trop Dis.* 2019;13:e0007614.
39. Urbanowicz RA, McClure CP, Sakuntabhai A, et al. Human adaptation of Ebola Virus during the West African outbreak. *Cell.* 2016;167:1079–1087, e1075.
40. Allela L, Boury O, Pouillot R, et al. Ebola virus antibody prevalence in dogs and human risk. *Emerg Infect Dis.* 2005;11:385–390.
41. International Society for Infectious Diseases. Ebolavirus, animal reservoir (06): Spain, canine, official comment. *ProMed Mail*; 2014. Available at: https://promedmail.org/promed-post/?id=2917112.
42. American Veterinary Medical Association. *Ebola virus.* 2019. Available at: https://www.avma.org/ebola-virus.
43. Harvala H, Wong V, Simmonds P, et al. Acute viral hepatitis - should the current screening strategy be modified? *J Clin Virol.* 2014;59:184–187.
44. Dalton HR, Seghatchian J. Hepatitis E virus: Emerging from the shadows in developed countries. *Transfus Apher Sci.* 2016;55:271–274.
45. Doceul V, Bagdassarian E, Demange A, et al. Zoonotic hepatitis E virus: classification, animal reservoirs and transmission routes. *Viruses.* 2016;8:270.
46. Centers for Disease Control and Prevention. Hepatitis E Questions and Answers for Health Professionals. 2020. Available at: https://www.cdc.gov/hepatitis/hev/hevfaq.htm.
47. Borgen K, Herremans T, Duizer E, et al. Non-travel related hepatitis E virus genotype 3 infections in the Netherlands; a case series 2004 - 2006. *BMC Infect Dis.* 2008;8:61.
48. Lewis HC, Boisson S, Ijaz S, et al. Hepatitis E in England and Wales. *Emerg Infect Dis.* 2008;14:165–167.
49. Lyoo KS, Yang SJ, Na W, et al. Detection of antibodies against hepatitis E virus in pet veterinarians and pet dogs in South Korea. *Ir Vet J.* 2019;72:8.
50. Wang L, Zheng Y, Fu C, et al. Seroprevalence of hepatitis E virus infection among dogs in several developed cities in the Guangdong province of China. *J Med Virol.* 2016;88:1404–1407.
51. Liang H, Chen J, Xie J, et al. Hepatitis E virus serosurvey among pet dogs and cats in several developed cities in China. *PLoS One.* 2014;9:e98068.
52. Song YJ, Jeong HJ, Kim YJ, et al. Analysis of complete genome sequences of swine hepatitis E virus and possible risk factors for transmission of HEV to humans in Korea. *J Med Virol.* 2010;82:583–591.
53. Dong C, Meng J, Dai X, et al. Restricted enzooticity of hepatitis E virus genotypes 1 to 4 in the United States. *J Clin Microbiol.* 2011;49:4164–4172.

54. McElroy A, Hiraide R, Bexfield N, et al. Detection of hepatitis E virus antibodies in dogs in the United Kingdom. *PLoS One*. 2015;10:e0128703.
55. Mochizuki M, Ouchi A, Kawakami K, et al. Epidemiological study of hepatitis E virus infection of dogs and cats in Japan. *Vet Rec*. 2006;159:853–854.
56. Yonemitsu K, Terada Y, Kuwata R, et al. Simple and specific method for detection of antibodies against hepatitis E virus in mammalian species. *J Virol Methods*. 2016;238:56–61.
57. Vitral CL, Pinto MA, Lewis-Ximenez LL, et al. Serological evidence of hepatitis E virus infection in different animal species from the Southeast of Brazil. *Mem Inst Oswaldo Cruz*. 2005;100:117–122.
58. Arankalle VA, Joshi MV, Kulkarni AM, et al. Prevalence of anti-hepatitis E virus antibodies in different Indian animal species. *J Viral Hepat*. 2001;8:223–227.
59. Boomkens SY, Slump E, Egberink HF, et al. PCR screening for candidate etiological agents of canine hepatitis. *Vet Microbiol*. 2005;108:49–55.
60. Zhang W, Shen Q, Mou J, et al. Hepatitis E virus infection among domestic animals in eastern China. *Zoonoses Public Health*. 2008;55:291–298.
61. Mesquita JR, Valente-Gomes G, Conceicao-Neto N, et al. Pet veterinarians have no increased risk of hepatitis E compared to the general population. *J Med Virol*. 2014;86:954–956.
62. Meng XJ, Wiseman B, Elvinger F, et al. Prevalence of antibodies to hepatitis E virus in veterinarians working with swine and in normal blood donors in the United States and other countries. *J Clin Microbiol*. 2002;40:117–122.
63. Jamal SM, Belsham GJ. Foot-and-mouth disease: past, present and future. *Vet Res*. 2013;44:116.
64. World Organization for Animal Health. Foot and Mouth Disease (FMD). 2022. Available at: http://www.oie.int/en/animal-health-in-the-world/official-disease-status/fmd/en-fmd-carte/.
65. Galloway IA. Foot and Mouth Disease Research Committee. In: *Fourth Progress Report*. London, UK: HM Stationery Office; 1937:345–349.
66. The Center for Food Safety and Public Health, Iowa State University. Foot-and-Mouth Disease Prevention Practices. 2006. Available at: http://www.cfsph.iastate.edu/Infection_Control/FADs/FMD_PrevPrac.pdf.
67. Bankowski RA, Wood M. Experimental vesicular exanthema in the dog. *J Am Vet Med Assoc*. 1953;123:115–118.
68. Binn LN, Norby EA, Marchwicki RH, et al. Canine caliciviruses of four serotypes from military and research dogs recovered in 1963-1978 belong to two phylogenetic clades in the *Vesivirus* genus. *Virol J*. 2018;15:39.
69. Renshaw RW, Griffing J, Weisman J, et al. Characterization of a vesivirus associated with an outbreak of acute hemorrhagic gastroenteritis in domestic dogs. *J Clin Microbiol*. 2018;56:e01951-17.
70. Asin J, Nyaoke AC, Moore JD, et al. Outbreak of rabbit hemorrhagic disease virus 2 in the southwestern United States: first detections in southern California. *J Vet Diagn Invest*. 2021;33:728–731.
71. Williams LBA, Edmonds SE, Kerr SR, et al. Clinical and pathologic findings in an outbreak in rabbits of natural infection by rabbit hemorrhagic disease virus 2 in the northwestern United States. *J Vet Diagn Invest*. 2021;33:732–735.
72. Wildlife Health.org. Rabbit Hemorrhagic Disease Virus 2 in the U.S.: Current Updates – April 2022. Available at: https://wildlifehealth.org/rabbit-hemorrhagic-disease-virus/.
73. Zheng T, Lu G, Napier AM, et al. No virus replication in domestic cats fed with RHDV-infected rabbit livers. *Vet Microbiol*. 2003;95:61–73.
74. Stout AE, Andre NM, Jaimes JA, et al. Coronaviruses in cats and other companion animals: Where does SARS-CoV-2/COVID-19 fit? *Vet Microbiol*. 2020;247:108777.
75. Lopes LR, de Mattos Cardillo G, Paiva PB. Molecular evolution and phylogenetic analysis of SARS-CoV-2 and hosts ACE2 protein suggest Malayan pangolin as intermediary host. *Braz J Microbiol*. 2020;51:1593–1599.
76. Lui GC, Yip TC, Wong VW, et al. Significantly lower case-fatality ratio of coronavirus disease 2019 (COVID-19) than severe acute respiratory syndrome (SARS) in Hong Kong-a territory-wide cohort study. *Clin Infect Dis*. 2021;72:e466–e475.
77. Centers for Disease Control and Prevention. Revised U.S. surveillance case definition for severe acute respiratory syndrome (SARS) and update on SARS cases: United States and worldwide, December 2003. *Morb Mortal Wkly Rep*. 2003;52:1202–1206.
78. Pyrc K, Berkhout B, van der Hoek L. Identification of new human coronaviruses. *Expert Rev Anti Infect Ther*. 2007;5:245–253.
79. Martina BE, Haagmans BL, Kuiken T, et al. Virology: SARS virus infection of cats and ferrets. *Nature*. 2003;425:915.
80. Yu IT, Li Y, Wong TW, et al. Evidence of airborne transmission of the severe acute respiratory syndrome virus. *N Engl J Med*. 2004;350:1731–1739.
81. Zaki AM, van Boheemen S, Bestebroer TM, et al. Isolation of a novel coronavirus from a man with pneumonia in Saudi Arabia. *N Engl J Med*. 2012;367:1814–1820.
82. Paules CI, Marston HD, Fauci AS. Coronavirus infections-more than just the common cold. *JAMA*. 2020;323:707–708.
83. Centers for Disease Control and Prevention. Middle Eastern Respiratory Syndrome. 2019. Available at: https://www.cdc.gov/coronavirus/mers/us.html.
84. World Health Organization. Middle East Respiratory Syndrome Coronavirus (MERS-CoV). 2019. Available at: https://www.who.int/news-room/fact-sheets/detail/middle-east-respiratory-syndrome-coronavirus-(mers-cov).
85. Johns Hopkins Coronavirus Resource Center. COVID-19 Dashboard by the Center for Systems Science and Engineering (CSSE) at Johns Hopkins University (JHU). 2022. Available at: https://coronavirus.jhu.edu/map.html.
86. CDC COVID-19 Response Team. Severe outcomes among patients with coronavirus disease 2019 (COVID-19) - United States, February 12-March 16, 2020. *Morb Mortal Wkly Rep*. 2020;69:343–346.
87. Cui J, Li F, Shi ZL. Origin and evolution of pathogenic coronaviruses. *Nat Rev Microbiol*. 2019;17:181–192.
88. Tiwari R, Dhama K, Sharun K, et al. COVID-19: animals, veterinary and zoonotic links. *Vet Q*. 2020;40:169–182.
89. Lytras S, Xia W, Hughes J, et al. The animal origin of SARS-CoV-2. *Science*. 2021;373:968–970.
90. Holmes EC, Goldstein SA, Rasmussen AL, et al. The origins of SARS-CoV-2: a crtical review. *Cell*. 2021;184:4848–4856.
91. Goh GK, Dunker AK, Foster JA, et al. Computational, experimental, and clinical evidence of a specific but peculiar evolutionary nature of (COVID-19) SARS-CoV-2. *J Proteome Res*. 2022. acs.jproteome.2c00001.
92. Esselmani R, Jain J, Susan-Resiga D, et al. Distinctive roles of furin and TMPRSS2 in SARS-CoV-2 infectivity. *Moll Cell Biol*. 2022. https://doi.org/10.1128/jvi.00128-22.
93. Sun K, Gu L, Ma L, et al. Atlas of ACE2 gene expression reveals novel insights into transmission of SARS-CoV-2. *Heliyon*. 2021;7:e05850.
94. Shi J, Wen Z, Zhong G, et al. Susceptibility of ferrets, cats, dogs, and other domesticated animals to SARS-coronavirus 2. *Science*. 2020;368:1016–1020.
95. Bosco-Lauth AM, Hartwig AE, Porter SM, et al. Experimental infection of domestic dogs and cats with SARS-CoV-2: Pathogenesis, transmission, and response to reexposure in cats. *Proc Natl Acad Sci U S A*. 2020;117:26382–26388.
96. Richard M, Kok A, de Meulder D, et al. SARS-CoV-2 is transmitted via contact and via the air between ferrets. *Nat Commun*. 2020;11:3496.
97. Kim YI, Kim SG, Kim SM, et al. Infection and rapid transmission of SARS-CoV-2 in ferrets. *Cell Host Microbe*. 2020;27:704–709 e702.
98. Yen H, Sit THC, Brackman CJ, et al. Transmission of SARS-CoV-2 delta variant (AY,127) from pet hamsters to humans, leading to onward human-to-human transmission: a case study. *Lancet*. 2022;399:1070–1078.
99. United States Department of Agriculture. Cases of SARS-CoV-2 in animals in the United States. 2021. Available at: https://www.aphis.usda.gov/animal_health/one_health/downloads/sars-cov2-in-animals.pdf.
100. Newman A, Smith D, Ghai RR, et al. First reported cases of SARS-CoV-2 infection in companion animals - New York, March-April 2020. *MMWR Morb Mortal Wkly Rep*. 2020;69:710–713.
101. Sailleau C, Dumarest M, Vanhomwegen J, et al. First detection and genome sequencing of SARS-CoV-2 in an infected cat in France. *Transbound Emerg Dis*. 2020;67:2324–2328.
102. Musso N, Costantino A, La Spina S, et al. New SARS-CoV-2 infection detected in an Italian pet cat by RT-qPCR from deep pharyngeal swab. *Pathogens*. 2020;9:746.

103. Segales J, Puig M, Rodon J, et al. Detection of SARS-CoV-2 in a cat owned by a COVID-19-affected patient in Spain. *Proc Natl Acad Sci U S A.* 2020;117:24790–24793.
104. Hosie MJ, Epifano I, Herder V, et al. Detection of SARS-CoV-2 in respiratory samples from cats in the UK associated with human-to-cat transmission. *Vet Rec.* 2021;188:e247.
105. Carpenter A, Ghai RR, Gary J. Determining the role of natural SARS-CoV-2 infection in the death of domestic pets: 10 cases (2020-2021). *J Am Vet Med Assoc.* 2021;269:1032–1039.
106. Rotstein DS, Peloquin S, Proia K, et al. Investigation of SARS-CoV-2 infection and associated lesions in exotic and companion animals. *Vet Pathol.* 2022. 3009858211067467.
107. Ferasin L, Fritz M, Ferasin H, et al. Myocarditis in naturally infected pets with the British variant of COVID-19. *bioRxiv.* 2021. https://doi.org/10.1101/2021.03.18.435945.
108. Pickering B, Lung O, Maguire F, et al. Highly divergent white-tailed deer SARS-CoV-2 wiith potential deer-to-human transmission. *BioRxiv.* 2022. https://doi.org/10.1101/2022.02.22.481551.
109. Wei C, Shan K-J, Wang W, et al. Evidence for a mouse origin of the SARS-CoV-2 Omicron variant. *J Genet Genomics.* 2021;48:1111–1121.
110. Kormann C. Did Omicron come from mice? The New Yorker. February 10, 2022. Available at: https://www.newyorker.com/science/elements/did-omicron-come-from-mice.
111. United States Department of Agriculture. USDA Statement on the Confirmation of COVID-19 in a Tiger in New York. 2020. Available at: https://www.aphis.usda.gov/aphis/newsroom/news/sa_by_date/sa-2020/ny-zoo-covid-19.
112. Bartlett SL, Diel DG, Wang L, et al. SARS-CoV-2 infection and longitudinal fecal screening in Malayan tigers (*Panthera tigris jacksoni*), Amur tigers (*Panthera tigris altaica*), and African lions (*Panthera leo krugeri*) at the Bronx zoo, New York, USA. *J Zoo Wild Med.* 2021;51:733–744.
113. Grome HN, Meyer B, Read E, et al. SARS-CoV-2 outbreak among Malayan tigers and humans, Tennessee, USA, 2020. *Emerg Infect Dis.* 2022;28:833–836.
114. Koeppel KN, Mendes A, Strydom A, et al. SARS-CoV-2 reverse zoonosis to pumas and lions, South Africa. *Viruses.* 2022;14:120.
115. Barabiuk C. The rise of COVID-19 vaccines for animals. The Scientist. December 9, 2021. Available at: https://www.the-scientist.com/news-opinion/the-rise-of-covid-19-vaccines-for-animals-69503.
116. Michael HT, Waterhouse T, Estrada M, et al. Frequency of respiratory pathogens and SARS-CoV-2 in canine and feline samples submitted for respiratory testing in early 2020. *J Small Anim Pract.* 2021;62:336–342.
117. Hamer SA, Pauvolid-Correa A, Zecca IB, et al. SARS-CoV-2 infections and viral isolations among serially tested cats and dogs in households with infected owners in Texas. USA. *Viruses.* 2021;13:938.
118. Neira V, Brito B, Aguero B, et al. A household case evidences shorter shedding of SARS-CoV-2 in naturally infected cats compared to their human owners. *Emerg Microbes Infect.* 2021;10:376–383.
119. Barrs VR, Peiris M, Tam KWS, et al. SARS-CoV-2 in quarantined domestic cats from COVID-19 households or close contacts, Hong Kong, China. *Emerg Infect Dis.* 2020;26:3071–3074.
120. Meisner J, Baszler TV, Kuehl KH, et al. Household transmission of SARS-CoV-2 from humans to pets in Washington and Idaho: burden and risk factors. *BioRxiv.* 2022. https://doi.org/10.1101/2021.04.24.440952.
121. Calvet GA, Pereira SA, Ogrzewalska M, et al. Investigation of SARS-CoV-2 infection in dogs and humans diagnosed with COVID-19 in Rio de Janeiro, Brazil. *PLoS One.* 2021;16:e0250853.
122. Centers for Disease Control and Prevention. Interim infection prevention and control guidance for veterinary clinics treating companion animals during the COVID-19 response. 2021. Available at: https://www.cdc.gov/healthypets/covid-19/veterinarians.html.
123. Centers for Disease Control and Prevention. Evaluation for SARS-CoV-2 Testing in Animals. 2022. Available at: https://www.cdc.gov/coronavirus/2019-ncov/animals/animal-testing.html.
124. American Veterinary Medical Association. SARS-CoV-2 in Animals. 2022. Available at: https://www.avma.org/resources-tools/animal-health-and-welfare/covid-19/sars-cov-2-animals-including-pets.
125. Biryukov J, Boydston JA, Dunning RA, et al. SARS-CoV-2 is rapidly inactivated at high temperature. *Environ Chem Lett.* 2021;19:1–5.
126. Centers for Disease Control and Prevention. Science Brief: SARS-CoV-2 and surface (fomite) transmission for indoor community environments. 2021. Available at: https://www.cdc.gov/coronavirus/2019-ncov/more/science-and-research/surface-transmission.html.
127. Temmam S, Barbarino A, Maso D, et al. Absence of SARS-CoV-2 infection in cats and dogs in close contact with a cluster of COVID-19 patients in a veterinary campus. *One Health.* 2020;10:100164.
128. Grzelak L, Temmam S, Planchais C, et al. A comparison of four serological assays for detecting anti-SARS-CoV-2 antibodies in human serum samples from different populations. *Sci Transl Med.* 2020;12:eabc3103.
129. Sit THC, Brackman CJ, Ip SM, et al. Infection of dogs with SARS-CoV-2. *Nature.* 2020;586:776–778.
130. Chen J, Huang C, Zhang Y, et al. Severe acute respiratory syndrome coronavirus 2-specific antibodies in pets in Wuhan, China. *J Infect.* 2020;81:e68–e69.
131. Patterson EI, Elia G, Grassi A, et al. Evidence of exposure to SARS-CoV-2 in cats and dogs from households in Italy. *Nat Commun.* 2020;11:6231.
132. Ruiz-Arrondo I, Portillo A, Palomar AM, et al. Detection of SARS-CoV-2 in pets living with COVID-19 owners diagnosed during the COVID-19 lockdown in Spain: A case of an asymptomatic cat with SARS-CoV-2 in Europe. *Transbound Emerg Dis.* 2021;68:973–976.
133. Zhao Y, Yang Y, Gao J, et al. A serological survey of severe acute respiratory syndrome coronavirus 2 in dogs in Wuhan. *Transbound Emerg Dis.* 2022;69:591–597.
134. Zhang Q, Zhang H, Gao J, et al. A serological survey of SARS-CoV-2 in cat in Wuhan. *Emerg Microbes Infect.* 2020;9:2013–2019.
135. Michelitsch A, Hoffmann D, Wernike K, et al. Occurrence of antibodies against SARS-CoV-2 in the domestic cat population of Germany. *Vaccines (Basel).* 2020;8:772.

SECTION 2

Bacterial Diseases

Jane E. Sykes

This section covers a number of important vector-borne and zoonotic diseases including ehrlichiosis, anaplasmosis, and rickettsioses; Q fever; leptospirosis and borreliosis; bartonellosis; brucellosis; plague; and tularemia. Although previously thought to be transmitted by fleas, evidence has accumulated that feline hemotropic mycoplasmas are most likely transmitted primarily through aggressive interactions among cats and that vectors are not involved (Chapter 58). With the increasing use of more potent immunosuppressive drugs, especially in dogs, there is also more recognition of atypical bacterial diseases such as nocardiosis and mycobacteriosis; these are covered in Chapters 60 and 61.

The modern era of antimicrobial therapy began with the discovery of sulfonamides in 1936. This was followed in the 1940s by the discovery of the therapeutic value of penicillin and streptomycin, and by 1950, the "golden age" of antimicrobial therapy was underway, and well-intentioned academic leaders predicted the demise of bacterial infections. But after only a few decades, antimicrobials are now facing an uncertain future. By the late 1980s, methicillin-resistant staphylococci were widespread, and gram-negative rods emerged as important nosocomial pathogens in hospitals. Veterinarians face major challenges with the increasing prevalence of multidrug-resistant pathogens, such as methicillin-resistant *Staphylococcus pseudintermedius* (Chapter 51), *Bordetella bronchiseptica* (Chapter 55), and other gram-negative bacteria (Chapter 53), and few new drugs in the antibiotic pipeline. Some strains of drug-resistant bacteria that have the potential to cause disease in humans have been identified with increasing prevalence in dogs and cats, such as *Clostridioides difficile* (Chapter 64) and pathogenic *Escherichia coli* (Chapter 63). It is critical that we model good antibacterial stewardship if we are to preserve critical weapons against life-threatening bacterial infections.

44

Ehrlichiosis

Shimon Harrus, Trevor Waner, Mathios E. Mylonakis, Jane E. Sykes, Barbara Qurollo

KEY POINTS

- First Described: *Ehrlichia canis* was first described in 1935 (Algeria).[1] *Ehrlichia ewingii* was described in 1992 (United States).[2] *Ehrlichia chaffeensis* was described in 1991 (United States).[3] The first report of naturally occurring ehrlichiosis in a cat occurred in France in 1986.[4]
- Cause: The most important species causing disease in dogs are *E. canis* (canine monocytic ehrlichiosis) and *E. ewingii* (canine granulocytic ehrlichiosis).
- Affected Hosts: *Ehrlichia canis* causes disease in dogs, humans, and cats. *Ehrlichia ewingii* causes disease in dogs, humans, and goats and has been detected in a clinically ill cat. *Ehrlichia chaffeensis* causes disease in humans, possibly dogs and goats, and has been detected in a clinically healthy cat. *Ehrlichia muris* subsp. *eauclairensis* causes disease in humans and possibly dogs. Panola Mountain *Ehrlichia* causes disease in dogs, goats, and humans in the United States.
- Geographic Distribution: *Ehrlichia canis* is distributed worldwide, but is more prevalent in tropical and subtropical regions. *Ehrlichia ewingii* is primarily found in the south-central and southeastern United States. Most reports of *E. chaffeensis* infection are from the southern and south-central United States, but it has also been identified in Africa. *Ehrlichia muris* subsp. *eauclairensis* has been found in the Upper Midwest of the USA. Panola Mountain *Ehrlichia* has been found in the southeastern United States.
- Mode of Transmission: *Rhipicephalus sanguineus* ticks (*E. canis*); *Amblyomma americanum* ticks (*E. ewingii* and *E. chaffeensis*), *Ixodes scapularis* ticks (*E. muris* subsp. *eauclairensis*), and *A. americanum* and *Amblyomma maculatum* ticks (Panola Mountain *Ehrlichia*).
- Major Clinical Signs: Dogs—typical clinical signs of *E. canis* infection are fever, lethargy, inappetence, weight loss, cutaneous and mucosal petechial and/or ecchymotic hemorrhages, lymphadenomegaly, splenomegaly, and uveitis. *Ehrlichia ewingii* primarily causes fever, lethargy, inappetence, and signs of polyarthritis. Cats—typical clinical signs of *Ehrlichia canis* infection are fever, lethargy, inappetence, weight loss, hyperesthesia, and joint pain. *E. ewingii* was detected in a clinically ill cat with thrombocytopenia and anemia.
- Differential Diagnoses: Other tick-borne diseases (e.g., granulocytic anaplasmosis, Lyme borreliosis, babesiosis, and cytauxzoonosis [cats]), bartonellosis, hemotropic mycoplasmosis, leptospirosis, and other systemic non-vector-borne diseases such as lymphoma, multiple myeloma, and systemic primary immune-mediated disease.
- Public Health Aspects: All four *Ehrlichia* species can infect and cause disease in humans. The most virulent human pathogen is *E. chaffeensis* and results in the highest percentage of hospitalizations and death compared with the other North American *Ehrlichia* species.

Ehrlichioses are a group of tick-transmitted diseases caused by intracellular, gram-negative bacteria that include *Ehrlichia canis, Ehrlichia ewingii,* and *Ehrlichia chaffeensis.* An organism related to *Ehrlichia ruminantium,* the cause of heartwater disease in cattle, has also been detected in ill dogs from South Africa.[5] *Ehrlichia muris eauclairensis* has been detected in an ill dog and humans from Upper Midwest of the United States (formerly *E. muris*-like).[6] Panola Mountain *Ehrlichia* was detected in a dog with atypical lymphocytosis and clonal T-cell expansion.[7] These organisms form morulae (Latin for "mulberry"), clusters of bacteria, within phagosomes of circulating leukocytes. *E. canis* infects monocytes, macrophages, and less frequently lymphocytes (Fig. 44.1A–C), and causes canine monocytic ehrlichiosis (CME), one of the most important infectious diseases of domestic dogs that are exposed to ticks, worldwide. *Ehrlichia ewingii* infects granulocytes and causes canine granulocytic ehrlichiosis; the organism is very difficult to culture and only short-term maintenance in cultured cells has been documented to date.[8] *Ehrlichia chaffeensis* causes human monocytic ehrlichiosis (HME); dogs are a proposed reservoir for this organism. The geographic distribution of each pathogen is generally restricted to that of their vectors and mammalian reservoir hosts. According to one large study, the prevalence of exposure to *Ehrlichia* spp. in the United States in dogs has been increasing in both endemic and nonendemic areas.[9]

Organisms in the genus *Ehrlichia* are grouped within the family Anaplasmataceae. Also within this family are the bacteria *Anaplasma platys* and *Anaplasma phagocytophilum,* which cause canine thrombocytic and granulocytic anaplasmosis, respectively (see Chapter 45); and organisms belonging to the genera *Neorickettsia* (see Chapter 47). *Rickettsia rickettsii,* the cause of Rocky Mountain Spotted Fever (RMSF), and other spotted fever group rickettsiae belong to a separate family, the Rickettsiaceae (see Chapter 46). The families Rickettsiaceae and Anaplasmataceae are phylogenetically related through the order Rickettsiales (Table 44.1).

The severity of clinical signs in animals with ehrlichial infections depends on factors such as the organism species and strain, inoculum size, host immunity, and genetic factors. Because of shared arthropod vectors and/or concurrent exposure to multiple tick species, co-infections with more than one rickettsial pathogen, as well as other arthropod-borne pathogens (such as *Babesia* and *Bartonella* spp.) occur and may obscure the clinical picture.

EHRLICHIA CANIS

Shimon Harrus, Trevor Waner, Mathios E. Mylonakis

ETIOLOGY AND EPIDEMIOLOGY

Ehrlichia canis is transmitted primarily by the brown dog tick, *Rhipicephalus sanguineus* sensu lato (Fig. 44.2), one of the most widely

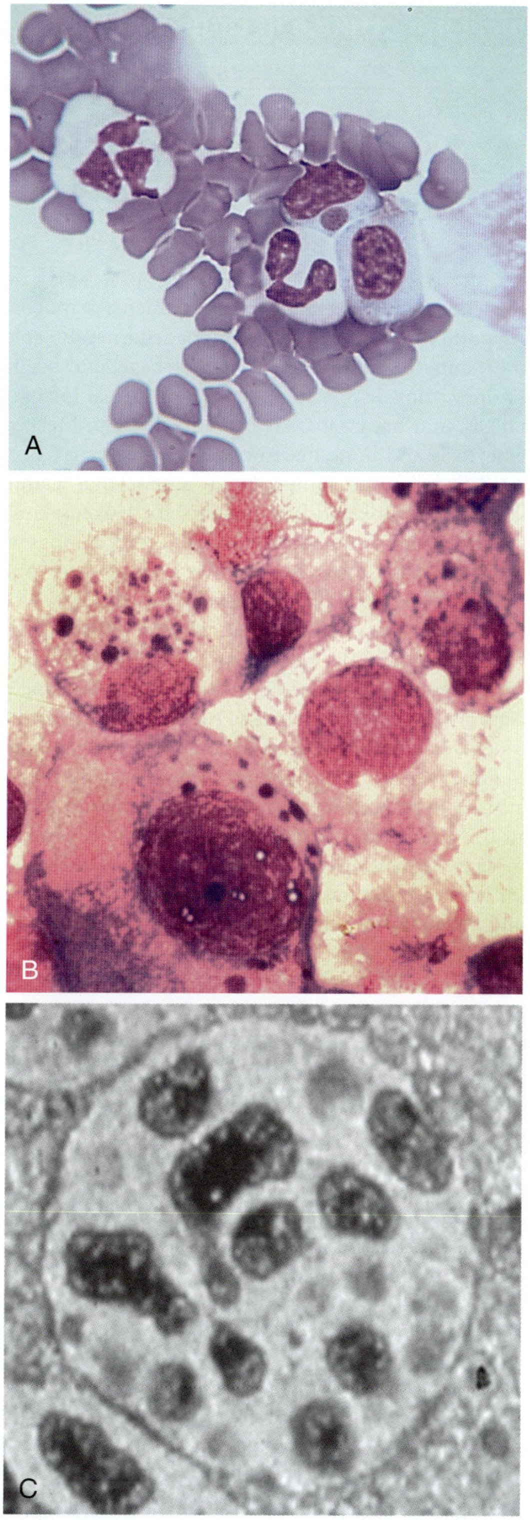

Fig. 44.1 (A) *Ehrlichia canis* morula in a peripheral blood mononuclear cell in a dog with experimental *E. canis* infection (buffy coat, Giemsa, originally photographed at ×1000). (B) Morulae within DH82 culture cells, as seen by light microscopy (originally photographed at ×400). (C) Morula within DH82 culture cell as seen by transmission electron microscopy (originally photographed at ×20,000). Note the multiple number of organisms within the morula. It can be seen that two of the organisms are undergoing binary fission.

distributed tick species, worldwide. In a transmission study, when *E. canis*-infected ticks were placed on naïve dogs, *E. canis* DNA could be detected in the dogs as early as 3 hours postexposure to the ticks.[10] Infection has been reported in dogs from Asia, Africa, Europe, the Americas, and most recently in Australia.[11] New Zealand appears to be free of *E. canis* infection. The DNA of *E. canis* has been detected in other tick species, which include other *Rhipicephalus* species (e.g., *Rhipicephalus turanicus* and *Rhipicephalus bursa*),[12,13] *Ixodes ricinus*,[14] and *Haemaphysalis*[15] and *Dermacentor* spp.[15,16] In one study, experimental transmission was accomplished with *Dermacentor variabilis* ticks.[17] Different strains of *E. canis* exist in different geographic regions and may vary in virulence. Although *Rh. sanguineus* is found throughout the United States (Fig. 44.3), it prefers warm climates, and so CME is diagnosed most frequently in dogs living in the southeastern and southwestern states. In Europe, *Rh. sanguineus* is primarily found in the Mediterranean basin, but its distribution appears to be moving northward, and CME has been reported in dogs that lack travel history as far north as the Netherlands.[18] Dogs can be persistent subclinical carriers for years.[19] Such dogs may be transported to nonendemic regions and subsequently develop the disease months or years later. Tick larvae or nymphs acquire infection when they feed on infected dogs and transmit the disease as nymphs or adults when feeding on naïve dogs. Jackals, foxes, and possibly coyotes may also act as reservoir hosts. *Ehrlichia canis* is transmitted transstadially (i.e., from larva to nymph to the adult tick) (Fig. 44.4).[20,21] Male ticks can also transmit the pathogen intrastadially.[22] No clear age or sex predilection for CME exists, but German shepherd dogs are reportedly more susceptible, and prognosis may be poorer in this breed. Cross-bred dogs may be less likely to develop CME.[23]

CLINICAL FEATURES

Pathogenesis and Clinical Signs

Ehrlichia canis multiplies by binary fission within vacuoles of mononuclear phagocytes (see Fig. 44.1A–C); rupture of infected host cells leads to infection of additional cells. Immune-mediated mechanisms are important in the pathogenesis of the disease, and the presence of the spleen appears to contribute to disease severity.[24]

Stages in the invasion and pathogenesis of *Ehrlichia* include adhesion, internalization, proliferation, and spreading. Outer membrane glycoproteins (e.g., gp19, gp36, and gp140kDa) are associated with adhesion and internalization.[25] The movement of *E. canis* through cells is dependent on polymerization of actin cytoskeleton and lysosomal evasion, and requires influx of iron and calcium ions.[26] The course of CME has been divided into acute, subclinical, and chronic phases. Clinical signs occur 8 to 20 days after infection. The clinical manifestations vary considerably among dogs, which may reflect factors such as *E. canis* strain variation, host immune response, stage of disease, and concurrent infections. Lethargy, inappetence, fever, and weight loss are the most common signs of the acute disease. Replication of the organism in reticuloendothelial tissues is associated with generalized lymphadenomegaly and splenomegaly. Ocular and nasal discharge and uveitis are common findings and are associated with lymphocytic-plasmacytic inflammation in these tissues. Retinal detachment may occur in rare cases due to serum hyperviscosity and subretinal hemorrhage. Bleeding tendencies occur in some dogs and may result from thrombocytopenia and platelet dysfunction.[24] Platelet dysfunction may at least in part be the result of immune-mediated platelet damage.[27] Experimentally infected dogs developed low platelet counts, activated platelets, and

TABLE 44.1 Members of the Order Rickettsiales of Clinical Importance in Dogs and Cats[a]

Family Anaplasmataceae			Family Rickettsiaceae
Ehrlichia canis	*Anaplasma phagocytophilium*	*Neoricketttsia helminthoeca*	*Rickettsia rickettsii*
Ehrlichia chaffeensis	*Anaplasma platys*	*Neoricketttsia risticii*	
Ehrlichia ewingii			

[a]Other species of *Ehrlichia* and *Rickettsia* may also cause disease in dogs, but their clinical significance is unclear.

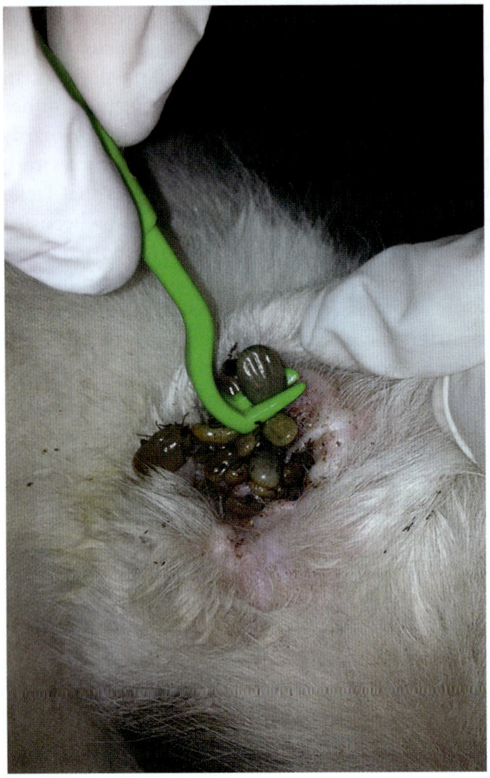

Fig. 44.2 The brown dog tick, *Rhipicephalus sanguineus* being removed from the ear of an infested dog.

antiplatelet antibodies.[28,29] The results of thromboelastography in one study revealed evidence of a hypercoagulable, hypofibrinolytic state.[28]

Neurologic signs may result from meningeal inflammation or hemorrhage. Dogs can recover spontaneously from the acute phase within 2 to 4 weeks, after which time they may eliminate the infection or remain subclinically infected. Sequestration of organisms within the spleen or other tissues may occur, and the organisms may evade the host immune system through modulation of the host immune response and by decreasing its antiehrlichial activities (i.e., decreased presentation by downregulation of MHC class II receptors, evasion of phagosome-lysosome fusion, decreased host cell apoptosis, recombination, and antigenic variation).[25,26] The subclinical phase of CME may persist for months to years.[19]

Chronic CME develops in only some infected dogs. Factors that influence the development of the chronic disease are unclear, but the pathogen, the host genetics, and the interrelations between them probably play their role. The presence of severe pancytopenia characterizes the severe chronic form of ehrlichiosis, and results from hypoplasia of all bone marrow cell lines.[30] Clinical signs at this stage are usually severe and include lethargy, inappetence, bleeding tendencies, mucosal pallor, fever or hypothermia, weight loss, lymphadenomegaly, splenomegaly, dyspnea, anterior uveitis, retinal hemorrhage, and edema.[23,31–33] Secondary opportunistic infections such as protozoal infections, viral papillomatosis, and bacterial UTIs can also develop. Marked granular lymphocytosis and bone marrow plasmacytosis may occur in all phases, sometimes accompanied by a monoclonal gammopathy, which may lead to misdiagnosis of lymphocytic leukemia or multiple myeloma. This has led to the recommendation that all dogs with well-differentiated lymphocytosis or otherwise unexplained monoclonal gammopathy be tested for *E. canis* infection.[34]

Common physical examination findings in dogs with CME include lethargy, fever, generalized peripheral lymphadenomegaly, and splenomegaly. Ocular and nasal discharge, cutaneous and mucosal petechial hemorrhages (Fig. 44.5A–C), peripheral edema, and/or neurologic signs may be evident. Ocular abnormalities include anterior uveitis, hyphema, scleral, conjunctival or retinal hemorrhage, retinal detachment, and optic neuritis, with anterior uveitis being most commonly reported (Fig. 44.6A and B).[32,33] Neurologic signs include twitching, ataxia, seizures, vestibular signs, hyperesthesia, and cranial nerve deficits. Dogs with chronic ehrlichiosis may have thin body condition or diffuse muscle atrophy and mucosal pallor in addition to the aforementioned signs.

DIAGNOSIS

Laboratory Abnormalities

Complete Blood Count

Thrombocytopenia is the most common hematologic abnormality of CME, occurring 1 to 4 weeks following infection with *E. canis*, in more than 90% of acutely infected dogs. Occasionally, mild leukopenia due to neutropenia, monocytopenia, and lymphopenia may occur, together with a mild left shift.[35] Nonregenerative anemia is usually present. During the subsequent subclinical phase, mild thrombocytopenia, with increased mean platelet volume, may persist.[36] Typically, dogs in the severe chronic phase of CME are profoundly pancytopenic.[30] Moderate to marked granular lymphocytosis may also occur in subclinically or chronically infected dogs.

In some acutely infected dogs, morulae are visualized within the circulating monocytes and less frequently in lymphocytes (see Fig. 44.1A). Examination of buffy coat smears, or lymph node or splenic aspirates increases the sensitivity for detection of morulae.[37] Cytology is notoriously insensitive for the detection of morulae in the subclinical and especially chronic infection, and it does not distinguish between *E. canis* and *E. chaffeensis* infection. In one study, morulae were found in only 2 of 19 dogs with chronic CME after careful screening.[30] Dogs with acute CME may have evidence of reactive lymphocytes, activated monocytes, mild left shift, erythrophagocytosis, metarubricytosis, thrombophagocytosis, phagocytosis of nuclear material, and megaplatelets in their blood smears.[12,35]

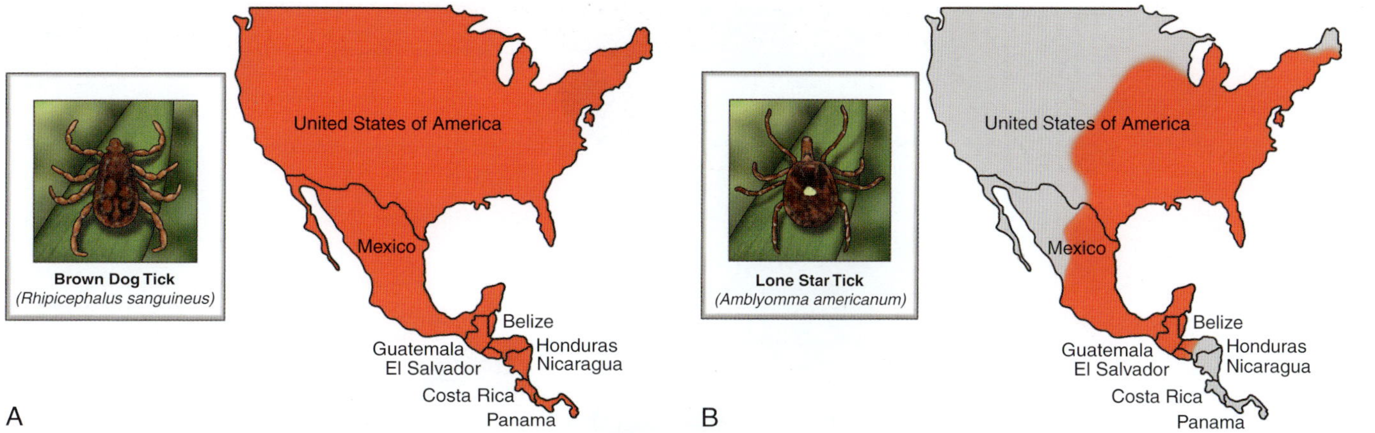

Fig. 44.3 (A) Distribution of *Rhipicephalus sanguineus*, which transmits *Ehrlichia canis*, in the United States and Central America. (B) Distribution of *Amblyomma americanum* in the United States and Central America. which transmits *Ehrlichia ewingii* and *Ehrlichia chaffeensis*. The distribution of *E. ewingii* infections in dogs more closely matches that of *A. americanum* than the distribution of *E. canis* matches that of *Rh. sanguineus* (highest prevalence in the southern states). This is because of chronic *E. canis* infections that occur in dogs with travel histories to southern states, where the climate is warmer and *Rh. sanguineus* is more prevalent.

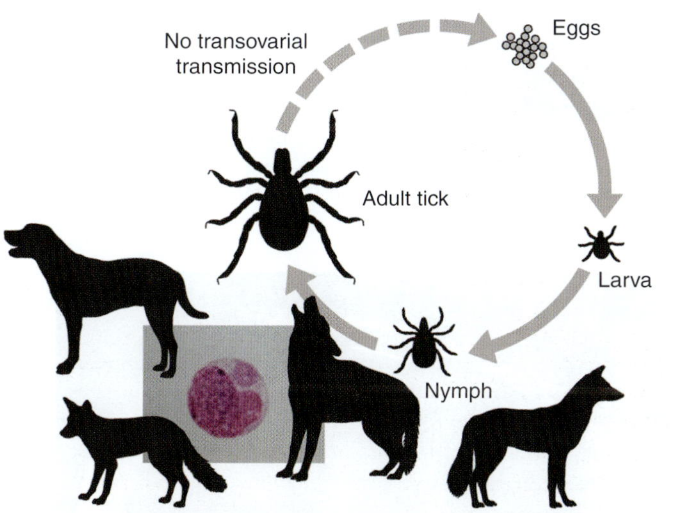

Fig. 44.4 Life cycle of *Ehrlichia canis*. The organism is transmitted only transstadially (from larva to nymph to adult) within the tick. Jackals, foxes, and possibly coyotes also act as reservoir hosts. A morula is shown within the cytoplasm of a monocyte as seen on a blood smear.

Serum Biochemical Tests

Serum chemistry abnormalities are seen during the acute and chronic phases and include hypoalbuminemia, hyperglobulinemia, hypergammaglobulinemia and elevated activities of serum ALT and ALP. Most often, hyperglobulinemia is due to polyclonal gammopathy.[23] Monoclonal gammopathy can also develop but is uncommon. Less frequently, increases in serum urea nitrogen and creatinine concentrations are present.[29]

Urinalysis

Transient proteinuria has been reported in dogs with acute CME.[38] Dogs with chronic CME may also have evidence of proteinuria.

Coagulation Profile

In addition to thrombocytopenia, coagulation abnormalities in dogs with CME include prolongation of the buccal mucosal bleeding time (BMBT), decreased platelet aggregation (thrombocytopathy), and prolongation of APTT.[29,39] Thromboelastography may reveal evidence of hypercoagulability and hypofibrinolysis.[28]

Cerebrospinal Fluid Analysis

Dogs with CNS involvement may have increased CSF protein concentrations and lymphocytic pleocytosis. Although rarely found, morulae may be detected in cells within the CSF.[40–42]

Bone Marrow Analysis

Bone marrow is commonly hypercellular in the acute phase but with chronic disease becomes hypoplastic and pale, which is the result of fatty infiltration, decrease of all bone marrow elements, decreased iron stores, and marrow plasmacytosis (Fig. 44.7). Bone marrow mastocytosis has also been described.[43] Myelofibrosis does not typically develop in chronic CME.[44]

Diagnostic Imaging

Sonographic Findings

Findings on abdominal ultrasonography in dogs with CME include splenomegaly, alterations in splenic echotexture, enlargement and hypoechogenicity of the abdominal lymph nodes, and scant peritoneal effusion.

Microbiologic Tests

Available diagnostic assays for ehrlichiosis in dogs are listed in Table 44.2.

Serologic Diagnosis

Most often, the diagnosis of CME is made using serology, which may be performed either by IFA testing, ELISA, or Western immunoblotting.[45] Using IFA testing, which is considered the gold standard serologic test, antibodies can be detected between 7 and 28 days after initial infection. Dogs with acute ehrlichiosis may have false-negative test results if sufficient time has not elapsed for antibody production to occur. PCR assays may be helpful for diagnosis in this situation. Use of a combination of serology with PCR is highly recommended as it allows better interpretation of the results and the animal health status. A positive initial serum antibody titer may reflect previous exposure and not necessarily active infection. Retesting should be performed 2 to 3 weeks later to demonstrate seroconversion and/or the possibility of an increase in the *E. canis* antibody titer. Serologic test results

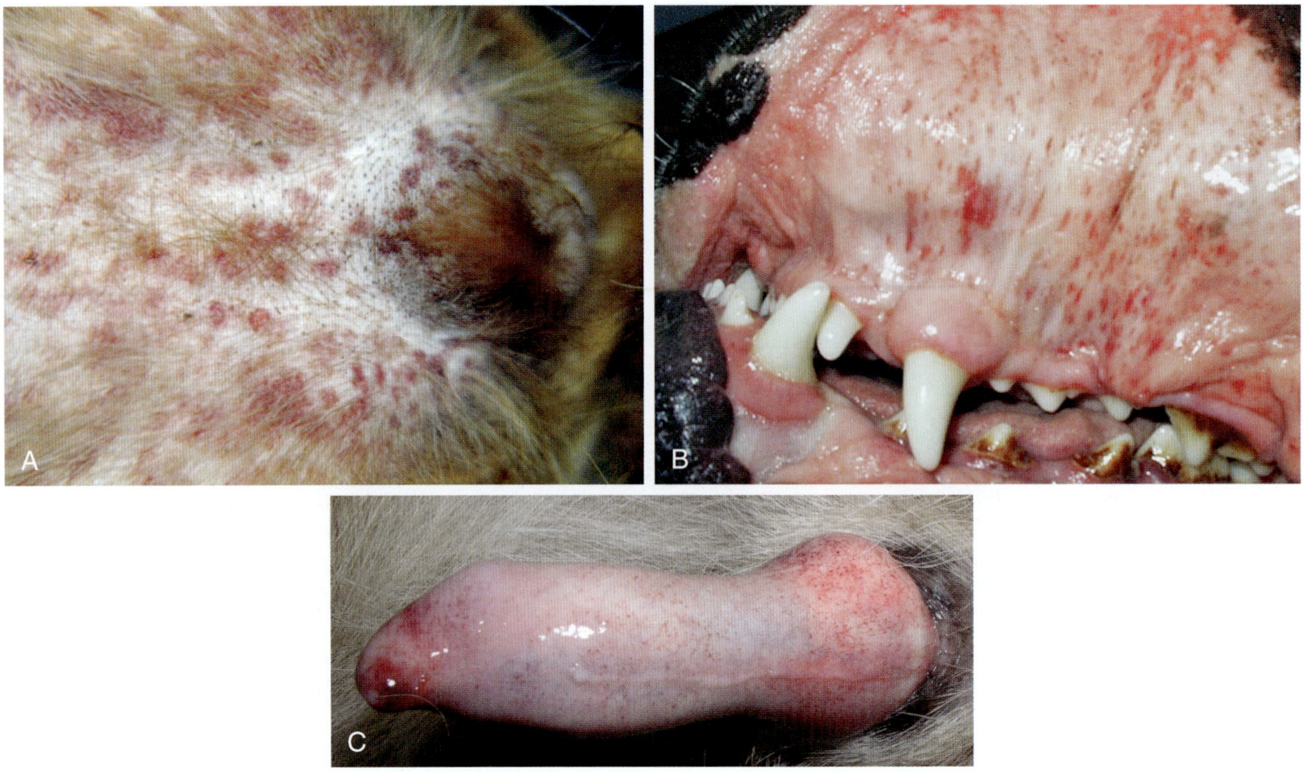

Fig. 44.5 (A) Ventral abdominal skin petechiation due to thrombocytopenia in a bitch infected with *Ehrlichia canis*. (B) Mucosal petechiae due to *E. canis* infection. (C) Numerous petechiae and ecchymoses in the penile mucosa of a dog with acute canine monocytic ehrlichiosis. (A,B courtesy Dr. Pedro Paulo Diniz, Western University of Health Sciences, Pomona, CA.)

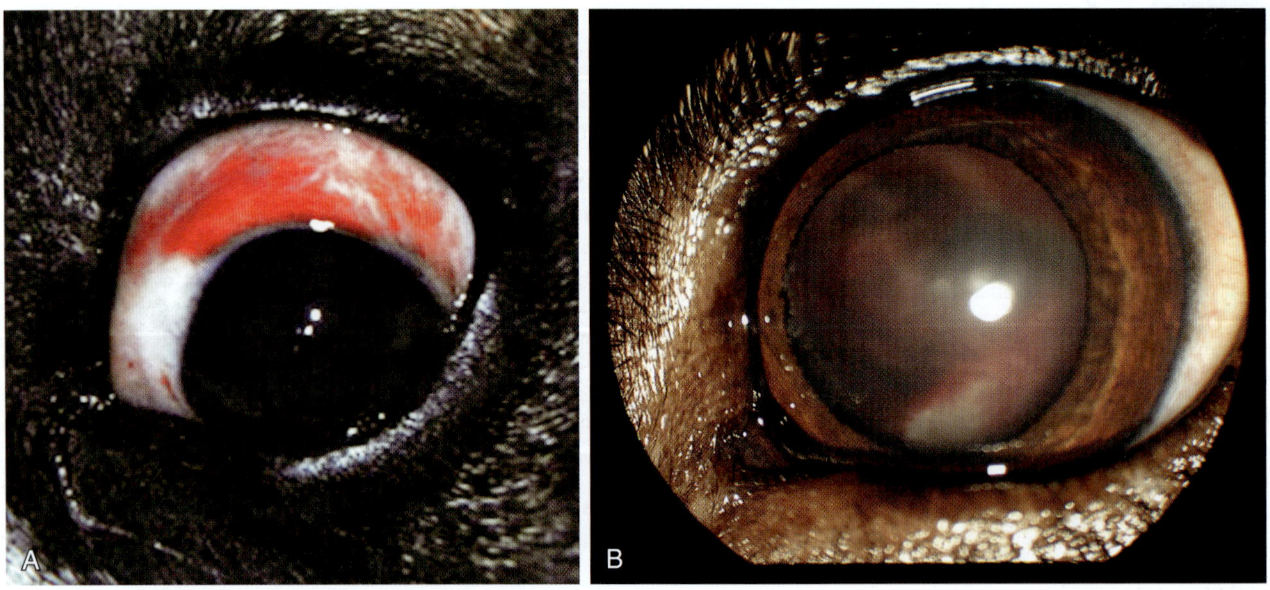

Fig. 44.6 (A) Scleral hemorrhage in a dog due to *Ehrlichia canis* infection. (B) Retinal hemorrhage and detachment in a 4-year-old female spayed Rhodesian ridgeback mix with canine monocytic ehrlichiosis. The dog also had thrombocytopenia (26,000 platelets/μL). Systolic blood pressure was within normal limits. (A, Courtesy Dr. Pedro Paulo Diniz, Western University of Health Sciences, Pomona, CA. B, Courtesy of University of California, Davis Veterinary Ophthalmology Service.)

should be interpreted in light of a dog's clinical signs and the results of testing for other potential causes of the dog's illness. Dogs with subclinical and chronic *E. canis* infection frequently have very high IFA titers (≥1:3,200), and these antibodies may persist in the face of treatment, suggesting persistence of the organism.[19] Antibody titers may decline in some dogs with treatment. High titers do not correlate with the severity of hyperglobulinemia, severity of disease, or duration of illness. A titer of 1:100 or greater is suggestive of exposure. Serologic cross-reactivity with other *Ehrlichia* species can occur, which includes *E. chaffeensis* and, less frequently, *E. ewingii*.[46] Variable cross-reactivity

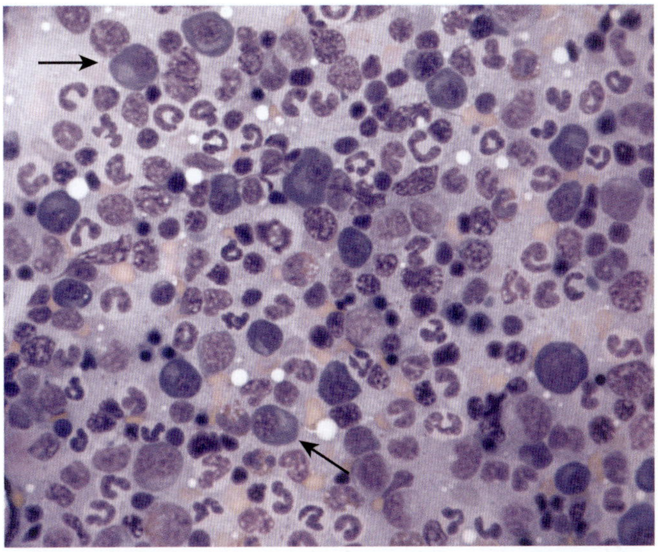

Fig. 44.7 Bone marrow plasmacytosis in an 8-year-old female spayed Labrador retriever with canine monocytic ehrlichiosis. Serum globulin was 12.1 g/dL (reference range, 2.3–4.4 g/dL), and serum protein electrophoresis revealed a polyclonal gammopathy. Plasma cells have a clock-faced nucleus, a clear area adjacent to the nucleus and a dark blue cytoplasm; two of the plasma cells in this figure are identified with black arrows. Mild to moderate megakaryocyte hyperplasia, mild erythroid hypoplasia, and mild mature granular lymphocytosis were also present. Romanowsky stain.

to *A. phagocytophilum* antigens can also occur.[45] In areas where other rickettsial agents are endemic, Western immunoblotting can be used to confirm that positive IFA antibody titers are truly reactive to *E. canis* antigens. However, Western blotting is laborious to perform and interpret, and not routinely available. As a result, Western immunoblotting has predominantly been used on a research basis. When *E. canis* antigens are used as target antigens, it may be difficult to distinguish between *E. canis* and *E. chaffeensis* infections.[47] Species-specific peptides in microtiter plate-based ELISA assays are highly specific for the detection of antibodies specific to *E. canis, E. ewingii,* and *E. chaffeensis* in experimentally and naturally infected dogs.[48,49]

In-clinic lateral-flow immunoassays, containing single or multiple antigens, have become popular rapid assays for detection of anti-*Ehrlichia* antibodies (e.g., SNAP 4Dx Plus, IDEXX Laboratories, Westbrook, ME, USA; Immunocomb, Biogal, Galed, Israel; Fastest, Megacor Diagnostik, Hoerbranz, Austria; FLEX4 Rapid Test, Abaxis, Union City, CA, USA). Some laboratories also offer ELISA-based assays that report the presence of antibodies to multiple vector-borne pathogens (e.g., Accuplex, Antech, USA). The results obtained from these assays are mostly qualitative, and semiquantitative in some. These tests can be sensitive and specific when compared with IFA, especially when the IFA titers are greater than 1:320.[50] However, variation in performance exists among assays; one study showed a low sensitivity of the FLEX4 Rapid test when compared with the SNAP test for detection of antibodies to *Borrelia burgdorferi*, and *Ehrlichia* and *Anaplasma* spp.[51] Practitioners should be aware that a positive result on these tests could reflect active infection or previous exposure, as is the case with IFA assays. If a positive result is obtained, determination of a quantitative titer using IFA may be helpful; high titers (e.g., greater than 1:800) may support chronic CME, and a fourfold rise in titer may support recent infection.

Molecular Diagnosis

Whole-blood PCR assays for detection of *E. canis* DNA are more sensitive than IFA or ELISA for early diagnosis of CME. PCR assays, targeting different genetic loci (16S rRNA, p28, p30, disulfide oxidoreductase, gp19, gp36, gp140), are widely available for routine diagnosis of *E. canis* infection.[12] Several laboratories offer panels that include real-time PCR assays for a variety of different vector-borne pathogens. The results of these assays should be interpreted in light of a dog's anamnesis (e.g., presence of ticks, trip to an endemic area), clinical signs, and the results of appropriate serologic assays; the latter should be performed to support the results of PCR testing. PCR assays for *E. canis* may be performed on blood, splenic aspirates, lymph nodes, or bone marrow specimens. IFA or ELISA testing is more sensitive than PCR assays for diagnosis of chronic CME.[30,52,53] The sensitivity of PCR assays for diagnosis of CME when performed on bone marrow in dogs with chronic ehrlichiosis has ranged from 25% to 68%, depending on the laboratory.[30] The use of PCR assays in the absence of serology is currently not suitable for screening potential blood donors for infection because of the lack of sensitivity of PCR. PCR assays may be useful to confirm infection in the first week of illness, when serologic assays are often negative. Real-time PCR assays are widely available which can distinguish *E. canis* from other *Ehrlichia* species. Clinicians should consult their diagnostic laboratory to ensure this is the case, especially in regions where multiple *Ehrlichia* species are present.

LAMP assays also have been developed for detection of *E. canis*.[54] These assays allow amplification under constant temperature (60°C to 65°C), allowing them to be performed in the clinic setting, as well as in a commercial diagnostic laboratory (see Chapter 6). LAMP assays are highly specific, efficient, and rapid (result available in less than an hour). In one study, the results of a LAMP-based POC assay for *Ehrlichia* spp. (PCRun, Biogal, Galed Laboratories, Israel) were equivalent to that of a TaqMan assay.[55] The study included 33 samples from dogs in the United Kingdom and 100 samples from dogs in Israel with a prevalence of infection as determined using TaqMan of 42% and 21%, respectively. The PCRun assay was shown to detect multiple species of *Ehrlichia* as well as *A. phagocytophilum* and *A. platys* without being able to distinguish among them, so more specific assays are required for an accurate diagnosis of CME.

Isolation in Culture

Ehrlichia canis can be cultured (e.g., from blood samples) in certain cell lines, such as DH82 and J774.A1 cells. Isolation is time-consuming and generally performed only on a research basis.[12]

Pathologic Findings

Gross pathologic findings in CME include widespread petechial and ecchymotic hemorrhages, generalized pallor, edema, lymphadenomegaly, and splenomegaly.[56,57] On histopathology, lymphoid and plasma cell hyperplasia and lymphoplasmacytic infiltrates may be present in numerous organs, such as the brain, eyes, spinal cord, spleen, liver, kidneys, lymph nodes, bone marrow, and lungs. Histiocytic infiltrates may be found in the lymph nodes. With chronicity, the proportion of plasma cells increases. Nonsuppurative meningitis and perivascular cuffing within the CNS can also occur.[56,57] Glomerulonephritis is rare in dogs with CME.[57] Interstitial renal plasmacytosis may occur in dogs with ehrlichiosis and may account for the proteinuria in some cases. Minimal histologic changes were noticed in the kidneys of dogs experimentally infected with *E. canis.* Ultrastructural examination showed fusion of podocyte processes that coincided with the development of proteinuria.[38]

TREATMENT AND PROGNOSIS

Antimicrobial Treatment

The treatment of choice for CME consists of antibacterial agents and supportive care (Table 44.3). Generally, the earlier the treatment of

TABLE 44.2 Diagnostic Assays Available for Ehrlichiosis in Dogs and Cats

Assay	Specimen Type	Target	Performance
Cell culture	Whole blood	*Ehrlichia canis*; *Ehrlichia ewingii* currently cannot be readily cultured	Not widely offered or utilized for routine diagnostic purposes. Requires several weeks' incubation and special laboratory facilities.
Morula detection	Blood smears, buffy coat smears, body fluids, tissue aspirates	*E. canis* or *E. ewingii* morulae	Low sensitivity (especially for chronic *E. canis* infection). *E. canis* morulae cannot be distinguished from those of *Ehrlichia chaffeensis*. *E. ewingii* morulae cannot be differentiated from those of *Anaplasma phagocytophilum*. Morulae may be confused with platelets, cytoplasmic granules, phagocytized nuclear material, and lymphoglandular bodies.
IFA serology	Serum	Antibodies to *E. canis*	Acute and convalescent serology is required for diagnosis of acute infection, because initial results may be negative in dogs with acute disease, and positive results can reflect previous exposure rather than active infection. Cross-reactivity occurs to other *Ehrlichia* species and occasionally to *A. phagocytophilum*.
ELISA serology	Serum	Antibodies to *E. canis* or *E. ewingii* antigens	Rapid, inexpensive, can be performed as an in-practice, POC test. Similar limitations as for IFA. Lack of quantitation in most commercial kits limits the ability to document seroconversion.
Western immuno-blotting	Serum	Antibodies to specific *E. canis* or *E. ewingii* antigens	Technically difficult; primarily used on a research basis to identify serologic responses to specific ehrlichial antigens. May be difficult to distinguish antibody responses to *E. canis* and *E. ewingii*.
PCR	Whole blood; spleen, lymph node or bone marrow aspirates	*E. canis*, *E. chaffeensis*, *Ehrlichia muris* subsp. *eauclairensis*, or *E. ewingii* DNA	Positive result confirms active infection. Negative results does not indicate absence of *Ehrlichia* spp. DNA. Sensitivity and specificity may vary depending on assay design and specimen type. Sensitivity for diagnosis of chronic CME may be low. The clinical significance of positive test results may be unclear as chronic subclinical infections occur (and whether *E. chaffeensis* causes disease in dogs is unclear). Assays that specifically detect *Ehrlichia muris* are not widely available on a commercial basis.

CME, Canine monocytic ehrlichiosis; *ELISA*, enzyme-linked immunosorbent assay; *IFA*, immunofluorescent antibody.

TABLE 44.3 Antimicrobial Drug Doses Used for Treatment of Ehrlichiosis in Dogs and Cats

Drug	Species	Dose (mg/kg)	Route (Alternative)	Interval (Hours)	Duration (Days)
Doxycycline	D, C	10	PO (IV)	24	21–28
	D, C	5	PO (IV)	12	21–28
Minocycline	D	10	PO	12	28
Oxytetracycline	D, C	7.5–10	IV	8	Until gastrointestinal signs abate, and then change to oral doxycycline as above

D, dogs; *C*, cats; *IV*, intravenous; *PO*, oral.

acutely infected dogs is initiated, the more favorable the prognosis and outcome. Dogs in the chronic phase that have severe myelosuppressive disease may be unresponsive to treatment.[58] Doxycycline (see Chapter 10) is considered the drug of choice for CME. It is readily absorbed to produce high blood, tissue, and intracellular concentrations. Given that *Ehrlichia* spp. can persist intracellularly, drug penetration into the cell is essential in eliminating infection. Doxycycline has the added advantages of a longer half-life and a higher CNS penetration when compared with other tetracyclines. A consensus statement of the ACVIM Infectious Disease Study Group suggested that dogs with CME should be treated with doxycycline (10 mg/kg daily) for a minimum of 28 days.[34] However, several studies have shown that shorter periods may be sufficient.[58] One study found that doxycycline (5 mg/kg twice daily) used for 14 days completely eliminated experimentally induced *E. canis* infection, as detected by PCR or blood cultures, from eight acutely infected dogs.[59] Other studies have shown that either 16 to 23 days or 21 to 28 days of treatment with doxycycline was sufficient to clear the organisms from all infected dogs.[28,60,61] However, in another study, a 6-week course of doxycycline (10 mg/kg, PO, daily) was not sufficient to clear *E. canis* bacteria from all subclinically experimentally infected dogs.[62] It is therefore currently recommended to treat acutely infected dogs with doxycycline (10 mg/kg, PO, daily) for 21 to 28 days.[58] Minocycline (10 mg/kg, PO, q12h) was also shown to clear infection as determined using whole-blood PCR in five naturally infected dogs, although the time to clearance (28 days) was longer than that for five dogs treated with doxycycline (10 mg/kg, PO, q24h) (21 days), with all dogs remaining PCR negative 7 days after discontinuing treatment.[63]

The efficacy of the "consensus doxycycline regimen" was investigated following experimental *E. canis* infection in the dog.[64] Despite clinical and hematologic recovery of the dogs and negative blood PCR results, *Rh. sanguineus* ticks fed on the dogs after doxycycline treatment became PCR positive for *E. canis* DNA, regardless of the phase during which the treatment was initiated. These results may imply that a very low level of infection, not detectable in whole blood using PCR, may persist in some cases following doxycycline treatment. Overall, noteworthy clinical improvement generally occurs within 24 to 48 hours after initiation of doxycycline therapy in dogs with acute-phase disease, as well as many dogs with mild chronic disease. The platelet count correspondingly begins to increase during this time and is usually in the reference range by 10 to 14 days after treatment initiation. Administration of glucocorticoids at standard immunosuppressive doses to a small number of dogs that had been experimentally infected with *E. canis* and treated with doxycycline was not found to be associated with recrudescence of infection.[65]

Rifampicin, an inhibitor of the B subunit of DNA-dependent RNA polymerase, has been assessed as a potential alternative drug to doxycycline for treatment of CME. In a recent experimental study, rifampicin (10 mg/kg, PO, q24h, for 21 days) hastened hematologic recovery in *E. canis* acutely infected dogs compared with untreated dogs, but achieved *E. canis* clearance in only two out of five dogs.[66]

Recovery is not equated with permanent immunity, and dogs can be reinfected with *E. canis* after a previously effective treatment. Moreover, experimental reinfection with heterologous strains has caused more severe disease manifestations than those with homologous strains.[59]

There is currently limited evidence-based justification for using other tetracyclines (e.g., tetracycline, oxytetracycline), or other drugs such as chloramphenicol, enrofloxacin, or imidocarb dipropionate in the treatment of CME. *Ehrlichia canis* appears to have intrinsic gyrase-mediated resistance to fluoroquinolones,[67] so although their use may be associated with clinical improvement,[68] they are not recommended. Imidocarb dipropionate, an antiprotozoal drug, has been used in the past in treating *E. canis* infections. *In vitro* and *in vivo* studies have shown that imidocarb (6.6 mg/kg, IM, two injections given 2 weeks apart) was not effective in clearing *E. canis* infection in dogs.[69] Because co-infection with *Babesia canis* and/or *Hepatozoon canis* (organisms transmitted by the same vector as for *E. canis*) may occur, imidocarb dipropionate may be used in conjunction with doxycycline when co-infections are identified.

Risk factors for mortality from CME in one study were severe leukopenia (WBC < 930 cells/μL), severe anemia (HCT < 11.5%), hypokalemia (<3.7 mmol/L), and prolonged APTT (>18.25 second).[70] After treatment, titers can decline and become negative in 6 to 9 months. Some dogs retain high titers for several years. Treatment for these dogs should be based on resolution of thrombocytopenia and improvement of hyperglobulinemia, although hyperglobulinemia may resolve over several months after treatment is discontinued. The use of PCR assays on splenic and/or bone marrow aspirates could be considered to determine if persistent infection is present in these dogs, but whether ongoing treatment with doxycycline changes the outcome for these dogs is unknown. Platelet counts should be reassessed 1 and 3 months after discontinuation of therapy, because of the potential for relapse or reinfection.[58]

Supportive Care

For dogs with CME that are dehydrated or anemic, intravenous fluids or blood products, respectively, may be required. In a nonseverely pancytopenic dog, if thrombocytopenia fails to resolve with doxycycline administration, a short course of therapy with immunosuppressive doses of glucocorticoids could be considered in addition to doxycycline. In one case report, use of high-dose filgrastim (50 μg/kg, SC, q48h for 4 days) together with glucocorticoids was followed by bone marrow recovery.[71]

IMMUNITY AND VACCINATION

A commercial vaccine for *E. canis* infection is currently not available, but in one study vaccination of dogs with an attenuated strain extensively reduced disease manifestations in dogs challenged with a virulent strain of *E. canis*.[72] The immune response to *E. canis* infection is not well understood. Because *E. canis* is an intracellular pathogen, cell-mediated immune response is required for pathogen elimination. In one study, dogs with acute infection developed CD8+ lymphocytosis that subsided after several weeks, despite organism persistence.[73] Cytokine studies suggest that the immune response may vary according to the strain of *E. canis* involved.[74,75] Genetic factors of the host are also likely to be important determinants of the immune response and outcome of infection.

PREVENTION

Avoidance of tick-infested areas and routine inspection of dogs for ticks after outdoor activities, especially in endemic areas, can help to prevent ehrlichiosis. Clients should be instructed to remove ticks properly and avoid handling ticks with bare hands or crushing them, to prevent exposure to infected hemolymph. A variety of devices are available to assist tick removal, which are placed around the area where the mouthparts enter the skin to avoid crushing or squeezing the tick and leaving the mouthparts behind (see Fig. 44.2). Fine-tipped tweezers can be used to grasp the tick as close to the skin as possible, followed by steady retraction to remove the tick. The bite wound should then be thoroughly cleaned with a suitable antiseptic solution (such as iodine or chlorhexidine-based antiseptics) or soap and water. Ticks can be disposed of in alcohol or tested for vector-borne pathogens using PCR assays.

The use of topical ectoparasiticides with activity against ticks also prevent tick-borne infectious diseases (see Chapter 13). Examples of effective canine products include those that contain amitraz, fipronil, pyrethroids (permethrin, etofenprox, pyrethrin, deltamethrin, flumethrin), sarolaner, afoxolaner, lotilaner, and fluralaner. Products that contain pyrethroids and amitraz have the most potent activity against ticks. In one field study, the use of monthly imidacloprid 10% and permethrin 50% effectively prevented infection with *E. canis* in kennel dogs.[76] In another study, the use of monthly (days 0, 28, and 56) topical imidacloprid 10% and permethrin 50% prevented tick transmission of *E. canis* to experimentally infected dogs, whereas use of monthly afoxolaner or a single dose of fluralaner did not completely prevent infection.[77] It was suggested that failure of isoxazolines to prevent transmission resulted from the slower speed of kill for these products, which was significantly lower than that for the imidacloprid/permethrin combination. Amitraz, a monoamine oxidase inhibitor, should not be used in dogs treated with selective serotonin reuptake inhibitors (SSRIs) such as fluoxetine, and pet owners who are receiving SSRIs should also use alternative preventatives for their dogs. Prophylactics should be applied consistently at the recommended interval for optimum activity. No preventatives completely protect dogs or cats from tick attachment, especially where tick infestation rates are high. Unfortunately, acaricide-resistant strains of *Rh. sanguineus* have been reported following the indiscriminate use of these drugs.[76]

Low-dose doxycycline (6.6 mg/kg, PO, q24h) has also been used to prevent infection in working dogs or those residing in kennels in which *E. canis* infection is a substantial problem. Resistance to doxycycline remains a theoretical concern in this situation.

Because of the potential persistent subclinical carrier state, blood donor dogs should be screened with serology and PCR for evidence of *E. canis* exposure or infection. All seropositive/PCR-positive dogs should be excluded as donors. Transport of persistent carrier dogs to nonendemic regions has the potential to introduce the infection or new strains of *E. canis* to these regions if the appropriate tick vectors are present.

PUBLIC HEALTH ASPECTS

Ehrlichia canis DNA has been detected in some human patients from Venezuela with clinical signs compatible with HME,[78] and in samples from blood bank donors in Costa Rica,[79,80] suggesting that strains closely related to *E. canis* might be a cause of monocytic ehrlichiosis in people in Central and South America. Appropriate precautions should be taken to prevent transmission when handling engorged ticks as well as blood and tissue specimens from infected dogs, and care should be taken to prevent needle-stick injuries.

EHRLICHIA CHAFFEENSIS

Shimon Harrus, Trevor Waner, Mathios E. Mylonakis

ETIOLOGIC AGENT AND EPIDEMIOLOGY

Ehrlichia chaffeensis, the cause of HME, can naturally infect dogs, based on molecular detection of the organism in southeastern Virginia, Oklahoma, North Carolina, Venezuela, and South Korea.[81–87] White-tailed deer (*Odocoileus virginianus*) serve as the principal reservoir host that sustains the enzootic cycle of *Ehrlichia chaffeensis* in North America.[88] *E. chaffeensis* is transstadially transmitted primarily by the lone star tick, *Amblyomma americanum*, but can also be transmitted by the gulf coast tick, *Amblyomma maculatum*. *Dermacentor variabilis* and possibly *Rh. sanguineus* and other tick species may also play a minor role in the transmission of this agent.[88–90]

CLINICAL FEATURES

Pathogenesis and Clinical Signs

Experimentally infected dogs develop mild and inconsistent clinical and clinicopathologic abnormalities, including fever, thrombocytopenia, and leukopenia.[82,91–94] Overall, the intensity of thrombocytopenia and histopathologic lesions in several organs tended to be less severe in dogs experimentally infected with *E. chaffeensis* compared with dogs inoculated at the same time with *E. canis*.[82,91] *Ehrlichia chaffeensis* DNA could be PCR amplified and antibody titers detected for up to 117 days and 180 days postinoculation, respectively,[93] while ticks could acquire the infection for up to 566 days following intradermal inoculation of a dog.[92] *Ehrlichia chaffeensis* infection in dogs may lead to a persistent carrier state, with localization in several tissues (e.g., bone marrow, spleen, liver, lymph nodes, lungs, kidneys, and brain).[91,92]

Physical Examination Findings

In naturally infected dogs, *E. chaffeensis* infection has been associated with lymphadenomegaly, anterior uveitis, and epistaxis,[82] but the clinical implications of this infection in dogs are still unclear.

DIAGNOSIS

Laboratory Abnormalities

Complete Blood Count and Serum Chemistry Profile

Anemia, thrombocytopenia, moderate pancytopenia, hyperproteinemia, and hypoalbuminemia have been reported in a limited number of naturally infected dogs.[81,86,87] However, as coinfections are common in naturally infected dogs, these findings should be interpreted with caution.

Microbiologic Tests

Cytologic Diagnosis

The diagnostic sensitivity of cytology for the confirmation of the *E. chaffeensis* infection has yet to be evaluated and to the best of the authors' knowledge, no microscopic visualization of *E. chaffeensis* morulae has been reported in experimentally or naturally infected dogs. Of note, the cytologic differentiation between *E. canis* and *E. chaffeensis* morulae in host cells is not possible.[95]

Serologic Diagnosis

Dogs experimentally infected with *E. chaffeensis* develop IgG antibody titres 7 to 23 days postinoculation, which remain detectable for at least 6 months postinoculation.[81,91,93] In the clinical setting, serologic diagnosis is complicated by strong cross-reactivity of *E. chaffeensis* antibodies with antigens of other *Ehrlichia* species.[12,81,83,84,96] Recently, species-specific peptides in microtiter plate-based ELISA assays have been shown to demonstrate very high specificity in the detection of antibodies specific to *E. ewingii*, *E. canis,* and *E. chaffeensis* in experimentally and naturally infected dogs.[46,49,81,83,84,96]

Molecular Detection Using Nucleic Acid–Based Testing

Real-time PCR assays for detection of *E. chaffeensis* have been applied mostly to whole blood and occasionally other tissues specimens.[85,91–93] Some commercial veterinary diagnostic laboratories offer vector-borne PCR panels that include an assay that specifically detects *E. chaffeensis*, with separate assays for *E. canis* and *E. ewingii.* The *16S rRNA* gene has been the major molecular target, but other genes including the *p28*, *gp120*, *homp*, and disulfide oxidoreductase have also been targeted.[81,83,85,92,93]

TREATMENT

In vitro susceptibility testing has indicated that doxycycline and rifampicin are the most active drugs against *E. chaffeensis* infection, but clinical trials are lacking for both antibiotic agents.[97]

PREVENTION

In endemic areas, the risk of acquiring *E. chaffeensis* infection can be lowered by implementing strict tick control programmes for dogs and premises. No vaccines are currently available for the protection of dogs against *E. chaffeensis* infection. However, vaccination with a live, attenuated *E. chaffeensis* mutant (Ech_0660) may have induced a pathogen-specific humoral and cellular immunity conferring protection in vaccinated dogs against tick-transmitted *E. chaffeensis* infection but not against a heterologous challenge with *E. canis*.[94]

PUBLIC HEALTH ASPECTS

In south-central and southeastern United States, *E. chaffeensis* is considered the major causative agent for HME, which is exhibited as an acute influenza-like illness characterized by fever, headache, malaise, and occasionally death in severely affected humans.[98] Dogs may be carriers of *E. chaffeensis* in endemic geographic regions and may be involved in transporting infected ticks to humans.

EHRLICHIA RUMINANTIUM

Shimon Harrus, Trevor Waner, Mathios E. Mylonakis

Ehrlichia ruminantium, the cause of heartwater in cattle, has been detected using PCR in the blood of dogs presenting with clinical signs suggestive of ehrlichiosis and also in clinically healthy dogs from countries in sub-Saharan Africa, including South Africa, Kenya, Uganda, Ethiopia, Nigeria, and Mali.[5,99] The organism has not been isolated from the blood of dogs in culture or tested for its infectivity to dogs; therefore, its virulence, potential vectors, and definitive classification are uncertain. Whether the clinical signs, which were similar to those of *E. canis* infection, were caused by or were incidental to the infection with this organism is uncertain.

EHRLICHIA MURIS SUBSPECIES *EAUCLAIRENSIS*

Shimon Harrus, Trevor Waner, Mathios E. Mylonakis, Jane E. Sykes

Ehrlichia muris was originally isolated from a wild mouse in Japan,[100] and later PCR amplified and sequenced.[101] *Ehrlichia muris* or a closely related organism was detected using molecular techniques in a febrile person in Russia,[102] and then in four people with febrile disease from Minnesota and Wisconsin.[103] The people from Minnesota and Wisconsin had clinical signs and laboratory abnormalities resembling those of human ehrlichiosis or granulocytic anaplasmosis, but no morulae were visualized in blood smears. They were seronegative to *A. phagocytophilum* and showed variable seroreactivity to *E. chaffeensis*.[103] The DNA of this organism was also detected in *Peromyscus leucopus* mice as well as *Ixodes scapularis* ticks from Minnesota and Wisconsin.[104] Subsequently, additional human cases were identified in the United States (at the time of writing, more than 100 cases according to the CDC), and multilocus sequence analysis led to the proposal that the organism from the United States be classified as a novel species, *E. muris* subsp. *eauclairensis*.[105]

Dogs experimentally infected with *E. muris* did not show clinical or hematologic abnormalities, did not seroconvert, and their PCR was negative for the duration of the follow-up period.[101] In 2012, the DNA of *E. muris* subsp. *eauclairensis* was identified in an ill dog from northern Minnesota that was seronegative for *E. canis* and seroreactive to *Anaplasma* spp., although the extent to which this organism contributed to the dog's clinical signs was unclear.[6] The extent to which *E. muris* subsp. *eauclairensis* can cause disease in dogs requires further investigation.

PANOLA MOUNTAIN *EHRLICHIA*

Jane E. Sykes

Panola Mountain *Ehrlichia* is a novel species of *Ehrlichia* that was identified in a goat in Georgia in the USA in 2006[106] and subsequently detected in a human from Atlanta with doxycycline-responsive neck pain. The person had been hiking 3 weeks previously in the Panola Mountain State Park in Georgia and had removed an *A. americanum* nymphal tick from his upper arm.[107] The organism is closely related to *E. ruminantium* and was subsequently detected in *A. americanum* ticks from all over the southeastern United States,[108] as well as *A. maculatum* ticks in the United States and *Amblyomma variegatum* ticks from the Caribbean and Africa.[109] Infections have been detected in white-tailed deer, which were also shown to be susceptible to experimental infection using infected *Amblyomma* ticks and may be reservoirs for the organism.[110] Panola Mountain *Ehrlichia* was also detected in a dog from Raleigh, North Carolina, with reactive lymphocytosis and clonal expansion of T cells, which appeared to respond to treatment with doxycycline.[7] The extent to which this organism causes disease in dogs and humans requires further study.

EHRLICHIA EWINGII

Barbara Qurollo

ETIOLOGIC AGENT AND EPIDEMIOLOGY

Ehrlichia ewingii, a gram-negative, obligate intracellular bacterium is the causative agent of canine and human granulocytic ehrlichiosis. To date, the organism has only been transiently cultured *in vitro*. *Ehrlichia ewingii* has been detected in dogs from North America, Cameroon, and Brazil.[2,79,111] In the south-central and southeastern states of the United States, *E. ewingii* may be the primary agent of canine ehrlichiosis. Of mostly healthy dogs from Oklahoma and Arkansas, 45% were seropositive for *E. ewingii*.[112] Furthermore, in two large-scale studies addressing healthy and sick dogs, the overall seroprevalence was 14.5% in the central states (Oklahoma, Arkansas, Missouri, and Kansas) and 5.9% in the southeastern states,[113] while seroprevalences of 5.7%, 5.2%, 3.4%, 1.2%, and 0.4% were reported in mid-Atlantic, south, northeast, midwest, and west, respectively.[49] The PCR-based prevalence of *Ehrlichia ewingii* infection ranges from 6% to 30% in ill or apparently healthy dogs.[83,84,112,114] The median age of 41 infected dogs in one study was 9 years, with most cases occurring in summer (39%), fall (27%), and winter (24%).[115] *E. ewingii* is transmitted transstadially by the lone star tick, *A. americanum*, which is the only proven vector, but the DNA of *E. ewingii* has also been detected in *D. variabilis*, *Rh. sanguineus*, and rarely *A. maculatum* ticks.[84,88,116] Infection and associated disease was identified for the first time in Texas in 2019, suggesting the presence of infected *Amblyomma* ticks in this region, and possibly an under-recognized disease.[117]

The white-tailed deer and possibly dogs are the major reservoir hosts of *E. ewingii* in nature.[114,118] One case report described evidence of vertical transmission of *Mycoplasma haemocanis* but not *E. ewingii* from an infected pregnant beagle.[119]

CLINICAL FEATURES

Pathogenesis and Clinical Signs

Dogs experimentally or naturally infected with *E. ewingii* can maintain the infection for at least 5 months or 2 years, respectively, possibly serving as reservoir hosts.[118,120–122] Like *A. phagocytophilum*, *E. ewingii* replicates in neutrophils and delays neutrophil apoptosis thus prolonging the life span of the host cells.[123] The course of infection is usually subclinical, or after an incubation period of 2–3 weeks may culminate in an acute disease with intermittent fever, lethargy, anorexia, lameness due to neutrophilic polyarthritis, and possibly neurologic manifestations.[122,124]

Physical Examination Findings

The most common clinical findings include fever and musculoskeletal signs. In dogs that are naturally infected with *E. ewingii*, physical examination may indicate a thin body condition, fever, lethargy, peripheral lymphadenopathy, splenomegaly or hepatomegaly, reluctance to move, lameness or stilted gait, joint swelling or pain on palpation, peripheral edema, and occasionally vomiting or diarrhea.[115,125] Joint pain was the most commonly reported sign in one study of 41 naturally infected dogs, and was present in over one third of the dogs.[115] Dogs that tested PCR positive for other vector-borne pathogens were excluded from this study, but other concurrent disorders were present in many of the dogs tested. Reported neurologic signs include proprioceptive deficits, paraparesis, ataxia, neck pain, anisocoria, tremors, and head tilt.[124] Importantly, an unknown proportion of dogs with spontaneous infection do not develop any clinical manifestations.[115,118]

DIAGNOSIS

Laboratory Abnormalities

Morulae may be cytologically detected in the peripheral blood, synovial fluid, or bone marrow in 1%–7% of granulocytes, but are morphologically indistinguishable from those of *A. phagocytophilum*.[115,125] In experimental infections, morulae have been seen in the peripheral blood of some dogs about 2 to 3 weeks PI, before the onset of clinical signs or seroconversion.[121,122] In the study of 41 infected dogs, morulae were reported in 6 (16%) of 37 dogs where CBC findings were available.[115]

Common hematologic abnormalities in dogs naturally infected with *E. ewingii* include thrombocytopenia (43% of dogs in one study), anemia, and mild to moderate neutrophilic leukocytosis with a left shift or rarely leukopenia.[111,115,124,125] Reactive lymphocytosis and mild neutrophil toxic changes may also occur.[115,124] Serum biochemistry may be unremarkable or show mild abnormalities such as hypoalbuminemia, hyperglobulinemia, and mildly elevated activities of serum ALP and ALT.[115,124,125] Increased serum urea nitrogen and symmetric dimethylarginine (SDMA) concentrations were detected in approximately one third of 41 infected dogs, and significant proteinuria in the face of inactive urine sediments was also frequently detected, suggesting the possibility of glomerulonephritis.[115] Synovial fluid analysis reveals neutrophilic polyarthritis (nucleated cell counts may range 16,000–125,000/μL).

Microbiologic Tests

Serologic Diagnosis

In experimentally infected dogs, antibodies appear approximately 1 month PI.[122] Serologic diagnosis of *E. ewingii* infection is currently limited to a POC ELISA assay that detects the presence of antibodies to a specific peptide of *E. ewingii* (SNAP 4Dx Plus, IDEXX Laboratories, Westbrook, ME, USA). Because this peptide is combined on a spot with a peptide that detects antibodies to *E. canis*, the antibody response to these pathogens cannot be distinguished from one another. Cross-reactions may also occur to other *Ehrlichia* species such as *E. chaffeensis*. Recently, species-specific peptides in microtiter plate-based ELISA assays have been shown to demonstrate very high specificity for the detection of antibodies specific to *E. ewingii*, *E. canis*, and *E. chaffeensis* in experimentally and naturally infected dogs.[46,48,49,112,113,118] Dogs with acute illness may initially test negative with serologic assays, and positive test results may reflect the presence of antibodies from previous exposure or subclinical infection.[48,122] A total of 83% of 41 infected dogs had antibodies to *Ehrlichia* species antigens using the SNAP 4Dx Plus assay.[115] Seroconversion from a negative to a positive result over a 2- to 4-week time period in paired serum samples may support a diagnosis of current active *E. ewingii* infection in endemic areas.

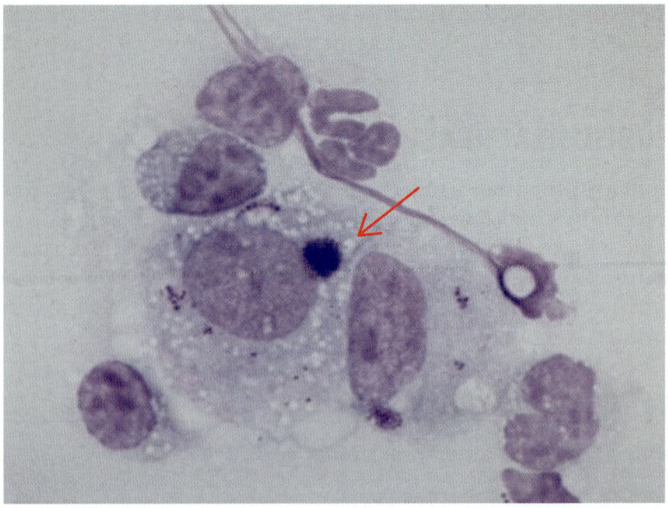

Fig. 44.8 *Ehrlichia* inclusion (arrow) in a mononuclear cell of a cat (Wright stain, ×1000). (Courtesy Michael Lappin, Colorado State University, Fort Collins, CO)

Molecular Diagnosis Using Nucleic Acid–Based Testing

Whole-blood PCR assays with variable sensitivities have been developed for the specific detection of *E. ewingii* DNA.[115,118,124,125] Taking into account the low specificity of serologic tests, *E. ewingii*-specific PCR assays are currently the only means to confirm active infection with this pathogen and to differentiate it from *A. phagocytophilum* infection. In experimental studies, PCR was shown to become positive as early as 4 days after inoculation.[122]

TREATMENT

Treatment with doxycycline results in rapid clinical improvement within 24 to 48 hours.[85,124] Subclinically infected dogs may spontaneously clear the infection within weeks to months.[118,121]

PREVENTION

In the endemic areas, the risk of acquiring *E. ewingii* infection can be lowered by implementing strict tick control programs for dogs and premises. Potential blood donor dogs should be screened for infection with *E. ewingii*-specific ELISA and PCR assays.

PUBLIC HEALTH ASPECTS

Human infection with *E. ewingii* has been rarely described in endemic regions of the United States.[85,126,127] In one study of 4,177 human patients that were tested using real-time PCR for *Ehrlichia* across 41 US states, 10 (9.2%) of 109 *Ehrlichia* infections were *E. ewingii*, with 2 patients from New Jersey and Indiana, where cases had previously not been described.[128] The remaining infections were caused by *E. chaffeensis* (99 cases) and none tested positive for *E. muris* subsp. *eauclairensis*. Affected humans show headache, nausea, fever, myalgia, and thrombocytopenia, with or without leukopenia, and respond to doxycycline treatment. Both immunocompetent and immunocompromised humans have reportedly been affected.[126] Although direct dog-to-human transmission does not occur, blood from affected dogs should be handled with caution.

FELINE EHRLICHIOSES

ETIOLOGIC AGENT AND EPIDEMIOLOGY

The species of *Ehrlichia* that infect cats after natural exposure have not been fully determined. Reports of *Ehrlichia*-like bodies or morulae have been detected in peripheral lymphocytes or monocytes of naturally exposed cats in the United States[129] (Fig. 44.8), Kenya,[130,131] France,[4,132–136] Brazil,[137] and Thailand.[138] Electron microscopic assessment of an isolate from feline mononuclear cells revealed organisms from 0.54 to 1.3 μm, intermediate in size between *E. canis* and *Neorickettsia sennetsu*.[130] Confirmation of feline ehrlichiosis on a molecular basis using PCR has improved our understanding of which species of *Ehrlichia* infect cats. Many recent studies in cats document PCR-amplified DNA from *Ehrlichia* spp. with similar, and in some cases identical, DNA sequence from those *Ehrlichia* spp. commonly detected in dogs.[139,139–151] In one North American report,[143] DNA most consistent with *E. canis* was documented in the blood of three clinically ill cats, and a second retrospective study[146] described *Ehrlichia* DNA in 6 of 331 (1.8%) feline whole blood samples that had been submitted for vector-borne disease testing. Of those six cats, sequence analysis identified one cat with *E. canis*, two cats with *E. chaffeensis* and three cats with *E. ewingii* infections. Prevalence studies of vector-borne pathogens in cats in Brazil have often yielded positive PCR results for *Ehrlichia*, whereas many studies from North America and Europe have been negative for *Ehrlichia* DNA, instead amplifying the DNA of *Anaplasma* or *Bartonella species*, or hemoplasmas. *Ehrlichia canis* DNA segments amplified from three cats in Brazil were 99% identical with each other and 100% identical with reported sequences from dogs in the area, suggesting that the same strain was infecting dogs and cats.[144] Furthermore, molecular studies from Brazil described amplified regions of the 16S rDNA and *dsb* gene from infected cats as 100% identical to *E. canis*.[139–141,149,151] In a Brazilian study of cats from Rio de Janeiro, investigators amplified 16S rRNA gene sequences with 100% identity to *E. canis*, but obtained negative *dsb* gene PCR results.[150] However, another study from Brazil identified 16S rDNA from *Ehrlichia* spp. that was 98% identical to *E. canis* in one cat and 97% identical to *E. chaffeensis* in another cat indicating the potential for a different species of *Ehrlichia* that infect cats.[142] In a French report,[132] the 16S rDNA *Ehrlichia* sequences obtained from two cats were 100% identical to those obtained from North American cats, and in two recent reports from Europe, *Ehrlichia* spp. DNA was amplified from 14 (5.4%) of 260 cats in Italy[148] and 35 (5.4%) of 649 domestic and stray cats in Portugal.[147] Sequence analysis was reported for one of the Portugal cats, which confirmed the presence of *E. canis* DNA. *Ehrlichia canis* DNA was amplified from blood of one cat in Trinidad, West Indies.[145] These reports support a conclusion that cats can be infected with the same or similar species of *Ehrlichia* commonly diagnosed in dogs and that veterinarians should consider molecular testing modalities in cats with clinical signs of ehrlichiosis. Most cats for which signalment was reported were domestic short-haired cats and 1 year or older. Both male and female cats were affected.

To the knowledge of the authors, only one experimental inoculation study of cats with *E. canis* has been conducted.[152] When cats were inoculated subcutaneously with an *E. canis* strain (North Carolina State University canine isolate) maintained in cell culture, *E. canis* DNA or antibodies that reacted to *E. canis* morulae were not detected in an 8-week follow-up period.[152] It is possible that: (1) subcutaneous inoculation is not an effective method for infecting cats with *E. canis*; (2) natural transmission via a tick species is necessary for infection; (3) the *E. canis* strain maintained after many passages through cell culture lost its natural virulence in a host animal; or (4) *Ehrlichia* species that replicate in cats are not identical to those infecting dogs.[143] Additional experimental infection studies in cats using different *Ehrlichia* spp. and transmission methods are warranted. In addition, whether *E. muris* can be transmitted to cats that ingest infected rodents requires further study.[100,101]

Sera from cats have been assessed for *Ehrlichia* spp. antibodies using IFA, ELISA, or Western immunoblot. By the use of IFA, serum antibodies that react with *E. canis* morulae have been detected in cats from multiple states of the United States,[129,146,153] France,[135,136] Italy,[154,155] Spain,[156–160] Kenya,[161] and Brazil.[140–142,150,162] In a neighborhood in Colorado from which a cat infected with a monocytic *Ehrlichia* was identified, 14 of 17 cats (82.4%) and 9 of 17 cats (52.9%) had serum antibodies detected by IFA against *E. canis* and *Neorickettsia risticii*, respectively.[129] Cats with antibodies against both species generally had higher titers to *E. canis* antigens. A recent serologic survey of 715 archived feline serum samples from client-owned cats in North America documented a low *Ehrlichia* seroprevalence.[146] The samples were screened with a qualitative ELISA with *Ehrlichia*-genus and species-specific peptides, and a subset of those were further analyzed by whole cell *E. canis* and *E. chaffeensis* IFA. *Ehrlichia* spp. antibodies to peptides were detected in 12 of 715 cats (0.14%), with species-specific seroreactivity to *E. canis*, *E. chaffeensis*, and *E. ewingii* documented in 5, 1, and 2 cats, respectively. Of the 59 cats screened by IFA, 5 cats had serum antibodies to *E. chaffeensis*, 1 of which was also seroreactive to *E. canis*, and 2 cats were seroreactive to *E. canis*.[146] Serosurveys performed in other countries using *E. canis* IFA documented *E. canis* antibodies in 67 of 680 client-owned and stray cats (9.9%) from Spain, 57 of 216 client-owned cats (26.4%) from Brazil, and 88 of 212 client-owned and stray cats (41.5%) from Brazil.[140,150,157] Recent serosurveys using *E. canis* or *Ehrlichia* spp. peptide ELISAs measured *Ehrlichia* antibodies in 73 of 624 (11.7%) client-owned cats from Germany and 2 of 100 (2%) stray cats from Bulgaria.[163,164] Overall, seroprevalence of *Ehrlichia* spp. in client-owned cats in North America was low, with potential epizootic areas such as the area in Colorado, while feline *Ehrlichia* seroprevalence was higher in Europe and South America. The differences in prevalence may be due to serologic testing modalities, lifestyle of the cats tested, and prevalence of *Ehrlichia* spp.

Many healthy cats have serum antibodies from exposure to other pathogens (e.g., *Bartonella henselae*)[160] that may cross-react with *E. canis* antigens, as observed for dogs.[153] Additionally, variable serologic cross-reactivity occurs among *Ehrlichia*, *Neorickettsia*, and *Anaplasma* spp.; therefore, seroreactivity to a specific test antigen does not definitely document exposure to the *Ehrlichia* spp. morulae or peptides used for testing.[34,152,165,166] Serologic cross-reactivity has been suspected in epidemiologic investigations in domestic or exotic cats, which likely overestimates infection prevalence.[146,156,159,160,162,167–169] For example, one study documented a cat with *A. phagocytophilum* DNA in blood that had serum antibodies to *E. chaffeensis* by IFA, and another cat with *E. chaffeensis* DNA in blood that did not have serum antibodies to *E. chaffeensis* by IFA but had antibodies to *E. canis* by IFA.[146] Standardization of *Ehrlichia* spp. serologic methodologies between laboratories has not been performed, and the most appropriate cutoff values have not been determined. Results of serologic tests performed by different laboratories have not shown 100% concordance.[143] Thus, results of antibody-based surveys should be interpreted with caution until such time as laboratories can better correlate serologic results with feline *Ehrlichia* spp. isolates or PCR assay findings.

The way in which the clinically ill, naturally exposed cats with ehrlichiosis described in the literature were infected remains unknown. Documentation of arthropod exposure in proven cases has been variable. A study in Brazil documented *Rh. sanguineus* sensu lato ticks parasitizing three cats infected with *E. canis,* where one of the attached ticks was also PCR positive for *E. canis.*[151] *Haemaphysalis leachi* was found on each of four cats with clinical ehrlichiosis in Kenya.[130,131] *Amblyomma aureolatum* was found on an infected cat in Brazil.[149] *Ctenocephalides felis* taken from cats in the United States and Australia were negative for *Ehrlichia* and *Anaplasma* spp. DNA.[170,171]

CLINICAL FEATURES

Pathogenesis, Clinical Signs and Physical Examination Findings

The pathogenesis of disease associated with ehrlichiosis in cats is unknown. Based on clinical, laboratory, and radiographic findings, pathogenesis of disease may be similar to that for *Ehrlichia* infection of dogs. In the three cats with *E. canis*-like DNA in blood, antinuclear antibodies were detected along with cytopenias, similar to results reported for infected dogs.[143] In one cat infected with *E. ewingii*, clinical signs were also similar to those seen in infected dogs, and consisted of anemia and thrombocytopenia.[146] Additional studies monitoring cats naturally or experimentally infected with *Ehrlichia* spp. are needed to better understand the pathogenesis of feline ehrlichiosis.

Clinical manifestations of ehrlichiosis have been described in 22 cats with suspected morulae in mononuclear cells,[4,129–131,134,135,137,172] and in 4 cats with *Ehrlichia* spp. DNA in blood (see Table 44.1).[143,146] Ehrlichiosis has also been suspected in 34 reported feline cases in which the diagnosis was presumptively based on the combination of positive *E. canis* or *N. risticii* serology results, clinical or laboratory findings consistent with ehrlichial infection, and response to known antiehrlichial drugs.[129,135,136,172–175] Furthermore, several studies that evaluated clinical signs in cats that were seropositive and/or PCR positive for *Ehrlichia* documented abnormalities consistent with ehrlichiosis, but results of treatment were not reported.[141,148,158] Some cats that tested positive for *Ehrlichia* using PCR have been apparently healthy. In other cats, co-morbidities such as lymphoma or concurrent infection with *Mycoplasma haemofelis, Cryptococcus neoformans*, FeLV, or FIV infections were detected.

When clinical signs are present, fever and nonspecific signs of lethargy, inappetence, and weight loss are common manifestations. Hyperesthesia, joint pain, dyspnea, vomiting, and diarrhea have also been described. Reported physical examination abnormalities include splenomegaly, lymphadenomegaly, dyspnea, petechiae, retinal detachments, vitreous hemorrhages, epistaxis, and pale mucous membranes.

DIAGNOSIS

Diagnostic tests used to detect *Ehrlichia* infections in cats are similar to those used in dogs (see Table 44.2). Assessment of regional and tick exposure, clinical signs, and characteristic laboratory abnormalities should prompt clinicians to proceed with diagnostic modalities such as PCR, IFA, ELISA, and cytologic examination of blood smears. Use of a combination of molecular and serologic modalities can improve evidence of infection or exposure to *Ehrlichia* spp.[176] Cytologic examination of blood, joint fluid, CSF, and tissue aspirates can identify active infections but is generally less sensitive than molecular techniques.

Laboratory Abnormalities

Anemia is most commonly nonregenerative and has been noted in cats with chronic disease histories. One cat with regenerative anemia was co-infected with a hemotropic *Mycoplasma* species.[4] Leukopenia, leukocytosis, neutrophilia, neutropenia, lymphopenia, lymphocytosis, monocytosis, and thrombocytopenia occur in some cats, alone or in combination. A Brazilian study documented thrombocytopenia and lymphopenia as the most common CBC abnormalities in eight cats with *E. canis* DNA in their blood[141]; the same study evaluated 42 cats seropositive to *E. canis* by IFA and documented anemia, leukocytosis, leukopenia, thrombocytopenia, lymphopenia, and monocytosis. A recent study of 57 cats from Brazil, either seropositive or PCR positive for *E. canis* reported anemia, thrombocytopenia, leukocytosis, left-shift neutrophilia, and hyperproteinemia as the most common abnormalites.[150] In contrast, 14 cats from Italy with *Ehrlichia* spp. in their blood,[148] 3 cats with *E. canis* in their blood,[151] and 1 cat in the southern United States with *E. chaffeensis* DNA in its blood had no CBC abnormalities.[146] Bone marrow evaluation of cats with cytopenias has revealed primarily hypoplasia of the affected cell line. However, one cat had bone marrow cytologic characteristics consistent with myeloid leukemia.[143] In regions where ticks are abundant, ehrlichiosis should be considered on the differential list for cats with unexplained leukocytosis or cytopenias.

Biochemical abnormalities have been infrequently reported in cats with suspected clinical ehrlichiosis and are nonspecific. Hyperproteinemia was the most consistent abnormality and polyclonal gammopathy was detected in five of the cats assayed by protein electrophoresis.[133,143,150,172] In a separate study, an epidemiologic association was made between monoclonal gammopathy and cats seropositive for *E. canis* antibodies.[153] Based on these results, in tick endemic regions, ehrlichiosis should be on the differential list for cats with hyperglobulinemia.

Cytologic Examination

Microscopic examination of stained blood smears may reveal *Ehrlichia* morulae in mononuclear cells or granulocytes. However, this method of diagnosis is not sensitive and cannot identify the *Ehrlichia* spp. present.

Organism Cultivation

Infection by *Ehrlichia* spp. can be confirmed by cell culture, but this is not routinely used in a clinical setting. Furthermore, not all *Ehrlichia* spp. can be grown in cell culture. Attempts to culture an *Ehrlichia* spp. from cats seropositive to *E. canis* were unsuccessful.[158] An *Ehrlichia*-like organism was isolated from whole blood from domestic cats on monocyte cultures[130] but not from a lioness from Kenya.[131] Although results of PCR assays will likely be used to help further define feline ehrlichiosis, clinicians should assist research laboratories in efforts to obtain feline *Ehrlichia* spp. isolates for comparative microbiologic studies.

Molecular Diagnosis Using Nucleic Acid–Based Testing

PCR assays have been used to successfully diagnose *Ehrlichia* infections in cats through the amplification of a variety of gene targets and comparison of DNA sequences with known *Ehrlichia* species.[132,139–149] The same assays used for dogs can be applied to cat blood and tissue specimens.

Serologic Testing

When antibodies are present, most cats with morulae in mononuclear cells have had antibodies in sera to *E. canis*, as detected using IFA. However, some cats with ehrlichiosis have been seronegative, and thus clinicians may have to obtain convalescent samples to document seroconversion. There has been poor correlation between the detection of *E. canis* DNA and seroreactivity. Of three cats with *E. canis*-like DNA in blood in one study, none had detectable antibodies to *E. canis* by IFA in two different laboratories, even though chronic disease existed.[143] Subsequent studies have examined the combination of serologic and molecular test results for detection of *Ehrlichia* spp. infection in cats.[140–142,146,156] Of eight cats from Brazil that were PCR positive for *E. canis*, six had serum antibodies to *E. canis* by IFA.[141] In another study, 12 of 20 cats that were PCR positive for *E. canis* had antibodies.[140] These results suggest that not all cats seroconvert when infected with *Ehrlichia* spp., that another *E. canis*-like organism that does not induce cross-reacting antibodies is present, or the sensitivity of currently available serologic assays is poor. In another study, five cats with presumed ehrlichiosis had serum antibodies that reacted with *N. risticii* but not to *E. canis*.[175] POC ELISAs designed to detect antibodies reactive to specific *Ehrlichia* spp. peptides are available for testing dog sera. Because these tests do not apply host species-specific conjugate, use of feline sera has been repo rted.[146,163,177] However, cats' immunologic reactivity to diagnostic peptides may differ from that of dogs. For example, one study reported that five cats seroreactive to the *E. canis* p16 peptide were not seroreactive to *E. canis* p30/p31-1 peptides or whole cell antigen from *E. chaffeensis* or *E. canis*.[146] Hence, a diagnosis of feline ehrlichiosis should never be based on positive serologic test results alone. Clinicians should always exclude other potential causes of the clinical syndrome.

Other Testing

Antinuclear antibody test results are positive in some cats with *Ehrlichia* spp. infection.[143] Coombs' test results have generally been negative. Neutrophilic polyarthritis and increased CSF protein concentrations were present in one cat.[143] Lymph node aspirates, when performed, show lymphoid or plasma cell hyperplasia.

Diagnostic Imaging

Of cats with ehrlichiosis that had historical or physical examination findings consistent with respiratory disease, interstitial lung patterns were the only abnormalities reported. Cardiomegaly was reported in two cats with *E. canis*-like DNA in their blood; however, most thoracic and abdominal radiographs were within normal limits.

Pathologic Findings

Before treatment, pyogranulomatous lymphadenitis was detected in a mesenteric lymph node from a cat from Colorado with antibodies against *E. canis* and *N. risticii*.[129] Perivascular plasma cell and lymphocyte infiltrates were detected in the lungs, kidneys, and liver of an untreated lioness in Kenya.[131] After doxycycline treatment in one cat, ARDS developed that was followed by death.[143] Neutrophilic and histiocytic myocarditis and pneumonia, multifocal lymphoplasmacytic nephritis, and multifocal lymphoplasmacytic pancreatitis were the predominant findings. However, *Ehrlichia* spp. or other infectious causes were not identified after death.

TREATMENT AND PROGNOSIS

Treatment of cats with monocytic ehrlichiosis is as recommended for dogs (see Table 44-3). Resolution of illness was seen in three cats following administration of doxycycline at 5 mg/kg, q12hr for 21 days and in one cat after treatment at 10 mg/kg, q24hr for 21 days.[129,173] One cat was seropositive 180 days after discharge but seronegative 1365 days after discharge, and another cat was seronegative 180 days after completing doxycycline therapy. Serologic follow-up was available for multiple presumptive cases in France,[135,136] where most cats became seronegative with time. However, increasing or persistently positive titers can occur as reported for the dog.[178] Imidocarb dipropionate administered at 5 mg/kg, intramuscularly, and repeated in 14 days was followed by resolution of disease in two cats in Kenya.[130] Although not effective in clearing *E. canis*, imidocarb diproprionate has been used for the treatment of infected dogs[161] and has been shown to be safe when administered to cats.[179] Enrofloxacin was used to treat two cats with suspected mononuclear ehrlichiosis[136]; however, this drug is considered to be inferior to tetracyclines for the treatment of ehrlichiosis in dogs.[34,69] The Infectious Disease Study Group of the ACVIM currently recommends treating cats with suspected clinical ehrlichiosis with doxycycline at 10 mg/kg, PO, q24h for a minimum of 28 days.[34] Whether the treatment protocols used to date eliminate the organism is currently unknown.[180,181]

Two cats with morulae in mononuclear cells were euthanized because of treatment failures with tetracycline[4] or doxycycline,[134] and death occurred in another.[143] Thrombocytopenia did not resolve until 7 months after doxycycline treatment in a cat infected with *E. ewingii*.[146]

IMMUNITY AND VACCINATION

Epidemiologic studies of tick-borne diseases in cats document a lower prevalence of *Ehrlichia* infections in cats than in dogs, and fewer tick-borne diseases are diagnosed in cats than in dogs. This may be due to environmental factors (many cats are strictly indoors), shorter periods of tick attachment in cats due to fastidious grooming, decreased testing of cats for vector-borne pathogens by veterinarians, and/or potential differences in canine and feline immune function.[184] Vaccines for feline ehrlichiosis are not available.

PREVENTION

Because routes of transmission for naturally infected cats are unknown, definitive statements concerning prevention cannot be made. Exposure of cats to potential arthropod vectors and ingestion of rodents should be avoided. Several topical ectoparasiticides with activity against ticks are available for cats. However, those with permethrin, deltamethrin, and amitraz cannot generally be used in cats (see Chapter 13), and use of these products should also be avoided on dogs that co-habitate with cats. Isoxazolines have been developed as oral ectoparasiticides and some formulations have been approved for use in cats.[185] *Ehrlichia* spp. can be transmitted by blood transfer, so cats used as blood donors that are in tick-endemic areas should be screened using both serology and PCR and excluded if positive.[184–186]

PUBLIC HEALTH ASPECTS

Human infection with *E. canis* has never been reported in association with cat contact. If cats are housed indoors and arthropod control is maintained, the risk to humans should be minimal. Appropriate precautions should be taken to prevent transmission when handling engorged ticks as well as blood and tissue specimens from infected cats.

CASE EXAMPLES

CANINE EHRLICHIOSIS

Signalment

"Dubi," a 7-year old, male, mixed breed dog from Tel Aviv, Israel.

History

Dubi was brought to the Koret School Veterinary Teaching Hospital, The Hebrew University, because of a 10-day history of lethargy and inappetence. Dubi had been drinking well and there was no history of vomiting or diarrhea. There was a history of exposure to ticks, and no history of trauma. Dubi's diet consisted of a commercial adult dry dog food.

Physical Examination

Body weight: 15.0 kg.

General: Quiet, depressed. T = 103.3°F/39.6°C, HR = 140 beats/minute, panting, mucous membranes pale pink with multiple mucosal petechiae, CRT < 2 seconds. Approximately 5% to 7% dehydrated.

Integument: No clinically significant abnormalities were noted. No ectoparasites were detected.

Musculoskeletal: BCS was 6/9.

Cardiovascular and respiratory systems: No clinically significant findings were present.

GI and urogenital systems: Cranial organomegaly was noted on abdominal palpation. Rectal examination revealed no significant abnormalities.

Lymph nodes: All peripheral lymph nodes were slightly enlarged.

Laboratory Findings

CBC: RBC 5.0 (5.5–8.7 × 10^6 cells/μL), HCT 32.0% (40%–55%), MCV 72 fL (65–75 fL), MCHC 34 g/dL (33–36 g/dL), WBC 9,400 cells/μL (6,000–13,000 cells/μL), neutrophils 6,400 cells/μL (3,000–10,500 cells/μL), lymphocytes 1,100 cells/μL (1,000–4,000 cells/μL), monocytes 1,680 cells/μL (150–1,200 cells/μL), eosinophils 220 cells/μL (0–1,500 cells/μL), basophils 0 cells/μL (0–50 cells/μL), platelets 65,000 platelets/μL (150,000–400,000 platelets/μL), MPV 16.5 fL (7–13 fL).

Serum chemistry profile: Sodium 151 mmol/L (145–154 mmol/L), potassium 4.5 mmol/L (3.6–5.3 mmol/L), chloride 110 mmol/L (108–118 mmol/L), bicarbonate 18 mmol/L (16–26 mmol/L), phosphorus 5.7 mg/dL (3.0–6.2 mg/dL), calcium 10.6 mg/dL (9.7–11.5 mg/dL), BUN 49 mg/dL (5–21 mg/dL), creatinine 1.3 mg/dL (0.3–1.2 mg/dL), glucose 85 mg/dL (64–123 mg/dL), total protein 7.7 g/dL (5.4–7.6 g/dL), albumin 2.4 g/dL (3.0–4.4 g/dL), globulin 4.2 g/dL (1.8–3.9 g/dL), ALT 53 U/L (19–67 U/L), AST 39 U/L (19–42 U/L), ALP 102 U/L (21–170 U/L), creatine kinase 355 U/L (51–399 U/L), GGT 5 U/L (0–6 U/L), cholesterol 255 mg/dL (135–361 mg/dL), total bilirubin 0.2 mg/dL (0–0.2 mg/dL), magnesium 2.4 mg/dL (1.5–2.6 mg/dL).

Urinalysis: SpG 1.022; pH 7.0; no RBC; no WBC.

Imaging Findings

Abdominal ultrasound: The spleen was enlarged with rounded edges and a heterogeneous, hypoechoic parenchyma. Abdominal lymph nodes were slightly enlarged. The liver had normal parenchymal architecture.

Microbiologic Testing

4Dx SNAP test serology (IDEXX Laboratories, ME, USA): Positive for antibodies to *E. canis*. Negative for antibodies to *Anaplasma* spp. and *B. burgdorferi* and negative for *Dirofilaria immitis* antigen.

Vector-borne disease serology (IFA): Positive for antibodies to *E. canis* at 1:1,280.

Vector-borne real-time PCR panel (whole blood): Positive for *E. canis* DNA. Negative for *A. phagocytophilum*, *A. platys*, *Bartonella* spp., *Rickettsia* spp., and *B. burgdorferi* DNA.

Diagnosis

CME, characterized by thrombocytopenia, hypoalbuminemia, hyperglobulinemia, generalized lymphadenopathy, splenomegaly, and mucosal petechiae.

Treatment

Dubi was initially treated with IV crystalloids (lactated Ringer's solution) and doxycycline (10 mg/kg, q24h). The dog was released home with instructions to continue the antibiotic treatment and report to the clinician on Dubi's condition after 72 hours, and to return for a recheck, CBC, and biochemistry panel after 21 days.

Three days later, the owners reported that the dog's attitude and appetite improved. After 21 days, the owners reported that Dubi was bright, alert, responsive, eating, and drinking well. On physical examination, no abnormalities were noted. CBC revealed no hematologic and biochemistry abnormalities. The spleen had returned to a sonographically normal appearance, and the abdominal lymph nodes were markedly reduced in size. Additional serology or follow-up PCR was not performed. He was subsequently lost to follow-up.

FELINE EHRLICHIOSIS[129]

Signalment

"Squirrel," a 10-year old female spayed domestic short-hair cat from Colorado.

History

"Squirrel" was brought to the College of Veterinary Medicine at Colorado State University because of a 2-week history of intermittent fever, anorexia, lethargy, and pain in the lumbar area. The referring veterinarian completed a CBC and serum biochemical analysis and reported abnormalities which included hyperproteinemia (8.9 g/dL; reference range, 5.4–8.4 g/dL), hyperglobulinemia (5.9 g/dL; reference range, 2.9–4.4 g/dL) and hypercholesteremia (263 mg/dL; reference range, 53–217 mg/dL). Serum antibodies for FeLV, FIV, *Toxoplasma gondii*, and FCoV were undetectable. The cat was treated with oral amoxicillin for 7 days with no improvement and then amoxicillin-clavulanic acid and subcutaneous fluids prior to presentation.

Physical Examination

Body weight: 3.1 kg.

General: Listless. T = 102°F (38.9°C), HR = 195 beats/minute, RR = 46 breaths/minute. Approximately 7% dehydrated.

Integument: No clinically significant findings.

Eyes, ears, nose, and throat: No clinically significant findings.

Musculoskeletal: Signs of pain upon palpation of the lumbar area.

Neurologic examination: No clinically significant findings.

Cardiovascular and respiratory systems: No clinically significant findings.

GI and urogenital systems: No clinically significant findings.

Lymph nodes: All peripheral lymph nodes were of normal size.

Laboratory Findings

CBC abnormalities: Normocytic, normochromic nonregenerative anemia: PCV 25%, MCV 43 fL, MCHC 32 g/dL. Neutrophilic leukocytosis: 23,700 nucleated cells/μL and 21,330 neutrophils/μL.

Serum chemistry profile: Hyperglobulinemia 4.6 g/dL (reference range, 2.9–4.4 g/dL)

Serum protein electrophoresis: Increased in β_1 fraction 0.9 g/dL (reference range, 0.23–0.84 g/dL)

Urinalysis: No clinically significant findings.

Cytologic Findings

Paracentesis was performed based on previous findings of fever and nonspecific hyperesthesia and showed a small amount of fluid with a large number of nondegenerate neutrophils, moderate numbers of large mononuclear cells, few eosinophils, and rare small mononuclear cells and basophils.

CASE EXAMPLES—cont'd

Exploratory Laparotomy

Exploratory laparotomy was performed because of concern for peritonitis. A 2- to 4-cm, irregular, raised mass was identified at the ileocecal junction. The liver was a mottled yellow, nutmeg color.

Postsurgical Histology and Cytology

Histopathology of the excised ileocecal mass was reported as inflammatory cell infiltration of a lymph node. The cells were primarily neutrophils and macrophages and a diagnosis of severe pyogranulomatous lymphadenitis was assigned. Liver tissue showed mild multifocal infiltration of bile ducts by neutrophils and lymphocytes and a diagnosis of mild cholangitis was assigned. Impression smears of mesenteric lymph nodes revealed clumps of intracellular gram-negative organisms in mononuclear cells, morphologically similar to *E. canis*.

Microbiologic Testing

All specimens were negative for routine aerobic bacterial culture.

No antibodies to *Chlamydia* spp. were detected (see Chapter 49).

Vector-borne disease serology (IFA): Positive for antibodies to *E. canis* at 1:80 and 1:160, 180 days following discharge. Positive for antibodies to *N. risticii* at 1:40, 180 days following discharge.

Diagnostic Imaging

Abdominal and thoracic radiographs were within normal limits.

Diagnosis

Suspected feline monocytic ehrlichiosis.

Treatment

At the referral hospital, Squirrel was initially treated with with cefoxitin (22 mg/kg, IV, q8h), crystalloids (lactated Ringer's solution), cat food puree administered via a gastrostomy tube. The antibiotic was changed to amoxicillin (22 mg/kg, PO, q12h) 4 days after surgery, upon release to the owner. At reexamination 4 days after release, Squirrel was lethargic and febrile (rectal temperature of 103.6°F). Doxycycline (5 mg/kg, PO, q12h) was administered via the gastrostomy tube. Two days later, the cat's attitude improved and fever was absent; treatment was continued for 21 days. The gastrotomy tube was removed 14 days following discharge and at that time the cat was clinically normal. *E. canis* and *N. risticii* antibody titers were negative 1,365 days after discharge.

Comments

In this cat, while organisms cytologically similar to *E. canis* were visualized and antibodies to *E. canis* detected by IFA, active infection with *E. canis* was not confirmed through culture or molecular testing. Where the cat became infected was unclear, but vector-borne disease testing performed on 17 cats living within a 2 mile radius of the infected cats identified 14 and 9 cats with antibodies to *E. canis* and *N. risticii*, respectively. The rationales for paracentesis and exploratory laparotomy were not completely clear. Two of the seropositive cats had a 2- to 4-month history of malaise and one cat lost weight during this time. All cats were apparently healthy at the time of blood collection and no abnormalities were detected by CBC, serum biochemistry panel, buffy coat films, urinalysis, or serology testing for other infectious agents. The two cats with malaise were treated with doxycycline (5 mg/kg, PO, q24h for 21 days) which was followed by resolution of illness within days after initiation of treatment.

SUGGESTED READINGS

Sainz Á, Roura X, Miró G, et al. Guideline for veterinary practitioners on canine ehrlichiosis and anaplasmosis in Europe. *Parasit Vectors*. 2015;8:75.

Qurollo B. Feline vector-borne diseases in North America. *Vet Clin North Am Small Anim Pract*. 2019;49:687–702.

REFERENCES

1. Donatien A, Lestoquard F. Existence en Algerie d'une Rickettsia du chien. *Bull Soc Pathol Exot*. 1935;28:418–419.
2. Anderson BE, Greene CE, Jones DC, et al. *Ehrlichia ewingii* sp. nov., the etiologic agent of canine granulocytic ehrlichiosis. *Int J Syst Bacteriol*. 1992;42:299–302.
3. Anderson BE, Dawson JE, Jones DC, et al. *Ehrlichia chaffeensis*, a new species associated with human ehrlichiosis. *J Clin Microbiol*. 1991;29:2838–2842.
4. Charpentier F, Groulade P. Probable case of ehrlichiosis in a cat. *Bull Acad Vet France*. 1986;59:287–290.
5. Allsopp MT, Allsopp BA. Novel *Ehrlichia* genotype detected in dogs in South Africa. *J Clin Microbiol*. 2001;39:4204–4207.
6. Hegarty BC, Maggi RG, Koskinen P, et al. *Ehrlichia muris* infection in a dog from Minnesota. *J Vet Intern Med*. 2012;26:1217–1220.
7. Qurollo BA, Davenport AC, Sherbert BM, et al. Infection with Panola Mountain *Ehrlichia* sp. in a dog with atypical lymphocytes and clonal T-cell expansion. *J Vet Intern Med*. 2013;27:1251–1255.
8. Killmaster LF, Levin ML. Isolation and short-term persistence of *Ehrlichia ewingii* in cell culture. *Vector Borne Zoonotic Dis*. 2016;16:445–448.
9. Gettings JR, Self SCW, McMahan CS, et al. Local and regional temporal trends (2013-2019) of canine *Ehrlichia* spp. seroprevalence in the USA. *Parasit Vectors*. 2020;13:153.
10. Fourie JJ, Stanneck D, Luus HG, et al. Transmission of *Ehrlichia canis* by *Rhipicephalus sanguineus* ticks feeding on dogs and on artificial membranes. *Vet Parasitol*. 2013;197:595–603.
11. ABC News. June 2, 2020. https://www.abc.net.au/news/2020-06-03/ehrlichiosis-detected-in-kimberley-dogs/12313052.
12. Harrus S, Waner T. Diagnosis of canine monocytotropic ehrlichiosis (*Ehrlichia canis*): an overview. *Vet J*. 2011;187:292–296.
13. Masala G, Chisu V, Foxi C, et al. First detection of *Ehrlichia canis* in *Rhipicephalus bursa* ticks in Sardinia, Italy. *Ticks Tick Borne Dis*. 2012;3:396–397.
14. Wielinga PR, Gaasenbeek C, Fonville M, et al. Longitudinal analysis of tick densities and *Borrelia*, *Anaplasma*, and *Ehrlichia* infections of *Ixodes ricinus* ticks in different habitat areas in The Netherlands. *Appl Environ Microbiol*. 2006;72:7594–7601.
15. Satta G, Chisu V, Cabras P, et al. Pathogens and symbionts in ticks: a survey on tick species distribution and presence of tick-transmitted micro-organisms in Sardinia, Italy. *J Med Microbiol*. 2011;60:63–68.
16. Sprong H, Fonville M, Docters van Leeuwen A, et al. Detection of pathogens in *Dermacentor reticulatus* in northwestern Europe: evaluation of a high-throughput array. *Heliyon*. 2019;5:e01270.
17. Johnson EM, Ewing SA, Barker RW, et al. Experimental transmission of *Ehrlichia canis* (Rickettsiales: Ehrlichieae) by *Dermacentor variabilis* (Acari: Ixodidae). *Vet Parasitol*. 1998;74:277–288.
18. Beugnet F, Marie JL. Emerging arthropod-borne diseases of companion animals in Europe. *Vet Parasitol*. 2009;163:298–305.
19. Harrus S, Waner T, Aizenberg I, et al. Amplification of ehrlichial DNA from dogs 34 months after infection with *Ehrlichia canis*. *J Clin Microbiol*. 1998;36:73–76.
20. Groves MG, Dennis GL, Amyx HL, et al. Transmission of *Ehrlichia canis* to dogs by ticks (*Rhipicephalus sanguineus*). *Am J Vet Res*. 1975;36:937–940.
21. Ipek NDS, Ozubek S, Aktas M. Molecular evidence for transstadial transmission of *Ehrlichia canis* by *Rhipicephalus sanguineus* sensu lato under field conditions. *J Med Entomol*. 2018;55:440–444.
22. Bremer WG, Schaefer JJ, Wagner ER, et al. Transstadial and intrastadial experimental transmission of *Ehrlichia canis* by male *Rhipicephalus sanguineus*. *Vet Parasitol*. 2005;131:95–105.
23. Harrus S, Kass PH, Klement E, et al. Canine monocytic ehrlichiosis: a retrospective study of 100 cases, and an epidemiological investigation of prognostic indicators for the disease. *Vet Rec*. 1997;141:360–363.

24. Harrus S, Waner T, Keysary A, et al. Investigation of splenic functions in canine monocytic ehrlichiosis. *Vet Immunol Immunopathol.* 1998;62: 15–27.
25. McBride JW, Walker DH. Molecular and cellular pathobiology of *Ehrlichia* infection: targets for new therapeutics and immunomodulation strategies. *Expert Rev Mol Med.* 2011;13:e3.
26. Alves RN, Levenhagen MA, Levenhagen MM, et al. The spreading process of *Ehrlichia canis* in macrophages is dependent on actin cytoskeleton, calcium and iron influx and lysosomal evasion. *Vet Microbiol.* 2014;168:442–446.
27. Waner T, Harrus S, Weiss DJ, et al. Demonstration of serum antiplatelet antibodies in experimental acute canine ehrlichiosis. *Vet Immunol Immunopathol.* 1995;48:177–182.
28. Shropshire S, Olver C, Lappin M. Characteristics of hemostasis during experimental *Ehrlichia canis* infection. *J Vet Intern Med.* 2018;32: 1334–1342.
29. Harrus S, Waner T, Eldor A, et al. Platelet dysfunction associated with experimental acute canine ehrlichiosis. *Vet Rec.* 1996;139:290–293.
30. Mylonakis ME, Koutinas AF, Breitschwerdt EB, et al. Chronic canine ehrlichiosis (*Ehrlichia canis*): a retrospective study of 19 natural cases. *J Am Anim Hosp Assoc.* 2004;40:174–184.
31. Gould DJ, Murphy K, Rudorf H, et al. Canine monocytic ehrlichiosis presenting as acute blindness 36 months after importation into the UK. *J Small Anim Pract.* 2000;41:263–265.
32. Komnenou AA, Mylonakis ME, Kouti V, et al. Ocular manifestations of natural canine monocytic ehrlichiosis (*Ehrlichia canis*): a retrospective study of 90 cases. *Vet Ophthalmol.* 2007;10:137–142.
33. Leiva M, Naranjo C, Pena MT. Ocular signs of canine monocytic ehrlichiosis: a retrospective study in dogs from Barcelona, Spain. *Vet Ophthalmol.* 2005;8:387–393.
34. Neer TM, Breitschwerdt EB, Greene RT, et al. Consensus statement on ehrlichial disease of small animals from the infectious disease study group of the ACVIM (American College of Veterinary Internal Medicine). *J Vet Intern Med.* 2002;16:309–315.
35. Gianopoulos A, Mylonakis ME, Theodorou K, et al. Quantitative and qualitative leukocyte abnormalities in dogs with experimental and naturally occurring acute canine monocytic ehrlichiosis. *Vet Clin Pathol.* 2016;45:281–290.
36. Waner T, Harrus S, Bark H, et al. Characterization of the subclinical phase of canine ehrlichiosis in experimentally infected beagle dogs. *Vet Parasitol.* 1997;69:307–317.
37. Mylonakis ME, Koutinas AF, Billinis C, et al. Evaluation of cytology in the diagnosis of acute canine monocytic ehrlichiosis (*Ehrlichia canis*): a comparison between five methods. *Vet Microbiol.* 2003;91:197–204.
38. Codner EC, Maslin WR. Investigation of renal protein loss in dogs with acute experimentally induced *Ehrlichia canis* infection. *Am J Vet Res.* 1992;53:294–299.
39. Cortese L, Pelagalli A, Piantedosi D, et al. Platelet aggregation and haemostatic response in dogs naturally co-infected by *Leishmania infantum* and *Ehrlichia canis*. *J Vet Med A Physiol Pathol Clin Med.* 2006;53:546–548.
40. Kaewmongkol G, Maneesaay P, Suwanna N, et al. First detection of *Ehrlichia canis* in cerebrospinal fluid from a nonthrombocytopenic dog with meningoencephalitis by broad-range PCR. *J Vet Intern Med.* 2016;30:255–259.
41. Meinkoth JH, Hoover JP, Cowell RL, et al. Ehrlichiosis in a dog with seizures and nonregenerative anemia. *J Am Vet Med Assoc.* 1989;195:1754–1755.
42. Lukács RM, Peters IR, Eminaga S, et al. *Ehrlichia canis* infection in the cerebrospinal fluid of a dog characterized by morulae within monocytes and neutrophils. *Vet Clin Pathol.* 2020;49:470–475.
43. Mylonakis ME, Koutinas AF, Leontides LS. Bone marrow mastocytosis in dogs with myelosuppressive monocytic ehrlichiosis (*Ehrlichia canis*): a retrospective study. *Vet Clin Pathol.* 2006;35:311–314.
44. Mylonakis ME, Day MJ, Siarkou V, et al. Absence of myelofibrosis in dogs with myelosuppression induced by *Ehrlichia canis* infection. *J Comp Pathol.* 2010;142:328–331.
45. Waner T, Harrus S, Jongejan F, et al. Significance of serological testing for ehrlichial diseases in dogs with special emphasis on the diagnosis of canine monocytic ehrlichiosis caused by *Ehrlichia canis*. *Vet Parasitol.* 2001;95:1–15.
46. Qurollo BA, Stillman BA, Beall MJ, et al. Comparison of *Anaplasma* and *Ehrlichia* species–specific peptide ELISAs with whole organism–based immunofluorescent assays for serologic diagnosis of anaplasmosis and ehrlichiosis in dogs. *Am J Vet Res.* 2021;82:71–80.
47. Rikihisa Y, Ewing SA, Fox JC. Western immunoblot analysis of *Ehrlichia chaffeensis, E. canis*, or *E. ewingii* infections in dogs and humans. *J Clin Microbiol.* 1994;32:2107–2112.
48. O'Connor TP, Saucier JM, Daniluk D, et al. Evaluation of peptide- and recombinant protein-based assays for detection of anti-*Ehrlichia ewingii* antibodies in experimentally and naturally infected dogs. *Am J Vet Res.* 2010;71:1195–1200.
49. Qurollo BA, Chandrashekar R, Hegarty BC, et al. A serological survey of tick-borne pathogens in dogs in North America and the Caribbean as assessed by *Anaplasma phagocytophilum, A. platys, Ehrlichia canis, E. chaffeensis, E. ewingii*, and *Borrelia burgdorferi* species-specific peptides. *Infect Ecol Epidemiol.* 2014;4.
50. Harrus S, Alleman AR, Bark H, et al. Comparison of three enzyme-linked immunosorbant assays with the indirect immunofluorescent antibody test for the diagnosis of canine infection with *Ehrlichia canis*. *Vet Microbiol.* 2002;86:361–368.
51. Liu J, Drexel J, Andrews B, et al. Comparative evaluation of 2 in-clinic assays for vector-borne disease testing in dogs. *Top Companion Anim Med.* 2018;33:114–118.
52. Gal A, Loeb E, Yisaschar-Mekuzas Y, et al. Detection of *Ehrlichia canis* by PCR in different tissues obtained during necropsy from dogs surveyed for naturally occurring canine monocytic ehrlichiosis. *Vet J.* 2008;175:212–217.
53. Seaman RL, Kania SA, Hegarty BC, et al. Comparison of results for serologic testing and a polymerase chain reaction assay to determine the prevalence of stray dogs in eastern Tennessee seropositive to *Ehrlichia canis*. *Am J Vet Res.* 2004;65:1200–1203.
54. Faggion S, Salvador A, Jacobino K, et al. Loop-mediated isothermal amplification assay for the detection of *Ehrlichia canis* DNA in blood samples from dogs. *Arch Vet Med.* 2013;45:197–201.
55. Thomson K, Yaaran T, Belshaw A, et al. A new TaqMan method for the reliable diagnosis of *Ehrlichia* spp. in canine whole blood. *Parasit Vectors.* 2018;11:350.
56. de Castro MB, Machado RZ, de Aquino LP, et al. Experimental acute canine monocytic ehrlichiosis: clinicopathological and immunopathological findings. *Vet Parasitol.* 2004;119:73–86.
57. Hildebrandt PK, Huxsoll DL, Walker JS, et al. Pathology of canine ehrlichiosis (tropical canine pancytopenia). *Am J Vet Res.* 1973;34:1309–1320.
58. Mylonakis ME, Harrus S, Breitschwerdt EB. An update on the treatment of canine monocytic ehrlichiosis (*Ehrlichia canis*). *Vet J.* 2019;246:45–53.
59. Breitschwerdt EB, Hegarty BC, Hancock SI. Doxycycline hyclate treatment of experimental canine ehrlichiosis followed by challenge inoculation with two *Ehrlichia canis* strains. *Antimicrob Agents Chemother.* 1998;42:362–368.
60. Eddlestone SM, Diniz PP, Neer TM, et al. Doxycycline clearance of experimentally induced chronic *Ehrlichia canis* infection in dogs. *J Vet Intern Med.* 2007;21:1237–1242.
61. Harrus S, Kenny M, Miara L, et al. Comparison of simultaneous splenic sample PCR with blood sample PCR for diagnosis and treatment of experimental *Ehrlichia canis* infection. *Antimicrob Agents Chemother.* 2004;48:4488–4490.
62. Harrus S, Waner T, Aizenberg I, et al. Therapeutic effect of doxycycline in experimental subclinical canine monocytic ehrlichiosis: evaluation of a 6-week course. *J Clin Microbiol.* 1998;36:2140–2142.
63. Jenkins S, Ketzis JK, Dundas J, et al. Efficacy of minocycline in naturally occurring nonacute *Ehrlichia canis* infection in dogs. *J Vet Intern Med.* 2018;32:217–221.
64. McClure JC, Crothers ML, Schaefer JJ, et al. Efficacy of a doxycycline treatment regimen initiated during three different phases of experimental ehrlichiosis. *Antimicrob Agents Chemother.* 2010;54:5012–5020.

65. Sato M, Veir JK, Shropshire SB, et al. *Ehrlichia canis* in dogs experimentally infected, treated, and then immune suppressed during the acute or subclinical phases. *J Vet Intern Med*. 2020;34:1214–1221.
66. Theodorou K, Mylonakis ME, Siarkou VI, et al. Efficacy of rifampicin in the treatment of experimental acute canine monocytic ehrlichiosis. *J Antimicrob Chemother*. 2013;68:1619–1626.
67. Maurin M, Abergel C, Raoult D. DNA gyrase-mediated natural resistance to fluoroquinolones in *Ehrlichia* spp. *Antimicrob Agents Chemother*. 2001;45:2098–2105.
68. Neer TM, Eddlestone SM, Gaunt SD, et al. Efficacy of enrofloxacin for the treatment of experimentally induced *Ehrlichia canis* infection. *J Vet Intern Med*. 1999;13:501–504.
69. Eddlestone SM, Neer TM, Gaunt SD, et al. Failure of imidocarb dipropionate to clear experimentally induced *Ehrlichia canis* infection in dogs. *J Vet Intern Med*. 2006;20:840–844.
70. Shipov A, Klement E, Reuveni-Tager L, et al. Prognostic indicators for canine monocytic ehrlichiosis. *Vet Parasitol*. 2008;153:131–138.
71. Palacios M, Arteaga R, Calvo G. High-dose filgrastim treatment of nonregenerative pancytopenia associated with chronic canine ehrlichiosis. *Top Companion Anim Med*. 2017;32:28–30.
72. Rudoler N, Baneth G, Eyal O, et al. Evaluation of an attenuated strain of *Ehrlichia canis* as a vaccine for canine monocytic ehrlichiosis. *Vaccine*. 2012;31:226–233.
73. Hess PR, English RV, Hegarty BC, et al. Experimental *Ehrlichia canis* infection in the dog does not cause immunosuppression. *Vet Immunol Immunopathol*. 2006;109:117–125.
74. Tajima T, Rikihisa Y. Cytokine responses in dogs infected with *Ehrlichia canis* Oklahoma strain. *Ann N Y Acad Sci*. 2005;1063:429–432.
75. Unver A, Huang H, Rikihisa Y. Cytokine gene expression by peripheral blood leukocytes in dogs experimentally infected with a new virulent strain of *Ehrlichia canis*. *Ann N Y Acad Sci*. 2006;1078:482–486.
76. Otranto D, Paradies P, Testini G, et al. Application of 10% imidacloprid/50% permethrin to prevent *Ehrlichia canis* exposure in dogs under natural conditions. *Vet Parasitol*. 2008;153:320–328.
77. Jongejan F, Crafford D, Erasmus H, et al. Comparative efficacy of oral administrated afoxolaner (NexGard) and fluralaner (Bravecto) with topically applied permethrin/imidacloprid (Advantix®) against transmission of *Ehrlichia canis* by infected *Rhipicephalus sanguineus* ticks to dogs. *Parasit Vectors*. 2016;9:348.
78. Perez M, Bodor M, Zhang C, et al. Human infection with *Ehrlichia canis* accompanied by clinical signs in Venezuela. *Ann N Y Acad Sci*. 2006;1078:110–117.
79. Ndip LM, Ndip RN, Esemu SN, et al. Ehrlichial infection in Cameroonian canines by *Ehrlichia canis* and *Ehrlichia ewingii*. *Vet Microbiol*. 2005;111:59–66.
80. Bouza-Mora L, Dolz G, Solorzano-Morales A, et al. Novel genotype of *Ehrlichia canis* detected in samples of human blood bank donors in Costa Rica. *Ticks Tick Borne Dis*. 2017;8:36–40.
81. Breitschwerdt EB, Hegarty BC, Hancock SI. Sequential evaluation of dogs naturally infected with *Ehrlichia canis, Ehrlichia chaffeensis, Ehrlichia equi, Ehrlichia ewingii,* or *Bartonella vinsonii*. *J Clin Microbiol*. 1998;36:2645–2651.
82. Dawson JE, Ewing SA. Susceptibility of dogs to infection with *Ehrlichia chaffeensis,* causative agent of human ehrlichiosis. *Am J Vet Res*. 1992;53:1322–1327.
83. Kordick SK, Breitschwerdt EB, Hegarty BC, et al. Coinfection with multiple tick-borne pathogens in a Walker Hound kennel in North Carolina. *J Clin Microbiol*. 1999;37:2631–2638.
84. Murphy GL, Ewing SA, Whitworth LC, et al. A molecular and serologic survey of *Ehrlichia canis, E. chaffeensis,* and *E. ewingii* in dogs and ticks from Oklahoma. *Vet Parasitol*. 1998;79:325–339.
85. Breitschwerdt EB, Hegarty BC, Qurollo BA, et al. Intravascular persistence of *Anaplasma platys, Ehrlichia chaffeensis,* and *Ehrlichia ewingii* DNA in the blood of a dog and two family members. *Parasit Vectors*. 2014;7:298.
86. Gutierrez CN, Martinez M, Sanchez E, et al. Cultivation and molecular identification of *Ehrlichia canis* and *Ehrlichia chaffeensis* from a naturally co-infected dog in Venezuela. *Vet Clin Pathol*. 2008;37:258–265.
87. Yu DH, Li YH, Yoon JS, et al. *Ehrlichia chaffeensis* infection in dogs in South Korea. *Vector Borne Zoonotic Dis*. 2008;8:355–358.
88. Yabsley MJ. Natural history of *Ehrlichia chaffeensis*: vertebrate hosts and tick vectors from the United States and evidence for endemic transmission in other countries. *Vet Parasitol*. 2010;167:136–148.
89. Long SW, Zhang X, Zhang J, et al. Evaluation of transovarial transmission and transmissibility of *Ehrlichia chaffeensis* (Rickettsiales: Anaplasmataceae) in *Amblyomma americanum* (Acari: Ixodidae). *J Med Entomol*. 2003;40:1000–1004.
90. Ndip LM, Ndip RN, Esemu SN, et al. Predominance of *Ehrlichia chaffeensis* in *Rhipicephalus sanguineus* ticks from kennel-confined dogs in Limbe, Cameroon. *Exp Appl Acarol*. 2010;50:163–168.
91. Nair AD, Cheng C, Ganta CK, et al. Comparative experimental infection study in dogs with *Ehrlichia canis, E. chaffeensis, Anaplasma platys* and *A. phagocytophilum*. *PloS One*. 2016;11:e0148239.
92. Stoffel RT, McClure JC, Butcher MM, et al. Experimental infection of *Rhipicephalus sanguineus* with *Ehrlichia chaffeensis*. *Vet Microbiol*. 2014;172:334–338.
93. Zhang XF, Zhang JZ, Long SW, et al. Experimental *Ehrlichia chaffeensis* infection in beagles. *J Med Microbiol*. 2003;52:1021–1026.
94. McGill JL, Wang Y, Ganta CK, et al. Antigen-specific CD4(+)CD8(+) double-positive T cells are increased in the blood and spleen during *Ehrlichia chaffeensis* infection in the canine host. *Front Immunol*. 2018;9:1585.
95. Allison RW, Little SE. Diagnosis of rickettsial diseases in dogs and cats. *Vet Clin Pathol*. 2013;42:127–144.
96. Starkey LA, Barrett AW, Chandrashekar R, et al. Development of antibodies to and PCR detection of *Ehrlichia* spp. in dogs following natural tick exposure. *Vet Microbiol*. 2014;173:379–384.
97. Branger S, Rolain JM, Raoult D. Evaluation of antibiotic susceptibilities of *Ehrlichia canis, Ehrlichia chaffeensis,* and *Anaplasma phagocytophilum* by real-time PCR. *Antimicrob Agents Chemother*. 2004;48:4822–4828.
98. Thomas RJ, Dumler JS, Carlyon JA. Current management of human granulocytic anaplasmosis, human monocytic ehrlichiosis and *Ehrlichia ewingii* ehrlichiosis. *Expert Rev Anti Infect Ther*. 2009;7:709–722.
99. Adamu M, Troskie M, Oshadu DO, et al. Occurrence of tick-transmitted pathogens in dogs in Jos, plateau state, Nigeria. *Parasit Vectors*. 2014;7:119.
100. Kawahara M, Suto C, Rikihisa Y, et al. Characterization of ehrlichial organisms isolated from a wild mouse. *J Clin Microbiol*. 1993;31:89–96.
101. Wen B, Rikihisa Y, Mott J, et al. *Ehrlichia muris* sp. nov., identified on the basis of 16S rRNA base sequences and serological, morphological, and biological characteristics. *Int J Syst Bacteriol*. 1995;45:250–254.
102. Nefedova VV, Korenberg EI, Kovalevskii Iu V, et al. Microorganisms of the order Rickettsiales in taiga tick (*Ixodes persulcatus* Sch.) from the Pre-Ural region. *Vestn Ross Akad Med Nauk*. 2008;47–50.
103. Pritt BS, Sloan LM, Johnson DK, et al. Emergence of a new pathogenic *Ehrlichia* species, Wisconsin and Minnesota, 2009. *N Engl J Med*. 2011;365:422–429.
104. Telford Iii SR, Goethert HK, Cunningham JA. Prevalence of *Ehrlichia muris* in Wisconsin deer ticks collected during the mid 1990s. *Open Microbiol J*. 2011;5:18–20.
105. Pritt BS, Allerdice MEJ, Sloan LM, et al. Proposal to reclassify *Ehrlichia muris* as *Ehrlichia muris* subsp. *muris* subsp. nov. and description of *Ehrlichia muris* subsp. *eauclairensis* subsp. nov., a newly recognized tick-borne pathogen of humans. *Int J Syst Evol Microbiol*. 2017;67:2121–2126.
106. Loftis AD, Reeves WK, Spurlock JP, et al. Infection of a goat with a tick-transmitted *Ehrlichia* from Georgia, U.S.A., that is closely related to *Ehrlichia ruminantium*. *J Vector Ecol*. 2006;31:213–223.
107. Reeves WK, Loftis AD, Nicholson WL, et al. The first report of human illness associated with the Panola Mountain *Ehrlichia* species: a case report. *J Med Case Rep*. 2008;2:139.
108. Loftis AD, Mixson TR, Stromdahl EY, et al. Geographic distribution and genetic diversity of the *Ehrlichia* sp. from Panola Mountain in *Amblyomma americanum*. *BMC Infect Dis*. 2008;8:54.
109. Loftis AD, Kelly PJ, Paddock CD, et al. Panola Mountain *Ehrlichia* in *Amblyomma maculatum* from the United States and *Amblyomma variegatum* (Acari: Ixodidae) from the Caribbean and Africa. *J Med Entomol*. 2016;53:696–698.

110. Yabsley MJ, Loftis AD, Little SE. Natural and experimental infection of white-tailed deer (*Odocoileus virginianus*) from the United States with an *Ehrlichia* sp. closely related to *Ehrlichia ruminantium*. *J Wildl Dis.* 2008;44:381–387.
111. Oliveira LS, Oliveira KA, Mourao LC, et al. First report of *Ehrlichia ewingii* detected by molecular investigation in dogs from Brazil. *Clin Microbiol Infect.* 2009;15(suppl 2):55–56.
112. Little SE, O'Connor TP, Hempstead J, et al. *Ehrlichia ewingii* infection and exposure rates in dogs from the southcentral United States. *Vet Parasitol.* 2010;172:355–360.
113. Beall MJ, Alleman AR, Breitschwerdt EB, et al. Seroprevalence of *Ehrlichia canis, Ehrlichia chaffeensis* and *Ehrlichia ewingii* in dogs in North America. *Parasit Vectors.* 2012;5:29.
114. Liddell AM, Stockham SL, Scott MA, et al. Predominance of *Ehrlichia ewingii* in Missouri dogs. *J Clin Microbiol.* 2003;41:4617–4622.
115. Qurollo BA, Buch J, Chandrashekar R, et al. Clinicopathological findings in 41 dogs (2008–2018) naturally infected with *Ehrlichia ewingii*. *J Vet Intern Med.* 2019;33:618–629.
116. Allerdice ME, Hecht JA, Karpathy SE, et al. Evaluation of Gulf Coast Ticks (Acari: Ixodidae) for *Ehrlichia* and *Anaplasma* species. *J Med Entomol.* 2017;54:481–484.
117. Modarelli JJ, Borst MM, Piccione J, et al. Molecular identification of *Ehrlichia ewingii* in a polyarthritic Texas dog. *Vet Clin Pathol.* 2019;48:96–99.
118. Starkey LA, Barrett AW, Beall MJ, et al. Persistent *Ehrlichia ewingii* infection in dogs after natural tick infestation. *J Vet Intern Med.* 2015;29:552–555.
119. Lashnits E, Grant S, Thomas B, et al. Evidence for vertical transmission of *Mycoplasma haemocanis,* but not *Ehrlichia ewingii*, in a dog. *J Vet Intern Med.* 2019;33:1747–1752.
120. Anziani OS, Ewing SA, Barker RW. Experimental transmission of a granulocytic form of the tribe Ehrlichieae by *Dermacentor variabilis* and *Amblyomma americanum* to dogs. *Am J Vet Res.* 1990;51:929–931.
121. Stockham SL, Tyler JW, Schmidt DA, et al. Experimental transmission of granulocytic ehrlichial organisms in dogs. *Vet Clin Pathol.* 1990;19:99–104.
122. Yabsley MJ, Adams DS, O'Connor TP, et al. Experimental primary and secondary infections of domestic dogs with *Ehrlichia ewingii*. *Vet Microbiol.* 2011;150:315–321.
123. Xiong Q, Bao W, Ge Y, et al. *Ehrlichia ewingii* infection delays spontaneous neutrophil apoptosis through stabilization of mitochondria. *J Infect Dis.* 2008;197:1110–1118.
124. Goodman RA, Hawkins EC, Olby NJ, et al. Molecular identification of *Ehrlichia ewingii* infection in dogs: 15 cases (1997–2001). *J Am Vet Med Assoc.* 2003;222:1102–1107.
125. Goldman EE, Breitschwerdt EB, Grindem CB, et al. Granulocytic ehrlichiosis in dogs from North Carolina and Virginia. *J Vet Intern Med.* 1998;12:61–70.
126. Buller RS, Arens M, Hmiel SP, et al. *Ehrlichia ewingii*, a newly recognized agent of human ehrlichiosis. *N Engl J Med.* 1999;341:148–155.
127. Nichols Heitman K, Dahlgren FS, Drexler NA, et al. Increasing incidence of ehrlichiosis in the United States: a summary of national surveillance of *Ehrlichia chaffeensis* and *Ehrlichia ewingii* infections in the United States, 2008–2012. *Am J Trop Med Hyg.* 2016;94:52–60.
128. Harris RM, Couturier BA, Sample SC, et al. Expanded geographic distribution and clinical characteristics of *Ehrlichia ewingii* infections, United States. *Emerg Infect Dis.* 2016;22:862–865.
129. Bouloy RP, Lappin MR, Holland CH, et al. Clinical ehrlichiosis in a cat. *J Am Vet Med Assoc.* 1994;204:1475–1478.
130. Buoro IB, Atwell RB, Kiptoon JC, et al. Feline anaemia associated with *Ehrlichia*-like bodies in three domestic short-haired cats. *Vet Rec.* 1989;125:434–436.
131. Buoro IBJ, Nyamwange SB, Kiptoon JC. Presence of *Ehrlichia*-like bodies in monocytes of an adult lioness. *Feline Pract.* 1994;22:36–37.
132. Beaufils JP, Breitschwerdt EB, Hancock SI, et al. Ehrlichiose feline: identification genetique de l'agent chez deux chats. *Prat Med Chir Anim Compagnie.* 2002;27:235–238.
133. Beaufils JP, Inokuma H, Martin-Granel J, et al. *Anaplasma platys* (*Ehrlichia platys*) infection in a dog in France: description of the case, and characterization of the agent. *Rev Med Vet.* 2002;153:85–90.
134. Beaufils JP, Martin-Granel J, Jumelle P. *Ehrlichia* infection in cats: a review of three cases. *Prat Med Chir Anim Compagnie.* 1995;30:397–402.
135. Beaufils JP, Martin-Granel J, Jumelle P. Ehrlichiose feline: a propos de deux cas. *Bull Acad Vet France.* 1997;70:73–80.
136. Beaufils JP, Martin-Granel J, Jumelle P, et al. Ehrlichiosis in cats. A retrospective study of 21 cases. *Prati Medi Chir Anim Compagnie.* 1999;34:587–596.
137. Almosny NRP, de Almeida LE, Moreira NS, et al. Ehrlichiose clinica em gato (*Felis catus*). *R Bras Ci Vet.* 1998;5:82–83.
138. Jittapalapong S, Jansawan W. Preliminary survey on blood parasites of cats in Bangkhen District Area. *Kasetsart J/Nat Sci.* 1993;27:330–335.
139. Andre MR, Herrera HM, Fernandes Sde J, et al. Tick-borne agents in domesticated and stray cats from the city of Campo Grande, state of Mato Grosso do Sul, midwestern Brazil. *Ticks Tick Borne Dis.* 2015;6:779–786.
140. Braga IA, dos Santos LG, de Souza Ramos DG, et al. Detection of *Ehrlichia canis* in domestic cats in the central-western region of Brazil. *Braz J Microbiol.* 2014;45:641–645.
141. Braga IA, dos Santos LG, Melo AL, et al. Hematological values associated to the serological and molecular diagnostic in cats suspected of *Ehrlichia canis* infection. *Rev Bras Parasitol Vet.* 2013;22:470–474.
142. Braga Mdo S, Andre MR, Freschi CR, et al. Molecular and serological detection of *Ehrlichia* spp. in cats on Sao Luis Island, Maranhao, Brazil. *Rev Bras Parasitol Vet.* 2012;21:37–41.
143. Breitschwerdt EB, Abrams-Ogg AC, Lappin MR, et al. Molecular evidence supporting *Ehrlichia canis*-like infection in cats. *J Vet Intern Med.* 2002;16:642–649.
144. de Oliveira LS, Mourao LC, Oliveira KA, et al. Molecular detection of *Ehrlichia canis* in cats in Brazil. *Clin Microbiol Infect.* 2009;15(suppl 2):53–54.
145. Georges K, Ezeokoli CD, Newaj-Fyzul A, et al. The application of PCR and reverse line blot hybridization to detect arthropod-borne hemopathogens of dogs and cats in Trinidad. *Ann N Y Acad Sci.* 2008;1149:196–199.
146. Hegarty BC, Qurollo BA, Thomas B, et al. Serological and molecular analysis of feline vector-borne anaplasmosis and ehrlichiosis using species-specific peptides and PCR. *Parasit Vectors.* 2015;8:320.
147. Maia C, Ramos C, Coimbra M, et al. Bacterial and protozoal agents of feline vector–borne diseases in domestic and stray cats from southern Portugal. *Parasit Vectors.* 2014;7:115.
148. Spada E, Proverbio D, Galluzzo P, et al. Molecular study on selected vector-borne infections in urban stray colony cats in northern Italy. *J Feline Med Surg.* 2014;16:684–688.
149. Pedrassani D, Biolchi J, Goncalves LR, et al. Molecular detection of vector-borne agents in cats in Southern Brazil. *Rev Bras Parasitol Vet.* 2019;28:632–643.
150. Guimaraes A, Raimundo JM, Rodrigues RB, et al. *Ehrlichia* spp. infection in domestic cats from Rio de Janeiro State, southeast Brazil. *Rev Bras Parasitol Vet.* 2019;28:180–185.
151. Braga IA, Taques IIGG, Costa JS, et al. *Ehrlichia canis* DNA in domestic cats parasitized by *Rhipicephalus sanguineus* sensu lato (sl) ticks in Brazil-case report. *Brazil J Vet Res Anim Sci.* 2017;54.4:412–415.
152. Lappin MR, Breitschwerdt EB. Unpublished observations. In: *Colorado State University (ML) and North Carolina State University (EB).* 2003.
153. Stubbs CJ, Holland CJ, Reif JS, et al. Feline ehrlichiosis; literature review and serologic survey. *Compend Contin Educ Pract Vet.* 2000;22:307–317.
154. Vita S, Santori D, Aguzzi I, et al. Feline leishmaniasis and ehrlichiosis: serological investigation in Abruzzo region. *Vet Res Commun.* 2005;29(suppl 2):319–321.
155. Ebani VV, Andreani E. Feline ehrlichiosis by *Ehrlichia canis*. Serological survey among cats of Tuscany. *Obiettivi Do Vet.* 2002;23:47–49.
156. Aguirre E, Tesouro MA, Amusategui I, et al. Assessment of feline ehrlichiosis in central Spain using serology and a polymerase chain reaction technique. *Ann N Y Acad Sci.* 2004;1026:103–105.
157. Ayllon T, Diniz PP, Breitschwerdt EB, et al. Vector-borne diseases in client-owned and stray cats from Madrid, Spain. *Vector Borne Zoonotic Dis.* 2012;12:143–150.
158. Ayllon T, Villaescusa A, Tesouro MA, et al. Serology, PCR and culture of *Ehrlichia/Anaplasma* species in asymptomatic and symptomatic cats from central Spain. *Clin Microbiol Infect.* 2009;15(suppl 2):4–5.

159. Ortuno A, Gauss CB, Garcia F, et al. Serological evidence of *Ehrlichia* spp. exposure in cats from northeastern Spain. *J Vet Med B Infect Dis Vet Public Health*. 2005;52:246–248.
160. Solano-Gallego L, Hegarty B, Espada Y, et al. Serological and molecular evidence of exposure to arthropod-borne organisms in cats from northeastern Spain. *Vet Microbiol*. 2006;118:274–277.
161. Matthewman LA, Kelly PJ, Wray K, et al. Antibodies in cat sera from southern Africa react with antigens of *Ehrlichia canis*. *Vet Rec*. 1996;138:364–365.
162. Filoni C, Catao-Dias JL, Bay G, et al. First evidence of feline herpesvirus, calicivirus, parvovirus, and *Ehrlichia* exposure in Brazilian free-ranging felids. *J Wildl Dis*. 2006;42:470–477.
163. Tsachev I, Baymakova M, Zlateva N, et al. Seroprevalence rates of tick-borne pathogens in cats from southern Bulgaria. *Vector Borne Zoonotic Dis*. 2020;20:864–867.
164. Schäfer I, Kohn B, Volkmann M, et al. Retrospective evaluation of vector-borne pathogens in cats living in Germany (2012–2020). *Parasites Vectors*. 2021;14:1–9.
165. Brouqui P, Dumler JS, Raoult D, et al. Antigenic characterization of Ehrlichiae: protein immunoblotting of *Ehrlichia canis, Ehrlichia sennetsu*, and *Ehrlichia risticii*. *J Clin Microbiol*. 1992;30:1062–1066.
166. Dumler JS, Asanovich KM, Bakken JS, et al. Serologic cross-reactions among *Ehrlichia equi, Ehrlichia phagocytophila*, and human granulocytic *Ehrlichia*. *J Clin Microbiol*. 1995;33:1098–1103.
167. Levy JK, Crawford PC, Lappin MR, et al. Infectious diseases of dogs and cats on Isabela Island, Galapagos. *J Vet Intern Med*. 2008;22:60–65.
168. Tabar MD, Altet L, Francino O, et al. Vector-borne infections in cats: molecular study in Barcelona area (Spain). *Vet Parasitol*. 2008;151:332–336.
169. Millan J, Candela MG, Palomares F, et al. Disease threats to the endangered Iberian lynx (*Lynx pardinus*). *Vet J*. 2009;182:114–124.
170. Barrs VR, Beatty JA, Wilson BJ, et al. Prevalence of *Bartonella* species, *Rickettsia felis, haemoplasmas* and the *Ehrlichia* group in the blood of cats and fleas in eastern Australia. *Aust Vet J*. 2010;88:160–165.
171. Lappin MR, Griffin B, Brunt J, et al. Prevalence of *Bartonella* species, *Hemoplasma* species, *Ehrlichia* species, *Anaplasma phagocytophilum* and *Neorickettsia risticii* DNA in the blood of cats and their fleas in the United States. *J Fel Med Surg*. 2006;8:85–90.
172. Beaufils JP. Ehrlichiosis: clinical aspects in dogs and cats. *Compend Contin Educ Pract Vet*. 1997;19:57–61.
173. Albay MK. The first report of ehrlichiosis in a cat in Turkey. *Veteriner Fakültesi Dergisi*. 2016;63:329–331.
174. Bjoersdorff A, Svendenius L, Owens JH, et al. Feline granulocytic ehrlichiosis: a report of a new clinical entity and characterisation of the infectious agent. *J Small Anim Pract*. 1999;40:20–24.
175. Peavy GM, Holland CJ, Dutta SK, et al. Suspected ehrlichial infection in five cats from a household. *J Am Vet Med Assoc*. 1997;210:231–234.
176. Maggi RG, Birkenheuer AJ, Hegarty BC, et al. Comparison of serological and molecular panels for diagnosis of vector-borne diseases in dogs. *Parasit Vectors*. 2014;7:127.
177. Levy SA, O'Connor TP, Hanscom JL, et al. Evaluation of a canine C6 ELISA Lyme disease test for the determination of the infection status of cats naturally exposed to *Borrelia burgdorferi*. *Vet Ther*. 2003;4:172–177.
178. Bartsch RC, Greene RT. Post-therapy antibody titers in dogs with ehrlichiosis: follow-up study on 68 patients treated primarily with tetracycline and/or doxycycline. *J Vet Intern Med*. 1996;10:271–274.
179. Lappin MR, Brewer M, Radecki S. Effects of imidocarb dipropionate in cats with chronic haemobartonellosis. *Vet Ther*. 2002;3:144–149.
180. Iqbal Z, Rikihisa Y. Application of the polymerase chain reaction for the detection of *Ehrlichia canis* in tissues of dogs. *Vet Microbiol*. 1994;42:281–287.
181. Schaefer JJ, Needham GR, Bremer WG, et al. Tick acquisition of *Ehrlichia canis* from dogs treated with doxycycline hyclate. *Antimicrob Agents Chemother*. 2007;51:3394–3396.
182. Day MJ. Cats are not small dogs: is there an immunological explanation for why cats are less affected by arthropod-borne disease than dogs? *Parasit Vectors*. 2016;9:507.
183. Cavalleri D, Murphy M, Seewald W, et al. A randomized, controlled field study to assess the efficacy and safety of lotilaner (Credelio™) in controlling ticks in client-owned cats in Europe. *Parasit Vectors*. 2018;11:411.
184. Hackett TB, Jensen WA, Lehman TL, et al. Prevalence of DNA of *Mycoplasma haemofelis, 'Candidatus* Mycoplasma haemominutum,' *Anaplasma phagocytophilum*, and species of *Bartonella, Neorickettsia*, and *Ehrlichia* in cats used as blood donors in the United States. *J Am Vet Med Assoc*. 2006;229:700–705.
185. Reine NJ. Infection and blood transfusion: a guide to donor screening. *Clin Tech Small Anim Pract*. 2004;19:68–74.
186. Wardrop KJ, Birkenheuer A, Blais MC, et al. Update on canine and feline blood donor screening for blood-borne pathogens. *J Vet Intern Med*. 2016;30:15–35.

45

Anaplasmosis

Jennifer Granick, Michael R. Lappin, Trevor Waner, Shimon Harrus, Mathios E. Mylonakis

KEY POINTS

- Cause: *Anaplasma phagocytophilum* (granulocytic anaplasmosis), *Anaplasma platys* (thrombocytotropic anaplasmosis).
- First Described: First reports of *A. phagocytophilum* infection came from sheep in 1951 (Scotland).[1–3] Canine infection was first reported in the United States (California) in 1982[4] and in domestic cats in 1999.[5] *Anaplasma platys* was first reported in the United States in dogs (Florida) in 1978[6] and in cats in Brazil in 2010.[7]
- Affected Hosts: *Anaplasma phagocytophilum* causes disease in dogs, cats, humans, ruminants (European strains), horses, and camelids. *Anaplasma platys* causes thrombocytopenia in dogs and cats.
- Geographic Distribution: In the United States, *A. phagocytophilum* is most prevalent in the upper midwestern, northeastern, and western states. Infection also occurs throughout continental Europe and the United Kingdom, Asia, and Russia. The organism has been detected in dogs from Africa and South America. *Anaplasma platys* occurs throughout the Americas, Europe, Asia, Australia, the Middle East, and Africa.
- Mode of Transmission: Tick vectors, primarily *Ixodes ricinus-persulcatus* complex ticks transmit *A. phagocytophilum. Rhipicephalus sanguineus* is suspected to be the major vector of *A. platys,* though this remains unconfirmed.
- Major Clinical Signs: The major clinical signs of *A. phagocytophilum* infection are fever, lethargy, inappetence, and lameness due to polyarthritis. Vomiting, diarrhea, cough, and neck pain may occur. Infection by *A. platys* is usually associated with no signs, but fever and lethargy are possible.
- Differential Diagnoses: Major differential diagnoses include other tick-borne diseases (such as ehrlichioses, rickettsioses, Lyme borreliosis, and babesiosis), bartonellosis, leptospirosis, primary immune-mediated disease, and lymphoma.
- Human Health Significance: *Anaplasma phagocytophilum* causes human granulocytic anaplasmosis. Dogs act as sentinels for human infection and may carry unfed ticks to humans on their coats.

ANAPLASMA PHAGOCYTOPHILUM INFECTION

Jennifer Granick, Michael Lappin

ETIOLOGIC AGENT AND EPIDEMIOLOGY

Canine and feline granulocytic anaplasmosis are caused by *Anaplasma phagocytophilum*, a tick-borne, obligately intracellular bacterium belonging to the family Anaplasmataceae. Based on DNA sequencing, the causative agent formerly called *Ehrlichia equi*, *Ehrlichia phagocytophila*, and, in humans, the human granulocytic ehrlichiosis (HGE) agent, was removed from the genus *Ehrlichia* in 2001 and placed into the genus *Anaplasma.*[8] *Anaplasma phagocytophilum* is tropic for granulocytes, primarily infecting neutrophils, where it forms host membrane-enclosed morulae. Ticks that belong to the *Ixodes ricinus-persulcatus* complex are the major vectors for *A. phagocytophilum.*

Rickettsiae of the family Anaplasmataceae are gram-negative, nonmotile, pleomorphic bacteria. They are obligate aerobes and obligate intracellular parasites.[9] All species in the genus *Anaplasma* inhabit cell membrane–derived vacuoles in immature or mature hematopoietic cells of mammalian hosts.[8] *Anaplasma phagocytophilum* preferentially infects cells of the myeloid lineage, predominantly neutrophils and rarely eosinophils.[8] Unlike other gram-negative bacteria, members of the family Anaplasmataceae lack a cell wall, and the absence of a peptidoglycan layer or LPS makes them dependent upon host cholesterol for survival but allows them to closely associate inside cellular inclusions.[9] Replication inside vacuoles results in the formation of morulae, which are basophilic structures detectable by light microscopy typically 1.5 to 2.5 μm (but up to 6 μm) in diameter, within the cytoplasm of granulocytes (Fig. 45.1).[10]

Anaplasma phagocytophilum causes granulocytic anaplasmosis in dogs, humans, horses, and, in Europe, domestic ruminants that include sheep, cattle, goats, and deer. Cats and camelids may also be affected. A variety of wild animal species, which include rodents and deer, act as reservoir hosts. For the midwestern and eastern United States, white-footed mice, the woodland deer mouse, and eastern chipmunks may act as reservoirs. Seroreactivity to *A. phagocytophilum* in white-footed mice in endemic areas of North America ranges from 10.1% to 85%.[11–14] In the western states, dusky-footed woodrats, gray squirrels, and chipmunks have all been implicated as reservoirs, but the dusky-footed woodrat is one of the most extensively exposed species (seroprevalence ranging from 17% to 80%),[15,16] followed by the western gray squirrel (70.7% seroprevalence and 12.1% PCR prevalence).[17] In Europe, bank voles, wood mice, yellow-necked mice, shrews, and roe and red deer are likely reservoirs.[18,19] In addition to mammals, birds likely play a role in the spread of infected ticks. Migratory birds in Europe and North America can be infected with *A. phagocytophilum* and evidence suggests that, in addition to spreading infection, they also can act as reservoirs by transmitting infection to tick larvae that co-feed with infected nymphs.[20,21] Dogs, cats, and humans are accidental hosts and are not important in the transmission of infection to other host species.

The geographic distribution of granulocytic anaplasmosis follows that of the *Ixodes* tick vectors and is expanding as vector ranges change, likely due to climate change (Fig. 45.2). Because *Ixodes* ticks are three-host ticks, and tick-to-tick transmission of *A. phagocytophilum* only occurs transstadially, nymph and adult stages are potential vectors.[8] In

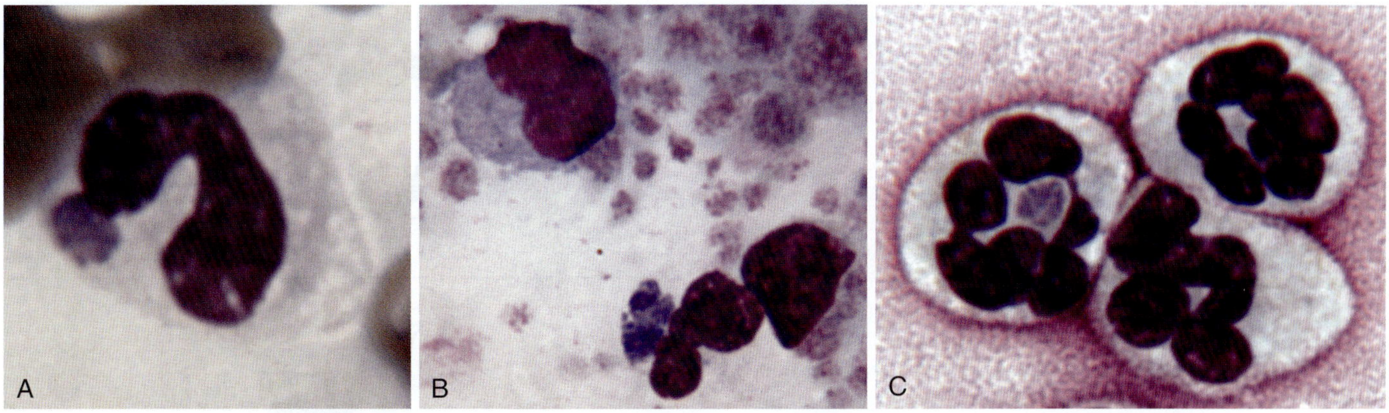

Fig. 45.1 *Anaplasma phagocytophilum* morulae in canine neutrophils. (A) Peripheral blood from a dog. A circular, stippled, deeply basophilic morula is present intracellularly within a band neutrophil. A few erythrocytes are densely clumped in the background (Wright Giemsa, ×100). (B) Buffy coat from a dog. Two abutting, large, circular, stippled, deeply basophilic morulae with irregular borders are present intracellularly within a neutrophil *(lower right)*. A lymphocyte and a monocyte are also present. A large number of platelets are seen in the background, which is expected in buffy coat direct smear preparations (Wright Giemsa, ×100). (C) Synovial fluid from a dog with inflammatory polyarthritis. A circular, stippled, basophilic morula is present intracellularly within a neutrophil *(left)*. Three neutrophils are present on a granular eosinophilic background, which reflects the mucin content of synovial fluid and is expected in such direct smear preparations (Wright Giemsa, ×100). (Courtesy Heather L. Wamsley, University of Florida, Gainesville, FL.)

the northeastern and upper midwestern United States, the tick vector of *A. phagocytophilum* is *Ixodes scapularis*, though recent extension into Ontario, Canada, has been reported.[22] Dispersal of *I. scapularis* ticks by ovenbirds and wood thrushes are responsible for the expanding range of these ticks both west and south.[23] *Ixodes pacificus* is the vector in the western United States. In Europe, the primary vector is *I. ricinus*, and the disease has been described in dogs throughout continental Europe and in the United Kingdom. *Ixodes persulcatus* and *Dermacentor silvarum* ticks transmit the organism in Asia and Russia. Other *Ixodes* spp. ticks have also been implicated in transmission. *Ixodes inopinatus* has been shown to carry *A. phagocytophilum* in Germany, though transmission has not been verified.[24] Evidence of *A. phagocytophilum* infection has been found in dogs from Brazil and Tunisia, and a closely related organism was found in dogs from South Africa.[25–27]

Many strains of *A. phagocytophilum* exist that differ in DNA sequence, geographic distribution, pathogenicity, and host tropism. For example, strains that infect domestic ruminants in Europe and white-tailed deer in the United States appear to be distinct from those that infect horses, humans, and dogs. Phylogenetic analyses have grouped strains into North American and European lineages,[28] though there is heterogeneity among lineages. Further analyses have separated the North American lineage into two clades, upper Midwest and Northeast,[29,30] and the European lineage into three other clades.[25,29] These differences likely have clinical implications. In the Netherlands and Belgium alone, four distinct and geographically separated ecotypes were identified, and only one of these was linked to human disease.[31] Higher morbidity and mortality rates in humans seem to be associated with American strains of *A. phagocytophilum* compared with those in Europe.[2,3] Conversely, in ruminants, *A. phagocytophilum* causes significant mortality in Europe but is considerably less pathogenic in North America.[32–35] There is a significant mismatch at the spatial scale between clinical cases in humans, dogs, and horses in the western United States and infection in the supposed reservoirs.[36] Similarly, the prevalence of strains causing disease in domestic animals and humans is decreased in eastern European locales in which roe deer are present versus those in which red deer predominate.[37] Taken together, these data suggest that multiple distinct *A. phagocytophilum* strains, which differentially infect various mammalian species, could circulate in endemic ecosystems.

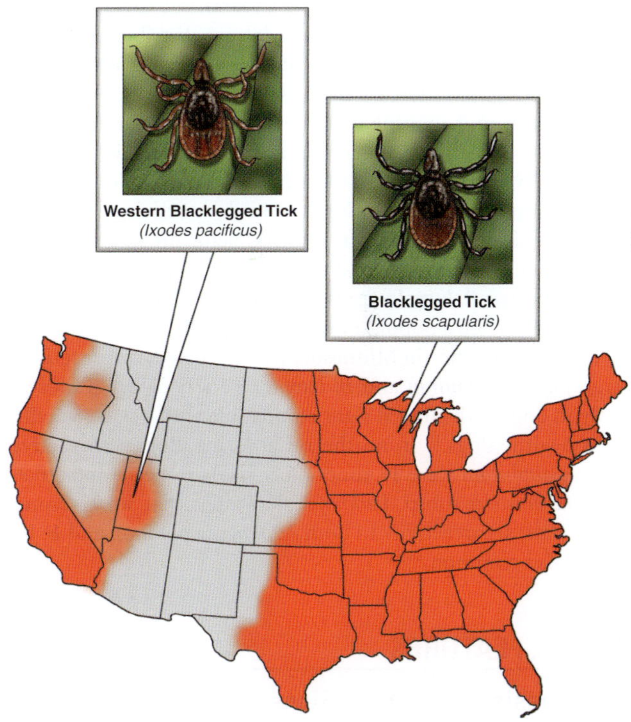

Fig. 45.2 Distribution of *Ixodes scapularis* and *Ixodes pacificus*, the vectors of *Anaplasma phagocytophilum*, in the United States. The distribution of granulocytic anaplasmosis follows that of the tick vectors.

Many seroprevalence studies of dogs and cats have been reported worldwide.[38,39] The seroprevalence varies with geographic location and whether the animals studied were clinically ill or healthy. The prevalence of positive antibody titers in dogs from some regions of Europe and North America exceeds 50%. A study that used a commercially available ELISA assay to determine the prevalence of seroreactivity to *A. phagocytophilum* in more than 400,000 dogs from the United States revealed wide variation in seroprevalence rates, with some counties in the upper midwestern and northeastern United States having seroprevalence rates that exceeded 40%.[40] A 2014 study found that the overall seroprevalence in these regions were 7.1% and 3.9%, respectively.[41] Interestingly, prevalence of seroreactivity to *A. phagocytophilum* in dogs appears to be increasing in some states and decreasing in others, which may reflect changes in ecosystems, testing, or tick prevention.[42] Less data exists for cats, though one study found that 3.7% of healthy cats and 21.7% of clinically ill cats presenting to one practice in Maine were seropositive for *A. phagocytophilum*.[43] In feral cats in the northeastern United States, *A. phagocytophilum* serum antibodies were detected in 17 of 175 cats (9.7%) and specific DNA was amplified from blood of 12 of 175 cats (6.9%).[44] Serologic cross-reactivity with *A. platys* may also influence these data in both dogs and cats, particularly in areas where *Rhipicephalus sanguineus* is endemic.

The seasonal pattern of disease reflects times of peak nymphal and adult tick activities, as well as periods when humans and their dogs are active outdoors. In the western United States, *A. phagocytophilum* infection occurs most frequently in dogs between April and July, when nymphal ticks are abundant. Some infections occur in October, during early questing of adult ticks. In Minnesota and Wisconsin, most cases are diagnosed in late spring (May, June) and fall (October, November).[45–47] In a study from Berlin, most cases occurred between May and September.[48] The median age of clinically affected dogs is 6 to 8 years (range, 6 months to 14 years).[46,47,49,50] In the upper Midwest of the United States, a bimodal age distribution has been recognized, with 25% of dogs 1 year of age or less, and 50% of dogs at least 8 years of age.[46] Affected cats in the northeastern United States have ranged from 4 months to 13 years of age (mean, 3.7 years).[51] Although no breed predispositions are recognized, in one study, golden retrievers comprised almost half of affected dogs; this may reflect the popularity of these dogs for outdoor activities.[52] Infection with other tick-borne pathogens is a risk factor for *A. phagocytophilum* infection. Evidence for co-infection with *Borrelia burgdorferi* is common because *B. burgdorferi* is transmitted by the same *Ixodes* tick species.[40,45,46] When a population of 731 naturally exposed dogs from one veterinary practice in Minnesota was evaluated, seroreactivity to both *A. phagocytophilum* and *B. burgdorferi* was detected more frequently in dogs with clinical signs compatible with tick-borne illness than in healthy dogs.[45] In northern California, dogs seroreactive to *A. phagocytophilum* were 18 times more likely to be seropositive for *Bartonella vinsonii* subsp. *berkhoffii* than dogs that were seronegative.[53] In cats, seroreactivity to both *A. phagocytophilum* and *B. burgdorferi* is also common.[43,44]

CLINICAL FEATURES

Pathogenesis and Clinical Signs

Anaplasma phagocytophilum is transmitted transstadially within the tick (i.e., from larva to nymph to adult), and not transovarially (from adult to egg). Dogs and cats thus become infected after exposure to infected nymphs or adult ticks, which acquire infection when they feed on wild animal reservoir hosts as larvae or nymphs (Fig. 45.3). Ticks must attach for 24 to 48 hours for transmission to occur.[54] Transmission could potentially occur more quickly, as *A. phagocytophilum* can reside in the salivary glands of unfed *Ixodes* spp. ticks.[55] Though the mechanisms of *A. phagocytophilum* entry into the bloodstream are unclear, *in vitro* infection of endothelial cells results in upregulation of cell adhesion molecules and inflammatory mediators

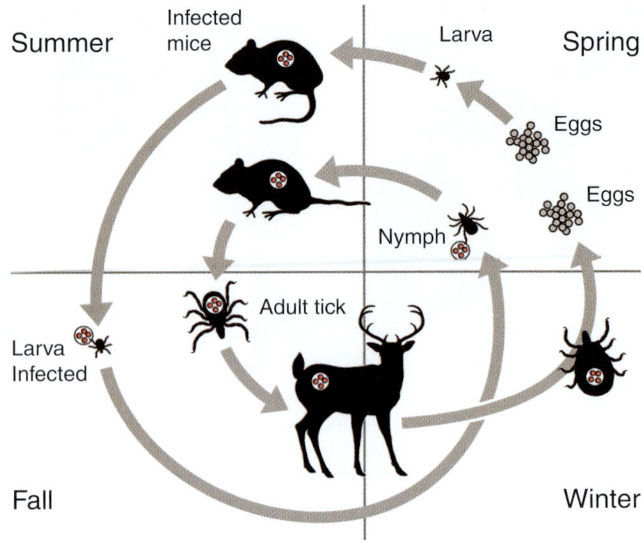

Fig. 45.3 Life cycle of *Ixodes scapularis* ticks and *Anaplasma phagocytophilum* infection. Uninfected larvae (top right) hatch in the late spring and acquire infection from small rodents in the summer. They then overwinter (often in protected mouse burrows) and then molt into nymphs the following spring. The nymphs feed in the late spring or early summer on a variety of animal species including rodents, humans, deer, and dogs. Nymphs molt into adults in the late summer to fall, which subsequently feed on large mammals such as deer, where they mate and drop off. The females then lay eggs and die. Dogs, cats, and humans become infected by nymphs or adult ticks.

that recruit and promote adhesion of neutrophils to the endothelial surface.[56] This may serve as a way for the bacteria to disseminate into the bloodstream. Furthermore, endothelial cells may serve as a reservoir for persistent infection, though this is controversial and may be strain dependent.

Once *A. phagocytophilum* enters the bloodstream, it attaches to the sialylated ligands on the surface of neutrophils, such as P-selectin glycoprotein ligand-1.[38] The organism then enters the neutrophil through caveolae-mediated endocytosis. *Anaplasma phagocytophilum* survives in the harsh neutrophil environment through dysregulation of neutrophil function and by bypassing phagolysosomal pathways. It inhibits neutrophil superoxide production and can reduce neutrophil motility and phagocytosis. *Anaplasma phagocytophilum* also reduces the adherence of infected neutrophils to endothelium and inhibits neutrophil transmigration into tissues, possibly through downregulation of selectin molecule expression.[38] This may promote its survival in peripheral blood. Normally, neutrophils circulate for 10 to 12 hours before they enter tissues and undergo death through apoptosis. *Anaplasma phagocytophilum* delays neutrophil apoptosis, which allows it to survive longer periods of time within the neutrophil.[38] *Anaplasma phagocytophilum* may also infect other cell types, such as bone marrow cells, endothelial cells, and megakaryocytes, although the importance of these cells in the pathogenesis of infection is not clear.

The clinical signs and laboratory abnormalities that occur in dogs and cats with granulocytic anaplasmosis probably vary somewhat in different geographic locations as a result of local strain variation. The vast majority of dogs and cats infected with *A. phagocytophilum* show no clinical signs. Some dogs and cats develop a self-limiting febrile illness, which in dogs occurs after an incubation period of 1 to 2 weeks. Lethargy occurs in almost all clinically affected cats and dogs. Fever and inappetence are also common findings. Lameness, reluctance to move, polydipsia, vomiting, diarrhea, and a soft cough can also occur. Generalized lymphadenopathy and splenomegaly develop as a result of reactive lymphoid hyperplasia and, in the spleen, concurrent extramedullary hematopoiesis.[57] Uncommonly, hemorrhage, manifested as mucosal petechiae, melena, or epistaxis, has been reported in naturally infected dogs, but co-infections with other tick-borne pathogens may contribute to these signs in some dogs.[47,49,50,58] Neurologic signs such as seizures, circling, cervical pain, and decreased placing reactions have been described in a few dogs from the upper Midwest with granulocytic anaplasmosis, but one dog with seizures had a history of idiopathic epilepsy.[47,58] Neurologic signs and detection of the organism in the CSF have been uncommonly reported in humans.[59,60]

Infection with *A. phagocytophilum* results in mild to moderate, and occasionally severe, thrombocytopenia, although other cytopenias may also occur (Table 45.1). The mechanism(s) of these hematologic abnormalities remain unclear. Though *A. phagocytophilum* are able to infect megakaryocytes, platelet production is not affected.[61] Antiplatelet antibodies occur in serum from humans and dogs with granulocytic anaplasmosis,[49,62] suggesting the possibility of immune-mediated mechanisms of thrombocytopenia. However, thrombocytopenia occurs in acute disease, before antibodies are noted, so other mechanisms may be important. Platelet destruction or consumption might be involved in the observed thrombocytopenia, as the bone marrow of infected dogs shows megakaryocyte hyperplasia.

Impaired neutrophil function as a result of *A. phagocytophilum* infection may predispose to development of secondary opportunistic infections or influence the outcome of co-infections with other tick-borne pathogens such as *B. burgdorferi*. Although uncommon, opportunistic infections have been occasionally documented in humans and dogs with granulocytic anaplasmosis and are well recognized in small ruminants.[63]

Infection with *A. phagocytophilum* appears to be self-limiting in many infected dogs and cats, with minimal fatality. Whether persistence of infection and chronic disease manifestations exist is controversial and may be dependent on the infecting strain and host immune response to infection. In one study, prednisolone treatment of three dogs that were experimentally inoculated with a Swedish strain of *A. phagocytophilum*, up to 6 months after infection was followed by the development of positive PCR results for the organism and, in some dogs, thrombocytopenia and reappearance of morulae on blood smears.[64] None of these dogs were treated with doxycycline. In another study, six dogs were inoculated with *A. phagocytophilum* via ticks harvested in the northeastern United States.[65] Prednisolone administration did not result in reactivation of infection regardless of whether or not the dogs were treated with doxycycline prior to immunosuppression. However, one dog's blood was positive for *A. phagocytophilum* via PCR 24 weeks after inoculation. Persistent infection is not recognized in humans,[66] and there is little evidence for persistent infection in naturally infected dogs; thus, the clinical significance of these experimental findings remains unclear.

Physical Examination Findings

The most common findings on physical examination in dogs include lethargy, fever (up to 106.7°F [41.5°C]), dehydration, tachypnea, mild peripheral lymphadenopathy, and splenomegaly.[38,61] Scleral injection in dogs and conjunctivitis in cats may be noted. Lameness, reluctance to move, swollen joints, and pain on joint manipulation may also be detected in some dogs. Increased lung sounds, abdominal pain, diarrhea, epistaxis, petechial hemorrhages, and neurologic signs such as circling, cervical pain, and decreased placing reactions occur uncommonly.

Physical examination findings reported in cats have been similar to those described in dogs, and include fever, lethargy, tachypnea, increased lung sounds, mild abdominal pain, hepatomegaly, splenomegaly, vomiting, ataxia, hyperesthesia, muscle and joint pain, lameness, conjunctivitis, and ocular discharge.[39,51,67–69]

DIAGNOSIS

Laboratory Abnormalities

Granulocytic anaplasmosis should be suspected in dogs and cats with acute febrile illness and thrombocytopenia that reside in endemic areas, regardless of tick exposure history. Diagnosis relies on detection of morulae within granulocytes, results of acute and convalescent serology, or molecular testing using PCR assays. The diagnostic criteria for confirmed human granulocytic anaplasmosis are clinical signs and laboratory findings suggestive of granulocytic anaplasmosis together with: (1) a fourfold rise in antibody titer to *A. phagocytophilum*; (2) presence of *A. phagocytophilum* antigen in tissue via immunofluorescence; (3) a positive PCR test result using specific *A. phagocytophilum* primers; or (4) isolation of *A. phagocytophilum* from blood.[66] Consistent clinical signs along with either detection of morulae in the blood or a single positive antibody titer of ≥ 640 is considered supportive of, but not diagnostic for, infection.[66] These criteria could also be applied to dogs. The use of multiple diagnostic modalities may be needed to confirm the diagnosis of granulocytic anaplasmosis in some dogs and cats.

TABLE 45.1 Hematologic Abnormalities in 10 Dogs with Granulocytic Anaplasmosis in Minnesota[a]

Test	Reference Range	Median	Range	Number Below Reference Range	Number Within Reference Range	Number Above Reference Range
Hematocrit (%)	37.5–60.3	39.8	34.7–48.9	3	7	0
Neutrophils (cells/μL)	2,100–11,200	6,180	2,870–7,540	0	10	0
Band neutrophils (cells/μL)	0–130	40	0–160	0	9	1
Monocytes (cells/μL)	0–1,200	150	0–490	0	10	0
Lymphocytes (cells/μL)	780–3,360	370	190–910	9	1	0
Eosinophils (cells/μL)	0–1,200	0	0	0	10	1
Platelets (cells/μL)	129,000–395,000	73,000	35,000–166,000	9	1	0

[a]Diagnosis was based on compatible clinical signs and morulae within circulating neutrophils.

Complete Blood Count

Thrombocytopenia occurs in approximately 90% of dogs with granulocytic anaplasmosis.[46,47,49,50,70] The platelet count in thrombocytopenic dogs is often mild to moderately decreased, though can occasionally be as low as 5,000 platelets/μL (see Table 45.1).[46,47,49,50,70] In one study of 54 thrombocytopenic dogs with PCR-confirmed granulocytic anaplasmosis, 39% had severe thrombocytopenia, with platelet counts below 30,000/μL.[70] The majority of affected dogs are lymphopenic, but lymphocytosis can occur.[47,49,50] Circulating reactive lymphocytes may be present. Anemia is common and typically mild and nonregenerative. In one study, a direct Coombs test was positive in 17% of dogs tested, suggesting a possible immune-mediated component to anemia in some dogs.[70] Both neutrophilia and neutropenia occur, but most dogs have neutrophil counts that lie in the lower half of the reference range. Low numbers of band neutrophils, as well as mild neutrophil toxicity, are often present. Monocytopenia or monocytosis can occur.[47,49,50] Cytologic examination of blood smears often reveals morulae within granulocytes (Fig. 45.4). Morulae were detected in neutrophils from 36%, 56%, 67%, and 100% of dogs in four respective case series.[47,49,50,52] Morulae appear as early as 4 days after experimental inoculation of dogs, well before seroconversion, and persist for 4 to 8 days.[57] The morulae are indistinguishable from those of *Ehrlichia ewingii*, so serology or PCR assays are needed to confirm *A. phagocytophilum* infection.

Presence of thrombocytopenia in cats with PCR-confirmed granulocytic anaplasmosis is variable and moderate in severity when it occurs. In two reports from the northeastern United States, 2 of 5 cats and 7 of 16 cats had thrombocytopenia at the time *A. phagocytophilum* DNA was amplified from blood.[69,71] In cats infected with *A. phagocytophilum* and *B. burgdorferi* after infestation with *I. scapularis* wild caught ticks from Rhode Island, lymphopenia was the only significant CBC finding. In one study of 16 cats, lymphopenia was detected in 7 of 11 cats with CBC results available for review.[71] In the same 11 cats, morulae were detected in neutrophils of three cats.

Serum Biochemical Tests

The most frequent serum biochemistry finding in dogs with granulocytic anaplasmosis is mild to moderate hypoalbuminemia (Table 45.2). Mild hyperglobulinemia, mild electrolyte abnormalities (hypokalemia, hyponatremia, and metabolic acidosis), and a mild increase in the activities of serum ALP and to a lesser extent ALT may occur.[47,50,52,61,70] Abnormalities in serum biochemical panel results from experimentally or naturally infected cats are uncommon.[39,69,71,72]

Urinalysis

Urinalysis in dogs with granulocytic anaplasmosis may reveal isosthenuria, hyposthenuria, and proteinuria. Increased urine protein-to-creatinine ratios were reported in two affected dogs from the United States (1.5 and 2.2),[61] but there is no evidence that *A. phagocytophilum* infection causes severe glomerulonephritis in dogs. Proteinuria was detected by dipstick in 2 of the 4 naturally infected cats tested in one report of 16 cases.[71]

Synovial Fluid Analysis

Dogs with granulocytic anaplasmosis can develop neutrophilic polyarthritis. In one study, 13 of 63 dogs had clinical signs and physical examination findings of lameness and 3 had synovial fluid cytologic findings consistent with immune-mediated polyarthritis.[70] Cytologic examination of synovial fluid in these dogs revealed increased numbers of nondegenerate neutrophils. In some affected dogs, morulae are found within these cells and the synovial fluid can be PCR positive (Fig. 45.4C).[70]

Diagnostic Imaging

Plain Radiography

Thoracic radiographs are usually normal in dogs with granulocytic anaplasmosis but may show a mild interstitial infiltrate. Focal alveolar infiltrates occur as well.[73]

Sonographic Findings

Abdominal ultrasound may reveal splenomegaly, with a hypoechoic spleen, or mild abdominal lymphadenomegaly.

Microbiologic Tests

Diagnostic assays available for anaplasmosis in dogs and cats are shown in Table 45.3.

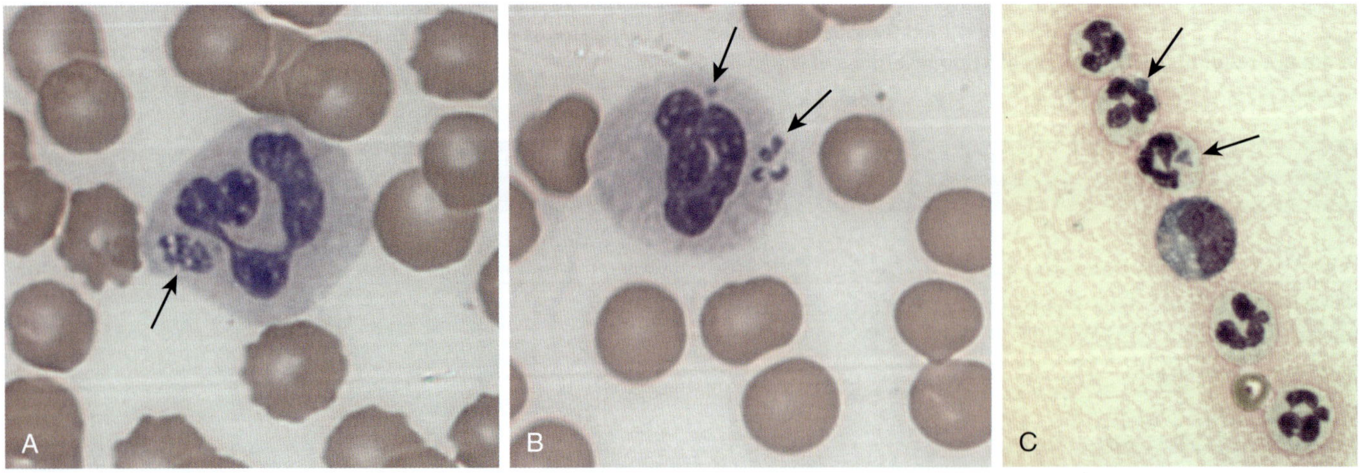

Fig. 45.4 (A) Intracytoplasmic morula and (B) cocci of *Anaplasma phagocytophilum (arrows)* within the neutrophils of an 8-year-old male neutered golden retriever with granulocytic anaplasmosis. (C) Morulae (*arrows*) are present in neutrophils within the synovial fluid of a 5-year-old curly-coated retriever that had polyarthritis.

TABLE 45.2 Findings on Serum Biochemistry Analysis in 10 Dogs with Granulocytic Anaplasmosis in Minnesota[a]

Test	Reference Range	Median	Range	Number Below Reference Range	Number Within Reference Range	Number Above Reference Range
Sodium (mmol/L)	145–153	144	137–147	8	2	0
Potassium (mmol/L)	3.6–5.3	4.0	3.7–4.4	0	10	1
Bicarbonate (mmol/L)	15–25	18.5	14.7–20.0	1	9	0
Albumin (g/dL)	2.7–3.7	2.8	2.1–3.5	3	7	0
Globulin (g/dL)	1.7–3.5	3.5	3.3–4.5	0	5	5
Total bilirubin (mg/dL)	0–0.3	0.2	0.2–0.3	0	10	0
Alanine aminotransferase (U/L)	22–92	43	17–97	3	6	1
Alkaline phosphatase (U/L)	8–139	107	30–544	0	8	2

[a]Diagnosis was based on compatible clinical signs and morulae within circulating neutrophils.

Serologic Diagnosis

Diagnosis of granulocytic anaplasmosis can be accomplished with acute and convalescent serology. Many veterinary laboratories perform serologic testing using IFA techniques. IgG antibodies are first detectable approximately 8 days after exposure, 2 to 5 days after morulae appear. As a result, early in the course of illness, antibodies may be undetectable. PCR assays may be more useful for diagnosis of acute infection in the absence of detectable morulae. Because positive titers can reflect previous exposure, demonstration of a fourfold rise in titer is required. Antibody titers may persist for many months.[52,64] In some human patients, antibody titers have persisted as long as 3 years.[63] In the United States, a silicon disc-based ELISA assay is available commercially for detection of antibodies to *A. phagocytophilum* (Accuplex 4, Antech Diagnostics, Irvine, CA, USA). The performance of this assay when compared with IFA requires further study. An in-clinic lateral-flow ELISA device (SNAP 4Dx Plus, IDEXX Laboratories, ME, USA), which uses a recombinant Msp2/p44 protein, is also available for the detection of antibodies to *Anaplasma* species in dog serum. Positive results obtained with these ELISA assays do not imply that *A. phagocytophilum* is the cause of illness, and as with IFA testing, negative results can occur in dogs with acute illness due to the lag in antibody production relative to the onset of clinical signs.

Serologic cross-reactivity between *Anaplasma* species occurs. Dogs infected with *A. platys* also seroreact to *A. phagocytophilum* antigen; this includes the recombinant Msp2 assay.[40] Serologic cross-reactivity between *A. phagocytophilum* and *Ehrlichia canis* also occurs, but is relatively uncommon and minor.[50,73,74] Dogs diagnosed with granulocytic anaplasmosis that have antibodies to *A. phagocytophilum* generally lack antibodies to *E. canis* using IFA testing.[38,40]

While not approved by the USDA for use with feline serum, one commercially available device (SNAP 4Dx Plus, IDEXX Laboratories, ME, USA) has been shown to detect *A. phagocytophilum* and *B. burgdorferi* antibodies in sera from naturally exposed and experimentally infected cats.[43,72] Antibodies against *A. phagocytophilum* in feline sera can also be detected by IFA.

Molecular Diagnosis Using Nucleic Acid–Based Testing

Several endpoint and real-time PCR assays for *A. phagocytophilum* exist for detection of *A. phagocytophilum* DNA in peripheral blood, buffy coat, bone marrow, or splenic tissue. These can be useful for early diagnosis of granulocytic anaplasmosis in dogs and cats. The sensitivity and specificity of PCR assays may vary depending on the assay design and the laboratory used. Most, but not all, assays detect either the 16S rRNA gene or the outer surface protein gene *msp2* (p44). Assays that detect the *msp2* gene are usually specific for *A. phagocytophilum*, whereas assays that detect the 16S rRNA gene may detect other *Anaplasma* species, and even other bacteria. *Anaplasma phagocytophilum* DNA has occasionally been amplified from healthy dogs, so results must be interpreted in light of the clinical signs.[45] In experimentally infected dogs, whole-blood PCR becomes positive several days before and after morulae appear on blood smears.[57,64]

In cats that are experimentally infected with *A. phagocytophilum* and *B. burgdorferi* following *I. scapularis* infestation, DNA can be amplified from blood up to 2 weeks before detection of antibodies.[72] This has also been documented in some field cases.[69]

Culture

Anaplasma phagocytophilum can be isolated in human promyelocytic leukemia cell lines (HL-60) and tick embryo cell lines. Culture is highly sensitive for diagnosis of acute infection in human patients,[75] but it is not routinely used in dogs for diagnostic purposes because it requires special facilities, technical expertise, and prolonged incubation.

Pathologic Findings

Little information is available regarding the pathology of granulocytic anaplasmosis in dogs or cats. Tissue injury appears to result from the host inflammatory response, rather than the bacterial infection itself.[76] In humans, splenic lymphoid depletion, macrophage aggregates and apoptosis within the liver, paracortical lymphoid hyperplasia, and hemophagocytic cells within reticuloendothelial tissues have been described.[77]

TREATMENT AND PROGNOSIS

The treatment of choice for granulocytic anaplasmosis in dogs and cats is doxycycline (5 mg/kg, PO, q12h).[39,78] In 16 naturally infected dogs, doxycycline therapy for 28 days resulted in clinical resolution in all dogs, and all dogs were negative by molecular testing of blood 1 and 2 months after initiation of therapy.[78] The optimum duration of

TABLE 45.3 Diagnostic Assays Available for Anaplasmosis in Dogs and Cats

Assay	Specimen Type	Target	Performance
Cell culture	Whole blood	*Anaplasma phagocytophilum*; *Anaplasma platys* cannot be cultured	Not widely offered or utilized for routine diagnostic purposes. Requires several weeks' incubation.
Cytology	Whole blood, buffy coat smears, body fluids, tissue aspirates	*A. phagocytophilum* or *A. platys* morulae	Low sensitivity (especially for *A. platys* infection). Morulae of *A. phagocytophilum* cannot be distinguished from those of *Ehrlichia ewingii*. Morulae may be confused with cytoplasmic granules or stain precipitate.
IFA serology	Serum	Antibodies to *Anaplasma* spp.	Acute and convalescent serology is required for diagnosis of acute infection, because initial results may be negative in dogs with acute disease and positive results may reflect previous exposure rather than active infection. Cross-reactivity occurs between *Anaplasma* spp.
ELISA serology	Serum	Antibodies to *Anaplasma* spp. antigens	Rapid, inexpensive, can be performed as an in-practice test. Similar limitations as IFA. Lack of quantitation limits ability to document seroconversion.
PCR	Whole blood, splenic or lymph node aspirates, bone marrow aspirates, buffy coat specimens, tissue specimens	*A. phagocytophilum* or *A. platys* DNA	Confirms active infection. Sensitivity and specificity may vary depending on assay design and specimen type. Because healthy animals may be PCR positive, positive PCR results must be interpreted in light of the clinical signs.

ELISA, enzyme-linked immunosorbent assay; *IFA*, immunofluorescent antibody; *PCR*, polymerase chain reaction.

therapy is unknown, but 2 weeks appears to be sufficient. The prognosis is excellent. Most dogs show clinical improvement within 24 to 48 hours of treatment, although some dogs require more than 1 week of treatment before clinical signs resolve.[46,50,78] Platelet counts often normalize 2 to 14 days after treatment is initiated, though in one study 4/16 dogs remained thrombocytopenic after a 4-week course of doxycycline.[46,78] In one study, 30% of 23 owners reported that their dog returned to normal activities in 1 to 2 days after treatment was initiated, 30% reported this took 3 to 5 days, 21% reported this took 1 to 3 weeks, and 17% reported that it took 1 month or longer for their dogs to return to normal activity.[46] Death due to granulocytic anaplasmosis has not been described in dogs or cats. Intravenous crystalloid fluids and antiemetics may be required for supportive care until clinical signs improve.

IMMUNITY AND PREVENTION

The immune response to *A. phagocytophilum* infection is not fully characterized. Both humoral and cell-mediated immune responses appear to be important in clearance of infection. Host cytokines such as IFN-γ may play a role in the initial control of *A. phagocytophilum* infection[79,80] but may also contribute to the inflammatory process associated with disease.[81] In lambs, *A. phagocytophilum* evades the host immune response through differential expression of MSP2, an outer surface protein involved in immune recognition.[82] Variation in MSP2 also occurs in chronically infected woodrats.[83] Further research is required to document whether persistence occurs through similar mechanisms in other host species. It is possible that recovery from natural infection confers long-term protection against development of disease. Reinfection has not been reported in dogs, but was described in one human patient.[84]

A vaccine for granulocytic anaplasmosis is not available for companion animals. There is one study of cats experimentally infested with *A. phagocytophilum* and *B. burgdorferi* containing ticks from Rhode Island, twice, 6 months apart.[85] In that study, repeated infection was documented in one of the four cats with primary *A. phagocytophilum* infection, suggesting that immunity against the agent was not permanent.

Infection may be prevented by avoidance of tick exposure, prompt tick removal, and use of topical ectoparasiticides (see Chapter 13). Although not a guaranteed protection, combinations of topical imidacloprid and permethrin; or fipronil, amitraz, and (*S*)-methoprene; and imidacloprid and flumetrin prevent transmission of *A. phagocytophilum* to dogs from infected ticks.[86–88]

PUBLIC HEALTH ASPECTS

Anaplasma phagocytophilum infection was first recognized in humans in the upper Midwest of the United States in the early 1990s and has since been increasingly recognized in humans from the United States, Europe, and Asia. Men are affected slightly more frequently than women. In Europe, the disease is most commonly reported in Sweden and Slovenia, where it was first reported in 1997, and those involved in forestry, hunting, farming, and veterinary care are at most risk.[89,90] Morulae are observed less often in humans with granulocytic anaplasmosis in Europe, and the disease may be milder than that described in humans from the United States.

Human granulocytic anaplasmosis closely resembles the disease in dogs, which has been described as an "influenza-like illness after a tick bite."[91] The most common clinical signs reported in human patients are myalgia, headache (which is often severe), malaise, and chills. Anorexia, nausea, arthralgias, and cough may also occur.[66,91,92] The disease typically resolves within 2 months in the absence of appropriate antibiotic treatment. Occasionally, more severe disease may occur. In one study, up to 17% of affected humans required admission to an intensive care unit.[91] Death occurs in 1% or fewer clinically affected humans, usually as a result of complications such as a septic or toxic shock–like syndrome, respiratory insufficiency, opportunistic fungal or viral infections, rhabdomyolysis, acute renal failure, hemorrhage, or neurologic disease.[66] Severe illness tends to occur in humans of advanced age or with concurrent immunosuppressive illness or drug therapy. Peripheral blood neutrophils containing morulae are present in 80% of cases, though only a low number of neutrophils may be infected.[91] Laboratory testing of peripheral blood typically reveals normal or slightly decreased white blood cell and platelet counts, sometimes with a neutrophilic left shift, and mild to moderate elevation of hepatic transaminase activities. In the United States, the disease is reportable to the CDC. Dogs act as sentinels for human exposure and may be a source of infection through mechanical carriage of infected ticks to humans.[93,94] Blood from affected dogs should be handled with caution, needle-stick injuries should be avoided, and precautions should always be taken when performing necropsies on an animal with suspected *A. phagocytophilum* infection.

ANAPLASMA PLATYS INFECTION

Trevor Waner, Shimon Harrus, Mathios Mylonakis

ETIOLOGIC AGENT AND EPIDEMIOLOGY

Anaplasma platys (previously *Ehrlichia platys*), is the cause of infectious canine cyclic thrombocytopenia (ICCT). The disease was first described by Harvey *et al.* in the United States in 1978[6] and since then it has been reported worldwide.[95] *Anaplasma platys* is an obligatory intracellular rickettsial organism which has a tropism for platelets (Figs. 45.5 and 45.6). To date, the organism has not been cultivated *in vitro*. The reclassification of the organism in 2001 as *Anaplasma* was based on nucleotide sequences of the heat shock protein gene (*groEL*), the heat shock operon (*groESL*), and the citrate synthase gene (*gltA*).[8]

Based on the identification of *A. platys* DNA in *Rh. sanguineus* (the brown dog tick) from different regions of the world, and the molecular evidence for transstadial transmission by *Rh. sanguineus* sensu lato, it is most likely that *A. platys* is transmitted by this tick species.[96,97] One study from Thailand identified *A. platys* DNA in *Dermacentor auratus* ticks from dogs.[98] Notwithstanding, no evidence was present that this tick species could potentially transmit the organism to dogs. The possibility that *D. auratus* ticks may have passively ingested *A. platys* while feeding on infected dogs is more likely.

Recent studies have suggested that vertical transmission of *A. platys* from pregnant bitches to their offspring (maternal transmission), during the first half of gestation, might occur.[99,100]

Although the disease has been identified as a disease of dogs, there is growing evidence that *A. platys* can infect a number of other animal species. Molecular evidence has identified the possibility of infection of cats with *A. platys*.[7,101] In both reports, the cats were thrombocytopenic. One of the cats had anorexia and inclusion bodies were observed in platelets.[7] In Portugal, *A. platys* has been reported in dogs, ticks, and red foxes, and recently in red deer and wild boars.[102] Other animals reported to be infected with *A. platys* include Bactrian camels in Xinjiang, China[103]; Arabian camels (*Camelus dromedarius*) in Tunisia[104]; and cattle in Algeria.[105] The ability of *A. platys* to cause disease in these host species has not been established. The importance of these findings lies in the possibility that these animals may serve as a reservoir for *A. platys*.

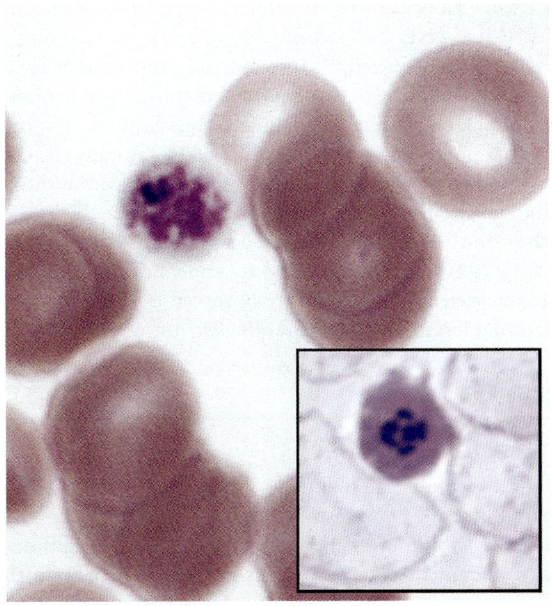

Fig. 45.5 *Anaplasma platys* in a platelet from a dog with infectious cyclic thrombocytopenia (Giemsa stain, ×2500). *Insert*, platelet containing morula of *A. platys* (new methylene blue, ×2300).

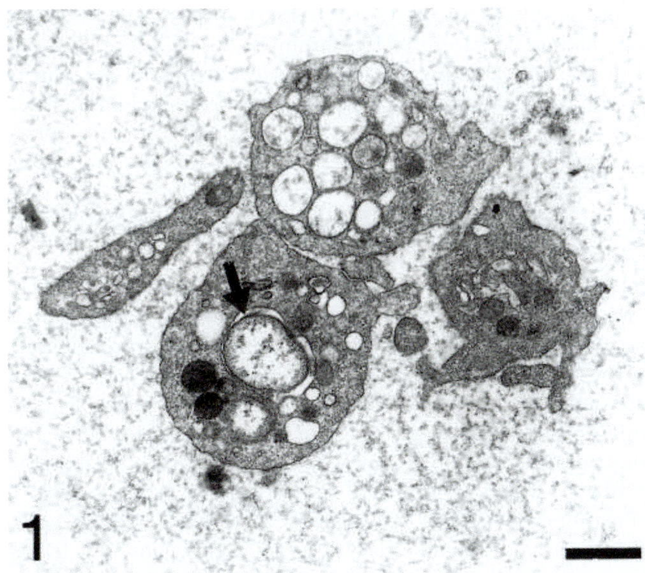

Fig. 45.6 Transmission electron micrograph of a platelet containing *Anaplasma platys* (arrow). The specimen examined was a peripheral blood platelet concentrate collected from a dog on day 18 after experimental infection. Bar = 1 µm. (From Arraga-Alvarado C, Palmar M, Parra O, Salas P. Ehrlichia platys (Anaplasma platys) in Dogs from Maracaibo, Venezuela: An Ultrastructural Study of Experimental and Natural Infections. *Veterinary Pathology*. 2003;40(2):149–156.)

CLINICAL FEATURES

Pathogenesis and Clinical Signs

There is some evidence that a variation in the virulence and pathogenesis of different *A. platys* strains exists between the United States and Australia compared with countries bordering the Mediterranean basin, suggesting that *A. platys* strains from the latter geographic locations are more pathogenic.[106] Co-infection with other vector-borne pathogens, which can modify or even exacerbate clinical signs, may also influence disease severity.[107] Increased intraoperative hemorrhage was described in dogs co-infected with *A. platys* and *E. canis*,[107] but this more likely reflects the influence of *E. canis*, which is the more pathogenic rickettsial species.

Dogs with milder forms of infection may show minimal clinical signs such as fever and hematochezia; rarely more severe clinical signs have been recognized.[108] These include anorexia, fever, cutaneous petechiae, ecchymoses, hyphema, hematuria, hematochezia, and epistaxis. Cutaneous signs including hyperkeratosis, alopecia, and erythema have been described in a study of 32 naturally infected dogs from the Mediterranean basin region.[109] However, the authors noted that although the prevalence of cutaneous signs was high (31.3% of dogs), the results should be interpreted carefully as other vector-borne diseases that cause cutaneous lesions are endemic in the area. Lethargy and musculoskeletal disorders were observed less often, and splenomegaly, ocular lesions, and dehydration were infrequently observed.[109]

DIAGNOSIS

Laboratory Abnormalities

Thrombocytopenia is the hallmark of *A. platys* infection. Mild nonregenerative anemia may also occur. Blood smear evaluation may reveal reactive lymphocytes and monocytes.[109] Morulae in the platelets have been documented to be present in dogs artificially infected IV with *A. platys* after 7 to 19 days.[110] Cycles of thrombocytopenia may occur at intervals of 1 to 2 weeks.[95]

Microscopic Detection in Blood Smears

Diagnosis can be made when the morulae are observed within platelets on blood smears (see Fig. 45.5); however, this is insensitive. The cyclic nature of the thrombocytopenia severely limits this diagnostic technique due to the low levels of bacteremia during thrombocytopenic episodes (Fig. 45.7); therefore, additional tests are recommended in order to confirm a diagnosis. Moreover, platelet inclusions such as dense bodies and alpha granules can be mistaken for morulae.

Serologic Testing

Serologic cross-reactivity exists between *A. platys* and *A. phagocytophilum*[111]; however, cross-reactivity between *A. platys* and *E. canis* is negligible.[112] Seroconversion of experimentally infected dogs occurs shortly after the first episode of bacteremia.[113] An immunoblot analysis based on recombinant *A. platys* major outer membrane proteins, P44 and Omp-1X, has been developed as a simple tool for the detection of antibodies against *A. platys*.[114] However, such assays require laboratory expertise.

Point-of-care (POC) ELISA test kits that detect *Anaplasma* antibodies are available commercially (e.g., SNAP 4Dx Plus Test, IDEXX Laboratories, Westbrook, ME, USA).[115,116] Due to the cross-reaction between *A. platys* and *A. phagocytophilum* antibodies, it is not possible to distinguish between the two, which can be problematic when both agents exist in the same geographic region. A positive result indicates exposure to either or both of the agents. It should also be taken into account that antibodies to *A. platys* only develop 1 to 2 weeks after infection; therefore, a recently infected dog might be seronegative to *A. platys*. A continuingly rising titer (paired titers) would indicate an active infection with either agent.

Molecular Detection

Considering the limitations of microscopy and serology in the diagnosis of *A. platys* infection, molecular detection is considered the most sensitive and specific diagnostic test. A number of PCR-based assays have been developed to detect *A. platys* in infected dogs and are offered by commercial veterinary diagnostic laboratories, often as part of vector-borne pathogen panels. A POC loop-mediated isothermal amplification (LAMP)-based assay has been developed.[117] Such assays may assist in rapid diagnosis, although further assessment of their clinical performance is required.

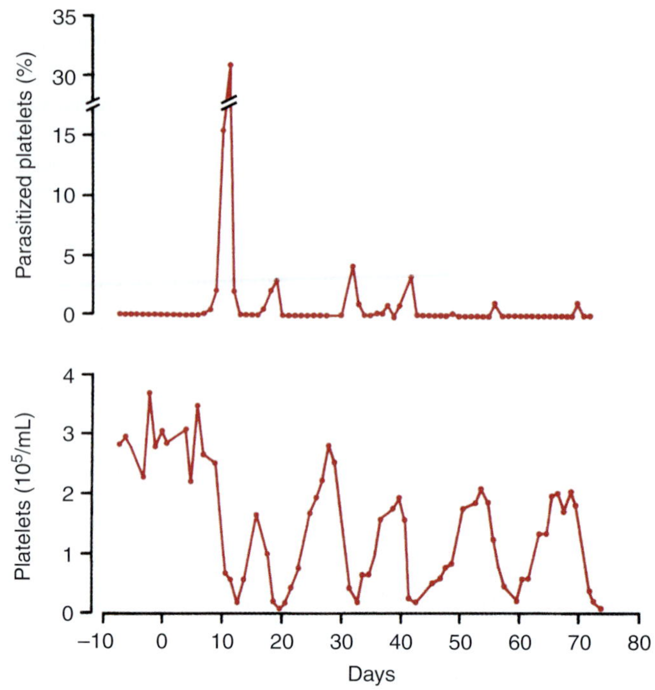

Fig. 45.7 Percentage of infected platelets and platelet counts from a dog inoculated intravenously with *Anaplasma platys*; 0 on the abscissa represents the day of inoculation. (From Harvey JW, Simpson CF, Gaskin JM. Cyclic thrombocytopenia induced by a *Rickettsia*-like agent in dogs. *J Infect Dis* 137:182–188. Reprinted with permission from the University of Chicago.)

TREATMENT AND PROGNOSIS

Although the optimal doxycycline dose and period of treatment of dogs with ICCT is unknown, a similar treatment protocol as recommended for *E. canis* (10 mg/kg doxycycline, PO, q24h) for 21 days is currently recommended.[118,119] However, some dogs with the more severe Mediterranean form of ICCT may not respond to 28 days of doxycycline at this dose.[109]

Infection with *A. platys* has also been documented to be a potential causative agent of secondary IMHA.[120] This should be considered in the course of the treatment and may affect the prognosis and the outcome of treatment.

As ticks are responsible for the natural transmission of *A. platys*, vector control prophylaxis is recommended to prevent the spread of ICCT (see Chapters 13 and 109).

PUBLIC HEALTH ASPECTS

Infection with *A. platys* was documented in two women from Venezuela.[121] In one case, *A. platys* morulae were identified ultrastructurally and in the second case *A. platys* DNA was amplified. In another report, a veterinarian with extensive animal and vector exposure in Grenada, Ireland, and South Africa was diagnosed with a coinfection of *A. platys, Bartonella henselae,* and a *Mycoplasma* species.[122] Furthermore, emphasizing the zoonotic potential of *A. platys*, sequential PCR testing has provided molecular evidence supporting intravascular persistence of *A. platys* and *Ehrlichia* spp. in two humans and their dog.[123]

CASE EXAMPLE

Signalment

"Loki," a 2-year-old male neutered Siberian Husky dog from Minneapolis, MN.

History

Loki's owner reported a 3-day history of inappetence and lethargy and a 2-day history of vomiting. Diarrhea was not observed. Loki continued to drink normally. Loki's owner also noted that he had been displaying some reluctance to lie down. The owner removed a tick from Loki about 1 week before presentation. He was up to date on core vaccines. Loki had no travel history outside of Minnesota.

Physical Examination

Body weight: 29.0 kg.

General: Quiet, alert, and responsive. Temperature = 104.3°F (40.2°C), HR = 130 beats/minute, RR = 32 breaths/minute, mucous membranes pink, CRT = 1 second.

Integument: Healthy haircoat was present. No ectoparasites observed. No evidence of petechiation or ecchymoses.

Eyes, ears, nose, and throat: No significant abnormalities were noted. Mild dental plaque and calculus of canine teeth, maxillary fourth premolars, and mandibular first molars. Mild amount of ceruminous debris was present within both ear canals.

Musculoskeletal: Normal gait and range of motion of joints in all limbs. Repeatedly painful on palpation of thoracolumbar spine. No pain on palpation of hips, stifles, tarsi, elbows, or carpi. No joint effusion detected.

Cardiovascular: Normal heart rhythm. Femoral pulses strong and synchronous. No murmurs detected.

Respiratory: Normal rate and effort. Normal bronchovesicular sounds. No crackles or wheezes on auscultation.

GI and genitourinary: Painful on palpation of mid to caudal abdomen (possibly referred back pain). No obvious masses, organomegaly, or fluid waves detected.

Lymph nodes: Peripheral lymph nodes small and symmetrical.

Laboratory Findings

CBC: HCT 37.0% (37.5%–60.3%), MCV 68.1 fL (63–75.3 fL), MCHC 34.7 g/dL (33.6–37.4 g/dL), WBC 6920 cells/μL (3,880–14,570 cells/μL), neutrophils 6,570 cells/μL (2,100–11,200 cells/μL), lymphocytes 280 cells/μL (780–3,360 cells/μL), monocytes 70 cells/μL (0–1200 cells/μL), platelets 65,000 platelets/μL (129,000–395,000 platelets/μL).

Blood smear findings: 1+ echinocytes, 1+ reactive lymphocytes, 1+ large platelets, few morulae present within neutrophils.

Serum chemistry profile: Sodium 137 mmol/L (145–153 mmol/L), potassium 4.1 mmol/L (3.6–5.3 mmol/L), chloride 105 mmol/L (109–118 mmol/L), bicarbonate 17.4 mmol/L (15–25 mmol/L), phosphorus 3.8 mg/dL (3.3–6.8 mg/dL), calcium 10.1 mg/dL (9.3–11.5 mg/dL), BUN 8 mg/dL (9–31 mg/dL), creatinine 0.9 mg/dL (0.6–1.6 mg/dL), glucose 107 mg/dL (75–117 mg/dL), total protein 6.6 g/dL (5.0–6.9 g/dL), albumin 3.0 g/dL (2.7–3.7 g/dL), globulin 3.6 g/dL (1.7–3.5 g/dL), ALT 48 U/L (22–92 U/L), AST 39 U/L (16–44 U/L), ALP 132 U/L (8–139 U/L), creatine kinase 115 U/L (36–348 U/L), GGT 3 U/L (0–6 U/L), cholesterol 440 mg/dL (143–373 mg/dL), total bilirubin 0.3 mg/dL (0–0.3 mg/dL), magnesium 2.2 mg/dL (1.7–2.4 mg/dL).

Urinalysis: SPG 1.007; pH 7.5, no protein (SSA), no bilirubin, no hemoprotein, no glucose, 0–1 WBC/HPF, occasional RBC/HPF, no crystals, 5–20 lipid droplets/HPF.

Imaging Findings

Abdominal radiographs: Serosal margin detail was good throughout the abdomen. The stomach was mildly distended with gas. Small intestinal size was diffusely normal, and the gas content of the small intestine was appropriate. No fecal material was identified in the colon, but there was no colonic distention. The liver, spleen, and kidneys appeared normal. The urinary bladder was moderately to markedly distended with fluid. Fluid was persistently present in the caudal portion of the intrathoracic esophagus. The caudal vena cava was mildly small. No musculoskeletal abnormalities were seen.

Serology

Negative for heartworm antigen, negative for antibodies to *Anaplasma, Ehrlichia,* and *Borrelia* (SNAP 4Dx Plus Assay, IDEXX Laboratories, ME, USA).

Diagnosis

Canine granulocytic anaplasmosis.

Treatment

Doxycycline, 5 mg/kg PO q12h for 14 days; maropitant 2 mg/kg PO q24hr for 3 days; carprofen 1.9 mg/kg PO q12hr for 5 days. Fever resolved and appetite improved within 24 hours after initiation of treatment. Loki was back to normal within 3 days.

Comments

This dog was diagnosed with granulocytic anaplasmosis based on the presence of characteristic cytologic findings of morulae within neutrophils on blood smear evaluation. The morulae were presumed to be due to *A. phagocytophilum* and not *E. ewingii,* which can have an identical cytologic appearance, due to the restricted geography of these infections. The thoracolumbar pain present in this dog was unusual, but could have been associated with polyarthritis, despite no obvious effusion of limb joints. The timing of clinical signs approximately 1 week after tick exposure is consistent with the acute nature of this infection. Loki was seronegative using the SNAP 4Dx Plus test (IDEXX Laboratories) as it was too early in the course of disease for seroconversion. This highlights the need for additional testing for diagnosis. In this case, morulae were present within granulocytes on blood smear evaluation, though this is not always the case. Additional testing could have included PCR of whole blood.

SUGGESTED READINGS

Carrade DD, Foley JE, Borjesson DL. Canine granulocytic anaplasmosis: a review. *J Vet Intern Med.* 2009;23:1129–1141.

Schafer I, Kohn B. *Anaplasma phagocytophilum* infection in cats: a literature review to raise clinical awareness. *J Feline Med Surg.* 2020;22:428–441.

Stillman BA, Monn M, Liu J, et al. Performance of a commercially available in-clinic ELISA for detection of antibodies against *Anaplasma phagocytophilum, Anaplasma platys, Borrelia burgdorferi, Ehrlichia canis,* and *Ehrlichia ewingii* and *Dirofilaria immitis* antigen in dogs. *J Am Vet Med Assoc.* 2014;245:80–86.

REFERENCES

1. Foggie A. Studies on the infectious agent of tick-borne fever in sheep. *J Pathol Bacteriol.* 1951;63:1–15.
2. Aguero-Rosenfeld ME, Horowitz HW, Wormser GP, et al. Human granulocytic ehrlichiosis: a case series from a medical center in New York State. *Ann Intern Med.* 1996;125:904–908.
3. Blanco JR, Oteo JA. Human granulocytic ehrlichiosis in Europe. *Clin Microbiol Infect.* 2002;8:763–772.
4. Madewell BR, Gribble DH. Infection in two dogs with an agent resembling *Ehrlichia equi. J Am Vet Med Assoc.* 1982;180:512–514.

5. Bjoersdorff A, Svendenius L, Owens JH, et al. Feline granulocytic ehrlichiosis-a report of a new clinical entity and characterisation of the infectious agent. *J Small Anim Pract.* 1999;40:20–24.
6. Harvey JW, Simpson CF, Gaskin JM. Cyclic thrombocytopenia induced by a *Rickettsia*-like agent in dogs. *J Infect Dis.* 1978;137:182–188.
7. Lima ML, Soares PT, Ramos CA, et al. Molecular detection of *Anaplasma platys* in a naturally-infected cat in Brazil. *Braz J Microbiol.* 2010;41:381–385.
8. Dumler JS, Barbet AF, Bekker CP, et al. Reorganization of genera in the families Rickettsiaceae and Anaplasmataceae in the order Rickettsiales: unification of some species of *Ehrlichia* with *Anaplasma, Cowdria* with *Ehrlichia* and *Ehrlichia* with *Neorickettsia*, descriptions of six new species combinations and designation of *Ehrlichia equi* and 'HGE agent' as subjective synonyms of *Ehrlichia phagocytophila. Int J Syst Evol Microbiol.* 2001;51:2145–2165.
9. Lin M, Rikihisa Y. *Ehrlichia chaffeensis* and *Anaplasma phagocytophilum* lack genes for lipid A biosynthesis and incorporate cholesterol for their survival. *Infect Immun.* 2003;71:5324–5331.
10. Popov VL, Han VC, Chen SM, et al. Ultrastructural differentiation of the genogroups in the genus *Ehrlichia. J Med Microbiol.* 1998;47:235–251.
11. Belongia EA, Reed KD, Mitchell PD, et al. Prevalence of granulocytic *Ehrlichia* infection among white-tailed deer in Wisconsin. *J Clin Microbiol.* 1997;35:1465–1468.
12. Magnarelli LA, Williams SC, Norris SJ, et al. Serum antibodies to *Borrelia burgdorferi, Anaplasma phagocytophilum,* and *Babesia microti* in recaptured white-footed mice. *J Wildl Dis.* 2013;49:294–302.
13. Stafford KC 3rd, Massung RF, Magnarelli LA, et al. Infection with agents of human granulocytic ehrlichiosis, Lyme disease, and babesiosis in wild white-footed mice (*Peromyscus leucopus*) in Connecticut. *J Clin Microbiol.* 1999;37:2887–2892.
14. Walls JJ, Greig B, Neitzel DF, et al. Natural infection of small mammal species in Minnesota with the agent of human granulocytic ehrlichiosis. *J Clin Microbiol.* 1997;35:853–855.
15. Drazenovich N, Foley J, Brown RN. Use of real-time quantitative PCR targeting the msp2 protein gene to identify cryptic *Anaplasma phagocytophilum* infections in wildlife and domestic animals. *Vector Borne Zoonotic Dis.* 2006;6:83–90.
16. Nieto NC, Madigan JE, Foley JE. The dusky-footed woodrat (*Neotoma fuscipes*) is susceptible to infection by *Anaplasma phagocytophilum* originating from woodrats, horses, and dogs. *J Wildl Dis.* 2010;46:810–817.
17. Nieto NC, Foley JE. Evaluation of squirrels (Rodentia: Sciuridae) as ecologically significant hosts for *Anaplasma phagocytophilum* in California. *J Med Entomol.* 2008;45:763–769.
18. Liz JS, Anderes L, Sumner JW, et al. PCR detection of granulocytic ehrlichiae in *Ixodes ricinus* ticks and wild small mammals in western Switzerland. *J Clin Microbiol.* 2000;38:1002–1007.
19. Petrovec M, Bidovec A, Sumner JW, et al. Infection with *Anaplasma phagocytophila* in cervids from Slovenia: evidence of two genotypic lineages. *Wien Klin Wochenschr.* 2002;114:641–647.
20. Daniels TJ, Battaly GR, Liveris D, et al. Avian reservoirs of the agent of human granulocytic ehrlichiosis? *Emerg Infect Dis.* 2002;8:1524–1525.
21. De La Fuente J, Naranjo V, Ruiz-Fons F, et al. Potential vertebrate reservoir hosts and invertebrate vectors of *Anaplasma marginale* and *A. phagocytophilum* in central Spain. *Vector Borne Zoonotic Dis.* 2005;5:390–401.
22. Nelder MP, Russell CB, Lindsay LR, et al. Recent emergence of *Anaplasma phagocytophilum* in Ontario, Canada: early serological and entomological indicators. *Am J Trop Med Hyg.* 2019;101:1249–1258.
23. Tonelli BA, Dearborn DC. An individual-based model for the dispersal of *Ixodes scapularis* by ovenbirds and wood thrushes during fall migration. *Ticks Tick Borne Dis.* 2019;10:1096–1104.
24. Hauck D, Springer A, Pachnicke S, et al. *Ixodes inopinatus* in northern Germany: occurrence and potential vector role for *Borrelia* spp., *Rickettsia* spp., and *Anaplasma phagocytophilum* in comparison with *Ixodes ricinus. Parasitol Res.* 2019;118:3205–3216.
25. Inokuma H, Oyamada M, Kelly PJ, et al.: Molecular detection of a new *Anaplasma* species closely related to *Anaplasma phagocytophilum* in canine blood from South Africa, *J Clin Microbiol* 2005;43:2934–2937.
26. M'Ghirbi Y, Ghorbel A, Amouri M, et al.: Clinical, serological, and molecular evidence of ehrlichiosis and anaplasmosis in dogs in Tunisia, *Parasitol Res* 2009;104:767–774.
27. Santos HA, Pires MS, Vilela JA, et al.: Detection of *Anaplasma phagocytophilum* in Brazilian dogs by real-time polymerase chain reaction, *J Vet Diagn Invest* 2011;23:770–774.
28. Alberti A, Zobba R, Chessa B, et al. Equine and canine *Anaplasma phagocytophilum* strains isolated on the island of Sardinia (Italy) are phylogenetically related to pathogenic strains from the United States. *Appl Environ Microbiol.* 2005;71:6418–6422.
29. Carpi G, Bertolotti L, Pecchioli E, et al. *Anaplasma phagocytophilum* groEL gene heterogeneity in *Ixodes ricinus* larvae feeding on roe deer in Northeastern Italy. *Vector Borne Zoonotic Dis.* 2009;9:179–184.
30. Massung RF, Owens JH, Ross D, et al. Sequence analysis of the ank gene of granulocytic ehrlichiae. *J Clin Microbiol.* 2000;38:2917–2922.
31. Jahfari S, Coipan EC, Fonville M, et al. Circulation of four *Anaplasma phagocytophilum* ecotypes in Europe. *Parasit Vectors.* 2014;7:365.
32. Gokce HI, Woldehiwet Z. Differential haematological effects of tick-borne fever in sheep and goats. *Zentralbl Veterinarmed B.* 1999;46:105–115.
33. Massung RF, Mather TN, Levin ML. Reservoir competency of goats for the Ap-variant 1 strain of *Anaplasma phagocytophilum. Infect Immun.* 2006;74:1373–1375.
34. Stuen S, Bergstrom K, Palmer E. Reduced weight gain due to subclinical *Anaplasma phagocytophilum* (formerly *Ehrlichia phagocytophila*) infection. *Exp Appl Acarol.* 2002;28:209–215.
35. van Miert AS, van Duin CT, Schotman AJ, et al. Clinical, haematological and blood biochemical changes in goats after experimental infection with tick-borne fever. *Vet Parasitol.* 1984;16:225–233.
36. Foley J, Nieto NC, Madigan J, et al. Possible differential host tropism in *Anaplasma phagocytophilum* strains in the Western United States. *Ann N Y Acad Sci.* 2008;1149:94–97.
37. Hamsikova Z, Silaghi C, Takumi K, et al. Presence of roe deer affects the occurrence of *Anaplasma phagocytophilum* ecotypes in questing *Ixodes ricinus* in different habitat types of Central Europe. *Int J Environ Res Public Health.* 2019;16.
38. Carrade DD, Foley JE, Borjesson DL. Canine granulocytic anaplasmosis: a review. *J Vet Intern Med.* 2009;23:1129–1141.
39. Schafer I, Kohn B. *Anaplasma phagocytophilum* infection in cats: a literature review to raise clinical awareness. *J Feline Med Surg.* 2020;22:428–441.
40. Bowman D, Little SE, Lorentzen L, et al. Prevalence and geographic distribution of *Dirofilaria immitis, Borrelia burgdorferi, Ehrlichia canis,* and *Anaplasma phagocytophilum* in dogs in the United States: results of a national clinic-based serologic survey. *Vet Parasitol.* 2009;160:138–148.
41. Little SE, Beall MJ, Bowman DD, et al. Canine infection with *Dirofilaria immitis, Borrelia burgdorferi, Anaplasma* spp., and *Ehrlichia* spp. in the United States, 2010-2012. *Parasit Vectors.* 2014;7:257.
42. Dewage BG, Little S, Payton M, et al. Trends in canine seroprevalence to *Borrelia burgdorferi* and *Anaplasma* spp. in the eastern USA, 2010-2017. *Parasit Vectors.* 2019;12:476.
43. Hoyt K, Chandrashekar R, Beall M, et al. Evidence for clinical anaplasmosis and borreliosis in cats in Maine. *Top Companion Anim Med.* 2018;33:40–44.
44. Galemore ER, Labato MA, O'Neil E. Prevalence of *Anaplasma phagocytophilum* infection in feral cats in Massachusetts. *JFMS Open Rep.* 2018;4. 2055116917753804.
45. Beall MJ, Chandrashekar R, Eberts MD, et al. Serological and molecular prevalence of *Borrelia burgdorferi, Anaplasma phagocytophilum,* and *Ehrlichia* species in dogs from Minnesota. *Vector Borne Zoonotic Dis.* 2008;8:455–464.
46. Granick JL, Armstrong PJ, Bender JB. *Anaplasma phagocytophilum* infection in dogs: 34 cases (2000-2007). *J Am Vet Med Assoc.* 2009;234:1559–1565.
47. Greig B, Asanovich KM, Armstrong PJ. Geographic, clinical, serologic, and molecular evidence of granulocytic ehrlichiosis, a likely zoonotic disease, in Minnesota and Wisconsin dogs. *J Clin Microbiol.* 1996;34:44–48.
48. Kohn B, Silaghi C, Galke D, et al. Infections with *Anaplasma phagocytophilum* in dogs in Germany. *Res Vet Sci.* 2011;91:71–76.
49. Kohn B, Galke D, Beelitz P, et al. Clinical features of canine granulocytic anaplasmosis in 18 naturally infected dogs. *J Vet Intern Med.* 2008;22:1289–1295.

50. Poitout FM, Shinozaki JK, Stockwell PJ. Genetic variants of *Anaplasma phagocytophilum* infecting dogs in western Washington state. *J Clin Microbiol.* 2005;43:796–801.
51. Savidge C, Ewing P, Andrews J. *Anaplasma phagocytophilum* in cats: a retrospective analysis and clinical evaluation of fifteen cases from the north eastern United States. *J Vet Intern Med.* 2011;25:706.
52. Egenvall AE, Hedhammar AA, Bjoersdorff AI. Clinical features and serology of 14 dogs affected by granulocytic ehrlichiosis in Sweden. *Vet Rec.* 1997;140:222–226.
53. Foley JE, Brown RN, Gabriel MW. Spatial analysis of the exposure of dogs in rural north-coastal California to vectorborne pathogens. *Vet Rec.* 2007;161:653–657.
54. des Vignes F, Piesman J, Heffernan R, et al. Effect of tick removal on transmission of *Borrelia burgdorferi* and *Ehrlichia phagocytophila* by *Ixodes scapularis* nymphs. *J Infect Dis.* 2001;183:773–778.
55. Kidd L, Breitschwerdt EB. Transmission times and prevention of tick-borne diseases in dogs. *Comp Cont Educ Pract.* 2003;25:742.
56. Wang J, Dyachenko V, Munderloh UG, et al. Transmission of *Anaplasma phagocytophilum* from endothelial cells to peripheral granulocytes in vitro under shear flow conditions. *Med Microbiol Immunol.* 2015;204:593–603.
57. Egenvall A, Bjoersdorff A, Lilliehook I. Early manifestations of granulocytic ehrlichiosis in dogs inoculated experimentally with a Swedish *Ehrlichia* species isolate. *Vet Rec.* 1998;143:412–417.
58. Eberts MD, Vissotto de Paiva Diniz PP, Beall MJ, et al. Typical and atypical manifestations of *Anaplasma phagocytophilum* infection in dogs. *J Am Anim Hosp Assoc.* 2011;47:e86–94.
59. Kim SW, Kim CM, Kim DM, et al. Manifestation of anaplasmosis as cerebral infarction: a case report. *BMC Infect Dis.* 2018;18:409.
60. Lee FS, Chu FK, Tackley M. Human granulocytic ehrlichiosis presenting as facial diplegia in a 42-year-old woman. *Clin Infect Dis.* 2000;31:1288–1291.
61. Granick JL, Reneer DV, Carlyon JA, et al. *Anaplasma phagocytophilum* infects cells of the megakaryocytic lineage through sialylated ligands but fails to alter platelet production. *J Med Microbiol.* 2008;57:416–423.
62. Wong SJ, Thomas JA J. Cytoplasmic, nuclear, and platelet autoantibodies in human granulocytic ehrlichiosis patients. *J Clin Microbiol.* 1998;36:1959–1963.
63. Bakken JS, Dumler S. Human granulocytic anaplasmosis. *Infect Dis Clin North Am.* 2008;22:433–448 (viii).
64. Egenvall A, Lilliehook I, Bjoersdorff A. Detection of granulocytic *Ehrlichia* species DNA by PCR in persistently infected dogs. *Vet Rec.* 2000;146:186–190.
65. Contreras ET, Dowers KL, Moroff S, et al. Clinical and laboratory effects of doxycycline and prednisolone in *Ixodes scapularis*-exposed dogs with chronic *Anaplasma phagocytophilum* infection. *Top Companion Anim Med.* 2018;33:147–149.
66. Bakken JS, Dumler JS. Human granulocytic anaplasmosis. *Infect Dis Clin North Am.* 2015;29:341–355.
67. Heikkila HM, Bondarenko A, Mihalkov A. *Anaplasma phagocytophilum* infection in a domestic cat in Finland: case report. *Acta Vet Scand.* 2010;52:62.
68. Tarello W. Microscopic and clinical evidence for *Anaplasma (Ehrlichia) phagocytophilum* infection in Italian cats. *Vet Rec.* 2005;156:772–774.
69. Lappin MR, Breitschwerdt EB, Jensen WA, et al. Molecular and serologic evidence of *Anaplasma phagocytophilum* infection in cats in North America. *J Am Vet Med Assoc.* 2004;225:893–896, 879.
70. Chirek A, Silaghi C, Pfister K, et al. Granulocytic anaplasmosis in 63 dogs: clinical signs, laboratory results, therapy and course of disease. *J Small Anim Pract.* 2018;59:112–120.
71. Savidge C, Ewing P, Andrews J, et al. *Anaplasma phagocytophilum* infection of domestic cats: 16 cases from the northeastern USA. *J Feline Med Surg.* 2016;18:85–91.
72. Lappin MR, Chandrashekar R, Stillman B, et al. Evidence of *Anaplasma phagocytophilum* and *Borrelia burgdorferi* infection in cats after exposure to wild-caught adult *Ixodes scapularis. J Vet Diagn Invest.* 2015;27:522–525.
73. Plier ML, Breitschwerdt EB, Hegarty BC. Lack of evidence for perinatal transmission of canine granulocytic anaplasmosis from a bitch to her offspring. *J Anim Hosp Assoc.* 2009;45:232–238.
74. Breitschwerdt EB, Hegarty BC, Hancock SI. Sequential evaluation of dogs naturally infected with *Ehrlichia canis, Ehrlichia chaffeensis, Ehrlichia equi, Ehrlichia ewingii*, or *Bartonella vinsonii. J Clin Microbiol.* 1998;36:2645–2651.
75. Aguero-Rosenfeld ME. Diagnosis of human granulocytic ehrlichiosis: state of the art. *Vector Borne Zoonotic Dis.* 2002;2:233–239.
76. Dumler JS, Barat NC, Barat CE. Human granulocytic anaplasmosis and macrophage activation. *Clin Infect Dis.* 2007;45:199–204.
77. Lepidi H, Bunnell JE, Martin ME. Comparative pathology, and immunohistology associated with clinical illness after *Ehrlichia phagocytophila*-group infections. *Am J Trop Med Hyg.* 2000;62:29–37.
78. Yancey CB, Diniz P, Breitschwerdt EB, et al. Doxycycline treatment efficacy in dogs with naturally occurring *Anaplasma phagocytophilum* infection. *J Small Anim Pract.* 2018;59:286–293.
79. Akkoyunlu M, Fikrig E. Gamma interferon dominates the murine cytokine response to the agent of human granulocytic ehrlichiosis and helps to control the degree of early rickettsemia. *Infect Immun.* 2000;68:1827–1833.
80. Birkner K, Steiner B, Rinkler C, et al. The elimination of *Anaplasma phagocytophilum* requires CD4+ T cells, but is independent of Th1 cytokines and a wide spectrum of effector mechanisms. *Eur J Immunol.* 2008;38:3395–3410.
81. De Martino SJ, Carlyon JA, Fikrig E. Coinfection with *Borrelia burgdorferi* and the agent of human granulocytic ehrlichiosis. *N Engl J Med.* 2001;345:150–151.
82. Granquist EG, Stuen S, Lundgren AM. Outer membrane protein sequence variation in lambs experimentally infected with *Anaplasma phagocytophilum. Infect Immun.* 2008;76:120–126.
83. Rejmanek D, Foley P, Barbet A. Antigen variability in *Anaplasma phagocytophilum* during chronic infection of a reservoir host. *Microbiology.* 2012;158:2632–2641.
84. Horowitz HW, Aguero-Rosenfeld M, Dumler JS. Reinfection with the agent of human granulocytic ehrlichiosis. *Ann Intern Med.* 1998;129:461–463.
85. Lappin MR, Huesken R, Stanneck D. *Anaplasma phagocytophilum* and *Borrelia burgdorferi* infections in cats exposed twice to *Ixodes scapularis. Top Companion Anim Med.* 2021 (Submitted for publication).
86. Blagburn BL, Spencer JA, Billeter SA. Use of imidacloprid-permethrin to prevent transmission of *Anaplasma phagocytophilum* from naturally infected *Ixodes scapularis* ticks to dogs. *Vet Ther.* 2004;5:212–217.
87. McCall JW, Baker CF, Mather TN. The ability of a topical novel combination of fipronil, amitraz and (S)-methoprene to protect dogs from *Borrelia burgdorferi* and *Anaplasma phagocytophilum* infections transmitted by *Ixodes scapularis. Vet Parasitol.* 2011;179:335–342.
88. Kramer F, Husken R, Krudewagen EM, et al. Prevention of transmission of *Borrelia burgdorferi* sensu lato and *Anaplasma phagocytophilum* by *Ixodes* spp. ticks to dogs treated with the Seresto® collar (imidacloprid 10% + flumethrin 4.5%). *Parasitol Res.* 2020;119:299–315.
89. Strle F. Human granulocytic ehrlichiosis in Europe. *Int J Med Microbiol.* 2004;293(suppl 37):27–35.
90. Matei IA, Estrada-Pena A, Cutler SJ, et al. A review on the eco-epidemiology and clinical management of human granulocytic anaplasmosis and its agent in Europe. *Parasit Vectors.* 2019;12:599.
91. Bakken JS, Krueth J, Wilson-Nordskog C. Clinical and laboratory characteristics of human granulocytic ehrlichiosis. *JAMA.* 1996;275:199–205.
92. Dumler JS, Madigan JE, Pusterla N, et al. Ehrlichioses in humans: epidemiology, clinical presentation, diagnosis, and treatment. *Clin Infect Dis.* 2007;45(suppl 1):S45–S51.
93. Cleaveland S, Meslin FX, Breiman R. Dogs can play useful role as sentinel hosts for disease. *Nature.* 2006;440:605.
94. Duncan AW, Correa MT, Levine JF, et al. The dog as a sentinel for human infection: prevalence of *Borrelia burgdorferi* C6 antibodies in dogs from southeastern and mid-Atlantic States. *Vector Borne Zoonotic Dis.* 2005;5:101–109.

95. Waner T, Harrus S. Infectious canine cyclic thrombocytopenia. In: Day MJ, ed. *Arthropod-borne Infectious Diseases of Dogs and Cats*. Boca Raton, FL: CRC Press; 2016:183–187.
96. Lappin MR. Update on flea and tick associated diseases of cats. *Vet Parasitol.* 2018;254:26–29.
97. Aktas M, Ozubek S. Molecular evidence for trans-stadial transmission of *Anaplasma platys* by *Rhipicephalus sanguineus* sensu lato under field conditions. *Med Vet Entomol.* 2018;32:78–83.
98. Parola P, Cornet JP, Sanogo YO, et al. Detection of *Ehrlichia* spp., *Anaplasma* spp., *Rickettsia* spp., and other eubacteria in ticks from the Thai-Myanmar border and Vietnam. *J Clin Microbiol.* 2003;41: 1600–1608.
99. Latrofa MS, Dantas-Torres F, de Caprariis D, et al. Vertical transmission of *Anaplasma platys* and *Leishmania infantum* in dogs during the first half of gestation. *Parasit Vectors.* 2016;9:269.
100. Matei IA, Stuen S, Modry D, et al. Neonatal *Anaplasma platys* infection in puppies: further evidence for possible vertical transmission. *Vet J.* 2017;219:40–41.
101. Qurollo BA, Balakrishnan N, Cannon CZ, et al. Co-infection with *Anaplasma platys, Bartonella henselae, Bartonella koehlerae* and '*Candidatus* Mycoplasma haemominutum' in a cat diagnosed with splenic plasmacytosis and multiple myeloma. *J Feline Med Surg.* 2014;16:713–720.
102. Pereira A, Parreira R, Nunes M, et al. Molecular detection of tick-borne bacteria and protozoa in cervids and wild boars from Portugal. *Parasit Vectors.* 2016;9:251.
103. Li Y, Yang J, Chen Z, et al. *Anaplasma* infection of Bactrian camels (*Camelus bactrianus*) and ticks in Xinjiang, China. *Parasit Vectors.* 2015;8:313.
104. Belkahia H, Ben Said M, Sayahi L, et al. Detection of novel strains genetically related to *Anaplasma platys* in Tunisian one-humped camels (*Camelus dromedarius*). *J Infect Dev Ctries.* 2015;9:1117–1125.
105. Dahmani M, Davoust B, Benterki MS, et al. Development of a new PCR-based assay to detect Anaplasmataceae and the first report of *Anaplasma phagocytophilum* and *Anaplasma platys* in cattle from Algeria. *Comp Immunol Microbiol Infect Dis.* 2015;39:39–45.
106. Harrus S, Aroch I, Lavy E, et al. Clinical manifestations of infectious canine cyclic thrombocytopenia. *Vet Rec.* 1997;141:247–250.
107. Lanza-Perea M, Zieger U, Qurollo BA, et al. Intraoperative bleeding in dogs from Grenada seroreactive to *Anaplasma platys* and *Ehrlichia canis.* *J Vet Intern Med.* 2014;28:1702–1707.
108. Wilson JF. *Ehrlichia platys* in a Michigan dog. *J Am Anim Hosp Assoc.* 1992;28:381–383.
109. Bouzouraa T, Rene-Martellet M, Chene J, et al. Clinical and laboratory features of canine *Anaplasma platys* infection in 32 naturally infected dogs in the Mediterranean basin. *Ticks Tick Borne Dis.* 2016;7:1256–1264.
110. Nair AD, Cheng C, Ganta CK, et al. Comparative experimental infection study in dogs with Ehrlichia canis, *E. chaffeensis, Anaplasma platys* and *A. phagocytophilum. PloS One.* 2016;11:e0148239.
111. Inokuma H, Fujii K, Matsumoto K, et al. Demonstration of *Anaplasma (Ehrlichia) platys* inclusions in peripheral blood platelets of a dog in Japan. *Vet Parasitol.* 2002;110:145–152.
112. Waner T, Harrus S, Jongejan F, et al. Significance of serological testing for ehrlichial diseases in dogs with special emphasis on the diagnosis of canine monocytic ehrlichiosis caused by *Ehrlichia canis. Vet Parasitol.* 2001;95:1–15.
113. French TW, Harvey JW. Serologic diagnosis of infectious cyclic thrombocytopenia in dogs using an indirect fluorescent antibody test. *Am J Vet Res.* 1983;44:2407–2411.
114. Lai TH, Parraga ME, Alvarez E, et al. *Anaplasma platys* immunoblot test using major surface antigens. *Vector Borne Zoonotic Dis.* 2016;16:581–587.
115. Liu J, Drexel J, Andrews B, et al. Comparative evaluation of 2 in-clinic assays for vector-borne disease testing in dogs. *Top Companion Anim Med.* 2018;33:114–118.
116. Stillman BA, Monn M, Liu J, et al. Performance of a commercially available in-clinic ELISA for detection of antibodies against *Anaplasma phagocytophilum, Anaplasma platys, Borrelia burgdorferi, Ehrlichia canis,* and *Ehrlichia ewingii* and *Dirofilaria immitis* antigen in dogs. *J Am Vet Med Assoc.* 2014;245:80–86.
117. Li HT, Sun LS, Chen ZM, et al. Detection of *Anaplasma platys* in dogs using real-time loop-mediated isothermal amplification. *Vet J.* 2014;199:468–470.
118. Chang WL, Su WL, Pan MJ. Two-step PCR in the evaluation of antibiotic treatment for *Ehrlichia platys* infection. *J Vet Med Sci.* 1997;59:849–851.
119. Gaunt S, Beall M, Stillman B, et al. Experimental infection and co-infection of dogs with *Anaplasma platys* and *Ehrlichia canis*: hematologic, serologic and molecular findings. *Parasit Vectors.* 2010;3:33.
120. Antognoni MT, Veronesi F, Morganti G, et al. Natural infection of *Anaplasma platys* in dogs from Umbria region (Central Italy). *Vet Ital.* 2014;50:49–56.
121. Arraga-Alvarado CM, Qurollo BA, Parra OC, et al. Case report: molecular evidence of *Anaplasma platys* infection in two women from Venezuela. *Am J Trop Med Hyg.* 2014;91:1161–1165.
122. Maggi RG, Mascarelli PE, Havenga LN, et al. Co-infection with *Anaplasma platys, Bartonella henselae* and '*Candidatus* Mycoplasma haematoparvum in a veterinarian'. *Parasit Vectors.* 2013;6:103.
123. Breitschwerdt EB, Hegarty BC, Qurollo BA, et al. Intravascular persistence of *Anaplasma platys, Ehrlichia chaffeensis,* and *Ehrlichia ewingii* DNA in the blood of a dog and two family members. *Parasit Vectors.* 2014;7:298.

46

Spotted Fever Rickettsioses, Flea-Borne Rickettsioses, and Typhus

Linda Kidd, Edward B. Breitschwerdt

KEY POINTS

- First Described: *Rickettsia rickettsii* was first described in Montana, United States, 1909[1] (Ricketts).
- Cause: *Rickettsia rickettsii*, a gram-negative, obligately intracellular bacteria. Other spotted fever group (SFG) *Rickettsia* spp., typhus group (TG) *Rickettsia* spp., and *Rickettsia felis* (a separate lineage designated ancestral group) are important causes of emerging infectious disease in people. *Rickettsia conorii*, a SFG *Rickettsia* spp., causes Mediterranean spotted fever (MSF) in people and a doxycycline-responsive disease in dogs that is similar to Rocky Mountain Spotted Fever (RMSF). A novel *Rickettsia* species causing a febrile illness similar to *R. rickettsii* and *R. conorii* has been more recently reported in dogs in the United States.
- Affected Hosts: Humans and dogs (*R. rickettsii*).
- Geographic Distribution: North, Central, and South America.
- Primary Mode of Transmission: Ticks (*Dermacentor* spp., *Rhipicephalus sanguineus, Amblyomma* spp.). Most affected dogs lack a history of a tick bite. *Rickettsia conorii* is transmitted by *Rh. sanguineus* in the Mediterranean basin.
- Major Clinical Signs: RMSF is generally an acute, febrile illness. Clinical signs are consistent with a vasculitis because *R. rickettsii* infects endothelial cells. Major clinical signs include fever, vomiting, ocular signs (retinal hemorrhage, uveitis, episcleral injection), lymphadenomegaly, splenomegaly, peripheral edema, cutaneous hyperemia and necrosis, polyarthritis, and neurologic signs. Signs may be complicated by prior or simultaneous infection with other tick-borne pathogens. The degree to which other SFG *Rickettsia*, TG *Rickettsia*, and *R. felis* cause illness in dogs and cats is being investigated.
- Differential Diagnoses: Infection with other tick-borne agents such as *Anaplasma phagocytophilum, Ehrlichia* spp., *Bartonella* spp., *Babesia* spp., and *Borrelia burgdorferi* should be considered. Other causes of severe systemic decompensation and vasculitis such as sepsis and SIRS due to other causes may mimic RMSF. Leptospirosis and other causes of vasculitis and thrombocytopenia may also mimic RMSF. Other differential diagnoses for the neurologic signs seen in RMSF must also be considered. Appropriate antimicrobial treatment with doxycycline must begin before the diagnosis is confirmed by laboratory testing. Misdiagnosis and delayed or inappropriate antimicrobial drug therapy increase morbidity and mortality.
- Human Health Significance: Owners and their physicians should be contacted whenever RMSF is diagnosed in any canine patient, because illness in dogs can coincide with or precede illness in humans. Dogs also are sentinels for MSF in people. Control of flea and tick vectors on dogs and cats is important to prevent rickettsioses in people.

ETIOLOGIC AGENTS AND EPIDEMIOLOGY

Rickettsial diseases are important causes of morbidity and mortality in dogs and humans worldwide. The terms "rickettsial disease," "rickettsioses," and even the term "*Rickettsia*" have been used to refer to several obligately intracellular organisms including *Rickettsia, Bartonella, Ehrlichia, Anaplasma, Coxiella,* and *Neorickettsia*. Previously, all of these organisms belonged to the order Rickettsiales and most were in the family Rickettsiaceae, based on their fastidious or intracellular nature and other characteristics. Therefore, members of these diverse genera were collectively referred to as "rickettsial organisms."[2,3] Advances in molecular biologic techniques have resulted in the reclassification of several of these organisms. Many have been moved out of the family Rickettsiaceae, and others have been moved out of the order Rickettsiales. Currently the order Rickettsiales includes only two families, the family Anaplasmataceae, which contains the genera *Anaplasma, Ehrlichia, Neoehrlichia, Wolbachia,* and *Neorickettsia*; and the family Rickettsiaceae, which includes the genera *Rickettsia* and *Orientia*.[3–6] The term "rickettsial" refers to diseases caused by organisms in the order Rickettsiales, "rickettsioses" refers to diseases caused by organisms in the family Rickettsiaceae (*Rickettsia* and *Orientia*), and "*Rickettsia*" refers specifically to members of the genus *Rickettsia*.[2,3,5]

The genus *Rickettsia* is divided into the SFG and the typhus group (TG) and an ancestral group based on phenotypic and, more recently, genotypic characteristics.[3,5–7] There is some evidence that *Rickettsia felis* and *Rickettsia akari* (currently classified as SFG *Rickettsia*) may have separate lineages.[6,8] Phenotypic characteristics that have historically been used to group the organisms into TG or SFG include the types of vectors that transmit them, their pathophysiologic manifestations of the disease, and serologic differences. Therefore, the division of *Rickettsia* into SFG and TG has clinical relevance.

SFG rickettsia species are transmitted by arthropod (primarily tick) vectors and infect endothelial cells in mammalian hosts.[3,6,7] The two most pathogenic and well-studied SFG rickettsiae that cause disease in humans and dogs are *Rickettsia rickettsii*, the cause of Rocky Mountain Spotted Fever (RMSF) in North, Central, and South America, and *Rickettsia conorii*, the cause of Mediterranean spotted fever (MSF) in Europe, Africa, Asia, and the Middle East. The first human case of RMSF was described in the late 1800s, and the first case of MSF was described in the 1920s.[9] Therefore, these organisms and their associated diseases are the most well characterized among the SFG rickettsiae.[5] Currently, there more than 20 species of tick-borne rickettsiae.[5,7] Some species appear to be nonpathogenic endosymbionts of ticks.[7] However, some SFG rickettsiae previously thought to be nonpathogenic, such as *Rickettsia parkeri* and *Rickettsia massiliae,* have more recently been associated with disease in humans.[10–12] Previously thought to have rather limited geographic boundaries, many SFG rickettsiae have also been detected in expanding geographic locales around the world.[7] Increasing travel and the effects of climate change on tick populations and habitat are thought to be partly responsible for this phenomenon.[13,14]

Dogs are sentinels for SFG rickettsioses in humans. Both *R. rickettsii* and *R. conorii* infect and cause disease in dogs.[15–21] *Rickettsia rickettsii* infection in dogs can occur before, or coincide with, outbreaks of RMSF in people in the same household or community.[22–26] Similarly, several serosurveys in endemic areas have shown an increased risk of MSF in people who live near dogs that are seropositive for SFG rickettsiae.[27–29] Other SFG rickettsial species infect dogs, but the extent to which they cause clinical disease has not yet been definitively established. Species implicated in natural infection in dogs include *R. massiliae, R. parkeri, R. felis, R. akari, Rickettsia amblyommii, Rickettsia montanensis, Rickettsia japonica,* and *Rickettsia australis.*[30–37] These rickettsial infections along with flea-borne rickettsioses are discussed further below. The DNA from SFG rickettsiae *R. massiliae* and *R. conorii* has been amplified from naturally infected cats, and cats in regions endemic to pathogenic and nonpathogenic SFG *Rickettsia* are seropositive to SFG rickettsiae.[38–41] The degree to which SFG rickettsiae cause illness in cats has yet to be defined.[38,39] Typhus group rickettsiae are a phenotypically and genotypically distinct group of rickettsiae that are described at the end of this chapter.

ROCKY MOUNTAIN SPOTTED FEVER

Young and purebred dogs are overrepresented in some but not other studies of RMSF in dogs.[18,19] Although some studies suggest that male dogs are at increased risk, no sex predilection has been definitively documented.[18,19,42] Severe disease has been reported in English springer spaniels with phosphofructokinase (PFK) deficiency and in German shepherd dogs.[19,42] Dogs that live outdoors, particularly those with access to shrubs and high grass, are at increased risk for RMSF.[18]

Rickettsia rickettsii is transmitted by several hard (ixodid) ticks including *Dermacentor variabilis* (the American dog tick) (Fig. 46.1A), *Dermacentor andersoni* (the Rocky Mountain wood tick) (Fig. 46.1B), *Amblyomma americanum* (the lone star tick), *Amblyomma cajennense sensu lato* (the Cayenne tick), *Amblyomma aureolatum* (the yellow dog tick), and *Rhipicephalus sanguineus* (the brown dog tick).[7,43–47] The primary vectors for *R. rickettsii* in the south-central and southeastern United States are *Dermacentor* ticks, whereas *Rh. sanguineus* is the primary vector in the southwest United States and Mexico. Tick species other than *D. variabilis, D. andersoni,* and *Rh. sanguineus* are also associated with *R. rickettsii* in the United States. For example, *A. americanum* transmitted RMSF to a person in North Carolina, and the organism has been isolated from *Dermacentor occidentalis* in California.[45,48] *Amblyomma cajennense sensu lato* species and to a lesser extent, *A. aureolatum* transmit this rickettsia in Brazil.[49]

Ticks that transmit *R. rickettsii* feed once during each life stage (Fig. 46.2). Both transstadial and transovarial transmission occurs in *Dermacentor* spp. infected with *R. rickettsii,* making them a reservoir as well as a vector of infection.[50,51] *Dermacentor* spp. and *Amblyomma* spp. are three-host ticks. Infection is transmitted among mammalian hosts and ticks when the tick feeds on different hosts during each stage

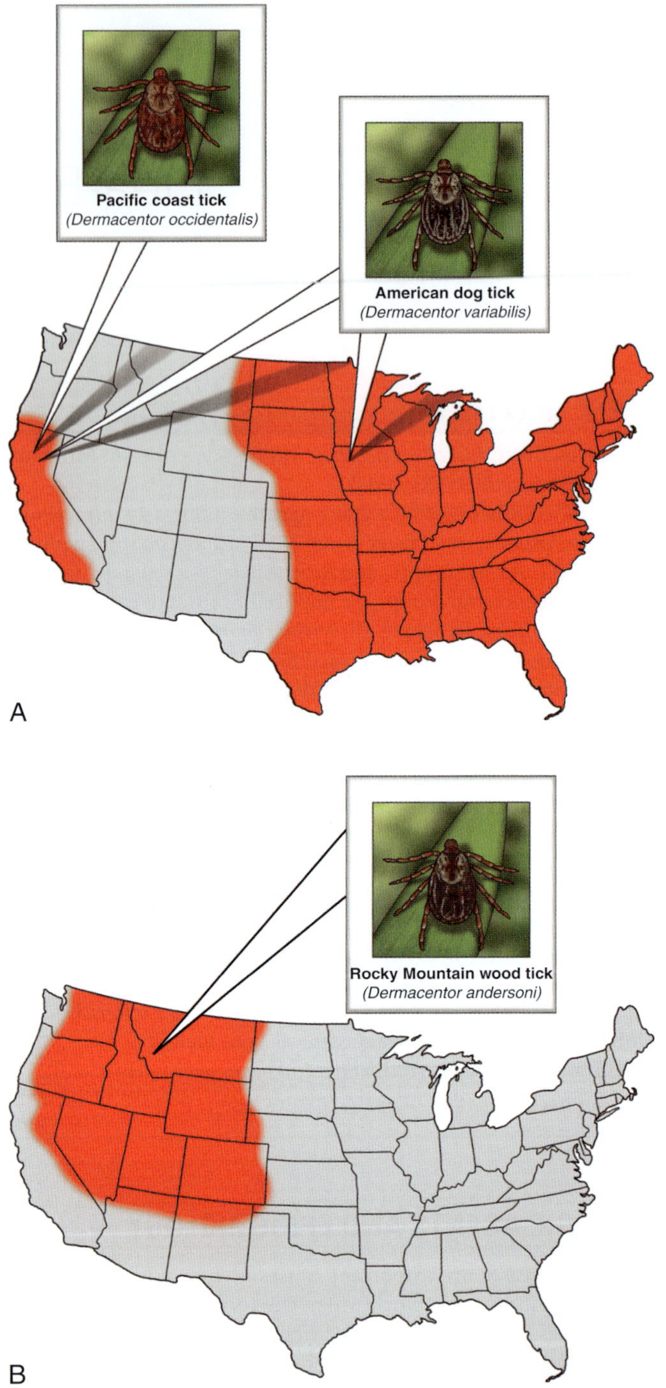

Fig. 46.1 (A) Distribution of *Dermacentor variabilis* and *Dermacentor occidentalis* ticks in the United States. (B) Distribution of *Dermacentor andersoni* ticks in the United States.

of molting. The sylvatic cycle for *Dermacentor* ticks involves small mammals, such as chipmunks, pine voles, mice, and ground squirrels. After organisms are ingested by the tick, SFG rickettsiae initially replicate in the epithelial cells of the tick midgut, enter the hemolymph and hemocytes, and then multiply in tissues.[51] Once in the salivary glands, the organism is transmitted to a naïve mammalian host on feeding. Transmission can occur within hours of attachment. However, transmission may be prolonged (up to 48 hours) when changes in virulence occur under conditions such as starvation of the tick. These "dormant" rickettsiae undergo a process called reactivation after the tick begins

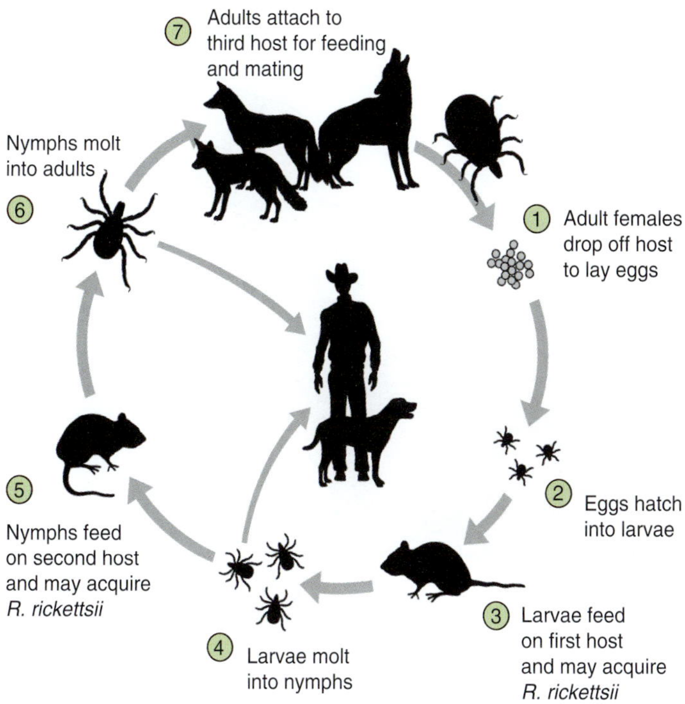

Fig. 46.2 Transmission cycle of *Rickettsia rickettsii* in tick populations, humans, and dogs. After adult female ticks lay eggs and they hatch *(1 and 2)*, *Dermacentor* spp. ticks acquire *R. rickettsii* upon feeding as larvae or nymphs on rodents *(3)*; they then transmit during subsequent feeding as nymphs or adults *(4 to 6)*. Adult ticks feed on a variety of canid species, such as foxes and possibly wolves and coyotes. In addition, *R. rickettsii* infection can be maintained transovarially in *Dermacentor* ticks, so some larvae that hatch from the egg mass already harbor an infection. (Redrawn from Nicholson WL, Allen KE, McQuiston JH, et al. The increasing recognition of rickettsial pathogens in dogs and people. *Trends Parasitol.* 2010;26:205–212.)

feeding.[52] Therefore, rapid tick removal can decrease the risk of transmission in many, but not all, circumstances.

Rhipicephalus sanguineus is a one-host tick, with dogs being the preferred host.[53] It can adapt to hot environments and commonly resides in walls of housing structures in close proximity to humans.[53] Increases in global temperature have been implicated in association with increased feeding on humans.[13,53] The role of this tick as a reservoir for *R. rickettsii* in nature has yet to be elucidated.

The role of dogs as a natural reservoir of infection for *R. rickettsii* is also unknown. Dogs are thought to act as incidental hosts when *Dermacentor* ticks are the vectors, because ticks rarely acquire the organism from rickettsemic dogs.[54] In contrast, all stages of *Rh. sanguineus* acquired infection at a high rate from experimentally infected dogs in one study, but this may have been related to the virulence of the rickettsial strain used.[47] A relatively high infection rate with SFG rickettsiae in naturally infected *Rh. sanguineus* has also been described.[7,46,48] Therefore, dogs may play a role in maintenance of a reservoir of *R. rickettsii* infection in endemic foci where *Rh. sanguineus* is the primary vector.

Direct transmission of *R. rickettsii* to humans has been described in laboratory settings through aerosolization. Direct transmission from tick blood or other contaminated biologic products also has the potential to occur. For example, in Portugal, a SFG rickettsia was directly transmitted to a human through conjunctival inoculation after a *Rh. sanguineus* tick removed from a dog was crushed.[55] Therefore, care should be taken when handling laboratory specimens and removing ticks.

RMSF occurs in North, Central, and South America (where it is known as Brazilian spotted fever). In North America, most cases of RMSF occur in the southeastern and south-central states. North Carolina, Oklahoma, Arkansas, Tennessee, and Missouri consistently have the highest reported number of human cases in the United States (Fig. 46.3). Disease distribution in the United States primarily follows the distribution of *D. variabilis*, the primary vector in this region; however, over the last decade the importance of *D. variabilis* as vectors in endemic areas has been questioned.[56] Although disease can occur at any time of the year, most cases of canine and human RMSF in the United States are reported from April through October, months of peak *Dermacentor* tick activity.[18,57–59] Interestingly, in contrast to the southern regions of the United States, a 2016 study showed no seasonality for the occurrence of human SFG rickettsioses in the western United States. The authors speculated that moderate temperatures and year-round activity of *Rh. sanguineus*, the vector for *R. rickettsii* in the southwest, might explain this finding.[58]

This tick also helps explain why the geographic distribution of RMSF in people in the United States has expanded beyond the distribution of *D. variabilis* and *D. andersoni*. Novel vectors, including *Rh. sanguineus*, have played a role in this phenomenon. This tick was associated with an outbreak of fatal human RMSF in a previously nonendemic area of Arizona.[24,60] Infection existed in the dog population before the fatal outbreak in people.[25,26] *Rhipicephalus sanguineus* is found throughout the United States, southern Canada, Mexico, and South America. Notably, *Rh. sanguineus* is the main vector for *R. rickettsii* in some parts of the Western Hemisphere.[7] Over the last decade, an outbreak in Mexicali, Mexico, just across the border from California and Arizona, was also attributed to *R. rickettsii* transmitted by *Rh. sanguineus* ticks associated with dogs.[61] This prompted ongoing surveillance efforts in ticks, dogs, and humans in southern California, a nonendemic area for RMSF. *Rickettsia rickettsii* was not found in *Rh. sanguineus* ticks removed from dogs residing in animal shelters located just across the United States border from the Mexican outbreak.[62,63] In addition, a 2020 study found increased exposure to SFG rickettsiae in dogs living in a California county that borders Mexico that had a history of traveling into Mexico, compared with dogs living in the same region that had not crossed the border.[64] These regional discrepancies in exposure risk may be due to subtle differences in microenvironment or other factors that affect regional infection rates in ticks and further emphasize the need for ongoing vigilance and surveillance for RMSF.[65]

Over the last decade, the incidence of SFG rickettsioses in people in the United States has increased.[58] There was a significant increase in the number of confirmed or suspected cases of SFG rickettsioses reported to the CDC in 2010–2014 as compared with 2005–2009 (Wilcoxon matched pairs signed-rank test P = .0058;) (Fig. 46.4). Some of the increase may be due to disease caused by species of SFG rickettsiae other than *R. rickettsii*.[58,66,67] Because the case definition of human spotted fever rickettsioses (SFR) can be based exclusively on serologic testing, which does not differentiate among species of SFG *Rickettsia*, the Council for State and Territorial Epidemiology changed the name RMSF to SFR for surveillance purposes in 2009. It is thought that up to one third of cases of SFG rickettsioses in the United States may actually have been caused by *R. parkeri* rather than *R. rickettsii*.[67] As is the case for humans, some dogs with positive titers to *R. rickettsii* may have been caused by exposure to other species of pathogenic or nonpathogenic SFG rickettsiae.

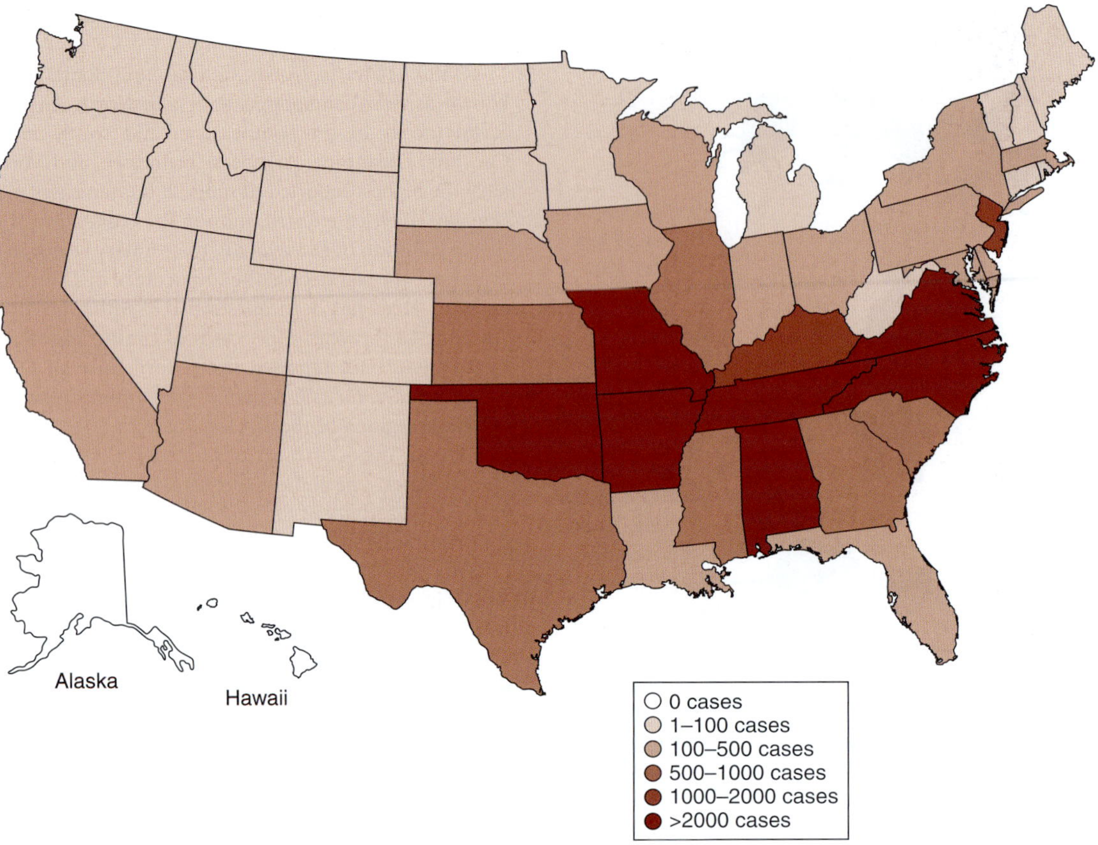

Fig. 46.3 Geographic distribution of the incidence of spotted fever group rickettsioses in people in the United States, 2010–2019. (Compiled from data from the Centers for Disease Control and Prevention, Morbidity and Mortality Weekly Reports: https://www.cdc.gov/mmwr/mmwr_nd/index.html.)

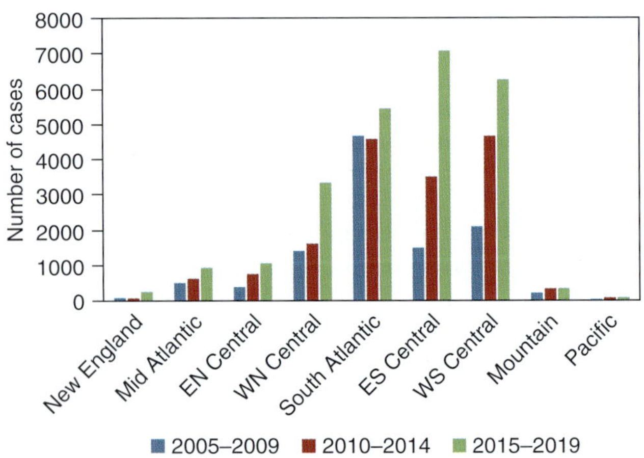

Fig. 46.4 Comparison of the incidence of confirmed and probable spotted fever rickettsioses in people in the United States during 2005–2009, 2010–2014, and 2015–2019. (Compiled from data from the Centers for Disease Control and Prevention, Morbidity and Mortality Weekly Reports (https://www.cdc.gov/mmwr/mmwr_nd/index.html). As defined by the CDC, NE = North-east States and includes CT, ME, MA, NH, RI, VT; Mid-Atlantic includes NJ, NY, PA; EN Central = East North-central states and includes IL, IN, MI, OH, and WI; WN Central = West North-central states and includes IA, KS, MN, MO, NE, ND, SD; WS Central = West South-central states and includes AR, LA, OK, TX; South-Atlantic includes DE, DC, FL, GA, MD, NC, SC, VA, WV; ES Central = East South-central and includes AL, KY, MS, TN; Mountain includes AZ, CO, ID, MT, NV, NM, UT and WY; and Pacific includes AK, CA, HI, OR and WA.)

CLINICAL FEATURES

Pathogenesis and Clinical Signs

The endotheliotropism of *Rickettsia* spp. infection results in the characteristic clinical sign of infection, which is disseminated vasculitis. In humans, cutaneous macules, papules, and petechiation that occur in association with vasculitis form a rash that looks like "spots," hence the name "spotted fever."[9] The clinical signs, time course of illness, and response to therapy for RMSF in dogs are very similar, if not identical, to those associated with RMSF in humans.[18–21] However, cutaneous lesions are not always present in dogs or humans ("RMSF"). In humans, SFR caused by organisms other than *R. rickettsii* are often associated with an eschar (an area of cutaneous necrosis) formation.[4,7,14] Clinicians should keep in mind that dogs from nonendemic areas that have classic signs of RMSF, or those that develop atypical clinical signs, may be infected with *R. rickettsii* or other SFG rickettsial species.

Once the organism is inoculated, it spreads through lymphatics or directly into the bloodstream to the small capillaries. *Rickettsia rickettsii* primarily infects endothelial cells, although smooth muscles and monocytes may also be infected.[4,68] The bacterial autotransporter outer membrane protein A (OmpA) and outer membrane protein B (OmpB), are important for attachment, adhesion, and virulence.[69–71] These proteins also account for differences in serotype, and antibodies to OmpB and OmpA contribute to immunity to reinfection. Other autotransporter proteins such as Sca1 and Sca2 are important for adhesion.[72] Phagocytosis is likely triggered by adhesion proteins interacting with host cell receptors.[72] Enzymes such as phospholipase

D and hemolysin C facilitate the release of the organisms into the host cell cytoplasm.[70,71] SFG *Rickettsia* live in both the cytoplasm and the nucleus, deriving nutrients and energy from the host cell.[4,6,69] They spread from cell to cell by inducing actin to polymerize, which transports the bacteria directly into adjacent cells.[70,73] This helps the bacteria to evade the immune response and to disseminate without rupturing the cell. They are also released into circulation when they exit the luminal surface of the cell membrane or when endothelial cell death or detachment occurs.[70] SFG rickettsiae activate the transcription factor NF-κB, which inhibits apoptosis, fosters further growth of the organism, and promotes inflammation.[69,70]

Damage to endothelial cells leads to vasculitis and an increase in microvascular permeability. Mechanisms of cellular damage include oxidative injury through the production of reactive oxygen species, cellular necrosis, and induction of endothelial apoptosis by CD8+ T cells.[68–70,72,74] Activation of PFK may be important in maintaining vascular integrity and energy metabolism in endothelial cells under hypoxic or oxidative stress,[75,76] which may explain the predisposition of English springer spaniels with PFK deficiency to severe disease. Vasculitis associated with *R. rickettsii* infection manifests as disordered primary hemostasis, tissue edema, hypovolemia, and microthrombosis.

Increased vascular permeability and the associated edema and hypovolemia results from disruption of adherens junctions, endothelial cell death, expression of inflammatory cytokines, such as IL1-β, IFN-γ, and TNF-α, and induction of COX-2 with subsequent prostaglandin production.[68,72] Microthrombosis results from altered platelet adherence to endothelium, increased tissue factor expression, increased plasminogen activator inhibitor, and thrombomodulin expression and the release of von Willebrand's factor.[68,72]

Low numbers of organisms circulate in blood for approximately 13 days after infection, which includes the time that clinical signs are observed.[20,77,78] Organisms are free and also contained within circulating endothelial cells, which are thought to be released from the vessels because of decreased adhesion after rickettsial invasion.[70] Thus, RMSF is primarily an *acute* disease. However, a 2014 study demonstrated a recurrence of clinical signs 44 days and circulating rickettsial organisms 60 days after experimental infection via *D. variabilis* ticks in a beagle.[79] Chronic infection has not been documented in naturally infected dogs or humans. Co-infection with other vector-borne agents is common. A 2014 serological survey involving dogs in the United States showed *R. rickettsii* and *Ehrlichia* spp. co-exposure to be the most common among vector-borne disease agents nationally.[59] Co-infection should be considered if the clinical signs are atypical, if there is an incomplete response to doxycycline therapy, or if clinical signs have been present chronically.[18,80]

Because of variation in the extent and severity of vascular injury among dogs, a range of signs can occur, and importantly, disease manifestations are initially mild and nonspecific.[16,18,19] Often, there is no known history of a tick bite. Therefore, the clinician (physician or veterinarian) must have a high index of suspicion in order to correctly diagnose and treat this disease. A delay in diagnosis and appropriate antimicrobial therapy dramatically increases morbidity and mortality in humans and dogs.[18,57] Lethargy and anorexia are common and may be the only clinical signs. Vomiting and diarrhea occur frequently in dogs and humans with RMSF. Melena may be observed, as may a variety of CNS abnormalities including vestibular disease and seizures.[18,19,21] Dramatic and rapid weight loss has been described.[21]

Physical Examination Findings

Fever is present in approximately 80% of naturally infected dogs. Ocular signs are also frequently observed and may include a mucopurulent discharge, scleral and conjunctival injection and hemorrhage, conjunctivitis,

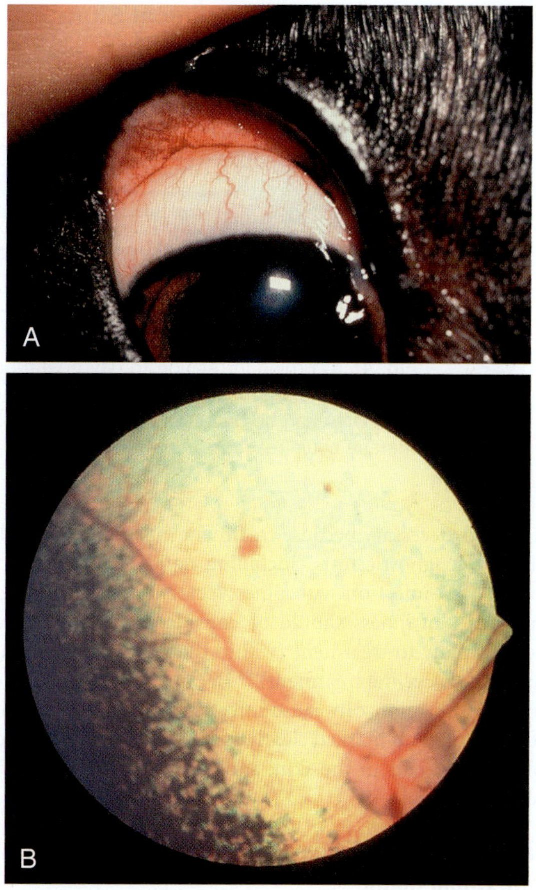

Fig. 46.5 Ocular complications in dogs with Rocky Mountain spotted fever. (A) Conjunctival hyperemia and scleral injection. (B) Retinal hemorrhages.

uveitis, retinal hemorrhage, and retinitis (Fig. 46.5). Lymphadenomegaly and splenomegaly also occur. Respiratory abnormalities include nasal discharge, epistaxis, and tachypnea. Mucocutaneous and cutaneous abnormalities include petechiae, ecchymosis, peripheral edema (which can be localized over a joint, the prepuce, or the mammary chain), hyperemia, and necrosis. Gangrenous necrosis can be so severe as to require reconstructive surgery after successful treatment of the acute febrile illness.[16–19,21,42,81] Orchitis and scrotal edema, hyperemia, and epididymal pain are common in intact male dogs and should prompt consideration of RMSF when present. Generalized myalgia and arthralgia can be observed. Arrhythmias may also be detected. CNS abnormalities can be focal or generalized and include paraparesis, tetraparesis, ataxia, hyperesthesia, ataxia, central or peripheral vestibular signs, stupor, seizures, and/or coma. Neurologic signs are more common in dogs with a high *R. rickettsii* antibody titer, which suggests a longer duration of illness or a delay in diagnosis.[18] Residual neurologic deficits may occur after infection in severely affected individuals. Microvascular hemorrhage, thrombosis, hypotension, oliguric renal failure, cardiovascular collapse, and coma can occur terminally.

DIAGNOSIS

Application of a combination of diagnostic tests is often necessary to confirm infection by SFG rickettsiae. Active infection is confirmed in a patient with compatible acute clinical signs and demonstration of the organism using PCR assays or IHC, or documentation of seroconversion (Fig. 46.6). Importantly, a high index of suspicion based on

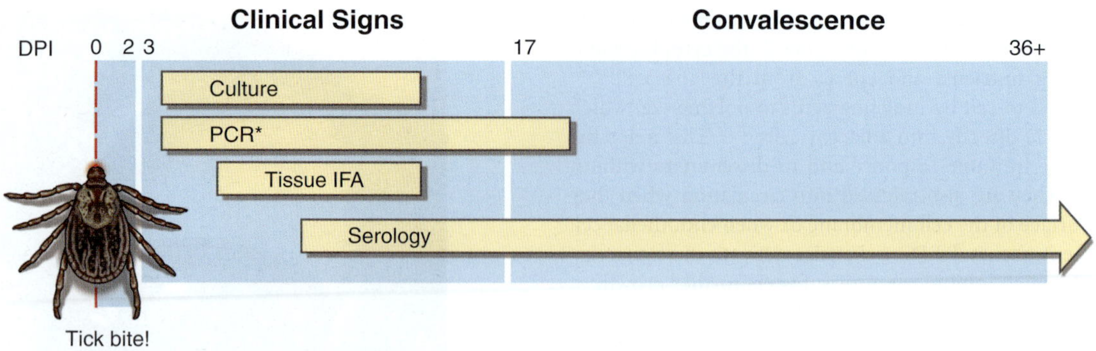

Fig. 46.6 Timing in relation to day postinfection *(DPI)* that clinical signs and diagnostic tests for *Rickettsia rickettsii* may be positive in an infected dog.[16,77–79,86,95] *Further studies are needed to determine exactly how DNA can be detected in peripheral blood after infection. *IFA*, immunofluorescent antibody; *PCR*, polymerase chain reaction.

clinical signs is necessary because treatment must be instituted before the results of diagnostic tests (including rapid PCR assays) confirm infection.[18,21] Co-infection with other vector-borne disease agents or alternate causes of illness should be considered in patients who fail to respond rapidly to treatment (within the first 24 to 48 hours after initiation of doxycycline treatment).[80] Because direct inoculation into blood or aerosolization can cause infection, all specimens should be handled with care and marked clearly as biohazards. Needle-stick injuries, contact with cuts in the skin, and aerosolization of rickettsemic blood should be avoided.

Laboratory Abnormalities

Complete Blood Count

Thrombocytopenia is common in RMSF and occurs due to vasculitis and immune-mediated platelet destruction.[82] However, thrombocytopenia does not occur in all dogs with RMSF.[18,21] The white blood cell count may initially decrease and then tends to increase with duration of illness.[19–21] Neutrophils may have toxic change.[18] Despite the acute nature of this severe illness, a nonregenerative anemia may be present and persist until the dog is treated appropriately and begins to recover.[16,18,21]

Serum Biochemical Tests

Serum biochemical abnormalities can include hypoalbuminemia (due to vasculitis or protein-losing nephropathy), increased serum ALP activity, hyponatremia, and mild hyperbilirubinemia.[16,18,21,83] Hyponatremia is thought to occur secondary to antidiuretic hormone secretion in response to hypovolemia in people with RMSF.[57]

Urinalysis

Urinalysis results in dogs with RMSF are variable and may include proteinuria, hematuria and bilirubinuria, and pyuria. Granular casts can be observed.[18,19]

Coagulation Profile

Coagulation abnormalities include prolonged APTT and increased serum fibrinogen concentration. Less commonly, prolonged PT and increased fibrin degradation products are observed. Although a prothrombotic state can occur during fulminant disease, disseminated intravascular coagulation is uncommon.[16,18]

Cytologic Examination of Tissue Aspirates and Body Fluids

Cytologic examination of aspirates from enlarged lymph nodes in dogs with RMSF is consistent with reactive lymphoid hyperplasia.[18,19] Arthrocentesis may reveal neutrophilic polyarthritis.[18,19] CSF analysis in dogs with neurologic signs may reveal a mixed cellular, neutrophilic, or lymphocytic pleocytosis.[18,19,21,84]

Diagnostic Imaging

Thoracic radiographs in dogs with RMSF may show an unstructured interstitial pattern.[19,85] Testicular ultrasound findings may be consistent with orchitis in intact males.[81]

Microbiologic Tests

Diagnostic assays available for RMSF in dogs are shown in Table 46.1. Because of the pathogenesis of the infection, laboratory diagnostics (including serology and PCR assays) may not indicate that infection is present at the time that clinical signs manifest (see Fig. 46.6). In addition, most diagnostic tests do not differentiate among species of SFG rickettsiae.

Culture

Because of the obligately intracellular and extremely pathogenic nature of *R. rickettsii,* cell culture is difficult to perform and processing of specimens for isolation is limited to BSL-3 facilities (see Table 46.1). Therefore, culture is not commonly used for routine diagnosis.

Serologic Diagnosis

Indirect microimmunofluorescence (MIF) assays that detect IgM and IgG antibodies are most commonly used to document seroconversion in dogs infected with *R. rickettsii*.[18] Because of a lack of specificity, assays that detect IgM alone cannot be used to accurately diagnose acute RMSF.[86] There is extensive serologic cross-reactivity among SFG rickettsiae, and thus a positive titer only indicates exposure to SFG rickettsial species. In general, the infecting species is presumed based on geographic locale, so RMSF is the presumptive diagnosis in dogs that seroconvert in the southeastern United States. However, other species of SFG rickettsiae may also be present and potentially induce disease.[30,87] Seropositivity that indicates exposure to SFG *Rickettsia* is common in dogs in the United States. Exposure to nonpathogenic SFG rickettsiae, some of which are common endosymbionts in ticks, may be a common cause of positive titers, particularly low and persistent titers, to *R. rickettsii* in healthy people and dogs.[67,88] Serologic cross-reactivity with SFG rickettsiae does not appear to occur in dogs infected with *Bartonella* spp.[89–91] In addition, previous infection with *R. rickettsii* may result in persistent antibody titers.[86] Thus, infection with *R. rickettsii* cannot be definitively diagnosed based on a single positive titer. However, a single high titer in the context of acute and

TABLE 46.1 Diagnostic Assays Available for Rocky Mountain Spotted Fever in Dogs

Assay	Specimen Type	Target	Performance
Indirect microimmuno-fluorescence assay (MIF)	Serum	IgM and IgG antibodies against *R. rickettsii*	Demonstration of a fourfold change in titer (seroconversion) is very sensitive. False-negative results are common during the acute phase of infection. A positive antibody response may reflect prior exposure to a nonpathogenic SFG rickettsia, or long-lived circulating antibody from previous infection with SFG rickettsiae. Cross-reactivity to other SFG rickettsiae occurs.
PCR	Whole blood	Gene target varies with testing laboratories	*In vitro* sensitivity may approach 100%; however, absolute (clinical) sensitivity is lower, approximately 60%, because organisms circulate in blood in low numbers and transiently during the acute phase of infection. Sensitivity is further reduced by antimicrobial drug treatment. Specificity approaches 100%, particularly if the laboratory sequences all PCR amplicons. PCR testing for other tick-borne organisms that cause similar clinical signs is available as PCR panels from some testing laboratories. Only a few PCR assays differentiate among *Rickettsia* species. Negative PCR assay results do not rule out infection.
Histopathology with direct IFA or Gimenez staining	Cutaneous biopsy (inguinal or flank targeting areas with lesions) or necropsy specimens	Characteristic perivascular inflammation and vasculitis with necrosis and presence of the organism	Direct IFA sensitivity is approximately 80% during acute infection. Biopsy of a petechial or ecchymotic lesion may increase sensitivity. False negatives occur if organisms are absent from the lesion because of random chance, timing of specimen collection, or prior antimicrobial treatment. Does not differentiate among species of SFG rickettsiae.

IFA, immunofluorescent antibody; *PCR*, polymerase chain reaction; *SFG*, spotted fever group.

compatible clinical signs and an appropriate response to therapy suggests infection.[18] Titers are commonly negative early in the course of infection, because clinical signs often occur before seroconversion in naturally and experimentally infected dogs.[21,86,92] Thus, acute and convalescent serology (run in the same laboratory and ideally in the same batch) and documentation of a fourfold change in titer is necessary to confirm acute SFG rickettsiae infection. The convalescent serum specimen should be drawn 2 to 3 weeks after the acute specimen.

Molecular Diagnosis Using Nucleic Acid–Based Testing

PCR testing of whole blood can be used to confirm infection in seronegative dogs during the acute phase of disease.[77,78,92] A sensitive PCR assay that detects and differentiates among SFG rickettsiae that infect dog blood has been described, and a variety of PCR assays are available through commercial veterinary diagnostic laboratories.[92] However, because *R. rickettsii* circulates in blood in low numbers and only transiently, the sensitivity of any diagnostic assay to detect infection in the bloodstream is limited. One real-time PCR assay, which could detect as few as five copies of organism DNA, had a sensitivity of only 53% for detection of *R. rickettsii* in acute samples from naturally infected dogs with signs of RMSF.[92] The sensitivity of another *R. rickettsii* PCR assay for detection of *R. rickettsii* in experimentally infected dogs ranged from 33% to 100% depending on the day of sample collection.[78] Furthermore, false negatives can occur after initiation of appropriate antimicrobial treatment. Therefore, although a positive PCR assay result confirms infection, a negative result does not exclude the diagnosis. Some PCR assays can differentiate among infecting *Rickettsia* species, whereas others only amplify conserved rickettsial DNA targets.[77,92] Clinicians should consult with laboratories to determine the *in vitro* (analytical) and *in vivo* (clinical) sensitivity of a PCR assay and its ability to differentiate among infecting *Rickettsia* species. Whenever possible, it is important for veterinary and human clinicians to submit specimens to laboratories that use PCR assays that differentiate among *Rickettsia* species.[58] Samples should be obtained before antirickettsial antibiotic therapy is administered. Combining PCR with serologic testing, repeating PCR assays on samples taken before treatment, and serologic testing of convalescent samples facilitates diagnosis.[92]

Pathologic Findings

Gross Pathologic Findings

Gross pathologic findings in dogs with RMSF are consistent with vasculitis and may include edema, particularly of the ears, muzzle, and scrotum; and ecchymosis, petechiae, and/or focal hemorrhages of the skin, mucous membranes, and viscera (including the brain). Lymphadenomegaly and splenomegaly are also common findings.[16,17,21,23]

Histopathologic Findings

Microscopically, the predominant lesion is vasculitis. Neutrophils, monocytes, and/or lymphoreticular cells predominate in the inflammatory lesions. Inflammatory cells may surround and invade large-, small-, and medium-size vessels of multiple organs and tissues and this is frequently accompanied by focal necrosis and hemorrhage. Meningoencephalitis, splenitis, myocardial necrosis, glomerulonephritis, and renal vasculitis have been described.[16,21,23]

Direct IFA can be used to detect organisms in skin and other organs. Identification of abundant SFG rickettsiae within and around small- to medium-size vessels and vascular endothelial cells can confirm infection.[21] In experimentally infected dogs, the sensitivity of IHC was 78.3%, and organisms could be visualized between days 7 and 12 of infection (days 3 to 8 of fever).[93] In that study, specimens collected from areas other than the central focus of vasculitis were negative. However, in naturally infected dogs, the sensitivity was 80% for skin specimens collected from the inguinal region. Half of those specimens lacked gross lesions.[19] Thus, the diagnostic sensitivity of IHC is most likely enhanced by obtaining lesional biopsies, but may not be decreased when a lesion is not biopsied. The sensitivity of direct IHC is decreased by antibiotic therapy. IHC does not differentiate between SFG rickettsial species. Gimenez stain can also be used to visualize rickettsial organisms

TABLE 46.2 Antimicrobials Used to Treat Rocky Mountain Spotted Fever in Dogs

Drug	Dose (mg/kg)	Route	Interval (Hours)	Duration (Days)
Doxycycline	5	PO, IV	12	7–14
Chloramphenicol[a]	30	PO, IV	8	7–14
Enrofloxacin	3[b] to 5	PO, IV	12	7–14

[a]May cause aplastic anemia in humans (wear gloves); may be less effective than doxycycline.
[b]Dose used in experimentally infected dogs.[95] Caution required in young animals (see Chapter 10).
IV, intravenous; *PO,* oral.

in tissues or tissue culture isolation attempts, but this stain is not rickettsia specific and does not allow for differentiation among species.

TREATMENT

Antimicrobial Treatment

Appropriate antibiotic therapy must be immediately instituted based on clinical suspicion for SFG rickettsiosis, and before diagnostic tests confirm infection. Inappropriate or delayed antibiotic therapy may increase morbidity and mortality.[18,57] Some antimicrobial drugs such as trimethoprim-sulfonamides may worsen disease progression of RMSF in human patients.[57] Doxycycline is the treatment of choice (Table 46.2). It effectively eliminates infection with *R. rickettsii* and also has activity against *A. phagocytophilum, Ehrlichia* spp., and *B. burgdorferi,* which may be present in co-infections or cause disease that resembles RMSF. In most cases, 7 days of treatment is adequate for RMSF. Treatment for a few days beyond defervescence is recommended. A longer course of treatment is recommended for dogs that are co-infected with *Ehrlichia* spp. or *B. burgdorferi* (see Chapters 44 and 69). Tooth discoloration and enamel hypoplasia, which are permanent adverse effects of tetracycline use in pediatric patients, has not been observed with short-term (7–10 days), low-dose (approximately 2.2 mg/kg q12h) doxycycline therapy in children less than 8 years of age.[57,94] Therefore, as is the case for adults, doxycycline is the treatment of choice for RMSF in children.[57] Chloramphenicol was effective for RMSF in experimentally infected dogs.[95] However, it may be less effective than doxycycline for treating RMSF in humans and has less activity *in vitro* against *Ehrlichia chaffeensis* and *A. phagocytophilum.*[57,96] Enrofloxacin was effective for treatment of RMSF in experimentally infected dogs.[95] However, enrofloxacin is not effective for treatment of *Ehrlichia canis* infections.[97] Use of parenteral antimicrobial drugs may be necessary in severely debilitated or vomiting patients.

Supportive Care

Many dogs with RMSF require hospitalization.[21] Aggressive supportive care for complications such as thrombosis, CNS deficits, and GI signs may be necessary. Because of the loss of vascular integrity, fluids should be administered with caution, and colloids may be warranted in some cases. The clinician should avoid exacerbation of interstitial edema, which can contribute to cerebral edema and death. The use of glucocorticoids in dogs with RMSF is controversial. Treatment with anti-inflammatory and immunosuppressive doses of glucocorticoids did not affect overall outcome in experimentally infected dogs, but rickettsemia was prolonged in dogs concurrently treated with immunosuppressive doses of glucocorticoids and doxycycline.[98] Anti-inflammatory doses of glucocorticoids have been used in dogs with severe CNS manifestations and may be necessary topically or systemically for treatment of ocular abnormalities.[84,99]

PROGNOSIS

The response to appropriate antibiotic therapy in dogs with RMSF is rapid (24 to 48 hours). Co-infection with *B. burgdorferi, Ehrlichia* spp., *Babesia* spp., and *Bartonella* spp. should be considered in dogs with severe or prolonged clinical signs or dogs that fail to respond to doxycycline. Residual CNS and other deficits may occur in severely affected patients.[18] The prognosis is good to excellent if the disease is diagnosed and treated with appropriate antibiotics and supportive care early in the course of illness.[18,84] Due to the potential clinical severity of RMSF, reactivation of occult *Bartonella* spp. infection is possible.[89] In contrast to most other canine vector-borne infections, doxycycline is not recommended as a sole treatment for bartonellosis.[100]

IMMUNITY AND VACCINATION

Innate and adaptive (primarily CMI) immunity are important in the clearance of SFG *Rickettsia* infections. Dendritic cells (DCs) serve as a bridge between innate and adaptive immunity. Binding of rickettsial LPS to DC TLR-4 causes DC activation and production of inflammatory cytokines; recruitment, activation, and expansion of NK cells and NK IFN-γ production; and DC-mediated induction of T-helper 1 and T-helper 17 adaptive immune responses.[72] CD4+ and CD8+ cells, along with macrophages and DCs, are believed to be sources of inflammatory cytokines such as IFN-γ, TNF-α, IL-1β, and RANTES (CCL5). These cytokines increase the production of nitric oxide synthetase and hydrogen peroxide by the endothelial cell, which helps to eliminate the organisms.[69,70] The endothelial cells themselves also produce cytokines such as IL-6, IL-8, and MCP-1 (CCL2) that recruit immune cells and combat infection. It is thought that endothelial cells present antigen to CD8+ T cells in the context of MHC I.[72] CD8+ cells appear to be particularly important in clearance of rickettsiae from the endothelium.[101] Antibodies are not thought to be important initially for clearance of infection because they form after the fulminant stages of disease.[70,72] However, antibodies are long-lived and together with CMI may prevent subsequent infection. Immunity to reinfection is thought to be lifelong in people, and experimentally infected dogs did not develop illness following rechallenge at 6 months and 3 years after the initial infection. Vaccination is not available for dogs or humans currently, but may be in the future.[102,103]

PREVENTION

The use of acaricides, avoidance of tick-infested areas, and routine inspection of dogs for ticks after outdoor activities can help to prevent RMSF. The reader is referred to Chapters 13 and 109 for information on tick prevention and safe tick removal. Safe tick removal is especially critical when exposure to *R. rickettsii* is a possibility. In cases where *Rh. sanguineus* is the vector, environmental control of ticks is particularly important.[104]

PUBLIC HEALTH ASPECTS

A "One Health" approach to the management of canine and human RMSF is important. It has been well established that people living near dogs and with dogs in endemic areas are at increased risk for acquiring RMSF. This results from increased human contact with ticks through interaction with tick-infested dogs. Interestingly, one 2019 study of personnel working in veterinary clinics showed that exposure risk was highest in groomers.[105] Dogs and humans can also independently acquire the infection from different ticks questing in the same environment, particularly as *R. rickettsii* is transmitted transovarially to offspring. Because dogs have higher exposure to ticks than their human counterparts, they serve as excellent environmental sentinels for RMSF.[22,23,25,87] In the United States, the diagnosis of SFG rickettsioses in humans is notifiable to public health authorities. Some counties in certain states also require reporting for dogs, particularly during suspected outbreaks.[106] From a public health standpoint, it is important for veterinarians to confirm a diagnosis of RMSF in a dog whenever possible, and to warn the family of the increased risk of acquiring a *R. rickettsii*–infected tick in the same location as the dog acquired the disease. Veterinarians must communicate with owners and physicians that infection in a dog may precede tick-transmitted infection to owners or neighbors. Clients should be instructed to remove ticks properly. Education of owners with regard to the importance of tick control and prevention for both people and pets and the environment is critical. Novel and well-characterized species of SFG rickettsiae are important causes of emerging infectious disease in humans. Because dogs are sentinels for infection, veterinarians play an important role in detection, definition, and prevention of illness in their canine patients and their human companions.

MEDITERRANEAN SPOTTED FEVER

Rickettsia conorii subsp. *conorii* is the cause of an endemic tick-borne rickettsial illness of people in the Mediterranean basin and Africa known as MSF (or boutonneuse spotted fever). Several other subspecies of *R. conorii* (*indica*, *caspia*, and *israelensis*) are responsible for clinical or subclinical infections in people in India, Eastern Europe, and the Middle East, respectively.[7] In humans, the clinical appearance of MSF is similar to RMSF, except that the presence of an eschar at the site of tick bite is common.

MSF is transmitted by *Rh. sanguineus*. It is suspected that this tick serves as a reservoir for the disease.[7] Whether dogs or other vertebrate hosts are also reservoirs is uncertain, but experimentally, dogs are able to transmit the organism to *Rh. sanguineus* ticks.[7,107] Serologic studies indicate a high rate of exposure among clinically healthy dogs[29,108] and cats in endemic areas.[108] However, seroconversion was associated with fever in a 2015 study of ill dogs in Italy.[35] Host immunity is likely important in determining if clinical illness develops in dogs with MSF. Like RMSF, dogs serve as sentinels for MSF in humans.[7] Interestingly, one study found that *R. conorii* survived 35 days in stored canine whole blood, suggesting that iatrogenic infection from transfused blood products is potentially possible.[109]

Male Yorkshire terriers were the only affected breed in the first clinical report of naturally occurring MSF in dogs.[15] This breed also had the highest rate of infection with *R. conorii* in another study testing for SFG rickettsemia in large numbers of dogs in Italy.[110] An inherent susceptibility to MSF in Yorkshire terriers is suspected, but uncertain.

Findings of clinical and pathologic studies in experimentally and naturally infected dogs with MSF are analogous to those described in RMSF. Clinical signs include lethargy and, less commonly, vomiting and diarrhea.[35] Physical examination abnormalities include elevated rectal temperature (generally 40.1°C to 41°C [104.2°F to 105.8°F]), hyperesthesia, peripheral edema, orchitis, erythema, stiff gait, lymphadenomegaly, splenomegaly, tachycardia, lameness, conjunctival swelling, and dehydration.[15,35,111]

Laboratory abnormalities associated with MSF in dogs include neutrophilic leukocytosis with a variable left shift, thrombocytopenia, hypoproteinemia and concurrent hypoalbuminemia, hyperglobulinemia, and increased serum urea nitrogen concentration, C-reactive protein (CRP) concentration, and hepatic aminotransferase activities. Although α-hyperglobulinemia is observed in RMSF in dogs as an acute-phase reaction, the additional observation of increased β- and γ-globulins in natural cases of MSF would suggest a longer-standing infection with *R. conorii* before the onset of clinical illness or coinfection with other vector-borne pathogens.

Diagnosis is made either by demonstrating seroconversion, or a positive PCR test, and a corresponding clinical improvement after antirickettsial therapy. Serologic cross-reactivity with other SFG *Rickettsia* preclude definitive speciation if diagnosis is based on serologic testing. Because of the high seroprevalance in dogs in endemic areas, a single positive titer does not confirm active infection.

Antimicrobial treatment is the same as for RMSF, and response to doxycycline appears to be rapid.[15] The public health risk of tick-infested dogs infected with *R. conorii* would be presumably high because *Rh. sanguineus* can become domiciled indoors in homes or kennels. This been demonstrated with *Rh. sanguineus*-associated RMSF in the United States and Mexico.[46,112] A higher association of MSF in people with dog ownership supports this contention.[113] Inadvertent tick bites and direct inoculation and subsequent infection sustained during removal of ticks from dogs have been associated with transmission to humans.[55,114] Tick control in dogs and the environment would have a likely beneficial effect of reducing the prevalence of this disease in both humans and dogs. Interestingly, a 2016 serosurvey showed a decrease of exposure to *R. conorii* in humans in an endemic area. It was suggested that widespread tick control in dogs contributed to the decline in human exposure.[115]

OTHER TICK-BORNE SPOTTED FEVER GROUP RICKETTSIAE

Although RMSF and MSF are the most well-characterized SFR in the world, serologically, genetically, and pathogenically distinct SFG rickettsiae have also been described as important disease-causing agents in humans.[7] Many closely related SFG rickettsial species of unknown pathogenicity have been detected in or isolated from ticks in the United States. Other than *R. rickettsii*, SFG species isolated from ticks associated with dogs in the United States include *R. parkeri*, *R. amblyommii*, *R. montanensis* (formerly *R. montana*), *Rickettsia rhipicephali*, *Rickettsia bellii*, *Rickettsia andeanae*, and *R. massiliae*.[30,83,116]

Rickettsia parkeri was previously considered to be a nonpathogenic SFG rickettsia. Its vector is *Amblyomma maculatum* (the Gulf Coast tick). *Rickettsia parkeri* has now been shown to cause clinical illness in humans in the United States.[117] It is suspected that many cases of human RMSF that are diagnosed in areas where *A. maculatum* is endemic are caused by *R. parkeri* rather than *R. rickettsii*.[58] *Rickettsia parkeri* also was associated with a spotted fever type of illness in hikers in Arizona. *Amblyomma triste* was the suspected vector.[118] Human disease associated with *R. parkeri* infection appears to be milder and is characterized by the presence of eschar and lymphadenomegaly, signs not commonly seen with RMSF.[14] In 2011, *R. parkeri* was amplified using PCR from overtly healthy shelter dogs in Louisiana.[34]

Rickettsia amblyommii, *R. montanensis*, *R. rhipicephali*, and *R. bellii* are thought to be of low pathogenicity or nonpathogenic in humans.[7] However, like *R. parkeri*, evidence suggests that *R. amblyommii* and *R. montanensis* may cause illness in people in the United States, and account for some of the reported SFR in areas endemic for RMSF.[119,120] In the last decade, DNA from *R. amblyommii* and *R. montanensis* has been amplified from the blood of naturally exposed, apparently healthy dogs.[37] The rickettsemia was short-lived. *Rickettsia rhipicephali*, *R. bellii*, and *R. andeanae* have not been shown to cause disease in dogs or humans to date.

Rickettsia massiliae has been characterized as a human pathogen in Europe, and was implicated as a cause of febrile illness in dogs and people living in a *Rh. sanguineus*-infested home in Los Angeles.[30,121] *Rickettsia massiliae* DNA has also been amplified from the blood of naturally infected cats and from the blood of a naturally infected dog.[38,122] *Rickettsia phillipii* (SFG *Rickettsia* strain 364D) is the cause of an emerging tick-borne disease known as Pacific Coast Fever. Pacific Coast Fever is transmitted by *D. occidentalis* ticks.[123] Although cases have been reported in California, cases could occur within the entire geographic range of this tick, which includes Oregon to Baja California, Mexico. Whether it causes disease in dogs has not been determined.

In a 2020 report, a novel, genetically well-characterized rickettsia species with 95% homology to both *R. massiliae* and *Rickettsia heilongjiangensis* was amplified from the blood of three different dogs in three different regions of the United States.[124] Clinical signs resembled RMSF and the dogs were seroreactive to *R. rickettsii*.

Diseases similar to MSF have also been described in people in the Eastern Hemisphere. Queensland tick typhus (*R. australis*), Flinders Island spotted fever (*Rickettsia honei*), Australian spotted fever (*Rickettsia marmionii*), African tick bite fever (*Rickettsia africae*), Astrakhan fever (*R. conorii* sub sp. *caspia*), Japanese spotted fever (*R. japonica*), Far Eastern spotted fever (*R. heilongjiangensis*), North Asian tick typhus (*Rickettsia sibirica*), and European tick-borne lymphadenopathy (*Rickettsia helvetica*, "*Rickettsia sibirica* sub sp. *mongolotimonae*," *Rickettsia slovaca*, *Rickettsia aeschlimannii*, *R. massiliae*) are analogous diseases of humans caused by other SFG rickettsiae and transmitted by arthropods in geographically distinct regions.[7] *Rickettsia helvetica* is found in *Ixodes* spp. ticks and has a wide distribution in Europe and the Far East. *Rickettsia helvetica* DNA, along with that from *R. japonica*, has been identified by PCR in ticks removed from dogs and cats in Japan.[125] Dogs and cats have had positive serologic reactions to this *Rickettsia*, indicating exposure, and DNA of *R. japonica* has been amplified from dog blood.[126,127] *Rickettsia japonica* causes transient clinical signs including fever, anorexia, and depression in immunosuppressed but not healthy experimentally infected dogs.[33] Antibodies to *R. australis* have been documented in dogs in southeastern Australia. Antibodies to SFG rickettsiae have been detected in the blood of dogs and cats in the Tasmanian region of Australia; however, there was no correlation between seroreactivity and the animal's health.[128] Experimental infection in dogs was subclinical, and although seroconversion occurred, *R. australis* could not be reisolated.[31] Taken together, these studies suggest that SFG rickettsiae other than *R. rickettsii* may cause milder disease in dogs, as is the case in humans, and that novel rickettsiosis should be considered in dogs with atypical clinical signs or those presenting in endemic or nonendemic areas. Some PCR assays and other molecular biological techniques may be used to differentiate among species in clinical cases. Whenever possible, it is important for veterinary and human clinicians to submit to laboratories that use PCR that can differentiate among SFG species.[58] Among other examples, determination of the infecting species resulted in the recognition of the novel *Rickettsia* sp. in dogs in the United States.[124] Antibodies to SFG rickettsiae that are nonpathogenic (or of low pathogenicity) cross-react with pathogenic SFG rickettsiae and therefore may make determining the meaning of a positive titer in an ill patient challenging.

RICKETTSIALPOX

Rickettsialpox is a nonfatal febrile zoonotic illness caused by *R. akari*, a SFG rickettsia that predominantly affects people in urban areas. Serum antibodies to *R. akari* were found in dogs examined during routine veterinary care in New York City.[129] The only possible source of exposure for a person in North Carolina who developed rickettsialpox was captured mice brought in by a pet cat.[130] An 8-month-old dog from Mexico was infected with *R. akari* and had hyporexia, fever, vomiting, and melena.[131] Physical examination abnormalities were weight loss, abdominal discomfort, suspected myalgia, and hepatosplenomegaly. Hematologic and biochemical abnormalities included neutrophilic leukocytosis, anemia, thrombocytopenia, increased hepatic aminotransferase activity, hypoalbuminemia, and hypoglobulinemia. Treatment was instituted with oral doxycycline for 7 days, and remission occurred in 48 hours. The organism was also detected by PCR in two *Rh. sanguineus* ticks found on the dog. The maintenance of *R. akari* involves horizontal transmission between the house mouse *(Mus musculus)* and its mite *(Liponyssoides sanguineus)*. Transovarial and transstadial transmission occurs in the mite. Seropositivity in dogs indicates that an alternative form of this transmission cycle might exist. It is presumed that mites feed on dogs; however, a tick such as *Rh. sanguineus*, or another tick vector as-yet unknown may be responsible for exposing dogs.

FLEA-BORNE SPOTTED FEVER (*RICKETTSIA FELIS* INFECTION)

A flea-borne typhus-like illness caused by *R. felis* has been reported in people from many countries worldwide.[132] *Rickettsia felis* shares some phenotypic characteristics with the TG *Rickettsia*. For example, *R. felis* is primarily flea-borne rather than tick-borne, and it is ultrastructurally indistinguishable from, and has extensive serologic cross-reactivity with, *Rickettsia typhi*. However, genotypic studies show that it is more closely related to SFG *Rickettsia*, or may be a part of a separate phylogenetic lineage.[8,133]

The cat flea *(Ctenocephalides felis)* is the primary vector for *R. felis*, although *R. felis* has been detected in other arthropod vectors including other flea species, ticks, and mites.[132] More than 90% of fleas purchased commercially for research purposes are infected, whereas the percentage in naturally infected fleas is much lower and depends on the geographic area. In the United States, the disease is endemic in southern Texas and California and overlaps that of human murine typhus caused by *R. typhi*.[134] Opossums and fleas have been found to be co-infected with both rickettsiae, and cat flea infection with *R. felis* is more common than with *R. typhi* in these regions.[134–139] Given the presence of both agents in fleas, some reports of murine typhus based on serology may have been caused by *R. felis*.[132] Indeed, PCR and restriction fragment length polymorphism identified *R. typhi* in four of five people from Texas who had typhus, and *R. felis* was found in the remaining person.[138] However, the importance of *R. felis* as a predominant cause of typhus-like illness in southern California has been questioned.[140] An infection cycle in people with *R. felis* and *C. felis* has been found in France, Germany, and Brazil.[141,142] The infection probably exists worldwide in areas where cat fleas are prevalent. In Africa, there is some evidence that additional vectors may play a role in human cases.[132]

Rickettsia felis is transmitted vertically through transovarial transmission and possibly through consumption of infected feces by larvae to successive generations of *C. felis*.[132,143,144] Infection can be maintained in cat fleas for up to 12 generations without the fleas having fed on an infected host. Therefore, it is also likely serves as a reservoir.[132] Horizontal transmission from vector to vector by a shared meal occurs, but whether mammalian blood or tissues serve as a source of infection for fleas has been questioned.[132] Infection with *R. felis* has been transmitted among cats by infected fleas, and cats are seropositive to *R. typhi* antigen in endemic areas.[137,145,146] Experimental infection of cats with *R. felis* produced subclinical infection with seroconversion between 2 and 4 months.[145] Fever was not associated with natural exposure to *R. felis* in one study.[39] Another study suggested that lymphadenopathy and polycythemia may be associated with infection.[147] In one study, neither the organism nor its nucleic acid was identified from blood of cats naturally infested with infected *C. felis*.[148] However, a 2018 study described amplification of *R. felis* DNA from the blood of a community cat in southern California.[135] Two additional cats in the California study had circulating DNA from the *R. felis*-like agent "*Candidatus* Rickettsia senegalensis." Out of 64 flea pools collected from community cats in that study, 12 were PCR positive for *R. felis*, 5 were PCR positive for "*Candidatus* R. senegalensis," and none were PCR positive for *R. typhi*.

Rickettsia felis was detected using PCR from dogs sampled in northern Cambodia and Queensland, Australia, and dogs have been shown to be seropositive in endemic areas in some but not other studies.[137,146,149–151] A recent study using PCR and cell culture demonstrated sustained *R. felis* rickettsemia in experimentally infected 14-week-old puppies.[152] Transmission of *R. felis* between infected and uninfected *C. felis* fleas also occurred. No changes in RBC or platelet count were documented in infected puppies, although some puppies developed transient leukocytosis, self-limiting diarrhea, and decreased appetite. One puppy demonstrated petechial hemorrhages. Whether clinical disease may occur in naturally infected puppies or adult dogs with or without co-morbidities is not known.

In the United States, *R. felis* has been detected in cat fleas taken from cats or dogs from states where sampling has been done.[135,144,148,153] Cats, dogs, and opossums may be likely hosts that transport infected fleas into human habitats.[154] Infection in humans is transferred by flea bites; however, flea feces contain viable organisms that might be inoculated into cutaneous bites or scratches similar to the suspected transmission of *Bartonella henselae*.[132] Clinical signs in humans include fever, headache, and rash. Fatigue, myalgia, photophobia, conjunctivitis, abdominal discomfort, vomiting, and diarrhea are also observed.[155] Doxycycline is the preferred treatment in humans, but many of the other drugs used to treat SFG rickettsial infections are also effective. Clearing of infection in cats or dogs by use of antimicrobials has not been determined. Flea control is essential to reduce the public health risk in endemic areas.

TYPHUS GROUP RICKETTSIAE

Typhus refers to diseases caused by TG rickettsiae. The TG *Rickettsia* spp. include *Rickettsia prowazekii* and *R. typhi*. TG rickettsiae are phenotypically and genotypically different than SFG rickettsiae. For example, they are serologically distinct, they reside in cytoplasm and not the nucleus, and they do not spread between cells through actin polymerization, but instead replicate until the cell bursts.[6,72] Humans are the primary reservoirs of *louse-borne typhus*, or *epidemic typhus*, a sporadic illness caused by *R. prowazekii*. It occurs when events favor proliferation and spread of the human body louse, such as unsanitary conditions and natural disasters. The organism infects the louse's alimentary tract and is excreted in its feces. Irritation from biting lice causes the person to scratch, thereby contaminating the abraded site with infected louse feces. Infection can also occur after rubbing contaminated hands on mucosal surfaces. Lice infected by *R. prowazekii* die within 1 to 3 weeks after ingestion of infected blood. Lice do not transmit the infection transovarially to their progeny. Another reservoir for this infection in humans in the United States appears to be the southern flying squirrel. The disease is referred to as "sylvatic epidemic typhus." The clinical signs in humans are generally similar to those of RMSF. Interestingly, in apparent contrast to infection with *R. rickettsii*, *R. prowazekii* can recrudesce years after initial infection in the same person.[156] This is referred to as "Brill-Zinsser disease" or recrudescent typhus. Antibody reactivity to TG rickettsiae has been observed in the sera of dogs suspected of having rickettsial disease.[157] *Rickettsia prowazekii* caused no illness or sustained infection in experimentally inoculated immunocompetent dogs.[157] No information clarifies whether this organism infects dogs or cats in nature.

Murine typhus, or *endemic typhus*, has a more worldwide distribution than louse-borne typhus. It is caused by *R. typhi*, which is transmitted by fleas. It is most prevalent in the temperate and subtropical climates where the reservoir rodent hosts and their fleas are found. The disease is transmitted by scratching of infected flea feces into a pruritic bite wound. Some transovarial transmission occurs, so direct bites from fleas can also produce illness in people. The clinical signs in people are very similar to those of RMSF. In the continental United States, murine typhus is endemic in southern California and South Texas. In this region, the natural host and vector system is the opossum and cat flea. It has also been isolated from cat fleas infesting dogs in Oklahoma.[153] In one study, dog and cat owners were no more likely to be seropositive than nonowners.[158] However, in another study, owning a dog was a significant risk factor for human exposure.[159] Because it is flea-transmitted, flea control on pets is important to help prevent human infection. *Rickettsia typhi* has been amplified from the blood of dogs[160] and from *Rh. sanguineus* ticks,[161] suggesting other vectors may play a role in transmission.

Scrub typhus is a rickettsial disease of humans caused by *Orientia* (previously *Rickettsia*) *tsutsugamushi* in southeastern Asia, the South Pacific, and Australia. It is transmitted by the chigger mite, and wild rodents and birds are reservoir hosts. Clinical signs are similar to those of RMSF. However, dogs have been experimentally infected with *O. tsutsugamushi* without signs of clinical illness. *Orentia tsutsugamushi* was amplified from the blood of a dog in Japan with clinical signs of rickettsial disease that responded to minocycline. Blood samples taken from 10 dogs fed in the same area as the ill dog were also PCR positive.[162] An *O. tsutsugamushi*-like organism has also been amplified from the blood of a naturally infected dog in South Africa.[163] The role of this organism as a disease-causing agent in dogs and cats requires further study.

CASE EXAMPLES

ROCKY MOUNTAIN SPOTTED FEVER IN A DOG

Signalment

A 5-year-old MC Australian shepherd from North Carolina.

History

The dog was examined by the North Carolina State University veterinary emergency service on April 11 because of recent onset of lethargy, fever, tachypnea, and a stiff gait when walking. Historically the dog had been healthy, had received routine vaccinations, heartworm preventative, and a flea preventative, and ran approximately 3 miles each evening with the owner, who was a veterinarian. On the day of examination and several hours after the evening run, the dog became lethargic, refused to eat dog food or treats, and seemed painful upon manipulation. The owner noticed that the dog's HR, which was normally 50 to 60 beats/minute, was 120 beats/minute at rest. Rectal temperature at home just prior to presentation was 104.4°F (40.2°C). Three days before the dog was evaluated, the owner had removed a nonengorged tick from the dog.

Physical Examination

Physical examination findings included a body weight of 21.3 kg, 3%–5% dehydration, pain score of 1 out of 4, rectal temperature of 103.7°F (39.8°C), HR 130 beats/minute, tachypnea (42 breaths/minute), and a normal CRT. The BCS was 5/9. The dog stood in a hunched position and had a stiff gait, but localizing pain was not elicited on palpation of the spine, joints, or long bones. There was no nasal or ocular discharge, no petechiae or rash, and no obvious swelling or joint effusion. Popliteal lymph nodes were prominent, but there were no other abnormalities noted on physical examination. Systolic blood pressure was 153 mmHg, and diastolic and mean blood pressures were 93 and 111 mmHg, respectively.

Laboratory Findings

The hematocrit was 42%, total plasma protein was 6.2 mg/dL, and the platelet count was 120,000/μL. A serum biochemical profile showed only hypoglobulinemia (1.7 g/dL).

Microbiologic Testing

A SNAP 4Dx Plus (IDEXX Laboratories, Portland, ME, USA) in-house ELISA assay was negative. Indirect IFA assays for *Babesia canis, B. henselae, Bartonella vinsonii* subsp. *berkhoffii*, and *E. canis* were negative (no detectable antibodies at a 1:16 screening dilution). The dog was seroreactive to *R. rickettsii* at a titer of 1:64. A PCR panel capable of detecting *Anaplasma* spp., *Babesia* spp., *Ehrlichia* spp., and *Rickettsia* spp. was negative on whole blood. A convalescent *R. rickettsii* antibody titer was 1:256, which supported a diagnosis of SFG rickettsiosis, most likely RMSF.

Treatment

Because of the acute onset of lethargy and fever, the history of recent tick attachment, the documentation of thrombocytopenia, and the relatively high frequency of RMSF in dogs and people in North Carolina, doxycycline (4.8 mg/kg, PO, q12h) was prescribed for 3 weeks before the results of microbiologic testing became available. The dog responded rapidly after doxycycline treatment, with appetite and behavior normalizing within 24 to 48 hours after the first dose.

Comment

Although the clinical signs in this dog were relatively nonspecific, the clinical presentation was very typical of RMSF. Because *R. rickettsii* causes generalized vascular injury resulting in increased vascular permeability, fluid and protein leakage out of the intravascular space, and an acute neutrophilic inflammatory response throughout tissue sites within the body, pain that appears to shift in location (back pain, joint pain, abdominal pain, and neck pain) is a typical disease manifestation. Also, the hunched appearance reported in this dog is commonly observed in dogs with RMSF. As this dog was owned by veterinarian and a tick had been removed a few days earlier, a clinical diagnosis and appropriate treatment were initiated earlier in the course of illness than is typical of most dogs with RMSF. The rapid initiation of doxycycline may have blunted the humoral antibody response and decreased the convalescent antibody titer to a level that is lower than expected in most cases of RMSF in dogs. It is important to note that PCR assay is insensitive in the early stages of RMSF, as there are often inadequate numbers of organisms in the blood to achieve successful amplification of rickettsial DNA. A very rapid response to doxycycline is expected, unless there has been a delay in diagnosis, accompanied by the onset of neurologic abnormalities. Dogs that develop neurologic complications experience a more prolonged recovery and can have residual neurologic deficits.

ROCKY MOUNTAIN SPOTTED FEVER IN A HUMAN PATIENT

On May 9, a 61-year-old man, who resided on a farm in Wake County, North Carolina, removed an embedded tick from the hairy portion of his right armpit. Although the duration of attachment was unknown, it was likely that the tick was acquired 2 to 3 days earlier while pulling weeds from a hay field. Using a tick identification key, an experienced research technician classified the tick as a male *A. americanum* and stored the tick in a vial containing alcohol. On May 16, while working on the farm, the patient experienced mild nausea after drinking water and became transiently dizzy. The next morning chills developed, and by the mid-afternoon the patient became febrile (101.2°F [38.4°C]), developed muscle pain, a mild headache, and remained in bed until the next morning. These symptoms became progressively more severe during the day and the tick attachment site had developed into an erythematous, circular lesion with induration and a necrotic center, consistent with a rickettsial eschar. Due to the history of tick attachment and fever (maximum temperature 102.9°F [39.4°C]), a SFR, such as RMSF, or neutrophilic or monocytic ehrlichiosis, caused by *Ehrlichia ewingii* or *E. chaffeensis*, respectively, was suspected. Neutropenia (2,553 cells/μL) was accompanied by a left shift (5% band neutrophils) and thrombocytopenia (148,000/μL). Doxycycline was dispensed with instructions to take 100 mg q12h for 7 days. That evening, after sleeping for 6 hours, the patient ate a small quantity of food, after which he became severely nauseated and fainted, and impact with the floor was associated with a severe blow to the back of the head. The next day (May 19) a maculopapular rash appeared that predominantly involved the inferior portions of the arms and legs. Throughout the day the distribution of the rash spread and the severity progressed from barely visible to obvious over most of the body. At no time did the rash involve the palms or plantar surface of the feet. Fever resolved within 36 hours after the initiation of doxycycline, and the rash began to fade gradually after 48 hours of treatment. Within a week after starting doxycycline, the patient was experiencing no symptoms and had no sequelae as a result of the infection or the fall. A repeat CBC (May 25) identified a normal neutrophil count (4,378 cells/μL), no band neutrophils, and a normal platelet count (320,000/μL). Acute-phase serum was collected and stored until the convalescent sample was obtained. *Rickettsia* and *Ehrlichia* spp. PCR was performed immediately. PCR amplicons, obtained from the patient's blood and from the tick, were sequenced, confirming the presence of *R. rickettsii* DNA. PCR for *Ehrlichia* spp. DNA was negative from both the tick and the patient. Subsequently, seroconversion to *R. rickettsii* antigens was identified (1:64 acute titer, convalescent titer 1:512 after 4 weeks). The patient did not seroconvert to *Ehrlichia* spp. antigens.

Comment

Historically, transmission of *R. rickettsii* in North America was attributed solely to *D. variabilis* in the eastern United States and to *D. andersoni* in the western United States. However, between 2002 and 2004, researchers at the CDC documented *Rh. sanguineus* transmission of *R. rickettsii* to people residing in Arizona. Although this is most likely an infrequent occurrence, this patient was infected with *R. rickettsii* by *A. americanum*. It is important to note the similarities between the historical, physical examination, and laboratory findings for the dog discussed previously and the human patient. In several published case reports, dogs develop RMSF before a family member contracts the infection from a tick. Thus, it is important for veterinarians to recognize and confirm a diagnosis of RMSF in dogs and to educate the client as to the risk of tick exposure within their local environment.

SUGGESTED READINGS

Biggs HM, Behravesh CB, Bradley KK, et al. Diagnosis and management of tickborne rickettsial, diseases: Rocky Mountain spotted fever and other spotted fever group, rickettsioses, ehrlichioses, and anaplasmosis - United States. *MMWR Recomm Rep (Morb Mortal Wkly Rep)*. 2016;65: 1–44.

Gasser AM, Birkenheuer AJ, Breitschwerdt EB. Canine Rocky Mountain spotted fever: a retrospective study of 30 cases. *J Am Anim Hosp Assoc.* 2001;37:41–48.

Elchos BN. Goddard J. Implications of presumptive fatal Rocky Mountain spotted fever in two dogs and their owner. *J Am Vet Med Assoc.* 2003;223:1450–1452.

Nicholson WL, Allen KE, McQuiston JH, et al. The increasing recognition of rickettsial pathogens in dogs and people. *Trends Parasitol.* 2010;26:205–212.

REFERENCES

1. Ricketts HT. Some aspects of Rocky Mountain spotted fever as shown by recent investigations. 1909. *Rev Infect Dis.* 1991;13:1227–1240.
2. Jensenius M, Davis X, von Sonnenburg F, et al. Multicenter GeoSentinel analysis of rickettsial diseases in international travelers, 1996-2008. *Emerg Infect Dis.* 2009;15:1791–1798.
3. Fournier PE, Raoult D. Current knowledge on phylogeny and taxonomy of *Rickettsia* spp. *Ann N Y Acad Sci.* 2009;1166:1–11.
4. Bechah Y, Capo C, Mege JL, et al. Rickettsial diseases: from *Rickettsia*-arthropod relationships to pathophysiology and animal models. *Future Microbiol.* 2008;3:223–236.
5. Raoult D, Fournier PE, Eremeeva M, et al. Naming of Rickettsiae and rickettsial diseases. *Ann N Y Acad Sci.* 2005;1063:1–12.
6. Yu X-J, Walker DH. *Rickettsia*. In: *Bergey's Manual of Systematics of Archaea and Bacteria*. Online: John Wiley and Sons Inc.; 2015.
7. Parola P, Paddock CD, Socolovschi C, et al. Update on tick-borne rickettsioses around the world: a geographic approach. *Clin Microbiol Rev.* 2013;26:657–702.
8. Shpynov S, Pozdnichenko N, Gumenuk A. Approach for classification and taxonomy within family Rickettsiaceae based on the formal order analysis. *Microbes Infect.* 2015;17:839–844.
9. Parola P, Paddock CD, Raoult D. Tick-borne rickettsioses around the world: emerging diseases challenging old concepts. *Clin Microbiol Rev.* 2005;18:719–756.
10. Goddard J. Historical and recent evidence for close relationships among *Rickettsia parkeri, R. conorii, R. africae*, and *R. sibirica*: implications for rickettsial taxonomy. *J Vector Ecol.* 2009;34:238–242.
11. Garcia-Garcia JC, Portillo A, Nunez MJ, et al. A patient from Argentina infected with *Rickettsia massiliae*. *Am J Trop Med Hyg.* 2010;82:691–692.
12. Cragun WC, Bartlett BL, Ellis MW, et al. The expanding spectrum of eschar-associated rickettsioses in the United States. *Arch Dermatol.* 2010;146:641–648.
13. Parola P, Socolovschi C, Jeanjean L, et al. Warmer weather linked to tick attack and emergence of severe rickettsioses. *PLoS Negl Trop Dis.* 2008;2:e338.
14. Parola P, Labruna MB, Raoult D. Tick-borne rickettsioses in America: unanswered questions and emerging diseases. *Curr Infect Dis Rep.* 2009;11:40–50.
15. Solano-Gallego L, Kidd L, Trotta M, et al. Febrile illness associated with *Rickettsia conorii* infection in dogs from Sicily. *Emerg Infect Dis.* 2006;12:1985–1988.
16. Keenan KP, Buhles Jr WC, Huxsoll DL, et al. Studies on the pathogenesis of *Rickettsia rickettsii* in the dog: clinical and clinicopathologic changes of experimental infection. *Am J Vet Res.* 1977;38:851–856.
17. Keenan KP, Buhles Jr WC, Huxsoll DL, et al. Pathogenesis of infection with *Rickettsia rickettsii* in the dog: a disease model for Rocky Mountain spotted fever. *J Infect Dis.* 1977;135:911–917.
18. Gasser AM, Birkenheuer AJ, Breitschwerdt EB. Canine Rocky Mountain spotted fever: a retrospective study of 30 cases. *J Am Anim Hosp Assoc.* 2001;37:41–48.
19. Greene CE, Burgdorfer W, Cavagnolo R, et al. Rocky Mountain spotted fever in dogs and its differentiation from canine ehrlichiosis. *J Am Vet Med Assoc.* 1985;186:465–472.
20. Breitschwerdt EB, Walker DH, Levy MG, et al. Clinical, hematologic, and humoral immune response in female dogs inoculated with *Rickettsia rickettsii* and *Rickettsia montana*. *Am J Vet Res.* 1988;49:70–76.
21. Breitschwerdt EB, Meuten DJ, Walker DH, et al. Canine Rocky Mountain spotted fever: a kennel epizootic. *Am J Vet Res.* 1985;46:2124–2128.
22. Elchos BN, Goddard J. Implications of presumptive fatal Rocky Mountain spotted fever in two dogs and their owner. *J Am Vet Med Assoc.* 2003;223:1450–1452. 1433.
23. Paddock CD, Brenner O, Vaid C, et al. Short report: concurrent Rocky Mountain spotted fever in a dog and its owner. *Am J Trop Med Hyg.* 2002;66:197–199.
24. Demma LJ, Eremeeva M, Nicholson WL, et al. An outbreak of Rocky Mountain Spotted Fever associated with a novel tick vector, *Rhipicephalus sanguineus*, in Arizona, 2004: preliminary report. *Ann N Y Acad Sci.* 2006;1078:342–343.
25. Nicholson WL, Gordon R, Demma LJ. Spotted fever group rickettsial infection in dogs from eastern Arizona: how long has it been there? *Ann N Y Acad Sci.* 2006;1078:519–522.
26. Nicholson WL, Paddock CD, Demma L, et al. Rocky Mountain spotted fever in Arizona: documentation of heavy environmental infestations of *Rhipicephalus sanguineus* at an endemic site. *Ann N Y Acad Sci.* 2006;1078:338–341.
27. Raoult D, Toga B, Dunan S, et al. Mediterranean spotted fever in the South of France; serosurvey of dogs. *Trop Geogr Med.* 1985;37:258–260.
28. Mannelli A, Mandola ML, Pedri P, et al. Associations between dogs that were serologically positive for *Rickettsia conorii* relative to the residences of two human cases of Mediterranean spotted fever in Piemonte (Italy). *Prev Vet Med.* 2003;60:13–26.
29. Segura-Porta F, Diestre-Ortin G, Ortuno-Romero A, et al. Prevalence of antibodies to spotted fever group rickettsiae in human beings and dogs from and endemic area of mediterranean spotted fever in Catalonia, Spain. *Eur J Epidemiol.* 1998;14:395–398.
30. Beeler E, Abramowicz KF, Zambrano ML, et al. A focus of dogs and *Rickettsia massiliae*-infected *Rhipicephalus sanguineus* in California. *Am J Trop Med Hyg.* 2011;84:244–249.
31. Sexton DJ, Banks J, Graves S, et al. Prevalence of antibodies to spotted fever group rickettsiae in dogs from southeastern Australia. *Am J Trop Med Hyg.* 1991;45:243–248.
32. Satoh H, Tsuneki A, Inokuma H, et al. Seroprevalence of antibodies against spotted fever group rickettsia among dogs and humans in Okinawa, Japan. *Microbiol Immunol.* 2001;45:85–87.
33. Inokuma H, Matsuda H, Sakamoto L, et al. Evaluation of *Rickettsia japonica* pathogenesis and reservoir potential in dogs by experimental inoculation and epidemiologic survey. *Clin Vaccine Immunol.* 2011;18:161–166.
34. Grasperge BJ, Wolfson W, Macaluso KR. *Rickettsia parkeri* infection in domestic dogs, Southern Louisiana, USA, 2011. *Emerg Infect Dis.* 2012;18:995–997.
35. Solano-Gallego L, Capri A, Pennisi MG, et al. Acute febrile illness is associated with *Rickettsia* spp. infection in dogs. *Parasit Vectors.* 2015;8:216.
36. Levin ML, Zemtsova GE, Montgomery M, et al. Effects of homologous and heterologous immunization on the reservoir competence of domestic dogs for *Rickettsia conorii* (*israelensis*). *Ticks Tick Borne Dis.* 2014;5:33–40.
37. Barrett A, Little SE, Shaw E. "*Rickettsia amblyommii*" and *R. montanensis* infection in dogs following natural exposure to ticks. *Vector Borne Zoonotic Dis.* 2014;14:20–25.
38. Segura F, Pons I, Miret J, et al. The role of cats in the eco-epidemiology of spotted fever group diseases. *Parasit Vectors.* 2014;7:353.
39. Bayliss DB, Morris AK, Horta MC, et al. Prevalence of *Rickettsia* species antibodies and *Rickettsia* species DNA in the blood of cats with and without fever. *J Feline Med Surg.* 2009;11:266–270.
40. Vilhena H, Martinez-Diaz VL, Cardoso L, et al. Feline vector-borne pathogens in the north and centre of Portugal. *Parasit Vectors.* 2013;6:99.

41. Case JB, Chomel B, Nicholson W, et al. Serological survey of vector-borne zoonotic pathogens in pet cats and cats from animal shelters and feral colonies. *J Feline Med Surg*. 2006;8:111–117.
42. Greene CE, ed. *Infectious Diseases of the Dog and Cat*. 4th ed. St. Louis: Elsevier Saunders; 2012.
43. Warner RD, Marsh WW. Rocky Mountain spotted fever. *J Am Vet Med Assoc*. 2002;221:1413–1417.
44. Guedes E, Leite RC, Prata MC, et al. Detection of *Rickettsia rickettsii* in the tick *Amblyomma cajennense* in a new Brazilian spotted fever-endemic area in the state of Minas Gerais. *Mem Inst Oswaldo Cruz*. 2005;100:841–845.
45. Breitschwerdt EB, Hegarty BC, Maggi RG, et al. *Rickettsia rickettsii* transmission by a lone star tick, North Carolina. *Emerg Infect Dis*. 2011;17:873–875.
46. Demma LJ, Traeger MS, Nicholson WL, et al. Rocky Mountain spotted fever from an unexpected tick vector in Arizona. *N Engl J Med*. 2005;353:587–594.
47. Piranda EM, Faccini JL, Pinter A, et al. Experimental infection of *Rhipicephalus sanguineus* ticks with the bacterium *Rickettsia rickettsii*, using experimentally infected dogs. *Vector Borne Zoonotic Dis*. 2011;11:29–36.
48. Wikswo ME, Hu R, Metzger ME, et al. Detection of *Rickettsia rickettsii* and *Bartonella henselae* in *Rhipicephalus sanguineus* ticks from California. *J Med Entomol*. 2007;44:158–162.
49. Campos-Calderon L, Abrego-Sanchez L, Solorzano-Morales A, et al. Molecular detection and identification of Rickettsiales pathogens in dog ticks from Costa Rica. *Ticks Tick Borne Dis*. 2016;7:1198–1202.
50. Chen LF, Sexton DJ. What's new in Rocky Mountain spotted fever? *Infect Dis Clin North Am*. 2008;22:415–432 (vii-viii).
51. Dantas-Torres F. Rocky Mountain spotted fever. *Lancet Infect Dis*. 2007;7:724–732.
52. Kidd LB. Transmission times and prevention of tick-borne diseases in dogs. *Compend Contin Educ Pract Vet*. 2003;25:742–751.
53. Dantas-Torres F. Biology and ecology of the brown dog tick, *Rhipicephalus sanguineus*. *Parasit Vectors*. 2010;3:26.
54. Norment BR, Burgdorfer W. Susceptibility and reservoir potential of the dog to spotted fever-group rickettsiae. *Am J Vet Res*. 1984;45:1706–1710.
55. Brissos J, de Sousa R, Santos AS, et al. Rickettsial infection caused by accidental conjunctival inoculation. *BMJ Case Rep*. 2015;2015.
56. Stromdahl EY, Jiang J, Vince M, et al. Infrequency of *Rickettsia rickettsii* in *Dermacentor variabilis* removed from humans, with comments on the role of other human-biting ticks associated with spotted fever group Rickettsiae in the United States. *Vector Borne Zoonotic Dis*. 2011;11:969–977.
57. Biggs HM, Behravesh CB, Bradley KK, et al. Diagnosis and management of tickborne rickettsial diseases: Rocky Mountain spotted fever and other spotted fever group rickettsioses, ehrlichioses, and anaplasmosis - United States. *MMWR Recomm Rep (Morb Mortal Wkly Rep)*. 2016;65:1–44.
58. Drexler NA, Dahlgren FS, Heitman KN, et al. National surveillance of spotted fever group rickettsioses in the United States, 2008-2012. *Am J Trop Med Hyg*. 2016;94:26–34.
59. Yancey CB, Hegarty BC, Qurollo BA, et al. Regional seroreactivity and vector-borne disease co-exposures in dogs in the United States from 2004-2010: utility of canine surveillance. *Vector Borne Zoonotic Dis*. 2014;14:724–732.
60. Diniz PP, Beall MJ, Omark K, et al. High prevalence of tick-borne pathogens in dogs from an Indian reservation in northeastern Arizona. *Vector Borne Zoonotic Dis*. 2010;10:117–123.
61. Eremeeva ME, Zambrano ML, Anaya L, et al. *Rickettsia rickettsii* in *Rhipicephalus* ticks, Mexicali, Mexico. *J Med Entomol*. 2011;48:418–421.
62. Tinoco-Gracia L, Quiroz-Romero H, Quintero-Martinez MT, et al. Prevalence of *Rhipicephalus sanguineus* ticks on dogs in a region on the Mexico-USA border. *Vet Rec*. 2009;164:59–61.
63. Fritz CL, Kriner P, Garcia D, et al. Tick infestation and spotted-fever group *Rickettsia* in shelter dogs, California, 2009. *Zoonoses Public Health*. 2012;59:4–7.
64. Estrada I, Balagot C, Fierro M, et al. Spotted fever group rickettsiae canine serosurveillance near the US-Mexico border in California. *Zoonoses Public Health*. 2020;67:148–155.
65. Telford SR. Status of the "east side hypothesis" (transovarial interference) 25 years later. *Ann N Y Acad Sci*. 2009;1166:144–150.
66. Moncayo AC, Cohen SB, Fritzen CM, et al. Absence of *Rickettsia rickettsii* and occurrence of other spotted fever group rickettsiae in ticks from Tennessee. *Am J Trop Med Hyg*. 2010;83:653–657.
67. Raoult D, Parola P. Rocky Mountain spotted fever in the USA: a benign disease or a common diagnostic error? *Lancet Infect Dis*. 2008;8:587–589.
68. Sahni SK, Rydkina E. Host-cell interactions with pathogenic *Rickettsia* species. *Future Microbiol*. 2009;4:323–339.
69. Walker DH, Valbuena GA, Olano JP. Pathogenic mechanisms of diseases caused by *Rickettsia*. *Ann N Y Acad Sci*. 2003;990:1–11.
70. Walker DH. Rickettsiae and rickettsial infections: the current state of knowledge. *Clin Infect Dis*. 2007;45(suppl 1):S39–S44.
71. Sahni SK, Narra HP, Sahni A, et al. Recent molecular insights into rickettsial pathogenesis and immunity. *Future Microbiol*. 2013;8:1265–1288.
72. Mansueto P, Vitale G, Cascio A, et al. New insight into immunity and immunopathology of rickettsial diseases. *Clin Dev Immunol*. 2012;2012:967852.
73. Balraj P, Renesto P, Raoult D. Advances in rickettsia pathogenicity. *Ann N Y Acad Sci*. 2009;1166:94–105.
74. Eremeeva ME, Liang Z, Paddock C, et al. *Rickettsia rickettsii* infection in the pine vole, *Microtus pinetorum*: kinetics of infection and quantitation of antioxidant enzyme gene expression by RT-PCR. *Ann N Y Acad Sci*. 2003;990:468–473.
75. Cummiskey JM, Simon LM, Theodore J, et al. Bioenergetic alterations in cultivated pulmonary artery and aortic endothelial cells exposed to normoxia and hypoxia. *Exp Lung Res*. 1981;2:155–163.
76. Asahina T, Kashiwagi A, Nishio Y, et al. Impaired activation of glucose oxidation and NADPH supply in human endothelial cells exposed to H2O2 in high-glucose medium. *Diabetes*. 1995;44:520–526.
77. Breitschwerdt EB, Papich MG, Hegarty BC, et al. Efficacy of doxycycline, azithromycin, or trovafloxacin for treatment of experimental Rocky Mountain spotted fever in dogs. *Antimicrob Agents Chemother*. 1999;43:813–821.
78. Piranda EM, Faccini JL, Pinter A, et al. Experimental infection of dogs with a Brazilian strain of *Rickettsia rickettsii*: clinical and laboratory findings. *Mem Inst Oswaldo Cruz*. 2008;103:696–701.
79. Levin ML, Killmaster LF, Zemtsova GE, et al. Clinical presentation, convalescence, and relapse of Rocky Mountain spotted fever in dogs experimentally infected via tick bite. *PloS One*. 2014;9. e115105.
80. Kordick SK, Breitschwerdt EB, Hegarty BC, et al. Coinfection with multiple tick-borne pathogens in a Walker Hound kennel in North Carolina. *J Clin Microbiol*. 1999;37:2631–2638.
81. Ober CP, Spaulding K, Breitschwerdt EB, et al. Orchitis in two dogs with Rocky Mountain spotted fever. *Vet Radiol Ultrasound*. 2004;45:458–465.
82. Grindem CB, Breitschwerdt EB, Perkins PC, et al. Platelet-associated immunoglobulin (antiplatelet antibody) in canine Rocky Mountain spotted fever and ehrlichiosis. *J Am Anim Hosp Assoc*. 1999;35:56–61.
83. Greene CE, Kidd L, Breitschwerdt EB. Rocky Mountain and Mediterranean spotted fevers, cat-flea typhuslike illness, rickettsialpox and typhus. In: Green CE, ed. *Infectious Diseases of the Dog and Cat*. 4th ed. St. Louis Missouri USA: Elsevier; 2012:259–276.
84. Mikszewski JS, Vite CH. Central nervous system dysfunction associated with Rocky Mountain spotted fever infection in five dogs. *J Am Anim Hosp Assoc*. 2005;41:259–266.
85. Drost WT, Berry CR, Breitschwerdt EB, et al. Thoracic radiographic findings in dogs infected with *Rickettsia rickettsii*. *Vet Radiol Ultrasound*. 1997;38:260–266.
86. Breitschwerdt EB, Levy MG, Davidson MG, et al. Kinetics of IgM and IgG responses to experimental and naturally acquired *Rickettsia rickettsii* infection in dogs. *Am J Vet Res*. 1990;51:1312–1316.
87. Nicholson WL, Allen KE, McQuiston JH, et al. The increasing recognition of rickettsial pathogens in dogs and people. *Trends Parasitol*. 2010;26:205–212.

88. Breitschwerdt EB, Moncol DJ, Corbett WT, et al. Antibodies to spotted fever-group rickettsiae in dogs in North Carolina. *Am J Vet Res.* 1987;48:1436–1440.
89. Lashnits E, Neupane P, Maggi RG, et al. Detection of *Bartonella* spp. in dogs after infection with *Rickettsia rickettsii. J Vet Intern Med.* 2020;34:145–159.
90. Neupane P, Sevala S, Balakrishnan N, et al. Validation of *Bartonella henselae* western immunoblotting for serodiagnosis of bartonelloses in dogs. *J Clin Microbiol.* 2020;58.
91. Solano-Gallego L, Bradley J, Hegarty B, et al. *Bartonella henselae* IgG antibodies are prevalent in dogs from southeastern USA. *Vet Res.* 2004;35:585–595.
92. Kidd L, Maggi R, Diniz PP, et al. Evaluation of conventional and real-time PCR assays for detection and differentiation of Spotted Fever Group *Rickettsia* in dog blood. *Vet Microbiol.* 2008;129:294–303.
93. Davidson MG, Breitschwerdt EB, Walker DH, et al. Identification of rickettsiae in cutaneous biopsy specimens from dogs with experimental Rocky Mountain spotted fever. *J Vet Intern Med.* 1989;3:8–11.
94. Todd SR, Dahlgren FS, Traeger MS, et al. No visible dental staining in children treated with doxycycline for suspected Rocky Mountain spotted fever. *J Pediatr.* 2015;166:1246–1251.
95. Breitschwerdt EB, Davidson MG, Aucoin DP, et al. Efficacy of chloramphenicol, enrofloxacin, and tetracycline for treatment of experimental Rocky Mountain spotted fever in dogs. *Antimicrob Agents Chemother.* 1991;35:2375–2381.
96. Chapman AS, Bakken JS, Folk SM, et al. Diagnosis and management of tickborne rickettsial diseases: Rocky Mountain spotted fever, ehrlichioses, and anaplasmosis, United States: a practical guide for physicians and other health-care and public health professionals. *MMWR Recomm Rep (Morb Mortal Wkly Rep).* 2006;55:1–27.
97. Neer TM, Eddlestone SM, Gaunt SD, et al. Efficacy of enrofloxacin for the treatment of experimentally induced *Ehrlichia canis* infection. *J Vet Intern Med.* 1999;13:501–504.
98. Breitschwerdt EB, Davidson MG, Hegarty BC, et al. Prednisolone at anti-inflammatory or immunosuppressive dosages in conjunction with doxycycline does not potentiate the severity of *Rickettsia rickettsii* infection in dogs. *Antimicrob Agents Chemother.* 1997;41:141–147.
99. Low RM, Holm JL. Canine Rocky mountain spotted fever. *Compend Contin Educ Pract Vet.* 2005;27:530–538.
100. Breitschwerdt EB. Bartonellosis, One Health and all creatures great and small. *Vet Dermatol.* 2017;28. 96–e21.
101. Walker DH, Dumler JS. The role of CD8 T lymphocytes in rickettsial infections. *Semin Immunopathol.* 2015;37:289–299.
102. Walker DH. The realities of biodefense vaccines against *Rickettsia. Vaccine.* 2009;27(suppl 4):D52–D55.
103. Alhassan A, Liu H, McGill J, et al. *Rickettsia rickettsii* whole-cell antigens offer protection against Rocky Mountain spotted fever in the canine host. *Infect Immun.* 2019;87:e00628–18.
104. Drexler N, Miller M, Gerding J, et al. Community-based control of the brown dog tick in a region with high rates of Rocky Mountain spotted fever, 2012-2013. *PloS One.* 2014;9:e112368.
105. Escarcega-Avila AM, de la Mora-Covarrubias A, Quezada-Casasola A, et al. Occupational risk for personnel working in veterinary clinics through exposure to vectors of rickettsial pathogens. *Ticks Tick Borne Dis.* 2019;10:299–304.
106. Tick Borne Disease Surveillance: Spotted Fever Group Rickettsia. Vol. 3. California Department of Public Health Vector Borne Disease Bulletin; 2009:4.
107. Levin ML, Killmaster LF, Zemtsova GE. Domestic dogs (*Canis familiaris*) as reservoir hosts for *Rickettsia conorii. Vector Borne Zoonotic Dis.* 2012;12:28–33.
108. Solano-Gallego L, Hegarty B, Espada Y, et al. Serological and molecular evidence of exposure to arthropod-borne organisms in cats from northeastern Spain. *Vet Microbiol.* 2006;118:274–277.
109. Lucchese L, Ravagnan S, Da Rold G, et al. Survival of *Rickettsia conorii* in artificially contaminated whole and leukoreduced canine blood units during the storage period. *Parasit Vectors.* 2020;13:118.
110. Solano-Gallego L, Trotta M, Caldin M, et al. Molecular survey of *Rickettsia* spp. in sick dogs in Italy. *Zoonoses Public Health.* 2008;55:521–525.
111. Kelly P, Matthewman L, Beati L, et al. African tick-bite fever: a new spotted fever group rickettsiosis under an old name. *Lancet.* 1992;340:982–983.
112. Straily A, Drexler N, Cruz-Loustaunau D, et al. Notes from the field: community-based prevention of Rocky Mountain spotted fever - Sonora, Mexico, 2016. *MMWR Morb Mortal Wkly Rep.* 2016;65:1302–1303.
113. Aharonowitz G, Koton S, Segal S, et al. Epidemiological characteristics of spotted fever in Israel over 26 years. *Clin Infect Dis.* 1999;29:1321–1322.
114. Oztoprak N, Celebi G, Aydemir H, et al. Mediterranean spotted fever due to contact with dog-tick. *Mikrobiyol Bul.* 2008;42:701–706.
115. Espejo E, Andres M, Perez J, et al. Prevalence of antibodies to *Rickettsia conorii* in human beings and dogs from Catalonia: a 20-year perspective. *Epidemiol Infect.* 2016;144:1889–1894.
116. Trout Fryxell RT, Steelman CD, Szalanski AL, et al. Molecular detection of *Rickettsia* Species within ticks (Acari: Ixodidae) collected from Arkansas, United States. *J Med Entomol.* 2015;52:500–508.
117. Paddock CD, Finley RW, Wright CS, et al. *Rickettsia parkeri* rickettsiosis and its clinical distinction from Rocky Mountain spotted fever. *Clin Infect Dis.* 2008;47:1188–1196.
118. Herrick KL, Pena SA, Yaglom HD, et al. *Rickettsia parkeri* rickettsiosis, Arizona, USA. *Emerg Infect Dis.* 2016;22:780–785.
119. Billeter SA, Blanton HL, Little SE, et al. Detection of *Rickettsia amblyommii* in association with a tick bite rash. *Vector Borne Zoonotic Dis.* 2007;7:607–610.
120. Delisle J, Mendell NL, Stull-Lane A, et al. Human infections by multiple spotted fever group rickettsiae in Tennessee. *Am J Trop Med Hyg.* 2016;94:1212–1217.
121. Vitale G, Mansuelo S, Rolain JM, et al. *Rickettsia massiliae* human isolation. *Emerg Infect Dis.* 2006;12:174–175.
122. Movilla R, Altet L, Serrano L, et al. Molecular detection of vector-borne pathogens in blood and splenic samples from dogs with splenic disease. *Parasit Vectors.* 2017;10:131.
123. Padgett KA, Bonilla D, Eremeeva ME, et al. The eco-epidemiology of Pacific Coast tick fever in California. *PLoS Negl Trop Dis.* 2016;10:e0005020.
124. Wilson JM, Breitschwerdt EB, Juhasz NB, et al. A novel *Rickettsia* species infecting dogs in the United States. *Emerg Infect Dis.* 2020;26:3011.
125. Hiraoka H, Shimada Y, Sakata Y, et al. Detection of rickettsial DNA in ixodid ticks recovered from dogs and cats in Japan. *J Vet Med Sci.* 2005;67:1217–1222.
126. Satoh H, Motoi Y, Camer GA, et al. Characterization of spotted fever group rickettsiae detected in dogs and ticks in Okinawa, Japan. *Microbiol Immunol.* 2002;46:257–263.
127. Tabuchi M, Jilintai, Sakata Y, et al. Serological survey of *Rickettsia japonica* infection in dogs and cats in Japan. *Clin Vaccine Immunol.* 2007;14:1526–1528.
128. Izzard L, Cox E, Stenos J, et al. Serological prevalence study of exposure of cats and dogs in Launceston, Tasmania, Australia to spotted fever group rickettsiae. *Aust Vet J.* 2010;88:29–31.
129. Comer JA, Diaz T, Vlahov D, et al. Evidence of rodent-associated *Bartonella* and *Rickettsia* infections among intravenous drug users from Central and East Harlem, New York City. *Am J Trop Med Hyg.* 2001;65:855–860.
130. Krusell A, Comer JA, Sexton DJ. Rickettsialpox in North Carolina: a case report. *Emerg Infect Dis.* 2002;8:727–728.
131. Zavala-Velazquez JE, Ruiz-Sosa JA, Sanchez-Elias RA, et al. *Rickettsia felis* rickettsiosis in Yucatan. *Lancet.* 2000;356:1079–1080.
132. Brown LD, Macaluso KR. *Rickettsia felis*, an emerging flea-borne rickettsiosis. *Curr Trop Med Rep.* 2016;3:27–39.
133. Reif KE, Macaluso KR. Ecology of *Rickettsia felis*: a review. *J Med Entomol.* 2009;46:723–736.
134. Boostrom A, Beier MS, Macaluso JA, et al. Geographic association of *Rickettsia felis*-infected opossums with human murine typhus, Texas. *Emerg Infect Dis.* 2002;8:549–554.
135. Mullins KE, Maina AN, Krueger L, et al. Rickettsial infections among cats and cat fleas in Riverside County, California. *Am J Trop Med Hyg.* 2018;99:291–296.

136. Maina AN, Fogarty C, Krueger L, et al. Rickettsial infections among *Ctenocephalides felis* and host animals during a flea-borne rickettsioses outbreak in Orange County, California. *PloS One*. 2016;11:e0160604.
137. Schriefer ME, Sacci Jr JB, Taylor JP, et al. Murine typhus: updated roles of multiple urban components and a second typhuslike rickettsia. *J Med Entomol*. 1994;31:681–685.
138. Schriefer ME, Sacci Jr JB, Dumler JS, et al. Identification of a novel rickettsial infection in a patient diagnosed with murine typhus. *J Clin Microbiol*. 1994;32:949–954.
139. Williams SG, Sacci Jr JB, Schriefer ME, et al. Typhus and typhuslike rick ettsiae associated with opossums and their fleas in Los Angeles County, California. *J Clin Microbiol*. 1992;30:1758–1762.
140. Billeter SA, Metzger ME. Limited evidence for *Rickettsia felis* as a cause of zoonotic flea-borne rickettsiosis in Southern California. *J Med Entomol*. 2017;54:4–7.
141. Raoult D, La Scola B, Enea M, et al. A flea-associated *Rickettsia* pathogenic for humans. *Emerg Infect Dis*. 2001;7:73–81.
142. Richter J, Fournier PE, Petridou J, et al. *Rickettsia felis* infection acquired in Europe and documented by polymerase chain reaction. *Emerg Infect Dis*. 2002;8:207–208.
143. Higgins JA, Sacci Jr JB, Schriefer ME, et al. Molecular identification of rickettsia-like microorganisms associated with colonized cat fleas (*Ctenocephalides felis*). *Insect Mol Biol*. 1994;3:27–33.
144. Azad AF, Radulovic S, Higgins JA, et al. Flea-borne rickettsioses: ecologic considerations. *Emerg Infect Dis*. 1997;3:319–327.
145. Wedincamp Jr J, Foil LD. Infection and seroconversion of cats exposed to cat fleas (*Ctenocephalides felis* Bouche) infected with *Rickettsia felis*. *J Vector Ecol*. 2000;25:123–126.
146. Sorvillo FJ, Gondo B, Emmons R, et al. A suburban focus of endemic typhus in Los Angeles County: association with seropositive domestic cats and opossums. *Am J Trop Med Hyg*. 1993;48:269–273.
147. Breitschwerdt EB, Levine JF, Radulovic S, et al. *Bartonella henselae* and *Rickettsia* seroreactivity in a sick cat population from North Carolina. *Intern J Appl Res Vet Med*. 2005;3:287–302.
148. Hawley JR, Shaw SE, Lappin MR. Prevalence of *Rickettsia felis* DNA in the blood of cats and their fleas in the United States. *J Feline Med Surg*. 2007;9:258–262.
149. Inpankaew T, Hii SF, Chimnoi W, et al. Canine vector-borne pathogens in semi-domesticated dogs residing in northern Cambodia. *Parasit Vectors*. 2016;9:253.
150. Hii SF, Kopp SR, Abdad MY, et al. Molecular evidence supports the role of dogs as potential reservoirs for *Rickettsia felis*. *Vector Borne Zoonotic Dis*. 2011;11:1007–1012.
151. Hii SF, Abdad MY, Kopp SR, et al. Seroprevalence and risk factors for *Rickettsia felis* exposure in dogs from Southeast Queensland and the northern Territory, Australia. *Parasit Vectors*. 2013;6:159.
152. Ng-Nguyen D, Hii SF, Hoang MT, et al. Domestic dogs are mammalian reservoirs for the emerging zoonosis flea-borne spotted fever, caused by *Rickettsia felis*. *Sci Rep*. 2020;10:4151.
153. Noden BH, Davidson S, Smith JL, et al. First detection of *Rickettsia typhi* and *Rickettsia felis* in fleas collected from client-owned companion animals in the Southern Great Plains. *J Med Entomol*. 2017;54:1093–1097.
154. Nelson K, Maina AN, Brisco A, et al. A 2015 outbreak of flea-borne rickettsiosis in san Gabriel valley, Los Angeles county, California. *PLoS Negl Trop Dis*. 2018;12:e0006385.
155. Kelly P, Roberts S, Fournier PE. A review of emerging flea-borne bacterial pathogens in New Zealand. *N Z Med J*. 2005;118:U1257.
156. McQuiston JH, Knights EB, Demartino PJ, et al. Brill-Zinsser disease in a patient following infection with sylvatic epidemic typhus associated with flying squirrels. *Clin Infect Dis*. 2010;51:712–715.
157. Breitschwerdt EB, Hegarty BC, Davidson MG, et al. Evaluation of the pathogenic potential of *Rickettsia canada* and *Rickettsia prowazekii* organisms in dogs. *J Am Vet Med Assoc*. 1995;207:58–63.
158. Wiggers RJ, Stewart RS. Ownership of cats or dogs does not increase exposure to *Rickettsia typhi*. *Tex Med*. 2002;98:56–57.
159. Devamani CS, Schmidt WP, Ariyoshi K, et al. Risk factors for scrub typhus, murine typhus, and spotted fever seropositivity in urban areas, rural plains, and peri-forest hill villages in South India: a cross-sectional study. *Am J Trop Med Hyg*. 2020;103:238–248.
160. Nogueras MM, Pons I, Pla J, et al. The role of dogs in the eco-epidemiology of *Rickettsia typhi*, etiological agent of Murine typhus. *Vet Microbiol*. 2013;163:97–102.
161. Dzul-Rosado K, Lugo-Caballero C, Tello-Martin R, et al. Direct evidence of *Rickettsia typhi* infection in *Rhipicephalus sanguineus* ticks and their canine hosts. *Open Vet J*. 2017;7:165–169.
162. Namikawa K, Tanabe A, Satake S, et al. Canine *Orientia tsutsugamushi* infection: report of a case and its epidemicity. *Southeast Asian J Trop Med Public Health*. 2014;45:395–401.
163. Kolo AO, Sibeko-Matjila KP, Maina AN, et al. Molecular detection of zoonotic rickettsiae and *Anaplasma* spp. in domestic dogs and their ectoparasites in Bushbuckridge, South Africa. *Vector Borne Zoonotic Dis*. 2016;16:245–252.

47

Neorickettsiosis

Jane E. Sykes

KEY POINTS

- Cause: *Neorickettsia helminthoeca*, the *Stellantchasmus falcatus* (SF) agent/Elokomin fluke fever (EFF) agent (salmon poisoning disease [SPD]) and *Neorickettsia risticii*. All are gram-negative, obligately intracellular bacteria that belong to the family Anaplasmataceae. A related organism, *Neorickettsia sennetsu*, causes febrile illness in humans who ingest raw fish in Asia (Sennetsu fever).
- First Described: The first reports of SPD were from northwestern Oregon, United States, in 1814 (Astoria).[1] Reports of natural infection of dogs with *N. risticii* first appeared from the United States in 1994.[2]
- Affected Hosts: *Neorickettsia helminthoeca* infects dogs, foxes, coyotes, raccoons, and captive bears. The SF agent infects dogs. *Neorickettsia risticii* infects horses (causing Potomac horse fever or equine neorickettsiosis), bats, and dogs. In addition, experimental transmission to dogs and cats has resulted in disease.
- Intermediate Hosts: The intermediate hosts for *N. helminthoeca* and probably the SF agent are aquatic snails (*Oxytrema silicula*) and fish (especially salmonids). For *N. risticii*, they are aquatic snails (*Juga* and *Elimia* spp.) and aquatic insects (caddisflies and mayflies).
- Geographic Distribution: The distribution of SPD is limited to the coastal areas of Washington, Oregon, northern California, British Columbia, and Brazil (2004). Infections with *N. risticii* have been documented in horses from the United States, Canada, and South America, including Uruguay and Brazil.
- Route of Transmission: SPD is transmitted to dogs by ingestion of the infected trematode vector *Nanophyetus salmincola*, most often in salmonid fish. *Neorickettsia risticii* is transmitted to horses by ingestion of the trematode vector *Acanthatrium oregonense* within aquatic insects. The mode of transmission of *N. risticii* to dogs is unknown, but they also may become infected through ingestion of infected aquatic snails or insects.
- Major Clinical Signs: SPD is often associated with fever, lethargy, anorexia, vomiting, diarrhea, and lymphadenomegaly. In the rare reports of *N. risticii* infection, dogs and cats have shown signs of lethargy, vomiting, hematemesis, petechial hemorrhages, fever, and polyarthritis.
- Differential Diagnoses: These include lymphoma, CPV infection, CDV infection, granulocytic anaplasmosis, ehrlichiosis, leptospirosis, septic shock, disseminated fungal disease (especially cryptococcosis), hemorrhagic gastroenteritis, dietary indiscretion, GI foreign body, pancreatitis, hypoadrenocorticism, and inflammatory bowel disease. For SPD, appropriate antimicrobial treatment with doxycycline must begin before the diagnosis is confirmed by laboratory testing. Misdiagnosis and delayed or inappropriate antimicrobial drug therapy increase morbidity and mortality.
- Human Health Significance: *Nanophyetus salmincola* can cause GI disturbances and eosinophilia in humans, but *N. helminthoeca* does not cause human disease. Similarly, *N. risticii* has not been reported to cause human disease. *Neorickettsia sennetsu* is a related pathogen that causes febrile illness in humans consuming raw fish in Asia.

SALMON POISONING DISEASE

ETIOLOGIC AGENT AND EPIDEMIOLOGY

Salmon poisoning disease (SPD) is primarily caused by the gram-negative, obligately intracellular rickettsial pathogen *Neorickettsia helminthoeca*, which, like other *Neorickettsia* spp., resides within a trematode (fluke) vector for the course of the trematode's life cycle from egg to adult. The complete genome of *N. helminthoeca* has been sequenced.[3]

The trematode vector of *N. helminthoeca* is *Nanophyetus salmincola*, thought to be the most common trematode species endemic to the United States. The disease occurs in dogs, foxes, and coyotes. In addition, two captive polar bears receiving long-term glucocorticoid therapy for skin conditions succumbed to an SPD-like disease after eating inadequately frozen salmon,[4] an SPD-like disease was also reported in two captive Malayan sun bears after they were fed live trout from a northern California reservoir,[5] and SPD was confirmed using molecular methods in a captive African lion (*Panthera leo krugeri*) from Oregon after it was fed raw salmon.[6] Domestic cats are not susceptible to SPD, but trematodes develop when infected fish are ingested.[7]

SPD is geographically restricted to coastal regions of northern California, Oregon, and Washington in the United States, and southern British Columbia in Canada. This reflects the distribution of an aquatic snail, *Oxytrema silicula* (also known as *Juga silicula*), which is an intermediate host of the trematode (Fig. 47.1). The snail is prevalent in coastal streams. A similar disease has been described in dogs from southern Brazil,[8–10] and infection with *N. helminthoeca* was detected in several dead coatis (*Nasua nasua*) from a wildlife sanctuary in Foz do Iguaçu (southern Brazil).[11] It was not clear whether the infection in the coatis was clinical or subclinical; two of the coatis had died as a result of vehicle trauma. The trematode host and intermediate hosts involved in southern Brazil remain unclear.[8]

Another related, yet antigenically distinct organism is capable of causing SPD in dogs, the Elokomin fluke fever (EFF) agent.[12–16] Discovered during attempts to understand the role of black bears as reservoirs for SPD, it was initially thought to be a less pathogenic strain of *N. helminthoeca*, because experimental infection of dogs with the agent resulted in only mild disease.[14] The EFF agent has never been sequenced. In 2020, an organism known as the *Stellantchasmus falcatus* (SF) agent was detected in three dogs from the Pacific Northwest with severe clinical signs of SPD.[17] This organism is so named because it was first detected in the metacercariae of the trematode SF in grey mullet fish in Japan.[18,19] Inoculation of the SF agent into a dog resulted in mild disease.[19] The 16S rRNA gene sequence of the SF agent was published in 1996,[20] and in

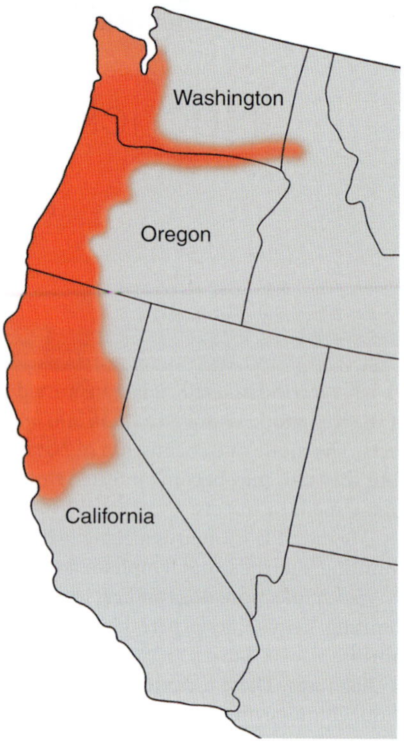

Fig. 47.1 Geographic distribution of salmon poisoning disease in dogs from the United States. The distribution also extends into the southern portion of British Columbia.

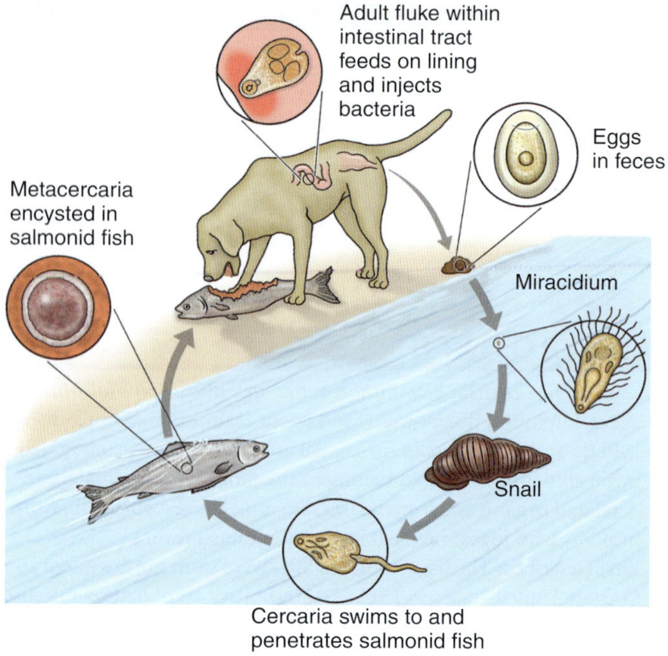

Fig. 47.2 Life cycle of *Nanophyetus salmincola*, the trematode vector of salmon poisoning disease. The fluke harbors the rickettsial organism throughout its lifecycle.

2016, an organism with the same 16S rRNA gene sequence was detected in *N. salmincola* metacercariae in Chinook salmon in the Willamette valley in Oregon.[21] It was then suggested that the EFF agent and the SF agent might be the same organism. The SF agent has also been detected in an adult fluke (*Metagonimoides oregonensis*) in Florida,[22] so there is the possibility that as-yet unrecognized disease occurs in dogs in Florida. The intermediate hosts for this fluke on the east coast are thought to be aquatic snails (*Pleurocerca* spp.) and the salamander (rather than salmonid fish), and so disease may be unrecognized on the east coast because intermediate hosts are infrequently consumed by domestic dogs. Raccoons are the primary definitive host for the fluke.

Dogs usually become infected with *N. helminthoeca* when they ingest encysted trematode metacercariae within uncooked or undercooked freshwater fish, most commonly salmonid fish. The Pacific giant salamander is also a competent second intermediate host. Ingestion of encysted metacercariae is followed by maturation of the trematode over a 6-day period, which feeds on the intestinal mucosa and inoculates the rickettsia into the host. The fluke has an oral sucker and a ventral sucker, which are used to grasp host intestinal tissue, although the fluke itself does not cause extensive damage to the intestinal wall.[23] Infected trematode ova are shed in the stool for 60 to 250 days.[24] After several months, miracidia develop within the eggs, hatch, swim away, and penetrate the snail. They then develop into rediae, each of which give rise to many free-swimming cercariae. Thousands of cercariae are released intermittently from the snail. These rapidly penetrate the skin of a fish (or are ingested by the fish), and encyst throughout the fish as metacercariae (Figs. 47.2 and 47.3). The metacercariae usually localize in the kidneys of fish, but can be found in any tissue, as well as slime on the skin of fish. Infected fish may contain more than 1,000 metacercariae. Infected fish may have visible damage to their skin, and the infection may also interfere with their swimming activity.[25] Fish are infected in freshwater and retain the trematode and the rickettsial infection throughout their ocean migration before

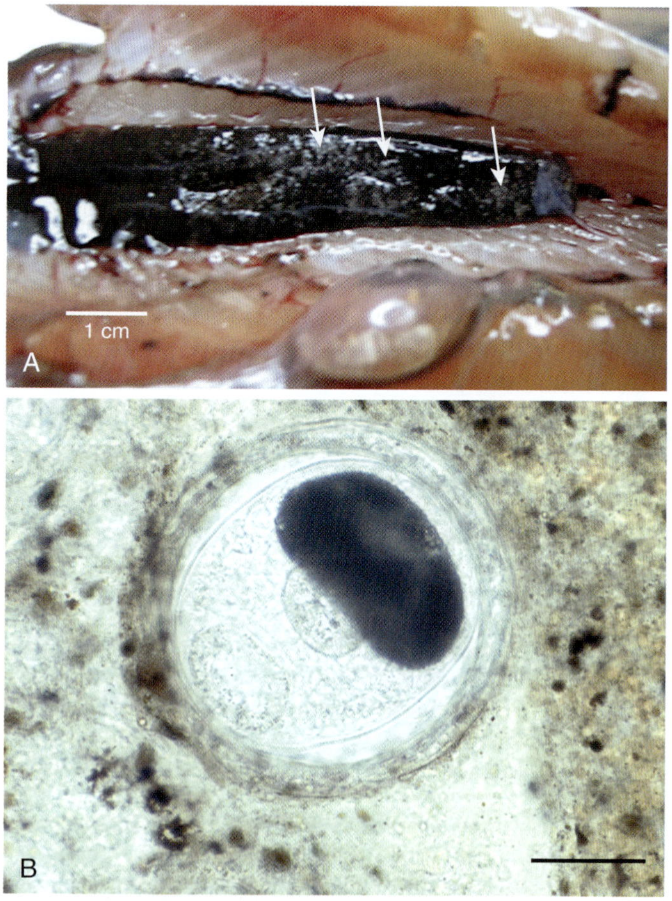

Fig. 47.3 (A) "Salt grain" appearance of metacercariae of *Nanophyetus salmincola (arrows)* in the kidneys of a Chinook salmon. (B) Wet mount squash of fresh kidney material from a Chinook salmon showing a metacercaria of *N. salmincola*. Bar = 100 μm. (A, Courtesy Craig Banner, Oregon Department of Fish and Wildlife. B,Courtesy Dr. Ronald Hedrick, University of California, Davis.)

returning to fresh water up to 3 years later.[26] Dog-to-dog transmission of *N. helminthoeca* has been demonstrated experimentally by mechanical aerosolization or rectal administration of lymph node suspensions or homogenates of rectal mucosa.[27] SPD also has been transmitted by parenteral injection of infected blood, spleen and lymph suspensions, adult flukes, helminth-infected snail livers, and helminth eggs. Partial transmission success was obtained by allowing ticks (*Haemaphysalis leachi* and *Rhipicephalus sanguineus*) that had fed on infected dogs to subsequently feed on susceptible dogs and by parenteral injection of suspensions of *Rh. sanguineus* into dogs.[28]

Intact male dogs and Labrador retrievers appear to be overrepresented among dogs with SPD,[29] possibly because they are popular with individuals engaged in fishing activities, although dogs of any sex and breed can be affected. Dogs of any age are affected; the median age in one study was 3 years.[29] Dogs develop SPD at any time of year. Occasionally, dogs from areas not endemic for SPD develop disease after they ingest fish that is exported from endemic areas.[30]

Most but not all infected dogs have a history of access to or consumption of raw or improperly cooked fish.[29,31] Consumption of any part of the fish, including the entrails and skin, may result in SPD. Supermarket-bought salmon may also be infected.[29] Infection has also been reported after swimming activity, without apparent exposure to fish.[29]

CLINICAL FEATURES

Pathogenesis and Clinical Signs

Neorickettsia helminthoeca replicates within macrophages. Rickettsiae enter the blood early in the course of the disease and spread to the lymph nodes, spleen, tonsils, thymus, liver, lungs, and brain.[32] This results in a granulomatous inflammatory response that is most profound in the stomach, intestines, lymph nodes, and spleen. Granulomatous meningitis has also been detected in dogs with SPD.[33,34] Affected dogs in southern Brazil have also had evidence of chronic interstitial pneumonia and choroid plexitis.[8]

The incubation period ranges from 2 to 14 days (median, 7 days), but may be as long as 33 days.[35] The severity of illness varies considerably (Box 47.1). Dogs with peracute infection may be found dead.[29] A marked febrile response is commonly detected (>70% of cases) (Box 47.2) and may reach 42°C (107.6°F).[29] A median rectal temperature of 40.6°C (105°F) was reported in one series of naturally infected dogs.[29] Rectal temperature gradually decreases to normal or below normal over the subsequent 4 to 8 days. Terminally ill dogs may be hypothermic. Some animals show only a mild increase in temperature or a brief period of fever; they may still die if left untreated. Virtually all dogs develop inappetence or anorexia, and lethargy is also common. Vomiting occurs in more than 80% of dogs, and rarely, hematemesis.[29] Diarrhea is also common (>70% of dogs) and may be semiformed to liquid in consistency, sometimes containing frank blood, melena, and, less commonly, mucus. Occasionally, a history of diarrhea and vomiting is absent. Other signs include serous nasal discharge, weight loss, and increased thirst and urination. Neurologic signs including mental obtundation, myoclonic twitching, seizures, and apparent neck pain have been reported in fewer than 20% of affected dogs, a primary differential diagnosis being CDV infection.[29] Dogs from southern Brazil have also shown neurologic signs and evidence of respiratory distress.[8]

Physical Examination Findings

Dehydration is frequently noted on physical examination and may be severe. More than 70% of dogs have peripheral lymphadenomegaly, which may be generalized or involve only some peripheral lymph nodes (see Box 47.2). Lymph nodes may be up to 4 cm in diameter and firm on palpation. Lack of lymphadenomegaly may be present occasionally, sometimes as a result of lymph node necrosis. Abdominal palpation may reveal pain, and splenomegaly may also be detected. Other abnormalities include tachypnea or labored respirations, tachycardia, scleral or conjunctival injection, serous nasal discharge, and edema that involves the limbs, face, or cervical region.[29] Mucosal pallor, tachycardia, and weak pulses may be present in dogs with hypovolemic shock. Cardiac arrhythmias such as ventricular premature contractions have also been noted, and signs of hemorrhage such as epistaxis and hyphema may also be present. Rectal examination may indicate the presence of liquid stool, sometimes accompanied by fresh blood or melena.

BOX 47.1 Signs in the Clinical History of 29 Dogs with Salmon Poisoning Disease from the United States

Inappetence or anorexia: 100%
Lethargy: 86%
Vomiting: 86%
Diarrhea: 72%
Hematochezia: 38%
Weight loss: 28%
Melena: 21%
Polyuria and polydipsia: 3%

BOX 47.2 Physical Examination Findings in 29 Dogs with Salmon Poisoning Disease from the United States

Peripheral lymphadenomegaly: 74%
Fever: 73%
Dehydration: 65%
Abdominal pain: 28%
Tachypnea or labored respirations: 24%
Tachycardia: 24%
Neurologic signs: 17%
Weak pulses: 17%
Splenomegaly: 14%
Scleral injection: 14%
Mucosal pallor: 10%
Hypothermia: 5%

DIAGNOSIS

Laboratory Abnormalities

Complete Blood Count

Thrombocytopenia is present in 90% of affected dogs. Anemia is present in up to 40% of dogs with SPD and generally occurs as a result of GI hemorrhage. More commonly, the CBC shows evidence of lymphopenia, thrombocytopenia, and neutrophilia, frequently with bandemia (Table 47.1). Uncommonly, neutropenia occurs.[29] Toxic changes may be present within neutrophils, and immature monocytes may occasionally be found in the peripheral blood. Despite the association with helminthiasis, eosinophilia is often not present.

Serum Chemistry Profile

Hyponatremia and hypokalemia are the most common electrolyte abnormalities in dogs with SPD and result from GI losses that occur with vomiting and diarrhea (Table 47.2). Low concentrations of ionized calcium may be detected in some dogs, possibly as a result of

TABLE 47.1 Hematologic Findings in 29 Dogs with Salmon Poisoning Disease from the United States

Test	Reference Range	Percent Below Reference Range	Percent Within Reference Range	Percent Above Reference Range	Range For Dogs With Salmon Poisoning Disease	Number of Dogs
Hematocrit (%)	40–55	39	61	0	22–53	23
Neutrophils (cells/μL)	3,000–10,500	4	53	43	728–26,224	23
Band neutrophils (cells/μL)	Rare	0	40	60	0–6,825	20
Monocytes (cells/μL)	150–1,200	9	61	30	42–3,290	23
Lymphocytes (cells/μL)	1,000–4,000	78	22	0	0–2,070	23
Eosinophils (cells/μL)	0–1,500	0	100	0	0–690	21
Platelets (cells/μL)	150,000–400,000	90	0	10	10,000–446,000	20

TABLE 47.2 Findings on Serum Biochemistry Analysis in 29 Dogs with Salmon Poisoning Disease from the United States

Test	Reference Range	Percent Below Reference Range	Percent Within Reference Range	Percent Above Reference Range	Range For Dogs With Salmon Poisoning Disease	Number of Dogs
Sodium (mmol/L)	145–154	59	36	5	133–161	22
Potassium (mmol/L)	4.1–5.3	41	59	0	3.7–5.0	22
Chloride (mmol/L)	105–116	9	77	14	98–118	22
Bicarbonate (mmol/L)	16–26	20	15	65	11–28	20
Calcium (mg/dL)	9.9–11.4	83	17	0	7.2–10.9	23
Phosphorus (mg/dL)	3.0–6.2	9	74	17	2.7–13.0	23
Creatinine (mg/dL)	0.5–1.6	4	4	13	0.4–3.3	23
BUN (mg/dL)	8–31	0	83	17	8–110	23
Albumin (g/dL)	2.9–4.2	83	17	0	0.9–3.8	23
Globulin (g/dL)	2.3–4.4	26	70	4	1.6–4.7	23
Cholesterol (mg/dL)	135–345	22	69	9	79–408	23
Total bilirubin (mg/dL)	0–0.4	0	83	17	0–3.1	23
ALT (U/L)	19–70	4	74	22	17–1,443	23
ALP (U/L)	15–127	0	39	61	29–985	23

ALP, alkaline phosphatase; *ALT,* alanine aminotransferase; *BUN,* blood urea nitrogen.

decreased intestinal absorption. Hypoalbuminemia is present in most (>80%) dogs. Hypoglobulinemia and hypocholesterolemia occur in fewer than 25% of dogs with SPD. Abnormal liver enzyme activities may be present, the most common of which is increased ALP activity,[29,34] but increases in the activity of ALT and AST may also occur, and hyperbilirubinemia is present in fewer than 20% of dogs. Azotemia can be evident in dogs with severe dehydration.

Urinalysis

Bilirubinuria and proteinuria are frequently detected on urinalysis in dogs with SPD.[29] Uncommonly, cylindruria and glucosuria are present, perhaps as a result of renal injury secondary to impaired renal perfusion. Microscopic hematuria occurs in some dogs, possibly reflecting underlying coagulopathies that can occur in dogs with SPD.

Clotting Function

Evaluation of clotting function in some dogs may show evidence of DIC. Abnormalities include increased PT or APTT, increased fibrin degradation products, and decreased antithrombin activity.[29]

Diagnostic Imaging

Plain Radiography

Abdominal radiographs may be unremarkable or reveal fluid-filled small intestines; focal areas of decreased serosal detail; and less frequently, hepatomegaly or splenomegaly. Thoracic radiographs are typically unremarkable or show reduction in size of the intrathoracic vasculature, consistent with hypovolemia.

Sonographic Findings

Abdominal ultrasound examination of dogs with SPD often shows mild or moderate generalized abdominal or mesenteric lymphadenomegaly, as well as splenomegaly with a mottled splenic echotexture. Some dogs that lack peripheral lymphadenomegaly have abdominal lymphadenomegaly on ultrasound examination,[29] and ultrasound-guided aspiration of enlarged abdominal lymph nodes can be helpful for diagnosis in dogs that lack peripheral lymphadenomegaly. Lymph nodes develop a rounded appearance with a hypoechoic or hypoechoic mottled echogenicity (Fig. 47.4). Fluid-distended intestinal loops, sometimes with wall thickening, corrugation, hypermotility, or hypomotility, may be documented. Uncommonly, hepatomegaly or a small amount of free peritoneal fluid is identified.

Microbiologic Tests (Table 47.3)

Diagnosis Using Fecal Examination

SPD can be confirmed when operculated trematode eggs are found in fecal samples of dogs with consistent clinical signs, which appear within 5 to 8 days after the ingestion of infected fish. The light brown eggs are approximately 87 to 97 µm long and 35 to 55 µm wide, with a small, blunt point on the end opposite the indistinct operculum (Fig. 47.5). Although the sensitivity of centrifugal zinc sulfate fecal flotation for detection of *N. salmincola* ova in dogs with SPD is similar to that of fecal sedimentation, some dogs that test negative by one method test positive using the other, so the sensitivity of fecal examination for diagnosis is maximized by performing both centrifugal zinc sulfate fecal flotations and fecal sedimentation together. In one study, 93% of dogs with SPD tested positive for *N. salmincola* ova using a combination of fecal flotation and fecal sedimentation.[29] False negatives may occur when the duration of illness is shorter than the prepatent period of *N. salmincola* or when light fluke burdens are present. The finding of fluke ova on fecal examination may not be diagnostic of SPD, because dogs may be infected with trematodes that do not harbor the rickettsia, and ova may be shed for months after recovery. Nevertheless, *N. salmincola* ova were detected in only 0.2% of more than 1,800 fecal flotations in dogs seen at a teaching hospital in an endemic area, and all positive test results were in dogs suspected to have SPD. Thus, the specificity of fecal examination for a diagnosis of SPD appears to be extremely high.[29]

Centrifugal zinc sulfate fecal flotation may reveal co-infections with other GI parasites, which can complicate the clinical picture. Co-infections with *Dipylidium caninum* and *Trichuris vulpis* have been reported in dogs with SPD.[29]

Cytologic Diagnosis

In addition to fecal examination for trematode ova, SPD can be diagnosed following cytologic examination of peripheral lymph node aspirates, or ultrasound-guided aspirates of abdominal lymph nodes or the spleen. Cytologic findings consist of histiocytic hyperplasia and lymphoid reactivity. Rickettsial organisms are 0.3-µm cocci or coccobacilli and may be seen in large numbers within the cytoplasm of macrophages. Pleomorphic rods up to 2 µm long, sometimes forming

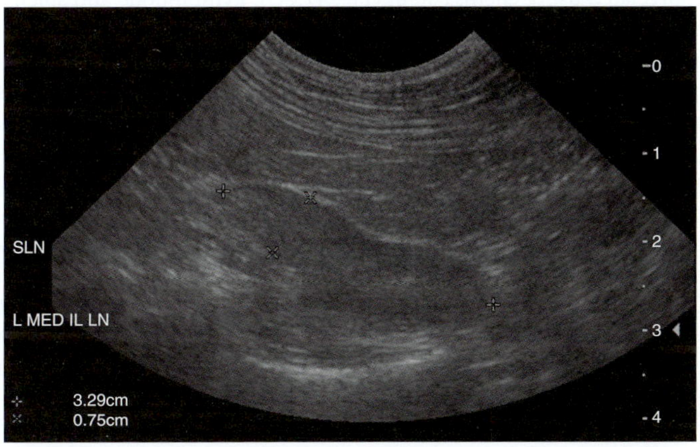

Fig. 47.4 Enlarged and hypoechoic abdominal (medial iliac) lymph nodes as detected using abdominal sonographic examination in a 9-year-old male German shepherd dog with salmon poisoning disease.

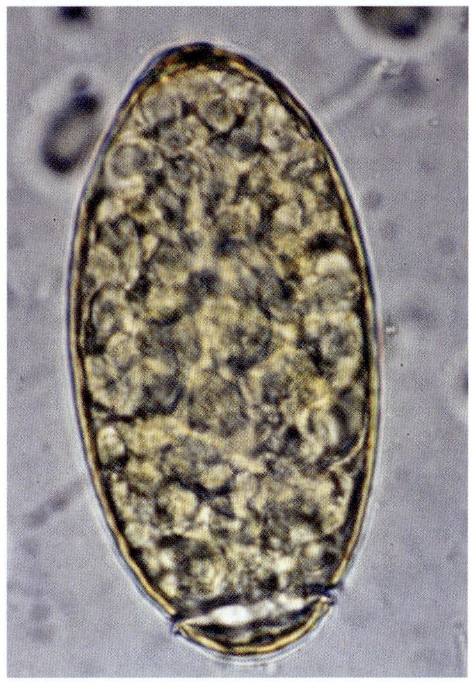

Fig. 47.5 Egg of *Nanophyetus salmincola* (×480).

TABLE 47.3 Diagnostic Assays Available for Salmon Poisoning Disease in Dogs

Assay	Specimen Type	Target	Performance
Fecal sedimentation combined with zinc sulfate centrifugal fecal flotation	Feces	*Nanophyetus salmincola* ova	Specificity nears 100% when performed by a parasitologist. Sensitivity probably > 90%. Eggs are light brown, ovoid, operculate at one end and measure 0.087–0.097 mm × 0.038–0.055 mm.
Cytology	Lymph node or splenic aspirates	Detection of *Neorickettsia* spp. within macrophages	Sensitivity > 70% when performed by a veterinary clinical pathologist. Sensitivity may be improved by examination of aspirates from multiple lymph node. Organisms within macrophages may be confused with debris or hemosiderin. Other changes include lymphocytic reactivity and histiocytic hyperplasia.
Histopathology	Biopsy or necropsy specimens, especially lymph nodes, spleen, gastrointestinal tissues	*Neorickettsia* spp. within macrophages	Organisms may be stained with Giemsa. Antimicrobial therapy can lead to false-negative results.
PCR	Blood, lymph node or splenic aspirates, tissue samples, feces	*Neorickettsia helminthoeca* DNA	Some assays may also detect other *Neorickettsia* spp., including the SF agent. Clinicians should consult with the laboratory. The optimum sample type is unknown. Antimicrobial therapy may lead to negative PCR results.

PCR, polyermase chain reaction; *SF*, *Stellantchasmus falcatus*.

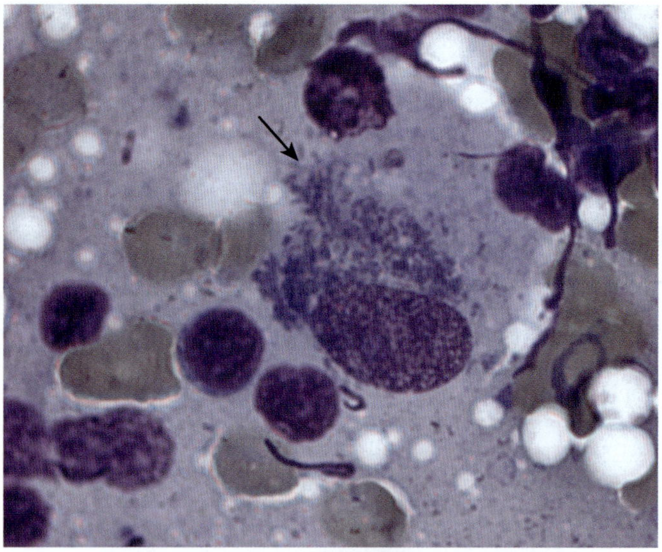

Fig. 47.6 Lymph node aspirate from a dog with salmon poisoning disease. Note the large histiocyte that contains granular coccoid organisms consistent with *Neorickettsia helminthoeca* (arrow).

rings or crescents, have also been observed. The organisms resemble granular to amorphous material of a uniform blue color using Wright stain, occasionally forming loose clusters of organisms (morulae) (Fig. 47.6).[29,35,36] Similar findings were described in dogs infected with the SF agent.[17] Extracellular organisms are not easily separated from artifacts and should not be considered diagnostic for SPD. In as many as one quarter to one third of dogs, rickettsial organisms are not identified. The presence of histiocytic hyperplasia should alert the clinician to the possibility of SPD. Organisms may also be absent in dogs with a recent history of antimicrobial therapy.

Serologic Diagnosis

Serologic tests for *N. helminthoeca* antibodies or antigen are not available on a commercial basis for veterinary practitioners. Antibodies to *N. helminthoeca* can cross-react serologically with those of *Ehrlichia* spp., so it is possible that dogs with SPD might test positive using serologic tests for *Ehrlichia* spp. (provided enough time had elapsed for antibody formation to occur).[37] In one study, most dogs with SPD that were tested for antibodies against other rickettsial pathogens did not seroreact to *Ehrlichia canis* or *Anaplasma phagocytophilum*.[29] Serologic cross-reactivity occurs among *N. helminthoeca*, the SF agent, *Neorickettsia risticii*, and *Neorickettsia sennetsu*.[38]

Molecular Diagnosis Using Nucleic Acid–Based Testing

Real-time PCR assays have been used to detect the DNA of *N. helminthoeca* in clinical specimens from affected dogs.[29] Real-time PCR assays for *N. helminthoeca* are available from some veterinary molecular diagnostic laboratories and can be performed on blood, lymph node or splenic aspirates, and possibly fecal samples from dogs with SPD in order to confirm the diagnosis. More research is required to understand the sensitivity and specificity of PCR assays for diagnosing SPD in dogs, including the optimum specimen type for testing. A broad-spectrum *Neorickettsia* spp. PCR assay was used to detect the SF agent in dogs.[17] Some real-time PCR assays designed to detect *N. helminthoeca* have the potential to also detect the SF agent and other *Neorickettsia* spp.[29] However, genetic differences between the SF agent and *N. helminthoeca* have been identified that would allow development of species-specific assays.[38] Clinicians should contact their laboratory to determine the specificity of the PCR assays offered.

Cell Culture

Neorickettsia helminthoeca has been grown in canine monocytes,[16] canine leukocytes and sarcoma cells, mouse lymphoblasts, and a macrophage cell line.[39,40] However, cell culture is not used for routine diagnosis.

Pathologic Findings

Gross Pathologic Findings

Gross necropsy findings in dogs with SPD consist of enlargement of lymphoid tissues, including the tonsils, thymus, lymph nodes, and spleen. Lymph nodes may be yellowish and edematous and may contain white foci that represent foci of granulomatous inflammation. Petechial hemorrhages may be noted on the lymph nodes, GI tract, pancreas, gallbladder, and urinary bladder. The GI tract may be thickened and contain white foci. The lumen of the intestinal tract may contain free blood (Fig. 47.7A). Intestinal intussusception has also been described in association with SPD.[4] Flukes are only 0.8 to 1.1 mm long and 0.3 to 0.5 mm wide[41] and may not always be visible grossly.

Histopathologic Findings

Lymphoid tissues show marked depletion of lymphoid follicles, and subcapsular and medullary sinuses are filled with histiocytes, the cytoplasm of which can contain numerous rickettsial organisms, which occasionally form clusters within vacuoles. Organisms are readily appreciated using Giemsa stain (Fig. 47.7C). Lymph node and splenic necrosis may also be present.[4,29] Inflammatory nodules that contain lymphocytes, plasma cells, and infected histiocytes expand the lamina propria of the GI tract and extend into the submucosa. Parasites consistent with *N. salmincola* may be found embedded in the mucosa, primarily within the duodenum (Fig. 47.7B).[27,33] Nevertheless, flukes are not always found using histopathology in dogs that die from SPD, even in the absence of anthelmintic therapy.

One dog that died of SPD had widespread and multiple thromboses involving numerous organs with associated tissue infarction. Granulomatous meningitis has been described at necropsy in dogs that were experimentally infected with *N. helminthoeca*.[34] In addition to having characteristic GI and lymphoid lesions described in dogs from the United States, dogs from southern Brazil have had evidence of choroid plexitis as well as chronic interstitial pneumonia, with marked accumulations of alveolar macrophages and thickening of alveolar septa due to hyperplasia of type II pneumocytes.[8] IHC was used to demonstrate intralesional *Neorickettsia* antigen within affected tissues.

TREATMENT AND PROGNOSIS

The treatment of choice for SPD is doxycycline, tetracycline, or oxytetracycline, which should be given for a minimum of 7 days. Administration of tetracyclines is generally associated with clinical improvement within 24 hours, and signs resolve within 1 to 4 days.[29] Dogs that are vomiting may require treatment with parenteral tetracyclines. Clinical improvement has also been reported following treatment with enrofloxacin and parenteral trimethoprim-sulfamethoxazole. Antimicrobials that do not appear to be effective include first-generation cephalosporins, penicillins, aminoglycosides, chloramphenicol, and metronidazole.[29] Although complete clinical recovery may occur without anthelmintic treatment, the fluke infection should be treated with praziquantel after initial recovery from SPD (Table 47.4).[42] Elimination of *N. salmincola* from infected animals minimizes the diarrhea associated with fluke infections alone and minimizes or eliminates fluke eggs from feces. Dogs should also be treated and evaluated for concurrent parasite infections of the GI tract.

Dogs with mild signs or infrequent vomiting may respond well to treatment with oral tetracyclines alone, whereas those with more severe disease often require hospitalization for IV antimicrobial and crystalloid fluid therapy (Table 47.4). Oral antimicrobial therapy can be continued once

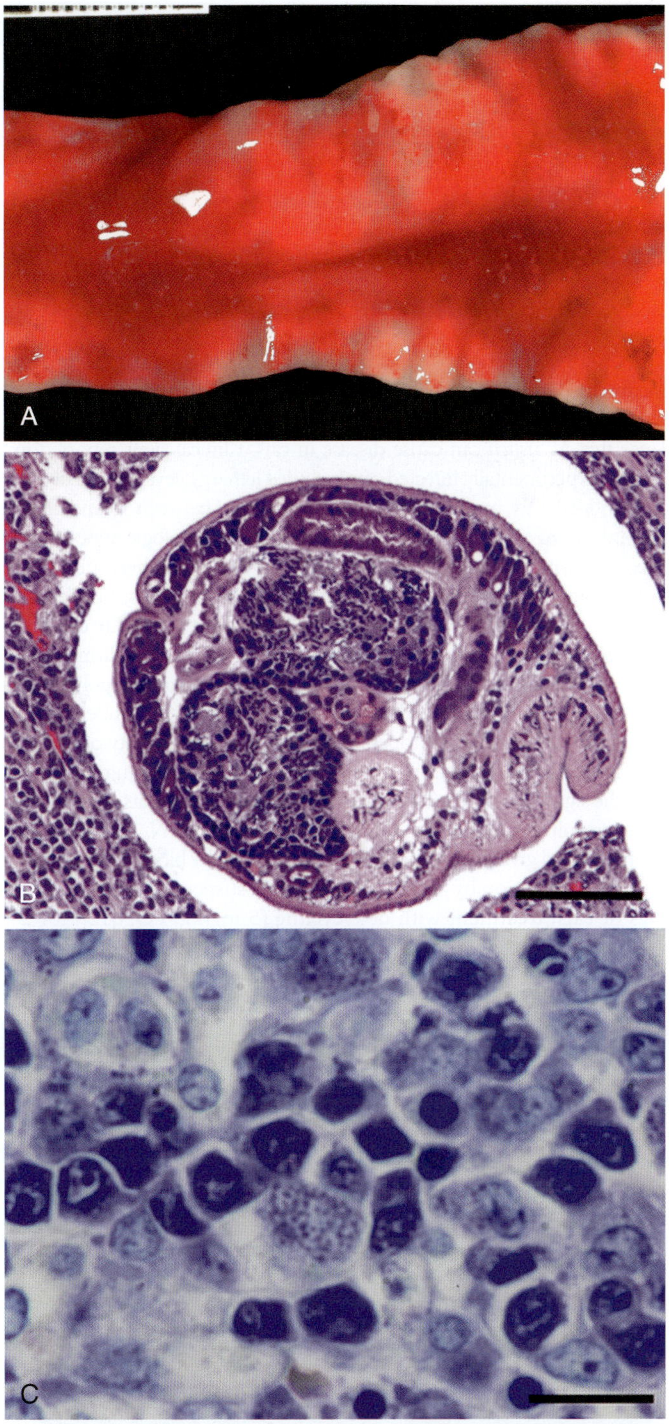

Fig. 47.7 (A) Intestinal mucosa of an 8-month-old female spayed Maltese mix dog that died of salmon poisoning disease. The intestinal wall was thickened and the contents were dark red and mucoid. (B) Duodenum. A transverse section of an adult *Nanophyetus* fluke is embedded within the intestinal villi. H&E stain. Bar = 200 μm. (C) Lymph node, medullary sinus from a dog with salmon poisoning disease. Many histiocytes have intracytoplasmic clusters of coccobacilli less than 1μm in diameter. Giemsa stain. Bar = 5 μm. (A, Courtesy University of California, Davis Veterinary Anatomic Pathology Service. B and C, From Sykes JE, Marks SL, Mapes S, et al. Salmon poisoning disease in dogs: 29 cases. *J Vet Intern Med.* 2010;24:504–513.)

vomiting ceases. The presence of severe hypovolemia or hypoalbuminemia may necessitate treatment with colloids such as fresh frozen plasma, dextrans, or hetastarch. Packed RBCs or whole blood may be required for dogs with severe anemia. Treatment with central or partial parenteral nutrition may also be required if vomiting is persistent and does not respond to antiemetics such as metoclopramide, maropitant, or ondansetron. Close monitoring of HCT, albumin, electrolytes, acid-base status, renal parameters, and coagulation parameters may be required in some severely affected dogs. Blood cultures should be considered in dogs with severe hemorrhagic diarrhea and abnormal perfusion parameters, after which treatment with broad-spectrum parenteral antimicrobial drugs should be commenced.

Prolonged hospitalization may be required for dogs that develop complications such as cardiac arrhythmias, intussusceptions, adverse reactions to tetracyclines, DIC, or bacteremia.[29,31] In a study of dogs evaluated at a tertiary referral hospital, death or euthanasia occurred in 14% of 29 dogs with SPD.[29] The mortality rate may be lower in dogs seen in primary care practice, so long as appropriate treatment can be administered. In general, early treatment is associated with an excellent prognosis. Without treatment, death can occur within 5 to 10 days. The exact cause of death in SPD is unknown. Bacterial sepsis may result from translocation of bacteria across the damaged intestinal wall. Severe hypoalbuminemia and anemia secondary to GI hemorrhage and fluid losses may contribute.

IMMUNITY AND VACCINATION

Animals that recover from SPD are immune to reinfection with the same strain of *N. helminthoeca*,[4,43,44] but challenge with an alternate strain (then the EFF agent) results in disease, and antibodies fail to cross-react with the alternate strain. Reinfection with the EFF/SF agent may explain why SPD has been reported to occur more than once in some dogs.[4,21,29] In an unpublished survey of 331 practitioners in endemic areas, 35% reported that they had diagnosed SPD in dogs that had been treated previously for SPD.[4] No vaccine is available.

PREVENTION

Nanophyetus salmincola metacercariae are effectively destroyed by proper cooking or freezing of infected fish at –20°C for 24 hours.[30] Ingestion of raw fish by dogs in endemic areas should be discouraged, and dog owners in endemic areas should be educated about the disease. Dogs that have eaten raw fish from an endemic area, or those swimming in rivers or lakes in these areas, should be watched carefully for signs of lethargy, vomiting, or decreased appetite that occur within 2 weeks of exposure. If multiple dogs are simultaneously exposed to a source of *N. helminthoeca*, and one dog develops SPD, treatment of the other dogs in the group with 7 days of doxycycline should be considered. Medical equipment used in the treatment of dogs with SPD should not be reused on other patients without proper sterilization.

PUBLIC HEALTH ASPECTS

Human infection with *N. helminthoeca* has not been reported. However, humans may become infected with the fluke, *N. salmincola*, after consumption of poorly cooked fish. Most humans are subclinically infected, although abdominal discomfort, diarrhea, vomiting, weight loss, nausea, and peripheral eosinophilia may occur.[45] The SF agent was discovered during a search for the cause of "Hyuga" fever, which was thought to be caused by *N. sennetsu*. However, only the SF agent, and not *N. sennetsu*, was discovered in metacercariae from grey mullet fish ingested raw by most people that developed the disease.[19] Therefore, it is possible that the SF agent may be able to cause febrile disease in people, but this requires further study.

TABLE 47.4 Antimicrobials Used to Treat Salmon Poisoning Disease in Dogs

Drug	Dose (mg/kg)	Route	Interval (Hours)	Duration (Days)
Doxycycline	5	PO, IV	12	7–14
Tetracycline	22[a]	PO	8	7
	7	IV	8	7
Oxytetracycline	7–10[a]	PO, IV	8	7
Praziquantel[b]	10–30	PO	24	1–2

[a]Reduce dose in renal failure; may cause teeth discoloration in young animals.
[b]For treatment of fluke infection.
IV, intravenous; *PO*, oral.

NEORICKETTSIA RISTICII INFECTION

Rarely, dogs have been reported to develop disease in association with infection by *N. risticii*, the cause of equine neorickettsiosis ("Potomac horse fever"), or a closely related organism.[2] The life cycle of this organism involves a trematode vector, which in the eastern United States is *Acanthatrium oregonense*.[46] The fluke miracidia infect aquatic snails (*Elimia virginica* and likely other species) and metacercariae can be found in aquatic insects (caddisflies and mayflies).[47] Adult trematodes also lay eggs in the intestinal tract of insectivorous bats.[46] Potomac horse fever has been reported from the United States, eastern Canada, and South America, with reports from Uruguay and southern Brazil.[48]

Horses are often infected in summer following ingestion of infected aquatic insects and develop a severe systemic illness with fever, lethargy, anorexia, dehydration, diarrhea, laminitis, or abortion. In one report, *N. risticii* or a closely related organism was detected using culture and PCR in a small number of dogs from the western and southwestern United States with signs of fever, lethargy, vomiting, hematemesis, petechial hemorrhages, edema, or polyarthritis.[2] These dogs were seroreactive to *N. risticii* antigens using IFA. Serologic evidence of exposure to *Neorickettsia* spp. has also been documented in dogs from Thailand and Spain.[49,50] Experimental infection of dogs did not result in development of clinical signs.[51] There is some evidence that *N. risticii* can cause disease in cats. Clinical signs reported in a study of experimentally infected cats included lethargy, fever, anorexia, diarrhea, and lethargy, and infected cats seroconverted between 10 and 23 days after infection.[52] There were no clearly defined hematologic abnormalities associated with the infection. To date, *N. risticii* has not been detected in naturally infected cats using culture or molecular methods, but serologic evidence of *Neorickettsia* spp. infection has been reported in cat populations from the United States[53] and Spain[54,55] and in a small number of cats with signs of anorexia, lethargy, fever, vomiting, diarrhea, polyarthritis, and ocular discharge.[56] Laboratory findings in these cats included anemia, leukopenia, and thrombocytopenia. Because of the possibility of serologic cross-reactivity with other organisms, further studies are required to determine the significance of this organism in dogs and also in cats. In the meantime, screening of blood donors using PCR assays for *N. risticii* has been recommended given the potential for transmission by blood transfusion.[57]

Should infection by *N. risticii* be strongly suspected or confirmed in dogs or cats, treatment with doxycycline (5 mg/kg, PO, q12h for 2–3 weeks) is recommended.

CASE EXAMPLE

Signalment

"Herman," 9-year-old male German shepherd dog from Sacramento, CA (Fig. 47.8).

History

Herman's owner reported a 2-day history of inappetence, lethargy, and one episode of vomiting. The dog had been drinking normally. There had been no diarrhea, coughing, sneezing, or increased thirst and urination. The owner also reported that Herman ate turkey and chicken that contained bones 3 days before the onset of illness. He was normally fed a strict diet of rabbit- and potato-based prescription dog food and grilled salmon because of atopic dermatitis. Herman was sometimes fed salmon scraps from the local supermarket, which the owner grilled briefly. He had not traveled out of his local area. He was up to date on vaccinations, which included vaccines for distemper, hepatitis, parvovirus, and rabies.

Current Medications

Lincomycin 29 mg/kg PO q12h; trimeprazine tartrate 0.2 mg/kg PO q48h; and prednisolone 0.1 mg/kg q48h for atopic dermatitis.

Other Medical History

Herman had been diagnosed with hip osteoarthritis using pelvic radiography 8 months earlier. Controlled weight loss was the recommended treatment. He was cryptorchid, and the abdominal testicle had been removed when he was a young dog. The descended testicle was still present.

Physical Examination

Body weight: 51.5 kg.

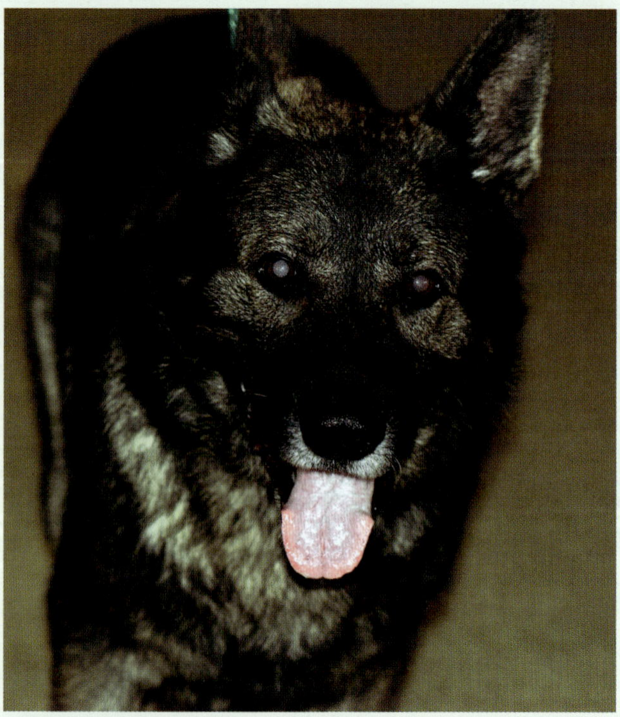

Fig. 47.8 "Herman," a 9-year-old male German shepherd dog with salmon poisoning disease.

CASE EXAMPLE—cont'd

General: Quiet, alert and responsive. Ambulatory on all four limbs. Temperature = 104.3°F (40.2°C), HR = 108 beats/minute, RR = 60 breaths/minute, mucous membranes pink, CRT = 1 second.

Integument: A full, shiny haircoat was present and there was no evidence of ectoparasites.

Eyes, ears, nose, and throat: No significant abnormalities were noted. A mild amount of brown waxy debris was present within both ear canals.

Musculoskeletal: A BCS of 6/9 with symmetrical muscling was noted. Mild to moderate pelvic limb weakness was identified.

Cardiovascular: Strong femoral pulses were noted. No murmurs or arrhythmias were detected on thoracic auscultation.

Respiratory: An increased RR with increased abdominal effort was present.

GI and genitourinary: Abdominal palpation revealed a tense abdomen, with abdominal splinting, and splenomegaly. There was one descended testicle, which was smooth with no masses. No abnormalities were detected on rectal examination. Soft feces were present in the rectum, and the prostate was palpable and symmetrical.

Lymph nodes: Marked peripheral lymphadenopathy was present. Mandibular, superficial cervical, and popliteal lymph nodes were all 3–4 cm in diameter and firm.

Laboratory Findings

CBC: HCT 40.4% (40%–55%), MCV 65 fL (65–75 fL), MCHC 36.6 g/dL (33–36 g/dL), WBC 4,240 cells/μL (6,000–13,000 cells/μL), neutrophils 3,689 cells/μL (3,000–10,500 cells/μL), lymphocytes 466 cells/μL (1,000–4,000 cells/μL), monocytes 42 cells/μL (150–1,200 cells/μL), platelets 74,000 platelets/μL (150,000–400,000 platelets/μL).

Serum chemistry profile: Sodium 141 mmol/L (145–154 mmol/L), potassium 4.0 mmol/L (3.6–5.3 mmol/L), chloride 112 mmol/L (108–118 mmol/L), bicarbonate 13 mmol/L (16–26 mmol/L), phosphorus 2.8 mg/dL (3.0–6.2 mg/dL), calcium 9.9 mg/dL (9.7–11.5 mg/dL), BUN 15 mg/dL (5–21 mg/dL), creatinine 1.1 mg/dL (0.3–1.2 mg/dL), glucose 86 mg/dL (64–123 mg/dL), total protein 6.9 g/dL (5.4–7.6 g/dL), albumin 3.6 g/dL (3.0–4.4 g/dL), globulin 3.3 g/dL (1.8–3.9 g/dL), ALT 108 U/L (19–67 U/L), AST 109 U/L (19–42 U/L), ALP 105 U/L (21–170 U/L), creatine kinase 381 U/L (51–399 U/L), GGT < 3 U/L (0–6 U/L), cholesterol 296 mg/dL (135–361 mg/dL), total bilirubin 0.4 mg/dL (0–0.2 mg/dL), magnesium 1.7 mg/dL (1.5–2.6 mg/dL).

Urinalysis: SpG 1.048; pH 6.0, 2+ protein (SSA), 1+ bilirubin, 1+ hemoprotein, no glucose, 0–1 WBC/HPF, 20–30 RBC/HPF, rare ammonium biurate crystals, many lipid droplets.

Imaging Findings

Thoracic radiographs: The cardiovascular and pulmonary structures appeared within normal limits. A mild diffuse bronchial pattern throughout all lung fields was considered consistent with the age of the patient. Marked spondylosis deformans was present throughout the thoracic spine.

Abdominal ultrasound: The liver had a diffuse, coarse echotexture. The spleen was markedly, diffusely enlarged and had a diffuse hypoechoic, mottled echotexture. The prostate gland was enlarged and had multiple small anechoic cysts within its parenchyma. One testicle was present in the scrotum and had a striated, heterogenous echotexture. A second inguinal or intra-abdominal testis was not observed. Multiple enlarged, hypoechoic inguinal lymph nodes were present (see Fig. 47.4). A large (2.5 cm), round, hypoechoic mass with a focal area of mineralization was present in the cranial abdomen caudal to the liver and most likely represented a lymph node. Multiple enlarged, hypoechoic sublumbar lymph nodes were observed. The splenic lymph nodes were enlarged and mildly hypoechoic.

Cytology Findings

Cytology of ultrasound-guided splenic aspirate: splenic stromal clumps contained increased numbers of plump histiocytes and many large clumps of hemosiderin. Histiocytes were also present in moderate numbers throughout the smear, often in clumps, and often mildly vacuolated. They were occasionally erythrophagocytic and often contained hemosiderin. Interpretation: moderate to marked histiocytic inflammation.

Cytology of popliteal lymph node aspirate (see Fig. 47.6): moderate reactive lymphoid hyperplasia with pyogranulomatous inflammation was identified. Rare histiocytes were present that contained intracellular small coccoid purple-blue structures that were organized individually and in clusters. These were consistent with *N. helminthoeca* organisms.

Fecal Examination

Fecal flotation: Negative for parasites.

Fecal sedimentation: *N. salmincola* ova, <1 per 10× field.

Diagnosis

SPD

Treatment

Doxycycline, 5 mg/kg PO q12h for 14 days. This was associated with resolution of fever and inappetence within 24 hours of starting treatment. By 7 days after diagnosis, Herman's owner reported that Herman was completely back to his normal self.

Comments

This dog was diagnosed with SPD based on the presence of characteristic cytologic findings on examination of a lymph node aspirate, together with the detection of *N. salmincola* ova in the stool. The case was unusual because the dog was infected after ingestion of incompletely cooked supermarket-bought salmon, which the dog had been fed for years without developing illness. Although the splenic aspirate contained inflammatory cells typical of those seen in SPD, organisms could not be convincingly documented.

SUGGESTED READINGS

Mack RE, Bercovitch MG, Ling GV, et al. Salmon poisoning disease complex in dogs—a review of 45 cases. *Calif Vet*. 1990;44:42–45.

Sykes JE, Marks SL, Mapes S, et al. Salmon poisoning disease in dogs: 29 cases. *J Vet Intern Med*. 2010;24:504–513.

Pastenkos G, Snekvik K, Bradway D, et al. A novel neorickettsial infection in 3 dogs in the Pacific Northwest. *Vet Pathol*. 2020;57:286–289.

REFERENCES

1. Millemann RE, Knapp SE. Biology of *Nanophyetus salmincola* and "salmon poisoning disease". In: Dawes B, ed. *Advances in Parasitology*. New York, NY: Academic Press; 1970:1–39.
2. Kakoma I, Hansen RD, Anderson BE, et al. Cultural, molecular, and immunological characterization of the etiologic agent for atypical canine ehrlichiosis. *J Clin Microbiol*. 1994;32:170–175.
3. Lin M, Bachman K, Cheng Z, et al. Analysis of complete genome sequence and major surface antigens of *Neorickettsia helminthoeca*, causative agent of salmon poisoning disease. *Microb Biotechnol*. 2017;10:933–957.
4. Gorham JR, Foreyt WJ, Sykes JE. *Neorickettsia helminthoeca* infection (salmon poisoning disease). In: Greene CE, ed. *Infectious Diseases of the Dog and Cat*. 4th ed. St Louis, MO: Elsevier Saunders; 2012: 219–226.
5. Gai JJ, Marks SL. Salmon poisoning disease in two Malayan sun bears. *J Am Vet Med Assoc*. 2008;232:586–588.
6. Thomas KS, Sykes JE, Hernandez BEA. Diagnosis of salmon poisoning disease in an African Lion (*Panthera leo krugeri*). In: *Proceedings of the*

2015 American Association of Zoological Veterinarians Conference. Portland, OR. 2015.
7. Knapp SE, Millemann RE. Salmon poisoning disease. In: Davis JW, ed. *Infectious Diseases of Wild Mammals*. Ames, IA: Iowa State University Press; 1981:376–387.
8. Headley SA, Viana NE, Michelazzo MMZ, et al. *Neorickettsia helminthoeca* associated lymphoid, enteric, and pulmonary lesions in dogs from Southern Brazil: an immunohistochemical study. *Transbound Emerg Dis*. 2020;67:49–59.
9. Headley SA, Kano FS, Scorpio DG, et al. *Neorickettsia helminthoeca* in Brazilian dogs: a cytopathological, histopathological and immunohistochemical study. *Clin Microbiol Infect*. 2009;15(suppl 2):21–23.
10. Headley SA, Scorpio DG, Barat NC, et al. *Neorickettsia helminthoeca* in dog, Brazil. *Emerg Infect Dis*. 2006;12:1303–1304.
11. Headley SA, de Oliveira TES, de Mello Zanim Michelazzo M, et al. Immunohistochemical and molecular evidence of putative *Neorickettsia* infection in coatis (*Nasua nasua*) from Southern Brazil. *J Zoo Wildl Med*. 2018;49:535–541.
12. Cordy DR, Gorham JR. The pathology and etiology of salmon disease. *Am J Pathol*. 1950;26:617–637.
13. Farrell RK. Transmission of two rickettsia-like disease agents of dogs by endoparasites in northwestern USA. In: *1st International Congress of Parasitology*. Vol. 438; 1966.
14. Farrell RK, Leader RW, Johnston SD. Differentiation of salmon poisoning disease and Elokomin fluke fever: studies with the black bear (*Ursus americanus*). *Am J Vet Res*. 1973;34:919–922.
15. Kitao T, Farrell RK, Fukuda T. Differentiation of salmon poisoning disease and Elokomin fluke fever: fluorescent antibody studies with *Rickettsia sennetsu*? *Am J Vet Res*. 1973;34:927–928.
16. Frank DW, McGuire TC, Gorham JR, et al. Cultivation of two species of *Neorickettsia* in canine monocytes. *J Infect Dis*. 1974;129:257–262.
17. Pastenkos G, Snekvik K, Bradway D, et al. A novel neorickettsial infection in 3 dogs in the Pacific Northwest. *Vet Pathol*. 2020;57:286–289.
18. Fukuda T, Sasahara T, Kitao T. Studies on the causative agent of Hyuganetsu disease. *J Japan Assoc Infect Dis*. 1962;36:235–241.
19. Fukuda T, Yamamoto S. *Neorickettsia*-like organism isolated from metacercaria of a fluke, *Stellantchasmus falcatus*. *Jpn J Med Sci Biol*. 1981;34:103–107.
20. Wen B, Rikihisa Y, Yamamoto S, et al. Characterization of the SF agent, an Ehrlichia sp. isolated from the fluke *Stellantchasmus falcatus*, by 16S rRNA base sequence, serological, and morphological analyses. *Int J Syst Bacteriol*. 1996;46:149–154.
21. Greiman SE, Kent ML, Betts J, et al. *Nanophyetus salmincola*, vector of the salmon poisoning disease agent *Neorickettsia helminthoeca*, harbors a second pathogenic *Neorickettsia* species. *Vet Parasitol*. 2016;229:107–109.
22. Greiman SE, Tkach VV, Pulis E, et al. Large scale screening of digeneans for *Neorickettsia* endosymbionts using real-time PCR reveals new *Neorickettsia* genotypes, host associations and geographic records. *PloS One*. 2014;9. e98453.
23. Bennington E, Pratt I. The life history of the salmon poisoning fluke, *Nanophyetus salmincola* (Chapin). *J Parasitol*. 1960;46:91–100.
24. Foreyt WJ, Thorson S, Gorham JR. Experimental salmon poisoning disease in juvenile coyotes (*Canis latrans*). *J Wildl Dis*. 1982;18:159–162.
25. Baldwin NL, Millemann RE, Knapp SE. "Salmon poisoning" disease. 3. Effect of experimental *Nanophyetus salmincola* infection on the fish host. *J Parasitol*. 1967;53:556–564.
26. Weiseth PR, Farrell RK, Johnston SD. Prevalence of *Nanophyetus salmincola* in ocean-caught salmon. *J Am Vet Med Assoc*. 1974;165:849–850.
27. Bosman DD, Farrell RK, Gorham JR. Non-endoparasite transmission of salmon poisoning disease of dogs. *J Am Vet Med Assoc*. 1970;156:1907–1910.
28. Philip CB. There's always something new under the parasitological sun (the unique story of helminth-borne salmon poisoning disease). *J Parasitol*. 1955;41:125–148.
29. Sykes JE, Marks SL, Mapes S, et al. Salmon poisoning disease in dogs: 29 cases. *J Vet Intern Med*. 2010;24:504–513.
30. Farrell RK, Dee JF, Ott RL. Salmon poisoning in a dog fed kippered salmon. *J Am Vet Med Assoc*. 1968;152:370–371.
31. Mack RE, Becovitch MG, Ling GV, et al. Salmon poisoning disease complex in dogs—a review of 45 cases. *California Veterinarian*. 1990;44:42–45.
32. Frank DW, McGuire TC, Gorham JR, et al. Lymphoreticular lesions of canine neorickettsiosis. *J Infect Dis*. 1974;129:163–171.
33. Hadlow WJ. Neuropathology of experimental salmon poisoning of dogs. *Am J Vet Res*. 1957;18:898–908.
34. Philip CB, Hadlow WJ, Hughes LE. *Neorickettsia helminthoeca*, a new rickettsialike disease agent of dogs in western United States transmitted by a helminth. In: *6th International Congress of Microbiology, Rome*. 1953:70–82.
35. Gorham JR, Foreyt WJ. Salmon poisoning disease. In: Greene CE, ed. *Clinical Microbiology and Infectious Diseases of the Dog and Cat*. 1st ed. Philadelphia, PA: WB Saunders; 1984:538–544.
36. Johns JL, Strasser JL, Zinkl JG, et al. Lymph node aspirate from a California wine-country dog. *Vet Clin Pathol*. 2006;35:243–246.
37. Rikihisa Y. Cross-reacting antigens between *Neorickettsia helminthoeca* and *Ehrlichia* species, shown by immunofluorescence and Western immunoblotting. *J Clin Microbiol*. 1991;29:2024–2029.
38. Rikihisa Y, Zhang C, Kanter M, et al. Analysis of p51, groESL, and the major antigen P51 in various species of *Neorickettsia*, an obligatory intracellular bacterium that infects trematodes and mammals. *J Clin Microbiol*. 2004;42:3823–3826.
39. Rikihisa Y, Stills H, Zimmerman G. Isolation and continuous culture of *Neorickettsia helminthoeca* in a macrophage cell line. *J Clin Microbiol*. 1991;29:1928–1933.
40. Noonan WE. *Neorickettsia helminthoeca in Cell Culture*. PhD Thesis. Corvallis, OR: Oregon State University; 1973.
41. Witenburg G. On the anatomy and systematic position of the causative agent of so-called salmon poisoning. *J Parasitol*. 1932;18:258–263.
42. Foreyt WJ, Gorham JR. Evaluation of praziquantel against induced *Nanophyetus salmincola* infections in coyotes and dogs. *Am J Vet Res*. 1988;49:563–565.
43. Donham CR, Simms BT, Miller FW. So-called salmon poisoning in dogs (progress report). *J Am Vet Med Assoc*. 1926;68:701–715.
44. Sakawa H, Farrell RK, Mori M. Differentiation of salmon poisoning disease and Elokomin fluke fever: complement fixation. *Am J Vet Res*. 1973;34:923–925.
45. Eastburn RL, Fritsche TR, Terhune Jr CA. Human intestinal infection with *Nanophyetus salmincola* from salmonid fishes. *Am J Trop Med Hyg*. 1987;36:586–591.
46. Gibson KE, Rikihisa Y, Zhang C, et al. *Neorickettsia risticii* is vertically transmitted in the trematode *Acanthatrium oregonense* and horizontally transmitted to bats. *Environ Microbiol*. 2005;7:203–212.
47. Chae JS, Pusterla N, Johnson E, et al. Infection of aquatic insects with trematode metacercariae carrying *Ehrlichia risticii*, the cause of Potomac horse fever. *J Med Entomol*. 2000;37:619–625.
48. Dutra F, Schuch LF, Delucchi E, et al. Equine monocytic ehrlichiosis (Potomac horse fever) in horses in Uruguay and southern Brazil. *J Vet Diagn Invest*. 2001;13:433–437.
49. Amusategui I, Tesouro MA, Kakoma I, et al. Serological reactivity to *Ehrlichia canis, Anaplasma phagocytophilum, Neorickettsia risticii, Borrelia burgdorferi* and *Rickettsia conorii* in dogs from northwestern Spain. *Vector Borne Zoonotic Dis*. 2008;8:797–803.
50. Suksawat J, Xuejie Y, Hancock SI, et al. Serologic and molecular evidence of coinfection with multiple vector-borne pathogens in dogs from Thailand. *J Vet Intern Med*. 2001;15:453–462.
51. Dawson JE, Abeygunawardena I, Holland CJ, et al. Susceptibility of cats to infection with *Ehrlichia risticii*, causative agent of equine monocytic ehrlichiosis. *Am J Vet Res*. 1988;49:2096–2100.
52. Ristic M, Dawson J, Holland CJ, et al. Susceptibility of dogs to infection with *Ehrlichia risticii*, causative agent of equine monocytic ehrlichiosis (Potomac horse fever). *Am J Vet Res*. 1988;49:1497–1500.
53. Stubbs CJ, Holland CJ, Reif JS, et al. Feline ehrlichiosis. *Comp Cont Ed Pract Vet*. 2000;22:307–317.

54. Aguirre E, Tesouro MA, Amusategui I, et al. Assessment of feline ehrlichiosis in central Spain using serology and a polymerase chain reaction technique. *Ann N Y Acad Sci*. 2004;1026:103–105.
55. Ayllon T, Diniz PP, Breitschwerdt EB, et al. Vector-borne diseases in client-owned and stray cats from Madrid, Spain. *Vector Borne Zoonotic Dis*. 2012;12:143–150.
56. Peavy GM, Holland CJ, Dutta SK, et al. Suspected ehrlichial infection in five cats from a household. *J Am Vet Med Assoc*. 1997;210:231–234.
57. Wardrop KJ, Birkenheuer A, Blais MC, et al. Update on canine and feline blood donor screening for blood-borne pathogens. *J Vet Intern Med*. 2016;30:15–35.

48

Coxiellosis and Q Fever

Jane E. Sykes, Jacqueline M. Norris

KEY POINTS

- First Described: Mid 1930s, Queensland, Australia, in slaughterhouse workers (Derrick).[1]
- Cause: *Coxiella burnetii,* an obligately intracellular gram-negative bacterial species that belongs to the family Coxiellaceae.
- Affected Hosts: Humans are most susceptible; reproductive disease can occur in farm animal species such as sheep, goats, and cattle, but the evidence for disease in cats and dogs is inconclusive.
- Geographic Distribution: Worldwide, with the exception of New Zealand and Antarctica.
- Major Clinical Signs: Dogs and cats are usually subclinically infected. Abortion, premature birth, and stillbirth have been reported in infected cats or dogs at the center of Q fever outbreaks in humans, but the role of *C. burnetii* in disease in cats and dogs is uncertain.
- Differential Diagnoses: Other infectious causes of reproductive disorders or pregnancy loss such as brucellosis, herpesviral infections, leptospirosis, neosporosis, CDV, and CPV infection. Noninfectious causes of pregnancy loss, such as endocrinopathies, genetic disorders, and nutritional deficiency, should also be considered.
- Human Health Significance: Q fever in humans results primarily from contact with infected sheep, goats, and cattle, or indirect contact with surfaces contaminated with secretions or excretions of these animals. However, contact with infected periparturient companion animals can also lead to transmission. Q fever in humans is most commonly an acute febrile illness, but pneumonia and chronic complications such as endocarditis, granulomatous hepatitis, and chronic fatigue can occur.

ETIOLOGIC AGENT AND EPIDEMIOLOGY

Coxiella burnetii is a gram-negative, obligately intracellular, small, pleomorphic rod that causes Q fever in humans, a significant zoonosis worldwide. Sheep, cattle, and goats are the most commonly reported reservoirs for the organism, but infected cats and less commonly dogs have also been implicated in transmission to humans.[2–7] Animals other than humans are often subclinically infected, although reproductive complications such as premature birth, abortion, and stillbirth may occur. In avian species, systemic illness has been associated with infection by other *Coxiella*-like organisms.[8–10] Reservoir hosts shed organisms in vaginal secretions and the products of parturition due to recrudescence of infection during pregnancy, with shedding in the urine, feces, saliva, and/or milk in some species. The placentas of infected animals are heavily infected (up to 10^9 organisms per gram of tissue). At parturition, aerosols are created, which are subsequently inhaled by other animals and humans (Fig. 48.1). Ingestion of unpasteurized contaminated milk is a less common and more controversial mode of transmission.[11,12] The term *Q fever* stands for *query* fever, the name it was given when it first emerged in Queensland, Australia, before the underlying cause had been identified. In humans, acute Q fever is characterized by a febrile "flu-like" illness, with headaches and profound fatigue, and sometimes pulmonary and hepatic involvement. However, infection is initially asymptomatic in 60% of those infected.[13] Persistent focal Q fever (previously known as chronic Q fever) can follow acute Q fever or asymptomatic infection and can be characterized by cardiac disease (endocarditis, pericarditis, myocarditis), fatigue syndromes, skin rash, and neurologic, pulmonary, and hepatic disease.

Unlike other obligate intracellular pathogens, *C. burnetii* survives prolonged periods in the environment, where it resists high temperature, a variety of disinfectants, and ultraviolet light. The organism exists in two forms: a small cell variant, which is a nonreplicating form that survives in the environment, and a large cell variant, which replicates within mononuclear phagocytes, especially alveolar macrophages (lung) and Kupffer cells (liver). Survival of the organism for up to 10 months on wool at 15°C to 20°C (59°F to 68°F) has been reported, and it can also survive in tissues that have been stored in formalin for several months. It is inactivated by 1% Lysol or 5% hydrogen peroxide.[14] Although originally classified within the order Rickettsiales, the availability of sequence information led to its reclassification as a gammaproteobacterium in the order Legionellales, which also includes *Legionella* species. *Coxiella burnetii* undergoes phase variation, which is associated with alterations in its cell wall components. The variants have nominally been called phase I and phase II.[15] The changes in cell surface antigens and the creation of phase variants have clinical implications for serologic testing in humans due to the production of phase I and phase II antibodies to the bacterium at different stages of natural infection (see Diagnosis, later). The whole genome of *C. burnetii* has been sequenced.[16]

Coxiella burnetii is extremely contagious, and only small numbers of organisms are required to cause disease in humans. The epidemiology of Q fever varies geographically. Because of its predilection for domestic ruminant species, Q fever is most commonly reported from rural areas although the potential role of wildlife continues to be explored. *Coxiella burnetii* has been detected within a huge variety of different tick and other arthropod species. Within ticks, it replicates in the midgut and it is shed in large quantities in tick feces. Although ticks have the potential to transmit the organism to domestic animal species, the most significant role of ticks appears to be in transmission to wildlife,[17] and molecular investigations question whether *C. burnetii* or other *Coxiella* spp. are involved.[18] Nevertheless, transstadial transmission of *C. burnetii* in *Ixodes ricinis* ticks has been accomplished under experimental conditions, supporting the role of *I. ricinus* as a vector.[19] *Coxiella burnetii* has been identified in fish, wild birds,

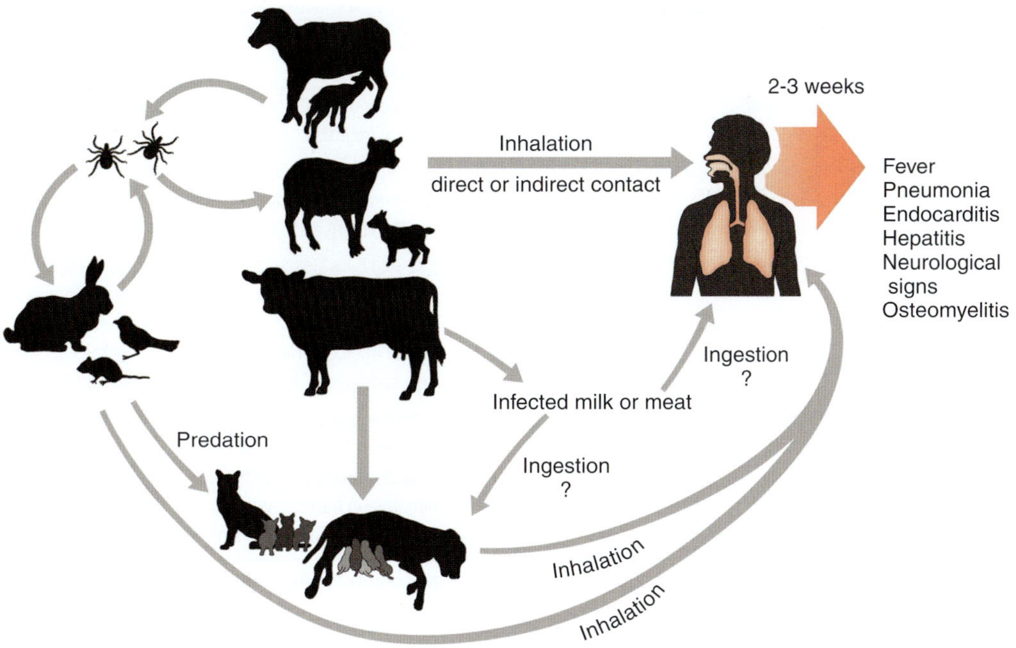

Fig. 48.1 Transmission of *Coxiella burnetii.* The organism is most often transmitted to humans when animals give birth. People become infected by inhalation when they directly contact the products of parturition or as a result of indirect contact with organisms that survive in the environment. Sheep, cattle, and goats are the most common reservoirs of the organism for human infection, but infected cats and less commonly dogs can also transmit the infection to humans. Although not a major mode of transmission, ticks can also harbor the organism and are thought to maintain transmission to wildlife species, especially rodents (such as small mice) and rabbits, and also birds. Dogs, cats, and humans can also become infected when they contact (or ingest) wildlife species. Ingestion of infected milk also may be a lesser mode of transmission.

rodents, marsupials, horses, swine, camels, marine mammals, ducks, turkeys, geese, cats, dogs, and rabbits. Although the mechanism is not clearly defined or established, cats and dogs could potentially become infected through exposure to infected sheep, cattle, and goats—possibly through ingestion of products from these species—and through contact with, or ingestion of, infected wildlife reservoir hosts such as rodents, birds, macropods, and rabbits.

Exposure to stillborn kittens or apparently healthy newborn kittens has been a risk factor for human infection in Africa, Japan, Korea, Canada, Australia, and the United States. In a study of intact female cats from Colorado, *C. burnetii* DNA was not detected in vaginal swab specimens or uterine biopsies from 50 shelter cats using a PCR assay, but 4 of 47 uterine biopsies from client-owned cats were positive.[20] Further molecular studies of uterine tissues of 26 normal cats and 11 cats with histopathologic evidence of uterine disease or other reproductive abnormalities identified three positive samples, two of which were from cats with normal reproductive systems.[21] In the Netherlands, following the largest Q fever outbreak in humans ever documented (2007 to 2010, approximately 4,000 cases), *C. burnetii* DNA was not detected in the placentas from 15 cats but was found in 4 of 54 (7%) dog placentas from veterinary clinical practices that focus their expertise on breeding animals. Some seroprevalence studies suggest that infection is more common in stray cats and dogs than in client-owned animals, while others suggest an increased prevalence in breeding cats or dogs from remote communities.[22–24] Further research is required to determine risk factors for exposure in dogs and cats including the role of ingestion of raw meat.[25–27] In one study from Australia, *C. burnetii* DNA was detected in 43% of 58 raw meat packages sold for companion animal consumption.[25] All of the positive samples contained meat of kangaroo origin amongst other things, whereas all the negative samples contained no kangaroo. No association has been found between prevalence of Q fever in humans and cat or dog ownership.[28] Laboratory-acquired infections have been described in humans, and infection can occur as a result of exposure to straw, manure, or dust, such as that from contaminated farm vehicles and contaminated clothing. Q fever has emerged as a disease of United States combat arms military personnel deployed to Iraq.[29] Studies of a large, 2-year outbreak in the Netherlands showed that dust-accumulating surfaces contained higher levels of *C. burnetii* DNA than vaginal swabs from sheep and goats.[30] The organism can travel for miles as a result of windborne transmission.

CLINICAL FEATURES

Pathogenesis and Clinical Signs

After inhalation (and to a lesser extent, ingestion), *C. burnetii* enters mononuclear phagocytes and survives within the harsh environment of the phagolysosome.[31] Remarkably, the acidic conditions of the lysosome appear to be a requirement for the metabolic functions of *C. burnetii.* Replication is prolonged, and minimal CPEs occur in infected cells. The organism appears to modulate apoptosis in order to inhibit cell death and promote its own replication.[31,32] Subsequently, infected cells enter the bloodstream. After experimental infection, bacteremia may be prolonged (up to 1 month) in cats.[33] The organism can persist in a variety of tissues, and in human patients, this contributes to chronic disease manifestations, such as prolonged fever, endocarditis, vasculitis, chronic fatigue, and immune-mediated consequences such as demyelinating polyradiculoneuritis.[34] Appropriate diagnosis and treatment at the acute stage of clinical illness is important in reducing the risk of postacute Q fever sequelae and development of chronic disease. Reactivation of shedding has been described during pregnancy in humans.[14] Infected cats and dogs usually show no clinical signs of infection, but stillbirth, abortion, and prolonged vaginal bleeding for 3 weeks before delivery have

TABLE 48.1 **Diagnostic Assays Available for Q Fever**

Assay	Specimen type	Target	Performance
Cell culture	Placental materials, vaginal swabs, blood, urine, feces, milk	*Coxiella burnetii*	Not widely offered or utilized for routine diagnostic purposes. Requires special facilities.
Histopathology	Placental materials	*C. burnetii*	Organisms may be seen when present in large numbers and stain with Gimenez stain. Immunohistochemistry and fluorescence *in situ* hybridization can be used to identify the organisms as *C. burnetii*.
Serology	Serum	Antibodies to phase I or phase II *C. burnetii*	Acute and convalescent serology is required for diagnosis of acute infection. At least 1 to 2 months may be required for seroconversion. Cross-reactivity may occur to related bacteria. IFA is considered the serologic test of choice in human patients. CFT is the OIE standard in animals but is less sensitive. IFA method has now been optimized for cats and dogs.
PCR	Whole blood, tissue specimens, vaginal swabs, milk, feces	*C. burnetii* DNA	Confirms active infection. Sensitivity and specificity may vary depending on stage of infection, assay design, and specimen type. PCR is most sensitive in acute infections (in the first 2 weeks of illness in humans), but is usually negative in humans with chronic infections. Subclinical shedding in animals is variable but is greatest during parturition.

CFT, complement fixation test; *IFA,* immunofluorescent antibody; *OIE,* World Organization for Animal Health; PCR, polymerase chain reaction.

been reported in cats.[7,35] The organism replicates in trophoblasts, and in experimentally infected goats, massive bacterial replication occurs in the placenta just before abortion.[36] An infected rabbit hound dog that transmitted *C. burnetii* to a family in Nova Scotia gave birth to four puppies, all of which died within 24 hours of birth.[2] The importance of *C. burnetii* in reproductive tract disease and chronic disease manifestations such as endocarditis in cats and dogs requires further investigation.

DIAGNOSIS

Microbiologic Tests

Diagnostic assays available for Q fever are listed in Table 48.1. In humans, a combination of serologic testing and molecular testing using PCR is recommended, especially in acute infections when serologic test results are often negative.[37]

Culture

Coxiella burnetii can be isolated in a variety of different cell lines. It has also been isolated in a cell-free medium that mimics the phagolysosome environment.[38] Because it is highly infectious to humans, most laboratories do not have the special facilities required to isolate *C. burnetii*. Thus, diagnosis of infection is usually performed using serology, PCR, or IHC.

Serologic Diagnosis

The World Organization for Animal Health (OIE) reference test for serologic diagnosis of *C. burnetii* infection in animals is ELISA.[39] A variety of serologic assays have been used to detect antibodies to phase I or phase II *C. burnetii* antigens in humans and other animals, including IFA assays, ELISA, and CFT. CFT is considered the least sensitive and specific method, but is still used for diagnosis.[40] In human patients, anti–phase II antibodies (IgG and IgM) are present in acute Q fever, whereas anti–phase I IgG antibodies predominate in chronic infection.[17,41] In humans, the use of IFA assays has been recommended for diagnosis of Q fever.[14,37,42] Acute and convalescent serology is required for diagnosis of acute Q fever in humans. It can take at least a month before seroconversion occurs; titers peak around 8 weeks after infection.[17] Diagnosis of focal persistent Q fever in humans is based on detection of an increased phase I IgG antibody titer (≥1:1024) and an identifiable persistent clinical manifestation, such as endocarditis.[37] Because infection is usually not clinically detected in dogs and cats, serologic assays have primarily been used in dogs and cats for epidemiologic studies or as part of import requirements to Q fever–free countries such as New Zealand. An IFA assay has been optimized for use in feline and canine serum and species-specific cutoff values have now been established that replace the less sensitive CFT used previously.[23,24]

Molecular Diagnosis Using Nucleic Acid–Based Testing

Both conventional and real-time PCR assays have been described for detection of *C. burnetii* DNA. PCR assays are the diagnostic test of choice for organism detection and have revolutionized knowledge of the epidemiology of *C. burnetii* infections. In animals, PCR assays have primarily been used on a research basis. In humans, PCR is typically performed on whole blood (acute infections) or heart valve tissue (endocarditis), and is almost always positive in acute infections before antibodies develop.[37] Negative results can occur with PCR assays in chronic infections or even as early as 2 weeks after onset of acute illness in humans, because of undetectable levels of the infection or absence of bacteremia. Because *C. burnetii* is highly infectious to humans, special handling (BSL-3) conditions are required for fresh specimens that are submitted for *C. burnetii* PCR assays. When infection by *C. burnetii* is suspected (such as in placentas or aborted material), the laboratory should be contacted in advance, and specimens should be labeled and transported appropriately.

Pathologic Findings

Little information is available about the pathology of *C. burnetii* infection in dogs and cats. In affected livestock, *C. burnetii* causes a necrotizing placentitis with mixed inflammatory cell infiltrate and nonsuppurative vasculitis. In some cases, small, basophilic intracytoplasmic organisms can be seen (Fig. 48.2). The organisms stain with Gimenez, Giemsa, and modified acid-fast stains, but not Gram, silver, or periodic acid–Schiff stains.[43] IHC and FISH[44] can be used to identify *C. burnetii* antigen within lesions.

TREATMENT

Many acute infections in humans are self-limiting (or even subclinical), and symptoms respond to nonspecific therapy such as antipyretics and rehydration. However, because of concerns related to the development of focal persistent Q fever, specific antimicrobial therapy is recommended regardless of the severity of acute Q fever. When antimicrobial

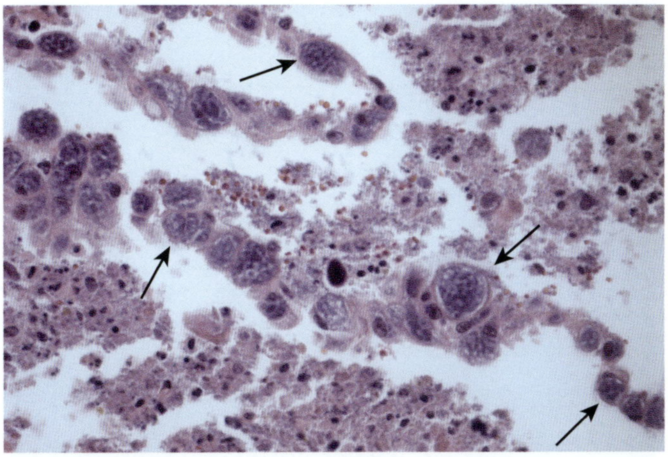

Fig. 48.2 Histopathology showing severe, acute necrotizing placentitis in the placenta of a goat from which dead fetuses were removed by caesarian section. Trophoblasts are distended with abundant basophilic bacterial organisms *(arrows)*. The organisms were subsequently identified as *Coxiella burnetii* with immunohistochemistry.

agents are required, doxycycline for at least 14 days or quinolones have been used successfully to treat pneumonia and hepatitis in human patients with *C. burnetii* infection. Combination therapy, such as doxycycline and hydroxychloroquine (which alkalinizes phagolysosomes) (as recommended by the CDC)[37] or doxycycline, ciprofloxacin, and rifampin for prolonged periods (e.g., 2 years), has been required for treatment of Q fever endocarditis, and valve replacement is frequently needed.[14,17] Antibody titers decrease with successful treatment. Q fever during pregnancy, which may result in abortion when infection occurs in the first trimester, is treated with trimethoprim-sulfamethoxazole for the duration of the pregnancy.[45] Treatment of an infected sheep herd with oxytetracycline on days 100 and 120 of gestation did not prevent shedding of *C. burnetii* in milk, vaginal swabs, or feces as assessed with PCR, nor did it affect the duration of shedding.[46]

PUBLIC HEALTH ASPECTS

In humans, asymptomatic infections with *C. burnetii* are probably widespread. When it occurs, Q fever is most often a systemic febrile illness. Because it mimics a variety of other illnesses, and confirmatory diagnostic tests require a specific index of suspicion by the medical clinician, Q fever is most likely under recognized. Veterinarians involved in mixed or farm animal practice, slaughterhouse workers, and workers in the livestock industry (farmers, shearers, transporters of animals) are most likely to develop Q fever as a result of direct contact with infected livestock. Person-to-person spread of Q fever is rarely reported, but humans can shed organisms during parturition, and infection of an obstetrician during delivery has been described.[47] Infection during pregnancy may also be associated with reproductive complications such as fetal death.[48,49] Transmission during necropsy examinations has also been reported. Between 2014 and 2017, approximately 160 to 190 cases of Q fever were reported to the CDC each year.[50] Approximately 80% of cases were acute and 20% were chronic, and more than one third of cases were from three states—California, Iowa, and Texas (Fig. 48.3). Peak months are in the spring and early summer, which correlates with the peak of the birthing season for cattle, sheep, and goats. In Australia where the disease

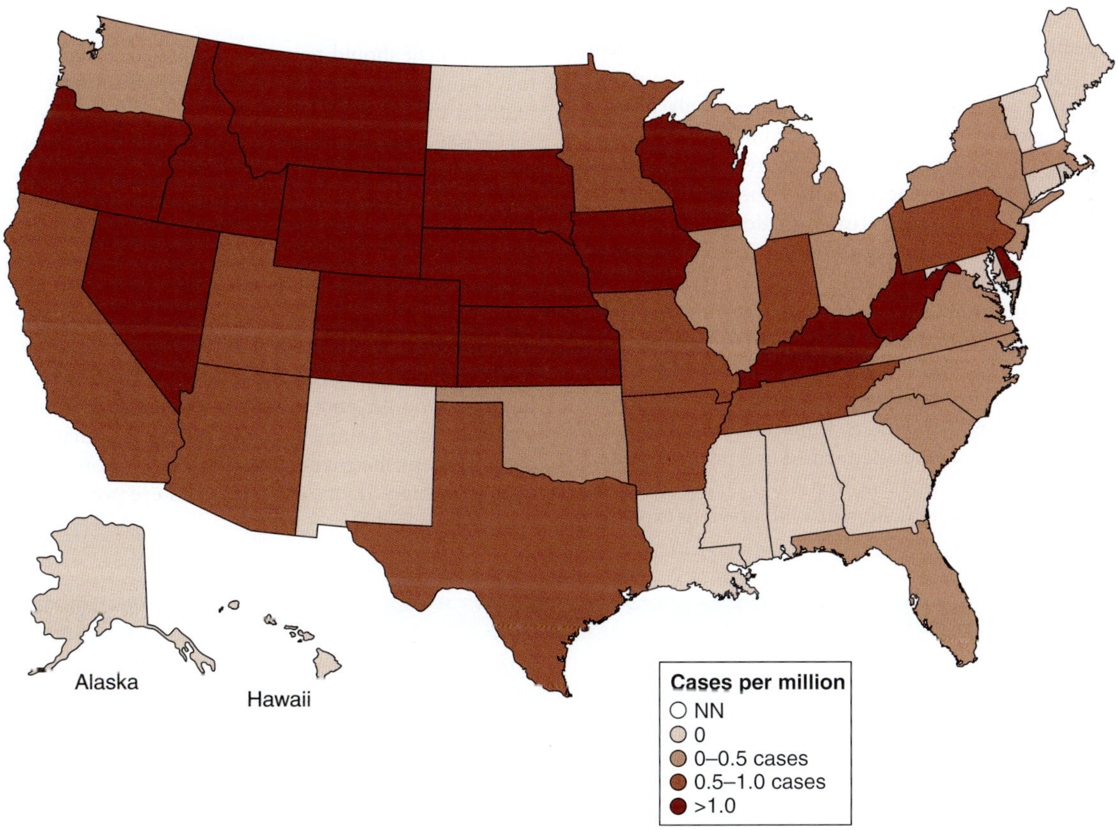

Fig. 48.3 Annual reported incidence (per million persons) for Q fever in the United States in 2017. Cases are most frequently reported from western and plains states where ranching and rearing of livestock are common. (From CDC, https://www.cdc.gov/qfever/stats/index.html)

is also notifiable, 300 to 500 cases are reported annually with most cases occurring in two states—Queensland and New South Wales.[51]

In humans, acute Q fever occurs after an incubation period that ranges from 9 to 39 days, although shorter incubation periods are possible with exposure to high doses of the agent.[14] The incubation period after exposure to an infected cat has ranged from 9 days to 4 weeks.[4,14] Males are predisposed, which relates to an increased likelihood of exposure to ruminants, the more common mode of exposure, and older men are more susceptible to disease.[37] Patients who develop pneumonia may also develop severe headache, as well as sweats, chills, fatigue, and myalgia. Other signs include cough, chest pain, nausea and vomiting, sore throat, diarrhea, a rash, and abdominal pain and hematuria.[14] Myocarditis and pericarditis can occur rarely. Blood work often shows a normal white cell count, and thrombocytopenia or marked thrombocytosis can occur. Serum biochemistry testing reveals mild to moderate increases in the activity of hepatic transaminases in almost all patients.[14] Pulmonary infiltrates are present on thoracic radiographs (Fig. 48.4), and in some cases, pleural effusion.[14,17] Q fever pneumonia is rarely fatal. Focal persistent Q fever may manifest as endocarditis, optic neuritis, osteomyelitis, granulomatous hepatitis, interstitial pulmonary fibrosis, and prolonged fever. In addition, a chronic fatigue syndrome, has been described in up to 10–15% of patients who develop acute infection with *C. burnetii*.[52] This syndrome appears to be due to cytokine dysregulation and may be characterized by incapacitating fatigue, nausea, headache, night sweats, myalgia, muscle fasciculations, lymphadenomegaly, disturbed sleep, irrational anger, and inability to concentrate. Endocarditis follows acute Q fever in fewer than 1% of cases,[41] and it may not become apparent for several years after acute illness. Approximately 3% to 5% of human endocarditis cases have been attributed to *C. burnetii*. Host factors seem to be important in whether chronic manifestations of Q fever occur. Cellular immunity and the production of IFN-γ appear to be required for resolution of infection.[41]

Because treatment with tetracyclines does not seem to reduce shedding by reservoir hosts, an emphasis has been placed on the development of effective vaccines for public health purposes. A phase I inactivated vaccine (Coxevac, Ceva, France) is commercially available in some parts of Europe to prevent shedding by reservoir livestock species, such as sheep and goats. Vaccination of sheep flocks led to a reduced number of abortions and decreased shedding, but did not completely prevent infection.[41] Vaccination was ineffective in previously infected cattle or naïve pregnant cattle.[53] Another phase I whole cell vaccine (Q-VAX, Commonwealth Serum Laboratories, Parkville, Australia) has also been used to protect naïve but at-risk humans, such as livestock workers (farmers, shearers, slaughterhouse workers, animal transporters), veterinarians, veterinary nurses, cat and dog breeders, wildlife carers, and laboratory workers, from infection. A Q-VAX skin test as well as serologic assays are performed as a prescreening of potential vaccine recipients for prior sensitization to Q fever antigens to minimize adverse vaccine reactions; humans with previous exposure to *C. burnetii* should never be vaccinated. It has been recommended that humans should not drink raw milk from infected farms. Aborted material and placentas can be buried with lime or incinerated.[41]

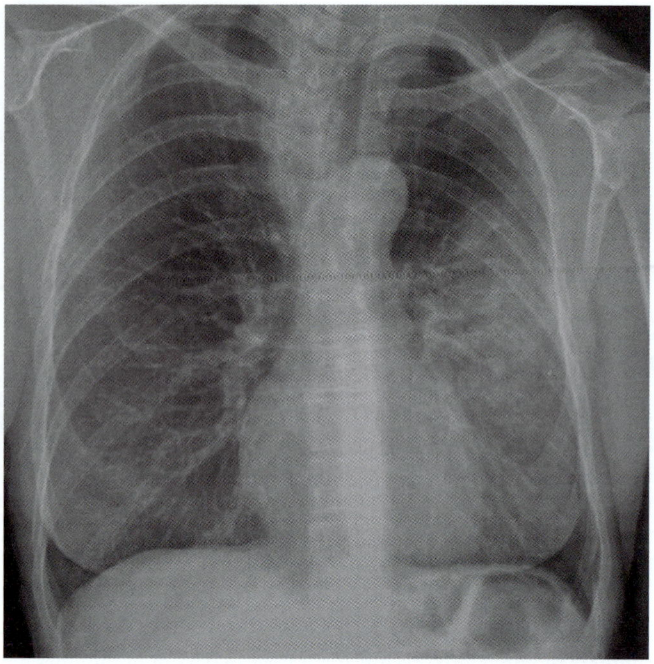

Fig. 48.4 Thoracic radiograph from a 49-year old female veterinarian with probable acute Q fever pneumonia. Left lobar consolidation is present. Cough, fever, myalgia and headache developed 2 weeks after running through a barn where lambing ewes with endemic coxiellosis were present. There was no response to amoxicillin and azithromycin, but treatment with 3 weeks of doxycycline led to gradual resolution of clinical signs. Phase I and Phase II acute titers were 1:256. Convalescent titers are pending at the time of writing.

Q fever has occurred in people exposed to periparturient cats. An outbreak in an Australian small animal veterinary hospital was linked to a cesarean section in a pregnant queen; nine veterinary personnel and the queen's owner had evidence of recent infection (see case example).[3] The most severely affected individuals had assisted in the surgery and performed mouth-to-mouth resuscitation on the newborn kittens. Small animal practices should incorporate measures into their infection control protocols to limit exposure to *C. burnetii*, including wearing appropriate PPE when around birth products and avoiding mouth-to-mouth and mouth-to-nose resuscitation of neonates. In mixed or large animal practices where veterinarians are exposed to periparturient sheep and goats, the use of proper PPE, including protective clothing (boots, coveralls) and eye protection and N95 masks, is recommended.[50]

CASE EXAMPLE

Signalment

A 50-year-old female veterinarian and a 23-year-old female veterinary technician from southeastern Australia.

History

A 3-year-old female British short-hair cat with dystocia was brought to a veterinary clinic by the breeder/owner at 8 o'clock in the morning. One kitten was stillborn in the home environment overnight. Safe delivery of the two remaining kittens required a cesarean section. Surgery was performed immediately, and the kittens were delivered and revived by vigorous rubbing with dry towels. The kittens were discolored by yellow-green placental material and were slow to revive. They were able to successfully suckle once the queen had recovered from general anesthesia. The queen and kittens were returned to the breeder's cattery the same afternoon.

CASE EXAMPLE—cont'd

Two weeks after the surgery, the veterinarian and the veterinary technician who had been involved in the cesarean section developed fever, severe headache, neck pain, chills, night sweats, myalgia, and stiffness. The veterinarian sought medical attention. Psittacosis was considered the most likely diagnosis by the attending physician, because psittacine birds were frequently treated in the clinic. A serologic test for chlamydiosis was negative, but nevertheless treatment with doxycycline was commenced. The veterinary technician's clinical signs were more severe and included cough, chest pain, nausea, and vomiting. As a result, she was hospitalized for 3 weeks for further diagnostic testing, treatment, and convalescence. When the technician tested positive by PCR assay for *C. burnetii* DNA on day 10 after the onset of illness, serial diagnostic tests for Q fever were also performed on the veterinarian. However, the veterinarian did not test positive until over a month after the day of the cesarean (Table 48.2).

Comments

Determination of the date of onset of illness is essential in any diagnostic investigation of Q fever in people for correct interpretation of diagnostic test results. In the first 8 to 10 days after the onset of illness, patients are frequently (80%) bacteremic (and therefore PCR positive) but still antibody negative. IgM class antibody to phase II antigens, as measured via IFA or ELISA assays, appear as early as 10 to 12 days after the onset of illness, but this may also be delayed, as occurred in the veterinarian in this example. IgM class antibody to phase I and IgG class antibody to phase II antigens often appear on day 15 to 20, but again this can be delayed. Small animal veterinarians and veterinary technicians or nurses who are exposed to kittens and placental secretions and subsequently develop illness should inform their practitioner of the possibility of exposure to *C. burnetii* because diagnosis requires a high index of suspicion and specific diagnostic assays. Fatigue often persists in patients for months after the onset of illness (as was the case for the veterinary technician in this example) and does not necessarily mean that focal persistent Q fever has developed.

TABLE 48.2 Results of Diagnostic Assays for Q fever in a Veterinarian and Veterinary Technician after Exposure to an Infected Cat's Reproductive Secretions

Days After Illness Onset	REAL-TIME PCR ON WHOLE BLOOD		SEROLOGY FOR IgM AND IgG TO PHASE I AND PHASE II ANTIGENS[a]	
	Veterinarian	Technician	Veterinarian	Technician
10	ND	Positive	ND	Negative for IgG and IgM to phase II antigen
14	Negative	ND	Negative	ND
20	Negative	Negative	Negative	Positive for IgM to phase I and phase II antigens, positive for IgG to phase II antigen. Positive CFT for antibodies to phase II antigen
35	ND	ND	Positive for IgM and IgG to phase II antigen. Positive CFT for antibodies to phase II antigens	ND

[a]Performed by immunofluorescent antibody unless otherwise specified.
CFT, complement fixation test; *ND,* not determined.

SUGGESTED READINGS

Anderson A, Bijlmer H, Fournier PE, et al. Diagnosis and management of Q fever–United States, 2013: recommendations from CDC and the Q fever working group. *MMWR Recomm Rep (Morb Mortal Wkly Rep).* 2013;62:1–30.

Porter SR, Czaplicki G, Mainil J, et al. Q Fever: current state of knowledge and perspectives of research of a neglected zoonosis. *Int J Microbiol.* 2011;2011:248418.

Kopecny L, Bosward KL, Shapiro A, et al. Investigating *Coxiella burnetii* infection in a breeding cattery at the centre of a Q fever outbreak. *J Feline Med Surg.* 2013;15:1037–1045.

REFERENCES

1. Derrick EH. "Q" fever, a new fever entity: clinical features, diagnosis and laboratory investigation. *Med J Aust.* 1937;2:281–299.
2. Buhariwalla F, Cann B, Marrie TJ. A dog-related outbreak of Q fever. *Clin Infect Dis.* 1996;23:753–755.
3. Kopecny L, Bosward KL, Shapiro A, et al. Investigating *Coxiella burnetii* infection in a breeding cattery at the centre of a Q fever outbreak. *J Feline Med Surg.* 2013;15:1037–1045.
4. Kosatsky T. Household outbreak of Q-fever pneumonia related to a parturient cat. *Lancet.* 1984;2:1447–1449.
5. Malo JA, Colbran C, Young M, et al. An outbreak of Q fever associated with parturient cat exposure at an animal refuge and veterinary clinic in southeast Queensland. *Aust N Z J Public Health.* 2018;42:451–455.
6. Marrie TJ, Langille D, Papukna V, et al. Truckin' pneumonia: an outbreak of Q fever in a truck repair plant probably due to aerosols from clothing contaminated by contact with newborn kittens. *Epidemiol Infect.* 1989;102:119–127.
7. Marrie TJ, MacDonald A, Durant H, et al. An outbreak of Q fever probably due to contact with a parturient cat. *Chest.* 1988;93:98–103.
8. Shivaprasad HL, Cadenas MB, Diab SS, et al. *Coxiella*-like infection in psittacines and a toucan. *Avian Dis.* 2008;52:426–432.
9. Vapniarsky N, Barr BC, Murphy B. Systemic *Coxiella*-like infection with myocarditis and hepatitis in an eclectus parrot (*Eclectus roratus*). *Vet Pathol.* 2012;49:717–722.
10. Woc-Colburn AM, Gamer MM, Bradway D, et al. Fatal coxiellosis in Swainson's Blue mountain Rainbow Lorikeets (*Trichoglossus haematodus moluccanus*). *Vet Pathol.* 2008;45:247–254.
11. Benson WW, Brock DW, Mather J. Serologic analysis of a penitentiary group using raw milk from a Q fever infected herd. *Public Health Rep.* 1963;78:707–710.
12. Fishbein DB, Raoult D. A cluster of *Coxiella burnetii* infections associated with exposure to vaccinated goats and their unpasteurized dairy products. *Am J Trop Med Hyg.* 1992;47:35–40.

13. Raoult D, Marrie T, Mege J. Natural history and pathophysiology of Q fever. *Lancet Infect Dis.* 2005;5:219–226.
14. Marrie TJ, Raoult D. *Coxiella burnetii* (Q fever). In: Bennett JE, Dolin R, Blaser MJ, eds. *Mandell, Douglas and Bennett's Principles and Practice of Infectious Diseases.* 8th ed. Philadelphia, PA: Elsevier Saunders; 2015: 2208–2216.
15. Jerrells TR, Hinrichs DJ, Mallavia LP. Cell envelope analysis of *Coxiella burnetii* phase I and phase II. *Can J Microbiol.* 1974;20:1465–1470.
16. Seshadri R, Paulsen IT, Eisen JA, et al. Complete genome sequence of the Q-fever pathogen *Coxiella burnetii. Proc Natl Acad Sci U S A.* 2003;100:5455–5460.
17. Angelakis E, Raoult D. Q Fever. *Vet Microbiol.* 2010;140:297–309.
18. Oskam CL, Gofton AW, Greay TL, et al. Molecular investigation into the presence of a *Coxiella* sp. in *Rhipicephalus sanguineus* ticks in Australia. *Vet Microbiol.* 2017;201:141–145.
19. Korner S, Makert GR, Mertens-Scholz K, et al. Uptake and fecal excretion of *Coxiella burnetii* by *Ixodes ricinus* and *Dermacentor marginatus* ticks. *Parasit Vectors.* 2020;13:75.
20. Cairns K, Brewer M, Lappin MR. Prevalence of *Coxiella burnetii* DNA in vaginal and uterine samples from healthy cats of north-central Colorado. *J Feline Med Surg.* 2007;9:196–201.
21. Fujishiro MA, Scorza AV, Gookin JL, et al. Evaluation of associations among *Coxiella burnetii* and reproductive abnormalities in cats. *J Feline Med Surg.* 2016;18:344–347.
22. Ma G, Norris JM, Mathews KO, et al. New insights on the epidemiology of *Coxiella burnetii* in pet dogs and cats from New South Wales, Australia. *Acta Trop.* 2020;205:105416.
23. Shapiro AJ, Bosward KL, Heller J, et al. Seroprevalence of *Coxiella burnetii* in domesticated and feral cats in eastern Australia. *Vet Microbiol.* 2015;177:154–161.
24. Shapiro AJ, Norris JM, Heller J, et al. Seroprevalence of *Coxiella burnetii* in Australian dogs. *Zoonoses Public Health.* 2016;63:458–466.
25. Shapiro A, Bosward K, Mathews K, et al. Molecular detection of *Coxiella burnetii* in raw meat intended for pet consumption. *Zoonoses Public Health.* 2020;67:443–452.
26. Komiya T, Sadamasu K, Kang MI, et al. Seroprevalence of *Coxiella burnetii* infections among cats in different living environments. *J Vet Med Sci.* 2003;65:1047–1048.
27. Willeberg P, Ruppanner R, Behymer DE, et al. Environmental exposure to *Coxiella burnetii*: a sero-epidemiologic survey among domestic animals. *Am J Epidemiol.* 1980;111:437–443.
28. Skerget M, Wenisch C, Daxboeck F, et al. Cat or dog ownership and sero-prevalence of ehrlichiosis, Q fever, and cat-scratch disease. *Emerg Infect Dis.* 2003;9:1337–1340.
29. Anderson AD, Baker TR, Littrell AC, et al. Seroepidemiologic survey for *Coxiella burnetii* among hospitalized US troops deployed to Iraq. *Zoonoses Public Health.* 2011;58:276–283.
30. de Bruin A, de Groot A, de Heer L, et al. Detection of *Coxiella burnetii* in complex matrices by using multiplex quantitative PCR during a major Q fever outbreak in The Netherlands. *Appl Environ Microbiol.* 2011;77:6516–6523.
31. Voth DE, Heinzen RA. Lounging in a lysosome: the intracellular lifestyle of *Coxiella burnetii. Cell Microbiol.* 2007;9:829–840.
32. Cordsmeier A, Wagner N, Luhrmann A, et al. Defying death - how *Coxiella burnetii* copes with intentional host cell suicide. *Yale J Biol Med.* 2019;92:619–628.
33. Gillespie JH, Baker JA. Experimental Q fever in cats. *Am J Vet Res.* 1952;13:91–94.
34. Lefebvre M, Grossi O, Agard C, et al. Systemic immune presentations of *Coxiella burnetii* infection (Q Fever). *Semin Arthritis Rheum.* 2010;39:405–409.
35. Nagaoka H, Sugieda M, Akiyama M, et al. Isolation of *Coxiella burnetii* from the vagina of feline clients at veterinary clinics. *J Vet Med Sci.* 1998;60:251–252.
36. Sanchez J, Souriau A, Buendia AJ, et al. Experimental *Coxiella burnetii* infection in pregnant goats: a histopathological and immunohistochemical study. *J Comp Pathol.* 2006;135:108–115.
37. Anderson A, Bijlmer H, Fournier PE, et al. Diagnosis and management of Q fever–United States, 2013: recommendations from CDC and the Q fever working group. *MMWR Recomm Rep (Morb Mortal Wkly Rep).* 2013;62:1–30.
38. Omsland A, Cockrell DC, Howe D, et al. Host cell-free growth of the Q fever bacterium *Coxiella burnetii. Proc Natl Acad Sci U S A.* 2009;106:4430–4434.
39. World Organisation for Animal Health. Q Fever. *In Manual of Diagnostic Tests and Vaccines for Terrestrial Animals*; 2019:560–577. Available at: https://www.oie.int/en/standard-setting/terrestrial-manual/access-online/.
40. Allan-Blitz LT, Sakona A, Wallace WD, et al. *Coxiella burnetii* endocarditis and meningitis, California, USA, 2017. *Emerg Infect Dis.* 2018;24.
41. Porter SR, Czaplicki G, Mainil J, et al. Q Fever: current state of knowledge and perspectives of research of a neglected zoonosis. *Int J Microbiol.* 2011;2011:248418.
42. Melenotte C, Million M, Raoult D. New insights in *Coxiella burnetii* infection: diagnosis and therapeutic update. *Expert Rev Anti Infect Ther.* 2020;18:75–86.
43. Moore JD, Barr BC, Daft BM, et al. Pathology and diagnosis of *Coxiella burnetii* infection in a goat herd. *Vet Pathol.* 1991;28:81–84.
44. Jensen TK, Montgomery DL, Jaeger PT, et al. Application of fluorescent in situ hybridisation for demonstration of *Coxiella burnetii* in placentas from ruminant abortions. *Apmis.* 2007;115:347–353.
45. Carcopino X, Raoult D, Bretelle F, et al. Managing Q fever during pregnancy: the benefits of long-term cotrimoxazole therapy. *Clin Infect Dis.* 2007;45:548–555.
46. Astobiza I, Barandika JF, Hurtado A, et al. Kinetics of *Coxiella burnetii* excretion in a commercial dairy sheep flock after treatment with oxytetracycline. *Vet J.* 2010;184:172–175.
47. Raoult D, Stein A. Q fever during pregnancy: a risk for women, fetuses, and obstetricians. *N Engl J Med.* 1994;330:371.
48. Ghanem-Zoubi N, Paul M: Q fever during pregnancy: a narrative review. *Clin Microbiol Infect*, 26:854–870, 2020.
49. Nielsen SY, Mølbak K, Henriksen TB, et al.: Adverse pregnancy outcomes and *Coxiella burnettii* antibodies in pregnant women, Denmark. *Emerg Infect Dis.* 20:925–931, 2014.
50. Centers for Disease Control and Prevention. Q Fever. www.cdc.gov/qfever/stats/index.html.
51. Australian Government Department of Health. Australia's notifiable disease status, 2013: Annual report of the National Notifiable Diseases Surveillance System: Part 8. https://www1.health.gov.au/internet/main/publishing.nsf/Content/cda-cdi3903i7.htm.
52. Marmion BP, Shannon M, Maddocks I, et al. Protracted debility and fatigue after acute Q fever. *Lancet.* 1996;347:977–978.
53. Guatteo R, Seegers H, Joly A, et al. Prevention of *Coxiella burnetii* shedding in infected dairy herds using a phase I *C. burnetii* inactivated vaccine. *Vaccine.* 2008;26:4320–4328.

Chlamydial Infections

Jane E. Sykes

KEY POINTS

- First Described in Cats: In 1944, United States.[1]
- Causes: *Chlamydia felis* (and possibly other chlamydiae such as *Chlamydia pneumoniae*) causes ocular disease in cats; *Chlamydia psittaci* and *Chlamydia abortus* have both rarely been detected in association with ocular and respiratory disease in cats and dogs.
- Geographic Distribution: Worldwide.
- Mode of Transmission: Direct contact with respiratory secretions and possibly also vaginal secretions and feces.
- Major Clinical Signs (Cats): Acute and chronic conjunctivitis, chemosis, serous to mucopurulent ocular discharge, blepharospasm, with or without sneezing and nasal discharge.
- Differential Diagnoses (Cats): FHV-1, FCV, *Mycoplasma* spp., *Bordetella bronchiseptica* infections.
- Human Health Significance: *Chlamydia felis* has rarely been documented as a cause of human conjunctivitis. The importance of cats and dogs as a source of other human chlamydial infections requires further investigation. *Chlamydia psittaci* is generally acquired from avian species and not from dogs and cats.

ETIOLOGY AGENT AND EPIDEMIOLOGY

Chlamydiae are obligately intracellular bacteria that belong to the order Chlamydiales and primarily cause conjunctivitis in cats, but may also play a role in other systemic and reproductive disorders in dogs and cats that remain poorly characterized. Most knowledge of chlamydial infections results from research on human chlamydial infections, such as *Chlamydia trachomatis*, *Chlamydia pneumoniae* and *Chlamydia psittaci*, which have significant clinical and public health importance (see Public Health Significance). Chlamydiae structurally resemble gram-negative bacteria, lack peptidoglycan, and have extremely small genomes; they depend on the host cell for many amino acids and nucleotides. They exist in two forms: an infectious elementary body (EB), which is 0.2 to 0.6 μm in diameter and exists outside the cell, and the reticulate body (RB), which is larger (0.5 to 1.5 μm), noninfectious, and replicates within the cytoplasm of host cells, before it matures and forms EBs (Fig. 49.1). The EBs survive only a few days in the environment at room temperature and are readily inactivated by most disinfectants. Transmission occurs via direct contact or, to a lesser extent, aerosols. Fomites are also likely to be an important means of transmission among group-housed cats in heavily contaminated environments. In one study of stray and pet cats from Switzerland, rectal shedding was documented using real-time PCR in 25% of infected cats; 22% of infected cats had both positive conjunctival and rectal swabs. Therefore, rectal shedding may also contribute to environmental contamination.[2] Although the chlamydiae at one time separated into two genera, *Chlamydia* and *Chlamydophila*, based on sequence analysis of the 16S rRNA and 23S rRNA genes, there has been disagreement in the field regarding this classification, and reversion to the single genus *Chlamydia* has since been recommended based on the availability of complete genome sequence information.[3,4]

Chlamydiae persistently infect epithelial cells of the ocular, respiratory, GI, and genitourinary systems; chlamydial infections of the synovium have also been reported in a number of different host species. Different chlamydial species tend to cause disease in certain hosts, although evidence has accumulated that some chlamydial species may be capable of causing disease in more than one host species (Table 49.1). Some disease manifestations in a single host species may be caused by more than one chlamydial species. For example, whilst the human ocular disease trachoma is caused primarily by *C. trachomatis*, it has now also been associated with infection by *C. pneumoniae* and *C. psittaci*.[5] *Chlamydia felis* is an important cause of conjunctivitis and possibly reproductive disease in domestic cats, but recently DNA that resembles that of the human pathogen *C. pneumoniae* has now also been detected in ocular swabs from cats with conjunctivitis from Europe.[6] *Chlamydia abortus* DNA was also detected in 4.3% of 69 Chlamydiaceae-infected cats from Switzerland[2] and was detected in histopathology specimens from 1 of 13 cats with arteriosclerosis.[7] There are rare reports of chlamydial infections in dogs, in association with ocular and respiratory disease, polyarthritis, and atherosclerosis.[8–13] However, chlamydiae were not detected with PCR in canine atherosclerotic lesions from 16 dogs in one study.[7] Respiratory disease associated with *C. psittaci* infection has been reported most frequently among dogs.

The most significant pathogen of cats is *C. felis*, which causes acute and chronic conjunctivitis in cats worldwide. Conjunctivitis due to *C. felis* infection has also been reported in a free-ranging Eurasian lynx (*Lynx lynx*).[14] Based on sequence information from outer membrane protein genes, all feline isolates appear to be genetically similar. However, the results of serologic methods and random amplification of polymorphic DNA (RAPD) fingerprinting suggest that more than one strain of *C. felis* might exist. The prevalence of infection varies from one group of cats to another, geographic location, age of the cat population sampled, and presence or absence of clinical illness. Infection is most commonly detected in multiple cat households, especially breeding catteries. *Chlamydia felis* DNA is uncommonly detected in conjunctival swabs from healthy cats. For example, in household cats, clinically healthy cats, those with a history of past conjunctivitis, and those with active conjunctivitis, positive PCR results were 0%, 4.6% and 7.3%, respectively.[15] Isolation rates of up to 30% of household cats have been reported.[16] In shelter cats, the prevalence of *C. felis* infection has ranged from 0% to 15%.[17–20] In cats from 218 European rescue shelters,

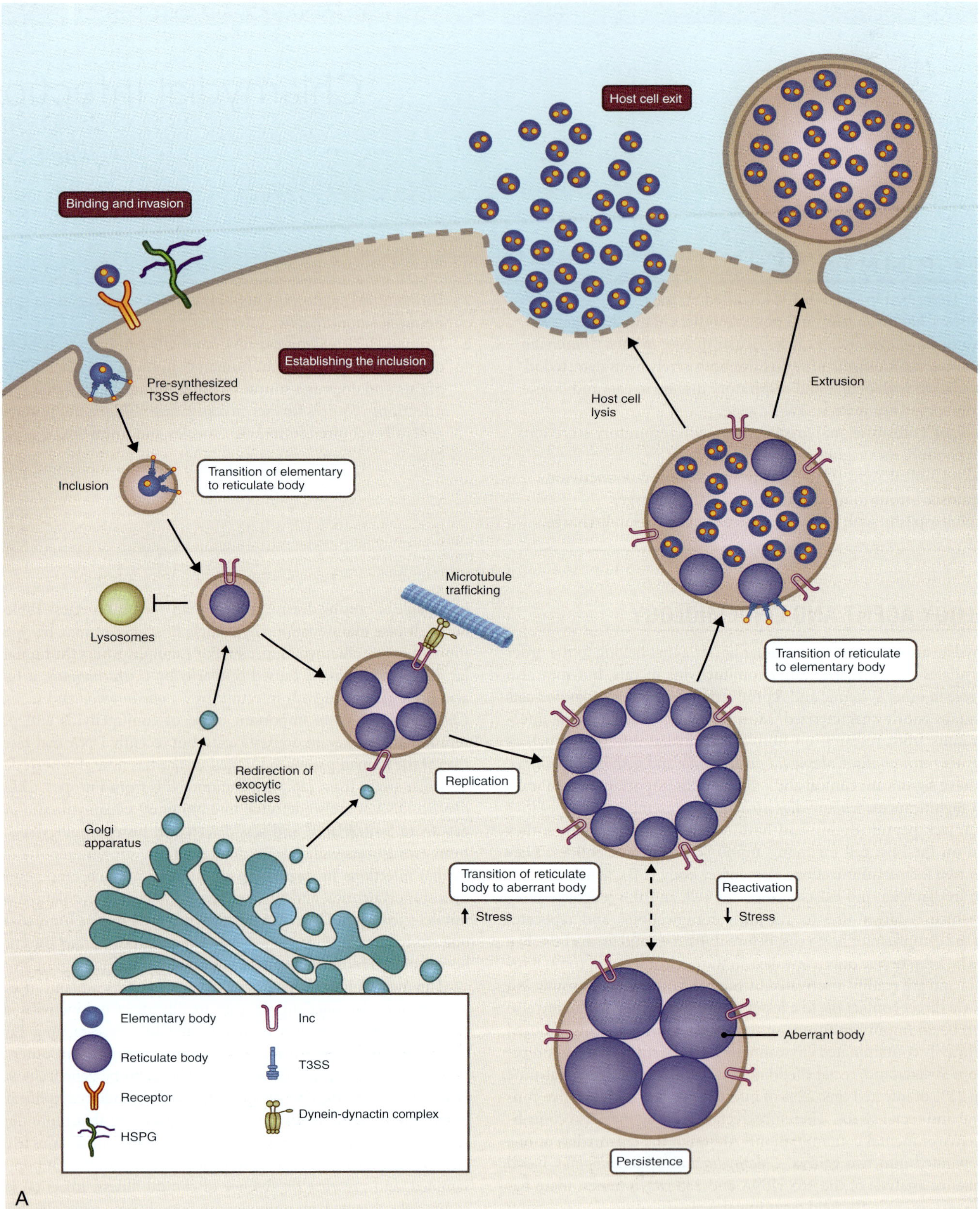

Fig. 49.1 (A) The binding of elementary bodies (EBs) to host cells is initiated by the formation of a trimolecular bridge between bacterial adhesins, host receptors, and host heparan sulfate proteoglycans (HSPGs). Next, pre-synthesized type III secretion system (T3SS) effectors are injected into the host cell, some of which initiate cytoskeletal rearrangements to facilitate internalization and creation of an anti-apoptotic state. The EB is endocytosed into a membrane-bound compartment (inclusion), which dissociates from the endolysosomal pathway. EBs convert to reticulate bodies (RBs) and newly secreted inclusion membrane proteins (Incs) promote nutrient acquisition by redirecting exocytic vesicles that are in transit from the Golgi apparatus to the plasma membrane. The RBs then replicate exponentially and secrete effectors that modulate processes in the host cell. Under stress, RBs enter a persistent state and transition to enlarged aberrant bodies. The bacteria can be reactivated upon removal of the stress. In late stages of infection, RBs synthesize EB-specific effectors before differentiating back to EBs. The EBs exit the host through lysis or extrusion. (Modified from Elwell C, Mirrashidi K, Engel J. *Chlamydia* cell biology and pathogenesis. *Nat Rev Microbiol.* 2016;14:385–400.)

Continued

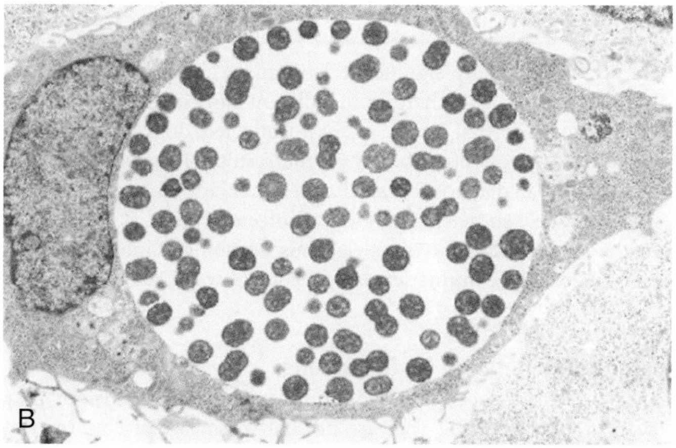

Fig. 49.1 cont'd. (B) Electron micrograph of chlamydial organisms growing in an inclusion in tissue culture. The larger RBs have more diffuse chromatin. One of the RBs appears to be dividing. The smaller dense bodies are EBs. (From Mandell GL, Bennett JE, Dolin R. *Principles and Practice of Infectious Diseases*. 7th ed. Philadelphia, PA: Elsevier: 2012;2:2440.)

breeding establishments, and private households, the prevalence of infection in cats without respiratory disease was 3% versus 10% in those with evidence of respiratory disease.[21] In this study, infection with *C. felis* was associated with suboptimal hygiene. Infection with *C. felis* is more commonly detected in young cats, especially those aged 2 to 12 months; kittens less than 2 months of age may be protected by maternal antibody, although neonatal infections have been described. Cats older than 5 years of age are very unlikely to be infected with *C. felis*. Co-infections with other respiratory pathogens, such as FHV-1 and FCV, are common and may contribute to increased severity of clinical signs.

The DNA of organisms that belong to the family Parachlamydiaceae has also been detected in cats with ocular disease. These organisms are *Chlamydia*-like organisms that reside symbiotically within amoebae. Parachlamydial species include *Neochlamydia*, *Parachlamydia*, *Protochlamydia*, *Rhabdochlamydia*, *Criblamydia*, *Simkania*, and *Waddlia*. DNA that closely resembles that of *Neochlamydia hartmanellae* has been detected in feline conjunctival specimens.[22] This organism is an endosymbiont of the amoeba *Hartmannella vermiformis*, which has been identified as a cause of ocular surface infection in humans and may play some role in feline ocular infections. The DNA of *Parachlamydia acanthamoebae* has also been detected with PCR in cats with keratitis and conjunctivitis.[23] As yet, amoebic co-infections have not been detected in cats. Further studies are required to determine the prevalence and clinical significance of these organisms.

CLINICAL FEATURES

Pathogenesis and Clinical Signs

Chlamydia felis infection is acquired by cats primarily through close contact, fomite, or, to a lesser extent, aerosol transmission. Kittens may be infected from the mother at birth. Whether venereal transmission occurs, as reported for other chlamydial species, is unknown, but in some infected cats, the organism is shed in vaginal discharges and from the rectum as well as in ocular discharges. After uptake of EBs, the EB transitions into the RB, which replicates by binary fission in a membrane-enclosed vacuole called an inclusion, and avoids lysosomal fusion. The RBs then transition back to the EB form, which is released into the extracellular milieu after cell lysis occurs and subsequently infect other host cells. The entire replication cycle takes about 2 days to complete (see Fig. 49.1).[24]

Chlamydiae primarily infect columnar epithelial cells, but they can also infect a variety of other cell types including endothelial cells,

TABLE 49.1 Chlamydial Species That Infect Animals and Humans

Species	Major Host(s)[a]	Major Clinical Manifestations
Chlamydia trachomatis	Humans	Conjunctivitis (serovars A–C); urethritis, cervicitis, proctitis (serovars D–K); lymphogranuloma venereum (serovars L1, L2, and L3)
Chlamydia pneumoniae	Humans	Upper respiratory infection, community-acquired pneumonia, possibly atherosclerosis and asthma
Chlamydia psittaci	Humans, a variety of bird species (e.g., parrots, finches, poultry, pigeons, pheasants, seagulls, egrets, puffins)	Pneumonia, systemic infection
Chlamydia felis	Cats	Conjunctivitis, upper respiratory infection, arthritis, reproductive disease
Chlamydia abortus	Sheep, cows, goats, cats, other mammals	Reproductive disease
Chlamydia pecorum	Cattle and sheep	Encephalomyelitis, pneumonia, reproductive tract disease, conjunctivitis, polyarthritis
Chlamydia caviae	Guinea pigs	Keratoconjunctivitis

[a]Infection may occasionally extend to other host species.

smooth muscle cells, lymphocytes, monocytes, and macrophages. *Chlamydia felis* replicates in the cytoplasm of conjunctival epithelial cells, and also spreads via the bloodstream to a variety of other tissues, such as the tonsil, lung, liver, spleen, GI tract, and kidney. Infection is typically followed 2 to 5 days later by the development of acute, chronic, or recurrent conjunctivitis, with or without signs of rhinitis, such as nasal discharge and sneezing. Most cats remain otherwise well and appetent. Lower respiratory tract signs such as cough and dyspnea rarely, if ever, occur. Corneal disease such as keratitis or corneal ulceration is rare, and if present, is likely caused by other or co-infecting pathogens such as FHV-1 or bacteria. Experimental inoculations have also been associated with fever, lethargy, lameness and joint pain (possibly due to polyarthritis), and weight loss.[25] There are also rare reports of gastritis and peritonitis in association with the detection of *Chlamydia*-like organisms in cats.[26,27]

After the initial episode of acute conjunctivitis, infection may persist for many months, and this may be accompanied by mild signs of conjunctivitis, or in some cases, no clinical signs of disease. Organisms have been isolated from the conjunctiva for up to 215 days after experimental infection.[28,29] Whether chronic disease is the result of repeated reinfection or the presence of persistent chlamydiae is unclear. Co-infections with other agents such as FCV, FHV-1, *Bordetella*, or *Mycoplasma* may increase the clinical severity of infection and duration of shedding. Other bacteria, including those that normally colonize the healthy conjunctival sac, can also act as secondary invaders and worsen the disease.

Whether *C. felis* can cause reproductive disease in cats remains unclear. The stage of pregnancy at which infection occurs, co-infection with other organisms such as FHV-1, concurrent immunosuppression, route of infection, and the strain involved may be important in determining the ability of *C. felis* to cause reproductive dysfunction, if this indeed occurs in cats.

Chlamydial infections are infrequently described in dogs. *Chlamydia psittaci* has been detected in dogs with respiratory disease, such as pneumonia and pleural effusion, and/or keratoconjunctivitis.[8–10] One group of bitches that had ocular and lower respiratory signs as well as stillbirths and low litter signs had nasal, conjunctival, and pharyngeal swab specimens that tested positive for *C. psittaci* infection with a nested PCR assay.[8] *Chlamydia abortus* was detected in a dog with keratoconjunctivitis.[11] The DNA of *C. pneumoniae* was detected in atherosclerotic lesions from dogs in Japan,[12] and *Chlamydia*-like organisms were found in a dog from South Africa with polyarthritis.[13]

Physical Examination Findings

Physical examination findings in cats with chlamydiosis include conjunctivitis, chemosis, serous to mucopurulent ocular discharge, and blepharospasm (Fig. 49.2). Signs of nasal involvement, such as stertorous respiration, serous or mucopurulent nasal discharge, and sneezing, may accompany conjunctivitis. Mucopurulent vaginal discharge has been reported in some cats that were experimentally infected by ocular inoculation.

Physical examination findings described in dogs with chlamydiosis have included fever, tachypnea, keratoconjunctivitis with mucopurulent ocular discharge, shifting leg lameness, and lymphadenopathy.[8–11,13]

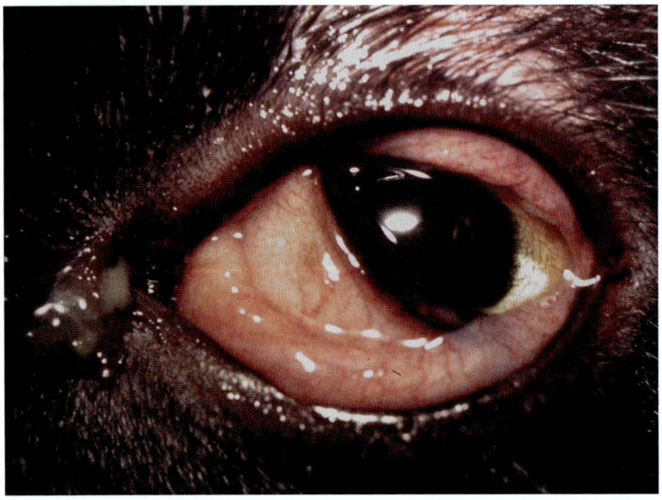

Fig. 49.2 Cat with acute chlamydial conjunctivitis. Note the intense hyperemia and chemosis.

DIAGNOSIS

There are no clinically significant laboratory abnormalities in cats with chlamydiosis, and there is insufficient information on laboratory abnormalities that might occur in affected dogs. Diagnosis of chlamydiosis is most often based on the results of molecular testing using PCR. For all diagnostic tests that detect chlamydial organisms, an attempt to collect sufficient numbers of infected epithelial cells should be made. This generally involves vigorous swabbing of infected mucosal sites such as the conjunctiva using a cotton swab (Table 49.2).

Microbiologic Tests

Cytologic Examination for Inclusions

Using light microscopy, chlamydial intracytoplasmic inclusions may be seen in epithelial cells that are present in smears of conjunctival scrapings. Inclusions comprise clusters of coccoid bacteria, and are usually 10 μm in diameter and stain basophilic (Fig. 49.3). Large inclusions adjacent to the nucleus can have a "cloak-like" appearance (hence the name *Chlamydia* which is derived from the Greek word meaning "cloak"). Giemsa is the preferred staining method. Inclusions are generally visible only early, if at all, during the course of infection, so this method is insensitive. Also, melanin granules in the cytoplasm of conjunctival epithelial cells can yield false-positive results. The use of direct FA staining or immunocytochemistry with antibodies directed to chlamydial antigens increases sensitivity and specificity.

ELISA Antigen Detection

A variety of commercial antigen detection enzyme immunoassay kits have been developed and marketed for diagnosis of human chlamydial infections in the past (e.g., Chlamydiazyme, Abbott Labs, Chicago, IL, USA). Nucleic acid amplification tests have now largely replaced the use of these assays for diagnosis of human infections. Reagents in ELISA used to detect the antigen of human chlamydial pathogens in swab specimens (such as conjunctival swabs) cross-react with *C. felis* antigen, so have also been used for diagnosis of feline chlamydiosis. Unfortunately, the kits vary considerably in their sensitivity and specificity. In general, ELISA methods that detect chlamydial antigen have lower sensitivity and specificity than cell culture, direct FA methods, and PCR for detecting feline infections.

Cell Culture

Culture of chlamydiae has traditionally been considered the gold standard for chlamydial diagnosis, but is now mostly performed on a research basis. Isolations from cats are usually highest from

TABLE 49.2 Diagnostic Assays Available for Chlamydiosis in Dogs and Cats

Assay	Specimen Type	Target	Performance
Cell culture	Conjunctival swabs	*Chlamydia* spp.	Not widely offered or utilized for routine diagnostic purposes. Requires special chlamydial transport media. False negatives may occur when organisms lose viability during transport or in chronic infections, when organism numbers are very low.
Cytology	Conjunctival smears	Chlamydial inclusions	Low sensitivity. Inclusions are most likely to be seen early in infection. False positives can occur when cytoplasmic granules are mistaken for inclusions. Fluorescent or immunoperoxidase antibody techniques may increase sensitivity and specificity.
Serology	Serum	Antibodies to *Chlamydia* spp.	Acute and convalescent serology is required for diagnosis of acute infection. Vaccination may interfere with interpretation of results. Not widely available worldwide.
Polymerase chain reaction (PCR)	Conjunctival swabs, scrapings or biopsies	*Chlamydia felis* DNA or *Chlamydia* spp. DNA	Confirms active infection. Assays may be genus- or species-specific. Sensitivity and specificity may vary depending on assay design and specimen type. Because healthy animals may be PCR-positive, positive PCR results must be interpreted in light of the clinical signs. Vaccination with modified live chlamydial vaccines has the potential to interfere with results.

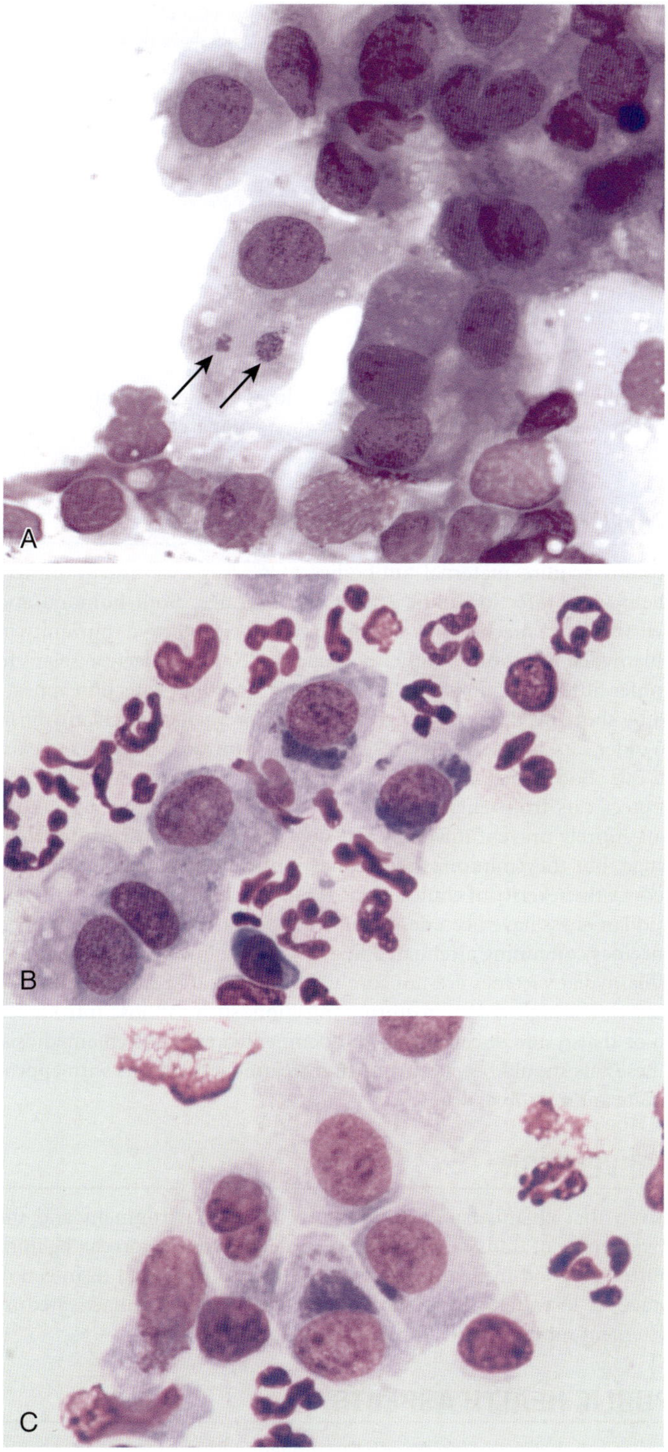

Fig. 49.3 Conjunctival scrapings from cats with chlamydial conjunctivitis. (A) Inclusions of *Chlamydia felis* are found in an epithelial cell *(arrows)* (Wright stain, original magnification 1000×). (B and C) Cloak-like inclusions adjacent to the nucleus of a conjunctival epithelial cell. (B and C, Courtesy of Dr. William Vernau, University of California, Davis.)

conjunctival swabs, although nasal and pharyngeal swab specimens may also contain infectious organisms. To enhance organism survival, swabs can be placed immediately in a chlamydial transport medium such as 2SP (0.2 M sucrose and 0.02 M phosphate). Routine viral transport medium contains antibiotics which will inactivate the organisms. The sample should be refrigerated (4°C) if it is not immediately

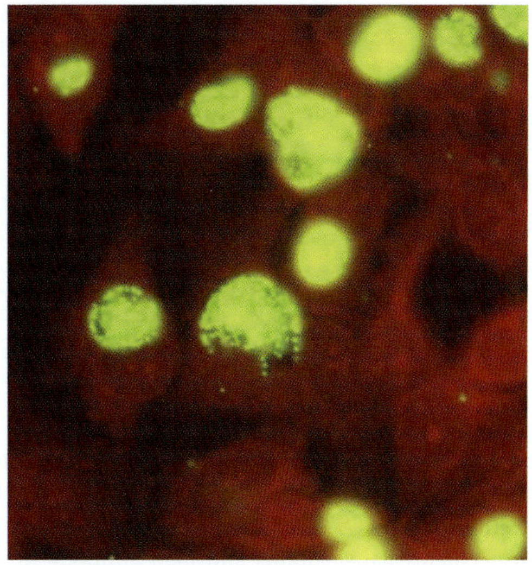

Fig. 49.4 Chlamydial inclusions stained with fluorescent antibody in a McCoy cell monolayer.

sent to the laboratory and ideally should reach the laboratory within 24 hours of specimen collection. In the laboratory, organisms can readily be grown in the yolk sac of embryonating eggs or in cell lines such as McCoy or HeLa cells. Incubation times are in the order of 2 to 3 days. Chlamydial inclusions within the infected cell culture are then identified using FA (Fig. 49.4).

Molecular Diagnosis Using Nucleic Acid–Based Testing

The use of molecular assays such as PCR has revolutionized the diagnosis of chlamydial infections in animals and humans, because these assays are rapid, sensitive, specific, and do not require special transport conditions. Sequence analysis of PCR products can be used to differentiate among species of chlamydiaceae. Both endpoint (conventional) and real-time PCR assays have been used to detect *C. felis* in conjunctival swab specimens from cats,[30–32] and real-time PCR assays that detect *C. felis* are offered by several commercial veterinary diagnostic laboratories worldwide. Unfortunately, considerable interlaboratory variation in assay performance can exist.[33] In addition, PCR assays for *C. felis* may not detect other chlamydial species, such as *C. pneumoniae*. Genus- or family-specific chlamydial PCR assays must be used to detect these organisms. The use of a DNA microarray assay for detection and identification of chlamydiae in cats was also reported.[7] The microarray assay consists of a chip that carries species- and genus-specific probes for identification purposes. DNA within the specimen is first amplified and biotin labeled with PCR, then reacted with the microarray probes.[34]

PCR assays for *C. felis* are usually more sensitive than culture in which comparisons have been made in naturally infected cats (see Table 49.2).[30] During antimicrobial treatment of infected cats, PCR results may continue to be positive for several days.[30,31] In one study, topical ophthalmic solutions such as proxymetacaine and fluorescein did not interfere with the ability of real-time PCR to detect *C. felis*, although there was a slight inhibitory effect when fusidic acid was used.[35] Because cats without signs of conjunctivitis have occasionally tested PCR positive for *C. felis*, the results of PCR must be interpreted in light of the history, clinical signs present, and response to appropriate treatment.

Serologic Testing

Serologic tests are not widely available for routine diagnosis of chlamydial infections. Assays for serum antibodies to chlamydiae, such

TABLE 49.3 Suggested Medications for Treatment of Cats with Ocular Chlamydiosis

Drug	Dose	Route	Interval (Hours)	Duration
Doxycycline[a]	10 mg/kg	PO	24	At least 4 weeks or 2 weeks after resolution of clinical signs
Amoxicillin-clavulanate	12.5	PO	12	4 weeks
Enrofloxacin	5	PO	24	3 weeks
Pradofloxacin	5	PO	24	6 weeks

[a]Doxycycline is the treatment of choice. For cats that fail to tolerate doxycycline, amoxicillin-clavulanate should be used. The fluoroquinolones enrofloxacin and pradofloxacin are an option for cats that do not tolerate either doxycycline or amoxicillin-clavulanate.

as IFA or ELISA, have been of limited benefit for detection of active infection because the IgG antibody titer increase is variable or prolonged, and IgM antibody titers are inconsistently increased. However, very high antibody titers (≥ 1:512) have been associated with clinical illness and/or chlamydial shedding, and high antibody titers among group-housed cats with conjunctivitis can suggest a role for *C. felis* in disease.[16,36,37] Chlamydial infections persist in the presence of high serum antibody levels, so serologic testing cannot be used to evaluate vaccine-induced protection. Serial titers may be needed to document active infections, and recent vaccination may interfere with interpretation of positive titer results. An ELISA that discriminates between the antibody response from vaccination and that from natural infection has been described.[38]

TREATMENT AND PROGNOSIS

Chlamydial infections are generally treated with tetracycline antibiotics. Oral administration of doxycycline at 5 to 10 mg/kg q12h, for 3 to 4 weeks results in clinical resolution in most cats. A dose of 10 mg/kg q24h can also be used.[37] Clinical improvement occurs within 24 to 48 hours after treatment is initiated. Treatment of all cats in a colony for 4 weeks is recommended, because in one study that used real-time PCR to detect infection, a 3-week course of treatment was insufficient to clear infection in some cats, but treatment for 28 days subsequently cleared infection in all cats.[31] Treatment may have to be continued for up to 6 to 8 weeks to ensure that all cats have been successfully treated. Regardless, treatment should continue for at least 2 weeks after the resolution of clinical signs.

Failure to respond completely may reflect the concurrent presence of viral causes of feline URTD. Because doxycycline hyclate administration can result in esophagitis and esophageal stricture formation, the administration of tablets should be followed by a bolus of water or food (see Chapter 10 for additional information on doxycycline). Ocular infections may initially respond to tetracycline eye ointment applied two or three times daily,[39] but recurrent infections have been documented,[40] possibly because systemic infection with chlamydiae can occur in cats with conjunctivitis.

For cats that do not tolerate doxycycline, 4 weeks of amoxicillin-clavulanate is a suitable alternative.[41] In experimentally infected cats, the efficacy of enrofloxacin (5 mg/kg, PO, q24h, for 14 days) was similar to that of doxycycline as determined with direct FA on conjunctival swabs, although a few cats in both the doxycycline and enrofloxacin groups had evidence of persistent infection at the end of the treatment period.[42] Doxycycline is the preferred antimicrobial drug because of concerns that relate to the possibility of retinal toxicity in cats treated with enrofloxacin. Doxycycline was more efficacious than pradofloxacin in experimentally infected cats that were monitored with PCR.[43] Sulfonamides or chloramphenicol are ineffective, and *in vitro*, penicillin is only inhibitory at higher doses. Treatment with azithromycin is also incompletely effective when compared with doxycycline (Table 49.3).[44]

IMMUNITY AND VACCINATION

Kittens acquire maternal antibodies to *C. felis* that usually protect them from infection until 7 to 9 weeks of age. Both humoral and cell-mediated mechanisms are important for protective immunity in chlamydial infections of other host species. Natural infection seems to confer little protection against reinfection, and this protection appears to be short-lived. However, given the low prevalence of chlamydiosis in older cats, an age-related resistance to chlamydiosis appears to exist in cats. Both inactivated and attenuated live vaccines are available to protect cats from chlamydial respiratory disease. These vaccines do not entirely prevent infection and shedding of chlamydiae after challenge, but they minimize the replication of the organism and hence reduce the severity of clinical signs. Transient fever, anorexia, lethargy, and lameness have been described 1 to 3 weeks after use of combined vaccines containing attenuated live *C. felis* in a low percentage of cats. Chlamydial vaccines are noncore vaccines that are recommended for cats with a high risk of acquiring infection, such as those introduced to or that reside in catteries with documented endemic chlamydiosis. These cats should be vaccinated after treatment of all cats with appropriate antimicrobial drugs.

PREVENTION

Given that chlamydiae survive poorly in the environment and the major route of transmission is close contact, transmission can be minimized by good hygiene, quarantine, single housing, and disinfection practices in cattery situations. Chlamydiae are readily inactivated by detergent solutions and common disinfectants.

PUBLIC HEALTH ASPECTS

The most significant chlamydial pathogens of humans are *C. trachomatis*, *C. pneumoniae*, and *C. psittaci*. *Chlamydia trachomatis* causes trachoma, the leading cause of infectious blindness worldwide, and it also is the most common bacterial cause of sexually transmitted diseases in humans. *Chlamydia pneumoniae* is extremely widespread, may infect nearly all humans, and is an important cause of community-acquired pneumonia worldwide. It has also been implicated in atherosclerotic cardiovascular disease, although its role in this condition remains unclear. *Chlamydia psittaci* is the cause of psittacosis in birds and humans, a potentially life-threatening zoonosis.

Chlamydia felis has long been suspected as a cause of conjunctivitis in humans. However, many of the reports of human infection with *C. felis* before the advent of genetic detection methods remain unconfirmed, because diagnosis was either based on culture without identification to the species level, or on serologic testing, which has the potential to cross-react with other chlamydiae and organisms such as *Bartonella*. Molecular assays have since been used to confirm the diagnosis of *C. felis* infection in humans. *Chlamydia felis* has rarely been detected in the conjunctiva of humans with conjunctivitis.[45,46] In these reports, the organism found in the humans was genetically indistinguishable from isolates recovered from the patients' cats. Although these associations have been difficult to document, routine precautions should be taken when handling cats with conjunctivitis, especially young cats with chronic conjunctivitis. Proper handwashing and routine cleaning and disinfection are likely to be sufficient to prevent transmission.

The identification of *C. psittaci* in dogs with respiratory disease and *C. pneumoniae* in cats with ocular disease suggests that dogs and cats may have the potential to be a source of these pathogens for humans, although avian species and other infected humans, respectively, are likely to be much more significant sources of infection.

CASE EXAMPLE

Signalment

"Sam," a 3-year-old male neutered domestic shorthair cat from Davis, CA.

History

Sam was brought to the University of California, Davis, by a veterinary student for evaluation of fever, right thoracic limb lameness, and bilateral conjunctivitis with mucopurulent ocular discharge of 2 days' duration. There had been no cough, sneezing, vomiting, diarrhea, or abnormal thirst or urination noted. Sam lived indoors with five other cats, three of which also had severe conjunctivitis, ocular discharge, fever, lethargy, and lameness for the last week. These three cats ranged in age from 8 months to 2.5 years. All of the cats had been vaccinated regularly for FHV-1, FCV, and FPV and tested negative for FeLV and FIV as kittens. They were all fed a commercial dry cat food.

Physical Examination

Body weight: 6.7 kg.

General: Bright, alert, responsive, and hydrated. T = 103.6°F, HR = 240 beats/minute, RR = 66 breaths/minute, mucous membranes pink, CRT = 1 second.

Eyes, ears, nose, and throat: No evidence of ocular discharge, mild conjunctival hyperemia; nasal planum clean and moist with no discharge; no oral erosions or ulcerations.

Musculoskeletal: BCS 7/9, decreased weight bearing on left thoracic limb, sometimes holds left thoracic limb up when sitting; possible mild effusion in the left elbow; resents flexion of the left carpus and left and right elbows.

Cardiovascular: No clinically significant abnormalities detected.

Respiratory: No clinically significant abnormalities.

GI and genitourinary: Nonpainful abdomen, no masses palpated, small-sized bladder.

Lymph nodes: No clinically significant abnormalities detected.

Laboratory Findings

CBC: HCT 46.3% (30%–50%), MCV 46.9 fL (42–53 fL), MCHC 30.7 g/dL (30–33.5 g/dL), WBC 10,500 cells/μL (4,500–14,000 cells/μL), neutrophils 7,455 cells/μL (2,000–9,000 cells/μL), lymphocytes 2,310 cells/μL (1,000–7,000 cells/μL), monocytes 525 cells/μL (50–600 cells/μL), eosinophils 210 cells/μL (150–1,100 cells/μL), basophils 0 cells/μL (0–50 cells/μL), platelets 174,000/μL (180,000–500,000 platelets/μL), with moderate macroplatelets.

Serum chemistry profile: Sodium 152 mmol/L (151–158 mmol/L), potassium 4.4 mmol/L (3.6–4.9 mmol/L), chloride 117 mmol/L (117–126 mmol/L), bicarbonate 18 mmol/L (15–21 mmol/L), phosphorus 4.0 mg/dL (3.2–6.3 mg/dL), calcium 9.5 mg/dL (9.0–10.9 mg/dL), BUN 21 mg/dL (18–33 mg/dL), creatinine 1.6 mg/dL (1.1–2.2 mg/dL), glucose 151 mg/dL (63–118 mg/dL), total protein 7.1 g/dL (6.6–8.4 g/dL), albumin 3.1 g/dL (2.2–4.6 g/dL), globulin 4.0 g/dL (2.8–5.4 g/dL), ALT 48 U/L (27–101 U/L), AST 8 U/L (17–58 U/L), ALP 31 U/L (14–71 U/L), GGT 0 U/L (0–4 U/L), cholesterol 154 mg/dL (89–258 mg/dL), total bilirubin 0.2 mg/dL (0–0.2 mg/dL).

Urinalysis: SpG 1.055; pH 6.5, trace protein, no hemoprotein, glucose, ketones, or bilirubin, 0–1 WBC/HPF, 0–2 RBC/HPF, few lipid droplets.

Synovial fluid cytology: Synovial fluid from the right stifle, right carpus, left carpus, and right tarsus was examined. All specimens apart from that from the left carpus were markedly blood contaminated and so could not be properly evaluated. The cell counts in these specimens ranged from 2,000 to 4,000 nucleated cells/μL, and consisted predominantly of neutrophils (66%–80%) and small mononuclear cells (7%–18%). The specimen from the left carpus had 2,000 nucleated cells/μL, of which 14% were neutrophils, 85% large mononuclear cells, and 1% small mononuclear cells. There were moderate numbers of erythrocytes and blood-associated leukocytes, as well as low numbers of large mononuclear cells of normal morphology, which was consistent with mild blood contamination and otherwise no cytologic abnormalities.

Conjunctival smear cytology: Chlamydial inclusions visualized within several epithelial cells.

Imaging Findings

Radiographs of the left radius and ulna, including carpus and elbow joints: No radiographic abnormalities.

Microbiologic Testing

FeLV antigen and FIV antibody serology: Negative

PCR for FCV (oropharyngeal swab specimens): Negative

Mycoplasma culture (conjunctival swab specimen): Negative

Diagnosis

A tentative diagnosis of chlamydial conjunctivitis and arthritis was made.

Treatment and Outcome

Treatment of all cats in the household with doxycycline (10 mg/kg, PO, q24h) was initiated. This was associated with rapid resolution of fever, ocular signs, and lameness.

Comments

The cats in this household may have had conjunctivitis and arthritis related to a chlamydial infection. The major differential diagnosis was FCV infection, which is more widespread than chlamydiosis and for which an association between lameness and infection has been widely documented. Infection with *Mycoplasma* spp. has also been associated with conjunctivitis as well as synovitis in cats (see Chapter 57). Infection with *C. felis* has been associated with development of lameness in experimentally infected cats, but there are no reports of lameness in association with natural infection. The negative PCR and culture results for FCV and *Mycoplasma* spp., respectively, could not definitively rule out infection with these agents. The presence of chlamydial inclusions in the conjunctival smear supported a diagnosis of chlamydiosis, but false positives can occur and unfortunately PCR was not performed to confirm the presence of a chlamydial agent. Nevertheless, the rapid response to doxycycline supported the possibility of a bacterial cause of the arthritis.

SUGGESTED READINGS

Gruffydd-Jones T, Addie D, Belak S, et al. *Chlamydophila felis* infection. ABCD guidelines on prevention and management. *J Feline Med Surg.* 2009;11:605–609.

Sibitz C, Rudnay EC, Wabnegger L, et al. Detection of *Chlamydophila pneumoniae* in cats with conjunctivitis. *Vet Ophthalmol.* 2011;14(suppl 1):67–74.

REFERENCES

1. Baker JA. A virus causing pneumonia in cats and producing elementary bodies. *J Exp Med.* 1944;79:159–172.
2. Bressan M, Rampazzo A, Kuratii J, et al. Occurrence of *Chlamydiaceae* and *Chlamydia felis pmp9* typing in conjunctival and rectal samples of Swiss stray and pet cats. *Pathogens.* 2021;10:951.
3. Sachse K, Bavoil PM, Kaltenboeck B, et al. Emendation of the family *Chlamydiaceae*: proposal of a single genus, *Chlamydia*, to include all currently recognized species. *Syst Appl Microbiol.* 2015;38:99–103.
4. Stephens RS, Myers G, Eppinger M, et al. Divergence without difference: phylogenetics and taxonomy of *Chlamydia* resolved. *FEMS Immunol Med Microbiol.* 2009;55:115–119.
5. Dean D, Kandel RP, Adhikari HK, et al. Multiple *Chlamydiaceae* species in trachoma: implications for disease pathogenesis and control. *PLoS Med.* 2008;5:e14.
6. Sibitz C, Rudnay EC, Wabnegger L, et al. Detection of *Chlamydophila pneumoniae* in cats with conjunctivitis. *Vet Ophthalmol.* 2011;14(suppl 1):67–74.
7. Sostaric-Zuckermann IC, Borel N, Kaiser C, et al. *Chlamydia* in canine or feline coronary arteriosclerotic lesions. *BMC Res Notes.* 2011;4:350.
8. Sprague LD, Schubert E, Hotzel H, et al. The detection of *Chlamydophila psittaci* genotype C infection in dogs. *Vet J.* 2009;181:274–279.
9. Gresham AC, Dixon CE, Bevan BJ. Domiciliary outbreak of psittacosis in dogs: potential for zoonotic infection. *Vet Rec.* 1996;138:622–623.
10. Arizmendi F, Grimes JE, Relford RL. Isolation of *Chlamydia psittaci* from pleural effusion in a dog. *J Vet Diagn Invest.* 1992;4:460–463.
11. Hoelzle K, Wittenbrink MM, Corboz L, et al. *Chlamydophila abortus*-induced keratoconjunctivitis in a dog. *Vet Rec.* 2005;157:632–633.
12. Sako T, Takahashi T, Takehana K, et al. Chlamydial infection in canine atherosclerotic lesions. *Atherosclerosis.* 2002;162:253–259.
13. Lambrechts N, Picard J, Tustin RC. *Chlamydia*-induced septic polyarthritis in a dog. *J S Afr Vet Assoc.* 1999;70:40–42.
14. Marti I, Pisano SRR, Wehrle M, et al. Severe conjunctivitis associated with *Chlamydia felis* infection in a free-ranging Eurasian lynx (*Lynx lynx*). *J Wildl Dis.* 2019;55:522–525.
15. Low HC, Powell CC, Veir JK, et al. Prevalence of feline herpesvirus 1, *Chlamydophila felis*, and *Mycoplasma* spp. DNA in conjunctival cells collected from cats with and without conjunctivitis. *Am J Vet Res.* 2007;68:643–648.
16. Wills JM, Howard PE, Gruffydd-Jones TJ, et al. Prevalence of *Chlamydia psittaci* in different cat populations in Britain. *J Small Anim Pract.* 1988;29:327–339.
17. Kang BT, Park HM. Prevalence of feline herpesvirus 1, feline calicivirus and *Chlamydophila felis* in clinically normal cats at a Korean animal shelter. *J Vet Sci.* 2008;9:207–209.
18. Veir JK, Ruch-Gallie R, Spindel ME, et al. Prevalence of selected infectious organisms and comparison of two anatomic sampling sites in shelter cats with upper respiratory tract disease. *J Feline Med Surg.* 2008;10:551–557.
19. Maggs DJ, Sykes JE, Clarke HE, et al. Effects of dietary lysine supplementation in cats with enzootic upper respiratory disease. *J Feline Med Surg.* 2007;9:97–108.
20. Bannasch MJ, Foley JE. Epidemiologic evaluation of multiple respiratory pathogens in cats in animal shelters. *J Feline Med Surg.* 2005;7:109–119.
21. Helps CR, Lait P, Damhuis A, et al. Factors associated with upper respiratory tract disease caused by feline herpesvirus, feline calicivirus, *Chlamydophila felis* and *Bordetella bronchiseptica* in cats: experience from 218 European catteries. *Vet Rec.* 2005;156:669–673.
22. von Bomhard W, Polkinghorne A, Lu ZH, et al. Detection of novel chlamydiae in cats with ocular disease. *Am J Vet Res.* 2003;64:1421–1428.
23. Richter M, Matheis F, Gonczi E, et al. *Parachlamydia acanthamoebae* in domestic cats with and without corneal disease. *Vet Ophthalmol.* 2010;13:235–237.
24. Saka HA, Thompson JW, Chen YS, et al. Quantitative proteomics reveals metabolic and pathogenic properties of *Chlamydia trachomatis* developmental forms. *Mol Microbiol.* 2011;82:1185–1203.
25. TerWee J, Sabara M, Kokjohn K, et al. Characterization of the systemic disease and ocular signs induced by experimental infection with *Chlamydia psittaci* in cats. *Vet Microbiol.* 1998;59:259–281.
26. Dickie CW, Sniff ES. *Chlamydia* infection associated with peritonitis in a cat. *J Am Vet Med Assoc.* 1980;176:1256–1259.
27. Hargis AM, Prieur DJ, Gaillard ET. Chlamydial infection of the gastric mucosa in twelve cats. *Vet Pathol.* 1983;20:170–178.
28. Wills JM. *Chlamydial Infection in the Cat.* PhD Thesis. University of Bristol; 1986.
29. O'Dair HA, Hopper CD, Gruffydd-Jones TJ, et al. Clinical aspects of *Chlamydia psittaci* infection in cats infected with feline immunodeficiency virus. *Vet Rec.* 1994;134:365–368.
30. Sykes JE, Studdert VP, Browning GF. Comparison of the polymerase chain reaction and culture for the detection of feline *Chlamydia psittaci* in untreated and doxycycline-treated experimentally infected cats. *J Vet Intern Med.* 1999;13:146–152.
31. Dean R, Harley R, Helps C, et al. Use of quantitative real-time PCR to monitor the response of *Chlamydophila felis* infection to doxycycline treatment. *J Clin Microbiol.* 2005;43:1858–1864.
32. Helps C, Reeves N, Tasker S, et al. Use of real-time quantitative PCR to detect *Chlamydophila felis* infection. *J Clin Microbiol.* 2001;39:2675–2676.
33. Sandmeyer LS, Waldner CL, Bauer BS, et al. Comparison of polymerase chain reaction tests for diagnosis of feline herpesvirus, *Chlamydophila felis*, and *Mycoplasma* spp. infection in cats with ocular disease in Canada. *Can Vet J.* 2010;51:629–633.
34. Borel N, Kempf E, Hotzel H, et al. Direct identification of chlamydiae from clinical samples using a DNA microarray assay: a validation study. *Mol Cell Probes.* 2008;22:55–64.
35. Segarra S, Papasouliotis K, Helps C. The in vitro effects of proxymetacaine, fluorescein, and fusidic acid on real-time PCR assays used for the diagnosis of feline herpesvirus 1 and *Chlamydophila felis* infections. *Vet Ophthalmol.* 2011;14(suppl 1):5–8.
36. Strom Holst B, Krook L, Englund S, et al. Shedding of chlamydiae in relation to titers of serum chlamydiae-specific antibodies and serum concentrations of two acute-phase proteins in cats without conjunctivitis. *Am J Vet Res.* 2011;72:806–812.
37. Gruffydd-Jones T, Addie D, Belak S, et al. *Chlamydophila felis* infection. ABCD guidelines on prevention and management. *J Feline Med Surg.* 2009;11:605–609.
38. Ohya K, Okuda H, Maeda S, et al. Using CF0218-ELISA to distinguish *Chlamydophila felis*-infected cats from vaccinated and uninfected domestic cats. *Vet Microbiol.* 2010;146:366–370.
39. Sparkes AH, Caney SM, Sturgess CP, et al. The clinical efficacy of topical and systemic therapy for the treatment of feline ocular chlamydiosis. *J Feline Med Surg.* 1999;1:31–35.
40. Donati M, Piva S, Di Francesco A, et al. Feline ocular chlamydiosis: clinical and microbiological effects of topical and systemic therapy. *New Microbiol.* 2005;28:369–372.
41. Sturgess CP, Gruffydd-Jones TJ, Harbour DA, et al. Controlled study of the efficacy of clavulanic acid-potentiated amoxycillin in the treatment of *Chlamydia psittaci* in cats. *Vet Rec.* 2001;149:73–76.
42. Gerhardt N, Schulz BS, Werckenthin C, et al. Pharmacokinetics of enrofloxacin and its efficacy in comparison with doxycycline in the treatment of *Chlamydophila felis* infection in cats with conjunctivitis. *Vet Rec.* 2006;159:591–594.
43. Hartmann AD, Helps CR, Lappin MR, et al. Efficacy of pradofloxacin in cats with feline upper respiratory tract disease due to *Chlamydophila felis* or *Mycoplasma* infections. *J Vet Intern Med.* 2008;22:44–52.
44. Owen WM, Sturgess CP, Harbour DA, et al. Efficacy of azithromycin for the treatment of feline chlamydophilosis. *J Feline Med Surg.* 2003;5:305–311.
45. Hartley JC, Stevenson S, Robinson AJ, et al. Conjunctivitis due to *Chlamydophila felis* (*Chlamydia psittaci* feline pneumonitis agent) acquired from a cat: case report with molecular characterization of isolates from the patient and cat. *J Infect.* 2001;43:7–11.
46. Wons J, Meiller R, Bergua A, et al. Follicular conjunctivitis due to *Chlamydia felis* – case report, review of the literature and improved molecular diagnostics. *Front Med.* 2017;4:105.

50

Streptococcal and Enterococcal Infections

John F. Prescott, Jane E. Sykes, Joshua B. Daniels

KEY POINTS

- First Described: Streptococci were first described in Germany in 1868 by Billroth.[1] Enterococci were separated from the genus *Streptococcus* in 1984.[2]
- Major Causes: In dogs and cats, the most common causes are *Streptococcus canis*, *Streptococcus equi* subsp. *zooepidemicus*, *Enterococcus faecium*, and *Enterococcus faecalis*, which are gram-positive coccoid bacteria.
- Geographic Distribution: Worldwide.
- Mode of Transmission: Direct contact usually; hospital environments can become contaminated with resistant enterococci. Organisms are usually commensals that invade opportunistically.
- Major Clinical Signs: Clinically highly variable opportunistic infection; includes arthritis, bacteremia and endocarditis, bronchopneumonia, cervical lymphadenitis, cholangiohepatitis, discospondylitis, keratitis, mastitis, meningoencephalitis, necrotizing fasciitis and toxic shock syndrome (primarily *S. canis*), neonatal bacteremia, osteomyelitis, otitis externa, peritonitis, pharyngitis, postoperative incision or wound infections, pyometra or metritis, pyothorax, rhinitis and necrotizing sinusitis, and UTIs. Inflammation associated with these infections tends to be very pyogenic. In the lungs, these organisms are frequent components of polymicrobial aspiration pneumonia.
- Differential Diagnoses: Primarily other gram-positive and gram-negative bacterial infections.
- Human Health Significance: The role of dogs and cats in the transmission of *Streptococcus pyogenes*, a major human pathogen, (Lancefield group A) is commonly exaggerated. Streptococcal species that infect dogs and cats occasionally infect human patients. Dogs and cats, or their contaminated environments, may also have the potential to serve as sources of MDR enterococcal infections for humans.

ETIOLOGY, EPIDEMIOLOGY, AND CLINICAL FEATURES

Streptococci are catalase-negative, gram-positive, nonmotile cocci that divide along a single axis, forming pairs and chains of organisms (Figs. 50.1 and 50.2). They are facultative-to-strict aerobes that require complex media for growth, preferably supplemented with blood for the β-hemolytic types. They cause localized to widespread pyogenic infections in animals and humans. Although numerous species are pathogenic, many are commensal microflora of the oral cavity, nasopharynx, skin, and genital and GI tracts. More than 115 species of streptococci have been described. Species of streptococci vary in host tropism and virulence properties, and so are discussed separately. There has been conflicting literature as to whether one of the most important streptococcal pathogens of humans, *Streptococcus pyogenes*, which causes human streptococcal pharyngitis ("strep throat"), can infect dogs and cats. Reports in the medical literature that pets may be a reservoir of infection for humans have frequently been based on erroneous identification studies (see Public Health Aspects). However, interspecies transmission has been reported for some pathogenic streptococci such as *Streptococcus pneumoniae, Streptococcus canis,* and *Streptococcus equi* subsp. *zooepidemicus*. As is the case in humans, streptococci that infect dogs and cats range from commensals of low virulence to highly virulent organisms that can cause severe disease manifestations and death.

Several classification systems exist for streptococci based on cultural characteristics, antigenic composition, and biochemical features. Streptococci have been classified based on their *in vitro* hemolytic properties as: β-hemolytic streptococci, which cause complete hemolysis when they grow on blood agar; α-hemolytic streptococci, which reduce hemoglobin to cause a greenish discoloration of the agar around bacterial colonies; and, rather strangely, "γ-hemolytic," which are actually nonhemolytic streptococci. The β-hemolytic strains tend to be most pathogenic. Organisms in the α-hemolytic and nonhemolytic (γ-hemolytic) categories are found on mucous membranes and skin of clinically healthy animals. If present in an infectious process, they are usually regarded as contaminants or unimportant invaders. When they do cause illness, it may take the form of valvular endocarditis or embolic abscess. The precise species classification of streptococci in numerous disease processes described next is in doubt, especially in the older literature. The lack of harmonization of methods used to speciate streptococci among veterinary diagnostic laboratories unfortunately perpetuates this uncertainty.

Streptococci are also classified from A through W based on their surface antigens (Lancefield classification system) and further classified based on phenotypic characteristics. The Lancefield classification system tends to correlate with pathogenicity. Lancefield groups A, B, C, E, G, L, and M are usually β-hemolytic. Major pathogenic streptococci of dogs and cats belong to Lancefield groups B, C, D, or G (Table 50.1). "Pyogenic streptococci" are β-hemolytic streptococci that belong to Lancefield groups A *(S. pyogenes)*, B *(Streptococcus agalactiae)*, C (includes *Streptococcus dysgalactiae* and *S. equi* subsp. *zooepidemicus*), and G (includes *S. canis*). "Viridans streptococci" is an archaic term for catalase-negative gram positive aerobic cocci that are either nonhemolytic or α-hemolytic (*viridis* = Latin for green) that tend to be commensals, have low virulence, and rarely invade tissues opportunistically. Many of these streptococci, which are also Lancefield group D, have now been classified as enterococci. Molecular typing schemes have revealed that hemolytic reactions, Lancefield antigens, and phenotypic characteristics do not necessarily predict genetic relatedness among streptococcal strains. Although these traditional classification

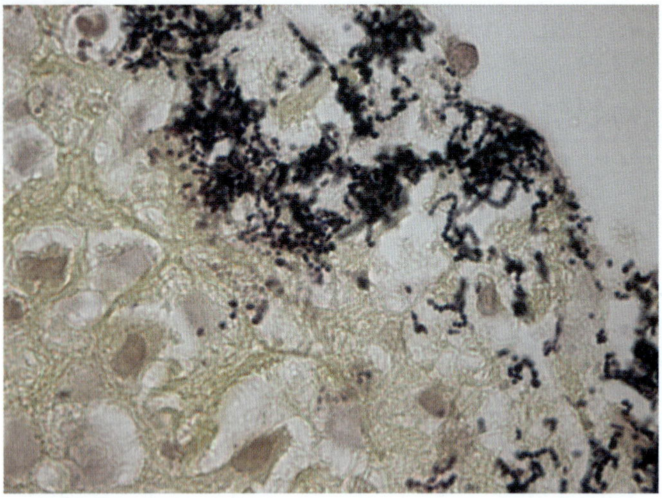

Fig. 50.1 Histopathology of the serosal surface of the liver of a 12-day-old domestic shorthair kitten that was euthanized after it was found hypothermic and tachypneic. Severe suppurative omphalophlebitis and peritonitis were present. Lesions contained numerous chains of gram-positive cocci. Brown and Benn stain, 1000× oil magnification.

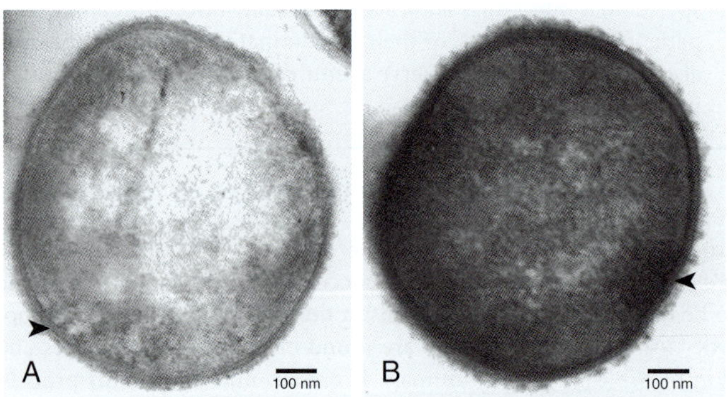

Fig. 50.2 Electron micrograph of (A) *Streptococcus pyogenes* and (B) *Streptococcus canis*. Proteinaceous cell surface fibrillae are present on *S. canis* that resemble the M-protein surface fibrils of the human pathogen *S. pyogenes*. The M protein is a key virulence factor of *S. pyogenes*. (From DeWinter LM, Low DE, Prescott JF. Virulence of *Streptococcus canis* from canine streptococcal toxic shock syndrome and necrotizing fasciitis. *Vet Microbiol*. 1999;70:95–110.)

methods are still in use by laboratory staff, microbiologists, and clinicians, most modern laboratories now use MALDI-TOF or possibly kit biochemical systems to identify these bacteria to their correct genus (*Enterococcus*, *Streptococcus*) and species.

Streptococci invade tissues opportunistically when there is a breach in normal host barriers. This leads to a wide variety of clinical disease manifestations, such as arthritis, cellulitis, endocarditis, meningoencephalitis, pyoderma, pneumonia, osteomyelitis, and UTIs. Severe and life-threatening manifestations of streptococcal infection include necrotizing fasciitis/myositis (NFM) and streptococcal toxic shock syndrome (STSS). The past decade has had a resurgence of severe invasive group A human streptococcal infections characterized by septic shock associated with multiple organ failure and with or without NFM.

Predisposing conditions for streptococcal infections in dogs and cats may include atopic dermatitis, wounds, foreign bodies (such as migrating grass awns), immunosuppressive drug treatment, and young age (especially neonates).[3] The most common clinical manifestation among fetuses and neonates is streptococcal bacteremia and sepsis, which can result in abortion and death. Streptococcal pneumonia may occur in association with infections with other respiratory pathogens, such as respiratory viruses, or occur secondary to bronchitis, hematogenous spread, or aspiration. In one study, streptococci were isolated from sick dogs more frequently in summer months.[3]

Streptococcus canis

Streptococcus canis is the streptococcal species most frequently isolated from dogs and cats.[3] It is a β-hemolytic, group G (pyogenic) streptococcus that colonizes the pharynx, GI tracts (especially the mouth), genital mucosa, and skin of healthy dogs and cats. It has also been isolated from other animal species, such as foxes, mice, mink, rabbits, and rats. Infection with *S. canis* may be associated arthritis, bacteremia, bronchopneumonia, cervical lymphadenitis, cholangiohepatitis, discospondylitis, endocarditis, ulcerative keratitis, mastitis, meningoencephalitis, NFM and STSS, neonatal bacteremia/sepsis, osteomyelitis, otitis externa, peritonitis, pharyngitis, postoperative incision or wound infections, pyometra or metritis, pyothorax, rhinitis and necrotizing sinusitis, and UTIs. Neonatal infections can occur when organisms are transmitted from the vaginal tract during parturition; they can also occur if organism accesses the systemic circulation via the umbilical vein. In juvenile kittens (3 to 7 months old), cervical lymphadenitis may follow a subclinical episode of pharyngitis and tonsillitis. Streptococcal meningitis results from direct extension from the sinuses or middle ear, or from bacteremia. Other embolic complications may accompany bacteremia with *S. canis*. Although opportunistic infections with *S. canis* occur sporadically, outbreaks of group G

TABLE 50.1 Classification of Streptococci Isolated from Dogs and Cats

Species	Lancefield Group	Hemolytic	Comments
S. canis	G	β	Most common. Dogs and cats are natural hosts. Causes a variety of clinical syndromes. Primary cause of streptococcal toxic shock syndrome and necrotizing fasciitis in dogs and cats.
S. equi subsp. *zooepidemicus*	C	β	Causes pneumonia and sinusitis, primarily in group-housed animals. Has also been associated with meningitis.
S. dysgalactiae	C	β	Uncommon. Has been isolated from dogs with bacteremia, dermatitis, or pneumonia.
S. bovis group (*S. gallolyticus* and *S. infantarius*)	D	α or γ	Uncommon. Has been isolated from dogs with urinary tract infections and endocarditis.
S. agalactiae	B	β or γ	Rare. Isolated from dogs and cats with endocarditis and neonatal bacteremia.

streptococcal infection have been reported in group-housed animals, which suggested spread of a virulent strain.[4–6]

Severe manifestations of *S. canis* infection, such as STSS and NFM, have been increasingly recognized in dogs and cats years, sometimes in the absence of obvious immunosuppressive underlying conditions or wounds.[7–10] In most cases, affected animals were previously healthy adult dogs or cats younger than 1 year of age. Although toxic shock syndrome can also be caused by staphylococci, STSS is defined as any streptococcal infection associated with the sudden onset of shock and organ failure. Mechanisms of shock and organ failure identified in human group A streptococcal infections include elaboration of pyrogenic exotoxins by streptococci, which act as superantigens. Superantigens stimulate T-cell responses through their ability to bind to, and cross-link, the MHC class II complex of antigen-presenting cells, and the T-cell receptor, which bypasses normal MHC-restricted antigen processing (Fig. 50.3). This leads to sudden and massive cascade of cytokine release, which in turn causes signs of fever, vomiting, and hypotension, together with tissue damage, DIC, and multiple organ dysfunction.[11] Cats with STSS had bacterial embolic localization with lesions in the lungs, heart, and liver.[12] Other streptococcal virulence factors also contribute to proinflammatory cytokine release and the development of hypotension. Laboratory abnormalities include thrombocytopenia, azotemia, hypoalbuminemia, and metabolic acidosis. Death can occur within 48 hours after the onset of illness. Specific criteria are used for diagnosis of STSS in human patients, and similar definitions could be used for diagnosis of STSS in dogs and cats (Box 50.1). Because relatively few dogs and cats with STSS have been described, predisposing factors have not been fully identified but in dogs include bites and use of anti-inflammatory drugs.[7,9] Importantly, there is also evidence that use of fluoroquinolones can predispose dogs with initially minor existing *S. canis* infections to developing STSS.[7,9] In humans, predisposing conditions include diabetes mellitus, alcoholism, surgical procedures, penetrating and nonpenetrating trauma, viral skin infections such as varicella, and possibly the use of NSAIDs. However as in dogs, predisposing factors are not always identified.

NFM is a bacterial infection of the deep subcutaneous tissues and fascia, characterized by extensive necrosis and gangrene of the skin and underlying tissues. It often begins as a minor wound and progresses rapidly over 24 to 72 hours, and it may be accompanied by STSS (Fig. 50.4). The popular term "flesh-eating bacteria" has been used to describe the organisms involved in "flesh-eating disease." Streptococcal NFM has been described in both dogs and cats. Bacteria at the inoculation site synthesize proteolytic enzymes and other products that facilitate the organism's spread via fascial planes and into muscles. Periosteal involvement, adjacent to involved muscle, has also been reported.[13] Lesions usually involve a limb (although have been described in one dog on the ventral thorax) and are intensely painful, with localized heat and swelling and accumulation of exudate along the fascial planes that requires drainage and debridement. In some dogs, extensive sloughing of necrotic skin occurs.[7] Bacteremia and complications that result from septic emboli may accompany NFM.[8] Outbreaks of NFM, arthritis, sinusitis, and meningitis caused by *S. canis* have been reported in cats in shelters,[4] breeding colonies,[14] and hoarding facilities.[6] In a spectacular report described in a grossly unhygienic and overcrowded institutional hoarding facility, the range of multiple

BOX 50.1 Criteria Used for Diagnosis of STSS in Human Patients, with Suggested Modifications for Diagnosis of STSS in Dogs and Cats

I. Isolation of *Streptococcus canis*

A. From a normally sterile site
B. From a nonsterile site

II. Clinical signs of severity

A. Hypotension: systolic blood pressure < 90 mmHg in dogs and < 80 mmHg in cats *and*
B. Two or more of the following signs:

1. Renal impairment: creatinine above the upper limit of the reference range
2. Coagulopathy: thrombocytopenia or DIC (prolonged clotting times, low serum fibrinogen concentration, and increased fibrin degradation products)
3. Liver involvement: serum AST, ALT, or total bilirubin concentrations at least twice the upper limit of the reference range
4. Acute respiratory distress syndrome defined as acute onset of diffuse pulmonary infiltrates and hypoxemia in the absence of cardiac failure, or evidence of diffuse capillary leak manifested as acute onset of pulmonary edema, or pleural or peritoneal effusions with hypoalbuminemia
5. A generalized erythematous macular rash that may desquamate
6. Soft tissue necrosis, including necrotizing fasciitis or myositis, or gangrene

ALT, Alanine aminotransferase; *AST,* aspartate aminotransferase; *DIC,* disseminated intravascular coagulation; *STSS,* streptococcal toxic shock syndrome.

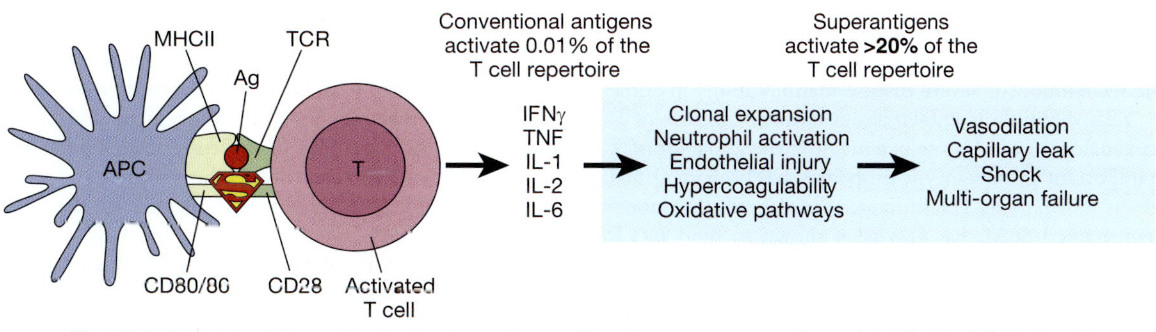

Fig. 50.3 Pathophysiology of toxic shock syndrome. *Streptococcus* superantigens bind first to MHC class II molecules on antigen-presenting cells, which stimulates cytokine expression and release, as well as expression of costimulatory molecules that promote T-cell receptor binding and activation. Subsequently, T-cell receptor binding occurs through the variable region on the receptor's beta chain (Vβ). Because superantigens can bind to multiple types of Vβ regions, a large proportion of the T-cell population can be simultaneously activated. For example, conventional antigens might activate < 0.1% of the T-cell population, whereas superantigens might activate > 20% of the population.

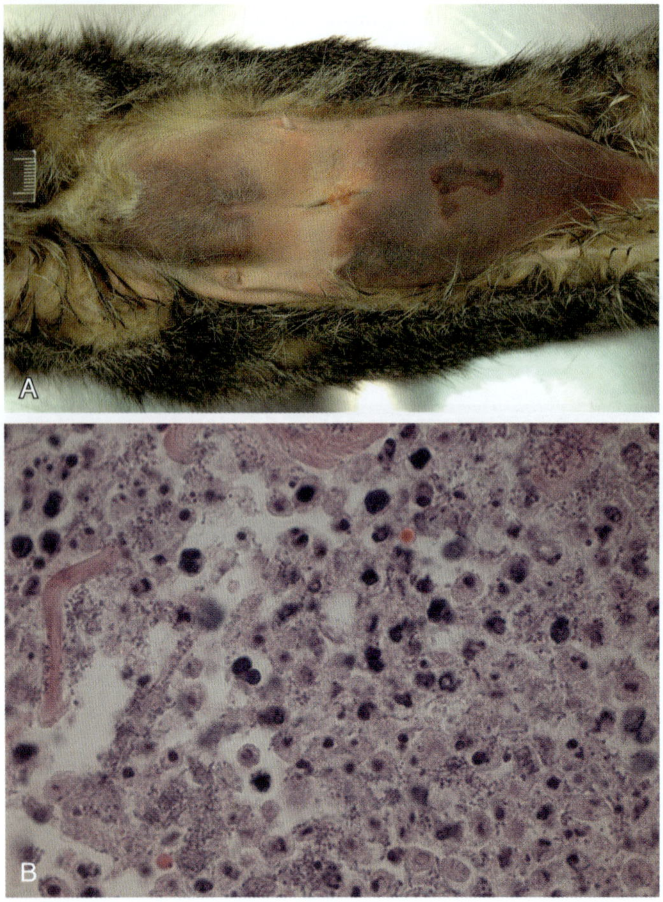

Fig. 50.4 (A) A 2-year-old female spayed domestic shorthair cat that was euthanized with necrotizing cellulitis, myositis and fasciitis, and peritonitis that developed after an ovariohysterectomy site became infected with *Streptococcus canis*. (B) Histopathology showed severe necrotizing cellulitis, myositis, and cellulitis with intralesional cocci that sometimes formed chains. Hematoxylin and eosin stain, 1000× oil magnification. (Courtesy of the University of California, Davis, Veterinary Anatomic Pathology Service.)

syndromes in numerous affected cats included acute rhinitis, cervical lymph node abscessation, severe septic arthritis, meningitis, otitis, STSS, and NFM.[6] Molecular typing (by pulsed-field gel electrophoresis) of isolates from one outbreak revealed that isolates were clonally related, which indicated spread of a virulent strain,[15] but another study of unrelated cases has not identified clonal spread[16] so that strain virulence may be less important than host predisposition.

Despite the recognition of severe disease manifestations in some dogs and cats, relatively little is known about virulence factors of *S. canis*. A protein analogous to M protein, a major virulence factor of *S. pyogenes* with important antiphagocytic properties, has been identified in *S. canis* and was shown to bind plasminogen and degrade thrombi.[17] This M protein, named SCM, has also been shown to bind IgG.[18] Genes that encode other virulence factors identified in *S. pyogenes*, such as pyrogenic exotoxins (*Spe* genes), streptococcal superantigen (SSA), streptokinase (Ska), and C5a peptidase (Scp, which cleaves the fifth component of complement), have not been detected.[19] However, one important study showed that exposure of *S. canis* to the fluoroquinolone antibiotic enrofloxacin caused bacterial cell lysis through inducing bacteriophage development, as a result of induction of the "SOS" response in strains containing these bacterial viruses, and the associated release of a bacteriophage-encoded lymphocyte mitogen related to pokeweed mitogen.[20] The presence of this mitogen gene on enrofloxacin-induced bacteriophages may explain the frequently noted association between fluoroquinolone treatment and the occurrence of STSS/NFM in dogs[7] because of a superantigen-like response of lymphocytes. Many of the dogs reported with STSS/NFM had received enrofloxacin in the early stages of disease, but the drug was not effective in halting the progression of the disease despite marginal *in vitro* susceptibility in some cases.[7] In fact, as suggested, enrofloxacin may have triggered the pathologic events caused by these virulent streptococci.[7,20] Fluoroquinolones are thus contraindicated in the treatment of dogs with *S. canis* infections.

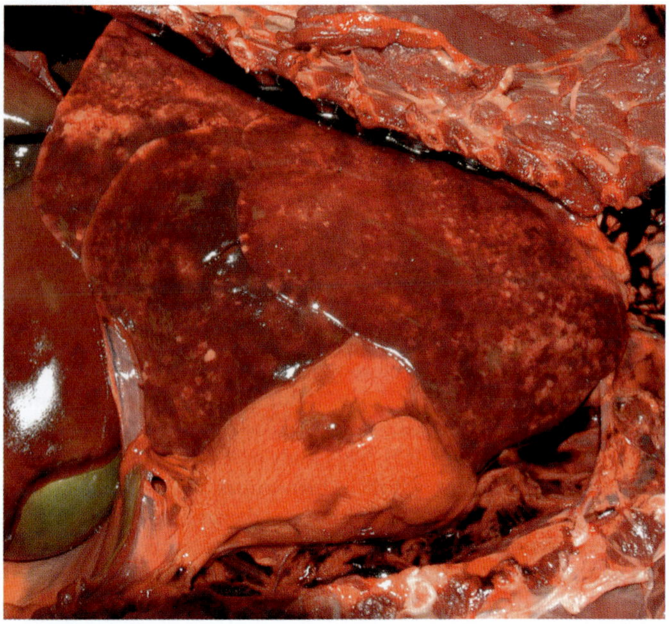

Fig. 50.5 Pneumonia in a shelter dog caused by *Streptococcus equi* subsp. *zooepidemicus*. The lungs are consolidated and dark red. (Courtesy of Dr. Patricia Pesavento, University of California, Davis.)

Streptococcus equi subsp. *zooepidemicus*

Streptococcus equi subsp. *zooepidemicus* is a β-hemolytic, group C streptococcus that is a commensal of the upper respiratory and lower genital tracts, and mouth, of many species including cats, dogs, guinea-pigs, horses, rabbits, seals, sheep, and swine. It is best known as the major opportunist pathogen of horses in which it causes wound infections, respiratory disease, endometritis, and abortion, among many other manifestations. Infections have also been reported in a variety of other animal species noted above but also less frequently in cattle, monkeys, seals, and humans. Different strains of *S. equi* subsp. *zooepidemicus* exist that may vary in pathogenicity and host tropism, and severe infections have been identified in several different host species, including the dog and cat. Infected horses can be a source of infection for dogs in some situations[21] but in most cases, there is no history of horse contact.

Several outbreaks of hemorrhagic, fibrinosuppurative, and necrotizing pneumonia associated with *S. equi* subsp. *zooepidemicus* infection have been described in group-housed dogs, such as those in kennels, research colonies, and shelter environments, from a variety of geographic locations worldwide and with an apparently increasing frequency (Fig. 50.5).[22–25] The pneumonia progresses rapidly in some dogs and may be accompanied by signs suggestive of STSS, such as fever and systemic hypovolemia. In some dogs, severe tachypnea and death occur within 24 to 48 hours of the first signs of respiratory disease, or dogs may be found dead without any preceding clinical signs. Other infected dogs show only mild signs of respiratory disease. Outbreaks of pneumonia, purulent rhinosinusitis, and meningoencephalitis have also been described in cats.[26–28] *Streptococcus equi* subsp. *zooepidemicus* meningoencephalitis occurred in a cat as a result of extension of otitis media/interna.[29]

The pathogenesis of infection with *S. equi* subsp. *zooepidemicus* in dogs and cats is unclear, but there is no doubt that this virulent organism can cause very severe disease, as it can in other species, including humans. Different strains are involved in outbreaks of severe disease in dogs and cats, so increasing reports cannot be attributed to clonal expansion of virulent clones. There is no evidence that there are differences in protective immunogenicity among these strains.[23] Co-infection with other contagious respiratory pathogens may initiate infection and can contribute to the severity of disease. Co-infections with CDV, CAdV-2, CHV-1, CIV, *Bordetella bronchiseptica*, or *Mycoplasma cynos* have been documented in some, but not all, affected dogs with *S. equi* subsp. *zooepidemicus* pneumonia.[22] Experimentally, co-infection of dogs with both CIV and *S. equi* subsp. *zooepidemicus* was associated with more severe clinical manifestations of disease than when either organism is inoculated alone.[30] Other environmental factors such as overcrowding may predispose to disease and its severity; in large prevalence surveys of respiratory pathogens in dogs with CIRD, *S. equi* subsp. *zooepidemicus* is rarely detected when compared with other pathogens in the complex.[31,32] Superantigen genes have been detected in some isolates of *S. equi* subsp. *zooepidemicus* from dogs,[33] but there has been no correlation between the presence of these genes and the severity of histopathologic lesions. However, expression of proinflammatory cytokines such as TNF-α, IL-6, and IL-8 in the lungs of affected dogs suggests that a potent inflammatory response is involved in the pathogenesis of disease.[24]

Other Streptococcal Species

Streptococci other than *S. canis* and *S. equi* subsp. *zooepidemicus* are of relatively minor significance in dogs and cats. *Streptococcus equi* subsp. *equi*, the etiologic agent of strangles, was isolated from a dog with tonsillar and submandibular lymphadenomegaly caused by pharyngeal foreign body penetration.[34] Genetic characterization confirmed the isolate as this usually highly equine-specific pathogen. The dog lived on premises where horses were kept; unexpectedly, no clinical cases of strangles had been identified in the horses in the local environment.

Group B streptococci (*S. agalactiae*) have been associated mainly with neonatal bacteremia and postpartum metritis in humans and mastitis in cows. Factors at the time of delivery, such as low birth weight or difficult delivery, precipitate the development of clinical illness. Skin, pharyngeal, and wound infections can occur. Immunosuppressed people can develop bacteremia, meningitis, and endocarditis as a result of infection. Group B streptococci are more frequently isolated than group G from people with these syndromes. *Streptococcus agalactiae* infections are rare in dogs and cats, although there are reports of involvement in bacteremia in a dog, in endocarditis, endometritis, and neonatal sepsis ("fading puppy syndrome"). Peritonitis with bacteremia and parturient endometritis and placentitis have been described in cats. Whether canine and feline strains are indigenous or of human or other animal origin is uncertain.

Streptococcus dysgalactiae is a β-hemolytic, group C streptococcus, like *S. equi* subsp. *zooepidemicus*. There are two subspecies, *S. dysgalactiae* subsp. *equisimilis* and *S. dysgalactiae* subsp. *dysgalactiae*. After *S. canis* and *S. equi* subsp. *zooepidemicus*, *S. dysgalactiae* subsp. *equisimilis* was the third most common β- or γ-hemolytic streptococcal species isolated from dogs at a veterinary teaching hospital in the United States, but was detected in only 13 of 393 dogs with streptococcal infections. Affected dogs had bacteremia and sepsis, dermatitis, or pneumonia.[3] *Streptococcus dysgalactiae* subsp. *dysgalactiae* has been reported in association with systemic neonatal infections and death in a litter of great Dane puppies.[35]

The porcine streptococcus, *Streptococcus suis*, has occasionally been isolated from cats with meningoencephalitis, pyothorax, or dermatitis.[36,37] *Streptococcus suis* was also isolated from the urine of a systemically unwell dog that had fever and bacteriuria in Canada.[38] The dog had no known exposure to swine; however, it had been allowed to chew on pig ear treats. It can be isolated from the anus, tonsils, and skin of healthy dogs and cats.[39] *Streptococcus suis* has been classified into serotypes, which have epidemiologic importance. Human infections are usually serotypes 2 and 14. The cases reported in dogs and cats have not belonged to these serotypes.

Other streptococcal species isolated from dogs and cats include the human pathogen *Streptococcus constellatus* (a *Streptococcus anginosus* group organism), which was isolated from a dog with pyoderma.[40] *Streptococcus bovis* group organisms are α- or nonhemolytic and usually possess Lancefield group D antigens. Biotypes that belong to this group, which differ in their biochemical characteristics, were reclassified as distinct species, *Streptococcus gallolyticus* and *Streptococcus infantarius*.[41] *Streptococcus bovis* group organisms are commensals of the GI tracts of humans and other animals, especially ruminants, and are important causes of bacteremia and endocarditis in humans, accounting for 11% to 17% of all endocarditis cases. They frequently affect multiple valves and are associated with embolic complications. For unknown reasons, fecal carriage of *S. bovis* group organisms by humans has been strongly associated with colorectal cancer. This especially seems to be true for *S. gallolyticus* subsp. *gallolyticus*.[42] Rarely, *S. bovis* group organisms are isolated from dogs and cats with UTIs. They have also been isolated from the blood of dogs with mitral valve endocarditis, one of which also had sternebral osteomyelitis.[43,44]

Enterococcus spp.

Enterococci are α- or nonhemolytic gram-positive bacteria that usually possess Lancefield group D antigens, and are commensals of the GI tracts of humans and other animals. In humans and pets, they have predominantly caused infections in hospitalized patients as nosocomial complications and are problematic in veterinary hospital settings because of their ability to persist in the environment as well as develop multiple antibacterial resistance. Enterococci form pairs or short chains of organisms that cannot morphologically be discriminated from streptococci. Enterococci can survive harsh environmental conditions, and are more likely than streptococci, especially β-hemolytic species, to survive in clinic and hospital settings. They are able to proliferate in medium that contains 6.5% NaCl, at temperatures that range from 10°C to 45°C (50°F to 113°F), and can be metabolically active in the presence of 40% bile salts, which in turn explains their improved ability to grow in the intestine when compared with the less robust genus *Streptococcus*. The genus *Enterococcus*, which contains 55 species, was separated from *Streptococcus* in the mid-1980s.[2]

Not only are enterococci environmentally hardy but they are often resistant to a wide variety of different antimicrobial drug classes. MDR enterococcal infections, especially those that are also resistant to vancomycin (vancomycin-resistant enterococci [VRE]), are a significant problem in human medicine. Of great clinical importance, resistance among enterococci occurs as a result of both intrinsic and acquired resistance mechanisms. Intrinsic resistance to low levels of most β-lactam antimicrobials occurs because enterococci possess low-affinity PBPs, making penicillins generally bacteriostatic, not bactericidal, against enterococci. Enterococci also have low-level intrinsic resistance to aminoglycosides, which results from decreased drug uptake. However, uptake of aminoglycosides is enhanced when enterococci are exposed to β-lactams, explaining the synergistic activity of this combination that is sometimes taken advantage of in treatment. Enterococci are resistant to trimethoprim-sulfamethoxazole because they utilize exogenously produced folate. Thus, even if the organisms appear susceptible to trimethoprim-sulfamethoxazole *in vitro* (when exogenous folate is lacking), the drug is not effective *in vivo*. Many laboratories therefore will not report MICs for this organism-drug combination. Enterococcal resistance to other antimicrobials, such as macrolides and vancomycin, results from acquired resistance mechanisms. Extensive multidrug resistance has been well documented in enterococci isolated from dogs and cats, but there are few reports of enterococci with acquired vancomycin resistance from dogs in the literature. These have been reports from the United Kingdom, New Zealand, and the United States.[45–47] All other isolates examined have been vancomycin susceptible. In contrast, in humans from Europe and North America, VRE account for up to 30% of enterococcal infections, notably in hospital-associated infections.[48]

Clinical microbiology laboratories should identify and distinguish between *Enterococcus faecalis* and *Enterococcus faecium*, the most prevalent species in humans. These two species differ in their epidemiology, antimicrobial susceptibility, and virulence properties. Since these are often hospital-associated infections, their identification to species may be a clue to their presence as contaminants in the environment, which may further be suggested if they have a common resistance profile. *Enterococcus faecium* is more likely to show high-level resistance (HLR) to penicillins, and to show multidrug resistance, than *E. faecalis*, and as a result, in humans, the prognosis for serious *E. faecium* infections may be worse than that for *E. faecalis* infections.[49] However, *E. faecalis* is more likely to produce biofilms than *E. faecium* and therefore are more likely to colonize catheters.[50] Although most infections in humans have been *E. faecalis*, an increase in the prevalence of MDR *E. faecium* infections has occurred, especially in hospitals. In particular, ampicillin- and fluoroquinolone-resistant *E. faecium* strains that belong to hospital-adapted strains of the clonal complex 17 (CC17) have emerged.[51] Strains belonging to this clade are a defined, globally disseminated population that is associated with hospitalized human patients but only rarely found in the community; it might be concluded that they have adapted to human hospitals. CC17 isolates have been found in dogs but belong to a different clade from those found in hospitalized humans. Their virulence gene profile and antimicrobial susceptibility profiles have differed from those of human isolates.[51–53] In contrast to *E. faecium*, clones of *E. faecalis* are not found only in hospitals but are also present in healthy humans and animals, and animals may therefore represent a source of infection for humans.[51,53] As in humans, the two most common species of *Enterococcus* associated with disease in dogs and cats are *E. faecalis* and *E. faecium*.[54]

In healthy dogs and cats, enterococci can be found on the skin and within the oral cavity, nasal cavity, and GI tract. In the United States, the most prevalent species in dogs appears to be *E. faecalis*, which comprised 68% of 155 isolates.[54] In the cat, in one study it was *Enterococcus hirae*, which comprised 52% of 121 isolates,[54] but in a more recent study it was *E. faecalis* (77%) followed by *E. faecium* (13%).[55] Other species isolated from sick dogs and cats include *Enterococcus casseliflavus*, *Enterococcus durans*, and *Enterococcus gallinarum*; *Enterococcus canintestini* has been isolated from healthy dogs.[56–58]

Although less pathogenic than many β-hemolytic streptococci, important virulence factors have been identified in enterococci that enable them to invade tissues and cause disease. These include a cytolysin, gelatinase, and a serine protease, as well as several surface proteins (e.g., the Ace protein, which allows the organism to adhere to connective tissue components, such as collagen). Enterococci also possess pili that play an important role in adherence. The ability of many enterococci to form biofilms means they can colonize catheters or other surfaces and be very difficult to eradicate, because in biofilms they are more likely to resist phagocytosis and antimicrobial drugs.[50] In addition, because enterococci are intrinsically resistant to a number of antimicrobials, treatment with broad-spectrum antibiotics (which destroy competing bacteria) selects for mucosal, including intestinal, colonization by enterococci. The development of enterococcal UTIs may be promoted by repeated use of antimicrobial drugs to treat recurrent UTIs if the underlying cause of infection is not identified or cannot be resolved. Because of these features and their robust nature, enterococci can contaminate the hospital environment and survive for long periods on fomites (door knobs, stethoscopes, monitoring devices), as well as be transmitted via the hands, gloves, and clothing of hospital personnel. Inoculation may occur via urinary, IV, or other invasive devices, or organisms may enter the body from a damaged GI tract.

Severe concurrent illness and immunosuppression may predispose to infection but is compounded by the resistance of these bacteria to antibiotics and their ability to proliferate in the large intestine and be shed in feces when the competing microflora has been removed by antibiotics. In addition to UTIs, enterococci may be isolated from dogs and cats with bacteremia and endocarditis, cholangiohepatitis, discospondylitis, hepatic abscesses, mastitis, pancreatitis, peritonitis, pyoderma, otitis externa, and wound infections. There have been rare reports of GI illness in association with enterococcal infection of the GI tract in dogs and cats. In affected cats, an association with diarrhea was supported by the presence of large mats of enterococci in association with the GI mucosa.[59,60] Frequently, enterococci are isolated from lesions in mixed infections with other GI microorganisms.

There is some evidence that *E. hirae*, a commensal species, plays a protective role in kittens infected with atypical enteropathogenic *Escherichia coli* (aEPEC).[61] Preparations that contain *E. faecium* strains have been investigated as probiotics in dogs and cats, with mixed results.[62–66]

Physical Examination Findings

Physical examination findings in dogs and cats with *Streptococcus* or *Enterococcus* infections vary with the anatomic site(s) of infection. Streptococcal infections are an important differential diagnosis in "fading" neonates; dogs with physical examination findings suggestive of endocarditis; dogs and cats with severe pneumonia and pyothorax; STSS and NF; rapid onset of systemic illness in association with a wound; or outbreaks of severe purulent upper respiratory disease, hemorrhagic pneumonia, and systemic illness in group-housed animals.

Findings suggestive of streptococcal or enterococcal endocarditis include fever, lethargy, tachycardia, joint pain and swelling, systolic heart murmurs, and signs of embolic complications such as lameness, limb edema, weak or absent pulses, or neurologic signs (see Chapter 122). Animals with streptococcal pneumonia may have a fever (up to 106.3°F or 41.3°C), cough, tonsillar enlargement and hyperemia, mucopurulent nasal discharge, and/or tachypnea with increased lung sounds. Lung sounds may be decreased if pleural effusion is present. Animals with NFM have variable extents of regional cutaneous erythema, sometimes in association with a wound; cutaneous ulceration, swelling, edema, intense pain, and warmth on palpation of the affected area. In human patients, the "finger test" has been used to assist recognition of NFM, whereby the area of suspected involvement is infiltrated with a local anesthetic, and a 2-cm incision is made in the skin and extended into the deep fascia. A lack of bleeding is a sign of NFM. A sterile double-gloved finger is then used to probe the incision, and the test is considered positive if tissues separate with little resistance.[67] In some animals, extensive skin sloughing can occur. In two dogs, acute onset of posterior paresis with lower motor neuron deficits developed because of the presence of septic emboli in blood vessels of the gray matter of the spinal cord and extension of infection into the surrounding connective tissue, muscle, and peripheral nerves.

Animals with STSS may be obtunded, with weak pulses, tachycardia, tachypnea, and prolonged CRT. Rectal temperatures may exceed 106°F (41.1°C), although the presence of fever is variable. Icterus may be present in animals that develop multiple organ dysfunction syndrome in association with STSS.

DIAGNOSIS

Laboratory Abnormalities

Complete Blood Count, Biochemistry, and Urinalysis Findings

Dogs and cats with severe manifestations of streptococcal infections (such as endocarditis, pneumonia, NF, and STSS) usually have a neutrophilic leukocytosis with a left shift, toxic neutrophils, lymphopenia, and monocytosis. A degenerative left shift or circulating metamyelocytes may be present. STSS may be accompanied by thrombocytopenia as a result of DIC, azotemia and/or increased liver enzyme activities, hypoalbuminemia, and hypoglycemia. Serum creatine kinase activity may be increased with muscle involvement. The urinalysis of dogs and cats with streptococcal or enterococcal UTIs may reveal pyuria, proteinuria, or hematuria, and cocci in pairs or chains may sometimes be evident on sediment examination.

Clotting Function

Dogs and cats with STSS that develop DIC may have clotting function abnormalities including prolonged coagulation times, increased fibrin degradation product and D-dimer concentrations, and decreased antithrombin concentrations.

Cytologic Abnormalities

Cytologic examination of specimens (respiratory lavage fluid, aspirates of affected tissues, or pus) from dogs and cats with streptococcal or enterococcal infections typically reveals large numbers of degenerate and nondegenerate neutrophils. Coccoid bacteria in pairs or characteristically in chains may also be seen. Cytologic examination of fine-needle aspirates from swollen areas in dogs and cats with NFM is essential to speed confirmation of infection and institute early appropriate antimicrobial therapy, because virulent strains of gram-negative bacteria can also cause this syndrome.

Microbiologic Tests

Isolation and Identification

Streptococci and enterococci that infect dogs and cats are readily isolated on routine bacteriologic media from aspirates, tissue biopsies, body fluids, and lavage specimens. Inoculation of complex solid media that contain blood is recommended and is the usual practice in laboratories. Streptococci may grow well in anaerobic incubation conditions, but these are not required because of their facultative nature. The laboratory may use selective media for specimens that are heavily contaminated with other bacteria. Species are identified based on their phenotypic characteristics (such as colony morphology and hemolytic properties), biochemical reactions, grouping with Lancefield antisera, and most frequently now by MALDI-TOF (see Chapter 3). Molecular typing methods such as pulsed-field gel electrophoresis or multilocus sequence typing may sometimes be done to investigate outbreaks in group-housed animals or hospital environments, largely for research purposes.

Antimicrobial susceptibility testing for β-hemolytic streptococci is often not performed by veterinary diagnostic laboratories, because virtually all such strains are penicillin (and amoxicillin) susceptible. This is also true for group A β-hemolytic streptococci (GAS, *S. pyogenes*) that infect humans. However, an increased prevalence of penicillin resistance, which occurs as a result of altered PBPs, has been detected in *S. pneumoniae*, which is primarily a human pathogen.[56] *Streptococcus pneumoniae* may also be resistant to other β-lactam drugs and macrolides. Acquired resistance may occur in non-β-hemolytic streptococci in dogs and cats, and so susceptibility testing is recommended for these bacteria. Some laboratories may falsely report β-hemolytic streptococci as resistant to trimethroprim-sulfamethazine because of the antagonistic effect of thymidine in bacteriologic media containing blood. Laboratory assessment of antimicrobial susceptibility is of critical importance for enterococci because of the high prevalence of resistance in this group, particularly among *E. faecium* isolates. Isolates with a consistent antibiotype (pattern of antimicrobial susceptibility) may indicate that a clinic or hospital has an *Enterococcus* contamination problem.

Pathologic Findings

Pathologic findings in *Streptococcus* infections vary depending on the organ system affected. Gross findings in *S. canis* sinusitis include accumulation of purulent material within the frontal sinus with osteolysis, and distortion of the nasal bridge in cats.[4] When meningitis is present, purulent material may be found in association with the meninges (Fig. 50.6). Lesions of NF in dogs and cats consist of edema, ecchymoses, and necrosis that extend within the fascia and subcutis in association with ulcerative skin lesions (see Fig. 50.4). An accumulation of pus may be found between fascial planes. Congestion of a variety of organs may be present in animals that have accompanying STSS. When *S. canis* or *Enterococcus* endocarditis is present, adherent and friable mass lesions may be seen in association with the mitral and/or, less commonly, the aortic valves. Dogs with streptococcal endocarditis are more likely to have concurrent polyarthritis than dogs with other bacterial causes of endocarditis.[43] On histopathology, valve lesions generally contain large numbers of degenerate and nondegenerate neutrophils, hemorrhage, necrosis, fibrin thrombi, and abundant gram-positive cocci (Fig. 50.7). Septic thromboemboli may be present in a variety of organs. Histopathologic lesions in neonates that die of sepsis include severe inflammation and necrosis, as well as septic emboli in a variety of tissues (see Fig. 50.1).

Grossly, the lungs of dogs with *S. equi* subsp. *zooepidemicus* pneumonia may be red, consolidated, and fail to collapse (see Fig. 50.5).

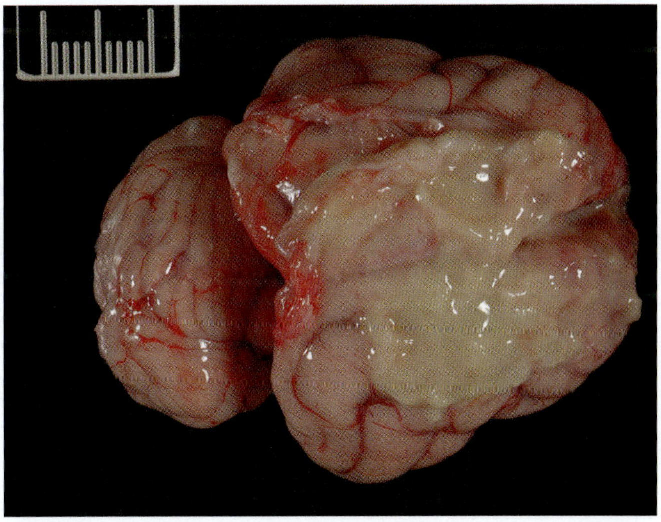

Fig. 50.6 Accumulation of purulent exudate over the meninges in a shelter cat that died of *Streptococcus canis* meningitis. (Courtesy of Dr. Patricia Pesavento, University of California, Davis.)

There may be variable quantities of hemorrhagic pleural effusion, petechial and ecchymotic hemorrhages on pleural surfaces, and bloody exudate within the airways and nasal cavity.[24] Typical histopathologic changes include fibrinous, necrotizing, and/or suppurative pneumonia or bronchopneumonia; fibrin thrombi; and intralesional clusters or chains of coccoid bacteria. Within lymph nodes, marked lymphoid depletion may be present, but lymphoid hyperplasia has also been reported. Occasionally, septic thromboemboli may be present in tissues or organs such as the lymph nodes, renal glomeruli, adrenal glands, brain, and splenic sinusoids.[68,69]

TREATMENT AND PROGNOSIS

In general, streptococcal infections should be treated with a β-lactam drug, preferably an aminopenicillin such as amoxicillin or a first-generation cephalosporin (Table 50.2). Early diagnosis and prompt treatment with appropriate antimicrobial drugs are essential to prevent more severe complications such as NF or STSS. In animals that present with severe signs such as septic shock or life-threatening pneumonia, initial treatment should be with a broad-spectrum antimicrobial drug combination, such as a β-lactam including amoxicillin and an aminoglycoside, which together commonly also has synergistic activity against streptococci, namely group C streptococci (*S. equi* subsp. *zooepidemicus*).

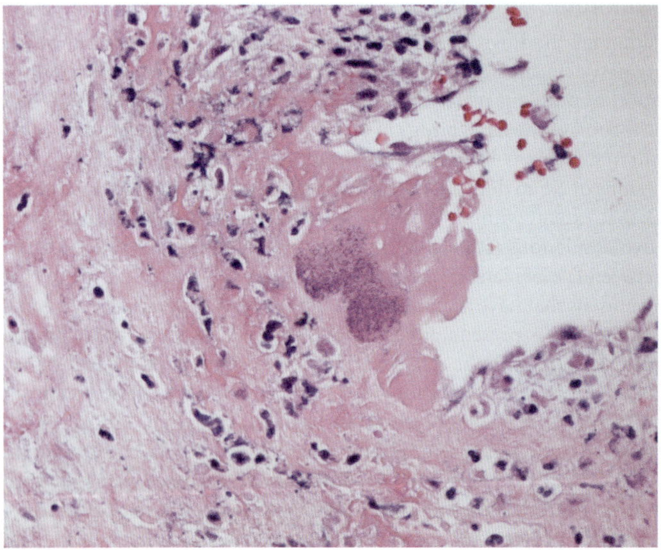

Fig. 50.7 Histopathology of the mitral valve of an 8-year-old male neutered springer spaniel that was seen for a 1-month history of right thoracic limb lameness, anorexia, and lethargy. There is severe, subacute, fibrinonecrotic endocarditis with intralesional cocci. When the dog was first evaluated, the platelet count was 9,000 platelets/μL and the dog was treated with vincristine for immune-mediated thrombocytopenia. Subsequently, the dog developed vomiting and diarrhea and became obtunded. Blood cultures grew *Streptococcus canis*. At necropsy, septic emboli were present in the kidneys, spleen, and lymph nodes. Necrotizing fasciitis was also present in multiple limbs, which was thought to have developed as a result of septic embolization.

Necrotizing Fasciitis and Streptococcal Toxic Shock Syndrome

Prompt surgical exploration and debridement is of critical importance in NF, because shock and organ failure will continue to progress in the face of antimicrobial treatment when necrotic tissue persists. Use of negative pressure wound therapy was associated with successful outcomes in three dogs.[10] Surviving animals often must have extensive skin grafting or dermoplasty to close open wounds created by the necrotic process. Imaging techniques such as ultrasound may be useful to help characterize the extent of lesions before surgery. Extremely aggressive fluid resuscitation with crystalloids and blood products may also be required, while blood pressure is monitored. STSS is a clinical emergency and requires IV benzyl penicillin as the drug of choice because of its exquisite activity.[70] In human patients, deep-seated streptococcal infections (NF and STSS) are often treated with *both* high-dose penicillin and clindamycin. This is because clindamycin suppresses exotoxin production by GAS, is more active than penicillin in experimental NF, and has a longer half-life than penicillin.[70,71] However, a low prevalence of clindamycin resistance exists in GAS, whereas all GAS are susceptible to penicillin.[70,71] Approximately 10% to 15% of contemporary *S. canis* isolates from dogs in Europe and nearly 18% of isolates from dogs in Japan have demonstrated clindamycin resistance.[72–74] Given this finding, the same combination could be used to treat NF in dogs and cats. In humans, IV immunoglobulin treatment is also recommended on the basis of clinical trials.[70] As noted earlier, fluoroquinolone antibiotics should be avoided in treatment of *S. canis* infections because they promote an endogenous bacterial mitogen production.[20] In addition, they are not of value in streptococcal infections because of their low activity.

Meningitis/Meningoencephalitis

High-dose penicillin or amoxicillin was the drug of choice for treatment of streptococcal meningitis in human patients caused by *S. pneumoniae* before the emergence of penicillin resistance in this species. It is the drug of choice for meningitis caused by β-hemolytic

TABLE 50.2 Suggested Antimicrobial Drugs for Treatment of Streptococcal Infections in Dogs and Cats

Drug	Dose mg/kg	Interval (Hours)	Route
Penicillin G potassium or sodium[a]	20,000–40,000 U/kg	6–8	IV, IM
Ampicillin sodium[a]	10–20	6–8	IV, IM, SC
Amoxicillin	6.6–20	8–12	PO
Cefazolin sodium	20-35	8	IV, IM
Cephalexin	10–30 (dogs), 15–20 (cats)	12	PO
Trimethoprim-sulfamethoxazole[b]	30	12	PO, IV

[a]Consider use with clindamycin, 10 mg/kg q12h IV or IM for necrotizing fasciitis or myositis; consider addition of gentamicin sulfate, 9–14 mg/kg q24h IV, IM, or SC for dogs with *S. equi* subsp. *zooepidemicus* pneumonia because of synergy of this combination for group C streptococci.
[b]Consider use for treatment of streptococcal meningitis as alternative to penicillin G.

TABLE 50.3 Suggested Medications for Treatment of Enterococcal Infections in Dogs and Cats

Drug	Dose mg/kg	Interval (Hours)	Route
Ampicillin sodium[a]	10–20	6–8	IV, IM, SC
Amoxicillin[a]	6.6–20	8–12	PO
Vancomycin[b]	15	8	IV
Linezolid[b]	10 (dogs)	8	PO
Chloramphenicol	40–50 (dogs), 12.5–20 (cats)	6–8 (dogs), 12 (cats)	PO, IV, IM
Nitrofurantoin[c]	2–3	8	PO

[a]In human patients, used with gentamicin sulfate, 1 mg/kg q12h IV for systemic enterococcal infections caused by enterococci susceptible to high-level aminoglycosides, because of the synergy of this combination.
[b]For enterococci that show high-level aminoglycoside resistance or when aminoglycosides cannot be used because of toxicity (animals with renal failure). Use in veterinary patients is controversial. Refer to Chapter 10 for additional information on the use of vancomycin. These drugs are critical human drugs and should be therefore used only after susceptibility testing and in the absence of any alternative treatments.
[c]For resistant urinary tract infections.

streptococci despite the relatively limited penetration of the CSF in uninflamed meninges; this is because of the strong susceptibility of these streptococci to penicillin and the greater penetration of penicillin in inflamed meninges. Trimethoprim-sulfamethoxazole has been used with apparent success to treat some dogs and cats with streptococcal meningitis.[27,75] See Chapter 129 for additional information on treatment of bacterial meningitis. Ceftriaxone has been used as an alternative to benzylpenicillin for treatment of human streptococcal meningitis and attains higher concentrations in the CSF with the advantage that its spectrum of activity covers gram-negative bacteria.

Bacteremia and Endocarditis

The reader is referred to Chapter 122 for information on treatment of bacteremia and endocarditis.

Enterococcal Infections

Suggested antimicrobial treatments for treatment of enterococcal infections in dogs and cats are shown in Table 50.3. Successful treatment of enterococcal infections requires awareness of the intrinsic resistance of enterococci to low levels of β-lactams and aminoglycosides, the synergistic effect of high doses of these drugs, the lack of efficacy of trimethoprim-sulfonamide combinations *in vivo*, and the ability of enterococci to acquire resistance genes to a large number of other antimicrobial compounds. Susceptibility testing is, therefore, always recommended when isolates are believed to be clinically relevant. Aminopenicillins such as amoxicillin generally have more activity against enterococci than penicillin or the carbapenems. Bactericidal regimens, which consist of a β-lactam and gentamicin, are used in human patients to treat systemic infections such as endocarditis or bacteremia. Enterococci are usually resistant to aminoglycosides at dilutions used in routine broth microdilution methods (low-level resistance). When the synergistic combination is indicated, but low-level resistance is present, isolates should be tested for HLR to aminoglycosides. Aminoglycoside HLR results from production of an aminoglycoside-modifying enzyme by enterococci. It emerged in the 1980s and has been a growing problem in both *E. faecium* and *E. faecalis* isolates from human patients. Aminoglycoside HLR has also been reported in *E. faecium* and *E. faecalis* isolated from dogs and cats,[45,46,76] but most isolates are susceptible to high concentrations of gentamicin. In human patients, a combination of ceftriaxone and ampicillin has been recommended to treat endocarditis caused by aminoglycoside HLR enterococci.[49] When enterococci show penicillin resistance, vancomycin can be substituted for penicillin, but this requires prolonged hospitalization for IV administration and is best avoided unless there is no alternative therapy, because vancomycin is a critical antimicrobial for treatment of resistant bacterial infections in humans. Single-agent treatment with linezolid (see Chapter 10) is an oral alternative for treatment of serious penicillin-resistant enterococcal infections, but in human patients it is recommended that this only be used when combinations of β-lactams and gentamicin cannot be used because of resistance, toxicity, or treatment failure.[48] Although most strains of enterococci isolated from humans are susceptible to linezolid, resistant strains have appeared.[77] Of concern, linezolid- and multidrug-resistant enterococci were described in raw commercial dog food in Europe in 2019 and 2020.[78] Use of linezolid may also be associated with adverse effects of anemia and gastrointestinal signs in dogs and cats.[79] Chloramphenicol may be successful for treatment of resistant enterococcal bloodstream infections when administered orally, but it is bacteriostatic, and concerns regarding adverse effects in humans exist (see Chapter 10).

Treatment of enterococcal UTIs with β-lactams such as ampicillin or amoxicillin may be successful even when resistance is documented in the susceptibility panel, because of the high concentrations that these drugs achieve in the urine.[48] Nitrofurantoin has also been useful for treatment of resistant enterococcal UTIs in humans, but routine treatment of subclinical bacteriuria caused by MDR enterococci is not recommended (see Chapter 127).[80] When enterococci are present with other bacteria, especially in the urinary tract, treatment of the nonenterococcal pathogen may be sufficient to resolve the infection.

PREVENTION

Because outbreaks of streptococcal infections in dogs and cats have been associated with overcrowding, co-infections, and other stressors, appropriate shelter and kennel management and hygiene, as well as vaccination against other respiratory pathogens, may help to prevent streptococcal infections. The predisposing factors may however not be clear. Proper wound care may prevent serious streptococcal infections such as bacteremia, endocarditis, NF, and STSS. Methods to reduce nosocomial infections by enterococci are outlined in Chapter 15. Resistant enterococcal infections may be prevented through restricted and appropriate use of antimicrobial drugs and proper management of underlying disorders that predispose to bacterial infections.

PUBLIC HEALTH ASPECTS

Streptococci include some of the most important bacterial pathogens of humans. The β-hemolytic GAS *S. pyogenes* causes streptococcal pharyngitis ("strep throat") and scarlet fever, as well as poststreptococcal rheumatic fever, rheumatic heart disease, and glomerulonephritis. In 2005, it was estimated that globally, GAS cause more than 616 million new cases of pharyngitis each year.[81] GAS have also been associated with other disease manifestations, which include NF, STSS, myositis, vaginitis, and bacteremia. As a result, *S. pyogenes* is the most extensively studied of all streptococci. There are more than 100 different serotypes, which are classified based on the sequence of the M protein gene (known as *emm* typing). M protein, a filamentous macromolecule that traverses the cell wall (see Fig. 50.2), is a key virulence factor of GAS. Chronic subclinical carriage of infection in the oropharynx occurs in some individuals. GAS can survive extremes in environmental temperature and humidity; however, most infections are associated with direct or close contact among susceptible individuals. Prevalence rates for GAS are higher in young children, especially those in daycare or classroom situations. The prevalence of positive throat culture findings in such circumstances may approach 50%, even in the absence of an obvious epidemic. Symptomatic, rather than carrier children, are most likely to bring infection into the home. Under such circumstances, the isolation rate in other people in the household approaches 25% to 50%. If the child is asymptomatic, the rate is only 9%. Although family pets have been implicated as a reservoir in households with recurrent streptococcal pharyngitis,[82–84] colonization or infection of dogs and cats with GAS appears to be rare or nonexistent when accurate streptococcal identification methods have been performed, although the idea that pets can be reservoirs seems to remain an enduring and unfortunate myth. One study found no evidence of oropharyngeal colonization by GAS in pets that were in contact with children with acute pharyngitis.[1] When domestic pets come into close contact with infected individuals, some pets may apparently develop pharyngeal colonization with GAS. Infected pets show no clinical illness or tonsillar enlargement and usually eliminate their infection within 2 to 3 weeks after they are removed from the household. Treatment of infected humans is generally limited to only those that are symptomatic, so it is not rational to screen pets for evidence of colonization.

Streptococcus pneumoniae is an important commensal of the human respiratory tract that causes a variety of diseases including bacteremia, meningitis, and pneumonia, otitis media, and sinusitis. Children are regarded as the most important reservoir. Although extremely rare in dogs and cats, infections with *S. pneumoniae* have been reported in a dog with meningoencephalitis,[64,85] a cat with arthritis,[72,86] and a cat with cellulitis.[73,87] It is likely that the dog and cats acquired the infection from humans, because humans are the natural hosts for *S. pneumoniae*.

Reports of human infection with *S. canis* and *S. equi* subsp. *zooepidemicus* exist, and represent a more genuine threat than the potential for zoonotic transmission of *S. pyogenes* or *S. pneumoniae* from companion animals discussed above. *Streptococcus canis* has increasingly been recognized as a cause of soft tissue infections in dog owners and has been isolated from humans with bacteremia, endocarditis, UTIs, osteomyelitis, and pneumonia.[88–92] Population genetic studies suggest that *S. canis* is a single population that can infect multiple animal species including humans, suggesting that the potential for human infection from dogs and cats is always present.[92] The situation can be complicated because human group G streptococci can be confused with *S. canis*, which is also Lancefield group G. Rarely, *S. equi* subsp. *zooepidemicus* has been isolated from humans with bacteremia, endocarditis, meningitis, acute nephritis, pneumonia, osteomyelitis, septic arthritis, or STSS. Most human infections with *S. equi* subsp. *zooepidemicus* have been traced to an animal source, such as contact with horses, or consumption of inadequately pasteurized milk products or pork. However, apparent transmission of *S. equi* subsp. *zooepidemicus* from a dog with *S. equi* subsp. *zooepidemicus* pneumonia to a handler, who developed severe systemic illness, has been described.[93] The sometimes very serious nature of *S. canis* and *S. equi* subsp. *zooepidemicus* infections in humans means that dogs or cats with severe streptococcal infections should be handled with appropriate precautions by anyone in contact with them. The risk can probably be contained by wearing gloves and protective clothing when handling dogs with STSS or NFM.

Dogs and cats are also a potential source for human infection by MDR enterococci. In one study, dogs that left a veterinary intensive care unit (ICU) were colonized with MDR enterococci with the capacity for biofilm formation and horizontal transfer of antimicrobial resistance genes.[94] Enterococcal infections in humans usually require significant host predisposition, although this is less the case for *S. canis* and *S. equi* subsp. *zooepidemicus* infections. Vancomycin-resistant enterococci with the same genotype as those found in people have been recovered from the feces of pet dogs and cats, and the discovery of linezolid- and multidrug-resistant enterococci in raw commercial dog food in Europe has significant public health implications.[79]

Because of the potential for transmission of streptococci and enterococci between dogs, cats, and humans, preventative measures such as hand washing after pets are handled, household disinfection, and avoidance of close contact (such as allowing pets to lick wounds or mucous membranes) should be considered, especially for immunocompromised pet owners. Dogs and cats should not be fed raw diets, even if commercially available as frozen raw food for pets. Veterinarians should also recognize the potential for clinics and hospital environments to become contaminated with *E. faecalis* and *E. faecium*, and take appropriate hygiene steps if this is recognized to have occurred.

CASE EXAMPLE 1

Signalment

"Rigby," an 8-year-old neutered Boston terrier from Central Ohio.

History

Rigby was evaluated by the emergency service of the Ohio State University Veterinary Medical Center for acute swelling of the entire left pelvic limb distal to the stifle. Two days prior to examination, he had been hospitalized in another facility where he was treated with activated charcoal, crystalloids, and GI protectants after ingestion of an unknown amount of deracoxib. Upon discharge from the other facility, the owner noticed a small swelling on the left hock which progressed rapidly towards the stifle during that day. The owner reported that Rigby had decreased energy and inappetence.

Physical Examination

Body weight: 10.9 kg.

General, cardiovascular, and respiratory: Bright, alert, and responsive. Hydrated. T = 103.5°F (39.7°C), HR = 112 beats/minute, II/VI left apical systolic murmur, strong femoral pulses, panting, BCS = 3/5, mucous membranes = pink, CRT < 2 seconds, BP = 195 mmHg (Doppler) right thoracic limb.

Integumentary and musculoskeletal: Ambulatory and weight-bearing on all limbs. The left pelvic limb was warm and erythematous with pitting edema that extended from the tarsus to the proximal tibia. The dog was able to fully flex the tarsal joint, however he was painful upon deep palpation.

Peripheral lymph nodes, external genital, neurologic, and ear/nose/throat examinations were all within normal limits.

CASE EXAMPLE 1—cont'd

Laboratory Findings

CBC, serum chemistries, and urinalysis were within normal limits.

Cytologic evaluation of an aspirate from a fluid pocket on the left tarsus revealed marked neutrophilic inflammation with both intracellular and extracellular cocci that occasionally formed chains.

Case Progression

Rigby was admitted to the ICU and managed with IV crystalloids and ampicillin/sulbactam with a differential diagnosis of severe cellulitis or NFM. Over the next several hours, the proximal left pelvic limb also became edematous and amputation was performed without complication (Fig. 50.8). The amputated limb revealed a positive finger test,[65] and subsequent histopathologic characterization of the tissue revealed extensive acute, diffuse, severe fibrinosuppurative cellulitis and dermatitis with hemorrhage and edema, compatible with NFM. The next morning, aerobic culture of the fluid aspirate yielded a pure, heavy growth of *S. canis*. Rigby's management in the ICU was continued for 2 additional days, and he was discharged on oral amoxicillin, tramadol, gabapentin, and douxo wipes for his amputation site. The heart murmur, which was appreciated on presentation and may have indicated concern for streptococcal endocarditis, was not recognized subsequently.

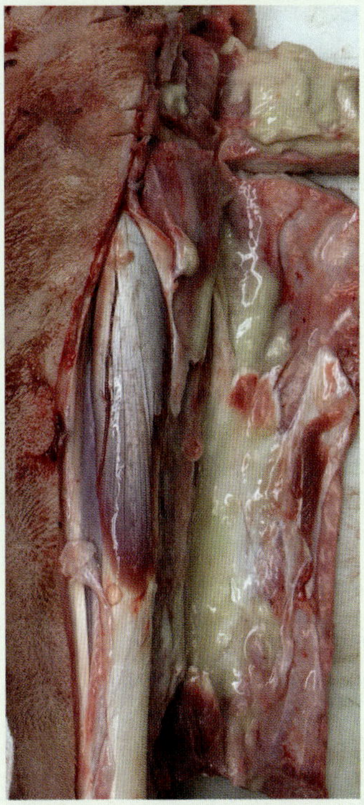

Fig. 50.8. Necrotizing fasciitis myositis of the proximal left pelvic limb caused by *Streptococcus canis* in an 8-year old male neutered Boston terrier. The limb was amputated and the image shows purulent material between fascial planes.

CASE EXAMPLE 2

Signalment

"Jazz," a 6-year-old female spayed miniature pinscher from Fairfield in northern California.

History

Jazz was brought to the University of California, Davis, Veterinary Medical Teaching Hospital, for evaluation of anorexia, lethargy, and diarrhea. Two days previously, the dog had been seen by the dermatology service for a focal area of alopecia and scaling on the dorsal midline in the thoracolumbar region that first appeared 7 months previously, enlarged to 6 × 4 cm in diameter over 2 months, and then remained static in size for the subsequent 5 months. Skin scrapings and fungal culture were performed, and four skin biopsies were obtained. An underlying vasculitis was suspected, and treatment with vitamin E (200 U, PO, q12h) and an oral fatty acid supplement was recommended pending the results of the diagnostic tests. The following day the owner noted edema of the right pelvic limb and discontinued the medications. Over the next 24 hours, Jazz became lethargic, inappetent, and developed liquid diarrhea and polydipsia. Jazz had been vaccinated regularly for canine distemper, adenovirus, and parvovirus infections and rabies and normally ate a commercial dry dog food. She was last vaccinated just after the skin lesion first appeared. The dog was mostly indoors, going outside on leash walks only, and there were no other pets in the household.

Other Medical History

Jazz had been spayed 5 weeks previously, at which time pyometra was an incidental finding and was treated with a 7-day course of amoxicillin.

Physical Examination

Body weight: 3.3 kg.

General: Lethargic, alert and ambulatory, but weak. Vocalized on palpation of the thorax and abdomen. T = 102.2°F (39.0°C), HR = 120 beats/minute, RR = 60 breaths/minute, mucous membranes pink, CRT = 1 second.

Eyes, ears, nose, and throat: Mild conjunctival hyperemia and bilateral serous ocular discharge were present.

Integument: There was mild subcutaneous edema and a small amount of serosanguinous fluid in the region of the skin biopsies, but sutures remained intact. There was a single, raised erythematous lesion adjacent to the skin biopsies that measured 0.5 × 0.5 cm in diameter. Severe edema was noted in the cranioventral thoracic region, which extended over an area that was 9 × 5 cm in diameter.

Other systems, including peripheral lymph nodes: No clinically significant findings.

Laboratory Findings

CBC: HCT 53.1% (40%–55%), MCV 71.2 fL (65–75 fL), MCHC 36.7 g/dL (33–36 g/dL), nucleated RBC 24/100 WBC, WBC 2,200 cells/μL (6,000–13,000 cells/μL), neutrophils 792 cells/μL (3,000–10,500 cells/μL), band neutrophils 740 cells/μL, metamyelocytes 88 cells/μL, myelocytes 44 cells/μL, lymphocytes 308 cells/μL (1,000–4,000 cells/μL), monocytes 220 cells/μL (150–1,200 cells/μL), platelets 97,000/μL (150,000–400,000 platelets/μL).

Markedly toxic band neutrophils, metamyelocytes, and myelocytes; moderately toxic neutrophils; and rare reactive lymphocytes were present.

Serum chemistry profile: Sodium 128 mmol/L (145–154 mmol/L), potassium 4.4 mmol/L (3.6–5.3 mmol/L), chloride 90 mmol/L (108–118 mmol/L), bicarbonate 21 mmol/L (16–26 mmol/L), phosphorus 8.7 mg/dL (3.0–6.2 mg/dL), calcium 10.0 mg/dL (9.7–11.5 mg/dL), BUN 63 mg/dL (5–21 mg/dL), creatinine 0.9 mg/dL

Continued

CASE EXAMPLE 2—cont'd

(0.3–1.2 mg/dL), glucose 75 mg/dL (64–123 mg/dL), total protein 5.6 g/dL (5.4–7.6 g/dL), albumin 2.2 g/dL (3.0–4.4 g/dL), globulin 3.4 g/dL (1.8–3.9 g/dL), ALT 185 U/L (19–67 U/L), AST 128 U/L (19–42 U/L), ALP 539 U/L (21–170 U/L), cholesterol 526 mg/dL (135–361 mg/dL), total bilirubin 0.5 mg/dL (0–0.2 mg/dL).

Urinalysis: SpG 1.021; pH 5.0, 1+ protein (SSA), 1+ bilirubin, 4+ hemoprotein, no glucose, no ketones, rare WBC/HPF, 0–2 RBC/HPF, few amorphous crystals, no bacteria seen.

Imaging Findings

Abdominal ultrasound: Enlargement of the uterine stump was present dorsal to the bladder. There were no cystic structures within the stump and no evidence of fluid in this region or lymphadenopathy.

Cytologic Findings

Needle aspiration of edema fluid from a region adjacent to the right axilla revealed large numbers of cocci, some in pairs, in the absence of significant numbers of leukocytes.

Microbiologic Testing

Aerobic bacterial culture (aspirate of edema fluid): Large numbers of *S. canis* colonies were isolated after overnight culture, and identified by MALDI-TOF the same day. A subsequent blood culture failed to yield any bacteria.

Treatment and Outcome

Treatment with IV fluids (0.9% NaCl with 20 mEq KCl/L) was initiated before the culture results were obtained. Ampicillin (20 mg/kg, IV, q6h), enrofloxacin (5 mg/kg, IV, q24h), and butorphanol were administered. The dog's body temperature subsequently dropped to 98.0°F (36.7°C) and blood glucose concentration dropped to 30 mg/dL. Fluids were supplemented with dextrose and a warming pad was used, and the dog's temperature returned to normal limits. Within hours, the edema had spread to the abdomen, and evidence of bruising appeared on the right thorax and ventrum. The raised erythematous lesion on the dorsum ulcerated, and dehiscence of the biopsy site adjacent to this region became apparent. Blood work showed a hematocrit of 39%, 2,700 WBCs/μL, 1,323 band neutrophils/μL, 702 neutrophils/μL, 162 lymphocytes/μL, 513 monocytes/μL, and 37,000 platelets/μL; serum sodium concentration was 142 mmol/L, potassium 3.7 mmol/L, creatinine 0.4 mg/dL, BUN 23 mg/dL, albumin 1.2 g/dL, globulin 3.1 g/dL, cholesterol 221 mg/dL, and total bilirubin 2.3 mg/dL. The activities of ALT, AST, and ALP were 79 U/L, 136 U/L, and 292 U/L, respectively. Treatment with dextran and plasma was initiated, but systolic blood pressure dropped to 80 mmHg, and the region adjacent to the biopsy sites became firm and painful and tore when palpated. Ampicillin was replaced by penicillin G (40,000 U/kg, IV, q6h), and enrofloxacin treatment was stopped. Forty-eight hours after admission, the dog was anesthetized and a large portion of necrotic skin was surgically debrided from the dog's dorsum. The debrided region was covered with a stent. During recovery, the dog was tachypneic, had increased lung sounds, and systolic blood pressure dropped to 50 mmHg. The dog developed respiratory arrest, and an endotracheal tube was placed, from which bloody fluid emanated. Cardiac arrest then ensued, and there was no response to closed cardiopulmonary resuscitation efforts.

Necropsy Findings

At necropsy, necrosis extended through the intercostal musculature of the right thoracic wall. Histopathologic lesions included severe, focally extensive, hemorrhagic and necrotizing panniculitis and fasciitis with intralesional bacteria and multifocal thrombi; diffuse necrotizing myositis of the right thoracic wall with intralesional bacteria; severe congestion and mild, multifocal hemorrhage and thrombosis within the kidneys; centrilobular congestion and severe bile stasis within the liver; congestion and hemorrhage within the lung; and generalized lymphoid depletion and sinusoidal histiocytosis within lymph nodes. Around the uterine stump, there was focal fibrosis and mild granulomatous serositis, but very few *S. canis* were cultured from the uterine stump. Histopathology of the biopsy specimens that had been collected before the onset of systemic illness showed severe, diffuse adnexal atrophy; mild, chronic, lymphoplasmacytic mural folliculitis; focal granulomatous furunculosis with hyperkeratosis; and mild, multifocal, perivascular neutrophilic dermatitis. No microorganisms were seen, although only special staining with PAS and Gomori's methenamine silver (GMS) was performed.

Diagnosis

NF, myositis, and STSS associated with *S. canis* infection.

Comments

This rare detailed case description illustrates how rapidly NF can progress and the ineffectiveness of antibiotic treatment in the presence of devitalized tissue. Clinical findings more than satisfied the criteria for diagnosis of STSS and NF in Box 50.1. The source of infection and the role that the uterine stump infection played was unclear. The effect of treatment of Jazz with the fluoroquinolone antibiotic, enrofloxacin, on development of STSS/NF is unclear, but this class of antibiotics is contraindicated in cases of *S. canis* infection since they may exacerbate disease as discussed earlier.[19]

SUGGESTED READINGS

Chung YS, Kwon KH, Shin S, et al. Characterization of veterinary hospital-associated isolates of *Enterococcus* species in Korea. *J Microbiol Biotechnol.* 2014;28:386–393.

Guzman Prieto AM, van Schaik W, Rogers MRC, et al. Global emergence and dissemination of enterococci as nosocomial pathogens: attack of the clones? *Frontiers Microbiol.* 2016;7:1–15.

Hammerum AM. Enterococci of animal origin and their significance for public health. *Clin Microbiol Infect.* 2012;18:619–625.

KuKanich KS, Lubbers BV. Review of enterococci isolated from canine and feline urine specimens from 2006 to 2011. *J Am Anim Hosp Assoc.* 2015;51:148–154.

Morrow BL, McNatt R, Joyce L, et al. Highly pathogenic beta-hemolytic streptococcal infections in cats from an institutionalized hoarding facility and a multi-species comparison. *J Fel Med Surg.* 2016;18:318–327.

Priestnall SL, Mitchell JA, Walker CA, et al. New and emerging pathogens in canine infectious respiratory disease. *Vet Pathol.* 2014;51:492–502.

Velineni S, Timoney JF, Russell K, et al. Clones of *Streptococcus zooepidemicus* from outbreaks of hemorrhagic canine pneumonia and associated immune responses. *Clin Vacc Immunol.* 2014;21:1246–1252.

REFERENCES

1. Wilson KS, Maroney SA, Gander RM. The family pet as an unlikely source of group A beta-hemolytic streptococcal infection in humans. *Pediatr Infect Dis J.* 1995;14:372–375.
2. Schleifer KH, Kilpper-Balz R. Transfer of *Streptococcus faecalis* and *Streptococcus faecium* to the genus *Enterococcus* nom. rev. as *Enterococcus faecalis* com. nov. and *Enterococcus faecium* com. nov. *Int J Syst Bacteriol.* 1984;34:31–34.
3. Lamm CG, Ferguson AC, Lehenbauer TW, et al. Streptococcal infection in dogs: a retrospective study of 393 cases. *Vet Pathol.* 2010;47:387–395.
4. Pesavento PA, Bannasch MJ, Bachmann R, et al. Fatal *Streptococcus canis* infections in intensively housed shelter cats. *Vet Pathol.* 2007;44:218–221.
5. Tillman PC, Dodson ND, Indiveri M. Group G streptococcal epizootic in a closed cat colony. *J Clin Microbiol.* 1982;16:1057–1060.
6. Morrow BL, McNatt R, Joyce L, et al. Highly pathogenic beta-hemolytic streptococcal infections in cats from an institutionalized hoarding facility and a multi-species comparison. *J Feline Med Surg.* 2016;18:318–327.
7. Prescott JF, Miller CW, Mathews KA, et al. Update on canine streptococcal toxic shock syndrome and necrotizing fasciitis. *Can Vet J.* 1997;38:241–242.

8. Sura R, Hinckley LS, Risatti GR, et al. Fatal necrotising fasciitis and myositis in a cat associated with *Streptococcus canis*. *Vet Rec*. 2008;162:450–453.
9. Miller CW, Prescott JF, Mathews KA, et al. Streptococcal toxic shock syndrome in dogs. *J Am Vet Med Assoc*. 1996;209:1421–1426.
10. Mastrocco A, Prittie J. Early and aggressive surgical debridement and negative pressure wound therapy to treat necrotizing fasciitis in three dogs. *Vet Surg*. 2021. Mar 16. Online ahead of print.
11. Walker MJ, Barnett TC, McArthur JD, et al. Disease manifestations and pathogenic mechanisms of Group A *Streptococcus*. *Clin Microbiol Rev*. 2014;27:264–301.
12. Taillefer M, Dunn M. Group G streptococcal toxic shock-like syndrome in three cats. *J Am Anim Hosp Assoc*. 2004;40:418–422.
13. Kulendra E, Corr S. Necrotising fasciitis with sub-periosteal *Streptococcus canis* infection in two puppies. *Vet Comp Orthop Traumatol*. 2008;21:474–477.
14. Iglauer F, Kunstyr I, Morstedt R, et al. *Streptococcus canis* arthritis in a cat breeding colony. *J Exp Anim Sci*. 1991;34:59–65.
15. Kruger EF, Byrne BA, Pesavento P, et al. Relationship between clinical manifestations and pulsed-field gel profiles of *Streptococcus canis* isolates from dogs and cats. *Vet Microbiol*. 2010;146:167–171.
16. DeWinter LM, Prescott JF. Relatedness of *Streptococcus canis* from canine streptococcal toxic shock syndrome and necrotizing fasciitis. *Can J Vet Res*. 1999;63:90–95.
17. Fulde M, Rohde M, Hitzmann A, et al. SCM, a novel M-like protein from *Streptococcus canis*, binds (mini)-plasminogen with high affinity and facilitates bacterial transmigration. *Biochem J*. 2011;434:523–535.
18. Bergmann S, Eichorn I, Kohler TP, et al. SCM, the M protein of *Streptococcus canis* binds immunoglobulin G. *Frontiers Cell Infect Microbiol*. 2017;7:80.
19. DeWinter LM, Low DE, Prescott JF. Virulence of *Streptococcus canis* from canine streptococcal toxic shock syndrome and necrotizing fasciitis. *Vet Microbiol*. 1999;70:95–110.
20. Ingrey KT, Ren J, Prescott JF. A fluoroquinolone induces a novel mitogen-encoding bacteriophage in *Streptococcus canis*. *Infect Immun*. 2003;71:3028–3033.
21. Acke E, Abbott Y, Pinilla M, et al. Isolation of *Streptococcus zooepidemicus* from three dogs in close contact with horses. *Vet Rec*. 2010;167:102–103.
22. Priestnall SL, Mitchell JA, Walker CA, et al. New and emerging pathogens in canine infectious respiratory disease. *Vet Pathol*. 2014;51:492–504.
23. Velineni S, Timoney JF, Russell K, et al. Clones of *Streptococcus zooepidemicus* from outbreaks of hemorrhagic canine pneumonia and associated immune responses. *Clin Vaccine Immunol*. 2014;21:1246–1252.
24. Priestnall SL, Erles K, Brooks HW, et al. Characterization of pneumonia due to *Streptococcus equi* subsp. *zooepidemicus* in dogs. *Clin Vaccine Immunol*. 2010;17:1790–1796.
25. FitzGerald W, Crowe B, Brennan P, et al. Acute fatal haemorrhagic pneumonia caused by *Streptococcus equi zooepidemicus* in greyhounds in Ireland with subsequent typing of the isolates. *Vet Rec*. 2017;181:119.
26. Blum S, Elad D, Zukin N, et al. Outbreak of *Streptococcus equi* subsp. *zooepidemicus* infections in cats. *Vet Microbiol*. 2010;144:236–239.
27. Britton AP, Davies JL. Rhinitis and meningitis in two shelter cats caused by *Streptococcus equi* subspecies *zooepidemicus*. *J Comp Pathol*. 2010;143:70–74.
28. Britton AP, Blum SE, Legge C, et al. Multi-locus sequence typing of *Streptococcus equi* subspecies *zooepidemicus* strains isolated from cats. *J Vet Diagn Invest*. 2018;30:126–129.
29. Martin-Vaquero P, da Costa RC, Daniels JB. Presumptive meningoencephalitis secondary to extension of otitis media/interna caused by *Streptococcus equi* subspecies *zooepidemicus* in a cat. *J Feline Med Surg*. 2011;13:606–609.
30. Larson LJ, Henningson J, Sharp P, et al. Efficacy of the canine influenza virus H3N8 vaccine to decrease severity of clinical disease after cochallenge with canine influenza virus and *Streptococcus equi* subsp. *zooepidemicus*. *Clin Vaccine Immunol*. 2011;18:559–564.
31. Maboni G, Seguel M, Lorton A, et al. Canine infectious respiratory disease: new insights into the etiology and epidemiology of associated pathogens. *PLoS One*. 2019;14. e0215817.
32. Day MJ, Carey S, Clercx C, et al. Aetiology of canine infectious respiratory disease complex and prevalence of its pathogens in Europe. *J Comp Pathol*. 2020;176:86–108.
33. Paillot R, Darby AC, Robinson C, et al. Identification of three novel superantigen-encoding genes in *Streptococcus equi* subsp. *zooepidemicus, szeF, szeN*, and *szeP*. *Infect Immun*. 2010;78:4817–4827.
34. Ladlow J, Scase T, Waller A. Canine strangles case reveals a new host susceptible to infection with *Streptococcus equi*. *J Clin Microbiol*. 2006;44:2664–2665.
35. Vela AI, Falsen E, Simarro I, et al. Neonatal mortality in puppies due to bacteremia by *Streptococcus dysgalactiae* subsp. *dysgalactiae*. *J Clin Microbiol*. 2006;44:666–668.
36. Devriese LA, Haesebrouck F. *Streptococcus suis* infections in horses and cats. *Vet Rec*. 1992;130:380.
37. Roels S, Devroye O, Buys H, et al. Isolation of *Streptococcus suis* from a cat with meningoencephalitis. *Vet Microbiol*. 2009;136:206–207.
38. Muckle A, Giles J, Lund L, et al. Isolation of *Streptococcus suis* from the urine of a clinically ill dog. *Can Vet J*. 2010;51:773–774.
39. Salasia SI, Lammler C, Devriese LA. Serotypes and putative virulence markers of *Streptococcus suis* isolates from cats and dogs. *Res Vet Sci*. 1994;57:259–261.
40. De Martino L, Nizza S, de Martinis C, et al. *Streptococcus constellatus*-associated pyoderma in a dog. *J Med Microbiol*. 2012;61:438–442.
41. Schlegel L, Grimont F, Ageron E, et al. Reappraisal of the taxonomy of the *Streptococcus bovis/Streptococcus equinus* complex and related species: description of *Streptococcus gallolyticus* subsp. *gallolyticus* subsp. nov., *S. gallolyticus* subsp. *macedonicus* subsp. nov. and *S. gallolyticus* subsp. *pasteurianus* subsp. nov. *Int J Syst Evol Microbiol*. 2003;53: 631–645.
42. Boleij A, van Gelder MM, Swinkels DW, et al. Clinical importance of *Streptococcus gallolyticus* infection among colorectal cancer patients: systematic review and meta-analysis. *Clin Infect Dis*. 2011;53:870–878.
43. Sykes JE, Kittleson MD, Pesavento PA, et al. Evaluation of the relationship between causative organisms and clinical characteristics of infective endocarditis in dogs: 71 cases (1992-2005). *J Am Vet Med Assoc*. 2006;228:1723–1734.
44. Tou SP, Adin DB, Castleman WL. Mitral valve endocarditis after dental prophylaxis in a dog. *J Vet Intern Med*. 2005;19:268–270.
45. Abbott Y, Kirby BM, Karczmarczyk M, et al. High-level gentamicin-resistant and vancomycin-resistant *Enterococcus faecium* isolated from a wound in a dog. *J Small Anim Pract*. 2009;50:194–197.
46. Manson JM, Keis S, Smith JM, et al. Characterization of a vancomycin-resistant *Enterococcus faecalis* (VREF) isolate from a dog with mastitis: further evidence of a clonal lineage of VREF in New Zealand. *J Clin Microbiol*. 2003;41:3331–3333.
47. Simjee S, White DG, McDermott PF, et al. Characterization of Tn1546 in vancomycin-resistant *Enterococcus faecium* isolated from canine urinary tract infections: evidence of gene exchange between human and animal enterococci. *J Clin Microbiol*. 2002;40:4659–4665.
48. Arias CA, Murray BE. *Enterococcus* species, *Streptococcus gallolyticus* group, and *Leuconostoc* species. In: Bennett JE, Dolin R, Blaser MJ, eds. *Mandell, Douglas and Bennett's Principles and Practice of Infectious Diseases*. Philadephia, PA: Elsevier Saunders; 2015:2328–2339.
49. Ghanem G, Hachem R, Jiang Y, et al. Outcomes for and risk factors associated with vancomycin-resistant *Enterococcus faecalis* and vancomycin-resistant *Enterococcus faecium* bacteremia in cancer patients. *Infect Control Hosp Epidemiol*. 2007;28:1054–1059.
50. Mohamed JA, Huang DB. Biofilm formation by enterococci. *J Med Microbiol*. 2007;56:1581–1588.
51. Guzman Prieto AM, van Schaik W, Rogers MR, et al. Global emergence and dissemination of enterococci as nosocomial pathogens: attack of the clones? *Front Microbiol*. 2016;7:788.
52. Damborg P, Top J, Hendrickx AP, et al. Dogs are a reservoir of ampicillin-resistant *Enterococcus faecium* lineages associated with human infections. *Appl Environ Microbiol*. 2009;75:2360–2365.
53. Hammerum AM. Enterococci of animal origin and their significance for public health. *Clin Microbiol Infect*. 2012;18:619–625.

54. Jackson CR, Fedorka-Cray PJ, Davis JA, et al. Prevalence, species distribution and antimicrobial resistance of enterococci isolated from dogs and cats in the United States. *J Appl Microbiol.* 2009;107:1269–1278.
55. KuKanich KS, Lubbers BV. Review of enterococci isolated from canine and feline urine specimens from 2006 to 2011. *J Am Anim Hosp Assoc.* 2015;51:148–154.
56. Delgado M, Neto I, Correia JH, et al. Antimicrobial resistance and evaluation of susceptibility testing among pathogenic enterococci isolated from dogs and cats. *Int J Antimicrob Agents.* 2007;30:98–100.
57. Naser SM, Vancanneyt M, De Graef E, et al. *Enterococcus canintestini* sp. nov., from faecal samples of healthy dogs. *Int J Syst Evol Microbiol.* 2005;55:2177–2182.
58. Ossiprandi MC, Bottarelli E, Cattabiani F, et al. Susceptibility to vancomycin and other antibiotics of 165 *Enterococcus* strains isolated from dogs in Italy. *Comp Immunol Microbiol Infect Dis.* 2008;31:1–9.
59. Helie P, Higgins R. Diarrhea associated with *Enterococcus faecium* in an adult cat. *J Vet Diagn Invest.* 1999;11:457–458.
60. Nicklas JL, Moisan P, Stone MR, et al. In situ molecular diagnosis and histopathological characterization of enteroadherent *Enterococcus hirae* infection in pre-weaning-age kittens. *J Clin Microbiol.* 2010;48:2814–2820.
61. Watson VE, Jacob ME, Bruno-Barcena JM. Influence of the intestinal microbiota on disease susceptibility in kittens with experimentally-induced carriage of atypical enteropathogenic *Escherichia coli. Vet Microbiol.* 2019;231:197–206.
62. Benyacoub J, Czarnecki-Maulden GL, Cavadini C, et al. Supplementation of food with *Enterococcus faecium* (SF68) stimulates immune functions in young dogs. *J Nutr.* 2003;133:1158–1162.
63. Bybee SN, Scorza AV, Lappin MR. Effect of the probiotic *Enterococcus faecium* SF68 on presence of diarrhea in cats and dogs housed in an animal shelter. *J Vet Intern Med.* 2011;25:856–860.
64. Veir JK, Knorr R, Cavadini C, et al. Effect of supplementation with *Enterococcus faecium* (SF68) on immune functions in cats. *Vet Ther.* 2007;8: 229–238.
65. Pilla R, Guard BC, Steiner JM, et al. Administration of a synbiotic containing *Enterococcus faecium* does not significantly alter fecal microbiota richness or diversity in dogs with and without food-responsive chronic enteropathy. *Front Vet Sci.* 2019;6:277.
66. Fenimore A, Martin L, Lappin MR. Evaluation of metronidazole with and without *Enterococcus faecium* SF68 in shelter dogs with diarrhea. *Top Companion Anim Med.* 2017;32:100–103.
67. Clark RR, McGill DJ. Necrotizing fasciitis: always use the finger. *Br Med J.* 2005;330:880.
68. Garnett NL, Eydelloth RS, Swindle MM, et al. Hemorrhagic streptococcal pneumonia in newly procured research dogs. *J Am Vet Med Assoc.* 1982;181:1371–1374.
69. Pesavento PA, Hurley KF, Bannasch MJ, et al. A clonal outbreak of acute fatal hemorrhagic pneumonia in intensively housed (shelter) dogs caused by *Streptococcus equi* subsp. *zooepidemicus. Vet Pathol.* 2008;45:51–53.
70. Parks T, Barrett L, Jones N. Invasive streptococcal disease: a review for clinicians. *Br Med Bull.* 2015;115:77–89.
71. Bisno AL, Stevens DL. Streptococcus pyogenes. In: Bennett JE, Dolin R, Blaser MJ, eds. *Mandell, Douglas and Bennett's Principles and Practice of Infectious Diseases.* 8th ed. Philadephia, PA: Elsevier Saunders; 2015:2285–2299.
72. Fukushima Y, Tsuyuki Y, Goto M, et al. Species identification of beta-hemolytic streptococci from diseased companion animals and their antimicrobial resistance data in Japan (2017). *Jpn J Infect Dis.* 2019;72:94–98.
73. Lyskova P, Vydrzalova M, Mazurova J. Identification and antimicrobial susceptibility of bacteria and yeasts isolated from healthy dogs and dogs with otitis externa. *J Vet Med A Physiol Pathol Clin Med.* 2007;54:559–563.
74. Pedersen K, Jensen H, Finster K, et al. Occurrence of antimicrobial resistance in bacteria from diagnostic samples from dogs. *J Antimicrob Chemother.* 2007;60:775–781.
75. Irwin PJ, Parry BW. Streptococcal meningoencephalitis in a dog. *J Am Anim Hosp Assoc.* 1999;35:417–422.
76. Harada T, Tsuji N, Otsuki K, et al. Detection of the *esp* gene in high-level gentamicin resistant *Enterococcus faecalis* strains from pet animals in Japan. *Vet Microbiol.* 2005;106:139–143.
77. Dowzicky MJ. Susceptibility to tigecycline and linezolid among gram-positive isolates collected in the United States as part of the tigecycline evaluation and surveillance trial (TEST) between 2004 and 2009. *Clin Ther.* 2011;33:1964–1973.
78. Chou PY, Yoon J, Hersh-Boyle RA, et al. Multidrug-resistant orthopaedic surgical site infections treated with linezolid in four dogs. *VCOT Open.* 2020;3:e72–e76.
79. Freitas AR, Finisterra L, Tedim AP, et al. Linezolid- and multidrug-resistant enterococci in raw commercial dog food, Europe, 2019-2020. *Emerg Infect Dis.* 2020;27:2221–2224.
80. Swaminathan S, Alangaden GJ. Treatment of resistant enterococcal urinary tract infections. *Curr Infect Dis Rep.* 2010;12:455–464.
81. Carapetis JR, Steer AC, Mulholland EK, et al. The global burden of group A streptococcal diseases. *Lancet Infect Dis.* 2005;5:685–694.
82. Falck G. Group A streptococci in household pets' eyes: a source of infection in humans? *Scand J Infect Dis.* 1997;29:469–471.
83. Mayer G, Van Ore S. Recurrent pharyngitis in family of four. Household pet as reservoir of group A streptococci. *Postgrad Med.* 1983;74:277–279.
84. Samir A, Abdel-Moein KA, Zaher HM. Emergence of penicillin-macrolide-resistant *Streptococcus pyogenes* among pet animals: an ongoing public health threat. *Comp Immunol Microbiol Infect Dis.* 2020;68:101390.
85. Irwin PJ, Parry BW. Streptococcal meningoencephalitis in a dog. *J Am Anim Hosp Assoc.* 1999;35:417–422.
86. Stallings B, Ling GV, Lagenaur LA, et al. Septicemia and septic arthritis caused by *Streptococcus pneumoniae* in a cat: possible transmission from a child. *J Am Vet Med Assoc.* 1987;191:703–704.
87. Zhang S, Wilson F, Pace L. *Streptococcus pneumoniae*-associated cellulitis in a two-month-old domestic shorthair kitten. *J Vet Diagn Invest.* 2006;18:221–224.
88. Galperine T, Cazorla C, Blanchard E, et al. *Streptococcus canis* infections in humans: retrospective study of 54 patients. *J Infect.* 2007;55:23–26.
89. Lam MM, Clarridge JE 3rd, Young EJ, et al. The other group G *Streptococcus*: increased detection of *Streptococcus canis* ulcer infections in dog owners. *J Clin Microbiol.* 2007;45:2327–2329.
90. Lacave G, Coutard A, Troche G, et al. Endocarditis caused by *Streptococcus canis*: an emerging zoonosis? *Infection.* 2016;44:111–114.
91. Ohtaki H, Ohkusu K, Ohta H, et al. A case of sepsis caused by *Streptococcus canis* in a dog owner: a first case report of sepsis without dog bite in Japan. *J Infect Chemother.* 2013;19:1206–1209.
92. Pinho MD, Matos SC, Pomba C, et al. Multilocus sequence analysis of *Streptococcus canis* confirms the zoonotic origin of human infections and reveals genetic exchange with *Streptococcus dysgalactiae* subsp. *equisimilis. J Clin Microbiol.* 2013;51:1099–1109.
93. Pinho MD, Foster G, Pomba C, et al. *Streptococcus canis* are a single population infecting multiple animal hosts despite the diversity of the universally present M-like protein SCM. *Frontiers Microbiol.* 2019;10:631.
94. Abbott Y, Acke E, Khan S, et al. Zoonotic transmission of *Streptococcus equi* subsp. *zooepidemicus* from a dog to a handler. *J Med Microbiol.* 2010;59:120–123.

51

Staphylococcal Infections

J. Scott Weese, John F. Prescott

KEY POINTS

- First Described: 1882, Scotland (Alexander Ogsten).
- Causes: In dogs and cats, the most common staphylococcal pathogens are *Staphylococcus pseudintermedius, Staphylococcus aureus,* and *Staphylococcus schleiferi.*
- Geographic Distribution: Worldwide.
- Mode of Transmission: Transmission is primarily through direct contact. Indirect transmission via fomites or the environment can occur.
- Major Clinical Signs: Pyoderma, otitis externa, surgical site infections, osteomyelitis, bacteremia and endocarditis, bronchopneumonia, urinary tract infections, ocular surface infections, rarely necrotizing fasciitis and toxic shock syndrome, pyothorax and peritonitis, discospondylitis, arthritis.
- Differential Diagnoses: Clinical signs are indistinguishable from infections caused by other opportunistic bacterial pathogens.
- Human Health Significance: Humans can become colonized or infected with staphylococcal isolates that colonize or infect dogs and cats. Methicillin-resistant *S. aureus,* which can persistently colonize humans, is of greatest concern, although human-pet transmission is probably much more common than pet-human transmission. *Staphylococcus pseudintermedius,* which can persistently colonize dogs, has occasionally been isolated from sick and healthy people who are in contact with dogs, and is of possible concern because of its tendency to show a high degree of MDR.

ETIOLOGIC AGENTS AND EPIDEMIOLOGY

The genus *Staphylococcus* contains a diverse genus of facultatively anaerobic bacteria that are widespread to ubiquitous commensals and opportunistic pathogens. They are gram-positive, catalase-positive cocci that tend to occur in clusters. As colonizers of mucous membranes and the skin, various *Staphylococcus* species can be found in or on most healthy animals. Widespread in healthy animals, staphylococci are classic opportunistic pathogens that can cause mild to life-threatening infections.

The clinical relevance of different staphylococcal species varies greatly. While virtually any species can cause disease, just a few species account for the vast majority of clinical infections. Staphylococcal species are divided into two main groups based on the production of the enzyme coagulase. Coagulase-positive staphylococci are the most virulent group and are most often associated with disease. The most important coagulase-positive species in dogs and cats are *Staphylococcus pseudintermedius*, *Staphylococcus aureus*, and *Staphylococcus schleiferi* subsp. *coagulans*. All can be found in healthy animals, but they account for a large percentage of opportunistic infections, including skin, ear, soft tissue, and urinary tract infections, and are leading causes of surgical site infections (SSIs).[1–5] *Staphylococcus intermedius* was previously considered the main *Staphylococcus* in dogs and cats, but it is now known that what was previously identified as *S. intermedius* is truly the closely related species *S. pseudintermedius*.[6,7]

Coagulase-negative staphylococci (CoNS) are common commensals that are often isolated as contaminants, but they can cause disease in certain situations. This group includes *Staphylococcus epidermidis*, *Staphylococcus haemolyticus*, *Staphylococcus xylosus*, *Staphylococcus sciuri*, *Staphylococcus schleiferi* subsp. *schleiferi*, and *Staphylococcus felis*, among others. Typically, CoNS infections involve compromised hosts and sites that have been injured by foreign bodies and invasive devices (e.g., IV catheters). Primary infections are uncommon, with the possible exception of *S. schleiferi* subsp. *schleiferi* pyoderma[8] and otitis and *S. felis* UTI.[9] Interpretation of the clinical relevance of CoNS is often complicated by their common presence at skin and mucosal surfaces and the corresponding potential for contamination during specimen collection.

There are differences in the epidemiology of staphylococcal colonization and infection between different staphylococcal species and between dogs and cats. Staphylococci have often been referred to as host-adapted species, but it is clear that dogs and cats can be infected by many different staphylococcal species. Regular transmission of staphylococci between species (e.g., human-pet) likely occurs and staphylococcal status is dynamic. While the term "colonization" is widely used to refer to the presence of staphylococci in or on healthy individuals, it is clear that there is no consistent "colonization" state. After exposure to a *Staphylococcus*, multiple outcomes may occur. The organism may be rapidly eliminated, reside in or on the haircoat or mucous membranes transiently (sometimes referred to as "contamination"), multiply and live on the host for a short period of time ("transient colonization"), or live on the host for prolonged periods of time. The degree of host adaptation of the *Staphylococcus* species and possibly the strain, and patient factors (e.g., immune status, commensal microbiota), presumably influence the outcome, although other factors such as genetics could also be involved. As a host-adapted *Staphylococcus*, *S. pseudintermedius* appears to be able to cause prolonged colonization in at least some dogs,[10] whereas, in contrast, *S. aureus* colonization in dogs appears to be more transient.[11,12]

The incidence of staphylococcal disease is poorly described, but staphylococci account for a large percentage of skin and soft tissue infections encountered in dogs and cats, along with a variety of less common conditions. Most, if not all, staphylococcal infections are secondary to an underlying cause (e.g. skin disease, wounds) and the constituents or basis of those underlying causes are the main factors associated with risk of staphylococcal infection.

Staphylococcus pseudintermedius

Staphylococcus pseudintermedius is a true canine commensal and is found on the skin or mucosal surfaces of a large percentage of dogs. Isolation rates of 31% to 68% have been reported in healthy dogs,[13–16] with higher rates (up to 100%) in puppies.[17] It is likely that the vast majority of dogs, if not all, harbor this species at least periodically. Colonization starts early in life, with puppies acquiring *S. pseudintermedius* from the dam within 8 hours after birth.[17] Various body sites can be colonized, particularly the nasal passages, oral cavity, skin, and perineal mucosa, although the pharyngeal mucosa seems to be a main colonization site.[18]

Staphylococcus pseudintermedius is less prevalent in cats, being reported in 6.8% to 22% of healthy cats.[15,19–21] As with dogs, opportunistic infections can develop, but the influence of long-term or transient colonization on risk of disease is unknown. In parallel with colonization rates, *S. pseudintermedius* infections are less common in cats than in dogs.[4]

Methicillin-resistant *S. pseudintermedius* (MRSP) has emerged as an important pathogen in veterinary medicine.

Staphylococcus aureus

Staphylococcus aureus is a well-recognized pathogen and common commensal, although it is less commonly found in dogs than *S. pseudintermedius*. It can be isolated from up to 12% to 14% of clinically healthy dogs and 4.3% to 20% of clinically healthy cats, but it may not truly be a commensal organism (at least in dogs) as carriage tends to be transient. Colonization may be highly human influenced, since the *S. aureus* strains found in dogs are often indistinguishable from those found in their human contacts.[15] It is possible that isolation of *S. aureus* often represents transient colonization or contamination acquired from humans. This appears to be particularly true with dogs. A study of dogs and their owners reported that in 50% of households where *S. aureus* was isolated from both a dog and family member, the *S. aureus* strains were indistinguishable, strongly suggesting interspecies transmission.[15] The situation with cats is less clear. Given the higher apparent prevalence of *S. aureus* colonization in cats in some studies and the lack of another predominant coagulase-positive *Staphylococcus* species commensal in cats, it is possible that *S. aureus* is a true feline commensal. Regardless, it can clearly be isolated from a small but still appreciable percentage of clinically healthy dogs and cats and can also cause disease in certain situations. The highest isolation rates are from skin and ear infections.[22] Risk factors for colonization have not been adequately investigated and may relate to the amount or degree of human contact.

Staphylococcus schleiferi subsp. *coagulans*

Staphylococcus schleiferi contains two subspecies; the coagulase-positive *S. schleiferi* subsp. *coagulans* and the coagulase-negative *S. schleiferi* subsp. *schleiferi*. *Staphylococcus schleiferi* subsp. *coagulans* is less commonly identified than *S. pseudintermedius* and *S. aureus*, but can be found in 0.8% to 4% of healthy dogs and 0% to 2% of healthy cats.[1,15,19,23,24] It is most commonly implicated in otitis externa and pyoderma,[8,19,25,26] but is rarely identified in other types of infections.[27] There appears to be prominent geographic variation in reports of this pathogen. Whether this is a result of true geographic variation or differences in laboratory identification is unknown. This species may be misidentified as *S. pseudintermedius* or *S. intermedius* group if methods aimed at differentiating it from those similar species are not used. This may be of little clinical consequence given the identical approach to management of infections caused by these species.

Coagulase-Negative Staphylococci

The coagulase-negative *Staphylococcus* spp. group contains a large number of species that are commonly found in healthy dogs and cats, along with virtually all other mammalian species. They are essentially ubiquitous inhabitants of the skin, nasal and oral cavities, pharynx, perineal mucosa, GI tract, and conjunctiva of dogs, cats, and other species. Commonly reported species from dogs include *S. epidermidis*, *S. xylosus*, *S. schleiferi* subsp. *schleiferi*, and *S. sciuri*, with *S. epidermidis*, *S. felis*, *S. haemolyticus*, *Staphylococcus saprophyticus*, and *Staphylococcus simulans* often reported in cats.[9,17,28–38] However, a broad range of other species can be encountered. As diagnostic laboratories rapidly move to methods such as MALDI-TOF MS that provide more accurate speciation (as opposed to the common generic identification of isolates as CoNS), the range of CoNS that are encountered will probably increase. Genus-level identification of CoNS has predominated in the past because of the effort required to speciate isolates, particularly when speciation would have little to no impact on diagnosis or management of cases. However, as more information about different species becomes available, it is likely that differences in the epidemiology and clinical relevance of different CoNS will be identified.

Despite widespread colonization, CoNS infections are uncommon. While most, if not all, CoNS are opportunistic pathogens with the potential to cause disease, virulence tends to be limited and CoNS are most often isolated as commensals or contaminants, not pathogens. In human medicine, CoNS are primarily a concern in hospitalized individuals, where skin, soft tissue, bloodstream, and invasive device infections predominate.[39–41] The role of CoNS in disease in dogs and cats is poorly investigated and complicated by studies that report any isolation of CoNS as "infection." Differentiation of infection versus contamination is a challenge, with most CoNS being of minimal concern, but some species (i.e., *S. schleiferi* subsp. *schleiferi*, *Staphylococcus lugdunensis*, and *S. felis*) are potentially important causes of community-onset disease. While rare, invasive *S. lugdunensis* infections have been reported in dogs,[42,43] and this may be a more virulent CoNS.

Methicillin-Resistant Staphylococci

While staphylococci are inherently susceptible to most antimicrobials, acquired resistance emerged as a concern shortly after the start of the "antibiotic era." Staphylococci have demonstrated an impressive ability to acquire new resistance genes in response to continued antimicrobial development, and resistant staphylococci have serious impacts on the health and welfare of both humans and animals.

Methicillin resistance is of particular concern. While methicillin is not used clinically in animals, the mechanism that confers resistance to methicillin (*mecA*) renders staphylococci resistant to virtually all beta-lactam antimicrobials—penicillins, cephalosporins, and carbapenems. This encompasses a large percentage of the antimicrobials that are used, particularly empirically. Additionally, methicillin-resistant staphylococci (MRS) commonly possess other resistance genes, further limiting effective antimicrobial options. Methicillin resistance has emerged in all clinically relevant staphylococci, and MRS have been isolated from a wide range of companion animal, food animal, exotic, and wildlife species.

As with methicillin-susceptible staphylococci, MRS can be found as part of the commensal microbiota of healthy individuals. Indeed, the majority of humans and animals that harbor MRS do so without any evidence of disease. Methicillin resistance is not, itself, a virulence factor, since it simply confers resistance to antimicrobials. Infections caused by MRS are the same as those caused by susceptible staphylococci, and occur in situations where secondary infections can develop. However, they are harder to treat because of the limited options and failure of empirical therapy can have a negative impact on outcome.

Much of the attention regarding MRS in dogs and cats initially focused on methicillin-resistant *S. aureus* (MRSA).[44–51] The emergence of MRSA in dogs and cats appears to be a direct reflection of the spread of MRSA in the human population; MRSA infections in pets were noted after MRSA emerged as an important cause of disease in the general human population and with MRSA strains from animals usually reflecting predominant human strains.[48,51–54] Whether MRSA is truly established in the dog and cat population, or whether colonization and infection of those species is a result of direct infection from humans is unclear. Regardless, MRSA can be isolated from a small percentage (e.g., 0% to 4%) of clinically healthy dogs cats.[48,55–63] Higher rates can be encountered periodically in animals in veterinary facilities; however, most instances of MRSA isolation are not associated with veterinary hospitals. Ownership by a human health care worker and participation in hospital visitation programs are risk factors for MRSA colonization in dogs,[11] as might be expected based on the increased likelihood of exposure to colonized people. Other risk factors for MRSA infection or colonization have been identified, with varying strength of evidence, particularly antimicrobial exposure and hospitalization.[22,59,64–66] Contact with children has also been identified as a risk factor.[11] Although these, and potentially other, risk factors should be considered, MRSA can be identified in any animal, and absence of known risk factors should not lead to excluding MRSA from consideration. In humans and horses, MRSA colonization is a risk factor for clinical MRSA infection in certain circumstances (e.g., after admission to the hospital).[67,68] It is reasonable to assume that this also applies to dogs and cats, yet this is not proven. Although MRSA colonization has zoonotic concerns (see below), the animal health implications of MRSA colonization in clinically healthy animals are likely minimal.

While MRSA was the first prominent methicillin-resistant *Staphylococcus* sp. in animals, MRSP has surpassed MRSA in its impact on dogs and cats. As with methicillin-susceptible strains, MRSP can be found in or on clinically healthy dogs and cats, with a wide range of reported prevalence (e.g., 0% to 17%).[29,61,63,69–76] MRSP is an opportunistic pathogen, and colonization does not necessarily lead to disease. Carriage of MRSP prior to tibial plateau leveling osteotomy (TPLO) was shown to be a risk factor for MRSP SSI,[77] but whether this applies to other surgical procedures or other diseases is unknown. It is reasonable to assume that colonization poses some degree of risk of subsequent infection in many situations, albeit presumably rather low and dependent on the presence of factors that predispose to development of an opportunistic infection. Reported risk factors for MRSP colonization or infection include antimicrobial exposure (particularly beta-lactams, immunosuppressive therapy, and hospitalization).[75,78–80] MRSP infections are not distinguishable clinically from those caused by susceptible strains, but are increasingly problematic because of the limited treatment options, particularly since MRSP isolates in many regions are commonly resistant to most available antimicrobials.

Methicillin resistance is not uncommon in commensal CoNS. Studies have reported prevalence ranging from 5% to 13% in clinically healthy dogs, and 5% in clinically healthy cats.[34,55,81] Methicillin-resistant strains are no more pathogenic than methicillin-susceptible strains, and the implications of colonization with methicillin-resistant CoNS are typically inconsequential although these strains are likely sources of acquired methicillin resistance for more virulent staphylococcal species.

CLINICAL FEATURES

Pathogenesis, Clinical Signs, and Physical Examination Findings

Staphylococci can possess a wide array of potential virulence factors; however, the role that many of these play in the actual development of disease is variable. Some virulence factors facilitate adhesion to, and colonization of host tissues. Others encode secreted enzymes and toxins that are responsible for invasion as well as local and distant disease. The pathophysiology of disease is complex and only superficially understood, reflecting the variable presence of numerous staphylococcal virulence determinants in different strains of the more pathogenic species. Interactions between various virulence factors are presumably critical, because no single virulence factor has been shown to be sufficient to establish an infection.

The ability to colonize body sites is a critical component of virulence, because it allows staphylococci to remain on or in the body waiting for an opportunity to cause an infection, particularly after an underlying insult such as a break in the body's physical or immunologic barriers. Important among these factors are surface adhesins, which do not directly result in damage to host tissues, but create an environment where staphylococci can persist. Adhesins may also facilitate evasion of the immune system. For *S. aureus*, the most important is probably protein A, which binds to the Fc portion of IgG.[82] Other surface proteins that include clumping factors, fibronectin-binding proteins, coagulase, and collagen-binding protein are important, since they each give pathogenic staphylococci the ability to readily colonize breaks in the skin or mucosal surfaces as the first part of the infection process. Once the organism reaches a sufficient density at this local site of infection, release of a peptide signal through the Agr quorum-sensing system activates many of the toxins and degradative enzymes while downregulating the numerous adhesion molecules. Various hemolysin toxins can lyse erythrocytes and other body cells. Proteases can cleave antibodies, play a role in protection against neutrophil defensins and platelet microbicidal peptides, contribute to destruction of tissue protein, and potentiate invasion.[83] Hyaluronidase and hyaluronate lysate may further contribute to virulence through digestion of hyaluronic acid in connective tissue and promoting degradation of tissues.[84,85] Lipase has a negative effect on the host's immune function and may help the bacterium harvest nutrients from the local environment. Alpha toxin is a potent membrane-damaging toxin that can produce local cell damage. Leukocidins damage leukocytes and lipid membranes. One, the Panton-Valentine leukocidin, has received much attention because of its apparent role in severe MRSA skin and soft tissue infections, as well as necrotizing fasciitis and necrotizing pneumonia in humans.[86–89] This leukocidin has been found in MRSA from dogs and cats,[90,91] but its role in disease is still unclear. Enterotoxin production is mediated by several staphylococcal enterotoxin genes, many of which can be found in *S. aureus* from dogs.[92,93] However, it is unclear whether staphylococcal enteric disease is of relevance in dogs and cats. Other toxins of note include exfoliative toxins A and B, which cause staphylococcal scalded skin syndrome, and toxic shock syndrome toxins, which cause toxic shock syndrome.

Less is known about *S. pseudintermedius*, but evidence indicates that this species has numerous virulence factors similar to those of *S. aureus*, such as protein A, leukocidins, exfoliative toxins, other exotoxins, fibronectin-binding protein, and biofilm-producing factors.[94,95] The exfoliative toxin of *S. intermedius* can be found in *S. pseudintermedius* isolates from a large percentage of dogs and cats,[96–100] and it may play a role in pyoderma and otitis, but that has not yet been proven.

Another potentially important aspect of staphylococcal virulence is the ability to form biofilms (see Chapter 121) (Fig. 51.1). Biofilm may be most relevant for infections of implants and invasive devices (e.g., IV catheters). Biofilm formation has been demonstrated for various staphylococci, including *S. pseudintermedius* and *S. aureus*.[95,101–103] The role of biofilm formation in disease is not well understood, but it probably plays an important role in development of chronic disease and resistance to treatment in certain situations, particularly surgical implant and invasive device infections.

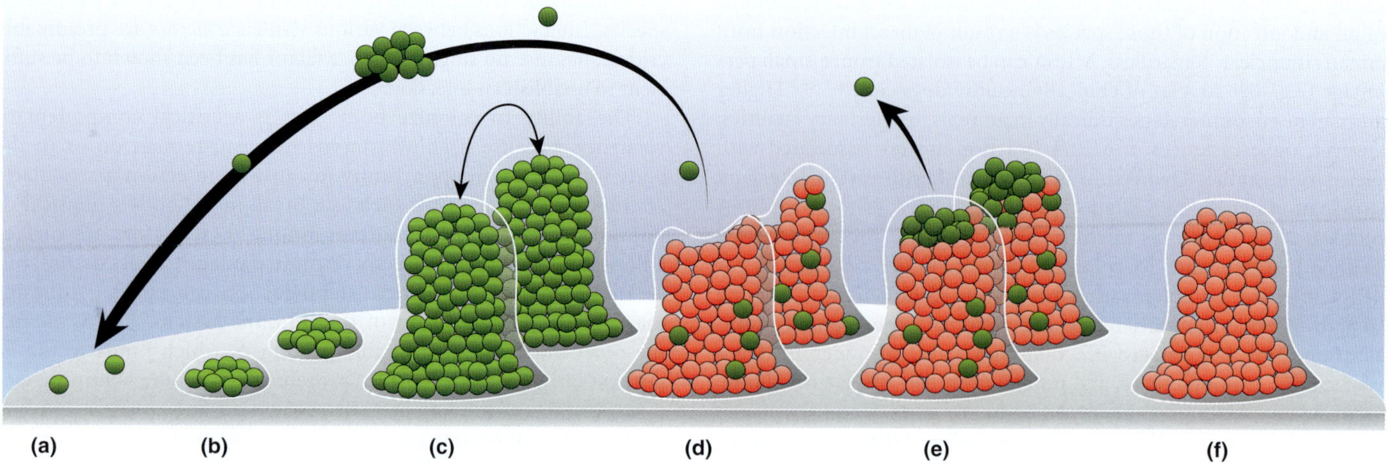

Fig. 51.1 Model of *agr* expression in staphylococcal biofilms. After initial colonization by individual cells *(a)*, microcolonies reach sufficient cell density for *agr*-dependent gene expression *(b)* and perhaps signaling between microcolonies *(c, arrows)*. Portions of the biofilm detach *(d)* as either large aggregates or individual cells. Simultaneously, parts of the biofilm population become metabolically inactive and lose membrane integrity. This is followed by new growth in the voids left by detached cells *(e)*, and the cycle is repeated. The microcolony finally reaches a relatively quiescent state where growth is slow and *agr* expression is undetectable *(f)*. Green = metabolically active bacteria that are producing virulence factors. Red = bacteria with states of relative inactivity.

Staphylococci cause a wide range of opportunistic infections, particularly acute bacterial skin and skin structure infections (also referred to as skin and soft tissue infections). Clinically, these can range from mild pyoderma to rapidly fatal necrotizing fasciitis. Any body system can be affected, including otherwise sterile sites (invasive infections). Severe manifestations of staphylococcal infection include staphylococcal toxic shock syndrome, bacteremia/sepsis, and necrotizing fasciitis (see Chapter 50). There is little to no difference in the clinical appearance of infections caused by different staphylococcal species, and no difference between methicillin-resistant and methicillin-susceptible infections. Additionally, staphylococcal infections cannot be differentiated from infections caused by other opportunistic pathogens without diagnostic testing.

Staphylococcus pseudintermedius

Staphylococcus pseudintermedius accounts for the vast majority of staphylococcal infections (and probably overall opportunistic infection) in dogs, and a lesser percentage in cats. The most common clinical manifestation of infection is pyoderma, including superficial and deep disease. *S. pseudintermedius* also causes a range of other infections including, in general order of occurrence, wound infections, SSIs, abscesses, UTIs, septic arthritis, osteomyelitis, discospondylitis, endocarditis, peritonitis, and ocular infections. The severity of disease is highly variable. Serious invasive infections including fatal toxic shock and cellulitis have been reported,[104,105] but these are rare. Most infections are mild to moderate in severity.

Staphylococcus aureus

A similar range of infections as produced by *S. pseudintermedius* can be produced by *S. aureus*. The main difference between *S. pseudintermedius* and *S. aureus* is the lower incidence of disease caused by the latter rather than disease location or severity. *S. aureus* infections may be more common in cats than in dogs, which probably relates to a lower prevalence of *S. pseudintermedius* colonization in cats. It is possible that infections more commonly associated with human contact (i.e., wound and SSIs contaminated by hands of owners or veterinary personnel) are more likely to be caused by *S. aureus* (including MRSA), but objective data are lacking.

Staphylococcus schleiferi subsp. *coagulans*

The main apparent difference in clinical expression of disease between *S. schleiferi* subsp. *coagulans* and other coagulase-positive staphylococcal infections is the rarity of infections beyond the skin and ears. However, the role of this staphylococcal species in disease may be underestimated because of the failure of many diagnostic laboratories to differentiate it from *S. pseudintermedius*. It has been suggested that *S. schleiferi* subsp. *coagulans* may tend to produce more superficial skin disease than *S. pseudintermedius* and *S. aureus*,[4] but supporting evidence is limited.

Coagulase-Negative Staphylococci

Interpretation of the role of CoNS in disease is difficult because they are often found in cultures as contaminants. Since most species are of limited virulence and often found at mucosal and skin sites, interpretation of the relevance of isolation of CoNS and the potential role in disease is a challenge. Further, as discussed above, while CoNS are generally considered as a group, it is possible that there are differences in clinical expression of disease among CoNS species. In particular, *S. schleiferi* subsp. *schleiferi* has been implicated as a cause of pyoderma and otitis.[8,19,27] A primary role of *S. felis* as an important cause of UTIs in cats has been suggested,[9] but remains unclear. *Staphylococcus lugdunensis* may also be a more pathogenic species. CoNS likely pose a greater risk for infections of invasive devices, surgical incisions, and other compromised sites.

DIAGNOSIS

There are no clinical, clinicopathologic, or diagnostic imaging results that are pathognomonic or even highly suggestive of staphylococcal infection.

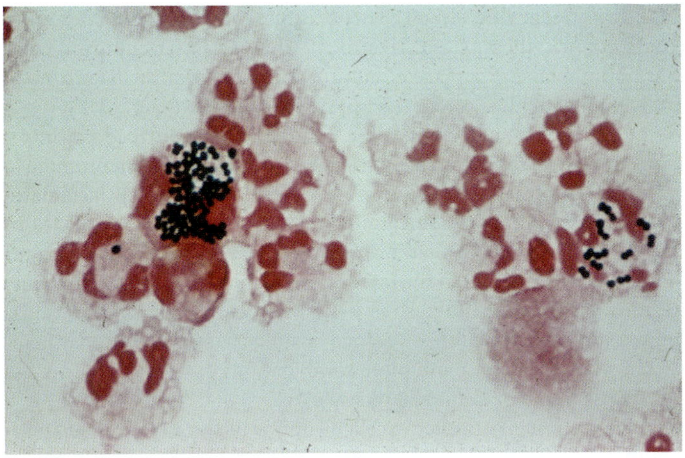

Fig. 51.2 *Staphylococcus aureus* engulfed in neutrophils. Note the "clumps" of gram-positive cocci characteristic of staphylococci.

Microbiologic Tests

Cytologic Diagnosis

Evaluation of smears or aspirates can indicate the presence of bacterial sepsis, and the presence of cocci, particularly clusters of gram-positive cocci, is suggestive of staphylococcal infection (Fig. 51.2). Cytologic evidence of an infectious inflammatory response, particularly an abundance of neutrophils and intracellular bacteria, is particularly suggestive.

Culture and Susceptibility Testing

Isolation of staphylococci from an infected site is the standard for diagnosis; however, whereas isolation of staphylococci tends to be relatively easy, interpretation of results can be challenging. Because staphylococci are common commensals, contamination of specimens, particularly those from skin and soft tissue infections, is a major problem in diagnosis. Care should, therefore, be taken to avoid contamination when collecting culture specimens. Particular care must be taken in diagnosing infections caused by CoNS, since they are common contaminants and are uncommonly pathogenic. This includes methicillin-resistant CoNS, which are not uncommonly isolated from healthy animals. Isolation of CoNS from a superficial site should be interpreted with caution. If a CoNS and another potential pathogen are identified concurrently, the CoNS is typically considered a contaminant. Isolation of CoNS from sterile sites (e.g., blood, pleural cavity) is more indicative of disease as long as samples were collected and handled properly; however, in human medicine, a single blood culture of CoNS is often dismissed as a likely contaminant.[106] If quantitative or semiquantitative culture results are provided, low growth (1+) of CoNS is of questionable relevance and quite possibly contamination, not infection.

Speciation of staphylococci is variably handled among diagnostic laboratories. Some laboratories provide only superficial identifications. However, speciation is required for proper antimicrobial susceptibility testing, as interpretive breakpoints differ among different species of *Staphylococcus* (see Chapter 3).[107,108] Speciation can also be useful for infection control purposes to help assess likely sources of infection and potential public health concerns, particularly when MRS are involved. It is also useful when trying to determine whether multiple culture results could indicate a cluster of hospital-associated infections, because infections with different species would rule out a common source exposure. It has often been considered that there is less need for speciation of CoNS because they are, in general, less pathogenic, with limited difference between species. However, if certain CoNS are potentially important primary pathogens (e.g., *S. schleiferi* subsp. *schleiferi* in pyoderma or *S. felis* in UTIs in cats), then speciation could be important for interpreting the relevance of isolation of CoNS.

Given the variability in susceptibility patterns among staphylococci and the emergence of MDR MRSP and MRSA, it is important that proper susceptibility testing be performed to guide treatment. Veterinarians should ensure that the diagnostic laboratory they use follow standard Clinical and Laboratory Standards Institute (CLSI) guidelines for performance and interpretation of susceptibility testing results.[109] In general, methods to detect antimicrobial susceptibility among staphylococci are well developed and validated. Problems with identification of methicillin resistance in *S. pseudintermedius* have been previously encountered,[107,108,110] although changes in CLSI guidelines for susceptibility testing of *S. pseudintermedius* have improved this situation. Problems with assessment of doxycycline susceptibility have also been identified, with use of human interpretative breakpoints leading to false reporting of doxycycline susceptibility in some *S. pseudintermedius* isolates.[111,112] Revised breakpoints have been recommended,[113] but these are not necessarily used by all diagnostic laboratories. Another area of concern is determination of clindamycin resistance because of inducible resistance, as is discussed under Systemic Antimicrobials.

Molecular Diagnosis Using Nucleic Acid–Based Testing

While the movement to rapid diagnostic testing will continue, there are currently no validated rapid tests for diagnosis of staphylococcal infections in dogs and cats. Although molecular assays based on PCR offer the potential for a rapid result, adequate test development and validation is required to ensure sensitivity and specificity. Of greater interest are assays that will rapidly identify MRSA or MRSP to guide initial treatment decisions. There are commercial assays for rapid detection of MRSA in humans; however, these have not been validated in animals, and investigation of one test in horses demonstrated poor performance.[114] A similar test for MRSP is not available, and clinicians must be aware that commercial veterinary "MRSA" PCR assays may simply be tests to detect *mecA,* the resistance gene that can be found in any MRS species, including CoNS.

TREATMENT AND PROGNOSIS

Management of staphylococcal infections is highly variable because of the diverse nature of disease. The general approach to treatment varies little between different staphylococcal species, and indeed between infections caused by staphylococci versus other opportunistic pathogens. Infection site and severity are key determinants of the required approach. Factors such as surgical intervention and supportive care may be required, and are sometimes the most important measures, but are not covered here.

Antimicrobials are not always needed for staphylococcal infections. In some situations, local approaches using biocides such as chlorhexidine or other antibacterial substances may be effective. The best example of this is superficial folliculitis, where topical therapy with chlorhexidine has been shown to be effective in the absence of concurrent systemic antimicrobials[115,116] and where topical therapy alone is the recommended first-line approach.[117] Other common situations may be amenable to nonantimicrobial approaches. Biocides as well as other substances with antibacterial activity (e.g., honey) can also be useful sole or adjunctive approaches to wound infections. Incision and drainage is the preferred approach for treatment of abscesses that are not associated with evidence of systemic infection or significant localized cellulitis. Similarly, mild superficial SSIs may be effectively managed through removal of skin sutures and cleaning of the site. Thus, while systemic antimicrobials are often required for the treatment of staphylococcal infections, there are many instances where other treatment approaches may be effective.

Systemic Antimicrobials

Treatment with systemic antimicrobials is ideally based on the results of culture and susceptibility testing. This has become particularly true as the prevalence of MDR staphylococci has increased. The prevalence of resistance to different antimicrobials varies between (and even within) regions, so knowledge of local susceptibility patterns is useful. Knowledge of typical clinical response to empirical antimicrobials can be useful to guide decisions, particularly in situations where culture specimens are uncommonly submitted. Published data from research papers or laboratory data compilations can provide interesting information but are potentially biased since, in most regions, culture specimens are disproportionately submitted from infections that are recurrent or have not responded to initial antimicrobial therapy. Therefore, these can be expected to over-represent (sometimes profoundly) the prevalence of antimicrobial resistance. Databases from referral institutions can have similar biases. Thus, care should be taken when making clinical decisions from such data sets, and thought must be given to how well the dataset represents the individual clinical case. Knowledge of resistance trends in the practice is more useful to guide empiric therapy and treatment while awaiting culture results, but nothing takes the place of culture and susceptibility data from an individual patient.

Drug options and dosages for treatment of staphylococcal infections are listed in Table 51.1. In general, resistance is uncommon to first-generation cephalosporins (e.g., cephalexin) or β-lactamase-resistant penicillins or penicillin/β-lactamase inhibitor combinations (e.g., amoxicillin-clavulanate), and these drugs are widely used as first-line treatments, although the increase in methicillin resistance in many regions has impacted the use of beta-lactams. In most situations, the prevalence of methicillin resistance is still sufficiently low that beta-lactams/beta-lactamase inhibitor combinations or cephalosporins can be used as initial or empirical therapy.

Clindamycin is another excellent option if the isolate is susceptible *in vitro*, and has been recommended as a first-line treatment for superficial folliculitis.[117] However, inducible clindamycin resistance must be considered, particularly in *S. aureus*.[118–120] With this phenomenon, isolates appear to be susceptible to clindamycin *in vitro*; however, resistance is induced on exposure *in vivo*, and treatment failure is expected. One study reported inducible resistance in 71% of MRSA strains from animals,[119] whereas another study reported that 55% of

TABLE 51.1 Selected Antimicrobial Options for the Treatment of *Staphylococcus* Infections

Drug	Dose (mg/kg)	Route	Interval (Hours)	Comments
Amoxicillin	22	PO	12	Only use based on culture and susceptibility testing because of the high prevalence of beta-lactamase production.
Amoxicillin-clavulanic acid	12.5–25	PO	8–12	Good empirical drug for suspected staphylococcal infections.
Cephalexin	22–25	PO	12	
Clindamycin	D: 10 C: 10–15	PO/SC	12	Excellent antistaphylococcal drug. D-test or equivalent must be used to rule out inducible resistance, particularly in MRSA.
Fluoroquinolones	Varies depending on specific drug			Avoid enrofloxacin in cats. Typically, the high end of the dosing range is preferred. Ciprofloxacin should be avoided because of unpredictable bioavailability.
Doxycycline	D: 5 C: 10	PO	12 24	Ensure that *S. pseudintermedius* testing is based on current interpretive breakpoints to avoid false indication of susceptibility.
Minocycline	D: 5 C: 8.8 or 50 mg/cat	PO	12 24	Useful if doxycycline is not available and for some doxycycline-resistant staphylococcal infections.
Trimethoprim-sulfamethoxazole or trimethoprim-sulfadiazine	15–30	PO	12	Schirmer's tear testing is recommended in dogs as a baseline and periodically if treatment of > 7-day duration is planned.
Chloramphenicol	D: 40–50 C: 12.5–20	PO/SC/IM/IV PO/SC/IV	8 12	Use with caution because of potential human exposure risks.
Amikacin	D: 15–30 C: 10–14	IV/IM/SC	24	Monitoring of renal function is advised.
Fosfomycin	D: 40	PO	12	Reserve for multidrug-resistant infections. Limited veterinary experience. Adverse gastrointestinal effects are not uncommon. Administer with food. Treatment should probably be limited to short durations. Should not be used in cats.
Nitrofurantoin	4–4.5	PO	8	Reserve for multidrug-resistant infections. Only for cystitis, not tissue-associated infections (including pyelonephritis).
Cefovecin	8	SC	Can be repeated in 7–14 days	Should be reserved for cases where the duration of treatment is required and when oral dosing with a first-line option such as amoxicillin +/– clavulanic acid, clindamycin or cephalexin is not possible.
Cefpodoxime	5–10	PO	24	Reserve for cases where oral dosing with a first-line option such as amoxicillin +/– clavulanic acid, clindamycin or cephalexin is not possible.

C, cats; *D*, dogs; *IM*, intramuscular; *IV*, intravenous; *MRSA*, methicillin-resistant *Staphylococcus aureus*; *PO*, oral; *SC*, subcutaneous.

erythromycin-resistant, clindamycin-susceptible MRSA from dogs were inducibly resistant.[118] Inducible resistance can be detected in the laboratory using a "D-test" and it is important to know what testing methods are used when diagnostic laboratories report clindamycin susceptibility. *S. aureus* isolates that are reported as erythromycin resistant but clindamycin susceptible should be considered resistant to clindamycin unless the D-test (or equivalent) has indicated the absence of inducible resistance. Inducible resistance is not a concern if erythromycin susceptibility is reported. Inducible resistance appears to be rare in *S. pseudintermedius* but, because it has been reported,[118,121] it is prudent to avoid clindamycin for the treatment of serious infections caused by erythromycin-resistant *S. pseudintermedius* without demonstration of absence of inducible clindamycin resistance. The same likely applies to other staphylococci as limited information is available.

Tetracyclines can be useful antistaphylococcal drugs, but resistance is not uncommon. Doxycycline is the most commonly used tetracycline and can be an effective treatment for various staphylococcal infections. Potential problems with the use of older doxycycline breakpoints for *S. pseudintermedius*, as discussed in more detail above, must be considered. If laboratories are using currently recommended breakpoints (susceptible if MICs are < 0.125 μg/mL or > 25 mm zone diameter),[113] doxycycline is a reasonable choice when *in vitro* susceptibility is reported. Minocycline has a somewhat broader spectrum of activity since some doxycycline-resistant staphylococci remain susceptible to minocycline.[111,112,122] This depends on the genetic mechanism of resistance, and the prevalence of minocycline susceptibility among doxycycline-resistant staphylococci varies depending on the *S. pseudintermedius* strain and the geographic region. Specific testing for minocycline is required when doxycycline-resistant isolates are encountered.

While most often used to target gram-negative pathogens, aminoglycosides can be excellent antistaphylococcal drugs, although the parenteral route of administration can be problematic and nephrotoxicity is a concern. Despite these concerns, amikacin has become a common treatment for MRSP infections because of the very limited options. Clinically relevant nephrotoxicity appears to be uncommon in systemically stable patients and is typically reversible if amikacin administration is stopped. Gentamicin can also be considered but is somewhat more toxic than amikacin, and lack of availability of amikacin would be the main reason to consider gentamicin.

Fluoroquinolones can have excellent intrinsic activity against staphylococci. Given their *in vitro* activity, their ability to penetrate the skin, the availability of oral formulations, and once-daily dosing requirement, fluoroquinolones have been popular choices for staphylococcal infections. They can be highly effective clinically, but concerns about fluoroquinolone resistance, in terms of both clinical treatment failure and public health consequences, have led to recommendations that they be reserved as second-line choices for many types of infections (e.g., bacterial cystitis, superficial folliculitis)[117,123] and be used only when resistance to other antimicrobials is present or likely. In humans, fluoroquinolones are not generally recommended as monotherapy for MRSA because of poor clinical response and rapid development of resistance.[124] This has not been objectively investigated in dogs and cats but there is no reason to suspect that it would be different in these species, so fluoroquinolones probably should be avoided whenever possible as treatments of resistant staphylococcal infections such as MRSA and MRSP when other viable alternatives exist. There has been less discussion about their indication in methicillin-susceptible infections. These should perhaps be approached with caution as well, because the presence or absence of methicillin resistance should be of limited relevance to the likelihood of treatment failure or emergence of resistance with quinolone treatment and because fluoroquinolone exposure is a well-documented risk factor for MRS infections in humans and dogs.[22,124,125] It is reasonable, therefore, to recommend prudent use of this drug class for any staphylococcal infection and to avoid empirical use of fluoroquinolones in any serious or life-threatening staphylococcal infection if possible.

Trimethoprim-sulfonamide is commonly active against MRS *in vitro*. Safety concerns exist, including keratoconjunctivitis sicca, arthropathy, and other idiosyncratic effects. These are most relevant with long durations of treatment but can occur with short-term therapy. Trimethoprim-sulfonamide can be used safely in most patients and is appropriate in situations with few other viable options. It should be avoided in animals with a history of/risk factors for keratoconjunctivitis sicca.

Chloramphenicol is also often active against staphylococci *in vitro* and anecdotally *in vivo*. There are human health concerns relating to fatal aplastic anemia from exposure to chloramphenicol, although this is an exceptionally rare idiosyncratic reaction. Careful drug handling instructions and client education as to its risks must be given. Chloramphenicol can also cause bone marrow suppression (particularly in cats) and is contraindicated in animals being treated with other myelosuppressive drugs. If chloramphenicol is to be used for a prolonged period of time, periodic (every 14 to 28 days) monitoring of a CBC count is advisable. Florfenicol might be a potential alternative to chloramphenicol, because it is not a health risk to humans. It can be administered orally, although it may be refused because of its taste. Although florfenicol has been used with anecdotal success in the treatment of MRSP and MRSA infections in dogs, treatment failure and development of resistance during treatment have been reported, and objective evaluation of efficacy is lacking.

Fosfomycin is uncommonly used in dogs, mainly as a treatment for resistant bacterial cystitis, but is a consideration for other staphylococcal infections. Fosfomycin resistance is currently uncommon in staphylococci[126] and fosfomycin represents a potential oral treatment option of MDR staphylococci. Clinical data are lacking and adverse GI effects are not uncommon. This drug should not be used in cats because of nephrotoxicity.[127]

Nitrofurantoin is a potential option for treatment of staphylococcal cystitis. While ineffective for infections other than cystitis (including pyelonephritis), nitrofurantoin is an option for some MDR staphylococcal cystitis cases. Resistance to nitrofurantoin is uncommon, but can occur.

As MRS become more prevalent and some strains become highly drug resistant, isolates that are resistant to almost all available drugs are being encountered in some regions. This has led to the consideration for use of antimicrobials that are critically important in human medicine, such as vancomycin and linezolid. Vancomycin, linezolid, tigecycline, and quinupristin-dalfopristin are drugs that are important for treatment of serious MDR infections in humans. Their use in animals raises many ethical questions that are difficult to answer. Concerns include increased pressure toward resistance of animal-harbored staphylococci and their subsequent transmission to humans. The concerns of public health risk are often opposed with concerns about animal health and welfare if proper treatment is not provided, and the fact that animal use makes up a minuscule percentage of overall use of these drugs. There is currently no consensus on the topic, but use of these drugs in animals is banned in some countries (e.g., The Netherlands, Sweden). At a minimum, these drugs should be reserved for situations where there are no other viable treatment alternatives, where the infection is not amenable to other (e.g., local) therapy, and where the infection is life threatening but potentially treatable. Before considering drugs such as these, all other therapeutic options should be considered and experts in infectious diseases should be consulted if possible. Currently, it is rare to require drugs such as these because there is almost always another treatment option.

Local Antimicrobial Therapies

Local or regional administration of antimicrobials can deliver high antimicrobial concentrations that can result in clinical efficacy even in the face of *in vitro* resistance. This is dependent on the amount of drug that reaches the site, the duration that those levels are achieved, and the MIC of the specific bacterial isolate. Various approaches can be used, most commonly involving concentration-dependent drugs (e.g., aminoglycosides). Intra-articular injection of antimicrobials (e.g., amikacin) can be considered in cases of septic arthritis to achieve high local concentrations. This approach is most commonly used in horses but is practical in many small animal patients, especially surgery-associated stifle infections in large-breed dogs. Local administration of antimicrobial-impregnated materials such as beads or collagen sponges[128–131] can sometimes produce sustained high drug levels (see Chapter 121). This approach can be particularly useful in implant-associated infections or infections of poorly vascularized sites such as bone. Other methods to deliver high drug levels to a site of infection are under investigation or development, and new options will likely be available in coming years.

Topical Antimicrobials

Topical antimicrobial therapy may be a useful adjunctive or sole therapy. The ability to deliver high concentrations of antimicrobial directly to the site of infection, with minimal systemic exposure, is a desirable approach. Clinically relevant resistance of staphylococci to topical antimicrobials such as mupirocin and fusidic acid is uncommon,[132–136] and the high local antimicrobial levels that can be achieved may largely offset acquired resistance.

The main limitations to topical therapy are potential difficulties getting topically applied antimicrobials to the infection site and providing an adequate duration of contact. Thus, topical therapy is best reserved as a sole method for treatment of very focal superficial infections, such as superficial wound infection and focal surface pyoderma, including otitis externa. Systemic therapy or a combination of systemic and topical therapy should be used for deeper infections or infections that do not respond completely to topical monotherapy. Whether topical antimicrobials offer any advantage over topical application of biocides (e.g., chlorhexidine) is unclear.

Other Topical Treatments

Direct topical application of biocides is a potential option for some skin and skin structure infections and is a preferred approach for the treatment of superficial pyoderma.[117] The potential efficacy of biocides involves a balance between the bactericidal activity of the compound and the tissue damage from biocide application. Some compounds have profound antibacterial properties but are not useful because of the degree of tissue damage that can ensue. For some biocides, the costs versus benefits of antibacterial properties and tissue damage are not well understood.[137]

As with topical antimicrobials, the ability of the biocide to reach the infection site and limited contact time are the main limitations. Biocides may be effective as the sole treatment of superficial infections, or as adjunctive therapy for deeper infections. Available options include chlorhexidine, povidone-iodine, and benzoyl peroxide gel. Topical use of chlorhexidine can be as effective as antimicrobials in resolving skin lesions in dogs with pyoderma, including infectious caused by MRSP,[115,116,138] and this is a recommended first-line approach for superficial folliculitis.[117] Other compounds such as accelerated hydrogen peroxide have also been proposed as topical therapies, but there is currently little information about their use. Silver-coated dressings may be useful for treatment of skin and wound infections. Essential oils are gaining popularity as topical therapies, although clinical efficacy data are limited. Various essential oils, including tea tree oil, geranium oil, lavender oil, and grapefruit seed extract, have been shown to possess antibacterial properties, including activity against MRSA and MRSP.[137,139,140] They may have an added effect whereby the vapor generated by their oils within bandage materials can penetrate more deeply into infected sites than the liquid form.[139,141] However, an overlooked aspect is the potential for tissue damage, because essential oils can have cytotoxic effects on mammalian cells.[142] Concerns about cytotoxicity have led to a recommendation that tea tree oil not be used in the treatment of burns.[141] Ingestion of a small volume of tea tree oil has caused neurologic disease in children,[143,144] and the risk to pets from licking topically applied oil or ingestion of treated bandage material is unclear. Further study of efficacy and safety are required.

Topical application of honey is another appealing alternative to antibiotic treatment that is safe. Honey has bactericidal effects against various bacteria, including staphylococci, *in vitro* and *in vivo*.[145–148] There are differences in bactericidal activity among different types of honey, and the best investigated honey has been Manuka honey, produced from the blossoms of *Leptospermum scoparium* (Manuka). Basic use of honey in dogs and cats simply involves direct application of food-grade honey to an infected site, covered by a bandage. A preferred method of application involves the use of dressings impregnated with Manuka honey because of the enhanced and more predictable bactericidal activity of this type of honey and pre-sterilization of the honey and dressing. There are theoretical concerns about bacterial contamination of honey, particularly with *Clostridium botulinum*. Although *C. botulinum* can be found in honey, honey-associated botulism in humans is almost invariably from ingestion of contaminated honey by infants. Tissue infection would require clostridial spores in honey reaching a deep, anaerobic site, something that is unlikely, and the authors are unaware of any infections linked to topical application of honey.

Other Considerations

Both *S. aureus* and *S. pseudintermedius* are important causes of surgical implant–associated infections.[5,149–152] These infections can be very difficult to treat because of the implant and its associated biofilm.[95,103,153] Antimicrobial therapy can often result in amelioration of clinical signs or initially apparent clinical cure; however, relapse is very common after cessation of antimicrobials. Elimination of infection can be difficult to impossible with implants in place, and removal of implants should be considered as soon as possible.

PREVENTION

Prevention of staphylococcal infections largely involves prevention or control of underlying risk factors (e.g., management of allergic skin disease), since staphylococcal infections are virtually always secondary, opportunistic infections. Measures to reduce SSIs and other hospital-associated infections are discussed further below and in Chapters 15 and 76.

Perioperative Prophylaxis

Staphylococci are leading causes of SSIs and perioperative antimicrobial prophylaxis, when indicated, should include excellent staphylococcal coverage. Most often, the first-generation cephalosporin cephazolin is used. Other options include clindamycin or ampicillin; however, the commonness of beta-lactamase–producing staphylococci may preclude use of ampicillin in many regions. When broad gram-negative coverage is needed, a second-generation (e.g., cefoxitin) or third-generation (e.g., cefotaxime) cephalosporin can be used, or a drug with better efficacy against gram-negative bacteria (e.g., aminoglycoside, fluoroquinolone) can be added. Routine use of third-generation cephalosporins and fluoroquinolones should be minimized because of the importance of those drug classes in human medicine. While MRS, particularly MRSP, are important causes of SSIs, routine prophylaxis targeting MRS is discouraged because of the limited treatment options and concerns that routinely using the few drugs available for therapy (e.g., amikacin) will increase the risk of resistance and even further treatment challenges. There may be limited situations where targeting MRS is indicated, such as when the patient has a concurrent or recent MRS infection, since MRSP colonization has been identified as predisposing to MRSP SSI.[77] More information on perioperative and postoperative prophylaxis for SSIs can be found in Chapter 76.

PUBLIC HEALTH ASPECTS

Staphylococcus aureus

Public health concerns regarding pets and *S. aureus* have almost exclusively involved MRSA, even though pet-to-human methicillin-susceptible *S. aureus* infections probably occur. Colonization of humans in contact with infected or colonized dogs and cats has been widely reported,[48,57,90,154–158] although the direction of transmission is usually unclear and it is likely that most pet-human pairs with MRSA reflect human-to-pet transmission since *S. aureus* seems to be more adapted to colonization of humans than colonization of dogs and cats. MRSA isolates from pets tend to reflect strains that predominate in people in any given geographic region, likely a testament to the human origin of MRSA in pets. Pets have been implicated as sources of infection for humans in households[15,159]; however, this has been based on circumstantial evidence. MRSA should be considered a potentially zoonotic pathogen and infection control measures should be instituted, as is discussed below. However, it should be realized that the incidence of pets being a source of human disease is probably low, and most instances of MRSA infection or colonization in pets are probably a result of the pet acquiring MRSA from a human source.

Notwithstanding the predominant association of MRSA with humans, there may be occupational health risks for veterinary personnel. Numerous studies of MRSA colonization in veterinary personnel have been performed, generally reporting colonization rates of up to 18% in small animal veterinary personnel.[160–166] It cannot be determined with certainty that these colonization rates reflect acquisition of MRSA from animals; however, identification of higher rates than present in the general population and similarity between human and animal strains support the possibility of occupational origin.

Infection Control Precautions in Veterinary Clinics

MRSA and MRSP pose challenges in veterinary clinics as they can be associated with clusters of infections in animals, as well as potential transmission to veterinary personnel. Infection control efforts need to be directed both at controlling the endemic level of disease and preventing outbreaks. The risks posed by MRSA and MRSP are poorly defined, as is the efficacy of different control measures. The response to MRSA and MRSP can vary among facilities based on the facility design, risk status of the patient population for MRSA/MRSP colonization, risk status of the patient population from MRSA/MRSP acquisition, risk adversity, and other aspects. While there is no standard approach, some basic concepts can be applied to all facilities and both MRSA and MRSP. These include the use of good general hygiene practices (especially handwashing), use of enhanced barriers (e.g., gown or dedicated protective outerwear, gloves) with animals that are known to be infected or colonized, routine and enhanced cleaning and disinfection, and the use of a variety of other standard infection control practices such as surgical asepsis (see Chapter 15).

When MRSA or MRSP infections are identified, a plan should be in place regarding how to handle that animal in the clinic and during subsequent examinations. All infected or colonized animals should be considered carriers until proven otherwise, and handled with contact precautions (gloves, dedicated protective outerwear). In clinics, they should be housed in isolation (or mini-isolation, with posted precautions and limited handlers) whenever possible and have no direct or indirect contact with other patients. Although there is little risk of aerosol transmission, housing infected animals in isolation decreases the likelihood of transmission via personnel or fomites. Infected or colonized outpatients should be admitted directly to an isolation area or examination room, rather than allowing them to remain in a waiting area. The practicality and impact of these approaches will vary between facilities. For example, in a dermatology practice, a large percentage of patients may be MRSP or MRSA carriers. Use of these measures on such a large number of animals may be impossible and the implications of MRSP/MRSA exposure of patients may not be as great as in a facility with a large elective orthopedic surgery caseload, where MRSP SSIs can be highly problematic. However, the higher likely MRSA and MRSP burdens in the patient population could pose increased risk to clinic personnel. Therefore, concurrent increases in hygiene and personal protective equipment use (e.g., handwashing and proper use of dedicated outerwear and gloves) may be more important than attempting to isolate potential animals infected and colonized with MRSA or MRSP. In contrast, in facilities with a greater population of patients with greater risk or implications of MRSA or MRSP infections (e.g., orthopedic surgery, immunosuppressed or critically ill patients), there may be more indication for isolation of known or high-risk patients infected or colonized with MRS.

MRSA in Clinic Personnel

MRSA exposure, colonization, or infection of veterinary hospital personnel can be a difficult area to address because of the general lack of understanding of the issues and the high-profile nature of MRSA. Concerns are often present when people realize that they have had contact with an MRSA-infected or -colonized animal, and the potential for occupational exposure is certainly present based on the high rates of MRSA colonization in veterinary personnel. Sometimes, people express a desire to have themselves or their staff tested for MRSA colonization. However, this is rarely indicated and is associated with many potential problems. Given the reported colonization rates of veterinarians and the presumably frequent exposure to colonized animals, routine infection control practices should be established to reduce the risk of MRSA transmission from unknown carriers (staff or pets). Testing of staff for MRSA colonization is not recommended. MRSA rates are high in veterinary personnel and it would not be surprising to find positive individuals in the absence of known MRSA transmission. Exclusion of colonized personnel from work is not reasonable considering the high MRSA colonization rates that have been identified and ongoing risk of exposure. Treatment directed at MRSA decolonization of involved humans is unlikely to be recommended by physicians, because it is uncommonly used in people in the general population in most regions. Furthermore, even with successful decolonization, there would be a continued risk of occupational exposure.

Veterinary personnel who become aware that they are colonized with MRSA should be especially diligent in following all hand hygiene protocols in the clinic and avoidance of hand-to-nose contact (because the nares are the most common site of colonization in humans, and hands are the prime source of transmission). There is no indication to remove a colonized individual from patient care duties, although restriction of contact with very high-risk patients (e.g., some surgical patients) could be considered. However, because the vast majority of veterinary personnel are not aware of their MRSA status, clinic personnel should assume that both they and their patients could be colonized. Employees who are concerned about MRSA colonization (e.g., those who have been working with an MRSA-positive animal) should be encouraged to see their physicians. Veterinary personnel should also be aware of their likely increased risk of MRSA infection and ensure that their physician knows that they may be at higher risk than the general population, something that might be important to consider when empirically treating infections or deciding whether preoperative MRSA screening is indicated.

Infection Control in Households

The principles of MRSA control for households are the same as those for veterinary clinics. Infected sites on pets should be covered with an impermeable barrier whenever possible. A key point is recognition of additional high-risk body sites (nose, mouth, and perineum) and avoidance of direct and indirect contact with those sites. Owners should be counselled on good household infection control practices, particularly regular hand hygiene. Infected or colonized pets should be prevented from having contact with pets outside the household until they are no longer infected or colonized. Although MRSA can be transmitted in households, the incidence is unclear, as are risk factors. Owners who have concerns, particularly if the concerns relate to the presence of high-risk people in the household (very young or very old, immunocompromised individuals), should be encouraged to seek advice from their physicians. Routine testing of clinically healthy pets whose owners have MRSA infection or of clinically healthy owners whose pets have MRSA is not indicated.

Pet Owners Diagnosed with MRSA Infection

Infected or colonized owners can be a source of infection for their pets, although the incidence of transmission from infected owners to pets is unknown. Owners diagnosed with MRSA infection should be told to wash their hands thoroughly before and after handling their pet, in order to prevent transmission of MRSA to the pet, and transmission from the pet should it subsequently become colonized. Owners should not kiss their pets or allow their pets to lick their faces or any broken skin. Screening of pets for MRSA carriage is rarely indicated, and should only be done if there is a clear plan to act on the results. Testing animals in the absence of testing all human contacts is illogical, and testing of animals can result in much confusion and the potential for poor decision-making if is it not conducted as part of a comprehensive household investigation with a plan of action in place to deal with the results. Pet screening may rarely be indicated as part of a whole-household intervention, which includes simultaneous screening and MRSA decolonization of all people.

Staphylococcus pseudintermedius

While *S. pseudintermedius* can cause infection in humans, the incidence of this appears to be very low. When one considers the high prevalence of *S. pseudintermedius* carriage by healthy dogs and the millions of dog-human contacts that occur on a daily basis, it is apparent that the risk posed by this bacterium is limited.

Colonization of humans with *S. pseudintermedius* occurs more often than overt clinical infection but is still uncommon, with reported rates of 1% to 4% in veterinary personnel and pet owners.[66,167,168] Presumably, this low rate of *S. pseudintermedius* carriage reflects pet-human transmission, as indistinguishable pet and human isolates are common in households where concurrent carriage is identified.[168] Like methicillin-susceptible strains, MRSP can be found in a small percentage of pet owners and veterinary personnel[66,167,169] and MRSP infections have been reported in humans.[170–172] The risk posed by MRSP should be considered low; however, given the highly drug-resistant nature (and associated treatment difficulty), care should be taken to use good infection control practices around infected animals in households and veterinary clinics. Good hygiene in households and veterinary clinics should greatly minimize the risk of MRSP transmission from colonized animals.

Other Staphylococci

Public health concerns regarding other staphylococci are currently limited. Since CoNS (including methicillin-resistant CoNS) are common in both animals and humans and tend to be of limited pathogenicity, they are not considered a relevant public health concern. Although many of the same CoNS species can cause disease in both humans and pets, it is unclear whether animals are a potential source of infection. Most human infections occur in hospitalized individuals, and there is currently no evidence suggesting that isolation or other enhanced infection control practices are required for pets with CoNS infections. Good general hygiene practices should be more than adequate in most, if not all, situations. This is probably most important as an act of prudence for infected pets that will potentially have contact with high-risk (very young, elderly, immunocompromised) individuals.

SCREENING FOR METHICILLIN-RESISTANT STAPHYLOCOCCI AND DECOLONIZATION

Carriage of MRSA or MRSP at colonization sites such as the nose, pharynx, GI tract, or skin may be found in a small percentage of healthy animals. Carriage is very common in animals with clinical MRS infections and may persist for some time after resolution of infection. MRSA carriage tends to be transient and self-limiting, but prolonged carriage of MRSP can occur in some dogs.[10] Because of the potential for transmission of these important staphylococci to other individuals and the role of these organisms in disease, measures to detect and eliminate screening would be desirable. In humans, MRSA screening is a key component of MRSA control in hospitals, but not the general population. Active decolonization, often using topical antimicrobials such as mupirocin or fusidic acid, sometimes with concurrent oral antimicrobial therapy, is used as a means of MRSA control in some situations in some regions, such as in individuals undergoing certain surgical procedures.[68,173] Even though long-term MRSA colonization can occur, the need for decolonization therapy in otherwise healthy individuals in the community is controversial and not universally performed because of variable efficacy,[174] questionable need, and concerns about development of further antibacterial resistance. Decolonization is most commonly used in specific populations, such as healthcare workers, patients undergoing surgical procedures, patients in intensive care units, or individuals in households with recurrent MRSA infections, and even in those situations, it is not universally applied and is not always effective when it is performed.

While active elimination of MRSP or MRSA colonization in dogs and cats could be desirable to reduce the risk of development of clinical infection or transmission to other individuals, there is no evidence that therapy to eliminate colonization is indicated or even potentially efficacious in dogs and cats. Adequate topical application of an antimicrobial to the entire nasal passages and pharynx of a dog or cat is not realistic, and incomplete treatment could lead to further antibacterial resistance. Because MRSA colonization appears to be transient in most if not all dogs and cats, and the use of good general hygiene measures to reduce reinfection almost invariably results in spontaneous decolonization, it is questionable whether active decolonization is even indicated. An active approach to MRSP decolonization would be more appealing because of the potential for long-term shedding in dogs. However, effective decolonization regimens have not been described.

CASE EXAMPLE

Signalment

"Meg," an 8-year-old FS Labrador retriever in southern Ontario, Canada.

History

This overweight but otherwise healthy dog was examined because of acute onset of left pelvic limb lameness. After being let out at night, Meg was heard barking and ran away, and was thought to be chasing a raccoon. Upon returning, she was non-weight bearing on the left pelvic limb. The next morning, the lameness was improved although still present. The dog would bear limited weight on the leg.

Upon initial examination, Meg was bright, alert, and responsive. She was overweight, with a BCS of 7/9. Grade 4/6 left pelvic limb lameness was present. Otherwise, physical examination was unremarkable. She resented manipulation of the left pelvic limb. A mild pain response was noted on palpation of the stifle. Moderate stifle effusion was noted. A positive cranial drawer sign and tibial thrust were noted. Radiographs of the stifle revealed moderate increase in soft tissue opacity within the joint, most consistent with joint effusion, and mild to moderate degenerative joint disease. Cranial cruciate ligament rupture was diagnosed and the dog underwent a TPLO procedure the following day. Cephazolin was administered approximately 30 minutes prior to incision, with one intraoperative dose 120 minutes after the initial dose and two postoperative doses (22 mg/kg, IV, q12h). A CBC, serum biochemistry profile, and urinalysis were performed for preoperative health screening, and no abnormalities were present. Surgery was without complication, and postoperative radiographs indicated appropriate tibial plateau leveling and appropriate positioning of the implant. The dog experienced a normal postoperative recovery and was treated with cephalexin (22 mg/kg, PO, q12h) for 48 hours after surgery. However, 14 days after surgery, the dog developed worsened lameness, with reluctance to bear weight on the surgically corrected limb.

Physical Examination Findings

On examination, Meg was bright, alert, and responsive. She would stand on the affected limb but exhibited grade 3-4/6 lameness. The surgical site was red and inflamed. It was noticeably warm on palpation and a mild amount of pus was extruded when the incision site was manipulated. The joint appeared stable.

Laboratory Findings

None were performed initially upon re-presentation.

Imaging Findings

Radiographic findings were consistent with those normally identified 2 weeks after a TPLO procedure.

Cytologic Findings

Using aseptic technique, an aspirate was collected from the soft tissue overlying the surgical implant site. Marked suppurative inflammation was noted, with abundant cocci within neutrophils.

Microbiologic Testing

Culture of the aspirate ultimately yielded MRSP. Beyond beta-lactams, the isolate was resistant to doxycycline, clindamycin, enrofloxacin, marbofloxacin, and trimethoprim sulfa. It was susceptible to amikacin and chloramphenicol. Minocycline MIC testing was requested, and the MIC was 0.125 μg/mL (susceptible).

Diagnosis

Results were consistent with a deep SSI caused by MRSP.

Treatment

The dog was anesthetized, and skin sutures were removed. Upon removal of the skin suture, it was apparent that there was substantial infection of the subcutaneous tissues (Fig. 51.3). In addition, the deep fascia overlying the implant had dehisced. The infected site was thoroughly lavaged and treatment with minocycline (5 mg/kg, PO, q12h) was started. Clinical signs improved over the next 3 days and the amount of discharge rapidly decreased. Antimicrobials were stopped after 28 days, at which point the dog was clinically normal with evidence of appropriate wound healing. However, 21 days after cessation of antimicrobials, mild (grade 1-2/6) lameness was noted. Mild stifle effusion was identified upon palpation. The surgical site looked unremarkable grossly. An aspirate from over the plate was collected and moderate suppurative inflammation was evident cytologically. Culture of the specimen yielded an MRSP isolate with an indistinguishable susceptibility pattern from that isolated previously. Radiographs were taken and complete healing of the osteotomy was evident. After discussion with the client, it was decided to remove the implant as it was suspected to be colonized with biofilm-embedded MRSP, with a poor prognosis for elimination of the infection with the implant left *in situ.* Amikacin (20 mg/kg IV) was administered preoperatively and implant removal was unremarkable. Amikacin was continued for 3 days (20 mg/kg, SQ, q24h) postoperatively. No subsequent problems were encountered with the limb.

Comments

MRSP is a leading cause of TPLO SSI, and TPLO infection rates can be high. MRSP isolates are often strong biofilm producers, and elimination of implant-associated infections can be difficult because of the ability of MRSP to elude the effects of antimicrobials and the immune system while embedded within biofilm on a surgical implant. While some infections are treatable with systemic antimicrobials, sometimes with adjunctive approaches such as antimicrobial-impregnated beads or gels, long-term cure is often not achieved. Removal of the implant is typically required for full resolution of the infection. In implant-associated infections, antimicrobials are sometimes required systemically until the time that bone healing permits implant removal. In this case, infection of the bone seemed to be limited and there was little apparent impact on bone healing. It is debatable whether antimicrobials are required after implant removal, but a short course (as was used here) is often administered.

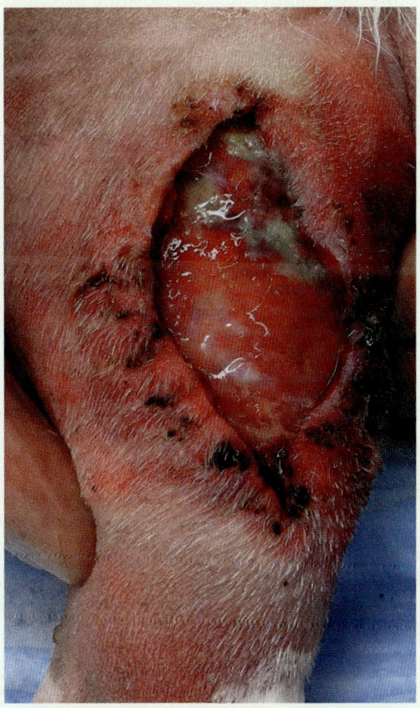

Fig. 51.3 Methicillin-resistant *Staphylococcus pseudintermedius* tibial plateau levelling osteotomy surgical site infection. (Courtesy of Dr. Ameet Singh.)

SUGGESTED READINGS

Frank LA, Loeffler A. Meticillin-resistant *Staphylococcus pseudintermedius*: clinical challenge and treatment options. *Vet Dermatol.* 2012;23:283–291.

Hillier A, Lloyd DH, Weese JS, et al. Guidelines for the diagnosis and antimicrobial therapy of canine superficial bacterial folliculitis (Antimicrobial Guidelines Working Group of the International Society for Companion Animal Infectious Diseases). *Vet Dermatol.* 2014;25:163–175.

Stull JW, Weese JS. Infection control in veterinary small animal practice. *Vet Clin North Am Small Anim Pract.* 2015;45:xi-xii.

Weese JS, van Duijkeren E. Methicillin-resistant *Staphylococcus aureus* and *Staphylococcus pseudintermedius* in veterinary medicine. *Vet Microbiol.* 2010;140:418–429.

REFERENCES

1. May ER, Hnilica KA, Frank LA, et al. Isolation of *Staphylococcus schleiferi* from healthy dogs and dogs with otitis, pyoderma, or both. *J Am Vet Med Assoc.* 2005;227:928–931.
2. Oliveira LC, Leite CA, Brilhante RS, et al. Comparative study of the microbial profile from bilateral canine otitis externa. *Can Vet J.* 2008;49:785–788.
3. Morris DO, Mauldin EA, O'Shea K, et al. Clinical, microbiological, and molecular characterization of methicillin-resistant *Staphylococcus aureus* infections of cats. *Am J Vet Res.* 2006;67:1421–1425.
4. Morris DO, Rook KA, Shofer FS, et al. Screening of *Staphylococcus aureus, Staphylococcus intermedius*, and *Staphylococcus schleiferi* isolates obtained from small companion animals for antimicrobial resistance: a retrospective review of 749 isolates (2003-04). *Vet Dermatol.* 2006;17:332–337.
5. Turk R, Singh A, Weese JS. Prospective surgical site infection surveillance in dogs. *Vet Surg.* 2015;44:2–8.
6. Devriese L, Hermans K, Baele M, et al. *Staphylococcus pseudintermedius* versus *Staphylococcus intermedius. Vet Microbiol.* 2009;133:206–207.
7. Devriese LA, Vancanneyt M, Baele M, et al. *Staphylococcus pseudintermedius* sp. nov., a coagulase-positive species from animals. *Int J Syst Evol Microbiol.* 2005;55:1569–1573.
8. Frank LA, Kania SA, Hnilica KA, et al. Isolation of *Staphylococcus schleiferi* from dogs with pyoderma. *J Am Vet Med Assoc.* 2003;222:451–454.
9. Litster A, Moss SM, Honnery M, et al. Prevalence of bacterial species in cats with clinical signs of lower urinary tract disease: recognition of *Staphylococcus felis* as a possible feline urinary tract pathogen. *Vet Microbiol.* 2007;121:182–188.
10. Laarhoven LM, de Heus P, van Luijn J, et al. Longitudinal study on methicillin-resistant *Staphylococcus pseudintermedius* in households. *PloS One.* 2011;6. e27788.
11. Lefebvre SL, Reid-Smith RJ, Waltner-Toews D, et al. Incidence of acquisition of methicillin-resistant *Staphylococcus aureus, Clostridium difficile*, and other health-care-associated pathogens by dogs that participate in animal-assisted interventions. *J Am Vet Med Assoc.* 2009;234:1404–1417.
12. Loeffler A, Pfeiffer D, Lindsay J, et al. Lack of transmission of methicillin-resistant *Staphylococcus aureus* (MRSA) between apparently healthy dogs in a rescue kennel. *Vet Microbiol.* 2010;141:178–181.
13. Fazakerley J, Nuttall T, Sales D, et al. Staphylococcal colonization of mucosal and lesional skin sites in atopic and healthy dogs. *Vet Dermatol.* 2009;20:179–184.
14. Fazakerley J, Williams N, Carter S, et al. Heterogeneity of *Staphylococcus pseudintermedius* isolates from atopic and healthy dogs. *Vet Dermatol.* 2010;21:578–585.
15. Hanselman BA, Kruth SA, Rousseau J, et al. Coagulase positive staphylococcal colonization of people and their household pets. *Can Vet J.* 2009;50:954–958.
16. Hartmann FA, White DG, West S, et al. Molecular characterization of *Staphylococcus intermedius* carriage by healthy dogs and comparison of antimicrobial susceptibility patterns to isolates from dogs with pyoderma. *Vet Microbiol.* 2005;108:119–131.
17. Saijonmaa-Koulumies LE, Lloyd DH. Colonization of neonatal puppies by *Staphylococcus intermedius. Vet Dermatol.* 2002;13:123–130.
18. Windahl U, Reimegard E, Strom Holst B, et al. Carriage of methicillin-resistant *Staphylococcus pseudintermedius* in dogs a longitudinal study. *BMC Vet Res.* 2012;8:34.
19. Abraham JL, Morris DO, Griffeth GC, et al. Surveillance of healthy cats and cats with inflammatory skin disease for colonization of the skin by methicillin-resistant coagulase-positive staphylococci and *Staphylococcus schleiferi* ssp. *schleiferi. Vet Dermatol.* 2007;18:252–259.
20. Lilenbaum W, Esteves AL, Souza GN. Prevalence and antimicrobial susceptibility of staphylococci isolated from saliva of clinically normal cats. *Lett Appl Microbiol.* 1999;28:448–452.
21. Lilenbaum W, Nunes EL, Azeredo MA. Prevalence and antimicrobial susceptibility of staphylococci isolated from the skin surface of clinically normal cats. *Lett Appl Microbiol.* 1998;27:224–228.
22. Faires MC, Traverse M, Tater KC, et al. Methicillin-resistant and -susceptible *Staphylococcus aureus* infections in dogs. *Emerg Infect Dis.* 2010;16:69–75.
23. Hanselman BA, Kruth S, Weese JS. Methicillin-resistant staphylococcal colonization in dogs entering a veterinary teaching hospital. *Vet Microbiol.* 2007;126:277–281.
24. Rich M, Roberts L, Jones M, et al. *Staphylococcus schleiferi* subspecies *coagulans* in companion animals. *Vet Rec.* 2007;161:107.
25. Bes M, Guérin-Faublée V, Freney J, et al. Isolation of *Staphylococcus schleiferi* subspecies *coagulans* from two cases of canine pyoderma. *Vet Rec.* 2002;150:487–488.
26. Hariharan H, Gibson K, Peterson R, et al. *Staphylococcus pseudintermedius* and *Staphylococcus schleiferi* subspecies *coagulans* from canine pyoderma cases in Grenada, West Indies, and their susceptibility to beta-lactam drugs. *Vet Med International.* 2014;2014:850126.
27. Cain CL, Morris DO, Rankin SC. Clinical characterization of *Staphylococcus schleiferi* infections and identification of risk factors for acquisition of oxacillin-resistant strains in dogs: 225 cases (2003-2009). *J Am Vet Med Assoc.* 2011;239:1566–1573.
28. Cox HU, Newman SS, Roy AF, et al. Species of *Staphylococcus* isolated from animal infections. *Cornell Vet.* 1984;74:124–135.
29. Davis JA, Jackson CR, Fedorka-Cray PJ, et al. Carriage of methicillin-resistant staphylococci by healthy companion animals in the US. *Lett Appl Microbiol.* 2014;59:1–8.
30. Stepanović S, Dimitrijević V, Vuković D, et al. *Staphylococcus sciuri* as a part of skin, nasal and oral flora in healthy dogs. *Vet Microbiol.* 2001;82:177–185.
31. Cox HU, Hoskins JD, Newman SS, et al. Temporal study of staphylococcal species on healthy dogs. *Am J Vet Res.* 1988;49:747–751.
32. Medleau L, Long RE, Brown J, et al. Frequency and antimicrobial susceptibility of *Staphylococcus* species isolated from canine pyodermas. *Am J Vet Res.* 1986;47:229–231.
33. Nagase N, Sasaki A, Yamashita K, et al. Isolation and species distribution of staphylococci from animal and human skin. *J Vet Med Sci.* 2002;64:245–250.
34. Bagcigil FA, Moodley A, Baptiste KE, et al. Occurrence, species distribution, antimicrobial resistance and clonality of methicillin- and erythromycin-resistant staphylococci in the nasal cavity of domestic animals. *Vet Microbiol.* 2007;121:307–315.
35. Kristensen S, Krogh HV. A study of skin diseases in dogs and cats. III. III. Microflora of the skin of dogs with chronic eczema. *Nord Vet Med.* 1978;30:223–230.
36. Krogh HV, Kristensen S. A study of skin diseases in dogs and cats. II. Microflora of the normal skin of dogs and cats. *Nord Vet Med.* 1976;28:459–463.
37. Penna B, Varges R, Martins R, et al. In vitro antimicrobial resistance of staphylococci isolated from canine urinary tract infection. *Can Vet J.* 2010;51:738–742.
38. Cox HU, Hoskins JD, Newman SS, et al. Distribution of staphylococcal species on clinically healthy cats. *Am J Vet Res.* 1985;46:1824–1828.
39. Adam HJ, DeCorby M, Rennie R, et al. Prevalence of antimicrobial resistant pathogens from blood cultures from Canadian hospitals: results of the CANWARD 2007-2009 study. *Diagn Microbiol Infect Dis.* 2011;69:307–313.

40. Rupp ME, Fey PD. *Staphylococcus epidermidis* and other coagulase negative staphylococci. In: Bennett JE, Dolin M, Blaser MJ, eds. *Principles and Practice of Infectious Diseases*. 8th ed. Philadelphia, PA: Saunders Elsevier; 2015:2272–2282.
41. Koksal F, Yasar H, Samasti M. Antibiotic resistance patterns of coagulase-negative *Staphylococcus* strains isolated from blood cultures of septicemic patients in Turkey. *Microbiol Res*. 2009;164:404–410.
42. Nakamura RK, Zimmerman SA, Lange AJ, et al. Isolation of methicillin-resistant *Staphylococcus lugdunensis* in a dog with endocarditis. *J Vet Cardiol*. 2012;14:531–536.
43. Rook KA, Brown DC, Rankin SC, et al. Case-control study of *Staphylococcus lugdunensis* infection isolates from small companion animals. *Vet Dermatol*. 2012;23:476–e490.
44. Manian FA. Asymptomatic nasal carriage of mupirocin-resistant, methicillin-resistant *Staphylococcus aureus* (MRSA) in a pet dog associated with MRSA infection in household contacts. *Clin Infect Dis*. 2003;36:e26–28.
45. Owen MR, Moores AP, Coe RJ. Management of MRSA septic arthritis in a dog using a gentamicin-impregnated collagen sponge. *J Small Anim Pract*. 2004;45:609–612.
46. van Duijkeren E, Box AT, Heck ME, et al. Methicillin-resistant staphylococci isolated from animals. *Vet Microbiol*. 2004;103:91–97.
47. van Duijkeren E, Wolfhagen MJ, Box AT, et al. Human-to-dog transmission of methicillin-resistant *Staphylococcus aureus*. *Emerg Infect Dis*. 2004;10:2235–2237.
48. Loeffler A, Boag AK, Sung J, et al. Prevalence of methicillin-resistant *Staphylococcus aureus* among staff and pets in a small animal referral hospital in the UK. *J Antimicrob Chemother*. 2005;56:692–697.
49. van Duijkeren E, Wolfhagen MJ, Heck ME, et al. Transmission of a Panton-Valentine leucocidin-positive, methicillin-resistant *Staphylococcus aureus* strain between humans and a dog. *J Clin Microbiol*. 2005;43:6209–6211.
50. Baptiste KE, Williams K, Willams NJ, et al. Methicillin-resistant staphylococci in companion animals. *Emerg Infect Dis*. 2005;11:1942–1944.
51. Weese JS, Dick H, Willey BM, et al. Suspected transmission of methicillin-resistant *Staphylococcus aureus* between domestic pets and humans in veterinary clinics and in the household. *Vet Microbiol*. 2006;115:148–155.
52. O'Mahony R, Abbott Y, Leonard FC, et al. Methicillin-resistant *Staphylococcus aureus* (MRSA) isolated from animals and veterinary personnel in Ireland. *Vet Microbiol*. 2005;109:285–296.
53. Strommenger B, Kehrenberg C, Kettlitz C, et al. Molecular characterization of methicillin-resistant *Staphylococcus aureus* strains from pet animals and their relationship to human isolates. *J Antimicrob Chemother*. 2006;57:461–465.
54. Davis MF, Misic AM, Morris DO, et al. Genome sequencing reveals strain dynamics of methicillin-resistant *Staphylococcus aureus* in the same household in the context of clinical disease in a person and a dog. *Vet Microbiol*. 2015;180:304–307.
55. Vengust M, Anderson ME, Rousseau J, et al. Methicillin-resistant staphylococcal colonization in clinically normal dogs and horses in the community. *Lett Appl Microbiol*. 2006;43:602–606.
56. Epstein CR, Yam WC, Peiris JS, et al. Methicillin-resistant commensal staphylococci in healthy dogs as a potential zoonotic reservoir for community-acquired antibiotic resistance. *Infect Genet Evol*. 2009;9:283–285.
57. Faires MC, Tater KC, Weese JS. An investigation of methicillin-resistant *Staphylococcus aureus* colonization in people and pets in the same household with an infected person or infected pet. *J Am Vet Med Assoc*. 2009;235:540–543.
58. Murphy C, Reid-Smith RJ, Prescott JF, et al. Occurrence of antimicrobial resistant bacteria in healthy dogs and cats presented to private veterinary hospitals in southern Ontario: a preliminary study. *Can Vet J*. 2009;50:1047–1053.
59. Loeffler A, Pfeiffer DU, Lindsay JA, et al. Prevalence of and risk factors for MRSA carriage in companion animals: a survey of dogs, cats and horses. *Epidemiol Infect*. 2010:1–10.
60. Kottler S, Middleton JR, Perry J, et al. Prevalence of *Staphylococcus aureus* and methicillin-resistant *Staphylococcus aureus* carriage in three populations. *J Vet Int Med*. 2010;24:132–139.
61. Gingrich EN, Kurt T, Hyatt DR, et al. Prevalence of methicillin-resistant staphylococci in northern Colorado shelter animals. *J Vet Diagn Invest*. 2011;23:947–950.
62. Ishihara K, Saito M, Shimokubo N, et al. Methicillin-resistant *Staphylococcus aureus* carriage among veterinary staff and dogs in private veterinary clinics in Hokkaido, Japan. *Microbiol Immunol*. 2014;58:149–154.
63. Wedley AL, Dawson S, Maddox TW, et al. Carriage of *Staphylococcus* species in the veterinary visiting dog population in mainland UK: molecular characterisation of resistance and virulence. *Vet Microbiol*. 2014;170:81–88.
64. Heller J, Innocent GT, Denwood M, et al. Assessing the probability of acquisition of meticillin-resistant *Staphylococcus aureus* (MRSA) in a dog using a nested stochastic simulation model and logistic regression sensitivity analysis. *Prev Vet Med*. 2011;99:211–224.
65. Soares Magalhães RJ, Loeffler A, Lindsay J, et al. Risk factors for methicillin-resistant *Staphylococcus aureus* (MRSA) infection in dogs and cats: a case-control study. *Vet Res*. 2010;41:55.
66. Walther B, Hermes J, Cuny C, et al. Sharing more than friendship: nasal colonization with coagulase-positive staphylococci (CPS) and co-habitation aspects of dogs and their owners. *PloS One*. 2012;7. e35197.
67. Weese JS, Rousseau J, Willey BM, et al. Methicillin-resistant *Staphylococcus aureus* in horses at a veterinary teaching hospital: frequency, characterization, and association with clinical disease. *J Vet Intern Med*. 2006;20:182–186.
68. Trautmann M, Stecher J, Hemmer W, et al. Intranasal mupirocin prophylaxis in elective surgery. A review of published studies. *Chemotherapy*. 2008;54:9–16.
69. Bean DC, Wigmore SM. Carriage rate and antibiotic susceptibility of coagulase-positive staphylococci isolated from healthy dogs in Victoria, Australia. *Aust Vet J*. 2016;94:456–460.
70. Han J-I, Yang C-H, Park H-M. Prevalence and risk factors of *Staphylococcus* spp. carriage among dogs and their owners: a cross-sectional study. *Vet J*. 2016;212:15–21.
71. Mouney MC, Stiles J, Townsend WM, et al. Prevalence of methicillin-resistant *Staphylococcus* spp. in the conjunctival sac of healthy dogs. *Vet Ophthalmol*. 2013;18:123–126.
72. Youn JH, Park YH, Hang'ombe B, et al. Prevalence and characterization of *Staphylococcus aureus* and *Staphylococcus pseudintermedius* isolated from companion animals and environment in the veterinary teaching hospital in Zambia, Africa. *Comp Immun Microbiol Infect Dis*. 2014;37:123–130.
73. Beck KM, Waisglass SE, Dick HLN, et al. Prevalence of meticillin-resistant *Staphylococcus pseudintermedius* (MRSP) from skin and carriage sites of dogs after treatment of their meticillin-resistant or meticillin-sensitive staphylococcal pyoderma. *Vet Dermatol*. 2012;23. 369–e367.
74. Feng Y, Tian W, Lin D, et al. Prevalence and characterization of methicillin-resistant *Staphylococcus pseudintermedius* in pets from South China. *Vet Microbiol*. 2012;160:517–524.
75. Grönthal T, Ollilainen M, Eklund M, et al. Epidemiology of methicillin resistant *Staphylococcus pseudintermedius* in guide dogs in Finland. *Acta Vet Scand*. 2015;57:37.
76. Morris DO, Boston RC, O'Shea K, et al. The prevalence of carriage of meticillin-resistant staphylococci by veterinary dermatology practice staff and their respective pets. *Vet Dermatol*. 2010;21:400–407.
77. Nazarali A, Singh A, Moens NMM, et al. Association between methicillin-resistant *Staphylococcus pseudintermedius* carriage and the development of surgical site infections following tibial plateau leveling osteotomy in dogs. *J Am Vet Med Assoc*. 2015;247:909–916.
78. Hensel N, Zabel S, Hensel P. Prior antibacterial drug exposure in dogs with meticillin-resistant *Staphylococcus pseudintermedius* (MRSP) pyoderma. *Vet Dermatol*. 2016;27. 72–8e20.
79. Lehner G, Linek M, Bond R, et al. Case-control risk factor study of methicillin-resistant *Staphylococcus pseudintermedius* (MRSP) infection in dogs and cats in Germany. *Vet Microbiol*. 2014;168:154–160.

80. Weese J, Faires M, Frank LA, et al. Factors associated with methicillin-resistant versus methicillin-susceptible *Staphylococcus pseudintermedius* infection in dogs. *J Am Vet Med Assoc*. 2012;240:1450–1455.
81. Baptiste KE, Williams K, Willams NJ, et al. Methicillin-resistant staphylococci in companion animals. *Emerg Infect Dis*. 2005;11:1942–1944.
82. Que Y, Moreillon P. *Staphylococcus aureus* (including staphylococcal toxic shock syndrome). In: Bennett JE, Dolin M, Blaser MJ, eds. *Principles and Practice of Infectious Diseases*. 8th ed. Philadelphia, PA: Saunders Elsevier; 2015:2237–2271.
83. Hermans K, Devriese LA, Haesebrouck F. Staphylococcus. In: Gyles C, Prescott J, Songer G, eds. *Pathogenesis of Bacterial Infections in Animals*. 3rd ed. Ames, IA: Blackwell; 2004:43–56.
84. Devriese LA, Oeding P. Characteristics of *Staphylococcus aureus* strains isolated from different animal species. *Res Vet Sci*. 1976;21:284–291.
85. Larkin EA, Carman RJ, Krakauer T, et al. *Staphylococcus aureus*: the toxic presence of a pathogen extraordinaire. *Curr Med Chem*. 2009;16:4003–4019.
86. Frazee BW, Salz TO, Lambert L, et al. Fatal community-associated methicillin-resistant *Staphylococcus aureus* pneumonia in an immunocompetent young adult. *Ann Emerg Med*. 2005;46:401–404.
87. Gilbert M, MacDonald J, Gregson D, et al. Outbreak in Alberta of community-acquired (USA300) methicillin-resistant *Staphylococcus aureus* in people with a history of drug use, homelessness or incarceration. *CMAJ (Can Med Assoc J)*. 2006;175:149–154.
88. Johnsson D, Mölling P, Strålin K, et al. Detection of Panton-Valentine leukocidin gene in *Staphylococcus aureus* by LightCycler PCR: clinical and epidemiological aspects. *Clin Microbiol Infect*. 2004;10:884–889.
89. Voyich JM, Otto M, Mathema B, et al. Is Panton-Valentine leukocidin the major virulence determinant in community-associated methicillin-resistant *Staphylococcus aureus* disease? *J Infect Dis*. 2006;194:1761–1770.
90. Boost MV, O'Donoghue MM, Siu KH. Characterisation of methicillin-resistant *Staphylococcus aureus* isolates from dogs and their owners. *Clin Microbiol Infect*. 2007;13:731–733.
91. Rankin S, Roberts S, O'Shea K, et al. Panton Valentine leukocidin (PVL) toxin positive MRSA strains isolated from companion animals. *Vet Microbiol*. 2005;108:145–148.
92. Abdel-Moein KA, Samir A. Isolation of enterotoxigenic *Staphylococcus aureus* from pet dogs and cats: a public health implication. *Vector Borne Zoonotic Dis*. 2011;11:627–629.
93. Adesiyun AA, Usman B. Isolation of enterotoxigenic strains of staphylococci from dogs. *Vet Microbiol*. 1983;8:459–468.
94. Couto N, Belas A, Oliveira M, et al. Comparative analysis of the virulence characteristics of methicillin-resistant and -susceptible *Staphylococcus pseudintermedius* isolates isolated from small animals: a RNA-Seq-based transcriptome analysis. *Antimicrob Agents Chemother*. 2015;30:962–967.
95. Singh A, Walker M, Rousseau J, et al. Characterization of the biofilm forming ability of *Staphylococcus pseudintermedius* from dogs. *BMC Vet Res*. 2013;9:93.
96. Bardiau M, Yamazaki K, Ote I, et al. Characterization of methicillin-resistant *Staphylococcus pseudintermedius* isolated from dogs and cats. *Microbiol Immunol*. 2013;57:496–501.
97. Iyori K, Hisatsune J, Kawakami T, et al. Identification of a novel *Staphylococcus pseudintermedius* exfoliative toxin gene and its prevalence in isolates from canines with pyoderma and healthy dogs. *FEMS Microbiol Lett*. 2010;312:169–175.
98. Lautz S, Kanbar T, Alber J, et al. Dissemination of the gene encoding exfoliative toxin of *Staphylococcus intermedius* among strains isolated from dogs during routine microbiological diagnostics. *J Vet Med B Infect Dis Vet Public Health*. 2006;53:434–438.
99. Ruzauskas M, Couto N, Pavilonis A, et al. Characterization of *Staphylococcus pseudintermedius* isolated from diseased dogs in Lithuania. *Polish J Vet Sci*. 2016;19:7–14.
100. Terauchi R, Sato H, Hasegawa T, et al. Isolation of exfoliative toxin from *Staphylococcus intermedius* and its local toxicity in dogs. *Vet Microbiol*. 2003;94:19–29.
101. Oliveira M, Bexiga R, Nunes SF, et al. Biofilm-forming ability profiling of *Staphylococcus aureus* and *Staphylococcus epidermidis* mastitis isolates. *Vet Microbiol*. 2006;118:133–140.
102. Osland AM, Vestby LK, Fanuelsen H, et al. Clonal diversity and biofilm-forming ability of methicillin-resistant *Staphylococcus pseudintermedius*. *J Antimicrob Chemother*. 2012;67:841–848.
103. Seo Y, Lee D, Rayamahji N, et al. Biofilm-forming associated genotypic and phenotypic characteristics of *Staphylococcus* spp. isolated from animals and air. *Res Vet Sci*. 2008;85:433–438.
104. Girard C, Higgins R. *Staphylococcus intermedius* cellulitis and toxic shock in a dog. *Can Vet J*. 1999;40:501–502.
105. Weese JS, Poma R, James F, et al. *Staphylococcus pseudintermedius* necrotizing fasciitis in a dog. *Can Vet J*. 2009;50:655–656.
106. Rahkonen M, Luttinen S, Koskela M, et al. True bacteremias caused by coagulase negative *Staphylococcus* are difficult to distinguish from blood culture contaminants. *Eur J Clin Microbiol Infect Dis*. 2012;31:2639–2644.
107. Bemis DA, Jones RD, Videla R, et al. Evaluation of cefoxitin disk diffusion breakpoint for detection of methicillin resistance in *Staphylococcus pseudintermedius* isolates from dogs. *J Vet Diagn Invest*. 2012;24:964–967.
108. Bemis DA, Jones RD, Frank LA, et al. Evaluation of susceptibility test breakpoints used to predict mecA-mediated resistance in *Staphylococcus pseudintermedius* isolated from dogs. *J Vet Diagn Invest*. 2009;21:53–58.
109. Clinical and Laboratory Standards Institute. Performance standards for antimicrobial disk and dilution susceptibility tests for bacteria isolated from animals; Approved standard. In: *CLSI Document VET01-A4*. 4th ed. Wayne, PA: Clinical and Laboratory Standards Institute; 2013.
110. Schissler JR, Hillier A, Daniels JB, et al. Evaluation of Clinical Laboratory Standards Institute interpretive criteria for methicillin-resistant *Staphylococcus pseudintermedius* isolated from dogs. *J Vet Diagn Invest*. 2009;21:684–688.
111. Hnot ML, Cole LK, Lorch G, et al. Evaluation of canine-specific minocycline and doxycycline susceptibility breakpoints for meticillin-resistant *Staphylococcus pseudintermedius* isolates from dogs. *Vet Dermatol*. 2015;26:334–338.
112. Weese JS, Sweetman K, Edson H, et al. Evaluation of minocycline susceptibility of methicillin-resistant *Staphylococcus pseudintermedius*. *Vet Microbiol*. 2012;162:968–971.
113. Maaland MG, Papich MG, Turnidge J, et al. Pharmacodynamics of doxycycline and tetracycline against *Staphylococcus pseudintermedius*: proposal of canine-specific breakpoints for doxycycline. *J Clin Microbiol*. 2013;51:3547–3554.
114. Anderson ME, Weese JS. Evaluation of a real-time polymerase chain reaction assay for rapid identification of methicillin-resistant *Staphylococcus aureus* directly from nasal swabs in horses. *Vet Microbiol*. 2007;122:185–189.
115. Borio S, Colombo S, La Rosa G, et al. Effectiveness of a combined (4% chlorhexidine digluconate shampoo and solution) protocol in MRS and non-MRS canine superficial pyoderma: a randomized, blinded, antibiotic-controlled study. *Vet Dermatol*. 2015;26:339–344. e372.
116. Loeffler A, Cobb MA, Bond R. Comparison of a chlorhexidine and a benzoyl peroxide shampoo as sole treatment in canine superficial pyoderma. *Vet Rec*. 2011;169:249.
117. Hillier A, Lloyd DH, Weese JS, et al. Guidelines for the diagnosis and antimicrobial therapy of canine superficial bacterial folliculitis (Antimicrobial Guidelines Working Group of the International Society for Companion Animal Infectious Diseases). *Vet Dermatol*. 2014;25:163–175.
118. Faires M, Gard S, Aucoin D, et al. Inducible clindamycin-resistance in methicillin-resistant *Staphylococcus aureus* and methicillin-resistant *Staphylococcus pseudintermedius* isolates from dogs and cats. *Vet Microbiol*. 2009;139:419–420.
119. Rich M, Deighton L, Roberts L. Clindamycin-resistance in methicillin-resistant *Staphylococcus aureus* isolated from animals. *Vet Microbiol*. 2005;111:237–240.
120. Rubin JE, Ball KR, Chirino-Trejo M. Antimicrobial susceptibility of *Staphylococcus aureus* and *Staphylococcus pseudintermedius* isolated from various animals. *Can Vet J*. 2011;52:153–157.
121. Chanchaithong P, Prapasarakul N. Occurrence and characterization of inducible clindamycin resistance in canine methicillin-resistant *Staphylococcus pseudintermedius*. *Vet J*. 2015;208:99–101.

122. Maaland MG, Guardabassi L, Papich MG. Minocycline pharmacokinetics and pharmacodynamics in dogs: dosage recommendations for treatment of meticillin-resistant *Staphylococcus pseudintermedius* infections. *Vet Dermatol.* 2014;25:182–190. e146–187.
123. Weese JS, Blondeau JM, Boothe D, et al. Antimicrobial use guidelines for treatment of urinary tract disease in dogs and cats: Antimicrobial Guidelines Working Group of the International Society for Companion Animal Infectious Diseases. *Vet Med International.* 2011;2011:1–9.
124. Liu C, Bayer A, Cosgrove SE, et al. Clinical practice guidelines by the Infectious Diseases Society of America for the treatment of methicillin-resistant *Staphylococcus aureus* infections in adults and children. *Clin Infect Dis.* 2011:1–38.
125. Zur G, Gurevich B, Elad D. Prior antimicrobial use as a risk factor for resistance in selected *Staphylococcus pseudintermedius* isolates from the skin and ears of dogs. *Vet Dermatol.* 2016;27. 468–e125.
126. Dicicco M, Weese S, Neethirajan S, et al. Fosfomycin susceptibility of canine methicillin-resistant *Staphylococcus pseudintermedius* isolates. *Res Vet Sci.* 2014;96:251–253.
127. Fukata T, Imai N, Shibata S. Acute renal insufficiency in cats after fosfomycin administration. *Vet Rec.* 2008;163:337–338.
128. Atilla A, Boothe HW, Tollett M, et al. In vitro elution of amikacin and vancomycin from impregnated plaster of Paris beads. *Vet Surg.* 2010;39:715–721.
129. Cribb NC, Bouré LP, Hanna WJ, et al. In vitro and in vivo evaluation of ferric-hyaluronate implants for delivery of amikacin sulfate to the tarsocrural joint of horses. *Vet Surg.* 2009;38:498–505.
130. Hayes GM, Gibson TWG, Moens NMM, et al. Intra-articular pharmacokinetics of a gentamicin impregnated collagen sponge in the canine stifle: an experimental study. *Vet Surg.* 2014;43:166–173.
131. Thomas LA, Bizikova T, Minihan AC. In vitro elution and antibacterial activity of clindamycin, amikacin, and vancomycin from R-gel polymer. *Vet Surg.* 2011;40:774–780.
132. Fulham KS, Lemarie SL, Hosgood G, et al. In vitro susceptibility testing of meticillin-resistant and meticillin-susceptible staphylococci to mupirocin and novobiocin. *Vet Dermatol.* 2011;22:88–94.
133. Godbeer SM, Gold RM, Lawhon SD. Prevalence of mupirocin resistance in *Staphylococcus pseudintermedius. J Clin Microbiol.* 2014;52:1250–1252.
134. Humphries RM, Wu MT, Westblade LF, et al. In vitro antimicrobial susceptibility of *Staphylococcus pseudintermedius* isolates of human and animal origin. *J Clin Microbiol.* 2016;54:1391–1394.
135. Matanovic K, Pérez-Roth E, Pintaric S, et al. Molecular characterization of high-level mupirocin resistance in *Staphylococcus pseudintermedius. J Clin Microbiol.* 2012;51:1005–1007.
136. Rubin JE, Chirino-Trejo M. Antimicrobial susceptibility of canine and human *Staphylococcus aureus* collected in Saskatoon, Canada. *Zoonoses Public Health.* 2011;58:454–462.
137. Valentine BK, Dew W, Yu A, et al. In vitro evaluation of topical biocide and antimicrobial susceptibility of *Staphylococcus pseudintermedius* from dogs. *Vet Dermatol.* 2012;23:493–e495.
138. Murayama N, Nagata M, Terada Y, et al. Efficacy of a surgical scrub including 2% chlorhexidine acetate for canine superficial pyoderma. *Vet Dermatol.* 2010;21:586–592.
139. Edwards-Jones V, Buck R, Shawcross SG, et al. The effect of essential oils on methicillin-resistant *Staphylococcus aureus* using a dressing model. *Burns.* 2004;30:772–777.
140. Kavanaugh NL, Ribbeck K. Selected antimicrobial essential oils eradicate *Pseudomonas* spp. and *Staphylococcus aureus* biofilms. *Appl Environ Microbiol.* 2012;78:4057–4061.
141. Faoagali J, George N, Leditschke JF. Does tea tree oil have a place in the topical treatment of burns? *Burns.* 1997;23:349–351.
142. Söderberg TA, Johansson A, Gref R. Toxic effects of some conifer resin acids and tea tree oil on human epithelial and fibroblast cells. *Toxicology.* 1996;107:99–109.
143. Del Beccaro MA. Melaleuca oil poisoning in a 17-month-old. *Vet Human Toxicol.* 1995;37:557–558.
144. Morris MC, Donoghue A, Markowitz JA, et al. Ingestion of tea tree oil (Melaleuca oil) by a 4-year-old boy. *Pediatr Emerg Care.* 2003;19: 169–171.
145. Alandejani T, Marsan J, Ferris W, et al. Effectiveness of honey on *Staphylococcus aureus* and *Pseudomonas aeruginosa* biofilms. *Otolaryngol Head Neck Surg.* 2009;141:114–118.
146. Jenkins R, Burton N, Cooper R. Manuka honey inhibits cell division in methicillin-resistant *Staphylococcus aureus. J Antimicrob Chemother.* 2011;66:2536–2542.
147. Kwakman PH, Van den Akker JP, Güçlü A, et al. Medical-grade honey kills antibiotic-resistant bacteria in vitro and eradicates skin colonization. *Clin Infect Dis.* 2008;46:1677–1682.
148. Maeda Y, Loughrey A, Earle JA, et al. Antibacterial activity of honey against community-associated methicillin-resistant *Staphylococcus aureus* (CA-MRSA). *Complement Ther Clin Pract.* 2008;14:77–82.
149. Arciola CR, Campoccia D, An YH, et al. Prevalence and antibiotic resistance of 15 minor staphylococcal species colonizing orthopedic implants. *IJAO.* 2006;29:395–401.
150. Montanaro L, Speziale P, Campoccia D, et al. Scenery of *Staphylococcus* implant infections in orthopedics. *Future Microbiol.* 2011;6:1329–1349.
151. Nicoll C, Singh A, Weese JS. Economic impact of tibial plateau leveling osteotomy surgical site infection in dogs. *Vet Surg.* 2014;43:899–902.
152. Trampuz A, Widmer AF. Infections associated with orthopedic implants. *Curr Opin Infect Dis.* 2006;19:349–356.
153. Mekni MA, Bouchami O, Achour W, et al. Strong biofilm production but not adhesion virulence factors can discriminate between invasive and commensal *Staphylococcus epidermidis* strains. *APMIS.* 2012;120: 605–611.
154. Daley P, Bajgai J, Penney C, et al. A cross sectional study of animal and human colonization with methicillin-resistant *Staphylococcus aureus* (MRSA) in an Aboriginal community. *BMC Publ Health.* 2016;16:595.
155. Drougka E, Foka A, Koutinas CK, et al. Interspecies spread of *Staphylococcus aureus* clones among companion animals and human close contacts in a veterinary teaching hospital. A cross-sectional study in Greece. *Prev Vet Med.* 2016;126:190–198.
156. Leonard FC, Abbott Y, Rossney A, et al. Methicillin-resistant *Staphylococcus aureus* isolated from a veterinary surgeon and five dogs in one practice. *Vet Rec.* 2006;158:155–159.
157. Loeffler A, McCarthy A, Lloyd DH, et al. Whole-genome comparison of meticillin-resistant *Staphylococcus aureus* CC22 SCCmecIV from people and their in-contact pets. *Vet Dermatol.* 2013;24. 538–e128.
158. Weese J, Dick H, Willey B, et al. Suspected transmission of methicillin-resistant *Staphylococcus aureus* between domestic pets and humans in veterinary clinics and in the household. *Vet Microbiol.* 2006;115: 148–155.
159. Morris DO, Lautenbach E, Zaoutis T, et al. Potential for pet animals to harbor methicillin-resistant *Staphylococcus aureus* when residing with human MRSA patients. *Zoonoses Public Health.* 2012;59:286–293.
160. Aklilu E, Zunita Z, Hassan L, et al. Molecular epidemiology of methicillin-resistant *Staphylococcus aureus* (MRSA) among veterinary students and personnel at a veterinary hospital in Malaysia. *Vet Microbiol.* 2013;164:352–358.
161. Anderson MEC, Lefebvre SL, Weese JS. Evaluation of prevalence and risk factors for methicillin-resistant *Staphylococcus aureus* colonization in veterinary personnel attending an international equine veterinary conference. *Vet Microbiol.* 2008;129:410–417.
162. Burstiner LC, Faires M, Weese JS. Methicillin-resistant *Staphylococcus aureus* colonization in personnel attending a veterinary surgery conference. *Vet Surg.* 2010;39:150–157.
163. Groves MD, Crouch B, Coombs GW, et al. Molecular epidemiology of methicillin-resistant *Staphylococcus aureus* isolated from Australian veterinarians. *PloS One.* 2016;11. e0146034.
164. Hanselman BA, Kruth SA, Rousseau J, et al. Methicillin-resistant *Staphylococcus aureus* colonization in veterinary personnel. *Emerg Infect Dis.* 2006;12:1933–1938.
165. Jordan D, Simon J, Fury S, et al. Carriage of methicillin-resistant *Staphylococcus aureus* by veterinarians in Australia. *Aust Vet J.* 2011;89: 152–159.
166. Zemlicková H, Fridrichová M, Tyllová K, et al. Carriage of methicillin-resistant *Staphylococcus aureus* in veterinary personnel. *Epidemiol Infect.* 2009;137:1233–1236.

167. Boost MV, So SY, Perreten V. Low rate of methicillin-resistant coagulase-positive staphylococcal colonization of veterinary personnel in Hong Kong. *Zoonoses Public Health*. 2011;58:36–40.
168. Hanselman BA, Kruth SA, Rousseau J, et al. Coagulase positive staphylococcal colonization of humans and their household pets. *Can Vet J*. 2009;50:954–958.
169. Frank LA, Kania SA, Kirzeder EM, et al. Risk of colonization or gene transfer to owners of dogs with methicillin-resistant *Staphylococcus pseudintermedius*. *Vet Dermatol*. 2009;20:496–501.
170. Börjesson S, Gómez-Sanz E, Ekström K, et al. *Staphylococcus pseudintermedius* can be misdiagnosed as *Staphylococcus aureus* in humans with dog bite wounds. *Eur J Clin Microbiol Inf Dis*. 2014;34:839–844.
171. Starlander G, Börjesson S, Grönlund Andersson U, et al. Cluster of infections caused by methicillin-resistant *Staphylococcus pseudintermedius* in a human hospital. *J Clin Microbiol*. 2014;52:3118–3120.
172. Somayaji R, Priyantha MA, Rubin JE, et al. Human infections due to *Staphylococcus pseudintermedius*, an emerging zoonosis of canine origin: report of 24 cases. *Diagn Microbiol Infect Dis*. 2016;85:471–476.
173. Murphy E, Spencer SJ, Young D, et al. MRSA colonisation and subsequent risk of infection despite effective eradication in orthopaedic elective surgery. *J Bone Joint Surg Br*. 2011;93:548–551.
174. Ammerlaan HSM, Kluytmans JAJW, Berkhout H, et al. Eradication of carriage with methicillin-resistant *Staphylococcus aureus*: effectiveness of a national guideline. *J Antimicrob Chemother*. 2011;66:2409–2417.

52

Miscellaneous Gram-Positive Bacterial Infections

Joshua B. Daniels, Jane E. Sykes

KEY POINTS

- Cause: Uncommon to rare gram-positive bacterial infections in dogs and cats include those caused by *Rhodococcus equi* (synonym *Rhodococcus hoagii*), *Corynebacterium* spp., *Listeria monocytogenes*, *Erysipelothrix* spp., and *Bacillus anthracis*.
- First Described: *Rhodococcus equi*: 1923, Sweden, in horses (Magnusson)[1]; *Corynebacterium urealyticum*: 1947, Spain, in humans (Cifuentes and Soriano)[2]; *L. monocytogenes*: 1927, England, in laboratory rabbits and guinea pigs (Murray)[3]; *Erysipelothrix* spp.: 1876, in mice (Koch)[4]; *B. anthracis*: 1850s, France, in sheep and cattle (Rayer, Devaine, Pollender).[5]
- Affected Hosts: *Rhodococcus equi* (horses, pigs, cattle, dogs, cats, humans), *C. urealyticum* (dogs, cats, humans), *L. monocytogenes* (many domestic mammals, poultry, humans), *Erysipelothrix* spp. (especially pigs, turkeys, and laying hens; but also other mammals including humans, dogs and cats; birds, fish and reptiles), and *B. anthracis* (primarily herbivorous mammals such as cattle, sheep and goats; but also humans and rarely dogs and possibly cats).
- Geographic Distribution: Worldwide; anthrax is most prevalent in Africa, the Middle East, and Latin America.
- Route of Transmission: Inhalation, inoculation, or ingestion (*R. equi*); invasion of normal microflora (*Corynebacterium* spp.); ingestion (*L. monocytogenes*); inoculation and possibly ingestion (*Erysipelothrix* spp.). Anthrax can be acquired through ingestion, inoculation, or inhalation; most cases in dogs result from ingestion, whereas humans are most commonly infected through cutaneous inoculation.
- Major Clinical Signs: *Rhodococcus equi*: cutaneous abscesses (cats), signs that depend on systemic organ involvement; *Corynebacterium* spp.: lower urinary tract signs (*C. urealyticum*), respiratory signs (*Corynebacterium ulcerans*), otitis externa (*Corynebacterium auriscanis*); *L. monocytogenes*: febrile gastroenteritis, neurologic signs, abortion, cholecystitis, abdominal lymphadenitis (*L. monocytogenes*); *Erysipelothrix*: fever, lameness, cardiac murmurs, spinal pain, erythematous cutaneous lesions (erysipelas); *B. anthracis*: fever, inappetence, edema of tissues surrounding the upper GI tract.
- Differential Diagnoses: Other gram-positive and gram-negative bacterial infections.
- Human Health Significance: All of these organisms are capable of causing disease in humans, and many infections in humans result from exposure to animals or animal products. Humans are not usually exposed as a result of contact with dogs and cats, but care should be taken when handling infected companion animals to avoid exposure through needle-stick injuries or ingestion (i.e., hand hygiene after handling infected animals). Isolation is not required. Companion animals exposed to *B. anthracis* should be decontaminated by thorough bathing.

RHODOCOCCUS EQUI (SYNONYM *RHODOCOCCUS HOAGII*) INFECTION

Rhodococcus equi is a pleomorphic, facultatively intracellular, gram-positive bacillus that has been primarily associated with pyogranulomatous pneumonia in foals, suppurative lymphadenitis in pigs, and granulomatous lymphadenitis in cattle. Although a revised name, *Rhodococcus hoagii,* has been proposed for this organism, this name has been disputed in the taxonomic literature, so the name *Rhodococcus equi* will continue to be used from this point forward.[6] It belongs to the Nocardiaceae family which also includes *Nocardia, Mycobacterium, Corynebacterium,* and *Gordonia.* Infection is acquired by inhalation from soil, inoculation into wounds or mucous membranes, or ingestion. Reports of infections in dogs and cats are rare, and are usually associated with immunosuppression such as that caused by chronic glucocorticoid administration[7] or retrovirus infection. *Rhodococcus equi* has rarely been cultured from the mucosal surfaces and skin of healthy dogs, as well as from dogs with myositis, hepatitis, osteomyelitis, dermatitis, endocarditis, pulmonary abscessation and pyothorax, endophthalmitis, and lymphadenitis.[7–9] *Rhodococcus equi* pneumonia was described in a dog from Brazil that was co-infected with *Toxoplasma gondii* and CDV.[9] Infection with CDV was thought to have led to immunocompromise and opportunistic infections with *T. gondii* and *R. equi.*

Rhodococcus equi is commonly recovered from soil that is enriched with herbivore manure and directly from feces of herbivores. The organism may enter the body through a contaminated penetrating wound and subsequently spread via lymphatics to regional lymph nodes and hematogenously to the liver, spleen, and visceral lymph nodes. Affected foals are typically infected through inhalation of dust. The organism then invades macrophages and inhibits phagolysosomal fusion by means of a complex cell wall, which results in pyogranulomatous to granulomatous inflammation. Dissemination occurs as a result of underlying immunosuppression. The virulence of *R. equi* has been related to plasmids that encode a virulence-associated protein (Vap), which allows it to persist in macrophages. Pathogenic strains of *R. equi* have been described as virulent or intermediately virulent based on carriage of host-adapted circular VAP plasmid types. The VAPA and VAPB plasmids have been associated with equine and porcine strains, respectively. The VAPA plasmid was detected in a cat with cutaneous rhodococcosis; the cat had a history of contact with horses.[10] A linear plasmid type, pVAPN, been associated with bovine and caprine strains. This plasmid type has been detected in *R. equi* isolates from two dogs,[7,9] as well as in immunocompromised humans.[11] A conserved conjugal transfer protein gene, *traA*, is present in all strains that carry plasmids. Strains that lack *VapA* or *VapB* genes (and are *traA*–) are considered avirulent, but have been associated with disease in immunocompromised animals.[7]

Most cats have abscesses or pyogranulomatous cellulitis that involve an extremity,[12–14] although a 2020 case series of 40 cats from Malaysia described pulmonary disease in 36 cats; 4 cats had only cutaneous lesions. Most of the cats in this study (25/40) were under 10 months of age.[15] Localized swelling with ulcerations or fistulas and purulent drainage have been found. Unlike typical bite wound abscesses, the lesions are generally not painful, and systemic signs of fever and anorexia are usually absent. Pyothorax and mediastinal lymphadenitis may be associated with anorexia, weight loss, and dyspnea.

Clinical findings in dogs and cats vary considerably depending on sites of dissemination, and have included abdominal distention with a palpable fluid wave, hepatomegaly, and mesenteric lymphadenomegaly; corneal ulceration; endophthalmitis; abscesses; cutaneous ulceration; cough, tachypnea and dyspnea (Fig. 52.1).[7] In one infected dog, generalized hyperesthesia was present.[8] Dissemination to many organs was associated with necrotizing pyogranulomatous hepatitis, osteomyelitis, and polymyositis.

Hematologic abnormalities may consist of leukocytosis with a left shift, monocytosis, and thrombocytopenia.[15] Hypoalbuminemia (22%) and hyperproteinemia (64%) were frequent findings in cats with rhodococcosis from Malaysia.[15] Radiographs have revealed soft tissue swelling; osteolytic and osteoproliferative changes in bones; thoracic lymphadenopathy; hepatomegaly; lung masses with pleural pneumothorax; effusion; and pulmonary interstitial or alveolar-interstitial patterns.[7,15]

Gram staining of aspirates or smear preparations of purulent discharge may reveal large, pleomorphic, gram-positive bacilli, which may be found inside macrophages. Thoracic or abdominal effusions are typically exudates with high protein (more than 3.5 g/dL) and nucleated cell counts (above 10,000 cells/μL); the majority of cells are lymphocytes or nondegenerate neutrophils. Organisms may not be apparent. Gross pathologic findings include peripheral abscesses, often with sinus tracts and purulent drainage; and enlarged and necrotic lymph nodes with a similar discharge on sectioning. Histologic examination reveals pyogranulomatous or granulomatous lesions with necrotic foci.[7] Macrophages contain phagocytized gram-positive bacteria. The organisms also stain positive with Fite's acid-fast stain. Pyogranulomatous to granulomatous lesions containing bacteria may be observed in a variety of parenchymal organs such as the liver, lung, and heart valves in animals with disseminated disease.

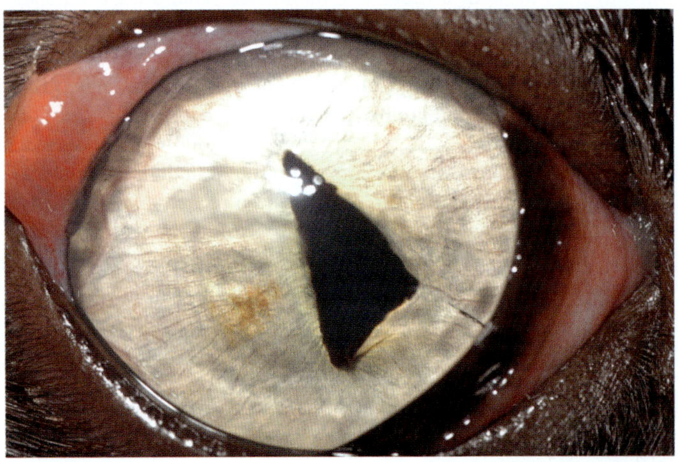

Fig. 52.1 Right eye of a 5-year-old female spayed domestic shorthair with dyscoria secondary to a retrobulbar abscess associated with *Rhodococcus equi* infection. The cat tested negative for feline leukemia virus and feline immunodeficiency virus. (Image courtesy University of California Davis Veterinary Ophthalmology Service.)

In the laboratory, *R. equi* grows readily in an aerobic environment and has distinctive colonial characteristics, but laboratories not familiar with equine isolates may fail to identify it correctly. The use of MALDI-TOF MS is likely to improve identification. Clinicians should communicate any suspicion for *R. equi* infection to the laboratory to ensure that proper microbiologic techniques are used to enhance colony growth. Culture of macerated tissue specimens appears to be more sensitive than culture of swabs of exudates or infected tissues.[14]

Surgical removal of extremity lesions is only temporarily effective, and new lesions commonly develop even after limb amputation. Surgical drainage of abscesses is an essential adjunctive procedure. Antimicrobial susceptibility testing should always be performed because resistant strains have been identified. In general, *in vitro* susceptibility is greatest to erythromycin, fluoroquinolones, rifampin, aminoglycosides, glycopeptides, and carbapenems.[16] In cats, treatment with lincomycin and gentamicin has been effective, and results with erythromycin have varied. Cats with disseminated lesions also respond poorly. Treatment with amoxicillin-clavulanate has been effective in reducing the size of lesions when used for a minimum of 14 to 16 days[13] but is a poor choice of antibacterials because of poor penetration of macrophages and common resistance to beta-lactams. In humans with pneumonia, only long-term treatment with erythromycin, combined with either rifampin or vancomycin, has been effective.[17] Monotherapy is not recommended.[18] As with treatment of other persistently intracellular organisms, combination treatment of lipophilic drugs that penetrate cells well is superior. The standard, highly effective treatment in foals is prolonged oral administration of erythromycin and rifampin. This combination can be recommended for cats, although greater toxicity may occur. However, the combination of clarithromycin-rifampin was superior to erythromycin-rifampin or azithromycin-rifampin in clinical improvement and radiographic resolution of pneumonia in infected foals.[19] Cats have been successfully treated with rifampin in combination with either clarithromycin, azithromycin, or a fluoroquinolone.[15,20] In humans, two- or three-drug combinations are recommended that include a macrolide, rifampin, carbapenem, fluoroquinolones, and/or an aminoglycoside.[18] Several months of treatment may be required, and in some cases, long-term treatment may be required to prevent relapse (Table 52.1).

Infections with *R. equi* are recognized in immunocompromised humans, including those infected with HIV (80% of cases), diabetics, organ transplant recipients, hemic neoplasia, lung cancer, and those with alcoholism. Infections in humans with HIV infection appear to be declining in incidence as a result of highly active antiretroviral therapy.[18] Pulmonary lobar infiltration with cavitation, similar to that observed with tuberculosis, has been the most frequently observed syndrome in human patients with AIDS[18]; *R. equi* was the most common microbiologically confirmed cause of pulmonary cavitation in HIV-infected humans in one study, accounting for 9% of cases.[17,18,21] Extrapulmonary lesions occur in about 20% of people with pulmonary infection. Infected cats or dogs have not been considered a major source of infection for people, who usually acquire the infection from environmental exposure. Nevertheless, infected pets with draining lesions could pose a minor theoretical risk to immunocompromised owners.

CORYNEBACTERIUM INFECTIONS

Corynebacteria are club-shaped, aerobic, gram-positive rods that are widely distributed in soil and water, and may contaminate the hospital environment. Numerous seemingly nonpathogenic corynebacteria have been isolated as microflora of dogs and cats. Some have been reported as causing otic infections or UTIs.[22,23] Many veterinary

TABLE 52.1 Antimicrobials Used To Treat Miscellaneous Gram-Positive Bacterial Infections

Drug	Indication	Species	Dose (mg/kg)	Route	Interval (Hours)
Penicillin G	A, L, E	D, C	20–40 × 10^3 U/kg	IV	8
Ampicillin sodium	A, L[a], E	D, C	20	IV	6
Amoxicillin	A, L[a], E	D, C	20	PO	8–12
Erythromycin	R[b]	D, C	10–20	PO	8
Clarithromycin	R[b]	D, C	7.5–12.5	PO	12
Rifampin[c]	R	D, C	15	PO	8
Doxycycline	CU, A[d]	D, C	5	PO	12
Gentamicin sulfate	L[e]	D	14 5–8	SC, IM, IV	24
Trimethoprim-sulfamethoxazole	L[e]	D, C	30[f]	PO, IV	12
Chloramphenicol	CU	D C[g]	40–50 12.5–20	PO, IV, IM	6–8 12
Ciprofloxacin	A	D, C	10	IV	12
Enrofloxacin	A	D	5–20	PO, IV[h], IM	24
Vancomycin	R, CU	D, C	15	IV[h]	8

[a]In combination with gentamicin or trimethoprim-sulfonamide.
[b]In combination with rifampin.
[c]Rifampin should be used only in combination with another drug such as erythromycin or clarithromycin. Adult cats have been treated with a total dose of 75 mg every 24 hours.
[d]For prophylaxis after exposure.
[e]In combination with ampicillin.
[f]Dose listed is for combined components, i.e., 5 mg of trimethoprim and 25 mg of sulfonamide.
[g]Avoid long-term use in cats. Monitor complete blood count with long-term use. Warn owners that human exposure to chloramphenicol may cause bone marrow disease. Avoid in animals with hepatic failure.
[h]Dilute in saline and give slowly over 30 minutes.
A, anthrax; *C*, cats; *CU*, *Corynebacterium urealyticum*; *D*, dogs, *E*, *Erysipelothrix*; *L*, *Listeria*; *R*, *Rhodococcus*.

diagnostic laboratories do not speciate *Corynebacterium* spp. isolated from dogs and only report them at the genus level. As molecular diagnostic instrumentation (e.g., MALDI-TOF) becomes more common in service laboratories, associations between members of *Corynebacterium* spp. and clinical syndromes will become more known to veterinarians.

Corynebacterium urealyticum has been occasionally associated with lower UTIs in dogs and cats with compromised urinary defense mechanisms,[24] including urinary retention secondary to compressive myelopathy, urethral obstruction, catheterization, and urologic surgery.[24–28] Anatomic defects, extensive antimicrobial use for other causes of UTI, immunosuppressive drugs, and foreign bodies have all been implicated as predisposing causes. The infection is uniquely characterized by the concurrent presence of alkaline urine, struvite, and calcium phosphate crystals that may precipitate to form calculi with or without encrusting urocystitis, which may be severe. Urinalysis typically reveals alkaline urine, struvite crystalluria, pyuria, hematuria, and variable bacteriuria.[24] Ultrasound examination of the urinary bladder may reveal thickening of the bladder wall, echogenic debris, and hyperechogenicity of the urinary bladder wall (encrusting cystitis) (Fig. 52.2). Urolithiasis may also be observed.[24] Findings suggestive of encrusting pyelitis have also been described. A cat with a *Corynebacterium jeikeium* UTI has been described with similar lesions.[29] Treatment involves appropriate antimicrobial therapy and thorough mechanical debridement of plaques associated with the bladder wall, which is essential for resolution. Cystoscopic debridement has been described as a minimally invasive treatment in veterinary patients.[30] In addition to these treatments, oral administration of urinary acidifiers has been used to treat human infections and may be beneficial. Many isolates are resistant to multiple antimicrobial drug classes, and so susceptibility testing is essential to guide therapy. In human patients, vancomycin is the treatment of choice. In order to preserve the use of vancomycin for serious human infections, doxycycline has been used in veterinary patients as an alternative. Doxycycline achieves concentrations in canine urine that exceed plasma concentrations and is likely appropriate for multiple uropathogens.[31] Susceptibility to chloramphenicol has been described in many isolates, and this also may represent an effective treatment.[24]

Corynebacterium ulcerans is capable of expressing diptheria toxins and has been associated with an exudative pharyngitis in humans that is indistinguishable from that caused by *Corynebacterium diphtheriae*.[18] Toxigenic strains *of C. ulcerans* have been isolated from clinically healthy dogs, which may serve as a source of infection for other dogs and animals.[32] *Corynebacterium ulcerans* was isolated, along with other bacteria, from transtracheal washings of a dog with suppurative bronchopneumonia.[33] It was also isolated from nasal swabs from two cats with nasal discharge.[34] These isolates were found to contain the bacteriophage that codes for diphtheria toxin and may have been responsible for the clinical illness in these cats. Isolates from cats and dogs are genetically similar to those from humans, and have been incriminated in zoonotic spread of infection to humans.[35–37] In one report, an immunocompromised person developed a diphtheria-like illness, and the organism was isolated from the throat and the tonsils, nose, and labial area of the person's dog that had chronic rhinorrhea.[36] However, consumption of raw milk or its unpasteurized products or close association with horses or cows is thought to be a more common source of infection for humans than exposure to dogs or cats.

Corynebacterium auriscanis has been implicated in polymicrobial otitis externa in the dog, usually as a mixed infection with *Staphylococcus pseudintermedius*.[22] Infection with *C. auriscanis* has

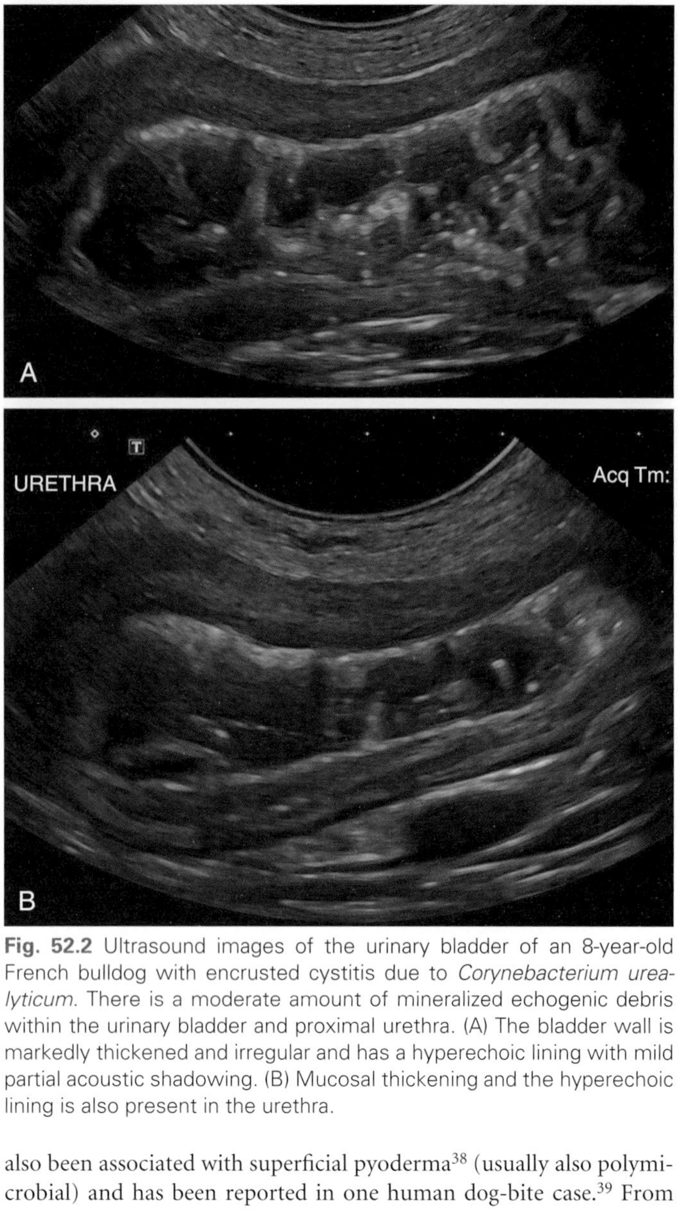

Fig. 52.2 Ultrasound images of the urinary bladder of an 8-year-old French bulldog with encrusted cystitis due to *Corynebacterium urealyticum*. There is a moderate amount of mineralized echogenic debris within the urinary bladder and proximal urethra. (A) The bladder wall is markedly thickened and irregular and has a hyperechoic lining with mild partial acoustic shadowing. (B) Mucosal thickening and the hyperechoic lining is also present in the urethra.

also been associated with superficial pyoderma[38] (usually also polymicrobial) and has been reported in one human dog-bite case.[39] From the limited antimicrobial susceptibility data that have been published about *C. auriscanis*, chloramphenicol, tetracyclines, macrolides, and amikacin are the most effective *in vitro*. However, because these infections are almost always polymicrobial, it is unclear how clinically relevant targeted antimicrobial therapy is for this organism when more virulent components of infections (e.g., coagulase-positive staphylococci, *Pseudomonas aeruginosa*) are adequately addressed by antibiosis.

LISTERIOSIS

Listeria monocytogenes is a pathogenic, partially β-hemolytic, gram-positive, rod-shaped facultative anaerobe that is morphologically indistinguishable from diphtheroids and may be mistaken for a contaminant in tissues, or misidentified as a diphtheroid, streptococcus, or enterococcus. It is motile as a result of possession of one to six polar flagellae. It is capable of growing in a wide range of temperatures, including refrigerator temperatures (4°C to 10°C), which have been used to select for its growth in the presence of contaminants. Although at least 16 serotypes of the organism exist based on H or O antigens, most disease is caused by types 4b, 1/2a, and 1/2b.[40] Isolates from companion animals, when typed, have also been 4b,[41] 1/2a,[42] or 1/2b.[43] As a ubiquitous saprophyte, *L. monocytogenes* can be isolated from soil, water, sewage, dust, and decaying vegetation. Pathogenic strains of *L. monocytogenes* can also be recovered from the stool of healthy animals, including humans. A study of fecal specimens from animals in Japan found a prevalence of 0.9% in dogs, but no bacteria were isolated from cats.[44] Commonly, *L. monocytogenes* can be found in farm animal feed and silage and in food products made from these animals. Recovery rates of 15 to 70% have been reported from raw vegetables, raw milk, cheese, and meats, including processed meats from delicatessen counters. Outbreaks of disease in humans have been associated with poor hygiene practices in the food production industry. Significant outbreaks have been associated with contaminated coleslaw,[45] turkey delicatessen meat (which resulted in the largest recall of meat ever in the United States),[46] chocolate milk,[47,48] and canteloupes.[49] Approximately one third of sporadic cases have been linked to ingestion of soft cheeses or delicatessen meats. Most humans that develop invasive disease are women in their third trimester of pregnancy (which may result in spontaneous abortion, stillbirth, premature labor, and neonatal infections), those over age 60, or those immunosuppressed due to hematologic malignancy, organ transplantation, HIV/AIDS, or glucocorticoid therapy. However, immunocompetent individuals may develop febrile gastroenteritis. A localized cutaneous infection was described in a veterinarian after contact with an aborted calf.[50] *Listeria monocytogenes* has also been isolated from raw pet foods, including those that include beef or chicken.[51] In one study from the Netherlands, 54% of raw food products for pets were contaminated with *L. monocytogenes*.[52] In a study from the United States, 12% of 576 raw pet food products tested positive.[53] In general, the source of infection in companion animals is not identified, but some cats have had a history of being fed raw food diets.[54] Underlying immunosuppressive illnesses identified in dogs have included endocrinopathies (diabetes mellitus and hyperadrenocorticism), hemic neoplasia,[42] and immunosuppressive drug therapy[42,43]; one affected cat tested positive for FeLV.

Natural infection usually results from ingestion of contaminated food; damage to the intestinal mucosal integrity is not necessary. More than 10^9 organisms are needed to infect healthy mammals. Alkalinization of the stomach by antacids may promote infection. Listeriosis in dogs and cats is uncommon; when it occurs, it is usually associated with ingestion of contaminated meat or meat by-products. The incubation period in humans ranges from 11 to 70 days. Reports of bacteremia due to *L. monocytogenes* in dogs and cats after oral ingestion of contaminated food have been rare. After penetration of the intestinal mucosa, *L. monocytogenes* localizes in mononuclear phagocytes. Resultant bacteremia may be associated with formation of septic emboli of many organs. The organism has a particular predilection for the CNS (especially the brainstem [rhombencephalitis] and meninges [meningitis]) and placenta. *Listeria* endocarditis has also been described in humans.

Vaccines have been developed that use attenuated strains of *L. monocytogenes* as a vector for expression of tumor antigens, which concurrently activate cytotoxic T cells. There are rare reports of such vaccines causing listeriosis in vaccinated humans. A conditionally licensed canine osteosarcoma vaccine with a live *Listeria* vector (COV-LLV, Aratana Therapeutics, Inc., KS, USA; at time of writing now owned by Elanco Animal Health) was shown in preliminary studies to significantly improve survival time when used in addition to standard-of-care amputation and chemotherapy.[55] One dog developed a cavitary rib mass following vaccination. The vaccine strain of *L. monocytogenes* was isolated from aspirates of the mass, and histopathology of the mass revealed metastatic osteoblastic osteosarcoma.[56] The dog remained alive over a year after removal of the mass with no further disease progression. A subsequent study described *Listeria* infections in 4 of 49 vaccinated dogs with osteosarcoma, and concerns were raised about the possibility of zoonotic transmission.[57]

Listeria monocytogenes can persist indefinitely in macrophages and escape humoral immune responses. A cell surface protein, internalin, interacts with E-cadherin on epithelial cells and macrophages, inducing phagocytosis (Fig. 52.3). The main virulence factor possessed by

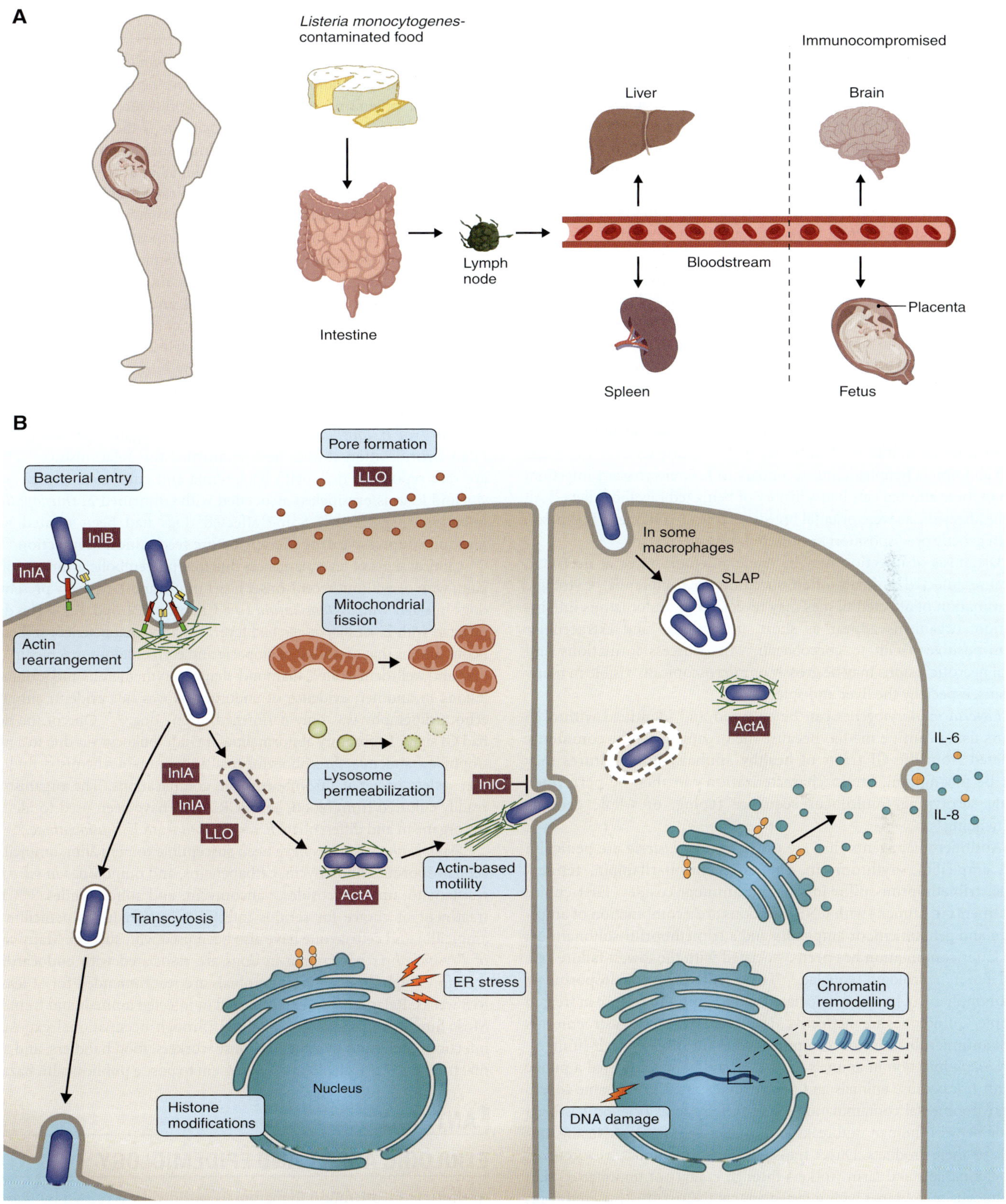

Fig. 52.3 Pathogenesis of *Listeria monocytogenes* infection. (A) After ingestion of contaminated food, *L. monocytogenes* can cross the intestinal barrier and spread into the bloodstream through the lymph nodes to disseminate to target tissues, such as the liver and spleen. In immunocompromised individuals, *L. monocytogenes* can cross the blood-brain barrier or placental barrier and cause meningitis, sepsis, premature birth, or abortion. (B) *Listeria monocytogenes* enters nonphagocytic cells, such as epithelial cells, through receptor-mediated endocytosis, and in most cases, it escapes from the vacuole. In some macrophages, it can replicate in spacious *Listeria*-containing phagosomes (*SLAPs*). Upon vacuolar escape, *L. monocytogenes* can polymerize actin and spread from cell to cell. Listeriolysin O (*LLO*), phospholipase A (PlcA), and PlcB mediate vacuolar escape. LLO also leads to changes in histone modification, mitochondrial fission, endoplasmic reticulum (*ER*) stress, and lysosomal permeabilization. Infection also leads to DNA damage, and the host cell combats infection by upregulating cytokine secretion. *ActA,* actin assembly-inducing protein; *IL,* interleukin; *Inl,* internalin. (Modified from Radoshevich L, Cossart P. *Listeria monocytogenes*: towards a complete picture of its physiology and pathogenesis. *Nature Rev Microbiol.* 2018;16:32–46. With permission.)

L. monocytogenes is listeriolysin O, which is a porin that induces T-cell unresponsiveness. This porin, together with phospholipases, enables the organism to escape phagosomes. In the cytoplasm, the organism pushes pseudopod-like projections outward (known as filopods), which are ingested by adjacent macrophages, enterocytes, or hepatocytes. The bacterial surface protein ActA is responsible for actin polymerization that promotes intercellular spread and evasion of the host immune response.[58]

Clinical signs are caused by the degree of intestinal inflammation and the sites of embolic microabscess formation. Fever, diarrhea, and vomiting have been most frequently reported. Neurologic signs, abortion, subclinical bacteriuria, and bacteremia have been apparent in some cases.[41,42,59] Localized infections can also occur.[42,60] Cholecystitis was described in one dog; *L. monocytogenes* was isolated from bile collected using cholecystocentesis.[43] Listerial myocarditis with congestive heart failure was reported in a 14-week old puppy from southeastern Australia that was evaluated for dyspnea, lethargy, and inappetence.[61] Cytologic evaluation of bone marrow from one dog with bacteremia revealed coccobacilli within macrophages and neutrophils.[62] In cats, peritonitis, pneumonia, hepatic involvement, encephalitis, and cutaneous abscesses have been described.[63–65] Systemic listeriosis in association with pleural mesothelioma was identified in one stray cat in the southern US at necropsy.[66] In a case series of three cats with abdominal lymphadenitis secondary to *L. monocytogenes* infection, two of three affected cats had a history of being fed raw food diets.[54] All of the affected cats were oriental breeds (Siamese, Tonkinese, Burmese), and a genetic predisposition for infection was speculated.

Diagnosis of infection may be made antemortem or at necropsy, because infected animals often succumb to bacteremia. Cytologic examination of affected tissues may reveal pyogranulomatous inflammation; organisms appear as short, intracellular and extracellular gram-positive bacilli to coccobacilli. Microabscess formations and focal necrotic lesions may be grossly or microscopically visible in many organs, especially the liver and spleen.

Listeria monocytogenes can be cultured and identified within 36 hours using routine media. Because the organism can be commonly isolated from the GI tracts of healthy animals, stool cultures may not be meaningful. Strain characterization can then be performed using serotyping, multilocus sequence typing, or whole genome sequencing.[67]

Antimicrobial agents that are active against *Listeria* are penicillin and ampicillin, erythromycin, chloramphenicol, rifampin, tetracycline, trimethoprim-sulfonamide, and aminoglycosides. First-choice treatments in humans with CNS infections are a combination of ampicillin and gentamicin, or ampicillin and a trimethoprim-sulfonamide; the latter combination has been associated with the lowest failure rate and fewer neurologic sequelae.[40] Treatment with cephalosporins or chloramphenicol has been associated with failure and relapse in treated people. Quinolones are ineffective. Treatment of *Listeria* gastroenteritis with antimicrobials is not recommended as the disease is self-limited.

Listeria infection in animals has not always been considered a public health risk because animals and people are exposed to the same source of environmental contamination. Nevertheless, an association has been made between human outbreaks and contact with food-producing animals or their products. Direct transmission from animals has occurred in veterinarians and farm workers through contact of unprotected skin or mucous membranes with infected animal tissues.[64,68] Most outbreaks occur in urban areas, where foodborne contamination is suspected. Infants, older adults, and pregnant women are most commonly affected. Recommendations for practices that prevent foodborne listeriosis have been developed,[40] including avoidance of certain foods (soft cheeses, delicatessen meats, smoked seafood) for people at higher risk. In a case of reverse zoonosis, listerial gastroenteritis was suspected in a litter of puppies and a newborn infant who received *Listeria*-infected milk discarded from the human mother's mammary gland.[69]

ERYSIPELOTHRIX INFECTIONS

Erysipelothrix rhusiopathiae and *Erysipelothrix tonsillarum* are small, gram-positive, nonmotile, nonsporulating pleomorphic facultatively anaerobic rods. These organisms, which are found worldwide, are associated with swine production. *Erysipelothrix rhusiopathiae* is the causative agent of swine erysipelas and other diseases in animals such as joint-ill in sheep and cattle and bacteremia in turkeys, ducks, and laboratory mice. The organism can be cultured from the tonsils of clinically healthy swine, the skin of freshwater and saltwater fish, and the decomposing plant and animal matter in their environments. Occupational exposure to these sources of bacteria may cause localized cutaneous or systemic infections in humans.

Initially, the genus *Erysipelothrix* was thought to have a single species—*rhusiopathiae*—but biochemical and genetic analyses have identified *E. tonsillarum*, a nonpathogenic commensal of the tonsils of swine.[70] In dogs, endocarditis, diskospondylitis, arthritis, and bacteremia were initially thought to be caused by *E. rhusiopathiae* after natural[71] and experimental[72] inoculation. However, all available isolates from these conditions reported in dogs have been now reclassified as serovar 7 of *E. tonsillarum*, which is nonpathogenic for swine.[70,73,74] DNA hybridization studies have confirmed this relationship.[75] There are rare reports of dogs with bacteremia and cutaneous lesions (erysipeloid lesions/erysipelas) associated with confirmed *E. rhusiopathiae* infection (Fig. 52.4).[76] Some affected dogs had been treated with immunosuppressive drug therapy before recognition of infection.[77,78]

Clinical signs of fever, lameness due to septic/embolic arthritis, spinal pain, with or without recent-onset heart murmur are typically present in dogs infected with *E. tonsillarum* (see Chapters 121 and 122). The dogs infected with *E. rhusiopathiae* had fever, lethargy, inappetence, and cutaneous lesions that consisted of alopecia and erythematous macules in one dog; and well-demarcated, diamond-shaped, erythematous and indurated lesions in another; evidence of endocarditis was not evident, although echocardiography was only performed in one dog.[76,77] One of the dogs had GI signs. Laboratory abnormalities include leukocytosis due to a neutrophilia, bandemia, thrombocytopenia, and serum biochemistry findings that reflect bacterial thromboembolic complications. The organism is readily cultured from blood, and PCR assays have been used to identify the organism and differentiate *E. tonsillarum* from *E. rhusiopathiae*.[76,79]

Erysipelothrix isolates have been susceptible to penicillin, ampicillin, cephalosporins, clindamycin, carbapenems, and quinolones *in vitro* but resistant to aminoglycosides, vancomycin, and sulfonamides.[70,80] The treatment of choice for serious infections in humans is penicillin G; ampicillin and ceftriaxone have also been used with success. Many cases of *Erysipelothrix* bacteremia in dogs are associated with endocarditis; therefore, high doses of antimicrobials are recommended for at least 6 to 8 weeks. Relapses are often reported in infected animals and humans. Most human infections are acquired through occupational exposure; infections are found in slaughterhouse workers, food handlers, and animal trappers.[68] Infected dogs do not seem to pose a public health hazard.

ANTHRAX

ETIOLOGIC AGENT AND EPIDEMIOLOGY

Anthrax, a disease found in mammals worldwide, is caused by *Bacillus anthracis*, a large (1 to 1.2 μm × 3–6 μm), gram-positive, aerobic, spore-forming bacillus. The disease and species name is derived from the black, charcoal-appearing cutaneous lesion it causes in humans (Greek *anthrakis*, meaning "coal"). Microscopically, the organisms may appear as long chains of gram-positive, square-ended bacteria, similar to a string of boxcars; shorter chains of two to three cells may be seen (Fig. 52.5). Vegetative *B. anthracis* cells produce a polypeptide capsule visible when the organism is stained with polychrome

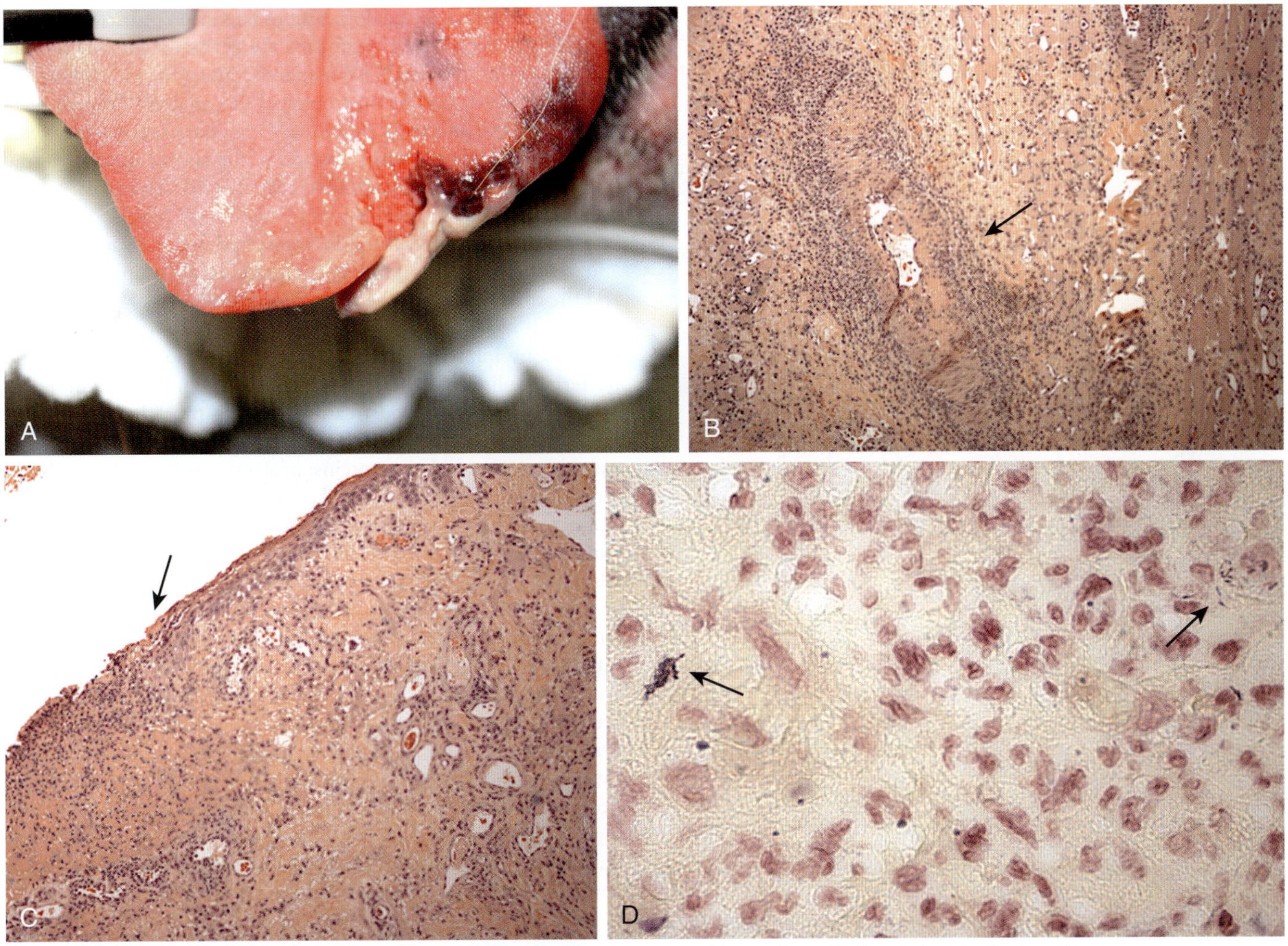

Fig. 52.4 (A) Necrotizing glossitis in a 2-year-old male neutered boxer dog with *Erysipelothrix rhusiopathiae* bacteremia. The dog also had focal dermatitis (6-cm elliptical plaque-like lesion over the left lumbar region) and septic polyarthritis. No evidence of infective endocarditis was found on echocardiography. (B) Histopathology of the tongue revealed severe multifocal subacute neutrophilic and histiocytic perivasculitis with necrotizing arteritis *(arrow)*; (C), glossitis with thrombosis and necrosis *(arrow)*; (D), intralesional gram-positive rods *(arrows)*. (B and C) Hematoxylin and eosin stain, 40× magnification. (D) Brown and Benn stain, 1000× oil immersion magnification. (Images courtesy University of California Davis Small Animal Internal Medicine and Anatomic Pathology services.)

methylene blue or Giemsa stains. Encapsulated anthrax organisms are refractory to phagocytosis, which enhances their ability to produce disease. Exotoxin production and capsule synthesis by the bacteria are mediated by plasmids pX01 and pX02, respectively.

Bacillus anthracis begins to sporulate at the end of the growth phase in its life cycle, an adaptation crucial to the perpetuation of the organism in nature. Spores are not seen on direct staining of specimens; however, they appear in culture when nutrients are depleted. Atmospheric oxygen is considered necessary for sporulation because sporulation does not occur in the unopened carcass of an animal succumbing to anthrax. Anthrax spores are very resistant to heat, radiation, disinfectants, and desiccation, resulting in their persistence for more than 40 years in certain soils and environments. However, in most soils, the organism has to compete with other soil bacteria, so survival is generally for months and rarely more than 4 years.[81]

Anthrax is most prevalent in Africa, the Middle East, and Latin America. Anthrax has been sporadically reported in livestock in the United States, most commonly in the central and the Mississippi Delta regions, from Texas and Louisiana north to the Dakotas and Minnesota (Fig. 52.6). Warm temperatures (above 18°C [60°F]), moisture, and alkaline soils with high nitrogen content allow vegetative growth and proliferation of spores that have been released into the soil from carcasses of animals that died of anthrax.[82] Epizootics tend to occur in summer or fall after heavy rainfall or flooding preceded by drought conditions. Livestock usually become infected by ingesting spores while grazing or by eating contaminated feed (Fig. 52.7). Isolated infections in dogs have been recorded during major anthrax outbreaks in farm animals. Based on evidence from natural and experimental infections, dogs and cats are considered relatively resistant,[83] humans have intermediate resistance, and ruminants and horses are most susceptible to infection. Many dogs and cats may experience subclinical infections. Domestic dogs have been used as a sentinel for surveillance efforts based on serologic surveys with ELISA assays.[84,85]

Naturally occurring anthrax in dogs is extremely rare and most commonly caused by ingestion of meat or hides from infected carcasses, or possibly ingestion of spores from grooming contaminated fur. There are no contemporary reports of anthrax in domestic cats, and older reports are poorly documented.[86] Infections in captive wild canids and felids have also been recorded after feeding on raw meat from contaminated carcasses. In 2001 in the United States, there was documented terrorist dissemination of anthrax spores to induce inhalation anthrax in humans (the anthrax attacks, or "Amerithrax" from its FBI case name).[87] Increased risk for inhalation anthrax may therefore exist for police, guide, or search-and-rescue dogs.

CLINICAL FEATURES

Pathogenesis, Clinical Signs, and Physical Examination Findings

Infection occurs after inert *B. anthracis* spores enter the host body by ingestion (typical route for dogs), by inhalation, or through a break in the skin. The incubation period is usually 3 to 7 days. At the point of entry in the GI mucosa, a primary focal hemorrhagic lesion is produced. Bacteria migrate to regional lymph nodes and the spleen.

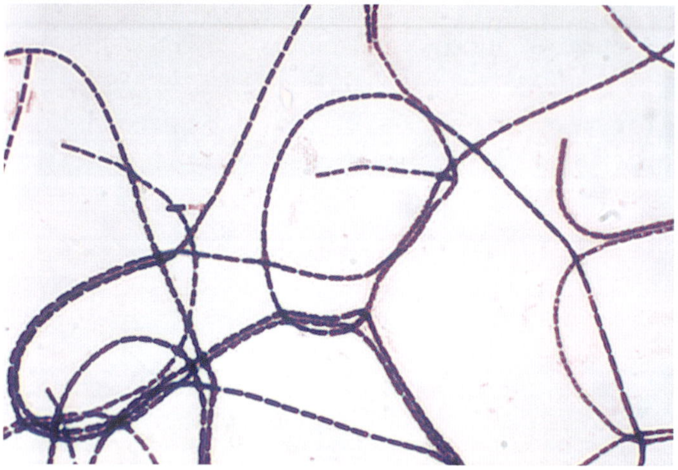

Fig. 52.5 Gram stain of *Bacillus anthracis* demonstrating long chains of bacilli that form when the organism is grown in culture. Prominent central or paracentral spores do not stain with Gram stain and appear as clear areas in many of the bacilli in chains. (From Centers for Disease Control and Prevention Public Health Image Library. ID 2105. https://phil.cdc.gov/Details.aspx?pid=2105.)

In experimentally infected dogs, lesions have been restricted to local foci in the lungs because the organisms are generally contained by fibrin and cellular infiltrations.[82] After spores contact the pulmonary alveoli, they are phagocytized by macrophages that migrate through the alveolar membrane and enter pulmonary lymphatics, eventually reaching hilar lymph nodes. Within host cells, the spores quickly germinate into fully encapsulated vegetative cells that release toxins. Vegetative cells respond to the host factors of high body temperature and carbon dioxide levels, resulting in transcriptional activation of capsule and toxin genes. The capsule is thought to be an antiphagocytic factor, and the toxin induces large-scale generation of cytokines such as IL-1 that result in septic shock.[88] Anthrax lethal toxin may also contribute to shock by inhibitory effects on glucocorticoid receptor function.[89] Bacterial replication results in death of the phagocytes, with release of organisms into the bloodstream. Although most *Bacillus* species are nonpathogenic to animals and humans, *B. anthracis*, through its pXO1 plasmid, expresses three proteins: protective antigen (PA), edema factor (EF), and lethal factor (LF). The three components are serologically distinct and cause no lesions when injected separately, but in binary combinations they produce edema toxin (PA and EF) and lethal toxin (PA and LF). PA mediates the entry of either EF or LF into the cytosol of host cells. EF is an adenylyl cyclase that inhibits TNF-α synthesis and impairs host defenses. LF, a metalloprotease, inhibits mitogen-activated protein kinases and induces macrophage lysis.

The clinical expression of anthrax may be peracute, acute, or subacute/chronic. In one report, the only clinical sign was anorexia.[90] After oral exposure, the infection in dogs and cats is usually manifest as fever (39.4°C to 40.5°C [103°F to 105°F]); anorexia; and local inflammation, necrosis, and edema of the upper GI tract—the first tissues to contact ingested bacteria. Swelling of head and neck tissues is usually apparent. Subsequent spread to the local and mesenteric lymph nodes, spleen, and liver typically occurs, causing enlargement of these organs. Acute

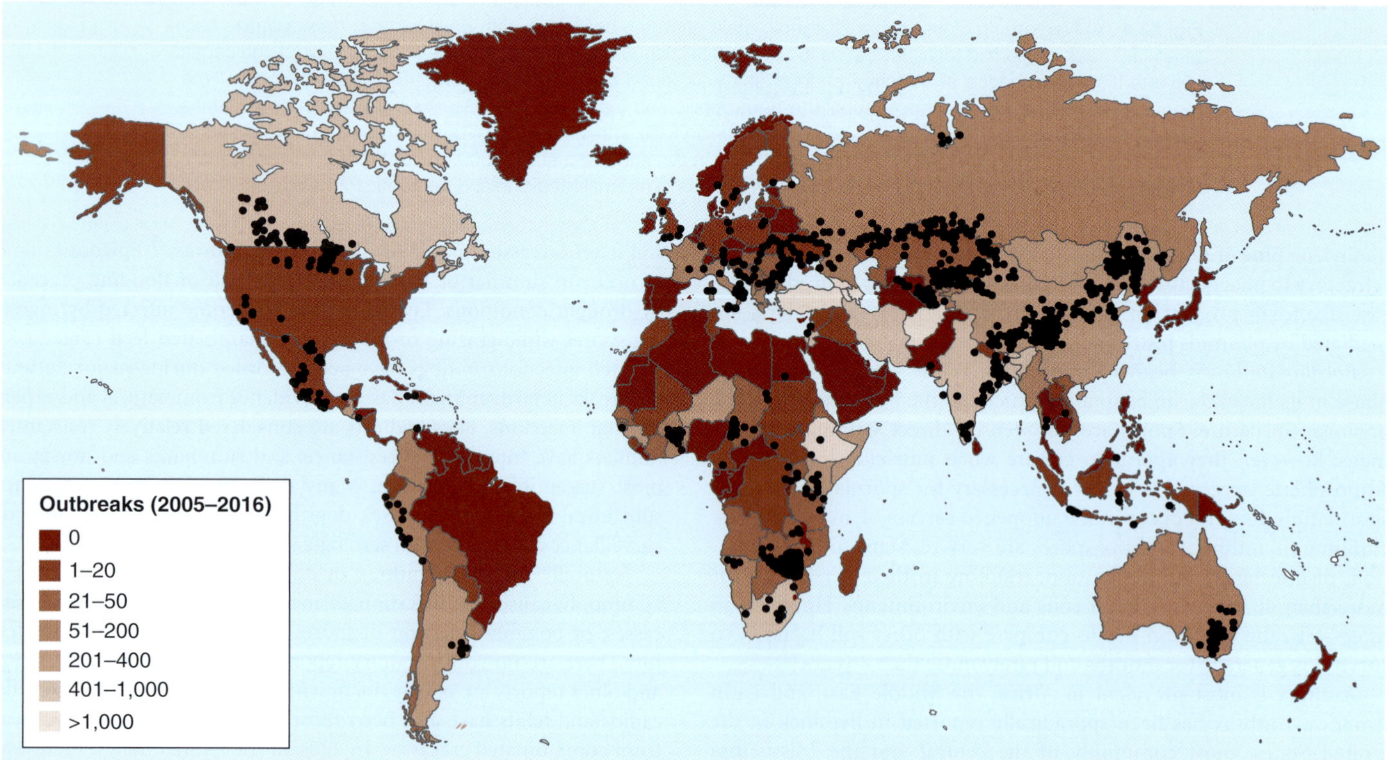

Fig. 52.6 Global distribution of anthrax outbreaks by country and geographic locations of anthrax events (January 2005 to August 2016). Black dots represent individual outbreak locations. (Modified from Carlson CJ, Kracalik IT, Ross N, et al. The global distribution of *Bacillus anthracis* and associated anthrax risk to humans, livestock and wildlife. *Nature Microbiol* 2019;4:1337–1343.)

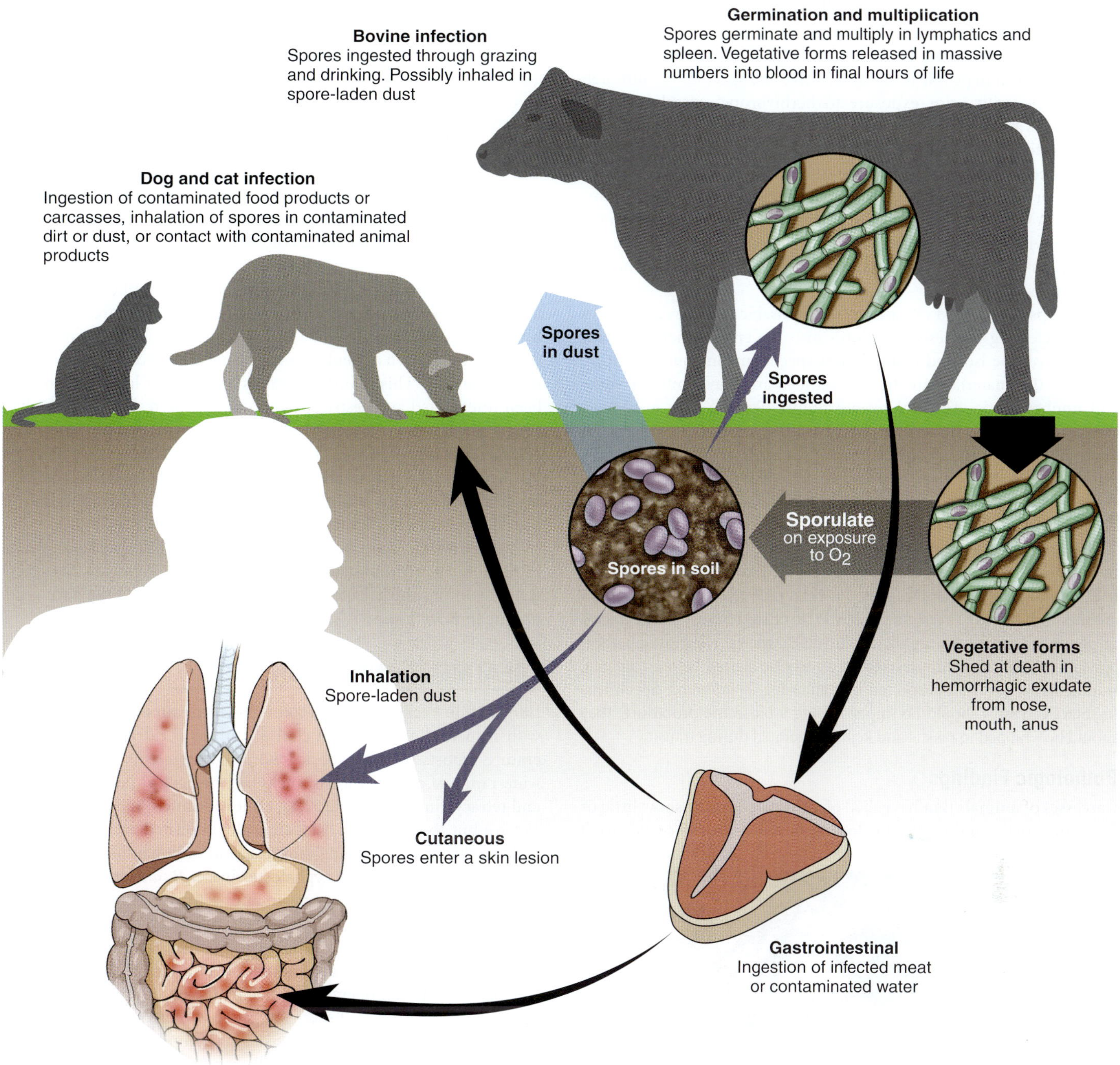

Fig. 52.7 Epidemiology of anthrax. Humans (and dogs and cats) become infected through ingestion of contaminated food products or carcasses, inhalation of spores in contaminated dirt or dust, or contact with contaminated animal products.

gastroenteritis, which is often hemorrhagic, can occur, as may sudden death, particularly in younger animals. Signs in younger or immunocompromised dogs and cats may resemble systemic anthrax in more susceptible species, described as fulminating bacteremia in which the principal lesions are edema, hemorrhage, and necrosis.

Cutaneous anthrax, the most common manifestation in humans worldwide, is rarely the primary clinical form in canids or felids. The initial cutaneous lesion at the site of inoculation appears first as a papule, progresses to a vesicle, ruptures, and develops into a black eschar secondary to focal necrosis. Experimental exposure of dogs to aerosolized anthrax spores did not reliably produce clinical disease other than short-term fever and anorexia.[82] In more susceptible species with suspected natural inhalational exposures, clinical signs include fever, lethargy, cough, and dyspnea, as well as signs that relate to bacteremia.

DIAGNOSIS

Anthrax is usually suspected based on history and clinical signs. Mild pulmonary infiltrates and pleural effusion may be detected radiographically in animals with inhalation anthrax.

Pus or tissue specimens from animals suspected of infection should be Gram stained to show gram-positive bacilli (which have the "boxcar" appearance) and stained with polychrome methylene blue to show the polypeptide capsule (which has the "string of pearls" appearance) (Fig. 52.8). Examination of stained smears of blood from a peripheral vein or of fine-needle aspirates is the most effective and safest means of making a diagnosis.

Serologic testing using ELISA to detect IgG to *B. anthracis* PA and capsular antigen in people is highly sensitive and specific,[91,92] although some people with prior exposure to herbivorous animals or their by-products have seropositive test results. A fourfold changing titer is needed to confirm active infection or recent exposure. Use of this test has been recommended because some cutaneous cases have been culture- or PCR-negative.[93] Few other antemortem tests are recommended. A skin test for diagnosis of anthrax in humans was used in the former Soviet Union. This anthrax skin test, which detects heightened CMI against the organism, was usually positive after 3 days of illness in 97% of those affected.[94]

Necropsy of affected carcasses is not advisable because sporulation occurs, releasing the resistant spores into the environment. *Bacillus anthracis* can be isolated from clinical specimens on routine culture media if the materials are fresh. Colonies are gray-white to white and nonhemolytic. The isolates are nonmotile and have a capsule. Vegetative cells may be isolated from blood, sputum, CSF, eschar, and feces (in gastrointestinal anthrax cases). In cases of suspected inhalation exposure, *B. anthracis* spores may be collected for culture using sterile water–moistened swabs taken from the nares and haired muzzle or face within 24 to 48 hours of exposure to aerosolized spores.[95]

Immunocytochemical direct FA examination of nasal swab specimens, pleural fluid smears, or pulmonary biopsy specimens using antibodies to *B. anthracis* cell wall and capsule has been used to diagnose inhalation anthrax in humans.[96] When available, PCR of sterile body fluids (blood or pleural effusion) can rapidly confirm a diagnosis. Diagnostic pathology laboratories and shippers should always be alerted before receiving shipments of materials suspected of containing *B. anthracis.* Specimens or intact carcasses should be shipped using a biosecure procedure; they should be wrapped in plastic and kept refrigerated during transit.

Pathologic Findings

Carcasses of animals that have died of anthrax generally show little or no rigor mortis, and dark, nonclotting blood is usually seen oozing from the oral and nasal cavities and anus. The carcass often is bloated and decomposes rapidly. If necropsy is inadvertently performed on an infected animal, characteristic lesions will be observed. Extensive gelatinous edema with focal areas of hemorrhage and necrosis is commonly seen at the site of GI entry, and may be present around lymph nodes and elsewhere in the GI tract. Diphtheritic membranes and ulceration may be present on tonsillar surfaces. Splenomegaly and a friable liver are often observed. Petechial hemorrhages may be noted on serosal surfaces. On histopathology, extensive areas of necrosis in submucosal tissues are accompanied by neutrophilic infiltrates. Gram-positive bacterial colonies may be identified in mucosal fibrinous exudates.

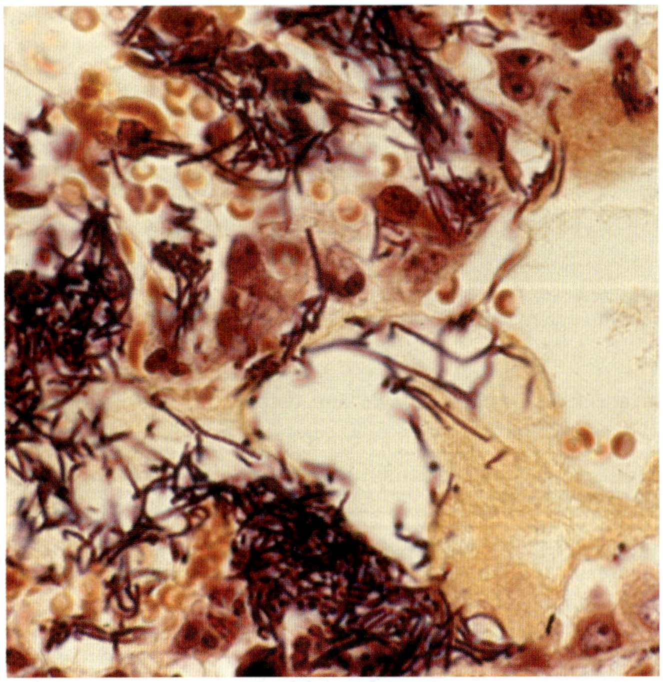

Fig. 52.8 Vegetative *Bacillus anthracis* with edema and hemorrhage in the lung of inhalation anthrax laboratory model (Brown and Hopps, ×400). (Courtesy Armed Forces Institute of Pathology, Washington, DC.)

Studies of inhalation anthrax lesions in dogs describe discrete, dark, firm pulmonary lesions, consisting of a hemorrhagic core surrounded by dense masses of fibrin and a highly cellular periphery formed from dense accumulation of neutrophils, plasma cells, monocytes, and large macrophages.[82] This intense fibrinous and cellular local response has been interpreted as a restrictive reaction by the resistant canine host to contain the *B. anthracis* invasion. Intrathoracic lymph nodes were enlarged because of reactive hyperplasia, but bacilli were not observed during histologic examination. In humans, lymph node enlargement causes mediastinal widening, a pathognomonic radiographic sign in the diagnosis of inhalation anthrax.

In pathologic specimens, anthrax can be confirmed by specific immunohistochemical staining with an antibody conjugate that specifically identifies the galactose-*N*-acetyl-D-glucosamine polysaccharide unique to *B. anthracis.*[97]

TREATMENT AND PROGNOSIS

Information regarding the recommended treatment of dogs or cats with suspected or confirmed clinical anthrax is extrapolated from literature reports of other species. *Bacillus anthracis* is susceptible to a wide range of antimicrobials, including penicillin, fluoroquinolones, and tetracyclines (see Table 52.1). Other antimicrobials that are active *in vitro* but that have not been clinically evaluated are chloramphenicol, erythromycin, aminoglycosides, and sulfonamides. Because of bacterial production of a cephalosporinase, *B. anthracis* isolates are typically resistant to cephalosporin antibacterials; potentiated sulfonamides are also ineffective. Initial doses of antimicrobials should be administered intravenously. The recommended treatment for people with systemic anthrax is a combination of a quinolone and a beta-lactam, such as meropenem; penicillin G could be used in dogs.[81] Although tissue cultures become negative within 24 hours after treatment is started, antibacterials are usually administered for 7 to 14 days. Although cutaneous infection usually resolves without medical treatment, antibacterials are recommended because cases may progress to systemic involvement (the fatality rate is 10% to 20% without treatment).[93] Humans with cutaneous anthrax are treated with doxycycline or ciprofloxacin monotherapy.

Additional supportive care may also be indicated. Animals with respiratory compromise from cervical edema may need treatment with glucocorticoids or tracheostomy. Pleural effusion may require drainage. Dressings with drainage from lesions should be incinerated, autoclaved, or disposed of as biohazardous waste. A dog or cat with suspected coat or skin exposure to anthrax aerosol should be thoroughly bathed with soap and water, as disinfectants that inactivate *Bacillus* spores are generally too caustic to use on skin. Use of accelerated hydrogen peroxide shampoos could also be considered. Persons decontaminating the haircoat of a pet should wear disposable gloves, mask, and gown. Isolation of affected animals is not required because anthrax is not transmissible after animals have been decontaminated.

IMMUNITY AND VACCINATION

If not superseded by bacteremia and death, the host response involves specific IgG antibodies against PA, with antibodies functioning to inhibit spore germination and stimulate phagocytosis by macrophages. Although livestock at risk should receive annual vaccinations, currently marketed, these have not been tested in companion animals, nor are they licensed or recommended for use in these species. Animal vaccines approved for large animals in endemic regions commonly use an avirulent nonencapsulated (pXO2-deficient) spore strain (Sterne strain). In contrast, an anthrax vaccine licensed in the United States for use in people is a cell-free filtrate containing protective antigen and alum. Five intramuscular injections (at 0 and 4 weeks and 6, 12, and 18 months) are required for immunity, and annual booster injections are recommended for maintenance.[93] An attenuated live vaccine for people, which was developed in the former Soviet Union, has been effective; however, it is not available in other countries.

PREVENTION

In endemic areas or during an outbreak, all meat fed to dogs and cats should be thoroughly cooked to eliminate the risk of exposure. To minimize environmental contamination by anthrax spores, carcasses of animals dying from anthrax should be destroyed by incineration or buried deep with a covering of quicklime (anhydrous calcium oxide). Decontamination involves a sporicidal solution of lye because ordinary disinfectants are ineffective (5% NaOH for 1.5 hours at 27.8°C or 3.6 hours at 21.1°C kills 99% of spores).[98] Soaking impervious articles in 10% formaldehyde or 4% glutaraldehyde for a minimum of 2 hours is sporicidal.[99] In the laboratory, surfaces can be decontaminated with 5% hypochlorite. Instruments used should be autoclaved or boiled at 100°C for 10 minutes.[98] All areas, equipment, and buildings that may have contacted infected animals should be cleaned and disinfected. Control of flying insects and scavenging insects and animals should be implemented. Personnel who are cleaning up after an outbreak or terrorist attack that kills livestock must wear protective clothing and respirators.

Postexposure prophylaxis protocols for people recommend at least 60 days of antibacterial administration because of concerns about environmental and pulmonary spore persistence.[100] Tetracyclines are preferred for postexposure prophylaxis, although amoxicillin or ampicillin may be substituted when the treatment course is prolonged or when contraindicated in pregnancy or lactation. The American Academy of Veterinary Pharmacology and Therapeutics and the American College of Veterinary Clinical Pharmacology have recommended that exposed working dogs be treated with doxycycline (5 mg/kg, PO, q24h) for 45 to 60 days.[101] Postexposure vaccination is also done for people using a CDC investigational drug protocol, at 0, 2, and 4 weeks SC.

PUBLIC HEALTH ASPECTS

Anthrax is a notifiable disease and should be reported to state and federal agencies. Care must be taken when handling infected tissues or carcasses because the organism can penetrate cuts in the skin, resulting in localized infection with subsequent dissemination. It has been estimated that between 2,000 and 20,000 cases occur worldwide each year.[93] In developed countries, 95% of naturally occurring cases in humans are cutaneous. They generally result from exposure to infected animals or contaminated animal products (wool, hair, bone, horns, hides).[93] Lesions are painless, pruritic papules, sometimes surrounded by vesicles, with an ulcerated, circular, black necrotic scab (Fig. 52.9). Although less common, inhalation or ingestion can result in either a highly fatal bacteremia caused by hemorrhagic pneumonitis or an oropharyngitis and gastroenteritis, respectively. Anthrax has been developed as a biologic warfare agent by Japan, the United Kingdom, the United States, Iraq, and the former Soviet Union. One millionth of a gram of inhaled anthrax spores is a lethal dose to a person. Apart from terrorist events, infection in people is almost always transmitted from infected animals or their by-products.

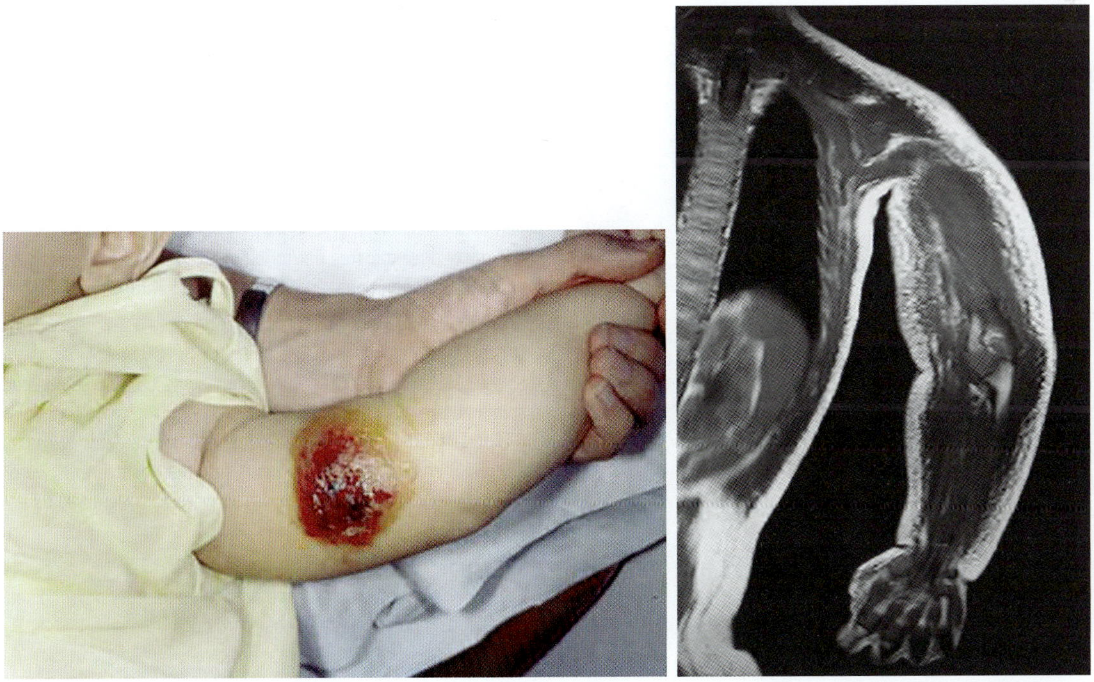

Fig. 52.9 Cutaneous anthrax in a 7-month-old child from New York (2001). (From Roche KJ, Chang MW, Lazarus H. Cutaneous anthrax infection: images in clinical medicine. *N Engl J Med.* 2001;345:1611. Copyright)

CASE EXAMPLE

Signalment

"Jimmy," a 4-year-old male neutered German shepherd (Fig. 52.10).

History

Jimmy was evaluated by the University of California-Davis VMTH Internal Medicine service for chronic weight loss, inappetence, and diarrhea that was refractory to medical therapy for inflammatory bowel disease. The clinical signs had been present for 13 months, and were first noticed shortly after Jimmy's owners moved from Hawaii to a 5-acre farm in northern California. The local veterinarian suspected inflammatory bowel disease or antibiotic-responsive diarrhea. Fecal flotations and a *Giardia* ELISA assay performed at that time were negative for parasites. Jimmy was treated with tylosin and a therapeutic diet trial with a prescription hydrolyzed protein diet. This was associated with moderate clinical improvement. Laboratory testing performed over the next 6 months revealed persistent mild hypoalbuminemia and severe hypocobalaminemia, which was treated with parenteral cyanocobalamin.

A year after the signs were first noted, the diarrhea recurred and weight loss was noted with mildly decreased appetite. The diarrhea was characterized by soft to liquid stool with increased frequency of defecation (3–4 times a day), some mucus and occasional mild hematochezia and tenesmus. Full thickness intestinal biopsies were obtained via exploratory laparotomy. Histopathology revealed chronic inflammatory gastroenteritis with a prominent eosinophilic component and mild lacteal dilation (suggestive of possible lymphangiectasia). Treatment with methylprednisolone (0.5 mg/kg, PO, q12h) and cyclosporine (5 mg/kg, PO, q24h) was not associated with clinical improvement. Around the same time, oral and nasal planum ulcerations were noted. Biopsy of these lesions was consistent with a diagnosis of cutaneous lupus erythematosus. Based on recommendations from a veterinary dermatologist, cyclosporine was substituted with leflunomide (5 mg/kg, PO, q24h), and the methylprednisolone dose was reduced (0.5 mg/kg, q24h). This was followed by improvement in the cutaneous lesions but the diarrhea continued. A second diet trial with a different commercial hydrolyzed diet was commenced.

From that point on, there was progressive weight loss, variable appetite, occasional urinary accidents in the house, and intermittent mixed large and small bowel-type diarrhea with hematochezia. The week before the dog was evaluated, the owner noted a marked decrease in Jimmy's energy and appetite.

Current Medications

Methylprednisone 0.5 mg/kg, PO, q24h and leflunomide 5 mg/kg, PO, q24h.

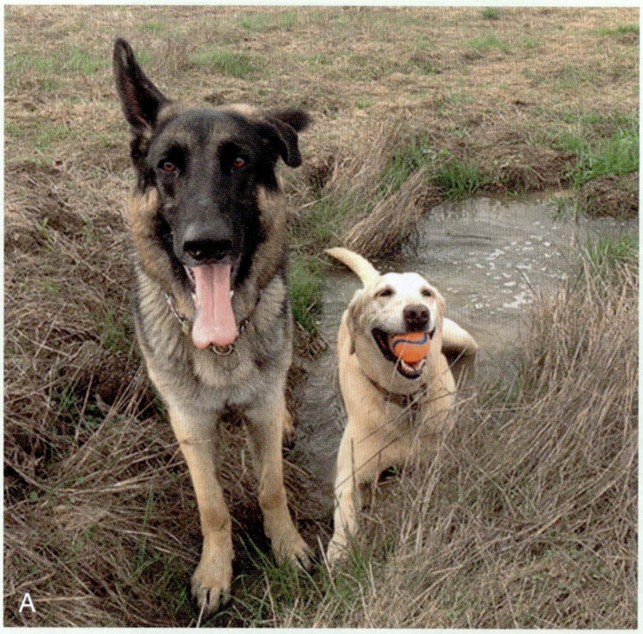

Fig. 52.10 "Jimmy," a 4-year-old male neutered German shepherd with chronic inflammatory bowel disease, cutaneous lupus, and listeriosis *(left)*.

Other Medical History

No significant previous medical history. Jimmy spent time both indoors and outdoors, with access to 5 acres of meadows, pastures of dairy cattle, sheep, goats, chicken, and geese. There was a Labrador retriever and another German shepherd on the ranch.

Physical Examination

Body weight: 23.8 kg.

General: Quiet, alert, responsive, hydrated. T = 103.3°F (39.6°C), HR = 110 beats/minute, RR = 24 breaths/minute.

Integument: Multiple 1-cm ulcerations were present on lateral metatarsus and carpus. There was a focal 6-cm area of alopecia and erythema over the left caudal dorsum.

Eyes, ears, nose, and throat: Mucous membranes pink, moist, CRT < 2 seconds. Multiple small depigmented ulcerative lesions on hard palate.

Musculoskeletal: Thin body condition, ambulatory, appeared weak in the pelvic limbs. Bilateral moderate temporal muscle atrophy.

Cardiovascular: No murmurs or arrhythmias noted. Moderate femoral pulses.

Respiratory: Panting, harsh lung sounds on auscultation of right thorax, referred to all lung fields.

GI and genitourinary: Moderate cranial organomegaly detected on abdominal palpation.

Lymph nodes: No peripheral lymphadenopathy.

Laboratory Findings

CBC: HCT 41.% (40%–55%), MCV 69 fL (65–75 fL), MCHC 34.7 g/dL (33–36 g/dL), WBC 22,170 cells/μL (6,000–13,000 cells/μL), neutrophils 19,288 cells/μL (3,000–10,500 cells/μL), band neutrophils 443 cells/μL, lymphocytes 1,109 cells/μL (1,000–4,000 cells/μL), monocytes 887 cells/μL (150–1200 cells/μL), platelets clumped. There was slight neutrophil toxicity and rare schistocytosis.

Serum chemistry profile: Sodium 140 mmol/L (145–154 mmol/L), potassium 4.1 mmol/L (3.6–5.3 mmol/L), chloride 106 mmol/L (108–118 mmol/L), bicarbonate 16 mmol/L (16–26 mmol/L), phosphorus 3.0 mg/dL (3.0–6.2 mg/dL), calcium 8.9 mg/dL (9.7–11.5 mg/dL), BUN 4 mg/dL (5–21 mg/dL), creatinine 0.3 mg/dL (0.3–1.2 mg/dL), glucose 83 mg/dL (64–123 mg/dL), total protein 4.7 g/dL (5.4–7.6 g/dL), albumin 2.6 g/dL (3.0–4.4 g/dL), globulin 2.1 g/dL (1.8–3.9 g/dL), ALT 514 U/L (19–67 U/L), AST 91 U/L (19–42 U/L), ALP 277 U/L (21–170 U/L), creatine kinase 138 U/L (51–399 U/L), GGT 9 U/L (0–6 U/L), cholesterol 237 mg/dL (135–361 mg/dL), total bilirubin 0.3 mg/dL (0–0.2 mg/dL), magnesium 1.4 mg/dL (1.5–2.6 mg/dL).

Urinalysis: SpG 1.011; pH 6.5, negative protein, 3 mg/dL bilirubin, 10 erythrocytes/μL, hemoprotein, no glucose, 0–3 WBC/HPF, 3–5 RBC/HPF, few lipid droplets.

Imaging Findings

Thoracic radiographs: The cardiovascular and pulmonary structures appeared within normal limits.

Abdominal ultrasound: Multiple fluid-filled small intestinal loops were identified with mucosal hyperechogenicity but normal wall layering. There was a scant volume of anechoic free peritoneal fluid. The liver was mildly hyperechoic. There was mild splenomegaly and prominent mesenteric lymph nodes.

Microbiologic Testing

Urine aerobic culture and susceptibility: 10^3 CFU/mL *L. monocytogenes* (identified using MALDI-TOF), susceptible to aminoglycosides, beta-lactams, trimethoprim-sulfamethoxazole, chloramphenicol.

Blood culture (aerobic and anaerobic): Blood samples were collected at times 0, 20, and 60 minutes. Large numbers of gram-positive rods were seen on a Gram-stained smear after incubation, which were also identified as *L. monocytogenes.*

Diagnosis

Listeria monocytogenes bacteremia.

Chronic enteropathy associated with inflammatory bowel disease.

Cutaneous lupus of German shepherd dogs.

Treatment

Leflunomide was discontinued and treatment with ampicillin (20 mg/kg, IV, q6h) and gentamicin (10 mg/kg, SC, q24h) was initiated. Methylprednisolone was continued.

CASE EXAMPLE—cont'd

Magnesium citrate was also administered (5 mg/kg, q24h) for hypomagnesemia that likely resulted from chronic malabsorption. At a recheck 1 week later, Jimmy's owners reported significant improvement in his activity level and appetite. His temperature had been normal at home and he was playing with the other dogs. He ate almost all of his food but did not ever seem very hungry, but his body weight increased by 0.6 kg. No urinary accidents in the house had occurred. Blood and urine cultures were negative. Although bandemia had resolved on the CBC, there was a persistent mature neutrophilia (27,245 cells/μL) and serum chemistry abnormalities persisted, with further increase in the serum ALT (1925 U/L). On physical examination, a new cardiac murmur was detected (grade II/VI systolic left apical). An echocardiogram revealed mild mitral valve regurgitation, reduced systolic function, and a 1-cm circular echogenic lesion that was adherent to the caudal apical surface of the left ventricular endomyocardium (Fig. 52.11A and B). This was suspected to be a mural thrombus. Serum troponin I concentration was increased (0.97 ng/mL, reference range: 0.09–0.17). Treatment with amoxicillin (20 mg/kg, PO, q8h) was continued and gentamicin was discontinued. Treatment with clopidogrel was considered, but withheld because of concerns that it might lead to dislodgement of a clot. However, approximately 1 week later, Jimmy developed acute onset of left thoracic limb lameness. On physical examination, his entire limb distal to the carpus was cool to the touch. No murmur was detected. A repeat echocardiogram showed that the mural mass was half the size it had previously been, with ragged edges. Abdominal ultrasound examination showed lesions consistent with multiple venous thrombi in the caudal vena cava, common iliac, hepatic, and renal veins. Wedge-shaped hypoechoic lesions were identified in the renal parenchyma and diffuse mixed echogenic regions were in the liver, suggestive of infarcts secondary to thromboemboli. Jimmy was treated with clopidogrel (1.5 mg/kg, PO, q24h), enoxaparin (1 mg/kg, SC, q8h), enalapril (0.5 mg/kg, PO, q12h) and pimobendan (0.3 mg/kg, PO, q12h). Amoxicillin was also continued.

One month later the lameness had resolved, there had been a 5-kg weight gain, and Jimmy's appetite and energy level were normal. Bloodwork showed resolution of laboratory abnormalities, including serum troponin I concentration, and echocardiography showed resolution of the mural lesion, persistent mild mitral regurgitation, and improved systolic function. Abdominal ultrasound examination showed resolution of thrombi within the major veins and static chronic renal changes consistent with infarcts. All medications except the clopidogrel and methylprednisolone were discontinued; at a recheck 2 months later, clopidogrel was discontinued and methylprednisolone dose was halved, and vitamin B12 supplementation was commenced (1500 μg, SC, q2weeks) because serum B12 concentration was low (219 ng/L, reference range 271–875 ng/L). Six months later, there was worsening of cutaneous lupus lesions, with appearance of multiple severe oral ulcerations (Fig. 52.11C). The inflammatory bowel disease was relatively well controlled with only mild intermittent diarrhea. Treatment with cyclosporine was commenced (5 mg/kg, PO, q24h), which was associated with resolution of the ulcers. However, 6 months later, Jimmy became hyporexic and weight loss was noted. The most significant finding on an extensive work-up that included bloodwork, blood cultures, echocardiography, and abdominal ultrasound was moderate thrombocytopenia (59,000 platelets/μL). Vector-borne disease serology was negative. Four months later (2 years after the diagnosis of listeriosis) he was brought to the UC Davis veterinary emergency service and was in cardiopulmonary arrest. A necropsy revealed disseminated, intravascular B-cell lymphoma in the lung, brain, kidney, pancreas, liver, small and large intestine, stomach, omentum, adrenal gland, heart, and periocular haired skin as well as moderate, chronic, diffuse, lymphoplasmacytic enteritis.

Comments

This dog likely developed *L. monocytogenes* bacteremia and mural endomyocarditis with thromboembolic complications secondary to immunosuppressive drug therapy and exposure to farm animal species. Although the listeriosis was treated successfully, ultimately persistence of immune-mediated disease necessitated ongoing immunosuppression with cyclosporine. It is possible that the use of cyclosporine predisposed to the ultimate cause of death, disseminated B-cell lymphoma.[102]

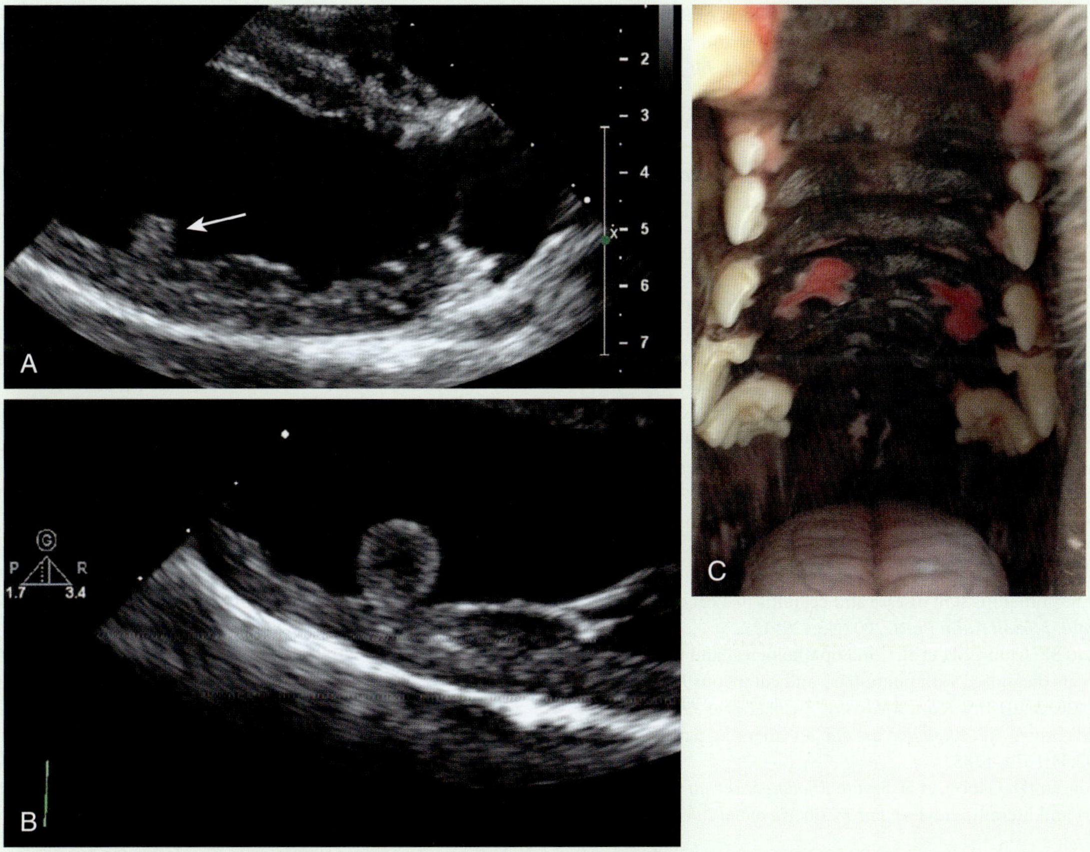

Fig. 52.11 (A) Right parasternal long-axis view of the heart of the dog in Fig. 52.10 showing a 1-cm circular mural lesion associated with the endomyocardium *(arrow)* that was thought to represent a clot or mass. (B) Close-up view of the mural lesion. (C) Oral ulcerations secondary to lupus. (Images courtesy of the University of California, Davis Veterinary Dermatology, Internal Medicine and Cardiology Services.)

SUGGESTED READINGS

Bryan LK, Clark SD, Diaz-Delgado J, et al. *Rhodococcus equi* infections in dogs. *Vet Pathol.* 2017;54:159–163.

Hanson H, Whitfield Y, Lee C, et al. *Listeria monocytogenes* associated with pasteurized chocolate milk, Ontario, Canada. *Emerg Infect Dis.* 2019;25:581–584.

Radoshevich L, Cossart P. *Listeria monocytogenes*: towards a complete picture of its physiology and pathogenesis. *Nat Rev Microbiol.* 2018;16:32–46.

Marshall KR, Walton SA, Boyd M, et al. Erysipeloid lesions caused by *Erysipelothrix rhusiopathiae* in a dog: clinical and histopathological findings, molecular diagnosis and treatment. *Vet Dermatol.* 2019,30:434. e134.

Decker RS. *Recounting the Anthrax Attacks: Terror, The Amerithrax Task Force, and the Evolution of Forensics in the FBI.* Lanham, MD: Rowman and Littlefield Publishing Group; 2018.

REFERENCES

1. Magnusson H. Spezifische infektiose pneumoniae beim fohlen. Ein neuer eiterreger beim pferd. *Arch Wiss Prakt Tierhelkd.* 1923;50:22–37.
2. Gonzalez-Enguita C, Vela-Navarrete R. *Corynebacterium urealyticum*: the historical importance of its discovery. *Actas Urol Esp.* 2017;41:140.
3. Murray EGD, Webb RA, Swann MBR. A disease of rabbits characterized by large mononuclear leucocytosis, caused by a hitherto undescribed bacillus, *Bacterium monocytogenes*. *J Pathol Bacteriol.* 1926;29:407–439.
4. Brooke CJ, Riley TV. *Erysipelothrix rhusiopathiae*: bacteriology, epidemiology and clinical manifestations of an occupational pathogen. *J Med Microbiol.* 1999;48:789–799.
5. Alibek K, Lobanova C, Popov S. Anthrax: a disease and a weapon. In: Fong IW, Alibek K, eds. *Bioterrorism and Infectious Agents: A New Dilemma for the 21st Century.* New York, NY: Springer; 2009:1–29.
6. Vázquez-Boland JA, Scortti M, Meijer WG. Conservation of *Rhodococcus equi* (Magnusson 1923) Goodfellow and Alderson 1977 and rejection of *Rhodococcus hoagii* (Morse 1912) Käparampfer et al 2014. *Int J Syst Evol Microbiol.* 2020;70:3572–3576.
7. Bryan LK, Clark SD, Diaz-Delgado J, et al. *Rhodococcus equi* infections in dogs. *Vet Pathol.* 2017;54:159–163.
8. Cantor GH, Byrne BA, Hines SA, et al. VapA-negative *Rhodococcus equi* in a dog with necrotizing pyogranulomatous hepatitis, osteomyelitis, and myositis. *J Vet Diagn Invest.* 1998;10:297–300.
9. Portilho FVR, Paes AC, Megid J, et al. *Rhodococcus equi* pVAPN type causing pneumonia in a dog coinfected with canine morbillivirus (distemper virus) and *Toxoplasma gondii*. *Microb Pathog.* 2019;129:112–117.
10. Rocha BZLL, Portilho FVR, Júnior FG, et al. Cellulitis-related *Rhodococcus equi* in a cat harboring VAPA-type plasmid pattern. *Microb Pathog.* 2021;160:105186.
11. Bryan LK, Alexander ER, Lawhon SD, et al. Detection of vapN in *Rhodococcus equi* isolates cultured from humans. *PLoS One.* 2018;13:e0190829.
12. Fairley CK, Yung A. *Rhodococcus equi* and HIV infection. *Aust N Z J Med.* 1990;20:99.
13. Farias MR, Takai S, Ribeiro MG, et al. Cutaneous pyogranuloma in a cat caused by virulent *Rhodococcus equi* containing an 87 kb type I plasmid. *Aust Vet J.* 2007;85:29–31.
14. Patel A. Pyogranulomatous skin disease and cellulitis in a cat caused by *Rhodococcus equi*. *J Small Anim Pract.* 2002;43:129–132.
15. Aslam MW, Lau SF, Chin CSL, et al. Clinicopathological and radiographic features in 40 cats diagnosed with pulmonary and cutaneous *Rhodococcus equi* infection (2012-2018). *J Feline Med Surg.* 2020;22:774–790.
16. Weinstock DM, Brown AE. *Rhodococcus equi*: an emerging pathogen. *Clin Infect Dis.* 2002;34:1379–1385.
17. Vestbo J, Lundgren JD, Gaub J, et al. Severe *Rhodococcus equi* pneumonia: case report and literature review. *Eur J Clin Microbiol Infect Dis.* 1991;10:762–768.
18. Kim R, Reboli AC. Other coryneform bacteria and rhodococci. In: Bennett JE, Dolin R, Blaser MJ, eds. *Mandell, Douglas, and Bennett's Principles and Practice of Infectious Diseases.* 8 ed. Philadelphia, PA: Elsevier Saunders; 2015:2373–2382.
19. Giguere S, Jacks S, Roberts GD, et al. Retrospective comparison of azithromycin, clarithromycin, and erythromycin for the treatment of foals with *Rhodococcus equi* pneumonia. *J Vet Intern Med.* 2004;18:568–573.
20. Hylton PK, Rizzi TE, Allison RW. Intracellular success: cytologic findings in an ulcerated submandibular mass from a cat. *Vet Clin Pathol.* 2006;35:345–347.
21. Takai S, Sasaki Y, Ikeda T, et al. Virulence of *Rhodococcus equi* isolates from patients with and without AIDS. *J Clin Microbiol.* 1994;32:457–460.
22. Aalbaek B, Bemis DA, Schjaerff M, et al. Coryneform bacteria associated with canine otitis externa. *Vet Microbiol.* 2010;145:292–298.
23. Collins MD, Hoyles L, Lawson PA, et al. Phenotypic and phylogenetic characterization of a new *Corynebacterium* species from dogs: description of *Corynebacterium auriscanis* sp. nov. *J Clin Microbiol.* 1999;37:3443–3447.
24. Maurey C, Boulouis HJ, Canonne-Guibert M, et al. Clinical description of *Corynebacterium urealyticum* urinary tract infections in 11 dogs and 10 cats. *J Small Anim Pract.* 2019;60:239–246.
25. Cavana P, Zanatta R, Nebbia P, et al. *Corynebacterium urealyticum* urinary tract infection in a cat with urethral obstruction. *J Feline Med Surg.* 2008;10:269–273.
26. Elad D, Aizenberg I, Shamir M, et al. Isolation of *Corynebacterium* group D2 from two dogs with urinary tract infections. *J Clin Microbiol.* 1992;30:1167–1169.
27. Gomez A, Nombela C, Zapardiel J, et al. An encrusted cystitis caused by *Corynebacterium urealyticum* in a dog. *Aust Vet J.* 1995;72:72–73.
28. Suarez ML, Espino L, Vila M, et al. Urinary tract infection caused by *Corynebacterium urealyticum* in a dog. *J Small Anim Pract.* 2002;43:299–302.
29. Puskar M, Lemons C, Papich MG, et al. Antibiotic-resistant *Corynebacterium jeikeium* urinary tract infection in a cat. *J Am Anim Hosp Assoc.* 2007;43:61–64.
30. Bailiff NL, Westropp JL, Jang SS, et al. *Corynebacterium urealyticum* urinary tract infection in dogs and cats: 7 cases (1996-2003). *J Am Vet Med Assoc.* 2005;226:1676–1680.
31. Wilson BJ, Norris JM, Malik R, et al. Susceptibility of bacteria from feline and canine urinary tract infections to doxycycline and tetracycline concentrations attained in urine four hours after oral dosage. *Aust Vet J.* 2006;84:8–11.
32. Dias AA, Silva Jr FC, Pereira GA, et al. *Corynebacterium ulcerans* isolated from an asymptomatic dog kept in an animal shelter in the metropolitan area of Rio de Janeiro, Brazil. *Vector Borne Zoonotic Dis.* 2010;10:743–748.
33. Sykes JE, Mapes S, Lindsay LL, et al. *Corynebacterium ulcerans* bronchopneumonia in a dog. *J Vet Intern Med.* 2010;24:973–976.
34. Taylor DJ, Efstratiou A, Reilly WJ. Diphtheria toxin production by *Corynebacterium ulcerans* from cats. *Vet Rec.* 2002;150:355.
35. Hogg RA, Wessels J, Hart J, et al. Possible zoonotic transmission of toxigenic *Corynebacterium ulcerans* from companion animals in a human case of fatal diphtheria. *Vet Rec.* 2009;165:691–692.
36. Lartigue MF, Monnet X, Le Fleche A, et al. *Corynebacterium ulcerans* in an immunocompromised patient with diphtheria and her dog. *J Clin Microbiol.* 2005;43:999–1001.
37. Katsukawa C, Kawahara R, Inoue K, et al. Toxigenic *Corynebacterium ulcerans* isolated from the domestic dog for the first time in Japan. *Jpn J Infect Dis.* 2009;62:171–172.
38. Boynosky NA, Stokking LB. Retrospective evaluation of canine dermatitis secondary to *Corynebacterium* spp. *J Am Anim Hosp Assoc.* 2015;51:372–379.
39. Bygott JM, Malnick H, Shah JJ, et al. First clinical case of *Corynebacterium auriscanis* isolated from localized dog bite infection. *J Med Microbiol.* 2008;57:899–900.
40. Lorber B. *Listeria monocytogenes*. In: Bennett JE, Dolin R, Blaser MJ, eds. *Mandell, Douglas, and Bennett's Principles and Practice of Infectious Diseases.* 8 ed. Philadelphia, PA: Elsevier Saunders; 2015:2383–2390.
41. Pritchard JC, Jacob ME, Ward TJ, et al. *Listeria monocytogenes* septicemia in an immunocompromised dog. *Vet Clin Pathol.* 2016;45:254–259.
42. Palerme JS, Pan PC, Parsons CT, et al. Isolation and characterization of atypical *Listeria monocytogenes* associated with a canine urinary tract infection. *J Vet Diagn Invest.* 2016;28:604–607.

43. Marien M. Isolation of *Listeria monocytogenes* from the gallbladder of a dog with liver insufficiency. *Vlaams Diergeneeskundig Tijdschrift.* 2007;76:352–354.
44. Iida T, Kanzaki M, Maruyama T, et al. Prevalence of *Listeria monocytogenes* in intestinal contents of healthy animals in Japan. *J Vet Med Sci.* 1991;53:873–875.
45. Schlech WF 3rd , Lavigne PM, Bortolussi RA, et al. Epidemic listeriosis: evidence for transmission by food. *N Engl J Med.* 1983;308:203–206.
46. Olsen SJ, Patrick M, Hunter SB, et al. Multistate outbreak of *Listeria monocytogenes* infection linked to delicatessen turkey meat. *Clin Infect Dis.* 2005;40:962–967.
47. Hanson H, Whitfield Y, Lee C, et al. *Listeria monocytogenes* associated with pasteurized chocolate milk, Ontario, Canada. *Emerg Infect Dis.* 2019;25:581–584.
48. Dalton CB, Austin CC, Sobel J, et al. An outbreak of gastroenteritis and fever due to *Listeria monocytogenes* in milk. *N Engl J Med.* 1997;336:100–105.
49. McCollum JT, Cronquist AB, Silk BJ, et al. Multistate outbreak of listeriosis associated with cantaloupe. *N Engl J Med.* 2013;369:944–953.
50. Zelenik K, Avbersek J, Pate M, et al. Cutaneous listeriosis in a veterinarian with the evidence of zoonotic transmission: a case report. *Zoonoses Public Health.* 2014;61:238–241.
51. Jones JL, Wang L, Ceric O, et al. Whole genome sequencing confirms source of pathogens associated with bacterial foodborne illness in pets fed raw pet food. *J Vet Diagn Invest.* 2019;31:235–240.
52. van Bree FPJ, Bokken G, Mineur R, et al. Zoonotic bacteria and parasites found in raw meat-based diets for cats and dogs. *Vet Rec.* 2018;182:50.
53. Nemser SM, Doran T, Grabenstein M, et al. Investigation of *Listeria, Salmonella*, and toxigenic *Escherichia coli* in various pet foods. *Foodborne Pathog Dis.* 2014;11:706–709.
54. Fluen TW, Hardcastle M, Kiupel M, et al. Listerial mesenteric lymphadenitis in 3 cats. *J Vet Intern Med.* 2019;33:1753–1758.
55. Mason NJ, Gnanandarajah JS, Engiles JB, et al. Immunotherapy with a HER2-targeting *Listeria* induces HER2-specific immunity and demonstrates potential therapeutic effects in a phase I trial in canine osteosarcoma. *Clin Cancer Res.* 2016;22:4380–4390.
56. Musser ML, Berger EP, Parsons C, et al. Vaccine strain *Listeria monocytogenes* abscess in a dog: a case report. *BMC Vet Res.* 2019;15:467.
57. Musser ML, Berger EP, Tripp CD, et al. Safety evaluation of the canine osteosarcoma vaccine, live *Listeria* vector. *Vet Comp Oncol.* 2021;19:92–98.
58. Radoshevich L, Cossart P. *Listeria monocytogenes*: towards a complete picture of its physiology and pathogenesis. *Nat Rev Microbiol.* 2018;16:32–46.
59. Sturgess CP. Listerial abortion in the bitch. *Vet Rec.* 1989;124:177.
60. Laikko T, Baverud V, Danielsson-Tham ML, et al. Canine tonsillitis associated with *Listeria monocytogenes. Vet Rec.* 2004;154:732.
61. Wong SA, Hugo TB. Myocarditis caused by *Listeria monocytogenes* in a dog. *Aust Vet J.* 2021. Online ahead of print.
62. Schroeder H, van Rensburg IB. Generalised *Listeria monocytogenes* infection in a dog. *J S Afr Vet Assoc.* 1993;64:133–136.
63. Jones BR, Cullinane LC, Cary PR. Isolation of *Listeria monocytogenes* from a bite in a cat from the common tree weta (*Hemideina crassidens*). *N Z Vet J.* 1984;32:79–80.
64. Raith K, Muntener T, Vandevelde M, et al. Encephalomyelitis resembling human and ruminant rhombencephalitis caused by *Listeria monocytogenes* in a feline leukemia virus-infected cat. *J Vet Intern Med.* 2010;24:983–985.
65. Turner T. A case of *Listeria monocytogenes* in the cat. *Vet Rec.* 1962;74:778.
66. Elbert JA, Rissi DR. Systemic *Listeria monocytogenes* infection and concurrent pleural mesothelioma in a cat. *J Vet Diagn Invest.* 2021;33:120–123.
67. Burall LS, Simpson AC, Chou L, et al. A novel gene, lstC, of *Listeria monocytogenes* is implicated in high salt tolerance. *Food Microbiol.* 2015;48:72–82.
68. McLauchlin J, Low JC. Primary cutaneous listeriosis in adults: an occupational disease of veterinarians and farmers. *Vet Rec.* 1994;135:615–617.
69. Svabic-Vlahovic M, Pantic D, Pavicic M, et al. Transmission of *Listeria monocytogenes* from mother's milk to her baby and to puppies. *Lancet.* 1988;2:1201.
70. Takahashi T, Fujisawa T, Tamura Y, et al. DNA relatedness among *Erysipelothrix rhusiopathiae* strains representing all twenty-three serovars and *Erysipelothrix tonsillarum. Int J Syst Bacteriol.* 1992;42:469–473.
71. Hoenig M, Gillette DM. Endocarditis caused by *Erysipelothrix rhusiopathiae* in a dog. *J Am Vet Med Assoc.* 1980;176:326–327.
72. Goudswaard J, Hartman EG, Janmaat A, et al. *Erysipelothrix rhusiopathiae* strain 7, a causative agent of endocarditis and arthritis in the dog. *Tijdschr Diergeneeskd.* 1973;98:416–423.
73. Kucsera G. Serological typing of *Erysipelothrix rhusiopathiae* strains and the epizootiological significance of the typing. *Acta Vet Acad Sci Hung.* 1977;27:19–28.
74. Swindle MM, Narayan O, Luzarraga M, et al. Contagious streptococcal lymphadenitis in cats. *J Am Vet Med Assoc.* 1980;177:829–830.
75. Takahasi T, Fujisawa T, Yamamoto K, et al. Taxonomic evidence that serovar 7 of *Erysipelothrix* strains isolated from dogs with endocarditis are *Erysipelothrix tonsillarum. J Vet Med B Infect Dis Vet Public Health.* 2000;47:311–313.
76. Marshall KR, Walton SA, Boyd M, et al. Erysipeloid lesions caused by *Erysipelothrix rhusiopathiae* in a dog: clinical and histopathological findings, molecular diagnosis and treatment. *Vet Dermatol.* 2019;30:434. e134.
77. Foster JD, Hartmann FA, Moriello KA. A case of apparent canine erysipeloid associated with *Erysipelothrix rhusiopathiae* bacteraemia. *Vet Dermatol.* 2012;23:528. e108.
78. Rhoades AC, Vernau W, Kass PH, et al. Comparison of the efficacy of prednisone and cyclosporine for treatment of dogs with primary immune-mediated polyarthritis. *J Am Vet Med Assoc.* 2016;248:395–404.
79. Yamazaki Y. A multiplex polymerase chain reaction for discriminating *Erysipelothrix rhusiopathiae* from *Erysipelothrix tonsillarum. J Vet Diagn Invest.* 2006;18:384–387.
80. Seelig U, Klopfleisch R, Weingart C, et al. Septic polyarthritis caused by *Erysipelothrix rhusiopathiae* in a dog. *Vet Comp Orthop Traumatol.* 2010;23:71–73.
81. Martin GJ, Friedlander AM. *Bacillus anthracis* (anthrax). In: Bennett JE, Dolin R, Blaser MJ, eds. *Mandell, Douglas, and Bennett's Principles and Practice of Infectious Diseases.* 8 ed. Philadelphia, PA: Elsevier Saunders; 2015:2391–2409.
82. Gleiser CA, Gochenour WS Jr, Ward MK. Pulmonary lesions in dogs and pigs exposed to a cloud of anthrax spores. *J Comp Pathol.* 1968;78:445–448.
83. Creel S, Creel NM, Matovelo JA, et al. The effects of anthrax on endangered African wild dogs (*Lycaon pictus*). *J Zool.* 1995;236:199–209.
84. Mukarati NL, Ndumnego O, van Heerden H, et al. A serological survey of anthrax in domestic dogs in Zimbabwe: a potential tool for anthrax surveillance. *Epidemiol Infect.* 2018;146:1526–1532.
85. Lembo T, Hampson K, Auty H, et al. Serologic surveillance of anthrax in the Serengeti ecosystem, Tanzania, 1996-2009. *Emerg Infect Dis.* 2011;17:387–394.
86. World Health Organization. *Anthrax in Humans and Animals.* 4 ed. 2008. Available at. https://www.ncbi.nlm.nih.gov/books/NBK310486/.
87. Jernigan JA, Stephens DS, Ashford DA, et al. Bioterrorism-related inhalational anthrax: the first 10 cases reported in the United States. *Emerg Infect Dis.* 2001;7:933–944.
88. Makino S, Watarai M, Cheun HI, et al. Effect of the lower molecular capsule released from the cell surface of *Bacillus anthracis* on the pathogenesis of anthrax. *J Infect Dis.* 2002;186:227–233.
89. Sherer K, Li Y, Cui X, et al. Lethal and edema toxins in the pathogenesis of *Bacillus anthracis* septic shock: implications for therapy. *Am J Respir Crit Care Med.* 2007;175:211–221.
90. Blackburn JK, Skrypnyk A, Bagamian KH, et al. Anthrax in a backyard domestic dog in Ukraine: a case report. *Vector Borne Zoonotic Dis.* 2014;14:615–617.
91. Harrison LH, Ezzell JW, Abshire TG, et al. Evaluation of serologic tests for diagnosis of anthrax after an outbreak of cutaneous anthrax in Paraguay. *J Infect Dis.* 1989;160:706–710.
92. Quinn CP, Semenova VA, Elie CM, et al. Specific, sensitive, and quantitative enzyme-linked immunosorbent assay for human immunoglobulin G antibodies to anthrax toxin protective antigen. *Emerg Infect Dis.* 2002;8:1103–1110.

93. Martin SW, Tierney BC, Aranas A, et al. An overview of adverse events reported by participants in CDC's anthrax vaccine and antimicrobial availability program. *Pharmacoepidemiol Drug Saf.* 2005;14:393–401.
94. Shlyakhov E, Rubinstein E. Evaluation of the anthraxin skin test for diagnosis of acute and past human anthrax. *Eur J Clin Microbiol Infect Dis.* 1996;15:242–245.
95. Hail AS, Rossi CA, Ludwig GV, et al. Comparison of noninvasive sampling sites for early detection of *Bacillus anthracis* spores from rhesus monkeys after aerosol exposure. *Mil Med.* 1999;164:833–837.
96. De BK, Bragg SL, Sanden GN, et al. A two-component direct fluorescent-antibody assay for rapid identification of *Bacillus anthracis. Emerg Infect Dis.* 2002;8:1060–1065.
97. McGee ED, Fritz DL, Ezzell JW, et al. Anthrax in a dog. *Vet Pathol.* 1994;31:471–473.
98. Spotts Whitney EA, Beatty ME, Taylor TH Jr, et al. Inactivation of *Bacillus anthracis* spores. *Emerg Infect Dis.* 2003;9:623–627.
99. Shadomy SV, Smith TL. Zoonosis update. Anthrax. *J Am Vet Med Assoc.* 2008;233:63–72.
100. Brookmeyer R, Johnson E, Bollinger R. Modeling the optimum duration of antibiotic prophylaxis in an anthrax outbreak. *Proc Natl Acad Sci U S A.* 2003;100:10129–10132.
101. Langston C. Postexposure management and treatment of anthrax in dogs-Executive Councils of the American Academy of Veterinary Pharmacology and Therapeutics and the American College of Veterinary Clinical Pharmacology. *AAPS J.* 2005;7:E272–E273.
102. Archer TM, Boothe DM, Langston VC, et al. Oral cyclosporine treatment in dogs: a review of the literature. *J Vet Intern Med.* 2014;28:1–20.

53

Gram-Negative Bacterial Infections

Virginia Sinnott-Stutzman, Jane E. Sykes

KEY POINTS

- First Described: Gram-negative bacteria were first described in Berlin by the Danish scientist Hans Christian Gram in 1884 when he used Gram stain to visualize *Klebsiella pneumoniae* in the lungs of people who died of pneumonia.[1]
- Causes: Examples include *Escherichia coli, Salmonella, Enterobacter, Citrobacter, Klebsiella, Campylobacter, Pseudomonas,* and *Acinetobacter.*
- Geographic Distribution: Worldwide.
- Mode of Transmission: Direct contact or contact with contaminated fomites; the bacteria often invade opportunistically.
- Major Clinical Signs: Affected sites include UTIs, wound infections, pneumonia, pyothorax, peritonitis, pyometra, ocular surface infections, otitis externa, pyoderma, bacteremia, and endocarditis, but virtually any body system can be affected.
- Differential Diagnoses: Infections with gram-positive bacteria such as *Staphylococcus* spp. and *Streptococcus* spp.; to a lesser extent, infections with nonbacterial pathogens such as fungi.
- Human Health Significance: Gram-negative bacteria shed by dogs and cats have the potential to colonize humans, especially those with impaired host defenses. They may also be responsible for infections of dog or cat bites. Infections caused by gram-negative pathogens resistant to all available antibiotics have resulted in the death of human patients.[2]

ETIOLOGIC AGENTS, EPIDEMIOLOGY, AND CLINICAL FEATURES

Gram-negative bacteria are ubiquitous agents of opportunistic infections in dogs and cats and primarily cause disease when host defenses are impaired. They are important causes of nosocomial disease; several species belong to the ESKAPE group of bacteria (*Enterococcus faecium, Staphylococcus aureus, Klebsiella pneumoniae, Acinetobacter baumannii, Pseudomonas aeruginosa* and *Enterobacter* spp.), a term that was developed to reflect the ability of these organisms to escape antimicrobial activity through resistance and highlight their importance as significant causes of morbidity and mortality in human healthcare facilities. Distinguishing the gram-negative species in this group from gram-positive bacteria is a complex outer membrane that contains LPS, as well as structures known as *porins* that regulate transport of molecules in and out of the cell including antimicrobial drugs. Between this outer membrane and the inner (cytoplasmic) membrane is a periplasmic space, which contains the structural polymer peptidoglycan (or *murein*) (Fig. 53.1). The peptidoglycan layer of gram-negative bacteria is much thinner than that of gram-positive bacteria, approximately one layer, or 7 to 8 nm thick (compared with many layers, or 20 to 80 nm thick for gram-positive bacteria). The inner cytoplasmic membrane contains many different proteins that are lipoproteins anchored into the outer lipid bilayer leaflet, transmembrane proteins, or peripheral membrane proteins that lie adjacent to the bilayer leaflets. Of particular clinical relevance are efflux pumps which can allow an organism to become resistant to multiple antibiotic classes. The pump type that most commonly causes such resistance is called the resistance-nodulation-cell division (RND) pump. This pump system, when active, can extrude a variety of molecules from gram-negative bacteria, including antimicrobial agents of various classes, conferring multidrug resistance to gram-negative organisms of several genera including *Escherichia coli, Klebsiella*, and *Pseudomonas* species.[3]

LPS is a large molecule that varies in composition from one bacterial species and strain to another. It contributes to the structural integrity of gram-negative bacteria and is a potent virulence factor. It consists of the *lipid A* backbone, a *core oligosaccharide,* and the *O antigen* side chain. Lipid A is a phosphorylated disaccharide to which long, hydrophobic fatty acid chains are attached, which anchor the LPS into the outer membrane (Figs. 53.1 and 53.2). The lipid A component is also known as *endotoxin* because it is the biologically active portion of the molecule, in that it stimulates a potent host inflammatory response (see Chapter 123). The core oligosaccharide connects lipid A to the O antigen side chain. Its composition differs between bacterial species. The O antigen is a repeating polysaccharide that projects from the surface of the bacterial cell and varies in length from 1 to 60 repeats. It is the antigenic portion of the molecule and is responsible for serogroup classification of gram-negative bacteria.

Gram-negative cocci, such as *Moraxella* or *Neisseria,* are not widely recognized as significant pathogens of dogs and cats. However, as commensals of the canine and feline oral cavity, they can cause bite wound infections in humans,[4] and *Neisseria canis* was isolated in pure culture from a deep mandibular abscess from one dog.[5] Gram-negative rods are classified into Enterobacterales (previously Enterobacteriaceae) and non-Enterobacterales species. Enterobacterales that cause disease in dogs and cats include *E. coli, Proteus, Salmonella, Enterobacter, Citrobacter, Serratia, Klebsiella*, and *Providencia*. Non-Enterobacterales species include the Pasteurellaceae *(Pasteurella multocida),* as well as *P. aeruginosa, Acinetobacter,* and *Ralstonia*. Other gram-negative bacteria are coccobacilli or spiral-shaped organisms and include *Bartonella, Bordetella, Campylobacter, Francisella, Helicobacter,* and *Brucella.*

Like gram-positive cocci, some gram-negative bacteria have tremendous ability to form biofilms, or bacterial aggregates that are embedded in a matrix of exopolysaccharide (bacterial slime), which form on living or nonliving surfaces. These protect the bacteria, and organisms in biofilms can resist the effect of antimicrobial drugs

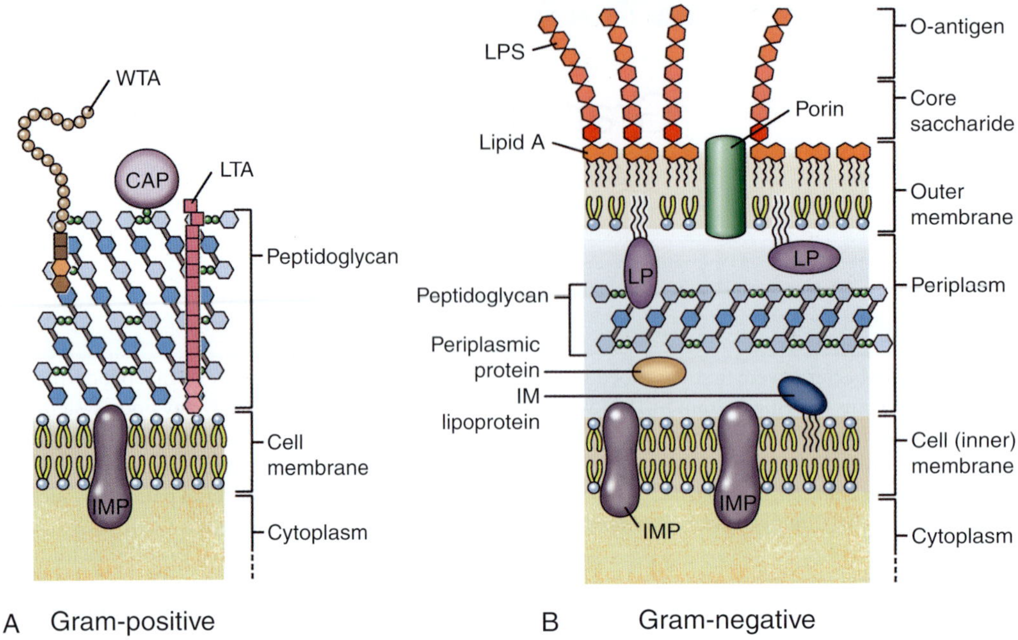

Fig. 53.1 Structure of the envelope of gram-positive (A) and gram-negative (B) bacteria. The thickness of the peptidoglycan layer is greater in gram-positive bacteria than in gram-negative bacteria. *WTA,* wall teichoic acid; *CAP,* covalently-attached protein; *LTA,* lipoteichoic acid; *LPS,* lipopolysaccharide; *IMP,* integral membrane protein; *IM,* inner membrane.

and disinfectants. In addition, expression of efflux pumps has been shown to be a key component of biofilm formation in gram-negative organisms.[6]

Virulence Factors

While the majority of gram-negative infections are caused by opportunistic pathogens that take advantage of weakened host immune systems, some gram-negative organisms have virulence factors which allow them to: (1) persist in host tissues that they do not normally colonize; (2) evade immune responses, and/or (3) adhere to, invade, or damage host cells. Different serotypes of the same species may vary greatly in their potential to cause disease. For example, *E. coli* O157:H7 is often isolated from cases of hemolytic uremic syndrome because it expresses two powerful virulence factors, Shiga toxin (Stx-2) and verocytotoxins (Shiga-like toxins). These induce necrosis of endothelial cells, which results in widespread thrombosis, thrombocytopenia, and often death. In contrast, *E. coli* strain VR50 is associated with asymptomatic bacteriuria in humans, and is currently being investigated as a therapeutic inoculum to prevent recurrent symptomatic UTIs in women.[7]

As whole genome sequencing is becoming an increasingly commonplace aspect of microbiology, hundreds of individual virulence factor genes across several genera of gram-negative organisms have been identified. These can be divided into several categories based on how they contribute to establishing infections and causing disease.

Adhesion Molecules

Adhesion mechanisms among gram-negative bacteria vary widely, but the general motif involves the interaction between bacterial surface organelles and either epithelium or an abiotic surface (i.e., surgical implant). Surface organelles include fimbriae, pili, and flagella. In most cases, genes involved in adhesion are regulated alongside genes that are involved with biofilm development. The virulence factor that allows *E. coli* VR50 to adhere to the mucosa of human bladders has been identified as the gene for afimbrial adhesion (*afa*).[8]

Invasion

Organisms that can cross epithelial barriers and/or invade host cells must possess enzymes that can break down membranes and connective tissue. As such, the host of invasion virulence factors include genes coding for various isoenzymes of phospholipase, collagenase, hyaluronidase, and lecithinase. In contrast to factors that mediate adhesion, invasion virulence factors generally cause some level of damage to target tissues. Genes that encode phospholipase D (*pld*) are key virulence factors that allow *A. baumannii* to penetrate the pulmonary epithelial barrier.[9]

Competition for Iron and Nutrients

Iron is tightly bound to proteins (such as hemoglobin) in mammals; free iron concentration in the host environment is minute. To facilitate survival, gram-negative bacteria express iron acquisition systems that are not required in iron-rich environments. Iron-sequestering proteins produced by gram-negative bacteria are among the most efficient iron chelators in the natural world. Examples of efficient bacterial iron chelators are enterobactin in *E. coli* and pyoverdine in *P. aeruginosa*.[10]

Resistance to Host Immunity

Microorganisms can evade host immunity in myriad ways. While most gram-negative organisms are not innately pathogenic and thus have little genome space dedicated to this task, pathogenic strains of *E. coli* modulate the host's response to endotoxin by inserting tyrosine-based inhibitory motifs into cell membranes which dampen the production of proinflammatory cytokines in response to the presence of endotoxin and other pathogen-associated molecular patterns. Additionally, *E. coli* can bind the Fc receptor of macrophages directly (without antibody present) and induce an inhibitory response, blocking phagocytosis.[11]

Toxin Secretion

Gram-negative pathogens can express genes which interrupt normal metabolic functions of host cells. In general, far greater numbers of gram-negative organisms possess these genes than express them, likely because there is a "fitness cost" (ATP cost) associated with their expression. These toxins are sometimes used to create a more favorable

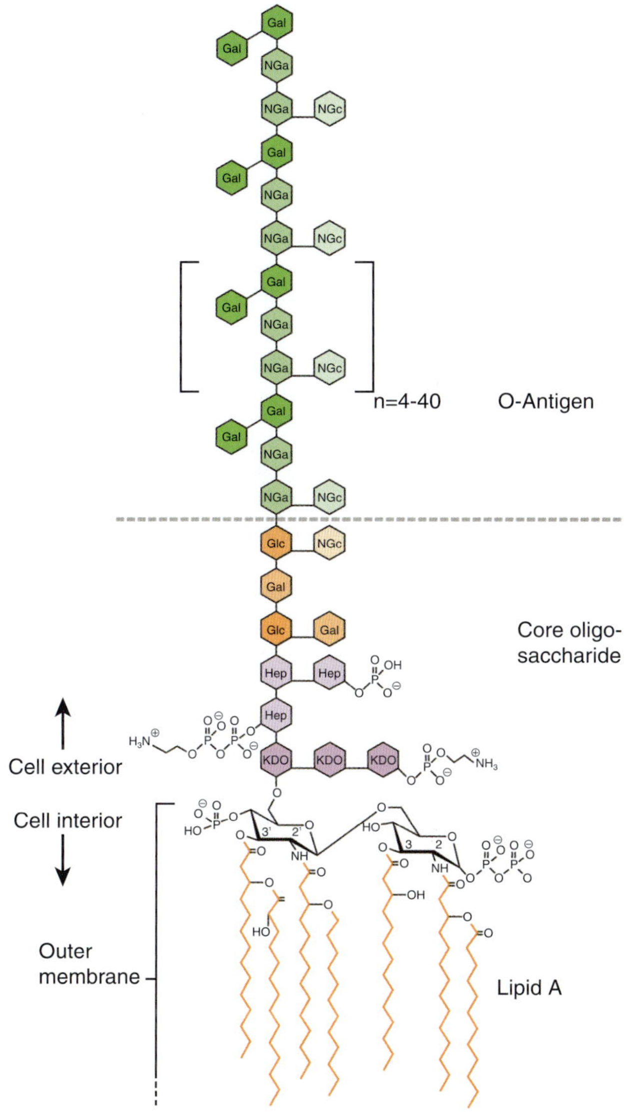

Fig. 53.2 Structure of bacterial lipopolysaccharide.

environment for bacterial replication. For example, in microanaerobic conditions, *P. aeruginosa* can produce exotoxin A, which inhibits protein synthesis by host cells, presumably so that competition for oxygen is reduced.[12]

Bacterial Motility

Gram-negative bacteria that possess flagella are not necessarily able to demonstrate coordinated motion. Motility patterns such as twitching, swimming, and swarming (which involves communication between organisms and activation of "quorum sensing" genes) are associated with ascending UTIs and medical device–related infections. Twitching is more commonly found in *Proteus* isolated from catheter-associated UTIs than in *Proteus* isolated from the feces of healthy individuals.[13]

Virulence Plasmids

Plasmids are packets of genetic material which bacteria can trade among one another. Many plasmids confer groups of potent virulence factors, often genes for cytotoxins, as well as antimicrobial resistance genes. In this way, an otherwise innocuous bacterial clone can quickly acquire both pathogenicity and antimicrobial resistance. Toxins associated with *E. coli* O157:H7 are largely encoded for on a virulence plasmid, *pO157*, and include enterohemolysin, serine protease, and catalase-peroxidase. Each of these enzymes alone is capable of interrupting cellular metabolism, initiating coagulation, or inducing apoptosis under certain conditions. Expression of all three as well as Shiga toxin can result in devastating diarrheal illness and hemolytic uremic syndrome.[14]

Enterobacterales

Many Enterobacterales contribute to the normal gastrointestinal flora of animals. Enterobacterales are non-spore forming, non-acid fast, facultative, anaerobic, gram-negative rods. They possess a capsule (*K antigen*) and may be motile via flagella (*H antigen*). Highly encapsulated species, such as *Klebsiella* and *Enterobacter,* have a mucoid appearance when they grow in culture. The flagella project from the bacterial cell and contain the filament-forming protein *flagellin,* which (with LPS) can stimulate the host inflammatory response. An internationally recognized classification system for Enterobacterales has been established based on differences in the antigen surface molecules, O (LPS), K (capsular), H (flagellar), with serotypes identified by a numerical assignment to each antigen they possess listed after the genus and species name (i.e., *E. coli* O157:H7). Additionally clonal strains of species of specific microbiologic or pathologic interest can be identified by serial alphanumeric designation (i.e., *E.coli* 83972 and *E. coli* VR50, two strains causing asymptomatic bacteriuria in women). The Enterobacterales also possess fimbriae or pili, which are thinner than flagella and play a role in adhesion and sometimes bacterial aggregation. Finally, they possess a variety of complex secretion systems (type I, II, III secretion systems). These facilitate export of toxins such as hemolysins, and molecules that are inserted into, and form pores in, host cell membranes.

Escherichia coli

More than any other species of Enterobacterales, *E. coli* possess the potential to be true pathogens, capable of causing communicable disease in otherwise healthy individuals. Diarrheagenic *E. coli* are a leading cause of human diarrheal disease in the developing world and a source of outbreaks in the developed world. Outbreaks of foodborne illness occur when produce becomes contaminated with animal (usually cattle) feces. Based on the virulence factors they express, enteropathogenic *E. coli* (EPEC) are classified into six major pathovars (i.e., groups defined by the specific pathologic lesions they produce). The reader is referred to Chapter 63 for more complete information on intestinal *E. coli* infections; however, those pathovars known to cause illness in dogs and cats are discussed below.

Enteropathogenic *Escherichia coli.* Organisms collectively called EPEC may comprise several serovars of *E. coli.* The group is defined by its pathogenesis, which is characterized by the distinctive lesions they create on the surface of intestinal epithelial cells. Termed "attaching and effacing," all EPEC express the *eae* gene for intimin, an adhesion protein partially responsible for the denuding of microvilli, but they do not express genes encoding for Shiga toxin. EPEC has been isolated from cats with and without diarrhea.[15] Dogs have long been implicated as carriers of EPEC, and healthy dogs without diarrhea can harbor EPEC.[16] This complicates the question of whether EPEC causes diarrhea in dogs. EPEC has been detected in dogs with diarrhea, but many of these dogs were also infected or colonized with other enteropathogens, so it was unclear if EPEC was a secondary pathogen or a primary cause of diarrhea.[17] In a case series in which a reasonable attempt was made to exclude other pathogens, EPEC were detected based on PCR analysis of *E. coli* isolated from all of seven dogs with hematemesis and/or hemorrhagic diarrhea.[18] Given the infrequency with which molecular diagnostics are performed in veterinary cases of diarrheal illness, EPEC may be underreported as a cause of diarrhea. EPEC should be among the differential diagnoses in cases where multiple members of a household or community of dogs are affected by diarrhea, keeping in mind the zoonotic potential of this pathogen.

Enterotoxigenic *Escherichia coli*. Enterotoxigenic *E. coli* (ETEC) produces either heat-stable toxin (ST), heat-labile toxin (LT), or both. There is little genomic homology among strains of ETEC and conserved genes do not encode proteins associated with pathogenesis. Instead, it is thought that the acquisition of plasmids that encode for colonization factors (to allow adhesion to intestinal epithelium) and ST, LT, or both define ETEC.[19] Diarrhea is induced by ST and LT, which stimulate secondary messenger systems that in turn open the cystic fibrosis transmembrane conductance regulator (CFTR) of enterocytes. The end result is bulk chloride loss into the intestinal lumen. As water and sodium follow, voluminous watery diarrhea results. ETEC has been identified in dogs with diarrhea.[20,21]

Adherent invasive *Escherichia coli*. Unlike most other pathovars of *E. coli*, adherent invasive *E. coli* (AIEC) is still defined by its phenotype because virulence genes associated with invasiveness have yet to be identified in this pathovar. An *E. coli* is defined as AIEC if it can invade and replicate within cell cultures efficiently enough to escape inactivation by gentamicin.[22] Adherent and invasive *E. coli* induce disease through a combination of host genetic predisposition and immune stimulation. These organisms adhere to and invade ileal cells (humans) and ileal and colonic cells (dogs), which is associated with Crohn's disease and granulomatous colitis, respectively. The microorganisms replicate within epithelial cells as well as macrophages, with inhibition of macrophage apoptosis. This results in high levels of TNF-α with associated intestinal inflammation and granuloma formation in patients with Crohn's disease.[19,23] Boxer dogs and French bulldogs with granulomatous colitis have AIEC associated with their lesions. Remission associated with fluoroquinolone administration suggests a similar pathogenesis.[24,25] Given the emergence of resistance and the microbiologically catastrophic effect of antibiotics on the gut microbiome, alternate therapies are being investigated in humans with Crohn's disease. Nonantibiotic therapies targeted at blocking AIEC adhesion and colonization are under investigation.[26]

Extraintestinal pathogenic *Escherichia coli*. Following the same nomenclature system used for EPEC, organisms that cause disease outside of the intestinal tract are often designated as extraintestinal pathogenic *E. coli* (ExPEC). An important subset of ExPEC, serovars or clones with virulence attributes that allow for urinary tract invasion, are often referred to as uropathogenic *E. coli* (UPEC). *Escherichia coli* is the most common cause of UTIs in dogs and cats and can also be isolated from dogs and cats with pyometra, prostatitis, peritonitis, cholangitis, cholecystitis, bacteremia and endocarditis, bronchopneumonia (such as that secondary to aspiration), and pyothorax.[27] There are two reports of severe soft tissue infections (necrotizing fasciitis) in dogs associated with *E. coli* infection.[28,29] Antimicrobial resistance in *E. coli* isolates from dogs and cats is an increasing problem; 51% of 376 isolates collected from sick dogs and cats in the United States in 2005 showed resistance to at least one drug, and 29% of the 376 isolates were MDR (defined as resistant to three or more classes of antimicrobial drugs).[30] Another investigation similarly found an increasing trend for resistance to fluoroquinolones, tetracyclines, and cephalosporins for nonurinary tract *E. coli* infections from 2002 to 2011.[31] A European investigation found that beta-lactamase production among *E. coli* respiratory infections in dogs was high, with only 37% of isolates sensitive to ampicillin but 83% susceptible to amoxicillin-clavulanic acid.[32] The prevalence of resistance in 395 isolates from healthy dogs and cats from Canada was lower (19%).[33] In a prevalence study in the United Kingdom, 1.9% of dogs visiting veterinary clinics had *E. coli* that expressed extended-spectrum beta-lactamase (ESBL) genes in their feces, and recent antibiotic use and being fed raw poultry were identified as risk factors for carrying resistant *E.coli*.[34] ESBL enzyme production has also been identified in *E. coli* isolates from dogs and cats in the United States,[35] and a few isolates were found to express New Delhi metallo-beta-lactamase (NDM-1), which hydrolyses carbapenems.[36] Nosocomial infections with MDR *E. coli* have also been described in dogs and cats.

In humans, strains of UPEC that cause UTIs differ from those that cause diarrhea, and there is some evidence that this may also be true for strains that cause UTIs versus pyometra in dogs and cats.[37–39] These strains possess a number of virulence factors, such as siderophores, type 1 and P fimbriae, hemolysin, and cytotoxic necrotizing factor. Specific virulence factors, as well as biofilm-forming capacity, have been associated with persistent or relapsing UTIs,[40,41] and UPEC can invade and persist within bladder epithelial cells. In a recent study of 194 UPEC specimens obtained from clinical human UTI cases, the most commonly expressed virulence genes (expressed in 58%–68% of strains) were two genes that permit adhesion to bladder epithelium (*fim, iha*), a gene coding for a capsule which may allow the organism to evade the immune system (*kpsMT*), and a gene for a toxin which is associated with the development of pyelonephritis (*usp*).[42] In one study, canine *E. coli* UTIs were more likely to be recurrent than those associated with other uropathogens.[43] Another investigation revealed that recurrent *E. coli* UTIs are more likely to be increasingly resistant to antibiotics.[31] There has been concern that dogs may act as a source of *E. coli* strains that are pathogenic for humans.[39,44] In other extraintestinal *E. coli* infections, *E. coli* more closely resemble commensal strains, and host factors may be more important than bacterial virulence factors.[45]

Proteus

Proteus mirabilis is a common cause of upper and lower UTIs in dogs as well as otitis externa and uncommonly pyoderma. It produces a potent urease and can contribute to development of struvite urolithiasis. Uroliths harbor bacteria that can emerge as the uroliths dissolve. *Proteus* has a characteristic swarming motility and may obscure the growth of other co-infecting microorganisms when grown in the laboratory on agar. Recently, highly resistant *P. mirabilis* isolates sharing some homology with human isolates have been identified in canine patients in France.[46] *Proteus penneri*, an uncommon cause of nosocomial infections and bacteremia in humans, has rarely been isolated from wound infections in dogs seen at the editor's hospital.[47]

Klebsiella

The most common species of *Klebsiella* that infects dogs and cats is *K. pneumoniae. Klebsiella oxytoca* is a nosocomial pathogen in humans and has been reported in association with IV catheter colonization in puppies with parvoviral enteritis.[48] *Klebsiella oxytoca* has also been isolated from clinical veterinary specimens (either cultures from patients or pathology specimens) in both Italy ($n = 24$) and Japan ($n = 14$, 7 of which were from urine).[49,50]

Klebsiella pneumoniae primarily causes upper and lower UTIs in dogs and cats, but can also cause pneumonia, sometimes with abscessation (Figs. 53.3 and 53.4). It has been isolated from dogs with hepatic abscesses.[51] *Klebsiella pneumoniae* is an important cause of nosocomial infections and may be associated with bacteremia, endocarditis, and postoperative skin and soft tissue infections. The capsule of *K. pneumoniae* is a major virulence factor. It inhibits phagocytosis and is responsible for the mucoid appearance of the organism in culture (Fig. 53.5A).

All strains of *K. pneumoniae* are resistant to ampicillin because they possess a chromosomal gene that encodes a penicillin β-lactamase. Some isolates, such as nosocomial isolates or those from persistent UTIs, possess plasmids that contain resistance genes for multiple antimicrobial drugs. Of greatest concern are *Klebsiella* isolates that express ESBL enzymes, which hydrolyze third-generation cephalosporins. The

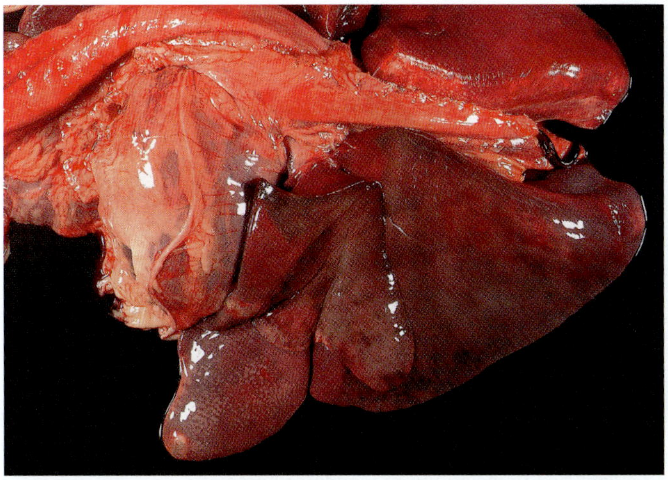

Fig. 53.3 Lungs of an 11-year-old intact male German shepherd dog with severe, acute, suppurative, necrotizing, and hemorrhagic bronchopneumonia due to *Klebsiella pneumoniae* infection. The lung lobes are severely congested. Five days before death, multiple laminectomies had been performed for intervertebral disc disease, and 2 days later the dog developed aspiration pneumonia that necessitated mechanical ventilation. Euthanasia was elected when there was further deterioration in the dog's condition, and bloody exudate was present in the endotracheal tube just before euthanasia.

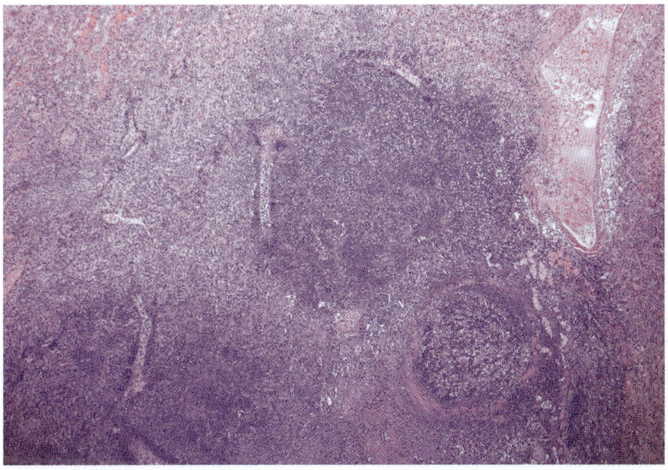

Fig. 53.4 Histopathology of the lung from a 4-month-old intact male Newfoundland dog with severe, multifocal, necrotizing lung abscesses. Intralesional rod-shaped bacteria were also present. *Klebsiella pneumoniae* was isolated from the lesions. Hematoxylin and eosin stain, 40× magnification.

genes that encode ESBLs are often located on plasmids that also contain genes for aminoglycoside resistance. Although MDR *K. pneumoniae* are not uncommonly isolated from dogs and cats, ESBL-producing *K. pneumoniae* isolates are rarely encountered but have recently been isolated from veterinary specimens in Switzerland.[52] Treatment options for MDR *K. pneumoniae* may be limited to aminoglycosides, carbapenems, and sometimes trimethoprim-sulfamethoxazole.

Serratia marcescens

Serratia marcescens is an important cause of nosocomial infections in both human and veterinary medicine. In human patients, infections with *S. marcescens* are often linked to IV drug use. The organism has a tremendous ability to survive in the environment and may contaminate and remain viable in disinfectant solutions.[53] It has been isolated from saline vials used in a multiple-dose fashion to dilute drugs in a veterinary hospital.[54] It sometimes grows as a contaminant, such as in blood cultures. Some, but not all, strains of *S. marcescens* produce a red pigment when grown in culture.[55]

In dogs, *S. marcescens* infection has been associated with UTIs, bacteremia and aortic valve endocarditis,[56] catheter-related infections in canine parvoviral enteritis,[43] and necrotizing fasciitis.[57] Contamination of blood products was linked to an outbreak of bacteremia in cats.[58] It has also caused severe necrosuppurative myositis in a young cat.[59] *Serratia* is resistant to ampicillin and first-generation cephalosporins as a result of a chromosomal β-lactamase. It may also acquire plasmid-mediated resistance to other antimicrobial drugs.

Enterobacter

Enterobacter cloacae and, to a lesser extent, *Enterobacter aerogenes* represent the majority of *Enterobacter* species isolated from clinical specimens from dogs and cats.[60] *Enterobacter* spp. are mainly isolated from dogs and cats with UTIs but occasionally cause wound or catheter-related infections and have been isolated from samples from the ear, skin, and eye.[60] They generally are intrinsically resistant to ampicillin and first-generation cephalosporins and may also be resistant to multiple other antimicrobial drug classes.

Citrobacter

Citrobacter species are named for their ability to use citrate as a sole carbon source. *Citrobacter freundii* is most commonly isolated from dogs and cats with UTIs but can also cause catheter-related infections, bacteremia, and endocarditis.[61,62] *Citrobacter koseri* was isolated from puppies with myocarditis.[63] Like *Enterobacter* and *Serratia, Citrobacter* are usually resistant to ampicillin and first-generation cephalosporins and may acquire a number of plasmid-mediated resistance genes, including those that encode ESBLs and resistance to fluoroquinolones.

Non-Enterobacterales

Pasteurella

Pasteurellaceae are small, fastidious, nonmotile bacilli or coccobacilli that are commensals of the oral cavities and upper respiratory tracts of dogs and especially cats. The most common species of *Pasteurella* associated with disease in dogs and especially cats is *P. multocida*. Other species include *Pasteurella canis, Pasteurella dagmatis,* and *Pasteurella stomatis. Pasteurella* spp. have been associated with a wide variety of disease manifestations that include pyothorax, upper respiratory tract infections (usually secondary to viral infections or chronic rhinosinusitis), bronchopneumonia, UTIs, ocular surface infections, wound infections, cutaneous abscesses, otitis externa, bacteremia, and, rarely, infective endocarditis. They may be found in mixed infections with other bacteria, such as *Streptococcus canis,* other gram-negative bacteria, or anaerobes. In humans, they are an important cause of animal bite wound infections.[4,64] *Pasteurella* spp. are usually broadly susceptible to antimicrobial drugs, and the treatment of choice is a penicillin such as penicillin G, ampicillin, or amoxicillin.

Pseudomonas aeruginosa

Pseudomonas aeruginosa is the main pathogenic species in the family Pseudomonadaceae. It is known for its ability to produce a variety of pigments when grown in culture, such as pyocyanin (blue), pyorubin (red), pyomelanin (black), and pyoverdin (yellow-green to yellow-brown and fluorescent), and for its characteristic "corn taco" or "grape"-like odor (Fig. 53.5B and C). *Pseudomonas aeruginosa* has one polar flagellum and is covered in thin, hair-like pili (Fig. 53.6). It can

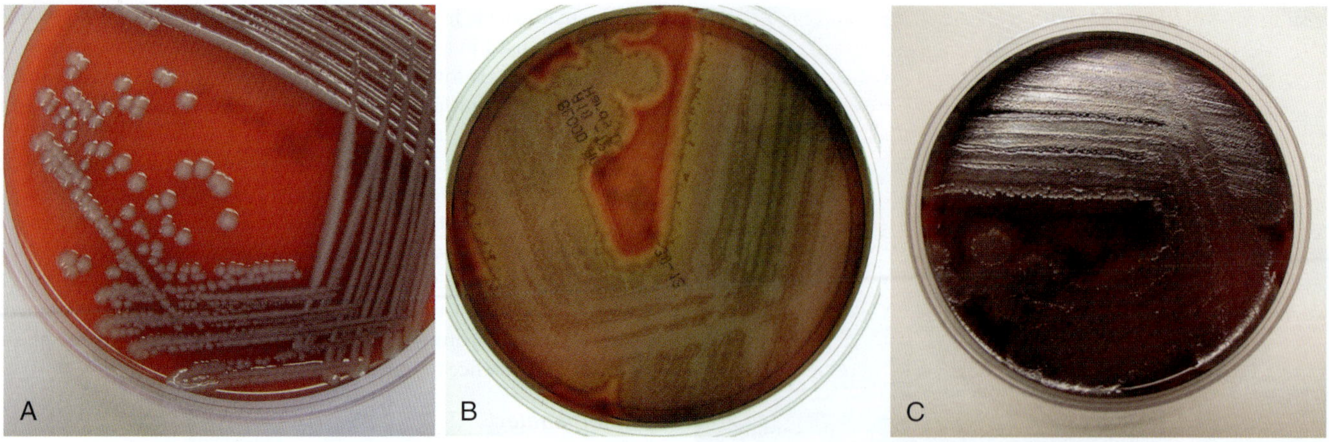

Fig. 53.5 Gram-negative aerobic bacteria growing on blood agar. (A) Mucoid colonies of *Klebsiella pneumoniae*. (B) *Pseudomonas aeruginosa*. Transillumination using a light box revealed the presence of hemolysis and production of a green pigment (pyoverdin). (C) The plate in (B) had a fruity odor and a "mother-of-pearl" appearance when not transilluminated.

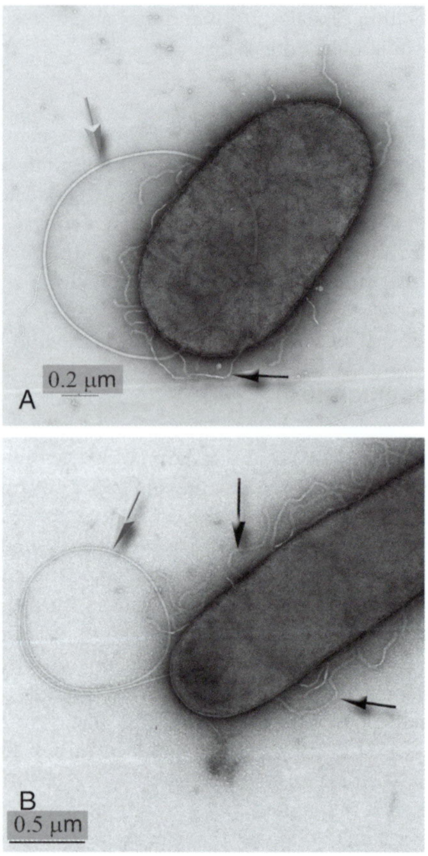

Fig. 53.6 Transmission electron micrograph image of Pseudomonas aeruginosa showing polar flagellum (gray arrows). (From Zaborina A, Holbrook C, Chen Y, et al. Structure-function aspects of PstS in multi-drug-resistant *Pseudomonas aeruginosa*. *PLoS Pathogens*. 2008;4:e43.)

also produce an extracellular polysaccharide known as *alginate,* which results in a mucoid colony appearance.

Pseudomonas aeruginosa is widespread in the environment and can grow in a huge variety of different conditions, reflecting its importance as a nosocomial pathogen. It is commonly found on plants, water, and soil. It can survive in disinfectants and grow in diesel and jet fuel. It is occasionally isolated from the skin, mucous membranes, and feces of healthy animals and humans. Almost any site of the body that is subject to injury can become colonized and subsequently infected. In humans, community-acquired infections can occur as a result of exposure to contaminated hot tubs, swimming pools, and contact lens solutions. In the hospital environment, *P. aeruginosa* often colonizes moist environments such as sinks, endotracheal tubes, and ventilator equipment. It also colonizes damp, macerated tissues such as the ear canals, damaged cornea, traumatized skin (such as wounds and burns), and the interdigital space. Because the organism can be resistant to a large number of different antimicrobial drugs, repeated treatment of secondary bacterial infections in sites where impaired host defenses exist with a variety of antimicrobials can select for MDR *P. aeruginosa* infection at these sites. Examples of such conditions in dogs and cats include recurrent aspiration pneumonia and/or bronchiectasis, cystitis, prostatitis, chronic feline rhinosinusitis, and otitis externa/media.

Pseudomonas aeruginosa possesses virtually every type of bacterial virulence factor, including exotoxins, a type III secretion system, LPS, pili, flagella, several proteases, phospholipases, iron-scavenging mechanisms such as pyoverdin production, and the ability to form extensive biofilms. Alginate protects the organism from phagocytosis, and the pigment pyocyanin produces reactive oxygen species, which in turn damage host cells. Multidrug resistance results from the production of specific β-lactamase enzymes (which can include ESBLs), antibiotic efflux pumps, enzymes that modify aminoglycosides or alter antibiotic-binding sites (such as DNA gyrase for fluoroquinolones), and decreased bacterial permeability.

Infections with broadly susceptible *P. aeruginosa* isolates could be treated with an antipseudomonal β-lactam (e.g., piperacillin, a carbapenem, cefepime, ceftazidime) alone or in combination with an aminoglycoside or a fluoroquinolone. As the MIC of most *P. aeruginosa* isolates is often closer to the breakpoint for fluoroquinolones than it is for other gram-negative organisms, it is wise to use the higher end of the dose range for fluoroquinolones with flexible dosing options.[65] The combination of an aminoglycoside and an antipseudomonal penicillin has synergistic activity against some *P. aeruginosa* infections. Currently, most MDR *P. aeruginosa* isolates from dogs and cats remain susceptible to carbapenems (such as meropenem) and aminoglycosides (especially amikacin), and so the usual treatment of choice is: (1) a combination of these two drugs, (2) removal of any foreign or necrotic material and, (3) if possible, resolution or management of any other underlying cause for impaired host defenses. Because parenterally administered aminoglycosides do not effectively penetrate airway mucus, nebulized tobramycin has been used to treat resistant *P. aeruginosa* infections of the airways in human patients, but these may not adequately penetrate consolidated lung tissue and the use of inhaled aminoglycosides is not recommended in the most recent guidelines for antimicrobial use in respiratory infections due to lack of evidence.[66] Effective treatment of MDR *P. aeruginosa* infections when they occur in locations such as the feline nasal cavity may be extremely difficult, if not impossible, because of irreversible turbinate loss, the requirement for injectable antimicrobial drugs, poor penetration of aminoglycosides to the site of infection, and an inadequate ability to effectively treat all surfaces of the nasal cavity with topical aminoglycosides.

Investigation of suspected nosocomial outbreaks of *P. aeruginosa* infection generally requires typing of isolates from affected animals and the environment with molecular methods such as pulsed-field gel electrophoresis or multilocus sequence typing. Use of antibiograms alone does not adequately discriminate between strains.

Acinetobacter

Like *P. aeruginosa*, *Acinetobacter* is an important nosocomial opportunistic pathogen. *Acinetobacter* is present in soil and water and can be found in frozen foods, pasteurized milk, and an enormous array of inert objects in the hospital environment, where it may persist for months. It colonizes the skin and mucous membranes of healthy humans as well as those of dogs and cats.[67,68] The main species that cause disease in animals are *A. baumannii* and, to a lesser extent, *Acinetobacter lwoffii* and *Acinetobacter calcoaceticus*. MDR isolates of *A. baumannii* have been responsible for outbreaks of nosocomial infections in veterinary hospitals[69,70] and, like MDR *P. aeruginosa*, may be resistant to a wide variety of antimicrobial drug classes. Carbapenem-resistant *A. baumannii* have been isolated from humans as well as animals.[70,71] Clinical manifestations of *Acinetobacter* infections in dogs and cats include nosocomial UTIs (e.g., after invasive urinary procedures such as catheterization), surgical wound infections, pneumonia, catheter-related bacteremia, and, rarely, endocarditis. Necrotizing fasciitis associated with *A. baumannii* infection was described in a cat.[72] When *Acinetobacter* is grown from a specimen, care should be taken to differentiate infection from contamination. Most veterinary isolates are susceptible to aminoglycosides and carbapenems; some are susceptible to trimethoprim-sulfamethoxazole and fluoroquinolones.[69]

DIAGNOSIS

Laboratory Abnormalities

Complete Blood Count, Biochemistry, and Urinalysis Findings

Dogs and cats with superficial gram-negative infections of sites that drain to the exterior, such as wounds, the external ear canal, the nasal cavity, and the lower urinary tract, often have no clinically significant laboratory abnormalities. Deep tissue or systemic infections with gram-negative bacteria may be associated with marked neutrophilia and a left shift, toxic neutrophils, or a degenerative left shift, sometimes with circulating metamyelocytes. Thrombocytopenia may be present in dogs and cats that develop disseminated intravascular coagulation (DIC). Anemia of inflammatory disease, lymphopenia, and monocytosis may be present. The urinalysis of dogs and cats with gram-negative bacterial UTIs may reveal pyuria, proteinuria, hematuria, and sometimes bacterial rods on sediment examination.

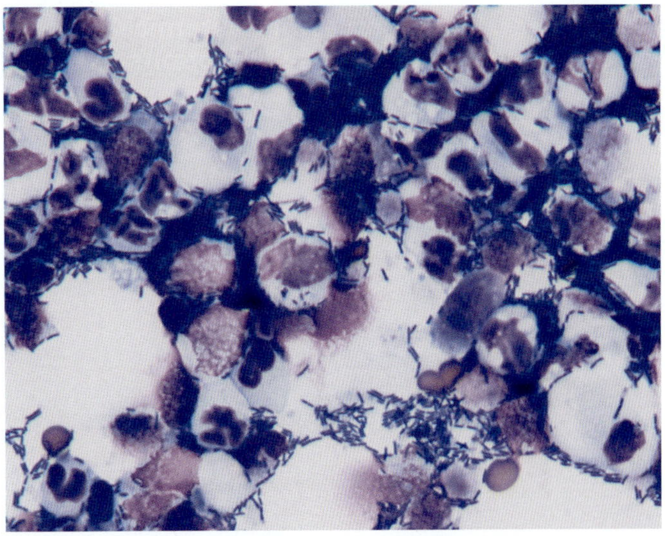

Fig. 53.7 Cytospin preparation of abdominal fluid from a dog with a traumatic bladder rupture and a concurrent *Escherichia coli* urinary tract infection. Note the numerous intracellular and extracellular blue-staining rod-shaped bacteria as well as numerous neutrophils and less abundant monocytes and macrophages. Diff-Quik stain, 1000x magnification. (Photo courtesy of Dr. Patricia Ewing, Angell Animal Medical Center.)

Clotting Function

Systemic gram-negative bacterial infections may be associated with evidence of DIC due to activation of the coagulation cascade by endotoxin. Elevations in PT, APTT, D-dimers, and reduced or falling platelet counts are common in DIC. Viscoelastic coagulometry (thromboelastography or thromboelastometry) in animals with sepsis often reveals a hypercoagulable state most noticeable in the maximum amplitude or maximum clot formation value, although in dogs with septic peritonitis (which commonly involves gram-negative infections), it was found that nonsurvivors were less likely to be hypercoagulable.[73]

Microbiologic Tests

Cytologic Diagnosis

The presence of rod-shaped bacteria on cytologic examination of Wright-Giemsa or Diff-Quik-stained smears of affected tissue aspirates, lavage fluid or purulent exudate suggests presence of a gram-negative organism in most cases of infection in the dog and cat, with Gram stain being confirmatory (Fig. 53.7). Large numbers of degenerate and/or nondegenerate neutrophils and lilac debris that suggests necrosis may be observed.

Isolation and Identification

Gram-negative bacteria are readily isolated from aspirates, tissue biopsies, body fluids, blood, and lavage specimens. MacConkey and blood agar are usually used to isolate gram-negative bacteria, which usually grow within 24 to 48 hours. *Pasteurella* spp. are more fastidious, and species that infect dogs and cats do not grow on MacConkey agar. Isolated organisms are traditionally then identified based on colony morphology and biochemical reactions. MALDI-TOF permits identification of rapid identification of organisms at the first sign of growth to the species level, and has the potential to rapidly identify genetic elements conferring resistance and thus informing antibiotic selection 24 to 48 hours before susceptibility results are available. Evaluation of antimicrobial susceptibility is important for all Enterobacterales, *P. aeruginosa*, and *Acinetobacter* spp., given their propensity to develop resistance to many antimicrobial drug classes.

TABLE 53.1 Examples of Systemic Antimicrobial Drugs That Could Be Selected for Treatment of Gram-Negative Bacterial Infections in Dogs and Cats

Infecting Species	Drug	Dose (mg/kg)	Interval (Hours)	Route
Pasteurella	Amoxicillin	20	8	PO
	Ampicillin	20	6–8	IV, IM, SC
	Penicillin G	20,000–40,000 U/kg	6–8	IV, IM
Susceptible Enterobacterales	Trimethoprim-sulfamethoxazole	30	12	PO, IV
	Amoxicillin–clavulanate potassium	20	8	PO
	Enrofloxacin	10–20	24	PO, IM, IV
MDR Enterobacterales, *Pseudomonas*, or *Acinetobacter*	Amikacin[a]	D: 15–30 C:10–14	24	IV, IM, SC
	Gentamicin[a]	D: 9–14 (dogs) C:5–8 (cats)	24	IV, IM, SC
	Piperacillin-tazobactam	50 Life-threatening infections: 4 mg/kg loading dose followed by 3.2 mg/kg/h IV	6 or constant rate infusion	IV
	Meropenem	12–25	88	SC, IV
	Ceftazidime	30	6	IV

[a]Use aminoglycosides in combination with an antipseudomonal β-lactam such as piperacillin, meropenem, or a third-generation cephalosporin.
C: cats; *D*: dogs; *IM*, intramuscular; *IV*, intravenous; *MDR*, multidrug resistant; *PO*, oral; *SC*, subcutaneous.

TREATMENT AND PROGNOSIS

The approach to treatment of gram-negative infections depends on patient history, the site of infection, and the severity of disease (Table 53.1). Identification and management of the underlying cause are also important to minimize selection for resistant organisms. Any foreign material (such as catheters or implants) must be removed, and necrotic tissue debrided. Biofilm-producing bacteria are more likely to be associated with deep tissue and bone infections, and higher doses and longer duration of therapy should be considered if biofilm is suspected.[74] When systemic antimicrobial drug treatment is required, it should preferably be based on the results of susceptibility testing. In cases of life-threatening infection, it is impractical to wait until such results return to commence therapy. Previous antibiotic therapy may select for resistant organisms and, given the ability of gram-negative organisms to rapidly acquire both multidrug resistance and virulence, a thorough consideration of the expectation of resistance is warranted prior to antibiotic selection. First, a thorough history which includes all antibiotics the patient has received in the last 6 months should be obtained, and inquiry into antibiotic use in co-habitating animals and humans is also reasonable. Avoidance of drugs of the same class as used previously is reasonable, especially in life-threatening infections. Second, consideration of whether the infection could be hospital acquired is indicated. A hospital-acquired infection should be considered if the patient shows signs of infection after admission to the hospital or within 2 to 3 days after discharge form the hospital. Additionally, if the region of infection was associated with a procedure or invasive device (i.e., signs of UTI after urinary catheterization), hospital-acquired organisms should be suspected. In such cases, treatment should also be based on knowledge of local resistance patterns among gram-negative bacteria, which may vary from region to region and practice to practice.

Pasteurella spp. are generally susceptible to penicillin or aminopenicillins such as amoxicillin. Because gram-negative bacteria have higher MICs to penicillins than do gram-positive bacteria, the high end of the dose range and more frequent administration may be necessary. In cases of severe infections, for time-dependent drugs of short half-life, a continuous infusion may be indicated at least for the first 2 to 3 days to allow drug concentrations to remain above the target MIC for 100% of the dosing interval. Some Enterobacterales are intrinsically resistant to ampicillin and first-generation cephalosporins, and initial treatment of serious infections while awaiting the results of susceptibility testing should include an aminoglycoside, a third-generation cephalosporin, or a fluoroquinolone. Trimethoprim-sulfamethoxazole, amoxicillin, or clavulanic acid–amoxicillin are reasonable initial choices for treatment of UTIs associated with bacterial rods.[75]

PREVENTION

Prevention of gram-negative infections involves resolution of impairment in host defenses and strict hospital infection control practices (see Chapter 15).

PUBLIC HEALTH ASPECTS

Strains of *E. coli* and other MDR gram-negative bacteria harbored by dogs resemble pathogenic strains isolated from humans.[44,71] As a result, concern has been raised that companion animals may be a source of organisms for human infection, especially those that reside with humans with compromised host defenses. It has been suggested through genomic sequencing of *phylogenetic group B2* infections in humans and companion animals that cats and dogs may be a spillover host for MDR *E. coli* (meaning pets are exposed to these strains by their owners but then the organism persists in the companion animal).[76,77]

Pasteurella multocida is the most commonly isolated organism from human dog and cat bite wounds.[4] *Pasteurella* spp. can also colonize the respiratory tracts of humans with underlying respiratory disease such as bronchiectasis or chronic sinusitis, and they occasionally have been reported in association with peritonitis, bacteremia, and endocarditis. Most of these humans have had contact with domestic animals in the household, and isolates from affected humans have been shown by molecular methods to be identical to those colonizing animals in the household.[78]

Thus, immunocompromised owners or those with impaired anatomic barriers should be instructed to wash their hands after handling their pet and perform regular household cleaning and disinfection. Companion animals should not be allowed to lick open wounds, the region that surrounds healing surgical incisions, or the owner's face.

CASE EXAMPLE

Signalment

"Lottie," a middle-aged, female spayed domestic shorthair from northern California.

History

Lottie was evaluated for chronic nasal discharge. Since her rescue as a stray 2.5 years earlier, intermittent sneezing and bilateral mucopurulent nasal discharge had been noted, and the discharge sometimes contained blood. Ten months before the evaluation, Lottie had been anesthetized for a nasal flush at a local veterinary clinic, but developed respiratory distress on recovery and was hospitalized with oxygen supplementation for 24 hours. She was ataxic, leaned to one side, and did not eat well for days, but over the subsequent months the ataxia and leaning gradually resolved. For the 2 weeks before the evaluation, Lottie had stertorous respiration and intermittent episodes of open-mouth breathing. For the past 9 months, Lottie had been treated with marbofloxacin and prednisolone. Before that, treatments for the nasal discharge included clavulanic acid–amoxicillin, doxycycline, or azithromycin, as well as L-lysine supplementation. Lottie lived with six other cats, all of which had access to the outdoors, and she was fed commercial canned and dry cat food. The FeLV and FIV status of these cats was unknown.

Current medications: marbofloxacin (5 mg/kg PO q24h) and prednisolone (1 mg/kg PO q24h).

Physical Examination

Body weight: 4 kg.

General: Bright, alert and responsive, hydrated. T = 100.3°F (37.9°C), HR = 220 beats/minute, purring, BCS 7/9.

Eyes, ears, nose, and throat: Mucopurulent nasal discharge was present that was most profuse on the left side. Nasal airflow was absent on the left side. Mild dental calculus was present, but there were no oral masses or ulceration.

Respiratory: An inspiratory stertor was present, and referred upper airway noises were detected on auscultation of the thorax.

Cardiovascular, GI and genitourinary, and lymph nodes: No clinically significant abnormalities were detected. It was difficult to palpate abdominal structures due to the presence of abdominal fat.

Neurologic examination: There was a mild, intermittent, left-sided head tilt. No other abnormalities were detected on full neurologic examination.

Laboratory Findings

CBC: HCT 39.1% (30–50%), MCV 44.7 fL (42–53 fL), MCHC 29.9 g/dL (30–33.5 g/dL), reticulocytes 111,400 cells/μL (7,000–60,000 cells/μL), WBCs 21,210 cells/μL (4,500–14,000 cells/μL), neutrophils 16,713 cells/μL (2,000–9,000 cells/μL), lymphocytes 4,115 cells/μL (1,000–7,000 cells/μL), monocytes 297 cells/μL (50–600 cells/μL), eosinophils 64 cells/μL (150–1,100 cells/μL), basophils 0 cells/μL (0–50 cells/μL), platelets 316,000/μL (180,000–500,000 platelets/μL).

Serum chemistry profile: Sodium 151 mmol/L (151–158 mmol/L), potassium 3.7 mmol/L (3.6–4.9 mmol/L), chloride 113 mmol/L (117–126 mmol/L), bicarbonate 19 mmol/L (15–21 mmol/L), phosphorus 5.8 mg/dL (3.2–6.3 mg/dL), calcium 10.2 mg/dL (9.0–10.9 mg/dL), BUN 49 mg/dL (18–33 mg/dL), creatinine 1.4 mg/dL (1.1–2.2 mg/dL), glucose 128 mg/dL (63–118 mg/dL), total protein 8.7 g/dL (6.6–8.4 g/dL), albumin 3.6 g/dL (2.2–4.6 g/dL), globulin 5.1 g/dL (2.8–5.4 g/dL), ALT 33 U/L (27–101 U/L), AST 21 U/L (17–58 U/L), ALP 36 U/L (14–71 U/L), GGT 0 U/L (0–4 U/L), cholesterol 192 mg/dL (89–258 mg/dL), total bilirubin 0.1 mg/dL (0–0.2 mg/dL).

Urinalysis: SpG 1.044, pH 6, 75 mg/dL protein, no glucose, bilirubin or ketones, 250 erythrocytes/μL hemoprotein, >100 RBC/HPF (traumatic cystocentesis), 0–1 WBC/HPF.

Imaging Findings

Thoracic radiographs: Cardiovascular structures were within normal limits. There was a small amount of air in the cervical esophagus (likely due to aerophagia) and a mild diffuse bronchointerstitial pattern that was attributed to an obese body condition.

Skull computed tomography scan: Contiguous transverse 0.6-mm collimated images of the skull were available for review without contrast administration. There was moderate turbinate destruction of both right and left nasal passages with lobular soft tissue attenuating material present along their length (Fig. 53.8A). There was stenosis of both frontal sinuses to the point where the left frontal sinus was completely occluded. The right frontal sinus was almost completely filled with soft tissue attenuating material. The ear canals were within

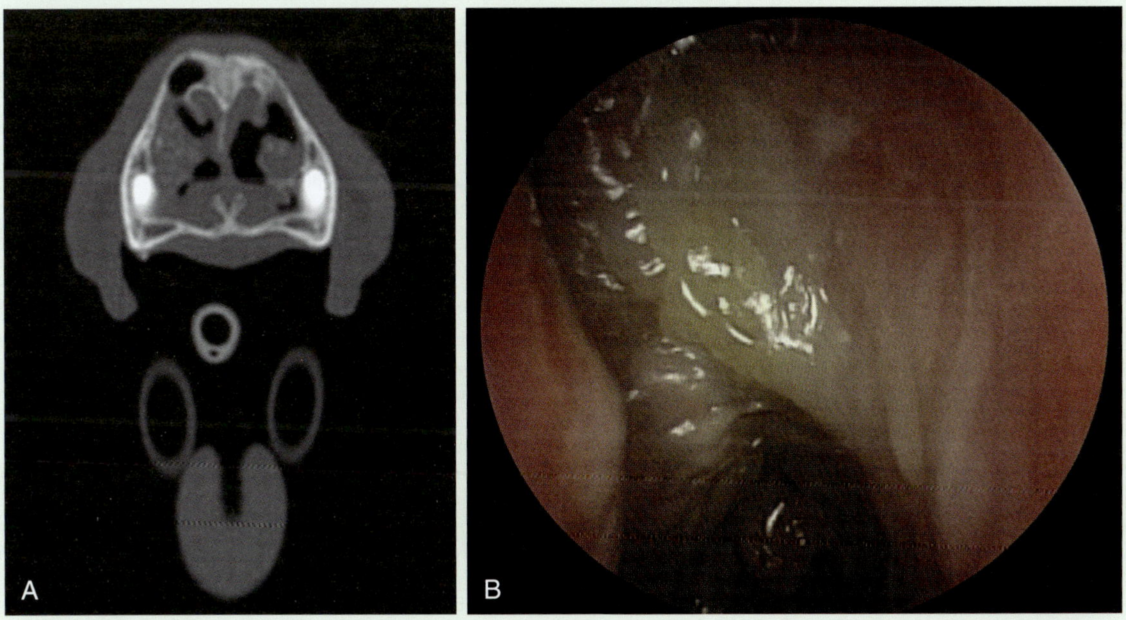

Fig. 53.8 Nasal cavity of a middle-aged, female spayed domestic shorthair with chronic rhinosinusitis and secondary infection with multidrug-resistant *Pseudomonas aeruginosa*. (A) Computed tomographic scan showing destruction of the turbinates of the left and right nasal passages. (B) Rhinoscopic findings included severe turbinate destruction, hyperemia, and accumulations of thick green mucus.

Continued

CASE EXAMPLE—cont'd

normal limits bilaterally. The mandibular lymph nodes were prominent but symmetrical.

Rhinoscopy: Severe turbinate destruction with diffuse hyperemia and large accumulations of inspissated green mucus was present throughout the nasal passages (Fig. 53.8B). Several biopsies of the right and left nasal cavities were obtained for histopathology.

Microbiologic Testing

Aerobic bacterial culture and *Mycoplasma* culture (nasal brush specimen): a direct smear showed moderate numbers of neutrophils, but no organisms were seen. Moderate numbers of *P. aeruginosa* were isolated. The *P. aeruginosa* was resistant to amoxicillin–clavulanic acid, ampicillin, cefazolin, cefovecin, cefoxitin, cefpodoxime, ceftiofur, chloramphenicol, doxycycline, enrofloxacin, marbofloxacin, ticarcillin, ticarcillin–clavulanic acid, and trimethoprim-sulfamethoxazole. It was susceptible only to amikacin (≤4 μg/mL), gentamicin (2 μg/mL), and imipenem (≤1 μg/mL).

Histopathology of Nasal Biopsy Specimens

The submucosa was markedly expanded and multifocally effaced by sheets of lymphocytes and plasma cells, with neutrophils and fewer numbers of mast cells surrounding irregular spicules of woven bone extending from primary turbinates. Less affected sections contained similar, predominately lymphoplasmacytic infiltrates that separated submucosal glands and elevated the superficial epithelium. Pathologic diagnosis: severe, chronic, and extensive lymphoplasmacytic and neutrophilic rhinitis with turbinate remodeling.

Diagnosis

Feline chronic rhinosinusitis with suspected opportunistic MDR *P. aeruginosa* infection.

Treatment and Outcome

The nasal cavity was lavaged. The prednisolone was tapered over 1 week, then discontinued, and 7 days later, treatment with piroxicam was commenced (0.3 mg/kg, PO, q24h for 7 days, then q48h thereafter). Other medications discussed with the owner were *N*-acetylcysteine and intranasal gentamicin drops, but the prognosis given for disease resolution was poor.

Comments

The underlying cause of feline chronic rhinosinusitis is poorly defined, but infection of kittens with respiratory viruses such as FHV-1 is suspected to play a role. Severe turbinate destruction predisposes to secondary opportunistic infections with a variety of bacteria, which include staphylococci, *Bordetella bronchiseptica, S. canis, Mycoplasma* spp., *E. coli, P. multocida,* and *P. aeruginosa.* In this cat, selection for MDR *P. aeruginosa* likely resulted from repeated and chronic use of a variety of antimicrobial drugs. The reticulocytosis and increased serum BUN concentration likely was secondary to chronic epistaxis and swallowed blood. The cat's neurologic signs and head tilt were thought to be due to peripheral vestibular disease, possibly due to otitis media, but there was no evidence of middle ear disease on the CT scan.

SUGGESTED READINGS

Gentilini F, Turba ME, Pasquali F, et al. Hospitalized pets as a source of carbapenem-resistance. *Front Microbiol.* 2018;9:2872.

Kukanich K, Lubbers B, Salgado B. Amoxicillin and amoxicillin-clavulanate resistance in urinary *Escherichia coli* antibiograms of cats and dogs from the midwestern United States. *J Vet Intern Med.* 2020;34:227–231.

Santaniello A, Sansone M, Fioretti A, Menna LF. Systematic review and meta-analysis of the occurrence of ESKAPE bacteria group in dogs, and the related zoonotic risk in animal-assisted therapy, and in animal-assisted activity in the health context. *Int J Environ Res Public Health.* 2020;17:3278.

REFERENCES

1. Gram C. Über die isolierte Färbung der Schizomyceten in Schnitt- und Trockenpräparaten. *Fortschr Med.* 1884;2:185–189.
2. Guh AY, Bulens SN, Mu Y, et al. Epidemiology of carbapenem resistant Enterobacteriaceae in 7 US communities, 2012-2013. *J Am Med Assoc.* 2015;314(14):1479.
3. Anes J, McCusker MP, Fanning S, et al. The ins and outs of RND efflux pumps in *Escherichia coli. Front Microbiol.* 2015;6:587.
4. Talan DA, Citron DM, Abrahamian FM, et al. Bacteriologic analysis of infected dog and cat bites. Emergency medicine animal bite infection study group. *N Engl J Med.* 1999;340:85–92.
5. Cantas H, Pekarkova M, Kippenes HS, et al. First reported isolation of *Neisseria canis* from a deep facial wound infection in a dog. *J Clin Microbiol.* 2011;49:2043–2046.
6. Kvist M, Hancock V, Klemm P. Inactivation of efflux pumps abolishes bacterial biofilm formation. *Appl Environ Microbiol.* 2008;74(23):7376–7382.
7. Wullt B, Svanborg C. Deliberate establishment of asymptomatic bacteriuria—a novel strategy to prevent recurrent UTI. *Pathogens.* 2016;5(3):52.
8. Beatson SA, Ben Zakour NL, Totsika M, et al. Molecular analysis of asymptomatic bacteriuria *Escherichia coli* strain vr50 reveals adaptation to the urinary tract by gene acquisition. *Infect Immun.* 2015;83(5):1749–1764.
9. Stahl J, Bergmann H, Göttig S, et al. *Acinetobacter baumannii* virulence is mediated by the concerted action of three phospholipases. *PloS One.* 2015;10(9). e0138360.
10. Holden VI, Bachman MA. Diverging roles of bacterial siderophores during infection. *Metallomics.* 2015;7(6):986–995.
11. Van Avondt K, van Sorge NM, Meyaard L. Bacterial immune evasion through manipulation of host inhibitory immune signaling. *PLoS Pathog.* 2015;11(3). e1004644.
12. Gaines JM, Carty NL, Tiburzi F, et al. Regulation of the *Pseudomonas aeruginosa* toxA, regA and ptxR genes by the iron-starvation sigma factor PvdS under reduced levels of oxygen. *Microbiology.* 2007;153(12):4219–4233.
13. Hola V, Peroutkova T, Ruzicka F. Virulence factors in *Proteus* bacteria from biofilm communities of catheter-associated urinary tract infections. *FEMS Immunol Med Microbiol.* 2012;65(2):343–349.
14. Schroeder M, Brooks B, Brooks A. The complex relationship between virulence and antibiotic resistance. *Genes.* 2017;8(1):39.
15. Morato EP, Leomil L, Beutin L, et al. Domestic cats constitute a natural reservoir of human enteropathogenic *Escherichia coli* types. *Zoonoses Public Health.* 2009;56(5):229–237.
16. Domingos MO, Melo KCM, Neves IV, et al. Potential for colonization of O111:H25 atypical enteropathogenic *E. coli. J Microbiol.* 2016;54(11):745–752.
17. Turk J, Maddox C, Fales W, et al. Examination for heat-labile, heat-stable, and Shiga-like toxins and for the eaeA gene in *Escherichia coli* isolates obtained from dogs dying with diarrhea:122 cases (1992–1996). *J Am Vet Med Assoc.* 1998;212:1735–1736.
18. Kjaergaard AB, Carr AP, Gaunt MC. Enteropathogenic *Escherichia coli* (EPEC) infection in association with acute gastroenteritis in 7 dogs from Saskatchewan. *Can Vet J.* 2016;57(9):964–968.
19. Croxen MA, Law RJ, Scholz R, et al. Recent advances in understanding enteric pathogenic *Escherichia coli. Clin Microbiol Rev.* 2013;26(4):822–880.
20. Drolet R, Fairbrother JM, Harel J, Hélie P. Attaching and effacing and enterotoxigenic *Escherichia coli* associated with enteric colibacillosis in the dog. *Can J Vet Res.* 1994;58(2):87–92.
21. Beutin L. *Escherichia coli* as a pathogen in dogs and cats. *Vet Res.* 1999;30(2):285–298.
22. Darfeuille-Michaud A, Boudeau J, Bulois P, et al. High prevalence of adherent-invasive *Escherichia coli* associated with ileal mucosa in Crohn's disease. *Gastroenterology.* 2004;127(2):412–421.
23. Dunne KA, Allam A, McIntosh A, et al. Increased S-nitrosylation and proteasomal degradation of caspase-3 during infection contribute to the

persistence of adherent invasive *Escherichia coli* (AIEC) in immune cells. *PloS One*. 2013;8(7):e68386.
24. Manchester AC, Hill S, Sabatino B, et al. Association between granulomatous colitis in French bulldogs and invasive *Escherichia coli* and response to fluoroquinolone antimicrobials. *J Vet Intern Med*. 2013;27(1):56–61.
25. Simpson KW, Dogan B, Rishniw M, et al. Adherent and invasive *Escherichia coli* is associated with granulomatous colitis in boxer dogs. *Infect Immun*. 2006;74(8):4778–4792.
26. Alvarez Dorta D, Sivignon A, Chalopin T, et al. The antiadhesive strategy in Crohn's disease: orally active mannosides to decolonize pathogenic *Escherichia coli* from the gut. *Chembiochem*. 2016;17(10):936–952.
27. Pekárková M, Lang J, Howard J. Infectious endocarditis caused by gas-producing *Escherichia coli* in a diabetic dog. *J Small Anim Pract*. 2008;49:44–46.
28. Worth AJ, Marshall N, Thompson KG. Necrotising fasciitis associated with *Escherichia coli* in a dog. *N Z Vet J*. 2005;53:257–260.
29. Buriko Y, Van Winkle TJ, Drobatz KJ, et al. Severe soft tissue infections in dogs: 47 cases (1996-2006). *J Vet Emerg Crit Care*. 2008;18(6):608–618.
30. Shaheen BW, Boothe DM, Oyarzabal OA, et al. Antimicrobial resistance profiles and clonal relatedness of canine and feline *Escherichia coli* pathogens expressing multidrug resistance in the United States. *J Vet Intern Med*. 2010;24:323–330.
31. Cummings KJ, Aprea VA, Altier C. Antimicrobial resistance trends among canine *Escherichia coli* isolates obtained from clinical samples in the northeastern USA, 2004–2011. *Can Vet J*. 2015;56(4):393–398.
32. Morrissey I, Moyaert H, de Jong A, et al. Antimicrobial susceptibility monitoring of bacterial pathogens isolated from respiratory tract infections in dogs and cats across Europe: ComPath results. *Vet Microbiol*. 2016;191:44–51.
33. Leonard EK, Pearl DL, Finley RL, et al. Comparison of antimicrobial resistance patterns of *Salmonella* spp. and *Escherichia coli* recovered from pet dogs from volunteer households in Ontario (2005-06). *J Antimicrob Chemother*. 2012;67:174–181.
34. Wedley AL, Dawson S, Maddox TW, et al. Carriage of antimicrobial resistant *Escherichia coli* in dogs: prevalence, associated risk factors and molecular characteristics. *Vet Microbiol*. 2017;199:23–30.
35. Shaheen BW, Nayak R, Foley SL, et al. Molecular characterization of resistance to extended-spectrum cephalosporins in clinical *Escherichia coli* isolates from companion animals in the United States. *Antimicrob Agents Chemother*. 2011;55:5666–5675.
36. Shaheen BW, Nayak R, Boothe DM. Emergence of a New Delhi metallo-β-lactamase (NDM-1)-encoding gene in clinical *Escherichia coli* isolates recovered from companion animals in the United States. *Antimicrob Agents Chemother*. 2013;57:2902–2903.
37. Chen YM, Wright PJ, Lee CS, et al. Uropathogenic virulence factors in isolates of *Escherichia coli* from clinical cases of canine pyometra and feces of healthy bitches. *Vet Microbiol*. 2003;94:57–69.
38. Freitag T, Squires RA, Schmid J, et al. Feline uropathogenic *Escherichia coli* from Great Britain and New Zealand have dissimilar virulence factor genotypes. *Vet Microbiol*. 2005;106:79–86.
39. Siqueira AK, Ribeiro MG, Leite Dda S, et al. Virulence factors in *Escherichia coli* strains isolated from urinary tract infection and pyometra cases and from feces of healthy dogs. *Res Vet Sci*. 2009;86:206–210.
40. Ejrnaes K, Stegger M, Reisner A, et al. Characteristics of *Escherichia coli* causing persistence or relapse of urinary tract infections: phylogenetic groups, virulence factors and biofilm formation. *Virulence*. 2011;2:528–537.
41. Soto SM, Smithson A, Horcajada JP, et al. Implication of biofilm formation in the persistence of urinary tract infection caused by uropathogenic *Escherichia coli*. *Clin Microbiol Infect*. 2006;12:1034–1036.
42. Paniagua-Contreras GL, Hernández-Jaimes T, et al. Comprehensive expression analysis of pathogenicity genes in uropathogenic *Escherichia coli* strains. *Microb Pathog*. 2017;103:1–7.
43. Ball KR, Rubin JE, Chirino-Trejo M, et al. Antimicrobial resistance and prevalence of canine uropathogens at the Western College of veterinary medicine veterinary teaching hospital, 2002-2007. *Can Vet J*. 2008;49:985–990.
44. Harada K, Okada E, Shimizu T, et al. Antimicrobial resistance, virulence profiles, and phylogenetic groups of fecal *Escherichia coli* isolates: a comparative analysis between dogs and their owners in Japan. *Comp Immunol Microbiol Infect Dis*. 2012;35:139–144.
45. Lara FBM, Nery DR, de Oliveira PM, et al. Virulence markers and phylogenetic analysis of *Escherichia coli* strains with hybrid EAEC/UPEC genotypes recovered from sporadic cases of extraintestinal infections. *Front Microbiol*. 2017. Available from: http://journal.frontiersin.org/article/10.3389/fmicb.2017.00146/full.
46. Schultz E, Haenni M, Mereghetti L, et al. Survey of multidrug resistance integrative mobilizable elements SGI1 and PGI1 in *Proteus mirabilis* in humans and dogs in France, 2010–13. *J Antimicrob Chemother*. 2015;70(9):2543–2546.
47. Nicolosi D, Nicolosi VM, Cappellani A, et al. Antibiotic susceptibility profiles of uncommon bacterial species causing severe infections in Italy. *J Chemother*. 2009;21(3):253–260.
48. Lobetti RG, Joubert KE, Picard J, et al. Bacterial colonization of intravenous catheters in young dogs suspected to have parvoviral enteritis. *J Am Vet Med Assoc*. 2002;220:1321–1324.
49. Donati V, Feltrin F, Hendriksen RS, et al. Extended-spectrum-beta-lactamases, ampC beta-lactamases and plasmid mediated quinolone resistance in *Klebsiella* spp. from companion animals in Italy. *PloS One*. 2014;9(3):e90564.
50. Harada K, Shimizu T, Mukai Y, et al. Phenotypic and molecular characterization of antimicrobial resistance in *Klebsiella* spp. isolates from companion animals in Japan: clonal dissemination of multidrug-resistant extended-spectrum β-lactamase-producing *Klebsiella pneumoniae*. *Front Microbiol*. 2016;7:1021.
51. Farrar ET, Washabau RJ, Saunders HM. Hepatic abscesses in dogs: 14 cases (1982-1994). *J Am Vet Med Assoc*. 1996;208:243–247.
52. Wohlwend N, Endimiani A, Francey T, Perreten V. Third-generation-cephalosporin-resistant *Klebsiella pneumoniae* isolates from humans and companion animals in Switzerland: spread of a dha-producing sequence type 11 clone in a veterinary setting. *Antimicrob Agents Chemother*. 2015;59(5):2949–2955.
53. Fox JG, Beaucage CM, Folta CA, et al. Nosocomial transmission of *Serratia marcescens* in a veterinary hospital due to contamination by benzalkonium chloride. *J Clin Microbiol*. 1981;14:157–160.
54. Sabino CV, Weese JS. Contamination of multiple-dose vials in a veterinary hospital. *Can Vet J*. 2006;47(8):779–782.
55. Mahlen SD. Serratia infections: from military experiments to current practice. *Clin Microbiol Rev*. 2011;24:755–791.
56. Perez C, Fujii Y, Fauls M, et al. Fatal aortic endocarditis associated with community-acquired *Serratia marcescens* infection in a dog. *J Am Anim Hosp Assoc*. 2011;47:133–137.
57. Plavec T, Zdovc I, Juntes P, et al. Necrotizing fasciitis caused by *Serratia marcescens* after tooth extraction in a Doberman pinscher: a case report. *Vet Med*. 2008;53:629–635.
58. Hohenhaus AE, Drusin LM, Garvey MS. *Serratia marcescens* contamination of feline whole blood in a hospital blood bank. *J Am Vet Med Assoc*. 1997;210:794–798.
59. Kelly EJ, Baldwin TJ, Chamberlain AP. Pathology in practice. *J Am Vet Med Assoc*. 2015;247(8):897–899.
60. Harada K, Shimizu T, Mukai Y, et al. Phenotypic and molecular characterization of antimicrobial resistance in *Enterobacter* spp. isolates from companion animals in Japan. *PloS One*. 2017;12(3):e0174178.
61. Galarneau JR, Fortin M, Lapointe JM, et al. *Citrobacter freundii* septicemia in two dogs. *J Vet Diagn Invest*. 2003;15:297–299.
62. Sykes JE, Kittleson MD, Pesavento PA, et al. Evaluation of the relationship between causative organisms and clinical characteristics of infective endocarditis in dogs: 71 cases (1992-2005). *J Am Vet Med Assoc*. 2006;228:1723–1734.
63. Cassidy JP, Callanan JJ, McCarthy G, et al. Myocarditis in sibling boxer puppies associated with *Citrobacter koseri* infection. *Vet Pathol*. 2002;39:393–395.
64. Philip WL, Page AV. Non-native joint infection after a dog lick: a case report describing a complicated two-stage revision and a comprehensive review of the literature. *Can J Infect Dis Med Microbiol*. 2015;26(4):212–217.

65. Boothe DM, Boeckh A, Simpson RB, Dubose K. Comparison of pharmacodynamic and pharmacokinetic indices of efficacy for 5 fluoroquinolones toward pathogens of dogs and cats. *J Vet Intern Med*. 2006;20:1297–1306.
66. Lappin MR, Blondeau J, Boothe D, et al. Antimicrobial use guidelines for treatment of respiratory tract disease in dogs and cats: Antimicrobial Guidelines Working Group of the International Society for Companion Animal Infectious Diseases. *J Vet Intern Med*. 2017;31:279–294.
67. Saphir DA, Carter GR. Gingival flora of the dog with special reference to bacteria associated with bites. *J Clin Microbiol*. 1976;3:344–349.
68. Krogh HV, Kristensen S. A study of skin diseases in dogs and cats. II. Microflora of the normal skin of dogs and cats. *Nord Vet Med*. 1976;28:459–463.
69. Zordan S, Prenger-Berninghoff E, Weiss R, et al. Multidrug-resistant *Acinetobacter baumannii* in veterinary clinics. Germany. *Emerg Infect Dis*. 2011;17:1751–1754.
70. Francey T, Gaschen F, Nicolet J, et al. The role of *Acinetobacter baumannii* as a nosocomial pathogen for dogs and cats in an intensive care unit. *J Vet Intern Med*. 2000;14:177–183.
71. Endimiani A, Hujer KM, Hujer AM, et al. *Acinetobacter baumannii* isolates from pets and horses in Switzerland: molecular characterization and clinical data. *J Antimicrob Chemother*. 2011;66:2248–2254.
72. Brachelente C, Wiener D, Malik Y, et al. A case of necrotizing fasciitis with septic shock in a cat caused by *Acinetobacter baumannii*. *Vet Dermatol*. 2007;18:432–438.
73. Bentley AM, Mayhew PD, Culp WTN, Otto CM. Alterations in the hemostatic profiles of dogs with naturally occurring septic peritonitis. *J Vet Emerg Crit Care*. 2013;23:14–22.
74. Sánchez CJ, Mende K, Beckius ML, et al. Biofilm formation by clinical isolates and the implications in chronic infections. *BMC Infect Dis*. 2013;13(1):47.
75. Weese JS, Blondeau JM, Boothe D, et al. Antimicrobial use guidelines for treatment of urinary tract disease in dogs and cats: Antimicrobial Guidelines Working Group of the International Society for Companion Animal Infectious Diseases. *Vet Med Int*. 2011;2011:263768.
76. Kidsley A, White RT, Beatson SA, et al. Companion animals are spillover hosts of the multidrug-resistant human extraintestinal *Escherichia coli* pandemic clones ST131 and ST1193. *Front Microbiol*. 2020;11:1968.
77. Kidsley A, O'Dea M, Saputra S, et al. Genomic analysis of phylogenetic group B2 extraintestinal pathogenic *E. coli* causing infection in dogs in Australia. *Vet Microbiol*. 2020;248:108783.
78. Sugino Y, Kato M, Yagi A, et al. *Pasteurella multocida* pneumonia with molecular evidence of zoonotic transmission. *Kansenshogaku Zasshi*. 2007;81:726–730.

54

Anaerobic Bacterial Infections

Dubraska Diaz-Campos, Jenessa A. Winston, Jane E. Sykes

KEY POINTS

- First Described: 1860s (Louis Pasteur).[1]
- Causes: *Bacteroides, Prevotella, Porphyromonas, Peptostreptococcus, Fusobacterium, Clostridium, Actinomyces, Propionibacterium*, other species.
- Geographic Distribution: Worldwide.
- Major Clinical Signs: Abscess formation in a variety of tissues, pyothorax, peritonitis, pyometra, periodontal disease, osteomyelitis, bacteremia.
- Differential Diagnoses: Bacterial infections caused by gram-positive and gram-negative aerobes.
- Human Health Significance: Anaerobes of the oral cavity of dogs and cats are an important component of animal bite wound infections in humans.

ETIOLOGIC AGENTS AND EPIDEMIOLOGY

Anaerobic infections are of great importance in human and veterinary medicine. Although anaerobic bacteria were discovered in the middle of the nineteenth century, the identification and isolation of these microorganisms were, and still are, a challenge. Obligate anaerobes are defined as microorganisms that require a reduced oxygen tension for growth and fail to form colonies on the surface of solid media in 10% CO_2, in air (18% oxygen).[2] They cannot grow in the presence of molecular oxygen because anaerobes do not make superoxide dismutase, and most do not produce catalase. These enzymes are necessary for the breakdown of reactive oxygen intermediates (e.g., superoxide anion, hydrogen peroxide) that are normally generated when bacteria grow in the presence of oxygen.[3] Species of obligate anaerobic bacteria and their morphology on Gram-stained smears are described in Table 54.1.

Normal host microbiota is responsible for a significant portion of innate immunity; however, some of these microorganisms also have the potential to become important opportunistic pathogens.[4,5] Anaerobes exist in the environment and make up a significant portion of the normal microbiota of dogs and cats.[6–9] The predominant microorganisms that colonize most mucosal surfaces are anaerobes, and metabolic by-products produced by this group are important in the regulation of the numbers of aerobic species (facultative and obligate) that also make up the normal microbiota. Thus, anaerobic bacteria play an important role in protection of mucosal surfaces from interactions involving other microorganisms with pathogenic potential.[7] For example, approximately 1 million salmonellae are needed to produce disease in animals with intact anaerobic gut microbiota, whereas fewer than 10 salmonellae are needed to produce disease in animals with few anaerobes. The importance of this observation is seen clinically; dogs are more susceptible to salmonellosis when they are medicated with antimicrobials, especially those effective in reducing the anaerobic component of the normal gut microbiota (e.g., ampicillin).[10]

Compromise of a mucosal surface or an adjacent area by perforation or other trauma may provide a portal of entry for the normal anaerobic microbiota into a normally sterile site. At this point, anaerobes and other members of the normal microbiota become opportunistic pathogens. These are important considerations because, to effectively prevent anaerobic infection, antibacterial therapy is commonly started before results of microbiologic analysis of collected clinical specimens are received. Knowledge of the normal microbiota at a specific site helps in making an educated guess about the microorganisms likely to be causing the infection. If anaerobic bacteria are involved in an infectious process, on average, two different species are almost always present with aerobic bacteria. The most commonly associated aerobic bacteria are enterics (mainly *Escherichia coli*), and members of the genus *Pasteurella, Staphylococcus* spp. and *Enterococcus* spp.[11]

If anaerobic bacteria possess appropriate virulence factors, they may also cause mucosal disease. In addition to periodontal disease, anaerobes are associated with disease in other regions of the GI tract; the most important of these anaerobes within the intestine are *Clostridioides difficile* (previously *Clostridium difficile)* and *Clostridium perfringens* (see Chapter 64).[12,13] Both of these species may be a part of the normal gut microbiota of dogs and cats, although evidence suggests that both may be passed to previously uncolonized animals.[14–16]

In human patients, infectious processes involving structures above the diaphragm are more likely to contain anaerobes originating in the mouth, whereas disease below the diaphragm usually involves anaerobes from the intestinal tract.[17] In dogs and cats, anaerobic bacteria are indigenous in different body sites. *Actinomyces* spp., *Porphyromonas* spp., and *Fusobacterium* spp. are the most prevalent genera of anaerobic bacteria in the oral microbiota of dogs.[6,9] In humans and in animals, bite wounds are frequently associated with polymicrobial infections with a component of anaerobic bacteria.[6,18]

The GI tract is loaded with a myriad of microorganisms, including anaerobic bacteria. Members of the order Clostridiales such as *C. perfringens* and *C. difficile* are also considered normal gut microbiota in dogs and cats. *Bacteroides* spp. and *Fusobacterium* spp. among other anaerobes are also found in the GI tract.[6,15,16,19–21]

Disease produced by *C. difficile* is the result of its proliferation in the enteric tract of the host after a trigger event (e.g., certain antimicrobial and chemotherapeutic agents). Epidemiologic evidence from human hospitals suggests that the agent can be spread from patient to patient, which results in outbreaks of *C. difficile*–associated disease.[22] Such observations imply that the organism either is, or has the

TABLE 54.1 Obligate Anaerobic Bacteria Most Commonly Isolated from Dogs and Cats, Source, and Gram-Stain Morphology

Microorganism	Source	Morphology
Gram-negative bacilli		
Bacteroides spp.	Important component of gut, genital tract, and other mucosal microbiota of mammals. Primarily cause abdominal infections, but also infections in different body sites	Pale rod
Porphyromonas spp.	In dogs and cats, part of the normal oral microbiota. Associated with periodontal disease and other conditions	Pale rod (coccobacillus)
Prevotella spp.	Indigenous microbiota in mucosa and gastrointestinal tract; associated with a variety of suppurative conditions	Pale rod (pairs or short chains)
Fusobacterium spp.	Normal oral and gut microbiota in mammals. In dogs and cats, *Fusobacterium* spp. have been associated with infections in body sites such as the bone, liver, gallbladder, among others	Negative (pale) Rod, usually thin
Gram-positive, non–spore-forming bacilli		
Actinomyces spp.	Colonize the oral cavity and gastrointestinal tract. After a break in the mucocutaneous barrier, infections occur in the oral cavity (abscesses) and other organs. *Actinomyces* spp. are frequently associated with bite wound infections	Positive Rod
Cutibacterium acnes (*Propionibacterium acnes*)	Skin and mucosal commensal. This is not considered an important pathogen and it is a contaminant in cultures	Positive Rod
Gram-positive cocci		
Peptostreptococcus spp.	Gastrointestinal tract, upper respiratory tract, urogenital tract, and skin of mammals. *Peptostreptococcus* have been linked to infections in multiple body sites.	Positive Cocci
Gram-positive, spore-forming bacilli		
Clostridium and *Clostridioides* spp.	Only species of this genus form endospores anaerobically. *Clostridium perfringens* produces enterotoxins, producing diarrhea or enterotoxaemia. Some strains are histotoxic and cause tissue infections (e.g., gas gangrene). *Clostridioides difficile* has been related to diarrhea in dogs and cats. Both microbes are considered normal inhabitants of the gastrointestinal tract in mammals. Other clostridiales are etiologic agents of infections in different body sites.	Positive Rod (spores)

potential to be, contagious. Determining whether *C. difficile* is truly a contagious pathogen is difficult because it is so prevalent in the enteric tract of clinically healthy animals.[12,15,16] There is evidence that the canine claw bed and nasal cavity can be colonized by toxigenic *C. difficile*; thus, they could disseminate this microorganism or its spores between households and environment and potentially contribute to community-relevant sources for *C. difficile* infection in humans.[15,23–25]

Although *C. perfringens* is commonly associated with GI infections, it has also been implicated in other clinical conditions in dogs and cats.[26,27] It is unclear whether toxigenic *C. perfringens* is contagious. It likely causes disease when it proliferates in the intestinal tract and produces enterotoxin. Novel pore-forming toxin genes (*netE* and *netF*) were identified in a *C. perfringens* type A strain associated with acute hemorrhagic diarrhea in dogs and foals.[28–30] Factors that stimulate proliferation of *C. perfringens* are unknown. It must also be determined whether the source of the agent is endogenous, acquired from another infected animal, or acquired from the environment. The report of outbreaks of *C. perfringens*–associated diarrhea in small animal hospital settings suggests that it may be contagious, although it is important to remember that some *C. perfringens* are present in the enteric tract of clinically healthy dogs.[13,31,32] Detectable levels of *C. perfringens* enterotoxin are not often found in the feces of clinically healthy animals.[33]

Bacteroides spp. represent an important component of the microbiome in dogs and cats.[34] In particular, *Bacteroides fragilis* frequently cause anaerobic infections in dogs and cats, often associated with the GI tract and abdominal fluid, body organs (lung, liver, kidney), abscesses, and subcutaneous tissues.[26,27,34] The genus *Fusobacterium* is also an important component of the oral mucosal and GI normal microbiota.[34,35] *Fusobacterium canifelium* is common in the oral cavity of dogs and cats and has been isolated from dog and cat bite wounds in humans.[36] Unfortunately, this organism is typically resistant to quinolones, unlike human isolates. Data compiled from 4,333 anaerobic cultures submitted to 10 institutions showed that *Clostridium*, *Bacteroides*, and *Peptostreptococcus* spp. were the three most frequently isolated species of obligate anaerobes from dogs and cats (Table 54.2).

Pathogenesis

Most commonly, obligate anaerobic bacteria cannot live in healthy tissue. On certain mucosal surfaces (e.g., intestinal tract, gingival crevices, genital tract), they live with other microorganisms (facultative anaerobes) that scavenge molecular oxygen, which generates a local environment with very low redox potential (E_h, a measure of oxygen tension). Likewise, in compromised tissue, inflammatory cells and co-inoculated aerobic microorganisms lower E_h sufficiently for anaerobes to grow. Factors that predispose to anaerobic infections are shown in Box 54.1.

Components of anaerobic bacteria elicit potent inflammatory responses. Gram-negative anaerobes possess LPS with endotoxic activity. The peptidoglycan of gram-positive anaerobes incites the same inflammatory response as gram-positive aerobic microorganisms. Some anaerobic bacteria have capsular antigens (e.g., *B. fragilis*, pigmented *Prevotella* spp., and *Porphyromonas* spp.), which incite inflammatory responses that result in abscess formation; capsules without viable bacteria can also induce abscess formation.[17,19,37] Some evidence

TABLE 54.2 Bacterial Species Isolated in Anaerobic Cultures from Dogs and Cats

Organism	Number of Positive Anaerobic Cultures[a,b] (%)
Clostridium spp.	1,332 (21.4)
Bacteroides spp.	1,202 (19.3)
Peptostreptococcus spp.	517 (8.3)
Fusobacterium spp.	501 (8.1)
Propionibacterium spp.	219 (3.5)
Prevotella spp.	217 (3.5)
Actinomyces spp.	178 (2.9)
Porphyromonas spp.	155 (2.5)
Unidentified anaerobic organisms	97 (1.6)
Miscellaneous anaerobic bacteria species[c]	957 (15.3)
Aerobic bacteria	846 (13.6)

[a]Total anaerobic culture performed: 4,333.
[b]Total isolates obtained: 6,221.
[c]Species accounting for < 1% of total cultures.
Data compiled from 10 veterinary institutions (CityU Hong Kong, Cornell University, Kansas State University, Missouri Veterinary Diagnostic Laboratory, The Ohio State University, University of Illinois, University of Nebraska Veterinary Diagnostic Laboratory, University of Guelph, Virginia Maryland College of Veterinary Medicine, Washington State University), 2009–2019.

BOX 54.1 Factors That Contribute to Development of Anaerobic Infections

Causes of Physiologic Injury
Immunosuppression
Cytotoxic chemotherapy
Glucocorticoid therapy
Malignancies
Neutropenia
Hypogammaglobulinemia
Narrow-spectrum aerobic antibacterial therapy
Diabetes mellitus

Altered Tissue Oxygenation
Vascular compromise
Hypotension
Tissue anoxia
Gastrointestinal obstruction

Tissue Trauma
Tissue Contamination
Gastrointestinal or urogenital perforation
Bite or puncture wounds of soft tissue
Foreign body migration

suggests that co-inoculated aerobic microorganisms induce anaerobe capsule formation. Capsules also play a more traditional role by inhibiting phagocytosis.[38]

Aerobic and anaerobic microorganisms have a synergistic relationship.[38,39] Anaerobes act with facultative aerobes such as *E. coli* to induce abscess formation more rapidly than either bacterial group alone. *Actinomyces*, a facultative anaerobe, is commonly found in association with foreign body migrations, pyothorax, or peritonitis.[40,41] Facultative bacteria lower the oxidation-reduction potential of the tissue environment, facilitating anaerobic bacterial proliferation. Necrotic and abscessed tissue protect facultative organisms and anaerobic bacteria from antimicrobials, as well as body defenses such as phagocytosis. Aerobic organisms also scavenge oxygen and curtail phagocytosis of anaerobes (and vice versa).[42] Enzymes such as β-lactamase produced by one member of the aerobic-anaerobic partnership protect susceptible microorganisms in the vicinity from being inactivated by β-lactam antibacterials. These synergistic interactions are important to keep in mind when designing therapeutic regimens, because antibacterial therapy should be directed at both populations for optimal resolution of the infection.

Some anaerobes produce toxins. *Fusobacterium necrophorum* produces a toxin that forms pores in leukocyte membranes.[43] *Clostridioides difficile* produces toxins (A and B) that disrupt the cytoskeletal elements of the intestinal epithelial cell, resulting in cell death.[15,22,31] *Clostridium perfringens* produces an enterotoxin that interacts with the target cell membrane, resulting in the formation of pores that are made partly by the enterotoxin and partly by the target cell. Electrolytes are lost through these pores, resulting in reversal of ion and water flow (diarrhea) and, finally, death of the cell.[32,33] A pore-forming toxin within the leukocidin/hemolysin superfamily family, NetF, has been associated with canine hemorrhagic gastroenteritis and foal necrotizing enteritis (see Chapters 64 and 125).[28] Other studies have also suggested that *C. perfringens* strains that possess *netE* and *netF* genes may play a role in dogs with acute hemorrhagic disease syndrome.[29,30]

Some species of anaerobes produce adhesins (pili or fimbriae), which have been associated with virulence.[44] However, adhesins probably do not play a major role in pathogenesis other than by way of their association with specific locations on mucosal surfaces. For example, blood or abscess isolates of *B. fragilis* are rarely piliated, whereas those found on mucosal surfaces almost always have pili.[38]

CLINICAL FEATURES

Anaerobic bacteria stimulate pyonecrotic inflammation in a variety of organs. This process stems primarily from the inflammatory response triggered by anaerobic capsule material, cell wall constituents of microorganisms, and thwarted attempts at phagocytosis (which leads to deposition of lysosomal contents into surrounding tissue). The prevalence of anaerobic bacterial infections varies depending on the anatomic site of infection. Most anaerobic bacteria cultured from dogs and cats are associated with GI tract disorders, followed by pleural or abdominal fluids, abscesses, or respiratory tract infections (Table 54.3).[45]

Clinical findings in anaerobic infections also depend on the affected body site (Table 54.4). Exudates from infectious processes that contain anaerobes often are malodorous and may be darkly discolored. Fever, leukocytosis, hypoglycemia, increased serum ALP activity, and hypoalbuminemia reflect the systemic manifestations of an acute-phase reaction to the anaerobic infection. Hypoalbuminemia may be compounded by loss of serum proteins into effusions or from draining wounds.[41]

Anaerobes of the oral cavity are important contributors to periodontal disease; tooth root abscessation and mandibular osteomyelitis; retrobulbar abscesses; and bite wound infections. Along with other bacteria, anaerobes may be isolated from the lungs and pleural cavity of dogs or cats with aspiration pneumonia and pyothorax, respectively. Intestinal anaerobes may be isolated from the abdominal cavity of animals with septic peritonitis that has resulted from intestinal or cecal rupture. The female genital tract is also heavily colonized with anaerobic bacteria, and pyometra may sometimes be associated with mixed

TABLE 54.3 Relative Frequency of Isolation of Obligate Anaerobic Bacteria with Respect to Disease Process or Site in Dogs and Cats

Specimen Source	Number of Positive Cultures[a] (%)	Number of Positive Cultures by Species[b,c] (%)
Miscellaneous	924 (21.3)	Dog: 780 (22.4) Cat: 144 (17.1)
Gastrointestinal tract	495 (11.4)	Dog: 395 (11.3) Cat: 100 (11.8)
Fluid	471 (10.9)	Dog: 341 (9.8) Cat: 130 (15.4)
Pleural	143 (3.3)	
Abdominal	137 (3.2)	
Unknown	105 (2.4)	
Other	86 (2.0)	
Abscess	372 (8.6)	Dog: 296 (8.5) Cat: 76 (9.0)
Respiratory tract	346 (8.0)	Dog: 253 (7.3) Cat: 93 (11.0)
Urinary tract	312 (7.2)	Dog: 231 (6.6) Cat: 81 (9.6)
Otic	275 (6.3)	Dog: 218 (6.2) Cat: 57 (6.7)
Wound	268 (6.2)	Dog: 222 (6.4) Cat: 46 (5.5)
Hepatobiliary tract	185 (4.3)	Dog: 142 (4.1) Cat: 43 (5.1)
Integument	148 (3.4)	Dog: 131 (3.8) Cat: 17 (2.0)
Ophthalmic	99 (2.3)	Dog: 86 (2.5) Cat: 13 (1.5)
Reproductive tract	83 (1.9)	Dog: 79 (2.3) Cat: 4 (0.5)
Musculoskeletal	81 (1.9)	Dog: 74 (2.1) Cat: 7 (0.8)
Surgical	81 (1.9)	Dog: 75 (2.1) Cat: 6 (0.7)
Oral cavity	59 (1.4)	Dog: 45 (1.3) Cat: 14 (1.7)
Draining tract	41 (0.9)	Dog: 40 (1.1) Cat: 1 (0.1)
Lymph nodes/spleen	35 (0.8)	Dog: 31 (0.9) Cat: 4 (0.5)
Neurologic	30 (0.7)	Dog: 24 (0.7) Cat: 6 (0.7)
Cardiovascular	13 (0.3)	Dog: 12 (0.3) Cat: 1 (0.1)
Subcutaneous masses	12 (0.3)	Dog: 11 (0.3) Cat: 1 (0.1)
Blood cultures	3 (0.07)	Dog: 3 (0.1) Cat: 0

[a]Total anaerobic cultures performed: 4,333.
[b]Total canine anaerobic cultures performed: 3,489.
[c]Total feline anaerobic cultures performed: 844.
Data compiled from 10 veterinary institutions (CityU Hong Kong, Cornell University, Kansas State University, Missouri Veterinary Diagnostic Laboratory, The Ohio State University, University of Illinois, University of Nebraska Veterinary Diagnostic Laboratory, University of Guelph, Virginia Maryland College of Veterinary Medicine, Washington State University), 2009–2019.

aerobic and anaerobic infections that include the anaerobic species *Bacteroides*, *Prevotella*, *Fusobacterium*, and *Peptostreptococcus*.

Plant awn migration in dogs and cats may lead to abscess formation in a variety of tissues, including retroperitoneal tissues and the brain. These abscesses usually contain a mixed population of aerobes and anaerobes, especially *Fusobacterium*, *Actinomyces*, and *Bacteroides* spp. Brain abscessation can follow direct extension of anaerobic bacterial infection from otitis, or tooth root infection. Alternatively, spread may occur via the hematogenous route (Fig. 54.1).

Periodontal Disease

Periodontal disease is one of the most common disorders seen in veterinary medicine and may result in chronic pain, decreased appetite, and loss of teeth. Periodontal disease begins with formation of dental plaque, a bacterial biofilm comprised primarily of gram-positive facultative aerobes, which occurs as a result of poor oral hygiene and other host factors. Subsequently there is proliferation of pathogenic bacteria, which include gram-negative rods and especially anaerobes, which secrete toxins and incite an inflammatory response. Anaerobes implicated in canine and feline periodontal disease (such as *Porphyromonas gulae*) appear to differ than those isolated from human periodontal disease (*Porphyromonas gingivalis*).[46–49] Periodontal disease is manifested as gingival erythema, edema, gingival bleeding, and halitosis, with accumulation of calculus, gingival recession, alveolar bone loss, and sometimes the presence of purulent exudate (Fig. 54.2).

Retrobulbar Abscesses

Retrobulbar or orbital abscesses may result from tooth root abscessation, penetrating foreign bodies such as grass awns, or penetrating trauma to the orbit. They are characterized by unilateral exophthalmos, protrusion of the third eyelid, conjunctival hyperemia, serous to mucopurulent ocular discharge, inappetence, fever, and pain on opening the mouth (Fig. 54.3). A fluctuant swelling or draining tract posterior to the last ipsilateral molar may be present on examination of the oral cavity. In one study, *Bacteroides* spp. and *Clostridium* spp. were the most frequent anaerobes isolated from 34 dogs with retrobulbar abscesses; other frequently isolated bacteria were *Staphylococcus*, *E. coli*, and *Pasteurella* spp. In cats, the most frequent anaerobe was *Bacteroides vulgatus*, and the most common non-anaerobe was *Pasteurella* spp.[50]

Skin and Soft Tissue Infections

Cat bite abscesses may be one of the most common reasons that cats are brought to veterinary clinics. Clinical signs include fever, lethargy, inappetence, pain, and firm or fluctuant subcutaneous swellings, which may rupture and drain purulent material. In addition to *Pasteurella multocida*, oral anaerobes are frequently isolated from these abscesses.[51] Anaerobic species involved include *Peptostreptococcus anaerobius*, *Porphyromonas* spp., *Clostridium* spp. (e.g., *Clostridium villosum*), *Fusobacterium* spp., *Bacteroides* spp. (especially *Bacteroides tectum*), and *Prevotella* spp.[52]

Other skin and soft tissue infections associated with a variety of anaerobes include foreign body penetrating wounds and dog bite wounds (see Chapter 75). Necrotizing fasciitis has generally been associated with toxigenic microaerophilic gram-positive bacterial infections in dogs and cats (Chapter 50), although gram-negative organisms may also be involved. Necrosis and spread of infection can be associated with co-infecting anaerobic bacteria that contaminate the site of infection. In some cases, anaerobic bacteria are isolated as the predominant organisms.[53]

TABLE 54.4 Comparative Clinical Features of Anaerobic Infections

Site	Clinical Features	Sources
Integument	Fever, firm subcutaneous swellings, fluctuance or gas pockets, ulceration with discharge	Puncture or bite wounds, hematogenous[84,85]
Head and Neck	Cranial or cervical abscesses: subauricular swelling, anorexia, odynophagia, gingivitis and stomatitis, para-aural abscesses, tonsillar abscesses, inner ear infections Meningoencephalitis, brain abscess: hyperesthesia, neurologic deficits, ataxia Orbital: exophthalmos, pain when opening mouth, ocular discharge, conjunctival hyperemia, panophthalmitis[50,93]	Traumatic ear canal separations,[86] pharyngeal foreign body penetration (stick injuries),[87,88] dental infections,[46,89] chronic sinusitis,[90] tonsillar or salivary gland abscesses, chronic otitis media,[91] bite wounds, meningitis[92]
	Corneal ulcers: miosis, lacrimation, photophobia, corneal opacity[93,94]	Preexisting corneal damage from ocular trauma or surgery, often mixed with aerobes
Intrathoracic		
Pulmonary	Cough, fever, dyspnea, lobar or multifocal consolidation (abscesses), hypertrophic osteopathy	Pneumonia, endocarditis,[95] aspiration pneumonia[45,96]
Intrapleural or mediastinal	Fever, dyspnea, muffled heart sounds, leukocytosis, pyothorax[41]	Penetrating chest injuries, inhaled foreign bodies, esophageal foreign body perforation[97–99]
Intra-Abdominal		
Peritoneal	Fever, abdominal distention, anorexia, intra-abdominal abscesses, adhesions[100]	Postoperative foreign suture materials (e.g., silk, multifilament nylon, braided material), ovariohysterectomy, migrating foreign bodies, bowel leakage, genital tract infections, actinomycosis
Hepatobiliary	Anorexia, lethargy, vomiting, diarrhea, fever, dehydration, hepatomegaly, icterus, mucosal bleeding	Bacteremia, hepatic trauma, necrosis or neoplasia, ascending biliary infection[20,21,101]
Enteric	Diarrhea, which may be hemorrhagic	Intestinal stasis, blind loop syndrome, colitis, colonic ulceration
Retroperitoneal	Swelling in lumbar flank, sinus tracts or drainage, pain, fever, anorexia, reluctance to walk	Osteomyelitis of lumbar vertebrae from plant awns, ovarian or uterine ligatures,[102] actinomycosis, ruptured urethra and perirenal abscess[103]
Paraspinal	Pain, reluctance to walk, fever, paraspinal hyperesthesia, paresis or paralysis	Usually epidural from local penetration or extension of paraspinal or nasopharyngeal infection, bite wounds. Meningitis: less likely anaerobic and often from hematogenous sources[104]
Musculoskeletal	Osteomyelitis, fever, lameness, limb swelling with variable fluctuance or gas pockets[105]	Bite or puncture wounds, compound fractures, hematogenous sources[106]
Urogenital		
Renal	Pyelonephritis[107]	Ascending bacterial infection from the distal urogenital tract
Genital	Pyometra[108]	

Pneumonia and Pyothorax

Anaerobic bacteria such as *Fusobacterium* spp., *Peptostreptococcus anaerobium, Prevotella* spp., and *Porphyromonas* spp. can be isolated from dogs and cats with aspiration pneumonia, foreign body pneumonia (especially that due to plant awn migration), and pyothorax.[54] Dogs with plant awn migration develop multifocal necrotizing pneumonia with abscess formation. Anaerobic bacterial pneumonia can also result from aspiration of anaerobes within the oral cavity. This usually occurs in animals with underlying esophageal or laryngeal defects, neurologic disorders, altered consciousness, or dysphagia. In some cases, aspiration pneumonia may be followed by lung abscess formation (Fig. 54.4). In human patients, a period of 6 to 7 days after aspiration is required for necrosis and abscess formation to occur, and so aspiration pneumonia with lung abscess formation is generally a chronic disease process.

Clinical signs of pulmonary infections include fever, lethargy, inappetence, cough, and tachypnea. The reader is referred to Chapter 124 for more detailed descriptions of bacterial pneumonia and pyothorax.

Peritonitis

Septic peritonitis that involves anaerobes may result from rupture of the intestinal tract, especially the cecum or colon. Anaerobes such as *Bacteroides* spp. and *Clostridium* spp. may be more likely to be isolated from these infections. Other anaerobes that may be present in dogs and cats with septic peritonitis include *Fusobacterium* spp. and *Propionibacterium* spp.[55] Disease that results from bowel perforation often contains a population of organisms that reflect the bowel microbiota at the site of perforation, which may include anaerobes, aerobic gram-positive bacteria (such as *Enterococcus* spp.), *Candida* spp., and gram-negative aerobes such as *E. coli.* Rupture of the female genital tract secondary to pyometra may also be associated with peritonitis that involves anaerobes.

Bacteremia

Anaerobic bacteremia in dogs and cats can be associated with seemingly localized anaerobic infections, such as peritonitis or pyothorax, although it is not often recognized.[56,57] When anaerobes are

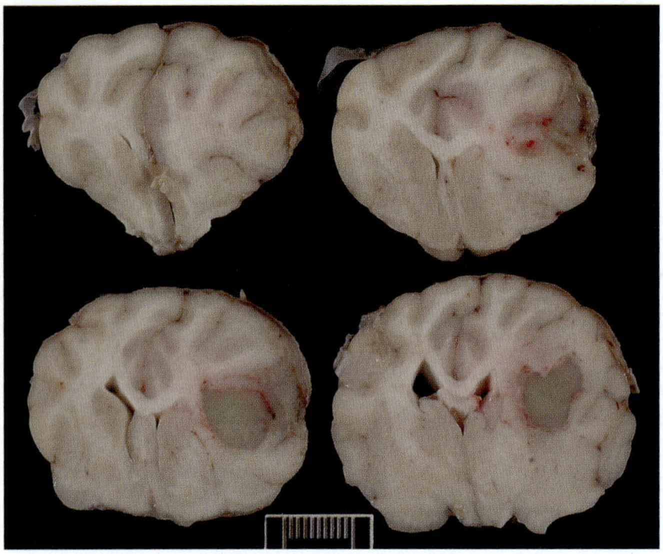

Fig. 54.1 Abscess in the white matter of the right frontal lobe of a 2-year-old female spayed Chihuahua that had a 1-month history of difficulty chewing food and lethargy and a 3-week history of progressive obtundation, neck pain, and tetraparesis. Signs initially improved following treatment with prednisone, but then recurred as the prednisone dose was reduced. The abscess in the frontal lobe communicated with the overlying meninges, which were expanded by a chronic and fibrosing suppurative inflammatory infiltrate. Another abscess was present in the midbrain, which suggested hematogenous spread of infection. Although no bacteria were seen within the lesions with special stains, *Actinomyces canis* and *Fusobacterium nucleatum* were cultured from the lesions. (Image courtesy of the University of California, Davis Veterinary Anatomic Pathology Service.)

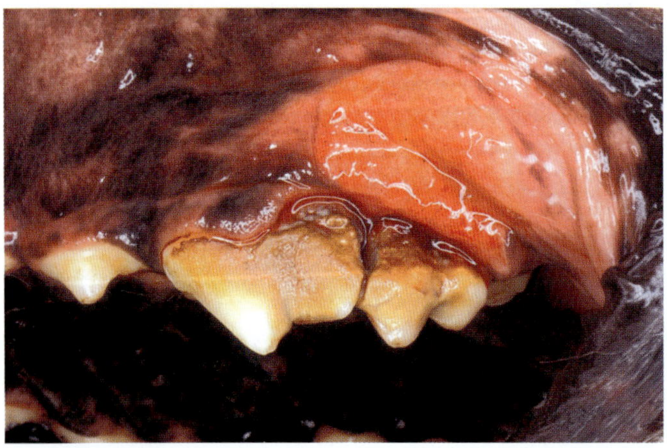

Fig. 54.2 Periodontitis in a dog. There is significant gingival inflammation, plaque and calculus accumulation, and purulent exudate. Gingival recession and contact ulceration of the buccal mucosa are also present. (Courtesy Frank J.M. Verstraete, UC Davis Dentistry and Oral Surgery Service.)

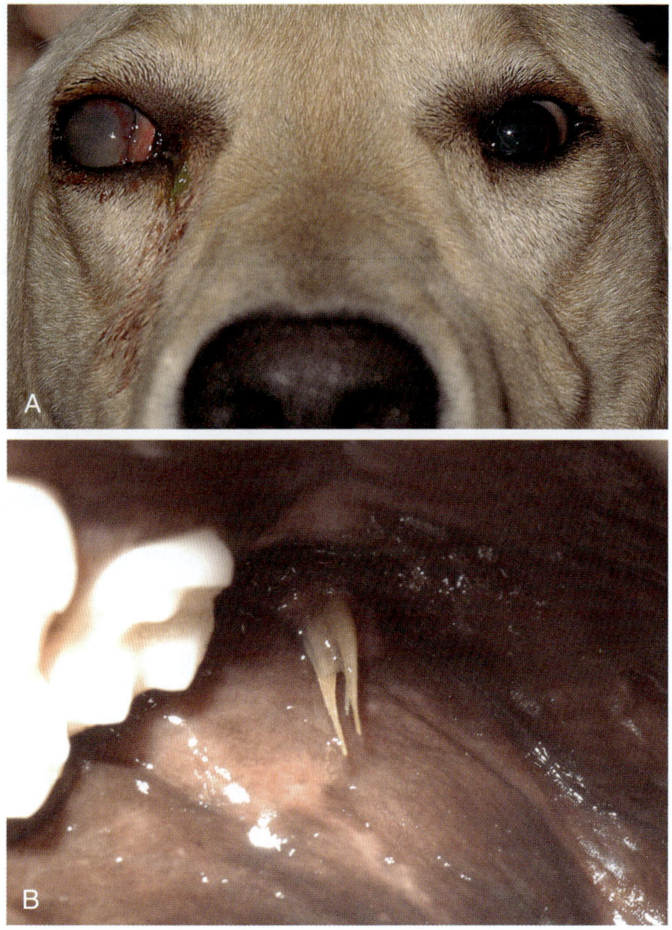

Fig. 54.3 Retrobulbar abscess and endophthalmitis secondary to a migrating grass awn foreign body in a 10-month-old intact male Labrador retriever. (A) Note the mucopurulent ocular discharge from the right eye, as well as buphthalmos (enlargement of the eye) and exophthalmos. The nictating membrane and conjunctiva are hyperemic and there is diffuse corneal edema. Hypopyon and iris bombe were also present. Globe retropulsion was reduced and painful on the right side. (B) Multiple grass awns were present all over the dog's hair coat and an awn (shown) was removed from the gingiva posterior to the last right maxillary molar tooth. The right eye was subsequently enucleated. No additional grass awns were found. Histopathology of the globe showed severe chronic fibrinosuppurative panophthalmitis with focal, 0.3 cm scleral rupture in the caudal sclera near the optic nerve, regional orbital granulation tissue, and rupture of the lens. (Images courtesy of the University of California, Davis Veterinary Ophthalmology Service.)

occasionally isolated from dogs and cats with bloodstream infections, they are usually polymicrobial infections together with aerobic bacteria. In a European study of 66 bacteremic cats, 12% of bacterial isolates from the bloodstream were obligate anaerobes.[56] In a study of 140 dogs with bacteremia, anaerobes comprised 9% of the isolates.[57] Of 39 dogs and 10 cats with critical illness and bacteremia from Colorado, anaerobes were isolated from 31% of the dogs and 40% (4 of 10) of the cats. The most common anaerobic bacterial species isolated from the dogs was *C. perfringens* (nine dogs), followed by *Bacteroides* species (two dogs).[58] The cats were infected with *Bacteroides* or *Fusobacterium* species. The possibility of bacteremia due to a mixed population of aerobic and anaerobic bacteria should be considered in dogs with systemic grass awn migration. Anaerobic bacteria appear to be a very rare cause of endocarditis in dogs (see Chapter 122).[59]

DIAGNOSIS

Abnormalities that suggest an anaerobic bacterial infection include a putrid odor, discolored purulent discharge, gas production within tissues (especially with *C. perfringens* infections) (Fig. 54.5), a bite or puncture wound, penetrating foreign bodies, abscessation, pyothorax, aspiration pneumonia, damage to mucosal surfaces with which anaerobes are usually associated, and/or necrotic or gangrenous tissue

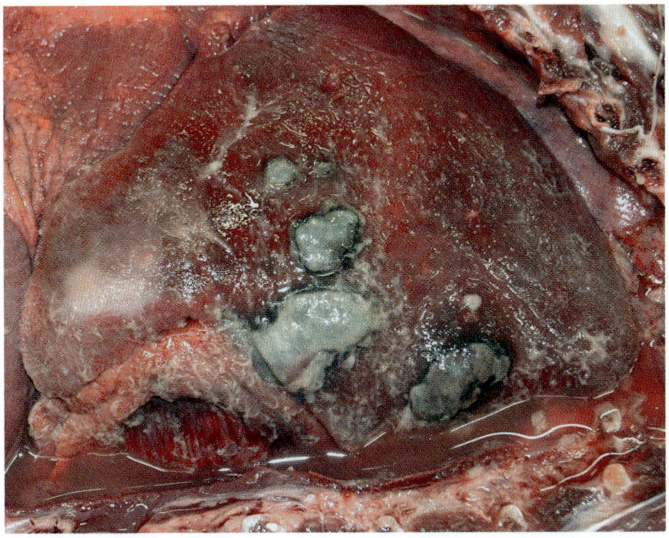

Fig. 54.4 Necropsy findings in an 11-year-old male neutered Labrador retriever with severe aspiration pneumonia secondary to laryngeal tie-back surgery for laryngeal paralysis, which occurred 2 months before death. Aspiration led to bronchopneumonia with multifocal abscessation, pleural rupture, pyothorax, and pneumothorax. There are multiple to coalescing black to dark gray, soft, irregular, foci that measured up to 4.5 cm in diameter at the level of the cardiac notch and caudal aspect of the right cranial lung lobe. On cut surface, dark gray to black material oozed from the parenchyma. Aerobic bacterial culture yielded large numbers of organisms that included *Streptococcus canis*, nonfermenter group 3 organisms, and *Pasteurella canis*. Anaerobic culture yielded large numbers of *Peptostreptococcus anaerobius*. (Image courtesy of the University of California, Davis Anatomic Pathology Service.)

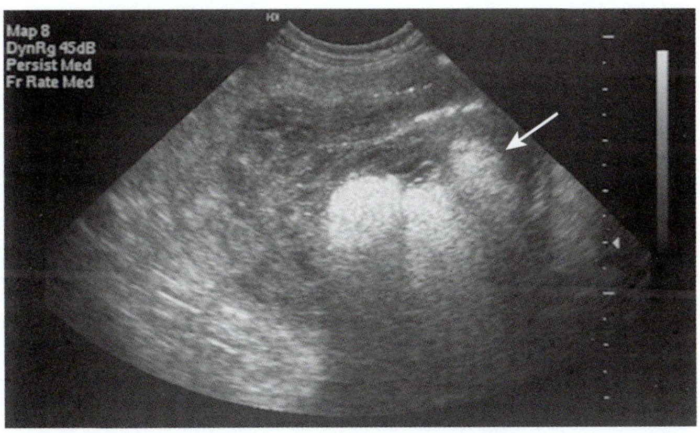

Fig. 54.5 Splenic abscess in an 11-year-old male neutered Labrador mix that also had duodenal lymphoma. Ultrasound image of a large splenic mass that contains numerous hyperechoic foci, consistent with the presence of gas. Necropsy showed severe, focally extensive, neutrophilic, and necrotizing splenitis. The duodenum was perforated at the site of the neoplasm. *Escherichia coli*, *Bacteroides tectus*, and a *Prevotella heparinolyticus*-like organism were cultured from the splenic abscess.

(Box 54.2). However, absence of these features does not rule out infection with anaerobes, and some of these abnormalities can occur in association with isolated aerobic bacterial infections. For example, although anaerobes such as *Clostridium* spp. may be involved in emphysematous cystitis in humans and dogs, the most common cause of emphysematous cystitis are gram-negative aerobes, especially *E. coli*.

BOX 54.2 Clinical Findings That Suggest Anaerobic Infection

Fever, pain, and swelling
Bite or puncture wound
Foul-smelling wounds or discharges
Unexpected gas in tissues or body cavities
Abscess formation
Contiguous infection to mucosal surface with anaerobic microflora
Necrotizing fasciitis (co-infection)
Necrotic or devitalized tissue
Gangrenous tissue
Dark, discolored exudates
Presence of sulfur granules in exudates
Mixed population of organisms or filamentous forms shown by microscopy
Failure to culture organisms with routine methods

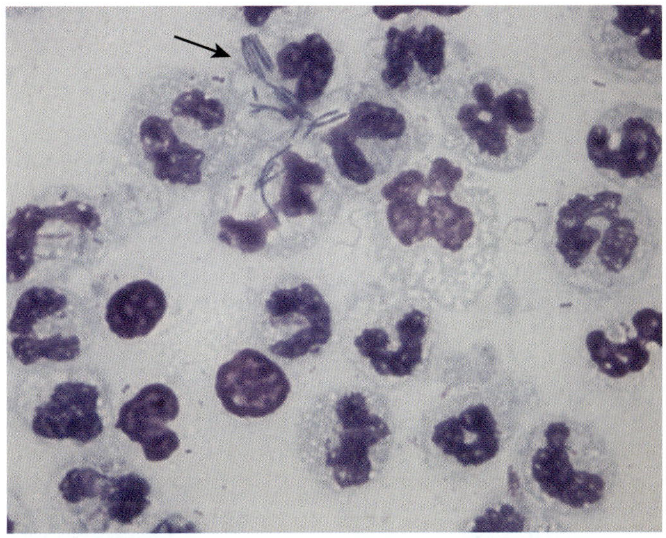

Fig. 54.6 Cytology of pleural fluid collected using thoracocentesis from an 8-year-old female spayed domestic shorthair cat with pyothorax that shows the presence of a mixed population of bacteria that includes filamentous organisms suggestive of anaerobes. Aerobic and anaerobic bacterial culture yielded a mixed growth of *Prevotella* spp., *Peptostreptococcus anaerobius*, *Fusobacterium* spp. and an unidentified anaerobic gram-positive rod *(arrow)*.

Laboratory Abnormalities

Complete Blood Count, Biochemistry, and Urinalysis Findings

No specific CBC, biochemistry, or urinalysis findings suggest anaerobic infection. Infections may be associated with leukocytosis due to a neutrophilia with a left shift and toxic neutrophils.

Microbiologic Tests

Cytologic Diagnosis

In addition to clinical features, cytologic analysis of specimens can help to determine whether an anaerobic infection is present. Abundant degenerative neutrophils are usually found with multiple and often morphologically diverse forms of intracellular and extracellular bacteria. Large and filamentous morphology is often typical of anaerobes (Fig. 54.6).[60,61] Some gram-negative anaerobic rods are pale-staining and they are often thin, can be sometimes misshapen, and occasionally have pointed ends.

Extracellular bacteria may result from bacterial contamination of a specimen or contamination of the staining solution. Microscopic evaluation for morphologic shape and Gram staining should be performed

TABLE 54.5 Acceptable and Unacceptable Specimens for Anaerobic Culture[45,109]

Body Site	Acceptable Specimens	Unacceptable Speciments
Abdominal cavity	Abdominal/peritoneal fluids; bile aspirates; surgical biopsies	Swabs
Abscesses	Closed abscess: needle aspirates collected after surface decontamination Open abscess: see Wounds	
Blood	Aseptically collected blood inoculated in blood culture bottles following the manufacturer recommendations	Catheter or catheter tips
Body organs (tissues)	Deep biopsy; percutaneous needle aspiration into deeper tissues	Swab
Bone	Deep aspirates of drainage; bone biopsies	Swab, soft tissue samples
Dental or respiratory sinus tissue	Biopsy or aspirate after decontamination	Swab
Feces	At least 2 g of stools only for screening fecal pathogens (*Clostridioides difficile* or *Clostridium perfringens*)	Swab
Female genital tract	Tissue biopsies; guarded uterine swab	Vaginal, cervical swab
Joint	Synovial fluid collected by arthrocentesis inoculated in blood culture bottles following the manufacturer recommendations	Surface swab
Wounds; soft tissues	Deep biopsy specimens; deep wound aspirates at the advancing wound edge after debridement and cleaning the surface	Surface swabs, pus, sinus tracts

when the specimen is collected so that the results can be compared with culture results or the type of organism can be predicted by its shape and staining properties (see Table 54.1). The prediction of an anaerobic infection based on cytologic (Gram stain) findings may guide the empiric use of therapeutic agents targeted for this class of microorganisms.[26,61]

Culture

Anaerobes are difficult to isolate in clinical practice unless precautions are taken. Errors in specimen collection, handling, and submission are the primary reasons anaerobes are not routinely isolated. Therefore, attention to collection practices, minimizing transport time, optimizing transport temperature, and use of appropriate transport media are fundamental if anaerobic culture is performed (see Chapter 3) (Table 54.5).[19,60,62,63] Anaerobes are sensitive to oxygen and because they grow slowly, they are also easily overgrown in specimens that contain aerobes; greater than 70% of cultures are mixed. In addition, multiple anaerobes are often found in the same specimen (Table 54.6). Because swabs tend to dry out and become oxygenated, their use is discouraged. If swabs are used, the tip should be moistened with a pre-reduced medium such as brain-heart infusion broth and maintained in anaerobic conditions. Refrigeration has been shown to be detrimental to the isolation of anaerobic bacteria; thus, specimens should not be held at temperatures lower than 4°C (see Table 54.5). In comparison, aerobes multiply at 25°C and in some cases overgrow the anaerobic component. At 15°C, aerobes do not multiply to any significant extent, and anaerobes remain viable. Acceptable time periods between specimen collection and culture depend on specimen type, volume, and whether transport medium is used. Anaerobic microorganisms in large pieces of tissue or quantities of fluid (greater than 2 mL) are relatively protected from toxic interaction with oxygen and can survive for up to 24 hours before culture, whereas anaerobes in smaller specimens or swabs usually cannot. Anaerobic transport media greatly increase the survival of anaerobes and discourage the growth of aerobes. Anaerobic media are available for transport of aspirated material, tissue or biopsy material, and material collected on swabs.[62,64] Culture of anaerobic bacteria

TABLE 54.6 Occurrence of Anaerobic Bacteria from Positive Cultures by Specimen

Number of Isolate(s) per Specimen[a]	Number of Positive Cultures[b] (%)	Number of Positive Cultures by Species[c,d] (%)
1	3076 (71)	Dog: 2,499 (71.6) Cat: 577 (68.4)
2	844 (19.5)	Dog: 668 (19.1) Cat: 176 (20.9)
3	284 (6.6)	Dog: 218 (6.2) Cat: 66 (7.8)
4	83 (1.9)	Dog: 72 (2.1) Cat: 11 (1.3)
5	24 (0.6)	Dog: 15 (0.4) Cat: 9 (1.1)
6	10 (0.2)	Dog: 6 (0.2) Cat: 4 (0.5)
7	7 (0.2)	Dog: 6 (0.2) Cat: 1 (0.1)
8	5 (0.1)	Dog: 5 (0.1) Cat: 0

[a]Indicates the number of anaerobic bacteria isolated from a single specimen from a total of 6,221 (including four unknowns).
[b]Total anaerobic cultures performed: 4,333.
[c]Total canine anaerobic cultures performed: 3,489.
[d]Total feline anaerobic cultures performed: 844.
Data compiled from 10 institutions (CityU Hong Kong, Cornell University, Kansas State University, University of Missouri Veterinary Diagnostic Laboratory, The Ohio State University, University of Illinois, University of Nebraska Veterinary Diagnostic Laboratory, University of Guelph, Virginia Maryland College of Veterinary Medicine, Washington State University), 2009–2019.

is laborious, expensive, and time consuming. At the laboratory, media must be inoculated with specimens as soon as they are received. Use of pre-reduced, anaerobically sterilized media improves the success of isolation. After inoculation, media is placed in an anaerobic chamber with an atmosphere of 5% carbon dioxide, 5% hydrogen, and 90% nitrogen, or in an oxygen-free carbon dioxide until it can be put in the chamber. During culture follow-up, culture plates must always be handled in an anaerobic hood or a chamber that has been flushed with anaerobic gas mix. Commonly, the isolation and identification of an anaerobe in a sample containing only one species takes 2–4 days.[60,62,63]

Anaerobic culture is costly and most infectious processes contain an average of two different species of anaerobes and at least one aerobe. This significantly increases the effort and cost associated with anaerobe isolation. Use of phenotypical and biochemical methods for identification is laborious and requires well-trained personnel. The adoption of MALDI-TOF MS has allowed laboratories to more accurately and rapidly identify new anaerobes (see Chapter 3).[65–67] However, the acquisition of this technology is cost prohibitive for small laboratories.

Mucosal disease produced by anaerobes is somewhat more difficult to diagnose. Isolation from sites where obligate anaerobes are part of the resident microbiota, such as the oral or pharyngeal cavity, vagina, external auditory meatus, conjunctiva, or skin, can be difficult to associate with pathogenicity. Diagnosis of GI disease caused by *C. difficile* and *C. perfringens* requires the use of specialized agar for isolation, immunologic tests to determine the presence of microorganism or toxin in feces or in broth culture, or molecular assays that detect toxin genes in feces or the isolates themselves.[60,68]

Few veterinary laboratories perform susceptibility testing for anaerobes because it is difficult and expensive. Guidelines for testing have been established by the CLSI.[69] The agar dilution assay has been considered the only validated and recommended method for all anaerobic organisms; however, this method can be labor intensive and the assay results have not always been repeatable or consistent for all anaerobic species.[63,69,70] The CLSI recommends broth microdilution method only for testing *Bacteroides* spp. and *Parabacteroides* spp.[69] Some laboratories use commercial gradient strips (E-testing) because these are more convenient for routine testing (see Chapter 3).[26] However, a lack of agreement when using this method has also been described.[63,71]

A disc test can be performed to determine whether an isolate produces β-lactamase (Nitrocefin Disc, B.D. Sparks, MD, USA). For this test, a portion of an isolated colony is smeared onto a disc that contains a substrate that changes color when a β-lactamase is present. The most common anaerobic β-lactamases are encoded by the *cepA* gene, and more than 97% of *B. fragilis* carry this gene.[72,73] These strains are resistant to penicillin, ampicillin, amoxicillin, and most of the cephalosporins, except cefoxitin. Clavulanate irreversibly binds to these enzymes. Cefoxitin resistance is most commonly due to a β-lactamase encoded by the *cfxA* gene. Cefoxitin resistance rates in *B. fragilis* group organisms range from 3.7% to 19% by species in the United States and 9.6% to 75% internationally.[72] The presence of *cepA* and *cfxA* have been reported in *Bacteroides* spp. isolated from domestic animals.[27] Table 54.7 summarizes the prevalence of β-lactamase production found among various anaerobes isolated from dogs and cats in one study.

Because of the cost and difficulties of culture and low sensitivity especially when specimens cannot reach the laboratory within hours, presumptive diagnoses of anaerobic infections are often made based on history, anatomic site, characteristics of the exudate (e.g., odor and sometimes color), and results of cytologic examination (see Box 54.2, Table 54.1, and Fig. 54.6). Antimicrobial treatment of a suspected anaerobic component is usually empiric.

TABLE 54.7 Prevalence of β-Lactamase-Producing Strains of Anaerobic Gram-Negative Bacteria Isolated from Dogs and Cats

Organism	Species	Number	β-Lactamase Positive (%)	β-Lactamase Negative (%)
Bacteroides fragilis	Dog	40	36 (90)	4 (10)
	Cat	18	16 (89)	2 (11)
B. fragilis group	Dog	26	19 (73)	7 (27)
	Cat	11	10 (91)	1 (9)
Other *Bacteroides*	Dog	22	11 (50)	11 (50)
	Cat	18	14 (78)	4 (22)
Porphyromonas spp.	Dog	21	7 (33)	14 (67)
	Cat	10	5 (50)	5 (50)
Prevotella spp.	Dog	46	21 (46)	25 (54)
	Cat	16	8 (50)	8 (50)
Fusobacterium nucleatum	Dog	4	0	4 (100)
	Cat	5	1 (20)	4 (80)
Fusobacterium spp.	Dog	1	0	1 (100)
	Cat	3	0	3 (100)
Miscellaneous species	Dog	48	19 (40)	29 (60)
	Cat	30	16 (53)	14 (47)

Data compiled from William R. Pritchard Veterinary Medical Teaching Hospital, University of California, Davis, CA, 1999–2008.

TREATMENT AND PROGNOSIS

Successful treatment of anaerobic infections may require medical and, on many occasions, surgical interventions combined with appropriate antimicrobial therapy. Antimicrobial therapy without surgical drainage is usually unsuccessful. Abscesses or pus-filled cavities have poor blood supply, and drainage allows for entrance of newly exuded fluids containing the antimicrobial agent. Furthermore, few antibacterial drugs work effectively in the presence of accumulated pus. Because anaerobic infections are often polymicrobial, antimicrobial therapy of infectious processes with an anaerobic component should focus on the anaerobic and the presumed aerobic components. In dogs and cats, the most commonly isolated aerobes are enterics (*E. coli*), *Pasteurella*, and *Staphylococcus pseudintermedius*.[5,26]

Anaerobic bacteria are inherently resistant to certain antibacterials (e.g., the aminoglycosides and the second-generation quinolones), although extended-spectrum (third- and fourth-generation) quinolones, such as pradofloxacin, have a reasonable activity against anaerobes at generally used therapeutic dosages.[74,75] Although there are reports of an increase in the prevalence of antimicrobial resistance in anaerobes isolated from humans, the use of empiric agents in veterinary medicine is still recommended.[26] The prevalence of resistance to β-lactams and fluoroquinolones is high among *Bacteroides* spp., but it is also observed in other anaerobes of the gram-negative group.[27,72,74]

The most active antimicrobials against anaerobes are metronidazole, amoxicillin-clavulanate, chloramphenicol, and clindamycin (Table 54.8). Numerous β-lactamase inhibitor combinations such as ampicillin-sulbactam, ticarcillin-clavulanate (if available), and piperacillin-tazobactam have been shown to be very active against human anaerobic isolates but have not been tested on veterinary isolates.[26,27,70] Factors such as tissue penetration should be considered

TABLE 54.8 Suggested Antimicrobial Drugs for Treatment of Anaerobic Bacterial Infections in Dogs or Cats[a]

Drug	Dose (mg/kg)	Interval (Hours)	Route
Amoxicillin-clavulanate potassium	12.5–25	12	PO
Ampicillin-sulbactam	10–20	8	IV, IM
Metronidazole	15	12	IV
	15	12 (dogs), 24 (cats)	PO
Clindamycin hydrochloride,	11	12 (dogs), 24 (cats)	PO
clindamycin phosphate[b]	10	12	IV, IM
Chloramphenicol, chloramphenicol sodium succinate	40–50 (dogs), 12.5–20 (cats)	6–8 (dogs), 12 (cats)	PO, IV, IM[c]
Pradofloxacin	3–5 (dogs), 5–10 (cats)	24	PO[d]

[a]The concurrent presence of aerobes should also be considered when selecting antimicrobial drugs.
[b]For intravenous administration, dilute 1:10 in 0.9% saline and administer over 30–60 minutes.
[c]See Chapter 10 for warnings about chloramphenicol use.
[d]In countries where available.

when selecting antimicrobial drugs, and the concurrent presence of aerobic bacteria must also be taken into account. A combination of a β-lactam/β-lactamase inhibitor drug or clindamycin and a drug with activity against gram-negative bacteria, such as a fluoroquinolone or an aminoglycoside, could be a reasonable choice for initial treatment of serious infections whilst awaiting the results of susceptibility testing for aerobic bacteria when mixed aerobic-anaerobic infections are suspected.

There are few studies published that report antimicrobial susceptibility data from veterinary anaerobe isolates. In the United States, a veterinary diagnostic laboratory reported that a few isolates were resistant against antimicrobials tested by the gradient strip method (amoxicillin-clavulanic [1/145], ampicillin [7/77], chloramphenicol [4/242], clindamycin [12/158], metronidazole [10/247] and penicillin [54/243]).[26] Collected unpublished data from anaerobes tested in 10 veterinary diagnostic laboratories shows that these bacteria were susceptible to most antimicrobial agents, with the exception of *B. fragilis*.

Strains of the *netF*-producing type A *C. perfringens* (which has been associated with necrotizing enteritis in neonatal foals and necrotizing and hemorrhagic enteritis in dogs) showed susceptibility to 12 antimicrobial agents, including all β-lactams tested (such as penicillin G and ampicillin), clindamycin, chloramphenicol, and metronidazole. However, these isolates consistently displayed a reduced susceptibility or resistance to tetracycline.[76]

Drugs in the broad-spectrum carbapenem group such as imipenem, meropenem, and ertapenem have been very effective in anaerobic infections associated with mixed aerobic populations. However, empiric use of these agents in veterinary medicine is not routinely recommended based on antimicrobial stewardship concepts. Although anaerobes may be susceptible to trimethoprim-sulfonamides *in vitro*, inhibitors (mainly thymidine) are found *in vivo* that make this drug combination an unpredictable treatment for anaerobic microorganism infections.[77] The response to tetracyclines is unpredictable as well.[4]

PREVENTION

Prevention of anaerobic bacterial infections involves management or prevention of underlying conditions that predispose to these infections (see Clinical Features). Vaccines for prevention of anaerobic bacterial infections are not available. An inactivated, whole cell vaccine preparation *Porphyromonas denticanis, P. gulae,* and *Porphyromonas salivosa* was available for several years for prevention of periodontal disease in dogs, but was withdrawn from the market due to apparent lack of efficacy when its conditional license expired.

PUBLIC HEALTH ASPECTS

It is estimated that 250,000 human bites, 400,000 cat bites, and 4.5 million dog bites occur in the United States each year in both adults and children.[18] Although most of the wounds resulting from animal bites contain aerobic microorganisms, approximately one third contain anaerobes. All are thought to be members of the normal oral cavity microbiota of dogs and cats. The most common anaerobes belong to the same genera as the anaerobes found in disease processes in dogs and cats.[18,78] Some members of the oral microbiota of dogs and cats produce serious disease in immunocompromised individuals and those that are asplenic or have liver disease (see Chapter 75).

Clostridioides difficile is an important cause of disease in humans and it has been found in food-producing animals and retail meats. *Clostridioides difficile* ribotypes in animals are associated with human infections; however, prevalence and spore numbers were low.[79–82] No association between *C. difficile* fecal carriage and raw meat consumption was noted in dogs[81]; however, other enteric pathogens such as *Salmonella* were detected.[83] *Clostridium perfringens* can be transmitted to people on contaminated foods from production animals. No data exist concerning the communicability of *C. perfringens* from dogs and cats to people. However, because it appears that this microorganism can be acquired from contaminated environments, it seems likely, but unproven, that *C. perfringens* from any source can infect dogs, cats, or people. Whether resulting disease depends on a trigger event remains undetermined (see Chapter 64).

CASE EXAMPLE

Signalment

"Cocoa," a 4-month-old intact female Labrador retriever from Gonzales, CA.

History

Cocoa was brought to the University of California, Davis, William R. Pritchard Veterinary Medical Teaching Hospital for evaluation of a history of seizures. Approximately 6 weeks before referral, the dog was seen for redness and protrusion of the left eye (exophthalmos). She was treated with amoxicillin-clavulanic acid for 1 week, and the left ocular exophthalmos resolved, but subsequently protrusion of the right eye was noted. A second 1-week course of amoxicillin-clavulanic acid was instituted, and the exophthalmos again resolved. One month later, Cocoa appeared painful on opening her mouth. She was treated with cephalexin and meloxicam with no apparent improvement. Two days later she was inappetent. When the owners offered her food by hand, she ate, became ataxic, fell over, her thoracic limbs stiffened, and foamy saliva was noted around her mouth. She was taken to an emergency clinic and she vomited in the car. At the emergency clinic, she had three generalized seizures that were treated with diazepam. She was also treated with enrofloxacin (5 mg/kg, IV, once).

CASE EXAMPLE—cont'd

Cocoa's diet normally consisted of commercial dog food and she had been vaccinated for distemper, hepatitis, parvovirus at 8 and 12 weeks of age. There had been no coughing, sneezing, diarrhea, exposure to ticks or toxins, trauma, or travel outside California.

Physical Examination

Body weight: 15.3 kg.

General: Quiet but alert and responsive. Hydrated. T = 102.8°F (39.3°C), pulse = 110 beats/minute, panting, mucous membranes pink, CRT = 1 second.

Eyes, ears, nose, and throat: No clinically significant abnormalities were noted. No evidence of pain on opening the mouth provided neck movement was prevented.

Integument: No abnormalities detected.

Musculoskeletal, cardiovascular, GI, genitourinary systems, and peripheral lymph nodes: No clinically significant findings.

Neurologic examination: Mild obtundation noted. The dog held her head down and was reluctant to move her neck. There was moderate to marked ataxia that involved all four limbs, with the pelvic limbs most severely affected, and the right pelvic and thoracic limbs more severely affected than the left. Cranial nerve examination revealed only a decreased corneal reflex on the right side. Conscious proprioceptive deficits were noted in all four limbs, with the right limbs more severely affected. There was severe pain on palpation of the cervical spine and moderate pain on palpation of the lumbosacral spine. Based on the neurologic examination, multifocal CNS lesions were suspected.

Laboratory Findings

CBC: HCT 34.4% (40%–55%), MCV 64.9 fL (65–75 fL), MCHC 34.9 g/dL (33–36 g/dL), reticulocytes 22,000 cells/μL (7,000–65,000 cells/μL), WBC 17,780 cells/μL (6,000–13,000 cells/μL), neutrophils 12,979 cells/μL (3,000–10,500 cells/μL), band neutrophils 533 cells/μL, lymphocytes 3,023 cells/μL (1,000–4,000 cells/μL), monocytes 1,245 cells/μL (150–1,200 cells/μL), platelets 392,000 platelets/μL (150,000–400,000 platelets/μL).

Serum chemistry profile: Sodium 143 mmol/L (145–154 mmol/L), potassium 4.6 mmol/L (3.6–5.3 mmol/L), chloride 102 mmol/L (108–118 mmol/L), bicarbonate 23 mmol/L (16–26 mmol/L), phosphorus 6.9 mg/dL (3.0–6.2 mg/dL), calcium 11.1 mg/dL (9.7–11.5 mg/dL), BUN 7 mg/dL (5–21 mg/dL), creatinine 0.4 mg/dL (0.3–1.2 mg/dL), glucose 95 mg/dL (64–123 mg/dL), total protein 6.1 g/dL (5.4–7.6 g/dL), albumin 2.8 g/dL (3.0–4.4 g/dL), globulin 3.3 g/dL (1.8–3.9 g/dL), ALT 35 U/L (19–67 U/L), AST 52 U/L (19–42 U/L), ALP 103 U/L (21–170 U/L), creatine kinase 556 U/L (51–399 U/L), GGT 4 U/L (0–6 U/L), cholesterol 262 mg/dL (135–361 mg/dL), total bilirubin 0.1 mg/dL (0–0.2 mg/dL).

Urinalysis: SpG 1.013; pH 6.5, negative for protein, glucose, ketones, bilirubin, hemoprotein, WBC, RBC, casts, and bacteria.

Imaging Findings

Thoracic radiographs: Cardiopulmonary structures were within normal limits.

Abdominal ultrasound: The gastric wall was mildly thickened with bright, echogenic speckles within the muscularis layer. The submucosa of the stomach was echogenic. Impressions: Changes associated with the stomach were suggestive of gastritis. The remainder of the abdominal ultrasound was unremarkable.

Spinal radiographs: Open physes were present within the vertebral column. No abnormalities were identified.

Brain MRI: In the pre-contrast brain study, a flattened, fusiform structure was identified in the dorsal part of the foramen magnum that caused moderate dorsoventral compression of the spinal cord (Fig. 54.7). This structure was hypointense to brain but hyperintense to CSF on the T1-weighted images and moderately hyperintense on dual echo and fluid-attenuated inversion recovery (FLAIR) images. The post-contrast brain study showed diffuse meningeal enhancement that involved the spinal cord and brain with the most prominent enhancement noted along the ventral brainstem and left cerebral hemisphere. The contrast enhancement pattern was consistent with meningitis. There was a discrete rim of enhancement surrounding the aforementioned fusiform structure, which gave it a cystic appearance. This structure appeared to be extradural in location. The structure in the foramen magnum had partial fluid characteristics, but was not consistent with pure fluid, and in light of the meningeal enhancement, was thought to most likely represent an abscess.

Analysis of CSF (Lumbar CSF)

CSF protein: 726 mg/dL (reference range, < 25 mg/dL)

Total RBCs: 5 cells/μL (reference range, 0 cells/μL)

Total nucleated cells: 7,500 cells/μL (reference range, < 2 cells/μL)

Differential: 88% neutrophils, 12% large mononuclear cells

Microscopic evaluation: The specimen was highly cellular and contained a large number of nondegenerate neutrophils. A few pyknotic forms were noted. Lower numbers of monocytoid cells, large reactive lymphocytes, and rare eosinophils also were observed. Interpretation: Marked neutrophilic pleocytosis (purulent inflammation).

Cytologic Analysis of CSF (Cisternal)

A direct smear of cisternal CSF was examined and found to contain disrupted cells and mildly to moderately degenerate neutrophils. These were admixed with low numbers of monocytoid cells and intermediate-sized reactive lymphocytes. Rare neutrophils were observed with intracellular rod-shaped bacteria. Few free rod-shaped bacteria were noted in the background.

Microbiologic Testing

Aerobic urine culture: No growth was detected.

Aerobic and anaerobic blood cultures: No growth was detected.

Aerobic and anaerobic CSF culture: Small numbers of *B. fragilis*, positive for β-lactamase production.

Diagnosis

Bacteroides fragilis meningitis with extradural abscess formation.

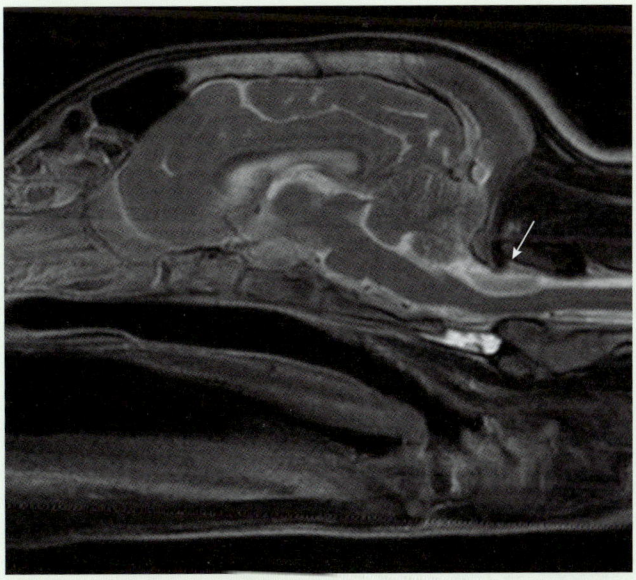

Fig. 54.7 Post-contrast brain magnetic resonance image (MRI) of a 4-month-old intact female Labrador retriever with *Bacteroides fragilis* meningitis and an epidural abscess located in the dorsal part of the foramen magnum. There is a flattened, fusiform structure in the dorsal part of the foramen magnum associated with moderate dorsoventral compression of the spinal cord *(arrow)*. Diffuse meningeal enhancement and a discrete rim of enhancement surrounding the fusiform structure are present.

Continued

CASE EXAMPLE—cont'd

Treatment and Outcome

Cocoa was treated with ticarcillin (50 mg/kg, IV, q6h), metronidazole (10 mg/kg, IV, q8h), and IV crystalloids (LRS with 20 mEq/L KCl at 50 mL/h, IV). The following day her mentation improved and she became more willing to move. On day 3 after starting antibiotics, treatment was changed to clavulanic acid-amoxicillin (16 mg/kg, PO, q8h) and metronidazole (16 mg/kg, PO, q12h). On day 4, Cocoa was less ataxic and had normal conscious proprioception, but had a seizure while on a walk outside. The seizure lasted 45 seconds and was manifested by jaw chomping and defecation, but Cocoa did not fall over or lose consciousness. Potassium bromide (40 mg/kg, PO, q8h for 4 days, then 40 mg/kg, PO, q24h) was added to the treatment regimen and Cocoa was discharged from the hospital.

At a recheck 3 weeks later, Cocoa's owners reported that she had shown steady clinical improvement and for the last week she had been acting like a normal puppy. There had been no seizures. She received her final series of vaccines 1 week ago. No abnormalities could be detected on full neurologic examination. A CBC showed persistent mild nonregenerative anemia (HCT 34.8%), 5,253 neutrophils/μL, and 228 band neutrophils/μL. A repeat MRI showed a marked decrease in the diffuse meningeal enhancement and marked reduction in the size of the cystic structure, although there was persistent mild spinal cord compression. Analysis of CSF revealed a CSF protein concentration of 37 mg/dL, < 1 RBC/μL, 24 nucleated cells/μL, with 12% neutrophils, 51% small mononuclear cells, and 37% large mononuclear cells. Microscopic examination revealed a heterogenous population of lymphocytes that included small mature lymphocytes, larger reactive lymphocytes, and many plasmacytoid lymphocytes along with mature plasma cells and moderately vacuolated macrophages. A few nondegenerate neutrophils were present. Antimicrobial drug treatment was continued and a recheck was recommended in 3 months, but the dog was subsequently lost to follow-up.

Comments

The history of exophthalmos increased suspicion for an anaerobic bacterial infection of the CNS in this dog; therefore, anaerobic culture of the CSF and blood was performed. Given the young age of this dog, a migrating foreign body was suspected. The history, together with the distribution of lesions in the CNS and the lack of lesions elsewhere, suggested direct extension of the infection from the retrobulbar location to the meninges, rather than hematogenous spread of infection. Because the dog was treated with antibiotics before culture was performed, the concurrent presence of other facultative organisms or other anaerobic species may have been obscured. The identification of β-lactamase production by the *B. fragilis* isolate was not surprising because of the high (> 90%) prevalence of β-lactamase production by this species. *B. fragilis* is also known for its propensity to form abscesses.

SUGGESTED READINGS

Brook I. Spectrum and treatment of anaerobic infections. *J Infect Chemother.* 2015;22:1–13.

Pence MA. Antimicrobial resistance in clinically important anaerobes. *Clin Microbiol News.* 2019;41:1–7.

REFERENCES

1. Sebald M, Hauser D. Pasteur, oxygen and the anaerobes revisited. *Anaerobe.* 1995;1:11–16.
2. Finegold SM. Anaerobic bacteria in humans: an overview. *Anaerobe.* 1995;1:3–9.
3. Hentges DJ. Anaerobes: General characteristics. In: Baron S, ed. *Medical Microbiology.* Galveston, TX: The University of Texas Medical Branch at Galveston; 1996. Accessible at https://www.ncbi.nlm.nih.gov/books/NBK7638/#top.
4. Hirsh D, Indiveri M, Jang S, et al. Changes in prevalence and susceptibility of obligate anaerobes in clinical veterinary practice. *J Am Vet Med Assoc.* 1985;186:1086–1089.
5. Jang S, Breher J, Dabaco L, et al. Organisms isolated from dogs and cats with anaerobic infections and susceptibility to selected antimicrobial agents. *J Am Vet Med Assoc.* 1997;210:1610–1614.
6. Oh C, Lee K, Cheong Y, et al. Comparison of the oral microbiomes of canines and their owners using next-generation sequencing. *PLoS One.* 2015;10.
7. Love DN, Vekselstein R, Collings S. The obligate and facultatively anaerobic bacterial flora of the normal feline gingival margin. *Vet Microbiol.* 1990;22:267–275.
8. Srečnik Š, Zdovc I, Javoršek U, et al. Microbiological aspects of naturally occurring primary endodontic infections in dogs. *J Vet Dent.* 2019;36:124–128.
9. Elliott DR, Wilson M, Buckley CMF, et al. Cultivable oral microbiota of domestic dogs. *J Clin Microbiol.* 2005;43:5470–5476.
10. Uhaa I, Hird D, Hirsh D, et al. Case-control study of risk factors associated with nosocomial *Salmonella krefeld* infection in dogs. *Am J Vet Res.* 1988;49:1501–1505.
11. Greene CE. *Infectious Diseases of the Dog and Cat.* WB Saunders, Elsevier Science; 2006.
12. Struble AL, Tang YJ, Kass PH, et al. Fecal shedding of *Clostridium difficile* in dogs: a period prevalence survey in a veterinary medical teaching hospital. *J Vet Diagn Invest.* 1994;6:342–347.
13. Sykes JE, Marks SL. Enteric Clostridial Infections. In: Sykes, JE (ed). *Canine and Feline Infectious Diseases.* Elsevier; 2013:458.
14. O'Neill G, Adams J, Bowman R, et al. A molecular characterization of *Clostridium difficile* isolates from humans, animals and their environments. *Epidemiol Infect.* 1993;111:257–264.
15. Alam MJ, McPherson J, Miranda J, et al. Molecular epidemiology of *Clostridioides difficile* in domestic dogs and zoo animals. *Anaerobe.* 2019;59:107–111.
16. Riley T, Adams J, O'Neill G, et al. Gastrointestinal carriage of *Clostridium difficile* in cats and dogs attending veterinary clinics. *Epidemiol Infect.* 1991;107:659–665.
17. Styrt B, Gorbach SL. Recent developments in the understanding of the pathogenesis and treatment of anaerobic infections. *New Engl J Med.* 1989;321:240–246.
18. Bula-Rudas FJ, Olcott JL. Human and animal bites. *Pediatr Rev.* 2018;39:490–500.
19. Noor A, Khetarpal S. *Anaerobic Infections.* Treasure Island (FL): StatPearls Publishing; 2018. Available at: https://europepmc.org/article/NBK/nbk482349.
20. Tamborini A, Jahns H, McAllister H, et al. Bacterial cholangitis, cholecystitis, or both in dogs. *J Vet Intern Med.* 2016;30:1046–1055.
21. Wagner KA, Hartmann FA, Trepanier LA. Bacterial culture results from liver, gallbladder, or bile in 248 dogs and cats evaluated for hepatobiliary disease: 1998–2003. *J Vet Intern Med.* 2007;21:417–424.
22. Silva Jr J, Tang YJ, Gumerlock PH. Genotyping of *Clostridium difficile* isolates. *J Infect Dis.* 1994;169:661–664.
23. Janezic S, Mlakar S, Rupnik M. Dissemination of *Clostridium difficile* spores between environment and households: dog paws and shoes. *Zoonoses Public Health.* 2018;65:669–674.
24. Weese J, Finley R, Reid-Smith R, et al. Evaluation of *Clostridium difficile* in dogs and the household environment. *Epidemiol Infect.* 2010;138:1100–1104.
25. Rodriguez C, Taminiau B, Bouchafa L, et al. *Clostridium difficile* beyond stools: dog nasal discharge as a possible new vector of bacterial transmission. *Heliyon.* 2019;5. e01629.
26. Lawhon S, Taylor A, Fajt V. Frequency of resistance in obligate anaerobic bacteria isolated from dogs, cats, and horses to antimicrobial agents. *J Clin Microbiol.* 2013;51:3804–3810.

27. Mayorga M, Rodríguez-Cavallini E, López-Ureña D, et al. Identification and antimicrobial susceptibility of obligate anaerobic bacteria from clinical samples of animal origin. *Anaerobe*. 2015;36:19–24.
28. Mehdizadeh Gohari I, Parreira VR, Nowell VJ, et al. A novel pore-forming toxin in type A *Clostridium perfringens* is associated with both fatal canine hemorrhagic gastroenteritis and fatal foal necrotizing enterocolitis. *PLoS One*. 2015;10. e0122684.
29. Sindern N, Suchodolski JS, Leutenegger CM, et al. Prevalence of *Clostridium perfringens* netE and netF toxin genes in the feces of dogs with acute hemorrhagic diarrhea syndrome. *J Vet Intern Med*. 2018;33:100–105.
30. Mehdizadeh Gohari I, Unterer S, Whitehead AE, et al. NetF-producing *Clostridium perfringens* and its associated diseases in dogs and foals. *J Vet Diagn Invest*. 2020;32:230–238.
31. Weese JS, Staempfli HR, Prescott JF, et al. The roles of *Clostridium difficile* and enterotoxigenic *Clostridium perfringens* in diarrhea in dogs. *J Vet Intern Med*. 2001;15:374–378.
32. Kruth S, Prescott J, Welch M, et al. Nosocomial diarrhea associated with enterotoxigenic *Clostridium perfringens* infection in dogs. *J Am Vet Med Assoc*. 1989;195:331–334.
33. Twedt D. *Clostridium perfringens*-associated enterotoxicosis in dogs. In: *Current Veterinary Therapy XI*. Philadelphia: WB Saunders Company; 1992:602–604.
34. Jha AR, Shmalberg J, Tanprasertsuk J, et al. Characterization of gut microbiomes of household pets in the United States using a direct-to-consumer approach. *PLoS One*. 2020;15. e0227289.
35. Reddy KE, Kim HR, Jeong JY, et al. Impact of breed on the fecal microbiome of dogs under the same dietary condition. *J Microbiol Biotechnol*. 2019;29:1947–1956.
36. Citron DM. Update on the taxonomy and clinical aspects of the genus *Fusobacterium*. *Clin Infect Dis*. 2002;35:S22–S27.
37. Tzianabos AO, Onderdonk AB, Rosner B, et al. Structural features of polysaccharides that induce intra-abdominal abscesses. *Science*. 1993;262:416–419.
38. Brook I. Pathogenesis and management of polymicrobial infections due to aerobic and anaerobic bacteria. *Med Res Rev*. 1995;15:73–82.
39. Brook I. Role of encapsulated anaerobic bacteria in synergistic infections. *Crit Rev Microbiol*. 1987;14:171–193.
40. Stillion JR, Letendre JA. A clinical review of the pathophysiology, diagnosis, and treatment of pyothorax in dogs and cats. *J Vet Emerg Crit Care*. 2015;25:113–129.
41. Epstein SE, Balsa IM. Canine and feline exudative pleural diseases. *Vet Clin North Am Small Anim Pract*. 2020;50:467–487.
42. Vel WA, Namavar F, Verweij-van Vught AM, et al. Killing of *Escherichia coli* by human polymorphonuclear leucocytes in the presence of *Bacteroides fragilis*. *J Clin Pathol*. 1985;38:86–91.
43. Pillai DK, Amachawadi RG, Baca G, et al. Leukotoxic activity of *Fusobacterium necrophorum* of cattle origin. *Anaerobe*. 2019;56:51–56.
44. Hofstad T. Virulence determinants in nonsporeforming anaerobic bacteria. *Scand J Infect Dis*. 1989;62:Suppl 15–24.
45. Dear JD. Bacterial pneumonia in dogs and cats: an update. *Vet Clin North Am Small Anim Pract*. 2020;50:447–465.
46. Hardham J, Dreier K, Wong J, et al. Pigmented-anaerobic bacteria associated with canine periodontitis. *Vet Microbiol*. 2005;106:119–128.
47. Kato Y, Shirai M, Murakami M, et al. Molecular detection of human periodontal pathogens in oral swab specimens from dogs in Japan. *J Vet Dent*. 2011;28:84–89.
48. Perez-Salcedo L, Herrera D, Esteban-Saltiveri D, et al. Comparison of two sampling methods for microbiological evaluation of periodontal disease in cats. *Vet Microbiol*. 2011;149:500–503.
49. Senhorinho GN, Nakano V, Liu C, et al. Detection of *Porphyromonas gulae* from subgingival biofilms of dogs with and without periodontitis. *Anaerobe*. 2011;17:257–258.
50. Wang AL, Ledbetter EC, Kern TJ. Orbital abscess bacterial isolates and in vitro antimicrobial susceptibility patterns in dogs and cats. *Vet Ophthalmol*. 2009;12:91–96.
51. Love DN, Jones RF, Bailey M, et al. Isolation and characterisation of bacteria from abscesses in the subcutis of cats. *J Med Microbiol*. 1979;12:207–212.
52. Love DN, Malik R, Norris JM. Bacteriological warfare amongst cats: what have we learned about cat bite infections? *Vet Microbiol*. 2000;74:179–193.
53. Hess MO. Necrotising fasciitis due to *Prevotella bivia* in a cat. *J Small Anim Pract*. 2009;50:558–560.
54. Walker AL, Jang SS, Hirsh DC. Bacteria associated with pyothorax of dogs and cats: 98 cases (1989-1998). *J Am Vet Med Assoc*. 2000;216: 359–363.
55. Culp WT, Zeldis TE, Reese MS, et al. Primary bacterial peritonitis in dogs and cats: 24 cases (1990-2006). *J Am Vet Med Assoc*. 2009;234: 906–913.
56. Greiner M, Wolf G, Hartmann K. Bacteraemia in 66 cats and antimicrobial susceptibility of the isolates (1995–2004). *J Fel Med Surg*. 2007;9:404–410.
57. Greiner M, Wolf G, Hartmann K. Bacteraemia and antimicrobial susceptibility in dogs. *Vet Rec*. 2007;160:529–530.
58. Dow SW, Curtis CR, Jones RL, et al. Bacterial culture of blood from critically ill dogs and cats: 100 cases (1985-1987). *J Am Vet Med Assoc*. 1989;195:113–117.
59. Sykes JE, Kittleson MD, Pesavento PA, et al. Evaluation of the relationship between causative organisms and clinical characteristics of infective endocarditis in dogs: 71 cases (1992-2005). *J Am Vet Med Assoc*. 2006;228:1723–1734.
60. Markey B, Leonard F, Archambault M, et al. *Clinical Veterinary Microbiology*. 2nd ed. Elsevier Health Sciences; 2013.
61. Johnson LR, Queen EV, Vernau W, et al. Microbiologic and cytologic assessment of bronchoalveolar lavage fluid from dogs with lower respiratory tract infection: 105 cases (2001–2011). *J Vet Intern Med*. 2013;27:259–267.
62. Barenfanger J, Drake CA, Lawhorn J, et al. Outcomes of improved anaerobic techniques in clinical microbiology. *Clin Infect Dis*. 2002;35:S78–S83.
63. Nagy E, Boyanova L, Justesen US. How to isolate, identify and determine antimicrobial susceptibility of anaerobic bacteria in routine laboratories. *Clin Microbiol Infect*. 2018;24:1139–1148.
64. Mangels J. Anaerobic transport systems: are they necessary? *Clin Micro News Letter*. 1994;16(13):101–104.
65. Barreau M, Pagnier I, La Scola B. Improving the identification of anaerobes in the clinical microbiology laboratory through MALDI-TOF mass spectrometry. *Anaerobe*. 2013;22:123–125.
66. Kim D, Ji S, Kim JR, et al. Performance evaluation of a new matrix-assisted laser desorption/ionization time-of-flight mass spectrometry, ASTA MicroIDSys system, in bacterial identification against clinical isolates of anaerobic bacteria. *Anaerobe*. 2020;61:102131.
67. Shannon S, Kronemann D, Patel R, et al. Routine use of MALDI-TOF MS for anaerobic bacterial identification in clinical microbiology. *Anaerobe*. 2018;54:191–196.
68. Stevens DL, Bryant AE, Carroll K. Clostridium. In: *Manual of Clinical Microbiology*. 11th ed. American Society of Microbiology; 2015:940–966.
69. CLSI. *Methods for Antimicrobial Susceptibility Testing of Anaerobic Bacteria: Approved Standard*. 9th ed. Wayne, PA: Clinical and Laboratory Standards Institute; 2018.
70. Hecht D. Evolution of anaerobe susceptibility testing in the United States. *Clin Infect Dis*. 2002;35:S28.
71. Rennie R, Turnbull L, Brosnikoff C, et al. First comprehensive evaluation of the MIC evaluator device compared to E-test and CLSI reference dilution methods for antimicrobial susceptibility testing of clinical strains of anaerobes and other fastidious bacterial species. *J Clin Microbiol*. 2012;50:1153–1157.
72. Pence MA. Antimicrobial resistance in clinically important anaerobes. *Clin Microbiol News*. 2019;41:1–7.
73. Nagy E, Urbán E, Nord CE, et al. Antimicrobial susceptibility of *Bacteroides fragilis* group isolates in Europe: 20 years of experience. *Clin Microbiol Infect*. 2011;17:371–379.
74. Rashid MU, Weintraub A, Nord CE. Development of antimicrobial resistance in the normal anaerobic microbiota during one year after administration of clindamycin or ciprofloxacin. *Anaerobe*. 2015;31:72–77.

75. Borobio MV, Conejo M, Ramirez E, et al. Comparative activities of eight quinolones against members of the *Bacteroides fragilis* group. *Antimicrobial Agents Chemother.* 1994;38:1442–1445.
76. Mehdizadeh Gohari I, Boerlin P, Prescott JF. Antimicrobial susceptibility and clonal relationship of tetracycline resistance genes in netF-positive *Clostridium perfringens. Microb Drug Resist.* 2019;25:627–630.
77. Indiveri MC, Hirsh DC. Tissues and exudates contain sufficient thymidine for growth of anaerobic bacteria in the presence of inhibitory levels of trimethoprim-sulfamethoxazole. *Vet Microbiol.* 1992;31:235–242.
78. Abrahamian FM, Goldstein EJ. Microbiology of animal bite wound infections. *Clin Microbiol Rev.* 2011;24:231–246.
79. Weese JS, Avery BP, Rousseau J, et al. Detection and enumeration of *Clostridium difficile* spores in retail beef and pork. *Appl Environ Microbiol.* 2009;75:5009–5011.
80. Von Abercron SM, Karlsson F, Wigh GT, et al. Low occurrence of *Clostridium difficile* in retail ground meat in Sweden. *J Food Prot.* 2009;72:1732–1734.
81. Shaughnessy MK, Snider T, Sepulveda R, et al. Prevalence and molecular characteristics of *Clostridium difficile* in retail meats, food-producing and companion animals, and humans in Minnesota. *J Food Prot.* 2018;81:1635–1642.
82. Thanissery R, McLaren MR, Rivera A, et al. *C. difficile* carriage in animals and the associated changes in the host fecal microbiota. *Anaerobe.* 2020;66:102279.
83. Lefebvre SL, Reid-Smith R, Boerlin P, et al. Evaluation of the risks of shedding *Salmonellae* and other potential pathogens by therapy dogs fed raw diets in Ontario and Alberta. *Zoonoses Public Health.* 2008;55:470–480.
84. Roy J, Messier S, Labrecque O, et al. Clinical and in vitro efficacy of amoxicillin against bacteria associated with feline skin wounds and abscesses. *Can Vet J.* 2007;48:607.
85. Hoshuyama S, Kanoe M, Amimoto A. Isolation of obligate and facultative anaerobic bacteria from feline subcutaneous abscesses. *J Vet Med Sci.* 1996;58:273–274.
86. McCarthy PE, Hosgood G, Pechman RD. Traumatic ear canal separations and para-aural abscessation in three dogs. *J Am Anim Hosp Assoc.* 1995;31:419–424.
87. Peeters ME. The treatment of recurrent abscessation in the neck region of the dog, evaluation of 35 patients. *Tijdschr Diergeneesk.* 1992;117(suppl 1):30s.
88. Hartley C, McConnell JF, Doust R. Wooden orbital foreign body in a Weimaraner. *Vet Ophthalmol.* 2007;10:390–393.
89. Gade-Neto CR, Rodrigues RR, Louzada LM, et al. Microbiota of periodontal pockets and root canals in induced experimental periodontal disease in dogs. *J Invest Clin Dent.* 2019;10:e12439.
90. Visser CJ. Chronic maxillary sinus abscessation in the canine. *J Vet Dent.* 1990;7:12–13.
91. Cook LB, Bergman RL, Bahr A, et al. Inflammatory polyp in the middle ear with secondary suppurative meningoencephalitis in a cat. *Vet Radiol Ultrasound.* 2003;44:648–651.
92. Radaelli ST, Platt SR. Bacterial meningoencephalomyelitis in dogs: a retrospective study of 23 cases (1990-1999). *J Vet Intern Med.* 2002;16:159–163.
93. Betbeze C. Management of orbital diseases. *Topics Companion Anim Med.* 2015;30:107–117.
94. Ledbetter EC, Scarlett JM. Isolation of obligate anaerobic bacteria from ulcerative keratitis in domestic animals. *Vet Ophthalmol.* 2008;11:114–122.
95. Forrester SD, Fossum TW, Miller MW. Pneumothorax in a dog with a pulmonary abscess and suspected infective endocarditis. *J Am Vet Med Assoc.* 1992;200:351–354.
96. Epstein SE, Mellema MS, Hopper K. Airway microbial culture and susceptibility patterns in dogs and cats with respiratory disease of varying severity. *J Vet Emerg Crit Care.* 2010;20:587–594.
97. Barrs VR, Allan GS, Martin P, et al. Feline pyothorax: a retrospective study of 27 cases in Australia. *J Feline Med Surg.* 2005;7:211–222.
98. Johnson MS, Martin MW. Successful medical treatment of 15 dogs with pyothorax. *J Small Anim Pract.* 2007;48:12–16.
99. Ottenjann M, Lubke-Becker A, Linzmann H, et al. Pyothorax in 26 cats: clinical signs, laboratory results and therapy (2000-2007). *Berl Munch Tierarztl Wochenschr.* 2008;121:365–373.
100. Swayne SL, Brisson B, Weese JS, et al. Evaluating the effect of intraoperative peritoneal lavage on bacterial culture in dogs with suspected septic peritonitis. *Can Vet J.* 2012;53:971.
101. O'Neill E, Day M, Hall E, et al. Bacterial cholangitis/cholangiohepatitis with or without concurrent cholecystitis in four dogs. *J Small Anim Pract.* 2006;47:325–335.
102. Johnston D, Christie B. The retroperitoneum in dogs: retroperitoneal infections. *Comp Cont Educ Pract Vet.* 1990;12:1035–1045.
103. Marvel SJ, MacPhail CM. Retroperitoneal abscesses in seven dogs. *J Am Anim Hosp Assoc.* 2013;49:378–384.
104. Allan R, Fenwick SG, Clark P, et al. Meningitis in a dog caused by *Prevotella oralis. J Small Anim Pract.* 2004;45:421–423.
105. Siqueira EG, Rahal SC, Ribeiro MG, et al. Exogenous bacterial osteomyelitis in 52 dogs: a retrospective study of etiology and in vitro antimicrobial susceptibility profile (2000-2013). *Vet Q.* 2014;34:201–204.
106. Cattin I, Liehmann L, Ammon P, et al. Subcutaneous abscess caused by *Clostridium perfringens* and osteomyelitis in a dog. *J Small Anim Pract.* 2008;49:200–203.
107. Bouillon J, Snead E, Caswell J, et al. Pyelonephritis in dogs: retrospective study of 47 histologically diagnosed cases (2005–2015). *J Vet Intern Med.* 2018;32:249–259.
108. Dhaliwal GK, Wray C, Noakes DE. Uterine bacterial flora and uterine lesions in bitches with cystic endometrial hyperplasia (pyometra). *Vet Rec.* 1998;143:659–661.
109. Coyner K. Distinguishing between dermatologic disorders of the face, nasal planum, and ears: great lookalikes in feline dermatology. *Vet Clin North Am Small Anim Pract.* 2020;50:823–882.

Bordetellosis

Krystle L. Reagan

KEY POINTS

- First Described: In 1911 (*Bacillus bronchicanis*).[1] The genus *Bordetella* was named after Bordet who first described *Bordetella pertussis*.[2]
- Cause: *Bordetella bronchiseptica*, an aerobic gram-negative motile coccobacillus (family Alcaligenaceae).
- Affected Hosts: Dogs, cats, wild carnivores, pigs, horses, rabbits, rodents, turkey, humans. Dogs and cats share the same strains.
- Geographic Distribution: Worldwide.
- Mode of Transmission: Aerosol, contact with contaminated fomites and water sources.
- Major Clinical Signs: Sneezing, serous to mucopurulent nasal discharge, harsh or honking cough (especially dogs). Dogs and cats with bronchopneumonia can develop fever, lethargy, inappetence, tachypnea, productive cough, and mucopurulent nasal and ocular discharge.
- Differential Diagnoses: Upper and lower respiratory diseases such as dynamic airway disease, viral respiratory infections, fungal pneumonia, protozoal pneumonia, respiratory tract neoplasia, airway foreign bodies, chronic bronchitis, eosinophilic bronchopneumopathy or granulomatosis, parasitic infections (such as *Filaroides, Oslerus, Capillaria, Paragonimus, Dirofilaria*), bronchopneumonias secondary to conditions such as laryngeal paralysis or ciliary dyskinesia, left-sided congestive heart failure.
- Human Health Significance: *Bordetella bronchiseptica* is closely related to *B. pertussis* and *Bordetella parapertussis*, which cause whooping cough in humans. Uncommonly, it has been associated with respiratory disease in humans and rarely systemic infections such as peritonitis, bacteremia, and meningitis. It primarily causes disease in the immunocompromised. Contact with dogs and cats has been associated with human infections, but host specificity may also be strain related.

ETIOLOGIC AGENT AND EPIDEMIOLOGY

Bordetella spp. are small, pleomorphic, gram-negative coccobacilli. There are at least nine different bacterial species in the genus *Bordetella* (Table 55.1).[3] The only species known to cause disease in dogs and cats is *Bordetella bronchiseptica*, but *B. bronchiseptica* is closely related to *Bordetella pertussis* and *Bordetella parapertussis*, which cause pertussis (whooping cough) in humans. *Bordetella* species possess fimbriae (pili), and *B. bronchiseptica* is motile by means of flagella, which is composed of flagellin. Other species in the genus do not express flagellin. Genetic studies have shown that there is wide genetic diversity among *B. bronchiseptica* isolates, whereas *B. pertussis* is relatively well conserved. There is evidence that *B. pertussis* evolved from a distinct, human-associated lineage of *B. bronchiseptica*,[4] and it has been recommended that *B. bronchiseptica, B. pertussis,* and *B. parapertussis* be reclassified as subspecies of the "*B. bronchiseptica* cluster."[5] *Bordetella pertussis* has been shown to be able to colonize puppies in the absence of clinical signs of respiratory disease.[6]

Worldwide, *B. bronchiseptica* is an important and prevalent cause of respiratory disease in dogs and cats; it also infects and causes respiratory illness in many different animal species including wild carnivores, pigs, rabbits, and occasionally horses, other herbivores, rodents, turkeys, and humans. There are a large number of different strains of *B. bronchiseptica* that vary in virulence and host specificity. Results of molecular typing efforts have shown that strains that infect dogs can be passed to cats and vice versa.[7–9] The whole genome of *B. bronchiseptica* has been sequenced.[10] Its genome is larger than that of its close relatives, and it possesses several plasmids, some of which mediate antimicrobial drug resistance.[11]

Like viral respiratory infections, bordetellosis is especially prevalent in dogs and cats in shelters, pet stores, boarding facilities, and other situations where large numbers of potentially stressed animals may have been in close contact with one another. Infections with *B. bronchiseptica* frequently occur in concert with respiratory viral and/or *Mycoplasma* spp. infections (see Chapters 26, 28, and 57).[12,13]

Unlike *B. pertussis* and *B. parapertussis*, *B. bronchiseptica* can persist in the environment for at least 10 days and can grow in natural water sources.[14] *Bordetella bronchiseptica* is susceptible to most disinfectants, including accelerated hydrogen peroxide or chlorhexidine cleaners.[15]

The prevalence of *B. bronchiseptica* infections in group-housed animals, including shelters, varies from group to group, even in the same geographic region. For example, between 2009 and 2016, the prevalence of detection of *B. bronchiseptica* in European dogs with respiratory disease varied from 3.3% to 78.7%.[16] *Bordetella bronchiseptica* can be isolated from apparently healthy cats and cats with respiratory disease, but is more likely to be isolated from cats with respiratory disease.[17] In one European study that included 1,748 cats from private multiple-cat households, shelters, and breeding catteries, the more cats in the group, the greater the chance that *B. bronchiseptica* would be detected.[18] In rescue shelters, increased seroprevalence has been associated with poor hygiene.[18] In a study of 742 cats in the United Kingdom, *B. bronchiseptica* was isolated from 0% of pet cats, 19.5% of cats from rescue shelters, and 13.5% of cats from research colonies.[19] *Bordetella bronchiseptica* was cultured from 3.1% of 614 cats from four shelters in Louisiana,[20] 5.1% of nasal swabs from 59 cats with acute respiratory disease in Colorado,[21] 2.4% of pharyngeal swabs from 250 cats at intake in a Canadian shelter,[22] and none of 22 cats with respiratory disease in a shelter in California.[23] However, the prevalence of infection was nearly 50% in nasal swabs from 40 cats with rhinitis from a shelter in Colorado.[24] Similarly, a high prevalence (26%) of infection was detected with a PCR assay in 100 cats with upper respiratory disease from central Italy.[25]

TABLE 55.1 Species That Belong to the Genus *Bordetella*

Species	Host(s)	Disease
Bordetella bronchiseptica	Dogs, cats, pigs, horses, rabbits, rodents, sheep, seals, humans	Rhinitis, tracheobronchitis, bronchopneumonia
Bordetella pertussis	Humans	Whooping cough
Bordetella parapertussis	Humans, sheep	Whooping cough (humans); ovine-adapted strains cause respiratory disease in sheep
Bordetella holmesii	Humans	Upper respiratory tract disease, bacteremia
Bordetella trematum	Humans	Otitis media and wound infections
Bordetella avium	Poultry (especially turkeys)	Rhinotracheitis
Bordetella hinzii	Turkeys, rabbits, rarely humans	Turkey, rabbit upper respiratory disease
Bordetella petrii	Environment, rarely humans	None, osteomyelitis
Bordetella ansorpii	Humans	Bacteremia, skin infection

In a case review from the eastern United States, *B. bronchiseptica* was isolated from 49% of 65 pet dogs under 1 year of age with radiographic and microbiologic evidence of bacterial bronchopneumonia. Most of these dogs had originated from breeders (40%) or pet stores (41%), and only 8% were from shelters. Dogs infected with *B. bronchiseptica* were younger (7–35 weeks of age), had been owned for a shorter period of time (median, 18 days), were more likely to have originated from a pet store, and were less likely to have originated from a breeder than dogs with pneumonia caused by other organisms.[26] *Bordetella bronchiseptica* was detected using PCR in 9% of respiratory specimens from client-owned dogs with and without respiratory tract disease that were submitted to the Athens Veterinary Diagnostic Laboratory (Athens, GA, USA). The prevalence of infection was significantly higher in the colder months than in the summer, in contrast to the other respiratory pathogens detected, and was more likely to be detected in dogs less than 12 months of age.[27] Of 2,054 specimens submitted to IDEXX laboratories for PCR detection of respiratory testing in 2020, 15% were positive for *B. bronchiseptica*, the most frequently detected pathogen after *Mycoplasma cynos*.[28] In a study of dogs with respiratory disease from the United Kingdom, *B. bronchiseptica* was detected in 14.5% of 1,602 respiratory specimens submitted to four different laboratories from 2016 to 2019.[29]

Bordetella bronchiseptica was isolated from dogs with respiratory disease as well as from healthy dogs in a rehoming kennel in the United Kingdom.[30] Of 138 dogs with acute upper respiratory tract disease or dogs that were directly exposed to dogs with respiratory signs from Italy, eight (10.3%) of the acutely ill dogs were positive using PCR for *B. bronchiseptica* versus one (1.3%) of the healthy exposed dogs.[31] Additionally, when a cohort of dogs with acute respiratory signs were assessed by PCR for *B. bronchiseptica,* it was found that 78% (48/61) of sick dogs were PCR positive, whereas 45.6% (41/90) of clinically healthy control dogs were positive.[12] In another study, *B. bronchiseptica* DNA was detected using PCR in 19.5% of apparently healthy dogs on entry to a shelter.[32]

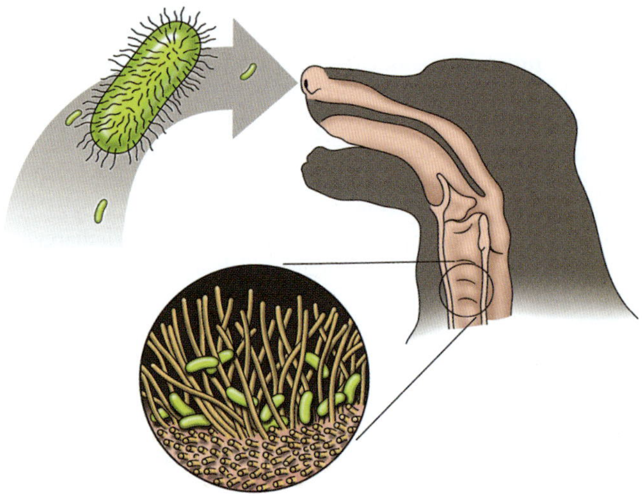

Fig. 55.1 *Bordetella bronchiseptica* infection. *Bordetella bronchiseptica* is inhaled, adheres to respiratory cilia by means of fimbrial adhesins, evades the immune system, and secretes a variety of toxins that damage the respiratory epithelium.

CLINICAL FEATURES

Pathogenesis and Clinical Signs

Transmission of *B. bronchiseptica* occurs primarily by the airborne route, but contact with contaminated fomites and water sources may also be important. The organism is highly contagious. Much of what is known about *B. bronchiseptica* pathogenesis is based on studies of infections in host species other than the dog or cat. *Bordetella bronchiseptica* is inhaled, adheres to respiratory cilia, evades the immune system, and secretes toxins that damage the respiratory epithelium (Figs. 55.1 and 55.2).

Adhesion of virulent strains of *B. bronchiseptica* to respiratory cilia occurs by means of fimbrial adhesins (FIM), a filamentous hemagglutinin (FHA), pertactin, and cell wall LPS. *Bordetella* colonization factor A (BcfA) is another outer membrane protein that appears to be important for tracheal colonization by *B. bronchiseptica*.[33] *Bordetella bronchiseptica* possesses genes that encode for pertussis toxin, an important adhesin in *B. pertussis*.[34] These genes are not expressed *in vitro*, but there is some evidence for pertussis toxin expression *in vivo*.[35]

Evasion of host defenses is mediated by the organism's outer capsular (O) antigens, adenylate cyclase toxin, type III secretion systems, and pertactin. The capsule and O antigen protect it from phagocytosis and destruction by complement. Adenylate cyclase toxin catalyzes the conversion of ATP to cAMP, which inhibits the migration and activation of phagocytes and T cells. Pertactin allows the organism to resist neutrophil-mediated clearance.[36] A type III secretion system was recently described with an *in vitro* model showing that it may prevent phagocytosis by macrophage and induces cellular necrosis.[37] A type VI secretion system also appears to play a key role in persistence of *B. bronchiseptica*.[38] Other virulence determinants present in the outer membrane include LPS and the Brk protein (Bordetella *r*esistance to *k*illing), which allow the organism to resist complement-mediated destruction. At least two other important exotoxins damage respiratory epithelial cells and cells of the immune system, and incite cytokine production: tracheal cytotoxin (TCT) and dermonecrotic toxin (DNT). TLR4 has been shown to play an important role in the innate immune response against *B. bronchiseptica*.[39] The flagellin of *B. bronchiseptica* has been shown to be a potent proinflammatory factor, and can signal through TLR5.[40]

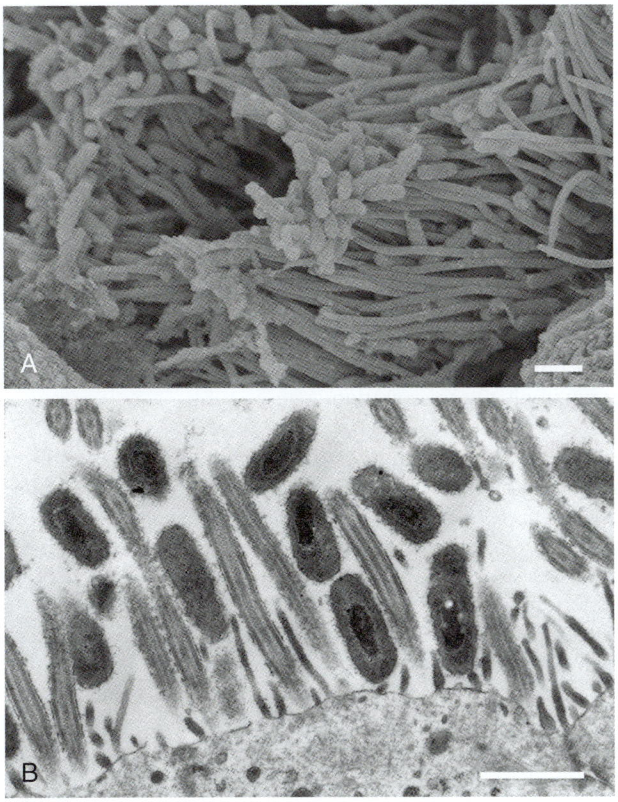

Fig. 55.2 (A) Scanning and (B) transmission electron microscopic images of *Bordetella bronchiseptica* in puppies that died from bronchopneumonia. Numerous piliated bacteria are seen adherent to cilia. (From Chambers JK, Matsumoto I, Shibahara T, et al. *J Comp Pathol.* 2019;167:41–45.)

The inflammation and altered cell function that occur as a result of *B. bronchiseptica* infection lead to increased fluid and mucus secretion, and impairment in host innate immune defenses predisposes to opportunistic viral and bacterial infections. Clinical signs vary in severity and may reflect factors such as the bacterial strain involved, host immunity, and the presence of co-infections. The incubation period ranges from 2 to 10 days. Rhinitis and tracheobronchitis may be associated with serous to mucopurulent nasal discharge, sneezing, stertor, and, especially in dogs, a persistent, often paroxysmal harsh cough. In some dogs, development of bronchopneumonia leads to fever, productive cough, lethargy, and decreased appetite. Bronchopneumonia may be due to *B. bronchiseptica* itself or it may result from co-infection with other respiratory pathogens, such as CDV. An outbreak of fatal *B. bronchiseptica* bronchopneumonia was described in 22 newborn puppies at a breeding facility in Japan; tests for other respiratory pathogens were negative.[41] In cats, infection is significantly associated with sneezing, and cough is uncommon.[19] Cats with pneumonia may develop tachypnea, cyanosis, and death.

Shedding of *B. bronchiseptica* by both dogs and cats can continue intermittently for at least a month and sometimes several months after infection. Evasion of the immune system through survival inside phagocytes may explain the persistent infection that occurs. In contrast, *B. pertussis* is rapidly destroyed by macrophages.[42]

Physical Examination Findings

On physical examination, dogs with uncomplicated bordetellosis are bright, alert, and active with a paroxysmal cough that can occur throughout the examination. The cough is often easily elicited on tracheal or laryngeal palpation. Conjunctivitis and serous to mucopurulent ocular and nasal discharge may be present in affected dogs and cats (Fig. 55.3). Dogs and cats with complicated *Bordetella* bronchopneumonia may be pyrexic, lethargic, and tachypneic with increased respiratory effort.

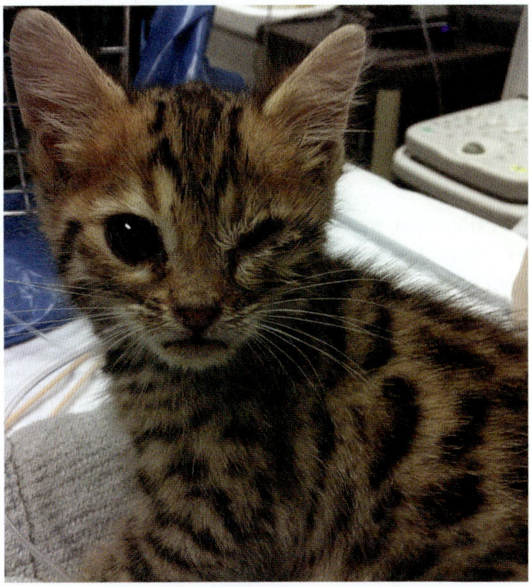

Fig. 55.3 Kitten with *Bordetella bronchiseptica* conjunctivitis and bronchopneumonia. The kitten was tachypneic and had mucopurulent ocular discharge.

There may also be increased lung sounds and/or referred upper airway noises on thoracic auscultation, and mucopurulent nasal discharge.

DIAGNOSIS

Laboratory Abnormalities

There are no specific laboratory abnormalities in uncomplicated bordetellosis. Usually the CBC is normal. Dogs with bronchopneumonia can also have a normal CBC,[26] or a mild to moderate neutrophilia, bandemia, and toxic neutrophils may be present. Cytologic examination of transtracheal lavage (TTL) or bronchoalveolar lavage (BAL) specimens may reveal a suppurative or mixed exudate, and sometimes intracellular and extracellular coccobacilli are visible (Fig. 55.4).

Diagnostic Imaging

Plain Radiography

Plain thoracic radiographs in dogs with uncomplicated bordetellosis may be unremarkable or show a mild diffuse interstitial or bronchointerstitial pattern. *Bordetella* bronchopneumonia may be characterized by development of peribronchial and alveolar infiltrates and lobar consolidation.

Microbiologic Tests

The main assays used for diagnosis of bordetellosis in dogs and cats are aerobic bacterial culture and PCR assays, which can be performed on nasal or oropharyngeal swabs, TTL or BAL specimens, or respiratory tract tissue collected at necropsy (Table 55.2). In some studies, *B. bronchiseptica* has been detected in nasal but not oropharyngeal swabs, but in other studies, the use of oropharyngeal swabs was more sensitive. Collection of swab specimens from the nasal cavity or posterior nasopharynx is preferred for diagnosis of pertussis in humans because these regions have ciliated epithelial cells, for which *B. pertussis* has affinity.[43] False-negative results occur when organism numbers in secretions are low, and depending on the sensitivity of the PCR assay used and the viability of the bacteria in the specimen, culture may be positive when PCR is negative and vice versa. Although the detection of *B. bronchiseptica* in TTL or BAL specimens is diagnostic for bordetellosis, it may be more difficult to interpret the significance of a positive culture or PCR assay result from nasal or oropharyngeal swabs, especially among group-housed dogs and cats when the background prevalence of infection is high. Co-infections with viral respiratory pathogens should always be considered when *B. bronchiseptica* is detected, as well as the presence of other comorbidities that suppress the innate or adaptive immune system that could predispose to bordetellosis (e.g., ciliary dyskinesia or brachycephalic obstructive syndrome in dogs, retroviral infections in cats).

Cytology

In 20 of 24 dogs that were diagnosed with bordetellosis in one study, organisms adherent to respiratory epithelial cilia were noted on cytologic examination of bronchoalveolar lavage fluid (BALF) or bronchial brush fluid (BBF).[44] The identification of bacteria on cytologic examination aided rapid diagnosis and was more sensitive than bacterial culture of BALF. Nevertheless, definitive identification of the bacteria using PCR or culture is still recommended to rule out the presence of other coccobacilli.

Bacterial Culture

Bordetella bronchiseptica can usually be isolated on routine aerobic bacterial culture media, such as MacConkey agar and blood agar.

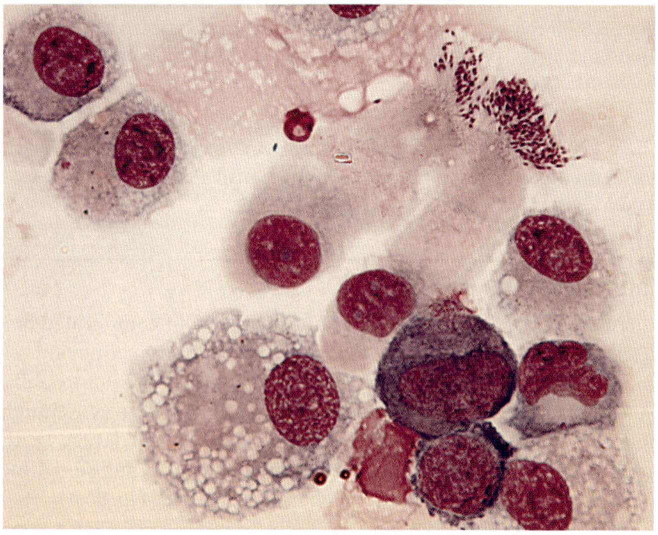

Fig. 55.4 Bronchoalveolar lavage cytology from a dog infected with *Bordetella bronchiseptica*. Numerous coccobacilli are adhered to the cilia of columnar epithelial cells. Wright stain, 1000× oil magnification. (Courtesy of Michael Scott, Michigan State University. In: Raskin RE, Meyer D, eds. *Canine and Feline Cytology: A Color Atlas and Interpretative Guide*. 2nd ed. St. Louis, MO: Saunders; 2010.)

Charcoal-based medium that is supplemented with cephalexin is preferred for isolation of *B. pertussis*, which is more fastidious. For *B. bronchiseptica*, use of methicillin or oxacillin in selective media can prevent overgrowth by contaminating microflora.[5] The laboratory should be informed when bordetellosis is on the differential diagnosis list. In one study, *B. bronchiseptica* was isolated from cats using nasal swabs but not oropharyngeal swabs.[21] The use of Dacron, rayon, or calcium alginate swabs is preferred for culture of *B. pertussis*, because growth is inhibited when cotton swabs are used.[43] Unlike PCR assays, successful detection of *B. bronchiseptica* using culture allows susceptibility testing, which assists in rational antimicrobial drug selection. It is also important to keep in mind that *B. bronchiseptica* can be detected in healthy animals, so its identification in specimens from a single animal does not imply disease causation.

Molecular Diagnosis Using Nucleic Acid–Based Testing

Sensitive and specific real-time PCR assays that detect *B. bronchiseptica* DNA have been described,[18,45] and assays are available through several commercial veterinary diagnostic laboratories. Some laboratories offer panels that also detect other respiratory pathogens, which can be useful for detection of co-infections. In cats, PCR was able to detect *B. bronchiseptica* DNA from conjunctival, nasal, and oropharyngeal swabs using a real-time PCR assay.[17]

As with culture, negative results can occur when organism numbers are low in the specimen, or when there has been recent antimicrobial drug use; however, PCR assays may be more likely to be positive than culture in these situations. Positive PCR assay results can occur for at least 4 weeks after intranasal vaccination.[46,47] A conventional PCR assay that differentiates between field strains and one vaccine strain of *B. bronchiseptica* has been described,[46] but commercially available real-time assays that distinguish between field and vaccine strains are needed. As for culture, the detection of *B. bronchiseptica* using PCR, especially in an individual animal, does not imply disease causation because the organism can be found in healthy animals.

Serologic Diagnosis

Antibodies to *B. bronchiseptica* can be detected using bacterial agglutination or recombinant or whole-cell ELISA assays, but serology is of limited use for diagnosis because of the high prevalence of antibodies in the dog and cat population and the influence of vaccination, which is routinely performed on entry to most shelters. Serology has primarily been used to study the epidemiology of infection and to examine immune responses as they relate to vaccination.

TABLE 55.2 Diagnostic Assays Available for Bordetellosis in Dogs and Cats

Assay	Specimen Type	Target	Performance
Aerobic bacterial culture	Nasal and oropharyngeal swabs, transtracheal and bronchoalveolar lavage specimens, airway and lung specimens collected at necropsy	*B. bronchiseptica*	False negatives can occur when specimens contain no or low numbers of organisms, or after antimicrobial treatment. Allows subsequent susceptibility testing. The clinical significance of positive culture results from nasal and oropharyngeal swab specimens may be difficult to interpret.
PCR assays	See Aerobic bacterial culture	*B. bronchiseptica* DNA	Sensitivity and specificity can vary depending on assay design. False negatives can occur when specimens contain no or low numbers of organisms, or after antimicrobial treatment. Testing specimens from multiple different anatomic sites or combining PCR assays with other diagnostic tests can increase sensitivity. Avirulent live vaccine organisms may be detected for several weeks after intranasal vaccination. Because of subclinical shedding, the clinical significance of a positive result may be difficult to interpret.
Serology	Serum	Antibodies against *Bordetella* antigens	Interpretation complicated by previous vaccination and widespread exposure.

Pathologic Findings

Gross Pathologic Findings

Gross pathologic findings in dogs with uncomplicated bordetellosis are usually minimal. There may be an accumulation of mucopurulent exudate in the airways. In more severely affected patients with *B. bronchiseptica* bronchopneumonia, lesions have been noted most commonly in the cranial and middle lung lobes, but consolidation may be diffuse (Fig. 55.5A). Fibrinous pleural fluid has also been reported in severely affected cats.[48]

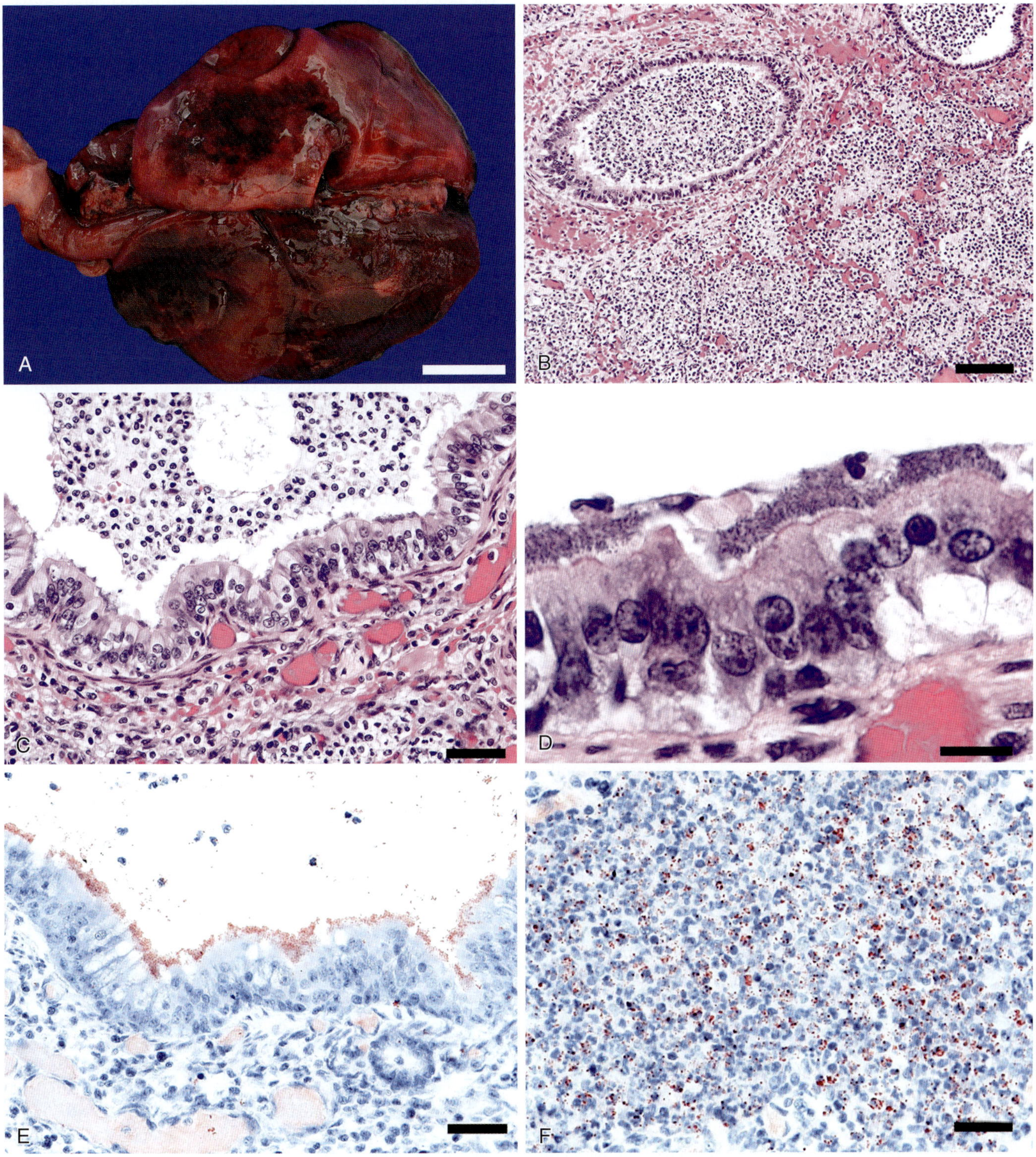

Fig. 55.5 Pathologic findings of *Bordetella bronchiseptica* bronchopneumonia. (A) Diffuse lung congestion. Bar, 1 cm. (B) Severe neutrophilic bronchitis. Bar, 200 μm. (C and D) Basophilic bacteria on the surface of bronchial epithelial cells. Bar, 50 μm (C) 20 μm (D). (E and F) Immunohistochemical staining for *B. bronchiseptica* antigen. Bacteria on the surface of bronchial epithelium, the cytoplasm of inflammatory cells in the bronchus, and bacteria in alveoli stain brown. Bar, 50 μm. (From Chambers JK, Matsumoto I, Shibahara T, et al. An outbreak of fatal *Bordetella bronchiseptica* bronchopneumonia in puppies. *J Comp Pathol.* 2019;167:41–45.)

Histopathologic Findings

Microscopic findings in dogs or cats with bordetellosis consist of a suppurative inflammatory response that is usually confined to the ciliated portions of the respiratory tract (Fig. 55.5B). Cilia are mostly intact, but regional bronchial epithelial necrosis may be present. Mild lymphoid hyperplasia may be present. Depending on the stage and severity of infection, aggregates of bacteria may be observed in association with the cilia (Fig. 55.5C and D).[48,49] IHC can be used to identify bacteria as *B. bronchiseptica* (Fig. 55.5E and F).

TREATMENT AND PROGNOSIS

Antimicrobial Treatment

Bordetella bronchiseptica isolates from dogs and cats have the propensity to exhibit multidrug resistance (i.e., resistance to three or more antimicrobial drug classes). Resistance to amoxicillin and trimethoprim-sulfamethoxazole is common. Widespread resistance to third-generation cephalosporins (cefovecin) has also been documented.[13] Many infections are mild or self-limiting, and so antimicrobial drug treatment should be reserved for animals with confirmed *B. bronchiseptica* infection that have persistent clinical signs (>7 to 10 days) or those with more severe clinical signs and radiographic abnormalities that suggest bronchopneumonia. Young kittens and puppies (<6 to 8 weeks of age) are candidates for early initiation of treatment because disease in neonates may progress rapidly to pneumonia and death. Treatment should be based, whenever possible, on the results of culture and susceptibility testing. When susceptibility results are not available, or when they are pending and bordetellosis is strongly suspected, the initial drug of choice is doxycycline. There is poor susceptibility of *B. bronchiseptica* to penicillins and first-generation cephalosporins, and beta-lactamase production is commonly present.[50,51] At the time of writing, doxycycline resistance is uncommon among isolates from dogs and cats,[52–55] and doxycycline effectively penetrates the lung tissue. Unfortunately, doxycycline is not the best choice for other secondary bacterial pneumonias because it is bacteriostatic, and parenteral doxycycline can be expensive and difficult to administer. This reinforces the need for culture whenever feasible in animals with evidence of pneumonia. Bacterial shedding may continue despite resolution of clinical signs, so affected dogs and cats should remain in isolation from other animals whenever possible for at least 2 months after treatment.

Rarely, treatment with systemic antimicrobial drugs fails to resolve clinical signs of bordetellosis, and the organism persists despite documented susceptibility to the antimicrobial drug selected. In this situation, the use of nebulized aminoglycosides has been suggested. In one retrospective study of 46 dogs with persistent bordetellosis that compared two different protocols for administration of nebulized gentamicin, administration of undiluted 5% gentamicin for 10 minutes q12h for several weeks (median, 4 weeks) appeared to be most efficacious.[56] A pediatric nebulizer was used to deliver the medication either via a face mask (dogs > 10 kg) or use of a cat carrier (dogs < 10 kg) covered with a blanket. The dogs in this study had disease that was refractory to oral antimicrobials, with a median duration of cough before aminoglycoside treatment of 2 months (range, 4 days to 2 years). For 36 dogs in the study, cough had been present since adoption from shelters, pet stores, or kennels. Limitations to this study were the use of historical controls and treatments with a variety of other medications based on clinician preference; because no saline control population was studied, it is possible that some dogs in the study recovered independent of the use of aminoglycosides. No adverse effects of nebulization were noted. However, because nebulization of aminoglycosides has the potential to cause airway irritation and select for resistant bacterial populations, its use should probably be restricted for dogs with refractory bronchopneumonia, or severe and persistent tracheobronchitis (e.g., >4 weeks in duration).

Supportive Care and Prognosis

The prognosis for dogs with uncomplicated bordetellosis is excellent. Cats and dogs with bronchopneumonia usually require other supportive treatments, such as IV fluid therapy, appropriate nutritional support, supplemental oxygen, and nebulization. In one study, bronchopneumonia associated with *B. bronchiseptica* infection was more severe than that associated with other bacterial agents, and affected dogs also had higher $PvCO_2$ values, were more likely to require supplemental oxygen, and had longer mean hospitalization times (7.2 days compared with 4.9 days).[26] In the study of dogs treated with nebulized gentamicin, dogs with a total cell count of less than 1000 cells/μL in BALF were more likely to be cured in 3–4 weeks than dogs with more than 1000 cells/μL.[56] The presence of other co-morbidities may also influence outcome.

IMMUNITY AND VACCINATION

Antibodies to outer surface molecules of *B. bronchiseptica,* especially IgA in mucosal secretions, are important for bacterial clearance. Several avirulent live, mucosal (intranasal or oral) *B. bronchiseptica* vaccines are available for dogs, some of which also contain CPIV with or without CAdV-2. These vaccines are designed to stimulate mucosal immunity and provide protection within 3 days after a single dose of vaccine.[57] Protection with intranasal vaccines also occurs in the face of maternal antibody and can last at least 1 year.[58,59] Inactivated parenteral *B. bronchiseptica* vaccines are also available for dogs, but two doses administered 3 to 4 weeks apart are required to optimize immunity, which occurs 1 week after the second dose. The rapid onset of protection that follows the use of intranasal vaccines makes them the vaccine type of choice for puppies and animals introduced into heavily contaminated environments, such as shelters, when immunization in advance of entry is usually not possible. Mucosal vaccines should not be given to animals treated with antimicrobial drugs (because they inactivate bacteria in the vaccine), and administration of intranasal vaccines to aggressive animals without sedation may not be feasible. Transient signs of mild to moderate respiratory disease occur in a small percentage of vaccinated dogs and cats several days after mucosal vaccination. In shelters, it may not be possible to differentiate between postvaccinal disease and infectious respiratory disease due to field pathogens, which complicates decisions that relate to isolation practices.

Administration of both intranasal and parenteral *B. bronchiseptica* vaccines is followed by the development of both serum IgG and nasal IgA responses, whereas serum IgA responses appear to be higher after intranasal vaccination.[60] Parenteral whole-cell vaccines, and more recently acellular vaccines that include virulence factors such as pertactin, FIM, FHA, and pertussis toxin, are widely used to prevent pertussis in humans.[26] Few scientific data are available on the efficacy of parenteral *B. bronchiseptica* vaccines in dogs when compared with intranasal vaccines. A 2007 study showed that an intranasal vaccine was more effective than a parenteral antigen extract vaccine.[61] In that study, cough scores of subcutaneously vaccinated dogs were not significantly different from placebo-vaccinated dogs. However, parenteral administration of a novel bacterial ghost vaccine, which is composed of the empty cell envelope of gram-negative bacteria, was shown to provide equivalent protection to a commercial parenteral antigen extract *B. bronchiseptica* vaccine (Bronchicine CAe, Zoetis). Use of both vaccines led to significant reduction in cough duration and score when compared with placebo-vaccinated control dogs ($P = .0001$).[62] Two doses of vaccine were given 3 weeks apart, and dogs were challenged 3 weeks later.

In addition, a limited number of studies have been performed that compare protection with oral versus intranasal vaccines. In a 2016 study, it was shown that research dogs vaccinated with an intranasal vaccine showed fewer clinical signs than those vaccinated with an oral vaccine,[63] whereas a more recent study that compared protection following challenge at 7 days after vaccination with an oral and an intranasal vaccine showed that both groups of dogs were equally protected from cough.[64]

Inadvertent parenteral administration of intranasal vaccines has the potential to lead to injection site reactions, hepatic necrosis, and even death in some dogs.[65] Subcutaneous fluids should be administered at the site of vaccination, and immediate treatment with antimicrobial drugs is indicated. It has been suggested that gentamicin sulfate solution be instilled into the affected area (2 to 4 mg/kg gentamicin sulfate in 10 to 30 mL of saline), and dogs should then be treated with oral doxycycline for 5 to 7 days.[66] Special packaging has been developed by some vaccine manufacturers in an attempt to prevent inadvertent parenteral administration of the intranasal vaccine.

Concerns have been raised that intranasal *B. bronchiseptica* vaccines may cause respiratory disease in immunosuppressed humans who inhale the vaccine during administration or who contact vaccine organisms shed by recently immunized dogs or cats.[67–69] However, as yet, there has been no molecular proof that the *B. bronchiseptica* strains isolated from affected human patients match vaccine strains. In fact, in one report of *B. bronchiseptica* pneumonia in an infant that was temporally related to intranasal vaccination of a pet dog, genetic analysis (ribotyping) showed that the vaccine was not the source of the infant's exposure.[70] The organism matched to another *B. bronchiseptica* strain that had previously been isolated from a human patient.

In some countries, intranasal *B. bronchiseptica* vaccines are available for cats, which can reduce signs of disease after challenge as long as 1 year after vaccination.[71] Because disease is rarely severe in cats more than 6 weeks of age, vaccination of cats has not been recommended on a routine basis,[71] but could be considered as an adjunct to management strategies such as reduction of overcrowding and proper disinfection if outbreaks of bordetellosis are a problem in group-housed cats. There is some evidence that vaccination of a FHV and FCV intranasal vaccine can convey some protection against a *B. bronchiseptica* infection.[72] Vaccination of immunocompromised cats is not recommended.[73]

PREVENTION

In the absence of management strategies to reduce stress, overcrowding, and comorbidities, vaccination is unlikely to completely prevent bordetellosis. The reader is referred to the sections on prevention in Chapters 16 (cats) and 17 (dogs) for additional information on prevention and management of outbreaks of respiratory infections in group-housed animals.

PUBLIC HEALTH ASPECTS

Bordetella bronchiseptica is an uncommon cause of respiratory disease in humans, but has been isolated from humans without clinical signs and humans with mild to severe respiratory disease, including pneumonia.[74–76] Most, but not all, affected humans have underlying immunosuppressive conditions that predispose them to infection. *Bordetella bronchiseptica* peritonitis has been reported in human patients receiving continuous peritoneal dialysis.[77,78] Bacteremia and meningitis have also been reported.[79,80] Bacteremia was described in an apparently immunocompetent patient from Greece with COVID-19.[81] Recent exposure to cats and to dogs with signs of "kennel cough" has been noted in most but not all human cases,[75,82] and airborne transmission between humans can occur in hospital settings.[83] At least in mouse models, human acellular pertussis vaccines appear to cross-protect against *B. bronchiseptica*.[84] Infections with *B. bronchiseptica* may be under recognized in people, because the direct fluorescent antibody test used for diagnosis of pertussis may not distinguish between *B. pertussis* and *B. bronchiseptica*. Clinically, recognition of *B. bronchiseptica* infections in humans is important, because *B. bronchiseptica* is resistant to macrolides, which are first-line agents for pertussis.[70] Until more is understood about the risks of canine mucosal *B. bronchiseptica* vaccines for immunocompromised humans, parenteral vaccination of at-risk dogs owned by seriously immunocompromised humans is probably warranted, and the owners of these dogs should be instructed to avoid or minimize situations in which their dogs could come into contact with large numbers of other dogs.

CASE EXAMPLE

Signalment

A 7-week-old intact female Persian kitten from California.

History

A research colony kitten was examined for a 3-day history of respiratory signs. Three days previously, sneezing was observed in this kitten and one of its littermates. A day later, the kitten developed lethargy, inappetence, and respiratory distress, and the littermate was found dead. The kitten had been treated with lactated Ringer's solution (LRS; 6 mL, SC, q24h) and azithromycin suspension (0.7 mg/kg, PO, q24h) since it became unwell. Two other kittens in the litter remained unaffected, and one had mild nasal discharge. All of the cats had tested negative for FeLV antigen and FIV antibody using a commercially available in-house ELISA kit.

Physical Examination

Body weight: 0.37 kg.

General: Alert, open-mouth breathing. T = 97.5°F (36.4°C), HR = 220 beats/minute, RR = 40 breaths/minute, mucous membranes pale pink.

Eyes, ears, nose, and throat: No abnormalities were noted.

Musculoskeletal: BCS 4/9.

Respiratory: Markedly increased inspiratory and expiratory effort, tachypnea, and open-mouth breathing were noted. Increased lung sounds were detected on auscultation.

Cardiovascular, GI, and genitourinary systems, and lymph nodes: No clinically significant abnormalities were detected.

Imaging Findings

Thoracic radiographs: There was collapse of the left cranial lung lobe and partial volume loss in the left caudal lung lobe with evidence of mediastinal shift to the left, possibly secondary to a bronchial mucus plug. A focal increase in opacity was noted in the area of the right middle lung lobe with hyperinflation of the right cranial and caudal lung lobes. There were regions of gas trapping, and the bronchi were enlarged. Emphysema was suspected, possibly congenital. Consolidation in the area of the right middle lung lobe was compatible with pneumonia.

Outcome

The kitten was treated with oxygen supplementation, terbutaline (0.01 mg/kg, SC, q6h), ticarcillin-clavulanate (50 mg/kg, IV, q8h), LRS with 5% dextrose (1 mL/hour

Continued

CASE EXAMPLE—cont'd

IV), a single dose of dexamethasone (1 mg/kg IV), and a single dose of furosemide (2 mg/kg IV). Euthanasia was performed 24 hours later due to lack of improvement and the poor prognosis.

Necropsy Findings

An endotracheal wash was performed immediately after euthanasia. This revealed marked, septic, suppurative inflammation and mild to moderate epithelial hyperplasia. Bacteria were present in large numbers extracellularly, within degenerate neutrophils, and in large mats.

Gross necropsy findings consisted of diffuse lung lobe collapse with multiple firm dark red areas throughout the parenchyma. On histopathology, there was severe, multifocal to coalescing, acute necrosuppurative bronchopneumonia with abundant clusters of gram-negative bacteria. Examination of the upper respiratory tract showed mild, multifocal neutrophilic rhinitis and mild, multifocal, lymphocytic tracheitis. The other kitten was also necropsied, with similar findings.

Microbiologic Testing (Endotracheal Wash Specimen)

Culture for aerobic bacteria, *Mycoplasma* spp., and virus isolation revealed only moderate numbers of *B. bronchiseptica*.

Diagnosis

Bordetella bronchiseptica bronchopneumonia.

Comments

This outbreak of severe bordetellosis in a research cat colony resulted in the death of several kittens, which deteriorated rapidly even in the face of supportive care. Co-infections were not detected, although PCR testing was not performed and the negative *Mycoplasma* culture and virus isolation results did not rule out the possibility of co-infection. Although susceptibility testing was not performed, resistance to the antimicrobials that were used can occur in *B. bronchiseptica*. Furthermore, the dose of azithromycin used as reported in the medical record was subtherapeutic.

LRS: Lactated Ringer's Solution

SUGGESTED READINGS

Berkelman RL. Human illness associated with use of veterinary vaccines. *Clin Infect Dis*. 2003;37:407–414.

Mattoo S, Cherry JD. Molecular pathogenesis, epidemiology, and clinical manifestations of respiratory infections due to *Bordetella pertussis* and other *Bordetella* subspecies. *Clin Microbiol Rev*. 2005;18:326–382.

REFERENCES

1. Ferry NS. Further studies on *Bacillus bronchisepticus*, the cause of canine distemper. *Am Vet Rev*. 1912;61:77–79.
2. Bordet J, Gengou O. Le microbe de la coqueluche. *Ann Inst Pasteur*. 1906;20:731–741.
3. Gross R, Keidel K, Schmitt K. Resemblance and divergence: the "new" members of the genus *Bordetella*. *Med Microbiol Immunol*. 2010;199: 155–163.
4. Diavatopoulos DA, Cummings CA, Schouls LM, et al. *Bordetella pertussis*, the causative agent of whooping cough, evolved from a distinct, human-associated lineage of *B. bronchiseptica*. *PLoS Pathog*. 2005;1:0373–0383.
5. Mattoo S, Cherry JD. Molecular pathogenesis, epidemiology, and clinical manifestations of respiratory infections due to *Bordetella pertussis* and other *Bordetella* subspecies. *Clin Microbiol Rev*. 2005;18:326–382.
6. Belcher KL, Wise DJ, Veit HP. Canine colonization and transmission of *Bordetella pertussis*. *Annals NY Acad Sci*. 2000:687–690.
7. Foley JE, Rand C, Bannasch MJ, et al. Molecular epidemiology of feline bordetellosis in two animal shelters in California, USA. *Prev Vet Med*. 2002;54:141–156.
8. Dawson S, Jones D, McCracken CM, et al. *Bordetella bronchiseptica* infection in cats following contact with infected dogs. *Vet Rec*. 2000;146:46–48.
9. Binns SH, Speakman AJ, Dawson S, et al. The use of pulsed-field gel electrophoresis to examine the epidemiology of *Bordetella bronchiseptica* isolated from cats and other species. *Epidemiol Infect*. 1998;120:201–208.
10. Parkhill J, Sebaihia M, Preston A, et al. Comparative analysis of the genome sequences of *Bordetella pertussis, Bordetella parapertussis* and *Bordetella bronchiseptica*. *Nat Genet*. 2003;35:32–40.
11. Speakman AJ, Binns SH, Osborn AM, et al. Characterization of antibiotic resistance plasmids from *Bordetella bronchiseptica*. *J Antimicrob Chemother*. 1997;40:811–816.
12. Schulz BS, Kurz S, Weber K, et al. Detection of respiratory viruses and *Bordetella bronchiseptica* in dogs with acute respiratory tract infections. *Vet J*. 2014;201:365–369.
13. Walter J, Foley P, Yason C, et al. Prevalence of feline herpesvirus-1, feline calicivirus, *Chlamydia felis*, and *Bordetella bronchiseptica* in a population of shelter cats on Prince Edward Island. *Can J Vet Res*. 2020;84:181–188.
14. Kirilenko NI. Survival of *Bordetella bronchiseptica* in the air and on some objects. *Zh Mikrobiol Epidemiol Immunobiol*. 1965;42:39–42.
15. Crawford S, Weese JS. Efficacy of endotracheal tube disinfection strategies for elimination of *Streptococcus zooepidemicus* and *Bordetella bronchiseptica*. *J Am Vet Med Assoc*. 2015;247:1033–1036.
16. Day MJ, Carey S, Clercx C, et al. Aetiology of canine infectious respiratory disease complex and prevalence of its pathogens in Europe. *J Comp Pathol*. 2020;176:86–108.
17. Litster A, Wu CC, Leutenegger CM. Detection of feline upper respiratory tract disease pathogens using a commercially available real-time PCR test. *Vet J*. 2015;206:149–153.
18. Helps CR, Lait P, Damhuis A, et al. Factors associated with upper respiratory tract disease caused by feline herpesvirus, feline calicivirus, *Chlamydophila felis* and *Bordetella bronchiseptica* in cats: experience from 218 European catteries. *Vet Rec*. 2005;156:669–673.
19. Binns SH, Dawson S, Speakman AJ, et al. Prevalence and risk factors for feline *Bordetella bronchiseptica* infection. *Vet Rec*. 1999;144:575–580.
20. Hoskins JD, Williams J, Roy AF, et al. Isolation and characterization of *Bordetella bronchiseptica* from cats in southern Louisiana. *Vet Immunol Immunopathol*. 1998;65:173–176.
21. Veir JK, Ruch-Gallie R, Spindel ME, et al. Prevalence of selected infectious organisms and comparison of two anatomic sampling sites in shelter cats with upper respiratory tract disease. *J Fel Med Surg*. 2008;10:551–557.
22. Gourkow N, Lawson JH, Hamon SC, et al. Descriptive epidemiology of upper respiratory disease and associated risk factors in cats in an animal shelter in coastal western Canada. *Can Vet J*. 2013;54:132–138.
23. Burns RE, Wagner DC, Leutenegger CM, et al. Histologic and molecular correlation in shelter cats with acute upper respiratory infection. *J Clin Microbiol*. 2011;49:2454–2460.
24. Spindel ME, Veir JK, Radecki SV, et al. Evaluation of pradofloxacin for the treatment of feline rhinitis. *J Fel Med Surg*. 2008;10:472–479.
25. Di Martino B, Di Francesco CE, Meridiani I, et al. Etiological investigation of multiple respiratory infections in cats. *New Microbiol*. 2007;30:455–461.
26. Radhakrishnan A, Drobatz KJ, Culp WTN, et al. Community-acquired infectious pneumonia in puppies: 65 cases (1993-2002). *J Am Vet Med Assoc*. 2007;230:1493–1497.
27. Maboni G, Seguel M, Lorton A, et al. Canine infectious respiratory disease: new insights into the etiology and epidemiology of associated pathogens. *PLoS One*. 2019;14. e0215817.
28. Michael HT, Waterhouse T, Estrada M, et al. Frequency of respiratory pathogens and SARS-CoV-2 in canine and feline samples submitted for respiratory testing in early 2020. *J Small Anim Pract*. 2021;62:336–342.
29. Singleton DA, Stavisky J, Jewell C, et al. Small animal disease surveillance 2019: respiratory disease, antibiotic prescription and canine infectious respiratory disease complex. *Vet Rec*. 2019;184:640–645.

30. Chalker VJ, Toomey C, Opperman S, et al. Respiratory disease in kennelled dogs: Serological responses to *Bordetella bronchiseptica* lipopolysaccharide do not correlate with bacterial isolation or clinical respiratory symptoms. *Clin Diag Lab Immunol.* 2003;10:352–356.
31. Decaro N, Mari V, Larocca V, et al. Molecular surveillance of traditional and emerging pathogens associated with canine infectious respiratory disease. *Vet Microbiol.* 2016;192:21–25.
32. Lavan R, Knesl O. Prevalence of canine infectious respiratory pathogens in asymptomatic dogs presented at US animal shelters. *J Small Anim Pract.* 2015;56:572–576.
33. Sukumar N, Mishra M, Sloan GP, et al. Differential Bvg phase-dependent regulation and combinatorial role in pathogenesis of two *Bordetella* paralogs, BipA and BcfA. *J Bacteriol.* 2007;189:3695–3704.
34. Linz B, Ivanov YV, Preston A, et al. Acquisition and loss of virulence-associated factors during genome evolution and speciation in three clades of *Bordetella* species. *BMC Genom.* 2016;17:767.
35. Stefanelli P, Mastrantonio P, Hausman SZ, et al. Molecular characterization of two *Bordetella bronchiseptica* strains isolated from children with coughs. *J Clin Microbiol.* 1997;35:1550–1555.
36. Inatsuka CS, Xu Q, Vujkovic-Cvijin I, et al. Pertactin is required for *Bordetella* species to resist neutrophil-mediated clearance. *Infect Immun.* 2010;78:2901–2909.
37. Kuwae A, Momose F, Nagamatsu K, et al. BteA secreted from the *Bordetella bronchiseptica* type III secetion system induces necrosis through an actin cytoskeleton signaling pathway and inhibits phagocytosis by macrophages. *PLoS One.* 2016;11:e0148387.
38. Weyrich LS, Rolin OY, Muse SJ, et al. A Type VI secretion system encoding locus is required for *Bordetella bronchiseptica* immunomodulation and persistence in vivo. *PLoS One.* 2012;7.
39. Rolin O, Smallridge W, Henry M, et al. Toll-like receptor 4 limits transmission of *Bordetella bronchiseptica. PLoS One.* 2014;9:e85229.
40. Lopez-Boado YS, Cobb LM, Deora R. *Bordetella bronchiseptica* flagellin is a proinflammatory determinant for airway epithelial cells. *Infect Immun.* 2005;73:7525–7534.
41. Chambers JK, Matsumoto I, Shibahara T, et al. An outbreak of fatal *Bordetella bronchiseptica* bronchopneumonia in puppies. *J Comp Pathol.* 2019;167:41–45.
42. Schneider B, Gross R, Haas A. Phagosome acidification has opposite effects on intracellular survival of *Bordetella pertussis* and *B. bronchiseptica. Infect Immun.* 2000;68:7039–7048.
43. Waters V, Halperin S. *Bordetella bronchiseptica.* Mandell GL, Bennett JE, Dolin R (eds). *Mandell, Douglas, and Bennett's Principles and Practice Of Infectious Diseases.* 7th ed. Churchill Livingstone; 2010:2955–2964.
44. Canonne AM, Billen F, Tual C, et al. Quantitative PCR and cytology of bronchoalveolar lavage fluid in dogs with *Bordetella bronchiseptica* infection. *J Vet Intern Med.* 2016;30:1204–1209.
45. Koidl C, Bozic M, Burmeister A, et al. Detection and differentiation of *Bordetella* spp. by real-time PCR. *J Clin Microbiol.* 2007;45:347–350.
46. Iemura R, Tsukatani R, Micallef MJ, et al. Simultaneous analysis of the nasal shedding kinetics of field and vaccine strains of *Bordetella bronchiseptica. Vet Rec.* 2009;165:747–751.
47. Ruch-Gallie R, Moroff S, Lappin MR. Adenovirus 2, *Bordetella bronchiseptica,* and parainfluenza molecular diagnostic assay results in puppies after vaccination with modified live vaccines. *J Vet Intern Med.* 2016;30:164–166.
48. Taha-Abdelaziz K, Bassel LL, Harness ML, et al. Cilia-associated bacteria in fatal *Bordetella bronchiseptica* pneumonia of dogs and cats. *J Vet Diagn Invest.* 2016;28:369–376.
49. Bemis DA, Greisen HA, Appel MJG. Pathogenesis of canine bordetellosis. *J Infect Dis.* 1977;135:753–762.
50. Prüller S, Rensch U, Meemken D, et al. Antimicrobial susceptibility of *Bordetella bronchiseptica* isolates from swine and companion animals and detection of resistance genes. *PLoS One.* 2015;10:e0135703.
51. Morrissey I, Moyaert H, de Jong A, et al. Antimicrobial susceptibility monitoring of bacterial pathogens isolated from respiratory tract infections in dogs and cats across Europe: ComPath results. *Vet Microbiol.* 2016;191:44–51.
52. Speakman AJ, Binns SH, Dawson S, et al. Antimicrobial susceptibility of *Bordetella bronchiseptica* isolates from cats and a comparison of the agar dilution and E-test methods. *Vet Microbiol.* 1997;54:63–72.
53. Speakman AJ, Dawson S, Corkill JE, et al. Antibiotic susceptibility of canine *Bordetella bronchiseptica* isolates. *Vet Microbiol.* 2000;71:193–200.
54. Johnson LR, Queen EV, Vernau W, et al. Microbiologic and cytologic assessment of bronchoalveolar lavage fluid from dogs with lower respiratory tract infection: 105 cases (2001-2011). *J Vet Intern Med.* 2013;27:259–267.
55. Rheinwald M, Hartmann K, Hähner M, et al. Antibiotic susceptibility of bacterial isolates from 502 dogs with respiratory signs. *Vet Rec.* 2015;176:357.
56. Morgane Canonne A, Roels E, Menard M, et al. Clinical response to 2 protocols of aerosolized gentamicin in 46 dogs with *Bordetella bronchiseptica* infection (2012-2018). *J Vet Intern Med.* 2020;34:2078–2085.
57. Gore T, Headley M, Larris R, et al. Intranasal kennel cough vaccine protecting dogs from experimental *Bordetella bronchiseptica* challenge within 72 hours. *Vet Rec.* 2005;156:482–483.
58. Lehar C, Jayappa H, Erskine J, et al. Demonstration of 1-year duration of immunity for attenuated *Bordetella bronchiseptica* vaccines in dogs. *Vet Ther.* 2008;9:257–262.
59. Jacobs AAC, Theelen RPH, Jaspers R, et al. Protection of dogs for 13 months against *Bordetella bronchiseptica* and canine parainfluenza virus with a modified live vaccine. *Vet Rec.* 2005;157:19–23.
60. Ellis JA, Gow SP, Lee LB, et al. Comparative efficacy of intranasal and injectable vaccines in stimulating *Bordetella bronchiseptica*-reactive anamnestic antibody responses in household dogs. *Can Vet J.* 2017;58:809–815.
61. Davis R, Jayappa H, Abdelmagid OY, et al. Comparison of the mucosal immune response in dogs vaccinated with either an intranasal avirulent live culture or a subcutaneous antigen extract vaccine of *Bordetella bronchiseptica. Vet Ther.* 2007;8:32–40.
62. Muhammad A, Kassmannhuber J, Rauscher M, et al. Subcutaneous immunization of dogs with *Bordetella bronchiseptica* bacterial ghost vaccine. *Front Immunol.* 2019;10:1377.
63. Ellis JA, Gow SP, Waldner CL, et al. Comparative efficacy of intranasal and oral vaccines against *Bordetella bronchiseptica* in dogs. *Vet J.* 2016;212:71–77.
64. Scott-Garrard MM, Chiang YW, David F. Comparative onset of immunity of oral and intranasal vaccines against challenge with *Bordetella bronchiseptica. Vet Rec Open.* 2018;5:e000285.
65. Toshach K, Jackson MW, Dubielzig RR. Hepatocellular necrosis associated with the subcutaneous injection of an intranasal *Bordetella bronchiseptica*-canine parainfluenza vaccine. *J Am Anim Hosp Assoc.* 1997;33:126–128.
66. Larson LJ, Newbury S, Schultz RD. Canine and feline vaccinations and immunology. In: Miller L, Hurley K (eds). *Infectious Disease Management in Animal Shelters.* Ames, IA: Wiley Blackwell; 2009:61–82.
67. Gisel JJ, Brumble LM, Johnson MM. *Bordetella bronchiseptica* pneumonia in a kidney-pancreas transplant patient after exposure to recently vaccinated dogs: case report. *Transplant Infect Disease.* 2010;12:73–76.
68. Berkelman RL. Human illness associated with use of veterinary vaccines. *Clin Infect Dis.* 2003;37:407–414.
69. Moore JE, Rendall JC, Millar BC. A doggy tale: risk of zoonotic infection with *Bordetella bronchiseptica* for cystic fibrosis (CF) patients from live licenced bacterial veterinary vaccines for cats and dogs. *J Clin Pharm Ther.* 2021. Jul 30. Online ahead of print.
70. Rath BA, Register KB, Wall J, et al. Persistent *Bordetella bronchiseptica* pneumonia in an immunocompetent infant and genetic comparison of clinical isolates with kennel cough vaccine strains. *Clin Infect Dis.* 2008;46:905–908.
71. Williams J, Laris R, Gray AW, et al. Studies of the efficacy of a novel intranasal vaccine against feline bordetellosis. *Vet Rec.* 2002;150:439–442.
72. Bradley A, Kinyon J, Frana T, et al. Efficacy of intranasal administration of a modified live feline herpesvirus 1 and feline calicivirus vaccine against disease caused by *Bordetella bronchiseptica* after experimental challenge. *J Vet Intern Med.* 2012;26:1121–1125.
73. Egberink H, Addie D, Belák S, et al. *Bordetella bronchiseptica* infection in cats ABCD guidelines on prevention and management. *J Fel Med Surg.* 2009;11:610–614.

74. Washington MA, Agee WA, Kajiura L, et al. A case of *Bordetella bronchiseptica* at a military medical facility in Hawai'i: phenotypic and molecular testing of an uncommon human pathogen. *Hawai'i J Med Public Health.* 2015;74:230–233.
75. Wernli D, Emonet S, Schrenzel J, et al. Evaluation of eight cases of confirmed *Bordetella bronchiseptica* infection and colonization over a 15-year period. *Clin Microbiol Infect.* 2011;17:201–203.
76. Clements J, McGrath C, McAllister C. *Bordetella bronchiseptica* pneumonia: beware of the dog! *BMJ Case Rep.* 2018;2018.
77. Hadley K, Torres AM, Moran J, et al. *Bordetella bronchiseptica* peritonitis - beware of the dog! *Perit Dial Int.* 2009;29:670–671.
78. Byrd LH, Anama L, Gutkin M, et al. *Bordetella bronchiseptica* peritonitis associated with continuous ambulatory peritoneal dialysis. *J Clin Microbiol.* 1981;14:232–233.
79. Woolfrey BF, Moody JA. Human infections associated with *Bordetella bronchiseptica. Clin Microbiol Rev.* 1991;4:243–255.
80. Powers HR, Shah K. *Bordetella bronchiseptica* bloodstream infection in a renal transplant patient. *Transpl Infect Dis.* 2017;19.
81. Papantoniou S, Tsakiris A, Ladopoulos T, et al. A case of *Bordetella bronchiseptica* bacteremia in a patient with COVID-19: brief report. *Cureus.* 2021;13:e15976.
82. Goldberg JD, Kamboj M, Ford R, et al. "Kennel cough" in a patient following allogeneic hematopoietic stem cell transplant. *Bone Marrow Transplant.* 2009;44:381–382.
83. Huebner ES, Christman B, Dummer S, et al. Hospital-acquired *Bordetella bronchiseptica* infection following hematopoietic stem cell transplantation. *J Clin Microbiol.* 2006;44:2581–2583.
84. Goebel EM, Zhang X, Harvill ET. *Bordetella bronchiseptica* infection or vaccination substantially protects mice against *B. bronchiseptica* infection. *PLoS One.* 2009;4.

56

L-Form Infections

Victoria J. Chalker

KEY POINTS

- First Described: In 1935, London (Klieneberger).[1]
- Causes: Cell wall-deficient variants of a variety of gram-positive and gram-negative bacteria.
- Geographic Distribution: Worldwide.
- Major Clinical Signs: Chronic draining or ulcerated soft tissue and skin lesions, polyarthritis, possibly other chronic pyogenic and pyogranulomatous lesions.
- Differential Diagnoses: Infections due to other fastidious bacteria such as *Mycoplasma*, *Nocardia*, *Mycobacterium*, *Bartonella*, and *Brucella* spp., nutritionally variant streptococci such as *Granulicatella*, *Borrelia burgdorferi* (in the case of polyarthritis); fungal infections (e.g., due to *Sporothrix* or *Coccidioides* spp.); persistence of a foreign body; neoplasia; congenital immunodeficiency; primary immune-mediated disease.
- Human Health Significance: Likely similar to that for the corresponding walled (or "normal") variant of the bacterial species involved.

ETIOLOGY AND EPIDEMIOLOGY

L-forms of bacteria, also known as cell wall-deficient bacteria, are morphologically similar to mycoplasmas. They are distinguishable from the latter by the variable size (1 to 4 μm diameter), their greater pleomorphism, and their penicillin-binding affinities. In addition, *Mycoplasma* spp. do not originate from bacteria that normally possess a cell wall. The term L-form was given to these bacteria because they were first discovered at the Lister Institute in London. Cell wall deficiencies can be induced *in vitro* or *in vivo* in many bacterial species (Box 56.1) through a variety of stressors, including exposure to chemicals that damage the cell wall, antimicrobials (e.g. beta-lactam drugs, and more rapidly with fosfomycin and D-cycloserine) or host immune responses.[2,3] The molecular events in the host that result in conversion to and from the L-form state are yet to be accurately defined. Proliferation of L-form bacteria occurs via an increased rate of membrane synthesis.[4] Lysozyme is found throughout the animal kingdom, produced by macrophages and can drive L-form formation, contributing to antibacterial intolerance (Fig. 56.1).[3] Once inside the host, L-forms can persist and remain viable, proliferating in the presence of antimicrobial drugs. On cessation of antimicrobial drug treatment they can revert to the walled state that can presumably cause further infection.[5–7]

CLINICAL FEATURES

In human patients, L-form bacteria have been implicated as causes of a variety of clinical syndromes that include culture-negative endocarditis, bacteremia, uveitis, pneumonia, osteomyelitis and arthritis, recurrent UTIs, soft tissue infections, and meningitis.[8–10] There are few reports of L-form infection in the literature in dogs and cats, and this area is understudied. The role of L-forms in chronic or recurrent infections is controversial. Demonstration of internalization, persistence, and potential for contribution to chronic infections has been demonstrated in infected rats.[11]

Cell wall-deficient bacteria have been isolated from cats with fever and persistently draining, spreading cellulitis and synovitis that often involve the extremities.[12,13] The usual source of infection has been contamination of penetrating bite wounds or surgical incisions. Infection begins at the point of inoculation and lesions spread, drain, dehisce, and do not heal. Bacteremia can occur and polyarthritis or distant abscess formation may develop as a sequela. Progressive polyarthritis that was unresponsive to antibacterials and glucocorticoids occurred in a dog infected with an L-form of *Nocardia*.[14] A *Pseudomonas aeruginosa* L-form was isolated from the blood of a dog after antibiotic treatment for *P. aeruginosa* endocarditis.[15]

DIAGNOSIS

Infection with L-forms should be considered a possibility in cats and dogs with culture-negative pyogranulomatous or suppurative inflammatory lesions, or when a bacterial etiology is suspected on the basis of clinical

BOX 56.1 Examples of Medically Important Bacteria That May Become Cell Wall-Deficient When Subjected to Appropriate Stressors

Actinomyces spp.
Enterococcus spp.
Escherichia coli
Bacillus spp.
Borrelia burgdorferi (also *Borreliella burgdorferi*)
Brucella spp.
Corynebacterium spp.
Lactobacillus spp.
Leptospira interrogans
Mycobacterium spp.
Nocardia spp.
Serratia marcescens
Pasteurella multocida
Pseudomonas aeruginosa
Proteus mirabilis
Salmonella typhimurium
Staphylococcus spp.
Streptococcus spp.

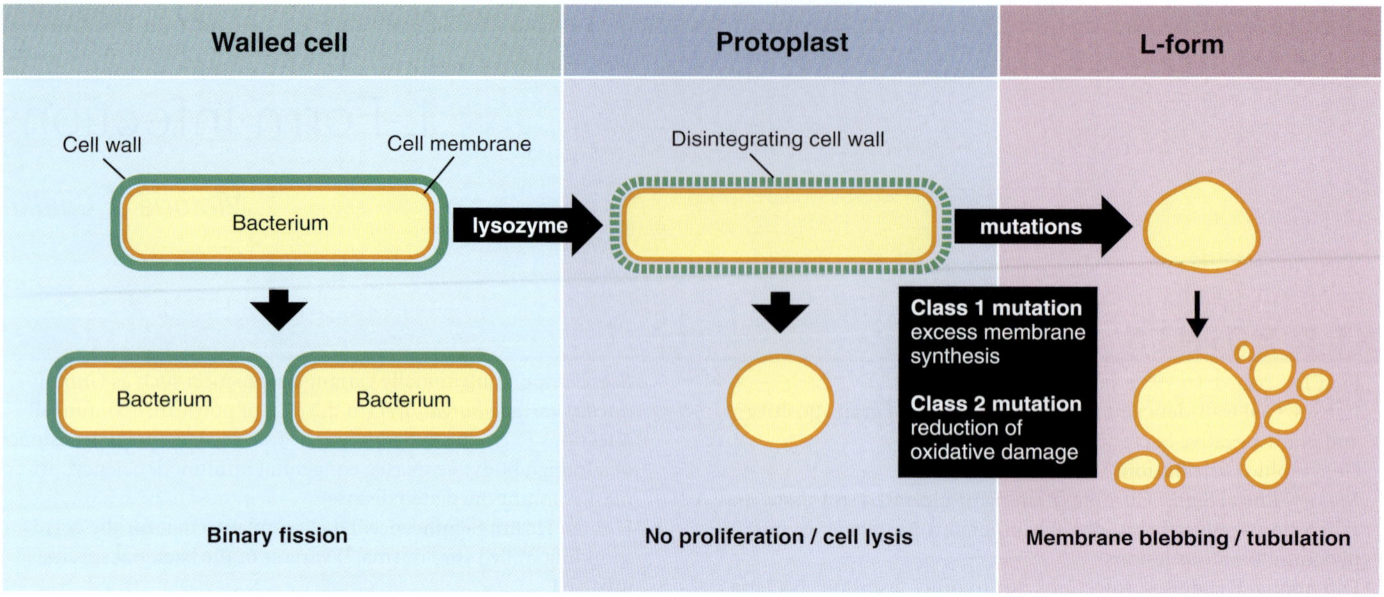

Fig. 56.1 Formation of L-form bacteria from walled bacterial cells. Walled cells of rod-shaped bacteria typically grow by elongation. Lysozyme removes the cell wall, with formation of protoplasts, but these are unable to grow due to oxidative damage. Subsequent mutations can allow the cell to grow as an L-form. (Adapted from Errington J, Mickiewicz K, Kawai Y, Wu LJ. L-form bacteria, chronic diseases and the origins of life. *Philos Trans R Soc B Biol Sci.* 2016;371:20150494.)

TABLE 56.1 Assays Available for Diagnosis of L-Form Bacterial Infections in Dogs and Cats

Assay	Specimen Type	Target	Performance
Culture	Biopsies, body fluids, wash specimens	L-form bacteria	Requires special L-form bacterial (hyperosmolar) media
Cytology or histopathology	Biopsies, smears of affected tissues	L-form bacteria	Organisms usually not visible owing to the lack of a cell wall, but may be Gram-variable. Low sensitivity and cannot be used to identify absence of a cell wall (although the presence of organisms that stain strongly with Gram stain indicates the presence of walled bacteria).
Electron microscopy	Biopsies	L-form bacteria	Confirms the presence of cell wall-deficient organisms in lesions. May not be possible to distinguish L-form bacteria from *Mycoplasma* spp. Often expensive and not readily available for routine diagnostic purposes.
Broad-range bacterial PCR and sequencing	Biopsies, body fluids, wash specimens	16S ribosomal subunit DNA of L-form bacteria	Confirms presence of bacteria in lesions when culture is negative. False positives may occur if contaminating bacteria are present. Does not distinguish between L-form bacteria and their walled counterparts. Sensitivity and specificity may vary between assays.

signs but routine cultures are negative. Physical examination and laboratory findings in cats and dogs infected with L-form bacteria may be similar to those in cats and dogs with other chronic, persistent bacterial infections.

Clinical laboratory abnormalities in cats with polyarthritis may include leukocytosis (over 25,000 cells/μL) with a mature neutrophilia and monocytosis, lymphocytosis, and eosinophilia.[12] Hyperfibrinogenemia and hyperglobulinemia may be found. Exudates contain predominantly macrophages and neutrophils with a few lymphocytes. Erythrophagia may be present; organisms cannot be detected by numerous cytologic stains. Radiographic abnormalities include periarticular soft tissue swelling and periosteal perforation.[12] In severe cases, damage occurs to the articular cartilage and subchondral bone.

Definitive diagnosis of L-form infection is difficult because the organisms are not visible using light microscopy and passage through special hypertonic laboratory media is required for growth of the organisms in culture. Traditional culture techniques may be negative. Infection has been transmitted experimentally by subcutaneous inoculation with cell-free material from tissues or exudates of infected cats. Other diagnostic tests are summarized in Table 56.1. Electron microscopic evaluation of tissues may show the characteristically pleomorphic, cell wall-deficient organisms in phagocytes (Fig. 56.2). The use of broad-range bacterial PCR assays that detect bacterial 16S ribosomal subunit DNA or metagenomics in tissues may be useful to detect L-form bacteria in tissues in the future when routine culture methods are negative, although this method does not distinguish between L-form bacteria and their walled counterparts. Infection with L-forms may also be suspected when lesions resolve in association with tetracycline antimicrobial drug treatment.

TREATMENT AND PROGNOSIS

Cell wall-deficient organisms found in cats have historically been most responsive to tetracyclines such as doxycycline; however, additional choices include macrolides, lincosamides, azalides, chloramphenicol, and fluoroquinolones. They are characteristically resistant to cell wall synthesis inhibitors such as the beta-lactam antibacterials or many other

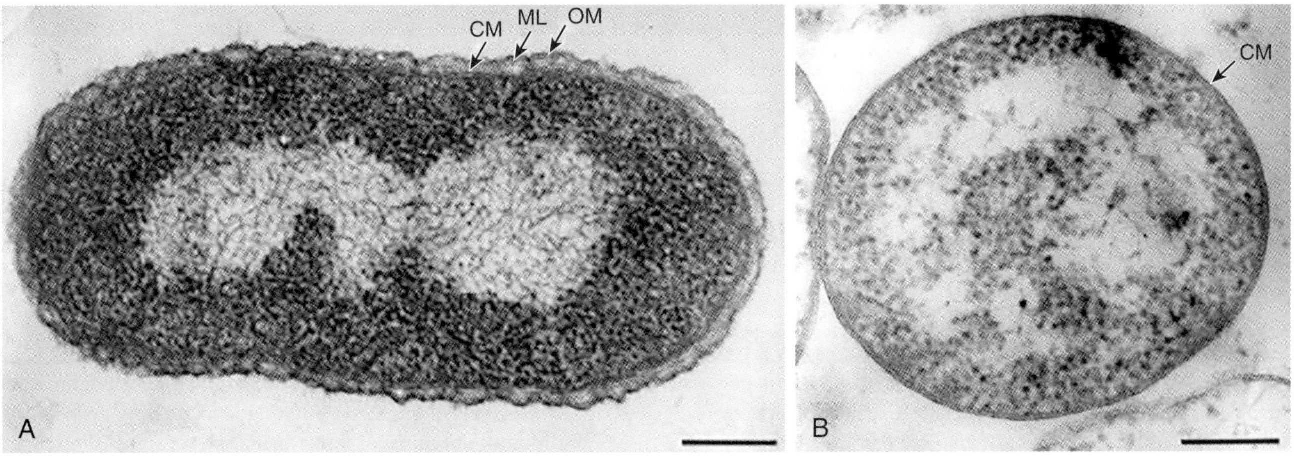

Fig. 56.2 Ultrathin sections of a cell of the N-form *Proteus mirabilis* VI (A) and its derived protoplast-type L-form *P. mirabilis* LVI (B). *CM*, cytoplasmic membrane; *ML*, peptidoglycan layer; *OM*, outer membrane. Bar: 0.2 μm. (From Allan, EJ, Hoischen, C, Gumpert, J. Bacterial L-Forms. *Advances in Applied Microbiology*. Volume 68, 2009; pp. 1–39. Copyright © 2009 Elsevier Inc. All rights reserved.)

broad-spectrum antimicrobials often chosen for persistent multifocal infections. Response to therapy should occur within 2 days, and therapy should continue for at least 1 week after discharges have stopped.[12,13]

PUBLIC HEALTH ASPECTS

The public health risk of L-form infections in dogs and cats is uncertain, because not all of the cell wall-deficient organisms have been adequately characterized. Instances of L-form infections in people are rare. A single report described isolation of an L-form of *Streptococcus sanguinis* from a vascular graft of a hemodialysis patient.[16] The L-form isolate was characterized as *S. sanguinis* of animal origin. The affected person's pet dog was reported to often lick the graft site, and *S. sanguinis* was also isolated from the dog's oral cavity. Although this was suggestive of zoonotic transmission, the identity of the isolates was not confirmed with molecular methods. L-form infections are not often considered or reported and the true extent of infections attributed to L-forms in humans and animals is not known.

SUGGESTED READINGS

Carro T, Pedersen NC, Beaman BL, et al. Subcutaneous abscesses and arthritis caused by a probable bacterial L-form in cats. *J Am Vet Med Assoc*. 1989;194:1583–1588.

Chmel H. Graft infection and bacteremia with a tolerant L-form of *Streptococcus sanguis* in a patient receiving hemodialysis. *J Clin Microbiol*. 1986;24:294–295.

REFERENCES

1. Kleineberger E. The natural occurrence of pleuropneumonia-like organisms in apparent symbiosis with *Streptobacillus moniliformis* and other bacteria. *J Pathol Bacteriol*. 1935;40:93–105.
2. Claessen D, Errington J. Cell wall deficiency as a coping strategy for stress. *Trends Microbiol*. 2019;27:1025–1033.
3. Kawai Y, Mickiewicz K, Errington J. Lysozyme counteracts beta-lactam antibiotics by promoting the emergence of L-form bacteria. *Cell*. 2018;172:1038–1049, e1010.
4. Mercier R, Kawai Y, Errington J. Excess membrane synthesis drives a primitive mode of cell proliferation. *Cell*. 2013;152:997–1007.
5. Domingue GJ,S, Woody HB. Bacterial persistence and expression of disease. *Clin Microbiol Rev*. 1997;10:320–344.
6. Mercier R, Kawai Y, Errington J. General principles for the formation and proliferation of a wall-free (L-form) state in bacteria. *Elife*. 2014;3.
7. Kawai Y, Mercier R, Errington J. Bacterial cell morphogenesis does not require a preexisting template structure. *Curr Biol*. 2014;24:863–867.
8. Markova ND. L-form bacteria cohabitants in human blood: significance for health and diseases. *Discov Med*. 2017;23:305–313.
9. Mickiewicz KM, Kawai Y, Drage L, et al. Author Correction: Possible role of L-form switching in recurrent urinary tract infection. *Nat Commun*. 2019;10:5254.
10. Onwuamaegbu ME, Belcher RA, Soare C. Cell wall-deficient bacteria as a cause of infections: a review of the clinical significance. *J Int Med Res*. 2005;33:1–20.
11. Michailova L, Kussovsky V, Radoucheva T, et al. Persistence of *Staphylococcus aureus* L-form during experimental lung infection in rats. *FEMS Microbiol Lett*. 2007;268:88–97.
12. Carro T, Pedersen NC, Beaman BL, et al. Subcutaneous abscesses and arthritis caused by a probable bacterial L-form in cats. *J Am Vet Med Assoc*. 1989;194:1583–1588.
13. Keane DP. Chronic abscesses in cats associated with an organism resembling *Mycoplasma*. *Can Vet J*. 1983;24:289–291.
14. Buchanan AM, Beaman BL, Pedersen NC, et al. *Nocardia asteroides* recovery from a dog with steroid- and antibiotic-unresponsive idiopathic polyarthritis. *J Clin Microbiol*. 1983;18:702–708.
15. Bone WJ. L-form of *Pseudomonas aeruginosa* the etiologic agent of bacterial endocarditis in a dog. *Vet Med Small Anim Clin*. 1970;65:224–227.
16. Chmel H. Graft infection and bacteremia with a tolerant L-form of *Streptococcus sanguis* in a patient receiving hemodialysis. *J Clin Microbiol*. 1986;24:294–295.

57

Mycoplasma Infections

Victoria J. Chalker, Jane E. Sykes

KEY POINTS

- First Described: Dogs, 1934 (Shoetensack, 1934).[1] Reports of human *Mycoplasma* infections also occurred around this time.[2]
- Causes: *Mycoplasma cynos* and *Mycoplasma felis* have been most commonly associated with disease, but many other mycoplasma species infect dogs and cats.
- Geographic Distribution: Worldwide.
- Mode of Transmission: Direct contact (respiratory/sexual), fomite transmission in overcrowded environments. Opportunistic invasion of commensal mycoplasmas also occurs.
- Major Clinical Signs: Conjunctivitis, sneezing, and nasal discharge (cats); cough, tachypnea, fever, weight loss (lower respiratory disease); swollen, painful joints (polyarthritis); subcutaneous abscesses; neurologic signs (meningoencephalitis); prostatitis, epididymitis-orchitis, or lower urinary tract signs (dogs).
- Differential diagnoses: Other gram-positive and gram-negative bacterial infections. Differential diagnoses for mycoplasma respiratory disease include viral infections, fungal and parasitic causes of pneumonia, aspiration pneumonia, and neoplasia.
- Human health significance: Canine and feline mycoplasma species have rarely been detected in immunocompromised humans with mycoplasmosis who have had contact with pet cats and dogs.

ETIOLOGIC AGENT AND EPIDEMIOLOGY

Mycoplasmas are fastidious bacteria that lack a cell wall. They belong to the class Mollicutes (which translates to "soft skin") and are the smallest known free-living organisms. Many require sterols for growth, and *Ureaplasma* species require urea for fermentation. They measure only 0.3 to 0.8 μm in size. More than 120 different species of *Mycoplasma* and 7 species of *Ureaplasma* have been identified. The range of mycoplasma species that infect dogs and cats is incompletely understood because precise species identification has been difficult (Box 57.1).[3–8] Additional mycoplasma species are likely to be discovered with the application of molecular methods in the future. Some *Mycoplasma* spp. infect multiple host species. Mycoplasmas are often difficult to grow on cell-free media, and some, such as the hemotropic mycoplasmas, have never been successfully cultured in the laboratory (see Chapter 58). The remainder of this chapter will refer only to the non-hemotropic mycoplasma species.

Mycoplasmas are commensal bacteria that are found widely in association with mucous membranes of all mammalian species. Simultaneous colonization with more than one *Mycoplasma* species is common. Mycoplasmas have also been associated with keratoconjunctivitis and/or URTD in cats; reproductive disease and UTIs in dogs; and lower respiratory tract disease, skin and soft tissue infections, meningoencephalitis, and arthritis in both cats and dogs (Box 57.2).[9–20] Because mycoplasmas are commonly isolated from the upper respiratory and genital tracts of healthy dogs and cats, their role in ocular, URTD, and urogenital tract disease has been difficult to determine. Several studies have now found an increased prevalence of mycoplasmas in cats with conjunctivitis or URTD when compared with healthy cats.[15,21,22] Mycoplasmas may act as secondary invaders when other pathogenic viruses and bacteria are present, or normal host defenses are impaired by other factors, such as underlying neoplasia or immunosuppressive drug therapy. When mycoplasmas are associated with systemic disease or pneumonia, young animals (less than 1 year of age) are often involved. Some mycoplasma species appear to be more pathogenic than others. For example, evidence has accumulated that *Mycoplasma cynos* is associated with lower respiratory tract disease in dogs, whereas *Mycoplasma canis* and *Mycoplasma edwardii* are not.[9,23,24] In one study, *M. cynos* infection was associated with increased severity of canine infectious respiratory disease (CIRD), younger age, and longer time spent in a kennel.[24] Experimental infection with *M. cynos* leads to respiratory disease in dogs, but infection with *Mycoplasma gateae, M. canis,* and *Mycoplasma spumans* does not.[25] CIRD clinical score with *M. canis* infection is significantly lower in dogs than that for *M. cynos* infection.[26] Cases with co-infection are more likely to develop severe clinical signs, and *M. cynos*, canine parainfluenza virus (CPIV), *M. canis*, and *Bordetella bronchiseptica* are the most common pathogens seen, with *M. cynos* and CPIV being the most frequent pathogen combination, with stronger association than with *B. bronchiseptica*.[26] The same authors found young age to be the most significant predictor of severity.[26] The role of mycoplasmas in feline lower urinary tract disease and lymphoplasmacytic pododermatitis has also been investigated using molecular techniques, but no association was found.[27,28]

CLINICAL FEATURES

Pathogenesis and Clinical Signs

In order to colonize mammalian hosts, mycoplasmas must adhere to host cells. *M. cynos* possesses an adhesin, HapA, that confers cytadherance.[29] Neuraminidases are present in dog and cat mycoplasmas, which may play a role in pathogenesis.[30] A number of pathogenic mycoplasma species of humans can invade cells, which may contribute to organism persistence and difficulties associated with isolation in the laboratory. Transmission of pathogenic mycoplasmas such as *M. cynos* may occur in overcrowded environments as a result of close contact or fomite spread. The finding of identical strains in multiple dogs from a kennel environment (by use of molecular typing methods) supports the concept of transmission between dogs in this environment.[31] The extent to which mycoplasmas can survive in the environment varies between mycoplasma species and has not been determined for mycoplasmas that infect dogs and cats.

BOX 57.1 Non-hemotropic Mycoplasma and Ureaplasma Species Infecting Dogs and Cats[3–8]

Dogs	Cats
M. cynos	*M. felis*
M. canis	*M. gateae*
M. molare	*M. arginini*
M. arginini	*M. feliminutum*
M. bovigenitalium	*M. canadense*[a]
M. edwardii	*M. cynos*[a]
M. feliminutum	*M. lipophilum*[a]
M. felis	*M. hyopharyngis*[a]
M. gateae	*U. felinum*
M. maculosum	*U. cati*
M. mucosicanis	*Acholeplasma laidlawaii*
M. opalescens	
M. spumans	
M. rosendalii (*M. mucosicanis*, HRC689)	
M. sp. VJC358	
U. canigenitalium	
Acholeplasma laidlawii	

[a] Identified on the basis of DNA sequencing of small segments of the 16S rRNA gene; sequence analysis of longer fragments may reveal these are in fact other mycoplasma species.

BOX 57.2 Diseases Associated with Mycoplasma Infections in Dogs and Cats

Disease	Species affected
Conjunctivitis	Cats
Upper respiratory tract disease	Cats
Pyothorax	Cats
Bronchopneumonia	Dogs, cats
Skin and soft tissue infections (abscesses)	Dogs, cats
Meningoencephalitis	Dogs, cats
Polyarthritis	Dogs, cats
Urinary tract infections	Dogs
Prostatitis	Dogs
Epididymitis and orchitis	Dogs

Conjunctivitis and Upper Respiratory Tract Disease

Mycoplasma spp. are commonly detected in cats in association with conjunctivitis and URTD. Concurrent infections with other upper respiratory pathogens (such as *B. bronchiseptica, Chlamydia felis*, and feline respiratory viruses) may contribute to clinical signs. Stressors such as overcrowding and unhygienic conditions may also promote proliferation of mycoplasmas and their transmission among cats. Ulcerative keratitis has been reported in association with mycoplasma infection, although the presence of corneal involvement may reflect the concurrent presence of FHV-1 or other factors that predispose to secondary invasion by *Mycoplasma* spp. (Fig. 57.1).

Pneumonia and Pyothorax

Virtually all dogs and cats can harbor mycoplasmas in their upper respiratory tract. Fewer than 25% of healthy dogs harbor mycoplasmas in their

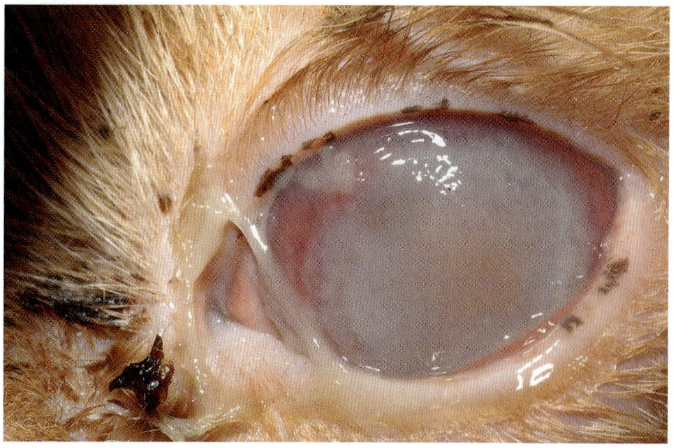

Fig. 57.1 Ulcerative keratitis in a 4-year-old female spayed Persian. Involvement of feline herpesvirus-1 was suspected, and *Mycoplasma* spp. was isolated from a corneal swab. The significance of the mycoplasma infection was unclear, but the ulcer healed after topical treatment with topical ofloxacin and azithromycin drops. (Image courtesy of the University of California, Davis Veterinary Ophthalmology service.)

trachea or lungs. In one study, mycoplasmas were detected in tracheobronchial lavage specimens from 21% of 28 cats with pulmonary disease, but not from 18 healthy cats.[32,33] Mycoplasmas may be isolated from the lower airways and lungs of dogs and cats with pneumonia, sometimes in pure culture.[34] Factors that predispose to the development of pneumonia are not always apparent.[35] Clinical signs of pneumonia are not specific for mycoplasma infection and include variable fever, cough, tachypnea, lethargy, and decreased appetite. Concurrent signs of URTD have been reported in some affected cats.[35] Rarely, mycoplasmas have been cultured from the pleural fluid of cats and dogs with pyothorax, both in pure culture as well as in mixed infections with other organisms.[36–38]

Urogenital Tract

Mycoplasma and *Ureaplasma* spp. have been found in the semen and urine of dogs with infertility and purulent epididymitis.[39] The role of mycoplasmas in reproductive tract disease in dogs and cats is unclear because of their frequent isolation from the urogenital tract of healthy dogs and cats. Large numbers of mycoplasmas (>10^5 CFU/mL) can occasionally be isolated in pure culture from urine collected by cystocentesis from dogs with prostatitis and LUTS.[16,39] Dogs with mycoplasma UTIs often have other comorbidities that impair normal urinary defenses, such as urinary tract neoplasia, calculi, or neurologic disease.[16]

Arthritis and Bacteremia

Isolated case reports of polyarthritis exist as a result of *M. spumans* and *M. edwardii* infections in dogs, and *M. gateae* and *Mycoplasma felis* infections in cats. Synovial fluid analysis usually reveals the presence of large numbers of neutrophils. This may lead to diagnostic confusion with primary immune-mediated polyarthritis. Systemic signs such as lethargy, fever, and inappetence usually accompany lameness. Evidence of immune compromise, such as underlying neoplasia or surgery, young age, or a history of glucocorticoid treatment, has generally been present in dogs and cats with mycoplasma polyarthritis. *Mycoplasma felis* has also been isolated from cats with monoarthritis, possibly secondary to bite wound infections.[19]

Meningoencephalitis

Mycoplasmas may gain access to the CNS as a result of penetrating wounds, ascending infection from the middle ear, or hematogenous spread. Meningoencephalitis associated with *M. felis* infection was described in a 10-month-old cat that showed signs of lethargy, fever, a head tilt, nystagmus, and tetraparesis.[14] *Mycoplasma felis* was isolated in pure culture from the CSF. The cat also had evidence of otitis media-interna at necropsy, but the role this played in development of the mycoplasma infection was unclear. *Mycoplasma edwardii* was isolated from the brain of a 6-week-old dog with a sudden onset of seizures.[10] Suppurative and histiocytic meningitis was detected at necropsy in conjunction with evidence of a possible penetrating wound to the skull. Infection with *M. canis* has been associated with some cases of granulomatous meningoencephalomyelitis and necrotizing meningoencephalitis in dogs, which requires further study.[40]

Physical Examination Findings

Physical examination findings in dogs and cats with mycoplasma infections depend on the organ affected, as well as underlying disease processes that facilitate opportunistic invasion by mycoplasmas. Ocular infections in cats are characterized by serous to mucopurulent ocular discharge, conjunctival hyperemia, and possibly keratitis. Upper respiratory tract infections may result in nasal discharge and sneezing, with or without conjunctivitis. Fever, tachypnea, and increased lung sounds may be present with pneumonia. Urinary tract infections may lead to clinical signs of lower urinary tract disease, such as hematuria or stranguria. *Mycoplasma* arthritis may be manifested by fever, joint pain and swelling, and sometimes local lymphadenopathy.[11–13]

DIAGNOSIS

Laboratory Abnormalities

Complete Blood Count, Serum Biochemical Tests, and Urinalysis

Findings on the CBC, serum biochemistry panel, and urinalysis in dogs or cats with mycoplasma infections are nonspecific and influenced by underlying disease processes. Dogs and cats with pneumonia, mycoplasma bacteremia, and polyarthritis may have a neutrophilia with a left shift and neutrophil toxicity, a degenerative left shift, mild nonregenerative anemia, hypoalbuminemia, and evidence of organ dysfunction such as increased serum liver enzyme activities and azotemia.[11,12,17]

Diagnostic Imaging

Plain Radiography

Mycoplasma pneumonia may be characterized by interstitial to alveolar patterns or lung lobe consolidation (Fig. 57.2); sometimes, mild pleural effusion is present. Radiographs of the joints of dogs and cats with mycoplasma polyarthritis may reveal periarticular soft tissue swelling. Erosive changes to the subchondral bone have also been described.[11]

Microbiologic Tests

Assays available for diagnosis of mycoplasma infections in dogs and cats are shown in Table 57.1.

Cytologic Examination

Mycoplasma spp. are often not visible with light microscopy because of their small size. They do not stain with Gram stain as a result of

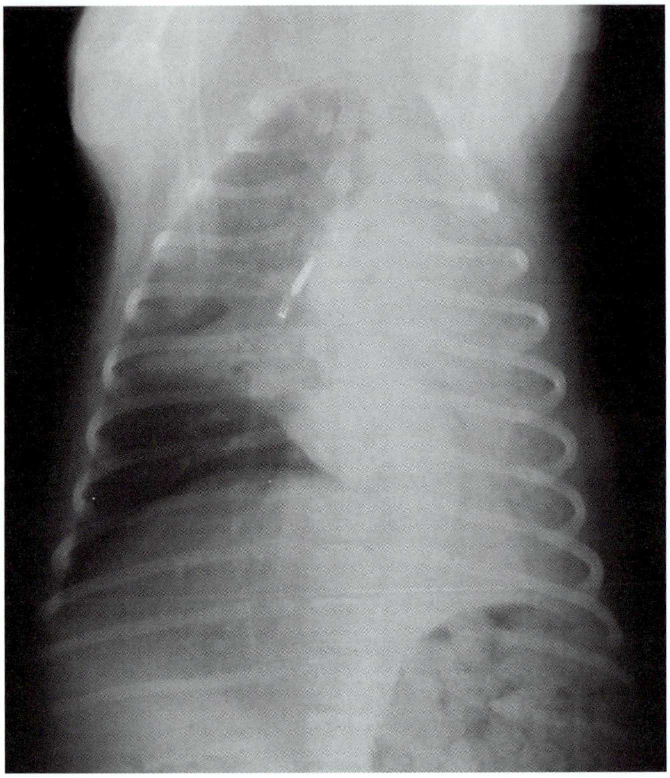

Fig. 57.2 Right lateral and ventrodorsal thoracic radiographs from a 3-month-old intact female pug with *Mycoplasma cynos* pneumonia. There is consolidation of the lung lobes associated with the left hemithorax and the right middle lung lobe. A diffuse interstitial pattern is present in the remainder of the right lung fields.

TABLE 57.1 Assays Available for Diagnosis of Mycoplasma Infections

Assay	Specimen Type	Target	Performance
Culture	Swabs, body fluids, wash specimens, tissue obtained at necropsy	Cultivable mycoplasma species	Some organisms grow on blood agar, but others require special mycoplasma media. Uncultivable mycoplasmas may also be present, which leads to false-negative results. Turnaround time may be slow (several days to weeks), species differentiation and antimicrobial drug susceptibility testing is often not performed. The significance of positive results from the upper respiratory and genital tract may be unclear.
PCR	Swabs, body fluids, wash specimens, tissue obtained at necropsy	*Mycoplasma* DNA	Allows rapid detection of the presence of mycoplasmas. More sensitive than culture for detection of fastidious or uncultivable mycoplasmas, although sensitivity and specificity may vary between assays. Some assays are designed to only detect certain pathogenic *Mycoplasma* species, such as *Mycoplasma cynos*. Sequencing of the PCR product may permit species identification. The significance of positive results may be unclear.

PCR, polymerase chain reaction.

the absence of a cell wall. Cytology of affected body fluids (such as bronchoalveolar lavage fluid, synovial fluid, and CSF) usually reveals a predominance of neutrophils with lesser numbers of histiocytes and lymphocytes.[11,12,14,34,35]

Isolation and Identification

Specimens suitable for culture of mycoplasmas include synovial fluid, blood, CSF, urine collected by cystocentesis, pleural fluid, semen, and tracheobronchial or bronchoalveolar lavage specimens. Swabs of the nasal cavity, conjunctiva, cornea, urethra, vagina, or cervix can also be submitted, but interpretation of results from these sites is difficult. If swabs are used, the swab should be rubbed vigorously on the mucosa because mycoplasmas are cell-associated. Rapid transport to the laboratory is important, because mycoplasmas are susceptible to deterioration with exposure to the environment. The use of special transport media (e.g., Stuart's medium or Amies medium without charcoal) for swab or tissue specimens may increase the yield of fastidious mycoplasma species if a delay of several hours is anticipated between collection of specimens and transport to the laboratory. Specimens should be refrigerated if delayed transport is unavoidable. If the delay is likely to be longer than 24 hours, specimens in transport media should ideally be frozen at –80°C.

Some mycoplasmas grow on blood agar under routine aerobic or anaerobic conditions. Others require special mycoplasma media, and some fail to grow under any laboratory conditions. The rate of growth in culture varies from one *Mycoplasma* species to another; for some mycoplasmas, colonies are visible in 2 or 3 days, whereas others require several weeks of incubation before colonies appear. Examination of plates under the light microscope may be required for detection of *Mycoplasma* colonies, because colonies range in size from 15 to 300 µm in diameter. The colonies of many mycoplasma species have a characteristic "fried egg" appearance (Fig. 57.3). Biochemical properties can be used to subgroup mycoplasmas, but species identification has traditionally required the use of species-specific antisera. Because cross-reactions can occur between species even when antisera are used, molecular typing methods (such as 16S rRNA gene or 16S/23S rRNA intergenic spacer region PCR and sequence analysis of the respective PCR products) or MALDI-TOF MS are now the method of choice for species identification.[7] Most veterinary diagnostic laboratories currently report only growth of a *Mycoplasma* spp., and do not identify organisms to the species level unless specifically requested. It is difficult

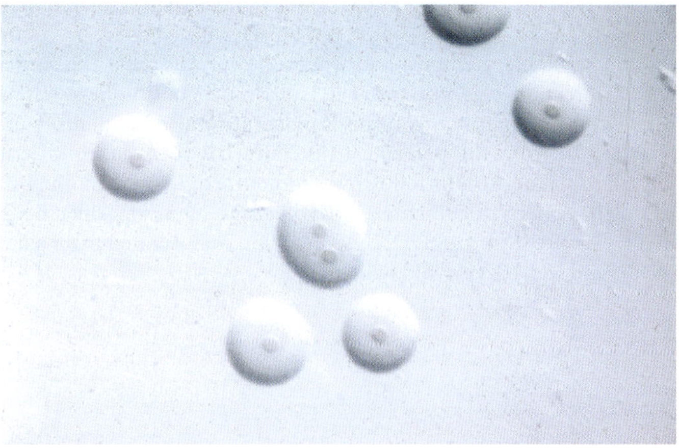

Fig. 57.3 Colonies of *Mycoplasma bovirhinis* showing the "fried egg" appearance that is typical of the growth of some *Mycoplasma* spp. in culture. (From The genera *Mycoplasma* and *Ureaplasma*. In: Songer JG Post KW, eds. *Veterinary Microbiology: Bacterial and Fungal Agents of Animal Disease*. 2nd ed. St. Louis, MO: Saunders; 2005.)

to interpret the significance of a positive mycoplasma culture from mucosal sites that are not normally sterile, including the lower respiratory tracts of dogs, so results must be interpreted in light of the clinical findings and the results of other diagnostic tests.

Antimicrobial susceptibility testing for mycoplasmas is labor intensive and not routinely performed, and established breakpoints are not available. The most widely used method is microbroth dilution (see Chapter 3).[41]

Molecular Diagnosis Using Nucleic Acid–Based Testing

Some veterinary diagnostic laboratories offer PCR assays that rapidly directly detect mycoplasma DNA in clinical specimens, without the need for culture. Several conventional and real-time PCR assays have been used to detect mycoplasmas of dogs and cats.[42–45] These assays may be specific for certain mycoplasma species (such as *M. cynos* or *M. felis*), or they may be genus-specific assays that detect a variety of mycoplasma species. PCR assays may be more sensitive than culture for detection of fastidious mycoplasma species. Sequencing of the PCR product generated from genus-specific PCR assays may be used to identify the infecting species present, provided the product is sufficiently long. As with culture, the significance of a positive PCR test result for *Mycoplasma* spp. may be unclear given the frequent colonization of healthy animals with mycoplasmas, so results must be interpreted with the underlying disease process and the results of other diagnostic tests.

Pathologic Findings

Gross pathology in dogs and cats with mycoplasmal diseases usually reveals the presence of purulent material in affected tissues. Histopathology shows predominantly neutrophilic inflammation within affected tissues, although histiocytes may also be present. Reactive lymphadenopathy may also be evident as a result of immune stimulation (Fig. 57.4).

TREATMENT AND PROGNOSIS

Treatment of mycoplasma infections involves specific antimicrobial therapy (Table 57.2) as well as management of other underlying disorders that may have predisposed to invasion by mycoplasmas. Tetracyclines or fluoroquinolones are active against most mycoplasma isolates. The optimal duration is unknown, but treatment for at least 2 weeks is reasonable. In a prospective study of shelter cats with URTD and *M. felis* infection, a 14-day course of doxycycline was more effective in causing reduction in *M. felis* load as determined with real-time PCR than a 7-day course, but there was no overall significant difference in the reduction in clinical signs between the two groups.[46] Nevertheless, 25% of the cats treated for 14 days were still infected after that time. In another study of cats with conjunctivitis, 3 weeks of treatment with pradofloxacin or doxycycline was required to eliminate infection as indicated by the detection of *Mycoplasma* DNA.[45] β-lactam drugs are not active against mycoplasmas because they lack peptidoglycan. Mycoplasmas are also intrinsically resistant to trimethoprim-sulfonamide combinations and rifampin. Some species are resistant to macrolides.

IMMUNITY AND VACCINATION

Mycoplasma spp. persist in tissues and epithelial cells despite the immune response. Mechanisms to evade the host immune response such as intracellular localization and antigenic variation of outer surface proteins have been identified in several mycoplasma species. Innate, humoral (especially IgA), and cell-mediated immune

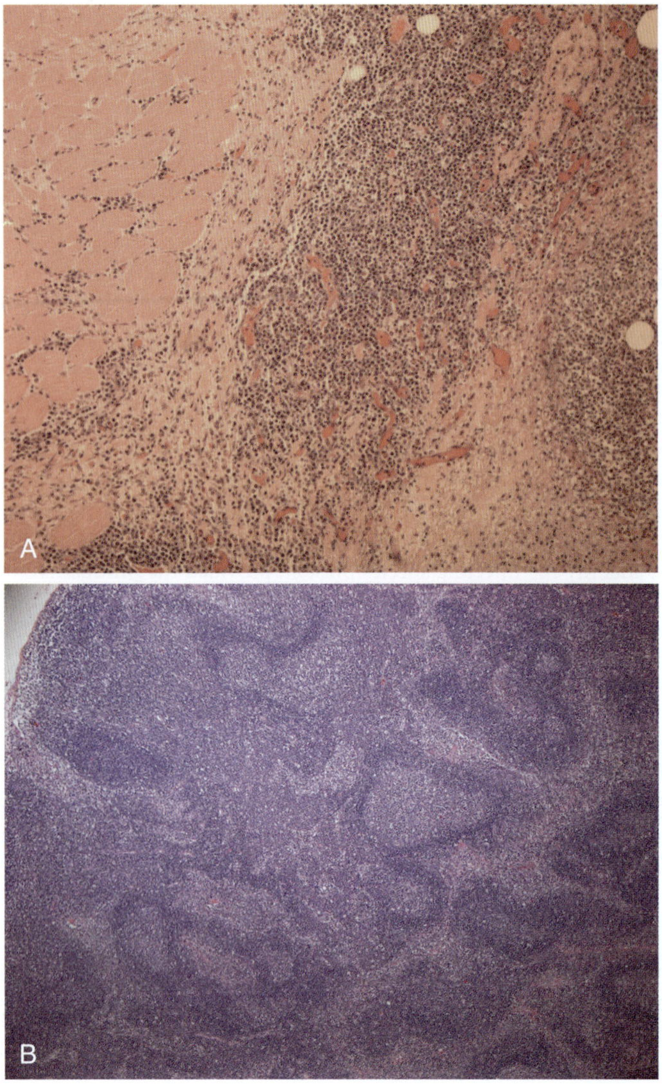

Fig. 57.4 Histopathology of the inguinal subcutaneous tissues (A) and sublumbar lymph node (B) from a 6 month-old, FIV-/FeLV-negative, male neutered domestic shorthair with severe suppurative cellulitis, steatitis, dermatitis, and myositis of the scrotal skin and subcutaneous tissue due to a *Mycoplasma* spp. infection. The cat had been neutered 13 days previously and was evaluated for a 2-day history of lethargy and reluctance to move. Physical examination revealed fever (104.6°F), severe conjunctivitis, generalized peripheral lymphadenomegaly, and firm mass lesions in the inguinal area. In addition to suppurative cellulitis and myositis, marked systemic lymph node hyperplasia was present. Hyperplasia was most profound in the sublumbar lymph nodes, which measured 4 cm in diameter.

responses may be required to clear mycoplasma infections, with humoral mechanisms of critical importance. Vaccines to limit disease caused by pathogenic mycoplasma species such as *M. cynos* are currently not available, although they have been used with success in food production animal species.

TABLE 57.2 Suggested Antimicrobial Drug Treatment for Mycoplasma Infections

Drug	Dose (mg/kg)	Route	Interval (Hours)
Doxycycline	5 to 10	PO or IV	12 to 24
Enrofloxacin[a]	5	PO or IV	24
Marbofloxacin	2 to 5.5	PO	24
Pradofloxacin[b]	5 to 10 (cats); 3 (dogs)	PO	24

[a]Use enrofloxacin only in cats when other alternatives are not possible due to risk for irreversible blindness.
[b]Use of pradofloxacin is extra-label in dogs in the United States (see Chapter 10). The dose for cats is for the oral suspension. The dose for the tablet formulation is 3 mg/kg.
IV, intravenous; *PO,* oral.

PREVENTION

Prevention of mycoplasma infections involves management or reversal of disorders that predispose to opportunistic invasion by mycoplasmas. Reduction of overcrowding and concurrent infections in shelter environments may also reduce the incidence and severity of mycoplasma infections (see Chapters 16 and 17). Routine disinfectants are sufficient to inactivate mycoplasmas that persist in the environment.

PUBLIC HEALTH ASPECTS

The vast majority of mycoplasma species associated with disease in humans are different to those found in dogs and cats. However, pharyngeal colonization with *M. canis* was also reported in a family and their pet dog.[47] *Mycoplasma felis* was isolated from multiple joints of a woman with common variable immunodeficiency who developed septic arthritis.[48] The woman had worked in an animal shelter, lived with a cat, and had been bitten on the hand by a healthy cat 6 months before she was evaluated. A mycoplasma was isolated from a cat scratch wound to the hand of a veterinarian.[49] Although *Staphylococcus aureus* was initially isolated from the wound, it failed to resolve completely after treatment with erythromycin. Subsequently the tenosynovitis developed, and a mycoplasma was isolated. The identity of the mycoplasma could not be determined using biochemical and serologic methods, and whether a cat was truly the source of this infection was not proven. Isolation of antibiotic-resistant *Mycoplasma maculosum* from immunocompromised patients[50] and *M. edwardii* from the peritoneal fluid of a 10-year-old child with polymicrobial peritonitis following a puncture of dialysis tubing by a pet dog have been documented.[51] *Mycoplasma canis*, identified using MALDI-TOF MS and 16S rDNA sequencing, was isolated from a dog bite wound in a 62-year-old woman.[52]

CASE EXAMPLE

Signalment

"Delilah," a 3-month-old intact female pug dog from Reno, NV.

History

Delilah was brought to the University of California, Davis VMTH, for evaluation of pneumonia. She had been purchased from a pet store 3 weeks before the date of evaluation. The owner noticed nasal and ocular discharge when the dog was brought home from the store, as well as a dry, nonproductive cough. Delilah was taken to a local veterinary clinic where she was diagnosed with "kennel cough" and treated with clavulanic acid-amoxicillin (15 mg/kg, PO, q12h) for 2 weeks. However, the cough persisted and Delilah's respiratory effort increased. She was then hospitalized at the local veterinary clinic and treated with ticarcillin-clavulanate (50 mg/kg, IV, q8h), supplemental oxygen, nebulization, and coupage. Radiographs showed infiltrates in the left lung lobes and right middle lung lobe that worsened over the course of hospitalization, so she was referred for further evaluation and treatment. There had been no decrease in appetite, vomiting, or diarrhea. She was fed a commercial puppy food and had no history of ticks, travel, trauma, or toxin exposure. The owner was not aware of previous vaccinations.

Physical Examination

Body weight: 2.2 kg.

General: Quiet, alert, hydrated. T = 101.0°F, pulse rate = 220 beats/min, respiratory rate = 60 breaths/min, slightly tacky mucous membranes with a normal capillary refill time.

Eyes, ears, nose, and throat: Mild serous ocular and nasal discharge bilaterally. Conjunctival hyperemia and chemosis was present, as well as scleral injection. No other clinically significant findings were present.

Musculoskeletal: BCS 4/9. Fully ambulatory with no evidence of muscle atrophy. Poor body conformation was present, characterized by medial deviation of the tarsi and hyperextension of the carpi.

Cardiovascular: No murmurs or arrhythmias were ausculted. Femoral pulses were strong and synchronous.

Respiratory: Tachypnea was present with marked abdominal effort. Lung sounds were markedly increased, especially on the left side. There were no crackles or wheezes. Coughing occurred several times during the examination.

GI: No abnormalities were detected on abdominal palpation, but abdominal palpation was difficult and brief because of the dog's compromised respiratory status.

Lymph nodes: All within normal limits of size.

Neurologic examination: No obvious neurologic deficits were present. A full neurologic examination was not performed.

Laboratory Findings

Venous blood gas: pH = 7.348, pCO_2 44 mmHg, pO_2 44.7 mmHg, HCO_3^- 23.2 mmol/L, base excess −1.4 mmol/L, ionized calcium 1.43 mmol/L, lactate 3.3 mmol/L.

CBC: HCT 35.4% (40%–55%), MCV 68.6 fL (65–75 fL), MCHC 31.1 g/dL (33–36 g/dL), WBC 31,580 cells/μL (6,000–13,000 cells/μL), neutrophils 6,948 cells/μL (3,000–10,500 cells/μL), band neutrophils 9,790 cells/μL, lymphocytes 9,158 cells/μL (1,000–4,000 cells/μL), monocytes 4,737 cells/μL (150–1,200 cells/μL), eosinophils 947 cells/μL (150–1,100 cells/μL), platelets 307,000 platelets/μL (150,000–400,000 platelets/μL). Band neutrophils and mature neutrophils had evidence of toxic changes.

Serum chemistry profile: anion gap 24 mmol/L (12–25 mmol/L), sodium 147 mmol/L (145–154 mmol/L), potassium 4.9 mmol/L (3.6–5.3 mmol/L), chloride 104 mmol/L (108–118 mmol/L), bicarbonate 24 mmol/L (16–26 mmol/L), phosphorus 8.0 mg/dL (3.0–6.2 mg/dL), calcium 10.5 mg/dL (9.7–11.5 mg/dl), BUN 10 mg/dL (5–21 mg/dL), creatinine 0.5 mg/dL (0.3–1.2 mg/dL), glucose 110 mg/dL (64–123 mg/dL), total protein 5.9 g/dL (5.4–7.6 g/dL), albumin 2.5 g/dL (3.0–4.4 g/dL), globulin 3.4 g/dL (1.8–3.9 g/dL), ALT 12 U/L (19–67 U/L), AST 38 U/L (19–42 U/L), ALP 144 U/L (21–170 U/L), GGT 0 U/L (0–6 U/L), cholesterol 188 mg/dL (135–361 mg/dL), total bilirubin concentration 0.0 mg/dL (0–0.2 mg/dL).

Urinalysis: SpG 1.045; pH 7.0, no protein, glucose, ketones, bilirubin, 0 WBC/HPF, rare RBC/HPF, rare triple phosphate and a few sodium urate crystals, rare lipid droplets.

Imaging Findings

Thoracic radiographs: There was complete consolidation of the lung lobes associated with the left hemithorax (see Fig. 57.2). Prominent air bronchogram formation was noted in these lung lobes and in the right middle lung lobe, which also appeared consolidated. Diffuse interstitial markings were present in the remainder of the right lung fields.

Thoracic ultrasound: Complete consolidation of the left lung was appreciated. Pleural effusion was not present. There was no evidence of lung lobe torsion.

Cytologic Findings

Transtracheal wash: One direct smear was evaluated that was highly cellular and contained a minimal amount of mucus. Cells were essentially all neutrophils, which were primarily nondegenerate but occasionally mildly to moderately degenerate. A single extracellular rod, and 2 neutrophils with intracellular structures that resemble bacteria were found.

Interpretation: Marked suppurative inflammation, suspicious for sepsis.

Microbiologic Testing

Gram-stained direct smear of transtracheal wash fluid: Large numbers of neutrophils. No organisms seen.

Aerobic and anaerobic bacterial culture and *Mycoplasma* culture (transtracheal wash fluid): Large numbers of *Mycoplasma* spp.; DNA sequence analysis revealed 100% identity to *M. cynos*. No other aerobic or anaerobic organisms isolated.

Direct FA for distemper virus antigen (conjunctival smear): Negative.

Centrifugal zinc sulfate fecal flotation: Negative.

Diagnosis

Mycoplasma cynos bronchopneumonia.

Treatment

Delilah was treated with supplemental oxygen, nebulization, coupage, and IV fluids. Treatment with ticarcillin-clavulanate was continued for 3 days, then changed to enrofloxacin (5 mg/kg PO q24h) and amoxicillin-clavulanate (19 mg/kg PO q12h), and nebulization with gentamicin was performed once daily, because there had been no improvement and persistent bordetellosis was considered a possibility. The following morning, lung sounds were improved and Delilah was very playful. Her nasal discharge resolved and the frequency of cough reduced. The CBC showed a regenerative anemia (HCT 33.2%, with 95,300 reticulocytes); 14,112 slightly toxic neutrophils/μL; 1,008 slightly toxic band neutrophils/μL; 5,796 lymphocytes/μL; and 3,780 monocytes/μL. Growth of *Mycoplasma* spp. was reported 5 days after specimens were submitted for culture. Oxygen supplementation was gradually reduced, and Delilah was discharged on day 8 of hospitalization, although significant radiographic improvement was not evident at that time and an occasional productive cough was still present. Treatment with enrofloxacin, amoxicillin-clavulanate, coupage, and exercise restriction was continued at home. At a recheck 3 weeks later, Delilah had gained weight (3.45 kg). An intermittent, moist but nonproductive cough was present only in the morning. Her appetite remained excellent, and there was no evidence of lethargy or exercise intolerance, and no evidence of ocular or nasal discharge. A physical examination was unremarkable, and Delilah's respiratory rate was 30 breaths/min. A CBC showed persistent mild regenerative anemia, with 7,260 neutrophils/μL and 330 band neutrophils/μL. Thoracic radiographs showed significantly improved aeration of the left cranial and caudal lung lobes, and near-complete resolution of the right-sided infiltrates. Treatment with amoxicillin-clavulanate was

Continued

CASE EXAMPLE—cont'd

then discontinued. Further improvement in the cough and pulmonary infiltrates were observed at a recheck 3.5 weeks later. After an additional 7 weeks of treatment, the cough had completely resolved, although partial atelectasis of the cranial portion of the left lung lobe persisted.

Comments

The isolation of a pure culture of *M. cynos* from this dog's transtracheal wash, together with the lack of response to β-lactam antimicrobial drugs and a prompt response once treatment with enrofloxacin was initiated, supported a diagnosis of mycoplasma pneumonia (and possibly also conjunctivitis) in this dog. The concurrent presence of respiratory viruses remains a possibility because other than direct FA testing for CDV, diagnostic tests for respiratory viruses were not performed, and co-infections with multiple respiratory pathogens in dogs from pet stores and shelter environments are common. Resolution of the cough and radiographic changes occurred over several months. There was concern expressed over the possibility of abnormal cartilage development in such a young dog due to prolonged treatment with enrofloxacin, but no adverse effects were reported. The optimum duration of treatment of mycoplasma pneumonia in dogs requires further study. The development of a regenerative anemia was interesting and may have reflected pulmonary hemorrhage or immune-mediated hemolysis. Reticulocytosis has been reported in human patients with community-acquired pneumonia due to *Mycoplasma pneumoniae.*

SUGGESTED READINGS

Klein S, Klotz M, Eigenbrod T. First isolation of *Mycoplasma canis* from human tissue samples after a dog bite. *New Microbes New Infect.* 2018;25:14–15.

Stenske KA, Bemis DA, Hill K, et al. Acute polyarthritis and septicemia from *Mycoplasma edwardii* after surgical removal of bilateral adrenal tumors in a dog. *J Vet Intern Med.* 2005;19:768–771.

Jambhekar A, Robin E, Le Boedec K. A systematic review and meta-analyses of the association between 4 mycoplasma species and lower respiratory tract disease in dogs. *J Vet Intern Med.* 2019;33:1880–1891.

REFERENCES

1. Shoetensack HM. Pure cultivation of filterable virus isolated from canine distemper. *Kitasako Archives Exp Med.* 1934;11:227–290.
2. Baseman JB, Tully JG. Mycoplasmas: sophisticated, reemerging, and burdened by their notoriety. *Emerg Infect Dis.* 1997;3:21–32.
3. Tallmadge RL, Mitchell PK, Anderson R, et al. Whole-genome sequence of the *Mycoplasma mucosicanis* type strain. *Microbiol Resour Announc.* 2019;8.
4. Chalker VJ. Canine mycoplasmas. *Res Vet Sci.* 2005;79:1–8.
5. Hartmann AD, Hawley J, Werckenthin C, et al. Detection of bacterial and viral organisms from the conjunctiva of cats with conjunctivitis and upper respiratory tract disease. *J Feline Med Surg.* 2010;12:775–782.
6. Heyward JT, Sabry MZ, Dowdle WR. Characterization of mycoplasma species of feline origin. *Am J Vet Res.* 1969;30:615–622.
7. Spergser J, Rosengarten R. Identification and differentiation of canine *Mycoplasma* isolates by 16S-23S rDNA PCR-RFLP. *Vet Microbiol.* 2007;125:170–174.
8. Tan RJ. Suceptibility of kittens to *Mycoplasma felis* infection. *Jpn J Exp Med.* 1974;44:235–240.
9. Jambhekar A, Robin E, Le Boedec K. A systematic review and meta-analyses of the association between 4 mycoplasma species and lower respiratory tract disease in dogs. *J Vet Intern Med.* 2019;33: 1880–1891.
10. Ilha MR, Rajeev S, Watson C, et al. Meningoencephalitis caused by *Mycoplasma edwardii* in a dog. *J Vet Diagn Invest.* 2010;22:805–808.
11. Zeugswetter F, Hittmair KM, de Arespacochaga AG, et al. Erosive polyarthritis associated with *Mycoplasma gateae* in a cat. *J Feline Med Surg.* 2007;9:226–231.
12. Stenske KA, Bemis DA, Hill K, et al. Acute polyarthritis and septicemia from *Mycoplasma edwardii* after surgical removal of bilateral adrenal tumors in a dog. *J Vet Intern Med.* 2005;19:768–771.
13. Barton MD, Ireland L, Kirschner JL, et al. Isolation of *Mycoplasma spumans* from polyarthritis in a greyhound. *Aust Vet J.* 1985;62:206–207.
14. Beauchamp DJ, da Costa RC, Premanandan C, et al. *Mycoplasma felis*-associated meningoencephalomyelitis in a cat. *J Feline Med Surg.* 2011;13:139–143.
15. Haesebrouck F, Devriese LA, van Rijssen B, et al. Incidence and significance of isolation of *Mycoplasma felis* from conjunctival swabs of cats. *Vet Microbiol.* 1991;26:95–101.
16. Jang SS, Ling GV, Yamamoto R, et al. *Mycoplasma* as a cause of canine urinary tract infection. *J Am Vet Med Assoc.* 1984;185:45–47.
17. Moise NS, Crissman JW, Fairbrother JF, et al. *Mycoplasma gateae* arthritis and tenosynovitis in cats: case report and experimental reproduction of the disease. *Am J Vet Res.* 1983;44:16–21.
18. Hooper PT, Ireland LA, Carter A. *Mycoplasma* polyarthritis in a cat with probable severe immune deficiency. *Aust Vet J.* 1985;62:352.
19. Liehmann L, Degasperi B, Spergser J, et al. *Mycoplasma felis* arthritis in two cats. *J Small Anim Pract.* 2006;47:476–479.
20. Gray LD, Ketring KL, Tang YW. Clinical use of 16S rRNA gene sequencing to identify *Mycoplasma felis* and *M. gateae* associated with feline ulcerative keratitis. *J Clin Microbiol.* 2005;43:3431–3434.
21. Low HC, Powell CC, Veir JK, et al. Prevalence of feline herpesvirus 1, *Chlamydophila felis*, and *Mycoplasma* spp. DNA in conjunctival cells collected from cats with and without conjunctivitis. *Am J Vet Res.* 2007;68:643–648.
22. Holst BS, Hanas S, Berndtsson LT, et al. Infectious causes for feline upper respiratory tract disease: a case-control study. *J Feline Med Surg.* 2010;12:783–789.
23. Rycroft AN, Tsounakou E, Chalker V. Serological evidence of *Mycoplasma cynos* infection in canine infectious respiratory disease. *Vet Microbiol.* 2007;120:358–362.
24. Chalker VJ, Owen WM, Paterson C, et al. Mycoplasmas associated with canine infectious respiratory disease. *Microbiology.* 2004;150:3491–3497.
25. Rosendal S. Canine mycoplasmas: pathogenicity of mycoplasmas associated with distemper pneumonia. *J Infect Dis.* 1978;138:203–210.
26. Maboni G, Seguel M, Lorton A, et al. Canine infectious respiratory disease: new insights into the etiology and epidemiology of associated pathogens. *PLoS One.* 2019;14:e0215817.
27. Abou N, Houwers DJ, van Dongen AM. PCR-based detection reveals no causative role for *Mycoplasma* and *Ureaplasma* in feline lower urinary tract disease. *Vet Microbiol.* 2006;116:246–247.
28. Bettenay SV, Lappin MR, Mueller RS. An immunohistochemical and polymerase chain reaction evaluation of feline plasmacytic pododermatitis. *Vet Pathol.* 2007;44:80–83.
29. Kastelic S, Cizelj I, Narat M, et al. Molecular characterisation of the *Mycoplasma cynos* haemagglutinin HapA. *Vet Microbiol.* 2015;175:35–43.
30. Bercic RL, Cizelj I, Bencina M, et al. Demonstration of neuraminidase activity in *Mycoplasma neurolyticum* and of neuraminidase proteins in three canine *Mycoplasma* species. *Vet Microbiol.* 2012;155:425–429.
31. Mannering SA, McAuliffe L, Lawes JR, et al. Strain typing of *Mycoplasma cynos* isolates from dogs with respiratory disease. *Vet Microbiol.* 2009;135:292–296.
32. Randolph JF, Moise NS, Scarlett JM, et al. Prevalence of mycoplasmal and ureaplasmal recovery from tracheobronchial lavages and of mycoplasmal recovery from pharyngeal swab specimens in cats with or without pulmonary disease. *Am J Vet Res.* 1993;54:897–900.

33. Randolph JF, Moise NS, Scarlett JM, et al. Prevalence of mycoplasmal and ureaplasmal recovery from tracheobronchial lavages and prevalence of mycoplasmal recovery from pharyngeal swab specimens in dogs with or without pulmonary disease. *Am J Vet Res*. 1993;54:387–391.
34. Chandler JC, Lappin MR. Mycoplasmal respiratory infections in small animals: 17 cases (1988-1999). *J Am Anim Hosp Assoc*. 2002;38: 111–119.
35. Foster SF, Barrs VR, Martin P, et al. Pneumonia associated with *Mycoplasma* spp. in three cats. *Aust Vet J*. 1998;76:460–464.
36. Malik R, Love DN, Hunt GB, et al. Pyothorax associated with *Mycoplasma* species in a kitten. *J Small Anim Pract*. 1991;32:31–34.
37. Gulbahar MY, Gurturk K. Pyothorax associated with a *Mycoplasma* sp. and *Arcanobacterium pyogenes* in a kitten. *Aust Vet J*. 2002;80: 344–345.
38. Walker AL, Jang SS, Hirsh DC. Bacteria associated with pyothorax of dogs and cats: 98 cases (1989-1998). *J Am Vet Med Assoc*. 2000;216:359–363.
39. L'Abee-Lund TM, Heiene R, Friis NF, et al. *Mycoplasma canis* and urogenital disease in dogs in Norway. *Vet Rec*. 2003;153:231–235.
40. Barber RM, Porter BF, Li Q, et al. Broadly reactive polymerase chain reaction for pathogen detection in canine granulomatous meningoencephalomyelitis and necrotizing meningoencephalitis. *J Vet Intern Med*. 2012;26:962–968.
41. Waites KB, Taylor-Robinson D. *Mycoplasma* and *Ureaplasma*. In: Versalovic J, Carroll KC, Funke G, et al., eds. *Manual of Clinical Microbiology*. Washington, D. C.: ASM Press; 2011:970–985.
42. Rebelo AR, Parker L, Cai HY. Use of high-resolution melting curve analysis to identify *Mycoplasma* species commonly isolated from ruminant, avian, and canine samples. *J Vet Diagn Invest*. 2011;23:932–936.
43. Soderlund R, Bolske G, Holst BS, et al. Development and evaluation of a real-time polymerase chain reaction method for the detection of *Mycoplasma felis*. *J Vet Diagn Invest*. 2011;23:890–893.
44. Chalker VJ, Owen WM, Paterson CJ, et al. Development of a polymerase chain reaction for the detection of *Mycoplasma felis* in domestic cats. *Vet Microbiol*. 2004;100:77–82.
45. Hartmann AD, Helps CR, Lappin MR, et al. Efficacy of pradofloxacin in cats with feline upper respiratory tract disease due to *Chlamydophila felis* or *Mycoplasma* infections. *J Vet Intern Med*. 2008;22:44–52.
46. Kompare B, Litster AL, Leutenegger CM, et al. Randomized masked controlled clinical trial to compare 7-day and 14-day course length of doxycycline in the treatment of *Mycoplasma felis* infection in shelter cats. *Comp Immunol Microbiol Infect Dis*. 2013;36:129–135.
47. Armstrong D, Yu BH, Yagoda A, et al. Colonization of humans by *Mycoplasma canis*. *J Infect Dis*. 1971;124:607–609.
48. Bonilla HF, Chenoweth CE, Tully JG, et al. *Mycoplasma felis* septic arthritis in a patient with hypogammaglobulinemia. *Clin Infect Dis*. 1997;24:222–225.
49. McCabe SJ, Murray JF, Ruhnke HL, et al. *Mycoplasma* infection of the hand acquired from a cat. *J Hand Surg Am*. 1987;12:1085–1088.
50. Heilmann C, Jensen L, Jensen JS, et al. Treatment of resistant mycoplasma infection in immunocompromised patients with a new pleuromutilin antibiotic. *J Infect*. 2001;43:234–238.
51. Lalan SP, Warady BA, Blowey D, et al. *Mycoplasma edwardii* peritonitis in a patient on maintenance peritoneal dialysis. *Clin Nephrol*. 2015;83:45–48.
52. Klein S, Klotz M, Eigenbrod T. First isolation of *Mycoplasma canis* from human tissue samples after a dog bite. *New Microbes New Infect*. 2018;25:14–15.

58

Hemotropic Mycoplasma Infections

Emi N. Barker, Séverine Tasker

KEY POINTS

- Cause: *Mycoplasma haemocanis* and "*Candidatus* Mycoplasma haematoparvum" in dogs, and *Mycoplasma haemofelis*, "*Candidatus* Mycoplasma haemominutum," and "*Candidatus* Mycoplasma turicensis" in cats. All are gram-negative, obligate epierythrocytic bacteria that belong to the family Mycoplasmataceae.
- First Described: *M. haemocanis* (basonym *Haemobartonella canis* [Benjamin and Lumb 1959][1] nom. rev. *Bartonella canis*, Germany [*ex.* Kikuth 1928])[2]; *M. haemofelis* (basonym *Haemobartonella felis* [Flint and Moss 1953][3] nom. rev. *Eperythrozoon felis*, South Africa [*ex.* Clark 1942]).[4]
- Affected Hosts: Domesticated dogs and cats, wild canidae, and wild felidae. Other hemoplasma species cause disease in a variety of other animal species.
- Intermediate Hosts: Unknown.
- Geographic Distribution: Worldwide; prevalence varies geographically.
- Primary Mode of Transmission: The mode of transmission in the field is uncertain. Ticks (*Rhipicephalus sanguineus* in particular) are suspected to transmit *M. haemocanis*. Other unidentified arthropod vectors may also be involved. Biting or aggressive interactions are a suspected mode, and possibly vertical transmission. Experimentally, transmission can occur through ingestion or injection of infected blood.
- Major Clinical Signs: Fever, lethargy, inappetence, weakness, pallor, and dehydration.
- Differential Diagnoses: Primary IMHA, other infectious diseases (e.g., cytauxzoonosis, FIV infection, FeLV infection, FIP), Heinz body anemia, and inherited erythrocyte disorders (e.g., pyruvate kinase deficiency, red cell fragility disorders).
- Human Health Significance: Infections have also been described in humans with novel hemoplasma species, as well as species that have possibly originated in animals such as the cat or dog, pigs, and sheep, raising the possibility of zoonotic infections.

ETIOLOGIC AGENT AND EPIDEMIOLOGY

Hemotropic mycoplasmas (hemoplasmas) are small (0.3–1.0 μm), wall-less bacteria that infect erythrocytes living on the surface of the erythrocyte membrane (Fig. 58.1). They infect a wide variety of mammalian species, including humans, as well as beetles. Infection can result in hemolytic anemia of variable severity, dependent on host and hemoplasma factors. Hemoplasma infections have been reported throughout the world.

Previously classified as rickettsial organisms within the *Haemobartonella* and *Eperythrozoon* genera, sequence analysis of the 16S rRNA genes resulted in their reclassification within the genus *Mycoplasma*, alongside species more commonly found on the mucosal surfaces of the respiratory and urogenital tracts (e.g., *Mycoplasma pneumoniae* and *Mycoplasma genitalium*).[5–7] Gene sequence analysis also revealed the existence of different species of hemoplasmas within individual host species. Hemoplasmas cannot be cultured in the laboratory, which limits full phenotypic characterization, so the "*Candidatus*" prefix is applied to newly described hemoplasmas until more information becomes available to support their classification. Because bacterial species cannot be demoted, those species previously defined and named cannot be assigned the *Candidatus* status. Similarities between the hemoplasmas and mucosal mycoplasmas are recognized, such as the absence of a cell wall, their small (physical and genomic) sizes, and fastidious growth requirements. However, the hemoplasmas' niche environment of the blood is not one that is commonly recognized for mucosal mycoplasmas. Non-16S rRNA gene-based phylogeny suggests that, although the hemoplasmas belong to the family Mycoplasmataceae, they should reside in a genus separate to that of the mucosal mycoplasmas.[8,9]

Three major hemoplasma species infect domestic cats as well as wild felids, *Mycoplasma haemofelis*, "*Candidatus* Mycoplasma haemominutum", and "*Candidatus* Mycoplasma turicensis." The whole genome sequences of two strains of *M. haemofelis* have been determined, as has the near-whole genome sequence of one strain of "*Ca.* M. haemominutum."[10–12] Prevalence studies for feline hemoplasma species have been performed worldwide with diverse results (Table 58.1); however, variation in population characteristics (from healthy to anemic, suspected of having hemoplasmosis or retrovirus-infected; and from client-owned to feral) and PCR methodology (with likely differing sensitivities and specificities) limits comparison between studies. Geographic variation in prevalence also appears to exist, with cats in warmer countries having a higher prevalence of infection. Mixed infections with one or both of the other feline hemoplasma species occur, with one study of Brazilian cats reporting that over 80% of hemoplasma-infected cats harbored more than one hemoplasma species.[13]

Mycoplasma haemofelis (previously the Ohio strain, or large form of *Haemobartonella felis*) is the most pathogenic feline hemoplasma and can cause moderate to severe hemolytic anemia in immunocompetent cats. Using cytologic evaluation of blood smears, *M. haemofelis* organisms are cocci that are usually found individually on RBCs, but sometimes they form short chains of three to six organisms (see Fig. 58.1). *Mycoplasma haemofelis* has been found using PCR in 0.4% to 14.0% of sick cats presented for veterinary care, although occasionally a higher prevalence is reported (see Table 58.1).

"*Ca.* M. haemominutum" (previously the California strain or small form of *H. felis*) is generally smaller than *M. haemofelis* and has not

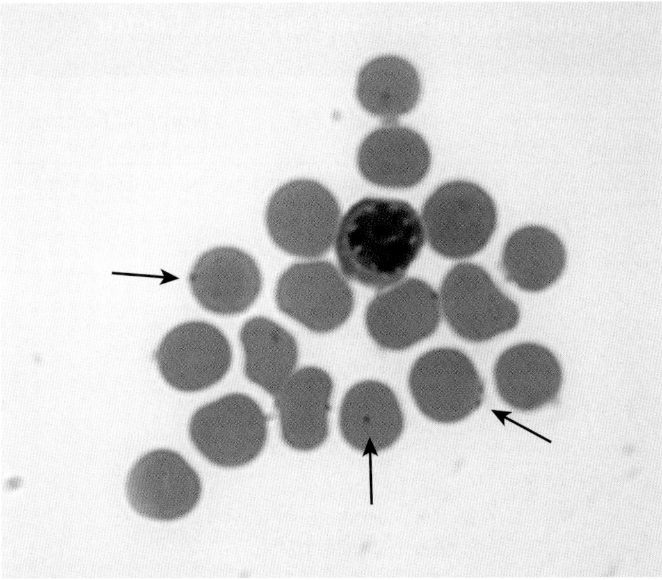

Fig. 58.1 Romanowsky-stained blood smear from an 8-year-old male neutered domestic shorthair cat showing epierythrocytic bacteria typical of *Mycoplasma haemofelis (arrows).*

clearly been associated with clinically significant disease in immunocompetent cats. Using cytologic evaluation of blood smears, "*Ca.* M. haemominutum" are small cocci, 0.3 to 0.6 μm in diameter, although *M. haemofelis* and "*Ca.* M. haemominutum" cannot be reliably distinguished by size alone. "*Ca.* M. haemominutum" is usually the most common species found in prevalence studies in the cat population worldwide, infecting typically 10% to 25%, although a higher prevalence is occasionally reported (see Table 58.1).

"*Ca.* M. turicensis" was first described in a cat from Switzerland that had severe intravascular hemolysis.[14] Infections with "*Ca.* M. turicensis" have since been detected worldwide (see Table 58.1). "*Ca.* M. turicensis" has not been identified using light microscopic examination of blood smears, and organism loads in infected cats are typically low. Infection with "*Ca.* M. turicensis" is usually slightly more prevalent in the cat population than infection with *M. haemofelis.* Most studies show a prevalence of 0% to 10% (see Table 58.1).

Infection of cats by hemoplasmas is strongly associated with male sex, nonpedigree status, and outdoor access.[13,15–28] Infection with "*Ca.* M. haemominutum" is more prevalent in older cats, presumably because of the cumulative risk of acquiring persistent subclinical infection over time. Young cats may be more likely to develop severe clinical disease due to *M. haemofelis* compared with older cats.[29,30] Epidemiologic studies have, however, only variably demonstrated

TABLE 58.1 Selected Prevalence Studies for Feline Hemoplasma Species and Risk Factor Analysis for Infection

				Prevalence					
Reference	Country	Number Of Cats	Health Status	All HP	Mhf	CMhm	CMt	Risk Factors For Infection[a]	Non-risk Factors For Infection[a]
Roura et al. (2010)[16]	Spain	191	61.3% sick	12.3%	3.7%	9.9%	0.5%	FIV infection; outdoor access; male	Age; breed; presence of anemia; FeLV status; health status; presence of other vector-borne infections
Tasker et al. (2003)[26]; Willi et al. (2006)[28]	UK	426	71.8% sick	18.5%	1.6%	17.1%	1.3%	Increased age (CMhm); male (CMhm)	
Martinez-Diaz et al. (2013)[42]	Portugal	320	60.5% sick	43.4%	12.8%	41.6%; 4.4% CMhp	1.3%	FeLV/FIV infection	Age; breed; sex; neuter status; health status; presence of ticks or fleas; outdoor access; presence of anemia
Willi et al. (2006)[27]	Switzerland	713	87.9% sick; 13.7% HP infection suspected	11.6%	1.5%	10.0%	1.3%	Increased age (CMhm); male (CMhm; Mhf); outdoor access (CMhm); geographic location (CMhm; Mhf); CMt infection (CMhm); ill and renal insufficiency (CMhm)	Health status; FeLV/FIV status (CMhm); presence of anemia (CMhm); PCV (CMhm/Mhf copy numbers)
Gentilini et al. (2009)[102]	Italy	307	Hospital population	18.9%	5.9%	17.3%	1.3%	FIV infection; summer season; low erythrocyte parameters (Mhf); increased WBC numbers (Mhf)	Age; breed; sex; presence of anemia; FeLV infection
Sykes et al. (2008)[25]	USA	310	Anemic/HP infection suspected	27.4%	4.8%	23.2%	6.5%	Male; FeLV/FIV infection (Mhf); reticulocytosis (Mhf); increased MCV (Mhf/CMhm); monocytosis (CMt)	FeLV/FIV infection (CMhm; CMt)

TABLE 58.1 Selected Prevalence Studies for Feline Hemoplasma Species and Risk Factor Analysis for Infection—cont'd

Reference	Country	Number Of Cats	Health Status	Prevalence: All HP	Mhf	CMhm	CMt	Risk Factors For Infection[a]	Non-risk Factors For Infection[a]
Sykes et al. (2007)[24]	USA	263	99.2% sick; 51.3% anemic	18.0%	0.4%	15.6%; 0.7% CMhp-like	0.4%	FeLV infection; increased HCT (CMhm); increased age (CMhm); outdoor access; FIV infection (CMhm); squamous cell carcinoma (CMhm)	FeLV status (CMhm)
Ghazisaeedi et al. (2014)[21]	Iran	100	100% sick	22.0%	14.0%	12.0%	4.0%	Male; age > 8 years; decreased erythrocyte parameters (HCT; RBC numbers)	
Lobetti et al. (2012)[20]	South Africa	102	100% sick	25.5%	3.9%	21.6%	0%	Lower HCT (Mhf); lower WBC numbers (Mhf); lower platelet numbers (Mhf); male (Mhf)	
Tasker et al. (2004)[19]; Willi et al. (2006)[28]	Australia	147	94.6% sick	32.0%	4.8%	23.8%	10.2%	Increased age (CMhm); non-pedigree (CMhm); lower HCT (CMhm); male (CMhm); HCT (inversely correlated with Mhf copy numbers)	
Tanahara et al. (2010)[22]	Japan	1770	66.4% sick	26.4%	5.1%	21.0%	6.7%	Male; age > 2 years; history of cat bite wounds; FIV infection	FeLV status
Georges et al. (2012)[23]	Trinidad and Tobago	152	42.7% sick (n = 50/117)	46.7%	27.0%	31.6%	2.0%	FeLV/FIV infection (any HP, CMhm); increased age (any HP, CMhm); male (CMhm)	Health status; presence of anemia; FeLV/FIV status (Mhf)
Walker Vergara et al. (2016)[103]	Chile	384	33.9% sick	15.1%	5.8%	10.2%; 0.6% CMhp	1.7%	Male; increased age; outdoor access; FIV infection; increased MCV (Mhf); Mhf vs. CMhm: younger, increased MCV (without anemia), and increased monocytes	Health status; erythrocyte parameters
Aquino et al. (2014)[13]	Brazil	432	Unknown	13.8%	11.1%	13.8%	4.4%	Male (any HP, Mhf, CMhm and CMt)	Hematologic variables; CMhm copy numbers were positively correlated with RBC numbers
Ravicini et al. (2016)[104]	Spain	116	Shelter population	7.8%	0.9%	6.9%	0.0%		
Attipa et al. (2017)[105]	Cyprus	174	75.3% sick	26.4%	7.5%	20.7%	6.9%	FeLV/FIV infection (any HP, CMhm, Mt); increased age (CMhm); shelter/feral vs. owned (CMhm); outdoor access; *Leishmania* infection (CMt)	
Bergmann et al. (2017)[106]	Germany	479	Unknown	9.4%	0.4% (0.2% Mhc)	8.8%	0.0%	Male; outdoor access; multi-cat households; FIV infection	Shelter vs. owned
Ravagnan et al. (2017)[107]	Italy	227	Free-roaming	13.2%	4.0%	12.3%	4.8%	Male; increased age; FIV infection	

TABLE 58.1 Selected Prevalence Studies for Feline Hemoplasma Species and Risk Factor Analysis for Infection—cont'd

Reference	Country	Number Of Cats	Health Status	Prevalence All HP	Mhf	CMhm	CMt	Risk Factors For Infection[a]	Non-risk Factors For Infection[a]
Diaz-Reganon et al. (2018)[108]	Spain	594	76.8% owned; 23.2% stray	10.6%	3.7%	8.1%	0.5%	Male (any HP, Mhf, CMhm); FeLV infection (any HP, CMhm); FIV infection (any HP, Mhf, CMhm); spring/summer months (any HP, CMhm), summer months (Mhf); anemia; stray vs. owned (any HP, Mhf); increased age in owned cats; outdoor access in owned cats	
Makino et al. (2018)[109]	Brazil	151	Unknown	25.8%	15.2%	14.6%	2.6%	Male (CMhm); nonpedigree (CMhm)	
Munhoz et al. (2018)[110]	Brazil	200	Healthy, owned	35.5%	15.5%	19.0%	9.0%	Suburban (Mhf); contact with other cats (CMhm); co-infection with Mt (CMhm)	Anemia
Persichetti et al. (2018)[111]	Italy	197	68% outdoor; 32% indoor only	18.3%	6.1%	13.2%	5.1%	Adult age; FIV positivity; presence of anemia; increased creatinine, increased creatine kinase	
Sarvani et al. (2018)[112]	Serbia	373		17.2%	5.4%	12.6%	6.2%	Male; FIV infection (any HP, CMhm); outdoor access (any HP, CMhm); nonpedigree; anemia, increased age (CMhm)	
Do et al. (2020)[113]	Thailand	473	Unknown	38.1%[b]	13.3%	83.3%	3.3%	Increased age	Sex; free-roaming status; presence of ectoparasites; endoparasite prophylaxis
Latrofa et al. (2020)[114]	Italy	958	Unknown	11.6%	1.5%	9.9%	0.2%	Male (any HP, CMhm)	Age group, geographical origin

[a]For infection with any hemoplasma species, unless indicated.
[b]Only 50% of positive samples were speciated, so estimates for overall prevalence of each species have been calculated and presented.
CMhm, "*Candidatus* Mycoplasma haemominutum"; *CMhp*, "*Candidatus* Mycoplasma haematoparvum"; *CMt*, "*Candidatus* Mycoplasma turicensis"; *FeLV*, feline leukemia virus; *FIV*, feline immunodeficiency virus; *HCT*, hematocrit; *HP*, hemoplasma; *MCV*, mean corpuscular volume; *Mhc*, *Mycoplasma haemocanis*; *Mhf*, *Mycoplasma haemofelis*; *PCV*, packed cell volume; *RBC*, red blood cell; *WBC*, white blood cell.

associations between anemia and *M. haemofelis* infection.[15,30] This may be because these studies usually include chronically and subclinically *M. haemofelis*–infected cats. Some studies, but not others, have shown an association between retrovirus and infection with any hemoplasma species. Studies that have examined the relationship between individual hemoplasma species infections and retroviral status have shown variable results (see Table 58.1).

Long-term carrier status can occur with feline hemoplasma infections, with infected cats often being subclinical.[26,31] This is particularly common with "*Ca.* M. haemominutum" infection, although suspected clearance of infection with this species has been reported by others with and without antibiotic treatment.[27] Some *M. haemofelis*–infected cats spontaneously clear infection from peripheral blood a few months following acute infection; this also has been reported with "*Ca.* M. turicensis" infection. However, generalized statements regarding long-term carrier status cannot be made since great variation exists, likely because of differences in the host-organism interaction and hemoplasma isolates. Carrier cats often have subclinical infections, but reactivation of infection can occur and may result in clinical disease[32,33]; however, this is uncommon in our experience.

Two major hemoplasma species infect dogs: *Mycoplasma haemocanis* and "*Candidatus* Mycoplasma haematoparvum." The whole genome sequence of one strain of *M. haemocanis* has been determined.[34] The reported prevalence for canine hemoplasma infection also varies widely in different studies (Table 58.2), with *M. haemocanis* generally being more prevalent. Geographic variation is marked, possibly due to the presence of the proposed canine hemoplasma tick vector *Rhipicephalus sanguineus*.[35,36] Kenneled dogs, young dogs, crossbreeds, and dogs with mange were more likely to be infected in one study,[35] whereas other studies found no association with age.[16,36,37] A high prevalence of hemoplasma infection has also been reported in fighting dogs,[38,39] which supports the possibility of ingestion of blood as a transmission route.

Infection with *M. haemocanis* has been associated with hemolytic anemia in splenectomized dogs, and rarely in dogs with other immunosuppressive disease or concurrent infections. The 16S rRNA gene sequence of *M. haemocanis* cannot be distinguished from that of *M. haemofelis*, but phylogenetic analyses of other genes, as well as whole genome sequence comparison, distinguishes them as separate species.[9,34,40] *Mycoplasma haemocanis* is a coccoid organism that often forms chains of organisms (Fig. 58.2). "*Ca.* M. haematoparvum" is a small (0.3 μm) coccoid organism that resembles "*Ca.* M. haemominutum" morphologically (Fig. 58.3). The 16S rRNA gene sequence of "*Ca.* M. haematoparvum" is most closely related to that of "*Ca.* M.

TABLE 58.2 Selected Prevalence Studies for Canine Hemoplasma Species and Risk Factor Analysis for Infection

Reference	Country	Number of Dogs	Health Status	Prevalence: All HP	Mhc	CMhp	Risk Factors For Infection[a]	Non-risk Factors For Infection[a]
Roura et al. (2010)[16]	Spain	182	Hospital population	14.3%	14.3%	0.6%	Other vector-borne infection	Age; sex; breed; presence of anemia; health status
Kenny et al. (2004)[115]	France	460	Sick	15.4%	5.9%	12.2%		
Wengi et al. (2008)[36]	Switzerland	889	99.2% sick	1.2%	0.9%	0.3%		Age; sex; presence of anemia
Novacco et al. (2010)[35]	Italy	600	24.0% sick and 76.0% healthy	9.5%	4.5%	5.8%	Nonpedigree; kenneled (vs. private owned); mange infection	Sex; PCV; health status
Novacco et al. (2010)[35]	Spain	200	64.0% sick, 30.5% healthy and 5.5% of unknown health status	2.5%	0.5%	2.0%		
Hetzel et al. (2012)[116]	Australia	251	Hospital population	1.6%	0.8%	0.8%		
Hii et al. (2012)[45]	Australia	100	Healthy	1.0% (1.0% CMhb)	0.0%	0.0%		
Hii et al. (2012)[45]	Australia	130	Healthy	20.0%	17.7%	2.3%	*Anaplasma platys* infection	
Barker et al. (2010)[37]	Trinidad	184	Sick	8.7%	6.0%	3.8%		Age; sex; hematologic parameters
Compton et al. (2012)[117]	USA	506	79.6% sick	1.3%	0.6%	0.8%		
Levy et al. (2011)[118]	USA	345	Unknown	11.9%	6.4%	5.2%		
Barker et al. (2010)[37]	Tanzania	100	Unknown	20.0%	19.0%	1.0%	Male (Mhc)	Age; presence of ticks
Inokuma et al. (2006)[119]	Sudan	78	Unknown	39.7%	9.0%	33.3%		
Aquino et al. (2016)[120]	Nigeria	245	65.4% sick	7.8%	7.3%	0.4%		Sex; breed; private owned vs. kenneled; health status; presence of ticks; ectoparasite prophylaxis; age; PCV; presence of anemia
Hasiri et al. (2016)[121]	Iran	53	49% anemic	13.2%	7.5%	5.7%	Platelet count (Mhc)	Presence of anemia; health status; age; breed; sex; indoor vs. outdoor housing; presence of other dogs
Bouzouraa et al. (2017)[122]	France	134	Anemic	7.5%	6.0%	1.5%		
Ravagnan et al. (2017)[107]	Italy	395	29.6% blood donors; 70.4% free-roaming	4.5%	3.5%	1.0%	Free-roaming (vs. blood donors)	Sex; age; origin in Italy
Aktas & Ozubek (2018)[123]	Turkey	621	Healthy	15.3%	11.0%	10.8%	Adult age; presence of ticks; co-infections with selected arthropod-borne pathogens; shelter/free-roaming vs. owned	Sex; shelter vs. free-roaming
Happi et al. (2018)[124]	Nigeria	89	Sick	13.5% (1.1% CMhb)	11.2%	0.0%	Presence of ticks	Sex; age; hematologic parameters; co-infections with selected arthropod-borne pathogens
Hofmann et al. (2019)[125]	Crete, Greece	103	Shelter	10.7%	10.7%	0%		

[a]For infection with any hemoplasma species, unless indicated.

CMhb, "*Candidatus* Mycoplasma haemobos"; *CMhp,* "*Candidatus* Mycoplasma haematoparvum"; *HP,* hemoplasma; *Mhc, Mycoplasma haemocanis*; *PCV,* packed cell volume.

haemominutum"; however, phylogenetic analysis of the *rnpB* gene has been used to distinguish them as separate species.[41]

Little work has been done regarding the time course of carrier status with canine hemoplasmas, but subclinical carrier dogs that are infected with *M. haemocanis* and "*Ca.* M. haematoparvum" exist.[36]

A "*Ca.* M. haematoparvum"–like organism has also been reported in a small number of cats in two studies.[24,42] In addition, "*Ca.* M. haemominutum" has been detected in several dogs using PCR assays. Organisms that resemble "*Ca.* M. haematoparvum" and "*Ca.* M. haemominutum" have been detected in European wolves and bush dogs from Brazil.[43] The ovine hemoplasma *Mycoplasma ovis* has been detected in a small number of dogs from the southeastern United States,[44] and the bovine hemoplasma "*Candidatus* Mycoplasma haemobos" was detected in a dog from northern Australia.[45] The clinical importance of these hemoplasma species in cats and dogs remains unclear.

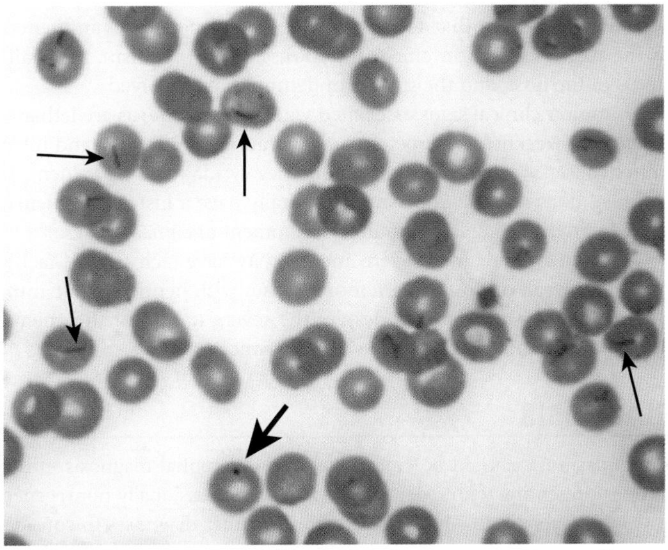

Fig. 58.2 Romanowsky-stained blood smear showing chains of epierythrocytic bacteria typical of *Mycoplasma haemocanis (thin arrows)*. A Howell-Jolly body is also present *(large bolded arrow)*.

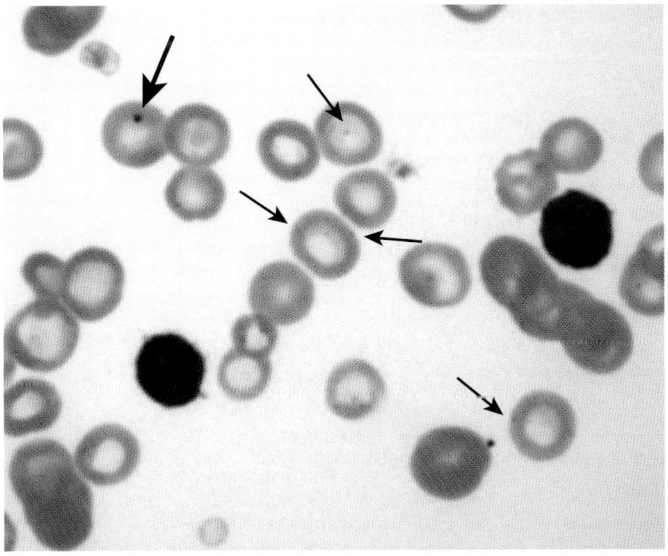

Fig. 58.3 Blood smear from a dog showing "*Candidatus* Mycoplasma haematoparvum" *(thin arrows)* and a Howell-Jolly body *(large bolded arrow)*.

Pathogenesis

Mycoplasma haemofelis is the most pathogenic of the feline hemoplasma species. Cats do not need to be immunocompromised or splenectomized to succumb to clinical disease with *M. haemofelis* (however, even splenectomized cats infected with "*Ca.* M. haemominutum" do not seem to develop disease).[46]

Acute infection often results in severe hemolytic anemia (primarily extravascular, but occasionally intravascular hemolysis is reported) although in some cases only mild anemia occurs. In experimental studies, clinical signs occur around 2 to 34 days after infection, and anemia lasts from 18 to 30 days. The onset of anemia is usually followed by a significant regenerative response with reticulocytosis. Chronic infection is not usually associated with significant anemia.[27] Experimental infections have shown that *M. haemofelis* blood organism numbers can fluctuate greatly over short periods of time, especially in the first few weeks of infection (Fig. 58.4). Antigenic variation, to evade the host immune system, may mediate these *M. haemofelis* organism number fluctuations,[47] as a very large portion (62%) of the genome encodes a set of uncharacterized hypothetical proteins arranged in series of paralogous repeats which could facilitate differing expression of hemoplasma surface proteins over time.

Persistent autoagglutination or a positive Coombs' test, indicating the presence of erythrocyte-bound antibodies, have been demonstrated in anemic cats with acute *M. haemofelis* infection.[48–50] One study[50] showed that erythrocyte-bound antibodies reactive at 4°C (cold reactive antibodies; both IgM and IgG) appeared a few days earlier than those reactive at 37°C (warm reactive antibodies; primarily IgG). However, in most cats, these antibodies appeared only after the development of anemia had started, and disappeared with antibiotic and supportive treatment alone, without the need for specific glucocorticoid treatment. The absence of erythrocyte-bound antibodies at the onset of development of anemia could reflect lack of sensitivity in their detection or that erythrocyte-bound antibodies appear as a result of hemoplasma-induced hemolysis rather than initiating it. Osmotic fragility[14,49] and reduced erythrocyte lifespan[51] have also been reported with *M. haemofelis* infection.

Although acute "*Ca.* M. haemominutum" infection is associated with a fall in RBC parameters,[50] anemia is not usually induced except in cats with concurrent diseases or infections (e.g., lymphoma or FeLV infection).[52,53] For example, cats that are co-infected with FeLV and "*Ca.* M. haemominutum" develop more significant anemia than cats infected with "*Ca.* M. haemominutum" alone, and progression to FeLV-induced myeloproliferative disease occurred more rapidly in one study of experimentally infected cats.[53] Although concurrent problems are usually present in "*Ca.* M. haemominutum"–infected cats that develop anemia, cases of so-called primary "*Ca.* M. haemominutum" anemia (i.e., without any apparent concurrent disease or infection present) have also been reported,[54] so infection with this species cannot be ruled out as a cause of anemia in an individual case. However, conflicting data exist as one US study documented that "*Ca.* M. haemominutum"–infected cats were less likely to be anemic than cats not infected with "*Ca.* M. haemominutum."[24]

The pathogenic potential of "*Ca.* M. turicensis" is not fully understood. Experimental infection has resulted in anemia[14] or a small decline in RBC parameters in some studies,[50] but generally anemia is uncommon following infection. Concurrent disease and immunosuppression are both thought to be involved in the pathogenesis of "*Ca.* M. turicensis" disease,[20] in a similar way to the pathogenesis described for "*Ca.* M. haemominutum." Inoculation of an immunosuppressed cat with "*Ca.* M. turicensis" resulted in severe anemia,[14] but little or no anemia occurred in immunocompetent cats after inoculation with "*Ca.* M. turicensis." Determination of the pathogenicity of "*Ca.* M. turicensis" in naturally infected cats has been difficult in epidemiologic studies as cats are often co-infected with other hemoplasma species, which confounds disease associations.

It is possible that different strains of each of the feline hemoplasma species reported exist, and that these also vary in pathogenicity. This might explain some of the conflicting data reported in different studies. However, other factors such as the underlying health status of the cat, and possibly even the transmission route of infection, may play a role in the outcome of hemoplasma infection. One isolate of the porcine hemoplasma *Mycoplasma suis* was able to penetrate porcine erythrocytes; its subsequent intracellular location was associated with marked pathogenicity and resistance to antimicrobial therapy.[55] It is possible that this could occur for hemoplasmas in other species.

Studies of the pathogenicity of canine hemoplasmas are sparse. Hemoplasma infection in dogs usually results in hemolytic anemia only in splenectomized or immunocompromised dogs,[56–59] and subclinical latent *M. haemocanis* infections can be reactivated following splenectomy. However, recognition of the possibility of hemoplasma infection is important to differentiate such cases from cases of primary IMHA as some infected dogs have a positive Coombs' test.[60,61]

The natural route of transmission of hemoplasma infection among cats and dogs in the field has not yet been determined, and it may be that different routes predominate for different hemoplasma species. Canine and feline hemoplasma DNA have been found in fleas, ticks, and mosquitoes.[30,62–69] However, this does not imply that these vectors mediate transmission, as the hemoplasma DNA could reflect their hematophagous activity on infected hosts. The clustered geographic distribution of infection in some studies supports the role of an arthropod vector in hemoplasma transmission.[24] Although *Ctenocephalides felis* has been implicated in hemoplasma transmission in cats, only very transient *M. haemofelis* infection has been reported in cats experimentally infected via the hematophagous activity of fleas, and clinical and hematologic signs of *M. haemofelis* infection were not induced in the recipient cat.[70] Additionally, there was no evidence of hemoplasma transmission when fleas were introduced into groups of cats housed together.[71] Transmission of *M. haemocanis* by the brown dog tick, *Rh. sanguineus*, in experimental infections has been reported, although this study was performed before the advent of molecular diagnostic methods to confirm infection.[64]

The association between hemoplasma infection and male sex and/or retrovirus (particularly FIV) infection status seen in some studies could suggest that cat fights could be involved in transmission of infection. Studies in Switzerland have found that subcutaneous inoculation of "*Ca.* M. turicensis"–containing blood resulted in infection transmission, whereas the same inoculation method using "*Ca.* M. turicensis"–containing saliva did not. This suggests that hemoplasma transmission by social contact (saliva via mutual grooming etc.) is less likely than transmission by aggressive interaction (blood transmission during a cat bite incident).[72] However, one study[71] found evidence of horizontal transmission of "*Ca.* M. haemominutum", but not *M. haemofelis*, by direct contact between cats in the absence of aggressive interaction and vectors. Vertical transmission for canine or feline hemoplasma infections has not been definitively proven using molecular methods, but has been strongly suggested for *M. haemocanis*[73] and hemoplasmas that infect other host species.[74] Blood transfusion is another route of transmission, and blood donors should be screened for hemoplasma infection.[75]

CLINICAL FEATURES

The clinical disease that follows hemoplasma infection is influenced by the stage of infection, the host response to the organism, the health status of the host, and the species of hemoplasma involved.

Common clinical signs associated with hemoplasmosis are lethargy, pallor, and weakness. Inappetence, dehydration, weight loss, and intermittent fever are also reported. Splenomegaly may also be evident. In contrast, dogs with hemoplasmosis typically have a history of splenectomy (a predisposing factor in the development of clinical disease).

Affected animals with severe anemia may have tachycardia, tachypnea, and weak or bounding femoral pulses with hemic cardiac murmurs. Icterus is uncommon despite the severe nature of the anemia involved. Moribund cats may be hypothermic.

DIAGNOSIS

Hemoplasmosis should be considered as a differential diagnosis in cats or dogs presenting with regenerative (although occasionally nonregenerative) anemia and possibly associated fever. Other diagnoses to consider are primary IMHA (less common in cats when compared with dogs),

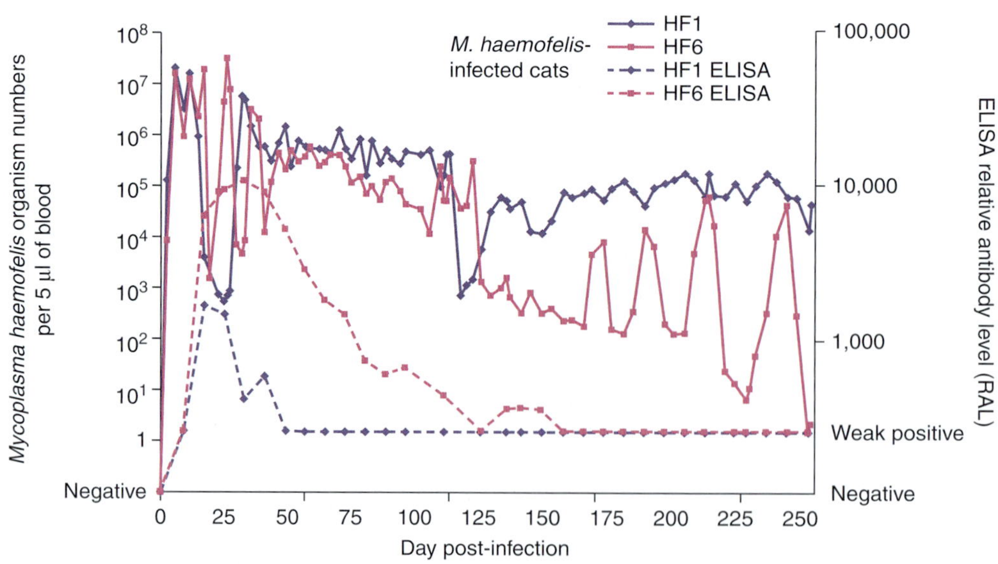

Fig. 58.4 *Mycoplasma haemofelis* copy number and *M. haemofelis* anti-DnaK ELISA following acute infection in two cats. HF1 = cat number 1 infected wtih *M. haemofelis;* HF6 = cat number 6 infected wtih *M. haemofelis. ELISA,* enzyme-linked immunosorbent assay. (From Barker EN, Helps CR, Heesom KJ, et al. Detection of humoral response using a recombinant heat shock protein 70, DnaK, of *Mycoplasma haemofelis* in experimentally and naturally hemoplasma-infected cats. *Clin Vaccine Immunol.* 2010;17:1926–32.)

secondary IMHA (e.g., secondary to drugs, neoplasia, or other infections), cytauxzoonosis (cats), retroviral infection (cats), babesiosis, Heinz body-associated hemolysis (cats), hypophosphatemia, and inherited RBC disorders (e.g., pyruvate kinase deficiency, and red cell fragility disorders).

Laboratory Abnormalities

Pathogenic hemoplasma infections typically cause a regenerative anemia that is macrocytic and hypochromic, although pronounced reticulocytosis is not always evident.[76] Normoblasts may be present. Manual reticulocyte counts should be interpreted with caution in *M. haemofelis*–infected cats, because hemoplasma-infected erythrocytes may have the same appearance as reticulocytes in blood smears stained with methylene blue. Occasionally, nonregenerative anemia can be present when insufficient time for a regenerative response has elapsed, or as a result of bone marrow suppression due to medication or concurrent disease such as FeLV infection. Neutrophil counts may be normal, elevated, or low, and lymphopenia may be present. Thrombocytopenia can also occur in affected dogs and cats, but the platelet count can also be within the reference range. Positive Coombs' test results, particularly with cold agglutinins, and persistent autoagglutination have been reported in acute hemoplasmosis. Hyperbilirubinemia is seen occasionally due to hemolysis. Hypoxic damage to the liver may result in increased activities of ALT and AST. Metabolic acidosis and prerenal azotemia may be noted. Hyperproteinemia, due to a polyclonal gammopathy, is sometimes seen in cats.[77] Urinalysis is usually unremarkable. Bilirubinuria may be present where hyperbilirubinemia is present. Soma cats may test positive for FIV or FeLV, which have been associated with infection (see Table 58.1).

Diagnostic Imaging

The most common radiographic or ultrasonographic finding in cats with hemoplasmosis is splenomegaly, due to a combination of increased splenic macrophage activity, splenic sequestration of erythrocytes, and extramedullary hematopoiesis (Fig. 58.5). The spleen may be absent in affected dogs because of splenectomy.

Microbiologic Tests

Assays available for diagnosis of hemoplasmosis in dogs and cats are listed in Table 58.3.

Cytologic Examination

Cytologic examination of blood smears may show hemoplasmas on the surface of erythrocytes (see Fig. 58.1) but this is very insensitive (0% to 37.5%)[21,26,29,78]; massive numbers of organisms must be present in blood before they can be visualized. Cytologic examination cannot easily differentiate between *M. haemofelis* and "*Ca.* M. haemominutum"[79]; "*Ca.* M. turicensis" has never been visualized by light microscopy. Specificity can also be an issue for cytologic diagnosis, as organisms need to be differentiated from stain precipitate, Howell-Jolly bodies, and basophilic stippling. As *M. haemocanis* organisms tend to form chains (see Fig. 58.2) and are visible in many clinically affected dogs, it is more readily differentiated from stain precipitate and erythrocyte morphologic changes. Hemoplasmas are not usually visible in chronically infected dogs or in dogs infected with "*Ca.* M. haematoparvum."

Culture

Attempts to isolate and grow feline hemotropic mycoplasmas in the laboratory have been unsuccessful.

Molecular Diagnosis Using Nucleic Acid–based Testing

PCR is now the diagnostic method of choice for hemoplasma infection. Numerous assays have been described to date, both conventional

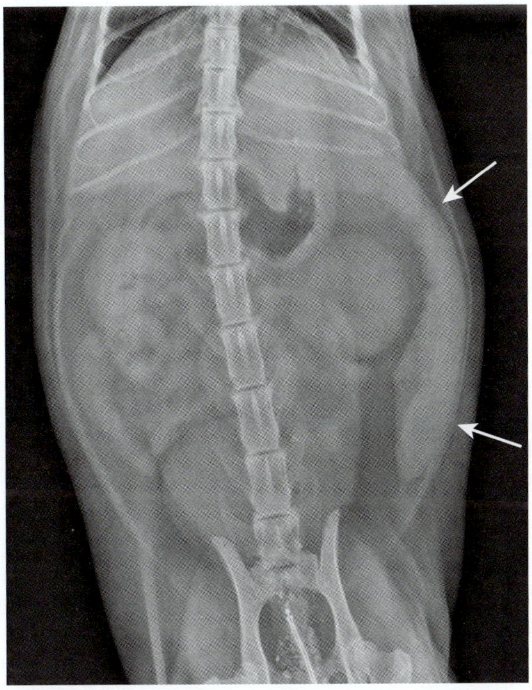

Fig. 58.5 Ventrodorsal abdominal radiograph from an 8-year-old male neutered domestic shorthair cat with hemolytic anemia secondary to *Mycoplasma haemofelis* infection. There is marked splenomegaly *(arrows)*.

TABLE 58.3 Assays Available for the Diagnosis of Hemoplasma Infection

Test	Specimen Required	Advantages	Disadvantages
Cytology	Thin blood smear of diagnostic quality stained with Diff-Quik, Wright stains, etc.	Results obtained very quickly Can be done at POC	Very limited sensitivity and specificity Requires PCR to confirm infecting species
PCR	EDTA-whole blood	High sensitivity and specificity Can identify infecting species If quantitative, may be used to monitor response to treatment	Expensive Not currently available as POC test with lag phase for results depending on turnaround time of PCR laboratory. (A POC test that uses isothermal non-quantitative amplification of DNA has been recently described to diagnose *Mycoplasma haemofelis* infection, but its sensitivity is variable)
Serology	Serum or plasma	May identify potential "carrier" cats May be more sensitive than PCR	Seropositive cats may not be actively infected with hemoplasmas Cross-reactivity between species Not currently available commercially

EDTA, ethylenediaminetetraacetic acid; *PCR,* polymerase chain reaction; *POC,* point of care.

and real-time quantitative PCR (qPCR), which are generally based on detection of segments of the 16S rRNA gene. When properly designed and executed, PCR is far more sensitive than cytology, although PCR may not detect organisms in some subclinical carrier cats that have very low numbers of organisms in the blood, below the detection limit of the PCR assay. Some hemoplasma PCR assays have been duplexed with a host housekeeping gene PCR, targeting the 28S rRNA gene[80] or glyceraldehyde-3-phosphate dehydrogenase gene[37]; the inclusion of such an internal control is important in order to identify false-negative results for hemoplasma infection due to the failure of DNA extraction, presence of PCR inhibitors, or setup errors. qPCR assays can enable the course of hemoplasma infection to be monitored, and permit evaluation of response to antimicrobial treatment. The fluctuations in blood organism numbers that can occur during acute *M. haemofelis* infection (see Fig. 58.4) should be considered when interpreting qPCR results, as decreases in organism number cannot always be deemed a consequence of effective antimicrobial treatment or host immune response. Because of the subclinical carrier state, a positive PCR result should be interpreted in light of clinical signs, clinicopathologic results, and any concurrent disease or immunosuppression present. The pathogenicity of the infecting hemoplasma detected should also be considered when deciding whether the positive PCR result represents the cause of the animal's signs.

A POC machine using isothermal nonquantitative amplification of DNA to diagnose *M. haemofelis* infection has been evaluated in a small study.[81] However, the technique requires in-house extraction of DNA from blood. The type of extraction kit used affects the sensitivity of the assay, which will need to be taken into account during interpretation.

TABLE 58.4 Suggested Antimicrobial Drug Dosages for Treatment of Hemoplasmosis in Cats[a]

Drug	Dose (mg/kg)	Route	Frequency	Notes/Comments
Doxycycline	5 10	PO PO	q12h q24h	First-line agent. Can be associated with gastrointestinal adverse effects, and esophagitis if incompletely swallowed
Marbofloxacin	2–5.5	PO	q24h	First-line agent. May be used in combination (sequentially) with doxycycline to clear *Mycoplasma haemofelis* infection[126]
Pradofloxacin	3–5	PO	q24h	Second-line agent. May be more efficacious at clearing *M. haemofelis* infection than doxycycline
Enrofloxacin	5	PO	q24h	Second-line agent. However, potential for irreversible retinal toxicity in cat as idiosyncratic reaction

[a]Drug availability and licensed dose rate may vary by country.

Serology

ELISAs that detect antibodies to an immunodominant protein of *M. haemofelis*, DnaK, have been developed (see Fig. 58.4).[82,83] Serologic cross-reactivity occurs to this antigen for all three feline hemoplasma species,[82] so the assay does not discriminate between infection with *M. haemofelis* and other hemoplasmas. Determination of acute and convalescent titers may be helpful to distinguish acute from chronic infection. Another study found that a similar serologic assay was more sensitive than PCR in detecting exposure to "*Ca.* M. turicensis."[83] Further work is required to determine the specificity of these assays before they can be made available commercially. Currently serologic assays are available only on a research basis.

Pathologic Findings

Generalized pallor, splenomegaly, and, in some cats, icterus are the main gross necropsy finding in cats that die or are euthanized as a result of hemoplasmosis. Histopathologic findings include extramedullary hematopoiesis, follicular hyperplasia, and splenic erythrophagocytosis.

TREATMENT

Both supportive and specific treatment is indicated for cats and dogs with clinical signs and clinicopathologic abnormalities consistent with hemoplasmosis. Clinical improvement usually occurs within 2–3 days of starting appropriate treatment. However, no antimicrobial treatment regimen exists that is known to predictably eliminate hemoplasma infection with any species.

Specific Therapy

The response of different hemoplasma species, and indeed different strains of the same species, to antimicrobials during infection varies. A number of antimicrobials (Table 58.4), notably tetracyclines[59,84] and fluoroquinolones,[84–88] can reduce hemoplasma organism numbers in cats and dogs, although the vast majority of studies published only examine *M. haemofelis* infection. Doxycycline is often used to treat hemoplasmosis as a first-line agent (see Chapter 10 for information on doxycycline). Because of the possibility of esophagitis in cats, administration of the hyclate preparation of doxycycline should always be followed by food or water. Fluoroquinolones are an alternative; marbofloxacin and pradofloxacin,[88] when available, are both efficacious. Enrofloxacin is also usually effective,[89] but caution must be exercised with its use in cats as it has been, rarely, associated with diffuse retinal degeneration and acute-onset irreversible blindness as an idiosyncratic reaction. Antimicrobials are typically given for 2–4 weeks, with longer treatment courses (e.g., 6–8 weeks) recommended by some to increase the likelihood of elimination of infection, although longer treatment courses still do not guarantee elimination. Azithromycin was not effective in one study of cats infected with *M. haemofelis* and/or "*Ca.* M. haemominutum."[78] Some cases appear to be refractory to standard antimicrobial treatments, and in one *M. haemocanis* case report[58] oxytetracycline, and subsequent enrofloxacin, treatment did not markedly reduce organism numbers, although clinical signs did improve.

A treatment protocol for clearance of chronic *M. haemofelis* infection has been described, with recrudescence of infection not induced following attempts at immunosuppression with methylprednisolone. The protocol comprised a course of doxycycline (5 mg/kg, PO, q12h for 4 weeks), followed by a course of marbofloxacin (2 mg/kg, PO, q24h for 2 weeks) for cats that remained positive by qPCR (as determined by repeated testing on multiple occasions). Treatment breaks of up to 4 weeks between the courses of antimicrobials did not influence the outcome.

Ideally, response to antimicrobials should be monitored by qPCR to ensure organism numbers are decreasing with therapy, or if clearance of infection is being attempted as described above, as response to treatment is not predictable. However, repeat qPCR may not be necessary if the patient shows a rapid and favorable clinical response to treatment. Repeat hematology profiles should also be performed.

Supportive Care

Affected dogs and cats may also require supportive treatment with IV fluid therapy to correct dehydration, or blood products to provide oxygen-carrying capacity. Anemic dogs and cats with signs consistent with decompensated anemia (tachycardia, weakness, tachypnea, metabolic acidemia) are best treated with a packed RBC, or whole blood, transfusion. Oxygen therapy can be provided pending stabilization of the patient's oxygen-carrying capacity.

Administration of glucocorticoids to cats and dogs with suspected hemoplasmosis is controversial. Their efficacy is unproven, they are not required for a clinical response, and immunosuppressive doses of glucocorticoids have been used experimentally to enhance bacteremia and induce reactivation of latent infection. However, they may be necessary in cats that fail to respond to antimicrobial therapy alone, or when the diagnosis is uncertain, and if erythrocyte-bound antibodies are identified.

PROGNOSIS

The prognosis for hemoplasmosis in cats and dogs is generally good if effective treatment is instigated promptly. Some cases are refractory to initial antimicrobial therapy, necessitating alternative antimicrobial treatments. Additionally, some animals remain hemoplasma carriers following recovery, and recrudescence of disease is possible months or years later.

IMMUNITY AND VACCINATION

Limited information is available in regard to the immune response to hemoplasma infection, and no vaccines are available. Studies of serum cytokine levels during acute infection have resulted in conflicting results regarding Th1 versus Th2 responses.[77,90,91] *M. haemofelis*– and "*Ca.* M. turicensis"–recovered cats are protected against rechallenge, but this protection is independent of an anti-DnaK humoral immune response.[90,91] "*Ca.* M. turicensis"–recovered cats are not protected against *M. haemofelis* challenge, and become PCR positive significantly earlier than the naïve cats, suggesting possible antibody-dependent enhancement.[77] The lack of cross-protection is supported by the frequent identification of co-infections with multiple hemoplasma species during prevalence studies. Furthermore, passive immunization via transfusion of a small volume of pooled plasma from *M. haemofelis*–recovered cats failed to provide immunity to infection with *M. haemofelis* and may exacerbate clinical disease.[92]

PREVENTION

Blood donors should be screened for hemoplasma infection by PCR to help prevent inadvertent transmission by blood transfusion from carrier cats or dogs. As the carrier status cannot be definitively eliminated, infected individuals should not be considered as potential future donors.

Avoidance of potential risk factors are also likely to prevent infection. This includes restriction of outdoor access; prevention of aggressive interactions among cats; and, in view of the potential for vector transmission, preventative flea and tick treatment.

PUBLIC HEALTH ASPECTS

Infections have been described in humans with novel hemoplasma species,[93,94] as well as species that have possibly originated in animals such as the cat,[95] pigs,[96–98] sheep,[93,99] or dogs,[100] raising the possibility of zoonotic infections. However, identification of the DNA of animal hemoplasmas in humans should be viewed cautiously in some of these studies because only a small portion or portions of the hemoplasma genome was detected. Furthermore, application of molecular diagnostic methods to archived human blood smears believed to contain hemoplasmas based on cytologic evaluation yielded negative results, suggesting the possibility of historical misdiagnosis.[101] Limited PCR-based human epidemiologic studies have failed to detect significant infections; although human hemoplasma infection has been reported in China, these studies have not described clinical disease.

Available case reports suggest that hemoplasma-associated disease is more likely in immunocompromised individuals. Until further information is available, veterinarians should handle blood from animals with caution, particularly those with impaired immune systems.

CASE EXAMPLE

Signalment

"Shadow," an 8-year-old male neutered domestic shorthair cat from Fairfield, CA.

History

Shadow was an indoor-outdoor cat that was acquired as a stray kitten from the owner's backyard. There had been no previous history of illness.

Shadow was brought to the University of California, Davis, Veterinary Medical Teaching Hospital emergency service for treatment of severe anemia. The owners reported that he had disappeared 5 days previously. He was found splayed across a fence and was unwilling to move, and vocalizing and salivating profusely. He was immediately taken to a local emergency clinic where he was found to be obtunded, pale, and severely dehydrated. His pulse was 180 beats/minute, respiratory rate was 60 breaths/minute, and temperature was 94.0°F (34.4°C). His systolic blood pressure was 80 mmHg. PCV was 12%. Shadow's condition was stabilized after treatment with supplemental oxygen, active warming, and IV crystalloid fluids (Normosol-R, 50 mL over 30 minutes, then 25 mL/hour). He tested negative for FIV antibody and FeLV antigen with an in-practice ELISA assay.

Physical Examination

Body weight/condition: 6 kg; BCS 7/9.

General: Obtunded, laterally recumbent. T = 97.8°F (36.6°C), HR = 150 beats/minute, RR = 60 breaths/minute, purring, pale and tacky mucous membranes with no detectable capillary refill, weak pulses.

Integument: No ectoparasites were noted. The pinnae and ventral abdominal skin were icteric.

Eyes, ears, nose, and throat: Moderate dental calculus was present. Pallor and mild icterus of the mucous membranes, nictitans, and sclera were noted (Fig. 58.6).

Cardiovascular: Weak pulses. No other clinically significant abnormalities were detected. No murmurs were detected, but the heart sounds were difficult to auscultate because of persistent purring.

Respiratory: Tachypneic; auscultation was limited because of purring.

GI and genitourinary: Nonpainful abdomen. Moderate cranial organomegaly. Urinary bladder not palpable.

Neurologic: A full neurologic examination was not performed, but no abnormalities were detected on examination of cranial nerve functions.

Lymph nodes: No clinically significant abnormalities detected.

Continued

CASE EXAMPLE—cont'd

Laboratory Findings

PCV/TPP: 14%/7.3 g/dL; icteric plasma.

Saline slide agglutination test: Negative.

Blood smear examination: Marked polychromasia, normoblastosis, and mild anisocytosis were present. Coccoid bodies that resembled hemoplasmas were present in association with erythrocytes (see Fig. 58.1).

Electrolyte/acid-base panel (venous blood): HCO_3 = 14 mmol/L, pH = 7.365, pCO_2 = 21.9 mmHg, pO_2 = 35.4 mmHg, Hb = 2.8 g/dL, O_2 – 59.5%, potassium = 4.0 mmol/L, sodium = 144 mmol/L, ionized calcium = 1.2 mmol/L, glucose = 157 mg/dL, lactate = 8.4 mmol/L, base excess = –12.2 mmol/L.

Imaging Findings

Thoracic radiographs: No clinically significant abnormalities were detected.

Abdominal radiographs: The spleen was markedly enlarged (see Fig. 58.5). The liver was mildly enlarged. Small mineral densities were present within ingesta and feces in the stomach and colon, respectively.

Treatment

The cat was placed on a heating pad and transfused with 1 unit of packed RBC, and supplemental oxygen was administered, after which HR increased to 200 beats/minute and RR decreased to 40 breaths/minute. Rectal temperature increased to 103.7°F (39.8°C) during the transfusion, and so dexamethasone was administered because of the concern for a transfusion reaction (0.2 mg/kg, IV, once). The cat was also treated with enrofloxacin (5 mg/kg, IV, q24h) (see Comments below) for suspected hemoplasmosis. The results of laboratory testing after transfer to the internal medicine service the day after admission are shown here.

CBC post-transfusion and antimicrobial treatment (reference interval): HCT 12.7% (30%–50%), MCV 76.5 fL (42–53 fL), MCHC 26.8 g/dL (30–33.5 g/dL), reticulocytes 155,600 cells/μL (7,000–60,000 cells/μL), nucleated RBC 39/100 WBC (0/100 WBC), corrected WBC 9,800 cells/μL (4,500–14,000 cells/μL), neutrophils 8,134 cells/μL (2,000–9,000 cells/μL), band neutrophils 98 cells/μL, lymphocytes 784 cells/μL (1,000–7,000 cells/μL), monocytes 784 cells/μL (50–600 cells/μL), eosinophils 0 cells/μL (150–1100 cells/μL), basophils 0 cells/μL (0–50 cells/μL), platelets 142,000/μL (180,000–500,000 platelets/μL).

Cytologic examination: Marked anisocytosis, marked polychromasia, few Howell-Jolly bodies, and many macrocytes and microcytes. No epierythrocytic organisms were identified.

Serum chemistry profile (reference interval): Sodium 143 mmol/L (151–158 mmol/L), potassium 5.2 mmol/L (3.6–4.9 mmol/L), chloride 107 mmol/L (117–126 mmol/L), bicarbonate 11 mmol/L (15–21 mmol/L), phosphorus 6.6 mg/dL (3.2–6.3 mg/dL), calcium 9.6 mg/dL (9.0–10.9 mg/dL), BUN 47 mg/dL (18–33 mg/dL), creatinine 1.2 mg/dL (1.1–2.2 mg/dL), glucose 98 mg/dL (63–118 mg/dL), total protein 7.2 g/dL (6.6–8.4 g/dL), albumin 3.0 g/dL (2.2–4.6 g/dL), globulin 4.2 g/dL (2.8–5.4 g/dL), ALT 166 U/L (27–101 U/L), AST 201 U/L (17–58 U/L), ALP 24 U/L (14–71 U/L), GGT 0 U/L (0–4 U/L), cholesterol 75 mg/dL (89–258 mg/dL), total bilirubin 6.1 mg/dL (0–0.2 mg/dL), magnesium 3.4 mg/dL (1.5–2.5 mg/dL), creatine kinase 446 U/L (73–260 U/L).

Urinalysis: SpG 1.040, pH 6, 75 mg/dL protein, no glucose, 5 mg/dL ketones, 6 mg/dL bilirubin, 250 erythrocytes/μL hemoprotein, 0-1 RBC/HPF, 0 WBC/HPF, rare transitional epithelial cells.

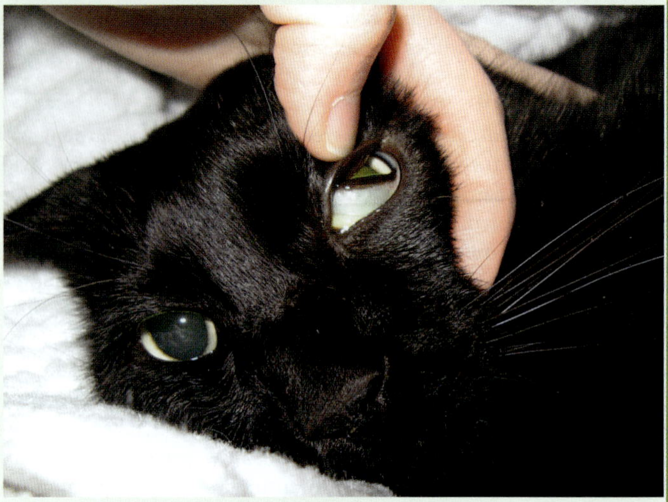

Fig. 58.6 Mild icterus of the nictating membrane in an 8-year-old male neutered domestic shorthair cat with hemolytic anemia secondary to *Mycoplasma haemofelis* infection.

Microbiologic testing: Real-time PCR (using blood smears on admission, pre-treatment) for *M. haemofelis*, "*Ca.* M. haemominutum", and "*Ca.* M. turicensis": positive for *M. haemofelis* DNA.

Diagnosis

Anemia due to *M. haemofelis* infection.

Additional Treatment and Outcome

Treatment was changed to doxycycline (10 mg/kg, PO, q24h, followed by 5 mL of water for 3 weeks). Treatment with IV crystalloid fluids was continued and oxygen supplementation was discontinued. Two days after admission, the PCV was 16% and the cat became fear aggressive and began eating. The cat was discharged the following day with a PCV of 18%, and a recheck at the local veterinary clinic that included a CBC was recommended 1 week later. The owner subsequently elected to house Shadow indoors.

Comments

This represents a typical case of hemoplasmosis in a male, neutered cat with access to the outdoors. Specific testing for hemoplasmas with PCR was performed on blood smears because treatment with packed RBC and antimicrobials had been initiated immediately on admission and whole blood was not saved before treatment was instituted. Although PCR on blood smears has lower sensitivity than when whole liquid blood is used, in this case sufficient organisms were present to generate a positive result, which confirmed the diagnosis of hemoplasmosis. Because the cat was hypovolemic on admission, parenteral antimicrobial treatment was chosen. Subsequently, treatment with oral doxycycline was initiated. Although continued treatment with oral enrofloxacin may have been a suitable alternative to doxycycline, retinal degeneration was a possible adverse effect of continued treatment with enrofloxacin, as well as enrofloxacin ideally being reserved as a second-line antimicrobial agent. Retesting for retroviruses was indicated 2 months after the first test was performed at the local veterinary clinic, as the cat may have been exposed to retroviruses but not yet have developed positive test results (see Chapters 32 and 33).

TPP, total plasma protein

SUGGESTED READINGS

Novacco M, Sugiarto S, Willi B, et al. Consecutive antibiotic treatment with doxycycline and marbofloxacin clears bacteremia in *Mycoplasma haemofelis*-infected cats. *Vet Microbiol*. 2018;217:112–120.

Tasker S, Hofmann-Lehmann R, Belak S, et al. Haemoplasmosis in cats: European guidelines from the ABCD on prevention and management. *J Fel Med Surg*. 2018;20:256–261.

REFERENCES

1. Benjamin MM, Lumb WV. *Haemobartonella canis* infection in a dog. *J Am Vet Med Assoc.* 1959;135:388–390.
2. Kikuth W. Über einen neuen Anämeerreger, *Bartonella canis*, nov. spec. *Klin Wochenschr.* 1928;7.
3. Flint JC, Moss LC. Infectious anaemia in cats. *J Am Vet Med Assoc.* 1953;122:45–48.
4. Clark R. *Eperythrozoon felis* (sp. Nov) in a cat. *J S Afr Vet Med Assoc.* 1942;13:15–16.
5. Messick JB, Walker PG, Raphael W, et al. '*Candidatus* Mycoplasma haemodidelphidis' sp. nov., '*Candidatus* Mycoplasma haemolamae' sp. nov and *Mycoplasma haemocanis* comb. nov., haemotrophic parasites from a naturally infected opossum (*Didelphis virginiana*), alpaca (*Lama pacos*) and dog (*Canis familiaris*): phylogenetic and secondary structural relatedness of their 16S rRNA genes to other mycoplasmas. *Int J Syst Evol Microbiol.* 2002;52:693–698.
6. Neimark H, Johansson KE, Rikihisa Y, et al. Proposal to transfer some members of the genera *Haemobartonella* and *Eperythrozoon* to the genus *Mycoplasma* with descriptions of '*Candidatus* Mycoplasma haemofelis', '*Candidatus* Mycoplasma haemomuris', '*Candidatus* Mycoplasma haemosuis' and '*Candidatus* Mycoplasma wenyonii'. *Int J Syst Evol Microbiol.* 2001;51:891–899.
7. Neimark H, Johansson KE, Rikihisa Y, et al. Revision of haemotrophic *Mycoplasma* species names. *Int J Syst Evol Microbiol.* 2002;52:683.
8. Guimaraes AM, Santos AP, do Nascimento NC, et al. Comparative genomics and phylogenomics of hemotrophic mycoplasmas. *PLoS One.* 2014;9:e91445.
9. Hicks CA, Barker EN, Brady C, et al. Non-ribosomal phylogenetic exploration of Mollicute species: new insights into haemoplasma taxonomy. *Infect Genet Evol.* 2014;23:99–105.
10. Barker EN, Darby AC, Helps CR, et al. Genome sequence for "*Candidatus* Mycoplasma haemominutum," a low-pathogenicity hemoplasma species. *J Bacteriol.* 2012;194:905–906.
11. Barker EN, Helps CR, Peters IR, et al. Complete genome sequence of *Mycoplasma haemofelis*, a hemotropic mycoplasma. *J Bacteriol.* 2011;193:2060–2061.
12. Messick JB, Santos AP, Guimaraes AM. Complete genome sequences of two hemotropic mycoplasmas, *Mycoplasma haemofelis* strain Ohio2 and *Mycoplasma suis* strain Illinois. *J Bacteriol.* 2011;193:2068–2069.
13. Aquino LC, Hicks CA, Scalon MC, et al. Prevalence and phylogenetic analysis of haemoplasmas from cats infected with multiple species. *J Microbiol Methods.* 2014;107:189–196.
14. Willi B, Boretti FS, Cattori V, et al. Identification, molecular characterisation and experimental transmission of a new hemoplasma isolate from a cat with hemolytic anemia in Switzerland. *J Clin Microbiol.* 2005;43:2581–2585.
15. Bauer N, Balzer HJ, Thure S, et al. Prevalence of feline haemotropic mycoplasmas in convenience samples of cats in Germany. *J Feline Med Surg.* 2008;10:252–258.
16. Roura X, Peters IR, Altet L, et al. Prevalence of hemotropic mycoplasmas in healthy and unhealthy cats and dogs in Spain. *J Vet Diagn Invest.* 2010;22:270–274.
17. Luria BJ, Levy JK, Lappin MR, et al. Prevalence of infectious diseases in feral cats in Northern Florida. *J Feline Med Surg.* 2004;6:287–296.
18. Stojanovic V, Foley P. Infectious disease prevalence in a feral cat population on Prince Edward Island, Canada. *Can Vet J.* 2011;52:979–982.
19. Tasker S, Braddock JA, Baral R, et al. Diagnosis of feline haemoplasma infection in Australian cats using a real-time PCR assay. *J Feline Med Surg.* 2004;6:345–354.
20. Lobetti R, Lappin MR. Prevalence of *Toxoplasma gondii, Bartonella* species and haemoplasma infection in cats in South Africa. *J Feline Med Surg.* 2012;14:857–862.
21. Ghazisaeedi F, Atyabi N, Zahrai Salehi T, et al. A molecular study of hemotropic mycoplasmas (hemoplasmas) in cats in Iran. *Vet Clin Pathol.* 2014;43:381–386.
22. Tanahara M, Miyamoto S, Nishio T, et al. An epidemiological survey of feline hemoplasma infection in Japan. *J Vet Med Sci.* 2010;72:1575–1581.
23. Georges K, Ezeokoli C, Auguste T, et al. A comparison of real-time PCR and reverse line blot hybridization in detecting feline haemoplasmas of domestic cats and an analysis of risk factors associated with haemoplasma infections. *BMC Vet Res.* 2012;8:103.
24. Sykes JE, Drazenovich NL, Ball LM, et al. Use of conventional and real-time polymerase chain reaction to determine the epidemiology of hemoplasma infections in anemic and nonanemic cats. *J Vet Intern Med.* 2007;21:685–693.
25. Sykes JE, Terry JC, Lindsay LL, et al. Prevalences of various hemoplasma species among cats in the United States with possible hemoplasmosis. *J Am Vet Med Assoc.* 2008;232:372–379.
26. Tasker S, Binns SH, Day MJ, et al. Use of a PCR assay to assess prevalence and risk factors for *Mycoplasma haemofelis* and '*Candidatus* Mycoplasma haemominutum' in cats in the United Kingdom. *Vet Rec.* 2003;152:193–198.
27. Willi B, Boretti FS, Baumgartner C, et al. Prevalence, risk factor analysis, and follow-up of infections caused by three feline hemoplasma species in cats in Switzerland. *J Clin Microbiol.* 2006;44:961–969.
28. Willi B, Tasker S, Boretti FS, et al. Phylogenetic analysis of '*Candidatus* Mycoplasma turicensis' isolates from pet cats in the United Kingdom, Australia and South Africa, with analysis of risk factors for infection. *J Clin Microbiol.* 2006;44:4430–4435.
29. Harvey JW, Gaskin JM. Feline haemobartonellosis: attempts to induce relapses of clinical disease in chronically infected cats. *J Am Anim Hosp Assoc.* 1978;14:453–456.
30. Shaw SE, Kenny MJ, Tasker S, et al. Pathogen carriage by the cat flea *Ctenocephalides felis* (Bouché) in the United Kingdom. *Vet Microbiol.* 2004;102:183–188.
31. Jensen WA, Lappin MR, Kamkar S, et al. Use of a polymerase chain reaction assay to detect and differentiate two strains of *Haemobartonella felis* infection in naturally infected cats. *Am J Vet Res.* 2001;62:604–608.
32. Novacco M, Boretti FS, Wolf-Jackel GA, et al. Chronic "*Candidatus* mycoplasma turicensis" infection. *Vet Res.* 2011;42:59.
33. Harvey JW, Gaskin JM. Experimental feline haemobartonellosis. *J Am Anim Hosp Assoc.* 1977;13:28–38.
34. do Nascimento NC, Guimaraes AM, Santos AP, et al. Complete genome sequence of *Mycoplasma haemocanis* strain Illinois. *J Bacteriol.* 2012;194:1605–1606.
35. Novacco M, Meli ML, Gentilini F, et al. Prevalence and geographical distribution of canine hemotropic mycoplasma infections in Mediterranean countries and analysis of risk factors for infection. *Vet Microbiol.* 2010;142:276–284.
36. Wengi N, Willi B, Boretti FS, et al. Real-time PCR-based prevalence study, infection follow-up and molecular characterization of canine hemotropic mycoplasmas. *Vet Microbiol.* 2008;126:132–141.
37. Barker EN, Tasker S, Day MJ, et al. Development and use of real-time PCR to detect and quantify *Mycoplasma haemocanis* and "*Candidatus* Mycoplasma haematoparvum" in dogs. *Vet Microbiol.* 2010;140:167–170.
38. Sasaki M, Ohta K, Matsuu A, et al. A molecular survey of *Mycoplasma haemocanis* in dogs and foxes in Aomori Prefecture, Japan. *J Protozool Res.* 2008;18:57–60.
39. Cannon SH, Levy JK, Kirk SK, et al. Infectious diseases in dogs rescued during dogfighting investigations. *Vet J.* 2016;211:64–69.
40. Birkenheuer AJ, Breitschwerdt EB, Alleman AR, et al. Differentiation of *Haemobartonella canis* and *Mycoplasma haemofelis* on the basis of comparative analysis of gene sequences. *Am J Vet Res.* 2002;63:1385–1388.
41. Sykes JE, Ball LM, Bailiff NL, et al. '*Candidatus* Mycoplasma haematoparvum', a novel small haemotropic mycoplasma from a dog. *Int J Syst Evol Microbiol.* 2005;55:27–30.
42. Martinez-Diaz VL, Silvestre-Ferreira AC, Vilhena H, et al. Prevalence and co-infection of haemotropic mycoplasmas in Portuguese cats by real-time polymerase chain reaction. *J Feline Med Surg.* 2013;15:879–885.
43. Andre MR, Adania CH, Allegretti SM, et al. Hemoplasmas in wild canids and felids in Brazil. *J Zoo Wildl Med.* 2011;42:342–347.
44. Varanat M, Maggi RG, Linder KE, et al. Molecular prevalence of *Bartonella, Babesia*, and hemotropic *Mycoplasma* sp. in dogs with splenic disease. *J Vet Intern Med.* 2011;25:1284–1291.
45. Hii SF, Kopp SR, Thompson MF, et al. Canine vector-borne disease pathogens in dogs from south-east Queensland and north-east Northern Territory. *Aust Vet J.* 2012;90:130–135.

46. Sykes JE, Henn JB, Kasten RW, et al. *Bartonella henselae* infection in splenectomized domestic cats previously infected with hemotropic *Mycoplasma* species. *Vet Immunol Immunopathol.* 2007;116:104–108.
47. Barker EN, Darby AC, Helps CR, et al. Molecular characterization of the uncultivatable hemotropic bacterium *Mycoplasma haemofelis. Vet Res.* 2011;42:83.
48. Zulty JC, Kociba GJ. Cold agglutinins in cats with haemobartonellosis. *J Am Vet Med Assoc.* 1990;196:907–910.
49. Maede Y, Hata R. Studies on feline haemobartonellosis. II. The mechanism of anemia produced by infection with *Haemobartonella felis. Jap J Vet Sci.* 1975;37:49–54.
50. Tasker S, Peters IR, Papasouliotis K, et al. Description of outcomes of experimental infection with feline haemoplasmas: copy numbers, haematology, Coombs' testing and blood glucose concentrations. *Vet Microbiol.* 2009;139:323–332.
51. Maede Y. Studies on feline haemobartonellosis. IV. Lifespan of erythrocytes of cats infected with *Haemobartonella felis. Jap J Vet Sci.* 1975;37:269–272.
52. De Lorimier LP, Messick JB. Anemia associated with '*Candidatus* Mycoplasma haemominutum' in a feline leukemia virus-negative cat with lymphoma. *J Am Anim Hosp Assoc.* 2004;40:423–427.
53. George JW, Rideout BA, Griffey SM, et al. Effect of preexisting FeLV infection or FeLV and feline immunodeficiency virus coinfection on pathogenicity of the small variant of *Haemobartonella felis* in cats. *Am J Vet Res.* 2002;63:1172–1178.
54. Reynolds CA, Lappin MR. "*Candidatus* Mycoplasma haemominutum" infections in 21 client-owned cats. *J Am Anim Hosp Assoc.* 2007;43:249–257.
55. Groebel K, Hoelzle K, Wittenbrink MM, et al. Unraveling a paradigm: *Mycoplasma suis* invades porcine erythrocytes. *Infect Immun.* 2009;77:576–584.
56. Sykes JE, Bailiff NL, Ball LM, et al. Identification of a novel hemotropic mycoplasma in a splenectomized dog with hemic neoplasia. *J Am Vet Med Assoc.* 2004;224:1946–1951.
57. Kemming G, Messick JB, Mueller W, et al. Can we continue research in splenectomized dogs? *Mycoplasma haemocanis*: old problem: new insight. *Eur Surg Res.* 2004;36:198–205.
58. Hulme-Moir KL, Barker EN, Stonelake A, et al. Use of real-time quantitative polymerase chain reaction to monitor antibiotic therapy in a dog with naturally acquired *Mycoplasma haemocanis* infection. *J Vet Diagn Invest.* 2010;22. 582-527.
59. Pitorri F, Dell'Orco M, Carmichael N, et al. Use of real-time quantitative PCR to document successful treatment of *Mycoplasma haemocanis* infection with doxycycline in a dog. *Vet Clin Pathol.* 2012;41:493–496.
60. Bundza A, Lumsden JH, McSherry BJ, et al. Haemobartonellosis in a dog in association with Coombs' positive anaemia. *Can Vet J.* 1976;17:267–270.
61. Bellamy JE, MacWilliams PS, Searcy GP. Cold-agglutinin hemolytic anaemia and *Haemobartonella canis* infection in a dog. *J Am Vet Med Assoc.* 1978;173:397–401.
62. Assarasakorn S, Veir JK, Hawley JR, et al. Prevalence of *Bartonella* species, hemoplasmas, and *Rickettsia felis* DNA in blood and fleas of cats in Bangkok, Thailand. *Res Vet Sci.* 2012;93:1213–1216.
63. Lappin MR, Griffin B, Brunt J, et al. Prevalence of *Bartonella* species, haemoplasma species, *Ehrlichia* species, *Anaplasma phagocytophilum*, and *Neorickettsia risticii* DNA in the blood of cats and their fleas in the United States. *J Feline Med Surg.* 2006;8:85–90.
64. Seneviratna P, Weerasinghe N, Ariyadasa S. Transmission of *Haemobartonella canis* by the dog tick, *Rhipicephalus sanguineus. Res Vet Sci.* 1973;14:112–114.
65. Taroura S, Shimada Y, Sakata Y, et al. Detection of DNA of '*Candidatus* Mycoplasma haemominutum' and *Spiroplasma* sp. in unfed ticks collected from vegetation in Japan. *J Vet Med Sci.* 2005;67:1277–1279.
66. Willi B, Boretti FS, Meli ML, et al. Real-time PCR investigation of potential vectors, reservoirs and shedding patterns of feline hemotropic mycoplasmas. *Appl Environ Microbiol.* 2007;73:3798–3802.
67. Barrs VR, Beatty JA, Wilson BJ, et al. Prevalence of *Bartonella* species, *Rickettsia felis*, haemoplasmas and the *Ehrlichia* group in the blood of cats and fleas in eastern Australia. *Aust Vet J.* 2010;88:160–165.
68. Lappin MR, Griffin B, Brunt J, et al. Prevalence of *Bartonella* species, haemoplasma species, *Ehrlichia* species, *Anaplasma phagocytophilum*, and *Neorickettsia risticii* DNA in the blood of cats and their fleas in the United States. *J Fel Med Surg.* 2008;8:85–90.
69. Reagan KL, Clarke LL, Hawley JR, et al. Assessment of the ability of *Aedes* species mosquitoes to transmit feline *Mycoplasma haemofelis* and '*Candidatus* Mycoplasma haemominutum'. *J Feline Med Surg.* 2017;19:798–802.
70. Woods JE, Brewer MM, Hawley JR, et al. Evaluation of experimental transmission of '*Candidatus* Mycoplasma haemominutum' and *Mycoplasma haemofelis* by *Ctenocephalides felis* to cats. *Am J Vet Res.* 2005;66:1008–1012.
71. Lappin MR. Feline haemoplasmas are not transmitted by *Ctenocephalides felis*. In: *9th Symposium of the CVBD World Forum*. Lisbon: Portugal; 2014:44–46.
72. Museux K, Boretti FS, Willi B, et al. *In vivo* transmission studies of '*Candidatus* Mycoplasma turicensis' in the domestic cat. *Vet Res.* 2009;40:45.
73. Lashnits E, Grant S, Thomas B, Qurollo B, Breitschwerdt EB. Evidence for vertical transmission of *Mycoplasma haemocanis*, but not *Ehrlichia ewingii*, in a dog. *J Vet Intern Med.* 2019;33(4):1747–1752.
74. Hornok S, Micsutka A, Meli ML, et al. Molecular investigation of transplacental and vector-borne transmission of bovine haemoplasmas. *Vet Microbiol.* 2011;152:411–414.
75. Tasker S. Haemotropic mycoplasmas: what's the real significance in cats? *J Feline Med Surg.* 2010;12:369–381.
76. Kewish KE, Appleyard GD, Myers SL, et al. *Mycoplasma haemofelis* and *Mycoplasma haemominutum* detection by polymerase chain reaction in cats from Saskatchewan and Alberta. *Can Vet J.* 2004;45:749–752.
77. Baumann J, Novacco M, Willi B, et al. Lack of cross-protection against *Mycoplasma haemofelis* infection and signs of enhancement in "*Candidatus* Mycoplasma turicensis"-recovered cats. *Vet Res.* 2015;46:104.
78. Westfall DS, Jensen WA, Reagan WJ, et al. Inoculation of two genotypes of *Haemobartonella felis* (California and Ohio variants) to induce infection in cats and the response to treatment with azithromycin. *Am J Vet Res.* 2001;62:687–691.
79. Tasker S, Helps CR, Belford CJ, et al. 16S rDNA comparison demonstrates near identity between a United Kingdom *Haemobartonella felis* strain and the American California strain. *Vet Microbiol.* 2001;81:73–78.
80. Peters IR, Helps CR, Willi B, et al. The prevalence of three species of feline haemoplasmas in samples submitted to a diagnostics service as determined by three novel real-time duplex PCR assays. *Vet Microbiol.* 2008;126:142–150.
81. Hawley J, Yaaran T, Maurice S, et al. Amplification of *Mycoplasma haemofelis* DNA by a PCR for point-of-care use. *J Vet Diagn Invest.* 2018;30:140-143
82. Barker EN, Helps CR, Heesom KJ, et al. Detection of humoral response using a recombinant heat shock protein 70, DnaK, of *Mycoplasma haemofelis* in experimentally and naturally hemoplasma-infected cats. *Clin Vaccine Immunol.* 2010;17:1926–1932.
83. Novacco M, Wolf-Jackel G, Riond B, et al. Humoral immune response to a recombinant hemoplasma antigen in experimental '*Candidatus* Mycoplasma turicensis' infection. *Vet Microbiol.* 2012;157:464–470.
84. Dowers KL, Olver C, Radecki SV, et al. Use of enrofloxacin for treatment of large-form *Haemobartonella felis* in experimentally infected cats. *J Am Vet Med Assoc.* 2002;221:250–253.
85. Ishak AM, Dowers KL, Cavanaugh MT, et al. Marbofloxacin for the treatment of experimentally induced *Mycoplasma haemofelis* infection in cats. *J Vet Intern Med.* 2008;22:288–292.
86. Tasker S, Caney SMA, Day MJ, et al. Effect of chronic FIV infection, and efficacy of marbofloxacin treatment, on '*Candidatus* Mycoplasma haemominutum' infection. *Microbes Infect.* 2006;8:653–661.
87. Tasker S, Caney SMA, Day MJ, et al. Effect of chronic FIV infection, and efficacy of marbofloxacin treatment, on *Mycoplasma haemofelis* infection. *Vet Microbiol.* 2006;117:169–179.
88. Dowers KL, Tasker S, Radecki SV, et al. Use of pradofloxacin to treat experimentally induced *Mycoplasma hemofelis* infection in cats. *Am J Vet Res.* 2009;70:105–111.
89. Tasker S, Helps CR, Day MJ, et al. Use of a Taqman PCR to determine the response of *Mycoplasma haemofelis* infection to antibiotic treatment. *J Microbiol Methods.* 2004;56:63–71.

90. Novacco M, Boretti FS, Franchini M, et al. Protection from reinfection in "*Candidatus* Mycoplasma turicensis"-infected cats and characterization of the immune response. *Vet Res.* 2012;43:82.
91. Hicks CA, Willi B, Riond B, et al. Protective immunity against infection with *Mycoplasma haemofelis. Clin Vaccine Immunol.* 2014;22:108–118.
92. Sugiarto S, Spiri AM, Riond B, et al. Passive immunization does not provide protection against experimental infection with *Mycoplasma haemofelis. Vet Res.* 2016;47:79.
93. Hattori N, Kuroda M, Katano H, et al. *Candidatus* Mycoplasma haemohominis in human, Japan. *Emerg Infect Dis.* 2020;26:11–19.
94. Alcorn K, Gerrard J, Cochrane T, et al. First report of *Candidatus* Mycoplasma haemohominis infection in Australia causing persistent fever in an animal carer. *Clin Infect Dis.* 2021;72:634–640.
95. Santos AP, Santos RP, Biondo AW, et al. Hemoplasma infection in HIV-positive patient, Brazil. *Emerg Infect Dis.* 2008;14:1922–1924.
96. Congli Y, Zhibiao Y, Ningyu Z, et al. The 1.8kb DNA fragment formerly confirmed as *Mycoplasma suis* (*M. suis*) specific was originated from the porcine genome. *Vet Microbiol.* 2009;138:197–198.
97. Yuan C, Liang A, Yu F, et al. *Eperythrozoon* infection identified in an unknown aetiology anaemic patient. *Ann Microbiol.* 2007;57:467–469.
98. Yuan CL, Liang AB, Yao CB, et al. Prevalence of *Mycoplasma suis* (*Eperythrozoon suis*) infection in swine and swine-farm workers in Shanghai, China. *Am J Vet Res.* 2009;70:890–894.
99. Sykes JE, Lindsay LL, Maggi RG, et al. Human co-infection with *Bartonella henselae* and two hemotropic mycoplasma variants resembling *Mycoplasma ovis. J Clin Microbiol.* 2010;48:3782–3785.
100. Maggi RG, Mascarelli PE, Havenga LN, et al. Co-infection with *Anaplasma platys, Bartonella henselae* and *Candidatus* Mycoplasma haematoparvum in a veterinarian. *Parasit Vectors.* 2013;6:103.
101. Tasker S, Peters IR, Mumford AD, et al. Investigation of human haemotropic *Mycoplasma* infections using a novel generic haemoplasma qPCR assay on blood samples and blood smears. *J Med Microbiol.* 2010;59:1285–1292.
102. Gentilini F, Novacco M, Turba ME, et al. Use of combined conventional and real-time PCR to determine the epidemiology of feline haemoplasma infections in northern Italy. *J Feline Med Surg.* 2009;11:277–285.
103. Walker Vergara R, Morera Galleguillos F, Gomez Jaramillo M, et al. Prevalence, risk factor analysis, and hematological findings of hemoplasma infection in domestic cats from Valdivia, Southern Chile. *Comp Immunol Microbiol Infect Dis.* 2016;46:20–26.
104. Ravicini S, Pastor J, Hawley J, et al. Prevalence of selected infectious disease agents in stray cats in Catalonia, Spain. *JFMS Open Rep.* 2016;2:2055116916634109.
105. Attipa C, Papasouliotis K, Solano-Gallego L, et al. Prevalence study and risk factor analysis of selected bacterial, protozoal and viral, including vector-borne, pathogens in cats from Cyprus. *Parasit Vectors.* 2017;10:130.
106. Bergmann M, Englert T, Stuetzer B, et al. Risk factors of different hemoplasma species infections in cats. *BMC Vet Res.* 2017;13:52.
107. Ravagnan S, Carli E, Piseddu E, et al. Prevalence and molecular characterization of canine and feline hemotropic mycoplasmas (hemoplasmas) in northern Italy. *Parasit Vectors.* 2017;10:132.
108. Diaz-Reganon D, Villaescusa A, Ayllon T, et al. Epidemiological study of hemotropic mycoplasmas (hemoplasmas) in cats from central Spain. *Parasit Vectors.* 2018;11:140.
109. Makino H, Jesus de Paula DA, Sousa VRF, et al. Natural hemoplasma infection of cats in Cuiaba, Mato Grosso, Brazil. *Semina: Ciências Agrárias.* 2018;39:875–880.
110. Munhoz AD, Simoes I, Calazans APF, et al. Hemotropic mycoplasmas in naturally infected cats in Northeastern Brazil. *Rev Bras Parasitol Vet.* 2018;27:446–454.
111. Persichetti MF, Pennisi MG, Vullo A, et al. Clinical evaluation of outdoor cats exposed to ectoparasites and associated risk for vector-borne infections in southern Italy. *Parasit Vectors.* 2018;11:136.
112. Sarvani E, Tasker S, Kovac evic Filipovic M, et al. Prevalence and risk factor analysis for feline haemoplasmas in cats from Northern Serbia, with molecular subtyping of feline immunodeficiency virus. *JFMS Open Rep.* 2018;4:2055116918770037.
113. Do T, Kamyingkird K, Bui LK, et al. Genetic characterization and risk factors for feline hemoplasma infection in semi-domesticated cats in Bangkok, Thailand. *Vet World.* 2020;13:975–980.
114. Latrofa MS, Iatta R, Toniolo F, et al. A molecular survey of vector-borne pathogens and haemoplasmas in owned cats across Italy. *Parasit Vectors.* 2020;13:116.
115. Kenny MJ, Shaw SE, Beugnet F, et al. Demonstration of two distinct hemotropic mycoplasmas in French dogs. *J Clin Microbiol.* 2004;42:5397–5399.
116. Hetzel N, Barker EN, Arteaga A, et al. Prevalence of canine haemotropic mycoplasma infections in Sydney, Australia. *Vet Rec.* 2012;171:126.
117. Compton SM, Maggi RG, Breitschwerdt EB. *Candidatus* Mycoplasma haematoparvum and *Mycoplasma haemocanis* infections in dogs from the United States. *Comp Immunol Microbiol Infect Dis.* 2012;35:557–562.
118. Levy JK, Lappin MR, Glaser AL, et al. Prevalence of infectious diseases in cats and dogs rescued following Hurricane Katrina. *J Am Vet Med Assoc.* 2011;238:311–317.
119. Inokuma H, Oyamada M, Davoust B, et al. Epidemiological survey of *Ehrlichia canis* and related species infection in dogs in eastern Sudan. *Ann N Y Acad Sci.* 2006;1078:461–463.
120. Aquino LC, Kamani J, Haruna AM, et al. Analysis of risk factors and prevalence of haemoplasma infection in dogs. *Vet Parasitol.* 2016;221:111–117.
121. Hasiri MA, Sharifiyazdi H, Moradi T. Molecular detection and differentiation of canine hemoplasma infections using RFLP-PCR in dogs in southern Iran. *Vet Arch.* 2016;86:529–540.
122. Bouzouraa T, Cadore JL, Chene J, et al. Implication, clinical and biological impact of vector-borne haemopathogens in anaemic dogs in France: a prospective study. *J Small Anim Pract.* 2017;58:510–518.
123. Aktas M, Ozubek S. A molecular survey of hemoplasmas in domestic dogs from Turkey. *Vet Microbiol.* 2018;221:94–97.
124. Happi AN, Toepp AJ, Ugwu CA, et al. Detection and identification of blood-borne infections in dogs in Nigeria using light microscopy and the polymerase chain reaction. *Vet Parasitol Reg Stud Rep.* 2018;11:55–60.
125. Hofmann M, Hodžić A, Pouliou N, et al. Vector-borne pathogens affecting shelter dogs in eastern Crete, Greece. *Parasitol Res.* 2019;118:1661–1666.
126. Novacco M, Sugiarto S, Willi B, et al. Consecutive antibiotic treatment with doxycycline and marbofloxacin clears bacteremia in *Mycoplasma haemofelis*-infected cats. *Vet Microbiol.* 2018;217:112–120.

59

Actinomycosis

Jane E. Sykes

KEY POINTS

- First Described: Actinomycosis was first described in cattle in 1877 (Otto Bollinger, Germany).[1]
- Causes: *Actinomyces* spp. (and to a lesser extent, other related species such as *Trueperella* spp. and *Arcanobacterium* spp.).
- Geographic Distribution: Worldwide, but especially from regions where grass awns are prevalent.
- Mode of Transmission: Opportunistic invasion of commensal bacteria following disruption of cutaneous or mucosal barriers.
- Major Clinical Signs: Subcutaneous masses and draining skin lesions (cervicofacial and cutaneous-subcutaneous disease); pulmonary nodules, masses and/or effusion with cough and tachypnea (thoracic disease); abdominal effusion or masses (abdominal disease); thoracolumbar pain or pelvic limb paresis/paralysis (retroperitoneal disease); rarely neurologic signs due to meningitis or brain abscesses (CNS disease).
- Differential Diagnoses: Infections caused by *Mycobacterium*, *Nocardia*, *Bartonella*, and fungal pathogens; chronic bacterial osteomyelitis caused by typical bacterial species; neoplasia.
- Human Health Significance: Direct transmission of disease from animals to humans does not occur, but humans have developed disease after bites from healthy dogs or cats.

ETIOLOGIC AGENTS AND EPIDEMIOLOGY

Actinomycosis is typically a slowly progressive infection caused by anaerobic or microaerophilic, filamentous, gram-positive bacteria that belong to the genus *Actinomyces,* and to a lesser extent, species that now have been recently assigned to genera such as *Arcanobacterium* and *Trueperella* (additional species that cause disease in humans belong to the genera *Actinobaculum* and *Cellulomonas*). *Actinomyces* spp. are normal inhabitants of mucous membranes, especially of the oropharynx, but also the genital and GI tracts, and cause opportunistic infections. Together with other oral commensal bacteria, actinomycetes colonize the periodontal mucosal surfaces and adhere to the tooth surface to form plaque. Numerous *Actinomyces* species have been cultured from the mucous membranes (e.g., gingiva, vaginal vault), dental plaque, and saliva of healthy dogs and cats. It is important to recognize that *Actinomyces* spp. have never been cultured from the environment, and disease is not transmitted from one animal to another.

Usually, actinomycosis develops when *Actinomyces* spp. that reside in association with mucous membranes are inoculated into tissues along with other bacteria, often as a result of a deeply penetrating wound or foreign body migration. Organisms isolated from lesions of dogs and cats with actinomycosis are shown in Table 59.1. Young adult to middle-aged large-breed dogs that have access to the outdoors are often affected, especially retriever and hunting breeds.[2,3] There is no clear sex predisposition, and the median age of dogs with actinomycosis is approximately 5 years.[4] Actinomycosis in outdoor dogs is often related to exposure to penetrating plant foreign bodies such as grass awns. In cats, actinomycosis usually follows bite wounds, and so is more commonly diagnosed in male cats.[4,5] In the author's hospital, 11 of 17 cats with actinomycosis were male. However, underlying retroviral infection is uncommonly present and does not appear to predispose to disease.

Because *Actinomyces* species are difficult to culture and are susceptible to antimicrobial drugs that are often used empirically, the prevalence of actinomycosis in dogs and cats has probably been underestimated.

CLINICAL FEATURES

Pathogenesis and Clinical Signs

Actinomycosis occurs following disruption of mucosal barriers. After ingestion or inhalation, plant awns may become contaminated with *Actinomyces* spp. and other bacteria from the oropharynx, after which the awns migrate to various sites and act as a nidus of infection. Alternatively, organisms may be introduced into tissues at the time of a bite wound injury. The latter is the most common route of infection in cats, and can manifest as pyothorax, peritonitis, or cellulitis.[4,5] The presence of associated aerobic and anaerobic bacteria from the oral cavity or intestinal tract ("companion microbes") undermines normal host defenses and reduces oxygen tension, which allows *Actinomyces* spp. to persist. *Actinomyces* spp. that possess fimbriae can bind to specific cell surface receptors on other bacteria, especially streptococci.

TABLE 59.1 *Actinomyces* and *Arcanobacterium* Species Isolated from Dogs and Cats with Actinomycosis

Dogs	Cats
Actinomyces viscosus[12,16,31]	*Actinomyces viscosus*[24,56]
Actinomyces bowdenii[46]	*Actinomyces bowdenii*[46]
Actinomyces hordeovulneris[54]	*Actinomyces hordeovulneris*[4,15]
Actinomyces canis[44]	*Actinomyces meyeri*[57]
Actinomyces odontolyticus[11]	*Actinomyces odontolyticus*[56]
Actinomyces catuli[43]	*Arcanobacterium pyogenes*[27]
Actinomyces turicensis[33]	
Actinomyces hyovaginalis[4]	
Actinomyces urogenitali[4]	
Arcanobacterium canis[4]	
Arcanobacterium pluranimalium[55]	
Trueperella pyogenes[a,27]	

[a]Previously *Arcanobacterium pyogenes*.

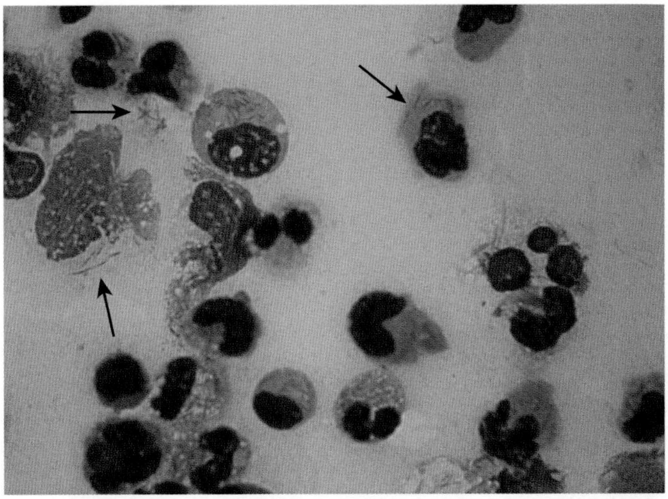

Fig. 59.1 Abdominal fluid cytology from a 3-year old male neutered domestic longhair cat with a 1-week history of progressive lethargy and anorexia, ascites, hyperbilirubinemia, and hypoproteinemia. Total protein was 2.2 g/dL and there were 75,500 nucleated cells/μL, with 92% neutrophils and 8% large mononuclear cells. High numbers of moderately degenerative neutrophils are present with low numbers of macrophages. Moderate numbers of filamentous beaded bacteria are present both in the background and within phagocytes *(arrows)*. *Actinomyces* spp. and *Fusobacterium nucleatum* were isolated from the peritoneal fluid. Necropsy revealed severe, chronic peritonitis with intralesional filamentous bacteria.

This bacterial co-aggregation inhibits the ability of neutrophils to phagocytize the organisms.[6] Dense colonies of *Actinomyces* spp. form, and these, together with other associated bacteria, are surrounded by neutrophils, macrophages, and plasma cells, with slowly progressive pyogranulomatous inflammation (Fig. 59.1). Large aggregations of organisms can lead to formation of "sulfur granules," tan to yellow colonies of actinomycetes, which may be microscopic or visible grossly. Proteolytic enzymes from the associated bacteria, macrophages, and degranulated neutrophils destroy connective tissue, which facilitates extension of the disease through normal tissue planes. Less often, organisms spread hematogenously to distant sites. In some cases, the inflammatory reaction is accompanied by mass formation and extensive fibrosis. The center of the lesions may eventually suppurate and soften, or draining tracts may develop. The tracts can close and reappear over weeks to months as infection gradually spreads through tissues.

The most common clinical forms of actinomycosis in cats and dogs involve the cervicofacial region, thorax, abdomen, and subcutaneous tissue, but CNS (meningitis and meningoencephalitis) and ocular infections (keratitis and endophthalmitis) can also occur.[7–9] *Cervicofacial actinomycosis* can follow bite wounds, perforation of the oropharynx by a foreign body, or chronic periodontal disease. The mandibular, submandibular, and ventral or lateral cervical areas are most frequently affected, but infections that involve the face, retrobulbar space, and temporal area can occur (Fig. 59.2A and B). *Cutaneous-subcutaneous actinomycosis* typically involves the lateral thoracic wall, flank region, and occasionally the limbs. Cutaneous lesions involving the thoracic or abdominal walls may represent extensions of thoracic, abdominal, or retroperitoneal actinomycosis.

Thoracic actinomycosis may be limited to the lung parenchyma but can involve other structures within the thorax, such as the mediastinum, pleura, pericardium, and chest wall. It follows aspiration of oropharyngeal material, often together with a contaminated grass awn. Alternative routes of thoracic infection include involvement of the mediastinum from esophageal perforation or direct extension of subcutaneous or abdominal disease. Clinical signs include cough and less commonly hemoptysis, tachypnea, dyspnea, decreased lung sounds (as a result of pyothorax or mass lesions), and subcutaneous soft tissue masses or draining skin lesions on the lateral thoracic wall. Sometimes there is a history of neck pain, gagging, or hypersalivation prior to the onset of tachypnea, possibly as a result of passage of a penetrating foreign body.

Abdominal actinomycosis develops when foreign bodies penetrate the GI mucosa, which leads to the formation of intraabdominal mass lesions and ascites.[2,10–12] Abdominal involvement may also follow direct extension from subcutaneous tissues or hematogenous spread of the organism to abdominal organs such as the liver. Although dogs are more often affected than cats, intraabdominal actinomycotic masses can occur in cats.[13–15] *Retroperitoneal actinomycosis* in dogs often follows the migration of plant awns through the lung and up the crus of the diaphragm to its dorsal attachment. Initially, fever of unknown origin may be the only clinical signs. Ultimately, progression can lead to osteomyelitis and compression fractures of the vertebral bodies, with spinal pain and paresis or paralysis of the pelvic limbs (Fig. 59.3).[16–18]

Actinomycosis of the brain and meninges in dogs can also occur (Fig. 59.4).[19–22] Brain abscesses may follow hematogenous dissemination from a distant site, or meningitis may result from extension of infection from an adjacent focus, such as the middle ear or skull.[21,23] In humans, risk factors for CNS actinomycosis include dental disease or tooth extraction, head trauma, GI tract surgery, and chronic otitis, mastoiditis, or sinusitis. CNS actinomycosis has been reported in dogs in association with concurrent otitis media/interna,[22] head trauma,[20] and in cats in association with retrobulbar abscesses[23] and cutaneous abscesses of the tail base.[24,25]

Rarely, infections of the urinary bladder,[26,27] gall bladder,[28,29] gastric wall,[15] and heart valve[30–33] have been recognized in dogs, cats, and human patients. One cat with actinomycotic rhinitis and optic neuritis was reported.[34]

Physical Examination Findings

Lesions in dogs and cats with cervicofacial or cutaneous-subcutaneous actinomycosis may be fluctuant or firm, indurated, have draining sinuses, and/or rarely be ulcerated. Pain and fever are variable. Thoracic or abdominal actinomycosis is often accompanied by a thin body condition and fever. Dogs and cats with thoracic actinomycosis may show tachypnea or dyspnea, and thoracic auscultation may reveal decreased lung sounds if pyothorax or severe pleuritis is present. Abdominal masses and/or ascites may be detected on abdominal palpation of dogs with abdominal actinomycosis. Dogs with retroperitoneal actinomycosis may show pain on palpation of the abdomen or lumbar spine, and when severe, signs of pelvic limb paralysis or paresis may be present, such as pelvic limb ataxia, deficits of conscious proprioception, increased segmental reflexes, and loss of pain sensation. Neurologic signs associated with *Actinomyces* meningitis or encephalitis include altered behavior, decreased consciousness, cervical pain, vision loss, ataxia, tetraparesis, and seizures.

DIAGNOSIS

It has been recommended that actinomycosis be considered as a diagnosis when one or more of three clinical features are present: (1) a combination of chronicity, progression across tissue boundaries, and mass-like features that resemble neoplasia; (2) the presence of a sinus tract, which may spontaneously resolve and reappear; (3) a refractory or relapsing infection after a short course of antimicrobial therapy, because cure requires prolonged treatment.[35] Historically, in the

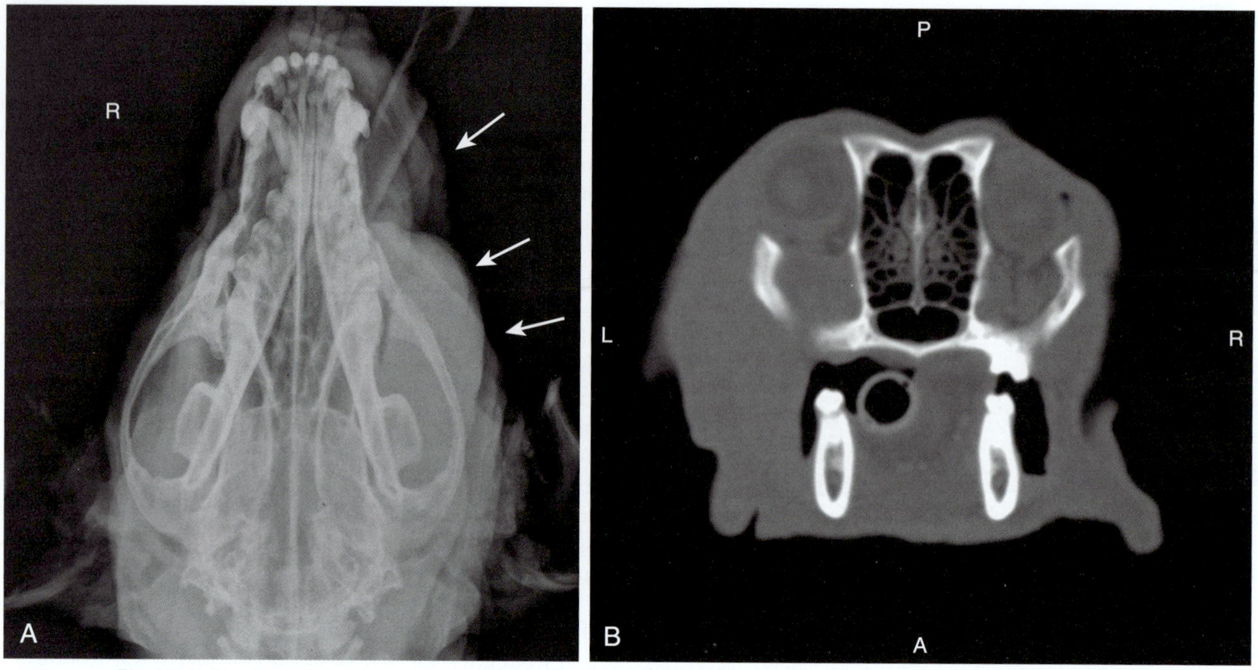

Fig. 59.2 Cervicofacial actinomycosis. (A) Skull radiograph and (B) computed tomography scan from an 8-year old female spayed Labrador retriever with slowly progressive, left-sided facial swelling. There is severe, regional soft tissue swelling over the left side of the face, which involved the left masseter muscle and zygomatic salivary glands, and extended into the retrobulbar space, with secondary exophthalmos *(arrows)*. Multiple premolars and molars of the left maxillary arcade were missing. Biopsy of the lesion revealed severe, diffuse, pyogranulomatous cellulitis with intralesional gram-positive, acid-fast negative bacilli. Culture yielded *Actinomyces hordeovulneris* (based on 16S rRNA gene sequencing), *Pasturella multocida* subsp. *multocida, Neisseria canis* (based on 16S rRNA gene sequencing), and an *Eikenella*-like organism.

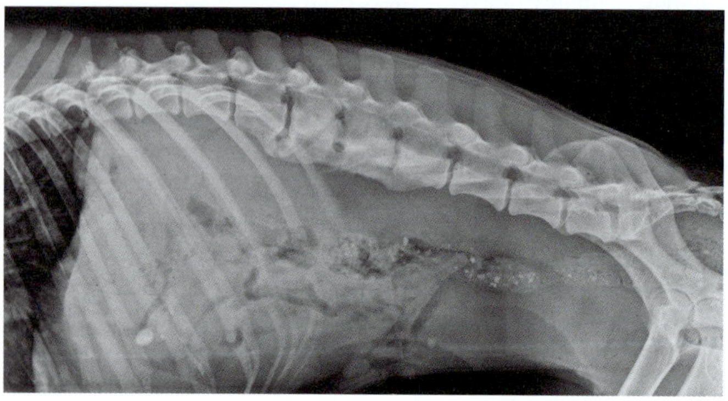

Fig. 59.3 Left lateral spinal radiograph from a 3-year-old female Border collie with retroperitoneal actinomycosis. The dog was seen for a 3-day history of lethargy, fever, apparent abdominal pain, and progressive pelvic limb paresis. Severe, smoothly marginated ventral spondylosis bridges the L1-L4 space. There is also marked irregular osteolysis of the 2nd, 3rd, and 4th lumbar vertebrae. There is destruction of the floor of the ventral canal. There is loss of visualization, narrowing, and irregularity of the intervertebral disc spaces at L2-3 and L3-4. There is marked loss of detail within the retroperitoneal space and the colon appears displaced slightly ventrally. Small irregular mineral foreign bodies are present within the stomach and colon.

human literature, actinomycosis has been referred to as the "most misdiagnosed disease."[36] Fibrous masses are frequently mistaken for neoplastic lesions, although reports of *Actinomyces* spp. infections that complicate neoplasia exist in human medicine.[37,38] Aspiration of firm lesions is often unrewarding, organisms are often difficult to isolate from lesions, and short periods of antimicrobial drug treatment are ineffective, which all serve to further mislead the clinician to a diagnosis of neoplasia. Actinomycosis should be considered on the list of differential diagnosis in any animal with a history of penetrating plant awn foreign bodies, draining skin lesions, chronic fibrous masses, persistent bite wounds, pyothorax, retroperitoneal abscesses, and focal neurologic signs, especially when young adult to middle-aged dogs are affected. Ultimately, diagnosis is based on clinical signs, identification of organisms with typical morphology with cytology or histopathology, and culture.

Laboratory Abnormalities

Complete Blood Count and Serum Biochemical Tests

Animals with extensive, chronic disease may have mild to moderate nonregenerative anemia, leukocytosis with a mild to moderate left shift and monocytosis, hypoalbuminemia, and hyperglobulinemia, which may be marked. Dogs with body cavity effusions may be hypoglycemic. There are usually no specific urinalysis findings.

Cytologic Examination of Body Fluids

Cytologic examination of aspirates of abscesses, effusions, or CSF typically reveals a suppurative to pyogranulomatous inflammatory response (>75% neutrophils). Total protein in pleural fluid is generally > 3.0 g/dL, with erythrocyte and nucleated cell counts often > 70,000 cells/μL. CSF from dogs and cats with cerebral actinomycosis may resemble pus grossly. Aspirates of firm masses may yield only blood. Sulfur granules may be visible in effusion fluid or draining purulent material from cutaneous lesions macroscopically, as white to tan to gray granules, or microscopically as dense clusters of organisms. When bacteria are visualized, they may be filamentous rods suggestive of *Actinomyces* spp., or "companion" microorganisms. The actinomycetes are gram-positive, non-acid-fast filamentous organisms that are

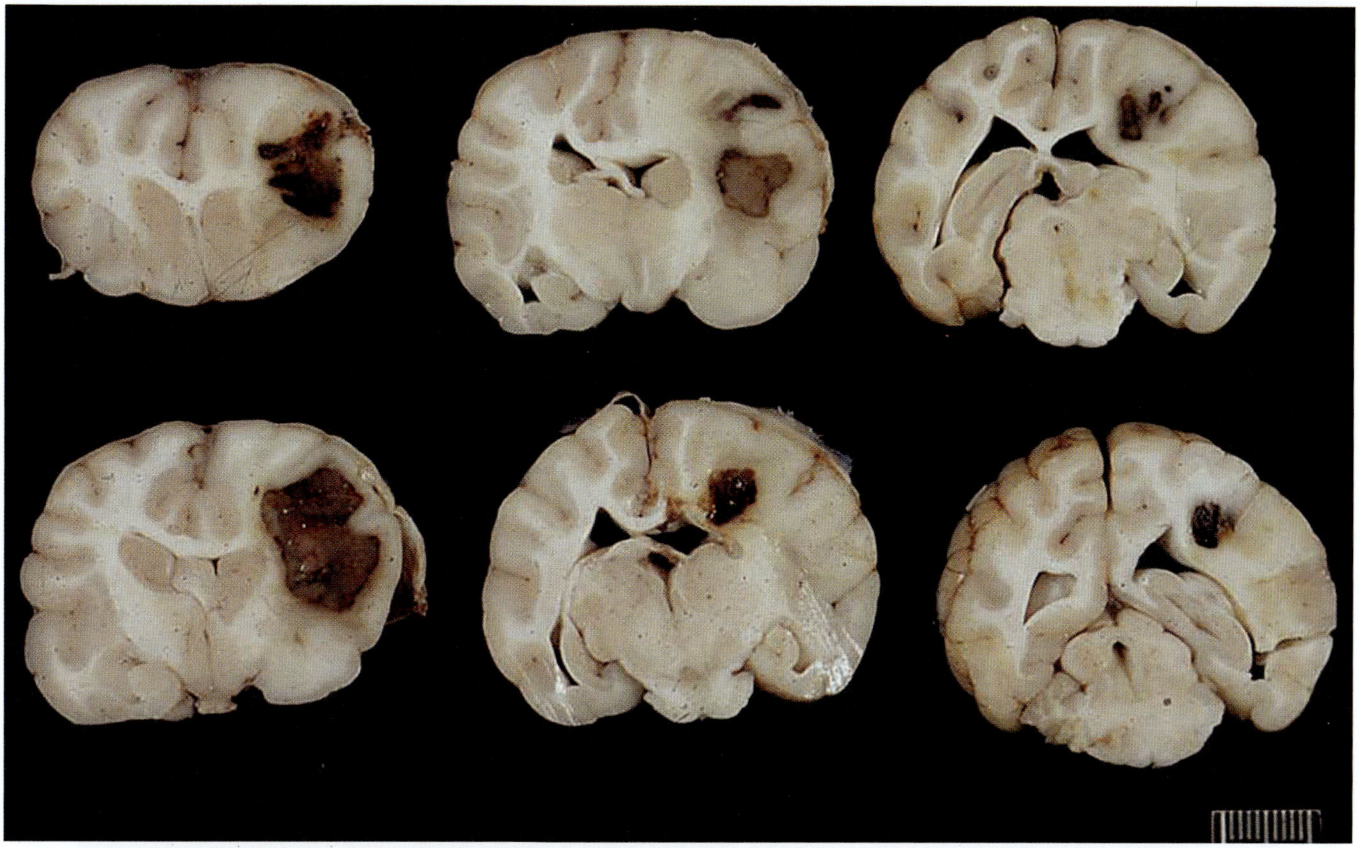

Fig. 59.4 Necropsy findings in a 1-year-old male neutered Yorkshire terrier with suspected CNS actinomycosis. Three weeks previously, surgery to correct an extrahepatic portosystemic shunt and remove a urate cystolith had been performed. The dog's appetite and activity level did not improve after the surgery, and for the week before the dog was reexamined, disorientation and weakness was noted. The dog deteriorated rapidly after it was hospitalized and euthanasia was performed. Osteogenesis imperfecta of the occipital bones was present and three separate abscesses were found in the left cerebral cortex. Histopathology revealed neutrophilic inflammation, hemorrhage, and granular mats of material that contained gram-positive, acid-fast negative branching bacteria (consistent with *Actinomyces* spp.), as well as a dense population of gram-negative, Giemsa-positive cocci. (Image courtesy University of California, Davis, Veterinary Anatomic Pathology Service.)

occasionally branched. The filaments are less than 1 μm wide, vary in length, and can stain irregularly, producing a beaded appearance (see Fig. 59.1). *Nocardia*, *Corynebacterium*, and *Mycobacterium* spp. can be confused with *Actinomyces* spp.

Diagnostic Imaging

Plain Radiography

Radiographs of cervicofacial or cutaneous-subcutaneous lesions may show lesions in adjacent bone, such as evidence of osteomyelitis and/or periosteal new bone formation. Pulmonary involvement may manifest as interstitial or alveolar infiltrates, sometimes with consolidation (Fig. 59.5A). Air bronchograms may be seen within mass lesions, suggesting the presence of a non-neoplastic process. Other variable findings include pleural thickening, pleural effusion, widening of the mediastinum, mass lesions, enlargement of the cardiac silhouette (with pericardial involvement), and periosteal new bone formation or osteomyelitis involving adjacent ribs, vertebral bodies, or sternebrae. Dogs with retroperitoneal actinomycosis may have evidence of periosteal new bone formation on the ventral aspects of two or three adjacent vertebral bodies (usually T13 through L4) on abdominal radiography; involvement of disc spaces is uncommon (see Fig. 59.3). Abdominal actinomycosis may be characterized by loss of abdominal detail due to peritoneal effusion and intraabdominal mass lesions.

Sonographic Findings

Ultrasonography can be useful to identify linear grass awn foreign bodies (see Fig. 59.5C).[39,40] Sonographic abnormalities in dogs with abdominal disease include variable amounts of flocculent ascites fluid, abdominal lymphadenopathy, and nodular or mass lesions that incorporate or displace adjacent structures. New bone formation may be detected on interrogation of the ventral aspects of the vertebral bodies during abdominal ultrasound in dogs with retroperitoneal disease.

Advanced Imaging

For animals with CNS involvement, MRI may reveal meningeal thickening, contrast enhancement, and/or intraparenchymal contrast-enhancing mass lesions.[4] MRI may also be useful for detection of grass awn foreign bodies. Advanced imaging allows assessment of the extent of actinomycosis (see Fig. 59.2) which may assist with surgical planning. In human cases, PET-CT with ^{18}F-fluorodeoxyglucose has been useful for diagnosis of actinomycosis and monitoring of response to treatment; evidence of intense hypermetabolism that resembles neoplasia has been associated with lesions.[41,42]

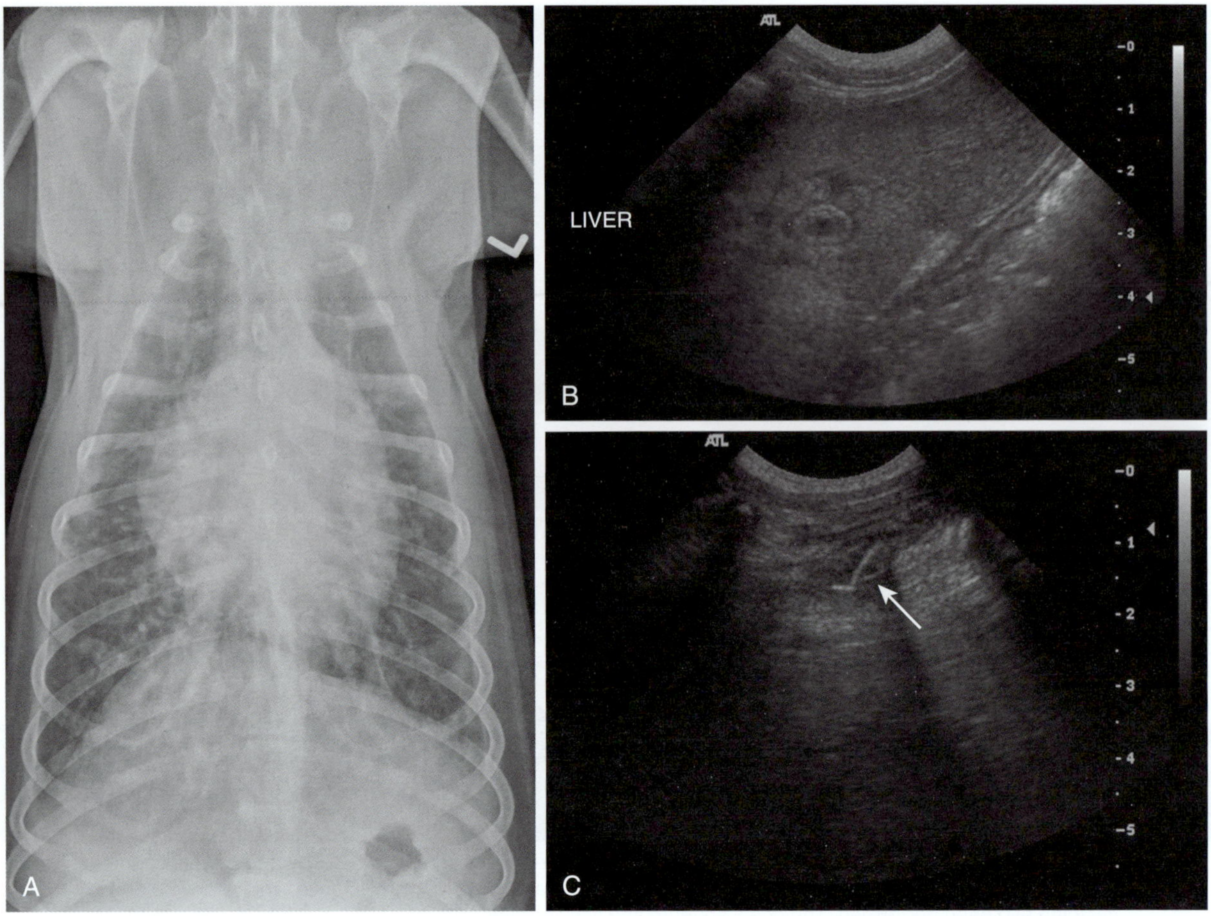

Fig. 59.5 Imaging findings in a 1-year-old female spayed Labrador retriever with systemic actinomycosis secondary to grass awn migration, which manifested as fever and lethargy. (A) Dorsoventral thoracic radiograph. Patchy diffuse interstitial opacities were present in all lung fields. (B) Ultrasound image of the liver. Within the left liver, there were focal, ill-defined heteroechoic or hypoechoic nodules. One of these areas (shown) had a well-demarcated, hyperechoic rim with irregular echogenic luminal contents. The nodules were consistent with multifocal hepatic abscesses. (C) Ultrasound image of the thoracic wall. A linear plant awn foreign body was identified *(arrow)*.

Microbiological Tests (Table 59.2)

Isolation and Identification

Because *Actinomyces* is a commensal of the oral cavity, it is commonly swallowed, inhaled, and transferred by licking; therefore, culture of the organism from the airways, GI tract, or skin does not necessarily constitute infection. Consistent cytologic or histopathologic findings (pyogranulomatous inflammation with or without the presence of filamentous bacteria) and the presence of companion microorganisms supports the diagnosis of actinomycosis.

Specimens for culture can be collected through fine-needle aspiration or, if possible, biopsy. Because *Actinomyces* spp. are exquisitely sensitive to many antimicrobial drugs, treatment of animals before obtaining specimens for culture can also prevent recovery of the organisms. Even a single dose of an antimicrobial can prevent successful isolation. Culture may be negative or yield only companion microorganisms, which may obscure the presence of *Actinomyces* spp.. As a result, diagnosis is often based on cytologic or histologic identification of the organism in specimens from animals with appropriate clinical signs.

Most *Actinomyces* spp. known to cause disease in dogs and cats are facultative anaerobes, but a few *Actinomyces* species are obligate anaerobes (*Actinomyces bovis, Actinomyces israelii, Actinomyces meyeri*).[43–46] Species that are facultatively anaerobic can grow aerobically, and some, such as *Actinomyces viscosus*, grow best in aerobic conditions. In addition, companion microorganisms are often obligate anaerobes or other aerobes, so both aerobic and anaerobic cultures should be requested when *Actinomyces* spp. infections may be present and the laboratory should be notified that *Actinomyces* spp. may be present. Tissue, aspirates of pus, or sulfur granules represent ideal specimens for anaerobic culture; swabs should be avoided.

Visible growth of *Actinomyces* spp. can occur within 48 hours but usually requires 5 to 7 days. It may be necessary to hold plates for 2 to 4 weeks. Species identification using traditional biochemical tests is difficult. PCR and sequence analysis of the 16S rRNA gene may be necessary for precise species identification. In the future, mass spectrometry (MALDI-TOF MS) may prove most useful for identification of *Actinomyces* species (see Chapter 3).[47]

In addition to actinomycetes, one to five other associated bacteria are often recovered from properly handled specimens. The most commonly isolated organisms are resident flora of the oral cavity or intestinal tract and include the anaerobes *Fusobacterium, Peptostreptococcus, Prevotella,* and *Bacteroides* spp.; and *Pasteurella multocida, Escherichia coli,* and *Streptococcus* spp.. Occasionally, pure cultures of *Actinomyces* spp. are isolated, but this does not exclude the concurrent presence of other organisms, especially strict anaerobes.

TABLE 59.2 Diagnostic Assays Available for *Actinomyces* Infection in Dogs and Cats

Assay	Specimen Type	Target	Performance
Culture	Aspirates of purulent material (e.g., abscesses, pleural effusion); whole blood; CSF; tissue specimens obtained by biopsy or at necropsy (e.g., subcutaneous tissue, heart valve, lung tissue); sulfur granules	*Actinomyces* spp.	Some organisms require anaerobic conditions. Requires several weeks' incubation and overgrowth by companion bacteria may occur. Because *Actinomyces* spp. are mucosal commensal bacteria, isolation from contaminated sites does not imply disease causation. PCR and sequencing may be required to identify the species present.
Cytology or histopathology with organism detection using special stains	Aspirates or tissue specimens	*Actinomyces* spp. organisms	Organisms are gram positive, do not take up acid-fast stain, and are often accompanied by other bacteria and sulfur granules. Definitive diagnosis requires culture because *Nocardia* can resemble *Actinomyces* spp.

CSF, cerebrospinal fluid; *PCR,* polymerase chain reaction.

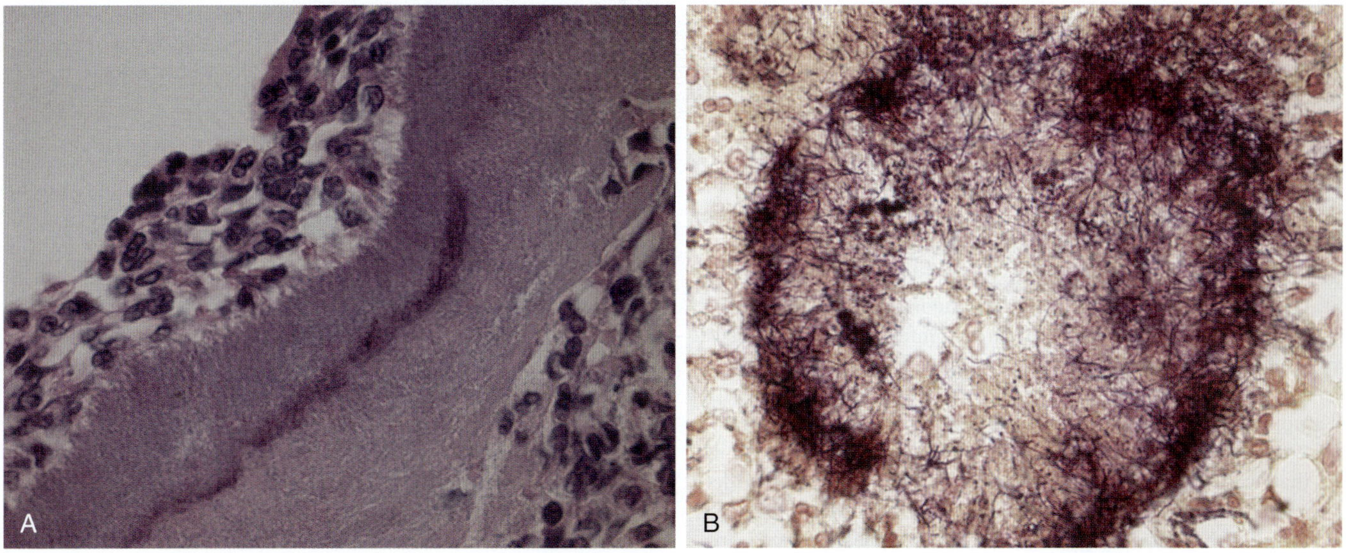

Fig. 59.6 Histopathology of a biopsy specimen from the xiphoid of a 10-year-old intact male English pointer dog with actinomycosis due to a migrating plant awn foreign body. The dog had 1-month history of a ventral thoracic wall mass. (A) Dense, granular mats of branching bacteria were present in a background of extensive granulation tissue and embedded plant material (not shown). H&E stain. (B) Brown and Benn (Gram) stain revealed colonies of gram-positive, filamentous, branching bacteria. *Actinomyces bowdenii* (based on 16S rRNA gene sequencing), *Pasteurella canis, Porphyromonas canoris, Cutibacterium acnes*, a *Bacteroides gingivalis*-like organism and a *Bacteroides ureolyticus*-like organism were isolated from the lesion.

Molecular Diagnosis Using Nucleic Acid–Based Testing

Specific assays for *Actinomyces* spp. have been developed and used for diagnosis of human actinomycosis[48] but are not commercially available for veterinary diagnosis.

Pathologic Findings

Gross lesions in animals with actinomycosis often consist of one or more poorly defined, indurated masses of the subcutaneous tissues, thoracic cavity, lungs, abdominal cavity, or retroperitoneal space, which incorporate adjacent structures. Masses may contain one or more pockets of a reddish-brown exudate. Fistulas, plant material, and sulfur granules may be found. Abdominal or thoracic effusions are often reddish-brown and may contain sulfur granules. Animals with thoracic and abdominal infections may also have a diffuse, red, velvety to granular thickening of the pleura or peritoneum and omentum. Rarely, abscesses may be present in the brain or there may be evidence of purulent meningitis.

Histopathology of affected tissues reveals abscesses with a core of neutrophils encapsulated by granulation tissue that contains macrophages, plasma cells, and lymphocytes in a dense, fibrous tissue matrix. Suppuration is always present in association with active disease, but some parts of lesions may lack neutrophil presence. When present, sulfur granules are generally in the center of microabscesses, but multiple tissue sections may be needed to find them. In tissue sections stained with H&E, the granules are round, oval, or scalloped amphophilic solid masses (Fig. 59.6A). The granules vary in size (from 30 to 3,000 μm in diameter) and often are rimmed by partially confluent radiating eosinophilic club-shaped structures collectively known as the *Splendore-Hoeppli phenomenon*. This phenomenon can also occur with zygomycosis, sporotrichosis, parasitic infections, foreign body reactions, and hypereosinophilic syndrome.[49,50] Antigen-antibody complexes, complement, and major basic protein of eosinophils have been detected within the Splendore-Hoeppli phenomenon. Special stains (Gram, Giemsa, and silver) are required to stain *Actinomyces* spp., and reveal clumps of tangled, intermittently branched, thin (<1 μm) filaments (Fig. 59.6B). Other nonfilamentous bacteria and/or plant material may also be present. *Actinomyces* are not acid fast. With the rare exception of some *Nocardia* spp. that

TABLE 59.3 Medications That Could Be Used to Treat *Actinomyces* spp. Infections in Dogs and Cats with Actinomycosis

Drug	Dose	Route	Interval (Hours)
Penicillin G	100,000 U/kg	IV, IM	6–8
Ampicillin sodium	20 mg/kg	IV, IM, SC	6–8
Amoxicillin	20 mg/kg	PO	8
Clindamycin[a]	11 mg/kg	PO	12 (dogs), 24 (cats)
Doxycycline[b]	5–10 mg/kg	PO	12–24

[a]For IV administration of clindamycin phosphate, see Chapter 10.
[b]10 mg/kg q12h preferred if tolerated without gastrointestinal adverse effects. Doxycycline or clindamycin should always be administered with a bolus of water to avoid esophagitis.
IM, intramuscular; *IV*, intravenous; *PO*, per os; *SC*, subcutaneous.

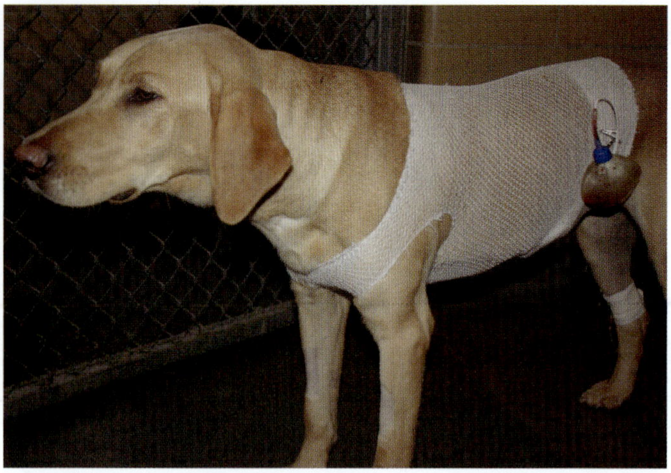

Fig. 59.7 A 1-year-old female spayed Labrador retriever with systemic actinomycosis secondary to a plant awn foreign body, after surgical removal of the plant awn and placement of a grenade drain.

are not acid fast, other fungi and bacteria that produce tissue granules can be distinguished from *Actinomyces* based on their staining and morphologic properties.

TREATMENT AND PROGNOSIS

Treatment of actinomycosis usually requires prolonged administration of antimicrobial drugs. Penicillin is the antimicrobial drug of choice because isolates are uniformly susceptible to penicillins (Table 59.3). High-dose therapy for prolonged periods (weeks to months) is generally required for animals with chronic infections and extensive fibrosis. In human patients with actinomycosis, high doses of penicillin are given parenterally for 2 to 6 weeks, followed by oral therapy with amoxicillin for 6 to 12 months.[35] If the animal is stable clinically, oral therapy can be tried from the outset,[11,51] but it should be recognized that weeks of parenteral treatment is strongly recommended for human infections.[35] Treatment must be extended significantly (weeks to months) beyond resolution of measurable disease to prevent relapse; in some cases, treatment for longer than a year may be required.[2,11] However, when actinomycosis is associated with foreign body migration, shorter durations of treatment may be possible if the foreign body is removed, drainage is established, and extensive scar tissue is not present. Alternative antimicrobial drug choices include clindamycin, doxycycline, chloramphenicol, imipenem-cilastatin, and ceftriaxone.[35] It has been recommended that cephalexin, metronidazole, and aminoglycosides be avoided for treatment of human actinomycosis.[35] Infections associated with companion microbes also usually resolve with penicillin, but on occasion they require broader-spectrum antibiotics during the initial treatment period followed by long-term administration of penicillin.

With the exception of foreign body material (Fig. 59.7), surgery has a controversial role in the treatment of actinomycosis, but may be required if there is extensive fibrous tissue formation or large accumulations of purulent material to facilitate drug penetration (see Chapter 124 for information on management of pyothorax). In human medicine, an initial attempt to control disease with aggressive medical therapy alone has been suggested, with surgical therapy if there is an inadequate response to therapy.[35] In animals with pulmonary abscesses, removal of affected lung lobes may be required. Fibrotic lesions are often extensively vascularized and may obliterate tissue planes, which complicates dissection. In dogs with solitary masses that involve the thoracic and abdominal walls, radical surgical excision is often curative, although repeat surgeries may be needed. An initial period of antibiotic therapy may reduce the size of lesions and improve lesion definition, which facilitates surgery followed by continued antimicrobial drug treatment at a later date. Surgery is also required if a nidus such as a grass awn is present.

Appropriate treatment of actinomycosis results in a cure rate of greater than 90%.[2,11,52] Cure rates with meningitis/meningoencephalitis and advanced thoracic or peritoneal disease with extensive mass lesions may be lower.

PREVENTION

Prevention of actinomycosis involves restriction of access to areas with extensive grass awn formation, and avoidance of fighting and biting activity between animals. When wounds occur, they should be carefully examined for foreign material and cleaned promptly. Plant awns found on animals' coats should also be removed and discarded as soon as possible.

PUBLIC HEALTH ASPECTS

No reports exist of actinomycosis being transmitted from clinically infected animals to humans or other animals; however, humans bitten by dogs, cats, or other humans can develop actinomycosis (see Chapter 75).[35,53] The most common species that infects humans is *A. israelii*.[35] This species is a commensal of the canine oral cavity but has not been isolated from dogs or cats with actinomycosis. Nevertheless, *A. viscosus*, *Actinomyces odontolyticus*, and *A. meyeri* are organisms that have been isolated from canine and feline as well as human actinomycosis cases.

CASE EXAMPLE

Signalment

"Penny," a 1-year old, female spayed Labrador retriever from Herald, CA.

History

Penny was evaluated by the UC Davis VMTH emergency service for a 1-week history of progressive inappetence, weight loss, lethargy, and fever. The inappetence was present for 7 days. Two days ago, Penny vomited up a small amount of kibble, and she had not eaten anything since. The owner reported that her feces had been formed and there were no changes in thirst or urination. Earlier in the day, Penny was evaluated at another veterinary clinic where a grade IV/VI left-sided cardiac murmur was auscultated and thoracic radiographs showed a bronchoalveolar and interstitial lung pattern. She was treated with cefazolin (27 mg/kg, IV) and furosemide (1 mg/kg, SC) and referred. Penny had been fully vaccinated for CDV, CPV, CAdV, and rabies. She missed some doses of heartworm prophylaxis medication recently, and otherwise receives no other medications. She lived with three other Labrador retrievers that were all well. She roamed on 8 acres of land and there was a pond on the property where she swam and had been known to eat small crayfish and frogs. Before she became inappetent, she was fed a commercial dry puppy food. Seven months ago she was evaluated at another veterinary clinic for vomiting and inappetence. At that time, she was moderately azotemic; an exploratory laparotomy was performed for a suspected foreign body, but no foreign body was found.

Physical Examination

Body weight: 22.5 kg.

General: Quiet, alert, responsive and wagging tail. Approximately 5% dehydrated. T = 105.2°F (40.7°C), HR 160 beats/minute, RR = 42 breaths/minute. Pink, slightly tacky mucous membranes, CRT < 2 seconds.

Integument: Full clean haircoat, no evidence of ectoparasites.

Eyes, ears, nose, and throat: No clinically significant abnormalities.

Musculoskeletal: BCS 3/9. Generalized mild muscle atrophy was present.

Cardiovascular: A grade II/VI left systolic murmur was auscultated. Femoral pulses were strong, regular, and synchronous.

Respiratory: Increased breath sounds were present bilaterally and diffusely. There was a mild increase in respiratory effort.

GI/genitourinary: No clinically significant abnormalities. Rectal palpation was unremarkable.

Lymph nodes: All within normal limits (approximately 1 cm).

Laboratory Findings

CBC: HCT 24.0% (40%–55%), MCV 65.6 fL (65–75 fL), MCHC 35.0 g/dL (33–36 g/dL), WBC 29,850 cells/μL (6,000–13,000 cells/μL), neutrophils 16,119 cells/μL (3,000–10,500 cells/μL), lymphocytes 2,985 cells/μL (1,000–4,000 cells/μL), monocytes 7,761 cells/μL (150–1,200 cells/μL), eosinophils 0 cells/μL (0–1,500 cells/μL), basophils 0 cells/μL (0–50 cells/μL), platelets 98,000 platelets/μL (150,000–400,000 platelets/μL), MPV 20.1 fL (7–13 fL). A few slightly toxic band neutrophils and moderate numbers of macroplatelets were present.

Serum chemistry profile: Sodium 144 mmol/L (145–154 mmol/L), potassium 4.3 mmol/L (3.6–5.3 mmol/L), chloride 114 mmol/L (108–118 mmol/L), bicarbonate 15 mmol/L (16–26 mmol/L), phosphorus 5.3 mg/dL (3.0–6.2 mg/dL), calcium 9.6 mg/dL (9.7–11.5 mg/dL), BUN 22 mg/dL (5–21 mg/dL), creatinine 0.8 mg/dL (0.3–1.2 mg/dL), glucose 44 mg/dL (64–123 mg/dL), total protein 7.8 g/dL (5.4–7.6 g/dL), albumin 2.5 g/dL (3.0–4.4 g/dL), globulin 5.3 g/dL (1.8–3.9 g/dL), ALT 31 U/L (19–67 U/L), AST 76 U/L (19–42 U/L), ALP 612 U/L (21–170 U/L), GGT 5 U/L (0–6 U/L), cholesterol 292 mg/dL (135–361 mg/dL), total bilirubin 0.8 mg/dL (0–0.2 mg/dL).

Urinalysis: SpG 1.016; pH 5.0, 1+ protein (SSA), 1+ bilirubin, 2+ hemoprotein, 1+ glucose, 0–1 WBC/HPF, 0–3 RBC/HPF, rare granular casts, many amorphous crystals, rare bilirubin crystals, many lipid droplets.

Coagulation panel: PT 7.7 seconds (7.5–10.5 seconds), APTT 15.2 seconds (9–12 seconds), fibrinogen 232 mg/dL (90–255 mg/dL), D-dimer 1.0–2.0 μg/mL (0–0.25 μg/mL).

Imaging Findings

Thoracic radiographs (three views): There were patchy diffuse unstructured interstitial opacities in all lung lobes (see Fig. 59.5A). The cardiovascular structures appeared within normal limits. The liver appeared markedly enlarged.

Echocardiography: The left ventricle was eccentrically hypertrophied. The papillary muscles had normal shape and echogenicity. There was no enlargement of the left atrium. There was no evidence of endocarditis. Decreased fractional shortening (26%; reference range, approximately 34%–46%) and increased end systolic diameter (3.9 cm; reference range, approximately 1.8–3.5 cm) and E-point septal separation (6.8 mm) were indicative of systolic dysfunction, which could also be appreciated subjectively. There was mild tricuspid regurgitation and trivial pulmonic insufficiency. Conclusions: moderate systolic dysfunction. It was recommended that the dog's diet and taurine blood/plasma levels be evaluated. It was also considered possible that the dog's febrile state was responsible for some of abnormalities observed on the echocardiogram.

Abdominal ultrasound: The liver appeared diffusely mottled, particularly in the left caudal region (see Fig. 59.5B). Within the left caudal liver, there was a focal, ill-defined heteroechoic area approximately 1 cm in diameter. Other smaller, ill-defined hypoechoic nodules were also present within the left liver. One of these areas in particular contained a well-demarcated, hyperechoic rim with irregular echogenic luminal contents and measured approximately 0.5 cm in diameter. Multiple large mesenteric lymph nodes were noted just caudal to the liver with the largest measuring approximately 1.3 cm by 4.5 cm. There was a mild amount of anechoic free abdominal fluid. The spleen was moderately enlarged, but the echotexture and echogenicity appeared within normal limits. There was mild renal pyelectasia bilaterally, but the associated renal papillae appeared within normal limits.

Microbiologic Testing

Aerobic and anaerobic blood cultures (five specimens): Negative.

IFA serology for serum antibody to *Ehrlichia canis*, *Anaplasma phagocytophilum*, *Rickettsia* , and *Babesia canis*: Negative.

IFA serology for serum antibody to *Bartonella vinsonii* subsp. *berkhoffii*, *Bartonella clarridgeiae*, and *Bartonella henselae*: Negative.

Bartonella culture (whole blood): Negative.

Serology for *Coccidioides* serum antibodies: Negative.

Cytologic Findings

Splenic aspirate (ultrasound-guided): Two smears were examined that contained a large amount of blood in the background and were highly cellular. Several small clumps of splenic stromal cells were noted. A large heterogeneous population of lymphocytes was found, with a moderate increase in plasma cells. A moderate number of hematopoietic cells also was observed, including megakaryocytes, myeloid, and erythroid precursors.

Interpretation: Moderate reactive lymphoid hyperplasia and extramedullary hematopoiesis.

Liver aspirate (ultrasound-guided): Two smears were examined that contained a diffusely stippled background containing abundant nuclear debris and were highly cellular. A large population of mildly to markedly degenerate neutrophils was observed. Degenerate cells ranged from highly pyknotic to severely karyolytic. A few neutrophils contained small intracellular bacterial rods.

Interpretation: Marked suppurative inflammation with bacterial sepsis.

CASE EXAMPLE—cont'd

Further Microbiologic Testing

Aerobic and anaerobic culture (ultrasound-guided liver aspirate): Small numbers of suspect *Actinomyces* spp. No anaerobes cultured. Partial 16S rRNA gene PCR and sequence analysis revealed 99% identity to *A. bowdenii.*

Diagnosis

Systemic *A. bowdenii* infection with hepatic involvement.

Treatment

Immediately upon admission, Penny was treated with IV lactated Ringer's solution with 20 mEq/L KCl and 5% dextrose at 75 mL/hour. After the specimens for blood culture were collected, treatment with enrofloxacin (10 mg/kg, IV, q24h) and ampicillin (22 mg/kg, IV, q8h) was initiated. Within 24 hours, the dog's rectal temperature had decreased to 101.3°F (38.5°C), the blood glucose had increased from 41 mg/dL to 107 mg/dL, and the dog began eating. A liver aspirate was submitted for culture on day 2 of hospitalization. A recheck abdominal ultrasound examination on day 3 showed progressive abscessation of the left liver and further enlargement of the gastrohepatic lymph nodes; the mesentery that surrounded the liver was mildly hyperechoic but less so than on the previous examination. By day 4 of hospitalization, growth of an *Actinomyces*-like organism was reported. On day 5, antimicrobial drug treatment was changed to clavulanic acid-amoxicillin (17 mg/kg, q8h). However, later in the day, Penny's temperature increased to 103.6°F (39.8°C), and so the initial antimicrobial drug prescription was reinstated. The dog's hematocrit had also dropped to 19%. Thoracic radiographs were repeated and showed almost complete resolution of the patchy pulmonary infiltrates. A follow-up echocardiogram was unchanged. An abdominal ultrasound examination was again repeated and showed persistent hypoechogenicity of the left liver lobe, but during the procedure a hyperechoic lesion that was consistent with a plant awn foreign body was discovered in the subcutaneous tissue in a caudoventral intercostal space. On day 6, surgery was performed to remove the plant awn. Packed red cells were administered during the procedure and a 16F chest tube was placed because the thoracic cavity was entered during the search for the foxtail, which, with the assistance of intraoperative ultrasound examination, was eventually located under the 13th rib just outside the pleural space. Sulfur granules were found embedded in the tissue during surgery. A closed suction grenade drain was also placed (see Fig. 59.7). The chest tube was removed later in the day. Treatment with enrofloxacin and ampicillin was continued, as well as with oxymorphone (0.04 mg/kg, SC, q6h) to control pain. On day 7, Penny's temperature was 100.7°F (38.2°C) and the drain was removed. Aerobic and anaerobic culture of the foxtail revealed small numbers of penicillin-susceptible *Enterococcus faecalis* and a *Streptomyces*-like organism. No anaerobes were cultured. Penny was discharged on day 8 with instructions to continue treatment with clavulanic-acid amoxicillin for an additional month. The dog subsequently did not return for a recheck examination but had no further clinical signs of illness.

Comments

This is an unusual case of disseminated *A. bowdenii* infection that led to hematogenous pneumonia and hepatic abscessation. Although there was an initial defervescence with antimicrobial drug treatment, anemia and pyrexia persisted, which led to a search for an abscess that might require drainage or a plant awn. Fortunately, a plant awn was ultimately identified with ultrasound, after which the dog's illness resolved completely. *E. faecalis* was isolated from the plant awn and represented a "companion microbe," but whether dissemination of this organism occurred was unclear. The *Streptomyces* spp. may have been a contaminant or the *Actinomyces* spp. may have been misidentified. Continuation of treatment with enrofloxacin and clavulanic acid after the culture results became available was probably unnecessary in this dog; amoxicillin would likely have been sufficient. The owner was warned that additional plant awns may still be present. The cause of the cardiomyopathy was not determined; plasma and whole blood taurine concentrations were within normal limits and follow-up examination was not performed.

SUGGESTED READINGS

Song RB, Vitullo CA, da Costa RC, et al. Long-term survival in a dog with meningoencephalitis and epidural abscessation due to *Actinomyces* species. *J Vet Diagn Invest.* 2015;27:552–557.

Kirpensteijn J, Fingland RB. Cutaneous actinomycosis and nocardiosis in dogs: 48 cases (1980-1990). *J Am Vet Med Assoc.* 1992;201:917–920.

Barnes LD, Grahn BH. *Actinomyces* endophthalmitis and pneumonia in a dog. *Can Vet J.* 2007;48:1155–1158.

REFERENCES

1. Bollinger O. Uber eine neue Pilmkrankheit beim Rinde. *Zbl Med Wissensch.* 1877;15:481–485.
2. Hardie EM, Barsanti JA. Treatment of canine actinomycosis. *J Am Vet Med Assoc.* 1982;180:537–541.
3. Kirpensteijn J, Fingland RB. Cutaneous actinomycosis and nocardiosis in dogs: 48 cases (1980-1990). *J Am Vet Med Assoc.* 1992;201:917–920.
4. Sykes JE. Actinomycosis and nocardiosis. In: Greene CE, ed. *Infectious Diseases of the Dog and Cat.* 4 ed. St. Louis: Elsevier Saunders; 2012:484–495.
5. Love DN, Jones RF, Bailey M, et al. Bacteria isolated from subcutaneous abscesses in cats. *Aust Vet Practit.* 1978;8:87–90.
6. Ochiai K, Kurita-Ochiai T, Kamino Y, et al. Effect of co-aggregation on the pathogenicity of oral bacteria. *J Med Microbiol.* 1993;39:183–190.
7. Ledbetter EC, Scarlett JM. Isolation of obligate anaerobic bacteria from ulcerative keratitis in domestic animals. *Vet Ophthalmol.* 2008;11:114–122.
8. Barnes LD, Grahn BH. *Actinomyces* endophthalmitis and pneumonia in a dog. *Can Vet J.* 2007;48:1155–1158.
9. Sherman A, Daniels JB, Wilkie DA, et al. *Actinomyces bowdenii* ulcerative keratitis in a dog. *Vet Ophthalmol.* 2013;16:386–391.
10. Chastain CB, Grier RL, Hogle RM, et al. Actinomycotic peritonitis in a dog. *J Am Vet Med Assoc.* 1976;168:499–501.
11. Edwards DF, Nyland TG, Weigel JP. Thoracic, abdominal, and vertebral actinomycosis. Diagnosis and long-term therapy in three dogs. *J Vet Intern Med.* 1988;2:184–191.
12. Georg LK, Brown JM, Baker HJ, et al. *Actinomyces viscosus* as an agent of actinomycosis in the dog. *Am J Vet Res.* 1972;33:1457–1470.
13. Kawamura N, Shimada A, Morita T, et al. Intraperitoneal actinomycosis in a cat. *Vet Rec.* 2005;157:593–594.
14. Sharman MJ, Goh CS, Kuipers von Lande RG, et al. Intra-abdominal actinomycetoma in a cat. *J Feline Med Surg.* 2009;11:701–705.
15. Pietra M, Zanoni RG, Peli A, et al. Gastric inflammatory pseudotumour secondary to *Actinomyces hordeovulneris* infection in a cat. *Ir Vet J.* 2015;69:12.
16. Davenport AA, Carter GR, Schirmer RG. Canine actinomycosis due to *Actinomyces viscosus*: report of six cases. *Vet Med Small Anim Clin.* 1974;69(1442):1444–1447.
17. Frendin J, Greko C, Hellmén E, et al. Thoracic and abdominal wall swellings in dogs caused by foreign bodies. *J Small Anim Pract.* 1994;35:499–508.
18. Johnson DE, Summers BA. Osteomyelitis of the lumbar vertebrae in dogs caused by grass-seed foreign bodies. *Aust Vet J.* 1971;47:289–294.
19. Song RB, Vitullo CA, da Costa RC, et al. Long-term survival in a dog with meningoencephalitis and epidural abscessation due to *Actinomyces* species. *J Vet Diagn Invest.* 2015;27:552–557.
20. Anvik JO, Lewis R. *Actinomyces* encephalitis associated with hydrocephalus in a dog. *Can Vet J.* 1976;17:42–44.

21. Couto SS, Dickinson PJ, Jang S, et al. Pyogranulomatous meningoencephalitis due to *Actinomyces* sp. in a dog. *Vet Pathol.* 2000;37:650–652.
22. Sturges BK, Dickinson PJ, Kortz GD, et al. Clinical signs, magnetic resonance imaging features, and outcome after surgical and medical treatment of otogenic intracranial infection in 11 cats and 4 dogs. *J Vet Intern Med.* 2006;20:648–656.
23. Barrs VR, Nicoll RG, Churcher RK, et al. Intracranial empyema: literature review and two novel cases in cats. *J Small Anim Pract.* 2007;48:449–454.
24. Bestetti G, Bühlman V, Nicolet J, et al. Paraplegia due to *Actinomyces viscosus* infection in a cat. *Acta Neuropathol.* 1977;39:231–235.
25. Stowater JL. Actinomycosis in the spinal canal of cat. *Feline Pract.* 1978;8:26–27.
26. Dhamborvorn T, Tritipsatit S, Meemongkoldilok S. Actinomycosis of the urinary bladder. *J Med Assoc Thai.* 2001;84:109–112.
27. Billington SJ, Post KW, Jost BH. Isolation of *Arcanobacterium* (*Actinomyces*) pyogenes from cases of feline otitis externa and canine cystitis. *J Vet Diagn Invest.* 2002;14:159–162.
28. Ormsby AH, Bauer TW, Hall GS. Actinomycosis of the cholecystic duct: case report and review. *Pathology.* 1998;30:65–67.
29. Harvey AM, Holt PE, Barr FJ, et al. Treatment and long-term follow-up of extrahepatic biliary obstruction with bilirubin cholelithiasis in a Somali cat with pyruvate kinase deficiency. *J Feline Med Surg.* 2007;9:424–431.
30. Balakrishnan N, Alexander K, Keene B, et al. Successful treatment of mitral valve endocarditis in a dog associated with *'Actinomyces canis*-like' infection. *J Vet Cardiol.* 2016;18:271–277.
31. Meurs KM, Heaney AM, Atkins CE, et al. Comparison of polymerase chain reaction with bacterial 16S primers to blood culture to identify bacteremia in dogs with suspected bacterial endocarditis. *J Vet Intern Med.* 2011;25:959–962.
32. Mardis JS, Many Jr WJ. Endocarditis due to *Actinomyces viscosus. South Med J.* 2001;94:240–243.
33. Junius G, Bavegems V, Stalpaert M, et al. Mitral valve endocarditis in a Labrador retriever caused by an actinomyces species identified as *Actinomyces turicensis. J Vet Intern Med.* 2004;18:899–901.
34. Moghaddam R, Jaffey JA, Hostnik ET, et al. Presumed primary bacterial rhinosinusitis-associated optic neuritis in a cat. *Front Vet Sci.* 2020;7:122.
35. Russo TA. Agents of actinomycosis. In: Mandell GL, Bennett JE, Dolin R, eds. *Principles and Practice of Infectious Diseases.* 7th ed. Philadephia, PA: Churchill Livingstone, Elsevier; 2010:3209–3219.
36. Cope VZ. Visceral actinomycosis. *Ann R Coll Surg Engl.* 1949;5:394–410.
37. Afolabi IR, Shashidhar VM. Carcinoma of the oesophagus masquerading as actinomycosis: a case report and a review of literature. *Pac Health Dialog.* 2004;11:94–95.
38. Batur Calis A, Ozbal AE, Basak T, et al. Laryngeal actinomycosis accompanying laryngeal carcinoma: report of two cases. *Eur Arch Oto-Rhino-Laryngol.* 2006;263:783–785.
39. Frendin J. Diagnostic imaging of back pain. *J Small Anim Pract.* 1999;40:278–285.
40. Sivacolundhu RK, O'Hara AJ, Read RA. Thoracic actinomycosis (arcanobacteriosis) or nocardiosis causing thoracic pyogranuloma formation in three dogs. *Aust Vet J.* 2001;79:398–402.
41. Qiu L, Lan L, Feng Y, et al. Pulmonary actinomycosis imitating lung cancer on (18)F-FDG PET/CT: a case report and literature review. *Korean J Radiol.* 2015;16:1262–1265.
42. Ha YJ, An JH, Shim JH, et al. A case of primary hepatic actinomycosis: an enigmatic inflammatory lesion of the liver. *Clin Mol Hepatol.* 2015;21:80–84.
43. Hoyles L, Falsen E, Pascual C, et al. *Actinomyces catuli* sp. nov., from dogs. *Int J Syst Evol Microbiol.* 2001;51:679–682.
44. Hoyles L, Falsen E, Foster G, et al. *Actinomyces canis* sp. nov., isolated from dogs. *Int J Syst Evol Microbiol.* 2000;50 Pt 4:1547–1551.
45. Hoyles L, Falsen E, Foster G, et al. *Actinomyces coleocanis* sp. nov., from the vagina of a dog. *Int J Syst Evol Microbiol.* 2002;52:1201–1203.
46. Pascual C, Foster G, Falsen E, et al. *Actinomyces bowdenii* sp. nov., isolated from canine and feline clinical specimens. *Int J Syst Bacteriol.* 1999;49 Pt 4:1873–1877.
47. Ng LS, Sim JH, Eng LC, et al. Comparison of phenotypic methods and matrix-assisted laser desorption ionisation time-of-flight mass spectrometry for the identification of aero-tolerant *Actinomyces* spp. isolated from soft-tissue infections. *Eur J Clin Microbiol Infect Dis.* 2012;32:1749–1752.
48. Fujita Y, Iikura M, Horio Y, et al. Pulmonary *Actinomyces graevenitzii* infection presenting as organizing pneumonia diagnosed by PCR analysis. *J Med Microbiol.* 2012;61(Pt 8):1156–1158.
49. Read RW, Zhang J, Albini T, et al. Splendore-Hoeppli phenomenon in the conjunctiva: immunohistochemical analysis. *Am J Ophthalmol.* 2005;140:262–266.
50. Sykes JE, Weiss DJ, Buoen LC, et al. Idiopathic hypereosinophilic syndrome in 3 Rottweilers. *J Vet Intern Med.* 2001;15:162–166.
51. Nelson JD, Hermann DW. Oral penicillin therapy for thoracic actinomycosis. *Pediatr Infect Dis.* 1986;5:594–595.
52. Frendin J. Pyogranulomatous pleuritis with empyema in hunting dogs. *Zentralbe Veterinary Med.* 1997;44:167–178.
53. Reiner SL, Harrelson JM, Miller SE, et al. Primary actinomycosis of an extremity: a case report and review. *Rev Infect Dis.* 1987;9:581–589.
54. Buchanan AM, Scott JL. *Actinomyces hordeovulneris*, a canine pathogen that produces L-phase variants spontaneously with coincident calcium deposition. *Am J Vet Res.* 1984;45:2552–2560.
55. Ulbegi-Mohyla H, Hassan AA, Alber J, et al. Identification of *Arcanobacterium pluranimalium* isolated from a dog by phenotypic properties and by PCR mediated characterization of various molecular targets. *Vet Microbiol.* 2010;142:458–460.
56. Love DN, Jones RF, Bailey M, et al. Isolation and characterisation of bacteria from abscesses in the subcutis of cats. *J Med Microbiol.* 1979;12:207–212.
57. Love DN, Jones RF, Bailey M, et al. Isolation and characterisation of bacteria from pyothorax (empyaemia) in cats. *Vet Microbiol.* 1982;7:455–461.

60

Nocardiosis

Jane E. Sykes

KEY POINTS

- First Described: In 1888, Alfort, France (Edmond Nocard).[1]
- Causes: *Nocardia* spp..
- Geographic Distribution: Worldwide, although infections in dogs and cats are most commonly reported from Brazil, the western United States, and Australia.
- Mode of Transmission: Inhalation or cutaneous inoculation of organisms in the environment, with opportunistic proliferation in the face of impaired host immune defenses.
- Major Clinical Signs: Lethargy, weight loss, inappetence; subcutaneous masses and nonhealing, crusted or draining skin lesions; pulmonary nodules, masses and/or effusion with cough and tachypnea; signs of dissemination (neurologic signs, chorioretinitis, abdominal effusion or masses, lameness).
- Differential Diagnoses: Actinomycosis, streptomycosis, mycobacteriosis, bartonellosis, fungal infections, neoplasia.
- Human Health Significance: Direct transmission of disease from animals to humans does not generally occur, but humans have developed disease after bites or scratches from healthy dogs or cats.

ETIOLOGIC AGENT AND EPIDEMIOLOGY

Nocardia are filamentous, branching, gram-positive bacteria that belong to the family Nocardiaceae (Fig. 60.1). Approximately 100 different *Nocardia* species have been recognized since the advent of molecular identification methods, half of which are human and animal pathogens.[2,3] The advent of molecular methods led to extensive revision of the taxonomy of *Nocardia* spp.[2] Species that belonged to the former *Nocardia asteroides* complex are now distinct species, and include *Nocardia cyriacigeorgica* (formerly *N. asteroides* sensu stricto), *Nocardia abscessus*, *Nocardia nova*, *Nocardia farcinica*, and *Nocardia otitidiscaviarum*.[2,4] Knowledge of the species involved is important because different *Nocardia* species differ in their antimicrobial susceptibility patterns, epidemiology, and pathogenicity. They also differ in the amount of mycolic acid in their cell wall, which affects their ability to stain with acid-fast stains.

Like actinomycosis, nocardiosis is a suppurative to granulomatous, localized or disseminated opportunistic infection caused by filamentous bacteria. However, unlike *Actinomyces* spp. (which are commensals of mucous membranes), *Nocardia* spp. are ubiquitous soil saprophytes that degrade organic matter. They are also found in fresh and salt water, dust, and on decaying plants and fecal matter.[4] They may be carried mechanically on the claws or skin. Infections are acquired via inhalation of organisms or inoculation via puncture wounds. Transfer of infection between animals does not occur.

Nocardiosis is much less frequently reported in dogs and cats than actinomycosis (which can have a similar clinical appearance), although nocardiosis is increasingly recognized in both human medicine and companion animals in association with a higher prevalence of immunocompromised hosts, such as those treated with potent immunosuppressive drugs (especially cyclosporine).[5–9] Where vaccination for CDV is inadequate or not widely instituted, nocardiosis in dogs has been associated with CDV-induced immunosuppression.[10–12]

The prevalence of nocardiosis and the prevailing *Nocardia* species that cause disease vary geographically. For example, within the United States, human nocardiosis has been most commonly reported from the southwestern states. Dry, dusty, and windy conditions in these areas may facilitate aerosolization and dispersal of nocardiae.[13] Dogs and cats from Australia and the western United States are most commonly infected with *N. nova*.[14–16] Other species isolated from dogs and cats are listed in Table 60.1. In humans, *Nocardia brasiliensis* is the most common species isolated from patients residing in tropical locations such as the southwestern United States, Central and South America, and Australia.

More than 60% of people with nocardiosis have underlying immunosuppressive disorders such as AIDS, COPD, autoimmune diseases that require immunosuppressive drug therapy, solid organ transplantation, diabetes mellitus, and hemic neoplasia.[17] Underlying immunosuppressive disease or drug treatment also seems to predispose dogs to nocardiosis. Nocardiosis has been documented in several dogs treated with cyclosporine and a dog with lymphoma.[5,7–9,15] Most affected cats have cutaneous infections that are associated with scratches or bite wounds.[14,18] Accordingly, > 75%–80% of affected cats are male; in the author's hospital, 9 of 10 affected cats were male.[14,15,18] Cats of any age can be affected and no breed predilection has been identified.[14] Some cats have underlying disorders that predispose them to nocardiosis, such as a history of renal transplantation, underlying retroviral infection, or glucocorticoid administration. Others have no obvious underlying immunosuppressive disease.

CLINICAL FEATURES

Pathogenesis and Clinical Signs

The pathogenicity of *Nocardia* spp. is influenced by the strain and growth phase of the organism, together with host susceptibility. Virulent strains of *Nocardia* are facultative intracellular pathogens that

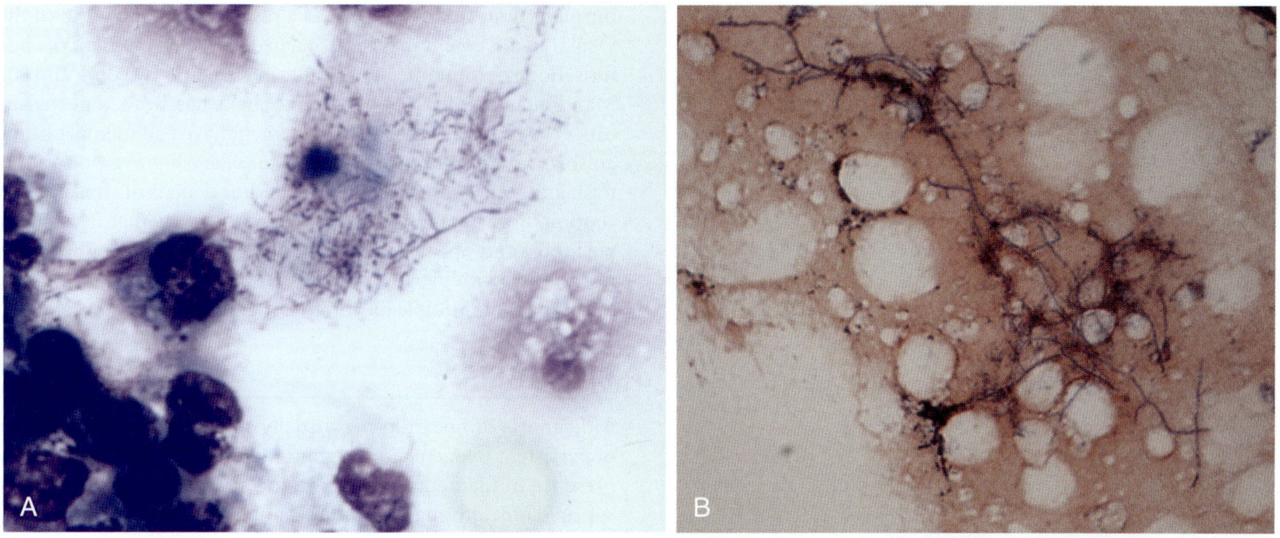

Fig. 60.1 (A) and (B) Gram-stained specimens showing *Nocardia* spp. The organisms are gram positive, filamentous, branching and slightly beaded. (A, Courtesy David F. Edwards, University of Tennessee, Knoxville, TN.)

TABLE 60.1 *Nocardia* Species Isolated from Dogs and Cats with Nocardiosis

Host Species	Dogs	Country
Dogs	*N. nova*	USA, Australia[14,15]
	N. paucivorans	USA[15]
	N. asiatica	USA, Brazil[10,15]
	N. abscessus	USA[9]
	N. otitidiscaviarum	Brazil[12]
	N. farcinica	Australia[14]
	N. brasiliensis	USA, Australia[5,42]
	N. niigatensis	USA[6]
	N. veterana	USA, Germany[11,34]
	N. cyriacigeorgica	Turkey[43]
	N. pseudobrasiliensis	USA[44]
Cats	*N. nova*	USA, Australia[15]
	N. cyriacigeorgica	Australia, West Indies (St Kitts)[14,30]
	N. africana	Japan, Brazil[29,45]
	N. elegans	Japan[46]
	N. brasiliensis	USA[42]
	N. otitidiscaviarum	Spain[47]
	N. jiangxiensis	West Indies (Nevis)[48]
	N. flavorosea/N. carnea	Japan[49]

inhibit phagosome-lysosome fusion, neutralize phagosomal acidification, resist oxidative burst, secrete superoxide dismutase, and alter lysosomal enzymes within neutrophils and macrophages.[17] These effects are partly related to the content and structure of mycolic acids within the bacterial cell wall, which vary among strains and throughout the growth phase. Filamentous log phase cells in the environment can be highly resistant to phagocytosis. Some strains have a greater propensity to invade the CNS.[19,20]

The normal host response to infection is characterized by an initial pyogenic inflammatory response, but a cell-mediated immune response is necessary to destroy the organisms. Diminished host resistance, especially in the form of impaired CMI, is a primary factor in susceptibility to nocardiosis and the extent to which dissemination occurs.

Cutaneous-subcutaneous nocardiosis, the most common form seen in cats (>75% of affected cats), is characterized by slow and progressive circumferential spread of a nonhealing, draining wound (Fig. 60.2). Lesions are typically subacute to chronic. Infections of feeding tube sites may also occur.[21] Mycetoma-like lesions in the inguinal area resemble those described for rapidly growing mycobacterial infections (see Chapter 61), with multiple draining sinuses. These may result from contamination of "raking" injuries inflicted by the hindlimbs during fighting behavior.[14] Alternatively, they might represent contamination of traumatic wounds from penetrating plant material. Cutaneous-subcutaneous nocardiosis was documented in eight of nine dogs from Brazil,[12] but represents the minority of nocardiosis cases in dogs from California, USA and Australia.[14,15] Dogs with cutaneous involvement typically develop draining wounds and masses, often on the head and limbs. Osteomyelitis can occur in association with cutaneous lesions.

The pathogenesis of *pulmonary or disseminated nocardiosis* is similar to that of the deep mycoses. Branching nocardial filaments fragment, which results in the formation of small, unicellular particles that are aerosolized and inhaled, possibly in dust. Once within the lung, *Nocardia* spp. proliferate in the face of immune suppression, which leads to formation of intrapulmonary masses or pneumonia, hilar lymphadenomegaly, and/or extrapulmonary masses and pleural effusion (pyothorax) (Figs. 60.3A and 60.4). Pulmonary nocardiosis is the most common form reported in humans, and also occurs in dogs and less commonly in cats. In dogs, it can have a peracute onset characterized by tachypnea, hemoptysis, hypothermia, collapse, and death; however, subacute to chronic clinical signs are more characteristic.[22–25] Co-infection with CDV is occasionally reported.[10–12,26,27] Disseminated nocardiosis occurs when organisms in the lung erode into blood vessels and spread systemically, with abscess formation in a variety of organs. This leads to signs of lethargy, fever, decreased appetite, and signs that relate to the location of the infectious process. Disseminated disease can occur in cats as well as in dogs. The most frequently involved extrathoracic organs are skin and subcutaneous tissue, kidney, liver, spleen, lymph nodes, CNS, eye, bone, and joints (see Fig. 60.3B). In dogs and cats, CNS lesions may cause seizures or a variety of other neurologic signs that relate to the local effects of abscesses or granulomas in the brain, meninges, or spinal cord. CNS

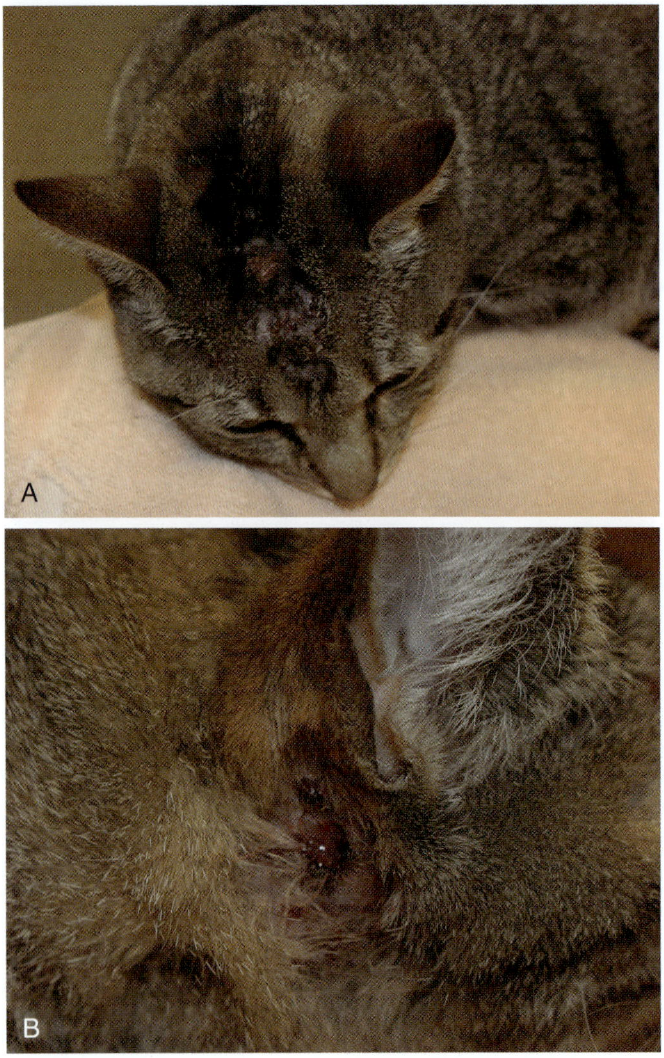

Fig. 60.2 A 6-year-old male neutered domestic shorthair cat with cutaneous-subcutaneous nocardiosis. The lesions progressed over at least a year after a cat bite abscess that was initially treated with clavulanic acid-amoxicillin, and consisted of nodular and crusted lesions on the head (A) and cervical region (B) that drained fluid and extended down the cervical region to the cranioventral thorax. The cat tested negative for feline immunodeficiency virus and feline leukemia virus. (Image courtesy University of California-Davis, Veterinary Dermatology Service.)

involvement is common in human nocardiosis. Peritoneal nocardiosis has also been rarely reported in cats, possibly as a result of penetrating wounds to the abdomen.[14,28]

Physical Examination Findings

Physical examination findings in animals with cutaneous-subcutaneous disease are similar to those in actinomycosis, with chronic, sometimes crusted, ulcerated, nonhealing draining wounds, and in cats may involve the extremities, inguinal area, flank, bridge of the nose, and neck (see Fig. 60.2). Animals with pulmonary or systemic involvement may have a thin body condition, lethargy, and fever. Tachypnea and cough may be present, and lung sounds may be increased (from bronchopneumonia) or decreased (from a mass lesion or pyothorax). Involvement of the liver, spleen, and lymph nodes may be associated with development of hepatomegaly, splenomegaly, and/or peripheral or abdominal lymphadenopathy. Subcutaneous mass lesions that sometimes drain purulent fluid may be present as a result of dissemination to the skin.[9] Ocular involvement may be associated with development of chorioretinitis. Bone or joint infection results in focal limb swelling and lameness. Mandibular involvement ("lumpy jaw") has been reported in some cats.[29,30] Animals with CNS involvement have had mental obtundation, anisocoria, decreased menace and pupillary light responses, head tilt, nystagmus, decreased gag reflexes, and/or deficits of conscious proprioception. Spinal pain, lower motor neuron signs that involved the pelvic limbs, and opisthotonus were described in one dog with suspected nocardiosis with pyogranulomas that involved the subdural and extradural space at multiple locations along the spinal cord.[7]

DIAGNOSIS

A diagnosis of nocardiosis is usually suspected based on the presence of persistent pyogenic to pyogranulomatous inflammatory lesions, the presence of filamentous bacteria, together with a history of immunosuppression, although the latter is not always present. Confirmation of the diagnosis generally requires culture.

Laboratory Abnormalities

Complete Blood Count and Serum Biochemical Tests

Laboratory abnormalities are similar to those with actinomycosis (nonregenerative anemia, neutrophilic leukocytosis with a left shift, monocytosis, and sometimes marked hyperglobulinemia). However, in immunosuppressed animals, lymphopenia, monocytopenia, and eosinopenia may be present. Hypercalcemia associated with granulomatous disease has been reported in a cat.[31]

Cytologic Examination of Body Fluids

Examination of pleural effusion, bronchial lavages, and aspirates of abscesses from animals with nocardiosis typically reveals suppurative to pyogranulomatous inflammation, with large numbers of degenerate neutrophils. Gram-positive, often partially or weakly acid-fast, beaded, filamentous organisms that branch at right angles may be observed individually or in loose aggregates (see Fig. 60.1). The filaments may also fragment to form rods and coccoid forms. *Actinomyces* spp. is not acid fast and *Mycobacterium* spp. do not branch. When the infecting *Nocardia* spp. is not acid fast, it may not be possible to distinguish it from an *Actinomyces* spp. organism. With Romanowsky-type stains, organisms may be eosinophilic or basophilic and have a beaded appearance. Organisms are usually around 0.5 μm in diameter and up to 30 μm long, but thicker organisms were described in one dog infected with *N. abscessus* (2 μm).[9] Macroaggregates (i.e., sulfur granules) have been noted infrequently in effusions. In contrast to actinomycosis, mixed bacterial populations in deep tissue sites are rarely present.

Diagnostic Imaging

Plain Radiography

Radiography of cutaneous-subcutaneous lesions may reveal soft tissue swelling with or without associated bone lysis and periosteal proliferation. The radiographic appearance of pulmonary lesions varies and includes multiple, diffuse pulmonary nodules, intrapulmonary or extrapulmonary solitary masses, focal or diffuse bronchointerstitial to alveolar infiltrates, lobar consolidations, pleural effusions, and often, dramatic hilar lymphadenopathy (Fig. 60.5).

Sonographic Findings

Abdominal ultrasound findings in dogs and cats with disseminated nocardiosis have not been described in detail because disseminated disease with abdominal organ involvement is rare. However, intraparenchymal mass lesions and flocculent ascites fluid may be noted.

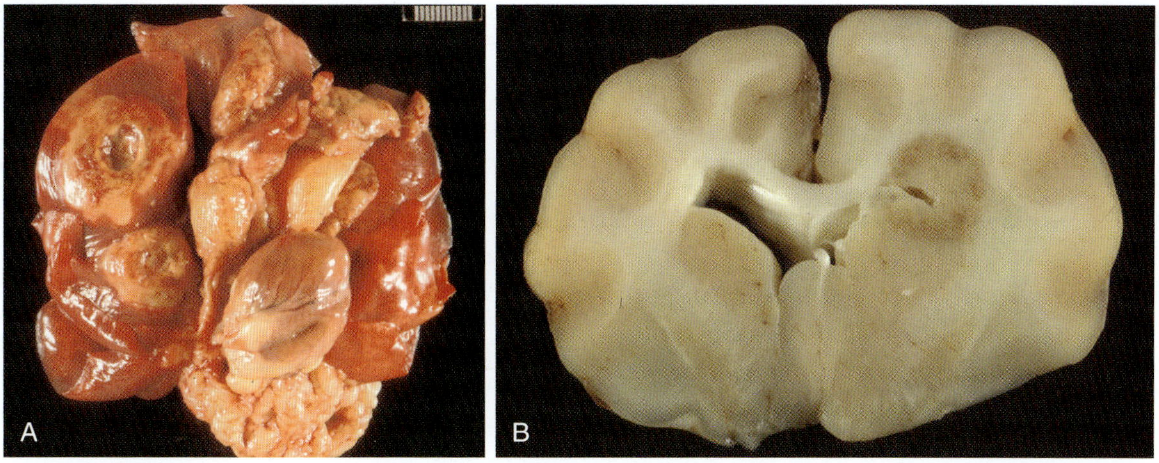

Fig. 60.3 Gross necropsy findings in a 4-year old male neutered domestic shorthair cat with disseminated nocardiosis caused by *Nocardia nova*. The cat was a renal transplant recipient. (A) Multifocal to coalescing large, white to grey, caseous pulmonary masses are present within the lungs. (B) The brain contained multifocal, white to grey foci that histologically consisted of large numbers of neutrophils and filamentous bacteria.

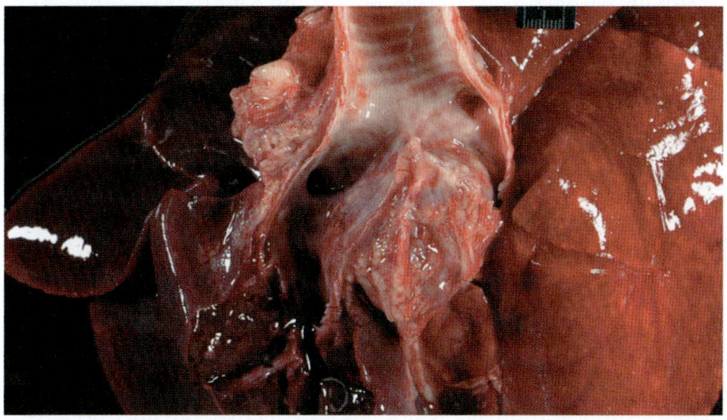

Fig. 60.4 Chronic abscess of the hilar lymph nodes and hilar soft tissue of a 5-year-old female spayed golden retriever. The lesion caused complete compressive occlusion of the left mainstem bronchus, with atelectasis of the left lung lobes. Histopathologic examination revealed pyogranulomatous and necrotizing cellulitis with intralesional filamentous bacteria. *Nocardia* spp. were isolated from the lesion. (Courtesy Chuck Mohr, University of California-Davis, CA)

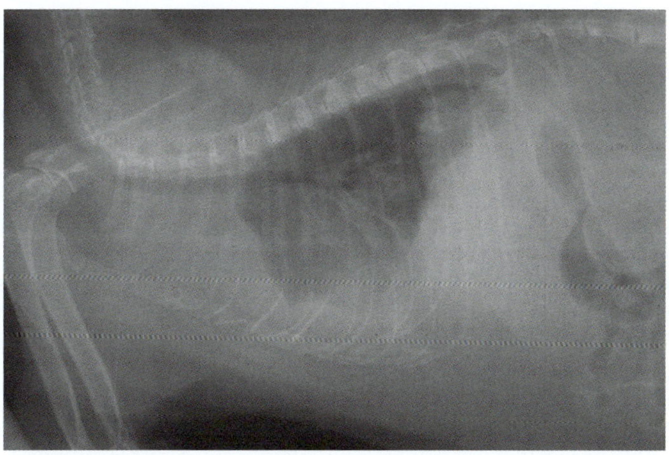

Fig. 60.5 Lateral thoracic radiograph of a 4-year-old male neutered domestic shorthair cat with disseminated nocardiosis. Pleural effusion is present and obscures the cardiac silhouette. A mass is associated with the caudal aspect of the left caudal lung lobe.

Advanced Imaging

Nodular lung lesions similar to those described in humans were identified with CT in one dog with disseminated nocardiosis.[9] CT and MRI abnormalities in dogs and cats with confirmed CNS nocardiosis have not been reported. One dog suspected to have nocardiosis had a large, T2-hyperintense circumscribed lesion in the occipital cortex that was consistent with a brain abscess, together with widespread cerebral edema and herniation of the cerebellum through the foramen magnum.[8]

Microbiologic Tests (Table 60.2)

Isolation and Identification

Nocardia spp. grow aerobically at a wide temperature range on simple media (e.g., Sabouraud's glucose agar, blood agar). Organisms are usually recovered in pure cultures, and colonies are often visible after 2 days. However, in some cases, 2 to 4 weeks of incubation may be necessary, and the organism may be overgrown by contaminating bacteria. Thus, the laboratory should be alerted if nocardiosis is suspected so that selective media and long incubation times are used. Colonies are smooth and moist, or rugose with a powdery surface due to aerial filamentation, and may be pigmented. Organisms may then be identified based on their microscopic appearance and their ability to take up acid-fast stains. However, not all pathogenic strains of *Nocardia* species are acid fast.[19,20,32] L-form *Nocardia* spp., cell wall-deficient variants, have been associated with clinical disease in humans and a dog.[33] These bacteria require special media for isolation and culture, similar to mycoplasmas (see Chapter 57).

Traditionally, *Nocardia* species have been distinguished based on growth characteristics and antibiotic susceptibility patterns; however, molecular methods provide a more reliable and rapid means of speciation. Biochemical methods of identification of *Nocardia* species are now considered inadequate. Sequence analysis of PCR products from the 16S rRNA gene identifies most pathogenic *Nocardia* spp., but differentiation of closely related species may require analysis of other genes or DNA-DNA hybridization.[4,17] The latter is considered the gold standard for *Nocardia* species determination.[4] MALDI-TOF MS permits rapid and reliable identification of *Nocardia* species in clinical microbiology laboratories.[34,35] PCR assays have also been used for direct detection of *Nocardia* spp. in clinical specimens, without prior isolation.[4]

TABLE 60.2 Diagnostic Assays Available for *Nocardia* Infection in Dogs and Cats

Assay	Specimen Type	Target	Performance
Culture	Aspirates of purulent material (e.g., abscesses, pleural effusion); whole blood; tissue specimens obtained by biopsy or at necropsy (e.g., subcutaneous tissue, lung tissue)	*Nocardia* spp.	Grows on most simple media. May require several weeks' incubation. Because *Nocardia* spp. are soil saprophytes, isolation from skin lesions does not imply disease causation. PCR and sequencing may be required to identify the species present.
Cytology or histopathology with organism detection using special stains	Aspirates or tissue specimens	*Nocardia* spp. organisms	Organisms are gram positive, variably acid fast, and not usually accompanied by sulfur granules or the Splendore Hoeppli phenomenon. Definitive diagnosis requires culture because non-acid-fast *Nocardia* can resemble *Actinomyces* spp.

PCR, polymerase chain reaction.

Because *Nocardia* organisms are ubiquitous in soil and may be inhaled by healthy animals, the isolation of small numbers of organisms from ulcerated skin lesions or the respiratory tract must be interpreted in conjunction with clinical signs and history of immune compromise. Repeated positive cultures or isolation of pure or large quantities of the organism are also suggestive of nocardiosis, and the isolation of a single colony from a normally sterile site is significant. Visualization of gram-positive filamentous bacteria in cytology specimens in association with acute inflammatory cells also assists in determination of clinical significance.

The susceptibility of *Nocardia* spp. to antimicrobial drugs varies considerably between different *Nocardia* species, and so species identification can guide appropriate antimicrobial drug selection (see Treatment, below, and Table 60.3). Susceptibility testing for *Nocardia* spp. is difficult and should be done by laboratories with special expertise. Susceptibility testing may be helpful when there is a failure to respond to initial therapy or relapse occurs from drug resistance. It may also be useful if there are concerns that relate to adverse drug reactions to sulfonamides, which are the initial treatment of choice (e.g., in dogs with immune-mediated disease that is complicated by cyclosporine-associated nocardiosis). Testing is also indicated when *N. farcinica* is present, which tends to be highly resistant to antimicrobial drugs, or when a *Nocardia* species with unpredictable susceptibility is isolated.

Pathologic Findings

Nocardiosis is characterized by suppurative necrosis and abscess formation and infrequently produces granulomas (see Figs. 60.3 and 60.5). Gross lesions in organs such as the spleen, lung, liver, and brain typically consist of numerous small (1 mm) to large (several centimeters), discrete or coalescing, intraparenchymal white or gray-white nodules. On cut section, nodules appear caseous to purulent. Lymph nodes are enlarged, often massively, and are firm to fluctuant with a caseous to purulent core. A reddish-brown exudate may be present in the pleural or peritoneal space or within abscesses. Although formation of sulfur granules by *Nocardia* spp. is uncommon compared with *Actinomyces* spp., small granules have occasionally been noted in skin lesions and pleural and peritoneal fluid.[16,22,28,36]

Histopathology usually reveals a central region of necrosis and suppuration, which, depending on the host immune response, may be surrounded by macrophages, lymphocytes, and plasma cells (Figs. 60.6A and 60.7A). In chronic cutaneous-subcutaneous infections, pyogranulomatous foci may be interspersed within dense fibrous tissue. Plant material may be observed if plants were involved in inoculation of *Nocardia* spp. into tissues, but the presence of plant material is more common with actinomycosis.

Nocardia are usually present in abundance within regions of necrosis and suppuration. *Nocardia* filaments are poorly visible in tissue sections stained with H&E or with Gridley's fungal or PAS. Organisms can be stained with Gram stain (Fig. 60.6B) or methenamine silver preparations,[9] especially with prolonged silver nitrate exposure. They are usually partially acid fast (Fig. 60.7B) and have the same appearance described in the Cytology section, earlier. In chronic skin infections, tissue granules characterized by colonies arranged in large, rosette-like arrays have been reported. In contrast to actinomycosis, other bacteria and the Splendore-Hoeppli phenomenon are not generally present.

TREATMENT AND PROGNOSIS

Treatment

Successful treatment of nocardiosis relies upon the combination of appropriate antimicrobial therapy combined with the use of surgical drainage or debridement. Chronic, extensive lesions may require surgical debridement or resection. Appropriate antimicrobial therapy that includes surgical drainage is not always effective, possibly because of an inadequate host immune response.[14] Existing immunosuppressive drug treatment should be discontinued or reduced, provided it does not cause relapse of a life-threatening underlying disease process.

The initial selection of an antimicrobial drug or drug combination should take into account the site of the infection, the host immune status, the infecting species of *Nocardia* (Table 60.3), and if available, susceptibility test results.[17] However, *in vitro* susceptibilities do not always translate into a clinical response *in vivo*. Sulfonamides, including trimethoprim-sulfonamide combinations (TMS), are the primary antimicrobial drugs for treating nocardiosis (Table 60.4). Treatment durations from 1 to 3 months are recommended in humans with cutaneous infections, up to 6 months for uncomplicated pulmonary infections, and 12 months or longer for systemic infections or infections in those who are immunocompromised.[17] Clinical improvement is generally observed within 7 to 10 days of starting treatment. High doses of TMS given for long periods to dogs (and to a lesser extent, cats) can produce a variety of adverse effects such as keratoconjunctivitis sicca and myelosuppression (see Chapter 10). If adverse drug reactions occur, selection of drugs other than TMS should ideally be based on susceptibility test results. If these are not available, choices should be made based on *in vitro* data (see Table 60.3). *Nocardia nova* is susceptible to amoxicillin but resistant to clavulanic acid-amoxicillin because of induction of chromosomal β-lactamase by clavulanic acid.[14,16] Substitution of antimicrobial drugs within a drug class may not provide effective treatment; for example, although sensitive to amikacin, *N. farcinica* isolates are resistant to gentamicin, and although sensitive to minocycline, *N. brasiliensis* isolates are mostly resistant to doxycycline.[37]

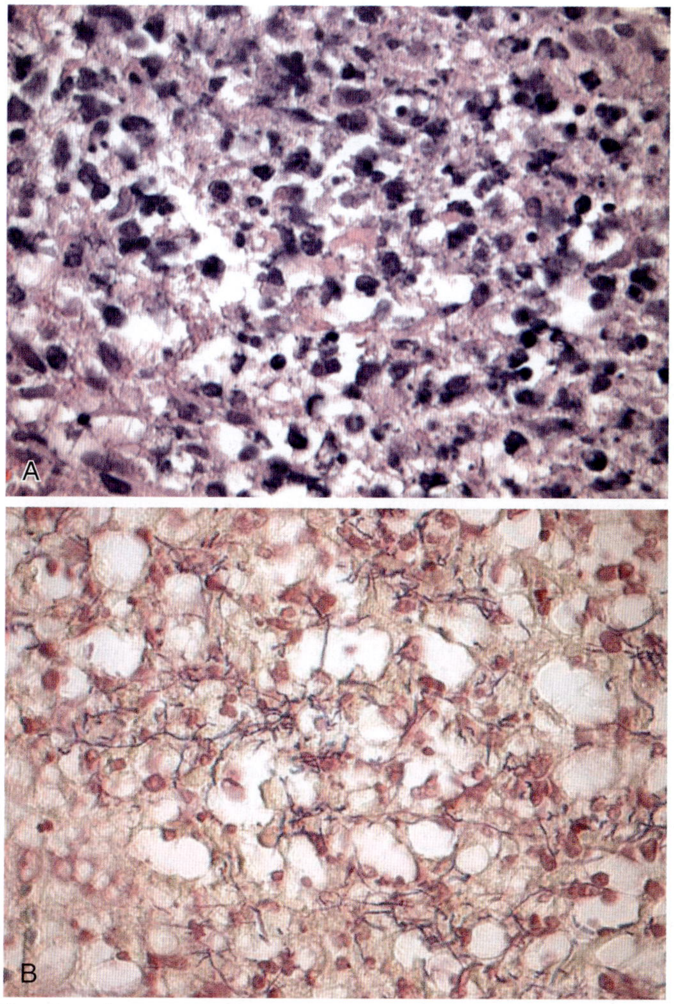

Fig. 60.6 Histopathologic findings in the cat described in Figs. 60.3 and 60.5. (A) Severe, necrotizing pyogranulomatous inflammation is present with intralesional bacteria, which are barely visible. H&E stain. (B) Gram staining revealed tangles of filamentous, branching gram-positive bacteria. Brown and Benn stain.

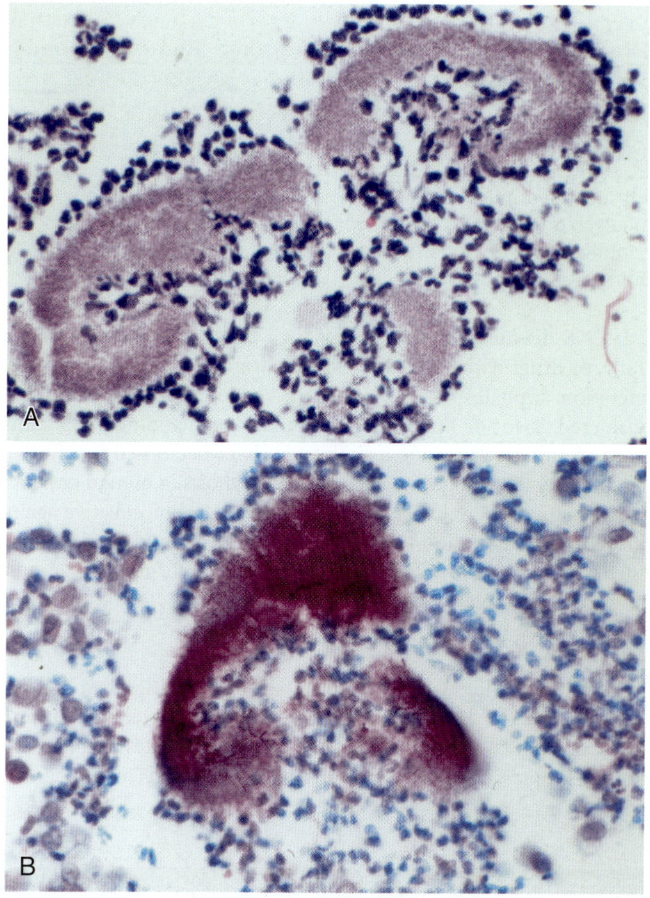

Fig. 60.7 (A) H&E-stained section of chronic, ulcerated cutaneous lesion on flank of 3-year-old male domestic longhaired cat. *Nocardia* tissue granules are surrounded by pyogranulomatous inflammatory reaction. (Long dimension of largest granule is 110 μm; ×66.). (B) Acid-fast stain (Fite-Faraco modification of Ziehl-Neelsen technique) of same tissue section (×132). (Courtesy David F. Edwards, University of Tennessee, Knoxville, TN.)

TABLE 60.3 Suggested Antimicrobial Drug Selection for Treatment of Pathogenic *Nocardia* spp. Based on Minimum Inhibitory Concentration Data[4]

Nocardia Species	Appropriate Antimicrobial Drug Choices	Antimicrobial Drugs To Avoid
N. abscessus	Ampicillin, amoxicillin-clavulanic acid, ceftriaxone, linezolid, amikacin and gentamicin, sulfamethoxazole	Imipenem, ciprofloxacin, clarithromycin
N. brevicatena/paucivorans complex	Ampicillin, amoxicillin-clavulanic acid, ceftriaxone, amikacin, sulfamethoxazole, ciprofloxacin	Gentamicin, clarithromycin
N. nova complex (includes *N. nova*, *N. africana*)	Ampicillin, sulfamethoxazole, erythromycin, clarithromycin, ceftriaxone, imipenem, amikacin	Amoxicillin-clavulanic acid
N. farcinica	Amikacin, sulfamethoxazole, ciprofloxacin (most isolates), imipenem (most isolates)	Ampicillin, broad-spectrum cephalosporins, clarithromycin, aminoglycosides other than amikacin
N. cyriacigeorgica	Ceftriaxone, amikacin, imipenem	Ampicillin, amoxicillin-clavulanic acid, clarithromycin, ciprofloxacin
N. brasiliensis	Minocycline, amoxicillin-clavulanic acid, sulfamethoxazole	Ampicillin, ciprofloxacin, clarithromycin
N. otitidiscaviarum	Gentamicin, amikacin, sulfamethoxazole, ciprofloxacin	All β-lactam antibiotics

TABLE 60.4 Medications that Could Be Used To Treat Dogs and Cats with Nocardiosis Pending Species Identification With or Without Susceptibility Testing

Drug	Dose (mg/kg)	Route	Interval (Hours)
Trimethoprim-sulfamethoxazole	30	PO, IV	12
Amikacin[a]	10–15	IV, IM, SC	24
Imipenem-cilastatin[a]	2–5	IV	8

[a]Amikacin and imipenem-cilastatin are generally used in combination with each other or with trimethoprim-sulfamethoxazole

IV, intravenous; *IM,* intramuscular; *PO,* oral or by mouth; *SC,* subcutaneous.

If CNS disease is present, either high doses of TMS given parenterally, or drugs with excellent CNS penetration, which include third-generation cephalosporins, imipenem, or meropenem, should be considered. Two- or three-drug combinations including TMS, amikacin, and either ceftriaxone or imipenem have been used pending the susceptibility test results to treat severe nocardiosis in human patients.[4] A combination of amikacin and imipenem should be effective against all isolates. Combination treatment with amikacin and TMS was suggested for cats with *N. farcinica* infections, which generally require aggressive, combination drug treatment.[14]

Prognosis

In a review of 53 dogs with nocardiosis, 50% of the dogs died and 39% were euthanized.[27] Of 36 cats with nocardiosis, 16 were either euthanized or died.[14] The high mortality rate may relate to underlying immunosuppressive disease and drug treatment, delayed diagnosis, and inappropriate treatment. With earlier diagnosis and more aggressive, multidrug therapy, mortality of nocardiosis in animals may decrease to the rate reported in humans. Only 20% of humans with primary infections died, whereas 42% of patients with predisposing conditions and more than 50% of patients with either systemic or CNS nocardiosis died.[19]

IMMUNITY AND VACCINATION

Immunity to nocardiosis is dependent on intact CMI, which is why infections often occur in animals and humans with conditions or drug treatment that compromise CMI. There are no vaccines for nocardiosis.

PREVENTION

Nocardiosis in cats may be prevented by housing cats indoors and limitation of fighting or biting activity. When wounds occur, they should be carefully examined for foreign material and cleaned promptly. Disease in both dogs and cats may be prevented by avoidance of excessive immunosuppression with potent drugs such as cyclosporine.

PUBLIC HEALTH ASPECTS

No cases of human nocardiosis acquired from direct contact with an animal have been reported; however, several cases of cutaneous nocardiosis transmitted to humans by cat scratches have been documented.[38–41] Humans with impaired CMI (such as those receiving immunosuppressive drug therapy or those with HIV infection) should wear gloves and practice hand washing after handling pets known to have nocardiosis, or another individual in the household should treat these animals.

CASE EXAMPLE

Signalment

"Bob," a 4-year-old male neutered domestic shorthair cat from San Francisco, CA.

History

Bob, a renal transplant recipient, was evaluated for a 2-week history of decreased activity and lethargy. Five days ago, the lethargy became more severe. Bob also stopped eating and urinated on himself several times. He was taken to a local emergency clinic where they noted mild hyponatremia (130 mmol/L) and a WBC count of 19,000 cells/μL, but there was no evidence of azotemia or elevated liver enzyme activities. No abnormalities were detected on abdominal ultrasound examination. Bob was treated overnight with IV fluids and sent home with instructions to administer clavulanic acid-amoxicillin (12.5 mg/kg, PO, q12h). However, the cat's condition failed to improve and so he was taken to a local veterinary clinic 3 days later. Further laboratory testing showed persistent hyponatremia, hypoalbuminemia, and mild hyperbilirubinemia. Urinalysis showed a specific gravity of 1.054, 3+ bilirubin, 1+hemoprotein, 0–2 WBC/HPF, 6–10 RBC/HPF, and no bacteria or casts. Aerobic bacterial urine culture was negative. The following day he became tachypneic and pleural effusion developed. In-house examination of the effusion fluid revealed cloudy fluid that contained large numbers of erythrocytes, degenerate neutrophils, and macrophages. No bacteria were seen with Gram stain. Bob was then referred to the University of California, Davis, VMTH, for further evaluation.

Bob received a renal transplant 2.5 years ago and had been treated with prednisone (0.5 mg/kg, PO, q12h) and cyclosporine (4 mg/kg, PO, q12h) since that time. A recent whole blood trough cyclosporine concentration was 1,100 ng/mL.

Physical and Neurologic Examinations

Body weight: 5.1 kg.

General: Severely obtunded, T = 100.8°F (38.2°C), HR = 240 beats/minute, RR = 55 breaths/minute, mild generalized icterus, mucous membranes pink to icteric, CRT = 1 second.

Integument: Clean coat, no evidence of ectoparasites.

Eyes, ears, nose, and throat: Anisocoria with the left pupil larger than the right, direct and consensual pupillary light reflexes were present, clear cornea and anterior chamber, no ocular discharge. Fundoscopic examination showed focal areas of tapetal hyperreflectivity and focal dark and dull lesions with peripheral hyperreflectivity.

Musculoskeletal: BCS 7/9, generalized weakness, recumbent, and unwilling to walk.

Cardiovascular: No murmurs or arrhythmias ausculted, pulses moderate and synchronous.

Respiratory: Tachypnea with a shallow respiratory pattern. Decreased lung sounds were present ventrally.

GI/genitourinary: No clinically significant abnormalities. The transplanted kidney could be palpated in the right abdomen. The bladder was small.

Lymph nodes: No clinically significant abnormalities.

Neurologic Examination

Mentation: Obtunded.

Gait/Posture: The cat had a tendency to lean to the right, but could not or would not walk more than a few steps.

CASE EXAMPLE—cont'd

Cranial nerves: Menace responses were absent bilaterally.

Postural reactions: Decreased conscious proprioception was present in all four limbs.

Spinal reflexes and panniculus reflex: Normal.

Neuroanatomic location: Cerebrothalamic, possibly right sided.

Laboratory Findings

CBC: HCT 30.4% (30%–50%), MCV 46.5 fL (42–53 fL), MCHC 32.6 g/dL (30–33.5 g/dL), reticulocytes 18,000 cells/μL (7,000–60,000 cells/μL), WBC 22,860 cells/μL (4,500–14,000 cells/μL), neutrophils 19,660 cells/μL (2,000–9,000 cells/μL), band neutrophils 2,286 cells/μL, lymphocytes 457 cells/μL (1,000–7,000 cells/μL), monocytes 229 cells/μL (50–600 cells/μL), eosinophils 229 cells/μL (150–1,100 cells/μL), basophils 0 cells/μL (0–50 cells/μL), platelets clumped but adequate. Neutrophils had slight toxic change and band neutrophils had marked toxic change.

Serum chemistry profile: Anion gap 24 mmol/L (15–28 mmol/L), sodium 136 mmol/L (151–158 mmol/L), potassium 3.5 mmol/L (3.6–4.9 mmol/L), chloride 98 mmol/L (113–121 mmol/L), bicarbonate 18 mmol/L (15–21 mmol/L), phosphorus 4.3 mg/dL (3.2–6.3 mg/dL), calcium 8.3 mg/dL (9.4–11.4 mg/dL), BUN 48 mg/dL (18–33 mg/dL), creatinine 0.8 mg/dL (1.1–2.2 mg/dL), glucose 140 mg/dL (73–134 mg/dL), total protein 4.8 g/dL (6.6–8.4 g/dL), albumin 1.4 g/dL (1.9–3.9 g/dL), globulin 3.4 g/dL (2.9–5.3 g/dL), ALT 19 U/L (28–106 U/L), AST 27 U/L (12–46 U/L), ALP 5 U/L (14–71 U/L), GGT 0 U/L (0–4 U/L), cholesterol 141 mg/dL (89–258 mg/dL), total bilirubin 1.5 mg/dL (0–0.2 mg/dL).

Imaging Findings

Thoracic radiographs (see Fig. 60.5): There was a moderate amount of pleural effusion present. There was a mass associated with the caudal aspect of the left caudal lung lobe. The cardiac silhouette was completely obscured on the lateral projection. On the VD projection, there appeared to be a mass effect superimposed over the caudal border of the cardiac silhouette that deformed the left and right caudal lung lobes.

Abdominal ultrasound: The native kidneys were markedly diminished in size, irregular in contour, and had a markedly irregular parenchyma with a lack of corticomedullary distinction. The transplanted kidney appeared within normal limits. The muscularis layer of the small intestine was mildly thickened diffusely. A Y-shaped region of mineralization is identified within the right liver lobes, which is likely associated with the biliary system.

Treatment and Outcome

Thoracocentesis was performed and 35 mL of turbid red fluid was removed. Preliminary examination of the fluid confirmed the referring veterinarian's findings. Unfortunately, the cat became progressively more agitated and tachypneic, thoracocentesis was aborted, and Bob was placed in a cage with oxygen supplementation. Treatment with IV crystalloid fluids (0.9% NaCl with 20 mEq/L KCl at 12 mL/hour), enrofloxacin (2.5 mg/kg, IV, q12h) and ampicillin (22 mg/kg, IV, q8h) was initiated and pleural fluid was submitted to the laboratory for cytologic examination and aerobic and anaerobic bacterial culture. The plan was to stabilize Bob with this treatment until additional thoracocentesis and chest tube placement could be performed, and specimens could be collected for additional diagnostic tests, if necessary. Differential diagnoses that were considered were cryptococcosis, toxoplasmosis, FIP, a systemic bacterial infection, and neoplasia. However, 10 hours after admission, at 2:00 AM, Bob developed respiratory and cardiac arrest. The owner elected euthanasia.

Necropsy Findings

Gross necropsy findings consisted of 120 mL of flocculent, serosanguinous fluid within the thoracic cavity and multifocal to coalescing, variably sized, white to grey, firm to caseous nodules that largely effaced the caudal lung lobes and extended through the pleural surface, with adhesions to the thoracic diaphragm and pleura (see Fig. 60.3A). A 2.5-mm nodule was also present in the wall of the left ventricle. The peritoneal cavity contained multiple adhesions from the small intestines to the omentum and the stomach to the left abdominal wall. The right medial liver lobe contained a focal, white to grey mass that was 10 cm in diameter and oozed purulent material when cut. The spleen contained multiple, white, raised, pinpoint foci. The native kidneys were shrunken, pale, irregular, and had loss of corticomedullary definition. The right transplanted kidney contained three to four, tan, firm, homogenous cortical nodules that ranged 2 to 4 mm in diameter. On cut section, the brain contained multifocal, randomly distributed, soft, white to grey, homogenous foci that measured 1 to 4 mm in diameter (see Fig. 60.3B). Histopathology of the lung, pleura, myocardium, thoracic diaphragm, spleen, liver, transplanted kidney, adrenal medulla, stomach, salivary gland, brain, and meninges revealed chronic, severe, necrotizing pyogranulomatous inflammation with intralesional branching filamentous bacteria. There was also chronic, moderate, multifocal, and necrotizing pyogranulomatous choroiditis and cyclitis in both eyes. The bacteria were gram positive but were not acid fast (see Fig. 60.6).

Microbiologic Testing

Aerobic and anaerobic bacterial culture (liver, lung specimens collected at necropsy): Small numbers of *N. nova*. No other bacteria were cultured.

Diagnosis

Disseminated *N. nova* infection.

Comments

In this case, disease followed a rapid clinical course, as can occur in human patients with severe immunodeficiency. The trough whole blood cyclosporine concentration was high; the goal of treatment is to obtain blood concentrations of approximately 300 to 500 ng/mL, although the optimum concentration that achieves adequate but not excessive immunosuppression in cats is not known.[21] Treatment with antimicrobial drugs was not effective given the advanced nature and severity of the disease in this cat.

SUGGESTED READINGS

Conville PS, Brown Elliott BA, Smith T, et al. The complexities of *Nocardia* taxonomy and identification. *J Clin Microbiol.* 2018;56.

MacNeill AL, Steil JC, Dossin O, et al. Disseminated nocardiosis caused by *Nocardia* abscessus in a dog. *Vet Clin Pathol.* 2010;39:381–385.

Malik R, Krockenberger MB, O'Brien CR, et al. *Nocardia* infections in cats: a retrospective multi-institutional study of 17 cases. *Aust Vet J.* 2006;84:235–245.

REFERENCES

1. Nocard ME. Note sur la maladie des boeufs de la Guadeloupe connue sous le nom de farcin. *Ann Inst Pasteur.* 1888;2:293–302.
2. Conville PS, Brown-Elliott BA, Smith T, et al. The complexities of *Nocardia* taxonomy and identification. *J Clin Microbiol.* 2018;56.
3. Mehta HH, Shamoo Y. Pathogenic *Nocardia*: a diverse genus of emerging pathogens or just poorly recognized? *PLoS Pathog.* 2020;16:e1008280.
4. Brown-Elliott BA, Brown JM, Conville PS, et al. Clinical and laboratory features of the *Nocardia* spp. based on current molecular taxonomy. *Clin Microbiol Rev.* 2006;19:259–282.
5. Siak MK, Burrows AK. Cutaneous nocardiosis in two dogs receiving ciclosporin therapy for the management of canine atopic dermatitis. *Vet Dermatol.* 2013;24:453–456. e102–453.
6. Strzok E, Siepker C, Armwood A, et al. Successful treatment of cutaneous *Curvularia geniculata, Nocardia niigatensis*, and viral papillomatosis in a dog during the therapeutic management of immune-mediated hemolytic anemia. *Front Vet Sci.* 2019;6:249.

7. Paul AE, Mansfield CS, Thompson M. Presumptive *Nocardia* spp. infection in a dog treated with cyclosporin and ketoconazole. *N Z Vet J.* 2010;58:265–268.
8. Smith PM, Haughland SP, Jeffery ND. Brain abscess in a dog immunosuppressed using cyclosporin. *Vet J.* 2007;173:675–678.
9. MacNeill AL, Steeil JC, Dossin O, et al. Disseminated nocardiosis caused by *Nocardia abscessus* in a dog. *Vet Clin Pathol.* 2010;39:381–385.
10. Teixeira Ribeiro AI, da Cruz Burema M, de Souza Borges AP, et al. Pyogranulomatous pleuropneumonia caused by *Nocardia asiatica* in a dog coinfected with canine morbillivirus (canine distemper virus). *Vet Med Sci.* 2020;6:25–31.
11. Uhde AK, Kilwinski J, Peters M, et al. Fatal nocardiosis in a dog caused by multiresistant *Nocardia veterana. Vet Microbiol.* 2016;183:78–84.
12. Ribeiro MG, Salerno T, Mattos-Guaraldi AL, et al. Nocardiosis: an overview and additional report of 28 cases in cattle and dogs. *Rev Inst Med Trop Sao Paulo.* 2008;50:177–185.
13. Saubolle MA, Sussland D. Nocardiosis: review of clinical and laboratory experience. *J Clin Microbiol.* 2003;41:4497–4501.
14. Malik R, Krockenberger MB, O'Brien CR, et al. *Nocardia* infections in cats: a retrospective multi-institutional study of 17 cases. *Aust Vet J.* 2006;84:235–245.
15. Sykes JE. Unpublished observations. University of California, Davis. 2012.
16. Hirsh DC, Jang SS. Antimicrobial susceptibility of *Nocardia nova* isolated from five cats with nocardiosis. *J Am Vet Med Assoc.* 1999;215:815–817. 795–796.
17. Sorrell TC, Mitchell DH, Iredell JR, et al. *Nocardia* species. In: Mandell GL, Bennett JE, Dolin R, eds. *Principles and Practice of Infectious Diseases.* Philadephia, PA: Churchill Livingstone, Elsevier; 2010:3199–3207.
18. Edwards DF. Actinomycosis and nocardiosis. In: Greene CE, ed. *Infectious Diseases of the Dog and Cat.* 3 ed. St Louis, MO: Saunders Elsevier; 2006:451–461.
19. Beaman BL, Beaman L. *Nocardia* species: host-parasite relationships. *Clin Microbiol Rev.* 1994;7:213–264.
20. McNeil MM, Brown JM. The medically important aerobic actinomycetes: epidemiology and microbiology. *Clin Microbiol Rev.* 1994;7:357–417.
21. Kadar E, Sykes JE, Kass PH, et al. Evaluation of the prevalence of infections in cats after renal transplantation: 169 cases (1987-2003). *J Am Vet Med Assoc.* 2005;227:948–953.
22. Campbell B, Scott DW. Successful management of nocardial empyema in a dog and cat. *J Am Anim Hosp Assoc.* 1975;11:769–773.
23. Cross RF, Nagao WT, Morrison RH. Canine nocardiosis; a report of two cases. *J Am Vet Med Assoc.* 1953;123:535–536.
24. Marino DJ, Jaggy A. Nocardiosis: a literature review with selected case reports in two dogs. *J Vet Intern Med.* 1993;7:4–11.
25. Lobetti RG, Collett MG, Leisewitz A. Acute fibrinopurulent pneumonia and haemoptysis associated with *Nocardia asteroides* in three dogs. *Vet Rec.* 1993;133:480.
26. Ackerman N, Grain E, Castleman W. Canine nocardiosis. *J Am Anim Hosp Assoc.* 1982;18:147–153.
27. Beaman BL, Sugar AM. *Nocardia* in naturally acquired and experimental infections in animals. *J Hyg.* 1983;91:393–419.
28. Tilgner SL, Anstey SI. Nocardial peritonitis in a cat. *Aust Vet J.* 1996;74:430–432.
29. de Farias MR, Werner J, Ribeiro MG, et al. Uncommon mandibular osteomyelitis in a cat caused by *Nocardia africana. BMC Vet Res.* 2012;8:239.
30. Soto E, Arauz M, Gallagher CA, et al. *Nocardia cyriacigeorgica* as the causative agent of mandibular osteomyelitis (lumpy jaw) in a cat. *J Vet Diagn Invest.* 2014;26:580–584.
31. Mealey KL, Willard MD, Nagode LA, et al. Hypercalcemia associated with granulomatous disease in a cat. *J Am Vet Med Assoc.* 1999;215:959–962. 946.
32. Lerner PI. *Nocardiosis. Clin Infect Dis.* 1996;22:891–903.
33. Buchanan AM, Beaman BL, Pedersen NC, et al. *Nocardia asteroides* recovery from a dog with steroid- and antibiotic-unresponsive idiopathic polyarthritis. *J Clin Microbiol.* 1983;18:702–708.
34. Yaemsiri S, Sykes JE. Successful treatment of disseminated nocardiosis caused by *Nocardia veterana* in a dog. *J Vet Intern Med.* 2018;32:418–422.
35. Verroken A, Janssens M, Berhin C, et al. Evaluation of matrix-assisted laser desorption ionization-time of flight mass spectrometry for identification of *Nocardia* species. *J Clin Microbiol.* 2010;48:4015–4021.
36. Davenport DJ, Johnson GC. Cutaneous nocardiosis in a cat. *J Am Vet Med Assoc.* 1986;188:728–729.
37. Gomez-Flores A, Welsh O, Said-Fernandez S, et al. In vitro and in vivo activities of antimicrobials against *Nocardia brasiliensis. Antimicrob Agents Chemother.* 2004;48:832–837.
38. Astudillo L, Dahan S, Escourrou G, et al. Cat scratch responsible for primary cutaneous *Nocardia asteroides* in an immunocompetent patient. *Br J Dermatol.* 2001;145:684–685.
39. Bottei E, Flaherty JP, Kaplan LJ, et al. Lymphocutaneous *Nocardia brasiliensis* infection transmitted via a cat scratch: a second case. *Clin Infect Dis.* 1994;18:649–650.
40. Freland C, Fur JL, Nemirovsky-Trebucq B, et al. Primary cutaneous nocardiosis caused by *Nocardia otitidiscaviarum*: two cases and a review of the literature. *J Trop Med Hyg.* 1995;98:395–403.
41. Sachs MK. Lymphocutaneous *Nocardia brasiliensis* infection acquired from a cat scratch: case report and review. *Clin Infect Dis.* 1992;15:710–711.
42. Ajello L, Walker WW, Dungworth DL, et al. Isolation of *Nocardia brasiliensis* from a cat with a review of its prevalence and geographic distribution. *J Am Vet Med Assoc.* 1961;138:370–376.
43. Eroksuz Y, Gursoy NC, Karapinar T, et al. Systemic nocardiosis in a dog caused by *Nocardia cyriacigeorgica. BMC Vet Res.* 2017;13:30.
44. Hilligas J, Van Wie E, Barr J, et al. Vertebral osteomyelitis and multiple cutaneous lesions in a dog caused by *Nocardia pseudobrasiliensis. J Vet Intern Med.* 2014;28:1621–1625.
45. Hattori Y, Kano R, Kunitani Y, et al. *Nocardia africana* isolated from a feline mycetoma. *J Clin Microbiol.* 2003;41:908–910.
46. Harada H, Endo Y, Sekiguchi M, et al. Cutaneous nocardiosis in a cat. *J Vet Med Sci.* 2009;71:785–787.
47. Luque I, Astorga R, Tarradas C, et al. *Nocardia otitidiscaviarum* infection in a cat. *Vet Rec.* 2002;151:488.
48. Silkworth A, Cavanaugh R, Bolfa P, et al. Cutaneous pyogranulomas associated with *Nocardia jiangxiensis* in a cat from the eastern Caribbean. *Trop Med Infect Dis.* 2019;4.
49. Nakanishi A, Mashita T, Akiyama K, et al. Suppurative granulomatous sinorhinitis associated with *Nocardia* spp. infection in a cat. *J Vet Med Sci.* 2015;77:597–599.

61

Mycobacterial Infections

Carolyn R. O'Brien, Conor O'Halloran, Danièlle A. Gunn-Moore, Jane E. Sykes

KEY POINTS

- First Described: Evidence of tuberculosis in humans dates back to between 2400 and 3400 B.C., but the causative agent was not demonstrated until 1882 (Robert Koch).[1]
- Cause: Companion animals can become infected by a number of different mycobacteria, including members of the *Mycobacterium tuberculosis* complex (MTBC) and non-tuberculous mycobacteria (NTM; family *Mycobacteriaceae,* order *Actinomycetales*). Mycobacteria belonging to the MTBC that have been detected in cats and dogs include *Mycobacterium bovis* and *Mycobacterium microti*; *M. tuberculosis* has also been detected in dogs. Many NTM are opportunistic pathogens of cats (and occasionally dogs); definitively identified species have been characterized as belonging to the *Mycobacterium leprae*-complex, *Mycobacterium avium*-complex, the rapid-growing mycobacteria (RGM), the slow-growing mycobacteria, and fastidious species with an enigmatic epidemiology.
- Affected Hosts: Mycobacteria can cause disease in almost all mammals. Each species within the MTBC is host adapted, and host species include humans, cattle, voles, goats, meerkats, mongoose, and deer. However, spillover from these hosts into other mammals is frequent, and infections have been identified in mammals as diverse as cats and dogs to lions and elephants. NTM have a host range that is even broader than the tuberculous mycobacteria, as they are also pathogens of fish and amphibians.
- Geographic Distribution: Mycobacterial infections are globally ubiquitous, but the relative frequency of infections with each species differs by location.
- Primary Mode of Transmission: The most frequent route of transmission to companion animals is thought to be inoculation of mycobacteria into the skin; less-frequent routes of transmission include the inhalation of aerosolized mycobacteria, ingestion of contaminated foodstuffs (e.g., raw milk, contaminated meat, or infected prey), direct contact of open wounds with contaminated environments, and, possibly, direct contact with an infected wildlife host, companion animal, or humans.
- Major Clinical Signs: Cutaneous nodular, ulcerated, or draining skin lesions; peripheral or internal lymphadenopathy; pneumonia with tachypnea and/or cough; osteomyelitis; granulomatous or pyogranulomatous infiltrates in a variety of abdominal organs; and, rarely, the CNS and/or eyes.
- Differential Diagnoses: Neoplasia (especially lymphoma and carcinoma), feline infectious peritonitis (cats), toxoplasmosis, tularemia, nocardiosis, actinomycosis, rhodococcosis, bartonellosis, leishmaniosis, and fungal infections.
- Human Health Significance: A third of the global human population is infected with an organism that belongs to the MTBC, while NTM are an emerging health risk for humans with comorbidities. The major zoonotic risk is associated with MTBC organisms, but there are only a small number of cases that have confirmed companion animals as the source of human infection, so the risk appears very low.

INTRODUCTION

Mycobacteria (genus *Mycobacterium,* family *Mycobacteriaceae,* order *Actinomycetales*) are aerobic (or in some cases, microaerophilic), non–spore-forming, non-motile, pleomorphic bacterial rods. They are more resistant to extremes of temperature and pH, and routine disinfection than most other bacteria, properties conferred by their notably thick, hydrophobic cell wall, which contains high concentrations of mycolic acids and lipids. This cell wall also confers resistance to decolorization with acid-alcohol. This acid-fast staining property, combined with their morphology, makes species of the genus recognizable microscopically, including in histopathologic and cytologic specimens.

The genus contains an increasing number of species that cause widely divergent clinical syndromes. At one extreme, these species have among them some of the most ancient, notorious, and arguably successful obligate pathogens of both people and animals. The most widely known and best characterized diseases of people are tuberculosis (most commonly caused by *Mycobacterium tuberculosis*) and leprosy (*Mycobacterium leprae*). Nine thousand-year-old human remains in the eastern Mediterranean contain evidence of the DNA of mycobacteria belonging to the *M. tuberculosis* complex (MTBC),[2] and MTBC DNA has been recovered from the diseased bones of a bison trapped in permafrost *circa* 17,000 years ago.[3] Nevertheless, strict criteria to exclude environmental contamination have only been validated in specimens that date from up to *circa* 5000 years ago.[4] The MTBC are of significant global concern; a third of the current global human population is estimated to be infected with an MTBC organism, of which 5% to 10% will eventually develop active clinical disease. It is estimated that up to 85% of all African bovids reside in areas with a high prevalence of poorly controlled bovine tuberculosis.[5]

At the other end of the spectrum are numerous potentially pathogenic environmental non-tuberculous mycobacteria (NTM). These opportunistic pathogens are also now recognized as a major global public health problem. Members of the *M. avium*-complex (MAC), in particular, are an emerging threat to human health. There is a growing body of evidence that hospital admissions due to associated pulmonary disease are increasing, particularly in countries with a low incidence of tuberculosis. This is ascribed to increased numbers of immunocompromised patients, the use of advanced diagnostic tools, and a larger awareness of the role of NTM in disease.[6]

The taxonomy of the genus is complex. Two primary systems exist for the taxonomic division of the genus. The Runyon scheme was developed in the latter half of the 20th century.[7] It is based on an isolate's laboratory growth characteristics, including substrate usage, growth time until colonies are visible, and colony phenotype. However, as it is not possible to grow all species under artificial conditions, with the advent of molecular techniques (such as whole-genome sequencing), there has been a departure from the Runyon system in favor of molecular phylogeny.

Mycobacteria can be divided into two main groups (Table 61.1):

1. The *Mycobacterium tuberculosis* complex (MTBC). The MTBC consists of 10 phylogenetically related species of mycobacteria associated with tuberculosis in man and/or other animals (*M. tuberculosis, Mycobacterium bovis, Mycobacterium africanum, Mycobacterium pinnipedii, Mycobacterium caprae, Mycobacterium canettii, Mycobacterium microti, Mycobacterium orygis, Mycobacterium suricattae*, and *Mycobacterium mungi*). These are obligate intracellular pathogens.
2. The NTM. These are opportunistic saprophytes, variably distributed in the environment, especially in soil and water systems (both natural and man-made). Of over 170 characterized NTM species, approximately 25 may be pathogenic in people and animals.[8] This group can be further subdivided into: (i) "slow-growing" (e.g., MAC), (ii) "rapid-growing", and (iii) "fastidious" mycobacteria. Slow-growing mycobacteria typically take longer than 7 days to culture in laboratory conditions.[9] RGM usually grow in the laboratory within 7 days at 24° to 45°C. Fastidious mycobacteria cannot be cultured by routine laboratory methods and have an enigmatic ecological niche.

MYCOBACTERIUM TUBERCULOSIS COMPLEX INFECTIONS

ETIOLOGY AND EPIDEMIOLOGY

Of the MTBC, only *M. tuberculosis*, *M. bovis*, and *M. microti* have been shown to infect dogs and cats (Table 61.2). *Mycobacterium africanum* and *M. canetti* are rare causes of human tuberculosis in Africa, *M. pinnipedii* infects seals, and *M. caprae* is primarily a ruminant pathogen. MTBC organisms share > 95% of DNA-DNA

TABLE 61.1 Mycobacterial Pathogens of Clinical Significance for Cats and Dogs

Group	Mycobacterial Species	Description
M. tuberculosis complex	*M. tuberculosis, M. bovis, M. microti*	Host-associated, slow-growing species. Cause cutaneous and disseminated granulomatous disease in dogs (all three species) and cats (*M. bovis* and *M. microti*)
Slow-growing non-tuberculous mycobacteria	*M. avium* subsp. *avium, M. avium* subsp. *hominissuis, M. avium* subsp. *paratuberculosis, M. kansasii, M. ulcerans, M. genavense, M. malmoense, M. celatum, M. terrae, M. simiae, M. nebraskense, "M. visibile"**	Opportunistic, environmental, slow-growing species. Cause pyogranulomatous cutaneous or disseminated disease in dogs or cats. Some may cause leprosy syndromes in cats
Rapidly growing non-tuberculous mycobacteria	*M. fortuitum, M. smegmatis, M. abscessus, M. chelonae, M. thermoresistibile, M. goodii, M. flavescens, M. alvei*	Opportunistic, environmental, rapidly growing species. Cause pyogranulomatous panniculitis, pneumonia, or disseminated infections in cats or dogs
Lepromatous mycobacteria	*M. lepraemurium*, the CLG organism, and other unnamed species, some with genetic resemblance to known non-tuberculous mycobacteria	Highly fastidious or unculturable mycobacteria. Cause nodular granulomatous to pyogranulomatous cutaneous disease in cats (all species) or dogs (CLG organism)

*The exact position of "*M. visibile*" is not clear; it has also been grouped within the lepromatous mycobacteria.
CLG, canine leproid granuloma.

TABLE 61.2 Organisms of the *Mycobacterium tuberculosis* Complex of Clinical Significance for Dogs and Cats

Species	Host(s)	Major Reservoir Hosts	Geographic Distribution of Reported Cases in Companion Animals	Clinical Signs	Human Health Significance
M. tuberculosis	Dogs	Humans	USA, Africa, southern Europe	Pneumonia and tracheobronchial lymphadenopathy; rarely dissemination to the CNS, liver, kidney	Primary cause of tuberculosis in humans. Reverse zoonosis. Transmission back to humans not reported but may be possible
M. bovis	Cats, dogs	Cattle, Eurasian badgers, other wildlife species	Southwestern England and Wales, New Zealand, Argentina, rarely USA	Cutaneous lesions, peripheral lymphadenopathy, occasionally dissemination to abdominal lymph nodes and other organs, osteomyelitis	Rare cause of tuberculosis in humans but transmission from animals to humans possible
M. microti	Cats, very rarely dogs	Voles, wood mice, shrews, camelids	Southwestern Scotland, northern and southern England, western Europe	Cutaneous lesions, peripheral lymphadenopathy, less often pneumonia, arthritis, osteomyelitis, ocular lesions	Very rare cause of tuberculosis in humans

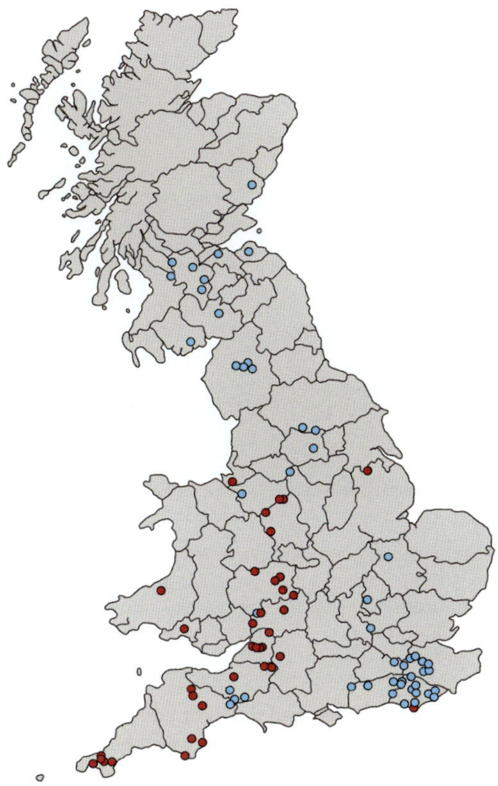

Fig. 61.1 Geographic distribution of *M. microti, M. bovis* and *M. avium* isolates from cats in the United Kingdom. (Redrawn from Gunn-Moore DA, McFarland SE, Brewer JI, et al. Mycobacterial disease in cats in Great Britain: I. Culture results, geographical distribution and clinical presentation of 339 cases. *J Feline Med Surg.* 2011;13:934-944.)

homology hence it is challenging to differentiate them from each other. Compared with other mycobacterial species, MTBC bacteria do not survive well in the environment, although *M. bovis* can survive months in feces, carcasses, or soil. Humans are the only reservoir host for *M. tuberculosis*, and *M. tuberculosis* is responsible for > 90% of tuberculosis in humans.

Cats

Only *M. bovis* and *M. microti* have frequently been detected in cats.[10-12] Rodents (especially voles and shrews) are reservoir hosts for *M. microti*, and cattle and a variety of wildlife species are reservoir hosts for *M. bovis*. The overwhelming majority of feline infections with *M. microti* and *M. bovis* have been reported from the United Kingdom (Fig. 61.1), where *M. microti* infection is endemic in voles, wood mice, and shrews, and *M. bovis* infection is endemic in Eurasian badgers and cattle. In one United Kingdom study, 19% of feline mycobacterial infections were caused by *M. microti* and 15% by *M. bovis* (Table 61.3).[13] Therefore any given cat with a mycobacterial infection in the United Kingdom has a greater than 1/3 probability of having tuberculosis. Similar data do not exist for other tuberculosis-endemic locations. Infection by *M. tuberculosis* is extremely rare in the cat; and it appears that cats have a natural resistance to this pathogen. Only very occasional infections are documented, generally through anthropozoonotic spread.[14]

In the United Kingdom, *M. bovis* infections occur where there are high levels of endemic infection in local bovine and wildlife populations such as the southwest of England.[13,15] In comparison, *M. microti* infections are much more common in areas with high prevalence of

TABLE 61.3 Mycobacterial Culture Results from United Kingdom Cats

Species	Number of Isolates	Percentage of Total Submissions	Percentage of Culture Positive
M. microti	63	19	40
M. bovis	52	15	33
M. avium	24	7	15
M. malmoense	4	1	3
M. fortuitum	4	1	3
M. celatum	1	<1	<1
M. intracellulare	1	<1	<1
Unclassified	10	2	6
No growth	180	53	-
Culture-positive total	159	47	-
Total	339	100	-

Specimens were from cats with histologic findings indicative of mycobacteriosis. Specimens were submitted to the Animal Health and Veterinary Laboratories Agency (now Animal and Plant Health Agency [APHA]) for mycobacterial culture between January 2005 and December 2008.[13,15]

this infection in the wild rodent population, typically southeast of London, the north of England, and throughout Scotland.[13]

Tuberculosis is most frequently diagnosed in adult male cats with a history of hunting.[13] The median age at diagnosis is 3 years for *M. bovis* and 8 years for *M. microti*. There is no link between MTBC infections and retrovirus infection in cats.

The distribution of lesions together with the facts that: (1) the highest incidence of infections occurs in young, male, active hunting cats (particularly those that prey on small rodents); (2) mice and voles are permissive hosts for *M. microti*[16]; and (3) mice, rats, stoats, mink, and ferrets (as well as a wide range of larger mammals) can harbor *M. bovis*,[17] suggests that cats are infected through injuries sustained while hunting. The geographic distribution of spoligotypes of *M. microti* and *M. bovis* aligns almost perfectly for feline, bovine, and wildlife mycobacterial strains. In the case of *M. bovis*, prey species likely act as intermediate hosts, and infection may also be acquired when wounds become contaminated by environmental sources, such as the areas around infected badger setts where *M. bovis* can persist for extended periods.[18]

Recently, the United Kingdom experienced an outbreak of *M. bovis* tuberculosis in cats that appeared to be associated with consumption of a commercial raw venison-based diet. Initially, six sick cats and seven cohabiting cats were identified with evidence of *M. bovis* infection. Five were either too sick to treat or deteriorated despite therapy. The cats were exclusively housed indoors and were fed the same commercially available raw food produced by a single manufacturer. Other possible sources of exposure to *M. bovis* were excluded. Infection with *M. bovis* genotype 10:a was confirmed by culture and DNA typing of isolates in five cats. Ultimately, infection was either confirmed or strongly suspected in more than 120 cats based on a positive immunological response in an IFN gamma-release assay (IGRA, see Diagnosis, below) with or without PCR-based confirmation of infection, 84 of which were subclinical contact cats. This outbreak demonstrated the critical nature of meat inspection procedures in the safe production of raw food diets for companion animals and also highlights the microbiologic risks that these diets can present.

The incidence of feline tuberculosis outside the United Kingdom appears to be lower. This may reflect differences in the epidemiology of these organisms—for example, *M. bovis* has been eliminated from much of central Europe, Australia, and some states in the United States. However, feline *M. bovis* infections have been reported from New Zealand, where brushtail possums act as reservoir hosts[19]; Argentina, where stray cats are often fed raw cattle lung[20]; and rarely the United States.[21] Major wildlife reservoirs in North America, which include the white-tailed deer, bison, and elk, are less likely to interact with cats compared with small mammals, which may explain why fewer *M. bovis* infections are reported in cats from the USA when compared with the United Kingdom. It is not known if *M. bovis* spreads from large herbivores to small rodents in the United States as it does in the United Kingdom, but that route of transmission remains possible. *Mycobacterium microti* infections occur in companion animals as well as species such as the wild boar in countries including France and Germany, where *M. bovis* is no longer a concern.

Tuberculosis has occurred where cats within the same household or in close geographical proximity develop signs within a short time of each other.[22,23] The epidemiological significance of such situations is unclear, as these cats may share a source of infected prey (e.g., local woodland); it is therefore possible that such infections are independently acquired rather than being representative of cat-to-cat transmission. However, multiple within-household cases have occurred where at least one cat has had no history of outdoor access (authors' unpublished observations). In these cases, cat-to-cat transmission is likely, probably as a result of close contact such as grooming. Cat-to-cat transmission was documented in an outbreak of *M. bovis* infection in a group of research cats in Australia,[24] after importing an infected kitten from the Ukraine into a cattery in Italy,[25] and was suspected in a household in Ireland.[26] It should be noted that the number of these cases remains small and the risk to healthy, immunocompetent cats in contact with an infected cat is low.

Nosocomial transmission of *M. bovis* has been reported.[26,27] In one outbreak, the index case, with a purulent ulcerated submandibular lesion, was euthanized and two cats that underwent elective surgery in the same practice developed tuberculosis. The subsequent cases developed severe systemic disease in a much shorter timescale than is typical of disease acquired through sylvatic infection.[21,26]

Although not definitively demonstrated, there is strong circumstantial evidence for transmission of tuberculosis from humans to pet cats.[28,29] This is unsurprising given the small infectious dose of *M. bovis* required to cause disease in mammals, including cats.[30,31]

Dogs

Most of the information about tuberculosis in dogs comes from sporadic case reports, mostly of *M. tuberculosis*[32-37] and *M. bovis* infections.[30,38-44] Dogs with tuberculous mycobacterial infections typically have either significant GI disease (weight loss, vomiting, and diarrhea; usually in association with *M. bovis* infection) or pulmonary pathology (Fig. 61.2). There are extremely rare reports of *M. microti* infection in dogs, to date exclusively reported in Europe.[45]

Dogs are uncommonly infected with *M. bovis*.[46-48] Wounds inflicted by badgers or a squirrel have preceded disease in affected dogs.[46] In the United Kingdom, disease in dogs has been restricted to southwestern England or Ireland. However, in 2016 and 2017 an outbreak of *M. bovis* tuberculosis affected a working pack of foxhounds in the United Kingdom.[49] The pack initially housed nearly 200 hounds and was located in the medium-risk area of the United Kingdom for endemic *M. bovis* infection (the "Edge area"). The pack were fed animal (beef or horse) by-products from local farms. Affected hounds showed signs of acute lethargy, hyporexia, marked polyuria and polydipsia, and then collapse and death or euthanasia within 48 hours of the onset of signs. Overall 164 clinically well hounds were tested for *M. bovis* infection with a combination of IGRA and antibody tests (DPP VetTB, Chembio); 59% responded positively to at least one of the tests. Infection was confirmed in three dogs at necropsy. Moderate to severe necrotizing granulomatous glomerulonephritis was identified in all affected animals, with rare intralesional acid-fast bacteria (AFB). Some dogs also had enlarged abdominal lymph nodes. This outbreak suggested that dog-to-dog transmission may be possible within certain epidemiological contexts and also that diagnostic tests used to identify infected individuals of other species can be useful in dogs.

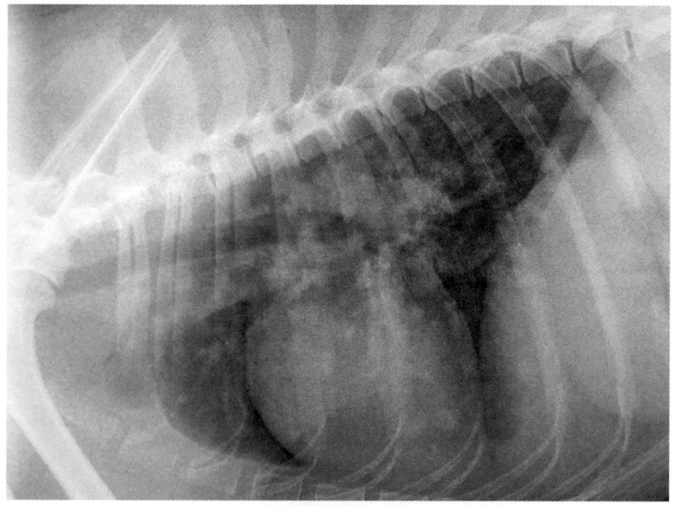

Fig. 61.2 Lateral thoracic radiograph from a 6-year-old, male, neutered, Jack Russell terrier dog infected with *M. bovis*. There are multifocal to coalescing areas of soft-tissue opacity (granulomas) distributed throughout the lung fields.

Disease due to *M. tuberculosis* has been reported in dogs worldwide.[32-34,40,44,50-53] Dogs are usually infected after prolonged aerosol exposure to contaminated human respiratory secretions, so the disease is a "reverse zoonosis" (*anthropozoonosis*). Thus, disease occurs in dogs in regions where tuberculosis occurs in humans. In the US, *M. tuberculosis* infection is most prevalent in humans from the northeast/mid-Atlantic states, southern states, Alaska, California, and Nevada (Fig. 61.3). Dogs have not been reported to spread *M. tuberculosis* infection to humans despite prolonged close contact in some situations,[34] possibly because the cavitary lesions that are required for transmission do not develop to the same extent in dogs as they do in humans. However, organisms have been detected in dogs' sputum, so transmission remains possible.

CLINICAL FEATURES

Pathogenesis and Clinical Signs

MTBC organisms are inhaled (*M. tuberculosis* and possibly *M. bovis*), ingested (*M. bovis* or *M. microti*), or inoculated into the skin (*M. bovis* or *M. microti*) and replicate locally. Organisms are then phagocytosed by macrophages but they survive and replicate within these cells, and macrophage destruction leads to recruitment of lymphocytes and additional monocytes, which initiates tubercle formation. Infected macrophages also travel to local lymph nodes, with development of a *primary complex* lesion. When CMI is either defective or actively subverted by mycobacteria, dissemination to distant sites occurs. Development of delayed-type hypersensitivity responses acts to control the initial infection, or

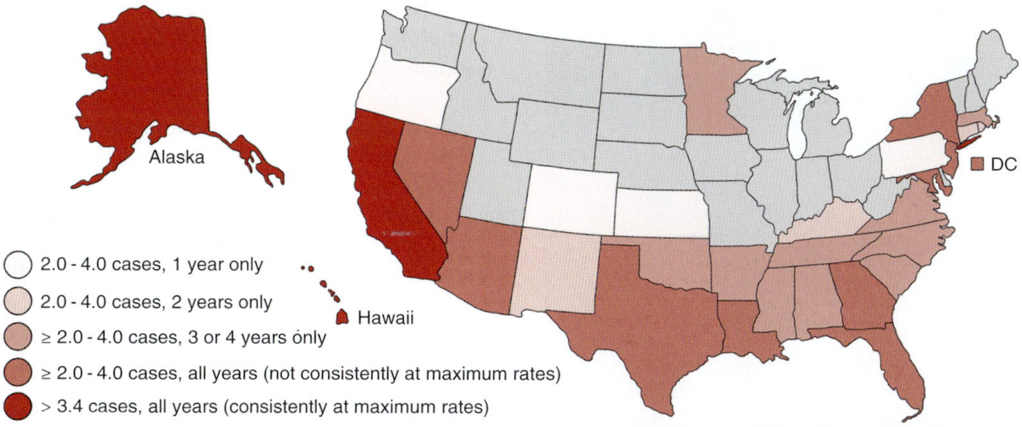

Fig. 61.3 Geographic distribution of human cases of *Mycobacterium tuberculosis* infection in the USA, 2005–2011. (Compiled from Morbidity and Mortality Weekly reports data on trends in human tuberculosis, years 2005, 2007, 2008, 2010, and 2011.)

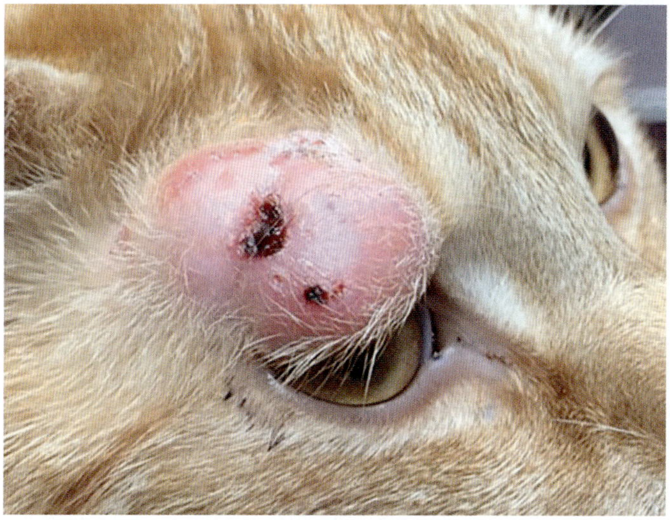

Fig. 61.4 Typical alopecic cutaneous nodule (granuloma) above the right eye of a 4-year-old, male, neutered, retrovirus-negative, domestic shorthair cat with *M. bovis* infection.

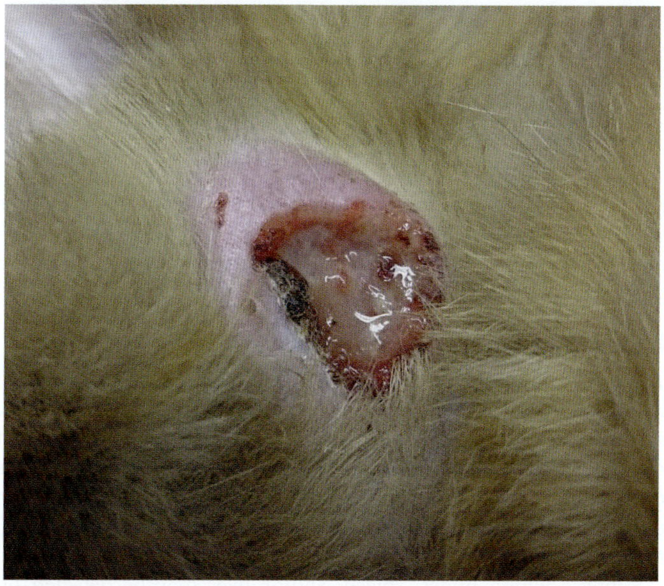

Fig. 61.5 A facial granuloma (a "fight and bite site") over the rostrolateral aspect of the temporomandibular joint of a 4-year-old, female, neutered, retrovirus-negative, domestic shorthair cat with *M. microti* infection.

may lead to central necrosis and calcification of the primary complex lesions, with persistence of organisms in the center of the lesions.

Most cats with tuberculosis have localized nodular cutaneous disease (Fig. 61.4), frequently with ulceration, and occasionally a draining sinus tract.[10,11,13] The lesions are typically distributed around the face, extremities, and tail base—the so-called "fight and bite sites" (Fig. 61.5). Skin lesions may be accompanied by a localized or even generalized lymphadenopathy. Lymphadenopathy, usually of the submandibular or popliteal nodes, may be the only sign (termed an *incomplete primary complex*). A predominately GI form of the disease exists, where granulomas form in the intestines.[30] Intestinal thickening, accompanied by multicentric abdominal lymph node involvement, almost always includes the mesenteric nodes. Subsequent intestinal malabsorption is associated with weight loss, diarrhea, vomiting, and anemia.[13] This form of the disease typically historically occurred in cats that drank tuberculous cows' milk. Since the introduction of pasteurization, this is less prevalent. More recently it occurred as a result of the ingestion of contaminated raw meat by cats in the United Kingdom.[49] Pulmonary lesions occur when bacteria are inhaled, with classic tubercle formation in lungs and hilar lymph nodes. Much more common, however, is pulmonary disease secondary to putative hematogenous spread of bacteria from the site of inoculation in the skin. This generates a diffuse interstitial pattern of disease (Fig. 61.6),[54] which eventually becomes bronchial and is clinically observable as progressive dyspnea followed by the development of a soft productive cough. Disseminated disease is associated with a range of clinical signs, including hepatosplenomegaly, pleural and pericardial effusions, generalized lymphadenopathy, weight loss, and pyrexia.[30] Ocular involvement (chorioretinitis,[55] conjunctivitis[47]) and tuberculous arthritis/osteomyelitis have been occasionally reported.[11,56]

Clinical signs in dogs with pulmonary tuberculosis due to *M. tuberculosis* are slowly progressive and consist of chronic, productive or non-productive cough, inappetence, weight loss, and lethargy.[34,51] Dissemination to non-pulmonary sites such as the CNS, liver, or kidney can result in neurologic signs,[50] weight loss, vomiting, or diarrhea.[44,52] Involvement of the lungs, liver, kidneys, and/or lymph nodes can occur in dogs infected with *M. bovis*.[46,48,57] Isolated lung and tracheobronchial node involvement similar to that often

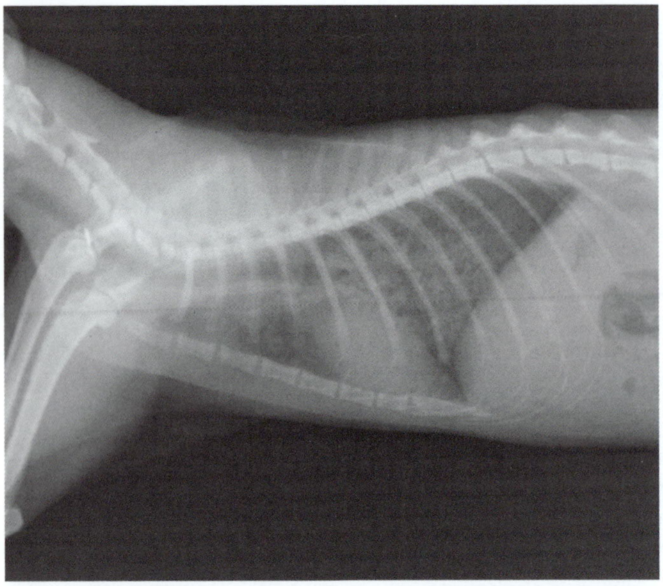

Fig. 61.6 Lateral thoracic radiograph from a 5-year-old, male, entire, retrovirus-negative, Egyptian Mau cat infected with *M. microti*. There is diffuse interstitial pathology with soft-tissue opacity and sternal lymphadenopathy; these are typical findings associated with secondary pulmonary dissemination of tuberculosis in the cat.

reported for *M. tuberculosis* was described in one dog.[48] Foxhounds with *M. bovis* infection had signs of lethargy, anorexia, polyuria/polydipsia, collapse, and death or euthanasia secondary to renal infection and necrosis.[49]

Physical Examination Findings

The most common physical examination findings in cats (and to a lesser extent in dogs) that are infected with *M. bovis* or *M. microti* include single or multiple firm cutaneous nodules, and enlargement of one or more peripheral lymph nodes. Cutaneous nodules may be mobile or fixed to underlying tissues (muscle and bone), and can ulcerate or drain purulent fluid. Skin lesions are most prevalent on the head, but can also occur on the limbs and the trunk.[10,11] Enlarged mesenteric lymph nodes, spleen, and/or liver may be detected on abdominal palpation. Involvement of internal lymph nodes is more common with *M. bovis* infections (21% of cats) than with *M. microti* infections (9% of cats).[13] Lameness may be present in cats with bone involvement.

Dogs with pulmonary involvement caused by *M. tuberculosis* may show fever, increased lung sounds, and cough. Other physical examination findings that relate to dissemination of infection may be present, such as thin body condition, neurologic signs, or hepatomegaly. Abnormal findings on examination of the respiratory tract and/or abdominal organs may also be detected in dogs with disseminated *M. bovis* or *M. microti* infection.

DIAGNOSIS

Diagnosis of MTBC infection usually relies on suggestive history, clinical signs, and radiographic abnormalities, combined with histopathology, molecular tests, and culture. When mycobacterial infection is suspected, specimens collected for analysis should be divided into two portions—one for histopathology (in formalin), one for mycobacterial culture, and/or mycobacterial PCR (fresh or frozen). The receiving laboratory should be informed that mycobacterial infection is a possibility.

Laboratory Abnormalities

Complete Blood Count, Serum Biochemical Tests, and Urinalysis

Laboratory abnormalities in dogs and cats infected with MTBC organisms are nonspecific. Mild anemia of inflammatory disease and neutrophilic leukocytosis, sometimes with a left shift, and monocytosis are occasionally present. The serum chemistry profile may show hypoalbuminemia and hyperglobulinemia. Increased serum liver enzyme activities have been reported in dogs with hepatic involvement.[44]

Hypercalcemia secondary to granulomatous disease can also occur in dogs or cats.[13,47] If total serum calcium concentration is elevated, then evaluation of serum ionized calcium concentration is recommended. Rates of hypercalcemia in *M. tuberculosis*-infected (human) adults vary from 6% to 48%.[58] Symptomatic hypercalcemia in human tuberculosis cases is uncommon, with rates of ~3% in adults.[59] Vitamin D concentrations are associated with mycobacterial immunity, and calcitriol has anti-mycobacterial activity *in vitro*. Macrophages produce calcitriol when they phagocytose mycobacteria following TLR2 stimulation. The serum concentration of 25(OH)D decreases, and ionized calcium concentration increases. These effects may manifest as hypovitaminosis D and hypercalcemia. This phenomenon has been long established in human medicine and more recently in cats with tuberculosis.[60,61] In both species, the presence of either factor at diagnosis is a poor prognostic indicator. It is unclear whether these findings are a marker of disseminated disease (and so will be harder to treat), or whether they inherently influence disease outcome. Clinical trials in humans have attempted to establish the benefit, if any, of treating with supplemental vitamin D to reduce subclinical hypercalcemia, but the results to date have been discordant, and its use is not currently included in any treatment guidelines.

Diagnostic Imaging

Plain Radiography

Findings on plain thoracic radiography in dogs infected with *M. tuberculosis* or *M. bovis* include tracheobronchial or mediastinal lymphadenopathy,[34,44,51] interstitial to alveolar infiltrates,[57] pleural effusion,[44] and lobar consolidation (Figs. 61.2 and 61.7).[34,57] Similar abnormalities may occur in cats infected with *M. microti* and *M. bovis* (see Fig. 61.6). Bronchial, alveolar, nodular interstitial, and unstructured interstitial patterns predominate in cats, and perihilar lymphadenopathy can be present.[10,12] Calcification of pulmonary lesions or lymph nodes may be evident in dogs or cats. Hepatomegaly, splenomegaly, or lymphadenopathy, with or without ascites, may be present on abdominal radiography, or abdominal radiographs may be unremarkable.[12] Radiographic evidence of osteomyelitis (especially osteolytic lesions) may occur in cats infected with *M. microti* or *M. bovis*, often in association with overlying cutaneous lesions.[12]

Computed Tomography

Thoracic CT findings have been reported for a dog infected with *M. tuberculosis*.[34] Lung lobe consolidation, multifocal stellate opacities, bronchial stenosis, bronchiectasis, tracheobronchial wall thickening, and partially mineralized masses consistent with enlarged mediastinal and tracheobronchial lymph nodes were present (see Fig. 61.7). In this dog, mineralization was not visible on plain thoracic radiographs. CT in human patients with tuberculosis is considered more sensitive than plain radiography for detection of pulmonary lesions and enlarged lymph nodes, and provides better visualization of calcifications.

In 20 cats from the United Kingdom with tuberculosis, CT abnormalities were most commonly seen in the thorax, and consisted of bronchial (n = 9), alveolar (n = 8), ground glass (n = 6), or structured interstitial (n = 15) lung patterns, which were often mixed. Tracheobronchial,

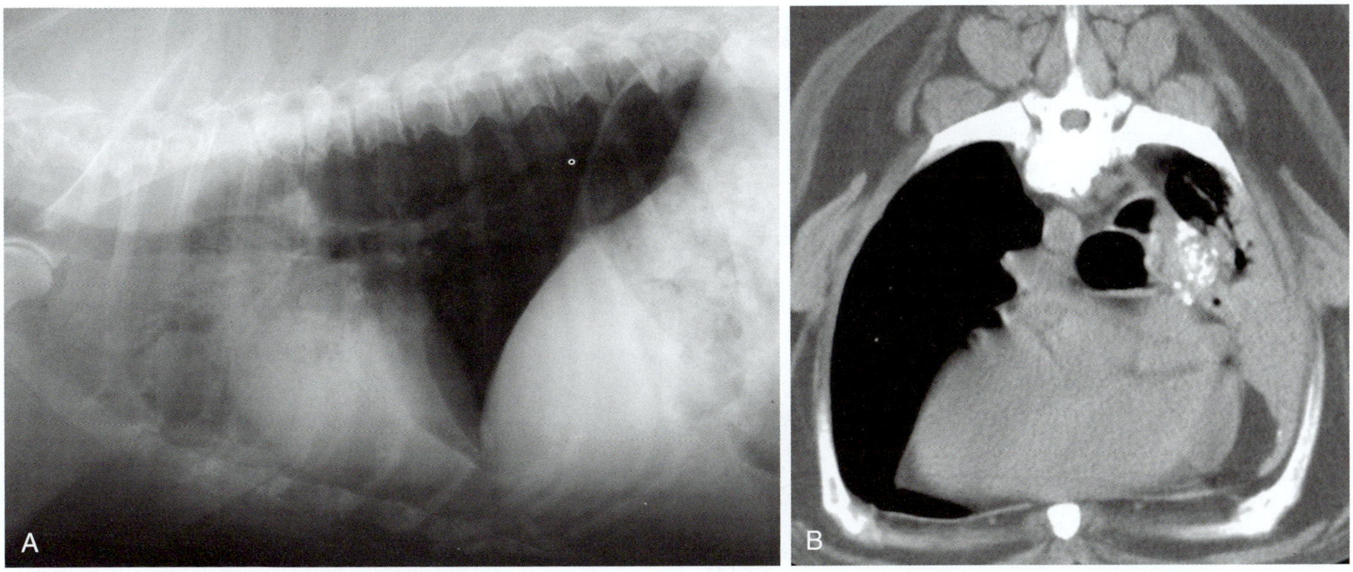

Fig. 61.7 Lateral thoracic radiograph (A) and 7-mm collimated CT image immediately cranial to the carina (B) from a 9-year-old female spayed golden retriever with pulmonary tuberculosis. (A) Consolidation of the right cranial lung lobe is present together with interstitial to alveolar infiltrates in the right middle lung lobe. (B) On the CT scan, the right cranial lung lobe is consolidated and markedly volume reduced. Air bronchograms are present centrally that extend dorsally toward a focal region of aerated lung. The granular mineral opacity adjacent to the right margin of the trachea represents mineralized lymphadenopathy of the right tracheobronchial lymph nodes. (From Sykes JE, Cannon AB, Norris AJ, et al. *Mycobacterium tuberculosis* complex infection in a dog. *J Vet Intern Med.* 2007;21:1108-1112.)

sternal, and cranial mediastinal lymphadenomegaly were common (n = 16). Other abnormalities included abdominal (n = 8) or peripheral (n = 18) lymphadenomegaly, hepatosplenomegaly (n = 7), mixed osteolytic/osteoproliferative skeletal lesions (n = 7), and cutaneous or subcutaneous soft-tissue masses/nodules (n = 4)[62] (Fig. 61.8).

Sonographic Findings

Abdominal sonography may be unremarkable or reveal hepatomegaly, splenomegaly, abdominal lymphadenopathy, and/or ascites. A dog with disseminated *M. tuberculosis* infection had multifocal hypoechoic masses within the kidneys and liver, and mineralization of the hepatic and renal parenchyma.[51]

Microbiologic Tests (Table 61.4)

Cytologic Diagnosis

Cytologic examination of bronchoalveolar lavage fluid is frequently unrewarding in cats with tuberculosis, whereas examination of aspirates from skin nodules can be very informative. Large numbers of activated macrophages as well as neutrophils are typically present.

Cytologic examination of aspirates, effusion, or lavage specimens from the respiratory tract of dogs with pulmonary tuberculosis typically reveals a mixed population of often heavily vacuolated histiocytes, and smaller numbers of degenerate or non-degenerate neutrophils and small lymphocytes.[34,44,57] Intracytoplasmic, nonstaining bacilli may be seen in macrophages (Fig. 61.9).[57] Moderate anisocytosis or anisokaryosis of exfoliated respiratory epithelial cells may be present, which might lead the clinician to suspect pulmonary neoplasia.[34] The presence of cholesterol crystals, caseous debris, and concentrically laminated crystalline structures known as calcospherite bodies can be a clue for the presence of MTBC infection.[34,57]

Acid-fast stains. Acid-fast stains can be applied to smears or tissue sections for detection of tuberculous mycobacteria (Fig. 61.10). Organisms are faintly beaded bacilli, and are often found within macrophages. The presence of AFB suggests mycobacterial infection, but is not specific for infection with MTBC organisms. Acid-fast staining of smear or cytospin preparations may be insensitive for detection of MTBC organisms and negative results do not rule out infection.

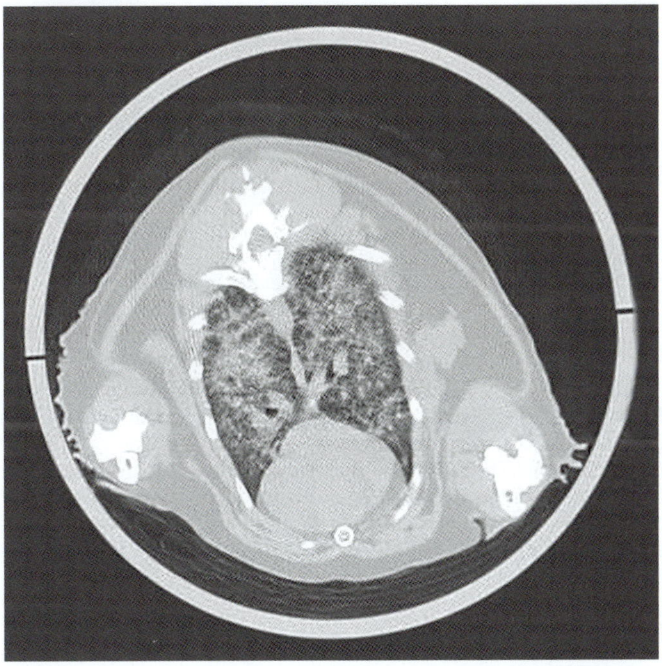

Fig. 61.8 A transverse CT-scanned section through the caudal thorax of a 3-year-old, male, neutered, retrovirus-negative, Oriental cat with *M. microti* infection. The scan reveals a diffuse-structured interstitial pattern comprising mixed nodular and linear structures, characteristic of a reticulonodular pattern which is typical of feline tuberculous pulmonary pathology.

TABLE 61.4 Assays Available for Diagnosis of Mycobacterial Infections in Dogs and Cats

Assay	Specimen Type	Target	Performance
Acid-fast staining	Tissue aspirates, buffy coat smears, body fluids, airway lavage specimens, tissues obtained at biopsy or necropsy	Acid-fast bacteria	Insensitive, especially for some mycobacterial species like MTBC bacteria. Other bacteria, such as *Rhodococcus* and *Nocardia* may also be acid-fast, so positive results are not specific for *Mycobacterium* spp.
Interferon gamma-release assay	Whole blood (peripheral blood mononuclear cells)	Cell-mediated immune response to mycobacterial antigens	Assists in discrimination between *M. bovis*, *M. microti*, and NTM infections, available in the United Kingdom
Mycobacterial culture	See acid-fast staining; avoid use of aspirates or swabs if possible	Culturable *Mycobacterium* spp	Some mycobacterial species are unculturable. Growth of MTBC organisms and slowly growing NTM may take weeks to months and identification requires special expertise. Allows molecular typing and susceptibility testing
PCR	See acid-fast staining	Mycobacterial DNA	Permits rapid identification of mycobacterial infection and differentiates MTBC from other mycobacteria, so appropriate precautions can be instituted. False-negative results can occur with insufficient specimen size, if there are very few bacteria present, or if degradation of DNA occurs. False-positive results are possible as a result of laboratory contamination

MTBC, *Mycobacterium tuberculosis* complex; NTM, non-tuberculous mycobacteria.

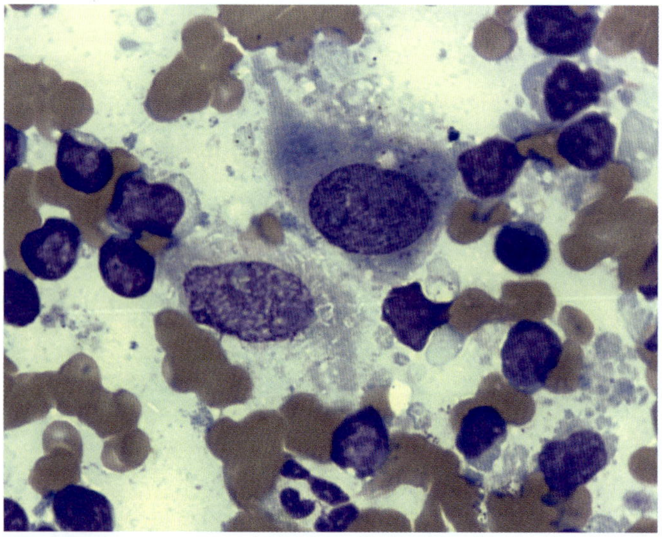

Fig. 61.9 Cytologic appearance of a fine-needle aspirate of a dermal granuloma in the skin of a 3-year-old domestic shorthair cat with *M. bovis* infection (Diff-Quik stain). Some reactive epithelioid macrophages contain intracytoplasmic negative-staining ("ghost") bacilli. Contributing to a pyogranulomatous inflammatory response were several mature and toxic neutrophils.

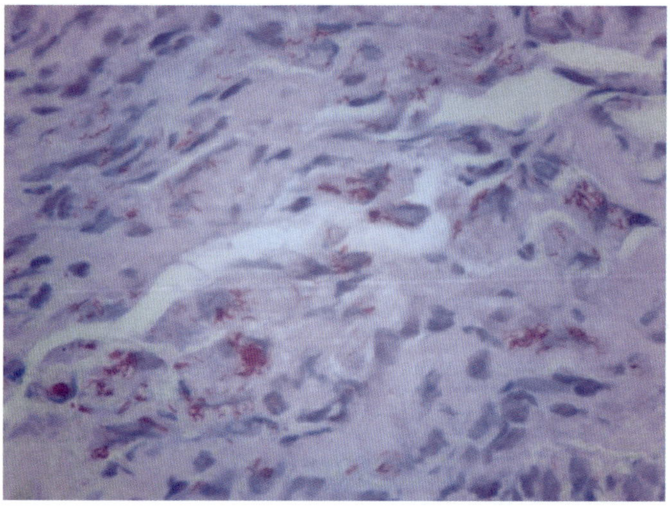

Fig. 61.10 A Ziehl-Neelsen-stained section of a granulomatous lesion biopsied from the nose of a 1-year-old, male, neutered, retrovirus-negative, domestic shorthair cat associated with *M. microti* infection. Staining reveals numerous positively stained (pink), slender, curved bacilli both intracellularly and in the extracellular space.

Immunologic Assays

Intradermal inoculation of tuberculin (a purified protein derivative from *M. tuberculosis*) is well validated and widely used for diagnosis of, and screening for, infection with MTBC organisms in humans. It is also known as the *Mantoux test*. Infected individuals develop a cutaneous delayed-type hypersensitivity reaction at the site of inoculation 48 to 72 hours later. False-negative test results can occur as a result of underlying immunosuppression. False-positive results occur as a result of non-tuberculous mycobacterial infection. Cats do not respond reliably to tuberculin skin testing. Tuberculin skin testing has been performed on the medial surface of the pinna of dogs, but false-positive results occur with a variety of other bacterial infections. Tests for anti-mycobacterial antibodies also appear to be nonspecific.[63]

IGRAs were developed on the principle of quantitatively evaluating IFN-γ production by peripherally circulating antigen-specific effector T-memory cells upon *in vitro* stimulation with mycobacterial antigens, to aid the diagnosis of both active and latent tuberculosis in cattle and, subsequently, human patients.[64] These assays have been widely adopted in the form of the QuantiFERON-TB Gold Test[65] and the T-SPOT.TB[66] as, in people, they have both greater sensitivity and specificity than the Mantoux test. Peripherally circulating blood mononuclear cells (PBMCs) are incubated *in vitro* in the presence of antigens that are present only on specific subsets of mycobacterial species, either in whole blood or as purified cell suspensions (depending on the assay used). Following a prescribed incubation period, either the number of

IFN-γ producing cells (T-SPOT.TB) or the amount of IFN-γ produced (QuantiFERON-TB Gold Test) is then quantified by ELISA.[64] This value is then interpreted to support a diagnosis, in the context of clinical signs and other diagnostic investigations. For example, in human diagnostics whole blood is incubated with the *M. tuberculosis*-specific antigen TB7.7, and two virulence-associated proteins— the 6-kDa early secretory antigenic target (ESAT-6) and the 10-kDa culture filtrate protein-10 (CFP-10). After 16 hours of incubation, the amount of IFN-γ is measured.[67]

IGRAs have several advantages over other diagnostic techniques; they generate results more rapidly than culture and even PCR methods, they are relatively noninvasive (requiring only a single peripheral blood sample), and they can be repeated if necessary as conducting the assay does not alter the systemic immune response (unlike the Mantoux test).

Since 2008, an adapted IGRA has been validated for use in cats, and since 2018 it has been used reliably in dogs.[49] For these assays, PMBCs are isolated from heparinized peripheral blood samples obtained from animals with clinical signs and/or histologic findings that strongly suggest mycobacterial disease. These cells are then incubated for 4 days *in vitro* under several conditions:

a) normal cell culture media (negative control),
b) a mitogen that stimulates IFN-γ production by αβT-cells (positive control),
c) purified protein derived from *M. avium*-complex (PPDA),
d) purified protein derived from *M. bovis* (PPDB), and
e) a combination of the peptides ESAT-6 and CFP-10.

After 4 days, the amount of IFN-γ in the cell culture supernatant is measured by ELISA. A response to the PPDB antigen that exceeds a response to PPDA is indicative of MTBC infection with a sensitivity of 100% in cats.[50,68] The response to ESAT-6 and CFP-10 can discriminate among MTBC as *M. microti* does not produce these molecules but all other members of the MTBC do.[69] Therefore in dogs the pattern "PPDB > PPDA, and ESAT-6/CFP-10 positive" would be generated in response to either *M. tuberculosis* or *M. bovis* infection. However, in cats this pattern suggests *M. bovis* infection, as cats are so rarely infected with *M. tuberculosis*. Unfortunately, some cats infected with *M. bovis* do not respond to the ESAT-6 and CFP-10 peptides; a small study showed that this occurred in 20% of infected cats, so this test does not always discriminate between *M. bovis* and *M. microti* infection.[68,70,71] Refinement of the cut-off values for cats increased test sensitivity for MTBC infections from 83.1% to 90.2%, and *M. bovis* infection from 43% to 68% while maintaining specificity at 100% for both pathogens.[72]

A response to PPDA peptide that exceeds that to PPDB supports a diagnosis of MAC infection. A lack of response to diagnostic peptides when mycobacteria have been identified through other methods (cytology, histopathology) suggests infection with another NTM organism.

IGRA tests can be used to test in-contact animals that have no clinical signs. However, the test must be interpreted with caution. The proportion of subclinical but IGRA-positive patients that go on to develop active clinical disease is unknown.

Bacterial Isolation and Identification

Mycobacterial culture is the "gold standard" for diagnosis of infection by MTBC. The use of laboratories with expertise in isolation of MTBC is recommended. Respiratory specimens such as respiratory washes are usually treated with the mucolytic N-acetylcysteine (NAC) and a sodium hydroxide solution to destroy contaminating bacteria. Specimens from normally sterile sites, such as pleural fluid, are not decontaminated in order to preserve viable mycobacteria as much as possible. Specimens are then inoculated onto special liquid or solid media for isolation of mycobacteria, such as 7H11 agar or Lowenstein-Jensen media (an egg-based medium). Modifications to the media composition may be required on the basis of the mycobacterial species suspected, so good communication between the clinician and the microbiology laboratory can optimize the chance of successful culture. Growth is occasionally evident only several weeks after inoculation of liquid media, and potentially months after inoculation of solid media. However, inoculation of solid media is required because some strains only grow on solid media and growth on solid media allows assessment of colony morphology. Once growth is evident, nucleic acid–based assays, mycolic acid analysis with high-performance liquid chromatography, or mass spectrometry (MALDI-TOF)[73] can be used to determine whether the organism belongs to the MTBC. Molecular mycobacterial antimicrobial drug susceptibility testing can also be performed.

Currently, performance of a series of phenotypic (biochemical) assays on cultured isolates is the gold standard method for differentiation of mycobacterial species that belong to the MTBC. Molecular techniques such as PCR-restriction endonuclease analysis, DNA probing, and 16S rRNA gene sequencing do not always differentiate between MTBC species. Specialized techniques for further typing of MTBC isolates include mycobacterial interspersed repetitive unit-variable-number tandem repeat (MIRU-VNTR) typing, and spoligotyping. Spoligotyping is a PCR-hybridization typing method that targets the direct repeat region of MTBC strains. This region contains multiple sequence repeats interspersed with nonrepetitive spacer sequences. MTBC species vary in the numbers of repeats and the presence or absence of some spacers, and can be differentiated on the basis of their hybridization patterns. Spoligotyping also allows identification of prevalent *M. tuberculosis* genotypes, such as the Beijing genotype, an aggressive, highly transmissible strain that has been associated with multiple drug resistance.[74] MIRU-VNTR is often combined with spoligotyping for identification of MTBC organism genotypes. Spoligotyping has been performed on several MTBC isolates from dogs and cats.

Molecular Diagnosis Using Nucleic Acid–Based Testing

Real-time PCR-based assays are available on a commercial basis for rapid detection of *Mycobacterium* spp. DNA in clinical specimens from dogs and cats in some countries. Genus-specific *Mycobacterium* spp. assays are available, as well as assays that detect mycobacteria other than tuberculosis (MOTT) organisms. These assays can be used in combination to determine whether an organism that belongs to the MTBC is present. A positive result with a genus-specific assay but a negative result with an assay for MOTT organisms implies the presence of an MTBC organism. The results of mycobacterial PCR assays should be interpreted in light of clinical findings, and PCR assays should ideally be used in conjunction with culture, which is the only way to confirm the mycobacterial species involved and allows antimicrobial drug susceptibility testing. The latter is important given the public health implications of MTBC infections.

Pathologic Findings

Gross Pathologic Findings

In addition to cutaneous lesions and peripheral lymphadenomegaly, cats with disseminated *M. bovis* or *M. microti* infections may have enlarged abdominal lymph nodes and multifocal tumor-like, greyish-white masses within parenchymal organs that may have hemorrhagic margins and/or a soft purulent or caseous center. Pulmonary lesions are often greyish-red and may be associated with serosanguineous pleural fluid.

The most frequent gross pathologic findings in dogs infected with *M. tuberculosis* include pulmonary congestion, lobar consolidation, or

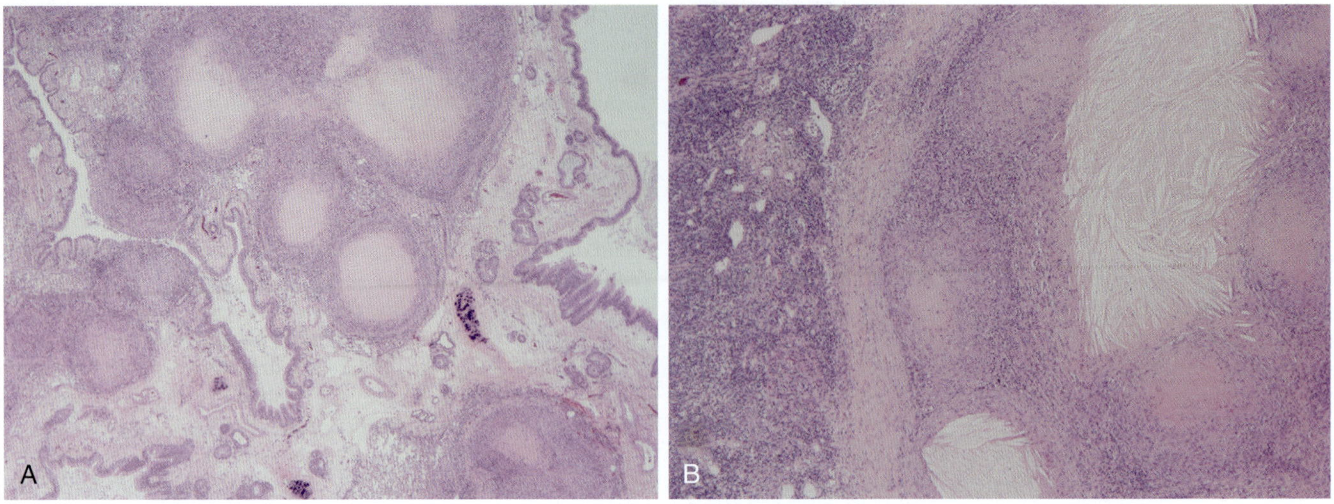

Fig. 61.11 Granulomatous inflammation associated *M. bovis* infection demonstrating a typical focal, subdermal organizing granuloma with a large area of central necrosis (hematoxylin and eosin stain, 10× magnification). Higher magnification revealed extensive effacement of the normal tissue architecture with numerous palisading macrophages with large nuclei and foamy cytoplasm infiltrating the tissue surrounding the necrotic area. Ziehl-Neelsen staining of the same biopsy (not shown) revealed moderate numbers of acid-fast bacteria within the area of necrosis.

granulomatous mass formation and sometimes massive enlargement of tracheobronchial and mediastinal nodes, which may contain multifocal gritty, yellow, caseous material.[34,51,57] Pleural effusion may also be present.[44] In dogs with dissemination, pale nodular lesions may be found in abdominal organs such the liver, peritoneal surfaces, and kidneys.[50,51,57] A dog from Africa that was infected with *M. tuberculosis* had nodular lesions that were confined to the liver and brain.[50] Dogs infected with *M. bovis* have abnormalities similar to those infected with *M. tuberculosis*.[46-48]

Histopathologic Findings

Histopathology may be performed on specimens obtained by excisional or incisional biopsy (e.g., nonhealing skin lesions, subcutaneous masses, or enlarged lymph nodes). In some cases, if there is only a single cutaneous lesion, excisional biopsy may be curative.[15] When specimens are submitted and mycobacteriosis is a differential diagnosis, this should be clearly stated on the submission form, along with a request for acid-fast staining of tissue sections; this will ensure that the samples are handled appropriately by the receiving laboratory. Direct communication with the laboratory about the suspicion for mycobacteriosis is also recommended, if possible.

Specimens collected for histopathology should be cut in half; one piece should be placed in formalin and the other frozen in a sterile container for subsequent culture or molecular testing should this be necessary. Histopathology alone cannot speciate mycobacteria, and is needed to establish the risk to owners and other animals in the household, potential treatment options, and prognosis.

Histopathologic findings are similar for all MTBC diseases. Characteristic tubercles or granulomas are present in tissues, which vary in size and may coalesce with one another (Fig. 61.11). Tubercles mostly consist of large numbers of epithelioid macrophages and a lesser numbers of neutrophils. Multinucleated giant cells are rarely identified in lesions from dogs or cats.[15,51] The inflammatory foci are surrounded by a layer of macrophages, neutrophils, lymphocytes and plasma cells, and an outer layer (or background) of granulation tissue. The center of the tubercle may be necrotic. Central mineralization and lipid accumulation have been described in some dogs infected with *M. tuberculosis*[34,57] but mineralization is rare in cats with *M. microti* or *M. bovis* infections. One study showed that in cats, *M. bovis* was associated with large multilayered granulomas that had central necrosis, whereas *M. microti* was more often found in small granulomas without central necrosis. For both pathogens, the presence of a fibrous capsule and the number of acid-fast bacilli were variable; some infections were associated with numerous acid-fast bacilli.[75] Acid-fast stains often reveal low numbers of centrally located AFB in most affected animals, but a careful search may be required, because organisms may be present in very low numbers.[34,51]

TREATMENT AND PROGNOSIS

Owners of animals with mycobacterial infections should be informed that a successful outcome requires a prolonged course of combination antibiotic therapy, and success is influenced both by owner and patient compliance. Drug toxicity, and the cost associated with treatment and monitoring can make optimal regimens difficult to maintain. For all mycobacterial infections, it is recommended that medical therapy be continued for at least 2 months past resolution of clinical signs or following resection of all visible lesions.

Drug-resistant tuberculosis with the detection of multidrug-, extensive drug-, or total drug-resistant isolates, as well as the human HIV pandemic, has dominated the focus of many of the recent changes to anti-mycobacterial drug therapies, and anti-tuberculosis therapy.[76–78] A fundamental goal of the management of mycobacterial infections is to avoid selection for drug-resistant isolates. This can only be achieved where clients understand the critical need to adhere to proper dosing protocols.

At the time of writing, treatment with rifampicin, isoniazid, pyrazinamide, and ethambutol (combined) for a minimum duration of 18 weeks is advocated for treatment of human tuberculosis by the CDC.[79] Unfortunately, isoniazid and ethambutol have been associated with severe nephrotoxicity, hepatotoxicity, and neurotoxicity in cats and dogs, and isoniazid has been associated with optic neuritis. Therefore these drugs should not be used as first-line therapies for companion animals.[80-85] Pyrazinamide is not active against *M. bovis*[86] and has also been associated with hepatotoxicity in cats, so is also not recommended.

TABLE 61.5 Anti-Tuberculosis Medications for Use in Cats and Dogs

Drug	Formulations	Dosing	Contraindications	Adverse Effects
Pradofloxacin	Suspension or tablets	5–7.5 mg/kg PO q24h	Not in dogs <12 months of age (18 months in giant breeds) or cats <6 weeks of age. Do not use in animals with epilepsy. See Chapter 10 for information on pradofloxacin in dogs	Neutropenia with high doses and/or long courses
Marbofloxacin	Tablets	2 mg/kg PO q24h	See pradofloxacin	Intermittent vomiting and transient diarrhea
Moxifloxacin	Tablets	10 mg/kg PO q24h	See pradofloxacin	Occasional vomiting. Potential for ocular toxicity unknown
Enrofloxacin (dogs only)	Tablets	5–20 mg/kg PO q24h	Not in dogs <12 months of age (18 months in giant breeds) due to potential adverse effects on cartilage. Avoid in animals with epilepsy	GI signs
Ciprofloxacin	Tablets	5–15 mg/kg PO q12h	See pradofloxacin	Occasional vomiting
Azithromycin	Capsule, suspension	5–15 mg/kg PO q24h	Pre-existing cardiomyopathy especially when arrhythmias are present. Pre-existing hepatopathy	Intermittent vomiting and diarrhea possible but uncommon
Clarithromycin	Tablets, suspension	7.5 mg/kg PO q12h	Concurrent use of NSAIDs or antacids. Pre-existing hepatopathy	Pinnal erythema. Generalized erythema. Hepatotoxicity
Rifampicin	Capsules, suspension	5–10 mg/kg PO q24h	Pre-existing hepatopathy. Pregnant queens	Hepatotoxicity; induction of liver enzymes, anorexia, generalized erythema, and pruritus. CNS signs. Discoloration of body fluids

A three-drug combination should be used (a fluoroquinolone, macrolide/azalide, and rifampicin).

Cats

Excisional biopsy can be curative for cats with single or small numbers of skin nodules caused by *M. bovis* or *M. microti*. Nevertheless, adjunctive medical therapy is recommended (Table 61.5). There is a significant risk of wound dehiscence following surgery. Currently, there is no evidence that surgery confers any additional benefit to rigorous medical management, so it is not widely advocated once a diagnosis has been obtained. The one possible exception is cats with intra-articular tuberculosis or significant osteomyelitis (Fig. 61.12).[86,87] For these cats, amputation of all or part (at least one joint above the lesion) of the limb with adjunctive medical therapy should be strongly considered.

A combination of a fluoroquinolone, a macrolide/azalide, and rifampicin is suggested for cats with tuberculosis. The fluoroquinolone of choice is pradofloxacin (where available) due to its excellent safety profile in the cat and its known activity against mycobacteria when compared to older fluoroquinolones.[88] Where this is not available, the use of moxifloxacin is advocated.[88] Less active alternatives are marbofloxacin or ciprofloxacin. The use of enrofloxacin in the cat is discouraged due to its association with acute irreversible retinopathy.[89] The macrolide/azalide of choice is azithromycin, because it requires only daily dosing and concentrates within pulmonary macrophages;[90,91] an alternative is clarithromycin.

Rifampicin has long been a cornerstone of anti-tuberculosis medical therapy, and anti-mycobacterial medical therapy in general. It should never be used as a monotherapy for mycobacterial disease as resistance develops rapidly.[92] Rifampicin has the potential to be significantly hepatotoxic when administered for long periods of time.[93,94] Liver function should, ideally, be monitored during treatment (days 0, 14, and then monthly or if clinical signs that might be due to liver disease develop). Treatment with rifampicin should be stopped if serum liver enzyme activities significantly exceed the upper reference interval, hyperbilirubinemia

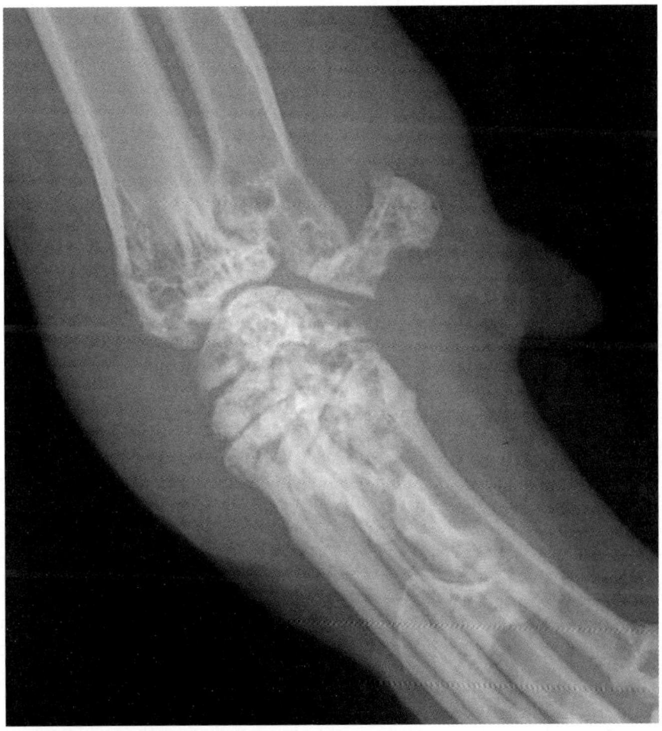

Fig. 61.12 Lateral radiograph of the right distal thoracic limb of a 4-year-old, male, neutered, retrovirus-negative Maine Coon cat with an intra-articular *M. microti* infection. There is severe osteolysis of the carpal bones as well as the distal radius and ulna surrounded by extensive soft-tissue swelling.

develops, or the patient develops clinical signs attributable to hepatic dysfunction. Use of medications that support liver function should be considered (e.g., S-adenosyl-L-methionine or NAC). Once recovered from apparent hepatotoxicity, rifampicin may be reintroduced at half of the initial dose, with close monitoring to ensure hepatopathy does not recur. Owners should be informed that rifampicin may cause urine, tears, and saliva to discolor to red-orange in color.[95] Deposition of the drug within the skin can cause skin discoloration, irritation erythema, and, occasionally, hyperesthesia. Premedicating with chlorpheniramine can help to reduce these problems in some cats. Rifampicin is teratogenic and so owners should be instructed to wear gloves when they handle it, and it should not be administered to pregnant queens.

Three months of combination therapy should be considered a minimum duration of treatment in all cases. Treatment should be extended for 2 months beyond the resolution of all clinical signs which includes any evidence of pulmonary dissemination detectable on plain radiography. Because of the sensitivity of CT imaging, subtle changes such as minor scars remain detectable and may persist indefinitely beyond the need for treatment.[96] Monitoring of IGRA results in cats did not appear to yield useful information for making treatment decisions.[97]

Drug administration to cats can be facilitated by drawing all medications into a single syringe for administration. Mixing liquid medications with food is typically unrewarding as many of these drugs are unpalatable to cats, especially rifampicin. The contents of reconstituted capsules plus split tablets can also be combined into a single gelatin capsule for daily administration. If oral dosing is not possible then drugs can be administered through an esophagostomy tube, which can significantly facilitate medicating these cats for a long duration of their treatment.

Therapy of refractory cases is more difficult as it requires more frequent drug administration and has the potential for more adverse effects. Rifampicin therapy should be maintained whenever possible and can be combined with isoniazid and ethambutol (Table 61.6). With good compliance, prognosis is fair. One review noted that 40% of treated cats reached and maintained complete clinical remission.[15] The remaining 60% of cats had temporary or partial remission, or no response to treatment.[98] However, many of the cats in this retrospective study were treated with sub-optimal therapies, such as short courses of a fluoroquinolone as monotherapy. With triple therapy, the authors' clinical experience suggests a positive prognosis for 70% to 80% of feline tuberculosis cases, particularly those with cutaneous and/or pulmonary involvement (Fig. 61.13).

Dogs

Dogs with pulmonary MTBC infections should be placed in isolation and aerosol precautions are indicated. Antimicrobial drug treatment of dogs (and cats) with confirmed *M. tuberculosis* infection is controversial and generally not recommended because of zoonotic concerns. Treatment of *M. bovis* cases should only be performed after owners have been fully educated about the potential risks of disease transmission.

As for feline MTBC infections, dogs undergoing therapy should be treated with a combination of rifampicin, a macrolide/azalide and a fluoroquinolone (see Table 61.5). Clarithromycin is the macrolide of choice based on evidence of efficacy and the greater ease of multi-day dosing in dogs when compared with cats. Treatment of a dog with *M. tuberculosis* infection was attempted with rifampin, isoniazid, and clarithromycin but the dog was euthanized after seizures developed.[34] Seizures in this case were suspected to be an adverse effect of isoniazid administration (see Table 61.6).

The prognosis for dogs with tuberculosis is considered guarded to poor. This is likely a reflection of the advanced degree of systemic disease that is typically present at the time of diagnosis and the high likelihood of adverse effects with more active anti-tuberculosis drugs used in humans (such as isoniazid). Early recognition and treatment of *M. bovis* or *M. microti* infections may yield similar outcomes as those seen for feline tuberculosis.

TABLE 61.6 Second-Line Anti-tuberculosis Medications for Use in Cats and Dogs as Part of Triple Therapy (Isoniazid, Ethambutol, and Rifampicin)

Drug	Dosing	Contraindications	Adverse Effects
Isoniazid	5–10 mg/kg PO q24h. Start at a low dose; do not exceed 300 mg/day.	Poorly evaluated in cats. Hepatic dysfunction. History of seizures	Hepatotoxicity; monitor liver enzymes. Peripheral neuritis. Seizures, especially in dogs (avoid use in dogs if possible). Acute kidney injury
Ethambutol	10–25 mg/kg PO q24h	Poorly evaluated in cats	Optic neuritis

See Table 61.5 for rifampicin dosing.

IMMUNITY AND VACCINATION

There are no vaccines available for prevention of mycobacterial disease in animals.

PREVENTION

In cats, prevention of *M. bovis* and *M. microti* infections can be achieved when cats are housed indoors and rodent populations are controlled. The feeding of raw cattle or game (e.g., deer, elk) also has the potential to transmit *M. bovis* to dogs or cats and should be discouraged.[99]

Prevention of *M. tuberculosis* infections in dogs relies on appropriate control and treatment of *M. tuberculosis* infections in affected humans that are in close contact with dogs. The possibility of serious zoonotic diseases such as tuberculosis should also be considered before stray dogs are adopted from countries where such infections are endemic.

PUBLIC HEALTH ASPECTS

Of all mycobacterial species that infect dogs and cats, the greatest risk to human health is posed by members of the MTBC. Confirmed disease by MTBC bacteria is usually notifiable to public health authorities. Over 90% of human tuberculosis is caused by *M. tuberculosis*. Only 1% of cases result from *M. bovis* infection, and human infection with *M. microti* is very rare.[100] Factors such as HIV infection, homelessness, and intravenous drug use predispose humans to *M. tuberculosis* infection. Tuberculosis continues to be an important public health problem worldwide, and drug resistance is emerging globally. Over the last 2 decades, case numbers have decreased to the lowest levels in history in the United States.[101] However, the incidence rate is highest among non-Hispanic Asian, non-Hispanic black, and Hispanic groups in the United States, which is 25, 8, and 7 times greater, respectively, than the rate for non-Hispanic whites.[101] Disease in immigrants to the United States results from reactivation of disease acquired in other countries.

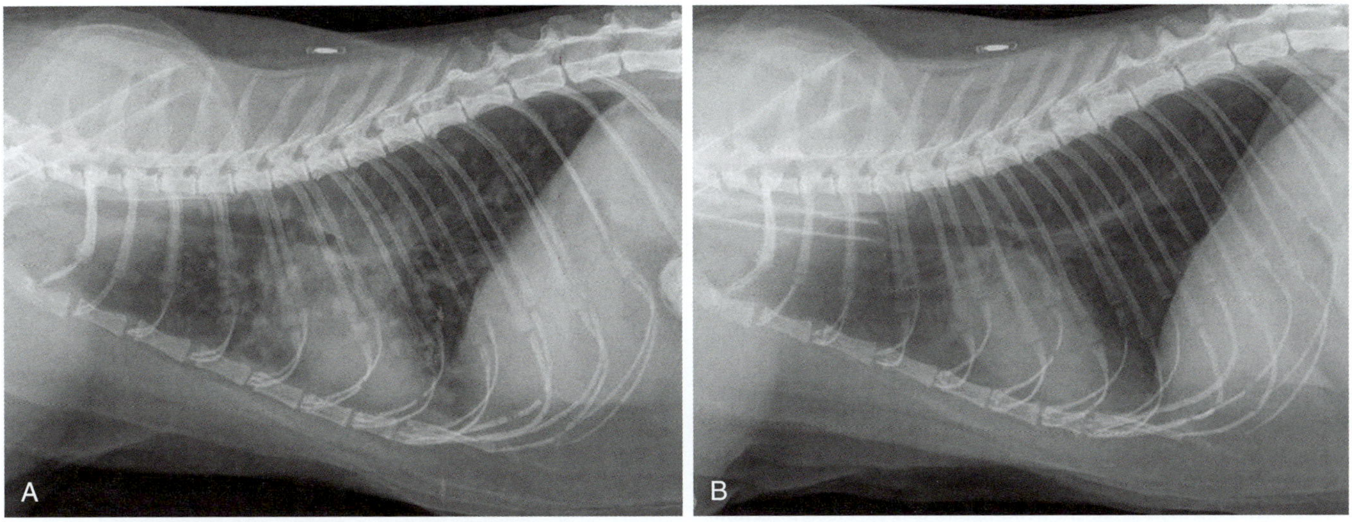

Fig. 61.13 (A) Lateral thoracic radiograph from a 3-year-old, female, intact, retrovirus-negative, domestic shorthair cat infected with *M. bovis*. The radiograph, taken at the time of diagnosis, shows multifocal to coalescing areas of soft-tissue opacity (granulomas) distributed throughout the lung fields. (B) Lateral thoracic radiograph taken from the same cat following 3 months of triple antibiosis consisting of rifampicin (10 mg/kg), azithromycin (10 mg/kg), and pradofloxacin (5 mg/kg) PO q24h.

Mycobacterium tuberculosis

If *M. tuberculosis* infection is suspected or confirmed in a dog, this should trigger a notification to the appropriate health care authorities for human testing. Euthanasia, rather than treatment, should always be undertaken for confirmed infected animals given the potential human health risk. However, it should be recognized that transmission of *M. tuberculosis* from dogs to humans has not been reported, and in one case report, no transmission to a diabetic child occurred despite extremely close and prolonged contact.[34] An investigation may be performed in order to identify the source of infection, and it may be necessary to perform one or more Mantoux tests on any individuals with significant contact with infected animals. Although transmission of *M. tuberculosis* from infected dogs to humans has not been reported as a result of direct contact, veterinary staff were infected when a necropsy of an infected dog was performed, possibly following aerosolization of infected brain tissue when the skull was sectioned with an electric saw.[50] High-density surgical masks (N95 masks) should be worn if surgery or necropsy is performed on a dog or cat suspected to have tuberculosis.

Mycobacterium bovis

Human disease resulting from exposure to companion animals infected with *M. bovis* is extremely rare. Globally, in the last 150 years, only six cases of human *M. bovis* tuberculosis have resulted from exposure to cats, and these cats had skin lesions that were draining pus that contained many Ziehl-Neelsen (ZN)-positive bacteria. As of September 2015, Public Health England, Public Health Wales, and Health Protection Scotland all consider the risks to humans to be "very low." That said, the risk should be considered seriously in the context of humans with specific risk factors for transmission (Box 61.1). Extensive and/or purulent lesions pose the greatest risk to human health and are generally less responsive to treatment. By comparison, single nonulcerated skin lesions and/or regional lymphadenopathy carry low zoonotic risk and may be very amenable to treatment.

Mycobacterium microti

The risk to humans for *M. microti* is significantly lower than that of *M. bovis*.[100] Fewer than 30 human cases of *M. microti* infection have been documented in published literature and 11 (~40%) of these had specific risk factors (see Box 61.1). None have resulted from exposure to an infected cat.

BOX 61.1 Risk Factors for Zoonotic Transmission of MTBC Infections

- Under 5 years old (some sources suggest 12 years)
- Pregnant
- HIV-positive
- Substance misuse
- Diabetes mellitus
- Severe kidney disease
- Solid organ transplant recipient
- Cancer patient receiving chemotherapy or radiation therapy
- Medical condition requiring treatment with systemic glucocorticoids
- Specialized treatment for rheumatoid arthritis or Crohn's disease
- On TNF-α inhibitors
- History of gastrectomy or jejunoileal bypass
- Silicosis

Compiled from advice published by United Kingdom public health organizations and WHO guidelines. Animal treatment should be discouraged when the above conditions are present in their owners, and at minimum, owners should be counseled on the potential for zoonotic transmission when the above conditions are present.

SLOW-GROWING NON-TUBERCULOUS MYCOBACTERIAL INFECTIONS

ETIOLOGY AND EPIDEMIOLOGY

Slow-growing NTM include organisms that belong to the MAC and a number of other fastidious mycobacterial pathogens that grow slowly in culture. Unlike organisms that belong to the MTBC, they are environmental saprophytes with a worldwide distribution. MAC organisms, for example, can be found in soil, dust, and aquatic environments that include showers, faucets, household drinking water, swimming pools, and hot tub spas.[102] The organisms also infect free-living amebae and form biofilms, which may promote environmental persistence. Subclinical infections with *M. avium* subsp. *avium* are common among birds, and *M. avium* subsp. *avium* is the main cause of avian tuberculosis.[103] Ingestion of infected birds or bird feces may be a route of transmission to dogs and cats.

The MAC consists of two closely related species, *M. avium* and *Mycobacterium intracellulare.* Four subspecies of *M. avium* have been described: subspecies *hominissuis*, *avium*, *paratuberculosis*, and *silvaticum*. It has been proposed that *M. avium* subsp. *hominissuis* and *M. avium* subsp. *silvaticum* be reclassified as variants of *M. avium* subsp. *avium*, and *M. lepraemurium* be reclassified as a new subspecies of *M. avium*, *M. avium* subsp. *lepraemurium* (see Fastidious NTM Infections, below),[104] leaving three subspecies of *M. avium*. However, this has not been universally adopted, and for the purpose of this chapter, the previous nomenclature will be used.

Mycobacterium avium subsp. *hominissuis* causes most infections in human patients, but the distribution of subspecies in affected dogs and cats is currently not fully understood, because molecular methods are required for identification at the subspecies level. *Mycobacterium avium* subsp. *hominissuis* infections have been identified in several dogs from continental Europe,[105,106] and *M. avium* subsp. *avium* was isolated from an affected cat.[107] The DNA of *M. avium* subsp. *paratuberculosis* was detected in intestinal biopsies from dogs with chronic GI signs, where it was of uncertain clinical significance.[108] More recently, it was cultured from enlarged mesenteric lymph nodes of a dachshund from South Africa that had evidence of disseminated infection with large numbers of intralesional AFB at necropsy.[109]

MAC organisms cause opportunistic infections in immunocompromised individuals. Most affected dogs and cats have been between 1 and 5 years of age. Infection is not directly transmissible from one infected individual to another, but disease may initially be indistinguishable from that caused by MTBC bacteria. In the US, although still rare, infection of cats and dogs with MAC organisms is more common than infection with MTBC organisms.

Cats

Slow-growing mycobacteria reported in association with disease in cats include organisms that belong to the MAC[110–129] (specifically, *M. avium* subsp. *avium*,[107–130] *M. avium* subsp. *hominissuis*,[131–133] and *M. intracellulare*[134,135]), *M. genavense*,[136] *M. malmoense*,[13,137] *Mycobacterium celatum*, *Mycobacterium terrae* complex,[138] *Mycobacterium simiae*,[139] *Mycobacterium xenopi*,[140–143] *Mycobacterium ulcerans*,[144] *Mycobacterium heckeshornense*,[145] *Mycobacterium nebraskense*,[146,147] and *Mycobacterium kansasii.*[147,148] Of all NTM, organisms that belong to the MAC were cultured most frequently from cats from the United Kingdom (see Table 61.3)[13]; however, in general, the culture data for NTM infections is inevitably skewed by the fact that fastidious organisms cannot be cultured. *Mycobacterium avium* accounted for 15% of 159 culturable mycobacterial infections in cats (73% were MTBC infections).[13] A spatial cluster of infection was identified in cats from eastern England.[13]

Advanced retrovirus infection or treatment with immunosuppressive drugs may predispose cats to MAC infection, although most affected cats have no identifiable immunodeficiency. A possible breed predisposition has been recognized in Siamese cats as well as Abyssinian and Somalis.[112,120] Diagnosis of *M. kansasii* infections in two indoor-only domestic shorthair cats from the same litter suggested a genetic predisposition to infection.[148] Other potential risk factors identified in cats with disease caused by slow-growing NTM include administration of exogenous glucocorticoids,[107] multidrug chemotherapy for lymphoma,[117] cyclosporine treatment in the context of renal transplantation,[114] retrovirus infection,[136,149] idiopathic αβ-T cell lymphopenia (particularly $CD4^+$ αβ-T-cells),[143] or concurrent comorbidities such as advanced chronic renal disease and cryptococcosis.[150]

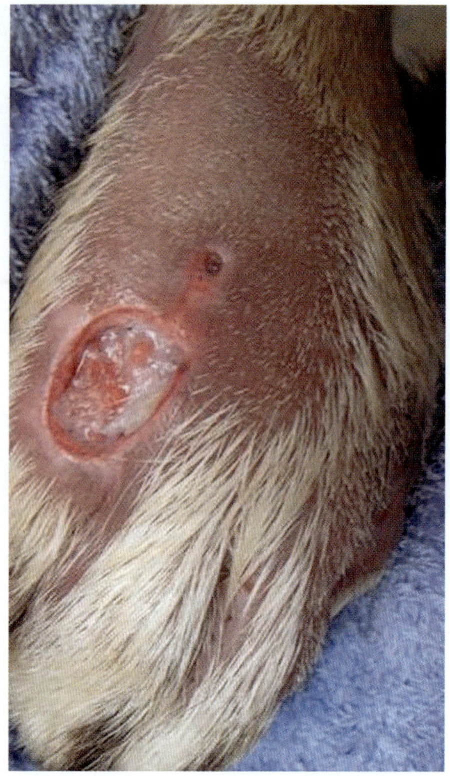

Fig. 61.14 Localized dermal infections in a dog due to *M. ulcerans*, the causative agent of Buruli ulcer. This organism produces a cytotoxic toxin, mycolactone, which is responsible for the deep skin ulcerations that are a hallmark of the disease.

Dogs

MAC organisms that have been associated with disease in dogs include *M. avium* subspecies *avium*,[151] *M. avium* subspecies *paratuberculosis* (MAP),[109] and *M. avium* subspecies *hominissuis.*[105,106,152,153] Disease occurs sporadically in any breed, but basset hounds, miniature schnauzers, and possibly Yorkshire terriers may be predisposed, possibly because of an inherited deficiency of CMI (see Chapter 130). Other slow-growing NTM isolated from dogs with mycobacterial infections are *M. kansasii*, *M. genavense*, *M. nebraskense*, and *M. ulcerans. Mycobacterium ulcerans* causes localized dermal infections in dogs (Buruli ulcer) in endemic areas of Victoria, Australia.[154] This organism produces a cytotoxic toxin, mycolactone, that is responsible for the deep skin ulcerations that are a hallmark of the disease (Fig. 61.14). Although the exact ecology of *M. ulcerans* has not been determined, it has a worldwide but highly focal endemicity, with most human infections occurring in West Africa and coastal southeastern Australia. It is suspected that the organism gains entry via breaches in the epidermis, possibly in some cases involving mechanical insect vectors.[155] Animal cases have only been reported from Australia, and also include possums[156,157], koalas,[158] a long-footed potoroo,[159] alpacas,[160] horses,[161] and a cat.[144]

CLINICAL FEATURES

Pathogenesis and Clinical Signs

In cats, disease caused by MAC organisms resembles that caused by *M. bovis* or *M. microti*. Some cats have cutaneous lesions (especially

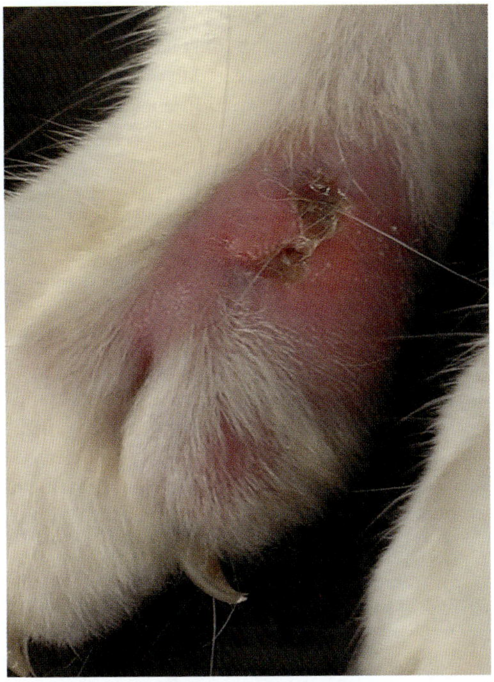

Fig. 61.15 An alopecic, erythematous granuloma on the medial aspect of the first digit of the right foot of a 6-year-old, male, neutered, retrovirus-negative, domestic shorthair cat caused by *M. avium* infection. The lesion is notable for its similarity in gross appearance to tuberculous lesions.

on the head and limbs) (Fig. 61.15). Other clinical abnormalities are osteomyelitis, pulmonary involvement with tachypnea or cough, peripheral and abdominal lymphadenomegaly, and GI, liver, splenic, renal, omental and uncommonly CNS or marrow involvement.[110,112–114,116,126,129,149,150] GI involvement may initially manifest as weight loss despite a good appetite.[112]

Canine MAC infection is typically associated with multisystemic disease, including any combination of generalized lymphadenopathy, anemia, weight loss, hepatopathy, and/or splenomegaly. Dogs with MAC infections often develop marked peripheral and abdominal lymphadenopathy, tonsillar enlargement, hepatosplenomegaly, and/or osteomyelitis. In some dogs, mandibular or cervical lymphadenopathy may be so severe that respiratory distress and dysphagia occur.[162] Less severe cases, with single cutaneous nodules have also been reported and should not be overlooked.[163] Secondary immune-mediated inflammatory disease, such as polyarthritis, has also been reported.[164] At necropsy, AFB and associated inflammatory lesions may also be found in the small and large intestines, liver, spleen, lung and pleura, bone marrow, and rarely the spinal cord.[105,165–169] Involvement of the GI tract may lead to chronic vomiting, diarrhea, hematochezia, melena, inappetence, and weight loss. Intestinal rupture in one dog led to bacterial peritonitis. Even though inflammatory lesions with intralesional AFB have been detected in the lung at necropsy, pulmonary involvement is not a prominent clinical feature of MAC infections in dogs, which may help distinguish the disease from *M. tuberculosis* infection.

Mycobacterium kansasii was isolated from a 3-year-old whippet with chronic pleural effusion[170] and also from a mammary mass of a 2-year-old Chihuahua.[171] The latter case also had chronic generalized demodicosis implying an underlying immune deficit was present, and it subsequently succumbed to the infection after prednisolone treatment for cutaneous lymphoma. Disseminated *M. genavense* infection was diagnosed in a 2-year-old pug with generalized lymphadenopathy, abdominal organomegaly, pyrexia, and limb pain.[172] *Mycobacterium ulcerans* is associated with localized ulcerative cutaneous disease (see Fig. 61.14). *Mycobacterium nebraskense* was isolated from a dog in Switzerland with multifocal cutaneous disease.[173]

Physical Examination Findings

Physical examination of cats with slow-growing NTM infections may reveal fever, a thin body condition, cutaneous lesions similar to those described for MTBC infection, peripheral or abdominal lymphadenopathy, renomegaly, hepatomegaly, tachypnea, and/or increased lung sounds. Rarely neurologic signs such as nystagmus occur.[112] Ocular involvement[174–176] as either a localized or systemic disease process has been reported.

In dogs, low-grade fever, a thin body condition, dehydration, mucosal pallor, tonsillar enlargement, lymphadenomegaly (especially of the mandibular or abdominal nodes), hepatosplenomegaly, and/or abdominal pain may be found. Melena or hematochezia may be detected on rectal examination. Osteomyelitis may be associated with lameness or mass lesions in association with underlying bone involvement. A dog with spinal cord involvement had pelvic limb paresis.[165] Other findings may be present depending on specific organ involvement.

DIAGNOSIS

Laboratory Abnormalities

Complete Blood Count, Serum Biochemical Tests, and Urinalysis

Findings on routine laboratory tests for cats and dogs with slow-growing NTM infections are similar to those described for MTBC infection. Most affected dogs or cats have had mild to moderate nonregenerative anemia, neutrophilia with mild to moderate bandemia, lymphopenia, hypoalbuminemia, hyperglobulinemia or hypoglobulinemia, and sometimes, hypercalcemia, hyperbilirubinemia and increased liver enzyme activities.[113,166,177] An absence of hematological or biochemical abnormalities has also been described.

Diagnostic Imaging

Plain Radiography

When radiographic abnormalities are present in cats infected with MAC, they often consist of diffuse interstitial or bronchointerstitial patterns.[112,113] Diffuse interstitial patterns may be present in the absence of clinical signs of respiratory involvement. Thoracic lymphadenopathy, mediastinal masses, or pleural effusion may be present in dogs.[106,170] Abdominal radiographs may show abdominal masses or hepatosplenomegaly in dogs as well as in cats. Radiographs of affected bone may reveal soft-tissue swelling and bony lytic lesions or periosteal proliferation.

Sonographic Findings

Abdominal sonography may be unremarkable or reveal hepatomegaly, splenomegaly, hypoechoic nodular lesions within the liver or spleen, a thickened intestinal wall, hyperechoic mesentery, or enlarged, hypoechoic or heteroechoic abdominal lymph nodes.[178]

Microbiologic Tests (see Table 61.4)

Cytologic Examination

Cytologic examination of aspirates from enlarged lymph nodes, abdominal organs, or lavage specimens from the respiratory tract of cats and dogs with MAC infections reveals large numbers of histiocytes with nonstaining intracellular bacteria (Fig. 61.16), and lower numbers of neutrophils.

Acid-fast stains. In general, AFB are identified more readily in smears or biopsies in slow-growing NTM infections when compared

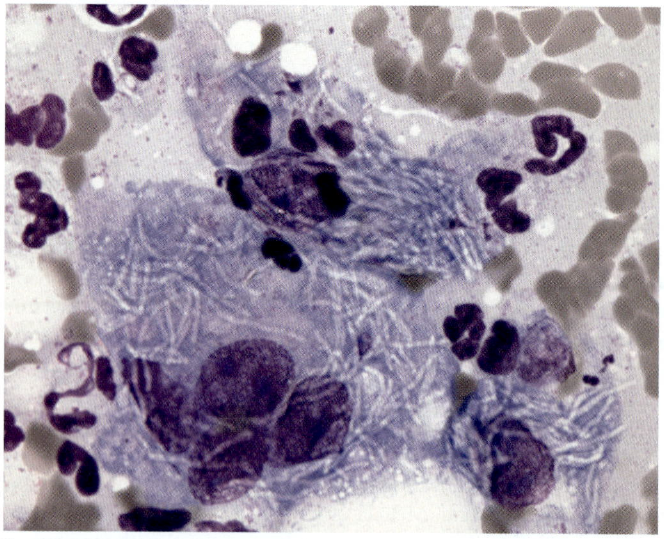

Fig. 61.16 Aspirate cytology from a cutaneous mass in a cat that developed after prolonged (> 1 year) treatment with cyclosporine. Large numbers of negatively stained mycobacterial organisms are present. (Image courtesy Dr. William Vernau, University of California-Davis Clinical Pathology Service.)

with MTBC infections and rapid-growing NTM infections, possibly because of the frequent presence of immunosuppression. Most reports of affected dogs and cats with either MAC or other slow-growing NTM show the detection of organisms in cytology specimens stained with acid-fast stains. One report described a dog with localized nasopharyngeal disease and absence of AFB, which was noted to be unusual.[163]

Bacterial Isolation and Identification

Up to 12 weeks of incubation may be required for visible growth of slow-growing NTM. Species can then be identified through the use of commercial DNA probe-based assays or PCR analysis. MAC subspecies determination requires specialized typing techniques such as IS*1245* restriction fragment length polymorphism typing, MIRU-VNTR, or the use of PCR assays that detect gene fragments present in some *M. avium* subspecies but not others.[105,107,178]

The CLSI criteria for the antimicrobial susceptibility testing of NTM recommends broth microdilution as the gold standard, preferably performed by a mycobacterial reference laboratory, or a similarly experienced facility.[180]

Molecular Diagnosis Using Nucleic Acid–Based Testing

PCR testing provides a rapid and typically accurate diagnosis and can be performed on fresh, frozen, or formalin-fixed paraffin-embedded tissue and Romanowsky-stained (but not ZN-stained) cytology slides.[181]

The most frequently utilized genes for mycobacterial identification are those which encode for 16S rRNA,[182] the 65-kDa heat shock protein (*hsp*65),[183] the β-subunit of bacterial RNA polymerase (*rpoB*),[184] 16-23S rRNA internal transcribed spacer ITS region,[185,186] and, less frequently, the DNA gyrases (*gyr*). Assays that target the IS*6110* element for MTBC,[187] IS*2404* for *M. ulcerans*,[188] and multiplex IS*901* and IS*1245* for differentiation of *M. avium* subsp. *avium* and M. *avium* subsp. *hominissuis*[189] have been utilized in the diagnosis of small animal infections.[131,144]

Although its popularity has reduced with the accessibility of genetic sequencing, PCR-restriction fragment analysis (PRA) (or restriction fragment length polymorphism [RFLP]) is a commonly used DNA profiling technique for identification of NTM. This technique involves amplification of a particular gene (e.g., ITS,[190] hsp65,[191,192] IS*1245* for *M. avium*[193]), and subsequent restriction enzyme digestion, followed by analysis via gel electrophoresis.

Pathologic Findings

In general, pathologic findings in cats or dogs with MAC infection consist of focal, multifocal, or generalized lymph node enlargement (up to 5 cm in diameter), and nodules in the spleen, liver, lungs, omentum, intestinal wall, and occasionally the kidneys. Nodules are white, grey, or yellow and may be caseous on cut section. Evidence of GI hemorrhage may be present in the intestine of affected dogs.[166]

Histopathology in slow-growing NTM infections typically reveals large numbers of histiocytes and lesser numbers of neutrophils, which in some cases may surround necrotic foci. Multinucleated giant cells are rarely seen, and mineralization has not been described. Moderate to large numbers of AFB are usually present within histiocytes (Fig. 61.17).

TREATMENT AND PROGNOSIS

Treatment of slow-growing NTM infections in dogs or cats is challenging. The majority of animals are euthanized as a result of their disease, but apparent cure has been reported in a few cats.[107,112,113,138] Successful treatment with a combination of enrofloxacin, clarithromycin, and rifampicin was reported in one dog with localized cutaneous lesions.[163] Another dog was successfully treated for disseminated *M. genavense* infection with clarithromycin, ethambutol, and enrofloxacin.[172] Treatment of *M. ulcerans* infection in dogs has typically involved 8 to 10 weeks of a third-generation fluoroquinolone (e.g., enrofloxacin) plus either clarithromycin or rifampicin.[194] Occasionally, surgical debridement has been helpful for recalcitrant lesions.

As for infection with MTBC organisms, the use of two or three drugs in combination is recommended to prevent emergence of resistance. The use of macrolides (especially clarithromycin) has greatly improved outcome for human patients with MAC infections, so inclusion of clarithromycin or azithromycin is recommended. The currently recommended treatment for humans with MAC infections consists of a rifamycin, ethambutol, and a macrolide such as clarithromycin. Combinations that include isoniazid have been used to treat other slow-growing NTM infections.[195]

Drug resistance patterns of slow-growing NTM vary widely, not just between species but also between isolates of the same species.[196] Furthermore, susceptibility test results do not always correlate with clinical outcome, as some of the genes that confer resistance (e.g., to macrolides) are inducible, especially for MAC.[197] Recommendations for susceptibility testing of uncommonly isolated species, which have been assessed to be clinically significant in people, may include testing against rifampicin, clarithromycin, amikacin, ciprofloxacin, ethambutol, linezolid, moxifloxacin, and trimethoprim-sulfamethoxazole.[179] MAC isolates are typically resistant to commonly used fluoroquinolones (e.g., enrofloxacin, marbofloxacin, orbifloxacin). The most successful protocols consist of triple therapy with a macrolide (clarithromycin or azithromycin), a fluoroquinolone (pradofloxacin, moxifloxacin, or possibly marbofloxacin [in the case of isolates other than *M. avium*]), rifampicin, or clofazimine. Some cats require extended (up to a year) or indefinite therapy. Relapses have been reported.[112] Various combinations of clarithromycin, clofazimine, doxycycline, rifamycins, and fluoroquinolones have been used to treat affected cats (Table 61.7). Clofazimine is an antimycobacterial drug with an

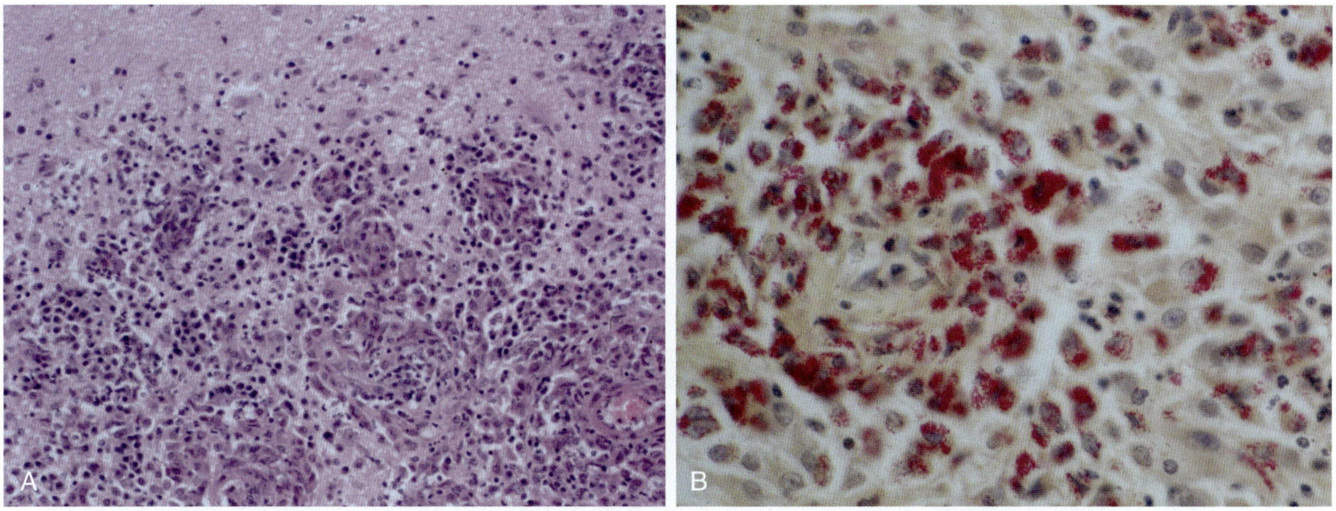

Fig. 61.17 (A) Granulomatous inflammation in the brain of a 10-year-old male neutered Siamese mix cat with disseminated *Mycobacterium avium* infection. Hematoxylin and eosin stain. (B) Section from the same cat stained with Ziehl-Neelsen (acid-fast) stain. There are large numbers of intracellular acid-fast bacteria.

unknown mechanism of action. In human patients, it has primarily been used to treat lepromatous or rapidly growing opportunistic mycobacteria, but may have some activity against MAC organisms.

PUBLIC HEALTH ASPECTS

As for dogs and cats, humans acquire slow-growing NTM infections from the environment; direct transmission from diseased animals to people has not been described. A *M. kansasii* infection in a person was associated with a dog bite to the hand,[197] although the infection occurred at the elbow 6 months later, so whether the dog was the source of infection remained unconfirmed. Ownership of caged birds by immunocompromised humans has been discouraged in the past because of the potential that these birds might shed MAC organisms. However, human disease is caused by *M. avium* subsp. *hominissuis* and not the avian organism (subsp. *avium*), so the feces of caged birds may not represent a significant source of infection. Three major clinical forms of MAC disease occur in people: localized pulmonary disease (which includes "hot tub lung disease", a hypersensitivity pneumonitis), cervicofacial lymphadenitis, and disseminated disease.[198] Rarely, cutaneous disease and disease in other locations occur. Disseminated disease occurs most often in humans with HIV infection, but children with congenital immunodeficiencies can also be affected. Prophylactic treatment with an antimycobacterial drug is recommended for HIV-infected humans with CD4+ T cell counts that are less than 50 cells/mm^3.[198] Cervicofacial lymphadenitis is an uncommon disease of children less than 3 years of age.

Although transmission of MAC organisms from diseased dogs and cats to humans should not, in theory, occur by direct contact, it may not be possible to distinguish MAC infection from infection with MTBC organisms (especially *M. bovis*) based on initial clinical findings. Veterinary staff should take care to avoid needle-stick injuries or cutaneous inoculation when collecting specimens (such as lymph node aspirates) from dogs and cats with NTM infections because of the possibility that disease might occur after cutaneous inoculation. Sedation is recommended whenever lymph node aspiration is indicated for an animal with an unknown cause of lymphadenopathy. Care should also be taken not to aerosolize tissues at necropsy when mycobacterial disease is suspected (such as that occurring with electric saws).

TABLE 61.7 Treatment of NTM Infections

Drug	Dosing	Contraindications	Adverse Effects
Clofazimine	4–10 mg/kg q24h PO *or* 25–50 mg/cat q24h PO	Poorly evaluated in cats	Hepatotoxicity GI signs Pitting corneal lesions Photosensitization (keep cats indoors during treatment)
Doxycycline monohydrate	10 mg/kg q12–24h PO	Concurrent barbiturate administration	GI signs; most frequently vomiting. Esophagitis with hyclate forms of the drug
Amikacin	10–15 mg/kg q24h IV, IM, or SC	Poorly evaluated in cats	Nephrotoxicity Ototoxicity

In addition to those in Table 61.5 *NTM*, non-tuberculous mycobacteria.

RAPID-GROWING NON-TUBERCULOUS MYCOBACTERIAL INFECTIONS

ETIOLOGY AND EPIDEMIOLOGY

Rapid-growing NTM grow in culture within 7 days and are responsible for most cutaneous mycobacterial disease in cats in the USA and Australia. Infections have also been described in the United Kingdom, Canada, western Europe, New Zealand, and South America.

Cats

Rapid-growing NTM that are pathogens in cats include members of the *Mycobacterium fortuitum* group[13,199–206] (*M. fortuitum*,[133,207] *Mycobacterium porcinum*,[88] and *Mycobacterium alvei*[88]), *Mycobacterium smegmatis* group[135,200,208,209] (*M. smegmatis sensu stricto*,[88,133] *Mycobacterium goodii*,[88,133,201] *Mycobacterium wolinskyi*[133]),

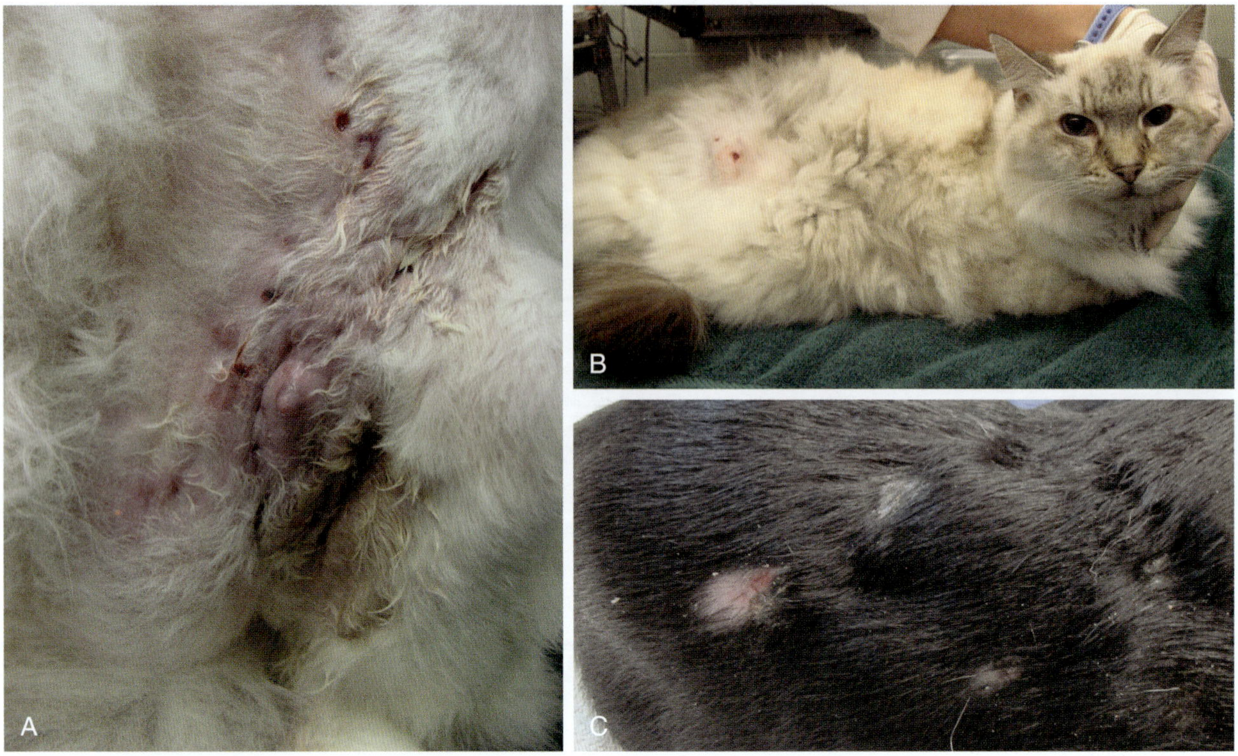

Fig. 61.18 Cutaneous-subcutaneous infections with rapidly-growing mycobacteria. A and B, Thirteen-year-old male neutered siamese cat with mycobacterial panniculitis. There are multiple nodular lesions in the inguinal region (A) and lateral flank and dorsal lumbar regions (B). In this cat, lesions progressed slowly over 8 years despite treatment with antimicrobial drugs. (C) Dorsum of an 8-year old dachshund mix with a multidrug resistant *Mycobacterium abscessus* infection. Multiple draining wounds and extensive scarring are present.

Mycobacterium chelonae/abscessus group[199,201,204,210] (*M. abscessus* subsp. *bolletti* [formerly *Mycobacterium massiliense*[211]]), *Mycobacterium mageritense* group,[88] *Mycobacterium mucogenicum* group,[135] *Mycobacterium falvenscens,*[199] *Mycobacterium phlei,*[212] and *Mycobacterium thermoresistibile.*[133,213–216] Cases have been reported from tropical (Brazil),[207] subtropical (southeastern and southwestern USA),[203,204,212] and temperate regions, including Australia,[88,209,214] New Zealand,[135] Canada,[135] Finland,[217] Germany,[215] United Kingdom,[13] and the Netherlands.[210,213] Geographical differences exist with respect to species distribution.

Dogs

Sporadic infections of dogs with rapid-growing NTM have been reported. *Mycobacterium goodii* was isolated from a dog with uncontrolled hyperadrenocorticism.[218] Systemic *M. smegmatis* infection was diagnosed in a young basset hound[219] (perhaps due to the same immunological defect that renders this breed susceptible to MAC infections). *Mycobacterium fortuitum* skin, bloodstream, and pulmonary infections have also been reported.[220–225]

CLINICAL FEATURES

Pathogenesis, Clinical Signs, and Physical Examination Findings

Rapid-growing NTM are thought to infect dogs and cats by cutaneous inoculation, which is reflected by the distribution of lesions. Inoculation of the organism directly into subcutaneous adipose tissue appears to increase the severity of disease in cats, to which overweight cats are predisposed.

Cats

Granulomatous panniculitis is the most common manifestation of disease caused by the rapid-growing NTM.[135,199,201–204,208–212,217,225–229] It is characterized by multiple punctate draining tracts and subcutaneous nodules which can coalesce to form large areas of typically non-painful, nonhealing ulcerated skin that overlies inflamed fat pads (Fig. 61.18). Initially, a circumscribed plaque or nodule of the skin and subcutis may be the only sign present. Later, subcutaneous tissue becomes thickened, and the overlying skin becomes adherent, alopecic, and punctuated with draining tracts. In cats, lesions often first appear in the inguinal region, although they can begin in the axillae, flanks, or dorsum. The disease may subsequently spread to contiguous areas of the lateral and ventral abdominal wall, perineum, and tail base. Severely affected cats may become pyrexic, anorexic, and reluctant to move, particularly if lesions are secondarily infected with skin commensals such as *Staphylococcus* and *Streptococcus* spp., but most cats are otherwise bright and appetent. Rarely, pneumonia caused by rapid-growing NTM has been described in cats. Lipoid mycobacterial pneumonia may arise in association with lactulose or paraffin treatment for furballs.[89] Pneumonia was also described in a cat infected with *M. thermoresistibile*; in one cat, infection followed a bath.[90] Clinical signs are typically cough, dyspnea, fever, malaise, and weight loss.

Dogs

In dogs, nodular lesions or nonhealing wounds with draining tracts often occur in the inguinal region, cervical region, and/or other proximal body locations.

Mycobacterium fortuitum also can cause pulmonary disease in dogs[85–89] as well as bacteremia.[81] Lipoid pneumonia was described in one young German shepherd from Louisiana.[230] Disseminated

RGM infections are very rare. Disseminated disease that resembled MAC infection was described in a basset hound infected with *M. smegmatis*.[91]

DIAGNOSIS

Laboratory Abnormalities

Complete Blood Count and Serum Chemistry Profile

Findings on the CBC, serum chemistry profile, and urinalysis in rapid-growing NTM infections are nonspecific. Cats with mycobacterial panniculitis may have no abnormalities.

Microbiologic Tests

Cytologic Diagnosis

Cytologic examination of aspirates from cutaneous lesions may reveal granulomatous to pyogranulomatous inflammation. Slides also should be stained with acid-fast stains (e.g., ZN or Fite's) to assist in identification of mycobacteria. A modified ZN-staining procedure may be needed for rapid-growing NTM, as they are not as acid-fast as other species. Although less invasive than biopsy, an FNA is likely to have lower sensitivity; panniculitis lesions frequently have few (if any) visible mycobacteria.

Bacterial Isolation and Identification

Isolation of mycobacteria in culture is currently the gold standard diagnostic test for confirmation of rapid-growing NTM infection. However, in some laboratories, it has a low sensitivity and may fail. MALDI-TOF can be used to identify rapid-growing NTM following culture (see Chapter 3). It is now also being used directly on clinical specimens, and the available spectral database for mycobacteria is steadily improving. Mycobacteria require prior inactivation and disruption of the mycolic acid-rich cell wall, both for biosafety reasons (in the case of the MTBC) and to liberate proteins within the cells. Success rates vary between 55% and 98% for correct species-level identification.[231]

Drug susceptibility testing of rapid-growing NTM is not only useful for clinical purposes, but historically has also been used to provide phenotypic data for typing of isolates (for example, susceptibility to trimethoprim, polymyxin B, and tobramycin). The National Committee for Clinical Laboratory Standards Mycobacterial Subcommittee has nominated broth dilution as the gold standard,[6] although this can be technically demanding and is not offered by many diagnostic laboratories.

Molecular Diagnosis Using Nucleic Acid–Based Testing

See slow-growing NTM infections. Molecular methods are rarely needed for diagnosis of rapid-growing NTM infections because they are often isolated readily in culture. PCR-sequencing may be used to identify rapid-growing NTM to the species level.

Pathologic Findings

Typical histopathologic findings in most cats with mycobacteriosis include granulomatous inflammation with foamy, epithelioid, and/or palisading macrophages, with significant infiltration of lymphocytes and/or neutrophils (pyogranulomatous inflammation).[15] With ZN stain, rapid-growing NTM infections generally have fewer AFB compared to slow-growing and fastidious NTM infections, though this is not always the case, and is not diagnostic. The use of modified Fite's or fluorescent Auramine-O stain may increase the sensitivity for detection of mycobacteria.[232]

TREATMENT AND PROGNOSIS

Infections caused by rapid-growing NTM can be successfully treated with lipophilic antimicrobial agents as directed by susceptibility data, together with surgical resection and reconstructive techniques. Because of the common presence of drug resistance, infections caused by rapid-growing NTM should undergo culture and susceptibility testing; however, the following information can be used to guide initial therapy. Based on the use of human breakpoints, members of the *M. smegmatis* complex are usually susceptible to doxycycline and fluoroquinolones but are often resistant to clarithromycin.[233,234] MICs tend to be higher for *M. fortuitum* in general, although it tends to be susceptible to fluoroquinolones and clarithromycin.[235,236] *Mycobacterium chelonae* tends to be resistant to all commonly used drugs except clarithromycin, gatifloxacin, and linezolid.[89,235–237] MICs for ciprofloxacin, enrofloxacin, moxifloxacin, and pradofloxacin using the broth microdilution method have been reported for feline *M. fortuitum*, *M. goodii*, and *M. smegmatis sensu stricto* isolates.[88,238] In areas where *M. smegmatis* and *M. fortuitum* complex infections predominate, treatment should commence empirically with a newer-generation fluoroquinolone (pradofloxacin or moxifloxacin). Where *M. chelonae* infections are more commonly diagnosed, the best first-line choice is clarithromycin or azithromycin. Multidrug therapy is recommended to reduce selection for resistant strains. In refractory cases, clofazimine, cefoxitin, linezolid, or amikacin may be used if indicated by drug susceptibility data. Cats should be reassessed every few weeks to monitor response to treatment. Cure may be achieved with medical therapy alone; however, some cases eventually become refractory to treatment, requiring wide, sometimes radical, surgical resection of residual infection, and then continuation of appropriate antibiotics for months. Referral to a board-certified surgeon is strongly recommended. The use of advanced reconstructive techniques and vacuum-assisted drainage may facilitate cure in some cases.[216] The total duration of therapy for mycobacterial panniculitis is usually 3 to 12 months. As for cats, panniculitis caused by rapid-growing NTM in dogs has been successfully treated using combination therapy combined with surgical excision of lesions, although relapse can occur.[201,239]

Empiric treatment of pneumonia caused by RGM should consist of either pradofloxacin or clarithromycin with adjustment based on susceptibility data. Pulmonary lesions that are refractory to appropriate medical therapy may need surgical resection, and antibiotic therapy should then be continued postoperatively for several months.

IMMUNITY AND VACCINATION

There are no vaccines for rapid-growing NTM infections.

PREVENTION

Because infections are associated with cutaneous inoculation of environmental organisms, housing cats indoors may reduce the risk of infection.

PUBLIC HEALTH ASPECTS

Rapid-growing NTM are opportunistic, environmental mycobacteria that are not usually transmitted from animals to humans. Disease in humans resembles that in dogs and cats. Localized cutaneous and soft-tissue infections with rapid-growing NTM have occurred after traumatic wounds and lacerations, including after dog and cat bites.[240,241] Infections with RGM have also occurred after surgical procedures like liposuction, LASIK surgery, and acupuncture.[242]

FASTIDIOUS NON-TUBERCULOUS MYCOBACTERIAL INFECTIONS

ETIOLOGY AND EPIDEMIOLOGY

Fastidious mycobacteria cannot be cultured by routine laboratory methods and have an enigmatic ecological niche. They generally cause nodular cutaneous lesions in dogs or cats. Genetic studies of fastidious mycobacteria typically group some of them amongst the slow growers, while others form a separate group containing *Mycobacterium leprae* and related bacteria.

Cats

To date, *Mycobacterium lepraemurium* (closely related to *M. avium*), "*Candidatus* Mycobacterium tarwinense" (related to the *M. simiae* group), *M. visibile*, and "*Candidatus* M. lepraefelis" (both related to *M. leprae* and *M. lepromatosis*) have been associated with feline leprosy syndrome (FLS). Infections have been reported from New Zealand,[243,244] eastern Australia,[245,246] western Canada,[247,248] the United Kingdom,[249,250] south-western USA,[251] the Netherlands,[252] France,[253,254] New Caledonia, Italy,[255] the Greek island of Kythira,[256] and Japan.[257] Affected cats have ranged in age from 1 year to 14 years and are often from rural or semi-rural environments. Inoculation of organisms into the skin through rodent bites or cat fight wounds is the suspected mode of transmission.

Historically, feline leprosy was divided into a tuberculoid form of disease which classically affected young cats with few mycobacteria being seen within the lesions, and a separate, leproid form which affected older cats, with numerous mycobacteria.[258] The pathologic picture now appears to depend more on the infective species rather than patient demographics, with most infections caused by "*Candidatus* M. tarwinense" and "*Candidatus* M. lepraefelis" being leproid in nature (91–95%), whereas just over half (58%) of the *M. lepraemurium* cases were of this pathologic type in one study.[259–261]

Dogs

Disease in dogs is known as canine leproid granuloma syndrome (CLGS). CLGS is caused by an as-yet uncharacterized, fastidious mycobacterium related to "*Candidatus* M. tarwinense" and *M. simiae*. Most reports have been from Australia,[262] New Zealand,[263,264] Brazil,[265–267] and the USA.[268] Zimbabwe[269] and Colombia have also reported cases. In 2014, a case was reported from Europe (Italy) for the first time[270] and cases have continued to be confirmed since.[271] Cases have also been suspected in dogs with a history of travel into the United Kingdom (authors' unpublished data). The mode of transmission to dogs is unknown. Transmission by biting insects has been hypothesized because most lesions occur on the pinnae and head. Possibly over-represented breeds include boxer and boxer mixes, Staffordshire bull terriers, German shepherd dogs, foxhounds, and Doberman pinschers. Short-coated hunting dogs, especially spaniels, may also be predisposed; active hunting work is a risk factor for infection.[264,268]

CLINICAL FEATURES

Pathogenesis, Clinical Signs, and Physical Examination Findings

Cats

In cats, infections caused by fastidious NTM typically manifest as single or multiple cutaneous and/or subcutaneous nodules on the head, limbs, or trunk and regional lymph nodes.[258,272] As with slow-growing NTM infections, nodules are typically non-painful and not adherent to underlying tissues. Skin over the lesions may be intact, alopecic, or ulcerated. Lesions caused by *M. lepraemurium* and "*Candidatus* M. lepraefelis" tend to be found on the head, limbs, and trunk; or may be widespread, involving many cutaneous sites.[258] Lesions caused by "*Candidatus* M. tarwinense" are mostly found on the head (particularly the eyes, lips, or mouth and thoracic limbs, and are not typically widespread.[272] Cats with *M. visibile* infection,[273] and at least one cat infected with "*Candidatus* M. lepraefelis",[260] have systemic involvement at necropsy.

Dogs

In dogs, firm cutaneous nodules are primarily localized on the head, especially the dorsal fold of the pinnae (Fig. 61.19), but may also be located on the lateral trunk, caudal dorsal area, and/or limbs. Nodules range in diameter from millimeters to several centimeters. Lesions may be singular or coalesce to cover large areas. As lesions get larger, they may ulcerate and can become pruritic if secondarily infected.[181] Affected dogs are typically systemically well; there is no involvement of draining lymph nodes, contiguous structures, or internal organs.

DIAGNOSIS

Diagnosis of fastidious NTM infections is based on the presence of consistent skin lesions, absence of signs of dissemination or systemic illness, suggestive cytologic and histopathologic findings, negative mycobacterial culture results, and positive 16S rRNA gene PCR assay results where PCR assays are available. Cytologic examination of fine-needle aspirates usually reveals pyogranulomatous inflammation with intracellular, negatively stained bacteria, which subsequently stain with acid-fast stains. Sequence analysis of PCR products that are generated from biopsy specimens is required to determine the likely species present.

TREATMENT

There have been rare instances of spontaneous resolution of feline leprosy, especially when *M. lepraemurium* is involved,[274] although most cases require treatment for cure. Viability assays that use *M. lepraemurium* grown in cell culture suggest a high degree of susceptibility to rifampicin and clofazimine.[275] Although *M. lepraemurium* appears to be somewhat susceptible to dapsone,[276] adverse effects of hepato- and neurotoxicity and blood dyscrasias limit the use of this drug in cats. Wide surgical resection of nodular skin lesions, plus clarithromycin combined with rifampicin, pradofloxacin, or moxifloxacin (with or without clofazimine) appears to be efficacious.[181,258]

CLGS typically resolves spontaneously within 1 to 3 months of diagnosis.[265,268,275] The efficacy of reported treatments is difficult to establish; however, occasionally persistent infections of greater than 3 to 6 months are observed, and in these instances treatment with antimycobacterial agents is probably warranted. Where lesions are localized, minimal surgical resection and then adjunctive medical therapy is frequently curative. Combination antibiotics with activity against slow-growing mycobacteria are appropriate choices, for example, pradofloxacin/moxifloxacin, rifampicin, clofazimine, and/or clarithromycin. Some authors report successful use of topical clofazimine in silver sulfasalazine, with or without dimethyl sulfoxide.[2]

IMMUNITY, VACCINATION, AND PREVENTION

See rapid-growing NTM infections.

PUBLIC HEALTH ASPECTS

There are no reports of transmission of fastidious NTM from companion animals to humans.

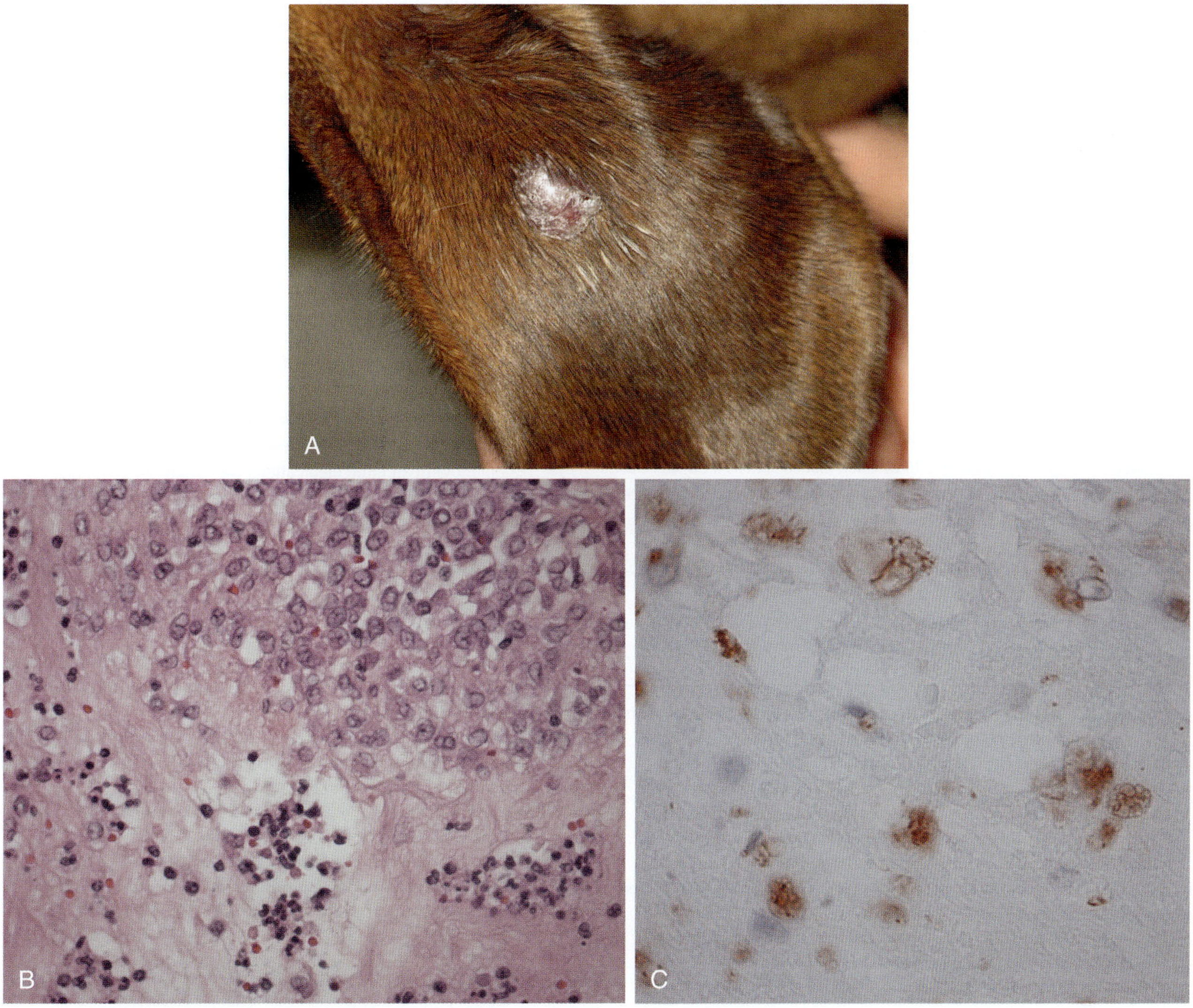

Fig. 61.19 Pinna of a 5-year-old male neutered boxer dog with canine leproid granuloma syndrome (CGLS). (A) A crusted lesion was present that measured 1 × 2 cm in diameter. (B) Histopathology of the CLGS lesions reveals pyogranulomatous inflammation. (C) A BCG immunostain (brown) identified the presence of intracellular *Mycobacterium* spp. organisms.

CASE EXAMPLE

Signalment

A 9-year-old, female neutered domestic shorthair cat that resided within the United Kingdom.

History

The cat was examined by a veterinarian for a mass on the left antebrachium. The owner reported the mass had been steadily increasing in size for 3 weeks. The cat was otherwise well. The cat had outdoor access and was a known avid hunter of local wildlife including birds and small rodents. There were no current medications or significant medical history.

Physical Examination

On physical examination, there was a raised, crusting, erythematous dermal nodular mass 2 cm in diameter over the cranial aspect of the left antebrachium, 3 cm proximal to the carpal joint. The left superficial cervical and left mandibular lymph nodes were mildly enlarged. Body weight was 4.4 kg with a body condition score of 5/9. No other abnormalities were present on the remainder of the clinical examination. The cat was prescribed a 7-day course of oral amoxicillin-clavulanate and meloxicam at standard doses.

On examination after the 7-day course of treatment, there was no change in the lesion or lymph nodes. The cat was anesthetized and incisional biopsies were taken from the lesion and both lymph nodes. The lesion biopsy was bisected and half was frozen in a sterile container while the remaining section and the sections of lymph node were fixed in formalin and submitted for histopathologic examination.

All specimens had multifocal, variably sized areas of necrosis with almost total effacement of the normal tissue. There was infiltration by large numbers of inflammatory cells comprising mostly of reactive (epithelioid) macrophages with enlarged nuclei and copious vacuolated cytoplasm. The macrophage infiltrate

Continued

CASE EXAMPLE—cont'd

was admixed with smaller numbers of mature and degenerate neutrophils and sparse numbers of lymphocytes, plasma cells, and reactive fibroblasts. Histologic diagnosis was chronic active necrotizing pyogranulomatous inflammation. ZN staining revealed rare, intracellular, slender, curved acid-fast bacilli that were consistent with mycobacteria.

Laboratory Findings

Hematology was unremarkable. On serum biochemistry, total serum calcium concentration was increased, but serum ionized calcium concentration was normal.

Imaging Findings

Thoracic radiographs were unremarkable.

Infectious Disease Testing

The cat was negative for both FeLV antigen and FIV antibody (SNAP, IDEXX Laboratories). IGRA revealed a significant response to all three test conditions (PPDA, PPDB, and ESAT-6/CFP-10) with a greater response to PPDB than PPDA; this suggested infection with a member of the MTBC other than *M. microti,* which in the United Kingdom was taken to be indicative of *M. bovis* infection.

To confirm the causative agent, the frozen section of the lesion biopsy was submitted to the Animal and Plant Health Agency for mycobacterial culture. After 8 weeks, *M. bovis* was isolated. Molecular typing resulted in identification of the isolate spoligotype, the same strain that had been isolated from infected cattle in the region.

Diagnosis

Mycobacterium bovis infection.

Treatment

Treatment with pradofloxacin (15 mg PO q24h), 50 mg azithromycin (50 mg PO q24h), and 50 mg rifampicin (50 mg PO q24h) was commenced.

After 1 month, repeat examination revealed resolution of all previously detectable gross abnormalities. Repeat hematology and serum biochemistry were unremarkable, showing only a mild increase in the activities of serum ALT and ALP. Treatment with all three medications was therefore continued for a further 2 months before cessation. The cat remained clinically normal one year after discontinuation of treatment.

SUGGESTED READINGS

Gunn-Moore DA, McFarland SE, Brewer JI, et al. Mycobacterial disease in cats in Great Britain: I. Culture results, geographical distribution and clinical presentation of 339 cases. *J Fel Med Surg.* 2011;13:934–944.

Gunn-Moore DA, McFarland SE, Schock A, et al. Mycobacterial disease in a population of 339 cats in Great Britain: II. Histopathology of 225 cases, and treatment and outcome of 184 cases. *J Fel Med Surg.* 2011;13:945–952.

Malik R, Smits B, Reppas G, Laprie C, O'Brien C, Fyfe J. Ulcerated and nonulcerated nontuberculous cutaneous mycobacterial granulomas in cats and dogs. *Vet Dermatol.* 2013;24:146–153.

Lloret A, Hartmann K, Pennisi MG, et al. Mycobacterioses in cats: ABCD guidelines on prevention and management. *J Fel Med Surg.* 2013;15:591–597.

REFERENCES

1. Sakula A. Robert Koch: centenary of the discovery of the tubercle bacillus. *Thorax.* 1882;1982(37):246–251.
2. Hershkovitz I, Donoghue HD, Minnikin DE, et al. Detection and molecular characterization of 9000-year-old *Mycobacterium tuberculosis* from a Neolithic settlement in the eastern Mediterranean. *PLoS One.* 2008;3:e3426.
3. Rothschild BM, Martin LD, Lev G, et al. *Mycobacterium tuberculosis* complex DNA from an extinct bison dated 17,000 years before the present. *Clin Infect Dis.* 2001;33:305–311.
4. Achtman M. How old are bacterial pathogens? *Proc R Soc B.* 2016; 20160990.
5. Cosivi O, Grange J, Daborn C, et al. Zoonotic tuberculosis due to *Mycobacterium bovis* in developing countries. *Emerg Infect Dis.* 1998;4:59.
6. Griffith DE, Aksamit T, Brown-Elliott BA, et al. An official ATS/IDSA statement: diagnosis, treatment, and prevention of nontuberculous mycobacterial diseases. *Am J Respir Crit Care Med.* 2007;175:367–416.
7. Runyon EH. Identification of mycobacterial pathogens utilizing colony characteristics. *Am J Clin Pathol.* 1970;54:578–586.
8. Jagielski T, Minias A, van Ingen J, et al. Methodological and clinical aspects of the molecular epidemiology of *Mycobacterium tuberculosis* and other mycobacteria. *Clin Microbiol Rev.* 2016;29:239–290.
9. Kim C-J, Kim N-H, Song K-H, et al. Differentiating rapid-and slow-growing mycobacteria by difference in time to growth detection in liquid media. *Diagn Microbiol Infect Dis.* 2013;75:73–76.
10. Rufenacht S, Bogli-Stuber K, Bodmer T, et al. *Mycobacterium microti* infection in the cat: a case report, literature review and recent clinical experience. *J Feline Med Surg.* 2011;13:195–204.
11. Gunn-Moore DA, Jenkins PA, Lucke VM. Feline tuberculosis: a literature review and discussion of 19 cases caused by an unusual mycobacterial variant. *Vet Rec.* 1996;138:53–58.
12. Bennett AD, Lalor S, Schwarz T, et al. Radiographic findings in cats with mycobacterial infections. *J Feline Med Surg.* 2011;13:718–724.
13. Gunn-Moore DA, McFarland SE, Brewer JI, et al. Mycobacterial disease in cats in Great Britain: I. Culture results, geographical distribution and clinical presentation of 339 cases. *J Feline Med Surg.* 2011;13:934–944.
14. Haligur M, Vural SA, Sahal M, et al. Generalised tuberculosis in a cat. *Bulletin-Veterinary Institute In Pulawy.* 2007;51:531.
15. Gunn-Moore DA, McFarland SE, Schock A, et al. Mycobacterial disease in a population of 339 cats in Great Britain: II. Histopathology of 225 cases, and treatment and outcome of 184 cases. *J Feline Med Surg.* 2011;13:945–952.
16. Cavanagh R, Begon M, Bennett M, et al. *Mycobacterium microti* infection (vole tuberculosis) in wild rodent populations. *J Clin Microbiol.* 2002;40:3281–3285.
17. Delahay RJ, Smith GC, Barlow AM, et al. Bovine tuberculosis infection in wild mammals in the South-West region of England: a survey of prevalence and a semi-quantitative assessment of the relative risks to cattle. *Vet J.* 2007;173:287–301.
18. Sweeney F, Courtenay O, Hibberd V, et al. Environmental monitoring of *Mycobacterium bovis* in badger feces and badger sett soil by real-time PCR, as confirmed by immunofluorescence, immunocapture, and cultivation. *Appl Environ Microbiol.* 2007;73:7471–7473.
19. de Lisle GW, Collins DM, Loveday AS, et al. A report of tuberculosis in cats in New Zealand, and the examination of strains of *Mycobacterium bovis* by DNA restriction endonuclease analysis. *N Z Vet J.* 1990;38:10–13.
20. Zumarraga MJ, Vivot MM, Marticorena D, et al. *Mycobacterium bovis* in Argentina: isolates from cats typified by spoligotyping. *Rev Argent Microbiol.* 2009;41:215–217.
21. Kaneene JB, Bruning-Fann CS, Dunn J, et al. Epidemiologic investigation of *Mycobacterium bovis* in a population of cats. *Am J Vet Res.* 2002;63:1507–1511.
22. Ramdas KE, Lyashchenko KP, Greenwald R, et al. *Mycobacterium bovis* infection in humans and cats in same household, Texas, USA. *Emerg Infect Dis.* 2012;2015(21):480–483.
23. Roberts T, O'Connor Ç, Nuñez-Garcia J, et al. Short communication: unusual cluster of *Mycobacterium bovis* infection in cats. *Vet Rec.* 2014;174:326.

24. Isaac J, Whitehead J, Adams JW, et al. An outbreak of *Mycobacterium bovis* infection in cats in an animal house. *Aust Vet J.* 1983;60:243–245.
25. Černá P, O'Halloran C, SjatkovskaJ O, Gunn-Moore DA. Outbreak of tuberculosis caused by *Mycobacterium bovis* in a cattery of Abyssinian cats in Italy. *Transbound Emerg Dis.* 2019;66(1):250–258.
26. Murray A, Dineen A, Kelly P, et al. Nosocomial spread of *Mycobacterium bovis* in domestic cats. *J Fel Med Surg.* 2015;17:173–180.
27. Murray A, Dineen A, Kelly P, et al. Nosocomial spread of *Mycobacterium bovis* in domestic cats. *J Feline Med Surg.* 2015;17:173–180.
28. Hawthorne VM, Lauder IM. Tuberculosis in man, dog, and cat. *Am Rev Respir Dis.* 1962;85:858–869.
29. Parodi A, Fontaine M, Brion A, et al. Mycobacterial infections of domestic carnivores. Present epidemiology of tuberculosis in dogs and cats. *Recl Med Vet.* 1965;141:421–432.
30. Snider WR, Cohen D, Reif JS, et al. Tuberculosis in canine and feline populations. Study of high risk populations in Pennsylvania, 1966-1968. *Am Rev Respir Dis.* 1971;104:866–876.
31. Saini D, Hopkins GW, Seay SA, et al. Ultra-low dose of *Mycobacterium tuberculosis* aerosol creates partial infection in mice. *Tuberculosis.* 2012;92:160–165.
32. Parsons SD, Gous TA, Warren RM, et al. Pulmonary *Mycobacterium tuberculosis* (Beijing strain) infection in a stray dog. *J S Afr Vet Assoc.* 2008;79:95–98.
33. Foster ES, Scavelli TD, Greenlee PG, et al. Cutaneous lesion caused by *Mycobacterium tuberculosis* in a dog. *J Am Vet Med Assoc.* 1986;188:1188–1190.
34. Sykes JE, Cannon AB, Norris AJ, et al. *Mycobacterium tuberculosis* complex infection in a dog. *J Vet Intern Med.* 2007;21:1108–1112.
35. Martinho AP, Franco MM, Ribeiro MG, et al. Disseminated *Mycobacterium tuberculosis* infection in a dog. *Am J Trop Med Hyg.* 2013;88:596–600.
36. Botelho A, Perdigao J, Canto A, et al. Pre-multidrug-resistant *Mycobacterium tuberculosis* Beijing strain associated with disseminated tuberculosis in a pet dog. *J Clin Microbiol.* 2014;52:354–356.
37. Engelmann N, Ondreka N, Michalik J, et al. Intra-abdominal *Mycobacterium tuberculosis* infection in a dog. *J Vet Intern Med.* 2014;28:934–938.
38. Aranaz A, Liébana E, Pickering X, et al. Use of polymerase chain reaction in the diagnosis of tuberculosis in cats and dogs. *Vet Rec.* 1996;138:276–280.
39. Clercx C, Coignoul F, Jakovljevic S, et al. Tuberculosis in dogs: a case report and review of the literature. *J Am Anim Hosp Assoc.* 1992;28:207–211.
40. Liu S, Weitzman I, Johnson GG. Canine tuberculosis. *J Am Vet Med Assoc.* 1980;177:164–167.
41. Lovell R, White E. Naturally occurring tuberculosis in dogs and some other species of animals. *Br J Tuberculosis.* 1940;34:117–133.
42. Une Y, Mori T. Tuberculosis as a zoonosis from a veterinary perspective. *Comp Immunol Microbiol Infect Dis.* 2007;30:415–425.
43. Rocha VC, Figueiredo SC, Rosales CA, et al. Infection by *Mycobacterium bovis* in a dog from Brazil. *Braz J Microbiol.* 2017;48:109–112.
44. Turinelli V, Ledieu D, Guilbaud L, et al. *Mycobacterium tuberculosis* infection in a dog from Africa. *Vet Clin Pathol.* 2004;33:177–181.
45. Deforges L, Boulouis HJ, Thibaud JL, et al. First isolation of *Mycobacterium microti* (Llama-type) from a dog. *Vet Microbiol.* 2004;103:249–253.
46. van der Burgt GM, Crawshaw T, Foster AP, et al. *Mycobacterium bovis* infection in dogs. *Vet Rec.* 2009;165:634.
47. Ellis MD, Davies S, McCandlish IA, et al. *Mycobacterium bovis* infection in a dog. *Vet Rec.* 2006;159:46–48.
48. Shrikrishna D, de la Rua-Domenech R, Smith NH, et al. Human and canine pulmonary *Mycobacterium bovis* infection in the same household: re-emergence of an old zoonotic threat? *Thorax.* 2009;64:89–91.
49. O'Halloran C, Hope JC, Dobromylskj M, et al. An outbreak of tubercu losis due to *Mycobacterium bovis* infection in a pack of English foxhounds (2016–2017). *Transbound Emerg Dis.* 2018;65:1872–1884.
50. Posthaus H, Bodmer T, Alves L, et al. Accidental infection of veterinary personnel with *Mycobacterium tuberculosis* at necropsy: a case study. *Vet Microbiol.* 2011;149:374–380.
51. Hackendahl NC, Mawby DI, Bemis DA, et al. Putative transmission of *Mycobacterium tuberculosis* infection from a human to a dog. *J Am Vet Med Assoc.* 2004;225:1573–1577. 1548.
52. Erwin PC, Bemis DA, McCombs SB, et al. *Mycobacterium tuberculosis* transmission from human to canine. *Emerg Infect Dis.* 2004;10:2258. 2210.
53. Vangone L, Cardillo L, Riccardi MG, et al. *Mycobacterium tuberculosis* SIT42 infection in an abused dog in southern Italy. *Front Vet Sci.* 2021;8:653360.
54. Talwar A, McGown A, Langham T, et al. A very strange tail. *Thorax.* 2014;69:1159–1160.
55. Formston C. Retinal detachment and bovine tuberculosis in cats. *J Small Anim Pract.* 1994;35:5–8.
56. Monti F. A clinical and radiological study of tuberculous osteo-arthritis (in a cat) treated with isoniazid. *Vet Ital.* 1956;7:871–884.
57. Bauer NB, O'Neill E, Sheahan BJ, et al. Calcospherite-like bodies and caseous necrosis in tracheal mucus from a dog with tuberculosis. *Vet Clin Pathol.* 2004;33:168–172.
58. Chan TY, Chan CH, Shek CC. The prevalence of hypercalcaemia in pulmonary and miliary tuberculosis—a longitudinal study. *Singapore Med J.* 1994;35:613–615.
59. Roussos A, Lagogianni I, Gonis A, et al. Hypercalcaemia in Greek patients with tuberculosis before the initiation of anti-tuberculosis treatment. *Resp Med.* 2001;95:187–190.
60. Morley J, Gunn-Moore D, Hope J. Investigating vitamin D metabolism in cats with tuberculosis caused by infection with *Mycobacterium bovis* and *Mycobacterium microti. J Small Anim Pract.* 2016;57:60.
61. Lalor S, Mellanby R, Friend E, et al. Domesticated cats with active mycobacteria infections have low serum vitamin D (25 (OH) D) concentrations. *Transbound Emerg Dis.* 2012;59:279–281.
62. Major A, Holmes A, Warren-Smith C, et al. Computed tomographic findings in cats with mycobacterial infection. *J Feline Med Surg.* 2016;18(6):510–517.
63. Greene CE, Gunn-Moore DA. Infections caused by slow-growing mycobacteria. In: Greene CE, ed. *Infectious Diseases of the Dog and Cat.* 4th ed. St Louis, MO: Elsevier Saunders; 2012:495–510.
64. Whitworth HS, Scott M, Connell DW, et al. IGRAs–the gateway to T cell based TB diagnosis. *Methods.* 2013;61:52–62.
65. Pollock NR, Kashino SS, Napolitano DR, et al. Evaluation of the effect of treatment of latent tuberculosis infection on QuantiFERON-TB gold assay results. *Infect Control Hosp Epidemiol.* 2009;30:392–395.
66. Bienek D, Chang C. Evaluation of an interferon-gamma release assay, T-SPOT®. TB, in a population with a low prevalence of tuberculosis. *Int J Tuberc Lung Dis.* 2009;13:1416–1421.
67. Khalili T, Nakhaee A, Salehi M, et al. A validity study of the QuantiFERON-TB Gold (QFT-TB) method for the diagnosis of pulmonary tuberculosis in a high risk population. *Swiss Med Wkly.* 2010;140:95–96.
68. Rhodes SG, Gruffydd-Jones T, Gunn-Moore D, et al. Adaptation of IFN-gamma ELISA and ELISPOT tests for feline tuberculosis. *Vet Immunol Immunopathol.* 2008;124:379–384.
69. Pym AS, Brodin P, Brosch R, et al. Loss of RD1 contributed to the attenuation of the live tuberculosis vaccines *Mycobacterium bovis* BCG and *Mycobacterium microti. Mol Microbiol.* 2002;46:709–717.
70. Rhodes SG, Gruffydd-Jones T, Gunn-Moore D, et al. Interferon-gamma test for feline tuberculosis. *Vet Rec.* 2008;162:453–455.
71. Rhodes SG, Gunn-Moore D, Boschiroli ML, et al. Comparative study of IFN-gamma and antibody tests for feline tuberculosis. *Vet Immunol Immunopathol.* 2011;144:129–134.
72. Mitchell JL, Stanley P, McDonald K, et al. Diagnostic accuracy of the interferon-gamma release assay (IGRA) for cases of feline mycobacteriosis. *Prev Vet Med.* 2021;193:10540.
73. Saleeb PG, Drake SK, Murray PR, et al. Identification of mycobacteria in solid-culture media by matrix-assisted laser desorption ionization-time of flight mass spectrometry. *J Clin Microbiol.* 2011;49:1790–1794.
74. Botelho A, Perdigão J, Canto A, et al. Pre-multidrug-resistant Mycobacterium tuberculosis Beijing strain associated with disseminated tuberculosis in a pet dog. *J Clin Microbiol.* 2014;52:354–356.
75. Mitchell JL, Del Pozo J, Woolley CSC, et al. Histological and immunohistochemical features suggesting aetiological differences in lymph node and (muco)cutaneous feline tuberculosis lesions. *J Small Anim Pract.* 2021;Jun 7. Online ahead of print.

76. Engel NC. The making of a public health problem: multi-drug resistant tuberculosis in India. *Health Policy Plan*. 2013;28:375–385.
77. Udwadia ZF. Totally drug-resistant tuberculosis in India: Who let the djinn out? *Respirology*. 2012;17:741–742.
78. Maeurer M, Schito M, Zumla A. Totally-drug-resistant tuberculosis: hype versus hope. *Lancet Resp Med*. 2014;2:256.
79. Nahid P, Dorman SE, Alipanah N, et al. Executive summary: official American Thoracic Society/Centers for Disease Control and Prevention/Infectious Diseases Society of America clinical practice guidelines: treatment of drug-susceptible tuberculosis. *Clin Infect Dis*. 2016;63:853–867.
80. Frank I, Lahav D, Aroch I. Myocardial necrosis and severe metabolic acidosis associated with isoniazid poisoning in a dog. *Vet Rec*. 2002;151:638–639.
81. Tateishi J. Comparative study of neurotoxicity of clioquinol, ethambutol, isoniazid and chloramphenicol in dogs. *Psychiatry Clin Neurosci*. 1974;28:11–17.
82. Haburjak J, Spangler W. Isoniazid-induced seizures with secondary rhabdomyolysis and associated acute renal failure in a dog. *J Small Anim Pract*. 2002;43:182–186.
83. Chin L, Sievers ML, Herrier RN, et al. Convulsions as the etiology of lactic acidosis in acute isoniazid toxicity in dogs. *Toxicol Appl Pharmacol*. 1979;49:377–384.
84. Doherty T. Isoniazid poisoning in a dog. *Vet Rec*. 1982;111:460. 460.
85. De Jong BC, Onipede A, Pym AS, et al. Does resistance to pyrazinamide accurately indicate the presence of. *Mycobacterium bovis? J Clin Microbiol*. 2005;43:3530–3532.
86. Yun J, Sung H, Kim T, et al. Comparison of the clinical characteristics of *Mycobacterium tuberculosis* and nontuberculous mycobacteria patients with joint involvement. *Infection*. 2015;43:207–209.
87. Vincent V. Bone and joint infections due to opportunistic mycobacteria, a review of French experience. *Int J Mycobacteriol*. 2015;4:8.
88. Govendir M, Hansen T, Kimble B, et al. Susceptibility of rapidly growing mycobacteria isolated from cats and dogs, to ciprofloxacin, enrofloxacin and moxifloxacin. *Vet Microbiol*. 2011;147:113–118.
89. Brown-Elliott BA, Wallace Jr RJ, Crist CJ, et al. Comparison of in vitro activities of gatifloxacin and ciprofloxacin against four taxa of rapidly growing mycobacteria. *Antimicrob Agents Chemother*. 2002;46:3283–3285.
90. Murphy BS, Sundareshan V, Cory TJ, et al. Azithromycin alters macrophage phenotype. *J Antimicrob Chemother*. 2008;61:554–560.
91. Baldwin D, Wise R, Andrews J, et al. Azithromycin concentrations at the sites of pulmonary infection. *Eur Resp J*. 1990;3:886–890.
92. Javid B, Sorrentino F, Toosky M, et al. Mycobacterial mistranslation is necessary and sufficient for rifampicin phenotypic resistance. *Proc Nat Acad Sci*. 2014;111:1132–1137.
93. Kyokawa Y, Nishibe Y, Wakabayashi M, et al. Induction of intestinal cytochrome P450 (CYP3A) by rifampicin in beagle dogs. *Chem Biol Interact*. 2001;134:291–305.
94. Reinach B, de Sousa G, Dostert P, et al. Comparative effects of rifabutin and rifampicin on cytochromes P450 and UDP-glucuronosyl-transferases expression in fresh and cryopreserved human hepatocytes. *Chem Biol Interact*. 1999;121:37–48.
95. de Sousa JS, Almeida V, Pinheiro JB. Red child syndrome. *Arch Dis Child*. 1987;62:1181. 1181.
96. Major A, O'Halloran C, Holmes A, et al. Use of computed tomography imaging during long-term follow-up of nine feline tuberculosis cases. *J Feline Med Surg*. 2017. 1098612X17699476.
97. Mitchell JL, O'Halloran C, Stanley P, et al. Serial interferon-gamma release assay (IGRA) testing to monitor treatment responses in cats with feline mycobacteriosis. *Pathogens*. 2021;10:657.
98. Thorel MF, Boisvert H. Abscess due to *Mycobacterium chelonei* in a cat. *Bull Acad Vet Fr*. 1974;47:415–422.
99. O'Halloran C, Tørnqvist-Johnsen C, Woods G, et al. Feline tuberculosis caused by Mycobacterium bovis infection of domestic UK cats associated with feeding a commercial raw food diet. *Transbound Emerg Dis*. 2021;68:2308–2320.
100. Xavier Emmanuel F, Seagar AL, Doig C, et al. Human and animal infections with *Mycobacterium microti*. Scotland. *Emerg Infect Dis*. 2007;13:1924–1927.
101. Schwartz NG, Price SF, Pratt RH, et al. Tuberculosis - United States, 2019. *MMWR*. 2020;69:286–289.
102. Whiley H, Keegan A, Giglio S, et al. *Mycobacterium avium* complex—the role of potable water in disease transmission. *J Appl Microbiol*. 2012;113:223–232.
103. Mijs W, de Haas P, Rossau R, et al. Molecular evidence to support a proposal to reserve the designation *Mycobacterium avium* subsp. *avium* for bird-type isolates and '*M. avium* subsp. *hominissuis*' for the human/porcine type of *M. avium*. *Int J Syst Evol Microbiol*. 52:1505–1518.
104. Tortoli E, Meehan CJ, Grottola A, et al. Genome-based taxonomic revision detects a number of synonymous taxa in the genus *Mycobacterium*. *Infect Genetics Evolution*. 2019;75:103983.
105. Haist V, Seehusen F, Moser I, et al. *Mycobacterium avium* subsp. *hominissuis* infection in 2 pet dogs. Germany. *Emerg Infect Dis*. 2008;14:988–990.
106. Campora L, Corazza M, Zullino C, et al. *Mycobacterium avium* subspecies *hominissuis* disseminated infection in a Basset hound dog. *J Vet Diagn Invest*. 2011;23:1083–1087.
107. de Groot PH, van Ingen J, de Zwaan R, et al. Disseminated *Mycobacterium avium* subsp. *avium* infection in a cat, The Netherlands. *Vet Microbiol*. 2010;144:527–529.
108. Glanemann B, Schonenbrucher H, Bridger N, et al. Detection of *Mycobacterium avium* subspecies *paratuberculosis*-specific DNA by PCR in intestinal biopsies of dogs. *J Vet Intern Med*. 2008;22:1090–1094.
109. Miller MA, Davey SC, Van Helden LS, et al. Paratuberculosis in a domestic dog in South Africa. *J S Afr Vet Assoc*. 2017;88:e1–e5.
110. Riviere D, Pingret JL, Etievant M, et al. Disseminated *Mycobacterium avium* subspecies infection in a cat. *J Feline Med Surg*. 2011;13:125–128.
111. Bukka A, Price CT, Kernodle DS, et al. *Mycobacterium tuberculosis* RNA expression patterns in sputum bacteria indicate secreted esx factors contributing to growth are highly expressed in active disease. *Front Microbiol*. 2011;2:266.
112. Baral RM, Metcalfe SS, Krockenberger MB, et al. Disseminated *Mycobacterium avium* infection in young cats: overrepresentation of Abyssinian cats. *J Feline Med Surg*. 2006;8:23–44.
113. Sieber-Ruckstuhl NS, Sessions JK, Sanchez S, et al. Long-term cure of disseminated *Mycobacterium avium* infection in a cat. *Vet Rec*. 2007;160:131–132.
114. Griffin A, Newton AL, Aronson LR, et al. Disseminated *Mycobacterium avium* complex infection following renal transplantation in a cat. *J Am Vet Med Assoc*. 2003;222:1097–1101. 1077-1098.
115. Knippel A, Hetzel U, Baumgartner W. Disseminated *Mycobacterium avium-intracellulare* infection in a Persian cat. *J Vet Med B Infect Dis Vet Public Health*. 2004;51:464–466.
116. Malik R, Gabor L, Martin P, et al. Subcutaneous granuloma caused by *Mycobacterium avium* complex infection in a cat. *Aust Vet J*. 1998;76:604–607.
117. Miller MA, Fales WH, McCracken WS, et al. Inflammatory pseudotumor in a cat with cutaneous mycobacteriosis. *Vet Pathol*. 1999;36:161–163.
118. Drolet R. Disseminated tuberculosis caused by *Mycobacterium avium* in a cat. *J Am Vet Med Assoc*. 1986;189:1336–1337.
119. Stewart L, White S, Kennedy F, et al. Cutaneous *Mycobacterium avium* infection in a cat. *Vet Dermatol*. 1993;4:87–90.
120. Jordan HL, Cohn LA, Armstrong PJ. Disseminated *Mycobacterium avium* complex infection in three Siamese cats. *J Am Vet Med Assoc*. 1994;204:90–93.
121. Suter MM, von Rotz A, Weiss R, et al. Atypical mycobacterial skin granuloma in a cat in Switzerland. *Zentralbl Veterinarmed A*. 1984;31:712–718.
122. Kaufman AC, Greene CE, Rakich PM, et al. Treatment of localized *Mycobacterium avium* complex infection with clofazimine and doxycycline in a cat. *J Am Vet Med Assoc*. 1995;207:457–459.
123. Perkins PC, Grindem CB, Levy JK. What is your diagnosis? An 11-year-old domestic longhaired cat with anemia. *Vet Clin Pathol*. 1995;24(77):97–98.
124. Kipar A, Schiller I, Baumgartner W. Immunopathological studies on feline cutaneous and (muco)cutaneous mycobacteriosis. *Vet Immunol Immunopathol*. 2003;91:169–182.
125. Matthews J, Liggitt H. Disseminated mycobacteriosis in a cat [*Mycobacterium avium*]. *J Am Vet Med Assoc*. 1983;6:701–702.
126. Barry M, Taylor J, Woods JP. Disseminated *Mycobacterium avium* infection in a cat. *Can Vet J*. 2002;43:369–371.
127. Hummel P. Occurrence of atypical mycobacteria in dogs and cats. *Zentralblatt fur Veterinarmedizin*. 1966;13B:51–61.
128. Hix JW, Jones TC, Karlson AG. Avian tubercle bacillus infection in the cat. *J Am Vet Med Assoc*. 1961;138:641–647.

129. Morita Y, Kimur H, Kozawa K, et al. Cutaneous infection in a cat caused by *Mycobacterium avium* complex serovar 6. *Vet Rec.* 2003;152:120.
130. Thegerstrom J, Marklund BI, Hoffner S, et al. *Mycobacterium avium* with the bird type IS1245 RFLP profile is commonly found in wild and domestic animals, but rarely in humans. *Scand J Infect Dis.* 2005;37:15–20.
131. Kriz P, Novakova B, Nagl I, et al. *Mycobacterium avium* subsp. *hominissuis:* generalized infection of cats. *Veterinarstvi.* 2012;62:680–684.
132. Buergelt C, Fowler J, Wright P. Disseminated avian tuberculosis in a cat [*Mycobacterium avium*]. *California Vet.* 1982;10:13–15.
133. Higgins J, Camp P, Farrell D, et al. Identification of *Mycobacterium* spp. of veterinary importance using *rpoB* gene sequencing. *BMC Vet Res.* 2011;7:1.
134. Deykin AR, Wigney DI, Smith JS, et al. Corneal granuloma caused by *Mycobacterium intracellulare* in a cat. *Aust Vet Practit.* 1996;26:23–26.
135. Davies JL, Sibley JA, Myers S, et al. Histological and genotypical characterization of feline cutaneous mycobacteriosis: a retrospective study of formalin-fixed paraffin-embedded tissues. *Vet Dermatol.* 2006;17:155–162.
136. Hughes MS, Ball NW, Love DN, et al. Disseminated *Mycobacterium genavense* infection in a FIV-positive cat. *J Feline Med Surg.* 1999;1:23–29.
137. Hetzel U, Dixon CE, Just AE, et al. *Mycobacterium malmoense* as an extrapulmonary pathogen of cats. *Vet Rec.* 2012;171:274.
138. Henderson SM, Baker J, Williams R, et al. Opportunistic mycobacterial granuloma in a cat associated with a member of the *Mycobacterium terrae* complex. *J Feline Med Surg.* 2003;5:37–41.
139. Dietrich U, Arnold P, Guscetti F, et al. Ocular manifestation of disseminated *Mycobacterium simiae* infection in a cat. *J Small Anim Pract.* 2003;44:121–125.
140. De Lorenzi D, Solano-Gallego L. Tracheal granuloma because of infection with a novel mycobacterial species in an old FIV-positive cat. *J Small Anim Pract.* 2009;50:143–146.
141. MacWilliams PS, Whitley N, Moore F. Lymphadenitis and peritonitis caused by *Mycobacterium xenopi* in a cat. *Vet Clin Pathol.* 1998;27:50–53.
142. Tomasovic AA, Rac R, Purcell DA. *Mycobacterium xenopi* in a skin lesion of a cat. *Aust Vet J.* 1976;52:103.
143. Meeks C, Levy JK, Crawford PC, et al. Chronic disseminated *Mycobacterium xenopi* infection in a cat with idiopathic CD4+ T lymphocytopenia. *J Vet Intern Med.* 2008;22:1043–1047.
144. Elsner L, Wayne J, O'Brien CR, et al. Localised *Mycobacterium ulcerans* infection in a cat in Australia. *J Feline Med Surg.* 2008;10:407–412.
145. Elze J, Grammel L, Richter E, et al. First description of *Mycobacterium heckeshornense* infection in a feline immunodeficiency virus-positive cat. *J Feline Med Surg.* 2013;15:1141–1144.
146. Niederhäuser S, Klauser L, Bolliger J, et al. First report of nodular skin lesions caused by *Mycobacterium nebraskense* in a 9-year-old cat. *JFMS Open Rep.* 2018;4: 2055116918792685. doi:.
147. Lee SH, Go DM, Woo SH, et al. Systemic *Mycobacterium kansasii* infection in a domestic shorthair cat. *J Comp Pathol.* 2017;157(2–3):215–219.
148. Černá P, Mitchell JL, Lodzinska J, et al. Systemic Mycobacterium kansasii infection in two related cats. *Pathogens.* 2020;9:959.
149. Latimer KS, Jameson PH, Crowell WA, et al. Disseminated *Mycobacterium avium* complex infection in a cat: presumptive diagnosis by blood smear examination. *Vet Clin Pathol.* 1997;26:85–89.
150. Graham KJ, Brain PH, Spielman D, et al. Concurrent infection with *Cryptococcus neoformans/gattii* species complex and *Mycobacterium avium* affecting the subcutis and bone of a pelvic limb in a cat. *J Feline Med Surg.* 2011;13:776–780.
151. Armas F, Furlanello T, Camperio C, et al. Molecular characterization and drug susceptibility profile of a *Mycobacterium avium* subspecies *avium* isolate from a dog with disseminated infection. *J Med Microbiol.* 2016;65:278–285.
152. Bende B, Jakab C, Balka G, et al. Systemic *Mycobacterium avium* subsp. *hominissuis* infection in a miniature schnauzer. *Magyar Allatorvosok Lapja.* 2013;135:138–148.
153. Hobi S, Bettenay S, Majzoub M, et al. *Mycobacterium avium* subspecies *hominissuis* infection in a dog from Germany with multifocal alopecia, exfoliative dermatitis, hypercalcaemia and subsequent sebaceous atrophy. *Vet Rec Case Reports.* 2015;3:e000168.
154. O'Brien CR, McMillan E, Harris O, et al. Localised *Mycobacterium ulcerans* infection in four dogs. *Aust Vet J.* 2011;89:506–510.
155. Merritt RW, Walker ED, Small PL, et al. Ecology and transmission of Buruli ulcer disease: a systematic review. *PLoS Negl Trop Dis.* 2010;4. e911.
156. Fyfe JAM, Lavender CJ, Handasyde KA, et al. A major role for mammals in the ecology of *Mycobacterium ulcerans. PLoS Negl Trop Dis.* 2010;4. e791.
157. O'Brien CR, Handasyde KA, Hibble J, et al. Clinical, microbiological and pathological findings of *Mycobacterium ulcerans* infection in three Australian possum species. *PLoS Negl Trop Dis.* 2014;8(1):e2666.
158. Mitchell PJ, Jerrett IV, Slee KJ. Skin ulcers caused by *Mycobacterium ulcerans* in koalas near Bairnsdale, Australia. *Pathology.* 1984;16:256–260.
159. Fyfe JA, Lavender CJ, Handasyde KA, et al. A major role for mammals in the ecology of *Mycobacterium ulcerans. PLoS Negl Trop Dis.* 2010;4:e791.
160. O'Brien C, Kuseff G, McMillan E, et al. *Mycobacterium ulcerans* infection in two alpacas. *Aust Vet J.* 2013;91:296–300.
161. van Zyl A, Daniel J, Wayne J, et al. *Mycobacterium ulcerans* infections in two horses in south-eastern Australia. *Aust Vet J.* 2010;88:101–106.
162. Miller MA, Greene CE, Brix AE. Disseminated *Mycobacterium avium—intracellulare* complex infection in a miniature schnauzer. *J Am Anim Hosp Assoc.* 1995;31:213–216.
163. Sharp E, Taylor S, O'Halloran C. Unusual presentation of canine *Mycobacterium avium* infection. *Vet Rec.* 2019;184:800.
164. Gelendi S, Taylor S, D'Aout C, et al. Mycobacterium avium infection associated with sterile polyarthritis in a dog. *J Small Anim Pract.* 2021; Sep 1. Online ahead of print.
165. Gow AG, Gow DJ. Disseminated *Mycobacterium avium* complex infection in a dog. *Vet Rec.* 2008;162:594–595.
166. Kim DY, Cho DY, Newton JC, et al. Granulomatous myelitis due to *Mycobacterium avium* in a dog. *Vet Pathol.* 1994;31:491–493.
167. Horn B, Forshaw D, Cousins D, et al. Disseminated *Mycobacterium avium* infection in a dog with chronic diarrhoea. *Aust Vet J.* 2000;78:320–325.
168. Bauer N, Burkhardt S, Kirsch A, et al. Lymphadenopathy and diarrhea in a miniature schnauzer. *Vet Clin Pathol.* 2002;31:61–64.
169. O'Toole D, Tharp S, Thomsen BV, et al. Fatal mycobacteriosis with hepatosplenomegaly in a young dog due to *Mycobacterium avium. J Vet Diagn Invest.* 2005;17:200–204.
170. Pressler BM, Hardie EM, Pitulle C, et al. Isolation and identification of *Mycobacterium kansasii* from pleural fluid of a dog with persistent pleural effusion. *J Am Vet Med Assoc.* 2002;220:1336–1340. 1313-1334.
171. Murai A, Maruyama S, Nagata M, et al. Mastitis caused by *Mycobacterium kansasii* infection in a dog. *Vet Clin Pathol.* 2013;42:377–381.
172. Kiehn TE, Hoefer H, Bottger EC, et al. *Mycobacterium genavense* infections in pet animals. *J Clin Microbiol.* 1996;34:1840–1842.
173. Timm K, Welle M, Friedel U, et al. *Mycobacterium nebraskense* infection in a dog in Switzerland with disseminated skin lesions. *Vet Dermatol.* 2019;30:262–e280.
174. Dietrich U, Arnold P, Guscetti F, et al. Ocular manifestation of disseminated *Mycobacterium simiae* infection in a cat. *J Small Anim Pract.* 2003;44:121–125.
175. Stavinohova R, O'Halloran C, Newton JR, et al. Feline ocular mycobacteriosis: clinical presentation, histopathological features, and outcome. *Vet Pathol.* 2019;56:749–760.
176. Deykin AR, Wigney DI, Smith JS, et al. Corneal granuloma caused by *Mycobacterium intracellulare* in a cat. *Aust Vet Practit.* 1996;26:23.
177. Eggers JS, Parker GA, Braaf HA, et al. Disseminated *Mycobacterium avium* infection in three miniature schnauzer litter mates. *J Vet Diagn Invest.* 1997;9:424–427.
178. Naughton JF, Mealey KL, Wardrop KJ, et al. Systemic *Mycobacterium avium* infection in a dog diagnosed by polymerase chain reaction analysis of buffy coat. *J Am Anim Hosp Assoc.* 2005;41:128–132.
179. Radomski N, Thibault VC, Karoui C, et al. Determination of genotypic diversity of *Mycobacterium avium* subspecies from human and animal origins by mycobacterial interspersed repetitive-unit-variable-number tandem-repeat and IS1311 restriction fragment length polymorphism typing methods. *J Clin Microbiol.* 2010;48:1026–1034.
180. Woods GL, Browm-Elliott BA, Conville PS. Susceptibility testing of *Mycobacteria, Nocardiae,* and other aerobic actinomycetes; Approved Standard—Second edition, CLSI document M24-A2. *Clinical and Laboratory Standards Institute (CLSI).* 2011. Wayne, PA.

181. Malik R, Smits B, Reppas G, et al. Ulcerated and nonulcerated non-tuberculous cutaneous mycobacterial granulomas in cats and dogs. *Vet Dermatol.* 2013;24:146–153. e132-143.
182. Tortoli E. Standard operating procedure for optimal identification of mycobacteria using 16S rRNA gene sequences. *Stand Genomic Sci.* 2010;3:145.
183. Dai J, Chen Y, Lauzardo M. Web-accessible database of hsp65 sequences from *Mycobacterium* reference strains. *J Clin Microbiol.* 2011;49:2296–2303.
184. Adekambi T, Colson P, Drancourt M. RpoB-based identification of nonpigmented and late-pigmenting rapidly growing mycobacteria. *J Clin Microbiol.* 2003;41:5699–5708.
185. Park H, Jang H, Kim C, et al. Detection and identification of mycobacteria by amplification of the internal transcribed spacer regions with genus- and species-specific PCR primers. *J Clin Microbiol.* 2000;38(11):4080–4085.
186. Roth A, Fischer M, Hamid ME, et al. Differentiation of phylogenetically related slowly growing mycobacteria based on 16S-23S rRNA gene internal transcribed spacer sequences. *J Clin Microbiol.* 1998;36:139–147.
187. Savelkoul PHM, Catsburg A, Mulder S, et al. Detection of *Mycobacterium tuberculosis* complex with Real Time PCR: comparison of different primer-probe sets based on the IS6110 element. *J Microbiol Methods.* 2006;66:177–180.
188. Fyfe JA, Lavender CJ, Johnson PD, et al. Development and application of two multiplex real-time PCR assays for the detection of *Mycobacterium ulcerans* in clinical and environmental samples. *Appl Environ Microbiol.* 2007;73:4733–4740.
189. Slana I, Kaevska M, Kralik P, et al. Distribution of *Mycobacterium avium* subsp. *avium* and *M. a. hominissuis* in artificially infected pigs studied by culture and IS901 and IS1245 quantitative real time PCR. *Vet Microbiol.* 2010;144:437–443.
190. Roth A, Reischl UDO, Streubel A, et al. Novel diagnostic algorithm for identification of mycobacteria using genus-specific amplification of the 16S-23S rRNA gene spacer and restriction endonucleases. *J Clin Microbiol.* 2000;38:1094–1104.
191. Telenti A, Marchesi F, Balz M, et al. Rapid identification of mycobacteria to the species level by polymerase chain reaction and restriction enzyme analysis. *J Clin Microbiol.* 1993;31:175–178.
192. Steingrube VA, Gibson JL, Brown BA, et al. PCR amplification and restriction endonuclease analysis of a 65-kilodalton heat shock protein gene sequence for taxonomic separation of rapidly growing mycobacteria. *J Clin Microbiol.* 1995;33:149–153.
193. van Soolingen D, Bauer J, Ritacco V, et al. IS1245 restriction fragment length polymorphism typing of *Mycobacterium avium* isolates: proposal for standardization. *J Clin Microbiol.* 1998;36:3051–3054.
194. Boyd SC, Athan E, Friedman ND, et al. Epidemiology, clinical features and diagnosis of *Mycobacterium ulcerans* in an Australian population. *Med J Aust.* 2012;196:341–344.
195. Southern PM. Tenosynovitis caused by *Mycobacterium kansasii* associated with a dog bite. *Am J Med Sci.* 2004;327:258–261.
196. Vernon A. Treatment of latent tuberculosis infection. *Semin Respir Crit Care Med.* 2013;34:67–86.
197. Doucet-Populaire F, Buriánková K, Weiser J, et al. Macrolide resistance in mycobacteria. *Med Chem Rev.* 2005;2:511–523.
198. Gordin FM, Horsburgh CR. *Mycobacterium avium* complex. In: Bennett JE, Dolin R, Blaser MJ, eds. *Principles and Practice of Infectious Diseases.* Philadephia, PA: Churchill Livingstone, Elsevier; 2015:2832–2843.
199. Jang SS, Hirsh DC. Rapidly growing members of the genus *Mycobacterium* affecting dogs and cats. *J Am Anim Hosp Assoc.* 2002;38:217–220.
200. Malik R, Shaw SE, Griffin C, et al. Infections of the subcutis and skin of dogs caused by rapidly growing mycobacteria. *J Small Anim Pract.* 2004;45:485–494.
201. Horne KS, Kunkle GA. Clinical outcome of cutaneous rapidly growing mycobacterial infections in cats in the south-eastern United States: a review of 10 cases (1996-2006). *J Feline Med Surg.* 2009;11:627–632.
202. Dewevre PJ, McAllister HA, Schirmer RG, et al. *Mycobacterium fortuitum* infection in a cat. *J Am Anim Hosp Assoc.* 1977;13:68–70.
203. Wilkinson GT, Kelly WR, O'Boyle D. Cutaneous granulomas associated with *Mycobacterium fortuitum* infection in a cat. *J Small Anim Pract.* 1978;19:357–362.
204. Kunkle GA, Gulbas NK, Fakok V, et al. Rapidly growing mycobacteria as a cause of cutaneous granulomas: report of five cases. *J Am Anim Hosp Assoc.* 1983;19:513–521.
205. Couto SS, Artacho CA. *Mycobacterium fortuitum* pneumonia in a cat and the role of lipid in the pathogenesis of atypical mycobacterial infections. *Vet Pathol.* 2007;44:543–546.
206. Michaud AJ. The use of clofazimine as treatment for *Mycobacterium fortuitum* in a cat. *Fel Pract.* 1994;22:7–9.
207. da Silva DA, Gremiao IDF, Menezes RC, et al. Autochthonous case of feline atypical cutaneous mycobacteriosis in the municipality of Rio de Janeiro-Brazil. *Acta Sci Vet.* 2010;38:327–331.
208. Wilkinson GT, Kelly WR, O'Boyle D. Pyogranulomatous panniculitis in cats due to *Mycobacterium smegmatis. Aust Vet J.* 1982;58:77–78.
209. Studdert VP, Hughes KL. Treatment of opportunistic mycobacterial infections with enrofloxacin in cats. *J Am Vet Med Assoc.* 1992;201:1388–1390.
210. Jassies-van der Lee A, Houwers DJ, Meertens N, et al. Localised pyogranulomatous dermatitis due to *Mycobacterium abscessus* in a cat: a case report. *Vet J.* 2009;179:304–306.
211. Albini S, Mueller S, Bornand V, et al. Cutaneous atypical mycobacteriosis due to *Mycobacterium massiliense* in a cat. *Schweizer Archiv fur Tierheilkunde.* 2007;149:553–558.
212. White SD, Ihrke PJ, Stannard AA, et al. Cutaneous atypical mycobacteriosis in cats. *J Am Vet Med Assoc.* 1983;182:1218–1222.
213. Willemse T, Groothuis DG, Koeman JP, et al. *Mycobacterium thermoresistibile*: extrapulmonary infection in a cat. *J Clin Microbiol.* 1985;21:854–856.
214. Foster SF, Martin P, Davis W, et al. Chronic pneumonia caused by *Mycobacterium thermoresistibile* in a cat. *J Small Anim Pract.* 1999;40:433–438.
215. Kirpal G, Merkt M, Rohde J. Dermatitis in a cat caused by mycobacteria. *Der Prakt Tierarzt.* 2010;91:472–476.
216. Vishkautsan P, Reagan KL, Keel MK, et al. Mycobacterial panniculitis caused by *Mycobacterium thermoresistibile* in a cat. *J Fel Med Surg Open Rep.* 2016;2. 2055116916672786.
217. Alander-Damsten YK, Brander EE, Paulin LG. Panniculitis due to *Mycobacterium smegmatis*, in two Finnish cats. *J Feline Med Surg.* 2003;5:19–26.
218. Bryden SL, Burrows AK, O'Hara AJ. *Mycobacterium goodii* infection in a dog with concurrent hyperadrenocorticism. *Vet Dermatol.* 2004;15:331–338.
219. Grooters AM, Couto CG, Andrews JM, et al. Systemic *Mycobacterium smegmatis* infection in a dog. *J Am Vet Med Assoc.* 1995;206:200–202.
220. Wylie KB, Lewis DD, Pechman RD, et al. Hypertrophic osteopathy associated with *Mycobacterium fortuitum* pneumonia in a dog. *J Am Vet Med Assoc.* 1993;202:1986–1988.
221. Fox LE, Kunkle GA, Homer BL, et al. Disseminated subcutaneous *Mycobacterium fortuitum* infection in a dog. *J Am Vet Med Assoc.* 1995;206:53–55.
222. Jang SS, Eckhaus MA, Saunders G. Pulmonary *Mycobacterium fortuitum* infection in a dog. *J Am Vet Med Assoc.* 1984;184:96–98.
223. Turnwald GH, Pechman RD, Turk JR, et al. Survival of a dog with pneumonia caused by *Mycobacterium fortuitum. J Am Vet Med Assoc.* 1988;192:64–66.
224. Malik R, Wigney DI, Dawson D, et al. Infection of the subcutis and skin of cats with rapidly growing mycobacteria: a review of microbiological and clinical findings. *J Feline Med Surg.* 2000;2:35–48.
225. Irwin PJ, Whithear K, Lavelle RB, Parry BW. Acute bronchopneumonia associated with *Mycobacterium fortuitum* infection in a dog. *Aust Vet J.* 2000;78(4):254–257.
226. Monroe WE, August JR, Chickering WR. Atypical mycobacterial infections in cats. *Comp Contin Educ Practit Vet.* 1988;10:1044–1048.
227. Malik R, Hunt GB, Goldsmid SE, et al. Diagnosis and treatment of pyogranulomatous panniculitis due to *Mycobacterium smegmatis* in cats. *J Small Anim Pract.* 1994;35:524–530.
228. Sameh Y, Archambault M, Parker W, et al. Pyogranulomatous panniculitis in a cat associated with infection by the *Mycobacterium fortuitum/peregrinum* group. *Can Vet J.* 2002;43:285–287.
229. Beccati M, Peano A, Gallo MG. Pyogranulomatous panniculitis caused by *Mycobacterium alvei* in a cat. *J Small Anim Pract.* 2007;48:664.
230. Leissinger MK, Garber JB, Fowlkes N, et al. *Mycobacterium fortuitum* lipoid pneumonia in a dog. *Vet Pathol.* 2015;52:356–359.

231. Ceyssens P-J, Soetaert K, Timke M, et al. MALDI-TOF for combined species identification and drug sensitivity testing in mycobacteria. *J Clin Microbiol.* 2017;55:624–634.
232. Ryan GJ, Shapiro HM, Lenaerts AJ. Improving acid-fast fluorescent staining for the detection of mycobacteria using a new nucleic acid staining approach. *Tuberculosis.* 2014;94:511–518.
233. Wallace RJ, Nash DR, Tsukamura M, et al. Human disease due to *Mycobacterium smegmatis. J Infect Dis.* 1988;158:52–59.
234. Brown BA, Springer B, Steingrube VA, et al. *Mycobacterium wolinskyi* sp. nov. and *Mycobacterium goodii* sp. nov., two new rapidly growing species related to *Mycobacterium smegmatis* and associated with human wound infections: a cooperative study from the International Working Group on Mycobacterial Taxonomy. *Int J Syst Bacteriol.* 1999;4:1493–1511.
235. Brown BA, Wallace Jr RJ, Onyi GO, et al. Activities of four macrolides, including clarithromycin, against *Mycobacterium fortuitum, Mycobacterium chelonae,* and *M. chelonae*-like organisms. *Antimicrob Agents Chemother.* 1992;36:180–184.
236. Swenson JM, Wallace Jr RJ, Silcox VA, et al. Antimicrobial susceptibility of five subgroups of *Mycobacterium fortuitum* and *Mycobacterium chelonae. Antimicrob Agents Chemother.* 1985;28:807–811.
237. Wallace RJ, Jr Brown-Elliott BA, Ward SC, et al. Activities of linezolid against rapidly growing mycobacteria. *Antimicrob Agents Chemother.* 2001;45:764–767.
238. Govendir M, Hansen T, Kimble B, et al. Clinical efficacy of moxifloxacin for treating rapidly growing mycobacteria (RGM) infections in cats. *J Vet Pharmacol.* 2009;32(S1):71.
239. Malik R, Shaw SE, Griffin C, et al. Infections of the subcutis and skin of dogs caused by rapidly growing mycobacteria. *J Small Anim Pract.* 2004;45:485–494.
240. Ariel I, Haas H, Weinberg H, et al. *Mycobacterium fortuitum* granulomatous synovitis caused by a dog bite. *J Hand Surg Am.* 1983;8:342–343.
241. Ngan N, Morris A, de Chalain T. *Mycobacterium fortuitum* infection caused by a cat bite. *N Z Med J.* 2005;118. U1354.
242. Brown-Elliott BA, Wallace RJ. Infections caused by non-tuberculous mycobacteria other than *Mycobacterium avium* complex. In: Bennett JE, Dolin R, Blaser MJ, eds. *Principles and Practice of Infectious Diseases.* Philadephia, PA: Churchill Livingstone: Elsevier; 2015:2844–2852.
243. Brown LR, May CD, Williams SE. A non-tuberculous granuloma in cats. *N Z Vet J.* 1962;10:7–9.
244. Thompson EJ, Little PB, Cordes DO. Observations of cat leprosy. *N Z Vet J.* 1979;27:233–235.
245. Allan GS, Wickham N. Mycobacterial granulomas in a cat diagnosed as leprosy. *Fel Pract.* 1976;6(33):35–36.
246. Lawrence WE, Wickham N. Cat leprosy: infection by a bacillus resembling. *Mycobacterium lepraemurium. Aust Vet J.* 1963;39:390–393.
247. Schiefer B, Gee BR, Ward GE. A disease resembling feline leprosy in western Canada. *J Am Vet Med Assoc.* 1974;165:1085–1087.
248. Gee BR, Schiefer B, Ward GE. Letter: disease resembling feline leprosy. *Can Vet J.* 1975;16:30.
249. Wilkinson GT. A non-tuberculous granuloma of the cat associated with an acid-fast bacillus. *Vet Rec.* 1964;76:777–778.
250. Robinson M. Skin granuloma of cats associated with acid-fast bacilli. *J Small Anim Pract.* 1975;16:563–567.
251. Frye FL, Carney JD, Loughman WD. Feline lepromatous leprosy. *Vet Med Small Anim Clin.* 1974;69:1272–1273.
252. Poelma FG, Leiker DL. Cat leprosy in The Netherlands. *Int J Lepr Other Mycobact Dis.* 1974;42:307–311.
253. Hughes MS, James G, Taylor MJ, et al. PCR studies of feline leprosy cases. *J Feline Med Surg.* 2004,6:235–243.
254. Laprie C, Duboy J, Malik R, et al. Feline cutaneous mycobacteriosis: a review of clinical, pathological and molecular characterization of one case of *Mycobacterium microti* skin infection and nine cases of feline leprosy syndrome from France and New Caledonia. *Vet Dermatol.* 2013;24:561–569. e133-564.
255. Lamagna B, Paciello O, Ragozzino M, et al. Isolated lepromatous conjunctivo-corneal granuloma in a cat from Italy. *Vet Ophthalmol.* 2009;12:97–101.
256. Courtin F, Huerre M, Fyfe J, et al. A case of feline leprosy caused by *Mycobacterium lepraemurium* originating from the island of Kythira (Greece): diagnosis and treatment. *J Feline Med Surg.* 2007;9:238–241.
257. Goto Y, Iwakiri A, Tabaru H, et al. Differential diagnosis of a case of feline leprosy. *J Japan Vet Med Assoc.* 2002;55:437–441.
258. Malik R, Hughes MS, James G, et al. Feline leprosy: two different clinical syndromes. *J Feline Med Surg.* 2002;4:43–59.
259. O'Brien CR, Malik R, Globan M, et al. Feline leprosy due to *Mycobacterium lepraemurium*: further clinical and molecular characterization of 23 previously reported cases and an additional 42 cases. *J Fel Med Surg.* 2017;19:737–746.
260. O'Brien CR, Malik R, Globan M, et al. Feline leprosy due to *Candidatus* 'Mycobacterium lepraefelis': further clinical and molecular characterisation of eight previously reported cases and an additional 30 cases. *J Fel Med Surg.* 2017;19:919–932.
261. O'Brien CR, Malik R, Globan M, et al. Feline leprosy due to *Candidatus* 'Mycobacterium tarwinense': further clinical and molecular characterization of 15 previously reported cases and an additional 27 cases. *J Fel Med Surg.* 2017;19:498–512.
262. Malik R, Love DN, Wigney DI, et al. Mycobacterial nodular granulomas affecting the subcutis and skin of dogs (canine leproid granuloma syndrome). *Aust Vet J.* 1998;76:403–407.
263. Smits B, Willis R, Fyfe J. Confirmation of canine leproid granuloma syndrome in New Zealand. *N Z Vet J.* 2011;59:153.
264. Smits B, Willis R, Malik R, et al. Case clusters of leproid granulomas in foxhounds in New Zealand and Australia. *Vet Dermatol.* 2012;23:465–e488.
265. Conceicao LG, Acha LM, Borges AS, et al. Epidemiology, clinical signs, histopathology and molecular characterization of canine leproid granuloma: a retrospective study of cases from Brazil. *Vet Dermatol.* 2011;22:249–256.
266. Maruyama S, Dias G, Otsuka M, et al. Canine leproid granuloma (clg) in São Paulo: a retrospective study of 37 cases (1990 to 2009). *J Vet Intern Med.* 2011;25:712.
267. Maruyama S. Clinical and epidemiological study of cases of canine leproid granuloma diagnosed by histopathology and by polymerase chain reaction (PCR). In: *Faculdade de Medicina Veterinária e Zootecnia. São Paulo.* Brazil: Universidade de São Paulo; 2010.
268. Foley JE, Borjesson D, Gross TL, et al. Clinical, microscopic, and molecular aspects of canine leproid granuloma in the United States. *Vet Pathol.* 2002;39:234–239.
269. Smith RLE. Canine skin tuberculosis. *Rhod Vet J.* 1973;3:63–64.
270. Dedola C, Zobba R, Pinna Parpaglia ML, et al. First report of canine leprosy in Europe: molecular and clinical traits. *Vet Rec.* 2014;174:120.
271. Jäger K, Gläsel A, Hilleman D, et al. First description of canine leproid granuloma in Germany: 2 case reports. *Tierarztl Prax Ausg K Kleintiere Heimtiere.* 2020;48:196–202.
272. Fyfe JA, McCowan C, O'Brien CR, et al. Molecular characterization of a novel fastidious mycobacterium causing lepromatous lesions of the skin, subcutis, cornea, and conjunctiva of cats living in Victoria, Australia. *J Clin Microbiol.* 2008;46:618–626.
273. Appleyard GD, Clark EG. Histologic and genotypic characterization of a novel *Mycobacterium* species found in three cats. *J Clin Microbiol.* 2002;40:2425–2430.
274. Roccabianca P, Caniatti M, Scanziani E, et al. Feline leprosy: spontaneous remission in a cat. *J Am Anim Hosp Assoc.* 1996;32:189–193.
275. Mendoza-Aguilar M, Almaguer-Villagrán L, Jiménez-Arellanes A, et al. The use of the microplate alamar blue assay (MABA) to assess the susceptibility of *Mycobacterium lepraemurium* to anti leprosy and other drugs. *J Infect Chemother.* 2012;18:652–661.
276. Malik R, O'Brien CR, Fyfe JA. Canine leproid granulomas (canine leprosy). In: Greene CE, ed. *Infectious Diseases of the Dog and Cat.* 4th ed. St Louis: Elsevier; 2011:513–515.

62

Salmonellosis

Jane E. Sykes, Patrick L. McDonough

KEY POINTS

- First Described: Washington, DC, United States, 1885 (Theobald Smith and Daniel Salmon).[1]
- Cause: *Salmonella* spp. (gram-negative rods that belong to the order Enterobacterales).[2]
- Affected Hosts: A large variety of warm-blooded animals and humans; cold-blooded animals may be subclinically to clinically infected.
- Geographic Distribution: Worldwide.
- Primary Mode of Transmission: Fecal-oral.
- Major Clinical Signs: Fever, lethargy, anorexia, diarrhea, vomiting, and less commonly reproductive failure, neurologic and/or respiratory signs.
- Differential Diagnoses: Differential diagnoses for suspected *Salmonella* enterocolitis include canine and feline parvovirus infection, canine distemper virus infection, other viral gastroenteritides, campylobacteriosis, clostridial diarrhea, salmon poisoning disease, giardiasis, tritrichomoniasis (cats), cryptosporidiosis, whipworms, leptospirosis, dietary indiscretion, gastrointestinal foreign body, pancreatitis, inflammatory bowel disease, lymphoma, hypoadrenocorticism, hyperthyroidism, toxins (including drugs).
- Human Health Significance: Important zoonosis. Dogs and cats may be a source of human infection with some *Salmonella* serotypes, some of which may be resistant to multiple antimicrobial drugs.

ETIOLOGY AND EPIDEMIOLOGY

Salmonella are gram-negative, motile, non–spore-forming facultative anaerobic rods that belong to the order Enterobacterales. Most *Salmonella* exist in two antigenic phases, which differ in composition of their flagellar antigens.

Salmonella are ubiquitous organisms that can be isolated from the intestinal tracts of an enormous variety of animal species and are a major cause of enterocolitis and sometimes severe systemic illness in humans and animals. Infections can be transferred among animal species and are zoonotic (Fig. 62.1). Many infections in humans are food-borne, especially in association with unpasteurized milk, meat (especially ground poultry meat), and eggs. *Salmonella* spp. have a remarkable ability to survive long periods of time (weeks to years) in the environment, and so fomite transmission is important. *Salmonella* thrive in moist environments (a good example is egg layer flock housing). In addition, *Salmonella* can multiply rapidly in contaminated food left at room temperature and can survive freezing for several weeks.[3]

The genus *Salmonella* comprises two species, *Salmonella enterica* and *Salmonella bongori*, each of which contains multiple serotypes.[4,5] Serotypes of *S. bongori* are generally associated with cold-blooded animals and rarely have been isolated from warm-blooded animals, including a dog with diarrhea.[6] There are six subspecies of *S. enterica* (Table 62.1) and approximately 2600 different serotypes. Before the availability of multiplex PCR assays, serotypes were identified on the basis of agglutination reactions of their O (somatic) and H (flagellar) antigens (see Chapter 53); most reference laboratories today have switched to commercial kits to identify *Salmonella* serotypes by multiplex PCR.[7] Subspecies I serotypes, which are responsible for almost all diseases in humans and warm-blooded animals worldwide, are assigned names such as *S.* ser. Typhimurium. Unless named before 1966, serotypes that belong to other subspecies are designated using antigenic formulas. The formulas describe the subspecies, O antigens: H antigens (phase 1): and if present, H antigens (phase 2) (e.g., *S.* IV 45:g,z_{51}:—).[5]

Certain serotypes of *Salmonella* are host restricted (also called host adapted), whereas others infect a broad range of host species (or called non–host adapted). *Salmonella* serotype Typhi, for example, is adapted to humans, causing typhoid fever, and does not infect animals. Other serotypes are adapted to certain host species (e.g., *S.* Pullorum and poultry), with rare transmission to other hosts. *Salmonella* Typhimurium is the most commonly isolated non–host adapted serotype from diseased humans and animals.

Infection of dogs and cats with *Salmonella* has been associated with the feeding of raw meat diets,[8-16] although commercial dry and raw dog food and pig ear pet treats have also become contaminated with the organism.[10,17-21] One study used whole genome sequencing to show that *Salmonella* infections in pets were associated with contaminated raw pet food diets.[11] The organism has been shown to survive weeks to months on pig ear treats, although viability over time decreases more rapidly at room temperature than under refrigeration.[22] Occasionally, co-infections with multiple *Salmonella* serotypes occur.[23] Outbreaks of *S.* Typhimurium infection in cats have been associated with seasonal bird migrations ("songbird fever").[24,25] An outbreak of salmonellosis was described in a colony of blood donor cats that developed severe enterocolitis; the source of infection was not identified.[26]

Salmonella is generally isolated less than 1% of the time from the feces of dogs and cats that are fed processed commercial pet foods,[27-31] although one study of household pet dogs in Ontario, Canada revealed a shedding prevalence of 23%[32] and a study from Thailand revealed a prevalence of 12.9%.[33] The highest rates of infection have been found in group-housed dogs, especially those fed raw meat diets, such as racing sled dogs and greyhound breeding facilities, where prevalences have exceeded 75%.[14,34,35] In South Africa, based on culture, the prevalence of *Salmonella* shedding in 74 hospitalized puppies with CPV-2 infection

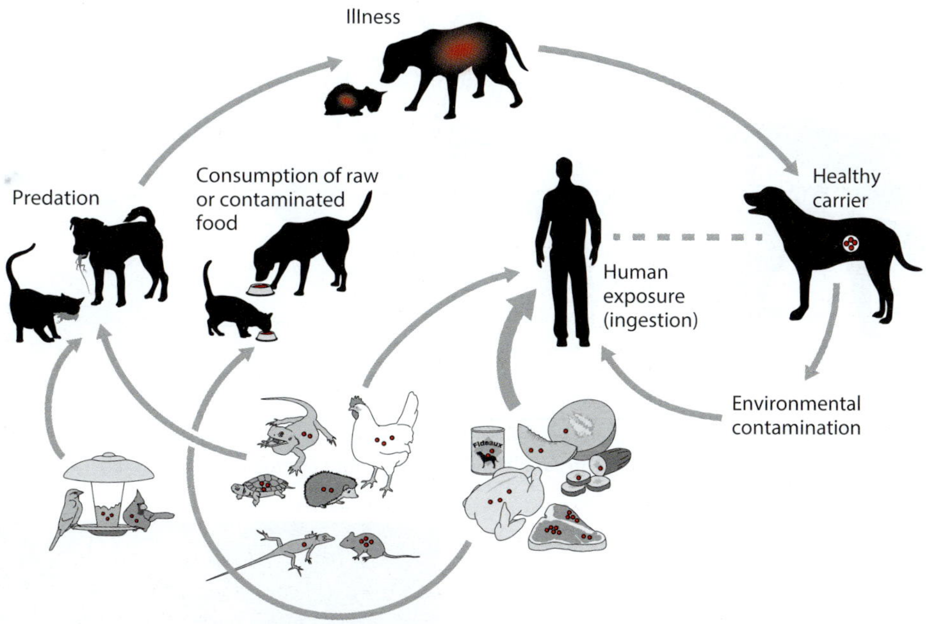

Fig. 62.1 Epidemiology of salmonellosis.

TABLE 62.1 Classification of Salmonellae

Species	Subspecies	Serotype Examples
Salmonella enterica	*enterica* (I)	*Salmonella* Typhimurium
		S. Typhi
		S. Choleraesuis
	salamae (II)	*S.* Greenside
	arizonae (IIIa)	*S.* IIIa 18:z_4,z_{23}:—
	diarizonae (IIIb)	*S.* IIIb 60:k:z
	houtenae (IV)	*S.* Marina
	indica (VI)	*S.* Srinagar
Salmonella bongori	V	*S.* Brookfield

was 22%, but this compared with a prevalence of 31% in a control group of 42 apparently healthy dogs.[36] *Salmonella* was isolated from the feces of 18 of 26 (69%) healthy pre-race Alaskan sled dogs, and 19 of 30 (63%) diarrheic racing Alaskan sled dogs, which underscored the lack of an association between the isolation of *Salmonella* and clinical diarrhea.[14] In one large study of dogs and cats visiting veterinary clinics from the United States between January 2012 and April 2014, *Salmonella* was isolated from 2.5% of 2,422 dogs and 0.06% of 542 cats.[37] Risk factors for infection based on univariate analysis were consumption of raw food, consumption of probiotics, administration of antimicrobial drugs, rural background (versus urban or suburban), and the presence of diarrhea; however, multivariate logistic regression analysis revealed that probiotic administration was associated with diarrhea, so it was no longer identified as a risk factor. The percentages of positive isolations were also highest in Georgia (8%) and Texas (10%). Coprophagic behavior may also contribute to salmonellosis in dogs. In cats, the feeding of raw poultry may increase risk for *Salmonella* infection,[38] and occasionally, high prevalences of infection have been detected in group-housed cats[31] and shelter cats. Ingestion of infected wild bird species by cats during seasonal bird migrations can also lead to salmonellosis.[24,25] In a study of diarrheic and nondiarrheic shelter cats in Florida, the prevalence of *Salmonella* shedding as determined by PCR assay was 6% and 4%, respectively.[39] In *Salmonella* isolates from dogs in Texas shelters, the most frequently identified serotypes were Newport and Javiana, for which there was evidence of within-shelter transmission in addition to introduction of new infections.[40] Susceptibility to shedding and disease is highest in immunosuppressed dogs and cats, including young animals, pregnant animals, those in overcrowded conditions, and those with underlying immunosuppressive illness (such as neoplasia, diabetes mellitus, retrovirus infection, and immune-mediated disease) or immunosuppressive drug therapy.[41-44]

CLINICAL FEATURES

Pathogenesis and Clinical Signs

After ingestion, salmonellae that survive the acidic environment of the stomach gain access to the intestine, where they disrupt tight junctions and, through a process known as bacteria-mediated endocytosis, they actively invade: (1) enterocytes; (2) M cells within the ileum (which sample luminal antigens); and (3) dendritic cells, which send protrusions into the gut lumen between intestinal epithelial cells (Fig. 62.2). As few as 200 organisms may be sufficient to produce nontyphoidal human disease, although the median dose required was 10^6 organisms.[45] A T3SS, together with other proteins encoded by *Salmonella* pathogenicity island 1 (SPI-1), is required for invasion of enterocytes, but invasion of dendritic cells is SPI-1-independent. Interaction of *Salmonella* with immune cells and epithelial cells within the gut leads to production of cytokines and chemokines, with massive influx of lymphocytes, macrophages, and neutrophils, sometimes with severe epithelial injury and mucosal sloughing.[46,47] This occurs in response to the presence of SPI-1 translocated proteins as well as activation of TLR4 by LPS and TLR5 by flagellin. Localization in the mesenteric lymph nodes, Peyer's patches, solitary intestinal lymphoid tissues, and intestinal epithelium, along with evasion of the host immune response, is followed by persistent shedding, often for several weeks, after which animals can become latently infected. Reactivation of shedding, with or without clinical illness, may occur, sometimes as a result of stress or immunosuppression.[48,49]

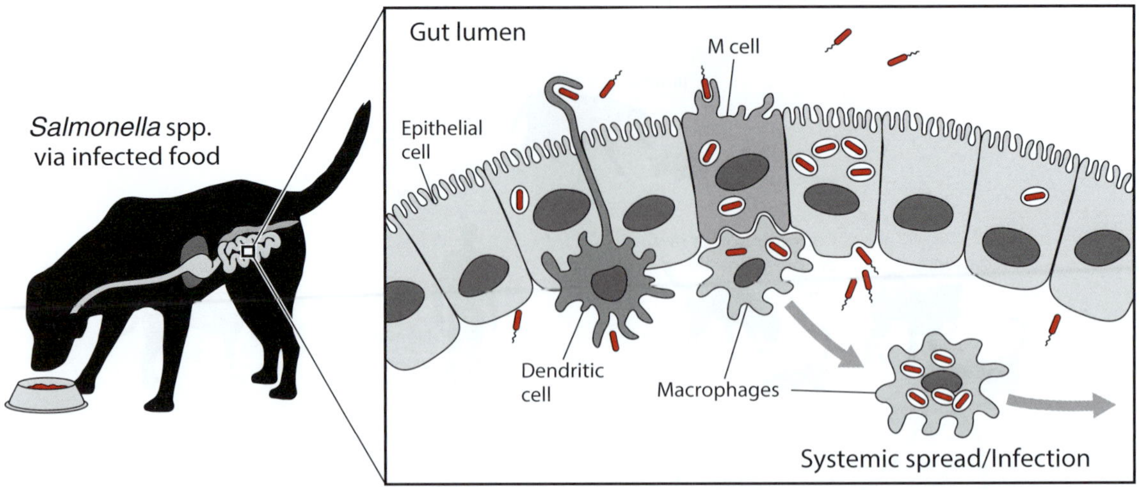

Fig. 62.2 The pathogenesis of *Salmonella* infection. (Modified from Hume PJ, Singh V, Davidson AC, et al. Swiss Army Pathogen: The *Salmonella* entry toolkit. *Front Cell Infect Microbiol.* 2017;7:348.)

If the organism has properties that allow it to spread systemically and host defenses are impaired, bacteremia and extraintestinal infection follow.[50] After crossing the intestinal barrier, *Salmonella* invade and replicate within macrophages using a second T3SS (present in SPI-2), which contributes to their dissemination and development of systemic infection. Virulent strains have a greater ability to multiply intracellularly in nonphagocytic cells.[46] Fever, hypoglycemia, and leukopenia occur. The *Salmonella* LPS can then induce endotoxic shock, with hypotension and activation of the complement and coagulation cascade. The coagulation cascade is also activated with exposure to *Salmonella* porins, which are hydrophobic outer membrane proteins. This is followed by DIC.

Dogs and cats infected with *Salmonella* spp. may show no signs or they may develop enterocolitis, focal suppurative infection, or severe systemic illness. The majority of dogs are chronically and subclinically infected. When disease occurs, signs often begin 3 to 5 days after infection or onset of immunosuppression. Fever (occasionally as high as 106°F [41°C]), lethargy, and anorexia may be followed by abdominal pain, vomiting, and watery to mucoid, often hemorrhagic, diarrhea and dehydration. Weight loss may be seen. Diarrhea may take several weeks to resolve. Rarely, chronic intermittent diarrhea that lasts up to 8 weeks develops.[51]

Severely affected animals develop signs of septic shock (see Chapter 123). Neurologic signs, and signs that relate to endocarditis, myocarditis, arthritis, pancreatitis, pneumonia, peritonitis, prostatitis, mesenteric lymphadenitis, and cholecystitis occur in some animals.[44,52-56] Infected cats may develop severe enterocolitis, with fever, pancytopenia, and hyperbilirubinemia. Some cats show persistent fever and anorexia with no diarrhea. Conjunctivitis has been described in cats in association with *Salmonella* infection.[57]

Occasionally salmonellae localize in a particular organ, such as the lungs, CNS, or urinary tract (Fig. 62.3). Signs of dysfunction of that organ system may follow, even when enteric signs or positive fecal culture results are absent.[58] Abortion and stillbirth can occur after transplacental infection, and the dam may also infect neonates, which leads to fading puppies.[59-61]

DIAGNOSIS

The traditional diagnosis of canine and feline salmonellosis is made based on culture of the organism in conjunction with clinical signs and assessment of potential risk factors, such as hospitalization, age, environmental exposure, and antibiotic administration. Diagnostic assays available for salmonellosis in dogs and cats are shown in Table 62.2.

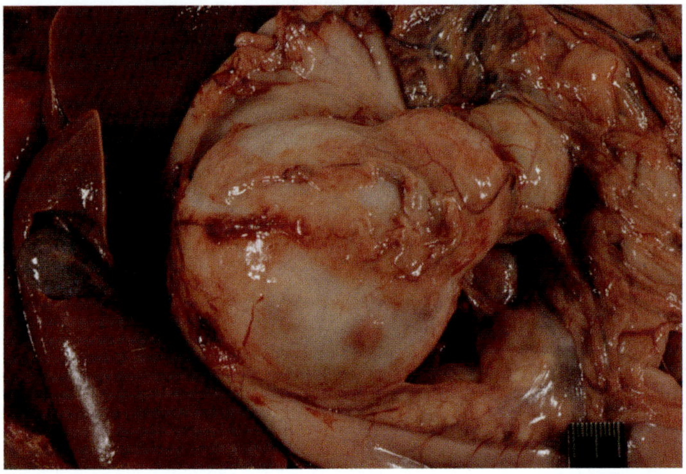

Fig. 62.3 Large, chronic pancreatic abscess due to *Salmonella* Typhimurium associated with a pancreatic adenocarcinoma in a 15-year-old castrated male domestic shorthair cat. The mass was multicystic and fluctuant, and when cut open was filled with cloudy fluid and lined by thick tan debris. (Courtesy University of California, Davis, Veterinary Anatomic Pathology Service.)

Laboratory Abnormalities

Complete Blood Count

The CBC in dogs or cats with salmonellosis may be unremarkable or may show a neutrophilia with a left shift; in bacteremic animals, anemia, a degenerative left shift, toxic neutrophils, lymphopenia, and thrombocytopenia are usually present. Rarely, intracellular bacteria are seen within neutrophils.

Serum Chemistry Profile

In animals with severe salmonellosis, changes in the serum chemistry profile include elevated liver enzyme activities, hyperbilirubinemia, azotemia, hypoalbuminemia, hypocholesterolemia, hypoglycemia, and electrolyte abnormalities.

Urinalysis

Salmonella spp. occasionally localize in the kidneys, with associated isosthenuria, pyuria, proteinuria, casts, and bacteriuria.

TABLE 62.2 Diagnostic Assays Available for Salmonellosis in Dogs and Cats

Assay	Specimen Type	Target	Performance
Bacterial isolation	Feces, blood, synovial fluid, tissue aspirates, bronchoalveolar lavage fluid, peritoneal or pleural effusions, urine, CSF, tissues obtained at necropsy	*Salmonella* species	Sensitive and specific. False negatives may occur, especially following antimicrobial therapy. Isolation from feces does not imply that *Salmonella* is the cause of disease. Allows subsequent antimicrobial susceptibility testing.
PCR	As for isolation	*Salmonella* DNA	Rapid (within hours); can be highly sensitive and specific. Positive results from feces do not imply that *Salmonella* is the cause of disease. Does not allow susceptibility testing or typing for epidemiologic purposes.

Clotting Function

Dogs and cats that develop DIC may have clotting function abnormalities that include prolonged coagulation times, increased fibrin degradation product concentrations, and decreased antithrombin concentrations.

Diagnostic Imaging

Plain Radiography

Thoracic radiographs may reveal bronchointerstitial to alveolar infiltrates in animals with pneumonia, or pleural effusion with pyothorax. Abdominal radiographs can reveal fluid-filled intestines, decreased serosal detail, and/or mild hepatomegaly.

Sonographic Findings

Depending on the severity of the infection, abdominal ultrasound may be unremarkable in dogs and cats with salmonellosis, or show changes that include abdominal lymphadenomegaly, intestinal wall thickening, fluid-filled bowel segments, hepatomegaly, splenomegaly, or ascites.

Microbiologic Testing

Bacterial Isolation

A diagnosis of salmonellosis can be made when *Salmonella* is isolated from a normally sterile site, such as the blood, bronchoalveolar lavage specimens, synovial fluid, or urine specimens collected by cystocentesis. Isolation of *Salmonella* from feces does not confirm that the organism is the cause of disease,[61] but it can raise suspicion that *Salmonella* may be playing a role in enterocolitis, and it has zoonotic significance (see Public Health Aspects, later). Isolation also allows antimicrobial susceptibility testing, which is important because many isolates of *Salmonella* are resistant to multiple antimicrobial drugs.

Salmonella grow readily at 37°C on routine bacteriologic media from specimens that have been collected from a normally sterile site. Selective broth enrichment followed by plating on selective media are required for specimens that are heavily contaminated with other bacteria such as feces. The best selective broth enrichment is Rappaport-Vassiliadis soya peptone broth (RVS) medium. After enrichment, subculturing is performed on media such as xylose lysine deoxycholate (XLD) and brilliant green (BG) agar media, which also favor growth of *Salmonella*. These methods have been used in veterinary microbiology laboratories to facilitate growth of more fastidious serotypes such as *S.* Dublin.[62] Many veterinary laboratories incorporate such protocols for isolation of *Salmonella* as part of a panel for detection of enteropathogenic bacteria. Once a *Salmonella* suspect colony appears, the organism can be identified to genus using MALDI-TOF MS. This allows identification of *Salmonella* at the species level within minutes.[63,64] It also can identify some important *S. enterica* subsp. *enterica* to the serovar level, and could reduce the need for laborious subtyping procedures.[63] Veterinary laboratories also retain the use of antisera to identify the major serogroups of *Salmonella* that may be of immediate veterinary and public health significance.

Molecular Diagnosis Using Nucleic Acid–Based Testing

Some veterinary diagnostic laboratories offer PCR assays for *Salmonella*, some of which are highly sensitive and specific when compared with culture.[62,65,66] PCR is more rapid than culture but currently does not provide information on antimicrobial susceptibility. It has been recommended that PCR assay after overnight enrichment in a nonselective broth be adopted as the gold standard for diagnosis, and that all specimens that test positive by PCR assay be cultured using selective enrichment to isolate and identify the infecting organism.[62,67] As with culture, detection of the organism in feces using PCR assays does not prove that it is the cause of gastrointestinal illness.

Pathologic Findings

Gross Pathologic Findings

Gross necropsy findings in dogs and cats with severe salmonellosis include widespread petechial and ecchymotic hemorrhages, hemorrhagic enteritis, abscesses within parenchymal organs, enlarged mesenteric lymph nodes, and fibrinohemorrhagic ascites fluid. Pulmonary consolidation and edema may also be present.

Histopathologic Findings

Histopathologic lesions in dogs and cats with salmonellosis are highly variable. Changes in severely affected animals may include suppurative pneumonia, necrotizing hepatitis, and necrotizing and fibrinohemorrhagic enterocolitis, typhlitis, and cholecystitis. More chronic lesions such as chronic cholecystitis have also been described.[68,69] Sometimes, gram-negative bacilli are identified within lesions with tissue Gram stains (Fig. 62.4).

TREATMENT AND PROGNOSIS

The movement of dogs and cats that test positive for *Salmonella* should be limited, and if possible, hospitalized animals should be isolated. The detection of *Salmonella* in the feces of dogs and cats with uncomplicated diarrhea does not warrant antimicrobial administration, and supportive care only is recommended. Most of these animals have self-limiting disease and shedding, and injudicious antimicrobial administration has the potential to prolong the carrier

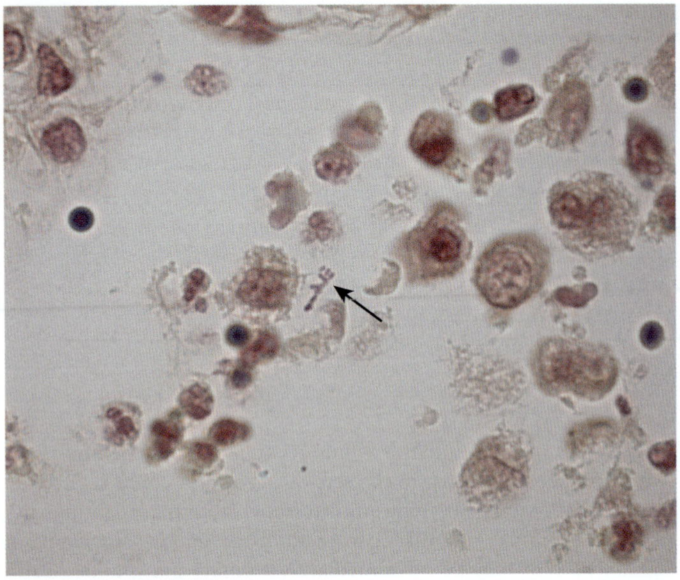

Fig. 62.4 Gram-negative bacilli (*arrow*) in the lungs of a cat with suppurative cholecystitis and pneumonia due to *Salmonella arizonae*. The cat had been treated with prednisone and cyclosporine for immune-mediated hemolytic anemia. Brown and Benn stain, 1000× magnification.

state and contribute to antimicrobial resistance. In humans, both short- and long-duration of antimicrobial treatment of uncomplicated non-typhoidal gastroenteritis did not reduce the duration of fever or diarrhea, and was associated with increased likelihood of positive fecal cultures 1 month after treatment as well as adverse drug reactions.[45] Treatment of an animal with uncomplicated diarrhea is also not advocated if the owner is immunocompromised, although appropriate husbandry recommendations and barrier control must be enforced.

Dogs and cats with systemic salmonellosis may require aggressive intravenous fluid therapy and colloidal support with hydroxyethyl starch or plasma, together with parenteral antimicrobial drugs. The choice of antimicrobial drugs should be based on the results of culture and susceptibility, because of the potential for resistance to multiple antimicrobial drugs through plasmid transfer. In the event of systemic disease, administration of a combination of ampicillin and a fluoroquinolone is advocated as empiric therapy while awaiting results of culture and susceptibility. Because of the importance of endotoxin in the pathogenesis of sepsis due to gram-negative bacteria such as *Salmonella*, considerable effort has been invested in development and application of drugs targeting endotoxin.[70] Clear benefit through reduction in mortality has not yet been demonstrated for these treatments, and to date they have not been widely used in dogs and cats. Several investigations have been focused on antagonists of TLR4, the LPS receptor.[71] Eritoran tetrasodium (E5564) and TAK-242 are examples of TLR4 antagonists that have been used in clinical trials involving septic humans, but no clear benefit has been shown.[71,72]

IMMUNITY AND VACCINATION

Salmonella spp. can persist in the host by interfering with dendritic cell function in the intestinal tract. The organism penetrates dendritic cells and avoids lysosomal degradation, which prevents subsequent antigen presentation by dendritic cells on molecules of the major histocompatibility complex.[73] Reduced intracellular proliferation of the organism within antigen-presenting cells may also limit antigen presentation and the development of an effective immune response.[74] Suppression and clearance of infection depends on the innate immune system, a Th1-type CD4 T-cell response, and production of antibodies by B cells. Although typhoid *Salmonella* vaccines have been developed for humans, none are available for dogs and cats.

PREVENTION OF ENTERIC BACTERIAL INFECTIONS

Prevention of enteric bacterial infections includes feeding dogs and cats properly cooked foods, hand washing before and after handling pets and pet food, and prevention of coprophagic behavior and predation. Proper handling and storage of pet foods can also limit the potential for food contamination during storage by rodents, insects, and human hands.

Within the hospital setting, fomites such as food dishes, endoscopes, proctoscopes, and rectal thermometers should be disinfected between uses, and single-use disposable thermometer covers should be used. Cages should be cleaned and properly disinfected (see Chapter 14) between animals. Blood donors should not be housed with the regular hospital population, as they may be a source of *Salmonella* infection.

Dogs and cats diagnosed with salmonellosis or *Salmonella* shedding should be isolated from other animals until shedding stops. Fecal cultures should be repeated every 2 weeks, and termination of shedding is identified when three successive negative cultures have been obtained.

PUBLIC HEALTH ASPECTS

All enteric bacterial infections of dogs and cats have the potential to infect and cause illness in humans. Nontyphoid salmonellosis (salmonellosis other than that caused by *S.* Typhi) can be transmitted from domestic animals to humans and cause serious enterocolitis, with fever, severe abdominal pain, diarrhea, nausea, inappetence, chills, and headache. Serious complications tend to occur in children, the elderly, or otherwise immunocompromised individuals such as those infected with HIV. The majority of cases result from ingestion of improperly cooked foods of animal origin, such as meat, milk, and eggs. Most, if not all, pet reptiles carry *Salmonella*, and there has been considerable effort to educate the public about the hazards of reptile-associated salmonellosis.[75] Dogs, and to a lesser extent cats, are less commonly incriminated as a source of *Salmonella*. Of particular concern, multidrug-resistant *Salmonella* strains, such as *S.* Typhimurium strain DT104, have been isolated from dogs, cats, and reptiles.[32,76] People exposed to dogs and cats that are fed raw meat diets are at increased risk of exposure. Nevertheless, there is a reasonable degree of mismatch between human and animal serotypes, which suggests that some serotypes are more likely to be transmitted to humans than others.

Proper hand washing after handling pets, pet food, and fomites such as bedding and food dishes can help prevent zoonotic transmission of *Salmonella*. Reptile ownership by families with children younger than 5 years of age or among the immunosuppressed is discouraged by public health authorities.[76] Proper food handling practices, including separating raw meat from vegetables and proper cooking of meat, can also reduce salmonellosis in humans.[19,77] Prevention of coprophagy and predation by dogs may also reduce the risk of human disease.

CASE EXAMPLE

Signalment

"Sampson," a 3-year-old male castrated shepherd mix from Fresno in southern California (Fig. 62.5).

History

Sampson was brought to a veterinarian for evaluation of a 3-month history of bilateral tarsal joint swelling. Some clinical improvement had been noted after treatment with oral tetracycline (28 mg/kg PO q8h) for 2 weeks. Subsequently, he was treated with oral prednisone (1.1 mg/kg PO q12h). Two weeks after the prednisone treatment was initiated, Sampson became nonambulatory in his pelvic limbs, and all of his peripheral joints became swollen and he was referred to the University of California, Davis, VMTH. A mass had been removed from his left dorsolateral thorax 3 weeks before referral that was assumed to be a foxtail abscess. Sampson had a good appetite. Increased thirst and urination had been noted after the prednisone treatment was initiated. There had been no coughing, sneezing, vomiting, or diarrhea. He was fed a duck- and potato-based diet for food allergy dermatitis and had been treated intermittently with prednisone, 4 mg PO q24h, for this condition since he was 6 months old. He had not traveled outside his local area, but he lived on a ranch and was known to consume horse feces and dead wild animals. There was no known tick exposure. He was up to date on vaccinations including canine distemper, adenovirus, parvovirus, and rabies vaccines.

Current medications: Prednisone 0.9 mg/kg PO q12h

Physical Examination

Body weight: 35.8 kg.

General: Quiet, alert, and responsive, 5% to 7% dehydrated. Recumbent. T = 102.9°F (39.4°C), HR = 140 beats/min, panting, mucous membranes pink and tacky, CRT = 1 s.

Integument: Multifocal epidermal collarettes were present and the haircoat was dry. A shaved area was present on the left lateral thoracic wall.

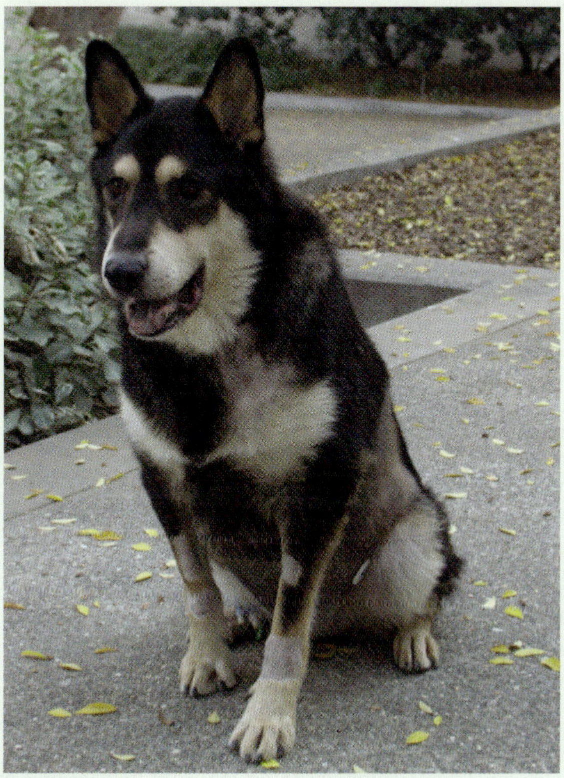

Fig. 62.5 "Sampson," a 3-year-old male castrated shepherd mix with salmonellosis.

Eyes, ears, nose, and throat: Moderate periodontal disease was present. A fundic examination was within normal limits.

Musculoskeletal: BCS was 5/9 with pelvic limb muscle atrophy. Pain and effusion of the carpi, tarsi, and stifles with decreased range of motion was noted. Spinal and pericervical pain was detected on palpation of these regions.

Cardiovascular: Weak but synchronous femoral pulses were noted. No murmurs or arrhythmias were auscultated.

Respiratory: There were moderately increased breath sounds in all lung fields.

GI/genitourinary: The abdomen was tense on palpation and moderate hepatomegaly was detected. The dog urinated a large amount of odiferous urine during the examination. No abnormalities were detected on rectal examination.

Lymph nodes: Moderate peripheral lymphadenopathy was present. Mandibular, superficial cervical, and popliteal lymph nodes were all 1.5 to 2.5 cm in diameter.

Laboratory findings

CBC: HCT 35.4% (40%–55%), MCV 67 fL (65–75 fL), MCHC 35.6 g/dL (33–36 g/dL), reticulocytes 101,200 cells/μL (7000–65,000 cells/μL), WBC 7870 cells/μL (6000–13,000 cells/μL), neutrophils 6139 cells/μL (3000–10,500 cells/μL), band neutrophils 1495 cells/μL, metamyelocytes 79 cells/μL, lymphocytes 0 cells/μL (1000–4000 cells/μL), monocytes 79 cells/μL (150–1200 cells/μL), platelets 419,000 platelets/μL (150,000–400,000 platelets/μL), neutrophils, band neutrophils, and metamyelocytes all showed moderate toxic changes.

Serum chemistry profile: Sodium 148 mmol/L (145–154 mmol/L), potassium 4.4 mmol/L (3.6–5.3 mmol/L), chloride 105 mmol/L (108–118 mmol/L), bicarbonate 14 mmol/L (16–26 mmol/L), phosphorus 5.8 mg/dL (3.0–6.2 mg/dL), calcium 10.3 mg/dL (9.7–11.5 mg/dl), BUN 10 mg/dL (5–21 mg/dL), creatinine 0.4 mg/dL (0.3–1.2 mg/dL), glucose 111 mg/dL (64–123 mg/dL), total protein 6.1 g/dL (5.4–7.6 g/dL), albumin 2.3 g/dL (3.0–4.4 g/dL), globulin 3.8 g/dL (1.8–3.9 g/dL), ALT 560 U/L (19–67 U/L), AST 72 U/L (19–42 U/L), ALP 3318 U/L (21–170 U/L), creatine kinase 197 U/L (51–399 U/L), GGT 59 U/L (0–6 U/L), cholesterol 212 mg/dL (135–361 mg/dL), total bilirubin 0.3 mg/dL (0–0.2 mg/dL).

Urinalysis: SpG 1.010; pH 8.0, 1+ protein (SSA), 3+ hemoprotein, no bilirubin or glucose, 25–35 WBC/HPF, 10–15 RBC/HPF, many rods.

Imaging Findings

Thoracic radiographs: The cardiovascular and pulmonary structures appeared within normal limits.

Right and left carpal, stifle, and tarsal radiographs: Intracapsular soft tissue swelling was associated with all joints.

Spinal radiographs: No abnormalities were detected.

Abdominal ultrasound: The liver was enlarged and hyperechoic. There was echogenic sediment in the urinary bladder.

Echocardiogram: Thickening and hyperechogenicity of the posterior leaflet of the tricuspid valve was noted which raised suspicion for endocarditis (Fig. 62.6).

Cytology Findings

Arthrocentesis of right and left carpi, right tarsus, and right stifle: Purulent inflammation was noted in the right tarsus, right stifle, and left carpus, with approximately 85% neutrophils and the remaining cells were a mixture of small and large mononuclear cells. In the right stifle, degenerate neutrophils are visualized, and some contained intracellular rod-shaped bacteria.

Microbiologic Testing

Serologic testing: An in-clinic ELISA for antibodies to *Borrelia burgdorferi*, *Anaplasma phagocytophilum*, and *Ehrlichia canis* was negative. Serum IFA for antibodies to *Bartonella vinsonii* subsp. *berkhoffii* was negative. Serology for *Coccidioides* spp. antibodies was also negative.

Continued

CASE EXAMPLE—cont'd

Aerobic bacterial culture of blood, joint fluid, and urine collected by cystocentesis: *Salmonella arizonae*, susceptible to all antimicrobials tested.

Diagnosis

Salmonella arizonae septic polyarthritis, bacteremia, and possible tricuspid valve endocarditis.

Treatment

Before obtaining susceptibility results, Sampson was treated with intravenous crystalloids, opioids for pain control, enrofloxacin (5 mg/kg IV q24h), and ampicillin (30 mg/kg IV q8h). The ampicillin was discontinued when the susceptibility results became available. The prednisone was tapered over a 3-day period and discontinued. The dog was moved to an isolation ward on diagnosis of salmonellosis. During hospitalization, Sampson's appetite declined initially, and he remained very painful for 6 days. After that time, he was able to sit up, began eating, and was discharged 8 days after admission.

Comments

Salmonella arizonae infections in humans have been associated with direct or indirect contact with reptiles. Reptile-associated salmonellosis is an increasing problem in humans in the United States and is especially a problem in infants and immunocompromised adults in contact with snakes and iguanas, or those who eat sun-dried rattlesnake meat for medicinal purposes. Horse feces from the farm were cultured for *Salmonella* and were negative. It is possible that the infection in this dog occurred as a result of ingestion of wild reptiles. The long history of glucocorticoid therapy for atopic dermatitis in this dog may have contributed to immunosuppression and predisposition to systemic salmonellosis.

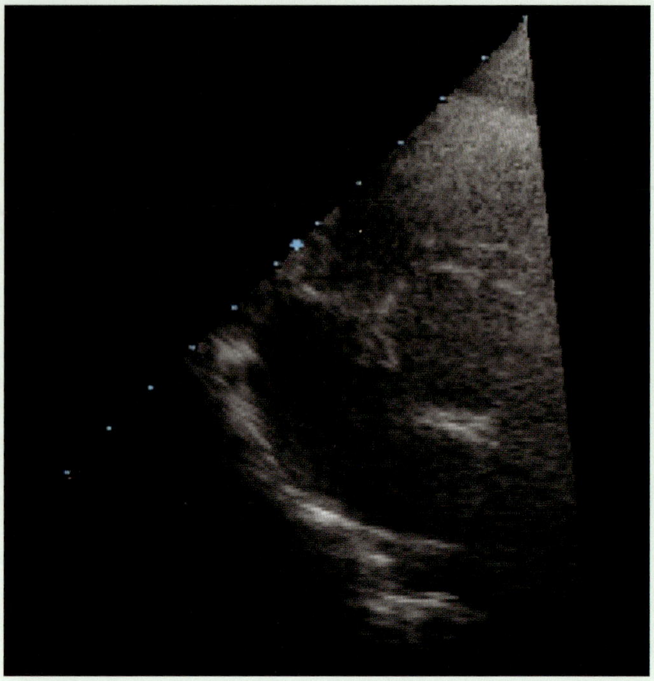

Fig. 62.6 Thickening and hyperechogenicity of the posterior tricuspid valve leaflet (*arrowhead*) in a dog with *Salmonella arizonae* bacteremia.

SUGGESTED READINGS

Behravesh CB, Ferraro A, Deasy M, et al. Human *Salmonella* infections linked to contaminated dry dog and cat food. *Pediatrics.* 2010;126:477–483. 2006-2008.

Crump JA, Sjolund-Karlsson, Gordon MA, et al. Epidemiology, clinical presentation, laboratory diagnosis, antimicrobial resistance, and antimicrobial management of invasive *Salmonella* infections. *Clin Microbiol Rev.* 2015;4:901–937.

REFERENCES

1. Salmon DE, Smith T. Investigations in swine plague. *USDA Bur Anim Indus Ann Rep.* 1885:184.
2. McAdam AJ. Enterobacteriaceae? Enterobacterales? What should we call enteric Gram-negative bacilli? A micro-comic strip. *J Clin Microbiol.* 2020;58. e01888-19.
3. Dominguez SA, Schaffner DW. Survival of *Salmonella* in processed chicken products during frozen storage. *J Food Prot.* 2009;72:2088–2092.
4. Brenner FW, Villar RG, Angulo FJ, et al. *Salmonella* nomenclature. *J Clin Microbiol.* 2000;38:2465–2467.
5. Centers for Disease Control and Prevention. Emerging Infectious Diseases. Scientific Nomenclature. Available from: https://wwwnc.cdc.gov/eid/page/scientific-nomenclature.
6. Foti M, Daidone A, Aleo A, et al. *Salmonella bongori* 48:z35:- in migratory birds, Italy. *Emerg Infect Dis.* 2009;15:502–503.
7. Herrera-Leon S, McQuiston JR, Usera MA, et al. Multiplex PCR for distinguishing the most common phase-1 flagellar antigens of *Salmonella* spp. *J Clin Microbiol.* 2004;42:2581–2586.
8. Davies RH, Lawes JR, Wales AD. Raw diets for dogs and cats: a review, with particular reference to microbiological hazards. *J Small Anim Pract.* 2019;60:329–339.
9. Finley R, Reid-Smith R, Ribble C, et al. The occurrence and antimicrobial susceptibility of salmonellae isolated from commercially available canine raw food diets in three Canadian cities. *Zoonoses Public Health.* 2008;55:462–469.
10. Finley R, Ribble C, Aramini J, et al. The risk of salmonellae shedding by dogs fed *Salmonella*-contaminated commercial raw food diets. *Can Vet J.* 2007;48:69–75.
11. Jones JL, Wang L, Ceric O, et al. Whole genome sequencing confirms source of pathogens associated with bacterial foodborne illness in pets fed raw pet food. *J Vet Diagn Invest.* 2019;31:235–240.
12. Lefebvre SL, Reid-Smith R, Boerlin P, et al. Evaluation of the risks of shedding salmonellae and other potential pathogens by therapy dogs fed raw diets in Ontario and Alberta. *Zoonoses Public Health.* 2008;55:470–480.
13. Lenz J, Joffe D, Kauffman M, et al. Perceptions, practices, and consequences associated with foodborne pathogens and the feeding of raw meat to dogs. *Can Vet J.* 2009;50:637–643.
14. McKenzie E, Riehl J, Banse H, et al. Prevalence of diarrhea and enteropathogens in racing sled dogs. *J Vet Intern Med.* 2010;24:97–103.
15. van Bree FPJ, Bokken G, Mineur R, et al. Zoonotic bacteria and parasites found in raw meat-based diets for cats and dogs. *Vet Rec.* 2018;182:50.
16. Viegas FM, Ramos CP, Xavier RGC, et al. Fecal shedding of *Salmonella* spp., *Clostridium perfringens*, and *Clostridiodes difficille* in dogs fed raw meat-based diets in Brazil and their owners' motivation. *PLoS One.* 2020;15:e0231275.
17. Behravesh CB, Ferraro A, Deasy 3rd M, et al. Human *Salmonella* infections linked to contaminated dry dog and cat food. *Pediatrics.* 2010;126:477–483. 2006-2008.
18. Centers for Disease Control and Prevention. Multistate outbreak of human *Salmonella* infections caused by contaminated dry dog food: United States, 2006-2007. *Morb Mortal Wkly Rep.* 2008;57:521–524.
19. Centers for Disease Control and Prevention. Notes from the field: human *Salmonella infantis* infections linked to dry dog food: United States and Canada, 2012. *Morb Mortal Wkly Rep.* 2012;61:436.

20. Selmi M, Stefanelli S, Bilei S, et al. Contaminated commercial dehydrated food as source of multiple *Salmonella* serotypes outbreak in a municipal kennel in Tuscany. *Vet Ital.* 2011;47:183–190.
21. Centers for Disease Control and Prevention. Outbreak of Multidrug-Resistant *Salmonella* Infections Linked to Contact with Pig Ear Pet Treats; 2019. https://www.cdc.gov/salmonella/pet-treats-07-19/index.html.
22. Taormina PJ. Survival rate of *Salmonella* on cooked pig ear pet treats at refrigerated and ambient temperature storage. *J Food Prot.* 2014;77: 50–56.
23. Morse EV, Duncan MA, Estep DA, et al. Canine salmonellosis: a review and report of dog to child transmission of *Salmonella enteritidis. Am J Public Health.* 1976;66:82–84.
24. Hernandez SM, Keel K, Sanchez S, et al. Epidemiology of a *Salmonella enterica* subsp. *enterica* serovar Typhimurium strain associated with a songbird outbreak. *Appl Environ Microbiol.* 2012;78:7290–7298.
25. Soderlund R, Jernberg C, Tronnberg L, et al. Linked seasonal outbreaks of *Salmonella* Typhimurium among passerine birds, domestic cats and humans, Sweden, 2009 to 2016. *Euro Surveill.* 2019;24. 1900074.
26. Koenig A, Cooper TL, Greene CE, et al. Clinical salmonellosis in a closed colony of blood donor cats. *Comp Med.* 2017;67:524–528.
27. Hill SL, Cheney JM, Taton-Allen GF, et al. Prevalence of enteric zoonotic organisms in cats. *J Am Vet Med Assoc.* 2000;216:687–692.
28. Murphy C, Reid-Smith RJ, Prescott JF, et al. Occurrence of antimicrobial resistant bacteria in healthy dogs and cats presented to private veterinary hospitals in southern Ontario: a preliminary study. *Can Vet J.* 2009;50:1047–1053.
29. Spain CV, Scarlett JM, Wade SE, et al. Prevalence of enteric zoonotic agents in cats less than 1 year old in central New York State. *J Vet Intern Med.* 2001;15:33–38.
30. Stavisky J, Radford AD, Gaskell R, et al. A case-control study of pathogen and lifestyle risk factors for diarrhoea in dogs. *Prev Vet Med.* 2011;99: 185–192.
31. Van Immerseel F, Pasmans F, De Buck J, et al. Cats as a risk for transmission of antimicrobial drug-resistant *Salmonella. Emerg Infect Dis.* 2004;10:2169–2174.
32. Leonard EK, Pearl DL, Finley RL, et al. Comparison of antimicrobial resistance patterns of *Salmonella* spp. and *Escherichia coli* recovered from pet dogs from volunteer households in Ontario (2005-06). *J Antimicrob Chemother.* 2012;67:174–181.
33. Wu X, Angkititrakul S, A LR, et al. Risk of antimicrobial resistant non-typhoidal *Salmonella* during asymptomatic infection passage between pet dogs and their human caregivers in Khon Kaen, Thailand. *Antibiotics (Basel).* 2020;9:477.
34. Morley PS, Strohmeyer RA, Tankson JD, et al. Evaluation of the association between feeding raw meat and *Salmonella enterica* infections at a Greyhound breeding facility. *J Am Vet Med Assoc.* 2006;228:1524–1532.
35. Viegas FM, Ramos CP, Xavier RGC, et al. Fecal shedding of *Salmonella* spp., *Clostridium perfringens*, and *Clostridioides difficile* in dogs fed raw meat-based diets in Brazil and their owners' motivation. *PLoS One.* 2020;15:e0231275.
36. Botha WJ, Schoeman JP, Marks SL, et al. Prevalence of *Salmonella* in juvenile dogs affected with parvoviral enteritis. *J S Afr Vet Assoc.* 2018;89: e1–e6.
37. Reimschuessel R, Grabenstein M, Guag J, et al. Multilaboratory survey to evaluate *Salmonella* prevalence in diarrheic and nondiarrheic dogs and cats in the United States between 2012 and 2014. *J Clin Microbiol.* 2017;55:1350–1368.
38. Philbey AW, Brown FM, Mather HA, et al. Salmonellosis in cats in the United Kingdom: 1955 to 2007. *Vet Rec.* 2009;164:120–122.
39. Sabshin SJ, Levy JK, Tupler T, et al. Enteropathogens identified in cats entering a Florida animal shelter with normal feces or diarrhea. *J Am Vet Med Assoc.* 2012;241:331–337.
40. Cummings KJ, Mitchell PK, Rodriguez-Rivera LD, et al. Sequence analysis of *Salmonella enterica* isolates obtained from shelter dogs throughout Texas. *Vet Med Sci.* 2020;6:975–979.
41. Hohenhaus AE, Rosenberg MP, Moroff SD. Concurrent lymphoma and salmonellosis in a cat. *Can Vet J.* 1990;31:38–40.
42. Moazed TC, Deeb BJ, DiGiacomo RF. Subcutaneous abscess due to *Salmonella adelaide* in a grey collie with cyclic hematopoiesis. *Lab Anim Sci.* 1990;40:639–641.
43. Cole SD, Palermo SM, Rankin SC. *Salmonella enterica* serovar Typhimurium isolated from the urine of a dog undergoing treatment for immune-mediated polyarthritis. *JMM Case Rep.* 2018;5:e005153.
44. Callegari C, Palermo G, Greco MF, et al. Pneumonia associated with *Salmonella* spp. infection in a cat receiving cyclosporine. *Schweiz Arch Tierheilkd.* 2014;156:499–503.
45. Pegues DA, Miller SI. *Salmonella* species. In: Bennett JE, Dolin R, Blaser MJ, eds. *Mandell, Douglas and Bennett's Principles and Practice of Infectious Diseases.* Philadelphia, PA: Elsevier Saunders; 2015:2559–2568.
46. Gal-Mor O. Persistent infection and long-term carriage of typhoidal and nontyphoidal salmonellae. *Clin Microbiol Rev.* 2019;32:e00088-18.
47. Grassl GA, Finlay BB. Pathogenesis of enteric *Salmonella* infections. *Curr Opin Gastroenterol.* 2008;24:22–26.
48. Delaloye J, Merlani G, Petignat C, et al. Nosocomial nontyphoidal salmonellosis after antineoplastic chemotherapy: reactivation of asymptomatic colonization? *Eur J Clin Microbiol Infect Dis.* 2004;23:751–758.
49. Lomborg SR, Agerholm JS, Jensen AL, et al. Effects of experimental immunosuppression in cattle with persistently high antibody levels to *Salmonella* Dublin lipopolysaccharide O-antigens. *BMC Vet Res.* 2007;3:17.
50. Fierer J, Guiney DG. Diverse virulence traits underlying different clinical outcomes of *Salmonella* infection. *J Clin Invest.* 2001;107:775–780.
51. Dow SW, Jones RL, Henik RA, et al. Clinical features of salmonellosis in cats: six cases (1981-1986). *J Am Vet Med Assoc.* 1989;194:1464–1466.
52. Vercelli A, Lo Cicero E, Pazzini L. *Salmonella typhimurium* endocarditis and myocarditis in a cat. *Case Rep Vet Med.* 2019;2019:7390530.
53. Krath ML, Hillhouse AE, Little SV, et al. MiSeq sequencing of *Salmonella enterica* subsp. *houtenae* isolates from a dog treated for hind-limb paresis. *Microbiol Resour Announc.* 2020;9:e00655-20.
54. Hertzer JN, Fujishiro M, Lawhon SD, et al. Treatment and management of *Salmonella* prostatitis in a heartworm-positive intact male dog: a case report. *BMC Vet Res.* 2021;17:135.
55. Andruzzi MN, Krath ML, Lawhon SD, et al. *Salmonella enterica* subspecies *houtenae* as an opportunistic pathogen in a case of meningoencephalomyelitis and bacteriuria in a dog. *BMC Vet Res.* 2020;16:437.
56. Binagla EM, Levy NA. *Salmonella* mesenteric lymphadenitis causing septic peritonitis in two dogs. *Vet Med (Auckl).* 2020;11:25–30.
57. Fox JG, Beaucage CM, Murphy JC, et al. Experimental *Salmonella*-associated conjunctivitis in cats. *Can J Comp Med.* 1984;48:87–91.
58. Rodriguez Jr CO, Moon ML, Leib MS. *Salmonella choleraesuis* pneumonia in a cat without signs of gastrointestinal tract disease. *J Am Vet Med Assoc.* 1993;202:953–955.
59. Caldow GL, Graham MM. Abortion in foxhounds and a ewe flock associated with *Salmonella montevideo* infection. *Vet Rec.* 1998;142:138–139.
60. Morse EV, Duncan MA. Canine salmonellosis: prevalence, epizootiology, signs, and public health significance. *J Am Vet Med Assoc.* 1975;167:817–820.
61. Redwood DW, Bell DA. *Salmonella panama*: isolation from aborted and newborn canine fetuses. *Vet Rec.* 1983;112:362.
62. Goodman LB, McDonough PL, Anderson RR, et al. Detection of *Salmonella* spp. in veterinary samples by combining selective enrichment and real-time PCR. *J Vet Diagn Invest.* 2017;29:844–851.
63. Dieckmann R, Malorny B. Rapid screening of epidemiologically important *Salmonella enterica* subsp. *enterica* serovars by whole-cell matrix-assisted laser desorption ionization-time of flight mass spectrometry. *Appl Environ Microbiol.* 2011;77:4136–4146.
64. Dieckmann R, Helmuth R, Erhard M, et al. Rapid classification and identification of salmonellae at the species and subspecies levels by whole-cell matrix-assisted laser desorption ionization-time of flight mass spectrometry. *Appl Environ Microbiol.* 2008;74:7767–7778.
65. Kurowski PB, Traub-Dargatz JL, Morley PS, et al. Detection of *Salmonella* spp. in fecal specimens by use of real-time polymerase chain reaction assay. *Am J Vet Res.* 2002;63:1265–1268.
66. Pusterla N, Byrne BA, Hodzic E, et al. Use of quantitative real-time PCR for the detection of *Salmonella* spp. in fecal samples from horses at a veterinary teaching hospital. *Vet J.* 2010;186:252–255.

67. Ward MP, Alinovi CA, Couetil LL, et al. Evaluation of a PCR to detect *Salmonella* in fecal samples of horses admitted to a veterinary teaching hospital. *J Vet Diagn Invest*. 2005;17:118–123.
68. Stiver SL, Frazier KS, Mauel MJ, et al. Septicemic salmonellosis in two cats fed a raw-meat diet. *J Am Anim Hosp Assoc*. 2003;39:538–542.
69. Timbs DV, Durham PJ, Barnsley DG. Chronic cholecystitis in a dog infected with *Salmonella* Typhimurium. *N Z Vet J*. 1974;22:100–102.
70. Opal SM, Gluck T. Endotoxin as a drug target. *Crit Care Med*. 2003;31:S57–S64.
71. Wittebole X, Castanares-Zapatero D, Laterre PF. Toll-like receptor 4 modulation as a strategy to treat sepsis. *Mediators Inflamm*. 2010;2010:568396.
72. Chen F, Zou L, Williams B, et al. Targeting Toll-like receptors in sepsis: from bench to clinical trials. *Antioxid Redox Signal*. 2021;35:1324–1339.
73. Bueno SM, Gonzalez PA, Carreno LJ, et al. The capacity of *Salmonella* to survive inside dendritic cells and prevent antigen presentation to T cells is host specific. *Immunology*. 2008;124:522–533.
74. Albaghdadi H, Robinson N, Finlay B, et al. Selectively reduced intracellular proliferation of *Salmonella enterica* serovar Typhimurium within APCs limits antigen presentation and development of a rapid CD8 T cell response. *J Immunol*. 2009;183:3778–3787.
75. Centers for Disease Control and Prevention. Healthy Pets, Healthy People. Reptiles and Amphibians. 2020. Available from: https://www.cdc.gov/healthypets/pets/reptiles.html.
76. Wright JG, Tengelsen LA, Smith KE, et al. Multidrug-resistant *Salmonella* Typhimurium in four animal facilities. *Emerg Infect Dis*. 2005;11:1235–1241.
77. Centers for Disease Control and Prevention. Information for Veterinarians. Multistate Outbreak of Human *Salmonella* Infantis Infections Linked to Dry Dog Food (Final Update); 2018. Available from: https://www.cdc.gov/salmonella/dog-food-05-12/vet-info.html.

63

Enteric *Escherichia coli* Infections

Jane E. Sykes

KEY POINTS

- First Described: Germany, 1885 (Theodor Escherich).[1]
- Cause: *Escherichia coli* (gram-negative rods that belong to the Enterobacterales).
- Affected Hosts: Humans and a large variety of animals.
- Geographic Distribution: Worldwide.
- Primary Mode of Transmission: Fecal-oral.
- Major Clinical Signs: Fever, lethargy, inappetence, diarrhea, vomiting.
- Differential Diagnoses: Differential diagnoses for suspected *E. coli* enterocolitis include canine and feline parvovirus infection, canine distemper virus infection, salmon poisoning disease, campylobacteriosis, clostridial diarrhea, salmonellosis, giardiasis, tritrichomoniasis (cats), cryptosporidiosis, whipworms, pythiosis, histoplasmosis, leptospirosis, dietary indiscretion, GI foreign body, pancreatitis, inflammatory bowel disease, lymphoma, hypoadrenocorticism, hyperthyroidism (cats), toxins (including drugs).
- Human Health Significance: Based on strain typing, dogs and cats have the potential to be a source of human infection by pathogenic *E. coli* strains capable of causing diarrhea. However, the vast majority of infections in humans occur in developing countries, in travelers, and are foodborne.

ETIOLOGY AND EPIDEMIOLOGY

Escherichia coli are pleomorphic gram-negative, non–spore-forming rods that belong to the family Enterobacterales. Like *Salmonella, E. coli* can survive long periods of time in feces, dust, and water. They are part of the normal flora of the GI tract but can be associated with enterocolitis in the presence of bacterial virulence factors and impaired local or systemic immunity. *Escherichia coli* infections can be transferred between animal species and some may be zoonotic; many infections are food borne.

There are more than 170 serogroups of *E. coli* based on the identity of the bacterial O (somatic) antigen, the sugar that is on the most external portion of the bacterial LPS (see Chapter 53). Organisms are also identified on the basis of their H (flagellar) antigens—for example, O157:H7 *E. coli*. Over 50 H antigens have been identified, but only a limited number of O and H combinations are associated with disease. Both the bacterial LPS (endotoxin) and the flagellar antigens are bacterial virulence factors. Other virulence factors in *E. coli* include adhesins, bacterial exotoxins such as cytotoxic necrotizing factor (CNF), hemolysins, heat-labile (LT) and heat-stable (ST) enterotoxins, and the capsular polysaccharide (K).

Escherichia coli strains that cause GI disease have been divided into distinct pathogenic categories (pathovars). Each pathovar is defined by a characteristic set of virulence factors that act in concert to determine the clinical, pathologic, and epidemiologic features of the disease they cause. However, it should also be noted that hybrid strains exist that possess features of multiple pathovars. The pathovars include enteropathogenic *E. coli* (EPEC), enterotoxigenic *E. coli* (ETEC), enterohemorrhagic *E. coli* (EHEC), enteroinvasive *E. coli* (EIEC), enteroaggregative *E. coli* (EAEC), adherent-invasive *E. coli* (AIEC), and possibly an additional group, diffusely adherent *E. coli* (DAEC) (Table 63.1 and Fig. 63.1). Currently, the epidemiology of many of these strains and their role in disease causation is not well defined in small animals, with most work having been done in humans and farm animal species. Many strains have been isolated from both nondiarrheic and diarrheic dogs and cats. An association between EPEC and EHEC (including H7:O157) infection and diarrhea in dogs has been detected.[2,3] In addition, AIEC strains have been well associated with granulomatous colitis in boxer dogs.[4,5]

CLINICAL FEATURES

Pathogenesis and Clinical Signs

EPEC strains carry the *eae*A gene on their chromosome (*E. coli* attaching effacing), which is located in a "pathogenicity island" referred to as LEE (locus of enterocyte effacement). The *eae*A gene encodes a 94-kDa protein, intimin, which allows the organism to adhere intimately to intestinal epithelial cells. This leads to local effacement of the microvilli and formation of numerous, actin-rich pedestals on which the bacteria reside (Fig. 63.2).[6] The bacteria secrete their own receptor using a T3SS, the Tir receptor, and Tir-intimin interactions are involved in pedestal formation. The pedestals may help the bacteria to remain extracellular and thus escape immune recognition by the host. The resulting characteristic histopathologic lesions on enterocytes have been referred to as "attaching and effacing lesions." Although the exact mechanism by which EPEC produce diarrhea is not known, several factors may be involved including loss of microvillous surface area, loss of tight junction integrity, and altered electrolyte transport, with associated secretory watery diarrhea.[7] Other effector proteins inoculated by the T3SS interrupt the NK-κB pathway to inhibit the host immune response. By definition, the EPEC pathovar does not produce Shiga toxin, Shiga-like toxin, or verotoxins. EPEC serotypes that have been associated with diarrhea in humans have been identified in dogs and cats.[2,8-12] EPEC strains have been divided into "typical" EPEC strains (tEPEC) and "atypical" EPEC strains (aEPEC); typical strains possess a plasmid known as the *E. coli* adherence factor (EAF) plasmid, which encodes the bundle-forming pilus (bfp) operon.[13] Typical EPEC strains are well recognized as a cause of diarrhea in humans, and aEPEC are emerging as a cause of diarrhea in children in developed countries.[14] In one study of kittens from shelters, aEPEC were isolated from both diarrheic and non-diarrheic kittens.[11] However, kittens with diarrhea harbored a greater load of aEPEC than those without, and kittens infected with

TABLE 63.1 Pathogenic Strains of *Escherichia coli* That Cause Enterocolitis

Strain	Lesion	Signs	Virulence Characteristic
Enteropathogenic *E. coli* (EPEC)	Attaching and effacing lesions (effacement of microvilli and pedestal formation)	Watery diarrhea	*eaeA* gene (encodes intimin). Typical EPEC (tEPEC) produce type IV bundle-forming pili
Enterotoxigenic *E. coli* (ETEC)	Adhere using fimbria (colonization factors) and produce heat-labile (LT) and/or heat-stable (ST) toxins	Diarrhea	LT and ST production
Shiga-toxin–producing *E. coli* (STEC); includes enterohemorrhagic *E. coli* (EHEC)	Produce Shiga-like toxins (verotoxins) that cause vascular endothelial damage, also produce attaching and effacing lesions	Diarrhea, hemorrhagic colitis, hemolytic-uremic syndrome	Shiga-like toxin production, EHEC also produce attaching and effacing lesions
Enteroinvasive *E. coli* (EIEC)	Actively invade colonic epithelial cells	Large bowel diarrhea	Plasmid-encoded invasion genes such as *ipaH*
Diffusely adherent *E. coli* (DAEC)	Uniform coverage of surface of epithelial cells rather than bricklike effect	Diarrhea in humans (children)	AIDA-1 (adhesin involved in diffuse adherence), *daaC* (fimbrial adhesin gene)
Adherent-invasive *E. coli* (AIEC)	Invade colonic epithelial cells using unknown virulence mechanisms	Granulomatous/histiocytic ulcerative colitis in dogs (especially boxers)	None known
Enteroaggregative *E. coli* (EAEC)	Adhere to intestinal epithelium via fimbriae and aggregate in bricklike fashion	Persistent watery diarrhea in humans	*aggR* gene; also produce toxins such as EAST-1

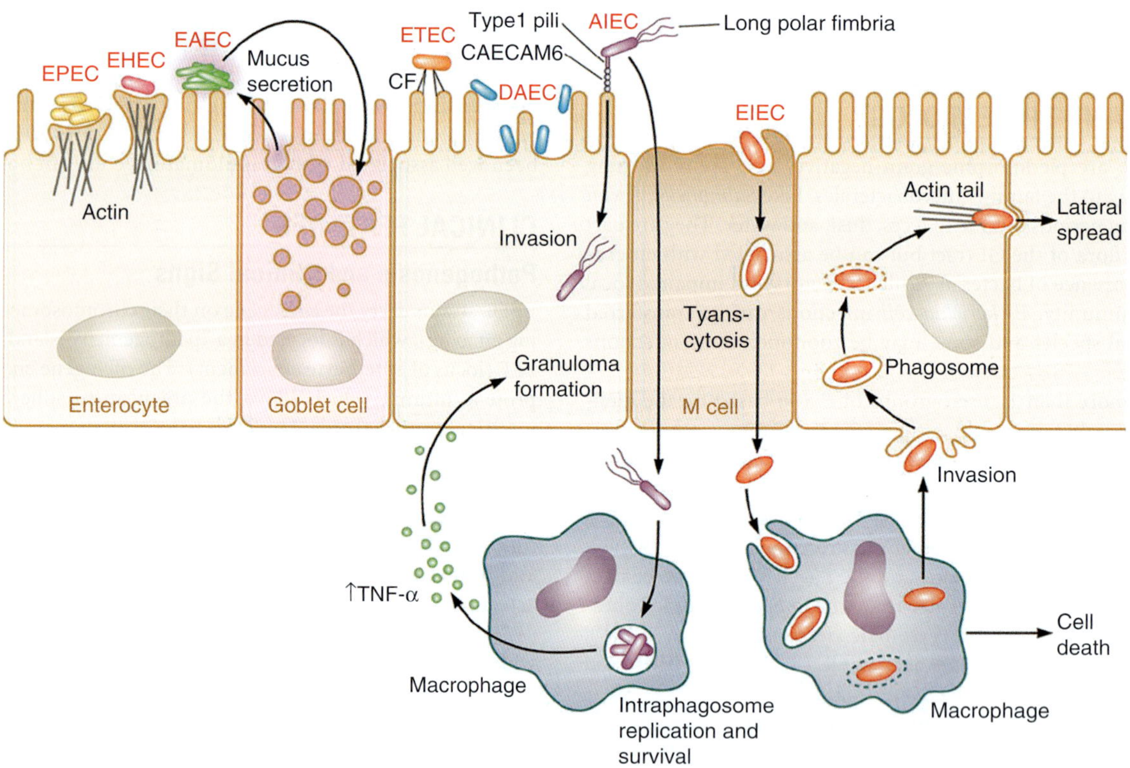

Fig. 63.1 Adherence patterns of enteric *Escherichia coli.* Pathogenic *E. coli* requires adherence to the host epithelium. Enteropathogenic *E. coli (EPEC) (yellow)* and enterohemorrhagic *E. coli (EHEC) (pink)* are extracellular pathogens that attach to the intestinal epithelium and efface microvilli, forming characteristic attaching and effacing lesions. Due to the presence of bundle-forming pili, EPEC is capable of forming microcolonies, resulting in a localized adherence (LA) pattern. Enterotoxigenic *E. coli (ETEC) (orange)* uses colonization factors *(CFs)* for attachment to host intestinal cells. Enteroaggregative *E. coli (EAEC) (green)* forms biofilms on the intestinal mucosa, and bacteria adhere to each other as well as to the cell surface to form an aggregative adherence pattern (AA) known as "stacked brick." Diffusely adherent *E. coli (DAEC) (blue)* is dispersed over the surfaces of intestinal cells, resulting in a diffuse adherence (DA) pattern. Adherent invasive *E. coli (AIEC) (purple)* colonizes the intestinal mucosa and is capable of invading epithelial cells as well as replicating within macrophages. AIEC uses type I pili to adhere to intestinal cells and long polar fimbriae that contribute to invasion. Enteroinvasive *E. coli (EIEC) (red)* are intracellular pathogens that penetrate the intestinal epithelium through M cells to gain access to the submucosa. EIEC escape submucosal macrophages by induction of macrophage cell death followed by basolateral invasion of colonocytes and lateral spread. (Modified from Croxen MA, Law RJ, Scholz R, et al. Recent advances in understanding enteric pathogenic *Escherichia coli. Clin Microbiol Rev.* 2013;26:822-880.)

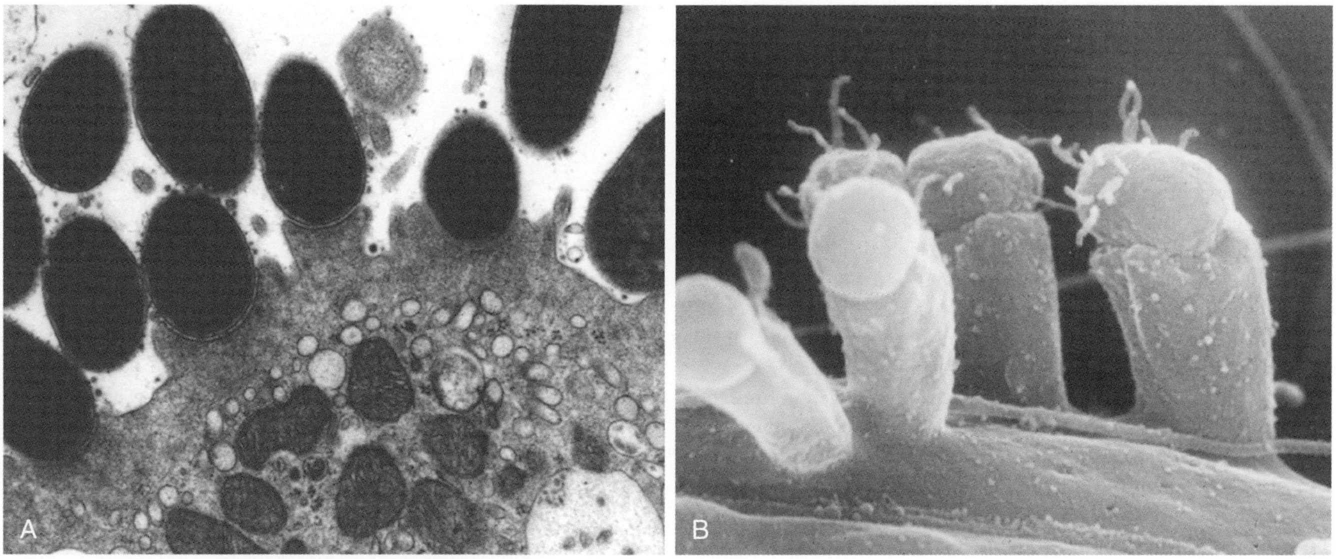

Fig. 63.2 Scanning and transmission electron micrographs showing actin pedestals induced by enteropathogenic and enterohemorrhagic *Escherichia coli* (EPEC and EHEC). (A) EPEC generates attaching and effacing (AE) lesions on the intestinal epithelium after infection of gnotobiotic piglets. Note the pedestal-like structures on host cells beneath attached bacteria. (From Campellone KG, Leong JM. Tails of two Tirs: actin pedestal formation by enteropathogenic *E. coli* and enterohemorrhagic *E. coli*. *Curr Opin Microbiol.* 2003;6(1):82-90.) (B) Actin pedestals that resemble AE lesions formed *in vivo* are also generated on cultured epithelial (HeLa) cells. (Courtesy of Knutton S. In: Knutton S, Rosenshine L, Pallen, MJ, et al. A novel EspA-associated surface organelle of enteropathogenic *Escherichia coli* involved in protein translocation into epithelial cells. *EMBO J.* 1998;17:2166-2176.)

aEPEC had more severe small intestinal and colonic lesions and were more likely to require subcutaneous fluid administration.[13]

ETEC are a major cause of diarrhea in human infants in developing countries and are the agents most frequently responsive for traveler's diarrhea. They are known for their ability to produce two broad types of virulence factors: adhesins (primarily fimbrial adhesins, also known as colonization factors) and enterotoxins. There are more than 20 different types of adhesins recognized. The enterotoxins are divided into high-molecular-weight labile toxins (LT), which are inactivated by heating at 60°C for 15 minutes; and low-molecular-weight stable toxins (ST), which are stable when exposed to a temperature of 100°C for 15 minutes.[15]

ETEC pathovars have been associated with up to 31% of cases of canine diarrhea, particularly in young dogs.[16-18] Most of the canine ETEC strains express ST enterotoxin, whereas ETEC strains that produce LT enterotoxin are rarely found. The bacteria adhere to the proximal small intestinal mucosa and produce plasmid-encoded LT and ST enterotoxins. LT is related to cholera toxin and is taken up by enterocytes. Once within intestinal epithelial cells, it activates adenylate cyclase, which leads to increased concentrations of intracellular cyclic AMP. This in turn activates protein kinase A, which activates the cystic fibrosis transmembrane conductance receptor (CFTR) with active secretion of chloride ions. Sodium and water follow, leading to diarrhea, hypovolemia, and metabolic acidosis. LT may also loosen intestinal epithelial cell tight junctions, further contributing to fluid loss.[19] It has been suggested that ST binds to the extracellular domain of guanylyl cyclase C, which leads to accumulation of intracellular cyclic guanosine monophosphate (GMP), activation of protein kinase C then the CFTR, and ultimately secretion of chloride, with resultant osmotic diarrhea. However, other mechanisms of action also likely operate, including inhibition of sodium uptake and increased intracellular calcium concentration, which opens a calcium-gated chloride channel and stimulates the arachidonic acid cascade.[20] Two different ST enterotoxins have been identified, STa and STb. STs also appear to be able to reduce the integrity of intestinal epithelial cell tight junctions.[19] ST-producing ETEC have been detected in young dogs with diarrhea.[16-18]

In addition to producing attaching and effacing lesions similar to those created by EPEC, STEC (Shiga-toxin–producing *E. coli*, which include EHEC) produce Shiga-like toxins (also known as verotoxins). They cause diarrhea, hemorrhagic colitis, and hemolytic-uremic syndrome (HUS) (e.g., *E. coli* strain O157:H7). The primary reservoir for these strains of *E. coli* are large herbivorous mammals, especially cattle, but the organisms can also persist for long periods of time in the environment. Shiga-like toxins are absorbed from the intestinal lumen and cause vascular endothelial damage, which may lead to a multiorgan thrombotic process in the absence of bacteremia. STEC can also produce other toxins that contribute to the pathogenesis of the disease. HUS in humans is characterized by renal failure, widespread microthrombotic damage to a variety of organs, hemolytic anemia, and sometimes diarrhea. Similar syndromes have been described in dogs, but an associated *E. coli* infection was not demonstrated.[21,22] In Argentina, STEC were detected in dogs that were contacts of humans with HUS.[23] HUS has been reproduced experimentally in dogs with a non-O157:H7 *E. coli* serotype.[24] Based on the similarity of renal lesions to those described in HUS, and the practice of feeding predominantly raw meat diets to greyhounds, it has been hypothesized that cutaneous and renal glomerular vasculopathy of greyhounds (also known as "Alabama rot" or "Greenetrack disease") may result from infection with STEC strains such as O157:H7.[25] A similar condition was described in a great Dane from Germany[26] and pet dogs in the United Kingdom.[27] Some dogs develop cutaneous lesions in the absence of renal failure; other dogs develop renal failure before the onset of cutaneous lesions.

EIEC actively invade colonic epithelial cells by way of a T3SS that allows them to escape macrophage phagocytosis and use the host actin-filament machinery to spread from cell to cell.[14] This, together with the associated inflammatory response, leads to hemorrhagic, large bowel diarrhea. In human patients, the EIEC pathovar is uncommonly detected compared with EPEC and ETEC. AIEC, which lack the virulence genes that identify EIEC, have been associated with granulomatous colitis in boxer dogs and infrequently in French bulldogs, Border collies, and breeds in the mastiff cluster.[28] This infection typically affects young adult boxer dogs that show signs of severe colitis, with colonic thickening and ulceration, and weight loss that is often marked.[5,29] Genetic susceptibility in boxer dogs and French bulldogs is associated with mutations in a region that encodes the CD48/SLAM family of genes on chromosome 48; mutations in this region have also been associated with inflammatory bowel disease in humans.[28,30]

The EAEC pathovar is considered an emerging pathogen in human patients. It adheres to epithelial cells of the terminal ileum and colon using fimbriae in a characteristic "stacked brick" pattern. Expression of these fimbriae is encoded by a plasmid gene known as *aggR*. Bacterial aggregation results in deposition of a thick biofilm on the gut mucosa, and this is followed by malabsorpsion and a subsequent inflammatory response, which leads to development of persistent watery diarrhea. Occasionally, EAEC strains also produce toxins, such as enteroaggregative heat-stable toxin-1 (EAST-1), which somewhat resembles the stable toxin of ETEC and can increase intracellular cyclic GMP.[31] There is also a diffusely adherent pathotype (DAEC) that uses a variety of adhesins to bind in a diffuse manner to enterocytes, interfering with microvillus function and stimulating an inflammatory response through activation of TLR5.[14] The role of EAEC and DAEC in dogs and cats requires further investigation.

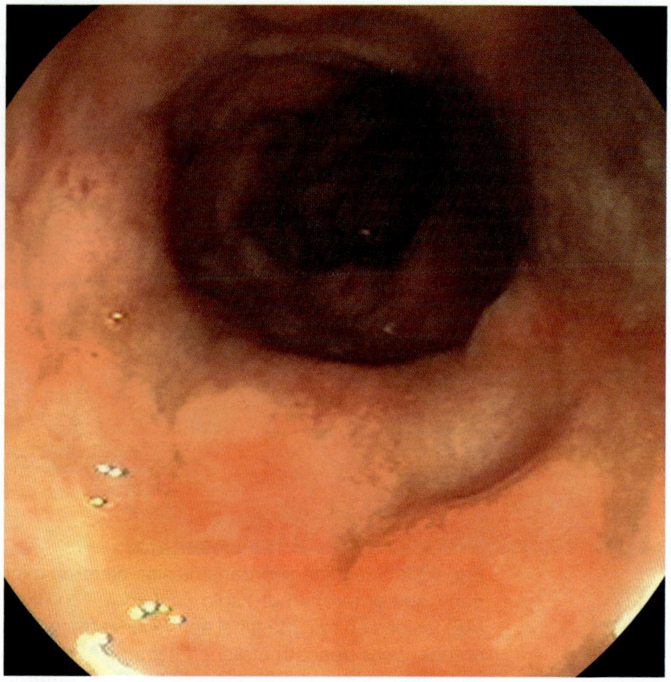

Fig. 63.3 Ulcerated and erythematous colon of a 2-year-old intact male boxer dog with granulomatous colitis as viewed during colonoscopy. The dog had a 7-month history of marked weight loss and severe diarrhea, with increased frequency of defecation and hematochezia.

Physical Examination Findings

Physical examination may reveal dehydration and abdominal pain in puppies or kittens with *E. coli* diarrhea. Dogs with HUS have had cutaneous erythema and well-demarcated, multifocal cutaneous ulcers of the limbs. Fever and peripheral edema have also been described. Dogs with granulomatous colitis may have poor body condition. A thickened and irregular rectal wall may be detected on rectal palpation, and the feces may contain fresh blood and mucus.

DIAGNOSIS

Diagnosis of intestinal *E. coli* infections, with the exception of granulomatous colitis of boxer dogs, is difficult or impossible with currently available diagnostic assays, because of the fact that healthy dogs and cats shed *E. coli*, and it is a combination of bacterial virulence factors and host immune competence that contributes to the development of clinical signs. This section therefore focuses primarily on the more specific clinical syndromes caused by EHEC and AIEC.

Laboratory Abnormalities

Complete Blood Count

CBC changes in dogs with *E. coli* diarrhea are generally mild and nonspecific. Leukocytosis may be present. Dogs infected with EHEC may be thrombocytopenic and have evidence of microangiopathic hemolysis. Microcytic anemia may be present in dogs with granulomatous colitis.

Serum Chemistry Panel and Urinalysis

Laboratory abnormalities in dogs with *E. coli* diarrhea could include electrolyte abnormalities and prerenal azotemia in dogs with severe diarrhea. Dogs infected with EHEC have had variable evidence of hypoalbuminemia, prerenal azotemia, increased activities of ALT and creatine kinase, hematuria, proteinuria, and isosthenuria. Boxer dogs with granulomatous colitis are commonly hypoalbuminemic.

Diagnostic Imaging

Findings on abdominal radiography and abdominal ultrasound are typically unremarkable or show fluid-filled intestinal loops. Abdominal ultrasound examination in dogs with granulomatous colitis often reveals mild or moderate mesenteric or sublumbar lymphadenomegaly, and the colonic wall can appear thickened.

Endoscopic Findings

Proctoscopy or colonoscopy is usually performed in order to obtain colonic biopsies from boxer dogs suspected to have granulomatous colitis. Proctoscopy requires less fastidious colonic preparation compared to colonoscopy, can be performed under heavy sedation, and is more cost-effective compared to colonoscopy. Most dogs with granulomatous colitis have involvement of the descending colon, underscoring the diagnostic utility of proctoscopy. Common changes in appearance to the colonic wall include erythema, irregularity, and ulceration of the rectal wall (Fig. 63.3).

Microbiologic Testing

Bacterial Isolation and Typing

Escherichia coli is commonly isolated on routine bacteriologic media from feces of both healthy and diarrheic dogs. A differential medium such as MacConkey agar is often used. Apart from dogs with granulomatous colitis, attempts to specifically identify *E. coli* as a cause of diarrhea are generally performed only by reference or public health laboratories when an outbreak has occurred, or for research purposes. *Escherichia coli* can be isolated from colonic biopsies of dogs with granulomatous colitis, which permits subsequent antimicrobial susceptibility testing.[32] Serologic identification, which is performed using specific O and H antisera, can be costly and is generally performed by large public health laboratories in epidemiologic investigations.

Virulence Assays

Immunoassays are available for detection of Shiga toxin, ST, and LT. A Vero cell cytotoxicity assay has been used to detect verocytotoxin. Identification of EPEC and AIEC often relies on assays that assess adherence in tissue culture. In research settings, molecular diagnostic techniques using DNA probes or PCR assays (including MLST) have revolutionized the ability to detect and differentiate between pathogenic and nonpathogenic strains of *E. coli*. EPEC characteristically possess the *eaeA* gene. Detection of genes that encode LT, ST, and Shiga-like toxin allows identification of ETEC and STEC. EIEC are identified based on the presence of invasion-associated genes such as *ipaH*.[31]

Pathologic Findings

The most significant pathologic findings in intestinal *E. coli* infections occur with EHEC and AIEC infections.

EHEC Infections

Cutaneous ulcerative lesions in dogs with suspected HUS are characterized histopathologically by fibrinoid vascular necrosis, with dermal thrombosis and leukocytoclastic vasculitis. Grossly, the kidneys may be swollen and have cortical petechiae. Histopathology reveals hyaline fibrinous thrombi in glomerular capillaries and afferent arterioles, glomerular and multifocal tubular necrosis, and leukocytoclastic vasculitis with fibrinoid necrosis.

AIEC Infections

Histopathologic lesions in dogs with granulomatous colitis are pathognomonic and include neutrophilic inflammation, epithelial ulceration, crypt hyperplasia and distortion, decreased goblet cell numbers, and abundant macrophages that stain positive with PAS stain (Fig. 63.4). The presence of *E. coli* within macrophages can be confirmed using fluorescence in situ hybridization, which has been recommended as part of the diagnostic workup of dogs suspected to have histiocytic ulcerative colitis.[6,30]

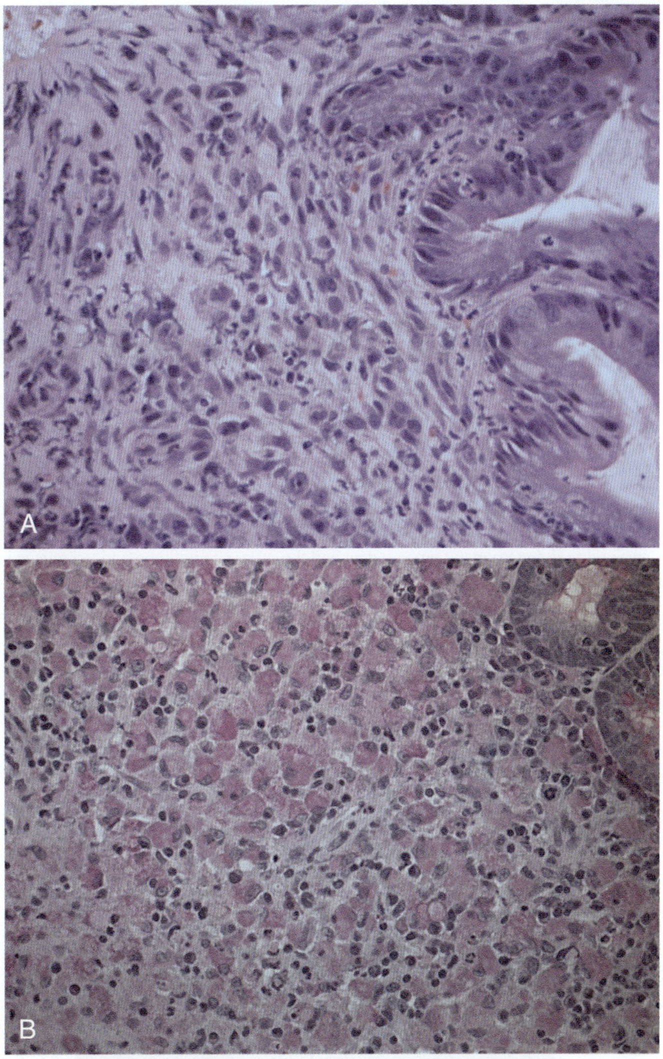

Fig. 63.4 (A) Histopathology showing severe, chronic, histiocytic colitis in a 2-year-old male boxer dog. The inflammatory infiltrate is comprised of large, epithelioid macrophages and lesser numbers of neutrophils, plasma cells, and lymphocytes. (B) Histiocytes in the lamina propria contain PAS-positive material.

TREATMENT AND PROGNOSIS

Dogs and cats with severe diarrhea due to pathogenic *E. coli* may require intravenous fluid therapy. With the exception of granulomatous colitis, antimicrobial therapy is generally not indicated unless there is fever and evidence of sepsis (see Chapter 125). Dogs with granulomatous colitis can show dramatic responses to treatment with enrofloxacin (10 mg/kg PO q24h), and a minimum treatment duration of 8 weeks is recommended.[30] Administration of fluoroquinolones is usually associated with rapid resolution of clinical signs and resolves cellular infiltration characteristic of this disorder on colonic biopsy. Because multidrug resistance has been documented in some isolates from dogs with granulomatous colitis, attempts to isolate *E. coli* from colonic biopsies before treatment are recommended so that antimicrobial susceptibility testing can be performed.[28,32] Antimicrobials that penetrate intracellularly, such as fluoroquinolones, chloramphenicol, rifampin, or trimethoprim-sulfonamides, should be chosen for treatment based on the results of susceptibility testing. For some isolates, carbapenems were the only drugs that penetrate intracellularly for which susceptibility was identified.[28]

IMMUNITY AND VACCINATION

Currently, no vaccines for *E. coli* infections are available for dogs and cats. Vaccines for EPEC, ETEC, and EHEC have been investigated for animals and humans on a research basis,[33-35] including a transdermal LT vaccine for prevention of travelers' diarrhea, although this was not shown to be effective in Phase III clinical trials.[36]

PUBLIC HEALTH ASPECTS

Pathogenic *E. coli* that cause diarrhea have been particularly prevalent in children in developing countries and in travelers to developing countries. STEC can be acquired following ingestion of undercooked ground hamburger meat, vegetables, and nonchlorinated drinking and swimming water that have been contaminated with fecal material, and as few as 100 organisms are required for infection. Infection has also been reported following contact with animals housed in petting zoos.[37] In a 2021 study from Switzerland, STEC were identified in 41% of commercially available raw meat-based diets for pets; of 28 strains identified, 29% carried genes linked to STEC of high pathogenic potential.[38] HUS is reported as the most common cause of acute renal failure in children. Clinical signs in humans consist of GI signs, often with profuse, bloody diarrhea, abdominal cramps, pallor, weakness, and oliguria or anuria.[39] Dogs have been suggested as a source of human infection with EPEC and EHEC.[8,10,11,40,41]

The possibility of zoonotic transmission of multidrug-resistant *E. coli* that are shed by dogs and cats is an emerging concern. A variety of resistance mechanisms have been identified in *E. coli* isolates from dogs and cats, which include production of efflux pumps and extended-spectrum and AmpC β-lactamase enzymes. There is some evidence that *E. coli* strains shed by healthy companion animals can be shared with humans that reside in the same household,[9,42-44] but more studies are required to determine the extent to which this occurs and its zoonotic significance. Transfer of plasmids that carry resistance genes from canine or feline *E. coli* isolates and those of humans also has the potential to occur.

For hospitalized animals, staff should use contact precautions for any dog or cat suspected to have enteropathogenic illness, including the use of warning signs, gloves and gowns, hand washing, and cleaning with bleach-based or accelerated hydrogen peroxide–based disinfectants. Endoscopes should be disinfected thoroughly between uses. Veterinarians should discuss the zoonotic implications of enteropathogenic bacterial infection with pet owners, especially in relation to the presence of young children or otherwise immunocompromised individuals in the household.

CASE EXAMPLE

Signalment

"Caesar," a 2-year-old male boxer dog from Tulare, CA (Fig. 63.5).

History

Caesar was evaluated for chronic diarrhea, which had been present since he was 6 months of age. His feces were loose and contained a small amount of frank blood. He strained to defecate many times a day, and the owner sometimes noticed mucus in the diarrhea. Every few months, Caesar's appetite and energy level declined and the diarrhea became more severe. His signs transiently improved after treatment with subcutaneous fluids and metronidazole. The owners had tried a variety of different diets such as fiber-supplemented diets and elimination diets that contain novel, single protein sources, but these strategies did not help. His current diet was a digestible commercial diet, and his appetite was good. He was up to date on vaccinations, including those for rabies, canine distemper, canine parvovirus, canine adenovirus, and *Bordetella bronchiseptica*. He was primarily an indoor dog with access to a suburban backyard.

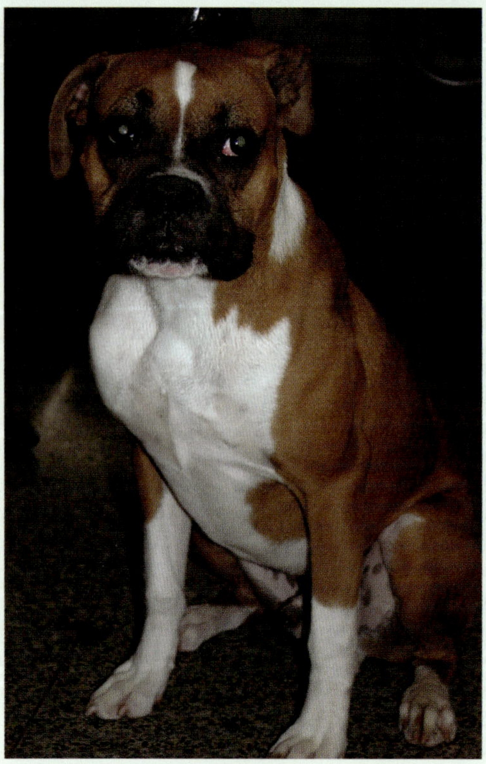

Fig. 63.5 "Caesar," a 2-year-old male boxer dog from Tulare, CA, that was diagnosed with granulomatous colitis following colonoscopy and biopsy.

Physical Examination

Body weight: 23.4 kg

General: Bright, alert, and responsive. Ambulatory on all four limbs. T = 102.5°F (39.2°C), HR = 102 beats/min, panting, mucous membranes pink, CRT = 1 s.

Integument, eyes, ears, nose, and throat: No significant abnormalities were noted. A moderate amount of dental calculus was present.

Musculoskeletal: Body condition score was 3/9 with symmetrical muscling.

All other systems: On rectal examination, the walls of the rectum were smooth. There was fresh blood on the glove following palpation. No other clinically significant abnormalities were noted.

Laboratory Findings

CBC: HCT 54.4% (40%–55%), MCV 76.8 fL (65–75 fL), MCHC 32.9 g/dL (33–36 g/dL), WBC 12,590 cells/μL (6000-13,000 cells/μL), neutrophils 9631 cells/μL (3000–10,500 cells/μL), lymphocytes 1674 cells/μL (1000–4000 cells/μL), monocytes 781 cells/μL (150–1200 cells/μL). Platelets were clumped but appeared adequate in number.

Serum chemistry profile: Sodium 155 mmol/L (145–154 mmol/L), potassium 4.2 mmol/L (3.6–5.3 mmol/L), chloride 116 mmol/L (108–118 mmol/L), bicarbonate 23 mmol/L (16–26 mmol/L), phosphorus 4.4 mg/dL (3.0–6.2 mg/dL), calcium 10.4 mg/dL (9.7–11.5 mg/dL), BUN 18 mg/dL (5–21 mg/dL), creatinine 1.1 mg/dL (0.3–1.2 mg/dL), glucose 105 mg/dL (64–123 mg/dL), total protein 6.5 g/dL (5.4–7.6 g/dL), albumin 2.9 g/dL (3.0–4.4 g/dL), globulin 3.6 g/dL (1.8–3.9 g/dL), ALT 68 U/L (19–67 U/L), AST 46 U/L (19–42 U/L), ALP 86 U/L (21–170 U/L), GGT 5 U/L (0–6 U/L), cholesterol 200 mg/dL (135–361 mg/dL), total bilirubin 0.1 mg/dL (0–0.2 mg/dL).

Fecal Examination

Centrifugal fecal flotation: Negative for parasites.

Colonoscopy: The entire mucosal surface of the colon was erythematous and irregular, with multifocal areas of mucosal ulceration (see Fig. 63.3).

Histopathology of colonic biopsies: Severe, chronic, histiocytic, and ulcerative colitis. Histiocytes in the lamina propria contained PAS-positive material (see Fig. 63.4).

Diagnosis

Granulomatous colitis of boxer dogs.

Treatment

Enrofloxacin, 6 mg/kg PO q24h for 8 weeks and a commercial low-residue dry and canned dog food. This was associated with clinical improvement within a week after starting the medication. At a recheck 4 weeks later, the owner reported that Caesar's feces were completely normal in consistency and frequency.

Comments

In this dog, the diagnosis of granulomatous colitis was made solely based on histopathologic findings. Culture of a biopsy specimen could also have been performed and is now recommended given the emergence of fluoroquinolone-resistant AIEC strains of *E. coli*.

SUGGESTED READINGS

Croxen MA, Law RJ, Scholz R, et al. Recent advances in understanding enteric pathogenic *Escherichia coli*. *Clin Microbiol Rev*. 2013;26:822–880.

Watson VE, Jacob ME, Flowers JR, et al. Association of atypical enteropathogenic *Escherichia coli* with diarrhea and related mortality in kittens. *J Clin Microbiol*. 2017;55:2719–2735.

REFERENCES

1. Escherich T. Die Darmbakterien des Neugeborenen und Säuglings. *Fortschr Med*. 1885;3:547–554. 515-522.
2. Morato EP, Leomil L, Beutin L, et al. Domestic cats constitute a natural reservoir of human enteropathogenic *Escherichia coli* types. *Zoonoses Public Health*. 2009;56:229–237.
3. Sancak AA, Rutgers HC, Hart CA, et al. Prevalence of enteropathic *Escherichia coli* in dogs with acute and chronic diarrhoea. *Vet Rec*. 2004;154:101–106.
4. Dogan B, Zhang S, Kalla SE, et al. Molecular and phenotypic characterization of *Escherichia coli* associated with granulomatous colitis of boxer dogs. *Antibiotics (Basel)*. 2020;9:540.
5. Simpson KW, Dogan B, Rishniw M, et al. Adherent and invasive *Escherichia coli* is associated with granulomatous colitis in boxer dogs. *Infect Immun*. 2006;74:4778–4792.
6. Celli J, Deng W, Finlay BB. Enteropathogenic *Escherichia coli* (EPEC) attachment to epithelial cells: exploiting the host cell cytoskeleton from the outside. *Cell Microbiol*. 2000;2:1–9.
7. Croxen MA, Law RJ, Scholz R, et al. Recent advances in understanding enteric pathogenic *Escherichia coli*. *Clin Microbiol Rev*. 2013;26:822–880.
8. Takagi H, Yamane K, Matsui M, et al. Pathotypes and drug susceptibility of *Escherichia coli* isolated from companion dogs in Japan. *Jpn J Infect Dis*. 2020;73:253–255.
9. Arais LR, Barbosa AV, Andrade JRC, et al. Zoonotic potential of atypical enteropathogenic *Escherichia coli* (aEPEC) isolated from puppies with diarrhoea in Brazil. *Vet Microbiol*. 2018;227:45–51.
10. Kjaergaard AB, Carr AP, Gaunt MC. Enteropathogenic *Escherichia coli* (EPEC) infection in association with acute gastroenteritis in 7 dogs from Saskatchewan. *Can Vet J*. 2016;57:964–968.
11. Watson VE, Jacob ME, Flowers JR, et al. Association of atypical enteropathogenic *Escherichia coli* with diarrhea and related mortality in kittens. *J Clin Microbiol*. 2017;55:2719–2735.
12. de Almeida PM, Arais LR, Andrade JR, et al. Characterization of atypical enteropathogenic *Escherichia coli* (aEPEC) isolated from dogs. *Vet Microbiol*. 2012;158:420–424.
13. Teixeira NB, Rojas TC, da Silveira WD, et al. Genetic analysis of enteropathogenic *Escherichia coli* (EPEC) adherence factor (EAF) plasmid reveals a new deletion within the EAF probe sequence among O119 typical EPEC strains. *BMC Microbiol*. 2015;15:200.
14. Nelson GE, Greene MH. Enterobacteriaceae. In: Bennett JE, Dolin R, Blaser MJ, eds. *Mandell, Douglas and Bennett's Principles and Practice of Infectious Diseases*. 9th ed. Philadelphia, PA: Elsevier Saunders; 2020:2669–2685.
15. Dubreuil JD. The whole shebang: the gastrointestinal tract, *Escherichia coli* enterotoxins and secretion. *Curr Issues Mol Biol*. 2012;14:71–82.
16. Beutin L. *Escherichia coli* as a pathogen in dogs and cats. *Vet Res*. 1999;30:285–298.
17. Drolet R, Fairbrother JM, Harel J, et al. Attaching and effacing and enterotoxigenic *Escherichia coli* associated with enteric colibacillosis in the dog. *Can J Vet Res*. 1994;58:87–92.
18. Hammermueller J, Kruth S, Prescott J, et al. Detection of toxin genes in *Escherichia coli* isolated from normal dogs and dogs with diarrhea. *Can J Vet Res*. 1995;59:265–270.
19. Dubreuil JD, Isaacson RE, Schifferli DM. Animal enterotoxigenic *Escherichia coli*. EcoSal Plus. 2016;7:10.1128/ecosalplus.
20. Butt S, Saleh M, Gagnon J. Impact of the *Escherichia coli* heat-stable enterotoxin b (STb) on gut health and function. *Toxins*. 2020;12:760.
21. Chantrey J, Chapman PS, Patterson-Kan JC. Haemolytic-uraemic syndrome in a dog. *J Vet Med A Physiol Pathol Clin Med*. 2002;49:470–472.
22. Dell'Orco M, Bertazzolo W, Pagliaro L, et al. Hemolytic-uremic syndrome in a dog. *Vet Clin Pathol*. 2005;34:264–269.
23. Alconcher LF, Rivas M, Lucarelli LI, et al. Shiga toxin-producing *Escherichia coli* in household members of children with hemolytic uremic syndrome. *Eur J Clin Microbiol Infect Dis*. 2020;39:427–432.
24. Wang JY, Wang SS, Yin PZ. Haemolytic-uraemic syndrome caused by a non-O157 : H7 *Escherichia coli* strain in experimentally inoculated dogs. *J Med Microbiol*. 2006;55:23–29.
25. Cowan LA, Hertzke DM, Fenwick BW, et al. Clinical and clinicopathologic abnormalities in greyhounds with cutaneous and renal glomerular vasculopathy: 18 cases (1992-1994). *J Am Vet Med Assoc*. 1997;210:789–793.
26. Rotermund A, Peters M, Hewicker-Trautwein M, et al. Cutaneous and renal glomerular vasculopathy in a great Dane resembling 'Alabama rot' of greyhounds. *Vet Rec*. 2002;151:510–512.
27. CountryFile. *Alabama Rot Dog Disease: How to Spot the Signs and Protect Your Dog*; 2021. https://www.countryfile.com/news/guide-to-alabama-rot-dog-disease-how-to-spot-the-signs-and-protect-your-dog/.
28. Manchester AC, Dogan B, Guo Y, et al. *Escherichia coli*-associated granulomatous colitis in dogs treated according to antimicrobial susceptibility profiling. *J Vet Intern Med*. 2021;35:150–161.
29. Van Kruiningen HJ, Civco IC, Cartun RW. The comparative importance of *E. coli* antigen in granulomatous colitis of boxer dogs. *APMIS*. 2005;113:420–425.
30. Mansfield CS, James FE, Craven M, et al. Remission of histiocytic ulcerative colitis in boxer dogs correlates with eradication of invasive intramucosal *Escherichia coli*. *J Vet Intern Med*. 2009;23:964–969.
31. Scavia G, Staffolani M, Fisichella S, et al. Enteroaggregative *Escherichia coli* associated with a foodborne outbreak of gastroenteritis. *J Med Microbiol*. 2008;57:1141–1146.
32. Craven M, Dogan B, Schukken A, et al. Antimicrobial resistance impacts clinical outcome of granulomatous colitis in boxer dogs. *J Vet Intern Med*. 2010;24:819–824.
33. Gu J, Liu Y, Yu S, et al. Enterohemorrhagic *Escherichia coli* trivalent recombinant vaccine containing EspA, intimin and Stx2 induces strong humoral immune response and confers protection in mice. *Microbes Infect*. 2009;11:835–841.
34. Keller R, Hilton TD, Rios H, et al. Development of a live oral attaching and effacing *Escherichia coli* vaccine candidate using *Vibrio cholerae* CVD 103-HgR as antigen vector. *Microb Pathog*. 2010;48:1–8.
35. Rojas RL, Gomes PA, Bentancor LV, et al. *Salmonella enterica* serovar Typhimurium vaccine strains expressing a nontoxic Shiga-like toxin 2 derivative induce partial protective immunity to the toxin expressed by enterohemorrhagic *Escherichia coli*. *Clin Vaccine Immunol*. 2010;17:529–536.
36. Behrens RH, Cramer JP, Jelinek T, et al. Efficacy and safety of a patch vaccine containing heat-labile toxin from *Escherichia coli* against travellers' diarrhoea: a phase 3, randomised, double-blind, placebo-controlled field trial in travellers from Europe to Mexico and Guatemala. *Lancet Infect Dis*. 2014;14:197–204.
37. Sherman PM, Ossa JC, Wine E. Bacterial infections: new and emerging enteric pathogens. *Curr Opin Gastroenterol*. 2010;26:1–4.
38. Treier A, Stephan R, Stevens MJ, et al. High occurrence of Shiga toxin-producing *Escherichia coli* in raw meat–based diets for companion animals – a public health issue. *Microorganisms*. 2021;9:1556.
39. Scheiring J, Andreoli SP, Zimmerhackl LB. Treatment and outcome of Shiga-toxin-associated hemolytic uremic syndrome (HUS). *Pediatr Nephrol*. 2008;23:1749–1760.
40. Hogg RA, Holmes JP, Ghebrehewet S, et al. Probable zoonotic transmission of verocytotoxigenic *Escherichia coli* O 157 by dogs. *Vet Rec*. 2009;164:304–305.
41. Nakazato G, Gyles C, Ziebell K, et al. Attaching and effacing *Escherichia coli* isolated from dogs in Brazil: characteristics and serotypic relationship to human enteropathogenic *E. coli* (EPEC). *Vet Microbiol*. 2004;101:269–277.
42. Harada K, Okada E, Shimizu T, et al. Antimicrobial resistance, virulence profiles, and phylogenetic groups of fecal *Escherichia coli* isolates: a comparative analysis between dogs and their owners in Japan. *Comp Immunol Microbiol Infect Dis*. 2012;35:139–144.
43. Johnson JR, Clabots C, Kuskowski MA. Multiple-host sharing, long-term persistence, and virulence of *Escherichia coli* clones from human and animal household members. *J Clin Microbiol*. 2008;46:4078–4082.
44. Stenske KA, Bemis DA, Gillespie BE, et al. Comparison of clonal relatedness and antimicrobial susceptibility of fecal *Escherichia coli* from healthy dogs and their owners. *Am J Vet Res*. 2009;70:1108–1116.

64

Enteric Clostridial Infections

Jane E. Sykes, Stanley L. Marks

KEY POINTS

- First Described: 1978 (causative role of *Clostridioides difficile* in pseudomembranous colitis) (George et al., 1978);[1] 1892 (*Clostridium perfringens*, by Nuttall and Welch);[2] evidence for a role of *C. perfringens* in foodborne illness was gathered over 50 years later.[3]
- Cause: *Clostridioides difficile* (previously *Clostridium difficile*) and *Clostridium perfringens*.
- Affected Hosts: Humans and a variety of other animals.
- Geographic Distribution: Worldwide.
- Primary Mode of Transmission: Fecal-oral; disease may result from toxin production by bacteria resident in the GI tract.
- Major Clinical Signs: Lethargy, anorexia, diarrhea, occasionally fever.
- Differential Diagnoses: Differential diagnoses for hemorrhagic gastroenteritis include salmon poisoning disease, CDV infection, canine and feline parvovirus infection, campylobacteriosis, salmonellosis, giardiasis, tritrichomoniasis (cats), cryptosporidiosis, whipworms, leptospirosis, dietary indiscretion, GI foreign body, pancreatitis, inflammatory bowel disease, lymphoma, hypoadrenocorticism, toxins (including drugs).
- Human Health Significance: Dogs and cats have the potential to be a source of human infection with *C. perfringens* and *C. difficile*, some of which may be resistant to antimicrobial drugs. Transmission of *C. difficile* from animals to humans has not been documented. The vast majority of human infections are acquired through other routes.

ETIOLOGY AND EPIDEMIOLOGY

Clostridioides difficile (formerly *Clostridium difficile*) and *Clostridium perfringens* are gram-positive, spore-forming, obligately anaerobic rods that are capable of toxin production. Clostridial spores are spherical to oval and distend the bacterial cells when they form within them (Fig. 64.1). They are very resistant to disinfection and can persist in the environment, including that within hospitals, for years. Clostridial species are found in soil and the intestinal tracts of a variety of different animal species. Despite these similarities, many differences exist between *C. difficile* and *C. perfringens* that relate to epidemiology, interpretation of diagnostic test results and treatment.

Clostridioides difficile is the most common cause of hospital and antimicrobial-associated diarrhea in hospitalized humans and can cause nosocomial diarrhea in dogs and cats in veterinary hospitals.[4,5] In one study, living with an immunocompromised human was a risk factor for *C. difficile* infection in dogs, but strains present in dogs were different to those found in the household environment.[6] Dogs visiting human health care facilities have also been shown to be at risk of acquiring *C. difficile* infections.[7] The recent emergence of "hypervirulent" *C. difficile* strains in people has resulted in the increased incidence of disease, increased mortality rates, increased relapse rates and recognition of community-associated diseases.[8,9] A similar change has not been observed in animals; however, a hypervirulent strain (North American pulsotype 1 or NAP1) was identified in a dog.[10] Strains with ribotypes that match those found in humans were identified in the feces of dogs visiting dog parks in Denmark,[11] fecal specimens from dogs in Germany,[12,13] Spain,[14,15] Italy,[16] Texas, USA,[17] and in dogs and cats from Brazil[18,19] and China.[20] Multiple studies have identified antimicrobial-resistant strains of *C. difficile* in the feces of dogs and cats, including strains resistant to clindamycin or metronidazole .[14-16,18,20,21] While pets have been implicated as a reservoir for human infection with toxigenic strains,[22-24] the extent to which dogs and cats play a role in human infection remains unclear.

Clostridium perfringens is especially widespread in soil and dust, and is now classified into 7 toxinotypes, A to G, based on the possession of major toxin genes that permit production of the toxins CPA (alpha), CPB (beta), ETX (epsilon), ITX (iota), CPE (enterotoxin), and NetB (necrotizing enteritis B-like toxin) (Table 64.1).[25] All *C. perfringens* strains produce CPA, which is encoded by a gene located in a stable region on the chromosome.[26] The other toxin genes are located on plasmids. The majority of clostridial foodborne illness in humans is caused by Type F strains, which produce CPE but not CPB, ETX or ITX. Strains that produce CPB, ETX, ITX, and NetB have been associated with diarrhea in food-producing animals.[27]

In dogs, *C. perfringens* infection has been associated with nosocomial diarrhea,[28] hemorrhagic enteritis,[29,30] and acute and chronic large bowel diarrhea. *Clostridium perfringens*–associated diarrhea can manifest with small intestinal, large intestinal, or diffuse clinical signs.[29-31] However, the importance of *C. perfringens* and *C. difficile* as causes of diarrhea in dogs and cats has been controversial, because these organisms have been isolated from both diarrheic and healthy animals. For example, *C. perfringens* can be isolated using culture in up to 100% of both diarrheic and non-diarrheic dogs.[31-33] The prevalence of *C. perfringens* colonization in healthy cats appears lower than that in the dog, ranging from 20% to 63%. Toxigenic strains can be found in both healthy and diarrheic dogs, although most studies have shown a correlation between detection of certain clostridial toxins (CPE, *C. difficile* toxin A, NetF) and diarrhea.[32,34]

CLINICAL FEATURES

Pathogenesis and Clinical Signs

Both *C. difficile* and *C. perfringens* cause diarrhea as a result of toxin production. The diarrhea can be mild and self-limiting or severe, acute, and hemorrhagic, with life-threatening consequences relating to dehydration and hypovolemic shock. Decreased appetite, vomiting, fever, and abdominal pain have also been reported in cats in association with clostridial infection, although the prevalence of infection is far lower in cats when compared to dogs.[35] Vomiting may also occur in dogs. Although clostridial diarrhea is often described as a large bowel-type diarrhea, clinical manifestations of both small and large bowel diarrhea have been described.

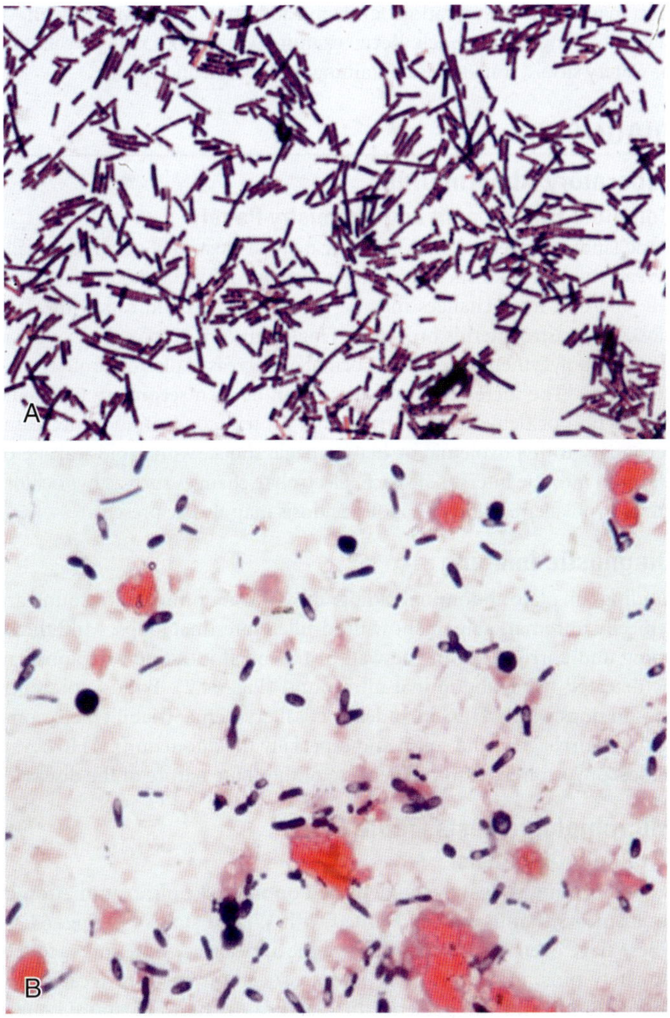

Fig. 64.1 (A) Gram stain of a pure culture of *Clostridium perfringens*. (From Onderdonk AB, Garrett WS. Diseases caused by *Clostridium*. In: Bennett JE, Dolin R, Blaser MJ (eds). *Mandell, Douglas, and Bennett's Principles and Practice of Infectious Diseases*, 9th ed. Philadelphia, PA: Elsevier; 2020:2960-2968. (B) Fecal smear from a dog with diarrhea showing spore-distended clostridial rods, leading to a characteristic "safety pin" and "tennis racquet" appearance.

Mechanism of Toxin Action

Clostridioides difficile *Toxins*. *Clostridioides difficile* can produce up to five toxins. The best studied are toxin A (TcdA), toxin B (TcdB), and *C. difficile* binary toxin (CDT, an ADP-ribosyltransferase which is made up of two components, hence the name binary). Studies suggest that strains that produce CDT in addition to TcdA and TcdB are more likely to be associated with severe disease in humans.[36] In contrast to humans, a history of antibiotic use does not always seem to be necessary for disease in dogs and cats. However, in one study, administration of antimicrobials prior to admission and the use of immunosuppressive drugs during hospitalization were risk factors for nosocomial colonization in both dogs and cats.[4] In another study of 136 fecal specimens from dogs in Texas, rates of colonization with toxigenic *C. difficile* increased significantly during antimicrobial therapy (to 33%) then declined to baseline (11%) when treatment was stopped.[17] Toxins A and B are large toxins that bind to small GTP-binding proteins (Rho, Rac, and Cdc42), which normally regulate intracellular actin dynamics. The result is a disruption of the cell cytoskeleton, with subsequent rounding and death of intestinal epithelial cells, and impairment of tight junctions, with resulting fluid accumulation and extensive damage, primarily to the large intestine. The two toxins also cause release of inflammatory cytokines from mast cells, macrophages, and epithelial cells.[37] The binary toxin CDT is composed of CDTb, which binds to a receptor on intestinal epithelial cells, and CDTa, which is then internalized and catalyzes the ADP-ribosylation of actin, resulting in its depolymerization and destruction of the cell cytoskeleton.[38]

Clostridium perfringens *toxins*. In addition to the toxins used for classification of toxinotypes, *C. perfringens* is capable of producing more than 20 other toxins or enzymes that can contribute to disease severity, such as perfringolysin O (PFO) and the pore-forming toxin NetF. CPE is a key toxin because it has been clearly associated with foodborne disease in humans.[27] It also has consistently been found in significantly more dogs with diarrhea than healthy dogs.[31-33] The gene for CPE (*cpe*) can be found on the chromosome or on plasmids, and expression occurs during sporulation. CPE causes pore formation and disrupts epithelial tight junctions by binding primarily to claudin, with increased paracellular permeability; large quantities of toxin can cause cell death.[27,39] CPE was detected with ELISA in 19.6% of 46 diarrheic dogs versus 2.1% of 48 healthy dogs, and in 8.3% of 48 diarrheic cats versus 0% of 39 healthy cats.[31,32,40] In another study, CPE was detected at a similar rate in 219 diarrheic and 54 non-diarrheic cats (4.1 versus 1.6%).[41] Strains of *C. perfringens* that possessed the *cpe* gene were identified in 32 (34%) of 95 healthy dogs and 50 (48%) of 104 dogs with GI disease.[33] In contrast, CPE was detected using ELISA in 1 (1%) of the healthy dogs and 17 (16%) of the diseased

TABLE 64.1 *Clostridium perfringens* Toxinotypes

Toxinotype	Alpha (CPA) (*cpa*)	Beta (CPB) (*cpb*)	Epsilon (ETX) (*etx*)	IOTA (ITX) (*iap* and *ibp*)[b]	Enterotoxin (*cpe*)	NetB (*netB*)
A	I	–	–	–	–	–
B	+	+	+	–	–	–
C	+	+		–	+/–	–
D	+	–	+	–	+/–	–
E	+	–	–	+	+/–	–
F[a]	+	–	–	–	+	–
G[a]	+	–	–	–	–	+

[a]Type F and G strains were classified as Type A before reclassification in 2018.[25]
[b]Binary toxin encoded by two genes, similar to that of *Clostridium botulinum*.

dogs. It should be emphasized that the commercially available ELISA test for detection of fecal CPE is a human-based immunoassay that has not yet been validated for use in the dog or cat. In addition, the mere detection of CPE using ELISA does not infer that the amount of toxin is sufficient to cause clinical signs. It is plausible that clinical signs only occur when a certain quantity of CPE is present, or only when it is produced in association with other virulence factors. CPE-associated *C. perfringens* diarrhea in dogs and cats is thought to occur subsequent to proliferation and sporulation of resident clostridial organisms in the intestinal lumen following an alteration in local intestinal conditions, with production of CPE. Decreased peristalsis, the effects of antimicrobial drugs on the resident intestinal microbiota, diet changes, or coinfections with other intestinal pathogens are factors that have the potential to lead to sporulation.

More recently, the *C. perfringens* toxin NetF has been recognized in association with disease in dogs and horses, specifically acute hemorrhagic diarrhea syndrome (AHDS) in dogs and foal necrotizing enterocolitis (see Chapter 125).[42-44] NetF can be found on a large plasmid together with NetE, another pore-forming toxin gene. NetF has sequence homology to the leukocidin/hemolysin family of pore-forming toxins which are able to permeabilize cell membranes through the formation of barrel-shaped pores.[45]

Canine AHDS, previously known as hemorrhagic gastroenteritis (HGE), is an acute syndrome of hemorrhagic diarrhea with dehydration and hemoconcentration that occurs worldwide.[46,47] The name was changed to AHDS because lesions are typically limited to the small and large intestines. However, vomiting precedes diarrhea in many dogs, and may contain blood.[46] Although any breed can be affected, in one large study, dogs with AHDS were smaller (median body weight 9.8 kg) and younger (median age 5 years) than dogs in the background hospital population, and Yorkshire terriers, miniature schnauzers, Maltese terriers and miniature pinschers were predisposed.[46] *Clostridium perfringens* can be detected in large numbers in association with necrotic small and large intestinal mucosal lesions of dogs with AHDS using immunohistochemistry.[47,48] Quantitative PCR also showed a significant increase in *C. perfringens* DNA copy number in dogs with AHDS when compared with healthy dogs and dogs with inflammatory bowel disease (IBD).[49] CPE was detected in 8/12 dogs (67%) with AHDS in one study.[16] A study from Germany evaluated the prevalence of clostridial toxin genes (using PCR) and toxin (using ELISA) in stool specimens from 54 dogs with idiopathic AHDS and 23 healthy control dogs. The toxin genes *tcdB* (*C. difficile*) and *cpe* were detected in 10/54 and 35/54 fecal specimens from dogs with AHDS and 3/23 and 9/23 healthy dogs, respectively. CDT A/B and CPE were detected in 2/54 and 13/54 fecal specimens from dogs with AHDS and none of the healthy dogs.[50] NetF appears to play a more important role than CPE in AHDS based on studies to date, but it is possible that other toxins may also be involved. In one study of dogs with AHDS associated with intralesional *C. perfringens* organisms on histopathology, the *netF* gene was detected in five of five *C. perfringens* isolates from duodenal biopsies of 10 dogs with AHDS, whereas *C. perfringens* was not detected in any duodenal biopsies from nine healthy control dogs.[48] In another study, *netF* was detected in 26 (48%) of 54 dogs with AHDS, 0 of 54 dogs with canine parvoviral enteritis, and 8 (12%) of 66 healthy dogs.[34] Studies based on detection of NetF itself (or NetF expression) are required, which has the potential to correlate to a greater extent with disease, as is the case with CPE. Pathogens other than *C. perfringens* may also play a role in some AHDS cases. For example, microbiome analysis of dogs with AHDS revealed not only a high proportion of *C. perfringens*, but also *Sutterella* spp.[49] *Sutterella* spp. play an uncertain role in GI disorders in humans, but have been implicated in IBD and treatment-resistant ulcerative colitis; some strains have the ability to degrade IgA.[51] However, their role as human commensals with potentially beneficial immunoregulatory properties has also been demonstrated.[52]

Physical Examination Findings

Physical examination findings in dogs and cats with severe clostridial diarrhea may include dehydration, fever, and abdominal pain, with or without signs of hypovolemic shock. Rectal examination in dogs may reveal loose or watery stools, sometimes containing fresh blood and mucus.

DIAGNOSIS

Laboratory Abnormalities

Complete Blood Count and Chemistry Panel

Basic laboratory testing in dogs and cats with clostridial diarrhea usually reveals mild and nonspecific changes. A neutrophilic leukocytosis with a left shift and toxic changes may be present in dogs and cats with acute clostridial gastroenteritis or AHDS. Dogs with AHDS may also have evidence of polycythemia despite a normal or decreased plasma protein concentration. The increase in hematocrit can be seen secondary to splenic contraction or dehydration, but plasma protein concentration decreases secondary to hypovolemic or hemorrhagic shock, with rapid leakage of albumin into the interstitial space. Electrolyte changes such as hypochloremia, hypokalemia, and metabolic acidosis may also be present.[46]

Diagnostic Imaging

Findings on plain abdominal radiography and abdominal ultrasound are typically unremarkable or show fluid-filled intestinal loops. Mild thickening and corrugation of the wall of the small intestine or colon may be detected using abdominal ultrasound (Fig. 64.2). Endoscopic findings in dogs with AHDS include mucosal erythema, friability, erosions, and hemorrhage in the colon and especially the duodenum.[47] However, endoscopy is rarely required because of the acute nature of the disease.

Microbiologic Tests (Table 64.2)

Cytologic Diagnosis

Spore-forming rods may be identified on microscopic examination of fecal smears that have been stained with Wright stains (see Fig. 64.1). These have been described as having the appearance of tennis racquets or safety pins. However, there is no association between fecal endospore counts and the presence of diarrhea, or between spore counts and the detection of CPE in fecal specimens. Detection of fecal endospores is thus an unreliable test for diagnosis of *C. perfringens* or *C. difficile* diarrhea in dogs and cats, and should not be used as a stand-alone test to make clinical inferences in diarrheic dogs and cats.[32,53]

Bacterial Isolation and Identification

Both *C. difficile* and *C. perfringens* can be isolated from the feces of both normal and diarrheic dogs and cats using strict anaerobic conditions for incubation. *Clostridium perfringens* is more tolerant of oxygen than *C. difficile*, and therefore may be easier to isolate (hence the name *difficile*, because of its difficulty to isolate in the laboratory).

Clostridioides difficile can be isolated from 0% to 58% of diarrheic and healthy dogs.[54] When fecal culture for *C. difficile* is performed on a viable fecal specimen by a reputable laboratory, a negative result strongly suggests that *C. difficile* is not present. In contrast, a positive culture does not differentiate between toxigenic and non-toxigenic strains, and further testing for the presence of toxin is warranted (see below).

Because of the high carriage rate of *C. perfringens* in both healthy and diarrheic dogs (> 70% in both groups), routine isolation of *C. perfringens* is not recommended for diagnosis, unless genetic typing of isolates is being performed, or epidemiologic studies are undertaken in outbreak situations. Use of culture to quantify organism burdens is recommended in conjunction with toxin gene detection to aid diagnosis of *C. perfringens* diarrhea in humans, with organism counts of $>10^6$ CFU per gram of feces together with toxin gene detection supportive of the diagnosis.[55,56] Spore counts involve treating stool with heat or alcohol before culturing it in an anaerobic environment and counting colonies. Such counts alone can still be detected in humans that have no signs of illness, and the method, when used without assessment of toxin production, has not proven useful for diagnosis of *C. perfringens* diarrhea in dogs.[31]

ELISA for *C. difficile* Antigen

Clostridioides difficile antigen ELISA can be useful as a screening test because it is easy to perform, rapid (< 1 hour to perform), and highly sensitive. The antigen test detects "common antigen" (glutamate dehydrogenase; GDH) that is predominantly present in toxigenic and non-toxigenic *C. difficile* strains and a few uncommon clostridial species. Although this test has the same limitations as culture in terms of detection of non-toxigenic strains and colonization, it is significantly more rapid and more practical to perform than culture, and given its sensitivity, a negative test allows the clinician to rapidly rule out *C. difficile* as a potential cause of diarrhea.

Assays for Toxin Production

Several commercial ELISAs are available for detection of *C. difficile* toxin A and toxin B in feces; however, none of these ELISAs have been validated for use in dogs and cats. Fecal swabs generally do not contain a sufficient quantity of stool for these assays. Even when performed on larger volumes of stool, the sensitivities and specificities of these assays may vary considerably. Importantly, a positive result does not prove that a clostridial infection is the cause of a dog or cat's diarrhea. Panels should include assays for both *C. difficile* toxin A and toxin B, because TcdA-negative, TcdB-positive strains have been documented in dogs, and production of both toxins is not needed for disease causation.[57] In humans, diagnosis is now accomplished by screening for the common antigen, and if positive, testing for toxin A and toxin B antigens. If those tests are negative, PCR assays can be done to detect toxin genes *tcdA* and *tcdB*. If the PCR assays are positive, a presumptive diagnosis of *C. difficile* infection is made. However, concerns have been raised that diagnosis on the basis of a positive PCR result does not imply toxin is being produced, and so other approaches that require toxin detection in conjunction with PCR have been recommended.[56]

Immunodetection for *C. perfringens* fecal enterotoxin is the most widely used diagnostic tool for *C. perfringens* in both humans and animals. Two commercially available immunoassays are currently used in veterinary diagnostic laboratories: a reverse passive latex agglutination assay (RPLA) and an ELISA. The assays have not been validated in animals to date. The RPLA has had poorer specificity when compared to several different ELISA methods, so ELISA assays are preferred.

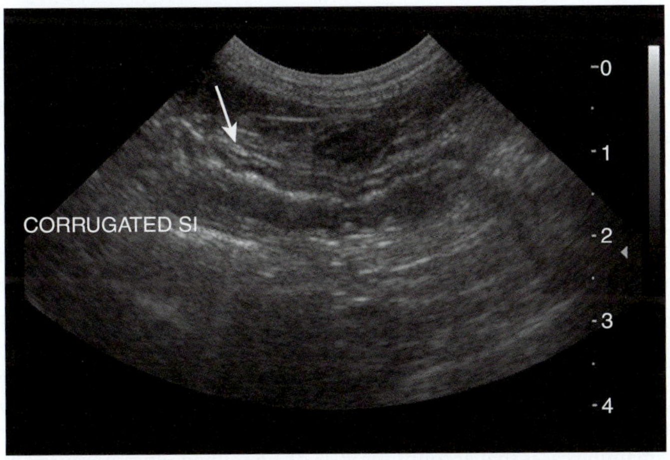

Fig. 64.2 Abdominal ultrasound image showing thickening and corrugation of the small intestinal wall (*arrow*) of a 2-year-old intact male Chihuahua with *Clostridium perfringens*–associated vomiting, hematemesis, diarrhea, and hematochezia. Large numbers of spore-forming gram-positive rods were seen on a fecal smear and *C. perfringens* enterotoxin (CPE) was detected in the feces using an ELISA assay.

Molecular Diagnosis Using Nucleic Acid–Based Testing

Real-time PCR assays are commercially available for detection of *C. perfringens* and *C. difficile* toxin genes in the feces of dogs and cats. It is important to recognize that the presence of clostridial toxin genes within fecal specimens does not prove that clostridia are the cause of an animal's diarrhea, because they do not prove that the organism can produce toxin within the intestinal tract of a patient. Conversely, negative PCR results for clostridial toxin genes do not rule out clostridial diarrhea, as clostridia lacking specific toxin genes may be present that possess other virulence factors, and inhibitors of PCR are common in fecal specimens. As mentioned earlier, real-time PCR assays for *C. difficile* toxin genes are used in conjunction with toxin antigen assays for diagnosis of *C. difficile* diarrhea in humans.[56] Similarly, detection of the *cpe* gene has been used to diagnose *C. perfringens* diarrhea in humans.[58] Fecal specimens from non-diarrheic dogs were less likely to be positive for CPE as detected using ELISA and PCR for the *cpe* gene (4%) when compared with diarrheic dogs (28%), and a combination of testing for the toxin (CPE) via ELISA and the enterotoxin gene (*cpe*) via PCR is likely superior to either test alone.[31] Some laboratories now offer PCR assays for detection of *netF* in fecal specimens from dogs.[34] Again, because the *netF* gene has been found in healthy dogs,[34] a positive result must be interpreted in light of clinical signs and other findings.

TABLE 64.2 Diagnostic Assays Available for Clostridial Enterocolitis in Dogs and Cats

Assay	Specimen Type	Target	Peformance
Bacterial isolation	Feces	*C. perfringens* and *C. difficile*	Isolation from feces does not imply that *Clostridium* is the cause of disease. Allows genotyping and subsequent antimicrobial susceptibility testing. False negatives may occur, especially for *C. difficile*, which requires strict anaerobic conditions
Common antigen test	Feces	*C. difficile*	Excellent negative predictive value for *C. difficile*
Toxin immunoassays	Feces	*C. perfringens* enterotoxin (CPE); *C. difficile* toxin A and toxin B	Positive test results may occur in dogs and cats that do not have diarrhea; negative results do not rule out clostridial diarrhea as other toxins may be involved and CPE is relatively labile
Polymerase chain reaction	Feces	*Clostridium perfringens* toxin genes (e.g., *cpe*, *netF*)	Rapid. Positive results from feces do not imply that *Clostridium* is the cause of disease. Toxin gene PCR may be useful in conjunction with positive ELISA results for toxin production. Negative results may occur if other toxin genes are important or if inhibitors of PCR are present

Pathologic Findings

Histopathologic findings in dogs with AHDS have been described and include acute necrosis of the mucosa with neutrophil infiltration.[47,48] A dense layer of bacteria on the surface of necrotic lesions can be identified, which stain gram positive using Brown and Benn stain.

TREATMENT AND PROGNOSIS

The mainstay of treatment is supportive care with aggressive crystalloid fluid therapy, antiemetics such as maropitant, and a diet formulated for GI disease that is fat-restricted. Although famotidine or omeprazole are often used for acid suppression, in humans their use has been associated with increased risk of *C. difficile* infection[59] and given the lack of gastric lesions in AHDS, their routine use is not warranted. Acid suppressant therapy should be considered in dogs and cats with intractable vomiting to reduce the likelihood of esophagitis. Only animals that are systemically ill merit appropriate antimicrobial therapy (Table 64.3). There is no documented evidence for the benefits of antimicrobial therapy in dogs with uncomplicated diarrhea associated with *C. perfringens* or *C. difficile* infection, even when hemorrhagic, and most of these animals can be managed supportively to ensure adequate hydration status without antimicrobial therapy. A prospective, blinded study that randomized dogs with *C. perfringens*–associated hemorrhagic gastroenteritis that showed no signs of sepsis to two groups, one treated with clavulanic acid-amoxicillin for 7 days and one treated with placebo, showed no difference in mortality rate, dropout rate, duration of hospitalization, or severity of clinical signs, either on any individual day or over the course of disease.[60] Importantly, the results of this study should be cautiously interpreted because dogs with other causes of hemorrhagic diarrhea (e.g., other infections, metabolic, drug-associated, neoplastic) were excluded. In addition, the prevalence of bacteremia in 87 dogs with idiopathic AHDS (11%) was not significantly different from the prevalence of bacteremia in healthy dogs (14%), and no difference in the severity of clinical signs, laboratory parameters, duration of hospitalization, or mortality between bacteremic and non-bacteremic dogs with AHDS was observed.[61]

Metronidazole (10–15 mg/kg PO q12h for 5 to 7 days) is the drug of choice for treatment of complicated *C. difficile* infections should they be suspected in dogs or cats. The vast majority of *C. perfringens* isolates from dogs have been susceptible to metronidazole, ampicillin, amoxicillin, tylosin, and macrolides such as erythromycin.[62] Because of the infrequency of resistance to these drugs, the lack of known breakpoints for veterinary anaerobes, and the lack of relationship between positive stool cultures and disease, antimicrobial susceptibilities are not performed on a routine basis for these organisms when isolated from dogs and cats. Most animals can be successfully treated with antimicrobials for 5 to 7 days, and appropriate treatment is generally associated with clinical improvement within 24 to 36 hours.

IMMUNITY AND VACCINATION

No vaccines are available to prevent clostridial diarrhea in dogs and cats.

PUBLIC HEALTH ASPECTS

Clostridioides difficile is an emerging pathogen and is increasingly recognized as an important cause of nosocomial diarrhea and pseudomembranous colitis in humans, especially the elderly, which is induced by antimicrobial treatment (especially ampicillin, amoxicillin, clindamycin, cephalosporins, and fluoroquinolones) or disruption of the normal GI flora. Humans with *C. difficile* infection develop bloating, and often foul-smelling diarrhea with abdominal pain, usually 5 to 10 days after starting antibiotics. Other signs include fever, nausea, anorexia, and malaise. Rare and life-threatening complications of pseudomembranous colitis include acute toxic megacolon, an acute dilatation of the colon with signs of obstruction, and colonic perforation. Hypervirulent strains (ribotypes O27 and O78) producing CDT, TcdA, and TcdB have been increasingly identified recently which cause a more severe disease, higher relapse rates, and increased mortality. Hypervirulent strains also have a deletion in the toxin C gene (*tcdC*), which normally downregulates toxin production.[56] Because of a high prevalence of metronidazole resistance in *C. difficile* isolates from humans, drugs such as vancomycin, the macrolide fidamoxacin, and fecal microbiota transplantation have been used for treatment.[63] It is theoretically possible that dogs may acquire *C. difficile* strains from humans; however, there has not been a documented case of zoonotic transmission from dogs to humans to date. Human colonization and disease usually occurs in hospital situations. However, in recent years, the importance of community-acquired infections has increased, comprising over 40% of cases reported, with concern about the role of companion animals as reservoirs.[24]

Clostridium perfringens infections are associated with sporadic and antimicrobial-associated diarrhea in humans and CPE is one of the most commonly identified causes of food poisoning in the industrialized world.[56,64] In Canada, it was identified as the second most common cause of foodborne illness (177,000 cases/year) after norovirus (1 million cases/year), with *Campylobacter* spp. (145,000 cases/year) and nontyphoidal *Salmonella* spp. (88,000 cases) accounting for the remaining cases that account for 90% of 1.6 million illnesses caused by known pathogens.[64] Clinical signs of infection include foul-smelling, frothy diarrhea, cramping and abdominal pain, and occasionally nausea and vomiting, usually 7 to 15 hours after eating suspected food, especially meat products that have been cooked with improper cooling and reheating. Vegetative cells are then ingested, and this can be followed by massive sporulation with toxin production in the intestinal tract. The zoonotic potential of *C. perfringens* isolates from dogs and cats requires further investigation.

TABLE 64.3 Antimicrobials That Can Be Used to Treat Complicated Clostridial Diarrhea* in Dogs and Cats

Drug	Dose (mg/kg)	Route	Interval (Hours)	Duration (Days)
Metronidazole	10	PO	12	5–7
Ampicillin	22	PO	8–12	5–7
Amoxicillin	22	PO	12	5–7
Tylosin	5–10	PO	24	5–7
Erythromycin	15	PO	8	5–7

*Accompanied by signs of sepsis.

CASE EXAMPLE

Signalment

"Bradley," 2-year-old male Chihuahua from Grass Valley, California.

History

Bradley was brought to an emergency clinic for a 12-hour history of hematemesis and diarrhea. He initially vomited up dog food, after which he continued to vomit hourly, the vomiting progressing to hematemesis. He also developed hemorrhagic diarrhea. He had been inappetent and not drinking, and the owner felt he was much quieter than usual. He primarily resided indoors and in the owner's backyard, and there was no travel history or history of access to toxins. There were two other dogs in the household that were apparently healthy. He was up to date on vaccinations for canine parvovirus, distemper virus, canine adenovirus, and rabies. His diet consisted of commercial dry dog food and table scraps.

Physical Examination

Body weight: 3.4 kg

General: Quiet, alert, and responsive, 5% to 7% dehydrated. Recumbent. Temperature = 100.0°F (37.8°C), heart rate = 100 beats/min, respiratory rate = 30 breaths/min, mucous membranes pink and tacky, CRT = 2 s.

Integument: Full coat with a small amount of flea excrement present. Diarrhea that contained fresh blood contaminated the hair in the perianal region.

Eyes, ears, nose, and throat: No abnormalities noted.

Musculoskeletal: Body condition score 4/9. Ambulatory.

Cardiovascular: Fair, synchronous femoral pulses. No murmurs or arrhythmias auscultated.

Respiratory: Normal breath sounds in all lung fields.

GI: Nonpainful on abdominal palpation, but defecated red, jelly-like material several times in the room following the examination.

Genitourinary: Urinated a large amount of odiferous urine during the examination.

Rectal examination: No abnormalities detected.

Lymph nodes: All within normal limits.

Laboratory Findings

CBC: HCT 46% (40%–55%), MCV 68 fL (65–75 fL), MCHC 36.3 g/dL (33–36 g/dL), WBC 11,030 cells/μL (6000–13,000 cells/μL), neutrophils 7280 cells/μL (3000–10,500 cells/μL), band neutrophils 1324 cells/μL, lymphocytes 1655 cells/μL (1000–4000 cells/μL), monocytes 772 cells/μL (150–1200 cells/μL), eosinophils 0 cells/μL (0–1500 cells/μL), platelets 273,000/μL (150,000–400,000 platelets/μL), TPP 5.5 g/dL (6.0–8.0 g/dL). Neutrophils and band neutrophils showed mild to moderate toxic changes.

Serum chemistry profile: Sodium 147 mmol/L (145–154 mmol/L), potassium 4.5 mmol/L (3.6–5.3 mmol/L), chloride 111 mmol/L (108–118 mmol/L), bicarbonate 29 mmol/L (16–26 mmol/L), phosphorus 3.9 mg/dL (3.0–6.2 mg/dL), calcium 9.6 mg/dL (9.7–11.5 mg/dl), BUN 15 mg/dL (5–21 mg/dL), creatinine 0.4 mg/dL (0.3–1.2 mg/dL), glucose 123 mg/dL (64–123 mg/dL), total protein 5.1 g/dL (5.4–7.6 g/dL), albumin 3.1 g/dL (3.0–4.4 g/dL), globulin 2.0 g/dL (1.8–3.9 g/dL), ALT 68 U/L (19–67 U/L), AST 31 U/L (19–42 U/L), ALP 30 U/L (21–170 U/L), GGT < 3 U/L (0–6 U/L), cholesterol 168 mg/dL (135–361 mg/dL), total bilirubin 0.1 mg/dL (0–0.2 mg/dL).

Urinalysis: SpG 1.042, pH 6.0, 1+ protein (SSA), 1+ bilirubin, no hemoprotein, no glucose, 1-2 WBC/HPF, 0 RBC/HPF, rare granular casts.

Coagulation panel: Prothrombin time 8.9 s (7.5–10.5 s), partial thromboplastin time 18.1 s (9–12 s); fibrinogen 349 mg/dL (90–255 mg/dL).

Imaging Findings

Abdominal ultrasound: Mild mesenteric and sublumbar lymphadenopathy was identified. Echogenicity of all lymph nodes was within normal limits. The small intestines had mild wall thickening and a corrugated appearance (see Fig. 64.2). The colon was fluid-filled.

Fecal Examination

Fecal centrifugation flotation: Negative for parasites.

Fecal sedimentation: Negative for parasites.

Microbiologic Testing

Parvovirus fecal antigen ELISA: Negative.

Fecal enteric panel: *Clostridioides difficile* TcdA and TcdB common antigen ELISA negative. ELISA positive for *Clostridium perfringens* enterotoxin A (CPE). No *Salmonella* spp. cultured. No *Clostridioides difficile* cultured. No *Campylobacter* spp. cultured.

Diagnosis

Suspected *C. perfringens*–associated acute hemorrhagic diarrhea syndrome.

Treatment

Bradley was initially hospitalized and treated with intravenous fluids, nil per os, and metronidazole, 7.5 mg/kg IV q12h. Vomiting did not continue, but red gelatinous diarrhea continued every hour for the next 12 hours. Within 24 hours, he had become bright and alert and was offered a fat-restricted bland diet, which he ate well. He was discharged and treated with metronidazole for an additional 5 days, with gradual reintroduction of his regular food.

Comments

Infection by *C. perfringens* was strongly suspected in this case based on the combination of consistent clinical signs, negative assay results for other pathogens, a positive toxin ELISA assay, and response to treatment. However, because the feces of healthy dogs can contain *C. perfringens* enterotoxin, a definitive diagnosis of *C. perfringens* enterocolitis could not be made. The use of antibiotics in this case was controversial; the dog was systemically unwell, but one could also argue that most dogs with AHDS have evidence of systemic illness, and use of antimicrobials to treat these dogs may represent suboptimal antimicrobial stewardship.

SUGGESTED READINGS

Weese JS, Armstrong J. Outbreak of *Clostridium difficile*-associated disease in a small animal veterinary teaching hospital. *J Vet Intern Med.* 2003;17(6):813–816.

Leipig-Rudolph M, Busch K, Prescott JF, et al. Intestinal lesions in dogs with acute hemorrhagic diarrhea syndrome associated with netF-positive *Clostridium perfringens* type A. *J Vet Diagn Invest.* 2018;30:495–503.

Hernandez BG, Vinithakumari AA, Sponseller B, et al. Prevalence, colonization, epidemiology, and public health significance of *Clostridioides difficile* in companion animals. *Front Vet Sci.* 2020;7:512551.

REFERENCES

1. George RH, Symonds JM, Dimock F, et al. Identification of *Clostridium difficile* as a cause of pseudomembranous colitis. *Br Med J.* 1978;1:695.
2. Welch WH, Nuttall GHF. A gas-producing bacillus (*Bacillus aerogenes capsulatus*, nov. spec.) capable of rapid development in blood vessels after death. *Bull Johns Hopkins Hosp.* 1892;3:81–91.
3. Hobbs BC, Smith ME, Oakley CL, et al. *Clostridium welchii* food poisoning. *J Hyg.* 1953;51:75–101.
4. Weese JS, Armstrong J. Outbreak of *Clostridium difficile*-associated disease in a small animal veterinary teaching hospital. *J Vet Intern Med.* 2003;17:813–816.

5. Clooten JK, Kruth SA, Weese JS. Genotypic and phenotypic characterization of *Clostridium perfringens* and *Clostridium difficile* in diarrheic and healthy dogs. *J Vet Intern Med.* 2003;17:123. ; author reply 123.
6. Weese JS, Finley R, Reid-Smith RR, et al. Evaluation of *Clostridium difficile* in dogs and the household environment. *Epidemiol Infect.* 2010;138:1100–1104.
7. Lefebvre SL, Reid-Smith RJ, Waltner-Toews D, et al. Incidence of acquisition of methicillin-resistant *Staphylococcus aureus, Clostridium difficile*, and other health-care-associated pathogens by dogs that participate in animal-assisted interventions. *J Am Vet Med Assoc.* 2009;234:1404–1417.
8. Cheng YW, Fischer M. Treatment of severe and fulminant *Clostridioides difficile* infection. *Curr Treat Options Gastroenterol.* 2019;17:524–533.
9. Pepin J, Alary ME, Valiquette L, et al. Increasing risk of relapse after treatment of *Clostridium difficile* colitis in Quebec, Canada. *Clin Infect Dis.* 2005;40:1591–1597.
10. Lefebvre SL, Arroyo LG, Weese JS. Epidemic *Clostridium difficile* strain in hospital visitation dog. *Emerg Infect Dis.* 2006;12:1036–1037.
11. Bjoersdorff OG, Lindberg S, Kiil K, et al. Dogs are carriers of *Clostridioides difficile* lineages associated with human community-acquired infections. *Anaerobe.* 2021;67:102317.
12. Rabold D, Espelage W, Abu Sin M, et al. The zoonotic potential of *Clostridium difficile* from small companion animals and their owners. *PLoS One.* 2018;13:e0193411.
13. Schneeberg A, Rupnik M, Neubauer H, et al. Prevalence and distribution of *Clostridium difficile* PCR ribotypes in cats and dogs from animal shelters in Thuringia, Germany. *Anaerobe.* 2012;18:484–488.
14. Andres-Lasheras S, Martin-Burriel I, Mainar-Jaime RC, et al. Preliminary studies on isolates of *Clostridium difficile* from dogs and exotic pets. *BMC Vet Res.* 2018;14:77.
15. Orden C, Blanco JL, Alvarez-Perez S, et al. Isolation of *Clostridium difficile* from dogs with digestive disorders, including stable metronidazole-resistant strains. *Anaerobe.* 2017;43:78–81.
16. Barbanti F, Spigaglia P. Microbiological characteristics of human and animal isolates of *Clostridioides difficile* in Italy: results of the Istituto Superiore di Sanita in the years 2006-2016. *Anaerobe.* 2020;61:102136.
17. Alam MJ, McPherson J, Miranda J, et al. Molecular epidemiology of *Clostridioides difficile* in domestic dogs and zoo animals. *Anaerobe.* 2019;59:107–111.
18. Rainha K, Fernandes Ferreira R, Trindade CNR, et al. Characterization of *Clostridioides difficile* ribotypes in domestic dogs in Rio de Janeiro, Brazil. *Anaerobe.* 2019;58:22–29.
19. Silva ROS, Ribeiro MG, de Paula CL, et al. Isolation of *Clostridium perfringens* and *Clostridioides difficile* in diarrheic and nondiarrheic cats. *Anaerobe.* 2020;62:102164.
20. Wei Y, Sun M, Zhang Y, et al. Prevalence, genotype and antimicrobial resistance of *Clostridium difficile* isolates from healthy pets in Eastern China. *BMC Infect Dis.* 2019;19:46.
21. Spigaglia P, Drigo I, Barbanti F, et al. Antibiotic resistance patterns and PCR-ribotyping of *Clostridium difficile* strains isolated from swine and dogs in Italy. *Anaerobe.* 2015;31:42–46.
22. Loo VG, Brassard P, Miller MA. Household transmission of *Clostridium difficile* to family members and domestic pets. *Infect Control Hosp Epidemiol.* 2016;37:1342–1348.
23. Stoesser N, Eyre DW, Quan TP, et al. Epidemiology of *Clostridium difficile* in infants in Oxfordshire, UK: risk factors for colonization and carriage, and genetic overlap with regional *C. difficile* infection strains. *PLoS One.* 2017;12:e0182307.
24. Hernandez BG, Vinithakumari AA, Sponseller B, et al. Prevalence, colonization, epidemiology, and public health significance of *Clostridioides difficile* in companion animals. *Front Vet Sci.* 2020;7:512551.
25. Rood JI, Adams V, Lacey J, et al. Expansion of the *Clostridium perfringens* toxin-based typing scheme. *Anaerobe.* 2018;53:5–10.
26. Forti K, Ferroni L, Pellegrini M, et al. Molecular characterization of *Clostridium perfringens* strains isolated in Italy. *Toxins.* 2020;12:650.
27. Navarro MA, McClane BA, Uzal FA. Mechanisms of action and cell death associated with *Clostridium perfringens* toxins. *Toxins.* 2018;10:212.
28. Kruth SA, Prescott JF, Welch MK, et al. Nosocomial diarrhea associated with enterotoxigenic *Clostridium perfringens* infection in dogs. *J Am Vet Med Assoc.* 1989;195:331–334.
29. Sasaki J, Goryo M, Asahina M, et al. Hemorrhagic enteritis associated with *Clostridium perfringens* type A in a dog. *J Vet Med Sci.* 1999;61:175–177.
30. Cave NJ, Marks SL, Kass PH, et al. Evaluation of a routine diagnostic fecal panel for dogs with diarrhea. *J Am Vet Med Assoc.* 2002;221:52–59.
31. Marks SL, Kather EJ, Kass PH, et al. Genotypic and phenotypic characterization of *Clostridium perfringens* and *Clostridium difficile* in diarrheic and healthy dogs. *J Vet Intern Med.* 2002;16:533–540.
32. Weese JS, Staempfli HR, Prescott JF, et al. The roles of *Clostridium difficile* and enterotoxigenic *Clostridium perfringens* in diarrhea in dogs. *J Vet Intern Med.* 2001;15:374–378.
33. Minamoto Y, Dhanani N, Markel ME, et al. Prevalence of *Clostridium perfringens, Clostridium perfringens* enterotoxin and dysbiosis in fecal samples of dogs with diarrhea. *Vet Microbiol.* 2014;174:463–473.
34. Sindern N, Suchodolski JS, Leutenegger CM, et al. Prevalence of *Clostridium perfringens* netE and netF toxin genes in the feces of dogs with acute hemorrhagic diarrhea syndrome. *J Vet Intern Med.* 2019;33:100–105.
35. Weese JS, Weese HE, Bourdeau TL, et al. Suspected *Clostridium difficile*-associated diarrhea in two cats. *J Am Vet Med Assoc.* 2001;218:1436–1439. 1421.
36. Del Prete R, Ronga L, Addati G, et al. *Clostridium difficile.* A review on an emerging infection. *Clin Ter.* 2019;170:e41–e47.
37. Carter GP, Rood JI, Lyras D. The role of toxin A and toxin B in *Clostridium difficile*-associated disease: past and present perspectives. *Gut Microb.* 2010;1:58–64.
38. Gerding DN, Johnson S, Rupnik M, et al. *Clostridium difficile* binary toxin CDT: mechanism, epidemiology, and potential clinical importance. *Gut Microb.* 2014;5:15–27.
39. McClane BA. The complex interactions between *Clostridium perfringens* enterotoxin and epithelial tight junctions. *Toxicon.* 2001;39: 1781–1791.
40. Leutenegger CM, Marks SL, Robertson J. Toxin quantification of *Clostridium perfringens* is a predictor for diarrhea in dogs and cats. *J Vet Intern Med.* 2012;26:794 (abstr).
41. Queen EV, Marks SL, Farver TB. Prevalence of selected bacterial and parasitic agents in feces from diarrheic and healthy control cats from Northern California. *J Vet Intern Med.* 2012;26:54–60.
42. Lacey JA, Johanesen PA, Lyras D, et al. In silico identification of novel toxin homologs and associated mobile genetic elements in *Clostridium perfringens. Pathogens.* 2019;8:16.
43. Mehdizadeh Gohari I, Parreira VR, Nowell VJ, et al. A novel pore-forming toxin in type A *Clostridium perfringens* is associated with both fatal canine hemorrhagic gastroenteritis and fatal foal necrotizing enterocolitis. *PLoS One.* 2015;10:e0122684.
44. Kiu R, Caim S, Alexander S, et al. Probing genomic aspects of the multi-host pathogen *Clostridium perfringens* reveals significant pan-genome diversity, and a diverse array of virulence factors. *Front Microbiol.* 2017;8:2485.
45. Mehdizadeh Gohari I, Brefo-Mensah EK, Palmer M, et al. Sialic acid facilitates binding and cytotoxic activity of the pore-forming *Clostridium perfringens* NetF toxin to host cells. *PLoS One.* 2018;13:e0206815.
46. Mortier F, Strohmeyer K, Hartmann K, et al. Acute haemorrhagic diarrhoea syndrome in dogs: 108 cases. *Vet Rec.* 2015;176:627.
47. Unterer S, Busch K, Leipig M, et al. Endoscopically visualized lesions, histologic findings, and bacterial invasion in the gastrointestinal mucosa of dogs with acute hemorrhagic diarrhea syndrome. *J Vet Intern Med.* 2014;28:52–58.
48. Leipig-Rudolph M, Busch K, Prescott JF, et al. Intestinal lesions in dogs with acute hemorrhagic diarrhea syndrome associated with netF-positive *Clostridium perfringens* type A. *J Vet Diagn Invest.* 2018;30:495–503.
49. Suchodolski JS, Markel ME, Garcia-Mazcorro JF, et al. The fecal microbiome in dogs with acute diarrhea and idiopathic inflammatory bowel disease. *PLoS One.* 2012;7:e51907.
50. Busch K, Suchodolski JS, Kuhner KA, et al. *Clostridium perfringens* enterotoxin and *Clostridium difficile* toxin A/B do not play a role in acute haemorrhagic diarrhoea syndrome in dogs. *Vet Rec.* 2015;176:253.
51. Kaakoush NO. *Sutterella* species, IgA-degrading bacteria in ulcerative colitis. *Trends Microbiol.* 2020;28:519–522.

52. Hiippala K, Kainulainen V, Kalliomaki M, et al. Mucosal prevalence and interactions with the epithelium indicate commensalism of *Sutterella* spp. *Front Microbiol.* 2016;7:1706.
53. Marks SL, Melli A, Kass PH, et al. Evaluation of methods to diagnose *Clostridium perfringens*-associated diarrhea in dogs. *J Am Vet Med Assoc.* 1999;214:357–360.
54. Marks SL, Rankin SC, Byrne BA, et al. Enteropathogenic bacteria in dogs and cats: diagnosis, epidemiology, treatment, and control. *J Vet Intern Med.* 2011;25:1195–1208.
55. Birkhead G, Vogt RL, Heun EM, et al. Characterization of an outbreak of *Clostridium perfringens* food poisoning by quantitative fecal culture and fecal enterotoxin measurement. *J Clin Microbiol.* 1988;26: 471–474.
56. Onderdonk A, Garrett WS. Diseases caused by *Clostridium*. In: Bennett JE, Dolin R, Blaser MJ, eds. *Mandell, Douglas, and Bennett's Principles and Practice of Infectious Diseases.* 9th ed. Philadelphia, PA: Elsevier; 2020:2960–2968.
57. Kuehne SA, Cartman ST, Heap JT, et al. The role of toxin A and toxin B in *Clostridium difficile* infection. *Nature.* 2010;467:711–713.
58. Loh JP, Liu YC, Chew SW, et al. The rapid identification of *Clostridium perfringens* as the possible aetiology of a diarrhoeal outbreak using PCR. *Epidemiol Infect.* 2008;136:1142–1146.
59. Park YH, Seong JM, Cho S, et al. Effects of proton pump inhibitor use on risk of *Clostridium difficile* infection: a hospital cohort study. *J Gastroenterol.* 2019;54:1052–1060.
60. Unterer S, Strohmeyer K, Kruse BD, et al. Treatment of aseptic dogs with hemorrhagic gastroenteritis with amoxicillin/clavulanic acid: a prospective blinded study. *J Vet Intern Med.* 2011;25:973–979.
61. Unterer S, Lechner E, Mueller RS, et al. Prospective study of bacteraemia in acute haemorrhagic diarrhoea syndrome in dogs. *Vet Rec.* 2015;176:309.
62. Marks SL, Kather EJ. Antimicrobial susceptibilities of canine *Clostridium difficile* and *Clostridium perfringens* isolates to commonly utilized antimicrobial drugs. *Vet Microbiol.* 2003;94:39–45.
63. Kampouri E, Croxatto A, Prod'hom G, et al. *Clostridioides difficile* infection, still a long way to go. *J Clin Med.* 2021;10:389.
64. Thomas MK, Murray R. Canadian burden of food-borne illness estimates working group. Estimating the burden of food-borne illness in Canada. *Can Commun Dis Rep.* 2014;40:299–302.

65

Campylobacteriosis

Els Acke

KEY POINTS

- First Described: In Germany, 1886, by Theodor Escherich, noted in stool specimens and intestinal mucus from human neonates with diarrhea.[1]
- Cause: *Campylobacter* spp. (*Campylo* meaning curved, *bacter* meaning rod), microaerophilic gram-negative bacteria belonging to the family Campylobacteraceae.
- Affected Hosts: A large variety of animal species, humans.
- Geographic Distribution: Worldwide.
- Route of Transmission: Fecal-oral.
- Major Clinical Signs: Lethargy, anorexia, small and large bowel diarrhea, vomiting, fever.
- Differential Diagnoses: Differential diagnoses for suspected *Campylobacter* enteritis include GI causes of diarrhea (other infections like salmonellosis, giardiasis, tritrichomoniasis (cats), or other disorders like intestinal lymphoma, inflammatory bowel disease, foreign body ingestion), dietary indiscretion, toxin/drug ingestion, but also extra-GI causes of diarrhea such as endocrine, hepatic disease, pancreatitis.
- Human Health Significance: Important zoonosis. Dogs and cats are a potential source of infection for human campylobacteriosis, and resistance to antimicrobials has been reported.

ETIOLOGY AND EPIDEMIOLOGY

Campylobacter organisms are gram-negative rods (0.2–0.8 μm wide by 0.5–5 μm long) with a polar flagellum giving them the characteristic "cork-screw" motility. Some species are nonmotile or have multiple flagella. They can occur singularly, in pairs (resulting in the typical "gull-winged" appearance), or in chains as long spirals (Fig. 65.1).[2,3] Degenerative coccoid forms can exist in adverse conditions, described as "viable but nonculturable" forms.[4] The first successful isolation of *Campylobacter* was in 1906, when the organism became established as a pathogen of veterinary importance in farm animals, causing infertility, abortion, and dysentery.[5] In 1963, Sebald and Véron proposed the formation of the genus *Campylobacter* and subsequently, different species were named.[3,6] Following the development of a selective culture medium,[7] *Campylobacter* became recognized as a common cause of acute diarrhea in humans.[6,8] Dogs[7] and cats[9] were confirmed to carry *Campylobacter* organisms in their feces, which implicated companion animals in the epidemiology of campylobacteriosis, and *Campylobacter* spp. as possible pathogens for dogs and cats. The organisms are considered commensals in many host animals, but especially in avian species, and campylobacteriosis is the leading cause of bacterial foodborne enteritis in humans worldwide with the major source of infection being the consumption of contaminated poultry meat.[10] The genus *Campylobacter* currently accounts over 30 different species and subspecies isolated from humans and animals; many of these are considered nonpathogenic (http://www.bacterio.net/campylobacter.html). A closely related and clinically important genus previously belonging to the family Campylobacteraceae is the genus *Helicobacter*.[11,12]

Campylobacter organisms are spread by the fecal-oral route with the main sources of infection for pet animals being undercooked/raw food and unpasteurized milk, water, and direct (fresh feces from infected animals) or indirect (fomites, vectors, and environment) contact with other animals including other cats and dogs, farm animals, poultry, ferrets, and hamsters.[13] Commercially available raw meat-based diets for cats and dogs were recently identified as a potential source of *Campylobacter* spp. infection with 28% (14/50) of collected meat samples testing positive, the majority in this study for *Campylobacter jejuni*.[14] The main *Campylobacter* species isolated in companion animals to date include *C. jejuni*, *Campylobacter upsaliensis*, and *Campylobacter helveticus*, with *C. upsaliensis* more frequently isolated from dogs and *C. helveticus* from cats.[14–23] Detection methods in the laboratory diagnosis of *Campylobacter* spp. infection are biased towards confirmation of *C. jejuni* and *Campylobacter coli* as these are considered the main species causing clinical *Campylobacter* infections in humans. However, the importance of "emerging" (or previously unidentified) *Campylobacter* species has become a major research field in human and veterinary medicine since the development of improved culture-based and molecular detection methods.[24–26] *Campylobacter upsaliensis*, *Campylobacter lari*, *Campylobacter concisus*, *Campylobacter ureolyticus*, and several other species are considered "emerging" species and have been implicated in human cases of campylobacteriosis with a range of clinical presentations (Table 65.1).[25,27,28] *Campylobacter ureolyticus* was recently identified in 10/31 and 4/44 fecal specimens collected from cats and dogs, respectively, in a study in Ireland where *C. ureolyticus* was confirmed to be an important cause of human campylobacteriosis,[29] and several potentially zoonotic "emerging" *Campylobacter* spp. were confirmed in fecal specimens from dogs with diarrhea by quantitative PCR.[26] An overview of *Campylobacter* species reported in dogs and cats is given in Table 65.1.

The detection rates of *Campylobacter* spp. from rectal swabs or fecal specimens obtained from dogs and cats vary depending on the age of the animals, animal species tested, housing, concomitant infection with other enteropathogenic organisms, the presence of enteric or other disease, the sampling season, the geographic region where the study was performed, and the study design.[14,18,30–37] Numerous prevalence studies have been published since the first isolation of *Campylobacter* spp. from domestic dogs and cats, with overall prevalences of *Campylobacter* spp. ranging 0%–87% for dogs and 0%–75% for cats.[9,14–17,19–22,31–57] Accurate speciation with use of molecular methods has been performed since the 21st century,[58] and study results are method dependent, which complicates comparison among studies. Higher prevalences were obtained when a combination of culture methods was used to optimize the recovery of a range of species.[36,59] A direct fecal quantitative PCR technique applied to specimens from healthy and diarrheic pet dogs showed an unprecedented number of positive detections with a significantly higher number of detectable species (up to 12) in diarrheic dogs when compared with healthy dogs (up to 7), demonstrating increased *Campylobacter* spp. richness in the diarrheic dog population.[26] Application of real-time PCR assays to feces from healthy and diarrheic cats also revealed a significantly higher prevalence of infection and a wider range of species when compared with a single culture method.[23]

A review and meta-analysis of 34 *Campylobacter* spp. prevalence studies reported a mean prevalence of 24.7% in household pets. Because of the lack of standardization of methods and reporting, several knowledge gaps still exist on the significance of *Campylobacter* spp. infections in companion animals and their risk to human health.[60] However, several factors have been significantly associated with *Campylobacter* spp. detection in dogs and cats. The prevalence in dogs and cats living as single household pets is lower than for in animals living in groups (e.g., in pounds and kennels), and intensive housing of dogs and cats is a risk factor for infection.[18,30,32,33,36,42,45,61–63] The higher isolation rate in intensively housed animals can be explained by increased likelihood of exposure due to horizontal spread arising from the living conditions with close contact between animals, stress, dietary changes, and increased incidence of GI disease from other pathogens. In the majority of studies, immature dogs and cats have higher prevalences than adult animals,[9,16,20,22,31,32,35–37,46,48,50,55,64–67] suggesting an age-related immunity.[13] This acquired gut immunity may also explain the lower incidence of campylobacteriosis observed in older animals and adult humans. The link between the presence of intestinal signs in pets and different *Campylobacter* species has been investigated, but adequate pathogenicity studies are needed. Several studies suggested an association between *C. jejuni* detection and signs of diarrhea in dogs and cats.[9,19,31,39,44,46,48,55,64,67,68] In addition, a wider range of *Campylobacter* species was detected in dogs with diarrhea than in those without diarrhea.[26] However, a significant association between clinical signs and detection of *Campylobacter* spp. in dogs or cats was not shown in other studies.[9,22,23,33,34,36,41–43,45,46,49,50,69–74] Co-infecting pathogens, and other pre-existing or concurrent disease may also predispose to *Campylobacter* spp. infection and the development of clinical signs.[49,75,76]

The prevalence of *Campylobacter* spp. infection is higher in dogs than in cats in the majority of studies,[14,22,33–35,42,44,58,64,77] suggesting that cats may be less susceptible to infection. However, similar prevalences have also been found in dogs and cats,[37] and higher prevalences were identified in shelter cats.[36] Compared with dogs, fewer studies have been performed in cats.

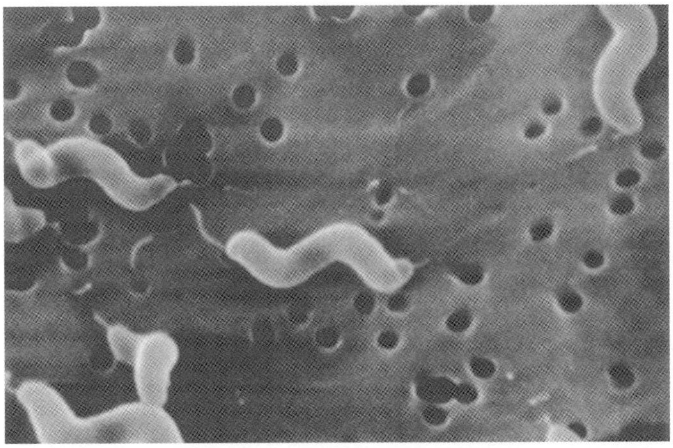

Fig. 65.1 Scanning electron micrograph of *Campylobacter*. (From Centers for Disease Control and Prevention, Atlanta, GA.)

TABLE 65.1 *Campylobacter* Species Reported in Dogs and/or Cats and Humans, and Possible Clinical Manifestations Reported.[a]

	POSSIBLE CLINICAL MANIFESTIONS REPORTED[b]	
***Campylobacter* spp.**	**Dogs and/or Cats**	**Humans**
C. coli	None, enteritis, IBD	Enteritis, bacteremia, meningitis, cholecystitis
C. concisus	Enteritis, oral disease	Enteritis, IBD, Barrett's esophagitis, bacteremia, periodontal disease, abscesses
C. curvus	None, enteritis	Enteritis, ulcerative colitis, Barrett's esophagitis, bacteremia, abscesses
C. fetus	None, enteritis	Enteritis, bacteremia, abscesses, cellulitis, endocarditis, mycotic aneurysm, peritonitis
C. gracilis	Enteritis	Periodontal disease, IBD, head and neck infections, abscesses
C. helveticus	None, enteritis	Enteritis
C. hyointestinalis	None, enteritis	Enteritis and bacteremia
C. jejuni	None, enteritis, bacteremia and cholangiohepatitis/cholecystitis, abortion, acute polyradiculoneuritis	Enteritis, bacteremia, myocarditis, meningitis, cholecystitis, UTI, IBD, Guillain-Barré syndrome, etc.
C. lari	None, enteritis, oral disease	Enteritis, bacteremia
C. mucosalis	Enteritis	Enteritis
C. rectus	None, enteritis, oral disease	Periodontal disease, enteritis, IBD, abscesses, bacteremia, tissue infections
C. showae	None, enteritis, oral disease	IBD, abscesses, bacteremia, periodontal disease
C. sputorum	None, enteritis	Enteritis, abscesses, bacteremia
C. upsaliensis	None, enteritis, acute polyradiculoneuritis	Enteritis, bacteremia, abscesses, placentitis
C. ureolyticus	None	Enteritis, IBD, abscesses, tissue or bone infections
C. volucris	None	Bacteremia

[a]See references 14, 28, 29, 37, 56, 81, 84, 87, 98, 101, 104, 105, 156, 157. The most commonly detected species are in bold.
[b]"Clinical manifestations" imply confirmed presence of *Campylobacter* spp. and not confirmed causation of clinical signs in dogs and cats.
IBD, Inflammatory bowel disease; *UTI,* urinary tract infection.

Campylobacter spp. were isolated more frequently from dogs sampled in the spring,[19,56] autumn,[32] or summer[34] and in cats in the summer[50] and autumn.[34,50] This may relate to the increased population of young susceptible puppies and kittens in the warmer months, or other season-related changes.

Raw meat-based diets (RMBD) are popular but are commonly contaminated with enteropathogens, which could pose a risk to animals consuming the diets, humans handling the diets, and to the environment.[78,79] A recent study confirmed 12/25 dogs fed RMBD and only 4/25 dogs fed dry kibble excreted *Campylobacter* spp.[80] However, two other studies have failed to confirm a significant association between raw meat feeding and fecal shedding of *Campylobacter* spp. in dogs.[79,81] Raw chicken consumption was a risk factor in the development of acute polyradiculoneuritis (APN) in a case-control study of Australian dogs, with a significantly higher number of APN cases testing positive for *C. upsaliensis* or *C. jejuni* on fecal culture and PCR within 7 days after developing lower motor neuron signs compared with healthy control dogs.[82] Further work is needed to evaluate the risk of feeding these diets to dogs and cats, and their association with shedding of zoonotic enteropathogens.

Multiple *Campylobacter* species can be simultaneously present in feces[14,21,23,26,37,83,84] and genetic heterogeneity has been detected in several *Campylobacter* species isolated from dogs and cats via molecular subtyping.[14,52,85–87] Also, the presence of co-infections with other organisms such as *Helicobacter* spp.,[73,88,89] endoparasites, and CPV-2[22,47,49,90] suggests that *Campylobacter* spp. may be a secondary or synergistic pathogen. In dogs that frequented dog parks in northern California, co-infections of *Campylobacter* spp. with *Clostridium* spp., coronavirus, circovirus, and *Cryptosporidium* spp. were identified.[57] In this study, enteropathogens were detected in 114 of 300 dogs using a large commercial fecal PCR panel. Co-infections with other organisms were confirmed in four of eight dogs that tested positive for *C. jejuni* and/or *C. coli*.[57] PCR assays that detected other *Campylobacter* spp. were not used in this study, which may have resulted in the low prevalence of *Campylobacter* spp. detection. Many animals excrete *Campylobacter* spp. intermittently or transiently, and a single animal will shed one or several different *Campylobacter* spp. and strains at some stage or stages in its life. Collection of multiple specimens increases the recovery rate of *Campylobacter* spp.[30,83,91] All healthy domestic dogs monitored by monthly fecal swab culture until 2 years of age excreted *Campylobacter* spp. at some stage in one longitudinal study, with 67% of the dogs testing positive at conclusion. The highest prevalence of shedding was in dogs under 1 year of age.[83] *Campylobacter upsaliensis* was shed more continuously and for longer duration than *C. jejuni*, which suggested that dogs may be a reservoir for *C. upsaliensis* or that the organism is a commensal in dogs.[62,83] In cats, the median duration of *Campylobacter* carriage in feces was 44 days and a small number of cats shed *Campylobacter* spp. over 5 months.[50]

CLINICAL FEATURES

Pathogenesis and Clinical Signs

The complete mechanisms by which *Campylobacter* spp. induce illness still remain unclear even after many years of human campylobacteriosis research. *Campylobacter jejuni* colonizes the jejunum, ileum, and colon, and the severity of infection and development of clinical signs are dependent on factors such as age, previous exposure, immune status, number and virulence of ingested organisms, environmental and physiological stressors, and the presence of other enteric pathogens or disease.[4,13] The virulence and survival of campylobacters involves motility, adhesion, invasion, and toxin production. Motility of the organisms relies on the presence of one or two polar flagella and chemotaxis. The *FlaA* and *FlaB* genes, which encode the major flagellin proteins, are highly conserved among campylobacters and have been used in molecular typing schemes.[92] The most important chemo-attractants are mucins and glycoproteins in the intestinal tract mucus.[93] *Campylobacter* organisms have several surface adhesins, which are necessary to establish colonization. CadF, an outer membrane adhesin, and CapA (*Campylobacter* adhesion protein A) are the most studied adhesins. Several invasion virulence factors have also been identified. Campylobacters produce several toxins, of which the cytolethal distending toxin (CDT) is the best characterized. In addition, several multidrug resistance and stress response genes have been identified.[4] *Campylobacter* multidrug efflux pumps are also important in the pathogenesis of clinical campylobacteriosis, and antimicrobial resistance rates for *Campylobacter* are rising.[4]

Pathogenicity and experimental studies in companion animals are scarce and have only involved a limited number of animals, challenge strains, and challenge dosages. In one third of *C. jejuni*–infected dogs, clinical signs of diarrhea were present after experimental infection, and soft feces developed in one of three *C. upsaliensis*–infected dogs.[49] Mild signs of enteric disease occurred after oral inoculation of puppies with *C. jejuni*.[94] Enteritis with histopathologic evidence of typhlitis and colitis was reported after oral infection of gnotobiotically raised beagle puppies with *C. jejuni*.[95] In a small number of young kittens and puppies experimentally infected with a *C. jejuni* strain associated with gastroenteritis in children, shedding without clinical signs occurred.[96]

In both dogs and cats, *Campylobacter* infections are usually subclinical and many animals carry *Campylobacter* spp. in their intestinal tract. Clinical signs typically occur in immature animals and where predisposing factors are present.[18] The incubation period is short; in experimental infection, signs of enteritis appeared within 3 days of oral challenge with *C. jejuni*.[95]

Mild to watery diarrhea (occasionally bloody or mucoid with tenesmus), lethargy, anorexia, and, less commonly, vomiting and fever have been reported in dogs and cats with natural infections.[13,18,97] Infection is self-limiting in most cases and affected animals recover within 2 weeks.[13,97] Extra-intestinal infections with *C. jejuni* bacteremia and cholangiohepatitis/cholecystitis have been described.[97,98] Campylobacteriosis may be associated with reproductive disorders[99]; *C. jejuni* was isolated from vaginal discharge in three bitches after they aborted,[100] was implicated in fetal bacteremia following *C. jejuni* infection and diarrhea in a bitch,[101] and perinatal death with infection of fetoplacental organs.[99] Chronic and intermittent diarrhea has been reported in dogs[46,76,102] and cats.[46,103] In a retrospective study where FISH was applied to intestinal histopathology samples of cats with inflammatory bowel disease (IBD), significantly higher numbers of *C. coli* were identified in cats with neutrophilic compared with lymphoplasmacytic IBD.[104] Some "emerging" *Campylobacter* spp. have been identified in saliva samples from pets with oral disease (see Table 65.1) but no definitive association with oral disease has been made, and the zoonotic risk from exposure to *Campylobacter* spp. in oral secretions is unknown.[105,106] Table 65.1 provides an overview of *Campylobacter* spp. detected in dogs and cats and possible clinical manifestations of infection.

Physical Examination Findings

Findings on physical examination of dogs and cats with campylobacteriosis are nonspecific and depend on severity and extent of infection. In animals with severe enteritis, signs of dehydration, lethargy, abdominal pain, and fever can be present, with evidence of melena and hematochezia in some patients.[18,97] Hepatic involvement may be associated with icterus and other signs of liver disease.[97]

DIAGNOSIS

Detection of *Campylobacter* spp. in dogs and cats does not necessarily confirm a diagnosis of campylobacteriosis. Possible underlying or concurrent diseases should always be considered taking signalment, history, clinical signs, and other differential diagnoses into consideration. Further diagnostic work-up should include testing for other infectious causes of enteritis and a broader evaluation for causes of GI disease. These tests might include a CBC and serum biochemistry panel and imaging studies. Complicated cases may require collection of other body fluid specimens for cytologic examination and culture (e.g., blood, bile).[18,97]

Laboratory Abnormalities

Findings on analysis of blood samples for CBC and serum chemistry, if present, are nonspecific. The CBC may reveal a leukocytosis. Regenerative anemia would be uncommon but may be present in animals with blood loss. Animals with bacteremia may have a left shift neutrophilia and thrombocytopenia. Serum chemistry may demonstrate the effects of dehydration associated with diarrhea and associated electrolyte abnormalities. When extra-intestinal infection is present, other changes can be detected such as elevated liver parameters.[97,98]

Diagnostic Imaging

Abdominal radiography and ultrasound in animals with enteritis often reveals only nonspecific changes. Animals with enteritis may have thickened intestinal mucosa, abnormal motility, reduced wall layering, and abdominal lymphadenopathy detected on abdominal ultrasonography.[107] Depending on the presence of extra-intestinal infection, involvement of other organs can be present (e.g., evidence of cholecystitis such as a thickened gall bladder wall) (Fig. 65.2).[97,98]

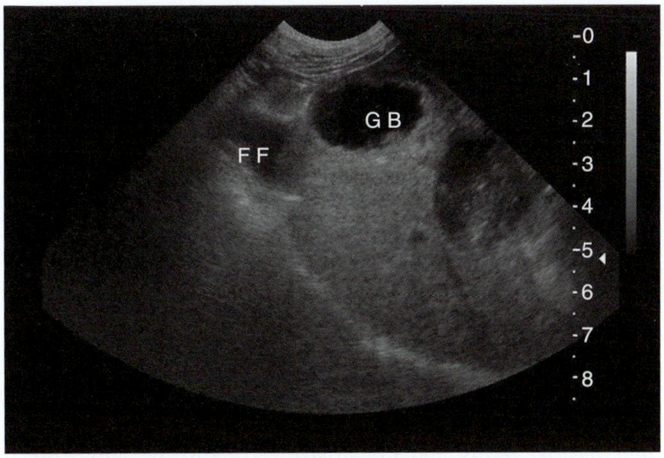

Fig. 65.2 Abdominal ultrasound image from a 10-year-old intact male Brittany spaniel with *Campylobacter* bacteremia, gastroenteritis, and probable cholecystitis, showing thickening of the gall bladder *(GB)* wall and free abdominal fluid *(FF)*.

Microbiologic Tests

Microscopic Examination

Based on microscopic morphology alone, a diagnosis of campylobacteriosis cannot be confirmed. On fecal Gram stains, large numbers of faintly staining gram-negative, slender, gull-wing-shaped rods may be present in animals with *C. jejuni* enteritis (Fig. 65.3).[18] Using dark field or phase contrast microscopy on fresh feces mixed with saline, curved bacteria that are highly motile and show the characteristic darting motion of *C. jejuni* may be detected. However, this technique is not routinely available in veterinary diagnostic laboratories and also lacks specificity.[13,108] Detection by microscopy only suggests the presence of *Campylobacter*-like organisms and should *not* be used to diagnose campylobacteriosis because of the inability to differentiate between similar-appearing organisms such as *Arcobacter* or nonpathogenic campylobacters (Table 65.2).

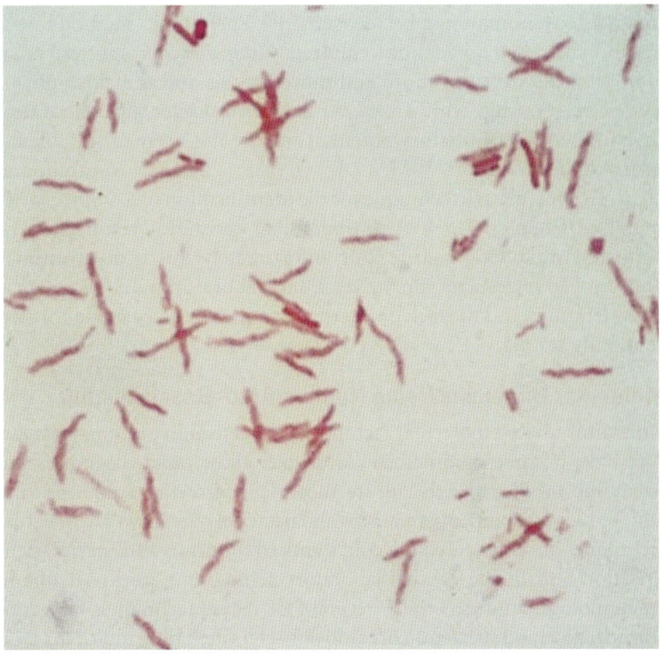

Fig. 65.3 Cytology showing *Campylobacter* organisms. Gram stain, 1000× magnification.

Isolation and Identification

For animals with enteritis, submission of 2–3 g of fresh feces in a sealed sterile container to a laboratory as soon as possible is advised for bacterial culture. If rectal swabs are collected, sterile swabs with Amies or Cary-Blair transport medium are recommended.[18] Certain *Campylobacter* spp. have a reduced viability when stored. For example, *C. concisus* should be cultured within 1 day of specimen collection. *Campylobacter jejuni* and *C. coli* are more resistant and can survive in refrigerated fecal samples up to 2 weeks.[109] Isolation rates of specific *Campylobacter* spp. strongly depend on the isolation techniques used. *Campylobacter* spp. culture is complicated due to the slow growth of some species; the requirement of a microaerophilic environment with an atmosphere of 5% to 10% oxygen and 1% to 10% carbon dioxide at 37°C to allow recovery of a range of thermotolerant *Campylobacter* species; and of selective culture media as antimicrobials present in conventional selective media inhibit growth.[10,28,110] The modified charcoal cefoperazone deoxycholate agar (mCCDA) medium was developed specifically and is still most widely used for the recovery of *Campylobacter* spp. in diagnostic laboratories.[111,112] Subsequently, a basal agar that contains cefoperazone, amphotericin, and teicoplanin (CAT) selective agents was developed for improved detection of *C. upsaliensis*.[113] For the isolation of a range of *Campylobacter* spp. from rectal swabs collected from cats and dogs, a combination of culture methods significantly improved the recovery rate and more accurately reflected the prevalence of *Campylobacter* spp. As a single method in the culture for *C. jejuni, C. upsaliensis, C. helveticus, C. lari* and *C. coli* from rectal swabs, CAT agar was most suitable.[14,59] Membrane filtration, a passive filtration culture method (the motile campylobacters pass through the filter to blood agar), with incubation

TABLE 65.2 Diagnostic Assays Available for Campylobacteriosis in Dogs and Cats

Assay	Specimen Type	Target	Performance
Bacterial isolation	Feces, blood, bile, intestinal tissues	*Campylobacter* organism	False negatives may occur, especially following antimicrobial therapy, and some species may not grow under routine conditions used to isolate *Campylobacter*. Isolation from feces does not imply that *Campylobacter* is the cause of disease. Allows subsequent antimicrobial susceptibility testing if available.
Polymerase chain reaction	As for isolation	*Campylobacter* DNA	Rapid, can be highly sensitive and specific. Positive results from feces do not imply that *Campylobacter* is the cause of disease.

in hydrogen-enriched microaerophilic atmosphere, also known as the "Cape Town protocol," proved successful in the isolation of several of the "emerging" species such as *C. concisus*, *Campylobacter sputorum*, *Campylobacter rectus*, and *Campylobacter curvus*, the prevalence of which is underestimated where traditional methods are used.[28,114,115] Incubation for 6 days for these species is recommended while examining the plates every 2 days with subculturing of morphologically different colonies. *Campylobacter jejuni* and *C. coli* grow relatively rapidly and if plates are not re-incubated, slower-growing and "emerging" campylobacters may not be recovered.[109] Phenotypic methods were traditionally used to identify cultured *Campylobacter* species; however, with discovery of more and more species and the close phylogenetic relationship with *Arcobacter* and *Helicobacter* spp., these tests have limited discriminatory potential and are not deemed suitable for accurate identification.[116] MALDI-TOF MS is a superior, rapid, and relatively inexpensive technique for the identification of *Campylobacter* spp. (see Chapter 3).[117,118] Antimicrobial resistance testing can be performed following culture, but unfortunately this is not routinely done for *Campylobacter* spp. by veterinary laboratories due to practical considerations and the lack of internationally accepted criteria for susceptibility testing.

Molecular Diagnosis Using Nucleic Acid–Based Testing

Nonculture-based molecular techniques for detection of *Campylobacter* spp. have become commercially available, allow rapid diagnosis, and overcome problems with culture media and growth conditions, and with reduced viability of organisms and bacterial overgrowth. Molecular techniques are considered the gold standard for genus and species identification also in the routine laboratory setting and are invaluable in epidemiologic studies.[28,116,119] Several PCR-based techniques for genus confirmation and speciation of campylobacters including multiplex PCR have been described.[116,120–122] Direct fecal real-time PCR techniques have been developed to detect a wide range of species.[26,123] Significantly improved diagnostic accuracy was reported using a real-time fecal PCR for four *Campylobacter* spp. versus bacterial isolation using one single culture method in cats with and without signs of diarrhea.[23] Other work reported improved sensitivity when a direct fecal PCR was used compared with culture; however, some isolates had negative PCR results which could be explained by degradation of bacterial DNA and presence of inhibitory substances in feces.[16] A PCR-denaturing gradient gel electrophoresis (PCR-DGGE) method for the detection and identification of *Campylobacter*, *Helicobacter*, and *Arcobacter* species has been applied to saliva specimens from humans and pets.[105]

Investigation of the significance of *Campylobacter* spp. as a cause of zoonotic disease, assessment of the importance of different sources of *Campylobacter* infection (e.g., animal, food, or environmental reservoirs), and development of measures to prevent transmission from animals to humans requires reliable and highly discriminatory subtyping methods.[119] Initial subtyping techniques were based on detection of variation in the flagellin (*fla*A) gene, but the need for more discriminatory techniques led to application of pulsed field gel electrophoresis (PFGE) in epidemiologic investigations (see Chapter 7).[124] Because PFGE is time-consuming, cumbersome, and costly, multilocus sequence typing (MLST) has become the subtyping gold standard due to its excellent discriminatory potential, portability, and reproducibility. MLST was initially developed for *C. jejuni* subtyping and then also described for several other species including *C. coli*, *C. upsaliensis*, and *C. helveticus*.[119,124,125] Whole genome sequencing has become widely available and allows not only superior strain differentiation but also identification of virulence and antimicrobial resistance determinants in *C. jejuni* and *C. coli*,[126,127] and further research applications are rapidly evolving.

Serology

Serologic assays are used in human medicine in epidemiologic investigations to confirm exposure and to investigate some of the long-term sequelae associated with *Campylobacter* spp. infections such as Guillain-Barré syndrome and reactive arthritis.[128] The use of antibody testing in clinical *Campylobacter* infections of dogs and cats has not been investigated extensively and serologic testing is not commercially available. Enzyme immunoassays have been developed for human fecal specimens. These are rapid, simple, and low-cost fecal antigen tests developed specifically to detect *C. jejuni* and *C. coli* with performance reported to be comparable with culture.[129] One study revealed significant cross reactivity with *C. upsaliensis*, *C. helveticus*, and *Campylobacter hyointestinalis* isolates from dogs, cats, and deer for one of the commercial fecal antigen tests, questioning the accuracy of results in the diagnosis of *C. jejuni* and *C. coli* enteritis in humans.[24] With refinement, these tests may be useful for future investigations of a wide range of *Campylobacter* spp. infections in humans and animals.

Pathologic Findings

Changes described on necropsy of dogs with campylobacteriosis include grossly abnormal small and large intestines[76] with thickening of mucosa of the ileum[130] and enlargement of mesenteric lymph nodes.[94,130] On histopathology, laboratory dogs with *Campylobacter* spp. enterocolitis had changes especially in the distal jejunum and ileum with fusion or blunting of the villi, rare crypt epithelial cell degeneration, and lymphoplasmacytic infiltration into the lamina propria. In the colon, superficial erosions were described, lymphoplasmacytic infiltration of the lamina propria, crypt epithelial hyperplasia, and *Campylobacter* spp. were confirmed by IHC.[76] One report described proliferative enteritis associated with *Campylobacter* spp. infection in two pups with marked hyperplasia of the ileal mucosa, elongated glandular crypts, inflammatory infiltrate in the lamina propria, and hyperplastic regions in the colonic mucosa.[130] Silver staining has shown filamentous bacteria in crypts (Fig. 65.4) and IHC can be used to confirm *Campylobacter* spp. infiltration.[76] Application of FISH to identify *Campylobacter* spp. on biopsy specimens from animals with neutrophilic IBD has suggested an association with *C. coli* infection in cats.[104]

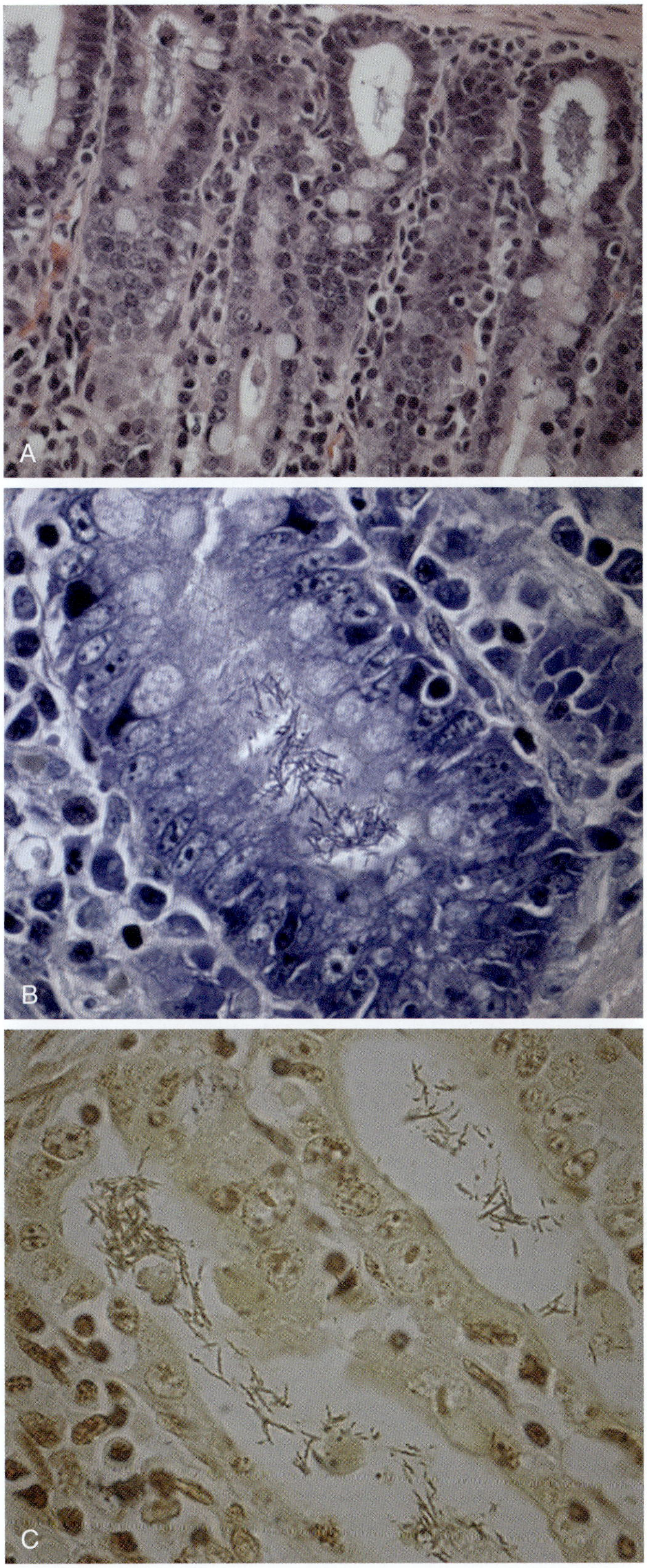

Fig. 65.4 Histopathology of an intestinal section from a 3-month-old Chihuahua puppy with *Campylobacter jejuni*–associated diarrhea. Abundant filamentous, spiral bacteria pack the crypts and there is an associated lymphoplasmacytic enterocolitis. (A) Hematoxylin and eosin stain. (B) Giemsa stain. (C) Warthin-Starry silver stain.

TREATMENT AND PROGNOSIS

As in humans, the majority of *Campylobacter* spp. infections in dogs and cats with signs of enteritis are self-limiting and only require supportive treatment. Antimicrobial therapy should be reserved for patients that are immunocompromised, febrile, or who have severe clinical signs, with or without extra-intestinal signs.[18] Also in clinical cases where shedding is confirmed and there is possible increased infectious risk (e.g., young children or immunocompromised people in the household, other animals), antimicrobial therapy should be considered if isolation of the animals is not possible. Few data are available on the efficacy of antimicrobial therapy of *Campylobacter* spp. enteritis in cats and dogs. There is increasing evidence that *Campylobacter* spp. isolated from dogs and cats show significant antimicrobial resistance to commonly used antimicrobial drugs, thus the judicious use of antibiotics is advised.[131–134] The macrolide and fluoroquinolone groups of antimicrobials have been traditionally recommended, but with the increasing resistance to enrofloxacin and ciprofloxacin, fluoroquinolones should not be considered first choice where results of susceptibility testing are unavailable.[18,135] In addition, this group of antimicrobials is not recommended for prolonged use in young animals due to possible adverse effects on cartilage development.[18,136] An overview of antimicrobial therapy options for enteric *Campylobacter* infections in dogs and cats is given in Table 65.3. Duration of therapy should be based on clinical response. Reported cases of *C. jejuni*–associated bacteremia and cholangiohepatitis or cholecystitis in dogs have been successfully treated with cefoxitin, erythromycin, or enrofloxacin.[97,98] Reinfection, intermittent excretion, specific *Campylobacter* species and strain variation, and the development of antimicrobial resistance have to be taken into account when evaluating therapeutic success. Incorrect diagnosis with subclinical *Campylobacter* spp. infection or carrier state should also be considered in cases with a poor response to therapy. The prognosis for campylobacteriosis in dogs and cats with self-limiting disease, and in those treated with appropriate antimicrobials if indicated, is excellent in the absence of systemic complications.

IMMUNITY AND VACCINATION

Clearance of *Campylobacter* infection depends on adequate innate, humoral, and cell-mediated immune responses. Short-term immunity develops after infection, but reinfection, colonization and development of long-term sequelae are possible.[137] Work in human campylobacteriosis has focused on intestinal microbiota shifts and how *C. jejuni* organisms could overcome intestinal colonization resistance following ingestion.[138] Vaccination of humans and especially poultry, as birds are the main reservoir for human *C. jejuni* infections, has been researched for many years but none of the vaccines developed have succeeded in induction of prolonged immunity, or in complete prevention of intestinal colonization in chickens.[137,139]

PREVENTION

Isolation of animals with confirmed clinical campylobacteriosis and fecal shedding is advised to minimize the risk of environmental contamination and of infection of other animals and humans predisposed to developing clinical signs. *Campylobacter* spp. are susceptible to routinely used disinfectants, and adequate hygiene measures should be communicated and implemented especially where animals are from intensive housing backgrounds,[140,141] and when raw meat-based diets are fed.[78,81]

TABLE 65.3 Drug Therapy for *Campylobacter* spp. Infections in Dogs and Cats[a,b]

Drug	Species	Dose[c] (mg/kg)	Route	Interval (Hours)
Erythromycin	B	10–15	PO	8
Azithromycin	B	5–10	PO	24
Enrofloxacin[d]	B	5	PO, SC, IV	24
Chloramphenicol	D	25–50	PO, SC, IM, IV	8
	C	10–25	PO	12
Tetracycline	B	10–20	PO	8
Tylosin	B	10	PO	12
Cefoxitin	B	15–20	SC, IM, IV	8

[a]See references 13, 18, 158.
[b]Duration of treatment should be based on clinical response.
[c]Dose per administration at specified interval.
[d]Other quinolones such as ciprofloxacin, difloxacin, or marbofloxacin are alternatives, although dosages vary.
B, both dog and cat; *C*, cat; *D*, dog; *IM*, intramuscular; *IV*, intravascular; *PO*, by mouth; *SC*, subcutaneous.

PUBLIC HEALTH ASPECTS

Campylobacter spp. remain the most significant cause of bacterial gastroenteritis in humans, and campylobacteriosis is a notifiable disease in many countries.[28,142] The main *Campylobacter* spp. isolated in enteritis patients worldwide remains *C. jejuni* followed by other species including *C. coli*, *C. concisus*, and *C. ureolyticus*.[28] Asymptomatic *C. jejuni* infections are rare in humans in developed countries. Children under the age of 5 years, young adults, and immunosuppressed or elderly people are most commonly affected. The handling or consumption of contaminated or undercooked meat and, less commonly, contaminated water or unpasteurized milk and dairy products, other foods, international travel, and contact with animals have been confirmed risk factors for human campylobacteriosis.[28,143] The mean incubation period is 3.2 days, with a range from 18 hours to 8 days. Clinical signs range from mild self-limiting enterocolitis to severe watery or bloody diarrhea with abdominal cramping, nausea, vomiting, and headache and fever. Patients usually improve after a few days of illness, although abdominal pain can persist for longer. Weight loss is common and some patients will relapse. Excretion of *Campylobacter* spp. can occur for weeks after clinical recovery, unless the infection has been treated with antimicrobials.[28,144] Bacteremia, extra-intestinal, and complicated or chronic disease may develop, and *Campylobacter* spp. have been associated with abscess formation, hepatic disease, meningitis and abortion, IBD, esophageal and periodontal diseases, the polyneuropathy Guillain-Barré syndrome, reactive arthritis, and many other disorders (see Table 65.1).[28] Contact with dogs and cats (especially immature and diarrheic animals) is a significant risk factor for *C. jejuni* and *C. coli* infection in humans, especially infants and children.[145–151] Clinical cases with confirmed identical subtypes of *Campylobacter* spp. in pets and humans from the same household have been reported,[152,153] and several studies applying MLST or whole genome sequencing to *C. jejuni* isolates from pets have identified identical sequence types in pets compared with those commonly found in human campylobacteriosis, suggesting common sources of infection and zoonotic risk from contact with dogs and cats.[14,52,79,87,154] As *C. upsaliensis* and *C. helveticus* isolates have mostly been confirmed in dogs and cats, respectively, and no other possible animal reservoir has been identified to date, cats and dogs may play an important role in the epidemiology of these species.[16,24,62,79,155] People living or working in close contact with cats and dogs should be aware of the potentially zoonotic organisms these animals may carry. Families with young children and immunocompromised people should be informed about the risks and recommended hygiene measures when handling puppies or kittens, animals with signs of gastroenteritis, and particularly when an animal is newly obtained from a shelter environment.[140,141]

CASE EXAMPLE

Signalment

"Maurice," a 4-month-old male entire Keeshond puppy from Flanders, Belgium.

History

Maurice was evaluated on an emergency basis with a 3-day history of inappetence, lethargy, vomiting, and hemorrhagic diarrhea. He had been purchased 5 weeks before from a local breeder, and routine vaccination and anthelmintic treatments were current. He was fed a dry puppy diet and had not traveled out of his local area. Other puppies from the litter were healthy, except for one that had signs of diarrhea which had responded to antimicrobial therapy prescribed by a veterinarian. There were no other animals in the household and none of the family members were ill. Maurice had free access to a large garden and went on walks.

Physical Examination

Body weight: 2.3 kg (BCS 3/9).

Abnormalities detected: Severely lethargic, 7% dehydrated, HR = 200 beats/minute with weak femoral pulses, RR = 36 breaths/minute, mucous membranes slightly pale, CRT > 2 seconds. Rectal temperature = 102.9°F (39.4°C). Maurice was uncomfortable on abdominal palpation.

Laboratory Findings

CBC: HCT 37.5% (37.3%–61.7%), Hgb 12.6 g/dL (13.1–20.5 g/dL), MCV 63.1 fL (61.6–73.5 fL), MCHC 33.6 g/dL (32–37.9 g/dL), reticulocytes 38,000/μL (10,000–110,000/μL), red cell distribution width 16.7% (13.6%–21.7%), WBC 4.24 × 10^9 cells/L (5.05–16.76 cells/L), neutrophils 1.13 × 10^9 cells/L (2.95–11.64 cells/L), lymphocytes 2.90 × 10^9 cells/L (1.05–5.10 cells/L), monocytes 0.18 × 10^9 cells/L (0.16–1.12 cells/L), eosinophils 0.03 × 10^9 cells/L (0.06–1.23 cells/L), platelets 169,000/μL (148,000–484,000/μL). Blood smear examination revealed thrombocyte aggregates and neutropenia.

Serum chemistry profile: Sodium 147 mmol/L (145–154 mmol/L), potassium 3.2 mmol/L (3.6–5.3 mmol/L), chloride 109 mmol/L (108–118 mmol/L), bicarbonate 13 mmol/L (16–26 mmol/L), phosphorus 3.0 mg/dL (3.0–6.2 mg/dL), calcium 9.9 mg/dL (9.7–11.5 mg/dL), BUN 12 mg/dL (5–21 mg/dL), creatinine 1.2 mg/dL (0.3–1.2 mg/dL), glucose 86 mg/dL (64–123 mg/dL), total protein 4.0 g/dL (4.8–7.2 g/dL),

CASE EXAMPLE—cont'd

albumin 1.9 g/dL (2.1–3.6 g/dL), globulin 2.1 g/dL (2.3–3.8 g/dL), ALT 102 U/L (19–67 U/L), AST 36 U/L (19–42 U/L), ALP 189 U/L (21–170 U/L), creatine kinase 280 U/L (51–399 U/L), GGT 2 U/L (0–6 U/L), cholesterol 292 mg/dL (135–361 mg/dL), total bilirubin 0.1 mg/dL (0–0.2 mg/dL), magnesium 1.4 mg/dL (1.5–2.6 mg/dL).

Imaging Findings

Abdominal ultrasound: The stomach was moderately distended with anechoic fluid, the duodenum and jejunum were diffusely and moderately distended with fluid and the mucosa was hyperechoic. There was decreased peristalsis. The colon was distended and fluid filled with a thickened hyperechoic wall. The jejunal lymph nodes were prominent with irregular shape but normal echogenicity and length/width ratio. Conclusion: signs of severe gastroenteritis with ileus and mucosal edema. Reactive lymphadenopathy.

Fecal Examination

Fecal real-time PCR panel was positive for CPV-2 (confirmed as CPV-2a), but negative for CCoV, CDV, and *Clostridium perfringens* toxin genes.

Screening for bacterial enteropathogens, parasites, giardiasis, and cryptosporidiosis revealed only positive *Campylobacter* spp. culture. Susceptible to ampicillin, amoxicillin clavulanate, erythromycin, tetracycline, and ciprofloxacin. PCR confirmed the presence of *C. jejuni.*

Diagnosis

Parvovirus enteritis combined with *C. jejuni* infection.

Treatment and Follow-Up

Maurice was kenneled in isolation and treated with crystalloid and colloid IV fluid therapy supplemented with potassium. Serum total protein, electrolytes, glucose, and CBC were monitored. Initial treatments consisted of amoxicillin clavulanate (20 mg/kg, IV, q8h for 3 days then switch to oral), enrofloxacin (5 mg/kg, IV, q24h for 5 days), maropitant (1 mg/kg, SC, q24h), metoclopramide CRI (1 mg/kg, IV, per 24h), and pantoprazole (1 mg/kg, IV, q24h). Fever resolved and there was clinical improvement, but nasoesophageal tube feeding was initiated on day 2 due to persistent anorexia. Within 1 week of hospitalization, he improved dramatically; vomiting, hemorrhagic diarrhea, and neutropenia resolved, and he started eating spontaneously. Maurice was discharged with treatment with oral amoxicillin clavulanate (20 mg/kg, PO, for 1 week), omeprazole (1 mg/kg, PO) and ranitidine (2 mg/kg, PO, q12h for 5 days). Fenbendazole was administered at 50 mg/kg, PO, q24h for 3 days. Repeat *Campylobacter* culture 1 week after discontinuing antibiotic treatment was negative.

Comments

This is a typical case of concomitant parvovirus and *Campylobacter* spp. infection. Broad-spectrum antimicrobial therapy was indicated with the presence of parvovirus-induced neutropenia, fever, hemorrhagic diarrhea, and suspected sepsis in this case. Choice was based on the clinical status of the patient, and antibiogram results were available 3 days after sample collection. Almost 50% of dogs with parvovirus enteritis had co-infection with *Campylobacter* spp. in one report,[90] and appropriate antimicrobial therapy is indicated in severely affected cases to reduce the risk of systemic complications and improve outcome.

SUGGESTED READINGS

Joseph LA, Francois Watkins LK, Chen J, et al. Comparison of molecular subtyping and antimicrobial resistance detection methods used in a large multistate outbreak of extensively drug-resistant *Campylobacter jejuni* infections linked to pet store puppies. *J Clin Microbiol.* 2020;58. e00771–20.

LaLonde-Paul D, Cummings KJ, Rodriguez-Rivera LD, et al. Ciprofloxacin resistance among *Campylobacter jejuni* isolates obtained from shelter dogs in Texas. *Zoonoses Public Health.* 2019;66:337–342.

Procter TD, Pearl DL, Finley RL, et al. A cross-sectional study examining *Campylobacter* and other zoonotic enteric pathogens in dogs that frequent dog parks in three cities in south-western Ontario and risk factors for shedding of *Campylobacter* spp. *Zoonoses Public Health.* 2014;61:208–218.

REFERENCES

1. Escherich T. Über das vorkommen von vibrionen im darmkanal und den stuhlgängen der säuglinge. *Munch Med Wochenschr.* 1886;33:815–817. 833-835.
2. Corry JE, Post DE, Colin P, et al. Culture media for the isolation of campylobacters. *Int J Food Microbiol.* 1995;26:43–76.
3. Vandamme P. Taxonomy of the family *Campylobacteraceae*. In: Nachamkin I, Blaser MJ, eds. *Campylobacter*. 2nd ed. Washington DC: ASM Press; 2000:3–27.
4. Bolton DJ. *Campylobacter* virulence and survival factors. *Food Microbiol.* 2015;48:99–108.
5. Skirrow MB. John McFadyean and the centenary of the first isolation of *Campylobacter* species. *Clin Infect Dis.* 2006;43:1213–1217.
6. Moore JE, Matsuda M. The history of *Campylobacter*: taxonomy and nomenclature. *Irish Vet J.* 2002;55:495–501.
7. Skirrow MB. *Campylobacter* enteritis: a "new" disease. *Br Med J.* 1977;2:9–11.
8. Dillon AR, Boosinger TR, Blevins WT. *Campylobacter* enteritis in dogs and cats. *Comp Contin Educ Practit Vet.* 1987;20:1176–1183.
9. Blaser MJ, LaForce FM, Wilson NA, et al. Reservoirs for human campylobacteriosis. *J Infect Dis.* 1980;141:665–669.
10. Silva J, Leite D, Fernandes M, et al. *Campylobacter* spp. as a foodborne pathogen: a review. *Frontiers Microbiol.* 2011;2:200.
11. Vandamme P, Falsen E, Rossau R, et al. Revision of *Campylobacter, Helicobacter*, and *Wolinella* taxonomy: emendation of generic descriptions and proposal of *Arcobacter* gen. nov. *Int J Syst Bacteriol.* 1991;41:88–103.
12. Goodwin CS, Armstrong JA, Chilvers T, et al. Transfer of *Campylobacter pylori* and *Campylobacter mustelae* to *Helicobacter* gen. nov. as *Helicobacter pylori* comb. nov. and *Helicobacter mustelae* comb. nov., respectively. *Int J Syst Evol Microbiol.* 1989;39:397–405.
13. Fox JG. *Campylobacter* infections. In: Greene CE. *Infectious Diseases of the Dog and Cat.* 4th ed. Elsevier Saunders; 2012:370–374.
14. Bojanić K, Midwinter AC, Marshall JC, et al. Isolation of *Campylobacter* spp. from client-owned dogs and cats, and retail raw meat pet food in the Manawatu, New Zealand. *Zoonoses Public Health.* 2017;64:438–449.
15. Westgarth C, Porter CJ, Nicolson L, et al. Risk factors for the carriage of *Campylobacter upsaliensis* by dogs in a community in Cheshire. *Vet Rec.* 2009;165:526–530.
16. Parsons BN, Porter CJ, Ryvar R, et al. Prevalence of *Campylobacter* spp. in a cross-sectional study of dogs attending veterinary practices in the UK and risk indicators associated with shedding. *Vet J.* 2010;184:66–70.
17. Parsons BN, Porter CJ, Williams NJ, et al. Prevalence of *Campylobacter* spp. infection in a cross-sectional study of dogs attending veterinary practices. *Zoonoses Public Health.* 2007;54. 137-137.
18. Marks SL, Rankin SC, Byrne BA, et al. Enteropathogenic bacteria in dogs and cats: diagnosis, epidemiology, treatment, and control. *J Vet Intern Med.* 2011;25:1195–1208.
19. Carbonero A, Torralbo A, Borge C, et al. *Campylobacter* spp., *C. jejuni* and *C. upsaliensis* infection-associated factors in healthy and ill dogs from clinics in Cordoba, Spain. Screening tests for antimicrobial susceptibility. *Comp Immunol Microbiol Infect Dis.* 2012;35:505–512.
20. Holmberg M, Rosendal T, Engvall EO, et al. Prevalence of thermophilic *Campylobacter* species in Swedish dogs and characterization of *C. jejuni* isolates. *Acta Vet Scand.* 2015;57:19.
21. Wieland B, Regula G, Danuser J, et al. *Campylobacter* spp. in dogs and cats in Switzerland: risk factor analysis and molecular characterization with AFLP. *J Vet Med Series B.* 2005;52:183–189.
22. Workman SN, Mathison GE, Lavoie MC. Pet dogs and chicken meat as reservoirs of *Campylobacter* spp. in Barbados. *J Clin Microbiol.* 2005;43:2642–2650.

23. Queen EV, Marks SL, Farver TB. Prevalence of selected bacterial and parasitic agents in feces from diarrheic and healthy control cats from Northern California. *J Vet Intern Med.* 2012;26:54–60.
24. Bojanić K, Midwinter AC, Marshall JC, et al. Variation in the limit-of-detection of the ProSpecT *Campylobacter* microplate enzyme immunoassay in stools spiked with emerging *Campylobacter* species. *J Microbiol Methods.* 2016;127:236–241.
25. Man SM. The clinical importance of emerging *Campylobacter* species. *Nature Rev Gastroenterol Hepatol.* 2011;8:669–685.
26. Chaban B, Ngeleka M, Hill JE. Detection and quantification of 14 *Campylobacter* species in pet dogs reveals an increase in species richness in feces of diarrheic animals. *BMC Microbiol.* 2010;10:73.
27. Nielsen HL, Ejlertsen T, Engberg J, et al. High incidence of *Campylobacter concisus* in gastroenteritis in North Jutland, Denmark: a population-based study. *Clin Microbiol Infect.* 2013;19:445–450.
28. Kaakoush NO, Castano-Rodriguez N, Mitchell HM, et al. Global epidemiology of *Campylobacter* infection. *Clin Microbiol Rev.* 2015;28:687–720.
29. Koziel M, Corcoran GD, Sleator RD, et al. Detection and molecular analysis of *Campylobacter ureolyticus* in domestic animals. *Gut Pathog.* 2014;6:9.
30. Malik R, Love DN. The isolation of *Campylobacter jejuni/coli* from pound dogs and canine veterinary patients in a veterinary hospital. *Aust Vet Practit.* 1989;19:16–18.
31. Burnens AP, Angeloz-Wick B, Nicolet J. Comparison of *Campylobacter* carriage rates in diarrheic and healthy pet animals. *Zentralbl Veterinarmed B.* 1992;39:175–180.
32. Torre E, Tello M. Factors influencing fecal shedding of *Campylobacter jejuni* in dogs without diarrhea. *Am J Vet Res.* 1993;54:260–262.
33. Baker J, Barton MD, Lanser J. *Campylobacter* species in cats and dogs in South Australia. *Aust Vet J.* 1999;77:662–666.
34. Lopez CM, Giacoboni G, Agostini A, et al. Thermotolerant *Campylobacters* in domestic animals in a defined population in Buenos Aires, Argentina. *Prev Vet Med.* 2002;55:193–200.
35. Sandberg M, Bergsjo B, Hofshagen M, et al. Risk factors for *Campylobacter* infection in Norwegian cats and dogs. *Prev Vet Med.* 2002;55:241–253.
36. Acke E, Whyte P, Jones BR, et al. Prevalence of thermophilic *Campylobacter* species in cats and dogs in two animal shelters in Ireland. *Vet Rec.* 2006:51–54.
37. Acke E, McGill K, Golden O, et al. Prevalence of thermophilic *Campylobacter* species in household cats and dogs in Ireland. *Vet Rec.* 2009;164:44–47.
38. Hastings DH. *Campylobacter* enteritis in pets. *Lancet.* 1978;2:1249–1250.
39. Ferreira MC, Ribeiro VL, Ricciardi ID. *Campylobacter*, dogs and human enteritis. *Vet Rec.* 1979;105:451.
40. Holt PE. Incidence of *Campylobacter, Salmonella* and *Shigella* infections in dogs in an industrial town. *Vet Rec.* 1980;107:254.
41. Hosie BD, Nicolson TB, Henderson DB. *Campylobacter* infections in normal and diarrhoeic dogs. *Vet Rec.* 1979;105:80.
42. Bruce D, Zochowski W, Fleming GA. *Campylobacter* infections in cats and dogs. *Vet Rec.* 1980;107:200–201.
43. Bruce D, Ferguson IR. *Campylobacter jejuni* in cats. *Lancet.* 1980;13:595–596.
44. McOrist S, Browning JW. Carriage of *Campylobacter jejuni* in healthy and diarrhoeic dogs and cats. *Aust Vet J.* 1982;58:33–34.
45. Bruce D, Fleming GA. *Campylobacter* isolations from household dogs. *Vet Rec.* 1983;112:16.
46. Fleming MP. Association of *Campylobacter jejuni* with enteritis in dogs and cats. *Vet Rec.* 1983;113:372–374.
47. Fox JG, Moore R, Ackerman JI. *Campylobacter jejuni*-associated diarrhea in dogs. *J Am Vet Med Assoc.* 1983;183:1430–1433.
48. Nair GB, Sarkar RK, Chowdhury S, et al. *Campylobacter* infection in domestic dogs. *Vet Rec.* 1985;116:237–238.
49. Olson P, Sandstedt K. *Campylobacter* in the dog: a clinical and experimental study. *Vet Rec.* 1987;121:99–101.
50. Bender JB, Shulman SA, Averbeck GA, et al. Epidemiologic features of *Campylobacter* infection among cats in the upper midwestern United States. *J Am Vet Med Assoc.* 2005;226:544–547.
51. Ogden ID, Dallas JF, MacRae M, et al. *Campylobacter* excreted into the environment by animal sources: prevalence, concentration shed, and host association. *Foodborne Pathogens Dis.* 2009;6:1161–1170.
52. Amar C, Kittl S, Spreng D, et al. Genotypes and antibiotic resistance of canine *Campylobacter jejuni* isolates. *Vet Microbiol.* 2014:168.
53. Procter TD, Pearl DL, Finley RL, et al. A cross-sectional study examining *Campylobacter* and other zoonotic enteric pathogens in dogs that frequent dog parks in three cities in south-western Ontario and risk factors for shedding of *Campylobacter* spp. *Zoonoses Public Health.* 2014;61:208–218.
54. Ramonaite S, Kudirkiene E, Tamuleviciene E, et al. Prevalence and genotypes of *Campylobacter jejuni* from urban environmental sources in comparison with clinical isolates from children. *J Med Microbiol.* 2014;63.
55. Verma AK, Amit K, Singh SK, et al. Prevalence and resistance to antimicrobial agents of *Campylobacter* sp. isolated from dogs in India. *J Biol Sci.* 2014;14:142–148.
56. Selwet M, Clapa T, Galbas M, et al. The prevalence of *Campylobacter* spp. and occurrence of virulence genes isolated from dogs. *Polish J Microbiol.* 2015;64:73–76.
57. Hascall KL, Kass PH, Saksen J, et al. Prevalence of enteropathogens in dogs attending 3 regional dog parks in Northern California. *J Vet Intern Med.* 2016;30:1838–1845.
58. Steinhauserova I, Fojtikova K, Klimes J. The incidence and PCR detection of *Campylobacter upsaliensis* in dogs and cats. *Letters Appl Microbiol.* 2000;31:209–212.
59. Acke E, McGill K, Golden O, et al. A comparison of different culture methods for the recovery of *Campylobacter* species from pets. *Zoonoses Public Health.* 2009;56:490–495.
60. Pintar KDM, Christidis T, Thomas MK, et al. A systematic review and meta-analysis of the *Campylobacter* spp. prevalence and concentration in household pets and petting zoo animals for use in exposure assessments. *PLoS One.* 2015;10. e0144976.
61. Fox JG, Krakowka S, Taylor NS. Acute-onset *Campylobacter*-associated gastroenteritis in adult beagles. *J Am Vet Med Assoc.* 1985;187:1268–1271.
62. Parsons BN, Williams NJ, Pinchbeck GL, et al. Prevalence and shedding patterns of *Campylobacter* spp. in longitudinal studies of kennelled dogs. *Vet J.* 2011;190:249–254.
63. Giacomelli M, Follador N, Coppola LM, et al. Survey of *Campylobacter* spp. in owned and unowned dogs and cats in Northern Italy. *Vet J.* 2015;204:333–337.
64. Fox JG, Moore R, Ackerman JI. Canine and feline campylobacteriosis: epizootiology and clinical and public health features. *J Am Vet Med Assoc.* 1983;183:1420–1424.
65. Engvall EO, Brandstrom B, Andersson L, et al. Isolation and identification of thermophilic *Campylobacter* species in faecal samples from Swedish dogs. *Scand J Infect Dis.* 2003;35:713–718.
66. Leonard EK, Pearl DL, Janecko N, et al. Factors related to *Campylobacter* spp. carriage in client-owned dogs visiting veterinary clinics in a region of Ontario, Canada. *Epidemiol Infect.* 2011;139:1531–1541.
67. Malayeri HZ, Jamshidi S, Salehi TZ, et al. Identification of *Campylobacter* spp. with multiplex PCR assay in healthy and diarrheic dogs. *Res Opin Anim Vet Sci.* 2014;4.
68. Sokolow SH, Rand C, Marks SL, et al. Epidemiologic evaluation of diarrhea in dogs in an animal shelter. *Am J Vet Res.* 2005;66:1018–1024.
69. Jorgensen K. Prevalence of *Campylobacter fetus* spp. *jejuni* in Danish dogs. *Nordisk Vet Med.* 1981;33:42–48.
70. Prescott JF, Bruin-Mosch CW. Carriage of *Campylobacter jejuni* in healthy and diarrheic animals. *Am J Vet Res.* 1981;42:164–165.
71. Gondrosen B, Knaevelsrud T, Dommarsnes K. Isolation of thermophilic *Campylobacters* from Norwegian dogs and cats. *Acta Vet Scand.* 1985;26:81–90.
72. Cave NJ, Marks SL, Kass PH, et al. Evaluation of a routine diagnostic fecal panel for dogs with diarrhea. *J Am Vet Med Assoc.* 2002;221: 52–59.
73. Rossi M, Hanninen ML, Revez J, et al. Occurrence and species level diagnostics of *Campylobacter* spp., enteric *Helicobacter* spp. and *Anaerobiospirillum* spp. in healthy and diarrheic dogs and cats. *Vet Microbiol.* 2008;129:304–314.
74. Duijvestijn M, Mughini-Gras L, Schuurman N, et al. Enteropathogen infections in canine puppies: (Co-)occurrence, clinical relevance and risk factors. *Vet Microbiol.* 2016;195:115–122.

75. Fox JG, Maxwell KO, Ackerman JI. *Campylobacter jejuni* associated diarrhea in commercially reared beagles. *Lab Anim Sci.* 1984;34:151–155.
76. Brown C, Martin V, Chitwood S. An outbreak of enterocolitis due to *Campylobacter* spp. in a beagle colony. *J Vet Diagn Invest.* 1999;11:374–376.
77. Hald B, Madsen M. Healthy puppies and kittens as carriers of *Campylobacter* spp., with special reference to *Campylobacter* upsaliensis. *J Clin Microbiol.* 1997;35:3351–3352.
78. Bojanic K, Midwinter AC, Marshall JC, et al. Isolation of *Campylobacter* spp. from client-owned dogs and cats, and retail raw meat pet food in the Manawatu, New Zealand. *Zoonoses Public Health.* 2017;64:438–449.
79. Olkkola S, Kovanen S, Roine J, et al. Population genetics and antimicrobial susceptibility of canine *Campylobacter* isolates collected before and after a raw feeding experiment. *PLoS One.* 2015;10. e0132660.
80. Runesvärd E, Wikström C, Fernström LL, Hansson I. Presence of pathogenic bacteria in faeces from dogs fed raw meat-based diets or dry kibble. *Vet Rec.* 2020;187:e71.
81. Fredriksson-Ahomaa M, Heikkila T, Pernu N, et al. Raw meat-based diets in dogs and cats. *Vet Sci.* 2017;4:33.
82. Martinez-Anton L, Marenda M, Firestone SM, et al. Investigation of the role of *Campylobacter* infection in suspected acute polyradiculoneuritis in dogs. *J Vet Intern Med.* 2018;32:352–360.
83. Hald B, Pedersen K, Waino M, et al. Longitudinal study of the excretion patterns of thermophilic *Campylobacter* spp. in young pet dogs in Denmark. *J Clin Microbiol.* 2004;42:2003–2012.
84. Koene MG, Houwers DJ, Dijkstra JR, et al. Simultaneous presence of multiple *Campylobacter* species in dogs. *J Clin Microbiol.* 2004;42:819–821.
85. Koene MGJ, Houwers DJ, Dijkstra JR, et al. Strain variation within *Campylobacter* species in fecal samples from dogs and cats. *Vet Microbiol.* 2009;133:199–205.
86. Acke E, McGill K, Lawlor A, et al. Genetic diversity among *Campylobacter jejuni* isolates from pets in Ireland. *Vet Rec.* 2010:166:102–106.
87. Parsons BN, Cody AJ, Porter CJ, et al. Typing of *Campylobacter jejuni* isolates from dogs by use of multilocus sequence typing and pulsed-field gel electrophoresis. *J Clin Microbiol.* 2009;47:3466–3471.
88. Shen Z, Feng Y, Dewhirst FE, et al. Coinfection of enteric *Helicobacter* spp. and *Campylobacter* spp. in cats. *J Clin Microbiol.* 2001;39:2166–2172.
89. Misawa N, Kawashima K, Kondo F, et al. Isolation and characterization of *Campylobacter, Helicobacter*, and *Anaerobiospirillum* strains from a puppy with bloody diarrhea. *Vet Microbiol.* 2002;87:353–364.
90. Sandstedt K, Wierup M. Concomitant occurrence of *Campylobacter* and parvoviruses in dogs with gastroenteritis. *Vet Res Comm.* 1981;4:271–273.
91. Newton CM, Newell DG, Wood M, et al. *Campylobacter* infection in a closed dog breeding colony. *Vet Rec.* 1988;123:152–154.
92. Lertsethtakarn P, Ottemann KM, Hendrixson DR. Motility and chemotaxis in *Campylobacter* and *Helicobacter*. *Annual Rev Microbiol.* 2011;65:389–410.
93. Hermans D, Pasmans F, Messens W, et al. Poultry as a host for the zoonotic pathogen *Campylobacter jejuni*. *Vector Borne Zoonotic Dis.* 2012;12:89–98.
94. Macartney L, Al-Mashat RR, Taylor DJ, et al. Experimental infection of dogs with *Campylobacter jejuni*. *Vet Rec.* 1988;122:245–249.
95. Prescott JF, Barker IK, Manninen KI, et al. *Campylobacter jejuni* colitis in gnotobiotic dogs. *Can J Comp Med.* 1981;45:377–383.
96. Prescott JF, Karmali MA. Attempts to transmit campylobacter enteritis to dogs and cats. *J Can Med Assoc.* 1978;119:1001–1002.
97. Marks S. Campylobacteriosis. In: Sykes J. *Canine and Feline Infectious Diseases*. 1st ed. Elsevier; 2013.
98. Oswald GP, Twedt DC, Steyn P. *Campylobacter jejuni* bacteremia and acute cholecystitis in two dogs. *J Am Anim Hosp Assoc.* 1994;30:165–169.
99. Sahin O, Burrough ER, Pavlovic N, et al. *Campylobacter jejuni* as a cause of canine abortions in the United States. *J Vet Diagn Invest.* 2014;26:699–704.
100. Odendaal MW, de Cramer KG, van der Walt ML, et al. First isolation of *Campylobacter jejuni* from the vaginal discharge of three bitches after abortion in South Africa. *Onderstepoort J Vet Res.* 1994;61:193–195.
101. Bulgin MS, Ward AC, Sriranganathan N, et al. Abortion in the dog due to *Campylobacter* species. *Am J Vet Res.* 1984;45:555–556.
102. Davies AP, Gebhart CJ, Meric SA. *Campylobacter*-associated chronic diarrhea in a dog. *J Am Vet Med Assoc.* 1984;184:469–471.
103. Fox JG, Claps M, Beaucage CM. Chronic diarrhea associated with *Campylobacter jejuni* infection in a cat. *J Am Vet Med Assoc.* 1986;189:455–456.
104. Maunder CL, Reynolds ZF, Peacock L, et al. *Campylobacter* species and neutrophilic inflammatory bowel disease in cats. *J Vet Intern Med.* 2016;30:996–1001.
105. Petersen RF, Harrington CS, Kortegaard HE, et al. A PCR-DGGE method for detection and identification of *Campylobacter, Helicobacter, Arcobacter* and related Epsilobacteria and its application to saliva samples from humans and domestic pets. *J Appl Microbiol.* 2007;103:2601–2605.
106. Yamasaki Y, Nomura R, Nakano K, et al. Distribution of periodontopathic bacterial species in dogs and their owners. *Arch Oral Biol.* 2012;57:1183–1188.
107. Penninck D, Smyers B, Webster CRL, et al. Diagnostic value of ultrasonography in differentiating enteritis from intestinal neoplasia in dogs. *Vet Radiol Ultrasound.* 2003;44:570–575.
108. McDonough PL, Simpson KW. Diagnosing emerging bacterial infections: salmonellosis, campylobacteriosis, clostridial toxicosis, and helicobacteriosis. *Sem Vet Med Surg (Small Anim).* 1996;11:187–197.
109. Lastovica AJ. Emerging *Campylobacter* spp.: the tip of the iceberg. *Clin Microbiol News.* 2006;28:49–56.
110. Newell DG, Frost JA, Duim B, et al. New developments in the subtyping of *Campylobacter* species. In: Nachamkin I, Blaser MJ, eds. *Campylobacter*. 2nd ed. Washington DC: ASM Press; 2000:27–44.
111. Hutchinson DN, Bolton FJ. Improved blood free selective medium for the isolation of *Campylobacter jejuni* from faecal specimens. *J Clin Pathol.* 1984;37:956–957.
112. Gun-Munro J, Rennie RP, Thornley JH, et al. Laboratory and clinical evaluation of isolation media for *Campylobacter jejuni*. *J Clin Microbiol.* 1987;25:2274–2277.
113. Aspinall ST, Wareing DR, Hayward PG, et al. A comparison of a new campylobacter selective medium (CAT) with membrane filtration for the isolation of thermophilic campylobacters including *Campylobacter upsaliensis*. *J Appl Bacteriol.* 1996;80:645–650.
114. Engberg J, On SL, Harrington CS, et al. Prevalence of *Campylobacter, Arcobacter, Helicobacter*, and *Sutterella* spp. in human fecal samples as estimated by a reevaluation of isolation methods for *Campylobacters*. *J Clin Microbiol.* 2000;38:286–291.
115. Lastovica AJ, le Roux E. Efficient isolation of campylobacteria from stools. *J Clin Microbiol.* 2000;38:2798–2799.
116. Engvall EO, Brandstrom B, Gunnarsson A, et al. Validation of a polymerase chain reaction/restriction enzyme analysis method for species identification of thermophilic campylobacters isolated from domestic and wild animals. *J Appl Microbiol.* 2002;92:47–54.
117. Cheng K, Chui H, Domish L, et al. Recent development of mass spectrometry and proteomics applications in identification and typing of bacteria. *Proteomics Clin Appl.* 2016;10:346–357.
118. Kiehntopf M, Melcher F, Hanel I, et al. Differentiation of *Campylobacter* species by surface-enhanced laser desorption/ionization-time-of-flight mass spectrometry. *Foodborne Pathogens Dis.* 2011;8:875–885.
119. On SLW. Isolation, identification and subtyping of *Campylobacter*: where to from here? *J Microbiol Methods.* 2013;95:3–7.
120. Fermer C, Olsson Engvall E. Specific PCR identification and differentiation of the thermophylic campylobacters, *Campylobacter jejuni, C. coli, C. lari, C. upsaliensis*. *J Clin Microbiol.* 1999;37:3370–3373.
121. Wang G, Clark CG, Taylor TM, et al. Colony multiplex PCR assay for identification and differentiation of *Campylobacter jejuni, C. coli, C. lari, C. upsaliensis*, and *C. fetus* subsp. *fetus*. *J Clin Microbiol.* 2002;40:4744–4747.
122. Neubauer C, Hess M. Detection and identification of food-borne pathogens of the genera *Campylobacter, Arcobacter* and *Helicobacter* by multiplex PCR in poultry and poultry products. *J Vet Med B, Infect Dis Vet Public Health.* 2006;53:376–381.

123. Chaban B, Musil KM, Himsworth CG, et al. Development of cpn60-based real-time quantitative PCR assays for the detection of 14 *Campylobacter* species and application to screening of canine fecal samples. *Appl Environ Microbiol.* 2009;75:3055–3061.
124. Taboada EN, Clark CG, Sproston EL, et al. Current methods for molecular typing of *Campylobacter* species. *J Microbiol Methods.* 2013;95:24–31.
125. Dingle KE, Colles FM, Wareing DR, et al. Multilocus sequence typing system for *Campylobacter jejuni. J Clin Microbiol.* 2001;39:14–23.
126. Cantero G, Correa-Fiz F, Ronco T, et al. Characterization of *Campylobacter jejuni* and *Campylobacter coli* broiler isolates by whole-genome sequencing. *Foodborne Pathogens Dis.* 2017:145–152.
127. Joseph LA, Francois Watkins LK, Chen J, et al. Comparison of molecular subtyping and antimicrobial resistance detection methods used in a large multistate outbreak of extensively drug-resistant *Campylobacter jejuni* infections linked to pet store puppies. *J Clin Microbiol.* 2020;58. e00771–20.
128. Tuuminen T, Lounamo K, Leirisalo-Repo M. A review of serological tests to assist diagnosis of reactive arthritis: critical appraisal on methodologies. *Frontiers Immunol.* 2013;4:418.
129. Granato PA, Chen L, Holiday I, et al. Comparison of premier CAMPY enzyme immunoassay (EIA), ProSpecT *Campylobacter* EIA, and ImmunoCard STAT! CAMPY tests with culture for laboratory diagnosis of *Campylobacter* enteric infections. *J Clin Microbiol.* 2010;48:4022–4027.
130. Collins JE, Libal MC, Brost D. Proliferative enteritis in two pups. *J Am Vet Med Assoc.* 1983;183:886–889.
131. Rodrigues CG, Melo RT, Fonseca BB, et al. Occurrence and characterization of *Campylobacter* spp. isolates in dogs, cats and children. *Pesqui Vet Brasil.* 2015;35:365–370.
132. Tsai HJ, Huang HC, Lin CM, et al. Salmonellae and campylobacters in household and stray dogs in northern Taiwan. *Vet Res Comm.* 2007;31:931–939.
133. Acke E, McGill K, Quinn T, et al. Antimicrobial resistance profiles and mechanisms of resistance in *Campylobacter jejuni* isolates from pets. *Foodborne Pathogens Dis.* 2009;6:705–710.
134. Cho H, Kim S, Min W, et al. Characterization of antimicrobial resistance and application of RFLP for epidemiological monitoring of thermophilic *Campylobacter* spp. isolated from dogs and humans in Korea. *Korean J Vet Res.* 2014;54.
135. Moser S, Seth-Smith H, Egli A, et al. *Campylobacter jejuni* from canine and bovine cases of campylobacteriosis express high antimicrobial resistance rates against (fluoro)quinolones and tetracyclines. *Pathogens.* 2020;9:691.
136. Burkhardt JE, Forster C, Lozo E, et al. Immunohistochemistry of articular cartilage from immature beagle dogs dosed with difloxacin. *Toxicol Pathol.* 1997;25:475–480.
137. Janssen R, Krogfelt KA, Cawthraw SA, et al. Host-pathogen interactions in *Campylobacter* infections: the host perspective. *Clin Microbiol Rev.* 2008;21:505–518.
138. Masanta WO, Heimesaat MM, Bereswill S, et al. Modification of intestinal microbiota and its consequences for innate immune response in the pathogenesis of campylobacteriosis. *Clin Development Immunol.* 2013;2013:10.
139. Kobierecka PA, Wyszyńska AK, Gubernator J, et al. Chicken anti-*Campylobacter* vaccine – comparison of various carriers and routes of immunization. *Frontiers Microbiol.* 2016;7:740.
140. Pena A, Abarca K, Weitzel T, et al. One Health in Practice: a pilot project for integrated care of zoonotic infections in immunocompromised children and their pets in Chile. *Zoonoses Public Health.* 2016;63:403–409.
141. Campagnolo ER, Philipp LM, Long JM, et al. Pet-associated campylobacteriosis: a persisting public health concern. *Zoonoses Public Health.* 2018;65:304–311.
142. Moore JE, Corcoran D, Dooley JSG, et al. Campylobacter. *Vet Res.* 2005;36:351–382.
143. Adak GK, Meakins SM, Yip H, et al. Disease risks from foods, England and Wales, 1996-2000. *Emerg Infect Dis.* 2005;11:365–372.
144. Skirrow MB, Blaser MJ. Clinical aspects of *Campylobacter* infection. In: Nachamkin I, Blaser MJ, eds. *Campylobacter.* 2nd ed. Washington DC: ASM Press; 2000:69–88.
145. Deming MS, Tauxe RV, Blake PA, et al. *Campylobacter* enteritis at a university: transmission from eating chicken and from cats. *Am J Epidemiol.* 1987;126:526–534.
146. Tenkate TD, Stafford RJ. Risk factors for Campylobacter infection in infants and young children: a matched case-control study. *Epidemiol Infect.* 2001;127:399–404.
147. Carrique-Mas J, Andersson Y, Hjertqvist M, et al. Risk factors for domestic sporadic campylobacteriosis among young children in Sweden. *Scand J Infect Dis.* 2005;37:101–110.
148. Saeed AM, Harris NV, DiGiacomo RF. The role of exposure to animals in the etiology of *Campylobacter jejuni/coli* enteritis. *Am J Epidemiol.* 1993;137:108–114.
149. Adak GK, Cowden JM, Nicholas S, et al. The Public Health Laboratory Service national case-control study of primary indigenous sporadic cases of campylobacter infection. *Epidemiol Infect.* 1995;115:15–22.
150. Davis MA, Moore DL, Baker KNK, et al. Risk factors for campylobacteriosis in two Washington state counties with high numbers of dairy farms. *J Clin Microbiol.* 2013;51:3921–3927.
151. Mughini Gras L, Smid JH, Wagenaar JA, et al. Increased risk for *Campylobacter jejuni* and *C. coli* infection of pet origin in dog owners and evidence for genetic association between strains causing infection in humans and their pets. *Epidemiol Infect.* 2013;141:2526–2535.
152. Wolfs TF, Duim B, Geelen SP, et al. Neonatal sepsis by *Campylobacter jejuni*: genetically proven transmission from a household puppy. *Clin Infect Dis.* 2001;32:E97–E99.
153. Damborg P, Olsen KE, Moller Nielsen E, et al. Occurrence of *Campylobacter jejuni* in pets living with human patients infected with *C. jejuni. J Clin Microbiol.* 2004;42:1363–1364.
154. Mughini-Gras L, Pijnacker R, Coipan C, et al. Sources and transmission routes of campylobacteriosis: A combined analysis of genome and exposure data. *J Infect.* 2021;82:216–226.
155. Parsons BN, Porter CJ, Stavisky JH, et al. Multilocus sequence typing of human and canine *C. upsaliensis* isolates. *Vet Microbiol.* 2012;157:391–397.
156. Chaban B, Links MG, Hill JE. A molecular enrichment strategy based on cpn60 for detection of epsilon-proteobacteria in the dog fecal microbiome. *Microbial Ecol.* 2012;63:348–357.
157. Bojanić K, Midwinter AC, Marshall JC, et al. Isolation of emerging Campylobacter species in working farm dogs and their frozen home-killed raw meat diets. *J Vet Diagn Invest.* 2019;31:23–32.
158. Weese JS. Bacterial enteritis in dogs and cats: diagnosis, therapy, and zoonotic potential. *Vet Clin North Am Small Anim Practit.* 2011;41:287–309.

66

Helicobacter Infections

Jane E. Sykes

KEY POINTS

- First Described: 1881 by Rappin (France),[1] who observed spiral bacteria in a dog's stomach; the association between *Helicobacter pylori* infection and disease in humans was made in 1983.[2]
- Cause: Various species of non-*H. pylori* helicobacters, rarely *H. pylori.*
- Primary Mode of Transmission: Fecal-oral and oral-oral transmission proposed, possibly water-borne. Transmission through contact with vomitus may also occur.
- Affected Hosts: Humans and a variety of other animals.
- Geographic Distribution: Worldwide.
- Major Clinical Signs: Possibly associated with chronic vomiting (gastric helicobacters) or diarrhea (intestinal helicobacters), although evidence for a causative role in disease is weak.
- Differential Diagnoses: Dietary indiscretion, gastrointestinal foreign body, chronic pancreatitis, inflammatory bowel disease, food-responsive enteropathy, eosinophilic fibrosing gastritis (cats), bilious vomiting syndrome, gastrointestinal neoplasia (lymphoma, mast cell neoplasia, gastric adenocarcinoma), chronic infiltrative infectious diseases of the gastrointestinal tract (including FIP, mycobacteriosis, canine cryptococcosis, pythiosis), hypoadrenocorticism, hyperthyroidism (cats), toxins (including drugs), gastric helminthiasis (e.g., *Physaloptera* and *Ollulanus* spp.).
- Human Health Significance: Dogs and cats may be a source of human infection with non-*H. pylori* helicobacters that have been associated with gastritis, gastroduodenal ulceration, and low-grade MALT lymphoma in humans.

ETIOLOGIC AGENT AND EPIDEMIOLOGY

Helicobacter spp. are flagellate, gram-negative, microaerophilic, curved to spiral-shaped motile bacteria (Figs. 66.1 and 66.2). They are grouped into oral, gastric, hepatic, and intestinal *Helicobacter* species, with intestinal species residing primarily in the large intestine.[3-5] In humans, gastric *Helicobacter* spp. are an important cause of gastritis and gastroduodenal ulceration, and increase the risk for development of gastric adenocarcinoma and lymphoma. However, they have also been associated with positive health effects, such as decreased gastroesophageal reflux and protection from some gastrointestinal neoplasms. In contrast, the extent to which *Helicobacter* spp. are capable of causing disease in dogs and cats is not fully understood, and newly discovered organisms in dogs and cats have drawn most attention with regard to their zoonotic potential.[6]

Helicobacter pylori is the type organism, and the most important organism infecting humans. *Helicobacter pylori* infection is rare in cats and dogs, and has been identified in one colony of cats and rarely in domestic pet and stray cats, usually in mixed infections with other *Helicobacter* species.[7-10] In 2021, infection with *H. pylori* was reported in two dogs and their owner in Japan.[11] Dogs and cats are generally infected with gastric non-*H. pylori* helicobacters[6] (also referred to as gastric *Helicobacter*-like organisms, or GHLOs). These are much larger than *H. pylori* (5 to 10 μm long versus 1.5 to 3 μm long for *H. pylori*) and species cannot be differentiated from one another based on their light or electron microscopic appearance alone. The nomenclature of non-*H. pylori* helicobacters is complicated, and species that have been identified in dogs and cats are listed in Table 66.1. Before they were characterized genetically, non-*H. pylori* helicobacters were originally referred to as "*Gastrospirillum hominis*" and later "*Helicobacter heilmannii.*" Subsequent analysis of multiple gene sequences from a variety of "*H. heilmannii*" from dogs and cats has revealed that "*H. heilmannii*"

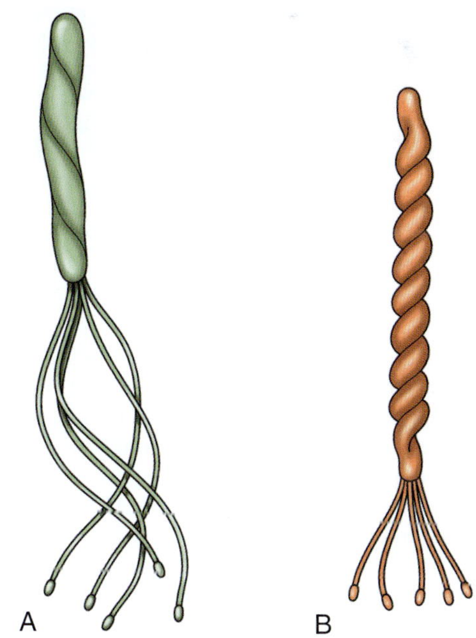

Fig. 66.1 Structure of gastric *Helicobacter* species. Note the terminal bunches of flagellar filaments. (A) *Helicobacter pylori.* (B) Gastric helicobacter-like organism.

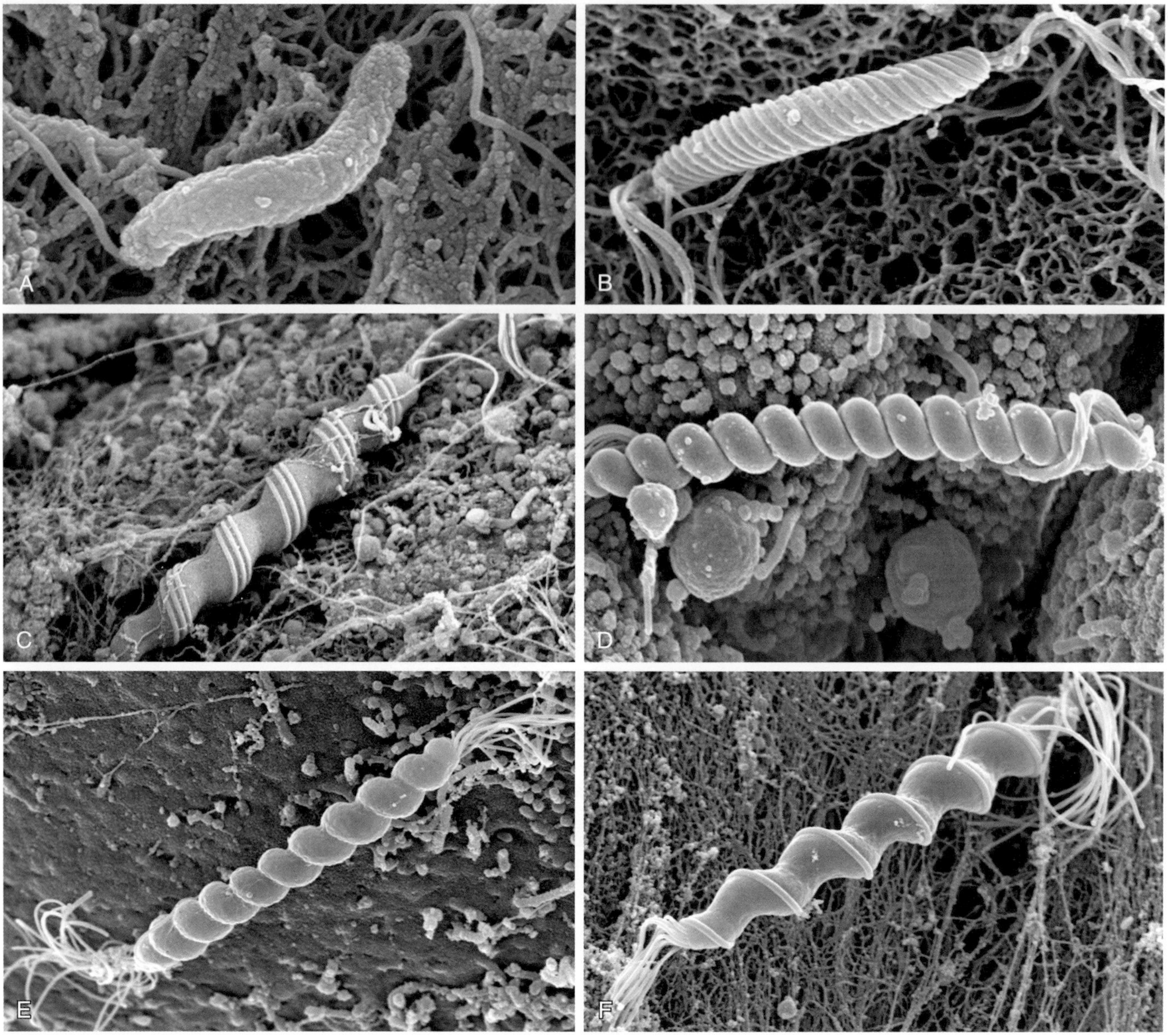

Fig. 66.2 Scanning electron micrographs of (A) *Helicobacter pylori*; (B) *Helicobacter rappini*; (C) *Helicobacter felis*; (D) *Helicobacter heilmannii*; (E) *Helicobacter bizzozeronii*; and (F) *Helicobacter salomonis*. (Courtesy M. H. Stoffel, University of Bern, Bern, Switzerland.)

is not one but a group of organisms that includes *Helicobacter felis*, *Helicobacter bizzozeronii*, *Helicobacter salomonis*, and an unculturable organism that has been confusingly named "*Candidatus* Helicobacter heilmannii." These organisms have also been implicated in human disease, albeit less commonly than *H. pylori*.[6]

Depending on the study, between 35% and 100% of dogs and cats have been found to be infected with non-*H. pylori* helicobacters, and gastric *Helicobacter* spp. can be found in apparently healthy animals and dogs and cats without signs of vomiting.[6,12-19] *Helicobacter* spp. infection has shown an association with gastric pathology in dogs and cats in some studies[13,20] but not in others.[12,21]

Dogs and cats are probably infected shortly after birth, as a result of fecal-oral and oral-oral transmission.[22] Transmission through contact with vomitus may also occur. Water-borne transmission has been hypothesized to play a role in spread of *H. pylori* to humans.[23] Shelter and colony dogs and cats appear to have a higher prevalence of infection, most likely due to the close proximity of animals to one another. One *Helicobacter* species may be able to suppress the presence of another, so that dogs and cats are primarily colonized with a single species, although in some animals the simultaneous presence of multiple species has been found.[8,24] The organisms have a remarkable ability to survive the low pH of the stomach, which they resist by living deep in the mucus glands of the stomach and through production of the enzyme *urease* (Fig. 66.3). The urease catalyzes the hydrolysis of urea to carbon dioxide and ammonia, thus raising the pH of the organism's milieu. In dogs and cats, the organisms can also be found inside parietal cells.[22,25]

CLINICAL FEATURES

Pathogenesis and Clinical Signs

The majority of dogs and cats infected with gastric helicobacters show no clinical signs. *Helicobacter* infection of some dogs and cats has been hypothesized to cause chronic intermittent vomiting, inappetence, pica, belching, weight loss, fever, and polyphagia.[25,26] Unfortunately, strong evidence supporting an association with such disease in dogs and cats is lacking. Some animals with biopsy-confirmed infection develop resolution of clinical signs following specific therapy for gastric helicobacter infection,[27-29] although the results of one study were difficult to interpret because of the concurrent administration of an elimination diet.[28] Experimental and natural infections of dogs and cats with non-*H. pylori* helicobacters have been associated with chronic lymphoplasmacytic gastritis and lymphoid follicular hyperplasia. Gastroduodenal ulceration and marked alterations in the gastric acid secretory axis have not been observed.[21,29,30] However, not all animals infected with non-*H. pylori* helicobacters have histopathologic evidence of gastritis, and there has been no correlation observed between the severity of gastric pathology and the degree of colonization by helicobacters.[31] More severe gastritis with marked lymphoid follicular hyperplasia and neutrophilic inflammatory infiltrates has been reported in cats and acutely in puppies experimentally infected with *H. pylori*.[32,33] The puppies developed gastrointestinal signs, including vomiting and loose stool shortly after inoculation. One cat was described with severe atrophic gastritis and linear gastric tears in association with a possible *H. pylori* infection.[27] It is conceivable that the degree of gastritis in dogs and cats may vary with the *Helicobacter* species or even strain, but this requires further study. In humans, gastric pathology has been associated with possession of a number of pathogenicity genes by *H. pylori*, including *cag*A (cytotoxin-associated gene A), *vac*A (vacuolating cytotoxin), and *ice*A (induced by contact with epithelium) (see Fig. 66.3).[34] The degree of vacuolating cytotoxin production can also vary between strains.[35]

In human patients, *H. pylori* infection has been well associated with gastric low-grade, B cell, MALT lymphoma. Clinical studies have documented that *H. pylori* eradication can achieve complete remission in some patients with *H. pylori*–positive early-stage gastric MALT lymphoma.[36] One study suggested a possible association between *Helicobacter* spp. infection and gastric lymphoma in cats.[37] In another report of 55 cats with nonhematopoietic intestinal carcinomas, helicobacters were detected using FISH in 56% of cases; furthermore, there was an association with large intestinal location (68% of tumors) and mucinous adenocarcinomas (92% of tumors).[38] More studies are required to confirm whether an association exists between intestinal neoplasia in cats and *Helicobacter* spp. infection.

Some evidence exists that colonization of the gall bladder by *H. pylori* in humans is associated with an increased risk of chronic cholecystitis and cholelithiasis.[39] Non-*H. pylori* helicobacters were reported in the hepatobiliary system of 2 of 32 cats with cholangiohepatitis.[9] *Helicobacter* spp. were also detected in the liver of 21% of 33 dogs with hepatic disease and none of 17 dogs that had normal liver pathology.[40] *Helicobacter canis* was detected in the liver of a 2-month-old puppy with multifocal necrotizing hepatitis that had acute weakness, vomiting, and death within hours.[41] *Helicobacter canis* was also detected in a colony of Bengal cats with diarrhea, but its role as a causative agent was uncertain.[42] Abundant organisms that genetically resembled *H. canis* were detected microscopically throughout the large intestine of a 2-month-old kitten with severe diarrhea, vomiting, dehydration, weight loss, and inappetence.[3]

DIAGNOSIS

Microbiologic Tests (Table 66.2)

Clinical diagnosis of *Helicobacter* infection in dogs and cats has most commonly been based on histopathology, cytology, rapid urease testing, and, to a lesser extent, PCR on gastric biopsies. Other tests such as the urea breath and blood tests, fecal PCR, and serological tests are primarily used in human patients and in the research arena.

Diagnosis Using Cytology and Histopathology

Spiral organisms can be readily detected using touch impressions of gastric tissue obtained following biopsy or necropsy, after staining with Gram or Diff-Quik stains, even when low numbers of organisms are present (Fig. 66.4). A cytology brush can also be used to obtain a specimen during endoscopy. Several biopsies or brush specimens may need to be evaluated from different regions of the stomach (fundus, cardia, antrum/pylorus) when the distribution of organisms is patchy. When organism burdens are high, the organisms can be detected using histopathology, which allows assessment of concurrent gastric pathology (Figs. 66.5 and 66.6). The use of silver stains (such as Warthin-Starry stain or Steiner stain), Giemsa, or toluidine blue stain, as well as immunostaining can dramatically increase sensitivity for organism detection, especially when low numbers of organisms are present (Figs. 66.5C and 66.6C).[43]

Bacterial Isolation

Isolation of gastric helicobacters can be difficult and as a result can have low sensitivity. Growth typically requires incubation on selective media in microaerobic conditions for 5 to 10 days. Isolation may be advantageous in research settings because it allows subsequent identification of the organism using conventional biochemical testing, whole-cell protein profiling, and DNA analysis.[18,44] It also allows antimicrobial susceptibility testing, which has recently been recommended before treating humans for *H. pylori* infection because of the increasing prevalence of antimicrobial resistance.[45] Resistance to antimicrobials has also been documented in non-*H. pylori* helicobacters isolated from dogs and cats.[46]

TABLE 66.1 *Helicobacter* Species That Have Been Identified in Dogs, Cats, and Humans[a]

Helicobacter Species	Location	Host Species
H. bizzozeronii	Stomach	Dog, humans
H. salomonis	Stomach	Dog
H. cynogastricus	Stomach	Dog
"*Candidatus* H. heilmannii"	Stomach	Dog, cat, humans
H. felis	Stomach	Dog, cat, humans
H. pametensis	Stomach	Cat
H. baculiformis	Stomach	Cat
H. pylori	Stomach	Cat
"*Flexispira rappini*"	Stomach, intestine	Dog, cat
H. bilis	Stomach, intestine	Dog, cat
H. canicola (H. cinaedi)	Intestine	Dog, cat
H. finneliae	Intestine	Dog, cat
"*H. colifelis*"	Intestine	Cat
H. marmotae	Intestine	Cat
H. canis	Intestine, liver	Dog, cat, human

[a]See references 4, 66, 74–83.

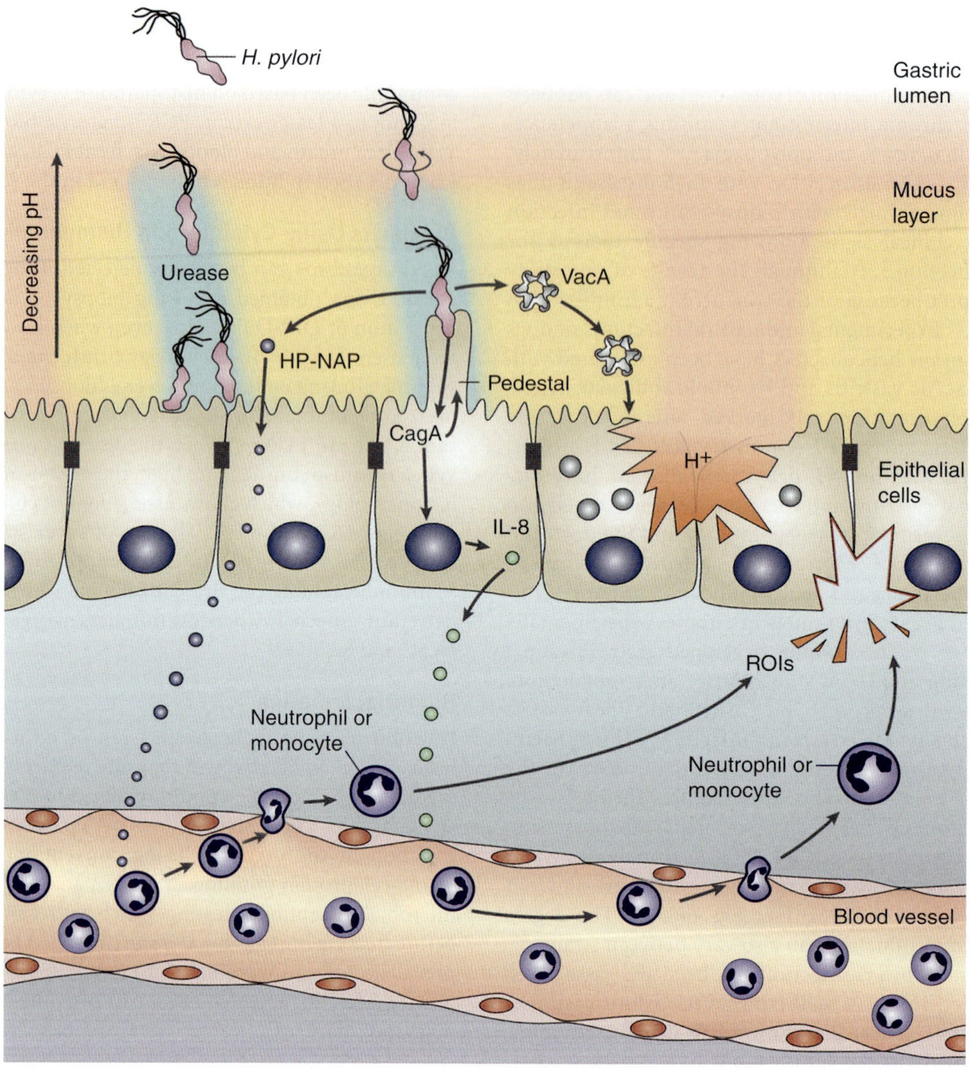

Fig. 66.3 Pathogenesis of *Helicobacter pylori* infection. During infection, *H. pylori* enters the gastric lumen where urease allows survival in the acidic environment (pink indicates a strongly acidic environment, yellow a mildly acidic one) by producing ammonia that buffers cytosolic and periplasmic pH as well as the surface layer around the bacterium (light blue). The flagella propel the organism into the mucus layer and allow it to reach the apical domain of gastric epithelial cells, to which it adheres using adhesins. The organism then injects the cagA protein into host cells with a type IV secretion system and releases other toxic factors such as VacA and a neutrophil activating protein (*HP-NAP*). VacA induces tight junction alterations, and HP-NAP crosses the epithelial lining and recruits neutrophils and monocytes. CagA causes alteration of the cytoskeleton, pedestal formation, and stimulates release of proinflammatory lymphokines, with release of reactive oxygen intermediates (*ROIs*). The combined toxic activity of VacA and ROIs leads to tissue damage that is enhanced by loosening of the protective mucus layer and acid permeation. (From Montecucco C, Rappuoli R. Living dangerously: how *Helicobacter pylori* survives in the human stomach. *Nature Rev Mol Cell Biol.* 2001;2:457-465. Figure 1)

Rapid Urease Testing

The rapid urease test involves incubating a gastric biopsy in a urea broth that contains the pH indicator phenol red. If gastric helicobacters are present in the biopsy, helicobacter urease breaks down the urea in the broth, with the release of ammonia, a rise in pH, and a color change occurs. The change in color can occur within 1 to 3 hours, although the broth is generally incubated at room temperature for 24 hours. The test is very sensitive, although false-negative results can occur if the distribution within the stomach is patchy or if organism loads are low. False-positive results have rarely been reported when other urease-producing bacteria are present in the stomach, such as *Proteus* spp.

Molecular Diagnosis Using Nucleic Acid-Based Testing

PCR assays have been used extensively to detect *Helicobacter* species in tissues, including those from dogs and cats. Sequence analysis of the PCR products can allow identification of the species present, which has been important in epidemiologic studies. FISH has also been used to detect, localize, and identify *Helicobacter* species infection in tissues from dogs and cats.[4,5,28,37,47]

Serologic Diagnosis

A variety of serum ELISA and immunoblotting assays have been used extensively in humans for screening for *H. pylori* infection, and some can be used to some extent to monitor the success of

TABLE 66.2 Diagnostic Assays Available for Gastric *Helicobacter* Infection in Dogs and Cats

Assay	Specimen Type	Target	Performance
Bacterial isolation	Gastric biopsies	*Helicobacter* organisms	Can take up to 10 days. Low sensitivity for non-*H. pylori* helicobacters, which can be difficult to culture. Patchy distribution may also lead to false negatives. Allows typing and antimicrobial susceptibility testing
Cytology	Impression smears of gastric biopsies or cytology brush specimens	*Helicobacter* organisms	Rapid and sensitive, but false negatives can occur rarely. Patchy distribution may also lead to false negatives. No information on inflammatory or architectural changes in underlying tissue
Histopathology	Gastric biopsies	*Helicobacter* organisms	Less sensitive than cytology. Patchy distribution may also lead to false negatives. Use of silver stains increases sensitivity when organism numbers are low. Allows determination of associated gastric histopathology
Rapid urease testing	Gastric biopsies	*Helicobacter* urease	Rapid and very sensitive. Patchy distribution and low organism loads may lead to false negatives. Very rare false positives with other urease-producing organisms
Fluorescence in situ hybridization	Gastric or intestinal biopsies	*Helicobacter* DNA	Allows visualization of organisms within lesions
Polymerase chain reaction	Gastric or intestinal biopsies	*Helicobacter* DNA	Rapid (within hours), can be highly sensitive and specific. Sequence analysis can determine the species involved
Serology	Serum	Antibodies to *Helicobacter* spp.	Moderate sensitivity in dogs and cats. Results do not correlate well with gastric histopathology. Does not always correlate with active infection. Has been primarily used in research settings to date
Urea breath and blood testing	Breath, blood	Radiolabelled carbon dioxide derived from the activity of *Helicobacter* urease	Requires specialized detection equipment. Although sensitive, false negatives may occur, such as following acid suppression. In dogs and cats, has been primarily used in research settings to date.

For all tests, positive results do not imply that *Helicobacter* is the cause of disease.

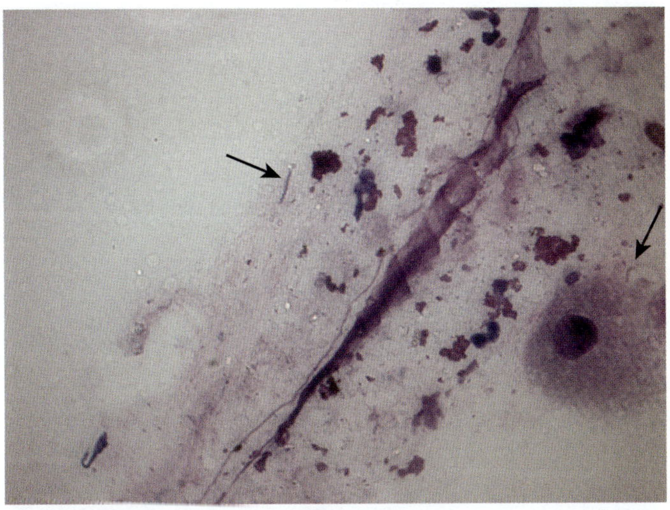

Fig. 66.4 Spiral-shaped gastric *Helicobacter*-like organisms visible in a Diff-Quik–stained smear *(arrows)* of a gastric biopsy from a 2-year-old male neutered Cavalier King Charles spaniel with chronic vomiting and regurgitation for which no other cause was apparent (1000× magnification).

therapy.[48,49] Serologic assays have been used on a research basis to noninvasively detect non-*H. pylori* helicobacter infection in dogs and cats, in some studies demonstrating moderate sensitivity and good specificity.[50-52]

Urea Breath and Blood Testing

Diagnosis and monitoring of the extent of *H. pylori* infection in human patients can also be accomplished noninvasively using urea breath and blood testing, which involves oral administration of urea that contains ^{14}C or the stable isotope ^{13}C. After ingestion, the labeled urea is converted to ammonia by *Helicobacter* urease, and the released carbon is absorbed systemically, where it can be measured in the blood. Subsequently, the labeled carbon dioxide is exhaled, and can be measured in the breath. Acid suppression may interfere with test results by decreasing *Helicobacter* urease activity, and so testing is generally performed several days after discontinuing treatment. False positives can also occur with the test.[53] Urea breath and blood testing has been used with success in dogs,[54] and breath testing has been used in cats[17,55] both before and following specific treatment for *Helicobacter* infection.

Fecal Antigen Assays

Assays detecting *H. pylori* infection in feces have been used for diagnosis in human patients[53] but their use in dogs and cats has not been described.

Pathologic Findings

Infection with non-*H. pylori* helicobacters in dogs and cats has been primarily associated with chronic lymphocytic or lymphoplasmacytic gastritis, with lymphoid follicular hyperplasia (Figs. 66.5A and 66.6A), although the extent of inflammation can vary dramatically from absent to severe.[16,56,57] Some extent of eosinophil infiltration has been described in some cats.[56] Neutrophil and eosinophil infiltrates may

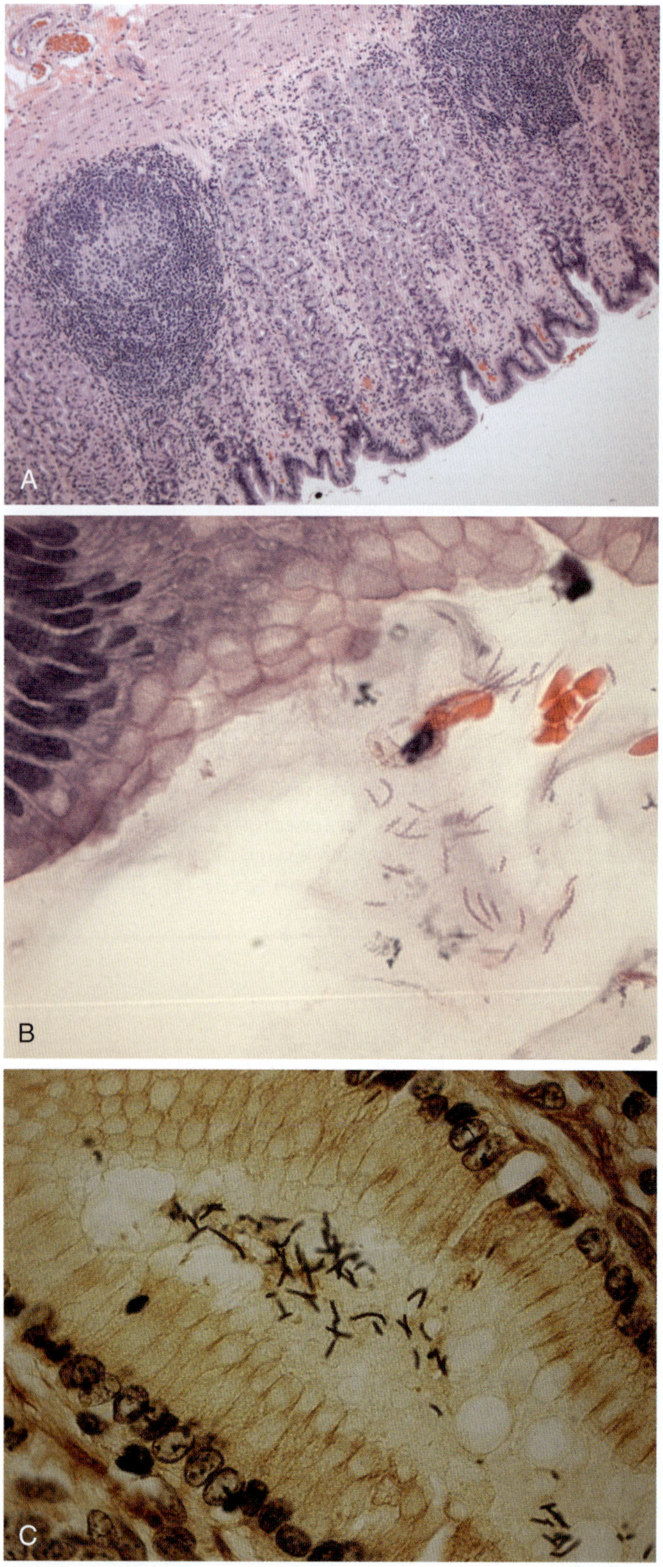

Fig. 66.5 Histopathology of the stomach of a 2-year old female spayed Maltese terrier with chronic vomiting and regurgitation. (A) Lymphoid follicular nodules. The remaining lamina propria was infiltrated by small numbers of eosinophils, neutrophils, lymphocytes, and plasma cells. H&E stain, 40× magnification. (B) Large numbers of spiral-shaped bacteria were visible in the superficial mucus and gastric glands. H&E stain, 1000× magnification. (C) Warthin-Starry stain showing agyrophilic intralesional spiral-shaped bacteria within the gastric glands (1000× magnification).

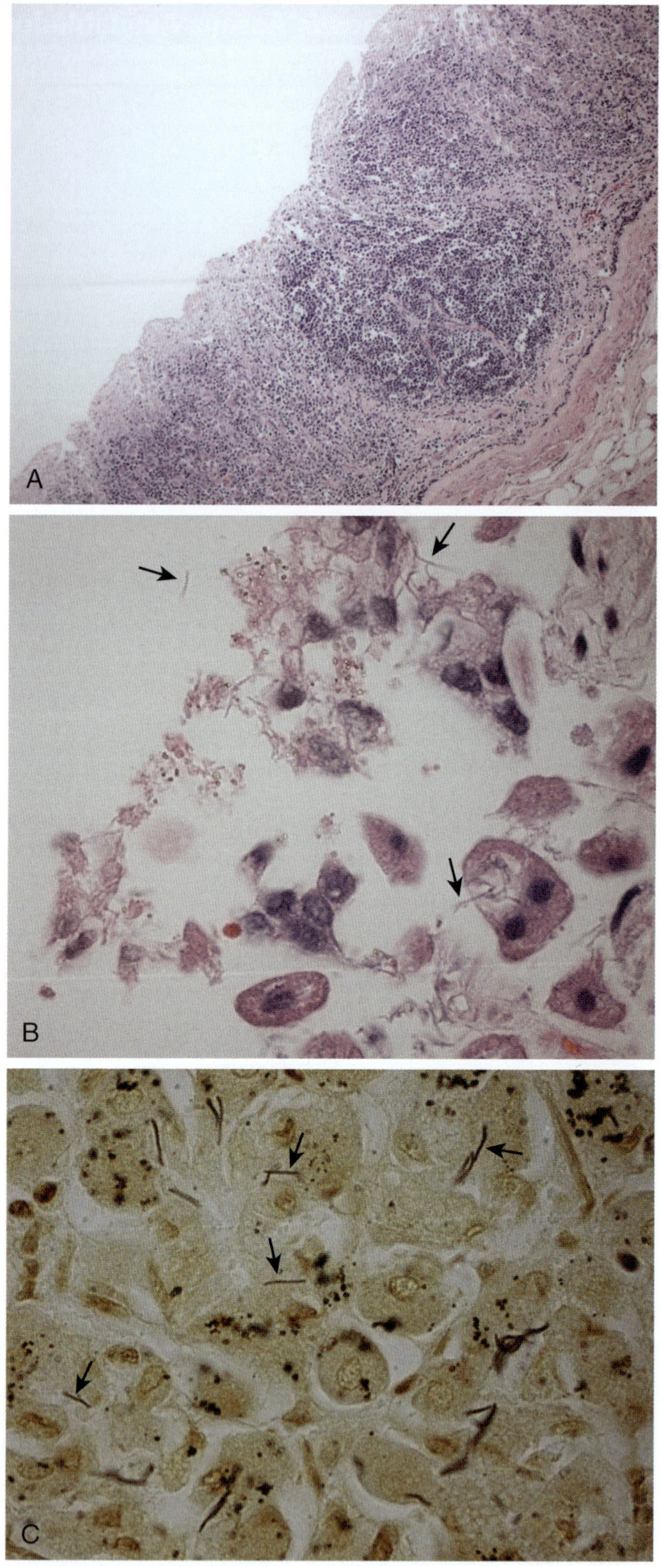

Fig. 66.6 Histopathology of the stomach of a 14-year-old male neutered domestic shorthair that was infected with feline immunodeficiency virus and was euthanized because of squamous cell carcinoma. Gastrointestinal signs were not reported. H&E stain. (A) Severe, chronic, lymphofollicular gastritis. H&E stain, 40× magnification. (B) Abundant fine, spiral-shaped bacteria were visualized in the superficial mucus and within parietal cells *(arrows)*. H&E stain. (C) Warthin-Starry stain showing intracellular agyrophilic spiral-shaped bacteria *(arrows)*; 1000× magnification.

accompany mononuclear inflammation in some cats infected with *H. pylori*.[56,58] Organisms may be found in the superficial mucus and crypts, and sometimes within parietal cells (Fig. 66.6).

Histopathologic findings in a cat infected with an intestinal helicobacter included large numbers of densely packed spiral bacteria covering the intestinal mucosa and present within the crypts, and minimal inflammatory changes. Hepatic changes in a dog with *H. canis* infection consisted of randomly distributed and coalescing hepatocellular necrosis with associated neutrophilic and mononuclear infiltrates.[41]

TREATMENT AND PROGNOSIS

Whether antimicrobial treatment should be used for gastric *Helicobacter* infections in dogs and cats is unknown. Humans with *H. pylori* infections are typically treated with a combination of a proton pump inhibitor, amoxicillin, and clarithromycin, with or without bismuth salicylate. An alternative treatment option is triple therapy with a proton pump inhibitor, fluoroquinolone (typically levofloxacin), and amoxicillin for 14 days, which is recommended when treatment failure occurs. Treatment of humans is reserved for symptomatic individuals, and the development of antimicrobial resistance by *H. pylori* is increasingly of concern.[59]

If instituted, treatment should be reserved for dogs and cats with gastrointestinal signs that have no other identifiable cause of illness, after a diagnosis of gastritis and *Helicobacter* infection has been confirmed using biopsy. A 2-week course of combination therapy with antimicrobials and a proton pump inhibitor or an H2 antagonist has not reliably eliminated gastric helicobacters in dogs and cats, although clinical signs often resolve.[29,54,60,61] It is possible that reinfection may occur in some animals after treatment. This theory is underscored by a study of 20 dogs that were naturally infected with *Helicobacter* spp. and treated with triple therapy (clarithromycin, amoxicillin, and lansoprazole) for 7 days. The dogs were then randomized into a control group, which was kept in isolation, and an experimental group, which was placed in contact with *Helicobacter*-positive dogs for 60 days. Triple therapy was effective in 100% of the dogs; however, recurrence of infection occurred in 80% of dogs in the experimental group, and in none of the dogs in the control group after 60 days.[62] A 3-week course of amoxicillin, metronidazole, and bismuth salicylate (Table 66.3) was efficacious in clearing gastric helicobacters in dogs and cats as determined using FISH, with resolution of associated vomiting, although histopathologic evidence of gastritis did not resolve.[28] Clarithromycin could be substituted for metronidazole.[18] One study showed that concurrent use of an H2 antagonist in dogs did not change outcome.[29] This is consistent with the observation that abnormalities in the gastric acid secretory axis, which occur in humans infected with *H. pylori*, do not appear to occur in dogs infected with non-*H. pylori* helicobacters.[21,30]

TABLE 66.3 Antimicrobials Used with Success to Treat *Helicobacter* spp. Infection in Dogs and Cats

Drug	Dose (mg/kg)	Route	Interval (Hours)	Duration (Days)
Metronidazole	11–15	PO	12	14–21
Amoxicillin	22	PO	12	14–21
Clarithromycin	5–10	PO	12	14–21
Bismuth salicylate	0.22 mL/kg	PO	6–8	14–21
Omeprazole	0.7–1.0	PO	24	14–21
Famotidine	0.5–1.0	PO	12	14–21

The first three drugs are administered as a combination. Alternatively, clarithromycin can be combined with amoxicillin and administered with either omeprazole or famotidine.

IMMUNITY AND VACCINATION

Gastric helicobacters are able to persist in the stomach despite a vigorous humoral immune response to the organism. Research has been underway to develop an effective vaccine for *H. pylori* infection in humans, and a variety of *H. pylori* antigens have been shown to induce protection in healthy human volunteers or mouse models.[63] No vaccine is available for *Helicobacter* infection in dogs and cats, and a greater understanding of the role of gastric helicobacters in canine and feline disease will be required in order to assess the need for effective vaccines against these organisms.

PUBLIC HEALTH ASPECTS

At least 50% of the world's human population is infected with *H. pylori*, although the prevalence of infection has been decreasing in developed countries.[64] In the Western world, 1 to 10% of people develop gastroduodenal ulceration as a result of chronic *H. pylori* infection. A smaller percentage of infected people (< 3%) develop gastric adenocarcinoma or MALT lymphoma in association with infection. Duodenal ulceration results from increased gastrin release in response to *H. pylori*-induced gastric antral inflammation. The factors influencing outcome are not well understood, but an individual's immune response to the organism, as well as the possession of virulence factors by *H. pylori* strains, appear to play an important role.[64] Eradication of infection using antimicrobial therapy can cure gastroduodenal ulceration and MALT lymphoma, but gastric adenocarcinoma generally persists despite treatment.[65] Although *H. pylori* has been documented to infect a colony of cats, infection of cats with this species is extremely rare and exposure to pets is not a risk factor for *H. pylori* infection in humans. However, in a 2021 study from Japan, *H. pylori* DNA was detected in two related dogs in a household as well as the owner of the dogs, and partial sequencing of the *ureAB* gene suggested the strains were identical.[11]

Non-*H. pylori* gastric helicobacter infection is uncommon in humans compared with *H. pylori* infection. Nevertheless, these helicobacters have also been associated with chronic active gastritis, gastroduodenal ulceration, and MALT lymphomas in people, although disease is generally less severe than that caused by *H. pylori*.[6] Clinical signs in humans may be absent or consist of nausea, epigastric pain, vomiting, hematemesis, heartburn, and decreased appetite. Treatment with triple antibiotic therapy and bismuth salicylate has led to resolution of infection and gastritis. Pets have been suggested as a source of these helicobacters for humans,[6,66-67] with close contact with dogs and cats being a risk factor for infection.[71] Licking has been suggested as a mode of transmission, based on the presence of non-*H. pylori* helicobacter DNA in the oral cavity of dogs.[22] Pigs are thought to play an even more important role in zoonotic transmission of non-*H. pylori* gastric helicobacters, with the swine *Helicobacter suis* being the most prevalent species identified in humans.[6]

Helicobacter cinaedi is an intestinal helicobacter associated with enteric disease and bacteremia in immunocompromised humans.[72] Although this organism has been described in dogs and cats, and nosocomial spread of *H. cinaedi* was suggested in one report,[73] further analysis of strains isolated from dogs suggested that they belonged to a distinct species, with the proposed name *Helicobacter canicola* sp. nov.[74]

CASE EXAMPLE 1

Signalment

"Mocha," 2-year-old female spayed Maltese terrier from Dixon, California.

History

Mocha had been vomiting and regurgitating intermittently since she was 1 year of age. As a puppy, the owner (a veterinary student) reported intermittent episodes of "burping." Mocha had a history of vomiting anywhere from 2 to 5 times a day. The vomiting was not associated with eating, drinking, or exercise, and occurred at random times throughout the day. The vomitus usually consisted of brown fluid and there were generally no recognizable food particles. Treatment with dietary changes that included a digestible elimination diet containing a novel, single protein source followed by a fat-restricted prescription diet had not resulted in improvement in her clinical signs. In addition, therapy with cisapride (3 mg PO q8h) and famotidine (2.5 mg PO q24h) or omeprazole (3.5 mg PO q24h) resulted in only slight improvement in the frequency of vomiting. Her appetite was appropriate and there had been no weight loss or diarrhea. She primarily lived indoors and there was a cat in the household. The dog was up to date on vaccinations, which included those for rabies, distemper, parvovirus, and canine adenovirus.

Physical Examination

Body weight: 3 kg.

General: Bright, alert and responsive, hydrated, nervous. Ambulatory on all four limbs. Temperature = 100.4°F (38.0°C), heart rate = 120 beats/min, respiratory rate 28 breaths/min, mucous membranes pink and moist, CRT = 1 s.

Integument: Full, clean hair coat.

Eyes, ears, nose, and throat: The only abnormality noticed was a left maxillary persistent deciduous canine tooth with calculus between the deciduous and adult teeth only.

Musculoskeletal: Body condition score 4/9 with symmetrical muscling.

Cardiovascular: Strong and synchronous femoral pulses. No murmurs or arrhythmias were detected.

Respiratory: Eupneic with normal breath sounds.

Gastrointestinal and genitourinary: Unremarkable abdominal palpation. "Burping" behavior was observed in the room, which occurred without any prodromal signs or abdominal effort. Lip-smacking behavior was noticed immediately afterwards.

Rectal examination: No abnormalities detected.

Lymph nodes: All within normal limits.

Laboratory Findings

CBC: HCT 46.5% (40–55%), MCV 64.4 fL (65–75 fL), MCHC 35.9 g/dL (33–36 g/dL), WBC 5,700 cells/μL (6,000–13,000 cells/μL), neutrophils 3,112 cells/μL (3,000–10,500 cells/μL), lymphocytes 1,830 cells/μL (1,000–4,000 cells/μL), monocytes 257 cells/μL (150–1,200 cells/μL), eosinophils 479 cells/μL (0–1,500 cells/μL), platelets 277,000/μL (150,000–400,000 platelets/μL).

Serum chemistry profile: sodium 147 mmol/L (145–154 mmol/L), potassium 4.4 mmol/L (3.6–5.3 mmol/L), chloride 111 mmol/L (108–118 mmol/L), bicarbonate 23 mmol/L (16–26 mmol/L), phosphorus 5.3 mg/dL (3.0–6.2 mg/dL), calcium 10.6 mg/dL (9.7–11.5 mg/dL), BUN 22 mg/dL (5–21 mg/dL), creatinine 1.1 mg/dL (0.3–1.2 mg/dL), glucose 95 mg/dL (64–123 mg/dL), total protein 5.7 g/dL (5.4–7.6 g/dL), albumin 4.0 g/dL (3.0–4.4 g/dL), globulin 1.7 g/dL (1.8–3.9 g/dL), ALT 42 U/L (19–67 U/L), AST 45 U/L (19–42 U/L), ALP 52 U/L (21–170 U/L), GGT < 3 U/L (0–6 U/L), cholesterol 241 mg/dL (135–361 mg/dL), total bilirubin 0.2 mg/dL (0–0.2 mg/dL).

Urinalysis: SpG 1.040, pH 7.0, no protein, glucose, or ketones, trace hemoprotein, 0–1 WBC/HPF, 0–1 RBC/HPF, moderate lipid droplets.

Serum pancreatic lipase immunoreactivity: < 30 μg/L (reference range 0–200 μg/L).

Imaging Findings

Abdominal radiographs: A moderate amount of gas was identified within multiple small intestinal loops, but an obstructive pattern was not identified. There was mildly decreased serosal detail, consistent with patient age and body condition score. A moderate amount of feces was present within the descending colon.

Thoracic radiographs: The cardiopulmonary structures were within normal limits. A small amount of gas was visualized within the esophagus on the left lateral projections.

Esophagram: Unremarkable study.

Abdominal ultrasound: No abnormalities identified.

Gastroduodenoscopy: Gross findings were suggestive of diffuse lymphoid follicular hyperplasia, with a mild "goose pimple" appearance to the gastric mucosa (Fig. 66.7). Multiple biopsies of all regions of the stomach, as well as multiple duodenal biopsies were obtained.

Stomach: Moderate, lymphofollicular, eosinophilic, and lymphoplasmacytic gastritis with intralesional spiral bacteria (see Fig. 66.5). Duodenum: mild, chronic, lymphofollicular, eosinophilic, and lymphoplasmacytic duodenitis and ileitis. Jejunum: diffuse, mild, eosinophilic, and lymphoplasmacytic enteritis.

Diagnosis

Eosinophilic and lymphoplasmacytic enteritis; chronic gastritis associated with *Helicobacter* spp. infection.

Treatment

Treatment for the *Helicobacter* infection was initiated with metronidazole (30 mg PO q12h), amoxicillin (60 mg PO q12h), and bismuth salicylate for 2 weeks. The owner reported almost complete resolution of the vomiting following treatment, but signs returned after they were discontinued and an additional course of treatment was instituted. Treatment with a fat-restricted prescription diet was continued. The frequency of vomiting has decreased to once a week.

Comments

Whether the *Helicobacter* spp. infection in this dog contributed to clinical signs or was an incidental finding in a dog with underlying eosinophilic and lymphoplasmacytic enteritis was not clear. The failure to respond to multiple diet changes, including an elimination diet, and the dramatic response to triple therapy supported a possible role for *Helicobacter* spp. infection, or a diagnosis of antibiotic-responsive gastroenteropathy unrelated to *Helicobacter* spp.

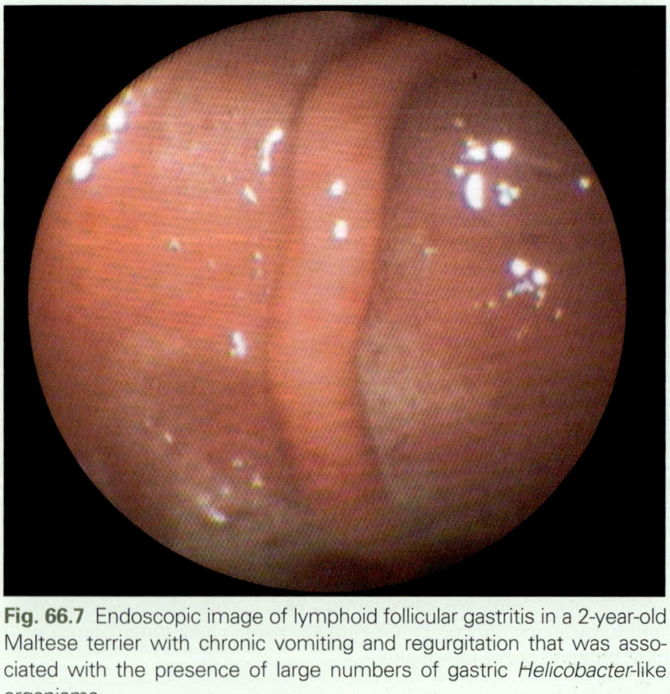

Fig. 66.7 Endoscopic image of lymphoid follicular gastritis in a 2-year-old Maltese terrier with chronic vomiting and regurgitation that was associated with the presence of large numbers of gastric *Helicobacter*-like organisms.

CASE EXAMPLE 2

Signalment

"Poppy," a 2-year-old female spayed Australian shepherd mix from northern California.

History

Poppy was evaluated at the University of California-Davis Small Animal Internal Medicine Service for a history of chronic intermittent large bowel diarrhea for the last 18 months. The diarrhea was watery to soft, and contained mucus and frank blood. Frequent straining had been noted when Poppy was attempting to defecate and only small quantities of feces were passed. Treatment with fenbendazole, metronidazole, or tylosin had resulted in temporary cessation of diarrhea, but the diarrhea returned after the medications were discontinued; during this period, tylosin treatment had been administered for 2 months. The owners noted that the diarrhea also resolved when Poppy was treated for a dog bite wound 2 months previously with cephalexin and carprofen, but returned when the drugs were discontinued 10 days later. A potato and whitefish prescription diet was fed exclusively for several months but the diarrhea persisted.

Current medications

Prescription low-fat, digestible diet; metronidazole 15 mg/kg PO q12h.

Other medical history

Poppy had been adopted as a puppy and was up to date on vaccinations.

Physical Examination

Body weight: 16 kg.

General: Bright, alert and responsive, hydrated. Ambulatory on all four limbs. Temperature = 102.1°F (38.9°C), heart rate = 96 beats/min, panting, mucous membranes pink and moist, CRT = 1–2 s.

Integument: Full, clean hair coat, no ectoparasites noted.

Eyes, ears, nose, and throat: No clinically significant abnormalities.

Musculoskeletal: Body condition score 4/9 with symmetrical muscling.

Cardiovascular: Strong and synchronous femoral pulses. No murmurs or arrhythmias were detected.

Respiratory: Eupneic with normal breath sounds.

Gastrointestinal and genitourinary: Mildly tense abdomen on abdominal palpation.

Rectal examination: No abnormalities detected.

Lymph nodes: All within normal limits.

Laboratory Findings

PCV 57%, TP 7.2 g/dL, SpG 1.042.

Serum chemistry profile: All values within reference ranges.

Vitamin B12: 764 ng/L (RR, 271–875 ng/L).

Fecal flotation: Negative for parasites.

Giardia and *Cryptosporidium* direct FA: Negative.

Imaging Findings

Abdominal ultrasound: The mesenteric lymph nodes were prominent measuring up to 8 mm in thickness. The stomach, small intestine, and colon were ultrasonographically normal with normal wall layering and thickness. The remainder of the complete abdominal ultrasound examination was within normal limits.

Gastroduodenoscopy and ileocolonoscopy: Mild hyperemia of the duodenal and colonic mucosa (Fig. 66.8A) was identified. Biopsy specimens from the stomach (9), duodenum (9), ileum (3), and colon (12) were collected for histopathology.

Histopathology Findings

Stomach: mild, chronic, lymphofollicular gastritis with luminal spiral bacteria (consistent with *Helicobacter* spp.)

Duodenum and ileum: Moderate, acute neutrophilic, and eosinophilic enteritis with mild central lacteal dilation.

Colon: Severe, acute neutrophilic, and eosinophilic colitis with epithelial necrosis, crypt hyperplasia, and abundant beaded bacteria (Fig. 66.8B). The luminal surface and mucosal crypts contained large numbers of thin beaded bacterial rods that did not stain with Brown and Brenn stain. Silver staining highlighted the bacteria and identified small numbers of bacteria within mucosal epithelial cells (Fig. 66.8C). These bacteria were frequently curved, and occasionally a spiral structure was discernable. Based on the number of bacteria and the associated damage and inflammation within the mucosa, these bacteria are likely to be the cause of pathology.

Fecal enteric panel: Direct smear: rare, wavy, gram-negative rods. Negative for *Clostridioides difficile* toxins type A and B by enzyme immunoassay, *Clostridium perfringens* enterotoxin type A by immunoassay, no *Salmonella* spp. cultured. No *Campylobacter* spp. cultured. Anaerobic culture: moderate numbers of *Clostridium sordellii*, small numbers of *Fusobacterium* spp.

FISH (Simpson Laboratory, CVM, Cornell University) (colonic biopsy specimen): With a eubacterial probe, in multiple regions there were adherent and

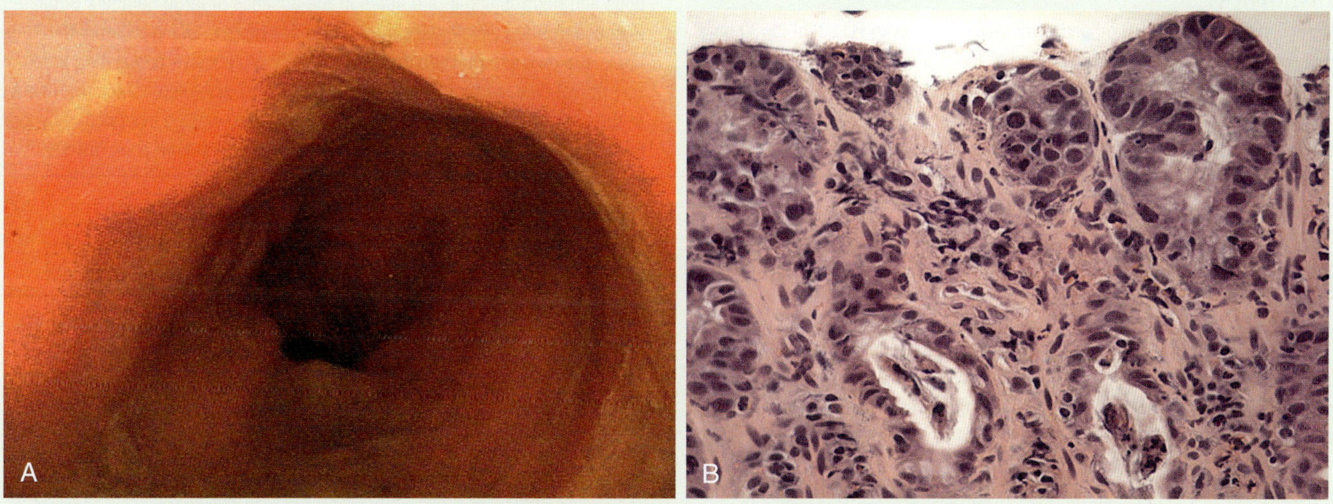

Fig. 66.8 (A) Endoscopic image of colitis in a 2-year-old Australian cattle dog with chronic intermittent large bowel diarrhea that was associated with neutrophilic and eosinophilic colitis with large numbers of intralesional spiral-shaped bacteria. (B) Histopathology image of a colonic biopsy showing neutrophilic and eosinophilic colitis (hematoxylin & eosin stain, 40× magnification). (A, Courtesy University of California-Davis Small Animal Internal Medicine Service; B, courtesy University of California-Davis Veterinary Anatomic Pathology Service.)

Continued

CASE EXAMPLE 2—cont'd

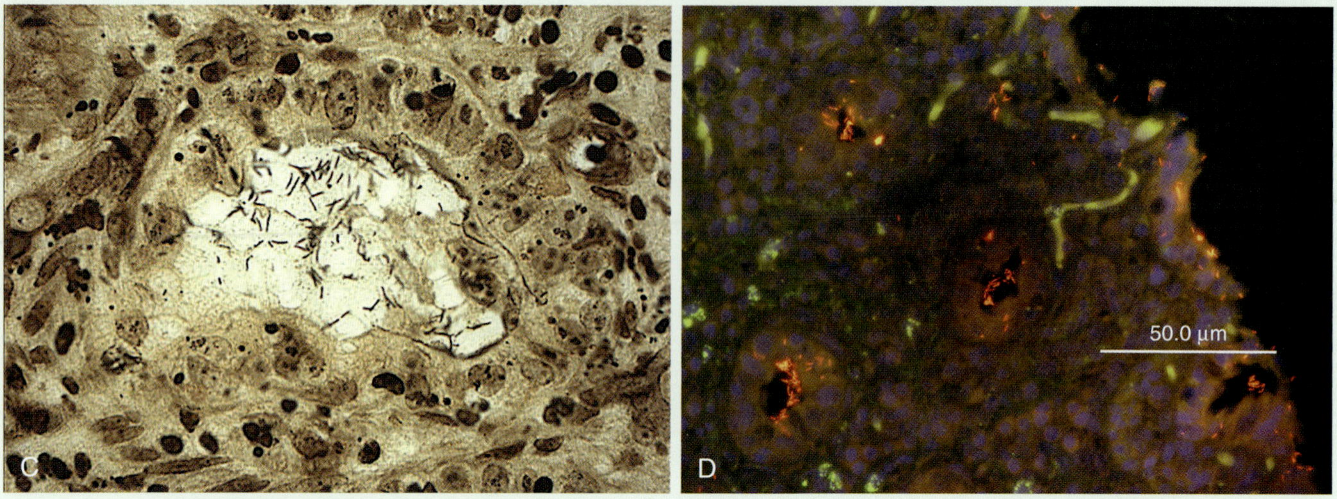

Fig. 66.8, cont'd (C) Warthin-Starry stain. There are numerous spiral-shaped bacteria within crypts (100× magnification). (D) FISH using a *Helicobacter* spp.-specific probe. The bacteria stain red with the probes and can be seen within crypts and the crypt epithelium, and adherent to colonic mucosa. (C, Courtesy University of California-Davis Veterinary Anatomic Pathology Service; D courtesy the Simpson Laboratory, Cornell University College of Veterinary Medicine.)

invasive bacteria that ranged from fat rods to long and slender to variegated/beaded rods within crypts that were invading the crypt epithelium. When a *Helicobacter* spp. probe was applied, fluorescence was associated with masses of bacteria within the crypts that were also invading the crypt epithelium and areas adjacent to the crypts (Fig. 66.8D).

Helicobacter spp. PCR-Sequencing (University of California-Davis molecular core facility) (colonic biopsy specimen): A 400-base pair amplicon was amplified with a *Helicobacter*-specific 16S rRNA gene PCR assay. When sequenced, the amplicon had 100% sequence identity to the 16S rRNA gene of *Helicobacter bilis* and 99% sequence identity (two base pair mismatches) to that of *H. canis*.

Diagnosis

Neutrophilic and eosinophilic colitis, likely secondary to infection by a *H. bilis*–like organism.

Treatment

Amoxicillin (19 mg/kg PO q12h) and enrofloxacin (8.5 mg/kg PO q24h) for 30 days. Treatment was associated with resolution of the diarrhea for 3 years. However, 3 years later Poppy was seen for acute onset of large bowel diarrhea, vomiting, and decreased appetite, and was found to have panhypoproteinemia (albumin 2.8 g/dL, globulin 1.4 g/dL). A serum cobalamin concentration and adrenocorticotropic hormone stimulation test were normal. The owner declined additional endoscopic biopsies and she was treated with another course of amoxicillin and enrofloxacin for 30 days, as well as a hydrolyzed protein diet. Her clinical signs resolved and at recheck appointments over the following 3 months, her hypoproteinemia resolved. A diagnosis of food-responsive enteropathy was made.

Comments

This was an unusual case of *Helicobacter*-associated colitis where disease association was implied by large numbers of curved to spiral-shaped organisms invading the mucosa together with inflammation, and a long-lasting response to antimicrobial therapy as the sole therapy. In addition to *Helicobacter* spp., differential diagnoses for the curved to spiral bacteria were *Campylobacter* spp., *Arcobacter* spp., *Anaerobiospirillum* spp., and *Brachyspira* spp. (see Chapter 67). Use of the FISH assay allowed specific identification of *Helicobacter* spp. within lesions. An alternative treatment would have been to use clarithromycin or azithromycin together with amoxicillin.

Interestingly, there was evidence of a similar inflammatory response (eosinophils and neutrophils) in the ileum in the absence of large numbers of bacteria. Because this dog developed clinical signs of a protein-losing enteropathy 3 years later, it is possible that the dog had a slowly progressive preexisting inflammatory bowel disease that predisposed it to *Helicobacter* spp. infection. However, at the time of diagnosis of helicobacteriosis, there was no evidence of hypoproteinemia, so the clinical expression of disease at each time point differed.

SUGGESTED READINGS

Haesebrouck F, Pasmans F, Flahou B, et al. Gastric helicobacters in domestic animals and nonhuman primates and their significance for human health. *Clin Microbiol Rev*. 2009;22(2):202–223.

Swennes AG, Parry NMA, Feng Y, et al. Enterohepatic *Helicobacter* spp. in cats with non-haematopoietic intestinal carcinoma: a survey of 55 cases. *J Med Microbiol*. 2016;65:814–820.

Giaretta PR, Suchodolski JS, Jergens AE, et al. Bacterial biogeography of the colon in dogs with chronic inflammatory enteropathy. *Vet Pathol*. 2020;57:258–265.

Montecucco C, Rappuoli R. Living dangerously: how *Helicobacter pylori* survives in the human stomach. *Nature Rev Mol Cell Biol*. 2001;2:457–466.

REFERENCES

1. Rappin JP. Contre l'etude de bacterium de la bouche etat normal. In: College de France, Nantes; 1881.
2. Warren JR, Marshall BJ. Unidentified curved bacilli on gastric epithelium in active chronic gastritits. *Lancet*. 1983;1:1273–1275.
3. Foley JE, Solnick JV, Lapointe JM, et al. Identification of a novel enteric *Helicobacter* species in a kitten with severe diarrhea. *J Clin Microbiol*. 1998;36:908–912.
4. Recordati C, Gualdi V, Craven M, et al. Spatial distribution of *Helicobacter* spp. in the gastrointestinal tract of dogs. *Helicobacter*. 2009;14:180–191.
5. Giaretta PR, Suchodolski JS, Jergens AE, et al. Bacterial biogeography of the colon in dogs with chronic inflammatory enteropathy. *Vet Pathol*. 2020;57:258–265.

6. Haesebrouck F, Pasmans F, Flahou B, et al. Gastric helicobacters in domestic animals and nonhuman primates and their significance for human health. *Clin Microbiol Rev*. 2009;22:202–223.
7. Elyasi B, Rezaie A, Moori Bakhtiari N, et al. *Helicobacter* genus in the intestine and liver of stray cats: the molecular, histopathological, and immunohistochemical study. *Braz J Microbiol*. 2020;51:2123–2132.
8. Canejo-Teixeira R, Oliveira M, Pissarra H, et al. A mixed population of *Helicobacter pylori, Helicobacter bizzozeronii* and "Helicobacter heilmannii" in the gastric mucosa of a domestic cat. *Ir Vet J*. 2014;67:25.
9. Greiter-Wilke A, Scanziani E, Soldati S, et al. Association of *Helicobacter* with cholangiohepatitis in cats. *J Vet Intern Med*. 2006;20:822–827.
10. Handt LK, Fox JG, Dewhirst FE, et al. *Helicobacter pylori* isolated from the domestic cat: public health implications. *Infect Immun*. 1994;62:2367–2374.
11. Kubota-Aizawa S, Matsubara Y, Kanemoto H, et al. Transmission of *Helicobacter pylori* between a human and two dogs: a case report. *Helicobacter*. 2021;26:e12798.
12. Kubota-Aizawa S, Ohno K, Kanemoto H, et al. Epidemiological study on feline gastric *Helicobacter* spp. in Japan. *J Vet Med Sci*. 2017;79:876–880.
13. Kubota-Aizawa S, Ohno K, Fukushima K, et al. Epidemiological study of gastric *Helicobacter* spp. in dogs with gastrointestinal disease in Japan and diversity of *Helicobacter heilmannii* sensu stricto. *Vet J*. 2017;225:56–62.
14. Eaton KA, Dewhirst FE, Paster BJ, et al. Prevalence and varieties of *Helicobacter* species in dogs from random sources and pet dogs: animal and public health implications. *J Clin Microbiol*. 1996;34:3165–3170.
15. Happonen I, Linden J, Saari S, et al. Detection and effects of helicobacters in healthy dogs and dogs with signs of gastritis. *J Am Vet Med Assoc*. 1998;213:1767–1774.
16. Hermanns W, Kregel K, Breuer W, et al. *Helicobacter*-like organisms: histopathological examination of gastric biopsies from dogs and cats. *J Comp Pathol*. 1995;112:307–318.
17. Neiger R, Dieterich C, Burnens A, et al. Detection and prevalence of *Helicobacter* infection in pet cats. *J Clin Microbiol*. 1998;36:634–637.
18. Neiger R, Simpson KW. *Helicobacter* infection in dogs and cats: facts and fiction. *J Vet Intern Med*. 2000;14:125–133.
19. Otto G, Hazell SH, Fox JG, et al. Animal and public health implications of gastric colonization of cats by *Helicobacter*-like organisms. *J Clin Microbiol*. 1994;32:1043–1049.
20. Lee A, Krakowka S, Fox JG, et al. Role of *Helicobacter felis* in chronic canine gastritis. *Vet Pathol*. 1992;29:487–494.
21. Simpson KW, McDonough PL, Strauss-Ayali D, et al. *Helicobacter felis* infection in dogs: effect on gastric structure and function. *Vet Pathol*. 1999;36:237–248.
22. Recordati C, Gualdi V, Tosi S, et al. Detection of *Helicobacter* spp. DNA in the oral cavity of dogs. *Vet Microbiol*. 2007;119:346–351.
23. Travis PB, Goodman KJ, O'Rourke KM, et al. The association of drinking water quality and sewage disposal with *Helicobacter pylori* incidence in infants: the potential role of water-borne transmission. *J Water Health*. 2010;8:192–203.
24. Wiinberg B, Spohr A, Dietz HH, et al. Quantitative analysis of inflammatory and immune responses in dogs with gastritis and their relationship to *Helicobacter* spp. infection. *J Vet Intern Med*. 2005;19:4–14.
25. Lecoindre P, Chevallier M, Peyrol S, et al. Gastric helicobacters in cats. *J Feline Med Surg*. 2000;2:19–27.
26. Hong S, Chung Y, Kang WG, et al. Detection of *Helicobacter felis* in a cat with gastric disease in laboratory animal facility. *Lab Anim Res*. 2016;32:122–127
27. Gualtieri M, Olivero D, Costa Devoti C. Spontaneaous linear gastric tears in a cat. *J Small Anim Pract*. 2015;56:581–584.
28. Jergens AE, Pressel M, Crandell J, et al. Fluorescence in situ hybridization confirms clearance of visible *Helicobacter* spp. associated with gastritis in dogs and cats. *J Vet Intern Med*. 2009;23:16–23.
29. Leib MS, Duncan RB, Ward DL. Triple antimicrobial therapy and acid suppression in dogs with chronic vomiting and gastric *Helicobacter* spp. *J Vet Intern Med*. 2007;21:1185–1192.
30. Simpson KW, Strauss-Ayali D, McDonough PL, et al. Gastric function in dogs with naturally acquired gastric *Helicobacter* spp. infection. *J Vet Intern Med*. 1999;13:507–515.
31. Suarez-Esquivel M, Alfaro-Alarcon A, Guzman-Verri C, et al. Analysis of the association between density of *Helicobacter* spp. and gastric lesions in dogs. *Am J Vet Res*. 2017;78:1414–1420.
32. Perkins SE, Fox JG, Marini RP, et al. Experimental infection in cats with a cagA+ human isolate of *Helicobacter pylori*. *Helicobacter*. 1998;3:225–235.
33. Rossi G, Rossi M, Vitali CG, et al. A conventional beagle dog model for acute and chronic infection with *Helicobacter pylori*. *Infect Immun*. 1999;67:3112–3120.
34. Ramis IB, Fonseca TL, de Moraes EP, et al. Molecular basis of pathogenicity in *Helicobacter pylori* clinical isolates. *J Clin Microbiol*. 2010;48:3776–3778.
35. Atherton JC, Cao P, Peek Jr RM, et al. Mosaicism in vacuolating cytotoxin alleles of *Helicobacter pylori*. Association of specific vacA types with cytotoxin production and peptic ulceration. *J Biol Chem*. 1995;270:17771–17777.
36. Chen LT, Lin JT, Tai JJ, et al. Long-term results of anti-*Helicobacter pylori* therapy in early-stage gastric high-grade transformed MALT lymphoma. *J Natl Cancer Inst*. 2005;97:1345–1353.
37. Bridgeford EC, Marini RP, Feng Y, et al. Gastric *Helicobacter* species as a cause of feline gastric lymphoma: a viable hypothesis. *Vet Immunol Immunopathol*. 2008;123:106–113.
38. Swennes AG, Parry NMA, Feng Y, et al. Enterohepatic *Helicobacter* spp. in cats with non-haematopoietic intestinal carcinoma: a survey of 55 cases. *J Med Microbiol*. 2016;65:814–820.
39. Wang L, Chen J, Jiang W, et al. The relationship between *Helicobacter pylori* infection of the gallbladder and chronic cholecystitis and cholelithiasis: a systematic review and meta-analysis. *Can J Gastroenterol Hepatol*. 2021;2021:8886085.
40. Takemura LS, Marcasso RA, Lorenzetti E, et al. *Helicobacter* infection in the hepatobiliary system and hepatic lesions: a possible association in dogs. *Braz J Microbiol*. 2019;50:297–305.
41. Fox JG, Drolet R, Higgins R, et al. *Helicobacter canis* isolated from a dog liver with multifocal necrotizing hepatitis. *J Clin Microbiol*. 1996;34:2479–2482.
42. Foley JE, Marks SL, Munson L, et al. Isolation of *Helicobacter canis* from a colony of bengal cats with endemic diarrhea. *J Clin Microbiol*. 1999;37:3271–3275.
43. Prachasilpchai W, Nuanualsuwan S, Chatsuwan T, et al. Diagnosis of *Helicobacter* spp. infection in canine stomach. *J Vet Sci*. 2007;8:139–145.
44. Jalava K, On SL, Vandamme PA, et al. Isolation and identification of *Helicobacter* spp. from canine and feline gastric mucosa. *Appl Environ Microbiol*. 1998;64:3998–4006.
45. Wenzhen Y, Yumin L, Quanlin G, et al. Is antimicrobial susceptibility testing necessary before first-line treatment for *Helicobacter pylori* infection? Meta-analysis of randomized controlled trials. *Intern Med*. 2010;49:1103–1109.
46. Van den Bulck K, Decostere A, Gruntar I, et al. In vitro antimicrobial susceptibility testing of *Helicobacter felis, H. bizzozeronii*, and *H. salomonis*. *Antimicrob Agents Chemother*. 2005;49:2997–3000.
47. Priestnall SL, Wiinberg B, Spohr A, et al. Evaluation of "Helicobacter heilmannii" subtypes in the gastric mucosas of cats and dogs. *J Clin Microbiol*. 2004;42:2144–2151.
48. Herbrink P, van Doorn LJ. Serological methods for diagnosis of *Helicobacter pylori* infection and monitoring of eradication therapy. *Eur J Clin Microbiol Infect Dis*. 2000;19:164–173.
49. Talebkhan Y, Ebrahimzadeh F, Esmaeili M, et al. *Helicobacter pylori* Omp18 and its application in serologic screening of infection. *Curr Microbiol*. 2011;62:325–330.
50. Seidel KE, Stolte M, Lehn N, et al. Antibodies against *Helicobacter felis* in sera of cats and dogs. *Zentralbl Veterinarmed B*. 1999;46:181–188.
51. Strauss-Ayali D, Scanziani E, Deng D, et al. *Helicobacter* spp. infection in cats: evaluation of the humoral immune response and prevalence of gastric *Helicobacter* spp. *Vet Microbiol*. 2001;79:253–265.
52. Strauss-Ayali D, Simpson KW, Schein AH, et al. Serological discrimination of dogs infected with gastric *Helicobacter* spp. and uninfected dogs. *J Clin Microbiol*. 1999;37:1280–1287.
53. Calvet X, Sanchez-Delgado J, Montserrat A, et al. Accuracy of diagnostic tests for *Helicobacter pylori*: a reappraisal. *Clin Infect Dis*. 2009;48:1385–1391.
54. Cornetta AM, Simpson KW, Strauss-Ayali D, et al. Use of a [13C]urea breath test for detection of gastric infection with *Helicobacter* spp in dogs. *Am J Vet Res*. 1998;59:1364–1369.

55. Neiger R, Seiler G, Schmassmann A. Use of a urea breath test to evaluate short-term treatments for cats naturally infected with *Helicobacter heilmannii*. *Am J Vet Res*. 1999;60:880–883.
56. Scanziani E, Simpson KW, Monestiroli S, et al. Histological and immunohistochemical detection of different *Helicobacter* species in the gastric mucosa of cats. *J Vet Diagn Invest*. 2001;13:3–12.
57. Simpson KW, Strauss-Ayali D, Scanziani E, et al. *Helicobacter felis* infection is associated with lymphoid follicular hyperplasia and mild gastritis but normal gastric secretory function in cats. *Infect Immun*. 2000;68:779–790.
58. Simpson KW, Strauss-Ayali D, Straubinger RK, et al. *Helicobacter pylori* infection in the cat: evaluation of gastric colonization, inflammation and function. *Helicobacter*. 2001;6:1–14.
59. Graham DY, Fischbach L. *Helicobacter pylori* treatment in the era of increasing antibiotic resistance. *Gut*. 2010;59:1143–1153.
60. Happonen I, Linden J, Westermarck E. Effect of triple therapy on eradication of canine gastric helicobacters and gastric disease. *J Small Anim Pract*. 2000;41:1–6.
61. Perkins SE, Yan LL, Shen Z, et al. Use of PCR and culture to detect *Helicobacter pylori* in naturally infected cats following triple antimicrobial therapy. *Antimicrob Agents Chemother*. 1996;40:1486–1490.
62. Anacleto TP, Lopes LR, Andreollo NA, et al. Studies of distribution and recurrence of *Helicobacter* spp. gastric mucosa of dogs after triple therapy. *Acta Cir Bras*. 2011;26:82–87.
63. Velin D, Michetti P. Advances in vaccination against *Helicobacter pylori*. *Expert Rev Gastroenterol Hepatol*. 2010;4:157–166.
64. Herrera V, Parsonnet J. *Helicobacter pylori* and gastric adenocarcinoma. *Clin Microbiol Infect*. 2009;15:971–976.
65. McColl KE. Clinical practice. *Helicobacter pylori* infection. *N Engl J Med*. 2010;362:1597–1604.
66. Alon D, Paitan Y, Ben-Nissan Y, et al. Persistent *Helicobacter canis* bacteremia in a patient with gastric lymphoma. *Infection*. 2010;38:62–64.
67. Dieterich C, Wiesel P, Neiger R, et al. Presence of multiple "Helicobacter heilmannii" strains in an individual suffering from ulcers and in his two cats. *J Clin Microbiol*. 1998;36:1366–1370.
68. Lavelle JP, Landas S, Mitros FA, et al. Acute gastritis associated with spiral organisms from cats. *Dig Dis Sci*. 1994;39:744–750.
69. Thomson MA, Storey P, Greer R, et al. Canine-human transmission of *Gastrospirillum hominis*. *Lancet*. 1994;344:1097–1098.
70. van Loon S, Bart A, den Hertog EJ, et al. *Helicobacter heilmannii* gastritis caused by cat to child transmission. *J Pediatr Gastroenterol Nutr*. 2003;36:407–409.
71. Meining A, Kroher G, Stolte M. Animal reservoirs in the transmission of *Helicobacter heilmannii*. Results of a questionnaire-based study. *Scand J Gastroenterol*. 1998;33:795–798.
72. De Groote D, Ducatelle R, Haesebrouck F. Helicobacters of possible zoonotic origin: a review. *Acta Gastroenterol Belg*. 2000;63:380–387.
73. Minauchi K, Takahashi S, Sakai T, et al. The nosocomial transmission of *Helicobacter cinaedi* infections in immunocompromised patients. *Intern Med*. 2010;49:1733–1739.
74. Kawamura Y, Tomida J, Miyoshi-Akiyama T, et al. Proposal of *Helicobacter canicola* sp. nov., previously identified as *Helicobacter cinaedi*, isolated from canines. *Syst Appl Microbiol*. 2016;39:307–312.
75. Baele M, Decostere A, Vandamme P, et al. *Helicobacter baculiformis* sp. nov., isolated from feline stomach mucosa. *Int J Syst Evol Microbiol*. 2008;58:357–364.
76. De Groote D, Van Doorn LJ, Van den Bulck K, et al. Detection of non-pylori *Helicobacter* species in "Helicobacter heilmannii"-infected humans. *Helicobacter*. 2005;10:398–406.
77. Fox JG, Shen Z, Xu S, et al. *Helicobacter marmotae* sp. nov. isolated from livers of woodchucks and intestines of cats. *J Clin Microbiol*. 2002;40:2513–2519.
78. Hanninen ML, Happonen I, Saari S, et al. Culture and characteristics of *Helicobacter bizzozeronii*, a new canine gastric *Helicobacter* sp. *Int J Syst Bacteriol*. 1996;46:160–166.
79. Jalava K, Kaartinen M, Utriainen M, et al. *Helicobacter salomonis* sp. nov., a canine gastric *Helicobacter* sp. related to *Helicobacter felis* and *Helicobacter bizzozeronii*. *Int J Syst Bacteriol*. 1997;47:975–982.
80. Kiehlbauch J.A., Brenner D.J., Cameron D.N., et al. Genotypic and phenotypic characterization of Helicobacter cinaedi and Helicobacter fennelliae strains isolated from humans and animals. *J Clin Microbiol*. 1995;33:2940–2947.
81. Kivisto R, Linros J, Rossi M, et al. Characterization of multiple *Helicobacter bizzozeronii* isolates from a Finnish patient with severe dyspeptic symptoms and chronic active gastritis. *Helicobacter*. 2010;15:58–66.
82. Rossi M, Hanninen ML, Revez J, et al. Occurrence and species level diagnostics of *Campylobacter* spp., enteric *Helicobacter* spp. and *Anaerobiospirillum* spp. in healthy and diarrheic dogs and cats. *Vet Microbiol*. 2008;129:304–314.
83. Van den Bulck K, Decostere A, Baele M, et al. *Helicobacter cynogastricus* sp. nov., isolated from the canine gastric mucosa. *Int J Syst Evol Microbiol*. 2006;56:1559–1564.

67

Miscellaneous Enteric Bacterial Infections

Jane E. Sykes

KEY POINTS

- Several bacterial species have been implicated in gastrointestinal disease with or without extraintestinal disease in dogs and cats, but have uncertain clinical significance or are uncommon to rare.
- *Anaerobiospirillum* spp., *Brachyspira* spp., and *Arcobacter* spp. are fastidious spiral bacteria that can be found in the intestinal tracts of healthy dogs and cats. They resemble *Campylobacter* spp. and *Helicobacter* spp. and some species have been reported to cause diarrhea and extraintestinal disease in humans. Their association with diarrhea in dogs and cats is unclear. There are rare reports of disease associated with *Anaerobiospirillum succiniciproducens* in dogs and cats.
- *Shigella* spp. is a nonmotile gram-negative bacteria that is one of the leading causes of bacterial diarrhea in humans worldwide. It can uncommonly cause subclinical infection in dogs and has not been reported to infect cats.
- *Pleisiomonas shigelloides* is a motile gram-negative bacterial pathogen that can cause gastrointestinal illness in humans (large-bowel diarrhea and vomiting). Risk factors for infection are consumption of raw or undercooked shellfish, traveling to tropical destinations, or exposure to reptiles and tropical fish. *Lawsonia intracellularis* is a gram-negative obligately intracellular bacteria that causes proliferative enteropathy in pigs and occasionally other species. These organisms have rarely been isolated from the feces of healthy and diarrheic dogs and cats; whether they cause diarrhea in dogs and cats is uncertain.
- *Clostridium piliforme* is a filamentous, spore-forming, motile, gram-negative rod that causes Tyzzer's disease in a variety of animal species, most commonly rodents and rabbits. Tyzzer's disease is an acute necrotizing enterocolitis that may also be associated with hepatitis and myocarditis. Rare cases in dogs and cats typically occur in puppies and kittens with concurrent viral diseases or animals that are immunosuppressed for other reasons.

This chapter covers miscellaneous enteric bacterial species that have been associated with disease in dogs and cats, or that have been isolated from the gastrointestinal tract of healthy dogs and cats but are associated with disease in humans. Pathogens covered are *Anaerobiospirillum* spp., *Arcobacter* spp., *Brachyspira* spp., *Shigella* spp., *Pleisomonas shigelloides*, *Lawsonia intracellularis*, and *Clostridium piliforme*. *Anaerobiospirillum succiniciproducens*, *Arcobacter* spp., and *Brachyspira pilosicoli* should be considered along with *Campylobacter* spp. and *Helicobacter* spp. in animals with disease caused by spiral or curved bacteria.

Anaerobiospirillum spp.

Anaerobiospirillum spp. are motile, gram-negative spiral-shaped anaerobic bacteria that are considered to be normal fecal flora of dogs and cats, but not humans. They have been reported to cause diarrhea, bacteremia, or prosthetic joint infections in humans, especially *A. succiniciproducens*[1-4] and to a lesser extent, *Anaerobiospirillum thomasii*.[5,6] Some affected humans have reported no history of animal contact.[7]

No significant statistical correlation has been found between the presence or absence of diarrhea in dogs or cats and infection with *Anaerobiospirillum*.[8] However, organisms closely related to *A. succiniciproducens* were identified in intestinal lesions of six cats with ileocolitis.[9] *Anaerobiospirillum succiniciproducens* was identified in peritoneal fluid of a dog with septic peritonitis,[10] and the sternal lymph node of a cat with ileocolic B-cell lymphoma.[11] In the latter case, the sternal node was markedly enlarged, and organisms were visible together with pyogranulomatous inflammation on cytological examination of a fine-needle aspirate. *Anaerobiospirillum* spp. resemble *Campylobacter* spp. and *Helicobacter* spp. using light microscopy and Gram staining, but do not grow on media for *Campylobacter* spp. and have a corkscrew-like motility as a result of a unique tuft of multiple flagella at one pole (lophotrichous morphology).[12] The organism can be identified using 16S rRNA gene broad-spectrum PCR and sequencing[11] or MALDI-TOF mass spectrometry.[4] It is generally resistant to metronidazole and clindamycin, variably susceptible to penicillin, but susceptible to beta lactam-beta lactamase inhibitors (e.g., clavulanic acid-amoxicillin), fluoroquinolones, carbapenems, and third-generation cephalosporins.[7]

Arcobacter spp.

Arcobacter spp. are gram-negative, motile, aerotolerant, spiral-shaped bacteria that are thought to be a cause of diarrhea, endocarditis, bacteremia, and peritonitis in humans. They can be found in feces of humans and other animals, as well as food products (especially poultry, pork, and beef), and other environmental sources.[5,13] *Arcobacter* spp. have been identified in the feces and saliva of dogs[14,15] and the oral cavity of cats,[16] but have not been reported in association with disease in dogs or cats.

Brachyspira spp.

Brachyspira spp. are flagellated, slow-growing, gram-negative spirochetes found in the large intestinal tract and feces of a variety of animal species, including humans, nonhuman primates, dogs, pigs, and avian species. The genus includes 16 species, some previously known as *Serpulina* spp. or *Treponema* spp.[17] *Brachyspira pilosicoli* and *Brachyspira hyodysenteriae* are established pathogens of pigs, causing porcine colonic spirochetosis and swine dysentery, respectively.

Brachyspira pilosicoli also causes disease in poultry (avian intestinal spirochetosis). *Brachyspira pilosicoli* and *Brachyspira aalborgi* have been reported as a cause of human intestinal spirochetosis (HIS), especially in immunocompromised individuals, although the association of *B. aalborgi* with disease is more tenuous.[18-21] In severe cases, large numbers of spirochetes can be seen using light microscopy attached to the luminal aspect of the colonic epithelium, creating a "false brush border."[18] The organisms can be visualized more readily using Warthin-Starry stains. Because of the slow growth of *B. pilosicoli* in culture, specialized selective media are generally required for isolation.[21]

Several *Brachyspira* species have been detected in healthy and diarrheic dogs, including *B. pilosicoli*, *Brachyspira canis*, *Brachyspira intermedia*, and *Brachyspira alvinipulli*.[22-24] In one study of dogs from Spain, *Brachyspira* spp. were detected using PCR in the feces of 41 (13%) of 311 dogs, including *B. pilosicoli* (5%), *B. canis* (8%), and one *B. intermedia*-like organism. Infection with *B. pilosicoli* was significantly associated with diarrhea, and dogs were more likely to be infected with *B. pilosicoli* if they were under one year of age.[24] However, because of intestinal adherence, spirochetes are not shed in formed feces of dogs and cats, and during large-bowel diarrheal episodes, especially in puppies, they dislodge from the epithelia and appear in large numbers in feces. Therefore a higher prevalence of detection of spirochetes in diarrheic stool does not necessarily imply disease causation. However, diarrheic dogs have been described where large numbers of organisms have been found in association with colonic mucosal lesions.[25,26] An SPF beagle pup with a history of chronic diarrhea and concurrent giardiasis had suspected colonic spirochetosis.[25] The treatment of choice in human patients with HIS is metronidazole for 10 to 14 days.[18,21] Routine disinfectants are sufficient to inactivate *Brachyspira* spp. in the environment.[27]

Shigella spp.

Shigella is a genus of nonmotile gram-negative bacteria that are morphologically indistinguishable from other enterobacteria and cause bacillary dysentery in apes and humans. On the basis of biochemical and serologic properties, *Shigella* are divided into four species: *Shigella dysenteriae*, *Shigella flexneri*, *Shigella boydii*, and *Shigella sonnei*. Each group is further divided into numerous subserotypes that vary in pathogenicity. Shigellae are not as environmentally resistant as salmonellae; they survive best in dried fecal matter on cloth that is kept in a dark, moist place. Because of their short survival time, the carrier host is most important in maintaining these organisms in nature. Dogs may become infected after contamination of their food or water supplies with infected human feces. Because of their coprophagous habits, some pets may become exposed in areas with improper sewage disposal. Dogs only transiently excrete the organisms. Cats have not been reported to be naturally infected.

Shigella spp. produce diarrhea by intestinal epithelial cell invasion and production of Shiga toxin (see also Shiga toxin–producing *Escherichia coli*, Chapter 63). Systemic manifestations of the toxin in infected humans include DIC with renal failure, thrombocytopenia, and microangiopathic hemolytic anemia. In primates the organism causes severe hemorrhagic, mucoid, large-bowel diarrhea. Lesions are usually ulcerative, and they spread from the distal to the proximal colon with time. In children and (although rarely) in adults, bacteremia may develop with or without diarrhea. Organisms have been isolated from a small number of clinically normal dogs, but they have not been directly implicated as a cause of diarrhea in this species.

Plesiomonas shigelloides

Plesiomonas shigelloides is a motile, gram-negative, rod-shaped facultatively anaerobic bacteria in the family Vibrionaceae. In humans, infection can result in diarrhea that can vary from mildly self-limiting to diarrhea that is severe and has a bloody mucoid consistency. Bacteremia, which can result in embolic spread to many organs, generally occurs in immunocompromised humans. Human infection usually follows consumption of poorly cooked or uncooked shellfish, but can also occur in individuals traveling to tropical regions and following exposure to reptiles and tropical fish. Feeding of fish, shellfish, or aquatic foodstuffs to dogs or cats may be a source for infection.[28]

Diarrheic illness has sometimes been attributed to *P. shigelloides* in dogs and cats.[29,30] However, the organism has rarely been reported in the feces of healthy dogs and cats.[31-33] Given this and the lack of evidence for an association with diarrhea, should the organisms be found in the feces of a diarrheic dog or cat, other diagnoses should be considered.

Lawsonia intracellularis

Lawsonia intracellularis is a gram-negative, anaerobic, obligate intracellular bacterium that occupies the distal portion of the small intestine of a variety of animal species. *Lawsonia intracellularis* infection has been associated with acute and chronic proliferative enteropathies in pigs[34] and other species.[35,36] There are rare reports of its detection using molecular methods in dogs with and without enteropathies.[37-41] As with *P. shigelloides*, its clinical significance in dogs remains unclear.

Clostridium piliforme

Clostridium piliforme causes *Tyzzer's disease*, a bacterial disease that occurs in a variety of mammalian and avian species including dogs and cats. Rodents and rabbits are most often affected. It is a long (0.5 μm × 10 to 40 μm), filamentous, spore-forming, gram-negative obligate intracellular bacterial species that moves by means of peritrichous flagella. Clinical disease in rodents appears to be precipitated by stress, such as crowding, unsanitary conditions, weaning, or transportation and irradiation, concurrent infections, glucocorticoid therapy, or other forms of immunosuppression.

The organism is ingested and replicates in the ileocecocolic region; with host immunocompromise, systemic dissemination can occur, with necrotizing enterocolitis, hepatitis, and myocarditis. Reports of spontaneous disease in dogs and cats have been described, usually in puppies and kittens and often in association with co-infections such as canine distemper virus infection or feline panleukopenia virus infection.[42-46] One group of affected kittens had familial lipoprotein lipase deficiency and were persistently lipidemic.[47]

Affected dogs and cats typically have rapid onset of lethargy, depression, anorexia, and abdominal discomfort. Hepatomegaly and abdominal distention are followed by hypothermia, with the animal becoming moribund very rapidly, with death within 24 to 48 hours. Diarrhea may not be evident. Icterus has been apparent in some animals, especially cats.

Because of the rapidly fatal course of Tyzzer's disease, diagnosis is usually made at necropsy. Laboratory abnormalities that may be apparent before death include bandemia with neutrophil toxicity, lymphopenia, hypoalbuminemia, and moderate to severe increases in the activity of serum liver enzymes. Characteristic findings at necropsy are multiple whitish-gray to hemorrhagic foci, 1 to 2 mm in diameter, on the capsule and cut surface of the liver. Similar lesions may be apparent on other viscera. The intestinal mucosa may be thickened and congested in the region of the terminal ileum and proximal colon.

Histologic findings usually include multifocal periportal hepatic necrosis with or without necrotic enterocolitis; other tissues, such as the myocardium, may be affected in some animals. Infiltrates of neutrophils and mononuclear cells are usually present at the margins of necrotic lesions. Numerous intracellular filamentous organisms are only faintly visible by

H&E stain in the hepatocytes at the margins of necrotic lesions and in the intestinal epithelial cells. Special stains such as Giemsa stain or Warthin-Starry or Gomori silver stain must be used to confirm the morphology of the organisms, which have a characteristic beaded appearance in a "pick-up sticks" arrangement (Fig. 67.1). Immunochemical stains can also be used to detect specific antigens of *C. piliforme*.[43] Nucleic acid hybridization or PCR can be used to demonstrate organism-specific nucleic acid in tissues.[48] *Clostridium piliforme* cannot be isolated on cell-free medium and so far has been cultured only in eggs or cell cultures.[49] Because *C. piliforme* can be found in the feces of clinically healthy animals, care should be taken not to make a diagnosis of Tyzzer's disease based on a positive result from feces or intestinal specimens alone.

Treatment of Tyzzer's disease has not been reported in dogs or cats, because diagnosis has always been made at necropsy, and infection tends to be overwhelming and associated with rapid mortality. Antibacterial efficacy is undetermined. In naturally infected foals, successful antibacterial treatment has been reported using ampicillin, aminoglycosides (amikacin or gentamicin), or penicillin.[48] Aggressive parenteral fluid therapy was also used. Prevention in puppies and kittens involves reducing factors such as overcrowding, unsanitary conditions, and poor nutrition.

Infection with *C. piliforme* has only been reported once in a person in 1996, and manifested as chronic verrucous cutaneous lesions in association with HIV–acquired immunodeficiency syndrome.[50] The source of infection of this person was not determined. Because transmission of the disease between hosts appears uncommon and the disease is so rare, cats and dogs would be expected to be an unlikely source of infection for humans.

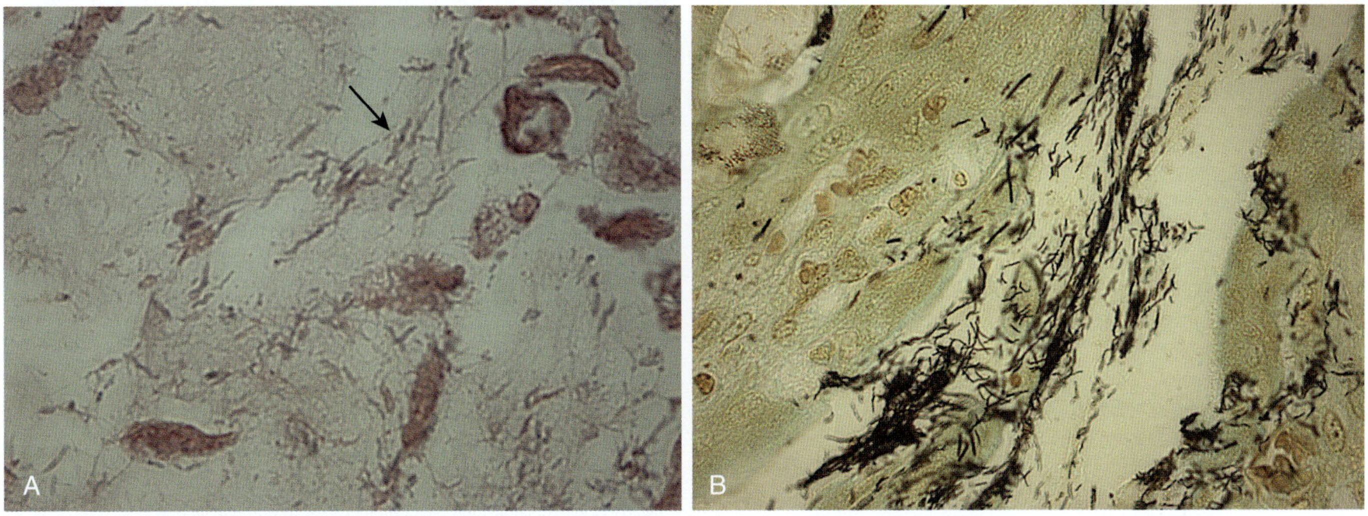

Fig. 67.1 Histopathology images of *Clostridium piliforme* enterocolitis (Tyzzer's disease) in a 5-week-old intact male domestic shorthair kitten that had a 3-day history of mucoid hemorrhagic diarrhea, inappetence, lethargy, and weight loss. A parvovirus fecal antigen test was negative. (A) Large numbers of pale basophilic filamentous rods *(arrow)* can be seen in the lumen of the colon. Hematoxylin and eosin stain, 1000× magnification. (B) The bacteria stain black with Warthin-Starry stain, demonstrating the characteristic "pick-up sticks" appearance that occurs with Tyzzer's disease. (Images courtesy University of California-Davis VMTH Anatomic Pathology Service.)

CASE EXAMPLE

Signalment:
"Callie," a 10-year-old female spayed Brittany spaniel from northern California.

History:
Callie was seen by the University of California-Davis Small Animal Emergency and Critical Care Service for a 10-day history of progressive lethargy, intermittent vomiting, and bleeding from the mouth. The oral bleeding began the day before the examination and was thought to be precipitated by a vomiting episode when Callie bit her cheek and had continued since then. Callie had shown no interest in food for the last 24 hours and had some intermittent yellow diarrhea. Two months previously, Callie had been diagnosed with IMHA/ITP which was initially detected as an incidental finding on routine bloodwork. At that time, her platelet count was < 5,000 platelets/μL, she had a hematocrit of 34% with 638,900 reticulocytes/μL, and neutrophilia (16,640 cells/μL), bandemia (208 cells/μL) and hypoalbuminemia were present (2.6 g/dL; RR, 2.8–4.2 g/dL). Thoracic radiographs were unremarkable, and the only finding on abdominal ultrasound examination was a slightly small liver. No spherocytes were seen, Coombs' test was negative, an antinuclear antibody test was negative, and an antimegakaryocyte antibody test on a bone marrow aspirate was negative. Cytologic examination of bone marrow showed mild myeloid hyperplasia and moderate megakaryocyte and erythroid hyperplasia. She was treated with prednisone, 1.25 mg/kg PO q12h as well as famotidine and sucralfate. Two weeks later, because the platelet count had not increased and she was experiencing significant adverse effects of prednisone administration, she was also treated with azathioprine for 2 weeks (2.5 mg/kg PO q48h), then cyclophosphamide (200 mg/m^2 PO, once), then cyclosporine for 2 weeks, and her prednisone dose was reduced.

Current medications:
Prednisone 0.6 mg/kg PO q12h; cyclosporine (5 mg/kg PO q12h), famotidine (0.5 mg/kg PO q24h), sucralfate (1 g PO q8h), levothyroxine (0.01 mg/kg PO q24h), monthly heartworm prophylaxis.

Other medical history:
Callie had been diagnosed with hypothyroidism several years previously and was well managed with levothyroxine.

Continued

CASE EXAMPLE—cont'd

Physical Examination

Body weight: 19.8 kg.

General: Severely obtunded, 5% dehydrated, nonambulatory. Mucous membranes pink and tacky, CRT 4 s, T = 104.5°F (40.3°C), P = 160 beats/min, R = 60 breaths/min, BCS 4/9.

Integument: Full clean haircoat. Fresh blood was identified around the mouth as a result of buccal bleeding, and there were multiple ecchymoses on the ventral abdomen and around the eyes.

Eyes, ears, nose, and throat: Bilateral epistaxis was identified with normal nasal airflow. Multiple ulcers were identified in the oral cavity, and there was evidence of mild periodontal disease.

Musculoskeletal: Moderate peripheral muscle atrophy, especially in the pelvic limbs.

Cardiovascular: Grade III/VI left systolic heart murmur, sinus tachycardia.

Respiratory: Mildly increased lung sounds.

Gastrointestinal and genitourinary: No clinically significant abnormalities. Rectal examination revealed melena.

Lymph nodes: All < 1 cm in diameter.

Laboratory Findings

CBC: HCT 29.7% (40–55%), MCV 74 fL (65–75 fL), MCHC 31.6 g/dL (33–36 g/dL), WBC 9310 cells/μL (6000–13,000 cells/μL), neutrophils 6587 cells/μL (3000–10,500 cells/μL), bands 1405 cells/μL (slight toxicity), lymphocytes 351 cells/μL (1000–4000 cells/μL), monocytes 176 cells/μL (150–1200 cells/μL), eosinophils 263 cells/μL (0–1500 cells/μL), platelets 8,000 platelets/μL (150,000–400,000 platelets/μL), mean platelet volume 7.5 fL (7–13 fL), reticulocytes 90,000/μL, nucleated RBC 6 cells/μL.

Serum chemistry profile: Sodium 142 mmol/L (145–154 mmol/L), potassium 4.9 mmol/L (3.6–5.3 mmol/L), chloride 103 mmol/L (108–118 mmol/L), bicarbonate 14 mmol/L (16–26 mmol/L), phosphorus 5.8 mg/dL (3.0–6.2 mg/dL), calcium 8.7 mg/dL (9.7–11.5 mg/dL), BUN 20 mg/dL (5–21 mg/dL), creatinine 1.1 mg/dL (0.3–1.2 mg/dL), glucose 97 mg/dL (64–123 mg/dL), total protein 3.7 g/dL (5.4–7.6 g/dL), albumin 1.7 g/dL (3.0–4.4 g/dL), globulin 2.0 g/dL (1.8–3.9 g/dL), ALT 1902 U/L (19–67 U/L), AST 489 U/L (19–42 U/L), ALP 1548 U/L (21–170 U/L), GGT 229 U/L (0–6 U/L), cholesterol 163 mg/dL (135–361 mg/dL), total bilirubin 2.0 mg/dL (0–0.2 mg/dL).

Urinalysis (postfluid bolus): SpG 1.024; pH 7.5, 2+ protein (SSA), 1+ bilirubin, 1+ hemoprotein, no glucose, 15–25 WBC/HPF, 2–5 RBC/HPF, 0–3 granular cases/HPF, many bacterial rods.

Aerobic bacterial urine culture: *Escherichia coli*, susceptible to amoxicillin-clavulanic acid, cephalexin, and enrofloxacin but resistant to amoxicillin and trimethoprim-sulfamethoxazole.

Treatment

Callie was treated for shock with aggressive fluid therapy, supplemental oxygen, and intravenous broad-spectrum antimicrobial drugs. However, she became progressively more obtunded and vomited multiple times. Epistaxis and additional cutaneous ecchymoses were noted. An activated clotting time was 163 s (normal < 75 s) and blood lactate was 9.0 mmol/L (normal < 2.5 mmol/L). The owner elected euthanasia.

Necropsy Findings:

A cosmetic necropsy was performed. Grossly, the main findings were multifocally extensive areas of ecchymoses and petechiation over the distal pelvic limbs extending into the inguinal region and caudal abdomen. The perineal region was stained with tarry fecal material. The liver was markedly enlarged and pale tan with a prominent reticular pattern and numerous pinpoint red foci. There was extensive serosal and mucosal petechial hemorrhage throughout the entire length of the intestinal tract. Histopathology revealed a severe, multifocal, acute, necrotizing hepatitis with numerous intrahepatocellular filamentous rod-shaped bacteria consistent with infection by *Clostridium piliforme*. No enterocolitis was identified, the melena likely being associated with microvascular hemorrhage.

Diagnosis

Tyzzer's disease.

Comments

Reported cases of Tyzzer's disease in dogs and cats in the literature have been puppies or kittens, often with co-infections (distemper, panleukopenia virus). This case was unusual in that it was an adult dog treated with immunosuppressive drugs for suspected primary immune-mediated thrombocytopenia and anemia. A whole blood cyclosporine concentration was obtained before euthanasia and was 280 ng/mL, in the range recommended for initial immunosuppression. The use of multiple different immunosuppressive drugs in sequence may have been a factor that predisposed to Tyzzer's disease. The *E. coli* lower urinary tract infection may also have occurred secondary to treatment with prednisone.

SUGGESTED READINGS

Johnston AR, Al Saghbini S, Wu ML, et al. Photo quiz: false intestinal brush border. Intestinal spirochetosis. *J Clin Microbiol*. 2015;53:3711–3956.

Hampson DJ. The spirochete *Brachyspira pilosicoli*, enteric pathogen of animals and humans. *Clin Microbiol Rev*. 2017;31:e00087-17.

Neto RT, Uzal FA, Hodzic E, et al. Coinfection with *Clostridium piliforme* and Felid herpesvirus 1 in a kitten. *J Vet Diagn Invest*. 2015;27:547–551.

REFERENCES

1. Alguacil-Guillen M, Ramos-Ruperto L, Ramos Ramos JC, et al. MALDI-TOF MS for rapid diagnosis of *Anaerobiospirillum succiniciproducens*, an unusual causative agent of bacteraemia in humans. Two case reports and literature review. *Anaerobe*. 2019;55:130–135.
2. Kelesidis T. Bloodstream infection with *Anaerobiospirillum succiniciproducens*: a potentially lethal infection. *South Med J*. 2011;104:205–214.
3. Schaumburg F, Dieckmann R, Schmidt-Brakling T, et al. First description of an *Anaerobiospirillum succiniciproducens* prosthetic joint infection. *New Microbes New Infect*. 2017;18:1–2.
4. Fox B, Berger MA, Roncallo M, et al. MALDI-TOF MS in *Anaerobiospirillum succiniciproducens* bacteremia: a report of 4 cases in different hosts. *Anaerobe*. 2018;54:267–270.
5. Streitenberger ER, Chavez CM, Rizzo MS, et al. *Anaerobiospirillum thomasii* bacteremia with fatal outcome. *Rev Argent Microbiol*. 2015;47:328–330.
6. Malnick H. *Anaerobiospirillum thomasii* sp. nov., an anaerobic spiral bacterium isolated from the feces of cats and dogs and from diarrheal feces of humans, and emendation of the genus *Anaerobiospirillum*. *Int J Syst Bacteriol*. 1997;47:381–384.
7. Epstein DJ, Ernst K, Rogers R, et al. The Brief Case: *Anaerobiospirillum succiniciproducens* bacteremia and pyomyositis. *J Clin Microbiol*. 2017;55:665–669.
8. Rossi M, Hanninen ML, Revez J, et al. Occurrence and species level diagnostics of *Campylobacter* spp., enteric *Helicobacter* spp. and *Anaerobiospirillum* spp. in healthy and diarrheic dogs and cats. *Vet Microbiol*. 2008;129:304–314.
9. De Cock HE, Marks SL, Stacy BA, et al. Ileocolitis associated with *Anaerobiospirillum* in cats. *J Clin Microbiol*. 2004;42:2752–2758.
10. Courtman NF. Septic peritonitis in a dog caused by *Anaerobiospirillum succiniproducens*. *Vet Clin Pathol*. 2016;45:352–355.
11. Conrado FO, Fox-Alvarez SA, Williams ML. What is your diagnosis? Fine-needle aspirate of an enlarged sternal lymph node in a cat. *Vet Clin Pathol*. 2019;48:137–139.
12. Wecke J, Horbach I. Ultrastructural characterization of *Anaerobiospirillum succiniciproducens* and its differentiation from *Campylobacter* species. *FEMS Microbiol Lett*. 1999;170:83–88.

13. Rivas L, Fegan N, Vanderlinde P. Isolation and characterisation of *Arcobacter butzleri* from meat. *Int J Food Microbiol.* 2004;91:31–41.
14. Houf K, De Smet S, Bare J, et al. Dogs as carriers of the emerging pathogen *Arcobacter. Vet Microbiol.* 2008;130:208–213.
15. Chaban B, Links MG, Hill JE. A molecular enrichment strategy based on cpn60 for detection of epsilon-proteobacteria in the dog fecal microbiome. *Microb Ecol.* 2012;63:348–357.
16. Fera MT, La Camera E, Carbone M, et al. Pet cats as carriers of *Arcobacter* spp. in Southern Italy. *J Appl Microbiol.* 2009;106:1661–1666.
17. Casas V, Vadillo S, San Juan C, et al. The exposed Proteomes of *Brachyspira hyodysenteriae* and *B. pilosicoli. Front Microbiol.* 2016;7:1103.
18. Johnston AR, Al Saghbini S, Wu ML, et al. Photo quiz: false intestinal brush border. Intestinal spirochetosis. *J Clin Microbiol.* 2015;53:3711–3956.
19. Chatani M, Kishita M, Inatomi O, et al. Severe colitis with portal venous gas caused by *Brachyspira pilosicoli* infection. *Intern Med.* 2019;58:3409–3413.
20. Eguchi T, Inoue K, Horino T, et al. Intestinal spirochetosis caused by *Brachyspira pilosicoli* in a systemic lupus erythematosus patient. *J Clin Rheumatol.* 2019;25:e142–e145.
21. Hampson DJ. The spirochete *Brachyspira pilosicoli*, enteric pathogen of animals and humans. *Clin Microbiol Rev.* 2017;31:e00087-17.
22. Razmyar J, Ghavidel M, Salari Sedigh H. Polymerase chain reaction assay targeting nox gene for rapid identification of *Brachyspira canis* in dogs. *Vet Res Forum.* 2019;10:67–72.
23. Oxberry SL, Hampson DJ. Colonisation of pet shop puppies with *Brachyspira pilosicoli. Vet Microbiol.* 2003;93:167–174.
24. Hidalgo A, Rubio P, Osorio J, et al. Prevalence of *Brachyspira pilosicoli* and "Brachyspira canis" in dogs and their association with diarrhoea. *Vet Microbiol.* 2010;146:356–360.
25. Duhamel GE, Hunsaker BD, Mathiesen MR, et al. Intestinal spirochetosis and giardiasis in a beagle pup with diarrhea. *Vet Pathol.* 1996;33:360–362.
26. Fellstrom C, Pettersson B, Zimmerman U, et al. Classification of *Brachyspira* spp. isolated from Swedish dogs. *Anim Health Res Rev.* 2001;2:75–82.
27. Corona-Barrera E, Smith DG, Murray B, et al. Efficacy of seven disinfectant sanitisers on field isolates of *Brachyspira pilosicoli. Vet Rec.* 2004;154:473–474.
28. Jagger T, Keane S, Robertson S. *Plesiomonas shigelloides*: an uncommon cause of diarrhoea in cats? *Vet Rec.* 2000;146:296.
29. Foster G, Patterson T, Pennycott T, et al. *Plesiomonas shigelloides*: an uncommon cause of diarrhoea in cats? *Vet Rec.* 2000;146:411.
30. Gonzalez-Rey C, Svenson SB, Bravo L, et al. Serotypes and anti-microbial susceptibility of *Plesiomonas shigelloides* isolates from humans, animals and aquatic environments in different countries. *Comp Immunol Microbiol Infect Dis.* 2004;27:129–139.
31. Sparkes AH, Papasouliotis K, Sunvold G, et al. Effect of dietary supplementation with fructo-oligosaccharides on fecal flora of healthy cats. *Am J Vet Res.* 1998;59:436–440.
32. Aldova E. Serotyping of *Plesiomonas shigelloides* strains with our own antigenic scheme. An attempted epidemiological study. *Zentralbl Bakteriol Mikrobiol Hyg.* 1987;265:253–262.
33. Youssef NM, El-Shamy HA, Abou-Donia HA, et al. A study of *Plesiomonas shigelloides* from human, pets and aquatic environments. *J Egypt Public Health Assoc.* 1993;68:293–308.
34. Karuppannan AK, Opriessnig T. *Lawsonia intracellularis*: revisiting the disease ecology and control of this fastidious pathogen in pigs. *Front Vet Sci.* 2018;5:181.
35. Feary DJ, Gebhart CJ, Pusterla N. *Lawsonia intracellularis* proliferative enteropathy in a foal. *Schweiz Arch Tierheilkd.* 2007;149:129–133.
36. Ohta T, Kimura K, Katsuda K, et al. Proliferative enteropathy caused by *Lawsonia intracellularis* in chickens. *J Comp Pathol.* 2017;156:158–161.
37. Herbst W, Hertrampf B, Schmitt T, et al. Diagnosis of *Lawsonia intracellularis* using the polymerase chain reaction (PCR) in pigs with and without diarrhea and other animal species. *Dtsch Tierarztl Wochenschr.* 2003;110:361–364.
38. Collins JE, Libal MC, Brost D. Proliferative enteritis in two pups. *J Am Vet Med Assoc.* 1983;183:886–889.
39. Husník R, Klimes J, Tomanová K, et al. *Lawsonia intracellularis* in a dog with inflammatory bowel disease. *Vet Med Czech.* 2003;5:141–145.
40. Tomanová K, Klimes J, Smola J, et al. Detection of *Lawsonia intracellularis* in a dog with inflammatory bowel disease using nested PCR and serology. *Vet Med Czech.* 2003;48:108–112.
41. Klimes J, Dezorzova K, Smola J, et al. Prevalence of antibodies against *Lawsonia intracellularis* in dogs with and without gastrointestinal disease. *Vet Med Czech.* 2007;52:502–506.
42. Neto RT, Uzal FA, Hodzic E, et al. Coinfection with *Clostridium piliforme* and Felid herpesvirus 1 in a kitten. *J Vet Diagn Invest.* 2015;27:547–551.
43. Headley SA, Shirota K, Baba T, et al. Diagnostic exercise: Tyzzer's disease, distemper, and coccidiosis in a pup. *Vet Pathol.* 2009;46:151–154.
44. Young JK, Baker DC, Burney DP. Naturally occurring Tyzzer's disease in a puppy. *Vet Pathol.* 1995;32:63–65.
45. Iwanaka M, Orita S, Mokuno Y, et al. Tyzzer's disease complicated with distemper in a puppy. *J Vet Med Sci.* 1993;55:337–339.
46. Ikegami T, Shirota K, Goto K, et al. Enterocolitis associated with dual infection by *Clostridium piliforme* and feline panleukopenia virus in three kittens. *Vet Pathol.* 1999;36:613–615.
47. Jones BR, Johnstone AC, Hancock WS. Tyzzer's disease in kittens with familial primary hyperlipoproteinaemia. *J Small Anim Pract.* 1985;26:411–419.
48. Borchers A, Magdesian KG, Halland S, et al. Successful treatment and polymerase chain reaction (PCR) confirmation of Tyzzer's disease in a foal and clinical and pathologic characteristics of 6 additional foals (1986-2005). *J Vet Intern Med.* 2006;20:1212–1218.
49. Spencer TH, Ganaway JR, Waggie KS. Cultivation of *Bacillus piliformis* (Tyzzer) in mouse fibroblasts (3T3 cells). *Vet Microbiol.* 1990;22:291–297.
50. Smith KJ, Skelton HG, Hilyard EJ, et al. *Bacillus piliformis* infection (Tyzzer's disease) in a patient infected with HIV-1: confirmation with 16S ribosomal RNA sequence analysis. *J Am Acad Dermatol.* 1996;34:343–348.

68

Leptospirosis

Simone Schuller, George E. Moore, Jane E. Sykes

KEY POINTS

- First Described: Heidelberg, Germany, 1886 (Adolf Weil).[1]
- Cause: *Leptospira* spp. (a spirochete bacterial pathogen, phylum Spirochaetes).
- Affected Hosts: Dogs, rarely cats, more than 150 other mammalian species.
- Geographic Distribution: Worldwide.
- Major Clinical Signs: Fever, lethargy, reluctance to move, anorexia, polyuria and polydipsia, vomiting, diarrhea, icterus, abnormal respiratory function.
- Major Differential Diagnoses: Nephrotoxicoses (e.g., NSAIDs, grapes and raisins, ethylene glycol), Lyme nephritis, acute glomerulonephritides, bacterial pyelonephritis, cholangiohepatitis, acute pancreatitis, canine monocytic ehrlichiosis, Rocky Mountain spotted fever, bacterial sepsis, leishmaniosis.
- Human Health Significance: Zoonosis. Human infection results from direct or indirect contact with contaminated urine. Mild influenza-like illness to severe illness with multiorgan failure (Weil's disease) have the potential to occur.

ETIOLOGIC AGENT AND EPIDEMIOLOGY

Leptospirosis is a zoonotic disease of worldwide significance affecting most mammalian species. It is caused by infection with spirochetes of the genus *Leptospira*. *Leptospira* spp. are thin, flexible, motile, spiral-shaped bacteria with hook-shaped ends, measuring 0.1 µm in width and 6 to 12 µm in length (Fig. 68.1). The organism owes its name to this specific morphology (*leptos* = "thin," *spira* = "coil"; *interrogans* = "question mark shape"). Leptospires are gram negative and have a double membrane structure consisting of cytoplasmic and outer membranes enclosing the periplasmic space. *Leptospira* are motile due to two periplasmic endoflagellae, which are inserted subterminally and wrapped around an internal protoplasmic cylinder. The leptospiral outer membrane contains LPS, multiple antigenic lipoproteins (e.g. LipL21, LipL32, LipL36, LipL41) and integral transmembrane proteins (e.g., porin OmpL1), and secretins (e.g., GspD).[2] Despite intensive research, the function of the majority of these proteins is incompletely understood. For example, much research has been conducted to show a relationship of LipL32, a major outer membrane protein present only in pathogenic *Leptospira* species, with clinical illness. However, pathogenic lesions with LipL32 mutants were indistinguishable from those produced with wild-type infections.[3]

Leptospira species have been grouped into pathogenic (group I, of which there are nine), intermediately pathogenic (group II, of which there are five), and six saprophytic species based on their 16S rRNA gene sequences. Saprophytic leptospires, such as *Leptospira biflexa*, grow at lower temperatures (11°C to 13°C) and in the presence of 8-azaguanine. These cultural criteria can be used to differentiate them from pathogenic leptospires, which have their growth optimized at 28°C to 30°C. More extensive phenotypic criteria commonly used for further subclassification of bacteria such as chemical properties and activities are largely unsuitable for *Leptospira*. Before the development of molecular typing methods, further subclassification was therefore almost exclusively based on serologic techniques.[2] Serovars are distinct by differences in their LPS antigens, which can be detected by specific monoclonal antisera. More than 250 serovars of *Leptospira interrogans* have been described and further classified into antigenically related serogroups. The term "serogroup" refers to serovars that share common antigens that often lead to serologic cross-reactions. Although serogroups currently have no taxonomic basis, they have been historically useful for epidemiologic tracking and understanding of the disease.[4] Each serovar is adapted to one or more wild or domestic animal reservoir host species (e.g., Icterohaemorrhagiae and rats, Ballum and mice), although molecular typing methods have revealed that there may be tighter associations between different sequence types (STs) and specific reservoir host species. The arrival of molecular typing methods has introduced further complexity, as serovars within the same serogroup can belong to multiple different *Leptospira* species (different species but similar LPS antigens). For example, serovars within the serogroup Grippotyphosa can be found in both *L. interrogans* and *Leptospira kirschneri*[5] (Table 68.1).

Leptospira spp. have a complex life cycle inside and outside of the host. Host-adapted serovars colonize the kidneys of infected wild and domestic mammalian *reservoir hosts* which shed leptospires in their urine. *Incidental hosts* become infected either by direct contact with infected urine, ingestion of reservoir hosts, or indirectly through exposure to contaminated water or soil. Lacking co-evolutionary adaptation, infected incidental hosts develop more severe clinical illness and shed organisms for shorter periods than reservoir hosts.

Pathogenic *Leptospira* spp. are readily inactivated in the environment when exposed to excessive heat, ultraviolet radiation, desiccation, a variety of disinfectants, and freezing conditions. Their association with stagnant water may relate to inactivation by mechanical damage, although cases have occurred after exposure to rapidly moving water sources such as waterfalls and following white-water rafting. However, in moist, warm, and neutral or slightly alkaline pH conditions, pathogenic leptospires can survive for weeks to months and successfully infect new hosts.[6] Current evidence suggests that leptospires do not multiply in the environment. They can be detected using molecular methods in water sources, but a number of studies have found them more prevalent in soil from the same geographic region. When conditions are optimal, it appears they can survive weeks

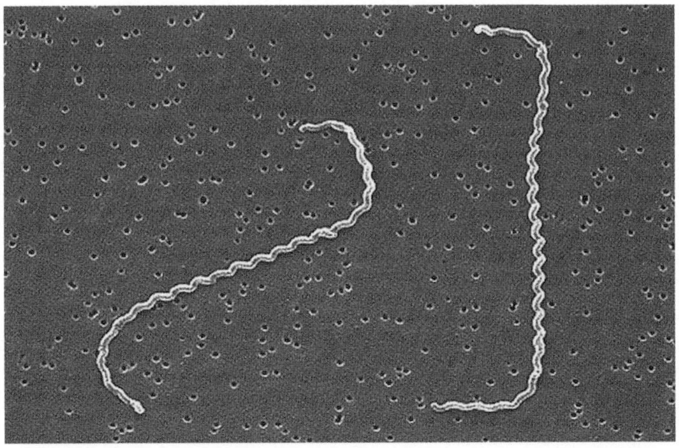

Fig. 68.1 Scanning electron micrograph of *Leptospira* spp. spirochetes showing helical structure and curved (hooked) ends (original magnification ×60,000). (Courtesy of Rob Weyant, Centers for Disease Control and Prevention.)

TABLE 68.1 Selected Serovars of *Leptospira interrogans* and *Leptospira kirschneri* that Infect Dogs*

Species	Serogroup	Serovar
Leptospira interrogans	Icterohaemorrhagiae	Icterohaemorrhagiae
	Canicola	Canicola
	Pomona	Pomona
	Australis	Bratislava
	Sejroe	ND
	Ballum	Ballum
Leptospira kirschneri	Grippotyphosa	Grippotyphosa

*Isolated from dogs with naturally occurring leptospirosis, or that induce disease in dogs after experimental inoculation.
ND, not determined.

to months in water-saturated soil.[7] The ability of leptospires to survive in the environment under different conditions appears to be somewhat strain dependent. One study showed that *L. kirschneri* serovar Grippotyphosa could survive 1 hour to 3 days (although generally up to 4 hours) in dog or cattle urine that had been diluted with distilled water or phosphate-buffered saline, but was unable to survive even for periods as short as 1 minute in undiluted dog urine (pH 5.8) and undiluted cow urine (pH 8.4) (across a range of temperatures from 15°C to 37°C); another study showed survival of *L. interrogans* serovar Hardjo in undiluted cow urine for 0 to 6 hours; survival was again promoted by dilution of the urine.[8]

Reservoir Hosts

Worldwide, small rodents are considered the most important reservoir hosts of pathogenic *Leptospira* spp. However, it is likely that every known mammalian species, including humans, and even reptiles can act as reservoir hosts for pathogenic *Leptospira* strains.[9] Multiple wildlife species were documented to show seroreactivity (up to 60% seropositive) to *Leptospira* serovars in a large multiyear national review in the United States.[10] Raccoons have been implicated as a source of serogroup Icterohaemorrhagiae in the northeastern United States[11] and Grippotyphosa infections in the midwest and northeastern regions of the United States and eastern Canada.[12-15] Raccoons might also be involved in serogroup Autumnalis, Bratislava, or Pomona infections in Washington state.[16] In the past, most of our knowledge about serovars in reservoir hosts has been based on serologic studies, which do not accurately reflect the epidemiology of infecting serovars.[17] Isolation of *Leptospira* spp. is generally necessary for accurate serovar identification or molecular typing. Isolation of *Leptospira* spp., however, is not straightforward. As molecular methods are being refined, limited typing of leptospires without prior culture is becoming feasible.[18] The use of PCR on kidney tissue and urine specimens collected from a variety of wildlife species worldwide is shedding light on the diversity of potential reservoir hosts of *Leptospira* spp. Several studies have shown a high prevalence of positive test results in small rodents,[19-24] supporting their role as a major reservoir. Other investigators have identified a high prevalence of urinary colonization in unexpected animal populations, such as wild hedgehogs in Europe,[25,26] Blanding's turtles in Illinois, USA,[27] and mountain lions in northern California.[28] Striped skunks, raccoons, and gray squirrels were also found to be reservoirs in northern California.[29]

California sea lions are infected with a specific molecular type of serovar Pomona, which is adapted to sea lions and causes episodic outbreaks of disease in juvenile sea lions.[30] The identification of a high prevalence of urinary colonization in feral cats in Western Australia has led to interest in the role of feral cats as reservoir hosts for leptospirosis.[31] In limited studies from Réunion Island[32] and east-central Illinois,[33] there was no evidence that feral cats played a role as reservoirs.

The simple detection of pathogenic leptospires in domestic and wildlife reservoir hosts in a geographic region does not necessarily imply that those *Leptospira* strains infect and cause disease in humans and domestic dogs in that region. Using molecular typing methods, it has been possible to show that strains of *Leptospira* identified in reservoir hosts do not always correlate with strains found in humans with leptospirosis.[34] In a study from French Polynesia, *Leptospira* strains detected using molecular methods in 244 human patients were compared with those found in several potential reservoir hosts.[35] The main source of infection for *Leptospira borgpetersenii* serovar Ballum and *L. interrogans* serovar Icterohaemorrhagiae was rats, for *L. interrogans* serovar Australis was dogs, and for *L. interrogans* serovar Pomona or Canicola was farmed pigs. *Leptospira interrogans* was associated with the most severe infections in humans, with 10 and 5 fatal cases being associated with serovars Icterohaemorrhagiae and Australis, respectively. More studies like this will be required to gain a better understanding of the link between animal reservoirs and human infections.

Factors that might influence transmission include strain virulence, the number of organisms shed/mL of urine by a reservoir host, the density and distribution of the reservoir host population (including their proximity to water sources that might be contaminated and their proximity to incidental hosts), and the volume of urine to which an incidental host is exposed. One study showed that of cows, deer, dogs, humans, mice, and rats, rats excreted the highest quantity of spirochetes/mL (median, 5.7×10^6 cells), but large mammals excrete a larger volume of urine and shed more organisms/day (5.1×10^8 to 1.3×10^9 cells).[36]

Dogs and Cats as Incidental Hosts

Both dogs and cats can contract leptospirosis and can shed leptospires in their urine, but cats appear to be relatively resistant to development of clinical illness. As a result, leptospirosis is uncommonly described in cats.[37-48] Cats may be infected after ingestion of infected prey, so outdoor exposure and hunting behavior may be risk factors for cats.[37] In experimentally and naturally infected cats, interstitial nephritis is the most consistent histopathological finding.[37,39,42,47]

Disease in dogs is primarily caused by the pathogenic (group I) species *L. interrogans* and *L. kirschneri.* Within these two species, more than 10 different serovars have been associated with disease in dogs worldwide, although the exact serovars causing disease in dogs in different geographic locations remains poorly understood, in part because of the difficulties associated with culture of leptospires. The most common serovars thought to infect dogs before the introduction of canine *Leptospira* vaccines several decades ago belonged to the serogroups Icterohaemorrhagiae and Canicola. Since that time, widespread seroconversion to other serogroups, especially Grippotyphosa and Pomona in North America, and Grippotyphosa and Australis in Europe has been noted in sick dogs. This apparent serovar shift could be due to the inclusion of additional serovars into the serologic testing panels (based on the microscopic agglutination test [MAT]), as well as increased contact between dogs, wildlife, and farm animal reservoir hosts for these serovars. Most of our knowledge regarding the *Leptospira* serogroups that infect dogs is derived from MAT results, but these do not accurately indicate the infecting serovar. However, with the advent of molecular methods such as multilocus sequence typing (MLST) and variable-number tandem repeat (VNTR) analysis, we are beginning to understand the true identity of serovars and strains of *Leptospira* spp. that cause disease in domestic dogs from different geographic locations, and typing may be possible in some circumstances following amplification of DNA directly from clinical specimens, without previous culture.[49] At the time of writing, only a small number of studies have been published that report serovars and strains infecting dogs. In Japan, the predominant serovars associated with diseased dogs in one study were Australis, Autumnalis, and Hebdomadis.[50] Furthermore, strains from humans clustered with those detected in dogs but not mice, and the profile of one human isolate was identical to that from a dog.[51] In northeast Italy, six STs were detected in 193 dogs with leptospirosis that belonged to *L. interrogans* (3 STs), *L. kirschneri* (2 STs), and *L. borgpetersenii* (1 ST), and the organisms detected belonged to serogroups Icterohaemorrhagiae, Australis, Sejroe, and Pomona.[25] Sequence types detected in the dogs were compared with STs in an Italian database and matched STs identified in rats, mice, cats, hedgehogs, horses, and one each of a goat, cow, pig, wild boar, and a wolf. Because vaccine-derived immunity to leptospirosis is considered serogroup specific, improved understanding of serogroups infecting dogs has the potential to lead to more protective vaccines.

Leptospirosis is considered a seasonal disease, with human and animal outbreaks often linked to heavy rainfall or flooding.[2,52] The peak seasonal distribution in parts of North America where freezing winters occur is late fall,[53-55] but in more temperate regions, peak seasonal distribution occurs after months of high rainfall (such as in late winter in northern California).[55,56] In parts of the United States where rainfall occurs throughout the year, there may be no seasonality to infections. Similarly, the number of acute leptospirosis cases per month was strongly correlated with the average monthly temperature and moderately correlated with the average rainfall in a cohort of 256 dogs from Switzerland presented to a referral hospital.[57] However, despite its seasonality, leptospirosis can be diagnosed at any time during the year. Outbreaks of leptospirosis in dogs can also occur in relatively arid regions, possibly because of predation of infected wildlife by dogs, or factors such as irrigation. An outbreak of leptospirosis in dogs in Arizona, for example, was reported and investigated by the CDC.[58,59] In late 2021, an outbreak in dogs occurred in Los Angeles, and was monitored by the Los Angeles county Department of Public Health.

Consistent with the transmission cycle of leptospires, dogs with leptospirosis in the United States were more likely to be living in the proximity of outdoor water, swimming or drinking from outdoor water sources, and having indirect exposure to wildlife.[60] Risk factors identified for age, sex, and breed of dogs with acute leptospirosis have yielded conflicting results and might be subject to temporal changes.[61] Males, herding dogs, hounds, working dogs, and mixed breeds have previously been reported to be at increased risk in the United States.[62] In a cohort of dogs from Switzerland, puppies (<1 year) and male dogs were significantly overrepresented compared to the general dog population.[57] However, in other studies, neither sex, age, nor breed predispositions were confirmed.[61,63] In a study in the United States using the Veterinary Medical DataBase (VMDB), dogs weighing less than 6.8 kg (15 lbs), and in particular, Yorkshire terriers, had the highest hospital prevalence for leptospirosis between 2000 and 2009.[61] This may be because small breeds are less likely to be vaccinated because of the perception that they are at increased risk for adverse effects following vaccination.[64] Over the past decade, residence in urban areas has emerged as a risk factor for *Leptospira* infection in dogs in some parts of North America, possibly due to exposure to urban wildlife species.[65,66]

CLINICAL FEATURES

Pathogenesis and Clinical Signs

Infection with pathogenic leptospires can lead to a wide range of clinical manifestations from subclinical to severe, and potentially lethal disease. The outcome of acute infection depends on the age and immune response of the host, the virulence and inoculum size of the pathogen, and the degree of co-adaptation of host and infecting serovar.[1] Further genetic analysis of isolates from natural disease outbreaks will be needed to determine if clinical signs can be linked to genetic features of specific strains. Pathogenic leptospires possess several virulence factors that help them to invade and establish infection in the mammalian host. These include leptospiral immunoglobulin-like proteins, adhesins, hemolysins, LPS, and a variety of other outer membrane proteins that may contribute to tissue injury and promote the inflammatory response.[67]

Hosts become infected when mucous membranes or abraded, scratched, or macerated skin come into contact with infected urine, tissues (such as following predation), or contaminated water or soil. After entering the warmer mammalian body environment, transcriptional changes occur that enhance the spirochete's pathogenicity.[68–70] Leptospires quickly establish a systemic infection via hematogenous spread. Unlike bloodstream infections with other gram-negative bacteria, leptospires do not cause fulminant disease shortly after the onset of infection. This has been attributed to the low endotoxic potential of leptospiral LPS.[71] The leptospires then spread and further replicate in many tissues, including the kidney, liver, spleen, CNS, pancreas, GI tract, eyes, and genital tract. Through numerous mechanisms, pathogenic leptospires are able to evade destruction by complement, as well as killing by neutrophils through inhibition of myeloperoxidase activity.[67] Leptospiral PAMPs stimulate the innate immune system by interacting with a number of pattern recognition receptors (PRRs), such as TLRs and nucleotide oligomerization domain (NOD)-like receptors (NLRs), which can then trigger a proinflammatory "cytokine storm" that contributes to tissue damage and organ dysfunction.[72] In particular, animals with severe leptospirosis have significant increases in TNF-α and IL-10, considered hallmarks of a cytokine storm. Interestingly, IL-10 may contribute either to inflammatory or anti-inflammatory responses to infection, depending on the stage and severity of disease.[72] It has been suggested that TGF-β1 may contribute to renal injury and fibrosis in incidental hosts. Virulence factors such as hemolytic toxins also may contribute to tissue damage, and surface lipoproteins such as LipL32 appear to be important in the pathogenesis of renal injury.[73]

Leptospiremia continues until the host mounts an effective acquired immune response, which clears the organism from bloodstream and most tissues. Thereafter, leptospires can persist in immune-privileged sites, such as the renal tubules and the eye.[1]

Differential expression of surface antigens of the spirochete may be responsible for its ability to evade host immune responses during the chronic shedding period.[74] Downregulation of TGF-β1 may lead to persistence of the organism in the absence of renal injury.[72]

The incubation period for acute leptospirosis is approximately 7 days, but may be shorter or longer depending on the dose and strain virulence, and the host immune response.[75]

Leptospirosis should be suspected in dogs that develop signs of acute febrile illness, kidney and/or hepatic injury, uveitis, pancreatitis in conjunction with kidney injury, or pulmonary hemorrhage; it should also be suspected in breeding dogs with abortion, stillbirths, or neonatal deaths.[76] In a study from Switzerland assessing the main organ manifestations (renal, hepatic, pulmonary, hemorrhagic) in 298 dogs with acute leptospirosis, 99.7% showed renal involvement, 35.4% showed hepatic involvement (as indicated by hepatic hyperbilirubinemia), 68.8% showed pulmonary involvement, and 18.4% signs were consistent with DIC. While most dogs (43.6%) demonstrated involvement of two different systems, 24.5% had involvement of only one organ, 23.2% of three, and 8.7% of all four systems.[57]

Fever, if present, occurs only at the onset of illness and is often accompanied by shivering, reluctance to move, and generalized muscle tenderness that may result from myositis. This may be followed by signs of lethargy, polyuria and polydipsia, inappetence, vomiting, and diarrhea.[77–87] GI signs in some dogs may result from pancreatitis and enteritis, in addition to acute renal and liver damage. Intestinal intussusception as a complication of acute leptospirosis, presumably associated with GI inflammation and motility disorders (paralytic ileus), has been described in several case reports.[88,89]

Polyuria and polydipsia may be the only initial sign and results from tubular dysfunction or a decreased responsiveness of the inner medullary connecting ducts to antidiuretic hormone (acquired nephrogenic diabetes insipidus). Oliguric/anuric renal failure was reported in 30% of dogs with acute leptospirosis from Switzerland.[57] During the acute phase, the predominant renal lesions are those of an acute interstitial nephritis, with tubular cell necrosis, apoptosis, and regeneration.[90,91] However, glomerular abnormalities have been described in both naturally infected dogs and experimentally infected animals with leptospirosis and indicate structural and functional glomerular involvement.[84,92] Tubular lesions are assumed to be due to direct effects of the organisms because renal lesions are generally associated with the presence of *Leptospira*,[90] and *Leptospira* outer membrane components can induce cell damage and inflammation in tubular epithelial cells *in vitro*[93] and *in vivo* using a zebrafish model.[94] During this phase of infection, a clinically significant reduction in renal function is present in most, but not all, patients with leptospirosis.[57,85]

Hepatic involvement can vary from mild liver enzyme elevations with or without hyperbilirubinemia to severe liver failure with signs of hepatic encephalopathy (Fig. 68.2). In human patients, both icteric and non-icteric forms of leptospirosis have been described, the icteric form being considered more severe and rapidly progressive.[1] This may also be true in dogs. In a cohort of 254 dogs with acute leptospirosis, a serum bilirubin of ≥10 μmol/L (reference range 0.5–4.0 μmol/L) was strongly associated (odds ratio 16.3; $P < 0.001$) with a negative outcome (death or euthanasia).[55] Hyperbilirubinemia coincided with the invasion of hepatic intercellular junction by migrating leptospires and disruption of bile canaliculi in experimentally infected hamsters.[95] In infected human and guinea pig livers, reduced staining for the cell-cell adhesion molecule E-cadherin was associated with liver plate disarray.[90] Hyperbilirubinemia and a cholestatic pattern of liver injury may be exacerbated by the presence of pancreatitis in some dogs.

Respiratory signs such as tachypnea and mild to severe dyspnea can occur in dogs with leptospirosis for many reasons, such as pulmonary edema due to overhydration, aspiration pneumonia, pain, or acidosis; however, clinicians should also consider leptospiral pulmonary hemorrhage (LPHS) as a cause of respiratory dysfunction. LPHS has been increasingly commonly reported in humans and animals with severe leptospirosis and has become a major cause of mortality.[56,57,96] Patients with LPHS can develop rapidly progressive intraalveolar pulmonary hemorrhage with cough, dyspnea, hemoptysis, and respiratory failure.

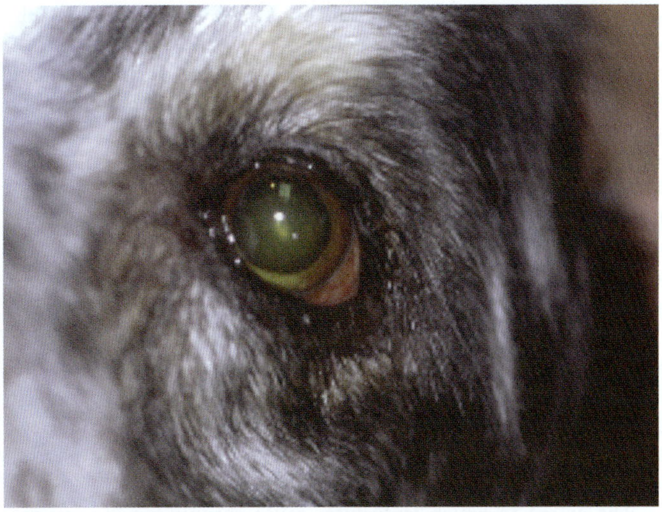

Fig. 68.2 Uveitis in an Australian shepherd with leptospirosis with leakage of serum bilirubin into the aqueous humor. (From Sykes JE. *Canine and Feline Infectious Diseases*. Elsevier; 2014.)

The pathogenic mechanisms of LPHS are poorly understood. Several hypotheses, including systemic inflammatory,[97,98] immune-mediated,[91,99,100] and direct leptospiral effects,[92,101] are under investigation. It is likely that the pathogenic mechanisms of LPHS are multifactorial, with both host- and pathogen-related factors playing a role.[102] The prevalence of LPHS in dogs appears to be particularly high in parts of continental Europe, with pulmonary complications reported in approximately two-thirds of dogs with leptospirosis in Berlin and a cohort from Switzerland.[57,87,96] It has therefore been hypothesized that LPHS may be linked to infection with specific regionally prevalent serovars or strains. However, the prevalence of LPHS may also be underrecognized in other parts of the world.

Bleeding tendencies in dogs with leptospirosis may be manifested as petechial hemorrhages, hematuria, hematemesis, epistaxis, hematochezia, punctate retinal hemorrhages, or melena.[79,84,103] Most dogs with leptospirosis in the United States show no evidence of bleeding diatheses. Although the precise mechanisms are unknown, bleeding tendencies may reflect endothelial damage and/or disordered coagulation.[104] Importantly, animals with LPHS can show severe intraalveolar hemorrhage in the absence of a systemic hemostatic disorder.[91]

Vasculitis can also contribute to the development of peripheral edema and mild pleural and peritoneal effusions. Electrocardiographic abnormalities, such as ventricular tachyarrhythmias, and elevations of serum troponin concentrations in some dogs suggest myocardial damage.[84,105] In human patients, aseptic meningitis is a common complication of leptospirosis and results in severe headache, delirium, and less commonly seizures or altered sensory perception.[1] Whether meningitis occurs in infected dogs is unknown, but mental dullness is often described in affected dogs, the severity of which may not be reflected by laboratory abnormalities.

Abortion is associated with leptospirosis in mares, cows, and sows; however, there are few reports in dogs. *Leptospira* serovar Buenos Aires (serogroup Djasiman) was isolated from an aborted fetus of a seropositive bitch.[106] Abortion and infertility was associated with a serogroup Batavia infection in a dog.[107]

Clinical signs in affected cats resemble those in dogs, although some cats have lacked evidence of hepatic injury and may show effusive disease.[37,38,45]

The role of persistent *Leptospira* infection as a cause of chronic kidney disease (CKD) in both cats and dogs requires more study. Progression of tubulointerstitial nephritis to tubular atrophy and renal fibrosis has been described in dogs infected with serovar Canicola[108] and rats infected with serovar Icterohaemorrhagiae.[109] A study from an endemic region in Brazil detected subclinical shedding of leptospires using PCR in 75% of 16 dogs with CKD and 21% of 48 healthy dogs.[110] In one study, cats with kidney disease (acute and chronic) were more likely to have antibodies against *Leptospira* spp. and to shed pathogenic leptospires in their urine than cats without kidney disease.[44] However, the prevalence of *Leptospira* antibodies in domestic cats is low and the vast majority of cats with kidney disease are seronegative.

The extent to which leptospires cause chronic hepatic injury in dogs is also unknown. In one report from France, leptospires were detected in bile canaliculi of young dogs with chronic hepatitis using immunohistochemistry and electron microscopy. These dogs showed signs of poor growth, weight loss, and ascites.[111] Chronic active hepatitis was associated with rising titers to serogroup Grippotyphosa in four of five American foxhounds living in a kennel.[112] Although noted as a cause of chronic hepatitis in dogs, attempts to detect *Leptospira* DNA in liver tissue from dogs with chronic hepatitis have generally been unrewarding.[112]

Physical Examination Findings

Findings on physical examination of dogs with leptospirosis vary with disease severity, chronicity, and possibly the infecting *Leptospira* strain. Severely affected dogs may show fever, dull mentation, dehydration, mild generalized peripheral lymphadenopathy, diffuse muscle pain, and pain on palpation of the abdomen or kidneys. Fever is typically only present early in the course of infection. In oliguric or anuric dogs that have been treated aggressively with intravenous fluids, evidence of overhydration may be present. Rarely, arrhythmias are detected on cardiac auscultation. Careful ophthalmologic examination may reveal conjunctivitis, scleral injection, and occasionally uveitis. Mild pallor, petechial or ecchymotic hemorrhages, and, less commonly, epistaxis may be present, although these findings appear to be rare in dogs from the United States and more commonly described in dogs from Europe. Respiratory difficulty, tachypnea, and harsh lung sounds may be evident in dogs that develop pulmonary complications. Dogs with liver involvement may be icteric. Rectal examination occasionally reveals melena or hematochezia. Young dogs with leptospirosis have been reported to develop severe systemic or skin calcifications in isolated case reports.[113,114]

DIAGNOSIS

Laboratory Abnormalities

Complete Blood Count

The hemogram in dogs with leptospirosis may reveal neutrophilia, sometimes with a left shift; nonregenerative anemia; lymphopenia; and/or thrombocytopenia (Table 68.2). Approximately half of dogs with leptospirosis have anemia, which is mostly mild to moderate. Causes of anemia can be blood loss via the respiratory or GI tract, vasculitis, and anemia of inflammatory disease. Hemolysis due to the effect of *Leptospira* toxins on erythrocytic membranes appears to be rare in dogs when compared to cattle or sheep, but rare cases of hemolytic anemia have been described in dogs.[115,116]

During the course of disease, leukemoid reactions with WBC counts $> 80 \times 10^9$/L have been rarely reported.[96] Thrombocytopenia occurs in up to 63% of dogs and can raise the level of suspicion for leptospirosis in dogs with acute kidney injury (AKI) with or without hepatic injury.[77,78,84,87,96] The mechanism is unclear. Consumption due to activation, adhesion, and aggregation to a stimulated vascular endothelium,[117] Kupffer cell phagocytosis,[118] immune-mediated platelet destruction,[119] or splenic sequestration could play variable roles.

Serum Biochemical Tests

Findings on the serum chemistry panel are shown in Tables 68.3 and 68.4. Azotemia is present in more than 80% to 90% of dogs,[57,77-79] although in two European studies, increased serum creatinine concentration was present in only 55% and 57% of affected dogs.[83,85] Hepatic injury, as evidenced by increases in the activities of serum ALT, AST, ALP, and hyperbilirubinemia, almost exclusively occur in conjunction with azotemia,[82,85] although isolated hepatic injury can occur. Typically a cholestatic pattern is present where there are mild to moderate increases in serum activity of ALP and total bilirubin, and mild increases in serum ALT activity. Dogs with very high serum liver enzyme activities (e.g., ALT in the thousands) and evidence of hepatic failure (i.e., hypocholesterolemia, hypoglycemia) are unlikely to have leptospirosis. Severe increases in serum total bilirubin concentration may reflect concurrent presence of *Leptospira*-induced pancreatitis.

Other findings on the serum chemistry panel include hypoalbuminemia and a variety of electrolyte abnormalities. Hyponatremia, hypochloremia, or hyperphosphatemia occur in most dogs. Decreased expression of sodium transporters by proximal convoluted tubule cells contributes to impaired sodium resorption, increased distal sodium delivery, and potassium wasting.[120] As a result, dogs with acute oliguric renal failure may have paradoxical hypokalemia or normokalemia rather than hyperkalemia.

Moderately and occasionally markedly increased serum CK activity is present in some dogs due to myositis. Increased serum troponin concentrations have been found in some dogs with leptospirosis, which suggests myocardial damage.[84,105] Increased serum pancreatic lipase immunoreactivity may occur, probably as a result of pancreatitis, or decreased renal excretion.[77,84]

Coagulation Function

In experimentally and naturally occurring leptospirosis in dogs, varying degrees of thrombocytopenia, reduced fibrinogen concentration, prolonged activated partial thromboplastin and prothrombin time values, reduced antithrombin activity, increased D-dimer concentration, and increased fibrinogen degradation products have been found, presumably as a result of excessive intravascular coagulation.[84,96,104,121] In many dogs, clotting parameters are within reference limits, or variable thrombocytopenia may be the only abnormality, suggesting compensated hemostatic mechanisms. The degree of thrombocytopenia in dogs with leptospirosis has been correlated with the severity of pulmonary manifestations and higher mortality.[96]

Urinalysis

Findings on urinalysis in dogs with leptospirosis include isosthenuria, occasionally hyposthenuria, and variable glucosuria, proteinuria, pyuria, cylindruria, and bilirubinuria.[82,84] UPCRs may be increased, although typically not as high as that occurring in dogs with Lyme nephritis (which is primarily a glomerulonephritis rather than an interstitial nephritis). Urine protein electrophoresis revealed that both high-molecular-weight proteins consistent with glomerular damage and/or low-molecular-weight proteins consistent with a tubular origin can be present.[84,122]

TABLE 68.2 Clinical Findings in Dogs with Leptospirosis

	USA (MA)[77]	USA (NJ)[78]	USA (NY)[79]	USA (NY)[82]	USA (CA)[80]	USA (LA)[86]	Canada (Ontario)[81]	Switzerland[83]	Italy[84]	South Germany[85]	Northeast Germany[96]
Number of dogs	17	17	36	55	36	51	31	11	16	42	50
Anorexia % (n)	NR	NR	67 (24)	75 (41)	68 (24)	57 (29)	81 (25)	73 (8)	69 (11)	76 (32)	84 (42)
Vomiting % (n)	NR	NR	50 (18)	64 (35)	88 (33)	41 (21)	81 (25)	82 (9)	81 (13)	57 (24)	72 (36)
Lethargy % (n)	24 (4)	88 (15)	58 (21)	78 (43)	65 (23)	43 (22)	90 (28)	18 (2)	87.5 (14)	81 (42)	90 (45)
Abdominal pain % (n)	29 (5)	35 (6)	33 (12)	22 (12)	42 (15)	NR	65 (20)	45 (5)	37.5 (6)	19 (8)	36 (18)
Diarrhea % (n)	24 (4)	6 (1)	33 (12)	29 (16)	NR	12 (6)	NR	36 (4)	38 (6)	40 (17)	50 (25)
Icterus % (n)	NR	35 (6)	11 (4)	13 (7)	NR	NR	29 (9)	36 (4)	17 (2)	45 (18)	10 (5)
Dehydration % (n)	NR	NR	36 (13)	26 (14)	NR	NR	52 (16)	27 (3)	NR	31 (13)	6 (3)
Stiffness / musculoskeletal pain % (n)	12 (2)	17 (3)	25 (9)	NR	23 (9)	2 (1)	35 (11)	NR	44 (7)	NR	8 (4)
Fever (rectal temp. ≥39.5°C) % (n)	6 (1)	6 (1)	11 (4)	9 (5)	15 (4)	NR	13 (4)	18 (2)	19 (3)	36 (15)	8 (4)
Hypothermia (rectal temp <38°C) % (n)	12 (2)	12 (2)	NR	NR	22 (8)	NR	NR	36 (4)	38 (6)	17 (7)	6 (3)
Oliguria/anuria % (n)	NR	NR	6 (2)	NR	39 (14)	4 (2)	NR	18 (2)	44 (7)	NR	20 (10)
Dyspnea/ tachypnea % (n)	6 (1)	NR	3 (1)	NR	NR	2 (1)	35 (11)	NR	44 (7)	NR	38 (19)
Weakness % (n)	NR	NR	39 (14)	NR	NR	NR	NR	18 (2)	NR	52 (21)	NR
Polyuria/ polydipsia % (n)	NR	NR	50 (18)	31 (17)	NR	NR	NR	27 (3)	NR	NR	NR
Weight loss % (n)	NR	NR	44 (16)	35 (19)	NR	NR	NR	9 (1)	NR	17 (7)	NR

NR, not reported.

TABLE 68.3 Selected Hematological Alterations in Dogs with Leptospirosis

	USA (MA)[77]	USA (NJ)[78]	USA (NY)[79]	USA (NY)[82]	USA (CA)[80]	USA (LA)[86]	Canada (Ontario)[81]	Canada (Saskatchewan)[14]	Switzerland[83]	Italy[84]	South Germany[85]	Northeast Germany[96]
Number of dogs	17	17	36	54	31	51	31	15	11	16	42	50
Anemia % (n)	24 (4)	18 (3)	33 (12)	53 (29)	NR	NR	45 (14)	NR	NR	38 (6)	45 (19)	50 (25)
Leukocytosis % (n)	47 (8)	53 (9)	31 (11)	37 (20)	55 (17)	NR	58 (18)	27 (4)	81 (9)	63 (10)	81 (34)	68 (34)
Leukopenia % (n)	NR	NR	NR	NR	NR	NR	NR	7 (1)	9 (1)	6 (1)	NR	NR
Neutrophilia % (n)	65 (11)	53 (9)	31 (11)	50 (27)	52 (16)	NR	61 (19)	27 (4)	NR	63 (10)	65 (25)	68 (30/44)
Left shift % (n)	NR	NR	6 (2)	NR	3 (1)	NR	NR	NR	81 (9)	NR	65 (25)	25 (11/44)
Monocytosis % (n)	29 (5)	NR	NR	NR	NR	NR	42 (13)	NR	NR	NR	NR	68 (30/44)
Lymphopenia % (n)	NR	NR	NR	NR	NR	NR	NR	NR	NR	NR	NR	2 (1/44)
Thrombocytopenia % (n)	56 (5/9)	24 (4)	14 (5)	30 (13/44)	55 (17)	51 (26)	35 (11)	NR	NR	7 (44)	53 (21/40)	58 (29)

NR, not reported

TABLE 68.4 Selected Biochemical Alterations in Dogs with Leptospirosis												
	USA (MA)[77]	USA (NJ)[78]	USA (NY)[79]	USA (CA)[80]	Canada (Ontario)[81]	Canada (Saskatchewan)[14]	USA (NY)[82]	Switzerland[83]	Italy[84]	South Germany[85]	Northeast Germany[96]	USA (LA)[86]
Number of dogs	17	17	36	31	31	15	54	11	16	42	50	51
Increased creatinine % (n)	100 (17)	82 (14)	83 (30)	100 (36)	87(27)	80 (12)	93 (50)	55 (6)	100 (16)	57 (24)	88 (44) 92 (46)*	71 (36)
Increased urea % (n)	100 (17)	82 (14)	81 (29)	100 (36)	94 (29)	73 (11)	93 (50)	54 (6)	100 (16)	62 (26)	88 (44)	75 (38)
Increased ALT % (n)	35 (6)	35 (6)	33 (12)	NR	26 (8)	33 (5)	32 (17)	55 (6)	69 (11)	74 (31)	78 (37/48)	51 (26)
Increased AST % (n)	29 (5)	NR	39 (14)	NR	NR	NR	56 (30)	55 (6)	69 (11)	61 (22/36)	NR	47 (24)
Increased ALP % (n)	59 (10)	65 (11)	56 (20)	19 (7)	58 (18)	33 (5)	57 (31)	55 (6)	63 (10)	69 (29)	90 (42/47)	59 (30)
Hyperbilirubinemia % (n)	24 (4)	42 (7)	17 (6)	22 (8)	68 (21)	33 (5)	41 (22)	55 (6)	56 (9)	79 (34)	73(35/48)	37 (19)
Hyperkalemia % (n)	17 (3)	12 (2)	NR	NR	NR	NR	NR	NR	31 (5)	12 (5/41)	NR	NR
Hypokalemia % (n)	17 (3)	NR	NR	NR	NR	NR	41 (22)	NR	NR	NR	NR	NR
Hyperphosphatemia % (n)	42 (7)	47 (8)	50 (18)	NR	NR	NR	78 (42)	55 (6)	94 (15)	45 (18/40)	NR	55 (28)
Hypophosphatemia % (n)	12 (2)	NR	NR	NR	NR	NR	NR	NR	NR	NR	NR	NR
Hypochloremia % (n)	12 (2)	NR	NR	NR	NR	NR	46 (25)	NR	25 (4)	NR	NR	NR
Hyponatremia % (n)	12 (2)	NR	NR	NR	NR	NR	17 (9)	NR	19 (3)	NR	NR	NR
Hypoalbuminemia % (n)	13 (3)	NR	NR	NR	NR	NR	35 (19)	64 (7)	75 (12)	NR	NR	NR

NR, not reported

Leptospires are not visible in routine urine sediment examination because the width of the organism is below the resolution of light microscopy.

Diagnostic Imaging

Plain thoracic radiography in dogs with leptospirosis may show no abnormalities, or mild to severe, diffuse interstitial pulmonary patterns may be present. Thoracic radiographs from dogs with LPHS can show severe focal to diffuse interstitial and alveolar patterns (Fig. 68.3). Initially, radiographic pulmonary changes typically appear in the caudodorsal parts of the lung fields.[96] Uncommonly, mild pleural effusion is present. Thoracic radiography might underestimate the lesion type and the severity in dogs with leptospirosis as compared with thoracic CT.[123]

Findings on abdominal sonography in dogs with leptospirosis include mild renomegaly, increased renal cortical echogenicity, cortical thickening, mild pyelectasia, perirenal fluid accumulation or mild ascites, a medullary band of increased echogenicity within the kidneys, and reduced corticomedullary definition (Fig. 68.4A).[124,125] None of these signs are specific for leptospirosis. Ultrasonographic changes suggestive of pancreatitis are occasionally present, such as enlargement and hypoechogenicity of the pancreas (Fig. 68.4B). Thickening of the gastric and, less commonly, small intestinal wall may also be present. Mild to moderate hepatomegaly, hypoechoic hepatic echotexture, and splenomegaly with mottling of the splenic echotexture may be detected, with or without evidence of mild abdominal lymphadenomegaly.

Microbiologic Tests

Diagnostic assays available for leptospirosis in dogs are summarized in Table 68.5.

Darkfield Microscopy

Examination of voided urine using darkfield microscopy is insensitive for diagnosis of leptospirosis. Considerable experience is required to accurately identify the spirochetes, so false positives also have the potential to occur.

Culture

Culture of leptospires is not routinely performed, because it is often slow, insensitive, and not widely available. Special *Leptospira* growth medium, such as Ellinghausen-McCullough-Johnson-Harris (EMJH) or Hornsby-Alt-Nally (HAN) medium, is required.[126] Cultures may require incubation for weeks, and overgrowth with other bacteria can occur if cultures become contaminated. Venous blood and/or urine should be collected using aseptic technique before initiating antimicrobial drug treatment. Ideally, a few drops of blood or urine are inoculated directly into culture medium alongside the patient. In humans, blood is optimally collected during the initial febrile period; urine can be collected after the first week of illness. Because the exact time of infection may be unknown, submission of both blood and urine can increase the chance of a positive test result.

Only certain reference laboratories have expertise in culture of leptospires and the ability to identify leptospires to the serovar level, which is performed using a cross agglutinin absorption test. Molecular typing methods can also be performed. Despite the difficulties associated with culture and identification of leptospires, a proper understanding of the epidemiology of leptospirosis depends on the use of these methods.

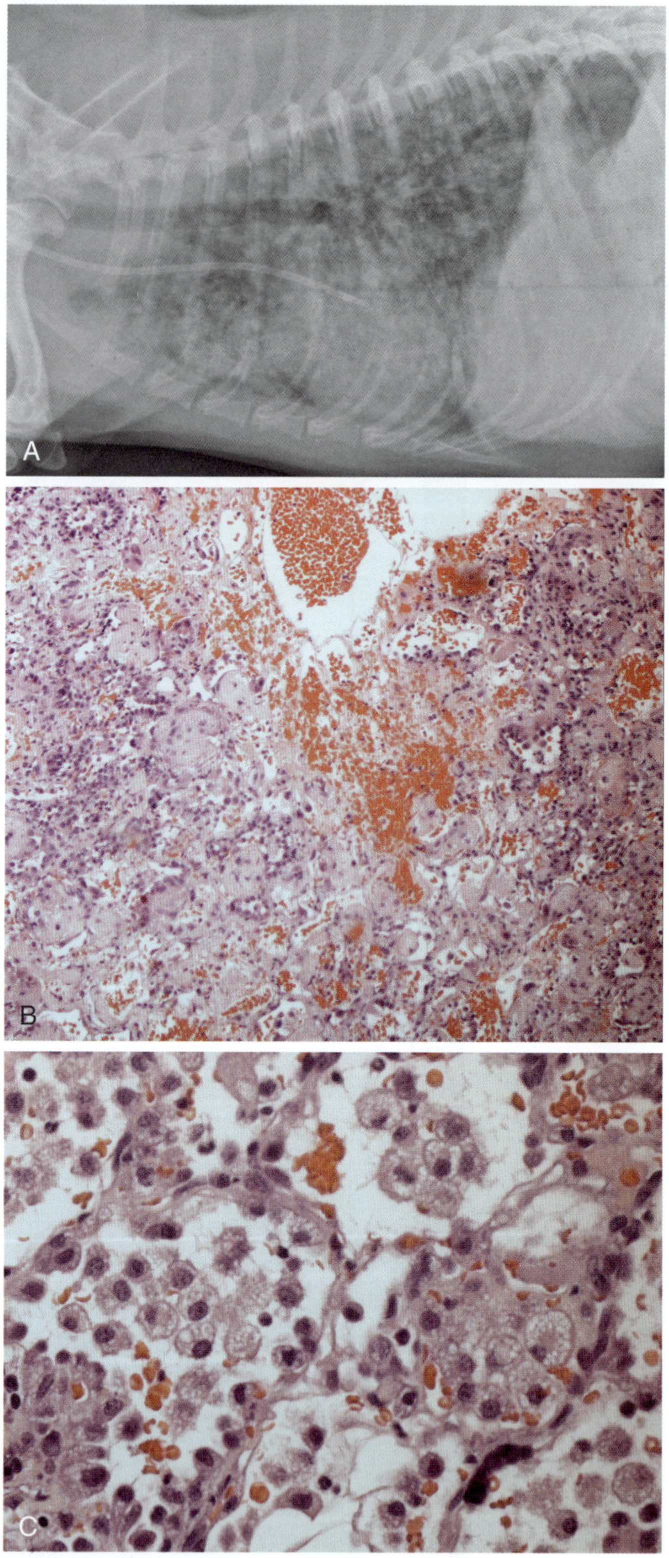

Fig. 68.3 Images from a 4-year-old male neutered Havanese terrier with severe leptospiral pulmonary hemorrhage syndrome and anuric renal failure. (A) Right lateral thoracic radiograph. A severe, diffuse alveolar pattern is present. Mechanical ventilation was needed and ultimately euthanasia was performed because of respiratory failure. Histopathology of a lung biopsy showed severe pulmonary hemorrhage (B) and marked alveolar histiocytosis (C). (From Sykes JE. *Canine and Feline Infectious Diseases*. Elsevier; 2014.)

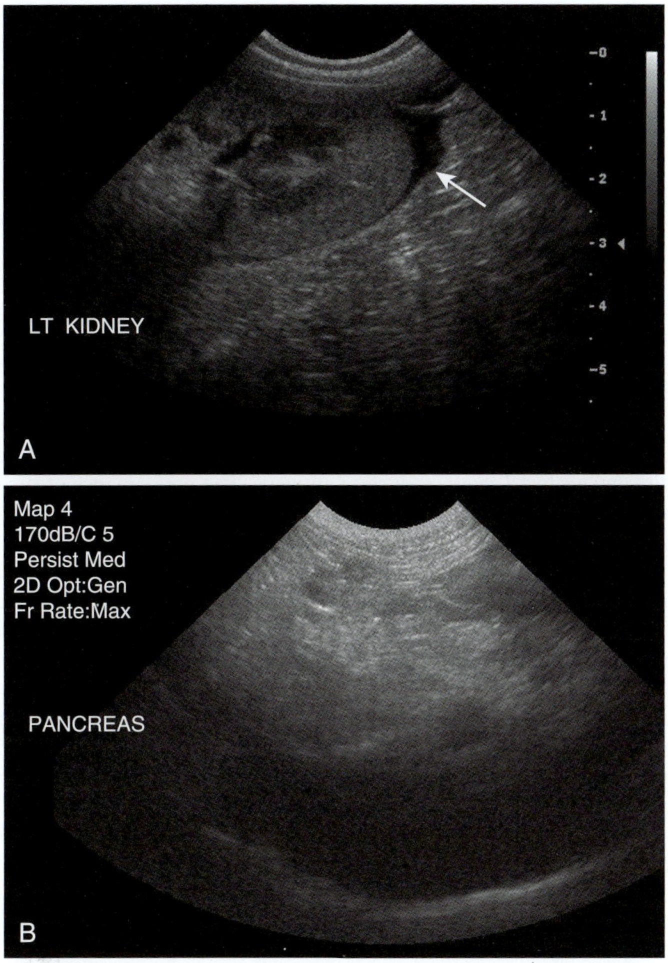

Fig. 68.4 (A) Abdominal sonogram image showing perirenal fluid accumulation in a 1.5-year-old male neutered kelpie with renal failure due to acute leptospirosis. (B) Abdominal sonogram image showing evidence of pancreatitis in a 6-year-old male neutered Australian cattle dog with leptospirosis. (Courtesy of University of California-Davis VMTH Diagnostic Imaging Service.)

Serologic Diagnosis

When performed properly, serologic diagnosis of leptospirosis is retrospective, and so dogs that are suspected to have leptospirosis should be treated as such until the results of serologic testing are available. Currently the test of choice for diagnosis of leptospirosis is serology using the MAT.[76,127] In this assay, serial dilutions of patient sera are incubated with a panel of live *Leptospira* serovars. This serovar panel should be defined based on the antibody prevalence data for the host species in the relevant geographic location, as failure to include the infecting serogroup can lead to false-negative results. Agglutination of leptospires by serum anti-*Leptospira* IgM and IgG is then assessed using darkfield microscopy (Fig. 68.5). The highest dilution of serum that causes ≥50% of the organisms of each serovar to agglutinate is reported either as titer (i.e., 100) or as reciprocal titer (i.e., 1:100).

The MAT has marked limitations with regard to sensitivity, specificity, and repeatability, especially if only single titers are interpreted.[128,129] Infected dogs are often antibody negative or have low titers early on in the course of illness, because of the relatively short incubation period and the normal delay in appearance of serum antibodies. On the other hand, noninfected dogs vaccinated with whole-cell *Leptospira* vaccines can have post-vaccinal titers of 1:6400 or higher to both vaccinal and nonvaccinal serovars.[130–132] While the majority of vaccinated dogs become antibody negative by week 15 post vaccination, vaccinal titers can persist for 12 months in a small percentage of dogs.[131] In addition, dogs evaluated for illness other than leptospirosis may possess antibodies from previous subclinical infection. A moderate to high titer very early in the course of illness (when most dogs are negative or have low titers) may actually be a clue to these confounders. Reactivity of anti-*Leptospira* antibodies with multiple serogroups and inclusion of only a limited number of serovars in the panel typically prevents determination of the infecting serogroup. Moreover, the serogroup with the highest MAT titer can vary over time ("paradoxical seroreactivity"), and the MAT does not reliably predict the infecting serogroup in acutely infected animals.[129]

Because a positive MAT can result from recent subclinical exposure or vaccination, the most reliable means to confirm a recent infection by MAT is to test paired samples, collected 10 to 14 days apart.[128,129] Waiting much longer than 2 weeks to collect the convalescent specimen is not recommended as the titer may begin to decline, so any change in

TABLE 68.5 Diagnostic Assays Available for Leptospirosis in Dogs

Assay	Specimen Type	Target	Performance
Darkfield microscopy	Urine	Leptospires	Low sensitivity and specificity. Requires technical expertise to interpret correctly.
Culture	Whole blood, urine	Leptospires	Low sensitivity. Special media and prolonged incubation times required. Difficult and not widely available. Antimicrobial therapy may lead to false-negative results.
Microscopic agglutination test	Serum	Antibodies against various *Leptospira* serovars	False negatives can occur early in the course of illness or with immunosuppression. False positives can occur with a history of vaccination or with previous exposure. Paired titers performed at the same laboratory generally required for diagnosis. Inter-laboratory variation in results may occur.
Rapid diagnostic chromatographic or ELISA-based tests	Serum or plasma	IgM or IgG against *Leptospira*	False negatives can occur early in the course of illness or with immunosuppression. False positives can occur with a history of vaccination or with previous exposure.
Histopathology	Kidney tissue collected via biopsy or necropsy	Leptospires	Organisms may be visualized with silver stains, immunohistochemistry, or FISH. Antimicrobial therapy may lead to false-negative results.
PCR	Blood, urine, tissue specimens	*Leptospira* DNA	Sensitivity and specificity unclear and may vary between assays offered by different laboratories. Antimicrobial therapy may lead to negative PCR results.

titer could be missed. The rise in titer may also be somewhat blunted by early antimicrobial treatment, and delayed responses have also been documented in humans (Fig. 68.6). Obtaining a serum sample for a follow-up titer at the time of discharge from the hospital (or at the first recheck appointment after discharge) could be a practical approach. A fourfold or greater rise in MAT is highly suggestive of leptospirosis (e.g., a titer of 1:200 rises to 1:800, corresponding to the fact that the serum is positive for two more consecutive dilutions—this represents a significant change in titer) or when an initially antibody-negative dog exhibits a convalescent titer ≥ 800 to one or multiple serovars.

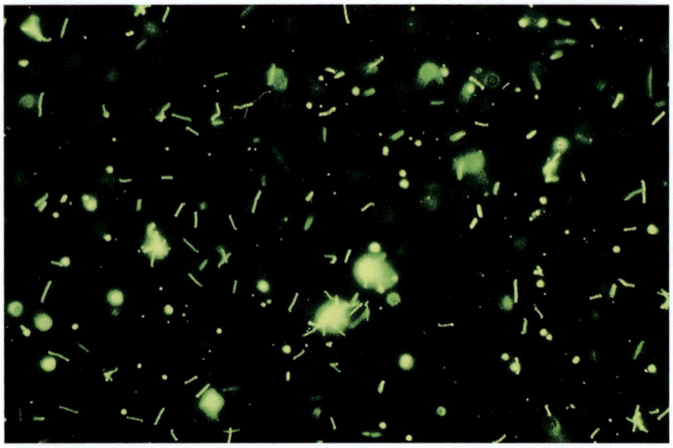

Fig. 68.5 Leptospires viewed using darkfield microscopy (original magnification ×100). (Courtesy of Mildred Galton, Public Health Image Library, Centers for Disease Control and Prevention. In: Bennett JE, Dolin R, Blaser MJ, eds. *Mandell, Douglas and Bennett's Principles and Practice of Infectious Diseases*. Philadelphia, PA: Elsevier; 2020:2898–2905.)

The MAT is widely available and relatively inexpensive in the United States, but is complex to perform and interpret. Performance of the test is hazardous to laboratory workers because live serovars are used, and the test is difficult to standardize. The identity of serovars used in the assay must be verified periodically to ensure that cross-contamination or culture deterioration has not occurred. A leptospirosis proficiency testing scheme is offered by the International Leptospirosis Society (ILS) to assist laboratories in the maintenance of quality assurance for the MAT.[133] Veterinarians should strive to use laboratories that participate in this quality assurance scheme, and should use the same laboratory on a regular basis.

Other serologic assays available for diagnosis of leptospirosis include ELISAs and chromatographic assays for IgG and IgM antibodies that are directed against *Leptospira* surface antigens. The performance of such assays have the potential to vary geographically based on the serogroups that are prevalent in the region. In Europe and in the United States, lateral-flow chromatographic assays detecting canine anti-*Leptospira* antibodies are commercially available (e.g., Test-it *Leptospira* Canine IgM Lateral Flow Assay, Life Assay; WITNESS Lepto Rapid Test, Zoetis; SNAP Lepto, IDEXX Laboratories; Immunocomb Canine *Leptospira* Antibody Test Kit, Biogal Galed Laboratories). At the time of writing, only the SNAP Lepto and WITNESS assays are available in the United States. The Test-it and WITNESS assays are IgM-based assays based on antigen from *L. interrogans* serovar Copenhageni strain Wijnberg or filtered whole-cell extracts of serovars Grippotyphosa and Bratislava,

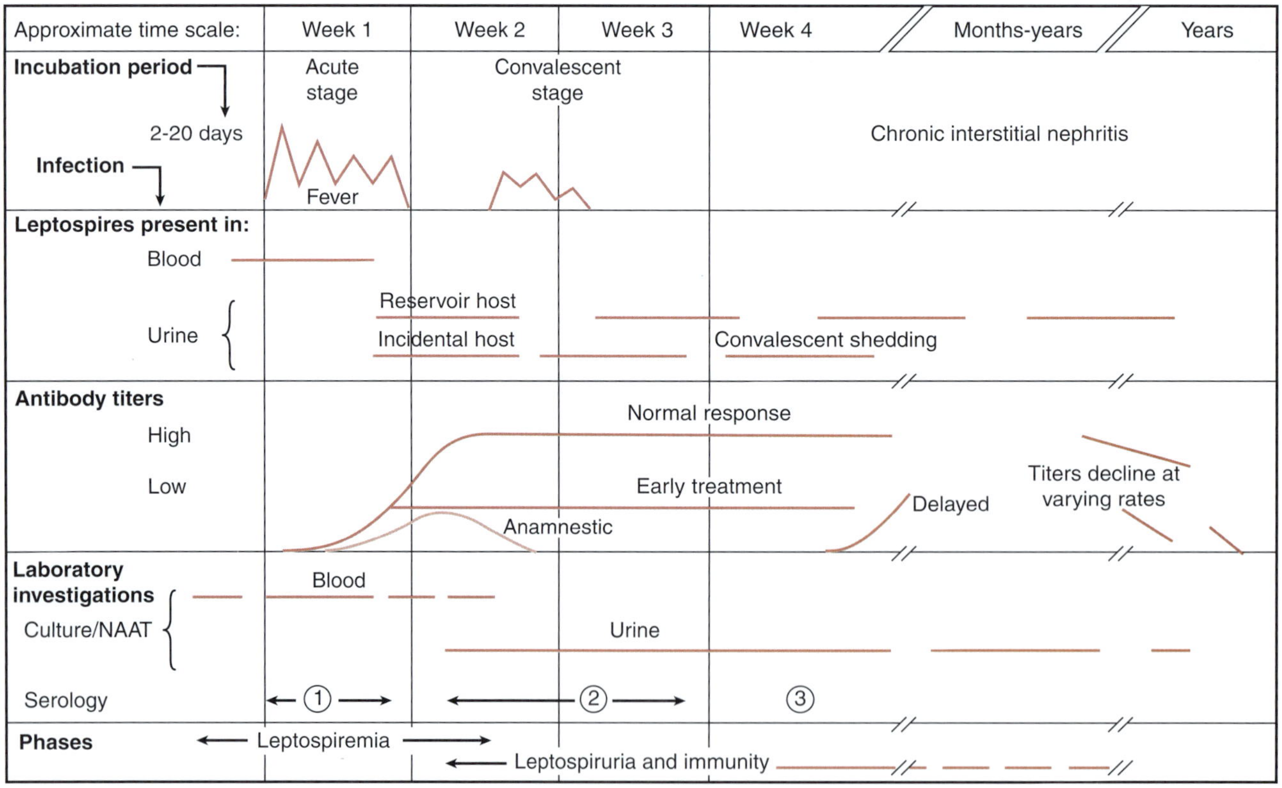

Fig. 68.6 Biphasic nature of leptospirosis and relevant investigations at different stages of disease. Specimens 1 and 2 for serology are acute and early convalescent phase specimens; 3 is a late convalescent phase specimen. (Modified from Turner LH. Leptospirosis. *Br Med J*. 1969;1:231-235; Levett PN. Leptospirosis. *Clin Microbiol Rev*. 2001;14:296-326; and Haake DA, Levett PN. *Leptospira* species (Leptospirosis). In: Bennett JE, Dolin R, Blaser MJ, eds. *Mandell, Douglas and Bennett's Principles and Practice of Infectious Diseases*. Philadelphia, PA: Elsevier; 2020:2898-2905.)

respectively, which are proteolytically digested and heat treated to make them broadly reactive with antibodies raised in response to infection with a wide range of serogroups. The SNAP Lepto assay uses a recombinant LipL32 antigen, found only in pathogenic leptospires, as the basis for detection of IgG and IgM antibodies to *Leptospira*, and is available as a diagnostic laboratory-based ELISA assay as well as a POC lateral-flow assay. The Immunocomb kit is a POC-modified ELISA assay designed to detect IgM and IgG antibodies to *L. interrogans* serovars Icterohaemorrhagiae, Canicola, Pomona, and Grippotyphosa. The performance of these assays when compared to acute and convalescent MAT serology requires further validation using a large number of dogs from a broad range of geographic locations. Because these are antibody assays, dogs may test negative early in the course of illness. In one study of experimentally infected beagle dogs, positive test results were more prevalent at day 10 after challenge with the WITNESS assay (100% of 32 dogs) and MAT (80–100% of dogs) when compared with the SNAP Lepto (10%).[134] These rapid POC assays may be useful to rapidly screen for an *absence* of antibodies as an alternative to relying on MAT, which is more expensive and has a slower turnaround time.[135] A negative test result could be followed with a second POC test 1 to 2 weeks later (to show a change from negative to positive should seroconversion have occurred). Positive results may reflect the presence of antibodies due to previous vaccination or exposure, so in this situation a titer should be immediately determined using MAT, with a convalescent titer performed 1 to 2 weeks later to demonstrate a fourfold rise in titer. Because the WITNESS and Test-it assays are IgM-based assays, they are less likely to be influenced by previous exposure and vaccination. However, one study showed that 12 weeks after vaccination of 25 healthy beagle dogs with a 4-serovar *Leptospira* vaccine, 6 dogs still tested positive with the WITNESS assay.[136] Therefore, even 3 months after vaccination or previous exposure, IgM-detection assays have the potential to remain positive, further underscoring the importance of obtaining quantitative acute and convalescent phase titers to confirm recent exposure.

Molecular Diagnosis Using Nucleic Acid–Based Testing

Several veterinary diagnostic laboratories in the United States and Europe offer real-time PCR assays for the detection of the DNA of pathogenic leptospires in blood and/or urine, or tissue specimens collected at necropsy such as liver and kidneys. The assays are commonly based on the amplification of segments of the 16S or 23S ribosomal RNA gene sequences[137] or the LipL32 gene, which is specific for pathogenic *Leptospira* spp.[138-140] The sensitivity and specificity of these assays in dogs with leptospirosis have not been thoroughly assessed. However, positive results were documented in 13% of free catch canine urine specimens in one study due to amplification of contamination of random bacterial DNA by a 16S rDNA PCR method.[141] Thus, assay performance likely varies from one laboratory to another. In-clinic PCR assays have also been developed to detect pathogenic leptospires in dogs (e.g., PCRun, Biogal Galed Laboratories, Israel),[142] although the clinical sensitivity and specificity of these assays require further study.

PCR assays have the potential to be advantageous for rapid diagnosis early in the course of illness, when serologic tests are negative and organism numbers in the blood are high. In a study in dogs experimentally infected with *L. interrogans* serovar Canicola, both culture and *lipL32* PCR in blood were positive on day 4 and negative thereafter, whereas urine culture and *lipL32* PCR were negative on day 4 and positive on day 8, 19, and 26.[139] Findings in this untreated cohort reflect the classic concept of an initial leptospiremic phase followed by urinary shedding. However, in naturally infected dogs, the exact time of infection is typically unknown, therefore testing of both blood and urine collected before initiation of antimicrobial drug treatment should be submitted in order to optimize sensitivity. The use of stabilizers to neutralize the urine pH and to inactivate DNases in order to preserve *Leptospira* DNA might be advantageous.[143] Even with sensitive PCR assays, negative results do not rule out a diagnosis of leptospirosis because dogs may shed very low numbers of organisms or shedding may be intermittent. Because subclinically infected dogs can shed leptospires, a positive PCR test result on urine may not necessarily correlate with illness. The prevalence of urinary shedding as detected using PCR was 0% of 100 dogs seen at the University of California-Davis VMTH with problems other than leptospirosis[144]; 13% of 198 shelter dogs from Tennessee, Virginia, and Kentucky[145]; 7.1% of 525 dogs from shelters and a veterinary teaching hospital in Ireland[138]; 1.5% of 200 healthy pet dogs in Germany[146]; 4.4% of dogs from New Caledonia[147]; 4.4% of 273 dogs from Thailand[148]; and 10.6% of 123 stray and shelter dogs in Brazil.[149] Vaccination of healthy dogs with inactivated *Leptospira* vaccines should not lead to positive PCR assay results,[132] so a history of *Leptospira* vaccination should not interfere with PCR diagnosis. Available PCR assays do not provide information on the infecting serovar or serogroup. However, techniques such as MLST and VNTR can be applied to PCR products for typing of the infecting strain, and in some cases this can be correlated to a serotype identity.[18] Correlation to the serovar level is not straightforward, and can require isolation and accurate serotyping and molecular typing of leptospires infecting dogs in the region, which can then be used as a reference for comparison.

Ultimately, application of a combination of serologic assays and PCR may optimize diagnosis of leptospirosis in dogs.[150] Figure 68.7 illustrates a possible approach to diagnosis through the use of a combination of MAT, POC assays, and PCR.

Machine Learning

Because of the characteristic patterns of laboratory abnormalities in leptospirosis, the disease lends itself well to diagnosis using machine learning. An algorithm for early diagnosis of leptospirosis that took into account CBC, serum biochemistry, and urinalysis findings had a sensitivity of 94% and a specificity of 98% when applied to the hospital population at the University of California-Davis. An algorithm that also included the results of an acute MAT had a sensitivity of 92% and specificity of 90%.[151]

Pathologic Findings

Gross Pathologic Findings

Gross pathologic findings in dogs with leptospirosis include jaundice, petechial and ecchymotic hemorrhages, and sometimes fibrin thrombi throughout the body. The lungs of dogs with LPHS may be wet, mottled, heavy, and dark-pink to red in color.[152] Ascites and/or pleural or pericardial effusion may be present, and the intestinal lumen may be filled with blood or contain melena. The kidneys of dogs with acute disease may be mildly enlarged, pale, and sometimes mottled or petechiated; they may also contain infarcts. Dogs with chronic renal injury secondary to leptospirosis can have kidneys that are shrunken and irregular (Fig. 68.8).

Histopathologic Findings

Infection of the kidneys by leptospires leads to an interstitial nephritis, with mixed inflammatory infiltrates. Acute tubular necrosis can also occur as a result of vasculitis and renal ischemia (Fig. 68.9A).[36]

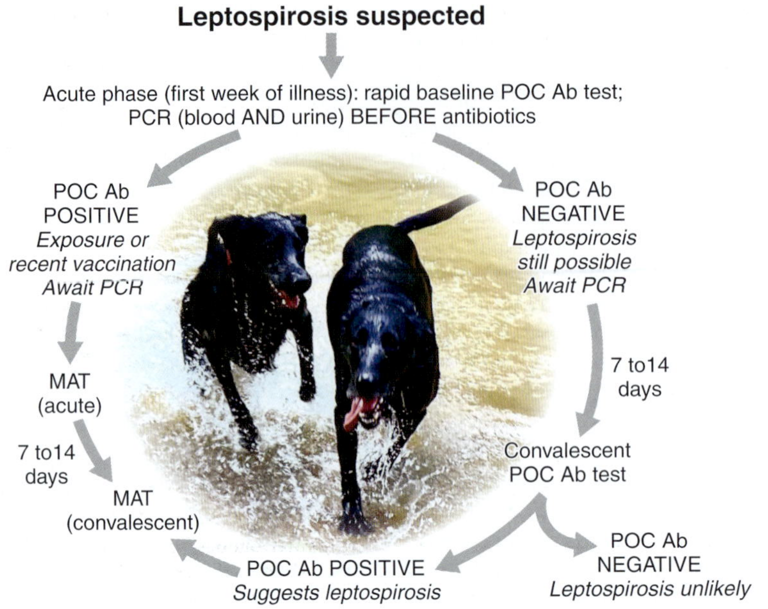

Fig. 68.7 Diagnostic algorithm that could be used to optimize diagnosis of leptospirosis using a combination of POC lateral-flow assays, PCR, and MAT.

Histopathologic changes in the liver are often mild and include mild random hepatic necrosis, mild neutrophilic periportal hepatitis, cholestasis, or liver plate disarray (Fig. 68.10). Multifocal, random, neutrophilic, and necrotizing myocarditis can also occur; myonecrosis is occasionally described in skeletal muscle. Histopathologic lesions of LPHS are similar across species and are characterized by various degrees of intraalveolar hemorrhage in the absence of a marked inflammatory cell infiltrate or vasculitis. Intraalveolar edema, fibrin, and hyaline membranes which are characteristic of disorders with diffuse alveolar damage can be present, but are not a predominant feature.[91,152,153] In contrast to liver and kidney, few organisms are present in lung tissue of immunocompetent hosts and do not co-localize with the pulmonary lesions.[91,100]

Silver stains such as Warthin-Starry stain and immunohistochemistry can be used to visualize bacteria within tissue specimens (see Fig. 68.9B). Direct fluorescent antibody staining and FISH (see Fig. 6.1B) have also been used to identify and localize leptospires within the kidneys. However, the number of organisms in incidental hosts is typically low and if antimicrobials were administered, spirochetes may be absent.

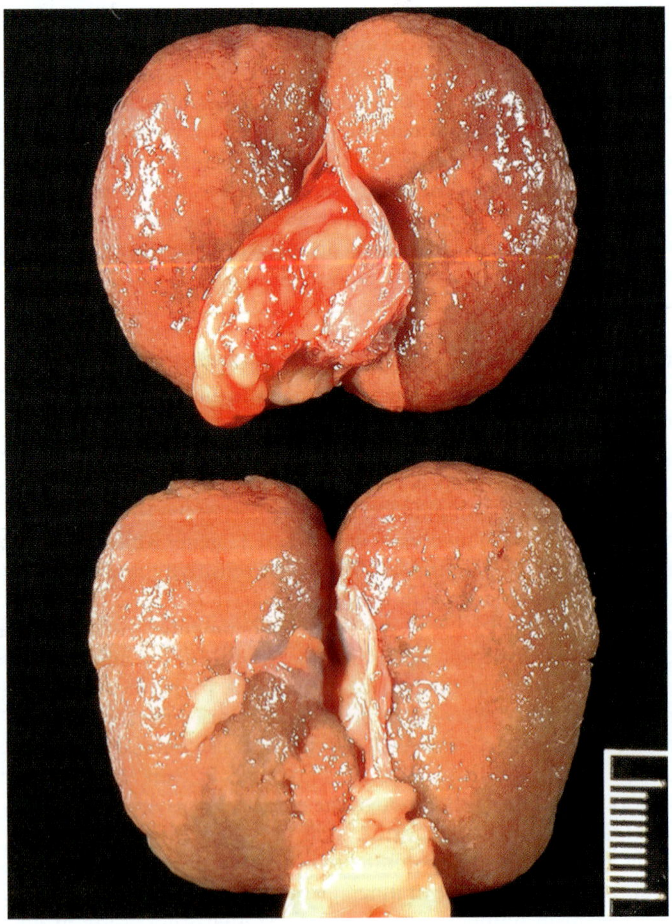

Fig. 68.8 Shrunken, irregular kidneys from a 16-year-old male neutered Jack Russell terrier. The dog was treated for severe acute leptospirosis at 12 years of age. At that time, after six dialysis treatments, the dog was discharged from the hospital with a creatinine of 4.2 mg/dL. Four years later, the dog died for reasons unrelated to renal injury but had evidence of chronic renal injury at necropsy. (Courtesy of UC Davis Veterinary Anatomic Pathology Service.)

TREATMENT

Effective treatment of acute leptospirosis involves appropriate antimicrobial therapy and supportive therapy for involved organ systems.

Antimicrobial Drugs

Leptospires are susceptible to a wide range of antibiotics. Treatment should be initiated as early as possible, before the results of diagnostic assays become available. In hamster models, doxycycline clears spirochetes from all tissues, including the kidney, within 3 days of infection; ampicillin is less effective at clearing organisms from the kidney.[154] Based on current evidence, current consensus statements on leptospirosis in dogs recommend that all dogs with leptospirosis should be treated with doxycycline, 5 mg/kg q12h or 10 mg/kg q24h for 2 weeks.[76,127] If vomiting or other adverse reactions preclude the

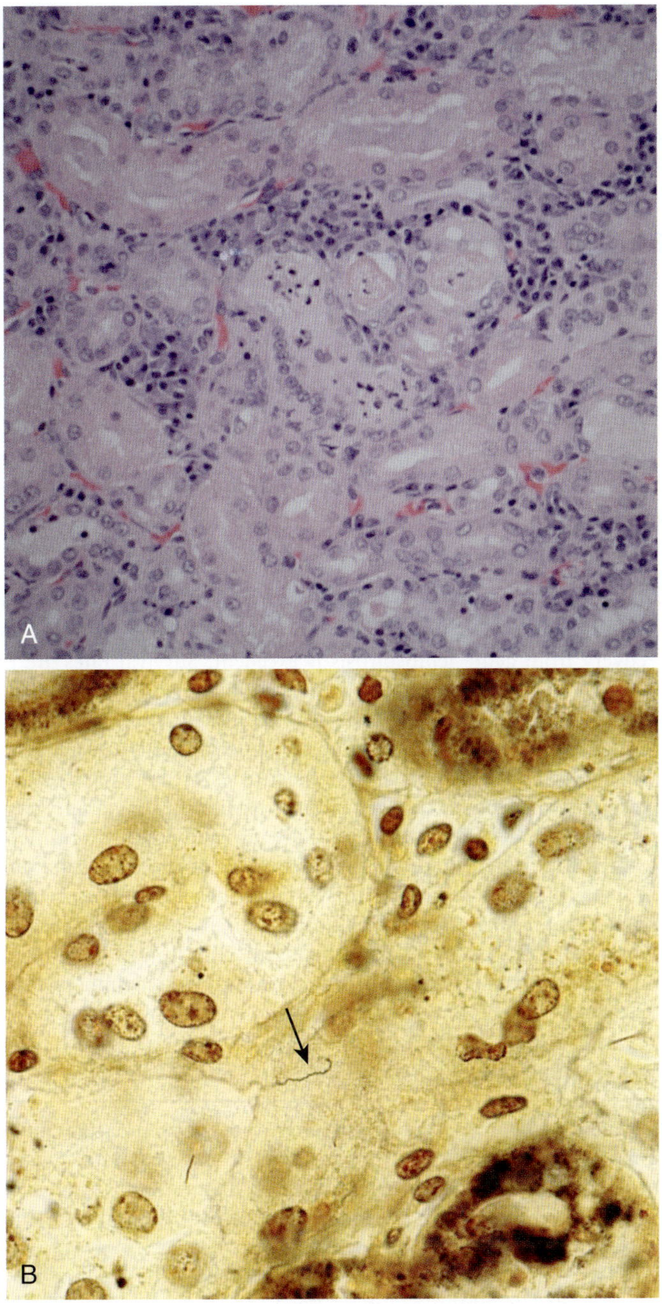

Fig. 68.9 (A) Histopathology of the kidney of a dog that died of leptospirosis. Acute tubular necrosis and interstitial nephritis is present. Hematoxylin and eosin stain. (B) Warthin-Starry stain showing low numbers of leptospires in the renal interstitium *(arrow)*. (Courtesy of Dr. Patricia Pesavento, University of California, Davis Veterinary Anatomic Pathology Service.)

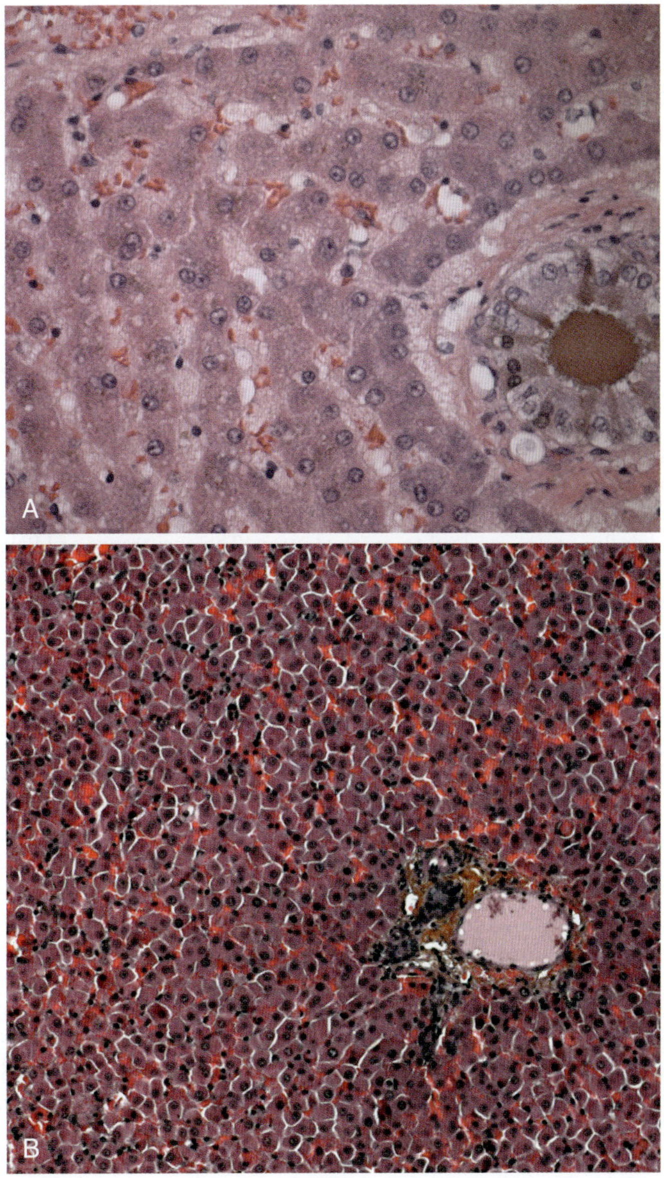

Fig. 68.10 Histopathology of the liver in leptospirosis. (A) Minimal hepatic changes and severe cholestasis in an 8-year-old male neutered Australian shepherd mix that was euthanized because of anuric leptospirosis. The activity of serum ALP and the serum total bilirubin concentration were mildly increased, and the dog seroconverted with the highest titer to serovar Pomona (1:400 to >1:3200 12 days later). (B) Liver plate disarray with hepatocellular dissociation in a dog with leptospirosis. (B, Courtesy of John Cullen, North Carolina State University and Jean-Jacques Fontaine, École Nationale Vétérinaire d'Alfort.)

use of doxycycline, parenteral ampicillin or penicillin G can be used (Table 68.6). The dosage should be adapted in dogs with decreased renal function. A safe and practical approach would be to double the administration interval in dogs with AKI Grade 4 and higher (creatinine > 440 μmol/L). Dogs initially treated with a penicillin derivative should be treated with doxycycline for 2 weeks after GI signs resolve. Fluoroquinolones are not highly efficacious for clearance of leptospires from tissues.[155] Other antimicrobials that have been efficacious in clinical trials involving human patients with leptospirosis include

TABLE 68.6 Antimicrobials Recommended for Treatment of Leptospirosis in Dogs

Drug	Dose	Route	Interval (Hours)	Duration (Days)
Doxycycline	5 mg/kg	PO, IV	12	14
Ampicillin	20 mg/kg*	IV	6	Variable
Penicillin	25,000–40,000 U/kg	IV	12	Variable

*Reduce dose in renal failure.

ceftriaxone, cefotaxime, and azithromycin,[156,157] but clinical trials of these drugs in canine leptospirosis are lacking.

Supportive Care

Treatment of dogs with AKI from leptospirosis generally follows the therapeutic recommendations for AKI from other etiologies. Correction of fluid, electrolyte, and acid-base disorders with appropriate fluid therapy remains the mainstay of the treatment, together with treatment of systemic hypertension and GI complications, pain management, and active nutritional support. Referral to a 24-hour care facility, ideally with access to dialysis, should be considered for severely ill dogs because of the need for intensive monitoring and close observation. Electrolyte and acid-base status may require frequent monitoring.

Fluid therapy is critical and should be calculated based on measurement of "outs and ins," together with careful attention to body weight, respiratory rate, lung sounds, blood pressure, and if possible, central venous pressure. For dogs with oliguric or anuric renal failure, high fluid rates can lead to overhydration. The occurrence of LPHS or vasculitis further limits the tolerance of patients to iatrogenic fluid excess. Diuretics such as furosemide or mannitol may be indicated. Failure of urine production after adequate hydration is achieved is an indication for hemodialysis. Dogs with polyuric renal failure may require extremely high fluid rates. Once recovery of kidney function has occurred, fluids should be tapered slowly before they are discontinued to ensure that proper hydration status is maintained. Treatment of dogs with GI signs includes a combination of antiemetics and gastroprotectants. Intussusceptions should be considered in dogs with persistent vomiting before antiemetics are contemplated.[88,89] In some dogs, possibly because of enteritis or pancreatitis, inappetence persists for several days after kidney and liver values normalize. The use of enteral feeding tubes is strongly advocated in dogs with anorexia as they allow efficient and early nutritional support with minimal risk of complications. Parenteral nutrition can be necessary in dogs with persistent vomiting. Pain management is particularly important in the early phases of the disease when painful swelling of the kidney, added to muscle, joint, pancreatitis, and GI pain can contribute markedly to the disease manifestations. Opioids, including buprenorphine or fentanyl, are usually recommended.

The treatment of LPHS is mainly supportive because the pathogenesis of this disease manifestation is poorly understood. Systematic radiographic screening even in the absence of respiratory signs allows early precautionary measures to be adopted. These include minimization of manipulations and stress and avoidance of systemic hypertension, overhydration, or hypervolemia. Dogs with LPHS may require oxygen therapy and, in severe cases, mechanical ventilation. Humans with LPHS have poor lung compliance, and ventilator treatment for ARDS is recommended, with low tidal volumes to prevent alveolar damage secondary to high ventilation pressures.[73] Treatment of active hemorrhage with desmopressin has yielded controversial results in humans[158,159] and did not appear to improve outcome in dogs, at least when administered as ocular drops.[160] Plasma or whole blood transfusions are only indicated in dogs with associated systemic disorders of hemostasis. Based on the hypothesis of an immune-mediated mechanism, immunomodulation has been investigated in humans with LPHS with promising preliminary results. Combination of cyclophosphamide, pulse glucocorticoid therapy, and therapeutic plasma exchanges to remove potentially autoreactive antibodies improved survival.[161–164] However, considering their complexity and the risk for complications, these therapies still need to be further investigated before they can be recommended for clinical practice.

Hemostatic disorders in dogs with leptospirosis vary widely in severity and they are multifactorial in origin. Both hyper- and hypocoagulable states have been shown to occur. DIC was described in 23% of dogs in one study, but was not associated with a negative outcome.[104] In dogs with DIC, plasma transfusions are indicated. Thrombocytopenia is common in dogs with leptospirosis, but rarely necessitates specific therapy.

Renal Replacement Therapy

Early hemodialysis results in improved survival and shorter hospital stays in human patients with leptospirosis.[165] Renal replacement therapy is indicated for dogs with inadequate urine output that develop volume overload, hyperkalemia, or uremia that do not respond to medical management. Approximately 50% of 89 dogs with leptospirosis at the University of California, Davis, VMTH over a 10-year period received hemodialysis; the median number of hemodialysis treatments required was 3 (range, 1–14). Recovery of adequate renal function usually occurs within 2 to 4 weeks of starting dialysis.

PROGNOSIS

When treatment is initiated early and aggressively, the prognosis for recovery from acute leptospirosis is excellent. Survival rates are in excess of 50%, and in centers where hemodialysis is available, survival rates can exceed 80%. Successful treatment is associated with normalization of the platelet count, serum BUN and creatinine concentrations, and serum liver enzyme activities within 10 to 14 days. Icterus may be slow to resolve, and urine-concentrating ability may not return for at least 4 weeks. A follow-up study of dogs with leptospirosis indicated that approximately 50% of the dogs surviving the acute phase of the disease displayed impairment of their renal function more than 1 year after hospital discharge,[166] thus chronic renal failure can be a sequela of acute infection/injury. Long-term monitoring of renal function is therefore strongly recommended in these dogs.

IMMUNITY AND VACCINATION

Recurrence of leptospirosis in dogs after recovery from natural infection appears to be rare, but the duration of immunity after natural infection is unknown. Immunity after vaccination with inactivated vaccines is serogroup specific and possibly serovar specific, with only partial immunity to heterologous serogroups.[167]

Current vaccines for dogs are inactivated bacterins that have been purified to optimize safety. Bivalent vaccines that contained only serovars Icterohaemorrhagiae and Canicola were first introduced for prevention of leptospirosis in dogs. Canine leptospirosis has been reported widely in dogs after vaccination with bivalent Icterohaemorrhagiae and Canicola vaccines,[96] thus bivalent vaccines do not sufficiently cross-protect against serovars responsible for the majority of current infections in dogs. Quadrivalent vaccines that contain Canicola, Icterohaemorrhagiae, Grippotyphosa, and Pomona have been available in the United States since 2001. Trivalent and quadrivalent vaccines are also available in Europe (Icterohaemorrhagiae, Canicola, and Grippotyphosa; Icterohaemorrhagiae, Canicola, Grippotyphosa, and Bratislava; and Icterohaemorrhagiae, Canicola, Grippotyphosa, and Australis) and increasingly in other parts of the world. One study showed that the trivalent vaccine was able to provide protection against challenge with serovar Copenhageni (serogroup Icterohaemorrhagiae) 2 weeks after vaccination.[168] Anecdotally, in the United States and Europe, quadrivalent vaccines appear to protect dogs from leptospirosis because the disease is now almost exclusively diagnosed in unvaccinated dogs.[13] In a retrospective case-control study in a Swiss cohort of 469 dogs with AKI, vaccination with a quadrivalent *Leptospira* vaccine including serogroups Icterohemorrhagiae, Canicola, Grippotyphosa, and Australis was associated with significantly lower odds to be diagnosed with leptospirosis.[169] However, one study from Italy reported instances of vaccine failure.[25] The duration of immunity following vaccination with bacterins is at least 12 months, with some studies showing protection from challenge 15 months after vaccination.[170–173]

Leptospira vaccines effectively prevent disease and reduce shedding after challenge with the serovar included in the vaccine. In preapproval vaccine trials, in order to produce a high incidence of clinical disease, dogs are challenged with conjunctival and intraperitoneal injection of $>10^6$, often $>10^9$, live leptospires.[170,171,174] As the quantity and nature of this experimental challenge does not truly mimic natural exposure, interpretation should be made cautiously of experimentally induced post-challenge urine shedding of leptospires in vaccinated dogs. Documentation of urine shedding in vaccinated dogs following natural exposure is very limited.

In the past, vaccination with *Leptospira* vaccines has been associated with type I hypersensitivity reactions such as anaphylaxis, especially in small-breed dogs. Anecdotal evidence from industry and veterinary practitioners in North America suggests that the prevalence of these reactions has considerably reduced in recent years (to <1%, with the majority of reactions being local reactions at the site of vaccination, rather than anaphylaxis) following efforts from industry to remove residual cell culture constituents, for example, excipient bovine proteins that have been associated with vaccine reactivity.[76,175]

Immunization is recommended for all dogs at risk of exposure. In some regions, this may be dogs that contact wildlife or farm animals, or dogs that swim, wade, or drink from environmental water sources. However, dogs in urban or suburban backyards may be at risk if there is exposure to wildlife or rodents in the immediate home environment; in other words all dogs may be at risk. A study of vaccination compliance in dogs from Germany revealed that only 50.1% of 3874 dogs had been vaccinated for leptospirosis, and the primary risk factor for lack of vaccination was recommendation from a veterinarian not to vaccinate for leptospirosis.[176] Evidence to show the protective effect of currently available leptospirosis vaccines beyond 12 or 15 months is lacking. Until more data become available, it has been recommended to restart a basic vaccination schedule with two doses administered 3 or 4 weeks apart in dogs that have not been revaccinated against leptospirosis for more than 18 months.[127] However, it is possible that a single booster at this time would restore immunity, as is generally recommended for even delays of many years in vaccination with bacterins for humans. Because positive titers do not indicate protection, antibody testing cannot be used to make decisions about need for vaccination.

For dogs that experience natural infection, immunization could commence after recovery, assuming that natural immunity is also serogroup specific and the possibility of exposure to other serovars exists. However, the duration of immunity after natural infection and the degree and duration of cross-protection to heterologous serovars that follows natural infection requires further investigation.

PREVENTION

Leptospirosis can be prevented by restricting dogs' access to potential reservoir host species or environmental water sources. Access to wildlife and farm animals can be reduced through fencing and rodent control. These measures, however, do not replace vaccination.

PUBLIC HEALTH ASPECTS

Leptospirosis is one of the most common zoonotic diseases worldwide. In humans, leptospirosis occurs after an incubation period of 2 to 20 days (mean, 10 days). In 90% of infections, it is a mild, influenza-like illness. Less commonly, it is manifested by severe multiorgan failure, with renal failure, hepatic failure, or LPHS. Abortion can occur during pregnancy. Weil's disease, which is characterized by impaired renal and hepatic function, usually occurs a week after an initial illness characterized by fever, myalgia, headache, chills, and conjunctivitis.[1]

In developed countries, most human leptospirosis cases follow recreational activities that involve water, such as houseboating or participation in triathlons, canoeing, kayaking, caving, adventure racing, or white-water rafting.[177] Individuals who contact or work with farm animals, for example, veterinarians, or wildlife can also develop leptospirosis. Contact with wild rodents adopted as pets has also led to human disease.[68] In developing countries, stray dogs may be a source of human infection, although rodents are likely also important.[69] The extent to which domestic cats might serve as reservoir hosts is not understood.

Reports of transmission from clinically affected incidental hosts (as opposed to subclinically infected reservoir hosts) to other animals are rare, and there are no reports that document transmission of leptospires from pet dogs to humans with the support of molecular typing methods. Humans are more likely to acquire leptospirosis from contact with subclinically infected reservoir hosts than from incidental hosts. Appropriate antimicrobial therapy may also reduce the possibility of transmission to humans. In an outbreak of leptospirosis in dogs in Arizona, no evidence of transmission to caregivers or owners was identified in an investigation by the CDC, despite significant contact with infected dogs with insufficient infection control protocols.[59] Nevertheless, precautions should be taken in the hospital environment to minimize zoonotic transmission (see Chapter 15). All dogs with AKI should be handled as leptospirosis suspects until an alternative diagnosis is established. Suggested precautions are shown in Box 68.1. Urine from dogs with leptospirosis can be inactivated with a variety of disinfectant solutions, including iodine-based disinfectants, quaternary ammonium solutions, and accelerated hydrogen peroxide. Large

BOX 68.1 Suggested In-Hospital Precautions for Dogs with Known or Suspected Leptospirosis*

- Warning signage on the cage or run
- Minimize movement around the hospital, avoiding transport along common hallways
- Wear gloves and disposable gowns
- Protective eyewear and face shields if aerosolization of urine likely
- Handwashing before and after handling
- No pregnant or immunocompromised staff to work with the patient
- Prompt disinfection of urine and urine spills
- Treatment with appropriate antimicrobial drugs
- Indwelling rather than intermittent urinary catheterization for monitoring urine output
- Dogs walked or gurneyed outside to urinate frequently if urinary catheter not in place
- Urination outside in a designated area that can be easily disinfected
- Warnings to others who handle the dog or specimens from the dog

*Precautions can be removed following 48–72 hours of ampicillin or doxycycline treatment.

volumes of urine can be inactivated by a 1:1 dilution with a 10% solution of household bleach. In dogs with indwelling urinary catheters, 10% bleach should be injected directly into the collection bag before disposal. All blood, urine, and tissues from dogs should be treated as medical waste. If a dog dies or is euthanized, individuals who are to handle the remains should be alerted of the possibility of leptospirosis.

Owners of affected dogs should be educated with regard to the zoonotic nature of the disease. The risk of infection to owners is probably low, because urinary shedding generally does not occur until 7 to 10 days after the onset of illness, and doxycycline treatment likely results in clearance of bacteria from the kidneys and urine within 2 to 3 days. Nevertheless, until antimicrobial therapy is completed, owners should avoid contact with their dog's urine. Thus, owners or family members may have unknowingly been exposed during pre-treatment at-home-care of their sick dog. Routine household disinfectants and gloved hands should be used to clean up urinary accidents that occur indoors. Dogs should be taken to urinate in a place that is away from water and away from other pets and people, especially children. Owners should wash their hands after they handle their pets. Veterinarians should recommend that owners seek medical attention if illness occurs around the time their dog is diagnosed with leptospirosis, or if they have any questions about the disease in humans. Immunocompromised humans should be referred to their medical practitioners for advice. Owners should also be informed that environmental sources of infection may represent an ongoing risk, not only to other dogs in the household but also to humans. If other dogs in the household had the same exposure history as a dog diagnosed with leptospirosis (e.g., they all went on a hike or swam in a lake), treatment of those dogs with 2 weeks of doxycycline should be considered, because subclinical infection and shedding may have occurred.[76,127]

Veterinarians should contact their local or state health department or the CDC if additional questions arise regarding the public health risks and zoonotic transmission of leptospirosis.

CASE EXAMPLE

Signalment

"Makalu," a 1.5-year-old male neutered kelpie dog from Dixon, California (Fig. 68.11).

History

Makalu had a 1-day history of lethargy and inappetence. The owner, a veterinarian, took his temperature at home and it was > 104°F (40°C). There had been no evidence of vomiting, diarrhea, coughing, sneezing, or increased thirst and urination. He lived on a property with another dog, three cats, sheep, goats, and a pot-bellied pig. He normally ate a commercial dry dog food, and was observed to eat a rawhide the day before he became ill. There was no history of previous travel, toxins, trauma, or tick exposure. He was 3 months overdue for vaccination, but was vaccinated as a puppy for distemper, hepatitis, parvovirus, rabies, and leptospirosis. The owner did not recall which *Leptospira* vaccines he received.

Current Medications

None.

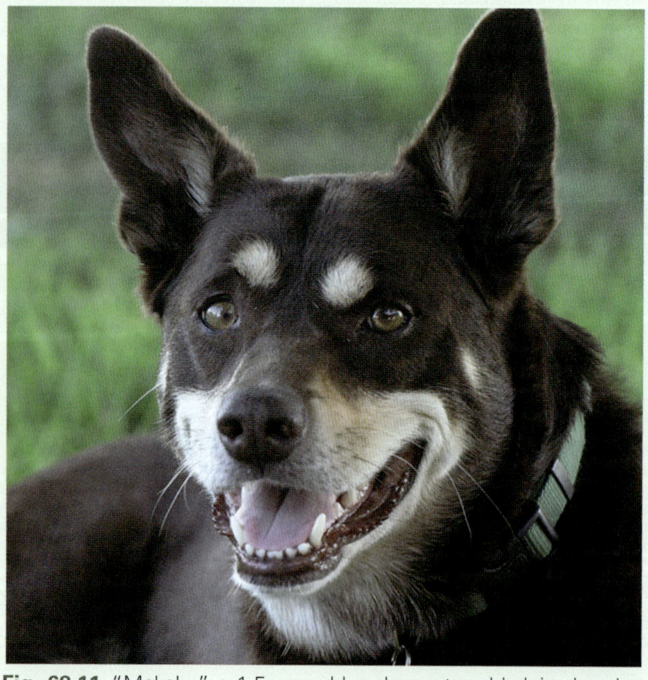

Fig. 68.11 "Makalu," a 1.5-year-old male neutered kelpie dog that developed leptospirosis. (From Sykes JE. *Canine and Feline Infectious Diseases.* Elsevier; 2014.)

Physical Examination

Body weight: 22.4 kg.

General: Quiet, alert, and responsive. Ambulatory on all four limbs, temperature = 103.7°F, heart rate = 80 beats/min, respiratory rate = 20 breaths/min, mucous membranes pink, CRT = 1 sec. Estimated to be 7 to 8% dehydrated based on skin turgor.

Integument: Full, shiny hair coat. No evidence of ectoparasites.

Eyes, ears, nose, and throat: Mild scleral injection and chemosis bilaterally. No other abnormalities noted.

Musculoskeletal: Appeared stiff, but no evidence of synovial effusion. Vocalized upon flexion of the right thoracic limb.

Cardiovascular: Strong femoral pulses. No murmurs or arrhythmias ausculted. Systolic blood pressure 145 mmHg.

Respiratory: Quiet bronchovesicular sounds in all fields.

GI: Tense abdomen, with abdominal splinting noted on palpation.

Rectal examination: No abnormalities detected. Prostate palpable and symmetrical.

Lymph nodes: No abnormalities detected.

Laboratory Findings

CBC: HCT 41.4% (40–55%), MCV 70.2 fL (65–75 fL), MCHC 36.0 g/dL (33–36 g/dL), WBC 8820 cells/μL (6000–13,000 cells/μL), neutrophils 7673 cells/μL (3000–10,500 cells/μL), lymphocytes 353 cells/μL (1000–4000 cells/μL), monocytes 441 cells/μL (150–1200 cells/μL), platelets 74,000 platelets/μL (150,000–400,000 platelets/μL).

Serum chemistry profile: Sodium 143 mmol/L (145–154 mmol/L), potassium 3.7 mmol/L (4.1–5.3 mmol/L), chloride 104 mmol/L (105–116 mmol/L), bicarbonate 17 mmol/L (16–26 mmol/L), phosphorus 5.1 mg/dL (3.0–6.2 mg/dL), calcium 9.6 mg/dL (9.9–11.4 mg/dL), BUN 90 mg/dL (8–31 mg/dL), creatinine 4.6 mg/dL (0.5–1.6 mg/dL), glucose 110 mg/dL (70–118 mg/dL), total protein 5.1 g/dL (5.4–7.4 g/dL), albumin 2.4 g/dL (2.9–4.2 g/dL), globulin 2.7 g/dL (2.3–4.4 g/dL), ALT 42 U/L (19–67 U/L), AST 146 U/L (21–54 U/L), ALP 73 U/L (15–127 U/L), creatine kinase 1387 U/L (46–320 U/L), GGT 2 U/L (0–6 U/L), cholesterol 189 mg/dL (135–345 mg/dL), total bilirubin 0.4 mg/dL (0–0.4 mg/dL).

Urinalysis: SpG 1.013; pH 7.5, 2+ protein (SSA), 1+ bilirubin, 3+ hemoprotein, 2+ glucose, 0 WBC/HPF, 20–30 RBC/HPF, rare transitional epithelial cells.

Coagulation profile: PT 8.8 (7.5–10.5), PTT 16.8 (9–12), fibrinogen 280 (90–255).

Serum ethylene glycol assay: Negative.

Imaging Findings

Thoracic radiographs: The cardiovascular and pulmonary structures were within normal limits.

CASE EXAMPLE—cont'd

Abdominal ultrasound: The liver and spleen were both enlarged. The tail of the spleen had a mildly mottled echotexture. Both kidneys were mildly enlarged, and approximately 8 cm in length. The renal cortices were mildly echogenic. Both kidneys were associated with a small amount of subcapsular and retroperitoneal fluid. The mesenteric lymph nodes were prominent.

Microbiologic Testing

Aerobic bacterial culture of blood and urine: No growth.

Serologic testing (MAT): Day 2 after the onset of illness, negative for antibodies to *Leptospira* serovars Canicola, Grippotyphosa, Hardjo, Icterohaemorrhagiae, and Pomona @ 1:100. Positive for antibodies to serovar Bratislava @ 1:100. Day 10 after the onset of illness, negative for antibodies to serovar Canicola. Positive for antibodies to serovars Grippotyphosa (1:400), Hardjo (1:100), Icterohaemorrhagiae (1:800), Pomona (1:12800), and Bratislava (1:3200).

Diagnosis

Leptospirosis.

Treatment

Makalu was treated aggressively with intravenous fluids, mannitol, famotidine, antiemetics, and ampicillin (20 mg/kg IV q6h). Despite treatment with fluids, mannitol, and furosemide, urine output remained at < 0.8 mL/kg per hour. After 18 hours of hospitalization, dialysis was initiated. A second dialysis treatment was given 2 days later, after which polyuria ensued (Table 68.7). On day 3, evidence of DIC developed, which included further prolongation of the PT (14.3 s) and PTT (21.1 s), hypofibrinogenemia (< 90 mg/dL), and a positive D-dimer assay, and he was treated with multiple units of fresh frozen plasma. Treatment with ondansetron was also initiated on day 3 because of persistent vomiting, and central parenteral nutrition was instituted on day 4. Makalu's mentation improved on day 5 and he began eating on day 8.

Comments

Liver enzyme activities were not increased in this dog on admission, but increased subsequently.

TABLE 68.7 Changes in Clinicopathologic Variables Over Time in a Dog Hospitalized with Leptospirosis that Was Treated with Hemodialysis

Variable	Day 1	Day 3	Day 4	Day 5	Day 8	Day 10
ALT	62	ND	105	110	82	71
ALP	83	ND	97	97	79	75
Bilirubin	0.4	ND	0.5	0.8	0.3	0.3
BUN	105 (27)*	144 (30)	54	47	35	27
Creatinine	5.6 (2.2)	12.9 (3.1)	4.8	3.3	2.1	1.6
Albumin	2.2	2.4	2.5	2.9	3.0	3.1
Platelets	74	ND	26	91	92	Clumped
Urine output	< 0.8	0.25	10	10	7	ND

*Values in parentheses are post-dialysis values.

SUGGESTED READINGS

Bertasio C, Boniotti MB, Lucchese L, et al. Detection of new *Leptospira* genotypes infecting symptomatic dogs: is a new vaccine formulation needed? *Pathogens.* 2020;9(6):484.

Sykes JE, Hartmann K, Lunn KF, et al. 2010 ACVIM small animal consensus statement on leptospirosis: diagnosis, epidemiology, treatment, and prevention. *J Vet Intern Med.* 2011;25:1–13.

Schuller S, Francey T, Hartmann K, et al. European consensus statement on leptospirosis in dogs and cats. *J Small Anim Pract.* 2015;56:159–179.

Levett PN. *Leptospirosis. Clin Microbiol Rev.* 2001;14:296–326.

Sykes JE, Reagan KL, Nally JE, et al. Role of diagnostics in epidemiology, management, surveillance, and control of leptospirosis, *Pathogens.* 2022;11:395.

REFERENCES

1. Levett PN. *Leptospirosis. Clin Microbiol Rev.* 2001;14:296–326.
2. Adler B (ed). *Leptospira and Leptospirosis.* Springer, Berlin, Heidelberg; 2015.
3. Murray GL, Srikram A, Hoke DE, et al. Major surface protein LipL32 is not required for either acute or chronic infection with *Leptospira interrogans. Infect Immun.* 2009;77:952–958.
4. Cerqueira GM, Picardeau M. A century of *Leptospira* strain typing. *J Mol Epidemiol Evol Genetics Infect Dis.* 2009;9:760–768.
5. Ahmed N, Devi SM, de los Á Valverde M, et al. Multilocus sequence typing method for identification and genotypic classification of pathogenic *Leptospira* species. *Annals Clin Microbiol Antimicrob.* 2006;5:28.
6. Thibeaux R, Geroult S, Benezech C, et al. Seeking the environmental source of leptospirosis reveals durable bacterial viability in river soils. *PLoS Negl Trop Dis.* 2017;11:e0005414.
7. Bierque E, Thibeaux R, Girault D, et al. A systematic review of *Leptospira* in water and soil environments. *PLoS One.* 2020;15:e0227055.
8. Khairani-Bejo S, Bahaman AR, Zamri-Saad M, et al. The survival of *Leptospira interrogans* serovar Hardjo in the Malaysian environment. *J Anim Vet Advances.* 2004;3:123–129.
9. Ganoza CA, Matthias MA, Saito M, et al. Asymptomatic renal colonization of humans in the peruvian Amazon by *Leptospira. PLoS Negl Trop Dis.* 2010;4:e612.
10. Pedersen K, Anderson TD, Maison RM, et al. *Leptospira* antibodies detected in wildlife in the USA and the US Virgin Islands. *J Wildl Dis.* 2018;54:450–459.
11. Richardson DJ, Gauthier JL. A serosurvey of leptospirosis in Connecticut peridomestic wildlife. *Vector Borne Zoonotic Dis.* 2003;3:187–193.
12. Mitchell MA, Hungeford LL, Nixon C, et al. Serologic survey for selected infectious disease agents in raccoons from Illinois. *J Wildl Dis.* 1999;35:347–355.
13. Prescott JF, Key D, Osuch M. Leptospirosis in dogs. *Can Vet J.* 1999;40:430–431.
14. Boutilier P, Carr A, Schulman RL. Leptospirosis in dogs: a serologic survey and case series 1996 to 2001. *Vet Ther.* 2003;4:387–396.
15. Tan CG, Dharmarajan G, Beasley J, et al. Neglected leptospirosis in raccoons (*Procyon lotor*) in Indiana, USA. *Vet Q.* 2014;34:1–10.
16. Davis MA, Evermann JF, Petersen CR, et al. Serological survey for antibodies to *Leptospira* in dogs and raccoons in Washington State. *Zoonoses Public Health.* 2008;55:436–442.
17. Levett PN. Usefulness of serologic analysis as a predictor of the infecting serovar in patients with severe leptospirosis. *Clin Infect Dis.* 2003;36:447–452.

18. Zilber AL, Picardeau M, Ayral F, et al. High-resolution typing of *Leptospira interrogans* strains by multispacer sequence typing. *J Clin Microbiol.* 2014;52:564–571.
19. Mayer-Scholl A, Hammerl JA, Schmidt S, et al. *Leptospira* spp. in rodents and shrews in Germany. *Int J Environ Res Public Health.* 2014;11:7562–7574.
20. Kudo Y, Vansith K, Rin E, et al. Molecular epidemiological survey of *Leptospira* infection of wild rodents in the urban settlement of Cambodia. *Vector Borne Zoonotic Dis.* 2018;18:144–150.
21. Rahelinirina S, Bourhy P, Andriamiaramanana F, et al. High prevalence of *Leptospira* spp. in rodents in an urban setting in Madagascar. *Am J Trop Med Hyg.* 2019;100:1079–1081.
22. Plata-Luis J, Foronda P, Martin-Alonso A, et al. *Leptospira interrogans* in rodents from Cape Verde. *Vector Borne Zoonotic Dis.* 2016;16:731–733.
23. Cosson JF, Picardeau M, Mielcarek M, et al. Epidemiology of *Leptospira* transmitted by rodents in southeast Asia. *PLoS Negl Trop Dis.* 2014;8:e2902.
24. Tadin A, Turk N, Korva M, et al. Multiple co-infections of rodents with hantaviruses, *Leptospira*, and *Babesia* in Croatia. *Vector Borne Zoonotic Dis.* 2012;12:388–392.
25. Bertasio C, Boniotti MB, Lucchese L, et al. Detection of new *Leptospira* genotypes infecting symptomatic dogs: is a new vaccine formulation needed? *Pathogens.* 2020;9:484.
26. Ayral F, Djelouadji Z, Raton V, et al. Hedgehogs and mustelid species: major carriers of pathogenic *Leptospira*, a survey in 28 animal species in France. *PLoS One.* 2016;11:e0162549.
27. Rockwell KE, Thompson D, Maddox C, et al. Blanding's turtles (*Emydoidea blandingii*) as a reservoir for *Leptospira* spp. *PLoS One.* 2019;14:e0210688.
28. Straub MH, Foley JE. Cross-sectional evaluation of multiple epidemiological cycles of *Leptospira* species in peri-urban wildlife in California. *J Am Vet Med Assoc.* 2020;257:840–848.
29. Straub MH, Church M, Glueckert E, et al. Raccoons (*Procyon lotor*) and striped skunks (*Mephitis mephitis*) as potential reservoirs of *Leptospira* spp. in California. *Vector Borne Zoonotic Dis.* 2020;20:418–426.
30. Wu Q, Prager KC, Goldstein T, et al. Development of a real-time PCR for the detection of pathogenic *Leptospira* spp. in California sea lions. *Dis Aquat Organ.* 2014;110:165–172.
31. Dybing NA, Jacobson C, Irwin P, et al. *Leptospira* species in feral cats and black rats from Western Australia and Christmas Island. *Vector Borne Zoonotic Dis.* 2017;17:319–324.
32. Gomard Y, Lagadec E, Humeau L, et al. Feral cats do not play a major role in leptospirosis epidemiology on Reunion Island. *Epidemiol Infect.* 2019;147:e97.
33. Grimm K, Rivera NA, Fredebaugh-Siller S, et al. Evidence of *Leptospira* serovars in wildlife and leptospiral DNA in water sources in a natural area in east-central Illinois, USA. *J Wildl Dis.* 2020;56:316–327.
34. Biscornet L, Dellagi K, Pages F, et al. Human leptospirosis in Seychelles: a prospective study confirms the heavy burden of the disease but suggests that rats are not the main reservoir. *PLoS Negl Trop Dis.* 2017;11:e0005831.
35. Grillova L, Angermeier H, Levy M, et al. Circulating genotypes of *Leptospira* in French Polynesia: a 9-year molecular epidemiology surveillance follow-up study. *PLoS Negl Trop Dis.* 2020;14:e0008662.
36. Barragan V, Nieto N, Keim P, et al. Meta-analysis to estimate the load of *Leptospira* excreted in urine: beyond rats as important sources of transmission in low-income rural communities. *BMC Res Notes.* 2017;10:71.
37. Arbour J, Blais MC, Carioto L, et al. Clinical leptospirosis in three cats (2001-2009). *J Am Anim Hosp Assoc.* 2012;48:256–260.
38. Bryson DG, Ellis WA. Leptospirosis in a British domestic cat. *J Small Anim Pract.* 1976;17:459–465.
39. Fessler JF, Morter RL. Experimental feline leptospirosis. *Cornell Vet.* 1964;54:176–190.
40. Luciani O. Receptivité et sensibilité du chat aux leptospires. Thesis/dissertation. *Ecole Nationale Vétérinaire de Nantes*; 2004.
41. Mason RW, King SJ, McLachlan NM. Suspected leptospirosis in two cats. *Aust Vet J.* 1972;48:622–623.
42. Rees HG. Leptospirosis in a cat. *New Zealand Vet J.* 1964;12:64.
43. Fenimore A, Carter K, Lunn K. Detection of leptospiruria in shelter cats in Colorado. In: *Proceedings of the 30th Annual Forum of the American College of Veterinary Internal Medicine.* 2012:783.
44. Rodriguez J, Blais MC, Lapointe C, et al. Serologic and urinary PCR survey of leptospirosis in healthy cats and in cats with kidney disease. *J Vet Intern Med.* 2014;28:284–293.
45. Agunloye CA, Nash AS. Investigation of possible leptospiral infection in cats in Scotland. *J Small Anim Pract.* 1996;37:126–129.
46. Weis S, Rettinger A, Bergmann M, et al. Detection of *Leptospira* DNA in urine and presence of specific antibodies in outdoor cats in Germany. *J Feline Med Surg.* 2016;19:470–476.
47. Hemsley LA. *Leptospira* Canicola and chronic nephritis in cats. *Vet Rec.* 1956;68:300–301.
48. Murillo A, Goris M, Ahmed A, et al. Leptospirosis in cats: current literature review to guide diagnosis and management. *J Fel Med Surg.* 2020;22:216–228.
49. Le Guyader M, Fontana C, Simon-Dufay N, et al. Successful *Leptospira* genotyping strategy on DNA extracted from canine biological samples. *J Microbiol Methods.* 2020;176:106007.
50. Koizumi N, Muto MM, Izumiya H, et al. Multiple-locus variable-number tandem repeat analysis and clinical characterization of *Leptospira interrogans* canine isolates. *J Med Microbiol.* 2015;64:288–294.
51. Koizumi N, Izumiya H, Ohnishi M. Genetic relatedness of *Leptospira interrogans* serogroup Autumnalis isolated from humans, dogs, and mice in Japan. *BMC Res Notes.* 2020;13:369.
52. Ward MP. Seasonality of canine leptospirosis in the United States and Canada and its association with rainfall. *Prev Vet Med.* 2002;56:203–213.
53. Gautam R, Guptill LF, Wu CC, et al. Spatial and spatio-temporal clustering of overall and serovar-specific *Leptospira* microscopic agglutination test (MAT) seropositivity among dogs in the United States from 2000 through 2007. *Prev Vet Med.* 2010;96:122–131.
54. Prescott J. Canine leptospirosis in Canada: a veterinarian's perspective. *Can Med Assoc J.* 2008;178:397–398.
55. Lee HS, Levine M, Guptill-Yoran C, et al. Regional and temporal variations of *Leptospira* seropositivity in dogs in the United States, 2000-2010. *J Vet Intern Med.* 2014;28:779–788.
56. Hennebelle JH, Sykes JE, Carpenter TE, et al. Spatial and temporal patterns of *Leptospira* infection in dogs from northern California: 67 cases (2001-2010). *J Am Vet Med Assoc.* 2013;242:941–947.
57. Major A, Schweighauser A, Francey T. Increasing incidence of canine leptospirosis in Switzerland. *Int J Environ Res Public Health.* 2014;11:7242–7260.
58. LaFerla Jenni M, Woodward P, Yaglom H, et al. Knowledge, attitudes, and practices among veterinarians during an outbreak of canine leptospirosis-Maricopa County, Arizona. 2017. *Prev Vet Med.* 2019;172:104779.
59. Guagliardo SAJ, Iverson SA, Reynolds L, et al. Despite high-risk exposures, no evidence of zoonotic transmission during a canine outbreak of leptospirosis. *Zoonoses Public Health.* 2019;66:223–231.
60. Ghneim GS, Viers JH, Chomel BB, et al. Use of a case-control study and geographic information systems to determine environmental and demographic risk factors for canine leptospirosis. *Vet Res.* 2007;38:37–50.
61. Lee HS, Guptill L, Johnson AJ, et al. Signalment changes in canine leptospirosis between 1970 and 2009. *J Vet Intern Med.* 2014;28:294–299.
62. Ward MP, Glickman LT, Guptill LE. Prevalence of and risk factors for leptospirosis among dogs in the United States and Canada: 677 cases (1970-1998). *J Am Vet Med Assoc.* 2002;220:53–58.
63. Alton GD, Berke O, Reid-Smith R, et al. Increase in seroprevalence of canine leptospirosis and its risk factors, Ontario 1998-2006. *Can J Vet Res.* 2009;73:167–175.
64. Moore GE, Guptill LF, Ward MP, et al. Adverse events diagnosed within three days of vaccine administration in dogs. *J Am Vet Med Assoc.* 2005;227:1102–1108.
65. Raghavan R, Brenner K, Higgins J, et al. Evaluations of land cover risk factors for canine leptospirosis: 94 cases (2002-2009). *Prev Vet Med.* 2011;101:241–249.
66. Azocar-Aedo L, Monti G. Meta-Analyses of factors associated with leptospirosis in domestic dogs. *Zoonoses Public Health.* 2016;63:328–336.

67. Chin VK, Basir R, Nordin SA, et al. Pathology and host immune evasion during human leptospirosis: a review. *Int Microbiol.* 2020;23:127–136.
68. Nally JE, Whitelegge JP, Bassilian S, et al. Characterization of the outer membrane proteome of *Leptospira interrogans* expressed during acute lethal infection. *Infect Immun.* 2007;75:766–773.
69. Lo M, Bulach DM, Powell DR, et al. Effects of temperature on gene expression patterns in *Leptospira interrogans* serovar Lai as assessed by whole-genome microarrays. *Infect Immun.* 2006;74:5848–5859.
70. Matsunaga J, Werneid K, Zuerner RL, et al. LipL46 is a novel surface-exposed lipoprotein expressed during leptospiral dissemination in the mammalian host. *Microbiol.* 2006;152:3777–3786.
71. Werts C, Tapping RI, Mathison JC, et al. Leptospiral lipopolysaccharide activates cells through a TLR2-dependent mechanism. *Nature Immunol.* 2001;2:346–352.
72. Cagliero J, Villanueva S, Matsui M. Leptospirosis pathophysiology: into the storm of cytokines. *Front Cell Infect Microbiol.* 2018;8:204.
73. Haake DA, Levett PN. *Leptospira* species (leptospirosis). In: Bennett JE, Dolin R, Blaser MJ, eds. *Mandell, Douglas and Bennett's Principles and Practice of Infectious Diseases.* Philadelphia, PA: Elsevier Saunders; 2020:2898–2905.
74. Monahan AM, Callanan JJ, Nally JE. Proteomic analysis of *Leptospira interrogans* shed in urine of chronically infected hosts. *Infect Immun.* 2008;76:4952–4958.
75. Greenlee JJ, Alt DP, Bolin CA, et al. Experimental canine leptospirosis caused by *Leptospira interrogans* serovars Pomona and Bratislava. *Am J Vet Res.* 2005;66:1816–1822.
76. Sykes JE, Hartmann K, Lunn KF, et al. 2010 ACVIM small animal consensus statement on leptospirosis: diagnosis, epidemiology, treatment, and prevention. *J Vet Intern Med.* 2011;25:1–13.
77. Rentko VT, Clark N, Ross LA, et al. Canine leptospirosis. A retrospective study of 17 cases. *J Vet Intern Med.* 1992;6:235–244.
78. Harkin KR, Gartrell CL. Canine leptospirosis in New Jersey and Michigan: 17 cases (1990-1995). *J Am Anim Hosp Assoc.* 1996;32:495–501.
79. Birnbaum N, Barr SC, Center SA, et al. Naturally acquired leptospirosis in 36 dogs: serological and clinicopathological features. *J Small Anim Pract.* 1998;39:231–236.
80. Adin CA, Cowgill LD. Treatment and outcome of dogs with leptospirosis: 36 cases (1990-1998). *J Am Vet Med Assoc.* 2000;216:371–375.
81. Prescott JF, McEwen B, Taylor J, et al. Resurgence of leptospirosis in dogs in Ontario: recent findings. *Can Vet J.* 2002;43:955–961.
82. Goldstein RE, Lin RC, Langston CE, et al. Influence of infecting serogroup on clinical features of leptospirosis in dogs. *J Vet Intern Med.* 2006;20:489–494.
83. Steger-Lieb A, Gerber B, Nicolet J, et al. An old disease with a new face: canine leptospirosis does not lose its relevance. *Schweiz Arch Tierheilkd.* 1999;141:499–507.
84. Mastrorilli C, Dondi F, Agnoli C, et al. Clinicopathologic features and outcome predictors of *Leptospira interrogans* Australis serogroup infection in dogs: a retrospective study of 20 cases (2001-2004). *J Vet Intern Med.* 2007;21:3–10.
85. Geisen V, Stengel C, Brem S, et al. Canine leptospirosis infections - clinical signs and outcome with different suspected *Leptospira* serogroups (42 cases). *J Small Anim Pract.* 2007;48:324–328.
86. Tangeman LE, Littman MP. Clinicopathologic and atypical features of naturally occurring leptospirosis in dogs: 51 cases (2000-2010). *J Am Vet Med Assoc.* 2013;243:1316–1322.
87. Knopfler S, Mayer Scholl A, Luge E, et al. Evaluation of clinical, laboratory, imaging findings and outcome in 99 dogs with leptospirosis. *J Small Anim Pract.* 2017;58:582–588.
88. Schweighauser A, Burgener IA, Gaschen F, et al. Small intestinal intussusception in five dogs with acute renal failure and suspected leptospirosis (L. australis). *J Vet Emerg Crit Care.* 2009;19:363–368.
89. Schulz BS, Seybold N, Adamik KN, et al. Ileocolic intestinal intussusception in a dog with leptospirosis. *Tierarztl Prax Ausg.* 2010;38:403–405.
90. De Brito T, Menezes LF, Lima DM, et al. Immunohistochemical and in situ hybridization studies of the liver and kidney in human leptospirosis. *Virchows Arch.* 2006;448:576–583.
91. Nally JE, Chantranuwat C, Wu XY, et al. Alveolar septal deposition of immunoglobulin and complement parallels pulmonary hemorrhage in a Guinea pig model of severe pulmonary leptospirosis. *Am J Pathol.* 2004;164:1115–1127.
92. Schuller S, Sergeant K, Renaut J, et al. Comparative proteomic analysis of lung tissue from Guinea pigs with leptospiral pulmonary haemorrhage syndrome (LPHS) reveals a decrease in abundance of host proteins involved in cytoskeletal and cellular organization. *J Proteomics.* 2015;122:55–72.
93. Yang CW, Wu MS, Pan MJ, et al. *Leptospira* outer membrane protein activates NF-kappaB and downstream genes expressed in medullary thick ascending limb cells. *J Am Soc Nephrol.* 2000;11:2017–2026.
94. Chang MY, Cheng YC, Hsu SH, et al. Leptospiral outer membrane protein LipL32 induces inflammation and kidney injury in zebrafish larvae. *Sci Rep.* 2016;6:27838.
95. Miyahara S, Saito M, Kanemaru T, et al. Destruction of the hepatocyte junction by intercellular invasion of *Leptospira* causes jaundice in a hamster model of Weil's disease. *Int J Exp Pathol.* 2014;95:271–281.
96. Kohn B, Steinicke K, Arndt G, et al. Pulmonary abnormalities in dogs with leptospirosis. *J Vet Intern Med.* 2010;24:1277–1282.
97. Fujita R, Koizumi N, Sugiyama H, et al. Comparison of bacterial burden and cytokine gene expression in golden hamsters in early phase of infection with two different strains of *Leptospira interrogans. PLoS One.* 2015;10:e0132694.
98. Maissen-Villiger CA, Schweighauser A, van Dorland HA, et al. Expression profile of cytokines and enzymes mRNA in blood leukocytes of dogs with leptospirosis and its associated pulmonary hemorrhage syndrome. *PLoS One.* 2016;11:e0148029.
99. Croda J, Neto AN, Brasil RA, et al. Leptospirosis pulmonary haemorrhage syndrome is associated with linear deposition of immunoglobulin and complement on the alveolar surface. *Clin Microbiol Infect.* 2010;16:593–599.
100. Schuller S, Callanan JJ, Worrall S, et al. Immunohistochemical detection of IgM and IgG in lung tissue of dogs with leptospiral pulmonary haemorrhage syndrome (LPHS). *Comp Immunol Microbiol Infect Dis.* 2015;40:47–53.
101. Martinez-Lopez DG, Fahey M, Coburn J. Responses of human endothelial cells to pathogenic and non-pathogenic *Leptospira* species. *PLoS Negl Trop Dis.* 2010;4:e918.
102. Medeiros Fda R, Spichler A, Athanazio DA. Leptospirosis-associated disturbances of blood vessels, lungs and hemostasis. *Acta Trop.* 2010;115:155–162.
103. Violette NP, Ledbetter EC. Punctate retinal hemorrhage and its relation to ocular and systemic disease in dogs: 83 cases. *Vet Ophthalmol.* 2018;21:233–239.
104. Barthelemy A, Magnin M, Pouzot-Nevoret C, et al. Hemorrhagic, hemostatic, and thromboelastometric disorders in 35 dogs with a clinical diagnosis of leptospirosis: a prospective study. *J Vet Intern Med.* 2017;31:69–80.
105. Keller SP, Kovacevic A, Howard J, et al. Evidence of cardiac injury and arrhythmias in dogs with acute kidney injury. *J Small Anim Pract.* 2016;57:402–408.
106. Rossetti CA, Liem M, Samartino LE, et al. Buenos Aires, a new *Leptospira* serovar of serogroup Djasiman, isolated from an aborted dog fetus in Argentina. *Vet Microbiol.* 2005;107:241–248.
107. Ellis WA. *Leptospirosis. J Small Anim Pract.* 1986;27:683–692.
108. McIntyre WIM, Montgomery GL. Renal lesions in *Leptospira* Canicola infection in dogs. *J Pathol Bacteriol.* 1952;64:145–160.
109. Sterling CR, Thiermann AB. Urban rats as chronic carriers of leptospirosis: an ultrastructural investigation. *Vet Pathol.* 1981;18:628–637.
110. Sant'Anna R, Vieira AS, Oliveira J, et al. Asymptomatic leptospiral infection is associated with canine chronic kidney disease. *Comp Immunol Microbiol Infect Dis.* 2019;62:64–67.
111. Adamus C, Buggin-Daubie M, Izembart A, et al. Chronic hepatitis associated with leptospiral infection in vaccinated beagles. *J Comp Pathol.* 1997;117:311–328.
112. Bishop L, Strandberg JD, Adams RJ, et al. Chronic active hepatitis in dogs associated with leptospires. *Am J Vet Res.* 1979;40:839–844.

113. Michel E, Kook PH, Voss K, et al. Generalized metastatic intestinal and cutaneous calcinosis in a Hovawart puppy with leptospirosis. *Schweiz Arch Tierheilkd*. 2011;153:27–31.
114. Munday JS, Bergen DJ, Roe WD. Generalized calcinosis cutis associated with probable leptospirosis in a dog. *Vet Dermatol*. 2005;16:401–406.
115. Beck A, Huber D, Antolic M, et al. Retrospective study of canine infectious haemolytic anaemia cases reveals the importance of molecular investigation in accurate postmortal diagnostic protocols. *Comp Immunol Microbiol Infect Dis*. 2019;65:81–87.
116. Furlanello T, Reale I. Leptospirosis and immune-mediated hemolytic anemia: a lethal association. *Vet Res Forum*. 2019;10:261–265.
117. Nicodemo AC, Del Negro G, Amato Neto V. Thrombocytopenia and leptospirosis. *Rev Inst Med Trop Sao Paulo*. 1990;32:252–259.
118. Yang HL, Jiang XC, Zhang XY, et al. Thrombocytopenia in the experimental leptospirosis of Guinea pig is not related to disseminated intravascular coagulation. *BMC Infect Dis*. 2006;6:19.
119. Davenport A, Rugman FP, Desmond MJ, et al. Is thrombocytopenia seen in patients with leptospirosis immunologically mediated? *J Clin Pathol*. 1989;42:439–440.
120. Araujo ER, Seguro AC, Spichler A, et al. Acute kidney injury in human leptospirosis: an immunohistochemical study with pathophysiological correlation. *Virchows Arch*. 2010;456:367–375.
121. Navarro CE, Kociba GJ. Hemostatic changes in dogs with experimental *Leptospira interrogans* serovar Icterohaemorrhagiae infection. *Am J Vet Res*. 1982;43:904–906.
122. Zaragoza C, Barrera R, Centeno F, et al. Characterization of renal damage in canine leptospirosis by sodium dodecyl sulphate-polyacrylamide gel electrophoresis (SDS-PAGE) and Western blotting of the urinary proteins. *J Comp Pathol*. 2003;129:169–178.
123. Gendron K, Christe A, Walter S, et al. Serial CT features of pulmonary leptospirosis in 10 dogs. *Vet Rec*. 2014;174:169.
124. Forrest LJ, O'Brien RT, Tremelling MS, et al. Sonographic renal findings in 20 dogs with leptospirosis. *Vet Radiol Ultrasound*. 1998;39:337–340.
125. Sonet J, Barthelemy A, Goy-Thollot I, et al. Prospective evaluation of abdominal ultrasonographic findings in 35 dogs with leptospirosis. *Vet Radiol Ultrasound*. 2018;59:98–106.
126. Hornsby RL, Alt DP, Nally JE. Isolation and propagation of leptospires at 37 degrees C directly from the mammalian host. *Sci Rep*. 2020;10:9620.
127. Schuller S, Francey T, Hartmann K, et al. European consensus statement on leptospirosis in dogs and cats. *J Small Anim Pract*. 2015;56:159–179.
128. Fraune CK, Schweighauser A, Francey T. Evaluation of the diagnostic value of serologic microagglutination testing and a polymerase chain reaction assay for diagnosis of acute leptospirosis in dogs in a referral center. *J Am Vet Med Assoc*. 2013;242:1373–1380.
129. Miller MD, Annis KM, Lappin MR, et al. Variability in results of the microscopic agglutination test in dogs with clinical leptospirosis and dogs vaccinated against leptospirosis. *J Vet Intern Med*. 2011;25:426–432.
130. Barr SC, McDonough PL, Scipioni-Ball RL, et al. Serologic responses of dogs given a commercial vaccine against *Leptospira interrogans* serovar Pomona and *Leptospira kirschneri* serovar Grippotyphosa. *Am J Vet Res*. 2005;66:1780–1784.
131. Martin LE, Wiggans KT, Wennogle SA, et al. Vaccine-associated *Leptospira* antibodies in client-owned dogs. *J Vet Intern Med*. 2014;28:789–792.
132. Midence JN, Leutenegger CM, Chandler AM, et al. Effects of recent *Leptospira* vaccination on whole blood real-time PCR testing in healthy client-owned dogs. *J Vet Intern Med*. 2012;26:149–152.
133. Chappel RJ, Goris M, Palmer MF, et al. Impact of proficiency testing on results of the microscopic agglutination test for diagnosis of leptospirosis. *J Clin Microbiol*. 2004;42:5484–5488.
134. Lizer J, Velineni S, Weber A, et al. Evaluation of 3 serological tests for early detection of *Leptospira*-specific antibodies in experimentally infected dogs. *J Vet Intern Med*. 2018;32:201–207.
135. Gloor CI, Schweighauser A, Francey T, et al. Diagnostic value of two commercial chromatographic "patient-side" tests in the diagnosis of acute canine leptospirosis. *J Small Anim Pract*. 2017;58:154–161.
136. Lizer J, Grahlmann M, Hapke H, et al. Evaluation of a rapid IgM detection test for diagnosis of acute leptospirosis in dogs. *Vet Rec*. 2017;180:517.
137. Harkin KR, Roshto YM, Sullivan JT. Clinical application of a polymerase chain reaction assay for diagnosis of leptospirosis in dogs. *J Am Vet Med Assoc*. 2003;222:1224–1229.
138. Rojas P, Monahan AM, Schuller S, et al. Detection and quantification of leptospires in urine of dogs: a maintenance host for the zoonotic disease leptospirosis. *Eur J Clin Microbiol Infect Dis*. 2010;29:1305–1309.
139. Branger C, Blanchard B, Fillonneau C, et al. Polymerase chain reaction assay specific for pathogenic *Leptospira* based on the gene hap1 encoding the hemolysis-associated protein-1. *FEMS Microbiol Lett*. 2005;243:437–445.
140. Stoddard RA. Detection of pathogenic *Leptospira* spp. through real-time PCR (qPCR) targeting the LipL32 gene. *Methods Mol Biol*. 2013;943:257–266.
141. Fink JM, Moore GE, Landau R, et al. Evaluation of three 5' exonuclease-based real-time polymerase chain reaction assays for detection of pathogenic *Leptospira* species in canine urine. *J Vet Diagn Invest*. 2015;27:159–166.
142. Thiel BE, Larson LJ, Okwumabua O, et al. R048P - Comparison of a novel point-of-care diagnostic, PCRun, with real time *Leptospira* PCR for detection of *Leptospira* antigen in canine samples. 2014. Available at: https://www.biogal.com/wp-content/uploads/2019/05/PCRun-CRWAD-Lepto-Abstract.pdf.
143. Delaude A, Rodriguez-Campos S, Dreyfus A, et al. Canine leptospirosis in Switzerland-A prospective cross-sectional study examining seroprevalence, risk factors and urinary shedding of pathogenic leptospires. *Prev Vet Med*. 2017;141:48–60.
144. Sykes JE. Unpublished observations.
145. Spangler D, Kish D, Beigel B, et al. Leptospiral shedding and seropositivity in shelter dogs in the Cumberland Gap region of Southeastern Appalachia. *PLoS One*. 2020;15:e0228038.
146. Llewellyn JR, Krupka-Dyachenko I, Rettinger AL, et al. Urinary shedding of leptospires and presence of *Leptospira* antibodies in healthy dogs from Upper Bavaria. *Berl Munch Tierarztl Wochenschr*. 2016;129:251–257.
147. Gay N, Soupe-Gilbert ME, Goarant C. Though not reservoirs, dogs might transmit *Leptospira* in New Caledonia. *Int J Environ Res Public Health*. 2014;11:4316–4325.
148. Altheimer K, Jongwattanapisan P, Luengyosluechakul S, et al. *Leptospira* infection and shedding in dogs in Thailand. *BMC Vet Res*. 2020;16:89.
149. Miotto BA, Guilloux AGA, Tozzi BF, et al. Prospective study of canine leptospirosis in shelter and stray dog populations: identification of chronic carriers and different *Leptospira* species infecting dogs. *PLoS One*. 2018;13:e0200384.
150. Miotto BA, Tozzi BF, Penteado MS, et al. Diagnosis of acute canine leptospirosis using multiple laboratory tests and characterization of the isolated strains. *BMC Vet Res*. 2018;14:222.
151. Reagan KL, Wang A, Huebner SN, et al. Development of machine learning algorithm model to predict leptospirosis diagnosis in dogs from hematologic, serum biochemical and urinalysis results. In: *Proceedings of the 11th International Leptospirosis Conference*. 2019.
152. Klopfleisch R, Kohn B, Plog S, et al. An emerging pulmonary haemorrhagic syndrome in dogs: similar to the human leptospiral pulmonary haemorrhagic syndrome? *Vet Med Int*. 2010;2010:928541.
153. Nicodemo AC, Duarte MI, Alves VA, et al. Lung lesions in human leptospirosis: microscopic, immunohistochemical, and ultrastructural features related to thrombocytopenia. *Am J Trop Med Hyg*. 1997;56:181–187.
154. Truccolo J, Charavay F, Merien F, et al. Quantitative PCR assay to evaluate ampicillin, ofloxacin, and doxycycline for treatment of experimental leptospirosis. *Antimicrob Agents Chemother*. 2002;46:848–853.
155. Griffith ME, Moon JE, Johnson EN, et al. Efficacy of fluoroquinolones against *Leptospira interrogans* in a hamster model. *Antimicrob Agents Chemother*. 2007;51:2615–2617.
156. Panaphut T, Domrongkitchaiporn S, Vibhagool A, et al. Ceftriaxone compared with sodium penicillin G for treatment of severe leptospirosis. *Clin Infect Dis*. 2003;36:1507–1513.
157. Phimda K, Hoontrakul S, Suttinont C, et al. Doxycycline versus azithromycin for treatment of leptospirosis and scrub typhus. *Antimicrob Agents Chemother*. 2007;51:3259–3263.
158. Niwattayakul K, Kaewtasi S, Chueasuwanchai S, et al. An open randomized controlled trial of desmopressin and pulse dexamethasone as

adjunct therapy in patients with pulmonary involvement associated with severe leptospirosis. *Clin Microbiol Infect.* 2010;16:1207–1212.
159. Pea L, Roda L, Boussaud V, et al. Desmopressin therapy for massive hemoptysis associated with severe leptospirosis. *Am J Resp Crit Care Med.* 2003;167:726–728.
160. Schweighauser ATF. Treatment of pulmonary haemorrhage in canine leptospirosis with desmopressin and dexamethasone. In: *Proceedings of the European College of Veterinary Internal Medicine.* 2008:206.
161. Meaudre E, Asencio Y, Montcriol A, et al. Immunomodulation in severe leptospirosis with multiple organ failure: plasma exchange, intravenous immunoglobulin or corticosteroids? *Ann Fr Anesth Reanim.* 2008;27:172–176.
162. Taylor D, Karamadoukis L. Plasma exchange in severe leptospirosis with multi-organ failure: a case report. *J Med Case Rep.* 2013;7:169.
163. Trivedi SV, Chavda RK, Wadia PZ, et al. The role of glucocorticoid pulse therapy in pulmonary involvement in leptospirosis. *J Assoc Physicians India.* 2001;49:901–903.
164. Trivedi SV, Vasava AH, Bhatia LC, et al. Plasma exchange with immunosuppression in pulmonary alveolar haemorrhage due to leptospirosis. *Indian J Med Res.* 2010;131:429–433.
165. Cerqueira TB, Athanazio DA, Spichler AS, et al. Renal involvement in leptospirosis: new insights into pathophysiology and treatment. *Braz J Infect Dis.* 2008;12:248–252.
166. Kis I, Schweighauser A, Francey T. Long-term outcome of dogs with acute kidney injury. In: *Proceedings of the American College of Veterinary Internal Medicine Forum.* 2012:798.
167. Sonrier C, Branger C, Michel V, et al. Evidence of cross-protection within *Leptospira interrogans* in an experimental model. *Vaccine.* 2000;19:86–94.
168. Bouvet J, Lemaitre L, Cariou C, et al. A canine vaccine against *Leptospira* serovars Icterohaemorrhagiae, Canicola and Grippotyphosa provides cross protection against *Leptospira* serovar Copenhageni. *Vet Immunol Immunopathol.* 2020;219:109985.
169. Francey T, Schweighauser A, Reber A, et al. Evaluation of changes in the epidemiology of leptospirosis in dogs after introduction of a quadrivalent anti-leptospiral vaccine in a highly endemic area. *J Vet Intern Med.* 2020;34:2405–2417.
170. Minke JM, Bey R, Tronel JP, et al. Onset and duration of protective immunity against clinical disease and renal carriage in dogs provided by a bivalent inactivated leptospirosis vaccine. *Vet Microbiol.* 2009;137:137–145.
171. Klaasen HL, van der Veen M, Sutton D, et al. A new tetravalent canine leptospirosis vaccine provides at least 12 months immunity against infection. *Vet Immunol Immunopathol.* 2014;158:26–29.
172. Grosenbaugh DA, Pardo MC. Fifteen-month duration of immunity for the serovar Grippotyphosa fraction of a tetravalent canine leptospirosis vaccine. *Vet Rec.* 2018;182:665.
173. Esteves SB, Santos CM, Salgado FF, et al. Efficacy of commercially available vaccines against canine leptospirosis: a systematic review and meta-analysis. *Vaccine.* 2022;40:1722–1740.
174. Schreiber P, Martin V, Najbar W, et al. Prevention of renal infection and urinary shedding in dogs by a *Leptospira* vaccination. *Vet Microbiol.* 2005;108:113–118.
175. Yao PJ, Stephenson N, Foley JE, et al. Incidence rates and risk factors for owner-reported adverse events following vaccination of dogs that did or did not receive a *Leptospira* vaccine. *J Am Vet Med Assoc.* 2015;247:1139–1145.
176. Eschle S, Hartmann K, Rieger A, et al. Canine vaccination in Germany: a survey of owner attitudes and compliance. *PLoS One.* 2020;15:e0238371.
177. Monahan AM, Miller IS, Nally JE. Leptospirosis: risks during recreational activities. *J Appl Microbiol.* 2009;107:707–716.

69

Borreliosis

Meryl P. Littman, Reinhard K. Straubinger, Jane E. Sykes

KEY POINTS

- First Described: Lyme disease (LD) – Connecticut, United States, 1982 (Burgdorfer)[1]; tick-borne relapsing fever (TBRF) – Colorado, United States, 1915.[2]
- Cause: Spirochetal bacteria of the genus *Borrelia* (and *Borreliella*); LD – *Borrelia burgdorferi* sensu lato,[3] *Borrelia mayonii.*[4] TBRF – *Borrelia hermsii*,[5–7] *Borrelia turicatae*,[7–9] *Borrelia persica*,[10–12] *Borrelia parkeri*,[7] *Borrelia miyamotoi*,[13,14] and others. At the time of writing, the taxonomy of *Borrelia* is in flux; the genus name *Borreliella* has been proposed for organisms other than relapsing fever borreliae.
- Primary Mode of Transmission: LD – *Ixodes* spp. ticks; TBRF – *Ornithodoros* spp. ticks for most, except *Ixodes* spp. for *B. miyamotoi.*
- Affected Hosts: LD – Humans and a large variety of animals; disease occurs in dogs, cats, humans, horses; TBRF – humans, dogs, cats, many reservoir and end hosts.
- Geographic Distribution: LD – North America, Europe, Asia; TBRF – North America, Europe, Middle East, Asia, Africa.
- Major Clinical Signs: LD – Fever, lethargy, inappetence, lameness due to oligoarthritis or polyarthritis; Lyme nephritis – vomiting, weight loss, signs of protein-losing nephropathy (PLN; thromboembolic events, effusions/edema, hypertension, eventual renal failure); TBRF – fever, lethargy, anorexia, neurologic signs, thrombocytopenia; anemia in cats.
- Differential Diagnoses: Lyme arthritis – lameness due to cruciate ligament rupture, primary immune-mediated polyarthritis, septic polyarthritis, and polyarthritis secondary to infection with other pathogens such as *Anaplasma* spp., *Ehrlichia* spp., *Bartonella* spp., *Rickettsia rickettsii*, and fungal organisms. Lyme nephritis – leptospirosis, bacterial pyelonephritis, primary immune-complex glomerulonephritis, familial nephropathies, amyloidosis, and glomerulonephritis secondary to other chronic infections such as dirofilariasis, babesiosis, ehrlichiosis, hepatozoonosis, leishmaniosis, and endocarditis. TBRF – fever of unknown origin, ITP, neurologic diseases.
- Human Health Significance: Dogs and cats are not a direct source of human infection but may bring unfed infected ticks into the house. Evidence of canine exposure to borreliosis is a sentinel for human exposure.

INTRODUCTION

The borrelioses are vector-borne infections that affect mammalian and avian hosts. Members of the genus *Borrelia*, which contains a large variety of species,[15] are usually categorized into one of two groups: the Lyme borreliosis organisms or the relapsing fever borreliae (Table 69.1). Both groups contain pathogenic species in addition to other borreliae that have been isolated only from ticks or non-clinical animals.

Lyme borreliosis is the most commonly diagnosed vector-borne disease of humans. It has been reported from North America, Europe, and Asia. Spontaneous and experimentally induced Lyme borreliosis has been described in dogs, cats, and other animals. Because of the difficulty in confirming a diagnosis and the diversity of borrelial species being isolated from ticks, controversy still exists regarding the exact prevalence and geographic distribution of infection. The relapsing fever borreliae affect humans and domestic animals. There are a few confirmed cases in which these organisms were isolated from sick dogs.

LYME BORRELIOSIS

ETIOLOGY AND EPIDEMIOLOGY

Like most spirochetes, borreliae are thin and elongated spiral-shaped bacteria (0.2 μm × 30 μm), consisting of a protoplasmic cylinder wound around an axial filament composed of multiple periplasmic endoflagella (Fig. 69.1). Dark-field, phase microscopy, or special staining techniques are needed for proper visualization of organisms. *Borrelia burgdorferi* sensu lato (s.l.; "in the broad sense") is a group of more than 20 accepted and proposed species.[15,16] Disease-relevant genospecies are listed in Table 69.1.[15,17] At the time of writing, the taxonomy of *Borrelia* is in flux and the name *Borreliella* has been proposed for non-relapsing fever borreliae; the relapsing fever borreliae would retain the genus name *Borrelia.* Because this has not been widely accepted, the name *Borrelia* will be used for both relapsing and non-relapsing fever organisms in this chapter. *Borrelia burgdorferi* sensu stricto (s.s.; "in the narrow sense") is the primary species responsible for Lyme disease in the United States. In humans, it is associated with annular skin lesions, oligo- or polyarthritis, meningitis, and carditis. In the United States, *Borrelia mayonii* in the upper midwest[4] and other borrelial species have been isolated from humans and *Ixodes* ticks on rabbits, rodents, and birds; their pathogenic significance for companion animals is uncertain.

In Eurasia, there are four main *Borrelia* genospecies: *Borrelia afzelii*, *Borrelia bavariensis*, *Borrelia garinii*, and *B. burgdorferi* s.s. Other species in Eurasia include *Borrelia lusitaniae*, *Borrelia valaisiana*, and *Borrelia japonica*. These appear to have common rodent and avian hosts, and many hosts harbor multiple infectious agents.[18–20] The greater diversity among species in Eurasia suggests that this complex of organisms originated in this region.[16,21] In Eurasia, meningopolyneuritis (Bannwarth syndrome) is the primary clinical sign in humans infected with *B. garinii* and *B. bavariensis*, whereas seropositivity due to infection with *B. afzelii* has been associated with chronic arthritis and acute and chronic dermatitis (erythema migrans and acrodermatitis chronica atrophicans, respectively).[22] *Borrelia lusitaniae* was isolated from a person in Portugal with an erythema migrans and produced experimental infection in mice.[23,24] *Borrelia valaisiana* has been isolated from *Ixodes ricinus* ticks on vegetation and birds; its DNA was also found in a human with meningoencephalitis.[25] *Borrelia afzelii* has been isolated from a naturally infected dog,[26] and mixed infections

TABLE 69.1 ***Borrelia* Species of Medical and Veterinary Importance**[a,b]

Species	Disease	Geographic Location	Vector	Wild Animal Reservoir	Domestic Hosts
***Borrelia burgdorferi* sensu lato**					
Borrelia burgdorferi sensu stricto	Lyme borreliosis. Humans: erythema migrans (annular skin lesions), polyarthritis, meningitis, carditis. Dogs: Lyme arthritis, Lyme nephritis	North America	*Ixodes scapularis, Ixodes pacificus*, and *Ixodes neotomae*	Larvae and nymphs: rodents, small mammals, birds Adults: deer, larger mammals, birds	Human, dog, cat, horse
	Lyme borreliosis	Europe	*Ixodes ricinus*	Same as above, except birds more prevalent for all stages	Human, dog, horse
Borrelia bavariensis *Borrelia garinii*	Erythema migrans, meningopolyneuritis, arthritis	Europe, Asia	*I. ricinus, Ixodes persulcatus*	Birds, small mammals	Human, dog?, cat?
Borrelia mayonii	Fever, headache, rash, neck pain, vomiting, spirochetemia	Upper Midwestern United States	*I. scapularis*	Small mammals	Human, other?
Borrelia afzelii	Erythema migrans, meningopolyneuritis, arthritis, ACA	Europe, Asia	*I. ricinus, I. persulcatus*	Small mammals	Human, dog?, cat?
Borrelia japonica	Unknown	Japan	*Ixodes ovatus, I. persulcatus*	Rodents, birds	Unknown
Borrelia bissettii[c]	Erythema migrans, lymphocytoma	Slovenia	*I. ricinus*	Rodents, birds	Human
	Unknown	North America	*I. neotomae, I. scapularis*	Rodents, birds?	Rodent[d]
Borrelia valaisiana	Meningoencephalitis	Europe, Asia	*I. ricinus*	Birds	Human
Borrelia spielmanii	Meningoencephalitis	Germany, Slovenia	*I. ricinus*	Birds?	Human
Borrelia lusitaniae	Erythema migrans	Europe, North Africa	*I. ricinus*	Rodents, lizards	Human, rodent[e]
Relapsing Fever Borreliae					
Borrelia turicatae	Spirochetemia, lymphadenomegaly, lameness, anterior uveitis, fever	Florida, Texas	*Ornithodoros turicata*	Unknown	Dog
Borrelia lonestari	STARI	Southeastern and south central United States	*Amblyomma americanum*	Deer	Human
Borrelia miyamotoi sensu lato	Fever, chills, headache, joint pain, fatigue, spirochetemia, possible neurologic signs	North America, Japan, Europe	*Ixodes* spp.	Rodents?	Human, other?
Borrelia recurrentis	Epidemic louse-borne relapsing fever	Central and East Africa, South America, Europe, Asia	*Pediculus humanus* (body louse)	None	Human
Borrelia anserine	Avian spirochetosis	Worldwide	*Argas persicus*	Birds	Poultry
Borrelia hermsii, Borrelia parkeri	Endemic tick-borne relapsing fevers, visible spirochetemia	North America (northwest, west)	*Ornithodoros* spp.	Rodents, small mammals	Human, dog
Borrelia persica	As above	Asia, Middle East	As above	As above	Human, dog, cat
Borrelia hispanica	As above	Spain	As above	As above	As above
Borrelia duttonii	As above	East Africa	As above	As above	As above
Borrelia coriaceae	Enzootic abortion	Western United States	*Ornithodoros coriaceus*	Deer	Cow

[a]Other species isolated from ticks or their reservoir hosts, but not established to infect domestic hosts include: *Borrelia andersonii* in *Ixodes dentatis*, United States; *Borrelia californiensis.*, western United States; *B. carolinensis.* southeastern United States; *Borrelia americana.*, southeastern and western United States; *Borrelia tanukii* in *I. tanuki*, Japan; *Borrelia turdi* in *I. turdis*, Japan; *Borrelia sinica* in *Ixodes ovatus* and *Niviventer confucianus*, China.
[b]At the time of writing, the taxonomy of borreliae is in flux; the genus name *Borreliella* has been proposed for species belonging to *Borrelia burgdorferi* sensu lato; relapsing fever borreliae would retain the genus name *Borrelia.*
[c]Isolated reports exist for infection of humans with these *Borrelia* species.
[d]Experimental infection.
[e]Experimental infection.
ACA, acrodermatitis chronica atrophicans; *STARI*, southern tick-associated rash illness; *?*, uncertain involvement.

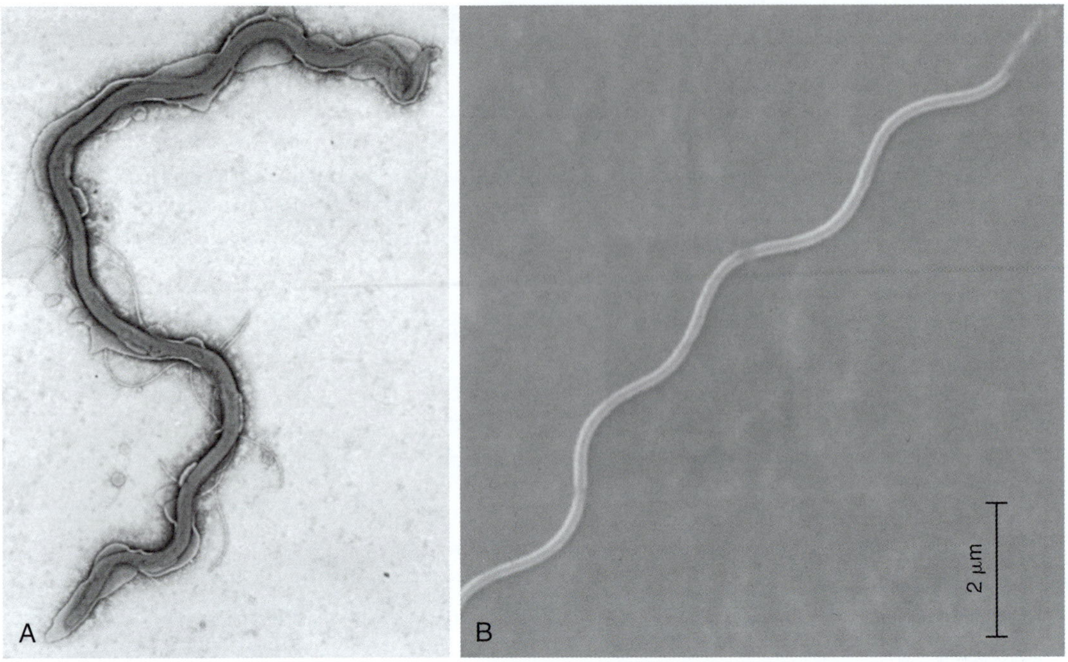

Fig. 69.1 (A) Transmission electron micrograph of *Borrelia burgdorferi* showing periplasmic flagella that have been released from the confines of the outer membrane secondary to specimen preparation (phosphotungstic acid, ×7100). (B) Scanning microscopic view of *B. burgdorferi* (×15,000). (Courtesy of R. Straubinger, LMU Munich, Germany.)

with this and other European species have been described. *Borrelia japonica* has been isolated from ticks found on dogs and humans in Japan.[27] In the same region, additional borrelial species have been isolated from ticks from small mammals; however, their pathogenic significance is uncertain.

Borreliae cannot survive as free-living organisms in the environment. They are host-associated, being transmitted between vertebrate reservoir hosts (mammals, birds, and lizards) and hematophagous arthropod vectors. *Borrelia burgdorferi* s.l. infections are geographically dispersed (see Table 69.1). In general, Lyme borreliosis occurs in the northern hemisphere in temperate latitudes with cooler climatic conditions. In North America, the majority of canine and human cases occur in the mid-Atlantic to New England coastal states, northeastern states into southern Canada, and upper midwestern states. Ecology supporting Lyme disease exists in adjacent states and also on the west coast down into northeastern Mexico (and especially just north of San Francisco),[28–30] and the areas affected are expanding as tick populations, reservoir hosts, and white-tailed deer populations expand (Fig. 69.2). In North America, evidence of exposure in dogs is often detected earlier and to a greater extent than in humans in areas of Lyme emergence. In a serosurvey of dogs in the United States, overall positive prevalence rates were highest in the northeast (11.6%), followed by the midwest (4.0%), west (1.4%), and southeast (1%) in decreasing order.[31,32] These data mirror the human prevalence data for disease prevalence.[33] Analysis of over 20 million antibody test results in dogs from 2010 to 2017 in 25 states from the eastern United States showed a trend for declining seroprevalence in 8 states along the mid-Atlantic coast from Virginia to New Hampshire, and Wisconsin; an increasing seroprevalence in 5 northeastern states and midwestern states where Lyme is endemic or emerging; and an increasing seroprevalence in 3 southern states that are not considered endemic regions.[34] In Canada, Lyme borreliosis in humans is endemic in southeastern Ontario. In a study that included 753,468 C_6 antibody test results from 2008 to 2015, there was a significant increase in seroprevalence (144%) over the course of the study, from 0.9% to 2.2%.[35] The risk of seropositivity

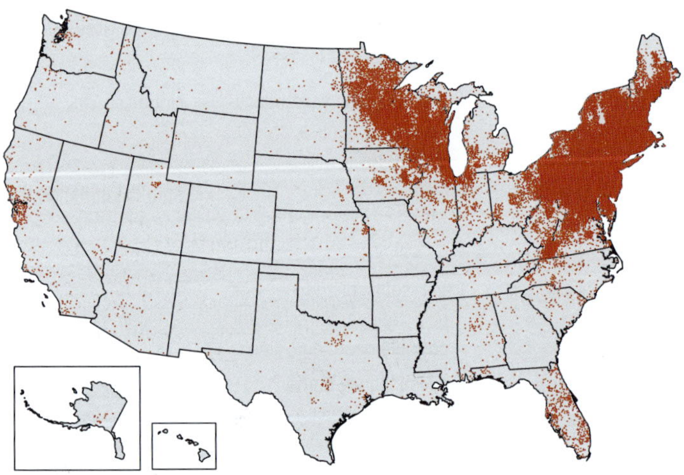

Fig. 69.2 Approximate geographic distribution of Lyme borreliosis in humans (and dogs) in the United States.

was greater in Manitoba (2.4%), Quebec (2.3%), Nova Scotia (9.5%), and New Brunswick (7.4%) than in the reference province of Ontario (1.8%), and lower in Alberta (0.8%) and British Columbia (0.5%). The seroprevalence in 199 dogs from Prince Edward Island was 3%, where 10% of *Ixodes scapularis* ticks were found to be infected.[36]

The principal vectors of *B. burgdorferi* s.l. are various species of slow-feeding hard ticks of the *Ixodes* spp. complex, the distribution of which reflects disease prevalence (Table 69.2). In the United States and Canada, closely related black-legged ticks, *I. scapularis* (in the northeastern, midwestern, and southeastern states to northeastern Mexico, and southern Canada) and *Ixodes pacificus* together with *Ixodes neotomae* (in the western states) appear to be involved.[37] Two major clades of *I. scapularis* have been identified in the United States, the American (northern) clade and the Southern clade.[38] *Ixodes scapularis* ticks found on dogs and cats in the northeast and midwest are almost exclusively of

TABLE 69.2 Selected Vectors of *Borrelia burgdorferi*[a]

Species	Geographic Location	FEEDING PREFERENCE		Infection Prevalence
		Larvae, Nymphs	Adults	
Ixodes scapularis American clade	United States (mid- and north-Atlantic coast, northern Midwest)	White-footed mouse (*Peromyscus leucopus*), small mammals, birds	Deer, larger mammals	<1% larvae 10%–25% nymphs 10%–80% adults
Ixodes scapularis Southern clade	United States (southeastern)	Lizards	Lizards (occasionally mammals)	<1% larvae <1% nymphs <1% adults
Ixodes pacificus, Ixodes neotomae	United States (western)	Lizards	Lizards (occasionally mammals)	1%–5%
Ixodes ricinus	Europe (western and central)	Small mammals, birds, mice (*Apodemus flavicollis, Apodemus sylvaticus, Clethrionomys glareolus*)	Deer, larger mammals	10%–25%
Ixodes persulcatus	Europe through central and northern Asia to China and Japan	Small mammals, birds	Deer, larger mammals	10%–25%

[a]*Borrelia burgdorferi* or related organisms have been recovered from numerous other ticks and arthropods in nature, but the significance is uncertain. Many sylvan cycles exist in nature in which tick vectors do not feed on large mammals. Only the established vectors for humans or domestic animals are listed here.

the American clade; two thirds of *I. scapularis* found on dogs and cats in the southeast were of the American clade and one third was of the Southern clade.[38] Ticks in the north central United States prefer deciduous, dry to mesic forests and sandy or loamy soils overlying sedimentary rock.[39] Ticks are not associated with grasslands, conifer forests, or acidic soils with low fertility or a claylike consistency. In the coastal states, tick infection and dog seroprevalence are greatest in the coastal counties,[40] presumably reflecting the tick's preference for moisture.[41]

These small (less than 3 mm) ixodid ticks generally feed on more than one host during their life cycle (Figs. 69.3 and 69.4). The number of hosts varies depending on the tick species. In North America, where approximately 50 to 80 vertebrate species serve as hosts, larvae and nymphs of *I. scapularis* in the north and parts of the south generally feed on small mammals and birds, whereas immature stages of *I. scapularis* in the south often feed on a variety of hosts including lizards.[42,43] Adults of these ticks feed on deer or larger mammals. Reptiles and other preferential hosts of *I. scapularis* in the southern and western regions are not competent reservoir hosts, and differences in the timing of feeding on these hosts do not allow for efficient transfer of infection for its overwintering in ticks. Therefore, the infection rate of southern *I. scapularis* ticks (less than 1%) is much lower than that of *I. scapularis* ticks in the northeastern United States (10% to 50%).[44] At least one lizard species possesses a borreliacidal substance in its blood similar to complement that reduces or prevents infection with *B. burgdorferi*.[45] Furthermore, because the southern *I. scapularis* ticks do not always feed on mammals, the prevalence of Lyme borreliosis in humans and domestic animals is low in the south.[46] Infected *Ixodes* ticks may be dispersed to new areas by feeding on migratory birds.[47–52]

In Europe, *B. afzelii, B. bavariensis, B. garinii*, and *B. burgdorferi* s.s. are responsible for the majority of infections. Most cases occur in the Scandinavian countries and in central Europe in areas with moderate temperature and moderate humidity (Austria, Belgium, Croatia, Czech Republic, parts of France, Germany, Hungary, Netherlands, Portugal, Slovenia, Switzerland etc.), with the prevalence tending to increase from west to east in association with *I. ricinus* activity (Fig. 69.5). *Ixodes ricinus* ticks, across the Mediterranean Sea in northern Africa, are also infected with *B. burgdorferi* s.l.[53] *Ixodes ricinus* ticks have also been infected with other *Borrelia* spp., including *Borrelia bissettii, B. valaisiana*, and *B. lusitaniae*.[54–56] In these cases, the infection is being maintained in nature; however, the clinical significance of such infections in humans or domestic animals is unknown. The distribution of infection stretches eastward across Eurasia, corresponding to the habitat of the tick *Ixodes persulcatus*, which transmits *B. bavariensis, B. garinii*, and *B. afzelii*.[57] Whereas *B. burgdorferi* s.s., *B. bavariensis*, and *B. afzelii* are associated with rodent reservoirs, *B. garinii* and *B. valaisiana* are associated with bird reservoirs.[58] *Ixodes ricinus* and *I. persulcatus* parasitize more than 200 vertebrate species. Several species of mice, voles, and rats are important reservoir hosts. Squirrels,

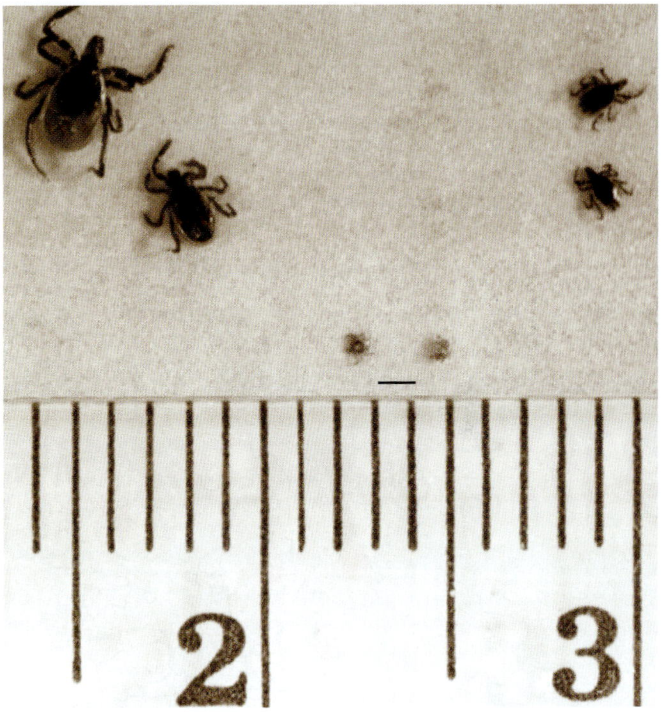

Fig. 69.3 *Ixodes scapularis* ticks. From largest to smallest, two adults (male, female), two nymphs, two larvae (bar = 1 mm). (Courtesy of Mike DeRosa, West Somerville, MA.)

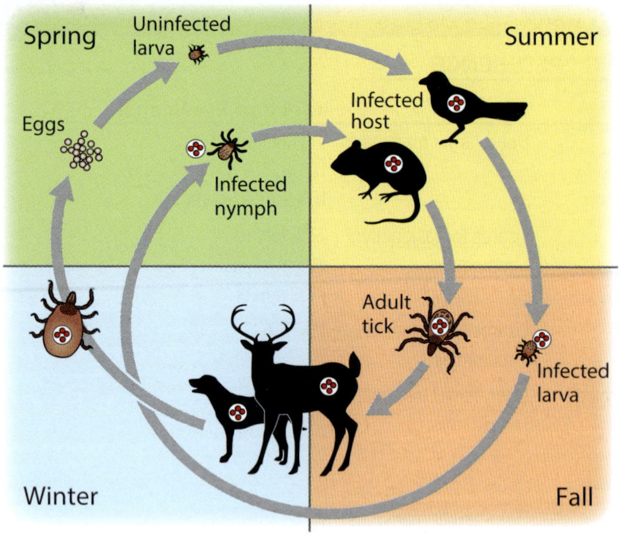

Fig. 69.4 Life cycle of *Ixodes scapularis*. The life cycle lasts a minimum of 2 years. Eggs are oviposited in the spring, and the larvae emerge approximately 1 month later. They feed once in the summer, usually on birds and small mammals, and then overwinter. The following spring, the larvae molt into nymphs, which then feed in late spring or early summer. The nymphs feed on mice or larger mammals such as dogs, deer, or humans and are considered the most likely source of *Borrelia burgdorferi* (and/or *Anaplasma phagocytophilum*) infection for dogs and people. Nymphs then molt into adults in the fall. The adults usually feed on larger mammals (often white-tailed deer), where they mate. The females die after laying their eggs, and the 2-year cycle is repeated. Circles that contain red dots represent infection with *B. burgdorferi* and/or *A. phagocytophilum*.

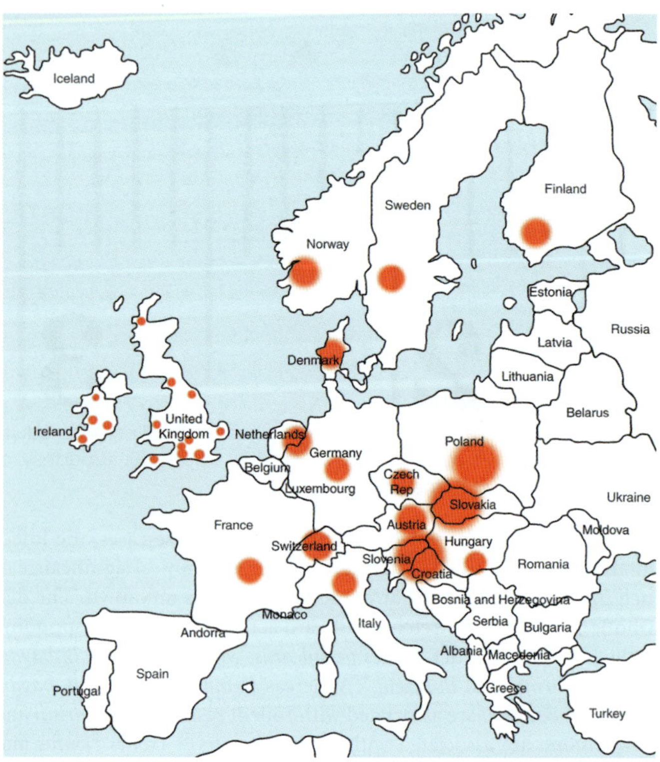

Fig. 69.5 Countries and regions where Lyme borreliosis occurs in Europe. The size of the red dot correlates with the relative prevalence of the infection in those areas.

hedgehogs, shrews, and birds are also involved in the maintenance of the infection cycle.

On the North American and Eurasian continents, larger ungulates such as deer and moose are important in the life cycle because adult *Ixodes* ticks feed on them and are carried for long distances. However, the level of infection in these large mammals is insufficient to transmit to feeding ticks, making them unsuitable reservoir hosts.[59–61] The *Ixodes* ticks that transmit Lyme borreliosis normally have a minimum 2-year life cycle and maintain infection in nature by harboring the organism over the winter period (see Fig. 69.4). In the northeastern and upper midwestern United States, *I. scapularis* primarily becomes infected when immature stages (especially larvae) feed on infected white-footed mice (*Peromyscus leucopus*) and birds.

Direct transmission of borreliae between reservoir hosts is unlikely, and transovarial transmission in ticks that carry Lyme borreliosis organisms is practically nonexistent, except for *Borrelia miyamotoi*.[62,63] Larvae, which have become infected by feeding in the summer and fall, harbor the organism over the winter and molt to infected nymphs.[64] When these nymphs feed in the spring, they transmit organisms to competent reservoir hosts. Nymphs, which feed on a wide variety of animals, are primarily responsible for the transmission of infection to domestic animals and humans, as well as infecting new rodent reservoir hosts.

Larvae and other tick stages can become infected from previously uninfected hosts by co-feeding with infected ticks that have attached in close temporal and spatial proximity.[65,66] However, co-feeding of infected and noninfected *I. ricinus* ticks was not as efficient in transmitting *B. afzelii* infection as was the transmission of the organism from previously infected mice to uninfected larvae.[19] Adult female ticks feed on larger mammals such as white-tailed deer, dogs, and livestock. Although feeding on deer is necessary to maintain the tick population, deer and cattle are not effective reservoir hosts for infection.[67] Nymphs are more likely to cause human infections because they remain undetected due to their small size (see Fig. 69.3). This allows them to remain attached for sufficient periods for successful transmission of spirochetes. Despite the zoonotic risk from nymphal ticks, adult ticks appear to have the highest rate of infectivity among stages, presumably because of repeated exposure to infected mammals and birds.

In the western United States, immature *I. pacificus* become infected by feeding primarily on western gray squirrels (*Sciurus griseus*), and the adult ticks transmit the infection to larger mammals during subsequent feedings. As occurs in Eurasia, birds may be more important in the sylvatic cycle of infection in the western United States.[68] *Ixodes trianguliceps* may also play an analogous but lesser role in Eurasia of maintaining infection in nature, similar to that of *I. spinipalpis* in the western United States, by feeding exclusively on rodent reservoirs.[69]

Ixodes ticks can be simultaneously infected with additional animal and human pathogens, including *Ehrlichia* spp. and *Rickettsia* spp. (e.g., *Ehrlichia muris* in the upper midwest),[70] *Anaplasma phagocytophilum* (see Chapter 45), *Babesia* spp. (*Babesia microti*, *Babesia odocoilei*, and *Babesia gibsoni*) (see Chapter 97), multiple *Borrelia* spp. (e.g., *B. miyamotoi* in the east, *B. mayonii* in the upper midwest), and tick-borne encephalitis viruses.[71–74] Diagnosis and interpretation of serologic tests, and correlating them with specific signs of clinical illness, are problematic when a co-infection exists (see Diagnosis).

Numerous hematophagous arthropods, including other tick species, fleas, flies, mites, and mosquitoes, carry *Borrelia* organisms in nature. These findings most likely indicate accidental contamination, and arthropods do not transmit infection. Contamination from feeding on infected vertebrates is suspected; accordingly, these other arthropods have not been documented to transfer infection to new hosts.[75] Only *I. scapularis*—and not *Amblyomma americanum* or *Dermacentor variabilis*—has effectively transmitted *B. burgdorferi* in North America.[75]

Although Lyme borreliosis is generally associated with mice and small mammals in forests, bordering shrubs of backyards, and gardens, it may be acquired in parks in major metropolitan centers where rats appear to be the effective reservoir host for feeding ticks.[76–78] In the northern midwestern United States, seropositivity among dogs was positively associated with numerous risk factors including increased tick exposure, time spent outdoors, and living in forested or urban wooded habitats and on sandy, fertile soils.[79]

In a natural infection model study with ticks, control dogs that were in direct contact with infected dogs for up to a year did not undergo seroconversion, and organisms could not be isolated from the urine or urinary bladder of infected dogs.[80] Canine urine is an unlikely source of infection. After natural infection, *in utero* spread to pups did not occur from seropositive dams. *Borrelia burgdorferi* can survive in blood processed for transfusion and stored under blood bank conditions,[81,82] but they do not induce infection after blood transfusion.[83] However, not a single case of *B. burgdorferi* infection caused by blood transfusion has been documented in humans[84,85] or animals, and no animal model exists in which Lyme borreliosis can be induced by artificial insemination or by IV injection of *B. burgdorferi* organisms.[83]

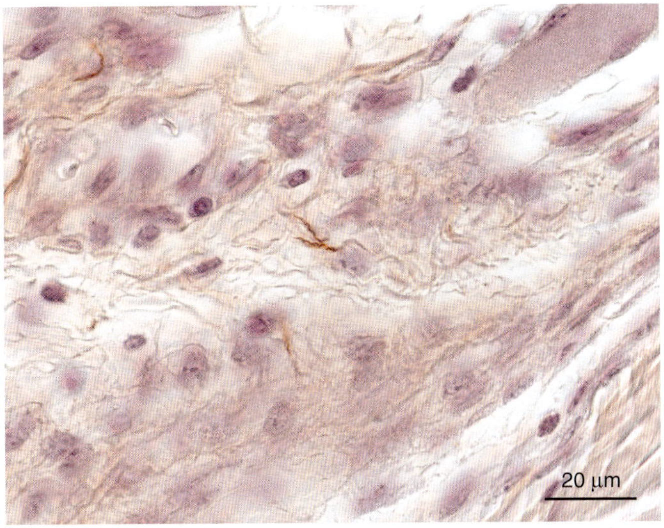

Fig. 69.6 *Borrelia burgdorferi* in the metatarsal tendon sheath of a research mouse with severe combined immunodeficiency. The spirochetes are stained brown using immunohistochemistry. (Courtesy of Dr. Stephen Barthold, University of California-Davis)

CLINICAL FEATURES

Pathogenesis and Clinical Signs

Borrelia burgdorferi carries up to 12 linear and 9 circular plasmids. The plasmid genome codes largely for outer surface proteins responsible for survival and persistence in vertebrate hosts and successful transmission by tick vectors.[86–88] Borreliae grown *in vitro* can lose plasmids and hence pathogenic potential.

The onset of spirochete transmission requires 12 to 24h (average 18h) of tick attachment, during which organisms multiply and cross the gut epithelium into the hemolymph, disseminate to the salivary glands, and infect the host through tick saliva.[89,90] Outer surface protein A (OspA), the predominant surface protein, is expressed on the outer surface of borreliae in the midgut of infected ticks and allows the spirochetes to adhere to the midgut by attaching to a receptor known as TROSPA.[91,92] In unfed ticks, virtually all spirochetes reside in the midgut. During feeding and because of the warmth of the new environment (skin surface temperature of the host), spirochetes begin to express OspC, which correlates with the migration of the spirochetes from the midgut into the hemolymph and finally to the salivary glands of the feeding tick.[86,87,89,93–98] Although originally thought that OspA is downregulated during feeding, more recent studies suggest that strong OspA expression is maintained throughout the tick feeding process; expression decreases only after infection of the mammalian host occurs.[92]

After dermal inoculation into the mammalian host, aided by tick salivary protein 15 (Salp15), OspC inhibits phagocytosis and promotes spirochete dissemination.[97–101] Salp15 binds to OspC and protects it from immune recognition; it also inhibits adaptive immune responses against Borrelia and tick antigens.[97] The expression of OspC allows the organism to become established in the host; however, it is not required for persistence beyond several weeks.[102] Levels of the immunodominant variable surface lipoprotein component (VlsE; variable major protein-like sequence, expressed) increase during the last 2 days of tick engorgement; the increase continues after OspC production ceases.[103] VlsE and other proteins are involved in chronic persistence of the spirochete and its avoidance of the host immune response. A genetically conserved, invariable region of VlsE protein is strongly immunodominant and important in serodiagnosis (see below, Serologic Testing).

Despite the numerous humans and animals that are bitten by infected ticks, only a few develop clinical disease. Host immune reactions are likely involved in preventing many of these infections. Studies show that the percentage of dogs that develop severe clinical signs of the disease is low when compared with the frequency of exposure based on seropositivity (3%–10% in central Europe; 70%–90% in highly endemic areas in the United States) and the rate of infection demonstrated in ticks.[104–109] Part of this seropositivity in dogs may indicate exposure to low numbers of *B. burgdorferi* organisms in a host with an efficient immune system or represent an exposure to infectious but nonpathogenic isolates of *Borrelia*.[110] Even among genetically similar *B. burgdorferi* s.s. strains, pathogenicity may vary based on plasmid content. Based on OspC genotyping, over 30 strains of *B. burgdorferi* s.s. have been identified. In the New England region of northeastern United States, OspC types A, B, I, K, and N were most common in humans, whereas infected dogs showed types A, B, F, I, and N; strains may differ in geological areas, hosts, pathogenicity, and tissue tropism.[111–115] Lack of cross-reactive immunity allows for multiple strain infections and reinfection.[116]

From the site of the tick bite, spirochetes replicate and migrate through the skin and connective tissues (Fig. 69.6). Later, they colonize many tissues, including the joints. Active migration in tissues is the likely route of dissemination as opposed to passive dissemination via the blood,[85] although spirochetemia occurs with *B. mayonii*.[4] This has implications for diagnosis. The spirochetes' requirement for N-acetyl-glucosamine, a component of collagen synthesis, may explain tissue tropism.[117]

Once in the body, *B. burgdorferi* acts as a persistent pathogen. The host immune response is capable of reducing spirochete numbers, and although the spirochete is not eliminated from the host after a few weeks of infection, *B. burgdorferi* is virtually undetectable in body fluids or internal organs, and exceedingly few spirochetes are found in other tissues.[80,118,119] The organism can evade host antibody and exist extracellularly by varying or masking its immunoreactive proteins,[86,87,99,120,121] and by changing its shape. Spiral, motile borreliae can convert into spherical life forms within minutes after they have encountered unfavorable environmental conditions (Fig. 69.7).[122,123] In this form, they survive for days without nutrition and without metabolic activity and revert into the well-known spiral form when conditions improve. These spherical forms are able to infect mice.[124,125] This may explain why *B. burgdorferi* can persist and be detected in tissue specimens by PCR or occasionally by culture even after months of antibacterial treatment.[125] Spirochete antigen has also been found in joints after treatment in mice.[126] Clinical illness results from the host's

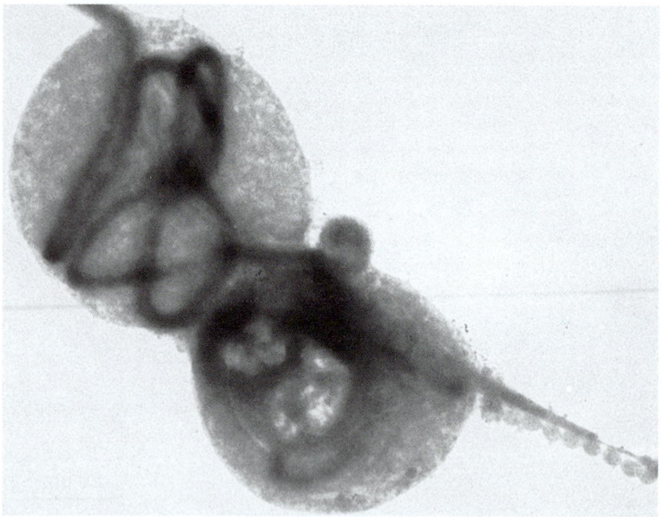

Fig. 69.7 Transmission electron microscopic (×12,000) appearance of the cystic form of *Borrelia burgdorferi*, a defense mechanism of the organism for survival under adverse conditions such as antimicrobial therapy or host immune defenses. (Courtesy of R. Straubinger, LMU Munich, Germany.)

own inflammatory response. Some of the immunopathologic events in joint, cardiac, or nervous tissue may be related to immune responses generated against specific borrelial antigens.[127] One of the most immunogenic proteins, flagellin, can elicit production of an antibody that binds to host neuroaxonal proteins. This sequence may in turn stimulate the inflammatory response in nervous tissue.[128] Clonal analysis indicates that the immune response in nervous tissue may be directed at the pathogen and neural self-antigens.[129]

Cytokine release results in damage to the surrounding tissue. In the joints, upregulation of IL-8, which recruits neutrophils to inflammatory sites, has been found in the synovial membranes of experimentally infected dogs.[130] This may contribute to the development of suppurative polyarthritis. In a few animals, the development of arthritis is probably related to pathologic perpetual host immune reactions. Humans with certain MHC haplotypes are prone to more severe, treatment-resistant clinical manifestations of the disease in which *B. burgdorferi* cannot be detected.[131]

The tissues of preferential localization may vary by *Borrelia* species and determine pathogenicity and, therefore, differences in clinical manifestations seen in various geographic regions. *Borrelia garinii* was found in the liver of dogs having elevated serum liver enzyme activities, a finding not associated with *B. burgdorferi* s.s. infection.[132] Despite the presence of glomerulonephritis in seropositive dogs, evidence of the presence of spirochetes has not been found in renal lesions.[133,134] The glomerular injury may relate to deposition of circulating immune complexes (CICs) secondary to infection rather than primary spirochetal localization. *Borrelia burgdorferi*–specific CICs have been found in the serum of infected dogs and elution studies of kidneys taken from suspect dogs after death showed *B. burgdorferi*–specific complexes in the glomerular deposits.[135,136]

Clinical Signs in Humans When Compared with Dogs

Clinical features of Lyme borreliosis in humans include an acute phase within a week of exposure with dermatitis (erythema migrans, an expanding bull's eye rash at the site of the tick bite) and influenza-like signs, followed weeks to months later by oligoarthritis in 60% of untreated cases (usually of the knee), or possibly (more common in Europe) neurologic manifestations (e.g., cranial nerve palsy, polyradiculitis, meningitis), myocarditis, or chronic dermatitis.[3,137] In contrast to humans in which asymptomatic seroconversion is uncommon in North America,[138] the vast majority of exposed dogs experience subclinical seroconversion.[104,106,107,139] Experimentally, no acute signs of illness occur in dogs, and signs of arthritis are not noted until at least 2 months post-exposure, well after seroconversion.[80,104,107,139] Erythema migrans is not reported in dogs, and neurologic,[140–144] cardiac,[145,146] or dermal signs are rare or poorly documented. However, perhaps 2% of naturally exposed dogs develop Lyme nephritis (immune-complex glomerulonephritis), which is rarely seen in humans.[147,148] Co-infections in both dogs and humans are common, especially with other tick-borne pathogens that are transmitted simultaneously and may precipitate or exacerbate clinical signs.[149]

Lyme Borreliosis in Dogs

Experimental infections. Initial attempts to recreate experimental Lyme borreliosis in dogs using laboratory-derived strains were unsuccessful, as they were in cats.[150,151] However, fever and lameness due to oligo- or polyarthritis have been experimentally produced after dermal inoculation or natural exposure to tick-derived *B. burgdorferi*.[80,130,152–155] Inoculation of spirochetes using field-collected ticks has been most successful; however, co-infections are common, especially with *A. phagocytophilum* (see Chapter 45). Clinical illness in experimentally infected young puppies occurred 2 to 9 months after tick exposure, well after seroconversion, and the severity and propensity to develop signs of illness seem to vary inversely with the animal's age and immune status. Exposed 6- to 12-week-old puppies had a self-limiting 4-day illness starting 2 to 5 months after exposure, consisting of fever and lameness due to acute arthritis in the limb closest to where ticks fed, sometimes with several similar relapses at 2-week intervals in the same or different limb. Exposed 13- to 26-week-old puppies had milder signs, and adult dogs seroconverted but showed no signs of illness.[80,155] Interestingly, about half of the experimental dogs were inadvertently co-infected with *A. phagocytophilum* and some were weakly positive for antibodies to *Babesia microti*. Signs of experimental disease appear milder than those in the field, possibly due to multiple tick exposures in the field (times and sites).

Systemic signs. Acute signs of fever (103.1°F to 104.9°F [39.5°C to 40.5°C]), shifting leg lameness, articular swelling, lymphadenomegaly, anorexia, and general malaise, all of which are responsive to antimicrobials, may be seen in experimentally[80,130,155] and in naturally exposed dogs.[102,104,105,139,156–158] The accuracy of diagnosis in natural infection is difficult to determine because limb and joint signs (swelling, lameness, and pain) with fever and inappetence have been observed with equal frequency in dogs with and without *B. burgdorferi*–specific antibodies.[159–161] One study found that 40% of dogs initially diagnosed with Lyme borreliosis were eventually found to have other causes for their clinical signs.[162]

Arthritis. Oligo- or polyarthritis is the most overt syndrome caused by acute *B. burgdorferi* infection in dogs. The first limb affected is usually closest to the site of tick attachment.[80] The onset of lameness can correspond to an increased body temperature. Lameness often lasts for a few days and then may shift to another limb or disappear. Despite the transient nature of the arthritis, inflammatory changes may persist in the joint.[152] Microscopic lesions have been most consistently found in the skin, lymphatic tissues, and joints, even though the organism can be isolated from other tissues.[163] Dogs with naturally occurring cranial cruciate ligament arthropathy in a Lyme borreliosis endemic area had a higher prevalence of *B. burgdorferi* and other bacterial gene sequences within synovial biopsy tissue than dogs with clinically healthy stifle joints and those with experimental cranial cruciate ligament rupture.[164,165] These bacteria may be important in the causation and pathogenesis of the inflammatory arthritis.

Glomerulonephritis (Lyme nephritis). Although an experimental model is lacking, protein-losing glomerulonephritis has been described in naturally infected dogs, mostly in Labrador and golden retrievers.[134,166–169] Even among retrievers, Lyme nephritis is uncommon and seropositivity is neither predictive nor associated with proteinuria.[170] Lyme nephritis is characterized by protein-losing nephropathy (PLN) in a seropositive dog, e.g., as a progressive or acute renal failure associated with proteinuria, azotemia/uremia, hypertension, thromboembolic events, peripheral edema, body cavity effusions, and occasionally neurologic signs.[104,107,167,171] The duration of clinical illness before evaluation has varied from 24 hours to 8 weeks, with a sudden onset of anorexia, vomiting, and lethargy. Dogs with more chronic progression show weight loss. About a third of dogs exhibit recent or concurrent lameness. Many dogs with advanced disease when first evaluated die or are euthanized as a result of renal failure. Since *B. burgdorferi* seropositivity is a marker for tick and wildlife exposure, it is important that other causes of renal proteinuria are ruled out (e.g., dirofilariasis, other tick-borne diseases, leptospirosis).[172,173] Renal biopsies of dogs with suspected Lyme nephritis do not show spirochetal invasion but rather immune-complex glomerulonephritis, tubular necrosis/regeneration, and interstitial nephritis.[134,166,167] Bernese mountain dogs in Europe have an increased prevalence of antibodies against *B. burgdorferi* s.l. compared with other breeds; however, seropositivity was not associated with proteinuria or lameness over a 2.5- to 3-year observation period.[174–179] Another case-control study also found no association between proteinuric kidney disease and *Borrelia* spp. seropositivity in Bernese mountain dogs.[180] Therefore, glomerular disease in this breed may be due to genetic and other causes. A genetic predisposition for resistance to *B. burgdorferi* infection was noted in purpose-bred beagles.[181]

Meningitis. Neurologic signs are later manifestations of Lyme borreliosis in humans, especially in *B. garinii* infections, which was reproducible in primate models.[182,183] Experimentally, young infected dogs developed mild focal meningitis, encephalitis, and perineuritis; however, neurologic signs were not observed.[155] Neurologic signs were not associated with seropositivity to *B. burgdorferi* in naturally infected dogs.[142–144] Nucleic acids of *B. burgdorferi* were not found in the CNS of dogs with a variety of natural CNS diseases.[141]

Other manifestations. A small, erythematous skin lesion (not the dramatic erythema migrans seen in humans) may develop at the site of tick attachment in dogs but disappears within the first week (Fig. 69.8). Spirochetes can be isolated from the skin for extended periods. Other syndromes rarely or poorly documented, and possibly circumstantial in seropositive dogs, include carditis,[145,146,184] rheumatoid arthritis,[185] or myositis.[186] In one dog with myocarditis from Poland, intralesional *Borrelia* DNA was detected at necropsy.[184]

Lyme Borreliosis in Cats

Despite the evidence of seropositivity for *B. burgdorferi* in cats, evidence of natural disease is relatively lacking when compared with dogs. Cats in endemic areas of the northeastern United States can become infested with *Ixodes* ticks. Reported prevalence rates of exposure to *B. burgdorferi* have ranged from 13% to 47% based on seropositive results by IFA, ELISA, immunoblotting, or C_6 peptide[187] antibody testing. In some studies, no difference in seroreactivity was found between cats with or without lameness, even if infected twice.[188–190] Cats in these studies were seroreactive to *A. phagocytophilum*, suggesting co-infection exposure.[189] Because anaplasmosis in cats may mimic signs of Lyme borreliosis, it is difficult to ascribe signs to Lyme borreliosis in co-infected cats.[190–192] However, in a study of 117 apparently healthy cats and 42 with clinical signs consistent with anaplasmosis or borreliosis from a single clinic in Maine, cats with signs of disease were fourfold more likely to be seropositive to *Anaplasma* spp. (9.5%), *Borrelia* C_6 antigen (23.8%), or both agents (7.1%) than healthy cats.[193] Based on serologic testing, clinical information, and response to treatment, *B. burgdorferi* was thought to be the most likely cause of illness. Lameness,

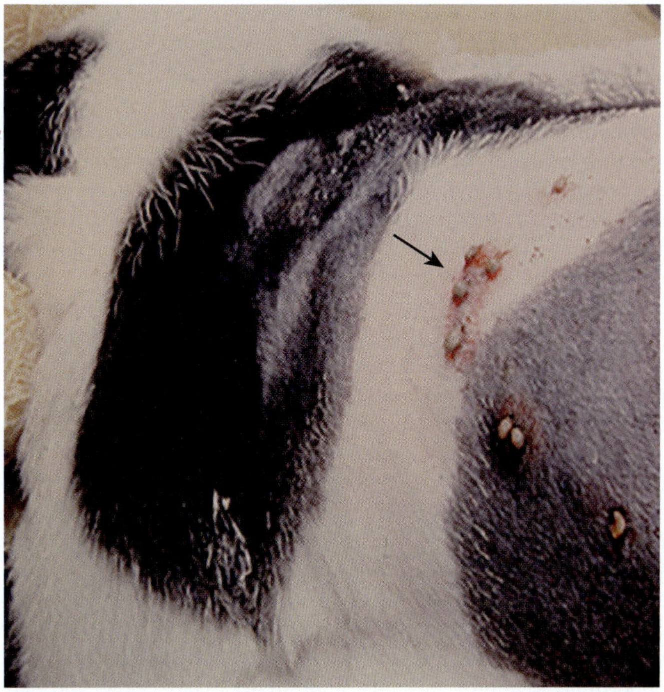

Fig. 69.8 Erythematous skin lesions *(arrow)* in a dog surrounding attached *Ixodes scapularis* ticks 4 days after experimental *Borrelia burgdorferi* inoculation. (Image courtesy of Reinhard Straubinger.)

lethargy, anorexia, and/or fever were the main signs described in cats seropositive for *B. burgdorferi* but seronegative for *A. phagocytophilum*. Sick cats in the United Kingdom had a low rate (4.2%) of *B. burgdorferi* seroreactivity, and clinical signs in the seropositive cats in that study did not include lameness.[194] *Borrelia burgdorferi* was suspected as a cause of bradyarrhythmia in two cats from the United Kingdom (in one cat, the spirochete was detected in blood using PCR),[195] and two cats with recurrent fever.[196] In Germany and European endemic areas, 2.2% (6/271) cats had C_6 peptide antibodies (5 with clinical signs); it was suggested that cats with shifting leg lameness or neurologic signs of unknown cause be tested.[197] Cats may be more resistant than dogs to the development of Lyme borreliosis. When cats were inoculated with organisms directly from arthropods, they developed multiple-limb lameness and had joint, pulmonary, lymphoid, and CNS inflammation at necropsy.[198,199] Arthritis or meningitis seems to be the predominant manifestation that would warrant investigation of Lyme borreliosis in cats, but it should also be considered as a cause of bradyarrhythmias/carditis in cats from endemic areas when other causes have been excluded.

DIAGNOSIS

There is no test that definitively confirms Lyme borreliosis; however, dogs with compatible clinical signs in endemic areas that have been exposed to ticks bear the highest consideration. Overestimation of case numbers may result from cross-reactivity to other infectious agents in older tests with low specificity (e.g., IFA), serologic test inaccuracies, and the fact that dogs with seropositive test results can have other illnesses that cause signs similar to Lyme borreliosis.[162,200,201] Furthermore, the interpretation of serologic results may be hampered by the existence of co-infections with other vector-borne pathogens.[74] In a survey from Baxter, MN, where *I. scapularis* is endemic, sick dogs were more likely to have positive antibody and PCR test results for both *A. phagocytophilum* and *B. burgdorferi* (than to either alone), compared to clinically healthy dogs in the same clinic population.[149] Therefore, co-infections may be important in determining whether infected animals develop clinical illness. Diagnosis of Lyme borreliosis should be based on known tick exposure in the endemic region, compatible clinical signs, and laboratory findings with exclusion of other diseases and favorable response to selective antimicrobial administration (although Lyme nephritis may not respond as readily). Major differential diagnoses for Lyme arthritis include trauma, other tick-borne diseases, immune-mediated arthritis, and degenerative joint disease; major differentials for Lyme nephritis are other causes of renal proteinuria such as leptospirosis, other tick-borne diseases, dirofilariasis, leishmaniosis, chronic infections, immune-complex glomerulonephritis, glomerulosclerosis, amyloidosis, and genetic glomerular diseases. Treatment response could be due to treatment of other unidentified causative pathogens or spontaneous resolution of signs; therefore, the diagnosis of Lyme borreliosis can be difficult.

Serologic screening of clinically healthy dogs for infection with *B. burgdorferi* is controversial.[104,107,202] From a positive standpoint, infection or exposure might be found at a preclinical stage of illness before immunopathologic consequences such as renal dysfunction occur; screening for occult proteinuria has been recommended for all seropositive dogs.[104,107,202] Conversely, should proteinuria be detected first, a diagnostic workup should include testing for antibodies to *B. burgdorferi* in dogs from endemic areas.[203,204] Detection of seropositive dogs is an opportunity to improve tick prevention strategies (see below) and alerts owners of their own potential exposure to ticks. On the negative side, routine testing can lead to overdiagnosis, overtreatment, or unnecessary owner concerns. Four of six panelists in the updated ACVIM consensus statement did not routinely recommend antimicrobial treatment for nonclinical nonproteinuric *B. burgdorferi* seropositive dogs.[104]

Laboratory Abnormalities

Complete Blood Count, Serum Biochemistry Profile, and Urinalysis

No specific hematologic or biochemical changes are pathognomonic for borreliosis. The presence of leukopenia or thrombocytopenia in tick endemic areas may be more likely to be caused by infection or co-infection with other vector-borne pathogens (especially *A. phagocytophilum*). Laboratory blood abnormalities in dogs with Lyme nephritis include hypoalbuminemia, azotemia, and hypercholesterolemia, and may include nonregenerative anemia, stress leukogram, mild/moderate thrombocytopenia, hyperphosphatemia, and variable hyperkalemia.[166] Urinalysis abnormalities in dogs with Lyme nephritis include proteinuria, with variable loss of concentrating ability, and possible hemoglobinuria, hematuria, glucosuria, and pyuria. However, other causes of renal disease such as leptospirosis and babesiosis were not always ruled out in studies that reported these findings in dogs suspected to have Lyme nephritis.[167] UPCRs are often greater than 5 and may be above 15 in some dogs. In one study from northern California, 40 dogs with positive C_6 serology and PLN were more likely to have thrombocytopenia, anemia, neutrophilia, azotemia, hyperphosphatemia, hematuria, glucosuria, and pyuria than 78 C_6-seronegative dogs with PLN. The prevalence of polyarthritis was not significantly different between groups. Of interest, pyuria was detected in 12/39 seropositive dogs but none of the seronegative dogs.[166]

Cytology of Synovial and Cerebrospinal Fluid

Synovial fluid changes in dogs with Lyme borreliosis consist of increased cell counts (5,000 to 100,000 cells/μL) with neutrophils predominating (up to 95%). Because not all joints may be affected, synovial fluid should be collected from at least three and preferably four peripheral joints. Protein concentration and turbidity are increased. CSF from humans with neuroborreliosis demonstrates lymphocytic pleocytosis and a mild protein increase. Consistent CSF values have not been found in dogs with suspected neurologic dysfunction.

Diagnostic Imaging

Plain Radiography

Radiographs of involved joints may show increased periarticular soft tissue opacity. Erosive arthritis has not been described.

Sonographic Findings

Abdominal sonographic findings in dogs with Lyme arthritis are unremarkable. In dogs with nephritis, the kidneys may look normal, or there may be thickening and increased echogenicity of the renal cortices, decreased renal corticomedullary distinction, and peritoneal effusion.

Microbiologic Tests

Serologic Testing

The presence of antibodies to *B. burgdorferi* signifies exposure but does not prove that clinical signs are caused by the organism. In endemic areas, apparently healthy dogs are often seropositive, possibly as a result of adequate host immune responses or, with less specific assays, from exposure to nonpathogenic forms of *B. burgdorferi* or other closely related spirochetes.[205] The diagnosis of Lyme borreliosis involves serologic testing because it is difficult to detect the organism in specimens of tissue samples or body fluids. However, seropositivity should be viewed as determining "seroreactivity to *B. burgdorferi*" and not evidence of causation. Paired sera (acute and convalescent) are not needed for Lyme disease since dogs typically seroconvert before clinical signs develop (in contrast to humans when seen for acute Lyme borreliosis). Paired serologic testing, however, may be needed to rule out other acute vector-borne diseases that cause signs similar to Lyme borreliosis (e.g., anaplasmosis, ehrlichiosis, RMSF, leptospirosis). Serial quantitative serologic testing may be helpful to determine a new baseline after antimicrobial therapy, which is associated with a reduction in C_6 antibody levels (clearance or decreased antigenic load). Subsequent rises in quantitative levels from the post-treatment baseline may signal relapse or reinfection, which may warrant further treatment and monitoring for proteinuria.

Antibody detection (whole cell). The first available immunodiagnostic tests for Lyme borreliosis used antigens from whole spirochete preparations. These methods were not standardized and had a high level of cross-reactivity with other bacteria such as *Leptospira* and *Borrelia turicatae*, the cause of TBRF in dogs from Florida and Texas.[9,158,201,206–213] With these assays, experimentally infected dogs developed positive IgG-ELISA-titers by 4 to 6 weeks after exposure.[80,152] Titers peaked 3 months after exposure and lasted for at least 2 years.[214] ELISA assays that detect only IgM are not useful in dogs since they only show signs once an IgG response has occurred. Antibody titers do not decline rapidly after treatment and IgG titers can remain positive for many years. An increase in titer that occurs 6 months or later after termination of antimicrobial therapy has been interpreted as proliferation of surviving spirochetes,[130,215] but may also result from reinfection. Dogs vaccinated with *Borrelia* vaccines may remain seroreactive for months to years after vaccination, making a diagnosis of *B. burgdorferi* infection based only on ELISA with whole cell preparations difficult.[216] Because of the shortcomings of antibody measurements with whole cell antigens, serologic tests of this type have been largely discontinued.

Immunoblotting, line immunoassay (LIA). Rarely used for initial screening, immunoblotting or LIA may be employed as a second-tier test to help confirm positive results, to differentiate infected from vaccinated animals, and to detect reactivity to other *Borrelia* spp. that may be missed by recombinant protein-based ELISA methods. The pattern of antibody reactivity after natural infection differs from that following vaccination. The size of bands on immunoblots varies in different investigations depending on techniques and strain differences and so the following information should only be used as a guideline. After natural exposure to *B. burgdorferi*, antibodies develop to proteins in the range of 100/83, 75, 66, 60, 58, 43, 41 (flagellin), 39, 30, 23 (OspC), and 21 kDa[139,217]; a diversity of antibody responses were found in experimentally exposed beagles.[218] Strong reactivity to OspA (31 kDa) occurs in vaccinated dogs[80,219–222] Reactivity to OspC (23 kDa) was generally useful as a marker for recent exposure; however, Lyme bacterins and the chimeric recombinant vaccine stimulate production of OspC-specific antibodies. Depending on the vaccine used, the interpretation of band patterns can be difficult.[139,221,223] Assays that incorporate recombinant VlsE antigen (see below) are useful because antibodies to this antigen only result from natural exposure (Fig. 69.9).

VlsE and C6-based assays. During the course of infection, *B. burgdorferi* evades the host immune response by varying the genes that encode for the immunodominant VlsE surface lipoprotein. One immunodominant region of VlsE, IR_6, is genetically, structurally, and antigenically highly conserved among many *B. burgdorferi* strains and genospecies. The genes that encode IR_6 are expressed only during infection of and replication in the mammalian host and not in culture (which is required for vaccine production) or in the arthropod vector. Therefore, antibodies to these genes signify natural exposure. The synthetically produced peptide C_6 is encoded by the IR_6 gene sequence. The C_6 peptide has been used for serodiagnostic testing of humans and animals as a marker for host invasion and infection. C_6-based assays have been substituted for conventional whole cell ELISA and immunoblotting in clinical diagnosis of human borreliosis.[224–228]

A commercially available POC test, SNAP 4Dx Plus (IDEXX Laboratories, Westbrook, ME), and the diagnostic laboratory-based Accuplex 4 assay (Antech Laboratories) detect serum antibody to the C_6 peptide (as well as heartworm antigen and antibodies to common *Anaplasma* spp. and *Ehrlichia* spp.). The C_6 assay can be used to more accurately differentiate between vaccinated and infected dogs compared with whole spirochete and immunoblot test methods (Table 69.3). C_6-based ELISA has been used to evaluate serologic responses in experimentally[229,230] and naturally[231,232] infected dogs. The C_6 antibody response increased 3 to 5 weeks after experimental infection, before antibody increases with conventional assays and before onset of lameness. C_6 antibody titers decreased more quickly after treatment than the antibody response measured by whole cell ELISA.[230] C_6 antibody levels were not increased in sera from healthy, uninfected dogs, those with other infections (e.g., dirofilariasis, babesiosis, ehrlichiosis, RMSF, leptospirosis), or those vaccinated with OspA, whole spirochete vaccines, or commonly used vaccines for other diseases.[229,233] When compared with immunoblotting, the sensitivity and specificity of the C_6 POC test in dogs were 98.8% and 100%, respectively.[234] Because not all dogs infected with spirochetes become ill, and because species and strains within *B. burgdorferi* s.l. complex vary in pathogenicity, the C_6 antibody response does not always correlate with clinical illness in dogs in North America or Europe.[104,107,235] Caution in overinterpreting the significance of a positive test result in a clinically healthy dog has been addressed by the initial and updated ACVIM consensus statement on Lyme borreliosis in dogs and cats.[104,107] Positive results may be observed in young pups as a result of *in utero* or colostral antibody transfer.[236] These results will become negative on subsequent evaluation through the postnatal period.

A quantitative C_6 antibody test (Quant C6, IDEXX Laboratories, Westbrook, ME) is available for monitoring the level and changes in antibody response after treatment. C_6 antibody concentrations remained high for 69 weeks in untreated, experimentally infected dogs.[230] If treated at

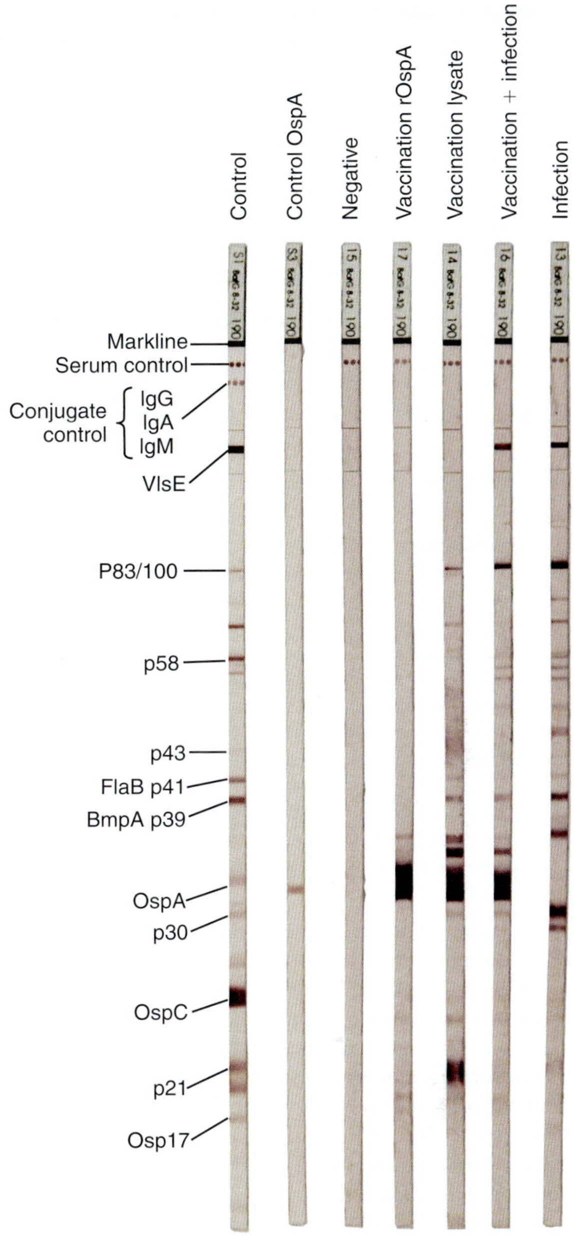

Fig. 69.9 Immunoblots of sera from dogs not infected with *Borrelia burgdorferi* (negative); immunized with recombinant OspA (vaccination rOspA); immunized with a lysate vaccine (vaccination lysate); immunized and infected with *B. burgdorferi* (vaccination + infection); and infected with *B. burgdorferi* (infection); the left strip shows all major signals available on the blot (control); the second strip from the left is stained with a monoclonal antibody against OspA (control OspA). (Courtesy of R. Straubinger, LMU Munich, Germany.)

week 31 with doxycycline for 28 days, C_6 antibody concentrations declined 12 weeks after beginning treatment from 63% to 92% (mean 81%) relative to pre-treatment values.[234] In treated, naturally infected, clinically healthy dogs with moderate-to-high C_6 antibody levels, titers declined over a period of 12 months.[232] This decline was more dramatic than that of clinically healthy untreated control dogs (also originally with moderate-to-high C_6 titers) at 6- and 12-month intervals. Generally, at least a 50% decline was noted after treatment, although there was minimal change in C_6 antibody levels in dogs with low initial values. Therefore, determination of baseline and follow-up titers at 3- to 6-month intervals may be beneficial in monitoring treatment efficacy.[237] Others argue that if clinical

TABLE 69.3 Comparative Serologic Test Results for Lyme Borreliosis in Dogs

Serologic Test	Naturally Infected Via Tick Exposure	Vaccinated with Whole Cell Bacterins	Vaccinated with rOspA Subunit	Vaccinated with crLyme (OspA and 7 Types of OspC)
IgM whole cell ELISA or IFA[a]	Positive within first 60–90 days for a transient duration	Positive within 2–4 weeks, can last for months to years	Positive within 2–4 weeks, can last for months to years	As for other vaccines
IgG whole cell ELISA or IFA[b]	After 60–90 days, positive for months or years	Detectable antibody levels starting at 4–6 weeks, will last for months to years	Detectable antibody levels starting at 4–6 weeks, will last for months to years	As for other vaccines
Immunoblot/LIA[c]	Numerous bands but generally *not* OspA or OspB; positive VlsE if that line is included	Predominant OspA; some also produce OspC bands; numerous other bands	OspA and few bands in the lower molecular range	OspA and OspC bands
C_6 ELISA assay[d]	Positive, even after treatment; months to years	Negative	Negative	Negative
VETSCAN Canine Lyme Rapid (Zoetis)	Positive	Possibly positive (OspC and flagellin)	Negative	Possibly positive (OspC)
Multiplex antibody testing	Positive OspC (>2–3 weeks, wanes in 3–5 months) Positive OspF (>6–8 weeks); possible positive OspA	Positive OspA; possibly positive OspC	Positive (OspA)	Positive OspA; possibly positive OspC

[a]IgM whole cell assays are the most nonspecific.
[b]IgG whole cell false-positive results can be caused by previous infections in recovered animals, vaccine, and reactions to many other closely related spirochetes. IFA is more specific in this regard but not as specific as specific protein-based assays.
[c]Immunoblot false-positive results include reactions with pathogenic and nonpathogenic isolates. Positive results can persist even after infection has been eliminated.
[d]Subclinical infection occurs with *Borrelia burgdorferi* strains when host immunity is adequately controlling infection. Qualitative C_6 assay is very sensitive and may be positive for months to years, even after treatment, so quantitative testing after treatment is preferred.
ELISA, enzyme-linked immunosorbent assay; *IFA*, indirect fluorescent antibody; *LIA*, line immunoassay; *Osp*, outer surface protein.

signs resolve, there is no value in monitoring C_6 antibody levels as there is no evidence that continuing treatment beyond resolution of clinical signs improves outcomes, and may contribute to antimicrobial resistance. In addition, increases in antibody titers may reflect continued exposure rather than treatment failure. The updated ACVIM consensus statement provides panelist perspectives on this issue.[104] Antimicrobial treatment for reasons other than Lyme borreliosis, or before its confirmation by serologic means, may reduce spirochetal burden and blunt the C_6 antibody response to *Borrelia*. This situation would limit the use of C_6 ELISA as a tool for monitoring. There have not been similar studies with ill dogs to allow association of serologic findings with clinical disease parameters.

The C_6 ELISA has also been evaluated in cats on a limited basis since the technology does not use species-specific reagents.[187,190] In experimentally tick-exposed cats, 8 of 13 seroconverted, but duration of positive results varied, as short as 1 week in one cat.[187,190] Of 24 cats tested in an endemic area, 17 had positive C_6 antibody test results that matched those obtained by a whole spirochete IFA assay.[187] Five cats had negative antibody test results on both assays, and two C_6-negative test results were positive at low serum dilutions with IFA; one of these was also positive using immunoblotting. No correlation was made with clinical illness. As with dogs, if a cat is evaluated with clinical signs such as fever and joint swelling, the C_6 assay may be helpful as an adjunctive test for diagnosis of Lyme borreliosis; however, co-infections with *A. phagocytophilum* or other diseases must also be considered. Caution is advised when interpreting the results of the C_6 assay in cats as further optimization experiments may be needed.[104]

Antibodies to other outer surface proteins—OspA, OspC, and OspF. During tick feeding, OspC begins to be expressed as the spirochetes lose their attachment to the midgut. Thus, OspC is presented early to the host's immune system; antibodies rise in 2–3 weeks, and are a marker for recent natural exposure in unvaccinated dogs. Without continued exposure, OspC antibodies wane in 3–5 months. Eventually OspF is expressed, with antibodies detected later at 6–8 weeks which remain elevated in untreated dogs. The Multiplex test (Cornell University Animal Health Diagnostic Center) offers quantitative testing of OspA, OspC, and OspF antibodies via the use of a fluorescent bead assay.[222,238,239] The interpretation of the OspA and OspC antibody test results may be difficult since 17% of nonvaccinated dogs were reactive to OspA.[221] There may be transient reactivity against OspA early after infection.[222] Humans with chronic Lyme disease (in North America but not Europe)[240] have high levels of anti-OspA antibodies (possibly due to expression of OspA during chronic infection as the organism goes through its antigenic repertoire),[131] and OspC-specific antibodies may be produced after vaccination with the newer bacterins and recombinant chimeric vaccines that contain OspC. The VETSCAN Lyme Rapid Test (Zoetis, Parsippany, NJ)[201,241] is a POC assay that tests for antibodies against proprietary synthetic chimeric recombinant peptides (VlsE, OspC, flagellin) as markers for natural exposure. As above, OspC antibodies may be induced by the newer bacterins and the recombinant chimeric vaccine. Canine OspC antibodies differ in intensity, frequency, and antigenicities when compared with those of humans.[242]

Measurement of CSF antibody. In humans, CSF antibody titers have been compared with those of serum in an attempt to diagnose neuroborreliosis.[243,244] Intrathecal production of specific antibodies to *B. burgdorferi* can be demonstrated if the ratio of CSF to serum *B. burgdorferi* antibody is greater than the CSF to serum albumin, total IgG, or specific IgG to another infectious agent. When the same assay method is used to measure specific IgG, the specific method has the most reliability.[245,246] In humans with neuroborreliosis, antibodies to both OspA and OspC have been found at higher titers in CSF than in serum.[247]

An increased intrathecal antibody concentration was demonstrated in dogs with neurologic dysfunction.[248,249] These results are difficult to assess because the dogs were from endemic areas and no supporting histopathologic or culture findings were supplied. The older (nonspecific) antibody tests were used, with possible cross-reactions from TBRF *Borrelia* spp. infections, which can cause neurologic signs in dogs. Lyme neuroborreliosis has not been well documented in dogs.[141–143]

Microscopic Detection of Spirochetes

Borrelia species that cause Lyme disease are rarely, if ever, visualized in body fluids such as synovial fluid using phase or dark-field microscopy or in tissues after nonspecific silver or specific immunologic staining methods. The spirochete density in clinical specimens is low, as is the specificity and sensitivity of microscopy.[250,251] Microscopy is best used to detect organisms in tick preparations (ticks squashed between microscope slides).

Culture

Culture of spirochetes from specimens collected from dogs with signs consistent with Lyme borreliosis is the most definitive means of documentation but is often difficult because of the low numbers of organisms present. The probability of isolating Lyme disease borreliae from blood is extremely low because these spirochetes (in contrast to the relapsing fever borreliae, see below) migrate through connective tissues and only incidentally enter the circulatory system, with the exception of *B. mayonii*.[4,252] A special medium, Barbour-Stoenner-Kelly (BSK) medium, is required for isolation. Skin and collagen-rich connective tissues (fascia, pericardium, peritoneum, meninges, synovium) are the most reliable tissues for culture from dogs when specimens are taken at or near the site of tick attachment.[252,253] Biopsy is performed using a 6-mm punch, and the specimens are placed in sterile tubes after removing the haired skin using a sterile technique. Specimens are processed with sterile pestles in medium, sequentially transferred to larger volumes of media, cultured at 33°C, and microscopically examined at 2-week intervals for 6 weeks. Culture may be more sensitive than PCR before antimicrobial therapy[215]; however, the turnaround time for culture results is longer than for PCR.

Molecular Diagnosis Using Nucleic Acid–Based Testing

PCR primers that target conserved DNA sequences can be used to detect various genospecies and strains of *Borrelia* spp. Primers that target plasmid (*OspA*) DNA are thought to be much more sensitive than chromosomal DNA because multiple copies of plasmids can be present in a single bacterium; however, the detection of plasmid DNA does not translate to the presence of viable spirochetes.[139,217,254] PCR should be performed on skin or synovial tissue (or affected tissue) biopsy rather than on body or synovial fluids because they are more likely to contain the organism in chronically infected, treated, or untreated dogs.[215] With respect to these concerns, PCR results of CSF and blood from dogs with neurologic disease have been negative.[143] PCR-positive results on blood have been found in dogs with suspected clinical borreliosis[255,256]; however, corresponding studies of control dogs were not reported to confirm a correlation with disease. Because of extremely low organism numbers, even with sensitive PCR assays, *B. burgdorferi* DNA is rarely found in tissues of naturally infected dogs.[139] Real-time quantitative PCR assays have been developed to detect spirochetal DNA in human clinical specimens.[257] By itself, detection of *B. burgdorferi* by PCR may be misleading, and its presence should always be correlated with clinical illness and serologic findings.[196]

Detection of Borreliae by Other Techniques

Tissue specimens can be examined microscopically for pathogenic spirochetes using direct FA, FISH, IHC, or gold particles that are visible on transmission electron microscopy. Xenodiagnosis, in which naïve ticks become infected after feeding on suspect infected hosts, has proved very reliable in the research laboratory setting but is expensive and time consuming.

Pathologic Findings

Gross Pathologic Findings

On gross necropsy, severely affected animals have swollen joints with synovial effusion. The synovial fluid may be yellow-tinged and cloudy, with decreased viscosity. Peripheral lymphadenomegaly may be present, especially in nodes draining the affected limbs. In dogs with nephritis, the kidneys are diffusely light tan and may have pinpoint red foci over cortical surfaces.[167] In addition, evidence of systemic edema, thrombosis and infarction, and uremia (parathyroid hyperplasia, ulcerative stomatitis, and gastritis) may be present.

Histopathologic Findings

In experimentally infected dogs (puppies more than adults), inflammation within the synovial membrane and the effusion consists of fibrin and neutrophils in acute cases. In more chronic infections, dogs develop nonsuppurative, predominantly lymphoplasmacytic, inflammation within the synovial membrane and joint capsule.[163,258] Some dogs that never develop lameness still have histologic evidence of arthritis. Histologic lesions may be present in the lymph nodes, joints, pericardium, and skin.[80] In addition, vasculitis, arteritis, perineuritis, and meningitis may be evident (Fig. 69.10).[259] Follicular enlargement and increased size of parafollicular areas in lymph nodes has been documented. Skin biopsy specimens have superficial perivascular lymphoplasmacytic infiltrates with mast cell accumulations.

Renal lesions have not been found in experimentally infected dogs but were evident in naturally diseased dogs (especially retrievers) with suspected Lyme nephritis.[167] Silver staining and PCR testing of the kidneys of dogs with suspected Lyme nephritis revealed rare spirochetes unrelated to lesion development,[133,134,167] but histologically immune-complex (membranoproliferative) glomerulonephritis, dilation of cortical renal tubules, diffuse tubular necrosis with regeneration, and interstitial lymphoplasmacytic inflammation have been found (Fig. 69.11). Elution studies on necropsy samples showed a variety of *B. burgdorferi*–specific antigen-antibody complexes.[135] Renal core biopsies are recommended as part of the diagnostic work-up for PLN to document immune-complex disease using electron microscopy and immunofluorescence studies[203,204,260]; however, there are no validated stains to use on antemortem specimens to prove that complexes are directed to *Borrelia* spp. antigens.

In experimentally infected cats, hepatic degeneration, splenic hyperplasia, regional lymph node plasmacytosis, nonsuppurative meningoencephalitis, pneumonitis, and renal lesions were noted.[198,199]

TREATMENT AND PROGNOSIS

Lyme Arthritis

Because of the difficulty in obtaining an accurate diagnosis, antibacterials are often given empirically in an attempt to make a therapeutic diagnosis. Many reports exist of successful recovery after administration of antimicrobial drugs in dogs with suspected Lyme arthritis. Improvement often occurs within 24 to 48 hours after antimicrobial therapy is initiated. The greatest success is achieved with treatment in the initial phases of clinical illness. Clinical improvement after any therapeutic intervention should be viewed with caution, because the acute limb and joint dysfunction is intermittent and often resolves after several days to weeks regardless of whether antimicrobials are given.[160] Treatment response may also reflect response to treatment of overlooked co-infections. In addition, doxycycline can cause nonspecific anti-inflammatory changes in injured joints and may have chondroprotective activity in noninfectious arthritis in dogs.[261] The lipid-soluble tetracyclines may inhibit inflammation associated with *B. burgdorferi* infection.[262] Should a response to treatment not occur in a 3-day time period, antimicrobial treatment should be discontinued and other causes of the clinical signs should be considered.

Early treatment is associated with a reduction in antibody titers and organisms in tissues and prevention or cure of clinical lameness and joint lesions.[252,259] Most treatment schemes are instituted for a minimum of 30 days. Amoxicillin, azithromycin, cefovecin, ceftriaxone, doxycycline, and minocycline have all been used. A 30-day treatment duration has been recommended based on the spirochete's generation time and to mimic treatment protocols for people with chronic infection.[253] However, on the basis of research studies, clearance of the organism after 30 days of treatment in dogs and rodents is not guaranteed, and relapse and recrudescence of infection can occur after antimicrobial therapy is discontinued.[156,214,215,252,259,263–268] Similar treatment outcomes have sometimes been reported for human patients,[269] although most people with chronic disease clear infection.[3,137,270] Clinical relapse may reflect reinfection with another strain

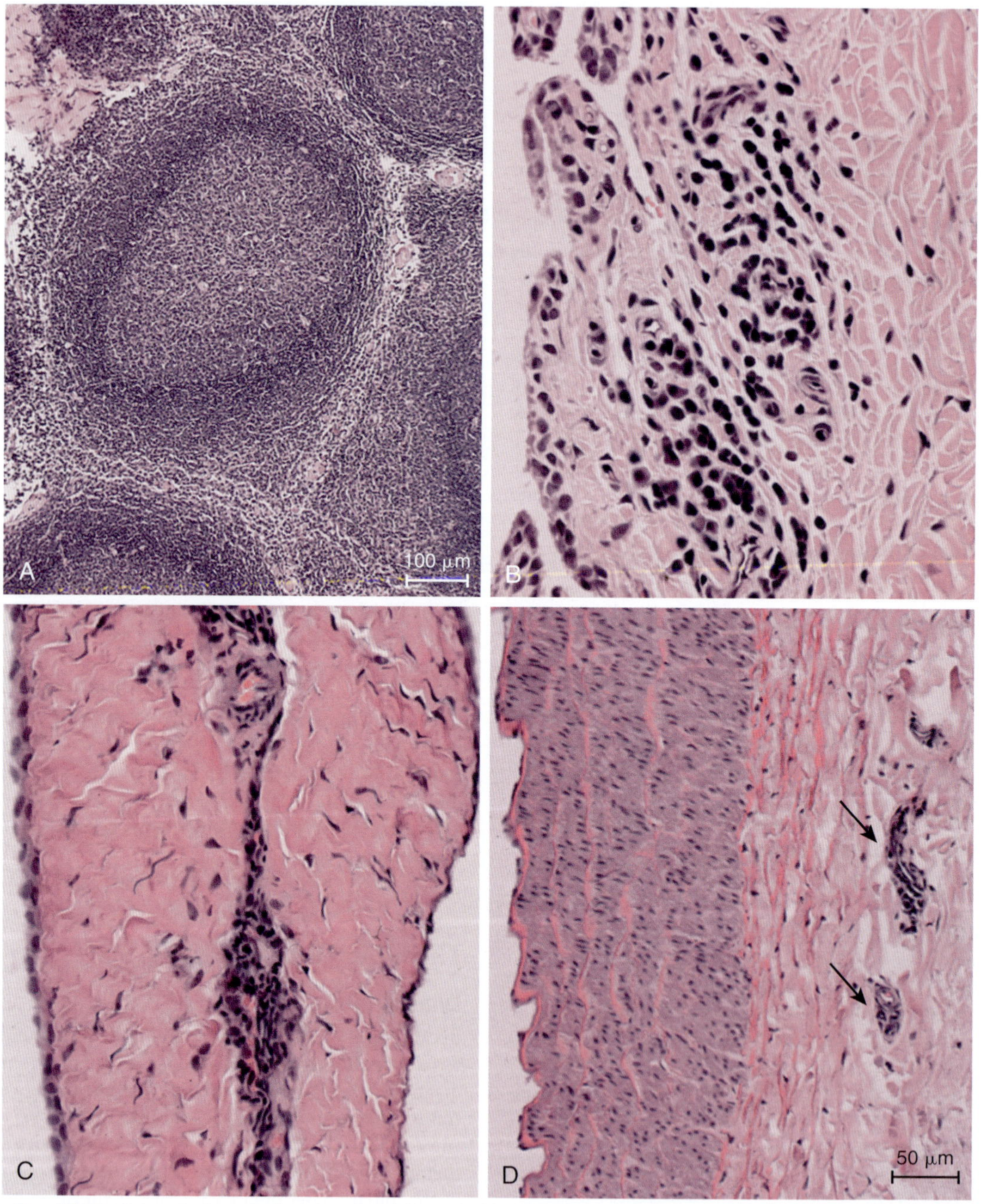

Fig. 69.10 Histopathologic lesions in a dog infected with *Borrelia burgdorferi*. Representative tissue sections of inflammatory lesions (hematoxylin and eosin stain). (A) Severe follicular hyperplasia of left axillary lymph node. (B) Synovial membrane of the left elbow with moderate nonsuppurative arthritis. Note accumulation of plasma cells in subsynovial tissue. (C) Mild nonsuppurative pericarditis with several cellular aggregates—mostly mononuclear cells in tissue. (D) Tunica media and tunica adventia of artery with small cuffs of mononuclear cells around the branch of vasa vasorum *(arrows)*. (Courtesy of R. Straubinger, LMU Munich, Germany.)

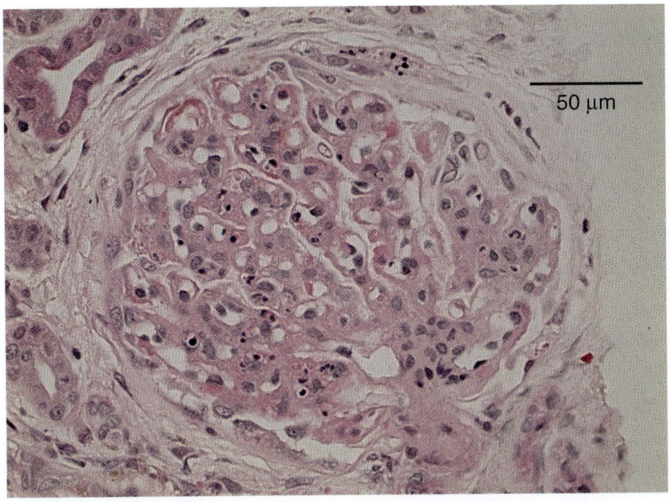

Fig. 69.11 Membranoproliferative glomerulonephritis in a 6-year-old, intact male golden retriever dog that was seropositive for *B. burgdorferi* C_6 protein antibodies and had clinical and biochemical evidence of protein-losing nephropathy. The morphologic diagnosis was moderate to severe, diffuse, global membranoproliferative glomerulonephritis with moderate chronic-active tubulointerstitial nephritis. The capillary walls are thickened and there is mesangial cell proliferation. There was also evidence of focal arteriolar mural disorganization, lamination, and sclerosis in this biopsy specimen. (Courtesy Dr. George Lees, Texas A&M University.)

of *B. burgdorferi.*[116,271] In addition to possible inability to clear all organisms or remnants, chronic inflammatory changes that occur in tissues such as the joints may become self-perpetuating. Intra-articular persistence of metabolically inactive spirochetes may occur even though the organisms cannot be cultured.[259,272] Persistence may stimulate chronic immune and inflammatory processes. Dogs with more chronic Lyme borreliosis are less likely to improve or more likely to have relapses, even if treatment continues for weeks or months.

Nevertheless, antimicrobial therapy is still the mainstay for treatment of borreliosis (Table 69.4). Antimicrobial susceptibility testing has shown ceftriaxone, erythromycin or its derivatives, amoxicillin, cefuroxime, doxycycline, tetracycline, and penicillin G to range from most to least effective.[81] Tetracyclines, ampicillin, and erythromycin have been used to treat human and animal patients. Cefovecin was shown to be efficacious in dogs, but may not have activity against other co-pathogens such as *Anaplasma.*[273] Newer erythromycin derivatives, such as azithromycin, or third-generation cephalosporins, such as ceftriaxone, have been administered for more refractory human cases.[274] High-dose IV penicillin G has been advocated in an attempt to treat unresponsive animals. Borreliae are not responsive to aminoglycosides and quinolones.[275]

Doxycycline is considered the drug of choice because it is a lipid-soluble tetracycline and is relatively inexpensive. The advantages of lipid solubility are that a lower dosage is needed, tissue distribution is greater, and intracellular penetration is better than that achieved with conventional tetracycline. Doxycycline is also active against common co-infecting organisms (*Rickettsia, Anaplasma, Ehrlichia, Leptospira,* or *Bartonella* spp.). For growing animals, amoxicillin is usually recommended because tetracyclines may stain dentition; however, doxycycline is less likely to cause this when compared with other tetracyclines.[276,277] Ceftriaxone is reserved as parenteral therapy for parenchymal CNS inflammation (encephalitis) in humans.[278,279] Oral doxycycline (3 weeks to 2 months), however, is effective and still recommended in treating peripheral CNS inflammation (meningitis and neuritis).[278,280–282]

In experimentally infected dogs, doxycycline, amoxicillin, azithromycin, or ceftriaxone have been administered for 1 month with resolution of clinical signs. There is inconsistent evidence for persistence of viable spirochetes after treatment in dogs.[139] In one study, positive tissue cultures, PCR, and rising ELISA titers were found months after treatment.[259] Later studies showed negative skin cultures, persistent *Borrelia* DNA, but lowered ELISA and C_6 peptide antibody titers, which did not rise at least 35 weeks after treatment.[214,215,230,252]

Treatment of clinically healthy seropositive dogs with antimicrobial therapy is controversial.[104,107,202,283] The existence or magnitude of a positive antibody titer does not predict illness.[104,107,235] Those opposing empiric antimicrobial therapy argue that, even though seroconversion occurs, many infected hosts have a natural immunity that prevents the organism from causing clinical disease. Furthermore, treatment of dogs in endemic areas that might have antibody titers could lead to the development of resistant strains of spirochetes and other resident bacterial microflora. Adverse reactions might also result from antimicrobial therapy. Finally, the carrier status may be somewhat protective. Arguments for treatment of apparently healthy seropositive dogs are that the incubation period can be prolonged and immunopathologic consequences of infection develop; treatment may help to prevent progression of these events during a subclinical period. Furthermore, even though dogs appear healthy, they can still have subclinical manifestations, such as proteinuria from immune-complex disease and associated renal inflammation. The level of quantitative C_6 antibody titer seems to correlate with levels of CICs. Quantitative C_6 and possibly OspF antibody titers and corresponding CICs seem to decrease after therapy.[136,222,284] At a minimum, preventive measures (tick control and possibly vaccination) should be recommended for seropositive dogs to prevent reinfection. The effect of vaccination in proteinuric dogs is unknown and some have recommended that it be avoided.[284]

In addition to antimicrobials, dogs with signs of arthritis may be treated with NSAIDs or analgesics. NSAIDs are not preferred should steroids become necessary (to avoid a wash-out period or potential GI irritation). Glucocorticoids are not recommended for Lyme arthritis, but seropositive dogs that are nonresponsive to antimicrobial therapy may have immune-mediated polyarthritis which is responsive to immunosuppressive therapy. Experimentally, dogs treated with high doses of antibiotics for 1 month and then high-dose prednisone (2 mg/kg, q12h, 2 weeks) showed no clinical signs of lameness while being treated, but after therapy was discontinued, signs of arthritis or reactivation of disease developed within 1 week.[214] This finding has not been reported in field cases. Immunosuppressive doses of glucocorticoids should be avoided in chronically infected dogs because of possible infection exacerbation, or they should be given in combination with antibacterials.

Lyme Nephritis

Treatment and prognosis of renal dysfunction associated with Lyme borreliosis varies according to the stage and severity of the illness at the time diagnosis is made. Without an experimental model, it is unknown whether prompt treatment with antibiotics can be curative, and the correct duration of antimicrobial treatment is unknown (some clinicians choose to treat 3–6 months, until the C_6 antibody level has waned). With progression, glomerular proteinuria can be associated with complications such as hypertension, thromboembolic events, nephrotic syndrome, and/or renal failure. In the early stages, standard treatments for PLN are recommended: angiotensin-converting enzyme inhibitors and/or angiotensin II receptor blockers, antithrombotics, omega-3 fatty acid supplement, renal diet (restricted in protein, phosphorus, and salt), and as indicated, antihypertensives, IV colloids/crystalloids, spironolactone, phosphate binders, antacids, and other

TABLE 69.4 Suggested Antibacterial Regimens for Lyme Borreliosis in Dogs

Drug[a]	Dose[b]	Route[b]	Interval (Hours)[b]	Duration (Days)[b]	Preferred Uses in Humans
Doxycycline or minocycline[d]	10 mg/kg	PO, IV	12–24	30–42[c]	Early disease, arthritis or neurologic manifestations, children ≥ 8 years old
Amoxicillin	20 mg/kg	PO	8	30	Early, arthritis or neurologic manifestations, children < 8 years old
Azithromycin	25 mg/kg	PO	24	10–20	Early disease
Clarithromycin	7.5–12.5 mg/kg	PO	12	30	
Cefovecin	8 mg/kg	SC	2 doses, 14 days apart	28	
Penicillin G	22,000 U/kg	IV	8	(14–)30	Persistent arthritis, neurologic manifestations, or carditis
Ceftriaxone	25 mg/kg	IV, SC	24	(14–)30	Late neurologic or cardiac manifestations, persistent arthritis
Cefotaxime	50 mg/kg or 20 mg/kg	IV	12 8	(14–)30	Neurologic manifestations

[a]See Chapter 10. Information on many drugs is based on extrapolation from literature on humans. Use of some drugs may be restricted depending on geographic location.
[b]Dose per administration at specified interval and duration are given for dogs.
[c]Proteinuric dogs may need longer treatment duration (see text) as well as appropriate medication and diet for protein-losing nephropathy.
[d]Doxycycline (or minocycline) is the preferred treatment for dogs with suspected Lyme disease (see text). Doxycycline may cause gastric or esophageal irritation, leading to vomiting or inappetence, and should be given with food.
IM, intramuscular; *IV*, intravenous; *PO*, oral; *SC*, subcutaneous.

renal failure support.[104,148,171,285] Immunosuppressive drug therapy is recommended if renal biopsy confirms immune-complex disease[286] or in cases that are deteriorating even without confirmation, since about half of all dogs with renal proteinuria have immune-complex glomerulonephritis.[204,287,288] Although the best protocol is unknown, current recommendations include mycophenolate or cyclophosphamide, sometimes with glucocorticoid treatment. The IRIS Study Group recommends mycophenolate as the first-choice immunosuppressive drug, perhaps with a tapering dose of prednisolone for dogs with acute rapidly progressive glomerular disease.[286] However, it should be kept in mind that glucocorticoids also may exacerbate hypertension, thromboembolic events, GI ulceration, and proteinuria. For dogs with stable disease, a combination of mycophenolate or chlorambucil alone or in combination with azathioprine on alternating days may be used. As the disease progresses, dogs may develop severe hypoproteinemia and decreased renal perfusion, which necessitates volume expanders, vasoactive agents, and osmotic diuresis. Plasmapheresis to remove CICs may be tried. Unfortunately, chronic renal manifestations are usually progressive despite therapy.

IMMUNITY AND VACCINATION

Controversy exists about the need for vaccination even in Lyme endemic areas (Table 69.5). The efficacy and safety profiles of the first available vaccines were disappointing.[104,107] While the results of field studies appear promising, they do not control for the use of tick prevention products, and experimental models use small numbers of dogs with tick challenges at less than 1 month to 1 year.[289–296]

A number of vaccines are commercially available in North America to prevent borreliosis in dogs.[118,289,294,297–303] In Europe, whole cell bacterins are available. The multiplicity of infecting species of *Borrelia* in Europe complicates vaccine-induced protection. In dogs, heterologous vaccines produce weak antibody cross-reactivity,[281] suggesting that *Borrelia* species–specific vaccines are necessary for adequate protection.[304] At the time of writing, a recombinant chimeric OspA Lyme vaccine for humans (Valnerva/Pfizer) that exhibits cross-species protection has advanced to Phase 3 clinical studies.

Vaccines for Lyme borreliosis are available for use beginning at 6 to 12 weeks of age, depending on the product. Primary vaccination schedules consist of two inoculations 3 weeks apart. Vaccination is not a replacement for adequate tick control measures. Dogs should be selected for vaccination based on the geographic location where they reside or travel and by the geographic location of their activities and habits. Outdoor, hunting, or field-trial dogs that frequent known tick-infested areas should be prioritized for vaccination. Dogs vaccinated with adjuvanted whole cell vaccines or recombinant OspA (rOspA) vaccines before infection develop enhanced resistance to infection.[289,290,294,301–303] This type of protection does not appear to develop in naturally infected animals. Reinfection by other strains is possible in animals that are treated or recover from natural infections.[116,305]

Lyme vaccines have a unique mechanism of action. Vaccination induces production of antibodies by the host, which are ingested by the tick and immobilize spirochetes in the tick gut during tick feeding. Because the vaccine-induced antibodies to OspA (and for some vaccines, to OspC variants) act within the tick, natural boostering can be limited and so frequent boostering with vaccines may be needed to maintain effective titers.[306] The protective titer levels are unknown. Protection was demonstrated following vaccination with an OspA/OspC bacterin at a 1-year tick challenge despite low titers,[289,294] but in another study, vaccine failure occurred in the face of positive titers.[300] Production of OspA and OspC antibody levels is highest with recombinant vaccines (rOspA and crLyme, respectively),[307,308] but even these vaccines may not yield full protection, therefore tick control is still recommended.

In the presence of complement, host antibodies to OspA cause an arrest of growth and prevention of salivary gland invasion in the ticks that feed on previously vaccinated animals.[89,302] Vaccination of an already infected animal does not clear infection.[303] Variable efficacy (50%–100%) has been noted for the commercial rOspA vaccine.[301,302,311] In a field study, infection rate was 25% in vaccinates versus 63% in non-vaccinates with a preventive fraction of 60.3%.[304]

TABLE 69.5 Vaccination for Prevention of Lyme Borreliosis: Pros and Cons

Pros	Cons
Tick control does not always work due to lack of compliance and misuse or failure of the product. Vaccines are an additional safety net when tick control fails.	Tick control is recommended anyway in endemic areas due to other tick-borne diseases. When used properly, tick control may be more efficacious than vaccination.
In endemic areas, 5%–10% is still a very high number of affected dogs.	The vast majority (90%–95%) of seropositive dogs do not become ill.
Histopathologic evidence of chronic arthritis may be an additive factor to arthritis later in life, although this is unproven.	Lyme arthritis is self-limiting or responds quickly to antibiotics.
Even though there is no experimental model for Lyme nephritis to study this question, evidence for postvaccinal sensitization or aggravation of Lyme nephritis is lacking or anecdotal at best. Decreasing exposure and infection will decrease the number of carriers with circulating immune complexes and perhaps lessen the opportunity for glomerular deposition.	There is no experimental model for Lyme nephritis, an immune-mediated illness. We do not know if Lyme vaccine prevents, aggravates, or may sensitize for it. OspA is an inflammatory protein. Other Lyme antigens may have molecular mimicry with cardiolipin, myelin, myosin, etc. The most severe cases of Lyme disease are immune-mediated and theoretically vaccination may sensitize for it.
Giving an extra booster vaccine at 6 months of age will help to increase protection. Vaccines can be given every 6–12 months, especially just before tick season.	Vaccines have inconsistent efficacy and duration of immunity.
Use of C_6 and OspF serologic tests can differentiate between vaccinal and natural antibodies.	Vaccination can interfere with interpretation of some serologic diagnostic test results.
Correctly applied vaccination aids in the prevention of *B. burgdorferi* infection.	Vaccine expense and possible adverse events in genetically predisposed individuals.

In another study, dogs were given the rOspA vaccine at 0 and 3 weeks, again at 6 months and then annually.[295] Using C_6 ELISA, 99% of seropositive dogs in that clinic were non-vaccinated, incompletely vaccinated, or previously seropositive dogs. However, this percentage decreased over a 33-month follow-up period in those dogs that received the complete vaccination series. In humans, immunity was often much stronger after a third vaccine was added to the series.[305,306] Regardless of the product used, when a third dose was given to dogs, a higher antibody titer was induced compared to the titer in dogs immunized only twice at the beginning of the vaccination schedule.[291] Therefore, extra-label recommendations in highly endemic areas might be to use a third immunization 6 months after the two initial doses. There was no consensus reached about the need to administer Lyme borreliosis vaccines on a 6-monthly basis among consensus statement panelists.[104]

OspC antigens are present, in lower levels than those of OspA, in all whole cell bacterins.[233,307] Monovalent bacterin studies showed a 78% preventive fraction for illness[308] and 90%–92% preventive fraction for seroconversion[304,309]; however field studies did not control for use of tick prevention measures. In a parenteral challenge study in mice, protection was not afforded by previous immunization with vaccines based on OspC, whereas it was with an OspA product.[310] However, in dogs, addition of a bacterin strain that induced antibodies to OspC offered protection even when OspA antibodies were not identified.[289,294,311] Use of a bivalent bacterin in dogs that stimulated both OspA and OspC borreliacidal antibodies protected dogs, after an infected tick-feeding challenge, against clinical illness and serologic or PCR evidence of infection.[289,294] Although OspC is highly immunogenic, considerable variation in OspC among strains of *B. burgdorferi* and other species such as *B. afzelii* makes heterologous protection with this antigen difficult.[271,319–321] This is the rationale for the development of the chimeric recombinant OspA-OspC vaccine (Vanguard crLyme, Zoetis, Parsippany, NJ, USA) available at the time of wrting. This vaccine consists of a chimeric OspC construct comprised of seven different OspC peptides. Whether inclusion of OspC in vaccines increases protection remains unknown, especially as more contemporary studies have suggested that expression of OspA is present throughout the bloodmeal, and OspA is only down-regulated after the spirochete enters the host.[92]

In one study, after vaccination with each of three vaccine types (Recombitek, Nobivac, and LymeVax), dogs were challenged with infected ticks.[300] Six of 18 vaccinated dogs became infected (based on DNA amplification of skin biopsies at the tick bite site and seroconversion against C_6, OspC, OspF, p39, and SLP). At the time of tick exposure, three dogs that subsequently became infected had evidence of vaccine-induced OspA-specific antibodies and one dog had both OspA- and OspC-specific antibodies. Not included in this study was the chimeric recombinant vaccine (Vanguard crLyme, Zoetis).[297,304] Dogs vaccinated with this chimeric vaccine were less likely than control dogs to develop serologic evidence of infection after tick challenge at 21 days after vaccination (7/16 dogs versus 14/16 dogs, respectively).[322] A 1-year challenge study is needed.

Since the most serious forms of Lyme borreliosis involve immune-complex deposition, the possibility that vaccination might trigger formation of CICs has raised concern.[323] In a preliminary study, when dogs with positive C_6 antibody titers were vaccinated, those with the highest titers and those given whole cell bacterins had the highest levels of CICs after vaccination compared with those with lower titers or given recombinant OspA vaccine.[136,237,284] These findings require confirmation and their clinical significance is unknown. An additional theoretical concern is the possibility that a hypersensitivity reaction may occur if a whole cell vaccine is given to a dog that harbors large quantities of the spirochete.[216] Although such an organism-specific reaction has not been substantiated, a whole cell *Borrelia* spp. vaccine was more likely to induce vaccine-induced adverse events than any other canine vaccine.[324] Nevertheless, the prevalence rate for such reactions is relatively low[324] and in accordance with that for bacterins in general.

PREVENTION

In humans, a single dose of doxycycline given within 72 hours of identified engorged *I. scapularis* attachment was 87% effective in preventing Lyme borreliosis,[325] although this has been controversial because of concerns that ticks are often misidentified and because the chance of infection even after a known tick bite is extremely low.[326] Regardless, in dogs and cats, high tick exposure rates probably preclude the usefulness of this concept. At the time of writing (2022), a human monoclonal antibody directed against OspA (2217LS) has entered Phase 1 clinical trials for prophylaxis of Lyme disease in humans (Lyme PrEP). The antibody is designed to be administered to at-risk humans just before the onset of the tick season, and like vaccine-induced antibodies, would act within the tick after the tick ingests a blood meal. This intriguing approach has the potential to be associated with a lower risk of adverse effects than vaccination, but whether protective antibody levels can be maintained for an entire tick season remains to be determined.[327]

Vector Control

Products for vector control in pets have included collars, topical powders, shampoos, dips or foams, sprays, spot applications, and new oral products (see Chapters 13 and 109). Amitraz-impregnated tick collars have prevented transmission of *Borrelia* spp. organisms to vector-exposed dogs[328] but are toxic to cats. Topical solutions that control, and in some cases repel, ticks are also available.[329–331] Fipronil may prevent Lyme borreliosis but may not kill ticks fast enough to prevent exposure to other tick-borne pathogens. Oral oxazolines (afoxolaner, fluralaner, lotilaner, sarolaner)[332] do not prevent tick attachment but produce a fast kill (< 8 hours) by binding to insect/tick-specific GABA-gated chloride channels. Even though transmission of *B. burgdorferi* requires at least 24 hours of tick attachment, products should be selected that reduce transmission of co-pathogens such as *A. phagocytophilum*, which can occur more rapidly. Daily examination and combing to remove attached ticks on animals should be done; however, ticks are considerably more difficult to find on animals than on humans.

Vector Control in the Environment

Landscaping techniques help to reduce tick exposure.[333] Application of acaricides to relatively large environmental areas is expensive, logistically difficult, and raises concerns about negative environmental impacts. The 2-year life cycle of *Ixodes* species and the redistribution of ticks by various hosts make it difficult to treat all stages simultaneously.

Removal of leaves and of bordering shrubs and bushes in backyards and gardens reduces the risk of tick exposure because *Ixodes* ticks need a humid, texture-rich environment to quest for prey. The efficacy of a rodent- or deer-targeted acaricide (fipronil) was assessed in various studies.[334,335] Host-targeted intervention was an efficacious, economical, safe, and environment-friendly alternative to area-wide spraying of acaricide to control free-living populations of ticks. However, from a practical management perspective, effective acaricide programs for wildlife are difficult, if not impossible, to implement.

Orally administered vaccines, containing *Escherichia coli* or vaccinia virus expressing OspA, have been used experimentally to protect mice against challenge infection with *B. burgdorferi*.[336–338] When combined in a bait delivery system, such a vaccine might be helpful in disrupting transmission of this infection. Even if effective, vaccination of sufficient numbers of reservoir species would be impossible. Reduction of the deer population might help to decrease the number of ixodid ticks, but other mammalian hosts could still propagate the vectors. Continual depopulation would be required to remove deer migrating back into the area. In the future, the possibility exists that islands in the northeast United States could study the effect of the release of genetically engineered mice (using CRISPR to induce resistance to infection), which may interrupt the transmission cycle.[339]

PUBLIC HEALTH ASPECTS

The case definition of human Lyme borreliosis is: (1) an erythematous rash or one objective sign of musculoskeletal, neurologic, or cardiovascular disease, and (2) laboratory confirmation of infection.[3,137] In the United States in 2015, roughly 30,000 cases were reported from 50 states and the District of Columbia.[340] However, it is estimated that 476,000 cases occur annually.[341] The distribution of endemic infection is limited to certain geographic areas (Northeast/mid-Atlantic/upper Midwest) and 90% of the cases are seen in just 14 states (PA, NY, MA, NJ, CT, WI, MD, MN, VA, ME, RI, VT, NH, and DE).[340] The sylvan cycle in nature appears limited to these areas. However, these regions may be redefined as a result of future climate changes affecting ticks, migration of reservoir hosts, and further investigation of tick-borne illnesses. Errors in reporting disease outside of these regions (other than from host movement) have probably been due to misclassification and overdiagnosis. For example, antibodies to *Borrelia hermsii*, the cause of TBRF in humans, cross-reacted with older whole spirochete antigen tests and likely overestimated the prevalence of Lyme disease.[342–344]

The highest annual incidence of Lyme borreliosis is among children younger than 14 years and adults older than 30 years. Clinical signs usually begin from several days to 1 month after a tick bite. Erythema migrans, an expanding nonpruritic ring-like erythematous lesion of at least 5 cm, may develop in the vicinity of the bite. Fever, myalgia, arthralgia, and headache (influenza-like symptoms) may accompany the lesion. Erythema migrans lesions can be found on individuals in nonendemic regions and may be associated with organisms inoculated by bites of ticks that are not competent vectors of *B. burgdorferi* (e.g., *A. americanum* transmitting *Borrelia lonestari*). These humans have mild constitutional symptoms but have seronegative test results for *B. burgdorferi*. In contrast, humans who become ill from *B. burgdorferi* infection may develop recurrent joint swelling and musculoskeletal soreness. Meningeal signs include pain, sensory loss, behavioral changes, and recurrent headaches. Peripheral neurologic signs can mimic multiple sclerosis. Myocarditis is characterized by development of symptoms characteristic of atrioventricular conduction disturbances. Subclinical infections are also thought to occur.[138] Treatment of Lyme borreliosis in humans is most rewarding during the early phases of illness. In 10%–20% of humans treated that are still ill with chronic Lyme borreliosis (e.g., musculoskeletal or neurocognitive impairments), antimicrobial therapy is no more effective than placebo.[3,137,270,345–349]

The most effective precautions include avoidance of tick habitats, wearing long pants and long-sleeved shirts, taping socks over cuffs, tucking pants into socks, wearing light-colored clothing (to help identify ticks for early removal), and treating clothing and exposed skin with repellents. These may be cumbersome in hot weather.[350,351] Agents that contain DEET repel ticks and can be applied to clothing or exposed skin. Those containing permethrin kill ticks on contact but can only be applied to clothing (caution near cats). Inspection for, and removal of ticks soon after leaving tick-infested areas helps prevent transmission of infection. Studies in animals show that little risk of infection exists within the first 24 hours of attachment, and a maximum rate of infection occurs between 48 and 72 hours of attachment or if the infected tick feeds until engorgement.[352] Prompt tick removal is best,[353] but removal up to 60 hours later may still reduce transmission.[354] The incidence of disease is also greater in humans when ticks are attached for 72 hours or more.[355]

Dogs and cats do not appear to be a source for infection in humans because they do not excrete infectious organisms in their body fluids (including urine) to any appreciable extent.[80] No evidence proves that infected pet dogs or cats pose a direct risk to humans other than that they introduce unfed ticks in various life cycle stages into a household. The ticks do not survive long indoors, and if they are attached to a pet, they do not reattach without molting. Most ticks do not partially feed, and if they are disengaged from their first host during feeding, their mouthparts are usually damaged so that they will not refeed on a second host. As with other tick-borne illnesses, improper handling of ticks resulting in release of midgut or salivary contents onto abraded skin or mucous membranes might allow percutaneous penetration of infectious material, although this has never been reported.

Dogs and cats appear to be sentinel hosts but not reservoir hosts for human infection.[33,40,189,356–358] In the same environment, dogs and cats have a greater risk of exposure than their human counterparts because of their greater likelihood of contacting the tick vector.[339] Even in areas where Lyme borreliosis is endemic, the risk of infection from a recognized ixodid tick bite is so low that prophylactic antimicrobial therapy of exposed humans is not routinely recommended.[326,360] A human rOspA vaccine was marketed in the United States, but its use was limited because of concerns about potential but unproven side effects, and the product was withdrawn from the market in 2002.[3,361] At the time of writing, a recombinant OspA chimeric vaccine is in clinical trials for prevention of Lyme borreliosis in humans; this is a multivalent vaccine that provides protection against OspA types in US and European *Borrelia* species. Future vaccine targets may also include tick salivary proteins required for infection (Salp15) or other antigens.[99,362–367]

TICK-BORNE RELAPSING FEVER (TBRF) BORRELIOSIS

ETIOLOGY AND EPIDEMIOLOGY

Numerous *Borrelia* species comprise the relapsing fever group of vector-borne agents that cause disease in domestic animals and people (see Table 69.1).[15] Except for *Borrelia recurrentis*, which is a louse-borne relapsing fever agent, all others are transmitted by ticks (often the soft tick, *Ornithodoros*, which only feeds for 15–90 minutes, so transmission of these borreliae is quite rapid). *Borrelia lonestari* has been associated with erythema migrans lesions in humans in southeastern and south central United States (Fig. 69.12).[368] The illness has been labeled southern tick-associated rash illness (STARI) although the true cause of this condition remains unknown. *Borrelia lonestari* is thought to be transmitted by *A. americanum* (the lone star tick).[367–371] Differences in strains or species may account for the regional differences in clinical findings that have been reported. White-tailed deer (*Odocoileus virginianus*) became infected experimentally and developed spirochetemia, whereas infections of dogs were unsuccessful, although an increase in their antibody titers was observed.[372] *Borrelia miyamotoi* is an emerging TBRF disease in humans (but not known to occur in pets) in the Northeast and mid-Atlantic regions of the United States.[13–15] It is transmitted by *Ixodes* spp. ticks and can mimic Lyme borreliosis. Differences include spirochetemia, faster transmission of the organism after tick attachment, and transmission by all tick stages, including larvae, since there may be transovarial tick transmission.[62]

Relapsing fever spirochetoses have been found in sick dogs and cats. Microscopically visible spirochetemia accompanied by clinical illness has been observed in dogs in Texas and Florida infected with *B. turicatae*.[7–9,211] Using recombinant ELISA and immunoblot assays, the prevalence of antibodies to *B. turicatae* in 878 dogs from Texas was 2%, with the majority of positive dogs being from southern and central Texas; 2 of 17 seroreactive dogs also seroreacted to *B. burgdorferi*.[373] *Borrelia hermsii* has been identified in sick dogs in northwestern states.[5,6,374] *Borrelia persica* is a TBRF spirochete that is found in southern countries of the former USSR, Iran, Iraq, Syria, Jordan, Turkey, Israel, Egypt, and Cyprus and is transmitted by *Ornithodoros tholozani*. It is known to infect humans, dogs, and cats.[10–12,375–377] *Borrelia hispanica* was detected in two dogs and a cat from Spain with nonspecific clinical illness, thrombocytopenia with or without anemia, and spirochetemia.[378] In Spain, Portugal, Morocco, and Tunisia, TBRF borreliae (especially *B. hispanica*) have been isolated from *Ornithodoros erraticus*, an important vector that feeds on rats, mice, gerbils, and other small mammals.[379] *Borrelia hispanica* can also be transmitted by *Ornithodoros occidentalis*. *Ornithodoros tholozani*, which transmits *B. persica*, inhabits the Middle East, the Balkans, and southern countires of the former USSR. It dwells in man-made shelters and caves while feeding on various wild and domestic animal hosts and humans.

Relapsing fever spirochetes are maintained in nature between susceptible reservoir hosts and competent soft ticks (except for *B. miyamotoi*, which is transmitted by *Ixodes* spp. ticks). Soft (argasid) ticks prefer a variety of burrow-inhabiting mammals as hosts. Thus, relapsing fever borreliae have more restricted geographic ranges and niche vectors than those causing Lyme borreliosis (see Table 69.1). *Borrelia hermsii* is the most common cause of TBRF in North America in humans and involves at least three main vectors. In the western United States and Mexico, *Ornithodoros turicata* infests burrows of rodents, terrapins, and snakes, as well as domestic habitats of people and animals. Also in the western United States, *Ornithodoros hermsi* and *Ornithodoros parkeri* feed on rodents and squirrels and live in dead trees, fallen logs, and in cabins and homes. Unlike the *Ixodes* ticks, *Ornithodoros* ticks harbor spirochetes for extended periods because their life cycle takes years to complete. Mammalian hosts may harbor persistent infections but are only intermittently spirochetemic for 14 to 30 days; thus, the ticks are most responsible for maintaining the infection in nature. TBRF has not been reported east of Texas and Oklahoma; however, sporadic isolations of these spirochetes have been made from ticks and humans outside endemic regions. In the southern United States, *B. lonestari* may be associated with seropositivity to *Borrelia* spp. in humans and animals in areas where *Ixodes* ticks are not found.[380,382] Deer may be reservoir species for this organism. In addition to *B. lonestari*, *A. americanum* can be co-infected with *Ehrlichia ewingii*, *Ehrlichia chaffeensis*, and *Rickettsia* spp., which are all capable of causing disease in humans. With the exception of *E. ewingii*, the clinical significance of these organisms in dogs is unknown.

In the southern hemisphere, a Lyme borreliosis-like disease (Baggio-Yoshinari syndrome), has been discovered in people in Brazil.[382] Symptoms in people include fever, erythema migrans, shifting intermittent lameness, and joint swelling. Visible spirochetemia, more typical of the relapsing fever spirochetoses, is apparent in the peripheral blood of affected humans. Dogs in the region are antibody-positive in *Borrelia* spp. assays; however, the incriminated spirochetes have not been isolated by cultivation or genetically identified in affected humans or seropositive dogs. A relapsing fever-like spirochete (*Borrelia brasiliensis*) has been isolated from the soft tick *Ornithodoros brasiliensis*, which predominantly infests dogs. Further study is needed to determine if it is the cause of this infection.

CLINICAL FEATURES

Pathogenesis and Clinical Signs

Borrelia hermsii causes the model spirochetal disease of the relapsing fever group. Unlike other *Ornithodoros* species, *O. hermsi* does not excrete coxal fluid while feeding; it must transmit the organism while biting the host. Whereas *B. burgdorferi* in *Ixodes* ticks migrate from the midgut to the salivary gland, the salivary gland, midgut, and other

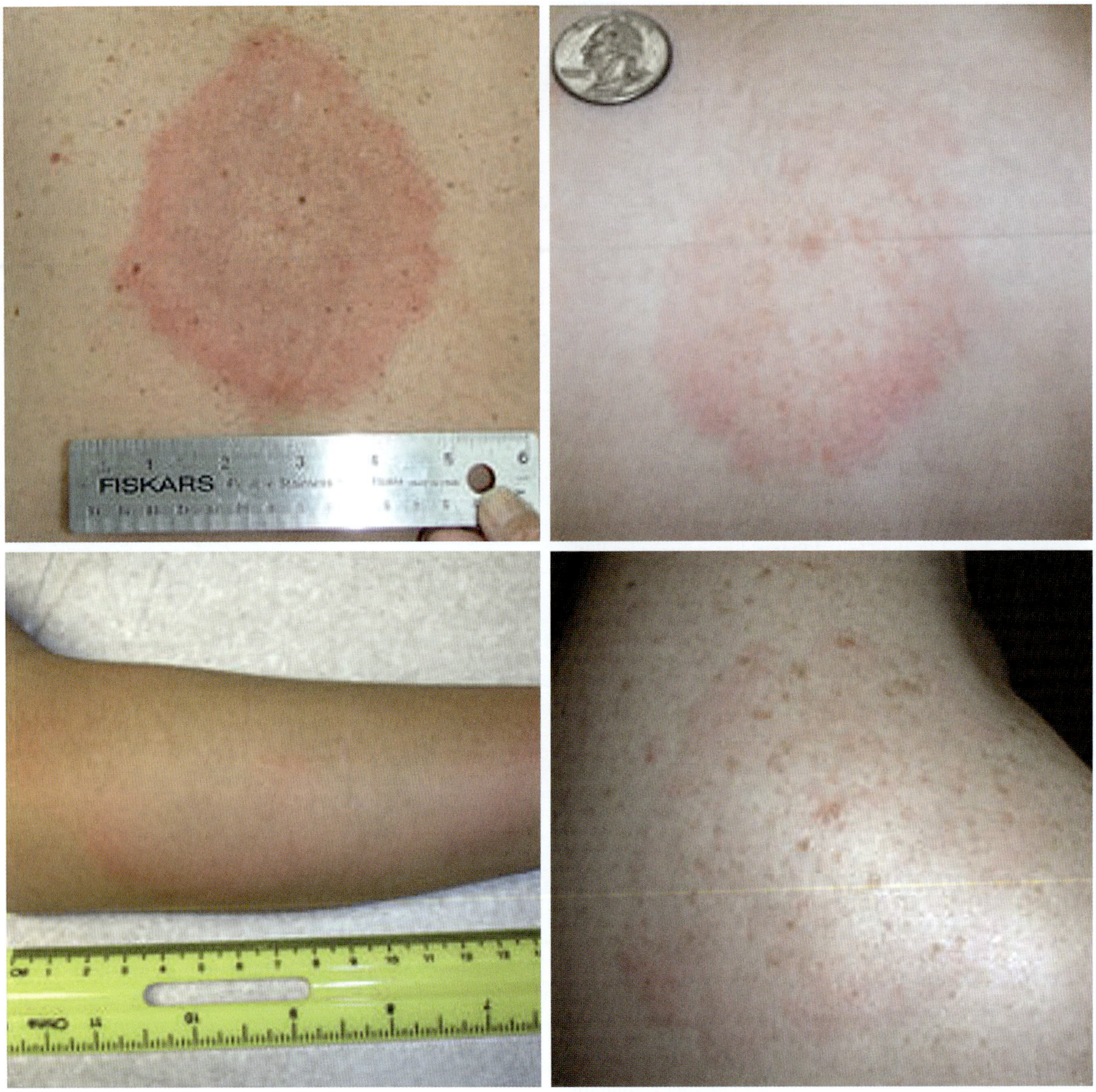

Fig. 69.12 Erythematous lesions at the site of *Amblyomma americanum* attachment (southern tick-associated rash illness, STARI). Once thought to be caused by *Borrelia lonestari*, the cause of the rash remains unclear. (From Centers for Disease Control and Prevention.)

tissues of *O. hermsi* are permanently contaminated with *B. hermsii* organisms, which allows for rapid transfer of the spirochetes during the short feeding times (minutes to hours).

In the mammalian host, *B. hermsii* has developed highly adapted mechanisms to evade the immune system.[120,383] Each inoculated spirochete may produce 30 unique antigenic variants, each expressing a major immunodominant protein that defines a specific serotype. In the mammalian host, episodes of cyclic spirochetemia are caused by waves of replicating spirochetes with relatively homogeneous serotypes. As the immune system responds to each new wave of replication, antigenic variation results in clinical relapse. The organism expresses variable major proteins, such as Vsp 33; however, after ingestion by the tick, a new major protein is upregulated on the cell surface and confers the unique serotype. Vsp 33 is homologous to OspC of *B. burgdorferi* and allows the organism to maintain its infectivity within the nonfeeding tick. Similar to the VlsE in *B. burgdorferi* organisms, rearrangement of silent genetic cassettes in the *vmp* gene accounts for antigenic variation and immune evasion.[120,384]

Clinical signs in dogs from Florida and Texas infected with *B. turicatae* included pyrexia, shifting leg lameness, hepatosplenomegaly, visible spirochetemia, anterior uveitis, and thrombocytopenia.[8,9,211] Many of the other relapsing fever spirochetes may infect dogs and cats as incidental hosts in the same way they are known to infect humans (see Table 69.1). The two dogs and cat infected with *B. hispanica* had nonspecific signs of inappetence and thrombocytopenia, with or without anemia.[378] However, co-infecting vector-borne pathogens may have also contributed to clinical signs in these animals.

DIAGNOSIS

As a result of the lack of serologic tests for TBRF, diagnosis is made by visualization of the spirochetes in blood smears using dark-field microscopy, Wright-Giemsa, acridine orange, silver, or Gram stain (Fig. 69.13). The presence of visible spirochetes differentiates relapsing fever from Lyme borreliosis, because the latter rarely, if ever, is associated with visible spirochetemia (except in the case of *B. mayonii* infection). Fresh blood smears are superior to those prepared from EDTA-preserved

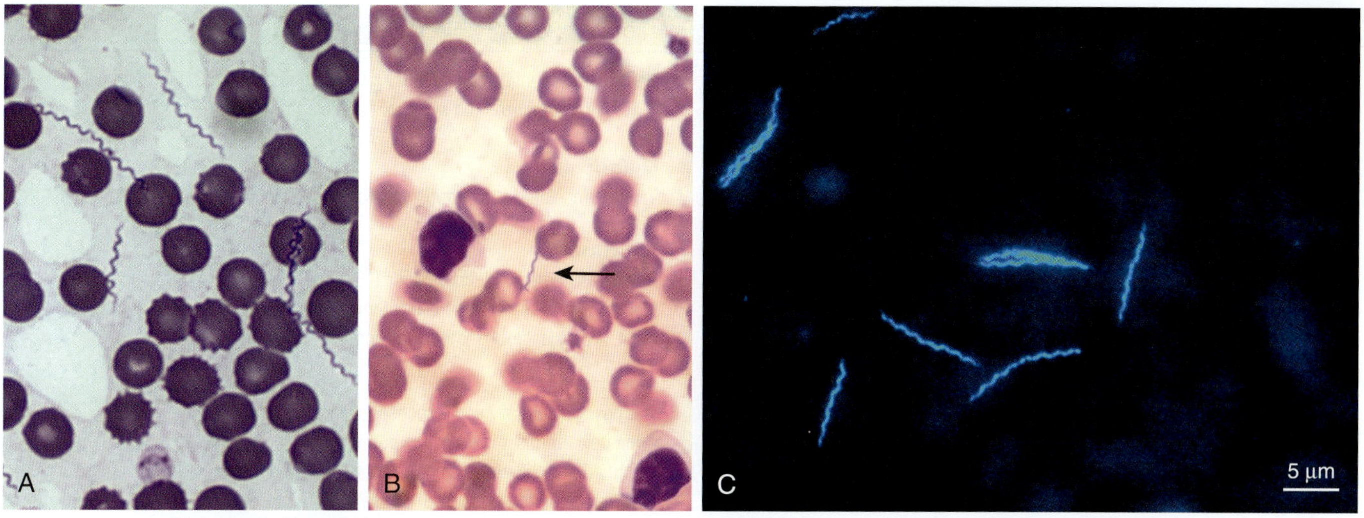

Fig. 69.13 *Borrelia hispanica* spirochetes from two dogs and a cat from Spain. (A) Blood smear from a 6-year-old male hound from Seville, Spain, with lethargy, anemia, and thrombocytopenia (Giemsa stain, 150× magnification). (B) Blood smear from a dog from Valencia, Spain, with anorexia and thrombocytopenia (100× magnification, *arrow* directed at spirochete). (C) 4′,6-diamidino-2-phenylindole (DAPI)-stained spirochetes cultured from the blood of a 1-year-old male cat with cachexia and regenerative anemia. (From Margos G, Pantchev N, Globokar M, et al. First cases of natural infections with *Borrelia hispanica* in two dogs and a cat from Europe. *Microorganisms.* 2020;8:1251.)

blood.[9] Sensitivity can be improved by buffy coat examination or inoculation of the blood into mice and subsequently into spirochete media. PCR-based methods can be used to identify the spirochetes.

TREATMENT AND PREVENTION

Therapy for relapsing fever spirochetosis is similar to that for Lyme borreliosis and involves treatment with doxycycline. The Jarisch-Herxheimer reaction, a severe febrile reaction to released bacterial endotoxins seen in some humans after treatment of TBRF, has not been documented in dogs. Clinical improvement after treatment was noted in most dogs infected by *B. turicatae*.[9,211] Prevention involves fast-kill tick-control since transmission is much faster than for Lyme borreliosis. Vaccines for Lyme disease would not be expected to prevent infection with *B. turicatae* or with other TBRF spirochetes.

CASE EXAMPLE

Signalment

"Dako," a 7-year-old MC Doberman pinscher from Amador County, CA.

History

Dako was evaluated for a 2-day history of lethargy, apparent blindness, inappetence, and inability to walk. He was taken to a local emergency clinic within 24 hours of illness where a neurologic examination was considered abnormal and an intracranial lesion was suspected. He was treated with IV fluids and given a single dose of ampicillin (1 g). The following day his mentation and thoracic limb strength had improved, but he remained unable to walk and had evidence of urinary incontinence. He lived on a farm and had contact with sheep, horses, llamas, chickens, geese, cats, and four other dogs, all of which were currently healthy, although one additional dog had died of acute renal failure 1 month ago. There was no travel history or toxin exposure, but frequent exposure to ticks occurred. Dako's diet consisted of commercial dry dog food, and occasionally pieces of cooked steak and raw goose eggs. He had not received a Lyme vaccine in the past but had been vaccinated regularly for CDV, CAdV, CPV2, and CPI3.

Current Medications

Monthly topical flea and tick preventative (fipronil and s-methoprene), monthly oral heartworm preventative (ivermectin and pyrantel).

Other Medical History

Color dilution alopecia.

Physical Examination

Body weight: 43.1 kg.

General: Quiet, alert, and responsive. Hydrated. Ambulatory on all four limbs but appeared very painful. Temperature = 101.9°F (38.8°C), HR = 78 beats/minute, RR = 24 breaths/minute, mucous membranes pink, CRT = 1 second. BCS = 5/9.

Integument: A thin haircoat with scaling was noted.

Eyes, ears, nose, and throat: Mild episcleral injection was present bilaterally. Moderate dental calculus and gingivitis were also present.

Musculoskeletal: Symmetrically well-muscled. Multiple distal joints were severely swollen and painful on palpation, including both carpi, tarsi, stifle, and elbow joints. The dog appeared painful when rising from recumbency and when walked, with pronounced right pelvic limb lameness.

Cardiovascular: No abnormalities detected.

Respiratory: No abnormalities detected.

GI: No abnormalities detected. Large bladder, actively urinated a large amount during the examination.

Rectal examination: No abnormalities detected.

Lymph nodes: Bilateral popliteal lymphadenomegaly (3 cm in diameter). Remaining peripheral lymph nodes measured 2 cm in diameter. All nodes were soft on palpation.

Neurologic examination: No neurologic abnormalities detected.

Laboratory Findings

CBC: HCT 48.4% (40%–55%), MCV 69.6 fL (65–75 fL), MCHC 34.9 g/dL (33–36 g/dL), WBC 17,100 cells/μL (6,000–13,000 cells/μL), neutrophils 15,561 cells/μL (3,000–10,500 cells/μL), lymphocytes 171 cells/μL (1,000–4,000 cells/μL), monocytes 1,026 cells/μL (150–1,200 cells/μL), eosinophils 342 cells/μL (0–1,500 cells/μL), platelets clumped (150,000–400,000 platelets/μL).

Continued

CASE EXAMPLE—cont'd

Serum chemistry profile: Sodium 148 mmol/L (143–151 mmol/L), potassium 3.5 mmol/L (3.6–4.8 mmol/L), chloride 115 mmol/L (108–116 mmol/L), bicarbonate 20 mmol/L (20–29 mmol/L), phosphorus 3.1 mg/dL (2.6–5.2 mg/dL), calcium 10.0 mg/dL (9.6–11.2 mg/dL), BUN 11 mg/dL (11–33 mg/dL), creatinine 0.8 mg/dL (0.8–1.5 mg/dL), glucose 102 mg/dL (86–118 mg/dL), total protein 6.1 g/dL (5.4–6.9 g/dL), albumin 3.6 g/dL (3.4–4.3 g/dL), globulin 2.5 g/dL (1.7–3.1 g/dL), ALT 17 U/L (21–72 U/L), AST 36 U/L (20–49 U/L), ALP 60 U/L (14–91 U/L), creatine kinase 217 U/L (55–257 U/l), GGT 1 U/L (0–6 U/L), cholesterol 167 mg/dL (139–353 mg/dL), total bilirubin 0.1 mg/dL (0–0.2 mg/dL), magnesium 1.8 mg/dL (1.9–2.5 mg/dL).

Urinalysis: SpG 1.018; pH 8.0, negative protein (SSA), negative bilirubin, negative glucose, 0–1 WBC/HPF, 0–2 RBC/HPF.

Cytology of synovial fluid obtained via arthrocentesis (see table below): Negative for morulae in WBC.

Imaging Findings

Thoracic radiographs: Unremarkable.

Abdominal ultrasound: The liver was diffusely hypoechoic but was normal in size. There was mild bilateral adrenomegaly (0.9 cm). The urinary bladder was very large and was in a pelvic location.

Microbiologic Testing

SNAP 4Dx Plus test (IDEXX Laboratories, ME): Positive for *B. burgdorferi* C_6–specific antibodies; negative for antibodies to *Anaplasma* spp. and *Ehrlichia* spp. and negative for *Dirofilaria immitis* antigen.

Lyme C6 Quant antibody ELISA (IDEXX Laboratories, ME): 153 U/mL (normal, <30 U/mL).

PCR for *B. burgdorferi* on synovial fluid: Negative.

Diagnosis

Immune-mediated polyarthritis; possibly secondary to *B. burgdorferi* infection.

Treatment

Dako was treated with doxycycline (10 mg/kg, PO, q12h) and tramadol (2 mg/kg, PO, q8h) and showed dramatic clinical improvement within 24 hours of initiating treatment. A physical examination was normal 2 weeks later.

Comments

The positive serology and response to doxycycline was suggestive of a diagnosis of Lyme polyarthritis, although it is possible there was some other cause that was not identified and the presence of C_6 antibodies was not related to this dog's illness. It may have been too early in the course of illness for this dog to have seroconverted to other vector-borne pathogens such as *A. phagocytophilum*. Other diagnostic assays that may have been useful in this dog (and in this geographic location) are serology for *Bartonella* spp.; PCR on blood for vector-borne pathogens such as *A. phagocytophilum*, *Rickettsia* spp., and *Ehrlichia canis*; aerobic bacterial culture of the synovial fluid; and convalescent serology for the vector-borne pathogens above. The negative synovial fluid PCR result does not rule out the possibility of Lyme arthritis because organism numbers within the synovial fluid of animals with Lyme arthritis may be extremely low. Furthermore, the dog had been treated with ampicillin before it was seen, which may have reduced organism numbers further.

	Right carpus	Left carpus	Right tarsus	Left stifle
Cell count (cells/μL)	23,730	29,370	ND	1,020
Neutrophils (%)	85	94	76	12
Small mononuclear cells (%)	2	0	1	41
Large mononuclear cells (%)	13	6	23	47
Interpretation	Marked purulent inflammation with non-degenerate neutrophils	Marked purulent inflammation with non-degenerate neutrophils	Marked purulent inflammation with non-degenerate neutrophils	Very mild purulent inflammation with non-degenerate neutrophils

SUGGESTED READINGS

Littman MP, Gerber B, Goldstein RE, et al. ACVIM consensus update on Lyme borreliosis in dogs and cats. *J Vet Intern Med*. 2018;32:887–903.

Piccione J, Levine GJ, Duff CA, et al. Tick-borne relapsing fever in dogs. *J Vet Intern Med*. 2016;30:1222–1228.

Kurokawa C, Lynn GE, Pedra JHF, et al. Interactions between Borrelia burgdorferi and ticks. *Nature Rev Microbiol*. 2020;18:587–600.

Vogt NA, Stevens CPG. Why the rationale for canine *Borrelia burgdorferi* vaccination is unpersuasive. *Front Vet Sci*. 2021;8:719060.

REFERENCES

1. Burgdorfer W, Barbour AG, Hayes SF, et al. Lyme disease-a tick-borne spirochetosis? *Science*. 1982;216:1317–1319.
2. Meader CN. Five cases of relapsing fever originating in Colorado, with positive blood findings in two. *Colorado Med*. 1915;12:365–368.
3. Steere AC, Strle F, Wormser GP, et al. Lyme borreliosis. *Nature Rev*. 2016;2:1–18.
4. Pritt BS, Mead PS, Johnson DKH, et al. Identification of a novel pathogenic *Borrelia* species causing Lyme borreliosis with unusually high spirochaetaemia: a descriptive study. *Lancet Infect Dis*. 2016;16:556–564.
5. Kelly AL, Raffel SJ, Fischer RJ, et al. First isolation of the relapsing fever spirochete, *Borrelia hermsii*, from a domestic dog. *Ticks Tick Borne Dis*. 2014;5:95–99.
6. Schwan TG, Policastro PF, Miller Z, et al. Tick-borne relapsing fever caused by *Borrelia hermsii*, Montana. *Emerg Infect Dis*. 2003;9:1151–1154.
7. Schwan TG, Raffel SJ, Schrumpf ME, et al. Phylogenetic analysis of the spirochetes *Borrelia parkeri* and *Borrelia turicatae* and the potential for tick-borne relapsing fever in Florida. *J Clin Microbiol*. 2005;43:3851–3859.
8. Piccione J, Levine GJ, Duff CA, et al. Tick-borne relapsing fever in dogs. *J Vet Intern Med*. 2016;30:1222–1228.
9. Whitney MS, Schwan TG, Sultemeier KB, et al. Spirochetemia caused by *Borrelia turicatae* infection in 3 dogs in Texas. *Vet Clin Pathol*. 2007;36:212–216.
10. Baneth G, Nachum-Biala Y, Halperin T, et al. *Borrelia persica* infection in dogs and cats: clinical manifestations, clinicopathological findings and genetic characterization. *Parasit Vectors*. 2016;9:244.
11. Schwarzer S, Margos G, Overzier E, et al. *Borrelia persica*: In vitro cultivation and characterization via conventional PCR and multilocus sequence analysis of two strains isolated from a cat and ticks from Israel. *Ticks Tick Borne Dis*. 2015;6:751–757.
12. Shirani D, Rakhshanpoor A, Cutler SJ, et al. A case of canine borreliosis in Iran caused by *Borrelia persica*. *Ticks Tick Borne Dis*. 2016;7:424–426.
13. Gugliotta JL, Goethert HK, Berardi VP, et al. Meningoencephalitis from *Borrelia miyamotoi* in an immunocompromised patient. *N Engl J Med*. 2013;368:240–245.

14. Krause PJ, Narasimhan S, Wormser GP, et al. Human *Borrelia miyamotoi* infection in the United States. *N Engl J Med*. 2013;368:291–293.
15. Cutler SJ, Ruzic-Sabljic E, Potkonjak A. Emerging borreliae - Expanding beyond Lyme borreliosis. *Mol Cell Probes*. 2017;31:22–27.
16. Castillo-Ramirez S, Fingerle V, Jungnick S, et al. Trans-Atlantic exchanges have shaped the population structure of the Lyme disease agent *Borrelia burgdorferi* sensu stricto. *Sci Rep*. 2016;6:22794.
17. Filipuzzi-Jenny E, Blot M, Schmid-Berger N, et al. Genetic diversity among *Borrelia burgdorferi* isolates: more than three genospecies? *Res Microbiol*. 1993;144:295–304.
18. Margos G, Wilske B, Sing A, et al. *Borrelia bavariensis* sp. nov. is widely distributed in Europe and Asia. *Int J Syst Evol Microbiol*. 2013;63:4284–4288.
19. Richter D, Allgower R, Matuschka FR. Co-feeding transmission and its contribution to the perpetuation of the Lyme disease spirochete *Borrelia afzelii*. *Emerg Infect Dis*. 2002;8:1421–1425.
20. Saint Girons I, Gern L, Gray JS, et al. Identification of *Borrelia burgdorferi* sensu lato species in Europe. *Zentralbl Bakteriol*. 1998;287:190–195.
21. Wang G, van Dam AP, Schwartz I, et al. Molecular typing of *Borrelia burgdorferi* sensu lato: taxonomic, epidemiological, and clinical implications. *Clin Microbiol Rev*. 1999;12:633–653.
22. Dressler F, Ackermann R, Steere AC. Antibody responses to the three genomic groups of *Borrelia burgdorferi* in European Lyme borreliosis. *J Infect Dis*. 1994;169:313–318.
23. Collares-Pereira M, Couceiro S, Franca I, et al. First isolation of *Borrelia lusitaniae* from a human patient. *J Clin Microbiol*. 2004;42:1316–1318.
24. Zeidner NS, Nuncio MS, Schneider BS, et al. A Portuguese isolate of *Borrelia lusitaniae* induces disease in C3H/HeN mice. *J Med Microbiol*. 2001;50:1055–1060.
25. Diza E, Papa A, Vezyri E, et al. *Borrelia valaisiana* in cerebrospinal fluid. *Emerg Infect Dis*. 2004;10:1692–1693.
26. Speck S, Reiner B, Wittenbrink MM. Isolation of *Borrelia afzelii* from a dog. *Vet Rec*. 2001;149:19–20.
27. Azuma Y, Isogai E, Isogai H, et al. Canine Lyme disease: clinical and serological evaluations in 21 dogs in Japan. *Vet Rec*. 1994;134:369–372.
28. Gordillo-Perez G, Vargas M, Solorzano-Santos F, et al. Demonstration of *Borrelia burgdorferi* sensu stricto infection in ticks from the northeast of Mexico. *Clin Microbiol Infect*. 2009;15:496–498.
29. Guzmàn-Cornejo C, Robbins RG, Pérez TM. The *Ixodes* (Acari: Ixodidae) of Mexico: parasite-host and host-parasite checklists. *Zootaxa*. 2007;1553:47–58.
30. Gordillo-Perez G, Torres J, Solorzano-Santos F, et al. *Borrelia burgdorferi* infection and cutaneous Lyme disease, Mexico. *Emerg Infect Dis*. 2007;13:1556–1558.
31. Bowman D, Little SE, Lorentzen L, et al. Prevalence and geographic distribution of *Dirofilaria immitis, Borrelia burgdorferi, Ehrlichia canis,* and *Anaplasma phagocytophilum* in dogs in the United States: results of a national clinic-based serologic survey. *Vet Parasitol*. 2009;160:138–148.
32. Companion Animal Parasite Council. Parasite Prevalence Maps. 2020. Available at: https://capcvet.org/maps/#/2020/all-year/lyme-disease/dog/united-states and https://capcvet.org/maps/#/2020/all-year/lyme-disease/dog/canada.
33. Liu Y, Nordone SK, Yabsley MJ, et al. Quantifying the relationship between human Lyme disease and *Borrelia burgdorferi* exposure in domestic dogs. *Geospat Health*. 2019;14.
34. Dewage BG, Little S, Payton M, et al. Trends in canine seroprevalence to *Borrelia burgdorferi* and *Anaplasma* spp. in the eastern USA, 2010-2017. *Parasit Vectors*. 2019;12:476.
35. Evason M, Stull JW, Pearl DL, et al. Prevalence of *Borrelia burgdorferi, Anaplasma* spp., *Ehrlichia* spp. and *Dirofilaria immitis* in Canadian dogs, 2008 to 2015: a repeat cross-sectional study. *Parasit Vectors*. 2019;12:64.
36. Foley-Eby AH, Savidge C, Lloyd VK. *Ixodes scapularis* ticks and *Borrelia burgdorferi* on Prince Edward Island: Passive tick surveillance and canine seroprevalence. *Can Vet J*. 2020;61:1107–1110.
37. Brown RN, Lane RS. Lyme disease in California: a novel enzootic transmission cycle of *Borrelia burgdorferi*. *Science*. 1992;256:1439–1442.
38. Ghosh P, Saleh MN, Sundstrom KD, et al. *Ixodes* spp. from dogs and cats in the United States: diversity, seasonality, and prevalence of *Borrelia burgdorferi* and *Anaplasma phagocytophilum*. *Vector Borne Zoonotic Dis*. 2021;21:11–19.
39. Guerra M, Walker ED, Jones C, et al. Predicting the risk of Lyme disease: habitat suitability for *Ixodes scapularis* in the north central United States. *Emerg Infect Dis*. 2002;8:289–297.
40. Stone EG, Lacombe EH, Rand PW. Antibody testing and Lyme disease risk. *Emerg Infect Dis*. 2005;11:722–724.
41. Herrmann C, Gern L. Survival of *Ixodes ricinus* (Acari: Ixodidae) under challenging conditions of temperature and humidity is influenced by *Borrelia burgdorferi* sensu lato infection. *J Med Entomol*. 2010;47:1196–1204.
42. Oliver JH. *Borrelia*, tick vectors, and reservoir hosts in southern U. S. In: *Proceedings of the Annual Spring Symposium of Emerging Infectious Diseases. Threats to the Southeastern US*. 2004.
43. Oliver JH Jr, Cummins GA, Joiner MS. Immature *Ixodes scapularis* (Acari: Ixodidae) parasitizing lizards from the southeastern U.S.A. *J Parasitol*. 1993;79:684–689.
44. Oliver JH Jr. Lyme borreliosis in the southern United States: a review. *J Parasitol*. 1996;82:926–935.
45. Lane RS, Quistad GB. Borreliacidal factor in the blood of the western fence lizard (*Sceloporus occidentalis*). *J Parasitol*. 1998;84:29–34.
46. Wright JC, Chambers M, Mullen GR, et al. Seroprevalence of *Borrelia burgdorferi* in dogs in Alabama, USA. *Prev Vet Med*. 1997;31:127–131.
47. Humair PF. Birds and *Borrelia*. *Int J Med Microbiol*. 2002;291(Suppl 33):70–74.
48. Keirans JE, Hutcheson HJ, Durden LA, et al. *Ixodes scapularis* (Acari: Ixodidae): redescription of all active stages, distribution, hosts, geographical variation, and medical and veterinary importance. *J Med Entomol*. 1996;33:297–318.
49. Kurtenbach K, De Michelis S, Sewell HS, et al. The key roles of selection and migration in the ecology of Lyme borreliosis. *Int J Med Microbiol*. 2002;291(Suppl 33):152–154.
50. Ogden NH, Trudel L, Artsob H, et al. *Ixodes scapularis* ticks collected by passive surveillance in Canada: analysis of geographic distribution and infection with Lyme borreliosis agent *Borrelia burgdorferi*. *J Med Entomol*. 2006;43:600–609.
51. Scott JD, Fernando K, Banerjee SN, et al. Birds disperse ixodid (Acari: Ixodidae) and *Borrelia burgdorferi*-infected ticks in Canada. *J Med Entomol*. 2001;38:493–500.
52. Smith RP Jr, Rand PW, Lacombe EH, et al. Role of bird migration in the long-distance dispersal of *Ixodes dammini,* the vector of Lyme disease. *J Infect Dis*. 1996;174:221–224.
53. Sarih M, Jouda F, Gern L, et al. First isolation of *Borrelia burgdorferi* sensu lato from *Ixodes ricinus* ticks in Morocco. *Vector Borne Zoonotic Dis*. 2003;3:133–139.
54. Derdakova M, Lencakova D. Association of genetic variability within the *Borrelia burgdorferi* sensu lato with the ecology, epidemiology of Lyme borreliosis in Europe. *Ann Agric Environ Med*. 2005;12:165–172.
55. Richter D, Schlee DB, Matuschka FR. Relapsing fever-like spirochetes infecting European vector tick of Lyme disease agent. *Emerg Infect Dis*. 2003;9:697–701.
56. Schneider BS, Schriefer ME, Dietrich G, et al. *Borrelia bissettii* isolates induce pathology in a murine model of disease. *Vector Borne Zoonotic Dis*. 2008;8:623–633.
57. Mukhacheva TA, Kovalev SY. *Borrelia* spirochetes in Russia: Genospecies differentiation by real-time PCR. *Ticks Tick Borne Dis*. 2014;5:722–726.
58. Gern L. Life cycle of *Borrelia burgdorferi* sensu lato and transmission to humans. *Curr Probl Dermatol*. 2009;37:18–30.
59. Jaenson TG, Talleklint L. Incompetence of roe deer as reservoirs of the Lyme borreliosis spirochete. *J Med Entomol*. 1992;29:813–817.
60. Nelson DR, Rooney S, Miller NJ, et al. Complement-mediated killing of *Borrelia burgdorferi* by nonimmune sera from sika deer. *J Parasitol*. 2000;86:1232–1238.
61. Telford SR 3rd, Mather TN, Moore SI, et al. Incompetence of deer as reservoirs of the Lyme disease spirochete. *Am J Trop Med Hyg*. 1988;39:105–109.
62. Rollend L, Fish D, Childs JE. Transovarial transmission of *Borrelia* spirochetes by *Ixodes scapularis*: a summary of the literature and recent observations. *Ticks Tick Borne Dis*. 2013;4:46–51.
63. Patrican LA. Absence of Lyme disease spirochetes in larval progeny of naturally infected *Ixodes scapularis* (Acari:Ixodidae) fed on dogs. *J Med Entomol*. 1997;34:52–55.

64. Bunikis J, Tsao J, Luke CJ, et al. *Borrelia burgdorferi* infection in a natural population of *Peromyscus leucopus* mice: a longitudinal study in an area where Lyme Borreliosis is highly endemic. *J Infect Dis.* 2004;189:1515–1523.
65. Ogden NH, Nuttall PA, Randolph SE. Natural Lyme disease cycles maintained via sheep by co-feeding ticks. *Parasitology.* 1997;115(Pt 6):591–599.
66. Randolph S, Gern L. Co-feeding transmission and its contribution to the perpetuation of the Lyme disease spirochete *Borrelia afzelii. Emerg Infect Dis.* 2003;9:893–894.
67. Richter D, Matuschka FR. Elimination of lyme disease spirochetes from ticks feeding on domestic ruminants. *Appl Environ Microbiol.* 2010;76:7650–7652.
68. Wright SA, Thompson MA, Miller MJ, et al. Ecology of *Borrelia burgdorferi* in ticks (Acari: Ixodidae), rodents, and birds in the Sierra Nevada foothills, Placer County, California. *J Med Entomol.* 2000;37:909–918.
69. Gorelova NB, Korenberg EI, Kovalevskii Iu V, et al. The isolation of *Borrelia* from the tick *Ixodes trianguliceps* (Ixodidae) and the possible significance of this species in the epizootiology of ixodid tick-borne borrelioses. *Parazitologiia.* 1996;30:13–18.
70. Hegarty BC, Maggi RG, Koskinen P, et al. *Ehrlichia muris* infection in a dog from Minnesota. *J Vet Intern Med.* 2012;26:1217–1220.
71. Holden K, Boothby JT, Kasten RW, et al. Co-detection of *Bartonella henselae, Borrelia burgdorferi*, and *Anaplasma phagocytophilum* in *Ixodes pacificus* ticks from California, USA. *Vector Borne Zoonotic Dis.* 2006;6:99–102.
72. Hovius KE, Beijer B, Rijpkema SG, et al. Identification of four *Borrelia burgdorferi* sensu lato species in *Ixodes ricinus* ticks collected from Dutch dogs. *Vet Q.* 1998;20:143–145.
73. Nadelman RB, Horowitz HW, Hsieh TC, et al. Simultaneous human granulocytic ehrlichiosis and Lyme borreliosis. *N Engl J Med.* 1997;337:27–30.
74. Nelder MP, Russell CB, Sheehan NJ, et al. Human pathogens associated with the blacklegged tick *Ixodes scapularis*: a systematic review. *Parasit Vectors.* 2016;9:265.
75. Piesman J, Happ CM. Ability of the Lyme disease spirochete *Borrelia burgdorferi* to infect rodents and three species of human-biting ticks (blacklegged tick, American dog tick, lone star tick) (Acari:Ixodidae). *J Med Entomol.* 1997;34:451–456.
76. Jobe DA, Lovrich SD, Nelson JA, et al. *Borrelia burgdorferi* in *Ixodes scapularis* ticks, Chicago area. *Emerg Infect Dis.* 2006;12:1039–1041.
77. Matuschka FR, Endepols S, Richter D, et al. Risk of urban Lyme disease enhanced by the presence of rats. *J Infect Dis.* 1996;174:1108–1111.
78. Smith RP Jr, Rand PW, Lacombe EH, et al. Norway rats as reservoir hosts for Lyme disease spirochetes on Monhegan Island, Maine. *J Infect Dis.* 1993;168:687–691.
79. Guerra MA, Walker ED, Kitron U. Canine surveillance system for Lyme borreliosis in Wisconsin and northern Illinois: geographic distribution and risk factor analysis. *Am J Trop Med Hyg.* 2001;65:546–552.
80. Appel MJ, Allan S, Jacobson RH, et al. Experimental Lyme disease in dogs produces arthritis and persistent infection. *J Infect Dis.* 1993;167:651–664.
81. Johnson RC, Kodner CB, Jurkovich PJ, et al. Comparative in vitro and in vivo susceptibilities of the Lyme disease spirochete *Borrelia burgdorferi* to cefuroxime and other antimicrobial agents. *Antimicrob Agents Chemother.* 1990;34:2133–2136.
82. Nadelman RB, Sherer C, Mack L, et al. Survival of *Borrelia burgdorferi* in human blood stored under blood banking conditions. *Transfusion.* 1990;30:298–301.
83. Liang L, Wang J, Schorter L, et al. Rapid clearance of *Borrelia burgdorferi* from the blood circulation. *Parasit Vectors.* 2020;13:191.
84. Bohme M, Schwenecke S, Fuchs E, et al. Screening of blood donors and recipients for *Borrelia burgdorferi* antibodies: no evidence of *B. burgdorferi* infection transmitted by transfusion. *Infusionsther Transfusionsmed.* 1992;19:204–207.
85. Gerber MA, Shapiro ED, Krause PJ, et al. The risk of acquiring Lyme disease or babesiosis from a blood transfusion. *J Infect Dis.* 1994;170:231–234.
86. Hyde JA. *Borrelia burgdorferi* keeps moving and carries on: a review of borrelial dissemination and invasion. *Front Immunol.* 2017;8:114.
87. Kenedy MR, Lenhart TR, Akins DR. The role of *Borrelia burgdorferi* outer surface proteins. *FEMS Immunol Med Microbiol.* 2012;66:1–19.
88. Strother KO, Broadwater A, De Silva A. Plasmid requirements for infection of ticks by *Borrelia burgdorferi. Vector Borne Zoonotic Dis.* 2005;5:237–245.
89. de Silva AM, Telford SR 3rd, Brunet LR, et al. *Borrelia burgdorferi* OspA is an arthropod-specific transmission-blocking Lyme disease vaccine. *J Exp Med.* 1996;183:271–275.
90. Ohnishi J, Piesman J, de Silva AM. Antigenic and genetic heterogeneity of *Borrelia burgdorferi* populations transmitted by ticks. *Proc Natl Acad Sci U S A.* 2001;98:670–675.
91. Pal U, de Silva AM, Montgomery RR, et al. Attachment of *Borrelia burgdorferi* within *Ixodes scapularis* mediated by outer surface protein A. *J Clin Invest.* 2000;106:561–569.
92. Kurokawa C, Lynn GE, Pedra JHF, et al. Interactions between *Borrelia burgdorferi* and ticks. *Nature Rev Microbiol.* 2020;18:587–600.
93. Pal U, Yang X, Chen M, et al. OspC facilitates *Borrelia burgdorferi* invasion of *Ixodes scapularis* salivary glands. *J Clin Invest.* 2004;113:220–230.
94. Schwan TG, Piesman J. Vector interactions and molecular adaptations of Lyme disease and relapsing fever spirochetes associated with transmission by ticks. *Emerg Infect Dis.* 2002;8:115–121.
95. Schwan TG, Piesman J, Golde WT, et al. Induction of an outer surface protein on *Borrelia burgdorferi* during tick feeding. *Proc Natl Acad Sci U S A.* 1995;92:2909–2913.
96. Carrasco SE, Troxell B, Yang Y, et al. Outer surface protein OspC is an antiphagocytic factor that protects *Borrelia burgdorferi* from phagocytosis by macrophages. *Infect Immun.* 2015;83:4848–4860.
97. Hovius JW, Schuijt TJ, de Groot KA, et al. Preferential protection of *Borrelia burgdorferi* sensu stricto by a Salp15 homologue in *Ixodes ricinus* saliva. *J Infect Dis.* 2008;198:1189–1197.
98. Tilly K, Krum JG, Bestor A, et al. *Borrelia burgdorferi* OspC protein required exclusively in a crucial early stage of mammalian infection. *Infect Immun.* 2006;74:3554–3564.
99. Dai J, Wang P, Adusumilli S, et al. Antibodies against a tick protein, Salp15, protect mice from the Lyme disease agent. *Cell Host Microbe.* 2009;6:482–492.
100. Radolf JD, Caimano MJ. The long strange trip of *Borrelia burgdorferi* outer-surface protein C. *Mol Microbiol.* 2008;69:1–4.
101. Ramamoorthi N, Narasimhan S, Pal U, et al. The Lyme disease agent exploits a tick protein to infect the mammalian host. *Nature.* 2005;436:573–577.
102. Tilly K, Rosa PA, Stewart PE. Biology of infection with *Borrelia burgdorferi. Infect Dis Clin North Am.* 2008;22:217–234.
103. Piesman J, Zeidner NS, Schneider BS. Dynamic changes in *Borrelia burgdorferi* populations in *Ixodes scapularis* (Acari: Ixodidae) during transmission: studies at the mRNA level. *Vector Borne Zoonotic Dis.* 2003;3:125–132.
104. Littman MP, Gerber B, Goldstein RE, et al. ACVIM consensus update on Lyme borreliosis in dogs and cats. *J Vet Intern Med.* 2018;32:887–903.
105. Krupka I, Pantchev N, Lorentzen L, et al. Durch Zecken übertragbare bakterielle Infektionen bei Hunden: Seroprävalenzen von *Anaplasma phagocytophilum, Borrelia burgdorferi* sensu lato und *Ehrlichia canis* in Deutschland. *Prakt Tierarzt.* 2007;88:776–788.
106. Levy SA, Magnarelli LA. Relationship between development of antibodies to *Borrelia burgdorferi* in dogs and the subsequent development of limb/joint borreliosis. *J Am Vet Med Assoc.* 1992;200:344–347.
107. Littman MP, Goldstein RE, Labato MA, et al. ACVIM small animal consensus statement on Lyme disease in dogs: diagnosis, treatment, and prevention. *J Vet Intern Med.* 2006;20:422–434.
108. Pantchev N, Pluta S, Huisinga E, et al. Tick-borne diseases (borreliosis, anaplasmosis, babesiosis) in German and Austrian dogs: status quo and review of distribution, transmission, clinical findings, diagnostics and prophylaxis. *Parasitol Res.* 2015;114(Suppl 1):S19–54.
109. Pantchev N, Schaper R, Limousin S, et al. Occurrence of *Dirofilaria immitis* and tick-borne infections caused by *Anaplasma phagocytophilum, Borrelia burgdorferi* sensu lato and *Ehrlichia canis* in domestic dogs in France: results of a countrywide serologic survey. *Parasitol Res.* 2009;105(Suppl 1):S101–114.

110. Anderson JF, Barthold SW, Magnarelli LA. Infectious but nonpathogenic isolate of *Borrelia burgdorferi*. *J Clin Microbiol.* 1990;28:2693–2699.
111. Brisson D, Baxamusa N, Schwartz I, et al. Biodiversity of *Borrelia burgdorferi* strains in tissues of Lyme disease patients. *PLoS One.* 2011;6:e22926.
112. Brisson D, Dykhuizen DE. OspC diversity in *Borrelia burgdorferi*: different hosts are different niches. *Genetics.* 2004;168:713–722.
113. Rhodes DV, Earnhart CG, Mather TN, et al. Identification of *Borrelia burgdorferi* OspC genotypes in canine tissue following tick infestation: implications for Lyme disease vaccine and diagnostic assay design. *Vet J.* 2013;198:412–418.
114. Wang G, Ojaimi C, Wu H, et al. Disease severity in a murine model of Lyme borreliosis is associated with the genotype of the infecting *Borrelia burgdorferi* sensu stricto strain. *J Infect Dis.* 2002;186:782–791.
115. Wormser GP, Liveris D, Nowakowski J, et al. Association of specific subtypes of *Borrelia burgdorferi* with hematogenous dissemination in early Lyme disease. *J Infect Dis.* 1999;180:720–725.
116. Nadelman RB, Hanincova K, Mukherjee P, et al. Differentiation of reinfection from relapse in recurrent Lyme disease. *N Engl J Med.* 2012;367:1883–1890.
117. Krupka I, Straubinger RK. Lyme borreliosis in dogs and cats: background, diagnosis, treatment and prevention of infections with *Borrelia burgdorferi* sensu stricto. *Vet Clin North Am Small Anim Pract.* 2010;40:1103–1119.
118. Coughlin RT, Fish D, Mather TN, et al. Protection of dogs from Lyme disease with a vaccine containing outer surface protein (Osp) A, OspB, and the saponin adjuvant QS21. *J Infect Dis.* 1995;171:1049–1052.
119. Greene CE, Appel MJG, Straubinger RK. Lyme borreliosis. In: Greene CE, ed. *Infectious Diseases of the Dog and Cat.* 2nd ed. Philadelphia, PA: WB Saunders; 1998:282–293.
120. Stone BL, Brissette CA. Host immune evasion by Lyme and relapsing fever borreliae: findings to lead future studies for *Borrelia miyamotoi*. *Front Immunol.* 2017;8:12.
121. Xu Q, McShan K, Liang FT. Essential protective role attributed to the surface lipoproteins of *Borrelia burgdorferi* against innate defences. *Mol Microbiol.* 2008;69:15–29.
122. Alban PS, Johnson PW, Nelson DR. Serum-starvation-induced changes in protein synthesis and morphology of *Borrelia burgdorferi*. *Microbiology (Reading).* 2000;146(Pt 1):119–127.
123. Brorson O, Brorson SH. Transformation of cystic forms of *Borrelia burgdorferi* to normal, mobile spirochetes. *Infection.* 1997;25:240–246.
124. Gruntar I, Malovrh T, Murgia R, et al. Conversion of *Borrelia garinii* cystic forms to motile spirochetes in vivo. *APMIS.* 2001;109:383–388.
125. Hodzic E, Imai D, Feng S, et al. Resurgence of persisting non-cultivable *Borrelia burgdorferi* following antibiotic treatment in mice. *PLoS One.* 2014;9:e86907.
126. Bockenstedt LK, Gonzalez DG, Haberman AM, et al. Spirochete antigens persist near cartilage after murine Lyme borreliosis therapy. *J Clin Invest.* 2012;122:2652–2660.
127. Raveche ES, Schutzer SE, Fernandes H, et al. Evidence of *Borrelia* autoimmunity-induced component of Lyme carditis and arthritis. *J Clin Microbiol.* 2005;43:850–856.
128. Sigal LH, Williams S. A monoclonal antibody to *Borrelia burgdorferi* flagellin modifies neuroblastoma cell neuritogenesis in vitro: a possible role for autoimmunity in the neuropathy of Lyme disease. *Infect Immun.* 1997;65:1722–1728.
129. Kuenzle S, von Budingen HC, Meier M, et al. Pathogen specificity and autoimmunity are distinct features of antigen-driven immune responses in neuroborreliosis. *Infect Immun.* 2007;75:3842–3847.
130. Straubinger RK, Straubinger AF, Harter L, et al. *Borrelia burgdorferi* migrates into joint capsules and causes an up-regulation of interleukin-8 in synovial membranes of dogs experimentally infected with ticks. *Infect Immun.* 1997;65:1273–1285.
131. Steere AC, Klitz W, Drouin EE, et al. Antibiotic-refractory Lyme arthritis is associated with HLA-DR molecules that bind a *Borrelia burgdorferi* peptide. *J Exp Med.* 2006;203:961–971.
132. Hovius KE, Stark LA, Bleumink-Pluym NM, et al. Presence and distribution of *Borrelia burgdorferi* sensu lato species in internal organs and skin of naturally infected symptomatic and asymptomatic dogs, as detected by polymerase chain reaction. *Vet Q.* 1999;21:54–58.
133. Chou J, Wunschmann A, Hodzic E, et al. Detection of *Borrelia burgdorferi* DNA in tissues from dogs with presumptive Lyme borreliosis. *J Am Vet Med Assoc.* 2006;229:1260–1265.
134. Hutton TA, Goldstein RE, Njaa BL, et al. Search for *Borrelia burgdorferi* in kidneys of dogs with suspected "Lyme nephritis". *J Vet Intern Med.* 2008;22:860–865.
135. Goldstein RE. Current understanding of Lyme nephropathy. *Proceedings of the 25th ACVIM Forum.* 2007:672–673.
136. Goldstein RE, Atwater DZ. Evaluation of serology and circulating immune complexes in dogs naturally infected with *Borrelia burgdorferi*. *J Vet Intern Med.* 2006;20:713.
137. Wormser GP, Dattwyler RJ, Shapiro ED, et al. The clinical assessment, treatment, and prevention of Lyme disease, human granulocytic anaplasmosis, and babesiosis: clinical practice guidelines by the Infectious Diseases Society of America. *Clin Infect Dis.* 2006;43:1089–1134.
138. Steere AC, Sikand VK, Schoen RT, et al. Asymptomatic infection with *Borrelia burgdorferi*. *Clin Infect Dis.* 2003;37:528–532.
139. Littman MP. Canine borreliosis. *Vet Clin North Am Small Anim Pract.* 2003;33:827–862.
140. Azuma Y, Kawamura K, Isogai H, et al. Neurologic abnormalities in two dogs suspected Lyme disease. *Microbiol Immunol.* 1993;37:325–329.
141. Barber RM, Li Q, Diniz PP, et al. Evaluation of brain tissue or cerebrospinal fluid with broadly reactive polymerase chain reaction for *Ehrlichia, Anaplasma*, spotted fever group *Rickettsia, Bartonella*, and *Borrelia* species in canine neurological diseases (109 cases). *J Vet Intern Med.* 2010;24:372–378.
142. Krimer PM, Miller AD, Li Q, et al. Molecular and pathological investigations of the central nervous system in *Borrelia burgdorferi*-infected dogs. *J Vet Diagn Invest.* 2011;23:757–763.
143. Jaderlund KH, Bergstrom K, Egenvall A, et al. Cerebrospinal fluid PCR and antibody concentrations against *Anaplasma phagocytophilum* and *Borrelia burgdorferi* sensu lato in dogs with neurological signs. *J Vet Intern Med.* 2009;23:669–672.
144. Jaderlund KH, Egenvall A, Bergstrom K, et al. Seroprevalence of *Borrelia burgdorferi* sensu lato and *Anaplasma phagocytophilum* in dogs with neurological signs. *Vet Rec.* 2007;160:825–831.
145. Levy SA, Duray PH. Complete heart block in a dog seropositive for *Borrelia burgdorferi*. Similarity to human Lyme carditis. *J Vet Intern Med.* 1988;2:138–144.
146. Detmer SE, Bouljihad M, Hayden DW, et al. Fatal pyogranulomatous myocarditis in 10 boxer puppies. *J Vet Diagn Invest.* 2016;28:144–149.
147. Rolla D, Conti N, Ansaldo F, et al. Post-infectious glomerulonephritis presenting as acute renal failure in a patient with Lyme disease. *J Renal Inj Prev.* 2014;3:17–20.
148. Littman MP. Lyme nephritis. *J Vet Emerg Crit Care.* 2013;23:163–173.
149. Beall MJ, Chandrashekar R, Eberts MD, et al. Serological and molecular prevalence of *Borrelia burgdorferi, Anaplasma phagocytophilum*, and *Ehrlichia* species in dogs from Minnesota. *Vector Borne Zoonotic Dis.* 2008;8:455–464.
150. Burgess EC. Experimental inoculation of dogs with *Borrelia burgdorferi*. *Zentralbl Bakteriol Mikrobiol Hyg A.* 1986;263:49–54.
151. Greene RT, Levine JF, Breitschwerdt EB, et al. Clinical and serologic evaluations of induced *Borrelia burgdorferi* infection in dogs. *Am J Vet Res.* 1988;49:752–757.
152. Greene CE, Straubinger RK, Levy SR. Borreliosis. In: Greene CE, ed. *Infectious Diseases of the Diseases of the Dog and Cat.* Elsevier Saunders; 2012:447–464.
153. Cerri D, Farina R, Andreani E, et al. Experimental infection of dogs with *Borrelia burgdorferi*. *Res Vet Sci.* 1994;57:256–258.
154. Wasmoen TL, Sebring RW, Blumer BM, et al. Examination of Koch's postulates for *Borrelia burgdorferi* as the causative agent of limb/joint dysfunction in dogs with borreliosis. *J Am Vet Med Assoc.* 1992;201:412–418.

155. Chang YF, Novosel V, Chang CF, et al. Experimental induction of chronic borreliosis in adult dogs exposed to *Borrelia burgdorferi*-infected ticks and treated with dexamethasone. *Am J Vet Res.* 2001;62:1104–1112.
156. Levy SA, Dombach DM, Barthold SW, et al. Canine Lyme borreliosis. *Compend Contin Educ Pract Vet Small Anim.* 1993;15:833–846.
157. Lissman BA, Bosler EM, Camay H, et al. Spirochete-associated arthritis (Lyme disease) in a dog. *J Am Vet Med Assoc.* 1984;185:219–220.
158. May C, Bennett D, Carter SD. Lyme disease in the dog. *Vet Rec.* 1990;126:293.
159. Cohen ND, Carter CN, Thomas MA Jr, et al. Clinical and epizootiologic characteristics of dogs seropositive for *Borrelia burgdorferi* in Texas: 110 cases (1988). *J Am Vet Med Assoc.* 1990;197:893–898.
160. Magnarelli LA, Anderson JF, Schreier AB. Persistence of antibodies to *Borrelia burgdorferi* in dogs of New York and Connecticut. *J Am Vet Med Assoc.* 1990;196:1064–1068.
161. Magnarelli LA, Anderson JF, Schreier AB, et al. Clinical and serologic studies of canine borreliosis. *J Am Vet Med Assoc.* 1987;191:1089–1094.
162. Speck S, Reiner B, Streich WJ, et al. Canine borreliosis: a laboratory diagnostic trial. *Vet Microbiol.* 2007;120:132–141.
163. Summers BA, Straubinger AF, Jacobson RH, et al. Histopathological studies of experimental Lyme disease in the dog. *J Comp Pathol.* 2005;133:1–13.
164. Muir P, Fox R, Wu Q, et al. Seasonal variation in detection of bacterial DNA in arthritic stifle joints of dogs with cranial cruciate ligament rupture using PCR amplification of the 16S rRNA gene. *Vet Microbiol.* 2010;141:127–133.
165. Muir P, Oldenhoff WE, Hudson AP, et al. Detection of DNA from a range of bacterial species in the knee joints of dogs with inflammatory knee arthritis and associated degenerative anterior cruciate ligament rupture. *Microb Pathog.* 2007;42:47–55.
166. Borys MA, Kass PH, Mohr FC, et al. Differences in clinicopathologic variables between *Borrelia* C6 antigen seroreactive and *Borrelia* C6 seronegative glomerulopathy in dogs. *J Vet Intern Med.* 2019;33:2096–2104.
167. Dambach DM, Smith CA, Lewis RM, et al. Morphologic, immunohistochemical, and ultrastructural characterization of a distinctive renal lesion in dogs putatively associated with *Borrelia burgdorferi* infection: 49 cases (1987-1992). *Vet Pathol.* 1997;34:85–96.
168. Grauer GF, Burgess EC, Cooley AJ, et al. Renal lesions associated with *Borrelia burgdorferi* infection in a dog. *J Am Vet Med Assoc.* 1988;193:237–239.
169. Sanders NA, Dambach DM, Littman MP. Clinical characterization of a rapidly progressive and fatal glomerulonephritis associated with *Borrelia burgdorferi* infection in the dog ("Lyme nephritis"). *J Vet Intern Med.* 1997;11:127.
170. Goldstein RE, Cordner AP, Sandler JL, et al. Microalbuminuria and comparison of serologic testing for exposure to *Borrelia burgdorferi* in nonclinical Labrador and golden retrievers. *J Vet Diagn Invest.* 2007;19:294–297.
171. Littman MP. Protein-losing nephropathy in small animals. *Vet Clin North Am Small Anim Pract.* 2011;41:31–62.
172. Slade DJ, Lees GE, Berridge BR, et al. Resolution of a proteinuric nephropathy associated with *Babesia gibsoni* infection in a dog. *J Am Anim Hosp Assoc.* 2011;47:e138–144.
173. Tangeman LE, Littman MP. Clinicopathologic and atypical features of naturally occurring leptospirosis in dogs: 51 cases (2000-2010). *J Am Vet Med Assoc.* 2013;243:1316–1322.
174. Gerber B, Eichenberger S, Haug K, et al. The dilemma with Lyme borreliosis in the dog with particular consideration of "Lyme nephritis". *Schweiz Arch Tierheilkd.* 2009;151:479–483.
175. Gerber B, Eichenberger S, Haug K, et al. Association of urine protein excretion and infection with *Borrelia burgdorferi* sensu lato in Bernese Mountain dogs. *Vet J.* 2009;182:487–488.
176. Gerber B, Eichenberger S, Joller-Jemelka HI, et al. Complement C3 in Bernese Mountain dogs. *Vet Clin Pathol.* 2010;39:164–168.
177. Gerber B, Eichenberger S, Wittenbrink MM, et al. Increased prevalence of *Borrelia burgdorferi* infections in Bernese Mountain dogs: a possible breed predisposition. *BMC Vet Res.* 2007;3:15.
178. Gerber B, Haug K, Eichenberger S, et al. Follow-up of Bernese Mountain dogs and other dogs with serologically diagnosed *Borrelia burgdorferi* infection: what happens to seropositive animals? *BMC Vet Res.* 2009;5:18.
179. Minkus G, Breuer W, Wanke R, et al. Familial nephropathy in Bernese Mountain dogs. *Vet Pathol.* 1994;31:421–428.
180. Preyss-Jageler C, Hartmann K, Dorsch R. Changes in renal parameters and their association with subclinical vector-borne infections in Bernese Mountain dogs. *BMC Vet Res.* 2020;16:285.
181. Contreras E, Moroff S, Lappin M. Evidence for genetic predisposition to *Borrelia burgdorferi* infection in purpose bred beagles. *J Vet Intern Med.* 2016;26:1473.
182. Pachner AR, Steiner I. Lyme neuroborreliosis: infection, immunity, and inflammation. *Lancet Neurol.* 2007;6:544–552.
183. Roberts ED, Bohm Jr RP, Lowrie RC Jr, et al. Pathogenesis of Lyme neuroborreliosis in the rhesus monkey: the early disseminated and chronic phases of disease in the peripheral nervous system. *J Infect Dis.* 1998;178:722–732.
184. Adaszek L, Gatellet M, Mazurek L, et al. Myocarditis secondary to *Borrelia* infection in a dog: a case report. *Ann Parasitol.* 2020;66:255–257.
185. Roush JK, Manley PA, Dueland RT. Rheumatoid arthritis subsequent to *Borrelia burgdorferi* infection in two dogs. *J Am Vet Med Assoc.* 1989;195:951–953.
186. Raya AI, Afonso JC, Perez-Ecija RA, et al. Orbital myositis associated with Lyme disease in a dog. *Vet Rec.* 2010;167:663–664.
187. Levy SA, O'Connor TP, Hanscom JL, et al. Evaluation of a canine C6 ELISA Lyme disease test for the determination of the infection status of cats naturally exposed to *Borrelia burgdorferi. Vet Ther.* 2003;4:172–177.
188. Magnarelli LA, Anderson JF, Levine HR, et al. Tick parasitism and antibodies to *Borrelia burgdorferi* in cats. *J Am Vet Med Assoc.* 1990;197:63–66.
189. Magnarelli LA, Bushmich SL, Ijdo JW, et al. Seroprevalence of antibodies against *Borrelia burgdorferi* and *Anaplasma phagocytophilum* in cats. *Am J Vet Res.* 2005;66:1895–1899.
190. Lappin MR, Chandrashekar R, Stillman B, et al. Evidence of *Anaplasma phagocytophilum* and *Borrelia burgdorferi* infection in cats after exposure to wild-caught adult *Ixodes scapularis. J Vet Diagn Invest.* 2015;27:522–525.
191. Lappin MR, Breitschwerdt EB, Jensen WA, et al. Molecular and serologic evidence of *Anaplasma phagocytophilum* infection in cats in North America. *J Am Vet Med Assoc.* 2004;225:893–896.
192. Savidge C, Ewing P, Andrews J, et al. *Anaplasma phagocytophilum* infection of domestic cats: 16 cases from the northeastern USA. *J Feline Med Surg.* 2016;18:85–91.
193. Hoyt K, Chandrashekar R, Beall M, et al. Evidence for clinical anaplasmosis and borreliosis in cats in Maine. *Top Companion Anim Med.* 2018;33:40–44.
194. May C, Carter SD, Barnes A, et al. *Borrelia burgdorferi* infection in cats in the UK. *J Small Anim Pract.* 1994;35:517–520.
195. Tornqvist-Johnsen C, Dickson SA, Rolph K, et al. First report of Lyme borreliosis leading to cardiac bradydysrhythmia in two cats. *JFMS Open Rep.* 2020;6:2055116919898292.
196. Shaw SE, Binns SH, Birtles RJ, et al. Molecular evidence of tick-transmitted infections in dogs and cats in the United Kingdom. *Vet Rec.* 2005;157:645–648.
197. Sigal LH. The polymerase chain reaction assay for *Borrelia burgdorferi* in the diagnosis of Lyme disease. *Ann Intern Med.* 1994;120:520–521.
198. Gibson MD, Omran MT, Young CR. Experimental feline Lyme borreliosis as a model for testing *Borrelia burgdorferi* vaccines. *Adv Exp Med Biol.* 1995;383:73–82.
199. Gibson MD, Young CR, Omran MT, et al. *Borrelia burgdorferi* infection of cats. *J Am Vet Med Assoc.* 1993;202:1786.
200. Foley J, Drazenovich N, Leutenegger CM, et al. Association between polyarthritis and thrombocytopenia and increased prevalence of vector-borne pathogens in Californian dogs. *Vet Rec.* 2007;160:159–162.
201. Gettings JR, Lopez JE, Krishnavahjala A, et al. Antibodies to *Borrelia turicatae* in experimentally infected dogs cross-react with *Borrelia burgdorferi* serologic assays. *J Clin Microbiol.* 2019;57.
202. Littman MP, Goldstein RE. A Matter of Opinion: Should we treat asymptomatic, nonproteinuric Lyme-seropositive dogs with antibiotics? *Clinician's Brief.* 2011;9:13–16.
203. Littman MP, Daminet S, Grauer GF, et al. Consensus recommendations for the diagnostic investigation of dogs with suspected glomerular disease. *J Vet Intern Med.* 2013;27:S19–S26.
204. Goldstein RE, Brovida C, Fernandez-Del Palacio MJ, et al. IRIS Glomerular Disease Study Group. Consensus recommendations for treatment

for dogs with serology positive glomerular disease. *J Vet Intern Med.* 2013;27(Suppl 1):S60–66.
205. Arteaga F, Golightly MG, Garcia Perez A, et al. Disparity between serological reactivity to *Borrelia burgdorferi* and evidence of past disease in a high-risk group. *Clin Infect Dis.* 1998;27:1210–1213.
206. Burgess EC, Schneider E, Bosler E. Testing for *Borrelia burgdorferi. J Am Vet Med Assoc.* 1989;195:844–846.
207. Frank JC. Taking a hard look at *Borrelia burgdorferi. J Am Vet Med Assoc.* 1989;194:1521.
208. Greene RT, Hirsch DA, Rottman PL, et al. Interlaboratory comparison of titers of antibody to *Borrelia burgdorferi* and evaluation of a commercial assay using canine sera. *J Clin Microbiol.* 1991;29:16–20.
209. Lindenmayer J, Weber M, Bryant J, et al. Comparison of indirect immunofluorescent-antibody assay, enzyme-linked immunosorbent assay, and Western immunoblot for the diagnosis of Lyme disease in dogs. *J Clin Microbiol.* 1990;28:92–96.
210. Schillhorn van Veen TW, Murphy AJ, Colmery B. False positive *Borrelia burgdorferi* antibody titres associated with periodontal disease in dogs. *Vet Rec.* 1993;132:512.
211. Breitschwerdt EB, Nicholson WL, Kiehl AR, et al. Natural infections with *Borrelia* spirochetes in two dogs from Florida. *J Clin Microbiol.* 1994;32:352–357.
212. Shin SJ, Chang YF, Jacobson RH, et al. Cross-reactivity between *B. burgdorferi* and other spirochetes affects specificity of serotests for detection of antibodies to the Lyme disease agent in dogs. *Vet Microbiol.* 1993;36:161–174.
213. Sugiyama Y, Sugiyama F, Yagami K. Comparative study on cross-reaction of leptospiral antibodies in several serological tests to detect antibodies to *Borrelia burgdorferi* in dogs. *J Vet Med Sci.* 1993;55:149–151.
214. Straubinger RK, Straubinger AF, Summers BA, et al. Status of *Borrelia burgdorferi* infection after antibiotic treatment and the effects of corticosteroids: An experimental study. *J Infect Dis.* 2000;181:1069–1081.
215. Straubinger RK. PCR-based quantification of *Borrelia burgdorferi* organisms in canine tissues over a 500-day postinfection period. *J Clin Microbiol.* 2000;38:2191–2199.
216. Jacobson RH, Chang YF, Shin SJ. Lyme disease: laboratory diagnosis of infected and vaccinated symptomatic dogs. *Semin Vet Med Surg Small Anim.* 1996;11:172–182.
217. Straubinger RK. Unpublished observations. Ithaca, NY: Cornell University; 1997.
218. Baum E, Grosenbaugh DA, Barbour AG. Diversity of antibody responses to *Borrelia burgdorferi* in experimentally infected beagle dogs. *Clin Vaccine Immunol.* 2014;21:838–846.
219. Greene RT, Walker RL, Burgess EC, et al. Heterogeneity in immunoblot patterns obtained by using four strains of *Borrelia burgdorferi* and sera from naturally exposed dogs. *J Clin Microbiol.* 1988;26:2287–2291.
220. Greene RT, Walker RL, Nicholson WL, et al. Immunoblot analysis of immunoglobulin G response to the Lyme disease agent (*Borrelia burgdorferi*) in experimentally and naturally exposed dogs. *J Clin Microbiol.* 1988;26:648–653.
221. Guerra MA, Walker ED, Kitron U. Quantitative approach for the serodiagnosis of canine Lyme disease by the immunoblot procedure. *J Clin Microbiol.* 2000;38:2628–2632.
222. Wagner B, Freer H, Rollins A, et al. Antibodies to *Borrelia burgdorferi* OspA, OspC, OspF, and C6 antigens as markers for early and late infection in dogs. *Clin Vaccine Immunol.* 2012;19:527–535.
223. Leschnik MW, Kirtz G, Khanakah G, et al. Humoral immune response in dogs naturally infected with *Borrelia burgdorferi* sensu lato and in dogs after immunization with a *Borrelia* vaccine. *Clin Vaccine Immunol.* 2010;17:828–835.
224. Bacon RM, Biggerstaff BJ, Schriefer ME, et al. Serodiagnosis of Lyme disease by kinetic enzyme-linked immunosorbent assay using recombinant VlsE1 or peptide antigens of *Borrelia burgdorferi* compared with 2-tiered testing using whole-cell lysates. *J Infect Dis.* 2003;187:1187–1199.
225. Marques AR, Martin DS, Philipp MT. Evaluation of the C6 peptide enzyme-linked immunosorbent assay for individuals vaccinated with the recombinant OspA vaccine. *J Clin Microbiol.* 2002;40:2591–2593.
226. Waddell LA, Greig J, Mascarenhas M, et al. The accuracy of diagnostic tests for Lyme disease in humans, a systematic review and meta-analysis of North American research. *PLoS One.* 2016;11:e0168613.
227. Wormser GP, Liveris D, Hanincova K, et al. Effect of *Borrelia burgdorferi* genotype on the sensitivity of C6 and 2-tier testing in North American patients with culture-confirmed Lyme disease. *Clin Infect Dis.* 2008;47:910–914.
228. Wormser GP, Schriefer M, Aguero-Rosenfeld ME, et al. Single-tier testing with the C6 peptide ELISA kit compared with two-tier testing for Lyme disease. *Diagn Microbiol Infect Dis.* 2013;75:9–15.
229. Liang FT, Jacobson RH, Straubinger RK, et al. Characterization of a *Borrelia burgdorferi* VlsE invariable region useful in canine Lyme disease serodiagnosis by enzyme-linked immunosorbent assay. *J Clin Microbiol.* 2000;38:4160–4166.
230. Philipp MT, Bowers LC, Fawcett PT, et al. Antibody response to IR6, a conserved immunodominant region of the VlsE lipoprotein, wanes rapidly after antibiotic treatment of *Borrelia burgdorferi* infection in experimental animals and in humans. *J Infect Dis.* 2001;184:870–878.
231. Gerber B, Haug K, Eichenberger S, et al. Comparison of a rapid immunoassay for antibodies to the C6 antigen with conventional tests for antibodies to *Borrelia burgdorferi* in dogs in Europe. *Vet Rec.* 2009;165:594–597.
232. Levy S, O'Connor TP, Hanscom JL, et al. Utility of an in-office C6 ELISA test kit for determination of infection status of dogs naturally exposed to *Borrelia burgdorferi. Vet Ther.* 2002;3:308–315.
233. O'Connor TP, Esty KJ, Hanscom JL, et al. Dogs vaccinated with common Lyme disease vaccines do not respond to IR6, the conserved immunodominant region of the VlsE surface protein of *Borrelia burgdorferi. Clin Diagn Lab Immunol.* 2004;11:458–462.
234. Chandrashekar R, Beall MJ, Thatcher B, et al. Serologic responses to peptides of *Anaplasma phagocytophilum* and *Borrelia burgdorferi* in dogs infested with wild-caught *Ixodes scapularis. Vet J.* 2017;226:6–11.
235. Barth C, Straubinger RK, Sauter-Louis C, et al. Prevalence of antibodies against *Borrelia burgdorferi* sensu lato and *Anaplasma phagocytophilum* and their clinical relevance in dogs in Munich, Germany. *Berl Munch Tierarztl Wochenschr.* 2012;125:337–344.
236. Eschner AK. Effect of passive immunoglobulin transfer on results of diagnostic tests for antibodies against *Borrelia burgdorferi* in pups born to a seropositive dam. *Vet Ther.* 2008;9:184–191.
237. Levy SA, O'Connor TP, Hanscom JL, et al. Quantitative measurement of C6 antibody following antibiotic treatment of *Borrelia burgdorferi* antibody-positive nonclinical dogs. *Clin Vaccine Immunol.* 2008;15:115–119.
238. Callister SM, LaFleur RL, Jobe DA, et al. Antibody responses to *Borrelia burgdorferi* outer surface proteins C and F in experimentally infected beagle dogs. *J Vet Diagn Invest.* 2015;27:526–530.
239. Wagner B, Freer H, Rollins H, et al. A fluorescent bead-based multiplex assay for the simultaneous detection of antibodies to *B. burgdorferi* outer surface proteins in canine serum. *Vet Immunol Immunopathol.* 2011;140:190–198.
240. Li X, Strle K, Wang P, et al. Tick-specific borrelial antigens appear to be upregulated in American but not European patients with Lyme arthritis, a late manifestation of Lyme borreliosis. *J Infect Dis.* 2013;208:934–941.
241. Abaxis. Peptides and methods for the detection of Lyme disease antibodies. US patent 9,201,071B2. December 2015.
242. Lovrich SD, La Fleur RL, Jobe DA, et al. Borreliacidal OspC antibody response of canines with Lyme disease differs significantly from that of humans with Lyme disease. *Clin Vaccine Immunol.* 2007;14:635–637.
243. Henriksson A, Link H, Cruz M, et al. Immunoglobulin abnormalities in cerebrospinal fluid and blood over the course of lymphocytic meningoradiculitis (Bannwarth's syndrome). *Ann Neurol.* 1986;20:337–345.
244. Wilske B, Schierz G, Preac-Mursic V, et al. Intrathecal production of specific antibodies against *Borrelia burgdorferi* in patients with lymphocytic meningoradiculitis (Bannwarth's syndrome). *J Infect Dis.* 1986;153:304–314.
245. Hansen K, Lebech AM. Lyme neuroborreliosis: a new sensitive diagnostic assay for intrathecal synthesis of *Borrelia burgdorferi*: specific immunoglobulin G, A, and M. *Ann Neurol.* 1991;30:197–205.
246. Steere AC, Berardi VP, Weeks KE, et al. Evaluation of the intrathecal antibody response to *Borrelia burgdorferi* as a diagnostic test for Lyme neuroborreliosis. *J Infect Dis.* 1990;161:1203–1209.

247. Schutzer SE, Coyle PK, Krupp LB, et al. Simultaneous expression of *Borrelia* OspA and OspC and IgM response in cerebrospinal fluid in early neurologic Lyme disease. *J Clin Invest.* 1997;100:763–767.
248. Feder BM, Joseph RJ, Moroff SD, et al. *Borrelia burgdorferi* antibodies in canine cerebrospinal fluid. *Proc ACVIM Annual Forum.* 1991:137.
249. Mandel NS, Senker EG, Bosler EM, et al. Intrathecal production of *Borrelia burgdorferi* specific antibodies in a dog with central nervous system Lyme borreliosis. *Compend Contin Educ Pract Vet Small Anim.* 1993;15:581–585.
250. Greene RT, Walker RL, Greene CE. Pseudospirochetes in animal blood being cultured for *Borrelia burgdorferi. J Vet Diagn Invest.* 1991;3:350–352.
251. Wang G. Direct detection methods for Lyme *Borrelia*, including the use of quantitative assays. *Vector Borne Zoonotic Dis.* 2002;2:223–231.
252. Straubinger RK, Straubinger AF, Summers BA, et al. Clinical manifestations, pathogenesis, and effect of antibiotic treatment on Lyme borreliosis in dogs. *Wien Klin Wochenschr.* 1998;110:874–881.
253. Callister SM, Jobe DA, Schell RF, et al. Detection of borreliacidal antibodies in dogs after challenge with *Borrelia burgdorferi*-infected *Ixodes scapularis* ticks. *J Clin Microbiol.* 2000;38:3670–3674.
254. Persing DH, Rutledge BJ, Rys PN, et al. Target imbalance: disparity of *Borrelia burgdorferi* genetic material in synovial fluid from Lyme arthritis patients. *J Infect Dis.* 1994;169:668–672.
255. Skotarczak B, Wodecka B, Rymaszewska A, et al. Prevalence of DNA and antibodies to *Borrelia burgdorferi* sensu lato in dogs suspected of borreliosis. *Ann Agric Environ Med.* 2005;12:199–205.
256. Wodecka B, Rymaszewska A, Sawczuk M, et al. Detectability of tick-borne agents DNA in the blood of dogs, undergoing treatment for borreliosis. *Ann Agric Environ Med.* 2009;16:9–14.
257. Ivacic L, Reed KD, Mitchell PD, et al. A LightCycler TaqMan assay for detection of *Borrelia burgdorferi* sensu lato in clinical samples. *Diagn Microbiol Infect Dis.* 2007;57:137–143.
258. Susta L, Uhl EW, Grosenbaugh DA, et al. Synovial lesions in experimental canine Lyme borreliosis. *Vet Pathol.* 2012;49:453–461.
259. Straubinger RK, Summers BA, Chang YF, et al. Persistence of *Borrelia burgdorferi* in experimentally infected dogs after antibiotic treatment. *J Clin Microbiol.* 1997;35:111–116.
260. Cianciolo RE, Brown CA, Mohr FC, et al. Pathologic evaluation of canine renal biopsies: Methods for identifying features that differentiate immune-mediated glomerulonephritides from other categories of glomerular diseases. *J Vet Intern Med.* 2013;27:S10–18.
261. Yu LP Jr, Smith GN Jr, Brandt KD, et al. Reduction of the severity of canine osteoarthritis by prophylactic treatment with oral doxycycline. *Arthritis Rheum.* 1992;35:1150–1159.
262. Bernardino AL, Kaushal D, Philipp MT. The antibiotics doxycycline and minocycline inhibit the inflammatory responses to the Lyme disease spirochete *Borrelia burgdorferi. J Infect Dis.* 2009;199:1379–1388.
263. Steere AC. Lyme disease (Lyme borreliosis) due to *Borrelia burgdorferi.* In: Bennett JE, Dolin R, Blaser MJ, eds. *Mandell, Douglas, and Bennett's Principles and Practice of Infectious Diseases.* Philadelphia, PA: Elsevier Saunders; 2015:2725–2735.
264. Bockenstedt LK, Mao J, Hodzic E, et al. Detection of attenuated, noninfectious spirochetes in *Borrelia burgdorferi*-infected mice after antibiotic treatment. *J Infect Dis.* 2002;186:1430–1437.
265. Levy SA, Dreesen DW. Lyme borreliosis in dogs. *Canine Pract.* 1992;17:5–13.
266. Malawista SE, Barthold SW, Persing DH. Fate of *Borrelia burgdorferi* DNA in tissues of infected mice after antibiotic treatment. *J Infect Dis.* 1994;170:1312–1316.
267. Pahl A, Kuhlbrandt U, Brune K, et al. Quantitative detection of *Borrelia burgdorferi* by real-time PCR. *J Clin Microbiol.* 1999;37:1958–1963.
268. Yrjanainen H, Hytonen J, Hartiala P, et al. Persistence of borrelial DNA in the joints of *Borrelia burgdorferi*-infected mice after ceftriaxone treatment. *APMIS.* 2010;118:665–673.
269. Donta ST. Tetracycline therapy for chronic Lyme disease. *Clin Infect Dis.* 1997;25(Suppl 1):S52–56.
270. Berende A, ter Hofstede HJ, Vos FJ, et al. Randomized trial of longer-term therapy for symptoms attributed to Lyme disease. *N Engl J Med.* 2016;374:1209–1220.
271. Golde WT, Robinson-Dunn B, Stobierski MG, et al. Culture-confirmed reinfection of a person with different strains of *Borrelia burgdorferi* sensu stricto. *J Clin Microbiol.* 1998;36:1015–1019.
272. Bradley JF, Johnson RC, Goodman JL. The persistence of spirochetal nucleic acids in active Lyme arthritis. *Ann Intern Med.* 1994;120:487–489.
273. Wagner B, Johnson J, Garcia-Tapia D, et al. Comparison of effectiveness of cefovecin, doxycycline, and amoxicillin for the treatment of experimentally induced early Lyme borreliosis in dogs. *BMC Vet Res.* 2015;11:163.
274. Dattwyler RJ, Luft BJ, Kunkel MJ, et al. Ceftriaxone compared with doxycycline for the treatment of acute disseminated Lyme disease. *N Engl J Med.* 1997;337:289–294.
275. Kim D, Kordick D, Divers T, et al. In vitro susceptibilities of *Leptospira* spp. and *Borrelia burgdorferi* isolates to amoxicillin, tilmicosin, and enrofloxacin. *J Vet Sci.* 2006;7:355–359.
276. Dotevall L, Hagberg L. Adverse effects of minocycline versus doxycycline in the treatment of Lyme neuroborreliosis. *Clin Infect Dis.* 2000;30:410–411.
277. Cross R, Ling C, Day NP, et al. Revisiting doxycycline in pregnancy and early childhood: time to rebuild its reputation? *Expert Opin Drug Saf.* 2016;15:367–382.
278. Halperin JJ, Shapiro ED, Logigian E, et al. Practice parameter: treatment of nervous system Lyme disease (an evidence-based review): report of the Quality Standards Subcommittee of the American Academy of Neurology. *Neurology.* 2007;69:91–102.
279. Logigian EL, Kaplan RF, Steere AC. Successful treatment of Lyme encephalopathy with intravenous ceftriaxone. *J Infect Dis.* 1999;180:377–383.
280. De Maria A, Primavera A. Possibility of the use of oral long-acting tetracyclines in the treatment of Lyme neuroborreliosis. *Clin Infect Dis.* 2000;31:848–849.
281. Dotevall L, Hagberg L. Successful oral doxycycline treatment of Lyme disease-associated facial palsy and meningitis. *Clin Infect Dis.* 1999;28:569–574.
282. Halperin JJ. Nervous system Lyme disease. *Curr Infect Dis Rep.* 2015;29:241–53.
283. Barr SC. Treating Lyme-seropositive dogs. *NAVC Clinician's Brief.* 2012;5:8.
284. Goldstein RE. Advances in the prevention and management of *Borrelia burgdorferi* infections in dogs. *Proc ACVIM Annual Forum.* 2010 and 2012.
285. Brown S, Elliott J, Francey T, et al. Consensus recommendations for standard therapy of glomerular disease in dogs. *J Vet Intern Med.* 2013;27:S27–S43.
286. Segev G, Cowgill LD, Heiene R, et al. IRIS Canine Glomerulonephritis Study Group Established Pathology Subgroup. Consensus recommendations for immunosuppressive treatment of dogs with glomerular disease based on established pathology. *J Vet Intern Med.* 2013;27(Suppl 1):S44–54.
287. Pressler B, Vaden S, Gerber B, et al. IRIS Canine Glomerulonephritis Study Subgroup on Immunosuppressive Therapy Absent a Pathologic Diagnosis. Consensus guidelines for immunosuppressive treatment of dogs with glomerular disease absent a pathologic diagnosis. *J Vet Intern Med.* 2013;27(Suppl 1):S55–59.
288. Schneider SM, Cianciolo RE, Nabity MB, et al. Prevalence of immune-complex glomerulonephritides in dogs biopsied for suspected glomerular disease: 501 cases (2007-2012). *J Vet Intern Med.* 2013;27(Suppl 1):S67–75.
289. LaFleur RL, Dant JC, Wasmoen TL, et al. Bacterin that induces anti-OspA and anti-OspC borreliacidal antibodies provides a high level of protection against canine Lyme disease. *Clin Vaccine Immunol.* 2009;16:253–259.
290. Wikle RE, Fretwell B, Jarecki M, et al. Canine Lyme disease: one year duration of immunity elicited with a canine OspA monovalent Lyme vaccine. *Intern J Appl Res Vet Med.* 2006;4:23–28.
291. Topfer KH, Straubinger RK. Characterization of the humoral immune response in dogs after vaccination against the Lyme borreliosis agent A study with five commercial vaccines using two different vaccination schedules. *Vaccine.* 2007;25:314–326.
292. Grosenbaugh DA, Rissi DR, Krimer PM. Demonstration of the ability of a canine Lyme vaccine to reduce the incidence of histological synovial lesions following experimentally-induced canine Lyme borreliosis. *Vet Immunol Immunopathol.* 2016;180:29–33.
293. Eschner AK, Mugnai K. Immunization with a recombinant subunit OspA vaccine markedly impacts the rate of newly acquired *Borrelia*

burgdorferi infections in client-owned dogs living in a coastal community in Maine, USA. *Parasit Vectors.* 2015;8:92.

294. LaFleur RL, Callister SM, Dant JC, et al. One-year duration of immunity induced by vaccination with a canine Lyme disease bacterin. *Clin Vaccine Immunol.* 2010;17:870–874.
295. Hebert D, Eschner A. Seroprevalence of *Borrelia burgdorferi*-specific C6 antibody in dogs before and after implementation of a nonadjuvanted recombinant outer surface protein A vaccine in a Rhode Island small animal clinic. *Vet Ther.* 2010;11:E1–9.
296. Vogt NA, Sargeant JM, MacKinnon MC, et al. Efficacy of *Borrelia burgdorferi* vaccine in dogs in North America: A systematic review and meta-analysis. *J Vet Intern Med.* 2019;33:23–36.
297. Ball EC. Vanguard crLyme: Chimeric recombinant vaccine technology for broad-spectrum protection against canine Lyme disease. In: *Zoetis Technical Bulletin.* 2015.
298. Keller D, Koster FT, Marks DH, et al. Safety and immunogenicity of a recombinant outer surface protein A Lyme vaccine. *JAMA.* 1994;271:1764–1768.
299. Ma J, Bulger PA, Dante S, et al. Characterization of canine humoral immune responses to outer surface protein subunit vaccines and to natural infection by Lyme disease spirochetes. *J Infect Dis.* 1995;171:909–915.
300. Moroff S, Woodruff C, Woodring T, et al. Multiple antigen target approach using the Accuplex4 BioCD system to detect *Borrelia burgdorferi* antibodies in experimentally infected and vaccinated dogs. *J Vet Diagn Invest.* 2015;27:581–588.
301. Straubinger RK, Dharma Rao T, Davidson E, et al. Protection against tick-transmitted Lyme disease in dogs vaccinated with a multiantigenic vaccine. *Vaccine.* 2001;20:181–193.
302. Conlon JA, Mather TN, Tanner P, et al. Efficacy of a nonadjuvanted, outer surface protein A, recombinant vaccine in dogs after challenge by ticks naturally infected with *Borrelia burgdorferi. Vet Ther.* 2000;1:96–107.
303. Straubinger RK, Chang YF, Jacobson RH, et al. Sera from OspA-vaccinated dogs, but not those from tick-infected dogs, inhibit in vitro growth of *Borrelia burgdorferi. J Clin Microbiol.* 1995;33:2745–2751.
304. Oliver LD Jr, Earnhart CG, Virginia-Rhodes D, et al. Antibody profiling of canine IgG responses to the OspC protein of the Lyme disease spirochetes supports a multivalent approach in vaccine and diagnostic assay development. *Vet J.* 2016;218:27–33.
305. Khatchikian CE, Nadelman RB, Nowakowski J, et al. Evidence for strain-specific immunity in patients treated for early Lyme disease. *Infect Immun.* 2014;82:1408–1413.
306. Barthold SW, Fikrig E, Bockenstedt LK, et al. Circumvention of outer surface protein A immunity by host-adapted *Borrelia burgdorferi. Infect Immun.* 1995;63:2255–2261.
307. Camire AC, Hatke AL, King VL, et al. Comparative analysis of antibody responses to outer surface protein (Osp)A and OspC in dogs vaccinated with Lyme disease vaccines. *Vet J.* 2021;273:105676.
308. Grosenbaugh DA, De Luca K, Durand PY, et al. Characterization of recombinant OspA in two different Borrelia vaccines with respect to immunological response and its relationship to functional parameters. *BMC Veterinary Research.* 2018;14:312–321.
309. de Silva AM, Fish D, Burkot TR, et al. OspA antibodies inhibit the acquisition of *Borrelia burgdorferi* by *Ixodes* ticks. *Infect Immun.* 1997;65:3146–3150.
310. Barthold SW, Levy SA, Fikrig E, et al. Serologic responses of dogs naturally exposed to or vaccinated against *Borrelia burgdorferi* infection. *J Am Vet Med Assoc.* 1995;207:1435–1440.
311. Levy SA, Clark KK, Glickman LT. Infection rates in dogs vaccinated and not vaccinated with an OspA *Borrelia burgdorferi* vaccine in a Lyme disease-endemic area of Connecticut. *Intern J Appl Res Vet Med.* 2005;3:1–5.
312. Sigal LH, Zahradnik JM, Lavin P, et al. A vaccine consisting of recombinant *Borrelia burgdorferi* outer-surface protein A to prevent Lyme disease. Recombinant Outer-Surface Protein A Lyme Disease Vaccine Study Consortium. *N Engl J Med.* 1998;339:216–222.
313. Steere AC, Sikand VK, Meurice F, et al. Vaccination against Lyme disease with recombinant *Borrelia burgdorferi* outer-surface lipoprotein A with adjuvant. Lyme Disease Vaccine Study Group. *N Engl J Med.* 1998;339:209–215.
314. Levy SA, Millership J, Glover S, et al. Confirmation of presence of *Borrelia burgdorferi* outer surface protein C antigen and production of antibodies to *Borrelia burgdorferi* outer surface protein C in dogs vaccinated with a whole-cell *Borrelia burgdorferi* bacterin. *J Appl Res Vet Med.* 2010;8:123–128.
315. Levy SA, Lissman BA, Ficke CM. Performance of a *Borrelia burgdorferi* bacterin in borreliosis-endemic areas. *J Am Vet Med Assoc.* 1993;202:1834–1838.
316. Levy SA. Use of a C6 ELISA test to evaluate the efficacy of a whole-cell bacterin for the prevention of naturally transmitted canine *Borrelia burgdorferi* infection. *Vet Ther.* 2002;3:420–424.
317. Probert WS, Crawford M, Cadiz RB, et al. Immunization with outer surface protein (Osp) A, but not OspC, provides cross-protection of mice challenged with North American isolates of *Borrelia burgdorferi. J Infect Dis.* 1997;175:400–405.
318. LaFleur RL, Callister SM, Dant JC, et al. Vaccination with the ospA- and ospB-negative *Borrelia burgdorferi* strain 50772 provides significant protection against canine Lyme disease. *Clin Vaccine Immunol.* 2015;22:836–839.
319. Barthold SW. Specificity of infection-induced immunity among *Borrelia burgdorferi* sensu lato species. *Infect Immun.* 1999;67:36–42.
320. Hodzic E, Feng S, Barthold SW. Stability of *Borrelia burgdorferi* outer surface protein C under immune selection pressure. *J Infect Dis.* 2000;181:750–753.
321. Zhong WM, Gern L, Sehle T, et al. Resolution of experimental and tick-borne *Borrelia burgdorferi* infection in mice by passive, but not active immunization using recombinant OspC. *Eur J Immunol.* 1999;29:946–949.
322. Marconi RT, Garcia-Tapia D, Hoevers J, et al. VANGUARD cr:Lyme: a next generation Lyme disease vaccine that prevents *B. burgdorferi* infection in dogs. *Vaccine: X.* 2020;6:100079.
323. Vogt NA, Stevens CPG. Why the rationale for canine *Borrelia burgdorferi* vaccination is unpersuasive. *Front Vet Sci.* 2021;8:719060.
324. Moore GE, Guptill LF, Ward MP, et al. Adverse events diagnosed within three days of vaccine administration in dogs. *J Am Vet Med Assoc.* 2005;227:1102–1108.
325. Nadelman RB, Nowakowski J, Fish D, et al. Prophylaxis with single-dose doxycycline for the prevention of Lyme disease after an *Ixodes scapularis* tick bite. *N Engl J Med.* 2001;345:79–84.
326. Shapiro ED. Doxycycline for tick bites–not for everyone. *N Engl J Med.* 2001;345:133–134.
327. Schiller ZA, Rudolph MJ, Toomey JR, et al. Blocking *Borrelia burgdorferi* transmission from infected ticks to nonhuman primates with a human monoclonal antibody. *J Clin Invest.* 2021;131:e144843.
328. Elfassy OJ, Goodman FW, Levy SA, et al. Efficacy of an amitraz-impregnated collar in preventing transmission of *Borrelia burgdorferi* by adult *Ixodes scapularis* to dogs. *J Am Vet Med Assoc.* 2001;219:185–189.
329. Endris RG, Cooke D, Amodie D, et al. Repellency and efficacy of 65% permethrin and selamectin spot-on formulations against *Ixodes ricinus* ticks on dogs. *Vet Ther.* 2002;3:64–71.
330. McCall JW, Baker CF, Mather TN, et al. The ability of a topical novel combination of fipronil, amitraz and (S)-methoprene to protect dogs from *Borrelia burgdorferi* and *Anaplasma phagocytophilum* infections transmitted by *Ixodes scapularis. Vet Parasitol.* 2011;179:335–342.
331. Spencer JA, Butler JM, Stafford KC, et al. Evaluation of permethrin and imidacloprid for prevention of *Borrelia burgdorferi* transmission from blacklegged ticks (*Ixodes scapularis*) to *Borrelia burgdorferi*-free dogs. *Parasitol Res.* 2003;90(Suppl 3):S106–107.
332. Honsberger NA, Six RH, Heinz TJ, et al. Efficacy of sarolaner in the prevention of *Borrelia burgdorferi* and *Anaplasma phagocytophilum* transmission from infected *Ixodes scapularis* to dogs. *Vet Parasitol.* 2016;222:67–72.
333. Centers for Disease Control and Prevention. Preventing ticks in the yard. 2019. https://www.cdc.gov/lyme/prev/in_the_yard.html.
334. Dolan MC, Maupin GO, Schneider BS, et al. Control of immature *Ixodes scapularis* (Acari: Ixodidae) on rodent reservoirs of *Borrelia burgdorferi* in a residential community of southeastern Connecticut. *J Med Entomol.* 2004;41:1043–1054.

335. Pound JM, Miller JA, George JE, et al. The United States Department of Agriculture's Northeast Area-Wide Tick Control Project: summary and conclusions. *Vector Borne Zoonotic Dis.* 2009;9:439–448.
336. Gomes-Solecki MJ, Brisson DR, Dattwyler RJ. Oral vaccine that breaks the transmission cycle of the Lyme disease spirochete can be delivered via bait. *Vaccine.* 2006;24:4440–4449.
337. Melo R, Richer L, Johnson DL, et al. Oral immunization with OspC does not prevent tick-borne *Borrelia burgdorferi* infection. *PLoS One.* 2016;11. e0151850.
338. Scheckelhoff MR, Telford SR, Hu LT. Protective efficacy of an oral vaccine to reduce carriage of *Borrelia burgdorferi* (strain N40) in mouse and tick reservoirs. *Vaccine.* 2006;24:1949–1957.
339. Swetlitz I. To halt the spread of Lyme, Nantucket residents consider genetically engineered mice. 2016. Available at: https://www.statnews.com/2016/06/07/nantucket-lyme-genetic-engineering/#:~:text=To%20halt%20the%20spread%20of%20Lyme%2C%20Nantucket%20residents%20consider%20genetically%20engineered%20mice&text=NANTUCKET%2C%20Mass.,modified%20mice%20on%20the%20island.
340. Centers for Disease Control and Prevention. Reported cases of Lyme disease by state or locality. 2010–2019. Available at: https://www.cdc.gov/lyme/stats/tables.html.
341. Kuehn BM. CDC estimates 300,000 US cases of Lyme disease annually. *JAMA.* 2013;310:1110.
342. Dworkin MS, Anderson DE Jr, Schwan TG, et al. Tick-borne relapsing fever in the northwestern United States and southwestern Canada. *Clin Infect Dis.* 1998;26:122–131.
343. Dworkin MS, Schwan TG, Anderson DE Jr. Tick-borne relapsing fever in North America. *Med Clin North Am.* 2002;86:417–433. viii-ix.
344. Dworkin MS, Schwan TG, Anderson DE Jr, et al. Tick-borne relapsing fever. *Infect Dis Clin North Am.* 2008;22:449–468. viii.
345. Aucott JN. Posttreatment Lyme disease syndrome. *Infect Dis Clin North Am.* 2015;29:309–323.
346. Klempner MS, Hu LT, Evans J, et al. Two controlled trials of antibiotic treatment in patients with persistent symptoms and a history of Lyme disease. *N Engl J Med.* 2001;345:85–92.
347. Lantos PM. Chronic Lyme disease. *Infect Dis Clin North Am.* 2015;29:325–340.
348. Melia MT, Auwaerter PG. Time for a different approach to Lyme disease and long-term symptoms. *N Engl J Med.* 2016;374:1277–1278.
349. Steere AC, Taylor E, McHugh GL, et al. The overdiagnosis of Lyme disease. *JAMA.* 1993;269:1812–1816.
350. Hayes EB, Piesman J. How can we prevent Lyme disease? *N Engl J Med.* 2003;348:2424–2430.
351. Centers for Disease Control and Prevention. Stop ticks to avoid Lyme and other tickborne diseases. Available at: https://www.cdc.gov/ncezid/dvbd/media/stopticks.html. 2019.
352. des Vignes F, Piesman J, Heffernan R, et al. Effect of tick removal on transmission of *Borrelia burgdorferi* and *Ehrlichia phagocytophila* by *Ixodes scapularis* nymphs. *J Infect Dis.* 2001;183:773–778.
353. Cook MJ. Lyme borreliosis: a review of data on transmission time after tick attachment. *Int J Gen Med.* 2015;8:1–8.
354. Piesman J, Dolan MC. Protection against Lyme disease spirochete transmission provided by prompt removal of nymphal *Ixodes scapularis* (Acari: Ixodidae). *J Med Entomol.* 2002;39:509–512.
355. Sood SK, Salzman MB, Johnson BJ, et al. Duration of tick attachment as a predictor of the risk of Lyme disease in an area in which Lyme disease is endemic. *J Infect Dis.* 1997;175:996–999.
356. Mather TN, Fish D, Coughlin RT. Competence of dogs as reservoirs for Lyme disease spirochetes (*Borrelia burgdorferi*). *J Am Vet Med Assoc.* 1994;205:186–188.
357. Johnson JL, Ginsberg HS, Zhioua E, et al. Passive tick surveillance, dog seropositivity, and incidence of human Lyme disease. *Vector Borne Zoonotic Dis.* 2004;4:137–142.
358. Duncan AW, Correa MT, Levine JF, et al. The dog as a sentinel for human infection: prevalence of *Borrelia burgdorferi* C6 antibodies in dogs from southeastern and mid-Atlantic States. *Vector Borne Zoonotic Dis.* 2005;5:101–109.
359. Eng TR, Wilson ML, Spielman A, et al. Greater risk of *Borrelia burgdorferi* infection in dogs than in people. *J Infect Dis.* 1988;158:1410–1411.
360. Shapiro ED, Gerber MA, Holabird NB, et al. A controlled trial of antimicrobial prophylaxis for Lyme disease after deer-tick bites. *N Engl J Med.* 1992;327:1769–1773.
361. Lathrop SL, Ball R, Haber P, et al. Adverse event reports following vaccination for Lyme disease: December 1998-July 2000. *Vaccine.* 2002;20:1603–1608.
362. Embers ME, Narasimhan S. Vaccination against Lyme disease: past, present, and future. *Front Cell Infect Microbiol.* 2013;3:6.
363. Plotkin SA. Need for a new Lyme disease vaccine. *N Engl J Med.* 2016;375:911–913.
364. Barrett PN, Portsmouth D. A novel multivalent OspA vaccine against Lyme borreliosis shows promise in Phase I/II studies. *Expert Rev Vaccines.* 2013;12:973–975.
365. Kaaijk P, Luytjes W. Vaccination against Lyme disease: Are we ready for it? *Hum Vaccin Immunother.* 2016;12:757–762.
366. Wressnigg N, Barrett PN, Pollabauer EM, et al. A novel multivalent OspA vaccine against Lyme borreliosis is safe and immunogenic in an adult population previously infected with *Borrelia burgdorferi* sensu lato. *Clin Vaccine Immunol.* 2014;21:1490–1499.
367. Wressnigg N, Pollabauer EM, Aichinger G, et al. Safety and immunogenicity of a novel multivalent OspA vaccine against Lyme borreliosis in healthy adults: a double-blind, randomised, dose-escalation phase 1/2 trial. *Lancet Infect Dis.* 2013;13:680–689.
368. Masters EJ, Grigery CN, Masters RW. STARI, or Masters disease: lone star tick-vectored Lyme-like illness. *Infect Dis Clin North Am.* 2008;22:361–376.
369. Bunikis J, Tsao J, Garpmo U, et al. Typing of *Borrelia* relapsing fever group strains. *Emerg Infect Dis.* 2004;10:1661–1664.
370. Castellaw AH, Showers J, Goddard J, et al. Detection of vector-borne agents in lone star ticks, *Amblyomma americanum* (Acari: Ixodidae), from Mississippi. *J Med Entomol.* 2010;47:473–476.
371. Varela AS, Luttrell MP, Howerth EW, et al. First culture isolation of *Borrelia lonestari*, putative agent of Southern tick-associated rash illness. *J Clin Microbiol.* 2004;42:1163–1169.
372. Moyer PL, Varela AS, Luttrell MP, et al. White-tailed deer (*Odocoileus virginianus*) develop spirochetemia following experimental infection with *Borrelia lonestari. Vet Microbiol.* 2006;115:229–236.
373. Esteve-Gasent MD, Snell CB, Adetunji SA, et al. Serological detection of tick-borne relapsing fever in texan domestic dogs. *PLoS One.* 2017;12:e0189786.
374. Schwan TG, Raffel SJ, Schrumpf ME, et al. Diversity and distribution of *Borrelia hermsii. Emerg Infect Dis.* 2007;13:436–442.
375. Assous MV, Wilamowski A. Relapsing fever borreliosis in Eurasia: forgotten, but certainly not gone. *Clin Microbiol Infect.* 2009;15:407–414.
376. Halperin T, Orr N, Cohen R, et al. Detection of relapsing fever in human blood samples from Israel using PCR targeting the glycerophosphodiester phosphodiesterase (GlpQ) gene. *Acta Trop.* 2006;98:189–195.
377. Hasin T, Davidovitch N, Cohen R, et al. Postexposure treatment with doxycycline for the prevention of tick-borne relapsing fever. *N Engl J Med.* 2006;355:148–155.
378. Margos G, Pantchev N, Globokar M, et al. First cases of natural infections with *Borrelia hispanica* in two dogs and a cat from Europe. *Microorganisms.* 2020;8:1251.
379. Dominguez MC, Vergara S, Gomez MC, et al. Epidemiology of tick-borne relapsing fever in endemic area, Spain. *Emerg Infect Dis.* 2020;26:849–856.
380. Moyer PL. Experimental animal infections with *Borrelia lonestari*, the putative cause of Southern Tick-Associated Rash Illness. Masters Thesis. 2005. University of Georgia, Athens, GA, USA. Available online at https://getd.libs.uga.edu/pdfs/moyer_patricia_l_200508_ms.pdf.
381. Shapiro ED, Gerber MA. Lyme disease. *Clin Infect Dis.* 2000;31:533–542.
382. Spolidorio MG, Labruna MB, Machado RZ, et al. Survey for tick-borne zoonoses in the state of Espirito Santo, southeastern Brazil. *Am J Trop Med Hyg.* 2010;83:201–206.
383. Rottgerding F, Kraiczy P. Immune evasion strategies of relapsing fever spirochetes. *Front Immunol.* 2020;11:1560.
384. Restrepo BI, Barbour AG. Antigen diversity in the bacterium *B. hermsii* through "somatic" mutations in rearranged vmp genes. *Cell.* 1994;78:867–876.

70

Bartonellosis

Pedro Paulo V.P. Diniz, Bruno B. Chomel, Lynn Guptill, Edward B. Breitschwerdt

KEY POINTS

- Bartonellosis is an emerging, zoonotic, vector-borne infectious disease of cats, dogs, other animals, and humans.
- Causes: The most common species reported in cats are *Bartonella henselae, Bartonella clarridgeiae,* and *Bartonella koehlerae,* whereas dogs are most often infected with *B. henselae* and *Bartonella vinsonii* subsp. *berkhoffii.*
- Geographic Distribution: Worldwide, with the highest prevalence in humid subtropical and tropical regions.
- Major Mode of Transmission: Fleas (*Ctenocephalides felis*) (through flea fecal contamination of wounds); possibly other flea species (such as *Pulex* spp.) and other vectors such as lice, biting flies, mites, and ticks. Blood transfusion transmission occurs experimentally.
- Clinical Signs: In dogs, signs that relate to infective endocarditis (lethargy, fever, cardiac murmur, cough, tachypnea, lameness, neurologic) are the most frequent and well understood. Cats are commonly healthy carriers; however, *Bartonella* can also cause fever, endocarditis, myocarditis, and transient lymphadenomegaly in cats and may cause (or contribute to) other systemic inflammatory disorders.
- Differential Diagnoses: Dogs: other bacterial causes of endocarditis; other vector-borne diseases such as ehrlichiosis, anaplasmosis, borreliosis, and babesiosis; and immune-mediated inflammatory diseases. Cats: major differential diagnoses are other bacterial causes of endocarditis, other systemic inflammatory diseases, and other causes of lymphadenomegaly.
- Human Health Significance: *Bartonella* causes cat scratch disease and other less common disorders, including endocarditis, in immunocompetent humans as well as vasoproliferative disorders (known as bacillary angiomatosis or peliosis) in immunocompromised humans.

ETIOLOGY AND EPIDEMIOLOGY

Bartonella spp. are fastidious, facultative intracellular gram-negative bacteria that infect a wide range of domestic and wild mammalian host species (Fig. 70.1). Different *Bartonella* species have adapted to specific mammalian reservoir hosts and can infect and occasionally cause disease in the reservoir or in incidental hosts. More than 10 species of *Bartonella* infect cats or dogs worldwide (Table 70.1). Cats are the principal reservoir host for *Bartonella henselae,* the main cause of cat scratch disease (CSD) in humans, and subclinical bacteremia in cats is widespread (8% to 56% of healthy cats worldwide).[1]

There is a wide diversity of *B. henselae* strains and at least two different 16S rRNA genotypes. Genotype I (Houston I) and some subgroups within Genotype II (Marseille) are more likely to be a source of human infection.[2,3] There are other methods of genetically classifying *B. henselae,* including multilocus sequence typing, amplified fragment length polymorphism, and more recently whole-genome sequencing; each identifies great genetic diversity within *B. henselae.*[4] Although additional data are needed, it is possible that the genotypes/strains most frequently isolated from bacteremic cats are relatively less virulent than the genotypes/strains that most often infect humans.[2]

Cat fleas (*Ctenocephalides felis*) play a major role in the transmission of feline *Bartonella* infections.[5] Experimentally, transmission among cats has not occurred in the absence of fleas and it is believed that the presence of cat fleas is essential for the maintenance of *Bartonella* infection within the cat population. *Bartonella henselae* can multiply in the digestive system of the flea and survive several days in flea feces.[6] The main source of infection appears to be flea feces that are inoculated by scratches from contaminated cat claws.[7] *Bartonella* DNA has been detected in cat saliva, possibly due to licking of *Bartonella*-contaminated flea feces or alternatively blood contamination of the oral cavity from dental disease or wounds. However, the transmission of *B. henselae* via cat saliva has not been documented experimentally. Other potential vectors, such as *Pulex* flea species, ticks, lice, mites, bedbugs, and biting flies also harbor *Bartonella* DNA, but vector competence remains to be confirmed. Experimental transmission of *Bartonella birtlesii* has been accomplished with *Ixodes ricinus* ticks,[8] and there is indirect epidemiologic evidence that ticks may transmit *Bartonella* to dogs.[9] Transmission via transfusion has not been documented in a client-owned dog or cat, but was documented experimentally in cats and mice[10–12] and has been suspected in human medicine.[13]

Because *Bartonella* infections are often subclinical in cats and dogs, the full extent to which *Bartonella* spp. cause disease in feline and canine species remains unclear. *Bartonella* spp. have been widely studied for their role in several idiopathic inflammatory disorders of cats, including uveitis, lymphadenopathy, caudal stomatitis, and rhinitis, but definitive evidence of disease causation has been difficult to clarify due to the high serologic and bacteremic prevalence in many cat populations studied. *Bartonella* spp. are important causes of endocarditis in dogs and occasionally cause endocarditis and myocarditis in cats (see Table 70.1).

Epidemiology of *Bartonella* Infection in Cats

Bartonella henselae and *Bartonella clarridgeiae* account for the majority of *Bartonella* spp. isolated from domestic cats in the United States (Fig. 70.2), Europe, the Philippines, the Middle East, and most other regions.[14,15] *Bartonella koehlerae* has been isolated from cats in Israel, the United States, and a few other countries; *Bartonella bovis* and *Bartonella quintana* have also been isolated from, or their DNA detected in, a few healthy domestic cats.[16–18] Domestic cats are considered an

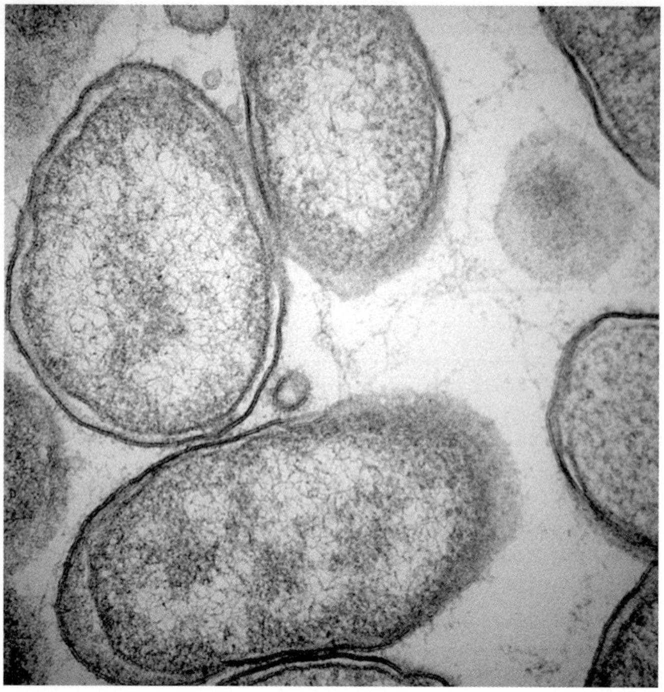

Fig. 70.1 Transmission electron photomicrograph of *Bartonella henselae* organisms in culture media (methanol uranyl acetate and then lead citrate, × 120,000). (Courtesy of Stanley Hayes, Rocky Mountain Laboratories, Hamilton, MT.)

important reservoir and vector for human infections with *B. henselae*, and cats are likely also reservoirs for *B. clarridgeiae and B. koehlerae*. Molecular methods have detected multiple *Bartonella* species in *Ct. felis*, the cat flea, along with other pathogens.[19,20] While these data suggest flea involvement in the transmission of several *Bartonella* species, competence for transmission for some *Bartonella* species by fleas has not yet been verified. Transplacental and transmammary transmissions from queens to kittens have not occurred when tested experimentally.[17,21] In addition to infection via fleas, cats have been infected experimentally via intravenous inoculation, as well as intradermal and oral routes.[5,7,11,22,23] Similar to domestic cats, wild felids, including bobcats, pumas, African lions, and cheetahs, can be infected with various *Bartonella* species.[24–27]

Young cats (≤1 year) are more likely than older cats to be bacteremic, and stray or feral cats infested with fleas are more likely to be bacteremic than pet cats that are not flea-infested.[6,28,29] Older cats are more likely to be seropositive than young cats, which likely reflects the increased chance of exposure over time. The prevalence of *Bartonella* bacteremia in cats is highest in warm, humid climates (e.g., 68% in the Philippines), and is low in colder climates (e.g., 0% in Norway).[3] *Bartonella henselae* type Marseille (type II) was more prevalent among cats in the western United States, western Europe, and Australia; type Houston-1 (type I) was more prevalent in Asia (Japan and the Philippines).[3] Some molecular typing methods reveal an even broader genetic diversity among feline strains, and most of the strains that infect humans cluster in a limited number of groups.[2,3] There is also evidence of genomic variation in *B. henselae* during the course of infection in cats.[30] The genetic diversity of *B. henselae* likely plays a role in the persistence of feline *B. henselae* infections, and has made vaccine development challenging. An improved understanding of genetic diversity among *B. henselae* isolates for cats, dogs, and humans may in turn lead to a better understanding of the differing pathogenicity of these isolates. Cats may be co-infected with multiple *B. henselae* genotypes/strains, and can also be concurrently infected with multiple *Bartonella* species.[31,32] Strain variation has important implications for diagnosis, treatment, and vaccine development to prevent infection in cats.

Epidemiology of *Bartonella* Infection in Dogs

Dogs are most commonly infected with *B. henselae* or *Bartonella vinsonii* subsp. *berkhoffii*; however, the frequency of infected dogs varies widely among regions and countries. Domestic and wild carnivores are thought to be the natural reservoir for *B. vinsonii* subsp. *berkhoffii* and *Bartonella rochalimae*, because these organisms establish prolonged bacteremia in these hosts.[24,33] For example, in California, 76% of coyotes *(Canis latrans)* were seropositive for *B. vinsonii* subsp. *berkhoffii*, with 28% of coyotes found to be bacteremic.[34] At least 14 *Bartonella* species have been detected in dogs, with 11 species capable of infecting both dogs and humans (see Table 70.1).

Because it is often difficult to culture *Bartonella* from domestic dog blood, prevalence studies in dogs have been primarily based on antibody detection. Unfortunately, *Bartonella* spp. seroreactivity correlates poorly with bacteremia and may underestimate the actual prevalence of *Bartonella* in dogs.[35] Also, variable serologic cross-reactivity occurs among *Bartonella* species, so seroprevalence studies cannot always be *Bartonella* species-specific. The prevalence of antibodies to *B. vinsonii* subsp. *berkhoffii* in dogs is highest in tropical or subtropical regions. For example, seroprevalence as high as 47% was detected in stray dogs from Morocco.[36] In the southeastern United States, the prevalence of *B. henselae* and *B. vinsonii* subsp. *berkhoffii* antibodies were 3.8% and 1.5%, respectively, in dogs tested for evidence of vector-borne disease exposure.[37] In another study of 15,451 serology specimens from dogs in North America between 2008 and 2014, 3.3% of dogs were *Bartonella* spp. seroreactive (*B. henselae* 2.1%, *B. koehlerae* 2.4%, and *B. vinsonii* subsp. *berkhoffii* 1.4%).[38] Studies based on enrichment culture coupled with molecular detection may provide a more sensitive indicator of bacteremia in dogs. In one study in the United States, 9.2% of 663 sick dogs were bacteremic for at least one species of *Bartonella*.[39] Risk factors identified in dogs from the southeastern and western United States are tick exposure, exposure to other vector-borne pathogens, residence in a rural environment, roaming, outdoor exposure, intact male sex, being of mixed breed, and being a herding or working dog.[9,38,40,41] The prevalence of *B. henselae* antibodies in sick dogs in the western region of the United States is less than 2%.[40] However, prevalence can be high in free-roaming dogs, as reported in Northern California, where 29% (54/184) of the dogs were seroreactive to *B. vinsonii* subsp. *berkhoffii*, *B. clarridgeiae*, and/or *B. henselae*.[42]

CLINICAL FEATURES

Pathogenesis and Clinical Signs

After infection (Fig. 70.3), *Bartonella* is found in erythrocytes and can also infect endothelial cells and bone marrow progenitor cells.[43] Inhibition of phagocytosis and pyroptosis (a highly inflammatory form of programmed cell death) of macrophages appears to promote *Bartonella* invasion into the bloodstream and potentially through lymphatic circulation.[44] The bacteria then establish a chronic, often subclinical, relapsing bacteremia that can last for weeks, months, or even years, which is likely an evolutionary adaptation that facilitates ongoing transmission by hematophagous arthropods.[1,20] Infection of endothelial cells appears to be necessary for the development of disorders such as vasculoproliferative disease and endocarditis.[15] *Bartonella* is thought to cause vasculoproliferative disease via cytokine-induced stimulation of endothelial cell proliferation and

TABLE 70.1 Comparison of Selected Disease-Producing Members of the Genus *Bartonella*

Common Pathogens for Dogs, Cats, or Humans (Alphabetical Order)

Organism (Classic Disease)	Geographic Occurrence	Confirmed Vector	Potential Vector	Reservoir Host	Incidental Host	Disease Associations
Bartonella bacilliformis (Oroya fever)	Andes Mountains	Sandfly (*Lutzomyia*)	Tick (*Dermacentor andersoni*)	Human	Human	Hemolytic anemia, fever, asymptomatic bacteremia, indolent angiomatous skin lesions (verruga peruana)[15]
Bartonella henselae (cat scratch disease)	Worldwide	Cat flea (*Ctenocephalides felis*), *Ixodes ricinus* ticks	Other ticks (*Ixodes* spp., *Dermacentor* spp., *Rhipicephalus* spp., *Haemaphysalis* spp.), deer keds (*Lipoptena mamazae*),[138] stable fly (*Stomoxys* spp.)[139]	Cat	Dog, human	Dog and human: peliosis hepatis,[71] granulomatous hepatitis,[97] generalized pyogranulomatous lymphadenitis,[140] panniculitis, polyarthritis,[141] endocarditis,[133,142,143] Dog: idiopathic effusions, hyperviscosity syndrome,[103] sielometaplasia,[102] hemangiopericytoma,[53] epistaxis,[86] necrotizing aural margin vasculitis[76] Human: localized tissue infection; angiomatosis, peliosis, granulomatous and pyogenic inflammation, lymphadenitis, endocarditis, neuroretinitis, focal retinochoroiditis, muscle pain, headache, fatigue[119] Cat: fever,[60] lymphadenomegaly,[62] endocarditis, myocarditis, diaphragmatic myositis, uveitis,[54,55] possibly caudal stomatitis,[56–59,62,63] possibly lower urinary tract disease, anemia, mild neurologic signs, and reproductive failure[17,56,59,93]
Bartonella quintana (trench fever)	Worldwide	Body louse (*Pediculus humanus*)	Cat flea (*Ctenocephalides felis*), bed bug (*Cimex lectularius*)[144]	Human, non-human primates (Rhesus macaques)[145]	Human, dog, cat	Dog and human: endocarditis.[96] Human: bacteremia, localized tissue infection, angiomatosis, peliosis, granulomatous and pyogenic inflammation, lymphadenitis[29,119]
Bartonella vinsonii subsp. *berkhoffii*	Worldwide	Likely fleas (*C. felis*)	Brown dog tick (*Rhipicephalus sanguineus*)	Dog, coyote, fox, wolf[146]	Dog, human	Dog: endocarditis,[69,113,142] cardiac arrhythmias, myocarditis, polyarthritis,[141] granulomatous rhinitis, anterior uveitis, chorioretinitis, meningoencephalitis, meningoradiculoneuritis,[147] anemia/thrombocytopenia, bacteremia, seroma,[85] hemangiopericytoma, granulomatous and pyogenic inflammation, panniculitis,[147] bacillary angiomatosis.[72] Human: endocarditis, fever, lymphadenopathy[20,137] Cat: osteomyelitis, systemic reactive angioendotheliomatosis[52,93]

Uncommon Pathogens for Dogs, Cats, or Humans (Alphabetical Order)

Organism (Classic Disease)	Geographic Occurrence	Confirmed Vector	Potential Vector	Reservoir Host	Incidental Host	Disease Associations
Bartonella alsatica	Europe	Rabbit flea (*Spilopsyllus caniculi*)	Unknown	Rabbit	Human	Endocarditis,[131] lymphadenitis[128]
Bartonella bovis (*Bartonella weissii*)	Worldwide	Unknown	Biting flies (*Haematobia* spp., *Hippobosca equina*)[14]	Ruminants (cattle, deer, moose[148])	Dog, cat	Dog: uveitis, hyperglobulinemia[38] Cattle: endocarditis[149]
Bartonella clarridgeiae	Worldwide	Cat flea (*Ctenocephalides felis*)	Unknown	Cat	Dog, human	Dog: endocarditis, chronic lymphocytic hepatitis with copper accumulation (Doberman pinscher)[97] Human: similar to *B. quintana*
Bartonella doshiae	Worldwide	Unknown	Unknown	Rodent	Human	Fatigue, blurred vision, arthralgia[150]

Continued

TABLE 70.1 Comparison of Selected Disease-Producing Members of the Genus *Bartonella*—cont'd

Organism (Classic Disease)	Geographic Occurrence	Confirmed Vector	Potential Vector	Reservoir Host	Incidental Host	Disease Associations
Bartonella elizabethae	Worldwide	Oriental rat flea (*Xenopsylla cheopis*)	Fleas	Rodent	Dog, human	Dog: possible opportunist, bacteremia, weight loss[151] Human: endocarditis, bacteremia[29]
Bartonella grahamii	Europe, United States	Rodent fleas (*Ctenophthalmus nobilis*)	Fleas	Rodent (wild mice)	Human, dog	Human: neuroretinitis[29] Dog: no signs reported[151]
Bartonella koehlerae	United States, Middle East, Australia, Thailand, Europe		Cat flea (*C. felis*)	Cat	Human, dog	Human and dog: endocarditis[143] Cat: endomyocarditis[152]
Bartonella melophagi	Africa, North America, Europe	Sheep ked (*Melophagus ovinus*)[153]	Unknown	Sheep	Human	Human: fatigue, muscle weakness[130]
Bartonella rochalimae	Worldwide	Human flea (*Pulex irritans*)	Other fleas	Gray fox, red fox, coyote, raccoon, jackal,[154] striped skunk, rodent, wolf[24,146,155]	Human, dog	Human: bacteremia and fever[156] Dog: endocarditis,[157] lameness, seizures[158]
Bartonella schoenbuchensis	Worldwide	Deer ked (*Lipoptena cervi*, *L. mazamae*)[138,159]	Unknown	Deer, elk, cattle, moose[160,161]	Human	Fatigue, muscle pain, fever[150]
Bartonella tamiae	Asia, North America, North Africa, Europe		Chigger mites (genera *Leptotrombidium*, *Schoengastia*, and *Blankarrtia*) Ticks (*Ixodes* sp., *Amblyomma* sp.)[162]	Rodent, bat[163]	Human	Headache, myalgia, anemia, maculopapular or petechial rash[129]
Bartonella taylorii	Worldwide	Rodent fleas (*Ctenophthalmus nobilis*)	Unknown	Rodent (wild mice)	Dog	No signs reported[151]
Bartonella tribocorum	Worldwide		Unknown	Rodent	Human	Fatigue, muscle pain, headache[150]
Bartonella vinsonii subsp. *arupensis*	United States		Deer tick (*Ixodes scapularis*) Rodent fleas	Rodent (white-footed mouse)	Human, dog	Human: bacteremia, fever, neurologic signs[29] Dog: no signs reported[147]
Bartonella washoensis	United States	Rodent fleas (*Oropsylla montana*) Tick?	Unknown	Rodent, ground squirrels	Human, dog	Cardiac disease, endocarditis[29]
Candidatus Bartonella ancashi	Andes Mountains	Unknown	Unknown	Rodent	Human	Verruga peruana[164]
Candidatus Bartonella mayotimonensis	North America, Europe	Unknown	Unknown	Bat	Human	Endocarditis[165]
Candidatus Bartonella merieuxii	Europe, Middle East, Mediterranean basin	Fleas?	Unknown	Dog, jackal, wolf[146]		Dog: mild nonregenerative anemia, neutrophilia[166]
Candidatus Bartonella volans (and volans-like)	North America	Fleas?	Unknown	Flying squirrels (*Glaucomys volans*)	Human, dog,[38] sea otter	Human: arthritis, memory loss, and encephalopathy[167] Dog: fever, lethargy, anorexia, weight loss, lameness, vomiting[83] Sea otter: endocarditis[20]

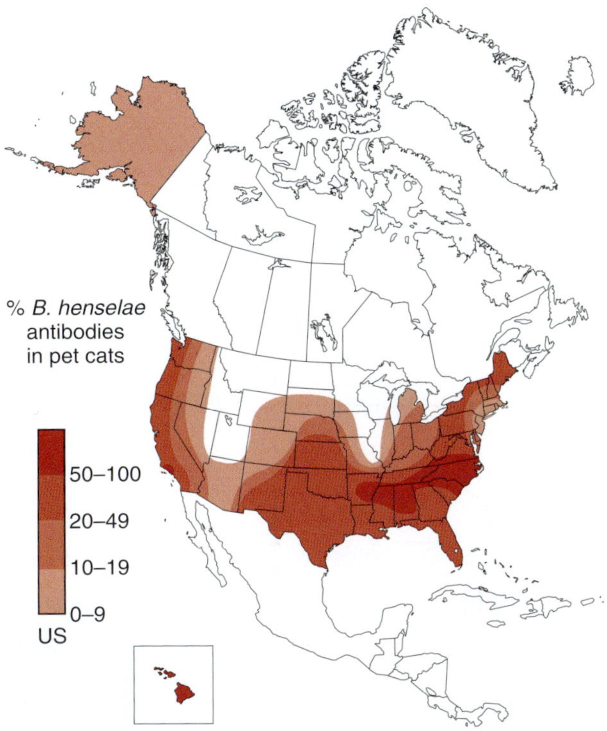

Fig. 70.2 Percentage of pet cats with *Bartonella henselae* antibodies throughout the United States based on samples received from 29 geographic regions. (Map data from Dehio C. Pathogenesis of *Bartonella* (*Rochalimaea*) infections. *Bull Inst Pasteur.* 1997;95:197–207; and Florin TA, Zaoutis TE, Zaoutis LB. Beyond cat scratch disease: widening spectrum of *Bartonella henselae* infection. *Pediatrics.* 2008;121:1413–1425.)

inhibition of endothelial cell apoptosis. Virulence factors characterized in *Bartonella* species include adhesins, heme acquisition mechanisms, type IV secretion systems, effector proteins (*Bartonella* effector proteins [BEPs]), and a low-potency lipopolysaccharide, among others.[15] Host immune status, related to elements such as breed-related immunodeficiency syndromes, other genetic idiosyncrasies, nutritional status, housing conditions, co-infections with other pathogens, immunosuppressive drug treatment or other medications, or defects in normal host barriers (such as congenital valvular disease in dogs with endocarditis), may also influence whether disease ultimately develops in *Bartonella*-infected cats and dogs.

Infected cats and dogs often show no overt clinical signs of illness. In some situations, disease manifestations that occur in *Bartonella*-infected dogs and cats are otherwise uncommon to rare and/or known to be associated with *Bartonella* infection in human patients. In other situations, nonspecific clinical signs are present and it has been impossible to clearly assign a disease causation role to *Bartonella* in an individual patient. Establishing a clear understanding of the role of *Bartonella* in disease causation has also been hindered primarily by limitations in diagnostic tests.

Clinical Manifestations in Cats

Experimental infections of specific pathogen free (SPF) cats with *Bartonella* have shed light on disease processes that can follow natural infection of cats with *Bartonella*. Cats inoculated intradermally with plate-grown *B. henselae* developed a small papule or abscess at the site of inoculation (Fig. 70.4), with concurrent transient fever and accompanying lethargy and inappetence. Lymphadenomegaly of the nodes draining the inoculation site lasted up to 6 weeks.[16–19] Transient mild neurologic signs (including nystagmus, whole body tremors, focal motor seizures, decreased or exaggerated responses to stimuli, and mild behavioral abnormalities) occurred in some cats.[16–19,45] Reproductive disorders, such as failed conception and fetal resorption, were also reported in multiple studies.[17,21,46] Most cats infected with *B. henselae* and/or *B. clarridgeiae* show no clinical signs, and gross lesions are lacking at necropsy. Cats infected with culture-grown *B. koehlerae, B. bovis, B. quintana, B. vinsonii* subsp. *berkhoffii*, or *B. rochalimae* also showed no clinical signs.[47] However, histopathology of cats infected by blood transfusion or culture-grown *B. henselae* or *B. clarridgeiae* showed peripheral or generalized lymph node hyperplasia, splenic follicular hyperplasia, and focal splenic microabscesses, lymphocytic cholangitis/pericholangitis, lymphocytic hepatitis, lymphoplasmacytic myocarditis, and/or interstitial lymphocytic nephritis.[16,18] Myocarditis was also reported in an experimentally infected cat.[48] Collectively, results from experimental infection studies involving cats suggest that the source of inoculum, the route of inoculation, and the virulence characteristics of the *Bartonella* species/strain can influence clinical, hematological, and pathological findings.

Bartonella also causes endocarditis or myocarditis in naturally infected cats, and was associated with feline endomyocarditis-left ventricular endocardial fibrosis complex in 18 of 36 cats evaluated.[49] *Bartonella henselae* DNA was amplified from aortic valvular vegetative lesions of cats, with visualization of the organism in lesions using silver stains.[20,50] Pyogranulomatous myocarditis and diaphragmatic myositis were associated with *B. henselae* infection in two cats, and organisms were detected in lesions with silver stains and IHC (Fig. 70.5).[51] *Bartonella vinsonii* subsp. *berkhoffii* DNA was detected in blood and bone lesions of a cat with carpal and metacarpal osteomyelitis (Fig. 70.6).[52] *Bartonella vinsonii* subsp. *berkhoffii* and *B. henselae* DNA was also PCR amplified and sequenced from cardiac tissues of several cats with systemic reactive angioendotheliomatosis, a vasculoproliferative disorder.[53]

The potential for *Bartonella* to be a contributor to chronic diseases seems likely given the prolonged bacteremia reported, and findings of inflammatory cell infiltrate in many tissues of experimentally infected cats. As a result, *Bartonella* has been investigated for a potential role in several idiopathic conditions of cats (see Table 70.1).[50–52,54–62] These include uveitis,[54–56] gingivostomatitis,[56–59,61,62] fever of unknown origin,[60] lower urinary tract disease,[56,59,63] hyperglobulinemia, anemia, inflammatory polyps, chronic kidney disease,[56,59] high serum pancreatic lipase immunoreactivity,[64] lymphadenopathy,[62] neurologic disease,[56,65,66] plasmacytic pododermatitis,[67] and chronic idiopathic rhinosinusitis.[68] There is currently no convincing and repeatable scientific evidence that *Bartonella* infection causes any of these conditions. Studies have varied in the methodology used to detect infection (serology, culture, and/or PCR assays). The utility of serology for establishing disease associations is limited, and studies that rely on *Bartonella* seroreactivity to evaluate disease association should be interpreted with caution. Finding *Bartonella* in tissues via PCR or culture should be evaluated carefully, as high proportions of cats may be infected with *Bartonella* species, and there may be other etiologies for clinical conditions being investigated. Because of the high prevalence of *Bartonella* exposure in domestic cats, an understanding of the significance of *Bartonella* in these conditions will require carefully controlled, long-term prospective study of large numbers of cats with clearly defined clinical conditions using *Bartonella* culture and/or PCR assays, along with investigation for other etiologies. It is important to consider that many of the conditions investigated likely have multifactorial etiologies, and cats exposed to *Bartonella* are likely exposed to other arthropod-vectored pathogens.

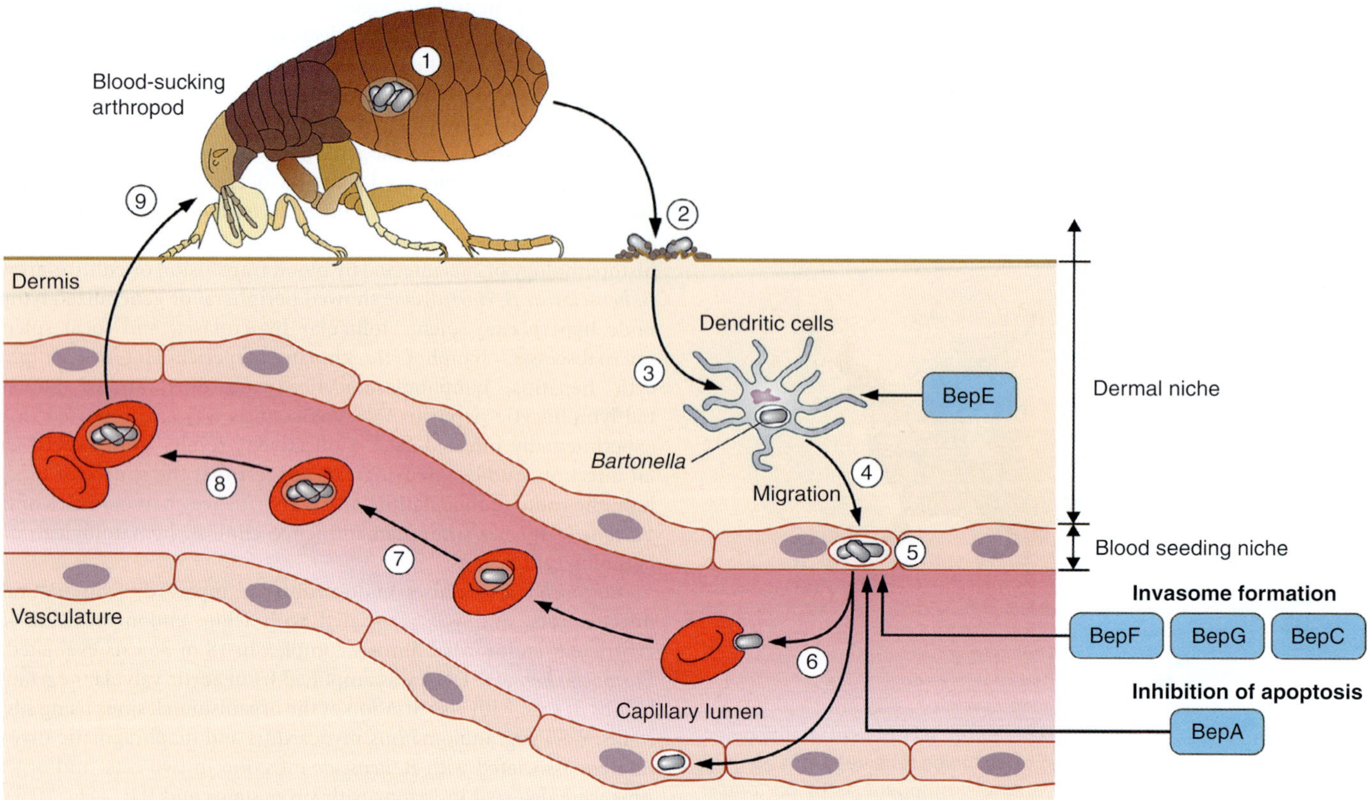

Fig. 70.3 Model of *Bartonella* infection in the reservoir host. (1) *Bartonella* replicate first in the midgut of the arthropod vector and are excreted in the feces. (2) Inoculation of *Bartonella*-containing insect feces into the dermis occurs by scratching. (3) *Bartonella* colonize cells of "dermal niche" such as dendritic cells. *Bartonella*-translocated effector protein E (*BepE*) facilitates the dissemination of *Bartonella* (4), while BepC, BepF, and BepG participate in the engulfment and internalization of the bacterial aggregate (invasome) by the targeted cell and BepA participates in the inhibition of apoptosis (5). *Bartonella* are periodically seeded into the bloodstream where they invade erythrocytes and endothelial cells at different organs (6). After limited replication inside the RBC (7), they persist for the remaining lifespan of the RBC (8) and are thus competent for transmission by a blood-sucking arthropod (9). (From Siamer S, Dehio C. New insights into the role of *Bartonella* effector proteins in pathogenesis. *Curr Opin Microbiol.* 2015;23:80-85.)

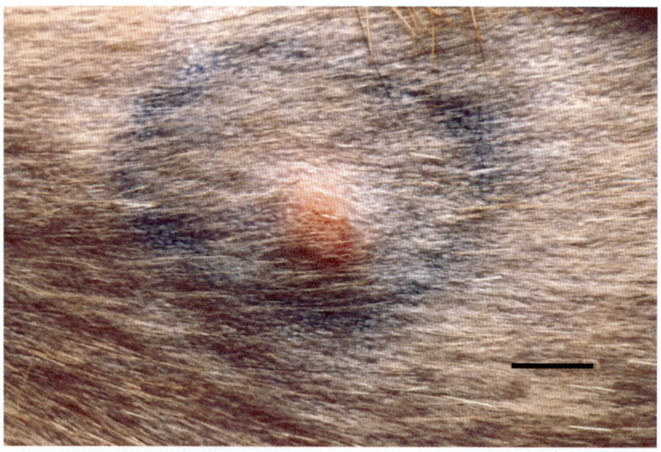

Fig. 70.4 Postinoculation papule 20 days after intradermal inoculation of *Bartonella henselae* in a cat. The size of the papule increased from the time of inoculation and only *B. henselae* was isolated from bacterial culture of an aspirate. (Bar =1 cm.) (Courtesy of Lynn Guptill, Purdue University, West Lafayette, IN.)

Clinical Manifestations in Dogs

Bartonella spp. are important causes of blood culture–negative endocarditis in dogs, but they have also been detected within lesions from many other pathologies using culture or PCR (see Table 70.1). Infection with *Bartonella* was identified from 19% to 28% of dogs with culture-negative endocarditis.[45,69] In United States military working dogs, 13 of 18 dogs with histologic diagnoses of culture-negative endocarditis, 3 of 5 dogs with endomyocarditis, and 3 of 3 dogs with endocardiosis tested positive for *Bartonella* using PCR; in contrast, only 1 of 28 control dogs without histologic evidence of cardiac lesions tested positive.[70] Worldwide, the DNA of several *Bartonella* species has been detected in the heart valves of dogs with endocarditis. The most common species identified has been *B. vinsonii* subsp. *berkhoffii*. In dogs, *Bartonella* endocarditis usually involves the aortic valve, although the mitral valve is occasionally affected, so the possibility of bartonellosis should not be ruled out in dogs with mitral valve endocarditis. Dogs with *Bartonella* endocarditis are more likely to be afebrile and more likely to have congestive heart failure than dogs with other causes of endocarditis, and their median survival time is shorter (Fig. 70.7).[45] Complications of *Bartonella* endocarditis include murmur, lameness,

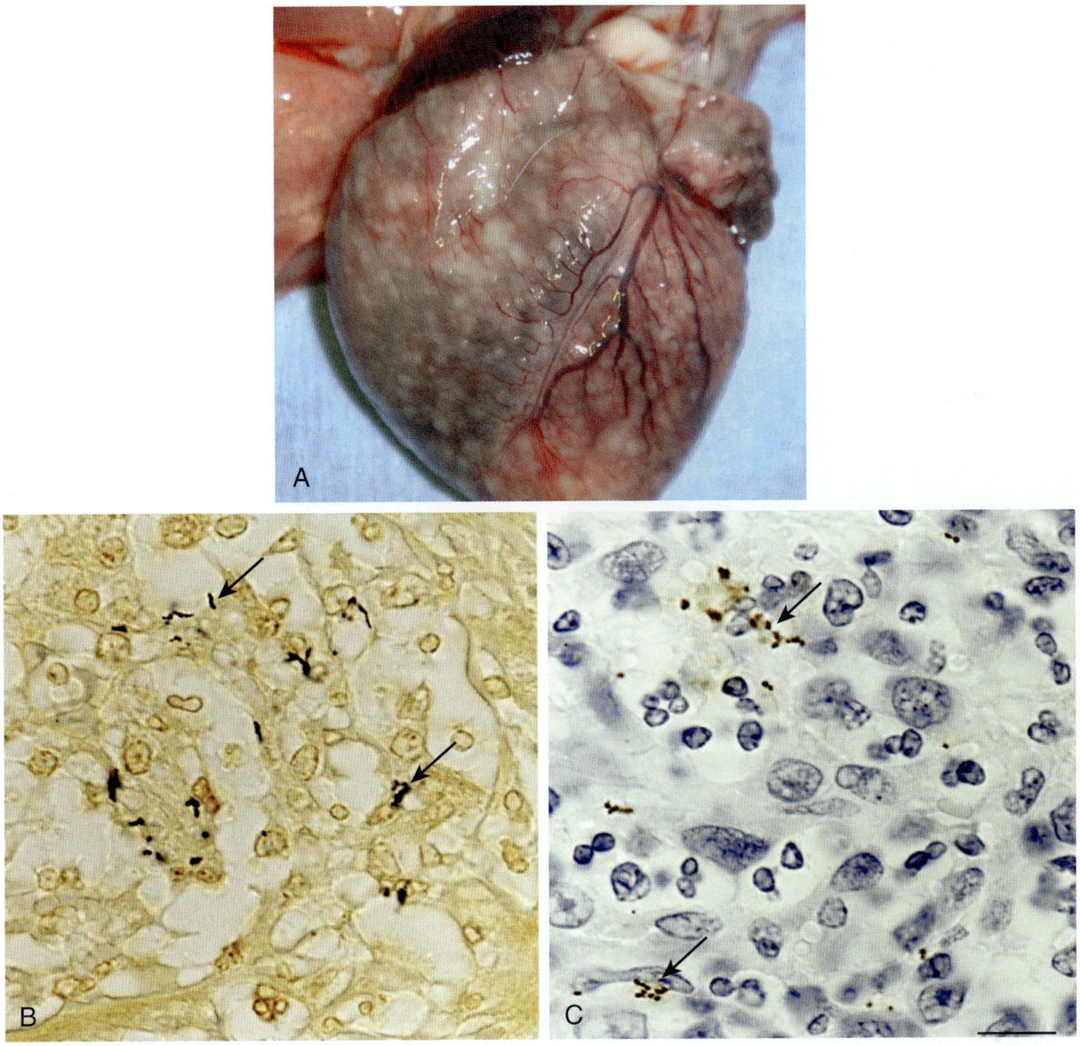

Fig. 70.5 (A) Granulomatous myocarditis associated with *Bartonella henselae* infection in an 8-week-old female domestic shorthair introduced to a shelter that was ridden with fleas. (B) Histopathology of the heart of the affected cat showing intralesional agyrophilic bacteria *(arrows)*. Warthin-Starry stain. (C) Short bacilli *(arrows)* in an inflammatory focus are immunoreactive (brown) for *Bartonella henselae*-specific monoclonal antibody. Immunohistochemistry with diaminobenzidine chromogen, hematoxylin counterstain. (A, courtesy of Drs. Jack Broadhurst and Edward Breitschwerdt. From Varanat M, Broadhurst J, Linder KE, et al. Identification of *Bartonella henselae* in 2 cats with pyogranulomatous myocarditis and diaphragmatic myositis. *Vet Pathol.* 2012;49:608-611.)

weakness, thromboembolic disease, neutrophilic polyarthritis, and collapse.

Bartonella isolates or *Bartonella* DNA have been detected in lesions from dogs with a variety of chronic pyogranulomatous or granulomatous inflammatory and vasculoproliferative diseases (Fig. 70.8). Consequently, the clinical manifestations vary over the time course of illness and in severity according to the organ or tissue most severely affected. *Bartonella henselae* was detected in a dog with peliosis hepatis and *B. vinsonii* subsp. *berkhoffii* in a dog with bacillary angiomatosis, both of which are rare conditions that are strongly associated with *Bartonella* infection in humans.[71–73] Peliosis hepatis and bacillary angiomatosis are vasculoproliferative diseases characterized by the presence of blood-filled proliferation of vascular tissue in the liver and skin, respectively. *Bartonella henselae* was also detected in an SPF beagle research dog that had aural vasculitis, with confirmation of intralesional infection using PCR amplification, DNA sequencing, and confocal immunostaining.[74] Based on case reports and seroprevalence studies, *Bartonella* has been associated with polyarthritis, epistaxis, and thrombocytopenia in dogs.[40] However, these associations could also reflect the presence of other detected or undetected diseases, including co-transmitted vector-borne pathogens that cause these disorders. *Bartonella* has been investigated for its potential role in lymphoma,[75] neurologic diseases,[76] idiopathic cavitary effusion,[77,78] idiopathic rhinitis,[79] and in splenic disorders including lymphoid nodular hyperplasia, hemangiosarcoma,[80] and fibrohistiocytic nodules.[81] *Bartonella* spp. DNA was amplified and sequenced from fresh frozen tissues from 73% of dogs diagnosed with hemangiosarcoma.[80] The clinical relevance of finding *Bartonella* infection in association with a neoplasm requires additional study.

Physical Examination Findings

Among 47 dogs confirmed to be infected with one or more *Bartonella* spp. in the United States, the most frequent signs were fever (40%), lethargy (40%), weight loss (34%), anorexia (32%), lymphadenopathy

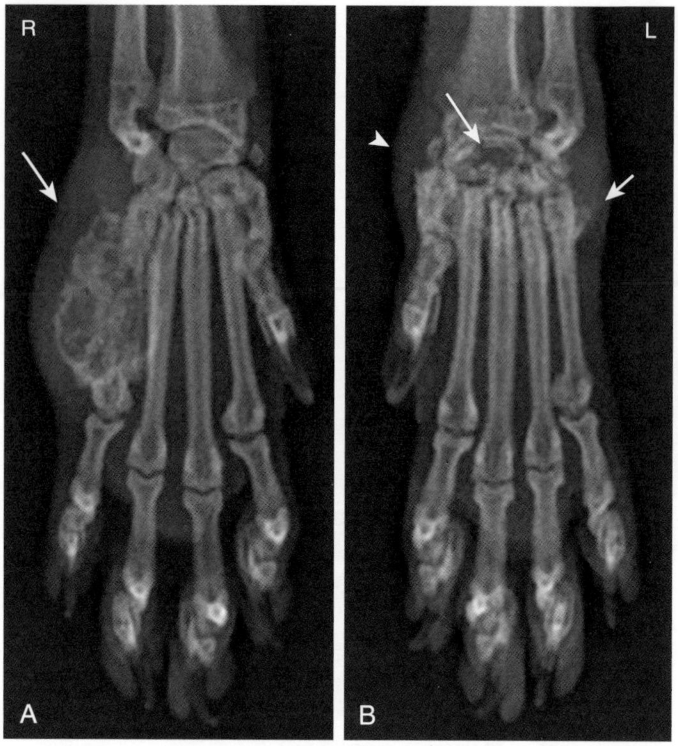

Fig. 70.6 Dorsopalmar radiograph of thoracic limbs. (A) Proliferative lesion of the right fifth metacarpal bone and adjacent soft-tissue swelling *(arrow)*. (B) Osteolysis of the radial carpal bone *(large arrow)*, osteoproliferation of the carpal and metacarpal bones *(small arrow)*, and carpal joint effusion *(arrowhead)*. (From Varanat M, Travis A, Lee W, et al. Recurrent osteomyelitis in a cat due to infection with *Bartonella vinsonii* subsp. *berkhoffii* genotype II. *J Vet Intern Med*. 2009;23:1273-1277.)

(30%), diarrhea (23%), neurological signs (21%), heart murmurs (21%), respiratory signs (21%), polyuria/polydipsia (21%), lameness (19%), vomiting (15%), and splenomegaly (13%).[82] When compared to dogs suspected of other tick-borne diseases, the presence of weight loss was more frequent in dogs infected with *Bartonella* species.[83] In dogs with *Bartonella* endocarditis, physical examination findings include lethargy, inappetence, and thin body condition; lameness or recumbency due to thromboembolic complications, weakness, or polyarthritis; joint effusion; and, uncommonly, fever (as high as 104.9°F [41°C]). Evidence of cardiac disease and congestive heart failure is often present, including respiratory distress, cough, increased lung sounds, and systolic and/or diastolic heart murmurs, cardiac arrhythmias, and pulse deficits. Neurologic signs such as anisocoria and obtundation can occur in dogs with thromboembolism that involves the CNS. There may also be evidence of flea or tick infestations in some dogs. Other physical examination findings that might be present in dogs with other manifestations of bartonellosis are mass lesions that involve lymph nodes or salivary glands; splenomegaly or hepatomegaly; cavitary effusions; peripheral edema; epistaxis; or nodular skin lesions (Fig. 70.9).[38,77,84–87]

Physical examination findings in cats with *Bartonella* endocarditis or myocarditis have included fever, lethargy, respiratory distress, cardiac murmurs, and arrhythmias.[50,51] Fever and lymphadenomegaly are common findings in experimentally infected cats, and *Bartonella* infection should be on the list of differential diagnoses for cats presenting with fever and/or lymphadenomegaly that cannot be otherwise explained, along with a history compatible with *Bartonella* exposure. In addition to endocarditis and myocarditis, *Bartonella* may contribute to acute-onset cardiac arrhythmias and sudden death.[49] *Bartonella* spp. DNA was amplified by PCR and sequenced from 18 of 36 cats (50%) with endomyocarditis and 1 of 12 (8.3%) cats with hypertrophic cardiomyopathy, whereas DNA was not amplified from any non-cardiac disease control hearts.

DIAGNOSIS

Most clinical signs or clinical pathologic abnormalities proposed to be attributable to bartonellosis are shared by conditions resulting from many other etiologies. Therefore determining which animals likely have clinical signs resulting from *Bartonella* infection can be difficult. Diagnostic testing should not be focused on *Bartonella* alone but should include evaluation for other potential causes of the clinical condition(s) being evaluated. Diagnosis of bartonellosis is based on the presence of consistent clinical abnormalities (especially endocarditis or myocarditis, but also other systemic inflammatory or vasculoproliferative diseases), a history of exposure to arthropod vectors, histopathologic findings, and positive culture or PCR assay results on blood or affected tissues (Table 70.2). It may be impossible to identify *Bartonella* as the cause of disease if the organism is not detected in the blood by PCR or enrichment blood culture/PCR and if affected tissues (e.g., valvular vegetations) cannot be obtained for analysis. Also, because healthy cats and dogs can be bacteremic, documentation of bacteremia must be viewed in the clinical context of the animal's illness. Similarly, visualizing organisms (or amplifying organism-specific DNA sequences) in tissue may not always confirm causation due to *Bartonella*, as this is distributed throughout many tissues because it is a blood-borne pathogen. Other possible causes of disease must also be investigated, and a response to antibiotic treatment could be evaluated (see Case Example). Finally, disease resolution in association with antibiotic administration may not indicate *Bartonella* as a cause, since other undocumented bacterial pathogens may be treated as a result of antibiotic therapy. Some antibiotics have anti-inflammatory and/or immune-modulating properties that make it difficult to differentiate whether a positive change in patient status is a result of antimicrobial properties of the drug, other properties of the drug, the host immune response having more time to address the pathogen, or a combination of factors.[88] Documentation of seroconversion and seroreversion in conjunction with antibiotic administration can be used to support a diagnosis of bartonellosis.[89] Increased documentation of seroconversion in dogs with an acute-onset illness will be important to better understand the extent to which acute versus chronic infections occur in dogs. In contrast, when dealing with a long-standing illness, serology (if positive) can only be used to implicate *Bartonella* exposure. As *Bartonella* seroprevalence is much lower in dogs compared to cats, positive serology is perhaps more diagnostically useful when evaluating a sick dog.[38] More specifically (and as occurs in humans), dogs with *Bartonella* endocarditis usually have high antibody titers to *Bartonella* spp. Conventional organism detection tests (blood culture and PCR) are insensitive because dogs tend to have very low levels of bacteremia when compared with cats. The sensitivity of *Bartonella* spp. detection has improved with the use of enrichment culture coupled with a highly sensitive PCR, which is the current recommended approach for confirming bacteremia in dogs.[85,90,91] Improved detection of *Bartonella* bacteremia in cats has also been demonstrated using methods combining enrichment culture and PCR assays.[92] Nonetheless, the prevalence rates of *Bartonella* spp. in cats and dogs do not correspond with the low number of reported clinical cases potentially because *Bartonella* infections are underdiagnosed in dogs and cats.[93]

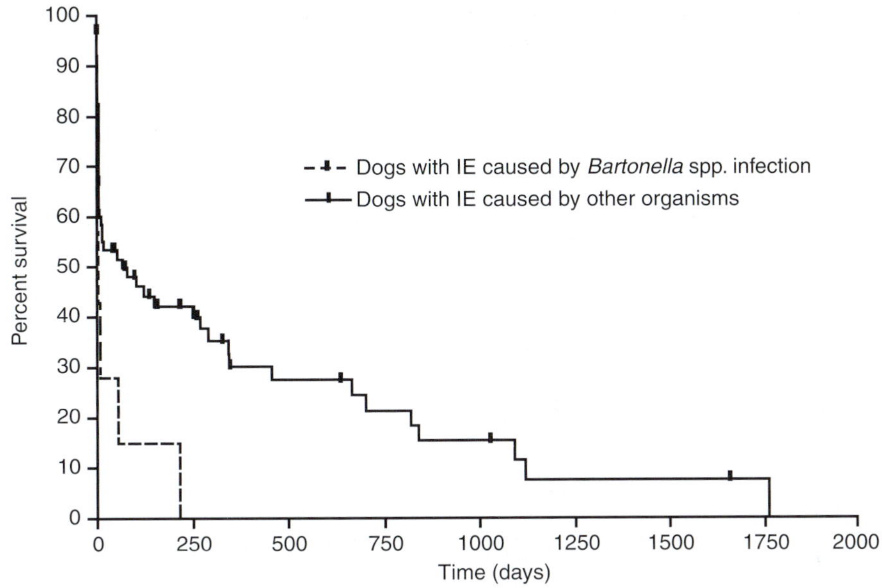

Fig. 70.7 Kaplan-Meier survival curve comparing survival of dogs with *Bartonella* infectious endocarditis (IE) with that of dogs with IE caused by other pathogens. (From Sykes JE, Kittleson MD, Pesavento PA, et al. Evaluation of the relationship between causative organisms and clinical characteristics of infective endocarditis in dogs: 71 cases (1992-2005). *J Am Vet Med Assoc.* 2006;228:1723-1734.)

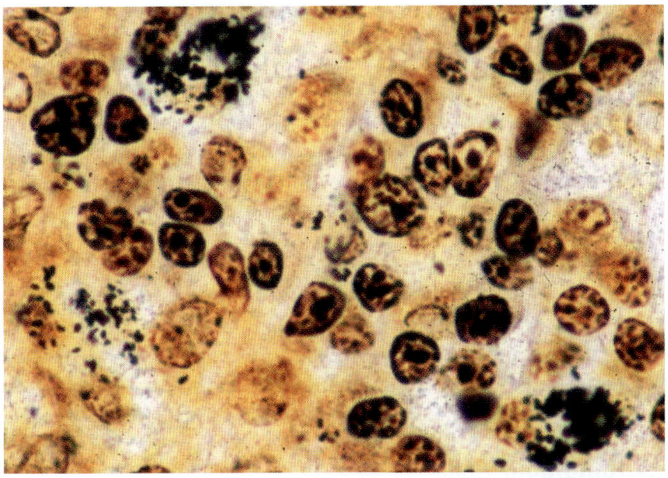

Fig. 70.8 Granulomatous lymphadenitis in a dog with *Bartonella vinsonii* ssp. *berkhoffii* infection. Coccobacilli are in clusters among lymphoid elements (Warthin-Starry silver, × 200). (Courtesy of T. Brown and E. Breitschwerdt, North Carolina State University, Raleigh, NC.)

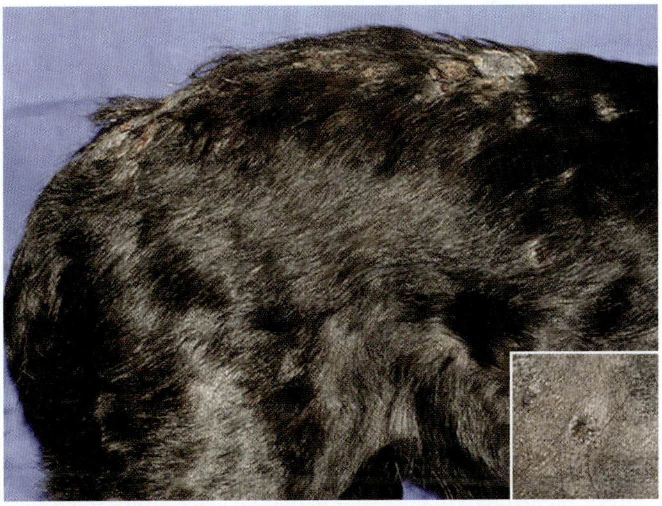

Fig. 70.9 An 8-year-old, spayed female Labrador retriever with panniculitis associated with *Bartonella henselae* infection. Lesions consisted of patchy to complete alopecia containing diffuse, palpable subcutaneous nodules with overlying hemorrhagic crusts. Several of the nodules were ulcerated, scarred, and crateriform in appearance (*inset*). (From Rossi MA, Balakrishnan N, Linder KE, et al. Concurrent *Bartonella henselae* infection in a dog with panniculitis and owner with ulcerated nodular skin lesions. *Vet Dermatol.* 2015;26(1):60-63, e21-62.)

Laboratory Abnormalities

Hematologic and biochemistry abnormalities in dogs and cats with *Bartonella* endocarditis are nonspecific and often mild. Most infected cats have no clinical pathologic abnormalities. Chronically infected dogs may also be hematologically unremarkable or have only mild nonregenerative anemia, neutrophilia, neutropenia, or thrombocytopenia. A few dogs have low to moderate numbers of circulating band neutrophils, lymphocytosis, and/or monocytosis.[94–96] Serum biochemical abnormalities can include azotemia, hypoalbuminemia, hypoglobulinemia, and hyperglobulinemia. Isosthenuria, proteinuria, cylindruria, and slightly increased urine protein-to-creatinine ratios have been present in the urine of some affected dogs. Dogs with hepatic involvement have had moderately increased serum ALT and/or ALP activities.[71,97] In one study from the United States, the most common laboratory abnormalities detected among *Bartonella*-bacteremic dogs were proteinuria (40%), anemia (38%), leukocytosis (36%), thrombocytopenia (34%), elevated liver enzymes (32%), hyperbilirubinemia (30%), hyperglobulinemia (26%), hypoglobulinemia (23%), azotemia (21%), monocytosis (17%), abnormal coagulation panel (PT/PTT) (13%), leukopenia (11%), and lymphocytosis (11%).[82,83] Ineffective erythropoiesis was diagnosed in a dog that failed immunosuppressive drug therapy, but had resolution of the anemia after documentation of *B. henselae* bacteremia, in association with antibiotic administration.[98]

TABLE 70.2 Diagnostic Assays Available for *Bartonella* Infection in Dogs and Cats

Assay	Specimen Type	Target	Performance
Culture	Whole blood, other tissue specimens	*Bartonella* spp.	Confirms infection and allows species identification. Specialized culture conditions required; best performed in laboratories with special expertise. Requires several weeks' incubation. Sensitivity is especially low in dogs because of low-level or intermittent bacteremia. The collection of serial samples and the use of BAPGM enrichment media followed by PCR may increase sensitivity but may increase the chance of false-positive results due to PCR-related contamination. Positive culture results alone do not imply disease causation, because healthy dogs and cats can have *Bartonella* in their tissues. Results must be interpreted in light of the clinical signs and history.
Histopathology with organism detecting using silver stains or IHC	Tissue specimens obtained by biopsy or necropsy	*Bartonella* spp. organisms	Low sensitivity, but supports disease causation when positive and properly performed and interpreted.
Serology	Serum	Antibodies to *Bartonella* spp.	Variable cross-reactivity between *Bartonella* species; species-specific assays are required. Immunofluorescent antibody and ELISA assays are best validated. Results correlate poorly with bacteremia. Positive results do not imply disease causation, because a significant proportion of healthy dogs and cats are seropositive. High positive titers are usually present in dogs and cats with endocarditis.
PCR	Whole blood, splenic or lymph node aspirates, other tissue specimens	*Bartonella* spp. DNA	Confirms active infection more rapidly than culture. Sensitivity and specificity may vary depending on assay design and specimen type; may not necessarily be more sensitive than culture. Positive results alone do not imply disease causation, because healthy dogs and cats can have *Bartonella* in their tissues. Results must be interpreted in light of the clinical signs and history. False-positive results may occur as a result of PCR-related contamination.

BAPGM, *Bartonella* alpha Proteobacteria growth medium.

A 2022 study found no clinically relevant laboratory abnormalities in cats infected with *Bartonella* other than neutrophilia.[99]

Cardiac biomarkers such as troponin I and natriuretic peptide (Nt-ProBNP) may be elevated in sick dogs with *Bartonella* endocarditis or myocarditis. Cardiac troponin I is a highly sensitive marker for myocardial damage, and was elevated (0.28 to 3.05 ng/mL, reference ≤0.11 ng/mL) in three out of eight *Bartonella* spp. infected or exposed dogs, lacking diagnostic indications of endocarditis.[100] Natriuretic peptides are a biomarker for stress or stretching of the myocardium, and are frequently elevated in patients with congestive heart failure, which can be caused by endocarditis or myocarditis.[101]

Diagnostic Imaging

Plain Radiography

Thoracic radiographs in dogs with *Bartonella* endocarditis often show evidence of congestive heart failure, with venous engorgement and pulmonary edema (Fig. 70.10). Lung lobe consolidation and hilar lymphadenopathy were described in a dog with systemic granulomatous disease and sialometaplasia.[102] Bilateral mandibular pyogranulomatous lymphadenitis and pulmonary nodules were found in a dog with *B. henselae* bacteremia.[103]

Abdominal Ultrasound

Ultrasound examination of dogs with systemic granulomatous or pyogranulomatous disease may reveal lymphadenomegaly and organomegaly,[104] and mixed echogenic patterns within the liver.[97] In two distinct reports, dogs with peliosis hepatis had ascites/hemoperitoneum and multiple, small nodular masses and hypoechoic cystic lesions within the liver (Fig. 70.11).[71,73]

Electrocardiography

Arrhythmias and conduction disturbances have been more frequently reported in patients with endocarditis or myocarditis, but occur in dogs without echocardiographic evidence of these disease processes. ECG findings are nonspecific and can vary from atrial, nodal, or ventricular conduction disturbances, including atrioventricular blocks and/or bundle branch blocks. In addition, supraventricular and/or ventricular premature complexes may be observed (Fig. 70.12).

Echocardiography

Echocardiography in dogs and cats with *Bartonella* endocarditis reveals oscillating valvular vegetations or thickened and hyperechoic valve leaflets, which usually involve the aortic valve (Fig. 70.13). There may be evidence of aortic regurgitation or insufficiency and eccentric hypertrophy of the left ventricle or decreased cardiac output.

Microbiologic Tests

Culture

Despite the limitations described earlier, culture of blood or other tissues for *Bartonella* facilitates a definitive diagnosis of infection. However, blood culture requires special techniques and can be insensitive because of the relapsing nature of bacteremia (see Fig. 70.3). Sensitivity can be improved by collecting serial blood samples (e.g., three blood draws within 7 days). Culture has especially low sensitivity in most dog populations because of the low level of bacteremia (especially when dogs are incidental hosts and develop the disease). Blood for culture should be obtained using aseptic collection and placed in EDTA-containing tubes, and then chilled or frozen during shipment. The collection of blood into plastic EDTA tubes allows the tubes to be frozen directly, which releases organisms from erythrocytes after which they are inoculated into optimized liquid growth media. Blood should be sent to laboratories familiar with the culture of these fastidious organisms, and the laboratories should be contacted for instructions regarding specimen collection and submission. Special media (such as fresh chocolate agar, or brain-heart infusion agar enriched with 5% to 10% blood) and culture conditions (5% CO_2, temperatures of 35°C to

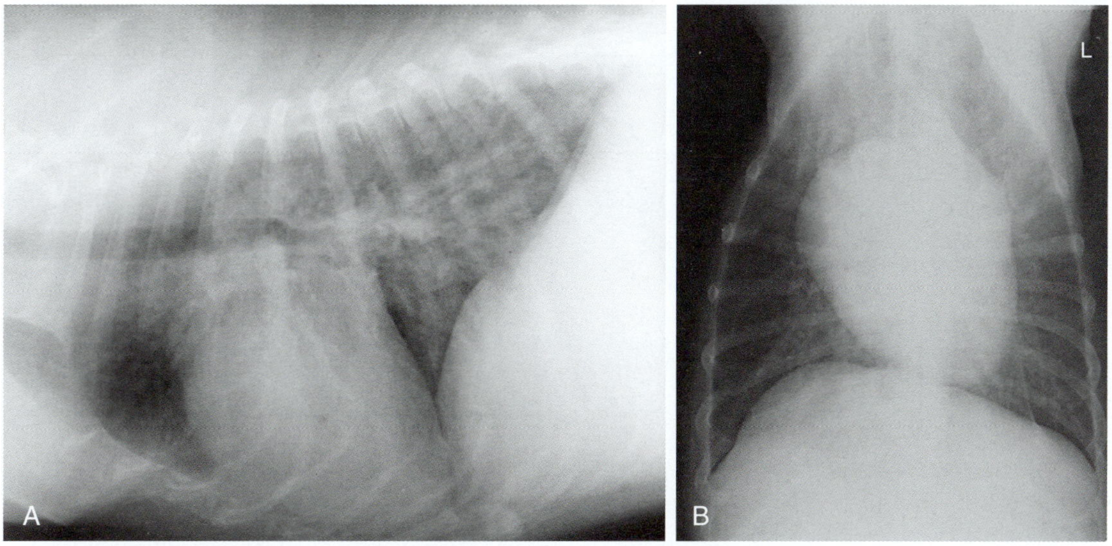

Fig. 70.10 Radiographs from a dog with acute aortic valve infective endocarditis associated with *Bartonella* spp. infection. The dog was evaluated for acute dyspnea. Thoracic radiographs show normal heart size and diffuse interstitial pulmonary infiltrates of the caudal lung lobes. Pulmonary veins were mildly distended. Because of the lack of cardiomegaly, there was debate whether the infiltrates were cardiogenic, and measurement of markedly elevated pulmonary capillary wedge pressure confirmed left heart failure as the cause of the infiltrates. (From MacDonald K. Infective endocarditis in dogs: diagnosis and therapy. *Vet Clin North Am Small Anim Pract.* 2010;40:665-684.)

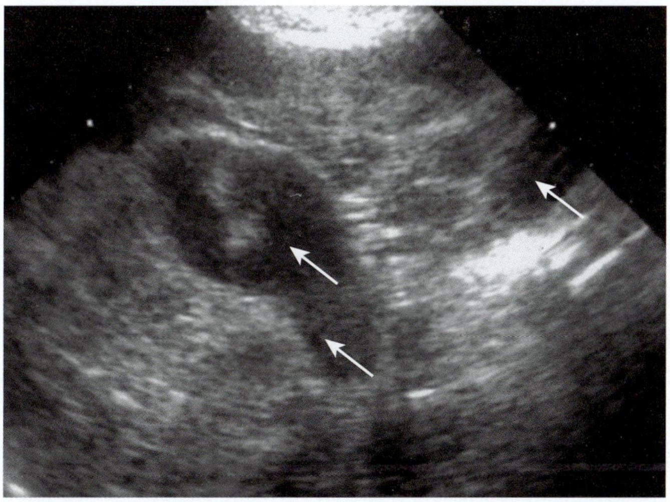

Fig. 70.11 Ultrasonographic appearance of the liver of a dog with peliosis hepatis, associated with *Bartonella henselae* infection showing hypoechoic areas *(arrows)* representing vascular peliosis. (Courtesy of Barbara Kitchell, University of Illinois, Urbana, IL.)

37°C) are used to enhance the likelihood of isolation of *Bartonella*.[75] Extended incubation times of up to 6 to 8 weeks can be required for successful isolation. The use of an insect growth medium (*Bartonella* alpha Proteobacteria growth medium, or BAPGM) that contains multiple micronutrients and defibrinated sheep blood for enrichment culture of blood, cerebrospinal and joint fluid, pathological effusions, and potentially other tissues, followed by PCR testing of the liquid culture at defined time points, in conjunction with sub-inoculation of the liquid culture medium onto agar plates, has enhanced culture sensitivity, compared to conventional microbiological approaches. It also has the potential to yield other fastidious organisms not cultured under routine conditions that may play a role in endocarditis.[105] Liquid culture did not significantly improve the isolation of *Bartonella* spp. in cats.[106]

Molecular Diagnosis Using Nucleic Acid–Based Testing

Many PCR-based assays have been developed for the rapid detection of *Bartonella* DNA in blood or other tissues.[100,107,108] Some veterinary diagnostic laboratories offer real-time PCR assays for the detection of *Bartonella* species as a component of vector-borne PCR panels. Some assays are designed to detect all *Bartonella* spp., whereas other assays are designed to be species-specific. Genetic analysis of PCR products by DNA sequencing or other modalities can be performed to identify the infecting *Bartonella* species. Diagnostic utilization of droplet digital PCR (ddPCR) has substantially improved the detection of *Bartonella* DNA while maintaining exceptional specificity.[109] The clinical performance of many of these assays, when compared among laboratories or compared with culture, has not been well studied. When used directly on blood specimens, PCR assays may be no more sensitive than conventional culture for the detection of *Bartonella*, and detection of DNA does not necessarily equate to the documentation of living organisms. However, the turnaround time for PCR assay results is typically much faster than for culture. False-positive PCR assay results due to laboratory contamination or sample contamination at the time of collection (of particular concern with tissues collected at necropsy) have the potential to occur. False-negative PCR results may occur due to DNA degradation or cross-linking secondary to formalin fixation or other factors. Whenever possible, clinicians should simultaneously collect and freeze tissues for PCR testing at the same time tissues are collected for histopathology. Reputable laboratories with experience in molecular diagnostics are recommended to achieve optimal sensitivity and specificity. Laboratories should be contacted before specimen submission for guidelines for specimen collection and shipment.

Serologic Testing

Immunofluorescent antibody (IFA), ELISA, and Western immunoblot assays are available for the detection of *Bartonella* spp. antibodies. Some degree of cross-reactivity occurs among *Bartonella* species, but multiple species-specific assays still should be performed to increase the chance of antibody detection. Cross-reactivity can be observed for endocarditis

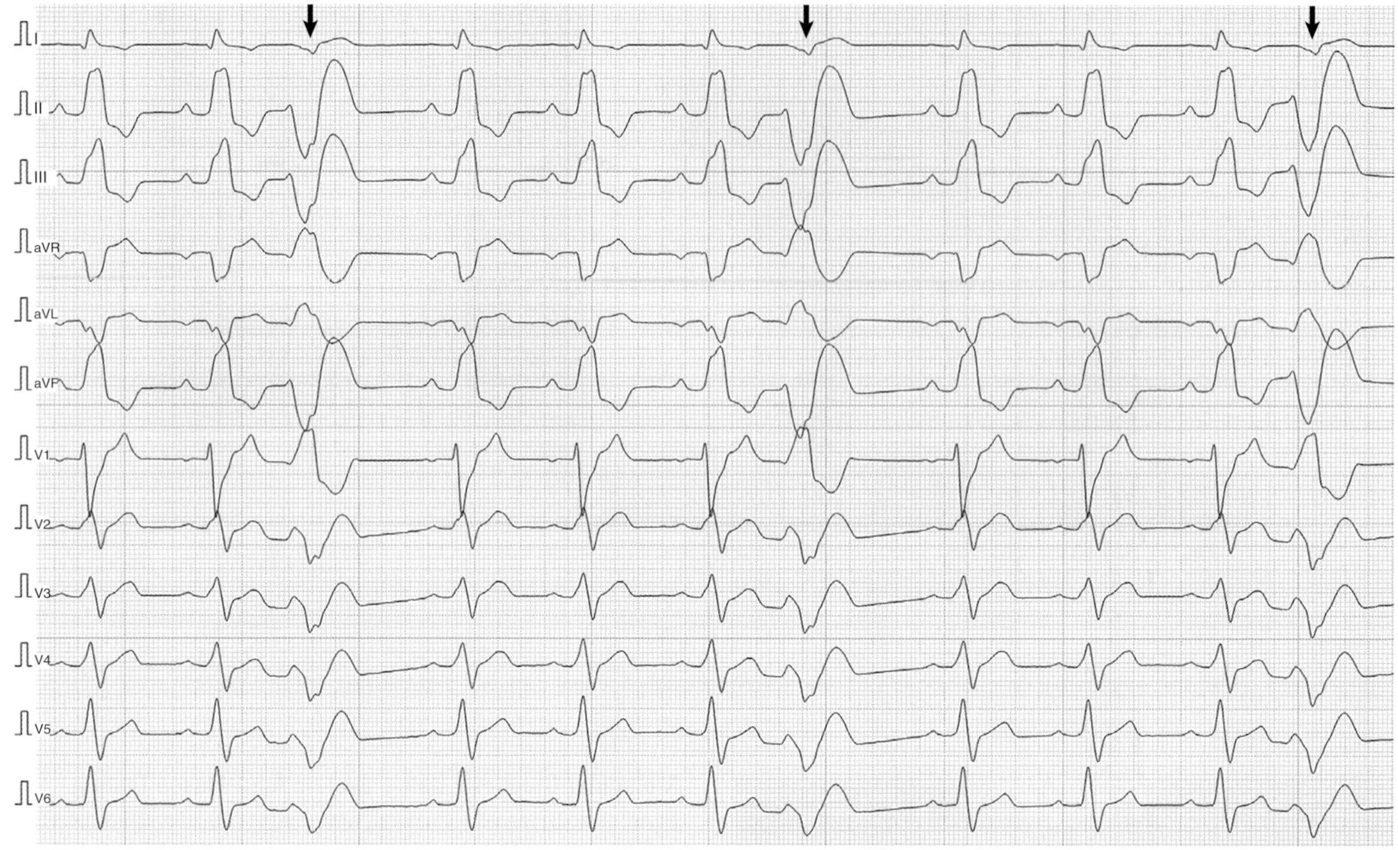

Fig. 70.12 Twelve-lead surface ECG recording of a dog with *Bartonella*-associated inflammatory cardiomyopathy, showing the presence of sinus rhythm conducted with left bundle branch block, interrupted by frequent ventricular ectopic beats with right bundle block morphology *(arrows)*. (From Santilli RA, et al. *Bartonella*-associated inflammatory cardiomyopathy in a dog. *J Vet Cardiol.* 2017;19(1):74-81.)

cases, where antibody titers can be quite high.[20,94] Experimentally, dogs generated a specific antibody response by IFA testing to each *Bartonella* species, without the development of cross-reactivity.[110] *Bartonella henselae* Western immunoblot was more sensitive than *B. henselae* IFA, but there were still infected dogs (PCR+) that were negative by both testing modalities.[111] In addition to the possibility of *Bartonella* spp. transmission by other arthropods, such as ticks, clinicians should be aware that dogs with flea infestations may be exposed to multiple *Bartonella* spp. as a result of a single or sequential flea exposures. Acute and convalescent titers can be used to assess a patient with an acute-onset illness, whereas paired titers are less likely to be valuable for patients with chronic and persistent infection. If serologic testing is performed in dogs, a panel that includes testing for *B. henselae, B. vinsonii* subsp. *berkhoffii, B. rochalimae, B. koehlerae,* and *B. clarridgeiae* would be optimal.[112] In cats, a serologic panel including *B. henselae, B. koehlerae,* and *B. clarridgeiae* should be considered. In the authors' experience, variability in the antigen of *Bartonella* species or strain used for testing may result in different results among laboratories. Measurement of *Bartonella* serum antibodies has a limited ability to help determine whether a sick animal has an active *Bartonella* infection. In both cats and dogs, bacteremia can occur in the absence of detectable antibodies, and seropositive cats and dogs are not always bacteremic. Some dogs that are chronically ill and *Bartonella* spp. nonseroreactive seroconvert after administration of antibiotics, potentially reflecting enhanced antigenic recognition. For example, in one study with 61 naturally infected and sick dogs, only 7 of 19 (36.8%) *B. henselae* and 4 of 10 (40%) *B. vinsonii* subsp. *berkhoffii* infected dogs for which sera were available were seroreactive to *B. henselae* and *B. vinsonii* subsp. *berkhoffii* antigens, respectively. Because of this, serology is not recommended as the sole diagnostic test for canine or feline bartonellosis and should be used and interpreted in conjunction with PCR testing or enrichment culture/PCR.[38]

Pathologic Findings

Gross necropsy of dogs and cats with *Bartonella* endocarditis may reveal evidence of congestive heart failure, with lung congestion and edema. Single or multiple nodules, variably sized, are typically present on the periphery of valvular leaflets, which may be small and firm or large, granular, and friable (Fig. 70.14). White plaques may be found adherent to the adjacent endocardial surfaces. Histopathology reveals chronic inflammation, with fibrous tissue and extensive mineral deposits. The presence of valvular mineralization should raise suspicion for *Bartonella* endocarditis because mineralization is uncommonly associated with endocarditis caused by other bacteria.[45] Small bacilli may be seen within lesions with silver stains or immunohistochemical stains for *B. henselae*.[50,51,72] Silver stains must be interpreted with caution because necrotic debris and nuclear material can mimic positive staining. Gross lesions in the dog with peliosis hepatis consisted of multiple, 0.1- to 0.3-cm cysts in the liver that were filled with cloudy, serosanguineous fluid (Fig. 70.15).[71,72] Nodular granulomatous or pyogranulomatous lesions in the myocardium, kidneys, lymphoid, or other tissues have also been described in animals with bartonellosis (Figs. 70.16 and 70.17),[97,113,114] and nodular pyogranulomatous inflammatory lesions with intralesional bacteria were described in the myocardium and diaphragm of cats with *Bartonella* myocarditis and diaphragmatic myositis (see Fig. 70.5).[51,115]

Cats with acute or chronic experimental *B. henselae* or *B. clarridgeiae* infections had hyperplasia of lymphoid organs, splenic microabscesses,

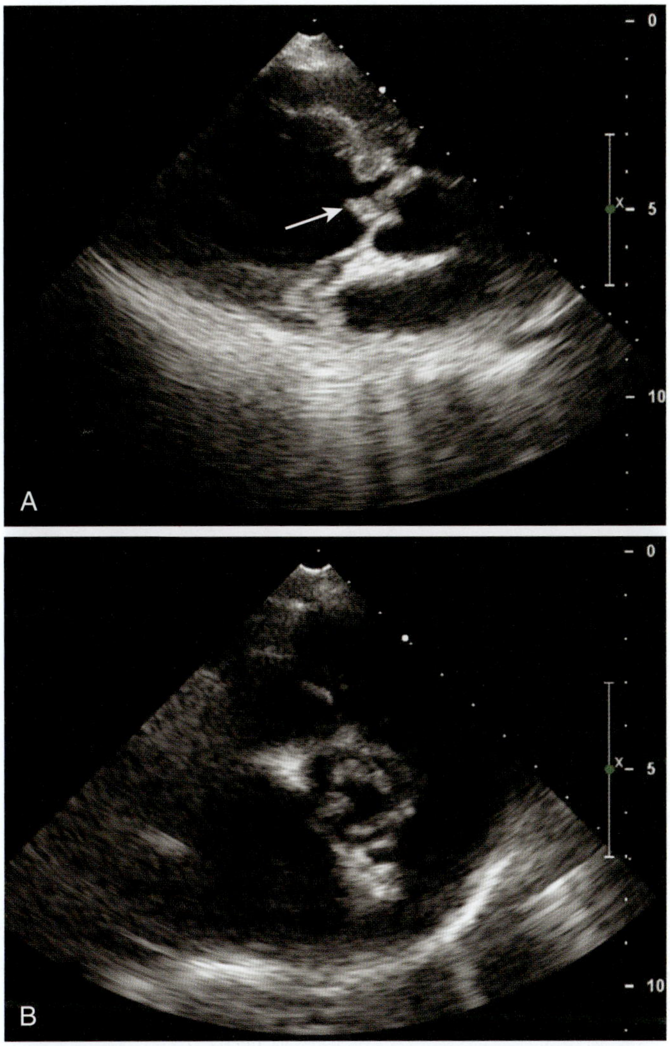

Fig. 70.13 Echocardiogram images from a 13-year-old German shepherd dog with blood culture–negative endocarditis. IFA serology for *Bartonella vinsonii* subsp. *berkhoffii*, *Bartonella clarridgeiae*, and *Bartonella henselae* were positive at titers of 1:512, 1:1024, and 1:128, respectively. On the long-axis view (A) there is an irregular hyperechoic lesion attached to the aortic valve cusps *(arrow)*, and the cusps appear thickened. On the short-axis view (B), the normal "Mercedes-Benz" sign has been destroyed by the aortic valvular thickenings. (From Sykes J. *Canine and Feline Infectious Diseases*. Elsevier; 2014.)

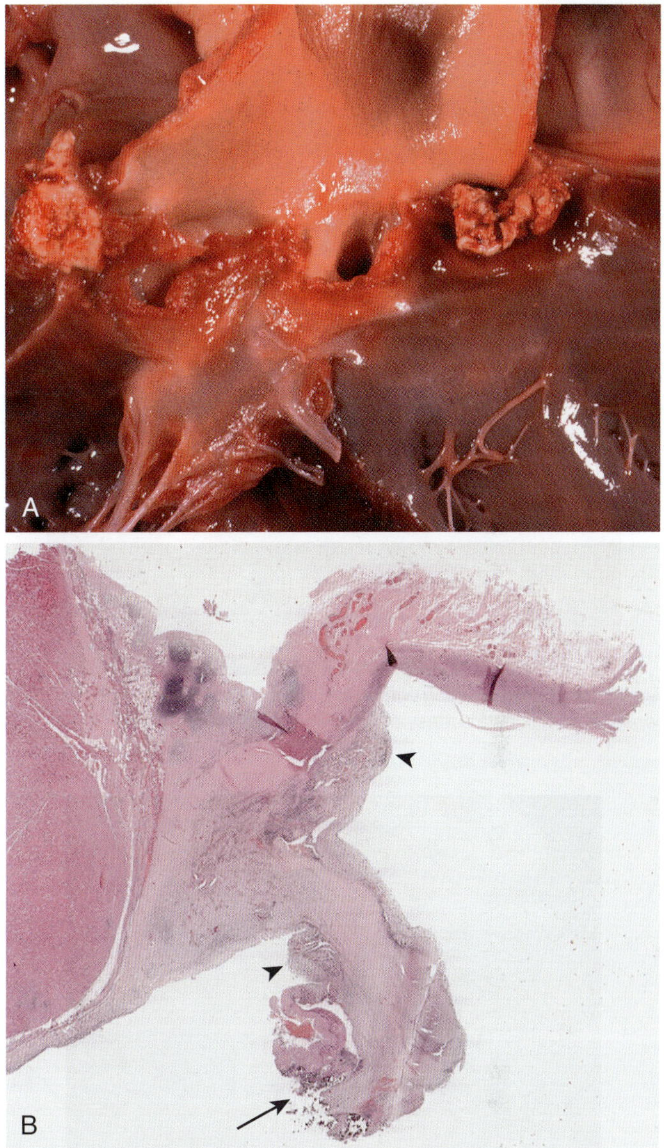

Fig. 70.14 Gross pathologic findings (A) and histopathology (B) of the aortic valve from a dog with *Bartonella* endocarditis. (A) The periphery of the valve is eroded. Variably sized, mineralized nodules expand the valve leaflet. There are multifocal, slightly raised, dull white plaques on the surface of the adjacent aorta and ventricular endocardium. (B) Aortic valve, aorta, and ventricular septum. The distal leaflet is fragmented and contains mineral deposits *(arrow)* and hemorrhage. At the base of the valve, the endothelial surface is lifted and there are broad bands of loose connective tissue, small vessels, and endothelial-lined clefts *(arrowheads)*. Hematoxylin and eosin stain, bar = 180 μm. (Reprinted from Pesavento PA, Chomel BB, Kasten RW, et al. Pathology of *Bartonella* endocarditis in six dogs. *Vet Pathol.* 2005;3:370-373.)

necrotizing granulomatous lesions in lymph nodes, and small foci of pyogranulomatous, neutrophilic, or lymphocytic inflammation in many tissues (including lung, liver, kidney, heart, and spleen) (Figs. 70.18 and 70.19).[16,22]

TREATMENT AND PROGNOSIS

Efficacy has not been established for any antimicrobial for the elimination of *Bartonella* infections in cats or dogs. In humans, the 2015 American and European guidelines for the management of infective endocarditis recommend the use of doxycycline combined with gentamicin for treatment of *Bartonella* infection,[116,117] but clinical improvement has been reported after the use of other antibiotics. A recommendation has been made to avoid the use of fluoroquinolones alone for treatment in humans.[118] Valve replacement is often indicated. Overall, treatment protocols for human *Bartonella* infections vary with clinical presentation and patient immune status.[107,119]

The prognosis for *Bartonella* endocarditis in dogs and cats is generally poor. Only a single case of successful treatment of suspected *B. henselae* endocarditis in a cat has been reported at the time of writing, where marbofloxacin and azithromycin were used for 6 weeks.[120] Supportive care and medications to manage congestive heart failure are often required. *Bartonella* spp. antibiotic resistance or treatment failures have been reported in association with the single use of azithromycin, doxycycline, and fluoroquinolones in dogs,[77,85,118] therefore monotherapy with these antimicrobials is no longer recommended. As bacterial isolation of *Bartonella* spp. is extremely difficult to achieve,

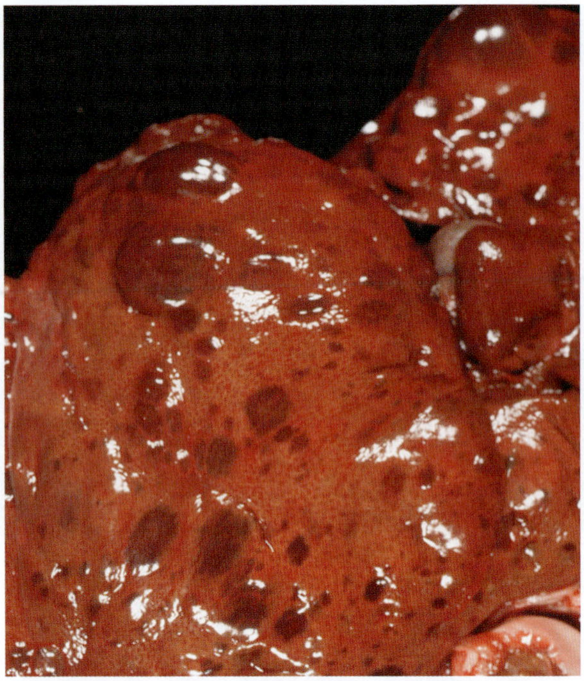

Fig. 70.15 Liver from a dog with peliosis hepatis associated with *Bartonella henselae* infection. (Courtesy of Tim Fan, University of Illinois, Urbana, IL.)

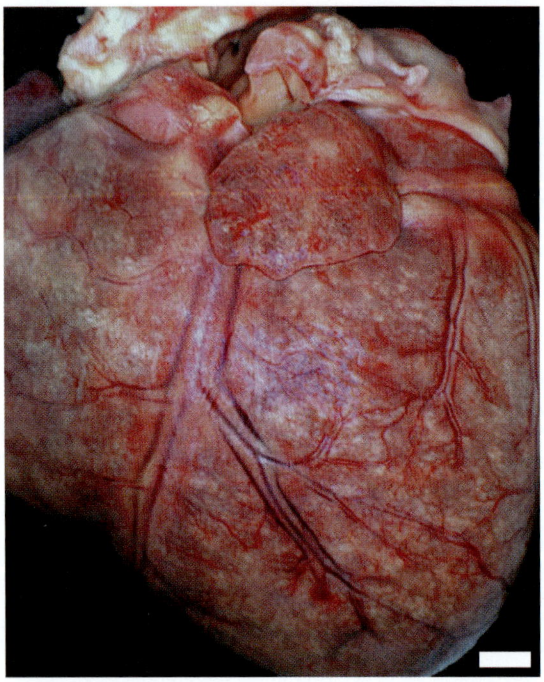

Fig. 70.16 Pyogranumolatous pancarditis associated with *Bartonella henselae* infection in a 6-year-old female spayed American pit bull terrier. Multifocal to coalescing white nodular foci are visible from the epicardium of the right and left ventricles and atria of a dog. Bar = 5 mm. (From Donovan TA, et al. Pyogranulomatous pancarditis with intramyocardial *Bartonella henselae* San Antonio 2 (Bh SA2) in a dog. *J Vet Intern Med.* 2017;31:142-148.)

determining antibiotic resistance patterns is often not possible. This greatly limits our ability to determine the mechanism(s) that are responsible for treatment failures. Oral antimicrobial alternatives for stable animals include high-dose doxycycline in combination with rifampin or fluoroquinolones, alone or in combination with

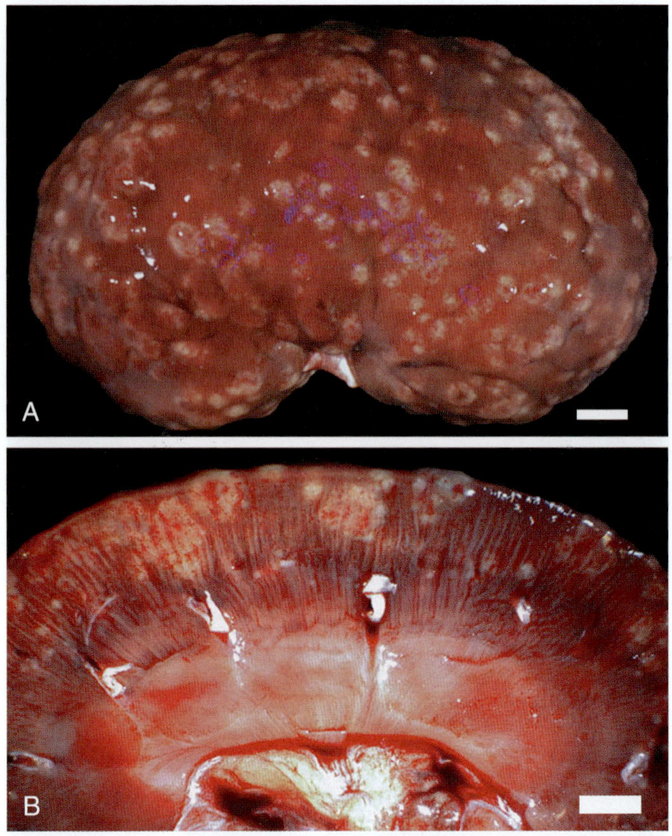

Fig. 70.17 Pyogranulomatous nephritis associated with *Bartonella henselae* infection in a 6-year-old female spayed American pit bull terrier. Visible from the renal cortex are dozens of multifocal to coalescing, tan nodular foci, which range from pinpoint to 1 cm in diameter. Bar = 5 mm. (From Donovan TA, et al. Pyogranulomatous pancarditis with intramyocardial *Bartonella henselae* San Antonio 2 (Bh SA2) in a dog. *J Vet Intern Med.* 2017;31:142-148.)

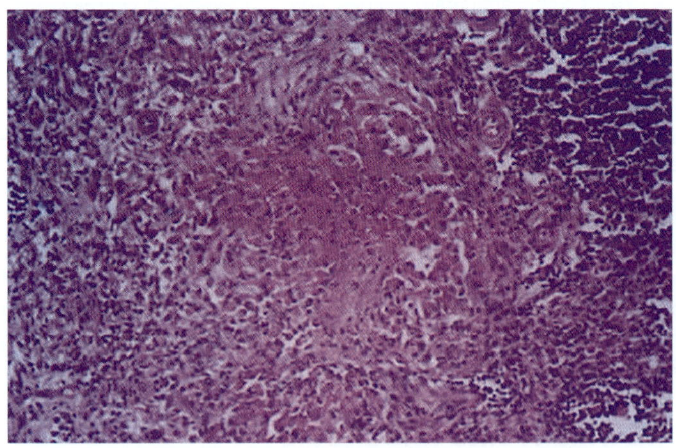

Fig. 70.18 Necrotizing granuloma in the lymph node of a cat infected with *Bartonella henselae*, 56 days following inoculation (hematoxylin and eosin stain, × 200). (Courtesy of Lynn Guptill, Purdue University, West Lafayette, IN.)

amoxicillin (Table 70.3).[121] To avoid a shock-like reaction (Jarisch-Herxheimer reaction) caused by the sudden release of bacterial endotoxins/antigens during the first days of antimicrobial treatment, it is recommended that antibiotics are not started concomitantly. Instead, the second antibiotic should be introduced at least 5 to 7 days after the first one.[121] Dogs with CNS signs have been empirically treated with

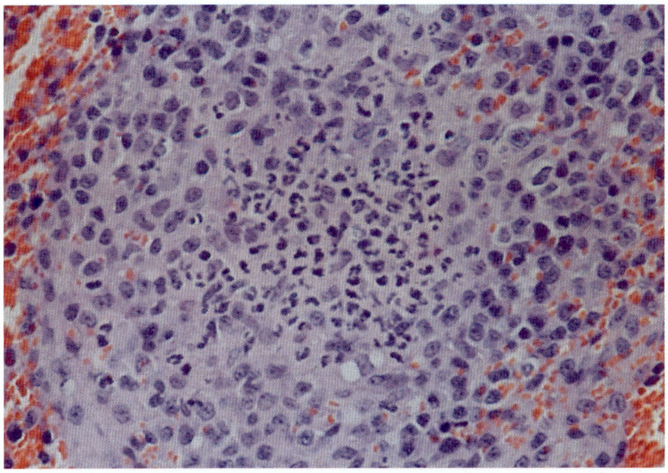

Fig. 70.19 Histologic section of feline spleen showing a microabscess 14 days following inoculation with *Bartonella henselae* (hematoxylin and eosin stain, × 400). (Courtesy of Lynn Guptill, Purdue University, West Lafayette, IN.)

doxycycline and rifampin; however, the use of rifampin in cats should be avoided if other alternatives are available.

Data from experimentally or naturally infected cats indicate that a high dose of doxycycline may be necessary to treat *Bartonella* infection in cats. There is no consensus regarding the best treatment for ill, infected cats, and data from randomized clinical trials are lacking. Initial treatment with doxycycline may be appropriate, with the addition of another antibiotic if this treatment does not appear to be effective. Antibiotic treatment may induce resistant strains of *Bartonella* and other resident microflora, therefore treatment should be reserved for use only in *Bartonella*-positive cats showing clinical signs. While antibiotic treatment reportedly decreases the level of bacteremia in cats, there is no evidence that treatment will decrease the probability of transmission of *Bartonella* to arthropod vectors, other cats, or humans. Care should be taken to avoid scratches or bites when administering drugs to bacteremic cats. Client education is necessary regarding the uncertainty of treatment efficacy, the advisability of long-term follow-up, and the chance for reinfection following treatment. The importance of flea control and other means of preventing transmission (see Prevention) should be strongly emphasized.

IMMUNITY AND VACCINATION

There are no vaccines available for the prevention of bartonellosis in cats or dogs. *Bartonella* evades the host immune system and establishes a persistent intracellular infection. Dogs and cats can be co-infected with multiple different *Bartonella* species, strains, or genotypes. Developing a vaccine is challenging because vaccination and challenge with the same or different *Bartonella* species/strains result in variable protection, and protection is generally specific to the infecting species or even the genotype.[122–124]

PREVENTION

Prevention of *Bartonella* infections in cats and dogs is best accomplished by avoiding exposure to arthropod vectors and infected animals. Vector control measures, such as the use of ectoparasiticides, can interrupt transmission of *B. henselae* among cats and should be maintained year-round for cats and dogs.[48,88] Housing cats indoors may also reduce exposure to fleas. To the extent possible, animal-to-animal contact should be restricted in shows and other group events.[125] *Bartonella* spp. can be transmitted by blood inoculation to cats and dogs, therefore blood donors should be screened for infection. The 2016 ACVIM guidelines on canine and feline blood donor screening recommend the optimal standard as to use dogs and cats that are seronegative and PCR assay or culture negative (Table 70.4). Because of the poor correlation between positive serology and bacteremia, and the high seroprevalence rates in cats, the minimal standard recommended by the ACVIM panel is to use a *Bartonella* spp. PCR-negative donor, regardless of the serology results.[10] However, because *Bartonella* spp. may reside within a healthy animal without evidence of bacteremia, it is important to remember that no currently available screening test can rule out *Bartonella* infection. It is not known how many *Bartonella* seropositive cats that have negative culture as well as PCR test results may be harboring *Bartonella* species. Therefore the most conservative protocol would be to avoid the use of any seropositive animal as a blood donor, even if PCR or BAPGM results are negative.

TABLE 70.3 Treatment Options for Sick Dogs and Cats with Suspected Bartonellosis

Antibiotic Drug	Dose (mg/kg)	Route	Interval (Hours)	Duration (Estimated)[a]
Doxycycline[b]	5–15 (dogs and cats)	PO	12	6 weeks
Amikacin[c]	15–30 (dogs), 10–14 (cats)	IM/IV/SC	24	7–21 days
Rifampin[d]	5 (dogs and cats)	PO	12	4–6 weeks
Enrofloxacin[e]	5 (cats), 5–20 (dogs)	PO	12–24	6 weeks
Pradofloxacin[f]	5–7.5 (cats, oral suspension) 3 (dogs and cats, tablets)	PO	12–24	6 weeks

[a]Longer duration of treatment may be required.
[b]Monotherapy is not recommended at doses below 10 mg/kg every 12h due to the risk of treatment failure. Recommended in combination with enrofloxacin or rifampin. See text for details.
[c]Use in combination with ampicillin (at 10–20 mg/kg every 6–8h) for the initial treatment of endocarditis. Monitor urine and renal values during treatment.
[d]Use in combination with doxycycline; do not treat with rifampin alone because of the likelihood of rapid selection for resistant bacteria. May cause GI adverse effects.
[e]Other fluoroquinolones are preferred in cats due to the higher risk of retinal toxicity with enrofloxacin. A dose of 5 mg/kg every 24h should never be exceeded in cats.
[f]Use in combination with doxycycline. Shorter interval (12h) is recommended. Tablet formulations are approved for dogs outside the United States. See Table 10.7 for details.
IM; intramuscular; IV; intravenous; PO, oral; SC, subcutaneous.

TABLE 70.4 2016 ACVIM Guidelines for *Bartonella* Screening of Blood Donors

Donor Species	Optimal Standard	Minimal Standard	Comments
Dog	Seronegative and BAPGM culture PCR-negative dogs[a]	PCR- negative dogs[a]	Serology results should not be used alone. Instead, they should be combined with PCR results if BAPGM culture is not practical. Conventional culture is not recommended due to poor sensitivity in dogs.
Cat	Seronegative and PCR- or culture-negative cats[a]	PCR- negative cats[a]	If a seronegative cat is difficult to find, a seropositive but PCR-negative cat may be used. Conventional culture can be used in cats.

[a]A broad PCR panel for multiple *Bartonella* spp. is recommended. The minimal standard is to test cats for *B. henselae* and dogs for *B. henselae* and *B. vinsonii* subsp. *berkhoffii*.

BAPGM, *Bartonella* alpha Proteobacteria growth medium.

Modified from Wardrop KJ, et al. Update on canine and feline blood donor screening for blood-borne pathogens. *J Vet Intern Med*. 2016;30:15-35.

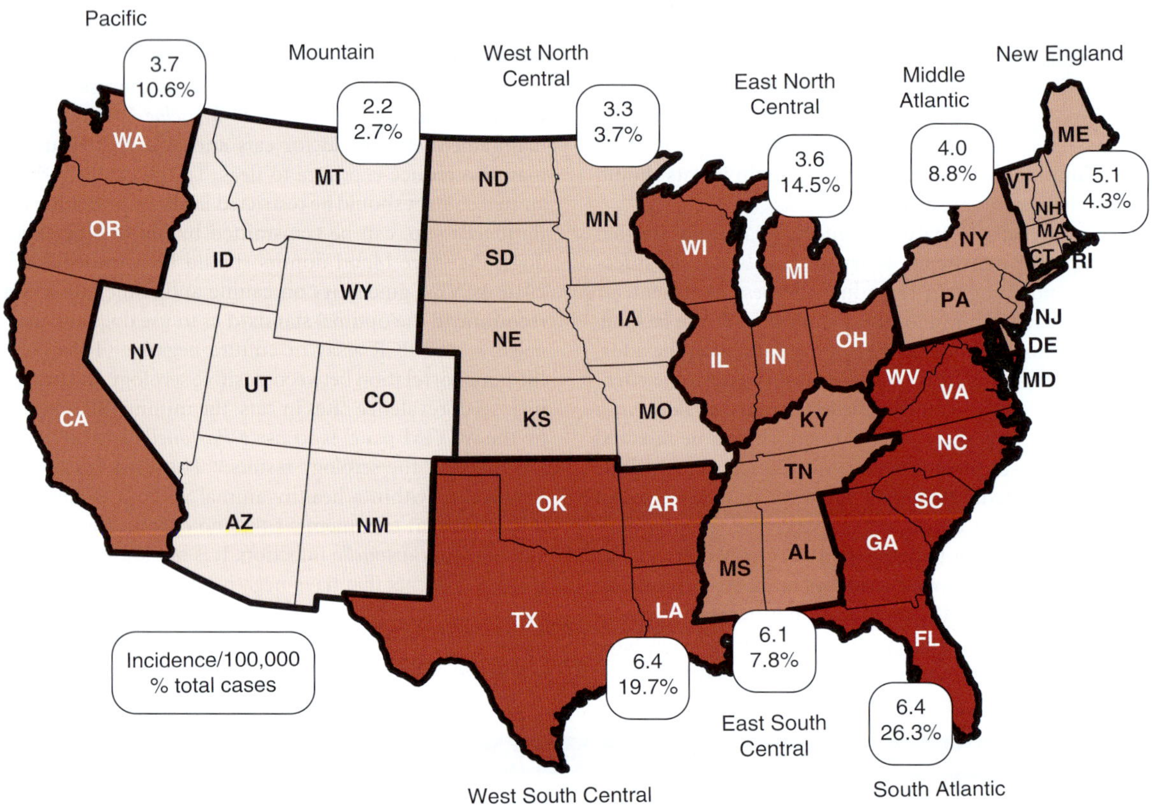

Fig. 70.20 Geographic distribution of cat scratch disease by US census division, United States, 2005–2013. Rates are reported as average incidence per 100,000 population per year. During the study period, there were <10 cases in Alaska and <10 cases in Hawaii. (Modified from Nelson CA, et al. Cat scratch disease in the United States, 2005-2013. *Emerg Infect Dis*. 2016;22:1741-1746.)

PUBLIC HEALTH ASPECTS

Dogs and cats are reservoirs for several zoonotic *Bartonella* species. Cats are a major reservoir for *B. henselae*, the principal cause of CSD in immunocompetent humans, and also serve as a vector for transmission. The average annual incidence of CSD in the United States is 4.5 outpatient diagnoses/100,000 population, with a higher incidence in the southern United States (Fig. 70.20).[126] CSD is characterized by the formation of a papule at the site of inoculation (a cat scratch) within 14 days, followed by the development of local lymphadenopathy (Fig. 70.21) and malaise 1 to 3 weeks after the scratch (or bite), which can persist for weeks to months. Most cases of CSD are self-limiting after several months and respond minimally to antimicrobial drug treatment. Occasionally, CSD is complicated by other disorders such as encephalopathy, relapsing bacteremia, osteomyelitis, neuroretinitis, endocarditis, glomerulonephritis, and other conditions, some of which require antimicrobial drug treatment.[29,116,127–132] Vasculoproliferative diseases such as bacillary peliosis (e.g., peliosis hepatis) and bacillary angiomatosis (Fig. 70.22) are among the most common complications in immunocompromised humans.[15,133] Children from 5 to 9 years of age have the highest incidence for outpatients and inpatients in the US.[126] Young cats are most often implicated in transmission to humans because young cats are more likely to be highly bacteremic than older cats. Dogs are less likely to act as vectors for *Bartonella* spp. when compared with cats, because the prevalence of *Bartonella* infection and the magnitude of bacteremia in dogs are lower than that in cats. Nevertheless, dogs have occasionally

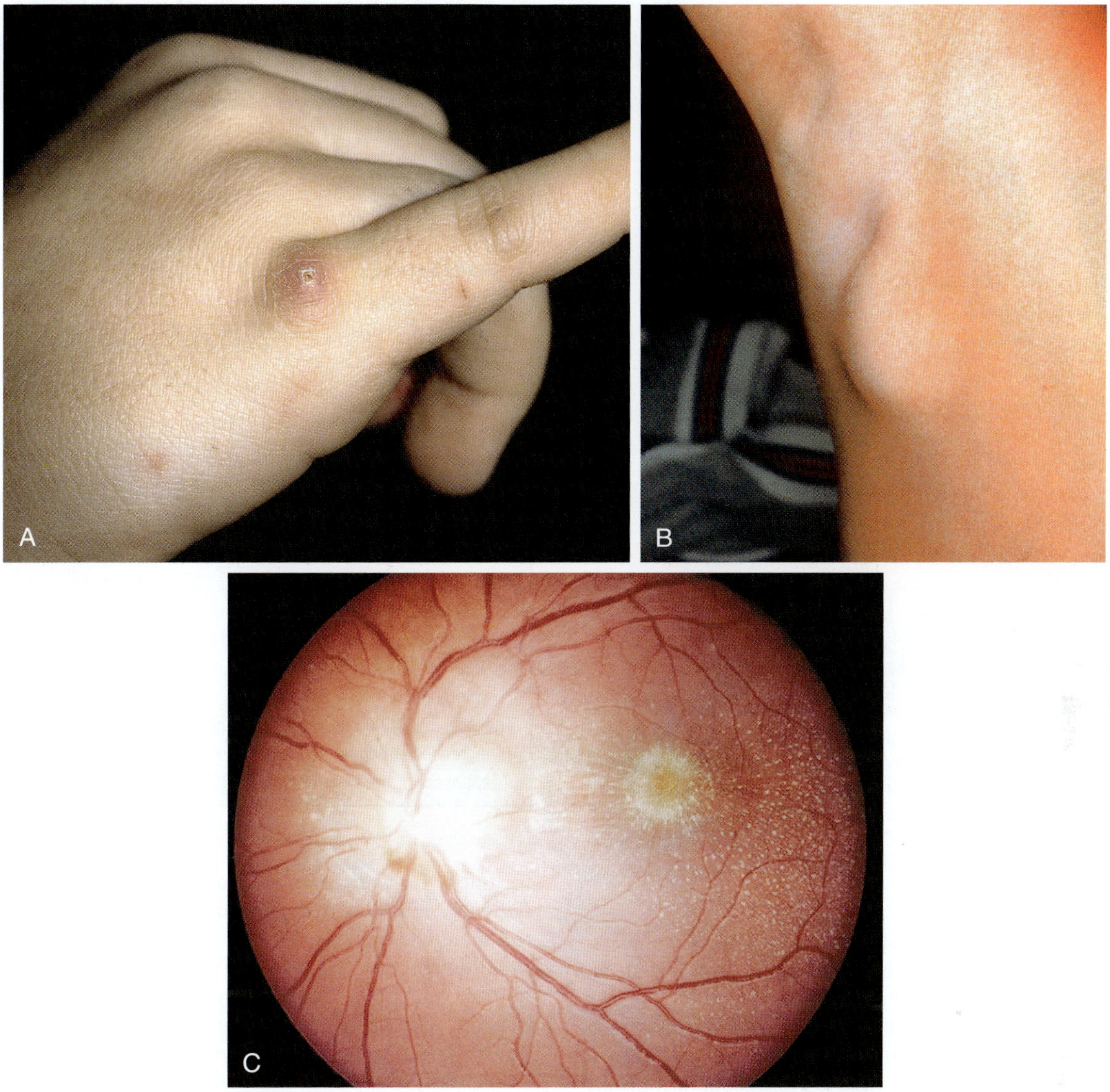

Fig. 70.21 Clinical features of cat scratch disease. (A) Cutaneous lesion at the site of inoculation in an immunocompetent host (7–10 days after a cat scratch and before the onset of local lymphadenopathy). (B) Regional lymphadenopathy in an immunocompetent host. (C) Cat scratch disease neuroretinitis. (A, From Dinulos J. *Habif's Clinical Dermatology: A Color Guide to Diagnosis And Therapy.* 7th ed. Philadelphia, PA: Elsevier; 2021. B, From Paller AS, Mancini AJ. *Hurwitz Clinical Pediatric Dermatology: A Textbook of Skin Disorders of Childhood and Adolescence.* 6th Ed. Philadelphia, PA: Elsevier; 2020. C, From Bennett JE, Dolin R, Nlaser MJ. *Mandell, Douglas, and Bennett's Principles and Practice of Infectious Diseases.* 9th Ed. Philadelphia, PA: Elsevier, 2020.)

been suspected as the source of transmission of *Bartonella* to humans through bite wounds or scratches, and to date, all *Bartonella* species identified in sick dogs are also pathogenic or potentially pathogenic in humans. Immunocompromised people should preferably choose healthy adult, well-socialized cats and dogs that have known health histories as pets over kittens and puppies, and should be properly educated in regard to the need for vector control. Cats' claws should be trimmed regularly, but there is no evidence that declawing prevents transmission. Animal scratches or bites should be avoided, and if they occur, the wounds should be washed thoroughly with soap and water, after which prompt medical attention should be sought. Children should be closely supervised when interacting with pet animals (see Chapter 75). The 2022 guidelines for preventing opportunistic infections among HIV-infected persons from the CDC, National Institutes of Health, and Infectious Diseases Society of America state: "No evidence indicates any benefits to cats or their owners from routine culture or serologic testing of the pet for *Bartonella* infection or from antibiotic treatment of healthy, serologically positive cats."[134] Because there is no antimicrobial drug treatment that is proven to reliably eliminate *Bartonella* infections from cats or dogs, treatment of healthy infected animals is not recommended. The administration of antimicrobial drugs to pets may cause a false sense of security and result in unnecessary bites or scratches. Owners should wear gloves when medicating sick pets. The pros and cons of the testing of healthy cats for *Bartonella* infection are shown in Box 70.1.[88]

Veterinarians and veterinary staff members are at risk for *Bartonella* exposure and infection.[135] *Bartonella* has the potential to be transmitted to veterinarians and staff as a result of scratches, less likely bite wounds as well as needle-stick injuries.[136,137] Veterinarians should avoid these injuries (consider the use of sedation whenever possible), wear gloves when handling any animal with fleas, thoroughly wash wounds that

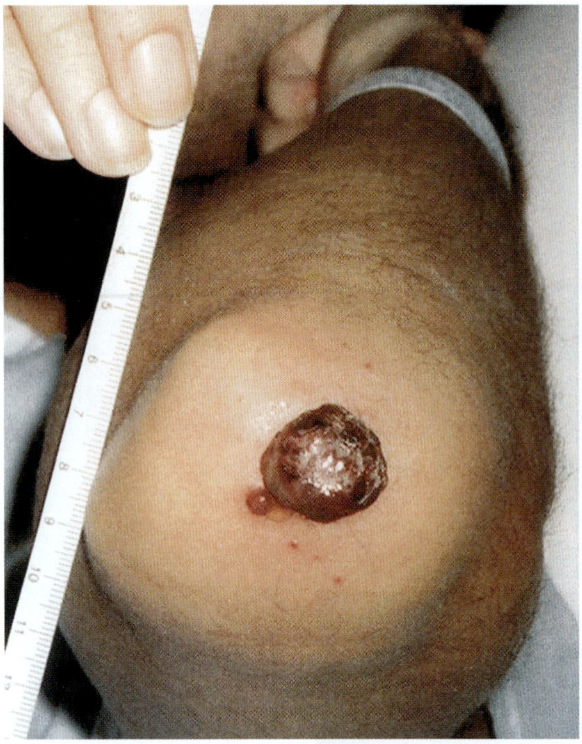

Fig. 70.22 Cutaneous bacillary angiomatosis lesions on the elbow of an AIDS patient. All lesions involuted with doxycycline treatment. (From Slater LN, Welch DF. *Bartonella,* including cat scratch disease. In: Mandell GL, Bennett JE, Dolin R, eds. *Mandell, Douglas and Bennett's Principles and Practice of Infectious Diseases*, 7th ed. Philadelphia, PA: Churchill Livingstone Elsevier; 2010:2995-3009.)

occur, and seek medical attention early if necessary. Gloves should also be worn if skin contact with animal blood or saliva is anticipated, and hand hygiene performed after all animal encounters.

Pet owners should receive printed information that provides a summary of the potential clinical conditions that *Bartonella* may cause in pet dogs and cats and common sense ways to avoid zoonotic transmission. A clear statement of the uncertainty of efficacy of antimicrobial treatment for *Bartonella*, the potential for reinfection of pets with *Bartonella* following treatment, and the need for excellent vector control should be included.

BOX 70.1 Advantages and Disadvantages of Routine Testing of Healthy Cats for *Bartonella* spp. Infection

Advantages

Cats with positive *Bartonella* test results can be eliminated as blood donors or breeding animals.

Compliance with client physician orders.

Disadvantages

Bartonella serology and PCR can be falsely positive or negative.

Some cats with positive serologic test results may have eliminated the infection.

Cats with negative test results may still be bacteremic, or become bacteremic within the near future.

Detection of positive *Bartonella* spp. test results in some situations may lead to needless administration of antibiotics or euthanasia.

A focus on testing may lead to lesser use of effective prevention methods such as flea control.

No treatment reliably eliminates bacteremia in healthy cats.

Antimicrobial drug treatment of cats has not been shown to prevent human infection or benefit healthy infected animals.

Treatment of positive cats may lead to unnecessary life-threatening adverse drug reactions, esophageal strictures (doxycycline), or blindness (fluoroquinolones).

The use of antimicrobials to treat healthy positive cats is likely to lead to increased antimicrobial resistance not just of *Bartonella*, but other microbes exposed to the administered antibiotics.

Although cats and dogs are important reservoirs of *Bartonella*, humans can also develop bartonellosis through other routes of transmission, such as via other arthropods and possibly through blood transfusions.[13] Human body lice primarily transmit *B. quintana* among humans (especially the homeless), which causes relapsing fever (trench fever) and endocarditis.[15]

CASE EXAMPLE

Signalment

"Piper," a 4-year-old neutered male domestic shorthair cat from north-central Indiana.

History

Piper was evaluated at the Purdue University Veterinary Teaching Hospital for ocular abnormalities, lethargy, decreased appetite, and occasional cough and sneezing over 1 week. Piper was obtained one year previously and had been a specific pathogen-free cat prior to adoption. Piper had shown signs of intermittent idiopathic cystitis and two instances of lower urinary tract obstruction/struvite crystalluria, for which he had been treated with catheterization to relieve the lower urethral obstruction, and was fed a prescription diet. Between episodes, he appeared healthy with no other clinical abnormalities. Piper had been housed indoors since adoption. He was neutered at 3 years of age without complication, just before adoption. Five weeks before evaluation, the family had acquired another cat from a pet store; this cat had fleas at the time of acquisition, but was otherwise healthy (Fig. 70.23). Piper was up to date on vaccinations for respiratory viruses, panleukopenia virus, and rabies. He was receiving heartworm preventative monthly and no other medications.

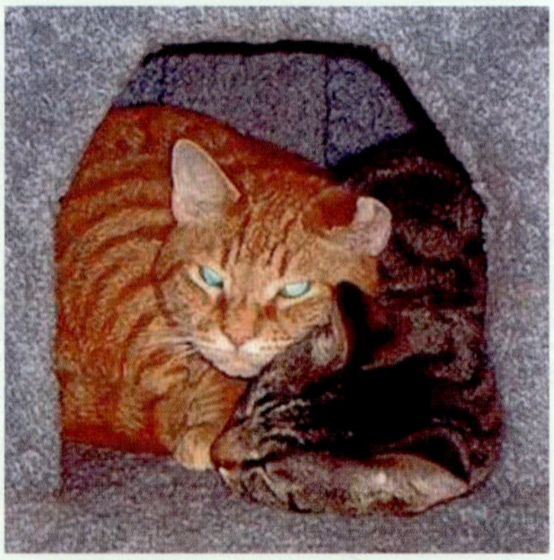

Fig. 70.23 Piper (left) shown in close contact with the newly acquired cat.

CASE EXAMPLE—cont'd

Physical Examination

Body weight: 5.1 kg.

Quiet, alert, responsive, and approximately 5% dehydrated. T = 103.8°F (39.5°C), HR = 160 beats/min, RR = 60 breaths/minute, mildly tacky and pink mucous membranes, CRT <2 s.

Body condition score 5.5/9, ambulatory, adequate muscle mass.

Marked chemosis with erythema, blepharospasm, and serous to mucoid discharge OU. Moderate gingivitis was noted with marked dental tartar. There was no evidence of nasal discharge or abnormal nasal airflow.

Ophthalmologic examination: Positive fluorescein-staining OS with small (1–2 mm) superficial ulcer; negative OD.

Laboratory Findings

CBC: Total protein 8.3 g/dL (6.0–8.0 g/dL), HCT 34% (30%–45%), MCV 41 fL (40–55 fL), MCHC 36 g/dL (30–36 g/dL), WBC 20,500 cells/μL (6000–18,000 cells/μL), neutrophils 18,040 cells/μL (3000–12,000 cells/μL), lymphocytes 1230 cells/μL (1500–7000 cells/μL), monocytes 410 cells/μL (50–850 cells/μL), eosinophils 820 cells/μL (100–1500 cells/μL), basophils 0 cells/μL (0–100 cells/μL), platelets 533,000 cells/μL (300,000–700,000 cells/μL)

Morphology: Enlarged platelets noted.

Treatment

Piper was discharged with oxytetracycline hydrochloride (5 mg/g)/polymyxin B sulfate (10,000 units/g) ophthalmic ointment, to be administered to the eyes q8h, and was treated with subcutaneous fluids.

Follow-Up

Two weeks later, Piper was evaluated again on an emergency basis in the evening for progressive lethargy and decreased appetite since the previous visit.

Physical examination findings were similar to the previous visit except that his eyes were markedly improved. He was more lethargic and was assessed as mildly dehydrated. Temperature was 104.0°F (40°C), pulse was 180 beats/minute, and respiratory rate was 40 breaths/minute. A fluorescein stain was negative OU. Piper received subcutaneous fluids and was discharged with oral amoxicillin, 20 mg/kg q8h, and returned the following day for reevaluation. His physical examination was unchanged (temperature, 104.3°F [40°C], pulse 170 beats/minute, respiratory rate: 20 breaths/minute).

A CBC at that time showed: Total protein 7.2 g/dL (6.0–8.0 g/dL), HCT 25% (30%–45%), MCV 42 fL (40–55 fL), MCHC 34 g/dL (30–36 g/dL), WBC 10,800 cells/μL (6000–18,000 cells/μL), neutrophils 10,040 cells/μL (3000–12,000 cells/μL), lymphocytes 320 cells/μL (1500–7000 cells/μL), monocytes 110 cells/μL (50–850 cells/μL), eosinophils 220 cells/μL (100–1500 cells/μL), basophils 110 cells/μL (0–100 cells/μL), platelets 351,000 cells/μL (300,000–700,000 cells/μL).

Morphology: Anisocytosis 1+, Dohle bodies 1+.

Piper's oral medication was empirically changed to doxycycline, 5 mg/kg PO q12h with water, to be given for 3 weeks, and the ophthalmic ointment was continued.

Piper improved initially, and his CBC results all were within reference ranges 1 week later. Doxycycline and the ophthalmic ointment were continued for the full 3 weeks. Piper did well until clinical signs reoccurred 6 weeks later and he was examined again.

Physical examination at that time showed: T = 104.6°F (40.3°C), pulse = 210 beats/min, RR = 40 breaths/min. Pale mucous membranes, CRT = 2 s. Enlarged popliteal lymph nodes, blood glucose 87 mg/dL via glucometer.

A CBC was repeated and showed: Total protein 7.2 g/dL (6.0–8.0 g/dL), HCT 30% (30%–45%), MCV 42 fL (40–55 fL), MCHC 33 g/dL (30–36 g/dL), WBC 19,600 cells/μL (6000–18,000 cells/μL), neutrophils 16,270 cells/μL (3000–12,000 cells/μL), lymphocytes 2350 cells/μL (1500–7000 cells/μL), monocytes 390 cells/μL (50–850 cells/μL), eosinophils 590 cells/μL (100–1500 cells/μL), basophils 0 cells/μL (0–100 cells/μL).

Platelets were too clumped to count; pathologist review showed adequate platelets, enlarged platelets.

Other morphology: Anisocytosis 1+, poikilocytosis 2+, Heinz bodies 2+, toxic neutrophils 1+, reactive lymphocytes noted; few with 1+ toxicity.

POC FeLV antigen and FIV antibody assay: Negative.

Because of the history of the onset of the febrile illness closely following the introduction of a new cat with fleas into the household, and the recurrence of fever following resolution of the ophthalmologic clinical signs, blood was collected for *Bartonella* culture, PCR, and serology, and doxycycline (5 mg/kg PO q12h, immediately followed by a bolus of water) was prescribed. Infection with *B. henselae* was confirmed by blood culture and PCR of blood. Piper was also seroreactive to *B. henselae*.

Outcome

Piper was evaluated again 2 weeks later and had improved, was no longer febrile or lethargic, and was eating well. Treatment was continued for 6 weeks, and a follow-up CBC showed all results within reference ranges.

Diagnosis

B. henselae bacteremia, likely a result of exposure to fleas from the newly introduced cat, was suspected to be the cause of the recurrent fever and peripheral lymphadenomegaly following resolution of the upper respiratory signs. The upper respiratory signs were suspected to be a result of feline upper respiratory disease, and could have been associated with pathogens such as FCV, FHV-1, *Mycoplasma*, and/or *Chlamydia*, but specific testing was not done for these infectious agents.

Comments

Bartonella infection in this cat was suspected because of fever and lethargy that occurred after the introduction of a new cat that had fleas. Whether the treatment with doxycycline contributed to the resolution of clinical signs cannot be determined. Cats that are experimentally infected with *Bartonella* show fever with lethargy approximately 2 to 4 weeks after inoculation, and this resolves without any treatment.

The owner was educated about the transmission of *Bartonella*, including the zoonotic potential, and the importance of treating flea infestations. Both cats were treated for fleas including preventive medications. The owners were advised to continue to keep the cats indoors, and to use flea preventative medications in the future if the cats' lifestyle changed.

SUGGESTED READINGS

Álvarez-Fernández A, Breitschwerdt EB, Solano-Gallego L. *Bartonella* infections in cats and dogs including zoonotic aspects. *Parasit Vectors.* 2018;11:624.

Nawrocki CC, Max RJ, Marzec NS, et al. Atypical manifestations of cat-scratch disease, United States, 2005-2014. *Emerg Infect Dis.* 2020;26:1438–1446.

Fleischman DA, Chomel BB, Kasten RW, et al. *Bartonella* infection among cats adopted from a San Francisco shelter, revisited. *Applied Environ Microbiol.* 2015;81:6446–6450.

REFERENCES

1. Breitschwerdt EB. Bartonellosis, one health and all creatures great and small. *Vet Dermatol.* 2017;28. 96-e21.
2. Arvand M, Feil EJ, Giladi M, et al. Multi-locus sequence typing of *Bartonella henselae* isolates from three continents reveals hypervirulent and feline-associated clones. *PLoS One.* 2007;2:e1346.
3. Bouchouicha R, Durand B, Monteil M, et al. Molecular epidemiology of feline and human *Bartonella henselae* isolates. *Emerg Infect Dis.* 2009;15:813–816.

4. Bouchouicha R, Boulouis HJ, Berrich M, et al. Comparison of the performances of MLVA vs. the main other typing techniques for *Bartonella henselae*. *Clin Microbiol Infect*. 2009;15(suppl 2):104–105.
5. Chomel BB, Kasten RW, Floyd-Hawkins K, et al. Experimental transmission of *Bartonella henselae* by the cat flea. *J Clin Microbiol*. 1996;34:1952–1956.
6. Boulouis HJ, Chang CC, Henn JB, et al. Factors associated with the rapid emergence of zoonotic *Bartonella* infections. *Vet Res*. 2005;36:383–410.
7. Foil L, Andress E, Freeland RL, et al. Experimental infection of domestic cats with *Bartonella henselae* by inoculation of *Ctenocephalides felis* (Siphonaptera: Pulicidae) feces. *J Med Entomol*. 1998;35:625–628.
8. Reis C, Cote M, Le Rhun D, et al. Vector competence of the tick *Ixodes ricinus* for transmission of *Bartonella birtlesii*. *PLoS Negl Trop Dis*. 2011;5:e1186.
9. Pappalardo BL, Correa MT, York CC, et al. Epidemiologic evaluation of the risk factors associated with exposure and seroreactivity to *Bartonella vinsonii* in dogs. *Am J Vet Res*. 1997;58:467–471.
10. Wardrop KJ, Birkenheuer A, Blais MC, et al. Update on canine and feline blood donor screening for blood-borne pathogens. *J Vet Intern Med*. 2016;30:15–35.
11. Kordick DL, Breitschwerdt EB. Relapsing bacteremia after blood transmission of *Bartonella henselae* to cats. *Am J Vet Res*. 1997;58:492–497.
12. Silva MN, Vieira-Damiani G, Ericson ME, et al. *Bartonella henselae* transmission by blood transfusion in mice. *Transfusion*. 2016;56:1556–1559.
13. Magalhaes RF, Urso Pitassi LH, Lania BG, et al. Bartonellosis as cause of death after red blood cell unit transfusion. *Ultrastruct Pathol*. 2009;33:151–154.
14. Chomel BB, Boulouis HJ, Breitschwerdt EB, et al. Ecological fitness and strategies of adaptation of *Bartonella* species to their hosts and vectors. *Vet Res*. 2009;40:29.
15. Pulliainen AT, Dehio C. Persistence of *Bartonella* spp. stealth pathogens: from subclinical infections to vasoproliferative tumor formation. *FEMS Microbiol Rev*. 2012;36:563–599.
16. Kordick DL, Brown TT, Shin K, et al. Clinical and pathologic evaluation of chronic *Bartonella henselae* or *Bartonella clarridgeiae* infection in cats. *J Clin Microbiol*. 1999;37:1536–1547.
17. Guptill L, Slater LN, Wu CC, et al. Evidence of reproductive failure and lack of perinatal transmission of *Bartonella henselae* in experimentally infected cats. *Vet Immunol Immunopathol*. 1998;65:177–189.
18. Guptill L, Slater L, Wu CC, et al. Experimental infection of young specific pathogen-free cats with *Bartonella henselae*. *J Infect Dis*. 1997;176:206–216.
19. Mikolajczyk MG, O'Reilly KL. Clinical disease in kittens inoculated with a pathogenic strain of *Bartonella henselae*. *Am J Vet Res*. 2000;61:375–379.
20. Chomel BB, Kasten RW, Williams C, et al. *Bartonella* endocarditis: a pathology shared by animal reservoirs and patients. *Ann N Y Acad Sci*. 2009;1166:120–126.
21. Fleischman DA, Chomel BB, Burgos K, et al. Impact of queen infection on kitten susceptibility to different strains of *Bartonella henselae*. *Vet Microbiol*. 2015;180:268–272.
22. Guptill L, Slater L, Wu CC, et al. Immune response of neonatal specific pathogen-free cats to experimental infection with *Bartonella henselae*. *Vet Immunol Immunopathol*. 1999;71:233–243.
23. O'Reilly KL, Bauer RW, Freeland RL, et al. Acute clinical disease in cats following infection with a pathogenic strain of *Bartonella henselae* (LSU16). *Infect Immun*. 1999;67:3066–3072.
24. Bai Y, Gilbert A, Fox K, et al. *Bartonella rochalimae* and *B. vinsonii* subsp. *berkhoffii* in wild carnivores from Colorado, USA. *J Wildl Dis*. 2016;52:844–849.
25. Molia S, Kasten RW, Stuckey MJ, et al. Isolation of *Bartonella henselae, Bartonella koehlerae* subsp. *koehlerae, Bartonella koehlerae* subsp. *bothieri* and a new subspecies of *B. koehlerae* from free-ranging lions (*Panthera leo*) from South Africa, cheetahs (*Acinonyx jubatus*) from Namibia and captive cheetahs from California. *Epidemiol Infect*. 2016;144:3237–3243.
26. Chomel BB, Molia S, Kasten RW, et al. Isolation of *Bartonella henselae* and two new *Bartonella* subspecies, *Bartonella koehlerae* subspecies *boulouisii* subsp. nov. and *Bartonella koehlerae* subspecies *bothieri* subsp. nov. from free-ranging Californian mountain lions and bobcats. *PLoS One*. 2016;11. e0148299.
27. Yamamoto K, Chomel BB, Lowenstine LJ, et al. *Bartonella henselae* antibody prevalence in free-ranging and captive wild felids from California. *J Wildl Dis*. 1998;34:56–63.
28. Chomel BB, Abbott RC, Kasten RW, et al. *Bartonella henselae* prevalence in domestic cats in California: risk factors and association between bacteremia and antibody titers. *J Clin Microbiol*. 1995;33:2445–2450.
29. Chomel BB, Boulouis HJ, Maruyama S, et al. *Bartonella* spp. in pets and effect on human health. *Emerg Infect Dis*. 2006;12:389–394.
30. Berghoff J, Viezens J, Guptill L, et al. *Bartonella henselae* exists as a mosaic of different genetic variants in the infected host. *Microbiol*. 2007;153:2045–2051.
31. Gurfield AN, Boulouis HJ, Chomel BB, et al. Epidemiology of *Bartonella* infection in domestic cats in France. *Vet Microbiol*. 2001;80:185–198.
32. Arvand M, Klose AJ, Schwartz-Porsche D, et al. Genetic variability and prevalence of *Bartonella henselae* in cats in Berlin, Germany, and analysis of its genetic relatedness to a strain from Berlin that is pathogenic for humans. *J Clin Microbiol*. 2001;39:743–746.
33. Chomel BB, Henn JB, Kasten RW, et al. Dogs are more permissive than cats or Guinea pigs to experimental infection with a human isolate of *Bartonella rochalimae*. *Vet Res*. 2009;40:27.
34. Chang CC, Kasten RW, Chomel BB, et al. Coyotes (*Canis latrans*) as the reservoir for a human pathogenic *Bartonella* sp.: molecular epidemiology of *Bartonella vinsonii* subsp. *berkhoffii* infection in coyotes from central coastal California. *J Clin Microbiol*. 2000;38:4193–4200.
35. Breitschwerdt EB, Maggi RG, Chomel BB, et al. Bartonellosis: an emerging infectious disease of zoonotic importance to animals and human beings. *J Vet Emerg Crit Care*. 2010;20:8–30.
36. Henn JB, Vanhorn BA, Kasten RW, et al. Antibodies to *Bartonella vinsonii* subsp. *berkhoffii* in Moroccan dogs. *Am J Trop Med Hyg*. 2006;74:222–223.
37. Yancey CB, Hegarty BC, Qurollo BA, et al. Regional seroreactivity and vector-borne disease co-exposures in dogs in the United States from 2004-2010: utility of canine surveillance. *Vector Borne Zoonotic Dis*. 2014;14:724–732.
38. Lashnits E, Correa M, Hegarty BC, et al. *Bartonella* seroepidemiology in dogs from North America, 2008-2014. *J Vet Intern Med*. 2018;32:222–231.
39. Perez C, Maggi RG, Diniz PP, et al. Molecular and serological diagnosis of *Bartonella* infection in 61 dogs from the United States. *J Vet Intern Med*. 2011;25:805–810.
40. Henn JB, Liu CH, Kasten RW, et al. Seroprevalence of antibodies against *Bartonella* species and evaluation of risk factors and clinical signs associated with seropositivity in dogs. *Am J Vet Res*. 2005;66:688–694.
41. Lashnits EW, Dawson DE, Breitschwerdt E, et al. Ecological and socioeconomic factors associated with *Bartonella henselae* exposure in dogs tested for vector-borne diseases in North Carolina. *Vector Borne Zoonotic Dis*. 2019;19:582–595.
42. Henn JB, Gabriel MW, Kasten RW, et al. Gray foxes (*Urocyon cinereoargenteus*) as a potential reservoir of a *Bartonella clarridgeiae*-like bacterium and domestic dogs as part of a sentinel system for surveillance of zoonotic arthropod-borne pathogens in northern California. *J Clin Microbiol*. 2007;45:2411–2418.
43. Mandle T, Einsele H, Schaller M, et al. Infection of human CD34+ progenitor cells with *Bartonella henselae* results in intraerythrocytic presence of *B. henselae*. *Blood*. 2005;106:1215–1222.
44. Hong J, Li Y, Hua X, et al. Lymphatic circulation disseminates *Bartonella* infection into bloodstream. *J Infect Dis*. 2017;215:303–311.
45. Sykes JE, Kittleson MD, Pesavento PA, et al. Evaluation of the relationship between causative organisms and clinical characteristics of infective endocarditis in dogs: 71 cases (1992-2005). *J Am Vet Med Assoc*. 2006;228:1723–1734.
46. Abbott RC, Chomel BB, Kasten RW, et al. Experimental and natural infection with *Bartonella henselae* in domestic cats. *Comp Immunol Microbiol Infect Dis*. 1997;20:41–51.
47. Chomel BB, Kasten RW, Stuckey MJ, et al. Experimental infection of cats with *Afipia felis* and various *Bartonella* species or subspecies. *Vet Microbiol*. 2014;172:505–510.

48. Bradbury CA, Lappin MR. Evaluation of topical application of 10% imidacloprid-1% moxidectin to prevent *Bartonella henselae* transmission from cat fleas. *J Am Vet Med Assoc.* 2010;236:869–873.
49. Donovan TA, Balakrishnan N, Carvalho Barbosa I, et al. *Bartonella* spp. as a possible cause or cofactor of feline endomyocarditis-left ventricular endocardial fibrosis complex. *J Comp Pathol.* 2018;162:29–42.
50. Chomel BB, Wey AC, Kasten RW, et al. Fatal case of endocarditis associated with *Bartonella henselae* type I infection in a domestic cat. *J Clin Microbiol.* 2003;41:5337–5339.
51. Varanat M, Broadhurst J, Linder KE, et al. Identification of *Bartonella henselae* in 2 cats with pyogranulomatous myocarditis and diaphragmatic myositis. *Vet Pathol.* 2012;49:608–611.
52. Varanat M, Travis A, Lee W, et al. Recurrent osteomyelitis in a cat due to infection with *Bartonella vinsonii* subsp. *berkhoffii* genotype II. *J Vet Intern Med.* 2009;23:1273–1277.
53. Beerlage C, Varanat M, Linder K, et al. *Bartonella vinsonii* subsp. *berkhoffii* and *Bartonella henselae* as potential causes of proliferative vascular diseases in animals. *Med Microbiol Immunol.* 2012;201:319–326.
54. Fontenelle JP, Powell CC, Hill AE, et al. Prevalence of serum antibodies against *Bartonella* species in the serum of cats with or without uveitis. *J Fel Med Surg.* 2008;10:41–46.
55. Lappin MR, Kordick DL, Breitschwerdt EB. *Bartonella* spp antibodies and DNA in aqueous humour of cats. *J Fel Med Surg.* 2000;2:61–68.
56. Sykes JE, Westropp JL, Kasten RW, et al. Association between *Bartonella* species infection and disease in pet cats as determined using serology and culture. *J Fel Med Surg.* 2010;12:631–636.
57. Belgard S, Truyen U, Thibault JC, et al. Relevance of feline calicivirus, feline immunodeficiency virus, feline leukemia virus, feline herpesvirus and *Bartonella henselae* in cats with chronic gingivostomatitis. *Berl Munch Tierarztl Wochenschr.* 2010;123:369–376.
58. Dowers KL, Hawley JR, Brewer MM, et al. Association of *Bartonella* species, feline calicivirus, and feline herpesvirus 1 infection with gingivostomatitis in cats. *J Fel Med Surg.* 2010;12:314–321.
59. Glaus T, Hofmann-Lehmann R, Greene C, et al. Seroprevalence of *Bartonella henselae* infection and correlation with disease status in cats in Switzerland. *J Clin Microbiol.* 1997;35:2883–2885.
60. Lappin MR, Breitschwerdt E, Brewer M, et al. Prevalence of *Bartonella* species antibodies and *Bartonella* species DNA in the blood of cats with and without fever. *J Fel Med Surg.* 2009;11:141–148.
61. Quimby JM, Elston T, Hawley J, et al. Evaluation of the association of *Bartonella* species, feline herpesvirus 1, feline calicivirus, feline leukemia virus and feline immunodeficiency virus with chronic feline gingivostomatitis. *J Fel Med Surg.* 2008;10:66–72.
62. Ueno H, Hohdatsu T, Muramatsu Y, et al. Does coinfection of *Bartonella henselae* and FIV induce clinical disorders in cats? *Microbiol Immunol.* 1996;40:617–620.
63. Breitschwerdt EB, Levine J, Radulovic S, et al. *Bartonella henselae* and *Rickettsia* seroreactivity in a sick cat population from North Carolina. *J Appl Res Vet Med.* 2005;3:287.
64. Bayliss DB, Steiner JM, Sucholdolski JS, et al. Serum feline pancreatic lipase immunoreactivity concentration and seroprevalences of antibodies against *Toxoplasma gondii* and *Bartonella* species in client-owned cats. *J Fel Med Surg.* 2009;11:663–667.
65. Leibovitz K, Pearce L, Brewer M, et al. *Bartonella* species antibodies and DNA in cerebral spinal fluid of cats with central nervous system disease. *J Fel Med Surg.* 2008;10:332–337.
66. Pearce LK, Radecki SV, Brewer M, et al. Prevalence of *Bartonella henselae* antibodies in serum of cats with and without clinical signs of central nervous system disease. *J Fel Med Surg.* 2006;8:315–320.
67. Bettenay SV, Lappin MR, Mueller RS. An immunohistochemical and polymerase chain reaction evaluation of feline plasmacytic pododermatitis. *Vet Pathol.* 2007;44:80–83.
68. Berryessa NA, Johnson LR, Kasten RW, et al. Microbial culture of blood samples and serologic testing for bartonellosis in cats with chronic rhinosinusitis. *J Am Vet Med Assoc.* 2008;233:1084–1089.
69. MacDonald KA, Chomel BB, Kittleson MD, et al. A prospective study of canine infective endocarditis in Northern California (1999–2001): emergence of *Bartonella* as a prevalent etiologic agent. *J Vet Intern Med.* 2004;18:56.
70. Davis AZ, Jaffe DA, Honadel TE, et al. Prevalence of *Bartonella* sp. in United States military working dogs with infectious endocarditis: a retrospective case-control study. *J Vet Cardiol.* 2020;27:1–9.
71. Kitchell BE, Fan TM, Kordick D, et al. Peliosis hepatis in a dog infected with *Bartonella henselae*. *J Am Vet Med Assoc.* 2000;216:519–523, 517.
72. Yager JA, Best SJ, Maggi RG, et al. Bacillary angiomatosis in an immunosuppressed dog. *Vet Dermatol.* 2010;21:420–428.
73. Berkowitz ST, Gannon KM, Carberry CA, et al. Resolution of spontaneous hemoabdomen secondary to peliosis hepatis following surgery and azithromycin treatment in a *Bartonella* species infected dog. *J Vet Emerg Crit Care.* 2016;26:851–857.
74. Southern BL, Neupane P, Ericson ME, et al. *Bartonella henselae* in a dog with ear tip vasculitis. *Vet Dermatol.* 2018;29:537-e180.
75. Duncan AW, Marr HS, Birkenheuer AJ, et al. *Bartonella* DNA in the blood and lymph nodes of golden retrievers with lymphoma and in healthy controls. *J Vet Intern Med.* 2008;22:89–95.
76. Barber RM, Li Q, Diniz PP, et al. Evaluation of brain tissue or cerebrospinal fluid with broadly reactive polymerase chain reaction for *Ehrlichia, Anaplasma*, spotted fever group *Rickettsia, Bartonella*, and *Borrelia* species in canine neurological diseases (109 cases). *J Vet Intern Med.* 2010;24:372–378.
77. Cherry NA, Diniz PP, Maggi RG, et al. Isolation or molecular detection of *Bartonella henselae* and *Bartonella vinsonii* subsp. *berkhoffii* from dogs with idiopathic cavitary effusions. *J Vet Intern Med.* 2009;23:186–189.
78. Weeden AL, Cherry NA, Breitschwerdt EB, et al. *Bartonella henselae* in canine cavitary effusions: prevalence, identification, and clinical associations. *Vet Clin Pathol.* 2017;46:326–330.
79. Hawkins EC, Johnson LR, Guptill L, et al. Failure to identify an association between serologic or molecular evidence of *Bartonella* infection and idiopathic rhinitis in dogs. *J Am Vet Med Assoc.* 2008;233:597–599.
80. Lashnits E, Neupane P, Bradley JM, et al. Molecular prevalence of *Bartonella, Babesia*, and hemotropic *Mycoplasma* species in dogs with hemangiosarcoma from across the United States. *PLoS One.* 2020;15:e0227234.
81. Varanat M, Maggi RG, Linder KE, et al. Molecular prevalence of *Bartonella, Babesia*, and hemotropic *Mycoplasma* sp. in dogs with splenic disease. *J Vet Intern Med.* 2011;25:1284–1291.
82. Perez C, Diniz PPVP, Maggi RG, et al. Canine bartonellosis mimics other tick-borne diseases. In: *Proceedings of the American College of Veterinary Internal Medicine Forum.* 2011:706–707.
83. Perez Vera C, Diniz PP, Pultorak EL, et al. An unmatched case controlled study of clinicopathologic abnormalities in dogs with *Bartonella* infection. *Comp Immunol Microbiol Infect Dis.* 2013;36:481–487.
84. Diniz PP, Billeter SA, Otranto D, et al. Molecular documentation of *Bartonella* infection in dogs in Greece and Italy. *J Clin Microbiol.* 2009;47:1565–1567.
85. Diniz PP, Wood M, Maggi RG, et al. Co-isolation of *Bartonella henselae* and *Bartonella vinsonii* subsp. *berkhoffii* from blood, joint and subcutaneous seroma fluids from two naturally infected dogs. *Vet Microbiol.* 2009;138:368–372.
86. Breitschwerdt EB, Hegarty BC, Maggi R, et al. *Bartonella* species as a potential cause of epistaxis in dogs. *J Clin Microbiol.* 2005;43:2529–2533.
87. Rossi MA, Balakrishnan N, Linder KE, et al. Concurrent *Bartonella henselae* infection in a dog with panniculitis and owner with ulcerated nodular skin lesions. *Vet Dermatol.* 2015;26(60–63):e21–62.
88. Brunt J, Guptill L, Kordick DL, et al. American Association of Feline Practitioners 2006 Panel report on diagnosis, treatment, and prevention of *Bartonella* spp. infections. *J Fel Med Surg.* 2006;8:213–226.
89. Golly E, Breitschwerdt EB, Balakrishnan N, et al. *Bartonella henselae, Bartonella koehlerae* and *Rickettsia rickettsii* seroconversion and seroreversion in a dog with acute-onset fever, lameness, and lymphadenopathy followed by a protracted disease course. *Vet Parasitol: Regional Studies Rep.* 2017;7:19–24.
90. Duncan AW, Maggi RG, Breitschwerdt EB. A combined approach for the enhanced detection and isolation of *Bartonella* species in dog blood samples: pre-enrichment liquid culture followed by PCR and subculture onto agar plates. *J Microbiol Methods.* 2007;69:273–281.

91. Perez C, Diniz PPVP, Maggi RG, et al. Diversity of *Bartonella* species in 62 dogs using the BAPGM pre-enrichment culture method. *J Vet Intern Med.* 2010;24. 759-759.
92. Drummond MR, Lania BG, Diniz P, et al. Improvement of *Bartonella henselae* DNA detection in cat blood samples by combining molecular and culture methods. *J Clin Microbiol.* 2018;56.
93. Alvarez-Fernandez A, Breitschwerdt EB, Solano-Gallego L. *Bartonella* infections in cats and dogs including zoonotic aspects. *Parasit Vectors.* 2018;11:624.
94. Chomel BB, Mac Donald KA, Kasten RW, et al. Aortic valve endocarditis in a dog due to *Bartonella clarridgeiae. J Clin Microbiol.* 2001;39:3548–3554.
95. Cockwill KR, Taylor SM, Philibert HM, et al. *Bartonella vinsonii* subsp. *berkhoffii* endocarditis in a dog from Saskatchewan. *Can Vet J.* 2007;48:839–844.
96. Kelly P, Rolain JM, Maggi R, et al. *Bartonella quintana* endocarditis in dogs. *Emerg Infect Dis.* 2006;12:1869–1872.
97. Gillespie TN, Washabau RJ, Goldschmidt MH, et al. Detection of *Bartonella henselae* and *Bartonella clarridgeiae* DNA in hepatic specimens from two dogs with hepatic disease. *J Am Vet Med Assoc.* 2003;222:47–51. 35.
98. Randell MG, Balakrishnan N, Gunn-Christie R, et al. *Bartonella henselae* infection in a dog with recalcitrant ineffective erythropoiesis. *Vet Clin Pathol.* 2018;47:45–50.
99. Williams M, Rao S, Braff J, et al. Associations between presence of *Bartonella* species deoxyribonucleic acid and complete blood cell count and serum biochemical changes in client-owned cats. *J Vet Intern Med.* 2022; 36:532–540.
100. Diniz PP, Maggi RG, Schwartz DS, et al. Canine bartonellosis: serological and molecular prevalence in Brazil and evidence of co-infection with *Bartonella henselae* and *Bartonella vinsonii* subsp. *berkhoffii. Vet Res.* 2007;38:697–710.
101. Oyama MA. Using cardiac biomarkers in veterinary practice. *Clin Lab Med.* 2015;35:555–566.
102. Saunders GK, Monroe WE. Systemic granulomatous disease and sialometaplasia in a dog with *Bartonella* infection. *Vet Pathol.* 2006;43:391–392.
103. Tucker MD, Sellon RK, Tucker RL, et al. Bilateral mandibular pyogranulomatous lymphadenitis and pulmonary nodules in a dog with *Bartonella henselae* bacteremia. *Can Vet J.* 2014;55:970–974.
104. Tabar MD, Maggi RG, Altet L, et al. Gammopathy in a Spanish dog infected with *Bartonella henselae. J Small Anim Pract.* 2011;52:209–212.
105. Fleischman DA, Chomel BB, Kasten RW, et al. *Bartonella* infection among cats adopted from a San Francisco shelter, revisited. *Appl Environ Microbiol.* 2015;81:6446–6450.
106. Davenport AC, Mascarelli PE, Maggi RG, et al. Phylogenetic diversity of bacteria isolated from sick dogs using the BAPGM enrichment culture platform. *J Vet Intern Med.* 2013;27:854–861.
107. Gutierrez R, Vayssier-Taussat M, Buffet JP, et al. Guidelines for the isolation, molecular detection, and characterization of *Bartonella* species. *Vector Borne Zoonotic Dis.* 2017;17:42–50.
108. Pitassi LH, de Paiva Diniz PP, Scorpio DG, et al. *Bartonella* spp. bacteremia in blood donors from Campinas, Brazil. *PLoS Negl Trop Dis.* 2015;9:e0003467.
109. Maggi RG, Richardson T, Breitschwerdt EB, et al. Development and validation of a droplet digital PCR assay for the detection and quantification of *Bartonella* species within human clinical samples. *J Microbiol Methods.* 2020;176:106022.
110. Balakrishnan N, Cherry NA, Linder KE, et al. Experimental infection of dogs with *Bartonella henselae* and *Bartonella vinsonii* subsp. *berkhoffii. Vet Immunol Immunopathol.* 2013;156:153–158.
111. Neupane P, Sevala S, Balakrishnan N, et al. Validation of *Bartonella henselae* western immunoblotting for serodiagnosis of bartonelloses in dogs. *J Clin Microbiol.* 2020;58:e01335-19.
112. Hegarty BC, Bradley JM, Lappin MR, et al. Analysis of seroreactivity against cell culture-derived *Bartonella* spp. antigens in dogs. *J Vet Intern Med.* 2014;28:38–41.
113. Breitschwerdt EB, Kordick DL, Malarkey DE, et al. Endocarditis in a dog due to infection with a novel *Bartonella* subspecies. *J Clin Microbiol.* 1995;33:154–160.
114. Pappalardo BL, Brown T, Gookin JL, et al. Granulomatous disease associated with *Bartonella* infection in 2 dogs. *J Vet Intern Med.* 2000;14:37–42.
115. Gulbahar MY, Karaca E, Ciftci A, et al. Pyogranulomatous myocarditis and diaphragmatic myositis associated with *Bartonella henselae* in a cat from Turkey. *Veteriner Faku¨ltesi dergisi.* 2019;66:103–107.
116. Habib G, Lancellotti P, Antunes MJ, et al. ESC Guidelines for the management of infective endocarditis: The Task Force for the Management of Infective Endocarditis of the European Society of Cardiology (ESC). Endorsed by: European Association for Cardio-Thoracic Surgery (EACTS), the European Association of Nuclear Medicine (EANM). *Eur Heart J.* 2015;36:3075–3128. 2015.
117. Baddour LM, Wilson WR, Bayer AS, et al. Infective endocarditis in adults: diagnosis, antimicrobial therapy, and management of complications: a scientific statement for healthcare professionals from the American Heart Association. *Circulation.* 2015;132:1435–1486.
118. Biswas S, Maggi RG, Papich MG, et al. Molecular mechanisms of *Bartonella henselae* resistance to azithromycin, pradofloxacin and enrofloxacin. *J Antimicrob Chemother.* 2010;65:581–582.
119. Prutsky G, Domecq JP, Mori L, et al. Treatment outcomes of human bartonellosis: a systematic review and meta-analysis. *Int J Infect Dis.* 2013; 17:e811–819.
120. Perez C, Hummel JB, Keene BW, et al. Successful treatment of *Bartonella henselae* endocarditis in a cat. *J Fel Med Surg.* 2010;12:483–486.
121. Breitschwerdt EB. Bartonellosis of the cat & dog. *Plumb's Therapeutics Brief.* 2015:18–23.
122. Greene CE, McDermott M, Jameson PH, et al. *Bartonella henselae* infection in cats: evaluation during primary infection, treatment, and rechallenge infection. *J Clin Microbiol.* 1996;34:1682–1685.
123. Regnery RL, Rooney JA, Johnson AM, et al. Experimentally induced *Bartonella henselae* infections followed by challenge exposure and antimicrobial therapy in cats. *Am J Vet Res.* 1996;57:1714–1719.
124. Yamamoto K, Chomel BB, Kasten RW, et al. Homologous protection but lack of heterologous-protection by various species and types of *Bartonella* in specific pathogen-free cats. *Vet Immunol Immunopathol.* 1998;65:191–204.
125. Stull JW, Kasten JI, Evason MD, et al. Risk reduction and management strategies to prevent transmission of infectious disease among dogs at dog shows, sporting events, and other canine group settings. *J Am Vet Med Assoc.* 2016;249:612–627.
126. Nelson CA, Saha S, Mead PS. Cat-scratch disease in the United States, 2005-2013. *Emerg Infect Dis.* 2016;22:1741–1746.
127. Ericson M, Balakrishnan N, Mozayeni BR, et al. Culture, PCR, DNA sequencing, and second harmonic generation (SHG) visualization of *Bartonella henselae* from a surgically excised human femoral head. *Clin Rheumatol.* 2017;36:1669–1675.
128. Angelakis E, Lepidi H, Canel A, et al. Human case of *Bartonella alsatica* lymphadenitis. *Emerg Infect Dis.* 2008;14:1951–1953.
129. Kosoy M, Morway C, Sheff KW, et al. *Bartonella tamiae* sp. nov., a newly recognized pathogen isolated from three human patients from Thailand. *J Clin Microbiol.* 2008;46:772–775.
130. Maggi RG, Kosoy M, Mintzer M, et al. Isolation of '*Candidatus* Bartonella melophagi' from human blood. *Emerg Infect Dis.* 2009;15:66–68.
131. Raoult D, Roblot F, Rolain JM, et al. First isolation of *Bartonella alsatica* from a valve of a patient with endocarditis. *J Clin Microbiol.* 2006;44:278–279.
132. Kaufman DL, Kogelnik AM, Mozayeni RB, et al. Neurological and immunological dysfunction in two patients with *Bartonella henselae* bacteremia. *Clin Case Rep.* 2017;5:931–935.
133. Nawrocki CC, Max RJ, Marzec NS, et al. Atypical manifestations of cat-scratch disease, United States, 2005-2014. *Emerg Infect Dis.* 2020; 26:1438–1446.
134. Clinical Info.HIV.gov. Guidelines for the Prevention and Treatment of Opportunistic Infections in Adults and Adolescents with HIV: Recommendations from the Centers for Disease Control and Prevention, the National Institutes of Health, and the HIV Medicine Association of the Infectious Diseases Society of America. 2022. Available at: https://clinicalinfo.hiv.gov/en/guidelines/adult-and-adolescent-opportunistic-infection/.

135. Lantos PM, Maggi RG, Ferguson B, et al. Detection of *Bartonella* species in the blood of veterinarians and veterinary technicians: a newly recognized occupational hazard? *Vector Borne Zoonotic Dis.* 2014;14:563–570.
136. Lin JW, Chen CM, Chang CC. Unknown fever and back pain caused by *Bartonella henselae* in a veterinarian after a needle puncture: a case report and literature review. *Vector Borne Zoonotic Dis.* 2011;11:589–591.
137. Oliveira AM, Maggi RG, Woods CW, et al. Suspected needle stick transmission of *Bartonella vinsonii* subspecies *berkhoffii* to a veterinarian. *J Vet Intern Med.* 2010;24:1229–1232.
138. Reeves WK, Nelder MP, Cobb KD, et al. *Bartonella* spp. in deer keds, *Lipoptena mazamae* (Diptera: Hippoboscidae), from Georgia and South Carolina, USA. *J Wildl Dis.* 2006;42:391–396.
139. Chung CY, Kasten RW, Paff SM, et al. *Bartonella* spp. DNA associated with biting flies from California. *Emerg Infect Dis.* 2004;10:1311–1313.
140. Morales SC, Breitschwerdt EB, Washabau RJ, et al. Detection of *Bartonella henselae* DNA in two dogs with pyogranulomatous lymphadenitis. *J Am Vet Med Assoc.* 2007;230:681–685.
141. Cadenas MB, Maggi RG, Diniz PP, et al. Identification of bacteria from clinical samples using *Bartonella* alpha-Proteobacteria growth medium. *J Microbiol Methods.* 2007;71:147–155.
142. Fenimore A, Varanat M, Maggi R, et al. *Bartonella* spp. DNA in cardiac tissues from dogs in Colorado and Wyoming. *J Vet Intern Med.* 2011;25:613–616.
143. Ohad DG, Morick D, Avidor B, et al. Molecular detection of *Bartonella henselae* and *Bartonella koehlerae* from aortic valves of Boxer dogs with infective endocarditis. *Vet Microbiol.* 2010;141:182–185.
144. Leulmi H, Bitam I, Berenger JM, et al. Competence of *Cimex lectularius* bed bugs for the transmission of *Bartonella quintana*, the agent of Trench Fever. *PLoS Negl Trop Dis.* 2015;9:e0003789.
145. Huang R, Liu Q, Li G, et al. *Bartonella quintana* infections in captive monkeys, China. *Emerg Infect Dis.* 2011;17:1707–1709.
146. Greco G, Zarea AAK, Sgroi G, et al. Zoonotic *Bartonella* species in Eurasian wolves and other free-ranging wild mammals from Italy. *Zoonoses Public Health.* 2021;68:316–326.
147. Cross JR, Rossmeisl JH, Maggi RG, et al. *Bartonella*-associated meningoradiculoneuritis and dermatitis or panniculitis in 3 dogs. *J Vet Intern Med.* 2008;22:674–678.
148. Korhonen E, Pérez Vera C, Pulliainen A, et al. Molecular detection of *Bartonella* spp. in deer ked pupae, adult keds and moose blood in Finland. *Epidemiol Infect.* 2015;143:578–585.
149. Maillard R, Petit E, Chomel B, et al. Endocarditis in cattle caused by *Bartonella bovis. Emerg Infect Dis.* 2007;13:1383–1385.
150. Vayssier-Taussat M, Moutailler S, Femenia F, et al. Identification of novel zoonotic activity of *Bartonella* spp., France. *Emerg Infect Dis.* 2016;22:457–462.
151. Bai Y, Kosoy MY, Boonmar S, et al. Enrichment culture and molecular identification of diverse *Bartonella* species in stray dogs. *Vet Microbiol.* 2010;146:314–319.
152. Donovan TA, Balakrishnan N, Carvalho Barbosa I, et al. *Bartonella* spp. as a possible cause or cofactor of feline endomyocarditis–left ventricular endocardial fibrosis complex. *J Comp Pathol.* 2018;162:29–42.
153. Kumsa B, Parola P, Raoult D, et al. *Bartonella melophagi* in *Melophagus ovinus* (sheep ked) collected from sheep in northern Oromia, Ethiopia. *Comp Immunol Microbiol Infect Dis.* 2014;37:69–76.
154. Marciano O, Gutierrez R, Morick D, et al. Detection of *Bartonella* spp. in wild carnivores, hyraxes, hedgehog and rodents from Israel. *Parasitology.* 2016;143:1232–1242.
155. Gerrikagoitia X, Gil H, Garcia-Esteban C, et al. Presence of *Bartonella* species in wild carnivores of northern Spain. *Appl Environ Microbiol.* 2012;78:885–888.
156. Eremeeva ME, Gerns HL, Lydy SL, et al. Bacteremia, fever, and splenomegaly caused by a newly recognized *Bartonella* species. *N Engl J Med.* 2007;356:2381–2387.
157. Gabriel MW, Henn J, Foley JE, et al. Zoonotic *Bartonella* species in fleas collected on gray foxes (*Urocyon cinereoargenteus*). *Vector Borne Zoonotic Dis.* 2009;9:597–602.
158. Ernst E, Qurollo B, Olech C, et al. *Bartonella rochalimae*, a newly recognized pathogen in dogs. *J Vet Intern Med.* 2020;34:1447–1453.
159. Dehio C, Sauder U, Hiestand R. Isolation of *Bartonella schoenbuchensis* from *Lipoptena cervi*, a blood-sucking arthropod causing deer ked dermatitis. *J Clin Microbiol.* 2004;42:5320–5323.
160. Dehio C, Lanz C, Pohl R, et al. *Bartonella schoenbuchii* sp. nov., isolated from the blood of wild roe deer. *Int J Syst Evol Microbiol.* 2001;51:1557–1565.
161. Adamska M. Wild ruminants in the area of the North-Western Poland as potential reservoir hosts of *Bartonella schoenbuchensis* and *B. bovis. Acta Parasitol.* 2008;53:407–410.
162. Billeter SA, Miller MK, Breitschwerdt EB, et al. Detection of two *Bartonella tamiae*-like sequences in *Amblyomma americanum* (Acari: Ixodidae) using 16S-23S intergenic spacer region-specific primers. *J Med Entomol.* 2008;45:176–179.
163. Leulmi H, Aouadi A, Bitam I, et al. Detection of *Bartonella tamiae, Coxiella burnetii* and rickettsiae in arthropods and tissues from wild and domestic animals in northeastern Algeria. *Parasit Vectors.* 2016;9:27.
164. Blazes DL, Mullins K, Smoak BL, et al. Novel *Bartonella* agent as cause of verruga peruana. *Emerg Infect Dis.* 2013;19:1111–1114.
165. Lin EY, Tsigrelis C, Baddour LM, et al. *Candidatus* Bartonella mayotimonensis and endocarditis. *Emerg Infect Dis.* 2010;16:500.
166. Samsami S, Ghaemi M, Sharifiyazdi H. Molecular detection and phylogenetic analysis of '*Candidatus* Bartonella merieuxii' in dogs and its effect on hematologic parameters. *Comp Immunol Microbiol Infect Dis.* 2020;72:101504.
167. Breitschwerdt EB, Maggi RG, Cadenas MB, et al. A groundhog, a novel *Bartonella* sequence, and my father's death. *Emerg Infect Dis.* 2009;15:2080–2086.

71

Canine Brucellosis

Autumn P. Davidson, Jane E. Sykes

KEY POINTS

- First Described: *Brucella canis* was first isolated from dogs by Leland Carmichael in 1966 (United States).[1]
- Causes: Most commonly *Brucella canis*; rarely *Brucella abortus, Brucella suis,* or *Brucella melitensis. Brucella* organisms are small (1.0 to 1.5 µm), gram-negative, non–spore-forming aerobic coccobacilli.
- Affected Hosts: The *Brucella* genus is composed of 12 classical species based on host preference, phenotypic characteristics, and genetic analysis: *B. abortus* (cattle), *B. canis* (dogs), *B. melitensis* (goats, sheep), *Brucella neotomae* (rodents), *Brucella ovis* (sheep), *Brucella pinnipedialis* (seals), *Brucella ceti* (porpoises, dolphins, whale), *Brucella microti* (voles), *Brucella inopinata* (unknown host), *Brucella papionis* (baboons), *Brucella vulpis* (foxes), and *B. suis* and its biovars (pigs, cattle, hares, rodents, and wild ungulates). Although most *Brucella*, with the exception of the biovars of *B. suis*, show host preference, they can also infect other host species. *Brucella canis* has a limited host range; only dogs and wild Canidae have been found to be susceptible. Rural dogs are susceptible to clinical infection with *B. abortus*, *B. suis*, and *B. melitensis.*
- Geographic Distribution: Worldwide, but infections are most often reported from the southwestern United States, Central and South America, China, and Japan. Sporadic reports have occurred in Canada and throughout Europe. Australia and New Zealand appear to be free of the disease.
- Route of Transmission: Direct mucosal exposure (oral, nasal, conjunctival, venereal) to contaminated body fluids (semen, vaginal discharge, urine, aborted fetuses, and their placentas).
- Major Clinical Signs: Most commonly infertility, abortion, scrotal enlargement secondary to epididymitis/orchitis, scrotal dermatitis, eventual testicular atrophy, lymphadenomegaly, splenomegaly, signs related to discospondylitis (spinal pain, pelvic limb paresis, or paralysis), uveitis, chorioretinitis, rarely osteomyelitis and meningoencephalitis. No signs may be present.
- Differential Diagnoses: Herpesvirus infection, bartonellosis, mycobacterial infections, chronic vector-borne diseases associated with splenomegaly such as ehrlichiosis and babesiosis, coxiellosis, other bacterial and fungal causes of metritis, orchitis/epididymitis, and discospondylitis, intervertebral disc disease, hemic neoplasia (such as lymphoma or multiple myeloma). Additional differential diagnoses for dogs with ophthalmitis include deep mycoses, rickettsial diseases, leptospirosis, and toxoplasmosis.
- Human Health Significance: *Brucella canis* can be transmitted to humans and most often causes mild, influenza-like illness.

ETIOLOGIC AGENT AND EPIDEMIOLOGY

Canine brucellosis is most commonly caused by *Brucella canis*, a small, gram-negative, non–spore-forming aerobic coccobacillus. The genus *Brucella* is named after Major General Sir David Bruce (1855–1931), an Australian-born British microbiologist. David Bruce discovered *Trypanosoma brucei* and worked in the Army Medical Service and the Royal Army Medical Corps. The *Brucella* genus is composed of 12 classical species based on host preference, virulence, phenotypic characteristics, and genetic analysis: *Brucella abortus* (cattle), *B. canis* (dogs), *Brucella melitensis* (goats, sheep), *Brucella neotomae* (rodents), *Brucella ovis* (sheep), *Brucella pinnipedialis* (seals), *Brucella ceti* (porpoises, dolphins, whale), *Brucella microti* (voles), *Brucella inopinata* (unknown host), *Brucella papionis* (baboons), *Brucella vulpis* (foxes), and *Brucella suis* and its biovars (pigs, cattle, hares, rodents, and wild ungulates).[2,3] Factors that define host preference are unknown despite remarkable (~97%) similarity at the genome level.

Members of the Canidae family are the natural hosts of *B. canis. Brucella abortus*, *B. suis*, and *B. melitensis* occasionally cause canine infections but are comparatively rare.[4–7] Even an attenuated vaccine strain of *B. melitensis* or *B. abortus*[8] can infect dogs. Cats can be infected experimentally with *B. canis*, with transient bacteremia, but are relatively resistant. Rabbits and nonhuman primates also have been found to be susceptible to experimental infections. No other animal species has developed significant agglutination titers.[9] Natural infection with non–*B. canis* species is thought to occur after ingestion of contaminated placentas and aborted fetuses from livestock; farm dogs may be predisposed.[10] In recent years, infection of dogs with *B. suis* has been associated with hunting activity and the feeding of raw meat diets[11–13]; a dog in the Netherlands became infected after being fed raw hare meat imported from Argentina. Dogs usually harbor the organisms in the lymph nodes of their GI tracts for extended periods. Dogs are not believed to be as important in the spread and maintenance of these non–*B. canis* infections as their respective farm animal or wildlife reservoirs. However, testing and removal of affected dogs from infected farms, in addition to affected livestock, have been considered the optimal preventive measures for eradication. *Brucella canis* infections are zoonotic, but other species of *Brucella* usually present a greater risk to human health (see Public Health Aspects).[2,14]

Brucellosis caused by *B. canis* is the primary contagious infectious venereal disease of concern in canine reproduction. *Brucella canis* causes reproductive failure in both male and female dogs. Screening for *B. canis* infection is an important part of the pre-breeding and pre-purchase evaluation of any dog (male or female) and should be included in the initial diagnostics in any case of canine abortion, orchitis, epididymitis, and apparent infertility in dogs (failure to conceive, change in semen quality). Because the incidence of canine brucellosis is low in many geographic locations, breeder compliance with regular screening can wane, which makes continued veterinarian vigilance important.[15] Notably, neutered and maiden or virgin dogs can also be infected. Interstate and international shipment of semen as well as dogs can result in brucellosis outside of its endemic regions.[16,17]

Brucella canis can cause systemic disease (often manifested as discospondylitis) in dogs not used for reproduction due to age or neutering status. Dogs with *B. canis* discospondylitis are typically medium- to large-breed dogs, with body weights that range from 14 to 64 kg; dogs have ranged in age from 1 to 8 years, with a median of 4 years in one study.[18,19] Of 22 dogs with *B. canis* discospondylitis known to the authors, 18 (82%) were intact male dogs, 3 (14%) were female spayed, and 1 (4%) was male neutered.[20] Three dogs described in the literature with *B. canis* ophthalmitis did not fit this signalment; one dog was a Pomeranian and none were intact males.[21]

Natural transmission of canine brucellosis occurs by several routes. Transmission of *B. canis* occurs through direct exposure to body fluids that contain sufficient numbers of the bacteria to cause infection (the minimum oral infectious dose for dogs is approximately 10^6 organisms, and the conjunctival dose is 10^4 to 10^5 organisms), most often in semen, lochia, aborted fetuses/placentas, urine, and, to a lesser extent, milk.[9] Mucosal transmission is therefore primarily oral, nasal, or conjunctival and secondarily venereal. Oronasal and conjunctival exposure follows the ingestion or aerosolization of infectious materials. The aerosol route is especially important in crowded kennel or benched dog show conditions.[22]

Infected bitches transmit *B. canis* during proestrus and estrus, at breeding, or after abortion through oronasal contact with vaginal discharges. Transmission is most common by oronasal contact with aborted materials because they contain up to 10^{10} organisms/mL. Shedding of *B. canis* may occur for periods up to 6 weeks after an abortion. Seminal fluid and urine have been incriminated as sources of infection from males that harbor organisms in the prostate and epididymides. The rate of isolation of *B. canis* from the semen of infected dogs is usually high for the first 6 to 8 weeks post inoculation (PI). Intermittent shedding of the organism in low numbers has been noted for up to 60 weeks PI and may continue for at least 2 years. Urinary excretion begins between 4 to 8 weeks after the onset of bacteremia and continues for at least 3 months. Concentrations of 10^3 to 10^6 organisms/mL of urine have been found in males, with lesser numbers of bacteria in the urine of females.[9] At one time, urine of infected males was thought to contain too few organisms to be infectious by the oronasal route; however, studies have demonstrated that *B. canis* can be transmitted from infected to uninfected mature male dogs after several weeks or months of close contact with infected dogs.[23,24] The propensity of males to shed the organism in the urine is probably related to the localization of *Brucella* in the prostate and epididymis, which are in close association with the urinary bladder. Neutering helps reduce this risk to a large extent but does not prevent shedding. Alternative means of transmission occur less frequently under natural circumstances; low numbers of organisms have been found in feces, nasal, and ocular secretions. Brucellae are stable in the environment for up to 2 months in the presence of cooler temperatures and organic debris.[9]

Transplacental transmission and direct cutaneous inoculation can also occur.[25] Although fomite-associated transmission can occur under appropriate circumstances (transmission has been reported after vaginoscopy), *B. canis* is short-lived outside the host and is readily inactivated by common disinfectants, including quaternary ammonium compounds, 1% sodium hypochlorite, 70% ethanol, iodine/alcohol solutions, and accelerated hydrogen peroxide.[9]

Canine brucellosis occurs most commonly as outbreaks in large commercial kennels, and less commonly in privately owned and housed dogs, although exceptions exist.[26–28] Determination of seroprevalence is strongly influenced by the method of testing used and its interpretation. The disease is endemic in the Americas, Africa, and Asia. Although the geographic distribution of canine brucellosis is not fully understood, increased incidence has been seen in the southern-most United States and commonly in Mexico, Central and South America, the People's Republic of China, and Japan.[29,30] These patterns may be associated with an increase in free-roaming, intact dogs. Among breeds in this region, beagles and Labrador retrievers have a higher prevalence of infection, as do feral dogs. Seroprevalence in an Indian reservation in South Dakota was 6.8%, with a gradual decrease in the prevalence over time.[31] Older dogs were more likely to be seropositive than younger dogs. Of 943 dogs entering a Minnesota shelter, 3.5% of owner-surrendered and 3.1% of strays were positive using the 2-mercaptoethanol rapid slide agglutination test (ME-RSAT) assay,[32] but only one positive dog, a dog from Texas, was also positive on AGID. Among Mississippi shelters, the seroprevalence using RSAT followed by ME-RSAT ranged from 0% to 8.6%.[33] In Michigan, prevalence of infection was low in dogs from noncommercial breeders, but infection appeared to be endemic in dogs being produced for pet ownership by commercial facilities.[34] Using a multilocus variable number of tandem repeats (VNTR) analysis (MLVA-13Bc method), 229 isolates of *B. canis* from the United States were grouped into three major clusters and 10 genotype groups.[35] Cluster A mainly contained genotype groups 1 and 2, with some 3 isolates; Cluster B contained group 6 isolates; and the remaining isolates were in Cluster C. Molecular typing methods such as VNTR and MLST are increasingly being applied to investigations of *B. canis* infections in dogs worldwide.[36,37]

There are sporadic reports of canine brucellosis in Canada and throughout continental Europe and the United Kingdom.[17,37–45] Australia and New Zealand appear to be free of the disease and have strict importation requirements in hopes of avoiding establishment of the disease.[46] Evidence of exposure to *B. suis* was detected in one in 10 eastern Australian dogs that had cointact with feral swine.[47] However, because infection with *B. canis* is chronic and subclinical, the organism can readily be imported into regions where the prevalence of disease is low through the movement of subclinically infected dogs. The increased practice and success of canine semen processing for exportation (chilling and cryopreservation) for the purpose of artificial insemination now makes canine brucellosis a concern worldwide, as direct mucosal contact among dogs is no longer necessary for transmission.[16]

CLINICAL FEATURES

Pathogenesis and Clinical Signs

The general sequence of events after infection by *Brucella* is summarized in Fig. 71.1. *Brucella* organisms attach to and penetrate mucous membranes; the severity of disease resulting is proportional to the infectious dose. Because they contain the highest concentration of organisms, vaginal discharge and semen of infected dogs are the most likely sources for infection by mucosal contamination. *Brucella* organisms have the ability to replicate intracellularly and be transmitted to new individuals, maintaining infection within the population of their respective reservoir host. Bacteria are phagocytized at contaminated mucosal sites by tissue macrophages and other phagocytic cells and transported to lymphatic and genital tract tissues where they multiply. After replication in regional lymph nodes, bacteremia occurs within 7 to 30 days after exposure and can persist up to 64 months. *Brucella canis* has a predilection for steroid-dependent (reproductive) tissues; subsequent dissemination to reticuloendothelial cells, the prostate, gravid uterus, testes, epididymides, and placenta occurs. The organism survives facultatively within monocytes and macrophages of the reticuloendothelial system, avoiding or suppressing host bactericidal

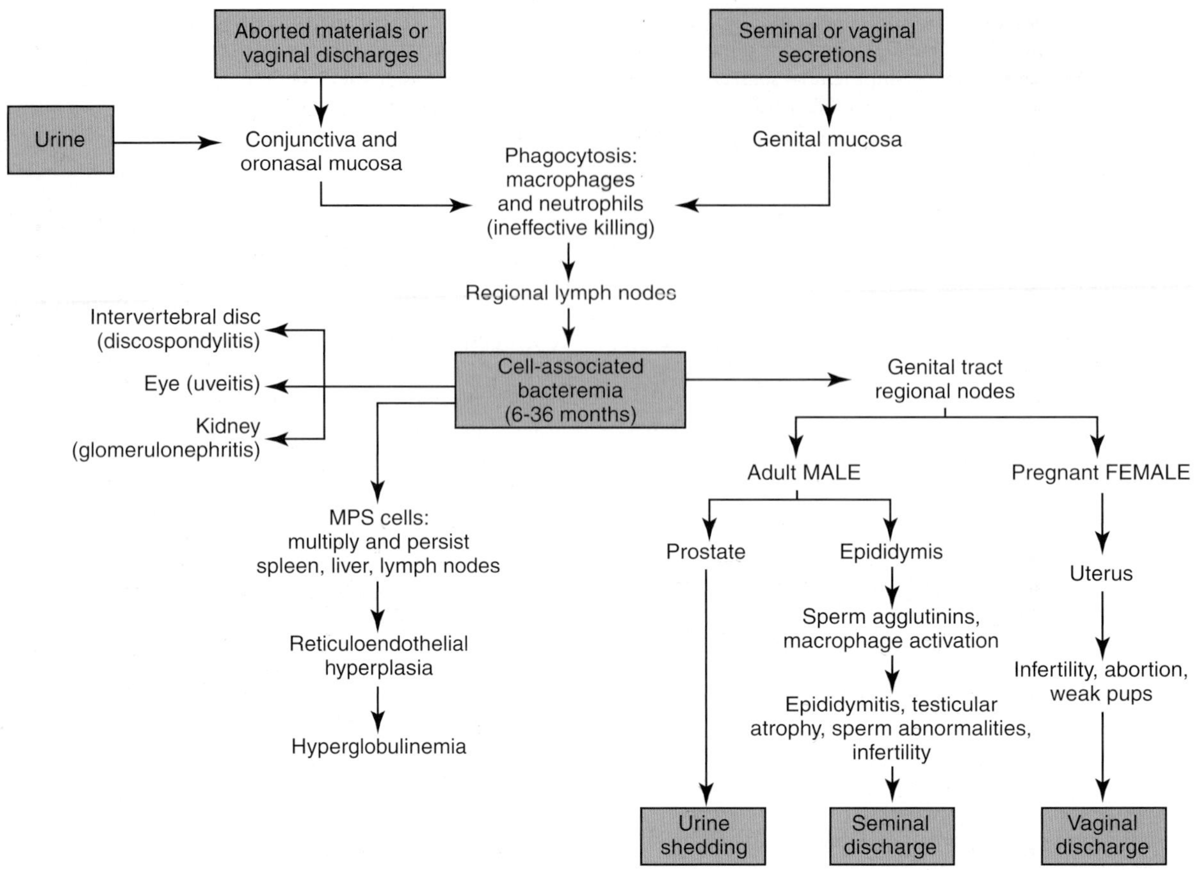

Fig. 71.1 Sequential pathogenesis of canine brucellosis. *MPS,* mononuclear phagocyte system.

mechanisms. *Brucella* organisms survive and multiply in reticuloendothelial cells because they inhibit the bactericidal myeloperoxidase-peroxide-halide system through the release of 5′-guanosine and adenine. The organism inhibits TNF-α, disrupting the bactericidal activity of natural killer cells and macrophages.[48] Early in infection, polymorphonuclear cells and macrophages kill intracellular *B. canis* relatively ineffectually. Generalized lymphoreticular hyperplasia (Fig. 71.2A) and hyperglobulinemia occur during the course of infection. As with other intracellular parasites, CMI is probably the most important defense mechanism against *B. canis.* Persistent, nonprotective antibody titers are characteristic of such infections and appear to have little influence on the level of bacteremia or number of organisms in tissues. The greatest numbers of *B. canis* organisms are found in the lymph nodes, spleen, and tissues of gonadal steroid dependency. Although usually confined to mononuclear phagocytes, they may enter other cells such as placental epithelium.

Brucella organisms can be found in the rough endoplasmic reticulum of placental trophoblastic giant cells in an infected dam's gravid uterus. Severe necrotizing placentitis with infarction of the labyrinth region, coagulation necrosis of the chorionic villi, and necrotizing arteritis result in fetal death. Embryonic death may occur as early as 20 days after mating. The organism can be found in the gastric contents of aborted fetuses. The uterus is not a favored site of growth in the nongravid or diestrual female.

The primary target of *Brucella* in the male dog are the portions of the reproductive tract that participate in the maturation, transport, and storage of spermatozoa. Pyospermia develops 3 to 4 months post infection. Necrotizing vasculitis and granulomatous inflammation results in epididymal and subsequent testicular pathology.[49,50] Microscopic epididymal inflammation usually develops beginning 5 weeks after infection (Fig. 71.2B). Granulomatous inflammation of the epididymides and testes in males causes sperm leakage, which provokes the immune system to produce a complex of anti-sperm agglutinating antibodies and DTH reactions against sperm that are unrelated to the antibodies against *B. canis.* The immune responses produced against spermatozoa further contribute to the epididymitis and orchitis resulting in eventual spermatogenic arrest and testicular atrophy seen in most infected males. Epididymitis and orchitis usually progress despite treatment because of their immunodestructive pathogenesis. The organism can be found in the prostate gland and urethra and is shed intermittently in the urine. The prostate gland may be a site of *Brucella* persistence in intact males for months to years.

Brucella canis, similar to other bloodborne bacteria, may localize in nonreproductive tissues such as the end-arterial circulation of the intervertebral disc, causing discospondylitis (see Chapter 121). Concurrent sacroiliitis was described in one dog.[51] Other tissues that filter bloodborne organisms or immune complexes may become involved, including the eye (anterior uveitis), kidney (glomerulopathy), and meninges (meningoencephalitis).

Spontaneous recovery from infection may occur within 1 to more than 5 years post infection; however, dogs with intervertebral disc or ocular infections, both sequestered from the immune system, usually develop progression of the disease unless it is treated. Antibacterial therapy may accelerate the clinical recovery of all dogs. Some dogs may have persistent bacteremia throughout this time, whereas others can harbor bacteria in tissues for several months after the bacteremia ceases. Despite tissue persistence, when *B. canis* is no longer detected in the blood, serum agglutination titers decrease (see Diagnosis).[52] Dogs that recover naturally have low or negative agglutination titers and yet are immune to reinfection, suggesting that protective immunity is cell

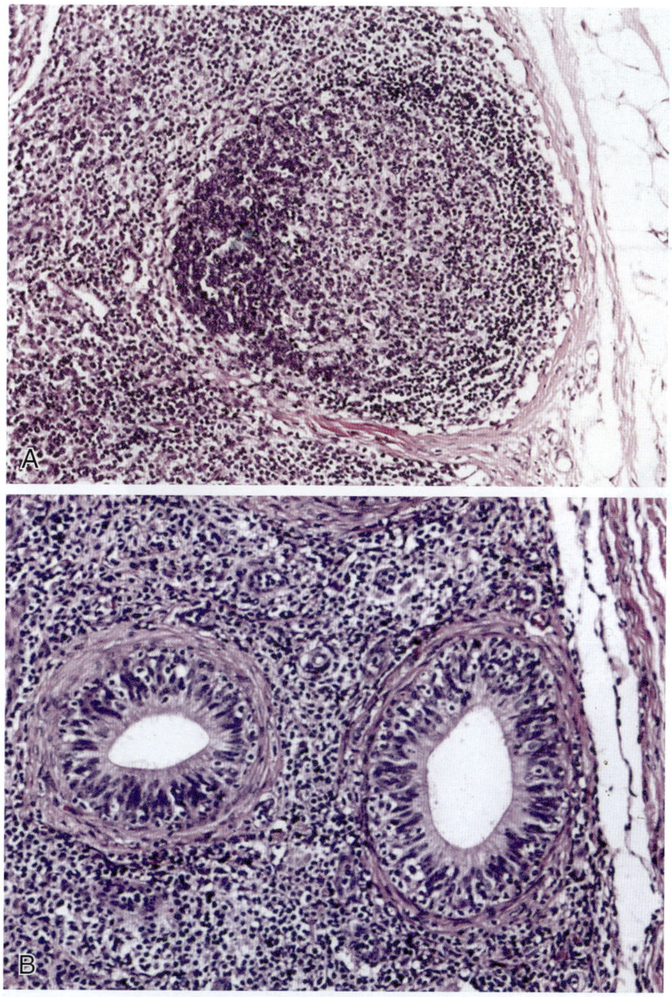

Fig. 71.2 (A) Follicular hyperplasia in the lymph node from a dog with chronic *Brucella canis* infection (hematoxylin and eosin stain, ×40). (B) Inflammatory cells in the head of the epididymis from a dog infected with *B. canis* (hematoxylin and eosin stain, ×40). (Courtesy of Leland Carmichael, Cornell University, Ithaca, NY.)

mediated. Recovered dogs that were challenged orally or IV as long as 4 years after spontaneous recovery from experimental infection were immune.[53] However, chronically infected dogs that were successfully treated with antibacterials were susceptible to oronasal challenge 12 weeks after treatment had been halted. Immunosuppression with glucocorticoids and antilymphocyte serum appears to increase the susceptibility of dogs to initial infection, but it does not augment the severity of the disease or alter the course of infection in experimentally infected dogs.[9]

Despite generalized systemic infection with *B. canis*, adult dogs rarely are seriously ill. The clinical systemic signs are often subtle or absent. Owners of working dogs have occasionally reported dry, lusterless coats, loss of vigor, and suboptimal athletic performance. Nongravid females show no signs of disease other than lymphadenomegaly (pharyngeal if orally acquired, inguinal and pelvic if venereally acquired), which occurs in both sexes. Ocular abnormalities and discospondylitis are frequently present in the absence of other systemic signs of illness. For unknown reasons, ocular abnormalities are often unilateral and include uveitis and multifocal granulomatous chorioretinitis. The most common finding in dogs with discospondylitis is episodic spinal pain resulting in gait abnormalities and lethargy. Meningoencephalitis may result in behavioral changes and neurologic deficits. Chronic multifocal pyogranulomatous

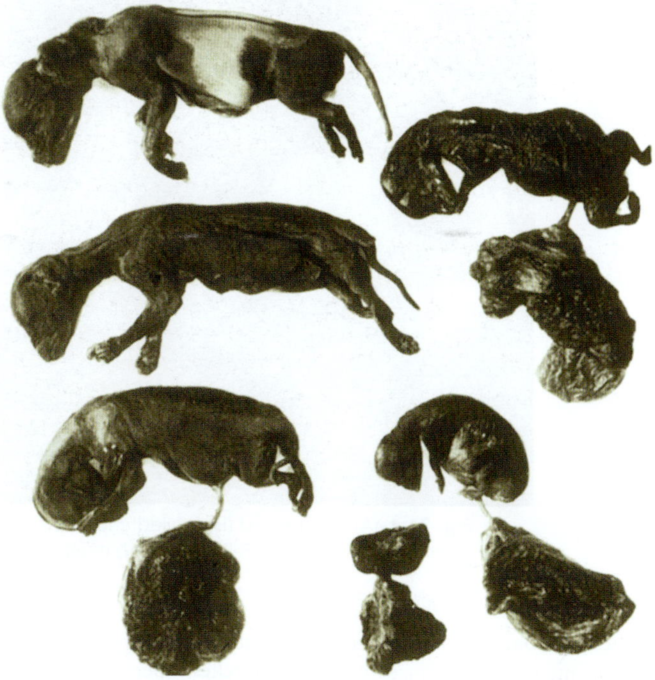

Fig. 71.3 Midterm abortion from a *Brucella canis*–affected bitch. Note the variation in fetal development indicating that death occurred at different stages. (Courtesy of Patricia Olson, DVM, PhD, DACT.)

dermatitis that resembled lick granuloma lesions has also been reported in an infected dog, but a direct causal relationship was not established.[54] Osteomyelitis or polyarthritis of the appendicular skeleton causes lameness of the affected limb. Infection of the bone that surrounded a total hip replacement was described in two dogs, 9 and 12 months after surgery.

Overt clinical signs usually involve reproductive disturbances in sexually mature animals. The primary clinical sign of canine brucellosis in the breeding bitch is pregnancy loss. Bitches usually abort dead pups between 45 and 60 days of gestation but show no other clinical signs. Pups are usually partially autolyzed, with subcutaneous edema and congestion and hemorrhage of the abdominal subcutaneous region. Moderate quantities of serosanguinous peritoneal effusions are found. Their appearance suggests fetal death *in utero* some time before abortion (Fig. 71.3). Decomposed fetuses are not usually found because the bitch ingests them. Abortion is typically followed by a brown or greenish-gray vaginal discharge that lasts for 1 to 6 weeks. Brucellosis should be suspected under any circumstance when apparently healthy bitches abort 2 weeks before term. Less commonly, bitches may carry infected puppies to term and whelp both live and dead puppies within a single litter. Most pups that are born alive will die within a few hours or days, but those that survive or that are infected as neonates usually have generalized peripheral lymphadenomegaly as the primary clinical manifestation of disease until they reach sexual maturity. Such puppies usually have persistent hyperglobulinemia, and some may have transient fever, leukocytosis, or seizures as the systemic manifestations of their infections.[9]

Although abortion of dead puppies is the primary clinical sign of reproductive failure reported with brucellosis, conception failures can occur at any time after breeding. Embryonic death may occur as early as 20 days after mating. Bitches with pregnancy loss early in gestation (resorption) can appear to be infertile (failure to conceive) unless early ultrasonographic pregnancy evaluation was performed to identify pregnancy. As with brucellosis in other species, infections with *B. canis* do not interfere with normal estrous cycles. A high proportion of

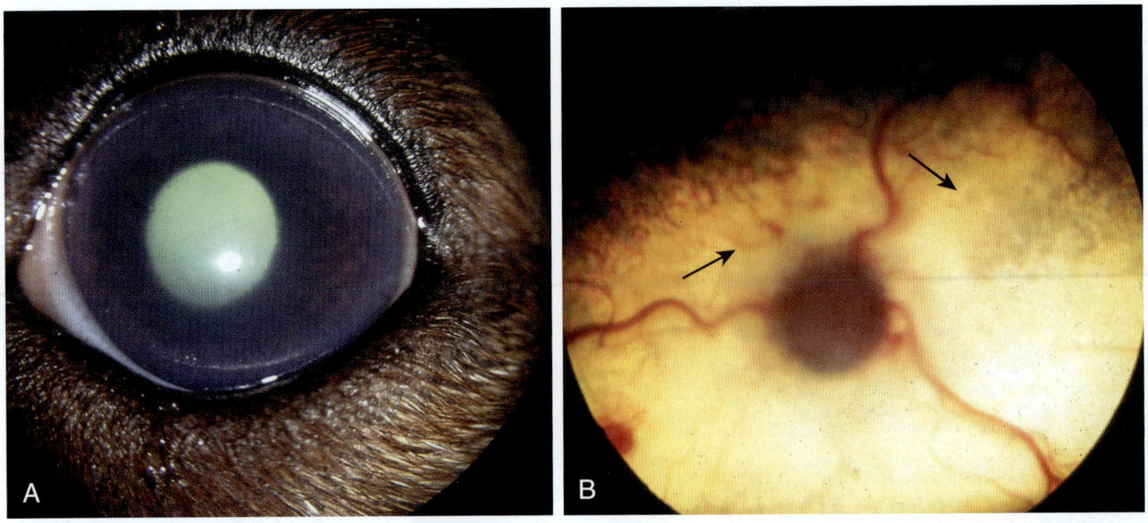

Fig. 71.4 (A) Uveitis and (B) healed chorioretinal lesions *(arrows)* from a dog with brucellosis. (Courtesy of Leland Carmichael, Cornell University, Ithaca, NY and University of Georgia, Athens, GA.)

bitches that abort may have normal litters subsequently. However, even after having normal litters, some infected bitches experience intermittent reproductive failures and remain infectious to their offspring.[55,56]

In male dogs, a variable degree of subfertility progressing to infertility exists in all cases. Small litter size or failure to produce pregnancy can be reported. Libido can be reduced and pain can be associated with ejaculation. A decreased volume of ejaculate is usually present. Clients are often unaware of the physical abnormalities of the epididymides or testes; in contrast, scrotal dermatitis is usually recognized because it causes self-excoriation.

Physical Examination Findings

Fever is uncommon and, with the exception of males, which commonly have physical changes to the external genitalia, most infections will not be diagnosed by routine history or physical examination. Generalized peripheral lymphadenomegaly can be present and splenomegaly may be detected on abdominal palpation. Dogs with meningoencephalitis can exhibit behavioral changes, anisocoria, ataxia, hyperesthesia, head tilt, and circling. Dogs with discospondylitis initially exhibit spinal pain and later paresis and ataxia if spinal cord compression develops. Delayed placing reactions, pelvic limb hyperreflexia, and, uncommonly, pelvic limb paresis or tetraparesis can occur. The presence of splenomegaly or abdominal lymphadenomegaly in dogs with discospondylitis should raise suspicion for *B. canis* infection.

Signs of ocular involvement include blepharospasm, conjunctival hyperemia, evidence of uveitis such as aqueous flare, iris hyperpigmentation, loss of the normal contour of the iris surface, hypopyon, posterior synechiae, and secondary glaucoma. Corneal edema, vitreous opacities, swelling and hyperemia of the optic disc, and evidence of multifocal granulomatous chorioretinitis have also been described (Fig. 71.4).[21,57] Polyarthritis secondary to immune stimulation can be evidenced by joint pain on palpation, decreased range of motion, or lameness.

Affected bitches in diestrus or anestrus can have normal physical examination findings. Because of the prominent testicular abnormalities, male dogs are presented for examination more often than are females. Males otherwise appear to be in good health. Affected dogs commonly have scrotal enlargement early in the course of disease due to epididymitis with or without orchitis (Fig. 71.5). Serosanguinous scrotal edema can be present, as well as scrotal erythema secondary to dermatitis from excoriation or a secondary bacterial dermatopathy (Fig. 71.6). Testicular atrophy and asymmetry are common chronic sequelae.[58]

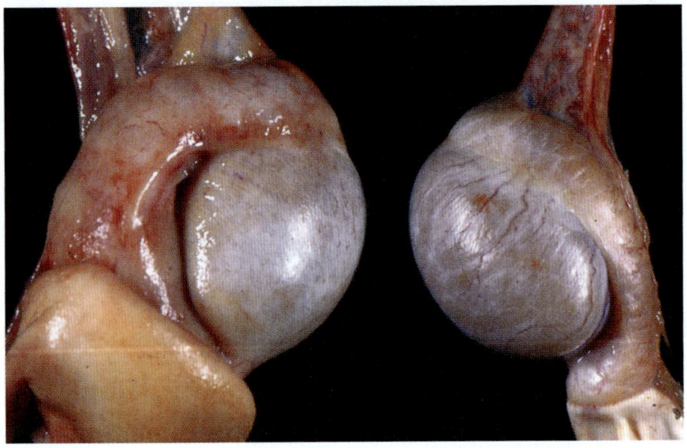

Fig. 71.5 Gross specimens; enlargement of the tail of the epididymis on the testicle from an experimentally infected dog 60 weeks post inoculation *(left)* compared with that of a noninfected dog. (Courtesy of Leland Carmichael, Cornell University, Ithaca, NY.)

DIAGNOSIS (TABLE 71.1)

Laboratory Abnormalities

Hematologic and biochemical values are either unaltered or nonspecific in canine brucellosis.

Complete Blood Count

The CBC may show leukocytosis due to a neutrophilia. Degenerate left shifts, monocytosis, and/or lymphopenia have been uncommonly reported. An increased incidence of positive Coombs' test findings in the absence of anemia has been reported.[9]

Serum Chemistry Profile

The chemistry panel is often normal, but hyperglobulinemia (β and γ) and hypoalbuminemia may be present, especially in chronically infected dogs.

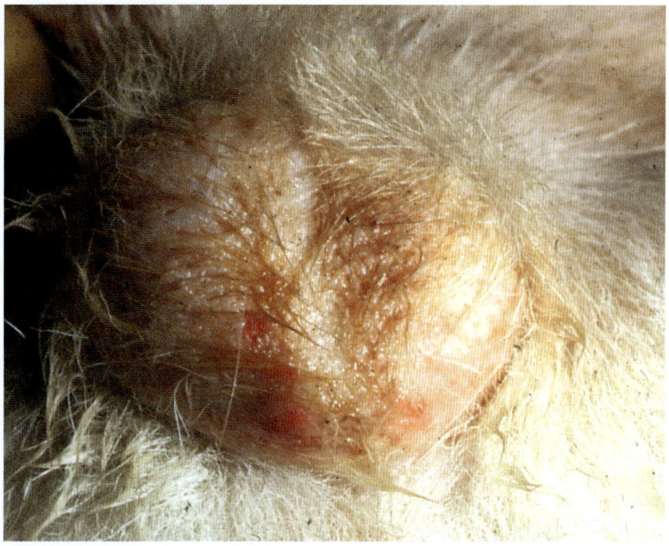

Fig. 71.6 Testicular enlargement and scrotal dermatitis in an experimentally infected dog 35 weeks post inoculation. (Courtesy of Leland Carmichael, Cornell University, Ithaca, NY.)

Urinalysis

The urinalysis is generally within normal limits, even when *B. canis* bacteriuria is present.

Diagnostic Imaging

Plain Radiography

Abdominal radiographs can show splenomegaly in dogs with systemic brucellosis. Plain radiography of the spine can show evidence of either multifocal or focal discospondylitis (Fig. 71.7). Advanced imaging (CT or MRI) may be more sensitive than plain radiography for detection of endplate lucency (Fig. 71.8); see also Chapter 121).

Sonographic Findings

Abdominal ultrasound examination of dogs with brucellosis can show no abnormalities, or abdominal lymphadenomegaly and splenomegaly can be present (Fig. 71.9A and B). Ultrasound of the prostate may reveal prostatic irregularity, hyperechogenicity, and parenchymal cysts typical of intact males. Ultrasound of the scrotum and scrotal contents can confirm the presence of edema of the tunics, epididymal enlargement with hyperechogenicity, testicular enlargement and hyperechogenicity, or atrophy and loss of parenchymal detail (Fig. 71.10).[59]

Microbiologic Tests

Cytologic Diagnosis

Aspirates of the spleen or lymph nodes of dogs with brucellosis reveal lymphoid reactivity on cytologic examination, sometimes with plasmacytosis. Scrotal edema is serosanguinous. Prostatic aspirates in one dog with prostatitis showed granulomatous inflammation with intracellular gram-negative coccobacilli.[42]

CSF analysis in dogs with *Brucella* discospondylitis is usually unremarkable. Pleocytosis, primarily consisting of neutrophils, and increased protein concentration can occur with meningoencephalitis, but they are unremarkable when discospondylitis alone is present.[8] Aspirates of ocular fluids (aqueous or vitreous humor) from a dog with panophthalmitis revealed pyogranulomatous inflammation with extracellular and intracellular small gram-negative cocci.[25]

Semen Examination

Sperm morphology should always be evaluated in dogs with infertility because of the obvious abnormalities that occur with brucellosis. Clinicians should keep in mind the potential infectious nature of semen during collection and evaluation. Semen abnormalities, evident by 5 weeks post infection, become pronounced by 8 weeks. Diminished sperm counts (oligospermia), poor motility (asthenospermia), and increased morphologic abnormalities (teratospermia) are characteristic of semen in dogs infected with *Brucella*, but are not specific for the disease. Detached sperm heads, proximal and distal cytoplasmic droplets, and acrosomal deformities are the most common morphologic abnormalities (Fig. 71.11). By week 15 post infection, sperm head-to-head agglutination suggests the presence of anti-sperm antibodies. Large aggregates of inflammatory cells, usually consisting of neutrophils, surround adherent macrophages containing phagocytized sperm. More than 90% of the sperm are abnormal by 20 weeks post infection. A lack of sperm cells (azoopermia) without inflammatory cells corresponds with the development of bilateral testicular atrophy.

Bacterial Isolation and Identification

Despite improvements in serologic diagnostic methods, blood cultures are still indicated to confirm infection if possible when brucellosis is suspected.[52] A positive *B. canis* culture has been advocated as the best diagnostic test in the first 2 months of the disease; however, dogs can be abacteremic 27 to 64 months after disease onset despite active infection. Isolation of *B. canis* is time consuming but not difficult because the organism grows well aerobically on conventional media used for other *Brucella* spp.. Only a positive result is definitive, because there are numerous reasons for isolation failure. Of the *Brucella* spp. that infect dogs or humans, *B. canis* is the only one with a consistent mucoid (rough) colonial morphology because its cell wall contains truncated LPS moieties. Isolation of the organism from blood, the most practical fluid for isolating the organism, is the most definitive diagnostic procedure. Blood culture should not be the sole test used to diagnose infection because bacteremia, although generally sustained, may be absent or intermittent in more chronically infected animals. Antibacterial administration may interfere with successful isolation of the organism. Blood culture can be helpful if serologic tests are ambiguous. Whole blood must be taken for culture because the organisms are associated with the leukocyte fraction. Bacteremia is detected 2 to 4 weeks after oronasal infection and, if untreated, persists for long periods (1 to 2 years or more). Urine culture is positive in some dogs, especially males, when blood culture is negative; however, unless cystocentesis is performed, urinary isolation of *B. canis* may be difficult because of overgrowth by urethral contaminants. However, urine collected via the urethra may have greater levels of semen, which is a predominant source of *B. canis* organisms. Collection of semen by ejaculation is valuable for culture during the first 3 months of infection, when the concentration of organisms is greatest. With discospondylitis, culture of disc or bone specimens removed at surgery, or material from needle aspiration of the disc space, may also be cultured. Of dogs with *Brucella* discospondylitis or ophthalmitis, 6 of 15 dogs tested positive by blood culture, 3 of 13 by urine culture, and 4 of 6 by culture of disc material or bone chips from the intervertebral disc space obtained at surgery.[19,49]

Brucella canis can be isolated from tissue specimens collected at surgery or necropsy. The lymph nodes, spleen, liver, bone marrow, and male reproductive organs are the most common sources even though gross lesions are seldom present in these organs. In the dam, post-abortion uterus, fetuses, placentas, and vaginal or uterine

TABLE 71.1 Diagnostic Tests Available for *Brucella* Infection in Dogs

Assay	Specimen Type	Target	Performance
Culture	Whole blood, urine, semen, disc aspirates or bone fragments (discospondylitis, osteomyelitis), tissue specimens obtained at laparotomy or necropsy (e.g., spleen, uterus, prostate, testes/epididymides), aborted fetuses and placental tissue	*Brucella* spp. organisms	Confirms infection but is insensitive. Antibiotic treatment can lead to false-negative results. Earliest positive at 2–4 weeks PI.
Histopathology with organism detection using IHC	Tissue specimens above obtained by surgical biopsy or at necropsy	*Brucella* spp. organisms	IHC may have low sensitivity depending on the tissue examined, but supports disease causation when positive and properly performed and interpreted. Earliest at 2–4 weeks PI.
Serology, rapid slide agglutination test (RSAT), and mercaptoethanol (ME-RSAT)	Serum	Antibodies to *Brucella* spp.	Rapid and inexpensive. False positives are common as a result of cross-reactivity with other bacterial species and require confirmation with an alternative test. Positive results do not imply active infection. False-negative results with RSAT can occur in dogs with sequestered infection; e.g., discospondylitis. The sensitivity of the RSAT may be higher than that of the ME-RSAT. ME-RSAT false-negatives 1%. Earliest at 3–4 weeks PI.
Serology, tube agglutination test (TAT), and mercaptoethanol (ME-TAT)	Serum	Antibodies to *Brucella* spp.	See RSAT. Usually positive by 3-6 weeks PI. Semi-quantitative. Titers ≥ 1:200 tend to correlate with bacteremia. ME-TAT usually positive by 5-8 weeks PI, somewhat increased specificity.
Serology, agar gel immunodiffusion (AGID); cell wall/somatic (AGID); internal cytoplasmic	Serum	Antibodies to *Brucella* spp.	Least sensitive for very early infection; very sensitive later. Detects chronic cases well, but can remain positive after recovery. Requires special expertise and is time-consuming to perform. AGID cell wall positive 5–10 weeks PI; cytoplasmic positive 8–12 weeks PI. Cytoplasmic antigen assays are more specific for *Brucella* spp. antigens.
Serology, indirect immunofluorescent antibody (IFA)	Serum	Antibodies to *Brucella* spp.	Requires expertise to perform and interpret. May have lower specificity and sensitivity when compared with TAT or ELISA assays.
Serology, ELISA	Serum	Antibodies to *Brucella* spp.	Has the potential to be sensitive and specific, but assays vary in performance. A standard, accepted assay is not currently available.
PCR	Whole blood, splenic or lymph node aspirates, disc aspirates, tissue specimens obtained at surgery or necropsy, vaginal swabs in proestrus/estrus or when aborting, semen, urine, placental materials, or fetuses.	*Brucella* spp. DNA	Confirms active infection and has the potential to be more sensitive than culture. Sensitivity and specificity may vary depending on assay design, specimen type, and quality assurance practices in the laboratory. Results should be interpreted with caution and in light of the clinical picture and the results of serologic tests and/or culture.

ELISA, enzyme-linked immunosorbent assay; *IHC,* immunohistochemistry; *PCR,* polymerase chain reaction; *PI,* post infection.

fluids most consistently yield positive cultures. False-negative results may occur in chronically infected animals because of extremely low numbers of organisms present. Centrifugation lysis methods may be advantageous under these circumstances because they increase the ability to culture intracellular pathogens.[39] Growth of *Brucella* can be identified on the basis of rough (as opposed to smooth) colony morphology, staining characteristics, and slide agglutination with anti-*Brucella* serum. Identification to the species level is best done by an experienced laboratory. Differentiation between *B. canis* and *B. suis* can be difficult. Recently, MALDI-TOF MS has been useful in assisting with rapid identification of *B. canis.*[60] In the United States, the New York State Diagnostic Laboratory at Cornell University, the Tifton Veterinary Diagnostic and Investigational Laboratory in Georgia, and the University of Florida are recognized to be reliable for definitive testing made necessary by positive *B. canis* screening tests in dogs intended for breeding, or for clinically affected dogs undergoing evaluation for infertility or abortion, or when outbreaks are being managed. Susceptibility testing can be performed, but *in vitro* test results may not correlate well with the *in vivo* treatment response.

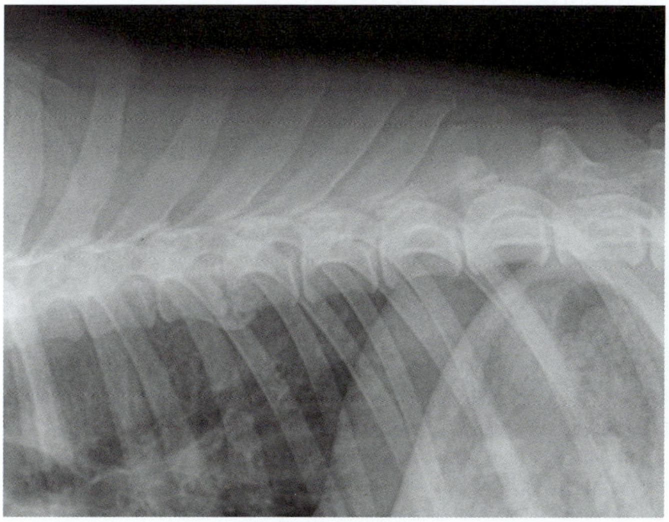

Fig. 71.7 Thoracic radiograph of *Brucella* discospondylitis at the T7-T8 junction with ventral spondylosis and collapse of the intervertebral disc space. (Courtesy of Anna Park, DVM, and James Lavely, DVM, DACVIM [Neurology].)

Serologic Diagnosis

Serologic testing is the most frequently used diagnostic method for detecting canine brucellosis. There are two reasons to perform serologic tests for brucellosis in dogs: (1) as part of a routine screening program in breeding kennels, whereby healthy dogs are screened for infection, and (2) for the initial diagnostics in sick dogs that are suspected to have brucellosis because of infertility, pregnancy loss, epididymitis/orchitis, discospondylitis, ophthalmitis or unexplained lymphadenopathy/splenomegaly.

Assays used for screening purposes are usually rapid and inexpensive, but can suffer from low specificity due to strong cross-reactivity between surface LPS antigens of *B. canis* and those of other less or nonpathogenic infectious agents. Up to 50% to 60% of dogs can have false-positive test results because of cross-reacting antibodies to microorganisms such as *Bordetella, Pseudomonas, Escherichia coli,* and *Moraxella* spp. All sera should be free of hemolysis because hemoglobin causes false-positive agglutination of the tube test antigen.

Even when antibodies detected truly represent anti-*Brucella* antibodies, the presence of these antibodies does not indicate active infection with *Brucella* because dogs can remain seropositive for months after they clear the infection. Antibodies to *Brucella* do not become detectable until 2 to 12 weeks after infection despite the presence of bacteremia at 2 weeks, so a window of time exists in which an infected dog eludes serologic diagnosis with any assay used. For this reason, newly acquired animals should be tested sequentially at least twice at 30-day intervals before introduction into a breeding kennel. Low or intermediate titers may reflect previous or very recent infection, and testing should be repeated, or attempts made to detect the organism by blood culutre or PCR.[60] Males may harbor the organism in the prostate glands and epididymides for extended periods after bacteremia ceases. In such instances, agglutination titers may decline naturally or as a result of treatment, yielding false-negative test results. Beyond the first 3 months of infection, the sensitivity of screening assays is generally believed to be high.

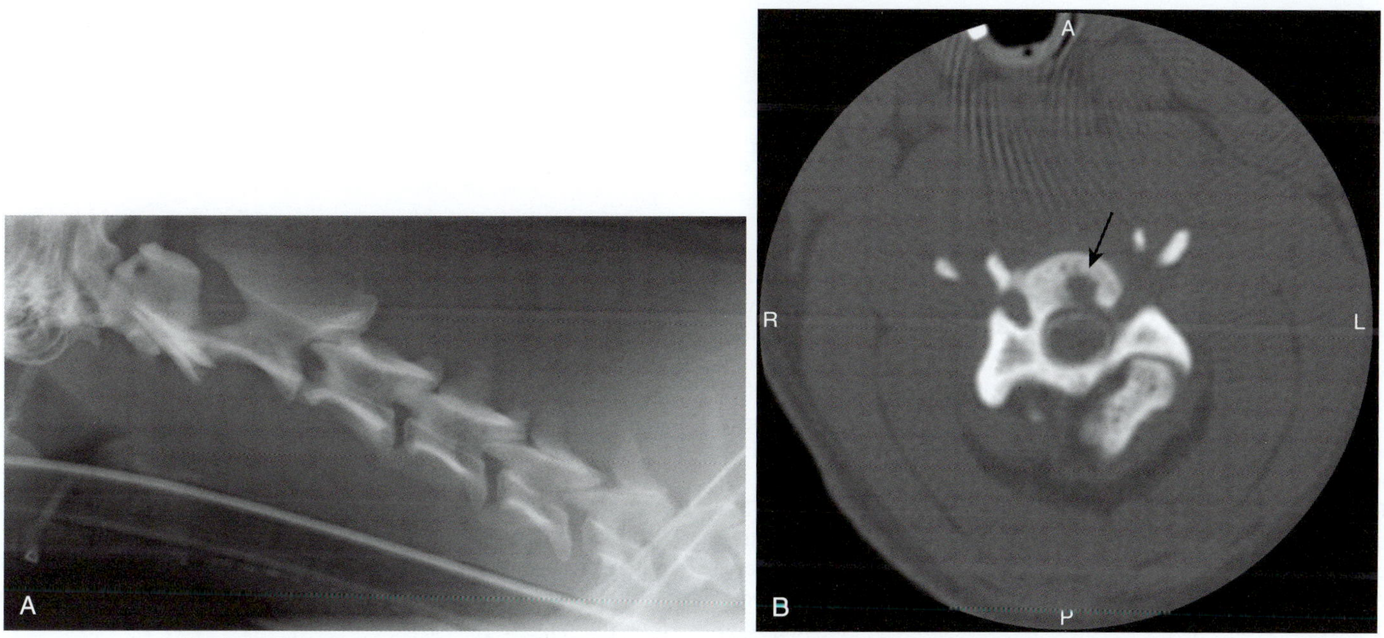

Fig. 71.8 Diagnostic images of a 1-year-old female spayed labradoodle with *Brucella canis* discospondylitis that was initially evaluated for cervical pain. Cerebrospinal fluid (CSF) analysis revealed a CSF protein concentration of 31 g/dL, with 3 nucleated cells/μL, 89% of which were small mononuclear cells and 11% of which were large mononuclear cells (marginal lymphocytic pleocytosis). *Brucella canis* was isolated from five of five blood culture specimens. Urine culture was negative. Of significance, a *B. canis* rapid slide agglutination test was negative. The dog was treated successfully with antimicrobial drugs (doxycycline and clavulanic acid–amoxicillin) and lesions resolved radiographically. (A) Plain lateral radiograph of the cervical spine; with endplate lucency associated with cranial endplate of C3 at the C2-3 articulation. The C2-3 disc space appears narrowed. (B) Computed tomography image; central lysis of the end plates at C2-3 is present *(arrow)*, compatible with discospondylitis at C2-3.

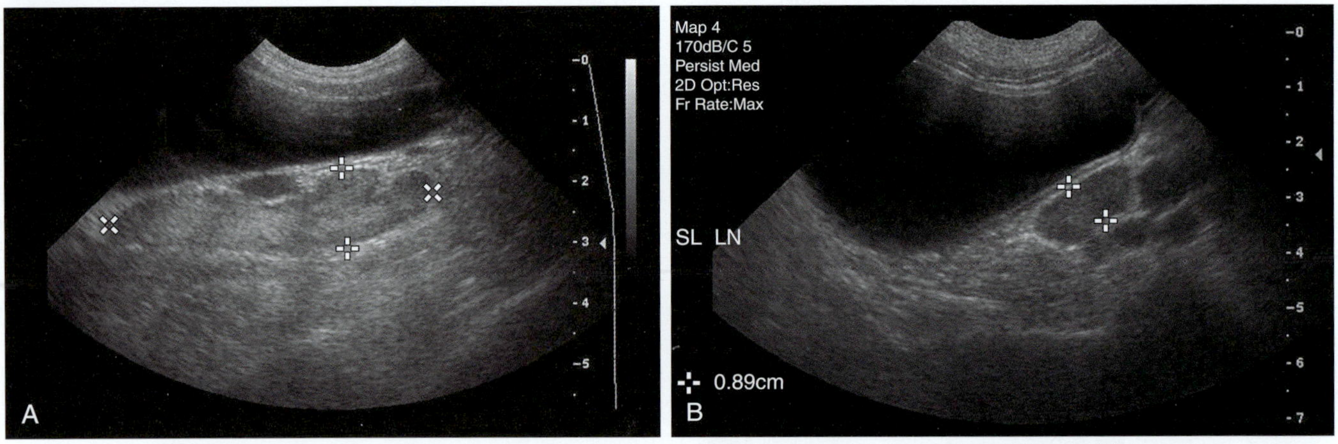

Fig. 71.9 (A) Sagittal ultrasound image of enlarged sublumbar lymph nodes *(cursors)* associated with acute *Brucella* epididymitis in a dog. The node is lobular and hyperechoic to the urinary bladder and blood vessel ventral to it. (B) Transverse ultrasound image of multiple enlarged sublumbar lymph nodes *(cursors)* in a dog with chronic *Brucella* prostatitis. (A,B courtesy of TW Baker.)

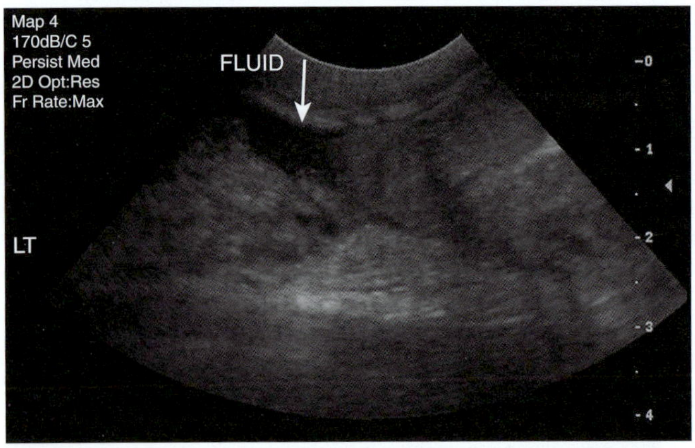

Fig. 71.10 Sagittal ultrasonographic image showing scrotal edema *(arrow)* just cranial to the epididymis and testis in a dog with *Brucella* epididymitis/orchitis. (Courtesy of TW Baker.)

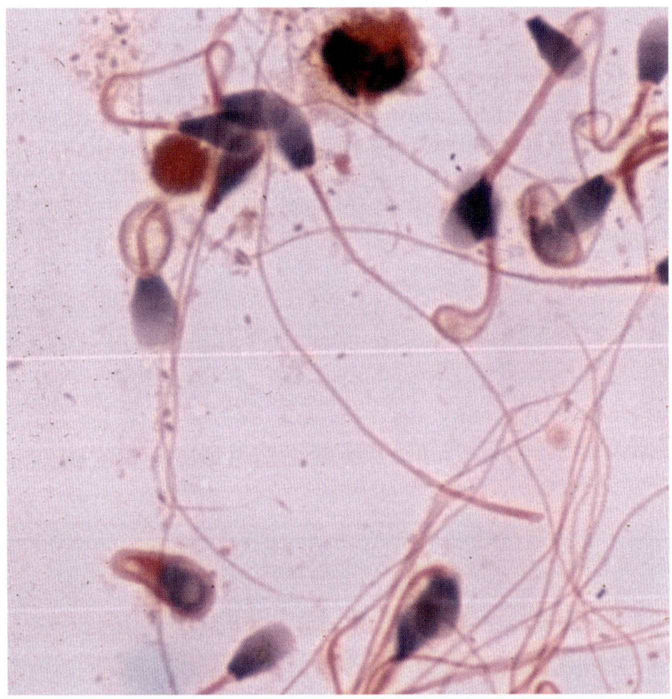

Fig. 71.11 Stained smear of semen specimen from a dog 35 weeks post inoculation. Multiple sperm morphologic abnormalities are present. (Courtesy of Leland Carmichael, Cornell University, Ithaca, NY.)

Examples of screening assays include the RSAT; the semiquantitative ME-RSAT; the semiquantitative tube agglutination test (TAT); AGID assays; and indirect IFA or ELISA assays. Veterinarians need to understand the limitations of the assays available to them through local veterinary diagnostic laboratories or in-house test kits. The RSAT uses *B. ovis* as the antigen, whereas the ME-RSAT uses *B. canis* antigen, which may improve specificity. However, in one study, the sensitivity of the ME-RSAT was only 32%, when compared with 71% for the RSAT, so the RSAT may be preferable for screening.[61] In the TAT, a titer of more than 1:200 correlates well with positive blood cultures, but lower titers are more difficult to interpret. The performance of AGID assays requires trained laboratory personnel and special media. Two AGID assays are available: an assay that uses cell wall antigens as the substrate (cell wall AGID assay) and an assay that uses cytoplasmic antigens of *Brucella* as the substrate (cytoplasmic AGID assay). The cell wall assay has the same low specificity as other assays that detect antibodies to *Brucella* LPS, and the sensitivity may be lower than that of the RSAT.[62] In contrast, the cytoplasmic assay is specific for antibodies to *Brucella*, so, when available, it is a useful confirmatory assay for dogs that test positive with other rapid serologic assays (Fig. 71.12).[63] Indirect IFA has lower sensitivity than many other serologic assays. A number of ELISA assays have been developed to overcome difficulties that relate to the low specificity of serologic assays for *B. canis* and the limited availability of other assays. The performance of these ELISA assays has varied, but sensitive and specific ELISA assays and a lateral flow immunoassay have been developed that may prove useful for rapid serologic testing in the future.[64]

In practice, for screening purposes, healthy bitches are tested at least 1 month before a planned breeding with a serologic assay of low specificity such as the RSAT because these assays are rapid, readily available, and inexpensive. Healthy, fertile stud dogs should be tested at least annually with the RSAT (and require that all bitches be screened and negative before contact breedings). A single high agglutination titer to *B. canis* usually indicates active infection, but this should be substantiated by additional tests. Dogs that are subclinical but have positive results on

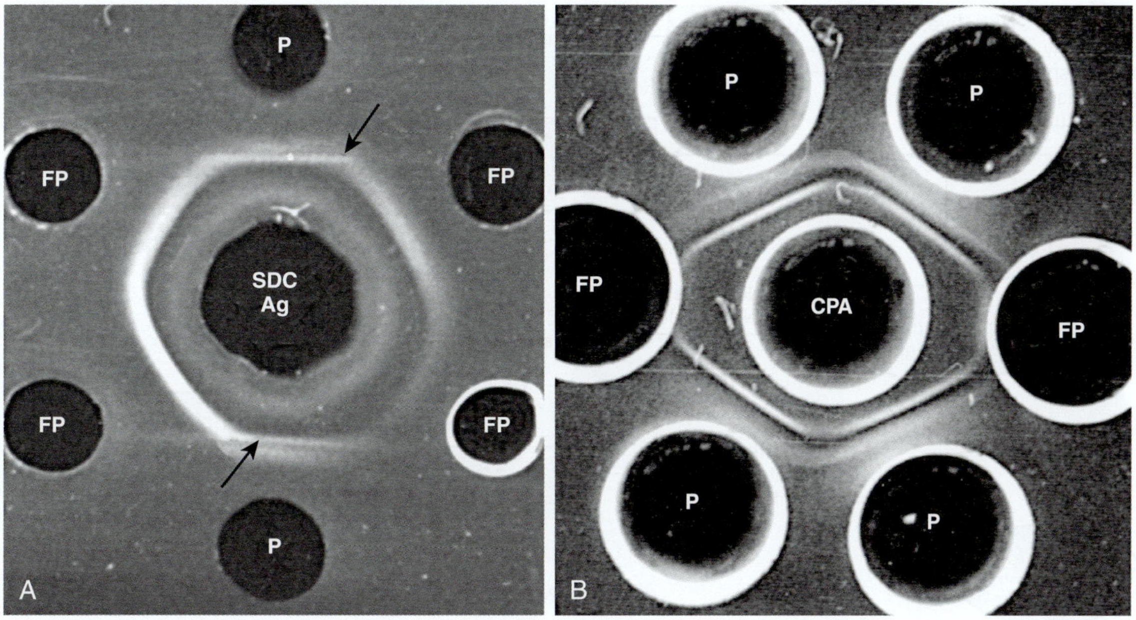

Fig. 71.12 Agar gel immunodiffusion patterns using sodium desoxycholate *(SDC)*-extracted somatic (lipopolysaccharide) antigens reacted with positive *(P)* and false-positive *(FP)* sera. (A) Cross-reactions are evident. *Arrows* indicate *Brucella canis*–specific precipitin line. (B) Cytoplasmic protein antigen *(CPA)*. Precipitin lines occur only with sera from *Brucella*-infected dogs using CPA.

agglutination procedures should never be condemned as infected until blood culture results or the more specific cytoplasmic protein antigen (CPAg) AGID or PCR test results confirm the positive findings.

In cases of subfertility or if recent exposure is suspected and the RSAT result is negative, a second test is performed a month later to assess for seroconversion (which would be expected if the dog was early in the course of infection when first tested); the dog should not be used for breeding in the interim. If the test result is then positive, a confirmatory assay should be performed. This could include the TAT or a more specific assay, such as the cytoplasmic AGID assay, a specific ELISA assay, blood or semen culture (although blood culture can lack sensitivity), or a nucleic acid-detection assay. The use of multiple assays may be required to confirm the diagnosis.

Chronically infected dams may have diagnostically equivocal antibody titers and negative blood cultures. In females, recrudescence of bacteremia and increased antibody titers develop during proestrus, estrus, pregnancy, or abortion. These are the most reliable times to screen subfertile or infertile dams for infection.

Serologic tests should be evaluated in light of clinical findings in the dog being evaluated (Fig. 71.13). Antibacterial therapy may suppress bacteremia and the associated serologic response, possibly contributing to false-negative serologic test results and failure to isolate the organism from infected dogs. Antibacterials should not be given until diagnostic testing has been completed.

Molecular Diagnosis Using Nucleic Acid–Based Testing

A variety of PCR assays have been developed for detection of *B. canis* DNA in clinical specimens. In one study, PCR on whole blood was more sensitive than blood culture or serology for detection of canine infection.[61] PCR assays have been used to successfully identify *B. canis* in semen from dogs with negative culture results, which suggests that this may ultimately be the most sensitive method of testing as part of the male dog pre-breeding evaluation, especially in cases where management of an outbreak is the concern. PCR testing of vaginal swab specimens was more sensitive than blood culture or blood PCR in dams suspected to be infected with *B. canis*.[62] PCR assays were also used to detect *B. canis* in the aqueous humor of dogs with endophthalmitis, and in lymph node aspirates.[21,58] *Brucella canis* DNA has also been detected in multiple tissues from stillborn fetuses and neonates at necropsy. Assays have been designed that differentiate among *Brucella* species.[57] A real-time PCR assay was used to detect *B. canis* in tissue specimens, urine, buffy coat, and intervertebral disc material of a dog with discospondylitis when culture of intervertebral disc material, blood, and urine was negative.[9]

Positive serologic test results in dogs with discospondylitis or other disease manifestations suggestive of brucellosis should be confirmed using culture or a NAAT whenever possible. Although uncommon, false-negative serologic test results can occur in dogs with discospondylitis, so attempts should also be made to detect the organism with culture or NAATs. Of various dogs with *B. canis* discospondylitis or ophthalmitis, 15 of 18 were positive with the RSAT, 16 of 16 were positive with the TAT, and 6 of 7 were positive with AGID assays. The three dogs that were negative with the RSAT had discospondylitis. One was positive by blood culture, and the other two dogs tested positive with the TAT at a later date.[19,21]

Further studies are needed in dogs to determine if PCR methods can be used as a predictor of successful eradication of the organism. Several veterinary diagnostic laboratories in the United States as well as veterinary academic laboratories now offer real-time PCR assays for detection of *B. canis* on a commercial basis.

Pathologic Findings

Gross Pathologic Findings

Macroscopic changes in adults or surviving pups are usually confined to lymphadenomegaly and splenomegaly.

Histopathologic Findings

Lymph node enlargement is the result of diffuse lymphoreticular hyperplasia. In dogs with chronic bacteremia, lymph node sinusoids and the spleen are filled with plasma cells and macrophages containing phagocytized bacteria. Diffuse submucosal lymphocytic infiltration occurs in

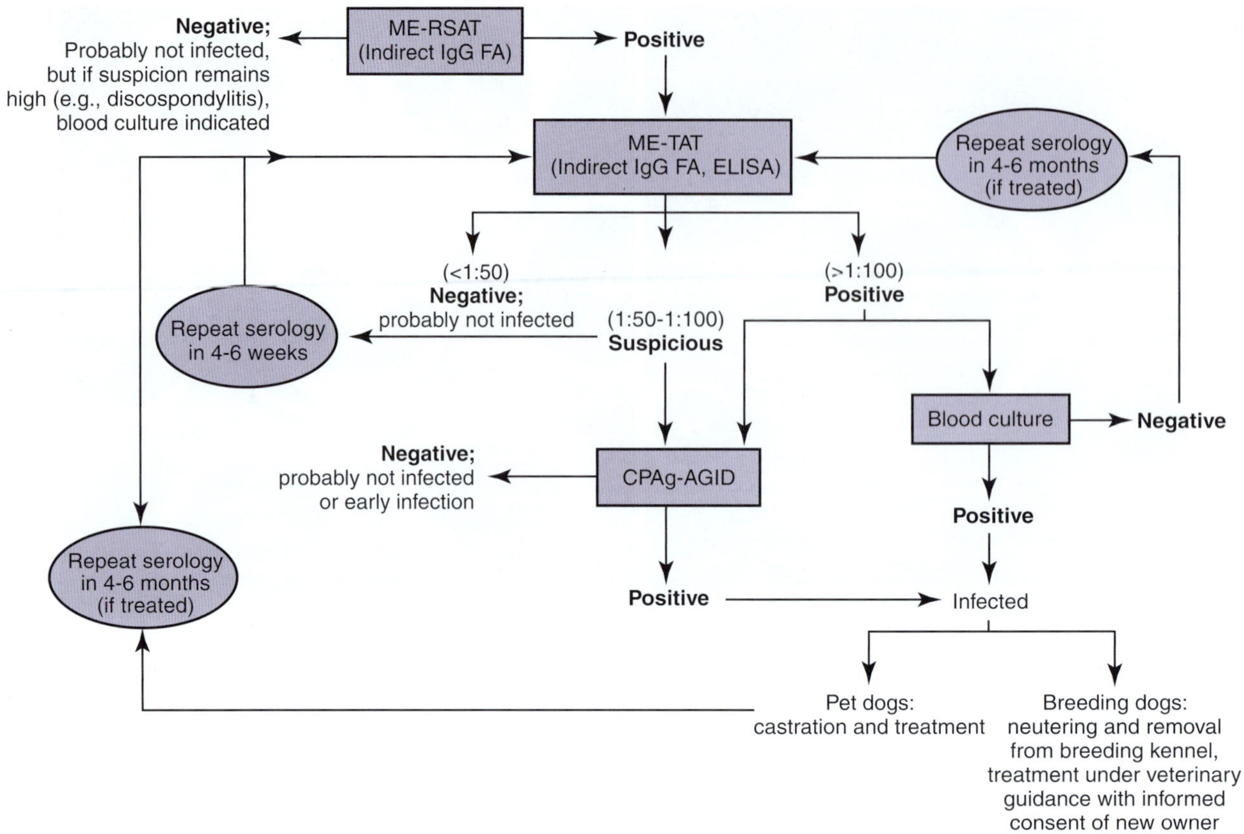

Fig. 71.13 Diagnostic algorithm for canine brucellosis. The indirect fluorescent antibody (*FA*) and enzyme-linked immunosorbent assay (*ELISA*) tests are alternative screening tests when there is unavailability of 2-mercaptoethanol rapid slide agglutination test (*ME-RSAT*) and 2-mercaptoethanol tube agglutination test (*ME-TAT*) antigens. Polymerase chain reaction (*PCR*) can be used as confirmation at various steps where uncertainty exists. See text for rationale in making these decisions. *CPAg-AGID,* cytoplasmic protein antigen-agar gel immunodiffusion.

all genitourinary organs. A necrotizing vasculitis occurs in the target tissues of gonadal steroids, including the prostate, scrotum, sheath, or vulva. Lesions are most prominent in the prostate, epididymides, and uterus, whereas milder changes are observed in the renal pelvis, testes, ductus deferens, urinary bladder, and ureters. Extensive necrosis of the prostatic parenchyma and seminiferous tubules is caused by inflammatory cell infiltration, which eventually results in atrophy or fibrosis. A chronic to subacute endometritis can be seen in the uterus, with glandular hyperplasia and reticular cell nodules (Fig. 71.14). Focal hepatic necrosis, myocarditis, and meningoencephalitis also have been described. Vertebral osteomyelitis and discospondylitis may be present in dogs with discospondylitis. Renal abnormalities occur in some dogs and consist of hyaline thickening of the basement membrane of glomeruli with minimal cellular infiltration or proliferation. A mild interstitial nephritis has been noted. Ocular disease includes granulomatous iridocyclitis and exudative retinitis, with diffuse infiltration by lymphocytes, plasmacytes, and neutrophils. Corneal endothelium has vacuolated cytoplasm with variable plasma cell infiltration; exudates with leukocytes are present in the anterior chamber. Placental trophoblasts can contain large numbers of gram-negative bacteria, and coagulative necrosis may be present. In male dogs, lesions are more likely to be restricted to the reproductive system. Special stains (e.g., Brown-Brenn stain) must be used to detect intracellular organisms. IHC has been used to confirm the presence of *Brucella* spp. in placental tissues (Fig. 71.15).

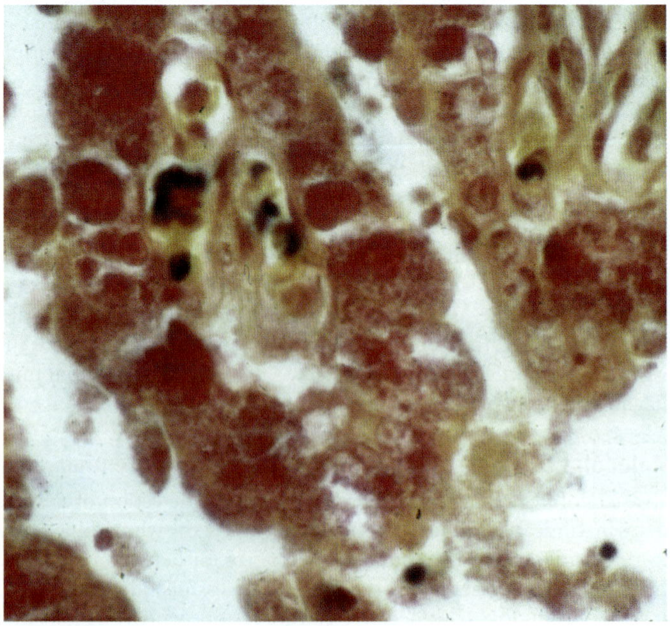

Fig. 71.14 Endometritis with glandular hyperplasia and multifocal inflammation from a dog with *Brucella canis* infection. (Courtesy of Leland Carmichael, Cornell University, Ithaca, NY.)

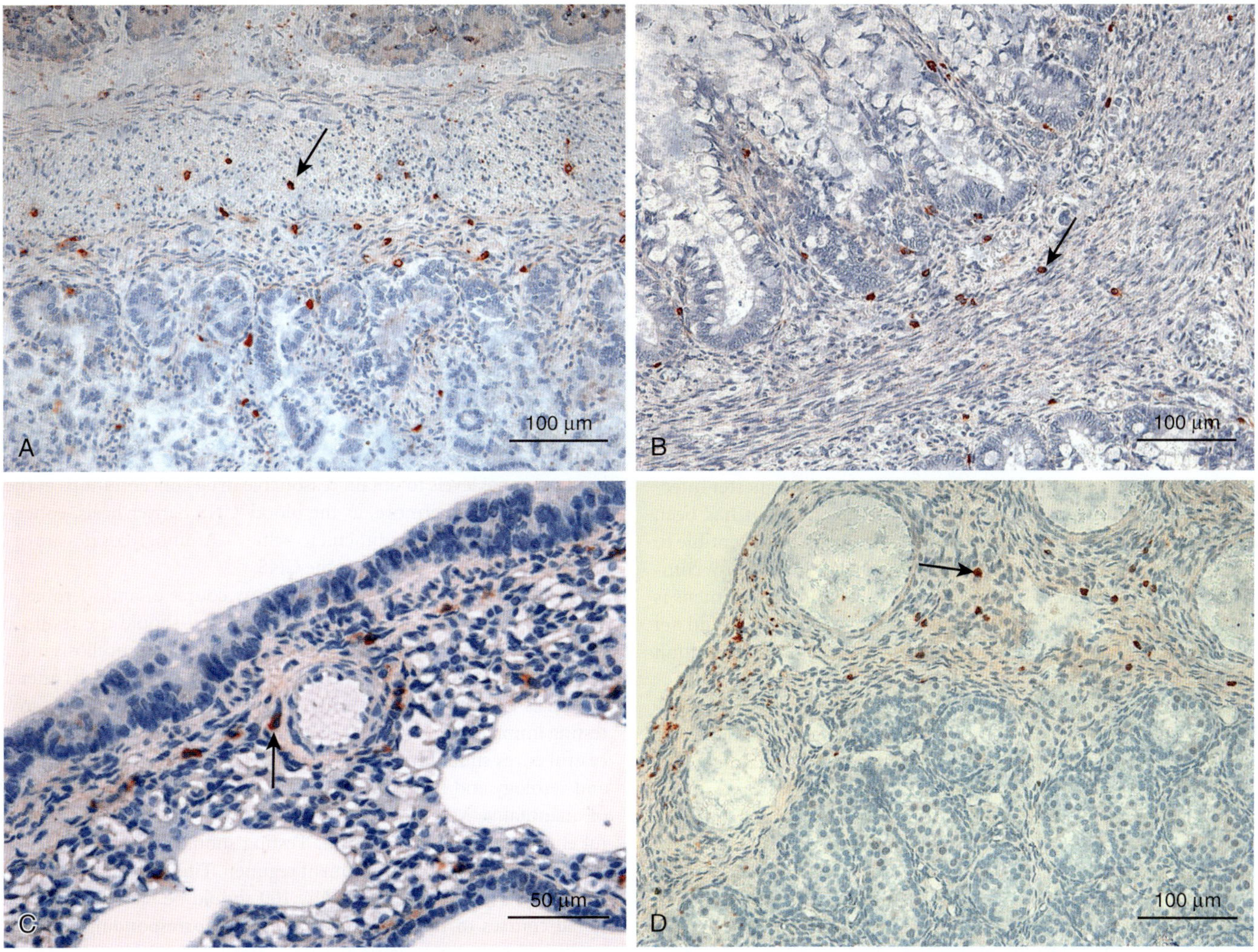

Fig. 71.15 Immunohistochemistry for detection of *Brucella* spp. in naturally infected canine stillborn and neonates. (A) Stillborn. Duodenum, with several diffusely distributed immunolabeled macrophages in the lamina propria and submucosa *(arrow)*. Bar = 100 µm. (B) Stillborn. Cecum, macrophages containing intracytoplasmic immunolabeled coccobacilli in lamina propria and muscle layer *(arrow)*. Bar = 100 µm. (C) Neonate, 10-day-old. Lung, with several interstitial immunostained macrophages around an arteriole and bronchioles *(arrow)*. Bar = 50 µm. (D) Neonate, 13-day-old. Testicle with several immunostained macrophages in the albuginea *(arrow)*. Bar = 100 µm. (From de Souza TD, de Carvalho TF, da Silva Mol, et al. Tissue distribution and cell tropism of *Brucella canis* in naturally infected canine foetuses and neonates. *Sci Rep*. 2018;8:7203.)

TREATMENT AND PROGNOSIS

In certain jurisdictions, brucellosis is a reportable disease in dogs or in humans; once a diagnosis is confirmed, proper authorities should be notified. Any dog in contact with the confirmed case should be quarantined and carefully evaluated for infection over a 60-day period. Infected dogs should be isolated from further contact with other dogs until they are less likely to be contagious. In breeding kennels, the infected dog should never be used for breeding again and should be removed from the breeding program. Infected males are very unlikely ever to regain fertility and should be neutered to reduce shedding. Infected females can regain fertility, but infection can persist. This means that they represent a source of infection for other dogs and that they are at risk for future loss of offspring; they also should be neutered. Eradication of the disease in breeding kennel situations has not been successful without removal of all current or historically infected dogs. Carrier dogs are important in maintaining *B. canis* infection in the dog population because its survival outside the host is short lived. Application of routine hospital disinfectants can inactivate the bacterium. The risk of infecting males when breeding with previously infected females can be minimized by judicious artificial insemination. Breeding of such animals should be done only under exceptional circumstances when it is considered essential (e.g., to prevent the loss of a valuable blood line) and after the risk is explained to an owner.

Because of the zoonotic potential of the disease and difficulty in eradicating the infection, euthanasia of affected dogs has been recommended; this is an unacceptable decision for many private breeders/hobby kennels or pet owners, leading to requests for therapy. Neutering is always indicated. Neutering decreases the number of organisms shed in semen, urine, and vaginal discharge, but does not eradicate infection.

Antibiotic therapy for treatment of brucellosis has historically not been rewarding, likely because the organism is intracellular and bacteremia is periodic. Antimicrobial drug treatment can reduce antibody titers without clearing infection. Relapses are common. Bacteremia often recurs days to months after treatment is discontinued, making

TABLE 71.2 Medications That Could Be Used To Treat Brucellosis in Dogs

Drug	Dose (mg/kg)	Route	Interval/Duration
Doxycycline or minocycline[a]	5–10	PO	q12h for 4 weeks
Streptomycin	5	IM or SC	q24h on weeks 1 and 4
Gentamicin sulfate	5	PO	q12h for 4 weeks
Enrofloxacin	10	PO	q24h for 4 weeks
Rifampin	5	PO	q24h

[a]Use in combination with one of the other drugs listed. Combinations of drugs are preferred for treatment where possible.

follow-up evaluation essential because animals can still sequester infection in tissues. Antibody titers can persist when infection has been cleared, making interpretation difficult. The organism is susceptible to several antibacterials, but the ineffectiveness of *in vivo* therapy commonly leads to failures or relapses. None of the treatment regimens is 100% successful. For greatest efficacy, dogs with brucellosis should *not* be treated with a *single* antibacterial regimen; in *all* cases, combination therapy should be used.

Combination therapy should be used whenever possible, preferably with tetracyclines (high-dose doxycycline or minocycline) for at least 1 to 2 months and an aminoglycoside (streptomycin or gentamicin) for the first 1 to 2 weeks of treatment (Table 71.2). Some also advocate use of two 1-week courses of aminoglycoside treatment spaced 1 month apart, or treatment with streptomycin every other week for 4–8 weeks. Combination therapy with tetracyclines and streptomycin is thought to be the most successful treatment, but unavailability of streptomycin, nephrotoxicity, parenteral therapy requirements, and expense may be problematic.[38,42,44] In addition, aminoglycosides do not provide adequate ocular or CNS penetration for dogs with ophthalmitis or meningitis. A combination of doxycycline and rifampin has been used to treat human brucellosis but may not be well tolerated by dogs because of GI adverse effects. The use of three or four drugs in combination (e.g., streptomycin, enrofloxacin, doxycycline with or without rifampin) was efficacious for treatment of ophthalmitis in dogs. Topical 1% prednisolone acetate and atropine ointment may be required for management of uveitis.[65–67]

One study reported a possible benefit of therapy with enrofloxacin (5 mg/kg, q12h, PO for 4 weeks, often for multiple courses) in a small group of infected dogs. Enrofloxacin did not completely eliminate *B. canis*, but it maintained fertility and avoided the recurrence of abortions, transmission of the disease to subsequently whelped puppies, and dissemination of microorganisms during parturition. Ultimately, however, most treated dogs remained culture positive. Clinical reproductive illness may have been prevented; however, confirmation of eradication of the organism could not be confirmed.[28] Combinations of enrofloxacin and doxycycline may be a more effective alternative for dogs unable to tolerate aminoglycoside or rifampin treatment and for dogs that have ocular or CNS involvement, but studies are lacking. Localized infections in hard-to-reach areas such as in the intervertebral disc should be treated with at least two or more sequential or intermittent 4-week courses of antimicrobial therapy after neutering. Treatment for 6 weeks or longer may be necessary and should be based on clinical, radiographic, and serologic monitoring.[22] Doxycycline and aminoglycoside combination is recommended for this treatment. Surgical intervention is rarely needed unless the diagnostic workup requires obtaining intervertebral tissues for culture. Decompressive surgery should be avoided in paraparetic dogs when possible by first evaluating the clinical response to antimicrobial therapy. Sequential radiography and titers at 3- to 6-month intervals are used to monitor progress. Serologic monitoring should be done with quantitative methods so that relative changes can be detected. Endophthalmitis with *B. canis* has been exceedingly difficult to treat and requires long courses of therapy with potent three- or four-drug combinations. There are few reports of successful elimination of ocular infection in dogs. The organism enters the eye,[68] and the ocular tissues are difficult to penetrate, especially with aminoglycosides. Enucleation is required if the eye has been severely damaged, because vision will never return and the eye acts as a persistent nidus for the organism. Even use of two antimicrobials is associated with relapse rates of ocular inflammation of 6% to 21%. Multiple-drug combination therapy with doxycycline, gentamicin, enrofloxacin, and subsequent addition of rifampin was successful in eliminating the ocular inflammation in one infected dog.[69] As with other CNS infections, therapy with antimicrobials must be at maximal levels to obtain reasonable drug concentrations at the site of infection. Furthermore, as the blood–CNS barrier heals, concentrations will be much more difficult to achieve. Aminoglycosides are of little use in clearing infections from the CNS.

Follow-up is always required after any course of antimicrobial therapy. Antimicrobial regimens must be repeated should the results indicate that infection has not been eliminated. Cures of brucellosis must not be assumed because bacteremia may recur weeks or months after antibacterials are discontinued. Attempted culture of bacteria or serologic testing immediately after treatment is halted is deceiving. Reports of successful cures should be viewed with caution unless subsequent cultures and serology and PCR have been performed for at least 6 months. Use of quantitative ME-TAT titers is the best means of monitoring successful elimination of the organism. Testing should be performed at 6- to 9-month intervals after a treatment regimen. Titer values should decrease if therapy is effective. Titers below 100 should be reached or else additional courses of treatment are indicated. Corresponding AGID titers results should also become negative. Persistence of increased (greater than 100) titers should evoke suspicion that the infection still exists.

Large commercial kennels (puppy mills) present the most challenging scenario. Owners are usually willing to euthanize confirmed positive cases but less willing to go through the expense and time required to eradicate the disease from the facility. Difficulties are compounded if antibacterial therapy is instituted when brucellosis is suspected but not confirmed, because isolation of *B. canis* becomes uncertain and serologic tests results are questionable. A kennel should be quarantined as soon as the diagnosis of *B. canis* is ascertained, and infected animals should be promptly eliminated. Appropriate disinfection procedures should be implemented to arrest the spread of infection via fomites. Persons working with infected dogs and their discharges or secretions should wear gloves until serotesting can be done to determine the extent of the infection. Animals should not be admitted to or released from the kennel until the disease is eradicated. Movement of dogs within a colony also should be restricted to removal of proven and suspect cases to isolation quarters. New additions are at high risk for infection, especially if dogs are not individually penned, which also increases the number of animals requiring repeated testing during the eradication process. Animals must not be released for sale or any other purpose because they may spread the disease. All dogs in an infected kennel should be serotested for at least 3 months after seronegative status is achieved, especially before each breeding, even if artificial insemination is used. If animals are retained as pets or working dogs, or if treatment is contemplated, they should be neutered and moved to separate housing. Although determining the origin of infections is important, this has proved difficult because of the reluctance of owners to reveal actual or suspected sources.

Preventive measures are particularly important in large breeding kennels or wherever a large number of dogs are kept, but no legally mandated control measures exist, and in the United States, canine brucellosis is not a reportable disease in most states. Prevention is accomplished by quarantine of all new acquisitions until two serotest results at a 1-month interval are negative. Animals from kennels known to have had breeding problems should be rejected unless test results are negative.[70] Animals with any clinical sign of canine brucellosis should be rejected. Animals used for breeding should be tested 3 to 4 weeks before each mating to allow time for test results to be reported. Dams should not be mated to stud dogs unless they have been tested and certified negative. If dogs leave a colony, they should be tested before readmission. All canine blood donors should be screened for brucellosis using serology because of the potential for transmission through transfusion of contaminated blood products.[71]

IMMUNITY AND VACCINATION

Serum agglutinating antibodies do not protect against infection in the dog as immunity likely depends on CMI. Presently, the development of a vaccine is considered undesirable because *Brucella* vaccines evaluated have offered only moderate protection, and immunized dogs develop antibodies that confound serodiagnosis. A promising vaccine candidate based on a *B. ovis* mutant was able to protect dogs against challenge with *B. canis*; dogs developed antibodies to rough *Brucella* spp.[72] Such a vaccine may be useful if the serologic response can be differentiated from that to *B. canis* through diagnostic test design.

PREVENTION

Prevention of infection and elimination of infected dogs should be the principal control strategy in kennels. Prevention requires at least yearly testing of all breeding stock and testing of all dogs to be introduced into a kennel. Ideally, two negative screening tests performed at least a month apart should occur before a dog or bitch is introduced into a breeding facility. *Confirmed* positive dogs should be isolated (euthanasia is advised by some), neutered, treated, and tested monthly (AGID, blood culture, or PCR assay on blood) until two consecutive negative tests occur, although occult infection can still be present.

Private breeders should require serologic screening of all female dogs offered for breeding. Should positive test results occur on screening, breeders should not accept dogs unless follow-up testing with confirmatory assays is negative. Artificial insemination without dog-to-dam contact should be used if any concern exists. Stud dogs should be screened at least annually. Because of the potential for non-venereal transmission, screening of maiden dogs and bitches before breeding is also recommended.[15,22]

Prevention of brucellosis in dogs caused by other species of *Brucella* involves avoidance of raw meat diets, hunting activities, and consumption of products of livestock parturition on farms.[11–13]

PUBLIC HEALTH ASPECTS

Humans can become infected with *B. canis*,[73,74] although they are relatively resistant to infection and other *Brucella* species account for the majority of human disease, especially *B. melitensis* (Fig. 71.16). The majority of human brucellosis cases in the United States caused by all

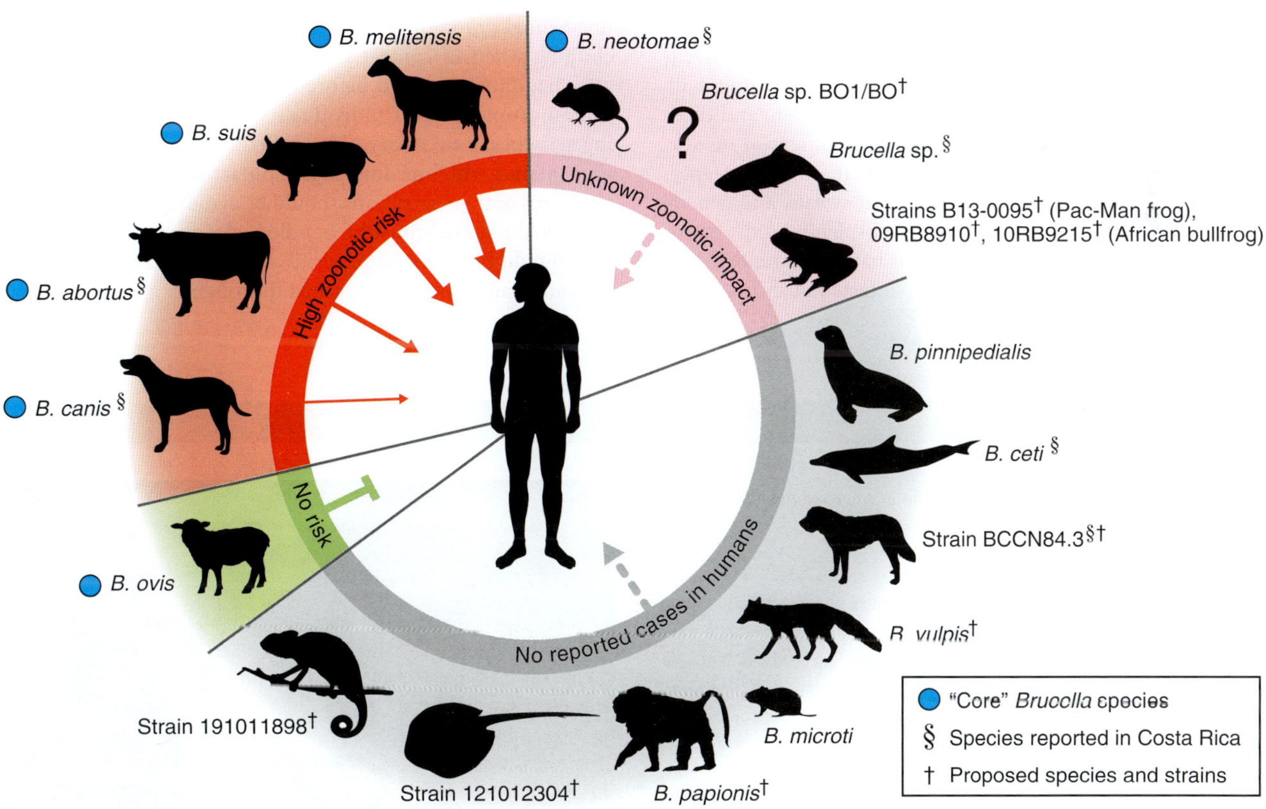

Fig. 71.16 Zoonotic potential of various *Brucella* species. The colors and arrow sizes represent the zoonotic risk displayed by each species isolated from its preferred host. (Modified from Suarez-Esquivel M, Chaves-Olarte E, Moreno E, et al. *Brucella* genomics: macro and micro evolution. *Int J Mol Sci.* 2020;21:7749.)

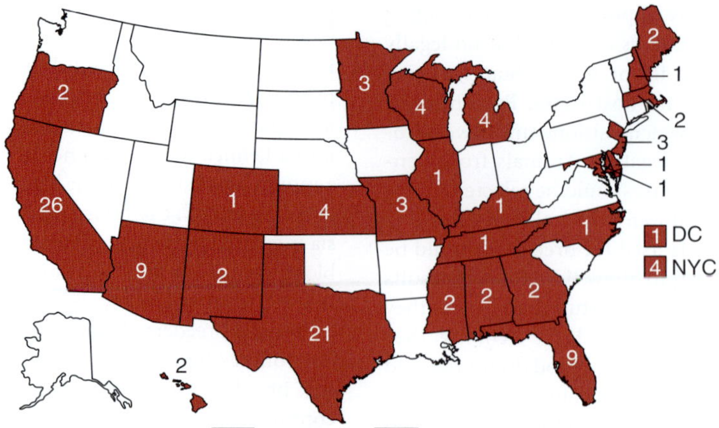

Fig. 71.17 Geographic distribution of reported human cases of brucellosis in 2010. Numbers represent the number of cases reported to the Centers for Disease Control and Prevention. DC, Washington DC; NYC, New York City (Modified from https://www.cdc.gov/brucellosis/resources/surveillance.html.)

species of *Brucella* are reported from California, Texas, Arizona, and Florida (Fig. 71.17). Approximately 40 cases of human infection with *B. canis* have been reported worldwide; however, the actual number is unknown, and the close contact that exists between humans and dogs increases the significance of the zoonotic risk posed. Brucellosis is the most commonly reported laboratory-acquired infection.[75] Serologic assays used for diagnosis of brucellosis in humans often do not detect antibodies to *B. canis*, so the disease may be overlooked. Transmission to humans most commonly occurs through contact with an infected dog's semen, vulvar discharge from an infected bitch, aborted fetuses or placentas, or through direct, accidental laboratory exposure. Thus, disease is more likely to occur in people who are in contact with breeding dogs, but disease occasionally occurs in the owners of pet dogs with discospondylitis. Immunocompromised humans, children, and those who are pregnant may be at greater risk for development of disease. Infection of humans with *B. canis* typically results in nonspecific, persistent clinical signs of fever, muscle aches, night sweats, and general malaise. Rarely, granulomatous hepatitis, hepatosplenomegaly, osteomyelitis, pulmonary disease, and endocarditis have been reported. In one case report, disease occurred in an HIV-infected dachshund dog breeder who reported infertility in one of the dogs, which had been tested by a veterinarian and was seropositive with a screening assay. Confirmatory testing with AGID performed at a university veterinary diagnostic laboratory yielded a negative result, so brucellosis was not thought to be present. However, subsequent blood culture of all the dogs in the household was positive in one other dog.[48,76] Affected humans are typically treated successfully with combinations of doxycycline and either aminoglycosides (for the first week) or rifampin, but monotherapy has been associated with unacceptable rates of relapse.

Prevention of human disease involves eradication of the disease in dog kennels; precautions such as the wearing of gloves and protective clothing when in contact with aborted material; and hand washing after handling dogs and before eating. Although it is preferable that immunocompromised individuals do not participate in dog breeding activities, if necessary, these individuals should take special care if they interact with breeding dogs. Contact with dogs with reproductive problems or their secretions should be avoided whenever possible, and if aborted material must be handled, gloves, gowns, and face protection should be worn, all protective wear should be disposed of properly, and hands should be washed thoroughly.[75,77,78–80]

CASE EXAMPLE

Signalment

"Sadie," a 6-year-old female spayed border collie mix from northern California (Fig. 71.18).

History

Sadie was brought to her local veterinarian for listlessness and reluctance to jump noted during the previous 48 hours. She had been adopted from a local humane shelter and had been ovariohysterectomized at 11 months of age. She lived in a rural agricultural area in northern California and was the only dog in the household; however, she was used for sheep herding with several other dogs.

Current Medications

Sadie was not on any medications.

Physical Examination

Sadie's vital signs were within normal limits, mucous membrane color was pink, and she was quiet and alert on physical examination. Body weight was 25 kg. Mild dental

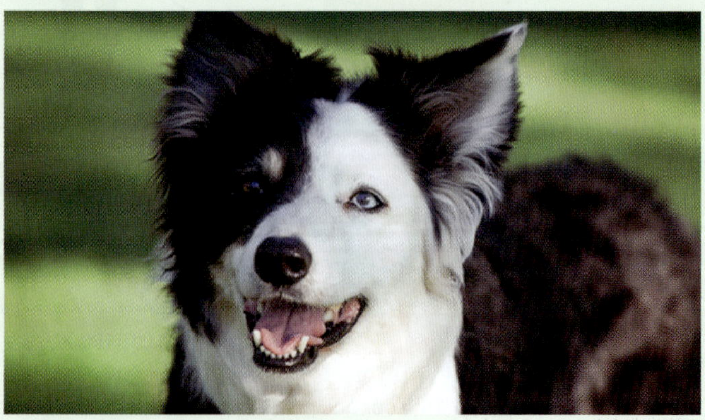

Fig. 71.18 Six-year-old female spayed border collie mix with brucellosis.

CASE EXAMPLE—cont'd

tartar was evident. Thoracic auscultation and abdominal palpation were unremarkable, pulses were synchronous, and no peripheral lymphadenomegaly was evident. Palpable dorsal thoracolumbar pain was demonstrated. She was reluctant to rise but was ambulatory. The neurologic examination including a funduscopic examination was normal.

Laboratory Findings

A CBC, chemistry panel, and urinalysis with aerobic culture were performed. Mild neutropenia (2,958 cells/μL; reference range, 3,000–11,500 cells/μL) was found; the chemistries and urinalysis were within normal limits with no proteinuria.

Imaging Findings

Radiographs of the spine revealed evidence of disc space collapse, spondylosis, and probable discospondylitis at the T7-T8 disc space (see Fig. 71.7).

Microbiologic Testing

A SNAP 4Dx Plus test (IDEXX Laboratories) for antigen of *Dirofilaria immitis* and antibodies to *Ehrlichia canis*, *Anaplasma phagocytophilum*, and *Borrelia (Borreliella* [incertae sedis]*) burgdorferi* was negative. Aerobic bacterial urine culture was negative. Serum was submitted for a *B. canis* IFA, which was positive at a titer of 1:200. A *B. canis* AGID was submitted and was also positive.

Treatment

Sadie was treated with tramadol (1–2 mg/kg, PO, q8h) and carprofen (3 mg/kg, PO, q12h). Once the serologic test results were available, a tentative diagnosis of *B. canis* discospondylitis was made, and she was treated with enrofloxacin (5.5 mg/kg, PO, q12h). Clinical improvement was reported in 2 weeks, and repeat radiographs were performed in 1 and 5 months. Equivocal change was reported in the appearance of T7-T8 at 1 month, but the 5-month radiograph showed no progression, suggesting the lesion was no longer active. The owners were advised of the zoonotic potential of this disease and the potential hazard of transmission to other dogs. The potential need for lifelong intermittent antibiotic therapy with risk of relapses was also discussed. Repeat AGID testing post therapy was advised. It was also advised that dogs in contact with Sadie be screened for brucellosis.

Comments

Dogs with *Brucella* discospondylitis frequently are brought to their veterinarian for clinical signs of spinal pain or lameness that resemble common musculoskeletal injuries such as intervertebral disc disease or rupture of the cranial cruciate ligament. Although not typical, this case illustrates the fact that *B. canis* disease can occur in a neutered female dog without any breeding history, and often occurs in the absence of fever or significant abnormalities on routine laboratory testing. A diagnosis of *Brucella* discospondylitis was strongly suspected based on positive serologic test results with multiple assays. Blood culture was not performed, but a urine culture was negative. Monotherapy with fluoroquinolones has been associated with high rates of relapse in human patients once antimicrobial drug treatment has been discontinued, so it is generally not recommended. Nevertheless, it can occasionally be successful.

SUGGESTED READINGS

Hensel ME, Negron M, Arenas-Gamboa A. Brucellosis in dogs and public health risk. *Emerg Infect Dis.* 2018;24:1401–1406.

Kauffman LK, Petersen CA. Canine brucellosis: old foe and re-emerging scourge. *Vet Clin North Am Small Anim Pract.* 2019;49:763–779.

REFERENCES

1. Carmichael LE. Abortion in 200 beagles. *J Am Vet Med Assoc.* 1966;149:1126.
2. Suarez-Esquivel M, Chaves-Olarte E, Moreno E, et al. *Brucella* genomics: macro and micro evolution. *Int J Mol Sci.* 2020:21:7749.
3. Foster JT, Beckstrom-Sternberg SM, Pearson T, et al. Whole-genome-based phylogeny and divergence of the genus *Brucella*. *J Bacteriol.* 2009;191:2864–2870.
4. Barr SC, Eilts BE, Roy AF, et al. *Brucella suis* biotype 1 infection in a dog. *J Am Vet Med Assoc.* 1986;189:686–687.
5. Forbes LB. *Brucella abortus* infection in 14 farm dogs. *J Am Vet Med Assoc.* 1990;196:911–916.
6. Hinic V, Brodard I, Petridou E, et al. Brucellosis in a dog caused by *Brucella melitensis* Rev 1. *Vet Microbiol.* 2010;141:391–392.
7. Alamian S, Dadar M. *Brucella melitensis* infection in dog: a critical issue in the control of brucellosis in ruminant farms. *Comp Immunol Microbiol Infect Dis.* 2020;73:101554.
8. Palmer MV, Cheville NF. Effects of oral or intravenous inoculation with *Brucella abortus* strain RB51 vaccine in beagles. *Am J Vet Res.* 1997;58:851–856.
9. Greene CE, Carmichael LE. Canine brucellosis. In: Greene CE, ed. *Infectious Diseases of the Dog and Cat.* 4 ed. St. Louis, MO: Elsevier Saunders; 2012:398–411.
10. Wareth G, Melzer F, El-Diasty M, et al. Isolation of *Brucella abortus* from a dog and a cat confirms their biological role in re-emergence and dissemination of bovine brucellosis on dairy farms. *Transbound Emerg Dis.* 2017;64:e27–e30.
11. Frost A. Feeding of raw *Brucella suis*-infected meat to dogs in the UK. *Vet Rec.* 2017;181:484.
12. van Dijk MAM, Engelsma MY, Visser VXN, et al. *Brucella suis* infection in dog fed raw meat, the Netherlands. *Emerg Infect Dis.* 2018;24:1127–1129.
13. Mor SM, Wiethoelter AK, Lee A, et al. Emergence of *Brucella suis* in dogs in New South Wales, Australia: clinical findings and implications for zoonotic transmission. *BMC Vet Res.* 2016;12:199.
14. Polt SS, Dismukes WE, Flint A, et al. Human brucellosis caused by *Brucella canis*: clinical features and immune response. *Ann Intern Med.* 1982;97:717–719.
15. Hollett RB. Canine brucellosis: outbreaks and compliance. *Theriogenology.* 2006;66:575–587.
16. Brower A, Okwumabua O, Massengill C, et al. Investigation of the spread of *Brucella canis* via the U.S. interstate dog trade. *Int J Infect Dis.* 2007;11:454–458.
17. Middlemiss C. *Brucella canis* in dogs in the UK. *Vet Rec.* 2021;188:155.
18. Henderson RA, Hoerlein BF, Kramer TT, et al. Discospondylitis in three dogs infected with *Brucella canis*. *J Am Vet Med Assoc.* 1974;165:451–455.
19. Kerwin SC, Lewis DD, Hribernik TN, et al. Diskospondylitis associated with *Brucella canis* infection in dogs: 14 cases (1980-1991). *J Am Vet Med Assoc.* 1992;201:1253–1257.
20. Sykes JE. Unpublished observations.
21. Ledbetter EC, Landry MP, Stokol T, et al. *Brucella canis* endophthalmitis in 3 dogs: clinical features, diagnosis, and treatment. *Vet Ophthalmol.* 2009;12:183–191.
22. Jones RL, Emerson JK. Canine brucellosis in a commercial breeding kennel. *J Am Vet Med Assoc.* 1984;184:834–835.
23. Carmichael LE, Joubert JC. Transmission of *Brucella canis* by contact exposure. *Cornell Vet.* 1988;78:63–73.
24. Serikawa T, Muraguchi T. Significance of urine in transmission of canine brucellosis. *Nihon Juigaku Zasshi.* 1979;41:607–616.
25. Pretzer SD. Bacterial and protozoal causes of pregnancy loss in the bitch and queen. *Theriogenology.* 2008;70:320–326.
26. Glynn MK, Lynn TV. *Brucellosis. J Am Vet Med Assoc.* 2008;233:900–908.
27. Gyuranecz M, Szeredi L, Ronai Z, et al. Detection of *Brucella canis*-induced reproductive diseases in a kennel. *J Vet Diagn Invest.* 2011;23:143–147.
28. Wanke MM, Delpino MV, Baldi PC. Use of enrofloxacin in the treatment of canine brucellosis in a dog kennel (clinical trial). *Theriogenology.* 2006;66:1573–1578.

29. Lopez G, Ayala SM, Escobar GI, et al. Use of *Brucella canis* antigen for detection of ovine serum antibodies against *Brucella ovis*. *Vet Microbiol.* 2005;105:181–187.
30. Baek BK, Lim CW, Rahman MS, et al. *Brucella abortus* infection in indigenous Korean dogs. *Can J Vet Res.* 2003;67:312–314.
31. Daly R, Willis KC, Wood J, et al. Seroprevalence of *Brucella canis* in dogs rescued from South Dakota Indian reservations, 2015-2019. *Prev Vet Med.* 2020;184:105157.
32. Whitten TV, Brayshaw G, Patnayak D, et al. Seroprevalence of *Brucella canis* antibodies in dogs entering a Minnesota humane society, Minnesota, 2016-2017. *Prev Vet Med.* 2019;168:90–94.
33. Hubbard K, Wang M, Smith DR. Seroprevalence of brucellosis in Mississippi shelter dogs. *Prev Vet Med.* 2018;159:82–86.
34. Johnson CA, Carter TD, Dunn JR, et al. Investigation and characterization of *Brucella canis* infections in pet-quality dogs and associated human exposures during a 2007-2016 outbreak in Michigan. *J Am Vet Med Assoc.* 2018;253:322–336.
35. Yang Y, Wang Y, Poulsen E, et al. Genotyping *Brucella canis* isolates using a highly discriminatory multilocus variable-number tandem-repeat analysis (MLVA) assay. *Sci Rep.* 2017;7:1067.
36. Yan G, Pang Z, Hu Y, et al. First isolation and multilocus sequence typing of *Brucella canis* from a subclinically infected pet dog in China. *Vet Sci.* 2022;9:22.
37. De Massis F, Sacchini F, Averaimo D, et al. First isolation of *Brucella canis* from a breeding kennel in Italy. *Vet Ital.* 2021;57:3.
38. Allen A, Ngeleka M, Parker K. Brucellosis in kennels in western Canada. *Can Vet J.* 2008;49:625.
39. Brennan SJ, Ngeleka M, Philibert HM, et al. Canine brucellosis in a Saskatchewan kennel. *Can Vet J.* 2008;49:703–708.
40. Corrente M, Franchini D, Decaro N, et al. Detection of *Brucella canis* in a dog in Italy. *New Microbiol.* 2010;33:337–341.
41. Dahlborn M, Johnsson M, Myllys V, et al. Seroprevalence of canine herpesvirus-1 and *Brucella canis* in Finnish breeding kennels with and without reproductive problems. *Reprod Domest Anim.* 2008;44:128–131.
42. Nockler K, Kutzer P, Reif S, et al. Canine brucellosis: a case report. *Berl Munch Tierarztl Wochenschr.* 2003;116:368–372.
43. Strom Holst B, Lofqvist K, Ernholm L, et al. The first case of *Brucella canis* in Sweden: background, case report and recommendations from a Northern European perspective. *Acta Vet Scand.* 2012;54:18.
44. Dunne J, Sehgal K, McMillan A, et al. Canine brucellosis in a dog imported into the UK. *Vet Rec.* 2002;151:247.
45. Second UK isolation of *Brucella canis*. *Vet Rec.* 2017;180:617.
46. Kneipp C, Malik R, Mor SM, et al. Commentary: retrospective and prospective perspectives on zoonotic brucellosis. *Front Microbiol.* 2019;10:1859.
47. Kneipp CC, Sawford K, Wingett K, et al. *Brucella suis* seroprevalence and associated risk factors in dogs in eastern Australia, 2016 to 2019. *Front Vet Sci.* 2021;8:727641.
48. Pappas G, Akritidis N, Bosilkovski M, et al. Brucellosis. *N Engl J Med.* 2005;352:2325–2336.
49. Anderson GI, Binnington AG. Discospondylitis and orchitis associated with high *Brucella* titre in a dog. *Can Vet J.* 1983;24:249–252.
50. Serikawa T, Takada H, Kondo Y, et al. Multiplication of *Brucella canis* in male reproductive organs and detection of autoantibody to spermatozoa in canine brucellosis. *Dev Biol Stand.* 1984;56:295–305.
51. Forbes JN, Frederick SW, Savage MY, et al. *Brucella canis* sacroiliitis and discospondylitis in a dog. *Can Vet J.* 2019;60:1301–1304.
52. Wooley RE, Hitchcock PL, Blue JL, et al. Isolation of *Brucella canis* from a dog seronegative for brucellosis. *J Am Vet Med Assoc.* 1978;173:387–388.
53. Moore JA, Gupta BN. Epizootiology, diagnosis, and control of *Brucella canis*. *J Am Vet Med Assoc.* 1970;156:1737–1740.
54. Dawkins BG, Machotka SV, Suchmann D, et al. Pyogranulomatous dermatitis associated with *Brucella canis* infection in a dog. *J Am Vet Med Assoc.* 1982;181:1432–1433.
55. Carmichael LE, Kenney RM. Canine abortion caused by *Brucella canis*. *J Am Vet Med Assoc.* 1968;152:605–616.
56. Johnson CA, Walker RD. Clinical signs and diagnosis of *Brucella canis* infection. *Compend Cont Educ Pract Vet.* 1992;14:763–772.
57. Gungur K, Bekir NA, Namiduru M. Ocular complications associated with brucellosis in an endemic area. *Eur J Ophthalmol.* 2002;12:232–237.
58. Schoeb TR, Morton R. Scrotal and testical changes in canine brucellosis: a case report. *J Am Vet Med Assoc.* 1978;172:598–600.
59. Davidson AP. Unpublished observations.
60. Purvis TJ, Krouse D, Miller D, et al. Detection of *Brucella canis* infection in dogs by blood culture and bacterial identification using matrix-assisted laser desorption/ionization time-of-flight mass spectrometry. *J Vet Diagn Invest.* 2017;29:586–588.
61. Keid LB, Soares RM, Vieira NR, et al. Diagnosis of canine brucellosis: comparison between serological and microbiological tests and a PCR based on primers to 16S-23S rDNA interspacer. *Vet Res Commun.* 2007;31:951–965.
62. Keid LB, Soares RM, Vasconcellos SA, et al. Comparison of agar gel immunodiffusion test, rapid slide agglutination test, microbiological culture and PCR for the diagnosis of canine brucellosis. *Res Vet Sci.* 2009;86:22–26.
63. Kustritz MV. Theriogenology question of the month. Agarose gel immunodiffusion (AGID) serologic testing for brucellosis. *J Am Vet Med Assoc.* 2000;216:181–182.
64. de Oliveira MZ, Vale V, Keid L, et al. Validation of an ELISA method for the serological diagnosis of canine brucellosis due to *Brucella canis*. *Res Vet Sci.* 2011;90:425–431.
65. Jennings PB, Crumrine MH, Lewis GE Jr, et al. The effect of a two-stage antibiotic regimen on dogs infected with *Brucella canis*. *J Am Vet Med Assoc.* 1974;164:513–514.
66. Johnson CA, Bennett M, Jensen RK, et al. Effect of combined antibiotic therapy on fertility in brood bitches infected with *Brucella canis*. *J Am Vet Med Assoc.* 1982;180:1330–1333.
67. Nicoletti P. Further studies on the use of antibiotics in canine brucellosis. *Compend Cont Educ Pract Vet.* 1991;13:944.
68. Roiz MP, Peralta FG, Valle R, et al. Microbiological diagnosis of brucellosis. *J Clin Microbiol.* 1998;36:1819.
69. Vinayak A, Greene CE, Moore PA, et al. Clinical resolution of *Brucella canis*-induced ocular inflammation in a dog. *J Am Vet Med Assoc.* 2004;224:1804–1807. 1788-1809.
70. Aras Z, Ucan US. Detection of *Brucella canis* from inguinal lymph nodes of naturally infected dogs by PCR. *Theriogenology.* 2010;74:658–662.
71. al-Kharfy TM. Neonatal brucellosis and blood transfusion: case report and review of the literature. *Ann Trop Paediatr.* 2001;21:349–352.
72. Eckstein C, Mol JPS, Costa FB, et al. *Brucella ovis* mutant in ABC transporter protects against *Brucella canis* infection in mice and it is safe for dogs. *PLoS One.* 2020;15:e0231893.
73. Hensel ME, Negron M, Arenas-Gamboa A. Brucellosis in dogs and public health risk. *Emerg Infect Dis.* 2018;24:1401–1406.
74. Cañario Viana MV, Wattam AR, Batra DG, et al. Genome sequences of three *Brucella canis* strains isolated from humans and a dog. *Genome Announc.* 2017;5:e01688–16.
75. Scheftel JM. *Brucella canis*: potential for zoonotic transmission. *Compend Cont Educ Pract Vet.* 2003;25:846–853.
76. Lawaczeck E, Toporek J, Cwikla J, et al. *Brucella canis* in a HIV-infected patient. *Zoonoses Public Health.* 2011;58:150–152.
77. Swenson RM, Carmichael LE, Cundy KR. Human infection with *Brucella canis*. *Ann Intern Med.* 1972;76:435–438.
78. Lucero NE, Corazza R, Almuzara MN, et al. Human *Brucella canis* outbreak linked to infection in dogs. *Epidemiol Infect.* 2010;138:280–285.
79. Lucero NE, Escobar GI, Ayala SM, et al. Diagnosis of human brucellosis caused by *Brucella canis*. *J Med Microbiol.* 2005;54:457–461.
80. Wallach JC, Giambartolomei GH, Baldi PC, et al. Human infection with M- strain of *Brucella canis*. *Emerg Infect Dis.* 2004;10:146–148.

72

Tetanus and Botulism

Jane E. Sykes, Jamie M. Burkitt Creedon

KEY POINTS

- First Described: The etiology of tetanus was identified in the late 1800s in Germany (Nicolaier).[1] *Clostridium botulinum* and its toxin were first described in Belgium in 1897 (van Ermengem).[2] Prior to that, descriptions of both tetanus and botulism had been recorded; tetanus was described by Hippocrates more than 2000 years ago.
- Causes: Tetanospasmin neurotoxin of *Clostridium tetani* (tetanus); and botulinal neurotoxin of *C. botulinum*, *Clostridium baratii*, or *Clostridium butyricum* (botulism).
- Affected Hosts: Both diseases affect humans and domestic animals, including dogs and cats.
- Geographic Distribution: Both are ubiquitous organisms that affect the worldwide population.
- Primary Mode of Transmission: Inoculation of spores into a wound (tetanus) or ingestion of preformed toxin (botulism).
- Major Clinical Signs: Spastic rigidity (tetanus) or flaccid paralysis (botulism).
- Differential Diagnoses: Differential diagnoses for tetanus include strychnine toxicosis, hypocalcemia, and masticatory muscle myositis. Differential diagnoses for botulism include causes of acute lower motor neuron disease such as idiopathic polyradiculoneuritis (coonhound paralysis), tick paralysis, coral snake envenomation, myasthenia gravis, ionophore toxicosis, and paralytic rabies.
- Human Health Significance: Botulism and tetanus are not directly transmissible from animals to humans, but care should be taken when handling specimens from animals with botulism.

ETIOLOGY: TETANUS AND BOTULISM

Tetanus and botulism are neurologic diseases caused by the toxins of *Clostridium tetani* and *Clostridium botulinum*, respectively. These environmentally ubiquitous organisms are gram-positive, anaerobic, spore-forming, rod-shaped bacteria, with worldwide distributions. The spores of *C. tetani* and *C. botulinum* are extremely hardy in the environment and resist boiling and disinfection with alcohol or formalin.

The vegetative form of *C. tetani* produces the two toxins *tetanospasmin* and *tetanolysin*. Botulism is caused by botulinal neurotoxins (BoNTs), which comprise a family of seven antigenically distinct toxins produced by *C. botulinum* (which produces all seven BoNT types A–G), *Clostridium butyricum* (type E only), and *Clostridium baratii* (type F only). Although these seven neurotoxins are produced by a variety of clostridial organisms and are themselves different, they have identical toxicologic effects, and are thus considered together. BoNT is produced by the sporulated or vegetative clostridial organism under anaerobic conditions. Species susceptibility to BoNT serotypes varies. For instance, most human cases of botulism are caused by BoNT types A, B, or E. All reported clinical feline[3] and most canine[4–10] cases of botulism have been caused by BoNT type C. Rare cases of botulism caused by BoNT type D,[11] one likely caused by type A,[7] and one caused by type B[12] have been reported in dogs.

Tetanospasmin and BoNT have similar structures and mechanisms of action even though they cause diseases that contrast sharply with one another. Both toxins are among the most potent toxins known with an LD_{50} of ≤ 1–5 ng/kg.[13,14] The toxins consist of two polypeptide chains, a heavy (H) chain and a light (L) chain, joined by a disulfide bond (Fig. 72.1). The H chain attaches to presynaptic nerve terminal membrane receptors, although the precise receptors have not been identified because of the extremely low concentrations at which these toxins act. Variation in receptor binding affinities may explain differences in species susceptibility to clostridial neurotoxins. The toxin is then internalized via receptor-mediated endocytosis into the presynaptic nerve terminal, where it has a local impact on nerve cell function (BoNT) or travels by retrograde axonal transport to the nerve cell body and diffuses into inhibitory interneurons, where it impacts CNS inhibitory interneuron function (tetanospasmin). The L chain, a zinc-dependent matrix metalloproteinase, is released from the vesicle and subsequently cleaves one or more *docking proteins.* These proteins are critical for the release of neurotransmitters from synaptic vesicles into the synaptic cleft and are located on the membrane of synaptic vesicles *(synaptobrevin)* or the presynaptic cell membrane (*syntaxin* and *SNAP-25*). Synaptobrevin binds to the docking proteins located on the presynaptic membrane. The resulting complex (the SNARE complex) docks the synaptic vesicle at the proper location for fusion and exocytosis of neurotransmitter molecules into the synaptic space (Fig. 72.2). Tetanospasmin cleaves synaptobrevin, whereas botulinum neurotoxin C cleaves syntaxin; other botulinum neurotoxins cleave synaptobrevin or SNAP-25. The process of recovery involves the sprouting of new presynaptic terminals, followed by recovery of the original synapse, after which new terminal outgrowths retract.[15]

TETANUS

EPIDEMIOLOGY

Humans and horses are most susceptible to tetanus, and so widespread vaccination against the disease is performed in these species. Disease occurs occasionally in dogs and is rare in cats. The development of tetanus in dogs and cats usually follows introduction of environmental spores into a penetrating wound, but more than one third of affected

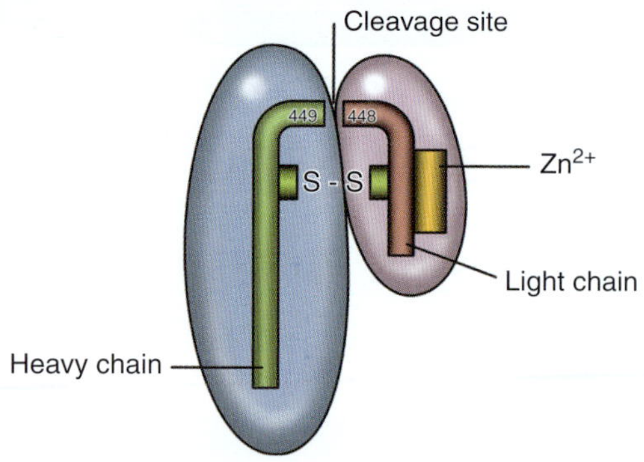

Fig. 72.1 Schematic of the structure of *Clostridium tetani* and *Clostridium botulinum* toxins.

dogs have no known wound history (*cryptogenic tetanus*)[16]; a similar prevalence of cryptogenic tetanus has been reported in humans.[17] Traumatic wounds of the feet, claws, or head; draining tracts associated with grass awn migration; animal bite wounds; tick bite wounds; bleeding claw trim wounds; wounds that result from chronic protozoal or fungal infections of the skin; teething wounds in dogs; and surgical wounds (particularly ovariohysterectomy and castration) have all been implicated.[16,18–20] One study in dogs suggests that tetanus occurs seasonally in the winter in England, though seasonality was not found in dogs in California.[21,22] Although dogs of any age, breed, or sex can develop tetanus, disease occurs most often in young, large-breed, active, intact male dogs.[16,18,19] Disease is seen in puppies as young as 8 weeks of age. Some studies describe a significant proportion of affected dogs as less than 1 year of age. Disease may be more severe in young than in mature dogs[16]; high mortality rates have been reported in the youngest people as well.[23] Cats are often young animals with outdoor access,[24] but cats of any age have been affected.[25]

CLINICAL FEATURES

Pathogenesis and Clinical Signs

Clostridium tetani spores are introduced into tissues where they germinate, replicate locally, and produce tetanospasmin toxin in anaerobic conditions. Ingestion is not a route of transmission because tetanospasmin is destroyed by GI secretions. Tetanolysin appears to promote local tissue degradation at the site of inoculation, which may optimize the tissue environment for organism growth. The toxin is produced as a single polyprotein that is cleaved extracellularly by a bacterial protease into the L and H chains, which remain connected by the disulfide bond. It then binds to presynaptic terminals of lower motor neurons and is internalized, travels up axons by retrograde axonal flow, and enters inhibitory interneurons in the brain and spinal cord, where it interferes with the release of inhibitory neurotransmitters γ-aminobutyric acid (GABA) and glycine (see Fig. 72.2). Toxin can also spread hematogenously to the CNS from the wound site. The result is unhindered excitation of motor neurons, spastic rigidity, and dysfunction of the sympathetic and parasympathetic nervous systems. Clinical signs occur 3 days to 3 weeks after a wound in both dogs and cats. Shorter incubation periods occur when the inoculation site is nearer the CNS and when a large amount of toxin is present. Paralysis may initially be localized to the wound site but can then generalize. Involvement of the head is common in dogs, and often owners of dogs with tetanus first notice an unusual appearance to their dog's eyes, a "swollen" face, or evidence of dysphagia.[16] Regurgitation or vomiting of food occurs in less than 20% of affected dogs, and a voice change or dysuria may be noted. Abnormal activity during sleep (twitching, running, vocalization) was documented in at least 46% of 50 surviving dogs with tetanus in the United Kingdom; these signs resolved in approximately half of these dogs within 6 months.[26] Death occurs in severely affected dogs due to paralysis of respiratory muscles; infectious complications such as pneumonia; upper airway obstruction; the development of severe hyperthermia with DIC, multiple organ failure, and/or pulmonary thromboembolism; and cardiac arrhythmias.[16,18,19] Hiatal hernia and coxofemoral joint luxations have also been described as complications of tetanus in dogs.[16,18,27,28] Disease in cats is usually localized to the limbs, but generalized tetanus can occur.[24,25,29–35] Many affected cats have an initial history of disappearance or a recognized wound, after which rigid lameness is noted.

Physical Examination Findings

Tetanus causes spastic muscle rigidity. *Generalized tetanus* involves spastic rigidity of all four limbs in addition to muscles of the head. *Localized tetanus* involves spasm in a single limb or region of the body. Like humans, dogs more often experience generalized tetanus; cats more often have localized tetanus, probably due to the feline species' relative resistance to tetanospasmin. Both species can experience either type. The cephalic form of tetanus is localized to the head secondary to a head wound; *cephalic tetanus* is seen in humans and involves flaccid facial paralysis that usually precedes generalized tetanus with spastic rigidity[36]; cephalic tetanus has not been described in dogs or cats.

Dogs and cats with *generalized tetanus* experience rigidly extended limbs. The tail is often held erect, or curved dorsally. Dogs that are ambulatory walk slowly with a stiff, stilted gait and can have a wide-based or "sawhorse" stance; voluntary movement of the head may occur slowly or appear difficult. Reflexes may be exaggerated or difficult to elicit due to excessive extensor tone. When muscles of the head are involved, tetanus causes globe retraction and thus third eyelid elevation, a wrinkled forehead and erect pinnae, retracted lips (*risus sardonicus*), and trismus—spasms of masticatory muscles that make it difficult to open the mouth (Fig. 72.3A). Cats with generalized tetanus may not have increased jaw tone.[33–35] Miosis may be present. Laryngeal spasm and hypersalivation occur in approximately half of affected dogs.[18,19]

Severely affected dogs are anxious and hypersensitive, develop opisthotonus, vocalize, or tremble, or can experience generalized seizures when stimulated. Patients are often hyperthermic due to increased muscle activity (up to 111°F [43.9°C]).[34] Moderate to severe obtundation can result. Abdominal palpation may reveal an enlarged bladder that is difficult to express, or palpation may be difficult because of abdominal muscle spasm. Tetanic spasms can lead to dyspnea and hypoventilation.[16,18] At least a third of dogs with generalized tetanus in a referral environment are bradycardic or have bradyarrhythmias (which include atrioventricular block or sinus arrest), with heart rates that range from 40 to 60 beats/minute; another one third of dogs are tachycardic (>150 beats/minute) or have variable heart rates, which may reflect autonomic dysfunction or pain.[16] The inciting wound that allowed introduction of *C. tetani* may or may not be found, particularly in dogs. In cats with tetanus, a wound is often identified.[29–33,37,38] Animals with generalized tetanus usually have a prolonged clinical course and require hospitalization for 1–2 weeks or more; median hospital stay for dogs has been reported to be 13–17 days.[18,19]

Localized tetanus usually involves rigid extension of the limb nearest or affected by the inoculating wound. Dogs with localized thoracic limb tetanus have caudal retraction of the limb with extension of both the elbow and carpus.[25] When a cat's thoracic limb is affected, spasm of the triceps muscle results in caudal extension of the limb with carpal flexion (in contrast to dogs) and elbow extension (Fig. 72.3B).[24,30] The head and neck may deviate toward the affected limb.[25] Localized tetanus can progress to generalized disease.

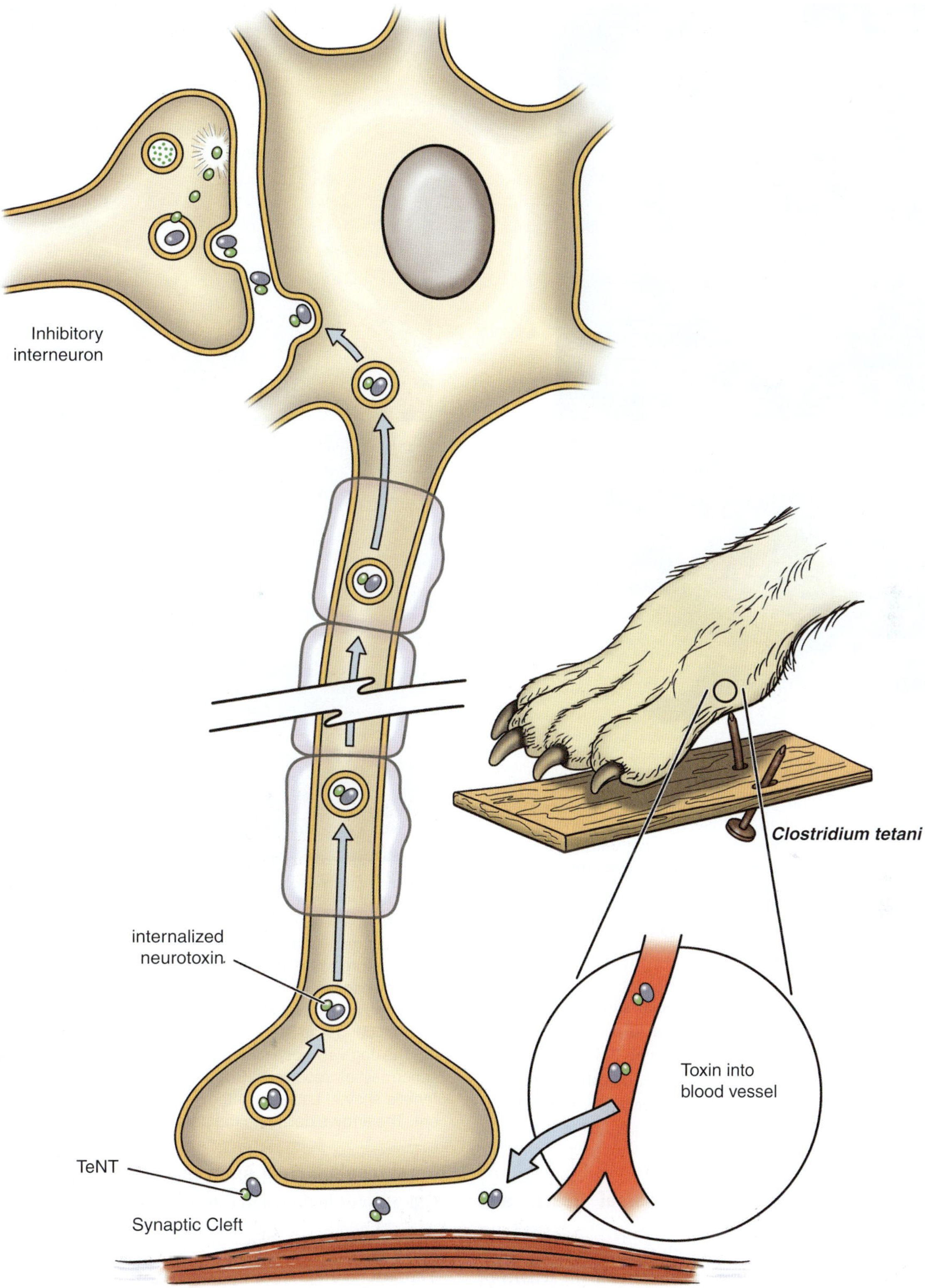

Fig. 72.2 Mechanism of action of tetanospasmin

DIAGNOSIS

Tetanus is a clinical diagnosis in all species. That is, there is no clinicopathologic, microbiologic, serologic, imaging, or other diagnostic test that is definitive for the disease; diagnosis is based on history and physical examination, and the exclusion of other rule-outs for the problem. The main rule-outs for generalized tetanus are hypocalcemic tetany, which is ruled out by a normal serum ionized calcium concentration, and strychnine toxicosis. Strychnine was historically used as a pesticide to kill small mammals, but has largely been replaced in the western world by other toxins. Thus, strychnine toxicosis is probably a less common clinical problem today than tetanus.

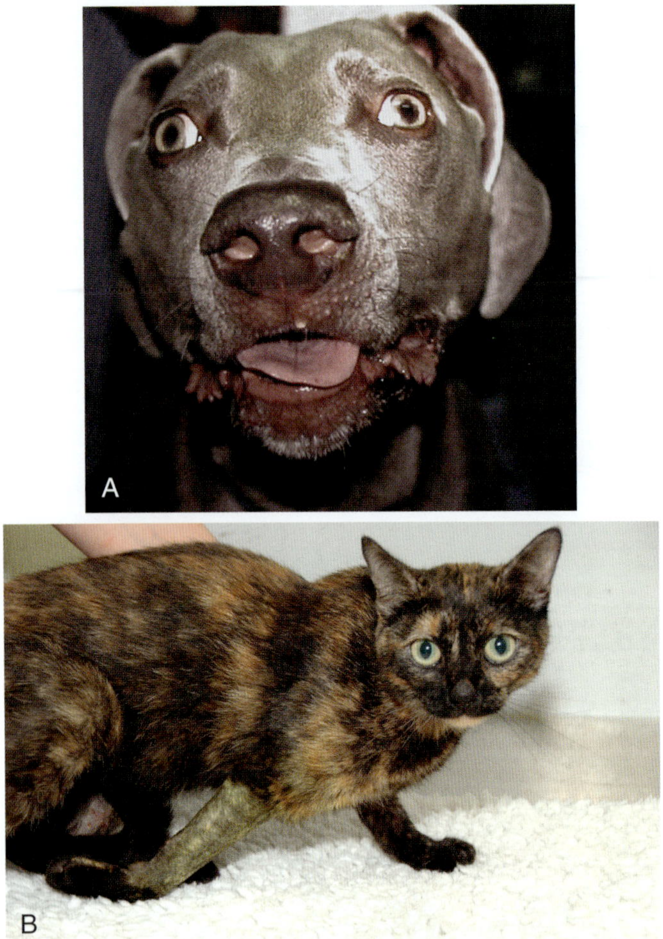

Fig. 72.3 (A) Weimaraner with generalized tetanus. The dog walked with a stiff gait and was salivating profusely. Risus sardonicus is evident. (B) A 3-year-old female domestic shorthair cat with localized tetanus that was seen for a 3-day history of right thoracic limb lameness. Extension of the shoulder and elbow and partial flexion of the carpal joint are present. (From Langner KFA, Schenk HC, Leithaeuser C, et al. Localised tetanus in a cat. *Vet Rec.* 2011;169:126.)

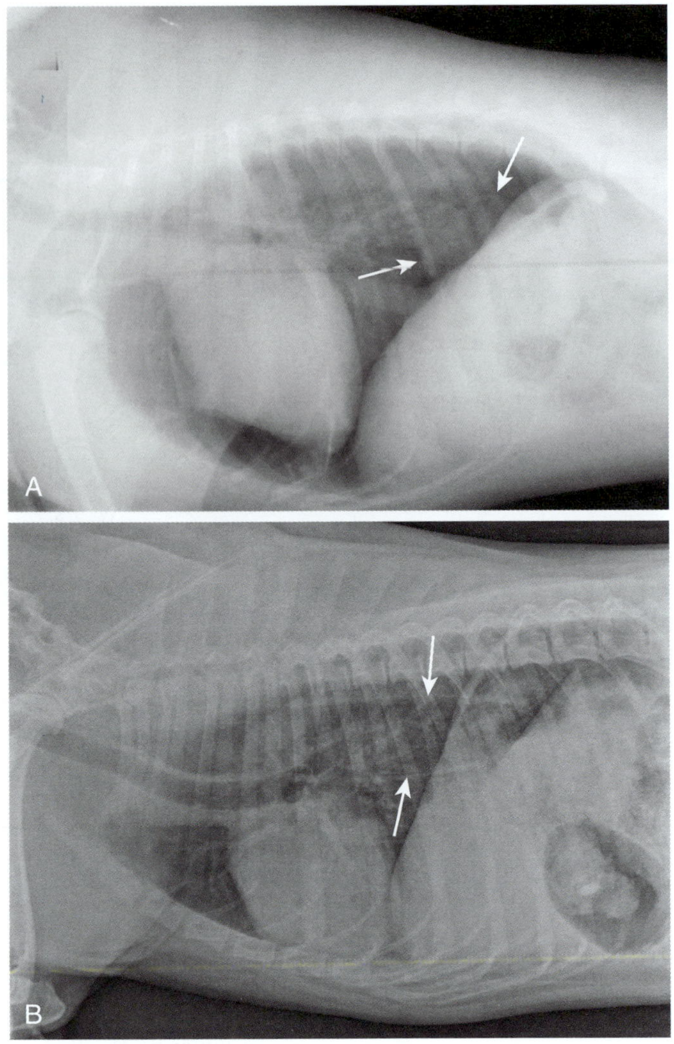

Fig. 72.4 Radiographic findings in dogs with tetanus (A) and botulism (B). (A) Lateral thoracic radiograph from a 3-year-old female spayed English springer spaniel with tetanus that was seen for vomiting, dysuria, respiratory distress, and a stiff gait. Pneumothorax and a hiatal hernia *(arrows)* can be appreciated. Before the radiographs were taken, an exploratory laparotomy had been performed because a foreign body was suspected. The pneumothorax developed postoperatively for reasons that were unclear. A foxtail wound was later found on the left distal pelvic limb between the digits. The dog was hospitalized for 19 days, during which time all radiographic abnormalities resolved. (B) Lateral thoracic radiograph from a 6-year-old female spayed Labrador retriever with botulism. Megaesophagus is present. The arrows delineate the dorsal and ventral esophageal wall.

The primary differential diagnosis for the facial signs of tetanus is masticatory muscle myositis, which is ruled out if nonfacial musculature is involved and by serologic testing for type 2M antibodies. A history of a traumatic event, surgical procedure, or other wound in the preceding 3 weeks, or of a period of disappearance, should raise suspicion for tetanus.

Laboratory Abnormalities

Complete Blood Count, Serum Biochemical Tests, and Urinalysis

Routine laboratory test results in animals with tetanus are often normal, but stress hyperglycemia, mild to severe increases in the activity of serum creatine kinase (usually < 20,000 U/L but sometimes > 200,000 U/L, reference range: 46–320 U/L), mildly increased AST activity, and myoglobinuria may be present.[16,18] Dehydration may result in hemoconcentration or prerenal azotemia. Animals with wounds or aspiration pneumonia may have an inflammatory leukogram. Severe hyperthermia in dogs with tetanus may lead to laboratory evidence of multiple organ dysfunction, with azotemia, increased liver enzyme activities, or hyperbilirubinemia. Thrombocytopenia and coagulation test abnormalities consistent with DIC may also be present in these dogs.

Cerebrospinal Fluid Analysis

CSF analysis in dogs and cats with tetanus is typically normal.

Diagnostic Imaging

Thoracic radiographs in animals with tetanus may reveal aspiration pneumonia.[16,18,19] Occasionally, dogs with generalized tetanus have evidence of a hiatal hernia on thoracic radiography,[16,27,39,40] which appears as a soft tissue mass in the caudal thorax (Fig. 72.4A). Abdominal ultrasound and advanced imaging modalities are generally noncontributory.

Electrodiagnostic Tests

Electrodiagnostic testing is not usually performed in animals with tetanus since the diagnosis can generally be made without it, and because electrodiagnostic findings in the disease are nonspecific.

Electromyography (EMG) evaluates the electrical activity in muscle while nerve conduction studies evaluate the quality and speed of nerve responses following stimulation. Animals with tetanus have had normal electrodiagnostic measurements[18] in some cases, and persistent electrical motor unit discharges in others.[24,41]

Microbiologic Tests

Isolation and Identification

Attempts to culture *C. tetani* from wounds are not recommended because the presence of *C. tetani* in a wound does not necessarily imply toxin production. In addition, culture for this organism is insensitive.[17]

Serologic Diagnosis

Serologic testing is not performed in cases of tetanus because it is a clinical diagnosis with so few rule-outs that it is a nearly pathognomonic presentation. Antibodies are produced to the toxin during natural infection,[42] but serology is generally neither available nor necessary for diagnosis.

Pathologic Findings

There are no specific gross or histopathologic findings associated with tetanus. Evidence of complications such as aspiration pneumonia, pulmonary thromboembolism, or DIC may be seen on necropsy in patients that die of severe cases.

TREATMENT AND PROGNOSIS

Specific Treatment

Tetanus antitoxin is widely available and should be administered as a single dose IV (equine antitoxin) or IM (human antitoxin) after an initial intradermal test dose to evaluate for an allergic reaction (Table 72.1). Dogs that react to the test dose can be premedicated with diphenhydramine and a low dose of dexamethasone. Adverse reactions to antitoxin include vomiting, retching, or tachypnea and may occur even in premedicated dogs.[16] Reduction in the rate of antitoxin administration or discontinuation of treatment leads to resolution of clinical signs. Administration of antitoxin does not reverse existing signs because it does not enter nerve terminals, but it may neutralize free toxin. A small amount of antitoxin can be administered locally if a wound is identified. The efficacy of tetanus antitoxin is controversial, and the optimal dose is not known. In one study, earlier IV administration of equine tetanus antitoxin did not influence disease progression or mortality as opposed to administration later in the course of disease.[16] Antitoxin administration may prevent localized tetanus from generalizing.

For animals with tetanus, treatment with antimicrobials that have activity against *C. tetani* is recommended. Appropriate antimicrobials for treatment of tetanus include IV metronidazole or penicillin G. Metronidazole is preferred because of its improved penetration into purulent material and the fact that penicillin can antagonize GABA. Studies in human patients have also shown improved outcome with metronidazole as opposed to procaine penicillin.[43] Once antitoxin has been administered and spasms are controlled (see Supportive Care), wounds should be managed appropriately. Earlier, appropriate antimicrobial treatment and wound debridement were not shown to influence progression or mortality in one small veterinary study in dogs.[16] However, early, definitive management with antitoxin, wound management, and appropriate antimicrobial therapy is a cornerstone of treatment in humans with tetanus,[44] and common sense suggests that veterinary patients would benefit from that same level of care.

Supportive Care

Supportive care is an essential part of management for patients with tetanus. The extent of care required depends on the severity of illness. IV fluids, soft bedding, frequent turning to prevent decubital ulcers, application of ocular lubricant to prevent corneal ulceration, bladder expression or urethral catheterization (ideally intermittent), enemas to relieve constipation, and nutritional support in the form of hand feeding, feeding tubes, or parenteral nutrition may be required. Force feeding is not recommended because it is unlikely to satisfy caloric needs and can contribute to the development of aspiration pneumonia.

To help minimize spasms, dogs or cats with generalized tetanus should be placed in a quiet, dimly lit environment away from excessive visual or auditory stimuli. Cotton balls can be used as earplugs. Sedatives and/or muscle relaxants such as acepromazine, benzodiazepines, dantrolene, or baclofen may be useful. Severely affected animals may require a constant-rate infusion of drugs such as pentobarbital, phenobarbital, or propofol. Barbiturates are no longer recommended for treatment of tetanus in humans, in whom benzodiazepines are the mainstay for sedation and relaxation.[45,46] If human disease is severe, drugs that cause neuromuscular blockade such as vecuronium are used, but this necessitates mechanical ventilation. Methocarbamol often appears ineffective and requires frequent administration,[16,19] and thus its use is not recommended because it may delay administration of more effective medications. Also, benzodiazepines are preferred to methocarbamol because they are GABA agonists and provide some sedation. Successful control of muscle spasms relieves pain and hyperthermia. If used, opioids should be administered with caution because they may contribute to constipation or GI adverse effects. Administration of magnesium sulfate infusions has also been associated with improvement in clinical signs; a dose of 70 mg/kg over 30 minutes followed by an initial CRI of 100 mg/kg/day has been recommended. Oral magnesium aspartate (12 mg/kg q12h) orally can be continued for 14 days once this is feasible.[47]

Fans and room temperature fluids may be beneficial for dogs with tetanus-induced heat injury. Administration of atropine may be required for animals with bradyarrhythmias (in dogs, HR < 60 beats/minute; in cats, HR < 120 beats/minute). Rarely, bradyarrhythmias have required temporary pacemaker placement.[16] Occasionally ($< 10\%$ of dogs with generalized tetanus in a referral population), mechanical ventilation is required to support respiration.[16] Temporary

TABLE 72.1 Suggested Dosages of Medication for Specific Treatment of Tetanus

Drug	Dose	Route	Interval (hours)	Duration (days)
Metronidazole	15 mg/kg	IV, PO	12	10
Tetanus equine antitoxin	100–1000 units/kg 500 units	IV, IM[a] SC near wound site	NA	Once
Human tetanus immune globulin	500 units	IM near wound if found	NA	Once

[a]IV use is preferred. Administer 0.1 mL intradermally as a test dose before infusion. The full dose should then be given slowly over 10 minutes. The maximum dose is 20,000 units/kg.

IM, intramuscular; *IV*, intravenous; *NA*, not applicable; *PO*, oral; *SC*, subcutaneous.

tracheostomy may be required to bypass the larynx in cases of severe upper airway obstruction.[18]

Prognosis

Provided complications do not occur, prognosis is generally good for animals with generalized tetanus. The overall 28-day survival rate for dogs with generalized tetanus in one study was around 80%,[16] whereas in another study of 20 dogs it was only 50%.[19] A classification system has been developed to assess the severity of tetanus in dogs for the purpose of prognostication (Table 72.2).[16] The survival rate for dogs that progressed to tetanus severity class I or II was 100%, but it dropped to 60% for dogs that progressed to tetanus severity class III or IV.[16] However, at the time of initial evaluation, only 11% of 37 dogs were in class III or IV, and dogs progressed to higher classes unpredictably, with 47% of the dogs categorized in class III or IV when the highest recorded class was assigned. Dogs with severe tetanus are more likely to develop complications such as aspiration pneumonia or multiple organ dysfunction than dogs with mild tetanus. In a few dogs that recover (< 10% of dogs that develop generalized tetanus), intermittent localized muscle spasm continues to occur for many months, which may be noticed by the owner during activities such as sleeping or eating.[16]

The prognosis for animals with localized tetanus is excellent with supportive care of wound management and antimicrobial treatment.

TABLE 72.2 Tetanus Severity Classification System for Dogs

Class	Clinical Signs
I	Absence of class II, III or IV signs *and* any or all of: • Miosis, enophthalmos, risus sardonicus, erect ears, or trismus • Hypersensitivity to noise, light or touch • Ambulatory
II	Absence of class III or IV signs *and* any or all of: • Dysphagia • Stiff gait, sawhorse stance, erect tail • Ambulatory
III	Class I or class II signs, absence of class IV signs, *and* any or all of: • Recumbency • Muscle fasciculations or spasms • Seizures
IV	Class I, II, or III signs *and* any or all of: • Bradycardia (HR ≤ 60 beats/minute) or bradyarrhythmia • Sinus tachycardia (HR ≥140 beats/minute) or tachyarrhythmia • Labile hypertension or hypotension (mean arterial blood pressure ≤60 mmHg or ≥ 130 mmHg, or systolic arterial blood pressure ≤ 80 mmHg or ≥150 mmHg) • Periods of apnea or respiratory arrest

Modified from Burkitt JM, Sturges BK, Jandrey KE, et al. Risk factors associated with outcome in dogs with tetanus: 38 cases (1987-2005). *J Am Vet Med Assoc.* 2007;230:76–83.

IMMUNITY AND VACCINATION

Given the relative rarity of tetanus in dogs and cats, vaccination is not recommended in these species. Recurrent tetanus has been documented in people, so recovery from natural disease does not necessarily result in protection from future episodes.[44] Thus, preventative measures should be discussed with owners of pets that recover from tetanus.

PREVENTION

Control of: (1) roaming, (2) exposure to plant awns, and (3) aggressive interactions with other animals may reduce the chance that wounds develop. If wounds are noticed, they should be cleaned promptly with soap and water. Surgical instruments should always be sterilized properly before use so that tetanus spores are inactivated, and needles should never be reused. Tetanus spores can be inactivated with iodine, glutaraldehyde, hydrogen peroxide, or autoclaving at 121°C and 15 psi for 15 minutes.

PUBLIC HEALTH ASPECTS

Animals with tetanus cannot transmit it directly to people who handle them. The main risk that dogs with tetanus pose to humans is through bite wounds, which can occur when owners attempt to administer oral medications to animals with increased jaw tone or spasm.

Tetanus in humans is rare in developed countries because most children are vaccinated against the disease. When it occurs, it is most often in people older than 65 years because of waning immunity, and in injection drug users.[48] Worldwide, the vast majority of cases occur in neonates from developing nations because of lack of immunization.

BOTULISM

EPIDEMIOLOGY

Botulism is rare in dogs and even rarer in cats. Clinical disease in dogs and cats follows ingestion of carrion that contains preformed neurotoxin. Botulism outbreaks in dogs have been reported in hunting foxhounds that have eaten domestic mammal or wild animal carcasses.[4,49] Maggots can vector *C. botulinum* and BoNT between bird carcasses,[50] and some cases of canine botulism have followed ingestion of bird carrion.[5,8,9,51] At least one case was associated with a botulism outbreak in waterfowl.[10] Most dogs reported have been medium- to large-breed, intact male or intact female dogs that vary in age; this finding is likely because the vast majority of botulism cases in dogs have been reported in foxhound packs. The only report of botulism in cats was an outbreak of disease that occurred after several cats were fed pelican carrion.[3] The relative resistance of dogs and cats to botulism has been hypothesized to reflect an adaptive response to a carnivorous lifestyle.

CLINICAL FEATURES

Pathogenesis and Clinical Signs

Clostridium botulinum spores germinate in anaerobic conditions and produce toxin. They grow best in temperatures that range from 30°C to 37°C, so carrion in warm conditions is ideal for BoNT production. The toxin is ingested, survives the acid stomach conditions, and is absorbed into the bloodstream from the small intestine. It then travels to peripheral cholinergic synapses, which include the neuromuscular junction and autonomic synapses, and inhibits release of acetylcholine (ACh) (Fig. 72.5). This leads to ascending, symmetrical flaccid paralysis, development of megaesophagus, and signs of autonomic dysfunction. Clinical signs usually occur within 12 to 72 hours after ingestion of botulinum toxin and may be complicated by signs from dietary indiscretion, although GI signs may also reflect the presence of autonomic derangement. Disease progresses rapidly over 1 or 2 days,

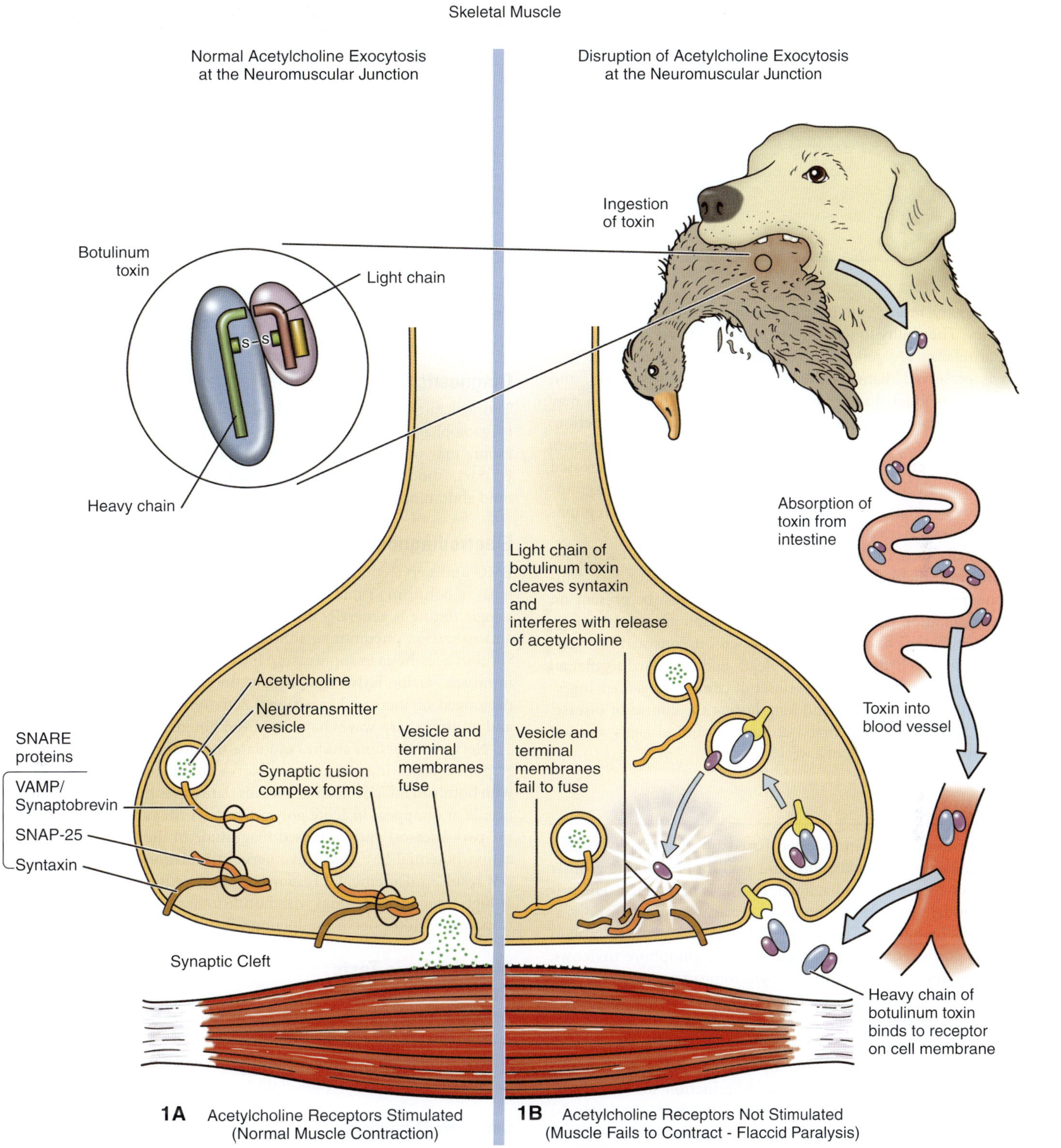

Fig. 72.5 Mechanism of action of botulinum toxin

and then begins to resolve with supportive care. Rapid development of signs after carrion ingestion is generally associated with a more severe course of disease. Death can result from respiratory muscle paralysis or aspiration of GI contents. Abnormalities in affected cats were ascending flaccid paralysis, lethargy, hypothermia, tachypnea, dehydration, and urinary incontinence.[3]

Physical Examination Findings

Botulism causes an acutely progressive, ascending, bilaterally symmetrical flaccid paralysis. Physical examination findings depend on the severity of intoxication. Fever is absent unless aspiration pneumonia has developed. Mildly affected animals show only ataxia or pelvic limb paresis, whereas those with severe intoxication are quadriplegic with

TABLE 72.3 Diagnostic Assays Available for Diagnosis of Botulism

Assay	Specimen Type	Target	Performance
Mouse inoculation bioassay	Feces, vomitus, intestinal contents, serum, foodstuffs	Botulinum toxin	Gold standard for diagnosis. False negatives can occur if toxin degradation occurs. Slow turnaround time means diagnosis is generally retrospective. Laborious and requires the use of laboratory animals.
ELISA toxin assays	Feces, vomitus, intestinal contents, serum, foodstuffs	Botulinum toxin	Rapid and inexpensive. Standard ELISA toxin assays have a lower sensitivity than the mouse inoculation assay.
ELISA assays that detect the antibody response to botulinum toxin	Serum	Anti–botulinum toxin antibodies	Negative antibody titers occur early in the course of disease, so acute and convalescent titers must be performed. Thus, diagnosis is retrospective.

absent voluntary motor activity and are unable to rise from lateral recumbency. The ability to wag the tail is often retained in dogs.[4,10,51] Segmental reflexes are generally decreased or absent, and pain perception is preserved. Patients usually experience constipation, and an "overflow" bladder due to lower motor neuron dysfunction may be present. Cranial nerve examination can reveal decreased function, especially facial nerve function and a decreased gag reflex, sometimes accompanied by ptyalism.[4,5,51,52] Dysphonia is common. Decreased blinking can result in corneal ulceration,[5,6] and concomitant keratoconjunctivitis sicca has been reported.[9] Mydriasis with sluggish pupillary light reflexes has been described.[4,52]

Occasionally tachycardia and tachypnea are present. Tachypnea may result from diaphragmatic muscle weakness or secondary aspiration pneumonia. Increased breath sounds may also be present on thoracic auscultation of dogs with secondary aspiration pneumonia. Physical examination findings in one affected cat consisted of hypothermia, lethargy, dehydration, quadriplegia, and decreased segmental reflexes.[3] In general, the sooner the onset of clinical signs after ingestion of toxin, the more severe and long-lasting the course of disease. Most cases worsen over the first 1–2 days of clinical signs and are markedly improved in less than a week.

DIAGNOSIS

Diagnosis of botulism is most often based on a history of recent exposure to carrion, clinical signs, and exclusion of the few other rule-outs; sometimes electrodiagnostic testing is performed. The primary differential diagnoses for botulism are acute idiopathic polyradiculoneuritis (coonhound paralysis), tick paralysis, acute fulminant myasthenia gravis, coral snake envenomation, ionophore toxicosis, and paralytic rabies. The intermediate syndrome of organophosphate intoxication and organophosphate-induced delayed neuropathy are also possible, though these syndromes are exceptionally rare in veterinary medicine. A full history should be obtained for vaccination status and possible exposure to organophosphate pesticides or ionophore antimicrobial agents, and a close examination should be performed for engorged ticks. An ACh receptor antibody assay can be performed to rule out fulminant myasthenia gravis. Serologic assays have been used to detect an antibody response to BoNT. Finally, specific assays that detect BoNT in serum, GI contents, or food can be performed (Table 72.3).

Laboratory Abnormalities

Complete Blood Count, Serum Biochemical Tests, and Urinalysis

Routine laboratory test results in animals with botulism are often normal. Dehydration may result in hemoconcentration or prerenal azotemia. Animals with aspiration pneumonia may have leukogram changes.

Cerebrospinal Fluid Analysis

CSF analysis in dogs and cats with botulism is typically normal.

Diagnostic Imaging

Thoracic radiographs in dogs with botulism may be unremarkable, or megaesophagus may be present (see Fig. 72.4B).[6,9,52] Aspiration pneumonia may occur.[4,9,52] Carrion bones are occasionally present in the GI tract. Abdominal ultrasonographic examination may be normal, or mild abdominal lymphadenopathy may be identified.

Electrodiagnostic Tests

EMG and nerve conduction studies can be useful to support a diagnosis of botulism (Table 72.4). Sedation or anesthesia for electrophysiologic testing is generally not advisable in dogs with megaesophagus and aspiration pneumonia, although this testing has been performed without anesthesia in some cases.[4] EMG evaluates the electrical activity in muscle. Using EMG, the primary finding in dogs with botulism is prolonged or increased insertional activity.[4,52] Fibrillation potentials and positive sharp waves have also been noted.[4,9]

Nerve conduction studies evaluate the quality and speed of nerve responses following stimulation. Nerve conduction findings in dogs with botulism include normal F waves (late waves that decrease in magnitude or disappear in acute polyradiculoneuritis, and thus distinguish the two diseases) and decreased magnitude of the compound muscle action potential.[4,9,52] Repetitive nerve stimulation at low frequencies can result in decremental responses, but repetitive nerve stimulation at high frequencies in dogs with botulism has no effect on the muscle response.[52] Motor nerve conduction velocity is normal[52] or decreased.[4]

Microbiologic Tests

Isolation and Identification

Detection of *C. botulinum*, *C. butyricum*, or *C. baratii* bacteria in source material,[3,6] or in the stomach contents,[3] vomitus, or feces[5,51] of affected animals helps support the diagnosis of botulism, but is neither sensitive nor specific for clinical disease.

Serologic Diagnosis

ELISA assays that detect the antibody response to botulinum neurotoxin are available and were used to confirm a diagnosis of botulism in one dog.[5] A convalescent specimen collected 3 weeks after the onset of illness was positive, but specimens collected at the time the dog was first evaluated and 10 days into the course of disease were negative. Thus, the diagnosis is generally retrospective with this method because most dogs have recovered by the time seroconversion occurs.

Toxin Detection

Botulinum toxin can be detected in feces,[4,7,9,51] vomitus,[8] GI contents collected at necropsy, source material (carrion),[3,9] or serum.[4,8–10,12,51]

TABLE 72.4 Pathophysiologic, Clinical, and Electrophysiologic Features of Botulism, Polyradiculoneuritis, and Myasthenia Gravis

	Pathophysiology	Neurologic Signs	Electrodiagnostic Findings	Time Course
Botulism	Botulinum toxin-induced inhibition of acetylcholine release	Ascending flaccid tetraparesis, autonomic signs (Mydriasis with incomplete/absent PLR, neurogenic KCS, urinary retention), dysphonia, decreased reflexes, respiratory muscle paralysis, facial nerve paralysis, megaesophagus, constipation, normal pain perception	EMG: prolonged or increased insertional activity; fibrillation potentials and positive sharp waves possible NCS: normal F waves, decreased magnitude of CMAP. Normal MNCV. Decremental response to repetitive nerve stimulation at low frequencies	Progresses over 1 to 2 days, then usually markedly improved within a week
Acute Canine Polyradiculoneuropathy	Lymphocytic radiculoneuritis and nerve root demyelination, mechanism unclear	Ascending flaccid tetraparesis, dysphonia, ventroflexion of the neck, variable hyperesthesia of distal limbs	EMG: Increased insertional activity, fibrillation potentials and positive sharp waves, complex repetitive discharges. Normal to decreased magnitude of CMAP with temporal disperson. Normal MNCV. (I think many cases have demyelination and reduced MNCV – most published cases report reduced MNCV and this is my personal experience). F waves may not be recordable or will be prolonged. Sensory nerve conduction and repetitive nerve stimulation normal.	Rapid progression over a few days, but progression may continue for 10 days. Time course to recovery weeks to months.
Acquired Myasthenia Gravis	Anti-acetylcholine receptor antibodies at the neuromuscular junction	Muscle weakness, exercise intolerance, regurgitation due to megaesophagus, rare facial nerve paralysis, normal reflexes	EMG: Normal CMAP, but with repetitive nerve stimulation, decremental CMAP response with improvement upon intravenous administration of edrophonium chloride (maybe – we don't routinely test post-edrophonium). Diagnosis is made by >10% decrement. Normal MNCV.	Variable progression, with acute fulminant and focal forms of disease.

CMAP, compound muscle action potential; *MNCV,* motor nerve conduction velocity.

Specimens should be held at 4°C, marked with a warning label, and shipped immediately to the laboratory. The most sensitive assay is a mouse inoculation assay, in which untreated mice and mice treated with serotype-specific antitoxin are inoculated with the specimen to determine if the antitoxin is protective.[53] However, several days are required to run this assay and it involves the sacrifice of laboratory animals. Toxin type-specific ELISA assays are available for rapid detection of BoNT C, but standard ELISA assays lack sensitivity when compared with mouse inoculation. Research efforts have been focused on the development of a variety of novel, rapid, highly sensitive, and inexpensive diagnostic assays that detect minute quantities of botulinum toxins.[53]

Pathologic Findings

There are no specific gross or histopathologic findings associated with botulism.

TREATMENT AND PROGNOSIS

Specific Treatment

There is no readily available specific treatment for botulism in dogs. In the United States, heptavalent equine antitoxin is available from the CDC for treatment of human botulism. However, its availability is tightly controlled, so it may be impossible to obtain for treatment of dogs and cats.[54] Antimicrobials are not indicated for the treatment of botulism, because the disease is due to the ingestion of preformed toxin.

Supportive Care

Supportive care is an essential part of management. The extent of care required depends on the severity of illness. IV fluids, soft bedding, frequent turning to prevent decubital ulcers, application of ocular lubricant to prevent corneal ulceration, bladder expression, enemas to relieve constipation, and nutritional support in the form of hand feeding, feeding tubes, or total parenteral nutrition may be required. Force feeding is not recommended because it is unlikely to satisfy caloric needs and can contribute to the development of aspiration pneumonia. Occasionally, intermittent positive pressure ventilation may be required to support ventilation. Antimicrobial drugs should only be used if secondary infection develops (e.g., bacterial pneumonia or UTI). Aminoglycosides should be avoided because they may contribute to neuromuscular blockade.

Prognosis

Provided complications do not occur, prognosis is generally good for animals with botulism. Most animals are markedly improved within a week of onset of clinical signs.

IMMUNITY AND VACCINATION

Botulism is so rare in dogs and cats that vaccination against it is considered unwarranted. Vaccination has been successful in other species, and BoNT vaccine development is an active area of research due to concerns about the toxin being used in bioterrorism.[55]

PREVENTION

Prevention of botulism involves limiting access to carrion and feeding heat-processed commercial diets that are unspoiled. Although BoNT can be denatured through boiling, spores can survive this treatment. Thus, cooked food should not be allowed to stand for long periods before it is fed to pets. The spores of *C. botulinum* are inactivated by pressure-cooking foods.

PUBLIC HEALTH ASPECTS

Animals with botulism cannot transmit the condition directly to people. Nevertheless, feces, tissues, or body fluids from animals with botulism should be handled with care and marked with warning labels before they are submitted to the laboratory because the toxin may be present in these items and only minute quantities are required to cause severe disease.

Three forms of botulism occur in people: infant botulism, wound botulism, and food botulism. Infant botulism occurs as a result of local production of botulinum toxin within the intestinal tract by *C. botulinum* in the absence of the competing intestinal microflora that are normally found in adults. Wound botulism occurs almost exclusively as a result of injection of contaminated heroin by IV drug users. Botulinum toxin preparations are used to treat conditions such as strabismus, esophageal achalasia, cervical dystonia, axillary hyperhydrosis (excessive sweating), or blepharospasm. There are rare reports of iatrogenic botulism after such use.[56,57] Life-threatening iatrogenic botulism has occurred after use of botulinum preparations that were unlicensed for cosmetic treatment of wrinkles.[58] Significant concerns have been raised about the possible use of botulinum toxin as an agent of bioterrorism. This has stimulated considerable research on the disease, which is otherwise very rare.

CASE EXAMPLE

Signalment

"Jenny," a 6-year-old female spayed Labrador retriever from Winters in northern California.

History

Jenny was brought to the University of California, Davis veterinary emergency service early in the morning for a 2-hour history of inability to stand. Her owners awoke to find her in another room, unable to get up for her morning walk. She appeared anxious and was breathing with increased effort, but was still wagging her tail. She also did not want to eat breakfast. There had been no known history of travel, toxins, trauma, or tick exposure. Over the past 2 months, she had been treated with prednisone (1 mg/kg, PO, daily for 5 days, followed by 0.74 mg/kg, PO, daily thereafter) for allergic dermatitis. Three weeks before the onset of illness, she was treated with a short course of cephalexin after an aural hematoma was repaired. Jenny had been regularly vaccinated with rabies, distemper, hepatitis, and parvovirus vaccines.

Physical Examination

Body weight: 27.2 kg.

General: Bright, alert, responsive, and hydrated. Laterally recumbent and anxious. T = 101.0°F, HR = 140 beats/minute, panting.

Integument, eyes, ears, nose, and throat: Sutures were present on the pinna of the right ear from the recent aural hematoma repair. Moderate dental calculus and gingivitis were present. There were no other abnormalities noted.

Musculoskeletal: BCS 5/9. The dog was unable to use the pelvic limbs to bear weight.

Cardiovascular, respiratory, GI, genitourinary, and lymph nodes: No clinically significant abnormalities were present.

Neurologic Examination

Mentation: Appropriate, anxious.

Gait/Posture: The dog was non-ambulatory, but voluntary movement was present in all four limbs. She was unable to stand and support weight, but could crawl and shuffle. She attempted to bear weight on her thoracic limbs and could maintain sternal recumbency. When supported to stand, the pelvic limbs collapsed and the thoracic limbs were minimally able to bear weight.

Cranial nerves: Slightly reduced palpebral reflexes and gag reflex. Absent corneal reflexes. No other deficits were noted.

Postural reactions: These were difficult to assess because of the dog's inability to stand, but appeared decreased.

Segmental reflexes: Reduced muscle tone was present in the thoracic limbs. Triceps, patella, and gastrocnemius reflexes were decreased. Reduced thoracic limb withdrawal reflexes were noted, but pelvic limb withdrawal reflexes were intact. Panniculus and perineal reflexes were also intact. Pain perception remained intact.

Spinal palpation: No apparent pain was present on palpation or cervical manipulation.

Neuroanatomic localization: Neuromuscular disease.

Laboratory Findings

CBC: HCT 41.0% (40%–55%), MCV 69 fL (65–75 fL), MCHC 36.6 g/dL (33–36 g/dL), WBC 5,800 cells/μL (6,000–13,000 cells/μL), neutrophils 3,671 cells/μL (3,000–10,500 cells/μL), lymphocytes 1,769 cells/μL (1,000–4,000 cells/μL), monocytes 197 cells/μL (150–1,200 cells/μL), eosinophils 145 cells/μL (0–1,500 cells/μL), platelets clumped but adequate (150,000–400,000 platelets/μL).

Serum biochemistry profile: Sodium 146 mmol/L (145–154 mmol/L), potassium 3.9 mmol/L (3.6–5.3 mmol/L), chloride 107 mmol/L (108–118 mmol/L), bicarbonate 21 mmol/L (16–26 mmol/L), phosphorus 2.3 mg/dL (3.0–6.2 mg/dL), calcium 11.4 mg/dL (9.7–11.5 mg/dL), BUN 15 mg/dL (5–21 mg/dL), creatinine 0.9 mg/dL (0.3–1.2 mg/dL), glucose 105 mg/dL (64–123 mg/dL), total protein 7.1 g/dL (5.4–7.6 g/dL), albumin 4.2 g/dL (3.0–4.4 g/dL), globulin 2.9 g/dL (1.8–3.9 g/dL), ALT 64 U/L (19–67 U/L), AST 25 U/L (19–42 U/L), ALP 129 U/L (21–170 U/L), creatine kinase 57 U/L (51–399 U/L), GGT 4 U/L (0–6 U/L), cholesterol 204 mg/dL (135–361 mg/dL), total bilirubin 0.2 mg/dL (0–0.2 mg/dL).

Urinalysis: SpG 1.025; pH 7.0, trace protein (SSA), 1+ bilirubin, no hemoprotein, glucose, ketones, WBC/HPF, RBC/HPF, bacteria or crystals in the sediment. Many lipid droplets were present.

Imaging Findings

Thoracic radiographs: The cardiopulmonary structures were within normal limits. There were mineralized opacities within the stomach. There was a small amount of gas in the midthoracic esophagus.

Abdominal ultrasound examination: Mild mesenteric lymphadenomegaly was identified. No other abnormalities were present.

Neuromuscular Testing

Edrophonium response test for myasthenia gravis: Negative.

Treatment

Jenny was admitted to the intensive care unit and treated with supportive care that included IV fluids (lactated Ringer's solution with 20 mEq/L KCl at 75 mL/hour),

CASE EXAMPLE—cont'd

soft bedding, intermittent manual bladder expression, physical therapy (massage and passive ROM exercises), and frequent turning. Treatment with prednisone was discontinued. Respiratory function was monitored continuously by observation, serial examination, and serial venous pCO_2 measurements. After repeated inspections for ticks, topical fipronil was applied in case the signs resulted from tick paralysis. Serum was submitted for an ACh receptor antibody titer, and feces were submitted for a botulinum toxin assay. Over the subsequent 12 to 18 hours, Jenny became anxious after she was fed canned food and began to retch and hypersalivate. Thoracic radiographs were repeated and showed megaesophagus (see Fig. 72.4B). Severe tachycardia also developed (HR = 210 beats/minute). An ECG showed ventricular tachycardia followed by supraventricular tachycardia. Systolic blood pressure was 145 mmHg. Acepromazine was administered (0.01 mg/kg, IV, once), after which her HR decreased to 90 beats/minute, with a normal sinus rhythm. A second neurologic examination showed progression of disease with reduced cervical tone and an inability to hold up the head, tetraplegia with absence of all segmental reflexes, and a reduced tail wag. The owners were warned that mechanical ventilation may be needed should the disease progress. Over the course of the next day, dysphonia and a mild cough developed, and Jenny regurgitated several times. Gastrostomy or jejunostomy tube feeding or parenteral nutrition were offered to the owner, but were declined. Four days after admission, improvement in the triceps reflex was noted, and on day 5, some voluntary movement was noted in the pelvic and thoracic limbs. At that time Jenny was successfully fed meatballs of canned dog food by hand. She was kept in sternal recumbency for 30 minutes after eating to minimize aspiration. On day 7, the ACh receptor antibody and botulinum toxin assay results became available.

Serum acetylcholine receptor antibody titer: 0.05 nmol/L (reference interval, < 0.6 nmol/L)

Botulinum toxin C mouse bioassay (fecal specimen): Positive for type C botulinum toxin. An extract from the fecal specimen was lethal in the bioassay. The effects were eliminated by heating the extract at 80°C for 10 minutes, which indicated that the toxic effects were due to a heat-labile toxin. Mice were also protected from the effects by anti–type C botulinum antisera but not by anti–type A botulinum antisera.

Diagnosis

Botulism.

Outcome

On day 8 after hospitalization, thoracic radiographs showed resolution of megaesophagus and no evidence of pneumonia. By day 10, Jenny began to shuffle along the floor. All segmental reflexes had returned but remained reduced. The dog was discharged from the hospital with instructions for continued care in the home environment. By day 15, Jenny's owners reported that her normal bark had returned, and she could walk 20 steps and defecate and urinate unassisted. A month after discharge she was re-examined and no abnormalities were detected.

Comments

The main differential diagnoses considered for this dog were myasthenia gravis and botulism. Initially, polyradiculoneuritis was also considered, but the subsequent development of megaesophagus was not consistent with this disorder. Ultimately, a diagnosis of botulism was confirmed through assay of the stool for botulinum toxin. A history of carrion ingestion was not known, but the dog lived in a semirural area, and the presence of mineralized stomach contents suggested that it had occurred. Prednisone administration may have contributed to polyphagia and ingestion of carrion by this dog.

SUGGESTED READINGS

Papageorgiou V, Kazakos G, Anagnostou T, et al. The role of magnesium in the management of acute and long-term symptoms caused by tetanus in two dogs. *Top Companion Anim Med*. 2021;44:100535.

REFERENCES

1. Nicolaier A. Ueber infectiösen tetanus. *Deut Med Wchnschr*. 1884;10:842–844.
2. Van Ermengem EP. Über einen neuen anaeroben Bacillus und seine Beziehung zum Botulismus. *Z Hyg Infektionskrankh*. 1897;26:1–56.
3. Elad D, Yas-Natan E, Aroch I, et al. Natural *Clostridium botulinum* type C toxicosis in a group of cats. *J Clin Microbiol*. 2004;42:5406–5408.
4. Barsanti JA, Walser M, Hatheway CL, et al. Type C botulism in American foxhounds. *J Am Vet Med Assoc*. 1978;172:809–813.
5. Bruchim Y, Steinman A, Markovitz M, et al. Toxicological, bacteriological and serological diagnosis of botulism in a dog. *Vet Rec*. 2006;158:768–769.
6. Darke PG, Roberts TA, Smart JL, et al. Suspected botulism in foxhounds. *Vet Rec*. 1976;99:98–99.
7. Marlow GR, Smart JL. Botulism in foxhounds. *Vet Rec*. 1982;111:242.
8. Richmond RN, Hatheway C, Kaufmann AF. Type C botulism in a dog. *J Am Vet Med Assoc*. 1978;173:202–203.
9. van Nes JJ, van der Most van Spijk D. Electrophysiological evidence of peripheral nerve dysfunction in six dogs with botulism type C. *Res Vet Sci*. 1986;40:372–376.
10. Wallace V, McDowell DM. Botulism in a dog: first confirmed case in New Zealand. *N Z Vet J*. 1986;34:149–150.
11. Doutre MP. 2nd case of botulism type D in the dog in Senegal. *Rev Elev Med Vet Pays Trop*. 1983;36:131–132.
12. Lamoureux A, Pouzot-Nevoret C, Escriou C. A case of type B botulism in a pregnant bitch. *J Small Anim Pract*. 2015;56:348–350.
13. Montecucco C, Molgo J. Botulinal neurotoxins: revival of an old killer. *Curr Opin Pharmacol*. 2005;5:274–279.
14. Rethy L, Rethy LA. Human lethal dose of tetanus toxin. *Lancet*. 1997;350:1518.
15. Meunier FA, Lisk G, Sesardic D, et al. Dynamics of motor nerve terminal remodeling unveiled using SNARE-cleaving botulinum toxins: the extent and duration are dictated by the sites of SNAP-25 truncation. *Mol Cell Neurosci*. 2003;22:454–466.
16. Burkitt JM, Sturges BK, Jandrey KE, et al. Risk factors associated with outcome in dogs with tetanus: 38 cases (1987-2005). *J Am Vet Med Assoc*. 2007;230:76–83.
17. Farrar JJ, Yen LM, Cook T, et al. Tetanus. *J Neurol Neurosurg Psychiatry*. 2000;69:292–301.
18. Adamantos S, Boag A. Thirteen cases of tetanus in dogs. *Vet Rec*. 2007;161:298–302.
19. Bandt C, Rozanski EA, Steinberg T, et al. Retrospective study of tetanus in 20 dogs: 1988-2004. *J Am Anim Hosp Assoc*. 2007;43:143–148.
20. Sykes JE. Tetanus and botulism. In: Sykes JE, ed. *Canine and Feline Infectious Diseases*. Elsevier; 2012:521–531.
21. Starybrat D, Burkitt-Creedon JM, Ellis J, et al. Retrospective evaluation of seasonality of canine tetanus in England (2006–2017): 49 dogs. *J Vet Emerg Crit Care*. 2021;31:541–544.
22. Burkitt-Creedon JM, Starybrat D, Humm K. Lack of seasonality of canine tetanus in California. *J Vet Emerg Crit Care*. 2021. In press.
23. Einterz EM, Bates ME. Caring for neonatal tetanus patients in a rural primary care setting in Nigeria: a review of 237 cases. *J Trop Pediatr*. 1991;37:179–181.
24. Polizopoulou ZS, Kazakos G, Georgiadis G, et al. Presumed localized tetanus in two cats. *J Feline Med Surg*. 2002;4:209–212.
25. Malik R, Church DB, Maddison JE, et al. Three cases of local tetanus. *J Small Anim Pract*. 1989;30:469–473.

26. Shea A, Hatch A, De Risio L, et al. Association between clinically probable REM sleep behavior disorder and tetanus in dogs. *J Vet Intern Med.* 2018;32:2029–2036.
27. Dieringer TM, Wolf AM. Esophageal hiatal hernia and megaesophagus complicating tetanus in two dogs. *J Am Vet Med Assoc.* 1991;199:87–89.
28. Goldhammer MA, Chapman PS, Grierson JM. Coxofemoral luxation in a border collie as a complication of a *Clostridium tetani* infection. *J Small Anim Pract.* 2008;49:159–162.
29. Baral RM, Catt MJ, Malik R. What is your diagnosis? Localised tetanus in a cat. *J Feline Med Surg.* 2002;4:221–224.
30. De Risio L, Gelati A. Tetanus in the cat: an unusual presentation. *J Feline Med Surg.* 2003;5:237–240.
31. Godwin RL. Tetanus in a cat. *Vet Rec.* 1985;116:574.
32. Langner KF, Schenk HC, Leithaeuser C, et al. Localised tetanus in a cat. *Vet Rec.* 2011;169:126.
33. Malik R, Simpson DJ, Church DB. What is your diagnosis? Tetanus. *J Small Anim Pract.* 1998;39:217–252.
34. Saranta JT. Tetanus in a cat. *J Am Vet Med Assoc.* 1977;170:3.
35. Tomek A, Kathmann I, Faissler D, et al. Tetanus in cats: 3 case descriptions. *Schweiz Arch Tierheilkd.* 2004;146:295–302.
36. Cook TM, Protheroe RT, Handel JM. Tetanus: a review of the literature. *Br J Anaesth.* 2001;87:477–487.
37. Goetz EF. Letter: tetanus in a cat. *J Am Vet Med Assoc.* 1976;169:174.
38. Robinson LR. Tetanus in a cat. *Vet Rec.* 1985;116:699.
39. Acke E, Jones BR, Breathnach R, et al. Tetanus in the dog: review and a case-report of concurrent tetanus with hiatal hernia. *Ir Vet J.* 2004;57:593–597.
40. Van Ham L, van Bree H. Conservative treatment of tetanus associated with hiatus hernia and gastro-oesophageal reflux. *J Small Anim Pract.* 1992;33:289–294.
41. De Risio L, Zavattiero S, Venzi C, et al. Focal canine tetanus: diagnostic value of electromyography. *J Small Anim Pract.* 2006;47:278–280.
42. Veronesi R, Bizzini B, Focaccia R, et al. Naturally acquired antibodies to tetanus toxin in humans and animals from the Galapagos Islands. *J Infect Dis.* 1983;147:308–311.
43. Ahmadsyah I, Salim A. Treatment of tetanus: an open study to compare the efficacy of procaine penicillin and metronidazole. *Br Med J.* 1985;291:648–650.
44. Attygalle D, Rodrigo N. New trends in the management of tetanus. *Expert Rev Anti Infect Ther.* 2004;2:73–84.
45. Okoromah CN, Lesi FE. Diazepam for treating tetanus. *Cochrane Database Syst Rev.* 2004:CD003954.
46. Rodrigo C, Fernando D, Rajapakse S. Pharmacological management of tetanus: an evidence-based review. *Crit Care.* 2014;18:217.
47. Papageorgiou V, Kazakos G, Anagnostou T, et al. The role of magnesium in the management of acute and long-term symptoms caused by tetanus in two dogs. *Top Companion Anim Med.* 2021;44:100535.
48. Centers for Disease Control and Prevention. Tetanus surveillance: United States, 2001-2008. *MMWR.* 2011;60:365–369.
49. Blakemore WF, Rees-Evans ET, Wheeler PEG. Botulism in foxhounds. *Vet Rec.* 1977;100:57–58.
50. Anza I, Vidal D, Mateo R. New insight in the epidemiology of avian botulism outbreaks: necrophagous flies as vectors of *Clostridium botulinum* type C/D. *Environ Microbiol Rep.* 2014;6:738–743.
51. Farrow BR, Murrell WG, Revington ML, et al. Type C botulism in young dogs. *Aust Vet J.* 1983;60:374–377.
52. Uriarte A, Thibaud JL, Blot S. Botulism in 2 urban dogs. *Can Vet J.* 2010;51:1139–1142.
53. Cai S, Singh BR, Sharma S. Botulism diagnostics: from clinical symptoms to in vitro assays. *Crit Rev Microbiol.* 2007;33:109–125.
54. Investigational heptavalent botulinum antitoxin (HBAT) to replace licensed botulinum antitoxin AB and investigational botulinum antitoxin E. *MMWR.* 2010;59:299.
55. Park JB, Simpson LL. Inhalational poisoning by botulinum toxin and inhalation vaccination with its heavy-chain component. *Infect Immun.* 2003;71:1147–1154.
56. Coban A, Matur Z, Hanagasi HA, et al. Iatrogenic botulism after botulinum toxin type A injections. *Clin Neuropharmacol.* 2010;33:158–160.
57. Ghasemi M, Norouzi R, Salari M, et al. Iatrogenic botulism after the therapeutic use of botulinum toxin-A: a case report and review of the literature. *Clin Neuropharmacol.* 2012;35:254–257.
58. Chertow DS, Tan ET, Maslanka SE, et al. Botulism in 4 adults following cosmetic injections with an unlicensed, highly concentrated botulinum preparation. *JAMA.* 2006;296:2476–2479.

73

Yersinia pestis (Plague) and Other Yersinioses

Bruno B. Chomel, Jane E. Sykes

KEY POINTS

- First Described: Descriptions of plague date back to around 1300 BC. The causative agent was isolated in 1894, in Hong Kong by Alexandre Yersin.[1,2]
- Cause: *Yersinia pestis*, a gram-negative coccobacillus (family Enterobacterales).
- Affected Hosts: *Yersinia pestis* causes disease in rodents, rabbits, wild carnivores, domestic dogs and cats, and humans. Wild felids (such as mountain lions or bobcats), goats, deer, antelope, camelids, and nonhuman primates can also develop illness.
- Geographic Distribution: USA: Southwestern United States; foci also exist in South East Asia, Africa (including the island of Madagascar), and South America (Peru, Brazil, Bolivia, and Ecuador).
- Major Mode of Transmission: Flea-borne, via an enormous variety of rodent flea species; ingestion of infected rodents or rabbits by cats and dogs. Human contamination reported by sleeping with flea-infested pets.
- Major Clinical Signs: Fever, lethargy, inappetence, lymphadenopathy, subcutaneous abscesses, hemoptysis (dogs).
- Differential Diagnoses: Tularemia, cat bite abscesses, *Streptococcus* spp. infections, feline infectious peritonitis, leptospirosis (dogs), aspiration or foreign body pneumonia (dogs).
- Human Health Significance: A small percentage (10%) of human plague cases result from exposure to infected cats, through bites, scratches, or respiratory droplet inhalation from cats with pneumonic plague. Dogs and cats can also expose humans through the carriage of infected fleas into households (especially when sleeping with owners).

ETIOLOGY AND EPIDEMIOLOGY

The genus *Yersinia* includes 11 different species, three of which are pathogenic in humans, cats, and dogs: *Yersinia pestis*, the agent of plague, and the two enteropathogenic species *Yersinia pseudotuberculosis* and *Yersinia enterocolitica*. Only *Y. pestis* is transmitted by arthropod vectors. Plague is caused by *Y. pestis*, a coccobacillus of the family Enterobacterales. It is a nonmotile, non–spore-forming, facultative anaerobic, gram-negative, bipolar-staining bacterium. The bacterium is non-saprophytic and sensitive to desiccation and temperatures ≥ 40°C. However, it can survive for several weeks to months in organic material such as infected carcasses, and survival in contaminated soil has been confirmed in natural conditions for at least 24 days and in experimental conditions for up to 40 weeks.[2,3] Cold temperatures or freezing may prolong the viability of this organism for years. The organism grows slowly in culture even at its optimum temperature (28°C on blood agar or MacConkey agar), so cultures should be held for at least 48 hours before being discarded. Colonies are much smaller than those of other Enterobacterales and may be overlooked. As recently as 1500 to 20,000 years ago, *Y. pestis* evolved from *Y. pseudotuberculosis*, a relatively benign enteric bacterium that is transmitted through contact with contaminated food and water.[3] As part of its transition from an enteric to vector-borne pathogen, *Y. pestis* has acquired two unique plasmids (pPla and pMT1), possesses genes required for persistence outside the vertebrate or vector, and gained apparently new functions for several chromosomal genes. *Yersinia pestis* produces a lipopolysaccharide endotoxin and a capsular envelope containing the antiphagocytic principal fraction I antigen. Three geographic variants of *Y. pestis* (*orientalis, antiqua*, and *mediaevalis*) have been distinguished biochemically but have identical virulence.

Yersinia pestis is maintained in wild burrowing rodents in rural regions of Asia (including the Middle East), Africa, and the Americas (Fig. 73.1). There is no plague in the Australian continent and New Zealand, Oceania, Japan, Taiwan, the Philippines, and Indonesia. The last case of plague in Europe was reported after World War II. The organism is transmitted between rodents by rodent fleas; humans, dogs, and cats are usually accidental and "dead-end" hosts (although direct transmission can occur through aerosols in humans and cats with pneumonic disease). Fleas become infected when they feed on heavily bacteremic rodents. The organism replicates in the flea gastrointestinal tract and creates in some flea species, such as *Xenopsylla cheopis*, the Oriental rat flea, a blockage of the proventriculus, located prior to the flea stomach, which causes the "starved" flea to repeatedly and aggressively feed and regurgitate bacteria into the bite site of a new host.[4,5] Infection is maintained by an obligatory flea-rodent-flea cycle involving bacteremic rodent hosts and their resident fleas (Fig. 73.2). More than 80 flea species have been found to be naturally infected with *Y. pestis*, and at least 28 flea species occurring in North America have been experimentally confirmed as vectors.[6] A large number of flea species can transmit *Y. pestis*, but some flea species, such as the Oriental rat flea *(X. cheopis)* worldwide and the ground squirrel flea *(Oropsylla montana)* in the western United States are particularly efficient vectors. Although nowhere near as efficient as these two fleas as a vector, the cat flea *(Ctenocephalides felis)*, for which the proventriculus blockage is usually absent, can infest rodent reservoirs and also has the potential to transmit *Y. pestis*.[7] However, the rapid transit of *Y. pestis* in the cat flea digestive tract makes the cat flea a poor plague vector. *Yersinia pestis* attains very high concentrations in rodent blood (108 organisms/mL) before the death of the rodent occurs, which allows fleas to acquire sufficient numbers of bacteria for efficient transmission to other rodents.[8] Fleas can remain infected for more than a year, which permits transmission long after the death of an infected rodent. Efficient transmission between rodents is enhanced by the fact that rodent fleas, which

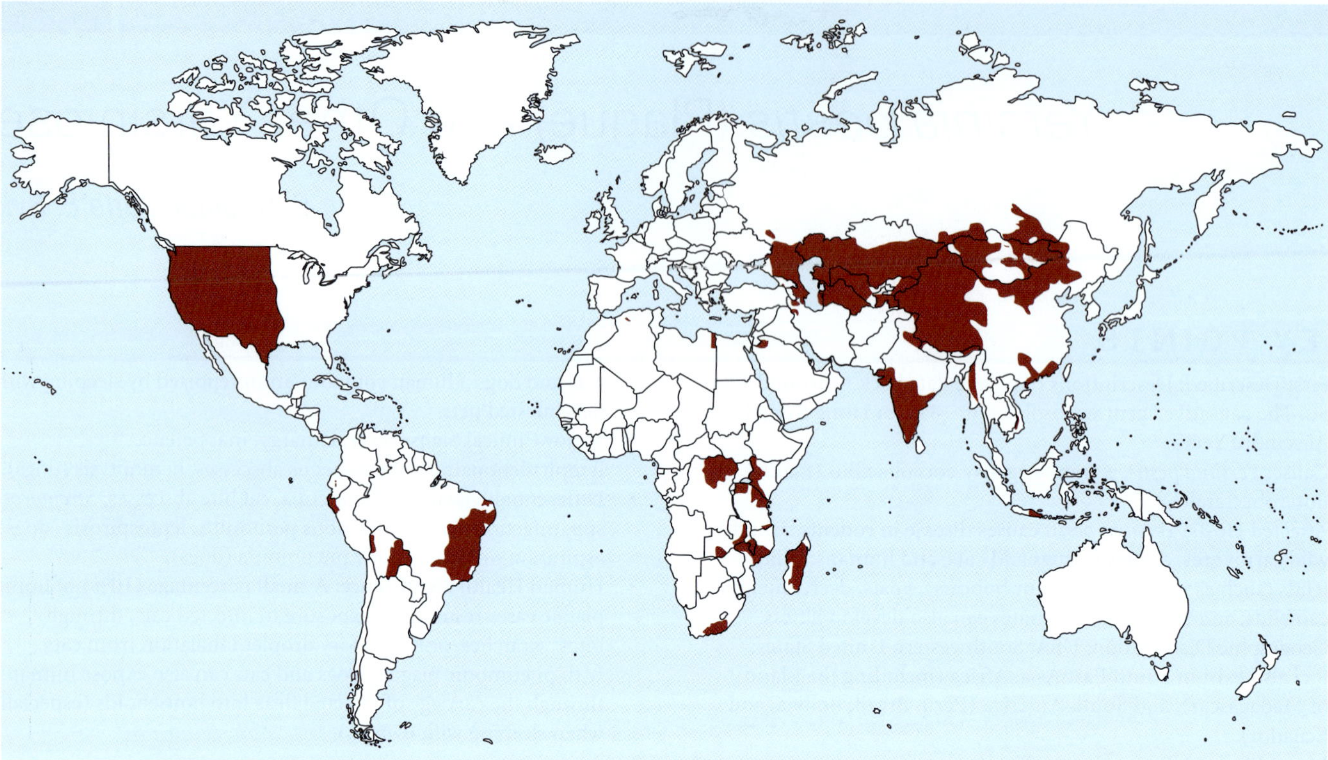

Fig. 73.1 Worldwide distribution of plague endemic areas. Data compiled from the World Health Organization, Centers for Disease Control and Prevention, and other sources. (From Centers of Disease Control and Prevention. Prevention of plague: recommendations of the Advisory Committee on Immunization Practices (ACIP). *MMWR Recomm Rep.* 1996;45:1-15. In: Mandell GL, Bennett JE, Dolin R, eds. *Mandell, Douglas and Bennett's Principles and Practice of Infectious Diseases,* 7th ed. Philadelphia, PA: Churchill Livingstone, Elsevier; 2011.)

are temperature sensitive, will search for a new warm-blooded host when their rodent host dies.

In the United States, plague foci are located throughout an area bounded on the east by the Rocky Mountains, with some incursions in the great Midwest plains, and on the west by the Pacific Ocean (Fig. 73.3). In North American carnivores, seroprevalence is highest in mustelids; intermediate in ursids (bears), felids, and canids; and lowest in procyonids.[9] Plague is transmitted to cats or dogs when they ingest or come into close contact with infected mammals (especially rodents or rabbits) or less commonly, after the bite of a rodent flea. Lesions of cats infected orally under experimental conditions were consistent with those in naturally infected cats. This corroborates the contention that cats most commonly contract plague through consumption of *Y. pestis*–infected rodents and not as a result of a flea bite. The histopathology of *Y. pestis* disease in these cats was comparable to that described for human plague.[10] Of 60 cats diagnosed with plague in one study, 75% had hunted rodents.[11]

Humans are infected by: (1) the bite of an infected flea (most common); (2) direct contact with contaminated tissues (such as handling dead rodents, rabbits, or other dead wild mammalian carnivores); or less frequently (3) inhalation of respiratory secretions by infected animals, especially cats (see Fig. 73.2). Death of a rodent from plague can cause the rodent's fleas to bite humans and other animals in a search for an alternative blood meal.

In the United States, plague in humans, dogs, and cats is now uncommon, although it is likely under-recognized in dogs and cats, and early recognition requires a high index of suspicion for the disease in endemic regions, because of the nonspecific nature of clinical signs.[12] Cats are more susceptible to disease than dogs. Affected dogs and cats can be of any age, breed, and sex, with a mean age of 3 years in one feline case series,[11] and 4 years in another.[13] Most plague cases in humans and cats occur in the southwestern United States, particularly northern New Mexico, but also southern Colorado, northern Arizona, and to a lesser extent California, southern Oregon, and western Nevada (especially in the Sierra Mountain ranges) (see Fig. 73.3). In 2016, plague was identified in six cats from Idaho; five were from southwestern Idaho, where dead ground squirrels with plague had been identified, and one was from eastern Idaho.[13] The probability of an area in the United States being a high-risk plague habitat increases with elevation up to 2300 meters and declines as elevation increases thereafter.[14]

Rodent or rabbit species associated with human cases include white-tailed antelope squirrels, ground squirrels, rock squirrels, cottontail rabbits, jack rabbits, prairie dogs, deer mice, Colorado chipmunks, and wood rats.[5] The prevalence of antibodies to *Y. pestis* in a survey of 4115 pet dogs and 466 pet cats from California in the mid-1990s was less than 5% in both species.[15]

In general, plague has a seasonal distribution that correlates with the timing of epizootics that lead to a die-off of susceptible rodents. In the United States, most plague cases occur from February through August, when rodents and their fleas are most active and humans and their companion animals are more likely to be outdoors. However, cases also occur outside these months, and so plague should not be

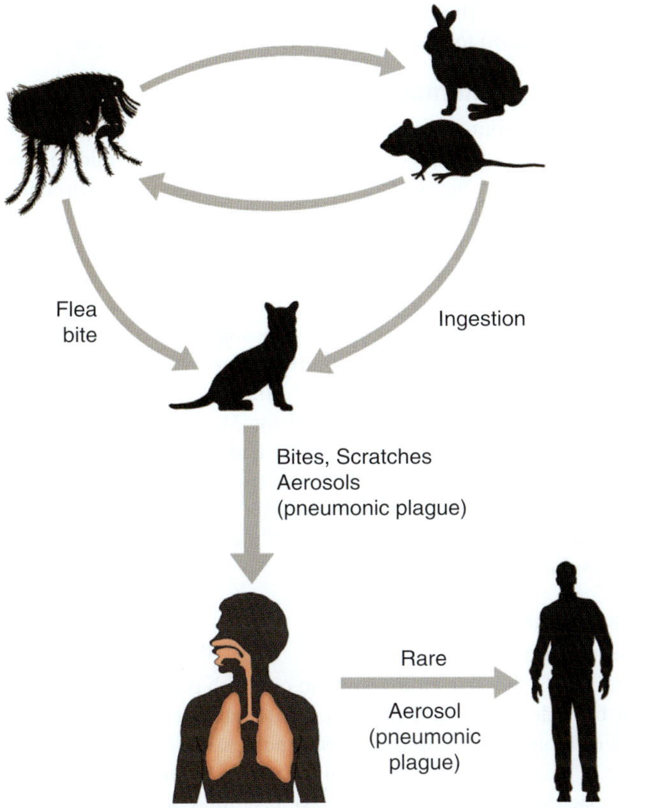

Fig. 73.2 The role of the cat in transmission of *Yersinia pestis* to humans. Most humans are infected by direct contact with wildlife reservoir hosts or a bite from an infected flea, but infections can also occur as a result of cat bites or direct exposure to cats that have pneumonic plague. Dogs can also be infected but are less susceptible than cats to disease and shedding. Direct aerosol transmission from one human to another is rare and only occurs in humans that have terminal pneumonic plague.

ruled out based on season. Interannual variability of plague incidence in endemic regions can be influenced by annual precipitation.[16] Summer soil moisture favors flea survival and vegetation growth for rodent populations. Global climate warming will likely influence the distribution of plague, with an expected shift of endemic regions away from the Equator.[17]

In general, the organism does not survive well in the environment outside infected hosts, with survival less than 72 hours on hard surfaces.[18] However, *Y. pestis* survived at least 24 days in blood-contaminated soil that was protected from UV light.[19] The extent to which environmental survival of *Y. pestis* contributes to the geographic distribution and epidemiology of the disease requires further clarification.

CLINICAL FEATURES

Pathogenesis and Clinical Signs

After inoculation into the mammalian host by fleas, *Y. pestis* is taken up by mononuclear cells, in which it survives, replicates, and produces F1 capsular envelope antigen. The envelope allows it to further resist phagocytosis, and a number of other virulence determinants including the *Yersinia* outer membrane proteins (Yomps), the Psa fimbriae antigen, and a broad-range protease known as Pla allow it to evade the immune system.[20] Cats and dogs usually become infected after they ingest or come into close contact with bacteremic rodents or other wildlife species that may have died of plague. In this situation, the organism has already produced a capsule and disseminates more rapidly than occurs after flea-borne transmission. Organisms are carried by lymphatics to regional lymph nodes. In more than half of affected cats, this results in an intense neutrophilic inflammatory response, variable fever, prostration, inappetence, and formation of the *bubo*, which is an enlarged and tender lymph node that occasionally forms an abscess and drains purulent material. This form of disease is known as *bubonic plague* and is the least fatal form of the disease. The location of

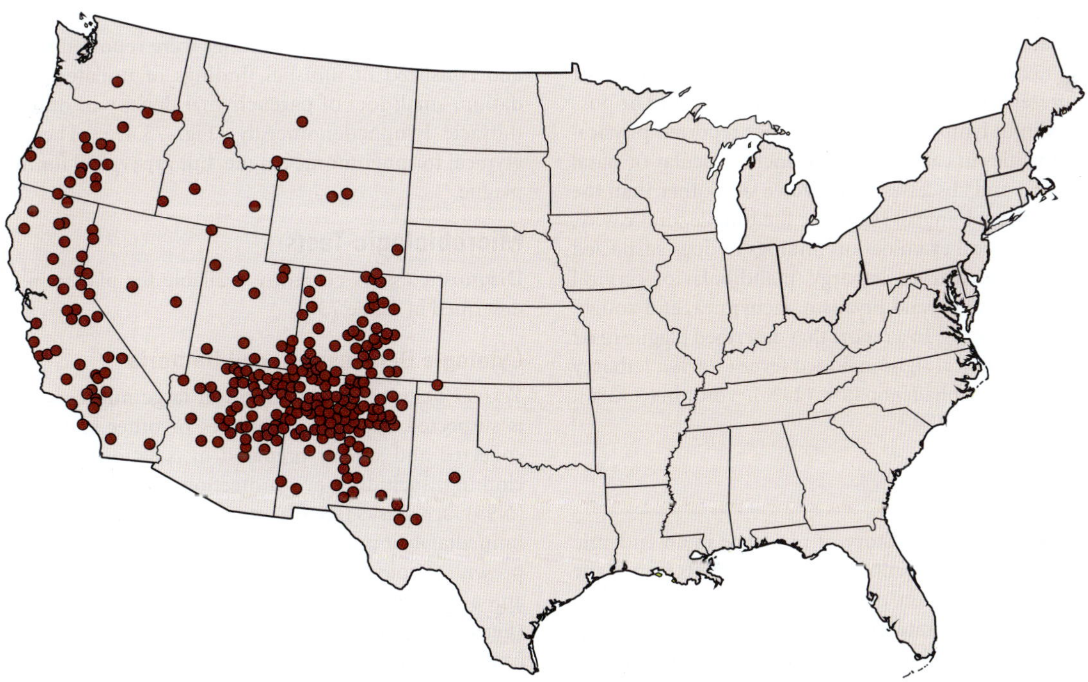

Fig. 73.3 Approximate distribution of human plague cases in western United States, 1970 to 2020. Each dot represents a case, with the dot placed randomly in the county of exposure. (Modified from Mead PS. *Yersinia* species (including plague). In: Bennett JE, Dolin R, Blaser MJ, eds. *Mandell, Douglas and Bennett's Principles and Practice of Infectious Diseases,* 8th ed. Philadelphia, PA: Elsevier Saunders, 2015. Data from 2007-2020 collated from ProMed-Mail reports, http://www.promedmail.org/.)

the bubo(es) depends on the initial site of infection. In cats that ingest infected rodents, the mandibular or retropharyngeal lymph nodes are usually involved, and affected cats shed bacteria from the oropharynx. Less often (around 20% of cats with bubonic plague), other peripheral lymph nodes are involved; this may follow flea-borne transmission that occurs at sites distant to the head.[11]

In some cats, bubo formation is accompanied by bacteremia, with associated endotoxemia and sepsis, and formation of hemorrhagic, neutrophilic, and necrotizing lesions in many organs. Disseminated intravascular coagulation and multiple organ failure can then ensue. Signs of severe sepsis or septic shock in affected cats include tachypnea, vomiting, tachycardia or bradycardia, and weak pulse quality. In some situations, bacteremia and multiple organ involvement occurs in the absence of identifiable buboes (*septicemic form*), which has a high mortality rate. *Pneumonic plague* occurs in about 10% of affected cats as a result of hematogenous spread of bacteria to the lungs or, less often, by inhalation of organisms and can result in dyspnea and cough. It has also been described in dogs.[12] The incubation period for plague is estimated to be 1 to 6 days, with shorter incubation periods after ingestion or inhalation of the organism, and death can occur within 2 to 3 days in the absence of appropriate treatment; occasionally the clinical course extends for 2 to 3 weeks. Some (<20%) cats show no signs of illness, or there may be transient fever, decreased appetite, and recovery. Transient febrile illness is also common in dogs.

Physical Examination Findings

Physical examination in cats with plague reveals lethargy (82% of cats), fever (71% of cats; mean rectal temperature of 40.5°C [105.1°F]), dehydration, a thin body condition, and lymphadenopathy. Lymphadenopathy most often involves the mandibular nodes. In one case series, 33% of 67 cats with bubonic plague had bilateral lymphadenopathy, 32% had left-sided lymphadenopathy, and 13% had right-sided lymphadenopathy; in the remainder of cats, the location was not known.[11] Bilateral disease occurred only when the mandibular and cervical nodes were involved. Lymph nodes may be markedly enlarged (up to 8 cm, with a mean of around 4 cm); may be edematous, abscessed, and painful on palpation; and may drain purulent material. Drainage was reported in 6 (15%) of 40 cats with bubonic plague. Dyspnea or tachypnea can be present in cats with pulmonary involvement or possibly as a result of painful lymphadenopathy. Other reported physical examination abnormalities in cats with plague include ocular or nasal discharge (14% of cats) and abscesses that involve sites other than the lymph nodes, such as the sublingual region or the tongue, oral cavity, face, limbs, or trunk. Physical examination findings in dogs suspected to have plague have included fever, lethargy, mandibular or cervical bubo formation, oral ulceration and ptyalism, tachypnea, and cough, sometimes with hemoptysis.[12,21] In a report that described plague in 62 dogs from New Mexico, clinical signs included fever (100%), lethargy (97%), anorexia (77%), lymphadenopathy (23%), vomiting (13%), diarrhea (8%), and abscesses (2%).[22]

DIAGNOSIS

Diagnosis of plague is based on a history of residence in an endemic area as well as contact with, or predation of, wild mammals (especially rodents or lagomorphs). Duration of illness, physical examination findings, and lymph node aspirate cytology also support the diagnosis. Clinicians should not exclude plague as a diagnosis based on season.[12] There is a relative lack of information available on laboratory abnormalities in dogs and cats with plague because the disease is rare. Ultimately, a diagnosis of plague can only be confirmed by culture, direct fluorescent antibody testing, and/or serologic testing. Confirmation of the diagnosis may ultimately take weeks, so a high level of suspicion for the disease is needed in endemic areas.

Laboratory Abnormalities

Hematologic abnormalities in naturally infected cats most often consist of mild to moderate neutrophilia, usually with a mild to moderate left shift, and occasionally lymphopenia and monocytopenia.[11,12] Leukopenia with a left shift can also occur in cats and dogs with pneumonic plague. Platelet counts have not been widely reported in naturally infected cats but may be low in cats with severe sepsis; thrombocytopenia has also been reported in dogs with pneumonic plague.[12] The serum biochemistry panel may show hypoalbuminemia, hyperglycemia, azotemia, electrolyte abnormalities, hyperbilirubinemia, and increased liver enzyme activities.[12,23] In the canine case series from New Mexico, a CBC was performed for 31 dogs; of these, 27 (87%) had a high WBC count and 18 (58%) had neutrophilia. The median WBC count was 21.6 × 10^3 WBCs/μL (range, 5.5 × 10^3 WBCs/μL to 38.1 × 10^3 WBCs/μL); median absolute neutrophil count was 16.5 × 10^3 neutrophils/μL (range, 1.8 × 10^3 neutrophils/μL to 24.5 × 10^3 neutrophils/μL).[22]

Diagnostic Imaging

Plain Radiography

Findings on thoracic radiography in cats with pneumonic plague have not been described in detail, but include diffuse interstitial, alveolar, and often nodular lung opacities. Findings in dogs with pneumonic plague have included lobar consolidation as well as patchy alveolar opacities.[12] Similar findings have been described in humans with pneumonic plague.[24]

Sonographic Findings

Abdominal ultrasound findings in cats with plague have not been reported. Based on pathologic findings, they might include abdominal lymphadenomegaly, splenomegaly, and hepatomegaly.

Computed Tomography

Computed tomography findings were reported for a dog with plague and consisted of unusual findings of unilateral lung lobe consolidation, small foci of parenchymal density in other lobes, and intrathoracic lymphadenomegaly (Fig. 73.4).[25] These were considered atypical for pneumonic plague, but are typical for human pneumonic plague.[24]

Microbiologic Tests

Diagnostic assays currently available for plague in dogs and cats are described in Table 73.1.

Cytologic Demonstration of Bacteria

Yersina pestis is usually found in large numbers in tissues. If plague is suspected, aspirates of buboes or other affected tissues should be collected and smears prepared in isolation while wearing protective clothing, including eye protection and properly fitted high-density (N95) face masks (see Chapter 15). The smears should be heat fixed or immediately immersed in fixative solution to inactivate any organisms present. Cytologic examination shows massive numbers of neutrophils and a monomorphic population of coccobacilli with bipolar staining (Fig. 73.5). This is in contrast to cat bite abscesses, where a mixture of bacteria is usually present.

Direct Immunofluorescent Antibody and Antigen ELISA Assays

Heat-fixed slides prepared from lymph node aspirates can be submitted to approved testing facilities for application of immunofluorescent

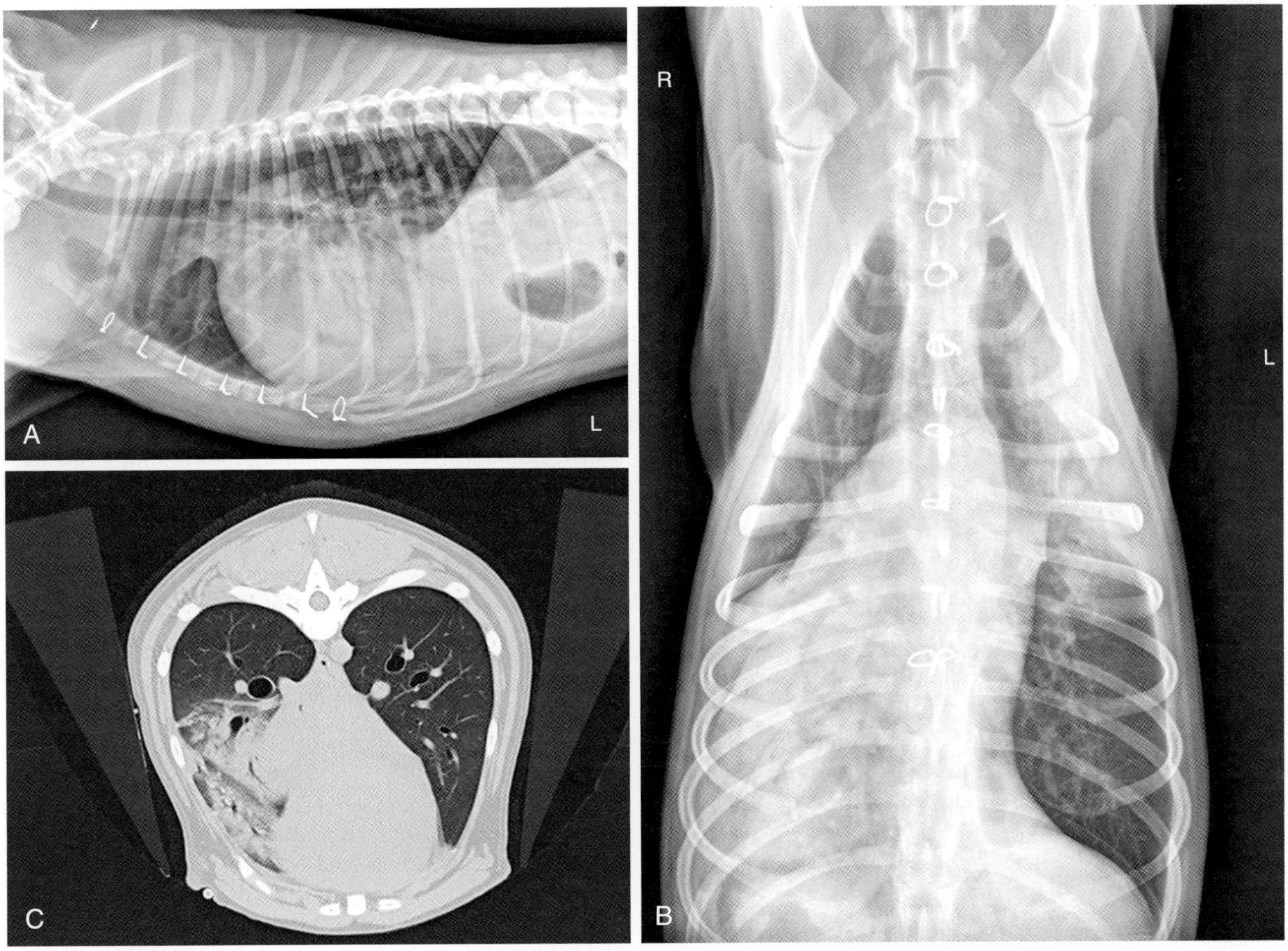

Fig. 73.4 Lateral (A) and ventrodorsal (B) thoracic radiographs and computed tomography scan (C) from a dog with plague showing severe lung consolidation and alveolar infiltrates. (A and B, from Schaffer PA, Hershkowitz CS, Dowers KL, et al. Delayed diagnosis of fatal pneumonic canine plague: clinical and pathologic features in two naturally infected Colorado dogs. *BMC Vet Res.* 2020;16(1):160. Published 2020 May 25. doi:10.1186/s12917-020-02361-z. C, from Schaffer PA, Brault SA, Hershkowitz C, et al. Pneumonic plague in a dog and widespread potential human exposure in a veterinary hospital, United States. *Emerg Infect Dis.* 2019;25:800-803.)

TABLE 73.1 Diagnostic Assays Available for Plague in Dogs and Cats

Assay	Specimen Type	Target	Performance
Culture	Lymph node aspirates, blood, tissues collected at necropsy	*Yersinia pestis*	Recent antibiotic treatment may cause false-negative results. May take 48 hours for colonies to appear. Hazardous to laboratory personnel and should be sent to laboratories with appropriate expertise when possible. MALDI-TOF may not accurately distinguish between *Y. pestis* and *Y. pseudotuberculosis*
Cytology	Lymph node aspirates	*Y. pestis* organisms (bipolar-staining bacilli)	Low sensitivity. Recent antibiotic treatment may cause false-negative results
Direct IFA	Lymph node aspirates, tissues collected at necropsy	*Y. pestis* F1 antigen	Increases sensitivity for detection of *Y. pestis* over cytology alone, but false negatives can still occur. Recent antibiotic treatment may cause false-negative results. Must be performed by laboratories with expertise in plague diagnosis
Serology	Serum	Antibodies to *Y. pestis*	Acute and convalescent serology is required for diagnosis of acute infection, because initial results may be negative, and positive results may reflect previous exposure rather than active infection
PCR-based assays	Lymph node aspirates, blood, tissues	*Y. pestis* DNA	Assays have not been validated in dogs and cats but several assays exist for diagnosis of human plague

antibody (direct IFA) against the F1 envelope antigen. Local public health authorities should be contacted for information on recommended testing facilities if direct IFA testing is required. IFA can also be applied to impression smears from tissues obtained at necropsy. Negative direct IFA results do not rule out plague, so culture and serology should also be considered.[11] A recombinant F1 antigen assay has been developed and offers advantages of lower biosafety requirements when compared to assays that use conventional F1

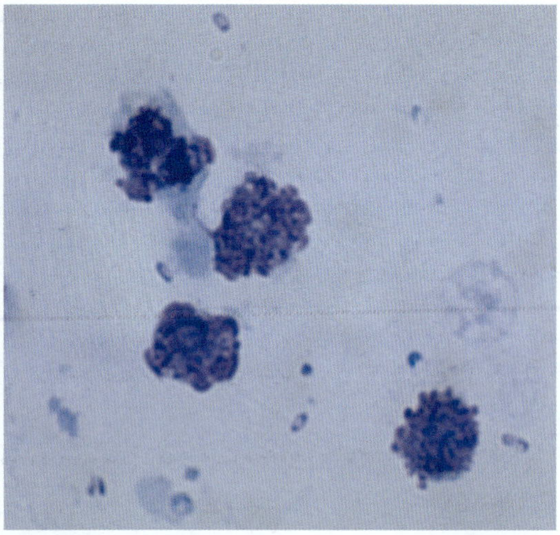

Fig. 73.5 Lymph node aspirate cytology from a cat with bubonic plague. Bipolar rods are scattered throughout the field. (From Nelson RW, Couto CG, eds. *Small Animal Internal Medicine,* 4th ed. St. Louis, MO: Mosby; 2009.)

antigen.[26] A lateral-flow dipstick assay has been described for rapid (within 15 minutes), sensitive, and specific POC diagnosis of plague in human patients, although false negatives may still occur.[27,28] This assay detects F1 antigen in body fluids such as sputum, lymph node aspirates, serum, and urine and has an estimated shelf life of about 2 years at room temperature. It has not been validated for diagnosis of plague in cats.

Isolation and Identification

Yersinia pestis can be grown from clinical specimens on routine media used for isolation of organisms that belong to the Enterobacterales. The organism grows slowly, and colonies are smaller than those of other Enterobacterales, so cultures must be held for at least 48 hours. If plague is suspected, specimens should never be shipped to routine veterinary diagnostic laboratories. Instead, local public health authorities should be contacted immediately for instructions regarding how and where to submit specimens for culture of *Y. pestis.* MALDI-TOF has been used to identify *Y. pestis*, but in the report that described the dog seen with plague at Colorado State University, the organism was incorrectly identified as *Y. pseudotuberculosis* with a high confidence score.[25] Because of concerns that the signs were not typical for *Y. pseudotuberculosis*, a PCR assay was done the following day (5 days after admission) that identified the organism as *Y. pestis.*

Serology

Acute and convalescent serology is required for serologic diagnosis of plague in cats and dogs. The most widely used serologic test is a passive hemagglutination inhibition (HI) assay (see Chapter 2), which is available through public health laboratories approved for plague diagnosis. Because of the extremely short incubation period, a significant proportion of affected cats and dogs may have negative titers when they first are brought to the veterinarian, so convalescent serum should be submitted at least 10 to 14 days after the initial titer request. Some cats may die before a rise in antibody titer occurs.[23] A fourfold increase in titer together with consistent clinical abnormalities confirms the diagnosis of plague. Titers in affected cats in one study ranged from less than 1:4 for acute specimens to 1:8192 for convalescent specimens.[11] In the case series of dogs from New Mexico, 54 plague cases had paired serologic samples tested, with 53 (98%) having positive test results on one or both samples, but only 2 (4%) dogs having positive results for the first serologic test. The median number of days between acute and convalescent serologic sample collection was 18 days, with a range of 10 to 54 days. Median convalescent antibody titer was 512 (range, 32 to 4,096).[22]

Molecular Diagnosis Using Nucleic Acid–Based Testing

PCR assays have been described for detection of *Y. pestis* DNA and are an attractive means of diagnosis because of their sensitivity and rapid turnaround time. In addition, the organism can be deliberately inactivated before specimens are submitted to the laboratory for PCR testing, which reduces the risk of laboratory-acquired infection. Real-time PCR assays have been validated for use on clinical specimens from humans,[28] but to date assays have not been validated for diagnosis of the disease in cats or dogs. The real-time PCR assay used to diagnose plague in a dog seen at Colorado State University was based on a CDC laboratory response network protocol (https://www.epa.gov/homeland-security-research/sam-and-us-centers-disease-control-and-prevention-cdc-laboratory-response).[25] Complex assays have been described that are able to accurately identify small sequence differences between *Y. pestis* and *Y. pseudotuberculosis.*[29] Real-time PCR was considerably more sensitive for diagnosis of human plague in Africa than the lateral-flow dipstick antigen assay or culture. A sensitive and specific isothermal amplification assay for rapid detection of *Y. pestis* has also been developed that could be used in field situations in highly endemic regions.[30]

Pathologic Findings

Gross pathologic findings in cats with plague include enlarged lymph nodes or abscesses with associated edema and hemorrhage, focal (up to 1 cm) lung lesions, and hemorrhages in a variety of organs. Histopathology in dogs and cats reveals hemorrhage, necrosis, neutrophilic infiltrates, fibrinopurulent pleuritis, and often very large numbers of small coccobacilli in tissues (although these are not always present) (Fig. 73.6).[12]

TREATMENT AND PROGNOSIS

Treatment of cats and dogs with plague involves supportive care, abscess drainage, and antimicrobial drug administration (Table 73.2). Animals suspected to have plague should be housed in isolation at least for the first 72 hours of antimicrobial drug therapy and handled by as few individuals as possible. Thoracic radiographs should be taken to assess for pulmonary involvement. Public health authorities should be notified immediately. Gowns, gloves, and suitable face protection (eye protection and a properly fitted high-density [N95] surgical mask) should be worn, and protective wear should be properly removed and disposed of after handling affected cats. Cats and dogs with plague should also be treated for fleas. Abscesses should be lanced and flushed with chlorhexidine solution. Any biohazardous waste should be double bagged and disposed of correctly. Routine disinfectants can be used to inactivate the organism in the environment. Antimicrobials with activity against most isolates of *Y. pestis* are aminoglycosides, tetracyclines such as doxycycline, chloramphenicol, and fluoroquinolones. In the New Mexico study, most plague-case dogs received enrofloxacin or doxycycline.[22,31-33] Trimethoprim-sulfamethoxazole and chloramphenicol also have activity against *Y. pestis.* Parenteral aminoglycosides such as gentamicin are preferred for seriously ill animals. Mortality rates in naturally infected cats that are not treated with antimicrobial drugs can reach 75%, but most (>90%) cats treated with antimicrobial drugs survive.[11] The time between antimicrobial drug treatment and recovery of affected cats ranged from 1 to 10 days in one study (mean, 4.4 days).[11]

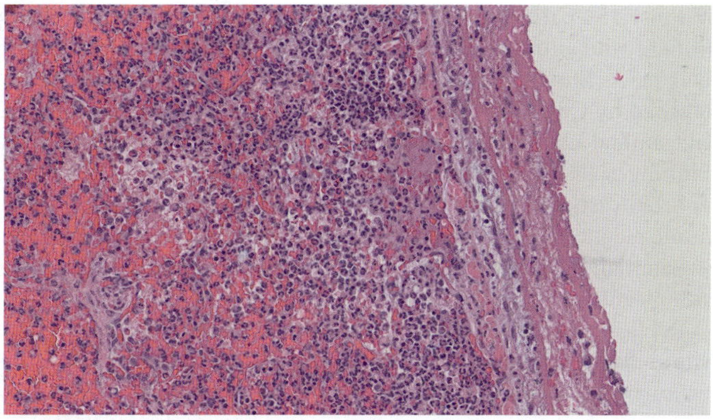

Fig. 73.6 Histopathology of the lung from a dog with pneumonic plague. There is severe necrotizing and suppurative pneumonia and pleuritis. (Image courtesy Paula Schaffer, Colorado State University.)

TABLE 73.2 Suggested Antimicrobial Drugs for Treatment of Plague in Cats and Dogs

Drug	Species	Dose (mg/kg)	Route	Interval (Hours)	Duration
Doxycycline	D, C	10	IV or PO*	24	10 days
Gentamicin	C	5–8	IV, IM, SC	24	10 days
	D	9–14	IV, IM, SC		
Enrofloxacin	D, C**	5	IV, IM, or PO	24	10 days

*Oral administration should be avoided for at least the first 72 hours of treatment to minimize exposure of the caregiver to *Y. pestis*. For IV doxycycline administration, dilute in 100 mL of lactated Ringer's saline and administer over 2 hours; if fluid overload is a concern, consider parenteral tetracycline or use of an aminoglycoside.

**The use of enrofloxacin to treat cats is controversial because of the potential for irreversible retinal toxicity and blindness. Do not exceed a dose of 5 mg/kg in cats. The use of alternative fluoroquinolones such as marbofloxacin, orbifloxacin, or pradofloxacin should be considered for cats.

IMMUNITY AND VACCINATION

There are no plague vaccines for dogs and cats. Although vaccines have been used to prevent plague in highly at-risk humans, these did not protect against pneumonic plague. Vaccine development for humans is continuing; for example, a vaccine based on a *Y. pseudotuberculosis* strain that produces an F1 pseudocapsule protected mice against both bubonic and pneumonic plague.[34] Currently there are no vaccines approved for use in the United States. Because *Y. pestis* is a potential agent of bioterrorism, efforts have been focused on development of subunit vaccines. However, *Y. pestis* has also been considered an unlikely agent of bioterrorism because in general it does not survive well in the environment, and person-to-person transmission requires close contact (1 m or less [3 feet]) with a dying person, usually on the last day of life.[5,22]

PREVENTION

Prevention of plague in dogs and cats involves housing cats indoors in endemic areas and discouragement of predation or exposure to/consumption of wild animals. Dogs should not be allowed to dig in endemic areas where rodent burrows exist. Flea preventatives should reduce the chance that dogs and cats will carry infected fleas into the house. Rodent control in the environment (e.g., removal of garbage and food scraps) should also be performed.

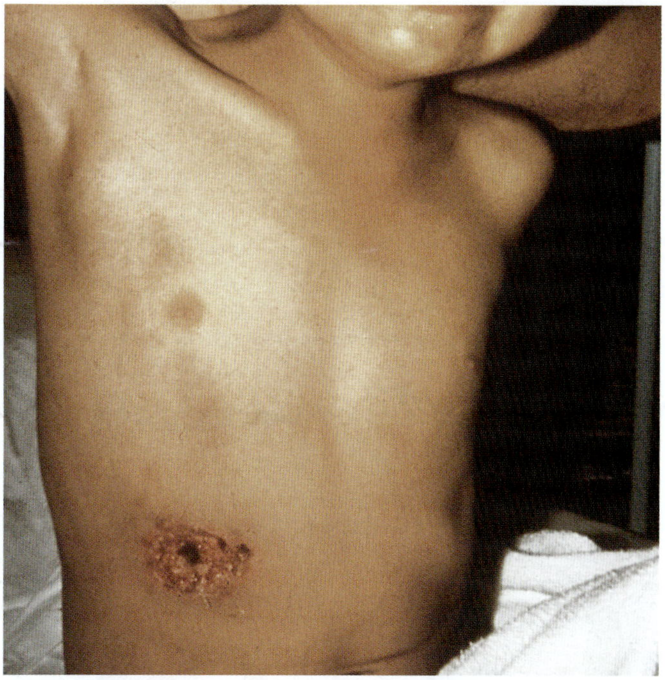

Fig. 73.7 Axillary bubo with ulceration and eschar formation at the site of an infected flea bite. (Courtesy Centers for Disease Control and Prevention. From Mead PS. Plague *(Yersinia pestis)*. In: Bennett JE, Dolin R, Blaser MJ, eds. *Mandell Douglas and Bennett's Principles and Practice of Infectious Diseases*, 9th ed. Philadelphia, PA: Elsevier, 2019:2783, Fig. 229A.6)

PUBLIC HEALTH ASPECTS

The clinical course of plague in humans closely resembles that in cats (Fig. 73.7). Three major pandemics of plague have occurred in humans: Justinian plague, which occurred in the Mediterranean basin during the sixth century Byzantine era; the "Black Death," which began in 1347 and spread throughout Europe; and modern plague, which began in China in the 1860s and was subsequently spread by rat-infested steamships to all continents inhabited by humans.[35] Interesting parallels have been drawn between the Black Death and the COVID-19 pandemic.[35] Currently, more than 80% of human plague cases reported to the WHO originate from sub-Saharan Africa and Madagascar. In the 1970s, Vietnam was the country reporting most human cases. From 1900 (when it first appeared) to 2015, 1036 cases were reported in the United States (www.cdc.gov). Between 2000 and 2019, 107 cases were reported to CDC with 11 deaths. The overall death rate in the United States for humans treated for plague is 15% to 22%. In endemic regions, humans who have close contact with rodents or their canine or feline predators are at risk. Most humans are infected as a result of contact with rodent fleas. Human disease has also been reported after skinning of rabbits or contact with wild carnivores (Fig. 73.8).[24,36] Fewer than 10% of human plague cases result from exposure to cats, with infection transmitted from cats to humans after a bite, scratch, or inhalation of respiratory droplets from cats with pneumonic plague.[37-39] However, exposure to cats often results in pneumonic plague, which has the worst prognosis and can progress to death within as little as 24 hours after the onset of symptoms. From 1977 to 1998, the CDC confirmed

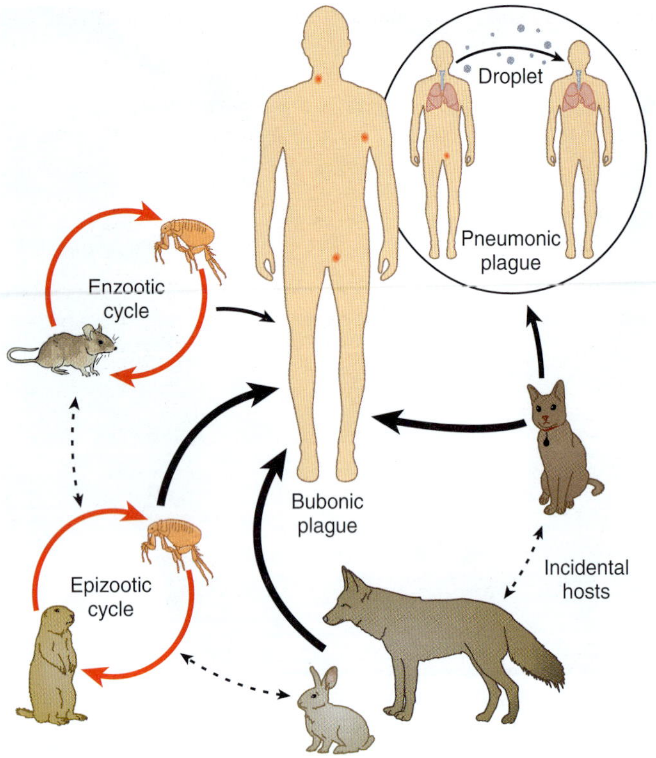

Fig. 73.8 Ecology and transmission of plague to humans. Red circles indicate zoonotic cycles. Wide solid arrows indicate common routes and thin arrows indicate uncommon routes of transmission to humans. (From Mead PS. Plague *(Yersinia pestis)*. In: Bennett JE, Dolin R, Blaser MJ, eds. *Mandell Douglas and Bennett's Principles and Practice of Infectious Diseases*, 9th ed. Philadelphia, PA: Elsevier, 2019:2781, Fig. 229A.3)

23 human plague infections acquired through inhalation of *Y. pestis*–infected droplets expelled from cats with secondary plague pneumonia.[40] Approximately one-fifth of those infected died, and one-fourth of those infected were veterinarians or their technicians. The remaining three-fourths of those infected were owners of or humans caring for sick cats. Approximately three-fourths of the humans developed bubonic plague, one person developed septicemic plague, and the remainder developed a pneumonic infection.[41] During 1926 to 2012, six (43%) of all primary pneumonic cases of human plague that occurred in the United States had contact with domestic cats.[42]

Occasionally, dogs or cats carry rodent fleas into the house, which may then transmit the infection to humans. Sleeping with a dog may also increase the risk of infection, and transmission of *Y. pestis* through contact with dogs has been increasingly recognized in recent years.[25,36,43,44] Exposure to infected fleas carried into a household by a dog was suspected in a report of two affected humans in Oregon, one of whom slept in the same bed with the pet dog during the 2 weeks before onset of illness.[43] The dog seroconverted to *Y. pestis*. Widespread exposure of 116 veterinary personnel at Colorado State University was reported in 2017 when a dog that had sniffed a dead prairie dog was seen for lethargy, fever, and hemoptysis.[25] In that dog, plague was initially not thought to be likely because the animal was a dog (rather than a cat), the season, a lack of peripheral lymphadenomegaly, and a radiographic imaging pattern suggestive of a foreign body. From 1970 to 2017, the proportion of plague cases associated with animal exposure in the United States increased over time, and 154 of 258 patients with animal exposure had contact with domestic animals before illness, including 121 with dogs and 102 with cats. Of those 154 patients, 42% had exposure to a domestic animal that brought wild animals into the house; 20% reported co-sleeping with their pet.[36] Most patients were reported from New Mexico (52%), followed by Colorado (14%) and Arizona (13%). Of those that had wild animal contact before development of plague, 40% reported skinning, 24% reported handling a sick or dead animal, and 22% reported casual handling or touching a wild animal.[36] Of six pneumonic plague cases associated with occupational exposure, five were veterinarians or veterinary technicians who were caring for animals with plague.

Pet flea control and reduction of exposure to rodents also serve to reduce plague in humans. Pet owners should be made aware that pets can carry fleas (and ticks) into the house and that flea control may reduce the chance of arthropod-transmitted human disease. Adoption of wild animals should be discouraged. In the veterinary hospital situation, plague can be prevented if there is a high index of suspicion for the disease and appropriate precautions are taken (see Treatment and Prognosis). Owners of pets suspected to have plague should be advised to contact their physicians without delay. Humans with exposure to affected animals are generally treated with prophylactic doxycycline or levofloxacin for 7 days.[24]

OTHER YERSINIOSES

Yersinia pseudotuberculosis and *Y. enterocolitica* are enteropathogenic bacteria that are distributed worldwide. They are classified into serotypes based on their O antigens, with different classification systems used for the two pathogens. Enteropathogenic yersiniae are maintained in a variety of food animals and wild animal reservoirs and are well-known causes of food-borne febrile gastrointestinal illness in humans; reactive arthritis may be a complication of infection in 15% of patients.[24] Pigs are a major reservoir for *Y. enterocolitica,* and outbreaks have primarily followed consumption of undercooked pork products.[24] *Yersinia enterocolitica* can also grow in food held at refrigeration temperatures. Affected human patients frequently exhibit right lower abdominal pain due to mesenteric adenitis or ileitis, which can mimic appendicitis. A small proportion of patients develop complications such as secondary polyarthritis and erythema nodosum (panniculitis).[24] Children are most susceptible. Immunocompromised humans (such as those with diabetes mellitus, malignancy, or immunosuppressive drug therapy) can occasionally develop bacteremia with systemic spread and abscesses in a variety of different organs. The mortality rate in this situation is at least 50%.[24] Dogs and cats can shed *Y. enterocolitica* and *Y. pseudotuberculosis* in their feces in the absence of clinical signs.[45,46] *Yersinia enterocolitica* was also isolated from 19% of 144 tonsils from stray dogs in Ireland.[47] Strains found in dogs can resemble those implicated in human disease,[48] and in several reports, dogs were suspected as a source for human infection and disease. *Yersinia enterocolitica* infection was associated with hepatitis in a 2-year-old Pekingese dog from Korea[49] and hepatitis and myocarditis in a 4-month-old Rottweiler.[47] It has also been isolated from young dogs with hemorrhagic diarrhea. There have been several reports of *Y. pseudotuberculosis* infection in cats, with microabscess formation in a variety of abdominal organs.[50-53] One cat from the United Kingdom was seen for acute-onset neurological signs, fever, increased serum liver enzyme activities, and leukopenia. Histopathology of liver biopsies showed severe necrotizing and pyogranulomatous hepatitis with intralesional gram-negative bacterial microcolonies.[53] A 7-year-old Labrador retriever search-and-rescue dog that was evaluated at the authors' hospital for hemoptysis, fever, and left cranial lung consolidation had pulmonary

Y. pseudotuberculosis infection; the clinical findings resembled those described for the dogs seen at Colorado State University for plague. Cases of human transmission from pets have also been reported, such as a diarrheic puppy dog which likely transmitted the infection to a 1-year-old girl.[54]

Enteropathogenic *Yersinia* species are usually susceptible to doxycycline, trimethoprim-sulfamethoxazole, chloramphenicol, aminoglycosides, and fluoroquinolones. Some organisms produce β-lactamase enzymes. Of concern, the mortality rate in *Y. pseudotuberculosis* bacteremia has been reported as 75% despite antimicrobial treatment.[24]

In dogs and cats, prevention of enteropathogenic yersiniosis involves feeding properly cooked foods and preventing predation. Other measures to reduce zoonotic transmission include hand washing after handling dogs and cats (especially before eating), wearing gloves when contact with saliva or feces is anticipated, and preventing dogs from licking the face or open wounds.

CASE EXAMPLE

Signalment

"Sam," a 5-year-old male neutered domestic shorthair cat from Woodland, CA.

History

Sam was brought to the UC Davis VMTH emergency service for evaluation of fever and inappetence. The owner first noticed he was ill 4 days previously, when he regurgitated a small amount of pink fluid about 1 hour after eating. The following day he was not eating, lethargic, and his water consumption was reduced. On day 3, he was taken to a local veterinary clinic where he was found to be febrile (105°F [40.5°C]), icteric, and had a mass on the left side of his neck. He was treated with enrofloxacin (1 mL SC, once), ketoprofen (0.1 mL SC), and clavulanic acid-amoxicillin (1 mL PO q12h), and blood was sent out for laboratory analysis. The results of a CBC showed a mild neutrophilia (13,083 cells/μL; reference range, 2,500–12,500 cells/μL) with slightly toxic neutrophils and a mild lymphopenia (1,176 cells/μL; reference range, 1,500–7,000 cells/μL). A biochemistry panel showed hyponatremia (133 mEq/L; reference range, 147–156 mEq/L), hypochloremia (99 mEq/L; reference range, 111–125 mEq/L), hypokalemia (3.4 mEq/L; reference range, 3.9–5.3 mEq/L), hyperglycemia (214 mg/dL; reference range, 70–150 mg/dL), hyperbilirubinemia (3.7 mg/dL; reference range, 0–0.4 mg/dL), increased serum CK activity (1858 U/L; reference range, 64–440 U/L), and a mild metabolic acidosis (bicarbonate 12 mEq/L; reference range, 13–25 mEq/L). ELISA serology for FeLV antigen and FIV antibody and IFA serology for FCoV antibody were negative. On receipt of the laboratory test results, the local veterinarian recommended referral.

Sam had been fed commercial dry and canned cat food and was treated monthly with fipronil. He was acquired at 6 weeks of age, at which time he was neutered. He had been vaccinated annually by the owner for feline herpesvirus-1, feline calicivirus, and feline panleukopenia virus, and was vaccinated for rabies for the first time 4 months ago. He had a history of intermittent inappropriate urination. He lived with three other cats, three dogs, and two rabbits, and the owner had brought home a wild mouse from the Lake Tahoe (Sierras) region several weeks ago. The rabbits were acquired by the owner 6 months ago, are kept indoors, and did not receive flea control. The owner fostered cats and occasionally dogs for the local animal shelter and cared for a colony of feral cats, which did not interact with the household cats. The household cats lived harmoniously indoors.

Physical Examination

Body weight: 5.4 kg

General: Lethargic but responsive. Resents handling. T = 105.9°F [41.1°C], R = 60 breaths/min, P = 176 beats/min, CRT < 2 s.

Integument: Mild scaling was present throughout the haircoat but no ectoparasites were visible.

Eyes, ears, nose, and throat: No significant clinical abnormalities. A small amount of dental calculus was present.

Musculoskeletal: Body condition score 6/9. There was a 2 × 2 × 6 cm firm subcutaneous mass alongside the trachea on the left side.

Cardiovascular: There were no murmurs or arrhythmias detected on cardiac auscultation. Pulses were strong and synchronous.

Respiratory: Tachypnea with a shallow respiratory pattern. Normal bronchovesicular sounds were present in all lung fields.

Abdominal palpation: No clinically significant abnormalities. Bladder palpable but small.

Lymph nodes: Left mandibular lymph node enlarged, 2 cm. All other lymph nodes appeared to be within normal limits.

Laboratory Findings

CBC: HCT 20.3% (30–50%), MCV 42.9 fL (42–53 fL), MCHC 33.0 g/dL (30–33.5 g/dL), reticulocytes 9,500 cells/μL (7,000–60,000 cells/μL), WBC 23,120 cells/μL (4,500–14,000 cells/μL), neutrophils 18,958 cells/μL (2,000–9,000 cells/μL), band neutrophils 3,699 cells/μL, lymphocytes 231 cells/μL (1,000–7,000 cells/μL), monocytes 231 cells/μL (50–600 cells/μL), eosinophils 0 cells/μL (150–1,100 cells/μL), basophils 0 cells/μL (0–50 cells/μL), platelets 102,000/μL (180,000–500,000 platelets/μL).

Serum chemistry profile: anion gap 18 mmol/L (13–27 mmol/L), sodium 143 mmol/L (151–158 mmol/L), potassium 3.2 mmol/L (3.6–4.9 mmol/L), chloride 110 mmol/L (117–126 mmol/L), bicarbonate 18 mmol/L (15–21 mmol/L), phosphorus 3.0 mg/dL (3.2–6.3 mg/dL), calcium 8.8 mg/dL (9.0–10.9 mg/dL), BUN 15 mg/dL (18–33 mg/dL), creatinine 0.8 mg/dL (1.1–2.2 mg/dL), glucose 151 mg/dL (63–118 mg/dL), total protein 6.6 g/dL (6.6–8.4 g/dL), albumin 2.5 g/dL (2.2–4.6 g/dL), globulin 4.1 g/dL (2.8–5.4 g/dL), ALT 30 U/L (27–101 U/L), AST 39 U/L (17–58 U/L), ALP 5 U/L (14–71 U/L), GGT < 3 U/L (0–4 U/L), cholesterol 134 mg/dL (89–258 mg/dL), total bilirubin 2.1 mg/dL (0–0.2 mg/dL), magnesium 2.0 mg/dL (1.5–2.5 mg/dL), creatine kinase 586 U/L (73–260 U/L).

Urinalysis: SpG 1.014; pH 8.0, trace protein (SSA), 1+ bilirubin, 2+ hemoprotein, 2+ glucose, rare WBC/HPF, 7–12 RBC/HPF, few lipid droplets.

Imaging Findings

Thoracic radiographs: No clinically significant abnormalities were present.

Abdominal ultrasound: No clinically significant abnormalities were present.

Neck ultrasound: There was moderate to severe enlargement of the retropharyngeal lymph nodes bilaterally and of the left mandibular salivary gland.

Microbiologic Testing

Cytologic examination of lymph node aspirates (mandibular and retropharyngeal): A slightly bloody background is admixed with markedly increased numbers of variably degenerate neutrophils. Low numbers of a mixed population of lymphocytes and scattered macrophages are also observed.

Interpretation: Marked suppurative inflammation.

Comments: Although no intracellular bacteria were seen, the number of neutrophils and their variably degenerate nature suggested sepsis as the primary differential diagnosis. The ability to observe bacteria cytologically and the results of bacterial culture may have been affected by recent antibiotic treatment.

Aerobic and anaerobic bacterial culture and susceptibility (lymph node aspirate): No growth.

PCR for *Francisella tularensis* DNA (lymph node aspirate): Negative.

Diagnosis

Severe suppurative lymphadenitis and fever, suspect plague or tularemia.

Treatment

Sam was transferred to isolation, during which time he bit a clinician, and was treated with intravenous fluids (lactated Ringer's solution and 20 mEq/L at 15 mL/h IV) and antimicrobial drugs (ampicillin, 20 mg/kg IV q8h and gentamicin, 5 mg/kg IV

Continued

CASE EXAMPLE—cont'd

q24h). Public health officials were contacted. The cat's rectal temperature initially increased to 107°F (41.6°C) and a bag of ice was placed beneath the cat's bedding; dark brown diarrhea was also noted. On the second day of hospitalization, Sam's rectal temperature was 105°F (40.5°C) and by day 3 it had normalized and Sam began to eat. It increased again to 103.9°F (40.0°C) the following day and the right mandibular and retropharyngeal lymph nodes became palpably enlarged. Subsequently the cat's rectal temperature normalized, laboratory abnormalities were improved, and the lymph nodes decreased in size and were soft on palpation. The cat was discharged with instructions to continue treatment with oral amoxicillin and subcutaneous gentamicin for 7 days, with a recheck planned at that time for an examination and convalescent *Y. pestis* and *F. tularensis* serology. The owner did not bring Sam back for a recheck examination, but a follow-up telephone conversation indicated that Sam had recovered completely.

Comments

A diagnosis of plague or tularemia was never confirmed in this cat although strongly suspected based on the history of wild rodent and rabbit exposure (with the rodent adopted from a plague endemic region) and the clinical abnormalities that were present. The findings of hyperbilirubinemia, thrombocytopenia, and increased serum CK activity were perhaps more suggestive of tularemia than plague, although hyperbilirubinemia and thrombocytopenia can occur in human plague. The history of antibiotic treatment may have contributed to the negative cytology, culture, and PCR results. Culture was requested on site shortly after admission because plague and tularemia were initially overlooked as likely diagnoses. Once these diseases were considered, an attempt was made to send specimens out to a public health laboratory for additional testing but this was complicated by concerns relating to the hazardous nature of the specimens. Handling of the cat was limited to as few individuals as possible and was difficult because the cat was aggressive. The clinician who was bitten by the cat immediately saw her physician who prescribed doxycycline for 7 days. Rabies quarantine was instituted because the cat was incompletely vaccinated for rabies. The owner was also educated about the possibility of plague or tularemia and the implications for human health. Although flea control was used, not all of the animals had flea prevention and there was significant turnover of a variety of wild and domestic animal species in the household. Continued adoption of wild animals by the owner was discouraged.

SUGGESTED READINGS

Glatter KA, Finkelman P. History of the plague: an ancient pandemic for the age of COVID-19. *Am J Med*. 2021;134:176–181.

Campbell SB, Nelson CA, Hinckley AF, et al. Animal exposure and human plague, United States, 1970-2017. *Emerg Infect Dis*. 2019;25:2270–2273.

Demeure C, Dussurget O, Mas Fiol G, et al. *Yersinia pestis* and plague: an updated view on evolution, virulence determinants, immune subversion, vaccination and diagnostics. *Microbes Infect*. 2019;21:202–212.

Kassem AM, Tengelsen L, Atkins B, et al. Notes from the field: plague in domestic cats—Idaho, 2016. *Morb Mortal Wkly Rep*. 2016;65:1378–1379.

Schaffer PA, Hershkowitz CS, Dowers KL, et al. Delayed diagnosis of fatal pneumonic canine plague: clinical and pathologic features in two naturally infected Colorado dogs. *BMC Vet Res*. 2020;16:160.

REFERENCES

1. Steensma DP, Kyle RA. Alexandre Yersin: discoverer of the plague bacillus. *Mayo Clin Proc*. 2020;95:e7–e8.
2. Yersin A. La peste bubonique a Hong Kong. *Ann Inst Pasteur (Paris)*. 1894;8:662–667.
3. Eisen RJ, Gage KL. Adaptive strategies of *Yersinia pestis* to persist during inter-epizootic and epizootic periods. *Vet Res*. 2009;40:1.
4. Dewitte A, Bouvenot T, Pierre F, et al. A refined model of how *Yersinia pestis* produces a transmissible infection in its flea vector. *PLoS Pathog*. 2020;16:e1008440.
5. Butler T. Plague into the 21st century. *Clin Infect Dis*. 2009;49:736–742.
6. Eisen RJ, Eisen L, Gage KL. Studies of vector competency and efficiency of North American fleas for *Yersinia pestis*: state of the field and future research needs. *J Med Entomol*. 2009;46:737–744.
7. Eisen RJ, Borchert JN, Holmes JL, et al. Early-phase transmission of *Yersinia pestis* by cat fleas (*Ctenocephalides felis*) and their potential role as vectors in a plague-endemic region of Uganda. *Am J Trop Med Hyg*. 2008;78:949–956.
8. Lorange EA, Race BL, Sebbane F, et al. Poor vector competence of fleas and the evolution of hypervirulence in *Yersinia pestis*. *J Infect Dis*. 2005;191:1907–1912.
9. Salkeld DJ, Stapp P. Seroprevalence rates and transmission of plague (*Yersinia pestis*) in mammalian carnivores. *Vector Borne Zoonotic Dis*. 2006;6:231–239.
10. Watson RP, Blanchard TW, Mense MG, et al. Histopathology of experimental plague in cats. *Vet Pathol*. 2001;38:165–172.
11. Eidson M, Thilsted JP, Rollag OJ. Clinical, clinicopathologic, and pathologic features of plague in cats: 119 cases (1977-1988). *J Am Vet Med Assoc*. 1991;199:1191–1197.
12. Schaffer PA, Hershkowitz CS, Dowers KL, et al. Delayed diagnosis of fatal pneumonic canine plague: clinical and pathologic features in two naturally infected Colorado dogs. *BMC Vet Res*. 2020;16:160.
13. Kassem AM, Tengelsen L, Atkins B, et al. Notes from the field: plague in domestic cats - Idaho, 2016. *Morb Mortal Wkly Rep*. 2016;65:1378–1379.
14. Eisen RJ, Enscore RE, Biggerstaff BJ, et al. Human plague in the southwestern United States, 1957-2004: spatial models of elevated risk of human exposure to *Yersinia pestis*. *J Med Entomol*. 2007;44:530–537.
15. Chomel BB, Jay MT, Smith CR, et al. Serological surveillance of plague in dogs and cats, California, 1979-1991. *Comp Immunol Microbiol Infect Dis*. 1994;17:111–123.
16. Ari TB, Gershunov A, Tristan R, et al. Interannual variability of human plague occurrence in the Western United States explained by tropical and North Pacific Ocean climate variability. *Am J Trop Med Hyg*. 2010;83:624–632.
17. Nakazawa Y, Williams R, Peterson AT, et al. Climate change effects on plague and tularemia in the United States. *Vector Borne Zoonotic Dis*. 2007;7:529–540.
18. Rose LJ, Donlan R, Banerjee SN, et al. Survival of *Yersinia pestis* on environmental surfaces. *Appl Environ Microbiol*. 2003;69:2166–2171.
19. Eisen RJ, Petersen JM, Higgins CL, et al. Persistence of *Yersinia pestis* in soil under natural conditions. *Emerg Infect Dis*. 2008;14:941–943.
20. Demeure C, Dussurget O, Fiol GM, et al. *Yersinia pestis* and plague: an updated view on evolution, virulence determinants, immune subversion, vaccination and diagnostics. *Microbes Infect*. 2019;21:202–212.
21. Orloski KA, Eidson M. *Yersinia pestis* infection in three dogs. *J Am Vet Med Assoc*. 1995;207:316–318.
22. Nichols MC, Ettestad PJ, Vinhatton ES, et al. *Yersinia pestis* infection in dogs: 62 cases (2003-2011). *J Am Vet Med Assoc*. 2014;244:1176–1180.
23. Gasper PW, Barnes AM, Quan TJ, et al. Plague (*Yersinia pestis*) in cats: description of experimentally induced disease. *J Med Entomol*. 1993;30:20–26.
24. Mead PS. *Yersinia* species (including plague). In: Bennett JE, Dolin R, Blaser MJ, eds. *Principles and Practice of Infectious Diseases*. 7th ed. Philadephia, PA: Elsevier Saunders; 2015:2607–2618.
25. Schaffer PA, Brault SA, Hershkowitz C, et al. Pneumonic plague in a dog and widespread potential human exposure in a veterinary hospital, United States. *Emerg Infect Dis*. 2019;25:800–803.
26. Tavares DHC, Bezerra MF, Magalhaes FB, et al. A new recombinant F1 antigen as a cost and time-effective tool for plague diagnosis. *J Microbiol Methods*. 2020;172:105903.

27. Chanteau S, Rahalison L, Ralafiarisoa L, et al. Development and testing of a rapid diagnostic test for bubonic and pneumonic plague. *Lancet.* 2003;361:211–216.
28. Riehm JM, Rahalison L, Scholz HC, et al. Detection of *Yersinia pestis* using real-time PCR in patients with suspected bubonic plague. *Mol Cell Probes.* 2011;25:8–12.
29. Papadopoulou E, Goodchild SA, Cleary DW, et al. Using surface-enhanced Raman spectroscopy and electrochemically driven melting to discriminate *Yersinia pestis* from *Y. pseudotuberculosis* based on single nucleotide polymorphisms within unpurified polymerase chain reaction amplicons. *Anal Chem.* 2015;87:1605–1612.
30. Randriantseheno LN, Rahantamalala A, Randrianierenana AL, et al. Development and evaluation of loop-mediated isothermal amplification for detection of *Yersinia pestis* in plague biological samples. *PLoS One.* 2020;15:e0237655.
31. Nelson CA, Fleck-Derderian S, Cooley KM, et al. Antimicrobial treatment of human plague: a systematic review of the literature on individual cases, 1937-2019. *Clin Infect Dis.* 2020;70:S3–S10.
32. Kugeler KJ, Mead PS, Campbell SB, et al. Antimicrobial treatment patterns and illness outcome among United States patients with plague, 1942-2018. *Clin Infect Dis.* 2020;70:S20–S26.
33. Scala G, Morrone G, Tamburrini M, et al. Autocrine growth function of human interleukin 1 molecules on ROHA-9, an EBV-transformed human B cell line. *J Immunol.* 1987;138:2527–2534.
34. Derbise A, Guillas C, Gerke C, et al. Subcutaneous vaccination with a live attenuated *Yersinia pseudotuberculosis* plague vaccine. *Vaccine.* 2020;38:1888–1892.
35. Glatter KA, Finkelman P. History of the plague: an ancient pandemic for the age of COVID-19. *Am J Med.* 2021;134:149–294.
36. Campbell SB, Nelson CA, Hinckley AF, et al. Animal exposure and human plague, United States, 1970-2017. *Emerg Infect Dis.* 2019;25:2270–2273.
37. Doll JM, Zeitz PS, Ettestad P, et al. Cat-transmitted fatal pneumonic plague in a person who traveled from Colorado to Arizona. *Am J Trop Med Hyg.* 1994;51:109–114.
38. Thornton DJ, Tustin RC, Pienaar BJ, et al. Cat bite transmission of *Yersinia pestis* infection to man. *J S Afr Vet Assoc.* 1975;46:165–169.
39. Werner SB, Weidmer CE, Nelson BC, et al. Primary plague pneumonia contracted from a domestic cat at South Lake Tahoe, Calif. *J Am Med Assoc.* 1984;251:929–931.
40. Gage KL, Dennis DT, Orloski KA, et al. Cases of cat-associated human plague in the Western US, 1977-1998. *Clin Infect Dis.* 2000;30:893–900.
41. Orloski KA, Lathrop SL. Plague: a veterinary perspective. *J Am Vet Med Assoc.* 2003;222:444–448.
42. Kugeler KJ, Staples JE, Hinckley AF, et al. Epidemiology of human plague in the United States, 1900-2012. *Emerg Infect Dis.* 2015;21:16–22.
43. Centers for Disease Control and Prevention. Notes from the field: two cases of human plague—Oregon, 2010. *Morb Mortal Wkly Rep.* 2011;60:214.
44. Gould LH, Pape J, Ettestad P, et al. Dog-associated risk factors for human plague. *Zoonoses Public Health.* 2008;55:448–454.
45. Fenwick SG, Madie P, Wilks CR. Duration of carriage and transmission of *Yersinia enterocolitica* biotype 4, serotype 0:3 in dogs. *Epidemiol Infect.* 1994;113:471–477.
46. Fukushima H, Nakamura R, Iitsuka S, et al. Prospective systematic study of *Yersinia* spp. in dogs. *J Clin Microbiol.* 1984;19:616–622.
47. Murphy BP, Drummond N, Ringwood T, et al. First report: *Yersinia enterocolitica* recovered from canine tonsils. *Vet Microbiol.* 2010;146:336–339.
48. Wang X, Cui Z, Wang H, et al. Pathogenic strains of *Yersinia enterocolitica* isolated from domestic dogs (*Canis familiaris*) belonging to farmers are of the same subtype as pathogenic *Y. enterocolitica* strains isolated from humans and may be a source of human infection in Jiangsu Province, China. *J Clin Microbiol.* 2010;48:1604–1610.
49. Byun JW, Yoon SS, Lim SK, et al. Hepatic yersiniosis caused by *Yersinia enterocolitica* 4:O3 in an adult dog. *J Vet Diagn Invest.* 2011;23:376–378.
50. Iannibelli F, Caruso A, Castelluccio A, et al. *Yersinia pseudotuberculosis* in a Persian cat. *Vet Rec.* 1991;129:103–104.
51. Obwolo MJ, Gruffydd-Jones TJ. *Yersinia pseudotuberculosis* in the cat. *Vet Rec.* 1977;100:424–425.
52. Spearman JG, Hunt P, Nayar PS. *Yersinia pseudotuberculosis* infection in a cat. *Can Vet J.* 1979;20:361–364.
53. Thompson D. Successful treatment of *Yersinia pseudotuberculosis* hepatitis in a cat presenting with neurological abnormalities. *JFMS Open Rep.* 2019;5:2055116919853644.
54. Hetem DJ, Pekelharing M, Thijsen SF. Probable transmission of *Yersinia enterocolitica* from a pet dog with diarrhoea to a 1-year-old infant. *BMJ Case Rep.* 2013:2013.

74

Tularemia

Jane E. Sykes, Bruno B. Chomel, Anne B. Nordstoga

KEY POINTS

- First Described: 1911, Tulare County, California.[1]
- Cause: Virulent strains of *Francisella tularensis*, a gram-negative coccobacillus (family Francisellaceae).
- Main Modes of Transmission: Inoculation, skin/mucosal contact, aerosol inhalation, ingestion, vector transmission.
- Major Vectors: Ticks (especially *Dermacentor andersoni, Dermacentor variabilis,* and *Amblyomma americanum* (eastern United States); and *Dermacentor reticulatus, Haemaphysalis concinna,* and *Ixodes ricinus* (Europe); biting flies (western United States); mosquitoes (Scandinavia).
- Affected Hosts: More than 300 animal species, which include rodents, rabbits, wild carnivores, domestic dogs and cats, sheep, horses, nonhuman primates, and humans.
- Geographic Distribution: Northern hemisphere between 30 degrees and 71 degrees of latitude; most severe disease cases in humans is reported from North America, especially the United States, where virulent strains are most prevalent.
- Major Clinical Signs: Fever, lethargy, inappetence, lymphadenopathy, subcutaneous abscesses, splenomegaly, hepatomegaly, GI signs such as vomiting and abdominal pain.
- Differential Diagnoses: Plague, cat bite abscess, *Streptococcus* spp. infections, feline infectious peritonitis, mycobacterial infections, lymphoma, sepsis caused by other gram-negative bacteria.
- Human Health Significance: Cats and less commonly dogs and wild canids (i.e., coyotes) can transmit tularemia to humans after they are exposed to infected rodents or rabbits. Cat bites are most commonly implicated.

ETIOLOGIC AGENT AND EPIDEMIOLOGY

Tularemia (also known as rabbit fever, hare fever, deerfly fever, and lemming fever) is an extremely infectious but uncommon zoonotic disease caused by *Francisella tularensis,* a small (0.2 × 0.2 × 0.7 μm), non-motile, aerobic, facultative intracellular gram-negative coccobacillus. The name "tularemia" comes from the first isolation of the organism from sick ground squirrels in Tulare County, California, in 1911 by McCoy and Chapin.[2] The first isolate from a human being was obtained in 1914 by Wherry and Lamb (OH, United States). Edward Francis extensively described the clinical, epidemiological, and diagnostic aspects of tularemia in the early 20th century.[3]

There are four subspecies of *F. tularensis: tularensis, holarctica, novicida,* and *mediasiatica*. Subspecies *tularensis* (also known as type A) and *holarctica* (type B) cause most disease in humans.[3] Subspecies *mediasiatica* is only found in Asia and the former Soviet Union. Subspecies *novicida* can cause illness in severely immunosuppressed humans and is widely studied as a model for tularemia because of its low virulence to laboratory workers.

Francisella tularensis subsp. *tularensis* has the greatest degree of virulence (for humans) and predominates in North America, whereas the less virulent subspecies *holarctica* predominates in Europe but is also present in North America. Additional genetic variation within type A and type B subpopulations of *F. tularensis* correlates with geographic distribution of cases and the severity of disease.[4] Molecular subtyping has further divided type A into subpopulations A1a, A1b, A2a, and A2b. The highest mortality rate (24%) in humans results from infections by A1b.[5] *Francisella tularensis* subsp. *holarctica* strains are typically separated into three biovars. Biovar 1 (erythromycin sensitive) is reported in western Europe and biovar 2 (naturally erythromycin resistant) is found in eastern European countries, although these strains overlap in their geographical spread. Biovar japonica (which ferments glycerol) is mainly found in Japan, but was also reported in China and Turkey, and more recently from Australia.[3,6]

Tularemia occurs primarily in the Northern Hemisphere, especially between 30 degrees and 71 degrees of latitude (Fig. 74.1). Human disease caused by a subsp. *novicida*–like organism was reported from the Northern Territory in Australia in 2003,[7] and subsp. *holarctica* was reported as the cause of disease in a woman from Tasmania, Australia after she was bitten by a ringtail possum.[8]

Even in North America, where *F. tularensis* subsp. *tularensis* predominates, tularemia is a rare disease, and most human cases occur in the central and north-central United States, especially Arkansas, Missouri, Kansas, South Dakota, and Oklahoma, with an additional focus in Massachusetts (especially Martha's Vineyard) (Fig. 74.2). Cases also occur in California. Type A1 is found in the central states endemic region and is the most virulent and invasive subtype, while type A2 is observed in the western United States and is less virulent. Type B is associated with water bodies especially the upper Mississippi and Missouri Rivers, high rainfall areas, rodents and ticks, whereas type A1 is associated with lagomorphs, cats, and ticks.[9] Despite its rarity, tularemia is a reportable disease in the United States because *F. tularensis* is considered a potential agent of bioterrorism. In Europe, *F. tularensis* subsp. *holarctica* is endemic in many countries ranging from Eastern to Western Europe. In Scandinavian countries, outbreaks in humans involving tens to hundreds of patients occur on a regular basis. Tularemia is considered a re-emerging zoonosis, with increasing numbers of reported cases in humans, in countries like Germany, France, Italy, and Spain.[3,10,11] Tularemia has been absent from the United Kingdom, with the exception of travel-related disease. It also occurs in Russia and Japan.[12]

Disease in cats and dogs due to *F. tularensis* has mainly been reported from the United States. Young adult cats and dogs are usually affected. As with plague, cats are more susceptible than

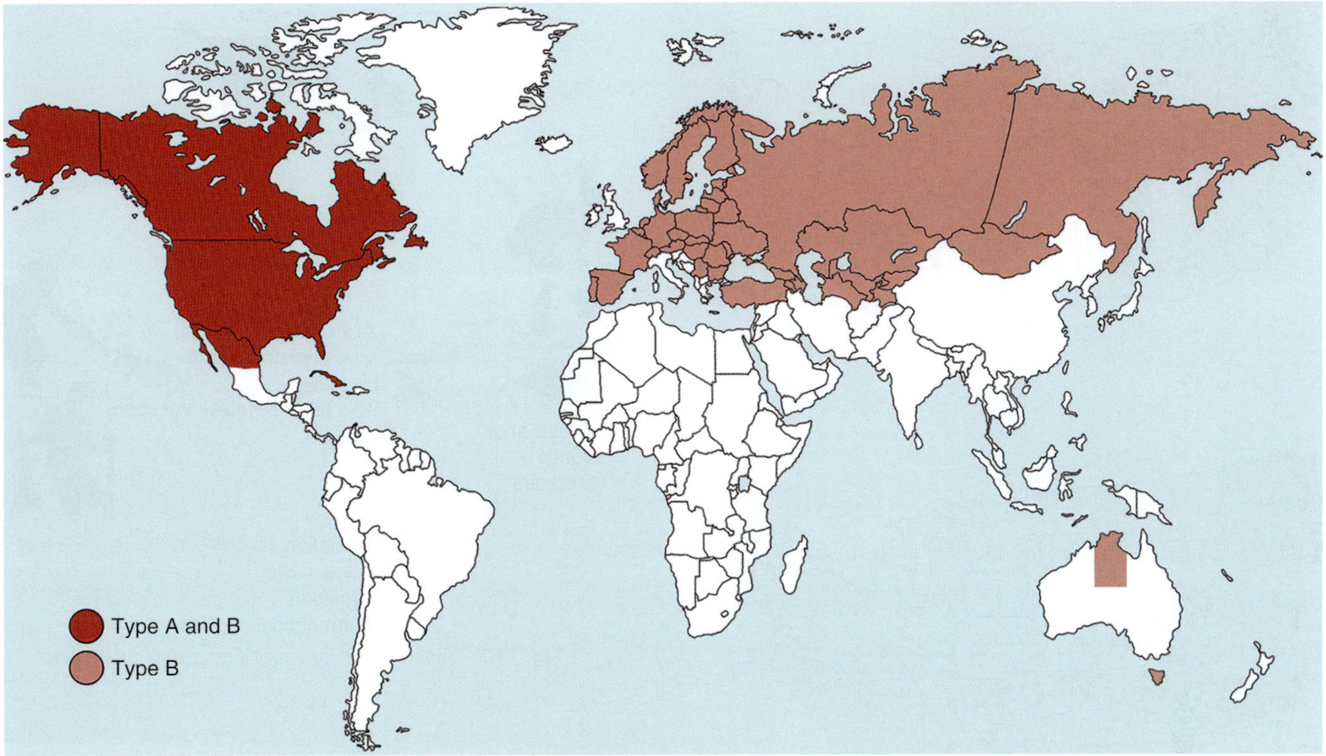

Fig. 74.1 Global distribution of tularemia. (Modified from Centers for Disease Control and Prevention).

dogs. Cases have been reported from Oklahoma[13-15] and Kansas,[16] but also from other locations that include Montana,[17] Missouri,[18] Massachusetts,[19] central Virginia,[20] and eastern Oregon,[21] which mirrors the distribution in humans. A case series of 88 dogs with tularemia was also described from New Mexico.[22] The median age of affected dogs in that study was 4 years and 8 months (range, 3 months to 14 years); 52% were neutered females, 33% were castrated male dogs, and 71% were medium- to large-breed dogs. Cases occurred every month of the year except December. In Oklahoma, feline tularemia has seasonal incidence peaks that occur from March to June and September to November.[8] In a review of 106 *F. tularensis* isolates collected mainly from Nebraska between 1998 and 2012, a strikingly high percentage (48%) were cat associated.[23] The highest number of feline-derived tularemia cases occurred in a city known to have multiple feral cat colonies and during a year with extended warm weather and extreme drought conditions.

Tularemia is likely underdiagnosed in cats and dogs because clinical signs are nonspecific. Many cats are diagnosed with tularemia at necropsy.[13,16] The seroprevalence in pet cats from Connecticut and New York state was 12%.[24] Feline tularemia seems to be mainly associated with *F. tularensis* subsp. *tularensis*, but *F. tularensis* subsp. *holarctica* is also found in cats.[13,15,25,26] However, in these studies, the focus has mainly been on zoonotic potential, and little is known about clinical disease in cats with *F. tularensis* subsp. *holarctica* infection. Tularemia was reported in a dog from Norway after hunting a mountain hare infected with *F. tularensis* subsp. *holarctica*.[27] Several additional cases of tularemia in dogs have been recognized in Norway and the United States in recent years.

Francisella tularensis is maintained in the environment by a huge variety of terrestrial and aquatic mammals, which include rabbits, hares, ground squirrels, prairie dogs, lemmings, voles, beavers, muskrats, water rats, ring tail possums, and other rodents.[12] It often causes severe disease in these species, although subclinical carriage may also occur. It can be transmitted by arthropod bites, inhalation or ingestion of the organism, and direct skin contact with infected tissues (probably when there are minute breaks in the skin) (Fig. 74.3). Inhalation of as few as 10 organisms can cause human disease, whereas larger numbers of organisms (10^8) must be ingested for disease to occur. Cats and dogs become infected when they hunt rodents or lagomorphs; a history of rabbit ingestion is most often described in association with reported feline and canine cases.[13-15,22,27] In a Norwegian study, antibodies to *F. tularensis* were found in 13 of 23 dogs exposed to lemmings, while all 10 dogs without exposure to hares or lemmings were seronegative.[27] The organism can also survive for years in frozen rabbit meat.

In the western United States (Utah, Nevada, and California), the most common arthropod vectors are biting flies, whereas ticks (especially *Dermacentor* spp. and *Amblyomma americanum*) are the most common vectors east of the Rocky Mountains.[28] In Europe, *Dermacentor* ticks and *Ixodes ricinus* are the main tick vectors; mosquitoes are important vectors in Scandinavia.[29] In Sweden, transstadial maintenance in mosquitoes and transmission to susceptible mammals have been documented.[29,30]

Francisella tularensis is well known for its ability to survive up to several months in fresh water sources, and survival in brackish water has also been demonstrated.[31] While *F. tularensis* contamination of water wells have resulted in several human outbreaks of oropharyngeal tularemia, transmission by vectors generally results in the ulceroglandular form.[32] Survival and replication of *F. tularensis* within free-living amebae such as *Hartmannella vermiformis* may contribute to the organism's ability to persist in water sources.[33]

CLINICAL FEATURES

Pathogenesis and Clinical Signs

The clinical manifestations of tularemia depend on the virulence of the infecting strain, the route of inoculation, and host immunity.

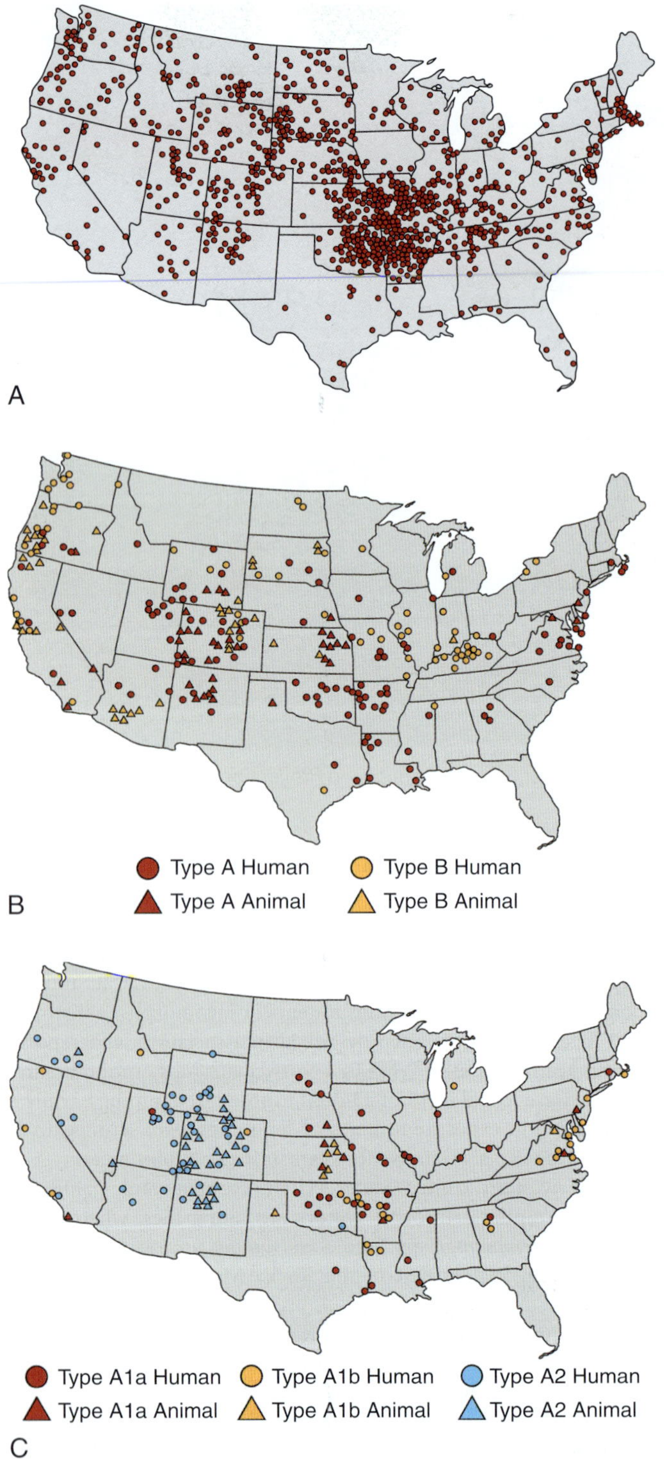

Fig. 74.2 Approximate geographic distribution of tularemia cases in the USA. Compare this with the geographic distribution of plague (Fig. 73.3). (A) Overall distribution of human tularemia cases. (B) Distribution of type A and type B isolates from humans and animals. (C) Distribution of isolates from humans and animals by molecular subtype. Note that the geographic distribution of human type A cases follows the distribution of subtype A1, the most virulent subtype being A1b. (A, compiled from data available from Kugeler et al.[5] and the Centers for Disease Control and Prevention through 2018; B, modified from Kugeler et al.[5])

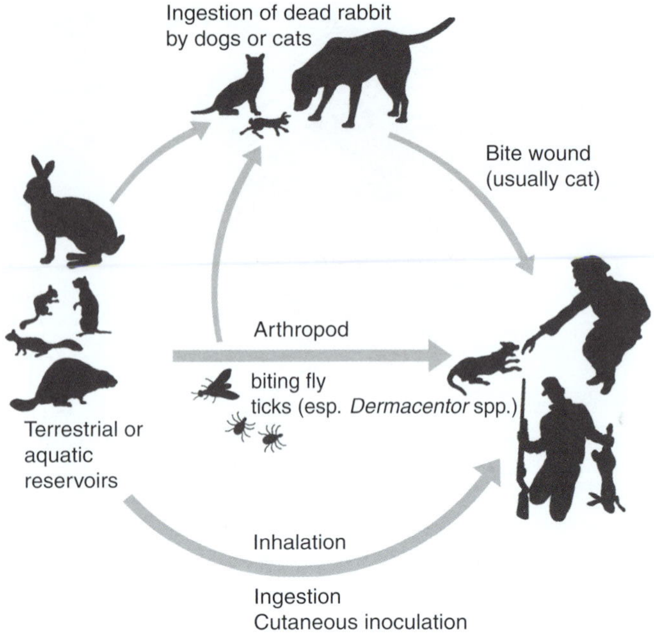

Fig. 74.3 Transmission cycle for *Francisella tularensis.*

Although tularemia may rapidly progress to death in cats, protracted illness has also been described.[21] Milder disease occurs in dogs when compared with cats.[22]

Francisella tularensis survives in macrophages through evasion of cellular destruction by phagosomes and inhibition of the respiratory burst. Several different virulence factors of *F. tularensis* have been identified, which include bacterial LPS, pili, a capsule, and a series of acid phosphatase enzymes. The endotoxic activity of the LPS of *F. tularensis* is 1000-fold less than that of *Escherichia coli.*[34,35] Production of acid phosphatase enzymes may be key to the organism's ability to inhibit the respiratory burst and survive in macrophages.[36] Many stages of the organism's intracellular lifestyle depend on a pathogenicity island (group of virulence genes) known as the *Francisella* pathogenicity island, which encodes a type VI–like secretion system associated with bacterial virulence.

For the first few days after cutaneous inoculation, *F. tularensis* replicates locally and can produce a papule that may then ulcerate. It then disseminates to local lymph nodes, which may be followed by bacteremia and sepsis, with infection of systemic, primarily reticuloendothelial tissues. The organism invades not only macrophages but also nonphagocytic cells such as hepatocytes and alveolar epithelial cells,[37] with induction of a profound inflammatory response and necrosis. Incubation periods that range from 1 to 5 days have been suspected in naturally occurring tularemia in dogs and cats, but longer incubation periods (up to 21 days) can occur in humans. Clinical signs typically manifest as a sudden onset of fever, lethargy, and inappetence. Other manifestations in affected cats have included a thin body condition, icterus, hepatomegaly, vomiting, dehydration, peripheral and/or abdominal lymphadenomegaly, splenomegaly, and oral and/or lingual ulceration. Hypothermia and bradycardia can occur in moribund cats;[13] one cat had seizures and was nonresponsive.[20] A single cat with localized cutaneous tularemia had a chronic (1-year duration) draining skin lesion in the region of (but not involving) the mandibular lymph nodes, in the absence of systemic signs.[21] Infection in dogs results in disease that is either subclinical or mild.[22,27] In reports of naturally affected dogs, clinical signs have included fever, lethargy, anorexia, and peripheral lymphadenopathy.[14,22,27,38] Other signs have included vomiting, diarrhea, respiratory signs, oculonasal discharge, and tonsillitis.[14,22,38]

Physical Examination Findings

Physical examination in cats with tularemia may reveal lethargy, fever (up to 40.5°C [105.1°F]) or hypothermia, a thin body condition, and dehydration.[13,15,17-19] Ulceration of the oral mucous membranes or tongue may be present.[13,19] Icterus may also occur.[36] Moribund cats may be hypothermic and bradycardic and may have weak pulse quality. Mild to marked peripheral lymphadenopathy is present in most but not all cats. Lymphadenopathy may be restricted to the lymph nodes of the head and neck[19] or may be generalized.[13,15] Abdominal palpation may reveal hepatomegaly or splenomegaly, or abdominal lymph nodes may be palpable. One or more signs of fever (up to 41.4°C [106.5°F]), lethargy, peripheral lymphadenopathy, mucoid ocular discharge, and tonsillitis may be present in dogs.[14,22,27,38]

DIAGNOSIS

Tularemia should be considered in cats and dogs with lymphadenopathy and fever that have a history of residence in or recent travel to an endemic area, as well as contact with or predation of wild mammals (especially lagomorphs). Plague is the major differential diagnosis of zoonotic importance in the southwestern United States (Table 74.1). Ultimately, the diagnosis can be confirmed by culture, PCR, and/or serologic testing. Access to approved laboratories that practice BSL 3 procedures is required to perform bacterial culture when tularemia is suspected. Local public health authorities should be contacted to report suspicion for the disease and for information on recommended testing facilities.

Laboratory Abnormalities

Complete Blood Count, Biochemistry Profile, and Urinalysis

Leukocyte counts in a limited number of cats with tularemia have been normal, decreased (as low as 1300 cells/μL), or increased with evidence of neutrophil toxicity.[13,15,19,20] Moderate to marked bandemia may be present.[15,19] Thrombocytopenia is a common finding (as low as 41,000 platelets/μL).[13,15] The serum biochemistry panel may show hypoglycemia, azotemia, and electrolyte abnormalities, increased liver enzyme activities, and hyperbilirubinemia (up to 7.6 mg/dL).[13,15,20] Bilirubinuria and hemoglobinuria may be present.[13] Leukocytosis due to a neutrophilia (just over 50% of dogs) and thrombocytopenia (38% of dogs) have been reported in infected dogs.[14,22]

Cytologic Examination of Lymph Node Aspirates

Cytologic examination of lymph node aspirates in cats with tularemia may reveal lymph node hyperplasia.[15] Lymph nodes may also contain necrotic debris and increased numbers of macrophages and/or degenerate neutrophils.[13,19] Because *F. tularensis* is tiny and stains only faintly, organisms are less likely to be visualized than those of *Yersinia pestis* (see Chapter 73).

Diagnostic Imaging

Plain Radiography

Findings on thoracic radiography in cats with tularemia have not been well described; one cat had normal thoracic radiographs.[15] Findings on abdominal radiography have included hepatomegaly and fluid-filled intestinal loops.[15]

TABLE 74.1 Differences and Similarities between Plague and Tularemia in Cats and Dogs in the United States

	Plague	Tularemia
Organism	Gram-negative bacillus (Enterobacterales). Survives relatively poorly in the environment. Grows on routine culture media used for gram-negative bacteria	Gram-negative coccobacillus (Francisellaceae). Can persist in the environment and water sources for months. Fastidious growth in culture; often requires special media and prolonged incubation
Major arthropod vectors	Diverse variety of rodent and rabbit fleas	*Dermacentor* spp. and *Amblyomma americanum* ticks
Geographic location	Southwestern United States	Western, southwestern, central, and eastern United States
Affected hosts	Cats > dogs	Cats > dogs
Usual history	Rodent contact or exposure to rodent fleas	Rodent and especially rabbit contact; ingestion often reported
Clinical signs	Acute disease with high fever and lymphadenopathy, most often of the mandibular and/or retropharyngeal lymph nodes. Hyperbilirubinemia and icterus do not appear to be common in affected cats	Acute or more chronic disease (sometimes associated with a thin body condition) with oral ulceration, lymphadenopathy of the mandibular and/or retropharyngeal lymph nodes, or generalized lymphadenopathy and abdominal organomegaly. Hyperbilirubinemia is frequent in affected cats, and icterus has been described
Lymph node aspirate cytology	Neutrophilic inflammation; monomorphic population of bipolar staining bacilli often present	Lymphoid reactivity or neutrophilic to pyogranulomatous inflammation and necrosis; bacteria often not visualized
Antimicrobial drugs	Aminoglycosides, doxycycline, chloramphenicol, trimethoprim-sulfamethoxazole	Aminoglycosides are the treatment of choice. Doxycycline, chloramphenicol, and fluoroquinolones may be effective but may be followed by relapse
Zoonotic potential	Exposure to cats with pneumonic plague can lead to human infection through aerosols; bites and scratches have also been implicated. Human pneumonic plague usually results from exposure to infected cats and can progress to death within a few days. Exposed humans may require prophylaxis with doxycycline	Most often follows bites from affected cats, less often scratches. Course of disease longer and mortality may be lower than occurs with pneumonic plague. Medical attention should be sought if bites or scratches occur

TABLE 74.2 **Diagnostic Assays Currently Available for Tularemia in Dogs and Cats**

Assay	Specimen Type	Target	Performance
Culture (not recommended)	Lymph node aspirates, blood, tissues collected at necropsy	*Francisella tularensis*	Recent antibiotic treatment may cause false-negative results. May require special media and takes at least 48 hours for colonies to appear. *Hazardous to laboratory personnel* and should be sent to laboratories with appropriate expertise when possible
Direct immunofluorescent antibody	Lymph node aspirates, tissues collected at necropsy	*F. tularensis* antigen	May be positive when culture is negative. False negatives can still occur. Recent antibiotic treatment may cause false-negative results
Serology	Serum	Antibodies to *F. tularensis*	Acute and convalescent serology is required for diagnosis, because initial results may be negative, and positive results may reflect previous exposure rather than active infection. Seroconversion may take up to 3 weeks
PCR	As for culture	*F. tularensis* DNA	Recent antibiotic treatment may cause false-negative results

Sonographic Findings

Abdominal ultrasound findings could include abdominal lymphadenomegaly, splenomegaly, and/or hepatomegaly. Abdominal lymphadenomegaly has been described in both a cat[15] and a dog.[27]

Microbiologic Tests

Diagnostic assays currently available for tularemia in dogs and cats are described in Table 74.2.

Direct Detection

Heat-fixed slides can be submitted to experienced laboratories for direct immunofluorescent antibody (IFA) staining for *F. tularensis*. Alternatively, IFA or immunoperoxidase stains can be applied to tissues obtained at necropsy.[16] Negative results do not rule out tularemia, but in some cases IFA may detect the organism when culture is negative.[39] Fluorescence in situ hybridization (FISH) has also been used to detect *F. tularensis* in tissues and differentiate between subspecies.[40] As for plague, lateral-flow assays have been described for rapid detection of *F. tularensis* LPS antigen in clinical specimens such as urine.[41] The use of these assays in dogs and cats has not been described.

Isolation and Identification

Francisella tularensis can be grown from clinical specimens, but it is very fastidious, grows slowly, is hazardous to laboratory personnel, and does not always grow on media used for routine isolation of gram-negative bacteria such as MacConkey agar (in contrast to *Y. pestis*). The use of cysteine-supplemented media (such as cysteine heart agar) and incubation in a CO_2-supplemented environment enhances recovery of the organism. Growth generally occurs 48 to 72 hours after inoculation, but cultures must be held for 7 to 10 days. Characteristic dewdrop colonies are isolated. Overgrowth of contaminating bacteria can occur unless the media is supplemented with antibiotics that inactivate these organisms. *Francisella tularensis* may grow from blood specimens after inoculation of routine blood culture media. Confirmation of the identity of the organism can be achieved with molecular methods. Whole-cell MALDI-TOF mass spectrometry has also been used for identification of *F. tularensis* isolates to the subspecies level (see Chapter 3).[42]

Serology

As for plague, acute and convalescent serology, with demonstration of a fourfold increase in titer, is required for serodiagnosis of tularemia in affected dogs and cats and is less hazardous to human health than culture. Tube agglutination and microagglutination assays are the standard methods for serodiagnosis, but ELISA assays have also been developed. Because of the extremely short incubation period, affected cats and dogs may have negative titers when they are first brought to the veterinarian, so convalescent serum should be submitted at least 2 to 3 weeks after the initial titer if the animal survives. Some cats die from the disease before a rise in antibody titer occurs. In addition, high titers may persist after recovery from infection, so a single positive titer is not diagnostic for tularemia.

Molecular Diagnosis Using Nucleic Acid–Based Testing

PCR assays that detect *F. tularensis* DNA represent an attractive means of diagnosis because of their sensitivity, rapid turnaround time, low risk to laboratory personnel, and the ability to differentiate between subspecies and genotypes of *F. tularensis*.[43,44] PCR assays have been used to detect *F. tularensis* in tissues at necropsy in cats.[18,45] A number of real-time PCR assays have been used to detect *F. tularensis* in human clinical specimens. Despite the sensitivity of PCR assays, false negatives can still occur. Real-time PCR assays for *F. tularensis* are offered on a commercial basis by some veterinary diagnostic laboratories in the United States.

Pathologic Findings

Gross pathologic findings in cats with tularemia include icterus, oral ulceration, lymphadenomegaly, splenomegaly, and hepatomegaly. Multifocal to coalescing irregular yellow, gray, or white foci (usually 1 to 5 mm in diameter) are present in these organs, and sometimes other organs such as the lung and myocardium.[13,18,19] When examined using histopathology, the nodules represent well-circumscribed but non-encapsulated masses of caseous necrosis, with abundant cellular debris, surrounded by infiltrates of degenerate neutrophils, macrophages, and/or fibroblasts. Lesions are centered on the splenic white pulp and cortical lymphoid follicles within lymph nodes. Necrosis and hemorrhage of lymphoid follicles within the GI tract may be present.[13,17] Organisms may be discernible with silver staining as tiny coccobacilli[17] or can be demonstrated with immunoperoxidase or immunofluorescence methods.[16,39]

TREATMENT AND PROGNOSIS

No substantial reports have been made on antimicrobial therapy of canine or feline tularemia. Treatment involves supportive care and antimicrobial drug administration (Table 74.3). As for plague, animals suspected to have tularemia should be housed in isolation at

TABLE 74.3 Suggested Antimicrobial Drugs for Treatment of Tularemia in Cats and Dogs

Drug	Dose (mg/kg)	Route	Interval (Hours)	Duration
Gentamicin	5–8	IV, IM, SC	24	14 days
Doxycycline	5	PO	12	2–3 weeks
Marbofloxacin	2.75–5.5	PO[a]	24	2–3 weeks

[a]Parenteral aminoglycosides are preferred for at least the first 72 hours of treatment to minimize exposure of the caregiver to *F. tularensis* during treatment.

least for the first 72 hours of antimicrobial drug therapy and handled by as few individuals as possible. Public health authorities should be notified. Gowns, gloves, and suitable face protection (eye protection and a properly fitted high-density surgical mask) should be worn, and protective wear should be properly removed and disposed of after handling affected animals. Any biohazardous waste should be double bagged and disposed of correctly. Routine disinfectants should be used to inactivate the organism in the environment. The drug of choice for initial treatment of tularemia in humans is a parenteral aminoglycoside such as streptomycin, with gentamicin as an alternative. Doxycycline can also be used but is associated with a higher relapse rate in humans than occurs with aminoglycosides.[44] Fluoroquinolones have the highest activity against *F. tularensis in vitro*,[46] but like tetracyclines, they may be associated with relapse *in vivo*.[44,47] Extension of the course of treatment from 2 weeks to 3 weeks when fluoroquinolones or doxycycline is used has been effective for treatment of human tularemia.[48] Other drugs with *in vitro* activity against *F. tularensis* include chloramphenicol and macrolides.[46]

IMMUNITY AND VACCINATION

Natural infection by *F. tularensis* is followed by protection against reinfection. Because *F. tularensis* is facultatively intracellular, cell-mediated immune responses are required for pathogen clearance, although humoral immunity is also important.[37] As a result, inactivated vaccines have not been effective for prevention of tularemia, because they primarily induce humoral immunity. An attenuated live vaccine that contained *F. tularensis* subsp. *holarctica* (live vaccine strain, or LVS) has been available for prevention of serious disease in people at high risk of exposure. However, this remains unlicensed because of concerns regarding efficacy and the route of administration, which was by scarification.[49] Since then there has been strong interest in vaccine development for prevention of human tularemia, because of concerns that the organism will be used as a weapon of bioterrorism.[37] Vaccines are not commercially available for dogs and cats given the rarity of disease in these species and the minor role that they play in transmission of disease to humans.

PREVENTION

Prevention of tularemia in dogs and cats involves housing cats indoors and discouragement of predation or exposure to dead wild rodents and rabbits. Use of tick preventatives also reduces the chance that dogs and cats will carry infected ticks into the house. Rodent control in the environment (e.g., removal of garbage) should also be performed.

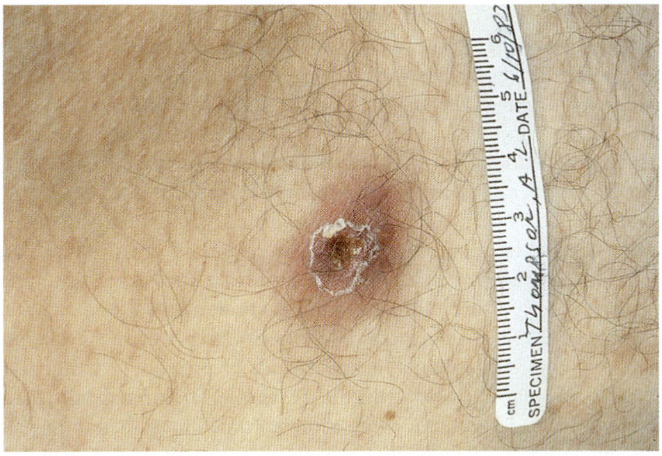

Fig. 74.4 Papule undergoing central necrosis with desquamation on the thigh of a middle-aged man infected with *Francisella tularensis*. (Courtesy of Dr. Joseph A. Bocchini, Louisiana State University Health Sciences Center, Shreveport, LA. In: Mandell GL, Bennett JE, Dolin R, eds. *Principles and Practice of Infectious Diseases*, 7th ed, Philadelphia, PA: Churchill Livingstone; 2010:2927-2937.)

PUBLIC HEALTH ASPECTS

In the United States, humans are most commonly infected by *F. tularensis* after arthropod bites (approximately half of the cases follow tick bites)[28] or handling infected wild animals. Common biological vectors are ticks, and in endemic areas in Sweden and Finland, mosquitoes play an important role in transmitting the bacteria.

Occupations associated with an increased risk of tularemia include farming, hunting, landscaping, meat handling, working with sheep, veterinary practice, and laboratory work. Severe illness is most often reported in young children (5 to 9 years) and the aged (>75 years). Men are more likely to be affected than women.[44]

Several overlapping forms of disease have been described in humans, the development of which depends on the route of inoculation and the virulence of the infecting strain: ulceroglandular, glandular, oculoglandular, oropharyngeal, typhoidal, and pneumonic.[44] Ulceroglandular tularemia results from cutaneous inoculation, oropharyngeal disease follows ingestion, and pneumonic tularemia can result from aerosol inhalation. Pneumonic tularemia has been described in people after activities such as lawn mowing or brush cutting in tick-infested areas. Infection of humans from cats and dogs (or wild canids, such as coyotes) can occur after these animals carry *F. tularensis* in their mouths after ingestion of wild prey.[50-52] Human-to-human transmission does not seem to occur.

Clinical signs in humans consist of acute onset of a flu-like illness, with fever, chills, and malaise after an average incubation period of 3 to 5 days. Sore throat, abdominal pain, vomiting, diarrhea, lymphadenopathy, rash, and a cough may also occur. Laboratory abnormalities include thrombocytopenia, elevated serum transaminase activities, increased serum creatine kinase activity, myoglobinuria, and pyuria.[44]

Infection with less virulent strains may result in transient flu-like illness followed by recovery. Without treatment, clinical signs can persist for several months, with chronic lymphadenopathy, weight loss, and debilitation.[44] Disease in chronically affected humans can resemble cat scratch disease.

Ulceroglandular tularemia is the most common form of human tularemia. It consists of a red and painful papule at the site of skin infection, with associated lymphadenopathy (Fig. 74.4). The papule then undergoes necrosis, forming an ulcer, which can take weeks to heal. In some individuals, lymph nodes may suppurate and become fluctuant. Multiple lesions can occur on the hands when infected animals have been handled, whereas tick bites typically result in single lesions elsewhere on the body.[44] Only lymphadenopathy may be present if the ulcer heals before the time of evaluation *(glandular tularemia). Oculoglandular tularemia* occurs when organisms gain access through the conjunctiva and is characterized by conjunctivitis, conjunctival ulceration, lacrimation, and associated lymphadenopathy.[44] *Oropharyngeal tularemia* is characterized by fever and severe throat pain; tonsillitis, oral ulceration, and associated lymphadenopathy may be present, which resembles the disease described in dogs and cats (which usually acquire infection via ingestion). Oropharyngeal tularemia tends to occur in children who ingest contaminated food or water and can resemble streptococcal pharyngitis (strep throat). *Typhoidal tularemia* is a febrile illness in the absence of prominent lymphadenopathy and may be associated with sore throat, abdominal pain, diarrhea, vomiting, icterus, and, with more chronic illness, hepatomegaly and splenomegaly. *Pneumonic tularemia* is the most severe form and results from inhalation of the organism or hematogenous spread of the organism to the lung, with clinical signs such as cough, chest pain, and hemoptysis. Thoracic radiographs can reveal lobar infiltrates, hilar lymphadenopathy, pleural effusion, and miliary infiltrates.[44] Changes resemble those seen in other chronic pneumonias, such as tuberculosis or fungal disease.

Although not the most common route of infection for humans, cat- and dog-bite–associated tularemia has been described (including among veterinary staff), and cats that live in rural endemic areas are important vectors of the most virulent strain of *F. tularensis*, type A1b.[48,52] Less commonly, human disease follows cat scratches or casual contact with cats.[39] In some cases, cats had recent contact with or ingested wild rabbits or rodents. Both apparently healthy and sick cats have been involved. Aerosol exposure to organisms on the coats of dogs (such as occurs when dogs shake their coats after contact with infected rabbits) has rarely been suspected in clusters of human disease.[51,53,54] In summary, tularemia should especially be considered in humans who develop illness in endemic areas within 3 weeks after a bite from a cat or dog that is a stray or that has had a recent history of wild rabbit or rodent contact. Following known exposure, prophylaxis with doxycycline has been used.[45] Disease in humans can mimic *Pasteurella multocida* cellulitis, the most common bacterial infection after a cat bite, but treatment with amoxicillin or clavulanic acid–amoxicillin is ineffective. It can also resemble cat scratch disease, and antibodies for *F. tularensis* may cross-react with *Bartonella* antigens, leading to diagnostic confusion.[2]

CASE EXAMPLE

Signalment

"Fido," an 8-month-old intact female, mixed-breed dog.

History

Fido was referred to Fredrikstad Small Animal Hospital, in the southeastern part of Norway, from a local animal clinic. Two days after a mountain hike, the dog became ill with lethargy and diarrhea. The owner had observed the dog eating lemmings. Over the next 3 days, the dog's condition worsened, with development of inappetence and vomiting 3 to 5 times daily.

On the day of the examination at Fredrikstad Small Animal Hospital, the dog had also developed hemorrhagic diarrhea; weight loss of 2 kg over a 1-week period was documented. The dog had been vaccinated for canine distemper, infectious canine hepatitis, parvovirus, and canine parainfluenza virus at 12 weeks of age, and had no previous history of illness.

Physical Examination

Body weight: 20 kg

General: Lethargic but responsive. T = 39.6°C [103.3°F], RR = 60 breaths/min, HR = 100 beats/min, CRT: 2 s.

Musculoskeletal: Body condition score 4/9.

Cardiovascular: No murmurs or arrhythmias were detected. Pulse quality was strong and synchronous.

Respiratory: No clinically significant findings.

Abdominal palpation: Mildly tense abdomen.

Lymph nodes: All peripheral lymph nodes appeared to be within normal limits.

Laboratory Findings

CBC: HCT 43.1% (37%–55%), MCV 61 fL (60–77 fL), MCHC 33.0 g/dL (30.0–37.5 g/dL), WBC 4140 cells/μL (5500–16,900 cells/μL), neutrophils 3060 cells/μL (2000–12,000 cells/μL), lymphocytes 640 cells/μL (500–4900 cells/μL), monocytes 310 cells/μL (300–2000 cells/μL), platelets 167,000 platelets/μL (175,000–500,000 platelets/μL).

Serum chemistry profile: Sodium 149 mmol/L (144–160 mmol/L), potassium 4.1 mmol/L (3.5–5.8 mmol/L), chloride 106 mmol/L (109–122 mmol/L), phosphorus 1.87 mmol/L (0.81–2.20 mmol/L), calcium 2.28 mmol/L (1.98–3.00 mmol/L), BUN 4.0 mmol/L (2.5–9.6 mmol/L), creatinine 68 μmol/L (44–159 μmol/L), glucose 5.83 mmol/L (4.11–7.95 mmol/L), total protein 70 g/L (52–82 g/L), albumin 27 g/L (23–40 g/L), globulin 43 g/L (25–45 g/dL), ALT 65 U/L (10–125 U/L), ALP 116 U/L (23–212 U/L), GGT 0 U/L (0–11 U/L), cholesterol 6.96 mmol/L (2.84–8.26 mmol/L), total bilirubin 6 μmol/L (0–15 μmol/L), amylase 330 U/L (500–1500 U/L).

Imaging Findings

Thoracic and abdominal radiographs: All structures appeared within normal limits.

Abdominal ultrasound: The mesenteric and iliac lymph nodes were enlarged and hypoechogenic, and measured up to 19 mm in diameter. Cytologic examination of fine-needle aspirate from an enlarged mesenteric lymph node showed mostly mature lymphocytes, with a few neutrophils and macrophages. Erythrocytes were present in moderate numbers. No bacteria or other infectious agents were seen in the aspirate. Conclusion: reactive lymphadenopathy.

Microbiologic testing:

PCR for *Francisella tularensis* DNA (swab specimen from the tonsils): negative.

Parvovirus antigen SNAP test (IDEXX Laboratories, Portland, ME): negative.

Fecal flotation: no parasites detected.

Serologic testing: Paired serum samples demonstrated a significant increase in antibody titer as determined using microagglutination test (MAT), from 1:20 on day 4 after exposure to lemmings to 1:640 on day 18.

Diagnosis

Tularemia.

Treatment

The dog was treated with IV fluids (128 mL/hour). Because of the high CRP, fever, lethargy, leukopenia, and bloody diarrhea, a decision to treat with antimicrobials was made (ampicillin, 20 mg/kg, IV, q8h). Two days later the dog had recovered, and had no diarrhea, no dehydration, or fever. Oral amoxicillin was continued for 3 more days.

Comments

In this case, a decision to pursue diagnostic testing for tularemia was made because of the history of exposure to lemmings, fever, and abdominal lymphadenopathy. The choice of antimicrobials was not optimal for treatment of tularemia but was initiated because of the concern for bacterial infection in light of the clinical findings. Most isolates of *F. tularensis* have shown *in vitro* resistance to penicillins,[46] so this dog likely recovered despite lack of specific antimicrobial therapy.

SUGGESTED READINGS

Kwit NA, Middaugh NA, VinHatton ES, et al. *Francisella tularensis* infection in dogs: 88 cases (2014-2016). *J Am Vet Med Assoc.* 2020;256:220–225.

Nordstoga A, Handeland K, Johansen TB, et al. Tularaemia in Norwegian dogs. *Vet Microbiol.* 2014;173:318–322.

Pennisi MG, Egberink H, Hartmann K, et al. *Francisella tularensis* infection in cats: ABCD guidelines on prevention and management. *J Feline Med Surg.* 2013;15:585–587.

Weinberg AN, Branda JA. Case records of the Massachusetts General Hospital. Case 31-2010. A 29-year-old woman with fever after a cat bite. *N Engl J Med.* 2010;363:1560–1568.

REFERENCES

1. McCoy GW, Chapin CW. *Bacterium tularense*, the cause of a plague-like disease in rodents. *Public Health Bulletin.* 1912;53:17–23.
2. Petersson E, Athlin S. Cat-bite-induced *Francisella tularensis* infection with a false-positive serological reaction for *Bartonella quintana. JMM Case Rep.* 2017;4:e005071.
3. Maurin M, Gyuranecz M. Tularaemia: clinical aspects in Europe. *Lancet Infect Dis.* 2016;16:113–124.
4. Petersen JM, Molins CR. Subpopulations of *Francisella tularensis* ssp. *tularensis* and holarctica: identification and associated epidemiology. *Future Microbiol.* 2010;5:649–661.
5. Kugeler KJ, Mead PS, Janusz AM, et al. Molecular epidemiology of *Francisella tularensis* in the United States. *Clin Infect Dis.* 2009;48:863–870.
6. Eden J-S, Rose K, Ng J, et al. *Francisella tularensis* ssp. *holarctica* in ringtail possums, Australia. *Emerg Infect Dis.* 2017;23:1198–1201.
7. Whipp MJ, Davis JM, Lum G, et al. Characterization of a *novicida*-like subspecies of *Francisella tularensis* isolated in Australia. *J Med Microbiol.* 2003;52:839–842.
8. Jackson J, McGregor A, Cooley L, et al. *Francisella tularensis* subspecies *holarctica*, Tasmania, Australia. *Emerg Infect Dis.* 2011;18:1484–1486. 2012.
9. Mani RJ, Morton RJ, Clinkenbeard KD. Ecology of tularemia in central US endemic region. *Curr Trop Med Rep.* 2016;3:75–79.
10. Hestvik G, Warns-Petit E, Smith LA, et al. The status of tularemia in Europe in a one-health context: a review. *Epidemiol Infect.* 2015;143:2137–2160.
11. Mahy S, Chavanet P, Piroth L, et al. Emergence of tularemia in France: paradigm of the Burgundy region. *Int J Infect Dis.* 2011;15:e882–883.
12. Ellis J, Oyston PC, Green M, et al. Tularemia. *Clin Microbiol Rev.* 2002;15:631–646.
13. Baldwin CJ, Panciera RJ, Morton RJ, et al. Acute tularemia in three domestic cats. *J Am Vet Med Assoc.* 1991;199:1602–1605.
14. Meinkoth KR, Morton RJ, Meinkoth JH. Naturally occurring tularemia in a dog. *J Am Vet Med Assoc.* 2004;225:545–547. 538.
15. Woods JP, Crystal MA, Morton RJ, et al. Tularemia in two cats. *J Am Vet Med Assoc.* 1998;212:81–83.
16. DeBey BM, Andrews GA, Chard-Bergstrom C, et al. Immunohistochemical demonstration of Francisella tularensis in lesions of cats with tularemia. *J Vet Diagn Invest.* 2002;14:162–164.
17. Rhyan JC, Gahagan T, Fales WH. Tularemia in a cat. *J Vet Diagn Invest.* 1990;2:239–241.
18. Spagnoli ST, Kuroki K, Schommer SK, et al. Pathology in practice. Francisella tularensis. *J Am Vet Med Assoc.* 2011;238:1271–1273.
19. Gliatto JM, Rae JF, McDonough PL, et al. Feline tularemia on Nantucket island, Massachusetts. *J Vet Diagn Invest.* 1994;6:102–105.
20. Inzana TJ, Glindemann GE, Snider G, et al. Characterization of a wild-type strain of *Francisella tularensis* isolated from a cat. *J Vet Diagn Invest.* 2004;16:374–381.
21. Valentine BA, DeBey BM, Sonn RJ, et al. Localized cutaneous infection with *Francisella tularensis* resembling ulceroglandular tularemia in a cat. *J Vet Diagn Invest.* 2004;16:83–85.
22. Kwit NA, Middaugh NA, VinHatton ES, et al. *Francisella tularensis* infection in dogs: 88 cases (2014-2016). *J Am Vet Med Assoc.* 2020;256:220–225.
23. Larson MA, Fey PD, Hinrichs SH, et al. *Francisella tularensis* bacteria associated with feline tularemia in the United States. *Emerg Infect Dis.* 2014;20:2068–2071.
24. Magnarelli L, Levy S, Koski R. Detection of antibodies to *Francisella tularensis* in cats. *Res Vet Sci.* 2007;82:22–26.
25. Staples JE, Kubota KA, Chalcraft LG, et al. Epidemiologic and molecular analysis of human tularemia, United States, 1964-2004. *Emerg Infect Dis.* 2006;12:1113–1118.
26. Yaqub S, Bjornholt JV, Enger AE. Tularemia from a cat bite. *Tidsskr Nor Laegeforen.* 2004;124:3197–3198.
27. Nordstoga A, Handeland K, Johansen TB, et al. Tularaemia in Norwegian dogs. *Vet Microbiol.* 2014;173:318–322.
28. Zellner B, Huntley JF. Ticks and tularemia: do we know what we don't know? *Front Cell Infect Microbiol.* 2019;9:146.
29. Lundström JO, Andersson AC, Backman S, et al. Transstadial transmission of *Francisella tularensis* holarctica in mosquitoes, Sweden. *Emerg Infect Dis.* 2011;17:794–799.
30. Backman S, Naslund J, Forsman M, et al. Transmission of tularemia from a water source by transstadial maintenance in a mosquito vector. *Sci Rep.* 2015;5:7793.
31. Berrada ZL, Telford SR Iii. Survival of *Francisella tularensis* type A in brackish-water. *Arch Microbiol.* 2011;193:223–226.
32. Afset JE, Larssen KW, Bergh K, et al. Phylogeographical pattern of *Francisella tularensis* in a nationwide outbreak of tularaemia in Norway, 2011. *Euro Surveill.* 2015;20:9–14.
33. Santic M, Ozanic M, Semic V, et al. Intra-vacuolar proliferation of *F. novicida* within *H. vermiformis. Front Microbiol.* 2011;2:78.
34. Ancuta P, Pedron T, Girard R, et al. Inability of the *Francisella tularensis* lipopolysaccharide to mimic or to antagonize the induction of cell activation by endotoxins. *Infect Immun.* 1996;64:2041–2046.
35. Gunn JS, Ernst RK. The structure and function of *Francisella* lipopolysaccharide. *Ann N Y Acad Sci.* 2007;1105:202–218.
36. Dai S, Mohapatra NP, Schlesinger LS, et al. The acid phosphatase AcpA is secreted in vitro and in macrophages by *Francisella* spp. *Infect Immun.* 2012;80:1088–1097.
37. Barry EM, Cole LE, Santiago AE. Vaccines against tularemia. *Hum Vaccin.* 2009;5:832–838.
38. Gustafson BW, DeBowes LJ. Tularemia in a dog. *J Am Anim Hosp Assoc.* 1996;32:339–341.
39. Capellan J, Fong IW. Tularemia from a cat bite: case report and review of feline-associated tularemia. *Clin Infect Dis.* 1993;16:472–475.
40. Splettstoesser WD, Seibold E, Zeman E, et al. Rapid differentiation of *Francisella* species and subspecies by fluorescent in situ hybridization targeting the 23S rRNA. *BMC Microbiol.* 2010;10:72.
41. Grunow R, Splettstoesser W, McDonald S, et al. Detection of *Francisella tularensis* in biological specimens using a capture enzyme-linked immunosorbent assay, an immunochromatographic handheld assay, and a PCR. *Clin Diagn Lab Immunol.* 2000;7:86–90.
42. Seibold E, Bogumil R, Vorderwulbecke S, et al. Optimized application of surface-enhanced laser desorption/ionization time-of-flight MS to differentiate *Francisella tularensis* at the level of subspecies and individual strains. *FEMS Immunol Med Microbiol.* 2007;49:364–373.
43. Molins CR, Carlson JK, Coombs J, et al. Identification of *Francisella tularensis* subsp. *tularensis* A1 and A2 infections by real-time polymerase chain reaction. *Diagn Microbiol Infect Dis.* 2009;64:6–12.
44. Penn RL. *Francisella tularensis* (tularemia). In: Bennett JE, Dolin R, Blaser MJ, eds. *Mandell, Douglas and Bennett's Principles and Practice of Infectious Diseases.* 8th ed. Philadephia, PA: Elsevier Saunders, 2015:2590–2602.
45. Stidham RA, Freeman DB, von Tersch RL, et al. Epidemiological review of *Francisella tularensis*: a case study in the complications of dual diagnoses. *PLoS Curr.* 2018;10.
46. Caspar Y, Maurin M. *Francisella tularensis* susceptibility to antibiotics: a comprehensive review of the data obtained in vitro and in animal models. *Front Cell Infect Microbiol.* 2017;7:122.
47. Steward J, Piercy T, Lever MS, et al. Treatment of murine pneumonic *Francisella tularensis* infection with gatifloxacin, moxifloxacin or ciprofloxacin. *Int J Antimicrob Agents.* 2006;27:439–443.

48. Weinberg AN, Branda JA. Case records of the Massachusetts General Hospital. Case 31-2010. A 29-year-old woman with fever after a cat bite. *N Engl J Med*. 2010;363:1560–1568.
49. Conlan JW, Shen H, Golovliov I, et al. Differential ability of novel attenuated targeted deletion mutants of *Francisella tularensis* subspecies *tularensis* strain SCHU S4 to protect mice against aerosol challenge with virulent bacteria: effects of host background and route of immunization. *Vaccine*. 2010;28:1824–1831.
50. Chomel BB, Morton JA, Kasten RW, et al. First pediatric case of tularemia after a coyote bite. *Case Rep Infect Dis*. 2016;2016:8095138.
51. Rumble CT. Pneumonic tularemia following the shearing of a dog. *J Med Assoc Ga*. 1972;61:355.
52. Kwit NA, Schwartz A, Kugeler KJ, et al. Human tularaemia associated with exposure to domestic dogs-United States, 2006-2016. *Zoonoses Public Health*. 2019;66:417–421.
53. Siret V, Barataud D, Prat M, et al. An outbreak of airborne tularaemia in France. *Euro Surveill*. 2006;11:58–60.
54. Teutsch SM, Martone WJ, Brink EW, et al. Pneumonic tularemia on Martha's Vineyard. *N Engl J Med*. 1979;301:826–828.

75

Bite and Scratch Wound Infections

Jane E. Sykes, Ellie J.C. Goldstein

KEY POINTS

- Causes: A variety of aerobic and anaerobic bacteria that include mycoplasmas and mycobacterial species. *Pasteurella* spp. are commonly isolated.
- Geographic Distribution: Worldwide.
- Major Clinical Signs: Fever, lethargy, hyperesthesia, puncture wounds, cutaneous swellings, lacerations, tissue avulsions, and signs that relate to damage and/or infection of other structures (such as the thorax, abdomen, and brain and spinal cord).
- Differential Diagnoses: Other traumatic injuries, cutaneous neoplasia, sterile nodular panniculitis (dogs), plague, tularemia.
- Human Health Significance: Cat and dog bite wound infections are common in humans and may be life-threatening in the immunocompromised. They also can be associated with transmission of potentially serious bloodborne bacterial pathogens such as *Bartonella, Francisella tularensis, Pasteurella multocida,* and *Capnocytophaga canimorsus.*

ETIOLOGY AND EPIDEMIOLOGY

Bite wounds are one of the most common reasons that dogs or cats are brought to veterinary hospitals for care. Despite this, there is surprisingly little information available on their epidemiology in comparison to the plethora of publications on animal bite wounds in people (see Public Health Aspects). Bite wounds often result in bacterial infection, but can also result in systemic viral infection (especially in the case of bitten cats), and less often, fungal or bloodborne protozoal infections such as babesiosis (Table 75.1).

Bacterial pathogens that cause bite wound infections are usually members of the normal oral cavity flora of the biting animal species, but organisms in the environment can also contaminate bite or scratch wounds (e.g., *Clostridium tetani, Mycobacterium* spp., *Nocardia* spp., *Bartonella* spp.). Bite wounds are instantly contaminated with a plethora of bacterial species from the oral cavity, but only a small proportion of these species possess virulence properties that allow them to proliferate within the wound and cause disease. The degree to which proliferation occurs also depends on host factors such as underlying immunocompromise. Although there are similarities that relate to the oral flora of the biting animal, the bacterial species that cause bite wound infections in dogs and cats can differ from those that cause dog or cat bite wound infections in human patients, so data from human studies should not be extrapolated to dog or cat bite wound infections.

Dogs

Bite wounds in dogs most often result from aggressive dog-dog interactions. The dog breeds affected depend on regional variation in dog breed popularity. Younger adult, male dogs and especially intact male dogs appear to be predisposed, but studies that compare affected dogs to a control (or "background") population have not been reported.[1–3] Bite wounds in dogs can also result from the bites of other domestic and wild animal species, but the epidemiology of infections that result from these wounds is not well described. One study described 154 dogs from southern California with coyote bite wounds; dogs < 10 kg were more likely to have wounds involving multiple body parts and abdominal penetrating wounds, and rib fractures were associated with mortality.[4]

Approximately 20% of dog-dog bite wounds become *infected,* as opposed to *contaminated.* The likelihood that a wound becomes infected increases with the time lag between the aggressive interaction and when veterinary attention is sought.[2,3] Infection develops 8 to 24 hours after the bite occurs and is less likely to develop if the wound is limited to the dermis.[3] The distribution of bacterial species involved varies from one study to another and may be influenced by whether infected or only contaminated wounds were evaluated. The most common bacterial species isolated from dog-dog bite wounds are *Staphylococcus pseudintermedius, Enterococcus* spp., *Pasteurella* spp., streptococci, and *Escherichia coli.*[1–3,5] *Staphylococcus aureus* and *Capnocytophaga canimorsus,* which are important pathogens in humans that are bitten by dogs, are rarely isolated from bitten dogs,[2,3] although the prevalence of *C. canimorsus* is probably underestimated because it is very difficult to grow in culture. In the author's hospital, *Pasteurella* spp. accounted for 17% of 41 bacterial species cultured from 33 dog bite wounds, followed by a variety of staphylococci (some methicillin-resistant) (15%), *E. coli* (12%), *Enterococcus* spp. (7%), and *Bacteroides* spp. (7%). Other organisms were *Peptostreptococcus* spp., *Clostridium* spp., and *Pseudomonas aeruginosa* (each 5%); and *Streptococcus viridans, Actinomyces* spp., *Acinetobacter* spp., *Serratia marcescens, Klebsiella pneumoniae, Myroides* spp., *Prevotella* spp., *Fusobacterium* spp., *Aeromonas* spp., *Mycobacterium smegmatis,* and *Mycoplasma* spp. (one isolate each or 2%). Obligate anaerobes were isolated from five dogs (15%), and in all five of these dogs, multiple bacterial species were isolated.

Cats

Most bite wounds in cats result from aggressive interactions with other cats, but nonfatal dog bite wounds can also occur. Occasionally, cats are bitten by a variety of other small wildlife species that vary geographically based on the local fauna present. In contrast to dogs, which often crush and tear tissues with their teeth, cats deliver deep puncture wounds that create an environment where obligate and facultative anaerobes flourish. Thus, anaerobic bacterial infections are more prevalent in cat bite abscesses than in dog bite wounds, and accordingly, polymicrobial infections are present more often in closed cat bite abscesses

TABLE 75.1 Pathogens that Cause Local or Systemic Infections in Dogs and Cats as a Consequence of Bite or Scratch Wounds from the Same or Another Animal Species[a]

Organism Class	Dogs	Cats
Viruses	Rabies	Rabies FeLV FIV
Mycoplasmas	Hemotropic mycoplasmas?	Nonhemotropic mycoplasmas Hemotropic mycoplasmas?
Gram-negative aerobes[b]	*Aeromonas* *Acinetobacter* *Capnocytophaga canimorsus* *Enterobacter* spp. *Escherichia coli* *Neissera (N. dumasiana)* *Pasteurella* *Proteus* *Pseudomonas aeruginosa* *Serratia marcescens*	*Escherichia coli* *Pasteurella*
Gram-positive aerobes[a]	*Actinomyces* *Corynebacterium* *Enterococcus* *Staphylococcus*, especially *S. pseudintermedius* *Streptococcus*	*Actinomyces* *Corynebacterium* *Enterococcus* *Lactobacillus* *Nocardia* *Streptococcus*
Anaerobes	*Bacteroides* *Clostridium* *Eubacterium* *Fusobacterium* *Peptostreptococcus* *Porphyromonas* *Prevotella* *Propionibacterium*	*Bacteroides* spp. *Clostridium* *Fusobacterium* *Porphyromonas* *Prevotella* *Propionibacterium* spp.
Mycobacteria	Rapid-growing mycobacteria Tuberculous mycobacteria (e.g., *M. bovis* in the United Kingdom)	Lepromatous mycobacteria (e.g., *M. lepraemurium*) Rapid-growing mycobacteria (e.g., *M. fortuitum*) Tuberculous mycobacteria (e.g., *M. microti* in the United Kingdom)
Fungi	*Sporothrix schenckii*	*Sporothrix schenckii* Opportunistic molds (e.g., *Paecilomyces* spp.), dematiaceous molds
Protozoa	*Babesia conradae*? *Babesia gibsoni* *Babesia vulpes*	None known

[a]When only a genus name is listed, multiple species from that genus have been isolated.
[b]The term "aerobe" refers to facultative anaerobes and obligate aerobes.

than in dog bite wounds. In a study of 36 closed cat bite abscesses, 168 bacterial strains were isolated, of which 72% were obligate anaerobes and 28% were facultative anaerobes.[6] The most prevalent anaerobes isolated from cat bite abscesses include *Porphyromonas, Bacteroides, Prevotella, Peptostreptococcus,* and *Fusobacterium*. *Pasteurella multocida,* a commensal of the oral cavity of virtually all cats, is the most common facultative anaerobe present.[6–8] *Porphyromonas* spp. appear to be particularly prevalent; in one study of 15 abscesses in Australian cats, they accounted for 92% to 99% of all the facultative and obligate anaerobes present.[9] Less often *Actinomyces*, β-hemolytic streptococci, lactobacilli, and *Propionibacterium* spp. have been isolated.

CLINICAL FEATURES

Dogs

Among dogs, dog bite wounds consist of abrasions, lacerations, avulsions (i.e., skin flaps), crushing injuries, and deep puncture wounds (Fig. 75.1). Abscesses can also develop. Dog bite wounds may also penetrate body cavities and cause pneumothorax, rib fractures, lung contusions or damage the esophagus, vertebral column, or GI tract. Pyothorax or bacterial peritonitis can also occur. Most dogs have between one and five wounds. Rarely, more than 10 wounds are present.[1–3] The majority of bite wounds occur cranial to the diaphragm, especially on the head and neck (Fig. 75.2). The location of the bite wounds also depends on the size of the bitten dog; large-breed dogs are more likely to have wounds on the neck and face, but small-breed dogs often have wounds on their dorsum or thorax. Injury to underlying tissue is frequently dramatically more severe than is apparent on the surface. Classification systems have been used to describe the severity of dog-dog bite wounds based on the type of injury (laceration vs. puncture wound) and the presence or absence of dead space or abscessation.[1–3] Abscessation is rarely associated with dog bite wounds as compared with cat bite wounds.[3] The presence of pus, fever, erythema, subcutaneous emphysema, and/or a foul odor suggests that infection has occurred. Uncommonly, hematogenous spread of bacteria leads to signs of severe sepsis or septic shock (see Chapter 123).

Cats

In cats, cat bite wounds may be difficult to identify on the surface or be undetectable, but infection can extend to penetrate bone, joints, tendon, and muscle.[8,10] Cat bite wounds are most often located on the thoracic limbs, lateral aspect of the face, and near the base of the tail (Fig. 75.3).[11] In contrast, scratches are often found on the bridge of the nose, pinna, and inguinal region. Cat bite abscesses are characterized by the presence of firm or fluctuant subcutaneous swellings or masses, with or without fever, lethargy, inappetence, and hyperesthesia. Some cats are brought to the veterinarian solely because of lethargy, and a careful physical examination is required before an abscess or cellulitis is detected. One or more scabs may be found on top of the abscess, or the overlying skin may lack hair and have a gray, necrotic appearance. If the abscess ruptures, cream-colored or red-brown purulent material may be identified on the haircoat, sometimes in association with a foul odor (Fig. 75.4). Alternatively, the haircoat may be matted over the site. Lameness may be apparent if the limbs are involved, and especially if there is extension to the bone or a joint. Involvement of the thoracic cavity may be associated with fever, lethargy, tachypnea, and decreased lung sounds due to pyothorax (see Chapter 124).[10] Bite wounds to the calvarium can result in neurologic signs such as circling, disorientation, head pressing, mental obtundation, delayed or absent placing reactions, tetraparesis, anisocoria, absent menace responses, and seizures.[12] Penetration of the caudal vertebral column and spinal cord can lead to vertebral fractures, osteomyelitis, bacterial meningitis, and signs of pelvic limb paralysis (Fig. 75.5). As in dogs, progression to severe sepsis or septic shock can occur, but most cat bite abscesses rupture and resolve spontaneously.

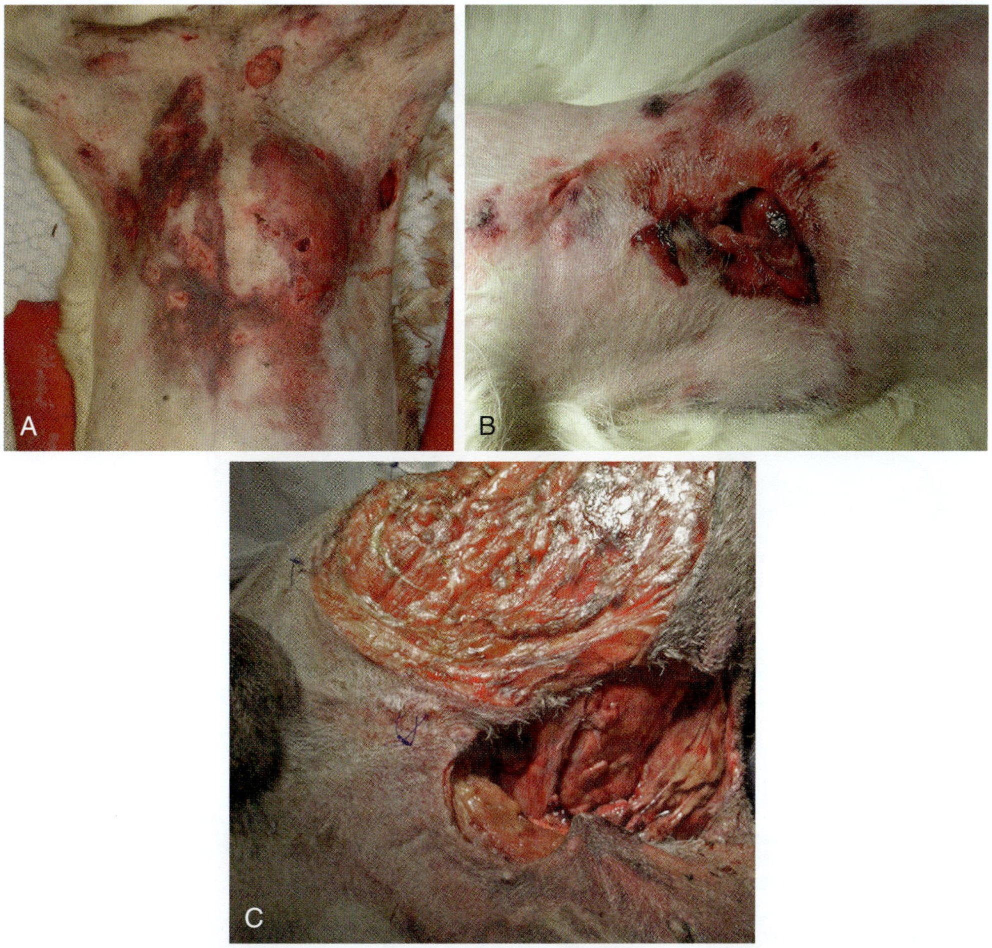

Fig. 75.1 Dog bite wounds. (A) Multiple puncture wounds, abrasions, and lacerations to the abdomen of a 10-year-old female spayed mixed-breed dog. A portion of the jejunum had perforated and had herniated into the subcutaneous tissue. The dog developed cardiac arrest after 2 days of aggressive treatment that included surgery and was euthanized. (B) Five-year-old male neutered Pomeranian dog with a bite wound to the lateral cervical region from a pit bull terrier dog that resulted in tissue avulsion. (C) Inguinal region of a 6-year-old intact male German shepherd dog with severe bite wounds and tissue avulsion that resulted in extensive exposure of muscle and bone. The dog had been attacked by four other dogs. The dog survived with aggressive medical treatment and surgery that included amputation of the right pelvic limb. (Courtesy of the University of California, Davis Veterinary Emergency and Critical Care Service.)

Cats with dog bite wounds often have life-threatening injuries.[10] Fractures, severe hemorrhage, and hypovolemic shock can dominate the clinical picture. Penetrating injury of cervical structures, the thorax, abdominal organs, brain, or spinal cord can occur (Fig. 75.6).[10] Thoracic wounds have been associated with a higher risk of mortality (27% in one study).[10] Death most often results from trauma rather than infection, but occasionally deep-seated infections or bacteremia develops if the cat survives the initial traumatic episode.

DIAGNOSIS

A diagnosis of bite wound infections is based on history of a fight or bite and physical examination findings that suggest that infection has developed. Cytologic examination of a wound may also assist in diagnosis of infection. The veterinarian should record whether the wound was provoked or unprovoked and note the time and location that the wound occurred and the biting animal species involved. Depending on the extent and location of bite wounds, radiographs of the affected region should be considered to assess for underlying damage to bone or body cavities. All cats with cat fight wounds should be tested for FeLV and FIV infection, and the test should be repeated 2 months later because transmission may have occurred at the time of the fight wound (see Chapters 32 and 33).

Laboratory Abnormalities

Laboratory abnormalities in cats or dogs with wound infections are variable and depend on the degree of tissue trauma, the underlying organs involved (if any), and the severity and type of infection. The CBC may show nonregenerative or regenerative anemia, neutrophilia with bandemia, toxic neutrophils, monocytosis, and lymphopenia or lymphocytosis. Animals with severe sepsis or septic shock may be thrombocytopenic. Findings on the chemistry panel include hypoalbuminemia and evidence of muscle damage (increased activities of CK, AST, and sometimes mild increases in serum ALT activity). Increased muscle enzyme activities may be a clue to an underlying cat bite wound in cats with fever of unknown origin. Prolongations of the PT and/or APTT may be present in animals with septic shock and disseminated intravascular coagulation.

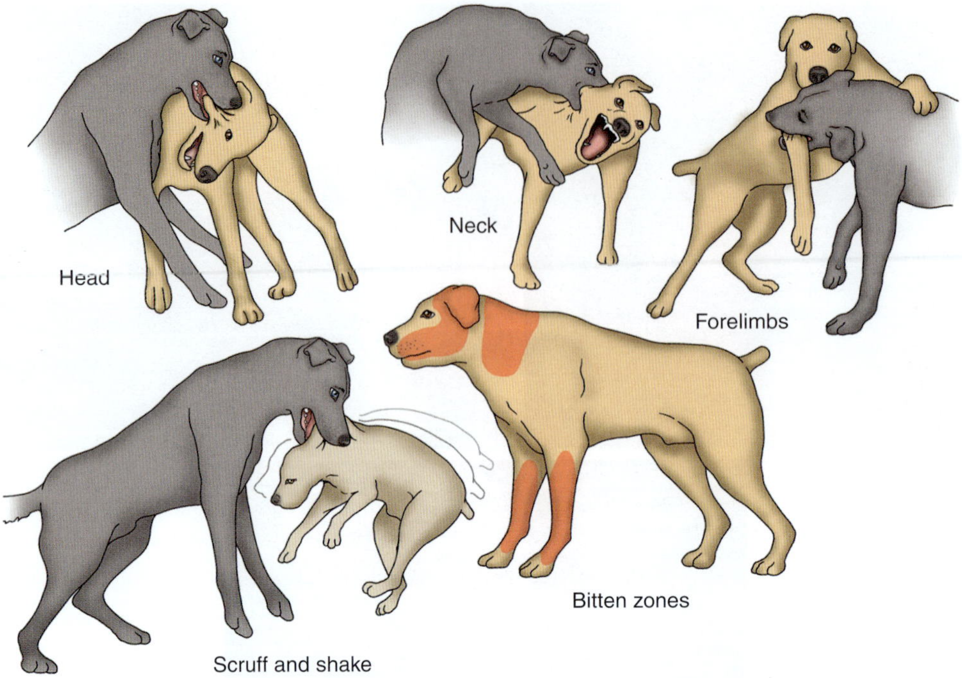

Fig. 75.2 Common anatomic distribution of dog-to-dog bite and fight wounds.

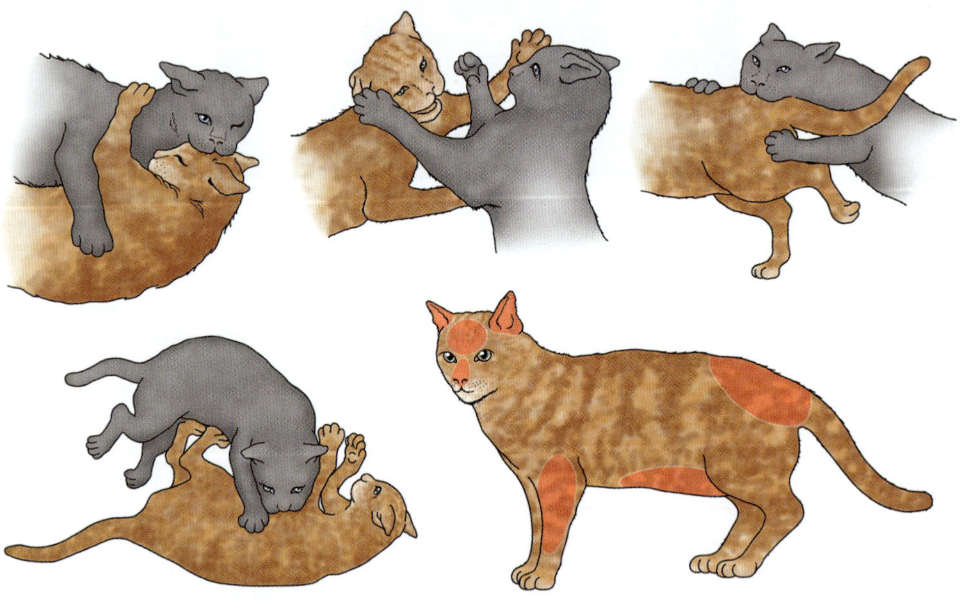

Fig. 75.3 Common anatomic distribution of cat-to-cat bite and fight wounds ("wound cat"). (Adapted from Malik R, Norris J, White J, et al. Wound cat. *J Feline Med Surg*. 2006;8:135-140.)

Diagnostic Imaging

Plain Radiography

Radiographs of the thorax in dogs or cats with bite wounds may show fractured ribs, pneumothorax, evidence of pulmonary contusions, mediastinal emphysema, diaphragmatic herniation, or pleural effusion due to hemothorax or pyothorax. Abdominal radiographs may show a lack of serosal detail due to hemoabdomen or bacterial peritonitis. Radiographs of the axial or appendicular skeleton may reveal fractures or tooth foreign bodies. In more chronic bite wound infections, evidence of osteomyelitis or septic arthritis may be present, with soft-tissue swelling and bony lysis (see also Chapter 121).

Sonographic Findings

Ultrasound of soft tissues can be useful to assess the extent of bite wound infections. Abdominal ultrasound is indicated for animals with bite wounds to the abdomen to assess for evidence of peritonitis or trauma to abdominal organs. Findings in dogs or cats with peritonitis include a hyperechoic mesentery with an irregular outline and free peritoneal fluid, which is typically echogenic (see Chapter 125).

Advanced Imaging

Findings on MRI in cats with brain abscesses secondary to cat bite wounds include space-occupying lesions with well-defined margins

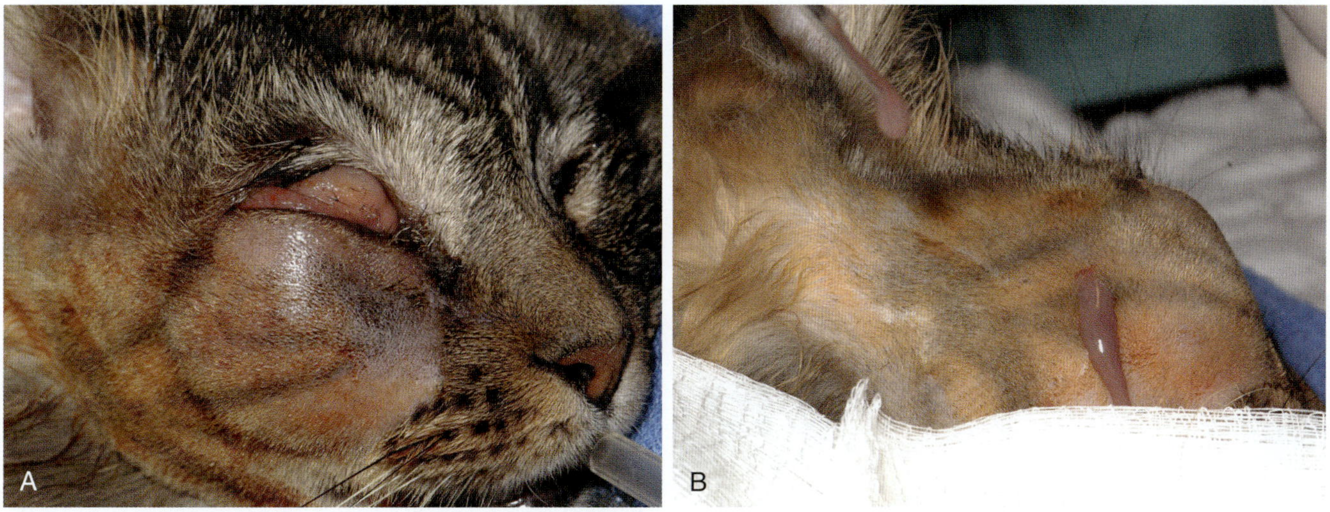

Fig. 75.4 (A) Six-year-old female spayed domestic shorthair cat with a cat bite abscess adjacent to the right eye that was associated with marked chemosis and periocular swelling. (B) Purulent material discharged from the abscess when it was drained surgically. (Images courtesy University of California, Davis Veterinary Ophthalmology service.)

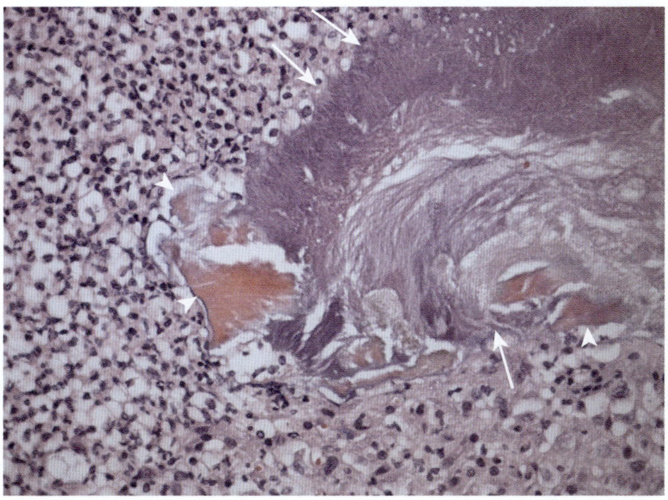

Fig. 75.5 Histopathology of the vertebral column of a young adult, male domestic shorthair that was found with a bite wound to the base of the tail that drained purulent material and pelvic limb paralysis with absent deep pain sensation. Multiple fractures of caudal vertebrae 4 and 5 were present in association with suppurative osteomyelitis *(arrowheads)*, cellulitis, ascending meningitis, and masses of intralesional bacteria *(arrows)*. Multiple anaerobes were cultured from the lesion. Hematoxylin and eosin stain.

that are hyperintense on T2-weighted images, and hypointense T1-weighted images.[12] Marked ring enhancement is usually present. Evidence of brain herniation may be detected.[12]

Cytologic Examination

Cytologic examination of swab or fluid specimens collected from infected wounds typically reveals large numbers of degenerate neutrophils with intracellular bacteria, which may include cocci, rods, or long, filamentous organisms (which are usually anaerobes).

Microbiologic Tests

Isolation and Identification

Dogs. Aerobic bacterial culture and susceptibility and anaerobic bacterial culture are indicated whenever possible from dogs that are suspected to have infected bite wounds. Routine culture lacks sensitivity for detection of anaerobes, and anaerobic bacterial infections respond predictably to treatment, so anaerobic culture could be considered optional if client finances are limited (see Chapter 54).

The skin around the wound should be clipped and cleaned with chlorhexidine solution, and an aspirate, swab, or devitalized tissue specimen should be collected from as deep within the wound as possible while the animal is sedated or anesthetized. When pockets of purulent material extend subcutaneously away from an open wound, collection of aspirates percutaneously with a needle and syringe can avoid contamination by surface bacteria. Because a positive culture from a wound does not imply infection, results must be interpreted in light of the physical examination and laboratory findings. Susceptibility test results for isolated bacteria can then be used to guide antimicrobial drug treatment. Blood cultures should be considered for dogs with evidence of severe sepsis or septic shock.

Cats. In general, culture of cat bite abscesses in cats is not routinely performed because they almost always respond to drainage with or without systemic antibacterial drug treatment. Cytologic examination and culture are indicated for cat bite abscesses/cellulitis if clinical signs of infection are persistent or recurrent in the face of treatment, or if severe infections that involve underlying bones, joints, or body cavities occur. Culture is also recommended for draining skin lesions in the inguinal region, which may result from infection with rapid-growing mycobacteria (see Chapter 61). Blood cultures are indicated for cats with signs of severe sepsis or septic shock.

TREATMENT

Surgical Management

Dogs

Dogs with dog bite wounds should be muzzled and the wound(s) covered with a clean, dry bandage immediately after the injury occurs to prevent further contamination of the wound until the animal's condition can be stabilized if necessary. If possible, the dog should then be sedated or anesthetized and a wide area of skin around the wound clipped in order to determine the extent of injury and prepare for surgery. Frequently, this leads to detection of additional full-thickness puncture wounds or lacerations. The skin around the wound should be scrubbed with chlorhexidine or povidone-iodine

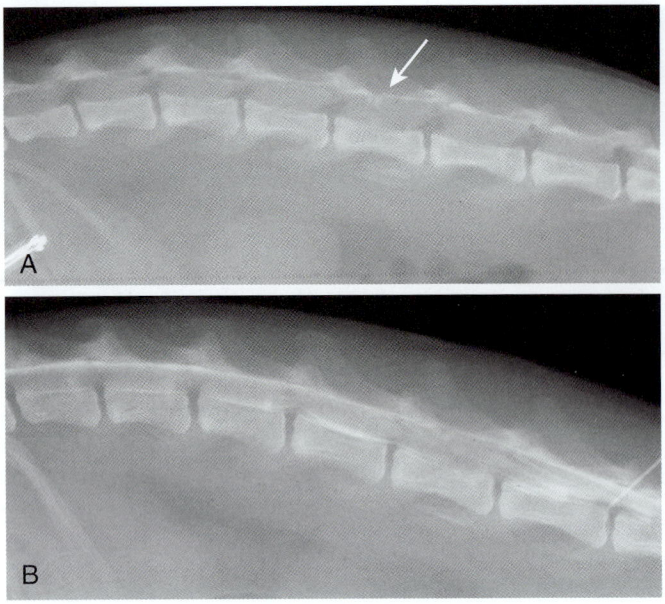

Fig. 75.6 (A) Lateral radiograph of the lumbar spine of a 3-year-old female Siamese cat with a dog bite wound to the lumbar spine. The cat was unable to stand and had absent placing reactions in the pelvic limbs. Patellar reflexes were also absent. Two osseous densities are superimposed at the level of the dorsal spinal canal at the level of the fourth lumbar vertebra (L4) *(arrow)*. The dorsoventral view showed deviation of the spinous process of L4 (not shown). CSF analysis revealed mild suppurative inflammation. (B) Myelogram. A spinal needle is inserted at L5-6 for injection of contrast agent. Spinal cord widening with associated thinning of the contrast column circumferentially is identified over the body of L4. Dorsal deviation and splitting of the ventral contrast column is present over L2-3 as a result of disc protrusion in this region. A decompressive hemilaminectomy over L4 to L6 was performed and a bone fragment was removed; the cat ultimately recovered.

solution. Full-thickness punctures and lacerations should then be explored, debris and devitalized tissue removed, and specimens collected for culture if infection is suspected. If the abdominal or thoracic cavity has been penetrated, surgical exploration of these cavities is typically required to identify and treat damaged viscera. Wounds should be lavaged extensively with copious quantities of sterile saline or lactated Ringer's solution under moderate pressure (such as using a 60-mL syringe attached to an 18-gauge needle). The use of antibiotics or antiseptics to lavage the wound is not generally recommended, as they can be toxic to tissue and provide minimal benefit for treatment of established wound infections. If used, 0.05% chlorhexidine diacetate (1 part 2% chlorhexidine to 39 parts water) is preferred because it has antibacterial activity in the presence of organic debris, residual antibacterial activity, and minimal systemic absorption and toxicity.

In general, infected wounds that are limited to the subcutaneous tissues and muscle are subsequently managed as open wounds in order to optimize drainage and debridement. Closure of infected wounds can lead to dehiscence and persistence of infection. Whenever possible, the wound is covered with bandages that absorb fluid, reduce dead space, prevent movement and contamination of the wound, and assist in debridement. Hydrophilic bandages are often used for the first 3 to 5 days. Wound closure is generally recommended for noninfected wounds that are in the "golden period" (first 6 to 8 hours after injury). The reader is referred to small animal surgical texts for more detailed information on surgical management of bite wound infections, including debridement, closure, reconstructive techniques, dressings, and bandaging (see Suggested Readings).[13]

TABLE 75.2 Suitable Antimicrobial Drugs for the Treatment of Bite Wound Infections in Dogs and Cats[a]

Drug	Species	Dose (mg/kg)	Interval (hours)	Route
Amoxicillin-clavulanic acid	D, C	12.5–20	8–12	PO
Ampicillin-sulbactam	D, C	10–20[b]	8	IV, IM
Pradofloxacin[c]	D	3	24	PO
	C	5–7.5	24	PO
Enrofloxacin	D	5–20	24	IV, IM, PO
Marbofloxacin	D	2.75–5.5	24	PO
Gentamicin	D	9–14	24	IV, IM
Amikacin	D	15–30	24	IV, IM
Metronidazole	D, C	10	8	PO, IV

[a]Doses of antimicrobial drugs that have activity primarily against gram-negative aerobes are listed for dogs, because isolation of gram-negative aerobes from cat bite abscesses is very rare.
[b]Dose according to ampicillin component.
[c]The pradofloxacin dose for dogs is for the tablet formulation available in Europe. The dose for cats is for the oral suspension. The use of pradofloxacin in dogs may be associated with myelosuppression and is off-label in some countries.
C, cat; *D*, dog.

Cats

As for open dog bite wounds, a wide area of skin around cat bite abscesses should be clipped and scrubbed. The abscess should then be lanced and specimens collected for culture if desired. The abscess cavity should then be lavaged, necrotic tissue debrided, and a placement of a drain should be considered to optimize drainage and prevent early wound closure. Whenever possible, the wound and drain should then be covered with a bandage. The drain is removed in 3 to 5 days. For cats with pyothorax, placement of chest tubes with or without surgical exploration may be required (see Chapter 124 and Suggested Readings for this chapter).[14] Cats with abscesses that involve the CNS have the potential to recover with craniectomy, drainage of purulent material within the abscess, removal of any tooth fragments present, and closure of subcutaneous tissue and the skin.[12]

Antimicrobial Treatment

Contaminated Wounds (First 8 Hours After Injury)

The need for antimicrobial treatment in contaminated, noninfected wounds is controversial, because there is no evidence that it prevents infection of the wound and it may select for infection with bacteria that are resistant to the antimicrobial drug used. Proper wound cleaning and debridement are likely to have the greatest impact on whether infection subsequently develops. Antimicrobial treatment could be considered for deep punctures or large, dirty wounds that require extensive debridement. If deemed necessary, the drug of choice for contaminated wounds is amoxicillin-clavulanic acid, because it has efficacy against most oral cavity commensals of the dog and cat mouth such as *Pasteurella* spp. and a variety of anaerobes, including those that produce β-lactamase enzymes.

Infected Wounds

For severely infected dog bite wounds, initial treatment should consist of parenteral antimicrobial drugs that have activity against gram-negative and gram-positive aerobic and anaerobic bacteria, which includes methicillin-resistant staphylococci (in regions where methicillin-resistant *S. pseudintermedius* is prevalent). Appropriate combinations include ampicillin-sulbactam and an aminoglycoside, or a combination of ampicillin, metronidazole, and an aminoglycoside (Table 75.2). Where methicillin-resistant *S. pseudintermedius* is not prevalent, a fluoroquinolone could be substituted for the aminoglycoside. Subsequent treatment should be based on the results of culture and susceptibility. Amoxicillin or amoxicillin-clavulanic acid are appropriate choices for treatment of cat bite abscesses once drainage has been established (although many cat bite abscesses will likely heal with drainage alone). Because *Pasteurella* spp. are not susceptible to clindamycin or first-generation cephalosporins, monotherapy with these drugs should be avoided. Pradofloxacin is also a suitable choice, because it has activity against anaerobes as well as a variety of aerobic bacterial species.

Antimicrobial drug treatment of infected bite wounds that are localized to the skin, subcutaneous tissue, and muscle should continue for 3 to 5 days after signs of infection are no longer evident. The reader is referred to Chapters 121, 124, and 125 for information on the management of osteomyelitis, septic arthritis, pyothorax, and peritonitis.

Rabies Prophylaxis

In regions where rabies occurs, bite wounds may need to be reported to local public health authorities. If the biting animal has an unknown vaccination history, or the bite was from a wild animal that was unavailable for testing, a rabies booster should be administered and the animal monitored for 45 days. If the bitten animal is unvaccinated or has a lapsed vaccination status, additional quarantine or euthanasia may be required (see Chapter 21).

PROGNOSIS

The odds of mortality for dogs that had bite wounds to the thorax were 23.4-fold higher when a positive bacterial culture was made and 12.1-fold higher when pleural effusion was present.[5] Mortality rate for cats with thoracic dog bite wounds was 27% at the same institution,[10] approximately double that for dogs. The prognosis for bite wound infections depends on the severity and extent of injury, the immune status of the host, and the organisms involved. Recurrent infections may result from underlying osteomyelitis, foreign bodies, immunodeficiency, or the presence of atypical organisms such as *Mycobacterium* spp., *Nocardia* spp., or *Mycoplasma* spp. (which do not respond to β-lactam drugs). Failure to respond to appropriate treatment should prompt a thorough physical examination; testing for retroviruses in cats; imaging of the affected area; and culture for aerobic and anaerobic bacteria and mycoplasmas. If the clinical picture is suggestive, culture for mycobacteria may also be indicated.

PREVENTION

Prevention of bite wounds involves education of pet owners with regard to housing cats indoors and use of secure collars and leashes for walking dogs (Box 75.1). Intact male dogs should be neutered if they are not to be used for breeding. Proper handling and socialization of puppies as well as behavior training should be encouraged. Pet owners should be instructed to avoid or closely supervise interactions between their dogs and unfamiliar dogs that are breeds of known aggressive tendency, such as American pit bull terriers, rottweilers, German shepherds, blue heelers, chow chows, and Jack Russell terriers, although mixed-breed dogs have also been identified in association with increased risk of bite injury.[15] Special caution is warranted for small-breed dogs, which may provoke larger breed dogs and are more likely to develop life-threatening injuries. Dogs that are unfamiliar with one another or dogs with a history of fighting with one another should never be left together without proper supervision.

BOX 75.1 Strategies to Prevent Dog Bites[24]

- Always supervise an infant or child who is near a dog (even your own or another known dog). Any dog can bite.
- Do not disturb any dog caring for puppies, eating, or sleeping.
- Never reach through or over a fence to pet a dog.
- Do not run past or from a dog.
- Teach children to move slowly around dogs.
- Do not encourage aggressive or rough play with any dog.
- Always ask permission from a dog's owner before petting a dog. Always let the dog sniff your hand before petting a dog.
- Never approach any unfamiliar dog. If an unfamiliar dog approaches, stand still with your arms to the side.
- Keep your dog healthy and provide routine veterinary care.
- Socialize and train your dog.

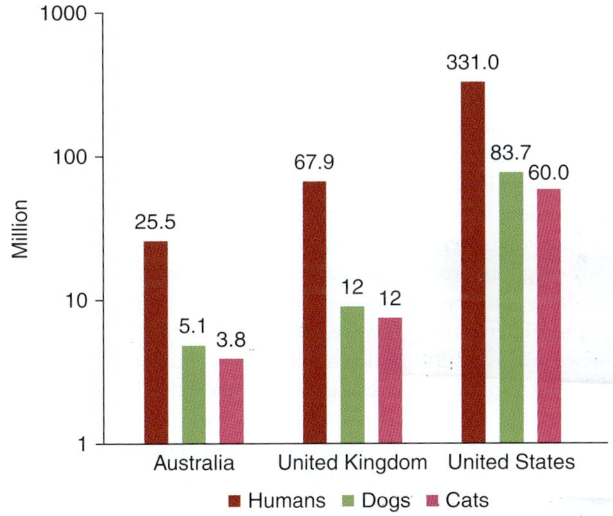

Fig. 75.7 Estimated absolute numbers of humans and owned dogs and cats in Australia, the United Kingdom, and the United States in 2020–2021 (data expressed in millions with a logarithmic scale on the y-axis).[16–18]

PUBLIC HEALTH ASPECTS

Epidemiology of Dog and Cat Bite Wounds

In 2021, the AVMA reported that in 2020, there were 83.7 million dogs and 60 million cats; 45% of households owned at least one dog and 26% of households owned cats.[16] This amounts to more dogs and cats than the combined human population in the United Kingdom and Australia in 2019 (Fig. 75.7). In the United Kingdom, the Pet Food Manufacturers' Association estimated that around 33% of households owned a dog and 27% owned a cat in 2021, with 59% of households owning pets.[17] In Australia in 2019, 40% of households owned dogs and 27% owned cats; the total pet population was estimated at 29 million, more than the estimated human population of 25 million.[18] Based on a survey conducted in 2018, fewer households in Japan owned dogs (11.5%) and cats (10.1%).[19] In the United States, German shepherds, rottweilers, and Jack Russell terriers are among the top 10 dog breeds owned. Dog and cat bite wounds account for approximately 1% of emergency department visits by humans in the United States, and similar numbers are reported in Europe. Dog bites accounted for more than 70% and cat bites accounted for 13% of animal bite visits to emergency rooms in New York City.[20] The median age of bitten people in one study was 15 years, in another study it was 28 years, and in a third study of facial dog bites from the Massachusetts General Hospital over a 20-year period (1997–2018) it was 29.5 years.[21–23]. Many bites occur in children, especially boys aged 5 to 9 years.[21,22,24–27] Children often have dog bites to the face, neck, and head.[28,29] Women and the elderly are at risk for cat bite injuries almost always to the hands. Patients who seek medical attention more than 8 hours after injury usually have infected wounds.

Dog Bite Infections

In the United States in 2018, dog bites accounted for 340,000 emergency department visits per year (900/day), and over 40% of those bitten were children or adolescents.[30] An analysis of police reports over an 8-year period in Detroit revealed that 83% of dog bite incidents were caused by a neighborhood dog, and most often occurred in the victim's yard by dogs that were found wandering-at-large or had escaped from their own yard.[31] Stay-at-home orders related to the COVID-19 pandemic have led to increased contact between children and their dogs, and one pediatric emergency department in Colorado reported a 3-fold rise in visit rates for dog bites (Fig. 75.8). In the case series of facial dog bites in Massachusetts, 88% of dogs were known, and provocation was reported in 65% of cases; pit bulls were responsible for most bites (8.5%). Behaviors described before the bite were playing with a dog, feeding a dog, or placing the face close to the dog. Pit bulls were also associated with most bites (36%) in case series of children and adolescents from central Texas[28] and people with orthopedic bite wound injuries in Fresno, California (50%).[32] A Canadian study found an association between dangerousness and increased body weight; entire male dogs were most dangerous despite absence in differences in body weight between neutered and non-neutered male dogs. In this study, dangerousness was categorized based on severity of injury and the appropriateness of aggressive behavior given the context.[33]

Between 3% and 20% of dog bite wounds in humans become infected.[34–36] The infecting organisms generally reflect the flora of the canine oral cavity, but may also derive from the environment or the bitten person's skin or oral cavity. Many infections are polymicrobial, but the organism that most often contributes to dog bite wound infections is *Pasteurella* spp., which is found in 50% of wounds (Table 75.3).[21,37–45] The most common species is *Pasteurella canis*, but *P. multocida* (subspecies *multocida*, *septica*, and *gallicida*), *Pasteurella stomatis*, and *Pasteurella dagmatis* may also be present.[46] Other common isolates from dog bite wounds include streptococci (especially the α-streptococcus *Streptococcus mitis* and *Streptococcus pyogenes*; *Streptococcus canis* is rarely isolated), staphylococci, *Corynebacterium* spp., *Neisseria* spp., and anaerobes.[37] Of the staphylococci, *S. aureus* is isolated most often (20% of infections). Infections with *S. pseudintermedius* occur rarely. Anaerobes are present in approximately 70% of infections and are almost always present in combination with other anaerobes and aerobic bacteria. Lethal outcomes of bite wound infections are rare but have been reported following infection by *C. canimorsus* and *P. multocida*.[47,48] *Pasteurella multocida* subsp. *septica* may have a greater predisposition to infect the CNS when compared with other *P. multocida* subspecies.[49]

Cat Bite Infections

Although cat bite wounds are less traumatic to tissue, they are more likely to become infected and progress to infection more rapidly than dog bite wounds.[14] Infection rates in children can be up to 50%.[34] The upper extremities are often affected. Most infections are polymicrobial. As in dog bite wounds, *Pasteurella* spp. are the most common organisms isolated and are present in 75% of wounds.[21,37] The predominant species are *P. multocida* subsp. *multocida* and *P. multocida* subsp. *septica*. Streptococci (including *S. pyogenes*) and staphylococci are also often present, but *S. aureus* is isolated less frequently from cat bite wounds than dog bite wounds. *Neisseria* and *Moraxella* are also often isolated from cat bite wounds (see Table 75.3). The prevalence of infection with anaerobes in cat bite wounds is similar to that in dog bite wounds.[21]

Clinical Manifestations of Human Infections

Infection of bite wounds in humans most often results in localized cellulitis, pain, purulent discharge, a black to gray appearance, and, less often, fever and local lymphadenopathy. Extension to underlying bones

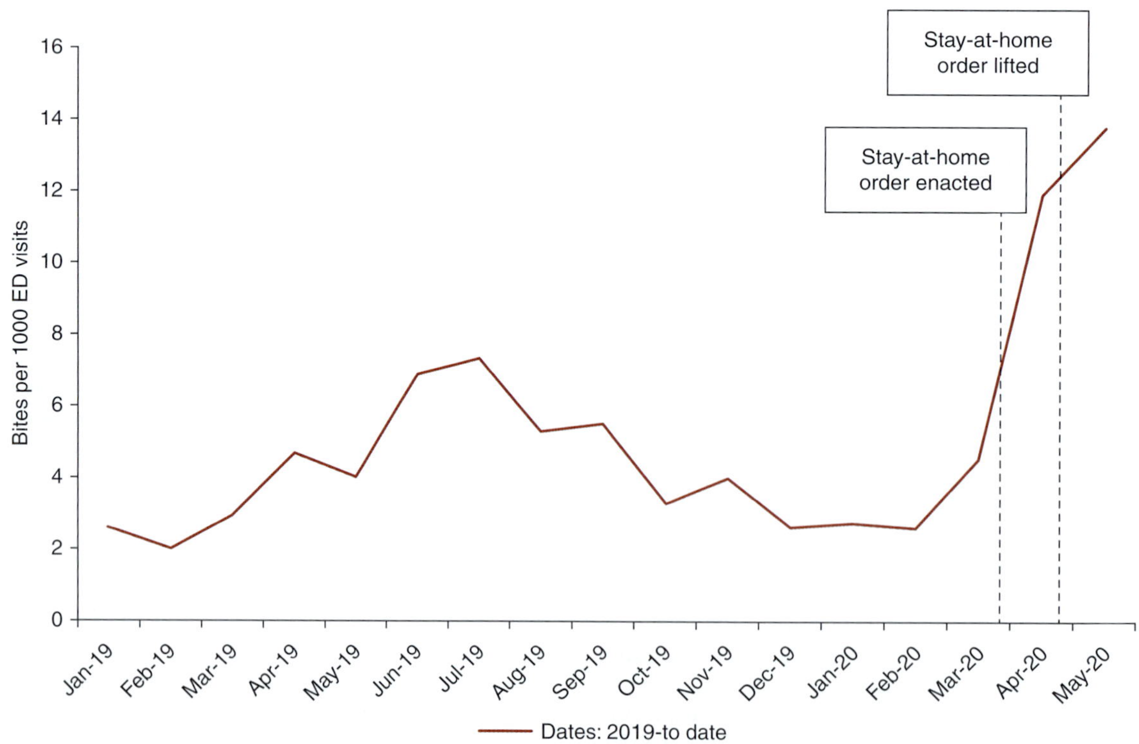

Fig. 75.8 Dog bite incidence before and after the COVID-19 pandemic. (Modified from Dixon CA, Mistry RD. Dog bites in children surge during coronavirus disease-2019: a case for enhanced prevention. *J Pediatr* 2020;225:231-232)

or joints can lead to osteomyelitis or septic arthritis, which is especially likely to occur after penetrating cat bite wounds to the hand (Fig. 75.9). Tenosynovitis is also common. Rarely, necrotizing fasciitis, bacteremia, meningitis, endocarditis, peritonitis, or brain abscesses develop.[28,50]

Most of the serious consequences of dog or cat bite wound infections occur in immunocompromised humans and involve *P. multocida* or *C. canimorsus.* Severe disease manifestations have also occurred after exposure of wounds to dog or cat saliva through licking, or after invasive medical supplies (such as dialysis tubing) were chewed or licked by a pet.[51] In a few cases, patients have had a history of contact with animals but no known bite or scratch wound.[52–57] Life-threatening infections with *P. multocida* tend to occur in infants, pregnant women with animal contact, patients on chronic glucocorticoid therapy, HIV-infected people, organ-transplant recipients, and patients with chronic liver disease.[50]

Capnocytophaga canimorsus is a capnophilic (carbon dioxide–loving), facultatively anaerobic, filamentous gram-negative bacterial rod that is found in the oral cavity of dogs and cats.[58] Although rarely reported as a cause of illness in dogs or cats, this organism can cause cellulitis, gangrene, bacteremia, meningitis, and endocarditis in humans.[50,58,59] *Capnocytophaga canimorsus* bacteremia is rare, but humans who are immunocompromised, especially those with chronic alcoholism, cirrhosis, or a history of splenectomy, are at risk for life-threatening *C. canimorsus* infections that progress rapidly, with a mortality of over 30%. However, severe infections have also been described in apparently immunocompetent humans.[60] The virulence factors that contribute to these severe infections are not well understood. The organism does not cause endotoxemia but appears to evade recognition by the immune system and resist phagocytosis.[50] In one series of humans with *C. canimorsus* sepsis, 56% of cases followed a dog bite and 10% of cases followed exposure of a wound to dog saliva by licking.[61] Veterinarians have also developed corneal infections with *C. canimorsus* when dog tooth fragments have struck them in the eye during dental extractions.[62,63] Most affected humans are older than 40 years of age. Clinical manifestations of *C. canimorsus* sepsis include fever, myalgia, and a petechial rash that involves the skin and mucous membranes, which may progress from purpura *(purpura fulminans)* to gangrene over a period of several days. Because *C. canimorsus* is very difficult to grow, early diagnosis and successful treatment require clinical suspicion and early treatment with effective antimicrobial drugs, such as β-lactam/β-lactamase inhibitor combinations, which are also active against *Pasteurella* spp.

Prevention of Bite Wounds in Humans

Veterinarians play an important role in educating the public about prevention of cat and dog bite wounds. Provision of information to clients who intend to purchase a new dog about dog breeds, puppy socialization, dog behavior training, and how to prevent and manage aggression and avoid bites or scratches (to themselves and to others) is encouraged. Dog owners should be instructed to always supervise children and infants when near a dog. Dog owners may have difficulty finding homeowners insurance if their dog bites someone. Many insurance companies will not insure a homeowner with certain breeds of dogs.

Veterinarians can also engage in community activities (especially in schools) where young children can be educated about pet ownership and how to avoid wounds and wound infections from their own or someone else's dog or cat. One report described a decrease in the severity of dog bite injury in children following implementation of an educational safety program for primary school children.[64] Immunocompromised individuals should be educated about the potential benefits and risks of pet ownership and precautions that can be taken to minimize infections. During 2015, 181 Los Angeles letter carriers were involved in dog attacks. Finally, care should be taken in the veterinary practice situation

TABLE 75.3 Pathogens that Can Infect Humans After a Bite or Scratch From a Dog or Cat[a]

	Dog	Cat
Viruses	Rabies	Rabies
Aerobic gram-positive bacteria	*Actinomyces viscosus* *Bacillus* *Corynebacterium* *Dietzia cinnamea* *Dermabacter hominis* *Enterococcus* *Gemella morbillorum* *Lactobacillus* *Leifsonia aquatica* *Micrococcus* *Oerskovia* *Pediococcus* *Staphylococcus* (including *S. pseudintermedius*) *Stomatococcus mucilaginosus* *Streptococcus* (*S. mitis*)[b]	*Actinomyces* *Bacillus* (*B. firmus*) *Enterococcus* (*E. durans*) *Erysipelothrix* spp. *Gemella morbillorum* *Lactobacillus* *Leifsonia aquaticum* *Rhodococcus* *Rothia dentocariosa* *Staphylococcus* (*S. epidermidis*) *Streptococcus* (*S. mitis*) *Streptomyces*
Aerobic gram-negative bacteria	*Aggregatibacter aphrophilus* *Bartonella*? *Bergeyella zoohelcum* *Bibersteinia* *Brevibacterium* *Capnocytophaga* *Cellulophaga lytica* *Citrobacter* *Comomonas* *Eikenella corrodens* *Escherichia coli* *Flavobacterium* *Frederiksenia canicola* *Klebsiella* *Luteimonas terricola* *Moraxella* *Neisseria* (especially *N. weaveri*) *Pasteurella* (*P. canis, P. dagmatis, P. stomatis*) *Pseudomonas* *Serratia marcescens* *Stenotrophomonas maltophilia* *Ralstonia pickettii* *Thermomonas haemolytica* *Xenophilus azovorans*	*Acinetobacter* *Actinobacillus* *Aeromonas hydrophila* *Alcaligenes* *Bartonella* *Bergeyella zoohelcum* *Brevibacterium* *Capnocytophaga* *Eikenella corrodens* *Enhydrobacter aerosaccus* *Enterobacter* *Flavimonas oryzihabitans* *Francisella tularensis* *Gemella morbillorum* *Klebsiella oxytoca* *Pasteurella* (*P. multocida*) *Pseudomonas* *Moraxella* (*M. catarrhalis*) *Neisseria* *Pantoea agglomerans* *Riemerella anatipestifer* *Ralstonia pickettii* *Yersinia pestis*
Anaerobic bacteria	*Alcaligenes faecalis* *Bacteroides* (*B. tectum*) *Campylobacter* *Canibacter oris* *Eubacterium* *Finegoldia magna* *Fusobacterium* (*F. nucleatum*) *Leptotrichia* *Peptostreptococcus* *Porphyromonas* *Prevotella* *Cutibacterium* (*C. acnes*) *Tannerella forsythia*	*Anaerobiospirillum succiniciproducens* *Bacteroides* (*B. tectum, B. pyogenes*) *Clostridium sordellii* *Eubacterium* *Filifactor villosus* *Fusobacterium* (*F. nucleatum*) *Peptostreptococcus* *Porphyromonas* (*P. gulae*) *Prevotella* *Cutibacterium* (*C. acnes*) *Veillonella*

Continued

TABLE 75.3 Pathogens that Can Infect Humans After a Bite or Scratch From a Dog or Cat[a]—cont'd

	Dog	Cat
Mycoplasmas	*Mycoplasma canis*	*Mycoplasma* spp.
Mycobacteria	*Mycobacterium fortuitum* *Mycobacterium kansasii*	*Mycobacterium fortuitum*
Fungi	*Blastomyces spp.* *Paecilomyces lilacinus*	*Sporothrix schenckii*

[a]See refs 21,37-45,67-75.
[b]For organisms that are present in >10% of cases, the most common species isolated is listed in parentheses.

to avoid bites or scratches to veterinary staff. Veterinary staff should be educated about the types of infections that can occur in the workplace; likelihood of these infections; risk factors for infection; appropriate preventative measures; and protocols to follow should a bite or scratch wound occur.[65] Immediate treatment of animal bite injuries has been shown to reduce complications and shorten hospitalization.[66] In general, antimicrobial preemptive treatment with activity against *Pasteurella* (i.e., not first-generation cephalosporins, dicloxacillin, erythromycin, clindamycin, or metronidazole unless in combination with antimicrobials active against *Pasteurella*, such as amoxicillin-clavulanic acid) is recommended for 3 to 5 days even in the first 24 hours after injury for moderate to severe bites, especially those to the hand or face, when a joint could be involved, when there is edema, or in an immunocompromised patient.[49] Primary closure is not recommended unless there are cosmetic or functional reasons that primary closure might be necessary. Routine hand-washing practices should be enforced, and licking by dogs or cats should be discouraged. Face protection should be worn by veterinary staff when dental procedures are performed. Bites and scratches may need to be reported to public health authorities, and all staff should be educated about the need to ensure that tetanus and rabies immunizations are not overdue.

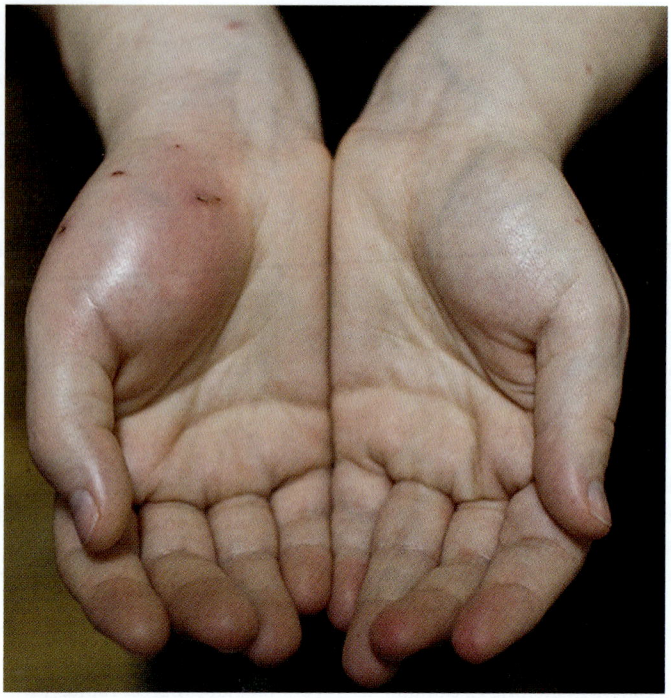

Fig. 75.9 Cat bite wounds to the base of the thumb of a veterinarian with associated cellulitis. Penetrating cat bite wounds of the hand have a tendency to extend to underlying bones and joints.

CASE EXAMPLE

Signalment

"Murphy," a 5-year-old intact male boxer dog from Vacaville in northern California.

History

Murphy was evaluated by the University of California, Davis Veterinary Emergency and Critical Care service for dog bite injuries after a fight with another dog in the household. The owner had returned home a few hours earlier to find Murphy bleeding from the neck. The other dog, a 5-year-old male neutered boxer mix, was found hiding and unable to stand with several "scratches" on his body. Murphy had a history of fights with other dogs. Both dogs in the household were fully vaccinated for CDV, parvovirus, adenovirus, and rabies. There was no other pertinent medical history.

Initial Physical Examination

Body weight: 46.2 kg.

General: Quiet, alert, responsive, and hydrated. T = 102.1°F (38.9°C), HR = 110, panting, pink and moist mucous membranes, CRT = 1 s.

Integument: The haircoat was full, thick, and dirty. There was a 1-cm superficial laceration on the ventral aspect of the pinna, and approximately 10 puncture wounds on the left ventral cervical region. A 2-cm superficial laceration was present at the cranial aspect of the dorsal midline, and a 5-cm superficial laceration was present on the left flank. No ectoparasites were seen.

Eyes, ears, nose, and throat: Bilateral conjunctival hyperemia and a mucoid ocular discharge were present. No other significant abnormalities were noted.

Musculoskeletal: BCS 6/9, ambulatory

Other systems: No clinically significant abnormalities were detected. Cranial nerve examination was unremarkable. A full neurologic examination was not performed.

Initial Treatment

Murphy was sedated with hydromorphone and dexmedetomidine. The left neck was clipped with a no. 40 clipper blade from the midpoint of the dorsal aspect of the head to the ventral aspect of the left ear and the thorax. The skin was cleaned with 0.05% chlorhexidine solution, and all puncture sites were probed and flushed with sterile saline. The sites were found to be relatively superficial. Drain sites were created with a no. 11 scalpel blade for three wounds, and a 3 × 0.75 inch Penrose drain was placed across a wound site that had the greatest amount of dead space and secured with a single interrupted suture. The dog was sent home with instructions for the owner to administer amoxicillin-clavulanic acid (16 mg/kg PO q12h) and tramadol (2.4 mg/kg PO q8-12h), to monitor the wound for development of excessive discharge, bleeding, swelling, or redness, and to keep the area clean with a washcloth soaked in warm water. Instructions were provided to return in 3 days to have the wound reevaluated and the drain removed.

The owners returned 7 days later for drain removal. At that time, they reported that Murphy had been eating normally, but had been drinking more than usual. His activity level had been normal, but they believed his neck had become swollen and tender. They had been administering the medications as directed.

CASE EXAMPLE—cont'd

Physical Examination (Day 7)

Body weight: 46.2 kg.

General: Quiet, alert, responsive, and hydrated but anxious. T = 103.1°F (39.5°C), HR = 114, RR = 36, pink and moist mucous membranes, CRT = 1 s.

Integument: There were marked crusts and scabs on the left lateral and ventral aspect of the neck. The Penrose drain was present with minimal amounts of discharge. Serous to purulent discharge was draining from the ventral puncture wounds. There was moderate crusting of the dorsal aspect of the left pinna.

Other systems: No change from the previous examination.

Treatment (Day 7)

The dog was again sedated and purulent material was collected for culture and susceptibility. The eschars were gently removed with forceps and the skin scrubbed with 0.05% chlorhexidine and water. Ultrasound of the neck region revealed pockets of hypoechoic material beneath the skin, and surgical debridement of the area under general anesthesia was recommended. Subsequently, Murphy was anesthetized and the wound was explored. No abscesses were found. The devitalized tissue was excised, the wounds flushed vigorously, and two Penrose drains were placed. The neck was bandaged initially, but this interfered with the dog's ability to breathe comfortably, so the bandage was removed. The dog was hospitalized overnight and treated with hydromorphone (0.05 mg/kg IV q4h) and warm compresses to the neck (q6h for 5 minutes). He was then sent home with instructions to administer tramadol as previously prescribed, clindamycin (20 mg/kg PO q12h), and enrofloxacin (10 mg/kg PO q24h), and to warm compress the neck every 4 to 6 hours for the next 3 days. They were also instructed to return in 3 to 5 days for reevaluation and drain removal.

Microbiologic Testing

Direct mear and Gram stain: Rare numbers of gram-positive cocci

Aerobic and anaerobic culture and susceptibility (swab from wound):

Isolate 1: Methicillin-resistant *Staphylococcus aureus,* resistant to all β-lactams and clindamycin; susceptible to amikacin (≤4 μg/mL), chloramphenicol (8 μg/mL), doxycycline (≤2 μg/mL), enrofloxacin (≤0.25 μg/mL), gentamicin (≤1 μg/mL), marbofloxacin (≤0.25 μg/mL), rifampin (≤1 μg/mL), and trimethoprim-sulfamethoxazole (≤0.50 μg/mL).

Isolate 2: *Enterococcus faecium* (intrinsic resistance to low-level aminoglycosides, cephalosporins, clindamycin, fluoroquinolones, trimethoprim-sulfamethoxazole), resistant to chloramphenicol and rifampin. Intermediate susceptibility to doxycycline (8 μg/mL), erythromycin (1 μg/mL), ticarcillin (64 μg/mL), and ticarcillin-clavulanate (64 μg/mL). Susceptible to ampicillin (1 μg/mL), clavulanic acid-amoxicillin (≤4 μg/mL), penicillin (4 μg/mL), and imipenem (≤1 μg/mL).

Isolate 3: *Pseudomonas aeruginosa,* resistant to ampicillin, amoxicillin-clavulanic acid, all cephalosporins tested, chloramphenicol, and doxycycline. Susceptibility to clindamycin was not reported because this species is usually resistant. Susceptible only to amikacin (≤4 μg/mL), gentamicin (2 μg/mL), enrofloxacin (0.50 μg/mL), imipenem (≤1 μg/mL), ticarcillin (16 μg/mL), ticarcillin-clavulanic acid (16 μg/mL). The MICs for trimethoprim-sulfamethoxazole and marbofloxacin were 2 μg/mL and ≤0.25 μg/mL, respectively.

Anaerobic culture: Moderate numbers of mixed growth that included *Bacteroides ureolyticus* group (β-lactamase negative), *Peptostreptococcus anaerobius,* and *Bacteroides* spp./*Prevotella* spp. (β-lactamase negative).

Diagnosis

Polymicrobial bite wound infection with anaerobes and multiple drug-resistant aerobic gram-positive and gram-negative bacteria.

Outcome

On receipt of the culture and susceptibility test results, the clindamycin was substituted with amoxicillin-clavulanic acid (16 mg/kg PO q12h). Treatment with enrofloxacin was continued and the owners were educated with regard to the public health significance of the infection and the need to wear gloves when handling the wound and for scrupulous hand-washing practices. The dog returned 4 days after surgery for drain removal. The owners reported that the drains had been producing considerable amounts of purulent material and that Murphy was doing well. He was afebrile and the wound was unchanged in appearance. He was again sedated, the area was scrubbed, and crusts were removed. The drains were removed. Murphy recovered uneventfully and the sutures were removed 10 days later at a local veterinary clinic. Five months later he was seen again for multiple bite wounds to the thoracic limbs and right thorax.

Comments

In this dog, bite wound injuries were complicated by infection with multiple gram-negative and gram-positive drug-resistant aerobic bacteria as well as anaerobes. The *S. aureus* and *P. aeruginosa* were resistant to amoxicillin-clavulanic acid, which had been used to prevent infection when the dog was first seen. In contrast, the anaerobes and the *E. faecium* were susceptible to amoxicillin-clavulanic acid, but presumably were able to proliferate and persist in the face of antimicrobial drug treatment as a result of the presence of the other drug-resistant bacteria, purulent material, and dead space. Bite wounds to the neck can be a challenge to manage because of the mobility of this area, which contributes to the maintenance of the dead space. The use of a bandage can reduce dead space, avoid further contamination, and reduce exposure to multidrug-resistant bacteria, but attempts to bandage the wound were not tolerated by this dog. Client education was an important part of management. The owners were instructed to separate the dogs when unattended to avoid further fights. Neutering may also have been of benefit.

SUGGESTED READINGS

Markewitz RDH, Graf T. *Capnocytophaga canimorsus* infection. *New Engl J Med.* 2020;383:1167.

McPhail C, Fossum TW. Surgery of the integumentary system. In: Fossum TW, ed. *Small Animal Surgery.* 3rd ed. St. Louis, MO: Mosby Elsevier; 2018:179–237.

Fossum TW. Surgery of the lower respiratory system: pleural cavity and diaphragm. In: Fossum TW, ed. *Small Animal Surgery.* St. Louis, MO: Mosby Elsevier; 2018:947–951.

Desai AN. Dog bites. *J Am Med Assoc.* 2020;323:2535.

Kannangara DW, Pandya D, Patel P. *Pasteurella multocida* infections with unusual modes of transmission from animals to humans: a study of 79 cases with 34 nonbite transmissions. *Vector Borne Zoonotic Dis.* 2020;20:637–651.

REFERENCES

1. Griffin GM, Holt DE. Dog-bite wounds: bacteriology and treatment outcome in 37 cases. *J Am Anim Hosp Assoc.* 2001;37:453–460.
2. Meyers B, Schoeman JP, Goddard A, et al. The bacteriology and antimicrobial susceptibility of infected and non-infected dog bite wounds: fifty cases. *Vet Microbiol.* 2008;127:360–368.
3. Mouro S, Vilela CL, Niza MM. Clinical and bacteriological assessment of dog-to-dog bite wounds. *Vet Microbiol.* 2010;144:127–132.
4. Frauenthal VM, Bergman P, Murtaugh RJ. Retrospective evaluation of coyote attacks in dogs: 154 cases (1997-2012). *J Vet Emerg Crit Care.* 2017;27:333–341.
5. Frykfors von Hekkel AK, Pegram C, Halfacree ZJ. Thoracic dog bite wounds in dogs: a retrospective study of 123 cases (2003-2016). *Vet Surg.* 2020;49:694–703.

6. Love DN, Jones RF, Bailey M, et al. Isolation and characterisation of bacteria from abscesses in the subcutis of cats. *J Med Microbiol.* 1979;12:207–212.
7. Love DN, Jones RF, Bailey M, et al. Bacteria isolated from subcutaneous abscesses in cats. *Aust Vet Pract.* 1978;8:87–90.
8. Love DN, Malik R, Norris JM. Bacteriological warfare amongst cats: what have we learned about cat bite infections? *Vet Microbiol.* 2000;74:179–193.
9. Norris JM, Love DN. The isolation and enumeration of three feline oral *Porphyromonas* species from subcutaneous abscesses in cats. *Vet Microbiol.* 1999;65:115–122.
10. Frykfors von Hekkel AK, Halfacree ZJ. Thoracic dog bite wounds in cats: a retrospective study of 22 cases (2005-2015). *J Feline Med Surg.* 2020;22:146–152.
11. Malik R, Norris J, White J, et al. Wound cat. *J Feline Med Surg.* 2006;8:135–140.
12. Costanzo C, Garosi LS, Glass EN, et al. Brain abscess in seven cats due to a bite wound: MRI findings, surgical management and outcome. *J Feline Med Surg.* 2011;13:672–680.
13. McPhail C, Fossum TW. Surgery of the integumentary system. In: Fossum TW, ed. *Small Animal Surgery*. 3rd ed. St. Louis, MO: Mosby Elsevier; 2018:179–237.
14. Fossum TW. Surgery of the lower respiratory system: pleural cavity and diaphragm. In: Fossum TW, ed. *Small Animal Surgery*. St. Louis, MO: Mosby Elsevier; 2018:947–951.
15. Essig Jr GF, Sheehan C, Rikhi S, et al. Dog bite injuries to the face: is there risk with breed ownership? A systematic review with meta-analysis. *Int J Pediatr Otorhinolaryngol.* 2019;117:182–188.
16. American Veterinary Medical Association. U.S. Pet Ownership Statistics; 2020. https://www.avma.org/javma-news/2021-12-01/pet-population-still-rise-fewer-pets-household.
17. Pet Food Manufacturer's Association. Pet Population; 2021. https://www.pfma.org.uk/statistics.
18. Animal Medicines Australia. Pets in Australia. A National Survey of Pets and People. https://animalmedicinesaustralia.org.au/report/pets-in-australia-a-national-survey-of-pets-and-people/. Last accessed April 21, 2022.
19. Statista. Distribution of Pet Ownership in Japan, by Species. https://www.statista.com/statistics/941746/japan-pet-ownership-distribution-by-species/#:~:text=The%20survey%20revealed%20that%20the,11.5%20and%2010.1%20percent%20respectively; 2018.
20. Bregman B, Slavinski S. Using emergency department data to conduct dog and animal bite surveillance in New York City, 2003-2006. *Public Health Rep.* 2012;127:195–201.
21. Talan DA, Citron DM, Abrahamian FM, et al. Bacteriologic analysis of infected dog and cat bites. Emergency medicine animal bite infection study group. *N Engl J Med.* 1999;340:85–92.
22. Weiss HB, Friedman DI, Coben JH. Incidence of dog bite injuries treated in emergency departments. *J Am Med Assoc.* 1998;279:51–53.
23. Zhu N, Cruz Walma A, Troulis MJ, et al. Facial dog bites treated at the Massachusetts General Hospital over a 20-year period. *Oral Surg Oral Med Oral Pathol Oral Radiol.* 2020;130:136–143.
24. Dixon CA, Mistry RD. Dog bites in children surge during Coronavirus Disease-2019: a case for enhanced prevention. *J Pediatr.* 2020;225:231–232.
25. Basco AN, McCormack ER, Basco Jr WT. Age- and sex-related differences in nonfatal dog bite injuries among persons aged 0-19 treated in hospital emergency departments, United States, 2001-2017. *Public Health Rep.* 2020;135:238–244.
26. Cook JA, Sasor SE, Soleimani T, et al. An epidemiological analysis of pediatric dog bite injuries over a decade. *J Surg Res.* 2020;246:231–235.
27. Nonfatal dog bite-related injuries treated in hospital emergency departments: United States, 2001. *Morb Mortal Wkly Rep.* 2003;52:605–610.
28. Abraham JT, Czerwinski M. Pediatric dog bite injuries in central Texas. *J Pediatr Surg.* 2019;54:1416–1420.
29. Mair J, Duncan-Sutherland N, Moaveni Z. The incidence and risk factors of dog bite injuries requiring hospitalisation in New Zealand. *N Z Med J.* 2019;132:8–14.
30. Centers for Disease Control and Prevention. Nonfatal Injury Data 2000-2018. https://wisqars.cdc.gov/nonfatal-reports.
31. Reese LA, Vertalka JJ. Preventing dog bites: it is not only about the dog. *Animals (Basel).* 2020;10:666.
32. Brice J, Lindvall E, Hoekzema N, et al. Dogs and orthopaeKdic injuries: is there a correlation with breed? *J Orthop Trauma.* 2018;32:e372–e375.
33. Frank D, Lecomte S, Beauchamp G. Behavioral evaluation of 65 aggressive dogs following a reported bite event. *Can Vet J.* 2021;62:491–496.
34. Bula-Rudas FJ, Olcott JL. Human and animal bites. *Pediatr Rev.* 2018;39:490–500.
35. Goldstein EJ. Bite wounds and infection. *Clin Infect Dis.* 1992;14:633–638.
36. Underman AE. Bite wounds inflicted by dogs and cats. *Vet Clin North Am Small Anim Pract.* 1987;17:195–207.
37. Abrahamian FM, Goldstein EJ. Microbiology of animal bite wound infections. *Clin Microbiol Rev.* 2011;24:231–246.
38. Ngan N, Morris A, de Chalain T. *Mycobacterium fortuitum* infection caused by a cat bite. *N Z Med J.* 2005;118:U1354.
39. Southern PM Jr. Tenosynovitis caused by *Mycobacterium kansasii* associated with a dog bite. *Am J Med Sci.* 2004;327:258–261.
40. Zendri E, Martignoni G, Benecchi M, et al. *Paecilomyces lilacinus* cutaneous infection associated with a dog bite. *J Am Acad Dermatol.* 2006;55:S63–S64.
41. McCabe SJ, Murray JF, Ruhnke HL, et al. *Mycoplasma* infection of the hand acquired from a cat. *J Hand Surg Am.* 1987;12:1085–1088.
42. Yuen JC, Malotky MV. *Francisella tularensis* osteomyelitis of the hand following a cat bite: a case of clinical suspicion. *Plast Reconstr Surg.* 2011;128:37e–39e.
43. Thornton DJ, Tustin RC, Pienaar BJ, et al. Cat bite transmission of *Yersinia pestis* infection to man. *J S Afr Vet Assoc.* 1975;46:165–169.
44. Gnann JW Jr, Bressler GS, Bodet CA 3rd, et al. Human blastomycosis after a dog bite. *Ann Intern Med.* 1983;98:48–49.
45. Ariel I, Haas H, Weinberg H, et al. *Mycobacterium fortuitum* granulomatous synovitis caused by a dog bite. *J Hand Surg Am.* 1983;8:342–343.
46. Vesza Z, Boattini M, Pinto M, et al. *Pasteurella* infections in a tertiary centre - from cellulitis to multiple-organ failure: retrospective case series. *SAGE Open Med Case Rep.* 2017;5. 2050313X17748286.
47. Markewitz RDH, Graf T. *Capnocytophaga canimorsus* infection. *N Engl J Med.* 2020;383:1167.
48. Byard RW, Langlois NEI. Variable mechanisms of dog-related deaths. *Am J Forensic Med Pathol.* 2020;41:287–290.
49. Goldstein EJ, Abrahamian FM. Bites. In: Bennett JE, Dolin R, Blaser MJ, eds. *Mandell, Douglas and Bennett's Principles and Practice of Infectious Diseases*. Philadelphia, PA: Elsevier Saunders; 2015:3510–3515.
50. Oehler RL, Velez AP, Mizrachi M, et al. Bite-related and septic syndromes caused by cats and dogs. *Lancet Infect Dis.* 2009;9:439–447.
51. Boinett C, Gonzalez A. *Pasteurella multocida* septicaemia in a patient on haemodialysis. *BMJ Case Rep.* 2009;2009. bcr01.2009.1492.
52. Jha P, Kalyoussef S. Fulminant septic shock with *Pasteurella multocida* in a young infant: no bite, scratch, or lick. *Vector Borne Zoonotic Dis.* 2021;21:59–62.
53. Mori J, Oshima K, Tanimoto T. Cat rearing: a potential risk of fulminant sepsis caused by *Capnocytophaga canimorsus* in a hemodialysis patient. *Case Rep Nephrol Dial.* 2020;10:51–56.
54. Kannangara DW, Pandya D, Patel P. *Pasteurella multocida* infections with unusual modes of transmission from animals to humans: a study of 79 cases with 34 nonbite transmissions. *Vector Borne Zoonotic Dis.* 2020;20:637–651.
55. Bryant BJ, Conry-Cantilena C, Ahlgren A, et al. *Pasteurella multocida* bacteremia in asymptomatic plateletpheresis donors: a tale of two cats. *Transfusion.* 2007;47:1984–1989.
56. Wade T, Booy R, Teare EL, et al. *Pasteurella multocida* meningitis in infancy - (a lick may be as bad as a bite). *Eur J Pediatr.* 1999;158:875–878.
57. Waghorn DJ, Robson M. Occupational risk of *Pasteurella multocida* septicaemia and premature labour in a pregnant vet. *Bjog.* 2003;110:780–781.
58. Gaastra W, Lipman LJ. *Capnocytophaga canimorsus*. *Vet Microbiol.* 2010;140:339–346.
59. Mader N, Luhrs F, Langenbeck M, et al. *Capnocytophaga canimorsus* - a potent pathogen in immunocompetent humans - systematic review and retrospective observational study of case reports. *Infect Dis (Lond).* 2020;52:65–74.

60. Bertin N, Brosolo G, Pistola F, et al. *Capnocytophaga canimorsus*: an emerging pathogen in immunocompetent patients: experience from an emergency department. *J Emerg Med*. 2018;54:871–875.
61. Pers C, Gahrn-Hansen B, Frederiksen W. *Capnocytophaga canimorsus* septicemia in Denmark, 1982-1995: review of 39 cases. *Clin Infect Dis*. 1996;23:71–75.
62. Chodosh J. Cat's tooth keratitis: human corneal infection with *Capnocytophaga canimorsus*. *Cornea*. 2001;20:661–663.
63. de Smet MD, Chan CC, Nussenblatt RB, et al. *Capnocytophaga canimorsus* as the cause of a chronic corneal infection. *Am J Ophthalmol*. 1990;109:240–242.
64. Kienesberger B, Arneitz C, Wolfschluckner V, et al. Child safety programs for primary school children decrease the injury severity of dog bites. *Eur J Pediatr*. 2021;Sep 17. Online ahead of print.
65. Desai AN. Dog bites. *J Am Med Assoc*. 2020;323:2535.
66. Seegmueller J, Arsalan-Werner A, Koehler S, et al. Cat and dog bite injuries of the hand: early versus late treatment. *Arch Orthop Trauma Surg*. 2020;140:981–985.
67. Pithadia DJ, Weathers EN, Colombo RE, et al. Severe and progressive cellulitis caused by *Serratia marcescens* following a dog scratch. *J Investig Med High Impact Case Rep*. 2019;7. 2324709619832330.
68. Klein S, Klotz M, Eigenbrod T. First isolation of *Mycoplasma canis* from human tissue samples after a dog bite. *New Microbes New Infect*. 2018;25:14–15.
69. Umemura H, Yamasaki O, Iwatsuki K. A cat bite-induced skin abscess associated with *Bacteroides pyogenes*, identified by mass spectrometry. *Eur J Dermatol*. 2018;28:392–393.
70. Lau JSY, Korman TM, Yeung A, et al. *Bacteroides pyogenes* causing serious human wound infection from animal bites. *Anaerobe*. 2016;42:172–175.
71. Gustavsson O, Johansson AV, Monstein HJ, et al. A wide spectrum of fastidious and ampicillin-susceptible bacteria dominate in animal-caused wounds. *Eur J Clin Microbiol Infect Dis*. 2016;35:1315–1321.
72. Chu AS, Harkness J. *Alcaligenes faecalis* cellulitis after a dog bite: case report and literature review. *Pediatr Emerg Care*. 2017;33:497–498.
73. Aravena-Roman M, Inglis TJJ, Siering C, et al. *Canibacter oris* gen. nov., sp. nov., isolated from an infected human wound. *Int J Syst Evol Microbiol*. 2014;64:1635–1640.
74. Eribe ERK, Olsen I. *Leptotrichia* species in human infections II. *J Oral Microbiol*. 2017;9. 1368848.
75. Hirvonen JJ, Lepisto I, Mero S, et al. First isolation of *Dietzia cinnamea* from a dog bite wound in an adult patient. *J Clin Microbiol*. 2012;50:4163–4165.

76

Surgical and Traumatic Wound Infections

J. Scott Weese, Ameet Singh

KEY POINTS

- Cause: Infection (typically bacterial) associated with breaches in normal host defenses, which are inherent risks with any surgical procedure.
- Geographic Distribution: Worldwide.
- Route of Transmission: Bacterial contamination can occur pre-, intra- or postoperatively. Contamination can come from the patient's microbiota, veterinary personnel, equipment, the environment (hospital and community), or owners.
- Major Clinical Signs: Most often, infections are superficial and are characterized by signs of inflammation at the superficial surgical site. Cardinal signs of inflammation and purulent discharge are typically present. Systemic signs of infection/inflammation are uncommon but can occur from deep or organ/space infections, or from bacterial translocation from an infected site.
- Differential Diagnoses: Surgical site inflammation is the main differential diagnosis.
- Human Health Significance: Some pathogens may pose a zoonotic risk, particularly methicillin-resistant *Staphylococcus aureus* (MRSA).

ETIOLOGY AND EPIDEMIOLOGY

The skin is a complex organ that serves as a barrier to the vast commensal and external microbiotas, which harbor a large collection of opportunistic pathogens. The skin microbiota has only recently been explored in detail in dogs and cats,[1–3] and it is still poorly understood. It contains a large and diverse population of bacteria, with smaller numbers of fungi, encompassing transient organisms from the environment or other individuals, and a more established resident population. Included in this is a range of harmless commensals and opportunistic pathogens, and it is reasonable to assume that all patients harbor multiple potential opportunistic pathogens on their skin and mucosal surfaces at any given time. Any traumatic injury to skin creates a potential portal for infection from those sites, other body sites (e.g., the GI tract), the environment, veterinary personnel, and owners. Factors such as wound size, depth, degree of contamination, presence of foreign material, degree of tissue damage, and compromise of vascular supply all play a role in whether infection develops.

A key concept in SSI prevention is consideration of the "period of risk." This is greatest during the time from first incision until some point at which healing of the surgical wound has formed an effective barrier. The starting point is the point at which the skin or mucosal barriers are breached. The end point is harder to discern. It presumably decreases greatly by the time of surgical wound closure, but is not complete until sometime (perhaps hours) after that, as an effective seal is created through the healing process.

While surgery is ideally performed in well-designed surgical suites, a sterile environment is not achievable. Risk from aerosolized bacteria and fungi exist in the best designed and maintained operating theatres, from pathogens in the environment, on surgical personnel, or on the patient. Surgical instruments are the main area where sterility can truly be achieved, yet these can carry pathogens into the wound once they are exposed to the external environment or patient.

Various studies have evaluated SSI rates in different patient populations, using different approaches. The use of active (e.g., patient examination, telephoning owners) versus passive (medical record review) approaches, and varying (or undescribed) definitions for SSI hamper comparisons between studies. Nevertheless, while the actual rates vary between and within procedures, the key aspect is that SSIs are uncommon on a percentage basis, but given the large number of surgical procedures that are performed, the impact of SSIs on the patient, owner, and clinician can be substantial.

Risk factors for SSIs have been studied in differing dog and cat populations, and results are somewhat inconsistent (Table 76.1). Various patient (e.g., breed, hypotension), procedure (e.g., dirty, procedures with implants), and surgeon (e.g., experience) risk factors have been reported, examples of which are presented in Table 76.2.

In humans, surgical wounds are classified as clean, clean contaminated, contaminated, and dirty.[4] This classification system also is commonly used in veterinary medicine, and while study of the impact of these categories on SSI risk has been limited, there is an association with increasing surgical risk class and SSI incidence.[5,6] Consideration of surgical wound category is useful when making decisions about antimicrobial prophylaxis, owner consultation about risk, and for surveillance purposes, albeit with some limitations (Table 76.3).

Clean surgical wounds are surgical incision sites with no prior trauma or inflammation; no breaks in sterile technique during surgery; and no contact with mucosal surfaces such as the respiratory, genitourinary, or GI tracts.

Clean contaminated surgical wounds are defined when there are minor breaks in surgical technique (such as a torn glove); contact with normal mucosae of the GI tract without spillage of visceral contents; or contact with uninfected genitourinary, biliary, or respiratory tracts. They also include otherwise clean procedures involving drain placement.

Contaminated surgical wounds have accidental GI tract spillage from penetration of an infected viscus or tissue, foreign bodies, devitalized tissue, or pus; or involve a break in sterile technique. Bacterial contamination is suspected, but purulent discharge is absent. Clean lacerations of the skin or subcutaneous tissues that are not already infected are often categorized as contaminated.

TABLE 76.1 Examples of Surgical Site Infections Surveillance Studies in Dogs and Cats

Population	n	SSI Rate
Dogs, TPLO[38]	437	2.3%
Dogs, TPLO[39]	134	14%
Dogs, TPLO[40]	145	8.4%
Dogs, TPLO[40]	155	7.1%
Dogs, TPLO[33]	549	6.7%
Dogs, TPLO[32]	226	13.3%
Dogs, TPLO[41]	242	10.8%
Dogs, TPLO[30]	902	6.1%
Dogs, TPLO[29]	1000	6.6%
Dogs, various procedures[6]	846	3%
Dogs and cats, various procedures[5]	1010	3%
Dogs and cats, various procedures[19]	1255	5.5%
Dogs, cranial crucial ligament rupture procedures[42]	811	3.2%
Dogs, hemilaminectomy[43]	154	0.6%
Dogs, laparoscopic ovariectomy or ovariohysterectomy[44]	224	1.3%
Dogs and cats, various procedures[7]	1143 dogs, 102 cats	2.8%
Dogs > 50 kg, TPLO and TTA[31]	91 TTA, 54 TPLO	TTA: 15.4% TPLO: 26%
Dogs, orthopedic implant procedures[45]	389	4.3%
Dogs, TTA[46]	224	5.3%
Dogs, TTA[47]	624	7.6%
Dogs, TTA[48]	1613	6.1%
Dogs, orthopedic implant procedures[34]	97	12.9%
Dogs, elbow arthroscopy[49]	750	0.2%
Dogs and cats, minimally invasive abdominal or thoracic procedures[50]	179	1.7%
Dogs and cats, open thoracic or abdominal procedures[50]	1255	5.5%
Dogs, total hip replacement[51]	100	1%

TPLO, tibial plateau levelling osteotomy; *TTA*, tibial tuberosity advancement.

Dirty surgical or traumatic wound infections are surgical wounds or nonsurgical defects that are already infected or have breaks in the skin associated with blunt trauma. Devitalized tissues, foreign bodies, or purulent discharges are often observed. Examples of dirty wounds include previously perforated viscera, devitalized wounds, compound fractures, foreign bodies, pus pockets, and acute cellulitis. Traumatic wounds are assumed to be contaminated and have a high risk of infection because microbes bypass the anatomic and immunologic barriers of the host. These wounds possess the highest risk of postoperative infection.

As indicated earlier, a variety of pathogens can cause SSIs, and these can originate in the patient's microbiota (e.g., *Staphylococcus pseudintermedius,* enterococci, Enterobacterales), the microbiota of veterinary personnel and owners (e.g., *S. aureus*), and the environment (e.g., Enterobacterales, *Serratia, Pseudomonas*). While a large number of pathogens can cause SSIs, a few species account for most infections. The most common tend to be coagulase-positive staphylococci, particularly *S. pseudintermedius,* which accounts for the majority of SSIs in many situations, and Enterobacterales (e.g., *Escherichia coli, Klebsiella, Enterobacter*).[6,7] The rise in methicillin-resistant staphylococci and extended-spectrum beta-lactamase (ESBL)–producing Enterobacterales, as well as frequent inherent and acquired resistance in other pathogens such as *Pseudomonas,* complicate treatment. *Streptococcus* spp. are sometimes involved, most commonly *Streptococcus canis.* This species is of particular relevance because of its potential to cause necrotizing fasciitis, most often as a consequence of enrofloxacin treatment.[8] Some bacteria are commonly identified but often of no or questionable clinical relevance, such as many coagulase-negative staphylococci and enterococci. Uncommon but important pathogens include *Serratia, Acinetobacter, Proteus, Actinomyces,* and *Stenotrophomonas.*[5–7]

Surveillance

Surveillance is an important component of SSI prevention. One cannot identify and define "abnormal" levels of infection without knowing "normal" levels. While large outbreaks are usually readily apparent, more subtle changes or rates that are higher than in comparable facilities may not be as obvious, leading to missed opportunities to intervene.

Identification of SSIs requires an understanding of SSI definitions, differentiation of inflammation and infection, and consistent assessment. Standard criteria for SSI identification in human surgery[4] are likely applicable to veterinary patients (Table 76.4). Consistent application of a definition for an SSI is critical because variable rigor can lead to spurious changes in apparent rates. Beyond definitions, the next important component is how SSIs are being investigated. SSI surveillance can involve review of medical records, prospective recording of complications as patients are identified with SSI at recheck examinations, or active surveillance through contacting owners at specific timepoints after surgery. These vary in their sensitivity and extent, and in general, the most active the approach, the more accurate the information. Reliance on medical records can markedly underestimate the true SSI rate,[6,7] particularly in referral facilities where patients with SSIs may be managed by a referring veterinarian and not reported to the surgical facility. Active methods such as direct examination or contact with owners at set timepoints can provide more accurate data but are more time-consuming.

Centralized reporting of SSIs within a facility is important, particularly in large facilities with many personnel. Reporting SSIs to a single person (e.g., infection control practitioner) or use of a centralized line-listing or similar document can help ensure that all SSIs are recorded and that changes in rates can be detected as early as possible. Determination of SSI rates is needed to put cases (numerators) into context. This requires an ability to determine the number of procedures (the denominator), something that can range from simple to almost impossible, depending on the records system. Ideally, there is an ability to readily report numerator and denominator, both overall and broken down by procedure, body system, or various other categories.

TABLE 76.2 Examples of Reported Risk Factors for Surgical Site Infection in Dogs

Population	Risk Factor	Odds Ratio
Dogs, TPLO[38]	Increasing weight	1.03
Dogs, TPLO[33]	MRSP carriage Bulldogs	6.7 11.1
Dogs, TPLO[41]	Increasing body weight	1.05 per 1kg
Dogs, TPLO[32]	Anesthesia time	1.01 per minute
Dogs, TPLO[29]	Intact male Increased body weight	1.85 1.02 per increased kg
Dogs, TPLO[40]	German shepherd Meniscectomy Attending surgeon having performed <20 procedures	9.7 2.5 3.0
Dogs, elbow dysplasia surgery[52]	Labrador retriever Rottweiler German shepherd Staffordshire bull terrier	5.7 5.6 3.3 3.1
Dogs undergoing surgery for cranial cruciate ligament disease[52]	Rottweiler	3.96
Dogs, various procedures[6]	Hypotension Surgical classification (compared to clean) Use of an implant	27.7 Dirty: 14.6 Clean contaminated: 2.2 5.6
Dogs, TTA[45]	Surgical time Anesthesia time	1.07 per minute increase 1.04 per minute increase
Dogs, orthopedic implant procedures[34]	Anesthesia time	1.02 per minute increase
Dogs and cats, abdominal and thoracic procedures[50]	Clipping >4h prior to surgery Surgical time	4.0 2.1 per every 90 minutes
Dogs and cats, various procedures[5]	Duration of surgery Number of personnel in the operating room Dirty wound	per minute 1.3 5.6
Dogs and cats, various procedures[19]	Clipping surgical site before induction Duration of surgery	3.0

MRSP, methicillin-resistant *Staphylococcus pseudintermedius; TPLO,* tibial plateau leveling osteotomy; *TTA,* tibial tuberosity advancement.

TABLE 76.3 Classification of Surgical Wounds and Indications for Prophylaxis

Clean	Contaminated
1. Wound from elective surgery 2. Nontraumatic 3. No entry into mucosal surface 4. No break in asepsis 5. No inflammation or drainage encountered	1. Fresh traumatic wound, infection likely 2. Break in sterile technique 3. Spillage from GI or urinary surface 4. Acute inflammation 5. Dental prophylaxis 6. Mucosal surgery
Clean Contaminated	**Infected (Dirty)**
1. Bacterial entry into GI, genitourinary, or respiratory tract mucosae with minimal spillage or simple laceration 2. No unusual contamination, no suppurative inflammation 3. Minor break in asepsis 4. Clean wound with drain placement	1. Abscessed or foreign material present 2. Viscus perforated or fecal contamination 3. Older (>4 hour) traumatic wound 4. Suppuration or necrotic tissue 5. Major break in asepsis

Some potentially biasing factors that must be considered when assessing SSI rates include:

- changes in caseload (e.g., increase or decrease in patient susceptibility, increased or decreased emergency procedures)
- changes in surgical procedures (e.g., addition of new procedures that have higher or lower inherent SSI rates)
- changes in personnel identifying or reporting SSIs
- surveillance bias when more attention is paid to SSIs and their documentation
- surveillance bias through introduction of active rather than just passive surveillance
- surveillance bias through change in SSI definition
- changes in apparent rates because of new records systems that allow for better data recovery.

Bacterial culture is important for diagnosis of SSI and determining optimal patient care, but is absolutely critical for SSI investigation. Knowing whether an increase is due to infections by the same organism or by different organisms can help infer the pathophysiology. For example, an increased rate by the same apparent organism (same species +/- same antibiogram) suggests a point source of infection. A clonal outbreak cannot be proven without additional testing (e.g., strain typing), something that is not often available, but knowing

TABLE 76.4 Definition of a Surgical Site Infection[4]

Surgical Site Infection	Criterion
Superficial incisional	Date of event for infection occurs within 30 days after any operative procedure *AND* involves only skin and subcutaneous tissue of the incision *AND* patient has at least ***one*** of the following: A. Purulent drainage from the superficial incision. B. Organisms identified from an aseptically obtained specimen from the superficial incision or subcutaneous tissue by a culture- or nonculture-based microbiologic testing method which is performed for purposes of clinical diagnosis or treatment. C. Superficial incision that is deliberately opened by a surgeon, attending physician, or other designee and culture- or nonculture-based testing is not performed *AND* patient has at least one of the following signs: pain or tenderness; localized swelling; erythema; or heat. D. Diagnosis of a superficial incisional SSI by the surgeon or attending physician or other designee.
Deep incisional	Date of event for infection occurs within 30 or 90 days after the operative procedure *AND* involves deep soft tissues of the incision (e.g., fascial and muscle layers) *AND* patient has at least ***one*** of the following: A. Purulent drainage from the deep incision. B. Deep incision that spontaneously dehisces, or is deliberately opened or aspirated by a surgeon, attending physician, or other designee *AND* organism is identified by a culture- or nonculture-based microbiologic testing method which is performed for purposes of clinical diagnosis or treatment or culture- or nonculture-based microbiologic testing method is not performed *AND* patient has at least ***one*** of the following signs: fever (>38°C); localized pain or tenderness. A culture- or nonculture-based test that has a negative finding does not meet this criterion. C. An abscess or other evidence of infection involving the deep incision that is detected on gross anatomical or histopathologic examination, or imaging test.
Organ/space	Date of event for infection occurs within 30 or 90 days after the operative procedure *AND* infection involves any part of the body deeper than the fascial/muscle layers that is opened or manipulated during the operative procedure. *AND* patient has at least ***one*** of the following: A. Purulent drainage from a drain that is placed into the organ/space (e.g., closed suction drainage system, open drain, T-tube, drain, CT-guided drainage). B. Organisms are identified from fluid or tissue in the organ/space by a culture- or nonculture-based microbiologic testing method that is performed for purposes of clinical diagnosis or treatment. C. An abscess or other evidence of infection involving the organ/space that is detected on gross anatomical or histopathologic examination, or imaging test evidence suggestive of infection. *AND* meets at least ***one*** criterion for a specific organ/space infection site listed in the Surveillance Definitions for Specific Types of Infections.

https://www.cdc.gov/nhsn/pdfs/pscmanual/17pscnosinfdef_current.pdf
SSI, surgical site infection.

whether the same or different organisms are involved can help target the investigation. The bacterial species involved in an outbreak can also be used to identify likely causes. For example, *S. aureus* is a largely human-associated organism, and a cluster of *S. aureus* (especially MRSA) infections would suggest a human source in the clinic and a need to investigate hygiene practices and postoperative wound care. As a common canine commensal, *S. pseudintermedius* exposure is exceedingly common, and clusters of infections can relate to various factors such as excessive skin trauma (e.g., clipper burn, excessive scrubbing), postoperative trauma or licks of the surgical wound by the patient, inadequate bandaging, and similar factors that allow for infection by a commensal organism. Enterobacterales (e.g., *E. coli, Klebsiella, Enterobacter*) are less common causes of SSI and a cluster of infections suggests a point source, which could involve personnel-based transmission from an index patient, inadequate cleaning and disinfection, and compromises in wound care. Organisms such as *Serratia, Acinetobacter, Pseudomonas,* and *Stenotrophomonas* are water-loving organisms that can persist in the environment and contaminate water sources, biocide solutions (e.g., pre-made surgical prep gauzes), endoscopy equipment, cold sterile solutions, and other clinic sites.[9–13] Identification of these should lead to a prompt investigation of the environment, cleaning and disinfection practices, biocide handling,

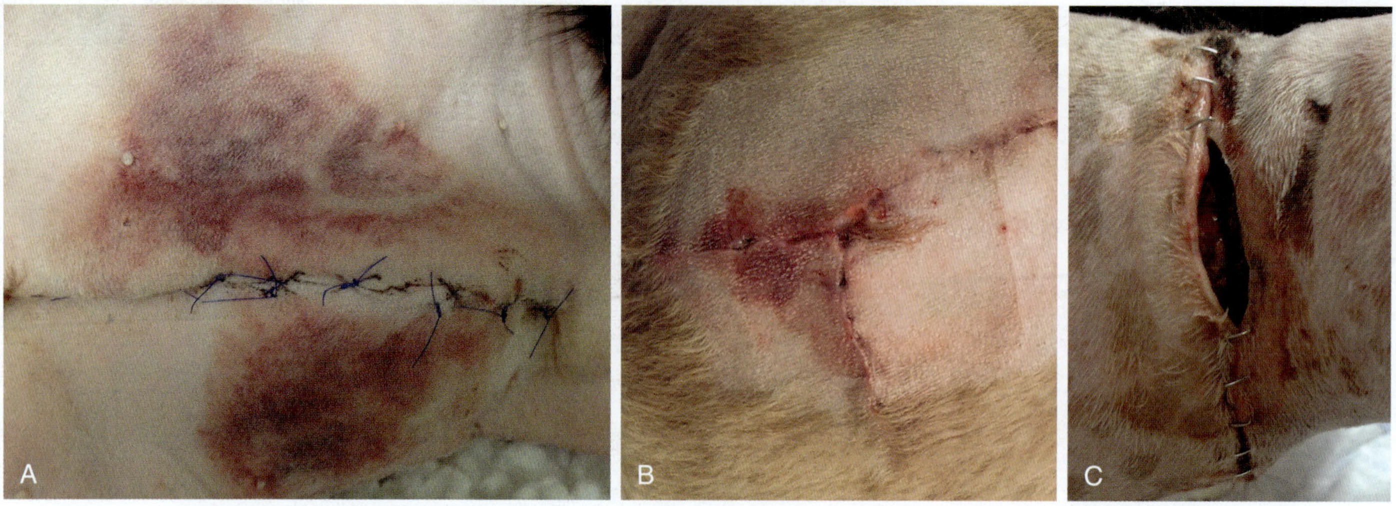

Fig. 76.1 (A) Surgical site undergoing normal healing. (B) Surgical site infection in a mixed-breed dog following internal plate fixation of a pelvic fracture. The dog was lame and the incision was red and draining purulent fluid. A methicillin-susceptible *Staphylococcus pseudintermedius* was cultured from the wound. (C) Severe surgical site infection in a dog; there is evidence of dehiscence and tissue necrosis. (B, Courtesy University of California-Davis Orthopedic Surgery Service.)

and equipment processing. Identification of even one infection caused by these should be of concern (as opposed to the more common staphylococcal SSIs) and more than one infection should be considered an outbreak until proven otherwise. These are just examples of how bacterial identification can be used to tailor the initial investigation.

CLINICAL FINDINGS

SSIs can range from readily apparent to occult. Most infections are superficial and are therefore readily identified by veterinary personnel or owners. The degree of discharge, pain, and systemic signs may be highly variable, and the onset may be gradual or peracute. Most often, initial signs relate to discharge from the surgical site. Changes in patient behavior, such as attempting to lick, scratch, or chew at the site may be noted. Those can also be normal responses to healing (and likely risk factors for inciting an infection), as inflammation is an inevitable response to surgery. Differentiation of SSI from surgical site inflammation is important, because the clinical implications, treatment plan, and infection control aspects of infection versus inflammation are different (Fig. 76.1). This is not always straightforward, and there may be situations where it is debatable whether mild infection or noninfectious inflammation are present. The use of standard definitions of classification of SSIs (see Table 76.4) is useful to facilitate proper diagnosis and differentiate infection and inflammation, as much as possible. Standard definitions also foster consistency between individuals and facilities.

Deep and organ/space SSIs may not be as readily apparent. Severe deep or organ/space infections can be present with little or no superficial component. Gross observation of the surgical site cannot be used to rule out an SSI. Signs of infection can also be masked in the traumatized patient and patients with important comorbidities, so complicating infection should be considered when any clinical signs worsen. Fever and leukocyte changes are not always predictive of infection. Some local inflammation or serous discharge should be expected at the incision site of any surgical procedure. Additional signs that may be associated with systemic infections are respiratory distress, hyperglycemia or hypoglycemia, acute kidney injury, thrombocytopenia, icterus, and mental obtundation. Any clinical abnormality developing in the postoperative period should prompt consideration of (and potentially investigation of) an SSI. Most SSIs develop within the first week or two postoperatively, but complications can develop later, particularly with implants. Current guidelines for human medicine recommend monitoring until 90 days postoperatively for certain procedures involving implants (https://www.cdc.gov/nhsn/pdfs/pscmanual/9pscssicurrent.pdf). Specific guidance for veterinary medicine is lacking but while infections occurring more than 30 days after the procedure are uncommon, infections linked to implant-associated procedures can be encountered months, or even years, after surgery. Whether this reflects a very slowly developing infection associated with the time of surgery or subsequent infection of the surgical site from later bacteremia or dispersion of biofilm-embedded bacteria is unknown. However, history of surgical implants is important to know, even well beyond the immediate postoperative period.

DIAGNOSIS

Clinically, diagnosis of SSI is usually straightforward, particularly superficial SSIs, where changes are grossly apparent. However, infection involving deep tissues without superficial involvement may not be obvious. Systemic manifestations of infection, such as rectal temperature elevations and leukocytosis or bandemia on a CBC, are more indicative of infection but are neither highly sensitive nor specific for SSI. A correlation has been made between elevation of rectal temperature 24 hours postoperatively and increased duration of surgical procedure.[14] However, an elevation of the rectal temperature the day after surgery does not always indicate the development of wound infection. With deeper wounds, diagnostic imaging (radiography, ultrasound, CT) may reveal deeper tissue damage, soft tissue swelling, or gas formation. With chronic orthopedic infections, bony lysis, bone proliferation, or sequestra may be observed.

Biomarkers such as CRP and postoperative neutrophil/lymphocyte ratio have been used in human medicine to distinguish between SSI and inflammation that is not associated with infection. A study of dogs undergoing tibial plateau leveling osteotomy (TPLO) used serum CRP and amyloid A concentrations to investigate early identification of SSI.[15] Significantly elevated concentrations of both markers at day 6 in dogs with SSI when compared to dogs with uncomplicated recovery were identified. However, whether this will be useful for clinical diagnosis and differentiation of infectious and noninfectious inflammation remains to be determined.

Diagnostic specimens should be collected in virtually all cases of suspected SSI, but there are situations where samples and testing are more important or more prone to error. In general, the more superficial the infection, the lower the value of culture because of the greater likelihood of contamination and the lesser need for systemic antimicrobial treatment. Culture is particularly important with severe infections, infections involving invasive devices, infections that are poorly responsive to antibiotics or developed during antibiotic treatment, and in other situations where resistant pathogens are more likely. In humans, culture of superficial wounds or draining tracts is not generally recommended because those specimens do not necessarily reflect the deeper, true component (see Chapter 3 and https://www.cdc.gov/antibiotic-use/healthcare/implementation/clinicianguide.html). There is no reason to think recommendations should be different in animals.

The main approaches to specimen collection for detection of SSIs are tissue biopsy, fine-needle aspirate, and swab. Properly collected tissue biopsy specimens are likely the most sensitive and specific, but they are uncommonly obtained because of invasiveness, time, and cost. If biopsy specimens are collected, they should be taken from viable tissue, not necrotic tissue. Fine-needle aspirates can obtain material from deep sites and limit contamination with superficial bacteria. Aspirates should be collected from affected areas, avoiding necrotic foci. Sampling from an abscess can be performed. Adequate material should be obtained for both cytology and culture. Multiple aspirates should be collected, when possible.

Swabs are most commonly obtained, as a cheap, easy, and generally effective approach. However, there are some limitations and the relative performance of swabs versus tissue specimens or aspirates is unknown. Swabs only sample surface organisms, not necessarily infected tissue. This can result in detection of secondary colonizers, missing the primary cause. The goal must be to limit the amount of surface contamination, to avoid sampling of obviously contaminated sites, and to carefully interpret results from swabs, considering the site and expected resident microbiota. In humans, the Levine technique is considered preferable to other methods (Box 76.1).[16,17]

Cytology is a cost-effective, easy, and overlooked diagnostic tool. It can provide rapid information to help make a diagnosis, to guide empirical therapy, to help assess unusual results (e.g., evidence of rods with a culture report indicating gram-negative rods such as *E. coli* from a site where staphylococcal infections dominate), and to presumptively identify organisms that may be difficult to culture (e.g. *Actinomyces, Nocardia, Mycobacterium*). Cytological specimens need to be collected with care, trying to obtain the most representative sample, but they are not subject to the same potential for contamination compared to culture because slight contamination from the commensal microbiota is less likely to be evident cytologically. Cytology can also help confirm the presence of a likely infectious disease and identify some noninfectious causes (e.g., neoplasia). Cytologic examination should be considered every time a diagnostic sample is obtained.

TREATMENT

Treatment of SSIs is highly variable and depends on the wound (e.g., location and severity of the infection), patient (e.g., comorbidities, allergies), and the offending pathogen (e.g., antimicrobial susceptibility). Superficial infections may be amenable to local therapy with cleaning and application of biocides (e.g., chlorhexidine) or topical antimicrobials (e.g., silver sulfadiazine, mupirocin, fusidic acid, bacitracin/neomycin/polymyxin B) or other therapies (e.g., honey). Suture removal may be indicated to remove a nidus of infection and to facilitate drainage. Deeper infections almost invariably require systemic antimicrobial therapy, which should be chosen based on culture and susceptibility testing, with exception of focal abscesses not accompanied by cellulitis or systemic signs such as fever.

BOX 76.1 Levine Technique for Wound Sampling

Clean wound with normal saline
Debride nonviable tissue
Wait 2–5 minutes
Moisten the swab with saline if site is dry
Culture the healthiest-looking tissue in the wound bed
Do not culture exudate, pus, eschar, or heavy fibrous tissue
Rotate the end of the swab over a 1 cm^2 area for 5 seconds
Apply sufficient pressure for tissue fluid to be expressed

When antimicrobials are indicated, empirical therapy is usually needed while awaiting culture and susceptibility results. The location of infection can indicate the most likely pathogens. Staphylococci are the most common causes of superficial infections and orthopedic infections, while Enterobacterales are more common in procedures associated with the gastrointestinal or urogenital tracts. Cytology can facilitate empirical therapy when an abundance of cocci (most commonly staphylococci), rods (most commonly Enterobacterales), or filamentous bacteria (e.g., *Actinomyces, Nocardia*) are observed. The use of a hospital antibiogram (see Chapter 8) can also assist with selection of appropriate empirical antimicrobials. Empirical therapy with a first-generation cephalosporin (e.g., cephalexin, cefazolin) or amoxicillin-clavulanic acid is commonly used for superficial infections. With more severe disease, where sepsis is of concern, broad-spectrum therapy (e.g., either amoxicillin/ampicillin or clindamycin, combined with a fluoroquinolone) is reasonable, with a plan to de-escalate once culture results are available.

Extensive debridement or surgical drainage of wounds may be required to prevent wound infection and reduce extensive swelling or abscess formation (Fig. 76.2). Wounds should be covered to prevent extensive drying of devitalized tissues, and drainage should be encouraged by incomplete closure or drain placement. Occlusive dressings containing adequate absorbent material should be changed whenever drainage is present. To encourage formation of sufficient granulation tissue, limbs should be immobilized or supported. Chronic nonhealing scar tissue should be resected from the wound. Surgical drains, intravenous catheters, and intubations in trauma patients also increase the risk of infections. See the Suggested Readings list for more information on the surgical approach to wound management following development of an SSI.

Systemic antimicrobials alone may be inadequate for treatment of many SSIs when they are complicated by bacterial biofilm formation, antimicrobial resistance, or difficulty delivering antimicrobials to the infection site at adequate levels. A variety of adjunct approaches may be required. These include surgical intervention to establish drainage, lavage, debride infected tissue, or to remove foreign material (e.g., implants, suture); surgical placement of antimicrobial-impregnated materials (e.g., beads, collagen sponges; see Chapter 121); injection of antimicrobial-impregnated gels; or intra-articular or regional limb perfusion as means of removing infectious foci and delivering high concentrations of antimicrobials to the site. The ability to deliver high antimicrobial concentrations with some approaches can potentially be effective for bacteria reported as resistant, as the determination of

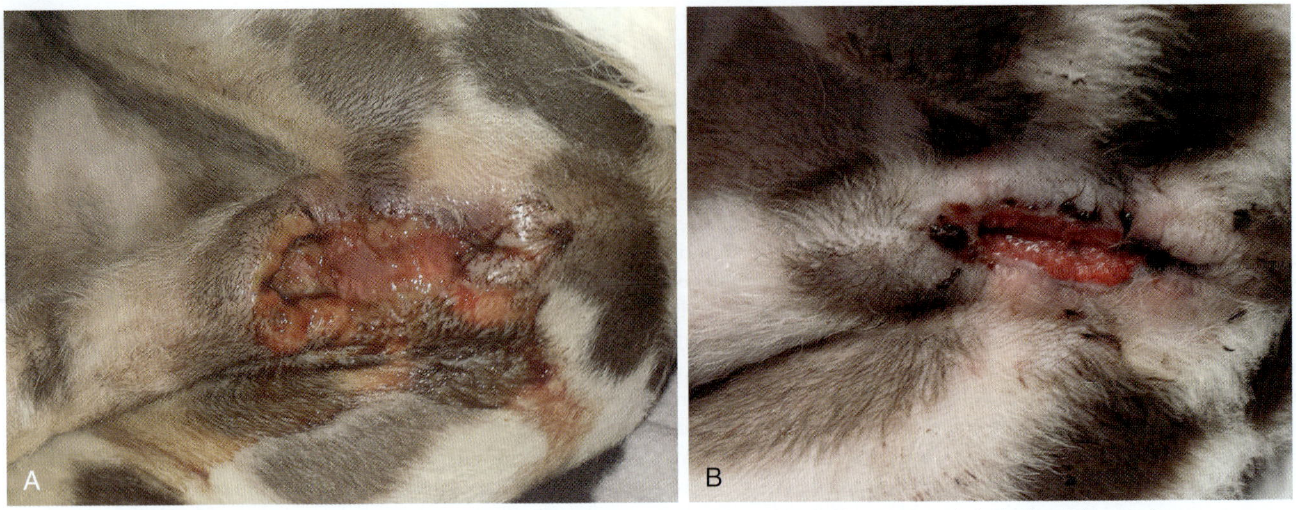

Fig. 76.2 (A) Scrotal urethrostomy site infection in a Dalmatian with dehiscence and devitalized tissue. A severely MDR, methicillin-resistant *S. pseudintermedius* (susceptible only to aminoglycosides) and small numbers of *Fusobacterium* spp. were cultured from the wound. (B) The wound healed with extensive debridement and lavage; a large hematoma was removed from a subcutaneous pocket at the left cranial aspect of the urethrostomy site. Resistance of the *S. pseudintermedius* to the empirically selected antimicrobial was predicted by susceptibility testing. However, because healing was progressing well, antimicrobial therapy was not adjusted. (Images courtesy University of California-Davis Soft Tissue Surgery Service.)

susceptibility or resistance is based on anticipated serum drug levels. If higher concentrations can be achieved (and sustained) at the site of infection, drugs to which the bacterial isolate is reported as resistant may be effective. Typically, antimicrobials used for these approaches are concentration-dependent drugs with long half-lives, such as aminoglycosides.

PREVENTION

Absolute prevention of SSIs is impossible. The nature of surgery will always predispose to some risk of infection. Accordingly, the key is to implement optimal practices to reduce the incidence and severity of SSIs. This is a complex area and one with a paucity of objective data; however, reasonable recommendations can be made based on data from human medicine, limited veterinary data, and general principles of surgery and infection control.

Surgical Site Antisepsis

Basic surgical aseptic technique is the cornerstone of SSI prevention.[18] At a fundamental level, SSI prevention can be thought of as a series of tools to reduce bacterial contamination, reduce tissue trauma, minimize surgical time, and prudently use foreign materials, while minimizing local (e.g., skin barrier damage) and systemic compromise (e.g., immunosuppression, hypoglycemia, hypotension, hypothermia).

Bacterial dose is a key determinant of the risk of infection, and measures to reduce bacterial contamination of the surgical site are a critical tool. The animal's hair should always be clipped (not shaved) and its skin prepared for surgery before it enters the operating room, as close to the time of surgery as is practical. Clipping before anesthesia was a risk factor in one study,[19] something that probably relates more to the ability to atraumatically clip an anesthetized animal. Care should be taken not to injure the skin during the clipping procedure, as skin integrity is probably one of the most important factors for SSI prevention. The goal is not to remove every remnant of hair. Rather, it is to reduce the impact of the hair coat on subsequent skin preparation and the surgical procedure. Leaving some remnants of hair is preferable to skin trauma from excessive clipping. Antisepsis of the skin at the incision site is designed to reduce the microbial burden, not sterilize the skin. A variety of approaches can be used, including the traditional three-step (chlorhexidine or iodine soap, alcohol, tincture of chlorhexidine or iodine) to one-step paint-on products. As with clipping, excessive scrubbing should be avoided in order to maintain skin integrity.

The two main perioperative and wound-care biocides are chlorhexidine and iodophors. Concentration is essential as higher concentrations result in more damage to host cells, while lower concentrations can limit antimicrobial efficacy. The relative efficacy of povidone iodine versus chlorhexidine is still somewhat unclear as conflicting data are available. The WHO has recommended alcohol-based chlorhexidine for surgical preparation,[18] but this recommendation has been challenged.[20] Chlorhexidine should be avoided when preparing sites around the eyes or ears because of ocular and ototoxicity concerns. In humans, it is also recommended to avoid chlorhexidine in the genital region because it can cause mucosal irritation. It is commonly stated that chlorhexidine may be preferable because of residual activity; however, the presence of a true residual effect in vivo has been challenged[21] and convincing evidence of a clinically relevant residual effect is lacking. The efficacy of chlorhexidine may be less impacted by organic debris such as blood. Chlorhexidine resistance has been identified;[22,23] however, there is little evidence that this currently poses a clinical risk as concentrations required to inhibit bacterial strains carrying resistance genes are still well below concentrations used clinically.

Disinfection and Sterilization

The sterilization of surgical instruments and facilities is an essential part of the operative procedure (see Chapter 15 for a review of hospital and equipment disinfection procedures). Surgical equipment should be appropriately sterilized using steam autoclaves or ethylene oxide, with appropriate quality-control practices, including routine use of biological indicators. Cold sterilization *should not* be used for any instruments that can undergo other forms of sterilization. Cold sterilization should be considered high-level disinfection at best, not sterilization as bacterial contamination of cold sterilization solutions is common.[24]

Procedure Factors

Use of proper surgical technique is perhaps the single most important factor in preventing postoperative infections. The risk of tissue infection is directly proportional to the increased amount of tissue handling, desiccation, and trauma. Foreign material and blood clots allow for adherence and replication of microorganisms and facilitate formation of biofilms. Bacterial contamination can lead to risk of infection in the immediate postoperative period or more insidious problems through colonization of implants.

The duration of the surgical procedure and anesthesia time are well established as risk factors for SSIs in both animals and humans. Surgical time should not be decreased at the expense of proper technique, but there are various measures that can be used to reduce anesthesia and surgical time, particularly those that relate to coordination and organization, to limit waiting time. There should be no delays between anesthetic induction and completion of the procedure. Proper coordination, including use of a surgical checklist,[25] can help reduce unnecessary delays.

Antimicrobial Prophylaxis

Perioperative antimicrobial administration can reduce the incidence of postoperative infection in certain procedures; however, objective evidence in small animal surgery is sparse and somewhat conflicting. Perioperative antimicrobials are most important for procedures where contamination is at increased risk of occurring or is unavoidable (e.g., dirty procedures), and potentially with procedures where the implications of an SSI can be devastating. Antimicrobials are not likely indicated for clean procedures that do not involve surgical implants.

When antimicrobials are indicated, the key concept is maintenance of therapeutic drug levels throughout the period of risk. This is typically achieved by administering the first dose intravenously 30 to 60 minutes prior to the first incision, with intraoperative dosing every 2 half-lives of the antimicrobial as long as the surgery is underway. For example, cefazolin is a commonly used antimicrobial and it has a half-life of 37 to 57 minutes,[26,27] meaning intraoperative redosing is indicated every 75 to 120 minutes.

Once the period of risk has ended, antimicrobials are presumably not indicated. Continuation of antimicrobials after surgery is rarely required. In humans, recommendations for most procedures are to not continue antimicrobials for longer than 24 hours after surgery.[28] In some situations, postoperative prophylaxis is continued, yet this rarely extends beyond 24 hours, a time at which it is reasonable to assume that any bacterial contaminants have been killed or are resistant and a relatively effective barrier to the outside microbiota has been established. In veterinary medicine, most of the available data pertain to TPLO, a procedure that is typically associated with a high infection rate. Numerous studies have reported a protective effect of postoperative antimicrobials for TPLO,[29–33] and another study of clean orthopedic implant procedures that was dominated by TPLOs also reported efficacy of postoperative antimicrobials.[34] However, what constitutes "postoperative" has not been adequately investigated. It is possible that antimicrobials only need to be continued for 24 hours postoperatively, as with most human procedures, but further study is required to determine the optimal regimen. There are no corresponding data supporting postoperative antimicrobial prophylaxis for other surgical procedures, and results from TPLO studies should not be extrapolated to other surgical procedures.

Wound Lavage

Contaminated cutaneous or soft tissue wounds should be lavaged with copious amounts of prewarmed saline, lactated Ringer's solution, or tap water. Pressure can be delivered with a 35-mL syringe and 18-gauge needle or similar size catheter or via a commercial device. Lavage without pressure is not as effective. It is debatable whether biocides are necessary in flush solutions versus sterile saline or running tap water, as physical flushing is more important in contaminated traumatic injuries or infected wounds to reduce bacterial levels. Lactated Ringer's solution has been reported to be less traumatic than normal saline or tap water to canine connective tissues *in vitro*,[35] so it might be the most desirable flush solution to preserve tissue healing. However, whether that corresponds to clinical wound lavage is debatable. When a biocide is desired, aqueous (as opposed to alcohol-based) formulations must be used and concentrations are typically lower than those used for intact skin, such as 0.05% for chlorhexidine.[36]

Engineered Devices

A variety of new approaches have been investigated to reduce the incidence of SSIs. There are abundant options in human medicine, some that have been explored in veterinary medicine, and many other potential options based on *in vitro* testing. These include approaches such as antimicrobial- or biocide-impregnated suture and devices (e.g., implants) coated with biocides, heavy metals, or other substances to inhibit bacteria. Results have been mixed and typically when an impact has been identified, it has been relatively modest. In companion animal veterinary medicine, limited data are available. Triclosan-impregnated suture had no discernable impact of TPLO SSI in one study.[37] However, it is a challenge to perform clinical SSI studies with sufficient statistical power to detect a difference, particularly if that difference is modest. Accordingly, this may be a scenario where it is better considered "absence of evidence of efficacy" versus "evidence of absence of efficacy." Despite the lack of good current efficacy data, there may be effective future options as new materials and approaches are studied.

CASE EXAMPLE

Signalment

"Edith," a 5-year-old female spayed bichon frise from Ontario, Canada.

History

Edith was brought for veterinary evaluation 5 days after a cystotomy to remove uroliths. The surgery was uneventful and normal recovery occurred. The dog was treated with preoperative cephazolin and discharged with instructions for exercise restriction and to ensure that an E-collar was worn at all times. The E-collar compliance was sporadic. The owner noticed the patient licking at the incision site the day before evaluation.

Current medications: None.

Other medical history: Nothing relevant.

Physical Examination

Body weight: 4.7 kg.

General: Unremarkable physical examination apart from the surgical site. Vital parameters and other physical examination findings were normal.

Surgical site: The suture line was intact but was inflamed, with a small amount of purulent debris and crusted material. The dog resented palpation of the site and a small amount of pus was expressed from the cranial aspect of the suture line.

Specimen collection: Two sutures were removed from the cranial aspect of the incision, where pus was expressed. The area was cleaned with sterile saline, and residual fluid was removed using sterile gauze. Avoiding contact with surrounding tissue, a sterile swab was pressed against the affected

Continued

CASE EXAMPLE—cont'd

subcutaneous tissues and rubbed back and forth for 5 seconds, to try to express fluid from the site. This was done twice to collect specimens for cytology and culture.

Cytology findings

Cytologic examination revealed suppurative inflammation, with approximately 90% neutrophils. Occasional intracellular cocci were evident.

Diagnosis

Superficial SSI, likely caused by self-trauma or licking the wound.

Treatment

Cephalexin, 26 mg/kg (125 mg) PO q12h for 5 days.

Strict compliance with E-collar use was emphasized.

Local treatment of the wound was considered but not deemed necessary based on the small size of the wound and relatively minor infection.

Comments

The diagnosis was straightforward given the clinical signs and recent surgery. Other antimicrobial options were considered initially, including amoxicillin-clavulanic acid and clindamycin. The cytology results allowed for confidence in targeting gram-positive bacteria, leading to a choice of cephalexin over the broader-potentiated penicillin. Clindamycin would have been an equivalent option to cephalexin in a gram-positive soft tissue infection such as this. *Staphylococcus pseudintermedius* that was susceptible to cephalexin, clindamycin, and amoxicillin-clavulanic acid was isolated from the specimen. The patient recovered uneventfully.

SUGGESTED READINGS

Verwilghen D, Singh A. Fighting surgical site infections in small animals: are we getting anywhere? *Vet Clin North Am Small Anim Pract*. 2015;45:243–276.

Turk R, Singh A, Weese JS. Prospective surgical site infection surveillance in dogs. *Vet Surg*. 2015;44:2–8.

Bratzler DW, Dellinger EP, Olsen KM, et al. Clinical practice guidelines for antimicrobial prophylaxis in surgery. *Surg Infect*. 2013;14:73–156.

REFERENCES

1. Ross AA, Müller KM, Weese JS, et al. Comprehensive skin microbiome analysis reveals the uniqueness of human skin and evidence for phylosymbiosis within the class Mammalia. *Proc Natl Acad Sci U S A*. 2018;115:E5786–E5795.
2. Pierezan F, Olivry T, Paps JS, et al. The skin microbiome in allergen-induced canine atopic dermatitis. *Vet Dermatol*. 2016;27:332-e82.
3. Rodrigues Hoffmann A, Patterson AP, Diesel A, et al. The skin microbiome in healthy and allergic dogs. *PLoS ONE*. 2014;9:e83197.
4. Mangram AJ, Horan TC, Pearson ML, et al. Guideline for prevention of surgical site infection, 1999. Centers for Disease Control and Prevention (CDC) Hospital Infection Control Practices Advisory Committee. *Am J Infect Control*. 1999;27:97–132.
5. Eugster S, Schawalder P, Gaschen F, et al. A prospective study of postoperative surgical site infections in dogs and cats. *Vet Surg*. 2004;33:542–550.
6. Turk R, Singh A, Weese JS. Prospective surgical site infection surveillance in dogs. *Vet Surg*. 2015;44:2–8.
7. Garcia Stickney DN, Thieman Mankin KM. The impact of postdischarge surveillance on surgical site infection diagnosis. *Vet Surg*. 2018;47:66–73.
8. Ingrey KT, Ren J, Prescott JF. A fluoroquinolone induces a novel mitogen-encoding bacteriophage in *Streptococcus canis*. *Infect Immun*. 2003;71:3028–3033.
9. Dolan SA, Littlehorn C, Glode MP, et al. Association of *Bacillus cereus* infection with contaminated alcohol prep pads. *Infect Control Hosp Epidemiol*. 2012;33:666–671.
10. Gleeson S, Mulroy E, Bryce E, et al. *Burkholderia cepacia*: an outbreak in the peritoneal dialysis unit. *Perit Dial Int*. 2019;39:92–95.
11. Kirschke DL, Jones TF, Craig AS, et al. *Pseudomonas aeruginosa* and *Serratia marcescens* contamination associated with a manufacturing defect in bronchoscopes. *N Engl J Med*. 2003;348:214–220.
12. Liu D, Zhang L-P, Huang S-F, et al. Outbreak of *Serratia marcescens* infection due to contamination of multiple-dose vial of heparin-saline solution used to flush deep venous catheters or peripheral trocars. *J Hosp Infect*. 2011;77:175–176.
13. Vonberg R-P, Gastmeier P. Hospital-acquired infections related to contaminated substances. *J Hosp Infect*. 2007;65:15–23.
14. Vasseur PB, Levy J, Dowd E, et al. Surgical wound infection rates in dogs and cats. Data from a teaching hospital. *Vet Surg*. 1988;17:60–64.
15. Löfqvist K, Kjelgaard-Hansen M, Nielsen MBM. Usefulness of C-reactive protein and serum amyloid A in early detection of postoperative infectious complications to tibial plateau leveling osteotomy in dogs. *Acta Vet Scand*. 2018;60:30.
16. Angel DE, Lloyd P, Carville K, et al. The clinical efficacy of two semi-quantitative wound-swabbing techniques in identifying the causative organism(s) in infected cutaneous wounds. *Int Wound J*. 2011;8:176–185.
17. Copeland-Halperin LR, Kaminsky AJ, Bluefeld N, et al. Sample procurement for cultures of infected wounds: a systematic review. *J Wound Care*. 2016;25. S4-6, S8.
18. Allegranzi B, Bischoff P, de Jonge S, et al. New WHO recommendations on preoperative measures for surgical site infection prevention: an evidence-based global perspective. *Lancet Infect Dis*. 2016;16:e276–e287.
19. Brown DC, Conzemius MG, Shofer F, et al. Epidemiologic evaluation of postoperative wound infections in dogs and cats. *J Am Vet Med Assoc*. 1997;210:1302–1306.
20. Maiwald M, Widmer AF. WHO's recommendation for surgical skin antisepsis is premature. *Lancet Infect Dis*. 2017;17:1023–1024.
21. Rutter JD, Angiulo K, Macinga DR. Measuring residual activity of topical antimicrobials: is the residual activity of chlorhexidine an artefact of laboratory methods? *J Hosp Infect*. 2014;88:113–115.
22. Correa JE, De Paulis A, Predari S, et al. First report of qacG, qacH and qacJ genes in *Staphylococcus haemolyticus* human clinical isolates. *J Antimicrob Chemother*. 2008;62:956–960.
23. Frosini SM, Bond R, Rantala M, et al. Genetic resistance determinants to fusidic acid and chlorhexidine in variably susceptible staphylococci from dogs. *BMC Microbiol*. 2019;19:81.
24. Murphy CP, Weese JS, Reid-Smith RJ, et al. The prevalence of bacterial contamination of surgical cold sterile solutions from community companion animal veterinary practices in southern Ontario. *Can Vet J*. 2010;51:634–636.
25. Weiser TG, Haynes AB, Lashoher A, et al. Perspectives in quality: designing the WHO Surgical Safety Checklist. *Int J Qual Health Care*. 2010;22:365–370.
26. Cagnardi P, Di Cesare F, Toutain PL, et al. Population pharmacokinetic study of cefazolin used prophylactically in canine surgery for susceptibility testing breakpoint determination. *Front Pharmacol*. 2018;9:1137.
27. Gonzalez OJ, Renberg WC, Roush JK, et al. Pharmacokinetics of cefazolin for prophylactic administration to dogs. *Am J Vet Res*. 2017;78:695–701.
28. Bratzler DW, Dellinger EP, Olsen KM, et al. Clinical practice guidelines for antimicrobial prophylaxis in surgery. *Surg Infect*. 2013;14:73–156.
29. Fitzpatrick N, Solano MA. Predictive variables for complications after TPLO with stifle inspection by arthrotomy in 1000 consecutive dogs. *Vet Surg*. 2010;39:460–474.
30. Frey TN, Hoelzler MG, Scavelli TD, et al. Risk factors for surgical site infection-inflammation in dogs undergoing surgery for rupture of the

cranial cruciate ligament: 902 cases (2005-2006). *J Am Vet Med Assoc.* 2010;236:88–94.
31. Hans EC, Barnhart MD, Kennedy SC, et al. Comparison of complications following tibial tuberosity advancement and tibial plateau levelling osteotomy in very large and giant dogs 50 kg or more in body weight. *Vet Comp Orthop Traumatol.* 2017;30:299–305.
32. Nazarali A, Singh A, Weese JS. Perioperative administration of antimicrobials during tibial plateau leveling osteotomy. *Vet Surg.* 2014;43:966–971.
33. Nazarali A, Singh A, Moens NM, et al. Association between methicillin-resistant *Staphylococcus pseudintermedius* carriage and the development of surgical site infections following tibial plateau leveling osteotomy in dogs. *J Am Vet Med Assoc.* 2015;247:909–916.
34. Pratesi A, Moores AP, Downes C, et al. Efficacy of postoperative antimicrobial use for clean orthopedic implant surgery in dogs: a prospective randomized study in 100 consecutive cases. *Vet Surg.* 2015;44:653–660.
35. Valente JH, Forti RJ, Freundlich LF, et al. Wound irrigation in children: saline solution or tap water. *Ann Emerg Med.* 2003;41:609–616.
36. Sanchez IR, Swaim SF, Nusbaum KE, et al. Effects of chlorhexidine diacetate and povidone-iodine on wound healing in dogs. *Vet Surg.* 1988;17:291–295.
37. Etter SW, Ragetly GR, Bennett RA, et al. Effect of using triclosan-impregnated suture for incisional closure on surgical site infection and inflammation following tibial plateau leveling osteotomy in dogs. *J Am Vet Med Assoc.* 2013;242:355–358.
38. Giannetto JJ, Aktay SA. Prospective evaluation of surgical wound dressings and the incidence of surgical site infections in dogs undergoing a tibial plateau levelling osteotomy. *Vet Comp Orthop Traumatol.* 2019;32:18–25.
39. Spencer DD, Daye RM. A prospective, randomized, double-blinded, placebo-controlled clinical study on postoperative antibiotherapy in 150 arthroscopy-assisted tibial plateau leveling osteotomies in dogs. *Vet Surg.* 2018;47:E79–E87.
40. Lopez DJ, VanDeventer GM, Krotscheck U, et al. Retrospective study of factors associated with surgical site infection in dogs following tibial plateau leveling osteotomy. *J Am Vet Med Assoc.* 2018;253:315–321.
41. Atwood C, Maxwell M, Butler R, et al. Effects of incision closure method on infection prevalence following tibial plateau leveling osteotomy in dogs. *Can Vet J.* 2015;56:375–381.
42. Stine SL, Odum SM, Mertens WD. Protocol changes to reduce implant-associated infection rate after tibial plateau leveling osteotomy: 703 dogs, 811 TPLO (2006-2014). *Vet Surg.* 2018;47:481–489.
43. Dyall BAR, Schmökel HG. Surgical site infection rate after hemilaminectomy and laminectomy in dogs without perioperative antibiotic therapy. *Vet Comp Orthop Traumatol.* 2018;31:202–213.
44. Corriveau KM, Giuffrida MA, Mayhew PD, et al. Outcome of laparoscopic ovariectomy and laparoscopic-assisted ovariohysterectomy in dogs: 278 cases (2003-2013). *J Am Vet Med Assoc.* 2017;251:443–450.
45. Aiken MJ, Hughes TK, Abercromby RH, et al. Prospective, randomized comparison of the effect of two antimicrobial regimes on surgical site infection rate in dogs undergoing orthopedic implant surgery. *Vet Surg.* 2015;44:661–667.
46. Yap FW, Calvo I, Smith KD, et al. Perioperative risk factors for surgical site infection in tibial tuberosity advancement: 224 stifles. *Vet Comp Orthop Traumatol.* 2015;28:199–206.
47. Wolf R, Scavelli T, Hoelzler M. Surgical and postoperative complications associated with tibial tuberosity advancement for cranial cruciate ligament rupture in dogs: 458 cases (2007-2009). *J Am Vet Med Assoc.* 2012;240:1481–1487.
48. Costa M, Craig D, Cambridge T, et al. Major complications of tibial tuberosity advancement in 1613 dogs. *Vet Surg.* 2017;46:494–500.
49. Perry KL, Li L. A retrospective study of the short-term complication rate following 750 elective elbow arthroscopies. *Vet Comp Orthop Traumatol.* 2014;27:68–73.
50. Mayhew PD, Freeman L, Kwan T, et al. Comparison of surgical site infection rates in clean and clean-contaminated wounds in dogs and cats after minimally invasive versus open surgery: 179 cases (2007-2008). *J Am Vet Med Assoc.* 2012;240:193–198.
51. Ireifej S, Marino DJ, Loughin CA, et al. Risk factors and clinical relevance of positive intraoperative bacterial cultures in dogs with total hip replacement. *Vet Surg.* 2012;41:63–68.
52. Boge GS, Moldal ER, Dimopoulou M, et al. Breed susceptibility for common surgically treated orthopaedic diseases in 12 dog breeds. *Acta Vet Scand.* 2019;61:19.

77

Miscellaneous Bacterial Infections

Carolyn R. O'Brien, Jane E. Sykes

KEY POINTS

Dermatophilosis

- First Described: 1915 in cattle from the Belgian Congo (Van Saceghem).[1]
- Cause: *Dermatophilus congolensis*, family Dermatophilaceae.
- Affected Hosts: Skin commensals on cattle, horses, small ruminants. Secondary hosts: humans, dogs, cats, platypus.
- Geographic Distribution: Worldwide, but infections are more common in humid environments.
- Primary Mode of Transmission: May be acquired by dogs and cats through contact with affected primary hosts or from contaminated fomites or soil.
- Major Clinical Signs: Exudative dermatitis (dogs), deep soft-tissue abscesses with fistulation (cats).
- Differential Diagnoses: Dogs: superficial pyoderma, mycobacteriosis, allergic dermatoses, immune-mediated dermatoses, drug eruptions, thermal or caustic skin damage. Cats: mycobacteriosis, nocardiosis, fungal infections, cutaneous neoplasia.
- Human Health Significance: Humans often develop infection as a result of contact with colonized or infected animals (especially horses, cattle, and elephants), although infections are very rare. No cases have been reported in association with contact with a dog or cat.

Melioidosis and Glanders

- First Described: *Burkholderia pseudomallei* was first described by Whitmore and Krishnaswami in 1912[2] in Burma. Glanders (*B. mallei*) was reported in ancient Greece by Hippocrates, c.450 BC; 100 years later Aristotle named the disease "meles." The organism was isolated for the first time by Loeffler and Schuetz in 1882.[3]
- Causes: *Burkholderia pseudomallei* (melioidosis) and *Burkholderia mallei* (glanders/farcy), gram-negative, aerobic, rod-shaped bacteria that belong to the family Burkholderiaceae.
- Affected Hosts: *Burkholderia pseudomallei*: Humans, non-human primates, captive marine mammals (e.g., dolphins, whales, sea lions), birds, reptiles, sheep, goats, cattle, alpaca, pigs, horses, mules, cats, dogs, and other wildlife (kangaroos, meerkats). *Burkholderia mallei*: Donkeys, mules, horses, camels, humans, cats, dogs, large carnivores (wolves, bears, lions, tigers, leopards, jackals, and hyenas).
- Geographic Distribution: *Burkholderia pseudomallei*: Tropics and subtropics. *Burkholderia mallei*: South America (Brazil), northern Africa, China, Iraq, Pakistan, India, Mongolia, Turkey, and United Arab Emirates.
- Primary Mode of Transmission: *Burkholderia pseudomallei*: Cutaneous inoculation via breaches in the integument; inhalation/aspiration of aerosols or muddy water, respectively; ingestion. *Burkholderia mallei*: Inhalation of aerosols, ingestion of contaminated water or feed, or via contact with fomites in solipeds, especially in situations where husbandry is substandard, and ingestion of infected meat in carnivores.
- Major Clinical Signs: Range from minor skin lesions, subacute to chronic pneumonia, to fulminant sepsis (*B. pseudomallei*).
- Differential Diagnoses: Mycobacteriosis, neoplasia, other saprophytic gram-negative infections, for example, *Chromobacterium violaceum*.
- Human Health Significance: *Burkholderia pseudomallei* is estimated to clinically affect approximately 165,000 people per year, 10% to 40% fatally. Both *B. pseudomallei* and *B. mallei* are classified as a Tier 1 Select biothreat agents by the United States CDC.

Chromobacteriosis

- First Described: Schroeter 1872.[4]
- Cause: *Chromobacterium violaceum*.
- Affected Hosts: Humans, pigs, cattle, dogs, non-human primates, water buffalo, Macquarie turtle, red panda, horse.
- Geographic Distribution: Worldwide but mostly tropical and subtropical regions.
- Primary Mode of Transmission: Cutaneous inoculation after exposure of wounds to contaminated water or soil.
- Major Clinical Signs: Localized cutaneous and regional lymph nodes, multi-systemic abscessation, pneumonia, and sepsis.
- Differential Diagnoses: *Burkholderia pseudomallei* infection, and other causes of gram-negative sepsis.
- Human Health Significance: Infections are acquired from the environment and are not transmitted between animals and humans. Infections in humans are often fatal.

DERMATOPHILOSIS

ETIOLOGY AND EPIDEMIOLOGY

Dermatophilus congolensis is a gram-positive, facultative anaerobic, branching filamentous, spore-forming actinomycete. The organism dimorphically exists as either a hyphal form or motile, flagellated cocci. During growth, hyphae branch, then undergo transverse and longitudinal division to produce packets of zoospores, consisting microscopically of three to eight paired rows of cocci. The organism is a normal component of the skin flora of cattle, horses, sheep, and goats. Numerous terrestrial and aquatic mammalian and reptilian host species can develop disease when infected as accidental hosts. Outbreaks in livestock can be associated with serious economic losses. Infections have been very rarely described in dogs,[5–7] cats,[8–14] and humans.[15] The prevalence of the disease in primary host species is increased by high environmental moisture levels (rainfall, humidity), and ambient temperatures, the presence of biting vectors and/or other causes of disruption of the dermis (e.g., thorns), as well as the presence of carrier animals.[16] The increased incidence in wet conditions can be attributed to two factors: (1) enhanced spread of infective zoospores and (2) compromise to the epidermal barrier.[17] Immunosuppressive therapy or concurrent illness may predispose animals to infection. There is also some evidence to suggest that host susceptibility may vary genetically.[17]

Dermatophilus congolensis is possibly a saprophyte, although attempts to culture it from the environment have proved unsuccessful and its environmental niche remains a mystery; in general, soil is not thought to be an important source of infection because the organism is not thought to survive long periods in the ground.[18] Spread between animals may occur due to direct contact, contact with contaminated fomites (e.g., horse rugs, brushes), or the environment (e.g., sheep dips, etc.). Chronic carrier animals are assumed to be the primary reservoir.[19] Arthropods such as fleas, ticks, and biting flies have been incriminated as possible mechanical vectors, but their role is not clear.

Dermatophilosis is variably or colloquially known as streptothricosis, "lumpy wool disease," "fleece rot," "strawberry foot rot," "mud fever," "rain-scald," "snuffleupagosis," and proliferative dermatitis, depending on the host species affected and the clinical picture. Experimental infection after inoculation onto damaged skin of dogs[20] and a kitten, and subcutaneous injection of an adult cat have been reported.[10]

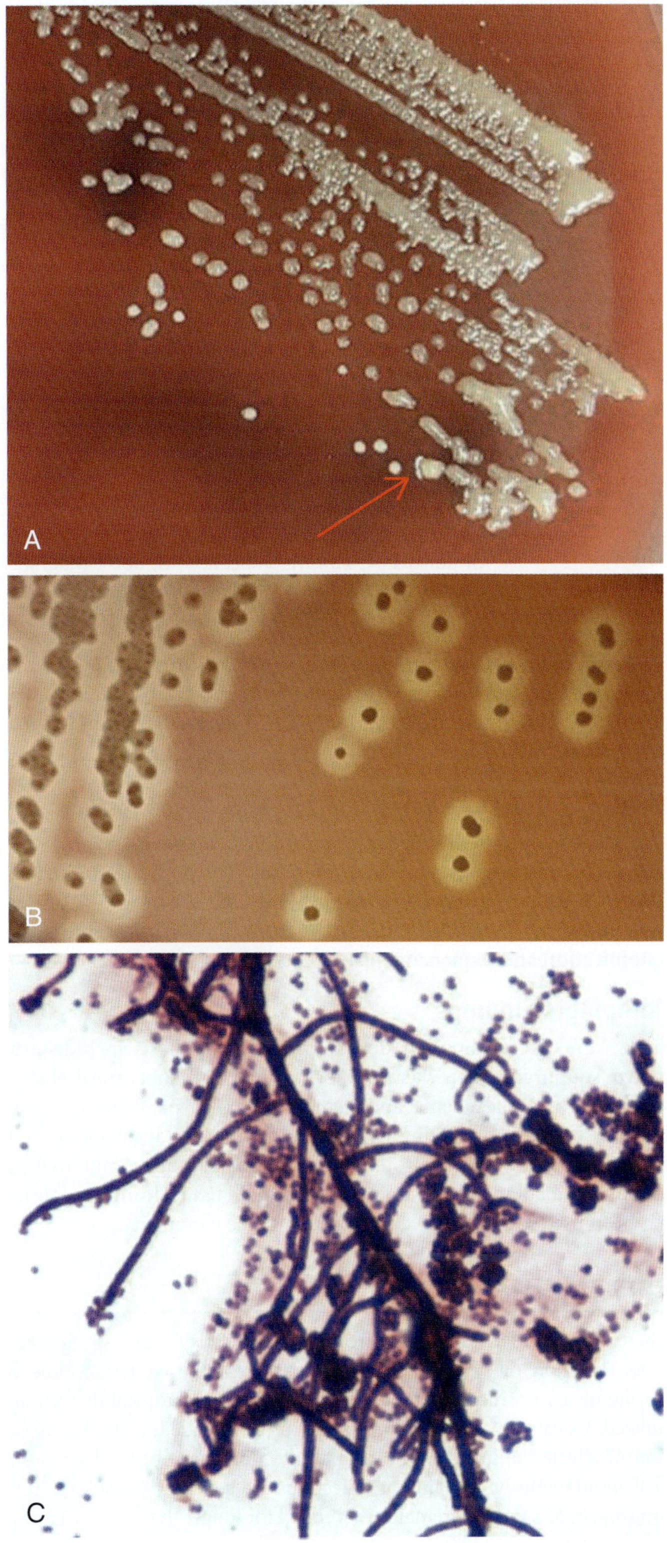

Fig. 77.1 *Dermatophilus congolensis* colonies on 5% sheep blood agar. Note pitting of the agar (A; *arrow*) by colonies and complete hemolysis of sheep erythrocytes (B). (C) Gram stain showing cocci individually and in paired rows ("railroad tracks") which are most commonly observed in patient specimens (see Fig. 77.2). (A and B, courtesy of Dr. Barbara Byrne, University of California-Davis Veterinary Microbiology Laboratory. C, from Alejo-Cancho I, Bosch J, Vergara A, et al. Dermatitis by *Dermatophilus congolensis*. *Clin Microbiol Infect*. 2015;21:e73-74.)

CLINICAL FEATURES

Pathogenesis and Clinical Signs

Dermatophilus congolensis is an opportunistic pathogen that invades skin that has been compromised by minor trauma (e.g., the bites of vectors) or maceration from prolonged contact with moisture. Once the infection becomes established, the exudative process results in separation of the epidermal layers, which allows filamentous hyphae to infiltrate tissues and flagellated cocci to migrate. Alternating layers of keratinized epidermis, vesicles containing exudate, pyogranulomatous inflammation, and bacteria result in development of scabs that are considered characteristic for the disease. Infected scabs can then flake off and become a potential source of infection for other animals and people. Cats develop nodular lesions with draining fistulas, usually with concurrent fever, anorexia, and lethargy. Oral[13,14] and urinary bladder[13] infections have also been reported in cats.

Physical Examination Findings

Dermatophilosis is typically confined to the skin in dogs and manifests as a non-pruritic, crusting dermatitis. Dry scabs are adherent to the hair in affected regions and underlying skin is ulcerated and erythematous. Systemic signs are typically minimal, unless the disease is associated with a comorbid, immunosuppressive condition. Cats may develop subcutaneous nodules[9] or deep abscesses, involving contiguous structures such as the subcutis, muscle, and lymph nodes, particularly in the popliteal region.[8–10]

DIAGNOSIS

Microbiologic Tests

Cytologic Diagnosis

Dermatophilus congolensis has a distinct appearance when examined using light microscopy of Romanowsky-stained preparations made from emulsified crusts or via impression smears collected from the base of freshly removed crusts.

Isolation and Identification

Dermatophilus congolensis grows best in microaerophilic culture conditions with 5% to 10% CO_2 on blood agar at 37°C. Inoculae derived from the underside of freshly removed crusts provide the best results. The organism forms small, grayish, wrinkled, raised colonies that exhibit β-hemolysis on blood agar (Fig. 77.1).[21] Due to the relatively slow growth of *D. congolensis,* culture of specimens contaminated with other skin bacteria can result in rapid overgrowth of the organism. Special techniques such as the use of selective media, 0.45 μm membrane filtration of material derived from the emulsion of crusts with distilled water, or

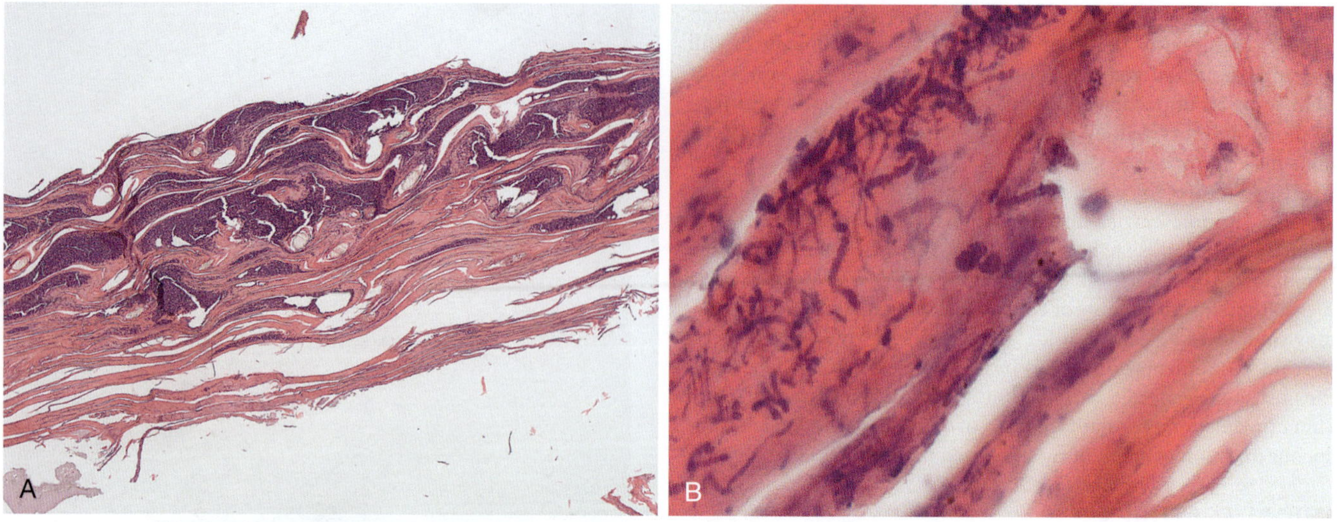

Fig. 77.2 Biopsy specimen showing many chains of *Dermatophilus congolensis* within a parakeratotic layer of dermis (A, 20× magnification; B, 600× magnification). Hematoxylin and eosin stain. (Courtesy of Dr. Verena Affolter, University of California-Davis, Anatomic Pathology Service.)

Haalstra's method (which monopolizes the chemoattractive effects of a carbon dioxide–rich environment on the motile cocci) may be employed to enhance the success of culture. MALDI-TOF mass spectrometry has been successfully used to rapidly identify *D. congolensis.*[21]

Molecular Diagnosis Using Nucleic Acid–Based Testing

Due to its economic importance, and the challenges associated with culture of this organism, several endpoint (conventional) and real-time PCR assays have been developed and used for diagnosis of dermatophilosis.[22–25] Infection in one cat from Illinois was identified by amplification and sequencing of 16S–23S rRNA gene DNA.[9]

Pathologic Findings

Histopathologic findings in dogs with dermatophilosis include exudative, suppurative hyperkeratotic dermatitis, with subcorneal abscessation, and dermal edema and hemorrhage. The parakeratotic layer typically contains branching hyphae containing characteristic coccoid zoospores (Fig. 77.2). Cats tend to have deeper pyogranulomatous lesions in subcutaneous or superficial lymphoid tissue. Immunostaining has been used to identify *D. congolensis* in tissue specimens.

TREATMENT

There are no widely established treatment protocols for any species, and a combination of systemic antimicrobials (typically oxytetracycline in ruminants and penicillin/streptomycin in horses) and topical therapy are utilized. Control of biting insects is also recommended, including isolation of affected animals. Some animal infections have been observed to heal spontaneously, and human infections are generally considered self-limiting, unless the skin remains macerated for longer than 10 to 16 hours a day.[18] Lesions should be kept clean and dry. Removal of adherent crusts via bathing with medicated shampoos (containing chlorhexidine or povidone iodine) is advocated and should be continued for at least 2 weeks. Lime sulfur dips (2%) may also be helpful in animals with superficial infections. The use of topical ointments is discouraged, as this promotes the moist, microaerophilic environment that the bacteria favors.

There are reports of successful treatment of dermatophilosis with a combination of penicillin and streptomycin in a dog[5] and ampicillin in a cat.[11] One cat was also successfully treated with doxycycline, where the organism was not susceptible to penicillin.[8] As there may be regional variations in drug susceptibility patterns, particularly to penicillins and fluoroquinolones, it is recommended that treatment be based on individual antibiogram data should culture be successful.[26,27]

PUBLIC HEALTH ASPECTS

Human dermatophilosis is rare and is, typically, but not always, associated with contact with animals (particularly cattle, horses, and elephants).[18,21,28] Affected humans often reside in or have a travel history to tropical locales (especially Africa, Australia, and Thailand). However, one case described lesions on the inner thigh in a 15-year-old girl who had been horseback riding in Michigan,[18] one case was described in an 8-year-old boy in Wisconsin without known animal contact,[29] and the first human cases ever reported were in four people from Orange County, NY who developed furunculosis after handling an infected deer in a wildlife reserve (1961).[30] Previous skin lesions are often reported (e.g., cuts, abrasions, psoriasis). There is a tendency for the legs of young women to be affected, and it has been proposed that shaving of the skin may lead to micro-abrasions that facilitate entry of the organism into the skin.[31] The handling of infected carcasses has also been associated with human infection. Most human cases have involved superficial cutaneous infections, manifesting as exudative pustular dermatitis, folliculitis, pitted keratolysis of the soles of the feet, subcutaneous nodules, or onycholysis; however, there are isolated reports of oral[32] and esophageal infections,[33] and one case of necrotizing granulomatous lymphadenopathy in an immunocompromised child. There are no reports of human infection secondary to contact with affected dogs or cats; however, precautions such as the wearing of personal protective equipment (e.g., disposable gowns and gloves) during handling of infected animals is recommended, including thorough hand washing after contact.

MELIOIDOSIS

ETIOLOGIC AGENT AND EPIDEMIOLOGY

Melioidosis is an infection caused by the facultative aerobic, gram-negative, motile, non-spore-forming beta-proteobacterium, *Burkholderia pseudomallei.* The bacterium is soil and water borne, and is mostly restricted to latitudes within 25 degrees north or south of the equator.[34] *Burkholderia pseudomallei* is estimated to cause disease in approximately 165,000 people

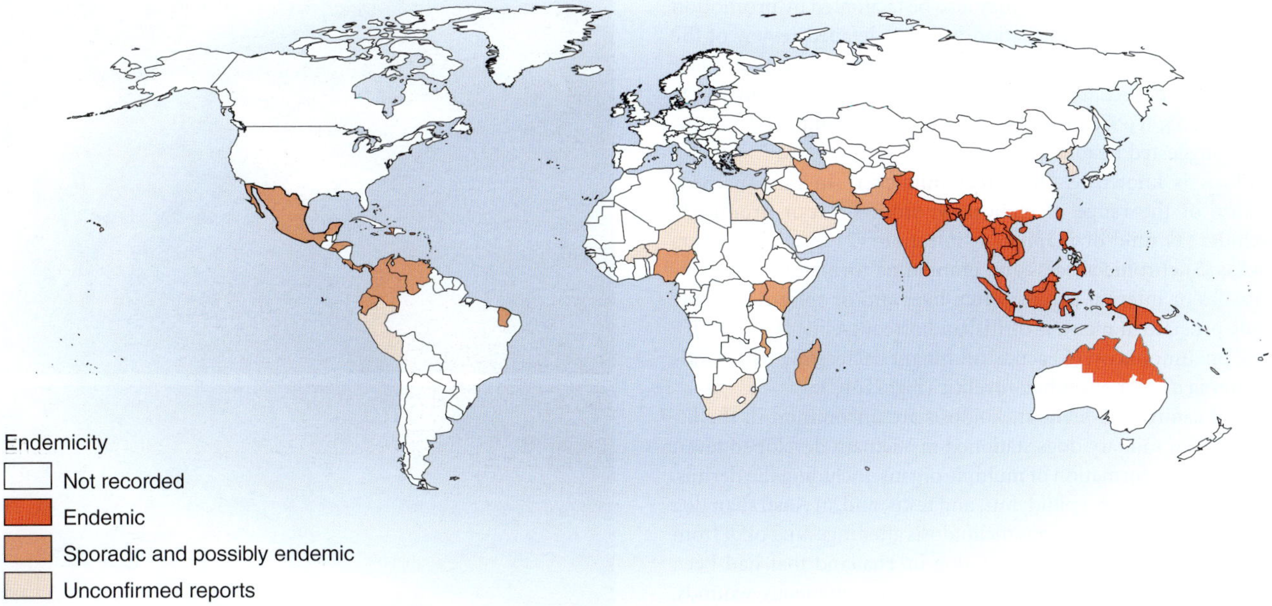

Fig. 77.3 The known geographic distribution of melioidosis. (From Currie BJ. *Burkholderia pseudomallei* and *Burkholderia mallei*: melioidosis and glanders. In: Bennett JE, Dolin R, Blaser MJ, eds. *Mandell, Douglas and Bennett's Principles and Practice of Infectious Diseases*. Philadelphia, PA: Elsevier; 2020:2707-2717.)

each year, with a mortality rate of 10% to 40%.[35] Most human cases are reported from Southeast Asia (particularly northeastern Thailand[36]) and Northern Australia (the "Top End" of the Northern Territory[37]), especially during the wet/monsoon seasons (Fig. 77.3).[38] Sporadic autochthonous cases are also reported outside of the area of high endemicity, including the Carribean,[39] Central and South America,[40] Africa,[41,42] the Indian subcontinent,[43] and the Middle East. Occasional cases of melioidosis have been reported in people from the southwestern United States, with no recent travel history to endemic regions.[44,45] Genetic analysis of strains involved has suggested that the organism may be present in the soil in Texas. Some of the affected individuals had histories of travel to endemic regions decades earlier, so it was felt that until the organism was isolated from the environment, it cannot be said that *B. pseudomallei* is endemic in the United States. Genetic analysis of worldwide strains implicates Australia as a likely geographical origin of the species with spread to Southeast Asia, thence to East Asia.[46,47] South American strains appear to have originated in Africa.[46]

Burkholderia pseudomallei can be isolated most reliably from moist clay soils and pooled surface water from endemic areas. Human infection numbers increase after heavy monsoonal rains and winds, presumably because of inhalation of organism-laden aerosols. Infection is thought to occur via cutaneous inoculation through open wounds contaminated with soil; bites of arthropod vectors; inhalation of dust, aerosols, or aspiration of muddy water (such as that occurs with near drowning); or ingestion of soil, contaminated infected carcasses, contaminated drinking water, or milk (following infection of the mammary gland). Because of the risks of inhalation or ingestion, the bacterium has been labeled as a biological weapon, and has been classified as a Tier 1 Select Agent by the CDC,[48] although its true potential in this scenario is unclear.

Burkholderia pseudomallei generally has a low propensity to cause disease in clinically healthy hosts, and infection mostly results in subclinical seroconversion. In humans, severe disease is almost always seen in individuals with compromised innate immunity, particularly those with impaired neutrophil function, such as with diabetes mellitus, alcohol abuse, chronic kidney or pulmonary disease, thalassemia, and cancer.[47,49] Smoking and/or glucocorticoid use are also associated with an increased risk of infection in people.[50] Major impairment of adaptive CMI, such as that seen in advanced HIV infection, does not appear to be a risk factor for disease in people.[51] Likewise, a high antibody titer does not protect against either primary infection or relapse.[52,53]

Geographical differences exist with regard to clinical manifestation and mortality, which is thought to be due to both regional access to adequate healthcare and, also host and bacterial genetics. The infecting dose, route of infection (particularly inhalation), and the duration of clinical signs prior to treatment also influence the severity of clinical disease.

Most cases in humans are acute infections that occur after short incubation periods (mean 9 days, range 1 to 21 days).[47] Although relatively uncommon, the infection may remain subclinical for long periods, with the sudden appearance of disease after many years of dormancy, like that seen with tuberculosis. The longest recorded incubation period was in a United States veteran of the Pacific theater of World War II, who was diagnosed 62 years after presumed exposure.[54] Because of concerns relating to reactivation of infection in soldiers returning from Vietnam, the disease was referred to as the "Vietnamese Time."[55,56]

Melioidosis is considered an emerging disease in humans and it has been proposed that the incidence of the disease in people is greatly under-reported in the developing world. This is likely to be even more the case for animal disease.

CLINICAL FEATURES

Pathogenesis, Clinical Signs, and Physical Examination Findings

Burkholderia pseudomallei is a facultative opportunistic intracellular organism, capable of replication within the cytosol of host cells (neutrophils, macrophages, and epithelial cells).[44] The bacteria are able to move within the cell to form protrusions of the cell membrane and result in cell-to-cell spread.[57] This may also be facilitated by promotion of multinucleated giant cell formation.[47,58,59] A detailed review of the pathogenesis of infection and the role of a vast array of virulence factors produced by *B. pseudomallei* (e.g., capsular polysaccharide, LPS, flagella, pili, T3SS, T6SS, proteases, lipases, phospholipases) is provided in the Suggested Reading list.[47]

Melioidosis is known as "the great mimicker" in human medicine because of the range of clinical syndromes it can produce.[60] These include: (1) mild or inapparent infection; (2) local skin ulcers (Fig. 77.4A); (3) chronic abscess and granuloma formation in subcutaneous tissues or internal organs (often liver and/or spleen, but may also include prostate in men), arthritis, and osteomyelitis (Fig. 77.4B); (4) chronic pneumonia or; (5) acute, fulminant bacteremia with resultant pneumonia and/or encephalomyelitis (Fig. 77.4C).

Reports of canine and feline melioidosis are uncommon in the literature.[61–66] Seven military dogs stationed in Vietnam developed fever, myalgia, and abscess formation of multiple organs, including the dermis, lung, liver, kidneys, spleen, epididymis, and testis, and an Australian dog developed disseminated cutaneous melioidosis after ingesting offal from a goat that had died of the disease. A dog in Thailand that had been trapped in a barbed wire fence developed severe cutaneous wounds, splenic abscessation, and bacteremia.[62] In 2016, *B. pseudomallei* was identified in a 4-year-old mixed-breed dog that had been admitted to a shelter in New York after spending 21 months in a dog shelter in Thailand. The dog was evaluated at the Cornell University Hospital for Animals for apparent spinal trauma, and during the clinical workup, *B. pseudomallei* was isolated from the dog's urine.[61] Of the six cats reported with melioidosis, three were presumed to have acquired the infection in Malaysia,[63] with the remaining three cases domiciled in Northern Australia.[63] Multifocal abscesses, lymphadenomegaly, hepatomegaly, and splenomegaly were most common in the affected cats.[63,65,66] Two cats had unilateral panophthalmitis and retrobulbar abscessation.[64]

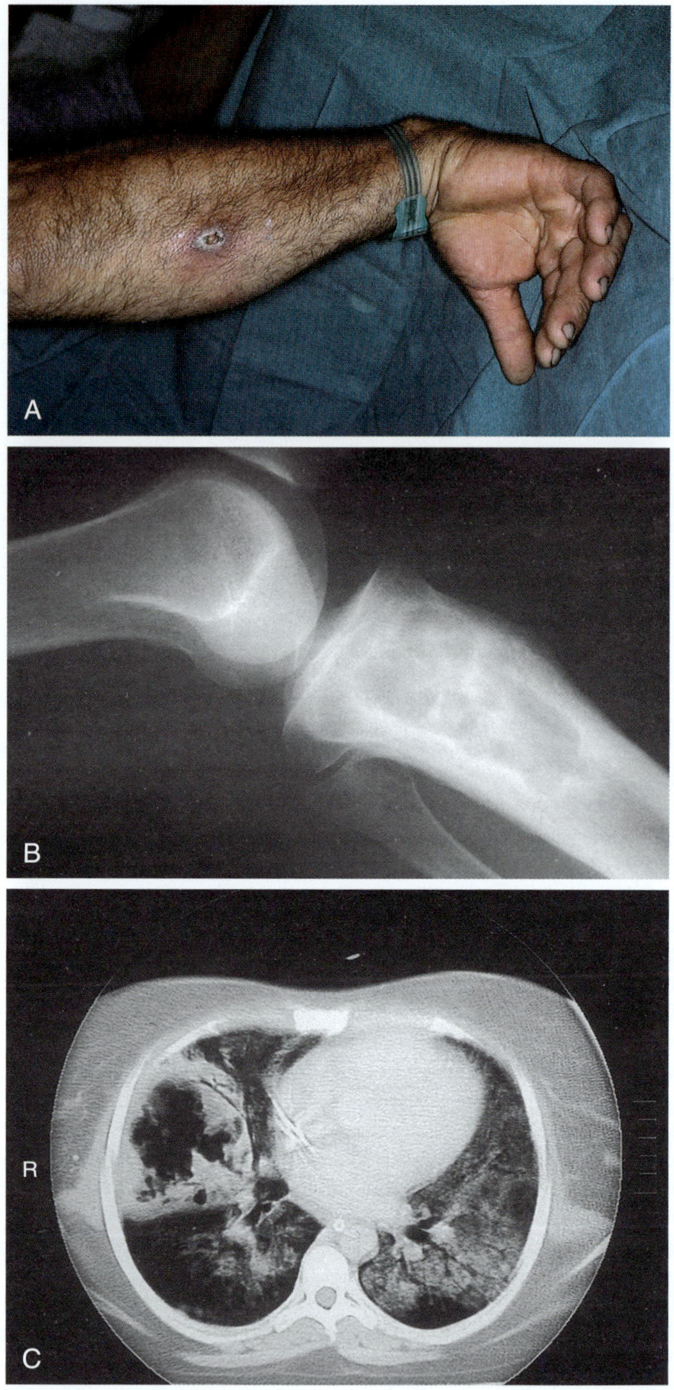

Fig. 77.4 (A) Cutaneous melioidosis on the right forearm of a 50-year-old man. (B) Radiograph of large radiolucency in the proximal tibia of a 43-year-old man with *Burkholderia pseudomallei* osteomyelitis. (C) CT scan of the thorax of a 26-year-old woman with fatal melioidosis, showing a large pulmonary abscess. (From Currie BJ. *Burkholderia pseudomallei* and *Burkholderia mallei*: melioidosis and glanders. In: Bennett JE, Dolin R, Blaser MJ, eds. *Mandell, Douglas and Bennett's Principles and Practice of Infectious Diseases*. Philadelphia, PA: Elsevier; 2020:2707-2717.)

DIAGNOSIS

The index of suspicion for melioidosis should be increased in animals that are domiciled in or have a travel history from areas of endemicity, especially Northern Australia and Thailand.

Microbiologic Tests

Cytologic Diagnosis

Thorough cytologic examination of Gram-stained smears of pus from lesions can sometimes reveal small numbers of bipolar-staining gram-negative rods (often described as having a "safety-pin" appearance); this should increase suspicion of the infection in endemic areas (Fig. 77.5). Immunofluorescent antibody staining is available in Thailand,[67] but access to this technique may be limited elsewhere.

Isolation and Identification

Although culture of the organism is considered the gold standard for diagnosis, results may take up to 7 days. This delay may contribute significantly to the high mortality rate in fulminant cases. Also, culture may have a low sensitivity.[68] Bacteremia occurs in between 38% and 73% of human cases, and blood culture systems typically result in successful isolation of the organism within 48 hours of incubation.[47] The isolate may also be erroneously identified as *Pseudomonas*, or dismissed as a contaminant in laboratories unfamiliar with the agent. Generally, *B. pseudomallei* is grown on routine bacteriologic media (blood, MacConkey), although selective media such as modified Ashdown's agar[69] incubated for 96 hours may be needed to isolate the organism from sites where contaminating microorganisms are present. *Burkholderia pseudomallei* may also be misidentified as less virulent *Burkholderia* species or as *Chromobacterium violaceum* with commercial bacterial identification kits.[70] The use of MALDI-TOF

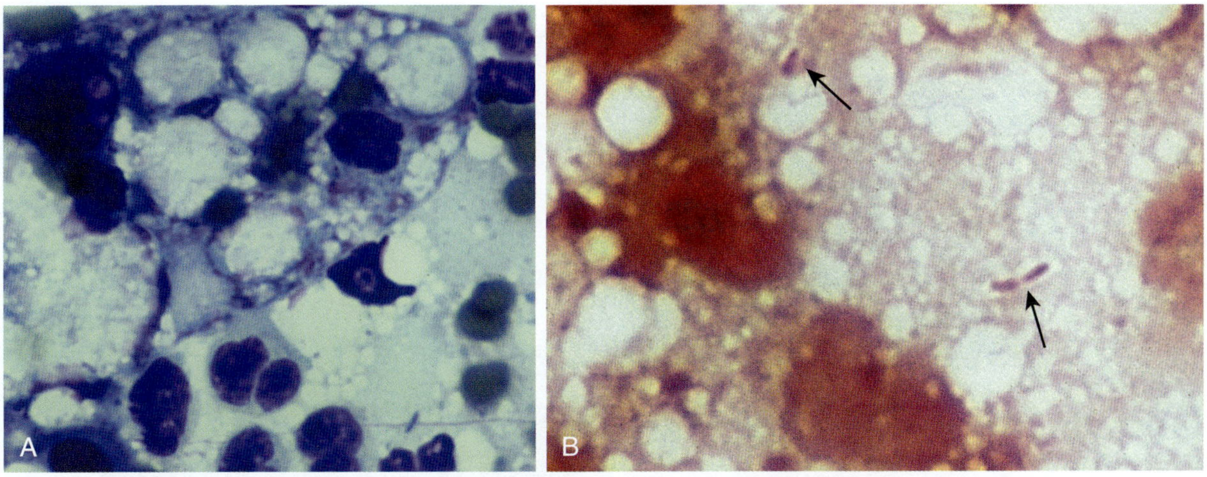

Fig. 77.5 Squash preparation of liver lesion from a cat with disseminated melioidosis obtained at necropsy. (A) Note the suppurative inflammation (Diff-Quik; original magnification ×330). (B) Extracellular gram-negative bacilli are present *(arrows)* (Burke's modification of the Gram stain; original magnification ×330). (From O'Brien CR et al. Disseminated melioidosis in two cats. *J Feline Med Surg.* 2003; 5:83-89; with permission from European Association of Feline Medicine.)

mass spectrometry by laboratories has allowed more rapid and accurate identification of *B. pseudomallei*.[47]

Serologic Diagnosis

Although indirect hemagglutination and enzyme-linked immunosorbent assays have been developed, they are of little clinical use, due to the high level of exposure in endemic areas. No serostudies have been published for dogs and cats to date.

Molecular Diagnosis Using Nucleic Acid–Based Testing

PCR and isothermal amplification assays can detect *B. pseudomallei* DNA in patient specimens; however, some of these assays have been found to have poor specificity and/or sensitivity.[71,72] Amplification and sequencing of the 16S rRNA gene is problematic as it does not reliably distinguish between *B. pseudomallei* and *Burkholderia thailandensis*.[73] The sequencing of the *groEL* gene may more reliably differentiate these two species.[74] A real-time PCR targeting the TTS1 gene cluster may also be used to identify the organism from culture systems[75]; however, the use of real-time assays on clinical samples has shown disappointing sensitivity.[76,77]

Antigen-Detection ELISA

A rapid, POC lateral-flow immunoassay has been developed to detect the presence of *B. pseudomallei* capsular antigen in sputum or pus.[76] It is not as sensitive as blood culture for detection of circulating organisms.

Pathologic Findings

Pathologic findings are microabscesses in affected organs and draining lymph nodes (Fig. 77.6). Immunohistochemical methods can detect the organism in affected tissues.[26]

TREATMENT AND PROGNOSIS

In people, treatment of melioidosis may be prolonged, is often unsuccessful, and relapses may occur. *Burkholderia pseudomallei* is resistant to many antimicrobial drugs, and successful treatment typically requires multidrug therapy for 12 to 20 weeks. There are few reports of successful treatment in animals and only one report of successful treatment of dogs and cats—the dog from Thailand that had been trapped in the barbed wire fence.[62] The dog introduced into New York was incontinent as a result of its spinal condition, and euthanasia was recommended because of public health concerns.[61] Surgical drainage of large abscesses may be required in conjunction with antimicrobial therapy. Antibacterial treatment is recommended for small or disseminated lesions.

The organism tends to be susceptible *in vitro* to trimethoprim-sulfonamides, amoxicillin-clavulanate, ticarcillin-clavulanate, some third-generation cephalosporins, tetracyclines, chloramphenicol, some fluoroquinolones, and carbapenems. It is generally resistant to penicillin G, aminopenicillins, first- and second-generation cephalosporins, most aminoglycosides (including gentamicin), most macrolides, quinolones, and rifampin.[79]

Current recommendations for treatment of acute melioidosis in human patients are an "intensive phase" of high doses of IV ceftazidime (+/− trimethoprim-sulfonamide) or meropenem (preferred if the patient has neurological involvement) for at least 10 to 14 days, and up to 4 to 6 weeks in patients with complicated pneumonia, deep organ abscesses, neurological, musculoskeletal, genitourinary, and/or extensive skin and soft-tissue involvement. This is followed by an "eradication" drug regimen of orally administered, high doses of trimethoprim-sulfonamide (plus folic acid supplementation) for 3 to 6 months.[47] Amoxicillin-clavulanate may be an alternative to trimethoprim-sulfonamide; however, acquired resistance is documented.[80] Following a response to treatment, affected animals should be closely monitored for signs of relapse. Melioidosis has a high rate of mortality in humans, with one study showing that 74% of patients with blood cultures that were positive after 24 hours of incubation died during their admission.[47] The dog from Thailand was treated with 2 weeks of meropenem (20 mg/kg IV q12h) followed by trimethoprim-sulfamethoxazole (25 mg/kg PO q12h) for 20 weeks.[62]

PUBLIC HEALTH ASPECTS

Generally, people in endemic areas become infected from the environment, as do animals. The organism has survived in a parenteral anesthetic solution and possibly an antiseptic cleaning agent containing cetrimide (3%) and chlorhexidine (0.3%). Zoonotic transmission is thought to be extremely rare, although anecdotal reports of animal-to-human transfer have been documented.[81] Identification of *B.*

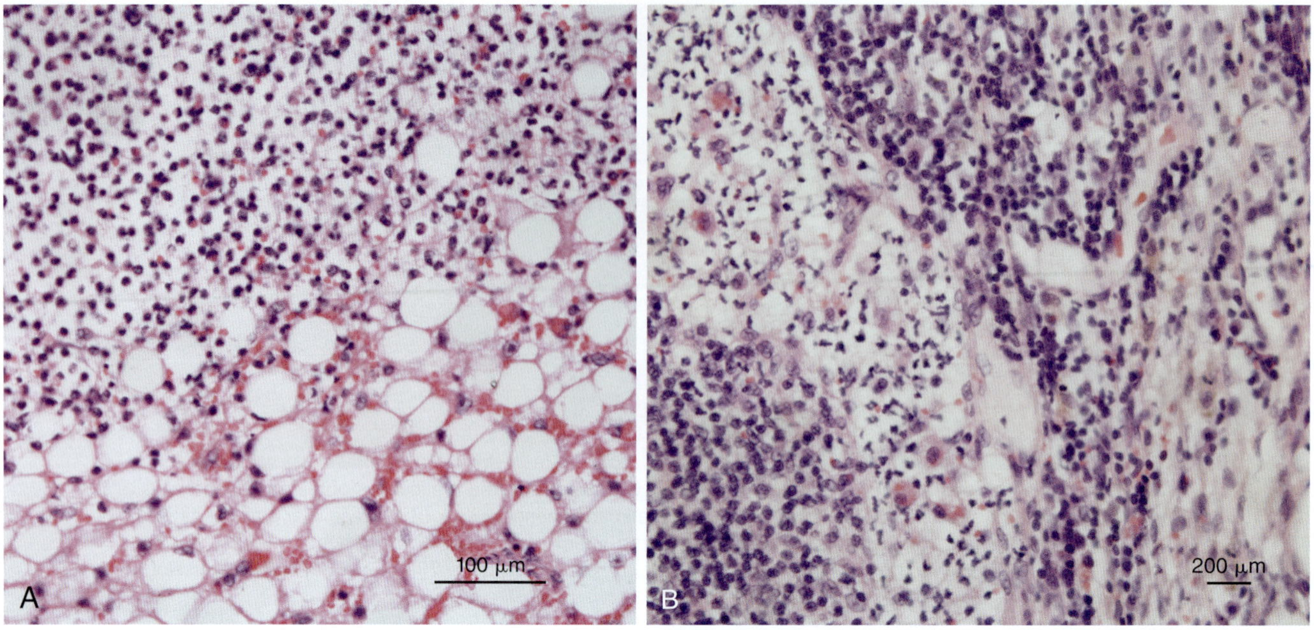

Fig. 77.6 (A) Histopathology of liver microabscesses from a 5-year-old domestic shorthair cat with melioidosis. Note the relatively well-circumscribed aggregation of the neutrophilic aggregation and the surrounding fatty degeneration of hepatocytes (hematoxylin and eosin stain, bar = 100 µm).(B) Histopathology of sternal lymph node from the same case. Note the neutrophilic exudate present in the cortical sinus. Involvement of the sternal lymph node was presumed secondary to the hepatitis observed in this case (hematoxylin and eosin stain, bar = 200 µm). (Courtesy of Mark Krockenberger, University of Sydney, Sydney, Australia.)

pseudomallei infection in companion animals in non-endemic regions should be reported to public health authorities. In the case of the dog introduced into the New York shelter, extensive contact tracing was performed, and it was recommended that highly exposed individuals be treated with prophylactic trimethoprim-sulfamethoxazole for 3 weeks.[61] Baseline and follow-up serologic testing indicated no significant evidence of human infection.

GLANDERS

ETIOLOGY AND EPIDEMIOLOGY

The causative agent of glanders, *Burkholderia mallei* (formerly *Pseudomonas mallei*), is a gram-negative, non-motile, non-spore-forming obligate intracellular bacterium. *Burkholderia mallei* has never been isolated from the environment,[82] instead being adapted to an equine host. It is estimated that approximately 3.5 million years ago, *B. mallei* evolved from the saprophytic organism *B. pseudomallei* through reductive evolution to become a specialist mammalian pathogen.[83,84]

Burkholderia mallei is susceptible to inactivation outside the host with heat (≥55°C/131°F for 10 min), ultraviolet light, and common disinfectants, although there have been reports of survival in tepid water for up to 1 month.

Glanders primarily affects solipeds (horses, donkeys, and mules) and these species are considered the natural reservoir of the organism, although it has been reported to occasionally occur in people and other animals, including dogs[85] and cats.[86] The disease is now very rare in the developed world; control programs eradicated it from Australasia in 1891, and the United States, Canada, and western Europe in 1965. It is now generally restricted to South America (Brazil), northern Africa, China, Iraq, Pakistan, India, Mongolia, Turkey, and United Arab Emirates.

Glanders is primarily transmitted from horse to horse via the inhalation of aerosols, ingestion of contaminated water or feed, or via contact with fomites, especially in situations where husbandry is substandard.[87] Transmission to non-equine species may occur via consumption of contaminated horsemeat, cutaneous inoculation, or inhalation. *Burkholderia mallei* has been used as a bioagent in numerous combat settings, being historically used to incapacitate warhorses in World War I and II, and more recently in the Afghan War.[88] The bacterium is classified as a Tier 1 Select Agent by the CDC,[48] and is also listed as a notifiable disease by the World Organization for Animal Health (OIE).

CLINICAL FEATURES

Pathogenesis and Clinical Signs

The organism may cause localized cutaneous disease (farcy) or acute bacteremia and pneumonia in both animals and people. After ingestion of infected horsemeat, cats were reported to develop nodules on the nasal mucosae and conjunctiva, as well as nasal discharge. The cats eventually developed dyspnea secondary to obstructive lymphadenopathy.[86] The affected dog, domiciled in Turkey and possibly fed infected horsemeat, was reported to have a non-healing cutaneous wound of the right gluteal region of approximately 18 months' duration.[85]

DIAGNOSIS

Diagnosis of glanders can be made via isolation and identification of the organism from lesions or exudates using routine laboratory techniques. MALDI-TOF mass spectrometry has been used to differentiate *B. mallei* from *B. pseudomallei*,[89] but incorrect identifications can still occur.[90] A variety of molecular assays (e.g., PCR and isothermal assays)[91,92] have also been developed for specific diagnosis of *B. mallei* infection that allow it to be differentiated from other *Burkholderia* species.

TREATMENT AND PROGNOSIS

Due to the risk of zoonotic transmission and the potential for ongoing subclinical infection and shedding despite antibiotic therapy, treatment of affected animals is often not advised. No documented treatment of cats or dogs exists.

Like *B. pseudomallei*, *B. mallei* is intrinsically resistant to many antibiotics. In consideration of treating infection in other hosts, *B. mallei* is susceptible *in vitro* to aminoglycosides, azithromycin, carbapenems, trimethoprim-sulfonamides, ceftazidime, doxycycline, amoxicillin-clavulanic acid, chloramphenicol, and piperacillin.[93,94] Treatment regimens recommended for people with glanders are virtually identical to those advocated for the management of melioidosis.[95]

PUBLIC HEALTH ASPECTS

Glanders can be transmitted directly to people from infected solipeds. Glanders is considered to be more zoonotic than melioidosis, and the risk of laboratory-acquired infections also appears to be higher with *B. mallei* infections.[55] For microbiology laboratory personnel, horse abattoir workers, veterinarians, and equine handlers in endemic regions, exposure to the organism may be a significant occupational hazard, and appropriate protective measures should be implemented if exposure is possible. In the laboratory, biosafety level 3 containment is recommended.

BURKHOLDERIA CEPACIA COMPLEX INFECTION

The *Burkholderia cepacia* complex (Bcc) is an emerging cause of opportunistic infections in dogs and cats. Organisms that belong to this complex are widely distributed in the environment and can be isolated from soil and aquatic environments, including drinking water. Infections by Bcc organisms are identified much more commonly than those with *B. pseudomallei* and *B. mallei*, and in human medicine they are known for their ability to cause disease in humans with cystic fibrosis.[56] The Bcc has been reported to cause deep pyoderma in dogs as well as sepsis in dogs on immunosuppressive drug treatment, especially cyclosporine, but oclacitinib in one dog.[96,97] In one study, four of six affected dogs were West Highland white terriers.[96] Physical examination findings have revealed multifocal irregular, erythematous to hemorrhagic alopecic papules, plaques, and nodules, with extensive crusting, draining tracts, and ulceration. These have been confined to the trunk and proximal limbs.

Skin biopsies from affected dogs have revealed neutrophilic to pyogranulomatous inflammation with intralesional gram-negative rod-shaped bacteria that stain with Warthin-Starry (silver) stain. Treatment with systemic fluoroquinolones, doxycycline, or trimethoprim-sulfamethoxazole, along with withdrawal of immunosuppressive drugs when possible, has been successful in almost all dogs, but one dog died as a result of *B. cepacia* sepsis.[96]

Between 1990 and 2020 at one of the authors' institutions (JS), *B. cepacia* was identified in one dog with cutaneous furunculosis that was being treated with cyclosporine for immune-mediated polyarthritis (IMPA), a male neutered miniature poodle (see Case Example). It was identified using culture as a secondary invader in six dogs with neoplasia that disrupted normal cutaneous and mucosal host defenses (cervical SCC, corneal SCC, osteosarcoma of the zygomatic arch and secondary otitis externa, nasal adenocarcinoma, and cutaneous T-cell lymphoma), and one dog with nasal aspergillosis. It was also isolated from the urine from one dog with atypical hypoadrenocorticism and a possible UTI; and a bronchoalveolar lavage specimen from a dog with bronchiectasis and secondary bacterial pneumonia. Treatment with enrofloxacin was generally used and resulted in elimination of the infection, but dogs continued to show clinical signs as a result of their underlying condition.

CHROMOBACTERIOSIS

ETIOLOGIC AGENT AND EPIDEMIOLOGY

Chromobacterium violaceum is a long, gram-negative, motile, facultatively anaerobic, non-spore-forming bacillus that belongs to the order Neisseriales. It exists as a saprophyte of soil and water in the tropics and subtropics, generally between latitudes 35 degrees north and south of the equator, although the geographical range may be expanding because of climate change.[98] In culture it is variably hemolytic, and produces the violet pigment, violacein, from the condensation of two tryptophan molecules.

Chromobacterium violaceum is a rare cause of disease in people and animals and infection is mostly acquired via inoculation of cutaneous wounds, although ingestion of contaminated water may be a possible source.[99,100] Fewer than 200 cases have been reported worldwide, with most cases coming from Southeast Asia; over 35 cases have been reported from the United States, mainly from Florida.[101] Most humans that develop disease are children or immunosuppressed adults, but some are apparently immunocompetent. Approximately 8% of the reported human cases have concurrent chronic granulomatous disease (CGD), a primary immune disorder in which neutrophils have an impaired respiratory burst due to defects in NADPH oxidase.[102] Glucose-6-phosphate deficiency also appears to predispose to the infection. A predisposition in young males was observed in one study,[98] possibly related to the mainly X-linked inheritance pattern of CGD.[102]

CLINICAL FEATURES

Pathogenesis and Clinical Signs

Cases often begin with localized skin or lymph node involvement and then may progress to widespread multi-systemic disease and fulminant bacteremia. Disease typically appears 1 day to 2 months after exposure. Infected people and animals are afflicted with abdominal organ and CNS abscessation, pneumonia, osteomyelitis, and necrotizing fasciitis.[98,103,104] A 60% mortality has been reported in affected humans in the United States.[101]

Four dogs have been reported with chromobacteriosis, including a dog from New South Wales, Australia with possible parvovirus infection[105]; two dogs from Florida,[106] and one from Poland.[107] One of the dogs from Florida (a 9-year-old beagle) was seen with signs of right-sided heart failure and evidence of pericarditis; culture of abdominal effusion yielded a heavy growth of *C. violaceum*. The dog's condition deteriorated, and after a subtotal pericardiectomy the dog developed cardiac arrest. Necropsy confirmed constrictive, effusive pericarditis but *C. violaceum* could no longer be isolated; the dog had been treated aggressively with parenteral antimicrobials during hospitalization (initially enrofloxacin and ampicillin followed by imipenem-cilastatin). The second dog from Florida was a 9-month-old Labrador retriever that developed necrotizing fasciitis at a surgical site after routine castration; the dog swam in a lake at a local park the night before the operation. The disease in this case was associated with a degenerative left shift, thrombocytopenia, hypoalbuminemia, mild hyperbilirubinemia and severe edema, and extensive necrosis and sloughing of the inguinal skin. *Chromobacterium violaceum* was isolated from the blood. Both of the dogs from Florida were afebrile at the time of initial evaluation. The dog from Poland also had a history of swimming in a lake, and was diagnosed with chronic bilateral otitis externa, from which *C. violaceum* was cultured.

DIAGNOSIS

Chromobacterium violaceum is readily cultured on MacConkey agar at 37°C, and is relatively easy to identify due to the characteristic violet-pigmented colonies (Fig. 77.7).[101,104] Not all isolates are pigmented, however, which may cause some confusion.[99] Because of the typically fulminant clinical progression, antemortem diagnosis hinges on a high index of suspicion and timely culture of blood, tissue, or exudates. Molecular identification via both single-target and multiplex PCR[108] have been reported.

TREATMENT AND PROGNOSIS

Most isolates are susceptible to fluoroquinolones, aminoglycosides, trimethoprim-sulfonamides, carbapenems, and tetracyclines.[98,109] The organism appears to be resistant to a relatively wide range of antibiotics including β-lactams, second-generation cephalosporins, rifampin, and vancomycin.[98] Because the infection is so rare, there are no firm guidelines to inform therapy. Therefore treatment should primarily be based on the results of antibacterial susceptibility data, although empiric therapy based on clinical suspicion, for example treatment with a fluoroquinolone, pending these results would be appropriate.[98,106]

The prognosis for the disease in people is historically poor, with approximately 60% mortality rates reported[98]; however, more recent studies describe a much more favorable outcome (7.1% mortality).[103] The authors of the latter study speculated that improved patient outcomes were possibly due to the early use of meropenem in cases managed at their institution.

Of the dogs with systemic infections, two succumbed to bacteremia.[105,106] The dog from Florida with necrotizing fasciitis and bacteremia was treated with aggressive supportive care, parenteral then oral enrofloxacin and amoxicillin-clavulanic acid, and multiple surgeries for debridement and drainage of the affected skin; on day 112 after initial admission, the wound had healed. The dog with otitis externa was treated successfully with a 2-week course of systemic enrofloxacin and a topical aural preparation containing marbofloxacin, clotrimazole, and dexamethasone acetate, applied deep into both ear canals once daily.[107]

Relapses have been reported in the human literature,[98] thus it would seem prudent to treat systemically affected animals with an oral drug regimen for an extended period (e.g., at least 1–2 months past resolution of illness), with close monitoring for any evidence of recrudescence.

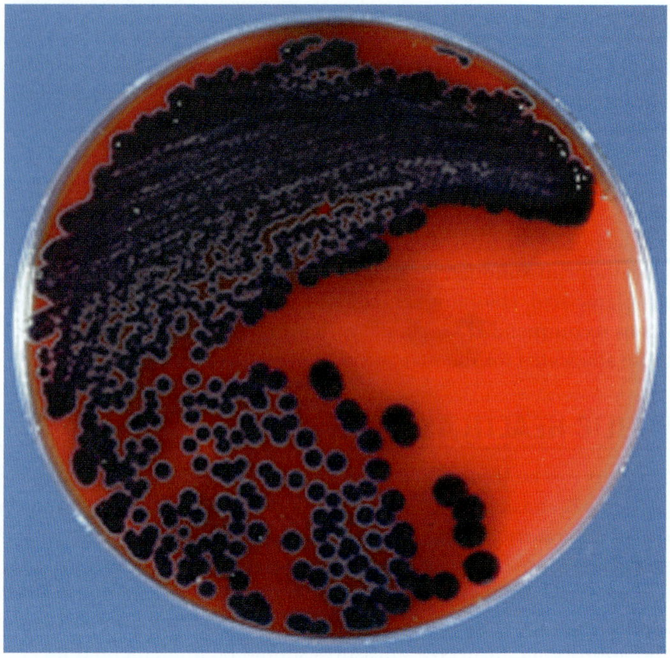

Fig. 77.7 Violet-black colonies of *Chromobacterium violaceum* from production of the pigment violacein. (From Steinberg JP, Lutgring JD, Burd EM. Other gram-negative and gram-variable bacilli. In: Bennett JE, Dolin R, Blaser MJ, eds. *Mandelll and Bennett's Principles and Practice of Infectious Diseases.* Philadelphia, PA: Elsevier; 2020:2847-2864.)

OTHER UNUSUAL BACTERIAL INFECTIONS

Streptomyces spp. and *Streptobacillus* spp. are filamentous bacteria that belong to the Actinomycetales and Leptotrichiaceae, respectively. *Streptomyces* spp. are gram-positive soil saprophytes that have rarely been reported as a cause of pyogranulomatous dermatitis and cellulitis in cats, with poor response to aggressive medical and surgical treatment.[110,111] *Streptobacillus moniliformis* is a gram-negative bacillus that is the cause of rat bite fever in humans, a rare but potentially lethal zoonosis that occurs worldwide, typically following the bite of a rat.[112] There is a single case report from 1961 of systemic disease associated with an organism resembling *S. moniliformis* in a dog from Canada.[113] The organism has also been detected in the oral cavity of healthy dogs, raising concern that humans may develop rat bite fever after a bite wound from a dog.[114] A *Streptobacillus* species was isolated from the lungs of a cat with pneumonia and characterized as *Streptobacillus felis* sp. nov. using molecular methods and mass spectrometry.[115]

CASE EXAMPLE

Signalment

"Jojo," an 8-year-old male neutered miniature poodle from Walnut Creek, California, USA.

History

Jojo was seen at a follow-up visit for IMPA, which had been diagnosed 16 months previously and treated with a tapering course of prednisone and cyclosporine. The owners reported that Jojo still occasionally exhibited lameness of the right thoracic limb, but otherwise was doing well at home and appeared to be bright and appetent. Two weeks before the examination, the owners noted that Jojo was developing some skin nodules on the dorsal aspect of his lumbar region. He was also showing some signs of pruritis in association with the lesions. They began treating him with topical mupirocin and cefpodoxime, which were left over from a previous episode of inguinal pyoderma. No improvement in the skin condition was noted.

Current Medications

Prednisone (0.25 mg/kg PO q48h), cyclosporine (5 mg/kg PO in the morning and 2.5 mg/kg in the evening), cefpodoxime 5 mg/kg PO q24h, cyclosporine ointment OU q24h, neomycin/polymyxin B/dexamethasone eye drops for keratoconjunctivitis sicca (KCS), monthly flea prevention (imidacloprid/pyriproxyfen topical), and heartworm prevention (monthly ivermectin).

CASE EXAMPLE—cont'd

Jojo had been diagnosed with KCS several years ago, which was adequately controlled with the topical ocular medications. Before he was diagnosed with IMPA, he had a history of recurrent superficial pyoderma and *Malassezia* infections that were secondary to allergic dermatitis. This had been managed with frequent bathing with topical shampoos, flea preventatives, mupirocin ointment, cefpodoxime, and fluconazole. He was fed a commercial chicken and rice dry diet.

Physical Examination

Body weight: 10 kg.

General: Bright, alert, responsive, and hydrated. T = 101.7°F, P = 96, mucous membranes pink, CRT < 1.5 s, panting, and very active in the examination room.

Integument: Short, clean haircoat with no evidence of ectoparasites. There were 10 to 15 prominent papules with crusting, scattered across the dorsum, with most lesions being present in the caudal dorsal region. The dermis beneath the papules appeared thickened in some areas.

Eyes, ears, nose, and throat: Mild bilateral nuclear sclerosis, mild bilateral mucoid ocular discharge, moderate generalized periodontal disease. No other clinically significant findings.

Musculoskeletal: Body condition score 5/9, with symmetrical musculature and no evidence of joint effusion, pain on palpation, or lameness.

Cardiovascular, respiratory, GI, and genitourinary: No clinically significant findings.

Lymph nodes: No lymphadenopathy evident.

Biopsy Findings

Multiple 0.5-cm punch biopsies were collected and submitted for histopathology and culture. Histopathology revealed severe, chronic, diffuse plasmacytic and neutrophilic dermatitis and folliculitis with furunculosis. Occasional gram-negative rods were observed within neutrophils and macrophages. A diffuse inflammatory infiltrate, composed of dense aggregates of primarily plasma cells and neutrophils, with fewer numbers of lymphocytes, macrophages, and mast cells, spanned the superficial to deep dermis of all sections. A nodular inflammatory infiltrate was present in the deep dermis to the subcutis of two sections. Multifocally scattered lymphocytes and neutrophils infiltrated the follicular epithelium, and there was focal rupture of the mid-portion of a hair follicle and the ruptured segment was surrounded by neutrophils (furunculosis). Rare neutrophils and macrophages contained intracellular clusters of intracytoplasmic bacterial rods measuring approximately 2 μm in length. The superficial dermis was edematous. Aggregates of neutrophils multifocally infiltrated the epidermis and there was multifocal epidermal ulceration. Gram staining highlighted the presence of clusters of intracellular gram-negative bacterial rods within occasional neutrophils and macrophages.

Aerobic and anaerobic bacterial culture: Culture of a macerated skin biopsy specimen yielded small numbers of *Burkholderia cepacia.* The isolate was susceptible to amikacin, amoxicillin-clavulanic acid, doxycycline, enrofloxacin, gentamicin, imipenem, and trimethoprim-sulfamethoxazole; and resistant to cefazolin, cefovecin, cefoxitin, cefpodoxime, erythromycin, and chloramphenicol.

Diagnosis

Burkholderia cepacia deep pyoderma.

Treatment and Outcome

Enrofloxacin, 10 mg/kg PO q12h for 4 weeks was prescribed. The owners were told to cease bathing/grooming during treatment. At a recheck examination 2 months later, no change in the skin lesions was identified. Another course of enrofloxacin was prescribed, and 2 weeks later the owners reported mild improvement in the skin lesions. Arthrocentesis was performed and cytologic examination of synovial fluid from the right carpus and tarsus showed no abnormalities. The cyclosporine dose was reduced to 2.5 mg/kg PO q12h. One month later, the skin lesions had reduced in size and Jojo was less pruritic. There had been no signs of lameness. Enrofloxacin treatment was continued for another month until the lesions had resolved. At a recheck examination 2 months later (5 months after diagnosis), there was no evidence of the skin lesions.

Comments

This dog had similar lesions to those reported in case series of dogs with *B. cepacia* furunculosis reported in the literature, which were also receiving cyclosporine treatment.[96,97] Ultimately, prolonged antimicrobial treatment was required, together with a reduction in the dose of cyclosporine. The organism was resistant to all cephalosporins tested, which explained the initial failure of the condition to respond to cefpodoxime. Fortunately, Jojo's polyarthritis remained in remission after the cyclosporine dose was reduced.

SUGGESTED READINGS

Burd EM, Juzych LA, Rudrik JT, et al. Pustular dermatitis caused by *Dermatophilus congolensis*. *J Clin Microbiol*. 2007;45:1655–1658.

Barger AM, Weedon GR, Maddox CW, et al. *Dermatophilus congolensis* in a feral cat. *J Feline Med Surg*. 2014;16:840–841.

Gassiep I, Armstrong M, Norton R. Human melioidosis. *Clin Microbiol Rev*. 2020;33:e00006–19.

O'Brien C, Krockenberger M, Martin P, et al. Disseminated melioidosis in two cats. *J Feline Med Surg*. 2003;5:83–89.

Ryan CW, Bishop K, Blaney DD, et al. Public health response to an imported case of canine melioidosis. *Zoonoses Public Health*. 2018;65:420–424.

Khan I, Wieler L, Melzer F, et al. Glanders in animals: a review on epidemiology, clinical presentation, diagnosis and countermeasures. *Transbound Emerg Dis*. 2013;60:204–221.

Crosse PA, Soares K, Wheeler JL, et al. *Chromobacterium violaceum* infection in two dogs. *J Am Anim Hosp Assoc*. 2006;42:154–159.

REFERENCES

1. Van Saceghem R. Dermatose contagieuse (impetigo contagieux). *Bull Soc Pathol Exot*. 1915;8:354–359.
2. Whitmore A, Krishnaswami C. An account of the discovery of a hitherto undescribed infective disease occurring among the population of Rangoon. *Indian Med Gaz*. 1912;47:262–267.
3. Van Arsdale II W. On the present state of knowledge in bacterial science in its surgical relations (concluded): actinomycosis—anthrax—glanders. *Ann Surg*. 1886;4:217.
4. Schroeter J. Ueber einige durch Bacterien gebildete Pigmente. *Beitr Biol Pflanz*. 1872;1:109–126.
5. Chastain C, Carithers R, Hogle R, et al. Dermatophilosis in two dogs. *J Am Vet Med Assoc*. 1976;169:1079–1080.
6. Hassan I. A case report of *Dermatophilus congolensis* in a dog at the Freetown Veterinary Clinic. *Beitr Trop Landwirtsch Veterinarmed*. 1982;20:409–411.
7. Blancou J. *Dermatophilus congolensis* infection in the dog (Van Saceghem, 1915). *Rev Elev Med Vet Pays Trop*. 1972;26:289–291.
8. Kaya O, Kirkan Ş, Ünal B. Isolation of *Dermatophilus congolensis* from a cat. *J Vet Med B Infect Dis Vet Public Health*. 2000;47:155–157.
9. Barger AM, Weedon GR, Maddox CW, et al. *Dermatophilus congolensis* in a feral cat. *J Feline Med Surg*. 2014;16:840–841.
10. Jones R. Subcutaneous infection with *Dermatophilus congolensis* in a cat. *J Comp Pathol*. 1976;86:415–421.
11. Carakostas M, Miller R, Woodward M. Subcutaneous dermatophilosis in a cat. *J Am Vet Med Assoc*. 1984;185:675.
12. Miller R, Ladds P, Mudie A, et al. Probable dermatophilosis in 2 cats. *Aust Vet J*. 1983;60:155–156.
13. O'hara P, Cordes D. Granulomata caused by *Dermatophilus* in two cats. *N Z Vet J*. 1963;11:151–154.
14. Baker G, Breeze R, Dawson CO. Oral dermatophilosis in a cat: a case report. *J Small Anim Pract*. 1972;13:649–653.

15. Towersey L, Martins ECS, Londero AT, et al. *Dermatophilus congolensis* human infection. *J Am Acad Dermatol.* 1993;29:351–354.
16. Zaria L. *Dermatophilus congolensis* infection (dermatophilosis) in animals and man! An update. *Comp Immunol Microbiol Infect Dis.* 1993;16:179–222.
17. Kagia K, Liu W-T. The family Dermatophilaceae. In: *The Prokaryotes.* Springer; 2014:317–325.
18. Burd EM, Juzych LA, Rudrik JT, et al. Pustular dermatitis caused by *Dermatophilus congolensis. J Clin Microbiol.* 2007;45:1655–1658.
19. Moriello K. Overview of dermatophilosis. In: *The Merck Veterinary Manual.* 2013.
20. Richard J, Pier A, Cysewski S. Experimentally induced canine dermatophilosis. *Am J Vet Res.* 1973;34:797–799.
21. Alejo-Cancho I, Bosch J, Vergara A, et al. Dermatitis by *Dermatophilus congolensis. Clin Microbiol Infect.* 2015;21:e73–74.
22. Aufox EE, Frank LA, May ER, et al. The prevalence of *Dermatophilus congolensis* in horses with pastern dermatitis using PCR to diagnose infection in a population of horses in southern USA. *Vet Dermatol.* 2018;29:435, e144.
23. Shaibu S, Kazeem H, Abdullahi U, et al. The use of polymerase chain reaction in the diagnosis of dermatophilosis from cattle, sheep and goats in Nigeria. *Asian J Anim Vet Adv.* 2010;9:1034–1036.
24. García A, Martínez R, Benitez-Medina JM, et al. Development of a real-time SYBR Green PCR assay for the rapid detection of *Dermatophilus congolensis. J Vet Sci.* 2013;14:491–494.
25. Frank LA, Kania SA, Weyant E. RT–qPCR for the diagnosis of dermatophilosis in horses. *Vet Dermatol.* 2016;27:431.
26. Tresamol P, Saseendranath M. Antibiogram of *Dermatophilus congolensis* isolates from cattle. *Int J Livest Res.* 2013;3:117–121.
27. Hermoso dMJ, Arenas A, Rey J, et al. In vitro studies of *Dermatophilus congolensis* antimicrobial susceptibility by determining minimal inhibitory and bacteriocidal concentrations. *Br Vet J.* 1993;150:189–196.
28. Aubin GG, Guillouzouic A, Chamoux C, et al. Two family members with skin infection due to *Dermatophilus congolensis*: a case report and literature review. *Eur J Dermatol.* 2016;26:621–622.
29. Albrecht R, Horowitz S, Gilbert E, et al. *Dermatophilus congolensis* chronic nodular disease in man. *Pediatrics.* 1974;53:907–912.
30. Dean DL, Gordon MA, Severinghaus CW, et al. Streptothricosis: a new zoonotic disease. *N Engl J Med.* 1961;61:1283–1287.
31. Aubin GG, Guillouzouic A, Chamoux C, et al. Two family members with skin infection due to *Dermatophilus congolensis*: a case report and literature review. *Eur J Dermatol.* 2016;26:621–622.
32. Bunker ML, Chewning L, Wang SE, et al. *Dermatophilus congolensis* and "hairy" leukoplakia. *Am J Clin Pathol.* 1988;89:683–687.
33. Ramanathan VS, Jahng AW, Shlopov B, et al. *Dermatophilus congolensis* infection of the esophagus. *Gastroenterology Res.* 2010;3:173–174.
34. Cheng AC, Currie BJ. Melioidosis: epidemiology, pathophysiology, and management. *Clin Microbiol Rev.* 2005;18:383–416.
35. Limmathurotsakul D, Golding N, Dance D, et al. Predicted global distribution of *Burkholderia pseudomallei* and burden of melioidosis. *Nat Microbiol.* 2016;1:15008.
36. Limmathurotsakul D, Wongratanacheewin S, Teerawattanasook N, et al. Increasing incidence of human melioidosis in Northeast Thailand. *Am J Trop Med Hyg.* 2010;82:1113–1117.
37. Currie BJ, Ward L, Cheng AC. The epidemiology and clinical spectrum of melioidosis: 540 cases from the 20 year Darwin prospective study. *PLoS Negl Trop Dis.* 2010;4:e900.
38. Currie BJ, Jacups SP. Intensity of rainfall and severity of melioidosis, Australia. *Emerg Infect Dis.* 2003;9:1538–1542.
39. Doker TJ, Sharp TM, Rivera-Garcia B, et al. Contact investigation of melioidosis cases reveals regional endemicity in Puerto Rico. *Clin Infect Dis.* 2015;60:243–250.
40. Inglis TJ, Rolim DB, Sousa ADQ. Melioidosis in the Americas. *Am J Trop Med Hyg.* 2006;75:947–954.
41. Katangwe T, Purcell J, Bar-Zeev N, et al. Human melioidosis, Malawi, 2011. *Emerg Infect Dis.* 2013;19:981–984.
42. Garin B, Djaomazala I, Dubois-Cauwelaert N. Autochthonous melioidosis in humans, Madagascar, 2012 and 2013. *Emerg Infect Dis.* 2014;20:1739.
43. Prakash A, Thavaselvam D, Kumar A, et al. Isolation, identification and characterization of *Burkholderia pseudomallei* from soil of coastal region of India. *Springerplus.* 2014;3:438.
44. Currie BJ. Melioidosis: evolving concepts in epidemiology, pathogenesis, and treatment. *Semin Respir Crit Care Med.* 2015;36:111–125.
45. Cossaboom CM, Marinova-Petkova A, Strysko J, et al. Melioidosis in a resident of Texas with no recent travel history, United States. *Emerg Infect Dis.* 2020;26:1295–1299.
46. Chewapreecha C, Holden MT, Vehkala M, et al. Global and regional dissemination and evolution of *Burkholderia pseudomallei. Nat Microbiol.* 2017;2:16263.
47. Gassiep I, Armstrong M, Norton R. Human melioidosis. *Clin Microbiol Rev.* 2020;33:e00006–19.
48. Centers for Disease Control and Prevention. Federal Select Agent Program. 2021. Available at: https://www.selectagents.gov/selectagentsandtoxinslist.html.
49. Wiersinga WJ, Currie BJ, Peacock SJ. Melioidosis. *N Engl J Med.* 2012;367:1035–1044.
50. Limmathurotsakul D, Kanoksil M, Wuthiekanun V, et al. Activities of daily living associated with acquisition of melioidosis in northeast Thailand: a matched case-control study. *PLoS Negl Trop Dis.* 2013;7:e2072.
51. Chierakul W, Wuthiekanun V, Chaowagul W, et al. Disease severity and outcome of melioidosis in HIV coinfected individuals. *Am J Trop Med Hyg.* 2005;73:1165–1166.
52. Sarovich DS, Ward L, Price EP, et al. Recurrent melioidosis in the Darwin Prospective Melioidosis Study: improving therapies mean that relapse cases are now rare. *J Clin Microbiol.* 2014;52:650–653.
53. Maharjan B, Chantratita N, Vesaratchavest M, et al. Recurrent melioidosis in patients in northeast Thailand is frequently due to reinfection rather than relapse. *J Clin Microbiol.* 2005;43:6032–6034.
54. Ngauy V, Lemeshev Y, Sadkowski L, et al. Cutaneous melioidosis in a man who was taken as a prisoner of war by the Japanese during World War II. *J Clin Microbiol.* 2005;43:970–972.
55. Currie BJ. *Burkholderia pseudomallei* and *Burkholderia mallei*: melioidosis and glanders. In: Bennett JE, Dolin R, Blaser MJ, eds. *Mandell, Douglas and Bennett's Principles and Practice of Infectious Diseases.* Philadelphia, PA: Elsevier Saunders; 2020:2706–2717.
56. Greenberg D. *Stenotrophomonas maltophila* and *Burkholderia cepacia* complex. In: Bennett JE, Dolin R, Blaser MJ, eds. *Mandell, Douglas and Bennett's Principles and Practice of Infectious Diseases.* Philadelphia, PA: Elsevier Saunders; 2020:2700–2705.
57. Allwood EM, Devenish RJ, Prescott M, et al. Strategies for intracellular survival of *Burkholderia pseudomallei. Front Microbiol.* 2011:37.
58. Stockton JL, Torres AG. Multinucleated giant cell formation as a portal to chronic bacterial infections. *Microorganisms.* 2020;8:1637.
59. Boddey JA, Day CJ, Flegg CP, et al. The bacterial gene lfpA influences the potent induction of calcitonin receptor and osteoclast-related genes in *Burkholderia pseudomallei*-induced TRAP-positive multinucleated giant cells. *Cell Microbiol.* 2007;9:514–531.
60. Khakhum N, Chapartegui-Gonzalez I, Torres AG. Combating the great mimicker: latest progress in the development of *Burkholderia pseudomallei* vaccines. *Expert Rev Vaccines.* 2020;19:653–660.
61. Ryan CW, Bishop K, Blaney DD, et al. Public health response to an imported case of canine melioidosis. *Zoonoses Public Health.* 2018;65:420–424.
62. Khrongsee P, Lueangthuwapranit C, Ingkasri T, et al. Successful treatments and management of a case of canine melioidosis. *Vet Sci.* 2019;6:76.
63. O'Brien C, Krockenberger M, Martin P, et al. Disseminated melioidosis in two cats. *J Felin Med Surg.* 2003;5:83–89.
64. Parkes HM, Shilton CM, Jerrett IV, et al. Primary ocular melioidosis due to a single genotype of *Burkholderia pseudomallei* in two cats from Arnhem Land in the Northern Territory of Australia. *J Felin Med Surg.* 2009;11:856–863.
65. Chooi K. Melioidosis and nymphal pentastomiasis in a cat. *Vet Rec.* 1986;119:311. 311.
66. Toh I, Heng HG, Zamri-Saad M, et al. Melioidosis in a kitten. *Malays J Vet Res.* 1998;10:73–76.
67. Wuthiekanun V, Desakorn V, Wongsuvan G, et al. Rapid immunofluorescence microscopy for diagnosis of melioidosis. *Clin Diagn Lab Immunol.* 2005;12:555–556.

68. Limmathurotsakul D, Jamsen K, Arayawichanont A, et al. Defining the true sensitivity of culture for the diagnosis of melioidosis using Bayesian latent class models. *PLoS One*. 2010;5:e12485.
69. Ashdown LR. An improved screening technique for isolation of *Pseudomonas pseudomallei* from clinical specimens. *Pathology*. 1979;11:293–297.
70. Inglis TJJ, Merritt A, Chidlow G, et al. Comparison of diagnostic laboratory methods for identification of *Burkholderia pseudomallei*. *J Clin Microbiol*. 2005;43:2201–2206.
71. Chantratita N, Meumann E, Thanwisai A, et al. Loop-mediated isothermal amplification method targeting the TTS1 gene cluster for detection of *Burkholderia pseudomallei* and diagnosis of melioidosis. *J Clin Microbiol*. 2008;46:568–573.
72. Chantratita N, Wuthiekanun V, Limmathurotsakul D, et al. Prospective clinical evaluation of the accuracy of 16S rRNA real-time PCR assay for the diagnosis of melioidosis. *Am J Trop Med Hyg*. 2007;77:814–817.
73. Lau SK, Sridhar S, Ho C-C, et al. Laboratory diagnosis of melioidosis: past, present and future. *Exp Biol Med*. 2015;240:742–751.
74. Woo PC, Woo GK, Lau SK, et al. Single gene target bacterial identification: groEL gene sequencing for discriminating clinical isolates of *Burkholderia pseudomallei* and *Burkholderia thailandensis*. *Diagn Microbiol Infect Dis*. 2002;44:143–149.
75. Novak RT, Glass MB, Gee JE, et al. Development and evaluation of a real-time PCR assay targeting the type III secretion system of *Burkholderia pseudomallei*. *J Clin Microbiol*. 2006;44:85–90.
76. Meumann EM, Novak RT, Gal D, et al. Clinical evaluation of a type III secretion system real-time PCR assay for diagnosing melioidosis. *J Clin Microbiol*. 2006;44:3028–3030.
77. Kaestli M, Richardson LJ, Colman RE, et al. Comparison of TaqMan PCR assays for detection of the melioidosis agent *Burkholderia pseudomallei* in clinical specimens. *J Clin Microbiol*. 2012;50:2059–2062.
78. Houghton RL, Reed DE, Hubbard MA, et al. Development of a prototype lateral flow immunoassay (LFI) for the rapid diagnosis of melioidosis. *PLoS Negl Trop Dis*. 2014;8:e2727.
79. Dance D, Wuthiekanun V, Chaowagul W, et al. The antimicrobial susceptibility of *Pseudomonas pseudomallei*. Emergence of resistance in vitro and during treatment. *J Antimicrob Chemother*. 1989;24:295–309.
80. Dance DA, Wuthiekanun V, Chaowagul W, et al. Development of resistance to ceftazidime and co-amoxiclav in *Pseudomonas pseudomallei*. *J Antimicrob Chemother*. 1991;28:321–324.
81. Choy JL, Mayo M, Janmaat A, et al. Animal melioidosis in Australia. *Acta Trop*. 2000;74:153–158.
82. Inglis TJJ, Sagripanti J-L. Environmental factors that affect the survival and persistence of *Burkholderia pseudomallei*. *Appl Environ Microbiol*. 2006;72:6865–6875.
83. Godoy D, Randle G, Simpson AJ, et al. Multilocus sequence typing and evolutionary relationships among the causative agents of melioidosis and glanders, *Burkholderia pseudomallei* and *Burkholderia mallei*. *J Clin Microbiol*. 2003;41:2068–2079.
84. Lin CH, Bourque G, Tan P. A comparative synteny map of *Burkholderia* species links large-scale genome rearrangements to fine-scale nucleotide variation in prokaryotes. *Mol Biol Evol*. 2008;25:549–558.
85. Keskin O, Ilhan Z. Isolation *of Pseudomonas mallei* from a dog. *Vet Fakultesi Dergisi Ankara Univ*. 2000;47:13–16.
86. Biberstein EL, Holzworth J. Bacterial diseases. In: *Diseases of the Cat: Medicine and Surgery Volume 1*. Philadelphia, PA: W.B. Saunders Company; 1987:279–319.
87. Dvorak GD, Spickler AR. Glanders. *J Am Vet Med Assoc*. 2008;233:570–577.
88. Khan I, Wieler L, Melzer F, et al. Glanders in animals: a review on epidemiology, clinical presentation, diagnosis and countermeasures. *Transbound Emerg Dis*. 2013;60:204–221.
89. Saxena A, Pal V, Tripathi NK, et al. A real-time loop mediated isothermal amplification assay for molecular detection of *Burkholderia mallei*, the aetiological agent of a zoonotic and re-emerging disease glanders. *Acta Trop*. 2019;194:189–194.
90. Rudrik JT, Soehnlen MK, Perry MJ, et al. Safety and accuracy of matrix-assisted laser desorption ionization-time of flight mass spectrometry for identification of highly pathogenic organisms. *J Clin Microbiol*. 2017;55:3513–3529.
91. Zakharova I, Teteryatnikova N, Toporkov A, et al. Development of a multiplex PCR assay for the detection and differentiation of *Burkholderia pseudomallei, Burkholderia mallei, Burkholderia thailandensis*, and *Burkholderia cepacia* complex. *Acta Trop*. 2017;174:1–8.
92. Pal V, Singh S, Tiwari AK, et al. Development of a polymerase chain reaction assay for detection of *Burkholderia mallei*, a potent biological warfare agent. *Defence Sci J*. 2016;66:458.
93. Kenny DJ, Russell P, Rogers D, et al. In vitro susceptibilities of *Burkholderia mallei* in comparison to those of other pathogenic *Burkholderia* spp. *Antimicrob Agents Chemother*. 1999;43:2773–2775.
94. Heine HS, England MJ, Waag DM, et al. In vitro antibiotic susceptibilities of *Burkholderia mallei* (causative agent of glanders) determined by broth microdilution and E-Test. *Antimicrob Agents Chemother*. 2001;45:2119–2121.
95. Van Zandt KE, Greer MT, Gelhaus HC. Glanders: an overview of infection in humans. *Orphanet J Rare Dis*. 2013;8:131.
96. Banovic F, Koch S, Robson D, et al. Deep pyoderma caused by *Burkholderia cepacia* complex associated with ciclosporin administration in dogs: a case series. *Vet Dermatol*. 2015;26:287, e264.
97. Cain CL, Cole SD, Bradley Ii CW, et al. Clinical and histopathological features of *Burkholderia cepacia* complex dermatitis in dogs: a series of four cases. *Vet Dermatol*. 2018;29:457. e156.
98. Yang C-H, Li Y-H. *Chromobacterium violaceum* infection: a clinical review of an important but neglected infection. *J Chin Med Assoc*. 2011;74:435–441.
99. Teoh AYB, Hui M, Ngo KY, et al. Fatal septicaemia from *Chromobacterium violaceum*: case reports and review of the literature. *Hong Kong Med J*. 2006;12:228–231.
100. Ponte R, Jenkins SG. Fatal *Chromobacterium violaceum* infections associated with exposure to stagnant waters. *J Pediatr Infect Dis*. 1992;11:583–586.
101. Steinberg JP, Lutgring JD, Burd EM. Other gram-negative and gram-variable bacilli. In: Bennett JE, Dolin R, Blaser MJ, eds. *Mandell, Douglas, and Bennett's Principles and Practice of Infectious Diseases*. Philadelphia, PA: Elsevier Saunders; 2020:2847–2864.
102. Meher-Homji Z, Mangalore RP, Johnson PD, et al. *Chromobacterium violaceum* infection in chronic granulomatous disease: a case report and review of the literature. *JMM Case Rep*. 2017;4:e005084.
103. dan Lin Y, Majumdar SS, Hennessy J, et al. The spectrum of *Chromobacterium violaceum* infections from a single geographic location. *Am J Trop Med Hyg*. 2016;94:710–716.
104. Markey B, Leonard F, Archambault M, et al. Miscellaneous gram-negative bacteria. In: Markey B, Leonard F, Archambault M, et al., eds. *Clinical Veterinary Microbiology*. 2nd ed. New York: Mosby/Elsevier; 2013:399–406.
105. Gogolewski R. *Chromobacterium violaceum* septicaemia in a dog. *Aust Vet J*. 1983;60:226.
106. Crosse PA, Soares K, Wheeler JL, et al. *Chromobacterium violaceum* infection in two dogs. *J Am Anim Hosp Assoc*. 2006;42:154–159.
107. Surma-Kurusiewicz K, Luft-Deptuła D, Adaszek Ł, et al. *Chromobacterium violaceum* infection in a dog. *Med Weter*. 2011;67:426–427.
108. Scholz HC, Witte A, Tomaso H, et al. Detection of *Chromobacterium violaceum* by multiplex PCR targeting the prgI, spaO, invG, and sipB genes. *Syst Appl Microbiol*. 2006;29:45–48.
109. Aldridge KE, Valainis GT, Sanders CV. Comparison of the in vitro activity of ciprofloxacin and 24 other antimicrobial agents against clinical strains of *Chromobacterium violaceum*. *Diagn Microbiol Infect Dis*. 1988;10:31–39.
110. Traslavina RP, Reilly CM, Vasireddy R, et al. Laser capture microdissection of feline *Streptomyces* spp. pyogranulomatous dermatitis and cellulitis. *Vet Pathol*. 2015;52:1172–1175.
111. Walton S, Martin P, Tolson C, et al. Orbital actinomycotic mycetoma caused by *Streptomyces cinnamoneus*. *JFMS Open Rep*. 2015;1. 2055116915589836.
112. Hryciw BN, Wright CP, Tan K. Rat bite fever on Vancouver Island: 2010-2016. *Can Commun Dis Rep*. 2018;44:215–219.
113. Ditchfield J, Lord LH, McKay KA. *Streptobacillus moniliformis* infection in a dog. *Can Vet J*. 1961;2:457–459.
114. Wouters EGH, Ho HTK, Lipman LJA, et al. Dogs as vectors of *Streptobacillus moniliformis* infection? *Vet Microbiol*. 2008;128:419–422.
115. Eisenberg T, Glaeser SP, Nicklas W, et al. *Streptobacillus felis* sp. nov., isolated from a cat with pneumonia, and emended descriptions of the genus *Streptobacillus* and of *Streptobacillus moniliformis*. *Int J Syst Evol Microbiol*. 2015;65:2172–2178.

SECTION 3

Fungal Diseases

Jane E. Sykes

Fungal diseases can be divided into superficial mycoses and deep mycoses. Superficial mycoses typically involve the skin and subcutis or mucosal surfaces, but rarely internal structures. Superficial mycoses include the most common fungal infections of dogs and cats such as dermatophytosis and *Malassezia* infections, which are addressed in this section in Chapters 78 and 79. Deep mycoses include the endemic mycoses caused by *Histoplasma* spp., *Blastomyces* spp., and *Coccidioides* spp.; cryptococcosis; sporotrichosis; and systemic mold infections.

For those with an interest in taxonomy, there have been significant changes in fungal nomenclature since the last edition, with the identification of new species of *Blastomyces* spp. in dogs, the proposed (and controversial) renaming of *Cryptococcus* spp. molecular types as separate species, the formal ("One Fungus, One Name") effort to use one name for mold pathogens rather than separate names for anamorphs and teleomorphs, and new names for *Pneumocystis* species. The chapter on sporotrichosis describes a major outbreak of zoonotic disease caused by *Sporothrix brasiliensis* in cats, dogs, and humans in Brazil, which involved thousands of cats and over 4,000 humans, the largest epidemic of this mycosis in the form of a zoonosis.

Although diagnosis and treatment of systemic mold infections used to be rare, with more widespread use of potent immunosuppressive drugs, veterinary practitioners are recognizing these infections more commonly. Many of these molds are resistant to commonly used antifungal drug treatments and have the potential to cause life-threatening disease. Other systemic fungal and algal infections that can be devastating if not recognized and treated early are candidiasis, oomycete infections (pythiosis and lagenidiosis), mucormycosis and entomophthoromycosis, and protothecosis. This section also includes chapters on organisms with unique classification, such as the "odd" fungus *Pneumocystis carinii* f. sp. *canis*, the aquatic protistan parasite (mesomycete) *Rhinosporidium seeberi*, and the mostly-fungus-somewhat-protozoan (microsporidian) parasite *Encephalitozoon cuniculi*.

Recent years have seen advancement in diagnostic testing capabilities for fungal infections, with an explosion in antigen detection tests, including point-of-care tests such as those for detection of cryptococcal polysaccharide antigen. Although the pace of advances in antifungal treatment has not been quite as fast, there is now more widespread use of newer azoles such as posaconazole and voriconazole, as well as improved understanding of the pharmacokinetics of azoles in dogs and cats. This has resulted in safer and more efficacious antifungal treatment regimens for dogs and cats. New azoles such as isavuconazole and antifungal drugs with novel mechanisms of action such as olorofim are now being used to treat refractory fungal infections in humans. We can look forward to further drug development activities and safety and pharmacokinetic studies so that similar drugs can be used to help companion animals in the future.

78

Dermatophytosis

Karen A. Moriello, Kimberly Coyner

KEY POINTS

- First Described: Clinical signs of dermatophytosis date back to the ancient Greek times.[1] One of the earliest texts describing the disease in animals was published in 1905.[2]
- Cause: There are over 30 species of dermatophytic fungi, but the most common dermatophytes that cause disease in dogs and cats are *Microsporum canis, Nannizzia gypsea* (previously *Microsporum gypseum*), *Trichophyton mentagrophytes*, and occasionally *Microsporum persicolor*. Most are zoophilic (and zoonotic) dermatophytes adapted for growth on keratinized structures of animals such as fur, skin cells, and toenails.
- Affected Hosts: *Microsporum canis* affects primarily dogs and cats, *T. mentagrophytes* commonly affects rodents, rabbits, and hedgehogs, and *M. persicolor* has been described in voles, but all dermatophyte species can infect any host. *Nannizzia gypsea* is a geophilic dermatophyte species which is usually found in decomposing fur/feathers present in the soil, but can infect living animals after contact with contaminated soil.
- Geographic Distribution: Dermatophytosis is present worldwide and is most common in warm climates.
- Route of Transmission: Exposure to spores is needed; dermatophytes are not part of the normal fungal biome. Dermatophytes are most commonly transmitted by direct contact between an infected and uninfected animal; fomite transmission via traumatic inoculation can occur via grooming equipment, bedding, collars, ectoparasites, and exposure to a contaminated environment. Successful fomite infection requires microtrauma to the skin in association with spore exposure.
- Major Clinical Signs: Clinical signs can be quite variable depending on animal and dermatophyte species involved, and chronicity and location of infection. Lesions commonly found include asymmetrical areas of papules, pustules, crusts, scaling, comedones, and alopecia. Erythema, hyperpigmentation, draining tracts, and nodular dermatitis can occur; as well as onychogryphosis. Pruritus is usually minimal but can sometimes be severe. Lesions can occur anywhere on the body but in cats tend to occur commonly on the face, ears, and paws, and then spread to other areas.
- Differential Diagnoses: Other causes for follicular infection including bacterial folliculitis and demodicosis, other ectoparasites, pemphigus foliaceus (in cases of severe facial or generalized crusting), and (in cases of nodular dermatitis), neoplasia, deep fungal infection, or mycobacterial granulomas. Dermatophytosis is most common in young animals, animals housed intensely, and/or animals under physiological stress.
- Human Health Significance: All dermatophytes are potentially zoonotic; *Microsporum canis* is the species most commonly transmitted from infected animals to humans. People handing infected animals should wear gloves. This is a low-level zoonotic disease and causes skin lesions in people; it is curable and infection is not life-threatening. Complications of animal-origin infections are rare, and when infection occurs in immunosuppressed people the most common potential adverse effects are those associated with prolonged treatment.[3-5] Most serious dermatophyte infections in people are of human origin and involve human pathogens.[3-5]

ETIOLOGIC AGENT AND EPIDEMIOLOGY

There are more than 30 species of dermatophytic fungal organisms; the dermatophytoses of veterinary importance are fungi in the genera *Microsporum* and *Trichophyton*.[6] Zoophilic dermatophyte species are adapted to living animal hosts; the most common species that affect dogs and cats are *Microsporum canis* and *Trichophyton mentagrophytes* (Table 78.1). Geophilic dermatophyte species such as *Nannizzia gypsea* (previously *Microsporum gypseum*) are usually found in fur, feathers, and horn present in the soil after the keratin products have been shed from the living animal. *Nannizzia gypsea* can also infect animals and humans after contact with contaminated soil. Anthropophilic dermatophytes species are adapted to humans and rarely infect dogs and cats; these include *Microsporum audouinii, Trichophyton tonsurans*, and *Epidermophyton floccosum*.

The classification of *Trichophyton* spp. and *Microsporum* spp. is evolving and species are being reclassified and renamed based on differing reproductive strategies.[7-9] There is a general consensus to move to a "one fungus-one name" classification system based on molecular typing; increasingly, clinicians will see the genus *Arthroderma* being used. Dermatophyte species can reproduce asexually (anamorphs) or sexually (teleomorphs, classified in the teleomorphic genus *Arthroderma*, phylum Ascomycota). The teleomorphic state of *Microsporum canis* is *Arthroderma otae*. The anamorphic species *Trichophyton mentagrophytes* can occur as a teleomorphic complex which includes *Arthroderma benhamiae* and *Arthroderma vanbreuseghemii*. Similarly, *N. gypsea* is now known to be a complex of the anamorphic phase *N. gypsea* and the teleomorphic *Arthroderma gypseum* and *Arthroderma incurvatum*. Risk factors for dermatophytosis include warm, humid environments, young age and group housing (such as shelters or catteries).[10-21] In a study of cats entering a northwestern animal shelter in the United States, owner-surrendered cats were half as likely to be diagnosed with *M. canis* dermatophytosis than transported cats.[21] Dermatophytosis is more common in cats than in dogs, but is still an uncommon disease even in cats; in one study of 1407 cats evaluated for skin disease, only 2.4% were diagnosed with dermatophytosis, far lower than the more common diagnoses of allergies/atopy (26%), bacterial skin infections (10%), ear mite infestation (6.1%), and flea infestation (5.2%).[22] Prevalence literature does

TABLE 78.1 Common Dermatophyte Species that Infect Dogs and Cats

Dermatophyte Species	Classification	Main Source
Microsporum canis (teleomorph *Arthroderma otae*)	Zoophilic	Cats, dogs, horses
Nannizzia gypsea (previously *Microsporum gypseum*) (teleomorphs *Arthroderma gypseum* and *A. incurvatum*)	Geophilic	Soil
Microsporum persicolor	Zoophilic	Voles, field mice
Trichophyton mentagrophytes (teleomorphs *Arthroderma benhamiae* and *A. vanbreuseghemii*)	Zoophilic	Rodents
Trichophyton verrucosum	Zoophilic	Cattle, other ruminants
Trichophyton erinacei	Zoophilic	Hedgehogs

not support the anecdotal comment that "it is ringworm until proven otherwise in cats." Infection with FeLV or FIV has not been shown to make cats more likely to develop dermatophytosis, but dermatophytosis has been described in cats and dogs with other immunosuppressive comorbidities.[23-26] There may be a genetic or breed predilection in some cases, as Persian cats and Yorkshire terriers are predisposed to dermatophytosis.[11,27-31] Terriers and hunting dogs are also over-represented for infection by *N. gypsea* and *M. persicolor*, likely due to skin abrasions and subsequent infection from contaminated soil while digging or hunting[32,33] (Fig. 78.1).

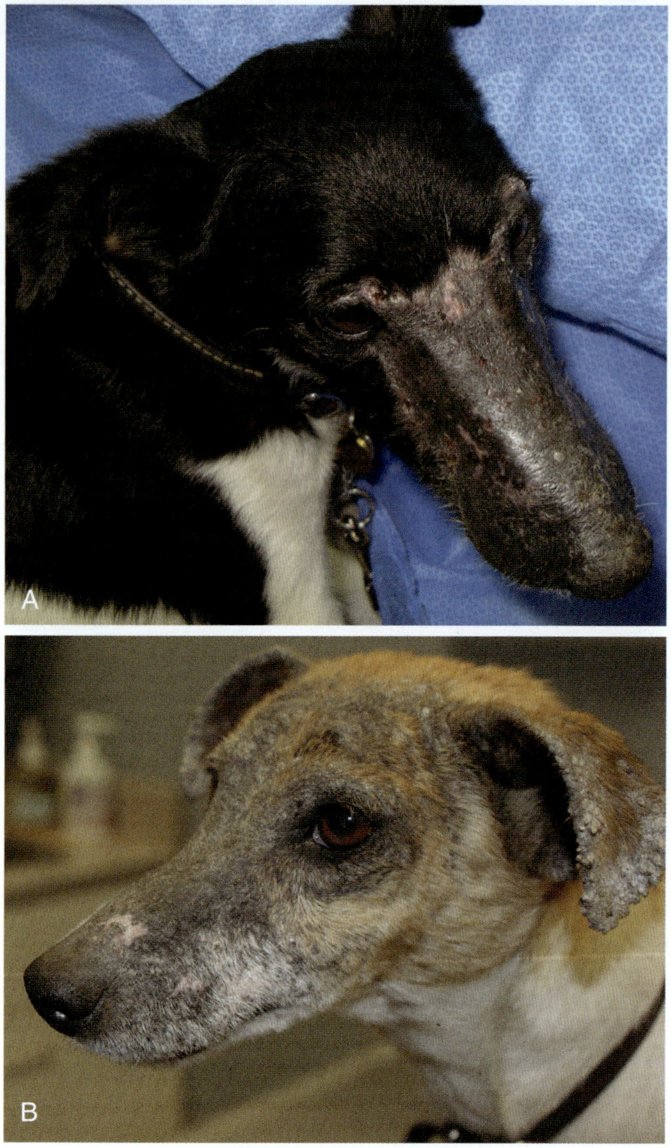

Fig. 78.1 Chronic *Trichophyton mentagrophytes* infections. There is alopecia, crusting, hyperpigmentation, and ulceration of the muzzle and periocular skin. (A) A 4.5-year-old male neutered fox terrier. (B) A 6-year-old female spayed Jack Russell terrier. (Courtesy University of California, Davis, Veterinary Dermatology Service.)

CLINICAL FEATURES

Pathogenesis and Clinical Signs

Dermatophyte infections are transmitted among animals or to people primarily through direct contact with infected hair, scale, and/or crusts. Concurrent microtrauma is needed to establish an active infection from contact with a contaminated environment. The infective form of the organism is the arthrospore, a very small spore formed from the segmentation and fragmentation of fungal hyphae in infected hair and keratin. The dose or quantity of naturally infective material needed to establish spontaneous infection is unknown; in an experimental model, 100 macroconidia spores from a culture plate were able to cause a lesion but only when coupled with microtrauma and occlusion for >72 hours.[34] *Microsporum canis* infections typically follow contact with an infected cat, while most *Trichophyton* infections are suspected to be due to contact with infected rodents or their nests. *Nannizzia gypsea* infections are contracted when the animals dig in contaminated soil.

Arthrospores adhere very strongly to keratin in skin cells, hairs, and toenails. A requirement for dermatophyte infection is damage to normal skin defense factors, which include fungistatic fatty acids in sebum and an intact epidermis. Microtrauma to the skin from pruritus or self-trauma, humidity, and ectoparasites all contribute to conditions optimal for dermatophyte infection.[34,35]

The infection process has three stages: 1) adhesion of arthroconidia to corneocytes, which occurs within 2 to 6 hours of exposure and is likely mediated by carbohydrate-specific adhesins expressed on the surface of arthroconidia as well as dermatophyte-secreted proteases such as subtilisins; 2) conidial germination, which occurs within 24 hours of infection and in which germ tubes emerge from the arthroconidia and penetrate the stratum corneum; and 3) fungal invasion of the keratin network.[36-39] Other proteolytic enzymes (keratinase, elastase, and collagenase) have been isolated from dermatophyte fungi and are likely involved in all three stages of the establishment and progression of an infection.[39,40] By 7 days of incubation, hyphae begin to form arthroconidia, completing the fungal life cycle. Lesions typically appear 1 to 3 weeks after exposure.[34]

Dermatophytes can counter the host immune response in a number of ways, including lymphocyte inhibition by fungal cell wall mannans, macrophage function alteration, and altered/slowed keratinocyte turnover.[37,41] Both humoral (Th2) and cellular (Th1) immune responses occur in dermatophyte-infected animals; however, clinical cure and protection against reinfection depends on a strong CMI response involving macrophages and cytokines such as IFN-γ.[37,42]

Dermatophytosis is primarily a follicular disease, and thus the most common clinical signs include asymmetrical hair loss, scaling, crusting, papules, comedones, and variable pruritus. Some patients develop a classic ring-like lesion with central healing with or without hyperpigmentation and fine follicular papules on the periphery

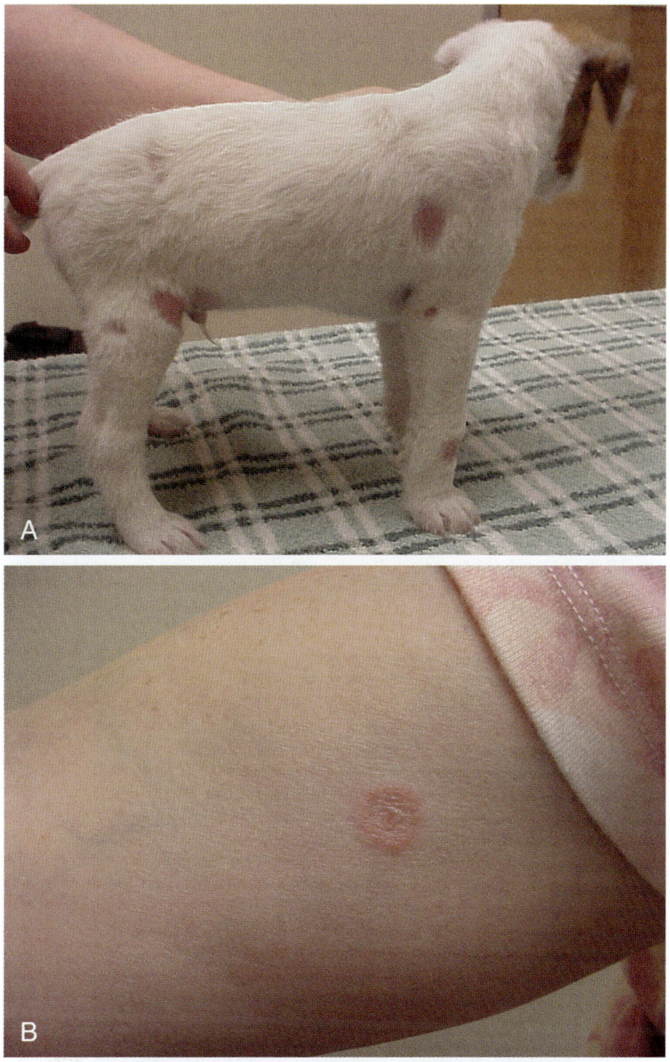

Fig. 78.2 (A) Jack Russell terrier puppy with multifocal classic well-circumscribed lesions caused by infection by *Microsporum canis.* (B) On questioning, the owner of the affected litter of puppies revealed that she also had a lesion on her arm. (Courtesy Dr. Terry Nagle.)

(Fig. 78.2). Generally, however, clinical signs are highly variable and depend on the degree of inflammation and hair shaft destruction. In cats, lesions tend to occur most commonly on the face, ears, and muzzle and then progress to paws and other body areas. Multifocal and diffuse lesions are most commonly seen in animals with concurrent immunosuppressive disease and/or physiological stress such as overcrowding. Hunting dogs often develop lesions on the muzzle and paws. Onychogryphosis may occur, which may involve one to multiple digits. Pustular dermatophytosis can histologically mimic pemphigus foliaceus. Both dogs and cats can develop nodular dermatophyte infections; Persian cats and Yorkshire terrier dogs are predisposed to such lesions. These include kerions (localized, raised, nodular, exudative inflammatory lesions), pseudomycetomas, and mycetomas (subcutaneous masses) and present as nodules that fistulate, ulcerate, and drain serous to purulent exudate. Mycetomas are characterized by the presence of: 1) tumefaction, 2) draining sinus tracts, and 3) tissue grains or granules. In contrast to true mycetomas (eumycetomas), which are localized lesions containing dense clusters of organisms, pseudomycetomas (also known as dermatophytic mycetomas) lack draining tracts, and consist of loosely compacted clusters of hyphae.

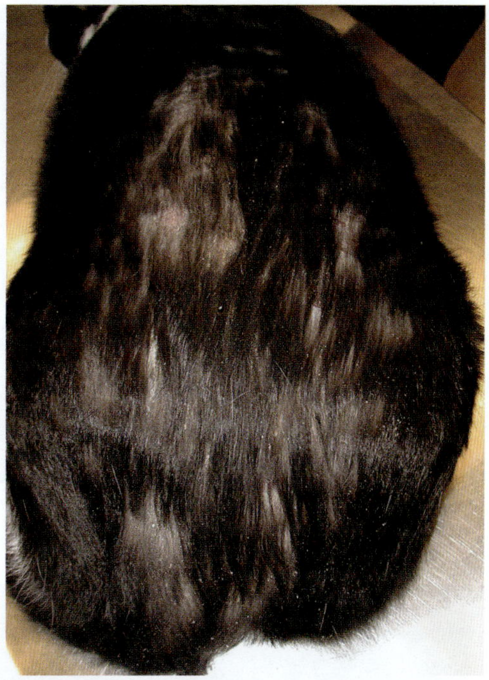

Fig. 78.3 Adult cat with pruritus and multifocal areas of hair loss, scales, and crusts associated with *Microsporum canis* infection.

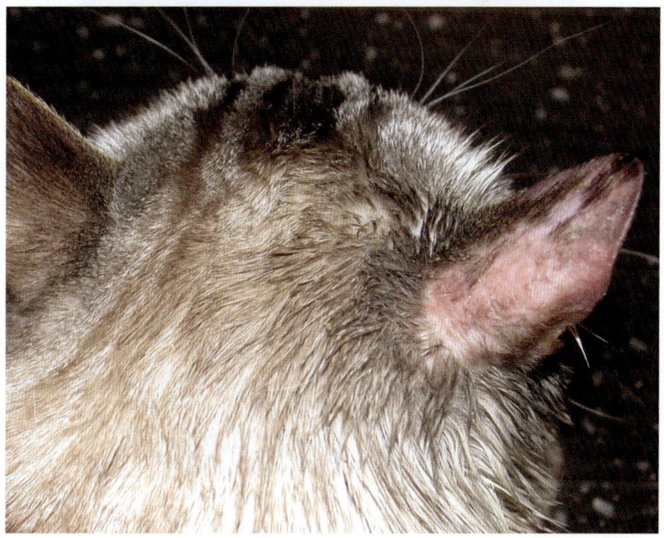

Fig. 78.4 Adult cat with unilateral otitis and hair loss on the ear pinnae associated with *Microsporum canis* infection.

Physical Examination Findings

Cats

Cats with dermatophytosis may develop focal to multifocal to extensive regional to generalized alopecia with variable crusting, scaling, erythema, follicular cast formation, comedones, and hyperpigmentation. Pruritus may range from none to severe, and in some cases miliary dermatitis, symmetrical alopecia, and eosinophilic plaques may develop. These lesions can resemble hypersensitivity dermatitis (Fig. 78.3). Lesions are commonly first noted on the face and limbs but can occur in any area. Alopecia, scaling, or crusting of one or both outer pinnae can occur (Fig. 78.4), as can chin dermatitis similar to feline acne. Uncommonly, lesions similar to pemphigus foliaceus such as bilaterally symmetrical facial, pinnal, nailbed, and footpad lesions can be seen. Dermatophyte

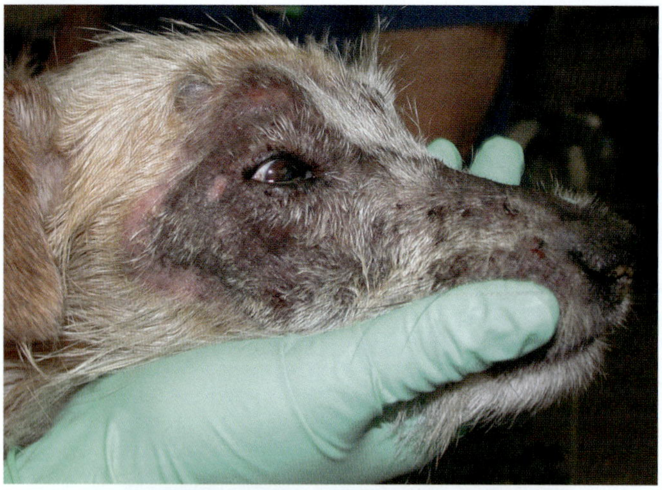

Fig. 78.5 Face of a 14-year-old dog infected with *Trichophyton mentagrophytes* (see Case Example).

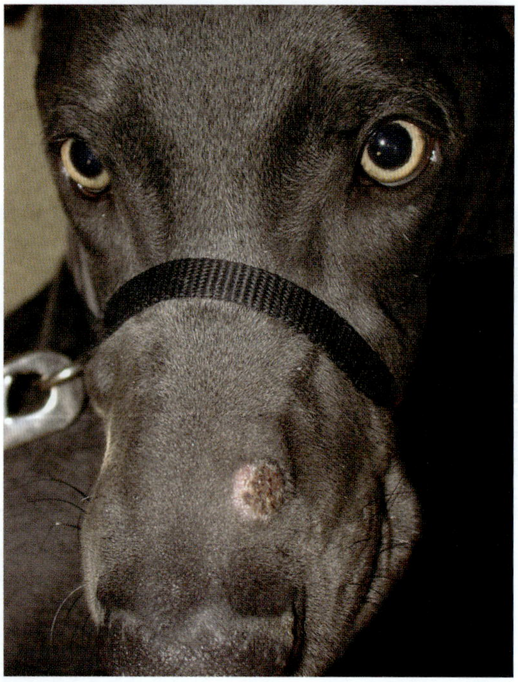

Fig. 78.6 A 5-year-old male neutered mixed-breed dog with a history of an acute development of a nodular lesion on the muzzle. The diagnosis was kerion reaction associated with *Microsporum canis* infection.

pseudomycetomas are uncommon and are characterized by dermal to subcutaneous granulomatous masses which can fistulate, ulcerate, and drain.

Dogs

Dogs most often develop focal to multifocal areas of alopecia with variable scaling, crusting, papules, and hyperpigmentation. These signs are clinically indistinguishable from more common causes of alopecia, bacterial pyoderma, and demodicosis. Crusting of the facial and muzzle skin (Fig. 78.5) and furunculosis can mimic immune-mediated diseases. Dermatophyte kerions (Fig. 78.6) are most commonly caused by *Trichophyton* spp. and *N. gypsea*, and dermatophyte pseudomycetomas have rarely been reported. Paw and claw involvement can be characterized by onychogryphosis involving one to multiple toenails, and occasionally all may be affected (Figs. 78.7 and 78.8).

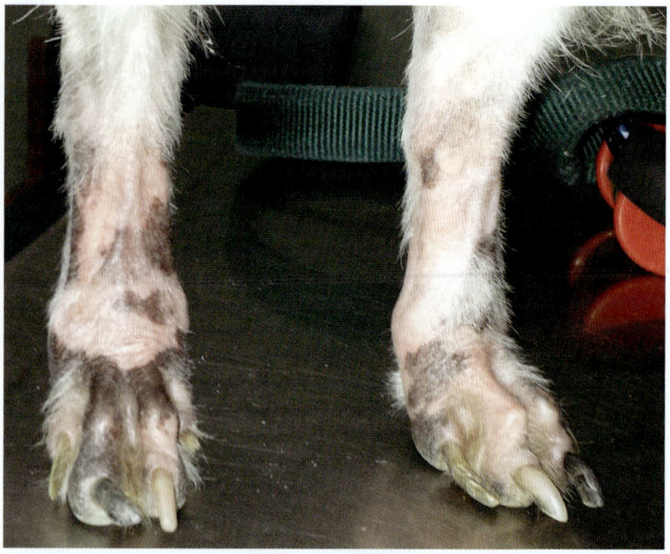

Fig. 78.7 Paw of a 14-year-old dog with *Trichophyton mentagrophytes* dermatophytosis (see Case *Example*).

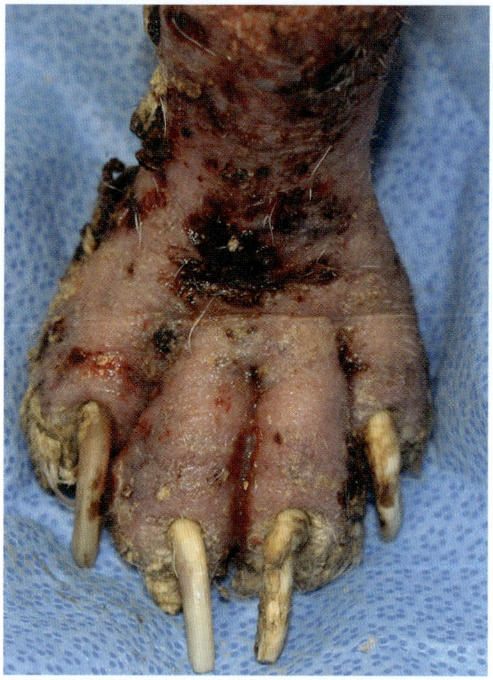

Fig. 78.8 Foot of a 9-year-old intact male terrier mix with dermatophytosis caused by *Nannizzia gypsea* (previously *Microsporum gypseum*). The dog competed in rodent hunting events that occurred in underground tunnels. Severe, chronic dermatitis with ulceration and alopecia that involved multiple distal limbs and claws was present. The claws were irregular and discolored. (Courtesy University of California, Davis, Veterinary Dermatology Service.)

DIAGNOSIS

The diagnosis of dermatophytosis relies not on any one single diagnostic test, but rather by clinical acumen and assimilation of available information. It is commonly stated that fungal culture is the "gold standard" diagnostic test; however, if the criterion is to demonstrate *infection*, that is invasion of the hair and skin by a dermatophyte, then the only tests that demonstrate this are direct examination of hairs and histological examination of skin biopsy specimens. The objectives of this section are to provide the clinician with recommendations for

TABLE 78.2 Diagnostic Tests Used for Dermatophytosis

Test	Type	Specimen/Purpose	Tool	Comments
Dermoscopy	POC tool	Identifies hairs for direct examination or culture. When used with direct examination can confirm infection	Handheld dermoscope	Provides excellent magnification of hairs; look for broken "comma" shaped hairs; pluck hairs for direct examination and/or culture
Wood's lamp examination	POC tool	Identifies hairs for direct examination and/or culture through detection of apple green fluorescence on hair shafts. When used in conjunction with direct examination can confirm infection	Plug-in Wood's lamp only, best with built-in magnification (e.g., Burton Wood lamp)	Reliably identifies hairs for direct examination and/or culture; over 90% of untreated *M. canis*–infected cats have positive fluorescence; requires good equipment and technique. Can be used to monitor response to treatment; loss of fluorescence at base of hair shaft indicates good response to treatment. *Nannizzia gypsea* and *Trichophyton* spp. do NOT fluoresce
Direct examination (cytologic examination)	POC	Identifies infected hairs to select for dermatophyte culture and species ID; confirm infection	Mineral oil, skin scraping-spatula, forceps	Permits identification of both *Microsporum* and *Trichophyton* infections. Entire edge and center of infected lesion should be scraped
Fungal culture	POC or commercial diagnostic laboratory	Hairs and/or scales	Dermatophyte test medium, toothbrushes, skin-scraping spatulas	Detects fungal spores on the haircoat; must be used in conjunction with clinical examination to confirm infection. False-positive tests can occur due to fomite contamination, false-negative tests occur due to poor sample selection. Test of choice for monitoring treatment
Skin biopsy	Diagnostic laboratory	Tissue; excisional biopsy specimen or deep wedge biopsy specimen from nodule, 6–8 mm skin biopsy specimen from other skin specimens	Skin biopsy punch, other surgical instruments/materials as appropriate	Surface pathology is important for diagnosis, do not scrub or prepare the skin before specimen collection. Special stains required to identify the dermatophytes, important to alert pathologist of differential diagnosis, cannot identify species unless specimen is submitted for tissue PCR
Molecular testing: real-time PCR	Diagnostic laboratory	Hairs, scales, and crusts	Large amounts of hair and/or crusts needed to ensure adequate specimen for testing	Negative test is suggestive that dermatophytosis is not present. Will detect viable and nonviable fungal DNA, false positives are common if fomite contamination is a possibility; cannot yet be used to monitor for mycological cure

POC, point of care.

what test(s) are most likely *to confirm the presence of disease* and what test(s) are most likely *to confirm the absence of an active infection in a treated animal* (i.e., cured, not a risk).

Diagnostic assays for dermatophytosis are divided into two major categories: point of care (POC) and commercial diagnostic laboratory assays (Table 78.2). POC diagnostics include dermoscopy, Wood's lamp examination, hair trichograms and skin scrapings, and in-house fungal culture. Diagnostic laboratory testing includes diagnostic laboratory fungal culture, nucleic acid amplification tests (PCR), and histopathology. CBCs, serum chemistry panels, urinalysis, and diagnostic imaging are not helpful for confirming either the presence or absence of dermatophytosis. These tests are helpful and indicated when concurrent illness is suspected to have predisposed an animal to widespread severe dermatophytosis.

Point-of-Care Diagnostic Assays and Tools

Dermoscopy

Dermoscopy is a POC tool used to identify hairs for direct examination and/or fungal culture. A dermascope is a noninvasive handheld tool that allows for illuminated magnification of the skin and hair. There are several studies in the veterinary literature describing normal cat skin and hair and dermoscopic examination of cats with dermatophytosis.[43-45] Infected hairs are opaque, slightly curved, or broken with a homogenous thickness. These infected hairs have been called "comma hairs" because of their appearance. Microscopic examination of hairs shows hyphae and spores. Dermoscopes vary in cost and their primary advantage is magnified illumination of broken hairs for the purpose of specimen collection for direct examination and fungal culture. Dermoscopes can be used with or without a Wood's lamp.

Wood's Lamp Examination

A Wood's lamp is a POC diagnostic tool used to identify hairs that are suitable for direct examination and/or fungal culture (Box 78.1). This is an ultraviolet light (320 to 400 nm wavelength, optimum 365 nm) that can detect microbial organisms that produce phosphors as a result of their growth on skin and/or hairs.[46] It is different from a "black light" which comprises a clear glass that filters medium- and short-wave ultraviolet light and emits a large amount of blue visible light. In veterinary medicine the primary pathogen of importance that fluoresces is *M. canis*. The characteristic green fluorescence of *M. canis*–infected hairs is due to a water-soluble pigment located within the cortex or medulla of the hair.[47-49] The fluorescence is the result of a chemical interaction that occurs as a result of the infection and is not associated with spores or infective material. *Nannizzia gypsea, M. persicolor*, and *Trichophyton* spp. do *not* fluoresce.

BOX 78.1 Practice Tips for Wood's Lamp Examination

1. Use a medical-grade, plug-in Wood's lamp with built-in magnification.[a] Handheld battery-operated devices should not be used. The lamp does not need to warm up before use.
2. Be sure the room is dark and that the animal can be safely restrained.
3. Allow adequate time for the examiner's eyes to adapt to darkness. To ensure this is the case, use a "positive" control if possible. A positive control can be prepared by mounting infected hairs between two glass slides. Fluorescence will remain positive for years.
4. Hold the lamp close to the skin (2 to 4 cm) and move very slowly over the haircoat. This greatly decreases false-positive findings from dust. Holding the lamp too far away is one of the most common mistakes made, and leads to false-negative results.
5. Start at the head and carefully inspect the haircoat. Infected hairs are often obscured by scale and crusts; it is important to gently lift crusts and scales and look under the crusts.
6. Fluorescence is present only on the hair shafts and not on skin, crusts, scales, or nail and is green in color (Fig. 78.9). One of the most common things mistaken for fluorescence is hair sebum which usually appears "yellow."
7. Clear acetate tape can be pressed against the skin and gently lifted off the skin and then mounted on a glass slide. This technique can be helpful to visualize short hairs that cannot be plucked easily. Alternatively, lesions can be gently scraped to collect hair, which is then mounted in mineral oil, cover-slipped, and then examined. A Wood's lamp can be held over this to identify fragments of fluorescing hairs, which then identifies areas to initiate microscopic examination. Do not use clearing agents such as KOH, as this will destroy the fluorescence and are not helpful in visualizing infected hairs.

[a]The authors recommend Burton UV light model UV 502 (https://www.burtonmedical.com/).

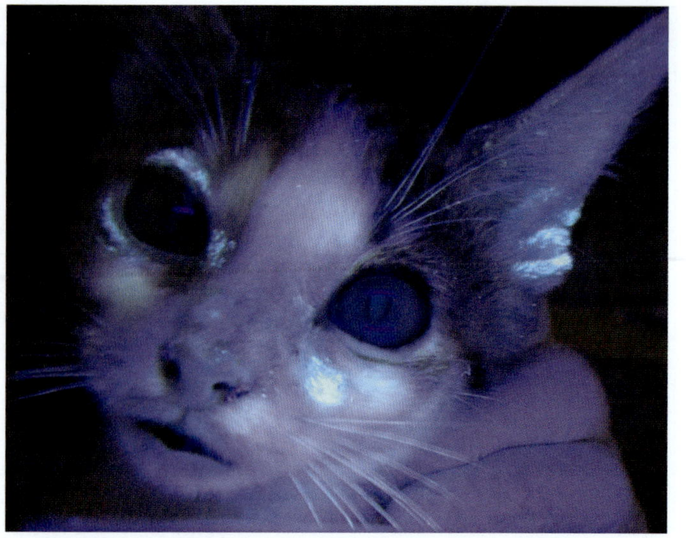

Fig. 78.9 Positive Wood's lamp examination on a kitten in a shelter. The kitten is being viewed through the magnifying glass of a medical-grade Wood's lamp from 18 inches away. The Wood's lamp bulbs can be seen on the top and bottom of the picture. This demonstrates the usefulness of a strong Wood's lamp coupled with magnification.

BOX 78.2 Practice Tips For Direct (Microscopic) Examination

1. Use both hair pluckings and skin scrapings.
2. Use mineral oil as a mounting medium; no studies show that clearing agents are superior to mineral oil. Clearing agents such as KOH can induce artifacts and damage the microscope lens.
3. Mineral oil does not destroy fluorescence on *M. canis*–infected hairs; a Wood's lamp can be held over the glass microscope slide to help locate hairs for examination.
4. Use a glass coverslip to enhance visualization of the specimen.
5. Examine the specimen at 4× and 10× magnification for abnormal hairs, which appear wider and paler than normal hairs even at low power (Fig. 78.10).
6. The addition of lactophenol cotton blue stain to the mineral oil can help visualize infected hairs.
7. Follicular casts (circumferential accumulations of keratin around the hairs) are common artifacts, which appear on focal areas of the shaft or around the hair root.

An evidence-based review found that commonly held beliefs about the usefulness of Wood's lamp examination are inaccurate.[50] Statements such as "less than 50% of strains fluorescence" are based upon retrospective studies of random-source diagnostic specimens.[11,51-53] When data from 30 experimental infection studies and spontaneous disease studies were examined, results were surprisingly different.[50] Experimental dermatophyte infection studies reported 100% fluorescence in cats, and studies involving spontaneous disease in untreated animals reported 91 to 100% fluorescence. In studies that reported on *M. canis* fluorescence in cats that previously received treatment (predominantly longhaired cats), the prevalence of fluorescence varied from 39% to 53%. Fluorescence disappears with successful treatment. In addition, baths and lime sulfur or enilconazole dips were not associated with any loss of fluorescence when used to monitor response to treatment. In small animal practice, Wood's lamp examination is likely to be positive in most animals with *M. canis* dermatophytosis. This also has been the experience of one of the authors (KAM) in animal shelters (Fig. 78.9). Fluorescing hairs are most likely to be found in untreated infections; fluorescence may be more difficult to identify in treated animals. False-positive and false-negative results are commonly due to inadequate equipment, lack of magnification, patient compliance, poor technique, or lack of training.[50] Wood's lamp examinations can be an important POC examination tool in shelters to screen cats for dermatophytosis. In one report of management of *M. canis* dermatophytosis in a shelter, 1226 cats were surrendered to the shelter in a 7-month period.[54] Of these cats, 273 (22.3%) were culture-positive; but only 60 of 273 had lesions, were positive on Wood's lamp, and were positive using direct (light microscopic) examination. The 213 remaining culture-positive cats lacked lesions and were Wood's lamp negative; these cats were determined to be fomite carriers. Infection from fomite carrier cats was not introduced into the facility as cats were housed in cages at intake until repeat fungal cultures were negative. The only intervention was allowing the cat to groom. The use of a Wood's lamp at intake allowed for rapid identification of infected cats (50 of 60 being kittens), and prevention of reintroduction of the contagion to the facility.

Direct Examination of Hairs and Scale

Direct (light microscopic) examination of hair and scale can confirm dermatophyte infection in the examination room (Box 78.2). Material can be collected with the aid of a dermoscope, Wood's lamp, or via a combination of skin scraping and plucking of hairs. The optimal way to collect specimens is by both superficial skin scraping and plucking of hairs from lesions. Use of this combined technique yielded positive results in 87.5% of cases in one study.[55] In this study, a Wood's lamp was not used and the authors confirmed *M. canis*, *Trichophyton*, and

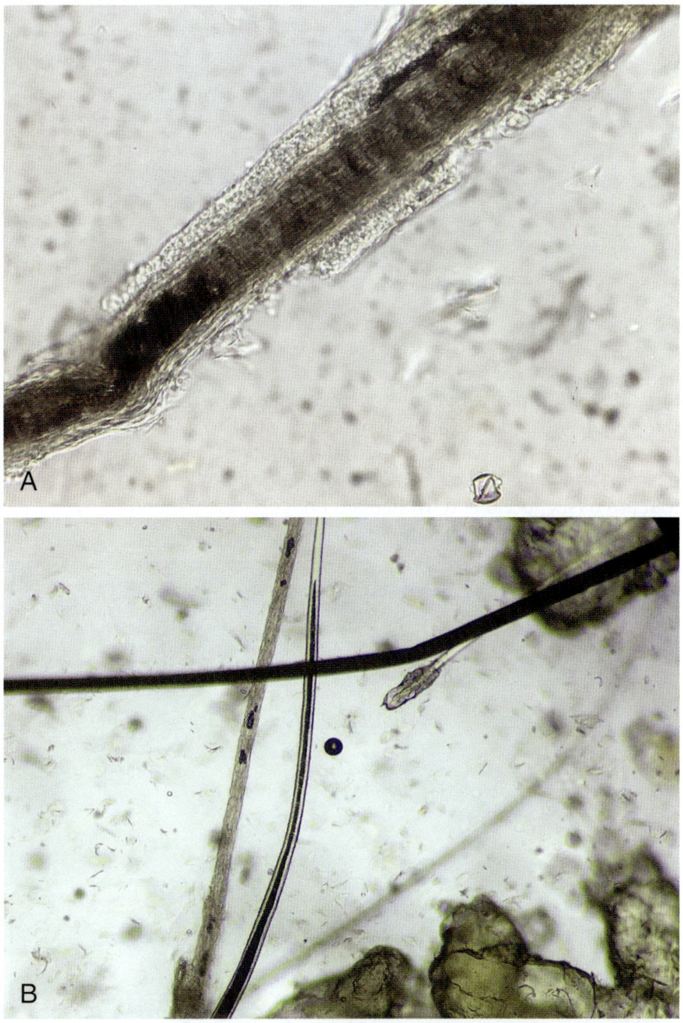

Fig. 78.10 (A) The infected hair is pale and shows disruption of the corticomedullary junction; dermatophyte arthroconidia are present encasing the cuticle of the hair (40x magnification). (B) In this trichogram cytology, the pale, fuzzy infected hair on the left side contrasts sharply with the normal hair in the center of the image (10x magnification).

N. gypsea based on culture of hairs determined to be infected on direct examination. Mounting specimens in mineral oil is time and cost-effective as it allows for concurrent microscopic examination for mites.

Dermatophyte Culture

Despite increased availability of molecular testing, fungal culture is still the most common method used to confirm a diagnosis of dermatophytosis and to identify the causative species (Box 78.3). It is also the only medical-legal test used to identify the fungal species. Fungal cultures may be performed as a POC in-clinic test or at a commercial diagnostic laboratory. A recent study revealed good correlation between POC cultures and diagnostic laboratories when both gross colony morphology along with microscopic features were used to identify colonies.[56] Importantly, there was a high error rate when culture media color change alone was used for diagnosis.

The POC procedure employs dermatophyte test medium (DTM), which consists of a nutrient medium, inhibitors of bacterial and saprophytic growth, and phenol red as a pH indicator. Several variations are available, some of which claim to speed growth of the culture, but this has not been found to be clinically significant and commercial media all appear to perform similarly.[57] Plates that have a large volume of medium and are easy to inoculate should be purchased. Plates are

BOX 78.3 Procedure for Point-of-Care Culture of Dermatophytes

1. Use a fungal culture medium that can easily be inoculated and allow it to warm to room temperature before inoculation.
2. Do not clean lesions with alcohol before specimen collection as this can result in a false-negative culture.
3. Collect specimens using a toothbrush. A new unopened toothbrush is mycologically sterile. Comb the target lesion approximately 20 times, or until the bristles are filled with hair. If lesions are not clearly visible, comb the entire haircoat. If lesions are heavily crusted, forceps or hemostats can be used to collect crusts and hairs for culture.
4. Stab bristles onto the surface of the plate with just enough pressure to turn the ends of the bristles yellow. Do no not pluck individual hairs from within toothbrush bristles for culture as this can lead to false-negative results. To inoculate hairs and/or crusts plucked directly from the lesions, press the hairs firmly onto the surface of the fungal culture plate. Do not embed them.
5. Store plates in clear plastic bags to keep media hydrated and prevent cross-contamination. It is not necessary to store plates in the dark.
6. Incubate at 25°C to 30°C (77°F to 86°F).
7. Examine the plates daily by holding the plate up to light to look for growth.
8. Colonies have pale, never heavily pigmented, colony growth and a red color change in the medium around them as they grow (Fig. 78.11). Red color change alone is never diagnostic. Microscopic confirmation is always required to confirm the presence of dermatophytes.
9. Make a clear acetate tape preparation using lactophenol cotton phenol blue stain and wait 15 minutes before microscopic examination to allow the stain to be absorbed by conidia and hyphae.[a] New methylene blue or Diff-Quik II solution (basophilic thiazine dye) can be used but may not be as effectively taken up by cells.
10. Key differentiating features of *Microsporum canis, Nannizzia gypsea*, and *Trichophyton* on cytologic examination using light microscopy are shown in Figures 78.12 to 78.15. If a suspected dermatophyte cannot be identified on in-house cytologic examination, submit the culture plate to a commercial diagnostic laboratory for definitive fungal identification.

[a] Lactophenol cotton blue stain can be purchased online.

preferable to vials because they permit inoculation with a toothbrush. For incubation, DTM containers should be loosely covered or capped at room temperature and protected from desiccation. Placement of individual cultures in a plastic self-closing bag will help prevent desiccation, cross-contamination, and mite infestation of the culture medium. Dermatophyte colonies appear as soon as 5 to 7 days after inoculation. In cultures of human dermatophyte infections, 98.5% of fungal cultures were positive before day 17.[58] When veterinary specimens were examined, 98.2% of fungal cultures for *M. canis* were positive by day 14 of incubation.[59] In a study of 202 diagnostic DTM plates from *M. canis*–infected shelter cats from a Pacific northwestern shelter, all had recognizable colony growth by day 7 (median 4 days), and 19 of 19 fomite carrier cat cultures exhibited growth by day 12.[21] A fungal culture can be considered negative if no pathogen has been isolated by day 14. Plates should be inspected daily for growth by holding the plate up to the light to look for colony growth. This avoids opening of culture plates until it is appropriate to do microscopic confirmation. Dermatophyte colonies are never green, gray, brown, or black. Pathogens are white, light tan, or buff in color and have a powdery to cottony mycelial growth. The red color change is caused by a change in the pH of the medium and is not diagnostic for dermatophytosis; it merely identifies colonies for microscopic sampling. The color change usually occurs at the time the colony is first visible, but may develop

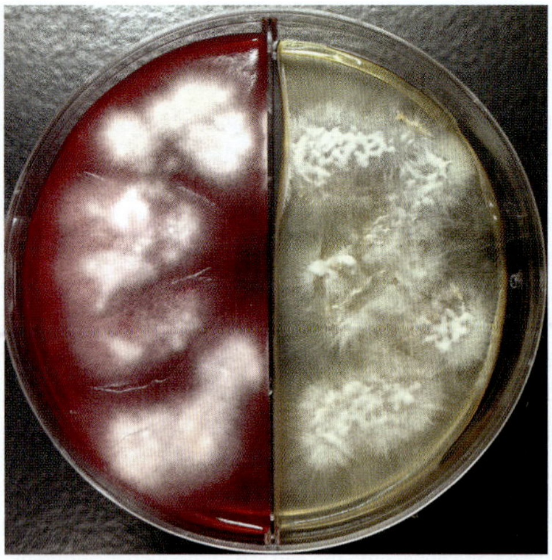

Fig. 78.11 Typical growth of *Microsporum canis* on DTM *(red)* and Sabouraud dextrose agar on dual growth plate. Note the pale colony growth. Dual plates are a good choice because they provide the "red flag" aid of the color indicator in DTM with a growth medium (Sabouraud). The phenol red in DTM can sometimes result in changes to the gross and microscopic features of dermatophytes, making in-clinic identification more difficult. This is avoided if dual plates are used, as this does not occur with Sabouraud medium.

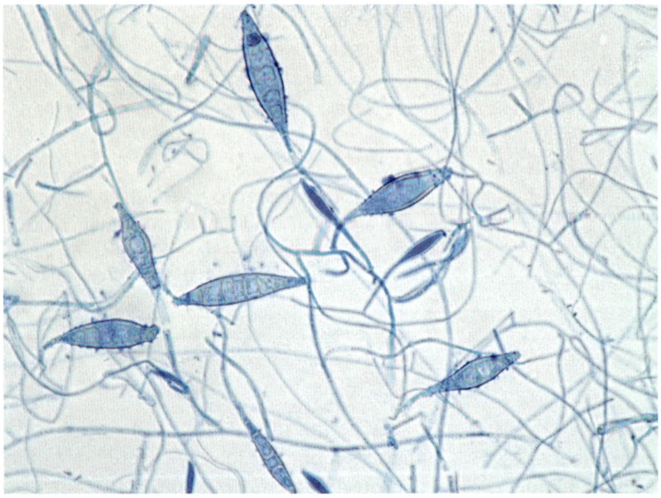

Fig. 78.12 *Microsporum canis* macroconidia stained with lactophenol cotton blue (40× magnification). The specimen was allowed to stand for 15 minutes before being examined. The stain has been absorbed intracellularly making the macroconidia more visible. Key characteristics are thick walls, tapered ends, rough walls and large amounts of hyphae and relatively few macroconidia compared to *N. gypsea.*

within 12 to 24 hours of fungal growth. Growth of any pathogenic or non-pathogenic fungus will eventually produce a red media color change after the colony has grown for several days to a week.

Unless there is a specimen collection error such as collection of only a few hairs rather than using a toothbrush for sampling lesions, large numbers of colonies of the dermatophyte will appear on the plate if dermatophytosis is present. The number of colonies decreases as the infection resolves spontaneously or with successful treatment. One of the most common problems with in-house culture is the lack of sporulation or growth, or both, of *M. canis* on DTM. A common cause of this is over-inoculation of the culture plates. This results in rapid swarming of the plate with fluffy colony growth but only unsporulated hyphae are noted on microscopic examination. Toothbrush specimens should be directly inoculated onto the surface of a plate to avoid overgrowth of contaminants. In one study that compared direct inoculation to the plucking of hairs from bristles that were then inoculated onto a plate, the latter technique resulted in marked contaminant growth.[60] The number of toothbrush inoculations on the plate should be limited to four to six, and individual impressions should be

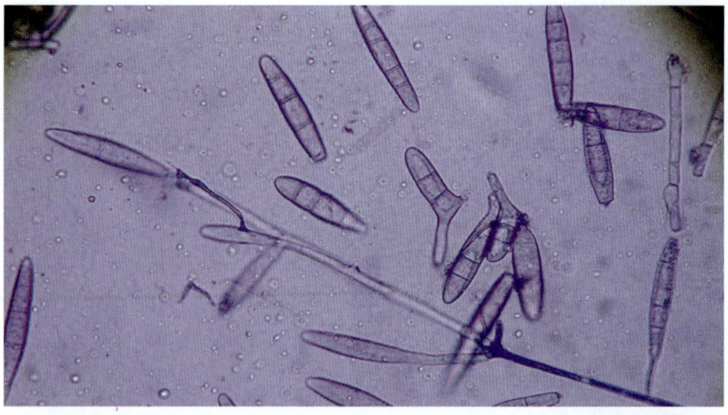

Fig. 78.13 *Nannizzia gypsea* macroconidia (40× magnification). Note the wider and blunted appearance compared to *Microsporum canis*, together with thin walls. A key differentiating feature on cytological examination is that *N. gypsea* produces large numbers of macroconidia that are easily found and hyphae are not commonly found.

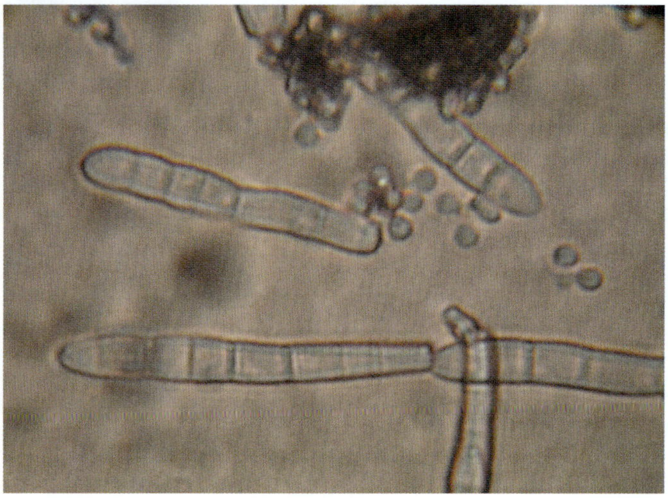

Fig. 78.14 Macroconidia of *Trichophyton* spp. The specimen appears pale; it was examined immediately after staining.

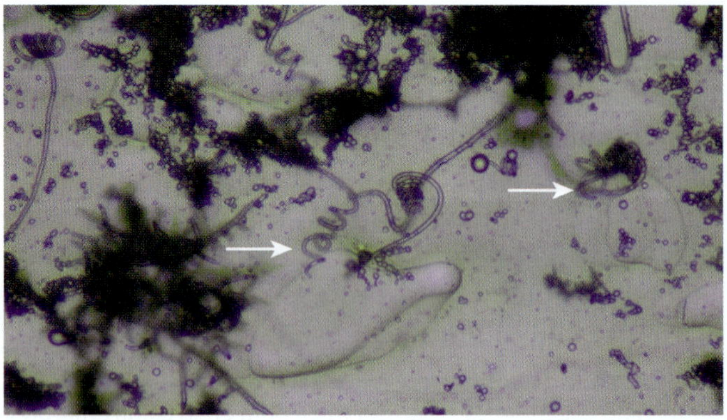

Fig. 78.15 Spiral hyphae most typical of *Trichophyton* spp. *(arrows)*. Note the large numbers of microconidia. Spiral hyphae are highly suggestive of *Trichophyton* spp.

clearly visible and not cover the entire plate surface. If the plate has been over-inoculated, a subculture can be performed to identify the pathogen. When evaluating fungal cultures in *treated* animals: 1) colony growth may be slower; cultures negative for growth at day 14 should be considered negative, 2) gross and microscopic fungal colony morphologies may appear abnormal, and 3) as dermatophytosis resolves, the number of dermatophyte CFU per plate should dramatically decrease, so this feature can be used to monitor response to treatment (see Box 78.3). If toothbrush specimens are sent to a human or veterinary diagnostic laboratory, clinicians should contact the laboratory to ensure they are familiar with toothbrush inoculation techniques and request weekly updates on growth. Quantification (CFU/plate) is important and should be reported as a 1-–10 count. MALDI-TOF mass spectrometry (see Chapter 3) has been used to successfully identify dermatophytes to the genus level; reliable species-level identification has been more challenging but shows promise as libraries improve.[61]

Skin Biopsy

Histological examination of skin biopsy specimens is indicated in three clinical situations in order to confirm the presence of true disease. The first is in the evaluation of nonhealing wounds or nodular lesions, because kerions and pseudomycetomas (dermatophytic mycetomas) often yield negative fungal cultures. The second is in the evaluation of dogs or cats with facial lesions where extensive crusting is present and/or if pemphigus foliaceus is suspected. In rare cases, dermatophytes can produce pustular histologic lesions with acantholysis. The third is in the workup of an animal with unusual skin disease not easily attributed to other causes. In all cases it is important to alert the pathologist that dermatophytes are suspected, because routine stains (i.e., H&E) are not as sensitive as PAS or Gomori's methenamine silver (GMS) for detection of fungal elements in tissue.

Specimen collection. The skin should not be prepared or disinfected before biopsy, as key diagnostic findings are present in the superficial crusts. It is critical to collect multiple (4–6) skin biopsy specimens no less than 6 mm in diameter, as tissue specimens shrink by 30% to 50% when placed in formalin. Deep wedge samples or excisional biopsies are preferred for nodular lesions. It is not uncommon for organisms to be scant in tissues, hence the need for multiple sections to increase the chance of making a diagnosis. Histopathology does not permit identification of the dermatophyte species present, and molecular testing on paraffin-embedded specimens is not widely available. In nodular lesions, submission of a wedge of tissue in sterile saline for a macerated fungal culture is ideal for identification of dermatophyte species present. Histological examination of skin biopsy specimens is not recommended as a basis to determine mycological cure.

Molecular Diagnosis Using Nucleic Acid–Based Testing

Reports on the use of PCR for the diagnosis of dermatophytosis in spontaneous skin disease are still relatively uncommon in the veterinary literature. One study reported 100% concordant results between PCR and culture for the diagnosis of nodular lesions in cats caused by *M. canis*.[62] A second study reported correct identification of *Trichophyton* infections in dogs (n = 7) and *M. canis* infections in cats (n = 8) in 15 specimens from animals with a diagnosis confirmed via both fungal culture and direct examination of hair.[63] In another study, 183 hair specimens from dogs and cats with suspected dermatophytosis were tested by PCR and fungal culture.[64] Fungal culture confirmed the diagnosis in 59 of 183 specimens, and endpoint (conventional) one-step PCR and nested PCR (see Chapter 6) were positive in 49 and 63 of 183 specimens, respectively. In this study, there were notable differences in the sensitivity and specificity of molecular assays used between dogs and cats. One-step testing was highly accurate for dogs (AUC > 90) but only mildly accurate for cats (AUC = 78.6). Nested PCR was accurate for cats (AUC = 93.6) and had a specificity and sensitivity of 94.4% and 94.9%, respectively, for both species.[64] Use of nested PCR is no longer recommended for routine molecular diagnosis because of its potential for false-positive test results due to contamination. In a field study of 132 cats, 21% of which were culture-positive for *M. canis*, there were no false-negative real-time PCR results.[65] False-positive real-time PCR results were common primarily from fomite carriage and real-time PCR was found to be inferior to fungal culture for determination of mycologic cure. PCR-based molecular methods have also been used to study the epidemiology of dermatophytosis and trace the source of human infections to animals; in one report, microsatellite-primed PCR fingerprinting was used to identify a carrier cat as a possible source of *M. canis* infection.[66]

In untreated animals, real-time PCR can be used to evaluate suspect skin lesions, and a negative test is highly suggestive that dermatophytosis is not present unless specimens of suboptimal quality are submitted. PCR assays, like toothbrush fungal cultures, cannot differentiate fomite carriers from truly infected animals, but with a toothbrush fungal culture, quantitative reporting (CFU/plate) helps to distinguish fomite carriage from active infection. Because PCR detects DNA from both viable and nonviable fungi, cured animals may have positive test results. A negative PCR test in an animal with apparent clinical cure also suggests mycological cure. However, if the PCR test is positive then a dermatophyte culture needs to be performed to determine if the PCR detected viable or nonviable fungal DNA. Pending the results of dermatophyte culture, topical antifungal therapy should be continued.

Specimen collection. Specimen quality is important for fungal PCR testing. The active infection is present in the hair follicle, making it important to submit a specimen that contains hair bulbs. A Wood's lamp or dermoscope can be used to identify suspect lesions or hairs. If crusted lesions are present, the crust should be gently lifted, taking care not to dislodge hairs. Hairs can be plucked with forceps and transferred to a sterile container. Alternatively, a target lesion can be aggressively combed with a toothbrush and then the entire toothbrush is submitted.

TREATMENT AND PROGNOSIS

Although dermatophytosis is a self-limiting disease in immunocompetent animals, treatment is recommended to shorten the course of infection because it is a contagious and zoonotic disease. Optimum treatment involves the use of a systemic antifungal drug to eradicate the infection in the hair follicle, topical therapy to disinfect the haircoat, and routine cleaning of the environment. The primary purpose of the environmental cleaning is to minimize problems associated with positive fungal cultures due to environmental contamination and not true disease during the treatment period. Recent treatment consensus guidelines state that "confinement needs to be used with care and for the shortest time possible". Dermatophytosis is a curable disease, but behavior problems and socialization problems can be lifelong if the young or newly adopted animals are not socialized properly. Veterinarians need to consider animal welfare and quality of life when making this recommendation.[50] Treatment is continued until there is both clinical and mycological cure.

Topical Antifungal Drug Treatment

Topical antifungal therapy is an equally important part of the treatment of dermatophytosis and is used in conjunction with a systemic antifungal drug (Box 78.4). Topical therapy removes dermatophytes from the haircoat, which is the source of infection for other animals and people. Topical therapy minimizes shedding of spores in the environment, minimizing the potential for false-positive fungal cultures and unnecessarily prolonged treatment. Haircoat disinfection is critical for mycological cure. The most common cause of a "persistent positive culture" in an animal that is otherwise clinically normal is a nidus

BOX 78.4 General Recommendations for Topical Antifungal Therapy

Clipping of haircoat not always indicated or possible; if done, use blunt-ended metal-tipped scissors.
Topical therapy should be continued until mycological cure is documented, even if systemic therapy has been completed.
Topical therapy with antifungal shampoos can be used on exposed but unaffected household pets.
Whole-body topical therapy is indicated to treat the haircoat; adjuvant focal therapy is recommended for hard-to-treat areas that might be inadequately treated by a client with a rinse or shampoo.
Whole-body topical therapy should be used concurrently with systemic antifungal therapy.

Whole-body therapy (twice weekly, wear gloves)

Leave-on rinses:
- Lime sulfur: 8 ounces (237 mL) in 120 ounces (3.55 L) of warm water for proper dilution. This is a 1:16 dilution and must be prepared just before use.[a]
- Enilconazole 100mg/mL (Imaverol, Austrazole): Dilute 1:50 or 20mL enilconazole with 1L water to make a 0.2% solution

Shampoo (no residual activity):
- Miconazole/chlorhexidine formulations are synergistic and recommended. Chlorhexidine alone is ineffective.
- Miconazole, ketoconazole, climbazole formulations are options.
- 3 to 10 minutes contact time, rinse coat thoroughly.

Adjuvant local therapy

For lesions and hard-to-treat areas such as face, periocular areas, or ears:
Apply once daily, wear gloves
1% terbinafine, 1 to 2% miconazole, 1% ketoconazole applied twice daily
1 to 2% vaginal miconazole can be used on periocular lesions
For ears, consider antibacterial drug-free otic preparations that contain ketoconazole or miconazole

Special cases

Shampoos can be used to treat the haircoat of exposed but unaffected housemates.
Leave-on mousse formulations can be used on pets initially if wetting is not possible.

[a] Lime sulfur veterinary products and lime sulfur agricultural products may be labeled differently. Agricultural products may list the active ingredient as 23% calcium polysulfide or 23% sulfur sulfide. These formulations are identical to veterinary-labeled products and should be diluted no differently, i.e., 1:16. It is very important to thoroughly shake lime sulfur containers as the ingredients will settle.

of infection on the face and/or in the ears. Maximum protection from exposure to spores is provided from products with residual activity, namely lime sulfur or enilconazole.

In general, clipping the entire haircoat is not recommended, as this may worsen clinical signs and spread infection. The use of electric clippers is strongly discouraged, as clippers can overheat and cause thermal injury. Electric clipper blades require meticulous gross decontamination before being sterilized. Disposal of electric clipper blades is an option, albeit an expensive one. Clipping of focal lesions or the whole haircoat should be performed with metal round-tipped children's scissors ("scissor clipping"). Animals should be clipped on newspaper to allow for easy disposal of infective material. Pretreatment with one or two lime sulfur rinses before clipping can minimize contamination of the environment. Longhaired adult cats and/or Yorkshire terriers may need to be clipped if the infection is not easily eradicated, recurrent, and/or if matted or thick fur make it difficult to thoroughly soak the haircoat and the surface of the skin.

Twice-weekly whole-body rinses or antifungal shampoos are recommended for the duration of therapy of infected animals. Additionally, topical whole-body rinses or antifungal shampoo treatments can be used to treat exposed uninfected animals and/or to minimize the risk of transmission to other animals in a household. A recent extensive evidence-based review of topical antifungal therapies found that products with documented clinical efficacy included lime sulfur dips (4–8 oz/gal or 15–30 mL/L), 0.2% enilconazole rinses (available in Canada and Europe), and combination miconazole/chlorhexidine shampoos.[50,67-72] *In vitro*, antifungal shampoos containing miconazole, ketoconazole, climbazole, or accelerated hydrogen peroxide are antifungal when used with a minimum of a 3-minute contact time.[73] Lime sulfur and enilconazole are fungicidal on contact and are leave-on, whole-body solutions with residual activity. Lime sulfur veterinary products and lime sulfur agricultural products may be labeled differently. Agricultural products may list the active ingredient as 23% calcium polysulfide or 23% sulfur sulfide. These formulations are identical to veterinary-labeled products and should be diluted no differently, that is, to 1:16. It is important to thoroughly shake lime sulfur containers prior to dilution as the ingredients will settle, and to freshly dilute the dip for each treatment.

Antifungal shampoos do not have any residual activity and so are a second-line treatment option to dips. In one author's experience (KAM), a leave-on climbazole mousse was effective as topical therapy in several situations where animals could not be wetted.

Local antifungal therapy (once or twice daily) with a topical azole or terbinafine cream as an adjunct therapy to whole-body rinses or shampoos is recommended for lesions in areas on the face and/or ears. Vaginal miconazole cream is a common ophthalmologic treatment for fungal keratitis and can be safely used to treat lesions around the eyes. Topical otic preparations containing miconazole, clotrimazole, or ketoconazole can be used daily to disinfect hairs within the ear.

TABLE 78.3 Systemic Antifungal Drugs for the Treatment of Dermatophytosis

Drug	Dose (mg/kg)	Route	Interval (Hours)	Comments
Itraconazole	5	PO	Cats: Alternating weekly schedule for three cycles Dogs: 24	Cycle may need to be repeated in cats with severe infections
Terbinafine	30–40	PO	24	
Ketoconazole	5	PO	Dogs: 24	Do not use in cats
Griseofulvin microsize	25–50	PO	24	Give with a fatty meal
Griseofulvin ultramicrosize	15	PO	q24h	Give with a fatty meal

Systemic Antifungal Drug Treatment

Systemic antifungal therapy eradicates the fungal infection within the hair follicle and is used in conjunction with topical antifungal therapy and environmental cleaning (Table 78.3). It is generally indicated in all animals with dermatophytosis as it is the only therapy that eradicates the infection within the hair follicle. Until infection is eradicated from within the hair follicle, the haircoat will be reseeded with spores.

Itraconazole is the drug of choice for the treatment of dermatophytosis. In cats, it is labeled for use at 5 mg/kg q24h on an alternating week-on/week-off treatment schedule for three cycles or until mycological cure. Similar studies have not been conducted in dogs. Itraconazole concentrates in the adipose tissue, sebaceous glands, and hair for weeks after administration.[74] The human brand name or generic 100 mg itraconazole capsules can be used at 5 mg/kg; however, capsules need to be reformulated. Compounded itraconazole in both dogs and cats has poor bioavailability and should not be used.[75,76] When 12 studies involving 316 animals treated with itraconazole for dermatophytosis were reviewed, adverse effects were rare and included salivation, mild anorexia, and vomiting.[50] No deaths were reported. In target animal safety studies in which cats were given 5, 15, and 25 mg/kg itraconazole q48h for 7 days for 17 weeks with an 8-week recovery period, the most common abnormal clinical observations noted were dose-related hypersalivation, vomiting, and loose stool, which were mild to moderate and self-resolving.[77] Elevations in the activity of serum hepatic enzymes above baseline were sporadic, dose related, and rarely above the reference range. In an extensive review of the literature, reports of severe adverse effects of itraconazole were in dogs or cats traced to studies where animals were treated for long periods with high doses for systemic fungal diseases, not dermatophytosis.[50] Itraconazole is safe in kittens as young as 10 days old.[74] Terbinafine has the lowest MIC for *Microsporum* and *Trichophyton* when compared to itraconazole, fluconazole, ketoconazole, or griseofulvin.[78-80] Terbinafine has been used to successfully treat *M. canis* dermatophytosis in experimentally induced infections and infections in laboratory cats, shelter cats, and pet cats.[54,81-85] Like itraconazole, terbinafine is highly concentrated in the hair of cats for several weeks after 14 days of continuous therapy[86]; however, similar studies have not been conducted on dog hair. In some countries, including the United States, terbinafine is available as a generic formulation, making it a cost-effective alternative to itraconazole for treatment of dermatophytosis. Doses of terbinafine in the literature range widely from 5 to 40 mg/kg per day; however, doses of 30–40 mg/kg have been reported to be most effective clinically. When 10 studies that included 284 animals treated with terbinafine were reviewed, the most common adverse effects associated with terbinafine treatment were occasional vomiting, diarrhea, and soft stools.[50] No deaths were reported. With the widespread availability of itraconazole and terbinafine, ketoconazole is not a first-choice systemic antifungal drug. The drug is not well tolerated in cats and more frequently causes vomiting, diarrhea, anorexia, and, with prolonged use, weight loss.[87] Griseofulvin was the first oral systemic antifungal drug for the treatment of dermatophytosis and for decades was the drug of choice. With respect to MIC, it is more active than fluconazole, similar to ketoconazole but less active than terbinafine or itraconazole.[78-80] It is only available in a human formulation. It is a known teratogen and should not be used in pregnant animals. It needs to be administered with a fatty meal to enhance absorption. Vomiting and diarrhea have consistently been reported as the most common adverse effects associated with administration. The most serious potential adverse effect is idiosyncratic bone marrow suppression.[88] Fluconazole has poor efficacy against dermatophytes and the highest MIC compared to itraconazole, terbinafine, ketoconazole, and griseofulvin for both *Microsporum* spp. and *Trichophyton* spp., so it should not be used for treatment of dermatophytosis.[78-80] Well-controlled *in vivo* studies have shown that lufenuron has no efficacy in the treatment of dermatophytosis and should not be used.[89-91]

BOX 78.5 Recommendations for Environmental Disinfection

Key Client Education Points

Dispel "Urban Myths"

Fungal spores do not multiply in the environment.

Fungal spores do not invade homes; they can grow in actively growing hairs and in skin.

Fungal spores do not cause respiratory disease; if they do cause disease it is a skin lesion.

Fungal spores are not "living" structures, it is a dormant stage of the life cycle.

Dermatophyte spores are present in many day-to-day environments.

Key Disinfection Points

If it can be washed, it can be disinfected.

Target areas are easy to detect, look for pet hair.

Mechanical cleaning and scrubbing with detergent are most important and often all that is needed.

Over-the-counter ready-to-use bathroom disinfectants labeled as active against *Trichophyton* spp. are active against animal pathogens. Products containing accelerated hydrogen peroxide are recommended.

Pre-moistened disinfectant wipes, such as accelerated hydrogen peroxide wipes, can be used on surfaces.

Avoid bleach as a disinfectant as it has no detergent properties, easily degrades, and is a human and animal health hazard.

Environmental sampling is not recommended unless there is concern that lack of a cure is due to false-positive fungal culture/PCR results.

Topical therapy on infected pets twice weekly minimizes contamination of the environment with spores.

Confine pet to easily cleaned areas of home.

General Recommendation

Clean as if "company is coming." Cleaning should be performed twice a week and clutter minimized. This is a good general recommendation for any situation where an infectious disease is present.

Specific Recommendations

Soft surfaces (laundry): Wash laundry until no pet hair is visible (1–2 washes); do not over-fill the laundry machine, use the longest agitation cycle available, hot water and/or bleach do not enhance disinfection.

Soft surfaces (carpet or upholstery): Keep pets off the carpet, vacuum daily to remove pet hair, disinfect using beater brush carpet scrubber with two washings. Pretreatment can be performed with an antifungal disinfectant, or an antifungal shampoo can be used as a carpet detergent. Disinfection is possible with hot water extraction.

Smaller hard surfaces (e.g., bowls, kitty litter boxes): Remove visible debris, wash repeatedly in detergent until clean, rinse. This may be all that is needed. Only use ready-to-use household disinfectants, spray surface thoroughly.

Larger hard surfaces (e.g., floor): Mechanically remove debris, especially hair (such as with disposable dust cloths), wash surface with a detergent until visibly clean, rinse, and remove excess water, use disinfectant to remove any remaining spores.

Hard surface furniture: Use commercial electrostatic dusting clothes to remove dust.

Discard disposable items such as collars, cloth or braided leashes, brushes, "clothing," doggie or kitty beds, soft toys.

Environmental Control

For more information on decontamination for dermatophytosis, the reader is referred to the Suggested Readings.[50,92] Cleaning and treatment recommendations are summarized in Box 78.5. Evidence-based studies on environmental decontamination have now shown that it is much easier to decontaminate an environment than past literature suggests and/or what clients may find on internet resources. In a study of 70 homes exposed to cats infected with *M. canis*, 69 of 70 were decontaminated with routine cleaning measures.[93] One home was not decontaminated due to admitted noncompliance with cleaning recommendations. Dermatophyte spores can only live and reproduce in keratin, hence they do not multiply in the environment. Dermatophyte spores are not the same as mildew or mold that overgrows in homes after water damage. Clients will report reading that "ringworm lives" in the environment up to 24 months. This comment stems from a laboratory study where specimens (n = 25 total) were stored and sampled at various time points. In that study, three of six specimens stored between 13 and 24 months were viable on fungal culture medium.[94] However, this study did not document that stored specimens were able to cause disease. In a different study, stored specimens were only viable for 13 months and it was not possible to induce infection in kittens.[95] Severely contaminated environments, such as might be present in hoarding situations, do represent a risk factor for infection in animals under physiological stress or animals that are predisposed to skin microtrauma (such as through flea infestation), or to people working in these types of environments without proper personal protective equipment. In a home, the major risk is false-positive fungal cultures that will lead to prolonged treatment.

The primary purpose of cleaning is to remove infective material from the environment and minimize the potential for false-positive fungal cultures that confound interpretation of post-treatment monitoring using fungal culture or PCR. The focus should be on mechanical cleaning and removal of debris, coupled with washing of the target surface until visibly clean. The surface needs to be rinsed of detergent as this will inactivate many disinfectants. In addition, the surface needs to be free of any excess water as this will dilute disinfectants. A recent study showed that household bathroom cleaners labeled as active against *Trichophyton* spp. are also active against *M. canis*.[96] In addition to systemic antifungal therapy, the most important additional aspect of treatment is to use topical antifungal therapy to disinfect the haircoat. In a recent study, proper cleaning combined with topical therapy removed infective material from homes within 1 week of treatment initiation.[97] The reader is referred to Suggested Readings for information on management and investigation of suspected outbreaks of dermatophytosis.[54,98,99]

Duration of Treatment

Treatment duration depends on the overall health of the patient. Simple infections in otherwise healthy animals resolve quickly. Complicated infections are those that occur in animals under physiological stress. These include more severe infections and infections in animals with comorbidities that necessitate modifications of treatment. Cats that are culture positive but lesion free at the time of sampling can also be considered "complicated" cases because they could represent simple fomite carriage or early infections that were not identified on initial examination. In studies of shelter cats that were intensely monitored via physical examinations, Wood's lamp examinations, and weekly fungal cultures treated with itraconazole (5–10 mg/kg q24h PO) for 21 days and concurrent twice-weekly lime sulfur rinses, found that the time to cure varied from 10 to 49 days in cats with simple infections and 23 to 80 in cats with more complicated infections.[67,100] The recommendation of two negative fungal cultures at 2-week intervals was based on a 1959 study using oral griseofulvin and no topical therapy or environmental disinfection in the treatment of Persian cats with dermatophytosis.[101] A recent study of 371

BOX 78.6 Recommendations for Monitoring Treatment of Dermatophytosis

1. Clinical cure will precede mycological cure and the first post-treatment examination should occur within 4 weeks. If new lesions develop, client compliance with treatment should be reviewed. Topical antifungal therapy should be performed the day before the examination.
2. In animals with *M. canis* infections, examinations should include a careful Wood's lamp examination, especially of sites where lesions were present and then ears, face, and fold areas (e.g., interdigital areas).
3. Treatment should be continued until the animal is culture-negative or is PCR-negative. In animals with simple infections, one negative culture should be sufficient. In animals with complicated infections, two negative fungal cultures may be needed, especially for long-haired animals. Topical therapy should be continued pending fungal culture or PCR results.
4. Animals can be considered mycologically cured if a PCR test is negative. If PCR is positive, fungal culture should be performed to determine if the test was detecting viable spores or nonviable fungal DNA.
5. Quantitative fungal culture is important in interpretation of response to treatment (Box 78.7). Simple results such as "positive" or "negative" are not adequate to determine cure.

BOX 78.7 Use of Quantitative Dermatophyte Culture to Monitor Treatment Success

A fungal culture plate that allows for toothbrush inoculation and easy visualization of colonies should be used. Standard Petri dish fungal culture plates or dual compartment plates are recommended.

Inoculate the plate with 4 to 7 stabs such that the bristles make a pattern on the plate; this ensures enough pressure was used.

Incubate plates in a plastic bag to retain moisture and minimize cross-contamination. Incubate plates at 25°C to 30°C.

No growth can be reported at 14 days.

Examine plates daily by holding them up the light to look for growth.

Record growth twice weekly as NG (no growth); C (contaminant growth, bacterial or fungal); S (suspect growth [early growth of a pale colony or early growth of pale colony with a red color change]); or Pathogen (requires microscopic identification).

In treated animals, the red color change may lag behind the colony growth, especially as the animal approaches cure.

The number of CFUs per plate can be used to monitor response to therapy, designated as a P or "pathogen score."

- P3: ≥10 CFU/plate (often too numerous to count): high-risk pet, active infection
- P2: 5–9 CFU/plate: continue treatment
- P1: 1–4 CFU/plate: most consistent with fomite exposure or exposure to another infected animal. Continue topical therapy, clean the environment, consider the possibility of exposure to an infected animal.

In most cases, animals with severe infections have a P3 score. As treatment progresses, the P score lowers. Cured animals have NG or C scores.

Treated pets that are exposed to fomite contamination commonly have cultures that fluctuate from negative to P1. When this pattern is seen, the owner should be instructed to address hygiene in the home. As fomite contamination is removed, fungal cultures become negative. In addition to identification of fomite exposure, this system rapidly alerts the clinician to animals that are failing therapy or are relapsing for one reason or another. Lack of response to therapy will be evident by a persistently high P score. Relapses will be represented by a sudden increase in CFU/plate.

shelter cats found that the first negative fungal culture was predictive of mycological cure in otherwise healthy cats where there has been good compliance with treatment recommendations[102] (Box 78.6).

Prognosis

Dermatophytosis is not a life-threatening or life-altering disease. It will spontaneously resolve without treatment, though resolution can take weeks to months. However, treatment is strongly recommended to shorten the course of the infection and prevent transmission to other susceptible animals and people. Spontaneous recovery will eradicate active infection in the hair follicle and clinical lesions, but infective spores will remain on the haircoat until removed via shedding of the hair or grooming. In otherwise healthy animals, the prognosis for rapid and complete recovery is good with treatment. This includes kerion reactions in hunting or working dogs. In 23 published cases of kerion reactions in dogs, all dogs recovered and there was no transmission to people. In dogs and cats with pseudomycetomas or mycetomas, prognosis is difficult to predict based upon published studies. Some animals responded to surgical excision with concurrent long courses of systemic antifungal treatment and others did not, relapsed, or were euthanized. The prognosis for resolution of dermatophytosis in animals with irreversible underlying illnesses or in immunocompromised animals is harder to determine and clients should be advised to expect longer treatment periods.

IMMUNITY AND VACCINATION

In cats, as in other species, recovery from dermatophyte infection is dependent upon the development of CMI, not of humoral immunity.[42,103-105] Any factors that impair CMI need to be mitigated. In a clinical situation, this means all aspects of pet health must be addressed (nutrition, parasite control, vaccination, etc.). Immunity from reinfection has been studied in an experimental infection model.[42] Five cats previously recovered from *M. canis* infection were rechallenged and only one cat was reinfected. This required clipping of the haircoat, scarification of the skin, and repeated (n = 3) direct applications of 1.5 mL of harvested *M. canis* macroconidia and hyphae to the scarified site of the skin. The lesion that developed was more inflammatory and of shorter duration than lesions in the control cats that were dermatophyte-naïve. This infection model was robust and not representative of natural infections. As with other infectious agents, recovery results in immunity but under extreme exposure and/or compromise of the host reinfection is possible. If reinfection of a previously treated and recovered animal is suspected, it should first be established that this is not due to fomite carriage. Studies in dogs and cats on the use of fungal vaccines have shown that vaccination is not protective against challenge exposure.[106,107] This makes sense, since recovery from infection is dependent upon cell-mediated immunity and not humoral immunity.

PREVENTION

As with most contagious diseases, prevention relies on avoiding contact with the infectious agent. In hunting and working dogs, it is impossible to prevent exposure to geophilic dermatophytes (*N. gypsea*) in the soil, or pathogens that are transmitted via rodents (e.g., *Trichophyton* spp.). It is not possible to prevent exposure of dogs and cats to dermatophytes of large animals if there is regular exposure. Risk factors for exposure of pet dogs include exposure to other infected dogs at "doggie day care," dog parks, behavior or activity classes, grooming facilities, and boarding facilities. All animals should receive year-round flea and tick preventatives, because skin microtrauma predisposes animals to many skin infections, one of which is dermatophytosis. In addition, dogs could be bathed in an antimicrobial shampoo containing chlorhexidine and miconazole or ketoconazole. This also minimizes the development of secondary bacterial infections which could be misdiagnosed as dermatophytosis.

The greatest risk for introduction of dermatophytosis into a home with an established pet population is the temporary or permanent introduction of a new animal. This includes not only dogs and cats but also small mammals. Any new addition to an established pet population should be isolated from other pets until that pet is examined by a veterinarian to rule out contagious disease. Pending this examination, the pet could be bathed in an antifungal shampoo to remove any fomite carriage of dermatophytes. Careful examination of the skin for lesions and examination with a Wood's lamp is especially important in animals adopted from shelters or rescue operations. Many shelters now have screening protocols in place, so adoptable animals may have already been screened for lesions and/or have had a toothbrush fungal culture. In any situation where there is a pending fungal culture, bathing two to three times weekly with an antifungal shampoo is recommended until fungal culture or PCR results are available.

In veterinary clinics, disease transmission is prevented through use of the same measures for any animal with a known or suspected contagious disease. Animals with known or suspect infectious diseases should remain out of the general waiting area until they can be transported directly to an examination room. During the visit, all procedures should be confined to the examination room to limit the areas hospital staff members need to clean and disinfect. If hospitalization is needed, animals with suspected or confirmed dermatophytosis should be housed in isolation. Antifungal therapy should be continued if possible, but at a minimum, topical therapy with an antifungal leave-on rinse or foam should be administered.

PUBLIC HEALTH ASPECTS

The word "tinea" refers to dermatophytosis in human medicine. The term is commonly used in conjunction with a modifier that designates its anatomic location. For example, "tinea pedis" means dermatophytosis of the feet. Tinea does not refer to any one particular species of dermatophyte; the predominant pathogen of people depends upon clinical localization and geographic area. The most commonly isolated pathogen from people is *Trichophyton rubrum.*[108] The classic dermatophyte lesion of people is commonly described as an erythematous, circular lesion with a raised crusted margin with variable pruritus. This lesion tends to be limited to the glabrous skin. Infections of feet, nails, hair, beards, inguinal areas, and hands have variable clinical presentations.

Dermatophyte species that cause disease in dogs and cats have the potential to cause human disease. *Microsporum canis* is the most common zoophilic dermatophyte. In general, zoophilic and geophilic (*N. gypsea*) species evoke a more profound inflammatory response than anthropophilic dermatophytes; the latter tend to cause more chronic infections in people.

Dermatophytosis is a common skin disease in immunocompromised people; however, the primary pathogen of concern is *T. rubrum*, not *M. canis*. Reports of *M. canis* infection are limited to single case reports of tinea capitis, pseudomycetoma, or mycetoma and were summarized in three reviews.[3-5] Two of the studies were reviews of humans with *M. canis* infections and of 21 cases, animal contact was confirmed in only 7 cases. None of the patients died from the dermatophyte infection and the disease was treatable, but required prolonged therapy. In another more extensive review on severe dermatophytosis and acquired or innate immunodeficiency in 84 patients, the most common pathogen was *T. rubrum* and only a few infections were due to *M. canis*. The most common underlying conditions associated with severe dermatophytosis were solid organ transplantation (n = 28), CARD9 (caspase recruitment domain-containing protein 9) deficiency (n = 19) (a rare immunodeficiency disorder), and HIV infection (n = 9).

People that handle infected animals should wear gloves and protective clothing. In confirmed cases, it is important to educate clients that the only way to treat the haircoat is via topical antifungal therapy. The topical therapy of choice for pets in homes with children and immunocompromised people is lime sulfur or enilconazole rinse applied two to three times weekly. Lime sulfur and enilconazole are immediately fungicidal and provide residual protection, unlike antifungal shampoos.

In the United States and in Europe, there are no regulations regarding isolation of children with tinea capitis. As a general recommendation, children infected by zoophilic dermatophytes may return to childcare facilities and/or school immediately after initiation of topical and systemic antifungal treatment. The recommendation for anthropophilic dermatophytes that are more contagious is at most a 1-week isolation at home.[109]

CASE EXAMPLE

Signalment

"Herman," a 14-year-old neutered male terrier cross dog from Tacoma, WA.

History

Herman had a 5-month history of progressive pruritic hair loss and crusting on three paws and the muzzle extending to the periocular region (see Fig. 78.5). Lesions persisted despite several courses of topical and oral antibacterial drug therapy, various combination topical corticosteroid/antibacterial ointments, and oral oclacitinib. The owner reported seeing scratches on the dog's nose that first appeared after the dog was seen to be digging in the woodbox. These were followed by the development of progressive crusting and hair loss on the muzzle followed by similar lesions on three of four paws (see Fig. 78.7). The dog required an Elizabethan collar to prevent self-trauma. Several other dogs and the owners were reportedly unaffected. The dog had not traveled out of the region. His vaccinations were current and included vaccines for distemper, canine infectious hepatitis, parvovirosis, and rabies.

Current Medications

Levothyroxine (0.02 mg/kg PO q12h), oclacitinib (0.5 mg/kg PO q24h), enrofloxacin (5 mg/kg PO q24h).

Other Medical History

The dog had received thyroid supplementation for the past 5 years with adequate serum post-pill T4 concentrations. The dog had a heart murmur, and was polyuric, polydipsic, and frequently incontinent for the past year. There has been a 1.4-kg weight loss in the past year. Laboratory work performed 2 years before examination was unremarkable.

Physical Examination

Body weight: 7.8 kg

General: Normal mentation. Ambulatory on all four limbs. Temperature = 100.2°F (37.9°C), heart rate = 140 beats/min, respiratory rate = 60 breaths/min, mucous membranes pink, CRT = 1 s.

Integument: Physical examination revealed alopecia, silvery adherent scaling, and crusting, which were present on both pelvic limb paws and the right front paw, with extension to the metatarsi and carpi (see Fig. 78.7). Similar alopecia and crusting were present on the dorsal and lateral aspects of the muzzle with extension to the periocular areas. The right side of the muzzle was more severely affected than the left side, and there was a thin ring of erythema and crusting with easily epilated hair on the periphery of the facial lesions (see Fig. 78.5). There were several spreading erythematous circular lesions on the inguinal area and medial aspect of the thighs.

Eyes, ears, nose, and throat: There was mild crusting present on the frontal and dorsal nasal planum, and the right side was more severely affected than the left side. The right upper and lower eyelids and periocular areas were alopecic, erythematous, patchily hyperpigmented, and mildly crusted. A mild amount of brown waxy debris was present within both ear canals.

Musculoskeletal: A body condition score of 4/9 with mild generalized muscle wasting was noted.

Cardiovascular: Strong femoral pulses were noted. A Grade III/VI left-sided systolic murmur was detected on thoracic auscultation.

Respiratory: No abnormalities were noted.

Gastrointestinal and genitourinary: Abdominal palpation revealed mild hepatomegaly.

Lymph nodes: Both popliteal and the right superficial cervical lymph nodes were mildly enlarged.

Laboratory Findings

CBC: HCT 45.0% (36–60%), MCV 74 fL (58–79 fL), MCHC 33 g/dL (30–38 g/dL), WBC 10,500 cells/μL (4000–15,500 cells/μL), neutrophils 8085 cells/μL (2060–10,600 cells/μL), lymphocytes 945 cells/μL (690–4500 cells/μL), monocytes 1155 cells/μL (0–840 cells/μL), platelets 213,000 platelets/μL (170,000–400,000 platelets/μL).

Serum chemistry profile: BUN 31 mg/dL (6–31 mg/dL), creatinine 0.7 mg/dL (0.5–1.6 mg/dL), glucose 109 mg/dL (70–138 mg/dL), total protein 7.0 g/dL (5.0–7.4 g/dL), albumin 2.8 g/dL (2.7–4.4 g/dL), globulin 4.2 g/dL (1.6–3.6 g/dL), ALT 69 U/L (12–118 U/L), ALP 186 U/L (5–131 U/L).

Urinalysis: SpG 1.012; pH 67.5, 3+ protein (SSA), negative bilirubin, glucose, ketones, WBC, casts, crystals, bacteria, 0–1 RBC/HPF, 2–3 fat droplets/HPF.

Dermatologic Diagnostics

Wood's lamp examination: Negative.

Trichogram for fungal organisms: Negative.

Skin scrapings for mites: Negative.

Cytology of crusted skin lesions: RBCs, neutrophils, macrophages, plasma cells, epithelial cells, scattered fungal hyphae.

Dermatophyte Culture

By day 7 after inoculation of dermatophyte culture, there were innumerable, small, raised, white, fluffy fungal colonies present with concurrent red media color change; microscopic examination of a tape preparation of fungal colonies showed hyphae and numerous small round microconidia. Repeat cytologic examination of fungal colonies on days 10 and 14 showed hyphae and microconidia but no macroconidia (which aid in species identification). Nevertheless, numerous spiral hyphae were noted that were consistent with *Trichophyton* hyphae (see Fig. 78.15). The dermatophyte culture was submitted to a commercial diagnostic laboratory for fungal identification, which confirmed the presence of *Trichophyton mentagrophytes*.

Diagnosis

Dermatophytosis caused by *T. mentagrophytes* and concurrent metabolic disease.

Treatment

Enrofloxacin and oclacitinib were discontinued and topical antifungal therapy was prescribed pending laboratory results based on the cytological findings. Specifically, twice-weekly lime sulfur dips and twice daily terbinafine cream were applied to paw and facial lesions. Environmental decontamination measures were discussed with the owner. The contagious and zoonotic nature of the infection was also discussed.

Once laboratory findings results were available, systemic antifungal therapy was prescribed (terbinafine 30 mg/kg PO q24h). Topical therapy and environmental cleaning were continued until repeat fungal culture (DTM) was negative.

Comments

Other diagnostic tests that were recommended but declined by the owner due to financial constraints included urine protein:creatinine ratio to quantitate proteinuria, a urine cortisol:creatinine ratio to evaluate for hyperadrenocorticism, and an abdominal ultrasound to screen for occult neoplasia if metabolic workup was unrevealing. The owner also declined 14-day dermatophyte recheck cultures but agreed to monthly cultures. At 4 and 8 weeks after treatment initiation the clinical signs were much improved, with resolved crusting/erythema and persistent scarring alopecia on the face and paws. Pruritus had improved to minor paw licking. Dermatophyte cultures at 4 and 8 weeks after treatment initiation were negative. Antifungal therapy was discontinued upon the second negative culture result with no relapse of dermatophytosis.

SUGGESTED READINGS

Newbury S, Moriello K. Feline dermatophytosis: steps for a suspected shelter outbreak. *J Fel Med Surg*. 2014;16:407–418.

Moriello K, Coyner K, Paterson S, et al. Diagnosis and treatment of dermatophytosis in dogs and cats. Clinical Consensus Guidelines of the World Association of Veterinary Dermatology. *Vet Dermatol*. 2017;28:266. e68.

Moriello K. Dermatophtyosis decontamination recommendations. In: Little S, ed. *August's Consultations in Feline Internal Medicine*. St. Louis MO: Elsevier Health Sciences; 2015:334–344.

Moriello K. Feline dermatophytosis aspects pertinent to disease management in single and multiple cat situations. *J Feline Med Surg*. 2014;16:419–431.

Food and Drug Administration. Freedom of information summary. Original new animal drug application: NADA 141-474 Itrafungol™ itraconazole oral solution, cats. For the treatment of dermatophytosis caused by Microsporum canis in cats. Sponsored by: Elanco US, Inc. 2016. Available at: https://animaldrugsatfda.fda.gov/adafda/app/search/public/document/downloadFoi/950.

REFERENCES

1. Negroni R. Historical aspects of dermatomycoses. *Clin Dermatol*. 2010;28:125–132.
2. Neumann G. Ringworm in domestic animals. *J Comp Pathol Ther*. 1905;18:193–207.
3. Rouzaud C, Hay R, Chosidow O, et al. Severe dermatophytosis and acquired or innate immunodeficiency: a review. *J Fungi (Basel)*. 2015;2:4.
4. Elad D. Immunocompromised patients and their pets: still best friends? *Vet J*. 2013;197:662–669.
5. Berg JC, Hamacher KL, Roberts GD. Pseudomycetoma caused by *Microsporum canis* in an immunosuppressed patient: a case report and review of the literature. *J Cutan Pathol*. 2007;34:431–434.
6. Weitzman I, Summerbell RC. The dermatophytes. *Clin Microbiol Rev*. 1995;8:240–259.
7. Taylor JW. One fungus = one name: DNA and fungal nomenclature twenty years after PCR. *IMA Fungus*. 2011;2:113–120.
8. Hawksworth DL, Crous PW, Redhead SA, et al. The Amsterdam declaration on fungal nomenclature. *IMA Fungus*. 2011;2:105–112.
9. Cafarchia C, Iatta R, Latrofa MS, et al. Molecular epidemiology, phylogeny and evolution of dermatophytes. *Infect Genet Evol*. 2013;20:336–351.
10. Lewis DT, Foil CS, Hosgood G. Epidemiology and clinical features of dermatophytosis in dogs and cats at Louisiana State University: 1981–1990. *Vet Dermatol*. 1991;2:53–58.
11. Cafarchia C, Romito D, Sasanelli M, et al. The epidemiology of canine and feline dermatophytoses in southern Italy. *Mycoses*. 2004;47:508–513.
12. Cafarchia C, Romito D, Capelli G, et al. Isolation of *Microsporum canis* from the hair coat of pet dogs and cats belonging to owners diagnosed with *M. canis* tinea corporis. *Vet Dermatol*. 2006;17:327–331.
13. Mancianti F, Nardoni S, Cecchi S, et al. Dermatophytes isolated from symptomatic dogs and cats in Tuscany, Italy during a 15-year-period. *Mycopathologia*. 2002;156:13–18.
14. Debnath C, Mitra T, Kumar A, et al. Detection of dermatophytes in healthy companion dogs and cats in eastern India. *Iran J Vet Res*. 2016;17:20.
15. Seker E, Dogan N. Isolation of dermatophytes from dogs and cats with suspected dermatophytosis in Western Turkey. *Prev Vet Med*. 2011;98:46–51.
16. McAleer R. Keratinophilic fungi on four animal groups. *Aust Vet J*. 1980;56:387–390.
17. Drouot S, Mignon B, Fratti M, et al. Pets as the main source of two zoonotic species of the *Trichophyton mentagrophytes* complex in Switzerland, *Arthroderma vanbreuseghemii* and *Arthroderma benhamiae*. *Vet Dermatol*. 2009;20:13–18.
18. Moriello KA, Kunkle G, DeBoer DJ. Isolation of dermatophytes from the haircoats of stray cats from selected animal shelters in two different geographic regions in the United States. *Vet Dermatol*. 1994;5:57–62.
19. Gordon E, Idle A, DeTar L. Descriptive epidemiology of companion animal dermatophytosis in a Canadian Pacific Northwest animal shelter system. *Can Vet J*. 2020;61:763–770.
20. Long S, Carveth H, Chang YM, et al. Isolation of dermatophytes from dogs and cats in the South of England between 1991 and 2017. *Vet Rec*. 2020;187:e87.
21. DeTar LG, Dubrovsky V, Scarlett JM. Descriptive epidemiology and test characteristics of cats diagnosed with *Microsporum canis* dermatophytosis in a Northwestern US animal shelter. *J Feline Med Surg*. 2019;21:1198–1205.
22. Scott DW, Miller WH, Erb HN. Feline dermatology at Cornell University: 1407 cases (1988–2003). *J Feline Med Surg*. 2013;15:307–316.
23. Sierra P, Guillot J, Jacob H, et al. Fungal flora on cutaneous and mucosal surfaces of cats infected with feline immunodeficiency virus or feline leukemia virus. *Am J Vet Res*. 2000;61:158–161.
24. Olivry T, Power H, Woo J, et al. Anti–isthmus autoimmunity in a novel feline acquired alopecia resembling pseudopelade of humans. *Vet Dermatol*. 2000;11:261–270.
25. Chen C, Su B. Concurrent hyperadrenocorticism in a miniature schnauzer with severe *Trichophyton mentagrophytes* infection. *Vet Dermatol*. 2002;13:211–229.
26. Hall E, Miller W, Medleau L. Ketoconazole treatment of generalized dermatophytosis in a dog with hyperadrenocorticism. *J Am Anim Hosp Assoc*. 1984;20:597–602.
27. Chang SC, Liao JW, Shyu CL, et al. Dermatophytic pseudomycetomas in four cats. *Vet Dermatol*. 2011;22:181–187.
28. de Oliveira Nobre M, Mueller EN, Tillmann MT, et al. Disease progression of dermatophytic pseudomycetoma in a Persian cat. *Rev Iberoam De Micol*. 2010;27:98–100.
29. Black SS, Abemethy TE, Tyler JW, et al. Intra–abdominal dermatophytic pseudomycetoma in a Persian cat. *J Vet Intern Med*. 2001;15:245–248.
30. Nuttall T, German A, Holden S, et al. Successful resolution of dermatophyte mycetoma following terbinafine treatment in two cats. *Vet Dermatol*. 2008;19:405–410.
31. Cerundolo R. Generalized *Microsporum canis* dermatophytosis in six Yorkshire terrier dogs. *Vet Dermatol*. 2004;15:181–187.
32. Carlotti DN, Bensignor E. Dermatophytosis due to *Microsporum persicolor* (13 cases) or *Microsporum gypseum* (20 cases) in dogs. *Canine Pract*. 1999;2:6.
33. Muller A, Guaguere E, Degorce-Rubiales F, et al. Dermatophytosis due to *Microsporum persicolor:* a retrospective study of 16 cases. *Can Vet J*. 2011;52:385–388.
34. DeBoer DJ, Moriello KA. Development of an experimental model of *Microsporum canis* infection in cats. *Vet Microbiol*. 1994;42:289–295.
35. Ogawa H, Summerbell R, Clemons K, et al. Dermatophytes and host defence in cutaneous mycoses. *Med Mycol*. 1997;36:166–173.
36. Zurita J, Hay RJ. Adherence of dermatophyte microconidia and arthroconidia to human keratinocytes in vitro. *J Invest Dermatol*. 1987;89:529–534.
37. Vermout S, Tabart J, Baldo A, et al. Pathogenesis of dermatophytosis. *Mycopathologia*. 2008;166:267–275.
38. Baldo A, Monod M, Mathy A, et al. Mechanisms of skin adherence and invasion by dermatophytes. *Mycoses*. 2012;55:218–223.
39. Duek L, Kaufman G, Ulman Y, et al. The pathogenesis of dermatophyte infections in human skin sections. *J Infect*. 2004;48:175–180.
40. Baldo A, Mathy A, Tabart J, et al. Secreted subtilisin Sub3 from *Microsporum canis* is required for adherence to but not for invasion of the epidermis. *Br J Dermatol*. 2010;162:990–997.
41. Dahl MV. Suppression of immunity and inflammation by products produced by dermatophytes. *J Am Acad Dermatol*. 1993;28:S19–S23.
42. Sparkes AH, Gruffydd-Jones TJ, Stokes CR. Acquired immunity in experimental feline *Microsporum canis* infection. *Res Vet Sci*. 1996;61:165–168.
43. Scarampella F, Zanna G, Peano A, et al. Dermoscopic features in 12 cats with dermatophytosis and in 12 cats with self–induced alopecia due to other causes: an observational descriptive study. *Vet Dermatol*. 2015;26:282. e263.
44. Zanna G, Auriemma E, Arrighi S, et al. Dermoscopic evaluation of skin in healthy cats. *Vet Dermatol*. 2015;26:14. e14.

45. Dong C, Angus J, Scarampella F, et al. Evaluation of dermoscopy in the diagnosis of naturally occurring dermatophytosis in cats. *Vet Dermatol.* 2016;27:275. e265.
46. Asawanonda P, Taylor CR. Wood's light in dermatology. *Int J Dermatol.* 1999;38:801–807.
47. Wolf FT. Chemical nature of the fluorescent pigment produced in *Microsporum*-infected hair. *Nature.* 1957;180:860–861.
48. Wolf FT, Jones EA, Nathan HE. Fluorescent pigment of *Microsporum. Nature.* 1958;182:475–476.
49. Foresman A, Blank F. The location of the fluorescent matter in microsporon infected hair. *Mycopathol Mycol Appl.* 1967;31:314–318.
50. Moriello KA, Coyner K, Paterson S, et al. Diagnosis and treatment of dermatophytosis in dogs and cats. Clinical Consensus Guidelines of the World Association for Veterinary Dermatology. *Vet Dermatol.* 2017;28:266–e268.
51. Sparkes A, Gruffydd-Jones T, Shaw S, et al. Epidemiological and diagnostic features of canine and feline dermatophytosis in the United Kingdom from 1956 to 1991. *Vet Rec.* 1993;133:57–61.
52. Wright A. Ringworm in dogs and cats. *J Small Anim Pract.* 1989;30:242–249.
53. Kaplan W, Georg LK, Ajello L. Recent developments in animal ringworm and their public health implications. *Ann N Y Acad Sci.* 1958;70:636–649.
54. Newbury S, Moriello K, Coyner K, et al. Management of endemic *Microsporum canis* dermatophytosis in an open admission shelter: a field study. *J Feline Med Surg.* 2015;17:342–347.
55. Colombo S, Cornegliani L, Beccati M, et al. Comparison of two sampling methods for microscopic examination of hair shafts in feline and canine dermatophytosis. *Vet (Cremona).* 2010;24:27–33.
56. Kaufmann R, Blum SE, Elad D, et al. Comparison between point–of–care dermatophyte test medium and mycology laboratory culture for diagnosis of dermatophytosis in dogs and cats. *Vet Dermatol.* 2016;27:284–e68.
57. Moriello KA, Verbrugge MJ, Kesting RA. Effects of temperature variations and light exposure on the time to growth of dermatophytes using six different fungal culture media inoculated with laboratory strains and samples obtained from infected cats. *J Feline Med Surg.* 2010;12:988–990.
58. Rezusta A, Gilaberte Y, Vidal–García M, et al. Evaluation of incubation time for dermatophytes cultures. *Mycoses.* 2016;59:416–418.
59. Stuntebeck R, Moriello KA, Verbrugge M. Evaluation of incubation time for *Microsporum canis* dermatophyte cultures. *J Feline Med Surg.* 2018;20:997–1000.
60. Di Mattia D, Fondati A, Monaco M, et al. Comparison of two inoculation methods for *Microsporum canis* culture using the toothbrush sampling technique. *Vet Dermatol.* 2019;30:60. e17.
61. da Cunha KC, Riat A, Normand AC, et al. Fast identification of dermatophytes by MALDI-TOF/MS using direct transfer of fungal cells on ground steel target plates. *Mycoses.* 2018;61:691. 69.
62. Nardoni S, Franceschi A, Mancianti F. Identification of *Microsporum canis* from dermatophytic pseudomycetoma in paraffin-embedded veterinary specimens using a common PCR protocol. *Mycoses.* 2007;50:215–217.
63. Brillowska-Dabrowska A, Michałek E, Saunte DML, et al. PCR test for *Microsporum canis* identification. *Med Mycol.* 2013;51:576–579.
64. Cafarchia C, Gasser RB, Figueredo LA, et al. An improved molecular diagnostic assay for canine and feline dermatophytosis. *Med Mycol.* 2013;51:136–143.
65. Jacobson LS, McIntyre L, Mykusz J. Comparison of real-time PCR with fungal culture for the diagnosis of *Microsporum canis* dermatophytosis in shelter cats: a field study. *J Feline Med Surg.* 2018;20:103–107.
66. Gnat S, Lagowski D, Nowakiewicz A, et al. Tinea corporis by *Microsporum canis* in mycological laboratory staff: unexpected results of epidemiological investigation. *Mycoses.* 2018;61:945–953.
67. Newbury S, Moriello K, Verbrugge M, et al. Use of lime sulphur and itraconazole to treat shelter cats naturally infected with *Microsporum canis* in an annex facility: an open field trial. *Vet Dermatol.* 2007;18:324–331.
68. Paterson S. Miconazole/chlorhexidine shampoo as an adjunct to systemic therapy in controlling dermatophytosis in cats. *J Small Anim Pract.* 1999;40:163–166.
69. Carlotti DN, Guinot P, Meissonnier E, et al. Eradication of feline dermatophytosis in a shelter: a field study. *Vet Dermatol.* 2010;21:259–266.
70. Jaham C, Page N, Lambert A, et al. Enilconazole emulsion in the treatment of dermatophytosis in Persian cats: tolerance and suitability. In: Kwochka KWWT, Von Tscharner C, eds. *Advances in Veterinary Dermatology.* Oxford: Butterworth Heinemann; 1998:299–307.
71. Hnilica KA, Medleau L. Evaluation of topically applied enilconazole for the treatment of dermatophytosis in a Persian cattery. *Vet Dermatol.* 2002;13:23–28.
72. Guillot J, Malandain E, Jankowski F, et al. Evaluation of the efficacy of oral lufenuron combined with topical enilconazole for the management of dermatophytosis in catteries. *Vet Rec.* 2002;150:714–718.
73. Moriello KA. In vitro efficacy of shampoos containing miconazole, ketoconazole, climbazole or accelerated hydrogen peroxide against *Microsporum canis* and *Trichophyton* species. *J Feline Med Surg.* 2016.
74. Food and Drug Administration. Freedom of information summary. Original new animal drug application: NADA 141-474 Itrafungol™ itraconazole oral solution, cats. For the treatment of dermatophytosis caused by Microsporum canis in cats. Sponsored by: Elanco US, Inc. 2016. Available at: https://animaldrugsatfda.fda.gov/adafda/app/search/public/document/downloadFoi/950.
75. Mawby D, Whittemore JC, Genger S, et al. Bioequivalence of orally administered generic, compounded, and Innovator–formulated itraconazole in healthy dogs. *J Vet Intern Med.* 2014;28:72–77.
76. Mawby DI, Whittemore JC, Fowler LE, et al. Comparison of absorption characteristics of oral reference and compounded itraconazole formulations in healthy cats. *J Am Vet Med Assoc.* 2018;252:195–200.
77. Food and Drug Administration. Freedom of information summary. Original new animal drug application: NADA 141-474 Itrafungol™ itraconazole oral solution, cats. For the treatment of dermatophytosis caused by *Microsporum canis* in cats. Sponsored by: Elanco US, Inc. 2016. Available at: https://animaldrugsatfda.fda.gov/adafda/app/search/public/document/downloadFoi/950.
78. Favre B, Hofbauer B, Hildering K-S, et al. Comparison of in vitro activities of 17 antifungal drugs against a panel of 20 dermatophytes by using a microdilution assay. *J Clin Microbiol.* 2003;41:4817–4819.
79. Brilhante RS, Cordeiro R, Medrano DJ, et al. Antifungal susceptibility and genotypical pattern of *Microsporum canis* strains. *Can J Microbiol.* 2005;51:507–510.
80. Perea S, Fothergill AW, Sutton DA, et al. Comparison of in vitro activities of voriconazole and five established antifungal agents against different species of dermatophytes using a broth macrodilution method. *J Clin Microbiol.* 2001;39:385–388.
81. Kotnik T. Treatment with terbinafine of experimentally infected cats with *M. canis*: tolerability and side effects of the drug. *Slov Vet Zb.* 2000;37:67–76.
82. Kotnik T. Drug efficacy of terbinafine hydrochloride (Lamisil®) during oral treatment of cats, experimentally infected with *Microsporum canis. J Vet Med B Infect Dis Vet Public Health.* 2002;49:120–122.
83. Kotnik T, Kožuh Eržen N, Kužner J, et al. Terbinafine hydrochloride treatment of *Microsporum canis* in experimentally-induced ringworm in cats. *Vet Microbiol.* 2001;83:161–168.
84. Mancianti F, Pedonese F, Millanta F, et al. Efficacy of oral terbinafine in feline dermatophytosis due to *Microsporum canis. J Feline Med Surg.* 1999;1:37–41.
85. Moriello K, Coyner K, Trimmer A, et al. Treatment of shelter cats with oral terbinafine and concurrent lime sulphur rinses. *Vet Dermatol.* 2013;24:618. e150.
86. Foust AL, Marsella R, Akucewich LH, et al. Evaluation of persistence of terbinafine in the hair of normal cats after 14 days of daily therapy. *Vet Dermatol.* 2007;18:246–251.
87. Medleau L, Chalmers S. Ketoconazole for treatment of dermatophytosis in cats. *J Am Vet Med Assoc.* 1992;200:77–78.
88. Kunkle G, Meyer D. Toxicity of high doses of griseofulvin in cats. *J Am Vet Med Assoc.* 1987;191:322–323.
89. DeBoer DJ, Moriello KA, Blum JL, et al. Effects of lufenuron treatment in cats on the establishment and course of *Microsporum canis* infection following exposure to infected cats. *J Am Vet Med Assoc.* 2003;222:1216–1220.

90. Moriello KA, Deboer DJ, Schenker R, et al. Efficacy of pre-treatment with lufenuron for the prevention of *Microsporum canis* infection in a feline direct topical challenge model. *Vet Dermatol.* 2004;15:357–362.
91. DeBoer D, Moriello K, Volk L, et al. Lufenuron and terbinafine for treatment of *Microsporum canis* infections in a feline model. *Vet Dermatol.* 2004;15:7–8.
92. Moriello K. Dermatophtyosis decontamination recommendations. In: Little S, ed. *August's Consultations in Feline Internal Medicine*. St. Louis MO: Elsevier Health Sciences; 2015:334–344.
93. Moriello KA. Decontamination of 70 foster family homes exposed to *Microsporum canis* infected cats: a retrospective study. *Vet Dermatol.* 2019;30:178-e55.
94. Sparkes AH, Werrett G, Stokes CR, et al. *Microsporum canis*: inapparent carriage by cats and the viability of arthrospores. *J Small Anim Pract.* 1994;35:397–401.
95. Keep JM. The viability of *Microsporum canis* on isolated cat hair. *Aust Vet J.* 1960;36:277–278.
96. Moriello KA, Kunder D, Hondzo H. Efficacy of eight commercial disinfectants against *Microsporum canis* and *Trichophyton spp.* infective spores on an experimentally contaminated textile surface. *Vet Dermatol.* 2013;24:621. e152.
97. Nardoni S, Giovanelli S, Pistelli L, et al. In vitro activity of twenty commercially available, plant-derived essential oils against selected dermatophyte species. *Nat Prod Commun.* 2015;10:1473–1478.
98. Newbury S, Moriello KA. Feline dermatophytosis: steps for investigation of a suspected shelter outbreak. *J Feline Med Surg.* 2014;16:407–418.
99. Moriello K. Feline dermatophytosis: aspects pertinent to disease management in single and multiple cat situations. *J Feline Med Surg.* 2014;16:419–431.
100. Newbury S, Moriello KA, Kwochka KW, et al. Use of itraconazole and either lime sulphur or Malaseb Concentrate Rinse (R) to treat shelter cats naturally infected with *Microsporum canis*: an open field trial. *Vet Dermatol.* 2011;22:75–79.
101. Kaplan W, Ajello L. Oral treatment of spontaneous ringworm in cats with griseofulvin. *J Am Vet Med Assoc.* 1959;135:253–261.
102. Stuntebeck LR, Moriello KA. One vs two negative fungal cultures to confirm mycological cure in 371 shelter cats treated for *Microsporum canis* dermatophytosis: a retrospective study. *J Feline Med Surg.* 2020;22:598-601.
103. DeBoer D, Moriello K. The immune response to *Microsporum canis* induced by a fungal cell wall vaccine. *Vet Dermatol.* 1994;5:47–55.
104. DeBoer DJ, Moriello KA. Humoral and cellular immune responses to *Microsporum canis* in naturally occurring feline dermatophytosis. *J Med Vet Mycol.* 1993;31:121–132.
105. Moriello KA, DeBoer DJ, Greek J, et al. The prevalence of immediate and delayed type hypersensitivity reactions to *Microsporum canis* antigens in cats. *J Feline Med Surg.* 2003;5:161–166.
106. DeBoer DJ, Moriello KA. Investigations of a killed dermatophyte cell-wall vaccine against infection with *Microsporum canis* in cats. *Res Vet Sci.* 1995;59:110–113.
107. DeBoer DJ, Moriello KA, Blum JL, et al. Safety and immunologic effects after inoculation of inactivated and combined live-inactivated dermatophytosis vaccines in cats. *Am J Vet Res.* 2002;63:1532–1537.
108. Nenoff P, Krüger C, Ginter–Hanselmayer G, et al. Mycology–an update. Part 1: dermatomycoses: causative agents, epidemiology and pathogenesis. *J Dtsch Dermatol Ges.* 2014;12:188–210.
109. Nenoff P, Krüger C, Paasch U, et al. Mycology–an update Part 3: dermatomycoses: topical and systemic therapy. *J Dtsch Dermatol Ges.* 2015;13:387–411.

79

Malassezia Dermatitis

Ross Bond

KEY POINTS

- First Described: *Malassezia pachydermatis* was first described in 1925 by Weidman in the skin scales of an Indian rhinoceros (*Rhinoceros unicornis*) with a generalized exfoliative dermatitis, kept in a zoological collection in Philadelphia, USA.[1]
- Causes: Dogs: *Malassezia pachydermatis*. Cats: *Malassezia pachydermatis*, occasionally other strictly lipid-dependent species.
- Affected Hosts: Mammals and birds.
- Geographic Distribution: Worldwide.
- Primary Mode of Transmission: Horizontal and vertical (at birth).
- Major Clinical Signs: *Malassezia* spp. invade opportunistically and cause a pruritic, greasy, malodorous, erythematous dermatitis commonly centered on folds or intertriginous areas.
- Differential Diagnoses: Hypersensitivity disorders, bacterial overgrowth and pyoderma, primary defects of cornification.
- Human Health Significance: *Malassezia pachydermatis* is a potential cause of fungemia in neonates in intensive care facilities. Other strictly lipid-dependent *Malassezia* spp. are commensal fungi of human skin that are implicated in various human skin diseases, including seborrheic dermatitis, pityriasis versicolor, and the "head-neck" form of atopic dermatitis.

ETIOLOGY AND EPIDEMIOLOGY

Malassezia spp. (previously *Pityrosporum* spp.) are lipophilic yeasts that reproduce asexually by monopolar or sympodial budding. These yeasts, classified within the class Malasseziomycetes in the subphylum Ustilaginomycotina of the phylum Basidiomycota, are most often isolated from the skin and mucosal sites of clinically healthy mammals and birds. The genus was traditionally divided into two groups based on their lipid dependency in culture media. *Malassezia pachydermatis* has long been regarded as unique within the genus in that it can be cultivated routinely on Sabouraud's dextrose agar without lipid supplementation (hence "lipophilic" but not "lipid-dependent"). *Malassezia pachydermatis* has remarkable genetic diversity.[2] This is apparently linked to evolutionary adaptation to the variety of its animal hosts, variation in distribution within those hosts,[3] and variable expression of putative virulence factors.[4]

The application of molecular biological techniques has led to substantial taxonomic revision amongst *Malassezia* spp., and 18 species are now recognized, namely *Malassezia furfur, Malassezia pachydermatis, Malassezia sympodialis, Malassezia globosa, Malassezia obtusa, Malassezia restricta, Malassezia slooffiae, Malassezia dermatis, Malassezia japonica, Malassezia yamatoensis, Malassezia nana, Malassezia caprae, Malassezia equina, Malassezia cuniculi, Malassezia arunalokei, Malassezia brasiliensis, Malassezia psittaci*, and *Malassezia verspertilionis*[5–9] (Table 79.1). Lipid dependence has recently been attributed to lack of the fatty acid synthase gene in the genome of all 14 species whose genome has been sequenced, including *M. pachydermatis*.[10–12] It is now clear that *M. pachydermatis* should be reconsidered as "lipid-dependent"; the ability to grow on Sabouraud's dextrose agar reflects a markedly enhanced ability to metabolize trace lipids derived from the peptone content of the Sabouraud's medium,[12] although this is somewhat academic given the widespread use of Sabouraud's medium in diagnostic veterinary laboratories.

In studies of the mycobiota of normal canine and feline skin, *Malassezia* spp. comprise a surprisingly small percentage of the fungal population[13,14]; instead, environmental molds such as *Alternaria* predominate. Dogs are very frequently colonized by *M. pachydermatis* but very rarely colonized by strictly lipid-dependent *Malassezia* spp.[15,16] Healthy cats are often colonized by *M. pachydermatis* and occasionally by strictly lipid-dependent species, including *M. sympodialis, M. globosa, M. furfur, M. slooffiae*, and *M. nana*.[17–20] *Malassezia nana* is the most common strictly lipid-dependent *Malassezia* sp. isolated from cats' ears. *Malassezia slooffiae* has been isolated from the claw folds of cats with seborrheic dermatitis.[21] The pathogenic potential of lipid-dependent *Malassezia* spp. in feline skin disease requires further assessment. Strictly lipid-dependent species are frequently isolated from human skin and are associated with a number of diseases,[22] but isolation of *M. pachydermatis* is rare.

In dogs, *M. pachydermatis* is frequently isolated from the haired skin of the chin and lips, interdigital skin, and external ear canal and less often from other intertriginous areas such as the axilla and groin.[23] Concentrations of organisms in healthy dogs are generally low but are markedly increased, often up to 10,000-fold, in many cases of *Malassezia* dermatitis, although overlap in organism densities can be found between some clinically healthy and affected dogs. The anatomic sites most often colonized in clinically healthy animals correlate with regions most often affected in dogs with skin disease caused by the yeast.

Malassezia dermatitis may be the only disease recognized in some dogs, but in others, concurrent disorders such as allergies, especially atopic disease, keratinization defects, endocrinopathies, and the presence of skin folds may be important in favoring proliferation of the yeast. *Malassezia pachydermatis* infection in dogs is an important "flare factor" for canine atopic dermatitis.[24] Breed predilections vary between geographic regions but may include basset hounds, West Highland white terriers, cocker spaniels, toy and miniature poodles, dachshunds, boxers, Cavalier King Charles spaniels, shih tzus, Australian silky terriers, and German shepherd dogs. Bull terriers with lethal acrodermatitis are known to have impaired immune function, and they harbor large numbers of *Malassezia* on their skin; *Candida albicans* co-infection may be partly responsible for lesions in the nails and footpads of these dogs. A seasonal increase in case numbers may

TABLE 79.1 Summary of the (2018) Taxonomy and Ecology of the Genus *Malassezia*

Species	Identified	Former Designations	Usual Source
M. furfur	1889	*Pityrosporum ovale*	Human PV
M. pachydermatis	1925	*Pityrosporum pachydermatis (Pityrosporum canis)*	Canids, rhinoceros
M. sympodialis	1990	*M. furfur* serovar A	Human PV
M. globosa	1996	*M. furfur* serovar B	Human PV/SD/AD
M. obtusa	1996		Humans (healthy)
M. slooffiae	1996		Humans + animals
M. restricta	1996	*M. furfur* serovar C	Human dandruff
M. dermatis	2002		Human AD
M. japonica	2003		Human AD
M. nana	2004		Cat (ears)
M. yamatoensis	2004		Human SD
M. caprae	2007		Goat
M. equina	2007	*Malassezia equi*	Horse
M. cuniculi	2011		Rabbit
M. arunalokei	2016		Human SD
M. brasiliensis	2016		Parrot
M. psittaci	2016		Parrot
M. verpertilionis	2018		Bat

AD, atopic dermatitis; *PV*, pityriasis versicolor; *SD*, seborrheic dermatitis.

be observed in geographic regions where a noticeable change to warm, humid climatic conditions is present.

Affected cats also may have underlying allergic and metabolic diseases, but immunosuppressive viruses such as FeLV and FIV, and paraneoplastic disorders (pancreatic paraneoplastic alopecia, exfoliative dermatitis with thymoma), may also favor infection. Devon Rex and Sphynx cats are predisposed to a seborrheic dermatitis associated with high *Malassezia* populations; Rex cats respond well to systemic therapy with itraconazole.[21,25–27] Molecular analysis of species colonizing Devon Rex cats showed a preponderance of *M. restricta* and *M. globosa*.[28]

CLINICAL FEATURES

Pathogenesis and Clinical Signs

The interactions between *Malassezia* yeasts and the skin of their mammalian hosts, and the factors which influence transition from commensal to pathogen, are the subject of intensive scientific endeavor, especially pertaining to the common skin pathogens of humans (*M. globosa, M. sympodialis, M. restricta*).[29] Adhesion of *Malassezia* cells to keratinocytes has the potential to modulate the expression of an array of cytokines, chemokines, and antimicrobial peptides, the outcome of which may be immune-stimulatory (as may occur in disease states) or immune-suppressive (promoting commensal carriage).[30] A change in host immunity, altered skin microclimate, or disruption in epidermal physiology associated with the diseases mentioned previously may predispose animals to clinical disease. Co-proliferation of staphylococci in the same lesions may exacerbate clinical signs and necessitates concurrent antibacterial therapy in some cases (Fig. 79.1).

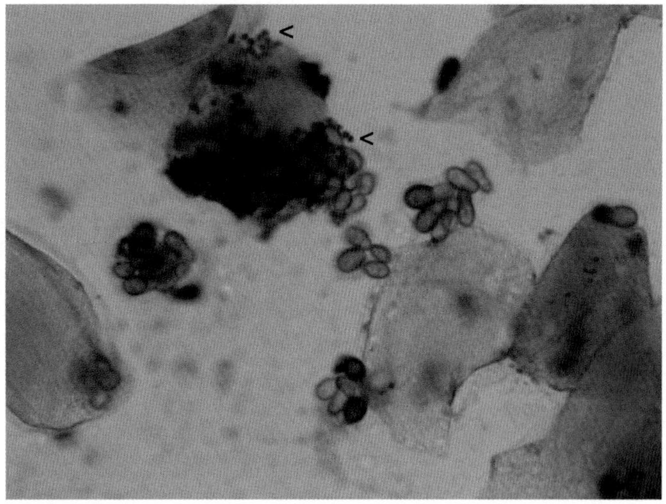

Fig. 79.1 Tape-strip cytologic specimen obtained from the ventral neck of a 4-year-old entire male basset hound with *Malassezia* dermatitis. Numerous aggregates of monopolar-budding yeasts with the typical morphology of *Malassezia pachydermatis* lying amongst or adherent to stratum corneum cells (squames) are accompanied by smaller numbers of coccoid bacteria *(black arrowheads)*. Diff-Quik stain, ×3000.

Comparative studies following the recent sequencing of 14 *Malassezia* species' genomes have significantly advanced opportunities for understanding of the adaption of the genus to its limited ecologic niches (mainly skin), elucidation of virulence factors necessary for colonization and infection, and identification of novel interventional targets for therapy.[12] The genus' evolution to lipid-dependency is associated with a wide expansion of lipase and phospholipase genes, and loss of carbohydrate metabolism genes. Lipases are highly expressed in the skin of human patients with seborrheic dermatitis and likely damage the epidermal barrier directly and by hydrolysis of triglycerides.[22,31] Phospholipase activity, modulated by the endogenous opioid peptide β endorphin,[32] was significantly higher amongst *M. pachydermatis* isolates derived from the dogs with otitis externa[33] or skin lesions[34] when compared with those obtained from the dogs with healthy external ears, or nonlesional skin, respectively. Other enzymes from *Malassezia* spp. such as aspartyl proteases and acid sphingomyelinases may also influence host-yeast inactions.

Malassezia spp. from human skin synthesize an array of indoles that act as potent ligands for the aryl hydrocarbon receptor (AhR), a nuclear receptor and transcriptional regulator with pleiotropic effects that include down-regulation of immune stimulation, modification of melanogenesis and epidermal cell function, and inhibition of antagonistic microbes.[22,35]

The *M. sympodialis* genome has a relative lack of genes encoding cell wall proteins that mediate adhesion.[36] However, *M. pachydermatis* can form biofilms *in vitro* and on catheters,[37] characterized by layers of adhering blastoconidia embedded in variable quantities of extracellular matrix.[38] This may reduce *in vivo* susceptibility to azole antifungal drugs[39] and act in synergism with phospholipase production to contribute to skin lesions in susceptible dogs.[38]

Whilst IgG serologic responses have been evaluated in dogs with *Malassezia*-associated skin diseases,[30] hypersensitivity responses to *Malassezia*-derived antigens are of greatest relevance to the clinician. Immediate, IgE-mediated reactivity to *M. pachydermatis,* identified by either intradermal or serologic testing,[40] may explain the marked exacerbation of the signs associated with yeast proliferation in sensitized dogs with underlying canine atopic dermatitis, and the associated clinical improvement when antifungal therapy is initiated.[24] Studies of the effectiveness of *Malassezia* allergen–specific immunotherapy with *Malassezia* allergens in atopic dogs with yeast sensitization are required. By contrast, basset hounds with *Malassezia* dermatitis usually show delayed rather than immediate intradermal test reactivity to *Malassezia* antigens,[41] although contact sensitization, as demonstrated by patch test reactivity, more closely correlates with disease status in this breed.[42] These data indicate that a spectrum of immunologic hyper-responsiveness is present in dogs with *Malassezia* dermatitis (none, immediate, delayed, contact), but since similar serologic and skin test reactivity is also seen in a proportion of unaffected dogs, these immunologic tests must be assessed in the context of clinical and cytologic data, and not used as stand-alone "diagnostic" tests.[40]

Dogs

Malassezia dermatitis lesions may be localized or generalized. In dogs, the disease is most often seen at anatomic sites that create a relatively warm, moist skin environment. Thus the interdigital skin, ventral neck, lip region, ear canal, axilla, groin, and folded areas are most often affected. Pruritus is normally reported and ranges in degree from mild to severe. Erythema accompanied by greasy exudation is commonly observed, especially in intertriginous areas where a brown exudate may mat the lower portion of the hair; malodor may be noted with extensive exudative lesions (Figs. 79.2 and 79.3). Traumatic alopecia, lichenification, and hyperpigmentation may develop in dogs with marked pruritus. *Malassezia* otitis externa is often characterized by brown cerumen, with varying levels of associated inflammation. Paronychia (nail-fold inflammation) associated with *M. pachydermatis* may lead to pedal pruritus accompanied by reddish-brown discoloration of the claw and or exudation in the nail fold. Dogs with frenzied facial pruritus associated with *M. pachydermatis* overgrowth of muzzle skin or lip-folds may be misdiagnosed as having neurologic disease. *Malassezia pachydermatis* is occasionally implicated as a cause of keratomycosis in dogs.[43,44]

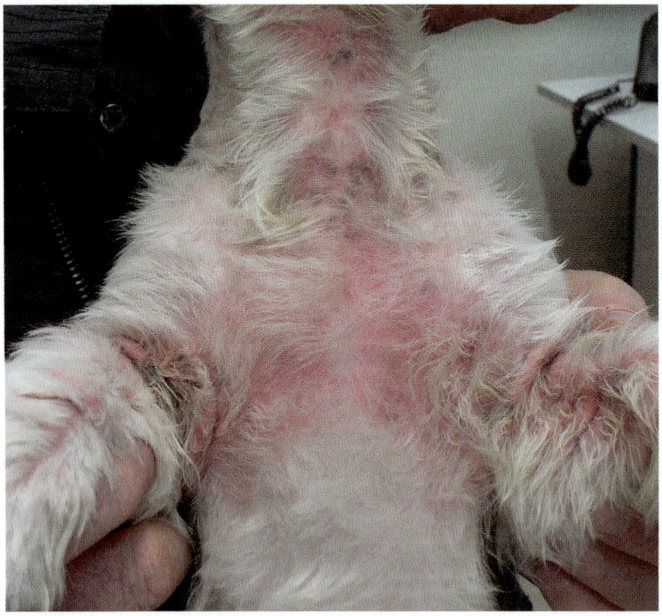

Fig. 79.2 A 4-year-old neutered male West Highland white terrier with severe *Malassezia* dermatitis. Lesions comprise intense erythema of the ventral neck, axillae, and medial aspect of the forelimbs with a rather demarcated and symmetric distribution. The hair overlying folded ridges of intensely inflamed and thickened skin is matted in a yellow, greasy, malodorous exudate. Focal areas of lichenification and hyperpigmentation are developing in the alopecic regions of the ventral neck.

Cats

Malassezia pachydermatis appears to be a relatively infrequent pathogen in cats, at least when compared with dogs. This finding may reflect the lower carriage rates of the yeast in the skin and ears of healthy cats. Ceruminous otitis externa responsive to topic otic antifungal medication is the most common clinical feature of *M. pachydermatis*–associated skin disease in cats, but occasional cases of localized or generalized *M. pachydermatis*–associated dermatitis have been described. Exfoliative erythroderma, greasy exudation, and varying degrees of pruritus may be seen. In Devon Rex cats with seborrheic dermatitis caused by *Malassezia* spp., greasy, tightly adherent, brown exudate on the claws or in the claw folds is often accompanied by a dark, greasy exudate that mats the hairs on the interdigital skin, axilla, and groin (Figs. 79.4 and 79.5). Cats with exfoliative dermatitis associated with thymoma and paraneoplastic alopecia may have concurrent proliferations of *Malassezia*.

DIAGNOSIS

The clinical signs of *Malassezia* dermatitis are not pathognomonic, and the disease should be routinely suspected in dogs with inflammatory skin diseases, especially those with erythema or greasy exudation as a dominant sign. *Malassezia* dermatitis may mimic or complicate both food-induced and nonfood-induced canine atopic dermatitis. Seborrheic presentations and fold-associated diseases should also prompt an evaluation of the presence and numbers of the yeast. The diagnosis is based on clinical signs, presence of elevated numbers of the yeast in lesional skin, *and* a clinical and mycologic response to antifungal therapy; it is important to recognize that high populations of *M. pachydermatis* can occur in clinically normal skin.

Microbiologic Tests

Cytologic Diagnosis

In clinical practice, yeast numbers are most usefully assessed by cytologic examination. Impression smears can be made directly onto glass slides, or exudate can be transferred to the slide using swabs. However, the author prefers the tape-strip method; clear cellophane tape is pressed on the surface of the skin, thus collecting the stratum corneum cells and any superficial microbes.[45] Unlike direct impressions, tape

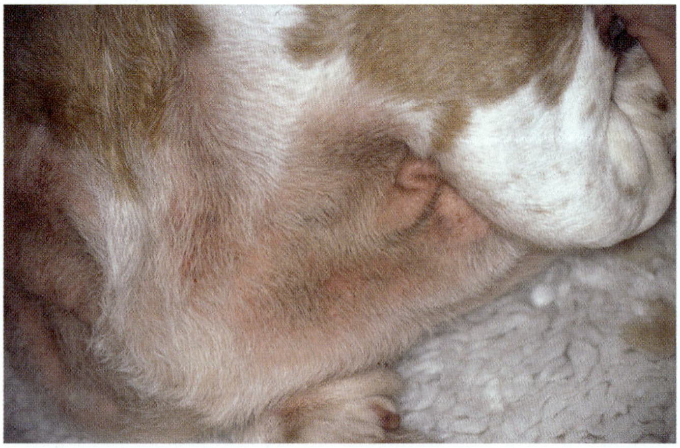

Fig. 79.3 A 2-year-old entire female basset hound with severe *Malassezia* dermatitis. Lesions comprise intense erythema and lichenification of the axillae, sternum, and ventral neck. The brown, greasy, malodorous exudate adherent to the lower portion of the hair shafts is clinically suggestive of microbial overgrowth (rather than an uncomplicated allergic dermatitis), most commonly associated with *Malassezia pachydermatis*, but also occasionally with bacterial overgrowth.

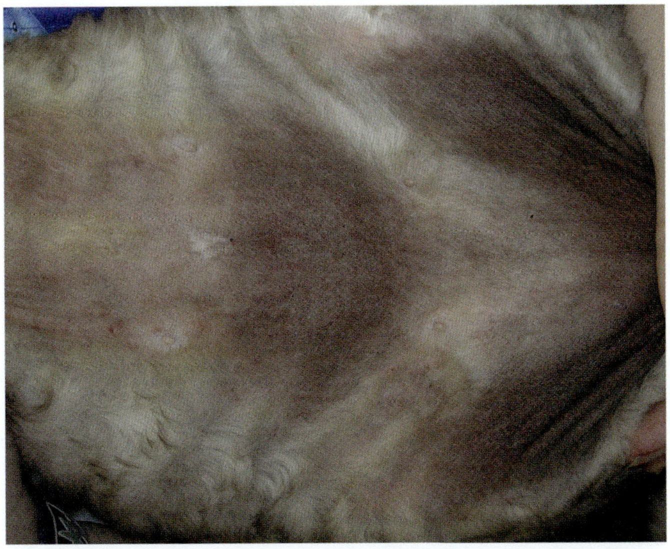

Fig. 79.4 *Malassezia* dermatitis in a 10-year-old female Devon Rex cat is manifest by alopecia, erythema, and demarcated, symmetric areas of brown discoloration of the skin of the ventral abdomen and medial thighs.

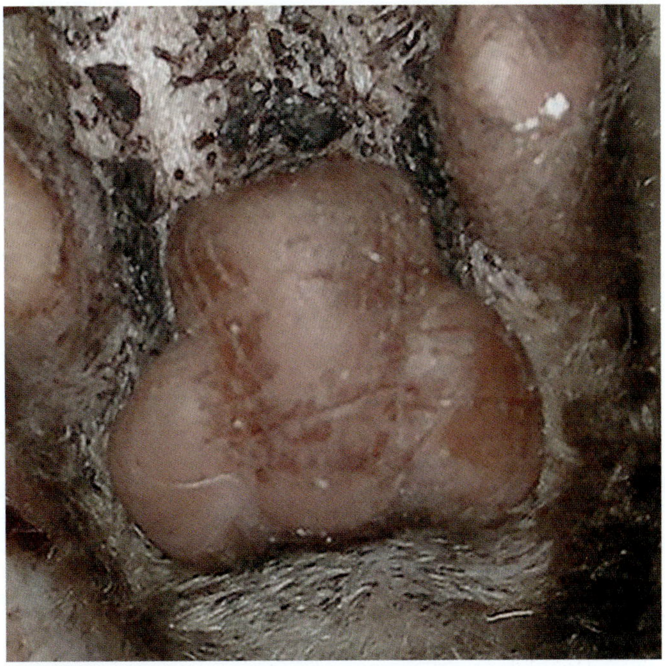

Fig. 79.5 *Malassezia* dermatitis in a 10-year-old female Devon Rex cat is manifest by a marked accumulation of a copious dark exudate adherent to the hairs of the palmar interdigital skin.

stripping can be used effectively in most anatomic sites and in dry or greasy lesions. The tape is stained, usually with a modified Wright stain, and examined using the light microscope (see Fig. 79.1). Characteristic peanut-shaped *Malassezia* spp. yeast cells are rarely seen in healthy skin but are usually readily identified in specimens from affected individuals. The use of swabs for cytology is best restricted to the ear canal.[23]

Although some authors have proposed guidelines on the number of yeasts needed for significance (e.g., one or more yeast per high-power field), this approach does not accommodate the overlap seen in yeast population densities in skin specimens from clinically healthy and diseased dogs. In addition, there are important breed and anatomic site differences in yeast population sizes in healthy dogs. In addition, hypersensitivity responses to yeast-derived allergens might enable a relatively small number of organisms to generate skin disease in sensitized individuals. Thus, a therapeutic trial is an important component in the diagnostic evaluation of *Malassezia* dermatitis. Treatment should be recommended whenever the yeast is readily identified in cytologic specimens obtained from consistent lesions.[23]

Culture

Culture of swab specimens is of limited diagnostic value because it merely confirms or refutes the presence of a commensal yeast. Cellophane tape-strip sampling just described for cytology can also be used to transfer cells to the surface of culture plates, although the potential for an antimicrobial effect of the adhesive tape should be considered. *Malassezia pachydermatis* can be isolated using Sabouraud's dextrose agar, modified Dixon's agar, or Leeming's medium, with optimal growth at temperatures between 32°C and 37°C. Lipid-supplemented media should be used when specimens are taken from cats because strictly lipid-dependent species may be present (Fig. 79.6); species identification of these yeasts is specialized and most reliably accomplished by molecular methods. The application of MALDI-TOF MS has led to improved and more rapid identification of *Malassezia* spp. following culture.[46–48]

Concerns have been raised about the increasing prevalence of antifungal drug resistance among pathogenic fungi. Treatment failures in human patients with *M. furfur* fungemia have suggested the possibility that resistance exists[49]; around the time of writing, multi-azole–resistant strains of *M. pachydermatis* have been isolated from dogs with refractory *Malassezia* dermatitis in Japan and Italy.[50,51] Genetic studies suggested that resistance in the isolate from the dog in Japan was due to overexpression of genes that encode ABC transporter proteins or mutations in *ERG11*. Unfortunately, susceptibility testing methods for *Malassezia* have not been standardized, and currently interpretive breakpoints for antifungal susceptibility testing of *Malassezia* species are not available. E-testing and broth microdilution methods have been used in the literature, and suspicion for resistance has been based on very high MICs (e.g., > 32) when compared with control isolates.

Molecular Diagnosis Using Nucleic Acid–Based Testing

At this time, molecular methods based on PCR are not in widespread use for diagnosis of *Malassezia* spp. infections in dogs and cats. However, a multiplex PCR method has been described for the detection of 11 *Malassezia* species in both samples obtained directly from skin and colonies in conventional culture systems.[52] A quantitative real-time PCR assay based on the β-tubulin gene appeared to be accurate and potentially more sensitive than cytologic examination when applied to swabs from dogs with otitis externa, which also has the potential to be used to monitor treatment response.[53] Molecular typing methods such as MLST, random amplified polymorphic DNA (RAPD), PFGE, and next-generation sequencing have been used as powerful tools for epidemiologic studies (see Chapter 7).[23]

Pathologic Findings

Skin biopsy specimens from animals with *Malassezia* spp. infections typically show marked irregular epidermal hyperplasia of the skin surface but extending to follicular infundibula, variable hyperkeratosis and parakeratosis, spongiosis especially of the deep one third of the epidermis, and a superficial perivascular or interstitial infiltrate of mononuclear cells, with focal accumulations of neutrophils, eosinophils, and mast cells (Fig. 79.7). Yeast cells may be seen in the stratum corneum, but the disruption of this layer that occurs during routine tissue processing may lead to an absence of the yeast; biopsy has a low sensitivity

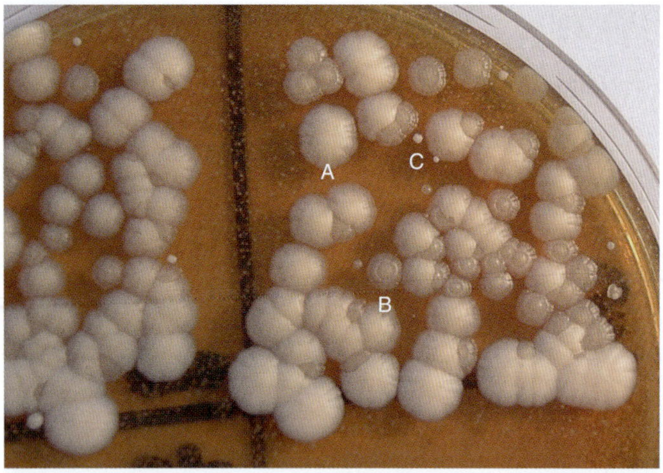

Fig. 79.6 Modified Dixon's agar plate inoculated with a swab from the claw fold of a 10-year-old female seborrhoeic Devon Rex cat. Two colony types of *Malassezia pachydermatis* are represented; large, domed, entire yellow colonies (above *A*) and smaller, buff-colored, domed or umbonate colonies (above *B*). The smaller yellow colonies are examples of *Malassezia slooffiae* (above *C*).

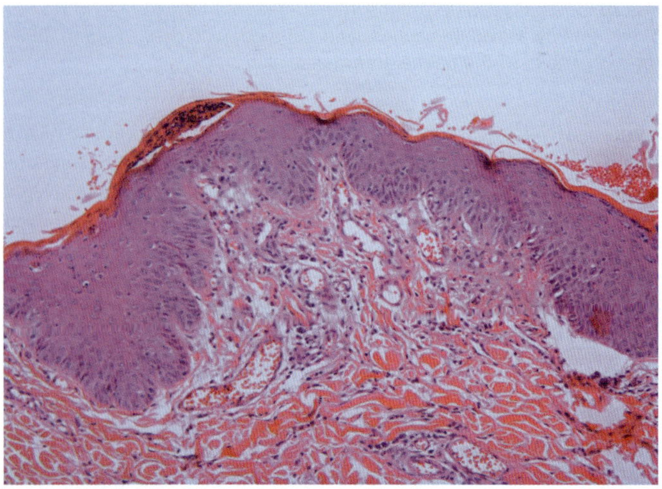

Fig. 79.7 Skin biopsy specimen from the axilla of a 6-year-old neutered female West Highland white terrier with *Malassezia* dermatitis. There is moderate-severe epidermal hyperplasia with "scalloping" and spongiosis of the deeper portion of the epidermis, along with an intra-corneal pustule. Dilation of the superficial dermal vasculature is accompanied by a moderate, predominately mononuclear cell, interstitial infiltrate. Hematoxylin and eosin, ×20.

for yeast detection when compared with cytologic examination (Fig. 79.8). The inflammatory pattern seen in *Malassezia* dermatitis is also commonly encountered in chronic allergic dermatitis.

TREATMENT

Treatment of *Malassezia* dermatitis is based on the use of topical and systemic antifungal treatments (Table 79.2), together with specific therapy for concurrent diseases that favor proliferation of the yeast, where possible.

Topical Therapy

Malassezia yeasts are located in the stratum corneum, and so topical therapy alone can be successful when potent antifungal agents are correctly applied. This approach depends on good compliance and

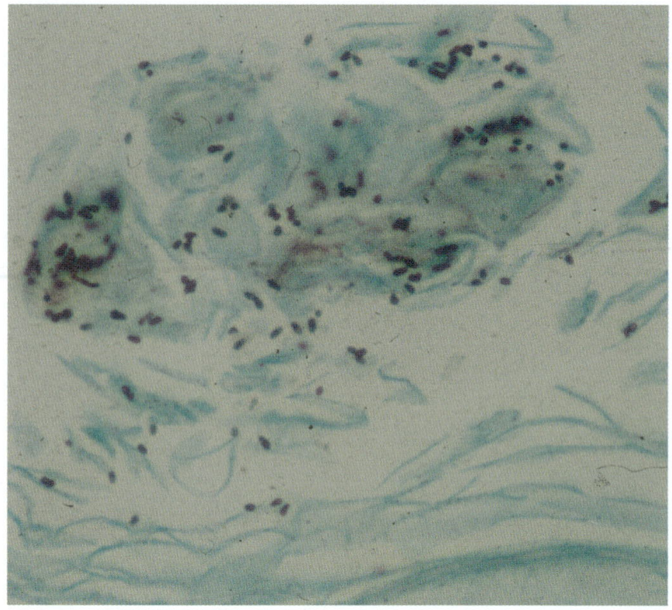

Fig. 79.8 Skin biopsy specimen from a dog with *Malassezia* dermatitis. Abundant *Malassezia pachydermatis* cells are evident within the stratum corneum, illustrating why topical therapy alone can be clinically effective in compliant dogs. Cytology, however, is generally superior to histopathology for the detection of the yeast in clinical cases. Methenamine silver, ×1000.

availability of effective products. Topical therapy avoids the expense and potential toxicity of systemic azole drugs but is more labor intensive for the owner. Evidence-based systematic reviews of antifungal treatments for *Malassezia* dermatitis in dogs support the recommendation of a 2% miconazole and 2% chlorhexidine shampoo twice weekly for 3 weeks as the sole treatment.[23,51,55] A prospective, randomized, and blinded field clinical trial showed that the clinical and cytologic efficacy of a 3% chlorhexidine shampoo was comparable to the miconazole–chlorhexidine product.[56] Maintenance treatment may be needed if an underlying cause cannot be identified and corrected. The anti-staphylococcal properties of shampoos containing miconazole and/or chlorhexidine[57] may also be advantageous in the event of concurrent bacterial overgrowth.

Clinical evidence that supports the use of a number of topical treatments with *in vitro* activity against *M. pachydermatis,* including acetic + boric acid, benzoyl peroxide, and other azoles is lacking.[55] Wipes that contain chlorhexidine, climbazole, and Tris-EDTA had clinical and mycological activity against *M. pachydermatis* in a small open study.[58] The use of wipes may be convenient for the local treatment of body folds and interdigital areas.

Reported efficacy of other topical substances for treatment of canine *Malassezia* dermatitis[59] and otitis externa[60] require further evaluation in blinded studies. These include honey-based gels, a variety of plant-derived essential oils, povidone-iodine, and agents used to treat human dandruff and seborrheic dermatitis (e.g., selenium sulfide).[23,61] A killer decapeptide (KP) engineered from the variable region of a single-chain recombinant anti-idiotypic antibody and representing the internal image of a yeast killer toxin (KT) with broad-spectrum antifungal activity was reportedly safe and effective in *Malassezia* otitis externa in four dogs over 8 days; with development, this approach may represent an alternative to current therapies.[62]

Systemic Therapy

There is fair evidence for use of ketoconazole (10 mg/kg, PO, q24h), and itraconazole (5 mg/kg, PO, q24h) for 3 weeks to treat *Malassezia*

TABLE 79.2 Recommended Treatments for *Malassezia* Dermatitis in Dogs and Cats

Species	Route	Product	Dose
Dog	Topical	2% miconazole + 2% chlorhexidine	Shampoo every 3 days
	Topical	3% chlorhexidine	Shampoo two-three times per week
	Systemic	Itraconazole	5 mg/kg q24h PO or 2 days on–5 days off for 21 days
Cat	Systemic	Itraconazole	5 mg/kg q24h PO or 7 days on–7 days off for 21 days

dermatitis in dogs.[54] Marketing authorization for oral ketoconazole in humans was suspended in Europe in 2013. Itraconazole is less toxic and has better tissue penetration than ketoconazole. A pulse-therapy regimen of itraconazole (5 mg/kg, PO, q24h) for 2 successive days each week has been described as an alternative to daily dosing.[63] Itraconazole has also been used to treat cats with *Malassezia* spp. overgrowth (5 mg/kg, PO, q24h),[64] or at 5 mg/kg on a 1 week on/1 week off pulse basis.[25] Reduced susceptibility to fluconazole *in vitro* is common in *M. pachydermatis*,[65,66] and clinical trial data for fluconazole is very limited.

While pilot studies have shown a potential role for daily or pulse oral dosing with terbinafine for treatment of canine *Malassezia* dermatitis (30 mg/kg, PO, q24h),[67–69] concentrations achieved in sebum and stratum corneum of dogs treated barely exceeded the MIC_{90} of field strains of *M. pachydermatis*, so further clinical and pharmacologic studies are required before use of this drug could be recommended for this indication.

Typically, the response to glucocorticoid therapy is poor. Griseofulvin is *not* effective in *Malassezia* infections. The reader is referred to Chapter 11 for detailed information on these antifungal drugs.

PREVENTION

Failure to identify and correct concurrent diseases may result in relapse of *Malassezia* infection. Intermittent or continuous maintenance therapy is often necessary in animals that experience relapsing disease, particularly in dogs with poorly controlled allergic disease or in dogs in which the reason for disease susceptibility cannot be identified. Although *Malassezia* allergens are now often included in intradermal allergen tests and IgE serology, at the time of writing there is little evidence to support the value of allergen-specific immunotherapy for prevention of *M. pachydermatis* hypersensitivity in dogs.[70]

PUBLIC HEALTH ASPECTS

A variety of *Malassezia* species have been associated with disease in humans, especially *M. restricta*, *M. furfur*, *M. globosa*, and *M. sympodialis*.[49] Yeast proliferation can lead to *Malassezia* folliculitis, seborrheic dermatitis, catheter-related fungemia, and a variety of other invasive infections.[71] Administration of lipid-containing total parenteral nutrition solutions are a risk factor for disseminated infections in humans, which often occur in neonates.[72,73]

Malassezia pachydermatis is rarely associated with diseases in humans. Owners of dogs (which are natural reservoirs for this yeast) with inflamed skin had a high rate of carriage of the organism.[74] A potentially fatal *M. pachydermatis* fungemia has been reported in premature babies and less often in immunocompromised adults.[75,76] Most of the affected neonates have been premature, had concurrent serious underlying disease, had central or peripheral catheters placed, and in some cases were receiving lipid emulsions as a component of parenteral nutrition. In some outbreaks, *M. pachydermatis* was thought to have been transmitted from neonate to neonate on the hands of health care workers; the original source of the yeast was not identified, but transfer from pet dogs has been suspected. These observations highlight the importance of hand washing by health care workers in the control of nosocomial infections.

CASE EXAMPLE

Signalment

"Basil," a 4-year-old neutered male West Highland white terrier from Hertfordshire, UK (see Fig. 79.2).

History

Basil's owner reported that skin disease had first developed at 12 months of age and had been continuous (unless treated) since then. Initial signs were foot-chewing (fore and hind feet), followed by progression to ventral and pinnal erythema, and bilateral erythema-ceruminous otitis externa. The dorsolumbar area had never been affected. These signs persisted in the face of routine ectoparasite control measures comprising monthly application of a spot-on formulation of imidacloprid and moxidectin, and annual spraying of the house with an insect growth regulator (pyriproxyfen). Parasites had never been seen by the owner and Basil was the only pet. Systemic antibiotic therapy was reportedly ineffective, but oral prednisolone rapidly and reproducibly resolved the lesions and pruritus. Signs were controlled for several years using prednisolone, usually at 0.25–0.5 mg/kg on an alternate day basis. Over the last few months, this regimen was no longer effective despite an increased daily dose of prednisolone, and progressive erythema, skin thickening and malodor had developed in parallel with intense pruritus. Apart from the skin disease, Basil was judged to be in good general health.

Current Medications

Prednisolone: 1.0 mg/kg, q24h, PO.
Cephalexin: 15 mg/kg, q12h, PO.
Imidacloprid: 100 mg/moxidectin 25 mg spot-on monthly.

Other Medical History

Dog lived indoors with daily exercise in the local park. Owners were not affected by skin disease. The dog had never travelled beyond the local area.

Physical Examination

Body weight: 10 kg.
General: Bright, alert and responsive.
Integument: Lesions comprised intense erythema of the ventral neck, axillae, and medial aspect of the forelimbs with a rather demarcated and symmetrical distribution. The hair overlying folded ridges of intensely inflamed and thickened skin was matted in a yellow, greasy, malodorous exudate. Focal areas of lichenification and hyperpigmentation were evident in the alopecic regions of the ventral neck. There was bilateral erythemato-ceruminous otitis externa with erythema, hyperpigmentation, and lichenification on the medial aspect of the pinnae, although pinnal margins were unaffected. Interdigital skin was intensely erythematous and brown exudate matted the lower portions of the hair. External parasites were not observed.
Lymph nodes: Moderate peripheral lymphadenopathy affecting superficial cervical and popliteal nodes.
Other organ systems: No abnormalities detected.

Continued

CASE EXAMPLE—cont'd

Laboratory Findings

Microscopy for parasites: Microscopic examination of coat brushings, hair plucks, and skin scrapings showed no pathogens.

Cytology findings: Cytologic examination of smears of ear wax from both ears showed squames and moderate numbers of *Malassezia* spp. yeasts. Tape-strip specimens from inflamed skin of the ventral neck, axillae, and interdigital skin showed large numbers of *Malassezia* spp. yeasts amongst squames, along with rare coccoid bacteria.

Working Diagnosis

Malassezia dermatitis secondary to canine atopic dermatitis.

Treatment

A 2% miconazole and 2% chlorhexidine shampoo was applied every 3 days (10-minute contact time with lather) to treat the *Malassezia* infection of the skin. A combination of miconazole, polymixin B, and prednisolone was applied to both ears twice daily for the *Malassezia* otitis externa. Cephalexin was withdrawn due to lack of cytologic and clinical evidence of pyoderma, but prednisolone was maintained on an alternate day basis in view of the severity of inflammation.

Follow-up

On re-examination after 4 weeks, an excellent response to therapy was observed, with resolution of erythema, malodor, and pruritus. The skin was much less thickened and hair regrowth was evident, and otitis externa had resolved. Cytologic examination showed only rare yeasts in skin and ear samples. Subsequent weekly use of the miconazole/chlorhexidine shampoo was sufficient to prevent relapse of the *Malassezia* dermatitis. Further investigation of the allergic phenotype by diet trialing with a commercial hydrolyzed soy and cornstarch product exclusively for 8 weeks did not influence the ongoing need for low alternate-day doses of prednisolone.

Final Diagnosis

The typical clinical signs and abundance of *Malassezia* yeasts at the first assessment, and subsequent excellent clinical and cytologic response to topical therapy fulfill the diagnostic criteria for *Malassezia* dermatitis.

Previous glucocorticoid responsive allergic skin disease starting before 3 years of age in an indoor dog with lesions affecting front feet and ears, with nonaffected ear margins and dorsolumbar skin, that persisted despite antimicrobial and antiparasitic measures and diet trialing also convincingly fulfill the diagnostic criteria developed[77] for underlying nonfood-induced canine atopic dermatitis. Owners declined IgE testing and allergen-specific therapy, preferring medical therapy alone.

Comments

Development of *Malassezia* dermatitis led to a dramatic progression of previously controlled allergic skin disease, illustrating the potential importance of this disease as a flare factor in canine atopic dermatitis. Topical therapy alone was sufficient in the hands of very motivated owners with a compliant pet. This case illustrates the importance of: (1) evaluating for underlying skin diseases in dogs and cats with infections caused by this commensal yeast, and (2) the need to consider potential complicating factors (primarily microbial infection and ectoparasitic infestation) in the management of allergic dogs.

SUGGESTED READINGS

Bond R, Morris DO, Guillot J, et al. Biology, diagnosis and treatment of *Malassezia* dermatitis in dogs and cats: Clinical Consensus Guidelines of the World Association for Veterinary Dermatology. *Vet Dermatol.* 2020;31:28–74.

Guillot J, Bond R. *Malassezia* yeasts in veterinary dermatology: an updated overview. *Front Cell Infect Microbiol.* 2020;10:79.

Theelen B, Cafarchia C, Gaitanis G, et al. *Malassezia* ecology, pathophysiology, and treatment. *Med Mycol.* 2018;56:S10–S25.

REFERENCES

1. Weidman FD. Exfoliative dermatitis in the Indian Rhinoceros (*Rhinoceros unicornis*) with description of a new yeast species, *Pityrosporum pachydermatis.* In: *Report of the Laboratory Museum Comparative Pathology.* Philadelphia: Zoological Society; 1925:36–45.
2. Sugita T, Takeo K, Hama K, et al. DNA sequence diversity of intergenic spacer I region in the non-lipid-dependent species *Malassezia pachydermatis* isolated from animals. *Med Mycol.* 2005;43:21–26.
3. Han SH, Chung TH, Nam EH, et al. Molecular analysis of *Malassezia pachydermatis* isolated from canine skin and ear in Korea. *Med Mycol.* 2013;51:396–404.
4. Buommino E, Nocera FP, Parisi A, et al. Correlation between genetic variability and virulence factors in clinical strains of *Malassezia pachydermatis* of animal origin. *New Microbiol.* 2016;39:216–223.
5. Cabanes FJ, Theelen B, Castella G, et al. Two new lipid-dependent *Malassezia* species from domestic animals. *FEMS Yeast Res.* 2007;7:1064–1076.
6. Cabanes FJ, Vega S, Castella G. *Malassezia cuniculi* sp. nov., a novel yeast species isolated from rabbit skin. *Med Mycol.* 2011;49:40–48.
7. Cabanes FJ, Coutinho SD, Puig L, et al. New lipid-dependent *Malassezia* species from parrots. *Rev Iberoam De Micol.* 2016;33:92–99.
8. Honnavar P, Prasad GS, Ghosh A, et al. *Malassezia arunalokei* sp. nov., a novel yeast species isolated from seborrheic dermatitis patients and healthy individuals from India. *J Clin Microbiol.* 2016;54:1826–1834.
9. Lorch JM, Palmer JM, Vanderwolf KJ, et al. *Malassezia vespertilionis* sp. nov.: a new cold-tolerant species of yeast isolated from bats. *Persoonia.* 2018;41:56–70.
10. Park M, Jung WH, Han SH, et al. Characterisation and expression analysis of mrlip1, a class 3 family lipase of *Malassezia restricta. Mycoses.* 2015;58:671–678.
11. Park M, Cho YJ, Lee YW, et al. Whole genome sequencing analysis of the cutaneous pathogenic yeast *Malassezia restricta* and identification of the major lipase expressed on the scalp of patients with dandruff. *Mycoses.* 2017;60:188–197.
12. Wu G, Zhao H, Li C, et al. Genus-wide comparative genomics of *Malassezia* delineates its phylogeny, physiology, and niche adaptation on human skin. *PLoS Genet.* 2015;11:e1005614.
13. Meason-Smith C, Diesel A, Patterson AP, et al. What is living on your dog's skin? Characterization of the canine cutaneous mycobiota and fungal dysbiosis in canine allergic dermatitis. *FEMS Microbiol Ecol.* 2015:91.
14. Meason-Smith C, Diesel A, Patterson AP, et al. Characterization of the cutaneous mycobiota in healthy and allergic cats using next generation sequencing. *Vet Dermatol.* 2017;28:71. e17.
15. Cafarchia C, Latrofa MS, Figueredo LA, et al. Physiological and molecular characterization of atypical lipid-dependent *Malassezia* yeasts from a dog with skin lesions: adaptation to a new host? *Med Mycol.* 2011;49:365–374.
16. Crespo MJ, Abarca ML, Cabañes FJ. Atypical lipid-dependent *Malassezia* species isolates from dogs with otitis externa. *J Clin Microbiol.* 2000;38:2383–2385.
17. Bond R, Howell SA, Haywood PJ, et al. Isolation of *Malassezia sympodialis* and *Malassezia globosa* from healthy pet cats. *Vet Rec.* 1997;141:200–201.
18. Crespo MJ, Abarca ML, Cabañes FJ. Isolation of *Malassezia furfur* from a cat. *J Clin Microbiol.* 1999;37:1573–1574.

19. Crespo MJ, Abarca ML, Cabañes FJ. Otitis externa associated with *Malassezia sympodialis* in two cats. *J Clin Microbiol.* 2000;38:1263–1266.
20. Hirai A, Kano R, Makimura K, et al. A unique isolate of *Malassezia* from a cat. *J Vet Med Sci.* 2002;64:957–959.
21. Åhman S, Perrins N, Bond R. Carriage of *Malassezia* spp. yeasts in healthy and seborrhoeic Devon Rex cats. *Med Mycol.* 2007;45:449–455.
22. Velegraki A, Cafarchia C, Gaitanis G, et al. *Malassezia* infections in humans and animals: pathophysiology, detection, and treatment. *PLoS Pathog.* 2015;11:e1004523.
23. Bond R, Morris DO, Guillot J, et al. Biology, diagnosis and treatment of *Malassezia* dermatitis in dogs and cats: clinical consensus guidelines of the World Association for Veterinary Dermatology. *Vet Dermatol.* 2020;31:28–74.
24. Olivry T, DeBoer DJ, Favrot C, et al. Treatment of canine atopic dermatitis: 2010 clinical practice guidelines from the international task force on canine atopic dermatitis. *Vet Dermatol.* 2010;21:233–248.
25. Åhman S, Perrins N, Bond R. Treatment of *Malassezia pachydermatis*-associated seborrhoeic dermatitis in Devon Rex cats with itraconazole - a pilot study. *Vet Dermatol.* 2007;18:171–174.
26. Åhman SE, Bergstrom KE. Cutaneous carriage of *Malassezia* species in healthy and seborrhoeic Sphynx cats and a comparison to carriage in Devon Rex cats. *J Feline Med Surg.* 2009;11:970–976.
27. Volk AV, Belyavin CE, Varjonen K, et al. *Malassezia pachydermatis* and *M nana* predominate amongst the cutaneous mycobiota of Sphynx cats. *J Feline Med Surg.* 2010;12:917–922.
28. Older CE, Diesel AB, Lawhon SD, et al. The feline cutaneous and oral microbiota are influenced by breed and environment. *PLoS One.* 2019;14:e0220463.
29. Grice EA, Dawson Jr TL. Host-microbe interactions: *Malassezia* and human skin. *Curr Opin Microbiol.* 2017;40:81–87.
30. Ashbee HR, Bond R. *Malassezia* species and immunity: host-pathogen interactions. In: Boekhout T, Gueho E, Mayser P, Velegraki A, eds. *Malassezia and the Skin. Science and Clinical Practice.* Heildelberg: Springer; 2010:139–174.
31. Patino-Uzcategui A, Amado Y, Cepero de Garcia M, et al. Virulence gene expression in *Malassezia* spp from individuals with seborrheic dermatitis. *J Invest Dermatol.* 2011;131:2134–2136.
32. Cafarchia C, Dell'Aquila ME, Traversa D, et al. Expression of the micro-opioid receptor on *Malassezia pachydermatis* and its effect in modulating phospholipase production. *Med Mycol.* 2010;48:73–78.
33. Teramoto H, Kumeda Y, Yokoigawa K, et al. Genotyping and characterisation of the secretory lipolytic enzymes of *Malassezia pachydermatis* isolates collected from dogs. *Vet Rec Open.* 2015;2:e000124.
34. Cafarchia C, Gasser RB, Latrofa MS, et al. Genetic variants of *Malassezia pachydermatis* from canine skin: body distribution and phospholipase activity. *FEMS Yeast Res.* 2008;8:451–459.
35. Magiatis P, Pappas P, Gaitanis G, et al. *Malassezia* yeasts produce a collection of exceptionally potent activators of the Ah (dioxin) receptor detected in diseased human skin. *J Invest Dermatol.* 2013;133:2023–2030.
36. Gioti A, Nystedt B, Li W, et al. Genomic insights into the atopic eczema-associated skin commensal yeast *Malassezia sympodialis. mBio.* 2013;4:00512. e00572.
37. Cannizzo FT, Eraso E, Ezkurra PA, et al. Biofilm development by clinical isolates of *Malassezia pachydermatis. Med Mycol.* 2007;45:357–361.
38. Figueredo LA, Cafarchia C, Desantis S, et al. Biofilm formation of *Malassezia pachydermatis* from dogs. *Vet Microbiol.* 2012;160:126–131.
39. Jerzsele A, Gyetvai B, Csere I, et al. Biofilm formation in *Malassezia pachydermatis* strains isolated from dogs decreases susceptibility to ketoconazole and itraconazole. *Acta Vet Hung.* 2014;62:473–480.
40. Oldenhoff WE, Frank GR, DeBoer DJ. Comparison of the results of intradermal test reactivity and serum allergen-specific IgE measurement for *Malassezia pachydermatis* in atopic dogs. *Vet Dermatol.* 2014;25:507–511. e584-505.
41. Bond R, Patterson-Kane JC, Lloyd DH. Intradermal test reactivity to *Malassezia pachydermatis* in healthy basset hounds and bassets with *Malassezia* dermatitis. *Vet Rec.* 2002;151:105–109.
42. Bond R, Habibah A, Patterson-Kane JC, et al. Patch test responses to *Malassezia pachydermatis* in healthy dogs. *Med Mycol.* 2006;44:175–184.
43. Prado MR, Brito EH, Girao MD, et al. Higher incidence of *Malassezia pachydermatis* in the eyes of dogs with corneal ulcer than in healthy dogs. *Vet Microbiol.* 2004;100:115–120.
44. Ledbetter EC, Starr JK. *Malassezia pachydermatis* keratomycosis in a dog. *Med Mycol Case Rep.* 2015;10:24–26.
45. Keddie F, Orr A, Liebes D. Direct staining on vinyl plastic tape, demonstration of the cutaneous flora of the epidermis by the strip method. *Sabouraudia.* 1961;1:108–111.
46. Julie D, Marie M, Florent M, et al. Performance of matrix-assisted laser desorption ionisation-time-of-flight mass spectrometry for identifying clinical *Malassezia* isolates. *J Clin Microbiol.* 2016;55:90–96.
47. Yamamoto M, Umeda Y, Yo A, et al. Utilization of matrix-assisted laser desorption and ionization time-of-flight mass spectrometry for identification of infantile seborrheic dermatitis-causing *Malassezia* and incidence of culture-based cutaneous *Malassezia* microbiota of 1-month-old infants. *J Dermatol.* 2014;41:117–123.
48. Denis J, Machouart M, Morio F, et al. Performance of matrix-assisted laser desorption ionization-time of flight mass spectrometry for identifying clinical *Malassezia* isolates. *J Clin Microbiol.* 2017;55:90–96.
49. Theelen B, Cafarchia C, Gaitanis G, et al. *Malassezia* ecology, pathophysiology, and treatment. *Med Mycol.* 2018;56:S10–S25.
50. Angileri M, Pasquetti M, De Lucia M, et al. Azole resistance of *Malassezia pachydermatis* causing treatment failure in a dog. *Med Mycol Case Rep.* 2019;23:58–61.
51. Kano R, Yokoi S, Kariya N, et al. Multi-azole-resistant strain of *Malassezia pachydermatis* isolated from a canine *Malassezia* dermatitis. *Med Mycol.* 2019;57:346–350.
52. Vuran E, Karaarslan A, Karasartova D, et al. Identification of *Malassezia* species from pityriasis versicolor lesions with a new multiplex PCR method. *Mycopathologia.* 2014;177:41–49.
53. Puig L, Castella G, Cabanes FJ. Quantification of *Malassezia pachydermatis* by real-time PCR in swabs from the external ear canal of dogs. *J Vet Diagn Invest.* 2019;31:440–447.
54. Negre A, Bensignor E, Guillot J. Evidence-based veterinary dermatology: a systematic review of interventions for *Malassezia* dermatitis in dogs. *Vet Dermatol.* 2009;20:1–12.
55. Mueller RS, Bergvall K, Bensignor E, et al. A review of topical therapy for skin infections with bacteria and yeast. *Vet Dermatol.* 2012;23:330–341. e362.
56. Maynard L, Reme CA, Viaud S. Comparison of two shampoos for the treatment of canine *Malassezia* dermatitis: a randomised controlled trial. *J Small Anim Pract.* 2011;52:566–572.
57. Clark SM, Loeffler A, Bond R. Susceptibility in vitro of canine methicillin-resistant and -susceptible staphylococcal isolates to fusidic acid, chlorhexidine and miconazole: opportunities for topical therapy of canine superficial pyoderma. *J Antimicrob Chemother.* 2015;70:2048–2052.
58. Cavana P, Peano A, Petit JY, et al. A pilot study of the efficacy of wipes containing chlorhexidine 0.3%, climbazole 0.5% and Tris-EDTA to reduce *Malassezia pachydermatis* populations on canine skin. *Vet Dermatol.* 2015;26:278. e261.
59. Nardoni S, Mugnaini L, Pistelli L, et al. Clinical and mycological evaluation of an herbal antifungal formulation in canine *Malassezia* dermatitis. *J Mycol Med.* 2014;24:234–240.
60. Nardoni S, Pistelli L, Baronti I, et al. Traditional Mediterranean plants: characterization and use of an essential oils mixture to treat *Malassezia* otitis externa in atopic dogs. *Nat Prod Res.* 2016:1–4.
61. Guillot J, Bond R. *Malassezia* yeasts in veterinary dermatology: an updated overview. *Front Cell Infect Microbiol.* 2020;10:79.
62. Cafarchia C, Immediato D, Paola GD, et al. In vitro and in vivo activity of a killer peptide against *Malassezia pachydermatis* causing otitis in dogs. *Med Mycol.* 2014;52:350–355.
63. Pinchbeck LR, Hillier A, Kowalski JJ, et al. Comparison of pulse administration versus once daily administration of itraconazole for the treatment of *Malassezia pachydermatis* dermatitis and otitis in dogs. *J Am Vet Med Assoc.* 2002;220:1807–1812.
64. Bensignor E. Treatment of *Malassezia* overgrowth with itraconazole in 15 cats. *Vet Rec.* 2010;167:1011–1012.

65. Cafarchia C, Figueredo LA, Iatta R, et al. In vitro evaluation of *Malassezia pachydermatis* susceptibility to azole compounds using E-test and CLSI microdilution methods. *Med Mycol.* 2012;50:795–801.
66. Cafarchia C, Figueredo LA, Favuzzi V, et al. Assessment of the antifungal susceptibility of *Malassezia pachydermatis* in various media using a CLSI protocol. *Vet Microbiol.* 2012;159:536–540.
67. Berger DJ, Lewis TP, Schick AE, et al. Comparison of once-daily versus twice-weekly terbinafine administration for the treatment of canine *Malassezia* dermatitis - a pilot study. *Vet Dermatol.* 2012;23:418–e479.
68. Rosales MS, Marsella R, Kunkle G, et al. Comparison of the clinical efficacy of oral terbinafine and ketoconazole combined with cephalexin in the treatment of *Malassezia* dermatitis in dogs: a pilot study. *Vet Dermatol.* 2005;16:171–176.
69. Guillot J, Bensignor E, Jankowski F, et al. Comparative efficacies of oral ketoconazole and terbinafine for reducing *Malassezia* population sizes on the skin of Basset Hounds. *Vet Dermatol.* 2003;14:153–157.
70. Aberg L, Varjonen K, Ahman S. Results of allergen-specific immunotherapy in atopic dogs with *Malassezia* hypersensitivity: a retrospective study of 16 cases. *Vet Dermatol.* 2017;28:633. e157.
71. Tragiannidis A, Bisping G, Koehler G, et al. Minireview: *Malassezia* infections in immunocompromised patients. *Mycoses.* 2010;53:187–195.
72. Dankner WM, Spector SA, Fierer J, et al. *Malassezia* fungemia in neonates and adults: complication of hyperalimentation. *Rev Infect Dis.* 1987;9:743–753.
73. Chryssanthou E, Broberger U, Petrini B. *Malassezia pachydermatis* fungaemia in a neonatal intensive care unit. *Acta Paediatr.* 2001;90:323–327.
74. Morris DO. *Malassezia pachydermatis* carriage in dog owners. *Emerg Infect Dis.* 2005;11:83–88.
75. Ilahi A, Hadrich I, Goudjil S, et al. Molecular epidemiology of a *Malassezia pachydermatis* neonatal unit outbreak. *Med Mycol.* 2018;56:69–77.
76. Larocco M, Dorenbaum A, Robinson A, et al. Recovery of *Malassezia pachydermatis* from eight infants in a neonatal intensive care nursery: clinical and laboratory features. *Pediatr Infect Dis J.* 1988;7:398–401.
77. Favrot C, Steffan J, Seewald W, et al. A prospective study on the clinical features of chronic canine atopic dermatitis and its diagnosis. *Vet Dermatol.* 2010;21:23–31.

Blastomycosis

Alyssa C. Mourning, Jane E. Sykes

KEY POINTS

- First Described: Blastomycosis was first described in the United States in 1894 by Thomas Casper Gilchrist.[1]
- Cause: *Blastomyces dermatitidis* and *Blastomyces gilchristii* are the main species that cause disease in humans and dogs in North America (family Ajellomycetaceae). *Blastomyces helices* was recently described in humans, dogs, and cats from western Canada and a variety of regions within the United States. Other species such as *Blastomyces percursus* cause disease in humans outside North America.
- Affected Hosts: Primarily humans and dogs, but also a variety of other domestic and wildlife mammalian species, including cats.
- Geographic Distribution: Blastomycosis is principally a disease of North America, but has been identified in Africa, the Middle East, India, Europe, and Central America. In North America, the endemic distribution includes the Mississippi, Missouri, and Ohio River valleys, the mid-Atlantic states, a small area of northeastern United States, as well as the Canadian provinces that border the Great Lakes (Quebec, Manitoba, and Ontario), Saskatchewan, and southeastern Canada near the St. Lawrence River.
- Primary Mode of Transmission: Inhalation of conidia from the environment. The spores enter the terminal airway and establish a primary infection in the lungs as a yeast form. In rare circumstances, cutaneous inoculation may occur. In most cases, cutaneous blastomycosis in the dog should be considered a manifestation of disseminated disease.
- Major Clinical Signs: Blastomycosis is often associated with fever, inappetence, weight loss, cough, tachypnea, respiratory difficulty, and nodular or ulcerative cutaneous lesions. Ocular lesions, lameness, and neurologic signs are also common.
- Differential Diagnosis: These include neoplasia, other deep mycoses, protothecosis, mycobacterial infections, systemic protozoal infections (leishmaniosis, toxoplasmosis, neosporosis), aspiration or foreign body pneumonia.
- Human Health Significance: *Blastomyces dermatitidis*, *B. gilchristii*, and *Blastomyces helicus* cause disease in humans, but direct transmission from animals to humans does not typically occur. There have been rare cases of transmission of infection after direct inoculation through bite wounds. Dogs are considered a sentinel for human exposure. At the time of writing, blastomycosis is reportable in Arizona, Louisiana, Michigan, Minnesota, and Wisconsin.

ETIOLOGY AND EPIDEMIOLOGY

Blastomycosis is a pulmonary or disseminated disease that is primarily caused by the dimorphic fungi *Blastomyces dermatitidis* and *Blastomyces gilchristii*. Humans and dogs appear to be most susceptible to disease, with rare disease reported in cats. Other mammalian species can also be affected, including cats, horses,[2,3] ferrets,[4] sea lions,[5] lemurs,[6] rhesus monkeys,[7] wolves,[8] foxes,[9] black bears,[10] as well as lions and other captive nondomestic felines such as tigers, cheetahs, and snow leopards.[11] *Blastomyces dermatitidis* and *B. gilchristii* are phenotypically identical but have been differentiated based on the use of genetic typing methods (microsatellite analysis).[12] It has been suggested that in humans, *B. gilchristii* may be less likely to disseminate from the lungs than *B. dermatitidis*, but infections with *B. gilchristii* may be more severe and more likely to present with acute lung disease that results in hospitalization.[13] Nevertheless, both species appear to be capable of causing pulmonary and disseminated disease, and the presence of certain alleles within each species may be associated with a greater likelihood of dissemination or mortality. Studies of the relative prevalence of these species in dogs and association with virulence are required. *Blastomyces helicus* was more recently recognized in dogs and cats from western Canada and the United States.[14]

Blastomycosis is principally a disease of North America, but has been identified in Africa, the Middle East, India, Europe, and Central America.[15–18] *Blastomyces dermatitidis* and *B. gilchristii* have overlapping distributions primarily in the Midwestern parts of the United States, especially around the Great Lakes, along the Ohio and Mississippi river valleys, and in the southeastern states (Fig. 80.1).[19–21] Another focus of endemicity exists in the St. Lawrence river region in the northeast, which extends up into Ontario, Canada.[22,23] Disease may also be seen in parts of Canada around the Great Lakes and has also been reported in dogs and humans from Saskatchewan.[24,25,26] An increase in pulmonary blastomycosis in humans has been reported over the last decade from upstate New York.[27] Occasionally, disease appears in nontraveled dogs that reside in nonendemic parts of the United States, such as in Wyoming, Colorado, and South Dakota.[28,29,30] Disease in humans associated with infection with *B. helicus* has been described in western Canada (Saskatchewan, Alberta) and in two dogs, two cats, and seven humans from scattered regions within the United States (human cases: Texas, northern California, Idaho, Utah, Nebraska; dogs and cats: Fort Collins, Colorado; Helena, Montana; and Atascadero, California).[14] Disease in humans was associated with underlying immunocompromise. A dog from Colorado was known to dig in prairie dog burrows, and one of the cats that was an indoor/outdoor cat from the mountains

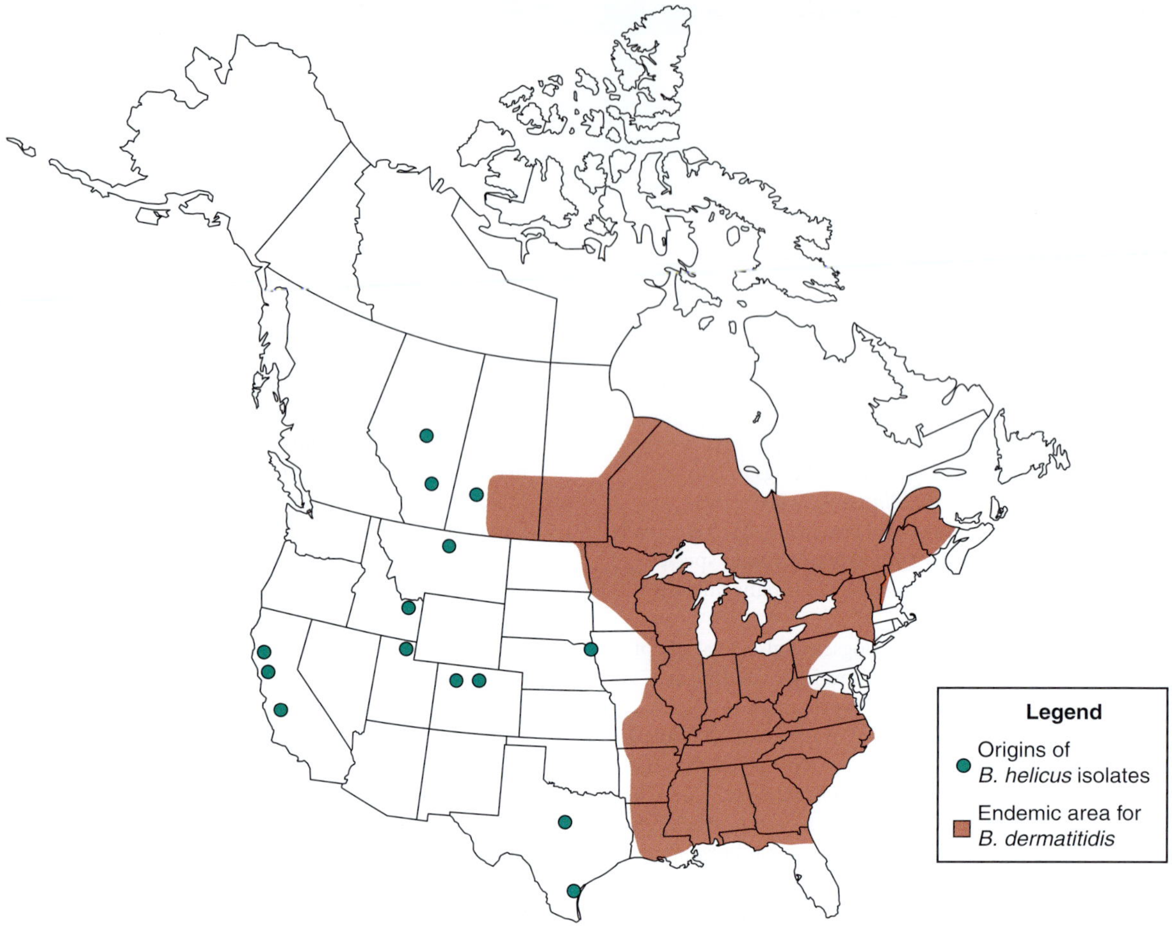

Fig. 80.1 Geographic distribution of blastomycosis in North America. The red shaded area represents the approximate distribution of *Blastomyces dermatitidis* and *Blastomyces gilchristii*. The blue dots represent reported cases of *Blastomyces helicus* in humans (southern Saskatchewan and Alberta, central and southern Texas, eastern Nebraska, southern Idaho, northern Utah, northern California); dogs (central Colorado, central coastal California); and cats (central Colorado, northern Montana).

west of Fort Collins was observed to play with potted plant soil. Canine blastomycosis has also been reported in India.[18] Human blastomycosis occurs in Africa, but reports of canine disease from Africa are absent from the literature. Species described in humans from Africa include *B. dermatitidis, B. gilchristii, Blastomyces percursus*, and *Blastomyces emzantsi* sp. nov.[21,31] Blastomycosis was described in Europe in a dog with a travel history to the United States.[16] However, travel-related disease occurs less often than other endemic mycoses that have longer incubation periods or more chronic, insidious disease courses, such as coccidioidomycosis.[32,33]

In the environment, *Blastomyces* grows in a saprophytic mycelial form that produces infective spores (conidia) that are 2–10 μm in diameter. The conidia are thought to be aerosolized and inhaled by the host. At body temperature (37°C) and in body tissues, the organism transforms into the yeast form and replicates asexually. Budding yeasts are 5–20 μm in diameter and have a thick, refractile double-contoured cell wall. The ecologic niche of *Blastomyces* spp. appears to be warm, moist, sandy soil that is rich in organic debris such as decaying vegetation and animal waste.[34] However, this has not been thoroughly defined because the fungus is difficult to isolate from the environment. No consistent seasonality has been linked to disease.

Living near a waterway is a risk factor for blastomycosis.[35] In Wisconsin studies, 95% of dogs with blastomycosis lived within 400 m (1,312 ft) of a body of water at altitudes less than 500 m (1,640 ft) above sea level.[36,37] Residence less than 400 m from a body of water increased the risk of blastomycosis by a factor of 10 in one study from Louisiana.[38] *Blastomyces dermatitidis* has been isolated from a woodpile near the Wisconsin River; over 14 years, four of nine dogs housed in a kennel close to the woodpile developed blastomycosis.[39] A study conducted in an endemic area of Tennessee also recognized the association of disease in dogs with proximity to water but did not find an association with soil type, soil pH, or amount of organic matter in the soil.[40] Although proximity to water is a risk factor, exposure to the outside environment is not necessary because blastomycosis can occur in strictly indoor dogs and cats.[38,41–43]

Rain or heavy dew appears to facilitate the release of infectious spores. In one study of 219 infected dogs over an 18-year period, increased rainfall and warmer temperatures preceded the highest incidence periods of infection.[44] The seasonal distribution rates of the cases were winter (24%), spring (18%), summer (36%), and fall (22%). No seasonal differences in disease are found in Tennessee, but more cases occur from late spring through late fall in Wisconsin.[45] In Louisiana, more cases were reported in August, September, October, and January than in the rest of the year.[38] Access to sites that have been excavated also increases the risk for infection because of exposure to organisms deep in the soil.[36] In humans, involvement in dirt-moving activities significantly increased the risk of developing blastomycosis.[43] In 1999, a large outbreak in humans and dogs in St. Louis county,

Minnesota, was associated with wet weather and an excavation site for a new neighborhood.[46]

Even within endemic regions, *Blastomyces* species are not widely distributed. Most humans and dogs living in such areas show no serologic or skin test evidence of exposure. A point source of exposure within an enzootic area is more likely. It is not unusual to find neighborhoods in which numerous dogs with blastomycosis are identified in a short time. In 14% of households in which blastomycosis has been diagnosed in humans or dogs, another case is diagnosed in the same household in the next several years.[41] Exposure of dogs and humans to a common source of infection while engaged in duck and raccoon hunting has been reported.[47,48] A study from Michigan showed that most dogs with blastomycosis were from the eastern half of the Upper Peninsula or the northern Lower Peninsula, and travel or residence north of the 45th parallel was a strong risk factor for infection.[20] The south-central portion of the state was a low-risk area. Hot spots for human blastomycosis have also been identified in northwestern Ontario, Canada, where disease incidence was over 12 times higher than for other regions in the province.[49]

Dogs appear to be more susceptible to infection than humans; in enzootic areas of Arkansas and Wisconsin, the incidence of blastomycosis is 10 times higher in dogs than in humans.[36] This may relate to greater exposure to the organism rather than a true genetic predisposition. The incidence in dogs was 1,420 per 100,000 dogs per year. Young age and proximity to a shoreline were risk factors.[50] Most affected dogs are immunocompetent. Blastomycosis is rarely reported in cats. A 5-year survey of the Veterinary Medical Data Program identified three infected cats, whereas 324 dogs with blastomycosis were found.[51] However, reports of multiple cases of blastomycosis in cats suggest that it may be more common than previously appreciated and possibly underdiagnosed.[42,52] As with other soil-borne mycoses such as histoplasmosis and cryptococcosis, blastomycosis can occur in cats that have been housed entirely indoors.[42,53] In one study, 10% of 41 cats affected with blastomycosis tested positive for FeLV antigen.[54]

Young adult, large-breed (>15 kg) dogs are predisposed, and a slight male predisposition has been identified in some studies, but not others.[20,29] Overrepresented breeds include coonhounds, pointers, Weimaraners, Labrador retrievers, golden retrievers, and Doberman pinschers.[29,38] This may reflect the increased likelihood of exposure of these dog types to organisms in the environment because they are more likely to be used in outdoor activities such as hunting.[20] Blastomycosis has also been diagnosed in strictly indoor dogs and cats.[41–43,53] Dogs younger than 6 months of age and as old as 17 years may be affected, but dogs in the 2- to 4-year age group have the highest risk of infection with the 4- to 6-year age group a close second.[29,38] No breed, age, or sex predisposition for blastomycosis has been recognized in the cat.

CLINICAL FEATURES

Pathogenesis and Clinical Signs

Blastomyces infection most often results from inhalation of conidia in the environment. Direct inoculation of organisms followed by localized cutaneous disease and/or osteomyelitis (inoculation blastomycosis) occurs rarely in dogs and humans.[33,55–57] After infection becomes established in the lungs, organisms may then disseminate systemically (Fig. 80.2). Dissemination is thought to occur via vascular and lymphatic routes. Although organisms enter the lung in almost all cases, lung lesions may resolve by the time the sites of disseminated infection become apparent. Occasionally, a focal lesion develops from a puncture wound,[55,56] but generally a solitary lesion should be considered part of a systemic process. *Blastomyces* spp. could not be isolated from the nares of any of 110 healthy dogs in a highly endemic region in

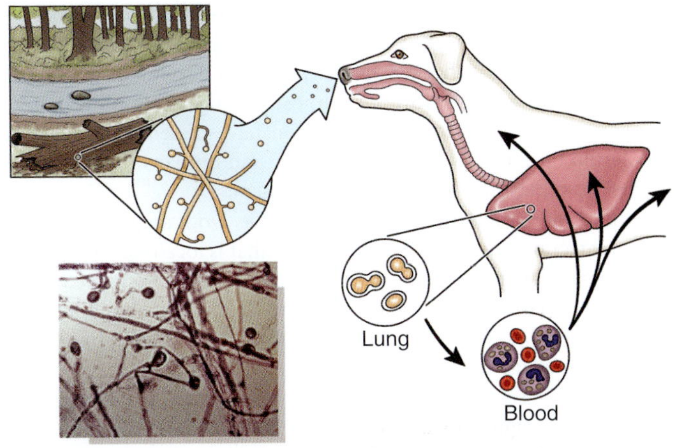

Fig. 80.2 Life cycle of *Blastomyces dermatitidis*. From the lung, the organism can disseminate to a variety of tissues, but especially the eye, lymph nodes, skin, and bones. (From Sykes JE. *Canine and Feline Infectious Diseases*. Elsevier; 2014.)

Wisconsin; of the 98 dogs with follow-up, one dog developed blastomycosis one month after culture was performed, 6 dogs died of other causes, and 91 dogs were healthy 3 years later.[58]

Blastomycosis may have a shorter incubation period in dogs than in humans.[47] Dogs may inhale a larger inoculum of organisms than humans because they are closer to the ground and actively sniffing the environment. Larger doses of inoculum may be associated with more rapid progression and earlier mortality.[59]

Once within the host, the conidia transform into yeasts that can resist destruction by neutrophils. The yeasts trigger a pyogranulomatous inflammatory response. Important virulence factors include a cell surface glycoprotein known as BAD-1 (previously known as WI-1), and other cell wall components such as α-1,3-glucan and possibly melanin.[60–62] The BAD-1 antigen is an adhesin that binds to host cell receptors on macrophages. It may also contribute to the yeast's ability to evade the host immune response by influencing cytokine secretion and impairing complement activation.[60,63–65] The thick cell wall of the yeast may be antiphagocytic. Melanin production by the yeast may influence the pathogenesis of blastomycosis.[61] In one study, it reduced susceptibility to amphotericin B (AMB), but not to itraconazole or voriconazole.

In some animals, the organism spreads hematogenously from the lungs to associated lymph nodes and other extrapulmonary sites. Extrapulmonary sites of predilection include the skin, eye, bone, lymph nodes, reproductive tissues (prostate and testes), and the CNS. However, virtually any tissue in the body may be affected, and infection has been reported in the mammary glands, nasal or oral cavities, larynx, cardiac tissues (myocardium, endocardium, and pericardium), and very rarely in the kidneys, liver, spleen, peritoneum, GI tract, and urinary bladder.[66–68] Skin involvement is very common with disseminated *B. dermatitidis* and *B. gilchristii* infections, whereas no evidence of skin involvement was noted for humans, dogs, and cats with *B. helicus* infections.[14] In the veterinary cases, organisms were identified in the lungs, but more detailed description of clinical signs was not reported.

Antibodies against the BAD-1 antigen produced no protection against infection in a mouse model,[69] which is consistent with high antibody concentrations specific for *Blastomyces* organisms in dogs with life-threatening, progressive blastomycosis. Many dogs experimentally infected by exposure to contaminated soil recover from blastomycosis without treatment.[70] It is likely that when naturally exposed, some dogs develop mild respiratory signs and recover spontaneously. Antibodies in 2 of 48 healthy dogs from an endemic area with no history of illness suggest that occasionally dogs do develop a subclinical, self-resolving disease.[71] However, almost all dogs with clinical signs that have warranted veterinary attention have disseminated disease and should be aggressively treated. Dogs[38] and humans[13] occasionally recover from blastomycosis without treatment.

Clinical signs of blastomycosis are variable. Dogs may develop subclinical infections, acute or chronic disease that is localized to the lungs and associated lymph nodes, or severe and progressive signs that result from dissemination of the organism to multiple extrapulmonary sites. The incubation period is variable and not precisely known, but is estimated to range from 5 to 12 weeks.

Nonspecific signs of illness such as lethargy, weakness, fever, inappetence, and weight loss are common. Other common clinical manifestations (between 20% and 50% of affected dogs) include signs of respiratory involvement (such as cough and increased respiratory rate), lymphadenopathy, ocular manifestations, cutaneous lesions, and lameness.[38,72] Lameness may result from fungal osteomyelitis, arthritis, or rarely, hypertrophic osteopathy.[73] GI signs (vomiting, diarrhea, hematemesis, and melena), polyuria or polydipsia, mammary gland masses, laryngeal masses, nasal discharge, sneezing and/or epistaxis, testicular masses, dysuria or hematuria secondary to prostatic involvement, cardiac arrhythmias, and neurologic signs due to meningoencephalitis or ependymitis occur less frequently.[38,68,74–78] Neurologic involvement secondary to extension of intranasal or retrobulbar *Blastomyces* granulomas through the calvarium can also occur.[75,79] Disseminated disease can also affect the brain without extension of granulomas.[80] There have also been reports of meningitis as the primary presentation of blastomycosis, without evidence of involvement outside the CNS.[81] Rarely, thromboembolic disease has been reported.[82]

Signs of disease usually have been present for a few days to a week before evaluation, but may have been apparent for up to a year. In some dogs the disease process seems to plateau; animals show few signs for weeks to months, but then suddenly progresses. Many dogs have a history of antibacterial therapy with minimal or temporary improvement.

Physical Examination Findings

Physical examination abnormalities in dogs with blastomycosis commonly include fever, thin body condition, dehydration, and signs of respiratory involvement. Fever is present in approximately 50% of affected dogs and is usually low grade (103°F to 104°F or 39.4°C to 40.0°C) but occasionally exceeds 106°F (41.1°C).[67,78] Respiratory signs include cough, tachypnea, increased respiratory effort, and increased lung sounds on thoracic auscultation. Other common findings on physical examination are firm cutaneous or subcutaneous masses, draining or ulcerated skin lesions, and peripheral lymphadenomegaly. Careful palpation of the entire skin surface can reveal small skin lesions. Cutaneous and subcutaneous lesions are frequently found on the trunk, limbs, and digits and can also involve the muzzle (Fig. 80.3A and B). Lesions of the tongue, gingiva, or mucocutaneous junctions may also be present (Fig. 80.4). Facial swelling, exophthalmos, or facial deformity has been described in some affected dogs.[75,83] Dogs with nasal cavity involvement can have stertorous respiration, decreased nasal airflow, or nasal discharge. Ocular signs may be unilateral or bilateral and include chorioretinitis (sometimes with retinal detachment) (Fig. 80.5); lesions consistent with optic neuritis; endophthalmitis or panophthalmitis; uveitis with aqueous flare, iris bombé, synechia, and miosis; cataract formation; conjunctivitis; keratitis; and photophobia.[84,85] Severe ocular involvement may result in increased intraocular pressures and/or loss of vision. Dogs with musculoskeletal involvement may be lame, have firm swellings associated with long bones, or exhibit joint swelling, warmth, and/or pain. Dogs with testicular blastomycosis may have scrotal swelling or palpable testicular masses. Neurologic signs are present in fewer than 5% of affected dogs and can include seizures, hypermetria, decreased placing reactions, tetraparesis, circling, ataxia, blindness, decreased or absent menace and/or pupillary light reflexes, nystagmus, and decreased facial sensation (Table 80.1).

Physical examination findings in cats with blastomycosis are similar to those described in dogs. These include fever, thin body condition, peripheral lymphadenopathy, tachypnea, increased or decreased lung sounds, ocular abnormalities (chorioretinitis with retinal detachment, uveitis, panophthalmitis, and secondary glaucoma), nodular or draining skin lesions (Fig. 80.6), and a variety of neurologic signs that include obtundation, ataxia, pelvic limb paresis, circling, hyperesthesia, decreased placing reactions, and blindness.[53,86–89]

DIAGNOSIS

A diagnosis of blastomycosis is usually suspected based on the presence of suspicious clinicopathologic abnormalities in a dog or cat from an endemic area. The diagnosis is usually confirmed through cytologic examination of fine-needle aspirates of affected tissues (especially skin lesions and lymph nodes), impression smears of draining skin lesions, respiratory lavage specimens (transtracheal washes or bronchoalveolar lavage), or body fluids (especially CSF or ocular fluid, but also synovial fluid, diagnostic peritoneal lavage, or urine sediment). Other methods of diagnosis include histopathology (e.g., of bone or tissue biopsies), fungal culture, PCR-based assays, and EIA antigen assays (Table 80.2).

Laboratory Abnormalities

Complete Blood Count

The hemogram of dogs or cats with blastomycosis can be unremarkable. However, a mild, normocytic, normochromic nonregenerative anemia is present in many affected animals likely due to chronic inflammation. Mild to moderate neutrophilia is also present in many dogs and may be accompanied by a mild to moderate bandemia.[38,90] Mild monocytosis, lymphocytosis, or lymphopenia may be detected.

Serum Biochemical Tests

Serum biochemistry findings in animals with blastomycosis include mild to moderate hyperglobulinemia due to a polyclonal gammopathy, hypoalbuminemia, and, uncommonly, mild hypercalcemia.[38,90,91] Hypoalbuminemia was present in 70 of 91 (77%) of dogs in one study, hyperglobulinemia in 58%, and hypercalcemia in 14% of dogs.[38] In one study, 22 dogs with blastomycosis had significantly higher serum ionized calcium concentrations than 35 healthy control dogs.[92] These dogs also had lower serum concentrations of 25-hydroxyvitamin D and parathyroid hormone, as has been described in patients with mycobacteriosis (see Chapter 61).

Urinalysis

The urinalysis is usually unremarkable in animals with blastomycosis, but occasionally proteinuria, pyuria, hematuria, or cylindruria are present. Rarely, *Blastomyces* spp. yeasts are identified in the sediment.

Cerebrospinal Fluid Analysis

CSF analysis in dogs with CNS blastomycosis can reveal increased total nucleated cell counts and increased CSF protein concentration.[93] Nucleated cells typically consist of a mixture of small and large

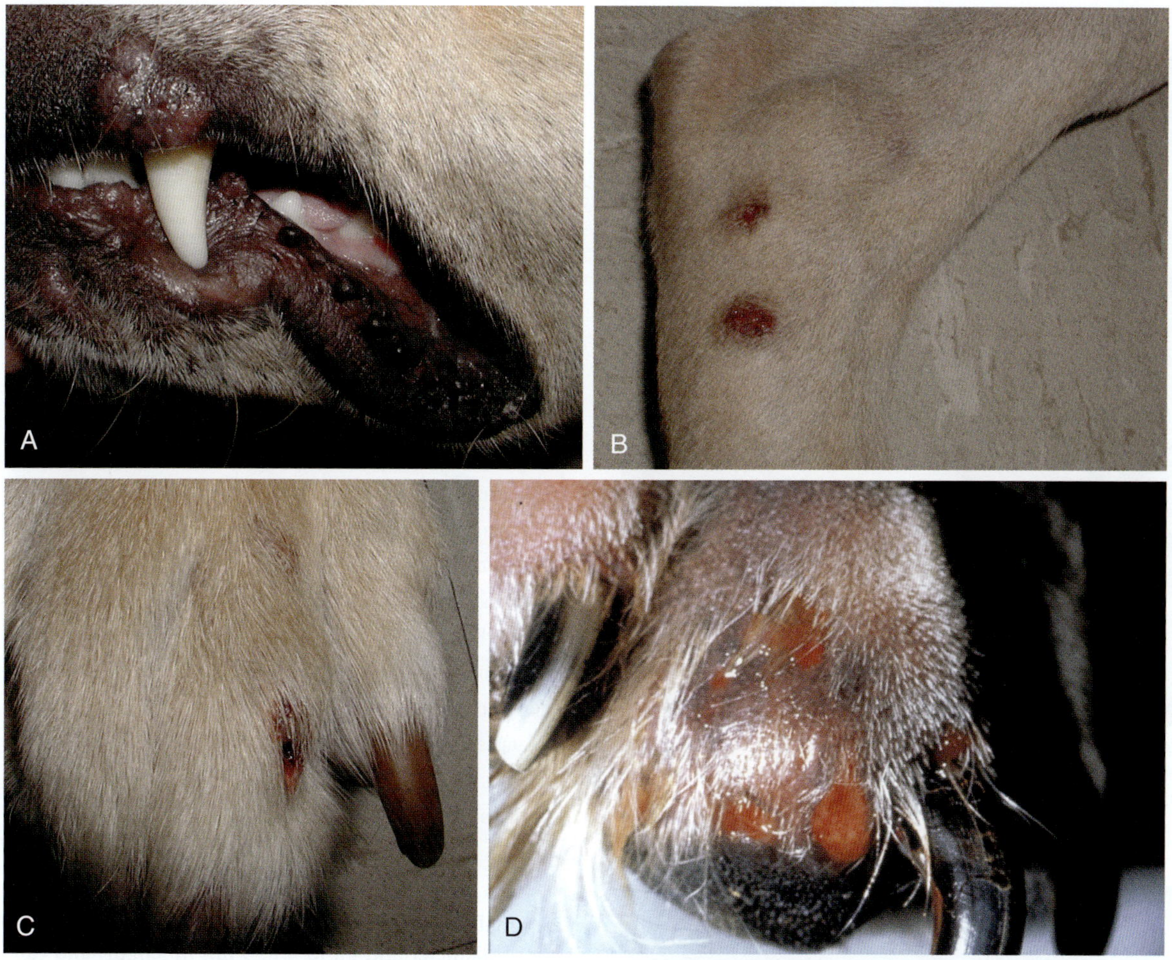

Fig. 80.3 (A-C) Disseminated blastomycosis in a Labrador retriever. (A) Nodular cutaneous lesions are present on the muzzle. There are also multiple, ulcerated, and draining skin lesions on the distal limbs (B) and digit (C). (D) Granulomatous lesion of nail bed associated with blastomycosis in a dog. (A-C, courtesy of Dr. Sheila Torres, University of Minnesota. D, courtesy of Linda Frank, University of Tennessee, Knoxville, TN.)

mononuclear cells and neutrophils. Although rare, in dogs with brain involvement, organisms may be found on cytological analysis.

Diagnostic Imaging

Plain Radiography

Radiographic patterns in dogs with blastomycosis vary considerably and include unstructured, miliary, or nodular interstitial patterns; a bronchointerstitial pattern; alveolar or mixed alveolar-interstitial patterns; pulmonary mass lesions (>3 cm in diameter); or single or multiple large (0.5 to 2.9 cm) pulmonary nodules that can resemble metastatic pulmonary neoplasia (Fig. 80.7).[38,94,95] Tracheobronchial lymphadenomegaly is present in approximately 25% of dogs.[94] Pleural thickening and mild pleural effusion are uncommonly identified (≤10% of affected dogs). Focal bronchiectasis has also been described. In one study, only 2 of 125 dogs with blastomycosis had no visible abnormalities on thoracic radiography. Findings in affected cats include diffuse miliary or nodular interstitial patterns, lobar consolidation, and/or pleural effusion.[53,86]

Radiographs of affected bone typically show osteolysis, often accompanied by periosteal proliferation and soft tissue swelling. Pathologic fractures may be identified (Fig. 80.8A and B). Evidence of hypertrophic osteopathy was present bilaterally along the humerus, radius, ulna, metacarpi, and phalanges of a dog with a mass lesion in the right middle lung lobe.[73]

Advanced Imaging

CT findings in dogs with CNS blastomycosis include intra-axial, intranasal, or retrobulbar mass lesions that are uniformly or heterogeneously contrast-enhancing.[75] An intra-axial contrast-enhancing mass lesion was also described in a cat.[96] Intranasal or retrobulbar mass lesions can invade the cribriform plate or other parts of the skull, with associated osteolysis. Meningeal or periventricular contrast enhancement may also be present.[75,76] MRI findings have not been extensively described in dogs. One dog had a retrobulbar mass lesion that extended through the calvarium; the lesion was iso- to hypointense on T2-weighted images, slightly hypointense on T1-weighted images, and showed strong homogenous contrast enhancement.[79] In addition to mass lesions, periventricular and meningeal contrast enhancement, as well as ventriculomegaly, have also been described.[97]

Microbiologic Tests

Cytologic Examination

Diagnosis has historically been made by identifying the organism through cytologic or histologic evaluation. Cytologic examination of

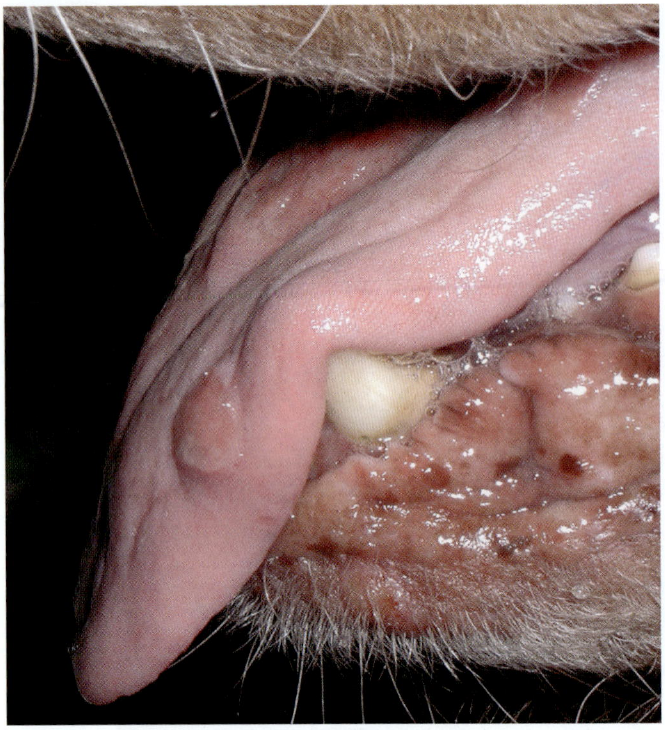

Fig. 80.4 Nodular and ulcerated lesions of the tongue in a dog with disseminated blastomycosis. (Courtesy of Dr. Sheila Torres, University of Minnesota.)

TABLE 80.1 Physical Examination Findings in 115 Dogs with Blastomycosis[29]

Clinical Sign	Percent of Dogs
Fever	62
Lymphadenopathy	56
Harsh lung sounds	50
Skin lesions	49
Chorioretinitis	43
Anterior uveitis	42
Cough	32
Emaciation	25
Retinal detachment	23
Cutaneous mass	16
Glaucoma	16
Tachypnea	16
Dehydration	15
Bony mass/swelling	14
Nasal discharge	8
Neurologic signs	6
Prostatomegaly	5
Mammary mass	3
Orchitis	2
Synovial effusion	2

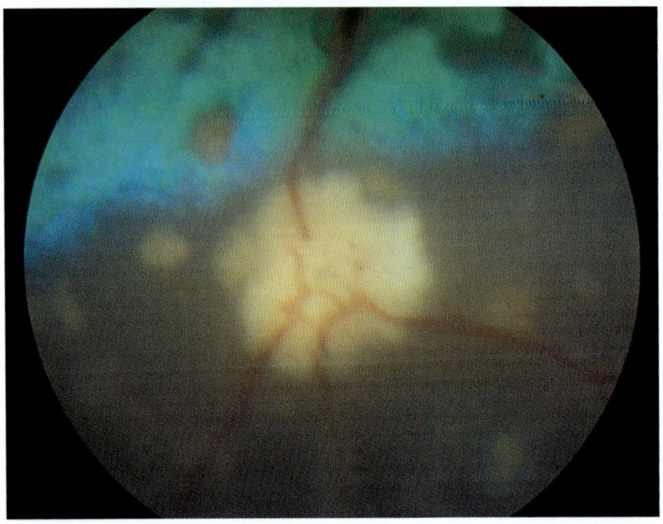

Fig. 80.5 Chorioretinitis and retinal detachment associated with blastomycosis in a dog. (Courtesy of Diane Hendrix, University of Tennessee, Knoxville, TN.)

fine-needle aspirates, respiratory wash specimens, or body fluids frequently reveals large numbers of *Blastomyces* spp. yeasts. The yeasts of *B. dermatitidis* and *B. gilchristii* are 8 to 15 μm in diameter, have a thick, refractile cell wall, and exhibit broad-based budding (Fig. 80.9A and B). Daughter cells are nearly as large as the parent cell when they detach. A pyogranulomatous inflammatory response is usually present. Occasionally, organisms are not seen; the sensitivity of transtracheal lavage for diagnosis of pulmonary blastomycosis in two studies of 17 and 39 dogs was 76% and 69%, respectively,[90,95] whereas the sensitivity of FNA of the lung was 46 of 57 (81%).[90] The yeasts of *B. helicus* are smaller than those of *B. dermatitidis* and *B. gilchristii* (2.5 to 6.5 μm in diameter and up to 4 to 9 μm in length) and can exhibit multiple budding with chains of organisms; hyphal forms also have been described.[14] These have the potential to be mistaken for *Candida* spp. and misidentification as *Histoplasma* spp. has been reported.

Serologic Diagnosis

Until recently, AGID was the most widely available antibody assay to detect antibodies to the *Blastomyces* spp. A antigen. Unfortunately, AGID assays have variable and generally unacceptable sensitivity for diagnosis of blastomycosis in dogs and cats, which has ranged from 17% to 91%.[38,71,86,90,98,99] An EIA that used crude mold-phase *Blastomyces* spp. as the antigen had a sensitivity of 76.1%,[99] and a radioimmunoassay designed to detect antibody responses to the BAD-1 antigen had a sensitivity of 92%.[71] The specificity of AGID assay exceeds 95% based on limited studies of healthy dogs or dogs with diagnoses other than blastomycosis.[71,98] Several other antigens have been studied for their potential to be used for antibody detection assays.[100] However, because false-positive test results have the potential to occur as a result of exposure and recovery in endemic areas or as a result of cross-reactivity to other infectious agents, diagnosis based on positive antibody serology alone is not recommended.

Higher sensitivities than AGID were reported with an EIA for antibodies to recombinant *Blastomyces* adhesion-1 repeat antigen (rBAD-1). The sensitivity of the antibody EIA was 95% in dogs versus 65% with the AGID assay. The specificity of the antibody EIA was 95% in healthy dogs, and 100% in dogs with nonfungal pulmonary disease.[101]

An assay that detects *Blastomyces* cell wall galactomannan antigen (MiraVista Diagnostics, Indianapolis, IN, USA) has largely replaced antibody assays for serologic diagnosis of canine blastomycosis. The *Blastomyces* antigen EIA is useful in the diagnosis of blastomycosis

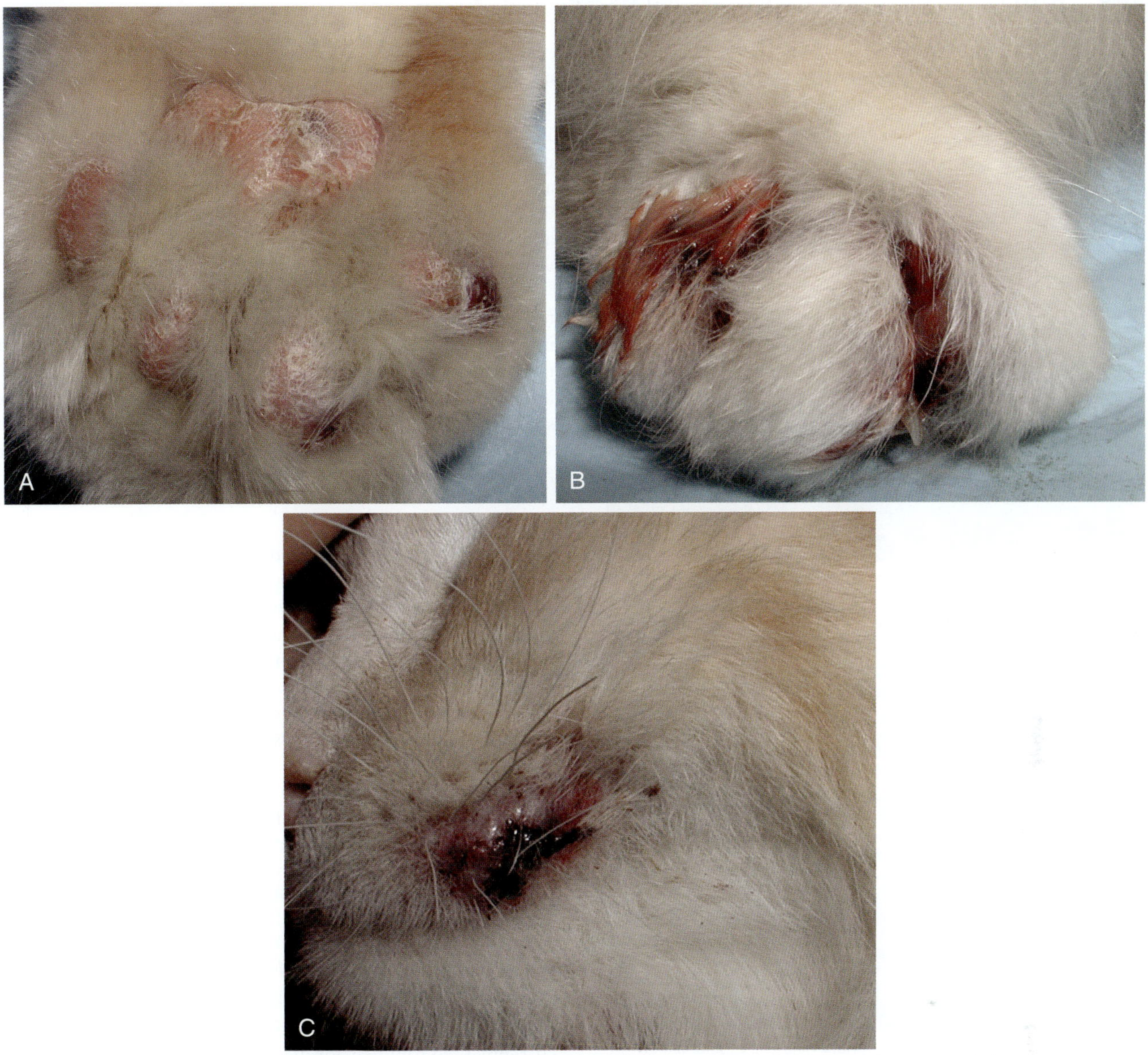

Fig. 80.6 Cutaneous lesions in a cat with disseminated blastomycosis that involved the footpads (A), interdigital folds (B), and lips (C). (Courtesy of Dr. Sheila Torres, University of Minnesota.)

TABLE 80.2 Diagnostic Assays Currently Available for Blastomycosis in Dogs and Cats

Assay	Specimen Type	Target	Performance
Cytologic examination	Aspirates of affected tissues, body fluids, impression smears of skin lesions	*Blastomyces* spp. yeasts	Organisms are usually present in variable numbers but occasionally may not be visualized. Organisms may appear disrupted after treatment with antifungal drugs.
Fungal culture	Aspirates or biopsies of affected tissues, body fluids	*Blastomyces* spp.	Rarely indicated. Sensitive and specific and may be required for animals when cytologic examination is negative. Risk of laboratory-acquired infections. Slow turnaround time (may require several weeks of incubation).
Antibody serology (gel immunodiffusion)	Serum	Antibodies to *Blastomyces* spp.	When present in conjunction with consistent clinical signs, positive test results usually indicate active infection, but the potential for false positives exists. Negative test results occur commonly in dogs and cats with blastomycosis (low sensitivity).
Antigen assay (ELISA)	Urine, serum	*Blastomyces* spp. antigen	Highly sensitive (>90%) when urine is used as the test specimen. False positives are extremely rare in dogs that lack fungal disease, but cross-reactivity with other fungal pathogens may occur (especially *Histoplasma*), so positive results are not diagnostic for blastomycosis.
Real-time PCR assays	Whole blood	*Blastomyces* spp. DNA	Not yet validated in adequate numbers of dogs or cats with blastomycosis; usefulness requires further evaluation.
Histopathology	Biopsy specimens from affected tissues	*Blastomyces* spp. yeasts	Sensitive, but yeasts may be difficult to find in some infections. Special stains may assist organism detection.

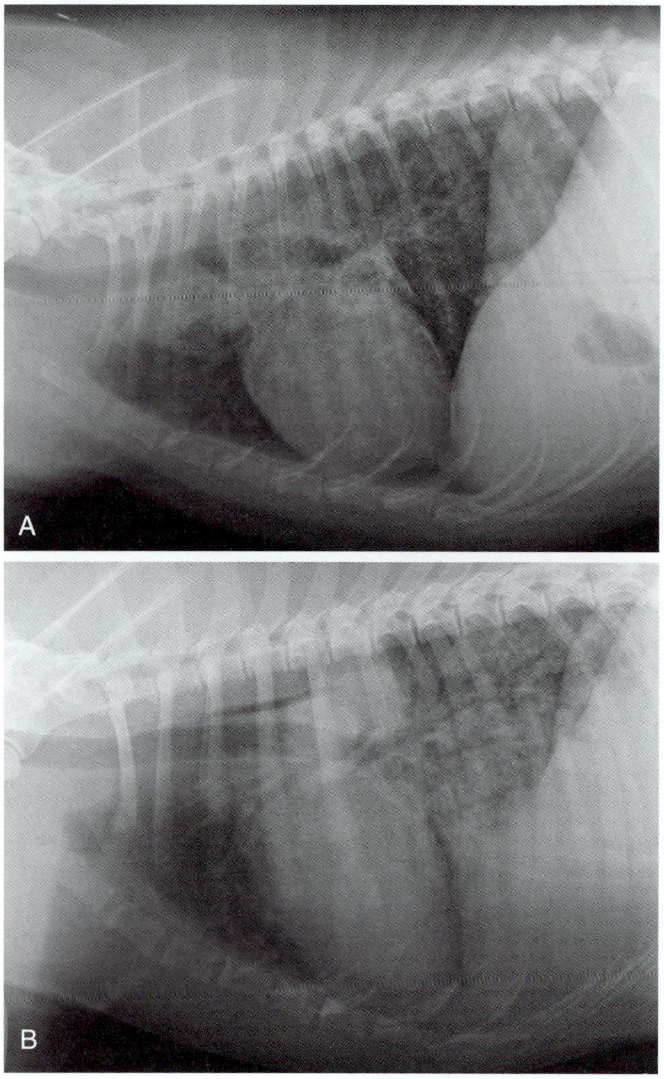

Fig. 80.7 Radiographic patterns in pulmonary blastomycosis. (A) Lateral thoracic radiograph from a 2-year-old female spayed Labrador retriever with a 1-week history of cough and inappetence. A diffuse miliary nodular interstitial pattern is present. (B) Lateral thoracic radiograph from a 5-year-old female spayed German shepherd dog with lethargy and inappetence. An alveolar pattern is present in the caudal lung lobes, along with marked hilar lymphadenopathy. There is also a nodular lesion in the cranial lung lobes just ventral to the trachea. (Courtesy of Daniel Cronk, University of Minnesota.)

(especially in cases lacking cytologic or histologic identification of the organism) and was first reported for use in dogs in 2008.[99] A *Blastomyces* antigen EIA has been available for diagnosis of blastomycosis in humans since 2004 and has since been modified to allow quantification.[102,103] In humans, the overall sensitivity of the quantitative *Blastomyces* antigen EIA was 90%, including 41/46 individuals (89%) with isolated pulmonary blastomycosis, 24/26 (92%) of those with pulmonary and extrapulmonary infection, and 15/17 (88%) of those with extrapulmonary involvement.[103] Equal sensitivity (79%) was reported for *B. dermatitidis* and *B. gilchristii* infections in humans, although there was a trend for antigen concentrations to be higher in *B. dermatitidis* infections.[104] Whether the same is true in dogs is unknown.

The performance of this assay was evaluated in 46 dogs with confirmed blastomycosis.[99] When urine was used, the sensitivity was 93.5%, whereas when serum was assayed, sensitivity was 87%. Only 1 of 43 control dogs without blastomycosis had a positive test result. In another study, 70 dogs with and without blastomycosis were evaluated using the MiraVista antigen EIA. Sensitivity was 100% in serum and urine specimens from dogs with blastomycosis, with specificity of 95% in urine specimens from dogs with nonfungal pulmonary disease and 100% in urine specimens from healthy dogs.[101] Positive test results were also reported for some *B. helicus* infections.[14]

In human patients, the sensitivity of urine galactomannan antigen testing was 90%, and specificity was 99% in patients without fungal infections. However, 96% of humans with histoplasmosis tested positive because of cross-reactivity.[99,103] Positive test results can also occur in dogs and cats that have histoplasmosis. The EIA antibody had 88% specificity when looking at dogs with blastomycosis and histoplasmosis, which indicates it may have a role in distinguishing blastomycosis from histoplasmosis.[101]

Fungal Culture

Blastomyces spp. can be isolated from clinical specimens on routine fungal media in the laboratory. Growth of a white mold typically appears after incubation for 1 to 3 weeks, but occasionally incubation periods of up to 5 weeks are required. The organism is identified based on the morphology of its conidia, which are round to oval and attached to hyphae. *Blastomyces dermatitidis* and *B. gilchristii* are morphologically indistinguishable, and differentiation requires molecular typing. This is typically not done (unless for epidemiologic studies) because of lack of known clinical significance. *Blastomyces helicus* can be identified based on its morphology in culture; unlike *B. dermatitidis*, it does not produce conidia. Because *Blastomyces* spp. grow as a mycelium in the laboratory, culture is a laboratory health hazard and should be performed only if necessary. The laboratory should be warned of the possibility of a dimorphic fungal infection so that appropriate precautions are taken.

Molecular Diagnosis Using Nucleic Acid–Based Testing

Real-time PCR assays have been developed that rapidly detect *Blastomyces* spp. in clinical specimens from humans,[105,106] but are not currently used routinely for diagnosis in dogs and cats. The sensitivity of one assay was 86% when compared with culture of clinical specimens.[106] PCR assays have not been widely applied to the diagnosis of blastomycosis in dogs and cats.

Pathologic Findings

Gross pathologic findings in dogs with blastomycosis include thin body condition; characteristic skin lesions; bony proliferations that may be accompanied by pathologic fracture; enlargement of the peripheral and/or tracheobronchial lymph nodes; ocular lesions; lung consolidation; and firm, pale, pulmonary nodules or masses that range in size from 1 mm to several centimeters in diameter. Masses may be caseous on cut surface. Animals with CNS involvement may have masses within the brain, secondary hydrocephalus, or retrobulbar or caudal nasal cavity granulomas that may invade the cribriform plate and extend along the optic nerves.[78,93] Rarely, pleural and/or peritoneal effusion and nodular lesions within abdominal viscera have been reported.[67] Testicular and prostatic masses can also be found.[78] Histopathology reveals granulomatous or pyogranulomatous inflammatory infiltrates in a variety of organs, often with intralesional budding yeasts (Fig. 80.10). Multinucleated giant cells, fibroblasts, and large numbers of lymphocytes may also be present. Ocular lesions include uveitis, choroiditis, retinal detachment, retinal degeneration, lens rupture, cataracts, optic neuritis, and vitritis.[78,84] Secondary hepatic and renal amyloidosis was described in one dog.[107]

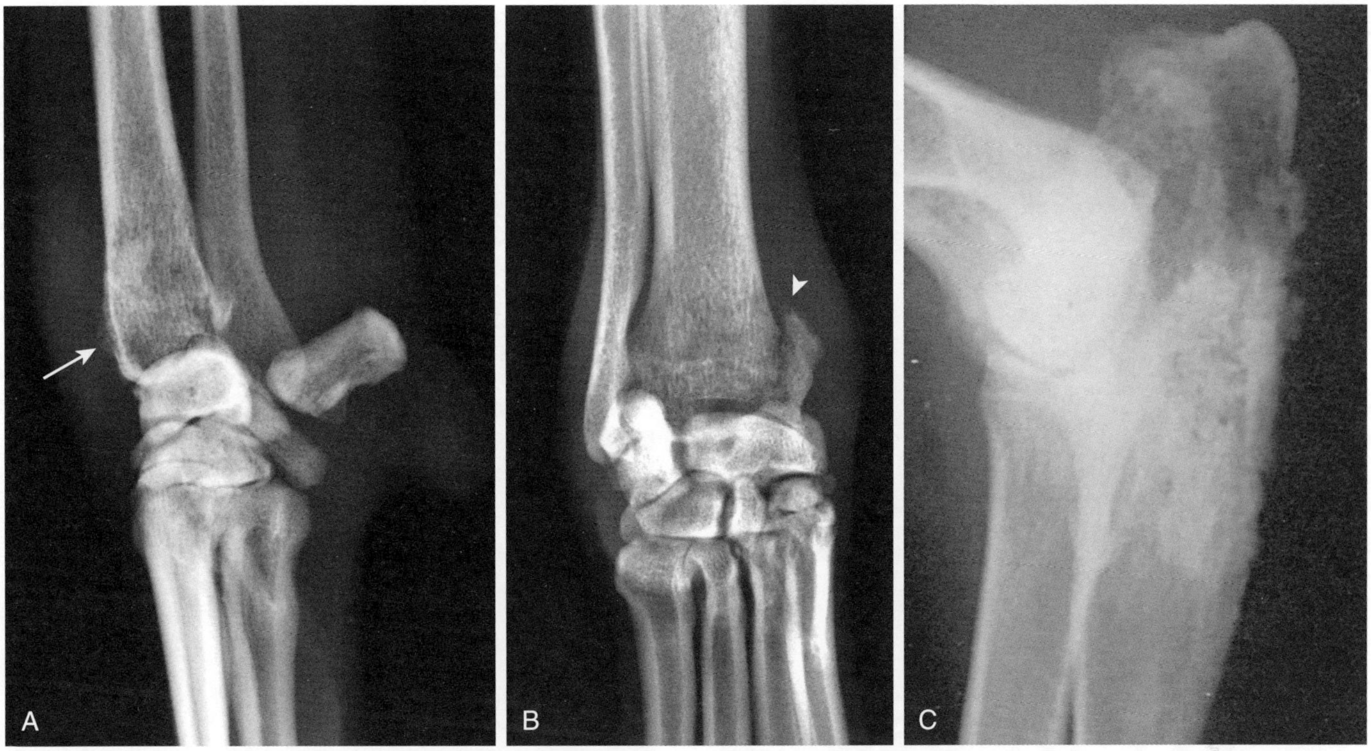

Fig. 80.8 Lateral (A) and anteropalmar (B) radiograph of the right carpus showing an osteolytic and osteoproductive *(arrow)* lesion with a pathologic fracture *(arrowhead)* and associated soft tissue swelling in the distal radius of a 6-year-old male neutered Labrador retriever with disseminated blastomycosis. (C) Semi-aggressive bone lesion characterized by osteolysis and amorphous bone production in the proximal tibia of a dog. (A and B, courtesy of Daniel Cronk, University of Minnesota.)

Organisms are not always detected in lesions, even in untreated dogs. Special stains such as silver stains, PAS, and immunohistochemical stains can assist in the identification of *Blastomyces* spp. yeasts within sections,[84,107,108] but failure to detect yeasts does not rule out blastomycosis.

TREATMENT AND PROGNOSIS

The most widely used treatment for blastomycosis in dogs is itraconazole, which is effective as a single agent in many dogs.[109] Itraconazole has largely replaced the use of ketoconazole for treatment of blastomycosis. The recommended dose of itraconazole for dogs is 5 mg/kg, PO, q24h. This dose has an equivalent efficacy as a dose of 5 mg/kg, PO, q12h and a lower rate of adverse effects such as anorexia.[109]

Seventy-four percent of dogs treated with 5 mg/kg q24h of itraconazole responded to treatment; a 77% response rate was found in a historic control group treated with AMB.[109] Of the dogs that responded initially, 20% of dogs treated with AMB and 20% of dogs treated with itraconazole had recurrence of disease after completing treatment.[109] In another study, 21 of 31 dogs (68%) responded to a 60- to 90-day course of itraconazole. Of those that responded, 5 of 21 dogs (24%) had a recurrence, and 4 of those dogs were successfully retreated with a second course of itraconazole.[38] The mortality rates of itraconazole- and AMB-treated dogs were similar (Table 80.3).

Itraconazole appears to penetrate the eye in dogs with active disease, because the dogs with ocular blastomycosis of the posterior chamber often respond to itraconazole treatment.[110] Twice-daily dosing with 5 mg/kg has been recommended for intraocular infections.[111] The bioavailability of compounded itraconazole is very low; therefore, use of compounded itraconazole is not recommended (see Chapter 11).[112]

The duration of azole treatment should be based on serial monitoring of clinical signs and radiographic lesions (e.g., every 4 to 8 weeks). Most dogs require at least 3 to 6 months of treatment. Some dogs require treatment for more than 1 year, especially those with osteoarticular infections or widespread dissemination. Because fluconazole is less active, its use is not recommended for treatment of human blastomycosis, unless itraconazole is not tolerated.[113–115]

Treatment with deoxycholate AMB or lipid-complexed AMB is also effective and should be considered for dogs with severe disease with widespread dissemination, dogs and cats with CNS involvement, for animals that do not respond to azole monotherapy, or for those that do not tolerate itraconazole.[90,116] Cats with blastomycosis have also been treated with variable success with combinations of AMB and azoles or AMB alone.[53,86] In human patients, the use of deoxycholate or lipid-complexed AMB is recommended for severe pulmonary or disseminated disease, followed by itraconazole therapy after there has been a satisfactory clinical response.[115] Whether protocols that include AMB offer a survival advantage over azole monotherapy for dogs or cats has not been well studied in a prospective fashion. Other drugs that have been used successfully to treat human blastomycosis include voriconazole and posaconazole.[114,117] Because of its ability to penetrate the CNS and eye, voriconazole has been recommended for treatment of human CNS blastomycosis after initial treatment with lipid-complexed AMB.[114,118]

Urine *Blastomyces* galactomannan antigen concentration declines with effective antifungal drug treatment.[99] Urine antigen testing has proven useful not only at the time of diagnosis but also when considering to discontinue treatment as well as documenting poor clinical

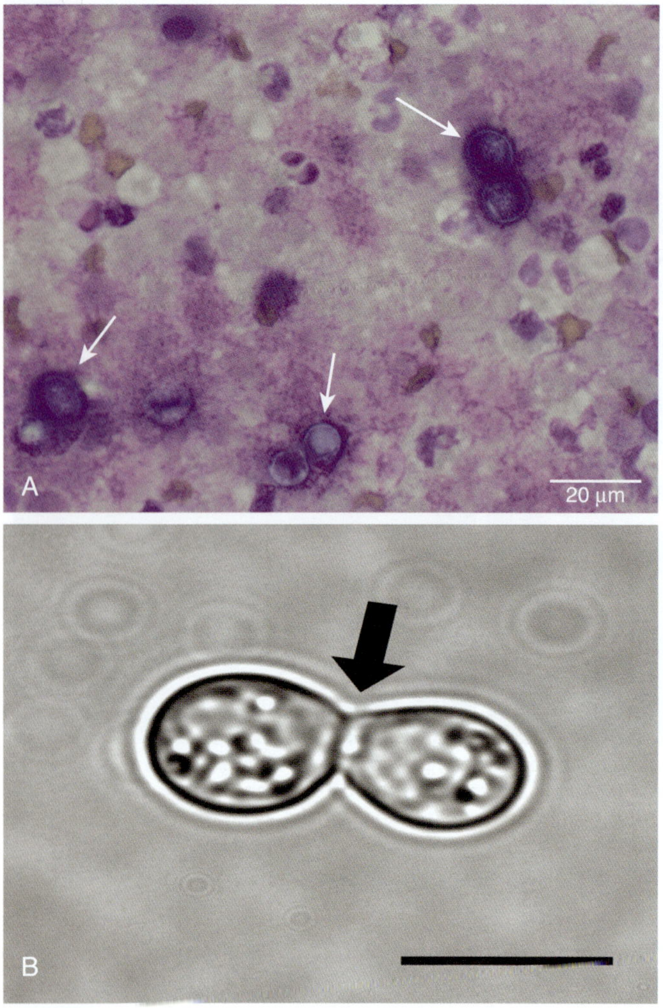

Fig. 80.9 (A) Cytology of a fine-needle aspirate of a skin lesion from a dog with blastomycosis. *Blastomyces* yeasts *(arrows)* have a thick wall and exhibit broad-based budding. A pyogranulomatous inflammatory response is also present. (B) B, *B dermatitidis* yeast. Broad-based budding yeast at 37°C. Arrow points to the broad-based bud between mother and daughter cells. Scale bar is 10 µm. (A, courtesy of Dr. Jed Overmann, University of Minnesota. B, From McBride JA, Gauthier GM, Klein BS. Clinical Manifestations and Treatment of Blastomycosis. *Clin Chest Med* 38 (2017) 435–449. Fig 1. http://dx.doi.org/10.1016/j.ccm.2017.04.006.)

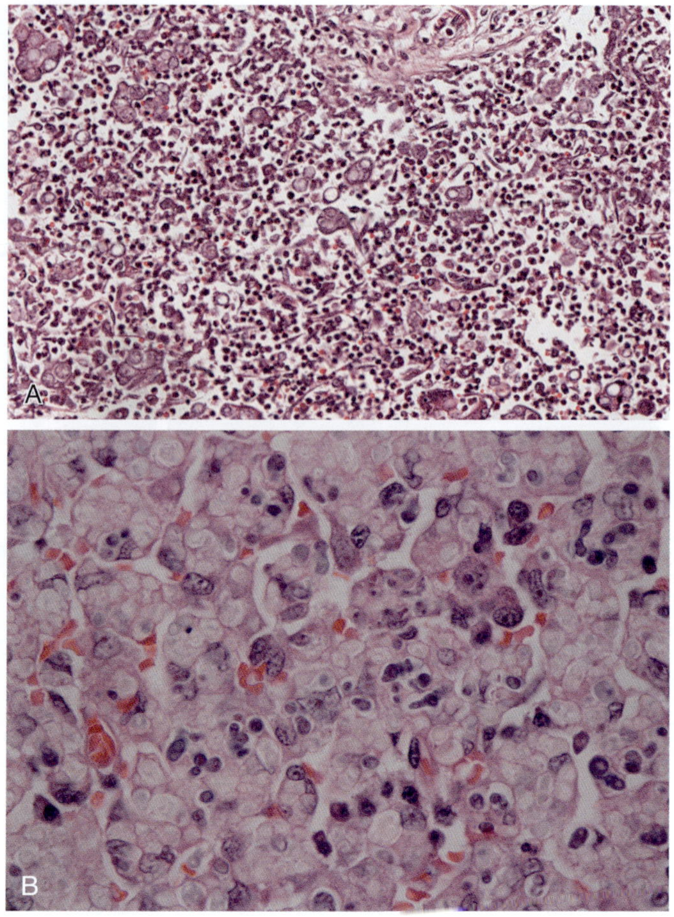

Fig. 80.10 Histopathologic findings in dogs with blastomycosis. (A) Histopathology of the lymph node from a 10-year-old female spayed Australian shepherd dog with blastomycosis. Severe pyogranulomatous lymphadenitis is present with moderate numbers of large yeast organisms. (B) Histopathology of the lung of another Australian shepherd dog that had a pulmonary and a mediastinal abscess due to *Blastomyces* spp. infection. Abundant yeast organisms are present. 1000× oil magnification. (A, courtesy of Dr. Catherine Benson, University of Minnesota. B, courtesy of Dr. Patricia Pesavento, University of California, Davis.)

response or relapse of disease.[119] A low *Blastomyces* galactomannan urine antigen concentration was positively correlated with survival in one retrospective study.[120] A common practice is to continue antifungal therapy until there have been two negative antigen tests at least 3 to 4 weeks apart.

Therapeutic drug monitoring should be considered should the response to treatment be inadequate (see Chapter 11).[109] The dose should be adjusted to achieve serum itraconazole concentrations of 2 µg/mL or greater.

Supportive Care

The severity of lung pathology increased in the initial week of treatment in 23% of dogs.[94] The worsening of signs has been attributed to an inflammatory response to killed yeasts in the lungs. The worsening of infiltrates seen radiographically was not associated with a less favorable outcome.[94] Death usually results from respiratory failure and occurs in 50% of the dogs with severe lung disease during the first 7 days of treatment. Mechanical ventilation was used to treat 5 (4%) of 125 dogs with pulmonary blastomycosis in one report, none of which survived.[90,94]

Dexamethasone (0.25 to 0.5 mg/kg, IV, for 2 to 3 days) can be given to dogs that develop life-threatening respiratory disease after starting antifungal drug treatment. Dogs that receive glucocorticoids for this purpose should be treated for at least 90 days with antifungal drugs.

Other treatments that may be required for treatment of dogs or cats with severe pulmonary blastomycosis are supplemental oxygen, nebulization and coupage, IV fluid therapy, and, in some cases, mechanical ventilation.[90] Dogs with CNS involvement may require treatment with anticonvulsants in order to control seizure activity. The concurrent use of systemic glucocorticoids should also be considered to control brain inflammation and edema, although whether this ultimately improves outcome is not known. For animals that lack CNS involvement, NSAIDs can be used to control pyrexia. Topical anti-inflammatory

TABLE 80.3 Drug Therapy for Blastomycosis

Drug	Species	Dose[a] (mg/kg)	Route	Interval (Hours)	Duration[b] (Days)
Itraconazole	Dog[c]	5	PO	24	60
	Cat	5	PO	12	60
Fluconazole	Dog	5	PO	12	60
Amphotericin B, lipid complex[d]	Dog	1	IV	3 times weekly	Varies[e]
Amphotericin B	Dog	0.5	IV	3 times weekly	Varies[f]
	Cat	0.25	IV	3 times weekly	Varies[g]

[a]Dose per administration at specified interval.
[b]Minimum duration of therapy. Ideally, therapy should continue for at least 1 month beyond the last detection of clinical illness/infection or two negative urine antigen tests at least 4 weeks apart.
[c]Itraconazole is preferred drug and dosage therapy. A 12-hour interval (10 mg/kg/day total dose) is recommended when intraocular involvement is present.[18] Fluconazole may also better penetrate the eye when treating intraocular infections; however, it is not as active as itraconazole. Enucleation may be needed.
[d]Three lipid formulations are available. Efficacy at this dose has been established for ABLC (Abelcet, Enzon Pharmaceuticals, Bridgewater, NJ).
[e]Stop when cumulative dose reaches 12 mg/kg.
[f]Stop when azotemic or cumulative dose reaches 4–6 mg/kg, then start azole, or when cumulative dose is 8–10 mg/kg when given alone.
[g]Stop when azotemic or cumulative dose reaches 4 mg/kg, then use itraconazole.
IV, intravenous; *PO*, oral.

and antiglaucoma agents may be indicated if ocular involvement is present. Enucleation may ultimately be required if endophthalmitis is present to control ocular pain and eliminate infection. Treatment of osteomyelitis or large pulmonary granulomas that are refractory to antifungal chemotherapy may require surgical treatment by amputation or lung lobectomy, respectively.

Cure rates of 50% to 75% have been reported in dogs with blastomycosis.[109,121] An additional 20%–24% of dogs experience relapse of disease after treatment is discontinued.[38,109,121] Recurrence after apparently successful treatment usually occurs in the first 6 months after completion of therapy, but recurrences can occur up to 3 years after completion of therapy.[38,109,121] As mentioned previously, clinical signs and radiographic lesions can worsen in the first few days of treatment in some affected dogs,[94] possibly due to the inflammatory response to dying organisms. The median time for resolution of primary radiographic patterns in dogs with pulmonary blastomycosis in one study was 186 days (range, 4 to >355 days).[94] Significantly longer mean treatment durations were required for radiographic improvement of large pulmonary masses when compared with alveolar and interstitial patterns. The most common radiographic sequela to pulmonary blastomycosis is development of one or more pulmonary bullae. Unstructured interstitial patterns may also persist, presumably as a result of pulmonary fibrosis.[94]

Involvement of the CNS, severe lung disease, and a high band neutrophil count have been identified as negative prognostic factors.[90,109,121] In another study where dogs with blastomycosis were followed for 5 years, serum 25-hydroxyvitamin D concentration and radiographic evidence of pulmonary involvement did not appear to influence prognosis,[97] but increased serum lactate concentration; bone, skin, and lymph node involvement; number of affected sites; and the presence of respiratory signs were associated with survival. In another study, the median band neutrophil count in dogs that did not survive was 1,200 cells/μL (range, 0 to 3,980 cells/μL), whereas that in survivors was 0 cells/μL (range, 0 to 2,380 cells/μL).[90] In that study, 63% of 125 dogs with blastomycosis survived. The prognosis for survival in animals with neurologic involvement is particularly poor. The prognosis for resolution of endophthalmitis is also poor; only 20% of eyes with endophthalmitis respond favorably to antifungal drug treatment.[85] Nevertheless, eyes that do not undergo enucleation can ultimately progress to phthisis bulbi after completion of treatment, without recurrence of systemic infection.[85]

IMMUNITY AND VACCINATION

Immunity to blastomycosis is initially dependent on phagocyte function, especially neutrophils and alveolar macrophages, which can clear conidia. However, once the organisms have transitioned to the yeast form, control of infection also depends on T cells, which stimulate macrophages to kill the yeasts.[115] Humoral immunity is not essential for resolution of infection.

An experimental vaccine that includes a genetically engineered, live-attenuated BAD-1 deletion mutant *B. dermatitidis* strain protected mice from experimental infection. This vaccine was documented as being safe in 25 beagles and 78 foxhounds in a field trial and induced specific immune responses to *B. dermatitidis* antigens.[122,123] Although further study is required, this vaccine holds promise for prevention of blastomycosis in dogs that reside in hyperendemic regions of the United States.

PREVENTION

Avoidance of specific foci of hyperendemicity where other dogs or humans have contracted blastomycosis may prevent blastomycosis, but this is not always possible.

PUBLIC HEALTH ASPECTS

Like dogs, humans acquire *Blastomyces* spp. infection from the environment. Dogs are considered sentinels for human exposure and infection,[17] although whether strains that infect dogs also infect humans requires further study. The incidence of blastomycosis in dogs is approximately eight times that in humans, and disease has been reported in humans and dogs that reside in the same household.[41,47] Approximately 50% of human infections are asymptomatic.[115] When illness develops, it typically occurs 30 to 45 days after exposure and is often a mild, self-limiting influenza-like illness with fever and cough. Blastomycosis is suspected in endemic areas when respiratory signs persist and fail to respond to treatment with antibacterial drugs. Radiographic abnormalities resemble those in dogs, although hilar lymphadenomegaly is not often seen. Chronic pulmonary blastomycosis can resemble pulmonary neoplasia or tuberculosis. Rarely, blastomycosis-associated ARDS develops, which is associated with a 75% mortality rate.[115,124] Dissemination to extrapulmonary sites similar to those involved in dogs occurs in 20% to 25% of affected humans. Skin lesions are common and are classified as either verrucous or ulcerative (Fig. 80.11A and B); bone involvement is reported in up to one fourth of cases. Although dissemination occurs equally among immunocompromised and immunocompetent humans, more severe infections with higher mortality rates can occur in immunocompromised patients such as those with AIDS, solid organ transplant recipients, and humans treated with TNF-α blockers (used to treat inflammatory diseases such as Crohn's disease, psoriasis, and rheumatoid arthritis).[115,124–127] Overall case fatality rates have ranged from 6% to 22%, and men are predisposed, possibly as a result of increased likelihood of exposure.[46] At the time of writing, blastomycosis is reportable in Arizona, Louisiana, Michigan, Minnesota, and Wisconsin.[128]

Inoculation blastomycosis that involves the skin and underlying bone has been described in veterinary personnel after sharps injuries or bite wounds from dogs with blastomycosis. One involved a needlestick injury after a lung aspirate in a dog with suspected blastomycosis, and another was an accident that occurred during a necropsy.[129,130] Bite wounds from dogs with blastomycosis can result in localized disease; disseminated disease occurred in a renal transplant recipient.[131–133] A veterinary technician developed pulmonary blastomycosis after *Blastomyces* spp. was cultured unexpectedly in a veterinary clinic in-house laboratory.[134] Although these routes of transmission are rare, prevention of sharps injuries, avoidance and proper management of bite wounds, and use of accredited veterinary laboratories for isolation of microorganisms from dogs and cats may reduce the risk of inoculation or laboratory-acquired blastomycosis in veterinary staff. The bandaging of skin lesions has been discouraged because it has the potential to promote transition of the organism to the mold form, but this has not been documented to occur. The body of deceased pets with blastomycosis should be disposed of promptly and by cremation.

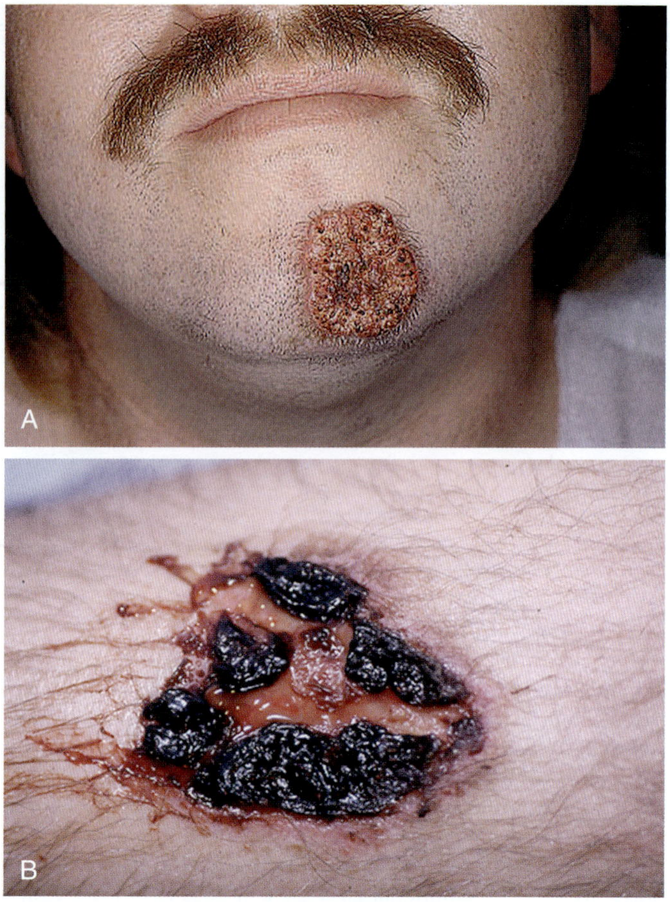

Fig. 80.11 Verrucous (A) and ulcerative (B) skin lesions in human patients with disseminated blastomycosis. (A, From Callen JP, Greer KE, Paller AS, Swinyer LJ. Color Atlas of Dermatology, ed 2, Philadelphia, 2000, Saunders. B, From Bradsher RW. Blastomycosis. In: Bennett JE, Dolin R, Blaser MJ, eds. *Mandell, Douglas and Bennett's Principles and Practice of Infectious Diseases*. Philadelphia, PA: Elsevier Saunders; 2015:2963–2973.)

CASE EXAMPLE

Signalment

"Sam," a 3-year-old male neutered golden retriever from Burlingame in northern California.

History

Sam was evaluated by the Veterinary Emergency and Critical Care Service at the University of California, Davis, for pulmonary blastomycosis, which had been diagnosed at a local veterinary clinic. Sam had a 1-week history of lethargy and inappetence. The day after illness was noted, Sam was taken to a local veterinary clinic. Routine blood work showed only anemia (hematocrit 34%), thrombocytosis (554,000 platelets/μL), and a mildly increased serum ALP activity (199 U/L). Thoracic radiographs showed hilar lymphadenomegaly, a mild diffuse miliary interstitial pattern, and focal alveolar infiltrates in the right cranial and left caudal lung lobe. Cytologic examination of a transtracheal lavage specimen showed pyogranulomatous inflammation with moderate numbers of yeasts that had morphology consistent with *Blastomyces* spp.. Serology (AGIG) for detection of antibodies to *Blastomyces* spp. was negative. Treatment with itraconazole (5 mg/kg, PO, q24h) was commenced, and after 2 days the dose was increased to 10 mg/kg, PO, q24h due to lack of clinical improvement. Subsequently, the dog's rectal temperature increased to 105°F (40.6°C) and a day later, radiographs showed an increase in the severity of the alveolar infiltrates. Treatment with carprofen (2.4 mg/kg, PO, q12h) was initiated, and subcutaneous fluids were administered. This was associated with resolution of pyrexia, but the dog remained lethargic and exercise intolerant, and the owners noted right pelvic limb lameness. The dog was referred for further evaluation.

Approximately 6 weeks before he became ill, Sam had been taken to Georgian Bay in Ontario, Canada, for 1 week. He had also been in the Vermont region for 2 months before that time. Other travel had been limited to various bayside and mountainous parts of northern California. The owner's brother's dog, which had traveled with Sam to Ontario and Vermont, had also been diagnosed with blastomycosis 3 weeks earlier.

Physical Examination

Body weight: 41.5 kg.

General: Quiet, alert, and responsive. T = 103.5°F (39.7°C), HR = 120 beats/minute, panting, CRT < 2 seconds, mucous membranes were moist and slightly cyanotic.

Eyes, ears, nose, and throat: No clinically significant abnormalities were detected. A fundoscopic examination with dilated pupils was unremarkable.

CASE EXAMPLE—cont'd

Musculoskeletal: BCS 4/9; no obvious lameness or pain on palpation was appreciated.

Respiratory: Increased respiratory effort was present. Lung sounds were increased diffusely on thoracic auscultation and partially obscured the heart sounds. Markedly increased respiratory effort was evident when the dog's gait was assessed as part of an orthopedic examination. An intermittent nonproductive cough was also appreciated.

All other systems: No clinically significant abnormalities were detected. No obvious neurologic deficits were noted, but a full neurologic examination was not performed.

Laboratory Findings

Blood oxygen saturation (pulse oximetry) = 91%, improved to 95% with flow-by supplemental oxygen.

CBC: HCT 37.3% (40%–55%), MCV 71.2 fL (65–75 fL), MCHC 35.1 g/dL (33-36 g/dL), WBC 14,640 cells/μL (6,000–13,000 cells/μL), neutrophils 11,273 cells/μL (3,000–10,500 cells/μL), band neutrophils 586 cells/μL, lymphocytes 1,318 cells/μL (1,000–4,000 cells/μL), monocytes 1,318 cells/μL (150–1,200 cells/μL), eosinophils 146 cells/μL (0–1,500 cells/μL), platelets 387,000 platelets/μL (150,000–400,000 platelets/μL).

Rare slight toxicity of band neutrophils was reported.

Serum chemistry profile: Sodium 148 mmol/L (145–154 mmol/L), potassium 5.0 mmol/L (4.1–5.3 mmol/L), chloride 116 mmol/L (105–116 mmol/L), bicarbonate 15 mmol/L (16–26 mmol/L), phosphorus 6.6 mg/dL (3.0–6.2 mg/dL), calcium 9.9 mg/dL (9.9–11.4 mg/dL), BUN 11 mg/dL (8–21 mg/dL), creatinine 0.5 mg/dL (0.5–1.6 mg/dL), glucose 81 mg/dL (60–104 mg/dL), total protein 5.6 g/dL (5.4–7.4 g/dL), albumin 1.8 g/dL (2.9–4.2 g/dL), globulin 3.8 g/dL (2.3–4.4 g/dL), ALT 15 U/L (19–67 U/L), AST 32 U/L (21–54 U/L), ALP 148 U/L (15–127 U/L), GGT 0 U/L (0–6 U/L), cholesterol 318 mg/dL (135–345 mg/dL), total bilirubin 0.4 mg/dL (0–0.4 mg/dL).

Urinalysis: SpG 1.015; pH 5.0, no protein (SSA), 1+ bilirubin, no hemoprotein, no glucose, no WBC, rare RBC/HPF, rare transitional epithelial cells, and a few amorphous crystals were seen.

Imaging Findings

Thoracic radiographs: A nodular soft tissue pattern was present diffusely throughout all lung lobes, which coalesced to alveolar infiltrates in the left caudal lung lobe and right cranial lung lobe (Fig. 80.12). The cardiac silhouette was mildly enlarged. Increased soft tissue opacity was noted in the perihilar region.

Abdominal ultrasound: The spleen was mildly enlarged, and there was mild mesenteric lymphadenopathy.

Diagnosis

Acute, severe pulmonary blastomycosis.

Treatment

Sam was placed in an oxygen cage with an inspired oxygen concentration (FiO_2) of 40% to 60%. An arterial blood gas revealed a pH of 7.301, pCO_2 of 36.6 mmHg, pO_2 of 79.1 mmHg, HCO_3 of 16.8 mmol/L, base deficit of 7.8 mmol/L, and measured O_2 saturation of 92.8%. The dog was also treated with crystalloid fluids (lactated Ringer's solution with 20 mEq/L KCl; 80 mL/hr, IV) and nebulization and coupage (q6h). For the first 24 hours, respiratory rate ranged from 90 to 105 breaths/minute and a nonproductive cough occurred every few hours. The dog drank water, but was inappetent. Treatment with lipid-complexed AMB was initiated (1 mg/kg, IV, on a Monday-Wednesday-Friday basis) and carprofen administration continued. By day 4, Sam was afebrile, eating, and oxygen saturation was 96% with FiO_2 of 46%. However, increased respiratory effort developed when oxygen supplementation was discontinued, and arterial blood gas analysis showed a pH of 7.335, pCO_2 of 27.2 mmHg, pO_2 of 65.8 mmHg, HCO_3 of 13.9 mmol/L, and base deficit of 10.6 mmol/L (room air). By day 5, Sam was playing with toys in the oxygen cage, and his appetite was excellent. Treatment with itraconazole (5 mg/kg, PO, q24h) was resumed in addition to the AMB. By day 8, oxygen saturation was 95% with FiO_2 of 30%. Thoracic radiographs showed persistent radiographic abnormalities, organization of the alveolar infiltrates, and apparent bronchiectasis. Survey radiographs of the appendicular skeleton showed no evidence of osteomyelitis. The dog was discharged after 11 days of hospitalization (cumulative AMB dose of 6 mg/kg). An additional seven treatments of AMB were then administered at the local veterinary clinic. Serial renal panels showed no evidence of nephrotoxicity.

At a recheck 1 month after the date of first evaluation, Sam remained somewhat lethargic and exercise intolerant, but had gained 3 kg. The frequency of cough had decreased from approximately eight times a day to once or twice daily over the previous 2 weeks. An arterial blood gas showed a pO_2 of 93.5

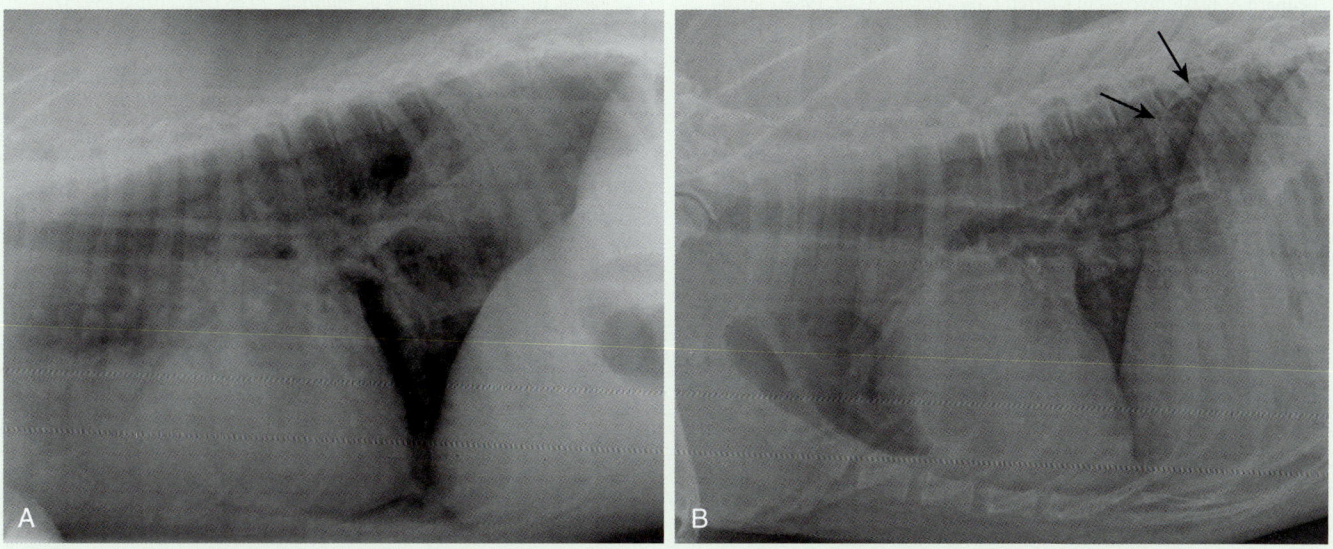

Fig. 80.12 Lateral thoracic radiographs from a young adult male neutered golden retriever with blastomycosis. (A) A nodular soft tissue pattern is present diffusely throughout all lung lobes, which coalesces to alveolar infiltrates in the left caudal lung lobe and right cranial lung lobe. (B) Residual pulmonary infiltrates are present in the right cranial lung lobe after 14 months of itraconazole treatment. There is also a large bulla in the left caudal lung lobe *(arrows)*. (From Sykes JE. *Canine and Feline Infectious Diseases*. Elsevier; 2014.)

Continued

CASE EXAMPLE—cont'd

mmHg, hematocrit was 27.8% with 39,400 reticulocytes/μL, and there was persistent hypoalbuminemia (2.0 mg/dL) and hyperglobulinemia (4.8 mg/dL). There was mild radiographic improvement in the pulmonary lesions. Treatment with itraconazole was continued for an additional 14 months, with serial monitoring of thoracic radiographs at 1, 2, 3, 8, and 14 months. At the 14-month time point, Sam had returned to his normal energetic self, weighed 45 kg, but had persistent mild infiltrates in the right cranial lung lobe on thoracic radiographs and a bulla in the left cranial lung lobe. There was also a mild to moderate generalized interstitial pattern with multiple small soft tissue opaque nodules that had not changed from the previous evaluation. One month after the itraconazole was discontinued, thoracic radiographs remained unchanged. Relapse did not occur. Sam was ultimately euthanized at 8 years of age as a result of an unrelated neoplastic disease.

Comments

This case is an example of acute pulmonary blastomycosis that followed travel to an endemic area. Another dog that traveled to the same area also developed disease. Sam appeared to require more aggressive therapy than itraconazole alone, so AMB was instituted, which was followed by gradual recovery from the infection. Although lipid-complexed AMB was used, treatment with deoxycholate AMB may also have led to cure. No evidence of dissemination was clearly identified. The lameness observed by the client may have represented weakness or exercise intolerance, but it is possible that bone involvement was present but not evident radiographically. The case also illustrates the residual pulmonary lesions that can develop in dogs with pulmonary blastomycosis, and the need for serial radiographic evaluations to assess these lesions. Although not performed in this dog, serial monitoring of antigenuria may also ultimately help determine the most appropriate time to discontinue therapy.

SUGGESTED READINGS

Schwartz IS, Wiederhold NP, Hanson KE, et al. *Blastomyces helicus*, a new dimorphic fungus causing fatal pulmonary and systemic disease in humans and animals in western Canada and the United States. *Clin Infect Dis.* 2019;68:188–195.

Ashraf N, Kubat RC, Poplin V, et al. Re-drawing the maps for endemic mycoses. *Mycopathologia.* 2020;185:843–865.

Centers for Disease Control and Prevention. Sources of Blastomycosis. 2020. Available at: https://www.cdc.gov/fungal/diseases/blastomycosis/causes.html; and: https://www.cdc.gov/fungal/pdf/more-information-about-fungal-maps-508.pdf.

Anderson JL, Frost HM, Meece JK. Spontaneous resolution of blastomycosis symptoms caused by *B. dermatitidis. Med Mycol Case Rep.* 2020;30:43–45.

REFERENCES

1. Gilchrist TC. Protozoan dermatitis. *J Cutan Gen Dis.* 1894;12:496–499.
2. Toribio RE, Kohn CW, Lawrence AE, et al. Thoracic and abdominal blastomycosis in a horse. *J Am Vet Med Assoc.* 1999;214:1357–1360, 1335.
3. Wilson JH, Olson EJ, Haugen EW, et al. Systemic blastomycosis in a horse. *J Vet Diagn Invest.* 2006;18:615–619.
4. Lenhard A. Blastomycosis in a ferret. *J Am Vet Med Assoc.* 1985;186:70–72.
5. Zwick LS, Briggs MB, Tunev SS, et al. Disseminated blastomycosis in two California sea lions (*Zalophus californianus*). *J Zoo Wildl Med.* 2000;31:211–214.
6. Rosser MF, Lindemann DM, Barger AM, et al. Systemic blastomycosis in a captive red ruffed lemur (*Varecia rubra*). *J Zoo Wildl Med.* 2016;47:912–916.
7. Wilkinson LM, Wallace JM, Cline JM. Disseminated blastomycosis in a rhesus monkey (*Macaca mulatta*). *Vet Pathol.* 1999;36:460–462.
8. Thiel RP, Mech LD, Ruth GR, et al. Blastomycosis in wild wolves. *J Wildl Dis.* 1987;23:321–323.
9. Nemeth NM, Campbell GD, Oesterle PT, et al. Red fox as sentinel for *Blastomyces dermatitidis*, Ontario, Canada. *Emerg Infect Dis.* 2016;22:1275–1277.
10. Dykstra JA, Rogers LL, Mansfield SA, et al. Fatal disseminated blastomycosis in a free-ranging American black bear (*Ursus americanus*). *J Vet Diagn Invest.* 2012;24:1125–1128.
11. Storms TN, Clyde VL, Munson L, et al. Blastomycosis in nondomestic felids. *J Zoo Wildl Med.* 2003;34:231–238.
12. Frost HM, Anderson JL, Ivacic L, et al. Development and validation of a novel single nucleotide polymorphism (SNP) panel for genetic analysis of *Blastomyces* spp. and association analysis. *BMC Infect Dis.* 2016;16:509.
13. Anderson JL, Frost HM, Meece JK. Spontaneous resolution of blastomycosis symptoms caused by *B. dermatitidis. Med Mycol Case Rep.* 2020;30:43–45.
14. Schwartz IS, Wiederhold NP, Hanson KE, et al. *Blastomyces helicus*, a new dimorphic fungus causing fatal pulmonary and systemic disease in humans and animals in western Canada and the United States. *Clin Infect Dis.* 2019;68:188–195.
15. Schwartz IS, Munoz JF, Kenyon CR, et al. Blastomycosis in Africa and the Middle East: a comprehensive review of reported cases and reanalysis of historical isolates based on molecular data. *Clin Infect Dis.* 2021;73:e1560–e1569.
16. Kucher I, Christiansen E, Schneider-Haiss M. Blastomykose bei einer Rottweiler-Hundin. *Kleinterpraxis.* 1998;43:627–631.
17. El Euch D, Cherif F, Aoun K, et al. Cutaneous blastomycosis: description of two cases in Tunisia. *Med Trop (Mars).* 2004;64:183–186.
18. Iyer PKR. Pulmonary blastomycosis in a dog in India. *Indian J Vet Pathol.* 1983;7:60–62.
19. Centers for Disease Control and Prevention. Sources of Blastomycosis. 2020. Available at: https://www.cdc.gov/fungal/diseases/blastomycosis/causes.html; and: https://www.cdc.gov/fungal/pdf/more-information-about-fungal-maps-508.pdf.
20. Shelnutt LM, Kaneene JB, Carneiro PAM, et al. Prevalence, distribution, and risk factors for canine blastomycosis in Michigan, USA. *Med Mycol.* 2020;58:609–616.
21. Brown EM, McTaggart LR, Zhang SX, et al. Phylogenetic analysis reveals a cryptic species *Blastomyces gilchristii*, sp. nov. within the human pathogenic fungus *Blastomyces dermatitidis. PLoS One.* 2013;8:e59237.
22. Cote E, Barr SC, Allen C, et al. Blastomycosis in six dogs in New York state. *J Am Vet Med Assoc.* 1997;210:502–504.
23. Morris SK, Brophy J, Richardson SE, et al. Blastomycosis in Ontario, 1994-2003. *Emerg Infect Dis.* 2006;12:274–279.
24. Harasen GL, Randall JW. Canine blastomycosis in southern Saskatchewan. *Can Vet J.* 1986;27:375–378.
25. Hoff B. North American blastomycosis in two dogs in Saskatchewan. *Can Vet J.* 1973;14:122–123.
26. Lohrenz S, Minion J, Pandey M, et al. Blastomycosis in Southern Saskatchewan 2000-2015: Unique presentations and disease characteristics. *Med Mycol.* 2018;56:787–795.
27. Bethuel NW, Siddiqui N, Edmonds L. Pulmonary blastomycosis in rural Upstate New York: A case series and review of literature. *Ann Thorac Med.* 2020;15:174–178.
28. De Groote MA, Bjerke R, Smith H, et al. Expanding epidemiology of blastomycosis: clinical features and investigation of 2 cases in Colorado. *Clin Infect Dis.* 2000;30:582–584.
29. Rudmann DG, Coolman BR, Perez CM, et al. Evaluation of risk factors for blastomycosis in dogs: 857 cases (1980-1990). *J Am Vet Med Assoc.* 1992;201:1754–1759.
30. Centers for Disease Control and Prevention. Blastomycosis acquired occupationally during prairie dog relocation: Colorado, 1998. *Morb Mortal Wkly Rep.* 1999;48:98–100.
31. Maphanga TG, Birkhead M, Munoz JF, et al. Human blastomycosis in South Africa caused by *Blastomyces percursus* and *Blastomyces emzantsi* sp. nov., 1967 to 2014. *J Clin Microbiol.* 2020;58:e01661–19.

32. Salzer HJF, Stoney RJ, Angelo KM, et al. Epidemiological aspects of travel-related systemic endemic mycoses: a GeoSentinel analysis, 1997-2017. *J Travel Med*. 2018;25:10.1093/jtm/tay055.
33. Sykes JE. Unpublished observations. 2020.
34. Baumgardner DJ, Laundre B. Studies on the molecular ecology of *Blastomyces dermatitidis*. *Mycopathologia*. 2001;152:51–58.
35. Reed KD, Meece JK, Archer JR, et al. Ecologic niche modeling of *Blastomyces dermatitidis* in Wisconsin. *PLoS One*. 2008;3:e2034.
36. Baumgardner DJ, Paretsky DP, Yopp AC. The epidemiology of blastomycosis in dogs: north central Wisconsin, USA. *J Med Vet Mycol*. 1995;33:171–176.
37. Baumgardner DJ, Steber D, Glazier R, et al. Geographic information system analysis of blastomycosis in northern Wisconsin, USA: waterways and soil. *Med Mycol*. 2005;43:117–125.
38. Arceneaux KA, Taboada J, Hosgood G. Blastomycosis in dogs: 115 cases (1980-1995). *J Am Vet Med Assoc*. 1998;213:658–664.
39. Baumgardner DJ, Paretsky DP. The in vitro isolation of *Blastomyces dermatitidis* from a woodpile in north central Wisconsin, USA. *Med Mycol*. 1999;37:163–168.
40. Chen T, Legendre AM, Bass C, et al. A case-control study of sporadic canine blastomycosis in Tennessee, USA. *Med Mycol*. 2008;46:843–852.
41. Baumgardner DJ, Paretsky DP. Blastomycosis: more evidence for exposure near one's domicile. *WMJ*. 2001;100:43–45.
42. Blondin N, Baumgardner DJ, Moore GE, et al. Blastomycosis in indoor cats: suburban Chicago, Illinois, USA. *Mycopathologia*. 2007;163:59–66.
43. Proctor ME, Klein BS, Jones JM, et al. Cluster of pulmonary blastomycosis in a rural community: evidence for multiple high-risk environmental foci following a sustained period of diminished precipitation. *Mycopathologia*. 2002;153:113–120.
44. Baumgardner DJ, Paretsky DP, Baeseman ZJ, et al. Effects of season and weather on blastomycosis in dogs: Northern Wisconsin, USA. *Med Mycol*. 2011;49:49–55.
45. Archer JR, Trainer DO, Schell RF. Epidemiologic study of canine blastomycosis in Wisconsin. *J Am Vet Med Assoc*. 1987;190:1292–1295.
46. Ireland M, Klumb C, Smith K, et al. Blastomycosis in Minnesota, USA, 1999-2018. *Emerg Infect Dis*. 2020;26:866–875.
47. Sarosi GA, Eckman MR, Davies SF, et al. Canine blastomycosis as a harbinger of human disease. *Ann Intern Med*. 1979;91:733–735.
48. Armstrong CW, Jenkins SR, Kaufman L, et al. Common-source outbreak of blastomycosis in hunters and their dogs. *J Infect Dis*. 1987;155:568–570.
49. Brown EM, McTaggart LR, Dunn D, et al. Epidemiology and geographic distribution of blastomycosis, histoplasmosis, and coccidioidomycosis, Ontario, Canada, 1990-2015. *Emerg Infect Dis*. 2018;24:1257–1266.
50. Baumgardner DJ, Turkal NW, Paretsky DP. Blastomycosis in dogs. A 15 year survey in a very highly endemic area near Eagle River, Wisconsin. *Wild Environ Med*. 1996:1–8.
51. Axtell RC, Scalarone GM. Serological differences in two *Blastomyces dermatitidis* isolates from different geographical regions of North America. *Mycopathologia*. 2002;153:141–144.
52. Gilor C, Graves TK, Barger AM, et al. Clinical aspects of natural infection with *Blastomyces dermatitidis* in cats: 8 cases (1991-2005). *J Am Vet Med Assoc*. 2006;229:96–99.
53. Breider MA, Walker TL, Legendre AM, et al. Blastomycosis in cats: five cases (1979-1986). *J Am Vet Med Assoc*. 1988;193:570–572.
54. Davies C, Troy GC. Deep mycotic infections in cats. *J Am Anim Hosp Assoc*. 1996;32:380–391.
55. Gray NA, Baddour LM. Cutaneous inoculation blastomycosis. *Clin Infect Dis*. 2002;34:E44–49.
56. Marcellin-Little DJ, Sellon RK, Kyles AE, et al. Chronic localized osteomyelitis caused by atypical infection with *Blastomyces dermatitidis* in a dog. *J Am Vet Med Assoc*. 1996;209:1877–1879.
57. Harris JR, Blaney DD, Lindsley MD, et al. Blastomycosis in man after kinkajou bite. *Emerg Infect Dis*. 2011;17:268–270.
58. Varani N, Baumgardner DJ, Czuprynski CJ, et al. Attempted isolation of *Blastomyces dermatitidis* from the nares of dogs: Northern Wisconsin, USA. *Med Mycol*. 2009;47:780–782.
59. Williams JE, Moser SA. Chronic murine pulmonary blastomycosis induced by intratracheally inoculated *Blastomyces dermatitidis* conidia. *Am Rev Respir Dis*. 1987;135:17–25.
60. Finkel-Jimenez B, Wuthrich M, Klein BS. BAD1, an essential virulence factor of *Blastomyces dermatitidis*, suppresses host TNF-alpha production through TGF-beta-dependent and -independent mechanisms. *J Immunol*. 2002;168:5746–5755.
61. Nosanchuk JD, van Duin D, Mandal P, et al. *Blastomyces dermatitidis* produces melanin in vitro and during infection. *FEMS Microbiol Lett*. 2004;239:187–193.
62. Klein BS. Role of cell surface molecules of *Blastomyces dermatitidis* in the pathogenesis and immunobiology of blastomycosis. *Semin Respir Infect*. 1997;12:198–205.
63. Wuthrich M, Finkel-Jimenez B, Brandhorst TT, et al. Analysis of non-adhesive pathogenic mechanisms of BAD1 on *Blastomyces dermatitidis*. *Med Mycol*. 2006;44:41–49.
64. Brandhorst T, Wuthrich M, Finkel-Jimenez B, et al. A C-terminal EGF-like domain governs BAD1 localization to the yeast surface and fungal adherence to phagocytes, but is dispensable in immune modulation and pathogenicity of *Blastomyces dermatitidis*. *Mol Microbiol*. 2003;48:53–65.
65. Klein BS. Molecular basis of pathogenicity in *Blastomyces dermatitidis*: the importance of adhesion. *Curr Opin Microbiol*. 2000;3:339–343.
66. Bateman BS. Disseminated blastomycosis in a German shepherd dog. *Can Vet J*. 2002;43:550–552.
67. Nielsen C, Olver CS, Schutten MM, et al. Diagnostic peritoneal lavage for identification of blastomycosis in a dog with peritoneal involvement. *J Am Vet Med Assoc*. 2003;223:1623–1627, 1600.
68. Van Vertloo LR, Gettinger MR, Naiman JH, et al. Upper airway obstruction due to primary laryngeal blastomycosis in a dog. *J Am Anim Hosp Assoc*. 2020;56:181.
69. Wuthrich M, Klein BS. Investigation of anti-WI-1 adhesin antibody-mediated protection in experimental pulmonary blastomycosis. *J Infect Dis*. 2000;181:1720–1728.
70. Smith SR, Pennline KJ, Bober LA, et al. Inhibition of collagen II-induced arthritis in mice: a comparison of the effects of Sch 24937, immunosuppressants and nonsteroidal antiinflammatory drugs on the clinical expression of disease. *Int J Immunopharmacol*. 1990;12:165–173.
71. Klein BS, Squires RA, Lloyd JK, et al. Canine antibody response to *Blastomyces dermatitidis* WI-1 antigen. *Am J Vet Res*. 2000;61:554–558.
72. Menges RW, Furcolow ML, Selby LA, et al. Clinical and epidemiologic studies on seventy-nine canine blastomycosis cases in Arkansas. *Am J Epidemiol*. 1965;81:164–179.
73. Brockus CW, Hathcock JT. Hypertrophic osteopathy associated with pulmonary blastomycosis in a dog. *Vet Radiol Ultrasound*. 1988;29:184–188.
74. Ditmyer H, Craig L. Mycotic mastitis in three dogs due to *Blastomyces dermatitidis*. *J Am Anim Hosp Assoc*. 2011;47:356–358.
75. Hecht S, Adams WH, Smith JR, et al. Clinical and imaging findings in five dogs with intracranial blastomycosis (*Blastomyces dermatitidis*). *J Am Anim Hosp Assoc*. 2011;47:241–249.
76. Saito M, Sharp NJ, Munana K, et al. CT findings of intracranial blastomycosis in a dog. *Vet Radiol Ultrasound*. 2002;43:16–21.
77. Totten AK, Ridgway MD, Sauberli DS. *Blastomyces dermatitidis* prostatic and testicular infection in eight dogs (1992-2005). *J Am Anim Hosp Assoc*. 2011;47:413–418.
78. Wilson RW, van Dreumel AA, Henry JN. Urogenital and ocular lesions in canine blastomycosis. *Vet Pathol*. 1973;10:1–11.
79. Baron ML, Hecht S, Westermeyer HD, et al. Intracranial extension of retrobulbar blastomycosis (*Blastomyces dermatitidis*) in a dog. *Vet Ophthalmol*. 2011;14:137–141.
80. Brick KE, Agger WA. Successful treatment of brainstem blastomycosis with fluconazole. *Clin Med Res*. 2012;10:72–74.
81. Dobre MC, Smoker WR, Kirby P. A case of solitary *Blastomyces dermatitidis* meningitis. *Clin Neurol Neurosurg*. 2011;113:665–667.
82. McGuire NC, Vitsky A, Daly CM, et al. Pulmonary thromboembolism associated with *Blastomyces dermatitidis* in a dog. *J Am Anim Hosp Assoc*. 2002;38:425–430.

83. Bromel C, Sykes JE. Epidemiology, diagnosis, and treatment of blastomycosis in dogs and cats. *Clin Tech Small Anim Pract*. 2005;20:233–239.
84. Hendrix DV, Rohrbach BW, Bochsler PN, et al. Comparison of histologic lesions of endophthalmitis induced by *Blastomyces dermatitidis* in untreated and treated dogs: 36 cases (1986-2001). *J Am Vet Med Assoc*. 2004;224:1317–1322.
85. Bloom JD, Hamor RE, Gerding PA Jr. Ocular blastomycosis in dogs: 73 cases, 108 eyes (1985-1993). *J Am Vet Med Assoc*. 1996;209:1271–1274.
86. Miller PE, Miller LM, Schoster JV. Feline blastomycosis: a report of three cases and literature review (1961 to 1988). *J Am Anim Hosp Assoc*. 1990;26:417–424.
87. McEwen SA, Hulland TJ. Cerebral blastomycosis in a cat. *Can Vet J*. 1984;25:411–413.
88. Meschter C, Heiber K. Blastomycosis in a cat in lower New York State. *Cornell Vet*. 1989;79:259–262.
89. Nasisse MP, van Ee RT, Wright B. Ocular changes in a cat with disseminated blastomycosis. *J Am Vet Med Assoc*. 1985;187:629–631.
90. Crews LJ, Feeney DA, Jessen CR, et al. Utility of diagnostic tests for and medical treatment of pulmonary blastomycosis in dogs: 125 cases (1989-2006). *J Am Vet Med Assoc*. 2008;232:222–227.
91. Dow SW, Legendre AM, Stiff M, et al. Hypercalcemia associated with blastomycosis in dogs. *J Am Vet Med Assoc*. 1986;188:706–709.
92. O'Brien MA, McMichael MA, Le Boedec K. 25-Hydroxyvitamin D concentrations in dogs with naturally acquired blastomycosis. *J Vet Intern Med*. 2018;32:1684–1691.
93. Nafe LA, Turk JR, Carter JD. Central nervous system involvement of blastomycosis in the dog. *J Am Anim Hosp Assoc*. 1983;19.
94. Crews LJ, Feeney DA, Jessen CR, et al. Radiographic findings in dogs with pulmonary blastomycosis: 125 cases (1989-2006). *J Am Vet Med Assoc*. 2008;232:215–221.
95. McMillan CJ, Taylor SM. Transtracheal aspiration in the diagnosis of pulmonary blastomycosis (17 cases: 2000-2005). *Can Vet J*. 2008;49:53–55.
96. Smith JR, Legendre AM, Thomas WB, et al. Cerebral *Blastomyces dermatitidis* infection in a cat. *J Am Vet Med Assoc*. 2007;231:1210–1214.
97. Bentley RT, Reese MJ, Heng HG, et al. Ependymal and periventricular magnetic resonance imaging changes in four dogs with central nervous system blastomycosis. *Vet Radiol Ultrasound*. 2013;54:489–496.
98. Legendre AM, Becker PU. Evaluation of the agar-gel immunodiffusion test in the diagnosis of canine blastomycosis. *Am J Vet Res*. 1980;41:2109–2111.
99. Spector D, Legendre AM, Wheat J, et al. Antigen and antibody testing for the diagnosis of blastomycosis in dogs. *J Vet Intern Med*. 2008;22:839–843.
100. RoyChowdhury M, Muzzall E, Baumgardner DJ, et al. Potential clinical utility of ERC-2 yeast phase lysate antigen for antibody detection in dogs with blastomycosis. *Med Mycol*. 2019;57:893–896.
101. Mourning AC, Patterson EE, Kirsch EJ, et al. Evaluation of an enzyme immunoassay for antibodies to a recombinant *Blastomyces* adhesin-1 repeat antigen as an aid in the diagnosis of blastomycosis in dogs. *J Am Vet Med Assoc*. 2015;247:1133–1138.
102. Durkin M, Witt J, Lemonte A, et al. Antigen assay with the potential to aid in diagnosis of blastomycosis. *J Clin Microbiol*. 2004;42:4873–4875.
103. Connolly P, Hage CA, Bariola JR, et al. *Blastomyces dermatitidis* antigen detection by quantitative enzyme immunoassay. *Clin Vaccine Immunol*. 2012;19:53–56.
104. Laux KL, Anderson JL, Bentivenga SP, et al. Urine antigen testing is equally sensitive to *B. dermatitidis* and *B. gilchristii* infections. *Clin Med Res*. 2020;18:133–139.
105. Sidamonidze K, Peck MK, Perez M, et al. Real-time PCR assay for identification of *Blastomyces dermatitidis* in culture and in tissue. *J Clin Microbiol*. 2012;50:1783–1786.
106. Babady NE, Buckwalter SP, Hall L, et al. Detection of *Blastomyces dermatitidis* and *Histoplasma capsulatum* from culture isolates and clinical specimens by use of real-time PCR. *J Clin Microbiol*. 2011;49:3204–3208.
107. Sherwood BF, LeMay JC, Castellanos RA. Blastomycosis with secondary amyloidosis in the dog. *J Am Vet Med Assoc*. 1967;150:1377–1381.
108. Sekhon AS, Marien GR, Easton B, et al. A canine case of North American blastomycosis in Alberta, Canada. *Mycoses*. 1988;31:454–458.
109. Legendre AM, Rohrbach BW, Toal RL, et al. Treatment of blastomycosis with itraconazole in 112 dogs. *J Vet Intern Med*. 1996;10:365–371.
110. Brooks DE, Legendre AM, Gunn GG, et al. The treatment of ocular blastomycosis with systemically administered itraconazole. *Prog Vet Comp Ophthalmol*. 1991;4:263–268.
111. Gionfriddo JR, Powell CC. Disseminated blastomycosis with ocular involvement in a dog. *Vet Med*. 2002;97:423–431.
112. Mawby DI, Whittemore JC, Genger S, et al. Bioequivalence of orally administered generic, compounded, and innovator-formulated itraconazole in healthy dogs. *J Vet Intern Med*. 2014;28:72–77.
113. Pappas PG, Bradsher RW, Kauffman CA, et al. Treatment of blastomycosis with higher doses of fluconazole. The National Institute of Allergy and Infectious Diseases Mycoses Study Group. *Clin Infect Dis*. 1997;25:200–205.
114. Bariola JR, Perry P, Pappas PG, et al. Blastomycosis of the central nervous system: a multicenter review of diagnosis and treatment in the modern era. *Clin Infect Dis*. 2010;50:797–804.
115. Smith JA, Kauffman CA. Blastomycosis. *Proc Am Thorac Soc*. 2010;7:173–180.
116. Krawiec DR, McKiernan BC, Twardock AR, et al. Use of an amphotericin B lipid complex for treatment of blastomycosis in dogs. *J Am Vet Med Assoc*. 1996;209:2073–2075.
117. Proia LA, Harnisch DO. Successful use of posaconazole for treatment of blastomycosis. *Antimicrob Agents Chemother*. 2012;56:4029.
118. Majdick K, Kaye K, Shorman MA. Central nervous system blastomycosis clinical characteristics and outcomes. *Med Mycol*. 2021;59:87–92.
119. Foy DS, Trepanier LA, Kirsch EJ, et al. Serum and urine *Blastomyces* antigen concentrations as markers of clinical remission in dogs treated for systemic blastomycosis. *J Vet Intern Med*. 2014;28:305–310.
120. Motchenbacher L, Furrow E, Rendahl AK, et al. Retrospecive analysis of the effects of *Blastomyces* antigen concentration in urine and radiographic findings with survival in dogs with blastomycosis. *J Vet Intern Med*. 2021;35:946–953.
121. Legendre AM, Selcer BA, Edwards DF, et al. Treatment of canine blastomycosis with amphotericin B and ketoconazole. *J Am Vet Med Assoc*. 1984;184:1249–1254.
122. Wuthrich M, Filutowicz HI, Klein BS. Mutation of the WI-1 gene yields an attenuated *Blastomyces dermatitidis* strain that induces host resistance. *J Clin Invest*. 2000;106:1381–1389.
123. Wuthrich M, Krajaejun T, Shearn-Bochsler V, et al. Safety, tolerability, and immunogenicity of a recombinant, genetically engineered, live-attenuated vaccine against canine blastomycosis. *Clin Vaccine Immunol*. 2011;18:783–789.
124. Carignan A, Denis M, Abou Chakra CN. Mortality associated with *Blastomyces dermatitidis* infection: A systematic review of the literature and meta-analysis. *Med Mycol*. 2020;58:1–10.
125. McBride JA, Sterkel AK, Matkovic E, et al. Clinical manifestations and outcomes in immunocompetent and immunocompromised patients with blastomycosis. *Clin Infect Dis*. 2021;72:1594–1602.
126. Pappas PG. Blastomycosis in the immunocompromised patient. *Semin Respir Infect*. 1997;12:243–251.
127. Gauthier GM, Safdar N, Klein BS, et al. Blastomycosis in solid organ transplant recipients. *Transpl Infect Dis*. 2007;9:310–317.
128. Ashraf N, Kubat RC, Poplin V, et al. Re-drawing the maps for endemic mycoses. *Mycopathologia*. 2020;185:843–865.
129. Ramsey DT. Blastomycosis in a veterinarian. *J Am Vet Med Assoc*. 1994;205:968.
130. Graham WR Jr, Callaway JL. Primary inoculation blastomycosis in a veterinarian. *J Am Acad Dermatol*. 1982;7:785–786.
131. Gnann JW Jr, Bressler GS, Bodet CA 3rd, et al. Human blastomycosis after a dog bite. *Ann Intern Med*. 1983;98:48–49.
132. Butka BJ, Bennett SR, Johnson AC. Disseminated inoculation blastomycosis in a renal transplant recipient. *Am Rev Respir Dis*. 1984;130:1180–1183.
133. Jaspers RH. Letter: Transmission of *Blastomyces* from animals to man. *J Am Vet Med Assoc*. 1974;164:8.
134. Cote E, Barr SC, Allen C. Possible transmission of *Blastomyces dermatitidis* via culture specimen. *J Am Vet Med Assoc*. 1997;210:479–480.

81

Histoplasmosis

Krystle L. Reagan, Jane E. Sykes

KEY POINTS

- Cause: *Histoplasma capsulatum* (phylum Ascomycetes).
- First Described: 1905, Panama (Samuel Darling), where it was initially mistaken for a protozoal pathogen in a person from Martinique.[1]
- Affected Hosts: Many mammals, including dogs, cats, and humans.
- Geographic Distribution: Worldwide, but especially the Ohio and Mississippi river valleys of the United States, and Latin America.
- Route of Transmission: Inhalation of microconidia in the environment.
- Major Clinical Signs: Cough, tachypnea, organomegaly, GI signs, pallor.
- Differential Diagnoses: Other deep mycoses, mycobacterial infections, hemic neoplasia, leishmaniosis.
- Human Health Significance: *Histoplasma capsulatum* also causes disease in humans, but direct transmission from animals to humans does not occur.

ETIOLOGIC AGENT AND EPIDEMIOLOGY

Histoplasma capsulatum is a dimorphic, soil-borne fungus that is found worldwide, but especially in the Mississippi and Ohio river valleys of the United States (Midwest and south-central) as well as in Latin America (Fig. 81.1). Disease has also been diagnosed in cats or dogs from other parts of the United States (northern and southern California, Texas, Colorado), Brazil, Thailand, Italy, Australia (Queensland), Japan, and eastern Canada (New Brunswick).[2–11] At least eight clades of the organism have been identified by genetic analysis: North American classes 1 and 2 (NAm1 and NAm2), Latin American groups A and B (LAmA and LAmB), and one each of Australian, Netherlands, Eurasian, and African, which appear to vary in virulence. A ninth clade, closely related to the North American class 1, was identified in cats with histoplasmosis from California, Texas, and Colorado.[2] Further divergent clades with the Latin American groups have also been described.[12] Three different variants have also been described based on pathogenicity and morphology, *H. capsulatum* var. *capsulatum*, *H. capsulatum* var. *duboisii*, and *H. capsulatum* var. *farciminosum*.[11,13] *Histoplasma capsulatum* var. *duboisii* occurs primarily in Africa and Japan. *Histoplasma capsulatum* var. *farciminosum* infections occur primarily in horses, but have also been reported in humans and dogs.

Histoplasma capsulatum grows best in soil as a mycelium (*Ajellomyces capsulatum*) where temperatures are between 22°C and 29°C, with an annual rainfall of 35 to 50 inches, and a relative humidity of 67% to 87%—conditions typically found between latitudes of 45° north to 30° south.[14] *Histoplasma capsulatum* can be found in the intestinal tract and guano of bats, which constitute the primary reservoir of the organism and serve to disseminate it geographically.[15] Bat caves can maintain perfect conditions for growth of *H. capsulatum*. Although *H. capsulatum* can be found in high concentrations in decaying avian guano (especially around blackbird or starling roosts and chicken coops), it is not found in fresh feces or shed in the feces of birds.

Cats appear to be as susceptible or slightly more susceptible to histoplasmosis than dogs. Affected cats can be as young as 2 months and in some cases, older than 15 years.[16] The mean age of affected cats in reported case series has ranged from 3.9 to 8.8 years.[17,18] For dogs, a mean age of 3 to 4.3 years has been reported,[19,20] and dogs in the 2- to 4-year and 4- to 7-year age groups were more likely to develop histoplasmosis than dogs less than 2 years of age.[21] Sporting or working dogs may be at greater risk of infection as a result of increased likelihood of exposure; in a study that utilized the Veterinary Medical Database, pointers were strongly over-represented.[21] Weimaraners and Brittany spaniels were also at increased risk. Persian cats were slightly over-represented in another study. A sex predisposition has not been clearly identified in dogs or cats, but more female than male dogs were affected in some case series.[18–20,22–24] This contrasts to human histoplasmosis, which tends to affect males. Most affected cats are retrovirus negative, but a significant percentage of cats in two studies (16% and 28%) were co-infected with FeLV.[16,18] A small percentage of affected cats have underlying comorbidities such as lymphoma, FIP, or a history of treatment with glucocorticoids.[16] Comorbidities described in dogs include dirofilariasis[19] and metastatic carcinoma.[11] Disease can occur in animals housed exclusively indoors.[25]

CLINICAL FEATURES

Pathogenesis and Clinical Signs

In the soil, the mycelial phase of *H. capsulatum* forms macroconidia and microconidia (Fig. 81.2), which are environmentally resistant. The microconidia are believed to be the form inhaled by mammalian hosts, because they are small enough (2 to 5 μm) to enter the terminal bronchioles and alveoli. Within the lungs (i.e., at a temperature of 37°C), the microconidia transition to a unicellular yeast phase, which replicates by budding. The incubation period is approximately 2 to 3 weeks.[26] Heat shock proteins on the fungus bind to CD11-CD18 integrins on alveolar macrophages, and receptor mediated phagocytosis results in fungal entry to pulmonary macrophages.[27,28] The organism then replicates within these cells through control of the phagolysosomal environment by raising the intracellular pH with urease, ammonia, and bicarbonate, and evades the host immune response.[29] The organism further evades detection of the host immune system by altering the cell membrane by synthesizing α-linked glucans to conceal β-glucans. The β-glucans are typically present at high levels within the fungal cell membrane and are PAMPs that trigger a proinflammatory response from the macrophage.[30,31] The organism ultimately destroys the cells, with subsequent replication in other resident alveolar macrophages and inflammatory phagocytes that are recruited to the lung.[28] Acquisition of iron by the fungus is essential for growth *in vivo*.[32]

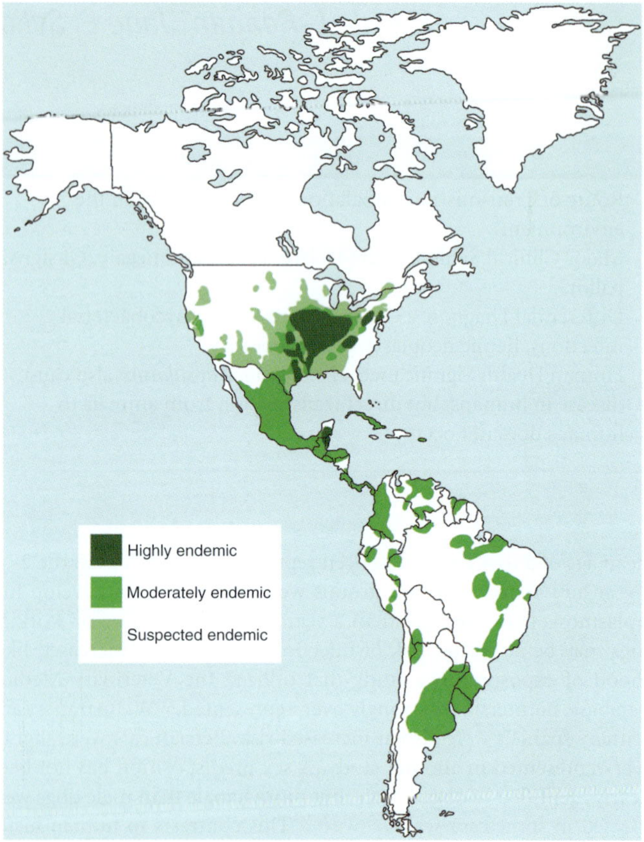

Fig. 81.1 Approximate geographic distribution of histoplasmosis in the Americas.

Cell-mediated immune responses (especially mediated by CD4+ cells, IFN-γ, and TNF-α) lead to the death of infected macrophages and are critical for early control and clearance of infection. There have been several reports of disseminated histoplasmosis in human patients in association with co-infections with HIV infection and COVID-19.[33,34]

Some animals control the initial infection but remain latently infected with small numbers of yeasts. Subsequent immune suppression with medications or secondary to other disease processes such as *Ehrlichia canis* infection or neoplasia can lead to reactivation of infection years later. Thus, the apparent incubation period may be as long as several years.

The clinical manifestations and rate of disease progression depend on the host immune response to infection, which varies both between and within host species (e.g., dog versus cat); the infectious dose; and the *Histoplasma* strain, which can vary geographically. The vast majority of infections are probably subclinical.[35] Replication of the organism leads to a granulomatous inflammatory response in the lungs, which consists primarily of macrophages and variable numbers of lymphocytes. Occasionally, the inflammatory response is followed by the development of fibrosis and scarring. Yeast forms migrate to local lymph nodes (such as the hilar lymph node) and other tissues that contain mononuclear cells, such as the liver and spleen. When CMI is defective or absent, this results in disseminated disease (referred to in human patients as *progressive disseminated histoplasmosis* [PDH]). PDH may be acute, subacute, or chronic.[36] In addition to lymph nodes, liver, and spleen, common sites of dissemination include the bone marrow, small and/or large intestinal tract, the skin, bones, central nervous system, and eye. Dogs with histoplasmosis in the United States appear to be particularly susceptible to intestinal involvement.

Clinical signs in cats are commonly vague and nonspecific, such as weight loss, decreased appetite, weakness, dehydration, and fever.[16–18] Approximately 40% of cats show respiratory signs due to pulmonary involvement such as dyspnea and tachypnea, and to a lesser extent cough and nasal discharge. However, respiratory signs may be absent in some cats with dissemination of infection to nonpulmonary sites. Tachypnea and dyspnea were also described in a cat with a cranial mediastinal mass.[37] Ocular signs occur in approximately one quarter

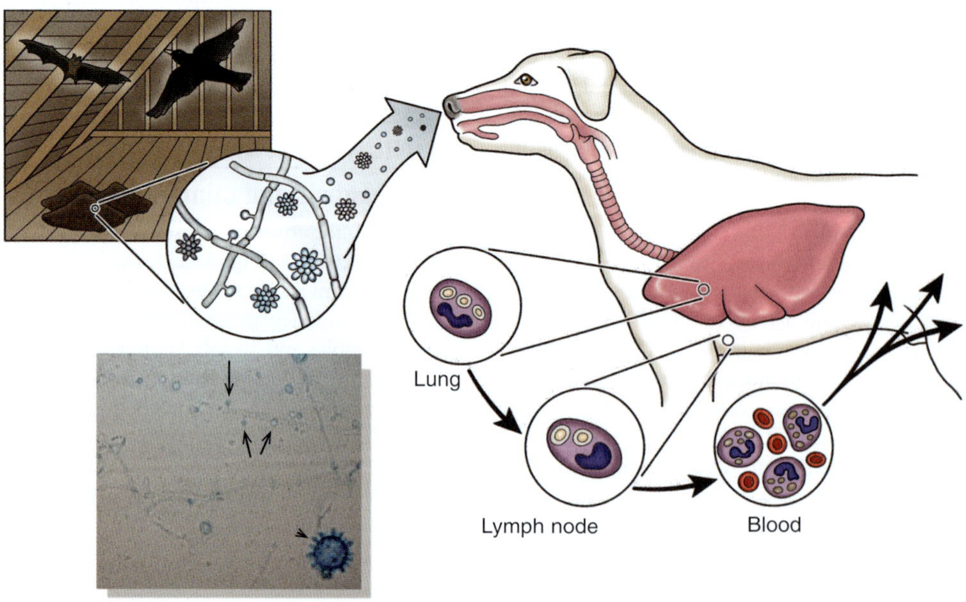

Fig. 81.2 Life cycle of *Histoplasma capsulatum*. In the environment, the organism forms macroconidia *(arrowhead, inset)* and microconidia *(arrows, inset)*. The microconidia are thought to be inhaled into the lungs of mammalian hosts. Within the lung, the organisms transform into yeasts that infect alveolar macrophages and then disseminate to the local lymph nodes and the systemic circulation.

of cats with histoplasmosis. Around 20% of cats have signs of skeletal involvement, usually lameness, which often involves multiple limbs.[16–18,22,38] Skin lesions, peripheral lymphadenopathy, vomiting, diarrhea, oral ulceration, myelopathy, and/or hematuria due to bladder wall involvement have also been reported.[15,17,18,22,39–45] A high proportion of affected cats that were necropsied had evidence of severe disseminated disease.[16]

In dogs, diarrhea, decreased appetite, weight loss, lethargy, fever (up to 40°C or 104°F), and mucosal pallor are the most common clinical signs.[9,10,19,20,23] In addition to decreased appetite, weight loss, and diarrhea, other clinical signs referable to the GI tract include melena, tenesmus, hematochezia, dyschezia, and/or increased frequency of defecation.[10,19,23] Profuse diarrhea may be chronic and may persist for several months. Hilar lymphadenomegaly may be severe and contribute to signs of cough in some dogs. Other signs include respiratory difficulty, icterus, vomiting, hepatomegaly, lymphadenomegaly, nasal discharge, epistaxis, ocular signs, polyuria and polydipsia, lameness due to osteomyelitis, and neurologic signs such as seizures.[10,19,20,46–48] Affected dogs in Japan have had chronic cutaneous or gingival lesions in the absence of pulmonary or GI involvement,[49–52] although disseminated disease has also been described.[11] Skin nodules were also reported in an Australian dog with histoplasmosis.[4] Varied clinical manifestations of histoplasmosis in different parts of the world have also been reported in humans as a result of strain variation in *H. capsulatum*.

Physical Examination Findings

Physical examination findings in affected cats include thin body condition or emaciation; fever; pale and/or rarely icteric mucous membranes; peripheral lymphadenopathy; respiratory signs such as respiratory distress, tachypnea, and increased or decreased lung sounds; single or multiple cutaneous nodules, ulcerations, and/or draining tracts; lameness; and detection of organomegaly, abdominal masses, and/or pain on palpation of the abdomen. Cats with musculoskeletal involvement may have evidence of swelling/effusion in one or more joints, especially the carpus and tarsus.[17] Ocular signs include blindness, masses, or thickening of the conjunctiva or nictating membrane, chorioretinitis, optic neuritis, anterior uveitis, retinal detachment, panophthalmitis, and glaucoma (Fig. 81.3).[53]

In dogs, lethargy, fever, thin body condition, and pale mucous membranes are found most often on physical examination. Other physical examination abnormalities include dehydration, hepatomegaly, icterus, and ascites; tachypnea, increased respiratory effort, and increased lung sounds; lymphadenomegaly that involves one or more peripheral lymph nodes; abnormal stool quality on rectal examination (diarrhea, hematochezia, or melena); nasal and ocular discharge; tachycardia; tongue lesions; and cutaneous nodules, ulceration, or draining tracts.[4,10,19,23,46,54,55] Ocular examination may reveal uveitis, evidence of optic neuritis, or chorioretinitis with retinal detachment.[23,56,57] One dog was seen for lameness, hyperemia, and edema of the left pelvic limb because of a sclerosing pyogranulomatous inflammatory mass in the inguinal region that resulted in venous occlusion.[54] Rarely neurologic signs such as ataxia, obtundation, head tilt, nystagmus, strabismus, seizures, facial paralysis, and tetraparesis may be present on physical examination as a result of hepatic encephalopathy or meningoencephalitis.[57–59]

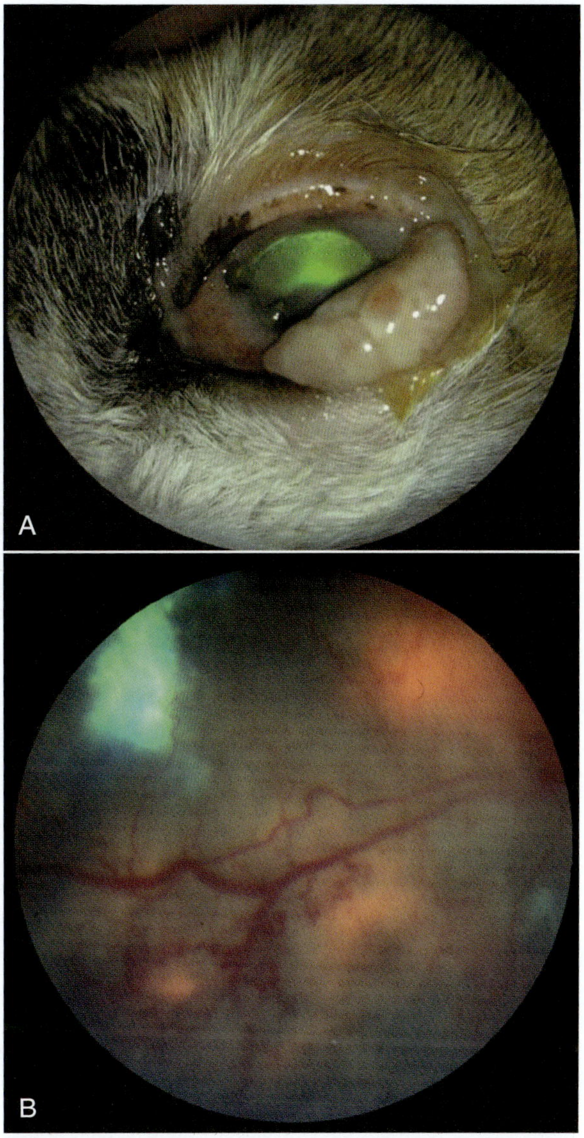

Fig. 81.3 Ocular changes in cats with histoplasmosis. (A) Blepharitis. (B) Granulomatous chorioretinitis with multifocal pigmented lesions. (A, From Ketring KL, Glaze MB. *Atlas of Feline Ophthalmology*. 2nd ed. Hoboken, NJ: Wiley-Blackwell; 2012. B, Courtesy of Dr. Mary Belle Glaze, Gulf Coast Animal Eye Clinic, Houston, TX.)

DIAGNOSIS

Laboratory Abnormalities

Complete Blood Count

The CBC in dogs and cats with histoplasmosis reflects the presence of systemic inflammation, GI hemorrhage, and/or bone marrow infiltration by fungal organisms. In both dogs and cats, anemia is a common abnormality on the CBC, may be mild to severe, and is usually normocytic, normochromic, and nonregenerative.[17–20,22,23,60,61] Increased numbers of nucleated erythrocytes have been reported in some affected dogs.[10,61] The total white cell count or neutrophil count may be normal, increased, or decreased.[19,22,23] Most affected cats have a normal or decreased white cell count,[18,60] but leukocytosis due to neutrophilia and monocytosis may be more common in affected dogs.[19,61] Increased numbers of band neutrophils with toxic neutrophils, lymphopenia, monocytopenia, and thrombocytopenia may be present in some severely affected animals.[17,18,22,23,60,62] Thrombocytopenia may be a result of platelet consumption, sequestration, and/or myelophthisis. Rarely, eosinophilia is present.[63]

Serum Chemistry Profile

Mild to severe hypoalbuminemia is present in most (>75%) of affected dogs and cats.[20] Cats with hepatic involvement may have

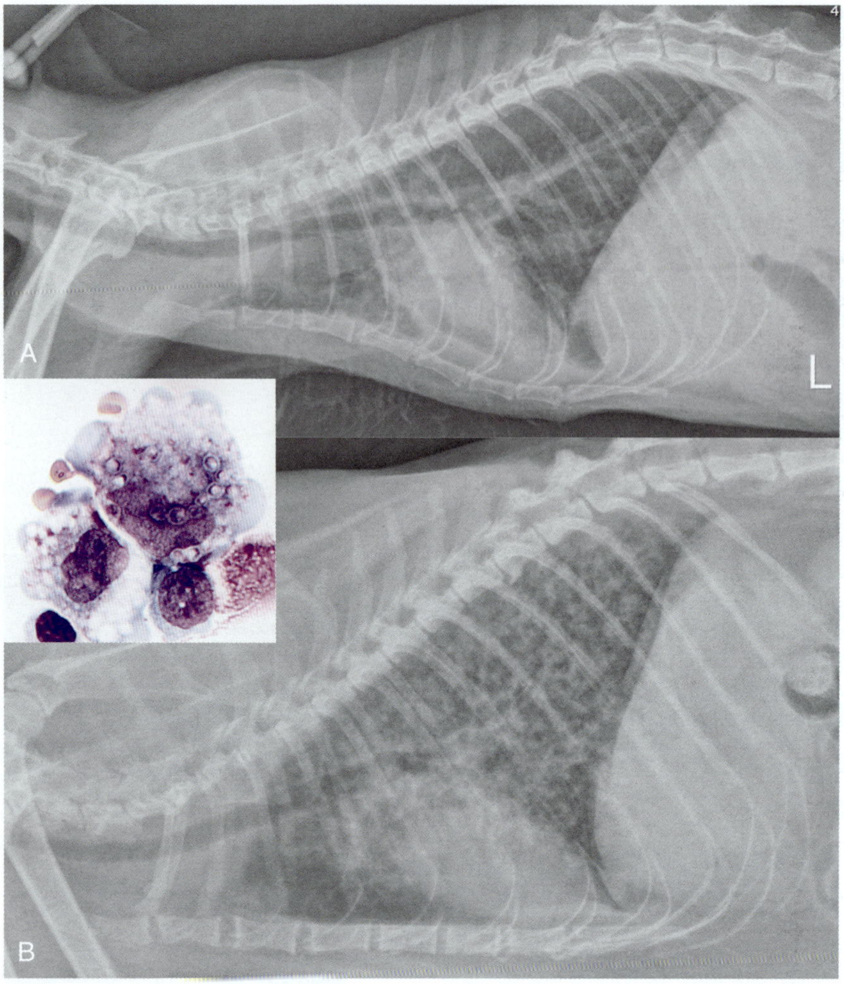

Fig. 81.4 Radiographic abnormalities in feline pulmonary histoplasmosis. (A) Lateral thoracic radiograph from a 12-year-old female spayed domestic longhair cat with disseminated histoplasmosis. There is a diffuse bronchointerstitial pulmonary pattern with an alveolar pattern ventrally, and bicavitary effusion. In the viewable abdomen, hepatomegaly can be appreciated. Cytologic analysis of pleural fluid revealed oval organisms consistent with *Histoplasma* spp. (inset). (B) Lateral thoracic radiograph from a 9-year-old male neutered Siamese cat with disseminated histoplasmosis that was evaluated for lethargy, inappetence, and weight loss of one-month duration. There is a diffuse, severe, nodular interstitial pattern. (Images courtesy University of California-Davis Veterinary Diagnostic Imaging, Small Animal Internal Medicine, and Clinical Pathology Services).

increased activities of serum ALT and AST.[22,60] Hyperbilirubinemia and increased ALP are sometimes reported.[17,22] Hypercalcemia and hyperglobulinemia have been described in a few affected cats.[17,22] Hyperglobulinemia, mild to moderate increases in the activity of serum ALT, AST, ALP, and GGT, and hyperbilirubinemia may be found in dogs.

Urinalysis

Results of urinalysis are usually within normal limits, but low urine specific gravity and bilirubinuria may be present in dogs with hepatic involvement.

Clotting Function

A few dogs with acute PDH have had coagulation abnormalities characterized by increased PT and PTT and fibrin degradation product or D-dimer concentrations.[47,61] Coagulation abnormalities in dogs with histoplasmosis may result from DIC and possibly severe hepatic involvement (see also Case Example).

Diagnostic Imaging

Plain Radiography

In cats, plain thoracic radiographic findings in histoplasmosis usually consist of diffuse, linear, nodular or miliary interstitial patterns, but mixed interstitial-alveolar-bronchial patterns and an absence of abnormal findings have also been described.[17,18,20,24,60,64] Plain thoracic radiographs in dogs may show an alveolar, interstitial, and/or bronchial patterns, tracheobronchial lymphadenomegaly, lung lobe consolidation, and/or rarely pleural effusion (Fig. 81.4).[47,62,64,65] Lesions can sometimes calcify, which does not seem to be the case in cats. Abdominal radiographs may show hepatomegaly, splenomegaly, or decreased serosal detail due to ascites. Radiographic evidence of osteomyelitis (usually osteolytic lesions) or joint involvement

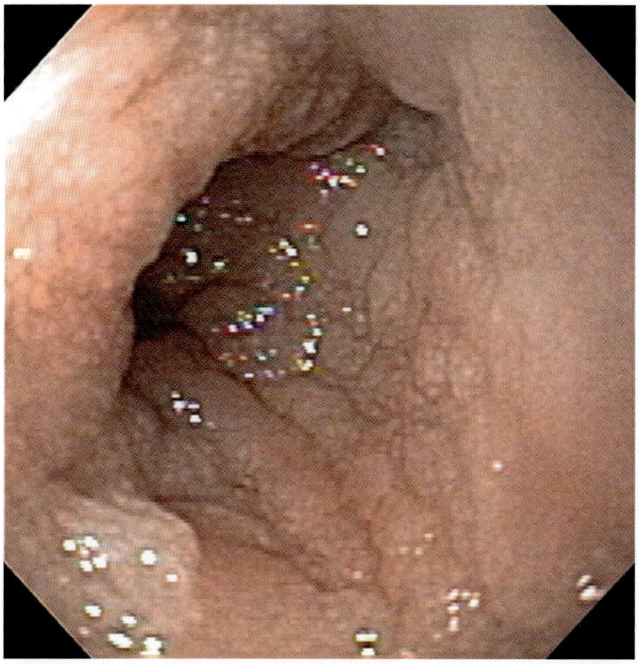

Fig. 81.5 Colonoscopy image from a dog with disseminated histoplasmosis with large intestinal involvement. The mucosa is thickened and granular. (Courtesy Dr. Michael Willard, Texas A&M University.)

(extracapsular and/or extracapsular swelling) may be present in cats, sometimes accompanied by pathologic fractures.[17] Osteomyelitis is rarely described in dogs.[46,48]

Sonographic Findings

Findings on abdominal sonographic examination of dogs with histoplasmosis have included enlargement and hypoechogenicity of the liver, abdominal lymphadenopathy, splenomegaly, and peritoneal effusion.[66] A thickened intestinal wall (most commonly the colon) may be present with disruption of bowel wall architecture.[66] Adrenomegaly, abdominal lymphadenomegaly, splenomegaly, and occasionally renomegaly have also been described in cats.[18,67]

Endoscopy

Colonoscopic findings in dogs with colonic histoplasmosis include irregularity, ulceration, increased granularity, and friability of the colonic wall (Fig. 81.5).

Magnetic Resonance Imaging

MRI may reveal mass lesions that are T1 and T2 isointense with contrast enhancement, as described in a dog with an extradural spinal cord lesion.[68]Although chronic meningitis is the most common manifestation of CNS involvement in humans,[36] ring-enhancing granulomatous mass lesions within the brain (histoplasmomas) have been described in affected people.[69]

Microbiologic Tests (Table 81.1)

Cytologic Examination

Histoplasma yeasts are usually seen extracellularly and intracellularly (usually within mononuclear phagocytes) on staining and cytologic examination of aspirates or impression smears of affected tissues (e.g., fine-needle aspirates of liver, spleen, lymph nodes, lung, bone marrow), rectal scrapings, or cytospin preparations of lung wash specimens or body fluids (e.g., CSF, synovial fluid, ascites, or pleural effusion). The accompanying inflammatory response may be pyogranulomatous, granulomatous, or suppurative. Occasionally one or more organisms are visualized in circulating monocytes, neutrophils, or eosinophils in severely ill animals with disseminated disease. Cytologic evidence of fungemia was detected in nearly 20% of affected cats in one study.[16] The yeasts are 2 to 4 μm in diameter, oval, have a basophilic center, and are surrounded by a clear halo, which results from shrinkage artifact (Fig. 81.6). A variety of stains can be used, such as Diff-Quik and Wright stains. The organism is not encapsulated, even though its name implies the presence of a capsule. Organisms may not be identified within chronic, fibrosing lesions.[54,70]

Serologic Diagnosis

Both antibody and antigen (ELISA) assays are available for serodiagnosis of histoplasmosis. Antibody assays for *H. capsulatum* are based on gel immunodiffusion or complement fixation and have poor diagnostic sensitivity.[16,19,22] False positives reportedly occur in recovered animals, although the specificity of antibody assays in dogs and cats is not well documented. In human patients, acute and convalescent antibody testing is useful for diagnosis of acute pulmonary histoplasmosis, and a single antibody titer is used as an aid for diagnosis of chronic forms of histoplasmosis. In particular, antibody assay of the CSF can be useful for diagnosis of culture-negative chronic *H. capsulatum* meningitis.

An ELISA assay for *H. capsulatum* antigen (MiraVista Diagnostics, Indianapolis, IN, USA) is widely used in human patients for diagnosis of histoplasmosis, and urine is the preferred specimen for testing because it results in a higher sensitivity than when serum is assayed.[70] The use of the antigen assay has been applied for the diagnosis of histoplasmosis in cats and dogs.[54,71] In one study, the urine of 17/18 cats with confirmed histoplasmosis was positive, whereas none of 26 cats with alternate diagnoses tested positive.[71] At the time of diagnosis, the sensitivity of the assay was 93% when urine was used, and 73% when serum was used.[38] There have been several reports of cats with biopsy- or culture-confirmed histoplasmosis with false-negative test results, including cats with ocular, joint, and renal involvement.[17,53,72,73]

The assay has also been used to monitor response to therapy in cats. Elimination of antigen is sensitive (urine 90%, serum 90.4%) for remission, but not specific (urine 64%, serum 52%).[38] Monitoring of antigenemia or antigenuria after discontinuation of treatment can be used to detect early relapse.[38]

In dogs, one study found that urine antigen testing had a sensitivity of 89.5% and specificity of 100%.[74] Two dogs with false-negative test results had disease restricted to the GI tract.[74]

False-positive test results using the *Histoplasma* antigen test occur in human patients with other disseminated mycoses, including blastomycosis, penicilliosis, and coccidioidomycosis,[75,76] so the assay must always be used in conjunction with other diagnostic assays.

An in-house, antibody-based *H. capsulatum* antigen assay (IMMY, Normon, OK) has been investigated for use in cats. This assay was compared to the commercially available ELISA antigen (MiraVista Diagnostics, Indianapolis, IN) on urine specimens. The POC assay has a sensitivity of 77% to 89% and specificity of 80% to 97% depending on the cut-point utilized.[77]

Culture

Histoplasma capsulatum can be isolated from clinical specimens on routine fungal media. There is a risk of laboratory-acquired infection when the organism grows in the mycelial form on artificial media, so culture should only be performed if necessary and the laboratory should be warned of the possibility that infection with a dimorphic fungus may be present so that appropriate precautions are taken. Although most

TABLE 81.1 Diagnostic Assays Available for Histoplasmosis in Dogs and Cats

Assay	Specimen Type	Target	Performance
Cytologic examination	Aspirates of affected tissues, sometimes blood smears or buffy coat preparations, body fluids	*Histoplasma capsulatum* organisms in mononuclear phagocytes and granulocytes	Organisms are usually present but in the absence of experience, they may be confused with protozoa such as *Leishmania* or other fungi such as *Sporothrix schenckii*. False negatives can occur in animals with very chronic clinical manifestations
Fungal culture	Aspirates or biopsies of affected tissues, body fluids	*H. capsulatum*	Sensitive and specific and may be required for animals with chronic histoplasmosis when cytologic examination is negative. Risk of laboratory-acquired infections. Slow turn-around time (several weeks of incubation may be required).
Antibody serology (CF or gel ID)	Serum	Antibodies to *H. capsulatum*	Positive test results indicate exposure but do not indicate active infection or correlate with clinical disease. Negative test results occur commonly in animals with histoplasmosis (low sensitivity).
Antigen assay (ELISA)	Urine, serum	*H. capsulatum* antigen	Commercial and in-house assays are available, and performance varies between the assays. The commercially available assay appears to be sensitive and specific in cats and dogs, but false-negative results can occur. An increased sensitivity is noted when urine is tested versus serum. Cross-reactivity with other fungal pathogens may occur, so positive results are not diagnostic for histoplasmosis.
Real-time PCR assays	Whole blood	*H. capsulatum* DNA	Not yet validated in adequate numbers of dogs or cats with histoplasmosis, usefulness requires further evaluation.
Histopathology	Biopsy specimens from affected tissues	*H. capsulatum* yeasts	Yeasts can be difficult to find in chronic infections. Special stains may assist organism detection.

CF, complement fixation; *ELISA*, enzyme-linked immunosorbent assay; *ID*, immunodiffusion; *PCR*, polymerase chain reaction.

cultures are positive within 2 or 3 weeks, growth may require up to 6 weeks of incubation. The organism is identified based on morphology.

Molecular Diagnosis Using Nucleic Acid–Based Testing

Real-time PCR assays have been developed for rapid detection of *H. capsulatum* in clinical specimens from affected humans,[78,79] but are not currently used routinely for diagnosis. The sensitivity of one assay was 73% when compared with culture of clinical specimens.[79] PCR assays have not been widely applied to the diagnosis of histoplasmosis in dogs and cats, and so further studies are required to determine their usefulness.

Pathologic Findings

Gross Pathologic Findings

Gross pathologic findings in dogs and cats with histoplasmosis consist of miliary nodules or larger focal lesions in the lungs and other organs, and enlarged lymph nodes, which may be mineralized in dogs with chronic disease. In dogs, the intestinal tract may be thickened and focal or diffuse hemorrhage may be present on the mucosal surface. The liver and spleen may be enlarged with rounded borders, and the liver may be mottled with a reticulated appearance. Pleural and peritoneal effusions are occasionally described.[62]

Histopathologic Findings

Histopathology yields pyogranulomatous or granulomatous inflammation with intralesional yeasts in a variety of organs (Fig. 81.7). Lymphocytes and plasma cells may be present, and in some dogs with chronic histoplasmosis, histologic evidence of fibrosis or calcification is apparent.[54,62] Special stains such as Gomori's methenamine silver or PAS may aid detection of the yeasts in tissues.

TREATMENT AND PROGNOSIS

Antimicrobial Treatment

Antifungal drugs with activity against *H. capsulatum* include the azole antifungal drugs ketoconazole, itraconazole, and fluconazole (see Chapter 11 for more information and dosing for antifungal drugs). Itraconazole and fluconazole are preferred to ketoconazole as they are more effective and less likely to cause toxicity.[22] In one study, remission rates in dogs were not different between those treated with fluconazole (64% remission) and itraconazole (71% remission)[20]; however, in human patients, itraconazole has consistently been more effective than fluconazole. Limited data suggest that posaconazole may be an effective salvage treatment in human patients with histoplasmosis that fails to respond to treatment with other antifungal drugs, which included

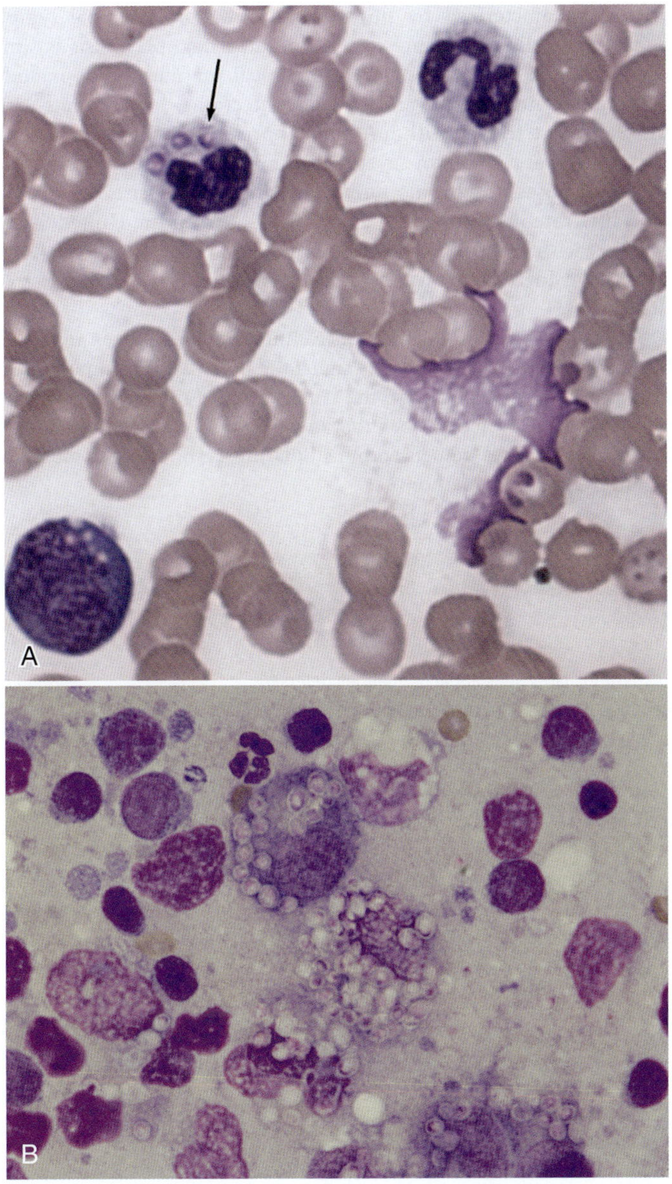

Fig. 81.6 (A) Blood smear from a dog with *Histoplasma capsulatum* fungemia. Three organisms can be seen in a circulating neutrophil *(arrow)*. Wright stain, 1000× magnification. (B) Fine-needle aspirate cytology from the right popliteal lymph node of the cat in Fig. 81.3A. There is pyogranulomatous inflammation with large numbers of intracellular yeast organisms with morphology consistent with that of *H. capsulatum*. Wright stain, 1000× magnification. (Courtesy Angela Royal, Louisiana State University.)

fluconazole, itraconazole, AMB, and voriconazole.[80] Development of resistance to fluconazole has been documented during treatment of cats and human patients with fluconazole.[81,82]

Deoxycholate or lipid AMB should be used initially to treat dogs or cats with severe acute pulmonary, acute disseminated, or CNS disease, after which treatment should be continued with itraconazole. If funds or patient factors do not permit itraconazole treatment, fluconazole can be used as a second-line agent.

The length of treatment and prognosis depends on the severity and chronicity of disease and the immune status of the host. At least 6 months of treatment is generally required. Many animals require treatment for 12 months or longer, and those with more chronic disease may require treatment for more than 2 years. The median duration of therapy for dogs in one study is 125 days for those treated with fluconazole and 182 days for those treated with itraconazole, which are not statistically different.[20] The decision to discontinue treatment should be based on lesion resolution (which may require serial imaging studies); resolution of positive urine antigen titers could also be used to decide when to discontinue treatment.[38] Relapse of disease after discontinuation of treatment is common, occurring in 10% to 40% of patients.[20,25,38]

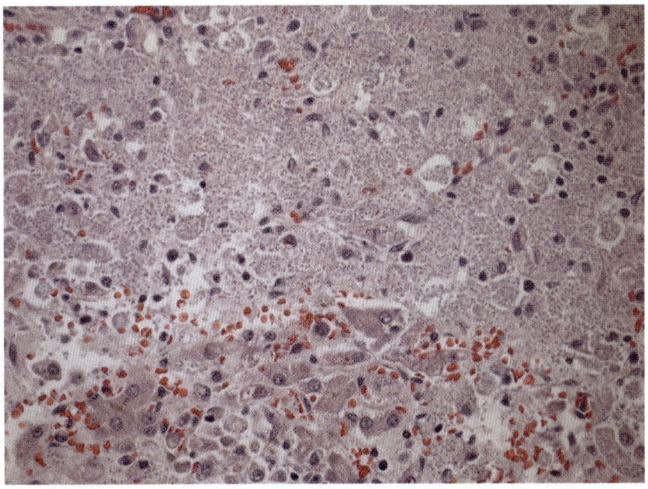

Fig. 81.7 Histopathology of the liver of a 5-month-old intact male redbone coonhound with disseminated histoplasmosis. There is severe granulomatous inflammation with massive numbers of intrahistiocytic yeast organisms.

Survival to hospital discharge for dogs and cats treated for histoplasmosis are 95% and 88% respectively.[20,83] Overall survival in cats treated for histoplasmosis is approximately 67%.[25,83] The need for supplemental oxygen delivery is a negative prognostic indicator in dogs and cats.[20,25] Additional negative prognostic indicators identified in dogs include hyperbilirubinemia, anemia, thrombocytopenia, and hypercalcemia.[20]

Supportive Treatment

Other supportive treatments that may be required depend on the extent of infection and include IV crystalloid fluids, supplemental oxygen, blood transfusions for severely anemic animals, nutritional support, antiemetics, and medications to manage consequences of hepatic failure such as hepatic encephalopathy. Enucleation may be required to manage persistent ocular infection and pain. The role of glucocorticoids for treatment of chronic manifestations of histoplasmosis is controversial, and they are not recommended for treatment of animals with active or disseminated histoplasmosis.

IMMUNITY AND VACCINATION

Immunity to *H. capsulatum* is dependent on a Th1 immune response. Production of IFN-γ and TNF α activates macrophages to destroy the fungus.[36,84] There is no vaccine for prevention of histoplasmosis, but there is interest in development of a vaccine for at-risk human patients because of increasing incidence of the disease.[36]

PREVENTION

Prevention of histoplasmosis involves avoidance of bat caves and areas previously inhabited by avian species in endemic areas. Nevertheless, histoplasmosis has occurred in animals housed exclusively indoors, and widespread exposure and recovery likely occurs in endemic areas.

PUBLIC HEALTH ASPECTS

As many as 80% of young adults in endemic areas have been previously infected by *H. capsulatum*, but less than 10% develop symptoms.[36,70] Risk factors identified for human histoplasmosis include exposure to soil disrupted as a result of excavation, exploration of caves inhabited by bats, or renovation of buildings inhabited by birds or bats. Males are predisposed.[36,85] Several forms of the disease have been described, which include acute pulmonary histoplasmosis, chronic pulmonary histoplasmosis (which may be cavitary or noncavitary), and acute or chronic PDH.[36] Complications of pulmonary histoplasmosis include granulomatous mediastinitis (characterized by enlargement and sometimes calcification of mediastinal lymph nodes, with compression of adjacent structures) or mediastinal fibrosis (characterized by fibrosis of caseous mediastinal lymph nodes). The clinical picture of disseminated histoplasmosis is similar to that described in dogs; rare clinical manifestations include meningitis, endocarditis, and vascular infections.[36,70] Humans with AIDS or those treated with immunosuppressive drugs (such as TNF antagonists) are at risk for severe, disseminated disease, and smokers are predisposed to chronic pulmonary histoplasmosis. The overall mortality rate in a 2018 study of 3,409 cases from the United States was 7%, with a hospitalization rate of 57%.[85] Itraconazole prophylaxis is considered for immunosuppressed patients who are at risk of the disease.[36]

Transmission from dogs or cats to humans has not been reported, but disease in dogs and cats may signal the potential for human infection as a result of exposure to the same source of infection in the soil; outbreaks have been described that involved both humans and dogs.[26] The bodies of deceased pets with histoplasmosis should be disposed of promptly and by cremation.

CASE EXAMPLE

Signalment

"Murphy," a 5-month-old intact male redbone coonhound from northern California.

History

Murphy was evaluated at the University of California, Davis Veterinary Medical Teaching Hospital, for a 1-week history of increased respiratory effort, hypersalivation, a single episode of vomiting, and lethargy. He was taken to a local veterinary clinic where he was found to have fever (103.2°F), pale mucous membranes, and a cranial abdominal mass on physical examination. Abdominal radiographs revealed moderate hepatomegaly and mild splenomegaly (available for review). He was treated with vitamin K, a single dose of injectable prednisone (2 mg/kg SC), and cephalexin (20 mg/kg, PO, q8h), and considerable improvement in his mentation was noted. However, after 5 days, anorexia, hypersalivation, vomiting, and liquid diarrhea developed and he returned to the local veterinary clinic where he was hospitalized and treated with IV fluids. The following day, obtundation and facial twitching developed and Murphy was referred for further diagnostics and treatment.

Current Medications

None

Other Medical History

Murphy was coughing 2 weeks ago but this subsequently resolved. He was also treated for a roundworm infection at that time, which was diagnosed by fecal flotation. Murphy was obtained from a breeder in Oklahoma. He had always appeared "slow" to the owner, his appetite had never been very good, and he seemed unthrifty. The other puppies in the litter were apparently healthy and there was no known exposure to toxins. The breeder had administered his first vaccines, and he was revaccinated for distemper, parvovirus, adenovirus, parainfluenza virus, and *Leptospira* by the referring veterinary clinic when he was acquired at 4 months of age.

Physical Examination

Body weight: 12.2 kg.

General: Obtundation was noted, the dog was in lateral recumbency and apparently unaware of his surroundings. Facial twitching occurred throughout the examination. T = 102.2°F, HR =140 beats/minutes, RR = 50 breaths/minute, mucous membranes moist and pink.

Eyes, ears, nose and throat: Moderate conjunctivitis was present. There was a mild bilateral serous nasal discharge. No other abnormalities were detected.

Musculoskeletal: Recumbent, appears small in stature, BCS 3/9.

Cardiovascular: No murmurs or arrhythmias were auscultated, strong pulse quality was present.

Respiratory: No significant abnormalities detected.

Abdominal palpation: Cranial organomegaly was present.

Lymph nodes: All were < 1.5 cm in diameter.

Laboratory Findings

Blood glucose: 70 mg/dL.

Plasma fasting ammonia concentration: 509 μg/dL (0–92 μg/dL).

Canine distemper virus immunofluorescent antibody (urine sediment): negative.

CBC: HCT 30.2% (40%–55%), MCV 61 fL (65–75 fL), MCHC 36.1 g/dL (33–36 g/dL), reticulocytes 49,200/μL (7,000–65,000/μL), WBC 22,000 cells/μL (6,000–13,000 cells/μL), neutrophils 10,340 cells/μL (3,000–10,500 cells/μL), band neutrophils 7,040 cells/μL, metamyelocytes 880 cells/μL, lymphocytes 1,100 cells/μL (1,000–4,000 cells/μL), monocytes 1,100 cells/μL (150–1,200 cells/μL), eosinophils 880 cells/μL (0–1,500 cells/μL), platelets 28,000 platelets/μL (150,000–400,000 platelets/μL). Moderately toxic neutrophils and markedly toxic band neutrophils and metamyelocytes were present. Occasional organisms with morphology consistent with *H. capsulatum* were seen within both neutrophils and monocytes. The myeloid series was shifted to the myelocyte stage with rare progranulocytes noted. Rare nucleated erythrocytes (metarubricytes) were also present. Many lymphocytes were reactive. Numerous macroplatelets were noted.

Serum chemistry profile: Sodium 143 mmol/L (145–154 mmol/L), potassium 4.7 mmol/L (4.1–5.3 mmol/L), chloride 108 mmol/L (105–116 mmol/L), bicarbonate 18 mmol/L (16–26 mmol/L), phosphorus 7.7 mg/dL (3.0–6.2 mg/dL), calcium 10.3 mg/dL (9.9–11.4 mg/dl), BUN 18 mg/dL (8–31 mg/dL), creatinine 0.4 mg/dL (0.8–1.6 mg/dL), glucose 117 mg/dL (70–118 mg/dL), total protein 5.8 g/dL (5.4–7.4 g/dL), albumin 2.1 g/dL (2.9–4.2 g/dL), globulin 3.7 g/dL (2.3–4.4 g/dL), ALT 31 U/L (19–70 U/L), AST 217 U/L (15–43 U/L), ALP 195 U/L (15–127 U/L), GGT 24 U/L (0–6 U/L), cholesterol 363 mg/dL (135–345 mg/dL), total bilirubin 1.1 mg/dL (0–0.4 mg/dL).

Urinalysis (cystocentesis): SpG 1.044; pH 5.0, 1+ bilirubin, no hemoprotein, no glucose, no protein, 0–1 RBC/HPF, rare WBC/HPF; no crystals, casts or bacteria seen.

Coagulation panel: PT 10.7 seconds (7.5–10.5 seconds), PTT 24.4 seconds (9–12 seconds), fibrin degradation products > 40 μg/mL (<10 μg/mL).

Imaging Findings

Thoracic radiographs: There was a diffuse bronchointerstitial pulmonary pattern especially in the region of the cranial right middle lung lobe. The heart and

CASE EXAMPLE—cont'd

pulmonary vasculature were slightly small. In the viewable abdomen, the liver was moderately enlarged.

Abdominal ultrasound: Severe hepatomegaly was present with normal hepatic echogenicity. A large, folded spleen and sublumbar and mesenteric lymphadenomegaly were present.

Microbiologic Testing

Fecal flotation: *Ancylostoma* ova.

Aspiration cytology (liver aspirate): The specimen was bloody and moderately cellular with numerous clusters of platelets and inflammatory cells. Occasional small clusters of hepatocytes were noted, which showed mild to moderate vacuolar degeneration. A few hepatocytes contained intracytoplasmic blue-green pigment consistent with bile. Inflammatory cells consisted primarily of activated macrophages which contained abundant intracellular yeast organisms consistent with *H. capsulatum*. Lower numbers of nondegenerate neutrophils, mixed lymphocytes, and occasional eosinophils and basophils were also found. Interpretation: *H. capsulatum* infection with marked pyogranulomatous inflammation. Mild to moderate hepatic vacuolar degeneration and cholestasis.

CSF analysis (cisternal): The fluid was clear and colorless. The protein concentration was 17 mg/dL (reference range, <25 mg/dL). There were < 1 RBC/μL (reference range, <1,200 RBC/μL) and 25 nucleated cells/μL (reference range, <2 cells/μL). The differential cell count consisted of 1% neutrophils, 6% lymphocytes, and 93% large mononuclear cells. The cytofuge specimen was cellular, and large, foamy macrophage-like cells predominated. Vacuoles within the cytoplasm contained digested debris, but no organisms could be discerned. Low numbers of small lymphocytes were also noted. Interpretation: Mononuclear pleocytosis.

Diagnosis

Acute PDH with suspected *H. capsulatum* meningitis; hookworm infestation.

Treatment

Murphy was hospitalized in the intensive care unit and treated with IV crystalloids (lactated Ringer's solution with 25 mEq/L KCl and 2.5% dextrose, 75 mL/hour), plasma, vitamin K, and heparin (100 U/kg, SC, q8h). The hookworm infection was treated with fenbendazole (50 mg/kg, PO, q24h for 3 days). Seizures were controlled with diazepam as needed and phenobarbital (2 mg/kg, IM, q12h). Hepatic encephalopathy was treated with a warm water enema, followed by a 3 mL/kg lactulose enema, and then oral lactulose (1 mL/kg, PO, q8h). Profuse watery diarrhea ensued. Treatment with lipid AMB was then initiated (2 mg/kg IV, over 2 hours, every other day). Initially, clinical signs improved and Murphy appeared brighter and began eating small amounts of a reduced protein diet. A CBC showed a HCT of 30%, 19,988 neutrophils/μL, 263 band neutrophils/μL with slight toxicity, 2,367 lymphocytes/μL, 2,367 monocytes/μL, 1,315 eosinophils/μL, and 65,000 platelets/μL. No *H. capsulatum* organisms were seen. The results of a biochemistry profile were similar to those reported at hospitalization, but electrolytes and glucose had normalized, and total bilirubin was 2.6 mg/dL.

On day 4 of hospitalization, he developed increased respiratory effort, weakness, and a head tremor. Thoracic radiographs showed a diffuse miliary interstitial infiltrate in the perihilar region and in the region of the right cranial lung lobe, which was slightly more severe that that seen at the time of hospitalization. By day 7 of hospitalization, he remained extremely weak and somewhat inappetent and the owners elected euthanasia due to financial limitations. At necropsy, there was severe hepatomegaly and splenomegaly, and the lungs were firm and mottled dark red to pink, and cut surfaces oozed white froth and blood. Histopathology revealed severe, diffuse, granulomatous inflammation with intrahistiocytic yeasts in the lungs, liver, spleen, bone marrow, sublumbar lymph nodes, and tracheobronchial lymph nodes (see Fig. 81.7). In the kidneys, there was severe, multifocal, granulomatous interstitial nephritis with intrahistiocytic yeasts. Multifocal granulomatous inflammation with intrahistiocytic yeasts was also seen in the pancreas, duodenum, jejunum, thyroid glands, and peritoneal fat. Within the brain there was minimal, focal, granulomatous meningitis.

Comments

In this dog, a diagnosis of disseminated histoplasmosis was straightforward because organisms were seen in a peripheral blood smear. The dog likely acquired infection in Oklahoma where the fungus is endemic. Overwhelming infection suggested a possible underlying immunodeficiency. The dog had evidence of DIC, hepatic encephalopathy, and granulomatous meningitis. Had treatment with AMB and additional supportive care continued, recovery might have occurred, but the costs of this treatment without guaranteed success led the owners to elect euthanasia. Clearly the burden of intact fungal organisms at necropsy was still massive despite several treatments with AMB. Even in human patients, overall cure rates for *H. capsulatum* meningitis are no better than 50%.

SUGGESTED READINGS

Lin Blache J, Ryan K, Arceneaux K, Histoplasmosis. *Compend Contin Educ Vet*. 2011;33:E1–E11.

Kroetz DN, Deepe GS. The role of cytokines and chemokines in *Histoplasma capsulatum* infection. *Cytokine*. 2012;58:112–117.

Wilson AG, KuKanich KS, Hanzlicek AS, Payton ME. Clinical signs, treatment, and prognostic factors for dogs with histoplasmosis. *J Am Vet Med Assoc*. 2018 Jan 15;252(2):201–209.

REFERENCES

1. Darling ST. A protozoal general infection producing pseudotubercles in the lungs and focal necrosis in the liver, spleen, and lymph nodes. *J Am Med Assoc*. 1906;46:1283–1285.
2. Arunmozhi Balajee S, Hurst SF, Chang LS, et al. Multilocus sequence typing of *Histoplasma capsulatum* in formalin-fixed paraffin-embedded tissues from cats living in non-endemic regions reveals a new phylogenetic clade. *Medical Mycology*. 2013;51:345–351.
3. Larsuprom L, Duangkaew L, Kasorndorkbua C, et al. Feline cutaneous histoplasmosis: the first case report from Thailand. *Med Mycol Case Rep*. 2017;18:28–30.
4. Mackie JT, Kaufman L, Ellis D. Confirmed histoplasmosis in an Australian dog. *Aust Vet J*. 1997;75:362–363.
5. Guerra BT, Almeida-Silva F, Almeida-Paes R, et al. Histoplasmosis outbreaks in Brazil: lessons to learn about preventing exposure. *Mycopathologia*. 2020;185:881–892.
6. Lomonaco L, Waller SB, Cleff MB, et al. Disseminated histoplasmosis in a cat rescued in Fortaleza, Brazil, and successfully treated with itraconazole - first case report identified molecularly. *Med Mycol Case Rep*. 2020;30:29–34.
7. Brilhante RS, Coelho CG, Sidrim JJ, et al. Feline histoplasmosis in Brazil: clinical and laboratory aspects and a comparative approach of published reports. *Mycopathologia*. 2012;173:193–197.
8. Johnson LR, Fry MM, Anez KL, et al. Histoplasmosis infection in two cats from California. *J Am Anim Hosp Assoc*. 2004;40:165–169.
9. Sanford SE, Straube U. Ontario. Disseminated histoplasmosis in a young dog. *Can Vet J*. 1991;32:692.
10. Tyre E, Eisenbart D, Foley P, et al. Histoplasmosis in a dog from new Brunswick. *Can Vet J*. 2007;48:734–736.
11. Murata Y, Sano A, Ueda Y, et al. Molecular epidemiology of canine histoplasmosis in Japan. *Med Mycol*. 2007;45:233–247.
12. Teixeira MM, Patané JSL, Taylor ML, et al. Worldwide phylogenetic distributions and population dynamics of the genus *Histoplasma*. *PLoS Negl Trop Dis*. 2016;10. e0004732-e0004732.

13. Kasuga T, White TJ, Koenig G, et al. Phylogeography of the fungal pathogen *Histoplasma capsulatum*. *Mol Ecol*. 2003;12:3383–3401.
14. Zeidberg LD, Ajello L, Webster RH. Physical and chemical factors in relation to *Histoplasma capsulatum* in soil. *Science*. 1955;122:33–34.
15. Taylor AR, Barr JW, Hokamp JA, et al. Cytologic diagnosis of disseminated histoplasmosis in the wall of the urinary bladder of a cat. *J Am Anim Hosp Assoc*. 2012;48:203–208.
16. Davies C, Troy GC. Deep mycotic infections in cats. *J Am Anim Hosp Assoc*. 1996;32:380–391.
17. Fielder SE, Meinkoth JH, Rizzi TE, et al. Feline histoplasmosis presenting with bone and joint involvement: clinical and diagnostic findings in 25 cats. *J Feline Med Surg*. 2019;21:887–892.
18. Aulakh HK, Aulakh KS, Troy GC. Feline histoplasmosis: a retrospective study of 22 cases (1986-2009). *J Am Anim Hosp Assoc*. 2012;48:182–187.
19. Mitchell M, Stark DR. Disseminated canine histoplasmosis: a clinical survey of 24 cases in Texas. *Can Vet J*. 1980;21:95–100.
20. Wilson AG, KuKanich KS, Hanzlicek AS, et al. Clinical signs, treatment, and prognostic factors for dogs with histoplasmosis. *J Am Vet Med Assoc*. 2018;252:201–209.
21. Selby LA, Becker SV, Hayes Jr HW. Epidemiologic risk factors associated with canine systemic mycoses. *Am J Epidemiol*. 1981;113:133–139.
22. Hodges RD, Legendre AM, Adams LG, et al. Itraconazole for the treatment of histoplasmosis in cats. *J Vet Intern Med*. 1994;8:409–413.
23. Clinkenbeard KD, Cowell RL, Tyler RD. Disseminated histoplasmosis in dogs: 12 cases (1981-1986). *J Am Vet Med Assoc*. 1987;193:1443–1447.
24. Wolf AM, Green RW. The radiographic appearance of pulmonary histoplasmosis in the cat. *Vet Radiol*. 1987;28:34–37.
25. Reinhart JM, KuKanich KS, Jackson T, et al. Feline histoplasmosis: fluconazole therapy and identification of potential sources of *Histoplasma* species exposure. *J Fel Med Surg*. 2012;14:841–848.
26. Davies SF, Colbert RL. Concurrent human and canine histoplasmosis from cutting decayed wood. *Ann Intern Med*. 1990;113:252–253.
27. Long KH, Gomez FJ, Morris RE, et al. Identification of heat shock protein 60 as the ligand on *Histoplasma capsulatum* that mediates binding to CD18 receptors on human macrophages. *J Immunol*. 2003;170:487–494.
28. Newman SL, Gootee L, Hilty J, et al. Human macrophages do not require phagosome acidification to mediate fungistatic/fungicidal activity against *Histoplasma capsulatum*. *J Immunol*. 2006;176:1806–1813.
29. Eissenberg LG, Goldman WE, Schlesinger P. *Histoplasma capsulatum* modulates the acidification of phagolysosomes. *J Exp Med*. 1993;177:1605–1611.
30. Garfoot AL, Shen Q, Wüthrich M, et al. The Eng1 β-glucanase enhances *Histoplasma* virulence by reducing β-glucan exposure. *mBio*. 2016;7:e01388-01315.
31. Garfoot AL, Rappleye CA. *Histoplasma capsulatum* surmounts obstacles to intracellular pathogenesis. *FEBS J*. 2016;283:619–633.
32. Hilty J, George Smulian A, Newman SL. *Histoplasma capsulatum* utilizes siderophores for intracellular iron acquisition in macrophages. *Med Mycol*. 2011;49:633–642.
33. Bertolini M, Mutti MF, Barletta JA, et al. COVID-19 associated with AIDS-related disseminated histoplasmosis: a case report. *Int J STD AIDS*. 2020;31:1222–1224.
34. Basso RP, Poester VR, Benelli JL, et al. COVID-19-associated histoplasmosis in an AIDS patient. *Mycopathologia*. 2021;186:109–112.
35. Emmons CW, Rowley DA, Olson BJ, et al. Histoplasmosis; proved occurrence of inapparent infection in dogs, cats and other animals. *Am J Hyg*. 1955;61:40–44.
36. Deepe GS. *Histoplasma capsulatum* (histoplasmosis). In: Bennett JE, Blaser MJ, Dolin R, eds. *Mandell, Douglas and Bennett's Principles and Practice of Infectious Diseases*. 7th ed. Philadephia, PA: Churchill Livingstone, Elsevier; 2015:2949–2962.
37. Boyd N, Thomason J, Pohlman L, et al. Mediastinal histoplasmosis with cardiac involvement in a cat. *J Vet Cardiol*. 2020;31:15–22.
38. Hanzlicek A, Meinkoth J, Renschler J, et al. Antigen concentrations as an indicator of clinical remission and disease relapse in cats with histoplasmosis. *J Vet Intern Med*. 2016;30:1065–1073.
39. Goad MEP, Roenick WJ. Osseous histoplasmosis in a cat. *Fel Pract*. 1983;13:32–36.
40. Tamulevicus AM, Harkin K, Janardhan K, et al. Disseminated histoplasmosis accompanied by cutaneous fragility in a cat. *J Am Anim Hosp Assoc*. 2011;47:e36–41.
41. Lamm CG, Rizzi TE, Campbell GA, et al. Pathology in practice. *Histoplasma capsulatum* infections. *J Am Vet Med Assoc*. 2009;235:155–157.
42. Vinayak A, Kerwin SC, Pool RR. Treatment of thoracolumbar spinal cord compression associated with *Histoplasma capsulatum* infection in a cat. *J Am Vet Med Assoc*. 2007;230:1018–1023.
43. Mavropoulou A, Grandi G, Calvi L, et al. Disseminated histoplasmosis in a cat in Europe. *J Small Anim Pract*. 2010;51:176–180.
44. Kobayashi R, Tanaka F, Asai A, et al. First case report of histoplasmosis in a cat in Japan. *J Vet Med Sci*. 2009;71:1669–1672.
45. Fischer NM, Favrot C, Monod M, et al. A case in Europe of feline histoplasmosis apparently limited to the skin. *Vet Dermatol*. 2013;24:635–638. e158.
46. Burk RL, Jones BD. Disseminated histoplasmosis with osseous involvement in a dog. *J Am Vet Med Assoc*. 1978;172:1416–1417.
47. Gilor C, Ridgway MD, Singh K. DIC and granulomatous vasculitis in a dog with disseminated histoplasmosis. *J Am Anim Hosp Assoc*. 2011;47:e26–30.
48. Lau RE, Kim SN, Pirozok RP. *Histoplasma capsulatum* infection in a metatarsal of a dog. *J Am Vet Med Assoc*. 1978;172:1414–1416.
49. Nishifuji K, Ueda Y, Sano A, et al. Interdigital involvement in a case of primary cutaneous canine histoplasmosis in Japan. *J Vet Med A Physiol Pathol Clin Med*. 2005;52:478–480.
50. Kagawa Y, Aoki S, Iwatomi T, et al. Histoplasmosis in the skin and gingiva in a dog. *J Vet Med Sci*. 1998;60:863–865.
51. Ueda Y, Sano A, Tamura M, et al. Diagnosis of histoplasmosis by detection of the internal transcribed spacer region of fungal rRNA gene from a paraffin-embedded skin sample from a dog in Japan. *Vet Microbiol*. 2003;94:219–224.
52. Sano A, Miyaji M. [Canine histoplasmosis in Japan]. *Nihon Ishinkin Gakkai Zasshi*. 2003;44:239–243.
53. Ewald MM, Rankin AJ, Meekins JM, et al. Disseminated histoplasmosis with ocular adnexal involvement in seven cats. *Vet Ophthalmol*. 2020;23:905–912.
54. Clemans JM, Deitz KL, Riedesel EA, et al. Retroperitoneal pyogranulomatous and fibrosing inflammation secondary to fungal infections in two dogs. *J Am Vet Med Assoc*. 2011;238:213–219.
55. Olson GA, Wowk BJ. Oral lesions of histoplasmosis in a dog. *Vet Med Small Anim Clin*. 1981;76:1449–1451.
56. Huss BT, Collier LL, Collins BK, et al. Polyarthropathy and chorioretinitis with retinal detachment in a dog with systemic histoplasmosis. *J Am Anim Hosp Assoc*. 1994;30:217–224.
57. Gwin RM, Makley Jr TA, Wyman M, et al. Multifocal ocular histoplasmosis in a dog and cat. *J Am Vet Med Assoc*. 1980;176:638–642.
58. Meadows RL, MacWilliams PS, Dzata G, et al. Diagnosis of histoplasmosis in a dog by cytologic examination of CSF. *Vet Clin Pathol*. 1992;21:122–125.
59. Schaer M, Johnson KE, Nicholson AC. Central nervous system disease due to histoplasmosis in a dog: a case report. *J Am Anim Hosp Assoc*. 1983;19:311–316.
60. Clinkenbeard KD, Cowell RL, Tyler RD. Disseminated histoplasmosis in cats: 12 cases (1981-1986). *J Am Vet Med Assoc*. 1988;190:1445–1448.
61. Carakostas MC, Miller RI, HGossett KA. Clinical laboratory evaluation of deep mycotic diseases in dogs. *J Small Anim Pract*. 1984;25:687–693.
62. Kowalewich N, Hawkins EC, Skowronek AJ, et al. Identification of *Histoplasma capsulatum* organisms in the pleural and peritoneal effusions of a dog. *J Am Vet Med Assoc*. 1993;202:423–426.
63. Clinkenbeard KD, Cowell RL, Tyler RD. Identification of *Histoplasma* organisms in circulating eosinophils of a dog. *J Am Vet Med Assoc*. 1988;192:217–218.
64. Burk RL, Corley EA, Corwin LA. The radiographic appearance of pulmonary histoplasmosis in the dog and cat: a review of 37 case histories. *J Am Vet Radiol Soc*. 1978;19:2–7.
65. Miller BM, Waterhouse G, Alford RH, et al. *Histoplasma* infection of abdominal aortic aneurysms. *Ann Surg*. 1983;197:57–62.

66. Chavez-Peon Berle E, KuKanich K, Biller D. Ultrasonographic findings of gastrointestinal histoplasmosis in dogs. *Vet Radiol Ultrasound.* 2021;62:108–115.
67. Atiee G, Kvitko–White H, Spaulding K, et al. Ultrasonographic appearance of histoplasmosis identified in the spleen in 15 cats. *Vet Radiol Ultrasound.* 2014;55:310–314.
68. Reginato A, Giannuzzi P, Ricciardi M, et al. Extradural spinal cord lesion in a dog: first case study of canine neurological histoplasmosis in Italy. *Vet Microbiol.* 2014;170:451–455.
69. Beekman R, Hu JM, Aronin SI, et al. Diagnosing ring-enhancing lesions in the brain of a patient with AIDS without brain biopsy: a case of central nervous system histoplasmoma. *Neurohospitalist.* 2018;8:86–91.
70. Kauffman CA. Histoplasmosis: a clinical and laboratory update. *Clin Microbiol Rev.* 2007;20:115–132.
71. Cook AK, Cunningham LY, Cowell AK, et al. Clinical evaluation of urine *Histoplasma capsulatum* antigen measurement in cats with suspected disseminated histoplasmosis. *J Fel Med Surg.* 2012;14:512–515.
72. Smith KM, Strom AR, Gilmour MA, et al. Utility of antigen testing for the diagnosis of ocular histoplasmosis in four cats: a case series and literature review. *J Feline Med Surg.* 2017;19:1110–1118.
73. Jarchow A, Hanzlicek A. Antigenemia without antigenuria in a cat with histoplasmosis. *J Fel Med Surg Open Reports.* 2015;1:2055116915618422.
74. Cunningham L, Cook A, Hanzlicek A, et al. Sensitivity and specificity of *Histoplasma* antigen detection by enzyme immunoassay. *J Am Anim Hosp Assoc.* 2015;51:306–310.
75. Wheat J, Wheat H, Connolly P, et al. Cross-reactivity in *Histoplasma capsulatum* variety *capsulatum* antigen assays of urine samples from patients with endemic mycoses. *Clin Infect Dis.* 1997;24:1169–1171.
76. Kuberski T, Myers R, Wheat LJ, et al. Diagnosis of coccidioidomycosis by antigen detection using cross-reaction with a *Histoplasma* antigen. *Clin Infect Dis.* 2007;44:e50–54.
77. Rothenburg L, Hanzlicek AS, Payton ME. A monoclonal antibody–based urine *Histoplasma* antigen enzyme immunoassay (IMMY®) for the diagnosis of histoplasmosis in cats. *J Vet Intern Med.* 2019;33:603–610.
78. Martagon-Villamil J, Shrestha N, Sholtis M, et al. Identification of *Histoplasma capsulatum* from culture extracts by real-time PCR. *J Clin Microbiol.* 2003;41:1295–1298.
79. Babady NE, Buckwalter SP, Hall L, et al. Detection of *Blastomyces dermatitidis* and *Histoplasma capsulatum* from culture isolates and clinical specimens by use of real-time PCR. *J Clin Microbiol.* 2011;49:3204–3208.
80. Restrepo A, Tobon A, Clark B, et al. Salvage treatment of histoplasmosis with posaconazole. *J Infect.* 2007;54:319–327.
81. Renschler JS, Norsworthy GD, Rakian RA, et al. Reduced susceptibility to fluconazole in a cat with histoplasmosis. *J Fel Med Surg Open Reports.* 2017;3:2055116917743364.
82. Wheat LJ, Connolly P, Smedema M, et al. Activity of newer triazoles against *Histoplasma capsulatum* from patients with AIDS who failed fluconazole. *J Antimicrob Chemother.* 2006;57:1235–1239.
83. Ludwig HC, Hanzlicek AS, KuKanich KS, et al. Candidate prognostic indicators in cats with histoplasmosis treated with antifungal therapy. *J Fel Med Surg.* 2018;20:985–996.
84. Kroetz DN, Deepe GS. The role of cytokines and chemokines in *Histoplasma capsulatum* infection. *Cytokine.* 2012;58:112–117.
85. Armstrong PA, Jackson BR, Haselow D, et al. Multistate epidemiology of histoplasmosis, United States, 2011-2014. *Emerg Infect Dis.* 2018;24:425–431.

82

Cryptococcosis

Krystle L. Reagan, Mark Krockenberger, Jane E. Sykes

KEY POINTS

- First Described: 1894, in a human patient in Germany (independently by Busse and Buschke).[1]
- Causes: *Cryptococcus gattii* species complex (SC), *Cryptococcus neoformans* SC, and rarely other cryptococcal species. The causative agents are basidiomycetes and usually referred to by their anamorph identification of *Cryptococcus* spp. (with the exception of *Papiliotrema laurentii*, formerly known as *Cryptococcus laurentii*), and the known teleomorphs (filamentous form) are *Filobasidiella* spp.
- Affected Hosts: Cats, dogs, humans, and a variety of other domestic and wild animal species.
- Geographic Distribution: Worldwide.
- Major Mode of Transmission: Inhalation of basidiospores from the environment.
- Major Clinical Signs: Nodular or ulcerative cutaneous lesions, upper respiratory tract signs, chorioretinitis, neurologic signs secondary to meningoencephalitis. In dogs, *Cryptococcus* can disseminate to abdominal organs and cause GI signs such as vomiting, diarrhea, and inappetence.
- Differential Diagnoses: For cats, differential diagnoses for cutaneous lesions include other deep mycoses (especially sporotrichosis), mycobacteriosis, nocardiosis, neoplasia (especially SCC), herpetic dermatitis, and eosinophilic granuloma complex. Differential diagnoses for suspected cryptococcal rhinitis include nasal lymphoma, foreign bodies, sinonasal/sino-orbital aspergillosis, oronasal fistulae, and neutrophilic rhinitis. For ocular and CNS lesions, differential diagnoses include neoplasia (especially lymphoma), toxoplasmosis, FIP, and otogenic bacterial meningitis. For dogs, differential diagnoses include other disseminated mycoses (especially histoplasmosis and blastomycosis), mycobacteriosis, actinomycosis and nocardiosis, other causes of rhinitis (such as foreign bodies, nasal aspergillosis, oronasal fistulas, lymphoplasmacytic rhinitis, and rhinosporidiosis), neoplasia (especially round cell neoplasia), toxoplasmosis, neosporosis, severe inflammatory bowel disease, and pancreatitis.
- Human Health Significance: Human infections occur as a result of exposure to organisms in the environment and are often associated with underlying immune compromise.

ETIOLOGIC AGENT AND EPIDEMIOLOGY

Cryptococcosis is an important fungal infection of humans and animals worldwide and the most common systemic mycosis of cats. The infection is acquired from the environment, and disease transmission from one animal to another has not been reported. Occasional outbreaks of cryptococcosis in humans and animals may result from exposure to common environmental sources.[2,3] Various domestic and native mammals may be infected, which include cats, dogs, ferrets, horses, camelids, goats, sheep, cattle, dolphins, birds, koalas, and other marsupials.[4–10] The incidence of cryptococcosis is eightfold higher in cats than in dogs.[11]

The genus *Cryptococcus* contains at least 37 yeast species. Organisms that belong to the *Cryptococcus neoformans* species complex (SC) and *Cryptococcus gattii* species complex (SC) cause the vast majority of infections in dogs, cats, and humans. *Cryptococcus gattii* SC organisms have emerged as pathogens of immunocompetent humans in temperate regions of North America, in particular on the west coast of the United States and in British Columbia, Canada. Other species, particularly *Papiliotrema laurentii* (previously *Cryptococcus laurentii*)[12] and *Cryptococcus albidus*, rarely cause disease in humans and animals, but may be emerging as a result of immunocompromise.[13–15] *Cryptococcus magnus* was isolated from the external ear canal of a cat with otitis externa,[16] and *Papiliotrema (Cryptococcus) laurentii* has been isolated from the external ear canal of dogs.[17] Molecular methods may be required to accurately identify these species; in one cat where classical phenotypic and biochemical methods led to identification of *C. albidus*, the organism was shown to be *C. neoformans* by 18S rRNA gene sequencing.[18]

Cryptococcus spp. are dimorphic, basidiomycetous fungi. The life cycle of the fungus is thought to involve growth in host tissues as an encapsulated haploid budding yeast, combined with the ability to undergo a transition to a filamentous form (or teleomorph) in the environment. Two mating types of *Cryptococcus* spp. exist, α and **a**. The α mating type is vastly more prevalent in environmental and clinical samples, with **a** mating type rarely found particularly in disease or even in the environment. Under appropriate laboratory conditions, the two mating types fuse and adopt a dikaryotic filamentous state, also known as the *perfect state*. This is followed by production of basidia, which are small, club-shaped structures on which basidiospores form (Fig. 82.1).[19] Cells of the α mating type can also undergo asexual reproduction via a process known as monokaryotic fruiting, which also involves filamentation and spore formation.[19–21] Although they have never been observed in nature, basidiospores (or possibly desiccated yeasts) are thought to be the main form that, when inhaled, gives rise to mammalian disease.[22] In animal tissues, basidiospores convert to the yeast form, which is round to oval with a variably sized capsule. The capsule is primarily (90% to 95%) composed of a polysaccharide known as glucuronoxylomannan (GXM), with smaller amounts of galactoxylomannan. The capsule enlarges after infection of mammalian hosts and protects the fungus from phagocytosis and environmental insults such as desiccation. Within tissues, *Cryptococcus* reproduces by forming one or two daughter cells (buds) that are connected to the parent cell by a narrow base (Fig. 82.2).

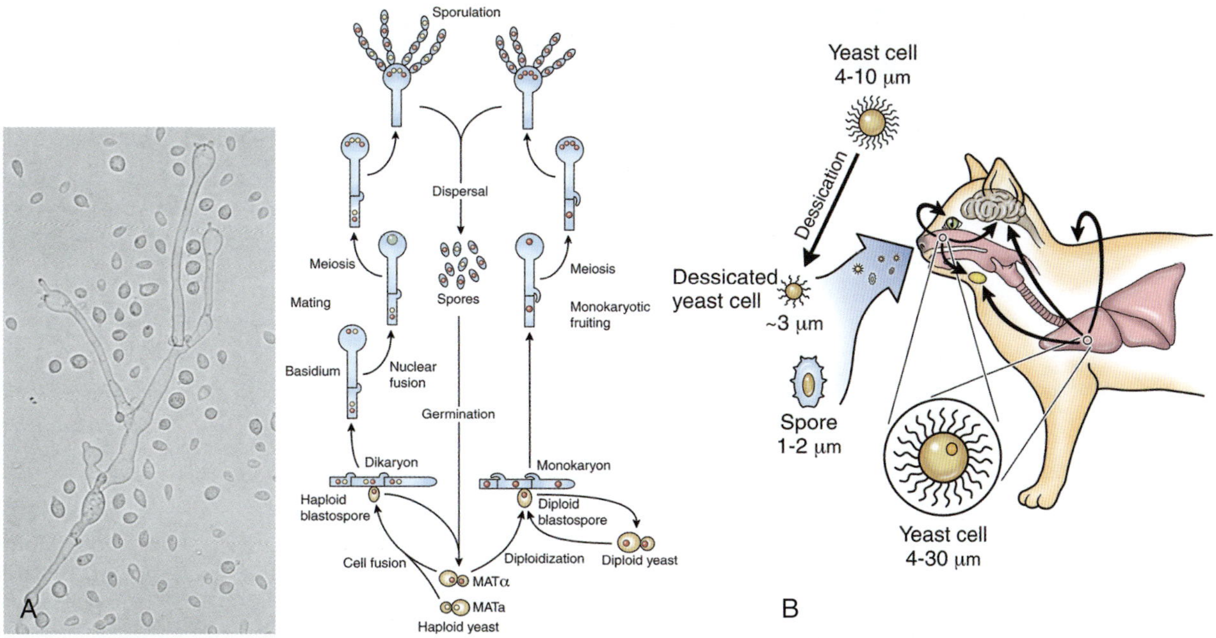

Fig. 82.1 Life cycle of *Cryptococcus* spp. (A) Spores result from either mating between cells of opposite mating types (*MATa* or *MATα*) and subsequent formation of dikaryotic hyphae or unisexual mating of MATα cells (monokaryotic fruiting). In both cases, sexual development within the filamentous form results in meiosis and basidiospore formation. The spores germinate to produce haploid, yeast-like cells that divide by budding. (B) Spores, and potentially desiccated yeast cells, are inhaled. Germination of spores or vegetative growth of yeast cells in the upper or lower respiratory tract results in the proliferation of budding yeasts. Dissemination to a variety of tissues can then occur, but especially to the lymph nodes, nasal cavity, skin, and central nervous system. (Modified from Kronstad JW, Attarian R, Cadieux B, et al. Expanding fungal pathogenesis: *Cryptococcus* breaks out of the opportunistic box. *Nat Rev Microbiol.* 2011;9:193–203. Basidiospore image courtesy Patrik Inderbitzen, University of California, Davis.)

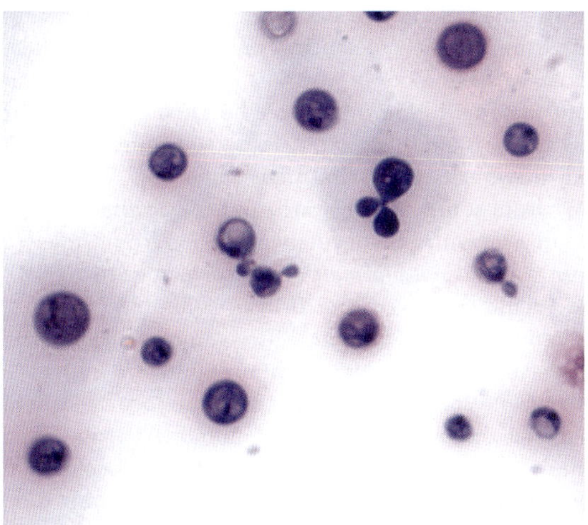

Fig. 82.2 Cerebrospinal fluid cytology from an 8-year-old male neutered domestic shorthair cat with cryptococcal meningitis. Large numbers of budding cryptococcal yeasts are present.

Historically, five serotypes of *Cryptococcus* (A, B, C, D, and AD) were recognized on the basis of antigenic differences in the capsular polysaccharide. Based on the results of molecular typing methods such as PCR fingerprinting, amplified fragment length polymorphism analysis, and restriction fragment length polymorphism analysis of the orotidine monophosphate pyrophosphorylase (URA5) and phospholipase genes, cryptococcal strains from around the world were divided into several major molecular types, some of which have been designated separate species names within *C. neoformans* SC and *C. gattii* SC:[23] VNI and VNII (*C. neoformans*), VNIII (*C. neoformans* × *Cryptococcus deneoformans* hybrid), VNIV (*C. deneoformans*), VGI (*C. gattii* sensu stricto), VGII (*Cryptococcus deuterogattii*), VGIII (*Cryptococcus bacillisporus*), VGIV (*Cryptococcus tetragattii*), and a VGIII/VGIV hybrid (*Cryptococcus decagattii*) (Table 82.1).[23–25] Differences in epidemiology, pathogenicity, clinical features, and drug susceptibility have been associated with each species.[26–29] Designation of separate species names for molecular types has been controversial because of the potential for this to cause confusion among clinicians,[30] but there is increasing use of these separate names in the literature. There will be a differential uptake of this nomenclature by diagnostic laboratories across the world, just as there was at the time that *C. gattii* was distinguished from *C. neoformans*. It emphasizes the need for clinicians to understand some of the history of nomenclature changes, not only when searching the literature for information about the causative organism but also when querying their laboratory about mycology results.

Cats of all ages may be affected,[31] but young adult cats appear to be at increased risk. In dogs, cryptococcosis is diagnosed predominantly in young adult dogs. In one study, the median age of cats and dogs was 6 and 4 years, respectively.[11] No clear sex predisposition exists. Siamese, birman, and ragdoll cats have been predisposed in Australian studies but were not found to be at risk in the United States.[11,32] Similarly, German shepherd dogs, Doberman pinschers, and great Danes appear to be predisposed in Australia, whereas in the United States, American cocker spaniel dogs were strongly predisposed with an odds ratio of 16.[8,11,31,33,34]

Most cats and dogs with cryptococcosis do not have identifiable underlying immunosuppressive illness. The prevalence of retrovirus infection in cat populations with cryptococcosis does not differ from that in cat populations without cryptococcosis.[11,31] However, some cats

TABLE 82.1 Relationships Between Phenotypes, Genotypes, and Species Belonging to *Cryptococcus neoformans* and *Cryptococcus gattii* Species Complexes

Serotype	Previous Species Name	Molecular Type	AFLP Genotype	New Species Name
A	*C. neoformans* var. *grubii*	VNI	1	*C. neoformans*
		VNII	1A/1B	
B + C	*C. gattii*	VGI	4	*C. gattii* sensu stricto
		VGII	6	*C. deuterogattii*
		VGIII	5	*C. bacillisporus*
		VGIV	7	*C. tetragattii*
		VGIIIc/VGIV hybrid	10	*C. decagattii*
D	*C. neoformans* var. *neoformans*	VNIV	2	*C. deneoformans*
AD		VNIII	3	*C. neoformans/C. deneoformans* hybrid

with cryptococcosis that are co-infected with FeLV appear to respond more slowly to treatment and may be more likely to have relapses.[35] Cats infected with FIV and cryptococcosis did not have an unfavorable prognosis in one study, and several were cured of the infection.[36] Cryptococcosis is occasionally reported in cats treated with immunosuppressive therapy or chemotherapy for malignancy.[11,37] Concurrent opportunistic infections have been reported in other cats (e.g., toxoplasmosis), as well as in dogs (e.g., neosporosis or papillomatosis), suggesting underlying immunodeficiency.[11,38] Administration of glucocorticoids to dogs and cats infected with *Cryptococcus* spp. can lead to the development of disseminated disease.

Cryptococcus neoformans Species Complex

Organisms that belong to the *C. neoformans* SC have a worldwide distribution. They primarily infect human patients who are immunocompromised, especially AIDS patients. The realized environmental niche for *C. neoformans* SC organisms is weathered bird (especially pigeon) guano which provides an alkaline, hyperosmolar, nitrogen-rich environment that allows prolific growth.[39] They can also be found in decaying plant matter in hollows of certain trees.[40] The organism can remain viable for at least 2 years in environments such as pigeon lofts. The majority of human cryptococcal infections result from infection with *C. neoformans* sensu stricto (ss) (VNI).[41] *C. neoformans* ss is the most common *Cryptococcus* species isolated from dogs and cats in southeastern Australia and accounts for more than 70% of infections.[31,32,34] Across the United States, most dogs with cryptococcosis are infected with *C. neoformans* SC organisms, but infection of cats with this species is rare.[11,42]

Cryptococcus gattii Species Complex

Organisms that belong to the *C. gattii* SC are endemic in Australia, New Zealand, Papua New Guinea, Southeast Asia, parts of Latin America, California, Mexico, Hawaii, Central and South Africa, and, to a lesser extent, certain parts of Europe (Austria, Germany, France, Italy, Greece, and Spain).[43,44] Since 1999, an epidemic of infections with *C. gattii* SC has occurred in humans and domestic and wild animals in British Columbia in Canada, especially Vancouver Island, and the Pacific Northwest of the United States, and infections have been occurring in humans at a rate higher than that in other endemic regions.[45–49] The main species identified in this epidemic has been *C. deuterogattii* (molecular types VGIIa and, to a much lesser extent, VGIIb and, in Oregon, also VGIIc). *Cryptococcus deuterogattii* (VGII) can be found on living tree bark (Garry oak, maple, cedar, and pine) and in air, and has also been found in freshwater and seawater. Proximity to areas with soil disturbance was a risk factor for dogs and cats.[48] In California, almost all cats appear to be infected with *C. bacillisporus* (VGIII), with occasional *C. deuterogattii* (VGII) infections.[11,42] The ecologic niche of *C. bacillisporus* (VGIII) in the United States remains somewhat unclear,[49] but it has recently been isolated from the bark of several tree species, including the Canary Island pine, American Sweetgum, Pohutukawa tree, Western Sycamore, and Blue Gum in southern California, as well as from soil in public parks and areas in the Los Angeles and San Diego regions.[50] However, as found for other endemic mycoses, approximately 25% of affected cats are housed exclusively indoors.[11]

In eastern Australia, 20% to 30% of human, feline, and canine cryptococcosis is caused by *C. gattii* SC organisms,[32,38] whereas in Western Australia, approximately 50% of cats and dogs with cryptococcosis are infected with *C. gattii* SC organisms.[8,49] Most *C. gattii* isolates from eastern Australia belong to *C. gattii* ss (VGI), whilst *C. deuterogattii* (VGII) is mostly seen in southwestern and northern Australia.[8,51] *Cryptococcus gattii* ss (VGI) in Australia is very strongly associated with dead plant material in *Eucalyptus* tree hollows.[5,52] Cats in rural environments are at risk of infection. Recently, *C. deuterogattii* (VGII) was identified in two cats with nasal signs[53] and dogs with disseminated disease[54,55] from southeastern Brazil, and *C. bacillisporus* (VGIII) was identified in a cat with a nasal cutaneous lesion from Chile.[56]

In contrast to *C. neoformans* ss, *C. deuterogattii* (VGII) isolates from the Pacific northwest and British Columbia can infect apparently immunocompetent humans.[57] *Cryptococcus bacillisporus* (VGIII) infections have been reported in immunosuppressed humans in southern California.[58] When disease occurs in immunocompetent hosts, it is often characterized by the presence of pulmonary mass lesions (cryptococcomas) and sometimes intracranial cryptococcomas.[59,60] As a result, pulmonary cryptococcomas are more commonly described in human patients infected with *C. bacillisporus* (VGIII) compared with those infected with *C. neoformans* ss.[60]

CLINICAL FEATURES

Pathogenesis and Clinical Signs

Based on the small size of basidiospores, the lung is thought to be the primary site of infection in humans. In cats, dogs, and koalas, the nasal cavity may be the primary site of infection (see Fig. 82.1). *Cryptococcus neoformans* ss has been shown to be a transient colonizer of the nasal mucus of cats, dogs, and koalas in Australia,[5,61] whereas *C. gattii* ss can be isolated in sufficient numbers and with sufficient frequency to potentially even be considered part of normal sinonasal flora of koalas in certain environments.[62] Significant pulmonary parenchymal involvement in these species is rare, although lesions can be detected on pulmonary CT scans and at necropsy. Importantly, the progression of disease from colonization to subclinical disease and clinical disease is best recognized in the koala.[5,62,63] Colonization of the nasal cavity may be followed by development of cryptococcal rhinitis in some (but not all) dogs and cats. However, some nasal cavity involvement may result from hematogenous dissemination, because injection of *Cryptococcus* spp. into the carotid artery of cats can lead to development of lesions on the bridge of the nose. Some localized cutaneous lesions may result from direct cutaneous inoculation (e.g., after a cat scratch), but skin lesions are usually interpreted as the result of dissemination or extension from the nasal cavity.

The pathogenesis of cryptococcosis depends on the size of the inoculum, virulence of the cryptococcal strain, and host immunity. *Cryptococcus* has been aptly described as "a sugar-coated killer with designer genes."[64] *Cryptococcus* has several important virulence factors, including its polysaccharide capsule, laccase (which makes melanin), mannitol, and other enzymes such as phospholipase, urease, and superoxide dismutase.[17,59,65] Capsular polysaccharide is continuously shed into the host's extracellular fluid, which includes blood, urine, and CSF. The capsule inhibits phagocytosis through its negative charge and via blockage of the Fc portion of bound antibodies from interacting with host phagocyte receptors. The capsule also depletes complement and interferes with migration of leukocytes from the bloodstream into infected tissues by causing them to shed selectin.[65,66] It also directly inhibits CMI by causing a shift from Th1 to a Th2 type immune response.[66] The ability of *C. neoformans* SC and *C. gattii* SC organisms to grow at mammalian body temperature is also an important virulence factor and is lacking in other species of *Cryptococcus*. Both *C. neoformans* SC and *C. gattii* SC organisms can undergo phenotypic switching by altering the cell membrane sterol composition and GXM structure allowing the organisms to evade the host immune response.[67]

The incubation period can range from 2 to 13 months.[68,69] Exposure and self-limiting infection may occur in some individuals, with reactivation of viable cryptococci in residual granulomatous foci months or years later with immunosuppressive drug therapy or illness.[59] Because of this delay, a travel history to areas where *Cryptococcus* is highly endemic (such as British Columbia or the west coast of the United States) may be present in animals and humans residing in nonendemic regions. After infection is established within the lung or nasal cavity, the organism can spread hematogenously via macrophages to other sites, particularly the lymph nodes, eye, skin, and CNS (see Fig. 82.1). *Cryptococcus* spp. can cross the capillary endothelium and enter the CNS by traveling within infected macrophages ("Trojan horse" mechanism). Free organisms may also be able to penetrate the blood-brain barrier by penetrating between damaged endothelial cells, or by transcytosis, whereby free organisms cross through capillary endothelial cells into the brain parenchyma, causing meningitis or meningoencephalitis.[30,70] In humans, cerebral cryptococcosis is often associated with increased intracranial pressure, and this probably also occurs in cats and dogs. Spread of infection to the eye, either along the optic nerves from the brain or as a result of hematogenous spread, may result in concurrent cryptococcal optic neuritis and chorioretinitis. In animals with nasal cavity involvement, extension of infection into the brain may also follow osteomyelitis of the cribriform plate or of the ventral wall of the frontal sinus. Middle ear involvement can also occur.[71] Infection also often spreads from the nasal cavity to the mandibular lymph nodes.

Multifocal cutaneous involvement in cats and dogs reflects hematogenous dissemination from the primary site of infection (usually respiratory tract), as do lesions in bone (e.g., digits) or periarticular soft tissues. Primary cutaneous lesions are rare, although occur more frequently in species like the koala, due to direct inoculation from heavily contaminated environments. Dogs infected with *C. neoformans* ss often develop widely disseminated disease, with involvement of sites such as the GI system, pancreas, mesenteric lymph nodes, kidneys, myocardium, and thyroid gland (Fig. 82.3).[11,33,72,73] In contrast, dogs infected with *C. deuterogattii* (VGII) in the United States tend to have isolated caudal nasal cavity cryptococcomas, which can extend through the cribriform plate into the brain (Fig. 82.4). Primary GI tract cryptococcosis is rare but does seem to occur and may be associated with *C. deuterogattii* (VGII).[74,75]

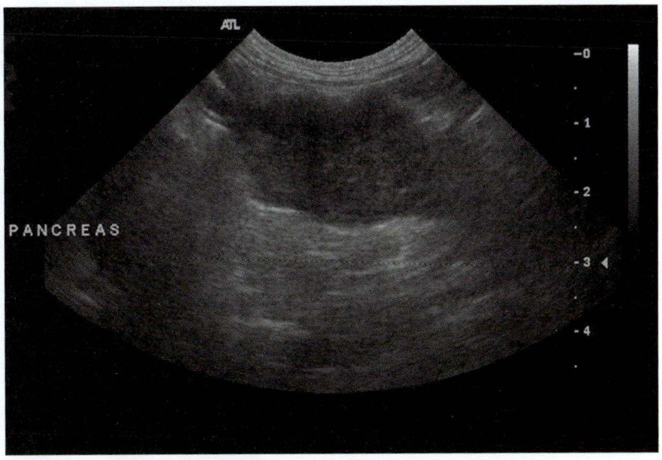

Fig. 82.3 Ultrasound image that shows an enlarged and hypoechoic pancreas in a 7-year-old female spayed basset mixed-breed dog with systemic cryptococcosis caused by *Cryptococcus neoformans* var. *grubii* (molecular type VNI). The dog was evaluated for gastrointestinal signs that were associated with severe cryptococcal pancreatitis and enteritis. The dog's lungs, heart, kidneys, liver, mesenteric lymph nodes, peritoneum, brain, and meninges were also involved at necropsy.

Clinical Features in Cats

Cryptococcosis is often a chronic infection in cats, and affected cats are usually otherwise well but occasionally have mild lethargy and inappetence. Fever is rare, and when it occurs, it tends to be of low grade. Upper respiratory tract signs due to nasal cavity involvement are common including sneezing and nasal discharge which can be mucopurulent, serous, or hemorrhagic in nature. A firm to fluctuant swelling over the bridge of the nose may be present with or without mandibular lymphadenopathy. Single or multifocal ulcerated or nonulcerated cutaneous masses may also be present (Fig. 82.5).[76]

Lower respiratory tract signs such as tachypnea are uncommon but can occur as a result of pleural effusion or severe mediastinal lymphadenomegaly. Neurologic signs vary depending on the location of lesions in and around the CNS (see Physical Examination Findings), and, rarely, cats with CNS involvement lack obvious neurologic signs. Optic neuritis and chorioretinitis develop in as many as one third of affected cats and almost always indicate CNS involvement.

Other signs include peripheral lymphadenomegaly (which may be unassociated with skin lesions and is often asymmetric), lameness due to osteomyelitis or cryptococcal arthritis, and swollen digits. Rarely, involvement of the abdominal lymph nodes, kidneys, lower urinary tract, spleen, liver, thyroid, and salivary glands occurs.

Clinical Features in Dogs

In contrast to cats, dogs frequently develop severe disseminated disease. In one study, 80% of dogs had involvement of multiple anatomic sites, and 50% of dogs had involvement of sites other than the nasal

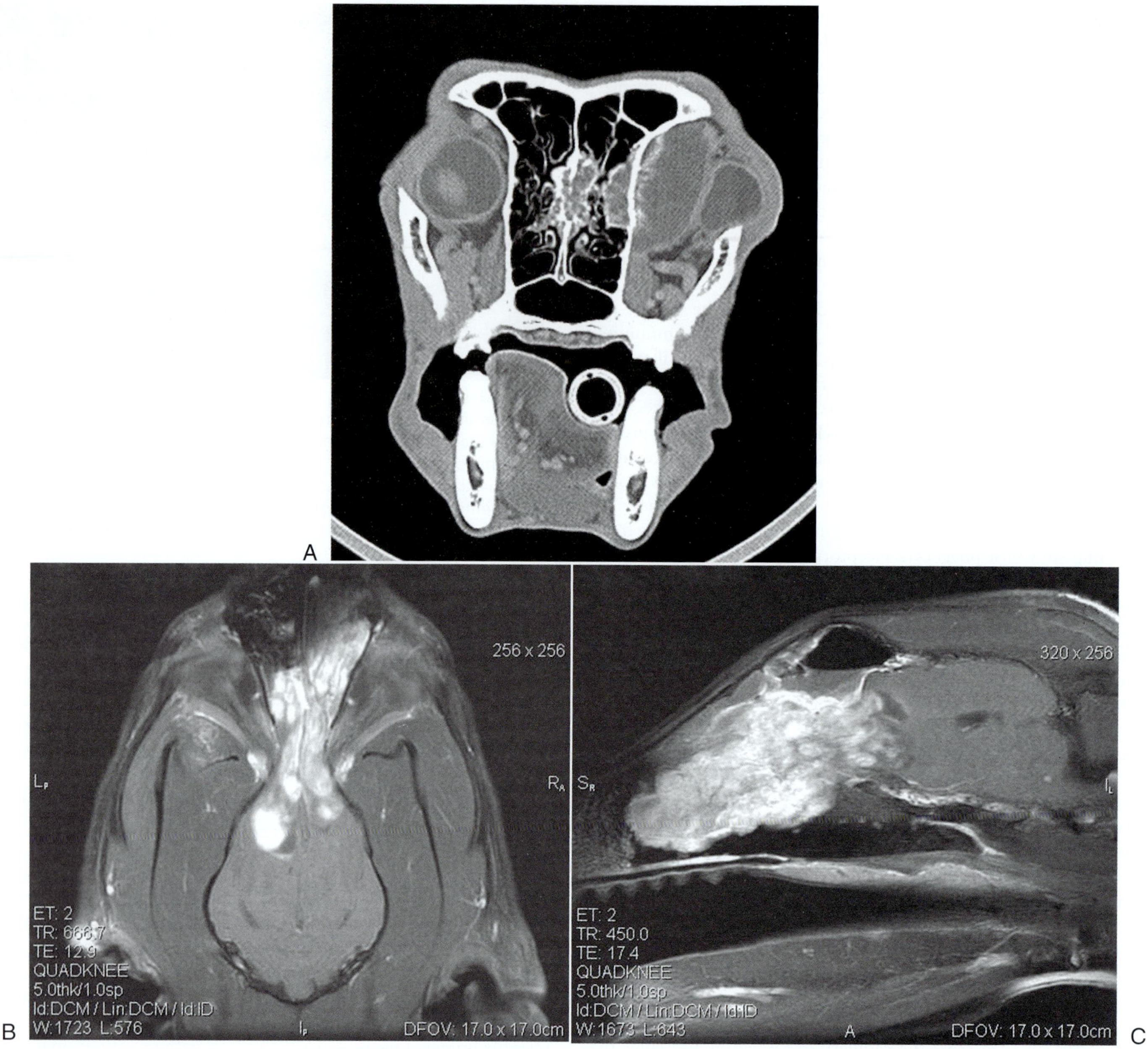

Fig. 82.4 Caudal nasal cryptococcosis in dogs infected with *Cryptococcus gattii.* (A) Computed tomography scan showing a large caudal nasal cavity cryptococcoma at necropsy that invaded the cribriform plate and retrobulbar space in a 5-year-old Doberman pinscher infected with *C. deuterogattii* (*C. gattii* molecular type VGIIa). There is a palisading periosteal response along the lateral margin of the right frontal and lacrimal bones. (B and C) Postcontrast magnetic resonance images of the head of a 2-year-old intact male malamute with a 1-week history of abnormal behavior and seizures. *Cryptococcus* was isolated from the nasal cavity. A large, contrast-enhancing mass is present in the caudal nasal cavity that invades the cribriform plate and extends into the brain. (Courtesy Dr. Stacey Hoffman.)

cavity, skin, lungs, lymph nodes, kidney, eye, and CNS.[11] Weight loss, lethargy, and inappetence are common nonspecific findings. Rhinosinusitis from cryptococcosis may be subclinical in dogs, so its incidence may be underestimated.[11,34] However, sneezing and mucopurulent nasal discharge can also occur. Neurologic signs were present in two thirds of affected dogs from California.[11] Dogs can also primarily show signs of GI or pancreatic involvement, such as vomiting, diarrhea, and abdominal pain.[54,74,75]

Cutaneous involvement is uncommon in dogs but, as in cats, may be a marker for disseminated disease. Although rarely detected antemortem, more than half of dogs have lower respiratory involvement at necropsy.[11] Other clinical signs that are infrequently present in dogs include peripheral lymphadenomegaly or lameness (due to osteomyelitis or arthritis) (Box 82.1).[77]

Physical Examination Findings

Cats

Upper respiratory tract signs are common physical examination findings in cats with cryptococcosis. These include sneezing; snuffling; and mucopurulent, serous, or hemorrhagic nasal discharge that is unilateral or bilateral. In some cats, a fleshy mass protrudes from the nostril. Other cats have one or more firm to fluctuant, ulcerated

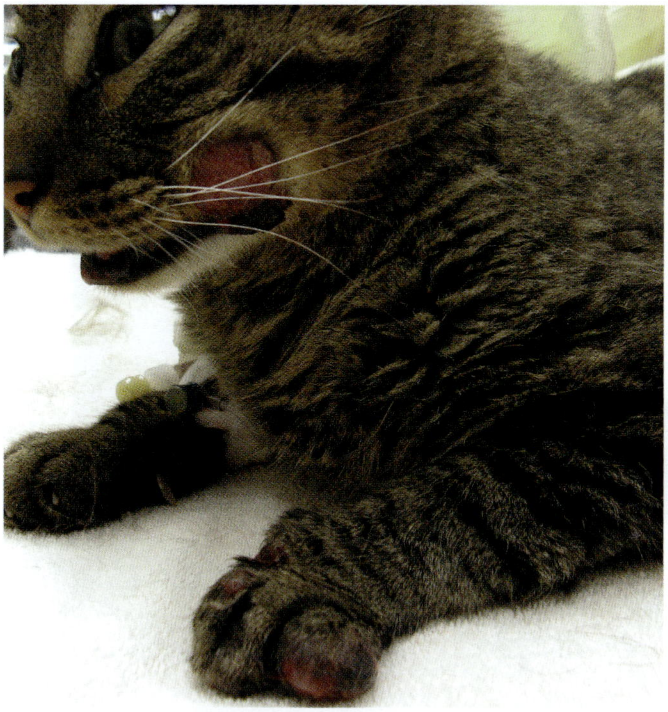

Fig. 82.5 Multiple ulcerated skin lesions in a cat from northern California with disseminated cryptococcosis caused by *Cryptococcus gattii* molecular type VGIII.

or nonulcerated, subcutaneous swellings over the bridge of the nose. These swellings may communicate with the frontal sinus or nasal cavity, and palpation of the lesions may reveal crepitus due to subcutaneous emphysema. Cats with nasopharyngeal cryptococcosis develop stertor, stridor, and, occasionally, otitis media. Mandibular lymphadenopathy is often present. Ulcerated or proliferative lesions of the buccal mucosa can also be found. Multifocal skin lesions consist of nodules or masses that are fluctuant to firm, up to several centimeters in diameter, and may ulcerate (see Fig. 82.5).

Neurologic examination abnormalities in cats with CNS involvement include obtundation; atypical behavior; slow menace, palpebral, or pupillary light responses; mydriasis or anisocoria (Fig. 82.6A); twitching or tremors; and seizures, circling, head pressing, ataxia, paresis, abnormal placing reactions, head tilt, nystagmus, and spinal pain.[10] Fundoscopic examination may reveal granulomatous chorioretinitis, exudative retinal detachment, papilledema, evidence of optic neuritis, and/or retinal hemorrhage (Fig. 82.6B). Severe ocular lesions or optic neuritis may result in blindness with dilated and unresponsive pupils.

Dogs

Many dogs with cryptococcosis are lethargic or obtunded because of disseminated disease and/or CNS involvement. When fever occurs, it is typically low grade. Other CNS signs in dogs include absent or slow menace, gag, or pupillary light responses, nystagmus, mydriasis, head tilt, strabismus, anisocoria, facial paralysis, paraparesis, abnormal placing reactions, ataxia, circling, seizures, twitching or tremors, reluctance to open the mouth, absent or decreased segmental reflexes, and, commonly, cervical hyperesthesia.[10,33] Some dogs show signs that resemble those of cervical disc herniation. The most common ocular abnormalities are chorioretinitis, papilledema, evidence of optic neuritis, and retinal detachment. Decreased nasal airflow may be present in dogs with nasal cavity cryptococcomas. Nodules, masses, or ulcers may involve any portion of the integument, and the nose, tongue, buccal mucosa, hard palate, lips, or nail beds.

BOX 82.1 Clinical Signs in Cats and Dogs with Cryptococcosis[a]

Nasal Cavity
Rhinitis (sneezing, nasal discharge), frontal sinusitis, deforming sinonasal disease, nasal planum disease, nasopharyngeal obstruction or dysfunction

Lung and Thoracic Cavity
Nodules (single or multiple), interstitial (miliary) or alveolar (fluffy) infiltrates, mediastinal lymphadenomegaly, hilar lymphadenomegaly, pleural effusion

Central Nervous System
Meningoencephalomyelitis, cryptococcomas of the brain or spinal cord, increased intracranial pressure, hydrocephalus

Skin and Subcutaneous Tissues
Papules, nodules, subcutaneous abscesses, draining lesions, ulcers, digital swellings, peripheral lymphadenopathy

Eye
Papilledema, chorioretinitis, optic neuritis, uveitis (miosis, aqueous flare, hypopyon), endophthalmitis, panophthalmitis

Genitourinary Tract
Prostatitis (prostatomegaly, dysuria), renal abscesses, bladder wall infection, funguria

Bone and Joints
Osteolytic lesions, arthritis

Heart
Myocarditis, pericarditis

Gastrointestinal Tract
Glossitis (lingual swelling, ulceration), gingivitis, gastritis, enteritis, typhlitis, hepatitis, mesenteric lymphadenomegaly, peritonitis, pancreatitis

Endocrine
Thyroiditis, adrenal gland granulomas

Musculoskeletal
Middle ear disease, arthritis, osteomyelitis

[a] Clinical abnormalities vary depending on the *Cryptococcus* species/molecular type, host species (dog versus cat) and level of immunocompromise. For example, widely disseminated disease that involves multiple parenchymal organs is most often seen in young adult, often purebred dogs with *Cryptococcus neoformans* sensu stricto (VNI) infection, resembling that in human AIDS patients. See text for more details.

DIAGNOSIS

Definitive diagnosis of cryptococcosis is usually straightforward and based on evaluation of representative tissue specimens with cytology, culture, and occasionally histopathology, with or without serologic detection of cryptococcal antigen in body fluids (Table 82.2). Suitable specimens include nasal swabs, nasal washings, needle aspirates from mass lesions or enlarged lymph nodes, bronchoalveolar lavage specimens, pleural fluid, CSF, and urine.

Laboratory Abnormalities

Complete Blood Count, Serum Chemistry Profile, and Urinalysis

Changes in the CBC, chemistry panel, and urinalysis in animals with cryptococcosis are generally mild and nonspecific. Mild to moderate

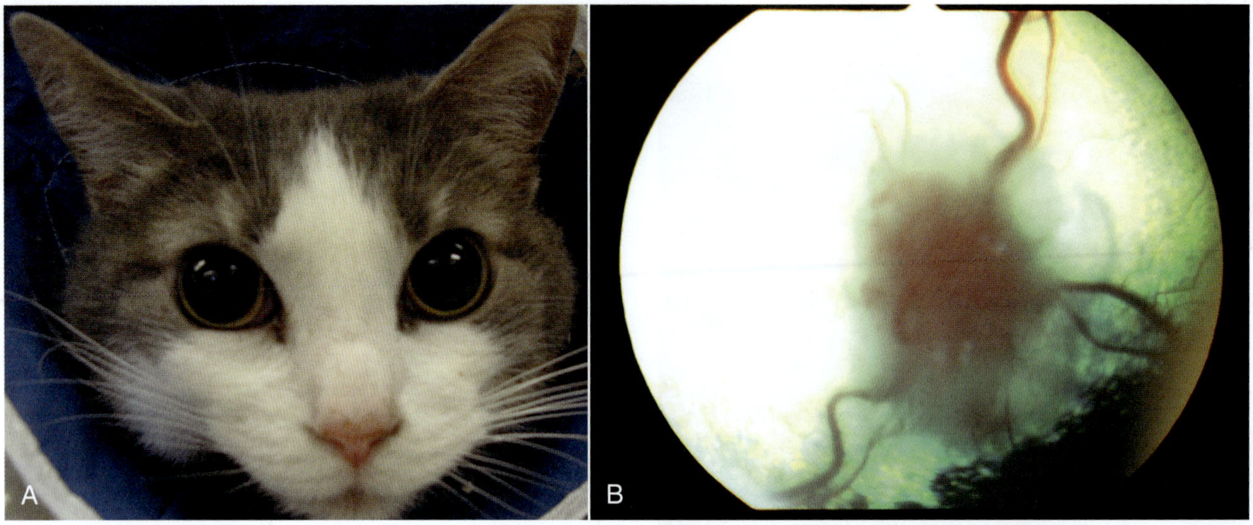

Fig. 82.6 Ocular abnormalities in cats with disseminated cryptococcosis. (A) Bilateral mydriasis in an 8-year-old male neutered domestic shorthair with cryptococcal meningoencephalitis. Fundoscopic examination was within normal limits. (B) Granulomatous chorioretinitis and retinal detachment in another cat with cryptococcosis. (Courtesy University of California, Davis, Veterinary Ophthalmology Service.)

TABLE 82.2 Diagnostic Assays Available for Cryptococcosis in Dogs and Cats

Assay	Specimen Type	Target	Performance
Cytologic examination	Aspirates of affected tissues, body fluids, impression smears of skin lesions or biopsies	*Cryptococcus* organisms	High sensitivity, but occasionally organisms are not visualized (such as in the CSF of some animals with CNS cryptococcosis).
Fungal culture	Aspirates or biopsies of affected tissues, body fluids such as CSF and urine	*Cryptococcus* spp.	Generally sensitive and specific, but false negatives are possible if specimen size is low. Requires several days' incubation. Allows species identification and antifungal drug susceptibility testing.
Cryptococcal antigen latex agglutination tests (LCAT)	Serum, CSF	*Cryptococcus* polysaccharide antigen	Sensitivity and specificity exceed 90%. False negatives can occur in dogs and with localized infections in cats. False positives are generally of low magnitude (<1:200 and usually <1:16). Titers vary between kits.
Immunochromatographic POC assays (IMMY Diagnostics, OK, USA and CryptoPS, Biosynex, Strasbourg, France)	Serum, CSF	*Cryptococcus* polysaccharide antigen	IMMY assay: Sensitivity greater than 90% and specificity 80%–85% on serum specimens in dogs and cats. CryptoPS assay: sensitivity approximately 80% and specificity 95%. Provide results in less than 15 minutes. Not yet validated for CSF in dogs and cats.
Real-time PCR assays	Biopsies, body fluids, aspirates	*Cryptococcus* DNA	Not yet validated in adequate numbers of dogs or cats with cryptococcosis; usefulness requires further evaluation.
Histopathology	Biopsy specimens from affected tissues	*Cryptococcus* spp. yeasts	High sensitivity, with rare false negatives. Special stains such as Mayer's mucicarmine and immunohistochemical stains facilitate organism detection and identification.

nonregenerative anemia; leukocytosis, often with monocytosis; and eosinophilia are the most common findings. Dogs with disseminated disease may have a neutrophilia with a left shift. The serum biochemical profile reflects specific organ involvement in animals with disseminated disease. Occasionally, cryptococcal yeasts are found on examination of the urine sediment.

Cerebrospinal Fluid Examination

The CSF in cats and dogs with neurologic signs due to cryptococcosis may have an increased protein concentration (usually between 10 and 140 mg/dL in cats, but may be several hundred or rarely more than 1,000 mg/dL in dogs).[10] Leukocyte counts can range from 2 to more than 1000 cells/μL in both dogs and cats. A mixed cellular pleocytosis is generally present, with neutrophils or large mononuclear cells generally outnumbering other cell types. Some dogs have a marked eosinophilic pleocytosis. Cryptococcal yeasts are visible in most but not all animals with cryptococcal meningitis (see Fig. 82.2).[10] Marked deterioration in neurologic status occasionally occurs in animals with CNS cryptococcosis immediately after CSF collection. Many animals have intracranial mass lesions or increased CSF pressure, which can increase the risk of cerebellar herniation following a cisternal tap. Wherever possible, attempts to make a diagnosis with serum antigen testing or collection of specimens from other anatomic sites should be considered as an alternative to diagnosis by CSF analysis.

Diagnostic Imaging

Plain Radiography

Thoracic radiographs in dogs and cats are often normal. In some animals, interstitial to alveolar infiltrates or small nodular lesions are present. Occasionally, large pulmonary nodules, hilar lymphadenopathy, a mediastinal granuloma, or pleural effusion are found.[58]

Computed Tomography

In cats with nasal cryptococcosis, CT of the nasal cavity can reveal soft tissue and fluid opacification of the nasal cavity or frontal sinus, peripherally contrast-enhancing mass lesions of the nasal planum, and lysis of the nasal bones or of the cribriform plate.[11] CT was used to document a contrast-enhancing right cranial lung lobe mass that invaded the distal trachea and right mainstem bronchus in a cat from Arizona.[78] In dogs, CT findings in the nasal cavity include peripherally contrast-enhancing mass lesions within the frontal sinuses, caudal nasal cavity, nasopharynx, or the retrobulbar space and associated osteomyelitis (see Fig. 82.4A). CNS abnormalities such as ventricular dilation and intra-axial contrast-enhancing mass lesions have been described in dogs using CT.[10] However, MRI is more sensitive for detection of CNS lesions in human patients,[59] and the same is probably true for dogs and cats.

Magnetic Resonance Imaging

MRI abnormalities in cats with CNS cryptococcosis consist of single or multifocal contrast-enhancing mass lesions that tend to be hyperintense on T2-weighted images and hypointense on T1-weighted images, as well as mild to moderate, diffuse or focal meningeal enhancement.[10] Some cats have lesions that appear fluid-filled on T2-weighted images but have a greater T1-weighted intensity than expected for acellular fluid ("high T2, low T1 lesions"; Fig. 82.7).[10] MRI in dogs may show contrast-enhancing mass lesions that are hyperintense on T2-weighted images and of variable intensity on T1-weighted images, as well as meningeal enhancement (see Fig. 82.4B). Ventriculomegaly and/or cribriform plate osteomyelitis may also be evident.

Sonographic Findings

Over 80% of cats with cryptococcosis have normal abdominal ultrasound examinations. Cats with kidney involvement can have iso- to hypoechoic intraparenchymal mass lesions on ultrasound, with or without associated renal failure. These sometimes involve the renal pelvis. However, cats with renal involvement can also have normal abdominal ultrasound examinations.[11]

Ultrasonographic findings in dogs include intra-abdominal lymphadenomegaly, multifocal gastric and small intestinal thickening, changes suggestive of pancreatitis, renal mass lesions, and/or ascites (see Fig. 82.3).[11,73]

Microbiologic Tests

Cytologic Examination

Cytologic examination can be performed on aspirates, body fluids, or impression smears of biopsy specimens. Romanowsky-type stains, new methylene blue, and Gram stain are all satisfactory for making a cytologic diagnosis. India ink can be used to examine CSF for cryptococcal yeasts, which appear unstained and silhouetted against a black background. India ink staining of CSF has been used in the diagnosis of human cryptococcal infections (Fig. 82.8).[59] However, lymphocytes and fat droplets can sometimes be confused with the organism.

Although cytologic examination of nasal or cutaneous exudates, aspirates, or body fluids for organisms is a rapid and sensitive test for cryptococcosis, negative test results do not eliminate the possibility of cryptococcosis. Generally, organisms are found only by cytologic examination of CSF in 60% to 80% of dogs and cats.[11] If a sufficient index of suspicion exists, additional diagnostic tests such as histopathology, antigen testing, and/or fungal culture are indicated.

Fungal Culture

Cryptococcus spp. are readily cultured from aspirates, exudate, CSF, urine, and tissue specimens. Attempts to culture the organism are recommended whenever possible before treatment is initiated, because isolation confirms the diagnosis, can be used to differentiate *C. gattii* SC from *C. neoformans* SC organisms, and permits antifungal susceptibility testing for cases that subsequently fail to respond adequately to antifungal drug treatment. Some veterinary diagnostic laboratories still report all *Cryptococcus* isolates as *C. neoformans* in the absence of tests to discriminate between *C. neoformans* SC and *C. gattii* SC organisms. If the report lists *C. neoformans* as the isolate, the laboratory must therefore be consulted to determine whether *C. neoformans* SC was differentiated from *C. gattii* SC. However, whether the clinician needs to know whether the isolate belongs to the *C. neoformans* SC or the *C. gattii* SC is debatable because at this time, species identification

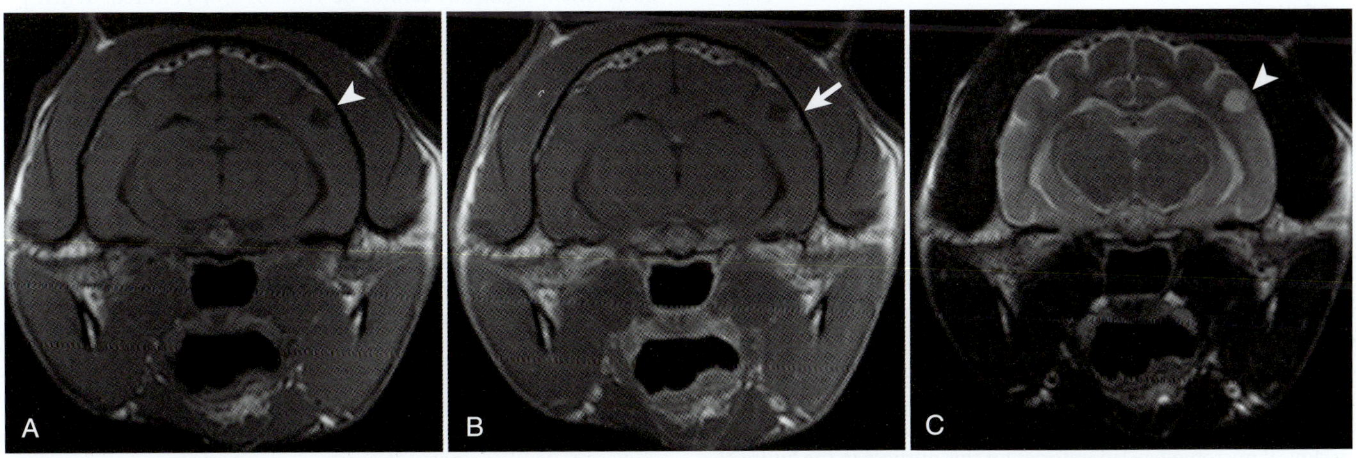

Fig. 82.7 Transverse T1-weighted pre-contrast (A), T1-weighted postcontrast (B), and T2-weighted (C) magnetic resonance imaging of the brain of an 8-year-old male neutered domestic shorthair with cryptococcosis. There is a focal lesion in the gray matter of the right cerebral cortex at the junction of the parietal and occipital lobes *(arrowhead)*. The lesion is T2 hyperintense, T1 hypointense, and rim-enhancing *(arrow)*. These signal characteristics were consistent with a pseudocyst lesion.

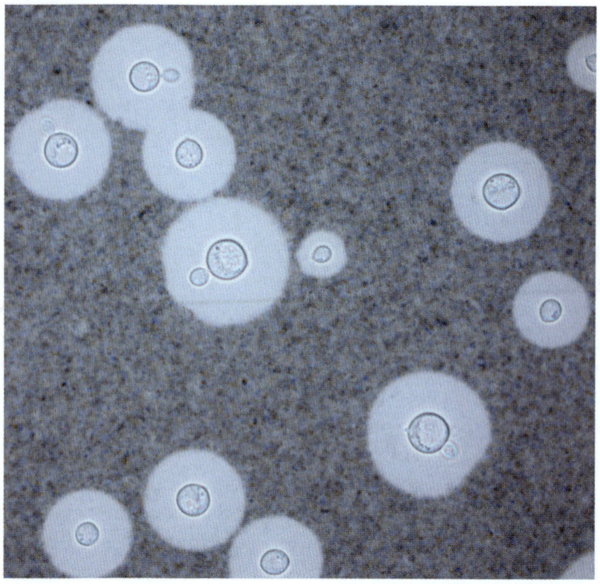

Fig. 82.8 India ink stained preparation of *Cryptococcus gattii* yeasts that had been grown in culture. 1000× oil magnification. (Courtesy Greg Hodges and George Thompson III, University of California, Davis.)

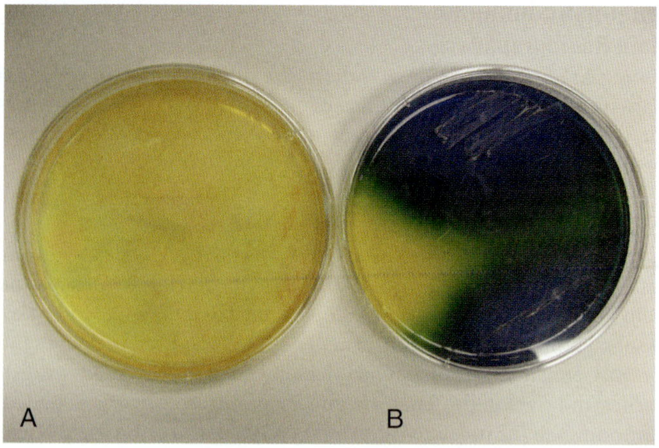

Fig. 82.9 Growth of *Cryptococcus neoformans* (A) and *Cryptococcus gattii* (B) on canavanine-glycine-bromothymol blue agar. *Cryptococcus neoformans* does not grow well in the presence of canavanine and does not utilize glycine, so the medium color remains unchanged. *Cryptococcus gattii* grows in the presence of L-canavanine and utilizes glycine as the sole carbon and nitrogen source, which raises the pH of the medium and causes the bromothymol blue indicator in the medium to turn the agar a vivid cobalt blue color.

does not clearly influence treatment recommendations or prognosis in dogs and cats. If *Cryptococcus* is isolated from a contaminated site such as the nasal cavity, a diagnosis of cryptococcosis should be supported with cytologic or histopathologic evidence of active infection. This is because subclinical colonization occurs in some animals.

Pathogenic *Cryptococcus* species grow on almost all laboratory media, but fungal isolation media (such as Sabouraud's dextrose agar) and incubation temperatures of 25°C or 30°C in addition to incubation at 37°C are preferred when fungi are being considered in the differential diagnosis. Antibiotics are added to the medium for isolation of *Cryptococcus* spp. from contaminated sites, such as the nasal cavity. Colonies usually are visible in 2 to 3 days, but sometimes incubation for up to 10 days is required. Unlike other dimorphic fungi, *Cryptococcus* grows as a yeast, rather than a mold, on routine fungal media and so is less likely to represent a laboratory hazard than organisms that grow as molds. The organisms form white, creamy colonies. Often colonies of the *C. gattii* SC are more mucoid than those of the *C. neoformans* SC. The organism is identified based on its microscopic morphology and either response to biochemical tests in commercial yeast identification kits or MALDI-TOF mass spectrometry (see Chapter 4). Canavanine-glycine-bromothymol blue (CGB) agar is used to differentiate between *C. neoformans* SC and *C. gattii* SC isolates.[79] Unlike *C. neoformans* SC organisms, *C. gattii* SC organisms grow on CGB agar and turn the media a brilliant deep blue (Fig. 82.9). Fungal culture of the CSF is frequently positive in patients with CNS cryptococcosis and should be performed even if the organism cannot be demonstrated cytologically or serologically. Culture of urine specimens collected using cystocentesis is also indicated when cryptococcosis is suspected, even when obvious renal involvement is not present and cytologic abnormalities are not present. Identification of molecular types for epidemiologic purposes requires specialized techniques such as multilocus sequence typing or PCR fingerprinting. However, MALDI-TOF mass spectrometry can also rapidly differentiate between *Cryptococcus* species, and may be used in veterinary clinical microbiology laboratories for this purpose in the future.[80]

Most cryptococcal isolates from dogs or cats are susceptible to amphotericin B (AMB), 5-flucytosine, and azoles. Rarely, resistance to 5-flucytosine and azole antifungal drugs (especially fluconazole) is detected. In general, MICs for fluconazole are higher than those for other azole drugs, and this does not imply resistance *in vivo*. In the human literature, it has been suggested that when the MIC rises during treatment, or if the initial MIC is at least 16 μg/mL for fluconazole, or at least 128 μg/mL for flucytosine, failure of antifungal drug treatment may result from drug resistance.[59] There is evidence that organisms that belong to the *C. gattii* SC may be more resistant to fluconazole than those that belong to the *C. neoformans* SC.[81]

Serologic Testing

Latex agglutination assays (referred to as the latex cryptococcal antigen test [LCAT]) for detection of cryptococcal polysaccharide capsular antigen are widely used for diagnosis of cryptococcosis in veterinary patients and are sensitive and specific.[11,82,83] (Note: the latex agglutination assay offered by Meridian Biosciences is known as the Cryptococcal Latex Agglutination System [CALAS]). Serologic assays detect the antigen of all species in the *C. neoformans* SC and *C. gattii* SC and can be used on serum or CSF. These can provide a rapid diagnosis when organisms cannot be visualized or cultured. When positive, serum cryptococcal antigen assays can be advantageous in animals with neurologic signs when CSF collection is unacceptably risky or if a diagnosis of cryptococcosis is unlikely but requires additional evidence for exclusion.

In human patients, commercial kits typically have at least 90% sensitivity and 97% to 100% specificity.[59] Results have been similar for small animal patients,[11,82,83] although false-negative results may be more common in dogs than in cats.[11] False-positive test results are reduced when test specimens are pretreated in the laboratory with pronase (a proteinase).[59] In human patients, titers below 1:8 can represent false-positive results, although false-positive titers of up to 1:200 have rarely been detected in cats.[11] These cats had other causative etiologies identified that explained their clinical signs. In some cats, these low positive titers may represent subclinical colonization. Attempts to obtain cytologic or histopathologic confirmation of infection in animals with titers of 1:200 or less are recommended.

Antigen titers are frequently extremely high (>1:65,536) in cats and dogs with cryptococcosis, but even a titer of 1:2 can indicate cryptococcal infection.[82] Titer results from different kits vary considerably; therefore, the methodology should not be altered when monitoring the response to treatment. A good prognosis is indicated by a decrease in antigen titer, whereas a persistent titer after treatment suggests continued infection. Reductions in the titer typically lag behind clinical improvement. No correlation has been found between pretreatment antigen titer and outcome.

Other detection methodologies exist including ELISA assays and immunochromatography. A POC dipstick cryptococcal antigen lateral flow assay (CrAg, IMMY Diagnostics, Norman, OK, USA) is one of the most reliable screening tests in human medicine and has the benefit of providing rapid test results.[84] It has been validated in cats and dogs from Australia with a sensitivity of 92% and 100% and specificity of 81% and 84%, respectively.[85] In the United States, the assay had a sensitivity of 92% and specificity of 93.2% compared with the LCAT when applied to cats and dogs with and without cryptococcosis. Another POC assay (CryptoPS, Biosynex, Strasbourg, France) correctly classified 8/10 tested LCAT-positive specimens and 56/59 LCAT-negative specimens (sensitivity 80%, specificity 94.9%). This latter assay is semiquantitative, with high titer and low titer bands, and offers greater ease of use in practice than the IMMY assay. However, suboptimal sensitivity of this assay when compared with the IMMY assay has also been documented in humans.[86] In animals recovering from cryptococcosis with treatment, sometimes the POC assays were positive when LCAT was negative, so these assays may be more sensitive for monitoring treatment.[87] Use of a combination of POC assays and LCAT may ultimately prove to offer the highest sensitivity for treatment monitoring, but whether this leads to reduced rates of relapse requires further study.

Because the sensitivity of cryptococcal antigen testing is not 100%, cryptococcosis should not be ruled out on the basis of a negative antigen titer alone. This is especially important in dogs, because false negatives are more common in dogs than in cats.[11] False negatives are most common in animals with localized ocular, CNS, or solitary cutaneous lesions. For dogs and cats suspected to have cryptococcal meningoencephalomyelitis that have negative serum antigen titers, CSF should be submitted for cytologic examination, antigen titers, and fungal culture.

Molecular Diagnosis Using Nucleic Acid–Based Testing

Real-time PCR assays for *Cryptococcus* spp. are offered on a commercial basis by some veterinary diagnostic laboratories. These assays can confirm the presence of *Cryptococcus* DNA in tissues or body fluids when other means fail. However, because a diagnosis of cryptococcosis is usually apparent based on the methods described earlier, PCR is currently not regarded as a routinely useful clinical tool. Because *Cryptococcus* DNA has been detected using PCR assays in small intestinal contents from healthy dogs and dogs with chronic enteropathies,[88] positive results on intestinal biopsies may not reflect cryptococcosis. Similarly, because subclinical nasal cavity colonization can occur, positive results on nasal biopsies may not represent invasive disease. Because false positives also have the potential to occur as a result of contamination in the PCR laboratory, a PCR diagnosis of cryptococcosis should always be supported by cytologic or histopathologic evidence of infection and/or culture of *Cryptococcus* spp. from a normally sterile site.

Pathologic Findings

Gross lesions associated with cryptococcosis vary from gelatinous masses that consist almost exclusively of organisms to well-ordered granulomas or pyogranulomas that typically occur in patients with improved CMI responses. The gelatinous appearance is a reflection of the large amount of capsular polysaccharide present in lesions. In sections stained with H&E, *Cryptococcus* yeasts are faint, eosinophilic, round to oval bodies that are surrounded by a clear halo (the unstained capsule). In fact, the histopathologic lesion is often dominated by the negative staining capsule, sometimes occupying most of the lesion. The organism's cell wall is more easily visualized with PAS, methenamine silver, or Fontana-Masson stain, although the capsule still does not stain well with these methods. With Mayer's mucicarmine stain, the cryptococcal capsule takes on a rose red color, and the organism appears pink against a blue background. Other fungi with similar morphologic features do not stain with Mayer's mucicarmine. Some *Cryptococcus* strains have poorly developed capsules. Infections with capsular-deficient organisms were described in four cats from the United States (Texas and upstate New York) with pyogranulomatous and eosinophilic dermatitis; in some of these cases, it was possible to identify infection with *C. neoformans* ss.[76] If necessary, IHC or the use of molecular methods (PCR) can be used to differentiate *Cryptococcus* from other fungi and molecular methods can provide information on the identity of the species complex present.[89]

Cats

In cats that die or are euthanized as a result of cryptococcosis, histopathology of lesions within the nasal cavity may reveal granulomatous rhinitis. CNS cryptococcosis consists of either meningitis[58] or meningoencephalomyelitis, with single or multiple cerebral granulomas (Fig. 82.10). Extension of infection from the meninges along perforating arteries into the Virchow-Robin spaces can result in cystic collections of yeast organisms sometimes referred to as "soap-bubble lesions" and known as gelatinous pseudocysts.[10] Ocular lesions include pyogranulomatous to granulomatous chorioretinitis, optic neuritis, uveitis, endophthalmitis, panophthalmitis, and retinal separation. Other affected organs include skin and subcutaneous tissues, kidneys, and lymph nodes. Renal granulomas have been found in some cats with disseminated disease. Granulomas can also occasionally be found in the spleen, adrenal glands, thyroid glands, and liver.

Dogs

Dogs that die or are euthanized because of cryptococcosis often have CNS infection, ocular involvement, or widely disseminated disease. The lesions consist of granulomatous or pyogranulomatous meningoencephalitis, sometimes with pseudocyst formation; neuritis of the optic, facial, or vestibular nerves; and pyogranulomatous or granulomatous chorioretinitis. Inflammatory lesions that contain *Cryptococcus* yeasts may also be present in the lungs, nasal cavity, kidneys, pancreas, liver, myocardium, GI tract, and spleen. Less commonly, involvement of the peritoneum, thyroid, tongue, prostate, pleura, joints, mediastinum, urinary bladder, and adrenal gland has been detected at necropsy.

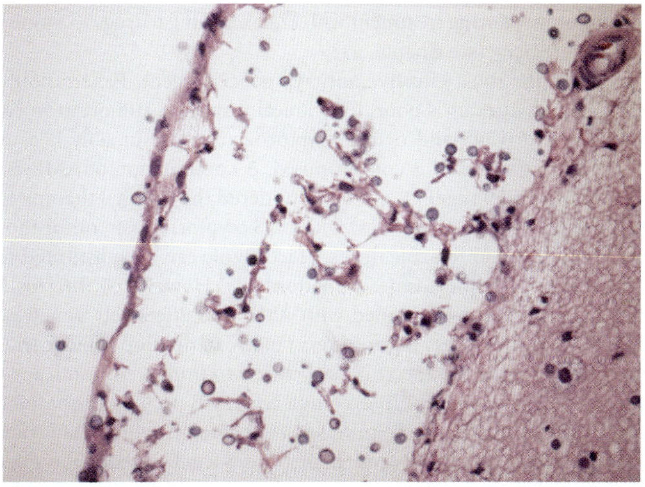

Fig. 82.10 Histopathology showing the meninges of a cat with cryptococcosis. Numerous round yeast organisms occupy the meningeal spaces. Hematoxylin and eosin stain.

TREATMENT

Treatment recommendations for dogs and cats with cryptococcosis have been based on evidence-based studies performed in human patients and clinical experiences; evidence-based studies are lacking for veterinary patients. The most common problems encountered are the high cost of therapy, requirement for multiple hospital visits, and the need for regular medication of pets for a protracted period. Resistance to antifungal medications is not common; however, development of fluconazole and flucytosine resistance has been reported.[90–92] Immunocompromised animals (which may include purebred dogs with no obvious underlying immunodeficiency) are especially likely to have persistent or progressive infection in the face of treatment. In many affected animals, treatment must be continued for years or the life of the animal. Surgical debulking could be considered before treatment for large cryptococcomas to improve drug penetration. However, even large cryptococcomas can resolve with medical treatment alone, and surgery should only be performed if lesions can be easily and safely resected. The reader is referred to Chapter 11 for detailed information on antifungal drugs.

Cats

Cats with localized cutaneous disease can sometimes be treated successfully with azole monotherapy. The initial drug of choice is fluconazole (10 mg/kg, PO, q12h), because of its good penetration of the brain, eye, and urinary tract; low cost; and minimal adverse effects.

Treatment should be continued until there is complete lesion resolution and the cryptococcal antigen titer becomes negative. A fourfold to fivefold reduction in the antigen titer suggests an adequate response. In cats with *C. gattii* ss or *C. neoformans* ss infections, this typically takes 2 to 12 months (median, 4 months),[32] although longer periods of therapy may be required for some cats. For recovered animals that achieve an antigen titer of 0, the titer can be monitored every 3 to 6 months so that any recurrence is diagnosed early. However, in the authors' experience, many cats with *C. deuterogattii* (VGII) and *C. bacillisporus* (VGIII) infections in North America fail to respond completely to fluconazole treatment, antigen titers persist at high levels, and relapse may ultimately occur after an initial treatment response. In some of these cats, treatment with itraconazole (5–10 mg/kg, PO, q24h [capsules] or 3–5 mg/kg, PO, q24h [solution]) can lead to clinical remission. Itraconazole does not have good penetration into the CNS; however, it has been used successfully to treat cryptococcal meningitis.[35,83,93] Ketoconazole has also been used with success when treating *C. deuterogattii* infections from the Vancouver Island region.[2] Serum liver enzyme activities should be monitored monthly during treatment with azole antifungal drugs to monitor for hepatotoxicity (see Chapter 11).

AMB is the most effective anticryptococcal agent. Penetration of the CNS and vitreous is poor, but clinical responses still occur in cats and dogs with CNS and ocular cryptococcosis, presumably because the blood-brain barrier is compromised. A combination of AMB and 5-flucytosine (250 mg, PO, q8h) is considered the optimal therapy for cats (and humans, but not dogs) with CNS cryptococcosis, or for those that fail to respond to azole drugs. Fluconazole can be substituted for 5-flucytosine if 5-flucytosine is unaffordable. However, 5-flucytosine shows synergy when combined with AMB and effectively penetrates the blood-brain barrier. Because resistance can develop rapidly when 5-flucytosine is used alone, it is used chiefly to improve the efficacy of other antifungal drugs.[92] Lipid-complexed AMB preparations are not necessarily more effective but are less nephrotoxic, which may translate into greater efficacy because higher doses can be used, although at a substantially increased cost. In human patients, higher doses of AMB more effectively sterilize the CSF. The reader is referred to Chapter 11 for dosing protocols for various formulations of AMB. Treatment with 5-flucytosine (or fluconazole) and AMB is continued for 2 to 4 weeks (ideally 4 weeks) or until azotemia develops, after which treatment is continued with azole monotherapy. Additional courses of AMB may be required to maintain clinical remission in some cats. Although controlled trials have not been performed, some cats with CNS cryptococcosis have shown apparent response to addition of terbinafine to the treatment regimen when other drugs failed to resolve clinical signs.[94]

Dogs

If affordable to the owner, dogs with disseminated disease or CNS involvement should be treated initially with deoxycholate or lipid-complexed AMB and fluconazole. Dogs treated with flucytosine frequently develop toxic epidermal necrolysis, typically 10 to 14 days after starting therapy, which precludes treatment with flucytosine in this species.[95] Some dogs with CNS involvement respond to azole monotherapy, although residual neurologic signs may persist.[10] Other potential outcomes include incomplete recovery, with persistent active infection despite therapy, or relapse after prolonged clinical remission. In one dog, surgical debridement of an extradural spinal cord granuloma combined with fluconazole treatment controlled spinal cord infection.[96] Again, azoles are fungistatic and rely on a CMI response and phagocytosis to remove cryptococcal yeasts from the host, which may be lacking in some dogs with cryptococcosis. Treatment of a dog with intestinal cryptococcosis with terbinafine was associated with long-term disease resolution when treatment with azoles, surgical debulking, and AMB failed.[73]

Other Antifungal Treatments

Other antifungal drugs that are effective for treatment of cryptococcosis include voriconazole and posaconazole. Both drugs penetrate the CNS and are therefore potentially advantageous for treatment of cryptococcal meningoencephalitis, but urinary concentrations are low. However, virtually all cats and some dogs do not tolerate voriconazole treatment because of GI, neurologic, and cardiac adverse effects.[97,98] In humans, posaconazole[99] is well tolerated, and it has been used to treat other fungal infections without complication in cats (see Chapter 11), so it could be an option for cats with refractory disease.[99] In the future, novel drugs such as the azole isavuconazole may offer promise for treatment of cryptococcal infections in dogs and cats,[100] but pharmacokinetic and toxicity studies will be required before agents used for humans can be considered safe and efficacious.

Supportive Care

Because many cats and dogs with CNS involvement deteriorate clinically during initial treatment with antifungal drugs as a result of the inflammatory response to dying yeasts, anti-inflammatory doses of short-acting glucocorticoids may be necessary to support animals with CNS cryptococcosis for the first few days to weeks of treatment and may increase survival rate at 10 days after initiation of treatment.[10] Deterioration of neurologic status in the first few days of treatment is not a negative prognostic indicator if the animal can be supported through this phase. Supportive care with IV fluid therapy, tube feeding, and antiseizure medications may be necessary. Rarely, dogs or cats require supplemental oxygen because of respiratory involvement.

PROGNOSIS

In general, cats show significant clinical improvement within 1 to 2 weeks of starting therapy. In studies from Australia, around 75% of cats were treated successfully.[8,32] As many as 60% of cats may be cured after an initial course of therapy, although some cats that show an initial favorable response to therapy can relapse, sometimes as long as 10 years after therapy is discontinued.[32] In one study, the median survival time of cats with CNS cryptococcosis was only 13 days (range, 0–4,050 days), but a median survival time was never reached if cats survived at least 3 days after diagnosis, so supportive care during this phase may be critical.[10]

The prognosis is more guarded for dogs. Six of 11 dogs with cryptococcosis in Australia were treated successfully.[32] In a study from the western United States[9] and another from southwestern Australia,[5] the success rate was lower, around 30%. The median survival time for dogs with CNS cryptococcosis was 7 days (range, 0–3,680 days).[10]

In human patients with cryptococcosis, negative prognostic indicators include underlying immunosuppressive disease or drugs, abnormal mental state, high organism burden at presentation (as defined by large numbers of yeasts in the CSF and/or high antigen titers), and a poor anti-inflammatory response in the CSF (<20 cells/μL).[101] The presence of CNS disease appears to negatively affect outcome in both cats and dogs.[102,103] In dogs and cats with CNS involvement, the presence of altered mental status at first evaluation was associated with increased mortality ($P = .03$).[10]

IMMUNITY AND VACCINATION

Cryptococcosis can occur in apparently immunocompetent or in immunodeficient individuals, although those with deficiencies of CMI are most commonly infected. Production of Th1-type cytokines such as IL-2, TNF-α, and IFN-γ and a granulomatous inflammatory response are important for elimination of infection, and decline in the CD4+ T-cell count to less than 50 to 100 cells/μL correlates well with the risk of infection in HIV-infected humans.[59] No vaccines are available.

PREVENTION

Prevention of cryptococcosis may be possible through avoidance of exposure to ecologic niches of the organism, such as pigeon feces. Nevertheless, cryptococcosis occurs in animals housed exclusively indoors, and widespread exposure and recovery likely occurs in endemic areas.

PUBLIC HEALTH ASPECTS

Cryptococcosis is an important opportunistic fungal infection of humans with AIDS, in particular those who are not treated with highly active antiretroviral therapy. Human infection is acquired from the environment and not by direct contact with infected animals, although intense exposure to avian excrement has been associated with some cryptococcosis cases in HIV-infected humans.[104] Malignancy, chemotherapy, immunosuppressive drug therapy, diabetes mellitus, splenectomy, cirrhosis, or sarcoidosis can also predispose to the disease. Severe meningitis and disseminated infections can develop in immunodeficient patients. Identification of *Cryptococcus* spp. infection or colonization of cats has been proposed as a sentinel for human infection in Italy and Brazil.[53,105]

The organism does not aerosolize from sites of tissue infection, so the disease cannot spread among humans or animals. The major public health significance of infected pets is that cats may act as a sentinel for infection of human beings, because of their susceptibility to infection. In the diagnostic laboratory, culture of *Cryptococcus* is not a significant health hazard, because only the yeast form is grown routinely, and this form does not aerosolize from media. During handling of infected tissues or cultures, precautions should be taken to prevent inadvertent cutaneous inoculation of the organism. Veterinarians should consider patient sedation for procedures that involve FNA in order to avoid inadvertent needle-stick injuries, which have caused localized cutaneous infection in the human health care setting.[106] Because sporotrichosis is a major differential diagnosis for cats with cutaneous lesions, gloves should always be worn and hand hygiene performed when handling cats with suspicious lesions (see Chapter 84).

CASE EXAMPLE

Signalment

"Simon," an 8-year-old male neutered domestic shorthair cat from northern California.

History

Simon was evaluated by the University of California, Davis, VMTH, for a 5-week history of progressive weakness, inappetence, and weight loss. Initially the owners noted that he was reluctant to jump and had a low tail carriage; intermittent episodes of head shaking and sneezing were also noted. He also had episodes of clenching the furniture with his claws. Three weeks before he was brought to the VMTH, Simon was seen at a local veterinary clinic where a physical examination was unremarkable. Broad-spectrum antimicrobial drugs were prescribed (amoxicillin-clavulanic acid and enrofloxacin for 7 days), and he was treated with subcutaneous fluids (lactated Ringer's solution, 150 mL, once). Over the following 5 days his clinical signs lessened, but then anorexia developed. Physical examination 2 days after the onset of anorexia revealed a rectal temperature of 102.5°F (39.2°C) and weight loss (from 3.7 kg at the previous visit to 3.2 kg). A CBC and biochemistry panel showed mild lymphopenia (1,157 cells/μL [reference range, 1500–7000 cells/μL]). Treatment with metronidazole (39 mg/kg, PO, q24h) and prednisone (3 mg/kg, PO, q24h) was instituted. Three days before he was brought to the VMTH, he began panting and vocalizing. The metronidazole was discontinued and the prednisone dose was reduced to 1.5 mg/kg, PO, q24h. The following day, the owners noted that Simon's eyelids were twitching, and he urinated and defecated on himself in the litter box. Clindamycin (6 mg/kg, PO, q12h) was prescribed for suspected toxoplasmosis, and Simon was referred for further evaluation.

Simon had no other previous medical or surgical history apart from being neutered as a kitten. He had access to the outdoors and there were no other cats in the household. There had been no changes in his thirst or urination, no vomiting or diarrhea, and he was last vaccinated at 5 years of age. He had killed a large rat approximately 5 weeks earlier and had not been himself since.

Physical Examination

Body weight: 2.9 kg.

General: Obtunded but responsive, estimated as 5% dehydrated. T = 100.2°F (37.9°C), HR = 200 beats/minute, RR = 60 breaths/minute, CRT < 2 seconds.

Eyes, ears, nose, and throat: Bilateral mydriasis and absent pupillary light reflexes were noted. There was no evidence of nasal discharge and nasal airflow was normal. Mucous membranes were pink and slightly tacky. Fundic examination was within normal limits.

Musculoskeletal: BCS 4/9, ambulatory. The cat had a slow gait with a short stride.

Respiratory: Tachypnea was present with a normal respiratory effort. Normal breath sounds were present on auscultation.

Cardiovascular, GI, genitourinary, and lymph nodes: No clinically significant abnormalities were detected. The urinary bladder was small.

Continued

CASE EXAMPLE—cont'd

Neurologic examination: The cat was mildly obtunded, walked with a crouched stance, and behaved as if nonvisual. Bilateral mydriasis and absent menace and pupillary light reflexes were confirmed. Intermittent horizontal nystagmus with the fast phase to the left was present. Cranial nerve examination was otherwise normal. Placing and hopping reactions were delayed in the left pelvic limb. There was a decreased left patellar reflex, but other segmental reflexes were intact. There was no apparent pain on spinal palpation, but the cat appeared painful when the tail was raised. Neuroanatomic location: multifocal CNS disease.

Laboratory Findings

CBC: HCT 27.2% (30%–50%), MCV 48.3 fL (42–53 fL), MCHC 29.8 g/dL (30–33.5 g/dL), reticulocytes 8,400 cells/μL (7,000–60,000 cells/μL), WBC 12,360 cells/μL (4,500–14,000 cells/μL), neutrophils 11,000 cells/μL (2,000–9,000 cells/μL), lymphocytes 828 cells/μL (1,000–7,000 cells/μL), monocytes 445 cells/μL (50–600 cells/μL), eosinophils 87 cells/μL (150–1,100 cells/μL), basophils 0 cells/μL (0–50 cells/μL), platelets 357,000/μL (180,000–500,000 platelets/μL).

Serum chemistry profile: Sodium 150 mmol/L (151–158 mmol/L), potassium 4.3 mmol/L (3.6–4.9 mmol/L), chloride 115 mmol/L (117–126 mmol/L), bicarbonate 19 mmol/L (15–21 mmol/L), phosphorus 5.4 mg/dL (3.2–6.3 mg/dL), calcium 10 mg/dL (9.0–10.9 mg/dl), BUN 21 mg/dL (18–33 mg/dL), creatinine 1.2 mg/dL (1.1–2.2 mg/dL), glucose 136 mg/dL (63–118 mg/dL), total protein 7.5 g/dL (6.6–8.4 g/dL), albumin 3.8 g/dL (2.2–4.6 g/dL), globulin 3.7 g/dL (2.8–5.4 g/dL), ALT 37 U/L (27–101 U/L), AST 28 U/L (17–58 U/L), ALP 8 U/L (14–71 U/L), GGT < 3 U/L (0–4 U/L), cholesterol 177 mg/dL (89–258 mg/dL), total bilirubin < 0.1 mg/dL (0–0.2 mg/dL).

Urinalysis: SpG 1.018; pH 7.0; 25 mg/dL protein; no bilirubin, hemoprotein, glucose; rare WBC/HPF, 0 RBC/HPF, few amorphous crystals, few lipid droplets.

ELISA for FeLV antigen and FIV antibody: Negative.

Latex agglutination for *Cryptococcus* antigen (LCAT): Positive at 1:32,768.

Imaging Findings

Plain thoracic and abdominal radiographs: The only abnormality present was mild lateral spondylosis of the caudal lumbar spine.

Abdominal ultrasonography: The liver was mildly enlarged and contained multiple small hyperechoic foci. In the kidneys, mild cortical hyperechogenicity and decreased corticomedullary distinction were present.

Magnetic resonance imaging (brain): Precontrast images showed a well-defined, round T2-hyperintense, T1-hypointense lesion in the gray matter of the right cerebral cortex at the junction of the parietal and occipital lobes (see Fig. 82.7). Postcontrast images showed moderate contrast enhancement of this lesion. There was mild contrast enhancement of the meninges ventral to the right preoptic area. There was moderate, focal contrast enhancement of the gray matter at the lateral aspect of the right pyriform lobe. There was contrast enhancement of the medial aspect of both pyriform lobes adjacent to the hypophysis. Impressions: multifocal contrast-enhancing lesions with T2 hyperintensity and a cystic lesion in the right cerebral cortex.

Cytologic Findings

CSF analysis (cisternal): Protein concentration 29 mg/dL (reference range, <25 mg/dL). The specimen had a moderate increase in cellularity with a low number of erythrocytes. Numerous thick-capsuled yeast organisms with frequent narrow budding forms were noted, consistent with *Cryptococcus* spp. Nucleated cells consisted of nondegenerate neutrophils admixed with low numbers of variably vacuolated macrophages and small lymphocytes. The differential cell count was 83% neutrophils, 7% small mononuclear cells, and 10% large mononuclear cells.

Microbiologic Testing

Fungal culture (CSF): *C. gattii* SC. Multilocus sequence typing revealed that the organism belonged to *C. deuterogattii* molecular type VGIIa.

Diagnosis

C. deuterogattii meningoencephalitis.

Treatment

Simon was treated with deoxycholate AMB (0.25 mg/kg in 30 mL 5% dextrose IV over 30 minutes on Monday, Wednesday, and Friday for five treatments). Before and after this treatment, 0.9% NaCl was administered at twice maintenance rate and kidney analytes were monitored. Flucytosine (62.5 mg, PO, q8h) and prednisone (2.5 mg, PO, q24h) were also administered. An esophagostomy tube was placed for enteral nutrition because of persistent inappetence. By day 7, Simon appeared more alert, pupillary light reflexes and menace responses were present but weak, and nystagmus had resolved. He was discharged from the hospital on day 12, with instructions to continue treatment with fluconazole (50 mg, PO, q12h) and prednisone (2.5 mg, PO, q48h), in addition to esophagostomy tube feeding. On day 24, he was reevaluated for lethargy of several days' duration. Physical examination showed resolution of cranial nerve abnormalities, but delayed hopping reactions in all limbs were present. He was treated with six additional AMB treatments over 2 weeks. He began eating, and the esophageal feeding tube was removed on day 40. Three months after diagnosis, his neurologic signs had almost completely resolved with the exception of occasional tremors, persistent mild placing reaction deficits, and lumbosacral pain. A cryptococcal antigen titer was positive at 1:65,536. The fluconazole was replaced with itraconazole solution (3 mg/kg, PO, q12h). After an additional month, the antigen titer was 1:1024, a serum chemistry profile was unremarkable, and the owners felt that Simon was a normal cat. The prednisone treatment was discontinued thereafter. A year later, the antigen titer was 1:20. At a recheck examination 2 years later, the cat was neurologically normal. The owner declined further antigen testing and chose to continue treatment with itraconazole.

Comments

This cat had CNS cryptococcosis caused by *C. deuterogattii* (molecular type VGIIa), a hypervirulent molecular type that emerged in British Columbia and the Pacific Northwest. The treatment plan was limited by client's financial concerns, which meant that the initial course of AMB and flucytosine treatment was short, and a second course of AMB was required. Subsequently, treatment with fluconazole was associated with limited improvement, but a change to itraconazole was followed by dramatic clinical improvement and reduction in antigen titers.

SUGGESTED READINGS

Datta K, Bartlett KH, Baer R, et al. Spread of *Cryptococcus gattii* into Pacific northwest region of the United States. *Emerg Infect Dis.* 2009;15:1185–1191.

Kronstad JW, Attarian R, Cadieux B, et al. Expanding fungal pathogenesis: *Cryptococcus* breaks out of the opportunistic box. *Nat Rev Microbiol.* 2011;9:193–203.

Trivedi SR, Malik R, Meyer W, et al. Feline cryptococcosis: impact of current research on clinical management. *J Feline Med Surg.* 2011;13:163–172.

REFERENCES

1. Knoke M, Schwesinger G. One hundred years ago: the history of cryptococcosis in Greifswald. Medical mycology in the nineteenth century. *Mycoses.* 1994;37:229–233.
2. Lester SJ, Kowalewich NJ, Bartlett KH, et al. Clinicopathologic features of an unusual outbreak of cryptococcosis in dogs, cats, ferrets, and a bird: 38 cases (January to July 2003). *J Am Vet Med Assoc.* 2004;225:1716–1722.
3. Stephen C, Lester S, Black W, et al. Multispecies outbreak of cryptococcosis on southern Vancouver Island, British Columbia. *Can Vet J.* 2002;43:792–794.

4. Datta K, Bartlett KH, Baer R, et al. Spread of *Cryptococcus gattii* into Pacific northwest region of the United States. *Emerg Infect Dis.* 2009;15:1185–1191.
5. Krockenberger MB, Canfield PJ, Barnes J, et al. *Cryptococcus neoformans* var. *gattii* in the koala (*Phascolarctos cinereus*): Serological evidence for subclinical cryptococcosis. *Med Mycol.* 2002;40:273–282.
6. Malik R, Alderton B, Finlaison D, et al. Cryptococcosis in ferrets: a diverse spectrum of clinical disease. *Aust Vet J.* 2002;80:749–755.
7. Malik R, Krockenberger MB, Cross G, et al. Avian cryptococcosis. *Med Mycol.* 2003;41:115–124.
8. McGill S, Malik R, Saul N, et al. Cryptococcosis in domestic animals in Western Australia: a retrospective study from 1995-2006. *Med Mycol.* 2009;47:625–639.
9. Rotstein DS, West K, Levine G, et al. *Cryptococcus gattii* VGI in a spinner dolphin (*Stenella longirostris*) from Hawaii. *J Zoo Wildl Med.* 2010;41:181–183.
10. Sykes JE, Sturges BK, Cannon MS, et al. Clinical signs, imaging features, neuropathology, and outcome in cats and dogs with central nervous system cryptococcosis from California. *J Vet Intern Med.* 2010;24:1427–1438.
11. Trivedi SR, Sykes JE, Cannon MS, et al. Clinical features and epidemiology of cryptococcosis in cats and dogs in California: 93 cases (1988-2010). *J Am Vet Med Assoc.* 2011;239:357–369.
12. Liu XZ, Wang QM, Goker M, et al. Towards an integrated phylogenetic classification of the Tremellomycetes. *Stud Mycol.* 2015;81:85–147.
13. Johnson LB, Bradley SF, Kauffman CA. Fungaemia due to *Cryptococcus laurentii* and a review of non-*neoformans* cryptococcaemia. *Mycoses.* 1998;41:277–280.
14. Kano R, Kitagawa M, Oota S, et al. First case of feline systemic *Cryptococcus albidus* infection. *Med Mycol.* 2008;46:75–77.
15. Labrecque O, Sylvestre D, Messier S. Systemic *Cryptococcus albidus* infection in a Doberman pinscher. *J Vet Diagn Invest.* 2005;17:598–600.
16. Kano R, Hosaka S, Hasegawa A. First isolation of *Cryptococcus magnus* from a cat. *Mycopathologia.* 2004;157:263–264.
17. Bernardo FM, Martins HM, Martins ML. A survey of mycotic otitis externa of dogs in Lisbon. *Rev Iberoam De Micol.* 1998;15:163–165.
18. Evans SJM, Jones K, Moore AR. Atypical morphology and disparate speciation in a case of feline cryptococcosis. *Mycopathologia.* 2018;183:479–484.
19. Kronstad JW, Attarian R, Cadieux B, et al. Expanding fungal pathogenesis: *Cryptococcus* breaks out of the opportunistic box. *Nature Rev Microbiol.* 2011;9:193–203.
20. Hull CM, Heitman J. Genetics of *Cryptococcus neoformans. Ann Rev Genetics.* 2002:557–615.
21. Wickes BL, Mayorga ME, Edman U, et al. Dimorphism and haploid fruiting in *Cryptococcus neoformans*: Association with the α-mating type. *Proc Nat Acad Sci USA.* 1996;93:7327–7331.
22. Velagapudi R, Hsueh YP, Geunes-Boyer S, et al. Spores as infectious propagules of *Cryptococcus neoformans. Infect Immun.* 2009;77:4345–4355.
23. Hagen F, Khayhan K, Theelen B, et al. Recognition of seven species in the *Cryptococcus gattii/Cryptococcus neoformans* species complex. *Fungal Genet Biol.* 2015;78:16–48.
24. Ngamskulrungroj P, Gilgado F, Faganello J, et al. Genetic diversity of the *Cryptococcus* species complex suggests that *Cryptococcus gattii* deserves to have varieties. *PLoS One.* 2009;4:e5862.
25. Kwon-Chung KJ, Boekhout T, Fell JW, et al. (1557) proposal to conserve the name *Cryptococcus gattii* against *C. hondurianus* and *C. bacillisporus* (*Basidiomycota, Hymenomycetes, Tremellomycetidae*). *Taxon.* 2002;51:804–806.
26. Singer LM, Meyer W, Firacative C, et al. Antifungal drug susceptibility and phylogenetic diversity among *Cryptococcus* isolates from dogs and cats in North America. *J Clin Microbiol.* 2014;52:2061–2070.
27. Thompson GR, Albert N, Hodge G, et al. Phenotypic differences of *Cryptococcus* molecular types and their implications for virulence in a *Drosophila* model of infection. *Infect Immun.* 2014;82:3058–3065.
28. Ashton PM, Thanh LT, Trieu PH, et al. Genomics of *Cryptococcus neoformans. BioRxiv.* 2018:356816.
29. G-hA L, Arthur I, Merritt A, et al. Molecular types of *Cryptococcus neoformans* and *Cryptococcus gattii* in Western Australia and correlation with antifungal susceptibility. *Med Mycol.* 2019;57:1004–1010.
30. Anjum S, Williamson PR. Clinical aspects of immune damage in cryptococcosis. *Curr Fungal Infect Rep.* 2019;13:99–108.
31. Malik R, Wigney DI, Muir DB, et al. Cryptococcosis in cats: clinical and mycological assessment of 29 cases and evaluation of treatment using orally administered fluconazole. *Med Mycol.* 1992;30:133–144.
32. O'Brien CR, Krockenberger MB, Wigney DI, et al. Retrospective study of feline and canine cryptococcosis in Australia from 1981 to 2001: 195 cases. *Med Mycol.* 2004;42:449–460.
33. Berthelin CF, Bailey CS, Kass PH, et al. Cryptococcosis of the nervous system in dogs, Part 1: epidemiologic, clinical, and neuropathologic features. *Prog Vet Neurol.* 1994;5:88–97.
34. Malik R, Dill-Macky E, Martin P, et al. Cryptococcosis in dogs: a retrospective study of 20 consecutive cases. *Med Mycol.* 1995;33:291–297.
35. Jacobs GJ, Medleau L, Calvert C, et al. Cryptococcal infection in cats: factors influencing treatment outcome, and results of sequential serum antigen titers in 35 cats. *J Vet Intern Med.* 1997;11:1–4.
36. Walker C, Malik R, Canfield P. Analysis of leucocytes and lymphocyte subsets in cats with naturally–occurring cryptococcosis but differing feline immunodeficiency virus status. *Aust Vet J.* 1995;72:93–97.
37. Kano R, Fujino Y, Takamoto N, et al. PCR detection of the *Cryptococcus neoformans* CAP59 gene from a biopsy specimen from a case of feline cryptococcosis. *J Vet Diagn Invest.* 2001;13:439–442.
38. Barrs VR, Martin P, Nicoll RG, et al. Pulmonary cryptococcosis and *Capillaria aerophila* infection in an FIV-positive cat. *Aust Vet J.* 2000;78:154–158.
39. Nielsen K, De Obaldia AL, Heitman J. *Cryptococcus neoformans* mates on pigeon guano: implications for the realized ecological niche and globalization. *Eukaryot Cell.* 2007;6:949–959.
40. Lazéra MS, Pires FDA, Camillo-Coura L, et al. Natural habitat of *Cryptococcus neoformans* var. *neoformans* in decaying wood forming hollows in living trees. *Med Mycol.* 1996;34:127–131.
41. Ashton P, Thanh L, Trieu P, et al. Three phylogenetic groups have driven the recent population expansion of *Cryptococcus neoformans. Nature Comm.* 2019;10:2035.
42. Trivedi SR, Malik R, Meyer W, et al. Feline cryptococcosis: impact of current research on clinical management. *J Feline Med Surg.* 2011;13:163–172.
43. Sorrell TC. *Cryptococcus neoformans* variety gattii. *Med Mycol.* 2001;39:155–168.
44. Viviani MA, Cogliati M, Esposto MC, et al. Molecular analysis of 311 *Cryptococcus neoformans* isolates from a 30-month ECMM survey of cryptococcosis in Europe. *FEMS Yeast Res.* 2006;6:614–619.
45. Bartlett KH, Cheng PY, Duncan C, et al. A decade of experience: *Cryptococcus gattii* in British Columbia. *Mycopathologia.* 2012;173:311–319.
46. MacDougall L, Kidd SE, Galanis E, et al. Spread of *Cryptococcus gattii* in British Columbia, Canada, and detection in the Pacific northwest, USA. *Emerg Infect Dis.* 2007;13:42–50.
47. Marr KA. *Cryptococcus gattii* as an important fungal pathogen of western North America. *Expert Rev Anti Infect Ther.* 2012;10:637–643.
48. Duncan CG, Stephen C, Campbell J. Evaluation of risk factors for *Cryptococcus gattii* infection in dogs and cats. *J Am Vet Med Assoc.* 2006;228:377–382.
49. Acheson ES, Galanis E, Bartlett K, et al. Searching for clues for eighteen years: Deciphering the ecological determinants of *Cryptococcus gattii* on Vancouver Island, British Columbia. *Med Mycol.* 2017;56:129–144.
50. Hurst S, Lysen C, Cooksey G, et al. Molecular typing of clinical and environmental isolates of *Cryptococcus gattii* species complex from southern California, United States. *Mycoses.* 2019;62:1029–1034.
51. Campbell LT, Currie BJ, Krockenberger M, et al. Clonality and recombination in genetically differentiated subgroups of *Cryptococcus gattii. Eukaryot Cell.* 2005;4:1403–1409.
52. Ellis DH, Pfeiffer TJ. Natural habitat of *Cryptococcus neoformans* var. *gattii. J Clin Microbiol.* 1990;28:1642–1644.
53. Brito-Santos F, Reis RS, Coelho RA, et al. Cryptococcosis due to *Cryptococcus gattii* VGII in southeast Brazil: the One Health approach revealing a possible role for domestic cats. *Med Mycol Case Reports.* 2019;24:61–64.

54. de Abreu DPB, Machado CH, Makita MT, et al. Intestinal lesion in a dog due to *Cryptococcus gattii* type VGII and review of published cases of canine gastrointestinal cryptococcosis. *Mycopathologia*. 2017;182:597–602.
55. Headley SA, Di Santis GW, de Alcantara BK, et al. *Cryptococcus gattii*-induced infections in dogs from Southern Brazil. *Mycopathologia*. 2015;180:265–275.
56. Vieille P, Cruz R, Leon P, et al. Isolation of *Cryptococcus gattii* VGIII from feline nasal injury. *Med Mycol Case Rep*. 2018;22:55–57.
57. Speed B, Dunt D. Clinical and host differences between infections with the two varieties of *Cryptococcus neoformans*. *Clin Infect Dis*. 1995;21:28–34.
58. Chaturvedi S, Dyavaiah M, Larsen RA, et al. *Cryptococcus gattii* in AIDS patients, southern California. *Emerg Infect Dis*. 2005;11:1686–1692.
59. Perfect JR. *Cryptococcus neoformans*. In: Mandell GL, Bennet JE, Dolin R, eds. *Mandell, Douglas, and Bennett's Principles and Practice of Infectious Diseases*, 7th edn. Elsevier; 2010:3287–3303.
60. Perfect JR. The triple threat of cryptococcosis: it's the body site, the strain and/or the host. *mBio*. 2012;3.
61. Malik R, Wigney D, Muir D, et al. Asymptomatic carriage of *Cryptococcus neoformans* in the nasal cavity of dogs and cats. *J Med Vet Mycol*. 1997;35:27–31.
62. Krockenberger MB, Canfield PJ, Malik R. *Cryptococcus neoformans* in the koala (*Phascolarctos cinereus*): colonization by C. n. var. *gattii* and investigation of environmental sources. *Med Mycol*. 2002;40:263–272.
63. Krockenberger MB, Canfield PJ, Malik R. *Cryptococcus neoformans* var. *gattii* in the koala (*Phascolarctos cinereus*): a review of 43 cases of cryptococcosis. *Med Mycol*. 2003;41:225–234.
64. Perfect JR. *Cryptococcus neoformans*: a sugar-coated killer with designer genes. *FEMS Immunol Med Microbiol*. 2005;45:395–404.
65. Alspaugh JA. Virulence mechanisms and *Cryptococcus neoformans* pathogenesis. *Fungal Genet Biol*. 2015;78:55–58.
66. Yauch LE, Lam JS, Levitz SM. Direct inhibition of T-cell responses by the *Cryptococcus* capsular polysaccharide glucuronoxylomannan. *PLoS Pathogens*. 2006;2:e120.
67. Jain N, Fries BC. Phenotypic switching of *Cryptococcus neoformans* and *Cryptococcus gattii*. *Mycopathologia*. 2008;166:181.
68. Georgi A, Schneemann M, Tintelnot K, et al. *Cryptococcus gattii* meningoencephalitis in an immunocompetent person 13 months after exposure. *Infection*. 2009;37:370–373.
69. MacDougall L, Fyfe M. Emergence of *Cryptococcus gattii* in a novel environment provides clues to its incubation period. *J Clin Microbiol*. 2006;44:1851–1852.
70. Casadevall A. Cryptococci at the brain gate: break and enter or use a Trojan horse? *J Clin Invest*. 2010;120:1389–1392.
71. Beatty JA, Barrs VR, Swinney GR, et al. Peripheral vestibular disease associated with cryptococcosis in three cats. *J Fel Med Surg*. 2000;2:29–34.
72. Malik R, Hunt GB, Bellenger CR, et al. Intra-abdominal cryptococcosis in two dogs. *J Small Anim Pract*. 1999;40:387–391.
73. Olsen GL, Deitz KL, Flaherty HA, et al. Use of terbinafine in the treatment protocol of intestinal *Cryptococcus neoformans* in a dog. *J Am Anim Hosp Assoc*. 2012;48:216–220.
74. Johnston L, Mackay B, King T, et al. Abdominal cryptococcosis in dogs and cats: 38 cases (2000-2018). *J Small Anim Pract*. 2021;62:19–27.
75. de Abreu DPB, Machado CH, Makita MT, et al. Intestinal lesion in a dog due to *Cryptococcus gattii* type VGII and review of published cases of canine gastrointestinal cryptococcosis. *Mycopathologia*. 2017;182:597–602.
76. Myers A, Meason-Smith C, Mansell J, et al. Atypical cutaneous cryptococcosis in four cats in the USA. *Vet Dermatol*. 2017;28:405–e497.
77. Headley SA, Mota FCD, Lindsay S, et al. *Cryptococcus neoformans* var. *grubii*-induced arthritis with encephalitic dissemination in a dog and review of published literature. *Mycopathologia*. 2016;181:595–601.
78. Schlacks S, Boozer T, Dial S, et al. CT identifies pulmonary cryptococcosis in a domestic feline. *Vet Radiol Ultrasound*. 2021;62:E54–E57.
79. Kwon-Chung KJ, Polacheck I, Bennett JE. Improved diagnostic medium for separation of *Cryptococcus neoformans* var. *neoformans* (serotypes A and D) and *Cryptococcus neoformans* var. *gattii* (serotypes B and C). *J Clin Microbiol*. 1982;15:535–537.
80. Firacative C, Trilles L, Meyer W. MALDI-TOF MS enables the rapid identification of the major molecular types within the *Cryptococcus neoformans/C. gattii* species complex. *PLoS One*. 2012;7:e37566.
81. Thompson GR, Wiederhold NP, Fothergill AW, et al. Antifungal susceptibilities among different serotypes of *Cryptococcus gattii* and *Cryptococcus neoformans*. *Antimicrob Agents Chemother*. 2009;53:309–311.
82. Malik R, McPetrie R, Wigney DI, et al. A latex cryptococcal antigen agglutination test for diagnosis and monitoring of therapy for cryptococcosis. *Aust Vet J*. 1996;74:358–364.
83. Medleau L, Marks MA, Brown J, et al. Clinical evaluation of a cryptococcal antigen latex agglutination test for diagnosis of cryptococcosis in cats. *J Am Vet Med Assoc*. 1990;196:1470–1473.
84. McMullan BJ, Halliday C, Sorrell TC, et al. Clinical utility of the cryptococcal antigen lateral flow assay in a diagnostic mycology laboratory. *PLoS One*. 2012;7:e49541.
85. Krockenberger MB, Marschner C, Martin P, et al. Comparing immunochromatography with latex antigen agglutination testing for the diagnosis of cryptococcosis in cats, dogs and koalas. *Med Mycol*. 2020;58:39–46.
86. Tenforde MW, Boyer-Chammard T, Muthoga C, et al. Diagnostic accuracy of the Biosynex CryptoPS cryptococcal antigen semi-quantitative lateral flow assay in patients with advanced HIV disease. *J Clin Microbiol*. 2020;59:e02307–e02320.
87. Reagan KL, McHardy I, Thompson GR 3rd, et al. Evaluation of the clinical performance of 2 point-of-care cryptococcal antigen tests in dogs and cats. *J Vet Intern Med*. 2019;33:2082–2089.
88. Suchodolski JS, Morris EK, Allenspach K, et al. Prevalence and identification of fungal DNA in the small intestine of healthy dogs and dogs with chronic enteropathies. *Vet Microbiol*. 2008;132:379–388.
89. Krockenberger MB, Canfield PJ, Kozel TR, et al. An immunohistochemical method that differentiates *Cryptococcus neofarmans* varieties and serotypes in formalin-fixed paraffin-embedded tissues. *Med Mycol*. 2001;39:523–533.
90. Kano R, Okubo M, Yanai T, et al. First isolation of azole-resistant *Cryptococcus neoformans* from feline cryptococcosis. *Mycopathologia*. 2015;180:427–433.
91. Sykes JE, Hodge G, Singapuri A, et al. In vivo development of fluconazole resistance in serial *Cryptococcus gattii* isolates from a cat. *Med Mycol*. 2017;55:396–401.
92. Vu K, Thompson GR III, Roe CC, et al. Flucytosine resistance in *Cryptococcus gattii* is indirectly mediated by the FCY2-FCY1-Fur1 pathway. *Med Mycol*. 2018;56:857–867.
93. Denning DW, Tucker RM, Hanson LH, et al. Itraconazole therapy for cryptococcal meningitis and cryptococcosis. *Arch Intern Med*. 1989;149:2301–2308.
94. Sykes JE. Personal observations 2012.
95. Malik R, Medeiros C, Wigney DI, et al. Suspected drug eruption in seven dogs during administration of flucytosine. *Aust Vet J*. 1996;74:285–288.
96. Kerwin SC, McCarthy RJ, VanSteenhouse JL, et al. Cervical spinal cord compression caused by cryptococcosis in a dog: successful treatment with surgery and fluconazole. *J Am Anim Hosp Assoc*. 1998;34:523–526.
97. Quimby J, Hoffman S, Duke J, et al. Adverse neurologic events associated with voriconazole use in 3 cats. *J Vet Intern Med*. 2010;24:647–649.
98. Vishkautsan P, Papich MG, Thompson GR III, et al. Pharmacokinetics of voriconazole after intravenous and oral administration to healthy cats. *Am J Vet Res*. 2016;77:931–939.
99. Mawby D, Whittemore J, Fowler L, et al. Posaconazole pharmacokinetics in healthy cats after oral and intravenous administration. *J Vet Intern Med*. 2016;30:1703–1707.
100. Rauseo AM, Coler-Reilly A, Larson L, et al. Hope on the horizon: novel fungal treatments in development. *Open Forum Infect Dis*. 2020;7:ofaa016.
101. Bicanic T, Harrison TS. Cryptococcal meningitis. *Br Med Bull*. 2004;72:99–118.

102. Duncan C, Stephen C, Campbell J. Clinical characteristics and predictors of mortality for *Cryptococcus gattii* infection in dogs and cats of southwestern British Columbia. *Can Vet J*. 2006;47:993–998.
103. O'Brien CR, Krockenberger MB, Martin P, et al. Long-term outcome of therapy for 59 cats and 11 dogs with cryptococcosis. *Aust Vet J*. 2006;84:384–392.
104. Fessel WJ. Cryptococcal meningitis after unusual exposures to birds. *New Engl J Med*. 1993;328:1354–1355.
105. Danesi P, Furnari C, Granato A, et al. Molecular identity and prevalence of *Cryptococcus* spp. nasal carriage in asymptomatic feral cats in Italy. *Med Mycol*. 2014;52:667–673.
106. Casadevall A, Mukherjee J, Yuan R, et al. Management of injuries caused by *Cryptococcus neoformans*-contaminated needles. *Clin Infect Dis*. 1994;19:951–953.

83

Coccidioidomycosis and Paracoccidioidomycosis

Polina Vishkautsan, Jane E. Sykes

KEY POINTS

- First Described: *Coccidioides* spp. was first described in 1892 (by the medical student Alejandro Posadas), in a person from Buenos Aires, Argentina, where it was initially mistaken for a protozoan (*Coccidia*).[1]
- Cause: Coccidioidomycosis is caused by *Coccidioides immitis* and *Coccidioides posadasii* (ascomycetes, no known teleomorph).
- Affected Hosts: Primarily humans and dogs, but also a variety of other animals that include cats, domestic farm animal species, and a variety of wildlife hosts.
- Geographic Distribution: Southwestern United States, northern Mexico, and parts of Central and South America (northeastern Brazil, Argentina, Paraguay, and Bolivia). Recently cases have also appeared in eastern Washington in the United States.
- Mode of Transmission: Inhalation of arthroconidia from the environment; rarely cutaneous inoculation.
- Major Clinical Signs: Cough, fever, inappetence, weight loss, tachypnea, increased respiratory effort, lameness, subcutaneous masses or draining skin lesions, lymphadenopathy, neurologic signs, ascites due to right-sided heart failure (pericarditis), ocular lesions (uveitis, chorioretinitis, endophthalmitis).
- Differential Diagnoses: Neoplasia, other deep mycoses, mycobacteriosis, actinomycosis or nocardiosis, toxoplasmosis or neosporosis, systemic immune-mediated disease.
- Human Health Significance: Direct transmission from animals to humans does not usually occur, although sharps injuries or bite wounds from affected animals may be a source of human infection. Dogs are a sentinel for human exposure.

COCCIDIOIDOMYCOSIS

ETIOLOGY AND EPIDEMIOLOGY

Coccidioides spp. are dimorphic, soil-borne fungi that exist in the environment as a mycelium and in tissues (at 37°C) as peculiar structures known as *spherules* (Fig. 83.1). The mycelium consists of chains of haploid, multinucleated, barrel-shaped arthroconidia (or arthrospores) that alternate with smaller, thin-walled, nonviable cells. The arthroconidia remain viable in the soil for long periods. They ultimately fragment from each other and are subsequently aerosolized and inhaled by animal hosts (Fig. 83.2). The inoculum needed for infection can be small, even a few arthroconidia.[2] This can be followed by the development of coccidioidomycosis, a localized pulmonary disease or a serious multisystemic disease if dissemination occurs in the face of an inadequate immune response.

In the environment, *Coccidioides* spp. are distributed in the lower Sonoran life zone, regions characterized by semi-arid to arid soils, low elevations above sea level, and hot summers. The organism has been aptly referred to as "the dust devil."[3] Worldwide, *Coccidioides* spp. are found in the southwestern Unites States, Mexico, and parts of Central and South America, specifically northeastern Colombia, Guatemala, Honduras, Venezuela, northeastern Brazil, the Chaco region in Argentina and Paraguay, and Bolivia (Fig. 83.3). In the southwestern United States, highly endemic regions are the south-central valley of California, especially Bakersfield ("valley fever") and Arizona, especially Tucson and Phoenix.[4] Other affected states in the United States are Utah, Nevada, New Mexico, and southwestern Texas. Since 2010, cases in non-traveled dogs and humans have been reported from Washington state.[5,6] Infections also occur in non-endemic regions in dogs and humans that have a travel history to endemic regions. Over the last two decades, the incidence of coccidioidomycosis in humans and likely also dogs has been on the rise (Fig. 83.4);[7,8] it has been speculated that this may be the result of population growth in endemic areas, climate change, a larger population of immunocompromised humans, and increased recognition and reporting.[9,10]

Two species of *Coccidioides* have been identified— *Coccidioides posadasii* and *Coccidioides immitis.* These appear to cause similar clinical manifestations and have similar antifungal drug susceptibilities, but further studies are required.[11] The geographic range of *C. immitis* is largely limited to endemic regions in California and eastern Washington state, whereas *C. posadasii* is found elsewhere.[7,12] However, there may be some overlap in the distribution of these organisms.[13]

Infection of animals and humans with *Coccidioides spp.* often follows a cycle of moist conditions (required for growth of the organism in the soil), a dry period, then soil disruption, such as that may occur with heavy rainfall, earthquakes, dust storms, prolonged droughts, or construction.[14–16] An association between the presence of *Coccidioides* in the soil and small desert mammal activity has been observed; these rodents may contribute to distribution of the fungus in the soil,[7] and it has been suggested that they may act as reservoirs of the fungus.

Dogs of any breed, age, or sex may be affected, although large-breed, young adult dogs predominate in some case series.[17,18] In dogs seen at the University of California-Davis VMTH, boxers, poodles, pointers, Labrador and golden retrievers, German shepherd dogs, Australian shepherds, Dalmatians, Scottish terriers, dachshunds, and beagles are over-represented when compared with the hospital patient population.[19] When compared with a control population of dogs with diseases other than coccidioidomycosis, risk factors for coccidioidomycosis among dogs seen at the University of California-Davis VMTH were younger age (young adult rather than older adult), digging behavior, and travel to Arizona or the California central valley.[20] In this study, predisposed breeds were viszlas, Dalmatians, weimaraners, greyhounds, English pointers, bull terriers, Brittany spaniels, and boxers. Risk factors for infection in dogs from Arizona included being housed outdoors during the day rather than indoors, roaming area more than 1 acre, and walking in the desert.[21] Latent infections may also occur in dogs and these can reactivate after treatment with immunosuppressive drugs, such as glucocorticoids and chemotherapeutic agents, including after previous recovery from coccidioidomycosis.

Although not as prevalent as in dogs, coccidioidomycosis also occurs in cats.[22,23] In two separate case series of cats from Arizona, cats ranged in age from 1 to 15 years (median, 5 years in one study and 6.8 years in another) and there was no obvious sex or breed predisposition.[22,23] Many cats were indoor only.[22] Only a small number of affected cats in the combined studies were co-infected with FIV or FeLV. Interestingly, a search of the UC Davis VMTH and pathology database from 1990 to 2015 revealed only one case of feline coccidioidomycosis, and that cat lived in Arizona, which might suggest cats are less susceptible to *C. immitis* infection than to *C. posadasii* infection.

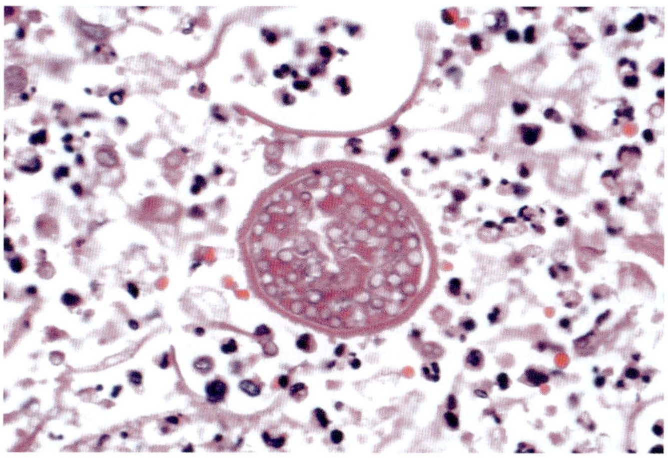

Fig. 83.1 Photomicrograph of a spherule in tissue. Hematoxylin and eosin stain. (Courtesy of Dr. Richard Sobonya, MD, University of Arizona.)

CLINICAL FEATURES

Pathogenesis and Clinical Signs

The clinical signs of coccidioidomycosis depend on factors such as the infectious dose and the immune status of the host. Arthroconidia are inhaled and are phagocytosed by alveolar macrophages. They then enlarge into a spherule, which measures 8 to 100 μm in diameter. Hundreds of endospores then develop within the spherule, which are released when the mature spherule ruptures. These attract neutrophils, which leads to a pyogranulomatous inflammatory response. Each released endospore that escapes immune destruction then enlarges into a new spherule, and the cycle continues. Endospores can also revert to mycelial growth when removed from the site of infection. In hosts that are unable to mount an effective immune response, endospores disseminate by lymphatics to tracheobronchial lymph nodes and hematogenously to a variety of body sites. Inoculation coccidioidomycosis can rarely occur, and generally results in lesions that are localized to the site of the wound. In one report, it followed removal of a foxtail from a wound.[24] Cutaneous coccidioidomycosis appears to be predominantly a sequela of disseminated infection, whereas primary cutaneous infection is a rare event.[25]

Most infections in endemic areas are subclinical.[26] Development of clinical signs often follows a subacute to chronic course, with variable and often mild systemic signs such as intermittent fever, lethargy, inappetence, and weight loss.[17,27] Many dogs otherwise appear healthy, with occasional periods of inappetence.[17] Clinical signs may be present for days to years before veterinary attention is sought.[18] Signs of respiratory tract involvement include a harsh cough, increased respiratory effort, tachypnea, and/or exercise intolerance.[18,27] Cough may be chronic and is sometimes associated with gagging or retching; occasionally it results from bronchial compression by enlarged tracheobronchial lymph nodes. Rarely, diffuse pneumonia follows a fulminant course, with signs that resemble acute bacterial pneumonia or septic shock, as reported in immunocompromised human patients.[4]

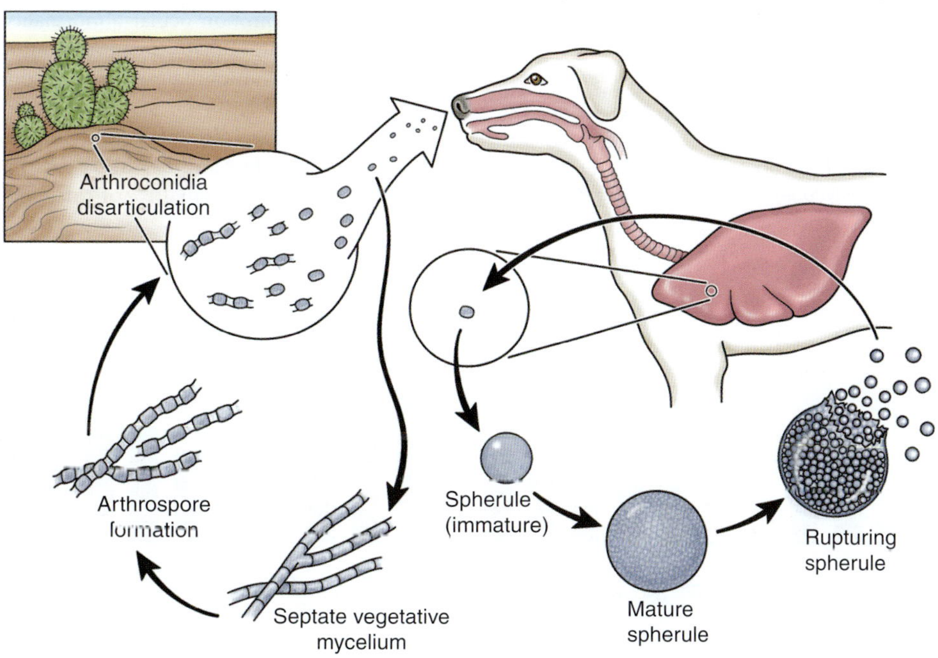

Fig. 83.2 Life cycle of *Coccidioides* spp. Hyphae fragment into arthroconidia, which are inhaled and form spherules in tissues. The spherules rupture and release endospores, which form new spherules. In some dogs, the organism disseminates from the lungs to a variety of other tissues, but especially local lymph nodes, bone, skin, the pericardium, the eye, and the CNS.

A smaller percentage of infected dogs develop disseminated infections. Sites of dissemination often include osteoarticular sites, the CNS, skin, peripheral lymph nodes, eye, reproductive organs (testes, prostate, and the uterus), and the pericardium.[18,19] Rarely, other sites such as the liver, spleen, GI tract, peritoneal cavity, and urinary system are affected.[17] Sometimes dissemination to only one anatomic site is evident; in other dogs multiple sites are involved. A history of respiratory signs may be absent.[17] Bone involvement may manifest as lameness and/or one or more firm swellings associated with the appendicular or axial skeleton. Dogs with skin involvement may have ulcerated skin lesions that drain serosanguinous fluid, or subcutaneous masses (Fig. 83.5).[17,25] Lesions are commonly located on the trunk for both dogs and cats, and in over 50% of cases lesions affect non-appendicular skeletal regions. In most cases, skin lesions should be considered separate sites of dissemination and not necessarily an extension of coccidioidal osteomyelitis.[25] Neurologic signs result from meningoencephalitis or mass lesions and include obtundation, blindness, nystagmus, absent menace reflexes, diminished gag responses, ataxia, abnormal placing reactions, pacing, circling, cervical pain, tetraparesis and seizures.[18,28–30] Ocular manifestations of coccidioidomycosis include chorioretinitis, uveitis, optic neuritis, and endophthalmitis.[18,31,32] Involvement of abdominal organs such as the liver and GI tract can lead to inappetence, vomiting, and/or diarrhea.[17] Pericarditis may lead to signs of right-sided cardiac failure, with ascites and pleural effusion.[17]

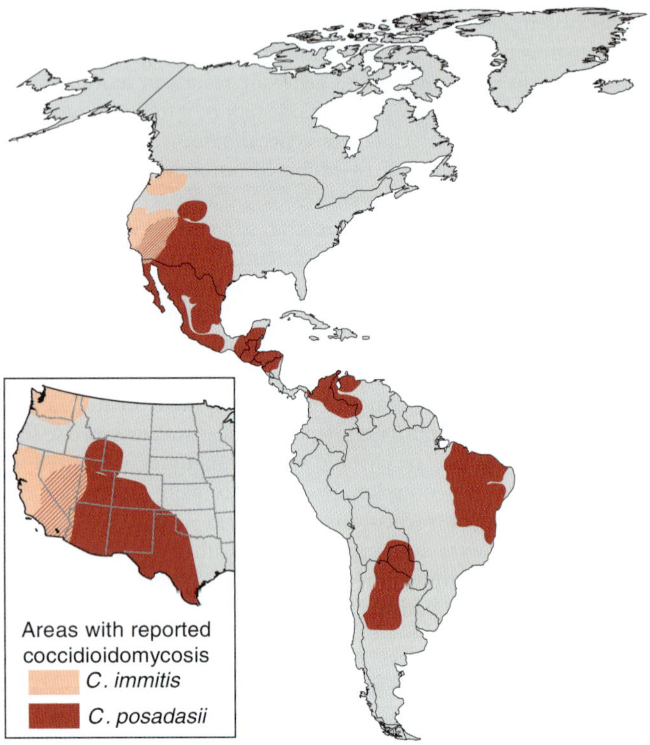

Fig. 83.3 Geographic distribution of *Coccidioides* spp. worldwide. The inset shows the distribution of *Coccidioides* species in southwestern United States. (Adapted from Ashraf N, Kubat RC, Poplin V. Re-drawing the maps for endemic mycoses. *Mycopathologica*. 2020;185:843-865)

Clinical signs in affected cats from Arizona have most often been respiratory signs (cough, tachypnea, dyspnea) and skin lesions, which may be nodular lesions, non-healing ulcers, or plaque-like crusting lesions.[22,25] In addition to those, nonspecific signs of weight loss, inappetence, and lethargy can be commonly seen. Fever and lameness due to bone involvement can also occur; lameness, paresis, or paraparesis was described in 22% of 51 cats in one case series.[22]

Physical Examination Findings

Fever is present in up to two-thirds of affected dogs with coccidioidomycosis (range, 103 to 106°F) on physical examination. Other common findings in dogs are lethargy, weakness, thin body condition or profound muscle atrophy, tachypnea, increased respiratory effort, inducible or spontaneous cough, and/or increased lung sounds.[18] Lameness and firm, often painful bony swellings with associated muscle atrophy may be present in dogs with osteomyelitis.[33] Less often, focal or (very rarely) generalized peripheral lymphadenomegaly, subcutaneous masses or draining skin lesions, or swollen joints are present. Dogs with pericardial coccidioidomycosis may have abdominal distention with a palpable fluid wave, tachycardia, tachypnea, jugular pulses, muffled breath and heart sounds due to pleural effusion, mucosal pallor, prolonged capillary refill time, and weak pulses.[34] Neurologic signs, when present, include seizures, obtundation, apparent blindness, ataxia, nystagmus, spinal pain, circling, and tetraparesis. The most common ocular abnormality is uveitis, but keratitis, conjunctivitis, granulomatous chorioretinitis, optic neuritis, retinal detachment, and endophthalmitis with secondary glaucoma have also been described.[18,31,32]

In cats with coccidioidomycosis, fever was reported in 31% of 48 cats in one study[23] and 8% of 51 cats in another.[22] Skin lesions were present in more than 40% of cats, and included draining skin

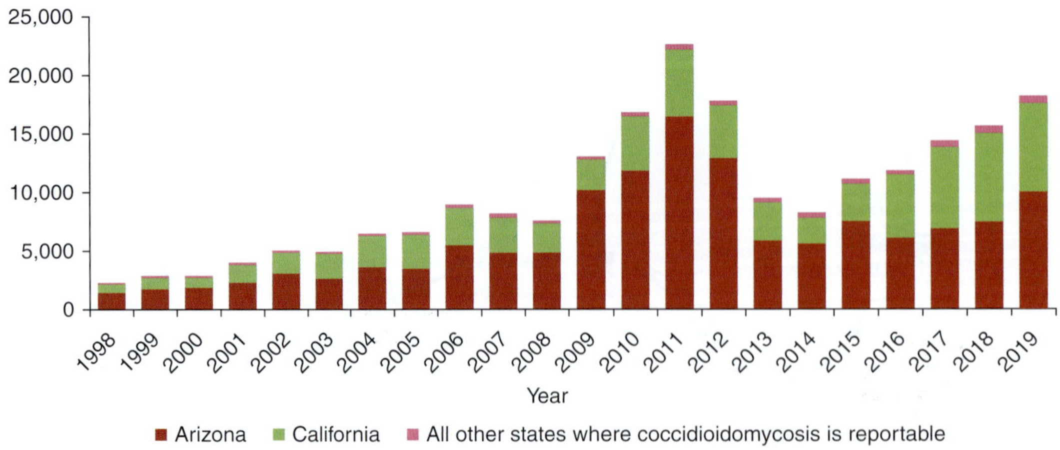

Fig. 83.4 Number of reported coccidioidomycosis cases in humans, 1998–2019. (From Centers for Disease Control and Prevention, Valley Fever (Coccidioidomycosis) Statistics. Available at https://www.cdc.gov/fungal/diseases/coccidioidomycosis/statistics.html.)

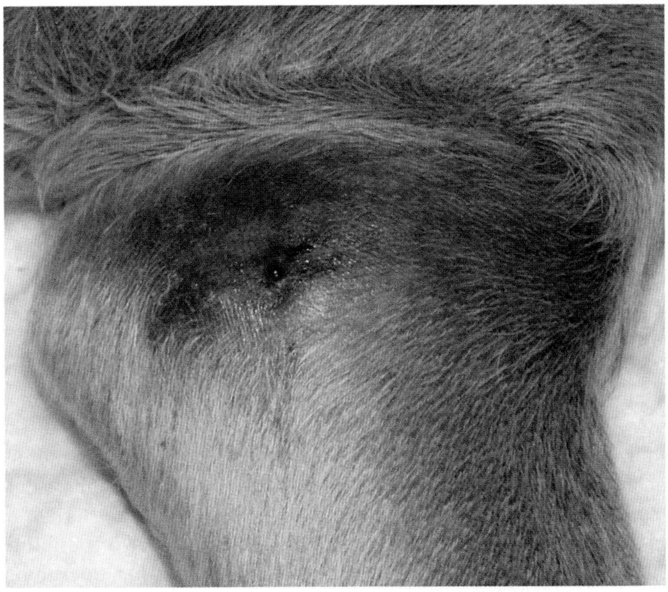

Fig. 83.5 Draining skin lesion on the left elbow of a 5-year-old shepherd mix with disseminated coccidioidomycosis. Radiography revealed a mixed productive and destructive lesion of the distal humerus and proximal ulna. Productive lesions of the sixth and seventh ribs were also present. Arthrocentesis revealed suppurative inflammation with no growth on culture. Diagnosis was ultimately made by biopsy of the synovium and serology. The *Coccidioides* antibody titer was 1:64.

lesions, subcutaneous granulomas, plaque-like crusting lesions, and abscesses.[23] Tachypnea or increased respiratory effort was present in 25% of affected cats in one study and in 39% in another; and lameness has been noted in approximately 20% of cats. Ocular abnormalities that include conjunctival masses, periorbital swellings, chorioretinitis, retinal detachment, endophthalmitis, and/or anterior uveitis have been described.[35,36] A small percentage of cats have neurological signs such as hyperesthesia, posterior paresis, seizures, and ataxia. Dissemination to abdominal organs such as the spleen can occur.[37]

DIAGNOSIS

Coccidioidomycosis is usually suspected based on a history of travel to or residence in an endemic region, and consistent clinical signs and radiographic findings. Coccidioidomycosis should be retained in the differential diagnoses for dogs and cats that have formerly lived in or traveled through endemic areas, for the rest of their lives and regardless of whether they have previously shown any sign of infection. Because the disease's geographic distribution is changing as a result of climate change, population shifts, and construction activity, early diagnosis requires a high index of suspicion in the regions where new reports of disease in people and animals become available. The diagnosis can be confirmed with cytologic examination of aspirates or body fluids, serologic assays that detect antibodies to *Coccidioides* spp., histopathology, and/or fungal culture (Table 83.1).

TABLE 83.1 Diagnostic Assays Currently Available for Coccidioidomycosis in Dogs and Cats

Assay	Specimen Type	Target	Performance
Cytologic examination	Aspirates of affected tissues, body fluids, impression smears of skin lesions	*Coccidioides* spherules and/or endospores	Low sensitivity and organisms may be difficult to accurately identify in some specimens. Immature spherules may be mistaken for other fungi or cellular aggregates or debris
Fungal culture	Aspirates or biopsies of affected tissues, body fluids such as CSF or pleural effusion, transtracheal, or bronchoalveolar lavage specimens	*Coccidioides* spp.	Generally sensitive and specific, but false negatives are possible if specimen size is low. Can require several weeks' incubation. A significant laboratory health hazard
Antibody serology (gel immunodiffusion [ID])	Serum, CSF	IgG or IgM antibodies to *Coccidioides* spp.	Sensitivity is close to 100%. Quantification of an IgG antibody titer is possible. Titers decline with successful treatment. In hyperendemic areas, titers as high as 1:16 have the potential to exist in subclinically infected or recovered dogs, so positive serology should be supported with other diagnostic tests for coccidioidomycosis. Serologic results may be negative in early infection or in animals with weak immune responses
Antibody-detection enzyme immunoassays (MiraVista Diagnostics, Indianapolis, IN, USA)	Serum	*Coccidioides* antibodies	Sensitivity of 89% and specificity 97% on serum specimens from dogs when compared with gel ID in one study of dogs from Arizona
Immunochromatographic POC assay (Sōna, IMMY Diagnostics, Oklahoma, USA)	Serum	*Coccidioides* antibodies	Sensitivity of 89% and specificity 100% on serum specimens from dogs when compared with gel ID in one study of dogs from California; agreement of 87.5% when applied to dogs from Arizona (see text). False-negative results may occur with low gel ID titers. Provides results in less than 15 minutes
Serology for *Coccidioides* antigen	Serum, urine	*Coccidioides* spp. galactomannan antigen	Low sensitivity (≤ 20%); false positives can occur in dogs with histoplasmosis or blastomycosis. Not recommended
Real-time PCR assays	Biopsies, body fluids, respiratory lavage specimens, aspirates	*Coccidioides* DNA	Not yet validated in adequate numbers of dogs or cats with coccidioidomycosis; usefulness requires further evaluation
Histopathology	Biopsy specimens from affected tissues, such as bone biopsies	*Coccidioides* spp. spherules	Limited sensitivity in dogs; submission of multiple biopsies is recommended when possible. Often only one or two spherules are visualized. Special stains such as PAS and silver stains facilitate organism detection

Laboratory Abnormalities

Complete Blood Count

CBC findings in dogs with coccidioidomycosis are nonspecific and resemble those of other deep mycoses. Most affected dogs have mild, normocytic, normochromic, non-regenerative anemia and mild leukocytosis. Leukocytosis results from a neutrophilia, occasionally with a left shift and evidence of neutrophil toxicity.[18,34] A monocytosis and lymphopenia may also be present, but in contrast to human infections, eosinophilia is not typically present. Neutrophilia and monocytosis have also been described in affected cats.[22]

Serum Biochemical Tests

Almost all dogs with coccidioidomycosis have hypoalbuminemia, and approximately half of affected dogs and cats have hyperglobulinemia (up to 7.8 mg/dL in one study).[18,22,23] Hypoalbuminemia is usually mild to moderate, but rarely may be more severe (< 1.5 g/dL). Uncommonly, mild hypercalcemia is present. Increased activity of serum ALP may be present in some dogs, possibly as a result of bone involvement.

Urinalysis

The urinalysis in dogs with coccidioidomycosis is often normal, but significant proteinuria (urine protein-to-creatinine ratios as high as 9.5, reference range < 1) has been reported in some dogs.[18] In a series of chronic canine coccidioidomycosis cases, glomerular lesions and proteinuria were documented.[38] Dogs with coccidioidomycosis should be carefully screened for proteinuria to initiate timely treatment. In addition, testing dogs with protein-losing nephropathies that have resided in *Coccidioides*-endemic areas for anti-*Coccidioides* antibodies has the potential to identify an underlying cause.

CSF Analysis

CSF analysis in dogs with CNS coccidioidomycosis usually reveals an increase in protein concentration (generally < 300 mg/dL, reference range < 25 mg/dL), and a mild to moderate increase in the nucleated cell count (usually < 50 cells/μL, reference range < 2 cells/μL).[18] The differential cell count may show mixed, predominantly lymphocytic, mixed mononuclear, or neutrophilic pleocytosis. Organisms are generally not observed.

Diagnostic Imaging

Plain Radiography

Thoracic radiographs in dogs with disseminated coccidioidomycosis are often unremarkable. The most common radiographic finding in dogs with pulmonary coccidioidomycosis is mild to severe hilar lymphadenomegaly (Fig. 83.6A), which was present in 10 of 19 dogs with coccidioidomycosis from California.[18] Hilar lymphadenomegaly can also be present in affected cats.[22,23] Although hilar lymphadenomegaly may be present as the only finding, most dogs with hilar lymphadenomegaly also have pulmonary infiltrates, which are usually mild to moderate and interstitial. Nodular interstitial, interstitial-alveolar, bronchointerstitial infiltrates, and/or sternal lymphadenomegaly can also be present (see Fig. 83.6B and C).[18,27] Dogs with pericarditis can have cardiomegaly and pleural effusion, with hepatomegaly and decreased abdominal detail. Findings in cats with pulmonary involvement have included bronchial, alveolar, and/or interstitial patterns, consolidation of one or more lung lobes, and less commonly solitary lung nodules or pleural effusion.[22]

Radiographs of affected bones in both dogs and cats with *Coccidioides* osteomyelitis reveal local periosteal proliferation as well as osteolysis and soft-tissue swelling. Lesions can resemble osteosarcomas (Fig. 83.7).[17,22,23,33]

Sonographic Findings

Abdominal ultrasound examination of dogs with coccidioidomycosis is typically unremarkable. Mild hepatosplenomegaly and abdominal lymphadenomegaly have been described in a small proportion of dogs.[18] Dogs with *Coccidioides* peritonitis may have echogenic, elongated plaques on serosal surfaces and peritoneal effusion. Ascites, hepatomegaly, and distended hepatic veins may be evident in dogs with pericarditis and right-sided heart failure.[34]

Echocardiography in dogs with *Coccidioides* spp. pericarditis can reveal thickening and mass lesions of the pericardium, adherence of the pericardium to the epicardium, pericardial and pleural effusion, and evidence of cardiac tamponade (see Fig. 122.3).[34] Detection of pleural effusion using thoracic ultrasound was described in 2 of 51 cats with coccidioidomycosis from Arizona.[22]

Advanced Imaging

Advanced imaging findings in dogs with coccidioidomycosis have not been extensively reported in the literature. Focal, contrast-enhancing intra-parenchymal mass lesions in the brain or osteomyelitis of the skull may be identified on CT of the head.[39] Thoracic CT findings include contrast-enhancing miliary nodular pulmonary lesions; single or multifocal larger nodules or masses; tracheobronchial, sternal, or mediastinal lymphadenopathy; focal regions of alveolar or peribronchial infiltrates; lobar consolidation; pleural or mediastinal thickening; and rarely pleural effusion (Fig. 83.8).

MRI of the brain in dogs with CNS coccidioidomycosis may show focal or multifocal lesions within the brain (Fig. 83.9).[40,41] While human patients typically develop meningitis, mass lesions may be more frequently identified in dogs. When granulomas are present, they can share multiple MRI features with CNS neoplasia or other infectious or inflammatory processes. Mass lesions may have indistinct borders on post-contrast T1-weighted images. The degree of intensity on T1- and T2-weighted images varies greatly.[30] Other findings include ventricular dilation and/or meningeal enhancement. Bilaterally symmetric T2 hyperintense lesions within the frontal lobes, caudate nuclei, and rostral internal capsule, with variable evidence of faint, wispy, contrast enhancement were described in a subpopulation of dogs with CNS coccidioidomycosis from Arizona; schnauzers were overrepresented.[41] Use of other diagnostic tests such as serology or demonstration of the organism are needed for definitive diagnosis of coccidioidomycosis.

Microbiologic Tests (see Table 83.1)

Cytologic Examination

Cytologic examination of aspirates of affected tissues, pleural effusion, or respiratory lavage specimens typically reveals granulomatous or pyogranulomatous inflammation, sometimes with rare multinucleated giant cells, scattered eosinophils, and/or a reactive lymphocyte population. However, occasionally a suppurative inflammatory response predominates. Fungal elements are often not found in fluid specimens. Fluid specimens should be centrifuged and multiple aspirates of masses or lymph nodes should be collected to increase chance of detection. The clinician should alert the laboratory if there is clinical suspicion of coccidioidomycosis since often there are only very few organisms on the slide; because of their large size, they have the potential to be overlooked. Spherules may be visualized as round, deeply basophilic, double-walled, slightly crinkled structures that range in diameter from 8 to 70 μm. Spherules are generally low in number, often associated with cellular aggregates, but often they are not evident or easily identified. Usually their internal structure is not easily discernable, but occasionally endospores are seen in association with ruptured spherules (Fig. 83.10). The endospores are 2 to 5 μm in diameter, are surrounded by a thin, non-staining halo, and have small, round to oval, densely aggregated, eccentric nuclei. Endospores may be found extracellularly or within phagocytes. In one report, endospores were visualized in a fine-needle aspirate from a bone lesion in the absence of spherules.[24]

Because cytology is relatively insensitive for diagnosis of coccidioidomycosis when compared with other deep mycoses, serologic testing for coccidioidomycosis should always be considered when cytology of

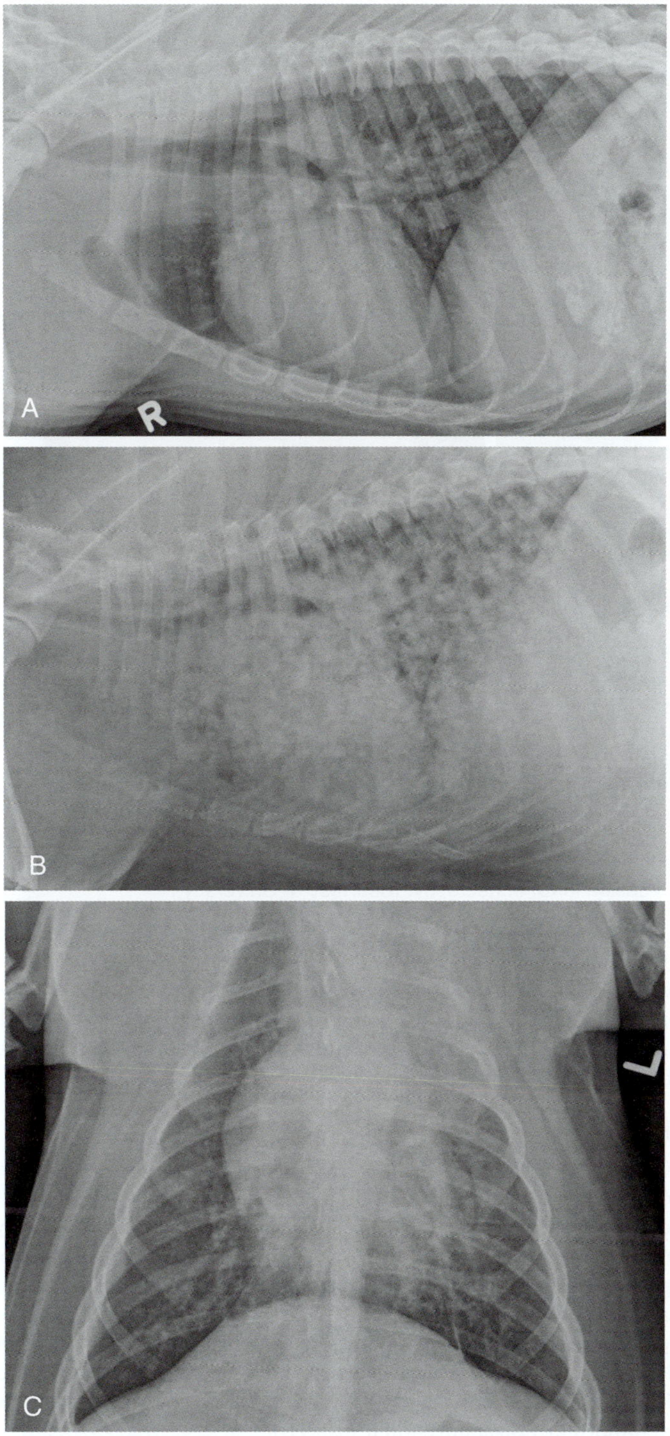

Fig. 83.6 Thoracic radiographic patterns in coccidioidomycosis. (A) Lateral thoracic radiograph from a 7-year-old intact male English pointer that shows severe tracheobronchial lymphadenomegaly and focal pulmonary infiltrates. (B) Lateral thoracic radiograph from a 3-year-old intact female Rottweiler with cough, anorexia, and respiratory distress. There are diffuse nodular and peribronchial infiltrates throughout the pulmonary parenchyma and possible hilar lymphadenopathy. Necropsy revealed necrogranulomatous interstitial pneumonia with intralesional spherules. The spleen, liver, and kidney were also involved. (C) Dorsoventral thoracic radiograph from a 2-year-old female spayed Labrador retriever with cough and inappetence. There is an alveolar pattern in the left cranial lung lobe.

tissue aspirates, body fluids, or lung washes reveals pyogranulomatous, suppurative, or granulomatous inflammation but organisms are not seen, and exposure to *Coccidioides* is possible based on the history.

Serologic Diagnosis

Serologic assays that detect antibodies to *Coccidioides* spp. are important diagnostic tests for coccidioidomycosis because organism detection assays have low sensitivity. Most diagnostic laboratories screen serum specimens with qualitative gel immunodiffusion (ID) assays for IgG or IgM antibodies (see Chapter 2). Detection of IgM (tube precipitin) or IgG (complement fixating) antibodies is reported, depending on the antigen preparation used in the assay. In dogs, IgM is detectable within 2 to 5 weeks of infection, and IgG appears after 8 to 12 weeks.[19] Quantification of an IgG antibody response can then be performed with quantitative ID, whereby serial dilutions of patient serum are subjected to gel ID.[26] In human patients, the complement fixation test is often used for quantification of IgG antibody, but frequent false-positive results have been described with this method in dogs as a result of anticomplementary properties of canine serum.[42] The complement fixation test is positive in most cats with coccidioidomycosis, with titers that range from 1:2 to 1:128.[23]

False-negative serologic test results are extremely rare in dogs with coccidioidomycosis tested at the author's institution,[18,34] but they have been described in dogs from Arizona[42–44] and rarely in cats.[22] False-negative results can occur in early infection and therefore sometimes a follow-up serologic test should be performed a few weeks later if clinical suspicion for coccidioidomycosis still remains. False-negative serologic test results can occur in immunocompromised patients. In people, false-negative results have been reported in forms of disease with a more benign clinical course, such as patients with isolated pulmonary nodules.

Positive antibody titers usually range from 1:2 to 1:256; the median titer was 1:32 in one study.[18] There appears to be no clear correlation between the magnitude of the IgG titer and the severity of illness in dogs. Dogs with active infection can have titers as low as 1:2, and healthy dogs in hyperendemic areas in Arizona can have titers as high as 1:16.[26] As a result, positive titers of 1:16 or lower should always be interpreted in light of clinicopathologic abnormalities and, in hyperendemic areas, other diagnostic tests (such as cytology or histopathology) should also be used to confirm the diagnosis if possible. Rapid antibody-detection assays have been developed, including enzyme immunoassays (EIAs) and an immunochromatographic lateral flow assay (LFA). A commercially available EIA (MiraVista Laboratories, Indianapolis, IN, USA) was evaluated in dogs compared to AGID and determined to have a sensitivity of 89.2% and specificity of 97.2%.[46] Although this assay is rapid compared to conventional gel ID, it requires shipment of specimens to a commercial laboratory, specialized training, and equipment to perform with delays in the time to diagnosis. A POC LFA for detection of antibodies to *Coccidioides* (Sōna LFA, IMMY Diagnostics, OK, USA), which received FDA approval for diagnosis of human coccidioidomycosis, has recently been assessed for the diagnosis of coccidioidomycosis in dogs. In a study from Arizona, an overall agreement of 87.5% was noted between the LFA and conventional gel ID.[47] Another study from the UC Davis VMTH revealed a sensitivity of 89% and a specificity of 100% when compared with conventional gel ID.[48] False negatives were observed in dogs with low gel ID titers, and so confirmatory testing is needed if the clinical suspicion for coccidioidomycosis remains. Otherwise, this assay represents an excellent rapid alternative to conventional gel ID.

A serologic assay that detects *Coccidioides* antigen in urine is available for diagnosis of coccidioidomycosis in human patients, such as in immunocompromised patients that lack the ability to produce significant quantities of antibody. However, preliminary data suggest that

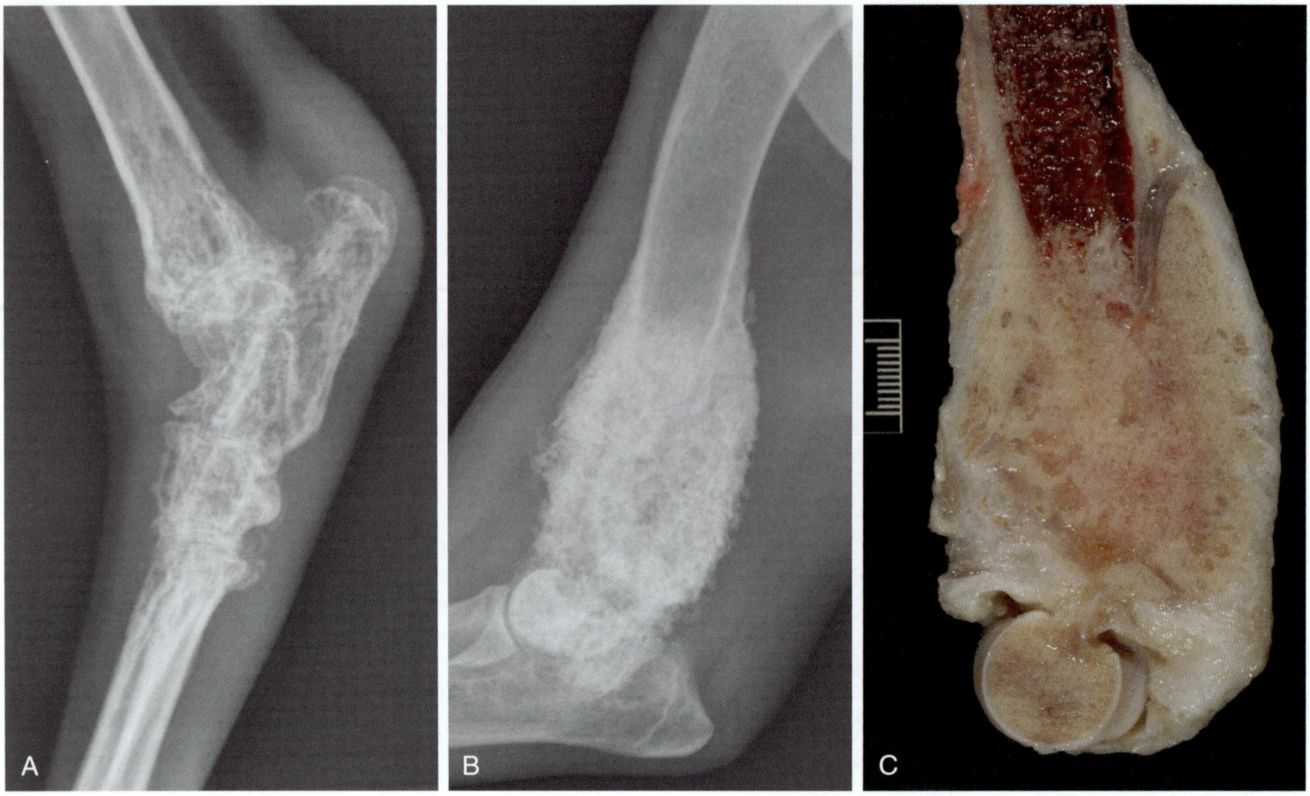

Fig. 83.7 Osteomyelitis caused by *Coccidioides* spp. (A) Left tarsus of a 4-year-old female spayed Dalmatian that was evaluated for signs of right-sided congestive heart failure due to pericarditis. Severe osteolysis is present. (B) Right humerus of a 4-year-old female spayed shepherd mix. There is a mixed productive and lytic lesion of the distal diaphysis of the right humerus. (C) Lesion in (B) at necropsy. (Courtesy of University of California, Davis Veterinary Anatomic Pathology Service.)

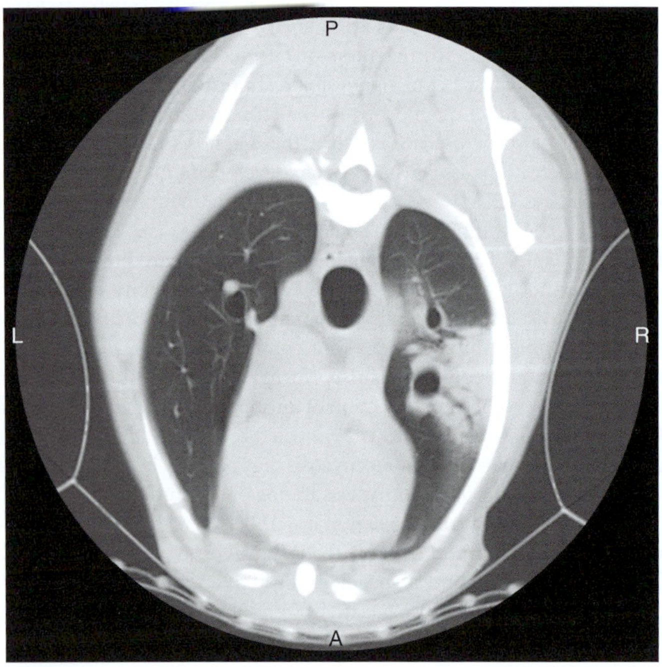

Fig. 83.8 CT scan of the thorax of a 2-year-old intact male Labrador retriever with coccidioidomycosis. There are infiltrates in the caudal aspect of the right cranial lung lobe which extend from the mediastinum to the pleural surface. The walls of the right cranial bronchus and associated airways are thickened. Bronchial lymphadenomegaly was also identified.

this assay has unacceptable sensitivity (≤ 20%) for diagnosis of canine coccidioidomycosis when serum, urine, or both specimens are tested, and false-positive reactions occur in a small proportion of dogs with blastomycosis or histoplasmosis.[49]

Fungal Culture

Coccidioides spp. can sometimes be isolated from clinical specimens on routine fungal media in the laboratory, but a negative culture result does not rule out coccidioidomycosis. Growth of a gray-white, downy mold that is tan to brown when visualized through the bottom of the plate usually appears after incubation for several days. The organism can be identified based on its light microscopic appearance, with or without molecular methods. Culture of *Coccidioides* spp. is a serious laboratory health hazard, and should be done by suitably equipped laboratories. The clinician should warn the laboratory of the possibility of dimorphic fungal infection if suspected.

Molecular Diagnosis Using Nucleic Acid–Based Testing

Real-time PCR assays have been used for rapid detection of *Coccidioides* spp. in respiratory specimens or CSF from affected humans, although sensitivity has been limited.[4,50] PCR assays have also been used in epidemiological studies to identify major growth sites for *Coccidioides* spp. in soil.[51] PCR assays have not yet been widely applied to the diagnosis of coccidioidomycosis in dogs and cats.

Pathologic Findings

Gross pathologic findings in dogs with coccidioidomycosis include mottling and consolidation of the pulmonary parenchyma; single

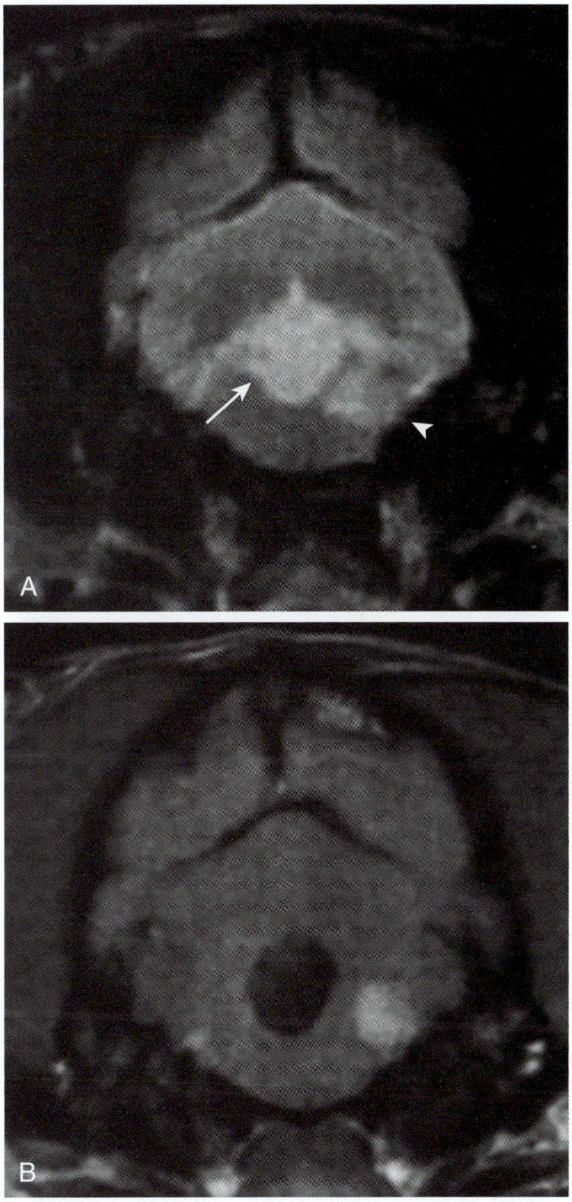

Fig. 83.9 MRI scan of the brain of a 7-year-old male neutered shih tzu with disseminated coccidioidomycosis. (A) A small focus of increased signal intensity on T2-weighting is present in the left lateral aspect of the brainstem *(arrowhead)*. Ventricular dilation is also present *(arrow)*. (B) T1-weighted image after administration of gadolinium. The lesion in the brainstem is contrast enhancing.

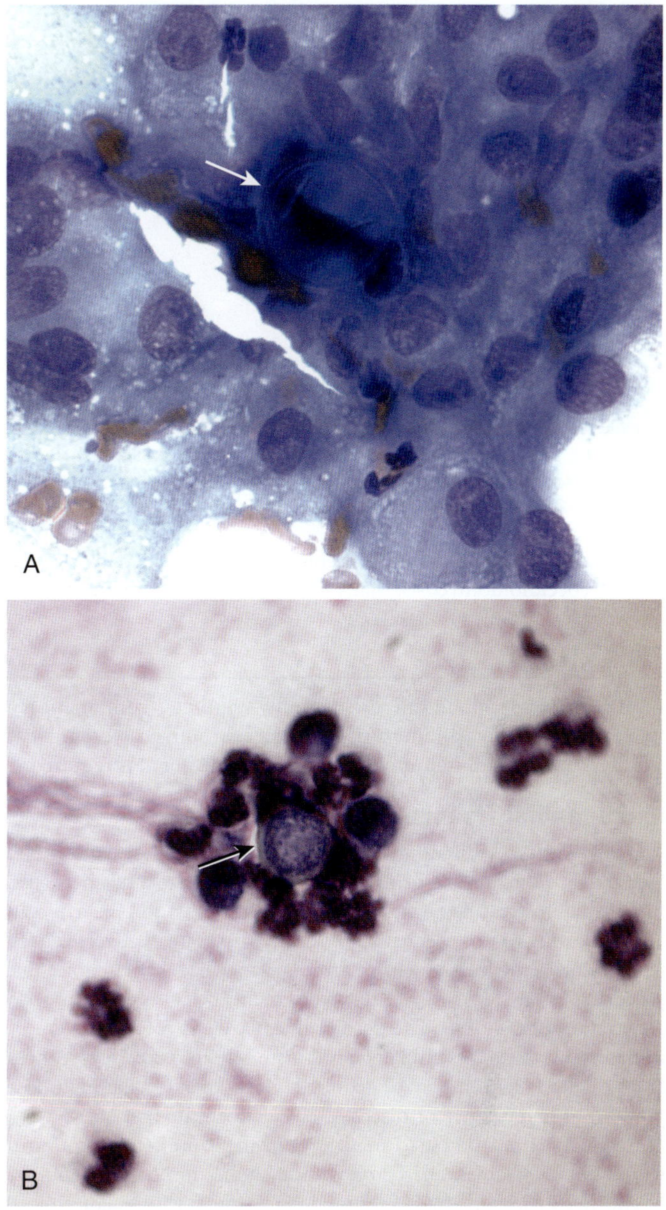

Fig. 83.10 Cytologic appearance of *Coccidioides* spp. spherules. (A) Spherules often appear as deeply basophilic, crinkled, intact, or ruptured ball-like structures *(arrow)*. (B) Sometimes, a refractile spherule wall is appreciated *(arrow)* and endospores are visualized within the spherule as granular material.

or multiple, pale masses, nodular lesions, or emphysematous bullae within the lungs (Fig. 83.11); enlarged and firm tracheobronchial, mediastinal or sternal lymph nodes; plaque-like lesions on the pleura; and pleural and pericardial effusion. The interior of masses or nodules may be firm, caseous, or liquefied. The pericardium and epicardium may be thickened with mass lesions and adhesions between the pericardium and epicardium.[34] Ascites may also be present in dogs with pericarditis. Dogs with disseminated disease may have diffuse muscle atrophy, one or more enlarged peripheral lymph nodes, irregular bony swellings with associated draining skin lesions, and/or evidence of arthritis and synovitis. Meningoencephalitis may be evident as mass lesions within the brain parenchyma, ventricular dilation secondary to obstruction of CSF flow by inflammatory lesions, regional discoloration within the brain, and/or discoloration and thickening of the meninges. Rarely prostatic enlargement, hepatic congestion and friability, multifocal nodular lesions within the myocardium or other parenchymal organs, and ocular lesions are present.

Histopathology of affected tissues reveals large numbers of neutrophils and macrophages and sometimes marked fibrosis, with occasional endosporulating or non-endosporulating spherules. Multinucleated giant cells may be present and can contain spherules.[41] Spherules have a thick wall and endospores may be visualized in mature spherules (Fig. 83.12). Often only one or two spherules are visualized, and in some cases they are not found at all. Use of special stains such as PAS and Gomori's methenamine silver can enhance organism identification within lesions. The presence of large numbers of spherules has been described in some affected cats.[37,52] Histopathologic lesions consistent

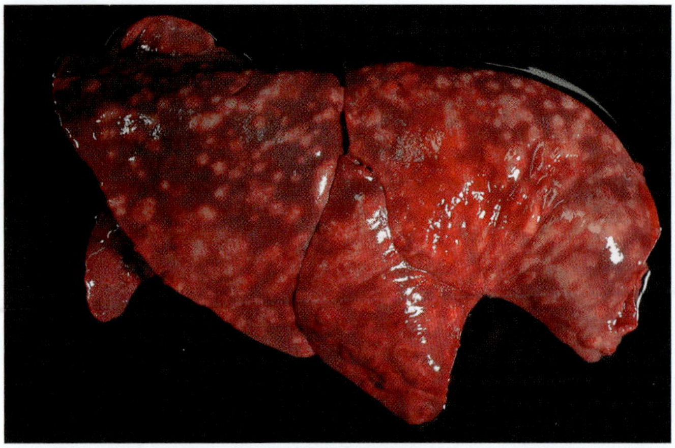

Fig. 83.11 Lungs of the dog in Figure 83.6B. Multiple pale nodules are present throughout the lung parenchyma.

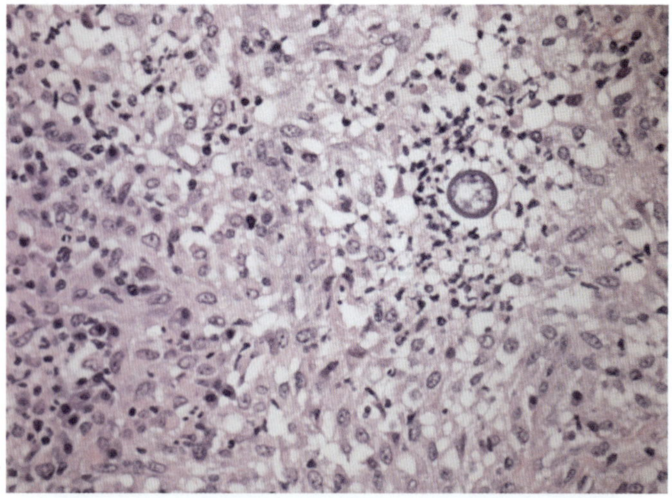

Fig. 83.12 Histopathology of the tarsus of the dog in Figure 83.7A. A single mature spherule is surrounded by a pyogranulomatous inflammatory response. The spherule contains large numbers of endospores.

with immune complex glomerulonephritis were described in dogs with chronic coccidioidomycosis. Many of those dogs had proteinuria.[38]

TREATMENT

Treatment of coccidioidomycosis typically requires a combination of antifungal drug therapy and supportive care; in some cases, surgery is required. Usually a minimum of 6 months of treatment is required.

Antimicrobial Treatment

Animals with coccidioidomycosis can respond well to azole monotherapy with fluconazole or itraconazole. Ketoconazole has been used successfully to treat dogs and cats in the past but is no longer recommended owing to its lower activity and increased rate of adverse effects. Fluconazole is the least expensive azole and may be a better choice than itraconazole for dogs with CNS involvement, because of its superior penetration of the CNS. The dose of fluconazole is 5 to 10 mg/kg PO q12h; for dogs with disseminated or refractory pulmonary disease, doses of 10 mg/kg PO q12h may be required. Occasionally, such high doses can lead to inappetence or diarrhea, especially in the first 1 to 2 weeks of treatment. Itraconazole (5 mg/kg PO q24h) is preferred for animals with bone involvement, based on clinical studies in people,[53] and may be effective in dogs that fail to respond to treatment with fluconazole. In human patients, itraconazole demonstrated a greater response rate in a blinded comparison with fluconazole.[53] Compounded formulations of itraconazole should be avoided. Small dogs are best treated with itraconazole suspension (10 mg/mL), which has higher bioavailability than the capsules (see Chapter 11). If capsules are used, they should be administered with food. If clinical signs do not improve with azole treatment, therapeutic drug monitoring could be considered to ensure serum drug concentrations are adequate. Periodic monitoring of liver enzymes is recommended for animals treated with azole antifungals.

Treatment with deoxycholate or lipid-complexed amphotericin B is recommended either alone or in combination with an azole for dogs with refractory disease or severe disease (see Chapter 11 for dosing protocols). However, studies that compare amphotericin B to azole therapy in dogs have not been performed. Combination therapy with an azole and terbinafine are anecdotally reported as beneficial in some dogs that become refractory to single azole treatment.[25] Controlled studies are lacking. Voriconazole and posaconazole have excellent *in vivo* activity against *Coccidioides* spp. Both have been used to treat refractory coccidioidomycosis in human patients.[4] These have been used to treat affected dogs[54,55] but use has been limited by expense. Voriconazole could be considered for treatment of refractory meningoencephalitis if client finances permit its use, because it has excellent penetration of the CNS.

Nikkomycin Z is a narrow-spectrum anti-fungal drug with potent *in vitro* activity against *Coccidioides* spp. It inhibits the synthesis of chitin, a fungal cell wall component which mammals lack. This drug is currently under development as an orphan drug for the treatment of coccidioidomycosis in people, but its prospects for commercial development are unclear.[56] It has shown efficacy in naturally affected dogs and experimentally infected mice.[57,58]

Surgical Management

Ultimately, some dogs with severe and persistent osteomyelitis require amputation to control the infection, and enucleation may be required for dogs with endophthalmitis. In some situations, spinal surgery is required in cases of discospondylitis or intra-spinal granulomas that cause spinal cord compression.[59,60] Successful treatment of *Coccidioides* pericarditis has been reported after subtotal pericardiectomy and epicardial excision, which should be performed in conjunction with antifungal drug therapy. The perioperative mortality rate in one study was reported as 24%, and the 2-year survival rate after discharge was 82%.[34]

Supportive Care

Other treatments that may be required for dogs with severe pulmonary coccidioidomycosis are similar to those described for blastomycosis, and include oxygen supplementation, nebulization and coupage, drainage of thoracic effusions, nutritional support, anti-inflammatory drugs, and intravenous fluid therapy. Concurrent treatment with glucocorticoids and anti-seizure medications may be necessary to reduce the severity of neurologic signs in dogs with CNS coccidioidomycosis. Topical prednisolone acetate solution and anti-glaucoma agents may be required for dogs with ocular lesions.

PROGNOSIS

The prognosis for resolution for coccidioidomycosis depends on the severity of infection and the extent of dissemination. The duration of treatment ranges from 6 months to many years, and in some cases (such as with bone or CNS involvement), life-long treatment is needed. IgG antibody titers decrease with successful treatment, which in general should be continued until lesions resolve and the titer is 1:2 or lower.

Residual radiographic opacities may be present in some dogs as a result of scar tissue formation. Dogs with localized pulmonary infection have the best prognosis; the prognosis is less predictable for dogs with CNS involvement. Long-term clinical remissions have been described in dogs treated with fluconazole for CNS coccidioidomycosis in two recent reports from Arizona.[40,41] A 2021 report of 45 client-owned dogs with suspected intracranial coccidioidomycosis described a mean duration of follow-up of 22.4 ± 20.5 months.[40] Some dogs with *Coccidioides* osteomyelitis may require life-long azole therapy.[33]

IMMUNITY AND VACCINATION

Immunity to *Coccidioides* spp. depends primarily on cell-mediated immunity, specifically T lymphocytes. No vaccine is currently available commercially for prevention of the disease, but the potential for effective immunization exists because recovered individuals rarely become reinfected. A variety of vaccine strategies have been examined for prevention of human coccidioidomycosis.[3] One candidate is a deletion mutant strain of *C. posadasii* that lacks a homolog of the gene *CPS1*, a virulence factor found in a maize pathogen. Vaccination of mice with this deletion mutant strain has protected mice from lethal infection with *C. posadasii* and *C. immitis*, and a vaccine based on this strain is currently under development for prevention of Valley fever in dogs.[3] An initial challenge study in a limited number of research beagles showed protection from disease following a prime followed by booster vaccination; subcutaneous swelling at the site of vaccination was the main adverse effect.[61] A single vaccination did not result in protection. Should this vaccine be successful, it may be a model for human vaccination.

PREVENTION

Prevention of coccidioidomycosis requires avoidance of hyperendemic areas (especially parts of Arizona and south-central California), which may not be possible. In endemic areas, dogs should be kept away from sites of soil disturbance (such as construction sites), and housed indoors during dust storms; digging should be discouraged. Housing dogs indoors during the day in endemic regions may reduce the chance of infection. Nevertheless, it should be remembered that clinical infections only develop in a minority of exposed dogs.

PUBLIC HEALTH ASPECTS

Coccidioidomycosis is a serious infection in human patients and has similar clinical manifestations to those described in dogs. As noted earlier in this chapter, coccidioidomycosis is considered an emerging infectious disease, and its incidence in people has increased in Arizona and California in the last decade, possibly as a result of population growth, immigration of immunologically naïve people, and construction. In an endemic area, construction and agricultural workers, archeologists, and excavators are at high risk for coccidioidomycosis.[2,4] African American and Filipino patients, as well as patients with AIDS and other causes of immunosuppression and women in the third trimester of pregnancy and immediately post-partum are at highest risk for disseminated disease, which occurs in approximately 1% to 3% of infected humans.[2]

Because of their susceptibility to infection, dogs have been used as a sentinel for human exposure to environmental sources of *Coccidioides* spp. in seroprevalence studies.[20,62] Direct transmission between infected veterinary patients and humans has not been reported. However, fatal disease occurred in a veterinary resident after necropsy of a horse with disseminated disease.[63] Inoculation coccidioidomycosis was reported in a veterinary technician from Arizona after a bite from a cat that was later diagnosed with disseminated disease.[37]

Inoculation coccidioidomycosis also has the potential to occur if sharps injuries occur during aspiration of affected tissues, surgical procedures, or necropsy examinations. Proper sedation or anesthesia should always be used if coccidioidomycosis is suspected in dogs or cats seen at veterinary clinics and the potential for a sharps injury exists. If accidental inoculation occurs, immediate attention should be sought from a physician. Prolonged fluconazole prophylaxis is generally recommended with monitoring of *Coccidioides* serology and liver function tests. Bandaging of skin lesions should be avoided because of a concern for conversion of the organism to a mycelial form in drying organic matter exposed to air, although no documented instances of transmission through exposure to bandages exist. Necropsies should be performed without delay with suitable protective clothing, and the carcasses of animals that die from coccidioidomycosis should immediately be incinerated. For the same reason, burial is not recommended because of the potential for contamination of the environment. Fluconazole prophylaxis is also indicated after accidental laboratory exposure to inocula.[64]

PARACOCCIDIOIDOMYCOSIS

Paracoccidioidomycosis is a severe systemic mycosis, almost exclusively of people, endemic in Latin America (Brazil, Argentina, Colombia, Ecuador, and Venezuela). The etiologic agents are organisms that belong to the *Paracoccidioides* species complex, such as *Paracoccidioides brasiliensis* and *Paracoccidioides lutzii*.[65,66] The eco-epidemiological niche of those fungi is not well characterized.[67] The main clinical characteristics in people are development of granulomatous lesions in the lungs, lymph nodes, liver, spleen, and skin.[68] Infections result from inhalation of conidia. *Paracoccidioides* spp. have been rarely recovered from animals. To date, the fungus has been isolated from a variety of avian and mammalian species, including three dogs and a cat.[49,52,69] Serologic studies have shown that other wild animals had contact with the fungus but did not develop signs of the disease. Serologic studies in Brazil showed seroprevalence of 31.6% in cats[67] and 14.8% to 80.5% in dogs.[70] Seropositivity was higher in dogs and cats living in rural areas.[70] There are only three case reports of clinical disease in dogs. The dogs all had peripheral lymphadenomegaly, and variable evidence of other organ involvement (pneumonia, hepatosplenomegaly, epididymitis, or pyogranulomatous dermatitis),[65,69,71] resembling clinical signs described in humans. The organism was found in peripheral lymph nodes using cytologic examination or histopathology and the organism was definitively identified using culture (which can take 20 to 30 days for growth to occur) and/or molecular methods.[65,69,71] In cytologic preparations, the organism is 10 to 20 µm in diameter, oval to elongated in shape, and has a thick cell wall; simultaneous side-by-side budding of two or more daughter cells from the parent cell has led to the description of a "Mickey Mouse" and "pilot-wheel" appearance in the literature (Fig. 83.13A and B).[69] There is a granulomatous inflammatory response, and multinucleated giant cells may be present.[69] On histopathology, the organism may be difficult to distinguish from other fungal pathogens when the characteristic budding pattern is not identified (Fig. 83.13C). Itraconazole is the drug of choice and was associated with good clinical responses in dogs.[65,69,71] Paracoccidioidomycosis was diagnosed in a cat that presented with general systemic and neurologic signs. The cat was treated successfully with fluconazole and amphotericin B.[72] Paracoccidioidomycosis should be considered as a differential diagnosis for dogs and cats that reside within endemic regions, and it should be considered when yeast-like structures that resemble organisms such as *Sporothrix*, *Cryptococcus*, or *Blastomyces* are seen in tissues on histopathology. Increased awareness of this disease in endemic regions may lead to recognition of more cases.

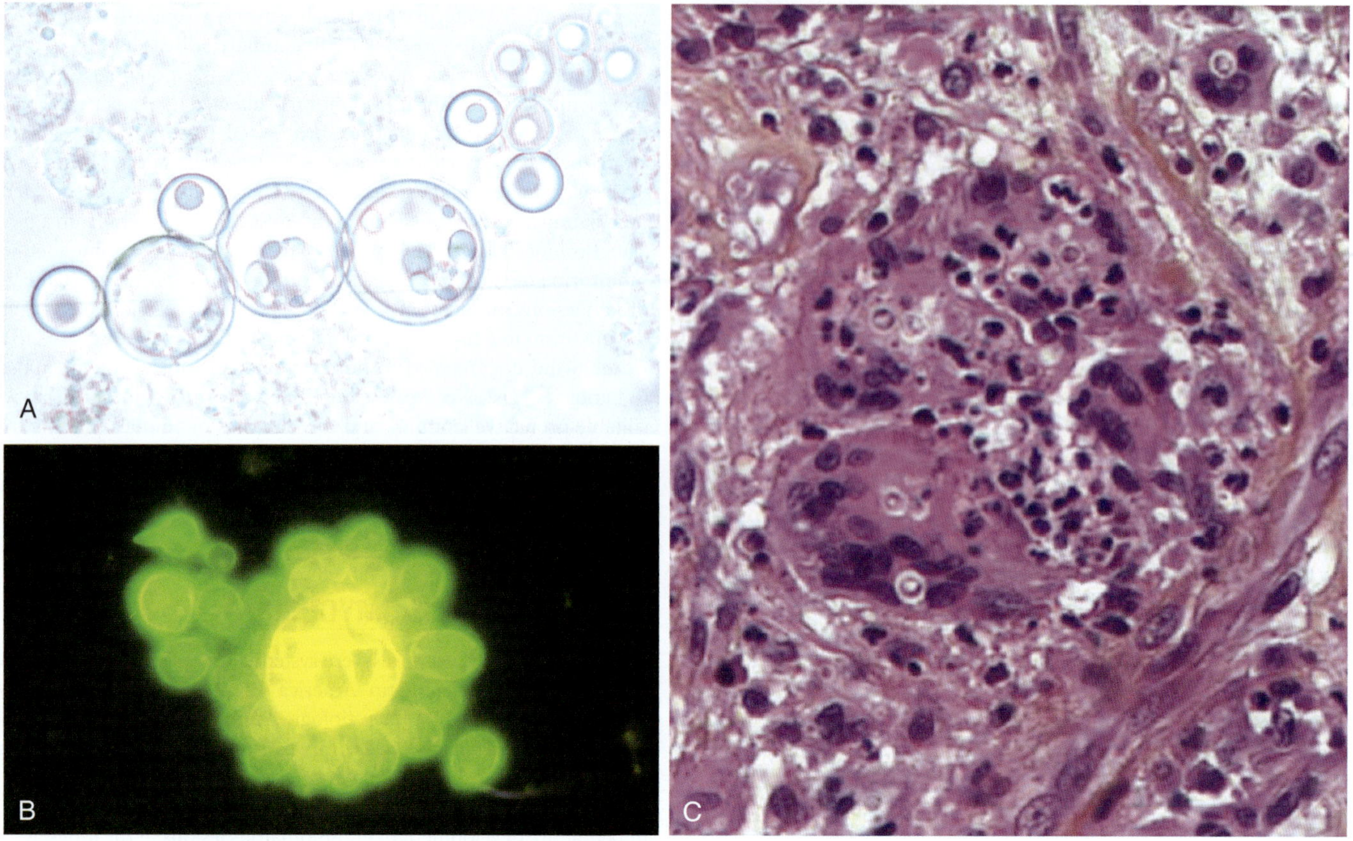

Fig. 83.13 *Paracoccidioides brasiliensis* in specimens from human patients. (A) Multiple budding and variation in cell size are apparent (potassium hydroxide preparation from purulent material, ×1000). Note the "Mickey Mouse" appearance of the organism on the left with two budding daughter cells at the 9 and 1 o'clock positions. (B) Multiple buds surrounding the parent cell are observed in a wet mount from a 36°C culture (calcofluor, ×1000). (C) Histopathologic appearance of yeast cells in tissue demonstrating multiple budding and mononuclear cell infiltration (hematoxylin and eosin stain, ×400). (From Restrepo-Moreno A, Tobón-Orozco AM, González-Marín A. Paracoccidioidomycosis. In: *Mandell, Douglas, and Bennett's Principles and Practice of Infectious Diseases*, 9th ed. Philadelphia: Elsevier; 2020:3211–3221.)

CASE EXAMPLE

Signalment

"Jenny," a 2-year-old female spayed Labrador retriever from Oxnard in southwestern California.

History

Jenny was evaluated for a 2-month history of cough, inappetence, and lethargy. For the first 3 days of illness, the owner noted only an intermittent harsh, nonproductive cough. On day 4 of illness, the dog became lethargic and inappetent, so she was taken to a local veterinary clinic. Thoracic radiographs revealed alveolar infiltrates in the left cranial lung lobe. A diagnosis of bacterial pneumonia was suspected, so Jenny was treated with enrofloxacin (6 mg/kg PO q24h), clavulanic acid-amoxicillin (12.5 mg/kg PO q12h), and metronidazole (8 mg/kg PO q12h) for 2 weeks. After the first week of treatment, there was no improvement, so a long-acting cephalosporin was administered (cefovecin, 8 mg/kg, SC, once). Two days later, treatment with prednisone (0.3 mg/kg PO q12h) was initiated which was followed by only mild improvement in the clinical signs. Jenny's owner then sought a second opinion on day 20 after onset of clinical signs, and *Coccidioides* serology was performed. The titer was positive for IgG at 1:64. The prednisone was discontinued and treatment was initiated with fluconazole (6.7 mg/kg PO q12h). However, after 1 month of treatment, there had been no clinical improvement and thoracic radiographs were unchanged. The fluconazole was substituted with a compounded itraconazole formulation (5 mg/kg PO q12h). However, after an additional 2 weeks of treatment there had been no further improvement in the cough, so the owner sought a third opinion at the University of California, Davis.

According to the owner, Jenny had a poor appetite for dog food but was eating home-cooked chicken, rice, and vegetables. Her activity level had been low. The cough occurred many times throughout the day and was unrelated to exercise and eating. Occasionally she had paroxysms of cough with a terminal retch. Other medical history included canine parvovirus infection when she was 8 weeks old and "kennel cough" when she was 9 months old, which resolved after 10 days. The owners lived in a semi-rural area just north of Los Angeles. The only travel had been to Atascadero further north on the California coast. She was the only animal in the household. There had been ongoing construction around the house to replace a septic system with a sewer, which began approximately 4 to 6 weeks before the onset of clinical signs.

Physical Examination

General: Quiet but alert and responsive, hydrated. T = 102.6°F (39.2°C), P = 100 beats/min, R = 24 breaths/min, CRT = 1 s.

Eyes, ears, nose, and throat: No ocular abnormalities noted. A dilated fundoscopic examination was unremarkable.

Musculoskeletal: BCS 4/9. The dog was ambulatory with no lameness or muscle atrophy.

Cardiovascular, GI, genitourinary, and lymph nodes: No clinically significant abnormalities were detected.

CASE EXAMPLE—cont'd

Imaging Findings

Thoracic radiographs were compared to the two-view thoracic study performed 2 weeks previously, which were available for review. The initial radiographs showed a dense alveolar pattern throughout the left cranial lung lobe and increased opacity in the region of the hilar lymph nodes with splaying of the mainstem bronchi (see Fig. 83.6C). These abnormalities improved slightly in the 10-day recheck interim, but alveolar infiltrates were still present throughout the left cranial lung lobe. There was a persistent, mild, diffuse pulmonary interstitial pattern in the remaining pulmonary parenchyma, which was most severe in the caudodorsal lung fields. This was considered excessive for the age of the patient. The cardiovascular structures were within normal limits.

Microbiologic Testing

Coccidioides serology: Positive by qualitative gel immunodiffusion for complement fixing antibody (IgG), negative for IgM. Quantitative immunodiffusion revealed an IgG titer of 1:128.

Serum itraconazole concentration: < 0.31 μg/mL (undetectable).

Diagnosis

Pulmonary coccidioidomycosis.

Treatment

The itraconazole capsules prescribed at the previous veterinary clinic were examined and found to contain a white powder rather than granules. Treatment was changed to brand name itraconazole (Sporonox), because compounded formulations can be unstable. Instructions were given to administer the itraconazole (5 mg/kg PO q24h) with food to improve absorption. Aspirin was also prescribed (12 mg/kg PO q12h). One month later, Jenny's cough and activity level had improved considerably. A CBC was within normal limits and a biochemistry panel showed hypoalbuminemia (3.3 g/dL, reference range 3.4–4.3 g/dL) and hyperglobulinemia (3.4 g/dL, reference range 1.7–3.1 g/dL). Liver enzyme activities were within reference ranges. Thoracic radiographs showed resolution of hilar lymphadenopathy with persistence of the alveolar infiltrates in the left cranial lung lobe. The IgG antibody titer to *Coccidioides* was 1:64. Three months later the cough had resolved completely, and after 6 months of treatment, there was complete resolution of thoracic radiographic abnormalities and the titer was 1:32. At this point, the owner switched to a generic formulation of itraconazole due to financial concerns. After an additional 3 and 6 months of treatment, the IgG titer was 1:16 and 1:8, respectively, with no further clinical signs. Treatment was continued for an additional 3 months (i.e., total of 15 months of treatment), and the dog remains alive at the time of writing.

Comments

This is an interesting case of pulmonary coccidioidomycosis that occurred outside the hyperendemic central valley region in California. Exposure may have resulted from soil disturbance as a result of sewer work. Because of the low suspicion for the disease, the disease was mistaken for bacterial pneumonia. The owner had limited financial resources, so an extensive respiratory workup (including respiratory lavage with cytology and culture) was declined. When *Coccidioides* serology was positive, fluconazole was prescribed, but there was no improvement. The decision to treat with a compounded formulation of itraconazole was made because of client financial limitations, but serum drug levels with this treatment were undetectable. Fortunately, disease ultimately resolved with a change to a noncompounded formulation, and there was progressive decline in serial IgG titers (which were always performed by the same laboratory). Whether treatment beyond complete resolution of the radiographic abnormalities was necessary is debatable.

SUGGESTED READINGS

Kollath DR, Miller KJ, Barker BM. The mysterious desert dwellers: *Coccidioides immitis* and *Coccidioides posadasii*, causative fungal agents of coccidioidomycosis. *Virulence*. 2019;10:222–233.

Mehrkens LR, Mohr FC, Sykes JE. Clinicopathologic and histopathologic renal abnormalities in dogs with coccidioidomycosis. *J Vet Intern Med*. 2016;30:1667–1671.

Headley SA, Pretto-Giordano LG, Di Santis GW, et al. *Paracoccidioides brasiliensis*-associated dermatitis and lymphadenitis in a dog. *Mycopathologia*. 2017;182:425–434.

REFERENCES

1. Hirschmann JV. The early history of coccidioidomycosis: 1892-1945. *Clin Infect Dis*. 2007;44:1202–1207.
2. Stockamp NW, Thompson GR. *Coccidioidomycosis. Infect Dis Clin North Am*. 2016;30:229–246.
3. Van Dyke MCC, Thompson GR, Galgiani JN, et al. The rise of *Coccidioides*: forces against the dust devil unleashed. *Front Immunol*. 2019;10:2188.
4. Thompson GR. Pulmonary coccidioidomycosis. *Semin Respir Crit Care Med*. 2011;32:754–763.
5. Litvintseva AP, Marsden-Haug N, Hurst S, et al. Valley fever: finding new places for an old disease: *Coccidioides immitis* found in Washington state soil associated with recent human infection. *Clin Infect Dis*. 2015;60. e1-3.
6. James AE, McCall JR, Petersen KR, et al. A survey of veterinarians' knowledge, attitudes and practices regarding an emerging disease: coccidioidomycosis in Washington state. *Zoonoses Public Health*. 2020;67:25–34.
7. Kollath DR, Miller KJ, Barker BM. The mysterious desert dwellers: *Coccidioides immitis* and *Coccidioides posadasii*, causative fungal agents of coccidioidomycosis. *Virulence*. 2019;10:222–233.
8. Centers for Disease Control and Prevention. Increase in reported coccidioidomycosis—United States, 1998-2011. *Morb Mortal Wkly Rep*. 2013;62:217–221.
9. Galgiani JN. Coccidioidomycosis (*Coccidioides* species). In: Bennett JE, Dolin R, Blaser MJ, eds. *Mandell, Douglas, and Bennett's Principles and Practice of Infectious Diseases*. Philadelphia, PA: Elsevier Saunders; 2020:3190–3200.
10. Benedict K, McCotter OZ, Brady S, et al. Surveillance for coccidioidomycosis—United States, 2011-2017. *MMWR Surveill Summ*. 2019;68:1–15.
11. Ramani R, Chaturvedi V. Antifungal susceptibility profiles of *Coccidioides immitis* and *Coccidioides posadasii* from endemic and non-endemic areas. *Mycopathologia*. 2007;163:315–319.
12. Fisher MC, Koenig GL, White TJ, et al. Molecular and phenotypic description of *Coccidioides posadasii* sp. nov., previously recognized as the non-California population of *Coccidioides immitis*. *Mycologia*. 2002;94:73–84.
13. Luna-Isaac JA, Muniz-Salazar R, Baptista-Rosas RC, et al. Genetic analysis of the endemic fungal pathogens *Coccidioides posadasii* and *Coccidioides immitis* in Mexico. *Med Mycol*. 2014;52:156–166.
14. Flynn NM, Hoeprich PD, Kawachi MM, et al. An unusual outbreak of windborne coccidioidomycosis. *N Engl J Med*. 1979;301:358–361.
15. Schneider E, Hajjeh RA, Spiegel RA, et al. A coccidioidomycosis outbreak following the Northridge, Calif, earthquake. *JAMA*. 1997;277:904–908.
16. Park BJ, Sigel K, Vaz V, et al. An epidemic of coccidioidomycosis in Arizona associated with climatic changes, 1998-2001. *J Infect Dis*. 2005;191:1981–1987.
17. Maddy KT. Disseminated coccidioidomycosis of the dog. *J Am Vet Med Assoc*. 1958;132:483–489.
18. Johnson LR, Herrgesell EJ, Davidson AP, et al. Clinical, clinicopathologic, and radiographic findings in dogs with coccidioidomycosis: 24 cases (1995-2000). *J Am Vet Med Assoc*. 2003;222:461–466.
19. Davidson AP, Pappagianis D. Canine coccidioidomycosis: 1970 to 1993. In: *5th International Conference on Coccidioidomycosis*. CA: Stanford University; 1994:155–162.

20. Grayzel SE, Martinez-Lopez B, Sykes JE. Risk factors and spatial distribution of canine coccidioidomycosis in California, 2005-2013. *Transbound Emerg Dis.* 2017;64:1110–1119.
21. Butkiewicz CD, Shubitz LE, Dial SM. Risk factors associated with *Coccidioides* infection in dogs. *J Am Vet Med Assoc.* 2005;226:1851–1854.
22. Arbona N, Butkiewicz CD, Keyes M, et al. Clinical features of cats diagnosed with coccidioidomycosis in Arizona, 2004-2018. *J Feline Med Surg.* 2020;22:129–137.
23. Greene RT, Troy GC. Coccidioidomycosis in 48 cats: a retrospective study (1984-1993). *J Vet Intern Med.* 1995;9:86–91.
24. Beaudin S, Rich LJ, Meinkoth JH, et al. Draining skin lesion from a desert poodle. *Vet Clin Pathol.* 2005;34:65–68.
25. Simoes DM, Dial SM, Coyner KS, et al. Retrospective analysis of cutaneous lesions in 23 canine and 17 feline cases of coccidioidomycosis seen in Arizona, USA (2009-2015). *Vet Dermatol.* 2016;27:346-e387.
26. Shubitz LE, Butkiewicz CD, Dial SM, et al. Incidence of *Coccidioides* infection among dogs residing in a region in which the organism is endemic. *J Am Vet Med Assoc.* 2005;226:1846–1850.
27. Millman TM, O'Brien TR, Suter PF, et al. Coccidioidomycosis in the dog: its radiographic diagnosis. *J Am Vet Radiol Soc.* 1979;20:50–65.
28. Burtch M. Granulomatous meningitis caused by *Coccidioides immitis* in a dog. *J Am Vet Med Assoc.* 1998;212:827–829.
29. Pryor WH Jr, Huizenga CG, Splitter GA, et al. *Coccidioides immitis* encephalitis in two dogs. *J Am Vet Med Assoc.* 1972;161:1108–1112.
30. Bentley RT, Heng HG, Thompson C, et al. Magnetic resonance imaging features and outcome for solitary central nervous system *Coccidioides* granulomas in 11 dogs and cats. *Vet Radiol Ultrasound.* 2015;56:520–530.
31. Angell JA, Merideth RE, Shively JN, et al. Ocular lesions associated with coccidioidomycosis in dogs: 35 cases (1980-1985). *J Am Vet Med Assoc.* 1987;190:1319–1322.
32. Shively JN, Whiteman CE. Ocular lesions in disseminated coccidioidomycosis in 2 dogs. *Pathol Vet.* 1970;7:1–6.
33. Shaver SL, Foy DS, Carter TD. Clinical features, treatment, and outcome of dogs with *Coccidioides* osteomyelitis. *J Am Vet Med Assoc.* 2022;260:63–70.
34. Heinritz CK, Gilson SD, Soderstrom MJ, et al. Subtotal pericardectomy and epicardial excision for treatment of coccidioidomycosis-induced effusive-constrictive pericarditis in dogs: 17 cases (1999-2003). *J Am Vet Med Assoc.* 2005;227:435–440.
35. Angell JA, Shively JN, Merideth RE, et al. Ocular coccidioidomycosis in a cat. *J Am Vet Med Assoc.* 1985;187:167–169.
36. Tofflemire K, Betbeze C. Three cases of feline ocular coccidioidomycosis: presentation, clinical features, diagnosis, and treatment. *Vet Ophthalmol.* 2010;13:166–172.
37. Gaidici A, Saubolle MA. Transmission of coccidioidomycosis to a human via a cat bite. *J Clin Microbiol.* 2009;47:505–506.
38. Mehrkens LR, Mohr FC, Sykes JE. Clinicopathologic and histopathologic renal abnormalities in dogs with coccidioidomycosis. *J Vet Intern Med.* 2016;30:1667–1671.
39. Sykes JE. Unpublished observations. 2020.
40. Kelley AJ, Stainback LB, Knowles KE, et al. Clinical characteristics, magnetic resonance imaging features, treatment, and outcome for presumed intracranial coccidioidomycosis in 45 dogs (2009-2019). *J Vet Intern Med.* 2021;35:2222–2231.
41. Spoor E, Stainback L, Plummer S, et al. A novel form of intracranial coccidioidomycosis is present in dogs and exhibits characteristic clinical and magnetic resonance imaging findings. *Vet Radiol Ultrasound.* 2019;60:47–55.
42. Gershman N, Villaba W, Neel K. Detection of canine IgG and IgM antibodies to *Coccidioides immitis* using a novel enzyme-linked immunosorbent assay (EIA) method. In: *5th International Conference on Coccidioidomycosis.* CA: Stanford University; 1994:137–146.
43. Gunstra A, Steurer JA, Seibert RL, et al. Sensitivity of serologic testing for dogs diagnosed with coccidioidomycosis on histology: 52 cases (2012-2013). *J Am Anim Hosp Assoc.* 2019;55:238–242.
44. Graupmann-Kuzma A, Valentine BA, Shubitz LF, et al. Coccidioidomycosis in dogs and cats: a review. *J Am Anim Hosp Assoc.* 2008;44:226–235.
45. Greene RT. Coccidioidomycosis and paracoccidioidomycosis. In: Greene CE, ed. *Infectious Diseases of the Dog and Cat.* 4th ed. St. Louis, MO: Elsevier Saunders; 2012:634–645.
46. Holbrook ED, Greene RT, Rubin SI, et al. Novel canine anti-*Coccidioides* immunoglobulin G enzyme immunoassay aids in diagnosis of coccidioidomycosis in dogs. *Med Mycol.* 2019;57:800–806.
47. Schlacks S, Vishkautsan P, Butkiewicz C, et al. Evaluation of a commercially available, point-of-care *Coccidioides* antibody lateral flow assay to aid in rapid diagnosis of coccidioidomycosis in dogs. *Med Mycol.* 2020;58:328–332.
48. Reagan KL, McHardy I, Thompson GR, et al. Clinical performance of a point-of-care *Coccidioides* antibody test in dogs. *J Vet Intern Med.* 2021;35:965–969.
49. Kirsch EJ, Greene RT, Prahl A, et al. Evaluation of *Coccidioides* antigen detection in dogs with coccidioidomycosis. *Clin Vaccine Immunol.* 2012;19:343–345.
50. Vucicevic D, Blair JE, Binnicker MJ, et al. The utility of *Coccidioides* polymerase chain reaction testing in the clinical setting. *Mycopathologia.* 2010;170:345–351.
51. Lauer A, Baal JD, Baal JC, et al. Detection of *Coccidioides immitis* in Kern County, California, by multiplex PCR. *Mycologia.* 2012;104:62–69.
52. Reed RE, Hoge RS, Trautman RJ. Coccidioidomycosis in two cats. *J Am Vet Med Assoc.* 1963;143:953–956.
53. Galgiani JN, Catanzaro A, Cloud GA, et al. Comparison of oral fluconazole and itraconazole for progressive, nonmeningeal coccidioidomycosis. A randomized, double-blind trial. Mycoses Study Group. *Ann Intern Med.* 2000;133:676–686.
54. Raghu C, Reagh C. Novel treatment of disseminated coccidioidomycosis in a dog with voriconazole. *Case Rep Vet Med.* 2018;2018:1785748.
55. Shubitz LF, Schlacks S, Vishkautsan P, et al. Posaconazole treatment of refractory coccidioidomycosis in dogs. *J Vet Intern Med.* 2021;35:2772–2777.
56. Larwood DJ. Nikkomycin Z ready to meet the promise? *J Fungi.* 2020;6:261.
57. Shubitz LF, Roy ME, Nix DE, et al. Efficacy of nikkomycin Z for respiratory coccidioidomycosis in naturally infected dogs. *Med Mycol.* 2013;51:747–754.
58. Shubitz LF, Trinh HT, Perrill RH, et al. Modeling nikkomycin Z dosing and pharmacology in murine pulmonary coccidioidomycosis preparatory to phase 2 clinical trials. *J Infect Dis.* 2014;209:1949–1954.
59. Foureman P, Longshore R, Plummer SB. Spinal cord granuloma due to *Coccidioides immitis* in a cat. *J Vet Intern Med.* 2005;19:373–376.
60. Dowdy H, Evans JE, Jaffey JE, et al. Case report: successful management of a compressive intraspinal *Coccidioides* species granuloma in a cat. *Front Vet Sci.* 2022;8:801885.
61. Shubitz LF, Robb EJ, Powell DA, et al. A *cps1* vaccine protects dogs against experimentally induced coccidioidomycosis. *Vaccine.* 2021;39:6894–6901.
62. Gautam R, Srinath I, Clavijo A, et al. Identifying areas of high risk of human exposure to coccidioidomycosis in Texas using serology data from dogs. *Zoonoses Public Health.* 2013;60:174–181.
63. Kohn GJ, Linne SR, Smith CM, et al. Acquisition of coccidioidomycosis at necropsy by inhalation of coccidioidal endospores. *Diagn Microbiol Infect Dis.* 1992;15:527–530.
64. Stevens DA, Clemons KV, Levine HB, et al. Expert opinion: what to do when there is *Coccidioides* exposure in a laboratory. *Clin Infect Dis.* 2009;49:919–923.
65. Ricci G, Mota FT, Wakamatsu A, et al. Canine paracoccidioidomycosis. *Med Mycol.* 2004;42:379–383.
66. de Oliveira HC, Assato PA, Marcos CM, et al. *Paracoccidioides*-host interaction: an overview on recent advances in the paracoccidioidomycosis. *Front Microbiol.* 2015;6:1319.
67. Oliveira GG, Belitardo DR, Balarin MR, et al. Serological survey of paracoccidioidomycosis in cats. *Mycopathologia.* 2013;176:299–302.
68. Restrepo A, Tobón-Orozco AM, González-Marin Á. Paracoccidioidomycosis. In: Bennett JE, Dolin R, Blaser MJ, eds. *Mandell, Douglas, and Bennett's Principles and Practice of Infectious Diseases.* Philadelphia, PA: Elsevier Saunders; 2020:3211–3221.
69. Headley SA, Pretto-Giordano LG, Di Santis GW, et al. *Paracoccidioides brasiliensis*-associated dermatitis and lymphadenitis in a dog. *Mycopathologia.* 2017;182:425–434.
70. Teles AJ, Klafke GB, Cabana AL, et al. Serological investigation into *Paracoccidioides brasiliensis* infection in dogs from Southern Rio Grande do Sul, Brazil. *Mycopathologia.* 2016;181:323–328.
71. de Farias MR, Condas LA, Ribeiro MG, et al. Paracoccidioidomycosis in a dog: case report of generalized lymphadenomegaly. *Mycopathologia.* 2011;172:147–152.
72. Gonzalez JF, Montiel NA, Maass RL. First report on the diagnosis and treatment of encephalic and urinary paracoccidioidomycosis in a cat. *J Feline Med Surg.* 2010;12:659–662.

84

Sporotrichosis

Luisa H.M. Miranda, Isabella D.F. Gremião, Sandro A. Pereira, Rodrigo C. Menezes, Tânia M.P. Schubach, Jane E. Sykes

KEY POINTS

- Cause: *Sporothrix* spp. (ascomycetes).
- First Described: *Sporothrix schenckii* was first described in 1896, in Maryland, United States, by Benjamin Schenk.[1]
- Affected Hosts: Infection has been reported principally in humans and cats, as well as in dogs and a variety of other mammalian and avian species.
- Geographic Distribution: Tropical, subtropical, and temperate zones worldwide.
- Route of Transmission: Cutaneous inoculation of conidia or yeasts, or less frequently, inhalation of conidia.
- Major Clinical Signs: Cutaneous nodules or ulcerated skin lesions, lymphangitis, lymphadenomegaly.
- Differential Diagnoses: Other systemic mycoses (especially cryptococcosis in cats), mycobacterial infections, nocardiosis or actinomycosis, cutaneous leishmaniosis, SCC, feline eosinophilic granuloma complex, feline herpesviral dermatitis, abscess, foreign body granulomas.
- Human Health Significance: Many human infections are acquired from the environment, but direct transmission can follow contact between infected cats and humans, and especially cat bites or scratches.

ETIOLOGIC AGENT AND EPIDEMIOLOGY

The fungal genus *Sporothrix* includes a group of thermodimorphic pathogens that cause human and animal infections.[1] These organisms are widespread in nature and have been isolated as a saprobe from senescent or dead vegetation, such as thorns, hay, straw, sphagnum moss, wood, and soil rich in decaying organic matter. *Sporothrix* sp. is most prevalent in warm, tropical, and subtropical climate regions. It grows in the environment or in culture at 25°C as a mycelium and converts to a small budding yeasts in mammalian host tissues or in culture at 37°C. Infectivity may result from selection of strains adapted to grow at temperatures higher than 35°C.[2] Although all *Sporothrix* isolates have in the past been grouped into the single species *Sporothrix schenckii*, multiple genotypes exist that vary in virulence and geographic distribution.[3–6] The classic agent *S. schenckii* now comprises several molecular siblings nested in a clinical clade with *Sporothrix globosa*, *Sporothrix luriei*, and *Sporothrix brasiliensis*,[7] with the latter being the most virulent.[8] The phylogenetically distant environmental species *Sporothrix mexicana*, *Sporothrix pallida*, *Sporothrix chilensis*, and *Sporothrix humicola* are rare agents of sporotrichosis in mammals being nested in the environmental clade.[8–13] However, the epidemiology of the various species of *Sporothrix* is incompletely understood. *Sporothrix brasiliensis* is so far restricted to Brazil, Argentina, and Paraguay.[14,15,16] Two different clusters of *S. schenckii sensu stricto* are prevalent in the Americas and Asia, and in the Americas and Africa, respectively. *Sporothrix globosa* is predominant in Asia and Europe, but rare in the Americas and Africa.[9] *Sporothrix schenckii, S. brasiliensis, S. humicola*,[17] and *S. albicans* have been isolated from cats, and *S. brasiliensis, S. schenckii*, and *S. luriei* have been isolated from dogs.[18]

Human sporotrichosis is distributed worldwide and is rare in Europe, with endemic areas in Brazil, Peru, Mexico, South Africa, China, and India. In Latin America, it is the most common subcutaneous mycosis in humans.[19] Feline sporotrichosis has been documented in the United States, Brazil, Mexico, Argentina, Spain, Germany, India, Malaysia, Japan, Australia, Paraguay, Thailand, and United Kingdom.[15,17,20–22] Reported cases of canine sporotrichosis are from the United States, Brazil, Canada, France, and Italy.[23–27] The classic infection results from direct inoculation of the fungus into skin via contact with contaminated plants or soil, or less frequently, by inhalation of conidia. Zoonotic transmission occurs through bites or scratches of animals. Infected cats are the main species implicated in the zoonotic transmission of *Sporothrix*. Additionally, there have been reports of this mycosis following bites or scratches by other animals,[28] such as armadillos, birds, and rodents, although without a significant zoonotic potential.[29] The oral cavity and claws of most animals are suggested to become contaminated from contact with the environment, which would allow the transmission of the fungus percutaneously through scratches or bites. However, the isolation of the agent from the oral cavity and claws has only been reported from cats.[30] Epidemics involving great numbers of people or wide geographic regions are rare and usually related to a common source of infection in the environment such as wood timbers and sphagnum moss.[2,31,32] *Sporothrix schenckii* has primarily been associated with sporadic transmission from the environment to humans, cats, and dogs in developed countries (Fig. 84.1). There were no reports of sporotrichosis epizootics before a cat-transmitted epidemic was reported in Rio de Janeiro, Brazil.[14,33] Between 1998 and 2015, approximately 5,000 human cases were recorded at Evandro Chagas National Institute of Infectious Diseases, Oswaldo Cruz Foundation, Rio de Janeiro, Brazil,[34] and most of them were related to zoonotic transmission by infected cats (Fig. 84.2A and B).[4] Most of the isolates from affected humans in Brazil were *S. brasiliensis*, but *S. schenckii sensu stricto* and *S. globosa* were also isolated.[7] It seems that *S. brasiliensis* is more likely associated with outbreaks of zoonotic sporotrichosis related to transmission by cats (see Fig. 84.1). Since 1998, 244 dogs were diagnosed through 2014[35] and 5,113 cats were diagnosed through 2018 at the same institution,[14] so far representing the largest outbreaks of this mycosis.[33] In Malaysia, cats seem to also take part in the transmission of *S. schenckii sensu stricto* to humans, as around 50% of the human cases from a case series reported a previous episode of scratches or bites from cats. Sporotrichosis due

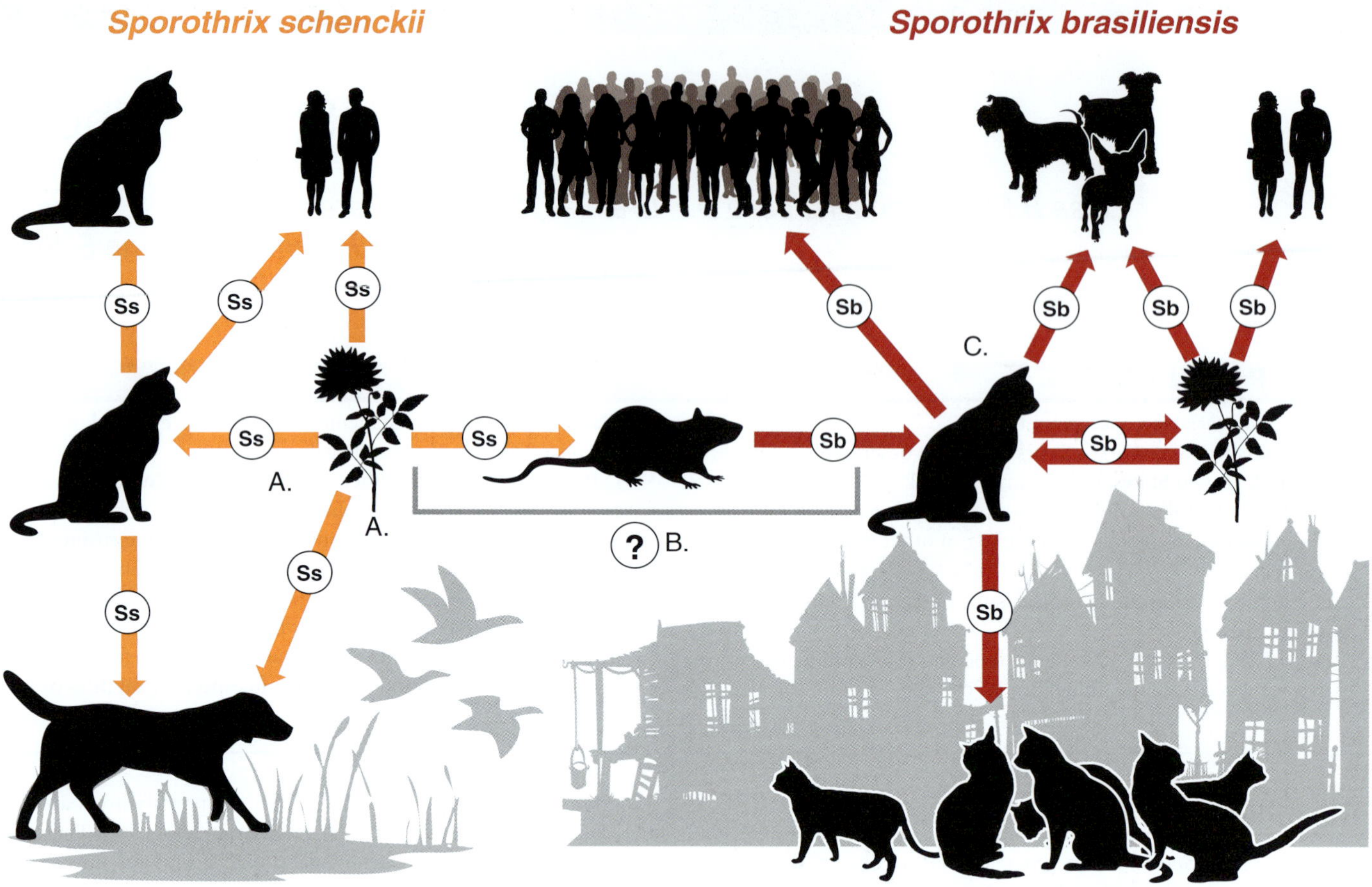

Fig. 84.1 Transmission of *Sporothrix schenckii* and *Sporothrix brasiliensis*. A, *Sporothrix schenckii* (*Ss*) is primarily transmitted through contact with environmental sources. The domestic cat may be infected and also be a source of infection to humans, dogs and other cats, primarily through scratches and bites. B, *Sporothrix brasiliensis* (*Sb*) is primarily a zoonotic pathogen that is transmitted from cats to humans. It is suggested to have shifted from an environment-adapted species to a feline-adapted species. In this scenario, the host-shifting steps are as-yet unsolved, but *Rattus norvegicus* has been hypothesized as a potential passage host (possibly through hunting behavior of cats). C, In the *Sb* zoonotic cycle, cats are the main source of infection for humans, dogs, and other cats, with resulting outbreaks most likely occurring in urban and periurban areas and affecting a larger number of individuals, in comparison with environment-acquired sporotrichosis. Likewise, *Sb*-infected cats may contaminate the environment not only through scratching but also through feces and following decomposition of their carcasses in the environment.

to *S. schenckii sensu stricto* was reported as the third principal cause of death in cats submitted to necropsy examination at a veterinary teaching hospital in Malaysia.[36–45]

Cats are the only species confirmed as a source of infection of *Sporothrix* sp., as demonstrated by isolation of fungus from skin lesions, which are rich in fungi, nasal and oral cavities, and claws of cats with sporotrichosis. The fungus isolation from the oral cavity of apparently healthy cats from Rio de Janeiro that were in contact with affected animals range from 1.5% to 3.6%.[46,47] In addition, in an endemic region in Peru, *Sporothrix* was isolated from the nasal cavity and/or nails of two cats (2.4%) without clinical signs of sporotrichosis.[48] The low prevalence of the isolation of *Sporothrix* spp. from apparently healthy cats suggests they contribute little to the transmission and maintenance of the disease. The mobility of cats in dwellings and surroundings, their habit of scratching vegetation, and their fighting behavior, especially in non-neutered male cats, may improve dispersal of the fungus in the environment.[49,50] Cats can be infected either through the classic route (environmental sources) or through scratches and bites during physical interaction with an infected cat. Direct contact with the exudate from infected cats' lesions is also a potential route of transmission, presumably facilitated by a previous breach in the skin integrity. Cat-to-cat transmission is the main route described in *S. brasiliensis* transmission.[13,14,22,47]

Canine sporotrichosis can be acquired during hunting activities with possible introduction of the organism through thorn injuries or wood splinters. However, in Brazil, the most frequent forms of transmission to dogs were through scratches, bites or contact with exudates from cutaneous lesions of cats.[23] No clear breed or sex predisposition has been identified, and dogs in the Rio de Janeiro epizootic ranged in age from 6 months to 12 years (median, 4 years). Mixed sporotrichosis and cryptococcosis was reported in a dog from Ontario, Canada.[51]

CLINICAL FEATURES

Pathogenesis and Clinical Signs

The transmission of *Sporothrix* classically results from cutaneous inoculation of organisms present in the environment, but can also result from inhalation of conidia. The cutaneous inoculation of the pathogen through scratches and bites by infected cats is also described and represents the major route of transmission of *S. brasiliensis*. Direct

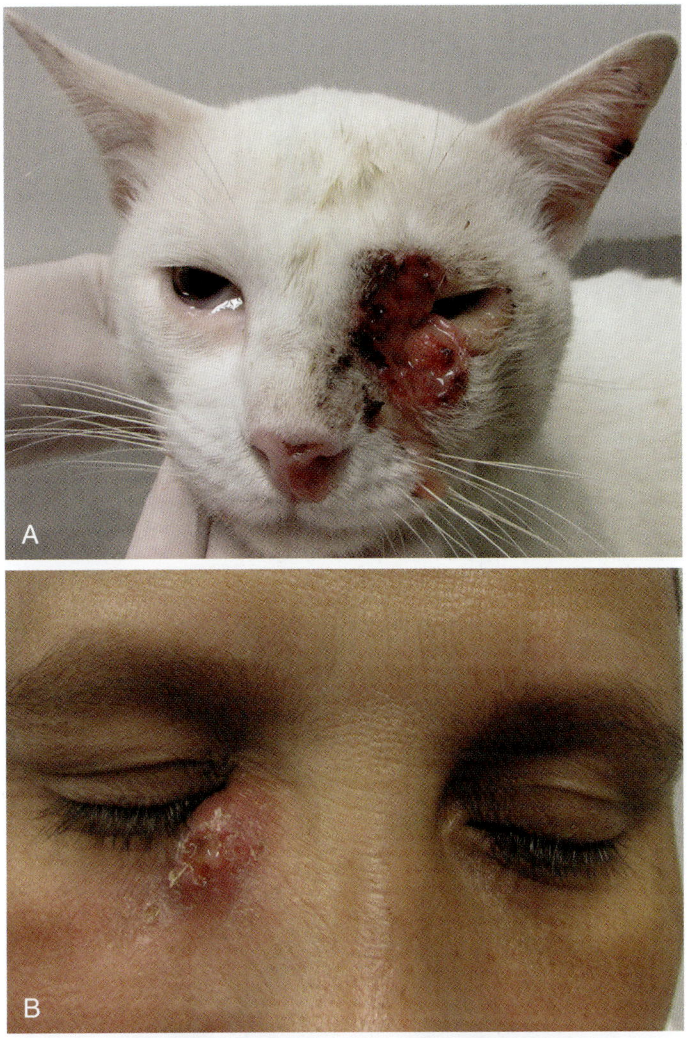

Fig. 84.2 Zoonotic transmission of *Sporothrix* spp. following exposure to feline cutaneous lesions. (A) Ulcerated lesions on the left pinna, face, nasal planum, nasal mucosa, and conjunctiva of the owner's cat from Brazil. (B) Ulcerated nodular lesion on the medial canthus of the right eye of the owner, which affected the lacrimal apparatus (fistulized dacryocystitis).

contact with cats that have sporotrichosis (even without a history of a previous break in the skin) can result in transmission.[46] Following inoculation, the fungus can remain in the dermis and subcutaneous tissue at the inoculation site, spread up regional lymphatics and produce lymphangitis and lymphadenitis, or disseminate systemically through blood vessels. The incubation time usually ranges from 3 to 30 days (within 14 days in average) in human and animal sporotrichosis, but can be months.[29] The initial skin lesions are firm subcutaneous nodules that slowly soften, generally draining purulent or hemorrhagic content, and progress to form exudative ulcers with slightly elevated well-defined rims.[23,46]

The optimal interaction of *Sporothrix* PAMPs and innate immunity receptors, such as Toll-like receptors (TLRs), has shown to be determinant for phagocytosis and cytokine production.[52,53] After phagocytosis, the fungus can evade oxidative damage, such as through production of melanin and mutations in stress-activated protein kinases.[54,55] The successful dissemination into host tissues is strongly related to the pathogen's ability of binding to proteins in the extracellular matrix. In this context, cell wall adhesins on the *Sporothrix* surface can bind to fibronectin.[56,57] Organisms that are thermotolerant (able to survive at temperatures closer to body temperature, or 37°C) may be more likely to cause invasive disease.[52,53,58]

The clinical form of the disease is determined principally by the immunologic status of the host, the load and depth of the inoculum, and the virulence of the infecting *Sporothrix* species.[59] *Sporothrix brasiliensis*, the principal species involved in zoonotic transmission and the causative pathogen of feline sporotrichosis in Brazil, is remarkably virulent,[60] and has been associated with disseminated and atypical presentations of sporotrichosis in humans.[61,62]

The classification of clinical forms used for humans includes several forms: lymphocutaneous, fixed cutaneous, mucocutaneous, extracutaneous, and disseminated. More than 50% of human patients develop the lymphocutaneous form and the infection spreads proximally along lymphatics, with formation of multiple secondary nodules that may ulcerate (Fig. 84.3). Among the extracutaneous forms in humans, osteoarticular and pulmonary involvement are the most common.[54,63] Co-infection with HIV and *Sporothrix* may be associated with disseminated cutaneous lesions, systemic sporotrichosis, and hospitalization.[64]

Dogs and cats frequently display more than one of these clinical forms simultaneously. The most common lesions in dogs and cats are cutaneous nodules and ulcers, sometimes with mucosal involvement. Although the cutaneous-lymphatic form is the most frequently seen in humans, this is not the case for cats, and possibly not for dogs.[23,46] In a retrospective study involving 347 cats with sporotrichosis, the cutaneous-lymphatic form was observed in only 19.3% of cats.[46]

Cats are highly susceptible to *Sporothrix* infection. The spectrum of clinical signs ranges from a single or multiple skin lesions to fatal systemic forms due to hematogenous dissemination. Multiple skin lesions in cats can occur because of multiple inoculation sites, self-trauma, grooming,[46] or they can be a manifestation of a systemic infection. Generalized disease is frequently reported in cats with sporotrichosis, with involvement of multiple organ systems.[65,66] The detection of the fungus by histopathologic examination and/or by culture is described in the lungs, heart, spleen, kidneys, lymph nodes, adrenal glands, and liver of naturally infected cats.[66–68] Hematogenous spread may be an early event and it was demonstrated by isolation of *Sporothrix* from the peripheral blood of cats with widespread cutaneous lesions as well as cats in good general condition with localized lesions, even when no clinical signs suggestive of a septic syndrome were observed.[30,69] Fatal disseminated cases are not described in Asia, which is suggested to be due to the lower thermotolerance of *S. schenckii sensu stricto* in comparison with *S. brasiliensis*.[45] Co-infection with FIV does not appear to be a risk factor for dissemination.[69]

The occurrence of respiratory signs may also precede the beginning of the cutaneous involvement and may be observed in cats without skin lesions.[44] The high frequency of these signs, and nasal mucosa and pulmonary lesions in cats with sporotrichosis, as well as the isolation of *Sporothrix* from bronchoalveolar lavage washings and from the lungs of necropsied cats, suggest that the inhalation route of entry may have epidemiologic importance in cats.[66,70]

Physical Examination Findings

The most common clinical signs in dogs and cats are cutaneous lesions. Extracutaneous signs are frequent, and primarily consist of lymphadenomegaly and respiratory signs, such as sneezing, nasal discharge, and dyspnea. Secondary bacterial infection may occur. Other clinical signs that may be observed are anorexia, hyporexia, vomiting, weight loss, and dehydration.[23,46] Hematologic and biochemical alterations observed in dogs and cats are nonspecific.[23,46]

Dogs

In dogs, as in humans, sporotrichosis is essentially a benign disease, although disseminated forms may rarely develop.[71–73] The most

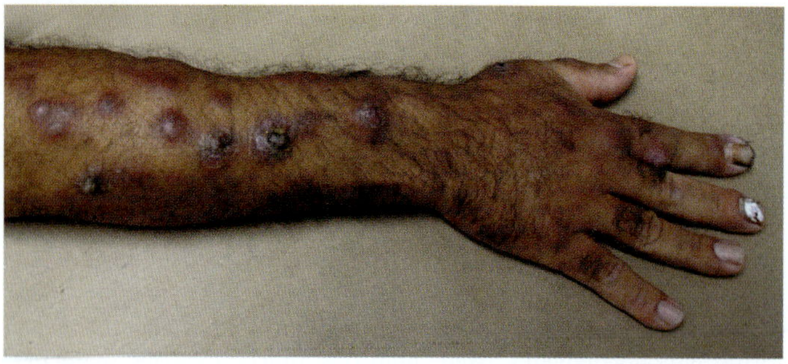

Fig. 84.3 Cutaneous lymphatic form of sporotrichosis on the right arm.

common lesions in dogs are skin nodules and ulcers, with frequent nasal mucosal involvement. Intranasal masses that protrude from the nostrils can be observed.[23,74] The skin lesions may be solitary or multiple and more frequently located on the head, especially on the nose (Fig. 84.4), followed by the limbs and thorax. Skin lesions on the nasal planum were observed in 56.8% of 44 dogs in one study, and 20.5% of dogs had nasal mucosal involvement, with isolated mucosal lesions in 3 (6.8%) dogs. The high frequency of lesions on the muzzle of dogs may be explained by injuries caused by cats that inhabit the same household environments.[23] Rarely, lesions course along lymphatics,[23,65,70,74] when they are usually associated with regional lymphadenomegaly.[23] Osteoarticular sporotrichosis occurs rarely in dogs and may manifest clinically as lameness and synovial effusion.[74,75] Disseminated cutaneous sporotrichosis in association with immunosuppressive therapy has been described in a dog.[76]

Canine sporotrichosis should be clinically differentiated from cutaneous neoplasia, cryptococcosis, histoplasmosis, blastomycosis, coccidioidomycosis, bacterial pyoderma, American tegumentary leishmaniosis, drug eruption, among others.[29,77]

Cats

The most frequent clinical forms of feline sporotrichosis are multiple skin lesions, usually in three or more anatomical sites, with involvement of nasal mucosa. Generally, cats with sporotrichosis exhibit good general health,[46] but lethargy, anorexia, and fever may occur in systemic infection.[78]

Skin lesions are characterized especially by nodules and ulcers. Plaques and tumor-like lesions are also observed.[29] The main affected site for skin lesions is the head (Fig. 84.5), especially the nasal region and the pinna. Other common sites are the distal limbs, digits, and tail, but lesions can also be found elsewhere on the body. Lesions of the conjunctiva (Fig. 84.6), and oral and genital mucosa can also be present in some affected cats. In addition to skin and mucosal lesions, lymphangitis, lymphadenomegaly, and extensive zones of necrosis that expose muscle and bone can be observed.[46]

Extracutaneous signs, particularly respiratory signs (sneezing, dyspnea, and nasal discharge) and nasal mucosa involvement, are frequent. Respiratory signs are observed in 42% of cats, mainly sneezing (39%).[79] Nasal mucosa lesions and respiratory signs can be associated with treatment failure and death.[79,80] The isolation of *Sporothrix* from nasal swab specimens and the occurrence of sneezing may precede appearance of skin lesions in some cases.[44]

Sporotrichosis differential diagnosis in cats includes neoplasia (mainly SCC), feline eosinophilic granuloma complex, bacterial pyoderma, mycobacteriosis, nocardiosis, actinomycosis, cryptococcosis, histoplasmosis, phaeohyphomycosis, American tegumentary leishmaniosis, feline herpesviral dermatitis, and severe allergic diseases (e.g., mosquito bites, flea allergy dermatosis), among others. The coexistence of sporotrichosis and other skin diseases, like neoplasia, eosinophilic

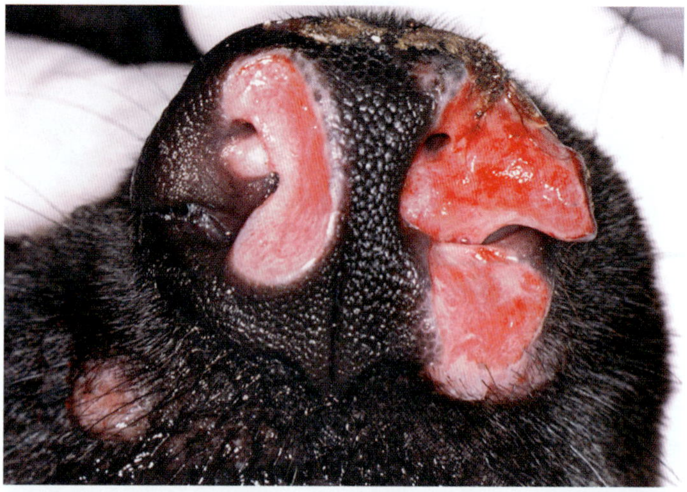

Fig. 84.4 Dog with *Sporothrix* spp. infection. There are ulcers on the muzzle and nasal planum with destruction of the nares, and mucosal involvement.

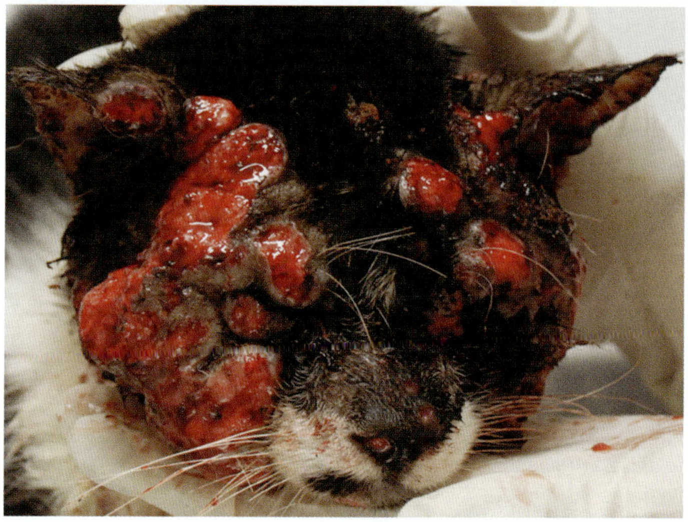

Fig. 84.5 Cat with *Sporothrix* spp. infection. There are multifocal to coalescing ulcerated nodules, on the head.

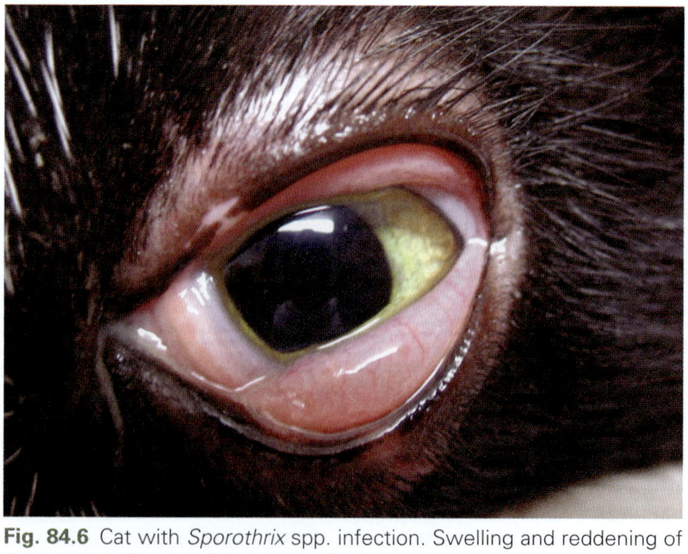

Fig. 84.6 Cat with *Sporothrix* spp. infection. Swelling and reddening of the lower and upper right conjunctival mucosa.

dermatosis, bacterial pyoderma, dermatophytosis, and demodicosis should be considered.[44,81]

DIAGNOSIS

A high degree of suspicion is required for the disease in non-endemic regions. Although clinical signs, patient history, and epidemiologic data can suggest sporotrichosis, definitive diagnosis depends on isolation of *Sporothrix* spp. in culture media. Cytology and histopathology are very useful routine tools for the preliminary diagnosis. IHC, serology and PCR are other options for the diagnosis of sporotrichosis.

Laboratory Abnormalities

Complete Blood Count

In many dogs and cats with sporotrichosis, the CBC is unremarkable. The most common abnormalities are mild anemia and leukocytosis due to a neutrophilia, sometimes with a mild left shift.[46,71] Monocytosis, eosinophilia, lymphocytosis, or lymphopenia may also be present. Approximately 50% of the dogs from the Rio de Janeiro epizootic were anemic, and around 20% had eosinophilia or neutrophilia.[23]

Serum Chemistry Profile

The most frequent serum biochemistry findings in cats and dogs with sporotrichosis are hyperglobulinemia and hypoalbuminemia. Increased liver enzyme activities can occur in affected cats and dogs.[23,46]

Urinalysis

Urinalysis in animals with sporotrichosis usually reveals no clinically significant abnormalities.

Diagnostic Imaging

Plain Radiography

A pulmonary interstitial infiltrate was described in one affected cat.[66] Thoracic radiographs on one dog and five cats seen at the author's teaching hospital revealed no radiographic abnormalities. Radiographs of bones that underlie skin lesions typically reveal only soft tissue swelling; rarely is underlying osteomyelitis detected.

Advanced imaging

CT of the nasal cavity in cats with lesions on the bridge of the nose may reveal masses within the nasal cavity that invade through nasal bones to involve the subcutaneous tissues (Fig. 84.7A and B). Severely thickened turbinate mucosa, an intranasal soft tissue density mass, and focal osteolysis were reported on nasal CT in a dog with signs of nasal cavity disease due to sporotrichosis.[82]

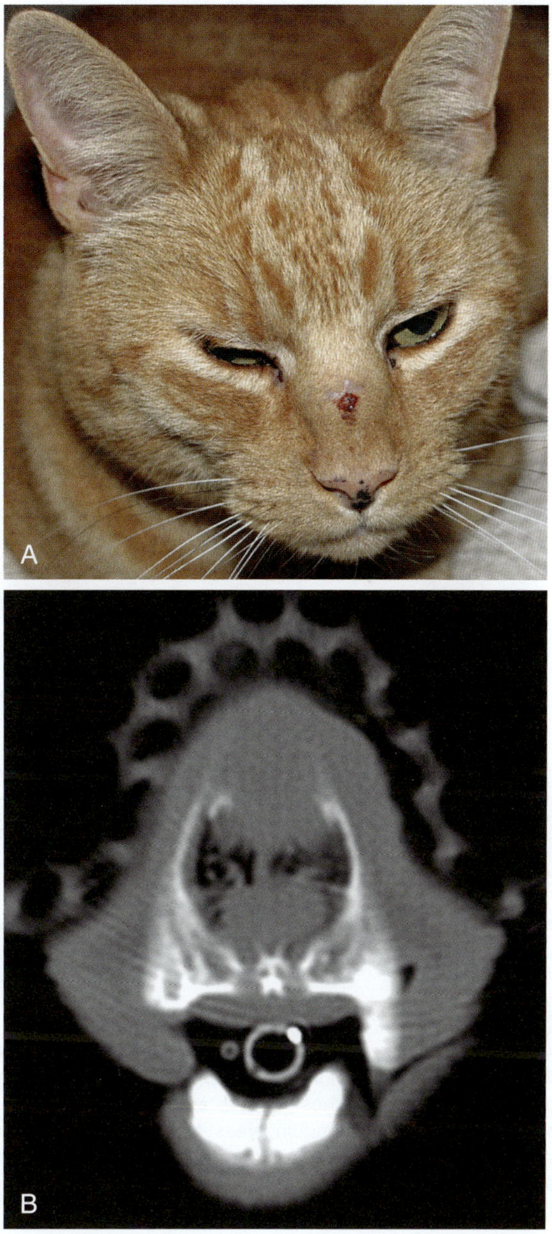

Fig. 84.7 Nasal sporotrichosis with communication to the overlying skin in a 14-year-old male neutered domestic shorthair cat. (A) The cat had a 1-year history of sneezing and a 2-month history of a mass on the bridge of the nose. (B) Computed tomography revealed a nasal cavity mass with nasal bone destruction and involvement of the subcutaneous tissues.

Microbiologic Tests

Specimens to be collected may include swab specimens of the nasal cavities, exudative lesions, and purulent or seropurulent content aspirated from nonulcerated nodular lesions, as well as incisional skin biopsy specimens.[46,83] In cats, swab specimens of exudative lesions are the recommended specimen for diagnosis of *Sporothrix* infection.[46]

Skin biopsies should be obtained from borders of active lesions with a 3- to 4-mm surgical punch. Two tissue specimens can be collected, one fixed in 10% buffered formalin for histopathology and immunohistochemical tests, and the second kept in a sterile glass flask with sterile saline and transported on ice to a diagnostic laboratory for fungal culture, preferentially within 8–10 hours.[59] In dogs, the best results for fungal isolation are from surgical skin biopsy specimens as they are more sensitive than swab specimens of exudative lesions.[23,46]

Suitable specimens for cytopathologic examination include impression smears of ulcerated skin, exudates or biopsy specimens (before placing in formalin), smears of swab specimens, skin scrapings, or fine-needle aspirates of abscesses and nodules.[84–86]

To diagnose dissemination, whole blood can be directly seeded in blood culture flasks.[69] BAL is useful for diagnosis of pulmonary involvement.[70] At necropsy, tissue specimens can be collected for mycology, cytology, histopathology, and immunohistochemical testing.

Cytopathologic Examination

The sensitivity of the cytopathologic examination of skin lesions of cats with sporotrichosis ranges from 79% to 87%.[85,87,88] This method is rapid, practical, and low cost, and a positive result can allow initiation of antifungal treatment while awaiting the results of culture.[87,89] However, despite cytopathology being highly sensitive for diagnosis of feline sporotrichosis, its sensitivity drops drastically after onset of antifungal treatment.[89] In dogs, a sensitivity of 32% was observed.[83,87]

Cytologic preparations stained with Wright or Romanowsky-type or Gomori's methenamine silver (GMS) stains permit good visualization of the yeast cells.[83,86] With Wright or Romanowsky-type staining, *Sporothrix* spp. appear as cigar-shaped to oval or round budding yeasts that are 3–5 μm by 5–9 μm in maximum length, with blue cytoplasm and a single round nucleus surrounded by a nonstaining cell wall (Fig. 84.8).[84,87] These organisms are seen mainly within the cytoplasm of macrophages, and neutrophils and also extracellularly.[76,84,85] *Sporothrix* spp. may be confused with *Histoplasma*, *Cryptococcus*, *Candida*, and *Leishmania* spp., and potentially other protozoan parasites such as *Toxoplasma gondii* and *Neospora caninum*.[29]

Fungal Culture

Fungal culture is the reference standard for the diagnosis of sporotrichosis in animals and humans due to its high sensitivity and specificity. The sensitivity of isolation from skin biopsies exceeds 95% in both dogs and cats.[23,46,65] In addition, fungal culture allows further identification of *Sporothrix* at species level by PCR.[7,8] However, it is time consuming, taking 10 to 15 days to obtain results. Other disadvantages of culture are that false-negative results can occur due to low fungal burden, prior treatment with topical or systemic antifungal agents, inadequate specimen size, deterioration of specimens during transport, and contamination with bacteria.

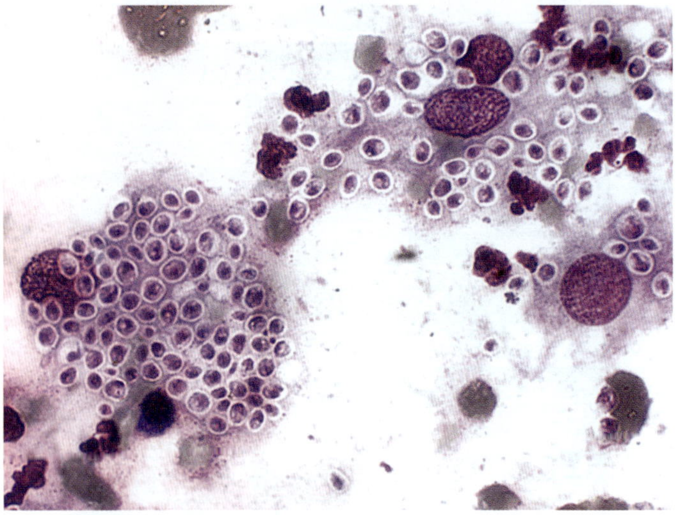

Fig. 84.8 Photomicrograph of impression smear from an ulcerated skin lesion in a cat with sporotrichosis. There are numerous oval to round and occasional cigar-shaped budding yeast-like forms. These have blue cytoplasm with a single nucleus, and are surrounded by a nonstaining cell wall. They are located within macrophages and extracellularly (panoptic stain, ×100).

Clinical material should be inoculated onto Sabouraud's dextrose agar with chloramphenicol and Sabouraud's dextrose agar with chloramphenicol plus cycloheximide and incubated at 25°C to 30°C. Mycelial growth of *Sporothrix* spp. can be observed in 3 to 5 days, although sometimes several weeks of incubation may be required.[58] Typical colonies are initially cream colored, smooth, and moist, gradually becoming dark brown or black, as a result of production of pigmented conidia, (Fig. 84.9A). However, much variation among isolates and even among subcultures of the same isolate can be observed. Various culture media can also influence the color and texture of colonies. Identification depends on the morphologic characteristics of the mycelial form and its conversion to the yeast form on blood agar or brain-heart infusion (BHI) agar plus yeast extract agar when incubated at 37°C. The microscopic characteristics of the mycelial form are slender, hyaline, septate, and branched hyphae measuring 1.5 to 2 μm in width. The conidia arise directly from the hyphae or from the apex of thin conidiophores, with conidia in a flowerlike arrangement. The intensity of colony color is directly proportional to the number of dark brown thick-walled conidia. The yeast phase is pleomorphic, showing oval or cigar-shaped cells and exhibiting single or multiple buds with elongated morphology. The organism can then be identified based on light microscopic appearance of the mold and yeast forms (see Fig. 84.9B and C).

Sporothrix species identification requires subsequent molecular analysis by specialized laboratories.[90] MALDI-TOF has also been successfully applied for the differentiation of *Sporothrix* species.[91]

Antifungal susceptibility testing can be performed, but established breakpoints are not available.

Serologic Diagnosis

ELISAs that detect antibody to *Sporothrix* cell wall antigens have been developed for diagnosis of human and feline sporotrichosis.[92–94] The best results for an ELISA's sensitivity and specificity for the diagnosis of feline sporotrichosis were 96% and 98%, respectively, using *S. schenckii* crude exoantigen, and 90% and 98%, respectively, using a cell wall antigen (SsCBF).[83]

ELISA and immunoblotting suggest 3-carboxymuconate cyclase (a 60-kDa protein in *S. brasiliensis* and a 70-kDa protein in *S. schenckii*) as

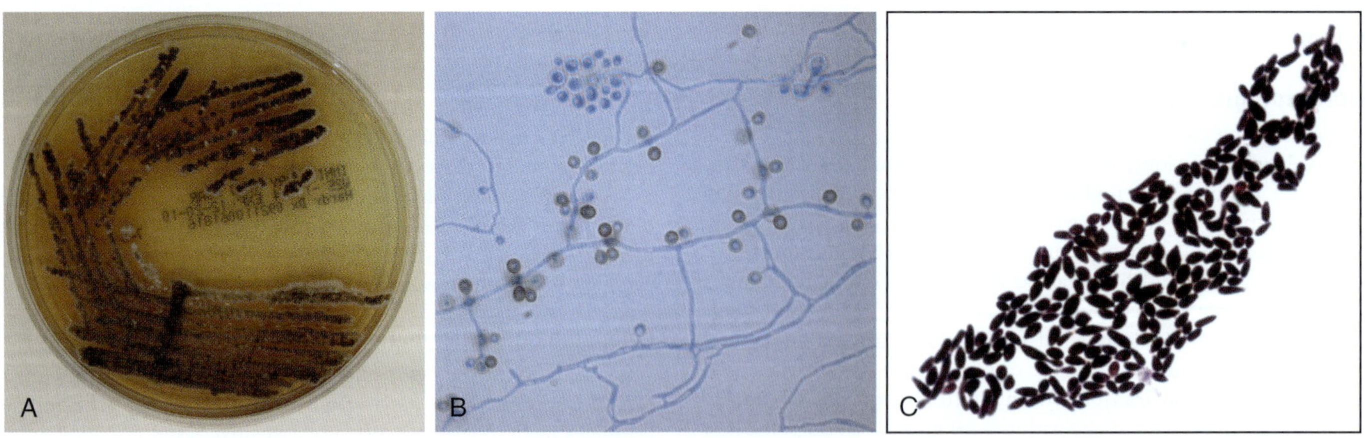

Fig. 84.9 *Sporothrix* sp. growing on laboratory media. (A) The fungus grows on fungal isolation media as a white mold at 30°C with production of pigmented conidia. (B) Using light microscopy, the mold form is characterized by the production of conidia in a flower-like arrangement and occasionally pigmented. Lactophenol cotton blue stain, 1000× oil magnification. (C) At 37°C, the organism converts to the yeast form. Gram stain, 1000× oil magnification.

the immunodominant antigen in feline sporotrichosis and a potential marker for serologic diagnosis. Although these methods do not distinguish between *S. brasiliensis* and *S. schenckii* infections, there is no reactivity when sera from healthy cats or from cats with other infections were used, so specificity appears to be promising.[94]

Recently, the ELISA test using SsCBF was adapted and validated for detecting IgG from sera of cats with sporotrichosis and is currently commercially available in private laboratories in Brazil.[22,95]

Molecular Diagnosis Using Nucleic Acid-Based Testing

Conventional identification methods are time consuming and prone to misidentification since there is an overlap of phenotypic characteristics among the species of *Sporothrix*. Therefore, rapid and accurate identification of *Sporothrix* relies on the use of molecular methods. PCR is an important tool used to identify *Sporothrix* species from animals and humans, especially when isolates are not identified by morphologic and physiologic phenotyping. PCR sequencing targeting the calmodulin gene is most used, but PCR sequencing targeting ITS1/2, large-subunit (LSU) ribosomal DNA, β-tubulin, chitin synthase,[9,96,97] and translation elongation factor[96,98] can also distinguish among species of *Sporothrix*. Recently, more rapid molecular assays that do not need sequencing for identification were developed. These include PCR fingerprinting based on random amplification of polymorphic DNA (RAPD) using the universal primer T3B,[99] amplified fragment length polymorphisms,[98] PCR-restriction fragment length polymorphisms (RFLPs),[100] species-specific PCR,[101] and rolling-circle amplification (RCA).[102–104] A PCR assay targeting the chitin synthase 1 gene was used with success for specific and rapid detection of *Sporothrix* DNA and identification at genus level in a biopsy specimen from a cat with sporotrichosis.[105] A species-specific PCR targeting calmodulin gene sequences has also been described, including its direct application in clinical specimens from cats with sporotrichosis.[101,106] In addition, RCA has been used to successfully detect and identify *Sporothrix* from both clinical and environmental specimens.[102]

Pathologic Findings

Gross Pathologic Findings

In addition to cutaneous and mucosal lesions, the main gross lesions in cats are small whitish nodular lesions measuring approximately 1 mm in diameter on the pleural surface and parenchyma of the lungs, and enlargement of lymph nodes.[65]

Histopathologic Findings

Histopathology of cutaneous lesions of feline and canine sporotrichosis is characterized by ulcerative and variable but usually intense pyogranulomatous inflammatory reaction in the dermis, which can reach the panniculus and subjacent skeletal muscles.[107,108] The inflammatory infiltrate usually reveals a predominance of neutrophils and macrophages, variable number of plasma cells and lymphocytes. Eosinophils and mast cells can be occasionally seen.[74,108,109] Multinucleated giant cells are infrequent in dogs and cats compared with their occurrence in humans.[108–110] The presence of Splendore-Hoeppli phenomenon ("asteroid bodies") around yeasts is commonly described in human infections,[111] but this is not typically observed in dogs or cats.[107,111]

There is a predominance of poorly formed granulomas (poorly delineated) in cutaneous lesions from cats, dogs, and humans with sporotrichosis.[23,107,108,110] Organized granulomas are less common (approximately 11%) in skin lesions of cats (Fig. 84.10) compared with dogs (38%–45%) and humans (38%).[23,107,108,110] Cats tend to have poorly formed granulomas composed of macrophages filled with yeast-like forms and a mild neutrophilic and lymphoplasmacytic surrounding reaction (Fig. 84.11).[108]

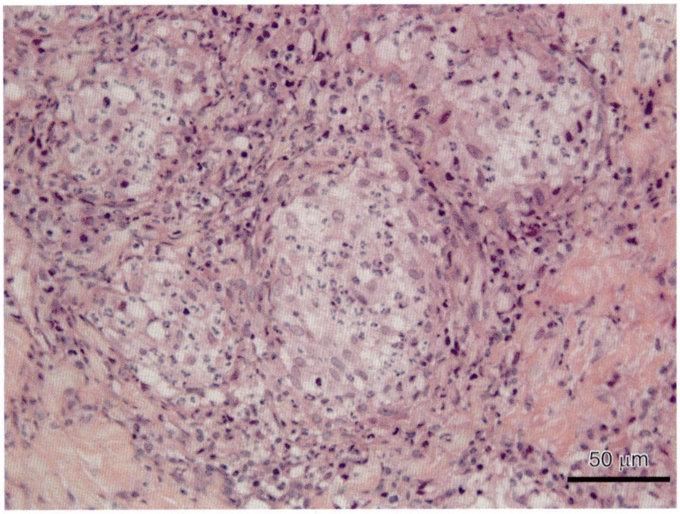

Fig. 84.10 Photomicrograph of a histologic section of a skin lesion of a cat with sporotrichosis showing multiple well delineated suppurative granulomas with a predominance of epithelioid cells (well-formed granuloma) (hematoxylin-eosin stain).

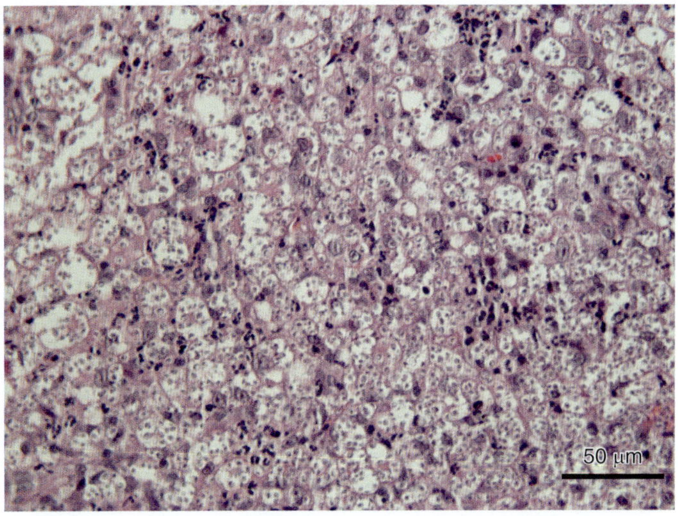

Fig. 84.11 Photomicrograph of a histologic section of a skin lesion of a cat with sporotrichosis showing poorly formed granulomas composed by macrophages filled with yeast-like forms (hematoxylin-eosin stain).

Systemic involvement is common in cats and a pyogranulomatous inflammatory reaction and yeasts can be observed in the lungs, spleen, lymph nodes, liver, kidneys, adrenal glands, eyes,[66–68] skeletal muscles, and tongue. Cats with intranasal sporotrichosis often have severe pyogranulomatous rhinitis with osteomyelitis, osteolysis, and necrosis of hyaline cartilage (Fig. 84.12).[44]

Histopathologic findings are nonspecific and similar to those of other pathogenic fungi and protozoans.[109] Therefore, histochemical stains such as GMS and PAS are needed to highlight *Sporothrix* spp. in tissues.[46,67] *Sporothrix* spp. yeasts are oval or cigar-shaped, range in size from 4 µm to 6 µm, generally exhibit a single bud with a narrow base, and are dark staining using GMS (Fig. 84.13A) and pink using PAS. Pseudohyphae, hyphae, and yeast-like forms with multiple budding are occasionally seen.[39,44,68] Yeast-like forms of *Sporothrix* spp. should be differentiated from those of *Histoplasma* spp., which are smaller (2 µm to 4 µm), do not present cigar-shaped forms, and are usually grouped in clusters inside macrophages.[112]

The yeast-like forms of *Sporothrix* can be seen inside neutrophils, macrophages, giant cells and osteoclasts, or extracellularly in purulent exudate and inflamed areas.[44] In cats with sporotrichosis, the number of *Sporothrix* organisms is usually high and can be detected in 94% of histopathologic examinations of skin biopsies stained by GMS.[46,67,68,108] Higher fungal loads in skin lesions detected by histopathology (GMS) were linked to young age and treatment failure with itraconazole (ITZ), as well as to poorly formed granulomas with fewer inflammatory cells and a longer time for wound healing.[80]

In dogs, as in humans, the yeast-like forms are usually rare, and the fungus is visualized in tissue specimens stained by PAS and GMS in approximately 17% and 44% of cases, respectively.[23,110,113] Use of GMS increases sensitivity when compared with PAS for diagnosis of canine sporotrichosis. Around 58% of cases show a maximum of five fungal elements in multiple histologic sections of skin biopsies.[108,113]

In order to increase the sensitivity of histologic diagnosis in formalin-fixed paraffin-embedded (FFPE) tissues from dogs, IHC is recommended. An IHC protocol using a rabbit anti-*Sporothrix* hyperimmune serum and an avidin-biotin detection system was described for the diagnosis of *Sporothrix* in FFPE skin samples of dogs (Fig. 84.13B) and cats.[113] The sensitivity of this assay was 65% in dogs and 88.6% in cats.[88,113] However, anti-*Sporothrix* antibodies are not commercially available.[114]

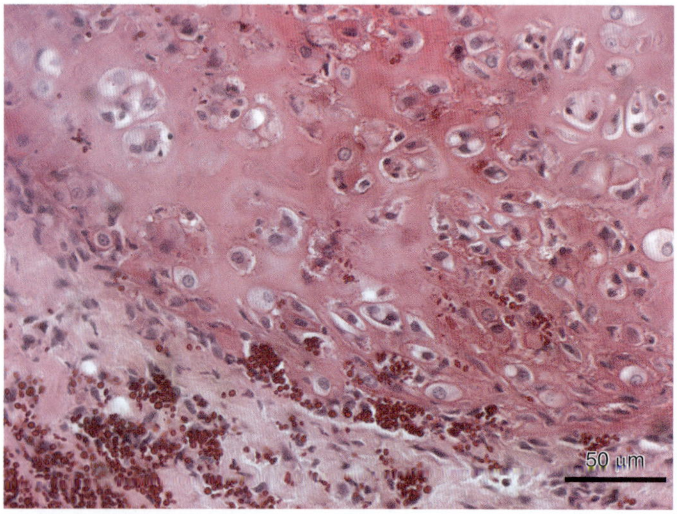

Fig. 84.12 Photomicrograph of a histologic section of the nasal mucosa and associated cartilage from a cat with intranasal sporotrichosis. There is a high load of yeast-like organisms that infiltrate cartilage (periodic acid–Schiff stain).

TREATMENT AND PROGNOSIS

Treatment of dogs and cats with sporotrichosis still represents a challenge for veterinarians.[115] The cost and availability of antifungal drugs vary and this often dictates the choices made.[74]

Antifungal drugs for sporotrichosis include ketoconazole (KTZ), ITZ, potassium iodide (KI), sodium iodide (NaI), terbinafine, fluconazole (FLZ), or AMB. Treatment of animal sporotrichosis should be continued for at least a month after complete resolution of clinical signs. Other therapeutic options are local thermotherapy, cryosurgery, and surgical resection of cutaneous lesions.[116–118] Clinical and biochemical monitoring is strongly recommended,[78] regardless of the prescribed treatment regimen. ITZ is considered the drug of choice in human, feline, and canine sporotrichosis treatment.[2,79,84,118] The recommended dosage of ITZ capsules for the treatment of feline or canine sporotrichosis is given with food to facilitate absorption (Table 84.1).[46,84] ITZ solution permits more accurate dose measurement and improved absorption and bioavailability at the recommended dose so that dosages per unit body weight are lower[46] (see Table 84.1); however, this formulation is not available in some countries. Compounded formulations are not recommended in substitution to the reference drug as they might not be bioequivalent, while generic formulations can be a suitable alternative (see Chapter 11).[22]

Concurrent bacterial infections should be simultaneously treated with an appropriate antibiotic/antibacterial agent.[119] Use of glucocorticoids or any immunosuppressive drug is contraindicated in dogs and cats during and after the treatment of the disease, because the disease can worsen or recur.[78,120] There are risks of fetal malformations associated with the use of KTZ and KI. Administration of any azole, terbinafine,[121] and KI[122] should be avoided during pregnancy.

Treatment response is assessed through clinical evaluation, and cure is defined as complete remission of cutaneous and extracutaneous

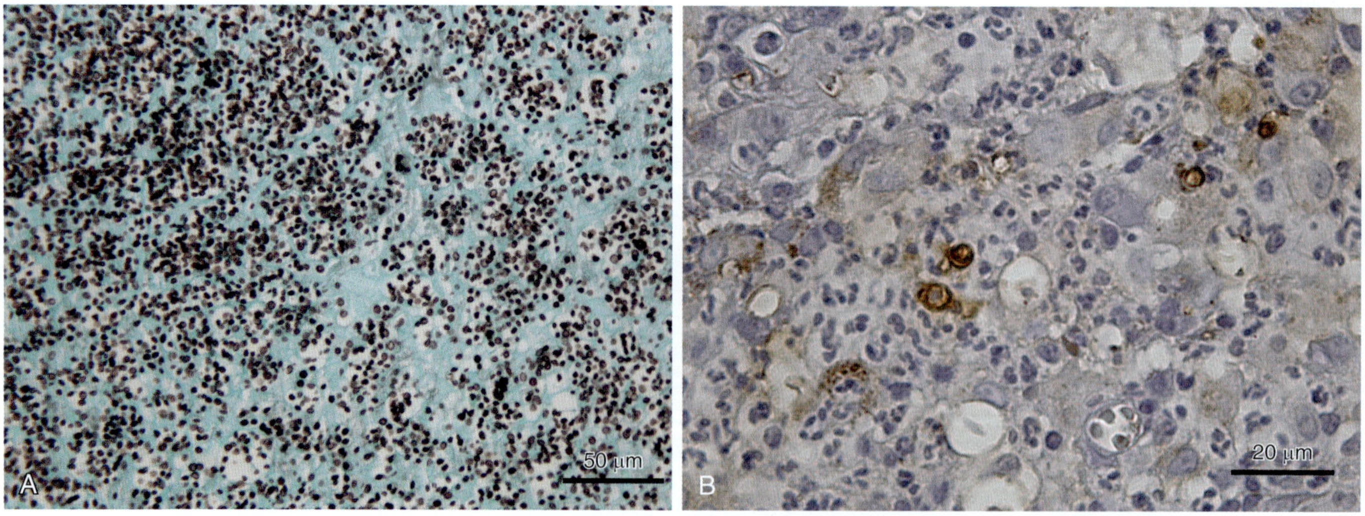

Fig. 84.13 Photomicrograph of a histologic section of a skin lesion of a cat with sporotrichosis following application of special stains and immunohistochemistry. (A) Large numbers of dark staining yeast-like forms are visualized with silver staining (Gomori's methenamine silver stain). (B) Dark brown yeast-like forms of *Sporothrix* are identified using immunohistochemistry using a rabbit anti-*Sporothrix* sp. hyperimmune serum and avidin-biotin detection system.

TABLE 84.1 Recommended Treatment for Sporotrichosis[a]

Drug	Species	Dose (mg/kg)[b]	Route	Interval (hours)
Supersaturated solution of potassium iodide	Dog	40	PO	8
	Cat	10–20	PO	12
Sodium iodide	Cat	10	PO	12
Potassium iodide (KI) capsules	Cat	2.5–20	PO	24
KI + itraconazole capsules	Cat[c]	KI 2.5–5.4	PO	24
	Dog	KI 4.5	PO	PO
Ketoconazole tablets	Dog	5–10	PO	24
	Cat	5–27.0	PO	12–24
Itraconazole capsules	Dog	5–10	PO	12–24
	Cat	5–27.7	PO	12–24
Itraconazole solution	Cat	1.25–3	PO	24
Terbinafine tablets	Cat	30	PO	24
	Dog	30	PO	24
Fluconazole capsules	Cat	10	PO	24

[a]Continue treatment at least 30 days beyond resolution of all clinical signs.
[b]Dose per administration at the specified interval.
[c]Itraconazole 100 mg/day.
PO, oral; *IL*, intralesional administration.

signs. The cooperation and persistence of the owners is instrumental in attempting a successful response to therapy. When sporotrichosis is not treated for an adequate time, it often recurs, usually with respiratory signs.

Importantly, in regions where zoonotic transmission of *Sporothrix* spp. occurs, the treatment of infected cats is one of the main control measures of this mycosis.

Cats

Sporotrichosis is more difficult to treat in cats than in dogs, generally requiring a prolonged period of therapy. Four to six months of treatment are usually necessary for a successful outcome, but in some cats, treatment may last more than a year.[86] Additionally, even when there is remission of clinical signs, fungal clearance cannot be confirmed and recrudescence may occur.[46]

In a retrospective study, the effectiveness and safety of ITZ and KTZ were assessed for the treatment of 773 *Sporothrix*-infected cats[79]: 598 cats received oral KTZ tablets and 175 cats received oral ITZ capsules at dosages listed in Table 84.1. Clinical cure was achieved in 238 (30.8%) cats, 171 (29%) with KTZ and 67 (38%) with ITZ. The median treatment time using either KTZ or ITZ was similar (26 to 28 weeks). Adverse effects were reported in 39.6% of the cats, with a higher occurrence in cats treated with KTZ. Hyporexia was the most frequent adverse effect, followed by vomiting and/or diarrhea. The high prevalence of adverse effects was attributed to the use of higher dosages than those usually employed for the treatment of feline sporotrichosis.[46,78,84] Higher doses were used because of the difficulty in achieving clinical cure with those recommended by the literature.[79] Nevertheless, the doses were similar to those used by other authors for the treatment of cats with systemic mycoses such as coccidioidomycosis and cryptococcosis.[123,124] When adverse GI effects related to KTZ and ITZ were observed, the total daily dose was split in two equal parts and given every 12 hours instead of every 24 hours.[78,84] Because of its effectiveness and safety in cats, ITZ has replaced KTZ in the treatment of feline sporotrichosis.

NaI or KI were otherwise considered the drugs of choice in human and canine sporotrichosis, but serious adverse effects have limited their use, especially in cats. Oral administration of supersaturated potassium iodide (SSKI) was used to treat sporotrichosis in cats, dogs (see Table 84.1 for doses), or humans in the past, before the widespread availability of ITZ. In the treatment of feline sporotrichosis, controversial results have been related with the use of SSKI or supersaturated sodium iodide (SSNaI). Some authors reported clinical cure and others the worsening of clinical condition and death.[125–127] Cats are very sensitive to iodides, and adverse effects can occur such as anorexia, depression, vomiting, hypothermia, hyperthermia, cardiovascular failure, cardiomyopathy, hyperexcitability, muscular spasms, ptyalism, and diarrhea.[128]

The use of KI capsules in lower doses than those previously employed (see Table 84.1) has re-emerged as an effective alternative for the treatment of feline sporotrichosis.[129,130] Because of its extremely bitter taste, a capsule formulation of KI has been used to treat affected cats, with a cure rate of 48% after 4 to 5 months (median time to achieve clinical cure was around 19 weeks).[130] Inappetence occurred in 52% of cats, and a smaller percentage of cats developed weight loss, diarrhea, or vomiting. Increased liver enzyme activities can also occur. The dose range used was 2.5 to 20 mg/kg, PO, q24h (median, 15 mg/kg). The dose was increased in 2.5 mg/kg increments every 5 days from the initial dose. Alterations in thyroid function can be an adverse effect of KI treatment in humans.[131]

Higher cure rates in feline sporotrichosis have resulted from use of a combination of KI capsules and ITZ.[129] The combination allowed the reduction of KI dose (see Table 84.1) compared with KI monotherapy, and led to a cure rate of 96.2% in a prospective cohort study (Fig. 84.14A and B). Dose increments of 2.5 mg/kg at every 30-day period were employed in those cats with worsening or persistence of clinical signs. Adverse effects were observed in 50% of the cats from this study and were managed with temporary treatment interruption and/or the introduction of hepatoprotective therapy with oral silymarin (30 mg/kg, PO, q24h). Clinical adverse effects, such as hyporexia, vomiting, and weight loss, were reported

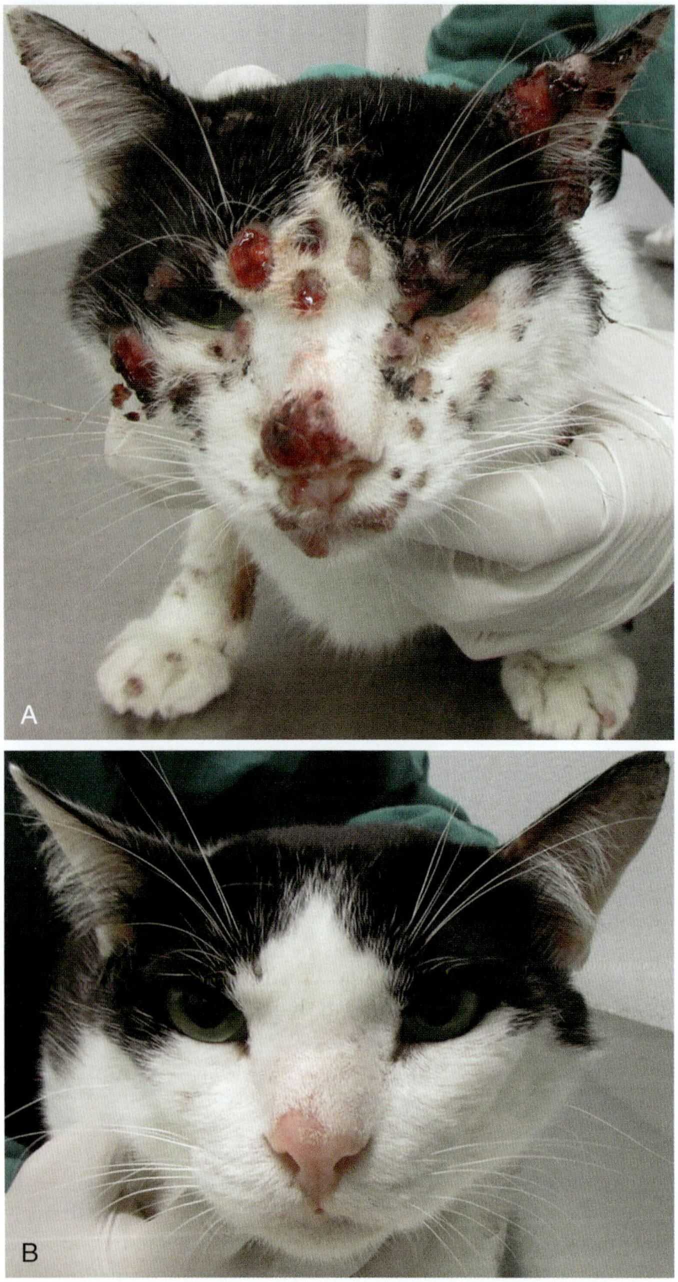

Fig. 84.14 Feline sporotrichosis during treatment. (A) Cat with multiple skin lesions on the head and thoracic limbs after 6 months of treatment with itraconazole. (B) Clinical cure after 6 additional months of therapy with a combination of itraconazole and potassium iodide.

in 20% of the cats, while a mild elevation in transaminase activities was detected in almost 17% of cats. The occurrence of clinical adverse effect was similar to that described for ITZ monotherapy and lower than that with the use of KI alone. This is likely to be explained by lower doses of KI when combined with ITZ, in comparison with KI monotherapy.[129]

Cats with ITZ-refractory sporotrichosis can be treated with the combination of ITZ and KI, notably when respiratory signs and nasal mucosa lesions are present.[132] The primary indication for AMB is the treatment of sporotrichosis refractory to ITZ.[116] Systemic administration of AMB by the IV route in cats is limited because of its adverse effects, mainly nephrotoxicity and thrombophlebitis.[36,67,127] Intralesional AMB administration in combination with ITZ was used successfully to treat fixed or multifocal cutaneous lesions in cats that were refractory to ITZ alone.[116,133] The solution was prepared by addition of 5 mL of 2% lidocaine and 5 mL of distilled water to a 50-mg vial of AMB (final concentration, 5 mg/mL). A total of 0.5 to 1.5 mL (median 0.7 mL) was administered intralesionally once a week to once every other week, and 73% of the cats were cured. The number of treatment sessions ranged from 1 to 5 (median, 2 treatment sessions per cat). Sterile abscess formation at the site of administration occurred in 15% of cats.[133]

Although terbinafine has been effective for treatment of cutaneous forms of human sporotrichosis,[134] and *in vitro* susceptibility studies have shown promising results,[135] its employment for the treatment of feline sporotrichosis is poorly described[46] and its effectiveness and safety in cats are not known.

FLZ is recommended for lymphocutaneous sporotrichosis in humans when the patient cannot tolerate other agents. In one cat with disseminated sporotrichosis, cutaneous lesions and respiratory signs resolved during treatment with FLZ, although an additional course of treatment was needed following relapse.[74] The effectiveness and safety of FLZ in the treatment of feline sporotrichosis needs to be further clarified.

Surgical resection of a lesion combined with antifungal therapy can be an alternative after failure of antifungal treatment in humans and cats, as long as the anatomic location of the lesions enables surgical intervention.[38,136–138]

Localized hyperthermia has been used as a safe and inexpensive method to treat fixed cutaneous and lymphocutaneous sporotrichosis in human patients and was used as the sole treatment in a cat with localized cutaneous disease.[139] In that case, a thermal bag that reached a temperature of 40°C to 42°C was applied twice daily for 15 minutes. When used alone, this method is not likely to be effective in animals with disseminated disease.

Lastly, cryosurgery was apparently effective in the treatment of 11 cats with sporotrichosis that were concurrently treated with ITZ,[140] initiated prior to the cryosurgical procedure. The treatment length until clinical cure ranged from 14 to 64 weeks (median 32 weeks), after starting ITZ therapy. Although the treatment duration until cure was longer than that reported with other schemes, this protocol can be an option for cats that do not tolerate higher doses of ITZ and in which systemic disease signs are not observed.

Despite the occurrence of treatment failure in cats, clinical cure may be achieved. The likelihood of cure is unrelated to the severity of the initial clinical findings. However, involvement of the nasal mucosa, respiratory signs, and high fungal loads detected by cytologic examination or histopathology in skin lesions are predictors of treatment failure with ITZ.[80,89] Co-infection with FIV does not seem to alter the likelihood of treatment success.[47] Clinical cure following treatment has been observed in the majority of the cats co-infected with FIV or FeLV. Moreover, the difference between the median treatment time to clinical cure in FIV-positive and FIV-negative cats was not statistically significant.[79]

Relapse can occur between 3 and 18 months after discontinuation of antifungal drug therapy. Spontaneous regression of a persistent cutaneous lesion was also described in a cat.[47] In animals with advanced disease, euthanasia may be indicated. This should also be regarded as a management alternative when long-standing clinical stagnation or progressive worsening of clinical condition is observed even under adequate therapeutic protocols. The expensive antifungal therapy and the concerns for zoonotic transmission are additional factors in which euthanasia is to be considered.

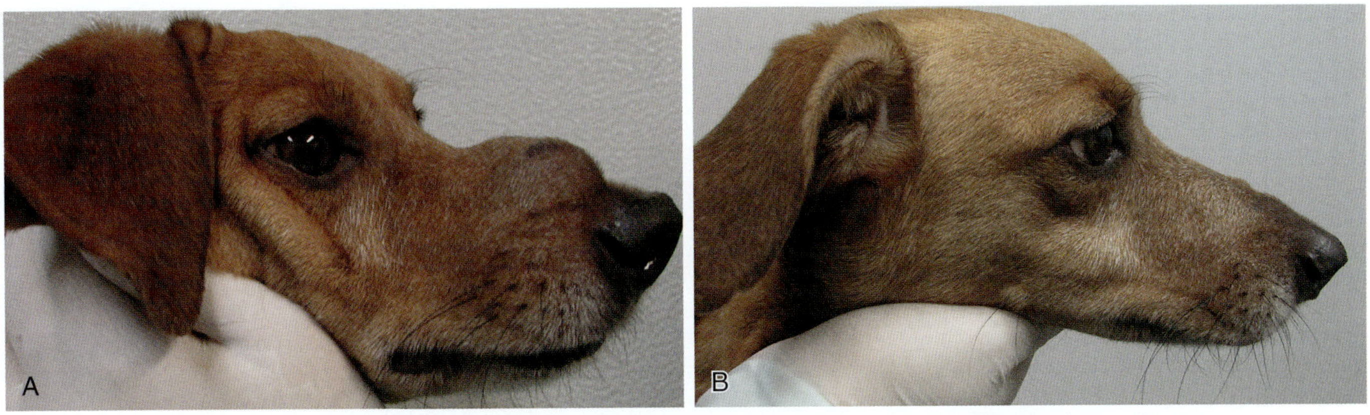

Fig. 84.15 Canine sporotrichosis during treatment. (A) Before treatment is initiated. There is a large subcutaneous mass lesion on the muzzle. (B) Clinical cure after 8 months of itraconazole therapy.

Dogs

Generally, canine sporotrichosis has a good prognosis and is easily treated. Spontaneous regression of cutaneous lesions has been described in a few cases[31] and dogs have remained lesion-free for 1 to 4 years on follow-up examinations.[23]

ITZ capsules can be used to treat canine sporotrichosis (Fig. 84.15A and B) at recommended dosages (see Table 84.1) for 2 to 5 months.[23] Adverse effects include anorexia, vomiting, diarrhea, elevated hepatic enzyme activities, and cutaneous vasculitis (see also Chapter 11).[141–143]

Although KTZ is not the first choice for treatment of canine sporotrichosis, clinical cure was obtained with the recommended dosage in Table 84.1 for 2 to 5 months.[23] Potential hepatotoxicity should be monitored during therapy.[119,144]

The treatment of canine sporotrichosis with oral administration of a SSKI is also described (see Table 84.1), but dogs should be monitored for any signs of iodism (mucopurulent oculonasal discharges, salivation, and weakness). If toxicity occurs, the medication should be discontinued for a week. If the adverse effects are mild, they may not recur, and therapy should then be reinstituted. If the adverse effects recur or the initial reactions were severe, another drug should be considered.[78] Although the effectiveness of KI capsules (see Table 84.1) for treating canine sporotrichosis is poorly known, a successful outcome was described in one dog with no reported adverse effects.[145]

Recently, terbinafine was described for the treatment of sporotrichosis in two dogs, being successful even in the presence of respiratory signs and nasal mucosa lesions. It may be a suitable alternative in animals that do not tolerate ITZ therapy.[146]

IMMUNITY AND VACCINATION

Most of the knowledge on the immune response to *Sporothrix* infection is derived from studies from human sporotrichosis and animal models.

The immune response to *Sporothrix* infection involves both innate and adaptive mechanisms. Elements from the *Sporothrix* cell wall function as PAMPs for recognition by pattern-recognition receptors (PRRs), such as TLRs and C-type lectin receptors (CLRs),[147] expressed by innate immune cells.[148] These contribute to the enhancement of a further adaptive response.[149,150] The generation of oxidative species during phagocytosis in the experimental model is also involved in fungicidal activities.[151]

Whether *Sporothrix* infection leads to a severe or a mild disease clearly is affected by the host's immune response in murine and human studies. Th1-dependent immunity, through $CD4^+$ cells and activated macrophages, persists as a required mechanism in the defense to *Sporothrix*,[152] while the response to more virulent strains of the fungus seem to be Th2-shifted.[153] Recently, Th17 also emerged as an important branch of immune response for fungal clearance in sporotrichosis.[154]

Cellular immunity is also recognized as important in the response to feline infections.[155] Cats with localized sporotrichosis that are in good general condition typically display well-organized granulomatous lesions with a lower fungal burden and a higher percentage of $CD4^+$ cells in their peripheral blood when compared with cats with disseminated sporotrichosis that exhibit a poor general condition. The latter group of cats have poorly organized granulomas and a high fungal burden, in association with a higher percentage of $CD8^{low}$ cells. Although the $CD8^{low}$ cells subset is connected to retroviral infections, such as HIV and FIV[156,157] in humans and cats, respectively, this subset was unrelated to FIV co-infection in the case of cats with sporotrichosis.

Some authors believe that the severity of feline sporotrichosis may be related to immunosuppression caused by co-infection with FIV or FeLV. In a recent study, a poor general condition in cats with sporotrichosis was correlated to FIV co-infection. Likewise, the evaluation of cytokine levels in cats with sporotrichosis revealed IL-10 expression to be significantly higher in FIV co-infected cats and in FeLV progressive infection than in retrovirus-negative cats.[158] Considering IL-10 is a key cytokine in the inhibition of Th1 immunity, its increase is believed to impair the host's optimal antifungal response. Still, severe sporotrichosis is increasingly reported in cats independently of retrovirus co-infection or other apparent immunosuppression, which supports the assumption that this disease develops in a different manner in cats.[46]

Despite the importance of cellular immunity in resolution of fungal infections, a humoral immune response contributes to the overall response in sporotrichosis and fuels further studies for the development of a vaccine.[159] Cell wall components have been studied as a promising source of vaccine candidate antigens. Passive immunization with antibodies to 3-carboxymuconate cyclase antibodies, a 70-kDa cell wall glycoprotein (gp70) that is important for fungal adherence to the extracellular matrix,[160] resulted in a protective effect in mice,[161] even when T-cell–deficient animals were used. Moreover, yeast opsonization with serum against cell wall proteins of *S. schenckii* markedly increases phagocytosis and strongly inhibits the adhesion of the fungus to fibroblasts. In a similar way, the opsonization of the fungus by antibodies anti-3-carboxymuconate cyclase enhanced phagocytic ability of macrophages and elicits the release of proinflammatory cytokines.[162] Carboxymuconate cyclase has been suggested as an antigen candidate for the further development of an effective vaccine for animal and human use.[94]

Another potential vaccine candidate from *Sporothrix* cell wall is the protein enolase. In conjunction with the adjuvant Montanide™ Pet Gel A (PGA), this protein has been shown to induce a strong Th1 reaction in addition to high antibody levels and decreased fungal load in the liver and spleen.[163] The use of a recombinant enolase-based PGA-adjuvanted vaccine demonstrated a protective effect in mice after challenge with virulent *Sporothrix* species.[164]

Despite the progress made in the past few years on the discovery of potential vaccine candidates, an effective vaccine for preventing sporotrichosis is still not commercially available.

PREVENTION

People handling cats with potential sporotrichosis should follow the biosafety measures listed in Box 84.1.[165] In addition, isolation of sick cats from other animals reared in the same environment is indicated. Care must be taken to avoid cuts or penetrating injuries when working with infected cats, and protective outerwear should be worn. Proper physical restraint or sedation of noncooperative animals must be done to allow complete examination of lesions and the collection of specimens for diagnosis.

Decontamination and cleaning of cages or transport containers can be achieved with sodium hypochlorite (1%), for at least 10 minutes. If possible, sun drying is also beneficial. After contact with infected animals, surfaces should be cleaned and disinfected with sodium hypochlorite solution (1%), for at least 10 minutes, followed by alcohol 70%, using disposable paper towels.[166] Accelerated hydrogen peroxide and polihexametilene biguanide (PHMB) are suitable alternatives to sodium hypochlorite.

An effective and viable therapeutic regimen applied to cats as well as public awareness programs on sporotrichosis prophylaxis are required in endemic areas, encouraging the following: responsible ownership, castration, cremation of dead cats, confinement of cats inside the home, limitation of the number of cats per household, regular cleaning of dwellings, and proper health care for cats. General public health measures such as basic sanitation, regular garbage collection, and cleaning of uninhabited lots are also required.[166]

BOX 84.1 Biosafety Measures for People Handling Cats with Suspected Sporotrichosis

Veterinary Clinics

- Personal protection equipment: disposable gloves, long-sleeved impermeable gowns, closed-toe footwear. In regions where epidemics occur, consider head covers, shoe covers, goggles, and N95 or surgical face masks.
- Hair should be tied back.
- After handling animals or contaminated equipment, remove gloves and wash hands with antiseptic (chlorhexidine, 2%; or povidone-iodine, 1%) and water.
- In case of injury through protective clothing by piercing, cutting, biting, or scratching, the wound must be immediately washed with soap and running water and professional medical advice obtained.
- Use experienced physical or preferably chemical restraint for examination of the animal or collection of specimens for laboratory evaluation.
- Dispose of animal waste in infectious waste labeled bags.
- After euthanasia, animals should be placed in infectious waste labeled bags and, after any necropsy examination, the final destination must be incineration.
- Needles and syringes and other disposable equipment used to collect specimens should be disposed of in labeled biohazard containers.
- Sharp items require approved rigid containers and soft items can be disposed of in infectious waste labeled bags.
- Soiled gauze squares should be treated as biohazardous and disposed of properly.
- Disposable gowns, gloves, and shoe and head covers should be treated as biohazardous and disposed of properly.
- Decontaminate and clean surfaces that were in contact with the animal, its tissues, or fluids using hypochlorite (1%) solution, accelerated hydrogen peroxide, or polihexametilene biguanide (PHMB) for 10 minutes. For impervious horizontal surfaces such as tables, alcohol (70% ethanol) can be applied for additional 10 minutes following a rinse of the hypochlorite solution. For smaller items, sun or ultraviolet (UV) light drying can facilitate decontamination and drying.

Owner

- Use disposable gloves when handling cats.
- Wash hands and arms after handling cats.
- Clothes should be washed in detergent and hot water and sun dried.
- Crate and dishes should be reserved exclusively for the infected pet and disinfected on a regular basis.
- Transport infected animals in plastic carriers instead of wood or cardboard to facilitate cleaning.

PUBLIC HEALTH ASPECTS

Sporotrichosis is classically associated with contact with contaminated plants or soil. Individuals with occupational risks are gardeners, florists, forestry workers, agricultural workers, farmers, hunters, fishers, and carpenters. Outbreaks have been reported after common exposure of multiple individuals to a source of contaminated plant material. Laboratory-acquired infections have also been described.[167,168]

Since the 1990s, zoonotic sporotrichosis, related to the direct transmission from infected cats, has emerged as an important alternative route for the infection. The first reported zoonotic epidemic of this mycosis was identified in 1998 in the city and surroundings of Rio de Janeiro, Brazil, and currently this region is considered hyperendemic for zoonotic sporotrichosis. Cases have occurred in an urban area mainly among people of underprivileged socioeconomic level. Taking care of diseased cats is the main factor associated with zoonotic transmission due to contact with infectious lesions and due to the higher risk of suffering scratches and bites when handling these cats.[6] Nearly 85% of affected humans reported contact with sick cats, and more than half of these individuals reported a history of a scratch or a bite. Housewives (30%), students (18%), and veterinarians (5%) were the primary at-risk populations.[5] Immunocompromised humans, such as HIV-infected patients, are a high-risk population and are susceptible to extracutaneous sporotrichosis with involvement of multiple organs.[64,169] Atypical clinical presentations as well as disseminated sporotrichosis in humans have been associated with *S. brasiliensis* infection, with no apparent connection to the host's immune status.[170]

The detection of *Sporothrix* strains on claws and in the oral cavities of cats that are genetically identical to those causing human disease provides evidence that zoonotic transmission can occur through scratches or bites.[171] Isolation of organisms from nasal secretions and cutaneous lesions implies the possibility of transmission through secretions and exudates. In contrast, no human cases were associated with a series of 23 veterinary cases from northern California.[74] This remarkable difference in the Brazilian zoonotic epidemic is probably due to the prevalence of the highly virulent *S. brasiliensis* in association with a successful route of transmission driven by cats.[172]

In contrast to feline sporotrichosis, canine sporotrichosis is of minimal zoonotic importance. Dogs are probably not directly involved in the transmission of sporotrichosis in view of the scarcity of yeasts in the lesions and the absence of *Sporothrix* in the oral cavity. In addition, there is no confirmation of human cases associated with transmission by dogs in the Brazilian epidemic.[49] Interhuman transmission is rare.[173,174]

CASE EXAMPLE

Signalment

"Milho," a 2-year-old mongrel intact male cat from Rio de Janeiro, Brazil.

History

Milho was examined at a reference center for diagnosis and treatment of sporotrichosis in Rio de Janeiro because of suspected sporotrichosis. The owner had observed skin lesions on the cat for a month before referral.

Physical Examination

The cat weighed 4.1 kg and was in a good overall condition. Clinical examination revealed multiple ulcerated skin lesions distributed over the face (Fig. 84.16A), nasal region, cervical region, hind limbs and fore limbs, as well as generalized lymphadenomegaly.

Laboratory Findings

Exudates from the ulcerated lesions (pelvic limbs, thoracic limbs, and cervical region) were collected under anesthesia before and during follow-up by sterile swab and seeded on to Sabouraud's dextrose agar, followed by incubation at 25°C. Suspected isolates were subcultivated on potato dextrose agar medium at 25°C for macroscopic and microscopic morphologic studies, and dimorphism (demonstration of both yeast and mold forms) was demonstrated by conversion to the yeast form on BHI agar medium at 37°C. For cytologic examination, impression smears of the same skin lesions were made.

Yeast-like cells were observed on cytologic examination, and *Sporothrix* spp. was isolated and identified from skin lesions using fungal culture. Alterations identified on routine hematology and serum biochemical panels were anemia, leukocytosis, and hypoalbuminemia. The cat was positive for FIV antibody and negative for FeLV antigen (SNAP Combo FeLV/FIV, IDEXX Laboratories, ME, USA).

Treatment

Oral ITZ capsules, at a dose of 100 mg, PO, q24 h (24.4 mg/kg), was prescribed. After 3 months of ITZ therapy, besides worsening of the initial skin lesions (Fig. 84.16B), new skin lesions and nasal mucosal involvement developed, together with respiratory signs (sneezing and nasal discharge).

Sporothrix continued to be isolated from exudates during the 3 months of ITZ monotherapy, and impression smears were still positive after 2 months, though with a progressive decrease in the number of yeasts present.

Due to poor clinical response, KI capsules at the dose of 15 mg, PO, q24h (3.65 mg/kg) were administered, while continuing ITZ (100 mg, PO, q24h). Both drugs were administered with food by the owner.

Two weeks after the ITZ+KI association had been initiated, the cat developed hyporexia. KI treatment was temporarily suspended for 3 days and oral silymarin 30 mg/kg, q24h, was administered. Within this period, the cat began eating normally, and KI was reintroduced at half the dose on alternate days for 15 days. After that, the full KI dose (15 mg, q24h) was again prescribed.

At the first follow-up visit, around 30 days after the introduction of KI, the cat had stopped sneezing and nasal discharge was not observed. Cutaneous lesions were healing, but lymphadenomegaly persisted.

At the following appointment, the owner reported hyporexia and weight loss was documented. A palpable soft mass on the left thoracic region (8 cm diameter) was detected on physical examination, and needle aspiration cytology confirmed abscess formation with polymorphonuclear leukocytes, necrotic cells, and numerous coccoid bacteria. After the drainage of the abscess, oral amoxicillin-clavulanic acid treatment was initiated (25 mg/kg, PO, q12h for 14 days).

Because of the inappetence, treatment with both antifungal drugs was temporarily suspended (15 days for ITZ and 20 days for KI). The drugs were reintroduced as follows: ITZ 100 mg PO q24h, and KI 7.5 mg PO q48h (1.8 mg/kg) for a week, then 15 mg PO q48h for a week, then 15 mg PO q24h. After 3 months of combination therapy, the cat was considered cured with complete healing of skin and mucosal lesions (Fig. 84.16C). After clinical cure, treatment was continued for an additional period of 4 weeks.

Comments

This cat demonstrated progression of clinical signs with the emergence of nasal mucosa involvement, even while receiving ITZ. *Sporothrix brasiliensis* is the most prevalent etiologic agent in Rio de Janeiro, Brazil, and is described as the most virulent among the *Sporothrix* species. A recent study demonstrated that none of the tested strains of *S. brasiliensis* recovered from cats were ITZ resistant.[175] Although antifungal susceptibility tests were not performed in this case, it should be considered that the causative strain may have exhibited some resistance to ITZ, or alternatively, there may have been problems related to absorption of ITZ. Therapeutic drug monitoring could have also been considered, although 100 mg PO q24h is a high dose of ITZ that can be associated with significant adverse effects in cats. Still, the high susceptibility of cats to *Sporothrix* species is not yet understood, but it is believed to be multifactorial.

The decrease in fungal burden during treatment suggests that in spite of the clinical failure, the potential of this cat as a source of infection was probably reduced. The use of KI capsules as a combined therapy led to a favorable outcome. Hyporexia and weight loss were managed as adverse effects of the therapy. However, the coincidental development of an abscess (presumably a cat-bite abscess) may have been the cause of hyporexia when they both occured at the same time.

Continued

CASE EXAMPLE—cont'd

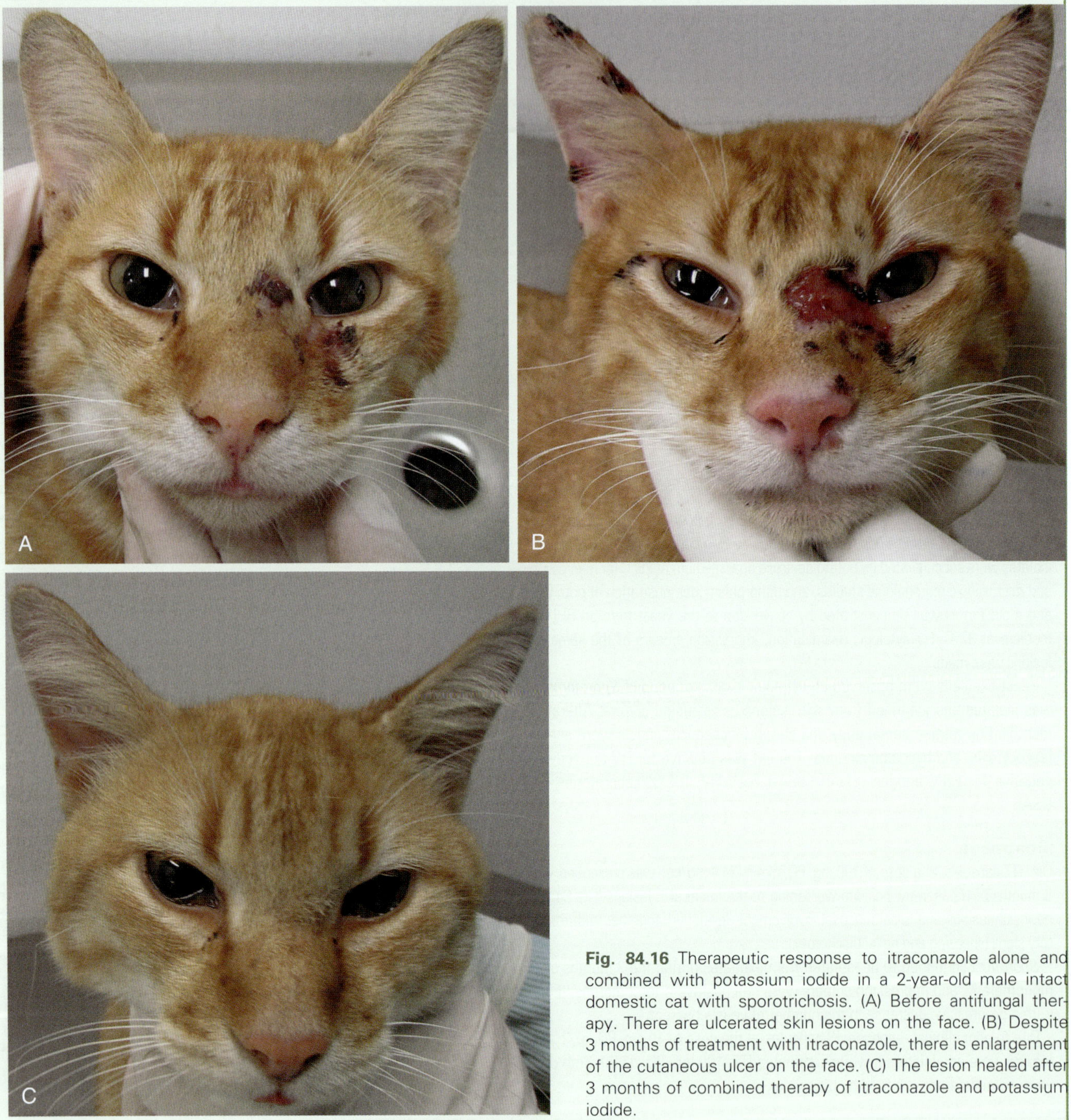

Fig. 84.16 Therapeutic response to itraconazole alone and combined with potassium iodide in a 2-year-old male intact domestic cat with sporotrichosis. (A) Before antifungal therapy. There are ulcerated skin lesions on the face. (B) Despite 3 months of treatment with itraconazole, there is enlargement of the cutaneous ulcer on the face. (C) The lesion healed after 3 months of combined therapy of itraconazole and potassium iodide.

SUGGESTED READINGS

Gremião IDF, Martins da Silva da Rocha E, et al. Guideline for the management of feline sporotrichosis caused by *Sporothrix brasiliensis* and literature revision. *Braz J Microbiol.* 2021;52:107–124.

Pereira SA, Passos SRL, Silva JN, et al. Response to azolic antifungal agents for treating feline sporotrichosis. *Vet Rec.* 2010;166:290–294.

Reis EG, Schubach TM, Pereira SA, et al. Association of itraconazole and potassium iodide in the treatment of feline sporotrichosis: a prospective study. *Med Mycol.* 2016;54(7):684–690.

REFERENCES

1. Rippon JW. Sporotrichosis. In: Rippon J, ed. *Medical Mycology: The Pathogenic Fungi and the Pathogenic Actinomycetes.* 3rd ed. Philadelphia, PA: WB Saunders; 1988:325–352.
2. Kauffman CA. Sporotrichosis. *Clin Infect Dis.* 1999;29:231–236.
3. Barros MB, Schubach A, Galhardo MC, et al. Sporotrichosis with widespread cutaneous lesions:report of 24 cases related to transmission by domestic cats in Rio de Janeiro, Brazil. *Int J Dermatol.* 2003;42:677–681.
4. Barros MB, Schubach TP, Coll JO, et al. Sporotrichosis: development and challenges of an epidemic. *Rev Panam Salud Publica.* 2010;27:459–460.
5. Barros MB, Schubach TM, Galhardo MC, et al. Sporotrichosis: an emergent zoonosis in Rio de Janeiro. *Mem Inst Oswaldo Cruz.* 2001;96:777–779.
6. Barros MBL, Schubach AO, Schubach TMP, et al. An epidemic of sporotrichosis in Rio de Janeiro, Brazil: epidemiological aspects of a series of cases. *Epidemiol Infect.* 2008;136:1192–1196.
7. Marimon R, Cano J, Gené J, et al. *Sporothrix brasiliensis, S. globosa*, and *S. mexicana*, three new *Sporothrix* species of clinical interest. *J Clin Microbiol.* 2007;45(10):3198–3206.
8. Rodrigues AM, de Hoog S, de Camargo ZP. Emergence of pathogenicity in the *Sporothrix schenckii* complex. *Med Mycol.* 2013;51(4):405–412.
9. Zhou X, Rodrigues AM, Feng P, et al. Global ITS diversity in the *Sporothrix schenckii* complex. *Fungal Divers.* 2014;66:153–165.
10. Govender NP, Maphanga TG, Zulu TG, et al. An outbreak of lymphocutaneous sporotrichosis among mine-workers in South Africa. *PLoS Negl Trop Dis.* 2015;9(9):e0004096.
11. Morrison AS, Lockhart SR, Bromley JG, et al. An environmental *Sporothrix* as a cause of corneal ulcer. *Med Mycol Case Rep.* 2013;2:88–90.
12. Rodrigues AM, Choappa RC, Fernandes GF, et al. *Sporothrix chilensis* sp. nov. (Ascomycota:Ophiostomatales), a soil-borne agent of human sporotrichosis with mild-pathogenic potential to mammals. *Fungal Biol.* 2016;120(2):246–264.
13. Rodrigues AM, Della Terra PP, Gremião ID, et al. The threat of emerging and re-emerging pathogenic *Sporothrix* species. *Mycopathologia.* 2020;185:813-842.
14. Gremião IDF, Oliveira MME, Monteiro de Miranda LH, et al. Geographic expansion of sporotrichosis, Brazil. *Emerg Infect Dis.* 2020;26(3):621–624.
15. Etchecopaz AN, Lanza N, Toscanini MA, et al. Sporotrichosis caused by *Sporothrix brasiliensis* in Argentina: case report, molecular identification and in vitro susceptibility pattern to antifungal drugs. *J Mycol Med.* 2020;30:100908.
16. Aldama A, Aldama AG, Pereira J. Value of molecular techniques and risk factors in the diagnosis and evolution of sporotrichosis. About 2 cases of *Sporothrix brasiliensis* and *S. globosa. An Fac Cienc Méd.* 2020;53:177–184.
17. Makri N, Paterson GK, Gregge F, et al. First case report of cutaneous sporotrichosis (*Sporothrix* species) in a cat in the UK. *JFMS Open Rep.* 2020;6(1):2055116920906001.
18. Oliveira DC, Lopes PG, Spader TB, et al. Antifungal susceptibilities of *Sporothrix albicans, S. brasiliensis*, and *S. luriei* of the *S. schenckii* complex identified in Brazil. *J Clin Microbiol.* 2011;49:3047–3049.
19. Chakrabarti A, Bonifaz A, Gutierrez-Galhardo MC, et al. Global epidemiology of sporotrichosis. *Med Mycol.* 2015;53(1):3–14.
20. Duangkaew L, Yurayart C, Limsivilai O, et al. Cutaneous sporotrichosis in a stray cat from Thailand. *Med Mycol Case Rep.* 2019;23:46–49.
21. Gremião ID, Miranda LH, Reis EG, et al. Zoonotic epidemic of sporotrichosis: cat to human transmission. *PLoS Pathog.* 2017;13:e1006077.
22. Gremião IDF, Martins da Silva da Rocha E, Montenegro H, et al. Guideline for the management of feline sporotrichosis caused by *Sporothrix brasiliensis* and literature revision. *Braz J Microbiol.* 2021;52:107–124.
23. Schubach TMP, Schubach A, Okamoto T, et al. Canine sporotrichosis in Rio de Janeiro, Brazil: clinical presentation, laboratory diagnosis and therapeutic response in 44 cases (1998–2003). *Med Mycol.* 2006;44:87–92.
24. Scott DW, Bentinck-Smith J, Haggerty GF. Sporotrichosis in three dogs. *Cornell Vet.* 1974;64(3):416–426.
25. Gougerot H & Caraven. Sporotrichose spontanée du chien. *Presse méd.* 1908;43:337.
26. Whittemore JC, Webb CB. Successful treatment of nasal sporotrichosis in a dog. *Can Vet J.* 2007;48(4):411–414.
27. Cafarchia C, Sasanelli M, Lia RP, et al. Lymphocutaneous and nasal sporotrichosis in a dog from southern Italy: case report. *Mycopathologia.* 2007;163(2):75–79.
28. Fichman V, Gremião IDF, Mendes-Júnior AAV, et al. Sporotrichosis transmitted by a cockatiel (*Nymphicus hollandicus*). *J Eur Acad Dermatol Venereol.* 2018;32(4):e157–e158.
29. Pereira SA, Gremião IDF, Menezes RC. Sporotrichosis in animals: zoonotic transmission. In: Carlos IZ, ed. *Sporotrichosis: New Developments and Future Prospects.* 1st ed. Cham, ZG: Springer International Publishing; 2015:83–102.
30. Schubach TM, de Oliveira Schubach A, dos Reis RS, et al. *Sporothrix schenckii* isolated from domestic cats with and without sporotrichosis in Rio de Janeiro, Brazil. *Mycopathologia.* 2002;153(2):83–86.
31. Dixon DM, Salkin IF, Duncan RA, et al. Isolation and characterization of *Sporothrix schenckii* from clinical and environmental sources associated with the largest U.S. epidemic of sporotrichosis. *J Clin Microbiol.* 1991;29:1106–1113.
32. The clinical, therapeutic and epidemiological features of sporotrichosis infection of the mines. In: Helm M, Berman C, eds. *Proceedings of the Transvaal Mine Medical Officers' Association Symposium on Sporotrichosis Infection on Mines of the Witwatersrand (Johannesburg).* Johannesburg: The Transvaal Chamber of Mines; 1947.
33. Schubach A, Barros MBL, Wanke B. Epidemic sporotrichosis. *Curr Opin Infect Dis.* 2008;21:129–133.
34. Silva MB, Costa MM, Torres CC, et al. Urban sporotrichosis: a neglected epidemic in Rio de Janeiro, Brazil. *Cad Saúde Pública.* 2012;28:1867–1880.
35. Viana PG, Pereira SA, Mutis MCS, et al. Clinical and epidemiological aspects of the largest epidemic of sporotrichosis in dogs: 203 cases [2004-2014]. In: Proceedings of the 7th Trends in Medical Mycology; Oct ;Lisbon, Portugal. *Mycoses.* 2015;58 (suppl 4):145.
36. Mackay BM, Menrath VH, Ridley MF, et al. Sporotrichosis in a cat. *Aust Vet Practit.* 1986;16:3–5.
37. Gonzalez Cabo JF, de las Heras Guillamon M, Latre Cequiel MV, et al. Feline sporotrichosis: a case report. *Mycopathologia.* 1989;108:149–154.
38. Hirano M, Watanabe K, Murakami M, et al. A case of feline sporotrichosis. *J Vet Med Sci.* 2006;68:283–284.
39. Scheufen S, Strommer S, Weisenborn J, et al. Clinical manifestation of an amelanotic *Sporothrix schenckii* complex isolate in a cat in Germany. *JMM Case Rep.* 2015;2. https://doi.org/10.1099/jmmcr.0.000039.
40. Reed KD, Moore FM, Geiger GE, et al. Zoonotic transmission of sporotrichosis: case report and review. *Clin Infect Dis.* 1993;16: 384–387.
41. Bove-Sevilla PM, Mayorga-Rodríguez J, Hernández-Hernández O. Sporotrichosis transmitted by a domestic cat. Case report. *Med Cutan Iber Lat Am.* 2008;36:33–35.
42. Zamri-Saad M, Salmiyah TS, Jasni S, et al. Feline sporotrichosis: an increasingly important zoonotic disease in Malaysia. *Vet Rec.* 1990;127:480.
43. Yegneswaran PP, Sripathi H, Bairy I, et al. Zoonotic sporotrichosis of lymphocutaneous type in a man acquired from a domesticated feline source: report of a first case in southern Karnataka, India. *Int J Dermatol.* 2009;48:1198–1200.

44. Gremião ID, Menezes RC, Schubach TM, et al. Feline sporotrichosis: epidemiological and clinical aspects. *Med Mycol.* 2015;53:15–21.
45. Han HS, Kano R. Feline sporotrichosis in Asia. *Braz J Microbiol.* 2021;52:125–134.
46. Schubach TMP, Schubach AO, Okamoto T, et al. Evaluation of an epidemic of sporotrichosis in cats: 347 cases (1998-2001). *J Am Vet Med Assoc.* 2004;224:1623–1629.
47. Macêdo-Sales PA, Souto SRLS, Destefani CA, et al. Domestic feline contribution in the transmission of *Sporothrix* in Rio de Janeiro State, Brazil: a comparison between infected and non-infected populations. *BMC Vet Res.* 2018;14:19.
48. Kovarik CL, Neyra E, Bustamante B. Evaluation of cats as the source of endemic sporotrichosis in Peru. *Med Mycol.* 2008;46:53–56.
49. Barros MB, Schubach AO, do Valle AC, et al. Cat-transmitted sporotrichosis epidemic in Rio de Janeiro, Brazil: description of a series of cases. *Clin Infect Dis.* 2004;38:529–535.
50. Freitas DF, do Valle AC, de Almeida Paes R, et al. Zoonotic sporotrichosis in Rio de Janeiro, Brazil: a protracted epidemic yet to be curbed. *Clin Infect Dis.* 2010;50:453.
51. Shany M. A mixed fungal infection in a dog: sporotrichosis and cryptococcosis. *Can Vet J.* 2000;41:799–800.
52. Rossato L, Santos SSD, Ferreira LG, de Almeida SR. The importance of Toll-like receptor 4 during experimental *Sporothrix brasiliensis* infection. *Med Mycol.* 2019;57(4):489–495.
53. Rossato L, Silvana Dos Santos S, Ferreira LG, Rogério de Almeida S. The impact of the absence of Toll-like receptor-2 during *Sporothrix brasiliensis* infection. *J Med Microbiol.* 2019;68:87–94.
54. Lopes-Bezerra LM, Schubach A, Costa RO. *Sporothrix schenckii* and sporotrichosis. *An Acad Bras Cienc.* 2006;78:293–308.
55. Ortega I, Soares Felipe MS, Vasconcelos AT, et al. Peroxide sensing and signaling in the *Sporothrix schenckii* complex: an in silico analysis to uncover putative mechanisms regulating the Hog1 and AP-1 like signaling pathways. *Med Mycol.* 2015;53:51–59.
56. Lima OC, Figueiredo CC, Previato JO, et al. Involvement of fungal cell wall components in adhesion of *Sporothrix schenckii* to human fibronectin. *Infect Immun.* 2001;69:6874–6880.
57. Teixeira PA, de Castro RA, Nascimento RC, et al. Cell surface expression of adhesins for fibronectin correlates with virulence in *Sporothrix schenckii. Microbiology.* 2009;155(Pt 11):3730–3738.
58. Barros MB, de Almeida Paes R, Schubach AO. *Sporothrix schenckii* and sporotrichosis. *Clin Microbiol Rev.* 2011;24:633–654.
59. Arrillaga-Moncrieff I, Capilla J, Mayayo E, et al. Different virulence levels of the species of *Sporothrix* in a murine model. *Clin Microbiol Infect.* 2009;15:651–655.
60. Clavijo-Giraldo DM, Matínez-Alvarez JA, Lopes-Bezerra LM, et al. Analysis of *Sporothrix schenckii* sensu stricto and *Sporothrix brasiliensis* virulence in *Galleria mellonella. J Microbiol Methods.* 2016;122:73–77.
61. Almeida-Paes R, de Oliveira LC, Oliveira MM, et al. Phenotypic characteristics associated with virulence of clinical isolates from the *Sporothrix* complex. *BioMed Res Int.* 2015;2015:212308.
62. Freitas DF, Santos SS, Almeida-Paes R, et al. Increase in virulence of *Sporothrix brasiliensis* over five years in a patient with chronic disseminated sporotrichosis. *Virulence.* 2015;6:112–120.
63. Aung AK, Teh BM, McGrath C, et al. Pulmonary sporotrichosis: case series and systematic analysis of literature on clinico-radiological patterns and management outcomes. *Med Mycol.* 2013;51:534–544.
64. Moreira JA, Freitas DF, Lamas CC. The impact of sporotrichosis in HIV-infected patients: a systematic review. *Infection.* 2015;43:267–276.
65. Madrid IM, Mattei AS, Fernandes CG, et al. Epidemiological findings and laboratory evaluation of sporotrichosis: a description of 103 cases in cats and dogs in southern Brazil. *Mycopathologia.* 2012;173:265–273.
66. Schubach TM, Schubach Ade O, Cuzzi-Maya T, et al. Pathology of sporotrichosis in 10 cats in Rio de Janeiro. *Vet Rec.* 2003;152:172–175.
67. Dunstan RW, Langham RF, Reinmann KA, et al. Feline sporotrichosis: a report of five cases with transmission to humans. *J Am Acad Dermatol.* 1986;15:37–45.
68. Werner RE, Levine BG, Kaplan W, et al. Sporotrichosis in a cat. *J Am Vet Med Assoc.* 1971;159:407–412.
69. Schubach TMP, Schubach A, Okamoto T, et al. Haematogenous spread of *Sporothrix schenckii* in cats with naturally acquired sporotrichosis. *J Small Anim Pract.* 2003;44:395–398.
70. Leme LRP, Schubach TMP, Santos IB, et al. Mycological evaluation of bronchoalveolar lavage in cats with respiratory signs from Rio de Janeiro, Brazil. *Mycoses.* 2007;50:210–214.
71. Sykes JE, Torres SM, Armstrong PJ, et al. Itraconazole for treatment of sporotrichosis in a dog residing on a Christmas tree farm. *J Am Vet Med Assoc.* 2001;9:1440–1443.
72. Iwasaki M, Hagiwara MK. Skeletal sporotrichosis in a dog. *Companion Anim Pract.* 1988;2:27–31.
73. Mascarenhas MB, Lopes NL, Pinto TG, et al. Canine sporotrichosis: report of 15 advanced cases. *Pesqui Vet Bras.* 2018;38:477–481.
74. Crothers SL, White SD, Ihrke PJ, et al. Sporotrichosis: a retrospective evaluation of 23 cases seen in northern California (1987-2007). *Vet Dermatol.* 2009;20:249–259.
75. Goad DL, Goad ME. Osteoarticular sporotrichosis in a dog. *J Am Vet Med Assoc.* 1986;189:1326–1328.
76. Bernstein JA, Cook HE, Gill AF, et al. Cytologic diagnosis of generalized cutaneous sporotrichosis in a hunting hound. *Vet Clin Pathol.* 2007;36:94–96.
77. Plotnick AN, Boshoven EW, Rosychuk RA. Primary cutaneous coccidioidomycosis and subsequent drug eruption to itraconazole in a dog. *J Am Anim Hosp Assoc.* 1997;33:139–143.
78. Rosser EJ, Dunstan RW. Sporotrichosis. In: Greene CE, ed. *Infectious Diseases of the Dog and Cat.* 3rd ed. Philadelphia, PA: WB Saunders; 2006:608–612.
79. Pereira SA, Passos SRL, Silva JN, et al. Response to azolic antifungal agents for treating feline sporotrichosis. *Vet Rec.* 2010;166:290–294.
80. de Souza EW, Borba CM, Pereira SA, et al. Clinical features, fungal load, coinfections, histological skin changes, and itraconazole treatment response of cats with sporotrichosis caused by *Sporothrix brasiliensis. Sci Rep.* 2018;8:9074.
81. Malik R, Vogelnest L, O'Brien CR, et al. Infections and some other conditions affecting the skin and subcutis of the naso-ocular region of cats—clinical experience 1987-2003. *J Feline Med Surg.* 2004;6:383–390.
82. Whittemore JC, Webb CB. Successful treatment of nasal sporotrichosis in a dog. *Can Vet J.* 2007;48:411–414.
83. Santos IB, Schubach TMP, Leme LRP, et al. Sporotrichosis—the main differential diagnosis with tegumentary leishmaniasis in dogs from Rio de Janeiro, Brazil. *Vet Parasitol.* 2007;143:1–6.
84. Welsh RD. Sporotrichosis. *J Am Vet Med Assoc.* 2003;223:1123–1126.
85. Pereira SA, Menezes RC, Gremião IDF, et al. Sensitivity of cytopathological examination in the diagnosis of feline sporotrichosis. *J Feline Med Surg.* 2011;13:220–223.
86. Clinkenbeard KD. Diagnostic citology: sporotrichosis. *Compend Contin Educ Pract Vet.* 1991;13(2):207–211.
87. Jessica N, Sonia RL, Rodrigo C, et al. Diagnostic accuracy assessment of cytopathological examination of feline sporotrichosis. *Med Mycol.* 2015;53(8):880–884.
88. Silva JN, Miranda LHM, Menezes RC, et al. Comparison of the sensitivity of three methods for the early diagnosis of sporotrichosis in cats. *J Comp Pathol.* 2018;160:72–78.
89. de Miranda LHM, Silva JN, Gremião IDF, et al. Monitoring fungal burden and viability of *Sporothrix* spp. in skin lesions of cats for predicting antifungal treatment response. *J Fungi (Basel).* 2018 Aug 7;4:92.
90. Oliveira MM, Almeida-Paes R, Muniz MM, et al. Phenotypic and molecular identification of *Sporothrix* isolates from an epidemic area of sporotrichosis in Brazil. *Mycopathologia.* 2011;172:257–267.
91. Oliveira MM, Santos C, Sampaio P, et al. Development and optimization of a new MALDI-TOF protocol for identification of the *Sporothrix* species complex. *Res Microbiol.* 2015;166:102–110.
92. Bernardes-Engemann AR, Costa RC, Miguens BR, et al. Development of an enzyme-linked immunosorbent assay for the serodiagnosis of several clinical forms of sporotrichosis. *Med Mycol.* 2005;43:487–493.
93. Fernandes GF, Lopes-Bezerra LM, Bernardes-Engemann AR, et al. Serodiagnosis of sporotrichosis infection in cats by enzyme-linked immuno-

sorbent assay using a specific antigen, SsCBF, and crude exoantigens. *Vet Microbiol.* 2011;147:445–449.
94. Rodrigues AM, Fernandes GF, Araujo LM, et al. Proteomics-based characterization of the humoral immune response in sporotrichosis: toward discovery of potential diagnostic and vaccine antigens. *PLoS Negl Trop Dis.* 2015;9:e0004016.
95. Baptista VS, Mothé GB, Santos GMP, et al. Promising application of the SsCBF ELISA test to monitor the therapeutic response of feline sporotrichosis caused by *Sporothrix brasiliensis* from Brazilian epidemics. *Braz J Microbiol.* 2021;52:145–153.
96. Rodrigues AM, Teixeira MM, de Hoog GS, et al. Phylogenetic analysis reveals a high prevalence of *Sporothrix brasiliensis* in feline sporotrichosis outbreaks. *PLoS Negl Trop Dis.* 2013;7:e2281.
97. Oliveira MME, Almeida-Paes R, Gutierrez-Galhardo MC, et al. Molecular identification of the *Sporothrix schenckii* complex. *Rev Iberoam De Micol.* 2014;31:2–6.
98. Zhang Y, Hagen F, Stielow B, et al. Phylogeography and evolutionary patterns in *Sporothrix* spanning more than 14,000 human and animal case reports. *Persoonia.* 2015;35:1–20.
99. de Oliveira MM, Sampaio P, Almeida-Paes R, et al. Rapid identification of *Sporothrix* species by T3B fingerprinting. *J Clin Microbiol.* 2012;50:2159–2162.
100. Rodrigues AM, de Hoog GS, Camargo ZP. Genotyping species of the *Sporothrix schenckii* complex by PCR-RFLP of calmodulin. *Diagn Microbiol Infect Dis.* 2014;78:383–387.
101. Rodrigues AM, De Hoog GS, Camargo ZP. Molecular diagnosis of pathogenic *Sporothrix* species. *PLoS Negl Trop Dis.* 2015;9:e0004190.
102. Rodrigues AM, Najafzadeh MJ, De Hoog GS, et al. Rapid identification of emerging human-pathogenic *Sporothrix* species with rolling circle amplification. *Front Microbiol.* 2015;6:1385.
103. Boechat JS, Oliveira MME, Almeida-Paes R, et al. Feline sporotrichosis: associations between clinical-epidemiological profiles and phenotypic-genotypic characteristics of the etiological agents in the Rio de Janeiro epizootic area. *Mem Inst Oswaldo Cruz.* 2018;113:185–196.
104. Boechat JS, Pereira SA, de Sá Machado AC, et al. Canine sporotrichosis: polyphasic taxonomy and antifungal susceptibility profiles of *Sporothrix* species in an endemic area in Brazil. *Braz J Microbiol.* 2021;52:135–143.
105. Kano R, Watanabe K, Murakami M, et al. Molecular diagnosis of feline sporotrichosis. *Vet Rec.* 2005;156:484–485.
106. Gonsales FF, Fernandes NCCA, Mansho W, et al. Direct PCR of lesions suggestive of sporotrichosis in felines. *Arq Bras Med Vet Zootec.* 2020;72:2001–2006.
107. Miranda LH, Quintella LP, dos Santos IB, et al. Histopathology of canine sporotrichosis: a morphological study of 86 cases from Rio de Janeiro (2001-2007). *Mycopathologia.* 2009;168:79–87.
108. Miranda LHM, Conceição-Silva F, Quintella LP, et al. Feline sporotrichosis: histopathological profile of cutaneous lesions and their correlation with clinical presentation. *Comp Immunol Microbiol Infect Dis.* 2013;36:425–432.
109. Miranda LHM, Quintella LP, Santos IB, et al. Comparative histopathological study of sporotrichosis and American tegumentary leishmaniosis in dogs from Rio de Janeiro. *J Comp Pathol.* 2010;143:1–7.
110. Quintella LP, Passos SRL, Galhardo ACF, et al. Histopathology of cutaneous sporotrichosis in Rio de Janeiro: a series of 119 consecutive cases. *J Cut Pathol.* 2011;38:25–32.
111. Rosa AC, Scroferneker ML, Vettorato R, et al. Epidemiology of sporotrichosis: a study of 304 cases in Brazil. *J Am Acad Dermatol.* 2005;52:451.
112. Guarner J, Brand ME. Histopathologic diagnosis of fungal infections in the 21st century. *Clin Microbiol Rev.* 2011;24:247.
113. Miranda LH, Quintella LP, Menezes RC, et al. Evaluation of immunohistochemistry for the diagnosis of sporotrichosis in dogs. *Vet J.* 2011;190:408–411.
114. Lopes-Alves L, Travassos LR, Previato JO, et al. Novel antigenic determinants from peptidorhamnomannans of *Sporothrix schenckii. Glycobiology.* 1994;4:281–288.
115. Pereira SA, Gremião ID, Kitada AA, et al. The epidemiological scenario of feline sporotrichosis in Rio de Janeiro, State of Rio de Janeiro, Brazil. *Rev Soc Bras Med Trop.* 2014;47:392–393.
116. Gremião IDF, Schubach TMP, Pereira SA, et al. Intralesional amphotericin B in a cat with refractory localized sporotrichosis. *J Feline Med Surg.* 2009;11:720–723.
117. Honse CO, Rodrigues AM, Gremião ID, et al. Use of local hyperthermia to treat sporotrichosis in cat. *Vet Rec.* 2010;166:208–209.
118. Pereira SA, Schubach TMP, Gremião IDF, et al. Therapeutic aspects of feline sporotrichosis. *Acta Sci Vet.* 2009;37:311–321.
119. Rosser EJ. Sporotrichosis. In: Griffin CE, Kwochka KW, MacDonald JM, eds. *Current Veterinary Dermatology: The Science and Art of Therapy.* St Louis, MO: Mosby; 1993:49–53.
120. MacDonald E, Ewert A, Reitmeyer JC. Reappearance of *Sporothrix schenckii* lesions after administration of Solu-Medrol R to infected cats. *Sabouraudia.* 1980;18:295–300.
121. Pilmis B, Jullien V, Sobel J, et al. Antifungal drugs during pregnancy: an updated review. *J Antimicrob Chemother.* 2015;70:14–22.
122. Moudgal VV, Sobel JD. Antifungal drugs in pregnancy: a review. *Expert Opin Drug Saf.* 2003;2:475–483.
123. Taboada J. Systemic mycoses. In: Ettinger S, Feldman E, eds. *Textbook of Veterinary Internal Medicine—Diseases of the Dog and Cat.* 5th ed. Philadelphia, PA: WB Saunders; 2000:453–476.
124. Medleau L, Marks MA, Brown J, et al. Clinical evaluation of a cryptococcal antigen latex agglutination test for diagnosis of cryptococcosis in cats. *J Am Vet Med Assoc.* 1990;196:1470–1473.
125. Anderson NV, Ivoghii D, Moore WE, et al. Cutaneous sporotrichosis in a cat: a case report. *J Am Anim Hosp Assoc.* 1973;9:526–529.
126. Nobre MO, Castro AP, Caetano D, et al. Recurrence of sporotrichosis in cats with zoonotic involvement. *Rev Iberoam De Micol.* 2001;18:137–140.
127. Nusbaum BP, Gulbas N, Horwitz SN. Sporotrichosis acquired from a cat. *J Am Acad Dermatol.* 1983;8:386–391.
128. Dunstan RW, Reimann KA, Langham RF. Feline sporotrichosis. *J Am Vet Med Assoc.* 1986;189:880–883.
129. Reis EG, Schubach TM, Pereira SA, et al. Association of itraconazole and potassium iodide in the treatment of feline sporotrichosis: a prospective study. *Med Mycol.* 2016;54:684–690.
130. Reis EG, Gremião ID, Kitada AA, et al. Potassium iodide capsule treatment of feline sporotrichosis. *J Feline Med Surg.* 2012;14:399–404.
131. Vasquez-del-Mercado E, Arenas R, Padilla-Desgarenes C. *Sporotrichosis. Clin Dermatol.* 2012;30:437–443.
132. da Rocha RFDB, Schubach TMP, Pereira SA, Dos Reis ÉG, Carvalho BW, Gremião IDF. Refractory feline sporotrichosis treated with itraconazole combined with potassium iodide. *J Small Anim Pract.* 2018 Nov;59:720–721.
133. Gremião I, Schubach T, Pereira S, et al. Treatment of refractory feline sporotrichosis with a combination of intralesional amphotericin B and oral itraconazole. *Aust Vet J.* 2011;89:346–351.
134. Francesconi G, Valle A, Passos S, et al. Terbinafine (250 mg/day):an effective and safe treatment of cutaneous sporotrichosis. *J Eur Acad Dermatol Venereol.* 2009;23:1273–1276.
135. Borba-Santos LP, Rodrigues AM, Gagini TB, et al. Susceptibility of *Sporothrix brasiliensis* isolates to amphotericin B, azoles, and terbinafine. *Med Mycol.* 2015;53:178–188.
136. Gremião IDF, Pereira SA, Rodrigues AM, et al. Combination of surgical treatment and conventional antifungal therapy in feline sporotrichosis. *Acta Sci Vet.* 2006;34:221–223.
137. Jung JY, Almond CH, Campbell DC, et al. Role of surgery in the management of pulmonary sporotrichosis. *J Thorac Cardiovasc Surg.* 1979;77:234–239.
138. Shinogi T, Misago N, Narisawa Y. Cutaneous sporotrichosis with refractory and reinfectious lesions in a healthy female. *J Dermatol.* 2004;31:492–496.
139. Kauffman CA, Bustamante B, Chapman SW, et al. Clinical practice guidelines for the management of sporotrichosis: 2007 update by the Infectious Diseases Society of America. *Clin Infect Dis.* 2007;45:1255–1265.
140. de Souza CP, Lucas R, Ramadinha RH, et al. Cryosurgery in association with itraconazole for the treatment of feline sporotrichosis. *J Feline Med Surg.* 2016;18:137–143.
141. Nichols PR, Morris DO, Beale KM. A retrospective study of canine and feline cutaneous vasculitis. *Vet Dermatol.* 2001;12:255–264.

142. Legendre AM. Antimycotic drug therapy. In: Bonagura JD, ed. *Kirk's Current Veterinary Therapy XII*. 12th ed. Philadelphia, PA: WB Saunders; 1995:327–331.
143. Legendre AM, Rohrbach BW, Toal RL, et al. Treatment of blastomycosis with itraconazole in 112 dogs. *J Vet Intern Med*. 1996;10:365–371.
144. Sherding RG, Johnson SE. Intestinal histoplasmosis. In: Kirk RW, Bonagura JD, eds. *Current Veterinary Therapy XI*. 11th ed. Philadelphia, PA: WB Saunders; 1992:610–611.
145. Grassani MH, Juppa ALCA, Silva DA, et al. Use of potassium iodide in the treatment of sporotrichosis in dog after failure treatment with ketoconazole and itraconazole – a case report. *Clin Vet*. 2012;101:116–120.
146. Viana PG, Figueiredo ABF, Gremião IDF, et al. Successful treatment of canine sporotrichosis with terbinafine: case reports and literature review. *Mycopathologia*. 2018;183:471–478.
147. Martínez-Álvarez JA, Pérez-García LA, Mellado-Mojica E, et al. *Sporothrix schenckii sensu stricto* and *Sporothrix brasiliensis* are differentially recognized by human peripheral blood mononuclear cells. *Front Microbiol*. 2017;8:843.
148. Carlos IZ, Sassá MF, da Graça Sgarbi DB, et al. Current research on the immune response to experimental sporotrichosis. *Mycopathologia*. 2009;168:1–10.
149. Sassá MF, Ferreira LS, Ribeiro LC, et al. Immune response against *Sporothrix schenckii* in TLR-4-deficient mice. *Mycopathologia*. 2012;174:21–30.
150. Negrini TC, Ferreira LS, Alegranci P, et al. Role of TLR-2 and fungal surface antigens on innate immune response against *Sporothrix schenckii*. *Immunol Invest*. 2013;42:36–48.
151. Kajiwara H, Saito M, Ohga S, et al. Impaired host defense against *Sporothrix schenckii* in mice with chronic granulomatous disease. *Infect Immun*. 2004;72:5073–5079.
152. Tachibana T, Matsuyama T, Mitsuyama M. Involvement of CD4+ T cells and macrophages in acquired protection against infection with *Sporothrix schenckii* in mice. *Med Mycol*. 1999;37:397–404.
153. Uenotsuchi T, Takeuchi S, Matsuda T, et al. Differential induction of Th1-prone immunity by human dendritic cells activated with *Sporothrix schenckii* of cutaneous and visceral origins to determine their different virulence. *Int Immunol*. 2006;18:1637–1646.
154. Ferreira LS, Gonçalves AC, Portuondo DL, et al. Optimal clearance of *Sporothrix schenckii* requires an intact Th17 response in a mouse model of systemic infection. *Immunobiology*. 2015;220:985–992.
155. Miranda LH, Santiago MA, Schubach TMP, et al. Severe feline sporotrichosis associated with an increased population of CD8low cells and a decrease in CD4$^+$cells. *Med Mycol*. 2016;54:29–39.
156. Ribba B, ElGarch H, Brunet S, et al. Time-course analysis of main markers of primary infection in cats with the feline immunodeficiency virus. *Comput Math Methods Med*. 2012;2012:342602.
157. Kundu SK, Merigan TC. Inverse relationship of CD8+CD11+ suppressor T cells with human immunodeficiency virus (HIV)- specific cellular cytotoxicity and natural killer cell activity in HIV infection. *Immunology*. 1991;74:567–571.
158. de Miranda LHM, Meli M, Conceição-Silva F, et al. Co-infection with feline retrovirus is related to changes in immunological parameters of cats with sporotrichosis. *PLoS One*. 2018;13:e0207644.
159. Nascimento RC, Almeida SR. Humoral immune response against soluble and fractionate antigens in experimental sporotrichosis. *FEMS Immunol Med Microbiol*. 2005;43:241–247.
160. Ruiz-Baca E, Toriello C, Perez-Torres A, et al. Isolation and some properties of a glycoprotein of 70 kDa (Gp70) from the cell wall of *Sporothrix schenckii* involved in fungal adherence to dermal extracellular matrix. *Med Mycol*. 2009;47:185–196.
161. Nascimento RC, Espíndola NM, Castro RA, et al. Passive immunization with monoclonal antibody against a 70-kDa putative adhesin of *Sporothrix schenckii* induces protection in murine sporotrichosis. *Eur J Immunol*. 2008;38:3080–3089.
162. Franco D de L, Nascimento RC, Ferreira KS, et al. Antibodies against *Sporothrix schenckii* enhance TNF-α production and killing by macrophages. *Scand J Immunol*. 2012;75:142–146.
163. Portuondo DL, Batista-Duharte A, Ferreira LS, et al. Comparative efficacy and toxicity of two vaccine candidates against *Sporothrix schenckii* using either Montanide™ Pet Gel A or aluminum hydroxide adjuvants in mice. *Vaccine*. 2017;35:4430–4436.
164. Téllez-Martínez D, Leandro Portuondo D, Loesch ML, et al. A recombinant enolase-Montanide™ PetGel A vaccine promotes a protective Th1 immune response against a highly virulent *Sporothrix schenckii* by toluene exposure. *Pharmaceutics*. 2019;11:144.
165. Gremião IDF, Pereira SA, Nascimento Jr A, et al. General instructions for handling cats which might have a sporotrichosis condition. *Clin Vet*. 2006;65:69–70.
166. Schubach A, Schubach TMP, Barros MBL, et al. Cat-transmitted sporotrichosis, Rio de Janeiro, Brazil. *Emerg Infect Dis*. 2005;11: 1952–1954.
167. Cooper CR, Dixon DM, Salkin IF. Laboratory-acquired sporotrichosis. *J Med Vet Mycol*. 1992;30:169–171.
168. Thompson DW, Kaplan W. Laboratory-acquired sporotrichosis. *Sabouraudia*. 1977;15:167–170.
169. Hardman S, Stephenson I, Jenkins DR, et al. Disseminated *Sporothrix schenckii* in a patient with AIDS. *J Infect*. 2005;51:e73–e77.
170. Almeida-Paes R, de Oliveira MM, Freitas DF, et al. Sporotrichosis in Rio de Janeiro, Brazil: *Sporothrix brasiliensis* is associated with atypical clinical presentations. *PLoS Negl Trop Dis*. 2014;8:e3094.
171. Reis RS, Almeida-Paes R, de Medeiros Muniz M, et al. Molecular characterization of *Sporothrix schenckii* isolates from humans and cats involved in the sporotrichosis epidemic in Rio de Janeiro, Brazil. *Mem Inst Oswald Cruz*. 2009;104:769–774.
172. Rodrigues AM, de Hoog GS, de Camargo ZP. *Sporothrix* species causing outbreaks in animals and humans driven by animal-animal transmission. *PLoS Pathog*. 2016;12:e1005638.
173. Jin XZ, Zhang HD, Hiruma M, et al. Mother and child cases of sporotrichosis infection. *Mycoses*. 1990;33:33–36.
174. Smith LM. Sporotrichosis: report of four clinically atypical cases. *J South Med Assoc Birmingham*. 1945;38:505–509.
175. Brilhante RS, Rodrigues AM, Sidrim JJ, et al. *In vitro* susceptibility of antifungal drugs against *Sporothrix brasiliensis* recovered from cats with sporotrichosis in Brazil. *Med Mycol*. 2016;54;275–259.

85

Candidiasis and Rhodotorulosis

Jane E. Sykes, Krystle L. Reagan

KEY POINTS

- First Described: The identification of *Candida* as a fungal pathogen was recognized in Stockholm around 1840 (Fredrik Berg),[1] but candidiasis was described as far back as around 400 BC by Hippocrates.
- Cause: *Candida* spp. (division Ascomycota, class Saccharomycetes).
- Affected Hosts: Dogs, cats, humans, and a variety of other animal species.
- Geographic Distribution: Worldwide.
- Mode of Transmission: Usually invasion of commensal yeasts secondary to immune suppression.
- Major Clinical Signs: Local dermatitis; otitis externa; keratitis; LUTS; abdominal pain, icterus, and/or ascites due to peritonitis; or severe systemic infections with fever, inappetence, ocular inflammation, lameness due to osteomyelitis, respiratory distress, icterus, vomiting.
- Differential Diagnoses: Other systemic fungal or bacterial infections.
- Human Health Significance: Human infections by *Candida* species result from invasion by normal flora, but human-to-human transmission of *Candida* strains can also occur. The potential for exchange of *Candida* species between animals and humans is not known.

CANDIDIASIS

ETIOLOGY AND EPIDEMIOLOGY

Candida species are yeasts that are typically benign counterparts of the normal GI, urogenital, and cutaneous flora but can invade tissues and cause disease as a result of disruption of normal host defenses. *Candida* species can also be isolated from soil, inanimate objects, and hospital environments. The yeasts are small (3 to 6 μm) and ovoid (blastospores) and reproduce by budding. Budding results in the formation of new yeast cells, pseudohyphae (chains of elongated yeast cells), and true septate hyphae. Disease syndromes caused by *Candida* species that occur in dogs and cats are listed in Box 85.1. More than 200 species of *Candida* exist, but only a few species have been identified as pathogens in dogs and cats (Table 85.1).[2–12] The most commonly isolated species is *Candida albicans,* and only *C. albicans* appears to cause disseminated disease in dogs and cats. However, an epidemiologic shift with increasing numbers of non-*C. albicans*–related infections in animals has been reported.[6,10,12,13] This change has also been documented in humans and is of significant concern as non-*C. albicans* species exhibit higher rates of fluconazole resistance.[14,15]

Local or disseminated infections where *Candida* is present with a mixture of bacterial species can occur. Local infections (such as UTIs) with two different *Candida* species have also been reported.[10,16]

When compared with human patients, candidiasis is uncommonly described in dogs and cats. Predisposing factors in dogs or cats with local or disseminated candidiasis have included diabetes mellitus,[5,10,17] treatment with immunosuppressive drugs or broad-spectrum antibacterial drugs,[10,12,18] a history of GI surgery,[8,11] lower urinary tract disease other than infection (e.g., urinary catheter placement, permanent stomata, atonic bladder),[12] parvoviral infections,[19–21] and/or underlying malignancy.[10,20] Often more than one of these factors is in the history. Disseminated candidiasis has most often been described in dogs, but also occurs in cats.[11,22] Although most animals have underlying immunocompromising conditions, disseminated candidiasis has been described in apparently immunocompetent animals,[23,24] which may reflect an unidentified underlying genetic immunodeficiency. Cats with FeLV or FIV infection do not have higher rates for *Candida* colonization,[25] and those with candidiasis usually test negative for FeLV and FIV.[16]

Analysis of the authors' hospital population suggests that cats are at least as likely as dogs to develop *Candida* UTIs.[16] In other studies, *Candida* species were isolated from the urine of 0.2% of more than 8,000 dogs with UTIs[26,27] and 0.2% of more than 2,000 dogs with persistent or recurrent UTIs.[27] Administration of antibacterial drugs is strongly associated with candiduria in dogs and cats.[12] Lower urinary tract disease other than infection, such as cystostomy tube placement, intermittent urinary catheterization, and perineal urethrostomy, has been reported in the history of some cats and dogs with *Candida* UTIs[6,10,12] and is significantly associated with candiduria in cats.[12] Local mucocutaneous infections can occur at the site of long-term placement of feeding tubes.[3]

CLINICAL FEATURES

Pathogenesis and Clinical Signs

A combination of disruption of normal host barriers and expression of virulence factors are likely necessary to allow *Candida* spp. to invade the host. Administration of antibacterials can lead to alterations in the normal bacterial flora, allowing *Candida* to proliferate.[28,29] Compromise to defenses of the lower urinary tract with urinary catheter placement or alterations to urine flow (e.g., perineal urethrostomies) are risk factors for the development of *Candida* UTIs.[6,12]

Candida can adhere to a variety of tissue components, such as epithelial and endothelial cells, as well as other bacteria and inanimate objects, such as catheters and stents, via integrin-like and carbohydrate adhesion molecules.[30,31] *Candida* yeasts produce many proteins that are associated with infection including hydrolases and heat shock proteins.[23] The yeasts readily form biofilms consisting of extracellular polymeric polysaccharides and budding, pseudohyphal, and hyphal

BOX 85.1 Disease Syndromes Associated with *Candida* Infections in Dogs and Cats

Keratitis
Cutaneous candidiasis
Otitis externa and otitis media
Urinary tract infections
Gastrointestinal candidiasis
Cholecystitis
Pancreatitis
Peritonitis
Disseminated infections

TABLE 85.1 *Candida* Species Associated with Disease in Dogs and/or Cats[2–12]

Species	Clinical Manifestations
Candida albicans	Dermatitis, UTI, otitis externa, keratitis, cholecystitis, disseminated infections
Candida glabrata (formerly *Torulopsis glabrata*)	UTI, feeding-tube site infections, pancreatitis
Candida krusei	UTI, feeding tube site infections
Candida guilliermondii	UTI, dermatitis
Candida parapsilosis	UTI, otitis, dermatitis
Candida tropicalis	UTI, otitis
Candida rugosa	UTI

forms.[32] Biofilm growth is enhanced by availability of carbon sources such as glucose (glucosuric patients) and on some substrates such as latex urinary catheter.[32] Formation of a biofilm confers resistance to antifungal drugs by allowing organisms at the center of the biofilm to slow growth rates, thus making cell cycle–dependent antifungal agents less effective. It also provides a physical barrier against antifungal penetration with the extracellular matrix and promotes the upregulation of drug efflux pumps.[32]

Within tissues, neutrophils are a key defense against *Candida*.[33] *Candida* blastospores are phagocytized and destroyed by neutrophils. Mononuclear cells play a less important role. Reactive oxygen species, hydrolytic enzymes, and antimicrobial peptides contribute to the intracellular destruction of blastospores by neutrophils. Thus, any condition that impairs neutrophil numbers or function, such as neutropenia or diabetes mellitus, predisposes dogs and cats to candidiasis. A large number of other cytokines, complement, dendritic cells, and lymphocytes are also involved in the immune response to *Candida*.[33] The formation of hyphae by *Candida* promotes tissue invasion, which may be followed by life-threatening fungemia and dissemination to multiple organs.[34] This ability of *Candida* to change its morphology ("morphologic dimorphism") is thought to be an important virulence factor.

Lower urinary tract candidiasis may be subclinical or associated with dysuria, stranguria, and/or hematuria. Systemic signs of pyrexia, lethargy, inappetence, and weight loss have also been described in affected dogs and cats,[6] but these signs may result from the presence of other predisposing diseases. Ascending infections may lead to development of *Candida* pyelonephritis.

Cutaneous candidiasis may manifest as erythema, scaling, alopecia, erosions, and crusting, often where disruption of cutaneous or mucocutaneous regions has occurred (such as a previous surgical site or a feeding tube or cystotomy stoma). Persistent disease in the face of systemic or topical treatment with broad-spectrum antibiotics should raise suspicion for candidiasis. Dogs with *Candida* otitis externa often have a history of chronic bacterial otitis externa that has been treated aggressively with systemic or topical antibacterials.

Overgrowth of *Candida* in the GI tract may occur in animals that are immunosuppressed or treated with glucocorticoids and/or broad-spectrum antibacterial drugs. In some cases, invasion of the mucosa into the lamina propria or deeper tissues occurs (e.g., intestinal candidiasis). A *Candida* GI granuloma was diagnosed in a cat after passage of an intestinal foreign body without previous antibacterial drug administration or known cause of immunosuppression.[35] Intestinal candidiasis is occasionally identified at necropsy in puppies that die after treatment for parvoviral enteritis and may be a reason for persistent vomiting, diarrhea, and death despite aggressive fluid and antibacterial drug therapy.[21] *Candida* spp. may also contribute to ulcerative glossitis in puppies with parvovirus infection (Fig. 85.1).

Candida albicans cholecystitis was reported in a 3-year-old cat from upstate New York.[36] Although no clear underlying cause could be identified, the cat had obstructive cholecystitis with what appeared to be an organizing mucocele, and a nematode of unknown identity was discovered in the cat's esophageal feeding tube during hospitalization. Another cat with diabetes mellitus was described with pancreatitis associated with a *Candida glabrata* infection.[37]

Candida peritonitis can occur after intestinal and/or biliary surgery or intestinal perforation secondary to NSAID administration.[8,11,38] Recent treatment with broad-spectrum antibacterial drugs is reported in most dogs that develop *Candida* peritonitis.[38] Mixed infections with *Candida* and intestinal flora may develop. Affected dogs are febrile, have abdominal pain, and may have other GI signs such as vomiting and diarrhea.

Disseminated candidiasis results from hematogenous spread of *Candida* from intestinal, urinary, or possibly corneal or cutaneous sites.[17,39,40] A diagnosis of disseminated candidiasis should be considered whenever *Candida* infections are identified in the eye, skin, or urinary tract of an animal that has (or subsequently develops) severe systemic illness. Clinical signs of disseminated candidiasis in dogs include fever, inappetence, anorexia, weight loss, and a variety of other clinical signs that reflect underlying immunosuppressive disease processes and specific organs involved. The latter can include the pancreas, liver, mesentery, spleen, kidneys, heart, lungs, lymph nodes, and, less often, the bone, intestinal tract, eyes, meninges, thyroid, and/or prostate gland.[5,17,20,23,39–44] Ocular signs in animals with disseminated disease include keratitis and corneal ulceration, uveitis, chorioretinitis, and endophthalmitis.[16,17,41,43] *Candida* keratitis may also occur as a localized process, sometimes secondary to aggressive treatment of corneal ulceration secondary to other disease processes with topical broad-spectrum antibacterial drugs. Thromboembolic disease may complicate disseminated infections. Pulmonary thromboembolism may result in respiratory distress and death.[5,16]

DIAGNOSIS

Laboratory Abnormalities

Laboratory abnormalities in dogs and cats with candidiasis result from the underlying disease process (such as diabetes mellitus or systemic neoplastic disease) as well as the location and severity of the fungal infection. Laboratory abnormalities in dogs or cats with *Candida* UTIs may be absent, or there may be evidence of renal failure with azotemia and isosthenuria. Grossly, urine may contain flocculent white debris. Urinalysis may reveal proteinuria, pyuria, and, in some cases, hematuria and/or *Candida* fungal elements (see Case Example). Dogs and cats with disseminated candidiasis or *Candida* peritonitis frequently have had nonregenerative anemia and mild to marked neutrophilia with bandemia and toxic neutrophil changes (in contrast to other deep mycoses, where hematologic abnormalities are often mild or absent).

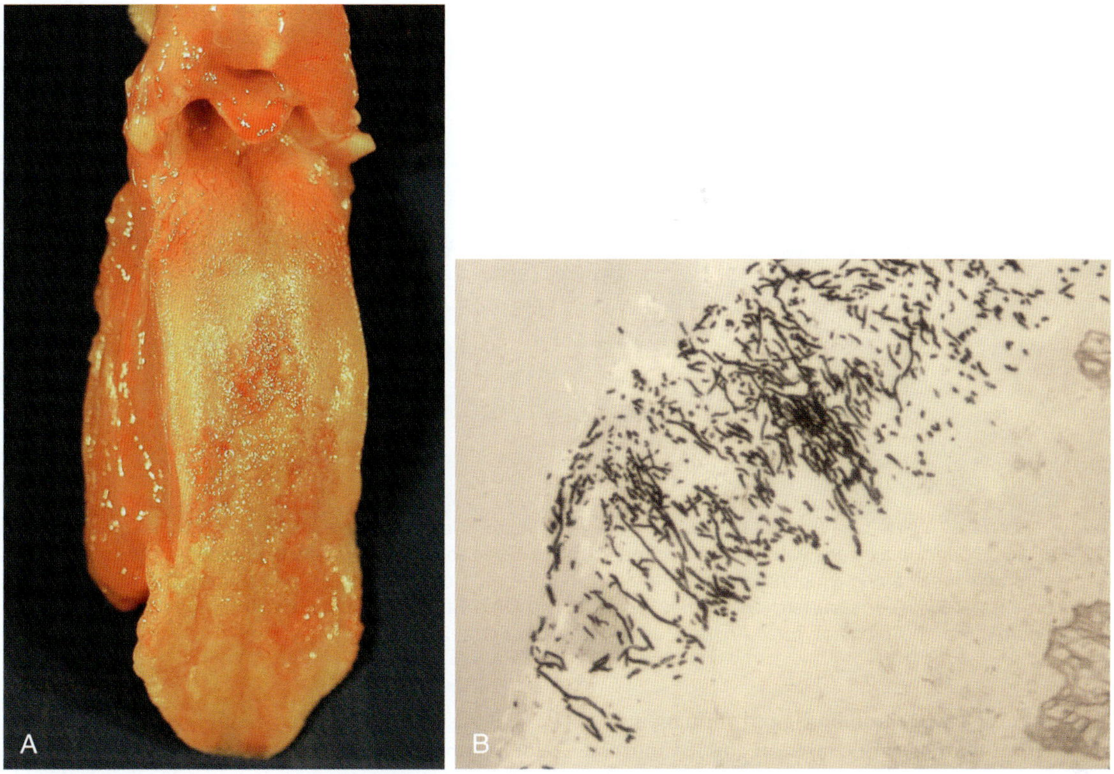

Fig. 85.1 (A) Tongue ulcerations at necropsy in a 2-month-old mixed-breed puppy that was euthanized because of canine parvoviral infection. (B) Histopathology revealed multifocal ulcerative glossitis, pharyngitis, and esophagitis with intralesional yeasts and pseudohyphae. Gomori's methenamine silver stain. (Courtesy University of California Davis Anatomic Pathology Service.)

Lymphopenia may be present as a result of underlying immunosuppressive illness or drug therapy. Some dogs are thrombocytopenic and have coagulation abnormalities consistent with DIC.[5] Findings on the serum biochemistry panel in dogs with disseminated candidiasis are variable and nonspecific but may include metabolic acidosis, moderate to severe hypoalbuminemia, and increased liver enzyme activities. The cat with *Candida* cholecystitis had marked hyperbilirubinemia (up to 33.8 mg/dL) and increased serum liver enzyme activities associated with a concurrent hepatitis.[36]

Diagnostic Imaging

Plain thoracic radiographs in dogs with disseminated candidiasis may be unremarkable or show increased pulmonary interstitial opacity, thoracic lymphadenomegaly, and/or pleural or pericardial effusion.[11,18,23] Abdominal ultrasound examination in dogs with *Candida* peritonitis or disseminated disease may reveal echogenic ascites fluid, mesenteric hyperechogenicity, changes consistent with pancreatitis, abdominal lymphadenomegaly, or increased echogenicity of the renal cortices or hepatic parenchyma. In animals with *Candida* UTIs, fungal balls may be detected as mobile, echogenic, spherical structures without distal acoustic shadowing within the lumen of the urinary bladder.[45]

Microbiologic Tests

Definitive diagnosis of candidiasis requires visualization of the organism within lesions by cytologic or histopathologic examination and confirmation of its identity using culture.

Cytologic Examination

Candida blastospores (5–7 μm), pseudohyphae, and true hyphae (3–5 μm-wide septate hyphae) can be visualized in swab specimens from the ear canal (ear cytology); tape preparations from the skin; urine sediment or other body fluids (Fig. 85.2); or ultrasound-guided aspirates of abdominal lesions.

Fungal Culture

Candida grows on routine bacteriologic media as well as fungal media such as Sabouraud dextrose agar. Creamy white colonies appear within 2 to 3 days, and so isolation of the yeast may be reported when it is present in specimens submitted for aerobic bacterial culture, which are typically incubated only for this period of time. If *Candida* is suspected based on the history, fungal culture (rather than bacterial culture alone) should be requested because *Candida* grows best on fungal isolation media. Because *Candida* can be isolated from the skin and mucous membranes of healthy dogs and cats, infection must be confirmed with cytology or histopathology when *Candida* is isolated from these sites.

Identification of *Candida* isolates is based on morphology and biochemical reactions. Preliminary differentiation of *C. albicans* from other *Candida* species can be made based on the ability of *C. albicans* to produce germ tubes when exposed to serum. MALDI-TOF MS (see Chapter 3) accurately and rapidly identifies *Candida* species[46] and may replace these methods in the future. Isolation of *Candida* allows not only definitive identification but also antifungal susceptibility testing (see Fig. 4.16). This is important for *Candida* because some isolates (especially *Candida glabrata* and *Candida krusei*) can exhibit antifungal drug resistance.

Pathologic Findings

Gross pathologic findings at necropsy in animals with disseminated candidiasis include peritoneal or pleural effusion, enlarged and edematous lymph nodes, congestion and necrotic whitish foci within

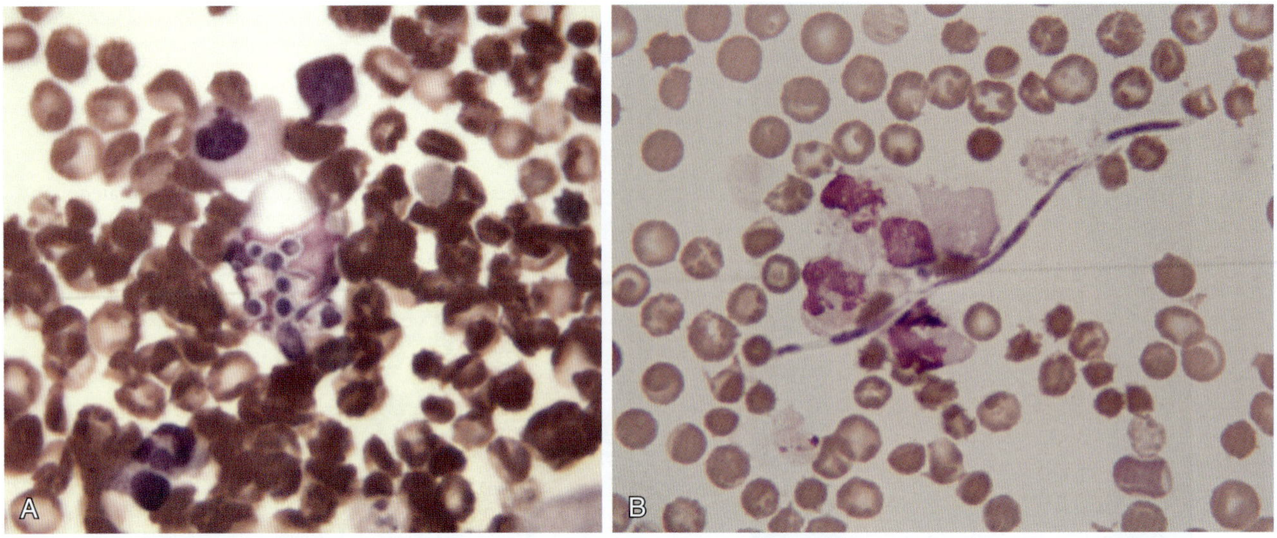

Fig. 85.2 *Candida albicans* within urine sediment from a 5-year-old female spayed Labrador retriever being treated for multicentric lymphoma and acute-onset hematuria. Both budding (A) and filamentous (B) fungal elements are visible. (Courtesy Dr. Barrak Pressler, The Ohio State University. From Bartges J, Polzin D. *Nephrology and Urology of Small Animals*. John Wiley and Sons; 2011.)

affected organs, evidence of tissue thrombosis, and formation of a gray-white or yellow-green fibrinonecrotic layer on affected mucosal surfaces.[5,11,21,23,40,44] Concurrent underlying disease processes are also often identified.

Histopathology of affected tissues reveals yeasts, pseudohyphae, and septate hyphae with an associated inflammatory response that is composed primarily of neutrophils, macrophages, and lymphocytes. Multinucleated giant cells may also be present.[23,40,44] Pseudohyphae and hyphae predominate in invasive infections (see Fig. 4.1). Evidence of blood vessel invasion, thrombosing vasculitis, and infarction may be seen, with multifocal mycotic granulomas in affected organs.[40] The organism is most readily visualized with special stains such as PAS and Gomori's methenamine silver. IHC has also been used to identify *Candida* within lesions.[23,40] When mixed infections with *Candida* and other bacteria are present, tissue Gram stains may reveal bacterial rods and/or cocci in addition to gram-positive fungal elements.

TREATMENT AND PROGNOSIS

Treatment of candidiasis should involve management of underlying immunosuppressive disorders, if possible, and specific antifungal drug treatment. Systemic antibacterial drugs should be discontinued if not clearly indicated, or the spectrum of activity should be narrowed as much as possible.

Cutaneous and corneal infections are usually treated with a combination of topical antiseptics or antifungal medications and systemic antifungal drugs until lesions resolve.[7]

Dogs and cats with candiduria should receive antifungal therapy as many of the underlying risk factors such as permanent urinary tract stomata or neoplasia cannot be easily corrected and ascending pyelonephritis has been reported.[5,10,17] Initial therapy should be with antifungal drugs that achieve high concentrations in the urine, such as fluconazole, for 4 to 6 weeks. Fungal urine culture should be used to confirm resolution of infection. Systemic antifungals alone may be adequate to resolve *Candida* UTIs in some animals, although resolution has been reported in some animals in the absence of antifungal drug therapy.[10]

Persistent infection may result from drug resistance, adverse effects of treatment that necessitate treatment discontinuation, or inadequate drug penetration into fungal masses that line the bladder wall (see Case Example). Intravesicular treatment with 1% clotrimazole may be effective in these cases.[47,48] Under anesthesia, the bladder is catheterized with a Foley catheter, emptied, and then lavaged with sterile saline. The bladder is then filled with 1% clotrimazole solution (e.g., 30 to 50 mL for a cat). The animal is rotated to promote contact of the solution with the uroepithelium, and after the solution has been in the bladder for an hour, the catheter is removed and the animal is allowed to recover. Treatment is continued weekly until *Candida* can no longer be isolated from the urine. Typically one to four treatments are required.[16,48] Ultrasound-guided administration of clotrimazole via cystocentesis to a dog with *Candida* cystitis was described in one report.[47]

Successful treatment of systemic candidiasis in dogs or cats is rarely described. One dog with *Candida* peritonitis was treated successfully by surgical exploration and lavage of the abdomen, placement of an abdominal drain, and IV fluconazole.[8] In addition, aggressive supportive measures were required that included IV fluid therapy, fresh frozen plasma, antiemetics, gastroprotectants, total parenteral nutrition, and antibacterial drugs for a suspected catheter-related infection. Antifungal drugs other than fluconazole used to treat invasive candidiasis in human patients include amphotericin B (AMB) or an echinocandin such as caspofungin,[49] both of which must be administered parenterally.

PREVENTION

Prevention of candidiasis involves avoidance of excessive immunosuppression, as well as discriminate use of antibacterial drugs, which should be tailored to the results of culture and susceptibility whenever possible.[12] Whether *Candida* species carried on the hands of humans can colonize dogs and cats is not known, but routine hand washing and the wearing of gloves when immunosuppressed animals are handled or intravascular devices are placed should minimize the chance of healthcare-associated infections. Although prophylactic antifungal drug treatment has been used to prevent invasive candidiasis in human high-risk groups, the low incidence of candidiasis in immunosuppressed dogs and cats does not warrant the use of prophylactic antifungal drugs in this group.

PUBLIC HEALTH ASPECTS

Candida species (especially *C. albicans*) are common causes of mucosal disease in humans. Since 2000, *Candida* has also emerged as an extremely important cause of invasive infections owing to the more widespread use of invasive medical devices and immunosuppressive drugs. In hospitalized human patients, *Candida* is reportedly the fourth most common organism isolated from the bloodstream.[50] Although many human infections result from invasion of tissues by commensal yeasts in the face of immune suppression, horizontal transmission of *Candida* and hospital-acquired infections have been described.[51] One *Candida* species of particular concern is *Candida auris*, a highly drug-resistant species of *Candida* that was first reported as a nosocomial pathogen in Japan in 2009 and has subsequently spread worldwide. Whether *Candida* isolates from dogs or cats colonize humans is not known. Zoonotic transmission of *Candida parapsilosis* from dogs was suggested by the authors of a case report that described two human cases of *C. parapsilosis* periorificial dermatitis (one periocular and another perioral).[52] This was on the basis of a history in both cases of volunteering in dog shelters, and historic evidence that dogs can be colonized by *C. parapsilosis*. However, the prevalence of *C. parapsilosis* colonization in dogs from the shelters was not investigated, and no molecular studies were performed to show that isolates colonizing the dogs were the same as those causing the two human infections.

RHODOTORULOSIS

Rhodotorula spp. are saprophytic yeasts within the division Basidiomycota (family Sporidiobolaceae). Previously thought to be nonpathogenic, they are now considered emerging opportunistic pathogens of humans and other animals.[53] *Rhodotorula* spp. are widespread in the environment and can be found in air, soil, lakes, ocean water, dairy products, and fruit juice. They are also commensal inhabitants of the skin, GI, and upper respiratory tracts of mammals, and are common contaminants of hospital surfaces, including endoscopes and dialysis equipment.[53] They may be isolated in low numbers from clinical specimens that may have become contaminated with environmental bacteria or fungi.

Opportunistic infections with *Rhodotorula* spp. in humans are very rare. When they occur, they most often are characterized by fungemia in patients with central venous catheters, including premature neonates, patients with hematologic malignancies, and patients receiving central parenteral nutrition.[53] However, they have also been identified as a cause of meningeal, skin, ocular, peritoneal, and prosthetic infections in humans with other immunocompromising conditions, including treatment with broad-spectrum antibacterials. The most common species isolated from humans is *Rhodotorula mucilaginosa* (approximately 70% of isolates), followed by *Rhodotorula glutinis* (approximately 7%).[54,55] In dogs, there have been fewer than five reports of *Rhodotorula* spp. infection in the literature. Associated conditions were granulomatous epididymitis, funguria, and pneumonia.[6,56,57] Care should be taken not to overinterpret light growth of *Rhodotorula* from potentially contaminated sites as clinically significant infection, especially in the absence of intralesional yeasts and when accompanied by mixed growth of bacterial organisms or other fungal contaminants.

AMB is the most common antifungal agent used for treatment of humans with *Rhodotorula* spp. infections, with a mortality rate of approximately 10%.[53] Although successful therapy with fluconazole has also been reported, *Rhodotorula* spp. are resistant to triazoles and echinocandins *in vitro*.[58] As with candidiasis, treatment of rhodotorulosis should likely include identification, and correction, if possible, of any predisposing local or systemic causes of altered immunity.

CASE EXAMPLE

Signalment

"Lizzie," an 18-year-old female spayed domestic shorthair cat from the San Francisco Bay area (Fig. 85.3A).

History

Lizzie was evaluated by the University of California, Davis, VMTH, for a 12-hour history of dysuria and hematuria. The owner described multiple episodes of urination and defecation outside the litter box with stranguria, hematuria, and tenesmus. Lizzie was also observed repeatedly grooming her perineum. The cat had been diagnosed with diabetes mellitus 10 years previously, and more recently with feline bronchial disease, a thoracolumbar (T3 to L3) myelopathy, generalized osteoarthritis, chronic constipation, bilateral cataracts, CKD, and recurrent bacteriuria (*Streptococcus bovis* group, *Escherichia coli*, *Enterococcus faecalis*, then *Aerococcus viridans*). She also had a cardiac murmur secondary to dynamic right ventricular outflow tract obstruction. Historic bacteriuria had been treated with a variety of antimicrobial drugs selected based on the results of aerobic bacterial urine culture and susceptibility (most recently doxycycline, but also amoxicillin-clavulanic acid or marbofloxacin in the past). Her current medications consisted of prozinc insulin (3.5 U, SC, q12h), lactulose (2 mL, PO, q12h), a soluble fiber supplement (1 teaspoon with food twice daily), inhaled fluticasone (110-μg puff, q12h), theophylline (12 mg/kg, PO, q24h), and doxycycline (5 mg/kg, PO, q12h). Her most recent blood work (collected 1 month previously) showed a creatinine of 1.8 mg/dL (reference range, 1.1–2.2 mg/dL) and a BUN of 34 (reference range, 18–33 mg/dL), which were similar to values obtained over the course of the previous 5 years. She was an indoor-only cat and was fed a commercial cat food with occasional turkey meat from the delicatessen. Her appetite was good, there had been no weight loss noted, her water consumption was unchanged, and there had been no vomiting or diarrhea. She had not been vaccinated for the past 4 years but was on regular flea preventative medication (nitenpyram as well as fipronil).

Physical Examination

Body weight: 4.1 kg.

General: Quiet, alert, and responsive, T = 100.5°F (38.1°C), HR = 170 beats/minute, RR = 28 breaths/minute, CRT <1 second, pale pink mucous membranes.

Integument: A dull, slightly unkempt haircoat with mild scale was noted.

Eyes, ears, nose, and throat: Immature cataracts were present bilaterally, and all teeth were absent on examination of the oral cavity. No other clinically significant abnormalities were detected.

Musculoskeletal: BCS was 4/9, and there was mild generalized muscle atrophy. The cat was reluctant to ambulate, and appeared painful on manipulation of the elbows, stifles, and coxofemoral joints bilaterally. Crepitus was detected on manipulation of the tarsus.

Cardiovascular and respiratory systems: A grade II/VI left parasternal heart murmur was auscultated. Pulses were strong and synchronous. No other abnormalities were detected.

Abdominal palpation: The abdomen was soft and nonpainful. Both kidneys were small (approximately 2 cm in diameter) and irregular. The urinary bladder was approximately 5 cm in diameter and soft. Severe erythema was noted around the vulva.

Lymph nodes: All were < 1 cm in diameter.

Continued

Laboratory Findings

Urinalysis: SpG 1.030; pH 6.0, 75 mg/dL protein, 1,000 mg/dL glucose, no ketones or bilirubin, 250 erythrocytes/μL hemoprotein, >100 WBC/HPF, >100 RBC/HPF, few transitional and squamous epithelial cells, many budding yeast organisms.

Microbiologic Testing

Aerobic bacterial urine culture: 10^5 *C. albicans*/mL were cultured.

Yeast antifungal drug susceptibility panel: Susceptible to 5-flucytosine (0.5 μg/mL), caspofungin (0.25 μg/mL), fluconazole (0.25 μg/mL), itraconazole (0.06 μg/mL), voriconazole (0.015 μg/mL). MICs for AMB and posaconazole were 0.5 μg/mL and 0.03 μg/mL, respectively (no interpretative criteria available).

Diagnosis

Susceptible *C. albicans* UTI.

Treatment

Lizzie was treated with fluconazole (50 mg, PO, q12h). At a recheck examination 10 days later, the owner reported ongoing pollakiuria and incontinence. A fungal urine culture again revealed 10^5 *C. albicans*/mL with a similar susceptibility profile. Addition of flucytosine was recommended (250 mg, PO, q8h) but was considered unaffordable to the owners. Treatment was continued for another month with little clinical improvement and persistence of infection. A blood glucose curve revealed 2-hourly blood glucose concentrations that were "high", 470, 368, 300, 383, and 423 mg/dL, respectively, so the insulin dose was increased to 4 U, q12h. Two weeks later, the owner described some improvement in the urinary incontinence and reduction in stranguria, but again 10^5 *C. albicans*/mL was cultured from the urine, and persistent urine scalding was noted around the perineum and on the pelvic limbs on physical examination. Body weight was 3.8 kg, and a blood glucose curve revealed 2-hourly blood glucose concentrations that were 457, 301, 209, 227, 300, and 296 mg/dL, respectively.

Topical treatment with clotrimazole was elected. Before the procedure was performed, a preanesthetic evaluation was done. A CBC showed a normocytic, normochromic, nonregenerative anemia (HCT 28.3%; reference range [RR]: 30%–50%), mature neutrophilia (15,206 cells/μL; RR; 2,000–9,000 cells/μL), lymphopenia (919 cells/μL; RR: 1,000–7,000 cells/μL), and monocytopenia (33 cells/μL; RR: 50–600 cells/μL). A serum biochemistry profile was unremarkable with the exceptions of a BUN concentration of 49 mg/dL (RR: 18–33 mg/dL) and a glucose concentration of 314 mg/dL (RR: 63–118 mg/dL). Urinalysis showed a specific gravity of 1.022; pH 6.0, 25 mg/dL protein, 1,000 mg/dL glucose, 0–2 WBC/HPF, 0–2 RBC/HPF, and moderate numbers of budding yeast organisms and fungal structures. Thoracic radiographs revealed mild cardiomegaly and a diffuse, static bronchial pattern consistent with the previous diagnosis of feline bronchial disease. Abdominal ultrasound findings included an enlarged and hyperechoic liver, mild diffuse thickening of the GI mucosa and submucosa, decreased renal corticomedullary distinction bilaterally with thickening of the renal cortices, a markedly thickened and irregular urinary bladder wall that contained hypoechoic, ill-defined nodules, and thick sediment within the urinary bladder lumen. Cystoscopy revealed a large amount of white, fluffy debris adherent to an edematous bladder wall as well as in the lumen (Fig. 85.3B). A 10F Foley catheter was placed over a 0.025-inch guidewire. The bladder was flushed and the majority of the debris removed. A total of 47 mL of 1% clotrimazole solution was infused into the bladder, and the solution was allowed to remain in place for 1 hour. The solution was removed, and Lizzie was allowed to recover from anesthesia. Treatment with fluconazole was continued, although the dose was lowered (25 mg, PO, q12h). At a recheck 2 weeks later, the owners reported that Lizzie was more active and was no longer pollakiuric, although she still urinated outside the litter box and intermittent vomiting had been noted. A CBC, biochemistry panel, and urinalysis revealed nonregenerative anemia (HCT 21.2%); lymphopenia (349 cells/μL); monocytopenia (70 cells/μL); increased activities of serum ALT (1028 U/L; RR: 27–101 U/L), AST (226 U/L; RR: 17–58 U/L), and ALP (223 U/L; RR: 14–17 U/L); hypercholesterolemia (324 U/L; RR: 89–258 U/L); and hyperbilirubinemia (0.7 mg/dL; RR: 0–0.2 mg/dL). Aerobic bacterial urine culture revealed more than 10^5 CFU/mL of hemolytic *E. coli*, and fungal culture of the urine was negative. The fluconazole was discontinued, after which the vomiting ceased and liver enzyme activities returned to reference ranges. Multiple bacterial UTIs were diagnosed over the following 6 months, but *Candida* was never again isolated from the urine.

Comments

In this cat, the *C. albicans* UTI may have occurred secondary to a combination of factors that likely included poorly controlled diabetes mellitus, CKD, neurologic disease, and repeated treatment with broad-spectrum antimicrobial drugs. Systemic antifungal drug treatment and improved control of diabetes mellitus were initially used as treatment strategies but failed, probably because of the large mats of fungus that were adherent to the bladder wall. Fortunately, a single topical clotrimazole treatment resulted in resolution of the yeast infection. The hepatopathy that developed was thought to be secondary to fluconazole toxicity since it resolved when the drug was discontinued.

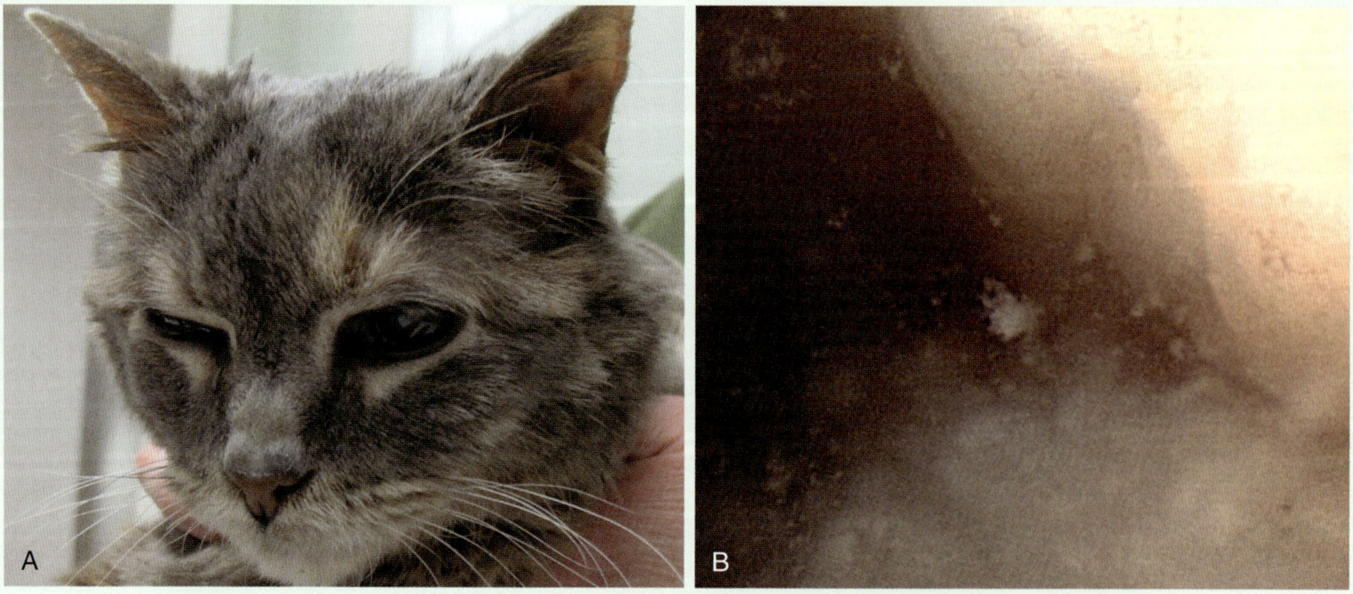

Fig. 85.3 (A) An 18-year-old female spayed domestic shorthair cat with a *Candida albicans* urinary tract infection, as well as diabetes mellitus, feline bronchial disease, a myelopathy, and generalized osteoarthritis. (B) Bladder lumen as viewed by cystoscopy. The urine contains large amounts of fluffy white debris that was loosely adherent to the bladder wall.

SUGGESTED READINGS

Cheng SC, Joosten LA, Kullberg BJ, et al. Interplay between *Candida albicans* and the mammalian innate host defense. *Infect Immun.* 2012;80:1304–1313.

Ong RK, Raisis AL, Swindells KL. *Candida albicans* peritonitis in a dog. *J Vet Emerg Crit Care (San Antonio).* 2010;20:143–147.

Reagan KL, Dear JD, Kass PH, Sykes JE. Risk factors for *Candida* urinary tract infections in dogs and cats. *J Vet Intern Med.* 2019:33 64–653.

REFERENCES

1. Barnett JA. A history of research on yeasts 12: medical yeasts part 1, *Candida albicans. Yeast.* 2008;25:385–417.
2. Bohm T, Parzefall B, Klinger CJ, et al. Recurrent polyp formation with *Candida tropicalis* infection and otitis in a dog. *Tierarztl Prax Ausg K Kleintiere Heimtiere.* 2020;48:365–368.
3. Boutilier P, Carr A. Fungal colonization and failure of a long-term gastrostomy tube in a cat. *Can Vet J.* 2005;46:709–710.
4. Dale JE. Canine dermatosis caused by *Candida parapsilosis. Vet Med Small Anim Clin.* 1972;67:548–549.
5. Heseltine JC, Panciera DL, Saunders GK. Systemic candidiasis in a dog. *J Am Vet Med Assoc.* 2003;223:821–824, 810.
6. Jin Y, Lin D. Fungal urinary tract infections in the dog and cat: a retrospective study (2001-2004). *J Am Anim Hosp Assoc.* 2005;41:373–381.
7. Mueller RS, Bettenay SV, Shipstone M. Cutaneous candidiasis in a dog caused by *Candida guilliermondii. Vet Rec.* 2002;150:728–730.
8. Ong RK, Raisis AL, Swindells KL. *Candida albicans* peritonitis in a dog. *J Vet Emerg Crit Care.* 2010;20:143–147.
9. Ozawa H, Okabayashi K, Kano R, et al. Rapid identification of *Candida tropicalis* from canine cystitis. *Mycopathologia.* 2005;160:159–162.
10. Pressler BM, Vaden SL, Lane IF, et al. *Candida* spp. urinary tract infections in 13 dogs and seven cats: predisposing factors, treatment, and outcome. *J Am Anim Hosp Assoc.* 2003;39:263–270.
11. Rogers CL, Gibson C, Mitchell SL, et al. Disseminated candidiasis secondary to fungal and bacterial peritonitis in a young dog. *J Vet Emerg Crit Care (San Antonio).* 2009;19:193–198.
12. Reagan KL, Dear JD, Kass PH, et al. Risk factors for *Candida* urinary tract infections in dogs and cats. *J Vet Intern Med.* 2019;33:648–653.
13. Yurayart C, Chindamporn A, Suradhat S, et al. Comparative analysis of the frequency, distribution and population sizes of yeasts associated with canine seborrheic dermatitis and healthy skin. *Vet Microbiol.* 2011;148:356–362.
14. Caston-Osorio J, Rivero A, Torre-Cisneros J. Epidemiology of invasive fungal infection. *Int J Antimicrob Agents.* 2008;32:S103–S109.
15. Diekema D, Arbefeville S, Boyken L, et al. The changing epidemiology of healthcare-associated candidemia over three decades. *Diagn Microbiol Infect Dis.* 2012;73:45–48.
16. Sykes JE. Unpublished observations. 2019.
17. Gerding PA Jr, Morton LD, Dye JA. Ocular and disseminated candidiasis in an immunosuppressed cat. *J Am Vet Med Assoc.* 1994;204:1635–1638.
18. Mohri T, Takashima K, Yamane T, et al. Purulent pericarditis in a dog administered immune-suppressing drugs. *J Vet Med Sci.* 2009;71:669–672.
19. Langheinrich KA, Nielsen SW. Histopathology of feline panleukopenia: a report of 65 cases. *J Am Vet Med Assoc.* 1971;158(suppl 2):863+.
20. Matsuda K, Sakaguchi K, Kobayashi S, et al. Systemic candidiasis and mesenteric mast cell tumor with multiple metastases in a dog. *J Vet Med Sci.* 2009;71:229–232.
21. Ochiai K, Valentine BA, Altschul M. Intestinal candidiasis in a dog. *Vet Rec.* 2000;146:228–229.
22. Miller WW, Albert RA. Ocular and systemic candidiasis in a cat. *J Am Anim Hosp Assoc.* 1988;71:521–524.
23. Brown MR, Thompson CA, Mohamed FM. Systemic candidiasis in an apparently immunocompetent dog. *J Vet Diagn Invest.* 2005;17:272–276.
24. Lorenzini R, De Bernardis F. Antemortem diagnosis of an apparent case of feline candidiasis. *Mycopathologia.* 1986;93:13–14.
25. Sierra P, Guillot J, Jacob H, et al. Fungal flora on cutaneous and mucosal surfaces of cats infected with feline immunodeficiency virus or feline leukemia virus. *Am J Vet Res.* 2000;61:158–161.
26. Ling GV, Norris CR, Franti CE, et al. Interrelations of organism prevalence, specimen collection method, and host age, sex, and breed among 8,354 canine urinary tract infections (1969-1995). *J Vet Intern Med.* 2001;15:341–347.
27. Norris CR, Williams BJ, Ling GV, et al. Recurrent and persistent urinary tract infections in dogs: 383 cases (1969-1995). *J Am Anim Hosp Assoc.* 2000;36:484–492.
28. Samonis G, Gikas A, Toloudis P, et al. Prospective study of the impact of broad-spectrum antibiotics on the yeast flora of the human gut. *Eur J Clin Microbiol Infect Dis.* 1994;13:665–667.
29. Spinillo A, Capuzzo E, Acciano S, et al. Effect of antibiotic use on the prevalence of symptomatic vulvovaginal candidiasis. *Am J Obstet Gynecol.* 1999;180:14–17.
30. Grubb SE, Murdoch C, Sudbery PE, et al. *Candida albicans*-endothelial cell interactions: a key step in the pathogenesis of systemic candidiasis. *Infect Immun.* 2008;76:4370–4377.
31. Karkowska-Kuleta J, Rapala-Kozik M, Kozik A. Fungi pathogenic to humans: molecular bases of virulence of *Candida albicans, Cryptococcus neoformans* and *Aspergillus fumigatus. Acta Biochim Pol.* 2009;56:211–224.
32. Seneviratne C, Jin L, Samaranayake L. Biofilm lifestyle of *Candida*: a mini review. *Oral Diseases.* 2008;14:582–590.
33. Cheng SC, Joosten LA, Kullberg BJ, et al. Interplay between *Candida albicans* and the mammalian innate host defense. *Infect Immun.* 2012;80:1304–1313.
34. Blanco JL, Garcia ME. Immune response to fungal infections. *Vet Immunol Immunopathol.* 2008;125:47–70.
35. Duchaussoy A-C, Rose A, Talbot JJ, et al. Gastrointestinal granuloma due to *Candida albicans* in an immunocompetent cat. *Med Mycol Case Rep.* 2015;10:14–17.
36. Palermo SM, Newman AW, Koch MW. *Candida albicans* cholecystitis with associated hepatitis in a cat. *JFMS Open Rep.* 2019;5. 2055116919854165.
37. Renner K, Hill S, Grinberg A, et al. Pancreatic candidiasis in a cat. *JFMS Open Rep.* 2021;7:20551169211052889.
38. Bradford K, Meinkoth J, McKeirnen K, et al. *Candida* peritonitis in dogs: report of 5 cases. *Vet Clin Pathol.* 2013;42:227–233.
39. Holoymoen JI, Bjerkas I, Olberg IH, et al. Disseminated candidiasis (moniliasis) in a dog. A case report. *Nord Vet Med.* 1982;34:362–367.
40. Rodríguez F, Fernández A, Espinosa de los Monteros A, et al. Acute disseminated candidiasis in a puppy associated with parvoviral infection. *Vet Rec.* 1998;142:434–436.
41. Enders A, van der Woerdt A, Donovan T. Endogenous mycotic endophthalmitis in a dog with candiduria and Evans syndrome. *Vet Ophthalmol.* 2017;20:84–88.
42. Kuwamura M, Ide M, Yamate J, et al. Systemic candidiasis in a dog, developing spondylitis. *J Vet Med Sci.* 2006;68:1117–1119.
43. Linek J. Mycotic endophthalmitis in a dog caused by *Candida albicans. Vet Ophthalmol.* 2004;7:159–162.
44. Skoric M, P F, Slana I. A case of systemic mycosis in a Hovawart dog due to *Candida albicans. Veterinarni Medicina.* 2011;56:260–264.
45. Choo D, Lee K, Yoon H. Fungal balls detected using ultrasonography in the urinary bladder of a dog. *Vet Radiol Ultrasound.* 2021;Oct 12: online ahead of print.
46. Rosenvinge FS, Dzajic E, Knudsen E, et al. Performance of matrix-assisted laser desorption-time of flight mass spectrometry for identification of clinical yeast isolates. *Mycoses.* 2013;56:229–235.
47. Forward ZA, Legendre AM, Khalsa HDS. Use of intermittent bladder infusion with clotrimazole for treatment of candiduria in a dog. *J Am Vet Med Assoc.* 2002;220:1496–1498.
48. Toll J, Ashe CM, Trepanier LA. Intravesicular administration of clotrimazole for treatment of candiduria in a cat with diabetes mellitus. *J Am Vet Med Assoc.* 2003;223:1156–1158.
49. Azie N, Neofytos D, Pfaller M, et al. The PATH (Prospective Antifungal Therapy) Alliance(R) registry and invasive fungal infections: update 2012. *Diagn Microbiol Infect Dis.* 2012;73:293–300.
50. Pappas PG, Lionakis MS, Arendrup MC, et al. Invasive candidiasis. *Nat Rev Dis Primers.* 2018;4:18026.

51. Ben Abdeljelil J, Saghrouni F, Emira N, et al. Molecular typing of *Candida albicans* isolates from patients and health care workers in a neonatal intensive care unit. *J Appl Microbiol.* 2011;111:1235–1249.
52. Pettit C, Diaz S, Kaffenberger B. Two cases of atypical periorificial dermatitis caused by *Candida parapsilosis* in patients volunteering in dog shelters. *Dermatol Online J.* 2019;25:13030/qt1t91k54q.
53. Wirth F, Goldani LZ. Epidemiology of *Rhodotorula*: an emerging pathogen. *Interdiscip Perspect Infect Dis.* 2012;2012:465717.
54. Tuon FF, de Almeida GM, Costa SF. Central venous catheter-associated fungemia due to *Rhodotorula* spp.: a systematic review. *Med Mycol.* 2007;45:441–447.
55. Tuon FF, Costa SF. *Rhodotorula* infection. A systematic review of 128 cases from literature. *Rev Iberoam Micol.* 2008;25:135–140.
56. Kadota K, Uchida K, Nagatomo T, et al. Granulomatous epididymitis related to *Rhodotorula glutinis* infection in a dog. *Vet Pathol.* 1995;32:716–718.
57. Spoor MS, Zigioli VA, Jacocks KA. What is your diagnosis? Bronchoalveolar wash fluid from a dog. *Vet Clin Pathol.* 2019;48:777–779.
58. Gomez-Lopez A, Mellado E, Rodriguez-Tudela JL, et al. Susceptibility profile of 29 clinical isolates of *Rhodotorula* spp. and literature review. *J Antimicrob Chemother.* 2005;55:312–316.

86

Aspergillosis and Penicilliosis

Vanessa R. Barrs, Jonathan D. Dear

KEY POINTS

- Cause: *Aspergillus* spp. and *Penicillium* spp., which are ascomycetes in the family Aspergillaceae, order Eurotiales.[1]
- First Described: Invasive aspergillosis was first described in 1815 in a jackdaw bird (Meyer).[2] Aspergillosis was first described in dogs in 1897 and in cats in 1982.[3]
- Affected Hosts: Dogs, cats, humans, and a variety of other animal species.
- Geographic Distribution: Worldwide.
- Primary Mode of Transmission: Inhalation of fungal spores (conidia) from the environment.
- Major Clinical Signs: Sinonasal aspergillosis and penicilliosis: nasal discharge, sneezing, epistaxis, depigmentation of the nares in dogs. Sino-orbital aspergillosis (cats): exophthalmos, third eyelid prolapse, and oral mass lesions or ulcers in the pterygopalatine fossa. Disseminated aspergillosis: inappetence, weight loss, spinal pain, lameness, pelvic limb paresis or paralysis, cough, vomiting, and tachypnea.
- Differential Diagnoses: Sinonasal aspergillosis: neoplasia, inflammatory rhinitis, oronasal fistulas, cryptococcosis, nasal mites (dogs), foreign bodies, and polyps (cats). Disseminated aspergillosis and penicilliosis: bacterial discospondylitis, bacterial pyelonephritis, and other systemic mold infections, especially paecilomycosis.
- Human Health Significance: Human *Aspergillus* infections are acquired from the environment. *Aspergillus fumigatus* is the most prevalent airborne fungal pathogen in developed countries. The global burden of aspergillosis is high; approximately 3 million people have chronic pulmonary aspergillosis and almost 5 million have allergic bronchopulmonary aspergillosis. Ten million immunocompromised patients per year are at risk of developing invasive aspergillosis, resulting in 200,000 new cases per annum, with a mortality rate of > 50%. Direct transmission from affected dogs and cats to humans does not occur.

Aspergillosis and penicilliosis are diseases caused by pathogenic fungi that belong to genus *Aspergillus* and *Penicillium*, respectively. These fungi are ubiquitous, saprophytic, hyaline molds that sporulate abundantly; their spores (conidia) can be found in soil, water, air, and decaying vegetation. Conidia become airborne after environmental disturbance and strong air currents. Their small size keeps them airborne both indoors and outdoors.[4] It is estimated that an individual person inhales several hundred *Aspergillus* conidia each day.[5] *Aspergillus* species, and very rarely *Penicillium* species, cause a variety of noninvasive and invasive forms of disease in dogs and cats that include keratomycosis, fungal otitis externa, fungal rhinosinusitis (FRS), bronchopulmonary aspergillosis, and disseminated invasive aspergillosis (DIA). *Aspergillus* species known to cause disease in dogs and cats are listed in Table 86.1.[6–23] The genus *Aspergillus* contains several hundred individual species and can be divided into six subgenera (*Aspergillus, Polypaecilum, Cremei, Fumigati, Nidulantes,* and *Circumdati*) comprising 27 sections and 75 series.[24] The subgenera most frequently implicated in canine and feline aspergillosis are *Fumigati, Circumdati,* and *Nidulantes*. Teleomorphs (sexual forms) have been identified for some *Aspergillus* and *Penicillium* species; the asexual state (anamorph) comprises hyphae with mitotic spores (conidia), while the teleomorph consists of fruiting bodies that contain meiotic spores (ascospores) (Fig. 86.1). Teleomorphs are likely to be present in the growth phase of these organisms, when growth has been long-term and the nutrients of the substrate favor sexual differentiation. Under the previous dual nomenclature system, the teleomorph of a fungus was assigned to a separate genus, which had taxonomic precedence over the anamorph name. Most species in section *Nidulantes* (one of nine sections in subgenus *Nidulantes*) have a sexual state and were named *Emericella*. Similarly, *Neosartorya* in section *Fumigati* (subgenus *Fumigati*) and *Eurotium* in section *Aspergilli* were teleomorph genus names of *Aspergillus* species with sexual states. In 2011, dual nomenclature was abandoned in favor of a "one-fungus, one-name" taxonomic rule in the International Code of Nomenclature for algae, fungi, and plants, under which teleomorph genus names have been transferred into *Aspergillus*; for example, *Neosartorya udagawae* is now *Aspergillus udagawae*.[25] This information is relevant for veterinarians and microbiologists since clinically relevant reports may have been published using either the anamorph or teleomorph name of the fungus.

Because accurate identification of *Aspergillus* and *Penicillium* species requires advanced molecular techniques, organisms can be misidentified based on their morphology in culture alone.

Because the etiology, epidemiology, clinical signs, diagnosis, and treatment of upper respiratory tract (URT) aspergillosis, DIA, and keratomycosis/otomycosis differ, they are considered separately in this chapter. The discussion is focused on aspergillosis because of the rarity of penicilliosis; however, clinical disease, diagnosis, and treatment are the same for penicilliosis.

UPPER RESPIRATORY TRACT ASPERGILLOSIS

ETIOLOGY AND EPIDEMIOLOGY

In dogs, sinonasal aspergillosis (SNA) is a subacute to chronic, noninvasive disease of the nasal cavity and sinuses. It is most often caused by *Aspergillus fumigatus*. Rarely, infection by other species, such as *Aspergillus niger* complex organisms (e.g., *Aspergillus tubingensis*) or *Aspergillus flavus* and the closely related fungus *Penicillium*, occurs

TABLE 86.1 *Aspergillus* Species Associated with Disease in Dogs and Cats[6–23]

Clinical Form	Host Species	*Aspergillus* Subgenus/Section/Series	*Aspergillus* Species[a]
Keratomycosis	Cats	*Fumigati/Fumigati/Fumigati*	*A. fumigatus*
		Circumdati/Flavi/Flavi	*A. flavus*
	Dogs		*Aspergillus* spp.[b]
Otomycosis	Cats	*Fumigati/Fumigati/Fumigati*	*A. fumigatus*
	Dogs	*Circumdati/Nigri/Nigri*	*A. niger*
			A. welwitschiae
		Cirdumdati/Terrei/Terrei	*A. terreus*
		Circumdati/Circumdati/Circumdati	*A. ochraceus*
		Fumigati/Fumigati/Fumigati	*A. fumigatus*
		Nidulantes/Nidulantes/Versicolores	*A. versicolor*
Sinonasal aspergillosis	Dogs	*Fumigati/Fumigati/Fumigati*	*A. fumigatus*
		Circumdati/Nigri/Nigri	*A. niger*
			A. tubingensis
		Circumdati/Nigri/Japonici	*A. uvarum*
		Circumdati/Flavi/Flavi	*A. flavus*
		Nidulantes/Nidiulantes/Nidulantes	*A. nidulans*
	Cats	*Fumigati/Fumigati/Fumigati*	*A. fumigatus*
			A. lentulus
		Fumigati/Fumigati/Thermomutati	*A. thermomutatus*
		Fumigati/Fumigati/Viridinutantes	*A. felis*
		Circumdati/Nigri/Nigri	*A. niger*
		Circumdati/Flavi/Flavi	*A. flavus*
Sino-orbital aspergillosis	Cats	*Fumigati/Fumigati/Viridinutantes*	*A. felis*
			A. udagawae
			A. wyomingensis
		Fumigati/Fumigati/Thermomutati	*A. thermomutatus*
		Fumigati/Fumigati/Fumigati	*A. fischeri*
Bronchopulmonary aspergillosis	Dogs and cats	*Fumigati/Fumigati/Fumigati*	*A. fumigatus*
		Circumdati/Flavi/Flavi	*A. flavus* (dog)
Disseminated invasive aspergillosis	Dogs	*Circumdati/Terrei/Terrei*	*A. terreus*
			A. alabamensis
		Circumdati/Terrei/Nivei	*A. carneus*
		Nidulantes/Flavipedes/Flavipedes	*A. flavipes*
		Circumdati/Nigri/Nigri	*A. niger*
		Nidulantes/Usti/Deflecti	*A. deflectus*
		Nidulantes/Nidulantes/Versicolores	*A. versicolor*
		Fumigati/Fumigati/Fumigati	*A. fumigatus*
		Fumigati/Fumigati/Fumigati	*A. lentulus*
		Fumigati/Fumigati/Viridinutantes	*A. felis*
	Cats	*Fumigati/Fumigati/Fumigati*	*A. fumigatus*
		Fumigati/Fumigati/Viridinutantes	*A. felis*

[a]Some isolates have not been identified beyond the series level level (including some *A. flavus*, *A. fumigatus*, and *A. niger*).
[b]Reported isolates have not been identified beyond genus level.

(see Table 86.1). SNA occurs worldwide, with cases most commonly reported from the United States and Australia. Any breed of dog can be affected, but disease is most common in large, nonbrachycephalic breeds, especially golden/Labrador retrievers, German/Belgian shepherd dogs, rottweilers, malamutes, and rough/Border collies.[26–40] Smaller breeds most frequently affected include bull terriers, Staffordshire terriers, and miniature schnauzers. Dogs of any age can be affected (median age around 6 years).[26,32,35,41–45] Males appear to be at greater risk of infection than females; of 459 reported cases, 62% were male.[27–42,44–46] Systemic immunodeficiency or concurrent systemic disease is rare in dogs with SNA. Local sinonasal cavity disease including foreign bodies, neoplasia, and trauma is occasionally identified.

Two forms of FRS occur in cats—SNA and sino-orbital aspergillosis (SOA). Similar to dogs, SNA is generally a noninvasive mycosis, with plaques or mats of hyphae that adhere to, but do not penetrate, the mucosal epithelium. By contrast, SOA is a deeply invasive mycosis that extends beyond the nasal cavity and paranasal sinuses to involve adjacent tissues including the orbit. The first case of feline FRS described was in a cat with SOA in 1982, more than a century

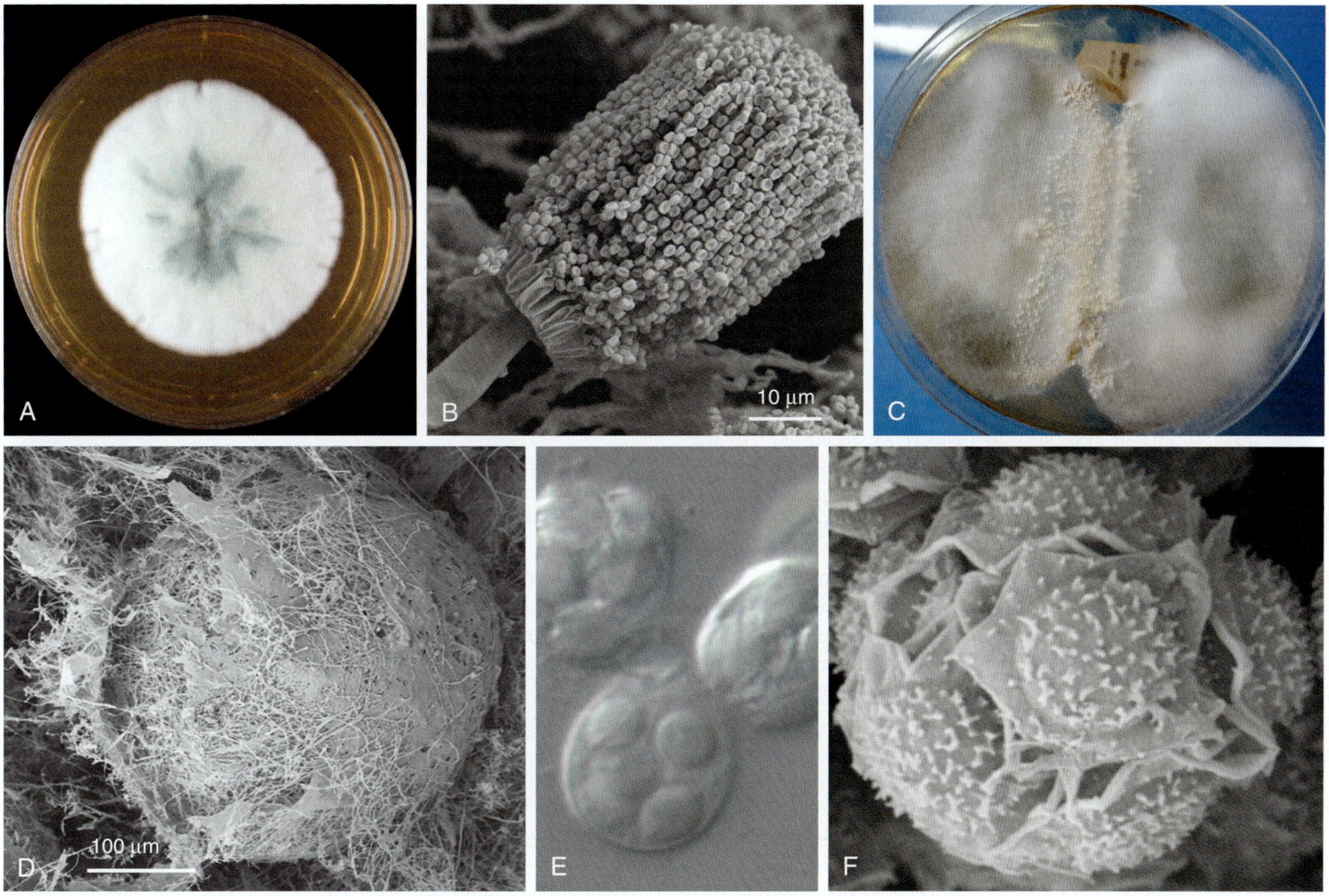

Fig. 86.1 Anamorph phase and teleomorph phase of *Aspergillus felis.* (A) Colony growth on malt extract agar comprising fungal hyphae *(white)* with green conidia centrally. (B) Scanning electron microscopic image of a conidiophore bearing chains of conidia. (C) At the intersection of growth of two colonies of *A. felis* of opposite mating type are multiple fruiting bodies or cleistothecia. (D) Scanning electron microscopic image of a single cleistothecium containing eight-spored asci. (E) Light microscopic image of an ascus containing 8 ascospores. (F) Scanning electron microscopic image of 8 ascospores inside an ascus.

after SNA was first described in dogs.[3] Since then over 70 cases of FRS have been reported in cats, mostly in the last decade.[3,6–9,11–13,47–62] Whether this increased reporting frequency is due to increased disease awareness or increased disease prevalence is not yet clear. Similar to canine SNA, the majority of cases in cats are from Australia or the United States, but cases from Japan, the United Kingdom, and mainland Europe reflect the global environmental presence of saprophytic *Aspergillus* species that cause these infections.

SNA in cats is most frequently caused by *A. fumigatus.* Other species within subgenus *Fumigati* such as *Aspergillus lentulus* and *Aspergillus thermomutatus* can also cause feline SNA (see Table 86.1). These closely related species are also called "cryptic" species because of their close morphologic resemblance to *A. fumigatus.* Accurate identification of cryptic species requires molecular techniques, and is important since antifungal resistance is common among these species. Species from other subgenera including *A. niger* and *A. flavus* can also cause feline SNA.

In early descriptions of SOA, causative organisms were not identified beyond the genus *Aspergillus*.[3,49] In several subsequent cases, *A. fumigatus* was identified, but identification was not definitive since it was morphological.[54] Where molecular methods have been used for definitive fungal identification (>25 cases), a novel species of *Aspergillus* discovered in affected cats, *Aspergillus felis*, was the most common cause of SOA, followed by *A. udagawae.* These species, in subgenus *Fumigati*, are cryptic species related to *A. fumigatus,* and even more closely related to *Aspergillus viridinutans.* There are currently 10 species in the *A. viridinutans* species complex, and of these, 3 have been detected in cats with SOA: *A. felis, A. udagawae,* and *Aspergillus wyomingensis.*[63]

Brachycephalic breeds of Persian and related lineage (Himalayans, exotic/British/Scottish shorthair cats, ragdolls) are predisposed to SNA and to SOA, but both conditions occur in any breed. Disease can occur in cats of any age (median, 5 years) and there is no sex predisposition. Most cats with URT aspergillosis test negative for FeLV or FIV infection. SNA and SOA occasionally occur in association with facial trauma, nasal neoplasia, and inhaled plant material, as has been reported in canine SNA.[64,65] Although cats with FRS are usually systemically immunocompetent, diabetes mellitus, a known risk factor for aspergillosis in humans, is likely also a risk factor for feline aspergillosis with upper or lower respiratory tract involvement.[11,51,57,66,67]

PATHOGENESIS

Sinonasal Aspergillosis

The pathogenesis of canine SNA is not fully understood despite investigations of innate and adaptive immune responses.[68–73] There are three lines of defense against fungal respiratory infection: (1) the respiratory mucosal epithelium traps and removes inhaled conidia via the mucociliary escalator and acts as an anatomic barrier to invasion; (2) fungal elements are phagocytosed by host cells (monocytes, macrophages, neutrophils, and respiratory epithelial cells) resulting in direct pathogen killing; and (3) dendritic cells respond to phagocytosis by promoting differentiation of naïve T cells into effector T-helper (Th) cell subtypes.

After inhalation, *Aspergillus* conidia that are not trapped and removed by mucociliary defenses germinate, if temperature and humidity are favorable, to form plaques of fungal hyphae that are adherent to the sinonasal mucosa. *Aspergillus* conidia are coated with hydrophobin proteins that facilitate mucosal adherence and protect conidia from recognition of PAMPs by innate and adaptive immune cells.[74] SNA is usually noninvasive; therefore, fungal hyphae do not penetrate the mucosal epithelium.

Dendritic cells express pattern recognition receptors (PRRs) including C-type lectin receptors, TLRs, NOD-like receptors (NLRs), and galectin family proteins that recognize specific fungal epitopes and induce specific Th responses, which are an essential determinant of host susceptibility or resistance to invasive aspergillosis.[75] In the immune response of humans to *A. fumigatus*, Th1 cytokine responses are generally protective, while Th2 cytokine responses increase susceptibility to invasive disease. Th17 responses are regulatory, promoting Th1 responses and suppressing Th2 responses. Th17 responses are implicated in the immunopathogenesis of chronic fungal infections by failure to restrain inflammation after IL-17A-dependent neutrophil recruitment.[75] T-regulatory (Treg) cells restrain exuberant immune reactivity and limit tissue damage in many chronic infections, but can handicap the effect of protective immunity. In addition to infected cells, or cells exposed to fungal PAMPs, Treg cells are a principal source of IL-10.

Cytokine profiling of dogs with SNA demonstrated upregulation of mRNA for cytokines associated with a Th1 response compared with normal controls or dogs with lymphoplasmacytic rhinitis.[68,69,72] In addition, there was upregulation of IL-10, which may limit the extent of local tissue destruction,[76] but paradoxically could also impede clearance of infection. Compared with normal dogs, dogs with SNA were found to have significantly higher expression of all 10 TLRs except for TLR5, and of NLR2, but not NLR1 in the nasal mucosa.[73] A subsequent mutational analysis of TLRs 2, 4 and 9 was performed,[70] since single-nucleotide polymorphism (SNPs) in these specific TLRs have been associated with higher risk of fungal disease in humans.[77] However, no SNPs associated with canine SNA were detected.

The functional phenotype of peripheral blood mononuclear cells (PBMCs) from normal dogs and dogs with SNA after challenge with heat-inactivated *A. fumigatus* conidia has also been determined.[71] There was significantly greater expression of IL-17A mRNA in PBMCs from affected dogs compared with controls, suggesting a role for a Th17-driven uncontrolled inflammatory response that could counteract the host's efforts to clear fungal infection through Th1-directed immunity.

Although SNA in dogs is noninvasive, it results in nasal turbinate and paranasal bony lysis, which can be severe. This is attributed to the inflammatory response of the host.[78] In addition, *A. fumigatus* synthesizes proteases, phospholipases, and toxic secondary metabolites, which may contribute to tissue destruction.[79] Other fungal metabolites unique to section *Fumigati* have one or more virulence properties including cytotoxicity (e.g., fumiquinazolines, trypacidin), ability to induce ciliastasis (e.g., verruculogen, helvolic acid) or apoptosis; and inhibition of immune responses, neutrophil responses, phagocytosis, and/or angiogenesis (e.g., gliotoxin, fumagillin, pyripyropenes).[79]

Sino-Orbital Aspergillosis

In SOA there is direct extension of a sinonasal infection to involve paranasal structures, usually via lysis of the thin orbital bone.[8] Cats with SOA have granulomatous invasive mycotic rhinosinusitis with submucosal hyphal invasion.[3,6,55] Once infection reaches the orbit, multilobulated fungal granulomas form in which hyphae are confined centrally.

As orbital granulomas expand, they cause dorsolateral displacement of the globe and bulge ventrally into the caudal oral cavity. In advanced disease, local extension to involve the CNS can occur, resulting in granulomatous mycotic meningitis. Hematogenous dissemination to involve other organs was reported in one case.[80] A role for species-specific fungal virulence factors in the development of disease is suspected since different fungal species cause SNA and SOA. The *A. felis* type strain, isolated from a cat with SOA, had significantly higher virulence in *Galleria melonella* larvae than *A. fumigatus*.[81] Whether unique fungal metabolites are involved in pathogenicity is not known, for example, viriditoxin is produced by all members of the *A. viridinutans* complex but not by *A. fumigatus*.[79]

CLINICAL FEATURES

Clinical Signs

Clinical signs of SNA in dogs include sneezing, reverse sneezing, chronic serous to mucopurulent nasal discharge, depigmentation, crusting or ulceration of the nasal planum, muzzle pain and, less commonly, epistaxis (Fig. 86.2). Clinical signs are subtle early in disease. Nasal discharge is initially unilateral but can become bilateral as the disease progresses. Signs in advanced disease may include lethargy, inappetence, and weight loss. Nasal pain can manifest as pawing at the face, hiding, or withdrawal when approached. Destruction or obstruction of the nasolacrimal duct can lead to epiphora. Osteolysis of the cribriform plate is often subclinical, but occasionally leads to meningitis with neurologic signs such as obtundation or seizures. Clinical signs of SNA in cats are similar although nasal depigmentation and signs of nasal pain have not been reported.

Cats with SOA are usually examined because of signs associated with a retrobulbar fungal granuloma including unilateral exophthalmos, a prolapsed, inflamed third eyelid, and blepharospasm or conjunctival discharge (Fig. 86.3). Exposure keratitis is common and uveitis is sometimes present. Nasal signs may be subtle or absent; however, the history usually reveals sneezing or nasal discharge in the 6 months before examination. In advanced disease, vision loss can occur due to severe ulcerative keratitis or infiltration of the optic nerve and/or optic chiasm.[6,49,50,55] Exophthalmos may become bilateral and neurologic signs may develop including seizures, nystagmus, circling, facial muscle fasciculation, and hyperesthesia.[6,58,59] Inappetence and dysphagia can also occur.[59]

Physical Examination Findings

Physical examination findings in dogs with SNA include unilateral or bilateral serous or mucopurulent nasal discharge, epistaxis, pain on palpation of the face, mild mandibular lymphadenomegaly, depigmentation, crusting or ulceration of the nares, and occasionally epiphora (see Fig. 86.2). Nasal airflow is usually normal or increased because of turbinate lysis. Sometimes palpation of the nasal bones or hard palate can reveal defects in the underlying bone. Dogs with cribriform plate involvement and meningitis may be obtunded or dehydrated. Dogs with severe epistaxis can have melena on rectal examination secondary to swallowed blood. Most affected dogs are afebrile.

Physical examination findings in cats with SNA consist of serous or mucopurulent nasal discharge, sneezing, stertor, epistaxis, and, in some cases, mandibular lymphadenomegaly, fever, or a discharging sinus over the nasal bridge or frontal sinus.[6] Cats with SOA most commonly have unilateral exophthalmos with dorsolateral

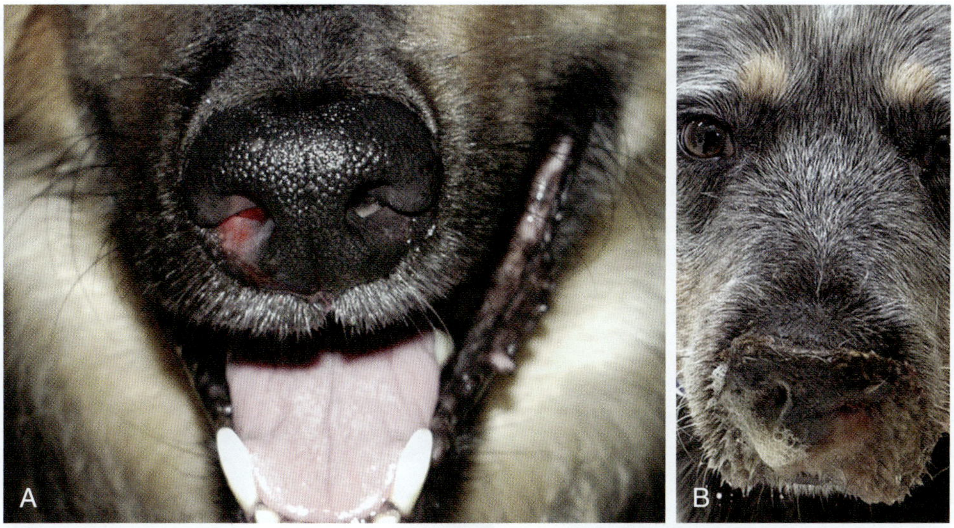

Fig. 86.2 (A) Unilateral depigmentation and ulceration of the nares of a 7-year-old shepherd mix with sinonasal aspergillosis (SNA). (B) Severe bilateral mucopurulent nasal discharge, crusting and ulceration, and unilateral depigmentation of the nares in a 6-year-old Australian cattle dog with SNA. (Courtesy Dr. Lynelle Johnson, Small Animal Internal Medicine Service, University of California, Davis & Dr. Natasha Evans, University of Sydney Veterinary Teaching Hospital.)

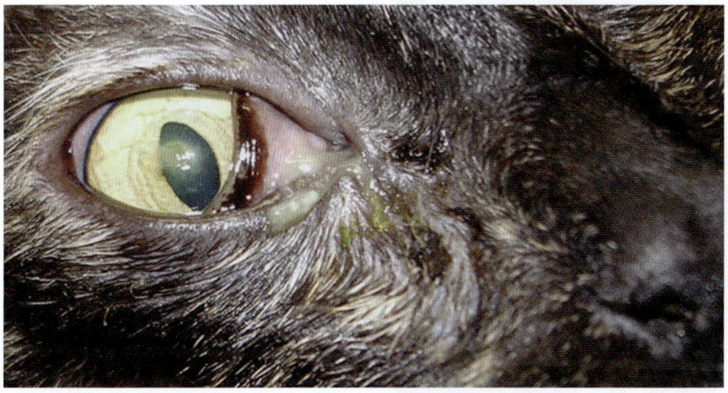

Fig. 86.3 A 2-year-old domestic shorthair cat with sino-orbital aspergillosis. Note the central corneal ulcer, conjunctival discharge, and prolapsed third eyelid caused by a right-sided orbital fungal granuloma.

deviation of the globe and prolapse of the third eyelid, which may also be inflamed. Corneal ulcers are usually central and are readily visualized with fluorescein stain (see Fig. 86.3). Other ocular signs variably present include miosis, an absent pupillary light response, an absent menace response, and signs of anterior or posterior uveitis. Resistance to retropulsion of the globe and normal intraocular pressure readings on tonometry enables differentiation of exophthalmos from buphthalmos.

Oral cavity involvement is first visible as a submucosal swelling in the pterygopalatine fossa adjacent to the last molar tooth, which may become ulcerated (Fig. 86.4). Ulceration of the hard palate occurs occasionally. Fungal invasion of maxillary subcutaneous tissues causes facial swelling, which may be subtle or severe and can ulcerate.[61] Fever and mandibular lymphadenomegaly are variably present. In most cases, there is no pain on opening of the mouth.

DIAGNOSIS

Early diagnosis of URT aspergillosis relies on a high degree of suspicion for the disease and availability of client financial resources because of a lack of uniformly available sensitive, noninvasive diagnostic tests for the disease. Serologic tests are performed early in investigation. Definitive diagnosis requires a combination of imaging, visualization of fungal plaques by rhinoscopy/sinuscopy (SNA), and identification of fungal elements on cytology or histopathology. Imaging should be performed before rhinoscopy to avoid the influence of iatrogenic hemorrhage on the results. Duplicate tissue or fungal plaques can be stored frozen, as well as submitted fresh for culture and in formalin for histopathology. If fungal cultures are negative, frozen tissues can be retrieved for molecular testing.

Laboratory Abnormalities

Dogs with SNA often have no abnormalities on CBC, serum chemistry profile, or urinalysis. Occasionally, mild nonregenerative anemia; mild neutrophilia, rarely with a left shift; mild eosinophilia; and/or mild hypoalbuminemia are present.[10] Cats with SOA may have a mild mature neutrophilia and sometimes mild to severe hyperglobulinemia.[6,49]

Diagnostic Imaging

Plain Radiography

Plain skull radiographs in dogs or cats with SNA may show unilateral or bilateral loss of turbinate detail, destruction of the nasal septum, and/or increased soft tissue opacity within the nasal cavity. The open-mouth view provides optimum evaluation of the turbinates (Fig. 86.5A). A "skyline" view of the nasal sinuses may show opacification of one or both sinuses and frontal bone hyperostosis (Fig. 86.5B).[33]

Advanced Imaging

Whenever possible, CT or MRI are preferred imaging modalities for the nasal cavity because of their increased sensitivity over plain radiography for evaluation of the nasal cavity, sinuses, and cribriform plate.[33] Bony changes are best appreciated on CT. Sinonasal cavity involvement can be unilateral or bilateral in dogs, and is usually bilateral and asymmetric in cats.[32,33] In some animals, lesions are limited to the frontal sinus.[8,45] Findings on CT or MRI in canine and feline SNA include moderate to severe "cavitated" nasal turbinate lysis and defects in the nasal septum; increased soft tissue opacity within the nasal cavity and/or sinuses due to mucosal inflammation, fluid accumulation, or fungal plaques; hyperostosis of the frontal

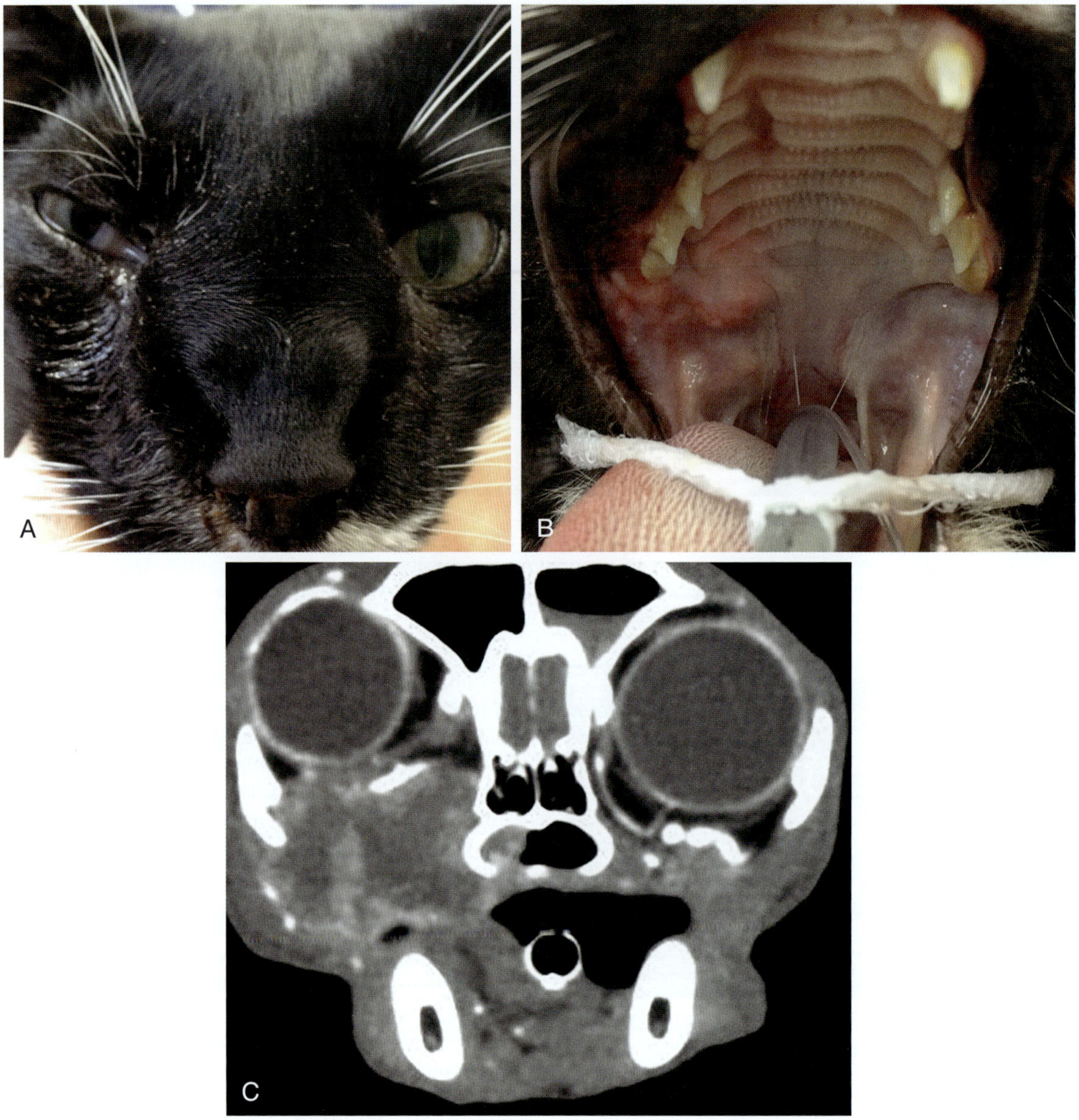

Fig. 86.4 A 3-year-old domestic shorthair cat with sino-orbital aspergillosis with unilateral right exophthalmos with prolapse of the third eyelid, blepharospasm, conjunctival discharge, and unilateral right nasal discharge (A); the orbital mass has extended into oral cavity in the right pterygopalatine fossa (B) and is visible on a post-contrast axial computed tomography scan in a soft tissue window as a heterogeneous mass with characteristic peripheral rim enhancement causing dorsolateral displacement of the globe and invasion into the oral cavity and subcutaneous maxillary tissues (C).

bones; and mandibular or retropharyngeal lymph node enlargement.[8,32,33,45] Nasal mucosal thickening is detected as a rim of soft tissue along the nasal bones, maxillary recess, and frontal bone. Osteolysis of the cribriform plate, orbital bone, frontal bones, and, rarely, the maxillary or palatine bones may be present (Fig. 86.5C). Meningeal enhancement is sometimes evident on contrast administration in dogs with cribriform plate destruction.[41] Fungal plaques and mucosal secretions fail to enhance with contrast and cannot be readily distinguished from each other. Deposits of calcium-containing fungal metabolites that aggregate to cause sinoliths are common in human maxillary sinus mycetomas, but have only been reported in one cat with SNA (rhinoliths),[50] one cat with SOA (sinolith),[8] and not in dogs.

Advanced imaging is recommended for all cases of suspected feline URT aspergillosis to differentiate SNA from SOA. In early disease, orbital involvement may not be apparent on clinical examination, and, if present, is an indication for systemic antifungal therapy as part of the management plan. CT findings in SOA include a retrobulbar mass in the rostral and ventromedial aspect of the orbit with indentation or dorsolateral displacement of the globe. In most cases, there is involvement of the ipsilateral paranasal maxillary soft tissues, and less commonly of the pterygopalatine fossa, either of which may cause a mass effect (see Fig. 86.4). There may also be a mass effect in the nasal cavity, nasopharynx, or paranasal sinuses. Orbital masses show heterogeneous contrast enhancement and often contain lobulated hypoattenuating foci with peripheral rim enhancement (see Fig. 86.4).[8,12,55,58,59] However, this

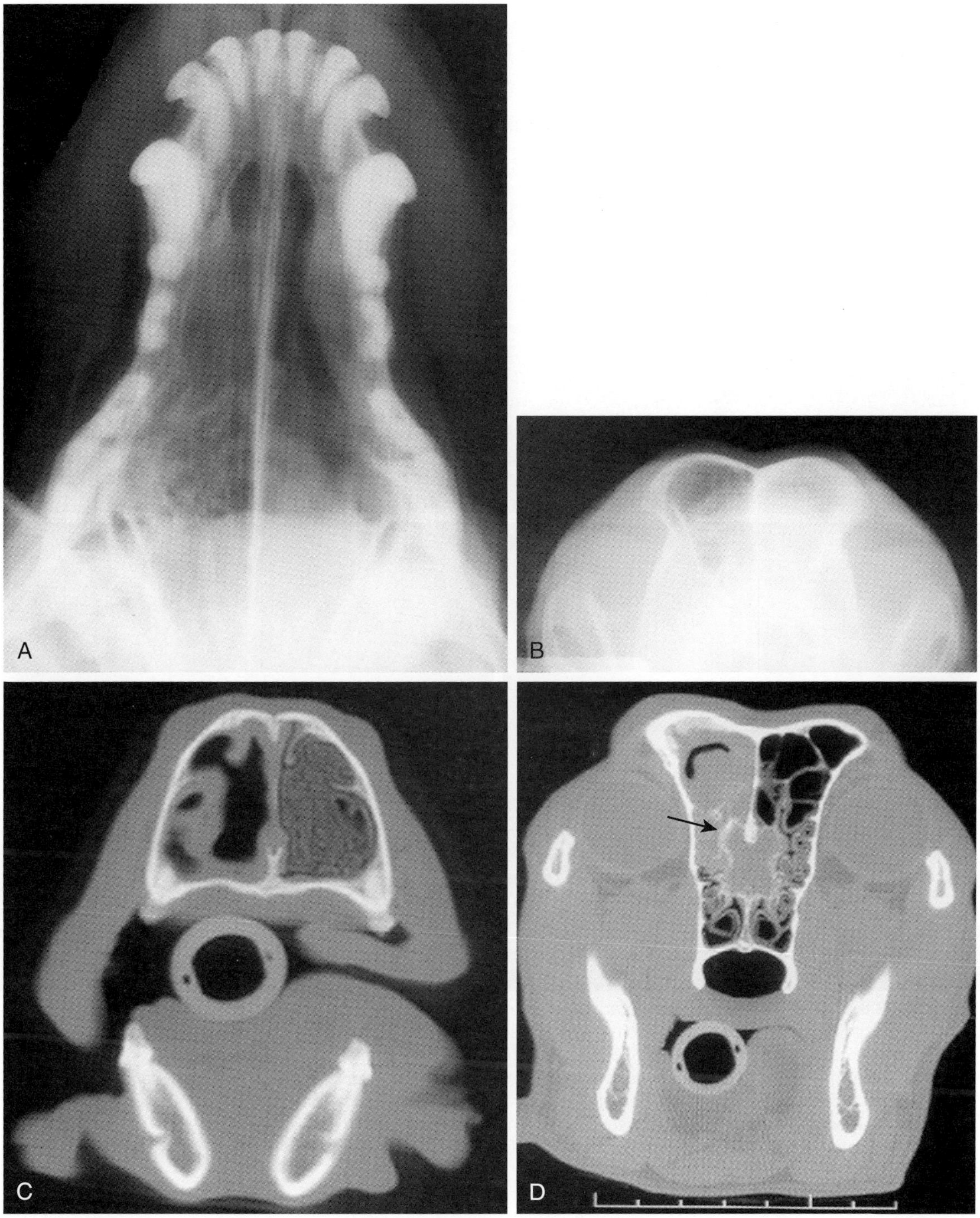

Fig. 86.5 Plain radiographs and computed tomography scan images of the nasal cavity of a 6-year-old female spayed golden retriever with sinonasal aspergillosis. (A) Open-mouth view. There is marked loss of detail in the left nasal cavity. (B) Skyline projection of the frontal sinuses. There is increased opacity in the left frontal sinus. (C) A transverse image through the nasal cavity shows marked turbinate loss on the left side. (D) Transverse image through the frontal sinuses and region of the cribriform plate. There is moderate fluid accumulation and irregular soft tissue structures in the left frontal sinus, and the frontal bone that overlies the sinus is thickened and irregular. Bony destruction at the level of the cribriform plate is present *(arrow)*.

pattern of enhancement is not specific for aspergillosis and can be seen with other mycoses (e.g., cryptococcosis) or neoplasia.[8] Sinonasal cavity involvement can almost always be detected in cats with SOA; changes are similar to SNA, but may be more subtle. With MRI, retrobulbar masses are T2-hyperintense. Invasion of temporal and masseter muscles by the mass may also be apparent on MRI (Fig. 86.6).[58]

Rhinoscopy and Sinuscopy

Visualization of fungal plaques by rhinoscopy and sinuscopy confirms the presence of mycotic rhinitis, and is a noninvasive, reliable method for obtaining fungal plaques and mucosal biopsies for cytology, histopathology, and fungal culture. Plaques are white, gray, yellow, black, greenish, or a mixture of these colors and are adhered to the nasal

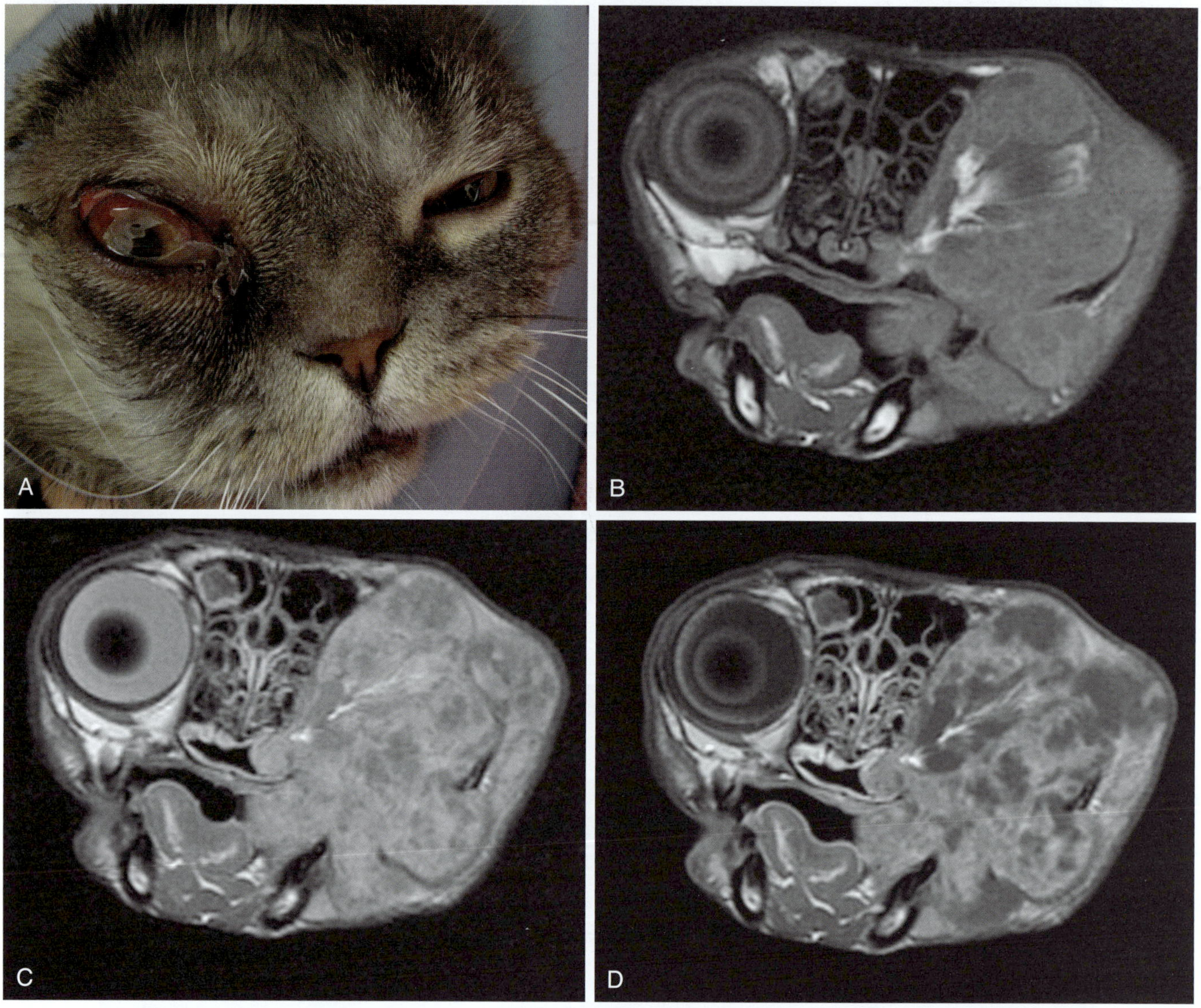

Fig. 86.6 (A) A 7-year-old male neutered Scottish fold cat with exophthalmos, conjunctivitis, and blindness of the right eye secondary to sino-orbital aspergillosis. A 1- to 2-cm mass was also identified in the pterygopalatine fossa on oral examination. (B–D) Magnetic resonance imaging of the head of the same cat. The right eye was displaced rostrally by a large retrobulbar mass that is (B) mildly, heterogeneously hyperintense on T1-weighted images, (C) hyperintense on T2-weighted images, and (D) enhanced with contrast. The mass extends medial to the ramus of the mandible and enters the nasopharynx as well as the oropharynx. A small T1-hyperintense structure is noted in the left frontal sinus.

mucosa or mucosa of the frontal sinus in cases of SNA. (Fig. 86.7). Cytologic examination is important to establish a diagnosis of SNA since there are other causes of mycotic rhinitis, and because mucopurulent exudates can occasionally be mistaken for fungal plaques.

In dogs, nasopharyngoscopy is performed with a flexible endoscope, after which a rigid telescope or flexible endoscope is used to examine the rostral portions of the nasal cavity. In some cases, extensive turbinate destruction allows a flexible endoscope to be passed directly into the frontal sinuses through the nasofrontal opening. If this is not possible, but CT or MRI findings suggest the possibility of frontal sinus lesions, trephination or surgical exploration of the frontal sinuses is necessary to visualize (and treat) this region. After trephination, a rigid endoscope can be used to examine the frontal sinus through the trephination site.

Nasopharyngoscopy using a flexible endoscope is useful in cats to identify choanal and nasopharyngeal fungal plaques or granulomas. In cats with SOA, although mycotic rhinitis is usually present, fungal plaques are not seen on rhinoscopy because of deep tissue invasion by fungal hyphae. The nasal cavity is examined using a rigid rhinoscope. Indications for sinus trephination are the same as for dogs.

Microbiologic Tests

Cytologic Examination

Cytologic examination of blind or rhinoscopy-directed mucosal swabs, brush specimens of the nasal cavity, or nasal biopsies from dogs or cats with SNA can reveal filamentous fungal hyphae and sometimes also conidia (Table 86.2). Hyphae stain well with Wright stain. They are septate and branch at 45-degree angles (see Fig. 4.3). Large numbers of degenerate neutrophils, ciliated epithelial cells, and/or bacteria are also usually present. In one study, the sensitivity of cytologic examination was 93% for endoscopic-guided cytology brush specimens, and 100% for squash preparations of biopsies of suspected mucosal fungal plaques, but it was only 20% or less for nasal discharge or smears made from blind swab specimens.[40]

TABLE 86.2 Diagnostic Assays Available for Aspergillosis in Dogs or Cats

Assay	Specimen Type	Target	Performance
Cytologic examination	Aspirates of affected tissues, body fluids, impression smears of biopsies	Fungal hyphae (with or without conidia in tissues exposed to air)	False negatives can occur when specimen size is small or low numbers of fungi are present. Cytology of brush specimens optimizes sensitivity for dogs with SNA. Identification to species level requires culture and molecular testing.
Fungal culture	Aspirates or biopsies of affected tissues, body fluids	*Aspergillus* species	Sensitivity for diagnosis of canine SNA is at least 75% when endoscopically guided nasal biopsies are cultured. Specificity is > 95%. Culture of a typical species (*A. terreus* or *A. deflectus*) from a dog with signs consistent with disseminated disease strongly suggests DIA. Molecular testing by PCR may be required to identify beyond the species complex level.
Antibody serology (AGID or ELISA)	Serum	Antibodies to *Aspergillus* species	Assays vary in sensitivity and specificity. In general, positive results support a diagnosis of canine SNA, but negative results do not rule out the disease. Insensitive for diagnosis of DIA.
Galactomannan antigen assay (ELISA)	Urine, serum	*Aspergillus* spp. galactomannan cell wall antigen	Insensitive for diagnosis of SNA, SOA, and probably bronchopulmonary disease. Very sensitive for diagnosis of DIA. Cross-reactivity with other fungal pathogens may occur (especially other molds). False positives also occur with Plasmalyte administration.
Real-time PCR assays	Whole blood	*Aspergillus* spp. DNA	Assays studied lack sensitivity or specificity for diagnosis of canine SNA. Usefulness for diagnosis of DIA requires further study.
Histopathology	Biopsy specimens from affected tissues	Fungal hyphae (with or without conidia in tissues exposed to air)	Sensitivity for diagnosis of canine SNA in rhinoscopically guided biopsies was 82%. Hyphae are usually visualized in biopsies from animals with DIA, but lesions may be difficult to access for biopsy. Special stains assist organism detection.

AGID, agar gel immunodiffusion; *DIA*, disseminated invasive aspergillosis; *ELISA*, enzyme-linked immunosorbent assay; *PCR*, polymerase chain reaction; *SNA*, sinonasal aspergillosis; *SOA*, sino-orbital aspergillosis.

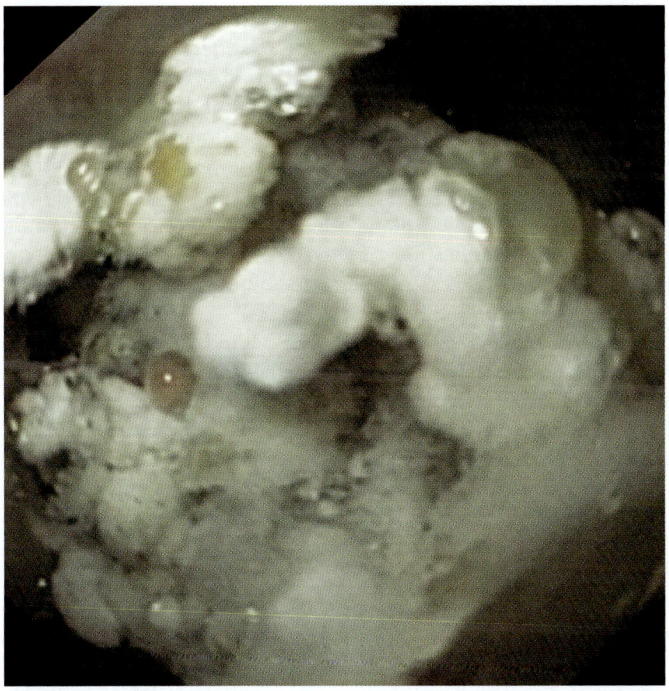

Fig. 86.7 Rhinoscopic view of white to gray fungal plaques in the nasal cavity of a 9-year-old male miniature schnauzer with sinonasal aspergillosis.

Fungal hyphae may be identified in cats with SOA on cytologic examination of fine-needle aspirates or squash preparations of nasopharyngeal or retrobulbar masses biopsied via the oral cavity or with ultrasound or CT guidance. However, because fungal hyphae are confined to central areas of granulomatous lesions, they may be missed.

Serologic Diagnosis

The sensitivity of serologic tests to detect the fungal cell wall antigen galactomannan (GM) or *Aspergillus*-specific antibodies in aspergillosis is heavily influenced by host immunocompetence (see Table 86.2). Antigen tests are affected by host ability to clear fungal antigen from the circulation, and antibody tests rely on an adequate humoral immune response. A commercial ELISA to detect GM in the serum (Platelia *Aspergillus* EIA, Bio-Rad) has a sensitivity of up to 90% in systemically immunocompromised patients, including neutropenic human patients with pulmonary aspergillosis and dogs with DIA.[82,83] However, in non-neutropenic patients with pulmonary aspergillosis, the assay sensitivity is < 30%.[82,84,85] Similarly, in dogs and cats with SNA, GM also performs poorly (23%–24% sensitivity).[43] In immunocompetent patients, GM is cleared by neutrophils, which possess mannose-binding receptors, or is complexed by antibody.[86,87] Also, lack of tissue invasion in noninvasive mycoses such as SNA may contribute to the lack of detectable circulating GM.

Assays to detect serum *Aspergillus*-specific antibodies include immunodiffusion (ID) assays that detect precipitins, such as AGID or counter immunoelectrophoresis (CIE) (see Fig. 2.7A), and ELISA assays. In general, ID assays have lower sensitivity and higher specificity than ELISAs for diagnosis of canine and feline URT aspergillosis. However, clinical performance data for some assays used in commercial veterinary diagnostic laboratories may not be available. The sensitivity of one ID assay (Meridian Bioscience, USA) for diagnosis was 57% to 77% for canine SNA[41–43] and 43% for feline URT aspergillosis.[9] The specificity for both assays was 98%–100%.The sensitivity and specificity of another ID assay (Immuno-Mycologics, OK, USA) for canine SNA was 31% and 97%, respectively.[88] The sensitivity and specificity of an ELISA assay that detects antibodies against a commercial *Aspergillus* antigen extract derived from *A. fumigatus, A. niger,*

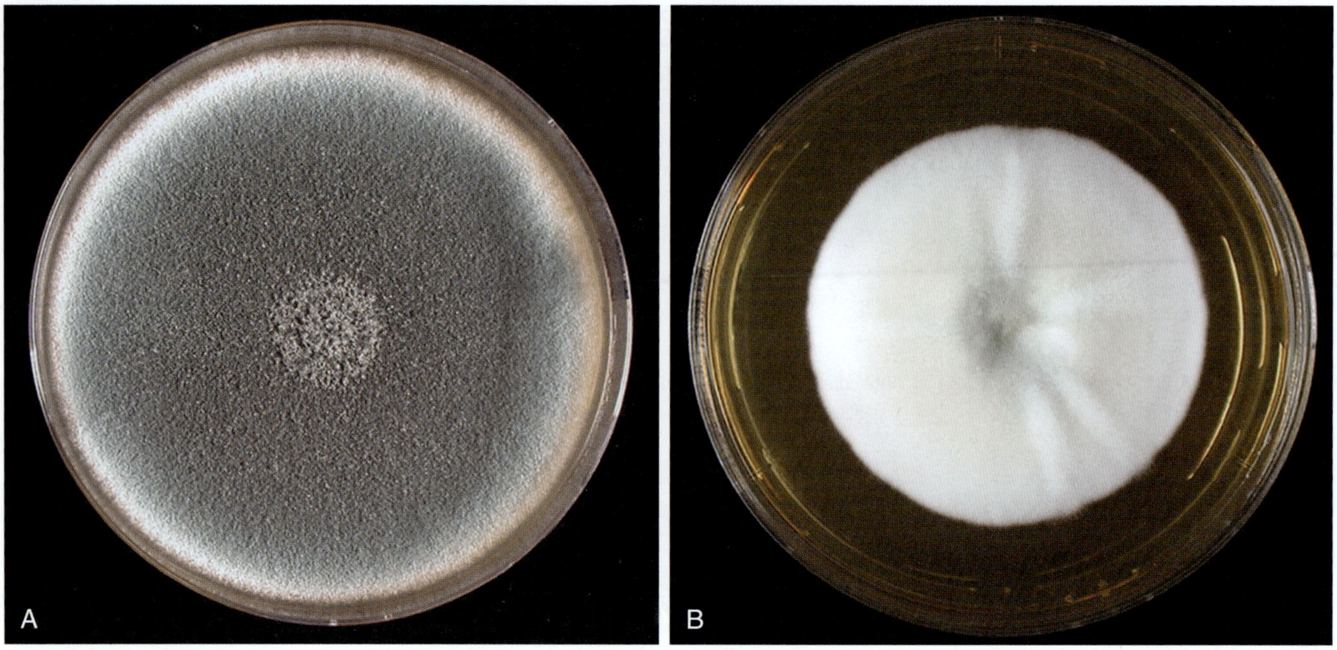

Fig. 86.8 Cultures of (A) *Aspergillus fumigatus* and (B) *Aspergillus felis* on malt-extract agar after 7 days of incubation at 27°C. Note the grey-green conidia of *A. fumigatus* which sporulates rapidly compared with *A. felis*.

and *A. flavus* was 88% and 97%, respectively, for canine SNA and 95% and 93%, respectively, for feline URT aspergillosis.[9,43] Thus, negative results with these antibody assays do not rule out SNA, but positive results strongly suggest the disease is present.

Fungal Culture

Aspergillus fumigatus can be readily grown on routine laboratory media. Colonies of mold generally appear within 96 hours, but occasionally longer incubation times are required.[44] In the absence of supportive rhinoscopic, cytologic, or histopathologic findings, positive cultures from the nasal cavity require cautious interpretation because *Aspergillus* may be found within the URT of healthy animals. Nevertheless, in two separate studies, no dogs with nonfungal nasal disorders had positive culture results for *Aspergillus*.[42,44] In one of these studies (which included 21 dogs with SNA and 37 dogs with nonfungal nasal disease), the sensitivity of fungal culture of endoscopic nasal tissue biopsies (including nasal mucosa and fungal plaques if visualized) for diagnosis of canine SNA was 81%.[42] In the other study, the sensitivity of fungal culture of nasal mucosal biopsies at 37°C was 75%, 88% for fungal plaques and < 19% for blindly collected nasal swab specimens (see Table 86.2).[44]

The fungal pathogens that cause feline URT aspergillosis can usually be isolated from tissue biopsies or fungal plaques on commercial culture media such as Sabouraud's dextrose agar or malt extract agar. Of 23 cases of feline SNA and SOA, 22 were culture-positive in one study.[6] One useful distinguishing feature of the cryptic species in *Aspergillus* subgenus *Fumigati* that cause URT aspergillosis in cats (e.g., *A. felis*) is their inability to grow at 50°C, in contrast to *A. fumigatus*, which does exhibit growth at 50°C. Fungal cultures from cats with URT aspergillosis can be subcultured and incubated at 50°C to determine whether a cryptic species is present. Fungal isolates that fail to grow at 50°C should be submitted for molecular testing for species identification. Cryptic species are also slower to sporulate than *A. fumigatus* and have white or cream-colored fungal colonies before sporulation in contrast to the rapidly sporulating grey-green colonies of *A. fumigatus* (Fig. 86.8).

Identification of *Aspergillus* species using macroscopic and microscopic morphologic features is inaccurate and many cryptic species within a complex cannot be reliably differentiated from each other. Morphologic features in combination with demonstration of fungal growth at 50°C is usually adequate to differentiate *A. fumigatus* from cryptic species.[21] Accurate identification of other species in *Aspergillus* subgenus *Fumigati* requires PCR and sequencing. Using DNA extracted directly from fungal cultures, longer gene targets can be amplified than from formalin-fixed paraffin-embedded tissues, and amplification of the ITS1-5.8S-ITS2 region of rDNA (751 bp) using primers ITS1 and ITS4 is standard. For some species, amplification of a secondary identification target such as calmodulin, β-tubulin, or the RNA polymerase II second largest subunit (*RPB2*) is required for definitive identification.[89]

MALDI-TOF MS is an alternative method for identification of *Aspergillus* species but has been limited by inadequate species and strain spectra representation in commercial libraries (see Chapter 3). For example, of 55 clinical *Aspergillus* isolates from Australia, 69% were correctly identified using the commercial database alone, but 93% were correctly identified when it was combined with an in-house database constructed from strains of *Aspergillus* circulating in Australia.[90]

Molecular Diagnosis Using Nucleic Acid–Based Testing

In veterinary medicine, the use of panfungal PCR assays for the diagnosis of mycotic disease is increasing. PCR can lack sensitivity for detection of fungi when compared with bacteria due to problems associated with fungal cell wall lysis in order to release DNA during the first step of DNA extraction. PCR assays targeting the ribosomal DNA (rDNA) gene cluster have the broadest application because this gene is multicopy (>50,000 copies per haploid fungal genome). It also contains regions that are highly conserved between fungal genera and that flank highly variable regions. Thus, universal primers can be designed based on the conserved regions, and the resulting sequences enable identification to at least genus or species complex level. The rDNA gene cluster comprises the small subunit rDNA (18*S*) gene, the 5.8*S* gene, and the large subunit (28*S*) gene. These regions are separated

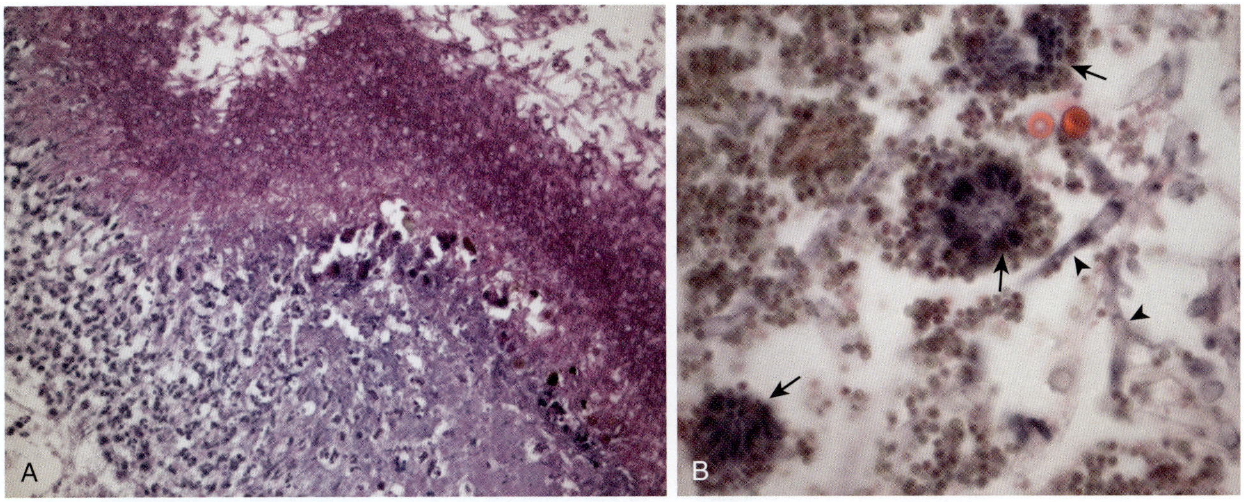

Fig. 86.9 Histopathology of a nasal biopsy from a 4-year-old intact male Border collie with sinonasal aspergillosis. (A) There is a profound neutrophilic inflammatory response beneath a thick mat of fungal hyphae, which stains magenta. Periodic acid-Schiff stain, 400× magnification. (B) *Aspergillus* hyphae *(arrowheads),* conidiophores *(small arrows),* and conidia *(spores)* can be seen on the surface of the lesion. Hematoxylin and eosin stain, 1000× oil magnification.

by the intergenic transcribed spacer (ITS) regions, ITS1 and ITS2, which are the most hypervariable regions. PCR assays that target the 361 bp ITS1 region (primers ITS1 and ITS2) or the 231 bp ITS2 region (primers ITS3 and ITS4) have been used to identify fungal pathogens in fresh, frozen, or formalin-fixed canine and feline tissues.[91,92] In two studies, the sensitivity of these PCR assays to correctly identify a fungal pathogen to genus or species level was approximately 65%.[91,92] Real-time PCR methods are increasingly used together with fungal antigen detection tests for the diagnosis of pulmonary aspergillosis in immunocompromised humans using blood (plasma or serum) or bronchoalveolar lavage fluid.[93] The use of real-time PCR assays to detect *Aspergillus* DNA in nasal biopsy specimens was evaluated for diagnosis of SNA in dogs, but assays evaluated had either unacceptably high rates of false-positive test results (PenAsp assay) or a low sensitivity (*Aspergillus* genus-specific PCR).[88] For both assays, dogs with SNA had higher DNA copy numbers than control dogs or dogs with lymphoplasmacytic rhinitis or neoplasia, but there was considerable overlap in copy numbers between dogs with SNA and those without SNA.

Pathologic Findings

The sensitivity of histologic examination of nasal mucosal biopsies for diagnosis of SNA was approximately 80% in two studies in which fungal plaques and adjacent mucosa were biopsied under endoscopic guidance (see Table 86.2).[41,42] Biopsy of the nasal mucosal tissue without the overlying fungal plaque can cause a false-negative result. Special fungal stains (e.g., PAS or GMS) increase the sensitivity of detection of fungal hyphae in histologic sections.

Histopathology of nasal biopsies from dogs and cats with SNA usually reveals mats of branching, septate fungal hyphae attached to nasal or sinus mucosa or within luminal exudates, in a background of lymphoplasmacytic and neutrophilic inflammation. Occasionally, the neutrophilic component predominates. Variable numbers of macrophages and eosinophils may also be present, as well as necrotic debris. Other findings include osteolysis, turbinate remodeling, and intralesional bacteria. Occasionally, intralesional plant material is detected. Conidiophores and conidia can be found because the fungus is exposed to air within the nasal cavity (Fig. 86.9).

In cats with SOA, retrobulbar fungal granulomas contain central areas of coagulative necrosis in which fungal hyphae are confined and surrounded by peripheral zones of inflammatory cells including neutrophils, eosinophils, macrophages, peripheral fibroblasts, lymphocytes, and plasma cells (Fig. 86.10A and B). Inflammatory lesions can also efface adjacent skeletal muscle and bone. The globe is resistant to fungal invasion, but may be affected by keratitis and anterior uveitis.[6,49,55,58] There may be invasion of adjacent structures including the nictitating membrane, eyelid, optic nerve, and optic chiasm.[6,49,54,55,59] Mycotic invasion of the sinus or nasal mucosa may also be evident (Fig. 86.10C).

TREATMENT AND PROGNOSIS

Successful treatment of SNA is challenging. Because of the large size of the nasal cavity and sinuses, clinical signs are often not apparent until disease is advanced. Delays in diagnosis can occur because of the costly and invasive nature of diagnosis and treatment and the need for specialized imaging techniques and endoscopic expertise. Owners of adult dogs that develop persistent nasal discharge (e.g., present for at least 1 week) should be encouraged to pursue advanced imaging and rhinoscopy as soon as possible so that the disease can be recognized and treated early, especially in regions such as California and Australia where there is a high disease incidence. Treatment with antibacterial drugs alone is discouraged because primary bacterial infection of the nasal cavity in adult dogs (in the absence of an underlying causes such as neoplasia or fungal infection) is extremely rare.

In general, treatment of canine and feline SNA requires thorough mechanical debridement of plaques with endoscopic biopsy forceps and copious irrigation until no visible fungus remains, which may necessitate extended anesthesia. In some cases, treatment is performed immediately after imaging and rhinoscopy, which further prolongs the period of anesthesia. If plaques within the frontal sinuses cannot be accessed by antegrade rhinoscopy through the nasofrontal opening, frontal sinus trephination and curettage or open surgical debridement of the frontal sinus may be required. Debridement of fungal plaques is followed by repeated lavage with 0.9% saline and suction, followed by topical antifungal drug therapy with clotrimazole or enilconazole. Additional systemic antifungal drug treatment could also be considered, but whether this improves the outcome over topical therapy alone is unknown.

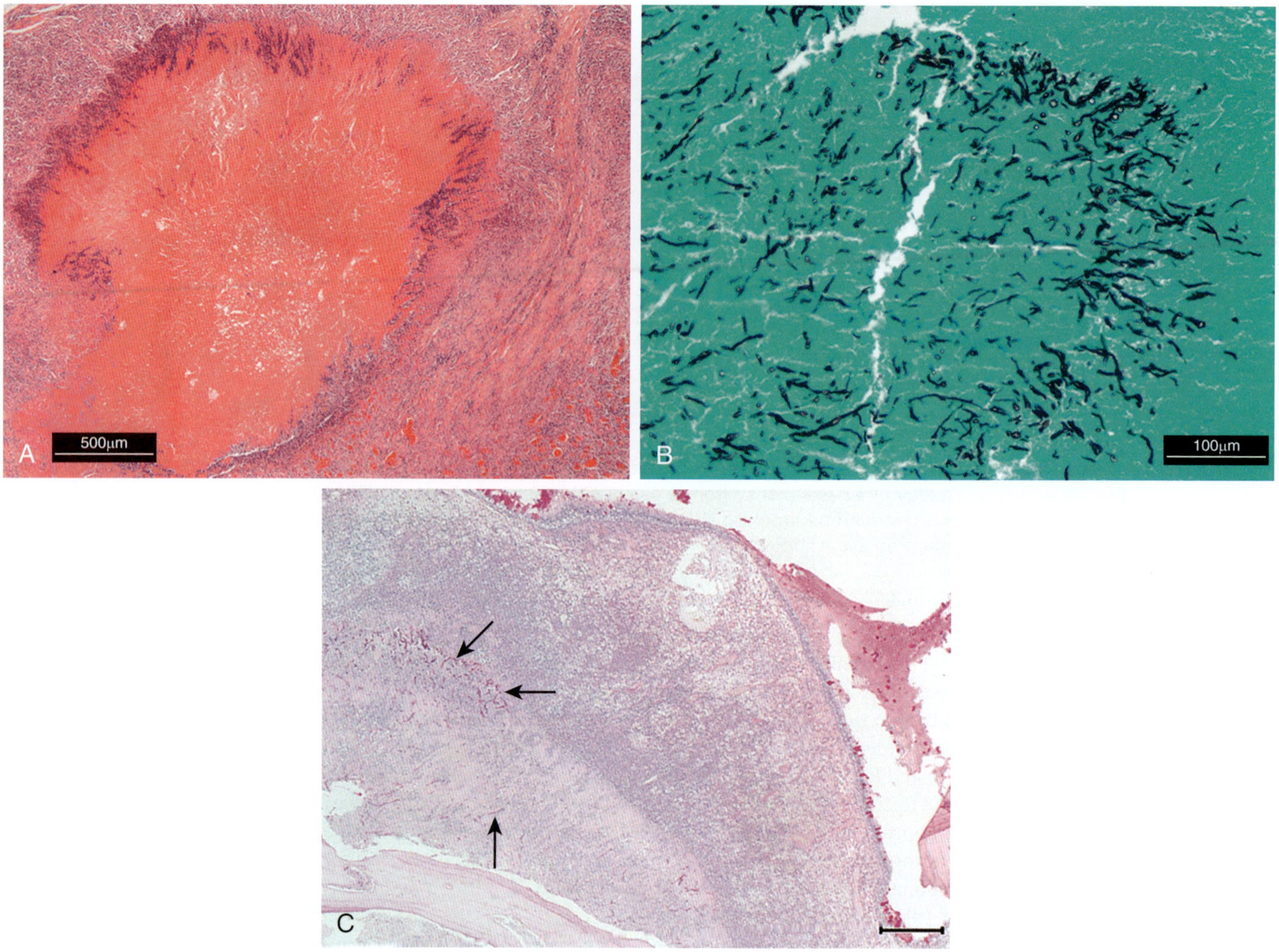

Fig. 86.10 Histopathology of (A and B) an orbital mass and (C) sinus mucosa from a 2-year-old domestic shorthair cat with sino-orbital aspergillosis, an invasive mycosis. (A) The orbital fungal granuloma contains central areas of coagulative necrosis in which fungal hyphae are confined and surrounded by peripheral zones of mixed inflammatory cells. (B) Septate, branching fungal hyphae are darkly stained with GMS stain. (C) Below the ciliated epithelium of the frontal sinus is an extensive inflammatory infiltrate and magenta-stained fungal hyphae *(arrows)*. Periodic acid-Schiff stain, scale bar 300 μm.

Canine Sinonasal Aspergillosis

A variety of noninvasive and invasive protocols for topical antifungal drug treatment of canine SNA after debridement of fungal plaques in the nasal cavity and frontal sinuses have been described, with varied rates of success. Currently, there is a lack of masked, randomized prospective clinical trials with consistent and long-term follow-up evaluation that indicate clear benefit of one treatment over another. Complete debridement of fungal plaques is associated with an improved first treatment success rate compared to partial debridement in dogs treated with topical antifungal azole infusions.[94] The protocol described here is used at the University of California Davis, Veterinary Medical Teaching Hospital (UCD VMTH). A similar protocol has been used successfully to treat SNA in cats.[57]

After thorough debridement of fungal plaques, a 24F Foley catheter is retroflexed over the soft palate and the balloon inflated until it can be palpated above the soft palate (Fig. 86.11). Placement of the catheter can be facilitated by insertion of a stiff guidewire into the catheter. Alternatively, a flexible catheter can be advanced from the rostrum through the nasal passage and into the oropharynx. The Foley catheter can then be sutured to this second catheter and be drawn into the nasopharynx by withdrawing the second catheter from the nasal folds. The tip of the catheter can then be bent into a U shape and hooked over the soft palate, after which the balloon is inflated. The nasopharynx is packed with moistened laparotomy pads, a gauze pad is placed over the incisive papilla, and the proximal end of the Foley catheter is clamped across the guidewire to prevent leakage of antifungal drug from the nasal cavity. The dog is then placed in dorsal recumbency with the skull positioned vertically (at 90 degrees to the tabletop), the eyes are lubricated and a protective wrap is placed around the muzzle to prevent spillage of medication into the eye. Clotrimazole (1%) or enilconazole (1% or 2%) solution is then administered into each nasal passage until full and a meniscus is visible. For large-breed dogs, 20 to 30 mL of solution is administered per side initially, and medication is dripped in to maintain filling of the nasal passage for 15 minutes.[94] The catheters and sponges are then removed with the dog's head tilted downward at an angle of 30 degrees, and the material is allowed to drain from the nasal cavity for 10 minutes. Debridement and a second treatment are then routinely performed 1 month later. Sometimes, a third treatment 1 month after that may be necessary. Clotrimazole can be irritating to tissues, and solutions with a propylene glycol vehicle can cause nasopharyngeal irritation and edema.[95,96] In general, however, clotrimazole solutions with a polyethylene glycol vehicle cause minimal adverse

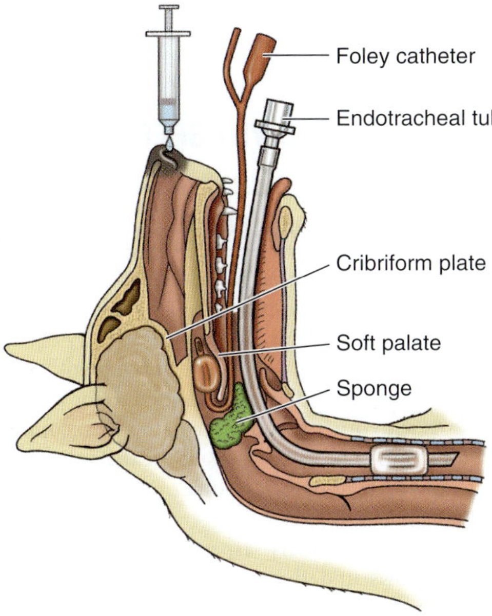

Fig. 86.11 Placement of catheter for topical treatment of canine sinonasal aspergillosis with clotrimazole or enilconazole.

effects. Enilconazole solutions may be less irritating, but there is no evidence that they are more effective than clotrimazole. They also tend to be less viscous, and may be more likely to be aspirated as a result.

One retrospective study compared two minimally invasive topical enilconazole infusion protocols after endoscopic plaque debridement.[94] One group of 24 dogs was treated with a 1-hour infusion of 2% enilconazole with rotation of the dog every 15 minutes by 90° to maximize sinonasal mucosal drug contact. After enilconazole drainage, 1% bifonazole cream was administered into the frontal sinuses. The second group of 24 dogs was treated with a simplified protocol using a 2% enilconazole infusion instilled for 15 minutes without rotation or addition of bifonazole cream. The simplified protocol was of much shorter duration (median 92 min compared to 201 min) and overall treatment success was 96% for both groups.[94]

Other studies describe administration of 1% clotrimazole cream into the nasal cavities and frontal sinuses after fungal plaque debridement with overall treatment success of 94% and 100%, respectively.[97,98] In one of these studies, sinus irrigation and topical application of clotrimazole was performed using a minimally invasive endoscopic approach to place a rigid urinary catheter over a guidewire into the frontal sinus.[98] This approach replaced the need for sinus trephination.

When cribriform plate lysis or lysis of the floor of a frontal sinus is present, topical treatment could potentially cause life-threatening neurologic signs or failure to recover from anesthesia. Chemical irritation from the topical azole drug could cause meningoencephalitis. Similarly, hyperosmolar carriers used in topical infusions (e.g., polyethylene glycol) could cause CNS injury.[99] Nevertheless, treatment has been performed without complication in some dogs with these defects.[41,98–100] Although their efficacy for treatment of SNA has been debated, oral azole antifungals with activity against molds (i.e., itraconazole, posaconazole, or voriconazole) have been used either as monotherapy for dogs with braincase lysis or in combination with terbinafine or topical antifungal drugs.[26,46,101,102] Debridement before commencing systemic antifungal drug treatment is strongly recommended, because effective drug concentrations are not likely to be obtained within fungal plaques. Antifungal susceptibility testing can

> **BOX 86.1 Therapeutic Approach for Feline Sinonasal Aspergillosis**
>
> 1. Determine whether infection is invasive or noninvasive based on histopathology and computed tomography (CT) findings.
> 2. Submit positive fungal culture to a mycology reference laboratory to determine species.
> 3. Identify and assess the presence of lysis of the cribriform plate or floor of the frontal sinuses on CT examination.
> 4. Debride fungal plaques from nasal cavity and frontal sinuses using endoscopy, suction, and copious saline irrigation.
> 5. Instill a 1% solution of clotrimazole solution in polyethylene glycol intranasally (1-hour soak under general anesthesia with 15-minute rotations).
> 6. If infection is invasive, or if cryptic species are identified, give additional systemic antifungal therapy.

also be considered for animals undergoing systemic therapy. Although there is no evidence of emerging azole resistance among *A. fumigatus* isolates from dogs and cats,[103] the prevalence of acquired azole resistance in environmental and human clinical isolates of *A. fumigatus* is increasing in many geographic regions.

The prognosis for canine SNA depends on the extent of disease at the time of diagnosis. Success rates vary from less than 30% to 100%, but methods to assess treatment success and follow-up times have not been consistent. Serial serologic testing by ID or ELISA is not useful to monitor treatment success since positive titers can persist for months to years beyond resolution of infection.[41] Response to treatment can only be assessed accurately by endoscopy. Even if infection is eliminated based on endoscopic reevaluation and biopsy, dogs with extensive turbinate loss are predisposed to recurrent bacterial infections of the nasal cavity, which result in persistent nasal discharge and sneezing. One study showed no difference in the prevalence of sneezing and nasal discharge between dogs that responded to initial treatment and dogs that failed to respond.[41] In studies where treatment protocols included debridement, a topical intranasal or intrasinusal azole (solution and/or cream), and endoscopic evaluation to confirm resolution of fungal plaques, 48% to 62.5% of dogs were clear of disease after one treatment, and 88% to 100% of dogs were clear of disease after at least one more treatment.[26,30,41,94,104] Relapse or re-infection occurs in 11–20% of treated dogs within 2 months to 2–3 years.[30,41,46,98] However, only two of these studies took into account relapse or reinfection, after the overall cure rate was reduced from 88% to 68% in one study[41] and from 100% to 89% in the other.[30] In another study, 11% (7/64) of dogs were diagnosed with relapse or reinfection 12 to 30 months after debridement and topical clotrimazole treatment, and all were successfully treated again.[46]

Feline Upper Respiratory Tract Aspergillosis

Evidence-based treatment protocols for feline SNA are not available due to a lack of prospective treatment trials. Successful treatment regimens reported in individual cases include oral azole therapy (itraconazole or posaconazole), oral azole therapy plus topical azole infusion (clotrimazole or enilconazole solution), or topical clotrimazole alone.[6,50,53,57,105] Similar to canine SNA, debridement of fungal plaques was an integral component of therapy for most successfully treated cases. A suggested strategy for treatment of feline SNA based on previous reports, treatment of canine SNA, and consideration of whether infection is invasive or noninvasive is outlined in Box 86.1. Overall, the prognosis for feline SNA appears similar to canine SNA, but a comparatively small number of cases has been evaluated.

Cats with SOA require treatment with systemic antifungal drugs. The results of antifungal susceptibility testing may be of value. One case that failed sequential treatment with itraconazole then amphotericin B (AMB) was cured with oral posaconazole.[54] The fungal isolate from that cat had high MICs for AMB and itraconazole and a low MIC for posaconazole. In one study, 12 cats with SOA were treated with an oral azole (itraconazole or posaconazole) alone or in combination with AMB and/or terbinafine, and 5 cats also had aggressive orbital debridement with enucleation. Treatment was successful in only one cat that did not have surgery.[6] Relapse of infection occurred 19 months after treatment was stopped but resolved after treatment with caspofungin and posaconazole. Results of antifungal susceptibility testing show that pathogenic species belonging to the *A. viridinutans* complex, including *A. felis, A. udagawae* and *A. wyomingensis* frequently have high MICs for itraconazole. A common method of antifungal susceptibility testing used in commercial laboratories, the Sensititre YeastOne method (Trek Diagnostic Systems Ltd., East Grinstead, UK) provides unreliable results for itraconazole compared with a reference broth microdilution method (EUCAST), but performs well for other antifungal drugs including azoles, AMB, and echinocandins, providing final results are reported at 72 hours of incubation, and not at 48 hours of incubation.[23] Overall the MICs of posaconazole and the echinocandins are usually low for these species, are higher for voriconazole, and variable for AMB. Thus, itraconazole is not recommended as a first-line therapy when these species are identified in cats with SOA. The combination of posaconazole and terbinafine is suggested as first-line therapy for cases of SOA and was effective in curing two cats with SOA caused by cryptic *Aspergillus* species.[106] In a previous study, isolates of *A. felis* were demonstrated to have low MICs for terbinafine.[7]

Posaconazole is well tolerated after oral and IV administration in cats, and hepatotoxicity is less common than with itraconazole.[6,23,107] Voriconazole administration has been associated with severe adverse effects in cats including paraplegia, blindness, anorexia, and cardiac arrhythmias (see Chapter 11).[6,58,60] In cats, voriconazole has a long oral half-life (>43 hours) and nonlinear pharmacokinetics are suspected to be the cause of toxicosis at higher drug doses due to saturation of metabolizing enzymes and decreased drug clearance.[108] The pharmacokinetics of caspofungin have been determined in cats; minimum effective concentrations appropriate for therapy can be reached using a loading dose of 1 mg/kg IV and subsequent daily doses of 0.75 mg/kg IV.[109] Overall, the prognosis for complete remission of SOA is guarded to poor.

Therapeutic Drug Monitoring

Therapeutic drug monitoring (TDM) is commonplace for human patients being treated for protracted periods with newer-generation antifungal azole drugs with low and/or highly variable oral bioavailability including posaconazole, voriconazole and isavuconazole.[110] TDM involves collection of a plasma sample from a patient immediately prior to the next dose of the drug. The most common and reliable method used for TDM is high-performance liquid gas chromatography (HPLC) combined with mass spectrometry.[111] TDM can be used in veterinary medicine using the same assays used for human patients since these assays are not species specific (see also Chapter 11).

PUBLIC HEALTH ASPECTS

There are no reports of transmission of SNA from affected dogs or cats to humans. Whether the handling of affected dogs by immunosuppressed humans poses a risk to their health is unknown, but such individuals should probably minimize close contact with affected animals. If contact is necessary, they should be encouraged to discuss the problem with their medical practitioner. At the least, gloves should be worn and proper hand washing practiced.

DISSEMINATED INVASIVE ASPERGILLOSIS AND PENICILLIOSIS

ETIOLOGY AND EPIDEMIOLOGY

DIA, formerly known as systemic aspergillosis, may involve the respiratory tract (bronchopulmonary aspergillosis) or may be a disseminated disease of multiple organ systems. The portal of entry of *Aspergillus* is thought to be via the respiratory tract with subsequent hematogenous spread, though rare cases of infection restricted to the lungs have been recorded.[112,113] As with other bloodborne pathogens, common sites of embolic dissemination of fungal organisms are the intervertebral discs, kidneys, brain, and eyes; nonetheless, other organs, muscles, and long bones may be affected.

Localized bronchopulmonary aspergillosis is rare in dogs and cats, and often follows underlying local or systemic immunodeficiency.[14,66,112,114] German shepherds appear to be predisposed to a form of bronchopulmonary aspergillosis characterized by the development of cavitary lung lesions.[14,115–117] These cases usually involve infection by *A. fumigatus* or cryptic species in subgenus *Fumigati*, whereas DIA in dogs is most often caused by *Aspergillus terreus* in subgenus *Circumdati*, or *Aspergillus deflectus* in subgenus *Nidulantes*. These findings contrast with SNA and SOA in dogs and cats (see previous section on Upper Respiratory Tract Aspergillosis) in which *A. fumigatus* and *A. felis* are most common. Other *Aspergillus* species have also been isolated from dogs with disseminated disease (see Table 86.1) In addition, fungal species from other families in order Eurotiales, including Trichocomaceae (including *Talaromyces* species and *Rasamsonia* species) and Thermoascaceae (*Paecilomyces* species) have been found to cause some cases of disseminated mold infections in dogs.[118–120].

In dogs, DIA may occur as a result of an uncharacterized genetic immunodeficiency, because female German shepherds are strongly predisposed to the disease, and immunosuppressive drug treatment is rarely present in the history of affected dogs.[15] Cases of DIA have been documented worldwide and the disease is likely ubiquitous, albeit underdiagnosed.[15,121–134] Two thirds of affected dogs seen at the UCD VMTH were German shepherds, and German shepherds were 43-fold more likely to develop the disease than other dog breeds.[15] Rhodesian ridgebacks also appear to be predisposed. Females are three times as likely to develop disseminated aspergillosis as males, and the median age of affected dogs is 4 years (range, 2 to 9 years). Concurrent or sequential infections with other opportunistic pathogens have been described in some dogs as in people.[135–137]

DIA in humans is usually secondary to immunodeficiency or immunosuppression, although invasive *Aspergillus* infections have been described in apparently immunocompetent individuals.[138] The most common underlying predisposing factors are leukemia (and subsequent hematopoietic stem cell transplant), neutrophil or macrophage dysfunction, neutropenia, acquired immunodeficiencies, and prior chronic antibacterial therapy.[139–141] The protective immune response to *Aspergillus* has been well characterized in murine models of infection and includes a variety of innate mechanisms (e.g., expression of TLR2 by pulmonary dendritic cells) in addition to Th1-regulated adaptive immunity characterized by the production of cytokines such as IL-18, IL-12, TNF-α, and IFN-γ.[142] Additionally, the protective immune response to *Aspergillus* in dogs is known to involve the activity of the Th17 subset of Th cells.[143] Individuals that have dominant Th2 immunity develop

TABLE 86.3 Historical Signs in 30 Dogs with Disseminated Invasive Aspergillosis

Signs	Percent of Dogs
Inappetence or anorexia	20
Pain	27
Lameness	13
Neurologic signs (especially pelvic limb ataxia and paresis)	20
Respiratory signs (especially cough)	13
Vomiting	7

From Schultz RM, Johnson EG, Wisner ER, et al. Clinicopathologic and diagnostic imaging characteristics of systemic aspergillosis in 30 dogs. *J Vet Intern Med.* 2008;22:851–859.

progressive disease, and glucocorticoid therapy is known to stimulate Th2-driven immune responses.[142,144,145] Hematopoietic stem cell transplant recipients have significantly greater risk of *Aspergillus* infection when donor stem cells carry the S4 TLR4 haplotype.[140]

Disseminated and bronchopulmonary aspergillosis are rare in cats.[66,80,146,147] Reported cases have occurred mostly in young cats, though one study documented infection in middle-age to older cats. No breed predispositions have been identified. Affected cats often have recognizable underlying immunosuppressive conditions such as diabetes mellitus, cancer chemotherapy, or severe viral infections (feline panleukopenia, FIP, or FeLV).[148] Aspergillosis has not been reported in cats with FIV infection, although such cats may have other opportunistic mycoses.[148]

CLINICAL FEATURES

Clinical Signs and Pathogenesis

Pulmonary aspergillosis or DIA is thought to develop after inhalation of *Aspergillus* conidia, which lodge in the alveoli and adhere to epithelial cells. In the absence of adequate local immune defenses, the conidia enlarge and germinate to form hyphae. Invasion of the bloodstream and dissemination to distant sites may occur because of systemic immunosuppression (either congenital or acquired). Fungal virulence factors are also likely to be important, although why *A. terreus* and *A. deflectus* are more likely than *A. fumigatus* to cause disseminated disease in dogs is unclear as DIA in humans is most frequently caused by subgenus *Fumigati* isolates.[149]

Anatomic sites of predilection in dogs with DIA are the vertebral endplates and discs, renal pelvis, spleen, long bones, and lymph nodes. However, any organ may be affected, including the liver, heart, cardiac valves, pancreas, eyes, lungs, brain, bone marrow, meninges, small intestine, skin, spinal cord, thyroid, adrenal glands, prostate, and trachea. Nasal cavity involvement is not generally a feature of the bronchopulmonary or disseminated forms, and dogs with DIA often lack evidence of pulmonary involvement. Disease involves multiple organ systems and develops over several months, but many dogs are terminally ill when first examined. The median reported duration of illness before admission in one study was 1 month (range, 2 days to 9 months).[15]

The most frequent clinical signs are lethargy, decreased appetite, pain, lameness, and neurologic signs secondary to discospondylitis (especially ataxia and paresis) (Table 86.3). A sudden onset of paraplegia may result from rupture of an infected intervertebral disc or vertebral subluxation from instability. Other signs include apparent blindness, ataxia, circling, head tilt, seizures, respiratory distress, and vomiting.[150] Cough, increased respiratory effort, and rarely hemoptysis

TABLE 86.4 Physical Examination Findings in 30 Dogs with Disseminated Invasive Aspergillosis

Finging	Percent of Dogs
Muscle wasting/thin body condition	40
Fever	27
Spinal pain	17
Vestibular signs	17
Peripheral lymphadenomegaly	17
Ocular abnormalities	13
Lameness	13
Ataxia	10
Paraparesis	10
Cough, increased breath sounds	10
Mental dullness	7
Vision impairment	7
Hemiparesis	7
Circling, seizures, arrhythmia	3

From Schultz RM, Johnson EG, Wisner ER, et al. Clinicopathologic and diagnostic imaging characteristics of systemic aspergillosis in 30 dogs. *J Vet Intern Med.* 2008;22:851–859.

may occur in dogs with bronchopulmonary aspergillosis.[14,117] Polyuria and polydipsia may develop as a consequence of renal insufficiency. Uveitis or endophthalmitis may be clinically apparent some months before generalized illness develops and thus may be an important clue to early diagnosis. Although uncommon, aspergillosis can also involve body cavities. Further systemic spread can occur from these sites. Pericarditis and associated effusion can result in signs of right-sided heart failure such as abdominal distention from a modified transudate peritoneal effusion.[151] It can also arise from rupture of a myocardial abscess, or from contiguous spread from the lung or hematogenous source. Fever, GI signs, abdominal distention, and anorexia are the most common findings with abdominal infections.

In the cat, clinical signs are generally referable to GI or pulmonary involvement, with nonspecific findings similar to those in dogs.

Physical Examination Findings

Physical examination findings in dogs with DIA are listed in Table 86.4. On physical examination, dogs with DIA may have muscle wasting and/or a thin body condition. Fever (up to 104.2°F or 40.1°C) was described in one quarter of affected dogs.[15] Musculoskeletal abnormalities include spinal pain, lameness, and, rarely, inability to stand. Neurologic signs include vestibular abnormalities, ataxia, mental dullness, paraparesis, vision impairment, hemiparesis, circling, and seizures. Dogs with respiratory involvement may cough and have harsh lung sounds and/or increased respiratory effort. Peripheral lymphadenomegaly may be detected. Ocular abnormalities include chorioretinitis, hyphema, and panophthalmitis.[15] Rarely, arrhythmias are detected secondary to myocardial involvement, but myocardial involvement is often subclinical.

DIAGNOSIS

Clinical Laboratory Findings

Complete Blood Count

Most dogs with DIA have leukocytosis due to a neutrophilia (Table 86.5).[15] A left shift with toxic neutrophils, eosinophilia,

TABLE 86.5 Selected Hematologic and Serum Biochemistry Analysis Results in 30 Dogs with Disseminated Invasive Aspergillosis

Variable	Median (Range)	No. (%) With Low Values	No. (%) With High Values	Reference Range
Hematocrit (%)	42 (14–46)	8 (31)	0	40–55
Neutrophils (cells/μL)	12,643 (7,584–28,321)	0	21 (81)	3,000–10,500
Band neutrophils (cells/μL)	0 (0–3,051)	0	10 (38)	Rare
Monocytes (cells/μL)	1,608 (499–3,760)	0	16 (62)	150–1,200
Lymphocytes (cells/μL)	1,566 (115–3,998)	4 (15)	0	1,000–4,000
Platelets (cells/μL)	262,000 (86,000–400,000)	1 (4)	0	150,000–400,000
Albumin (g/dL)	2.7 (1.3–3.6)	6 (24)	0	2.9–4.2
Globulin (g/dL)	4.4 (2.3–5.8)	0	12 (48)	2.3–4.4
Creatinine (mg/dL)	1.1 (0.5–7.8)	0	9 (36)	0.5–1.6
BUN (mg/dL)	19 (8–196)	0	9 (36)	8–31
Calcium (mg/dL)	10.8 (9.9–13.9)	0	8 (32)	9.9–11.4
ALT (IU/L)	37 (19–609)	0	3 (12)	19–67
ALP (IU/L)	78 (21–1,920)	0	3 (12)	15–127

ALP, alkaline phosphatase; *ALT,* alanine aminotransferase; *BUN,* blood urea nitrogen.

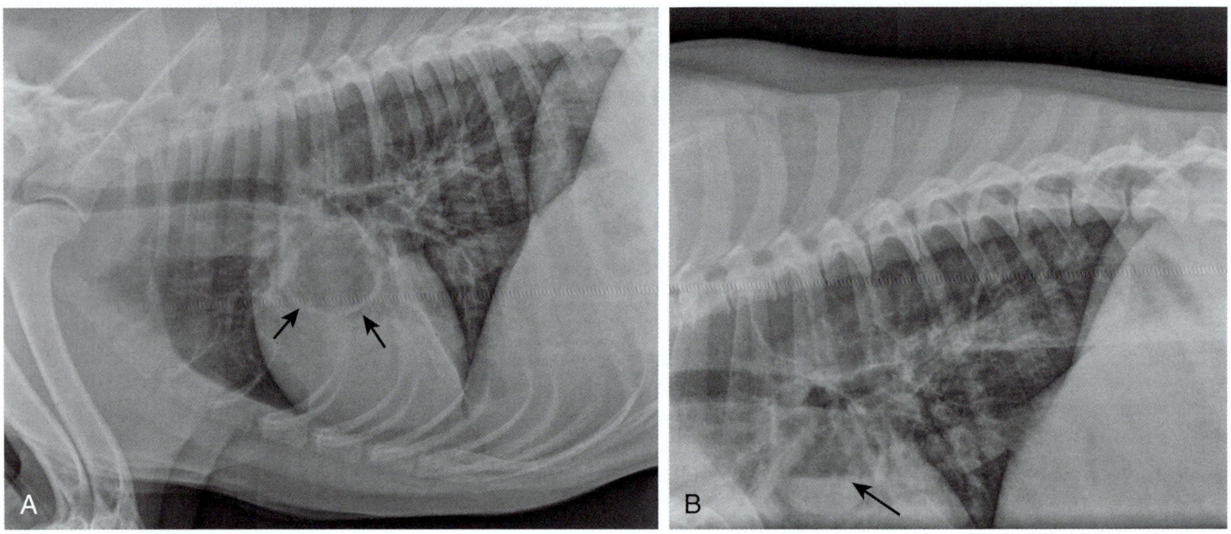

Fig. 86.12 Lateral thoracic radiograph of a 2-year-old male neutered German shepherd that had a 4-month history of cough and exercise intolerance. (A) A cavitary lesion *(arrows)* and alveolar infiltrates in the right middle lung lobe are present. (B) On a horizontal beam projection, a fluid line is present *(arrow)* within the dependent aspect of the lesion.

or monocytosis may also be present. Normocytic, normochromic nonregenerative anemia occurs in approximately one third of affected dogs and may be secondary to inflammatory or kidney disease.

Serum Biochemical Tests

Common abnormalities in the serum biochemical profiles of dogs with DIA include hyperglobulinemia, azotemia, hypercalcemia, and hypoalbuminemia (see Table 86.5).

Urinalysis

The urine specific gravity of azotemic dogs with DIA may be in the isosthenuric range because of renal insufficiency. Hematuria, proteinuria, and pyuria may also be detected. Fungal hyphae are rarely detected and were only identified in the urine sediment of 2 of 25 (8%) dogs with DIA in one study.[15]

Cerebrospinal Fluid Analysis

Analysis of the CSF in dogs with neurologic signs or spinal pain in affected dogs can be normal, or show an increased nucleated cell count and CSF protein concentration. The differential cell count reveals mixed or primarily mononuclear or neutrophilic pleocytosis.[150] Abnormalities of the CSF were identified in 8 of 10 dogs with DIA at the UCD VMTH.[135]

Diagnostic Imaging

Thoracic radiographs in dogs with bronchopulmonary aspergillosis may show a bronchial pattern or lung lobe consolidation.[112,127] Consolidation and cavitary lesions may be seen in the lungs of German shepherd dogs (Fig. 86.12).[115–117] Pulmonary cavitary lesions may be observed in dogs with chronic pulmonary localization.[115,116] Abnormalities in dogs with DIA include enlarged tracheobronchial and/or sternal lymph nodes, cranial mediastinal masses, pleural effusion, and/or pulmonary alveolar infiltrates.[15]

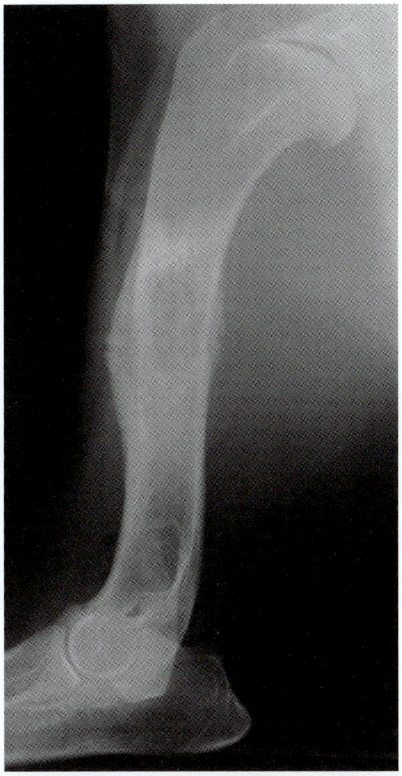

Fig. 86.13 Lateral radiograph of the left humerus of a 2-year-old male neutered German shepherd with disseminated aspergillosis. A primarily osteoproductive lesion is present in the mid-diaphysis.

Spinal radiographs reveal evidence of discospondylitis in approximately half of dogs with DIA, with a median of two sites affected (range, 1 to 9 sites).[15] Productive and destructive bony changes consistent with osteomyelitis may be present in other parts of the skeleton (Fig. 86.13). Most dogs have multiple affected sites, which include the vertebral bodies, sternebrae, ribs, scapula, humerus, and tibia.[15]

Sonographic Findings

Abdominal ultrasound abnormalities in dogs with DIA are most often in the kidneys, spleen, and abdominal lymph nodes.[15] Renal abnormalities include pyelectasia, a distorted and mottled architecture, decreased corticomedullary distinction, echogenic debris within the renal pelvis and proximal ureter, papillary blunting, and nodules or masses within the renal cortex (Fig. 86.14).[15] Occasionally, hydronephrosis is detected. Splenic abnormalities include hypoechoic nodules or masses, splenomegaly, changes consistent with infarction, or a mottled echotexture. Abdominal lymph nodes may be enlarged and/or hypoechoic. Other findings include diffuse hepatic or pancreatic hypoechogenicity, ascites, or evidence of venous thrombosis.

Advanced Imaging

MRI of the brain in dogs with *Aspergillus* infections that have disseminated to the CNS may reveal multifocal lesions that are hypointense to isointense and enhance with contrast on T1-weighted images. Three out of seven dogs with neurologic signs and confirmed *Aspergillus* infection had no identifiable MRI lesions in a recent case series.[150] Identified lesions are hyperintense or heterogenous on T2-weighted and fluid-attenuated inversion recovery (FLAIR) images. Mild or severe meningeal enhancement may also be present.

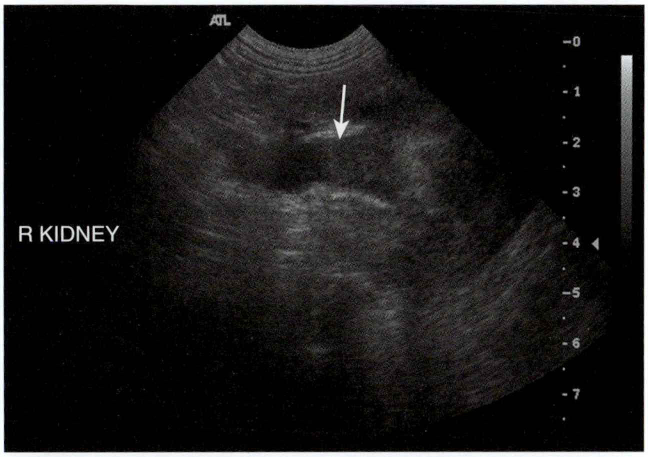

Fig. 86.14 Ultrasound image of the right kidney of a 6-year-old female spayed German shepherd dog with disseminated aspergillosis. There is dilation of the renal pelvis, which contains echogenic material *(arrow)*.

Cytologic Identification

Hyphae with morphology consistent with *Aspergillus* spp. may be present in aspirates of lymph nodes, kidney, lung tissue, or vertebral endplates or bone from dogs with systemic aspergillosis (see Fig. 4.3).[15] Cytologic examination of pleural effusion, airway lavage specimens, or urine may also reveal hyphae. False-negative results occur when organism numbers are low or specimen size is small. Accurate identification of the organism present requires fungal culture or molecular diagnosis (PCR) (see Table 86.2).

Microbiologic Testing

Aspergillus spp. are readily isolated on routine laboratory media. Isolation of *Aspergillus* spp. (especially *A. terreus* or *A. deflectus*) from normally sterile sites such as urine, blood, or aspirates of lymph node, bone, intervertebral disc, liver, or splenic tissue supports a diagnosis of DIA. Approximately 50% of dogs with DIA have positive urine cultures for *Aspergillus* spp., and around one third of dogs have positive blood or CSF cultures.[15] Isolation of *A. fumigatus* from airway washes should be interpreted more cautiously as it may represent contamination. Concurrent cytologic evidence of fungal hyphae is required for definitive diagnosis in this situation.

Once growth of mold occurs in culture, *Aspergillus* species can be identified to the subgenus and section level based on conidiophore morphology (Fig. 86.15). Accurate identification to the species level requires molecular techniques such as PCR, followed by sequencing, which can be performed by mycology reference laboratories (e.g., the Fungus Testing Laboratory at the University of Texas Health Science Center, San Antonio) (see Table 86.2). Such laboratories can also perform antifungal drug susceptibility testing. However, because clinical breakpoints have not been established for dogs or cats, the relevance of MICs for molds remains unclear.

Serologic Diagnosis

Assays that detect antibodies to *Aspergillus* species are insensitive for diagnosis of DIA.[15] This may reflect underlying host immunodeficiency (and hence inability to produce antibodies). Alternatively, antibodies in affected dogs may not cross-react with the antigens used in the test kits (see Table 86.2).

Antigen Detection

An *Aspergillus* GM antigen ELISA assay (Platelia, Bio-rad) has high sensitivity for diagnosis of disseminated aspergillosis in dogs when serum or urine specimens are tested.[83] In the author's hospital, all

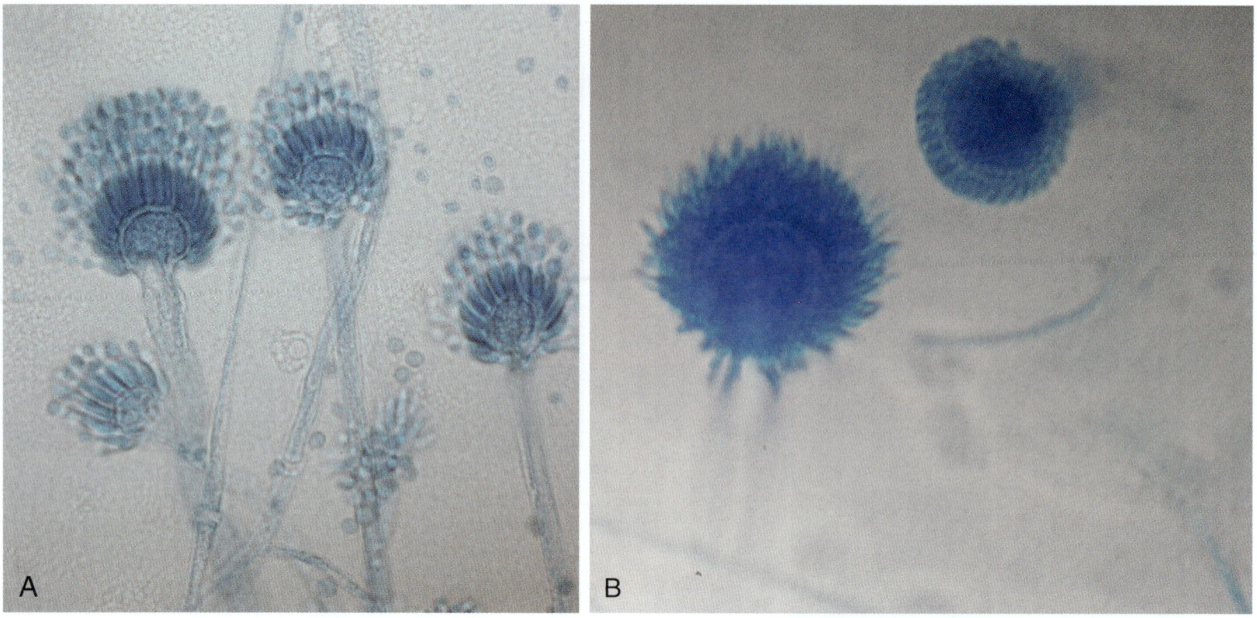

Fig. 86.15 (A) Morphology of *Aspergillus fumigatus*. (B) Morphology of *Aspergillus terreus,* which has an "upswept" appearance. The conidiophore is the specialized hyphal branch that bears the conidia (spores). The vesicle is the dilated top part of the conidiophore. Phialides are flask-shaped projections from the vesicle from which the conidia arise.

12 dogs with DIA had positive test results, with galactomannan indices (GMIs) that ranged from 6.4 to 12.2 (reference range, <0.5). Two dogs with localized pulmonary disease had serum GMIs of 0.14 and 0.77, which suggests that, as for SNA, the sensitivity of this assay for diagnosis of bronchopulmonary aspergillosis may be lower. High-level false-positive test results (GMIs > 1.5) appear to only occur in dogs with other fungal infections, especially those caused by *Penicillium*, *Rasamsonia* or *Paecilomyces*, and dogs treated with Plasmalyte IV fluid therapy. Plasmalyte contains sodium gluconate, which is produced by fermentation by *A. niger*; carry-over of small amounts of GM during production of the fermentation product is thought to occur.[152] Low-level false positives (0.5–1.5) can occur in dogs infected with other fungi (such as *Cryptococcus* spp.), some dogs with nonfungal disease such as neoplasia, some dogs treated with penicillin derivatives, and some dogs receiving oral probiotic nutraceuticals containing *Aspergillus*-derived ingredients.[153] A strong positive assay result in a dog with clinical abnormalities consistent with DIA and no history of Plasmalyte administration within the last 72 hours supports a diagnosis of a mold infection, but fungal culture or molecular identification is required to confirm that *Aspergillus* is the causative agent. A negative result in a dog with disseminated disease suggests that *Aspergillus* is not the cause, but it does not rule out the possibility of infection with another fungal species (see Table 86.2).

Molecular Diagnosis Using Nucleic Acid–Based Testing

Several real-time PCR assays have been developed and applied for the diagnosis of invasive aspergillosis in humans using blood or bronchoalveolar lavage fluid.[154–156] The sensitivity and specificity of these assays has varied, though they appear to be useful in monitoring response to therapy, becoming negative with successful treatment.[156,157] PCR assays have not been widely applied to diagnosis of DIA in dogs or cats. However, endpoint (conventional) PCR assays have been used for pathogen identification in cases where the organism cannot be cultured using fresh, frozen, or formalin-fixed tissue (see Table 86.2).[92]

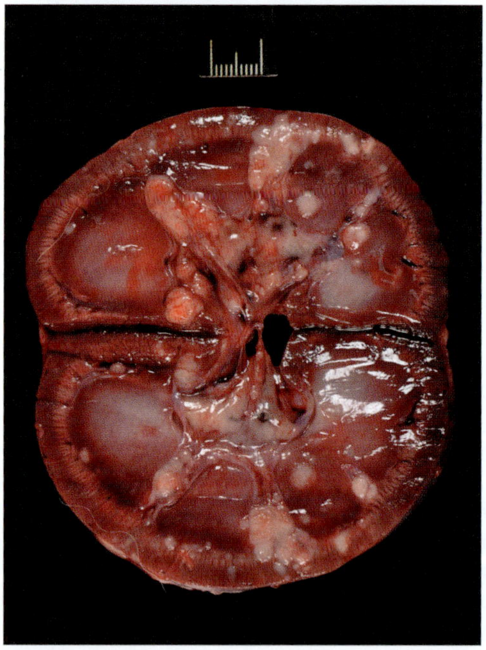

Fig. 86.16 Sagittal section of one kidney from a 2-year old female spayed Belgian Malinois with a disseminated Aspergillus deflectus infection. There were multifocal 0.3 to 0.5 cm tan firm nodules in the cortex and medulla. (Image courtesy University of California-Davis Veterinary Anatomic Pathology Service.)

Pathologic Findings

Gross pathologic findings in dogs with DIA include enlarged and/or congested lymph nodes; multifocal, pale, tan to white masses or nodules within a variety of parenchymal organs including the kidneys, liver, pancreas, or the pleura (Fig. 86.16); evidence of discospondylitis and/or osteomyelitis; serosanguinous pleural effusion; and/or mottled and congested lung lobes. Splenic infarction is also a common finding. The renal pelvis may be dilated and contain soft, granular material. Histopathology reveals granulomatous or pyogranulomatous inflammation with abundant intralesional fungal hyphae in a variety of tissues.[126,158] Infarcted areas secondary to thrombi containing fungal elements have been found in the spleen, kidneys, and liver. Some species, such as *A. terreus,* also produce accessory conidia (aleuriospores) in tissues, which may be free or extend from hyphae. Fibrinoid necrosis of blood vessels and associated hemorrhage may be present. Special stains such as GMS or PAS can delineate fungal hyphae in tissues. IHC and PCR on formalin-fixed tissues have also been used to identify *Aspergillus* (see Table 86.2).[92,126,128]

Diagnosis of DIA in cats is often made at necropsy, and findings may include pleural effusion, pulmonary granulomas, GI ulcers, or pseudomembranes, and involvement of urinary system or CNS.[66,159] The lesions are characterized by hemorrhage and necrosis, with variable numbers of inflammatory cells and fungal hyphae that may invade blood vessels, leading to thrombosis. Calcium oxalate crystals, a precipitate of oxalic acid produced by *Aspergillus* during the tricarboxylic acid cycle, have been identified in feline, human, and avian cases, though they are not reported often in dogs.[159,160]

TREATMENT AND PROGNOSIS

Many dogs with DIA have advanced disease at the time of evaluation, sometimes with respiratory distress, pathologic fractures, and vertebral subluxations resulting in cord compression. The prognosis for these dogs is poor. In one study, 57% of 30 dogs were euthanized within a week of examination (median, 3 days).[15] However, dogs that lack severe CNS signs, pain, or respiratory distress may enter remission for months and occasionally years when treated aggressively with antifungal drugs.[161,162] These dogs typically maintain high antigen titers or persistently positive urine cultures, and they ultimately relapse and die from the disease. Sometimes, euthanasia is performed earlier because of deteriorating quality of life or the unaffordable cost of treatment.

Since the disease was first documented in the 1970s, there have been progressive advances in the development of antifungal agents, and most of these human medications have been trialed in the treatment of small numbers of dogs with DIA. In many individual cases, a range of different drugs has been introduced sequentially as complications arose to specific agents. Overall, most agents are able to prolong the life of infected dogs only by months, with occasional individual animals surviving for up to 3 years.

The relative efficacy of different antifungal drug treatment regimens for DIA in dogs has not been studied prospectively. The most widely used treatments have been itraconazole, voriconazole, posaconazole, and/or AMB. Terbinafine has been used in addition to azole therapy with limited success in the authors' experience.[15] *Aspergillus* species are intrinsically resistant to fluconazole, so it should not be used.[163] Because azole-resistant strains of *Aspergillus* and other fungi are now recognized, a new generation of triazole drugs has now been developed for human medicine. Voriconazole, posaconazole, and isavuconazole all have activity against *Aspergillus* spp.[164,165] Although expensive, treatment with voriconazole or posaconazole can result in remissions of many months' duration in some dogs.[15,162,166] Posaconazole and isavuconazole in particular have shown promising activity in human patient and mouse models of invasive *A. terreus* infection.[167,168] Many dogs require treatment with multiple antifungal drugs to maintain remission, either in combination or in series. *A. terreus* strains from humans with invasive aspergillosis can become resistant to azoles during treatment and are also relatively resistant to AMB,[168,169] but clinical improvement can still occur after treatment of infected dogs with AMB (see Chapter 11).[15,170] The potential fungicidal and immunomodulatory effects of AMB are counterbalanced by its nephrotoxicity, which limits its use in patients with renal dysfunction. This problem has been addressed by the use of novel delivery systems that enhance uptake of the drug by reticuloendothelial cells at sites of inflammation and reduce accumulation in the kidneys. These formulations are: AMB-lipid complex (Abelcet, Liposome Co., Princeton, NJ); AMB-colloidal dispersion (Amphocil/Amphotec, Sequus Pharmaceuticals, Menlo Park, CA); and liposome-encapsulated AMB (AmBisome, Fujisawa Healthcare, Deerfield, IL, and Nexstar, San Dimas, CA).[171] AMB-lipid complex has been used to treat DIA in humans[172] and companion animals, but its use may be limited by its expense. An alternative IV lipid formulation has proven efficacious in the treatment of canine leishmaniosis but has not been evaluated for aspergillosis.[173]

Echinocandins selectively inhibit fungal β-glucan synthase (e.g., caspofungin). Caspofungin is efficacious in invasive aspergillosis of humans and is an attractive treatment due to its relatively low incidence of adverse events and drug interactions.[174,175] Expense and the need for IV administration has limited the use of echinocandins in dogs, but cost has decreased and is now more economical, though still incurs infusion-related costs.[176]

Dogs with localized bronchopulmonary aspergillosis have the best prognosis. These dogs are sometimes cured after treatment with itraconazole alone. Lung lobectomy may be required for successful treatment of German shepherds with cavitary lung lesions or dogs with pneumothorax resulting from their disease.[15,115,116,177]

Glucocorticoids should never be administered to dogs with aspergillosis, and their use has often inadvertently precipitated dissemination of the infection.

Feline DIA is so uncommon that treatment options have not been extensively reviewed. Rare cases of localized *Aspergillus* infection have recovered after complete surgical debridement of affected tissue. For example, fungal lobar pneumonia associated with pyothorax has been successfully managed by pulmonary lobectomy followed by systemic antifungal therapy.[66]

IMMUNITY AND VACCINATION

Immunity to disseminated aspergillosis is critically dependent on the function of neutrophils and dendritic cells, as well as effective T-cell function.[178] A vaccine to prevent the disease is not available. In an experimental system, mice vaccinated with *Aspergillus* antigens developed a protective Th1 immune response; however, vaccination for aspergillosis is unlikely to have a role in a clinical setting.[179] In experimental infections, a sonicate vaccine given before the administration of glucocorticoids protected mice against lethal pulmonary aspergillosis.[180]

PUBLIC HEALTH ASPECTS

In human patients, invasive aspergillosis primarily occurs in immunosuppressed humans with hematologic malignancy, or after solid organ or hematopoietic stem cell transplantation.[149] Infections are acquired from the environment. Transmission from affected dogs has not been described. Most cases (>70%) are caused by *A. fumigatus.* Infection with *A. terreus* is rare, and *A. deflectus* infection has not yet been described in humans.

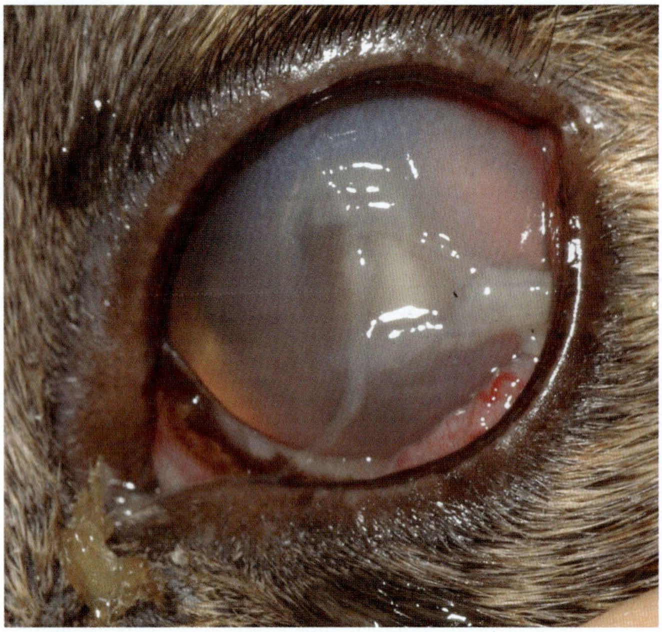

Fig. 86.17 Severe ulcerative keratitis in a 12-year-old spayed female domestic shorthair cat caused by an *Aspergillus fumigatus* complex organism. The condition was successfully treated using topical voriconazole and a conjunctival island graft. (Courtesy the University of California, Davis, Veterinary Ophthalmology Service.)

OCULAR AND OTIC DISEASE CAUSED BY *ASPERGILLUS* SPECIES

Infection of the cornea,[16,181,182] lens,[183] and ear canal[17–19] by *Aspergillus* species occur rarely in dogs and cats (see Table 86.1, Fig. 86.17). Diagnosis of these conditions requires visualization of hyphae on cytologic examination or histopathology of biopsy specimens in addition to fungal culture to rule out the possibility of contamination or colonization. One cat with *A. flavus* keratomycosis had a history of FHV-1-associated conjunctivitis and keratitis[16] and was successfully treated with 1% topical voriconazole (q2h to q4h). Similarly, a dog with *Aspergillus* keratoconjunctivitis was successfully treated with a corneal graft and 1% topical voriconazole.[182] Cats with *Aspergillus* otomycosis often have a history of diabetes mellitus or allergic dermatitis.[17,135] Dogs with otomycosis may have a history of grass awn foreign body, underlying allergic dermatitis, or otitis externa that has been extensively treated with topical and oral antibiotics.[17,18]

CASE EXAMPLE

Signalment

"Zach," a 2-year-old male neutered German shepherd from Roseville in northern California.

History

Zach was evaluated at the University of California, Davis, Veterinary Oncology Service for possible bone cancer. Two months previously, the owners noted that the dog vocalized when he stood up from rest. He was taken to a local veterinary clinic where he was diagnosed with lumbosacral pain and treated with carprofen (1.5 mg/kg, PO, q12h). Two weeks later, right pelvic limb lameness developed. Pelvic radiographs showed evidence of moderate osteoarthrosis of the left coxofemoral joint. Carprofen treatment was continued. After an additional 2 weeks, lethargy, inappetence, increased thirst and urination, and left thoracic limb lameness developed, and the dog began vomiting once daily. Radiographs of the left thoracic limb revealed an osteoproductive lesion in the mid-diaphysis of the left humerus, which was interpreted as a primary or metastatic bone tumor (see Fig. 86.13). Zach was one of two dogs in the household, was normally fed a dry commercial dog food diet, and was up to date on vaccinations, which included those for distemper, adenovirus, parvovirus, rabies, *Borrelia*, and *Bordetella*.

Physical Examination

Body weight: 33.5 kg.

General: Quiet, alert, and responsive. T = 103.4°F (39.7°C), HR = 120 beats/minute, panting, CRT < 2 seconds, mucous membranes moist and pink.

Eyes, ears, nose, and throat: No clinically significant abnormalities were detected. Fundoscopic examination revealed multiple hyporeflective regions, consistent with chorioretinitis, in the right fundus.

Musculoskeletal: BCS was 4/9, and generalized muscle wasting was present. There was no evidence of lameness or bone pain on orthopedic examination.

Cardiovascular, respiratory, GI, genitourinary, and lymph nodes: No clinically significant abnormalities were present.

Laboratory Findings

CBC: HCT 32.8% (40%–55%), MCV 65.2 fL (65–75 fL), MCHC 35.7 g/dL (33–36 g/dL), WBC 18,530 cells/μL (6,000–13,000 cells/μL), neutrophils 13,768 cells/μL (3,000–10,500 cells/μL), lymphocytes 2,087 cells/μL (1,000–4,000 cells/μL), monocytes 1,334 cells/μL (150–1,200 cells/μL), eosinophils 741 cells/μL (0–1,500 cells/μL), platelets 262,000 platelets/μL (150,000–400,000 platelets/μL).

Serum chemistry profile: Sodium 152 mmol/L (145–154 mmol/L), potassium 3.8 mmol/L (4.1–5.3 mmol/L), chloride 113 mmol/L (105–116 mmol/L), bicarbonate 24 mmol/L (16–26 mmol/L), phosphorus 5.7 mg/dL (3.0–6.2 mg/dL), calcium 11.8 mg/dL (9.9–11.4 mg/dL), BUN 31 mg/dL (8–21 mg/dL), creatinine 1.9 mg/dL (0.5–1.6 mg/dL), glucose 107 mg/dL (60–104 mg/dL), total protein 6.8 g/dL (5.4–7.4 g/dL), albumin 2.8 g/dL (2.9–4.2 g/dL), globulin 4.0 g/dL (2.3–4.4 g/dL), ALT 15 U/L (19–67 U/L), AST 27 U/L (21–54 U/L), ALP 28 U/L (15–127 U/L), GGT 2 U/L (0–6 U/L), cholesterol 205 mg/dL (135–345 mg/dL), total bilirubin 0.1 mg/dL (0–0.4 mg/dL).

Urinalysis: SpG 1.010; pH 7.0, 1+ protein (SSA), no bilirubin, 3+ hemoprotein, no glucose, 10–15 WBC/HPF, 50–60 RBC/HPF, 0–2 transitional epithelial cells, a few amorphous crystals, and a few budding organisms were seen.

Imaging Findings

Thoracic radiographs: The cardiopulmonary structures were unremarkable.

Bone survey radiographs: Single lateral radiographs of the distal left antebrachium, distal right antebrachium, and distal left and right pelvic limbs were performed. An additional lateral radiograph of the left humerus was also obtained and compared with referral radiographs taken 1 month previously. This showed progression of a primarily osteoproductive lesion in the mid-diaphysis of the left humerus. An additional site of chronic active periosteal reaction was noted along the distal caudal aspect of the left femur. Patchy increases in medullary density were identified in the distal diaphysis of both humeri.

CASE EXAMPLE—cont'd

Abdominal ultrasound: Hypoechoic mottling of the splenic hilus was identified. There was bilateral renal pyelectasia with echogenic material within the renal pelves bilaterally. There was marked blunting of the renal pelves bilaterally with mild hydroureter.

Microbiologic Findings

Cytologic examination of a fine-needle aspirate of lesion in the left humerus: Smears were moderately cellular with a dense, proteinaceous background and moderate amounts of cellular debris. Nucleated cells consisted of a population of numerous activated macrophages and variably degenerate neutrophils that were evenly distributed throughout the smear as well as in variably sized aggregates. Numerous multinucleated giant cells were noted. Throughout the specimen were moderate numbers of small, round, yeast organisms as well as numerous fungal hyphae, which were found intracellularly and extracellularly. The fungal hyphae were negative staining, branching, and septate, often with bulging ends.

Fungal culture and susceptibility (left humerus fine-needle aspirate, sent to University of Texas for molecular identification): Moderate numbers of *A. terreus.* MICs for AMB, itraconazole, and voriconazole were 2, 0.125, and 0.25 μg/mL, respectively.

Aerobic urine bacterial culture: Six colonies of *A. terreus.*

Aspergillus antibody serology (gel immunodiffusion): Negative.

Diagnosis

Disseminated invasive *A. terreus* infection.

Treatment

The dog was treated with IV fluids (lactated Ringer's solution with 20 mEq/L KCl at 75 mL/hour), lipid-complexed AMB (1 mg/kg IV on a Monday-Wednesday-Friday basis for 4 weeks), and itraconazole (5 mg/kg, PO, q12h). Over the course of AMB treatment, the dog's inappetence, lethargy, and lameness resolved and his serum creatinine and BUN concentrations remained stable with values of 2.1 mg/dL and 49 mg/dL, respectively, by the end of treatment. At a recheck 2 months after treatment was initiated, fungal culture of the urine revealed a single colony of *A. terreus*, and the creatinine was 1.7 mg/dL. After an additional month, bone survey radiographs showed significant remodeling of the left humeral and left femoral lesions. A serum biochemistry panel showed mildly increased creatinine concentration (1.8 mg/dL) and a serum ALT activity of 364 U/L; the increased serum ALT activity was thought to be secondary to itraconazole administration. Ultrasound of the abdomen showed mild renal pelvis dilatation, but the echogenic material within it had disappeared. Fungal culture of the urine was negative. Four months after treatment was initiated, intermittent vocalization and right pelvic limb lameness developed. Pain was detected only on lumbosacral palpation. Radiographs of this region revealed focal osteolysis of the ventral caudal aspect of the sixth lumbar vertebra. Clinical improvement did not occur after treatment with carprofen and tramadol.

Two weeks later, the dog developed respiratory distress and was seen by the Emergency and Critical Care Service. Mild dehydration, pyrexia (105.8°F or 41.0°C), gagging, and ptyalism were detected on physical examination. Thoracic radiographs were unremarkable, but a soft tissue density was seen in the pharyngeal region on cervical radiographs. Blood cultures were negative. The dog was sedated, and on oral examination, multiple large soft tissue masses were observed within the pharynx and around the rim of the epiglottis. Aspiration of the masses revealed suppurative inflammation and possible occasional fungal hyphae. Bronchoscopy was performed, and numerous yellow plaque-like lesions were visualized on the tracheal mucosa. Cytologic examination of biopsies of these lesions revealed fungal hyphae. The owner elected euthanasia. Necropsy findings included severe, locally extensive mural granulomas of the tracheal mucosa with intralesional fungal hyphae and suppurative and eosinophilic pharyngitis with necrosis and edema. There was evidence of healed pyelonephritis and granulomatous nephritis with intralesional fungal hyphae. Granulomatous osteomyelitis with intralesional hyphae was present in the left femur and humerus. There were multiple granulomas in the pancreas and spleen.

Comments

Disseminated aspergillosis in this dog was initially confused with bone neoplasia. An *Aspergillus* antibody titer was negative, which illustrates the lack of sensitivity of this assay for diagnosis of disseminated disease. GM antigen testing was not performed, but bone lesions were readily accessible for aspiration and culture. The small, round yeast organisms visualized together with the hyphae were likely accessory conidia, which can be found in *A. terreus* infections. Treatment with lipid-complexed AMB and itraconazole was initially associated with clinical remission, but infection was not eliminated. Based on necropsy examination, the cause of the suppurative pharyngeal masses that impaired respiration was not clear. Fungal cultures of the masses were negative.

SUGGESTED READINGS

Barrs VR, van Doorn TM, Houbraken J, et al. *Aspergillus felis* sp. nov., an emerging agent of invasive aspergillosis in humans, cats, and dogs. *PLoS One*. 2013;8:e64871.

Corrigan VK, Legendre AM, Wheat LJ, et al. Treatment of disseminated aspergillosis with posaconazole in 10 dogs. *J Vet Intern Med*. 2016;30:167–173.

Garcia RS, Wheat LJ, Cook AK, et al. Sensitivity and specificity of a blood and urine galactomannan antigen assay for diagnosis of systemic aspergillosis in dogs. *J Vet Int Med*. 2012;26:911–919.

REFERENCES

1. Houbraken J, Samson RA. Phylogeny of *Penicillium* and the segregation of *Trichocomaceae* into three families. *Stud Mycol*. 2011;70:1–51.
2. Page ID, Richardson M, Denning DW. Antibody testing in aspergillosis—quo vadis? *Med Mycol*. 2015:myv020.
3. Wilkinson GT, Sutton RH, Grono LR. *Aspergillus* spp. infection associated with orbital cellulitis and sinusitis in a cat. *J Small Anim Pract*. 1982;23:127–131.
4. Latge JP. *Aspergillus fumigatus* and aspergillosis. *Clin Microbiol Rev*. 1999;12:310–350.
5. Abad A, Fernandez-Molina JV, Bikandi J, et al. What makes *Aspergillus fumigatus* a successful pathogen? Genes and molecules involved in invasive aspergillosis. *Rev Iberoam Micol*. 2010;27:155–182.
6. Barrs VR, Halliday C, Martin P, et al. Sinonasal and sino-orbital aspergillosis in 23 cats: aetiology, clinicopathological features and treatment outcomes. *Vet J*. 2012;191:58–64.
7. Barrs VR, van Doorn TM, Houbraken J, et al. *Aspergillus felis* sp. nov., an emerging agent of invasive aspergillosis in humans, cats, and dogs. *PLoS One*. 2013;8:e64871.
8. Barrs VR, Beatty JA, Dhand NK, et al. Computed tomographic features of feline sino-nasal and sino-orbital aspergillosis. *Vet J*. 2014;201:215–222.
9. Barrs VR, Ujvari B, Dhand NK, et al. Detection of *Aspergillus*-specific antibodies by agar gel double immunodiffusion and IgG ELISA in feline upper respiratory tract aspergillosis. *Vet J*. 2015;203:285–289.
10. Sykes JE. Unpublished observations, 2017.
11. Kano R, Itamoto K, Okuda M, et al. Isolation of *Aspergillus udagawae* from a fatal case of feline orbital aspergillosis. *Mycoses*. 2008;51:360–361.
12. Kano R, Shibahashi A, Fujino Y, et al. Two cases of feline orbital aspergillosis due to *A. udagawae* and *A. virdinutans*. *J Vet Med Sci*. 2013;75:7–10.
13. Kano R, Takahashi T, Hayakawa T, et al. The first case of feline sinonasal aspergillosis due to *Aspergillus fischeri* in Japan. *J Vet Med Sci*. 2015;77:118–1185.

14. Southard C. Bronchopulmonary aspergillosis in a dog. *J Am Vet Med Assoc.* 1987;190:875–877.
15. Schultz RM, Johnson EG, Wisner ER, et al. Clinicopathologic and diagnostic imaging characteristics of systemic aspergillosis in 30 dogs. *J Vet Intern Med.* 2008;22:851–859.
16. Labelle AL, Hamor RE, Barger AM, et al. *Aspergillus flavus* keratomycosis in a cat treated with topical 1% voriconazole solution. *Vet Ophthalmol.* 2009;12:48–52.
17. Goodale EC, Outerbridge CA, White SD. *Aspergillus* otitis in small animals: a retrospective study of 17 cases. *Vet Dermatol.* 2016;27. e3–e2.
18. Coyner K. Otomycosis due to *Aspergillus* spp. in a dog: case report and literature review. *Vet Dermatol.* 2010;21:613–618.
19. Ghibaudo G, Peano A. Chronic monolateral otomycosis in a dog caused by *Aspergillus ochraceus. Vet Dermatol.* 2010;21:522–526.
20. Zhang S, Corapi W, Quist E, et al. *Aspergillus versicolor*, a new causative agent of canine disseminated aspergillosis. *J Clin Microbiol.* 2012;50:187–191.
21. Talbot JJ, Johnson LR, Martin P, et al. What causes canine sino-nasal aspergillosis? A molecular approach to species identification. *Vet J.* 2014;200:17–21.
22. Burrough E, Deitz K, Kinyon J, et al. Disseminated aspergillosis in a dog due to *Aspergillus alabamensis. Med Mycol Case Rep.* 2012;1:1–4.
23. Barrs VR. Unpublished observations, 2017.
24. Houbraken J, Kocsube S, Visage CM, et al. Classification of *Aspergillus, Penicillium, Talaromyces* and related genera (Eurotiales): An overview of families, genera, subgenera, sections, series and species. *Stud Mycol.* 2020;95:5–169.
25. Miller JS, Funk VA, Wagner WL, et al. Outcomes of the 2011 botanical nomenclature section at the XVIII International Botanical Congress. *Phytokeys.* 2011;5:1–3.
26. Billen F, Guieu LV, Bernaerts F, et al. Efficacy of intrasinusal administration of bifonazole cream alone or in combination with enilconazole irrigation in canine sino-nasal aspergillosis: 17 cases. *Can Vet J.* 2010;51:164–168.
27. Claeys S, Lefebvre JB, Schuller S, et al. Surgical treatment of canine nasal aspergillosis by rhinotomy combined with enilconazole infusion and oral itraconazole. *J Small Anim Pract.* 2006;47:320–324.
28. Lanthier T, Chalifoux A. Enilconazole as an adjunct to the treatment of four cases of canine nasal aspergillosis. *Can Vet J.* 1991;32:110–112.
29. Bray JP, White RA, Lascelles BD. Treatment of canine nasal aspergillosis with a new non-invasive technique. Failure with enilconazole. *J Small Anim Pract.* 1998;39:223–226.
30. Schuller S, Clercx C. Long-term outcomes in dogs with sinonasal aspergillosis treated with intranasal infusions of enilconazole. *J Am Anim Hosp Assoc.* 2007;43:33–38.
31. Sissener TR, Bacon NJ, Friend E, et al. Combined clotrimazole irrigation and depot therapy for canine nasal aspergillosis. *J Small Anim Pract.* 2006;47:312–315.
32. Saunders JH, Zonderland JL, Clercx C, et al. Computed tomographic findings in 35 dogs with nasal aspergillosis. *Vet Radiol Ultrasound.* 2002;43:5–9.
33. Saunders JH, Clercx C, Snaps FR, et al. Radiographic, magnetic resonance imaging, computed tomographic, and rhinoscopic features of nasal aspergillosis in dogs. *J Am Vet Med Assoc.* 2004;225:1703–1712.
34. Zonderland JL, Stork CK, Saunders JH, et al. Intranasal infusion of enilconazole for treatment of sinonasal aspergillosis in dogs. *J Am Vet Med Assoc.* 2002;221:1421–1425.
35. Sharman M, Paul A, Davies D, et al. Multi-centre assessment of mycotic rhinosinusitis in dogs: a retrospective study of initial treatment success (1998 to 2008). *J Small Anim Pract.* 2010;51:423–427.
36. Mortellaro CM, Franca PD, Caretta G. *Aspergillus fumigatus*, the causative agent of infection of the frontal sinuses and nasal chambers of the dog. *Mycoses.* 1989;32:327–335.
37. Lane JG, Warnock DW. The diagnosis of *Aspergillus fumigatus* infection of the nasal chambers of the dog with particular reference to the value of the double diffusion test. *J Small Anim Pract.* 1977;18:169–177.
38. Moore AH. Use of topical povidone-iodine dressings in the management of mycotic rhinitis in three dogs. *J Small Anim Pract.* 2003;44:326–329.
39. Sharman M, Lenard Z, Hosgood G, et al. Clotrimazole and enilconazole distribution within the frontal sinuses and nasal cavity of nine dogs with sinonasal aspergillosis. *J Small Anim Pract.* 2012;53:161–167.
40. De Lorenzi D, Bonfanti U, Masserdotti C, et al. Diagnosis of canine nasal aspergillosis by cytological examination: a comparison of four different collection techniques. *J Small Anim Pract.* 2006;47:316–319.
41. Pomrantz JS, Johnson LR. Repeated rhinoscopic and serologic assessment of the effectiveness of intranasally administered clotrimazole for the treatment of nasal aspergillosis in dogs. *J Am Vet Med Assoc.* 2010;236:757–762.
42. Pomrantz JS, Johnson LR, Nelson RW, et al. Comparison of serologic evaluation via agar gel immunodiffusion and fungal culture of tissue for diagnosis of nasal aspergillosis in dogs. *J Am Vet Med Assoc.* 2007;230:1319–1323.
43. Billen F, Peeters D, Peters IR, et al. Comparison of the value of measurement of serum galactomannan and *Aspergillus*-specific antibodies in the diagnosis of canine sino-nasal aspergillosis. *Vet Microbiol.* 2009;133:358–365.
44. Billen F, Clercx C, Le Garerres A, et al. Effect of sampling method and incubation temperature on fungal culture in canine sinonasal aspergillosis. *J Small Anim Pract.* 2009;50:67–72.
45. Johnson LR, Drazenovich TL, Herrera MA, et al. Results of rhinoscopy alone or in conjunction with sinuscopy in dogs with aspergillosis: 46 cases (2001-2004). *J Am Vet Med Assoc.* 2006;228:738–742.
46. Hazuchova K, Neiger R, Stengel C. Topical treatment of mycotic rhinitis-rhinosinusitis in dogs with meticulous debridement and 1% clotrimazole cream: 64 cases (2007-2014). *J Am Vet Med Assoc.* 2017;250:309–315.
47. Goodall SA, Lane JG, Warnock DW. The diagnosis and treatment of a case of nasal aspergillosis in a cat. *J Small Anim Pract.* 1984;25:627–633.
48. Halenda RM, Reed AL. Ultrasound computed tomography diagnosis: fungal, sinusitis and retrobulbar myofascitis in a cat. *Vet Radiol Ultrasound.* 1997;38:208–210.
49. Hamilton HL, Whitley RD, McLaughlin SA. Exophthalmos secondary to aspergillosis in a cat. *J Am Anim Hosp Assoc.* 2000;36:343–347.
50. Tomsa K, Glaus TA, Zimmer C, et al. Fungal rhinitis and sinusitis in three cats. *J Am Vet Med Assoc.* 2003;222:1380–1384.
51. Malik R, Vogelnest L, O'Brien CR, et al. Infections and some other conditions affecting the skin and subcutis of the naso-ocular region of cats - clinical experience 1987-2003. *J Feline Med Surg.* 2004;6:383–390.
52. Katz ME, Dougall AM, Weeks K, et al. Multiple genetically distinct groups revealed among clinical isolates identified as atypical *Aspergillus fumigatus. J Clin Microbiol.* 2005;43:551–555.
53. Whitney BL, Broussard J, Stefanacci JD. Four cats with fungal rhinitis. *J Feline Med Surg.* 2005;7:53–58.
54. McLellan GJ, Aquino SM, Mason DR, et al. Use of posaconazole in the management of invasive orbital aspergillosis in a cat. *J Am Anim Hosp Assoc.* 2006;42:302–307.
55. Barachetti L, Mortellaro CM, Di Giancamillo M, et al. Bilateral orbital and nasal aspergillosis in a cat. *Vet Ophthalmol.* 2009;12:176–182.
56. Karnik K, Reichle JK, Fischetti AJ, et al. Computed tomographic findings of fungal rhinitis and sinusitis in cats. *Vet Radiol Ultrasound.* 2009;50:65–68.
57. Furrow E, Groman RP. Intranasal infusion of clotrimazole for the treatment of nasal aspergillosis in two cats. *J Am Vet Med Assoc.* 2009;235:1188–1193.
58. Smith LN, Hoffman SB. A case series of unilateral orbital aspergillosis in three cats and treatment with voriconazole. *Vet Ophthalmol.* 2010;13:190–203.
59. Giordano C, Gianella P, Bo S, et al. Invasive mould infections of the naso-orbital region of cats: a case involving *Aspergillus fumigatus* and an aetiological review. *J Feline Med Surg.* 2010;12:714–723.
60. Quimby JM, Hoffman SB, Duke J, et al. Adverse neurologic events associated with voriconazole use in 3 cats. *J Vet Intern Med.* 2010;24:647–649.
61. Declercq J, Declercq L, Fincioen S. Unilateral sino-orbital and subcutaneous aspergillosis in a cat. *Vlaams Diergeneeskundig Tijdschrift.* 2012;81:357–362.
62. Taylor A, Peters I, Dhand NK, et al. Evaluation of serum *Aspergillus*-specific immunoglobulin A by indirect ELISA for diagnosis of feline

upper respiratory tract aspergillosis. *J Vet Intern Med.* 2016;30:1708–1714.

63. Hubka V, Barrs V, Dudova Z, et al. Unravelling species boundaries in the *Aspergillus viridinutans* complex (section *Fumigati*): opportunistic human and animal pathogens capable of interspecific hybrdization. *Persoonia.* 2018;41:142–174.
64. Barrs VR, Talbot JJ. Feline aspergillosis. *Vet Clin North Am Small Anim Pract.* 2014;44:51–73.
65. Sharp NJH, Harvey CE, Sullivan M. Canine nasal aspergillosis and penicilliosis. *Compend Contin Educ Pract Vet.* 1991;13:41–46.
66. Hazell KLA, Swift IM, Sullivan N. Successful treatment of pulmonary aspergillosis in a cat. *Aust Vet J.* 2011;89:101–104.
67. Davies C, Troy GC. Deep mycotic infections in cats. *J Am Anim Hosp Assoc.* 1996;32:380–391.
68. Peeters D, Peters IR, Helps CR, et al. Distinct tissue cytokine and chemokine mRNA expression in canine sino-nasal aspergillosis and idiopathic lymphoplasmacytic rhinitis. *Vet Immunol Immunopathol.* 2007;117:95–105.
69. Vanherberghen M, Bureau F, Peters IR, et al. Analysis of gene expression in canine sino-nasal aspergillosis and idiopathic lymphoplasmacytic rhinitis: a transcriptomic analysis. *Vet Microbiol.* 2012;157:143–151.
70. Mercier E, Peters IR, Farnir F, et al. Assessment of Toll-like receptor 2, 4 and 9 SNP genotypes in canine sino-nasal aspergillosis. *BMC Vet Res.* 2014;10.
71. Vanherberghen M, Bureau F, Peters IR, et al. Cytokine and transcription factor expression by *Aspergillus fumigatus*-stimulated peripheral blood mononuclear cells in dogs with sino-nasal aspergillosis. *Vet Immunol Immunopathol.* 2013;154:111–120.
72. Peeters D, Peters IR, Clercx C, et al. Quantification of mRNA encoding cytokines and chemokines in nasal biopsies from dogs with sino-nasal aspergillosis. *Vet Microbiol.* 2006;114:318–326.
73. Mercier E, Peters IR, Day MJ, et al. Toll- and NOD-like receptor mRNA expression in canine sino-nasal aspergillosis and idiopathic lymphoplasmacytic rhinitis. *Vet Immunol Immunopathol.* 2012;145:618–624.
74. Aimanianda V, Latge JP. Fungal hydrophobins form a sheath preventing immune recognition of airborne conidia. *Virulence.* 2010;1:185–187.
75. Romani L. Immunity to fungal infections. *Nat Rev Immunol.* 2011;11:275–288.
76. Romani L. Immunity to fungal infections. *Nat Rev Immunol.* 2004;4:1–23.
77. Carvalho A, Pasqualotto AC, Pitzurra L, et al. Polymorphisms in Toll-like receptor genes and susceptibility to pulmonary aspergillosis. *J Infect Dis.* 2008;197:618–621.
78. Peeters D, Day MJ, Clercx C. An immunohistochemical study of canine nasal aspergillosis. *J Comp Pathol.* 2005;132:283–288.
79. Frisvad JC, Larsen TO. Extrolites of *Aspergillus fumigatus* and other pathogenic species in *Aspergillus* Section *Fumigati. Front Microbiol.* 2016;6.
80. Cormack CA, Donahoe SL, Talbot JJ, et al. Disseminated invasive aspergillosis caused by *Aspergillus felis* in a cat. *J Vet Intern Med.* 2021;35:2395–2400.
81. Sugui JA, Peterson SW, Flgat A, et al. Genetic relatedness versus biological compatibility between *Aspergillus fumigatus* and related species. *J Clin Microbiol.* 2014;52:3707–3721.
82. Pfeiffer CD, Fine JP, Safdar N. Diagnosis of invasive aspergillosis using a galactomannan assay: A meta-analysis. *Clin Infect Dis.* 2006;42:1417–1427.
83. Garcia RS, Wheat LJ, Cook AK, et al. Sensitivity and specificity of a blood and urine galactomannan antigen assay for diagnosis of systemic aspergillosis in dogs. *J Vet Intern Med.* 2012;26:911–919.
84. Hachem RY, Kontoyiannais DP, Chemaly RF, et al. Utility of galactomannan enzyme immunoassay and (1,3) B-D-glucan in diagnosis of invasive fungal infections: low sensitivity for *Aspergillus fumigatus* infection in hematologic malignancy patients. *J Clin Microbiol.* 2009;47:129–133.
85. Kitasato Y, Tao Y, Hoshino T, et al. Comparison of *Aspergillus* galactomannan antigen testing with a new cut-off index and *Aspergillus* precipitating antibody testing for the diagnosis of chronic pulmonary aspergillosis. *Respirology.* 2009;14:701–708.
86. Mennink-Kersten M, Donnelly JP, Verweij PE. Detection of circulating galactomannan for the diagnosis and management of invasive aspergillosis. *Lancet Infect Dis.* 2004;4:349–357.
87. Herbrecht R, Letscher-Bru V, Oprea C, et al. *Aspergillus* galactomannan detection in the diagnosis of invasive aspergillosis in cancer patients. *J Clin Oncol.* 2002;20:1898–1906.
88. Peeters D, Peters IR, Helps CR, et al. Whole blood and tissue fungal DNA quantification in the diagnosis of canine sino-nasal aspergillosis. *Vet Microbiol.* 2008;128:194–203.
89. Samson RA, Visagie CM, Houbraken J, et al. Phylogeny, identification and nomenclature of the genus *Aspergillus. Stud Mycol.* 2014;78:141–173.
90. Sleiman S, Halliday CL, Chapman B, et al. Performance of matrix-assisted laser desorption ionization-time of flight mass spectrometry for identification of *Aspergillus, Scedosporium,* and *Fusarium* spp. in the Australian clinical setting. *J Clin Microbiol.* 2016;54:2182–2186.
91. Lau A, Chen S, Sorrell T, et al. Development and clinical application of a panfungal PCR assay to detect and identify fungal DNA in tissue specimens. *J Clin Microbiol.* 2007;45:380–385.
92. Meason-Smith C, Edwards EE, Older CE, et al. Panfungal polymerase chain reaction for identification of fungal pathogens in formalin-fixed animal tissues. *Vet Pathol.* 2017. 300985817698207.
93. Cruciani M, Mengoli C, Loeffler J, et al. Polymerase chain reaction blood tests for the diagnosis of invasive aspergillosis in immunocompromised people. *Cochrane Database Syst Rev.* 2015:CD009551.
94. Vangrinsven E, Girod M, Goossens D, et al. Comparison of two minimally invasive enilconazole perendoscopic infusion protocols for the treatment of sinonasal aspergillosis. *J Small Anim Pract.* 2018;59:777–782.
95. Caulkett N, Lew L, Fries C. Upper-airway obstruction and prolonged recovery from anesthesia following intranasal clotrimazole administration. *J Am Anim Hosp Assoc.* 1997;33:264–267.
96. Barr SC, Rishniw M, Lynch M. Questions contents of clotrimazole solution. *J Am Vet Med Assoc.* 2010;236:163–164.
97. Hazuchova K, Neiger R, Stengel C. Topical treatment of mycotic rhinitis-rhinosinusitis in dogs with meticulous debridement and 1% clotrimazole cream: 64% cases (2007-2014). *J Am Vet Med Assoc.* 2017;250:309–315.
98. Balber C, Hill TL, Bommer NX. Minimally invasive treatment of sino-nasal aspergillosis in dogs. *J Vet Intern Med.* 2018;32:2069–2073.
99. Stanton JA, Miller ML, Johnson P, et al. Treatment of canine sinonasal aspergillosis with clotrimazole in patients with cribriform plate lysis. *J Sm Anim Pract.* 2018;59:411–414.
100. Belda B, Petrovitch N, Matthews KG. Sinonasal aspergillosis: outcome after topical treatment in dogs with cribriform plate lysis. *J Vet Intern Med.* 2018;32:1353–1358.
101. Stewart J, Bianco D. Treatment of refractory sino-nasal aspergillosis with posaconazole and terbinafine in 10 dogs. *J Small Anim Pract.* 2017;58:504-509.
102. Bray RN, Raghu CL, Leuin AS, et al. Oral administration of voriconazole with surgical fungal plaque debridement for the treatment of sinonasal aspergillosis with cribriform plate lysis in three dogs. *J Am Vet Med Assoc.* 2020;256(1):111–116.
103. Talbot JJ, Kidd SE, Martin P, et al. Azole resistance in canine and feline isolates of *Aspergillus fumigatus. Comp Immunol Microbiol Infect Dis.* 2015;42:37–41.
104. Vedrine B, Fribourg-Blanc L-A. Treatment of sinonasal aspergillosis by debridement and sinonasal deposition therapy with clotrimazole under rhinoscopic guidance. *J Am Anim Hosp Assoc.* 2018;54:103–110.
105. Tamborini A, Roberston E, Talbot JJ, et al. Sinonasal aspergillosis in a British shorthair cat in the UK. *J Feline Med Surg Open Rep.* 2016;1:1–6.
106. Kay A, Boland L, Kidd SE, et al. Complete clinical response to combined antifungal therapy in two cats with invasive fungal rhinosinusitis caused by cryptic *Aspergillus* species in section *Fumigati. Med Mycol Case Rep.* 2021;34:13–17.
107. Mawby DI, Whittemore JC, Fowler LE, et al. Posaconazole pharmacokinetics in healthy cats after oral and intravenous administration. *J Vet Intern Med.* 2016;30:1703–1707.
108. Vishkautsan P, Papich MG, Thompson GR 3rd, et al. Pharmacokinetics of voriconazole after intravenous and oral administration to healthy cats. *Am J Vet Res.* 2016;77:931–939.
109. Leshinsky J, McLachlan A, Foster DJR, et al. Pharmacokinetics of caspofungin acetate to guide optimal dosing in cats. *PLoS One.* 2017;12:e0178783.

110. Dolton MJ, Ray JE, Chen SC-A, Ng K, Pont L, McLachlan AJ. Multicenter study of posaconazole therapeutic drug monitoring: exposure response relationship and factors affecting concentration. *Antimicrob Agents Chemother*. 2012;56:5503–5510.
111. Karthaus M, Lehrnbecher T, Lipp H-P, Kluge S, Buchheldt D. Therapeutic drug monitoring in the treatment of invasive aspergillosis with voriconazole in cancer patients – an evidence-based approach. *Ann Hematol*. 2015;94:547–556.
112. Adamama-Moraitou KK, Pardali D, Day MJ, et al. *Aspergillus fumigatus* bronchopneumonia in a Hellenic shepherd dog. *J Am Anim Hosp Assoc*. 2011;47:e13–e18.
113. Garcia ME, Caballero J, Cruzado M, et al. The value of the determination of anti-*Aspergillus* IgG in the serodiagnosis of canine aspergillosis: comparison with galactomannan detection. *J Vet Med B Infect Dis Vet Pub Health*. 2001;48:743–750.
114. Sykes JE, Mapes S, Lindsay LL, et al. *Corynebacterium ulcerans* bronchopneumonia in a dog. *J Vet Intern Med*. 2010;24:973–976.
115. Kulendra E, Halfacree Z, Goggs R, et al. Cavitary pulmonary lesion associated with *Aspergillus fumigatus* infection in a German shepherd dog. *J Small Anim Pract*. 2010;51:271–274.
116. Whitley NT, Cauvin A, Burton C, et al. Long term survival in two German shepherd dogs with *Aspergillus*-associated cavitary pulmonary lesions. *J Small Anim Pract*. 2010;51:561.
117. Guerin SR, Walker MC, Felly DF. Cavitating mycotic pneumonia in a German shepherd dog. *J Small Anim Pract*. 1993;34:36–39.
118. Whipple KM, Shmalberg JW, Joyce AC, et al. Cytologic identification of fungal arthritis in a Labrador retriever with disseminated *Talaromyces helicus* infection. *Vet Clin Pathol*. 2019;48:449–454.
119. Dear JD, Reagan KL, Hulsebosch SE, et al. Disseminated *Rasamsonia argillacea* species complex infection in 8 dogs. *J Vet Intern Med*. 2021;35:2232–2240.
120. Tappin SW, Ferrandis I, Jakovljevic S, et al. Successful treatment of bilateral *Paecilomyces* pyelonephritis in a German shepherd dog. *J Small Anim Pract*. 2012;53:657–660.
121. Day MJ, Penhale WJ, Eger CE, et al. Disseminated aspergillosis in dogs. *Aust Vet J*. 1986;63:55–59.
122. Kelly SE, Shaw SE, Clark WT. Long-term survival of four dogs with disseminated *Aspergillus terreus* infection treated with itraconazole. *Aust Vet J*. 1995;72:311–313.
123. Wigney DI, Allan GS, Hay LE, et al. Osteomyelitis associated with *Penicillium verruculosum* in a German-shepherd dog. *J Small Anim Pract*. 1990;31:449–452.
124. Kahler JS, Leach MW, Jang S, et al. Disseminated aspergillosis attributable to *Aspergillus deflectus* in a springer spaniel. *J Am Vet Med Assoc*. 1990;197:871–874.
125. Pastor J, Pumarola M, Cuenca R, et al. Systemic aspergillosis in a dog. *Vet Rec*. 1993;132:412–413.
126. Perez J, Mozos E, de Lara FC, et al. Disseminated aspergillosis in a dog: an immunohistochemical study. *J Comp Pathol*. 1996;115:191–196.
127. Clercx C, McEntee K, Snaps F, et al. Bronchopulmonary and disseminated granulomatous disease associated with *Aspergillus fumigatus* and *Candida* species infection in a golden retriever. *J Am Anim Hosp Assoc*. 1996;32:139–145.
128. Butterworth SJ, Barr FJ, Pearson GR, et al. Multiple discospondylitis associated with *Aspergillus* species infection in a dog. *Vet Rec*. 1995;136:38–41.
129. Booth MJ, van der Merwe LL. Opportunistic disseminated mycoses in dogs: 1993-2000. *J Vet Intern Med*. 2001;15:277.
130. Bruchim Y, Elad D, Klainbart S. Disseminated aspergillosis in two dogs in Israel. *Mycoses*. 2006;49:130–133.
131. Dallman MJ, Dew TL, Tobias L, et al. Disseminated aspergillosis in a dog with diskospondylitis and neurologic deficits. *J Am Vet Med Assoc*. 1992;200:511–513.
132. Gelatt KN, Chrisman CL, Samuelson DA, et al. Ocular and systemic aspergillosis in a dog. *J Am Anim Hosp Assoc*. 1991;27:427–431.
133. Kaufman AC, Greene CE, Selcer BA, et al. Systemic aspergillosis in a dog and treatment with hamycin. *J Am Anim Hosp Assoc*. 1994;30:132–136.
134. Perry JJ, Rech RR, Camus MS, et al. Pathology in practice. Disseminated aspergillosis. *J Am Vet Med Assoc*. 2010;236:173–175.
135. Sykes JE. Unpublished observations, 2012.
136. Krockenberger MB, Swinney G, Martin P, et al. Sequential opportunistic infections in two German shepherd dogs. *Aust Vet J*. 2011;89:9–14.
137. Watt PR, Robins GM, Galloway AM, et al. Disseminated opportunistic fungal disease in dogs: 10 cases (1982-1990). *J Am Vet Med Assoc*. 1995;207:67–70.
138. Karim M, Alam M, Shah AA, et al. Chronic invasive aspergillosis in apparently immunocompetent hosts. *Clin Infect Dis*. 1997;24:723–733.
139. Abbasi S, Shenep JL, Hughes WT, et al. Aspergillosis in children with cancer: A 34-year experience. *Clin Infect Dis*. 1999;29:1210–1219.
140. Bochud PY, Chien JW, Marr KA, et al. Toll-like receptor 4 polymorphisms and aspergillosis in stem-cell transplantation. *N Engl J Med*. 2008;359:1766–1777.
141. Guinea J, Torres-Narbona M, Gijon P, et al. Pulmonary aspergillosis in patients with chronic obstructive pulmonary disease: incidence, risk factors, and outcome. *Clin Microbiol Infect*. 2010;16:870–877.
142. Centeno-Lima S, Silveira H, Casimiro C, et al. Kinetics of cytokine expression in mice with invasive aspergillosis: lethal infection and protection. *FEMS Immunol Med Microbiol*. 2002;32:167–173.
143. Day MJ. Canine sino-nasal aspergillosis: parallels with human disease. *Med Mycol*. 2009;47:S315–323.
144. Blease K, Kunkel SL, Hogaboam CM. IL-18 modulates chronic fungal asthma in a murine model; putative involvement of Toll-like receptor-2. *Inflamm Res*. 2001;50:552–560.
145. Latge JP. The pathobiology of *Aspergillus fumigatus*. *Trends Microbiol*. 2001;9:382–389.
146. Fox JG, Murphy JC, Shalev M. Systemic fungal infections in cats. *J Am Vet Med Assoc*. 1978;173:1191–1195.
147. Ossent P. Systemic aspergillosis and mucormycosis in 23 cats. *Vet Rec*. 1987;120:330–333.
148. Callanan JJ. Feline immunodeficiency virus infection. In: Willett BJ, Jarrett O, eds. *Feline Immunology and Immunodeficiency*. Oxford, UK: Oxford University Press; 1995:111–130.
149. Steinbach WJ, Marr KA, Anaissie EJ, et al. Clinical epidemiology of 960 patients with invasive aspergillosis from the PATH Alliance registry. *J Infect*. 2012;65:453–464.
150. Taylor AR, Young BD, Levine GJ, et al. Clinical features and magnetic resonance imaging findings in 7 dogs with central nervous system aspergillosis. *J Vet Intern Med*. 2015;29:1556–1563.
151. Carpenter Jr DH, Mackin AJ, Gellasch KL. ECG of the month. Cardiac tamponade secondary to *A. niger*-induced constrictive pericarditis. *J Am Vet Med Assoc*. 2001;218:1890–1892.
152. Hage CA, Reynolds JM, Durkin M, et al. Plasmalyte as a cause of false-positive results for *Aspergillus* galactomannan in bronchoalveolar lavage fluid. *J Clin Microbiol*. 2007;45:676–677.
153. Reagan KL, Wheat LJ, Sykes JE. Effect of an oral probiotic nutraceutical containing *Aspergillus*-derived ingredients on a serum and urine galactomannan antigen assay in dogs. *Vet J*. 2020;265.
154. White D. Canine nasal mycosis: light at the end of a long diagnostic and therapeutic tunnel. *J Small Anim Pract*. 2006;47:307.
155. White PL, Linton CJ, Perry MD, et al. The evolution and evaluation of a whole blood polymerase chain reaction assay for the detection of invasive aspergillosis in hematology patients in a routine clinical setting. *Clin Infect Dis*. 2006;42:479–486.
156. Johnson GL, Bibby DF, Wong S, et al. A MIQE-compliant real-time PCR assay for *Aspergillus* detection. *PLoS One*. 2012;7:e40022.
157. Lass-Florl C, Aigner J, Gunsilius E, et al. Screening for *Aspergillus* spp. using polymerase chain reaction of whole blood samples from patients with haematological malignancies. *Br J Haematol*. 2001;113:180–184.
158. Day MJ, Penhale WJ. An immunohistochemical study of canine disseminated aspergillosis. *Aust Vet J*. 1991;68:383–386.
159. Leite-Filho RV, Fredo G, Lupion CG, et al. Chronic invasive pulmonary aspergillosis in two cats with diabetes mellitus. *J Comp Pathol*. 2016;155:141–144.
160. Payne CL, Dark MJ, Conway JA, et al. A retrospective study of the prevalence of calcium oxalate crystals in veterinary *Aspergillus* cases. *J Vet Diagn Invest*. 2017;29:51–58.

161. Dandrieux JRS, Mansfield CS, Stevenson M, et al. A retrospective multicentre study on treatment and outcome in disseminated aspergillosis in 41 dogs. *J Vet Intern Med.* 2020;34:372.
162. Corrigan VK, Legendre AM, Wheat LJ, et al. Treatment of disseminated aspergillosis with posaconazole in 10 dogs. *J Vet Intern Med.* 2016;30:167–173.
163. Marichal P, Vanden Bossche H. Mechanisms of resistance to azole antifungals. *Acta Biochim Pol.* 1995;42:509–516.
164. Walsh TJ, Lutsar I, Driscoll T, et al. Voriconazole in the treatment of aspergillosis, scedosporiosis and other invasive fungal infections in children. *Pediatr Infect Dis J.* 2002;21:240–248.
165. Maertens JA, Raad II , Marr KA, et al. Isavuconazole versus voriconazole for primary treatment of invasive mould disease caused by *Aspergillus* and other filamentous fungi (SECURE): a phase 3, randomised-controlled, non-inferiority trial. *Lancet.* 2016;387:760–769.
166. Legendre AM. Unpublished observations, 2012.
167. Salas V, Pastor FJ, Rodriguez MM, et al. In vitro activity and in vivo efficacy of posaconazole in treatment of murine infections by different isolates of the *Aspergillus terreus* complex. *Antimicrob Agents Chemother.* 2011;55:676–679.
168. Hachem RY, Kontoyiannis DP, Boktour MR, et al. *Aspergillus terreus*: an emerging amphotericin B-resistant opportunistic mold in patients with hematologic malignancies. *Cancer.* 2004;101:1594–1600.
169. Escribano P, Pelaez T, Recio S, et al. Characterization of clinical strains of *Aspergillus terreus* complex: molecular identification and antifungal susceptibility to azoles and amphotericin B. *Clin Microbiol Infect.* 2012;18:E24–E26.
170. Arendrup MC, Jensen RH, Grif K, et al. In vivo emergence of *Aspergillus terreus* with reduced azole susceptibility and a Cyp51a M217I alteration. *J Infect Dis.* 2012;206:981–985.
171. Dupont B. Overview of the lipid formulations of amphotericin B. *J Antimicrob Chemother.* 2002;49(suppl 1):31–36.
172. Chandrasekar PH, Ito JI. Amphotericin B lipid complex in the management of invasive aspergillosis in immunocompromised patients. *Clin Infect Dis.* 2005;40(Suppl 6):S392–S400.
173. Lamothe J. Activity of amphotericin B in lipid emulsion in the initial treatment of canine leishmaniasis. *J Small Anim Pract.* 2001;42:170–175.
174. Keating GM, Jarvis B. Caspofungin. *Drugs.* 2001;61:1121–1129. Discussion 1130-1121.
175. Chen SC, Slavin MA, Sorrell TC. Echinocandin antifungal drugs in fungal infections: a comparison. *Drugs.* 2011;71:11–41.
176. Ong V, James KD, Smith S, et al. Pharmacokinetics of the novel echinocandin cd101 in multiple animal species. *Antimicrob Agents Chemother.* 2017;61:e01626–16.
177. Trempala CL, Herold LV. Spontaneous pneumothorax associated with *Aspergillus* bronchopneumonia in a dog. *J Vet Emerg Crit Care (San Antonio).* 2013;23:624–630.
178. Park SJ, Burdick MD, Mehrad B. Neutrophils mediate maturation and efflux of lung dendritic cells in response to *Aspergillus fumigatus* germ tubes. *Infect Immun.* 2012;80:1759–1765.
179. Cenci E, Mencacci A, Bacci A, et al. T cell vaccination in mice with invasive pulmonary aspergillosis. *J Immunol.* 2000;165:381–388.
180. Ito JI, Lyons JM. Vaccination of corticosteroid immunosuppressed mice against invasive pulmonary aspergillosis. *J Infect Dis.* 2002;186:869–871.
181. Qualls Jr CW, Chandler FW, Kaplan W, et al. Mycotic keratitis in a dog: concurrent *Aspergillus* sp. and *Curvularia* sp. infections. *J Am Vet Med Assoc.* 1985;186:975–976.
182. Nevile JC, Hurn SD, Turner AG. Keratomycosis in five dogs. *Vet Ophthalmol.* 2016;19:432–438.
183. Wooff PJ, Dees DD, Teixeria L. *Aspergillus* spp. panophthalmitis with intralenticular invasion in dogs: report of two cases. *Vet Ophthalmol.* 2016.

87

Miscellaneous Fungal Diseases

Amy M. Grooters

KEY POINTS

Phaeohyphomycosis

- Causes: *Alternaria, Aureobasidium, Bipolaris, Cladophialophora, Cladosporium, Curvularia, Exophiala, Fonsecaea, Lecytophora, Microsphaeropsis, Moniliella, Mycoleptodiscus, Phialophora, Rhinocladiella, Scolecobasidium, Scytalidium*, and *Ulocladium*, among others.
- Affected Hosts: A variety of animal hosts that include cats, dogs, horses, and humans.
- Geographic Distribution: Worldwide.
- Mode of Transmission: Cutaneous inoculation of organisms from the environment.
- Major Clinical Signs: Localized cutaneous nodules that may appear pigmented, often on the nose or digits; occasionally meningoencephalitis, with associated neurologic signs.
- Differential Diagnosis: Neoplasia, cryptococcosis, blastomycosis, sporotrichosis, hyalohyphomycosis, mycobacterial infections, actinomycosis, nocardiosis.
- Human Health Significance: Direct transmission from animals to humans has not been described; humans develop infections from environmental sources.

Hyalohyphomycosis

- Causes: *Acremonium, Chrysosporium, Fusarium, Rasamsonia* (formerly *Geosmithia*), *Lomentospora, Oxyporus, Paecilomyces, Purpureocillium, Scedosporium* (*Pseudallescheria*), *Sagenomella, Talaromyces, Geomyces, Schizophyllum, Scopulariopsis, Lecythophora*, and *Westerdykella*, among others.
- Affected Hosts: A variety of animal hosts that include dogs, cats, and humans.
- Geographic Distribution: Worldwide.
- Mode of Transmission: Inhalation or cutaneous inoculation of organisms in the environment.
- Major Clinical Signs: Keratitis; lymphadenopathy; discospondylitis; osteomyelitis; pneumonia; cutaneous lesions; disseminated disease with involvement of kidneys, liver, spleen, bone marrow, heart, endocrine tissues, and/or CNS.
- Differential Diagnosis: Neoplasia, aspergillosis, penicilliosis, phaeohyphomycosis, sporotrichosis, cryptococcosis, blastomycosis, candidiasis, endemic mycoses, nocardiosis, actinomycosis, mycobacteriosis.
- Human Health Significance: Direct transmission from animals to humans has not been described; humans develop infections from environmental sources.

INTRODUCTION

In contrast to the well-recognized fungal pathogens that cause endemic mycoses (such as *Blastomyces, Histoplasma,* and *Cryptococcus*), miscellaneous fungal pathogens comprise large groups of fungi with unfamiliar names that traditionally have caused disease only sporadically. Although some of these fungi occasionally cause disease in immunocompetent patients, many cause infection only when normal host resistance mechanisms are compromised. Over the past 35 years, these opportunists have become increasingly important in human patients because immunocompromise associated with chemotherapy, organ transplantation, and HIV infection has become more prevalent. Similarly, over the past 15 years, the incidence of opportunistic fungal infections in dogs has increased substantially in association with the use of multiagent immunosuppressive therapy (especially with cyclosporine), with a 2017 study showing an incidence of 6.5% in dogs being treated for immune-mediated disease.[1] Thus, veterinarians are increasingly likely to encounter patients infected by an opportunistic fungal pathogen with which they are unfamiliar. Diagnosis of disseminated infections with these organisms in young, adult, purebred or inbred dogs with no evidence of underlying immunocompromising conditions may suggest the possibility of genetic immune defects. German shepherd dogs and anecdotally, Hungarian Vizslas appear to be at increased risk of disseminated aspergillosis (see Chapter 86), and some of the mold pathogens listed in this chapter have been reported as causes of disseminated disease in these breeds or their crosses.[2–6]

Unlike the common endemic fungal pathogens (for which a definitive diagnosis can often be made simply by visualizing the unique morphologic features of the organism in cytologic or histologic specimens), opportunistic fungi can only be identified to genus and species level by culture or molecular methods. However, they can be assigned to categories based on their morphologic features in tissue, such as pigmentation, hyphal diameter, and frequency of septation. These categories include *phaeohyphomycosis* (pigmented hyphal or yeast forms); *hyalohyphomycosis* (nonpigmented hyphal forms); *eumycotic mycetoma* (fibrosing granuloma with black or white tissue grains consisting of aggregates of pigmented or nonpigmented fungi, respectively); and *entomophthoromycosis* and *mucormycosis*, which together were previously termed zygomycosis (wide, infrequently septate, nonpigmented hyphae associated with pyogranulomatous and eosinophilic inflammation). Because of the similarities to pythiosis and lagenidiosis, entomophthoromycosis and mucormycosis are discussed in Chapter 88. Although identification of a specific organism after culture is ideal, classification of opportunistic mycoses based on the categories listed above is often sufficient to allow the clinician to make a reasonable prediction about clinical course and prognosis and to make appropriate treatment recommendations. This approach is perhaps most limiting for immunocompetent dogs with hyalohyphomycosis because some of the causative fungal agents (such as *Scedosporium boydii* [*Pseudallescheria boydii*] and *Paecilomyces variotii*) are inherently resistant to amphotericin B (AMB) and itraconazole, making genus- and species-level identification and sometimes antifungal susceptibility testing important.

When culture is performed, fresh tissue rather than swabs should be submitted to a laboratory with expertise in fungal culture. This author prefers to use a laboratory (Box 87.1) in which molecular identification of cultured isolates can routinely be performed when morphologic features alone are insufficient for definitive identification.

BOX 87.1 Diagnostic Laboratories with Expertise in Fungal Diagnostic Testing

Clinical Bacteriology and Mycology Laboratory, University of Tennessee College of Veterinary Medicine	https://vetmed.tennessee.edu/vmc/dls/bacteriology/
University of Florida Veterinary Diagnostic Labs, Molecular Fungal ID Lab	https://cdpm.vetmed.ufl.edu/services/diagnostic-labs/molecular-fungal-id-laboratory/
Fungus Testing Laboratory, University of Texas Health Science Center, San Antonio	https://lsom.uthscsa.edu/pathology/reference-labs/fungus-testing-laboratory/

An alternative to culture that has become more routinely available in recent years is extraction, amplification, and sequencing of fungal DNA from paraffin-embedded tissues, which is appealing because it does not require a second biopsy. Reported sensitivities for these assays have ranged from 54% to 94%.[7–10] Although a number of commercial laboratories now offer molecular diagnostics based on panfungal amplification and sequencing, use of a laboratory that interprets results in the context of histologic findings, and for which assay sensitivity and specificity have been described is preferred. Since many opportunistic fungi are common contaminants and can normally be found on skin, nasal mucosa, and other nonsterile sites, identification of a potential opportunistic fungal pathogen from a skin specimen, nasal swab, or exudate should not be considered evidence of fungal infection unless there is supportive histologic or cytologic evidence of tissue invasion by a morphologically compatible organism.

PHAEOHYPHOMYCOSIS

ETIOLOGY AND EPIDEMIOLOGY

The term "phaeohyphomycosis" refers to cutaneous, subcutaneous, cerebral, or disseminated infections caused by pigmented (also known as dematiaceous) hyphal or yeast forms that contain melanin in their cell walls.[10] Infection usually results from cutaneous

TABLE 87.1 Causative Agents and Histologic/Cytologic Characteristics Associated with Miscellaneous Fungal and Pseudofungal Pathogens

Disease	Causative Agents	Histologic and Cytologic Characteristics
Phaeohyphomycosis	*Alternaria, Aureobasidium, Bipolaris, Cladophialophora, Cladosporium, Curvularia, Exophiala, Fonsecaea, Lecytophora, Microsphaeropsis, Moniliella, Mycoleptodiscus, Phialophora, Rhinocladiella* (formerly *Ramichloridium*), *Scolecobasidium, Scytalidium, Ulocladium*, others	Pyogranulomatous inflammation associated with pigmented, irregularly septate hyphae or yeast-like cells that may be solitary or may cluster in small groups or chains. A beaded chain or toruloid appearance is supportive of a diagnosis of phaeohyphomycosis.
Hyalohyphomycosis	*Acremonium, Chrysosporium, Fusarium, Rasamsonia* (formerly *Geosmithia*), *Oxyporus, Paecilomyces, Purpureocillium, Scedosporium, Sagenomella, Geomyces, Schizophyllum, Scopulariopsis, Lecythophora, Westerdykella*, others	Pyogranulomatous inflammation associated with hyphal elements that have nonpigmented (transparent, hyaline) walls; *Aspergillus caninus (previously Phialosimplex caninus), Talaromyces spp., and Trichosporon asahii* may cause yeast-like forms in tissue
Mycetoma (black-grain)	*Curvularia, Cladophialophora, Madurella*	Pyogranulomatous inflammation associated with aggregates of pigmented fungal organisms (which appear grossly as pigmented tissue grains)
Mycetoma (white-grain)	*Scedosporium apiospermum, Acremonium*	Pyogranulomatous inflammation associated with aggregates of nonpigmented fungal organisms (which appear grossly as nonpigmented tissue grains)
Pythiosis	*Pythium insidiosum*	Pyogranulomatous and eosinophilic inflammation associated with broad (2–7 μm), infrequently septate hyphae (see Chapter 88)
Lagenidiosis	*Lagenidium giganteum* forma *caninum*	Pyogranulomatous and eosinophilic inflammation associated with broad (4–25 μm), infrequently septate hyphae (see Chapter 88)
Paralagenidiosis	*Paralagenidium karlingii*	Pyogranulomatous and eosinophilic inflammation associated with broad (2–11 μm), infrequently septate hyphae (see Chapter 88)
Entomophthoromycosis and mucormycosis (together previously termed zygomycosis)	Entomophthoromycosis: *Conidiobolus, Basidiobolus ranarum* Mucormycosis: *Rhizomucor, Mucor*, and *Cokeromyces*	Pyogranulomatous and eosinophilic inflammation associated with broad (5–20 μm), infrequently septate hyphae with thick prominent eosinophilic sleeve (see Chapter 88)
Aspergillosis	*Aspergillus terreus, A. deflectus, A. flavipes, A. fumigatus* species complex, others	Suppurative to granulomatous inflammation associated with multiple, nonpigmented, 2- to 6-μm, septate hyphae with parallel walls and 45-degree angle branching (see Chapter 86)
Candidiasis	*Candida albicans*, other *Candida* species	Suppurative inflammation with numerous 2- to 6-μm oval yeasts, pseudohyphae (chains of oval yeast cells), and true hyphae (see Chapter 85)

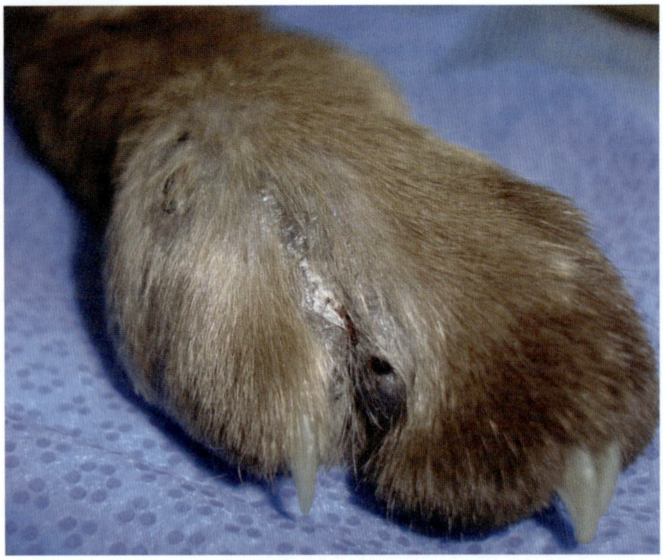

Fig. 87.1 Left distal thoracic limb of an 8-year-old male neutered Burmese cat with digital phaeohyphomycosis. (Courtesy University of California, Davis, Veterinary Dermatology Service.)

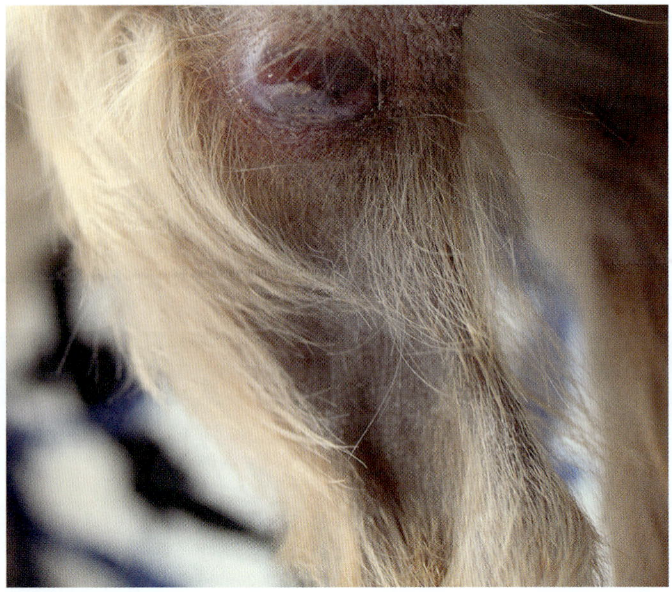

Fig. 87.2 Popliteal lymphadenopathy and abscessation caused by *Curvularia* spp. infection in a 1-year-old female Yorkshire terrier with cutaneous phaeohyphomycosis. (Courtesy Amy Grooters, Louisiana State University, Baton Rouge, LA.)

inoculation of organisms from the environment. For animals and humans with cerebral or disseminated infections, the route of infection is not always apparent. Fungal genera that have been identified as agents of phaeohyphomycosis in veterinary patients include *Alternaria, Aureobasidium, Bipolaris, Cladophialophora, Curvularia, Exophiala, Fonsecaea, Lecytophora, Microsphaeropsis, Moniliella, Mycoleptodiscus, Phialophora, Rhinocladiella* (formerly *Ramichloridium*),[11] *Scolecobasidium, Scytalidium*, and *Ulocladium*, among others (Table 87.1). In human patients, infections with some of these organisms occur more commonly in certain geographic locations where soil conditions may optimize their survival; for example, *Rhinocladiella mackenziei* and *Exophiala dermatitidis* infections predominate in the Middle East/India and East Asia, respectively.[12–14] In fact, infections with *R. mackenziei* account for the majority of fungal infections of the brain in the Middle East, and genomic analysis of this fungus suggests that the organism may be adapted to oil-polluted desert soil.[14]

CLINICAL FEATURES

The most common clinical manifestations of phaeohyphomycosis in immunocompetent small animal patients are lesions associated with the digits, pinnae, nasal planum, or nasal cavity in cats (Fig. 87.1).[15–24] Affected animals typically have cutaneous nodules or a visible nasal mass that may appear grossly pigmented, and thus may be confused with melanomas. Lesions tend to be locally invasive and may extend to involve regional lymph nodes (Fig. 87.2). Less commonly, granulomatous meningoencephalitis caused by pigmented fungi (especially *Cladophialophora* spp.) has been described in dogs and cats.[25–29] Systemic dissemination, as reported in two dogs with mycotic meningoencephalitis and nephritis, and in a cat with multiorgan involvement, is rare in the absence of immunosuppression and carries a poor prognosis.[28,30,31]

In immunocompromised patients, the most common presentation for phaeohyphomycosis is focal or multifocal cutaneous lesions in dogs treated with multiagent immunosuppressive therapy, especially which includes cyclosporine.[32–36] Dissemination to multiple cutaneous sites, lymph nodes, or even other organ systems seems to occur more often in immunocompromised than in immunocompetent patients.[37–39]

DIAGNOSIS

Laboratory and Imaging Abnormalities

Results of a CBC, biochemistry panel, and urinalysis in animals with cutaneous phaeohyphomycosis are typically unremarkable. Animals with disseminated disease can have abnormalities associated with underlying immunosuppressive illness or drug treatment. Imaging with CT or MRI in animals with CNS involvement may reveal focal or multifocal contrast-enhancing lesions that may be associated with hydrocephalus (Fig. 87.3).

Cytologic and Histologic Findings

On histologic or cytologic examination, dematiaceous fungi appear as dark-walled, irregularly septate hyphae of variable diameter, sometimes with bulbous ends, or as yeast-like cells, solitary or in small groups or chains (Fig. 87.4). Pigment may not always be apparent on cytologic examination (Fig. 87.5), or it may have a blue-green tint on Wright-Giemsa–stained specimens. On histologic examination, the presence of melanin in the walls of lightly pigmented hyphae can often be confirmed by the examination of unstained sections, by lowering the microscope condenser during examination, or by using a Fontana-Masson stain for melanin.

Isolation and Identification

Organisms that cause phaeohyphomycosis are readily isolated on routine fungal culture of infected tissue biopsies as well as from fine-needle aspirate specimens from infected lymph nodes. Further identification is based on colony and conidial morphology (see also Fig. 4.9B) and PCR and sequencing of ribosomal RNA genes. Identification of molds using MALDI-TOF MS has been challenging owing to the complex extraction protocols needed, but with refinement of protocols and libraries, this method shows great promise for reliable and rapid identification (see Chapter 4).[40] Because pigmented fungi are common laboratory contaminants and can sometimes be isolated from nonsterile sites on healthy animals (such as skin), positive cultures from potentially contaminated sites should only be considered significant if accompanied by cytologic or histologic evidence of fungal infection with a morphologically compatible organism.

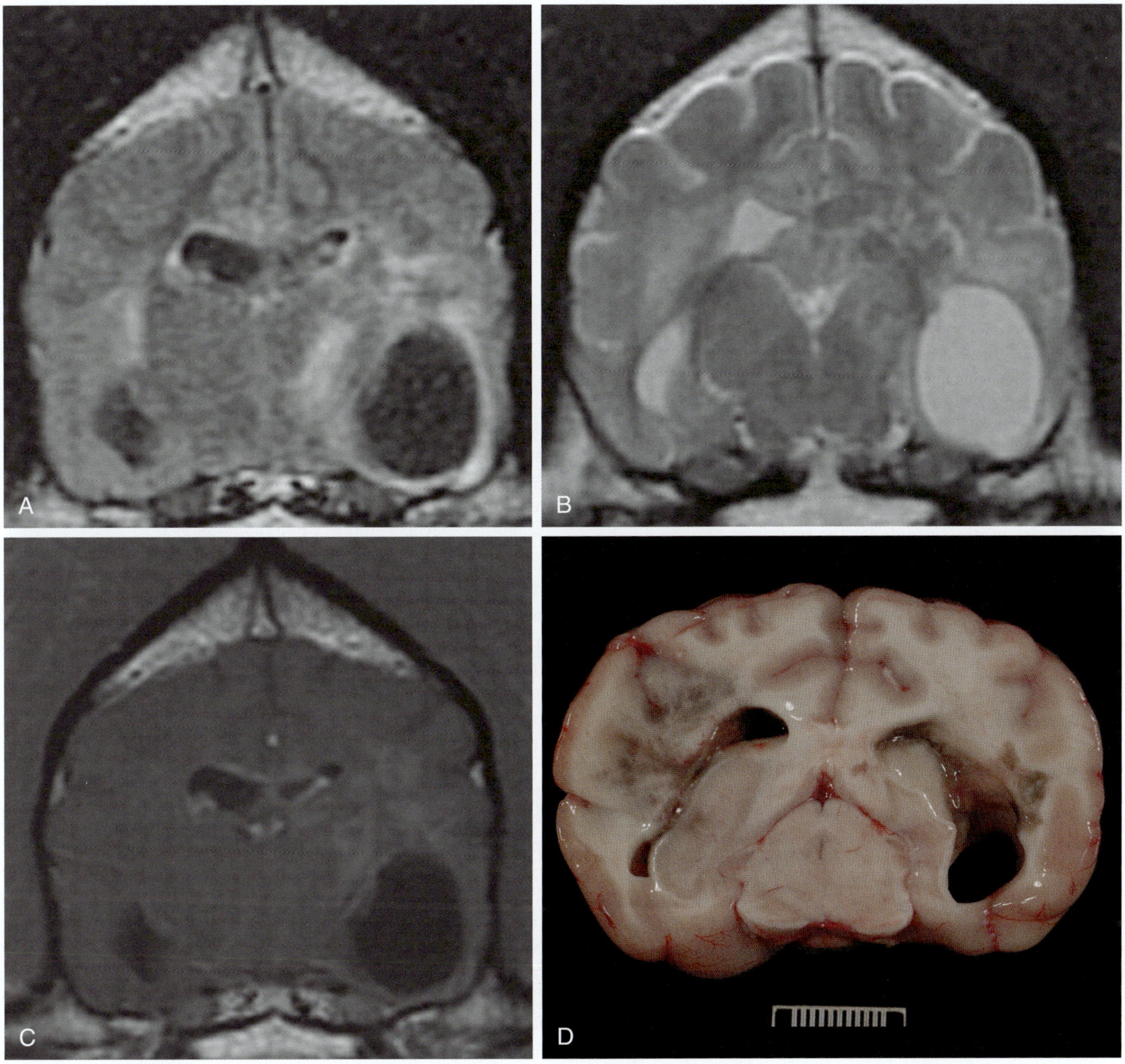

Fig. 87.3 Axial T1 postcontrast, T2, and FLAIR magnetic resonance images (A, B, and C, respectively) of the brain of a 6-year-old male neutered Border collie mix that was evaluated for neurologic signs including seizures and progressive obtundation. In the images shown, there is bilateral but asymmetric ventricular dilation that is severe on the right and mild to moderate on the left (asymmetric hydrocephalus). Multifocal regions of contrast enhancement are also present (A). Some of these regions appeared nodular; others had a ring-like appearance. There is also marked contrast enhancement of the ventricular ependymal lining. The regions of contrast enhancement correlate with regions of T2 and FLAIR hyperintensity (B and C) and were isointense on precontrast T1-weighted sequences (not shown). Meningoencephalitis caused by *Cladophialophora bantiana* and secondary hydrocephalus was diagnosed on brain biopsy and at necropsy (D). Olive-green pigmented masses can be seen on both the left and right sides of the brain. Interestingly, the dog also had cutaneous protothecosis. (Courtesy University of California, Davis, Veterinary Neurology and Anatomic Pathology Services.)

TREATMENT AND PROGNOSIS

Pigmented fungi are often poorly responsive to medical therapy, in part because melanin is a virulence factor. Aggressive surgical resection is the treatment of choice for solitary cutaneous phaeohyphomycosis lesions. The surgeon should attempt to obtain wide margins at the time of the initial surgery, submit the excised tissue for histopathology, and request that the margins be evaluated for evidence of incomplete resection. Digit amputation is usually indicated for lesions of the distal phalanx. If a full digit or more is involved, limb amputation should be considered. Medical therapy with itraconazole, posaconazole, or voriconazole (dogs only) is recommended for 3 to 6 months after surgery, because recurrence of disease at the surgical site is common.

Limited data are available regarding *in vitro* susceptibilities for isolates of pigmented fungi. Itraconazole, voriconazole, posaconazole, and AMB have the most consistent activity against pigmented fungi, whereas reported activities of fluconazole and ketoconazole have been poor.[41] For nonresectable lesions, treatment with itraconazole (10 mg/kg/day) often results in partial or complete resolution of cutaneous lesions, but recurrence is very common, so prolonged courses (9 to 12

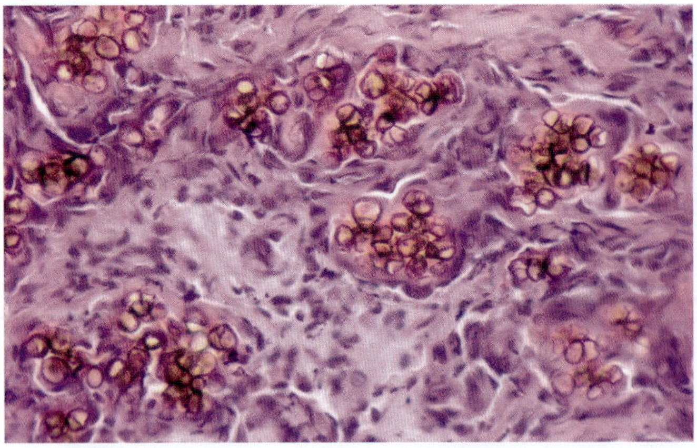

Fig. 87.4 Histopathology showing small groups of pigmented, yeast-like fungal organisms in tissue from a nasal mass in a cat with phaeohyphomycosis; hematoxylin and eosin stain. (Courtesy Amy Grooters, Louisiana State University, Baton Rouge, LA.)

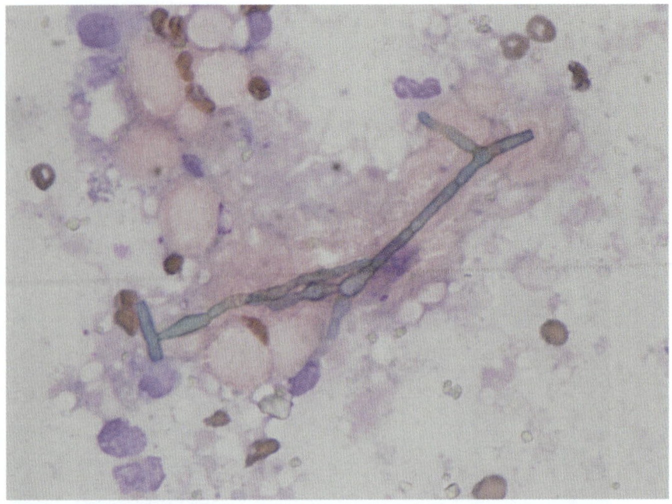

Fig. 87.5 Impression smear from the brain of the dog in Fig. 87.3. Septate, branching hyphae are present, but pigmentation is not clearly apparent. Wright stain, 1000× magnification. (Courtesy University of California, Davis, Veterinary Pathology Service.)

months) should be recommended. Posaconazole and voriconazole may be more effective than itraconazole for the treatment of phaeohyphomycosis. Posaconazole is typically easier to administer in cats because of its availability as a well-tolerated oral suspension. Voriconazole reaches high concentrations in the CNS, making it the drug of choice for treating intracranial phaeohyphomycosis. Long-term voriconazole therapy (7 to 10 mg/kg/day for 10 to 12 months) was used successfully to treat intracranial phaeohyphomycosis in one dog[26] and mycotic peritonitis caused by *Exophiala* in another.[37] Voriconazole has not been routinely used in cats because of associated neurotoxicity,[42] although the use of a lower dose in conjunction with therapeutic drug monitoring has recently been evaluated (see Chapter 11).[43]

In patients receiving immunosuppressive medications, cutaneous phaeohyphomycosis often responds more readily to medical therapy than does comparable disease that develops in an immunocompetent patient, but only if cyclosporine can be discontinued and other immunosuppressive medications can be rapidly tapered.[36] This author most often treats cutaneous phaeohyphomycosis that occurs in dogs receiving immunosuppressive therapy with itraconazole (10 mg/kg/day) for at least 6 months. If lesions are focal or otherwise amenable to wide surgical excision, a combination of medical and surgical therapy may be effective.[36] In one cat with a refractory *Cladophialophora* spp. infection that involved the dorsal aspect of the nose, rhinotomy with debulking together with topical malachite green and long-term oral itraconazole treatment was successful.[15] Although the author has observed two dogs in which lesions caused by cutaneous phaeohyphomycosis resolved without antifungal therapy after immunosuppressive drugs were discontinued, dissemination of disease despite therapy has also been observed. Therefore, the recommendation should be to discontinue immunosuppressive drugs as quickly as possible and also treat medically with itraconazole, posaconazole, or voriconazole (in dogs) for at least 2 months beyond lesion resolution.

PUBLIC HEALTH ASPECTS

Phaeohyphomycosis in humans clinically resembles that in dogs and cats and may include localized cutaneous lesions in immunocompetent hosts; life-threatening CNS infections in immunocompromised or apparently immunocompetent hosts; and, rarely, disseminated phaeohyphomycosis, primarily in immunocompromised hosts. The species most often associated with CNS infections are *Cladophialophora bantiana, Exophiala* (*Wangiella*) *dermatitidis*, and to a lesser extent, *Verruconis gallopava, R. mackenziei*, and *Fonsecaea monophora*.[12,44] A deficiency in CARD9, which leads to macrophage and microglial dysfunction, has been recognized in association with invasive *E. dermatitidis* in some human patients.[13] Infections caused by pigmented fungi are acquired from the environment. Although there is no evidence of transmission between mammalian hosts, routine precautions (such as wearing gloves when handling infected tissues or exudate) should be followed. Precautions should also be taken to prevent needle-stick injuries if phaeohyphomycosis is suspected.

HYALOHYPHOMYCOSIS

ETIOLOGY AND EPIDEMIOLOGY

The term "hyalohyphomycosis" refers to infections caused by fungi that are nonpigmented (hyaline or transparent) in tissue. Genera that have been described as agents of hyalohyphomycosis in dogs and cats include *Acremonium, Chrysosporium, Fusarium, Rasamsonia* (formerly *Geosmithia*), *Lomentospora, Oxyporus, Paecilomyces, Purpureocillium, Scedosporium, Talaromyces, Sagenomella, Geomyces, Schizophyllum, Scopulariopsis, Lecythophora,* and *Westerdykella,* among others (see Table 87.1). By convention, infections caused by *Aspergillus* and *Penicillium* species are not included in the term "hyalohyphomycosis," because aspergillosis and penicilliosis can usually be identified as such based on their clinicopathologic features in association with morphologic features that are fairly distinct (narrow, straight-walled septate hyphae that branch at acute angles, occasionally with conidia and conidiophores when lesions are in the nasal cavity).[45] Examples include sinonasal aspergillosis caused by *Aspergillus fumigatus*, and disseminated aspergillosis caused by *Aspergillus terreus* and *Aspergillus deflectus*. Other types of aspergillosis may be indistinguishable from hyalohyphomycosis without culture, and therefore may be grouped into the category of hyalohyphomycosis when culture or sequencing has not been performed. Examples include *Aspergillus caninus* (formerly *Phialosimplex caninus*), which produces scant irregular hyphae and numerous round to ovoid fungal structures in tissue, and *Aspergillus alabamensis*, both of which have been described to cause infection in dogs on immunosuppressive drug therapy.[46,47] As discussed in Chapter 4, fungal nomenclature can be confusing because of assignment of anamorph (asexual stage) and telomorph (sexual stage) names, and despite the move to the use of only one name, the use of older names still occurs in the published literature, and this, combined with changes in taxonomy related to analysis of sequence

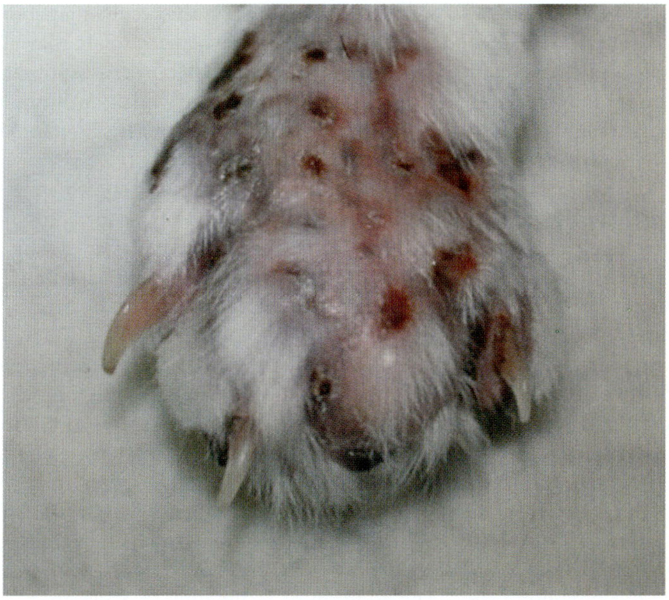

Fig. 87.6 *Scedosporium prolificans* infection in a domestic shorthair cat. There are multiple draining skin lesions and soft tissue swelling. (Courtesy Spencer Jang, University of California, Davis.)

data perpetuates confusion. For example, *Scedosporium apiospermum* was first isolated as a cause of white-grain mycetoma in humans in 1909, and was considered as the anamorph form of *S. boydii* (formerly *P. boydii*). Subsequently, analysis of molecular and phenotypic data indicated that *S. boydii* and *S. apiospermum* were two distinct species.[48,49] They are now grouped with three other *Scedosporium* species into the *S. apiospermum* species complex (sometimes also referred to as the *S. apiospermum/P. boydii* species complex)[50]; only *Scedosporium aurantiacum, S. boydii,* and *S. apiospermum* cause human disease. Similarly, *Rasamsonia argillacea*, formerly known as *Geosmithia argillacea*, is a complex that comprises four different species: *R. argillacea, Rasamsonia piperina, Rasamsonia eburnean,* and *Rasamsonia aegroticola*, all of which have been isolated from diseased humans.[51,52]

CLINICAL FEATURES

In general, hyalohyphomycosis occurs more often in dogs than in cats, with young adult, large-breed dogs most commonly affected. Clinical signs in immunocompetent animals are similar to those associated with systemic aspergillosis and include poor body condition, fever, lameness, and lymphadenomegaly, as well as CNS and ocular signs.[4] Although local disease confined to the skin (Fig. 87.6), nasal mucosa, or cornea can occur,[53–56] lymphadenopathy, osteomyelitis, discospondylitis, pneumonia, and chorioretinitis are more common manifestations.[57–59] Erosive polyarthritis and granulomatous lymphadenitis have been described in association with *Talaromyces* spp. infections in dogs (*Talaromyces georgiensis* and *Talaromyces helicus*).[6,60] Disseminated disease may also involve kidney, bone marrow, liver, spleen, heart, bladder, pancreas, thyroid, adrenal, and CNS, sometimes with associated fungemia.[6,61–63]

When hyalohyphomycosis develops in dogs receiving immunosuppressive medications, the clinical course may differ from that typically seen in immunocompetent dogs in two ways. First, the disease may be confined to the skin without evidence of systemic dissemination.[64] Second, like phaeohyphomycosis, hyalohyphomycosis that develops in animals on immunosuppressive therapy may respond more readily to medical therapy than disease that occurs in immunocompetent patients, but only if cyclosporine can be discontinued and other

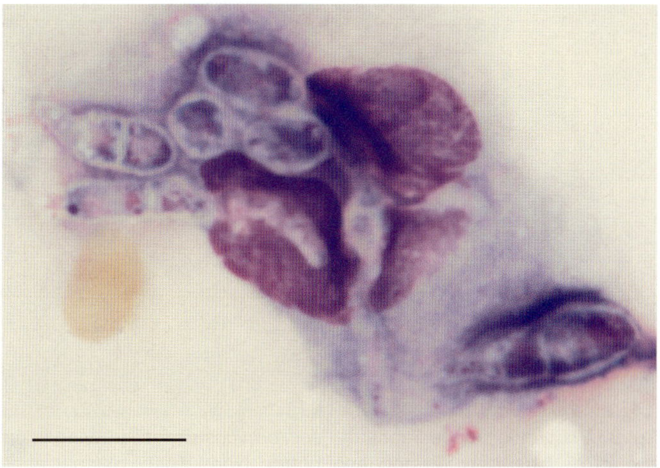

Fig. 87.7 Fine-needle aspirate cytology from a lytic bone lesion in a 4-year-old female spayed mixed-breed dog with hyalohyphomycosis. Note the septate, nonpigmented fungal hyphae present within the macrophage; Wright-Giemsa stain, bar =10 µm. (Courtesy Kaikhushroo Banajee, Louisiana State University, Baton Rouge, LA.)

immunosuppressive drugs can be tapered. Still, the prognosis for these patients should be considered guarded because of the potential for dissemination.[61,65]

DIAGNOSIS

Cytologic and Histologic Findings

Cytologically and histologically, fungi that cause hyalohyphomycosis are nonpigmented, frequently septate hyphae that typically branch at acute angles. They are often pleomorphic and may contain areas of globose swelling, especially at the end of the hyphae or between septations (Fig. 87.7 and see Fig. 4.8).[45] *Aspergillus caninus* (previously *Phialosimplex caninus*), *Talaromyces* spp., and *Trichosporon asahii* may cause yeast-like forms in tissue. Most of these organisms do not have other distinct morphologic characteristics, precluding further identification. Special stains such as PAS and Gomori's methenamine silver may be used to visualize organisms more readily.

Isolation and Identification

The fungi that cause hyalohyphomycosis are readily isolated by routine fungal culture methods from infected tissues as well as from fine-needle aspirate specimens from infected lymph nodes, bones, or abdominal organs. Because these fungi are common laboratory contaminants and can sometimes be isolated from the skin or hair of healthy animals, positive cultures from nonsterile sites should be considered significant only if accompanied by cytologic or histologic evidence of fungal infection with a morphologically compatible organism. Species identification is based on conidial morphology (Fig. 87.8) and may require PCR and sequencing of ribosomal RNA genes. As for phaeohyphomycosis, identification using MALDI-TOF MS may be useful in the future with refinement of methods and libraries. Genus and species identification may assist in selection of antifungal drug treatments, because some species are predictably less susceptible to conventional antifungal drugs (see Treatment and Prognosis).

Antigen Testing

Serology for detection of fungal galactomannan antigen is routinely included in the diagnostic evaluation of human patients suspected to have invasive aspergillosis or hyalohyphomycosis, but has only been evaluated in a limited number of veterinary patients.[66–69] In an investigation of galactomannan assay results in dogs with systemic

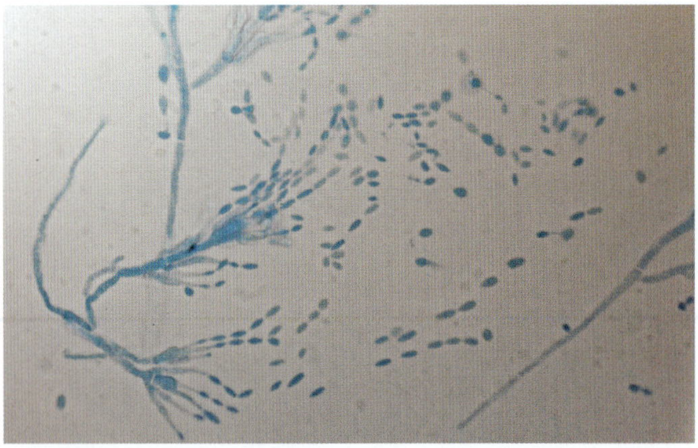

Fig. 87.8 Cytologic appearance of *Paecilomyces variotii* growing in culture in the laboratory. Lactophenol cotton blue, 1000× magnification. (Courtesy Spencer Jang, University of California, Davis.)

aspergillosis as well as those with other types of systemic fungal disease, the assay was found to be positive in two dogs with typical hyalohyphomycosis and negative in one dog that developed hyalohyphomycosis involving only skin and regional lymph nodes after immunosuppressive drug therapy.[67] In addition, positive galactomannan results have been observed in human patients with endemic mycoses (e.g., blastomycosis and coccidioidomycosis) as well as those receiving beta-lactam antibiotics.[70,71] Based on very limited information in dogs, it appears that a positive galactomannan assay may increase the index of suspicion for either hyalohyphomycosis or aspergillosis in animals with supportive clinical signs, but specificity for this purpose has not yet been adequately studied. False-negative results may also occur, especially in dogs without widespread disease.

TREATMENT AND PROGNOSIS

Treatment of hyalohyphomycosis has traditionally been challenging because many animals have disseminated disease. Drugs used most often to treat hyalohyphomycosis in small animals include AMB, itraconazole, voriconazole, posaconazole, and caspofungin. In human patients, *Scedosporium* spp., *Fusarium* spp., *P. variotii*, and *Purpureocillium lilacinum* (formerly *Paecilomyces lilacinus*) typically have highly resistant *in vitro* susceptibility patterns and are more difficult to treat successfully.[72] Specifically, *S. boydii* (previously *P. boydii*) is routinely resistant to AMB and has variable susceptibility to the triazoles, *P. lilacinum* is typically resistant to AMB, *P. variotii* is often resistant to voriconazole, and *Scopulariopsis* isolates are resistant to triazoles with variable susceptibility to AMB.[72–74] Voriconazole is considered the initial treatment of choice for several of these inherently resistant fungi, with posaconazole either as salvage therapy or as first-line therapy when *P. variotii* infection is identified.[72,73] The novel drug olorofim has recently shown considerable promise for treatment of refractory mold infections in humans based on *in vitro* susceptibility data, but the safety and efficacy of this drug in animals requires investigation.[75] The role of antifungal susceptibility testing for the treatment of hyalohyphomycosis is unclear, as clinical breakpoints have not been established for human or veterinary patients, and correlation between susceptibility results and clinical outcomes has not been demonstrated. However, one recent retrospective study of human isolates suggested that a lower MIC for the first drug used for treatment was associated with a better outcome, especially if that drug was AMB.[76] Susceptibility testing is often of limited value for veterinary cases because it requires culture, is expensive, requires submission of an isolate to an experienced reference laboratory (see Box 87.1), and many clients cannot afford the newer triazoles or echinocandins that the results may indicate are more likely to be effective. However, when an isolate is available and client finances do not limit choice of therapy, susceptibility testing may provide important information about which antifungals have a high MIC and thus are unlikely to result in a positive outcome, especially if used as a first-line therapy.

In animals with disseminated hyalohyphomycosis in which the specific pathogen is unknown, ideal therapy would typically combine a course of lipid-complexed AMB with a triazole, the latter of which is then continued indefinitely. Alternatively, when financial limitations preclude administration of AMB, patients who do not require hospitalization may be treated with a triazole alone. The efficacy of voriconazole and posaconazole is generally better than itraconazole for the treatment of hyalohyphomycosis, but the cost is significantly greater.[72] Posaconazole has been used successfully to resolve or reduce clinical signs in dogs with systemic aspergillosis, although relapse is common.[77] Similar results may be achieved in some dogs with hyalohyphomycosis. Although fluconazole is the least expensive of these medications, its efficacy for infections caused by molds is generally inferior to the newer triazoles, so its use is not recommended for the treatment of hyalohyphomycosis. The addition of terbinafine to azole antifungals has been recommended for the treatment of many opportunistic mycoses, but has not been well studied in dogs. Caspofungin may be used for the treatment of *Scedosporium* spp. infections in human patients, but no data regarding its use for treating hyalohyphomycosis in animals are available.[72] Although treatment of disseminated hyalohyphomycosis with antifungal drugs can prolong survival, clinical signs often recur even if signs initially resolve. Therefore, disseminated hyalohyphomycosis generally carries a guarded to poor prognosis.

Cutaneous hyalohyphomycosis that develops in an animal receiving immunosuppressive drug therapy may respond well to oral triazole therapy (assuming cyclosporine can be discontinued and other immunosuppressive drugs tapered)[78] or may rapidly disseminate. Therefore, fungal skin lesions that develop in immunocompromised patients should be treated aggressively, an attempt should be made to identify occult extracutaneous lesions, and a guarded prognosis should be offered. This author most often uses itraconazole (10 mg/kg/day) administered orally for at least 6 months. Other options include voriconazole, posaconazole, or AMB, the latter usually reserved for cases in which extracutaneous lesions are detected. Surgical removal of a focal lesion is rarely indicated and should only be considered if the lesion is confined to the skin and a thorough diagnostic evaluation has failed to find evidence of other organ involvement.

PUBLIC HEALTH ASPECTS

Hyalohyphomycosis in humans is acquired as a result of infection by fungi in the environment. Keratitis and nailbed infections (onychomycosis) can occur in immunocompetent humans. Invasive infections occur in immunocompromised patients such as transplant recipients, patients with AIDS, and leukemic or neutropenic patients. Although there is no evidence to suggest that transmission between mammalian hosts is possible, routine precautions (such as wearing gloves when handling infected tissues or exudate) should be followed. Precautions should especially be taken to prevent needle-stick injuries if hyalohyphomycosis is suspected.

EUMYCOTIC MYCETOMA

The term "mycetoma" refers to localized mycotic or actinomycotic infections of the skin, subcutaneous tissue, muscle, or bone that are characterized by the presence of colonies or aggregates of organisms that form "grains" in tissue. Actinomycotic mycetomas are caused by bacteria such as *Actinomyces* spp. or *Nocardia* spp. (see Chapters 59 and 60), dermatophytic mycetomas are caused by dermatophytes (see Chapter 78), and eumycotic mycetomas are caused by nondermatophyte fungi. Lesions result from traumatic implantation of soil organisms into tissue. The grains or granules of eumycotic mycetomas are pigmented (for black-grain mycetoma, caused by dematiaceous fungi) or hyaline (for white-grain mycetoma, caused by nonpigmented fungi), depending on the type of fungal pathogen involved (see Table 87.1).

Black-grain mycetomas are most often caused by *Madurella mycetomatis, Curvularia,* or *C. bantiana* and are typically associated with chronic nonhealing wounds and cutaneous nodules on the extremities.[79–82] Lesions often develop weeks to months after a traumatic incident in the same area. Draining tracts are often present, and black grains may be observed in the exudate. White-grain mycetomas, usually caused by *S. apiospermum* or *Acremonium* spp., most often occur as body-wall and/or intra-abdominal granulomas that develop subsequent to wound or incision contamination or postoperative dehiscence.[83–87] Interestingly, the lesions associated with white-grain mycetoma may not be evident until months or even a year or more after the surgical or traumatic event. Affected dogs may be evaluated for a draining mass on the body wall or clinical signs of peritonitis.

The treatment of choice for eumycotic mycetoma is aggressive surgical excision of infected tissues, including amputation if clinically indicated. Unfortunately, lesion location may preclude complete resection. Response to medical therapy is generally poor as the causative agents of eumycotic mycetoma are inherently resistant to most antifungals, but administration of itraconazole, voriconazole, or posaconazole may be considered as adjunctive therapy following surgical excision when wide margins cannot be achieved. Because the lesions are slowly growing, debulking the lesions followed by long-term triazole therapy may improve quality of life for a significant period of time.[86] Dissemination of eumycotic mycetoma beyond local tissues is rare, but disease within the abdomen or other local tissues may be extensive.

CASE EXAMPLE

Signalment

"CJ," a 1-year-old male intact boxer dog from central Louisiana.

History

CJ was initially evaluated for acute ataxia and abnormal limb placement. Based on results of CSF analysis as well as MRI of the brain and spinal cord, inflammatory CNS disease was diagnosed, and treatment with prednisone (1 mg/kg, PO, q12h) was initiated. Despite a good initial response, neurologic signs recurred 2 weeks later, at which time cytosine arabinoside (50 mg/m^2, SC, q12h, for four doses, repeated every 3 weeks) and azathioprine (1.6 mg/kg, PO, q48h) were added to the treatment protocol. Neurologic signs again improved, but 7 weeks later, the dog was evaluated for ulcerative lesions on the distal extremities that had been present for 1 week and lethargy that had been present for 3 days.

Physical Examination

Body weight: 29 kg.

General: Alert and responsive, but painful on ambulation because of ulcerative lesions on all four feet. Vital parameters were within normal limits. Peripheral lymph nodes were palpably normal.

Dermatologic examination: Pitting edema and multifocal ulcerative lesions were present on all four distal extremities, with sloughing of multiple footpads (Fig. 87.9A and B). Some of the pad lesions were proliferative and extended into the interdigital area (Fig. 87.9C). Multiple light brown–colored areas could be visualized within the fibrinonecrotic material that covered the area of the left metacarpal pad (see Fig. 87.9B). In addition, a 1-cm ulcerated lesion was present on the left pinna, a crusted lesion was present on the tip of the tail, and a small subcutaneous mass was present in the right saphenous area. Larger (3 cm) ulcerated lesions partially covered with eschar were present on the medial aspect of the right tarsus and the dorsal aspect of the left antebrachium. Major differential diagnoses considered were opportunistic fungal infection and drug eruption.

Cytology and Histology Findings

Cytologic evaluation of the left pinnal lesion, subcutaneous right saphenous mass, and right popliteal lymph node revealed septic neutrophilic to pyogranulomatous inflammation with septate, branching, 3- to 7-μm fungal hyphae, both extracellularly and within neutrophils. Pigmentation of hyphae was not observed.

Histologic evaluation of punch biopsies obtained from cutaneous lesions on the left front foot, right hind foot, and right forelimb revealed severe pyogranulomatous dermatitis with intralesional septate, pigmented hyphae.

Diagnosis

Disseminated cutaneous phaeohyphomycosis extending to regional lymphadenitis.

Treatment and Outcome

Pentoxifylline (30 mg/kg, PO, q24h) was administered because of suspected vasculitis associated with the cutaneous lesions. Antifungal therapy with itraconazole (10 mg/kg, PO, q24h) was initiated, but lesion progression was observed over the next several days, so lipid-complexed AMB treatment (2 mg/kg diluted in 5% dextrose, IV, over several hours three times weekly) was initiated. Unfortunately, 2 days later lesions had progressed rapidly with appearance of new draining tracts and abscess

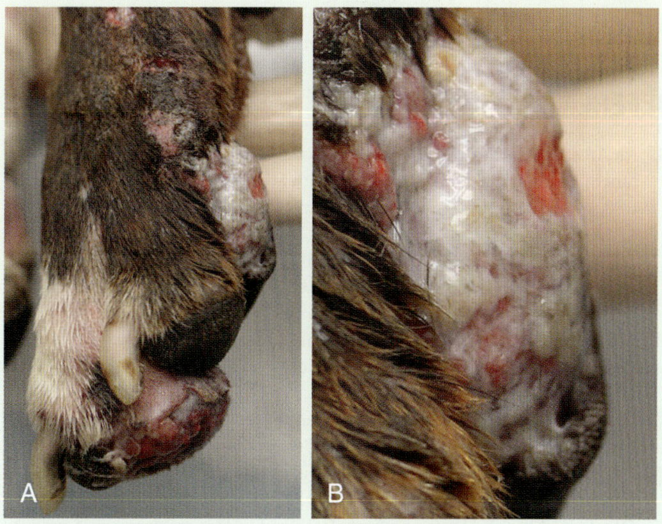

Fig. 87.9 (A–C) Phaeohyphomycosis of the left thoracic limb that developed after multiagent immunosuppressive therapy in 1-year-old boxer with inflammatory central nervous system disease. (Courtesy Amy Grooters, Louisiana State University, Baton Rouge, LA.) Continued

Continued

CASE EXAMPLE—cont'd

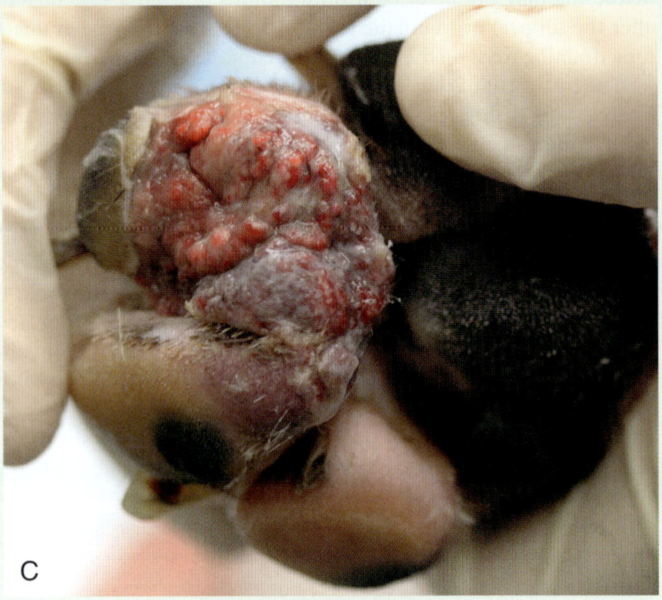

Fig 87.9–cont'd

formation. Because of the poor prognosis and pain associated with the lesions, the dog was euthanized.

Comments

As was noted here, pigmentation of hyphae may not always be visible on cytologic examination of lesions caused by phaeohyphomycosis, in part because hyphae and the cells that phagocytize them often take up enough color with the Wright-Giemsa stain to mask the pigmentation. Therefore, in this case, evaluation of histologic samples was important for differentiating phaeohyphomycosis from hyalohyphomycosis. Culture would have been ideal for definitive identification of the opportunistic fungal organism that caused the infection in this dog, but was not performed.

SUGGESTED READINGS

Dear JD, Reagan KL, Hulsebosch SE, et al. Disseminated *Rasamsonia argillacea* species complex infections in 8 dogs. *J Vet Intern Med*. 2021;35:2232–2240.

Dedeaux A, Grooters A, Wakamatsu-Utsuki N, et al. Opportunistic fungal infections in small animals. *J Am Anim Hosp Assoc*. 2018;54:327–337.

McAtee BB, Cummings KJ, Cook AK, et al. Opportunistic invasive cutaneous fungal infections associated with administration of cyclosporine to dogs with immune-mediated disease. *J Vet Intern Med*. 2017;31:1724–1729.

REFERENCES

1. McAtee BB, Cummings KJ, Cook AK, et al. Opportunistic invasive cutaneous fungal infections associated with administration of cyclosporine to dogs with immune-mediated disease. *J Vet Intern Med*. 2017;31:1724–1729.
2. Ballhausen BD, Geisweid K, Hartmann K, et al. Systemic *Acremonium* species infection in a dog. *Tierarztl Prax Ausg K Kleintiere Heimtiere*. 2016;44:424–428.
3. Lodzinska J, Cazzini P, Taylor CS, et al. Systemic *Rasamsonia piperina* infection in a German shepherd cross dog. *JMM Case Rep*. 2017;4:e005125.
4. Cook E, Meler E, Garrett K, et al. Disseminated *Chrysosporium* infection in a German shepherd dog. *Med Mycol Case Rep*. 2015;10:29–33.
5. Dunlap AE, Swinford AK, Wells KL. Disseminated *Scytalidium* infection in a German shepherd dog. *Med Mycol Case Rep*. 2015;7:20–22.
6. Okada K, Kano R, Hasegawa T, et al. Granulomatous polyarthritis caused by *Talaromyces georgiensis* in a dog. *J Vet Diagn Invest*. 2020;32:912–917.
7. Babouee Flury B, Weisser M, Prince SS, et al. Performances of two different panfungal PCRs to detect mould DNA in formalin-fixed paraffin-embedded tissue: what are the limiting factors? *BMC Infect Dis*. 2014;14:692.
8. Bernhardt A, von Bomhard W, Antweiler E, et al. Molecular identification of fungal pathogens in nodular skin lesions of cats. *Med Mycol*. 2015;53:132–144.
9. Meason-Smith C, Edwards EE, Older CE, et al. Panfungal polymerase chain reaction for identification of fungal pathogens in formalin-fixed animal tissues. *Vet Pathol*. 2017;54:640–648.
10. Revankar SG, Sutton DA. Melanized fungi in human disease. *Clin Microbiol Rev*. 2010;23:884–928.
11. Arzanlou M, Groenewald JZ, Gams W, et al. Phylogenetic and morphotaxonomic revision of *Ramichloridium* and allied genera. *Stud Mycol*. 2007;58:57–93.
12. Taj-Aldeen SJ, Almaslamani M, Alkhalf A, et al. Cerebral phaeohyphomycosis due to *Rhinocladiella mackenziei* (formerly *Ramichloridium mackenziei*): a taxonomic update and review of the literature. *Med Mycol*. 2010;48:546–556.
13. Wang C, Xing H, Jiang X, et al. Cerebral phaeohyphomycosis caused by *Exophiala dermatitidis* in a Chinese CARD9-deficient patient: a case report and literature review. *Front Neurol*. 2019;10:938.
14. Moreno LF, Ahmed AAO, Brankovics B, et al. Genomic understanding of an infectious brain disease from the desert. *G3 (Bethesda)*. 2018;8:909–922.
15. Brooks IJ, Walton SA, Shmalberg J, et al. Novel treatment using topical malachite green for nasal phaeohyphomycosis caused by a new *Cladophialophora* species in a cat. *JFMS Open Rep*. 2018;4. 2055116918771767.
16. Abramo F, Bastelli F, Nardoni S, et al. Feline cutaneous phaeohyphomycosis due to *Cladophyalophora bantiana*. *J Feline Med Surg*. 2002;4:157–163.
17. Beccati M, Vercelli A, Peano A, et al. Phaeohyphomycosis by *Phialophora verrucosa*: first European case in a cat. *Vet Rec*. 2005;157:93–94.
18. Dye C, Johnson EM, Gruffydd-Jones TJ. *Alternaria* species infection in nine domestic cats. *J Feline Med Surg*. 2009;11:332–336.
19. Fondati A, Gallo MG, Romano E, et al. A case of feline phaeohyphomycosis due to *Fonsecaea pedrosoi*. *Vet Dermatol*. 2001;12:297–301.
20. Knights CB, Lee K, Rycroft AN, et al. Phaeohyphomycosis caused by *Ulocladium* species in a cat. *Vet Rec*. 2008;162:415–416.
21. Krockenberger MB, Martin P, Halliday C, et al. Localised *Microsphaeropsis arundinis* infection of the subcutis of a cat. *J Feline Med Surg*. 2010;12:231–236.
22. Maeda H, Shibuya H, Yamaguchi Y, et al. Feline digital phaeohyphomycosis due to *Exophiala jeanselmei*. *J Vet Med Sci*. 2008;70:1395–1397.
23. Overy DP, Martin C, Muckle A, et al. Cutaneous phaeohyphomycosis caused by exophiala attenuata in a domestic cat. *Mycopathologia*. 2015;180:281–287.
24. Tennant K, Patterson-Kane J, Boag AK, et al. Nasal mycosis in two cats caused by *Alternaria* species. *Vet Rec*. 2004;155:368–370.

25. Anor S, Sturges BK, Lafranco L, et al. Systemic phaeohyphomycosis (*Cladophialophora bantiana*) in a dog: clinical diagnosis with stereotactic computed tomographic-guided brain biopsy. *J Vet Intern Med.* 2001;15:257–261.
26. Bentley RT, Faissler D, Sutherland-Smith J. Successful management of an intracranial phaeohyphomycotic fungal granuloma in a dog. *J Am Vet Med Assoc.* 2011;239:480–485.
27. Bouljihad M, Lindeman CJ, Hayden DW. Pyogranulomatous meningoencephalitis associated with dematiaceous fungal (*Cladophialophora bantiana*) infection in a domestic cat. *J Vet Diagn Invest.* 2002;14:70–72.
28. Giri DK, Sims WP, Sura R, et al. Cerebral and renal phaeohyphomycosis in a dog infected with *Bipolaris* species. *Vet Pathol.* 2011;48:754–757.
29. Velazquez-Jimenez Y, Hernandez-Castro R, Romero-Romero L, et al. Feline phaeohyphomycotic cerebellitis caused by *Cladosporium cladosporioides*-complex: case report and review of literature. *J Comp Pathol.* 2019;170:78–85.
30. Elies L, Balandraud V, Boulouha L, et al. Fatal systemic phaeohyphomycosis in a cat due to *Cladophialophora bantiana. J Vet Med A Physiol Pathol Clin Med.* 2003;50:50–53.
31. Poutahidis T, Angelopoulou K, Karamanavi E, et al. Mycotic encephalitis and nephritis in a dog due to infection with *Cladosporium cladosporioides. J Comp Pathol.* 2009;140:59–63.
32. Rajeev S, Clifton G, Watson C, et al. *Fonsecaea pedrosoi* skin infection in a dog. *J Vet Diagn Invest.* 2008;20:379–381.
33. Dedola C, Stuart AP, Ridyard AE, et al. Cutaneous *Alternaria infectoria* infection in a dog in association with therapeutic immunosuppression for the management of immune-mediated haemolytic anaemia. *Vet Dermatol.* 2010;21:626–634.
34. Herraez P, Rees C, Dunstan R. Invasive phaeohyphomycosis caused by *Curvularia* species in a dog. *Vet Pathol.* 2001;38:456–459.
35. Metry CA, Hoien-Dalen PS, Maddox CW, et al. Subcutaneous *Mycoleptodiscus indicus* infection in an immunosuppressed dog. *J Clin Microbiol.* 2010;48:3008–3011.
36. Swift IM, Griffin A, Shipstone MA. Successful treatment of disseminated cutaneous phaeohyphomycosis in a dog. *Aust Vet J.* 2006;84:431–435.
37. Murphy KF, Malik R, Barnes A, et al. Successful treatment of intra-abdominal *Exophiala dermatitidis* infection in a dog. *Vet Rec.* 2011;168:217.
38. Singh K, Flood J, Welsh RD, et al. Fatal systemic phaeohyphomycosis caused by *Ochroconis gallopavum* in a dog (*Canis familaris*). *Vet Pathol.* 2006;43:988–992.
39. Sutton DA, Wickes BL, Thompson EH, et al. Pulmonary *Phialemonium curvatum* phaeohyphomycosis in a standard poodle dog. *Med Mycol.* 2008;46:355–359.
40. Sanguinetti M, Posteraro B. Identification of molds by matrix-assisted laser desorption ionization-time of flight mass spectrometry. *J Clin Microbiol.* 2017;55:369–379.
41. Wong EH, Revankar SG. Dematiaceous molds. *Infect Dis Clin North Am.* 2016;30:165–178.
42. Quimby JM, Hoffman SB, Duke J, et al. Adverse neurologic events associated with voriconazole use in 3 cats. *J Vet Intern Med.* 2010;24:647–649.
43. Vishkautsan P, Papich MG, Thompson GR 3rd, et al. Pharmacokinetics of voriconazole after intravenous and oral administration to healthy cats. *Am J Vet Res.* 2016;77:931–939.
44. Velasco J, Revankar S. CNS infections caused by brown-black fungi. *J Fungi (Basel).* 2019;5.
45. Guarner J, Brandt ME. Histopathologic diagnosis of fungal infections in the 21st century. *Clin Microbiol Rev.* 2011;24:247–280.
46. Burrough E, Deitz K, Kinyon J, et al. Disseminated aspergillosis in a dog due to *Aspergillus alabamensis. Med Mycol Case Rep.* 2012;1:1–4.
47. Sigler L, Hanselman B, Ruotsalo K, et al. Cytological, microbiological and therapeutic aspects of systemic infection in a dog caused by the fungus *Phialosimplex caninus. Med Mycol Case Rep.* 2013;2:32–36.
48. Lackner M, de Hoog GS, Yang L, et al. Proposed nomenclature for *Pseudallescheria, Scedosporium* and related genera. *Fungal Diversity.* 2014;67:1–10.
49. Gilgado F, Cano J, Gene J, et al. Molecular phylogeny of the *Pseudallescheria boydii* species complex: proposal of two new species. *J Clin Microbiol.* 2005;43:4930–4942.
50. Luplertlop N. *Pseudallescheria/Scedosporium* complex species: From saprobic to pathogenic fungus. *J Mycol Med.* 2018;28:249–256.
51. Houbraken J, Giraud S, Meijer M, et al. Taxonomy and antifungal susceptibility of clinically important *Rasamsonia* species. *J Clin Microbiol.* 2013;51:22–30.
52. Babiker A, Gupta N, Gibas CFC, et al. *Rasamsonia* sp: An emerging infection amongst chronic granulomatous disease patients. A case of disseminated infection by a putatively novel *Rasamsonia argillacea* species complex involving the heart. *Med Mycol Case Rep.* 2019;24:54–57.
53. Caro-Vadillo A, Garcia-Real I, Paya-Vicens MJ, et al. Fungal rhinitis caused by *Scedosporium apiospermum* in a Labrador retriever. *Vet Rec.* 2005;157:175–177.
54. Rampazzo A, Kuhnert P, Howard J, et al. *Hormographiella aspergillata* keratomycosis in a dog. *Vet Ophthalmol.* 2009;12:43–47.
55. Marlar AB, Miller PE, Canton DD. Canine keratomycosis: a report of eight cases and literature review. *J Am Anim Hosp Assoc.* 1994;30:331–340.
56. Smith CG, Woolford L, Talbot JJ, et al. Canine rhinitis caused by an uncommonly-diagnosed fungus, *Scedosporium apiospermum. Med Mycol Case Rep.* 2018;22:38–41.
57. Erne JB, Walker MC, Strik N, et al. Systemic infection with *Geomyces* organisms in a dog with lytic bone lesions. *J Am Vet Med Assoc.* 2007;230:537–540.
58. Grant DC, Sutton DA, Sandberg CA, et al. Disseminated *Geosmithia argillacea* infection in a German shepherd dog. *Med Mycol.* 2009;47:221–226.
59. Hugnet C, Marrou B, Dally C, et al. Osteomyelitis and discospondylitis due to *Scedosporium apiospermum* in a dog. *J Vet Diagn Invest.* 2009;21:120–123.
60. Whipple KM, Shmalberg JW, Joyce AC, et al. Cytologic identification of fungal arthritis in a Labrador retriever with disseminated *Talaromyces helicus* infection. *Vet Clin Pathol.* 2019;48:449–454.
61. Armstrong PF, Sigler L, Sutton DA, et al. Fungal myelitis caused by *Phialosimplex caninus* in an immunosuppressed dog. *Med Mycol.* 2012;50:509–512.
62. Foley JE, Norris CR, Jang SS. Paecilomycosis in dogs and horses and a review of the literature. *J Vet Intern Med.* 2002;16:238–243.
63. Holahan ML, Loft KE, Swenson CL, et al. Generalized calcinosis cutis associated with disseminated paecilomycosis in a dog. *Vet Dermatol.* 2008;19:368–372.
64. Kano R, Maruyama H, Kubota M, et al. Chronic ulcerative dermatitis caused by *Fusarium sporotrichioides. Med Mycol.* 2011;49:303–305.
65. Ribas T, Pipe-Martin H, Kim KS, et al. Fungal myocarditis and pericardial effusion secondary to *Inonotus tropicalis* (phylum Basidiomycota) in a dog. *J Vet Cardiol.* 2015;17:142–148.
66. Taylor AR, Young BD, Levine GJ, et al. Clinical features and magnetic resonance imaging findings in 7 dogs with central nervous system aspergillosis. *J Vet Intern Med.* 2015;29:1556–1563.
67. Garcia RS, Wheat LJ, Cook AK, et al. Sensitivity and specificity of a blood and urine galactomannan antigen assay for diagnosis of systemic aspergillosis in dogs. *J Vet Intern Med.* 2012;26:911–919.
68. Mikulska M, Furfaro E, Del Bono V, et al. Galactomannan testing might be useful for early diagnosis of fusariosis. *Diagn Microbiol Infect Dis.* 2012;72:367–369.
69. Tortorano AM, Esposto MC, Prigitano A, et al. Cross-reactivity of *Fusarium* spp. in the *Aspergillus* galactomannan enzyme-linked immunosorbent assay. *J Clin Microbiol.* 2012;50:1051–1053.
70. Bart-Delabesse E, Basile M, Al Jijakli A, et al. Detection of *Aspergillus* galactomannan antigenemia to determine biological and clinical implications of beta-lactam treatments. *J Clin Microbiol.* 2005;43:5214–5220.

71. Xavier MO, Pasqualotto AC, Cardoso IC, et al. Cross-reactivity of *Paracoccidioides brasiliensis, Histoplasma capsulatum*, and *Cryptococcus* species in the commercial Platelia *Aspergillus* enzyme immunoassay. *Clin Vaccine Immunol.* 2009;16:132–133.
72. Tortorano AM, Richardson M, Roilides E, et al. ESCMID and ECMM joint guidelines on diagnosis and management of hyalohyphomycosis: *Fusarium* spp., *Scedosporium* spp. and others. *Clin Microbiol Infect.* 2014;20(suppl 3):27–46.
73. Feldman R, Cockerham L, Buchan BW, et al. Treatment of *Paecilomyces variotii* pneumonia with posaconazole: case report and literature review. *Mycoses.* 2016;59:746–750.
74. Lackner M, de Hoog GS, Verweij PE, et al. Species-specific antifungal susceptibility patterns of *Scedosporium* and *Pseudallescheria* species. *Antimicrob Agents Chemother.* 2012;56:2635–2642.
75. Kirchhoff L, Dittmer S, Buer J, et al. In vitro activity of olorofim (F901318) against fungi of the genus, *Scedosporium* and *Rasamsonia* as well as against *Lomentospora prolificans, Exophiala dermatitidis* and azole-resistant *Aspergillus fumigatus*. *Int J Antimicrob Agents.* 2020;56:106105.
76. Lamoth F, Damonti L, Alexander BD. Role of antifungal susceptibility testing in non-aspergillus invasive mold infections. *J Clin Microbiol.* 2016;54:1638–1640.
77. Corrigan VK, Legendre AM, Wheat LJ, et al. Treatment of disseminated *Aspergillosis* with posaconazole in 10 dogs. *J Vet Intern Med.* 2016;30:167–173.
78. Atencia S, Papakonstantinou S, Leggett B, et al. Systemic fungal infection in a dog: a unique case in Ireland. *Ir Vet J.* 2014;67:17.
79. Elad D, Orgad U, Yakobson B, et al. Eumycetoma caused by *Curvularia lunata* in a dog. *Mycopathologia.* 1991;116:113–118.
80. Guillot J, Garcia-Hermoso D, Degorce F, et al. Eumycetoma caused by *Cladophialophora bantiana* in a dog. *J Clin Microbiol.* 2004;42:4901–4903.
81. Sun PL, Peng PC, Wu PH, et al. Canine eumycetoma caused by *Cladophialophora bantiana* in a Maltese: case report and literature review. *Mycoses.* 2013;56:376–381.
82. Coyle V, Isaacs JP, O'Boyle DA. Canine mycetoma: a case report and review of the literature. *J Small Anim Pract.* 1996;25:261–268.
83. Toth EJ, Nagy GR, Homa M, et al. Recurrent *Scedosporium apiospermum* mycetoma successfully treated by surgical excision and terbinafine treatment: a case report and review of the literature. *Ann Clin Microbiol Antimicrob.* 2017;16:31.
84. Allison N, McDonald RK, Guist SR, et al. Eumycotic mycetoma caused by *Pseudallescheria boydii* in a dog. *J Am Vet Med Assoc.* 1989;194:797–799.
85. Jang SS, Popp JA. Eumycotic mycetoma in a dog caused by *Allescheria boydii*. *J Am Vet Med Assoc.* 1970;157:1071–1076.
86. Janovec J, Brockman DJ, Priestnall SL, et al. Successful treatment of intra-abdominal eumycotic mycetoma caused by *Penicillium duponti* in a dog. *J Small Anim Pract.* 2016;57:159–162.
87. Walker RL, Monticello TM, Ford RB, et al. Eumycotic mycetoma caused by *Pseudallescheria boydii* in the abdominal cavity of a dog. *J Am Vet Med Assoc.* 1988;192:67–70.

88

Pythiosis, Lagenidiosis, Paralagenidiosis, Entomophthoromycosis, and Mucormycosis

Amy M. Grooters

KEY POINTS

Pythiosis

- First Described: In 1884, India, in horses.[1]
- Cause: *Pythium insidiosum* (kingdom Stramenopila, class Oomycota), related to algae and *Prototheca* spp.
- Affected Hosts: Dogs and horses; less commonly cats, sheep, cattle, exotic species, and humans.
- Geographic Distribution: Tropical, subtropical, and some temperate regions worldwide, especially the Gulf Coast region of the United States.
- Mode of Transmission: Likely penetration of damaged skin or mucosa by motile zoospores, often after exposure to standing freshwater sources.
- Major Clinical Signs: Ulcerative, nodular, and mass-like cutaneous lesions with draining tracts (cutaneous form); weight loss, anorexia, vomiting, diarrhea, hematochezia (GI form).
- Differential Diagnosis: For suspected GI pythiosis, differential diagnoses include neoplasia, entomophthoromycosis, histoplasmosis, eosinophilic gastroenteritis, or chronic intestinal foreign bodies; for suspected cutaneous pythiosis, they include lagenidiosis, paralagenidiosis, entomophthoromycosis, phaeohyphomycosis, mycobacterial infections, actinomycosis, or furunculosis.
- Human Health Significance: *Pythium insidiosum* is a rare cause of disease in human patients; infection is not transmitted directly from affected animals to humans.

Lagenidiosis and Paralagenidiosis

- First Described: *Lagenidium giganteum* forma *caninum*: 2003, Louisiana, USA, in dogs.[2] *Lagenidium deciduum*: 2016, Louisiana, USA, in cats.[3] *Paralagenidium karlingii*: 2004, Louisiana, USA, in dogs; and Illinois, USA, in a human patient.[4]
- Geographic Distribution: Southeastern United States, Australia.
- Mode of Transmission: Likely penetration of damaged skin or mucosa by motile zoospores.
- Major Clinical Signs: *Lagenidium giganteum* forma *caninum*: Ulcerative, nodular, and mass-like cutaneous lesions with draining tracts; pelvic limb edema; local, thoracic, or abdominal lymphadenopathy; rupture of infected great vessels in the abdomen may result in hemoabdomen. *Paralagenidium karlingii* (dogs) and *L. deciduum* (cats): Nodular or ulcerative dermatopathy that may extend locally but rarely invades beyond cutaneous and subcutaneous tissues.
- Differential Diagnosis: Neoplasia, pythiosis, entomophthoromycosis, mucormycosis, mycobacterial infections, actinomycosis, snake bite.
- Human Health Significance: Infection is acquired from the environment; it is not transmitted from affected animals to humans.

Entomophthoromycosis and Mucormycosis (Together Previously Termed Zygomycosis)

- First Described: Reports of these infections in humans date back to the 1800s.
- Causes: *Basidiobolus* and *Conidiobolus* spp. (kingdom Fungi, order Entomophthorales); *Rhizopus, Absidia, Mucor* spp., and others (kingdom Fungi, order Mucorales).
- Affected Hosts: Dogs, cats, humans, horses, sheep, and other mammalian species.
- Geographic Distribution: Worldwide.
- Mode of Transmission: Inhalation, ingestion, or cutaneous exposure to organisms in soil and decaying organic matter.
- Major Clinical Signs: Entomophthoromycosis (also known as entomophthoramycosis) is associated with chronic, slowly progressive subcutaneous, GI, respiratory, retrobulbar, or nasal infections in immunocompetent animals; mucormycosis is associated with systemic (respiratory or GI) or cutaneous-subcutaneous infections in immunocompromised animals.
- Differential Diagnosis: Neoplasia, pythiosis, lagenidiosis, other deep mycoses, mycobacterial infections, actinomycosis.
- Human Health Significance: Disease in humans results from exposure to organisms in the environment, and direct transmission between animals has not been reported.

INTRODUCTION

Pythiosis, lagenidiosis, paralagenidiosis, entomophthoromycosis (also known as entomophthoramycosis), and mucormycosis are often grouped together because of similarities in their clinical presentations and histologic characteristics; all cause pyogranulomatous and eosinophilic inflammation associated with large, infrequently septate hyphae with nonparallel walls. Despite their clinicopathologic similarities, however, the pathogens that cause these infections are taxonomically diverse. *Pythium insidiosum, Lagenidium giganteum* forma *caninum, Lagenidium deciduum,* and *Paralagenidium karlingii* are water molds in the class Oomycetes. As such, they are more closely related to red algae and *Prototheca* spp. than to true fungi.[5] Important traits that distinguish oomycetes from fungi

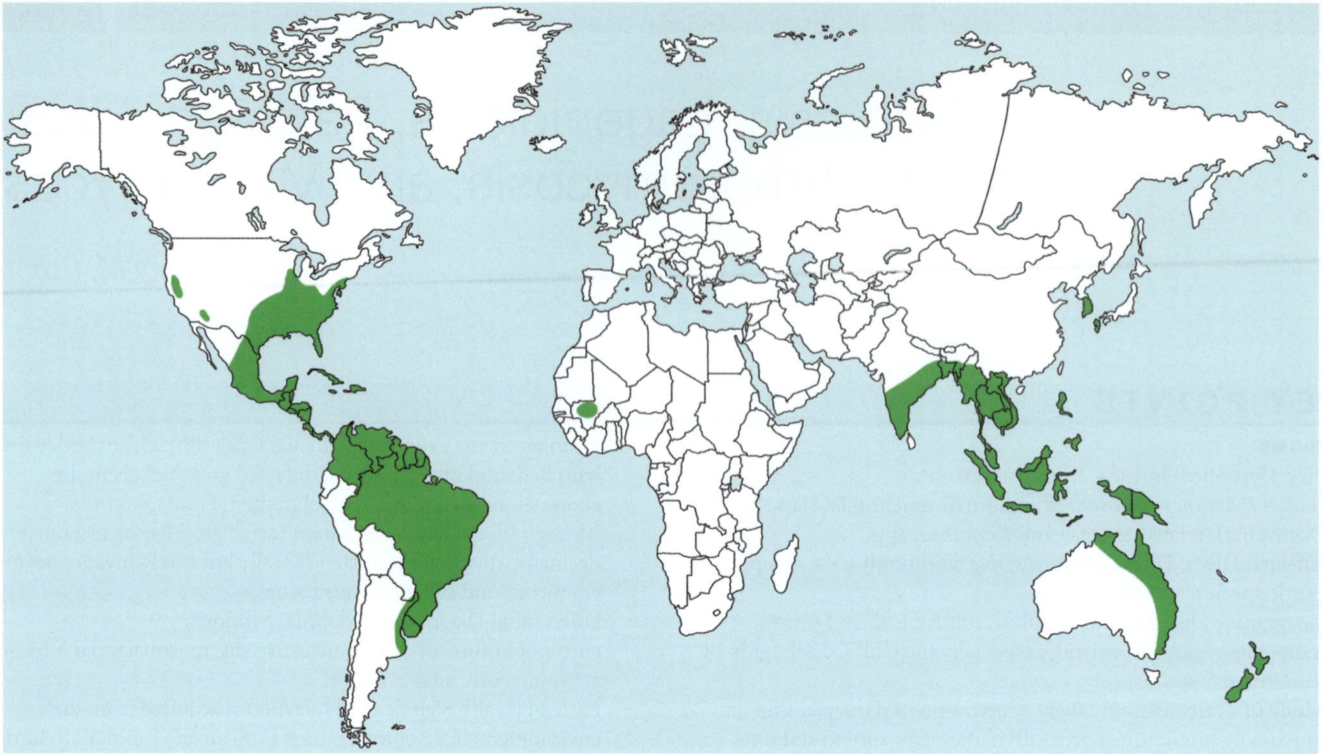

Fig. 88.1 Worldwide geographic distribution of pythiosis.

include the production of motile, flagellate zoospores that act as infective elements in wet environments, and the fact that the oomycete cell membrane generally lacks ergosterol.[6] In addition, there are clinically relevant differences in prognosis, recommended treatment, and epidemiology that make it important to distinguish among pythiosis, lagenidiosis, paralagenidiosis, entomophthoromycosis, and mucormycosis. Although *P. insidiosum* has been recognized as a pathogen in dogs and horses for more than 30 years, *Lagenidium* and *Paralagenidium* species have only been recognized as mammalian pathogens since 1999. In comparison to infections caused by the oomycetes, infections caused by fungi in the Entomophthorales and Mucorales in dogs and cats are rare. These organisms used to be referred to as zygomycetes, but molecular studies have led taxonomists to recommend abolishment of the class Zygomycota, instead placing the Entomophthorales within the phylum Zoopagomycota, and the Mucorales within the phylum Mucormycota.[7,8]

PYTHIOSIS

ETIOLOGY AND EPIDEMIOLOGY

Pythium insidiosum is an aquatic oomycete that causes severe, progressive GI or cutaneous disease that is often fatal. The infective form of *P. insidiosum* is thought to be the motile flagellate zoospore, which is an asexual reproductive structure produced in wet environments in association with plant material.[9] Zoospores of *P. insidiosum* are attracted to damaged tissue, and likely cause infection by encystation on and invasion of damaged skin or GI mucosa.[10] In support of this mechanism of infection, clinical reports have long suggested an association between pythiosis and frequent exposure to warm freshwater habitats. However, some infections occur in dogs with no history of access to lakes or ponds.

Globally, pythiosis occurs in tropical and subtropical climates, including Southeast Asia, eastern coastal Australia, and South America (Fig. 88.1). In the United States, the disease occurs most often in the Gulf Coast states, but it has also been recognized throughout the south; along the east coast as far north as Maryland and New Jersey; in the midwest including Missouri, Kansas, southern Illinois, and Indiana; and in the west in Arizona and California.[11,12]

Pythiosis is most common in young, large-breed dogs, especially Labrador retrievers and other outdoor working breeds. Infected dogs are typically evaluated by veterinarians in the fall, winter, and early spring.[13] Pythiosis is uncommon in cats compared with dogs, and specific breed and sex predilections have not been observed in the cases described to date. However, the development of cutaneous pythiosis in very young animals (less than 1 year of age) appears to occur more often in cats than in dogs. For both species, affected animals are typically immunocompetent.

CLINICAL FEATURES

The clinical signs associated with pythiosis are caused by GI or cutaneous lesions, or by extension of disease into regional lymph nodes or adjacent tissues. Generally, GI and cutaneous lesions do not occur together in the same animal. Rare cases of respiratory involvement with tracheobronchial lymphadenomegaly and disseminated pythiosis have been reported.[14,15]

Gastrointestinal Pythiosis

Gastrointestinal pythiosis in dogs is characterized by severe, segmental, transmural thickening of the stomach wall (Fig. 88.2), small intestine, colon, rectum, or, rarely, the esophagus.[13,16,17] It is not uncommon to find multiple segmental lesions in the same patient. The most commonly affected regions of the GI tract are the gastric outflow area, proximal duodenum, and ileocolic junction. Mesenteric lymphadenopathy is common but it is usually the result of reactive hyperplasia rather than infection. Extension of disease into the mesenteric root often causes severe mesenteric lymphadenomegaly,

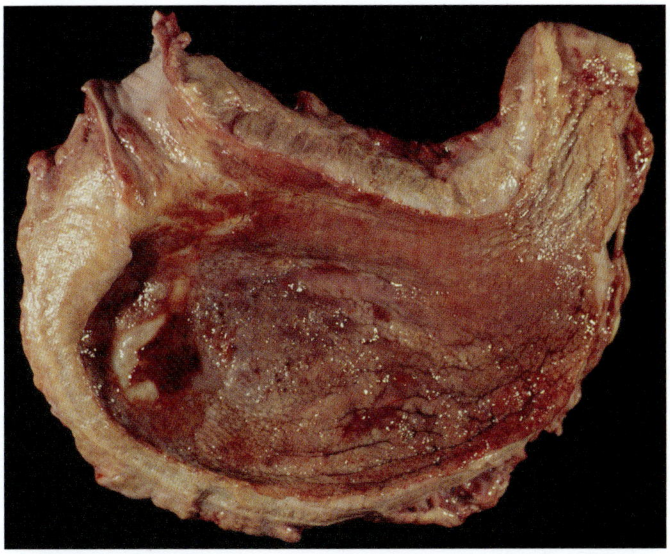

Fig. 88.2 Gastric pythiosis in a 1-year-old male neutered mixed-breed dog. Note extreme thickening of the gastric wall. (Courtesy Amy M. Grooters, Louisiana State University, Baton Rouge, LA.)

with the lymph nodes embedded in a single large, firm mass that is palpable in the cranial to midabdomen. Invasion of mesenteric vessels may result in bowel ischemia, infarction, perforation, or acute hemoabdomen. Rarely, infection may extend into adjacent tissues such as the pancreas or the uterus. Gastrointestinal pythiosis is rare in cats but has been described in two young adult male cats from the southeastern United States with focal intestinal lesions that were amenable to surgical resection,[18] a 2-year-old cat from Missouri, USA, with a sublingual mass,[19] and a cat from northeastern Brazil with a jejunal wall mass.[20]

Dogs with GI pythiosis typically have a history of chronic progressive weight loss, vomiting, diarrhea, anorexia, and sometimes hematochezia, depending on the location of the lesions. Regurgitation may be present in dogs with esophageal involvement. Physical examination usually reveals a poor body condition and often a palpable abdominal mass. Signs of systemic illness such as lethargy or depression are absent unless intestinal obstruction, infarction, or perforation occurs.

Cutaneous Pythiosis

Cutaneous pythiosis in dogs occurs most often at the base of the tail, or on the extremities, ventral neck, or perineum,[15,21,22] and is characterized by nonhealing wounds and invasive masses that contain ulcerated nodules and draining tracts (Fig. 88.3). In contrast to GI pythiosis, regional lymphadenopathy associated with cutaneous pythiosis often reflects extension of infection rather than just reactive hyperplasia. Extension of cutaneous disease to tissues other than regional lymph nodes is rare, but pulmonary lesions caused by *P. insidiosum* have been observed rarely in dogs.[14]

In cats, lesions associated with cutaneous pythiosis include cervical, inguinal, or truncal subcutaneous masses; draining nodular lesions or ulcerated plaque-like lesions on the tailhead or extremities[20,22]; and periorbital and nasopharyngeal lesions.[23]

DIAGNOSIS

Laboratory Abnormalities

The most common laboratory abnormalities associated with pythiosis are eosinophilia, anemia, hyperglobulinemia, and hypoalbuminemia. Hypercalcemia has been described once.[24]

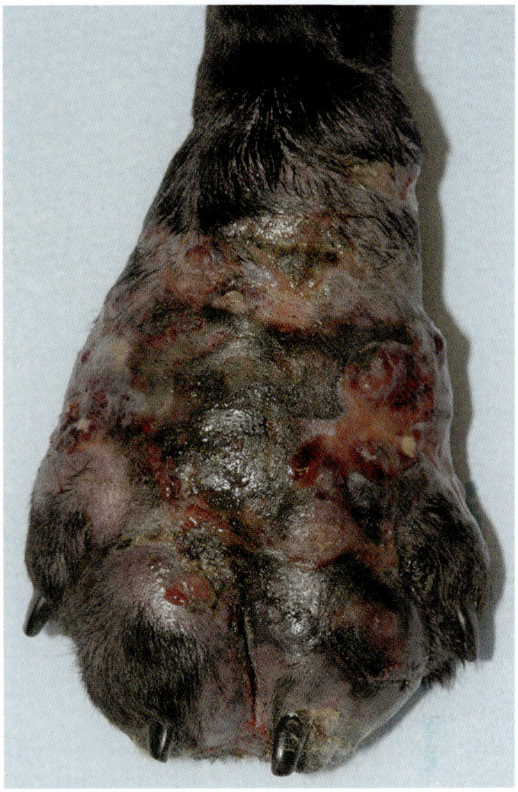

Fig. 88.3 Cutaneous pythiosis with paw involvement in a 6-month-old female Labrador retriever. Ulcerations, swelling, alopecia, and draining tracts are present. (Courtesy Amy M. Grooters, Louisiana State University, Baton Rouge, LA.)

Imaging Findings

In dogs with GI pythiosis, common radiographic findings include poor abdominal detail and the presence of an abdominal mass. Evidence of small bowel obstruction may also be observed. In rare cases of esophageal pythiosis, thoracic radiographs reveal increased soft tissue opacity in the region of the esophagus and deviation of the trachea. A dog with respiratory involvement had radiographic and CT evidence of severe tracheobronchial lymphadenomegaly with tracheal and mainstem bronchial compression.[14] Abdominal ultrasonography is the tool of choice for imaging animals suspected to have GI pythiosis and usually reveals severe segmental thickening of the GI tract, loss of normal wall layering, and mesenteric lymphadenomegaly, although lymphadenomegaly is not observed in all dogs.[25] Evidence of invasion of the pancreas and extrahepatic bile duct obstruction was described in one dog.[25] In addition, Doppler ultrasonography may identify the presence of vascular pathology (such as an aneurysm) that can result from invasion of mesenteric vessels. Abdominal ultrasonography is a critical tool for determining the location and extent of disease in dogs with GI pythiosis to determine the likelihood that surgical resection could be performed successfully and to assess prognosis. In addition, ultrasonography facilitates the acquisition of fine-needle aspirate specimens from affected segments of the GI tract and enlarged lymph nodes. In animals with cutaneous pythiosis, CT may provide information about the extent of disease and may assist with surgical planning when lesions are not located on an extremity.[26]

Microbiologic Tests

Diagnostic assays currently available for pythiosis, lagenidiosis, paralagenidiosis, entomophthoromycosis, and mucormycosis, in dogs and cats are described in Table 88.1.

TABLE 88.1 Diagnostic Assays Currently Available for Pythiosis, Lagenidiosis, Paralagenidiosis, Entomophthoromycosis and Mucormycosis in Dogs and Cats

Assay	Specimen Type	Target	Performance
Cytologic examination	Impression smears or aspirates of affected tissues	Negatively staining to rarely basophilic, broad, rarely septate fungal hyphae with tapered, rounded ends	Does not reliably differentiate among pythiosis, lagenidiosis, paralagenidiosis, entomophthoromycosis, and mucormycosis.
Culture	Biopsies of affected tissues	*Pythium insidiosum*, *Lagenidium* spp., *Paralagenidium* spp., *Conidiobolus* spp., *Basidiobolus* spp., and mucormycetes	Special tissue handling and expertise required for culture (see text). The use of swab specimens or aspirates may result in false negatives. Species identification requires the use of molecular techniques.
Antibody serology	Serum	Antibodies to *P. insidiosum*	Assays that detect anti-*Pythium* antibodies are sensitive and reasonably specific, although false-positive results can occur; titers fall with successful treatment. Assays that detect *Lagenidium* and *Paralagenidium* antibodies in dogs have poor specificity and should not be used.
Histopathology	Biopsies of affected tissues	Broad, rarely septate fungal hyphae with tapered, rounded ends	Does not reliably differentiate among pythiosis, lagenidiosis, paralagenidiosis, entomophthoromycosis, and mucormycosis. Use of special stains may facilitate detection.
PCR amplification and sequencing of rDNA	Biopsies of affected tissues	Oomycete, entomophthoramycete, or mucormycete DNA	Can be performed on cultured isolates (Box 88.1, *A*) or on formalin-fixed paraffin-embedded tissues (Box 88.1, *B*)

Cytologic Examination

Cytologically, pythiosis is characterized by pyogranulomatous and eosinophilic inflammation that can be visualized on impression smears made from firmly expressed exudate from draining tracts or fine-needle aspirates of subcutaneous lesions, thickened GI wall, or enlarged lymph nodes. Hyphae are observed occasionally in cytologic specimens, and their morphologic appearance (negatively staining to rarely basophilic, broad, pauciseptate hyphae with tapered, rounded ends) in conjunction with a typical inflammatory response can provide a tentative diagnosis of oomycosis, entomophthoromycosis, or mucormycosis.[24] Although a hyphal diameter > 7 μm makes a diagnosis of lagenidiosis or entomophthoromycosis more likely than pythiosis or paralagenidiosis, cytomorphologic features alone cannot provide a definitive diagnosis.

BOX 88.1 Laboratories with Expertise in Diagnosis of Pythiosis, Lagenidiosis, Paralagenidiosis, Entomophthoromycosis, and Mucormycosis

A. Clinical Bacteriology and Mycology Laboratory, University of Tennessee College of Veterinary Medicine: https://vetmed.tennessee.edu/vmc/dls/bacteriology/
B. University of Florida Veterinary Diagnostic Labs, Molecular Fungal ID Lab: https://cdpm.vetmed.ufl.edu/services/diagnostic-labs/molecular-fungal-id-laboratory/
C. Department of Pathobiology, College of Veterinary Medicine, Auburn University: https://www.vetmed.auburn.edu/academic-departments/dept-of-pathobiology/diagnostic-services/

Isolation and Identification

Isolation of *P. insidiosum* from infected tissues is not difficult but does require specific specimen handling and culture techniques. For best results, unrefrigerated tissue specimens should be wrapped in a saline-moistened gauze sponge and shipped at ambient temperature to arrive within 24 hours at a laboratory that has experience with culture of pathogenic oomycetes (Box 88.1, *A*). Small pieces of fresh, nonmacerated tissue are placed directly on the surface of vegetable extract agar supplemented with streptomycin and ampicillin (or an alternative selective medium) and incubated at 37°C.[27] Mycelial growth is typically observed within 12 to 24 hours. Isolation of *P. insidiosum* from swabs of exudate collected from draining skin lesions is generally unsuccessful. Because generation of the sexual reproductive structures that are necessary for definitive morphologic classification of pathogenic oomycetes rarely occurs in the laboratory, identification of *P. insidiosum* isolates is based on species-specific PCR amplification[28] or rRNA gene sequencing. Although production of zoospores is an important supporting feature for the identification of pathogenic oomycetes, it is not specific for *P. insidiosum*. MALDI-TOF MS has also shown promise for identification of *P. insidiosum*.[29,30]

Molecular Diagnosis Using Nucleic Acid–Based Testing

Species-specific PCR assays have been used to identify *P. insidiosum* DNA in fresh, frozen, or paraffin-embedded tissues from humans and animals, as well as DNA extracted directly from cultured isolates.[28,30–32] A sensitive isothermal PCR (LAMP) assay has also been developed; unlike PCR assays, this does not require a thermocycler and so is suited to low-resource settings.[33] In addition, amplification and sequencing of fungal and oomycete DNA from paraffin-embedded tissues using panfungal primers has recently become routinely available. Reported sensitivities for these panfungal assays have ranged from 54% to 94%.[34–36] Although a number of commercial laboratories now offer panfungal DNA amplification and sequencing, this author prefers to use a laboratory that interprets results in the context of histologic findings, and for which assay sensitivity and specificity have been described (Box 88.1, *B*).

Serologic Testing

ELISA detection of anti–*P. insidiosum* antibodies in dogs has been reported to be sensitive and specific for the diagnosis of pythiosis, and also allows response to therapy to be monitored.[37] Following complete surgical resection of infected tissues, a dramatic decrease in antibody levels is typically detected within 2 to 3 months. Although ELISA serology has been adapted for detection of anti–*P. insidiosum* antibodies in domestic and exotic cats, case numbers are too small to generate strong estimates of sensitivity and specificity. An ELISA-based serologic assay for anti–*P. insidiosum* antibodies is available at the time of writing through Auburn University (Box 88.1, *C*). Unfortunately, sensitivity and specificity for this assay have not been reported. A strongly false-positive result using the Auburn assay was reported in a dog with GI basidiobolomycosis,[38] and this author is aware of another false-positive result in a dog with hyalohyphomycosis. Therefore, the specificity of antibody serology for the diagnosis of pythiosis may be poorer than was previously thought, and positive results should always be interpreted in light of clinicopathologic findings.

Sensitive and specific ELISA or immunochromatographic assays that use the bacterial protein A/G as a conjugate have been reported.[39,40] This conjugate binds anti-*Pythium* antibodies from a variety of animal and human host species, which provides the potential for increased availability of serodiagnostic assays for dogs and cats, especially in parts of the world where more traditional assays are not available. Further clinical validation of these assays in dogs and cats with pythiosis is required, because of the low number of specimens from dogs and cats included in these studies.

Pathologic Findings

Histologically, pythiosis is characterized by eosinophilic pyogranulomatous inflammation, with multiple foci of necrosis that are surrounded and infiltrated by neutrophils, eosinophils, and macrophages. In addition, discrete granulomas composed of epithelioid macrophages, plasma cells, multinucleate giant cells, and fewer neutrophils and eosinophils are often observed. Organisms are typically found within areas of necrosis or at the center of granulomas. Vasculitis is occasionally present. In GI pythiosis, inflammation centers on the submucosal and muscular layers rather than the mucosa and lamina propria. Therefore, the diagnosis of pythiosis may be missed if endoscopic biopsies that fail to reach deeper tissues are submitted. Similarly, disease in animals with cutaneous pythiosis is typically found in the deep dermis and subcutis, necessitating deep wedge biopsies rather than punch biopsies for optimal evaluation. *Pythium insidiosum* hyphae are not routinely visualized on H&E–stained sections but may be identified as clear spaces surrounded by a narrow band of eosinophilic material. Hyphae are readily visualized in sections stained with Gomori's methenamine silver (GMS), but usually do not stain well with PAS. They are wide (mean, 4 μm; range, 2–7 μm), have nonparallel walls, are infrequently septate, and occasionally branch at right angles.[13,15]

TREATMENT AND PROGNOSIS

When lesion location allows resection with 5-cm margins, aggressive surgical resection of all infected tissues with wide margins is the treatment of choice for pythiosis. In animals with cutaneous lesions that are confined to a single distal extremity, amputation should be recommended unless there is evidence of regional lymph node infection. In patients with segmental GI pythiosis confined to the jejunum, ileocolic junction, or proximal colon, discrete lesions should be resected with 5-cm margins. Because mesenteric lymph nodes are usually reactive rather than infected, the presence of nonresectable mesenteric lymphadenopathy should not dissuade the surgeon from pursuing resection of a segmental bowel lesion, but enlarged lymph nodes should always be biopsied for prognostic information. In contrast to GI pythiosis, enlarged regional lymph nodes encountered in dogs with cutaneous pythiosis are often infected rather than reactive; therefore, they should be evaluated cytologically or histologically before amputation or other aggressive resection is attempted. In the author's experience, surgery is curative in a majority of animals with a distal limb lesion treated with amputation, or with a midjejunal lesion assessed as completely resected with 5-cm margins.

Historically, because of routinely poor responses of *P. insidiosum* to traditional antifungal drugs, very aggressive surgery such as a partial gastrectomy,[24] Billroth II procedure,[41] or massive resection of cutaneous lesions combined with reconstructive techniques[26] have been recommended for treatment of lesions in which optimal margins could not be obtained. Although these resections can sometimes result in a successful outcome, more often they are associated with lesion recurrence and/or significant postoperative morbidity. Surprisingly good outcomes have been observed using prednisone-containing medical protocols in dogs with GI pythiosis. These observations have led to recommendations that dogs with GI lesions that cannot be completely resected undergo medical therapy, rather than aggressive surgery that may not achieve 5-cm margins. In contrast, long-term positive responses to prednisone-containing medical protocols have not been observed in dogs with cutaneous pythiosis, so aggressive surgical resection remains the recommended therapy when skin margins of 5 cm and deep margins of two fascial planes may be achievable.[26] Local postoperative recurrence of disease is common in these patients, and can occur either at the site of resection or in regional lymph nodes. For this reason, postoperative therapy with itraconazole (10 mg/kg, PO, q24h) and terbinafine (5 to 10 mg/kg, PO, q24h) is often recommended for 2–6 months. To monitor for recurrence, ELISA serology can be performed at the time of surgery and 2 to 3 months later. In animals that have had a complete surgical resection and subsequently show no recurrence of disease, serum antibody levels usually drop 50% or more within 3 months. If this occurs, medical therapy can be discontinued. Unfortunately, if resection is incomplete, lesions often progress despite postoperative medical therapy, and clinical signs recur within weeks to months.

Medical therapy for nonresectable pythiosis has traditionally been unrewarding, likely because ergosterol (the target for most currently available antifungal drugs) is generally lacking in the oomycete cell membrane. Despite this fact, clinical and serologic cures have occurred in some patients treated with a combination of itraconazole (10 mg/kg, PO, q24h) and terbinafine (5 to 10 mg/kg, PO, q24h).[42] The addition of anti-inflammatory doses of prednisone to antifungal therapy significantly increases the likelihood of complete resolution of disease in dogs with nonresectable GI pythiosis.[12] As a result, this combination has become the treatment of choice in the author's practice for GI pythiosis when optimal margins may not be achievable. In addition, the author has observed complete resolution of GI pythiosis in a small number of dogs treated with prednisone alone. Current treatment recommendations for dogs with nonresectable GI pythiosis are: itraconazole (10 mg/kg, PO, q24h, usually FDA-approved generic capsules), terbinafine (5 to 10 mg/kg, PO, q24h), and prednisone (1 mg/kg, PO, q12h for 5–7 days, then q24h for 1 month). After the first 5 weeks of therapy, recheck ultrasonography is performed. At that time, lesions are typically either dramatically improved (in which case most patients go on to completely resolve their lesions) or unchanged (in which case lesions are very unlikely to improve). In patients that have improved, prednisone is continued at 1 mg/kg, q24h, for 1 additional month, and then slowly tapered if the patient is doing well clinically. Antifungals are usually administered for a total of at least 6 months. Although this protocol is not recommended for animals with lesions that are clearly resectable, it has substantially improved the prognosis for dogs with nonresectable GI pythiosis in the author's practice. Unfortunately, although the addition of prednisone to antifungal therapy for nonresectable cutaneous pythiosis may considerably improve lesions in the short term, the author has not observed complete long-term resolution of lesions in dogs with cutaneous pythiosis using medical therapy.

Mefenoxam, an agricultural fungicide used to treat oomycete pathogens that affect crops and ornamentals, has been used together with itraconazole and terbinafine to treat dogs with nonresectable or incompletely resected pythiosis.[42,43] However, there have been no evaluations of the efficacy of mefenoxam when used alone. Anecdotally, this author has found it to be ineffective in a very small number of dogs with pythiosis when used as sole therapy. Additional studies of the pharmacokinetics and safety of mefenoxam in dogs are required, as achievable tissue concentrations following oral administration are unknown. Therefore, at this time, its routine use cannot be recommended. An immunotherapy product derived from antigens of *P. insidiosum* has been used successfully to treat pythiosis in horses and humans.[44,45] Unfortunately, although controlled trials have not been completed, the efficacy of this product in dogs appears to be poor, and clinical improvement has not been observed in any of the author's patients.

PUBLIC HEALTH ASPECTS

Human infections caused by *P. insidiosum* are rare. Infections are acquired from the environment and have resulted in keratitis, periorbital cellulitis, and arteritis of the lower extremities. Most cases have been reported from Thailand, and almost all patients have thalassemia. Extremely rare reports of the disease exist from humans in North, South, and Central America, Australia, New Zealand, and other parts of Asia, many of whom are apparently healthy. Although there is no evidence to suggest that transmission between mammalian hosts is possible, routine precautions (such as wearing gloves when handling infected tissues or exudate) should be followed.

LAGENIDIOSIS AND PARALAGENIDIOSIS

ETIOLOGY AND EPIDEMIOLOGY

Most species in the genus *Lagenidium* are pathogens of insects, crustaceans, algae, and nematodes. The most well-studied species, *L. giganteum* f. *giganteum*, is a mosquito larval pathogen that was previously used as a biologic pesticide for control of mosquito populations. In the late 1990s, two novel oomycete pathogens that appeared to be members of the genus *Lagenidium* were recognized in dogs as causes of cutaneous lesions that resemble those associated with pythiosis. More recently, multigene phylogenetic analyses have allowed formal names to be published for these pathogens.[3] The first pathogen, which causes severe and often fatal progressive cutaneous disease, lymphadenopathy, pulmonary nodules, and great vessel invasion,[2] has been formally described as *L. giganteum* f. *caninum* because of its close phylogenetic relationship with *L. giganteum* f. *giganteum*. The second pathogen causes more slowly progressive disease that is limited to skin and subcutaneous tissues.[4] Although it shares many antigenic and morphologic similarities with *L. giganteum* f. *caninum* and other *Lagenidium* species, phylogenetic analyses support placement of this second novel pathogen in the new genus *Paralagenidium*.[3] Within *Paralagenidium*, phylogenetic analyses show two clades, one of which has the species name *Paralagenidium karlingii*.[3] Insufficient numbers of isolates from the second clade (AG-2015a) were available at the time of analysis to determine whether it falls within *P. karlingii* or represents a separate species within *Paralagenidium*.[3] The author has noted that dogs infected with isolates from *Paralagenidium* clade AG-2015a may have a more chronic clinical course than dogs infected with *P. karlingii*, with some dogs having very slowly progressive lesions for many years. In addition, the hyphae may exhibit some unique cytomorphologic features.[46] In addition to *L. giganteum* f. *caninum* and the *Paralagenidium* pathogens, a previously uncharacterized oomycete was isolated from chronic, ulcerative cutaneous lesions in two cats from Louisiana. Multigene phylogenetic analyses indicate that this pathogen is identical to *L. deciduum*, a novel oomycete isolated from nematodes in Taiwan.[3]

The epidemiologic features of lagenidiosis and paralagenidiosis are similar in many respects to those associated with cutaneous pythiosis. Sporulation and infectivity is thought to be similar to that associated with *P. insidiosum*, causing infection through production of motile aquatic zoospores that adhere to and encyst in damaged tissues. Affected animals are typically young to middle-aged dogs that live in the southeastern United States. Although most affected dogs have lived in Florida or Louisiana, cases in Texas, Tennessee, Alabama, Georgia, South Carolina, Maryland, Virginia, Indiana, and Illinois, as well as Australia have been identified. A number of infected dogs have had frequent exposure to lakes or ponds. None have had historic evidence of immunocompromise or were treated with immunosuppressive therapy before development of the infection.

CLINICAL FEATURES

Dogs with *L. giganteum* f. *caninum* infection are typically evaluated for progressive, multifocal or focal, cutaneous or subcutaneous lesions that involve the extremities, mammary region, perineum, or trunk.[2] These lesions may appear as firm dermal or subcutaneous nodules, or as ulcerated, thickened, edematous areas of deep cellulitis with regions of necrosis and numerous draining tracts (Fig. 88.4). As with cutaneous pythiosis, skin lesions in dogs with lagenidiosis tend to be progressive, locally invasive, and poorly responsive to medical therapy. In contrast to cutaneous pythiosis, dogs with lagenidiosis typically have regional lymphadenopathy and may also have occult lesions in the thorax or abdomen involving the great vessels, sublumbar and/or inguinal lymph nodes, lung, pulmonary hilus, or cranial mediastinum. Animals with great vessel or sublumbar lymph node involvement usually have cutaneous or subcutaneous lesions on the pelvic limbs and often develop pelvic limb edema. Sudden death caused by great vessel rupture and associated hemoabdomen may occur in these animals. A dog from Florida was described that had extension of a mass lesion that involved the right masseter muscle into the brain, with associated forebrain neurologic signs.[47]

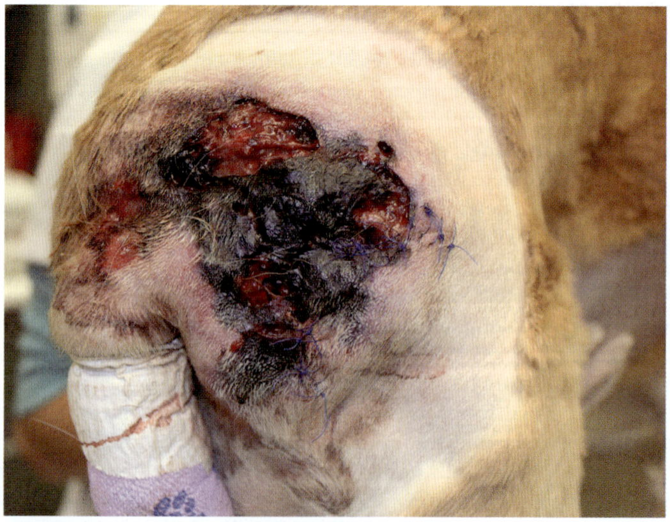

Fig. 88.4 Tailhead mass caused by lagenidiosis in a 9-year-old female spayed mixed-breed dog. Note the extensive tissue necrosis. (Courtesy Amy M. Grooters, Louisiana State University, Baton Rouge, LA.)

In dogs with paralagenidiosis, lesions are characterized by solitary or multifocal dermal nodules or nodular thickening (sometimes without alopecia) or an ulcerative, crusting dermatopathy that may become extensive but rarely invades beyond cutaneous and subcutaneous tissues. Distant lesions in the thorax and abdomen have not been identified, and the clinical course appears to be chronic and slowly progressive. The author observed one dog with paralagenidiosis caused by a clade AG-2015a isolate that had slowly extending, waxing and waning lesions for 8 years. In the one cat with *L. deciduum* infection for which detailed clinical information is available, there was a chronic, pruritic lesion over the caudodorsum that was characterized by miliary dermatitis, alopecia, and crusting that progressed to papules coalescing into erythematous to whitish plaques (personal communication, Drs. Laura Sickafoose and Sandra Merchant, Louisiana State University).

DIAGNOSIS

Because of their clinical, epidemiologic, and histologic similarities to pythiosis, lagenidiosis and paralagenidiosis are often misdiagnosed as pythiosis during routine histologic evaluation. Although there are subtle differences in hyphal size, morphology, and distribution among these infections, histologic lesions associated with lagenidiosis and paralagenidiosis are still often labeled as "suspected pythiosis" or "suspected zygomycosis" during routine evaluation. For this reason, clinicians should always attempt to confirm a suspected histologic diagnosis with culture or molecular diagnostic assays.

Laboratory Abnormalities

Laboratory abnormalities are often absent in dogs with lagenidiosis and paralagenidiosis; when present, they most often include hyperglobulinemia and eosinophilia. Hypercalcemia was associated with *L. giganteum* f. *caninum* infection in one dog with cutaneous lesions on all four limbs and severe lymphadenitis associated with popliteal, inguinal, and superficial cervical lymph nodes.[48]

Imaging Findings

Radiographic imaging of the thorax and sonographic imaging of the abdomen are essential parts of the diagnostic evaluation in dogs suspected to have *L. giganteum* f. *caninum* infection because of the potential for occult lesions in the thorax or abdomen. These may include solitary pulmonary nodules; sublumbar, inguinal, and medial iliac lymphadenopathy; thickening and invasion of the wall of the aorta or caudal vena cava (sometimes with associated aneurysm); and retroperitoneal or epaxial masses. MRI findings in the dog with right masseter muscle infection that extended into the brain included marked patchy hyperintense soft tissue lesions adjacent to the mandible (T1W, T2W, and FLAIR) that exhibited marked heterogeneous contrast enhancement, marked right-sided meningeal enhancement; T2W and FLAIR hyperintense, T1W hypointense, contrast-enhancing regions in the right piriform and temporal lobes; and a mass effect causing deviation of the falx cerebri and right lateral ventricle compression.[47]

Microbiologic Tests

Cytologic Examination

Cytologic examination of lymph node aspirates or impression smears made from draining lesions in dogs with lagenidiosis and paralagenidiosis reveal pyogranulomatous to eosinophilic inflammation with or without negatively staining to rarely basophilic, broad, poorly septate hyphae. Cytologic examination of impression smears from one dog infected with a clade AG-2015a *Paralagenidium* isolate showed hyphae that contained numerous colorless oval internal structures.[46]

Isolation and Identification

The diagnosis of lagenidiosis and paralagenidiosis can only be made by PCR amplification and rRNA gene sequencing performed on DNA extracted from either cultured isolates or infected tissue. Isolation techniques for *Lagenidium* and *Paralagenidium* species are similar to those described for *P. insidiosum*, but with peptone-yeast-glucose (PYG) agar. If PYG agar is not available, blood agar is a reasonable second choice. For best results, small pieces of fresh, nonmacerated tissue are placed directly on the surface of the agar and incubated at 37°C. Growth is typically observed within 24 to 48 hours. Because production of the sexual reproductive structures necessary for morphologic classification has not yet been possible, definitive identification of *Lagenidium* and *Paralagenidium* species is currently based on rRNA gene sequencing. Therefore, this author utilizes a laboratory that is experienced with both culture and amplification/sequencing of pathogenic oomycetes (see Box 88.1, *A*).

Serologic Testing

An ELISA for quantitation of anti–*L. giganteum* f. *caninum* antibodies has been described as a sensitive but nonspecific serologic test for the identification of *L. giganteum* f. *caninum*–infected, and to a lesser degree, *P. karlingii*–infected dogs.[49] Because of extensive cross-reactivity with anti–*P. insidiosum* and anti-*Paralagenidium* antibodies, positive ELISA results are often observed in dogs with pythiosis or paralagenidiosis in addition to those with lagenidiosis. In addition, some dogs with nonfungal dermatopathies have had false-positive results. Because of these limitations, serology should not be used as a basis for the diagnosis of lagenidiosis or paralagenidiosis.

Molecular Diagnosis Using Nucleic Acid–Based Testing

Amplification and sequencing of ribosomal DNA is currently the only diagnostic tool that allows differentiation among *L. giganteum* f. *caninum, P. karlingii*, clade AG-2015a *Paralagenidium* isolates, and *L. deciduum* (although it should be noted that *L. deciduum* infection has only been documented in cats). Molecular methods can be applied to DNA extracted from cultured isolates or from infected tissues.[31] Recently, amplification and sequencing of oomycete DNA from paraffin-embedded tissues using panfungal primers has become routinely available (see Box 88.1, *B*), which allows a diagnosis to still be made when culture was either not performed or was unsuccessful.

Pathologic Findings

Histologically, lagenidiosis and paralagenidiosis share many characteristics with pythiosis, entomophthoromycosis, and mucormycosis. All of these diseases are characterized by pyogranulomatous and eosinophilic inflammation associated with broad, irregularly branching, infrequently septate hyphae with nonparallel walls. Multinucleated giant cells and plasma cells are commonly present. In contrast to *P. insidiosum*, *L. giganteum* f. *caninum* and *Paralagenidium* spp. hyphae are often visible on H&E–stained sections. On GMS-stained sections, numerous broad, thick-walled, irregularly septate hyphae are easily recognized (Fig. 88.5), sometimes with visible round internal structures or a scant to thin eosinophilic sleeve noted around the hyphae. *Lagenidium giganteum* f. *caninum* hyphae typically demonstrate a great deal of variability in size, but in general are larger than *P. insidiosum* and *Paralagenidium* spp. hyphae (diameter range, 7–25 µm; mean, 12 µm).[2] In some sections, hyphae appear as round or bulbous structures, and right-angle branching is occasionally observed. *Paralagenidium* spp. hyphae are closer in diameter to *P. insidiosum*, with a mean diameter of 7.5 µm (range, 3–11 µm).[4,46]

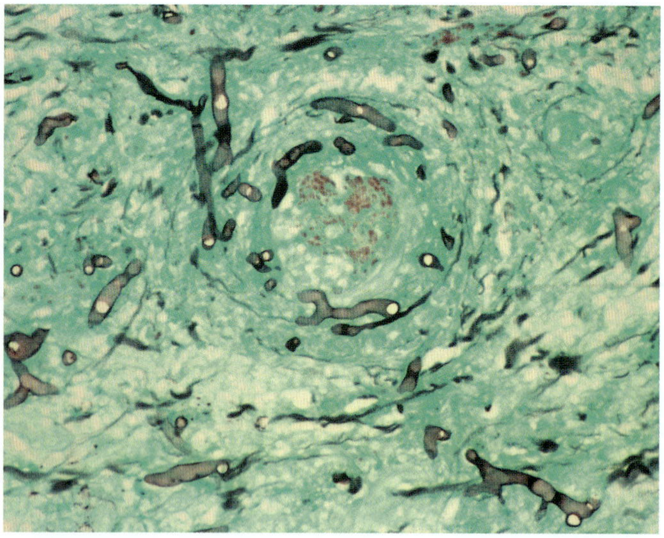

Fig. 88.5 Broad, thick-walled, infrequently septate hyphae associated with granulomatous vasculitis in a lymph node from a dog infected with *Lagenidium giganteum* forma *caninum*. (Courtesy Amy M. Grooters, Louisiana State University, Baton Rouge, LA.)

TREATMENT AND PROGNOSIS

As with pythiosis, aggressive surgical resection of infected tissues is the treatment of choice for lagenidiosis and paralagenidiosis when disease is confined to a resectable cutaneous lesion. For *L. giganteum* f. *caninum* infection, because occult systemic lesions are common, radiographic imaging of the chest and abdomen and sonographic imaging of the abdomen should be performed to determine the extent of disease prior to attempting surgical resection of cutaneous lesions. Unfortunately, the vast majority of dogs with lagenidiosis have nonresectable disease in the thorax, abdomen, or regional lymph nodes by the time the initial diagnosis is made. Because response to medical therapy is uniformly poor, the disease is routinely fatal.

In contrast, for dogs infected with paralagenidiosis, surgery that achieves 3- to 5-cm margins is often curative. As with pythiosis and lagenidiosis, medical therapy is usually ineffective in resolving lesions.[46] However, it may slow progression of the disease to a point that improves quality of life. The author is aware of one dog with recurrent multifocal cutaneous lesions due to paralagenidiosis in which treatment with a combination of itraconazole (10 mg/kg, PO, q24h) and terbinafine (5 to 10 mg/kg, PO, q24h) along with repeated aggressive surgical resection was curative. One dog with cutaneous *P. karlingii* infection of the perianal region was treated successfully with a combination of mefenoxam (8 mg/kg, PO, q24h; see Pythiosis), minocycline (10 mg/kg, PO, q12h), prednisone (0.5 mg/kg, q24h, tapered over 4 weeks), and hyperbaric oxygen therapy, followed by aggressive surgical resection.[50] The one cat with *L. deciduum* infection for which clinical information is available was poorly responsive to treatment in the short-term, but was not available for long-term follow-up, so no information about long-term response or prognosis is available.

PUBLIC HEALTH ASPECTS

Infections caused by *Lagenidium* and *Paralagenidium* species are acquired from the environment. Although there is no evidence to suggest that transmission between mammalian hosts is possible, routine precautions (such as wearing gloves when handling infected tissues or exudate) should be followed.

ENTOMOPHTHOROMYCOSIS AND MUCORMYCOSIS (PREVIOUSLY TOGETHER REFERRED TO AS ZYGOMYCOSIS)

ETIOLOGY AND EPIDEMIOLOGY

The term "zygomycosis" has been used to refer to disease caused by pathogenic fungi of the genera *Basidiobolus* and *Conidiobolus* (order Entomophthorales) and the genera *Rhizopus, Absidia, Mucor, Saksenaea, Cokeromyces*, and others (order Mucorales). These two orders were previously grouped in the phylum Zygomycota. Subsequent molecular studies led to reclassification of these fungi, placing the Entomophthorales within the phylum Zoopagomycota, and the Mucorales within the phylum Mucormycota. Therefore, although the term "zygomycosis" may continue to be used colloquially by pathologists and clinicians for some time, it is taxonomically obsolete, and should be replaced by the more specific and current terms "entomophthoromycosis" (also known as "entomophthoramycosis") and "mucormycosis."

In human patients, the Entomophthorales typically cause chronic localized infections in subcutaneous tissue or nasal submucosa of immunocompetent patients that reside in tropical or subtropical locations,[51] whereas the Mucorales tend to cause acute, rapidly progressive disease in debilitated or immunocompromised individuals or in immunocompetent individuals following trauma.[52] In veterinary patients, entomophthoromycosis is more common than mucormycosis, and is typically associated with infections caused by *Basidiobolus* and *Conidiobolus* spp., which are saprophytes commonly found in soil and decaying plant matter. Cutaneous infection with *Basidiobolus* or *Conidiobolus* spp. likely occurs by percutaneous inoculation of spores via minor trauma or insect bites. Infection may also result from inhalation or ingestion of spores. Culture-confirmed infections caused by pathogens in the order Mucorales have been described in only a small number of dogs and cats with a range of clinical presentations and underlying clinical conditions, making general characterizations of etiology difficult.

CLINICAL FEATURES

Entomophthoromycosis

In dogs, humans, horses, sheep, and other mammalian species, conidiobolomycosis occurs most often as a nasopharyngeal infection with or without local dissemination into tissues of the face, retropharyngeal region, and retrobulbar space. Manifestations of infection in dogs may include nasal or facial swelling or deformity, nasal discharge, ulceration of the nasal planum or hard palate, exophthalmos, chemosis, ocular discharge, and sometimes skin lesions near the eye (Fig. 88.6). In animals with retrobulbar disease that extends into the brain, neurologic signs may occur. *Conidiobolus* infection has been described in a single dog as a cause of multifocal nodular draining subcutaneous lesions and regional lymphadenopathy[53] and as a cause of pneumonia in a dog that was receiving chemotherapy.[54] Basidiobolomycosis is a rare cause of ulcerative skin lesions in dogs and has also been reported as a cause of respiratory disease in a dog.[55] It has also been reported to cause segmental GI disease with clinical features similar to those associated with GI pythiosis. *Basidiobolus ranarum* was described as a cause of a colonic mass in a shiba dog from Japan[56] and of colorectal disease in a French bulldog from central Louisiana.[38] *Basidiobolus microsporus* was identified in the feces of a boxer dog from Texas with colonic disease caused by *P. insidiosum*, but the clinical significance of the presence of *B. microsporus* was unclear.[57] Disseminated *Basidiobolus* infection involving the GI tract and other abdominal organs has been described in two dogs.[13,58]

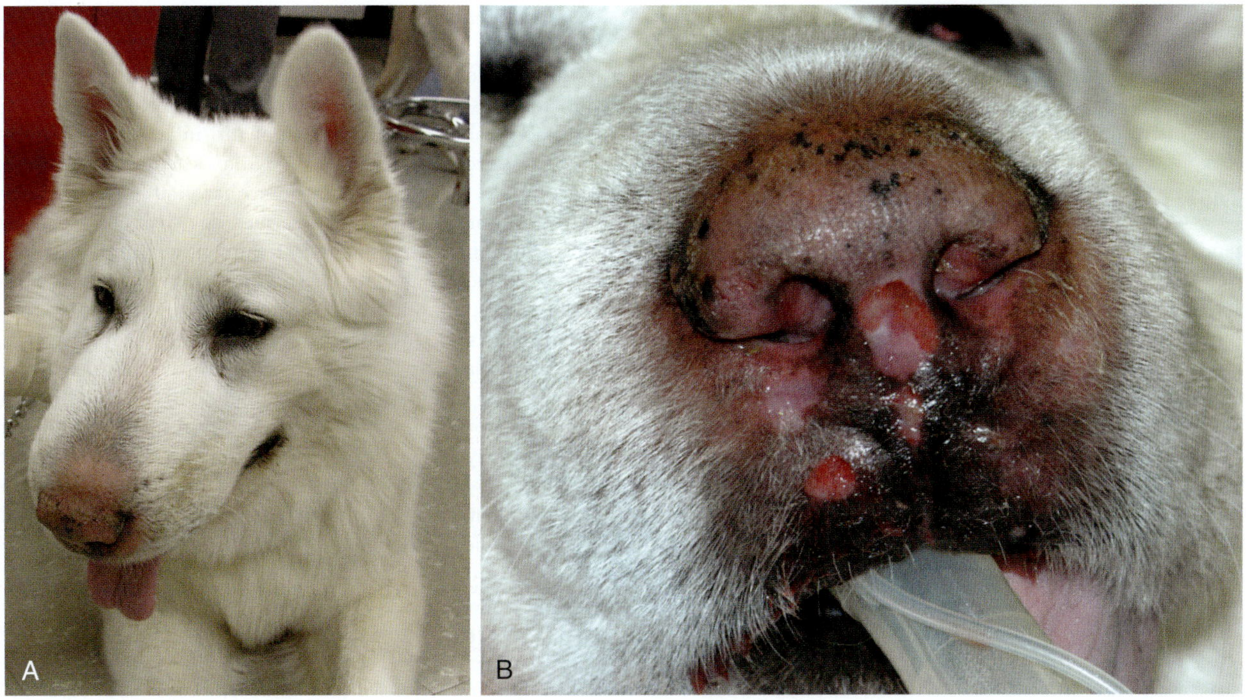

Fig. 88.6 (A) Nasopharyngeal *Conidiobolus* spp. infection in a 4-year-old male neutered German shepherd dog. (B) Note the severe swelling of the nose and muzzle and ulceration of the nasal planum. (Courtesy Amy M. Grooters, Louisiana State University, Baton Rouge, LA.)

Mucormycosis

In dogs and cats, culture-confirmed cases of mucormycosis are sparse and have been limited to single case reports. *Rhizomucor* was identified as the cause of duodenal perforation in a 7-month-old Persian cat,[59] and *Cokeromyces recurvatus* was isolated from abdominal fluid in a 16-year-old cat following jejunal perforation secondary to intestinal lymphoma.[60] *Rhizomucor pusillus* infection was associated with cerebral disease in a cat from France.[61] A subcutaneous mass caused by a *Mucor* species on the dorsum of the nose of a 14-year-old cat was treated successfully with posaconazole.[62] In dogs, infection by *Saksenaea vasiformis* was described in association with ulcerative cellulitis on the distal thoracic limb of a dog, and *C. recurvatus* was associated with the colonic mucosa in a dog with protein-losing enteropathy.[63]

DIAGNOSIS

Because of their histologic similarities, entomophthoromycosis and mucormycosis are often confused with pythiosis (which is much more common) when tissue biopsies are evaluated. Unfortunately, there are no serologic or immunohistochemical techniques that are routinely available for the differentiation of these infections, making identification of infected animals reliant on fungal culture of fresh tissues or ribosomal DNA amplification and sequencing from infected tissues.

Laboratory and Imaging Abnormalities

Laboratory abnormalities are not well described in animals with entomophthoromycosis or mucormycosis and would be expected to vary with the wide range of potential clinical presentations. Diagnostic imaging in the form of computed tomography often provides important information about the location and extent of disease in animals with nasopharyngeal and retrobulbar lesions caused by *Conidiobolus* spp. In addition, ocular ultrasonography may help to characterize the extent of disease in dogs with retrobulbar lesions.

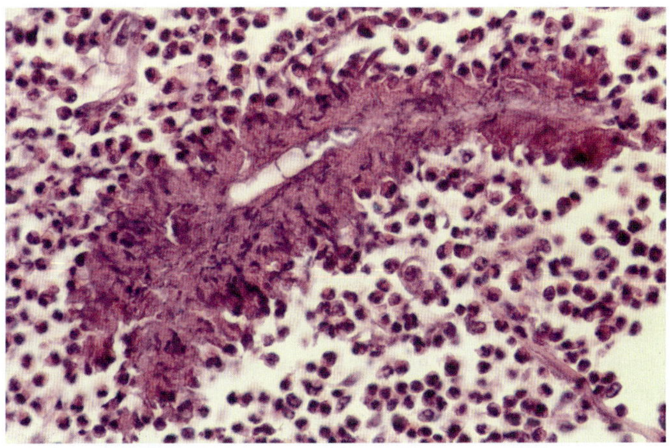

Fig. 88.7 *Conidiobolus* spp. hyphae in a tissue biopsy from an ulcerated palate lesion in a 3-year-old female boxer. Note the large amount of amorphous eosinophilic material (sleeve) surrounding the hyphal segment; hematoxylin and eosin stain. (Courtesy Amy M. Grooters, Louisiana State University, Baton Rouge, LA.)

Cytologic and Histologic Findings

The cytologic and histologic features of entomophthoromycosis and mucormycosis are similar to those associated with pythiosis and lagenidiosis. On GMS-stained sections, hyphae are broad, thin-walled, and occasionally septate. The histologic hallmark of entomophthoromycosis is the presence of a wide (2.5–25 μm) eosinophilic sleeve that surrounds the hyphae and makes them easily located on H&E-stained sections (Fig. 88.7). This finding may help to differentiate entomophthoromycosis from pythiosis and lagenidiosis, in which eosinophilic sleeves tend to be thin or absent. The hyphal diameter is also significantly larger for *Basidiobolus* spp. (mean 9 μm; range, 5–20 μm) and *Conidiobolus* spp. (mean 8 μm; range, 5–13 μm) than for *P. insidiosum* (mean, 4 μm; range, 2–7 μm).[64] Histologic features of mucormycosis vary because of the more numerous genera in this group. *Cokeromyces recurvatus* is a dimorphic fungus that may appear in cytologic or histologic specimens as unique, very large (30–90 μm), spherical, thick-walled yeasts that are often confused with *Coccidioides* spp. spherules.[60,63,65]

TREATMENT AND PROGNOSIS

Recommendations for the treatment of entomophthoromycosis and mucormycosis are not straightforward because attempted therapy has only been described in a few patients with culture-confirmed diagnoses. Although anecdotal information as well as a small number of cases in the literature suggest that cutaneous entomophthoromycosis may be less aggressive than cutaneous pythiosis or lagenidiosis, progression of lesions and sometimes even dissemination despite treatment have also been observed in *Conidiobolus* or *Basidiobolus*-infected dogs. The author's current recommendation for dogs with nasopharyngeal conidiobolomycosis is treatment with itraconazole (10 mg/kg, PO, q24h) for 12–18 months. Recurrence is common after medication is discontinued, so a prolonged course is usually prescribed. Newer oral azoles such as posaconazole would also be reasonable choices and may have better efficacy but may be more expensive. Cutaneous entomophthoromycosis in small animal patients should be treated with aggressive surgical resection of infected tissues whenever possible, followed by itraconazole therapy for at least 3 months, especially if 3- to 5-cm margins cannot be achieved. If resection is not possible, treatment with itraconazole, voriconazole, or posaconazole for 6 to 18 months should be recommended. In dogs with GI basidiobolomycosis, guidelines based on the human medical literature would suggest that resectable lesions should be treated with a combination of surgical resection with wide margins followed by itraconazole therapy for 6 months. For nonresectable lesions, a combination of anti-inflammatory doses of prednisone (as recommended for GI pythiosis) combined with long-term itraconazole, voriconazole, or posaconazole therapy is recommended by the author. The recently described dog with colorectal basidiobolomycosis initially responded to treatment with itraconazole, terbinafine, and prednisone, with nearly complete resolution of clinical signs and sonographic lesions.[38] However, therapy was discontinued after only 15 weeks and the dog died with metastatic neoplasia 3 weeks later. Despite the lack of gross lesions at necropsy, fungal organisms were identified on histopathologic examination of rectal tissues, emphasizing the importance of long-term antifungal therapy in these patients. For mucormycosis, lipid-complexed amphotericin B or posaconazole are generally recommended for treatment of human patients.[52,66] In veterinary patients, this author would consider posaconazole the treatment of choice, although data supporting this choice is largely based on information from human patients.

PUBLIC HEALTH ASPECTS

Entomophthoromycosis and mucormycosis are rare in human patients. Infections are acquired from the environment. There is no evidence to suggest that transmission between mammalian hosts occurs, provided normal precautions are followed.

CASE EXAMPLE

Signalment

"Jasper," an 18-month-old intact male Labrador retriever from central Louisiana.

History

Jasper was evaluated for a 1-month history of frequent vomiting and persistent diarrhea and a 2-week history of intermittent anorexia. In addition, the owner reported that the dog had lost approximately 6 kg. The diarrhea was watery and yellowish-brown and was produced in large quantity; hematochezia had not been noted. A fecal flotation and heartworm antigen test performed by the referring veterinarian 1 week before the dog was evaluated at the author's institution had been negative. Treatment with metronidazole (17 mg/kg, PO, q12h) and a change to an easily digestible prescription diet had failed to improve the vomiting and diarrhea. The patient was a field trial dog used for duck and dove hunting in central Louisiana. He frequently worked in rice fields and occasionally in bodies of fresh water and was generally housed in an outdoor kennel.

Physical Examination

Body weight: 30 kg.

General: Bright, alert, and responsive. Body temperature = 102.7°F (39.2°C), HR = 110 beats/minute, RR = 20 breaths/minute, mucous membranes pink, CRT ~ 2 seconds.

Eyes, ears, nose, and throat: No significant abnormalities were noted.

Musculoskeletal: The dog was underweight with a BCS of 3/9.

Cardiovascular and respiratory: Strong femoral pulses. No murmurs or arrhythmias were auscultated. Respiratory rate and effort were normal.

GI and genitourinary: The patient showed signs of discomfort during abdominal palpation; a large, firm, tubular mass was palpated in the midabdomen. Mild prostatomegaly was detected on rectal examination.

Lymph nodes: All palpable peripheral lymph nodes were normal in size and shape.

Laboratory Findings

CBC: HCT 33.7% (37%–55%), MCV 61.7 fL (62–77 fL), MCHC 20.8 g/dL (32–37 g/dL), WBC 10,600 cells/μL (8,000–14,500 cells/μL), neutrophils 6,200 cells/μL (3,000–11,500 cells/μL), lymphocytes 1,700 cells/μL (1,000–4,800 cells/μL), monocytes 1,100 cells/μL (100–1,400 cells/μL), platelets 254,000/μL (220,000–600,000 platelets/μL).

Serum chemistry profile: Sodium 142 mmol/L (140–153 mmol/L), potassium 4.4 mmol/L (3.8–5.5 mmol/L), chloride 110 mmol/L (107–115 mmol/L), bicarbonate 20 mmol/L (17–27 mmol/L), phosphorus 4.6 mg/dL (3.4–6.3 mg/dL), calcium 9.1 mg/dL (9.4–11.4 mg/dL), BUN 11 mg/dL (8–22 mg/dL), creatinine 0.7 mg/dL (0.5–1.7 mg/dL), glucose 96 mg/dL (80–115 mg/dL), total protein 5.7 g/dL (5.8–7.5 g/dL), albumin 2.0 g/dL (2.6–4.2 g/dL), globulin 3.7 g/dL (2.5–4.0 g/dL), ALT 34 U/L (0–60 U/L), AST 22 U/L (0–50 U/L), ALP 13 U/L (0–100 U/L), creatine kinase 134 U/L (0–200 U/L), cholesterol 158 mg/dL (150–240 mg/dL), total bilirubin 0.2 mg/dL (0–0.4 mg/dL).

Urinalysis: SpG 1.041, pH 7.5, 3+ protein, 3+ bilirubin, negative hemoglobin, negative glucose, negative ketones, 0–5 WBC/HPF, 0 RBC/HPF, many lipid droplets.

Imaging Findings

Plain abdominal radiographs: There was a generalized loss of serosal detail in the abdomen. Gas was present in the GI tract, but there was no evidence of abnormal intestinal tract dilation.

Abdominal ultrasound: A severely thickened segment of small bowel could be visualized extending from the cranial to the caudal abdomen. The wall of this bowel segment measured 1.1 cm in thickness and lacked normal layering (Fig. 88.8A). Mesenteric lymph nodes were enlarged and heterogeneous (Fig. 88.8B). There was a small amount of free abdominal fluid.

Cytologic Findings

Cytologic evaluation of ultrasound-guided mesenteric lymph node aspirates revealed reactive lymphoid hyperplasia. Examination of ultrasound-guided aspirates of

CASE EXAMPLE—cont'd

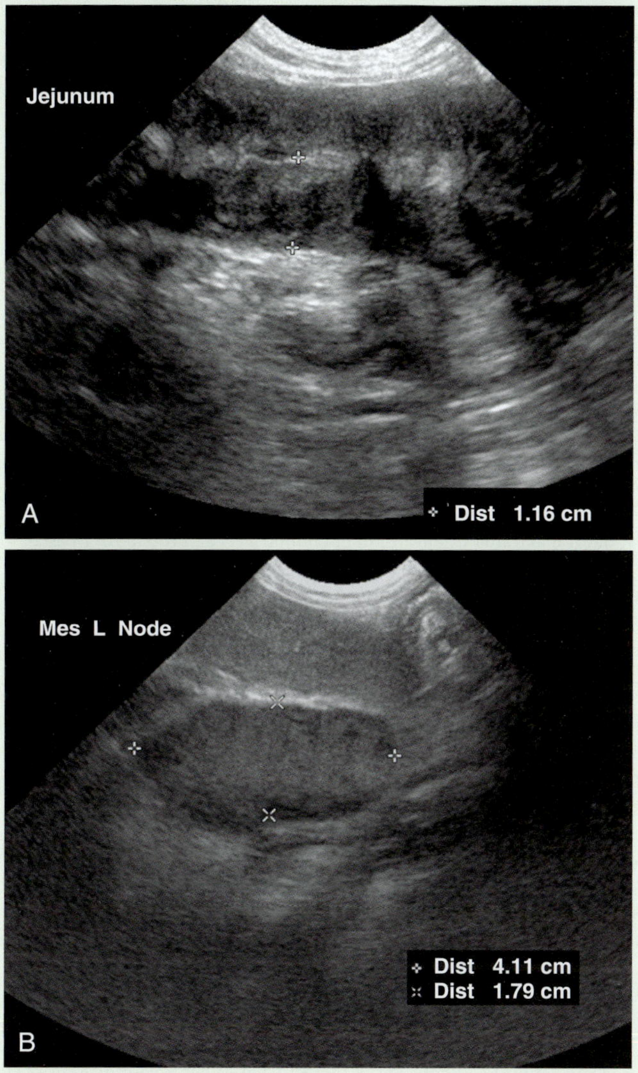

Fig. 88.8 Sonographic images of the abdomen of the dog described in the case example. Note the severe thickening and loss of layering in the wall of the jejunum (A) and the enlarged, heterogeneous appearance of the mesenteric lymph node (B).

the thickened segment of bowel showed that the cellularity was too low for cytologic evaluation.

Serologic Findings

ELISA serology for anti–*P. insidiosum* antibodies: Positive at 69%. Results of this assay are expressed as percent positivity in comparison with a strong positive control sample, with values > 40% positivity having been shown to be highly specific for pythiosis in dogs. Values in healthy dogs range from 3% to 15%.[37]

Diagnosis

Jejunal pythiosis.

Treatment

Abdominal exploratory examination revealed a 50-cm segment of the midjejunum that was severely thickened and firm. This segment was resected with 5-cm margins. After an uneventful postoperative recovery, the dog's vomiting, diarrhea, and anorexia resolved quickly. He was treated with itraconazole (10 mg/kg, PO, q24h) and terbinafine (8.3 mg/kg, PO, q24h) for 2 months in an effort to decrease the chance of recurrence of disease at the site of resection. Liver enzyme activities and serum bilirubin concentration were monitored during this time and remained within reference intervals.

Histopathologic Findings

Both the resected segment of jejunum as well as jejunal and ileocolic lymph nodes were submitted for histologic examination. Results revealed severe transmural eosinophilic pyogranulomatous enteritis and lymphoid hyperplasia. In the jejunal lesion, wide (3–8 μm), poorly septate hyphae with nonparallel walls were visualized on GMS-stained sections. No organisms were observed in the lymph node sections.

Follow-Up

At reevaluation 2 months after resection of the jejunal lesion, the dog remained free of clinical signs and had gained 3 kg body weight. Reevaluation of anti–*P. insidiosum* antibody serology at that time yielded a percent positivity of 20%. Because the rapid decrease in antibody levels from 69% to 20% was strongly suggestive of a surgical cure of GI pythiosis, oral antifungal medications were discontinued. Reevaluation of anti–*P. insidiosum* antibody serology 2 years later yielded results within the range observed in healthy dogs (6%).

Comments

Although most dogs with GI pythiosis have nonresectable lesions, those with midjejunal lesions can often be surgically cured. Preoperative abdominal ultrasound is essential since it helps to determine whether or not a GI lesion might be surgically resectable. Postoperative medical therapy was probably not necessary in the case described here since the postoperative clinical course and follow-up serology results strongly supported a surgical cure. In the author's experience, most dogs with a midjejunal lesion are surgically cured when the surgeon is confident that greater than 5-cm margins of healthy tissue were obtained with the resection and lymph node histology shows hyperplasia rather than infection. In such cases, medical treatment with itraconazole and terbinafine can be offered as optional but likely unnecessary therapy for 2 months until follow-up serology is performed.

SUGGESTED READINGS

Reagan KL, Marks SL, Pesavento PA, et al. Successful management of 3 dogs with colonic pythiosis using itraconzaole, terbinafine, and prednisone. *J Vet Intern Med*. 2019;33:1434–1439.

Marclay M, Langohr IM, Gaschen FP, et al. Colorectal basidiobolomycosis in a dog. *J Vet Intern Med*. 2020;34:2091–2095.

Dehghanpir SD, Bemis DA, Kania SA, et al. What is your diagnosis? Dermal nodules in a dog. *Vet Clin Pathol*. 2019;48:496–498.

REFERENCES

1. Smith F. The pathology of bursattee. *Vet J*. 1884;19:16–17.
2. Grooters AM, Hodgin EC, Bauer RW, et al. Clinicopathologic findings associated with *Lagenidium* sp. infection in 6 dogs: initial description of an emerging oomycosis. *J Vet Intern Med*. 2003;17:637–646.
3. Spies CFJ, Grooters AM, Levesque CA, et al. Molecular phylogeny and taxonomy of *Lagenidium*-like oomycetes pathogenic to mammals. *Fungal Biol*. 2016;120:931–947.

4. Grooters AM, Proia LA, Sutton D, et al. Characterization of a previously undescribed *Lagenidium* pathogen associated with soft tissue infection: initial description of a new human oomycosis. In: *Focus on Fungal Infections*. Vol. 14. ; 2004:174. New Orleans, LA.
5. Kwon-Chung KJ. Phylogenetic spectrum of fungi that are pathogenic to humans. *Clin Infect Dis*. 1994;19(suppl 1):S1–S7.
6. Grooters AM. Pythiosis, lagenidiosis, and zygomycosis in small animals. *Vet Clin North Am Small Anim Pract*. 2003;33:695–720.
7. Hibbett DS, Binder M, Bischoff JF, et al. A higher-level phylogenetic classification of the Fungi. *Mycol Res*. 2007;111:509–547.
8. Ibrahim AS, Edwards JEJ, Filler SG, et al. Mucormycosis and entomophthoramycosis (zygomycosis). In: Kauffman C, Pappas P, Sobel J, Dismukes W, eds. *Essentials of Clinical Mycology*. New York, NY: Springer; 2010.
9. Gaastra W, Lipman LJ, De Cock AW, et al. *Pythium insidiosum*: an overview. *Vet Microbiol*. 2010;146:1–16.
10. Mendoza L, Hernandez F, Ajello L. Life cycle of the human and animal oomycete pathogen *Pythium insidiosum*. *J Clin Microbiol*. 1993;31:2967–2973.
11. Berryessa NA, Marks SL, Pesavento PA, et al. Gastrointestinal pythiosis in 10 dogs from California. *J Vet Intern Med*. 2008;22:1065–1069.
12. Reagan KL, Marks SL, Pesavento PA, et al. Successful management of 3 dogs with colonic pythiosis using itraconzaole, terbinafine, and prednisone. *J Vet Intern Med*. 2019;33:1434–1439.
13. Miller RI. Gastrointestinal phycomycosis in 63 dogs. *J Am Vet Med Assoc*. 1985;186:473–478.
14. Kepler D, Cole R, Lee-Fowler T, et al. Pulmonary pythiosis in a canine patient. *Vet Radiol Ultrasound*. 2019;60:E20–E23.
15. Foil CSO, Short BG, Fadok VA, et al. A report of subcutaneous pythiosis in five dogs and a review of the etiologic agent *Pythium* spp. *J Am Anim Hosp Assoc*. 1984;20:959–966.
16. Fischer JR, Pace LW, Turk JR, et al. Gastrointestinal pythiosis in Missouri dogs: eleven cases. *J Vet Diagn Invest*. 1994;6:380–382.
17. Patton CS, Hake R, Newton J, et al. Esophagitis due to *Pythium insidiosum* infection in two dogs. *J Vet Intern Med*. 1996;10:139–142.
18. Rakich PM, Grooters AM, Tang KN. Gastrointestinal pythiosis in two cats. *J Vet Diagn Invest*. 2005;17:262–269.
19. Fortin JS, Calcutt MJ, Kim DY. Sublingual pythiosis in a cat. *Acta Vet Scand*. 2017;59:63.
20. Souto EPF, Maia LA, Virginio JP, et al. Pythiosis in cats in northeastern Brazil. *J Mycol Med*. 2020;30:101005.
21. Oldenhoff W, Grooters A, Pinkerton ME, et al. Cutaneous pythiosis in two dogs from Wisconsin, USA. *Vet Dermatol*. 2014;25:52. e21.
22. Thomas RC, Lewis DT. Pythiosis in dogs and cats. *Compend Contin Ed Pract Vet*. 1998;20:63–74.
23. Bissonnette KW, Sharp NJ, Dykstra MH, et al. Nasal and retrobulbar mass in a cat caused by *Pythium insidiosum*. *J Med Vet Mycol*. 1991;29:39–44.
24. LeBlanc CJ, Echandi RL, Moore RR, et al. Hypercalcemia associated with gastric pythiosis in a dog. *Vet Clin Pathol*. 2008;37:115–120.
25. Graham JP, Newell SM, Roberts GD, et al. Ultrasonographic features of canine gastrointestinal pythiosis. *Vet Radiol Ultrasound*. 2000;41:273–277.
26. Thieman KM, Kirkby KA, Flynn-Lurie A, et al. Diagnosis and treatment of truncal cutaneous pythiosis in a dog. *J Am Vet Med Assoc*. 2011;239:1232–1235.
27. Grooters AM, Whittington A, Lopez MK, et al. Evaluation of microbial culture techniques for the isolation of *Pythium insidiosum* from equine tissues. *J Vet Diagn Invest*. 2002;14:288–294.
28. Grooters AM, Gee MK. Development of a nested polymerase chain reaction assay for the detection and identification of *Pythium insidiosum*. *J Vet Intern Med*. 2002;16:147–152.
29. Mani R, Vilela R, Kettler N, et al. Identification of *Pythium insidiosum* complex by matrix-assisted laser desorption ionization-time of flight mass spectrometry. *J Med Microbiol*. 2019;68:574–584.
30. Bernheim D, Dupont D, Aptel F, et al. Pythiosis: case report leading to new features in clinical and diagnostic management of this fungal-like infection. *Int J Infect Dis*. 2019;86:40–43.
31. Znajda NR, Grooters AM, Marsella R. PCR-based detection of *Pythium* and *Lagenidium* DNA in frozen and ethanol-fixed animal tissues. *Vet Dermatol*. 2002;13:187–194.
32. Kulandai LT, Lakshmipathy D, Sargunam J. Novel duplex polymerase chain reaction for the rapid detection of *Pythium insidiosum* directly from corneal specimens of patients with ocular pythiosis. *Cornea*. 2020;39:775–778.
33. Htun ZM, Rotchanapreeda T, Rujirawat T, et al. Loop-mediated isothermal amplification (LAMP) for identification of *Pythium insidiosum*. *Int J Infect Dis*. 2020;101:149–159.
34. Babouee Flury B, Weisser M, Prince SS, et al. Performances of two different panfungal PCRs to detect mould DNA in formalin-fixed paraffin-embedded tissue: what are the limiting factors? *BMC Infect Dis*. 2014;14:692.
35. Bernhardt A, von Bomhard W, Antweiler E, et al. Molecular identification of fungal pathogens in nodular skin lesions of cats. *Med Mycol*. 2015;53:132–144.
36. Meason-Smith C, Edwards EE, Older CE, et al. Panfungal polymerase chain reaction for identification of fungal pathogens in formalin-fixed animal tissues. *Vet Pathol*. 2017;54:640–648.
37. Grooters AM, Leise BS, Lopez MK, et al. Development and evaluation of an enzyme-linked immunosorbent assay for the serodiagnosis of pythiosis in dogs. *J Vet Intern Med*. 2002;16:142–146.
38. Marclay M, Langohr IM, Gaschen FP, et al. Colorectal basidiobolomycosis in a dog. *J Vet Intern Med*. 2020;34:2091–2095.
39. Jaturapaktrarak C, Payattikul P, Lohnoo T, et al. Protein A/G-based enzyme-linked immunosorbent assay for detection of anti-*Pythium insidiosum* antibodies in human and animal subjects. *BMC Res Notes*. 2020;13:135.
40. Intaramat A, Sornprachum T, Chantrathonkul B, et al. Protein A/G-based immunochromatographic test for serodiagnosis of pythiosis in human and animal subjects from Asia and Americas. *Med Mycol*. 2016;54:641–647.
41. Dycus DL, Fisher C, Butler R. Surgical and medical treatment of pyloric and duodenal pythiosis in a dog. *J Am Anim Hosp Assoc*. 2015;51:385–391.
42. Hummel J, Grooters A, Davidson G, et al. Successful management of gastrointestinal pythiosis in a dog using itraconazole, terbinafine, and mefenoxam. *Med Mycol*. 2011;49:539–542.
43. Cridge H, Hughes SM, Langston VC, et al. Mefenoxam, itraconazole, and terbinafine combination therapy for management of pythiosis in dogs (six cases). *J Am Anim Hosp Assoc*. 2020;56:307.
44. Hubert JD, Grooters AM. Treatment of equine pythiosis. *Compend Contin Ed Pract Vet*. 2002;13:187–194.
45. Wanachiwanawin W, Mendoza L, Visuthisakchai S, et al. Efficacy of immunotherapy using antigens of *Pythium insidiosum* in the treatment of vascular pythiosis in humans. *Vaccine*. 2004;22:3613–3621.
46. Dehghanpir SD, Bemis DA, Kania SA, et al. What is your diagnosis? Dermal nodules in a dog. *Vet Clin Pathol*. 2019;48:496–498.
47. Shmalberg J, Moyle PS, Craft WF, et al. Severe meningoencephalitis secondary to calvarial invasion of *Lagenidium giganteum* forma *caninum* in a dog. *Open Vet J*. 2020;10:31–38.
48. Nett CS, Grooters AM, LeBlanc CJ, et al. Case Report: Hypercalcemia associated with disseminated *Lagenidium* sp infection in a dog. In: *5th World Congress of Veterinary Dermatology*; 2004. Vienna, Austria.
49. Hartfield JN, Grooters AM, Waite KJ. Development and evaluation of an ELISA for the quantitation of anti-*Lagenidium giganteum* forma *caninum* antibodies in dogs. *J Vet Intern Med*. 2014;28:1479–1484.
50. White AG, Smart K, Hathcock T, et al. Successful management of cutaneous paralagenidiosis in a dog treated with mefenoxam, minocycline, prednisone, and hyperbaric oxygen therapy. *Med Mycol Case Rep*. 2020;29:38–42.
51. Shaikh N, Hussain KA, Petraitiene R, et al. Entomophthoramycosis: a neglected tropical mycosis. *Clin Microbiol Infect*. 2016;22:688–694.
52. Bonifaz A, Tirado-Sánchez A, Calderón L, et al. Cutaneous mucormycosis: mycological, clinical, and therapeutic aspects. *Curr Fungal Infect Rep*. 2015;9:229–237.
53. Hillier A, Kunkle GA, Ginn PE, et al. Canine subcutaneous zygomycosis caused by *Conidiobolus* sp: a case report and review of *Conidiobolus* infections in other species. *Vet Dermatol*. 1994;5:205–213.
54. Hawkins EC, Grooters AM, Cowgill ES, et al. Treatment of *Conidiobolus* sp. pneumonia with itraconazole in a dog receiving immunosuppressive therapy. *J Vet Intern Med*. 2006;20:1479–1482.

55. Greene CE, Brockus CW, Currin MP, et al. Infection with *Basidiobolus ranarum* in two dogs. *J Am Vet Med Assoc.* 2002;221:528–532. 500.
56. Okada K, Amano S, Kawamura Y, et al. Gastrointestinal basidiobolomycosis in a dog. *J Vet Med Sci.* 2015;77:1311–1313.
57. Parambeth JC, Lawhon SD, Mansell J, et al. Gastrointestinal pythiosis with concurrent presumptive gastrointestinal basidiobolomycosis in a Boxer dog. *Vet Clin Pathol.* 2019;48:83–88.
58. Miller RI, Turnwald GH. Disseminated basidiobolomycosis in a dog. *Vet Pathol.* 1984;21:117–119.
59. Cunha SC, Aguero C, Damico CB, et al. Duodenal perforation caused by *Rhizomucor* species in a cat. *J Feline Med Surg.* 2011;13:205–207.
60. Nielsen C, Sutton DA, Matise I, et al. Isolation of *Cokeromyces recurvatus*, initially misidentified as *Coccidioides immitis*, from peritoneal fluid in a cat with jejunal perforation. *J Vet Diagn Invest.* 2005;17:372–378.
61. Ravisse P, Fromentin H, Destombes P, et al. Cerebral mucormycosis in the cat caused by *Mucor pusillus*. *Sabouraudia.* 1978;16:291–298.
62. Wray JD, Sparkes AH, Johnson EM. Infection of the subcutis of the nose in a cat caused by *Mucor* species: successful treatment using posaconazole. *J Feline Med Surg.* 2008;10:523–527.
63. Parker VJ, Jergens AE, Whitley EM, et al. Isolation of *Cokeromyces recurvatus* from the gastrointestinal tract in a dog with protein-losing enteropathy. *J Vet Diagn Invest.* 2011;23:1014–1016.
64. Miller RI, Campbell RS. The comparative pathology of equine cutaneous phycomycosis. *Vet Pathol.* 1984;21:325–332.
65. Ryan LJ, Ferrieri P, Powell Jr RD, et al. Fatal *Cokeromyces recurvatus* pneumonia: report of a case highlighting the potential for histopathologic misdiagnosis as coccidioides. *Int J Surg Pathol.* 2011;19:373–376.
66. Lamoth F, Kontoyiannis DP. Therapeutic challenges of non-aspergillus invasive mold infections in immunosuppressed patients. *Antimicrob Agents Chemother.* 2019;63:e01244-19.

89

Pneumocystosis

Remo Lobetti, Jane E. Sykes

KEY POINTS

- First Described: *Pneumocystis* was first discovered in Brazil in 1909 (Chagas), when it was initially mistaken for a trypanosome. It was first reported in dogs in the 1950s.
- Causes: *Pneumocystis* spp. (an Ascomycete).
- Affected Hosts: Dogs, humans, pigs, horses, goats, nonhuman primates.
- Geographic Distribution: Worldwide.
- Mode of Transmission: Opportunistic invasion of immunosuppressed hosts after aerosol transmission.
- Major Clinical Signs: Weight loss, respiratory distress, exercise intolerance, variable cough.
- Differential Diagnoses: Bacterial pneumonia, mycobacterial infections, other fungal causes of pneumonia, diffuse pulmonary neoplasia, parasitic lung disease.
- Human Health Significance: Severely immunocompromised humans are at risk for pneumocystosis, but only *Pneumocystis jirovecii* infects humans. Whether humans can become colonized with *Pneumocystis* strains that can infect dogs is not known.

ETIOLOGIC AGENT AND EPIDEMIOLOGY

Pneumocystis carinii, the etiologic agent of pneumocystosis, occurs worldwide and infects virtually all mammalian species, including humans. *Pneumocystis* is a saprophyte of low virulence that exists in temperate and tropical climates at altitudes up to 5,000 feet. Its primary habitat is the mammalian lung where it causes opportunistic pneumonia. Clinical pneumonia has been reported to occur spontaneously in dogs, pigs, horses, goats, primates, and humans. Subclinical or latent infections are common in rats, mice, guinea pigs, rabbits, cats, sheep, and various wild animals. Most reports of clinical *Pneumocystis* pneumonia are linked with documented or suspected immunodeficiency syndromes in the host. In humans with AIDS within the United States, it has been the most important opportunistic infection, occurring in 60% of patients over the course of disease.[1] With the availability of effective antiretroviral drugs but increased use of potent immunosuppressive drugs, *Pneumocystis* infections are now emerging as a serious problem in non-HIV-infected humans that are being treated with immunosuppressive or cytotoxic drugs.

Previously, *Pneumocystis* was classified as a unicellular protozoan (phylum Sarcomastigophora). However, ultrastructurally the reproductive behavior of *Pneumocystis* is similar to the ascospore formation of yeast cells, and its organelles and staining properties by light microscopy resemble those of pathogenic fungi. Phylogenetic classification based on 16S-like rRNA sequences indicates that *Pneumocystis* is most closely related to the fungi of the class Ascomycetes, especially *Saccharomyces cerevisiae*, and so it has been reclassified as a fungus, "albeit an odd one." Most recently, *Pneumocystis* has been assigned to the subphylum Taphrinomycotina within the division Ascomycota.[2] Biologically, however, *Pneumocystis* exhibits behavior that resembles a protozoan, because it is susceptible to drugs used to treat sporozoan infections but resistant to most antifungal drugs. Its cell wall contains cholesterol rather than ergosterol, which is the target of azole antifungals. The morphology of the organisms and the histopathology of the lesions produced by both human and animal isolates throughout the world are similar. Although controversial, five species of *Pneumocystis* have been described, which appear to be highly host-specific: *P. carinii* and *Pneumocystis wakefieldiae* that infect rats; *Pneumocystis murina* that infects mice; *Pneumocystis oryctolagi* that infects rabbits; and *Pneumocystis jirovecii* (pronounced "yee row vet zee") that infects humans.[1,3–5] The name *P. carinii* f. sp. *canis* was proposed for the organism that infects dogs.[6,7] Historically, *P. carinii* was thought to cause *Pneumocystis* pneumonia in humans, so *Pneumocystis* pneumonia has long been referred to as "PCP". Despite the name change to *P. jirovecii* in the 1970s, the term PCP has been retained because of familiarity. Biologic differences among isolates from different hosts are suggested by the relative difficulty of experimental cross–host species transmission. For purposes of this chapter, the organism that appears to be adapted to dogs will be referred to as *Pneumocytis canis*, which was also used in a large study that examined genomic relationships among different Pneumocystis species.[8]

Pneumocystis spp. appear to be maintained in nature by transmission from infected to susceptible animals within a species. The primary mode of spread is thought to be airborne droplet transmission among hosts, with neonates becoming colonized at birth.[9] Sporadic cases may represent an activation of latent infection by stress, crowding, and immunosuppressive therapy during hospitalization of latent carriers. Clinical disease has also been experimentally activated after glucocorticoid therapy and cytotoxic chemotherapy. A higher prevalence of infection has been reported in dogs with CDV infection compared with a corresponding control population,[10,11] and recently, a case was reported in a mix-breed dog (Maltese terrier-Papillon) that was treated with toceranib phosphate.[6] Genetic analysis of isolates in humans indicates that most infections are not previously acquired but rather result from an infected source that is likely of the same host species within a given geographic region.[12]

Most affected dogs have been miniature dachshunds younger than 1 year and adult Cavalier King Charles spaniels.[11,13–15] Cases also have occasionally been reported in other dogs, including a Pomeranian, Yorkshire terrier, a shih tzu, and a whippet.[16–18] The miniature dachshund, Cavalier King Charles spaniel, and Pomeranian had an underlying primary immune deficiency.[17,19,20] The shih tzu dog was found to have an X-linked CD40 ligand deficiency, a defect that impairs T cell costimulation and leads to a combined T cell and B cell immunodeficiency. It is possible that this mutation may have been present in other dogs with pneumocystosis, because genetic characterization at this level was not done.[18] Although the organism has been found in the lungs of cats, clinical disease has not been reported and thus in general, *Pneumocystis* infections of cats appear to be latent or subclinical. Cats that were experimentally infected with *P. carinii* isolated from mice developed a cough, tachypnea, and pneumonia if they were immunosuppressed with concurrent glucocorticoid administration.[21] In contrast, subclinical infections occurred in cats that did not receive immunosuppressive therapy.

CLINICAL FEATURES

Pathogenesis and Clinical Signs

Pneumocystis is inhaled from the environment and then can colonize the lower respiratory tract of clinically healthy mammals; however, they rarely multiply to large numbers in the lungs of clinically healthy hosts. Transmission of infection to neonates occurs almost ubiquitously during the birth process, with clearance and transient colonization over the course of a lifetime.[2] In conditions in which impaired host resistance (especially with reduced CD4 T-cell counts) or preexisting pulmonary disease is present, rapid proliferation of organisms can occur, either as a result of new infection or reactivation of "latent" infections.[1,2,22] The entire life cycle of *Pneumocystis* is completed within the alveolar spaces where organisms adhere in clusters to the lining cells (Fig. 89.1). In this location, two main forms, the haploid trophozoite (1–4 µm in diameter) and cyst (8 µm), are found. Trophozoites undergo sexual reproduction and pass through three stages (early, intermediate, and late sporocysts) to form a thick-walled mature cyst. The wall of these cysts is composed of the major surface glycoprotein (MSG), β-1,3 glucan, and β-1,6 glucan. The cyst contains eight ascospores, which form because of multiple nuclear division. The cyst ruptures, and the spores transform into trophozoites, which may replicate asexually to form more trophozoites, or sexually to form more cyst forms. The trophozoite form predominates in the lungs during infection, whereas cysts are responsible for propagation. The wall of the trophozoite contains MSG but not β-glucans.[2] Because β-glucans are essential for activating the dendritic cell and subsequent CD4+ T-cell immune response, the trophozoite form may be able to evade cellular recognition to a greater extent than the ascus form. Cells involved in the immune response to *Pneumocystis* are shown in Fig. 89.2. Existing studies in mice suggest that M2 macrophages are proinflammatory, and important in clearance of infection, whereas M1 macrophages exhibit defective clearance.[2]

The overgrowth and clustering of *Pneumocystis* within alveolar spaces leads to blockage of capillaries and decreased gaseous exchange. Intraalveolar organisms are often accompanied by thickening of alveolar septa, but they seldom invade the pulmonary interstitium and are rarely phagocytosed by alveolar macrophages. With an adequate immune response, the body usually eliminates the infection, but the removal of large numbers of organisms and cellular debris may take up to 8 weeks. Both the presence of the organisms and the minimal inflammatory response they provoke contribute to the pulmonary alveolar damage.

Although *Pneumocystis* infections are usually confined to the lungs, organisms have been reported in extra-pulmonary sites in humans and an infection in one dog. In humans, extra-pulmonary pneumocystosis is extremely rare and occurs primarily when accompanied by overwhelming pulmonary infection, profound underlying immunodeficiency, and long-term use of aerosolized pentamidine for prophylaxis against *P. jirovecii* pneumonia in individuals infected with HIV.[21] Sites of extra-pulmonary infection include the lymph nodes, spleen, liver, bone marrow, GI tract, eyes, thyroid gland, adrenal glands, kidneys, heart, pancreas, and external auditory canal.

The typical clinical history is that of gradual weight loss and respiratory difficulty that progresses over 1 to 4 weeks. Weight loss, which

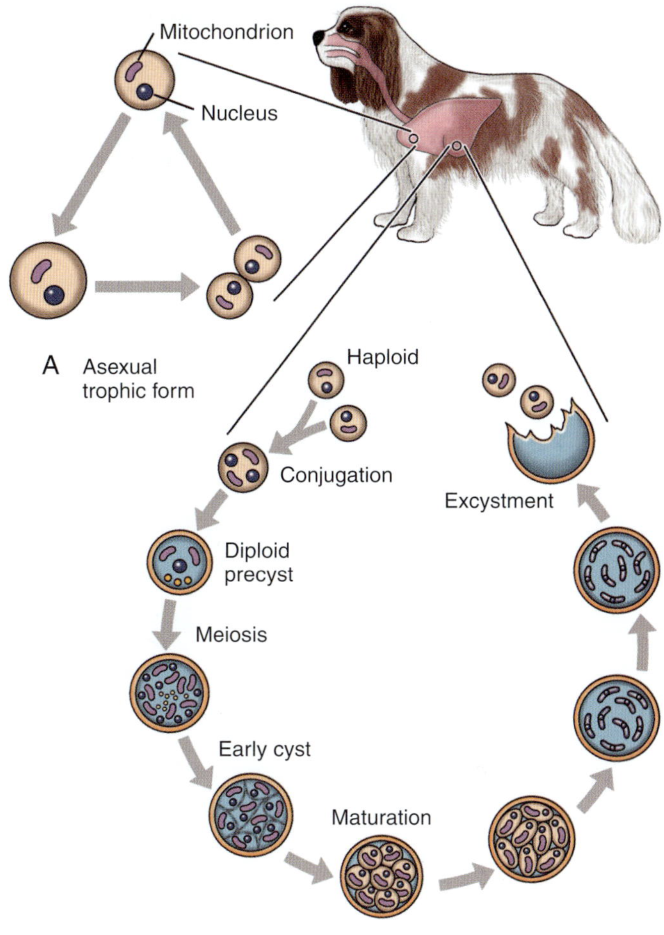

Fig. 89.1 Life cycle of *Pneumocystis* species. Trophozoites adhere to alveolar epithelial cells in the lungs and undergo both asexual (A) and sexual (B) reproduction. Sexual reproduction is initiated by conjugation, which results in formation of a zygote. Meiosis occurs followed by mitosis, which leads to the formation of eight ascospores within a mature cyst. The cyst ruptures, releasing spores that become trophozoites.

occurs despite a good appetite in most dogs, may be associated with diarrhea and occasional vomiting. Cough is not always reported, but reduced exercise tolerance is uniform. Infected animals often show a minimal or temporary response to antibiotic and glucocorticoid therapy.

Physical Examination Findings

Abnormalities on physical examination include dyspnea, tachypnea, increased breath sounds on thoracic auscultation, and variable cyanosis.[11] Animals are often in poor condition and cachectic, and can show dermatologic changes, as a result of superficial bacterial pyoderma and/or demodicosis (Fig. 89.3). Affected dogs remain relatively alert and fever is uncommon.

DIAGNOSIS

Laboratory Abnormalities

Complete Blood Count

Hematologic abnormalities are usually nonspecific, with neutrophilic leukocytosis being the most consistent finding.[11] Less frequently, eosinophilia and monocytosis are found. Lymphocyte numbers can be elevated, normal, or low. Polycythemia may occur secondarily to arterial hypoxemia from impaired gaseous exchange. Thrombocytosis is

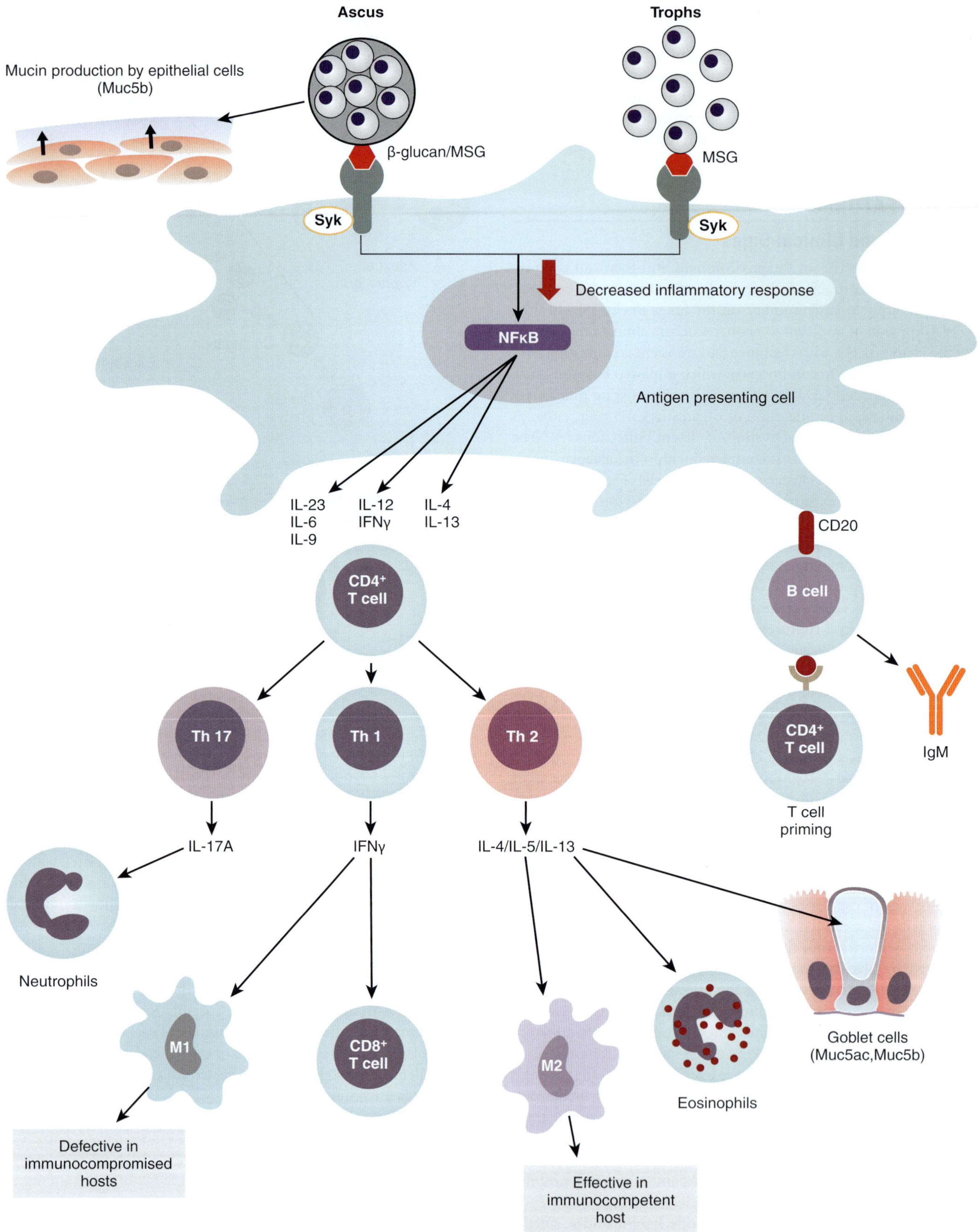

Fig. 89.2 Pathways involved in the immune response to *Pneumocystis* spp. *MSG,* major surface glycoprotein; *M1,* M1 type macrophage; *M2,* M2 type macrophage. (Modified from Walzer PD, Smulian AG. *Pneumocystis* species. In: Mandell GL, Bennett JE, Dolin R, eds. *Principles and Practice of Infectious Diseases.* 7th ed. Philadelphia: Elsevier; 2010:3377–3390.)

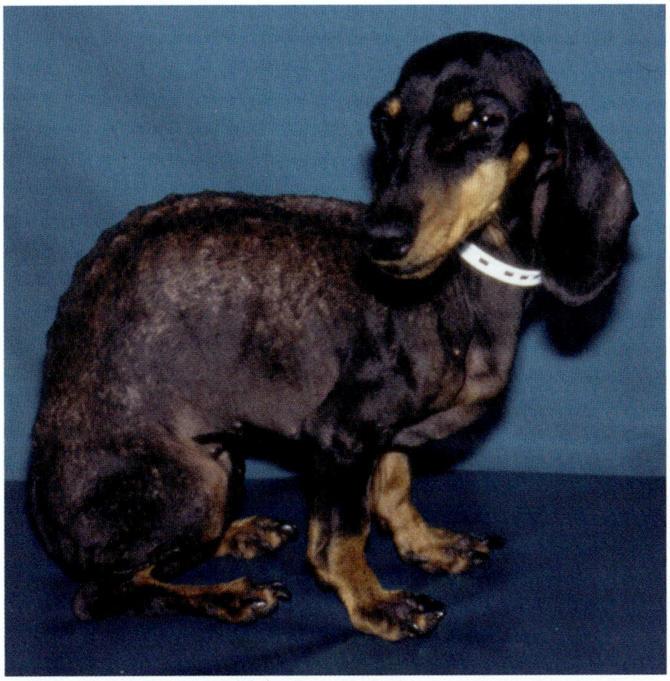

Fig. 89.3 A 1-year-old dachshund with pneumocystosis. Note the thin body condition and alopecia secondary to generalized demodectic mange.

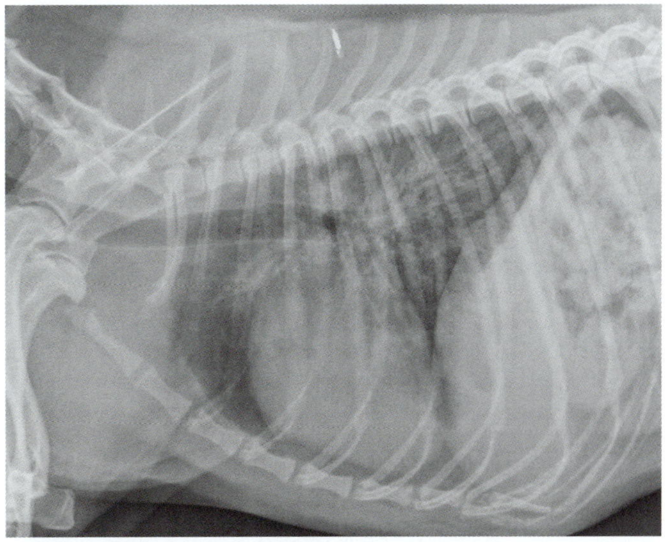

Fig. 89.4 Lateral thoracic radiographs from a 1-year-old male neutered Cavalier King Charles spaniel with pneumocystosis. A diffuse marked interstitial pattern is present. Mild right-sided cardiomegaly was also identified.

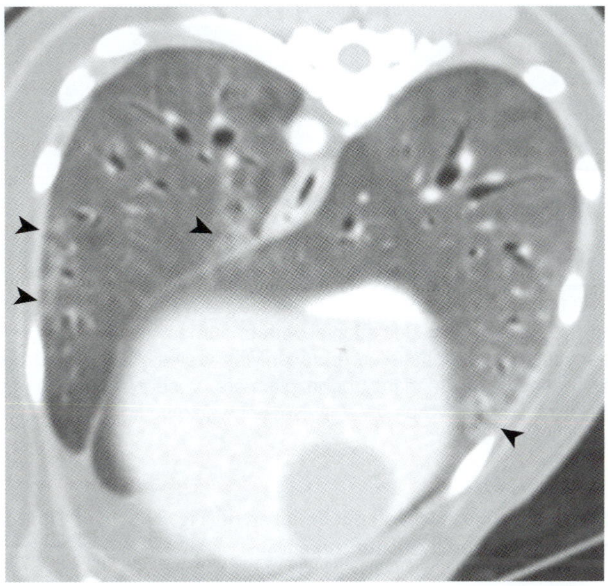

Fig. 89.5 Thoracic computed tomography scan from a 4-year-old female spayed Cavalier King Charles spaniel with pneumocystosis that was evaluated for lethargy, inappetence, and respiratory distress. There is a diffuse interstitial pattern and focal peripheral alveolar infiltrates *(arrowheads)*.

often present in miniature dachshunds. Artifactual thrombocytopenia and megathrombocytosis can occur in Cavalier King Charles spaniels, which is unrelated to the suspected immunodeficiency.

Serum Chemistry Profile

Biochemical alterations are usually nonspecific. Total serum proteins are usually within reference limits with a low to borderline-low globulin level, which correlates with low γ-globulin levels on serum protein electrophoresis.[11] Arterial hypoxemia, hypocapnia, and increased arterial blood pH indicate an uncompensated respiratory alkalosis. The pO_2 is often lower than would be expected from the clinical signs and thoracic radiographic findings.

Diagnostic Imaging

Findings on thoracic radiography are typically diffuse, bilaterally symmetric, granular or miliary-interstitial to alveolar changes (Fig. 89.4).[23] Solitary lesions, unilateral involvement, cavitary lesions, spontaneous pneumothorax, pneumomediastinum, and lobar infiltrates have also been described.[11,16,18] Additional findings in the dog may be tracheal elevation, right-sided heart enlargement, and pulmonary arterial enlargement secondary to pulmonary hypertension. CT findings in dogs with pneumocystosis reflect diffuse or multifocal pulmonary interstitial infiltrates ("ground glass appearance") and focal regions of increased opacity (Fig. 89.5).[6,18,24] Other reported CT findings are parenchymal bands, bronchiolar dilation, pleural thickening, and tracheobronchial lymphadenopathy.

Microbiologic Tests

Cytologic Diagnosis

The diagnosis of pneumocystosis requires direct demonstration of *Pneumocystis* in biopsy specimens, respiratory fluids, or occasional extrapulmonary sites (Table 89.1). Transtracheal, endotracheal, or bronchoalveolar washings; lung aspirates; and oropharyngeal secretions may contain organisms. Transtracheal washings have been effective for identification of organisms in dogs; however, cytologic examination of wash specimens can lack sensitivity.[25] Direct FA assays have been effective in increasing sensitivity for detection of organisms in sputum and respiratory lavage specimens from humans, and have been used as a gold standard.[26] None of the cytologic techniques are as reliable or as definitive as is histopathology examination of lung biopsy specimens for documenting active pneumocystosis. Lung biopsy is, however, more invasive, has potential complications of hemorrhage or pneumothorax, and associated with additional costs and hospitalization. *Pneumocystis* organisms are difficult to detect in respiratory secretions or washings, especially trophozoites, and success in finding them usually depends on the experience of the examiner and the collection and processing of specimens. Polychrome stains, such as Wright's, Giemsa, and methylene blue, will demonstrate nuclei of trophozoites and intracystic sporozoites in cytologic specimens, but the walls

TABLE 89.1 Diagnostic Assays Available for Pneumocystosis in Dogs or Cats

Assay	Specimen Type	Target	Performance
Cytologic examination	Lung aspirates; transtracheal, endotracheal, or broncho-alveolar lavage specimens	*Pneumocystis* trophozoites and cysts	False negatives can occur when specimen size is small or low numbers of organisms are present. Identification to the genus level requires immunostaining or PCR assay.
PCR assays	Lung aspirates; transtracheal, endotracheal, or broncho-alveolar lavage specimens	*Pneumocystis* spp. DNA	The sensitivity and specificity of assays may vary depending on assay design. Assays designed to detect *Pneumocystis jirovecii* may not detect organisms that infect dogs. In the absence of cytologic evidence of *Pneumocystis* infection, the significance of a positive PCR result must be interpreted in light of clinical findings, because of the potential for subclinical colonization.
Histopathology	Lung biopsy or necropsy specimens	*Pneumocystis* trophozoites and cysts	Large numbers of organisms are usually found filling alveolar spaces. Cyst forms are best demonstrated with silver stains or periodic acid–Schiff. The identity of the organisms can be confirmed with immunohistochemistry or PCR assay.

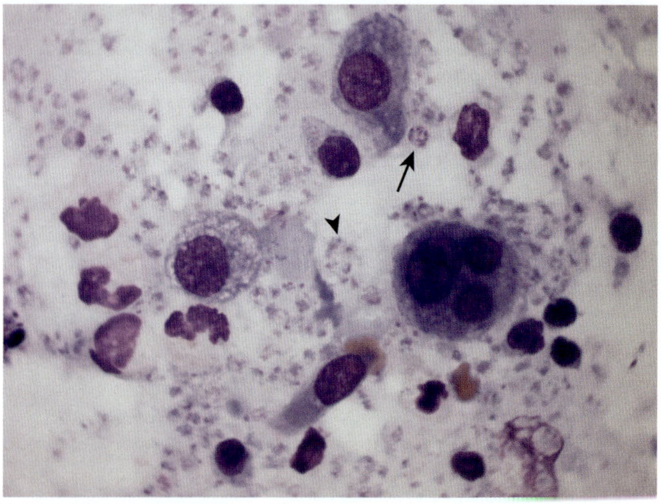

Fig. 89.6 Impression smear of lung tissue from a 1-year-old male neutered Cavalier King Charles spaniel with pneumocystosis. Large foamy and activated macrophages are present, as well as fewer neutrophils and lymphocytes. Abundant trophozoites are present and range in size from 1 to 2 μm *(arrowhead)*. Organisms can also be seen within a cyst *(arrow)*. Wright's stain.

of cysts and trophozoites will not be apparent (Fig. 89.6). Diff-Quik stain may be useful to rapidly identify organisms.[11,27]

Serologic Diagnosis

Serologic assays are available for detection of human infections with *P. jirovecii*; however, their diagnostic value is uncertain as many immunodeficient humans who develop pneumocystosis fail to produce antibody titers, and healthy individuals frequently have high titers. Increased antibody titers to *Pneumocystis* persist for long periods, offering a valuable index of infection in epidemiologic studies. However, they are of limited use for an immediate diagnosis.[28] Circulating *Pneumocystis* antigen has been detected in human serum by counterimmunoelectrophoresis and ELISA methods. However, antigenemia also is found in up to 15% of clinically normal humans who have been tested. Immunoperoxidase techniques have also been used to identify *Pneumocystis* spp. in impression smears and in formalin-fixed, paraffin-embedded lung sections.[11,29]

Culture

Pneumocystis spp. cannot be cultured in the laboratory from clinical specimens.

Molecular Diagnosis Using Nucleic Acid–Based Testing

PCR assays have been effective in the detection of *Pneumocystis* spp. in bronchoalveolar lavage specimens from humans[30] and in clinical specimens from dogs.[7,25] Assays designed to detect *P. jirovecii* typically do not detect *P. canis*, and so specific assays have been developed for diagnosis of pneumocystosis in dogs.[25] The sensitivity of PCR on bronchoalveolar lavage fluids from infected humans has been greater than that of conventional staining, but has the potential to detect both colonization as well as clinical infection, so results must be interpreted in light of clinical findings.[25,30,31] In human patients, use of quantitation in real-time PCR has shown potential for differentiation between colonization and pneumonia.[32] The same appears to be true in dogs.[25] DNA typing of *Pneumocystis* isolates using multilocus sequence typing has been used for epidemiologic studies of isolates from humans and dogs.[25,33]

Immunologic Findings

The majority of the immunologic studies in dogs have been performed in the miniature dachshund,[19] and a Pomeranian.[17] Lymphocyte stimulation assay results using phytohemagglutinin and pokeweed mitogen show severe immunosuppression, especially when compared with controls, even though a normal lymphocyte count can be present. Low globulin levels, immunoglobulin deficiencies, and decreased lymphocyte function have been reported in the Cavalier King Charles spaniel.[20,34] The absence of immunoglobulins in the presence of pathologic changes is a significant finding, as affected dogs have chronic persistent infections, which should result in an immunoglobulin response. Immunoglobulin deficiencies are still present after *P. canis* and skin infections have resolved, which suggests that the deficiency is a primary defect. From the lymphocyte transformation studies and the immunoglobulin fraction quantification, it would appear as though there are both T- and B-cell abnormalities in affected dogs. Serum complement activity measured in affected miniature dachshunds has been normal. CD3 and CD79a lymphocyte staining of lymph nodes and spleen shows marked absence of B cells with the presence of T cells.

The immunologic abnormalities in the miniature dachshund and Pomeranian are similar to what has been described in humans affected with common variable immunodeficiency syndrome, also known as acquired or adult-onset hypogammaglobulinemia. It is a primary immunodeficiency disease characterized by little or no antibody production by the B cells, normal or decreased numbers of B cells, and abnormal T-cell function.[35] In the shih tzu with CD40L deficiency, serum IgG and IgA concentrations were at the low end of the reference range, and the serum IgM concentration was in the middle of the reference range.[18] In humans, CD40L mutations are associated with hyper-IgM syndrome, where IgM concentrations are normal or increased, and IgG and IgA concentrations are low.

Pathologic Findings

Gross Pathological Findings

Pathologic findings in pneumocystosis are primarily confined to the lungs, although dissemination to regional lymph nodes, spleen, liver, bone marrow, and other organs has been reported. On gross examination, lungs are firm, consolidated, and pale brown or gray. The pulmonary and mediastinal lymph nodes are often enlarged. Despite the apparent lack of pleural inflammation, small amounts of fluid may be found in the pleural cavity. Cardiac enlargement, when present, has been right sided in all cases.

Histopathologic Findings

On histologic examination, alveolar spaces are filled with cohesive aggregates of amorphous, foamy, eosinophilic material that has a honeycomb-like pattern (Fig. 89.7). A few macrophages and detached alveolar lining cells also may be present, but polymorphonuclear leukocytes are generally absent. Special stains are needed to identify cyst forms (Fig. 89.8). Little or no phagocytosis of intact *Pneumocystis* organisms is present. However, nonviable organisms, such as those seen after treatment, are often phagocytosed, and macrophages may contain GMS-positive granular material that represents the residuum of cyst wall degradation. In some instances, alveolar septa are markedly thickened by dense accumulations of plasma cells, lymphocytes, and macrophages. The septa may be widened by fibrosis in chronic infections, especially after treatment. With GMS stain, cyst forms appear as black, spherical, ovoid, or crescent-shaped structures that range from 4 to 7 µm in diameter and have dot-like, argyrophilic, focal, cyst wall thickenings. Trophozoites in tissue sections and smears do not stain well with GMS or PAS and are best demonstrated with Giemsa or Gram stain. On ultrastructural examination, intact alveoli are filled with compact aggregates of trophozoite and cyst forms. Trophozoites commonly line alveoli. When compared with GMS, Gram stain and Giemsa have lower sensitivity, but molecular diagnosis has the highest sensitivity.

Appropriate histologic staining is essential to ensure detection of *Pneumocystis* spp. organisms. Various modifications of methenamine silver staining can be employed to stain the cyst walls brownish-black, but trophozoites will not be detected. The cysts of *Pneumocystis* spp. can be confused with small yeast-form fungi in GMS-stained tissue sections.

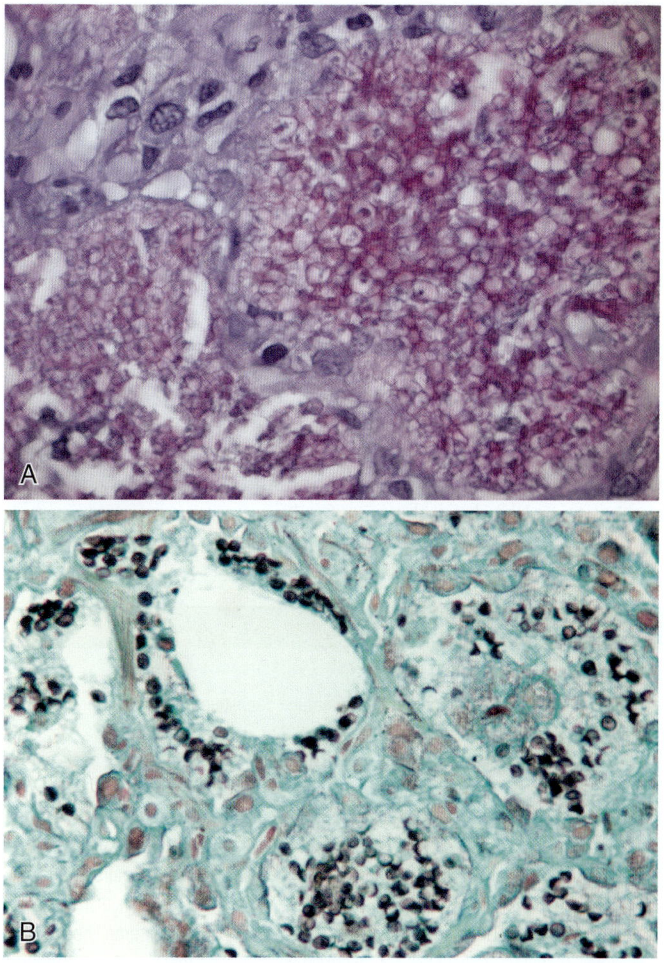

Fig. 89.7 Histopathology of the lung of an 18-month-old male neutered Cavalier King Charles spaniel with pneumocystosis. Foamy, honeycomb-like material fills the alveoli. (A) Periodic acid–Schiff stain. (B) Gomori's methenamine silver stain.

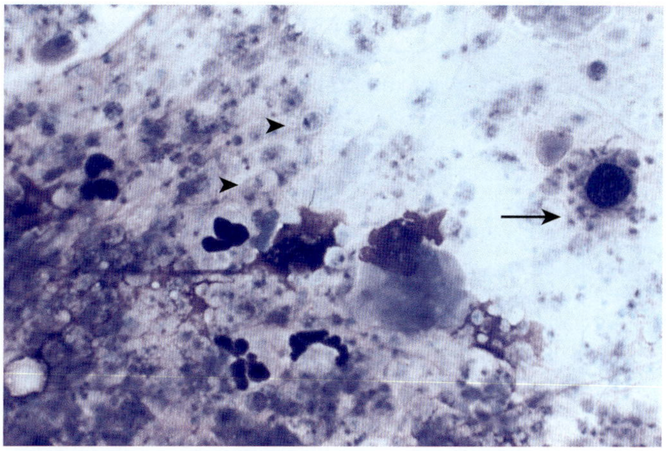

Fig. 89.8 Transtracheal aspirate cytology from a miniature dachshund showing *Pneumocystis* spp. organisms. Both free *(arrowheads)* and phagocytosed *(arrow)* organisms are evident (Diff-Quik stain, ×1000).

TREATMENT AND PROGNOSIS

Specific antimicrobial chemotherapy is most beneficial in cases in which the disease is suspected or diagnosed during its early stages (usually because of the affected dog breed). The two major chemotherapeutic agents that have successfully been used to treat pneumocystosis are TMS and pentamidine isethionate. Pentamidine isethionate is an aromatic diamidine that has been provided to reduce fatalities from the disease in humans.

TMS is more effective and less toxic than pentamidine for the treatment and prevention of PCP in immunodeficient humans. Most dogs in the literature have been treated with TMS,[11,18,23,36] and four were dachshunds that subsequently recovered.[23] The shih tzu with CD40L deficiency also recovered following treatment with TMS. A TMS dose of 15 mg/kg, every 8 hours, or 30 mg/kg, every 12 hours, for 3 weeks was used in these dogs; the longest reported follow-up in these studies was for 4 months, but the shi tzu was followed for 2 years. Folic acid supplementation should be given if adverse effects such as leukopenia and anemia are observed or if long-term therapy is required. In human infections, genotypic resistance to sulfonamides has been noted among some strains of *P. jirovecii*.[37]

Atovaquone is licensed for the treatment of humans with pneumocystosis;[38] it is not as effective against *Pneumocystis* as is pentamidine or TMS, but has lower toxicity. In humans, pentamidine and atovaquone have also been administered by aerosol and are well-tolerated alternatives for PCP prophylaxis.[39]

Combination therapy using clindamycin and primaquine also has been effective, but neither drug is effective alone. Further investigation on the effect of these treatments in naturally occurring disease is needed. Dapsone and trimethoprim or pyrimethamine, in combination, has been effective in experimental animals and clinical trials in immunosuppressed humans with pneumocystosis.[40,41] In experimentally infected animals, *P. carinii* is resistant to azole antifungal drugs and amphotericin B (because it lacks ergosterol in its cell wall).[42]

Supportive care is essential for any dog with *Pneumocystis* pneumonia because of disturbed alveolar gaseous exchange. Supplemental oxygen therapy may be needed, and ventilatory assistance may also be required. Immunosuppressive agents should be discontinued if possible. Antimicrobial chemotherapy of pulmonary pneumocystosis results in a decline in arterial oxygen related to the inflammatory reaction to dying organisms. Administration of anti-inflammatory doses of glucocorticoids has been shown to improve pulmonary function and survival in humans.[43–45] Medical management for pulmonary hypertension (e.g., sildenafil) may be required.

PUBLIC HEALTH ASPECTS

Pneumocystis organisms are ubiquitous in the environment. Humans and animals are exposed to the same environmental sources of *Pneumocystis.* Molecular and epidemiologic evidence suggests that spread may occur between humans because of localized outbreaks. Clinically affected humans and animals have the greatest concentrations of organisms in their airway secretions, and host immunocompetence is the most critical factor in determining whether illness develops. However, evidence suggests that the species of *Pneumocystis* that infects dogs is distinct from *P. jirovecii*, and so the risk of human infection with canine *Pneumocystis* strains may be negligible.[25]

CASE EXAMPLE

Signalment

"Tessa," a 1-year-old intact female miniature dachshund from the Johannesburg area, South Africa (see Fig. 89.3).

History

Tessa was evaluated for a history of tachypnea and weight loss that had been present over a 2-month period. The clinical signs had been nonresponsive to various treatments that had included multiple antibiotics, bronchodilators, mucolytics, multivitamins, and glucocorticoids. Additional history was that, since the age of 2 months, Tessa had had recurrent infections including otitis externa, hemorrhagic enteritis, tonsillitis, folliculitis, and pyogranulomatous dermatitis. These conditions had responded each time to supportive treatments.

Physical Examination

Body weight: 4.5 kg.

General: Quiet, alert, and responsive. Ambulatory on all four limbs. Rectal temperature = 101.8°F (38.8°C), HR = 138 beats/minute, RR = 129 breaths/minute, mucous membranes pink, CRT = 1 second.

Integument: Poor coat with focal alopecia on the head and back. No evidence of ectoparasites.

Eyes, ears, nose, and throat: No significant abnormalities noted. No evidence of ocular or nasal discharge.

Musculoskeletal: BCS 3/9 with symmetrical muscle wasting.

Cardiovascular: Strong femoral pulses. No murmurs or arrhythmias auscultated.

Respiratory: Increased respiratory rate with increased abdominal effort, tracheal palpation elicited a dry cough.

Abdomen: Normal abdominal palpation.

Rectal examination: No abnormalities detected. Normal feces in the rectum.

Lymph nodes: Normal mandibular, superficial cervical, and popliteal lymph nodes.

Laboratory Findings

CBC: HCT 54% (40%–55%), MCV 68 fL (65–75 fL), MCHC 35.7 g/dL (33–36 g/dL), WBC 34,600 cells/μL (6,000–15,000 cells/μL), neutrophils 23,200 cells/μL (3,000–11,000 cells/μL), band neutrophils 700 cells/μL (0–300 cells/μL), lymphocytes 5,500 cells/μL (1,000–4,800 cells/μL), monocytes 4,800 cells/μL (100–2,000 cells/μL), basophils 350 cells/μL (100 cells/μL), platelets 730,000 platelets/μL (200,000–500,000 platelets/μL).

Serum chemistry profile: Sodium 147 mmol/L (145–154 mmol/L), potassium 4.6 mmol/L (3.6–5.3 mmol/L), phosphorus 4.8 mg/dL (3.0–6.2 mg/dL), calcium 10.9 mg/dL (9.7–11.5 mg/dL), BUN 17 mg/dL (5–21 mg/dL), creatinine 0.5 mg/dL (0.3–1.2 mg/dL), glucose 132 mg/dL (64–123 mg/dL), total protein 5.1 g/dL (5.3–7.5 g/dL), albumin 3.5 g/dL (2.3–3.5 g/dL), globulin 1.6 g/dL (2–3.7 g/dL), α-globulins 0.8 (0.8–1.6 g/dL), β-globulins 0.6 (0.7–1.3 g/dL), γ-globulins 0.3 (0.4–1.1 g/dL), ALT 65 U/L (10–60 U/L), ALP 210 U/L (100–250 U/L), cholesterol 196 mg/dL (135–361 mg/dL), total bilirubin 0.1 mg/dL (0–0.2 mg/dL).

Urinalysis: SpG 1.045; pH 6.0, negative for protein, bilirubin, blood, and glucose. Inactive sediment.

Imaging Findings

On thoracic radiographs, the cardiovascular structures appeared within normal limits. A diffuse interstitial pulmonary pattern was present, similar to that shown in Fig. 89.4.

Cytology Findings

Transtracheal wash cytology demonstrated reactive alveolar macrophages with phagocytic vacuolization, large numbers of neutrophils, and many free and phagocytosed *Pneumocystis* organisms (see Fig. 89.8).

Aerobic Bacterial Culture

Culture of the transtracheal wash fluid yielded no growth after 48 hours' incubation.

Fecal Examination

Fecal flotation: Negative for parasites.

Diagnosis

Pneumocystis spp. pneumonia.

Treatment

Treatment instituted was a potentiated sulfonamide at 15 mg/kg, PO, q8h for 3 weeks, which resulted in a complete recovery.

Comments

This dog was diagnosed with *Pneumocystis* pneumonia as a result of a primary immune deficiency disease, most likely common variable immunodeficiency syndrome. The latter would also account for the chronic skin infections and gastroenteritis. CD3 and CD79a cell staining of a peripheral lymph node biopsy showed a marked absence of B cells with the presence of T cells.

SUGGESTED READINGS

1. Weissenbacher-Lang C, Fuchs-Baumgartinger A, Guija-De-Arespacochaga A, et al. Pneumocystosis in dogs: meta-analysis of 43 published cases including clinical signs, diagnostic procedures, and treatment. *J Vet Diagn Invest.* 2018;30:26–35.
2. Danesi P, Ravagnan S, Johnson LR, et al. Molecular diagnosis of *Pneumocystis* pneumonia in dogs. *Med Mycol.* 2017;55:828–842.

REFERENCES

1. Sokulska M, Kicia M, Wesolowska M, et al. *Pneumocystis jirovecii* – from a commensal to pathogen: clinical and diagnostic review. *Parasitol Res.* 2015;114:3577–3585.
2. Otieno-Odhiambo P, Wasserman S, Hoving JC. The contribution of host cells to *Pneumocystis* immunity: an update. *Pathogens.* 2019;8.
3. Chabe M, Aliouat-Denis CM, Delhaes L, et al. *Pneumocystis:* from a doubtful unique entity to a group of highly diversified fungal species. *FEMS Yeast Res.* 2011;11:2–17.
4. Hughes WT. *Pneumocystis carinii* vs. *Pneumocystis jiroveci*: another misnomer (response to Stringer et al.). *Emerg Infect Dis.* 2003;9:276–277. author reply 277–279.
5. Stringer JR, Beard CB, Miller RF, et al. A new name (*Pneumocystis jiroveci*) for *Pneumocystis* from humans. *Emerg Infect Dis.* 2002;8:891–896.
6. Best MP, Boyd SP, Danesi P. Confirmed case of *Pneumocystis* pneumonia in a Maltese Terrier x Papillon dog being treated with toceranib phosphate. *Aust Vet J.* 2019;97:162–165.
7. Petini M, Furlanello T, Danesi P, et al. Nested-polymerase chain reaction detection of *Pneumocystis carinii* f. sp. *canis* in a suspected immunocompromised Cavalier King Charles spaniel with multiple infections. *SAGE Open Med Case Rep.* 2019;7. 2050313X19841169.
8. Cissé OH, Ma L, Dekker JP, et al. Genomic insights into the host specific adaptation of the *Pneumocystis* genus. *Commun Biol.* 2021;4:305.
9. Bartlett MS, Smith JW. *Pneumocystis carinii*, an opportunist in immunocompromised patients. *Clin Microbiol Rev.* 1991;4:137–149.
10. Sukura A, Laakkonen J, Rudback E. Occurrence of *Pneumocystis carinii* in canine distemper. *Acta Vet Scand.* 1997;38:201–205.
11. Weissenbacher-Lang C, Fuchs-Baumgartinger A, Guija-De-Arespacochaga A, et al. Pneumocystosis in dogs: meta-analysis of 43 published cases including clinical signs, diagnostic procedures, and treatment. *J Vet Diagn Invest.* 2018;30:26–35.
12. Beard CB, Carter JL, Keely SP, et al. Genetic variation in *Pneumocystis carinii* isolates from different geographic regions: implications for transmission. *Emerg Infect Dis.* 2000;6:265–272.
13. Brownlie SE. A retrospective study of diagnosis in 109 cases of canine lower respiratory disease. *J Small Anim Pract.* 1990;31:371–376.
14. Canfield PJ, Church DB, Malik R. *Pneumocystis* pneumonia in a dog. *Aust Vet Practit.* 1993;23:150–154.
15. Ramsey IK, Foster A, McKay J, et al. *Pneumocystis carinii* pneumonia in two Cavalier King Charles spaniels. *Vet Rec.* 1997;140:372–373.
16. Weissenbacher-Lang C, Fuchs-Baumgartinger A, Klang A, et al. *Pneumocystis carinii* infection with severe pneumomediastinum and lymph node involvement in a Whippet mixed-breed dog. *J Vet Diagn Invest.* 2017;29:757–762.
17. Kanemoto H, Morikawa R, Chambers JK, et al. Common variable immune deficiency in a Pomeranian with *Pneumocystis carinii* pneumonia. *J Vet Med Sci.* 2015;77:715–719.
18. Merrill K, Coffey E, Furrow E, et al. X-linked CD40 ligand deficiency in a 1-year old male Shih Tzu with secondary *Pneumocystis* pneumonia. *J Vet Intern Med.* 2021;35:497–503.
19. Lobetti R. Common variable immunodeficiency in miniature dachshunds affected with *Pneumonocystis carinii* pneumonia. *J Vet Diagn Invest.* 2000;12:39–45.
20. Watson PJ, Wotton P, Eastwood J, et al. Immunoglobulin deficiency in Cavalier King Charles Spaniels with *Pneumocystis* pneumonia. *J Vet Intern Med.* 2006;20:523–527.
21. Yuezhong Y, Li Z, Baoping T. Pneumonia in cats caused by *Pneumocystis carinii* purified from mouse lungs. *Vet Parasitol.* 1996;61:171–175.
22. Kelly MN, Shellito JE. Current understanding of *Pneumocystis* immunology. *Future Microbiol.* 2010;5:43–65.
23. Kirberger RM, Lobetti RG. Radiographic aspects of *Pneumocystis carinii* pneumonia in the miniature Dachshund. *Vet Radiol Ultrasound.* 1998;39:313–317.
24. Schiborra F, Scudder CJ, Littler RM, et al. CT findings in *Pneumocystis carinii* pneumonia in five dogs. *J Small Anim Pract.* 2018;59:508–513.
25. Danesi P, Ravagnan S, Johnson LR, et al. Molecular diagnosis of *Pneumocystis* pneumonia in dogs. *Med Mycol.* 2017;55:828–842.
26. Moodley B, Tempia S, Frean JA. Comparison of quantitative real-time PCR and direct immunofluorescence for the detection of *Pneumocystis jirovecii. PLoS One.* 2017;12:e0180589.
27. Cregan P, Yamamoto A, Lum A, et al. Comparison of four methods for rapid detection of *Pneumocystis carinii* in respiratory specimens. *J Clin Microbiol.* 1990;28:2432–2436.
28. Daly KR, Huang L, Morris A, et al. Antibody response to *Pneumocystis jirovecii* major surface glycoprotein. *Emerg Infect Dis.* 2006;12:1231–1237.
29. Kondo H, Hikita M, Ito M, et al. Immunohistochemical study of *Pneumocystis carinii* infection in pigs: evaluation of *Pneumocystis* pneumonia and a retrospective investigation. *Vet Rec.* 2000;147:544–549.
30. Guegan H, Robert-Gangneux F. Molecular diagnosis of *Pneumocystis* pneumonia in immunocompromised patients. *Curr Opin Infect Dis.* 2019;32:314–321.
31. Flori P, Bellete B, Durand F, et al. Comparison between real-time PCR, conventional PCR and different staining techniques for diagnosing *Pneumocystis jiroveci* pneumonia from bronchoalveolar lavage specimens. *J Med Microbiol.* 2004;53:603–607.
32. Fauchier T, Hasseine L, Gari-Toussaint M, et al. Detection of *Pneumocystis jirovecii* by quantitative PCR to differentiate colonization and pneumonia in immunocompromised HIV-positive and HIV-negative patients. *J Clin Microbiol.* 2016;54:1487–1495.
33. Ricci G, Santos DW, Kovacs JA, et al. Genetic diversity of *Pneumocystis jirovecii* from a cluster of cases of pneumonia in renal transplant patients: cross-sectional study. *Mycoses.* 2018;61:845–852.
34. Hagiwara Y, Fujiwara S, Takai H, et al. *Pneumocystis carinii* pneumonia in a Cavalier King Charles Spaniel. *J Vet Med Sci.* 2001;63:349–351.
35. Cunningham-Rundles C, Knight AK. Common variable immune deficiency: reviews, continued puzzles, and a new registry. *Immunol Res.* 2007;38:78–86.
36. Lobetti RG, Leisewitz AL, Spencer JA. *Pneumocystis carinii* in the miniature dachshund: case report and literature review. *J Small Anim Pract.* 1996;37:280–285.
37. Calderon E, de la Horra C, Montes-Cano MA, et al. Genotypic resistance to sulfamide drugs among patients with *Pneumocystis jiroveci* pneumonia. *Med Clin (Barc).* 2004;122:617–619.
38. Stoeckle M, Tennenberg A. Atovaquone for *Pneumocystis carinii* pneumonia. *Ann Intern Med.* 1995;122:314. Author reply 314–315.
39. Kitazawa T, Seo K, Yoshino Y, et al. Efficacies of atovaquone, pentamidine, and trimethoprim/sulfamethoxazole for the prevention of *Pneumocystis jirovecii* pneumonia in patients with connective tissue diseases. *J Infect Chemother.* 2019;25:351–354.
40. Hughes WT. Use of dapsone in the prevention and treatment of *Pneumocystis carinii* pneumonia: a review. *Clin Infect Dis.* 1998;27:191–204.
41. Salzer HJF, Schafer G, Hoenigl M, et al. Clinical, diagnostic, and treatment disparities between HIV-infected and non-HIV-infected immunocompromised patients with *Pneumocystis jirovecii* pneumonia. *Respiration.* 2018;96:52–65.
42. Bartlett MS, Queener SF, Shaw MM, et al. *Pneumocystis carinii* is resistant to imidazole antifungal agents. *Antimicrob Agents Chemother.* 1994;38:1859–1861.
43. The National Institutes of Health-University of California Expert Panel for Corticosteroids as Adjunctive Therapy for *Pneumocystis* Pneumonia. Consensus statement on the use of corticosteroids as adjunctive therapy for *Pneumocystis* pneumonia in the acquired immunodeficiency syndrome. *N Engl J Med.* 1990;323:1500–1504.
44. Bozzette SA, Finkelstein DM, Spector SA, et al. A randomized trial of three antipneumocystis agents in patients with advanced human immunodeficiency virus infection. NIAID AIDS Clinical Trials Group. *N Engl J Med.* 1995;332:693–699.
45. Masur H. Prevention and treatment of *Pneumocystis* pneumonia. *N Engl J Med.* 1992;327:1853–1860.

90

Protothecosis and Chlorellosis

Jane E. Sykes

KEY POINTS

- First Described: *Prototheca* spp. was first isolated from tree slime in the 1880s. Naturally occurring protothecosis was not described until 1952, in cattle (mastitis). Canine disease was reported in 1969, 5 years after the first description of human protothecosis.[1]
- Cause: *Prototheca* spp. (belonging to the lower algae, *Chlorphyceae*).
- Affected Hosts: Dogs, cats, cattle, humans, other domestic and wild animal species.
- Geographic Distribution: Worldwide except Antarctica, but especially in warm, humid climates and where there is organic matter with a high water content.
- Mode of Transmission: Cutaneous inoculation of organisms into tissues, or possibly systemic invasion in the face of immunosuppression by organisms that have been ingested or colonize the intestinal tract.
- Major Clinical Signs: Cutaneous nodules or masses or systemic illness with weight loss, blindness due to ocular involvement, polyuria and polydipsia, hematochezia, vomiting, lameness, neurologic signs.
- Differential Diagnoses: Chlorellosis (a rare algal disease), a variety of fungal diseases (e.g., histoplasmosis, cryptococcosis, sporotrichosis), intestinal pythiosis, neoplasia (especially round cell neoplasia), toxoplasmosis, neosporosis, granulomatous colitis of boxer dogs, inflammatory bowel disease.
- Human Health Significance: Human infections occur as a result of exposure to organisms in the environment, and are often associated with underlying immune compromise.

PROTOTHECOSIS

ETIOLOGY AND EPIDEMIOLOGY

Protothecosis is an uncommon cutaneous or systemic disease caused by *Prototheca* species, which are unicellular algae. *Prototheca* spp. lack chlorophyll, and as a result they are dependent on a saprophytic lifestyle. Although ubiquitous in nature, they are especially prevalent in warm, humid climates (e.g., southern and southeastern USA, northeastern Australia, southern continental Europe, Japan) in aqueous environments where decaying organic matter is present. They have been isolated from tree slime, sewage, fresh and saltwater sources, fish tanks, soil, animal excrement, and foodstuffs. Routine water chlorination may not inactivate the organisms.[2] *Prototheca* spp. can also colonize the skin, GI, and respiratory tracts of humans.[3]

The algae are round to oval, 5 to 30 μm in diameter, have a thick cell wall, and reproduce asexually by endosporulation (internal division), which results in a sporangium that contains up to multiple sporangiospores. Rupture of the sporangium releases sporangia into tissues, and the cycle continues (Fig. 90.1). Although the classification of *Prototheca* species is still in flux, 15 species have recently been proposed based on analysis of partial *cytb* gene sequences (Table 90.1).[4] *Prototheca bovis*, *Prototheca wickerhamii*, *Prototheca cutis*, and *Prototheca miyajii* have been associated with human disease; over 200 human cases have been described in the literature and most human infections are characterized by localized cutaneous lesions. Disease in dogs has been associated with infections by *P. wickerhamii*, *Prototheca zopfii*, *Prototheca ciferrii*, and *P. bovis*,[4,5] although the *P. zopfii* cases may have been *P. bovis*. *Prototheca zopfii* genotypes 1 and 2 have been reclassified as *P. ciferrii* and *P. bovis*, respectively.

Prototheca ciferrii is weakly pathogenic and has been isolated from a minority of cases of protothecal mastitis in dairy cows.[6,7] In contrast, *P. bovis* is the most virulent species; it causes the vast majority of bovine mastitis cases worldwide and almost all disseminated cases of protothecosis in dogs.[6] *Protheca wickerhamii* has to date been isolated from all except one cat, some dogs, and almost all human patients, and is often associated with cutaneous disease (see Table 90.1).[5,8] Disseminated disease caused by *P. wickerhamii* infection in dogs may follow a less aggressive clinical course than that caused by *P. bovis*.[9]

Protothecosis is an uncommon and sporadic disease of dogs, with approximately 70 cases reported in the literature, and it is rarely reported in cats (less than 10 cases reported worldwide). In dogs, protothecosis is usually a serious disseminated disease but occasionally localized cutaneous disease occurs. Most affected dogs do not have a history of immunosuppressive drug therapy or illness. Boxer dogs and collies may be predisposed,[9,10] possibly secondary to an underlying genetic immunodeficiency, although a variety of other small and large breed dogs also can be affected.[5] Occasionally it occurs in dogs in conjunction with infection by other opportunistic pathogens such as *Neospora*,[11] which supports the likelihood that underlying immune deficiency is present. One report from Germany described disseminated disease in a Rhodesian ridgeback,[12] a breed predisposed to disseminated aspergillosis[13] and possibly neosporosis. One dog seen at the author's hospital was euthanized 4 years after renal transplantation and cyclosporine treatment because of disseminated protothecosis, and another dog with a lymphocutaneous *P. wickerhamii* infection had a history of treatment with chemotherapy for lymphoma.[11] The median age of affected dogs in one series of 17 dogs was 4 years (range, 18 months to 11 years), and approximately 70% of the affected dogs were female.[9]

In cats, protothecosis is manifested as single or multiple nodular skin lesions; disseminated disease has not been reported. As noted, almost all cats are infected with *P. wickerhamii*; there is one report of

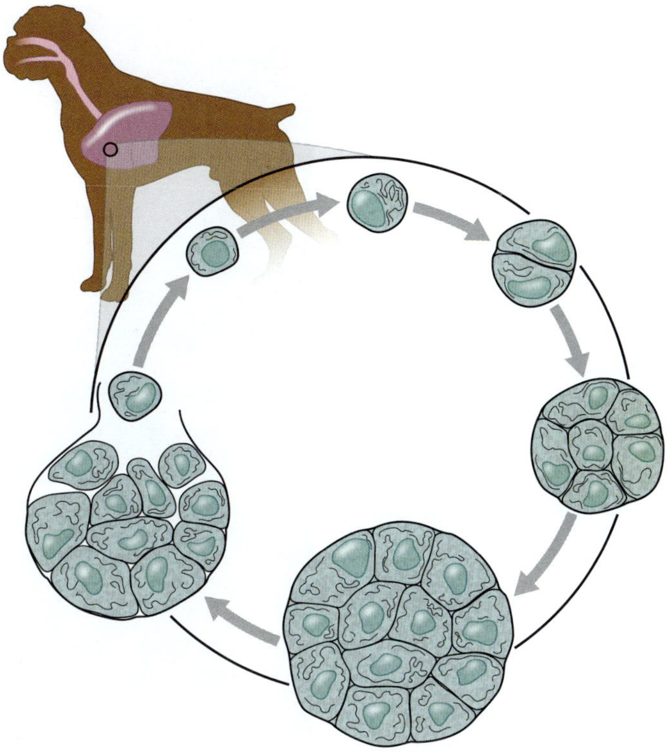

Fig. 90.1 Life cycle of *Prototheca*. The organism multiplies asexually by endosporulation, which results in a sporangium containing multiple sporangiospores. The sporangium ruptures, releasing spores into tissues, and the life cycle continues. (Redrawn from Klintworth GK, Fetter BF, Nielsen HS. Protothecosis, an algal infection: report of a case in man. *J Med Microbiol.* 1968;1:211–216.)

TABLE 90.1 **Major Species of *Prototheca* and Their Clinical Relevance**

Species	Host Species Infected	Clinical Manifestations
P. ciferrii (previously *P. zopfii* genotype 1)	Cattle, dogs	Mastitis (low pathogenicity), dogs (uncommon, disseminated infections or disseminated cutaneous infections)
P. bovis (previously *P. zopfii* genotype 2)	Dogs, humans, cattle, horses	Mastitis (cattle), disseminated infections (dogs)
P. wickerhamii	Dogs, cats, goats	Cutaneous and mucocutaneous disease
P. blaschkeae	Cattle, humans	Mastitis (cattle), cutaneous disease (humans)
P. cutis	Humans	Cutaneous disease
P. miyajii	Humans	Disseminated disease
P. zopfii[a]	Humans, dogs, cattle	Mastitis (cattle), cutaneous disease (humans), disseminated disease (dogs)
P. stagnora, P. ulmea, P. tumulicola, P. cerasi, P. cookei, P. pringsheimii, P. xanthoriae, P. paracutis	Nonpathogenic	NA

[a]Currently may refer to previously reported infections where genotyping was not performed, given that genotypes 1 and 2 were classified as *P. ciferrii* and *P. bovis*, respectively.
NA, not applicable.

a cat infected with *P. zopfii* genotype 2 (*P. bovis*), which had nodular lesions on the bridge of the nose and within the right nostril.[14] Affected cats are typically FIV and FeLV negative, otherwise in good health and have ranged in age from 3 to 16 years.[15-20] There is one report of an FIV-infected cat from Australia that developed multiple skin lesions; two of the lesions were associated with *P. wickerhamii* infection and the remaining were Bowenoid in situ carcinomas that contained *Felis catus* papillomavirus 2 sequences.[21]

CLINICAL FEATURES

Pathogenesis and Clinical Signs

The pathogenesis of protothecosis is not fully understood. Infection may occur secondary to cutaneous inoculation of organisms, which may be followed by development of localized cutaneous lesions or dissemination through lymphatic or hematogenous spread. It is also possible that systemic invasion occurs through organisms that are ingested or colonize the GI tract. *Prototheca* spp. were not detected using PCR in feces or rectal scrapings of 200 dogs from Italy, including stray dogs that roamed on dairy cattle farms (including farms where *Prototheca* mastitis had been diagnosed), and so it was suggested that invasion by commensals was an unlikely mode of infection.[5] An incubation period of 10 days to several weeks has been suggested for human protothecosis based on recollection of penetrating injuries before onset of disease.[2]

In dogs, *Prototheca* typically disseminates to a variety of tissues, but especially the colon, eyes, brain and meninges, kidneys, and long bones. This results in clinical signs of inappetence and weight loss; acute or chronic large bowel diarrhea (often accompanied by hematochezia and tenesmus); blindness; neurologic signs such as obtundation, seizures, or ataxia; polyuria and polydipsia; and sometimes lameness due to osteomyelitis.[9,20,22-24] Discospondylitis was reported in one dog with disseminated infection.[25] Deafness is often reported in association with disseminated protothecosis, and may occur as a result of CNS or inner ear involvement.[20,24,26] Ocular lesions include granulomatous chorioretinitis, uveitis, and panophthalmitis. Other affected organs include the liver, skeletal muscle, thyroid gland, lymph nodes, spleen, pancreas, stomach, small intestine, omentum, myocardium, aorta, spinal cord, and/or lungs.[24,26-28] Involvement of these organs may lead to other signs such as vomiting, small bowel diarrhea, and/or melena. Sudden death has also been reported, possibly secondary to myocardial involvement.[9,29,30] Cutaneous lesions in dogs with *P. wickerhamii* infection may be a manifestation of systemic infection rather than local inoculation; one dog with ulcerated lesions of the nares also had evidence of infection in multiple peripheral lymph nodes.[31]

Physical Examination Findings

Cutaneous lesions in dogs are alopecic, nodular, and may ulcerate. They often involve the footpads or distal limbs and associated draining lymph nodes, but involvement of other sites such as the trunk and planum nasale can also occur (Fig. 90.2A).[31] In cats, single or multiple firm and sometimes ulcerated cutaneous nodules may be present. Lesions may be located on the head, footpads, and distal limbs and tail base[15-17,21] and can resemble those caused by *Cryptococcus* or *Sporothrix* spp. (Fig. 90.2B).

Dogs with disseminated disease may be obtunded, dehydrated, and can have a thin body condition. Some dogs are febrile, but rectal temperature may also be normal. Ocular involvement may be manifested by blindness or evidence of conjunctivitis, hyphema, uveitis, cataract formation, panophthalmitis, or granulomatous chorioretinitis, often with retinal detachment.[32] Arrhythmias with pulse deficits may be present in dogs with protothecal myocarditis.[11] Neurologic signs that may be detected on physical or neurologic examination include obtundation, blindness, deafness, ataxia, deficits of conscious proprioception, circling, head tilt, nystagmus, strabismus, and abnormalities of cranial nerve function such as absent or decreased facial sensation, palpebral, menace, or gag reflexes.[9,22,33-36] Dried fecal material or blood may be present around the anus and rectal examination may reveal hematochezia, increased fecal mucus, or melena.

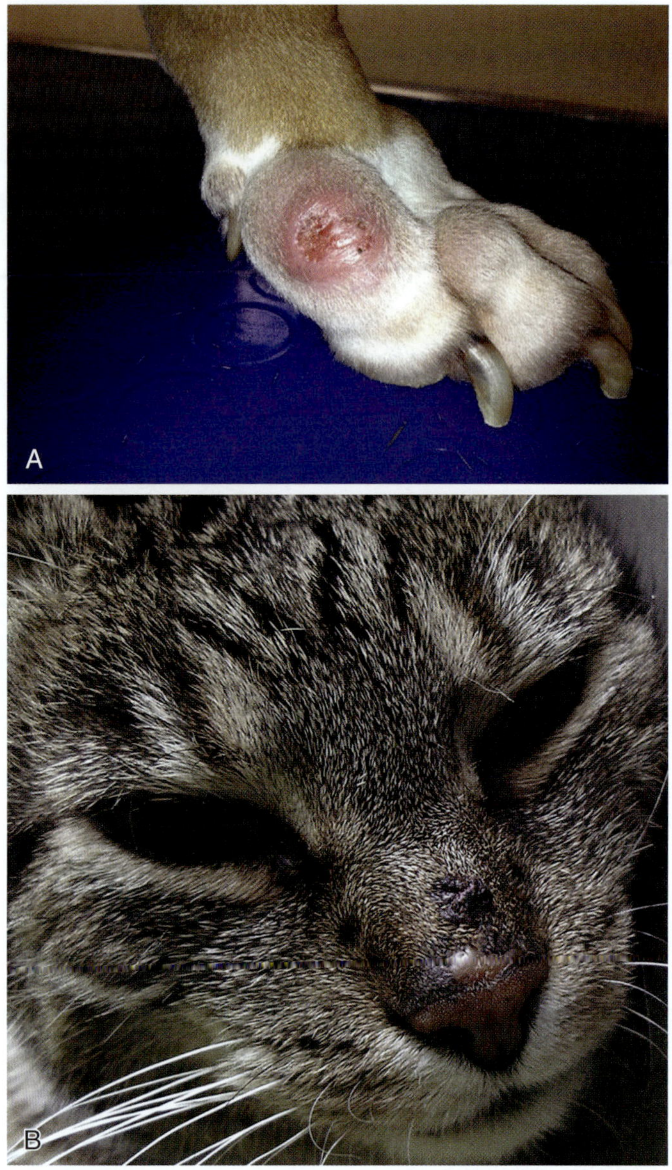

Fig. 90.2 Cutaneous manifestations of protothecosis. (A) *Prototheca wickerhamii* infection in a 6-year-old female boxer dog showing an ulcerated nodular lesion on the distal limb. The dog's footpads were also affected. (B) Nodular crusted lesions on the bridge of a 14-year-old female spayed domestic shorthair cat associated with a *Prototheca bovis* (previously *Prototheca zopfii* genotype 2) infection. (A, from Papadogiannakis EI, Velonakis EN, Spanakos GK, et al. Cutaneous disease as sole clinical manifestation of protothecosis in a boxer dog. *Case Rep Vet Med.* 2016;2016:2878751. B, from Huth N, Wenkel RF, Roschanski N, et al. *Prototheca zopfii* genotype 2-induced nasal dermatitis in a cat. *J Comp Pathol.* 2015;152:287–290.)

DIAGNOSIS

Laboratory Abnormalities

Complete Blood Count and Serum Biochemical Tests

The CBC in dogs with disseminated protothecosis is often normal. Occasionally it may show nonregenerative anemia and/or leukocytosis due to neutrophilia and sometimes monocytosis.[23,24,27] Mild bandemia and/or eosinophilia may be present in some dogs. The serum biochemistry panel may also be normal or reveal a mild hypoalbuminemia and hyperglobulinemia due to a polyclonal gammopathy. Mild to moderate azotemia may be evident in dogs with renal involvement.[23,27] More severe hypoalbuminemia and hypocholesterolemia may occur with diffuse small intestinal involvement.[9]

Urinalysis

The urinalysis may be unremarkable or show isosthenuria due to renal involvement. Other findings that may be present in dogs with urinary

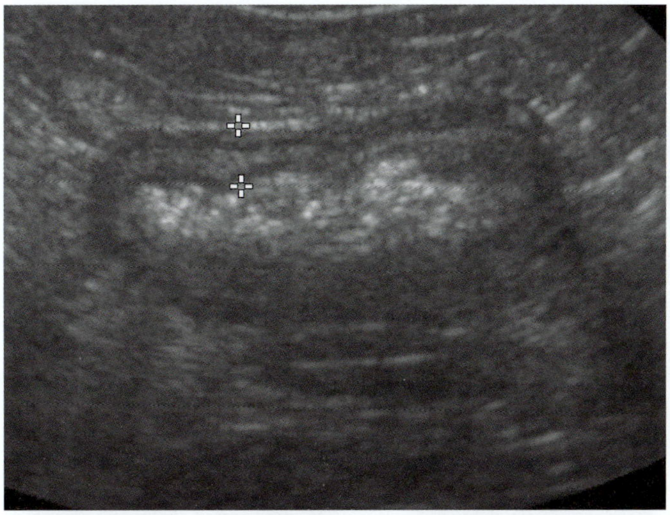

Fig. 90.3 Thickening and irregularity of the submucosal layer of the descending colon in a 2-year-old English springer spaniel with disseminated protothecosis. (Image courtesy University of California-Davis VMTH Diagnostic Imaging Service.)

tract involvement include hematuria, pyuria, proteinuria, and the presence of *Prototheca* organisms in the sediment.[23] Urinalysis and urine culture should be performed in all dogs suspected to have protothecosis, because more than half of affected dogs shed algae into the urine.

CSF Cytology

CSF analysis in dogs with CNS protothecosis may be normal or reveal markedly increased total nucleated cell count (sometimes > 1,000 cells/μL) and increased CSF protein concentration (often > 500 mg/dL).[27,33,34] Eosinophilic pleocytosis has been described in some dogs,[33,36] but eosinophils are not always present.[34] *Prototheca* algae may also be found in the CSF.[33,34]

Diagnostic Imaging

Plain Radiography

Thoracic radiographs in dogs with disseminated protothecosis are usually unremarkable.[23,27,28,30] Radiographs of affected long bones may reveal periosteal proliferative and/or osteolytic lesions due to osteomyelitis.[9] Bony lysis of lumbar vertebral endplates was described in one dog with *Prototheca* discospondylitis, with infection in this location confirmed at necropsy.[25]

Sonographic Findings

Findings described on abdominal ultrasound examination in dogs with disseminated protothecosis include hyperechogenicity of the renal cortices,[23] a thickened colonic wall with loss of normal bowel wall layering,[9] and abdominal lymphadenomegaly (Fig. 90.3). Some dogs have no abdominal sonographic abnormalities despite the presence of disseminated disease with colonic and renal involvement.[11]

Other Imaging

Colonoscopy in dogs with signs of large bowel diarrhea may reveal a hyperemic, friable, thickened, irregular, and ulcerated mucosa.[9] MRI of the brain of one dog with CNS involvement revealed mild to moderate ventriculomegaly, mild protrusion of the cerebellar vermis through the foramen magnum, syringomyelia, meningeal contrast enhancement, and a focus of increased signal intensity in the brain on T2-weighted and FLAIR sequences.[34] As it enlarged, the focus developed contrast enhancement and caused deformation of a lateral ventricle.

Microbiologic Tests

Cytologic Examination

Prototheca organisms may be seen using cytologic examination of rectal scrapings; fine-needle aspirates of lymph nodes, bone, or skin lesions; CSF, vitreal, or aqueous humor; and urine sediment. The organisms are spheroid, ovoid, bean-shaped, or elliptical and range in size from 1.5 to 30 μm in diameter (*P. bovis*) or up to 10 μm in diameter (*P. wickerhamii*).[31] They have a thick, hyaline cell wall that does not take up stain, and a basophilic, granular cytoplasm. Several daughter cells (usually < 10) may be seen inside the cell (Fig. 90.4). In the case of *P. wickerhamii* the endospores are arranged symmetrically like a daisy or soccer ball, whereas the endospores of *P. bovis* are distributed randomly.[2] The algae may be mistaken for fungi such as *Blastomyces*, *Coccidioides*, or *Cryptococcus*. Because large numbers of organisms are typically present, the sensitivity of cytological examination for diagnosis of algal infection is high. However, failure to find organisms does not rule out protothecosis.

Culture

Prototheca species can be readily cultured in the microbiology laboratory on standard media (such as blood agar and Sabouraud dextrose agar), and yeast-like colonies are usually visible within 7 days. Suitable specimens for culture include aspirates or biopsies of affected tissue and body fluids such as urine, CSF, and vitreous or aqueous humor. *Prototheca* was also cultured from the blood of a dog with disseminated disease.[30] Biochemical testing of isolates excludes other possible causes such as the green alga *Chlorella*, a very rare cause of disseminated disease in dogs that can closely resemble *Prototheca* in its microscopic appearance.[2,37] Differentiation of *Prototheca* species requires PCR and ribosomal RNA gene sequencing. MALDI-TOF MS has also been used for rapid identification of the species and genotype level.[6,12,38]

Antifungal susceptibility testing has been performed for *Prototheca* but has not been standardized, and the clinical relevance of the results is not clear.[2]

Molecular Diagnosis Using Nucleic Acid–Based Testing

Real-time PCR assays have been developed for detection and differentiation of *Prototheca* species,[39] but these are not available on a commercial basis for diagnosis of protothecosis in animals (Table 90.2).

PATHOLOGIC FINDINGS

Gross pathologic findings in dogs with disseminated infections include enlarged lymph nodes and gray, tan, or white nodular lesions or streaks in affected organs.[20,24,27,36] The colonic wall may be thickened and contain bloody fluid. Malacic foci may be present in the brain or the brain may appear normal grossly, even when meningoencephalitis is present.[11,35] Histopathologic examination of affected tissues typically reveals large numbers of sporulating and nonsporulating algal organisms (see Cytological Examination) accompanied by a mixed inflammatory response and foci of necrosis (Fig. 90.5). In some tissues the inflammatory response may be minimal to absent.[24,27] Organisms may be seen free and within macrophages. The cell wall stains well with Gomori's methenamine silver and PAS stain, but in contrast to *Chlorella*, cytoplasmic granules of *Prototheca* are PAS-negative. Cutaneous lesions in cats have been associated with a granulomatous inflammatory response with multinucleated giant cells and in some cases, necrosis and neutrophilic inflammation.[16,18] Because one cat had multiple skin lesions, some of which were Bowenoid in situ carcinomas and others associated with *Prototheca* spp. infection,[21] biopsy of multiple lesions is recommended.

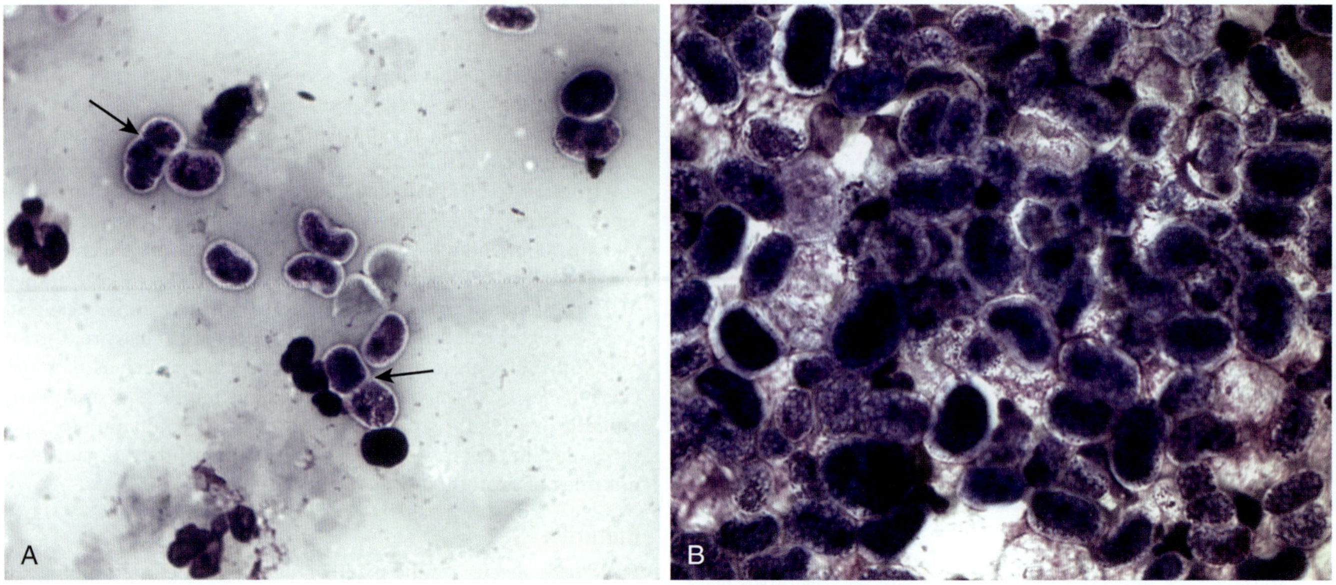

Fig. 90.4 (A) Cytology of a subretinal aspirate from an 8-year-old intact male mixed-breed dog with panophthalmitis due to *Prototheca* spp. infection. Moderate numbers of oval to bean-shaped organisms are present in a proteinaceous background that contained variably degenerate and ruptured neutrophils. The organisms have a thin clear capsule with deep purple cytoplasmic granulation. Sometimes endosporulation was evident *(arrows)*. Wright stain, 1000× oil magnification. (B) Cytology of a bone aspirate from a 2-year-old female mixed-breed dog that developed acute vision loss. Physical examination revealed bilateral retinal detachment and a nonpainful swelling of the right distal medial humerus. Abundant numbers of *Prototheca* algae are present. (Courtesy Dr. Emily Pieczarka.)

TABLE 90.2 Diagnostic Assays Available for Protothecosis

Assay	Specimen Type	Target	Performance
Cytologic examination	Aspirates of affected tissues, urine sediment, vitreous or aqueous humor, CSF	*Prototheca* algae	Usually large numbers of organisms are present, so sensitivity is high, but false negatives can occur (such as when urine sediment or fine-needle aspirates are examined). Organisms may be confused with other fungi or *Chlorella* species, so confirmation of the diagnosis requires culture.
Culture	Urine, blood, CSF, vitreous or aqueous humor, aspirates or biopsies of affected tissues	*Prototheca* species	*Prototheca* spp. grow rapidly (usually within 3 days) on routine media such as blood agar and Sabouraud dextrose agar. Species identification can be verified using nucleic acid–based methods and MALDI-TOF MS.
Histopathology	Skin or colonic biopsies, enucleated eyes, tissues collected at necropsy	*Prototheca* algae	Usually large numbers of organisms are present, so sensitivity is high. Organisms are highlighted with PAS or silver stains. Organisms may be confused with other fungi or *Chlorella* species, so confirmation of protothecosis requires culture. Grossly, tissues affected by *Chlorella* are green, and *Chlorella* infections in dogs are extremely rare.

TREATMENT AND PROGNOSIS

Where possible, surgical excision may be curative for localized cutaneous protothecosis.[16] However, even when lesions are solitary, cutaneous lesions may be a manifestation of disseminated disease, so medical therapy should also be used. Medical treatment of protothecosis is challenging. In human patients, treatment is generally with amphotericin B, which in some cases has resulted in complete cure. Addition of a tetracycline has also been associated with positive outcomes.[2,40] Azole antifungal drugs have also been tried but outcomes with azole antifungals alone are often poor, although clinical responses occur in some dogs with itraconazole alone.[11] In one human patient, a combination of amikacin and tetracycline led to cure.[41] Treatment of dogs with disseminated infections with amphotericin B has led to remission in some cases, but relapse occurs when the drug is discontinued, or dogs may fail to respond to treatment and ultimately die or be euthanized as a result of the disease.[9,30] One dog with protothecal meningoencephalitis appeared to improve clinically after treatment with systemic itraconazole and intrathecal amphotericin B (0.5 g q48h for five treatments), but was euthanized 4 weeks later due to progressive disease.[34]

Other treatments that may be required for protothecosis include IV fluid therapy, antiemetics, topical prednisolone acetate ophthalmic drops for uveitis, and ocular enucleation to control pain and/or remove

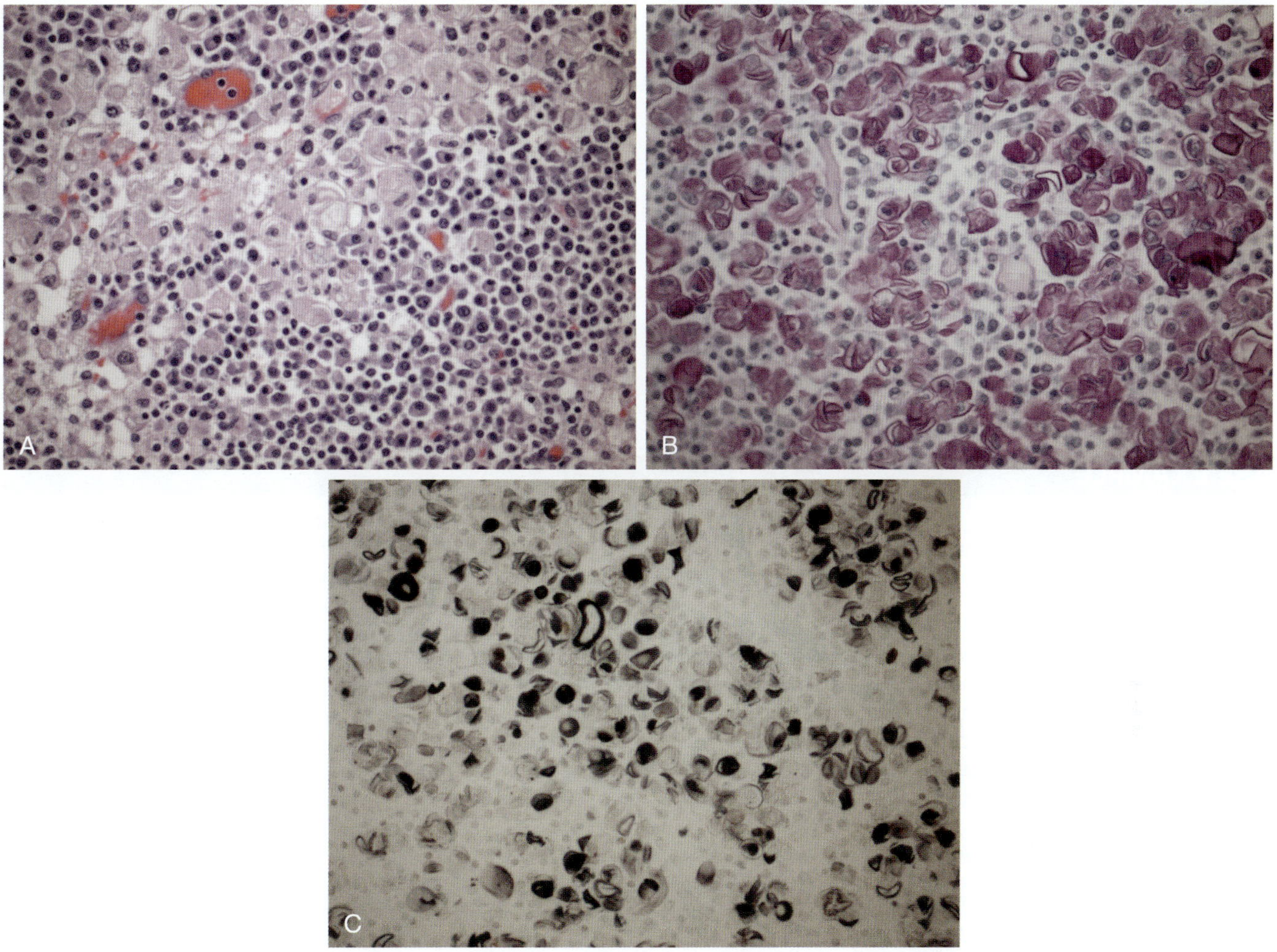

Fig. 90.5 Histopathology of the renal lymph node of a 6-year-old spayed female shih tzu with protothecosis that was being treated with cyclosporine after renal transplantation. Numerous *Prototheca* organisms are present. The organisms range in diameter from 5 to 15 μm and have several morphologic forms. Sporulating forms are up to 15 μm in diameter and contain two to four wedge-shaped endospores (daughter cells). Many of the organisms present as clear, refractile, oval to polyhedral bodies composed of a thick wall and devoid of cytoplasm and nuclei. (A) Hematoxylin and eosin stain. (B) PAS stain. (C) Gomori's methenamine silver.

a focus of infection that fails to respond to chemotherapy (see Case Example). Other treatments such as metronidazole, sulfasalazine, or dietary manipulation may help to control signs of protothecal colitis.

PUBLIC HEALTH APSECTS

Protothecosis is an uncommon disease of humans and most often caused by *P. wickerhamii*. Infection is acquired from environmental sources, and direct transmission from other animals or humans does not appear to be important. Mortality is low (< 5%) and two-thirds of infections are chronic infections that are localized to the skin.[2] Joint infections and tendonitis have been described after surgical or accidental wounds; some have been traced back to cleaning an aquarium.[42] Disseminated infections and a syndrome called olecranon bursitis (which follows elbow trauma) account for the remaining third of cases. Underlying local or systemic immune defects can be identified in many patients, and topical, local, or systemic glucocorticoid treatment is the most frequently identified risk factor. Other immunosuppressive disorders that may predispose humans to protothecosis include diabetes mellitus and malignancy. Severe disseminated disease has been described in bone marrow and kidney transplant recipients,[43,44] those with longstanding indwelling catheters or endotracheal tubes, and rarely in AIDS patients.[42,45] However, some severe infections have been reported in immunocompetent patients.[40]

CHLORELLOSIS

Chlorella spp. (order Chlorellales, family Chlorellaceae) are green (chlorophyll-containing) algae with an apparently identical ecologic niche and asexual reproductive cycle similar to *Prototheca* spp. The chlorophyll is contained within a single, large chloroplast. The precise relationship between these two genera is unclear, but similarities in morphology, life cycle, and environmental distribution suggest that *Prototheca* spp. may be achlorophyllous mutants of *Chlorella* spp. At necropsy, grossly affected tissues are bright green.[46] However, because chlorophyll is dissolved during tissue processing, formalin-fixed *Chlorella* spp. and *Prototheca* spp. are both colorless.[47] Therefore, *Prototheca* and *Chlorella* cannot be differentiated in H&E-stained tissues using standard light microscopy. Alternatively, when viewed under polarized light, large, irregular, birefringent starch granules are present within the cytoplasm of all *Chlorella* spp. endospores, whereas in *Prototheca* spp. these granules, if present, are smaller, less distinct, and present in only a minority of cells. These starch granules stain uniformly with PAS or Gomori's methenamine silver stains. Examination of ultrastructural features via transmission electron microscopy is likely the most reliable method for differentiating *Chlorella* spp. from *Prototheca* spp., because the large cytoplasmic chloroplast in the former organism is clearly visible.[46,47]

Disseminated chlorellosis has only been reported in one dog in 2009.[37] In that dog, which was from Michigan, USA, a granulomatous lingual mass with intralesional algal organisms was initially diagnosed as localized protothecosis. Over the course of 6 months of evaluation, the dog developed an extradural lumbar mass that resulted in caudal lower motor neuron signs, weight loss, and cough despite fluconazole treatment. Disseminated algal infection was confirmed on necropsy, including an exudative greenish mass infiltrating the epaxial musculature and contiguous with the adjacent lumbar extradural and intradural surfaces. Light and electron microscopy confirmed chlorellosis using the criteria described previously.

No information exists as to whether treatment options for chlorellosis differ from those previously discussed for protothecosis. A single case of *Chlorella* spp. infection was reported in 1983 in a 30-year-old woman from Nebraska, USA.[48] In that patient, localized cutaneous infection of the foot developed after exposure of a surgical wound to river water while canoeing. The infection was successfully managed with debridement and open-wound management until granulation occurred.

CASE EXAMPLE

Signalment

"Merlot," a 3-year-old female spayed Siberian husky dog from San Francisco, CA.

History

Merlot was evaluated at the University of California, Davis VMTH for a 1-month history of hemorrhagic diarrhea, decreased appetite, and weight loss. Initially the diarrhea contained fresh blood and mucus but more recently had contained only blood. The diarrhea occurred frequently and in small quantities, but hematochezia was not observed. The owner reported that Merlot had lost approximately 5 kg over the last month, and had increased thirst and urination. There had been no history of vomiting and Merlot's activity level was normal. Her diet consisted of a commercial dry dog food.

At a local veterinary clinic, multiple fecal flotations had been negative, and Merlot had been treated with metronidazole, aminopentamide, bismuth subsalicylate, enrofloxacin, loperamide, tetracycline, metoclopramide, and a highly digestible diet without clinical response. A barium series had been recently performed and findings were consistent with gastroenteritis.

Merlot moved to San Francisco from Massachusetts 4 months before the clinical signs began. On the way over the owner stopped in Texas, where Merlot became lost in a field for 30 minutes. The owner reported that Merlot was taken to a dog park in San Francisco several times a week. No other previous history of illness existed.

Physical Examination

Body weight: 18.2 kg

General: Bright, alert, responsive, and hydrated. T = 102.3°F (39.1°C), pulse = 80 beats/min, panting, mucous membranes pink, capillary refill time 1 s.

Eyes, ears, nose, and throat: Dried barium present on the lips. No other clinically significant findings. Fundoscopic examination revealed a region of retinal separation in the left ocular fundus that was adjacent to, dorsomedial to, and approximately the size of the optic disc. The lesion appeared to contain yellowish fluid.

Integument: Full haircoat.

Musculoskeletal: Thin but well-muscled.

Cardiorespiratory: No clinically significant findings.

Gastrointestinal/genitourinary: No masses palpated in the abdomen. Vocalized and appeared painful on caudal abdominal palpation. Frank blood was present on the glove after rectal examination.

Peripheral lymph nodes: No clinically significant findings.

Laboratory Findings

CBC: HCT 48.6% (40–55%), MCV 70.9 fL (65–75 fL), MCHC 34.6 g/dL (33–36 g/dL), WBC 12,100 cells/μL (6,000–13,000 cells/μL), neutrophils 9,438 cells/μL (3,000–10,500 cells/μL), lymphocytes 2,057 cells/μL (1,000–4,000 cells/μL), monocytes 363 cells/μL (150–1,200 cells/μL), eosinophils 242 cells/μL (0–1,500 cells/μL), platelets 259,000 platelets/μL (150,000–400,000 platelets/μL).

Serum chemistry profile: sodium 150 mmol/L (145–154 mmol/L), potassium 4.3 mmol/L (3.6–5.3 mmol/L), chloride 114 mmol/L (108–118 mmol/L), bicarbonate 28 mmol/L (16–26 mmol/L), phosphorus 4.2 mg/dL (3.0–6.2 mg/dL), calcium 9.8 mg/dL (9.7–11.5 mg/dl), BUN 21 mg/dL (5–21 mg/dL), creatinine 1.2 mg/dL (0.3–1.2 mg/dL), glucose 99 mg/dL (64–123 mg/dL), total protein 6.4 g/dL (5.4–7.6 g/dL), albumin 2.9 g/dL (3.0–4.4 g/dL), globulin 3.5 g/dL (1.8–3.9 g/dL), ALT 61 U/L (19–67 U/L), AST 42 U/L (19–42 U/L), ALP 126 U/L (21–170 U/L), cholesterol 145 mg/dL (135–361 mg/dL), total bilirubin 0 mg/dL (0–0.2 mg/dL).

Urinalysis: SpG 1.005; pH 6.0; no protein (SSA), bilirubin, hemoprotein, or glucose; 0–1 WBC/HPF, rare RBC/HPF, rare transitional epithelial cells; no crystals, casts, or bacteria. Moderate numbers of encapsulated organisms were present that measured 10 × 17 μm.

Imaging Findings

Abdominal ultrasound examination: No abnormalities were identified.

Microbiologic Testing

Centrifugal zinc sulfate fecal flotation: Negative, but yeast-like bodies observed.

Giardia and *Cryptosporidium* fluorescent antibody testing (fecal specimen): Negative

Cytologic examination of rectal scrapings: Moderate numbers of neutrophils, small numbers of gram-positive coccobacilli, and small numbers of what appeared to be algal organisms were present.

Aerobic bacterial urine culture: Small numbers of *Prototheca* spp.

Algal susceptibility testing: MICs for amphotericin B, fluconazole, and itraconazole were 0.5 μg/mL, > 64 μg/mL, and 1 μg/mL, respectively.

Histopathology (rectal biopsy obtained by proctoscopy): Erosive and hemorrhagic colitis, eosinophilic and lymphoplasmacytic, moderate, with marked expansion of the lamina propria by intralesional spherical organisms (protothecal colitis) (see Fig. 90.5).

Aerobic bacterial and fungal culture of a rectal biopsy: Small numbers of mixed enteric species and *Prototheca* spp.

Diagnosis

Disseminated *Prototheca* spp. infection with ocular and colonic involvement.

Treatment

Merlot was initially treated with lipid-complexed amphotericin B (3 mg/kg IV) on a Monday, Wednesday, and Friday basis for five doses, after which increased serum creatinine concentration was noted (1.7 mg/dL). She was also treated with oxytetracycline (21 mg/kg PO q8h) during this time. She was discharged

CASE EXAMPLE—cont'd

after 11 days with instructions to administer itraconazole (5 mg/kg PO q12h) and lufenuron (5 mg/kg PO q24h). At a recheck examination 2 weeks later, the owners reported Merlot's appetite had improved slightly and that she was having normal bowel movements once to twice a day. Each bowel movement was followed by a small amount of diarrhea at the end of defecation, with bloody mucoid material occasionally present. Since her previous visit, a foxtail had been removed from her right pelvic limb and she had been sprayed in the face by a skunk. Physical examination revealed a body weight of 19.2 kg, but aqueous flare and multifocal retinal separations were present in both eyes. Urinalysis was unremarkable and rectal scrapings showed no evidence of algal organisms. A biochemistry panel showed normalization of the creatinine and mildly increased activity of ALT, likely secondary to itraconazole administration. Topical prednisolone acetate ophthalmic drops and two additional lipid-complexed amphotericin B treatments were administered, but bilateral retinal detachment, blindness, then bilateral hyphema, and apparent ocular pain developed despite this treatment. Bilateral enucleation was performed. Histopathology of the enucleated globes showed bilateral granulomatous uveitis and retinitis with intralesional *Prototheca* organisms (see Fig. 90.5B). In the left eye, posterior synechiae, intraocular hemorrhage, and cataract formation were identified.

At a recheck examination 3 months after enucleation, Merlot was eating well and had no signs of large bowel diarrhea. Her body weight was stable and physical examination, a CBC, a biochemistry panel, and cytological examination of a rectal scraping were unremarkable. Itraconazole treatment was continued at a lower dose (5 mg/kg PO daily) and the lufenuron was discontinued. Two months later, and shortly after a new puppy was introduced, Merlot developed vomiting and diarrhea with small amounts of hematochezia, and her body weight dropped to 17.5 kg. A serum biochemistry panel showed mild hypoalbuminemia (2.6 g/dL). Cytologic examination of a rectal scraping again revealed *Prototheca* organisms, and a fecal flotation was negative. Merlot was treated with fenbendazole and the dose of itraconazole was increased to 7.5 mg/kg PO daily, after which diarrhea resolved. Four months later (14 months after initial diagnosis), the dog remained in remission but was subsequently lost to follow-up.

Comments

Diagnosis of protothecosis in this dog was straightforward and initially based on routine urine sediment examination and culture. Colonic involvement was confirmed using proctoscopy and biopsy. The most likely place that *Prototheca* infection was acquired was in Texas, but it is possible that infection was acquired elsewhere. Partial clinical remission was observed after treatment with lipid-complexed amphotericin B and itraconazole, but enucleation was required to control pain. Remission was prolonged (> 1 year) even though only seven amphotericin B treatments were administered in the first 2 months after diagnosis. Lufenuron is a chitin synthetase inhibitor. Chitin is present in the cell wall of some algae (including *Chlorella*), but whether *Prototheca* possess chitin in their cell wall is not clear.

SUGGESTED READINGS

Lass-Florl C, Mayr A. Human protothecosis. *Clin Microbiol Rev*. 2007;20:230–242.

Falcaro C, Furlanello T, Binanti D, et al. Molecular characterization of *Prototheca* in 11 symptomatic dogs. *J Vet Diagn Invest*. 2021;33:156–161.

Quigley RR, Knowles KE, Johnson GC. Disseminated chlorellosis in a dog. *Vet Pathol*. 2009;46:439–443.

REFERENCES

1. Van Kruiningen HJ, Garner FM, Schiefer B. Protothecosis in a dog. *Pathol Vet*. 1969;6:348–354.
2. Lass-Florl C, Mayr A. Human protothecosis. *Clin Microbiol Rev*. 2007;20:230–242.
3. Sonck CE, Koch Y. *Prototheca* as parasites of skin. *Mykosen*. 1971;14: 475–482.
4. Masuda M, Jagielski T, Danesi P, et al. Protothecosis in dogs and cats-new research directions. *Mycopathologia*. 2021;186:143–152.
5. Falcaro C, Furlanello T, Binanti D, et al. Molecular characterization of *Prototheca* in 11 symptomatic dogs. *J Vet Diagn Invest*. 2021;33:156–161.
6. Ahrholdt J, Murugaiyan J, Straubinger RK, et al. Epidemiological analysis of worldwide bovine, canine and human clinical *Prototheca* isolates by PCR genotyping and MALDI-TOF mass spectrometry proteomic phenotyping. *Med Mycol*. 2012;50:234–243.
7. Ricchi M, Goretti M, Branda E, et al. Molecular characterization of *Prototheca* strains isolated from Italian dairy herds. *J Dairy Sci*. 2010;93:4625–4631.
8. Papadogiannakis EI, Velonakis EN, Spanakos GK, et al. Cutaneous disease as sole clinical manifestation of protothecosis in a boxer dog. *Case Rep Vet Med*. 2016;2016:2878751.
9. Stenner VJ, Mackay B, King T, et al. Protothecosis in 17 Australian dogs and a review of the canine literature. *Med Mycol*. 2007;45:249–266.
10. Vince AR, Pinard C, Ogilvie AT, et al. Protothecosis in a dog. *Can Vet J*. 2014;55:950–954.
11. Sykes JE. Unpublished observations.
12. Geisen V, Mayer C, Harrer J, et al. Disseminated protothecosis with ulcerative granulomatous colitis in a Rhodesian ridgeback from Germany. *Tierarztl Prax Ausg K Kleintiere Heimtiere*. 2020;48:369–375.
13. Schultz RM, Johnson EG, Wisner ER, et al. Clinicopathologic and diagnostic imaging characteristics of systemic aspergillosis in 30 dogs. *J Vet Intern Med*. 2008;22:851–859.
14. Huth N, Wenkel RF, Roschanski N, et al. *Prototheca zopfii* genotype 2-induced nasal dermatitis in a cat. *J Comp Pathol*. 2015;152:287–290.
15. Coloe PJ, Allison JF. Protothecosis in a cat. *J Am Vet Med Assoc*. 1982;180:78–79.
16. Dillberger JE, Homer B, Daubert D, et al. Protothecosis in two cats. *J Am Vet Med Assoc*. 1988;192:1557–1559.
17. Endo S, Sekiguchi M, Kishimoto Y, et al. The first case of feline *Prototheca wickerhamii* infection in Japan. *J Vet Med Sci*. 2010;72:1351–1353.
18. Finnie JW, Coloe PJ. Cutaneous protothecosis in a cat. *Aust Vet J*. 1981;57:307–308.
19. Kaplan W, Chandler FW, Holzinger EA, et al. Protothecosis in a cat: first recorded case. *Sabouraudia*. 1976;14:281–286.
20. Migaki G, Font RL, Sauer RM, et al. Canine protothecosis: review of the literature and report of an additional case. *J Am Vet Med Assoc*. 1982;181:794–797.
21. Kessell AE, McNair D, Munday JS, et al. Successful treatment of multifocal pedal *Prototheca wickerhamii* infection in a feline immunodeficiency virus-positive cat with multiple Bowenoid in situ carcinomas containing papillomaviral DNA sequences. *JFMS Open Rep*. 2017;3. 2055116916688590.
22. Lane LV, Meinkoth JH, Brunker J, et al. Disseminated protothecosis diagnosed by evaluation of CSF in a dog. *Vet Clin Pathol*. 2012;41:147–152.
23. Pressler BM, Gookin JL, Sykes JE, et al. Urinary tract manifestations of protothecosis in dogs. *J Vet Intern Med*. 2005;19:115–119.
24. Gaunt SD, McGrath RK, Cox HU. Disseminated protothecosis in a dog. *J Am Vet Med Assoc*. 1984;185:906–907
25. Manino PM, Oliveira F, Ficken M, et al. Disseminated protothecosis associated with diskospondylitis in a dog. *J Am Anim Hosp Assoc*. 2014;50: 429–435.
26. Cook JR Jr, Tyler DE, Coulter DB, et al. Disseminated protothecosis causing acute blindness and deafness in a dog. *J Am Vet Med Assoc*. 1984;184:1266–1272.
27. Rakich PM, Latimer KS. Altered immune function in a dog with disseminated protothecosis. *J Am Vet Med Assoc*. 1984;185:681–683.
28. Buyukmihci N, Rubin LF, DePaoli A. Protothecosis with ocular involvement in a dog. *J Am Vet Med Assoc*. 1975;167:158–161.

29. Blogg JR, Sykes JE. Sudden blindness associated with protothecosis in a dog. *Aust Vet J*. 1995;72:147–149.
30. Moore FM, Schmidt GM, Desai D, et al. Unsuccessful treatment of disseminated protothecosis in a dog. *J Am Vet Med Assoc*. 1985;186:705–708.
31. Whipple KM, Wellehan JF, Jeon AB, et al. Cytologic, histologic, microbiologic, and electron microscopic characterization of a canine *Prototheca wickerhamii* infection. *Vet Clin Pathol*. 2020;49:326–332.
32. Shank AM, Dubielzig RD, Teixeira LB. Canine ocular protothecosis: a review of 14 cases. *Vet Ophthalmol*. 2015;18:437–442.
33. Gupta A, Gumber S, Bauer RW, et al. What is your diagnosis? Cerebrospinal fluid from a dog. Eosinophilic pleocytosis due to protothecosis. *Vet Clin Pathol*. 2011;40:105–106.
34. Young M, Bush W, Sanchez M, et al. Serial MRI and CSF analysis in a dog treated with intrathecal amphotericin B for protothecosis. *J Am Anim Hosp Assoc*. 2012;48:125–131.
35. Salvadori C, Gandini G, Ballarini A, et al. Protothecal granulomatous meningoencephalitis in a dog. *J Small Anim Pract*. 2008;49:531–535.
36. Tyler DE, Lorenz MD, Blue JL, et al. Disseminated protothecosis with central nervous system involvement in a dog. *J Am Vet Med Assoc*. 1980;176:987–993.
37. Quigley RR, Knowles KE, Johnson GC. Disseminated chlorellosis in a dog. *Vet Pathol*. 2009;46:439–443.
38. von Bergen M, Eidner A, Schmidt F, et al. Identification of harmless and pathogenic algae of the genus *Prototheca* by MALDI-MS. *Proteomics Clin Appl*. 2009;3:774–784.
39. Ricchi M, Cammi G, Garbarino CA, et al. A rapid real-time PCR/DNA resolution melting method to identify *Prototheca* species. *J Appl Microbiol*. 2011;110:27–34.
40. Samarasekara J, Mukherjee S, Ismail A, Corns R. Cerebral protothecosis mimicking high-grade glioma. *BMJ Case Rep*. 2021;14:e235362.
41. Zhao J, Liu W, Lv G, et al. Protothecosis successfully treated with amikacin combined with tetracyclines. *Mycoses*. 2004;47:156–158.
42. Pascual JS, Balos LL, Baer AN. Disseminated *Prototheca wickerhamii* infection with arthritis and tenosynovitis. *J Rheumatol*. 2004;31:1861–1865.
43. Lass-Florl C, Fille M, Gunsilius E, et al. Disseminated infection with *Prototheca zopfii* after unrelated stem cell transplantation for leukemia. *J Clin Microbiol*. 2004;42:4907–4908.
44. Mohd Tap R, Sabaratnam P, Salleh MA, et al. Characterization of *Prototheca wickerhamii* isolated from disseminated algaemia of kidney transplant patient from Malaysia. *Mycopathologia*. 2012;173:173–178.
45. Kaminski ZC, Kapila R, Sharer LR, et al. Meningitis due to *Prototheca wickerhamii* in a patient with AIDS. *Clin Infect Dis*. 1992;15:704–706.
46. Riet-Correa F, Carmo P, Uzal FA. Protothecosis and chlorellosis in sheep and goats: a review. *J Vet Diagn Invest*. 2021;33:283–287.
47. Chandler FW, Kaplan W, Callaway CS. Differentiation between *Prototheca* and morphologically similar green algae in tissue. *Arch Pathol Lab Med*. 1978;102:353–356.
48. Jones JW, McFadden HW, Chandler FW, et al. Green algal infection in a human. *Am J Clin Pathol*. 1983;80:102–107.

Rhinosporidiosis

Jane E. Sykes

KEY POINTS

- First Described: In the 1890s, in Argentina (Malbran and then Seeber).[1]
- Cause: *Rhinosporidium seeberi* (kingdom Protista, class Mesomycetozoea).
- Affected Hosts: Dogs, humans, horses, rarely cats, and other domestic animals.
- Geographic Distribution: Worldwide but especially in warm, wet environments such as the southeastern and southcentral United States.
- Mode of Transmission: Unclear, possibly exposure to contaminated water sources in association with trauma.
- Major Clinical Signs: Sneezing, epistaxis, mass protruding from nares.
- Differential Diagnoses: Nasal neoplasia, cryptococcosis, sinonasal aspergillosis, nasal mites, foreign bodies.
- Human Health Significance: Human infections by *R. seeberi* are likely acquired from the environment, and direct transmission from affected animals to humans has not been described.

ETIOLOGY AND EPIDEMIOLOGY

Rhinosporidiosis is caused by *Rhinosporidium seeberi*, which causes slow-growing tumor-like masses in the nasal cavity. Although once thought to be a fungus, molecular methods have identified this organism as an aquatic protistan parasite (class Mesomycetozoea) that is taxonomically located where animals and fungi diverge and is closely related to pathogens of fish.[2,3] The organism is difficult or impossible to culture. Rhinosporidiosis has been most widely reported in humans and dogs, but cats, horses, and other mammalian and avian species may also be affected. There is some evidence that host-specific strains of *R. seeberi* exist.[4]

Rhinosporidiosis is most prevalent in humans from southern India, Sri Lanka, and Argentina but also occurs in North America, Africa, Europe, and Asia. In dogs and cats, rhinosporidiosis has been reported from many regions of the United States, Ontario in Canada,[5] Argentina,[6] northern Brazil,[7] Paraguay,[2] Italy in continental Europe,[8] and the United Kingdom.[9] Within North America, the disease has most often been reported in dogs and cats from the southcentral and southeastern states (Fig. 91.1). The overwhelming majority of affected dogs have been young adult to middle-aged (with a range of 1 to 13 years of age), otherwise healthy, large-breed hunting dogs such as Labrador and golden retrievers, Doberman pinschers, Siberian huskies, German shepherds, and Rhodesian ridgebacks. However, small-breed dogs can also be affected.[9] No clear sex predisposition has been identified, but of cases reported in the literature, males have outnumbered females. Affected cats have been outdoor cats. One affected cat had concurrent nasal adenocarcinoma,[10] but other cats have had no reported comorbidities.

While the mode of transmission of *R. seeberi* is not precisely understood, disease often occurs in association with contact with aquatic or marshy environments. It is thought that spores are released into the environment, where they come into contact with susceptible human and animal hosts.[3] Spores may be introduced into tissues after trauma to the mucous membranes, where they form sporangia that produce new spores. Because disease in humans also occurs in arid regions, airborne spore transmission has also been suggested.

CLINICAL FEATURES

Pathogenesis and Clinical Signs

In dogs and cats, infection by *R. seeberi* leads to formation of pedunculate or sessile masses within the nasal cavity, usually in the rostral third.[8] The polyps can range in size from a few millimeters to several centimeters. Clinical signs consist of subacute (weeks) to chronic (> 1 year) sneezing with or without epistaxis, snuffling, and sometimes a serous to serosanguinous unilateral nasal discharge. Sneezing may be frequent and severe and associated with excitement or increased activity. In some dogs, a polypoid pink mass protrudes from the nasal cavity. The masses are often stippled with white-yellowish granules less than 1 mm in diameter, which represent mature sporangia.[8]

DIAGNOSIS

Most animals with rhinosporidiosis have no significant hematologic or biochemical abnormalities on blood work. Plain radiography is insensitive for detection of nasal masses caused by *R. seeberi*.[8] CT reveals soft tissue masses in the rostral third of the nasal cavity that can enhance with contrast (Fig. 91.2). In some cases, evidence of turbinate loss is present. The masses can be visualized directly using rostral rhinoscopy and are pink to gray and may be covered with miliary white to yellow foci (Fig. 91.3).

Definitive diagnosis requires cytology or histopathology of the masses, which reveal large numbers of organisms. Cytologic examination of smears from nasal swabs, cytology brush specimens, or impression smears made from biopsies of the polyps reveals suppurative to pyogranulomatous inflammation with dysplastic epithelial cells and numerous immature to mature *R. seeberi* endospores, which occur singly or in clusters.[11] Sometimes sporangia that contain hundreds of endospores are visualized. Mature endospores stain intensely, are round to oval and 10 to 15 μm in diameter, and have a thick cell wall (Fig. 91.4). Immature endospores are 2 to 4 μm in diameter, contain a paracentral, light pink-purple structure that may represent nuclear material, and 1 to 2 smaller, spherical, dark purple structures.[11]

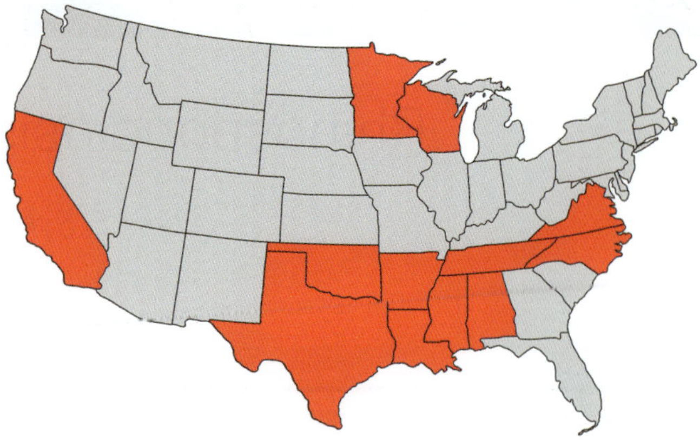

Fig. 91.1 States within the United States in which rhinosporidiosis has been reported in dogs and cats.

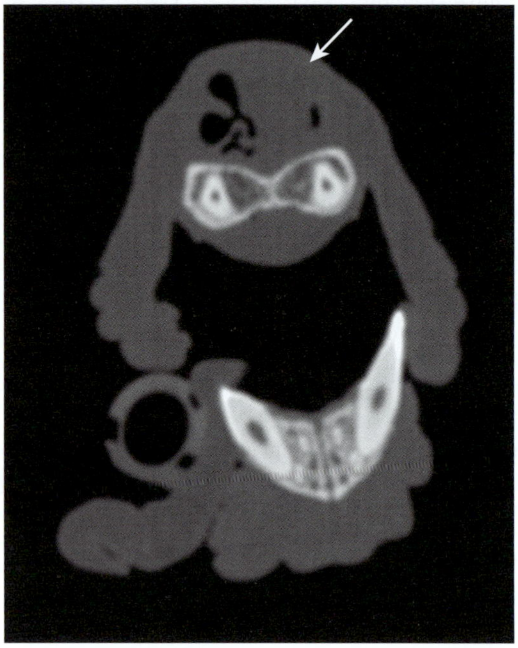

Fig. 91.2 Computed tomography scan of the nasal cavity of a 16-month-old female Labrador retriever with rhinosporidiosis. A soft tissue mass that enhanced with contrast is present in the rostral nasal cavity *(arrow)*.

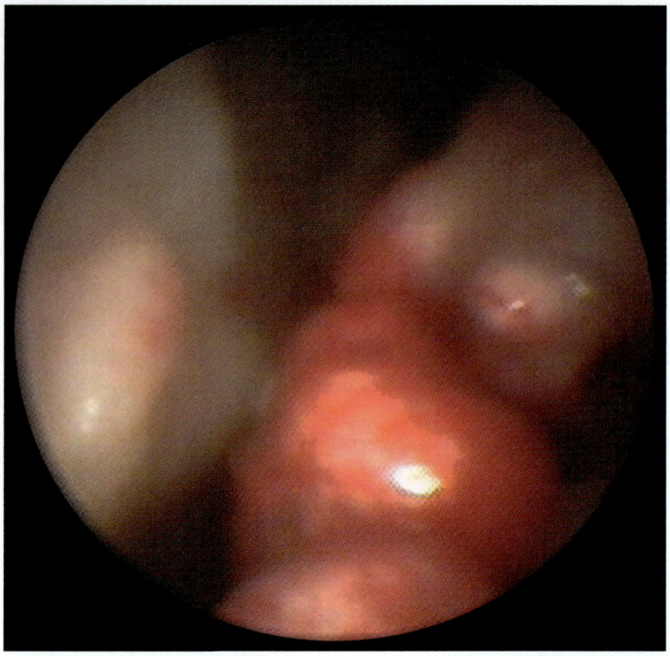

Fig. 91.3 Rhinoscopic image of a polypoid mass caused by *Rhinosporidium seeberi* in the nasal cavity of a 10-year-old intact female yellow Labrador retriever.

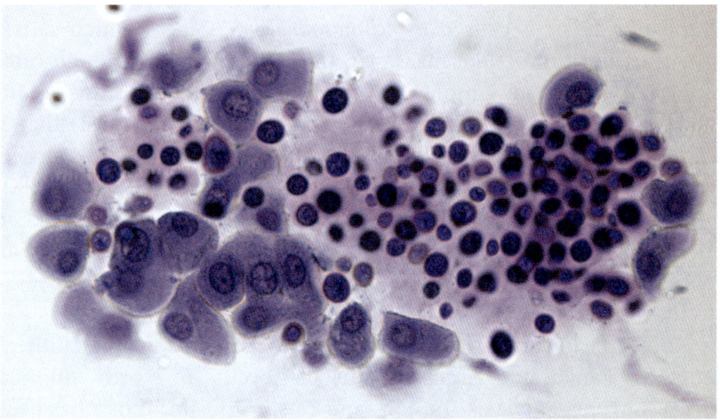

Fig. 91.4 Impression smear of a biopsy taken from the nasal cavity of a 6-year-old female spayed Labrador retriever with rhinosporidiosis. A large cluster of endospores is present together with several epithelial cells.

Histopathology reveals the presence of abundant sporangia in various stages of development and a mild to severe pyogranulomatous inflammatory response (Fig. 91.5). Lymphocytes, plasma cells, and in some cases, multinucleate giant cells and evidence of turbinate remodeling with activated osteoclasts and osteoblasts may be present. Juvenile sporangia are small (< 100 μm in diameter) and have a single nucleus that is surrounded by fibrillar material. Mature sporangia are up to 500 μm in diameter and may be seen releasing endospores at the polyp surface through a pore in the sporangial wall. Although the organisms stain well with special stains such as PAS, Gomori's methenamine silver, and Meyer's mucicarmine, these stains are usually not required for diagnosis.[8]

TREATMENT AND PROGNOSIS

The treatment of choice for dogs and cats is surgical removal of polyps, which generally requires rhinotomy. Because the polyps are often rostrally located, excisions can often be extended caudally from the nares. Many dogs have no recurrence of clinical signs thereafter, but some dogs experience disease recurrence within months of surgery.[6,12,13] The median time to recurrence in 4 dogs from Mississippi treated surgically was 749 days (range, 180-916 days).[14] Treatment of these dogs can be frustrating and costly. Povidone iodine is active *in vitro* against *R. seeberi* and could be applied in the form of gauze packs topically after surgery in an attempt to minimize the chance of recurrence (see Case Example).[15] Further study is required to determine if this changes outcome. In some dogs, apparent transient or long-term responses to treatment with ketoconazole[9,16] or dapsone (1.1 mg/kg, PO, q8–12h) have been described. Responses to dapsone have also been described in human patients. Dapsone could be used to treat dogs with refractory disease, but because both dapsone and ketoconazole have the potential to cause significant adverse effects, careful monitoring is required. Dapsone is a sulfur drug (diaminophenyl sulfone) that has been reported to cause leukopenia or thrombocytopenia in dogs.[17] Treatment of cats with dapsone is not recommended due to a high prevalence of adverse effects in this species, specifically neurotoxicosis and anemia.

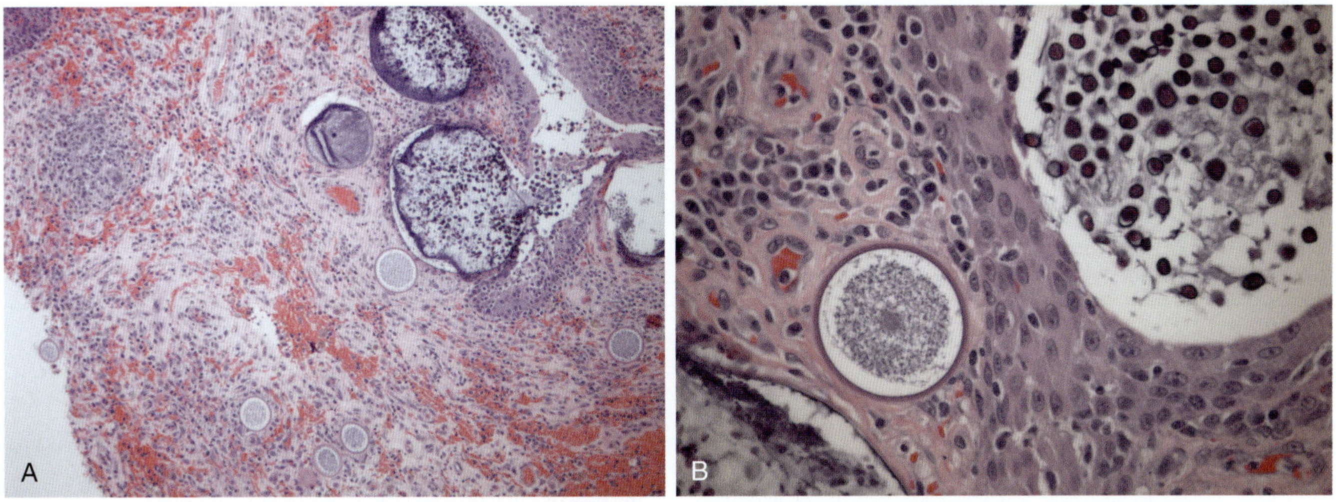

Fig. 91.5 Histopathology of a polyp caused by *Rhinosporidium seeberi.* (A) Low-power image that shows sporangia in various stages of development. (B) High-power image (1000× oil magnification) that shows a juvenile sporangium adjacent to a mature sporangium, which contains endospores *(right)*. Hematoxylin and eosin stain.

PUBLIC HEALTH ASPECTS

In humans, rhinosporidiosis usually involves the nasal cavity or nasopharynx, but involvement of the conjunctiva, genitalia or the skin, and rarely disseminated cutaneous disease, can occur.[2,18] Involvement of calvarial bones was described in one person who also had evidence of dissemination affecting the right lower limb.[19] Disease is most often reported in males with a male-to-female ratio of 3:1, and affected individuals are most often 15 to 40 years of age. Infection is likely acquired from the environment, and transmission from animals to humans has not been described. It is possible that strains of *R. seeberi* that infect humans may differ from those that infect dogs.

CASE EXAMPLE

Signalment

"Sarah," a 16-month-old intact female Labrador retriever from the central valley of northern California.

History

Sarah was evaluated by her local veterinary clinic for a 1-month history of sneezing, which occurred throughout the day and was more frequent and severe during periods of excitement. The owners had not noted any nasal discharge and were concerned about the possibility of a foreign body. A limited rhinoscopic examination with an otoscope cone at the local veterinary clinic revealed a large, fleshy, irregular mass in the dorsal meatus near the nares. A biopsy of the mass was consistent with a diagnosis of rhinosporidiosis, and Sarah was referred to the University of California, Davis Veterinary Internal Medicine service, for further evaluation and treatment.

Sarah was obtained from a breeder in Oregon as a puppy and since then has been used as a duck hunting dog in California. During the hunting season, she wades and swims in both stagnant and fresh water sources. The owners also have ponds in their backyard. She was otherwise healthy and was fed a dry commercial dog food diet.

Physical Examination

Body weight: 32.2 kg.

General: Excited, alert, responsive, and hydrated. T = 101.6°F (38.7°C), HR = 140 beats/minute, panting, CRT < 2 seconds, mucous membranes were moist and pink.

Eyes, ears, nose, and throat: Face was symmetrical with no pain on palpation, normal ocular retropulsion. No evidence of nasal discharge. Absent nasal airflow on the right side. Minimal dental calculus present. No other clinically significant findings.

Musculoskeletal: BCS 4/9. Adequate musculature, normal gait.

Cardiovascular: No murmurs or arrhythmias were auscultated. Pulses strong and symmetrical.

Respiratory: No significant abnormalities were detected.

Abdominal palpation and genitourinary examination: No significant abnormalities were detected.

Lymph nodes: All were < 1–1.5 cm in diameter and soft.

Laboratory Findings

Pre-anesthetic laboratory assessment: PCV 44%, total solids 6.6 g/dL. Serum urea nitrogen estimated at 15–26 mg/dL with a reagent strip.

Imaging Findings

CT of the head: A round, 0.9 × 1.7 × 2.3-cm, soft tissue mass was present in the rostral, dorsal right nasal cavity extending from the level of the incisors to the root of the right maxillary canine tooth. The mass was moderately, heterogeneously contrast enhancing. The superficial soft tissues overlying the mass were thickened and contrast enhancing. The remainder of the nasal cavities and sinuses appeared within normal limits. The mandibular and medial retropharyngeal lymph nodes appeared within normal limits.

Diagnosis

Nasal rhinosporidiosis.

Treatment

A rhinotomy was performed using an anterolateral approach, and a single 1.5 × 0.5-cm pedunculated mass was identified attached to the mucosal layer of the nasal septum. The mass was resected with sharp dissection and diathermy. A povidone

Continued

CASE EXAMPLE—cont'd

iodine-soaked gauze pad was placed on the site of resection for 7 minutes, and the nasal vestibule was packed with an iodine-soaked gauze pad for 1 hour after surgical closure. Histopathology confirmed the diagnosis of nasal rhinosporidiosis. The dog was discharged with instructions to administer tramadol (3 mg/kg, PO, q12h) for pain relief and dapsone (0.8 mg/kg, PO, q8h, for 2 weeks, then 0.8 mg/kg, PO, q12h, for 3 months). At a recheck 2 weeks later, the sneezing had reduced in frequency but vomiting was reported every 2 days approximately 2 hours after the morning dose of dapsone. A CBC and biochemistry panel were unremarkable. The frequency of dapsone administration was reduced to twice daily. Subsequently, Sarah did well with no recurrence of disease or adverse effects of medication.

Comments

In this dog, topical povidone iodine and dapsone were used after rhinotomy in an attempt to prevent recurrence, because the owners indicated that they would not have sufficient funds to repeat rhinotomy. The owners were warned about the possibility of re-infection if Sarah continued her hunting activities.

SUGGESTED READINGS

Caniatti M, Roccabianca P, Scanziani E, et al. Nasal rhinosporidiosis in dogs: four cases from Europe and a review of the literature. *Vet Rec.* 1998;142:334–338.

Cridge H, Mamaliger N, Baughman B, et al. Nasal rhinosporidiosis: clinical presentation, clinical findings, and outcome in dogs. *J Am Anim Hosp Assoc.* 2021;57:114–120.

Dewangan B, Naik R, Membally R, et al. Calvarial involvement in disseminated rhinosporidiosis: a case report and literature review. *J Postgrad Med.* 2020;66:38–41.

REFERENCES

1. Fredricks DN, Jolley JA, Lepp PW, et al. *Rhinosporidium seeberi*: a human pathogen from a novel group of aquatic protistan parasites. *Emerg Infect Dis.* 2000;6:273–282.
2. Arias Sanchez AF, Romero Arias SD, Garcés Samudio CG. Case report: rhinosporidiosis, case report, and literature review. *Am J Trop Med Hyg.* 2020;104:708–711.
3. Mendoza L, Vilela R, Rosa PS, et al. *Lacazia loboi* and *Rhinosporidium seeberi*: a genomic perspective. *Rev Iberoam Micol.* 2005;22:213–216.
4. Silva V, Pereira CN, Ajello L, et al. Molecular evidence for multiple host-specific strains in the genus *Rhinosporidium*. *J Clin Microbiol.* 2005;43:1865–1868.
5. Hoff B, Hall DA. Rhinosporidiosis in a dog. *Can Vet J.* 1986;27:231–232.
6. Castellano MC, Idiart JR, Martin AA. Rhinosporidiosis in a dog. *Vet Med Small Anim Clinician.* 1984;79:45.
7. Almeida FA, Feitoza Lde M, Pinho JD, et al. Rhinosporidiosis: the largest case series in Brazil. *Rev Soc Bras Med Trop.* 2016;49:473–476.
8. Caniatti M, Roccabianca P, Scanziani E, et al. Nasal rhinosporidiosis in dogs: four cases from Europe and a review of the literature. *Vet Rec.* 1998;142:334–338.
9. Miller RI, Baylis R. Rhinosporidiosis in a dog native to the UK. *Vet Rec.* 2009;164:210.
10. Brenseke BM, Saunders GK. Concurrent nasal adenocarcinoma and rhinosporidiosis in a cat. *J Vet Diagn Invest.* 2010;22:155–157.
11. Meier WA, Meinkoth JH, Brunker J, et al. Cytologic identification of immature endospores in a dog with rhinosporidiosis. *Vet Clin Pathol.* 2006;35:348–352.
12. Mosier DA, Creed JE. Rhinosporidiosis in a dog. *J Am Vet Med Assoc.* 1984;185:1009–1010.
13. Allison N, Willard MD, Bentinck-Smith J, et al. Nasal rhinosporidiosis in two dogs. *J Am Vet Med Assoc.* 1986;188:869–871.
14. Cridge H, Mamaliger N, Baughman B, et al. Nasal rhinosporidiosis: clinical presentation, clinical findings, and outcome in dogs. *J Am Anim Hosp Assoc.* 2021;57:114–120.
15. Arseculeratne SN, Atapattu DN, Balasooriya P, et al. The effects of biocides (antiseptics and disinfectants) on the endospores of *Rhinosporidium seeberi*. *Indian J Med Microbiol.* 2006;24:85–91.
16. Easley JR, Meuten DJ, Levy MG, et al. Nasal rhinosporidiosis in the dog. *Vet Pathol.* 1986;23:50–56.
17. Lees GE, McKeever PJ, Ruth GR. Fatal thrombocytopenic hemorrhagic diathesis associated with dapsone administration to a dog. *J Am Vet Med Assoc.* 1979;175:49–52.
18. Prasad K, Veena S, Permi HS, et al. Disseminated cutaneous rhinosporidiosis. *J Lab Physicians.* 2010;2:44–46.
19. Dewangan B, Naik R, Membally R, et al. Calvarial involvement in disseminated rhinosporidiosis: a case report and literature review. *J Postgrad Med.* 2020;66:38–41.

92

Microsporidiosis (Encephalitozoonosis)

Karen F. Snowden, Jane E. Sykes

KEY POINTS

- First Described: In 1922, the first reports described histologic lesions and organisms in the brains of rabbits.[1] A series of clinical papers authored by Levaditi, Nicolau, and Schoen describing lesions in rabbits followed in 1923, and the organism was named by that group in 1924.[2] Canine infections were first described as an encephalitis-nephritis syndrome in 1952 by Plowright.[3] *Encephalitozoon cuniculi* was first isolated from dogs in 1978 by Shadduck et al.[4]
- Cause: *Encephalitozoon cuniculi*, phylum Microsporidia, family Unikaryonidae. Microsporidia are eukaryotic, intracellular organisms related to fungi that are found in a wide range of invertebrate and vertebrate hosts including a limited number of species found in mammals.
- Affected Hosts: *Encephalitozoon cuniculi* infects a wide range of mammalian hosts including domestic rabbits, mice, rats, hamsters, guinea pigs, dogs, nonhuman primates, humans, and a number of wild rodent species; additional host species are described in miscellaneous reports.
- Geographic Distribution: *Encephalitozoon cuniculi* infections in rabbits, rodents, dogs, and other hosts are geographically widespread with reports from the United States, Europe, South America, Africa, and Asia.
- Primary Route of Transmission: *Encephalitozoon cuniculi* has a direct life cycle with the major route of transmission through the ingestion of infective environmentally resistant spores. Transplacental transmission has also been documented in rabbits, dogs, and blue foxes.
- Major Clinical Signs: Encephalitis-nephritis syndrome. Young animals demonstrate inappetence and depression with progressive neurologic signs such as incoordination and ataxia, circling, and central blindness leading to death. Chronic progressive renal disease and end-stage renal failure have also been documented in young adult animals.
- Differential Diagnoses: Clinical disease in dogs is most frequently confused with neurologic signs associated with CDV infections as well as rabies or systemic toxoplasmosis.
- Human Health Significance: Systemic, sometimes fatal, *E. cuniculi* infections have been reported in a small number of immunocompromised humans. Direct transmission of the pathogen from animals to humans has not been clearly documented, but it is likely that indirect transmission of the organisms may be related to animal shedding of infective spores into the environment with subsequent human exposure.

ETIOLOGY AND EPIDEMIOLOGY

Members of the phylum Microsporidia are eukaryotic obligate intracellular pathogens that occasionally cause infection and disease in mammalian hosts. Historically these organisms were taxonomically classified as protozoa, but molecular analysis has reclassified Microsporidia as more closely related to the fungi.[5–7] More than 1,200 species of microsporidia, grouped into approximately 100 genera, infect insects and members of all classes of vertebrates.[8,9]

Microsporidia have a unique mechanism for host cell invasion. They contain a distinctive coiled polar filament or tubule structure that acts as an extrusion apparatus (Figs. 92.1 and 92.2).[8,9] This polar filament is used to propel the sporoplasm (spore contents containing the microsporidian nucleus) into the host cell. The spore has a tri-layered coat which consists of an outer glycoprotein layer, a middle layer that contains chitin, and an internal plasma membrane; together these confer resistance to destruction by environmental factors. Spore infectivity is minimally affected by freezing and thawing, and spores survive at pH levels from 4 to 9. The infectivity of spores stored in neutral buffer at 4°C and 20°C persisted for more than 24 days.[9,10] However, spores can be inactivated by various disinfectants including 0.5%–30% hydrogen peroxide, 5% ammonium hydroxide, peroxyacetic acid, or didecyl dimethyl ammonium chloride with adequate contact time.[11,12] Similarly, spores were rapidly inactivated with 10% sodium hypochlorite (bleach) or 70% ethyl alcohol.[11,13]

Natural infections with microsporidia have been described in a wide range of mammalian hosts including domestic and wild rabbits, domestic and wild rodents, dogs, foxes, cats, nonhuman primates, and humans, with sporadic reports in other domestic animals and a variety of wildlife.[8,14,15] Several different microsporidial species infect humans, causing diarrhea, encephalitis, keratoconjunctivitis, respiratory, or disseminated disease primarily in immunocompromised hosts (Fig. 92.3). The most important is *Enterocytozoon bieneusi*, followed by *Encephalitozoon intestinalis*; others include *Encephalitozoon cuniculi* and *Encephalitozoon hellem*. From a veterinary perspective, the most important microsporidian pathogen is *E. cuniculi*, the primary focus of this chapter.

Infections with *E. cuniculi* have been described in rabbits, rodents, and dogs with occasional reports in cats, nonhuman primates, and a wide range of domestic and wild mammals.[8,14,15] Three genotypes (strains) of *E. cuniculi* have been identified.[16] Differences in these isolates have been confirmed by protein electrophoresis, Western blotting, and small-subunit rRNA (SSU rRNA) gene sequence analysis. Genotype I has been identified in rabbits and humans.[17] Genotype II has been identified in mice, rats, and blue foxes.[15,16] The only strain identified in dogs to date is genotype III, which has also been found in nonhuman primate and human infections.[18–21]

Infection of most mammalian hosts with *E. cuniculi* occurs following ingestion of spores shed in the urine or feces of infected hosts, which subsequently contaminate the environment (Fig. 92.4).[8,9,15] Transplacental

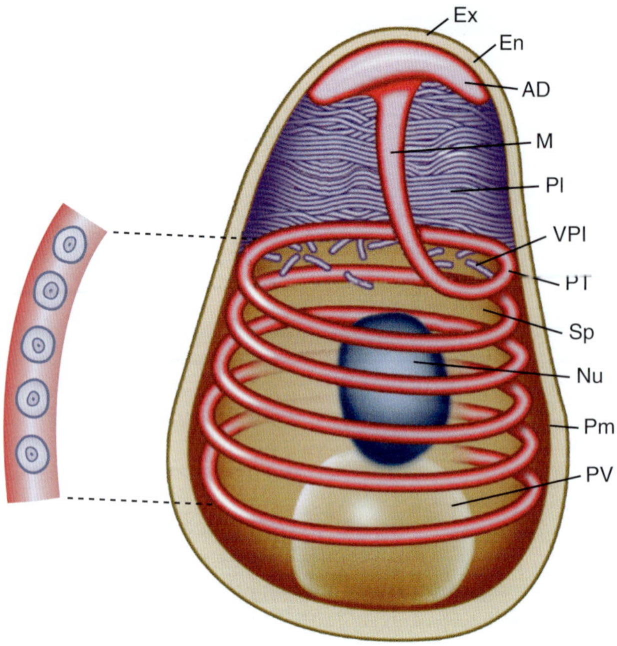

Fig. 92.1 Schematic diagram illustrating the structure of a microsporidian spore. The extrusion apparatus consists of the polar tube *(PT)*, vesiculotubular polaroplast *(VPl)*, lamellar polaroplast *(Pl)*, anchoring disc *(AD)*, and manubrium *(M)*. The inset shows a cross-section of the polar tube coils. The endospore *(En)* is an inner, thicker, electron-lucent region. The exospore *(Ex)* is an outer electron-dense region. The plasma membrane *(Pm)* separates the spore coat from the sporoplasm *(Sp)* which contains ribosomes in a coiled helical array. The posterior vacuole *(PV)* is a membrane-bound structure below the nucleus *(Nu)*. (Modified from Wittner M, Weiss LM, eds. *The Microsporidia and Microsporidiosis*. Washington, DC: American Society of Microbiology Press ©1999 American Society for Microbiology. Used with permission. No further reproduction or distribution is permitted without the prior written permission of American Society for Microbiology.)

transmission has been reported in rabbits and dogs.[22,23] Inhalation of spores is included in the literature as a route of transmission, but there is little evidence to confirm or refute that possibility for dogs.

Neurologic disease attributed to *E. cuniculi* was first described in rabbits in the early 1920s.[1,2] Histologically confirmed reports of microsporidial infections in dogs were published in the 1950s and 1960s that described an encephalitis-nephritis syndrome in puppies caused by *E. cuniculi*.[3,24] The scientific name *Nosema cuniculi* was also used in some scientific reports in the 1960s and 1970s.[24] The organism was first isolated from dogs in 1978.[4]

Microsporidial diseases are not well recognized in dogs. The prevalence of antibodies to *Encephalitozoon cuniculi* in domestic dogs has ranged from 0% in specimens submitted to diagnostic laboratories in Norway[25] to 70% in a South African dog kennel.[25] Other surveys report seroprevalence rates of 14.3% in Brazil,[26] 18% in South Africa,[25] 18.5% in Colombia,[26] 20.5% in the United Kingdom,[27] 21.8% in Japan,[28] 40% in Egypt,[29] and 29.8%, 37.8%, and 48.5% in three studies from Slovakia.[30–32] The wide range in seroprevalence can partly be explained by the use of different immunodiagnostic test methods (ELISA, IFA, direct agglutination) and evaluation of dogs from various sources (strays, kennels, veterinary clinics, or unknown) and from different geographic locations. These data suggest that exposure of dogs to microsporidia is frequent, and that subclinical infections are probably common but are unrecognized or undetected.

Microsporidial spores were detected microscopically in fecal specimens from 6 of 20 dogs in an urban animal shelter in the United States.[33] In a study from Egypt, spores were microscopically detected in trichrome-stained smears in 36 of 108 (33.3%) dog fecal specimens.[34] Using a fecal PCR test, 18 of 100 dog fecal specimens collected at a veterinary clinic in Iran were positive.[35] One of the difficulties in interpreting data from fecal microscopy is that the microsporidial species is not determined, and so the possibility that the dog ingested spores from environmental sources without being infected cannot be ruled out. Similarly, detection of microsporidial DNA in fecal specimens does not clearly confirm infection, but could result in ingestion of spores from food sources or environmental contamination, since microsporidia in general are ubiquitous.

Experimental infections have shown that cats may become infected with *E. cuniculi*; however, natural infections of cats are rare and epidemiologic information is minimal.[36] In a survey of 232 cats in Virginia, 15 animals were seropositive by IFA, and the prevalence of IgG antibodies to *E. cuniculi* was not significantly different between cats with or without CKD.[37] In a Swiss study, one of 45 cats were seropositive, and no microsporidial spores were detected in 45 cat fecal specimens.[38]

CLINICAL FEATURES

Pathogenesis and Clinical Signs

Once internalized, infectious spores invade host cells by propelling the sporoplasm through the everted polar filament by a process called "germination." The sporoplasm of *E. cuniculi* develops within a host cell–derived membrane-bound parasitophorous vacuole. The organisms undergo asexual replication and then sporogony to develop the spore coat and organelles, which are needed for infectivity and environmental resistance. Host cells eventually rupture and release organisms that infect new cells. Alternatively, environmentally resistant spores form, which are shed in the urine or feces. Typical organs of localized infection in dogs and cats include the kidney, liver, and brain.[15,36,39]

The development of clinical signs has been most commonly reported in domestic rabbits and dogs, with sporadic reports in other species.[15] Clinically significant *E. cuniculi* infections generally occur in neonatal and young puppies and are acquired by transplacental transmission or ingestion of spores shed from the mother.[18,23] Older dogs may become infected with microsporidia by ingestion of spores from contaminated urine or feces. Experimental canine infections have been documented after transmission by oral or intraperitoneal inoculation, or transplacentally from infected bitches.[39,40] Kittens have been infected experimentally by intracerebral, intraperitoneal, or oral inoculation.[36]

Dogs

The clinical presentation of *E. cuniculi* infection in dogs ranges from subclinical to fatal. Based on seroprevalence studies, exposure to the pathogen and subclinical infections are probably common, but undocumented. The most common clinical manifestation of encephalitozoonosis is an encephalitis-nephritis syndrome, which occurs in puppies from 4 to 10 weeks of age.[3,18,23,24,41–43] A single pup, several pups, or an entire litter may show signs of inappetence, stunted growth, and unthriftiness. As infection progresses, animals show neurologic abnormalities such as mental obtundation, loss of awareness of surroundings, incoordination progressing to pelvic limb ataxia, seizures, and blindness. Clinical disease is most frequently confused with neurologic signs associated with CDV infections as well as rabies, neosporosis, or

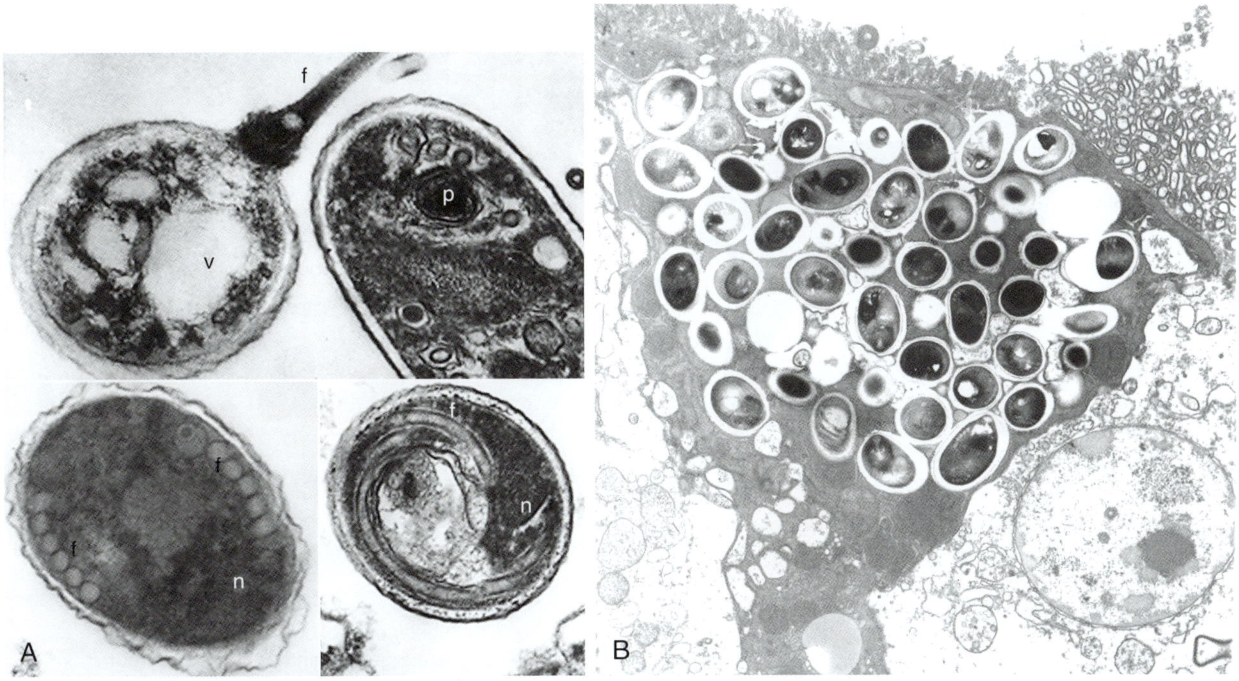

Fig. 92.2 (A) Electron microscopy of a mature *Encephalitozoon cuniculi* spore. Anterior polaroplast (*p*), loops of the polar filament (*f*) in longitudinal and cross-section views, nucleus (*n*), posterior vacuole (*v*), and electron-lucent spore wall are shown. (B) Transmission electron micrograph showing a cluster of *Encephalitozoon hellem* spores within an enterocyte of a hummingbird. (B, Courtesy Karen F. Snowden DVM, PhD, DACVM.)

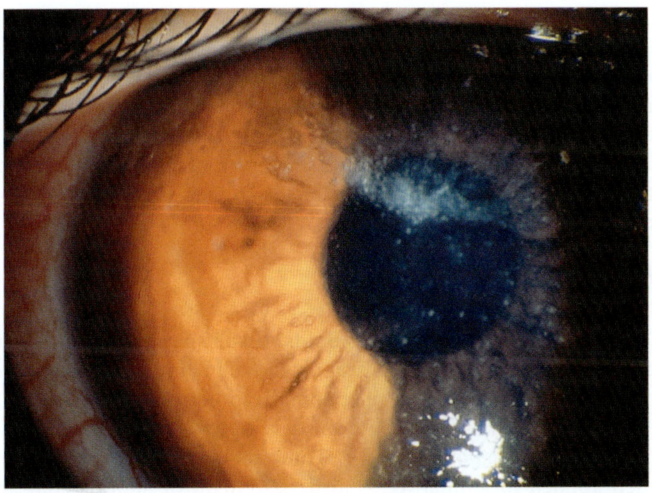
Fig. 92.3 Ocular slit lamp examination of a human patient with punctate keratoconjunctivitis caused by *Encephalitozoon hellem*. (From Weiss LM. Microsporidiosis. In: Bennett JE, Dolin R, Blaser MJ, eds. *Mandell, Douglas, and Bennett's Principles and Practice of Infectious Diseases*. Philadelphia: Elsevier Saunders; 2015:3031–3046.)

toxoplasmosis. Most puppies succumb to the infection over the course of a few days. Bitches that produce infected litters consistently exhibit subclinical infection.[18,23]

In addition to neurologic disease, chronic bilateral nephritis that culminates in renal failure has occasionally been reported in puppies and young adult dogs.[18,41,43] Bilaterally, the kidneys may be palpably enlarged or may be fibrotic and shrunken in size, and the dogs are usually emaciated.

Ocular lesions have also been described in dogs in one report from Europe.[44] Chronic anterior uveitis and focal cataracts were reported in three cases, and all three dogs had high titers against *E. cuniculi* with microsporidia identified microscopically or by PCR testing. The case descriptions are similar to ocular lesions that are more widely recognized in rabbits.[45–47] Ocular encephalitozoonosis has also been described in blue foxes raised for fur production in Scandinavia[48] and in cats (see below).

Cats

Naturally occurring feline encephalitozoonosis is not well described in veterinary literature. Neurologic disease was described in three Siamese cat littermates from South Africa.[49] Infected kittens exhibited lethargy, muscle twitching, and spasms. In another report, a young kitten with cerebellar hypoplasia was euthanized, and necropsy revealed generalized encephalitozoonosis. The intralesional presence of *E. cuniculi* was confirmed using molecular methods.[50]

Several additional reports describe ocular lesions in cats. In one report from the late 1970s, conjunctivitis, uveitis, and corneal opacities in a cat were attributed to *E. cuniculi*,[51] but in a later review, the morphologic features of the organisms in histologic sections were challenged, and a new scientific name was suggested.[8] More recently, uveitis and cataracts associated with *E. cuniculi* infection were described in 11 cats (19 eyes).[52] All cats were seropositive for *E. cuniculi*, and *E. cuniculi* was identified histologically or using molecular assays in surgically removed lenses. *Encephalitozoon cuniculi* was also detected by PCR in enucleated ocular material from a cat with chronic anterior uveitis and cataracts.[53] These lesions were similar to those described in rabbits infected with *E. cuniculi*.[45–47]

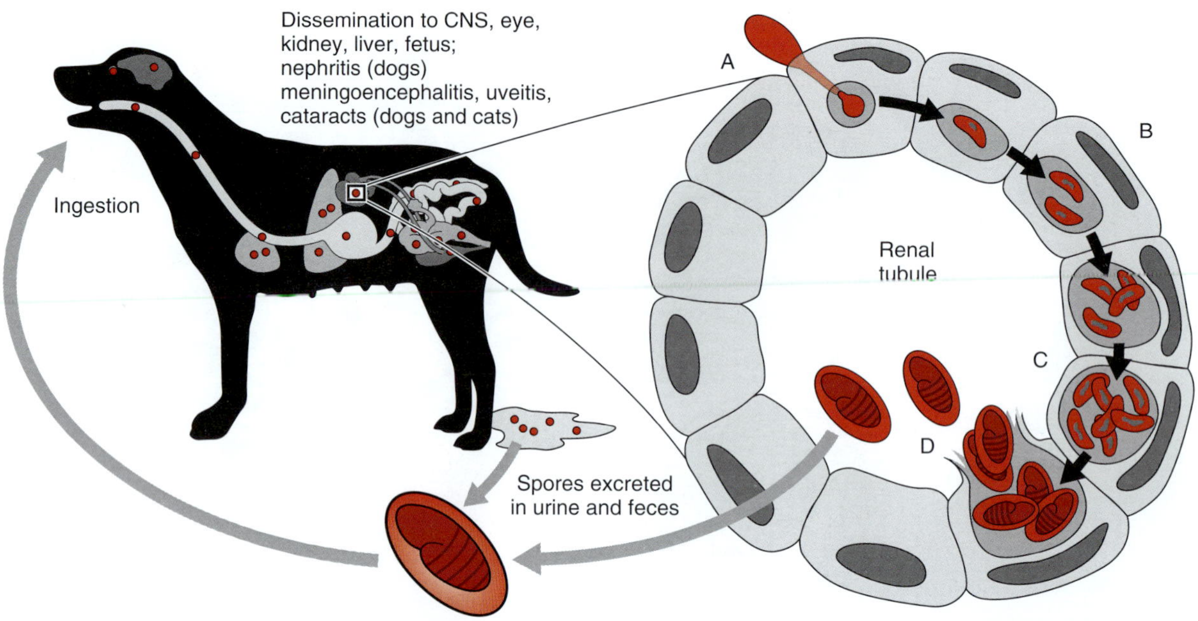

Fig. 92.4 Intracellular life cycle of *Encephalitozoon cuniculi* in the renal tubular epithelium. Diagram is based on light and electron microscopic examination of the organism. Spores are ingested and penetrate the gut wall, entering the systemic circulation. Spores can spread to many organs, such as the kidney shown here. *(A)* The mature spore uses a polar filament to propel its sporoplasm into the host cell. *(B)* Proliferative forms of pathogen (schizonts) replicate within a vacuole. Binary fission occurs during contact with membrane of intracellular vacuole. As maturation progresses, spores collect in the center of vacuole. (C) "Parasitophorous" vacuole containing spores and proliferative forms. These stages are visible under light microscope. (D) The vacuole ruptures, releases its spores into the renal tubular lumen, and the organism is excreted in urine.

Experimentally, infection was readily established in cats, but severe clinical disease was not noted.[36] Meningoencephalitis and nephritis of varying severity were noted on histopathology at necropsy, similar to lesions reported in dogs and other hosts. However, infection with *E. cuniculi* has not been associated with naturally occurring CKD in cats.[54]

DIAGNOSIS

Diagnosis of *E. cuniculi* infections can be challenging due to a lack of readily available commercial diagnostic testing options. Both microscopic and serologic methods have been used antemortem to facilitate the diagnosis of microsporidial infections in dogs. Frequently, a definitive diagnosis is made at necropsy based on histopathologic lesions and observation of intracellular parasites in multiple organs. Mature spores of *E. cuniculi* are small and oval, measuring approximately 1.5 μm wide and 2.5 μm long. Therefore, the small size and poor staining qualities of *Encephalitozoon* organisms make them difficult to visualize with routine microscopic and histologic techniques.

Laboratory Abnormalities

In one report documenting a litter of naturally infected puppies, no abnormalities were reported on CBCs, blood urea nitrogen tests, or urinalyses.[4] In other reports, anemia has been documented, with variable findings on the leukogram.[39,41] Increased serum urea nitrogen or creatinine concentrations have been reported in clinically ill puppies and subclinically infected bitches in association with impaired renal function.[23,41,55,56]

In experimentally infected animals, a normochromic, normocytic anemia is a consistent finding and may be secondary to kidney injury and impaired erythropoietin production.[39,40] Serum biochemical findings have been variable, and include increased activities of serum ALT and ALP along with variably increased serum urea nitrogen and creatinine concentrations, and sometimes increased serum total protein concentrations.[39,40,57]

Microbiologic Tests

Cytologic Diagnosis

Cytologic examination of body fluids, tissue specimens, or feces is important when making a clinical diagnosis in animals with disseminated infections. A variety of staining techniques for the detection of spores in body fluids have been developed for diagnostic use in human medical laboratories.[58,59] These methods work equally well when applied to animal feces, urine sediment, or sputum, but are not readily available in commercial veterinary diagnostic laboratories. Fee-for-service testing using these methods may be locally available through human hospital services. Spores shed into the urine from infected renal tubular epithelial cells are readily identifiable in urine sediment with Gram or Ziehl-Neelsen staining.[58,59] Spores may also be found in aqueous humor and phacoemulsified lens material from cats with uveitis and cataracts.[52] Stained spores are gram positive, whereas proliferative stages are gram negative. Microsporidia in stool specimens are sometimes more difficult to distinguish from other gram-positive bacteria than in urine sediment or other body secretions.[60]

Microsporidia stain with modified trichrome stain (e.g., StainQuick Microsporidia Kit, Scientific Device Laboratory, Des Plaines, IL, USA) and appear bright pink with a diagonal pink band and a clear posterior vacuole; bacteria stain with the counterstain (Fig. 92.5A).[61–64] Yeasts also stain bright pink but lack a posterior vacuole, they are usually larger and more round than the oval microsporidia, and they show budding characteristics.

Chitin-staining fluorochromes (e.g., calcofluor white) are useful for detecting microsporidia but require a microscope equipped with UV lighting and appropriate barrier filters.[61,62,65,66] Organisms stain as white to turquoise oval halos when viewed with UV microscopy (Fig. 92.5B). These staining methods do not distinguish species of microsporidia.

Indirect fluorescence assays using monoclonal antibodies or hyperimmune polyclonal antisera can specifically identify microsporidia spores to the genus or species level (Fig. 92.5C). However, this method is generally used in research settings or in epidemiologic surveys and is not readily available as a diagnostic test for use in clinical settings since reagents are not commercially available.[55,67]

Electron Microscopy

Transmission electron microscopy (TEM) has been considered a gold standard for the specific diagnosis of microsporidiosis in the medical field and in selected veterinary cases.[56,68–70] Microsporidial spores contain the distinctive coiled polar tubule organelle that distinguishes microsporidia from all other organisms (see Figs. 92.1 and 92.2A).[7] The number and organization of the polar tubule coils are important morphologic characteristics that aid in identifying the organisms to a genus or species level. However, TEM is relatively insensitive, costly, and time consuming and requires technical expertise.

Serologic Diagnosis

Immunocompetent hosts produce antibodies to *E. cuniculi*, which can be detected using IFA, ELISA, and direct agglutination.[27,36,57,71] However, serologic tests for dogs or cats are not readily available on a commercial basis. Also some concerns exist about the sensitivity of these serologic tests in immunologically immature puppies or in clinically normal exposed hosts where infection is not confirmed.

Molecular Diagnosis Using Nucleic Acid–Based Testing

Increasingly, microsporidia are diagnosed in body secretions, feces, or tissues from human patients using molecular methods.[72–75] Some of these methods have been utilized for diagnosis of encephalitozoonosis in animals.[18,68,69] Both endpoint (conventional) PCR and real-time PCR assays have been described in the literature but are not currently available on a commercial basis. Molecular assays may soon replace TEM as the method of choice for confirmation of microsporidiosis because of increased sensitivity, availability, and the ability to identify organisms to a species level.

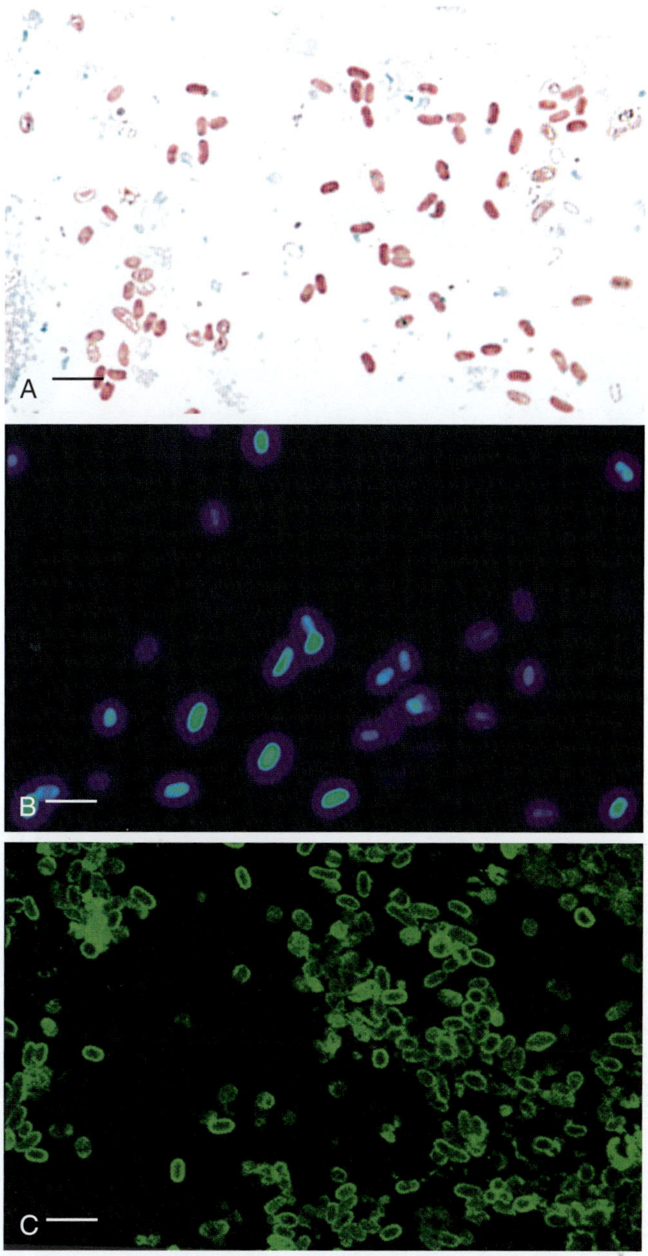

Fig. 92.5 Diagnostic assays for detection of *Encephalitozoon cuniculi* in urine and feces. (A) *E. cuniculi* spores stained with trichrome and viewed by brightfield microscopy. Of the three techniques, this provides the best demonstration of size and polar vacuole (bar = 5 μm). (B) *Encephalitozoon cuniculi* spores stained with calcofluor white. White organisms with blue halo viewed with ultraviolet microscopy. (C) *Encephalitozoon cuniculi* spores stained with rabbit polyclonal antiserum, secondary antibody linked to Alexa 468 fluorochrome, and visualized with fluorescence confocal microscopy.

Pathologic Findings

Gross Pathologic Findings

Descriptions of gross lesions are mostly based on necropsy evaluation of puppies with the encephalitis-nephritis syndrome.[18,23,41] Typically, puppies are in poor or emaciated condition with bilaterally enlarged, pale kidneys, sometimes with pale radiating streaks in the renal cortex. Brain congestion or swollen, edematous gyri, or hemorrhagic foci in meninges are sometimes observed. In older dogs, the kidneys are often shrunken with irregular cortical surfaces, and may contain mild petechiae or severe cortical cysts and infarcts (Fig. 92.6). Additional abnormalities sometimes reported include lymphadenopathy, splenomegaly, pinpoint white lesions in the hepatic parenchyma, patchy consolidation and edema of the lungs, fibrinous pericarditis, regional enteritis, and gastric mucosal petechiation. Gross lesions of encephalitozoonosis in experimentally infected dogs include hepatomegaly, petechiae on multiple organs, renomegaly, hemorrhagic cystitis, and splenomegaly.[39]

Histopathology

Histologically, dogs with encephalitozoonosis consistently have nonsuppurative meningoencephalitis (Fig. 92.7).[18,42,70] Fibrinoid necrosis of small- and medium-size arteries of the brain can result in vasculitis, thrombosis, encephalomalacia, and infarction. The kidneys of dogs and cats exhibit multifocal nonsuppurative interstitial nephritis.[76] Parasitophorous vacuoles with organisms are present in the renal tubular epithelia. Nonsuppurative vasculitis around small- and medium-sized arteries is often visualized in other tissues such as the heart or liver. Other nonspecific lesions include pulmonary edema, nonsuppurative interstitial pneumonia and enteritis, reticuloendothelial hyperplasia of the spleen, and hyperplasia of the bone marrow. Experimentally infected animals have had brain and kidney lesions similar to those described in natural infections.[39]

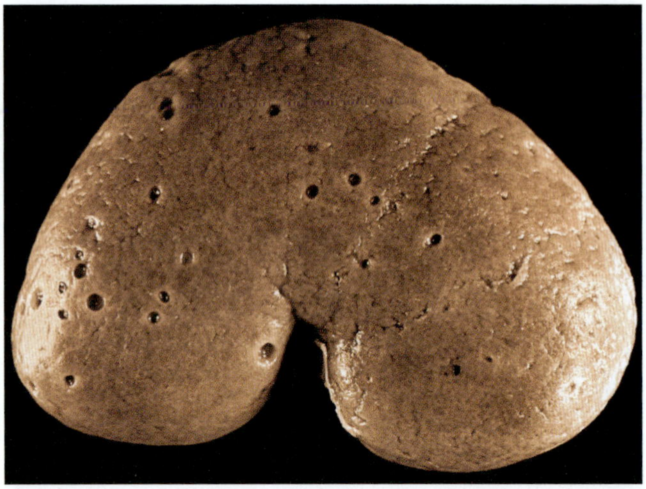

Fig. 92.6 Kidney with pale, firm cortex that has irregular-subcapsular surface and numerous projecting cysts filled with clear fluid.

Reported findings in cats with uveitis, cataracts, or both have included lymphoplasmacytic inflammation of the ciliary body and iris, and perivascular lymphoplasmacytic infiltrates within the retina.[52] Lenses have had evidence of liquefaction of lens fibers, deposition of calcium salts, epithelial hyperplasia, and fibrous metaplasia; organisms have been visible in liquefied lens fibers primarily adjacent to the anterior lens capsule, but in some cases, the posterior lens capsule as well. Rupture of the lens capsule was identified in one of 11 cats (19 eyes) with *E. cuniculi*–associated ocular disease.[52]

It should be noted that intracellular organisms are easily overlooked using microscopy with H&E staining, especially when few organisms are present. Tissue Gram stains such as Brown and Brenn stain can aid in visualization of gram-positive *E. cuniculi* organisms in histologic sections of host tissues.[18]

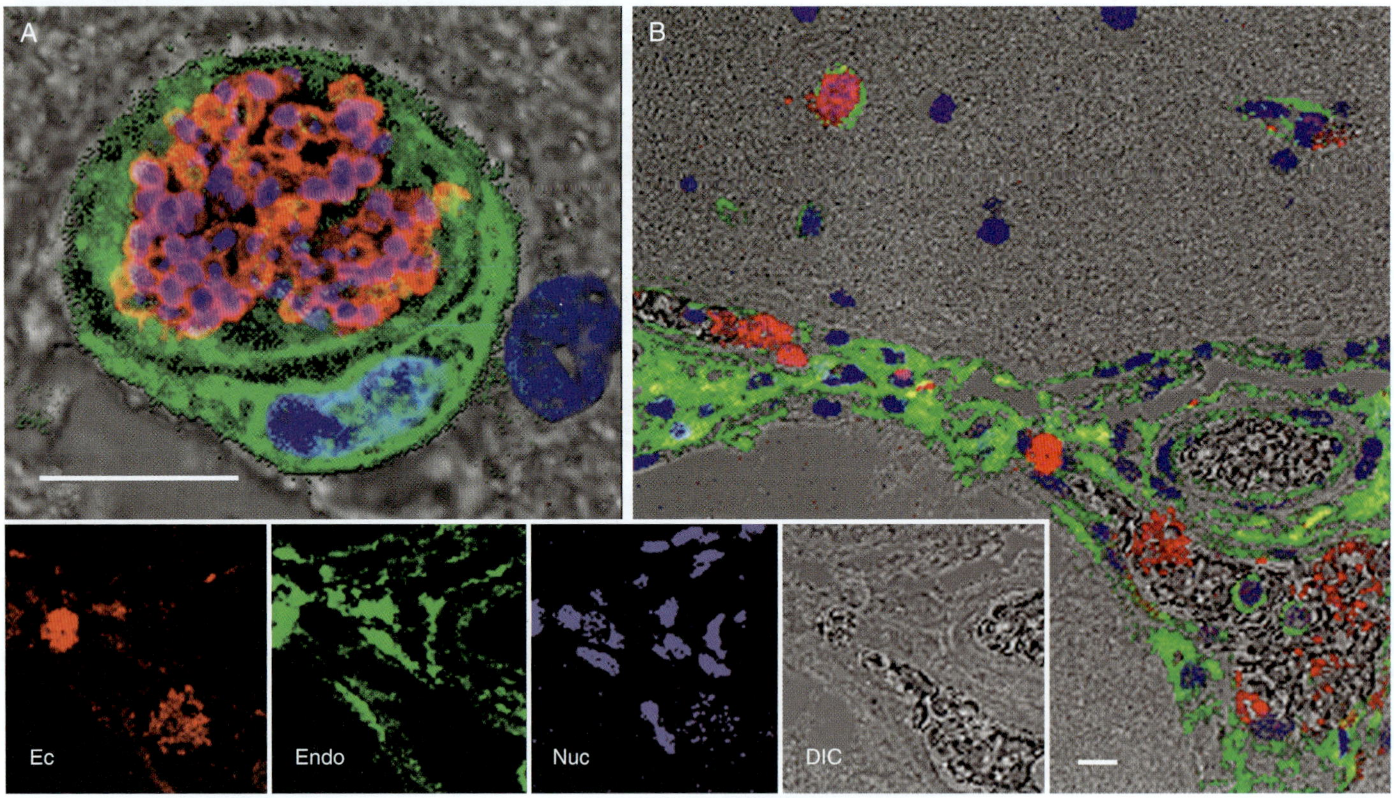

Fig. 92.7 (A) Parasitophorous vacuole packed with *Encephalitozoon cuniculi* (*red*) in endothelial cell (*green*) of nearly occluded cerebral capillary from fetal dog with transplacental infection. (B) Lower-power confocal image demonstrates *E. cuniculi* in and near cerebral vasculature. *Encephalitozoon cuniculi (Ec)* is stained with rabbit antiserum and secondary antibody linked to Alexa 468; endothelium (*Endo*) is marked with isolectin B4 and Alexa 568. Small numbers of inflammatory cell and resident nuclei (*Nuc*) are blue (TO-PRO-3 dye). Background (gray) is differential interference phase contrast (*DIC*). Bar = 5 μm.

TREATMENT AND PROGNOSIS

Although no treatment is currently recommended for either canine or feline encephalitozoonosis, some clinical and experimental therapies have been evaluated in humans, rabbits, and mice. The benzimidazoles have activity against *Encephalitozoon* spp. Albendazole has been used to successfully treat *Encephalitozoon* infections in humans and in domestic rabbits.[7,46,77–79] The related drug, fenbendazole, has been used with variable success in rabbits,[46,80,81] and was used successfully to treat a dog with nephritis caused by *E. cuniculi* genotype I.[82]

A second antimicrobial compound isolated from fungi, fumagillin, and its synthetic analogue, TNP-470, has been used to treat ocular disease caused by microsporidia.[79,83] Fumagillin is toxic for mammals, but its therapeutic use has been reported in selected human cases.[7,84,85] Fumagillin is not commercially available as a pharmaceutical product, but can be compounded from a product available for use with honeybees (Fumadil B, available from bee suppliers).

A number of additional antibiotic and antiprotozoal compounds have been explored for efficacy against microsporidia with variable or minimal success such as atovaquone, clindamycin, furazolidone, nikkomycin-Z, and nitazoxanide.[7,79] Clearly, better therapeutic products are still needed for microsporidiosis treatment in humans and animals.

TABLE 92.1 Major Genera of Microsporidia That Cause Disease in Humans

Microsporidia	Human Condition
Anncaliia spp.	Keratitis, myositis, cutaneous infections, disseminated infections
Enterocytozoon bieneusi	Diarrhea, cholangitis, rhinitis, bronchitis
Encephalitozoon cuniculi	Peritonitis, hepatitis, rhinosinusitis, seizures, nephritis, disseminated infection
Encephalitozoon hellem	Conjunctivitis, keratoconjunctivitis, rhinosinusitis, pneumonia, nephritis, cystitis, diarrhea, disseminated infection
Encephalitozoon intestinalis	Diarrhea, cholecystitis, cholangitis, nephritis, pneumonia, disseminated infection
Pleistophora spp.	Myositis
Trachipleistophora spp.	Myositis, keratoconjunctivitis, rhinosinusitis, encephalitis, disseminated infection
Tubulinosema spp.	Myositis, disseminated infection
Nosema ocularum	Keratoconjunctivitis
Vittaforma corneae	Keratoconjunctivitis, disseminated infection

PREVENTION

Since *Encephalitozoon* is primarily transmitted through the ingestion or possible inhalation of environmentally resistant spores that are shed in urine or feces, proper cleaning and disinfection of the environment is an often overlooked starting point at infection prevention. Maintaining sanitary conditions is also important when handling suspected cases of encephalitozoonosis.

PUBLIC HEALTH ASPECTS

Encephalitozoon cuniculi is generally considered an animal pathogen, but systemic, sometimes fatal, infections have been reported in humans.[86,87] The zoonotic potential of *E. cuniculi* remains unclear and needs to be explored. No direct evidence proves that dogs infect humans with microsporidia, or that humans infect dogs. One report suggested transmission of *E. cuniculi* to a dog groomer with AIDS.[87] Another report described a 10-year-old girl who underwent seroconversion to *E. cuniculi* after close contact with an infected puppy.[23] Relatively few isolates of *E. cuniculi* from a variety of host species are available for comparison, so the host predilection of the *E. cuniculi* strains is still unclear.

OTHER MICROSPORIDIAN SPECIES

Several additional microsporidian species have been identified in humans, dogs, and cats, suggesting zoonotic potential (Table 92.1). These organisms have not been associated with disease in dogs and cats. *Encephalitozoon intestinalis* is primarily recognized as a diarrhea-associated enteric pathogen in humans but has been sporadically reported in dogs in epidemiologic surveys.[88,89] In a small study of animal samples from Mexico, *E. intestinalis* spores were detected by PCR and IFA in one dog fecal specimen.[88] In Turkey, 12.4% of 282 fecal specimens from dogs tested positive for *E. intestinalis* using PCR, and 2.4% were positive for *E. cuniculi*.[90] Using light microscopy and a PCR assay, *E. intestinalis* was detected in feces of a pet cat and its owner, who was an AIDS patient with chronic diarrhea.[91] No clinical disease caused by *E. intestinalis* has been reported in dogs or cats. The potential for dogs or cats to serve as a reservoir host or to be a source of human exposure is unknown. It is also possible that these rare pet infections with *E. intestinalis* are examples of zooanthroponosis, where the parasite is transmitted from humans to animals.

Similarly, *E. bieneusi*, a common intestinal opportunistic parasite in human AIDS patients, has been identified in stool specimens from cats, dogs, and other domestic animals.[7,79,92–96] In a survey of stray and pet dogs and cats in China, *E. bieneusi* was detected by PCR in fecal specimens from 15.5% of 348 dogs and 11.7% of 96 pet cats.[97] In contrast, in Thailand, *E. bieneusi* was not detected by nested PCR in fecal specimens from 206 dogs, but was identified in 31.3% of 80 cat fecal specimens.[98] In a Japanese study that examined 104 animal fecal specimens by PCR, *E. bieneusi* was detected in two dogs and a cat.[92] *Enterocytozoon bieneusi* was also detected using PCR in 15% of 120 dog fecal specimens and 17% of 46 cat fecal specimens from Colombia,[99,100] and 4.9% of 82 dog fecal specimens and 9.1% of 44 cat fecal specimens from Poland.[96]

A number of genotypes of *E. bieneusi* have been described. Some strains have been found only in humans, others have only been described in domestic animals, and other genotypes have been documented in both human and animal hosts.[93–95,97] The zoonotic potential of these infections needs additional investigation.

CASE EXAMPLES

CASE 1

Signalment

"Zara," an approximately 15-year-old female spayed domestic shorthair cat from northern California, United States.

History

Zara was referred to a small animal internal medicine specialty service with a 1- to 2-week history of diarrhea and weight loss. A thin body condition was noted on physical examination. The only finding on blood work was mild hypoalbuminemia (2.4 g/dL). Abdominal ultrasound examination revealed mild diffuse small bowel wall thickening, with loss of normal wall layering and mild mesenteric lymphadenopathy. Serum cobalamin concentration was low. Histopathology on full-thickness biopsies of the stomach, duodenum, and jejunum, as well as a mesenteric lymph node, revealed a well-differentiated intestinal lymphoma that involved the duodenum and jejunum. The lymph node was reactive with no evidence of neoplasia. Zara was treated with prednisolone (5 mg, PO, q12h), chlorambucil (2 mg, PO, q48h), and cobalamin (250 μg, SC, weekly for 6 weeks, then once monthly). The diarrhea resolved, but inappetence continued and Zara failed to gain weight.

After 5 weeks, the owner then took Zara to a second specialty clinic. Zara had lost 0.5 kg (11% of body weight). A comprehensive profile was unremarkable, and abdominal ultrasound revealed resolved bowel wall thickening. The new internist altered the chlorambucil/prednisone dose regimen (chlorambucil: 2 mg, PO, q24h for 4 days once every 2 weeks; prednisolone: 5 mg, PO, q24h) in case the weight loss and persistent inappetence were adverse reactions to the medications. Four months later, the owner reported that Zara was eating well, with no diarrhea or vomiting, and she had gained 0.3 kg.

Three months later, Zara was seen again by the second internist for a sudden onset of vision loss and decreased appetite.

Current Medications

Prednisolone (5 mg, PO, q24h), chlorambucil (2 mg, PO, q24h for 4 days once every 2 weeks), and cobalamin (250 μg, SC, once monthly).

Other Medical History

Zara had been adopted as a stray 3 years previously and was housed exclusively indoors with several other indoor-only cats.

Physical Examination

Mild weight loss (0.3 kg) and bilateral mature cataracts were noted on physical examination. There were no other clinically significant findings.

Laboratory Findings

CBC and serum chemistry profile: The results of a CBC and serum chemistry profile were unremarkable.

Serologic testing: FeLV antigen and FIV antibody (SNAP FIV/FeLV Combo Test, IDEXX Laboratories): Negative.

FCoV IFA serology: Negative for antibodies.

Toxoplasma gondii ELISA serology: Negative for antibodies.

Imaging Findings

An abdominal ultrasound examination was unremarkable. There were no abnormalities of the bowel wall and lymph nodes.

Zara was referred to a veterinary ophthalmologist for cataract surgery. A PCR assay for *E. cuniculi* DNA on phacoemulsified lens material was positive. Serologic testing for IgG to *E. cuniculi* was positive at 1:64.

Diagnosis

Bilateral mature cataracts secondary to *E. cuniculi* infection.

Treatment

At the time of referral to the veterinary ophthalmologist, the prednisone dose was increased (5 mg, PO, q12h) and the chlorambucil was discontinued. When the results of the PCR assay for *E. cuniculi* were available, Zara was also treated with fenbendazole (20 mg/kg, PO, q24h for 3 weeks). Prednisolone and chlorambucil were discontinued. Two months later, she had regained 0.3 kg, and was feeling very well. However, because of recurrence of inappetence and weight loss, 16 months after diagnosis of encephalitozoonosis, biopsies of the stomach and intestines were repeated using gastroendoscopy and again revealed small cell lymphoma. Prednisolone and cyclophosphamide treatment was commenced. However, 18 months after the cataract surgery, she was evaluated by the emergency service at the second specialty practice for sudden-onset neurologic signs that included obtundation, circling, and pacing with pelvic limb paresis. The owner declined further work-up by the neurology service, and Zara was euthanized. A necropsy was not performed.

Comments

This cat was diagnosed with ocular encephalitozoonosis based on the rapid development of cataracts in the absence of diabetes mellitus, together with a positive PCR result for *E. cuniculi* on phacoemulsified lens material and a positive antibody test for *E. cuniculi*. The cause of the neurologic signs was unknown; given her advanced age, neoplasia is a likely differential diagnosis, but encephalitozoonosis also remains a possibility.

Acknowledgment

This case was courtesy of Dr. Marcia Smith, DVM DipACVIM, Loomis Basin Veterinary Clinic.

CASE 2

Signalment

"Pixie," a 24-day-old female Boston terrier puppy from Houston, Texas, United States.

History

Pixie was presented at her local veterinary clinic with a 2-day history of decreased activity and failure to nurse adequately. The puppy was one of a litter of two pups from a 3-year-old multiparous bitch, and the other puppy behaved normally according to the owner. Pixie came from a small breeding kennel with three Boston terrier females aged 2, 3, and 4 years old, and one 6-year-old male. The 2-year old bitch whelped 4 weeks ago, and all three pups from that litter died at 14 to 21 days old. No investigation of those neonatal deaths was requested by the kennel owner since it was the first litter for this recently purchased bitch.

Clinical Findings

On physical examination, Pixie was moribund with a body temperature of 96.8°F (36.0°C) and HR of 64 beats/minute. The owner declined further diagnostic testing, and since the prognosis was grave, the puppy was humanely euthanized. The body was submitted to the state veterinary medical diagnostic laboratory for necropsy. The pathologist made a presumptive diagnosis of disseminated microsporidiosis with histopathologic findings compatible with *E. cuniculi* infection.

Additional Diagnostic Testing

Serum was submitted from all four adult dogs to a research laboratory for IFA testing. The 2-year-old bitch had a high titer to *E. cuniculi* of 1:128, the 3-year-old dam of the puppy had a titer of 1:32, and the other two dogs from the kennel had no significant titer. These data suggest that the recently purchased 2-year-old bitch was infected with *E. cuniculi* that resulted in the death of her litter. It is likely that the 3-year-old periparturient bitch became infected through environmental contamination and passed that infection on to Pixie. The infection status of Pixie's littermate was unknown, but scientific reports have documented canine litters where some puppies were infected while littermates were not.

SUGGESTED READINGS

Snowden KF, Lewis BC, Hoffman J, et al. *Encephalitozoon cuniculi* infections in dogs: a case series. *J Am Anim Hosp Assoc.* 2009;45:225–231.

Benz P, Maass G, Csokai J, et al. Detection of *Encephalitozoon cuniculi* in the feline cataractous lens. *Vet Ophthalmol.* 2011;14(Suppl 1):37–47.

REFERENCES

1. Wright JH, Craighead EM. Infectious motor paralysis in young rabbits. *J Exp Med.* 1922;36:135–140.
2. Levaditi C, Nicolau S, Schoen R. *Encephalitozoon cuniculi*(nov. 'Spec) L'etiologie de l'encephalite epi-zootique du lapin, dans ses rapports avec l'etude experimentale de l'encephalite lethargique. *Ann Inst Pasteur.* 1924:651–712.
3. Plowright W. An encephalitis-nephritis syndrome in the dog probably due to congenital *Encephalitozoon* infection. *J Comp Pathol.* 1952;62:83–92.
4. Shadduck JA, Bendele R, Robinson GT. Isolation of the causative organism of canine encephalitozoonosis. *Vet Pathol.* 1978;15:449–460.
5. Fischer WM, Palmer JD. Evidence from small-subunit ribosomal RNA sequences for a fungal origin of Microsporidia. *Mol Phylogenet Evol.* 2005;36:606–622.
6. Lee SC, Corradi N, Byrnes EJ 3rd, et al. Microsporidia evolved from ancestral sexual fungi. *Curr Biol.* 2008;18:1675–1679.
7. Weiss LM. Microsporidiosis. In: Bennett JE, Dolin R, Blaser MJ, eds. *Mandell, Douglas, and Bennett's Principles and Practice of Infectious Diseases.* Philadelphia, PA: Elsevier Saunders; 2015:3031–3046.
8. Canning EU, Lom J. *The Microsporidia of Vertebrates.* New York: Academic Press; 1986.
9. Didier ES, Snowden KF, Shadduck JA. Biology of microsporidian species infecting mammals. *Adv Parasitol.* 1998;40:283–320.
10. Didier ES, Stovall ME, Green LC, et al. Epidemiology of microsporidiosis: sources and modes of transmission. *Vet Parasitol.* 2004;126:145–166.
11. Jordan CN, Dicristina JA, Lindsay DS. Activity of bleach, ethanol and two commercial disinfectants against spores of *Encephalitozoon cuniculi. Vet Parasitol.* 2006;136:343–346.
12. Ortega YR, Torres MP, Van Exel S, et al. Efficacy of a sanitizer and disinfectants to inactivate *Encephalitozoon intestinalis* spores. *J Food Prot.* 2007;70:681–684.
13. Johnson CH, Marshall MM, DeMaria LA, et al. Chlorine inactivation of spores of *Encephalitozoon* spp. *Appl Environ Microbiol.* 2003;69:1325–1326.
14. Mathis A, Weber R, Deplazes P. Zoonotic potential of the microsporidia. *Clin Microbiol Rev.* 2005;18:423–445.
15. Snowden KF. Microsporidia in higher vertebrates. In: Weiss LM, Becnel JJ, eds. *Microsporidia: Pathogens of Opportunity.* Ames, IA: Wiley & Sons; 2014:469–492.
16. Didier ES, Vossbrinck CR, Baker MD, et al. Identification and characterization of three *Encephalitozoon cuniculi* strains. *Parasitology.* 1995;111(Pt 4):411–421.
17. Deplazes P, Mathis A, Baumgartner R, et al. Immunologic and molecular characteristics of *Encephalitozoon*-like microsporidia isolated from humans and rabbits indicate that *Encephalitozoon cuniculi* is a zoonotic parasite. *Clin Infect Dis.* 1996;22:557–559.
18. Snowden KF, Lewis BC, Hoffman J, et al. *Encephalitozoon cuniculi* infections in dogs: a case series. *J Am Anim Hosp Assoc.* 2009;45:225–231.
19. Asakura T, Nakamura S, Ohta M, et al. Genetically unique microsporidian *Encephalitozoon cuniculi* strain type III isolated from squirrel monkeys. *Parasitol Int.* 2006;55:159–162.
20. Didier ES, Visvesvara GS, Baker MD, et al. A microsporidian isolated from an AIDS patient corresponds to *Encephalitozoon cuniculi* III, originally isolated from domestic dogs. *J Clin Microbiol.* 1996;34:2835–2837.
21. Snowden K, Logan K, Didier ES. *Encephalitozoon cuniculi* strain III is a cause of encephalitozoonosis in both humans and dogs. *J Infect Dis.* 1999;180:2086–2088.
22. Baneux PJ, Pognan F. In utero transmission of *Encephalitozoon cuniculis*-train type I in rabbits. *Lab Anim.* 2003;37:132–138.
23. McInnes EF, Stewart CG. The pathology of subclinical infection of *Encephalitozoon cuniculi* in canine dams producing pups with overt encephalitozoonosis. *J S Afr Vet Assoc.* 1991;62:51–54.
24. Basson PA, McCully RM, Warnes WEJ. Nosematosis: Report of a canine case in the Republic of South Africa. *J South Afr Vet Assoc.* 1966;37:3–9.
25. Stewart CG, van Dellen AF, Botha WS. Canine encephalitozoonosis in kennels and the isolation of *Encephalitozoon* in tissue culture. *J S Afr Vet Assoc.* 1979;50:165–168.
26. Lindsay DS, Goodwin DG, Zajac AM, et al. Serological survey for antibodies to *Encephalitozoon cuniculi* in ownerless dogs from urban areas of Brazil and Colombia. *J Parasitol.* 2009;95:760–763.
27. Hollister WS, Canning EU, Viney M. Prevalence of antibodies to *Encephalitozoon cuniculi* in stray dogs as determined by an ELISA. *Vet Rec.* 1989;124:332–336.
28. Sasaki M, Yamazaki A, Haraguchi A, et al. Serological survey of *Encephalitozoon cuniculi* infection in Japanese dogs. *J Parasitol.* 2011;97:167–169.
29. Abu-Akkada SS, Ashmawy KI, Dweir AW. First detection of an ignored parasite, *Encephalitozoon cuniculi*, in different animal hosts in Egypt. *Parasitol Res.* 2015;114:843–850.
30. Halanova M, Cislakova L, Valencakova A, et al. Serological screening of occurrence of antibodies to *Encephalitozoon cuniculi* in humans and animals in Eastern Slovakia. *Ann Agric Environ Med.* 2003;10:117–120.
31. Herich R, Levkutova M, Kokincakova T, et al. Prevalence of anti-microsporidial antibodies in randomly examined dogs in Eastern Slovakia. *Medycyna Weterynaryjna.* 2008;64:658–662.
32. Stefkovic M, Maslej P, Halanova M, et al. A study on antibody prevalence due to microsporidian *Encephalitozoon cuniculi* in dogs (*Canis familiaris*) using indirect immunofluorescence. *Folia Vet.* 2001;45:184–187.
33. Jafri HS, Reedy T, Moorhead AR, et al. Detection of pathogenic protozoa in fecal specimens from urban dwelling dogs. In: *42nd Annual Meeting of the American Society of Tropical Medicine and Hygiene*; 1993. Atlanta, GA.
34. Al-Herrawy AZ, Gad MA. Microsporidial spores in fecal samples of some domesticated animals living in Giza, Egypt. *Iran J Parasitol.* 2016;11:195–203.
35. Jamshidi S, Tabrizi AS, Bahrami M, et al. Microsporidia in household dogs and cats in Iran; a zoonotic concern. *Vet Parasitol.* 2012;185:121–123.
36. Pang VF, Shadduck JA. Susceptibility of cats, sheep, and swine to a rabbit isolate of *Encephalitozoon cuniculi. Am J Vet Res.* 1985;46:1071–1077.
37. Hsu V, Grant DC, Zajac AM, et al. Prevalence of IgG antibodies to *Encephalitozoon cuniculi* and *Toxoplasma gondii* in cats with and without chronic kidney disease from Virginia. *Vet Parasitol.* 2011;176:23–26.
38. Deplazes P, Mathis A, Muller C, et al. Molecular epidemiology of *Encephalitozoon cuniculi* and first detection of *Enterocytozoon bieneusi* in faecal samples of pigs. *J Eukaryot Microbiol.* 1996;43:93S.
39. Szabo JR, Shadduck JA. Experimental encephalitozoonosis in neonatal dogs. *Vet Pathol.* 1987;24:99–108.
40. Szabo JR, Shadduck JA. Immunologic and clinicopathologic evaluation of adult dogs inoculated with *Encephalitozoon cuniculi. J Clin Microbiol.* 1988;26:557–563.
41. Botha WS, van Dellen AF, Stewart CG. Canine encephalitozoonosis in South Africa. *J S Afr Vet Assoc.* 1979;50:135–144.
42. McCully RM, Van Dellen AF, Basson PA, et al. Observations on the pathology of canine microsporidiosis. *Onderstepoort J Vet Res.* 1978;45:75–91.
43. Stewart CG, Botha WS. Canine encephalitozoonosis. *Zimbabwe Vet.* 1989;20:89–93.
44. Nell B, Csokai J, Fuchs-Baumgartinger A, et al. *Encephalitozoon cuniculi* causes focal anterior cataract and uveitis in dogs. *Tierarztl Prax Ausg K Kleintiere Heimtiere.* 2015;43:337–344.
45. Giordano C, Weigt A, Vercelli A, et al. Immunohistochemical identification of *Encephalitozoon cuniculi* in phacoclastic uveitis in four rabbits. *Vet Ophthalmol.* 2005;8:271–275.
46. Kunzel F, Joachim A. Encephalitozoonosis in rabbits. *Parasitol Res.* 2010;106:299–309.
47. Stiles J, Didier E, Ritchie B, et al. *Encephalitozoon cuniculi* in the lens of a rabbit with phacoclastic uveitis: confirmation and treatment. *Vet Comp Ophthalmol.* 1997;7:233–238.

48. Arnesen K, Nordstoga K. Ocular encephalitozoonosis (nosematosis) in blue foxes. Polyarteritis nodosa and cataract. *Acta Ophthalmol (Copenh).* 1977;55:641–651.
49. van Rensburg IB, du Plessis JL. Nosematosis in a cat: a case report. *J S Afr Vet Med Assoc.* 1971;42:327–331.
50. Rebel-Bauder B, Leschnik M, Maderner A, et al. Generalized encephalitozoonosis in a young kitten with cerebellar hypoplasia. *J Comp Pathol.* 2011;145:126–131.
51. Buyukmihci N, Bellhorn RW, Hunziker J, et al. *Encephalitozoon (Nosema)* infection of the cornea in a cat. *J Am Vet Med Assoc.* 1977;171:355–357.
52. Benz P, Maass G, Csokai J, et al. Detection of *Encephalitozoon cuniculi* in the feline cataractous lens. *Vet Ophthalmol.* 2011;14(suppl 1):37–47.
53. Csokai J, Fuchs-Baumgartinger A, Maass G. Detection of *Encephalitozoon cuniculi* -infection (strain II) by PCR in a cat with anterior uveitis. *Weiner Tierarztliche Monatsschrift.* 2010;97:210–215.
54. Kunzel F, Rebel-Bauder B, Kassl C, et al. Meningoencephalitis in cats in Austria: a study of infectious causes, including *Encephalitozoon cuniculi. J Feline Med Surg.* 2017;19:171–176.
55. Zierdt CH, Gill VJ, Zierdt WS. Detection of microsporidian spores in clinical samples by indirect fluorescent-antibody assay using whole-cell antisera to *Encephalitozoon cuniculi* and *Encephalitozoon hellem. J Clin Microbiol.* 1993;31:3071–3074.67.
56. Gosh K, Schwartz D, Weiss LM. Laboratory diagnosis of microsporidia. In: *Microsporidia: Pathogens of Opportunity.* Ames, IA: Wiley & Sons; 2014:421–456.
57. Stewart CG, Collett MG, Snyman H. The immune response in a dog to *Encephalitozoon cuniculi* infection. *Onderstepoort J Vet Res.* 1986;53:35–37.
58. Garcia LS. Laboratory identification of the microsporidia. *J Clin Microbiol.* 2002;40:1892–1901.
59. Goodman DG, Garner FM. A comparison of methods for detecting *Nosema cuniculi* in rabbit urine. *Lab Anim Sci.* 1972;22:568–572.
60. Ignatius R, Henschel S, Liesenfeld O, et al. Comparative evaluation of modified trichrome and Uvitex 2B stains for detection of low numbers of microsporidial spores in stool specimens. *J Clin Microbiol.* 1997;35:2266–2269.
61. DeGirolami PC, Ezratty CR, Desai G, et al. Diagnosis of intestinal microsporidiosis by examination of stool and duodenal aspirate with Weber's modified trichrome and Uvitex 2B strains. *J Clin Microbiol.* 1995;33:805–810.
62. Didier ES, Orenstein JM, Aldras A, et al. Comparison of three staining methods for detecting microsporidia in fluids. *J Clin Microbiol.* 1995;33:3138–3145.
63. Ryan NJ, Sutherland G, Coughlan K, et al. A new trichrome-blue stain for detection of microsporidial species in urine, stool, and nasopharyngeal specimens. *J Clin Microbiol.* 1993;31:3264–3269.
64. Weber R, Bryan RT, Owen RL, et al. Improved light-microscopical detection of microsporidia spores in stool and duodenal aspirates. The Enteric Opportunistic Infections Working Group. *N Engl J Med.* 1992;326:161–166.
65. Luna VA, Stewart BK, Bergeron DL, et al. Use of the fluorochrome calcofluor white in the screening of stool specimens for spores of microsporidia. *Am J Clin Pathol.* 1995;103:656–659.
66. Vavra J, Chalupsky J. Fluorescence staining of microsporidian spores with the brightener Calcofluor White M2R. *J Protozool.* 1982;29(Suppl):503.
67. Aldras AM, Orenstein JM, Kotler DP, et al. Detection of microsporidia by indirect immunofluorescence antibody test using polyclonal and monoclonal antibodies. *J Clin Microbiol.* 1994;32:608–612.
68. Nimmo JS, Snowden K, O'Donoghue P. Fatal encephalitozoonosis in two koalas. *Aust Vet J.* 2007;85:428–432.
69. Snowden K, Daft B, Nordhausen RW. Morphological and molecular characterization of *Encephalitozoon hellem* in hummingbirds. *Avian Pathol.* 2001;30:251–255.
70. van Dellen AF, Botha WS, Boomker J, et al. Light and electron microscopical studies on canine encephalitozoonosis: cerebral vasculitis. *Onderstepoort J Vet Res.* 1978;45:165–186.
71. Jordan CN, Zajac AM, Snowden KS, et al. Direct agglutination test for *Encephalitozoon cuniculi. Vet Parasitol.* 2006;135:235–240.
72. De Groote MA, Visvesvara G, Wilson ML, et al. Polymerase chain reaction and culture confirmation of disseminated *Encephalitozoon cuniculi* in a patient with AIDS: successful therapy with albendazole. *J Infect Dis.* 1995;171:1375–1378.
73. Muller A, Stellermann K, Hartmann P, et al. A powerful DNA extraction method and PCR for detection of microsporidia in clinical stool specimens. *Clin Diagn Lab Immunol.* 1999;6:243–246.
74. Valencakova A, Balent P, Novotny F, et al. Application of specific primers in the diagnosis of *Encephalitozoon* spp. *Ann Agric Environ Med.* 2005;12:321–323.
75. Verweij JJ, Ten Hove R, Brienen EA, et al. Multiplex detection of *Enterocytozoon bieneusi* and *Encephalitozoon* spp. in fecal samples using real-time PCR. *Diagn Microbiol Infect Dis.* 2007;57:163–167.
76. Botha WS, Dormehl IC, Goosen DJ. Evaluation of kidney function in dogs suffering from canine encephalitozoonosis by standard clinical pathological and radiopharmaceutical techniques. *J S Afr Vet Assoc.* 1986;57:79–86.
77. Blanshard C, Ellis DS, Tovey DG, et al. Treatment of intestinal microsporidiosis with albendazole in patients with AIDS. *AIDS.* 1992;6:311–313.
78. Harcourt-Brown FM, Holloway HK. *Encephalitozoon cuniculi* in pet rabbits. *Vet Rec.* 2003;152:427–431.
79. Weiss LM. Clinical syndromes associated with microsporidiosis. In: Weiss LM, Becnel JJ, eds. *Microsporidia: Pathogens of Opportunity.* Ames, IA: Wiley & Sons; 2014:371–402.
80. Sieg J, Hein J, Jass A, et al. Clinical evaluation of therapeutic success in rabbits with suspected encephalitozoonosis. *Vet Parasitol.* 2012;187:328–332.
81. Suter C, Muller-Doblies UU, Hatt JM, et al. Prevention and treatment of *Encephalitozoon cuniculi* infection in rabbits with fenbendazole. *Vet Rec.* 2001;148:478–480.
82. Engelhardt S, Buder A, Pfeil K, et al. [Nephritis in a Staffordshire Terrier puppy caused by *Encephalitozoon cuniculi* genotype I]. *Tierarztl Prax Ausg K Kleintiere Heimtiere.* 2017;45.
83. Coyle C, Kent M, Tanowitz HB, et al. TNP-470 is an effective antimicrosporidial agent. *J Infect Dis.* 1998;177:515–518.
84. Mertens RB, Didier ES, Fishbein MC, et al. Disseminated *Encephalitozoon cuniculi* microsporidiosis: infection of the brain, heart, kidneys, trachea, adrenals, urinary bladder, spleen, and lymph nodes in an AIDS patient. *Mod Pathol.* 1997;10:68–77.
85. Molina JM, Goguel J, Sarfati C, et al. Trial of oral fumagillin for the treatment of intestinal microsporidiosis in patients with HIV infection. ANRS 054 Study Group. Agence Nationale de Recherche sur le SIDA. *AIDS.* 2000;14:1341–1348.
86. Tosoni A, Nebuloni M, Ferri A, et al. Disseminated microsporidiosis caused by *Encephalitozoon cuniculi* III (dog type) in an Italian AIDS patient: a retrospective study. *Mod Pathol.* 2002;15:577–583.
87. Weitzel T, Wolff M, Dabanch J, et al. Dual microsporidial infection with *Encephalitozoon cuniculi* and *Enterocytozoon bieneusi* in an HIV-positive patient. *Infection.* 2001;29:237–239.
88. Bornay-Llinares FJ, da Silva AJ, Moura H, et al. Immunologic, microscopic, and molecular evidence of *Encephalitozoon intestinalis* (*Septata intestinalis*) infection in mammals other than humans. *J Infect Dis.* 1998;178:820–826.
89. Cali A, Kotler DP, Orenstein JM. *Septata intestinalis* N. G., N. Sp., an intestinal microsporidian associated with chronic diarrhea and dissemination in AIDS patients. *J Eukaryot Microbiol.* 1993;40:101–112.
90. Duzlu O, Yildirim A, Onder Z, et al. Prevalence and genotyping of microsporidian parasites in dogs in turkey: zoonotic concerns. *J Eukaryot Microbiol.* 2019;66:771–777.
91. Velasquez JN, Chertcoff AV, Etchart C, et al. First case report of infection caused by *Encephalitozoon intestinalis* in a domestic cat and a patient with AIDS. *Vet Parasitol.* 2012;190:583–586.
92. Abe N, Kimata I, Iseki M. Molecular evidence of *Enterocytozoon bieneusi* in Japan. *J Vet Med Sci.* 2009;71:217–219.

93. Dengjel B, Zahler M, Hermanns W, et al. Zoonotic potential of *Enterocytozoon bieneusi*. *J Clin Microbiol.* 2001;39:4495–4499.
94. Lobo ML, Xiao L, Cama V, et al. Genotypes of *Enterocytozoon bieneusi* in mammals in Portugal. *J Eukaryot Microbiol.* 2006;53(suppl 1):S61–64.
95. Mathis A, Breitenmoser AC, Deplazes P. Detection of new *Enterocytozoon* genotypes in faecal samples of farm dogs and a cat. *Parasite.* 1999;6: 189–193.
96. Piekarska J, Kicia M, Wesolowska M, et al. Zoonotic microsporidia in dogs and cats in Poland. *Vet Parasitol.* 2017;246:108–111.
97. Karim MR, Dong H, Yu F, et al. Genetic diversity in *Enterocytozoon bieneusi* isolates from dogs and cats in China: host specificity and public health implications. *J Clin Microbiol.* 2014;52:3297–3302.
98. Mori H, Mahittikorn A, Thammasonthijarern N, et al. Presence of zoonotic *Enterocytozoon bieneusi* in cats in a temple in central Thailand. *Vet Parasitol.* 2013;197:696–701.
99. Santin M, Cortes Vecino JA, Fayer R. *Enterocytozoon bieneusi* genotypes in dogs in Bogota, Colombia. *Am J Trop Med Hyg.* 2008;79:215–217.
100. Santin M, Trout JM, Vecino JA, et al. *Cryptosporidium, Giardia* and *Enterocytozoon bieneusi* in cats from Bogota (Colombia) and genotyping of isolates. *Vet Parasitol.* 2006;141:334–339.

SECTION 4

Protozoal Diseases

Jane E. Sykes

Protozoa are unicellular eukaryotes that may be free-living or parasitic. Parasitic protozoa are the cause of important zoonotic diseases of dogs and cats worldwide, such as toxoplasmosis, leishmaniosis, giardiasis, and cryptosporidiosis. They also cause regional vector-borne systemic diseases such as babesiosis, hepatozoonosis, trypanosomiasis, rangeliosis, and cytauxzoonosis that can be associated with a high degree of morbidity and mortality in companion animals. With advancement in molecular techniques, there has been the recognition of new species and strains of many pathogens that cause these diseases in animals, as well as improved understanding of their epidemiology. For example, we now know that there are at least 15 different *Babesia* species that infect dogs and cats worldwide, we have seen expansion of the geographic range of *Cytauxzoon felis* infections, and we have a deeper understanding of the zoonotic potential of different *Giardia* and *Cryptosporidium* strains. However, even in this era of molecular pathogenesis studies, our knowledge of the basic life cycles and transmission dynamics of some protozoal pathogens of dogs and cats remains incomplete (such as for *Rangelia vitalii* and certain *Sarcocystis* species), and new drugs are needed in order to treat them effectively. Undoubtedly, more studies in the near future will shed light on these diseases with improved opportunity for intervention strategies to promote the health of not only dogs and cats but also other animal species that may be infected with these organisms.

93

Toxoplasmosis

Michael R. Lappin, Jitender P. Dubey

KEY POINTS

- First Described: The organism that was ultimately named *Toxoplasma gondii* was first described in France in 1908 (Nicolle and Manceaux).[1]
- Cause: *Toxoplasma gondii,* a coccidian protozoan parasite (phylum Apicomplexa).
- Affected Host Species: Cats are the definitive host and are the only species known to complete the sexual phase of *T. gondii* culminating in the passage of oocysts in feces. Cats and most other vertebrates can serve as intermediate hosts; invertebrates can serve as transport hosts by mechanical carriage of *T. gondii* oocysts.
- Geographic Distribution: *Toxoplasma gondii* has a worldwide distribution except in the absence of cats.
- Major Clinical Signs: Fever, ocular inflammation, ataxia, seizures, muscle pain, and respiratory distress are the most common clinical signs in cats; dogs have similar signs but develop illness less frequently than cats.
- Differential Diagnoses: In the dog, *Neospora caninum* induces the most similar clinical signs; many other chronic intracellular bacterial infections and fungal infections in dogs and cats need to be considered as differential diagnoses for many of the clinical and laboratory abnormities induced by *T. gondii.*
- Human Health Significance: There is significant risk to the fetus after transplacental infection and to any immunocompromised person; whether significant effects on human behavioral abnormalities are induced by infection is still debated.

ETIOLOGIC AGENT AND EPIDEMIOLOGY

Toxoplasma gondii is a coccidian that is one of the most prevalent parasites infecting warm-blooded vertebrates around the world.[2-5] Only cats complete the sexual phase in the GI tract (also known as the enteroepithelial cycle) and pass environmentally resistant oocysts in feces (Fig. 93.1). Sporozoites develop within oocysts after 1 to 5 days of exposure to oxygen and appropriate environmental temperature and humidity (Fig. 93.2). This process is known as sporulation. After a new potential host ingests sporulated oocysts, sporozoites are released that can penetrate the intestinal tracts of cats or intermediate hosts and disseminate in blood or lymph as tachyzoites (rapidly dividing) during active infection. *Toxoplasma gondii* tachyzoites can penetrate most mammalian cells and they replicate asexually within infected cells until the cell is destroyed. If an appropriate immune response occurs, replication of tachyzoites is attenuated and slowly dividing bradyzoites develop that persist within cysts in extraintestinal tissues. These tissue cysts form readily in the CNS, muscles, and visceral organs. Live bradyzoites may persist in tissue cysts for the life of the host. Ingestion of *T. gondii* bradyzoites in uncooked, infected tissues of prey species or species used for food in people is a common way to induce infection in cats, dogs, and people. Commercial raw meat diets for companion animals occasionally contain *T. gondii.*[6] Cats that ingest bradyzoites excrete more *T. gondii* oocysts than cats that ingest sporulated oocysts.[7]

It is likely that most *T. gondii*–infected cats and dogs harbor tissue cysts for life. Thus, the presence of serum antibodies is likely to indicate current infection. *Toxoplasma gondii* seroprevalence rates vary by the lifestyle of the cat or dog. In general, increased seroprevalence correlates with increased age as a result of increased risk of exposure over time. It also correlates with outdoor exposure, since animals with access to the outdoors are most likely to contact infected intermediate hosts. A meta-analysis of global feline *T. gondii* seroprevalence studies was published in 2020; the pooled global seroprevalence was estimated to be 35% (Fig. 93.3A).[8] In a study of clinically ill cats in the United States, *T. gondii* antibodies were detected in 31.6% of the 12,628 cats tested.[9] The seroprevalence was lowest in regions with low humidity (Fig. 93.3B). In another study of feral cats in Florida, *T. gondii* antibodies were detected in 12.1% of the cats.[10] Although *T. gondii* infection is common among cats, the oocyst excretion period is generally less than 21 days if the infection was initiated by ingestion of tissue cysts containing bradyzoites. Thus, detection of *T. gondii* oocysts in feline feces is uncommon. For example, in two studies in the United States, *T. gondii* oocysts were detected in feces of fewer than 1% of cats.[11,12] Cats allowed outdoors were shown to be 2.77 times more likely than indoor cats to be parasitized and *T. gondii* oocysts can be detected in the soil.[12-14] While the largest number of *T. gondii* oocysts excreted are after the first exposure to tissue cysts, repeat excretion can occur.[15]

Dogs do not produce *T. gondii* oocysts, but they can mechanically transmit oocysts after they ingest feline feces.[16] The tissue phases of *T. gondii* infection occur in dogs and may be associated with clinical disease. Approximately 20% of dogs in the United States are seropositive for *T. gondii* antibodies.[17] Before 1988, many dogs diagnosed with toxoplasmosis based on histologic evaluation were in fact infected with *Neospora caninum* (see Chapter 94).

CLINICAL FEATURES

Pathogenesis and Clinical Signs

Infection of warm-blooded vertebrates occurs after ingestion of any of the three life stages of *T. gondii* (sporozoite, tachyzoites, bradyzoites) or it can occur by transplacental transmission. Cats can also be infected through the transmammary route.[18] In dogs, evidence for venereal transmission also exists, and repeated transplacental infection has been documented.[19,20]

Most cats are not purposely coprophagic, so most are infected when they ingest *T. gondii* bradyzoites in tissue cysts during carnivorous

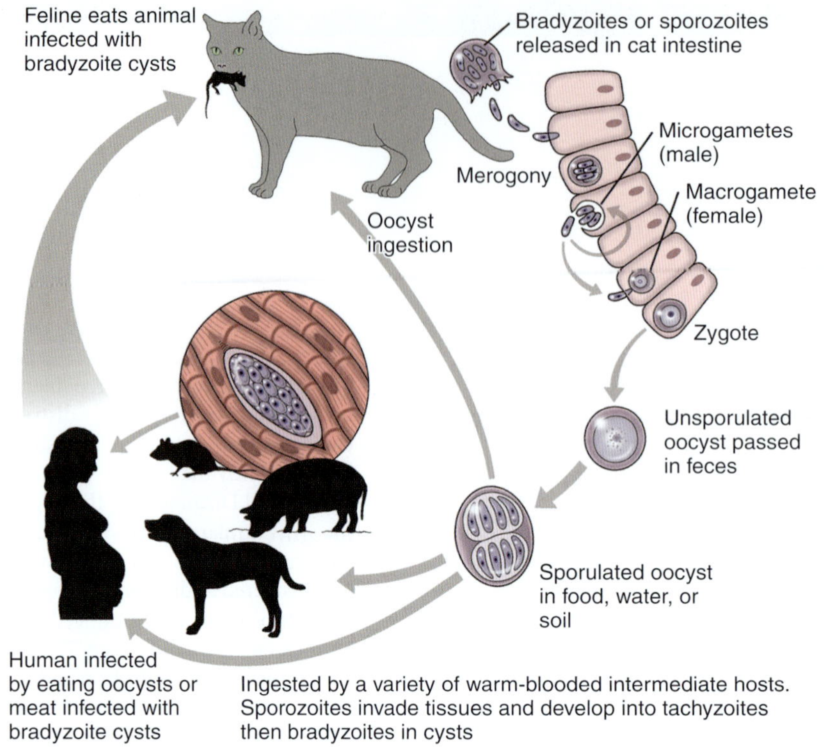

Fig. 93.1 Life cycle of *Toxoplasma gondii.* Cats are most often infected when they ingest tissue cysts in prey. The bradyzoites transform into merozoites and undergo repeated cycles of schizogony in the cat's intestinal tract. The merozoites then transform into microgametes (male) and macrogametes (female). When a microgamete penetrates a macrogamete, a zygote forms. The zygote is excreted as an unsporulated oocyst in the feces, which is not infectious. Sporulation occurs after 1 to 5 days. The extraintestinal cycle occurs in cats or other intermediate hosts after they ingest sporulated oocysts or tissue cysts. Sporozoites penetrate intestinal cells and transform into tachyzoites, which rapidly multiply in nucleated cells throughout the body in the face of immunosuppression. This can result in severe disease in the developing fetus. Ultimately, organisms are contained by the immune system within bradyzoite cysts in muscle, brain, and visceral organs (latent infection).

feeding. After ingestion, the bradyzoites transform into merozoites, which replicate in the epithelial cells of the intestinal tract, then transform into microgametes and macrogametes. When a microgamete penetrates a macrogamete, a zygote forms. The zygote then transforms into an unsporulated oocyst, which is excreted in feces for 3 to 21 days. After sporulation (formation of sporozoites within the oocyst), oocysts can survive in the environment for months to years and are resistant to most disinfectants. The *T. gondii* oocyst excretion prepatent period is stage dependent (ingestion of bradyzoites has a shorter prepatent period than ingestion of sporozoites) but is not dose dependent.[7] In addition, transmission of *T. gondii* is most efficient when cats consume tissue cysts (carnivorism) and when intermediate hosts consume oocysts (fecal-oral transmission). Infection of rodents with *T. gondii* leads to clinical signs of altered behavior, so the rodent becomes less fearful of cats.[21] This may increase the likelihood that the definitive host (cat) will become infected and potentiate the sexual phase of the organism. People and cats develop antibodies against sporozoites confirming infection after ingestion of sporulated oocysts.[22-24]

Whether clinical toxoplasmosis develops is dependent on both host and parasite effects. Some strains of *T. gondii* may be more pathogenic than others, and some genotypes may have specific tissue affinities, such as a tendency to cause ocular disease in cats or people.[25-30] If a poor immune response is mounted after primary infection, overwhelming tachyzoite replication that results in tissue necrosis is the major cause of disease.[2-5] This mechanism is also likely in cats or dogs with chronic (latent) toxoplasmosis that then become immune suppressed. One example is activation of *T. gondii* infection in cats or dogs after administration of immunosuppressive drugs such as cyclosporine.[31-34] Other immunosuppressive conditions such as FIV infection can also result in activation of toxoplasmosis.[35] The mechanisms for chronic clinical toxoplasmosis have not been fully determined. *Toxoplasma gondii* antigens and antigen-containing immune complexes have been documented in the serum of affected cats and so could play a role in some syndromes like uveitis.[36,37] However, persistent infection was not associated with chronic kidney disease in cats of one study.[38]

The large majority of cats infected with *T. gondii* never develop detectable clinical abnormalities. In general, the enteroepithelial cycle in the cat rarely leads to clinical signs. Only 10% to 20% of experimentally inoculated cats develop self-limiting, small bowel diarrhea for 1 to 2 weeks following primary oral inoculation with *T. gondii* tissue cysts; this is presumed to be from the enteroepithelial replication of the organism. *Toxoplasma gondii* enteroepithelial stages were found in intestinal tissues from two cats with inflammatory bowel disease that had positive response to administration of anti-*Toxoplasma* drugs.[39] Eosinophilic fibrosing gastritis was described in one *T. gondii*–infected cat.[40]

Fatal extraintestinal toxoplasmosis in cats can develop from overwhelming intracellular replication of tachyzoites following primary infection; hepatic, pulmonary, CNS, and pancreatic tissues are commonly involved.[2-5,41-43] Kittens infected by the transplacental or transmammary routes develop the most severe signs of extraintestinal toxoplasmosis and generally die of pulmonary or hepatic disease. Common clinical signs in cats with disseminated toxoplasmosis

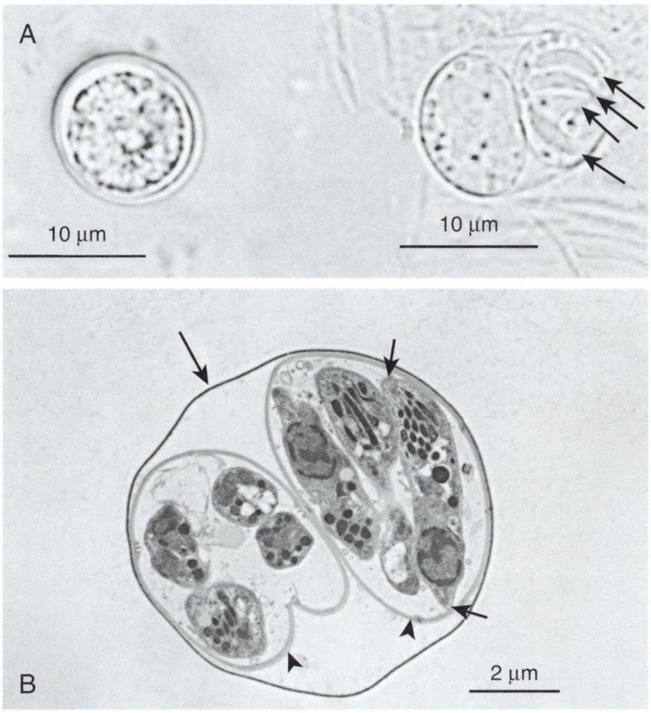

Fig. 93.2 (A) Unsporulated oocyst of *Toxoplasma gondii. (left).* Sporulated oocyst with two sporocysts *(right).* Four sporozoites *(arrows)* are visible within one of the sporocysts. (B) Transmission electron micrograph of a sporulated oocyst. Note the thin oocyst wall *(large arrow)*, two sporocysts (*arrowheads*, one of which is cut longitudinally), and sporozoites (short arrows, anterior and posterior end of one sporozoite). (A, From Dubey JP, Miller NL, Frenkel JK. The *Toxoplasma gondii* oocyst from cat feces. *J Exp Med.* 1970;132:636-662. B, From Dubey JP, Lindsay DS, Speer CA. Structure of *Toxoplasma gondii* tachyzoites, bradyzoites and sporozoites, and biology and development of tissue cysts. *Clin Microbiol Rev.* 1998;11:267-299.)

include lethargy, anorexia, and respiratory distress.[44] Disseminated toxoplasmosis has been documented in cats concurrently infected with FeLV, FIV, or FIP virus, as well as following cyclosporine administration for allergic dermatitis, immune-mediated disorders, or after renal transplantation.[31,32,45]

Chronic toxoplasmosis occurs in some cats and should be on the differential diagnosis list for cats with uveitis, chorioretinitis (Fig. 93.4), cutaneous lesions, fever, muscle hyperesthesia, myocarditis with arrhythmias, weight loss, anorexia, seizures, ataxia, icterus, diarrhea, respiratory distress, pyogranulomatous cystitis, or pancreatitis.[2-5,46-59] Toxoplasmosis appears to be a common infectious cause of uveitis in cats; anterior uveitis or posterior uveitis can occur, and the manifestations can be either unilateral or bilateral.[2,60,61] Kittens infected transplacentally or through the transmammary route commonly develop ocular disease.[25]

In dogs, respiratory, GI, or neuromuscular infection with associated signs of fever, vomiting, diarrhea, respiratory distress, ataxia, seizures, and icterus occurs most commonly with generalized toxoplasmosis.[2,62-68] Generalized toxoplasmosis is most common in immunosuppressed dogs, such as those with CDV infection or those that have been treated with cyclosporine to prevent renal transplant rejection. Neurologic signs depend on the location of the primary lesions and include ataxia, seizures, tremors, cranial nerve deficits, paresis, and paralysis. Dogs with myositis present with weakness, stiff gait, or muscle atrophy. Rapid progression to tetraparesis and paralysis with lower motor neuron dysfunction can occur. One study associated *T. gondii* antibodies with polyradiculoneuritis in dogs.[68] Some dogs with suspected neuromuscular toxoplasmosis probably have neosporosis. While *T. gondii* has been associated with retinitis, anterior uveitis, iridocyclitis, nodular conjunctivitis, and optic neuritis in some dogs with toxoplasmosis, these manifestations are less common than in cats.[2,69] One study of 51 dogs with uveitis and 84 dogs without uveitis failed to show an association with *T. gondii* antibodies in serum and the presence of uveitis.[70] *Toxoplasma gondii* was detected in 78.6% of 41 stillborn puppies in one study.[71] Myocardial infarction with ventricular arrhythmias occurs in some infected dogs and cutaneous disease manifested as pustules, pruritus, subcutaneous nodules, and/or alopecia can occur.[34,72]

DIAGNOSIS

Diagnosis of toxoplasmosis requires interpretation of specific microbiologic tests (Table 93.1) in light of the presence of consistent clinical abnormalities. No clinical abnormalities are specific for the disease.[2-5]

Laboratory Abnormalities

Complete Blood Count

Toxoplasma gondii should be on the differential diagnosis list for cats or dogs with appropriate clinical findings and nonregenerative anemia, neutrophilic leukocytosis or neutropenia, lymphocytosis or lymphopenia, monocytosis, and/or eosinophilia.

Serum Chemistry Profile

Depending on the organ system involved, cats with clinical toxoplasmosis may have increases in serum protein and bilirubin concentrations, as well as increased activities of creatine kinase, ALT, ALP, and lipase.[2-5] Findings are similar for dogs; dogs with chronic toxoplasmosis may develop hyperglobulinemia that is generally polyclonal.[73]

Urinalysis

Proteinuria and bilirubinuria have been detected in some dogs or cats with clinical toxoplasmosis.

Cerebrospinal Fluid Analysis

CSF protein concentrations and cell counts are often higher than normal, with the predominant white blood cells in CSF being small mononuclear cells. However, increased neutrophils also are commonly found in cats with acute CNS toxoplasmosis. Increased CSF protein concentrations and mixed inflammatory cell infiltrates occur in dogs with CNS toxoplasmosis.

Diagnostic Imaging

Plain Radiography

Pulmonary toxoplasmosis most commonly causes diffuse interstitial to alveolar patterns (Fig. 93.5); pleural effusion has rarely been documented.

Sonographic Findings

Ultrasound findings consistent with pancreatitis or diffuse hepatitis could be noted in dogs or cats with involvement of these tissues due to *T. gondii* infection. Intra-abdominal lymphadenomegaly may be noted in dogs or cats with polysystemic disease.

Advanced Imaging

MRI findings in dogs and cats with toxoplasmosis may be unremarkable, or focal or mass lesions may be identified in the brain and/or spinal cord. On MRI, lesions are often isointense on T1-weighted imaging and hyperintense on T2-weighted imaging, and they may enhance peripherally or uniformly with contrast (Fig. 93.6).[74-76]

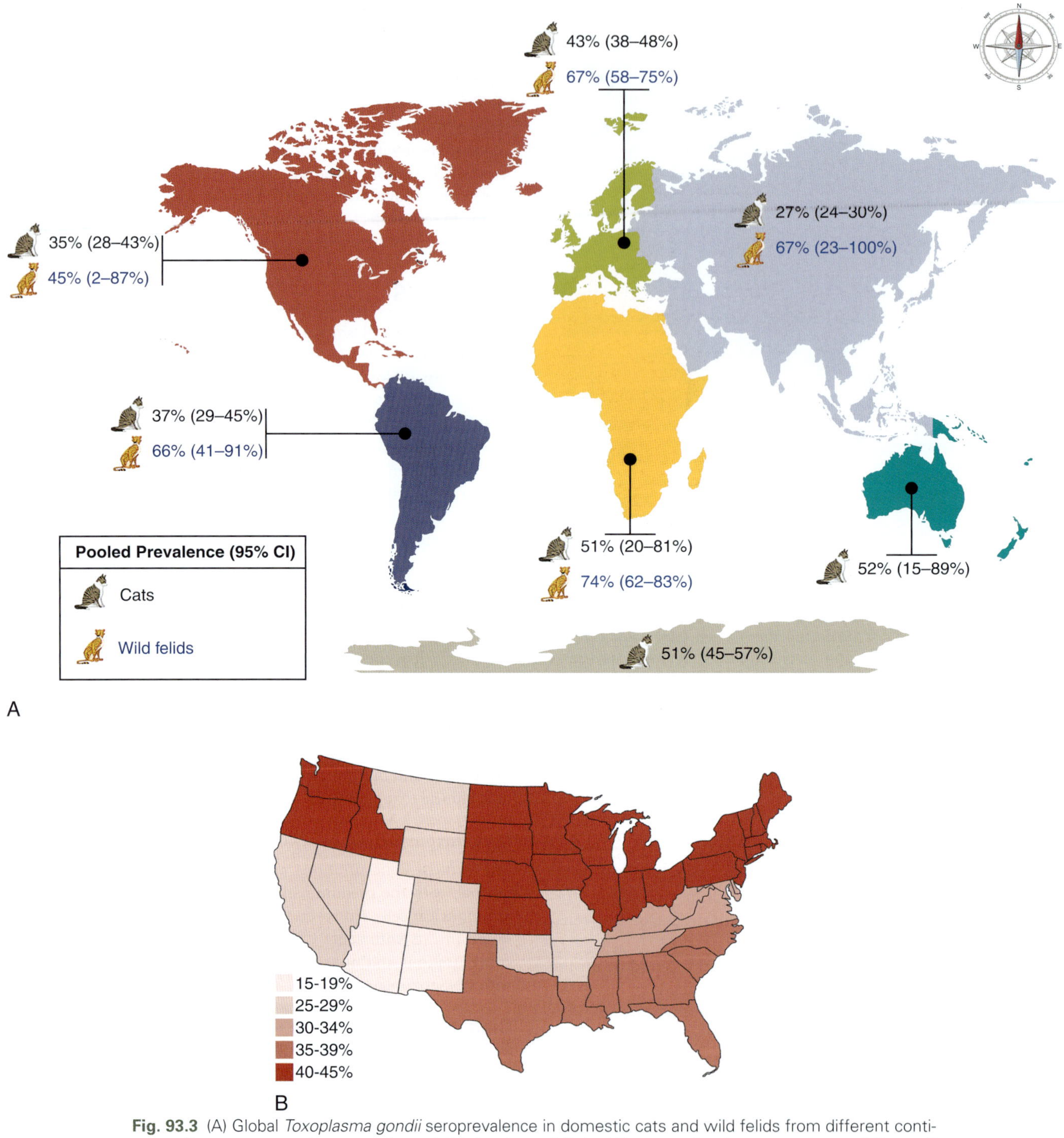

Fig. 93.3 (A) Global *Toxoplasma gondii* seroprevalence in domestic cats and wild felids from different continents. Data are reported as mean (range). (B) Continental United States regional seroprevalence of *T. gondii* antibodies in clinically ill cats. Results were based on the presence of *T. gondii*-specific IgG or IgM in serum. Information was available from 3,640 serum specimens. (A, Modified from Montazeri M, Galeh TM, Moosazadeh M, et al. The global serologic prevalence of *Toxoplasma gondii* in felids during five decades (1967-2017): a systematic review and meta-analysis. *Parasites Vectors*. 2020;13:82. B, From Vollaire MR, Radecki SV, Lappin MR. Seroprevalence of *Toxoplasma gondii* antibodies in clinically ill cats in the United States. *Am J Vet Res*. 2005;66:874-877.)

Microbiologic Tests

Cytologic Diagnosis

Using cytologic examination, *T. gondii* bradyzoites or tachyzoites can be detected in tissues, effusions, bronchoalveolar lavage fluids, aqueous humor, or CSF (Fig. 93.7).[47,51,52,54] A definitive antemortem diagnosis of toxoplasmosis can be made if the organism is identified; however, this is uncommon, particularly in association with sublethal disease. In the dog, *N. caninum* tachyzoites cannot be distinguished from those of *T. gondii* on cytologic examination, and so further diagnostics are needed to make a definitive

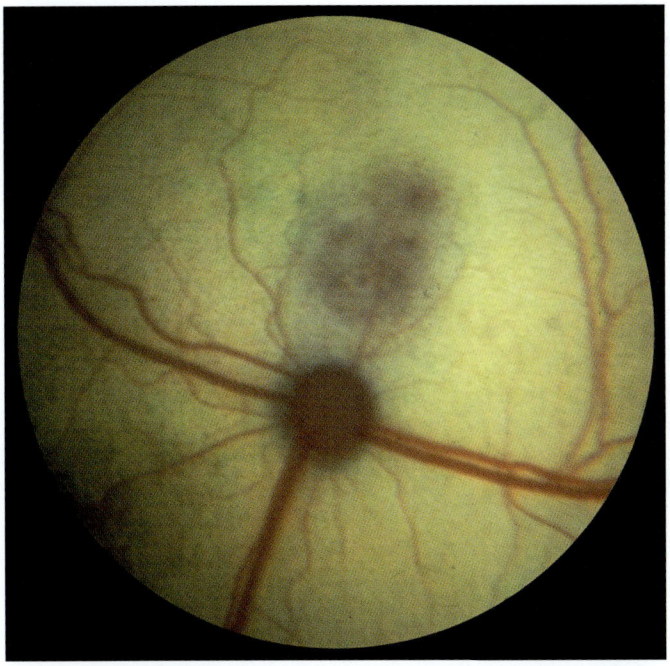

Fig. 93.4 *Toxoplasma gondii*–associated chorioretinitis in an experimentally inoculated cat.

diagnosis; results of PCR assays are used frequently to differentiate these pathogens.[2-5]

Fecal Flotation

Toxoplasma gondii oocysts measure 10 × 12 μm. When identified in feces of cats with diarrhea, this suggests infection by *T. gondii*.[2-4,77] However, *Besnoitia* and *Hammondia* infections of cats produce morphologically similar oocysts. If oocysts of this size are detected in feces of dogs, *N. caninum* infection is most likely if clinical disease is present.[2] However, *T. gondii* oocysts can be present if the dog has ingested infected feline feces. As discussed, PCR assays are available commercially to differentiate DNA of *T. gondii* and *N. caninum*. Alternately, serum antibody responses can be followed sequentially to attempt to determine the infecting genus. Overall, detection of oocysts in cats has a poor negative predictive value for clinical toxoplasmosis, because the signs that develop from disseminated infections occur after oocyst excretion has been completed.

Serologic Diagnosis

Cats. Detection of *T. gondii* antibodies in serum is used most frequently for the diagnosis of clinical toxoplasmosis in cats. A multitude of different techniques have been evaluated, including ELISA, IFA, Western blot immunoassay, and a variety of agglutination tests.[78-88] ELISA, IFA, and Western blot immunoassays have been adapted to detect IgM, IgG, and IgA antibody responses by using heavy-chain–specific secondary antibodies.[78,84,85] *Toxoplasma gondii*–specific serum IgA antibody responses are similar to IgG antibody responses, and this antibody class is usually measured only in research studies. Several commercial laboratories in the United States offer *T. gondii* IgM and IgG testing by ELISA.[89] The following are common findings concerning *T. gondii* IgM and IgG antibody test results in cats.

Toxoplasma gondii IgM antibody titers

- Using ELISA, approximately 80% of healthy, experimentally infected cats have detectable *T. gondii*–specific IgM in serum within 2 to 4 weeks after inoculation with *T. gondii*; these titers generally are negative within 16 weeks after infection.[78,79]
- As occurs in some healthy women, persistent IgM titers (>16 weeks) have been documented commonly in cats co-infected with FIV and in cats with ocular toxoplasmosis.[60,86] Because of these findings and the fact that some cats never have a detectable IgM response, IgM titers cannot accurately be used to predict when a cat is excreting oocysts. If a clinician is concerned that an individual cat is excreting *T. gondii* oocysts, fecal flotation or a fecal PCR assay should be performed.
- In one study of cats with clinical toxoplasmosis, *T. gondii* IgM titers were detected in the serum of 93% of the cats, whereas *T. gondii* IgG titers were detected in only 60% of the cats. Thus, IgM antibodies have a higher etiologic predictive value than IgG for clinical feline toxoplasmosis.[78,86]
- Some cats with chronic *T. gondii* infections that are initially IgM positive, but then become IgM negative, again became IgM positive after repeat inoculation with *T. gondii* in the face of FIV- or glucocorticoid-induced immunosuppression.[78,88] However, clinical signs of toxoplasmosis do not develop in these cats. Thus, presence of IgM antibodies in feline serum does not always mean that clinical toxoplasmosis is present.

Toxoplasma gondii IgG titers

- *Toxoplasma gondii*–specific IgG can be detected by ELISA in serum in the majority of healthy experimentally inoculated cats within 3 to 4 weeks after infection.[78,79]
- By the time IgG antibodies are detected, the oocyst excretion period has usually been completed. Thus, IgG-seropositive cats are of minimal public health risk.
- *Toxoplasma gondii* agglutinating antibody titers can be detected for at least 6 years after infection in experimentally inoculated cats. Because the organism probably persists in tissues for life, IgG antibodies probably do as well.[83]
- Single, high IgG titers do not necessarily suggest recent or active *T. gondii* infection; healthy cats can have titers that exceed 1:10,000 as long as 6 years after experimental induction of toxoplasmosis.[83]
- Some cats with low *T. gondii* antibody titers can become seronegative based on the cutoff value used in an individual assay even though *T. gondii* is still within tissues. Based on an approximately 10% interassay variation in the ELISA technique, some cats with low positive IgG titers (1:64) can be positive for IgG antibodies on one analysis and negative on a subsequent analysis or vice versa.
- An increasing *T. gondii* IgG titer documents recent or active infection, but in experimentally infected cats, the time span from the first detectable positive IgG titer to the maximal IgG titer is approximately 2 to 3 weeks. Thus, some cats with clinical toxoplasmosis will have reached their maximal IgG titer by the time they are evaluated serologically.
- Rising *T. gondii* IgG antibody titers occur in healthy infected cats as well as cats with clinical toxoplasmosis and so, when assessed alone, do not prove clinical toxoplasmosis.
- In humans and cats that reactivate chronic *T. gondii* infection after immune suppression, IgG titers only rarely increase.

Dogs. In dogs, assays that detect IgM and IgG titers are available in some commercial laboratories.[89] There have been very few research studies that assess canine serologic responses to *T. gondii* in different situations. However, most of the findings documented in cats appear to be true in dogs, based on the author's clinical experience.

For the reasons just discussed, antibody test results alone cannot be used to make a diagnosis of feline or canine toxoplasmosis. However,

TABLE 93.1 Microbiologic Assays for Diagnosis of *Toxoplasma gondii* Infection

Assay	Specimen Type	Assay Target	Comments
Fecal flotation	Feces	*T. gondii* oocysts	The negative predictive value of this assay is poor for clinical toxoplasmosis, since most cats cease excretion by the time illness occurs.
Fecal PCR assay	Feces	*T. gondii* DNA	As for fecal flotation.
Cytologic examination	Effusions, skin lesions, tissue aspirates	*T. gondii* tachyzoites and occasionally bradyzoites	Confirms current infection and is generally associated with disease. Organisms cannot be readily distinguished from *Neospora caninum*.
Histopathology	Multiple tissues	*T. gondii* tachyzoites and bradyzoites	If the organisms are detected in the presence of inflammation and necrosis, clinical toxoplasmosis is likely. Can be difficult to differentiate *T. gondii* from tissue protozoans such as *N. caninum* in dogs. Immunohistochemistry can be used to differentiate the two agents.
PCR assay	Effusions, blood, multiple tissues	*T. gondii* DNA	*T. gondii* DNA can be amplified from the blood of normal dogs and cats and so PCR on blood has a low positive predictive value. Amplification of specific DNA confirms infection, and if appropriate clinical signs and inflammation are present, positive results document clinical toxoplasmosis.
Serology for *T. gondii* IgM	Serum	*T. gondii* IgM antibodies	Most consistent with recent infection but can be induced during reinfection and by other immune drugs such as glucocorticoids. Positive results do not correlate with active disease.[a]
T. gondii IgG	Serum	*T. gondii* IgG antibodies	Most consistent with infection of > 10 days duration. Positive results do not correlate with active disease.[a]
Agglutination assays	Serum	*T. gondii* antibodies	Hypothetically detects all antibody classes but can be falsely negative in animals that only possess anti-*Toxoplasma* IgM antibody. Positive results do not correlate with active disease.[a]

[a]Results of serum antibody assays are combined with clinical findings to aid in making a diagnosis of clinical toxoplasmosis.

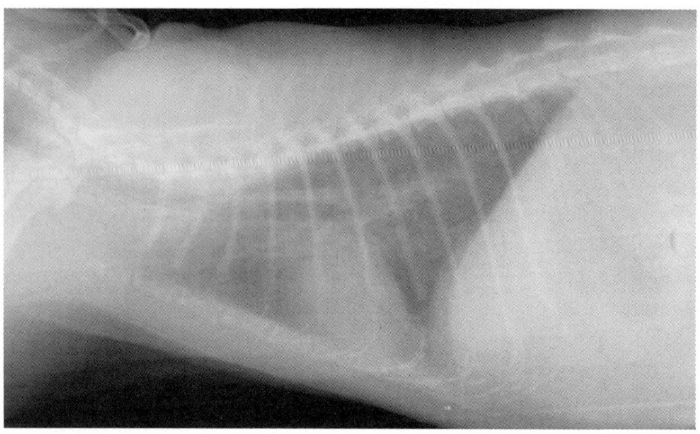

Fig. 93.5 Thoracic radiographs of a 7-year-old female spayed domestic shorthair cat with pulmonic toxoplasmosis that developed 1 month after renal transplantation. There is a diffuse interstitial pattern. The cat subsequently developed respiratory arrest, and tachyzoites were seen in fluid that was suctioned from the endotracheal tube used for resuscitation. Necropsy revealed severe, diffuse, necrotizing pneumonia with intralesional tachyzoites. Histiocytic, lymphoplasmacytic, and necrotizing lesions with intralesional tachyzoites were also seen in the renal allograft, ureter, bladder, liver, pancreas, peritoneum, muscularis mucosa of the stomach, and myocardium. Tachyzoites were not seen in the brain, but there was perivascular inflammation that suggested the possibility of infection. Immunohistochemistry confirmed that the tachyzoites were *T. gondii*.

the following combination can be used to make a presumptive antemortem diagnosis:

- Demonstration of antibodies in serum that suggest exposure to *T. gondii*.
- Demonstration of an IgM titer higher than 1:64, or a fourfold or greater rise in IgG titer, which suggests recent or active infection.
- Clinical signs of disease consistent with toxoplasmosis.
- Exclusion of other common causes of the clinical syndrome.

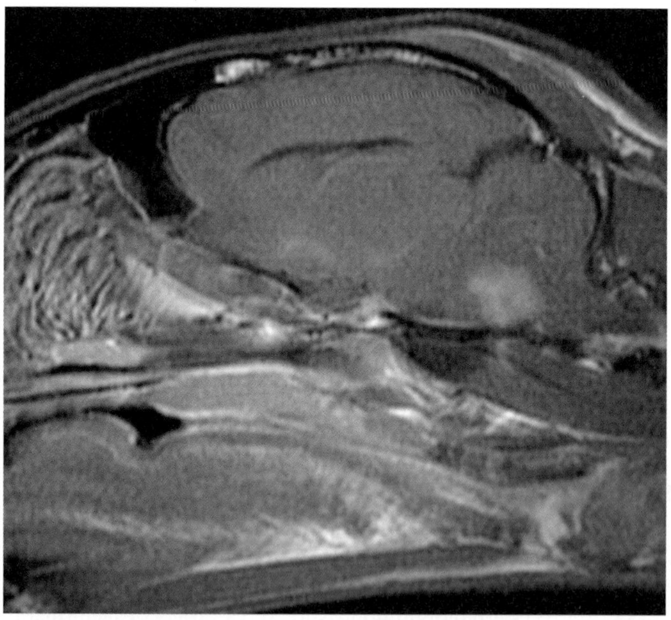

Fig. 93.6 T1-weighted postcontrast sagittal magnetic resonance image from an 11-year-old female spayed domestic longhair that was evaluated for a 5-day history of inappetence, ataxia, abnormal vocalization, and circling. The cat was FIV and FeLV negative and had no other immunosuppressive conditions. A contrast-enhancing lesion is present in the right brainstem. CSF analysis revealed a mixed monocytic (primarily lymphocytic) pleocytosis with a total nuclear cell count of 36 cells/μL and a total protein concentration of 78 mg/dL. Meningoencephalitis secondary to *T. gondii* infection was confirmed at necropsy.

- Positive response to appropriate treatment.

Because *T. gondii* infection cannot be eliminated from tissues, most cats and dogs will be antibody positive for life, so there is little reason to repeat serum antibody titers after the clinical disease has resolved or to

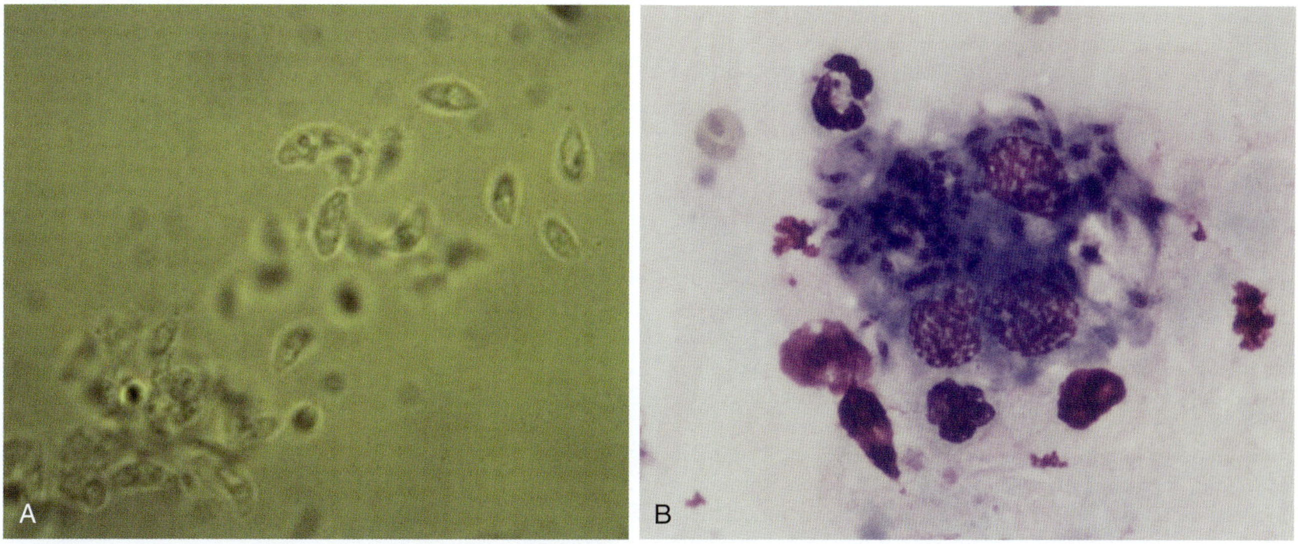

Fig. 93.7 (A) Tachyzoites of *Toxoplasma gondii* from the peritoneal cavity of a cat with fulminant toxoplasmosis. Unstained specimen. (B) Cluster of tachyzoites in a tracheobronchial lavage specimen from a 12-year-old male neutered cat that developed respiratory distress 3 weeks after renal transplantation. Wright stain, 1000× oil magnification.

administer drugs with *T. gondii* activity to cats or dogs without clinical signs of toxoplasmosis.

Other Serologic Assays. Assays that measure *T. gondii* antigens or immune complexes have been evaluated in some cats. However, as for antibody tests, antigen or immune complexes can be detected in cats with or without clinical illness. These assays are not offered commercially.[35,36,78]

Molecular Diagnosis Using Nucleic Acid–Based Testing

Recently, PCR assays have been used to document *T. gondii* DNA in feces and can be used to differentiate among *T. gondii* strains as well as to distinguish *T. gondii* from other organisms.[77] *Toxoplasma gondii* DNA can be amplified from the blood of healthy cats and dogs, and so positive PCR assay results do not correlate with clinical disease.[90,91] Thus, PCR assays are used most frequently with cytologic examination or histopathology to document that the organisms seen were *T. gondii*, or to detect *T. gondii* in aqueous humor or CSF in conjunction with serology.[61,63-65,91] The genotype of *T. gondii* can also be determined, and additional studies are needed to more closely correlate genotypes to clinical disease-inducing potential or manifestations in dogs and cats.[27-29]

The combination of detection of *T. gondii*–specific antibody in serum, blood, aqueous humor, or CSF and amplification of *T. gondii* DNA using NAATs the most accurate way to diagnose ocular or CNS toxoplasmosis. While *T. gondii*–specific IgA, IgG, and DNA can be detected in aqueous humor and CSF of both normal and clinically ill cats, *T. gondii*–specific IgM has only been detected in the aqueous humor or CSF of clinically ill cats and so may be the best indicator of clinical disease. Whether this is true for dogs has not been assessed to date.

Pathologic Findings

Gross Pathologic Findings

Infection with *T. gondii* generally induces pyogranulomatous reactions and necrosis. The pyogranulomas may be visualized grossly depending on the organ involved. Effusions that are characteristic of modified transudates or exudates may be found at necropsy.

Histopathologic Findings

Histopathology in animals with toxoplasmosis usually reveals pyogranulomatous inflammation with necrosis. *Toxoplasma gondii* tachyzoites or tissue cysts are commonly detected (Fig. 93.8A and B). However, if necrosis is severe, the organism may be obscured. In these cases, DNA can often be amplified from the tissues or the agent can be visualized after immunohistochemical staining (Fig. 93.8C). Because *T. gondii* and *N. caninum* induce similar syndromes in dogs, performance of PCR assays for both organisms in dogs is indicated in order to differentiate between them.

TREATMENT AND PROGNOSIS

Cats or dogs with suspected clinical toxoplasmosis should be administered supportive care as needed. Clindamycin hydrochloride or a trimethoprim-sulfonamide combination has been prescribed most frequently for the specific treatment of clinical toxoplasmosis (Table 93.2).[2-5,87] One of the drugs should be prescribed for 1 week, since most clinical signs of toxoplasmosis will begin to resolve within that time period. If a positive response is recognized, treatment should be continued for a total of 4 weeks if possible. If there is a poor response to therapy after the first 7 days, an alternative drug should be considered. Recurrence of clinical signs may be more common in cats or dogs treated for less than 4 weeks.[92]

Azithromycin has been used successfully in a limited number of cats, but the optimal duration of therapy is unknown. Pyrimethamine combined with sulfa drugs is effective for the treatment of human toxoplasmosis but commonly results in toxicity in cats. Pyrimethamine has been administered successfully with other drugs for the treatment of neosporosis in dogs and so may be effective for treatment of clinical toxoplasmosis in this species. Ponazuril has been used experimentally in *T. gondii* infected rodents and should be studied for the treatment of feline toxoplasmosis.[93,94] Currently, an optimal treatment regimen for the use of this drug for this purpose in cats is unknown. However, ponazuril (20 mg/kg PO q24h for 28 days) was apparently successful in the treatment of a dog with suppurative keratitis and necrotizing conjunctivitis due to *T. gondii* infection.[69] Addition of fluconazole to pyrimethamine and trimethoprim was also effective in rodent models of toxoplasmosis and requires further study.[95] Cats or dogs with suspected *Toxoplasma* uveitis should be treated with anti-*Toxoplasma* drugs in combination with topical or systemic glucocorticoids to avoid secondary lens luxations and glaucoma. Enucleation may be required if lens luxations and glaucoma develop from persistent uveitis.

The prognosis is poor for cats or dogs with hepatic, CNS, or pulmonary disease caused by tachyzoite replication, particularly in those that are immunocompromised by anti-inflammatory drugs or retrovirus co-infection. If they survive, cats or dogs with CNS involvement may not experience complete resolution of neurologic signs after treatment.

IMMUNITY AND VACCINATION

There is no evidence to suggest that any drug can eliminate *T. gondii* infection in dogs or cats. Thus, recurrence of disease is always possible, and infected dogs and cats often remain seropositive. Systemic reactivation of *T. gondii* infection after administration of immunosuppressive drugs can occur in both dogs and cats as discussed in the clinical features section. In cats, if repeat oocyst excretion occurs, the number of oocysts excreted is smaller than after the primary inoculation and excretion is of short duration.[18] However, it has been difficult to induce repeat oocyst excretion in chronically infected cats with clinical doses of cyclosporine.[33]

Several types of vaccines have been studied to block oocyst excretion in cats, but there is no vaccine for prevention of clinical toxoplasmosis in dogs or cats.[96]

PREVENTION

To avoid exposure to *T. gondii,* cats and dogs should not be allowed to hunt or be fed undercooked meats.[2,6,13,97,98] Care should be taken to control transport hosts such as cockroaches that have been shown to carry *T. gondii* oocysts. Cleaning cat litterboxes daily may lessen the risk of sporulated oocyst transmission between cats and between cats and their owners. Pallas cats are known to be very susceptible to *T. gondii*–associated illness. In a recent study, use of clindamycin prophylactically was shown to lessen neonatal mortality rates.[99]

PUBLIC HEALTH ASPECTS

Primary *T. gondii* infection in immunocompetent humans results in self-limiting fever, malaise, and lymphadenopathy that may not be recognized or is misdiagnosed. Primary infection of mothers by *T. gondii* during gestation can lead to clinical toxoplasmosis in the fetus; stillbirth, CNS disease, and ocular disease are common clinical manifestations (Fig. 93.9). As T-helper cell counts decline, approximately 10% of people with AIDS develop toxoplasmic encephalitis from reactivation of bradyzoites in tissue cysts.[100-104] Results of studies attempting to associate *T. gondii* infection with behavioral or mental abnormalities in people have variable results.[105,106] Since it is difficult or impossible to eliminate *T. gondii* from the tissues of people, avoiding exposure is optimal.[101,107-109]

People most commonly acquire toxoplasmosis by ingestion of sporulated oocysts or tissue cysts, or transplacentally (Fig. 93.10). To prevent toxoplasmosis, humans should avoid consumption of undercooked meats or ingestion of sporulated oocysts. In a study of 6,282 meat samples from 698 retail meat stores, using a feline bioassay, *T. gondii* was detected in none of the beef or chicken specimens tested and only a small number of pork specimens.[97] However, *T. gondii* has been detected in the tissues of free-ranging chickens.[98]

Although exposure to cats is epidemiologically associated with acquiring toxoplasmosis in some studies, touching individual cats is probably not a common way to acquire toxoplasmosis for the following reasons:[2-5,100,107]

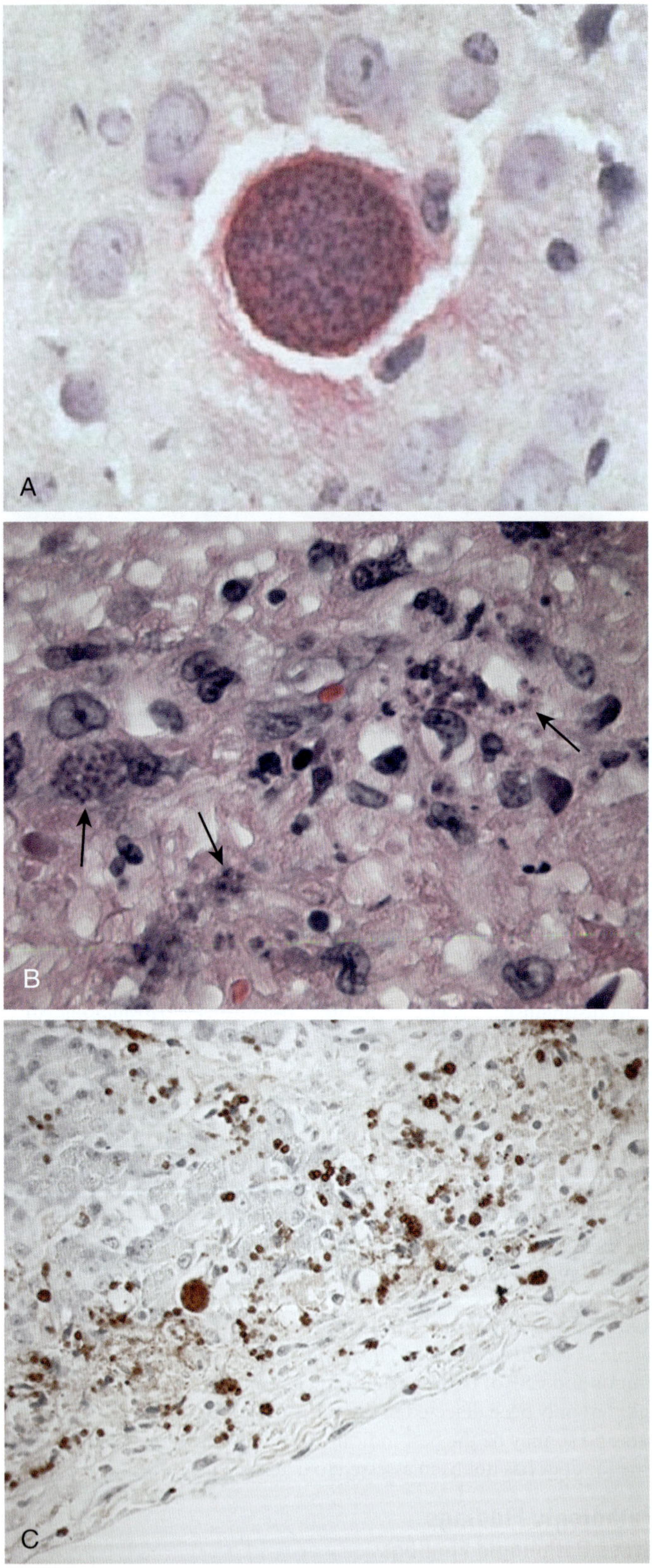

Fig. 93.8 Histopathologic findings in *Toxoplasma gondii* infections. (A) A tissue cyst filled with *T. gondii* bradyzoites in the brain tissues of an experimentally infected mouse. (B) Pancreas of the cat in Figure 93.4. There is pyogranulomatous inflammation with intralesional tachyzoites *(arrows)*; hematoxylin and eosin stain. (C) Immunohistochemistry clearly demonstrates the presence of *T. gondii* tachyzoites in the pancreas (brown staining).

TABLE 93.2 Antimicrobial Drugs That May Be Used to Treat Clinical Toxoplasmosis in Dogs and Cats

Drug	Dose	Route	Interval	Duration
Azithromycin	10 mg/kg	PO	q24h	4 weeks
Clindamycin	10–12 mg/kg	PO	q12h	4 weeks
Ponazuril	20 mg/kg	PO	q24h	4 weeks
Trimethoprim-sulfa	15 mg/kg	PO	q12h	4 weeks

If a positive response to treatment is achieved by week 4 but the animal is still improving slowly, continue treatment for 1 week past clinical resolution or when maximal response is recognized.

- Cats generally only excrete oocysts for days to several weeks after primary inoculation.
- Repeat oocyst excretion is rare and when it occurs, it is generally associated with smaller numbers of oocysts being excreted than after primary infection, even in cats receiving glucocorticoids or cyclosporine, or in those infected with FIV or FeLV.
- Cats are very fastidious and usually do not allow feces to remain on their skin for time periods long enough to lead to oocyst sporulation; the organism was not isolated from the hair of cats that had been excreting millions of oocysts 7 days previously.

However, because some cats will repeat oocyst excretion when exposed a second time, cat feces should always be handled carefully.[15] If a fecal specimen from a cat contains oocysts that measure 10 × 12 μm, it should be assumed that the organism present is *T. gondii*. The feces should be collected and removed daily until the oocyst excretion period is complete; administration of clindamycin (20 mg/kg PO daily) may shorten the oocyst excretion period if started after infection is documented.[2]

Because humans are not commonly infected with *T. gondii* through contact with individual cats, testing healthy cats for evidence of *T. gondii* infection is not recommended.[101,107] Fecal examination is an adequate procedure to determine when cats are actively excreting oocysts but cannot indicate when a cat has excreted oocysts in the past. There is no serologic assay that accurately indicates this, and most cats that are excreting oocysts are seronegative. Most seropositive cats have completed the oocyst excretion period and are unlikely to repeat excretion of large numbers of oocysts; most seronegative cats would excrete the organism if infected. If owners are concerned that they may have toxoplasmosis, they should see their physicians for testing.

Dogs do not complete the enteroepithelial phase of *T. gondii* but can mechanically transmit oocysts after ingesting feline feces.[16]

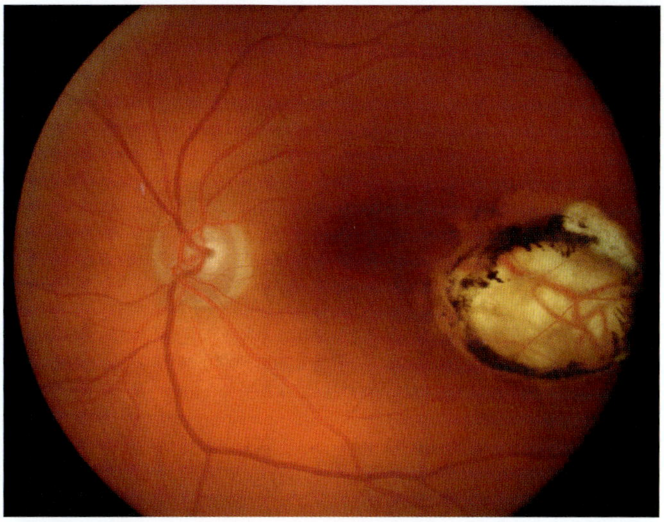

Fig. 93.9 Healed chorioretinitis in a 60-year-old woman who had recovered from congenital toxoplasmosis. The infection resulted in a permanent visual deficit. (Courtesy Mrs. Susan Sykes.)

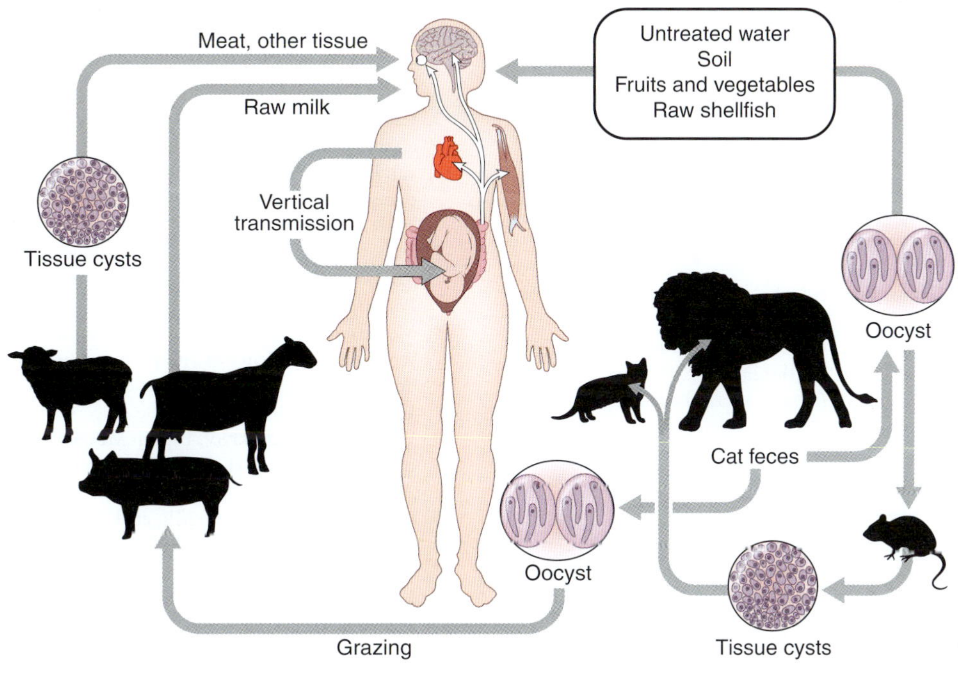

Fig. 93.10 Routes of zoonotic transmission of *Toxoplasma gondii*. (From Montoya JG, Boothroyd JD, Kovacs JA. *Toxoplasma gondii*. In Bennett JE, Dolin R, Blaser MJ, eds. *Mandell, Douglas, and Bennett's Principles and Practice of Infectious Diseases*. Philadelphia, PA: Elsevier; 2020:pp. 3355-3387.)

CASE EXAMPLE

Signalment

"Fluffy," a 3-year-old male neutered Siamese mix from Evans in northern Colorado.

History

Fluffy was referred after being treated for anterior uveitis and recurrent fever at another clinic. The clinical signs had been noted for approximately 1 month. Fluffy was entirely indoors in a suburban environment, but adopted from a humane society at around 6 months of age. His last vaccines (rabies, FHV1, FCV, and panleukopenia virus) were administered 6 months before the uveitis was first noted. He was fed a commercial processed food. There were no other animals at the house. He was treated with selamectin monthly but had not received his dose this month because of the fever. The fever seemed intermittent, and when normal, Fluffy had normal appetite and attitude. The uveitis persisted in spite of treatment with amoxicillin-clavulanic acid administered daily for 10 days and topical 1% prednisolone acetate applied three times daily.

Physical Examination

Body weight: 4.2 kg

General: Quiet, alert, and responsive. Ambulatory on all four limbs. T = 104.3°F (40.2°C), HR = 180 beats/min, RR = 30 breaths/min, mucous membranes pink, CRT = 1 s.

Integument: A dull haircoat was present. There was no evidence of ectoparasites.

Eyes: Bilateral anterior uveitis was present; fundoscopic examination was difficult due to aqueous flare.

Musculoskeletal: Body condition score was 4/9; possible discomfort was detected on muscle palpation.

Gastrointestinal: The cranial abdomen was tense with abdominal splinting noted on palpation.

All other systems: No significant abnormalities were noted.

Laboratory Findings

Complete blood count: All values were within reference ranges.

Serum biochemistry profile: All values were within reference ranges except for the activity of serum AST (190 U/L; reference range, 19–42 U/L) and the activity of serum CK (2000 U/L; reference range, 50–125 U/L).

Urinalysis: No significant abnormalities; SpG = 1.041.

Imaging Findings

Thoracic and abdominal radiographs and abdominal ultrasound were offered but declined by the owner.

Microbiologic Testing

Serologic testing: FeLV antigen negative; FIV antibody negative; serum *Bartonella* IgG negative; *Bartonella* PCR assay negative on whole blood; *T. gondii* serum IgM 1:256; *T. gondii* serum IgG 1:1024.

Diagnosis

Suspected chronic, and possibly recurrent, toxoplasmosis.

Treatment

Clindamycin (12 mg/kg PO q12h) was administered for 28 days; fever resolved on day 3 of treatment. Prednisolone acetate was continued every 6 hours topically bilaterally for the first 14 days and was discontinued after anterior uveitis resolved. Subsequently, chorioretinal scars were noted on fundoscopic examination.

Comments

The findings were suggestive of chronic recurrent toxoplasmosis, which does not respond to treatment with β-lactam antibiotics. Myositis or pancreatitis may have contributed to some of the clinical and laboratory findings. These tissues commonly contain tissue cysts with *T. gondii* bradyzoites that can repeatedly replicate as tachyzoites, which in turn results in acute disease. *Toxoplasma gondii* IgM can be detected in some cats with recurrent disease. Fluffy may have been infected with *T. gondii* when he was a stray and had an exacerbation or alternatively may have been infected more recently in the home environment by ingestion of a transport host (cockroach, etc.) or intermediate host (rodent).

SUGGESTED READINGS

Montazeri M, Mikaeili Galeh T, Moosazadeh M, et al. The global serological prevalence of *Toxoplasma gondii* in felids during the last five decades (1967-2017): a systematic review and meta-analysis. *Parasit Vectors.* 2020;13:82.

Lappin MR, Elston T, Evans L, et al. 2019 AAFP feline Zoonoses Guidelines. *J Feline Med Surg.* 2019;21:1008–1021.

Dubey JP, Cerqueira-Cézar CK, Murata FHA, et al. All about toxoplasmosis in cats: the last decade. *Vet Parasitol.* 2020;283:109145.

Dubey JP, Murata FHA, Cerqueira-Cézar CK, et al. *Toxoplasma* infections in dogs: 2009-2020. *Vet Parasitol.* 2020;287:109223.

Dubey JP. *Toxoplasmosis of Animals and Humans.* 3rd ed. Boca Raton, FL: CRC Press; 2022.

REFERENCES

1. Nicolle C, Manceaux L. Sur une infection à corps de Leishman (ou organismes voisins) du gondii. *C R Seances Acad Sci.* 1908;147:763–766.
2. Dubey JP, Lindsay DS, Lappin MR. Toxoplasmosis and other intestinal coccidial infections in cats and dogs. *Vet Clin North Am Small Anim Pract.* 2009;39:1009–1034.
3. Lappin MR. Update on the diagnosis and management of *Toxoplasma gondii* infection in cats. *Top Companion Anim Med.* 2010;25:136–141.
4. Lappin MR. Polysystemic protozoal infections. In: Couto G, Nelson R, eds. *Small Animal Internal Medicine.* 6th ed. St Louis, MO: Elsevier; 2019:1514–1531.
5. Calero-Bernal R, Gennari SM. Clinical toxoplasmosis in dogs and cats: an update. *Front Vet Sci.* 2019;6:54.
6. van Bree FPJ, Bokken GCAM, Mineur R, et al. Zoonotic bacteria and parasites found in raw meat-based diets for cats and dogs. *Vet Rec.* 2018;182(2):50.
7. Dubey JP. Comparative infectivity of oocysts and bradyzoites of *Toxoplasma gondii* for intermediate (mice) and definitive (cats) hosts. *Vet Parasitol.* 2006;140:69–75.
8. Montazeri M, Mikaeili Galeh T, Moosazadeh M, et al. The global serological prevalence of *Toxoplasma gondii* in felids during the last five decades (1967-2017): a systematic review and meta-analysis. *Parasit Vectors.* 2020;13(1):82.
9. Vollaire MR, Radecki SV, Lappin MR. Seroprevalence of *Toxoplasma gondii* antibodies in clinically ill cats in the United States. *Am J Vet Res.* 2005;66:874–877.
10. Luria BJ, Levy JK, Lappin MR, et al. Prevalence of infectious diseases in feral cats in Northern Florida. *J Feline Med Surg.* 2004;6:287–296.
11. Spain CV, Scarlett JM, Wade SE, et al. Prevalence of enteric zoonotic agents in cats less than 1 year old in central New York State. *J Vet Intern Med.* 2001;15:33–38.
12. Dabritz HA, Miller MA, Atwill ER. Detection of *Toxoplasma gondii*–like oocysts in cat feces and estimates of the environmental oocyst burden. *J Am Vet Med Assoc.* 2007;231:1676–1684.
13. Chalkowski K, Wilson AE, Lepczyk CA, Zohdy S. Who let the cats out? A global meta-analysis on risk of parasitic infection in indoor versus outdoor domestic cats (*Felis catus*). *Biol Lett.* 2019;15(4):20180840.

14. de Wit LA, Kilpatrick AM, VanWormer E, et al. Seasonal and spatial variation in *Toxoplasma gondii* contamination in soil in urban public spaces in California, United States. *Zoonoses Public Health*. 2020;67(1):70–78.
15. Zulpo DL, Sammi AS, Dos Santos JR, et al. *Toxoplasma gondii:* a study of oocyst re-shedding in domestic cats. *Vet Parasitol*. 2018;249:17–20.
16. Lindsay DS, Dubey JP, Butler JM, Blagburn BL. Mechanical transmission of *Toxoplasma gondii* oocysts by dogs. *Vet Parasitol*. 1997;73:27–33.
17. Levy JK, Lappin MR, Glaser AL, et al. Prevalence of infectious diseases in cats and dogs rescued following Hurricane Katrina. *J Am Vet Med Assoc*. 2011;238:311–317.
18. Powell CC, Brewer M, Lappin MR. Detection of *Toxoplasma gondii* in the milk of experimentally infected lactating cats. *J Vet Parasitol*. 2001;102:29–33.
19. Arantes TP, Lopes WD, Ferreira RM, et al. *Toxoplasma gondii*: evidence for the transmission by semen in dogs. *Exp Parasitol*. 2009;123:190–194.
20. Bresciani KD, Costa AJ, Toniollo GH, et al. Transplacental transmission of *Toxoplasma gondii* in reinfected pregnant female canines. *Parasitol Res*. 2009;104:1213–1217.
21. Vyas A, Kim SK, Giacomini N, et al. Behavioral changes induced by *Toxoplasma* infection of rodents are highly specific to aversion of cat odors. *Proc Natl Acad Sci U S A*. 2007;104:6442–6447.
22. Mangiavacchi BM, Vieira FP, Bahia-Oliveira LM, Hill D. Salivary IgA against sporozoite-specific embryogenesis-related protein (TgERP) in the study of horizontally transmitted toxoplasmosis via *T. gondii* oocysts in endemic settings. *Epidemiol Infect*. 2016;144:2568–2577.
23. Torrey EF, Yolken RH. *Toxoplasma* oocysts as a public health problem. *Trends Parasitol*. 2013;29:380–384.
24. Scott J, Morris A, Hawley J. Evaluating the significance of *Toxoplasma gondii* sporozoite antibodies in cats: a pilot study. In review. *J Fel Med Surg*. 2022.
25. Powell CC, Lappin MR. Clinical ocular toxoplasmosis in neonatal kittens. *Vet Ophthalmol*. 2001;4:87–92.
26. Spycher A, Geigy C, Howard J, et al. Isolation and genotyping of *Toxoplasma gondii* causing fatal systemic toxoplasmosis in an immunocompetent 10-year-old cat. *J Vet Diagn Invest*. 2011;23:104–108.
27. Amouei A, Sarvi S, Sharif M, et al. A systematic review of *Toxoplasma gondii* genotypes and feline: geographical distribution trends. *Transbound Emerg Dis*. 2020;67(1):46–64.
28. Crouch EEV, Mittel LD, Southard TL, et al. Littermate cats rescued from a shelter succumbed to acute, primary toxoplasmosis associated with TOXO DB genotype #4, generally circulating in wildlife. *Parasitol Int*. 2019;72:101942.
29. da Silva JR . Isolation and genotyping of *Toxoplasma gondii* in Brazilian dogs. *Korean J Parasitol*. 2017;55:239.
30. Shwab EK, Saraf P, Zhu XQ, et al. Human impact on the diversity and virulence of the ubiquitous zoonotic parasite *Toxoplasma gondii*. *Proc Natl Acad Sci U S A*. 2018;115(29):E6956–E6963.
31. Beatty J, Barrs V. Acute toxoplasmosis in two cats on cyclosporin therapy. *Aust Vet J*. 2003;81:339.
32. Bernsteen L, Gregory CR, Aronson LR, et al. Acute toxoplasmosis following renal transplantation in three cats and a dog. *J Am Vet Med Assoc*. 1999;215:1123–1126.
33. Lappin MR, VanLare KA, Seewald W, et al. Effect of oral administration of cyclosporine on *Toxoplasma gondii* infection status of cats. *Am J Vet Res*. 2015;764:351–357.
34. Webb JA, Keller SL, Southorn EP, et al. Cutaneous manifestations of disseminated toxoplasmosis in an immunosuppressed dog. *J Am Anim Hosp Assoc*. 2005;41:198–202.
35. Davidson MG, Rottman JB, English RV, et al. Feline immunodeficiency virus predisposes cats to acute generalized toxoplasmosis. *Am J Pathol*. 1993;143:1486–1497
36. Lappin MR, Cayatte S, Powell CC, et al. Detection of *Toxoplasma gondii* antigen containing immune complexes in the serum of cats. *Am J Vet Res*. 1993;54:415–419.
37. Lappin MR, Greene CE, Prestwood AK, et al. Enzyme-linked immunosorbent assay for the detection of circulating antigens of *Toxoplasma gondii* in the serum of cats. *Am J Vet Res*. 1989;50:1586–1590.
38. Hsu V, Grant DC, Zajac AM, et al. Prevalence of IgG antibodies to *Encephalitozoon cuniculi* and *Toxoplasma gondii* in cats with and without chronic kidney disease from Virginia. *Vet Parasitol*. 2011;176:23–26.
39. Peterson JL, Willard MD, Lees GE, et al. Toxoplasmosis in two cats with inflammatory intestinal disease. *J Am Vet Med Assoc*. 1991;99:473–476.
40. McConnell JF, Sparkes AH, Blunden AS, et al. Eosinophilic fibrosing gastritis and toxoplasmosis in a cat. *J Feline Med Surg*. 2007;9:82–86.
41. Dubey JP, Carpenter JL. Histologically confirmed clinical toxoplasmosis in cats: 100 cases (1952-1990). *J Am Vet Med Assoc*. 1993;203:1556–1566.
42. Dubey JP, Johnstone I. Fatal neonatal toxoplasmosis in cats. *J Am Anim Hosp Assoc*. 1982;18:461–467.
43. Dubey JP, Carpenter JLN. Toxoplasmosis in littermate cats. *J Am Vet Med Assoc*. 1993;203:1546–1549.
44. Evans NA. Acute respiratory distress syndrome and septic shock in a cat with disseminated toxoplasmosis. *J Vet Emerg Crit Care*. 2017;27:472.
45. Zandonà L, Brunetta R, Zanardello C, Vascellari M, Persico L, Mazzolini E. Cerebral toxoplasmosis in a cat with feline leukemia and feline infectious peritonitis viral infections. *Can Vet J*. 2018;59(8):860–862.
46. Nordquist BC, Aronson LR. Pyogranulomatous cystitis associated with *Toxoplasma gondii* infection in a cat after renal transplantation. *J Am Vet Med Assoc*. 2008;232:1010–1012.
47. Park CH, Ikadai H, Yoshida E, et al. Cutaneous toxoplasmosis in a female Japanese cat. *Vet Pathol*. 2007;44:683–687.
48. Kul O, Atmaca HT, Deniz A, et al. Clinicopathologic diagnosis of cutaneous toxoplasmosis in an Angora cat. *Berl Munch Tierarztl Wochenschr*. 2011;124:386–389.
49. Pfohl JC, Dewey CW. Intracranial *Toxoplasma gondii* granuloma in a cat. *J Feline Med Surg*. 2005;7:369–374.
50. Simpson KE, Devine BC, Gunn-Moore D. Suspected *Toxoplasma*-associated myocarditis in a cat. *J Feline Med Surg*. 2005;7:203–208.
51. Hawkins EC, Davidson MG, Meuten DJ, et al. Cytologic identification of *Toxoplasma gondii* in bronchoalveolar lavage fluid of experimentally infected cats. *J Am Vet Med Assoc*. 1997;210:648–650.
52. Brownlee L, Sellon RK. Diagnosis of naturally occurring toxoplasmosis by bronchoalveolar lavage in a cat. *J Am Anim Hosp Assoc*. 2001;37:251–255.
53. Alves L, Gorgas D, Vandevelde M, et al. Segmental meningomyelitis in 2 cats caused by *Toxoplasma gondii*. *J Vet Intern Med*. 2011;25:148–152.
54. Falzone C, Baroni M, De Lorenzi D, et al. *Toxoplasma gondii* brain granuloma in a cat: diagnosis using cytology from an intraoperative sample and sequential magnetic resonance imaging. *J Small Anim Pract*. 2008;49:95–99.
55. Lindsay SA, Barrs VR, Child G, et al. Myelitis due to reactivated spinal toxoplasmosis in a cat. *J Feline Med Surg*. 2010;12:818–821.
56. Butts DR, Langley-Hobbs SJ. Lameness, generalised myopathy and myalgia in an adult cat with toxoplasmosis. *JFMS Open Rep*. 2020;6(1): 2055116920909668.
57. Lo Piccolo F, Busch K, Palić J, Geisen V, Hartmann K, Unterer S. *Toxoplasma gondii*-associated cholecystitis in a cat receiving immunosuppressive treatment. *Tierarztl Prax Ausg K Kleintiere Heimtiere*. 2019;47(6):453–457.
58. Mari L. Distal polyneuropathy in an adult Birman cat with toxoplasmosis. *JFMS Open Rep*. 2016;2:2055116916630335.
59. Murakami M, Mori T, Takashima Y, et al. A case of pulmonary toxoplasmosis resembling multiple lung metastases of nasal lymphoma in a cat receiving chemotherapy. *J Vet Med Sci*. 2018;80(12):1881–1886.
60. Lappin MR, Roberts SM, Davidson MG, et al. Enzyme-linked immunosorbent assays for the detection of *Toxoplasma gondii*–specific antibodies and antigens in the aqueous humor of cats. *J Am Vet Med Assoc*. 1992;201:1010–1016.
61. Powell CC, McInnis CL, Fontenelle JP, et al. *Bartonella* species, feline herpesvirus-1, and *Toxoplasma gondii* PCR assay results from blood and aqueous humor samples from 104 cats with naturally occurring endogenous uveitis. *J Feline Med Surg*. 2010;12:923–938
62. Dubey JP, Carpenter JL, Topper MJ, et al. Fatal toxoplasmosis in dogs. *J Am Anim Hosp Assoc*. 1989;25:659–664.
63. Al-Qassab S, Reichel MP, Su C, et al. Isolation of *Toxoplasma gondii* from the brain of a dog in Australia and its biological and molecular characterization. *Vet Parasitol*. 2009;164:335–339.
64. da Silva AV, Pezerico SB, de Lima VY, et al. Genotyping of *Toxoplasma gondii* strains isolated from dogs with neurological signs. *Vet Parasitol*. 2005;127:23–27.

65. Langoni H, Matteucci G, Medici B, et al. Detection and molecular analysis of *Toxoplasma gondii* and *Neospora caninum* from dogs with neurological disorders. *Rev Soc Bras Med Trop*. 2012;45:365–368.
66. Plugge NF, Ferreira FM, Richartz RR, et al. Occurrence of antibodies against *Neospora caninum* and/or *Toxoplasma gondii* in dogs with neurological signs. *Rev Bras Parasitol Vet*. 2011;20:202–206.
67. Dubey JP, Chapman JL, Rosenthal BM, et al. Clinical *Sarcocystis neurona, Sarcocystis canis, Toxoplasma gondii*, and *Neospora caninum* infections in dogs. *Vet Parasitol*. 2006;137:36–49.
68. Holt N, Murray M, Cuddon PA, et al. Seroprevalence of various infectious agents in dogs with suspected acute canine polyradiculoneuritis. *J Vet Intern Med*. 2011;25:261–266.
69. Swinger RL, Schmidt Jr KA, Dubielzig RR. Keratoconjunctivitis associated with *Toxoplasma gondii* in a dog. *Vet Ophthalmol*. 2009;12:56–60.
70. Kosec G, Hacin B, Sansom PG, et al. Prevalence of antibody seroconversion to *Toxoplasma gondii* in uveitis and non-uveitis dogs. *Vet Rec Open*. 2019;6(1):e000318.
71. Taques IIGG, Barbosa TR, Martini AC, et al. Molecular assessment of the transplacental transmission of *Toxoplasma gondii, Neospora caninum, Brucella canis* and *Ehrlichia canis* in dogs. *Comp Immunol Microbiol Infect Dis*. 2016;49:47–50.
72. Hoffmann AR, Cadieu J, Kiupel M, et al. Cutaneous toxoplasmosis in two dogs. *J Vet Diagn Invest*. 2012;24:636–640.
73. Yarim GF, Nisbet C, Oncel T, et al. Serum protein alterations in dogs naturally infected with *Toxoplasma gondii*. *Parasitol Res*. 2007;101:1197–1202.
74. Pfohl JC, Dewey CW. Intracranial *Toxoplasma gondii* granuloma in a cat. *J Fel Med Surg*. 2005;7:369–374.
75. Falzone C, Baroni M, De Lorenzi D, et al. *Toxoplasma gondii* brain granuloma in a cat: diagnosis using cytology from an intraoperative sample and sequential magnetic resonance imaging. *J Small Anim Pract*. 2008;49(2):95–99.
76. Alves L, Gorgas D, Vandevelde M, et al. Segmental meningomyelitis in 2 cats caused by *Toxoplasma gondii*. *J Vet Intern Med*. 2011;25:148–152.
77. Salant H, Spira DT, Hamburger J. A comparative analysis of coprologic diagnostic methods for detection of *Toxoplasma gondii* in cats. *Am J Trop Med Hyg*. 2010;82:865–870.
78. Lappin MR. Feline toxoplasmosis: interpretation of diagnostic test results. *Semin Vet Med Surg*. 1996;11:154–160.
79. Lappin MR, Greene CE, Prestwood AK, et al. Diagnosis of recent *Toxoplasma gondii* infection in cats by use of an enzyme-linked immunosorbent assay for immunoglobulin M. *Am J Vet Res*. 1989;50:1580–1585.
80. Lappin MR, Bush DJ, Reduker DW. Feline serum antibody responses to *Toxoplasma gondii* and characterization of target antigens. *J Parasitol*. 1994;80:73–80.
81. Lappin MR, Powell CC. Comparison of latex agglutination, indirect hemagglutination, and ELISA techniques for the detection of *Toxoplasma gondii*-specific antibodies in the serum of cats. *J Vet Intern Med*. 1991;5:299–301.
82. Dabritz HA, Gardner IA, Miller MA, et al. Evaluation of two *Toxoplasma gondii* serologic tests used in a serosurvey of domestic cats in California. *J Parasitol*. 2007;93:806–816.
83. Dubey JP. Duration of immunity to shedding *Toxoplasma gondii* oocysts by cats. *J Parasitol*. 1995;81:410–415.
84. Cannizzo KP, Lappin MR, Cooper CM, et al. *Toxoplasma gondii* antigen recognition by serum IgM, IgG, and IgA of queens and their neonatally infected kittens. *Am J Vet Res*. 1996;57:1327–1330.
85. Burney DP, Lappin MR, Cooper CM, et al. Detection of *Toxoplasma gondii*-specific IgA in the serum of cats. *Am J Vet Res*. 1995;56:769–773.
86. Lappin MR, George JW, Pedersen NC, et al. Primary and secondary *Toxoplasma gondii* infection in normal and feline immunodeficiency virus-infected cats. *J Parasitol*. 1996;82:733–742.
87. Lappin MR, Greene CE, Dawe DL. Clinical feline toxoplasmosis: serologic diagnosis and therapeutic management of 15 cases. *J Vet Intern Med*. 1989;3:139–143.
88. Lappin MR, Dawe DL, Lindl PA, et al. The effect of glucocorticoid administration on oocyst shedding, serology, and cell-mediated immune responses of cats with recent or chronic toxoplasmosis. *J Am Anim Hosp Assoc*. 1992;27:625–632.
89. Colorado State University Veterinary Diagnostic Laboratories. http://www.dlab.colostate.edu.
90. Burney DP, Spilker M, McReynolds L, et al. Detection of *Toxoplasma gondii* parasitemia in experimentally inoculated cats. *J Parasitol*. 1999;5:947–951.
91. Lee JY, Lee SE, Lee EG, et al. Nested PCR-based detection of *Toxoplasma gondii* in German shepherd dogs and stray cats in South Korea. *Res Vet Sci*. 2008;85:125–127.
92. Lappin M. Unpublished observations.
93. Mitchell SM, Zajac AM, Kennedy T, et al. Prevention of recrudescent toxoplasmic encephalitis using ponazuril in an immunodeficient mouse model. *J Eukaryot Microbiol*. 2006;53:S164–S165.
94. Mitchell SM, Zajac AM, Davis WL, et al. Efficacy of ponazuril in vitro and in preventing and treating *Toxoplasma gondii* infections in mice. *J Parasitol*. 2004;90:639–642.
95. Martins-Duarte ES, de Souza W, Vommaro RC. *Toxoplasma gondii:* the effect of fluconazole combined with sulfadiazine and pyrimethamine against acute toxoplasmosis in a murine model. *Exp Parasitol*. 2013;133:294–299.
96. Ramakrishnan C, Maier S, Walker RA, et al. An experimental genetically attenuated live vaccine to prevent transmission of *Toxoplasma gondii* by cats. *Sci Rep*. 2019;9(1):1474.
97. Dubey JP, Hill DE, Jones JL, et al. Prevalence of viable *Toxoplasma gondii* in beef, chicken, and pork from retail meat stores in the United States: risk assessment to consumers. *J Parasitol*. 2005;91:1082–1093.
98. Gonçalves IN, Uzêda RS, Lacerda GA, et al. Molecular frequency and isolation of cyst-forming coccidia from free ranging chickens in Bahia State, Brazil. *Vet Parasitol*. 2012;190:74–79.
99. Girling SJ, Pizzi R, Naylor AD, et al. Use of clindamycin in Pallas' cats [*Otocolbus* (*felis*) *manul*] to reduce juvenile toxoplasmosis-associated mortality rates. *J Zoo Wildl Med*. 2020;51(1):39–45.
100. Angulo FJ, Glaser CA, Juranek DD, et al. Caring for pets of immunocompromised persons. *J Am Vet Med Assoc*. 1994;205:1711–1722.
101. Kaplan JE, Benson C, Holmes KK, et al. Guidelines for prevention and treatment of opportunistic infections in HIV-infected adults and adolescents. Recommendations from CDC, the National Institutes of health, and the HIV Medicine Association of the Infectious Diseases Society of America. *MMWR Recomm Rep*. 2009;58(RR04):1–198.
102. Wallace MR, Rossetti RJ, Olson PE, et al. Cats and toxoplasmosis risk in HIV-infected adults. *J Am Med Assoc*. 1993;269:76–77.
103. Safarpour H, Cevik M, Zarean M, et al. Global status of *Toxoplasma gondii* infection and associated risk factors in people living with HIV. *AIDS*. 2020;34(3):469–474.
104. Jones JL, Dargelas V, Roberts J, et al. Risk factors for *Toxoplasma gondii* infection in the United States. *Clin Infect Dis*. 2009;49:878–884.
105. Lindgren M, Torniainen-Holm M, Härkänen T, et al. The association between *Toxoplasma* and the psychosis continuum in a general population setting. *Schizophr Res*. 2018;193:329–335.
106. Nayeri Chegeni T, Sharif M, Sarvi S, et al. Is there any association between *Toxoplasma gondii* infection and depression? A systematic review and meta-analysis. *PLoS One*. 2019;14(6):e0218524.
107. Lappin MR, Elston T, Evans L, et al. 2019 AAFP Feline Zoonoses Guidelines. *J Feline Med Surg*. 2019;21(11):1008–1021.
108. Day MJ. Pet-related infections. *Am Fam Physician*. 2016;94:794–802.
109. Dabritz HA, Conrad PA. Cats and *Toxoplasma*: implications for public health. *Zoonoses Public Health*. 2010;57:34–52.

94

Neosporosis

Jane E. Sykes, Michael R. Lappin, Jitender P. Dubey

KEY POINTS

- First Described: In 1984, in boxer dogs in Norway (Bjerkas et al.).[1]
- Cause: *Neospora caninum,* a coccidial protozoan parasite (phylum Apicomplexa).
- Affected Hosts: Dogs are the definitive hosts, and canids are the only species known to complete the sexual phase of *N. caninum* replication with passage of oocysts in the feces. Clinical illness primarily occurs in dogs and cattle. Livestock and many other species of animals, including dogs, act as intermediate hosts.
- Geographic Distribution: Worldwide.
- Mode of Transmission: Dogs can be infected transplacentally. Postnatally, dogs may be infected after they ingest infected tissues of intermediate hosts, bovine fetal membranes, or sporulated oocysts in the environment.
- Major Clinical Signs: Stillbirth, abortion, ascending paralysis, muscle atrophy, neurologic (especially cerebellar) signs, nodular dermatitis, respiratory distress.
- Differential Diagnoses: Toxoplasmosis, sarcocystosis, hepatozoonosis, deep mycoses, protothecosis, rabies, CDV infection, West Nile virus infection, canine monocytic ehrlichiosis, migrating ascarid infections, neuronal storage diseases, granulomatous meningoencephalitis, immune-mediated neuromuscular disease, primary or metastatic neoplasia.
- Human Health Significance: *Neospora caninum* antibodies have been detected in some humans, but the parasite has not been detected in human tissues; therefore, zoonotic health consequences are still unclear.

ETIOLOGY AND EPIDEMIOLOGY

Neospora caninum is an obligately intracellular protozoan pathogen that closely resembles *Toxoplasma gondii*; before its description in 1984, it was misidentified as *T. gondii*.[2–4] Domestic dogs and wild canids (coyotes, dingoes, and wolves) act as definitive hosts of *N. caninum* and shed oocysts after ingestion of *N. caninum* tissue cysts (extraintestinal cycle) (Fig. 94.1).[5–7] Although antibodies against *N. caninum* have been detected in naturally exposed cats and cats have developed clinical neosporosis after experimental infection, neither the parasite nor clinical neosporosis has been detected in naturally exposed cats.[8–10] Clinical neosporosis results from systemic replication of *N. caninum* tachyzoites (which divide by a process known as endodyogeny) and has been described in dogs and certain domestic and wild herbivores such as cattle, sheep, goats, deer and other cervids, and marsupials. A related parasite, *Neospora hughesi,* sporadically causes myeloencephalitis in horses.[11] This organism has an unknown definitive host.[12]

Neospora caninum is one of the most important causes of infertility, abortion, and neonatal mortality in cattle worldwide. Sheep and goats can also develop reproductive and neonatal disease, but the economic importance of *N. caninum* in sheep and goats is less clear when compared with cattle.[13] Herbivores likely become infected when they ingest sporulated oocysts excreted in feces of canids or through transplacental transmission. Oocysts sporulate and become infective 24 to 72 hours after they are excreted in feces of canids and can survive in the environment for prolonged periods. After oocysts are ingested, sporozoites are released in the intestinal tract and penetrate intestinal epithelial cells. Organisms can then disseminate to a variety of tissues, where they transform into bradyzoites and become encysted (tissue cysts). In dogs, transplacental infection can occur when bitches acquire infection during pregnancy or when there is reactivation of infection in dams infected before pregnancy. Transplacental infections can occur in subsequent pregnancies from the same dam or repeated up to three generations, so that multiple litters of puppies can be affected. In one study, *N. caninum* DNA was amplified from the tissues of 52.4% of 41 stillborn puppies from five seropositive bitches.[14] Infection of immunologically naïve cattle late in pregnancy is most likely to lead to transplacental spread with abortion (also known as *exogenous* transplacental transmission).[15] However, transplacental transmission as a result of reactivation of latent infection during pregnancy (*endogenous* transplacental transmission) can also occur.[16] The pregnant cow typically shows no other overt clinical signs of infection.

Aside from transplacental transmission, dogs can become infected and excrete oocysts when they ingest bovine placental material as well as other bovine tissues, such as the muscle, liver, brain, and heart muscle.[5] This horizontal transmission is important and is thought to maintain infection in the dog population.[17] Antibodies or DNA of *N. caninum* has been found in birds, small rodents, and lagomorphs, but whether predation of these species leads to oocyst excretion by dogs is not clear.[13] Because birds can ingest *N. caninum* sporulated oocysts while feeding on the ground, a number of studies have evaluated the role of birds in this parasitism.[18] In one experimental study, chickens were resistant to *N. caninum* infection.[19] In another study, the evidence suggested that ingestion of infected chicken eggs by dogs may lead to oocyst excretion.[20] In dogs, carnivorism is considered the main route of postnatal transmission; dogs fed sporulated oocysts did not develop a patent infection.[21]

When dogs do excrete *N. caninum* oocysts, excretion begins 5 to 13 days after ingestion of infected tissues; oocysts can be excreted for several days but seroconversion does not always occur. Rarely, protracted oocyst excretion for several months has been described.[22] Generally, puppies excrete more oocysts than adult dogs,[23] and the number of oocysts shed decreases with repeated exposures to infected tissues.

In dogs, seroprevalence increases with age (because of an increased likelihood of exposure through horizontal transmission over time) and

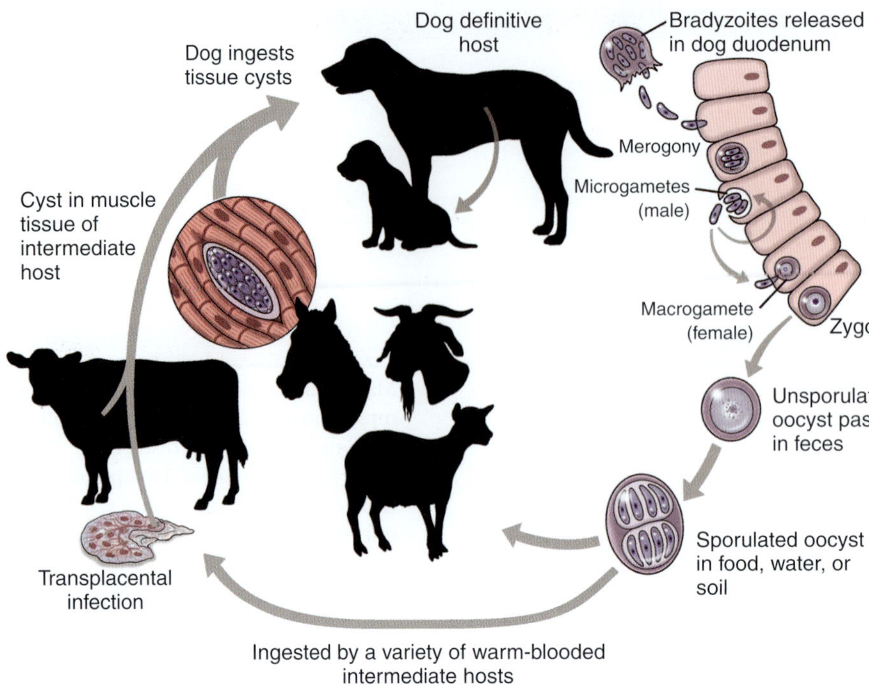

Fig. 94.1 Life cycle of *Neospora caninum*. Dogs become infected when they ingest tissue cysts in bovine placental material and other bovine tissues. Bradyzoites are released in the intestine and transform into merozoites, where they undergo merogony. A zygote forms and is shed in the feces as an unsporulated oocyst. In addition, organisms can penetrate the dog's intestinal tract and form tissue cysts. Reactivation of these cysts in pregnancy can result in repeated transplacental transmission to the fetus. Herbivores are infected when they ingest sporulated oocysts. Infection of cattle can lead to transplacental spread of tachyzoites and abortion.

is higher in free-roaming dogs than in pet dogs. Dogs that reside on cattle farms or dogs in rural areas are also more likely to be seropositive than dogs that reside in urban areas.[24–27] Introduction of infected dogs to a farm can lead to outbreaks of abortion in cattle on the farm,[28] and the more dogs present on a farm, the greater the chance that cattle will be exposed. In one study from Australia, the prevalence in dogs increased over a 20-year period.[29] Although mixed-breed dogs are more likely to be seropositive than purebred dogs, purebred dogs often develop clinical neosporosis,[30] possibly because of genetic defects in CMI. Commonly affected breeds in the literature and/or in the practices of the authors include boxers, Rhodesian ridgebacks, bull mastiffs, greyhounds, basset hounds, Labrador retrievers, Rottweilers, and West Highland white terriers.[13]

CLINICAL FEATURES

Pathogenesis and Clinical Signs

Although exposure to *N. caninum* is common, clinical disease (neosporosis) is uncommon in dogs. The development of neosporosis, the signs that develop, and their rate of progression may depend on the virulence of the infecting *N. caninum* strain and the age and immunocompetence of the host.[2,4,13,30,31] Many affected dogs are infected transplacentally, after which clinical signs usually become apparent from 4 weeks to 6 months of age. Up to 50% of puppies in a litter can be infected, but not all puppies develop signs simultaneously, and sometimes only one puppy in the litter develops clinical illness.[32] Stillbirths and neonatal deaths may also be reported.[30] Reactivation of subclinical infection can occur in older dogs after treatment with immunosuppressive drugs or chemotherapy.[33–35] Co-infection with *Ehrlichia canis* and *Hepatozoon canis* was recognized in one adult dog from Israel with meningoencephalitis.[36] In this dog, *E. canis* morulae and *N. caninum* tachyzoites were identified within CSF eosinophils (which is atypical for *E. canis*) and CSF monocytes, respectively; *H. canis* DNA was only detected in peripheral blood. Seven years before the onset of CNS signs, *E. canis* morulae and *H. canis* gamonts had been detected in peripheral blood. The dog had been treated with doxycycline and imidocarb dipropionate at that time, with normalization of CBC and disappearance of organisms. However, it is possible that persistent infection with *E. canis* contributed to immunosuppression and reactivation of neosporosis. Horizontal acquisition of *N. caninum* infection by adult dogs may occur through consumption of raw meat; one dog that developed neosporosis had a history of being fed raw elk meat.[34]

Transplacental infection of puppies usually leads to myositis and polyradiculoneuritis that initially involves the lumbosacral spinal nerve roots. This is manifested as ascending paralysis, muscle atrophy, and fibrous muscle contracture with arthrogryposis (joint contracture), hyperextension of the pelvic limbs, and loss of patellar reflexes.[30] Early signs of disease include exercise intolerance, ataxia, a high-stepping gait, splaying of the pelvic limbs, a "bunny hopping" gait, urinary incontinence, and/or muscle pain.[30,37–39] Clinical signs progress in some dogs to lethargy, tetraplegia, inability to fully open the mouth, dysphagia, and respiratory difficulty. Involvement of esophageal muscle may lead to megaesophagus.[40,41] Mandibular paralysis, vomiting, and lethargy were described as the only clinical signs in one affected dog.[41] Although ocular lesions are not a major clinical feature of neosporosis, focal chorioretinitis has been reported in some puppies.[42] Less often, young dogs develop signs of hepatitis; pneumonia; meningoencephalomyelitis; or myocarditis with arrhythmias, acute onset of respiratory distress, or sudden death.[39,40,43,44] Puppies with neuromuscular signs may have subclinical infection of other organ systems.[40]

In contrast to puppies, adult dogs typically develop polymyositis and/or meningoencephalomyelitis, with a variety of neurologic

TABLE 94.1 Diagnostic Assays Available for Neosporosis in Dogs

Assay	Specimen Type	Target	Performance
Fecal flotation	Feces	*Neospora caninum* oocysts	Dogs with clinical neosporosis typically are negative for oocysts in feces when tested, so this has a very low sensitivity and is not used routinely for diagnosis. Oocysts cannot be readily distinguished from those of *Hammondia heydorni* or *Toxoplasma gondii.*
Fecal PCR assay	Feces	*N. caninum* DNA	As for fecal flotation but additional data are needed.
Cytologic examination	CSF, aspirates of skin lesions, rarely specimens from the respiratory tract	*N. caninum* tachyzoites	Insensitive except in the case of skin lesions. Confirms active infection and is generally associated with disease. Organisms cannot be readily distinguished from *T. gondii.*
Serology (IFA or ELISA)	Serum or CSF	Antibodies to *N. caninum*	Assays can vary in performance between laboratories. A fourfold increase in titer is associated with recent infection. Dogs with chronic neosporosis may not show a rise in titer, but titers > 1:800 in conjunction with consistent clinical signs suggest neosporosis.
Histopathology	Muscle biopsies, multiple tissues collected at necropsy	*N. caninum* bradyzoites and tachyzoites	If organisms are detected in the presence of inflammation and necrosis, clinical neosporosis is likely. May be difficult to differentiate between *N. caninum* and *T. gondii.* Immunohistochemistry or PCR assay can aid in the differentiation of the two species.
PCR assay	CSF, bronchoalveolar lavage fluid, lymph node, liver, or lung aspirates, tissue biopsies (e.g., muscle, lung, liver, lymph node), or other tissues (CNS or ocular) collected at necropsy	*N. caninum* DNA	Assay performance may vary between laboratories. Because positive PCR results can occur in healthy dogs, they must be interpreted in light of clinical signs and detection of characteristic granulomatous infection in the specimens tested.

CNS, central nervous system; *CSF,* cerebrospinal fluid; *ELISA,* enzyme-linked immunosorbent assay; *IFA,* immunofluorescent antibody; *PCR,* polymerase chain reaction.

signs.[31,40,45] Although lesions can occur throughout the CNS,[40] *N. caninum* has a predilection for the cerebellum.[46] Some dogs can develop cerebellar atrophy. Disseminated infections that involve the myocardium, liver, lungs, skin, GI tract, pancreas, and/or eyes can also occur in adult dogs but are less common than encephalitis. Unusual cases are occasionally reported in the literature, including a dog with bacterial peritonitis and identification of *N. caninum* tachyzoites in peritoneal fluid.[47] In some cases, signs of localized neosporosis can occur before a disseminated infection is recognized. Examples include a 12-year-old schipperke dog with a 2-month history of severe colitis[48,49] and a 7-year-old boxer with an 8-day history of widespread ulcerated cutaneous nodules and lethargy. In both cases, treatment with systemic glucocorticoids was administered shortly before clinical deterioration in association with widespread disseminated infection.

Physical Examination Findings

Physical examination findings in puppies with polyradiculoneuritis-myositis vary from mild ataxia and muscle atrophy to tetraparesis with rigid extension of one or both pelvic limbs and arthrogryposis. Reduced patellar and sometimes other segmental reflexes (including the perianal reflex) are often present.[30,37,50,51] Severely affected dogs may be lethargic and exhibit respiratory difficulty, and it may only be possible to open the mouth a few centimeters. Fever is rare.[30]

Adult dogs with *N. caninum* meningoencephalitis may be obtunded and exhibit signs that include ataxia, circling, head tilt, nystagmus, hypermetria, head tremors, delayed placing reactions, abnormal cranial nerve function, anisocoria, depressed segmental reflexes, tetraparesis, cervical hyperesthesia, and seizures.

Dogs with myocardial involvement may develop acute onset of respiratory difficulty and cyanosis.[30] Cutaneous involvement is manifested as dermatitis with single or multifocal firm nodules, crusting, and/or ulceration, which can appear at additional sites over time and may or may not be accompanied by other systemic signs of infection.[33,52–55] Rarely, dogs with pulmonary involvement are evaluated for cough or respiratory difficulty.[56]

DIAGNOSIS

Neosporosis should be suspected in young dogs (<1 year of age) that develop ascending paralysis and muscle atrophy. It should also be suspected in dogs that develop neurologic (and especially cerebellar) signs or nodular dermatitis, especially in predisposed breeds or dogs treated with immunosuppressive drugs. Diagnosis most often relies on serology or detection of protozoal organisms in body fluids, aspirates, or tissues using light microscopy and/or PCR assays (Table 94.1). Often, antemortem diagnosis is based only on serologic testing because organisms are not easily found.

Laboratory Abnormalities

Complete Blood Count, Serum Biochemistry Panel, and Urinalysis

As for toxoplasmosis, there are no specific hematologic or biochemical abnormalities that suggest neosporosis. The CBC is often normal, but occasionally mild nonregenerative anemia, mild eosinophilia, or monocytosis is evident.[30] The serum biochemistry panel reveals increased CK and AST activity in dogs with myositis.[35,37,39,57] In a study from the UK of dogs with meningoencephalitis, increased activity of CK and AST could be used to raise suspicion for a diagnosis of neosporosis as opposed to noninfectious causes of meningoencephalitis.[58] Occasionally, increased activity of serum ALT (due to hepatitis or severe myositis) or hyperglobulinemia is evident.[35,57] The urinalysis is generally unremarkable.

Cerebrospinal Fluid Analysis

The CSF of dogs with *N. caninum* meningoencephalitis may be normal or show mild to markedly increased total nuclear cell count (sometimes > 1,000 cells/µL) and mild to markedly increased CSF protein concentration.[31,45] Usually, a mononuclear pleocytosis is present, but

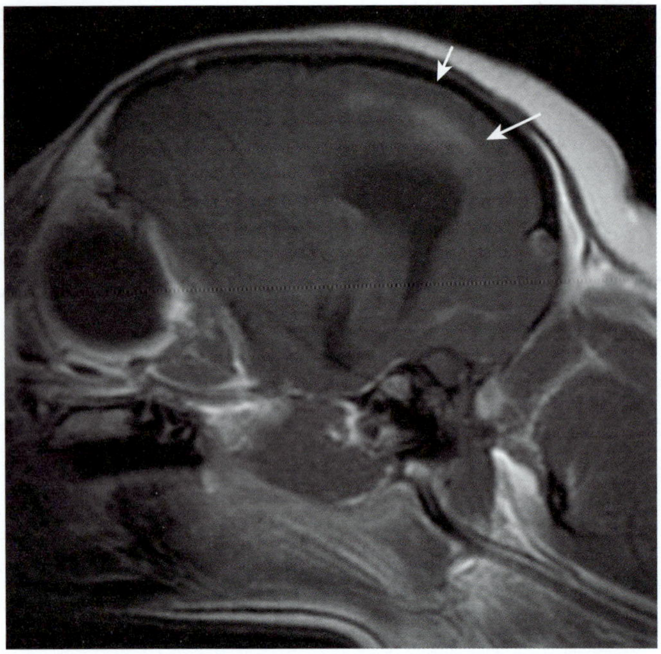

Fig. 94.2 Sagittal T1-weighted postcontrast MRI image from a 4-year-old female spayed Chihuahua with suspected *Neospora caninum* meningoencephalitis. Multiple poorly defined regions of contrast enhancement were identified in the cerebral cortices *(large arrow)*, and mild meningeal enhancement was evident *(small arrow)*. Cerebrospinal fluid (CSF) analysis revealed a mononuclear pleocytosis, and *Neospora* DNA was detected in the CSF using polymerase chain reaction.

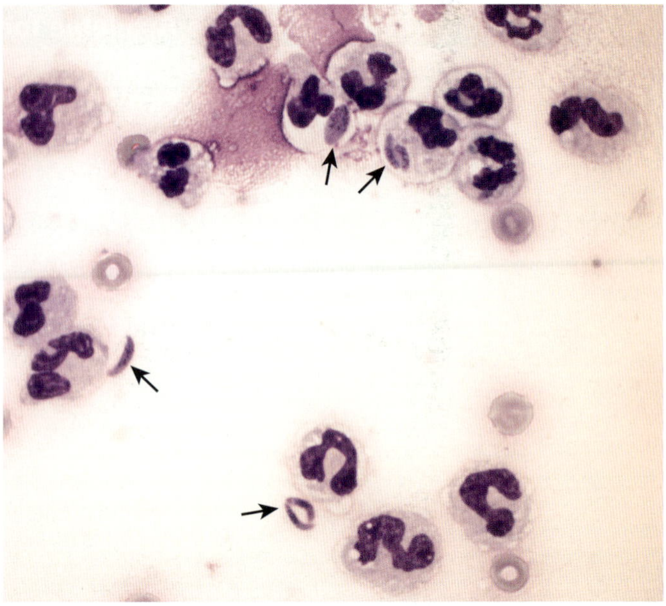

Fig. 94.3 Cytology of abdominal fluid sediment in a 7-year-old male neutered Rhodesian ridgeback showing intracellular and extracellular *Neospora caninum* tachyzoites *(arrows)*. Nucleated cells are predominantly nondegenerate to mildly degenerate neutrophils.

occasionally the response is mixed or primarily composed of neutrophils or eosinophils.[31,37,45,50] *Neospora caninum* tachyzoites are occasionally seen cytologically in CSF.[34,45]

Diagnostic Imaging

Plain Radiography

Thoracic radiographs in dogs with neosporosis are usually unremarkable but may show a diffuse interstitial pattern in dogs with pneumonia, or evidence of megaesophagus in dogs with neuromuscular signs.[30]

Sonographic Findings

Abnormalities are rarely detected on abdominal ultrasound examination of dogs with neosporosis.

Advanced Imaging

MRI of adult dogs with cerebellar signs associated with *N. caninum* infection may show moderate to marked bilateral cerebellar atrophy.[31] Meningeal contrast enhancement may be present.[31,45] Single or multifocal T2-weighted and FLAIR hyperintensities that enhance with contrast on T1-weighted images may be present within the cerebellum or other parts of the brain (Fig. 94.2). Mild to moderate heterogeneous T2-weighted and FLAIR hyperintensities can also be seen in the masseter and temporalis muscles, which may appear atrophied.

Electrodiagnostic Testing

Electromyography in dogs with neosporosis may reveal spontaneous fibrillation potentials, positive sharp waves, and repetitive discharges.[37,39] In some dogs, nerve conduction studies have revealed reduced conduction velocities and compound muscle action potentials.[37]

Microbiologic Tests

Cytologic Examination

The tachyzoites of *N. caninum* may be visualized within aspirates of skin lesions (which often contain many organisms) and rarely in CSF or other body fluids. They are approximately 6 × 1 μm and oval to crescent shaped.[34,45,47,50] They may be seen singly, in pairs, or in larger groups, extracellularly and intracellularly, and are often associated with a pyogranulomatous inflammatory response (Fig. 94.3). *Neospora caninum* tachyzoites cannot be distinguished from those of *T. gondii* on cytologic examination. Because some cross-reactivity between *N. caninum* and *T. gondii* can occur with immunocytochemistry depending on the antibodies used, the use of PCR assays is recommended to definitively identify organisms as *N. caninum*. For unknown reasons, such cross-reactivity may be most likely to occur in dermal neosporosis.[17]

Fecal Flotation

Microscopic examination of feces after use of centrifugal techniques with sugar or zinc sulfate solutions can be used to detect the oocysts of *N. caninum*. However, clinically affected dogs do not typically shed oocysts. When oocysts are seen, they are indistinguishable from those of *Hammondia heydorni* or *T. gondii*. While dogs do not complete the life cycle of *T. gondii*, the oocysts of *T. gondii* can be detected in feces transiently if a dog ingests positive cat feces.

Serologic Diagnosis

Serologic assays are available commercially that detect antibody to *N. caninum* in serum and/or in CSF. Titers are often higher in serum than in the CSF of affected dogs. Indirect IFA assays are widely used, but ELISA assays have also been developed and may be used to detect IgM and IgG antibodies. Seroconversion usually occurs within 2 to 3 weeks of infection, and a rising serum titer can be identified in acutely infected dogs.[39] This rise may not occur in chronically infected dogs, so in this case a single high titer in a dog with consistent clinical signs is suggestive of the diagnosis. The magnitude of titer should not be relied on for clinical diagnosis because congenitally infected sick puppies usually have low antibody titers.[13] Whether use of antibiotics during the acute phase of illness blunts antibody titer development is unknown. Some dogs with neosporosis have extremely high serum titers (e.g., in the tens of thousands), but others have only low antibody titers. The latter situation might reflect the presence of underlying immunodeficiency and inability to produce antibodies. Because interassay variation may cause results to differ between laboratories,[59] the same laboratory should always be used when paired titers are performed or when titers are monitored over time.

Some weak serologic cross-reactivity may occur between the antigens of *T. gondii* and *N. caninum*, so low titers to *T. gondii* may be present in dogs infected with *N. caninum*. Cross-reactivity appears to be less common when IFA assays are used.[59] Serologic cross-reactivity can also occur to *N. hughesi,* again at a slightly lower titer,[60] but the extent to which this organism infects dogs is not clear. Since many of the clinical manifestations of neosporosis and toxoplasmosis are similar, the authors recommend screening affected dogs for antibodies against both agents concurrently. If antibodies against both agents are present, the highest titer may indicate the infecting organism. However, it is also possible that dual infection could occur.

Molecular Diagnosis Using Nucleic Acid–Based Testing

Both endpoint (conventional) and real-time PCR assays are available to aid in the diagnosis of neosporosis.[61–64] Suitable specimens for testing include CSF, bronchoalveolar lavage fluid, lymph node, liver or lung aspirates, tissue biopsies (e.g., muscle, lung, liver, lymph node), or other tissues (CNS or ocular) collected at necropsy. If pyogranulomatous inflammation is detected but organisms are not seen cytologically or histopathologically, the use of PCR assays that detect both *N. caninum* and *T. gondii* should be considered. The sensitivity and specificity of these assays have the potential to vary considerably between laboratories, and more information is required on how these assays perform for antemortem diagnosis of clinical neosporosis in dogs. Because *N. caninum* DNA can be amplified in tissues from healthy dogs, PCR results must always be interpreted considering the clinicopathologic findings and serologic test results. In one study, *N. caninum* DNA was amplified from the liver and/or spleen of one third of shelter dogs that had been euthanized, and PCR assay results did not always correlate with the results of serology.[61] PCR assays can be used to confirm that organisms seen in tissues or body fluids are truly *N. caninum* and not another protozoan parasite such as *Sarcocystis* or *T. gondii*.[63]

Pathologic Findings

Gross pathologic findings may be absent in dogs with neosporosis, or foci of discoloration may be present in the brain and spinal cord, and/or there may be evidence of meningitis (e.g., meningeal thickening or adherence of the meninges to the brain or cranial vault). White streaks within muscle may be found in affected puppies.[37] Histopathology in these puppies reveals polyradiculoneuritis with myelin loss and axonal degeneration, and there may be evidence of muscle fiber degeneration and fibrosis.

Examination of the brain and spinal cord of dogs with CNS involvement usually reveals multifocal nonsuppurative meningoencephalitis and/or myelitis with neuronal degeneration and necrosis, perivascular cuffing, and gliosis. Both gray and white matter can be affected, and the cerebellum may be primarily involved. A mixed inflammatory response with myonecrosis and sometimes dystrophic mineralization may be seen in affected skeletal or cardiac muscle. Tissue cysts or tachyzoites may be evident (Fig. 94.4). Tissue cysts are up to 100 μm in diameter and have a wall that is 4 μm in diameter, which is thicker than that for *T. gondii*. Skin biopsies from dogs with dermal neosporosis contain tachyzoites and pyogranulomatous inflammation. Occasionally (such as in acute, fulminant infections in immunosuppressed dogs), tachyzoites are found in other tissues, including the peripheral nerves, the eye, reproductive tissues, adrenal glands, lung, liver, kidney, spleen, and esophageal muscle.[40] If intralesional protozoa are identified or suspected, IHC and PCR assays can be used to distinguish *N. caninum* from other protozoal species.[63] Although serologic cross-reactivity between *N. caninum* and *T. gondii* is uncommon, it can occur with some antibodies, so IHC is best performed with a panel of antibodies to each protozoan parasite.

In healthy dogs or dogs that die of other diseases, rare tissue cysts in the absence of an inflammatory response may be found at necropsy in skeletal muscle and the CNS.

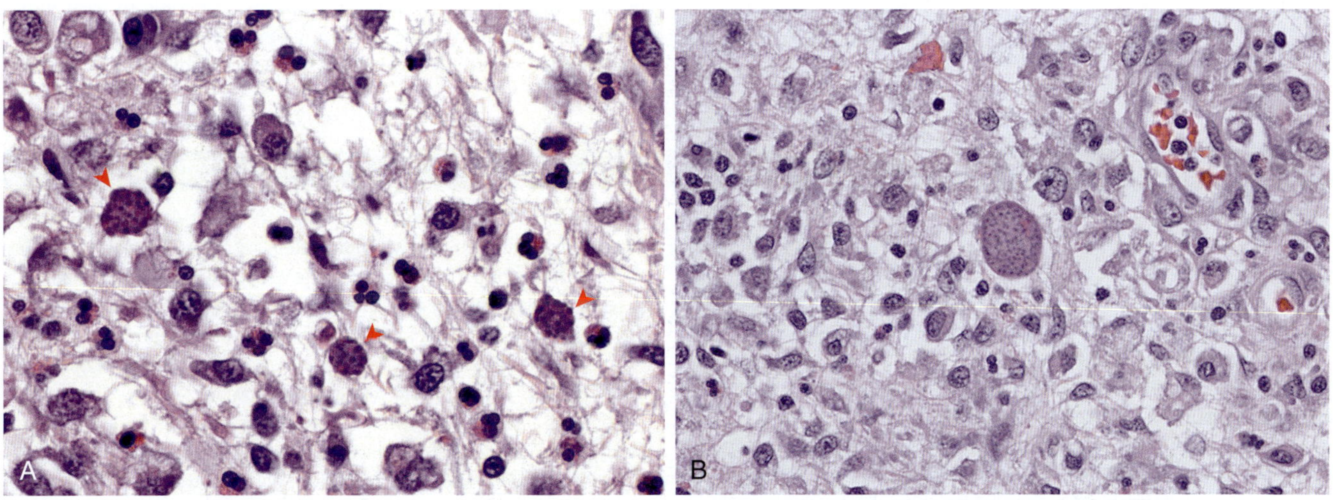

Fig. 94.4 Histopathology of the cerebellum from a 6-year-old intact male Rhodesian ridgeback with neosporosis. (A) Large areas of malacia were present admixed with a marked granulomatous inflammatory infiltrate and abundant protozoal cysts *(arrowheads)*. (B) The protozoal cysts had a thick wall and stained positive with anti-*Neospora* antibodies (not shown). (Courtesy Dr. Robert Higgins, University of California, Davis Veterinary Anatomic Pathology Service.)

TREATMENT AND PROGNOSIS

Several antimicrobial drugs have been prescribed in an attempt to treat neosporosis in dogs (Table 94.2). Historically, clindamycin has frequently been used in many cases because of potential activity against *T. gondii*.[30,64,65] Treatment is usually only temporarily, partially, or completely ineffective, and long periods (>8 weeks) of treatment may be required.[2,4,30,31] Tissue cysts persist despite treatment with clindamycin.[64] Other treatments that have been successful (or partially successful) are trimethoprim-sulfadiazine-pyrimethamine, combinations of clindamycin and trimethoprim-sulfadiazine, or combinations of clindamycin and pyrimethamine. Clindamycin and sulfa-drugs have static effects against *N. caninum*. Ponazuril and toltrazuril have cidal effects and show promise based on studies in *N. caninum*–infected mice.[66] Ponazuril was used safely for weeks in the treatment of keratoconjunctivitis due to *T. gondii* in a dog after treatment with clindamycin failed.[67] Treatment should be continued so long as clinical improvement is occurring. The prognosis for puppies once muscle contracture has developed is poor. It has been suggested that once neosporosis has been diagnosed in a puppy, all dogs in a litter should be treated, because the later the treatment is initiated after the onset of clinical signs, the worse the prognosis. However, without data to confirm that recommendation, veterinarians should at least consider checking the serum *N. caninum* antibody titers of puppies whose littermates have succumbed to neosporosis, and treatment should be considered for those with positive titers. The use of immunosuppressive drugs should be avoided in seropositive puppies.

TABLE 94.2 Antimicrobials Used To Treat Neosporosis in Dogs

Drug[a]	Dose (mg/kg)	Route	Interval (Hours)	Duration (Days)
Clindamycin	10–12	PO	q8h	At least 4 weeks
Trimethoprim-sulfa	15	PO	q12h	At least 4 weeks
Pyrimethamine	1	PO	q24h	At least 4 weeks
Ponazuril[b]	20	PO	q24h	At least 4 weeks

[a]Combinations of drugs are commonly prescribed to severely affected puppies.
[b]Ponazuril or toltrazuril have cidal effects and may be best for central nervous system lesions.[66]

A low dose of glucocorticoids (e.g., prednisone, 0.5 mg/kg, PO, q12h) in addition to anti-protozoal drugs is often used to treat *N. caninum* meningoencephalomyelitis, but no prospective controlled trials have been performed to determine if this alters outcome. Since latent *N. caninum* infection has been activated by the use of immunosuppressive drugs, the concurrent administration of glucocorticoids could promote a negative outcome.[33–35] Physiotherapy may also be beneficial for young dogs with polyradiculoneuritis-myositis.

IMMUNITY AND VACCINATION

Immunity to *N. caninum* is dependent on CMI responses. No vaccines for canine neosporosis exist.

PREVENTION

Neosporosis on farms can be prevented by not allowing dogs to access bovine placental materials, dead calves, or raw or undercooked meat and by preventing dogs from defecating around livestock. Predation should also be discouraged. The use of a muzzle for dogs that work on farms has been suggested to prevent *Neospora* abortions in cattle.[17] It may be necessary to stop the breeding of bitches that have puppies that develop neosporosis, and the owners of puppies that are diagnosed with neosporosis should be advised to inform the breeder of the diagnosis. No drugs are known to prevent transplacental transmission. Where possible, avoidance of excessive pharmacologic immunosuppression (e.g., with glucocorticoids, cyclosporine, azathioprine, or other immunosuppressive drugs) may help to prevent the disease in adult dogs. However, the relative rarity of reactivated neosporosis in adult dogs does not justify routine serologic screening of dogs for infection before commencing immunosuppressive drug treatment.

PUBLIC HEALTH ASPECTS

Antibodies against *N. caninum* have been detected in the serum of some humans, including those with current HIV antibodies.[68,69] However, in one small study of women with repeated abortion, no link to *N. caninum* was found.[70] Most recently, none of the 600 human clinical samples that were from people with signs of toxoplasmosis but negative for *T. gondii* were positive for DNA of *N. caninum*.[71] Overall, the evidence to date suggests that *N. caninum* is not a significant zoonosis. However, it is still prudent for pregnant or immunosuppressed people to wear gloves or wash hands carefully while gardening or cleaning up canine feces and to avoid undercooked meats, particularly beef for this agent.

CASE EXAMPLE

Signalment

"Lenny," a 6-year-old intact male Rhodesian ridgeback from coastal northern California.

History

Lenny was evaluated on a referral basis for a 1-week history of an abnormal gait. The owner first noticed that Lenny was not paying attention during an obedience show. Over the next few days, Lenny was observed to stumble on stairs, and he also fell from a bed. For the 3 days before evaluation, the owner had noted that Lenny appeared uncoordinated and off balance. There had been no changes in his mentation and no evidence of inappetence, vomiting, diarrhea, or changes in thirst or urination. A soft, intermittent nonproductive cough had been noted since the onset of the other clinical signs. Bloodwork at a local veterinary clinic showed a normal CBC, increased activity of serum CK (2,922 U/L, reference range [RR]: 10–200 U/L), ALT (155 U/L, RR: 5–60 U/L), and AST (135 U/L, RR: 5–55 U/L). Serum thyroxine concentration was within the reference range. A urinalysis was unremarkable and aerobic bacterial urine culture was negative. Serology for antibodies to *Borrelia burgdorferi*, *Anaplasma* spp., *Ehrlichia* spp., and antigen of *Dirofilaria immitis* (SNAP 4Dx Plus test, IDEXX Laboratories) was negative. A *T. gondii* titer was pending. Lenny was treated with clindamycin (7.5 mg/kg, PO, q12h) and doxycycline (5 mg/kg, PO, q12h) with no signs of improvement.

Lenny had traveled extensively to Iowa, Colorado, and Kentucky but had no history of toxin exposure or trauma. He was fed a raw diet that consisted of turkey necks, chicken meat, lamb, and vegetables. He was up to date on routine vaccinations (distemper, adenovirus, parvovirus, and rabies) and on heartworm prophylaxis, but did not receive flea or tick prophylaxis and had been exposed to ticks in the past. He had been bred once and only one of three puppies survived. There was no other significant medical history.

CASE EXAMPLE—cont'd

Physical Examination

Body weight: 40.2 kg.

General: Bright and alert, hydrated. T = 100.5°F (38.1°C), HR = 80 beats/minute, panting, mucous membranes pink and moist, CRT = 1 second.

Musculoskeletal: BCS was 4/9. Truncal ataxia was present with a wide-based stance (see Neurologic examination). There was no evidence of lameness or muscle atrophy.

All other systems: With the exception of the neurologic examination, no other clinically significant abnormalities were detected.

Neurologic examination: The dog was alert and responsive. Truncal ataxia was present with hypermetria that was most pronounced on the left side. Head tremors were also noted. A slight left-sided head tilt was present, together with a decreased to absent menace response on the left side. There was normal physiologic nystagmus and no evidence of spontaneous nystagmus. Delayed placing reactions were detected in all four limbs but were most pronounced on the right side. Spinal reflexes were within normal limits. Neuroanatomic location: cerebellar/vestibular disease.

Laboratory Findings

Muscle biochemistry panel: AST 85 U/L (21–54 U/L), CK 1,683 U/L (46–320 U/L).

Imaging Findings

Thoracic radiographs and abdominal ultrasound examination: No abnormalities were detected.

Magnetic resonance imaging (brain): On T2-weighted images, there was increased intensity of the vermis and left cerebellar hemisphere. The cerebellum appeared normal on T1-weighted images. Subtle regions of contrast enhancement were suspected in the left cerebellum on sagittal T1-weighted postcontrast images.

Other Testing

CSF analysis: Total nucleated cell count (TNCC) was 62 cells/μL (normal < 2 cells/μL); total protein was 75 mg/dL (normal < 25 mg/dL). There were 86% eosinophils, 8% small mononuclear cells, 5% large mononuclear cells, and 1% nondegenerate neutrophils. The large mononuclear cells were mostly of unremarkable morphology but occasionally had mildly increased cytoplasmic vacuolation. No infectious agents were seen.

Microbiologic Testing

Serologic testing (IFA): *Neospora caninum* serum antibody titer positive at 1:20,480; the CSF titer was 1:640.

Zinc sulfate fecal flotation: Negative for parasite ova.

Fecal Baermann examination: Negative for parasite larvae.

Treatment

Before the *Neospora* titers were available, a diagnosis of eosinophilic meningoencephalitis was made, and the dog was treated with prednisone (0.5 mg/kg, PO, q12h) but showed no clinical improvement over the subsequent 3 days. A second CSF specimen collected at that time had a cell count of 37 cells/μL and a total protein concentration of 59 mg/dL, with no change in the differential cell count. Lenny was discharged from the hospital, and once the *N. caninum* serology results became available (1 week later), treatment with trimethoprim-sulfamethoxazole (15 mg/kg, PO, q12h) and ponazuril (10 mg/kg, or 2.5 mL of 15% ponazuril paste, PO, q24h) was added. A baseline Schirmer tear test (performed to monitor for keratoconjunctivitis sicca secondary to sulfamethoxazole) was negative. At a recheck examination 3 weeks later, all neurologic signs were persistent but mildly improved. A CBC showed mild, nonregenerative anemia (34.9%) and mild bandemia (198 cells/μL). Serum CK activity was 88 U/L. CSF analysis showed a total protein concentration of 33 mg/dL and a TNCC of 2 cells/μL, with 0% eosinophils, 51% small mononuclear cells, and 49% mildly reactive large mononuclear cells. The serum and CSF antibody titers to *N. caninum* were both 1:5,120. A Schirmer tear test was normal. Two weeks later, the trimethoprim-sulfamethoxazole was discontinued. Neurologic signs persisted but continued to show mild but slow improvement over the next 3 weeks. The ponazuril was discontinued, but after an additional 3 weeks, the head tremors worsened slightly. Blood work was unchanged, CSF analysis (cisternal and lumbar) was within normal limits, and serum and CSF *N. caninum* antibody titers were 1:1,280 and 1:640, respectively. The prednisone was also discontinued. Two months later (4 months after initial diagnosis), severe ataxia and falling returned over a 2-week period. The owner declined reinstitution of antiprotozoal treatment and elected euthanasia. A complete necropsy revealed severe, locally extensive, necrotizing granulomatous encephalitis that was localized to the cerebellum. Abundant protozoal cysts were present within the cerebellar lesions, which were identified using immunohistochemical stains as *N. caninum*. Protozoa were not visualized in any other tissues.

Diagnosis

Granulomatous cerebellitis secondary to *N. caninum* infection.

Comments

Neosporosis in this dog resulted from cerebellar encephalitis, which illustrated the suggested predilection of *N. caninum* for the cerebellum. Development of encephalitis rather than polyradiculoneuritis-myositis is typical of neosporosis in adult dogs. It is possible this dog contracted neosporosis as a result of consumption of a raw food diet; tissue cysts have been identified in the CNS tissues of a lamb,[72] and chickens are possibly intermediate hosts based on seropositivity and positive PCR assay results on the brain tissue.[18–20] The inflammatory response in the CSF was profoundly eosinophilic, as previously reported in other dogs with neosporosis. Fecal flotation was negative for *N. caninum* oocysts, which is expected given the life cycle of the parasite and the short shedding period with low numbers of oocysts shed. The fecal examinations were performed to evaluate for the possibility of visceral larva migrans, given the CSF eosinophilia. Although treatment with trimethoprim-sulfamethoxazole and then ponazuril led to resolution of CSF abnormalities, clinical signs showed only mild improvement. Treatment of neosporosis with glucocorticoids remains controversial, but attempts to reduce the prednisone dose were associated with worsening of clinical signs. Ultimately, all treatment was discontinued because of minimal improvement in clinical signs but resolution of laboratory abnormalities. Relapse subsequently ensued, and the diagnosis was confirmed at necropsy.

SUGGESTED READINGS

Curtis B, Harris A, Ullal T, et al. Disseminated *Neospora caninum* infection in a dog with severe colitis. *J Vet Diagn Invest.* 2020;32:923–927.

Aroch I, Baneth G, Salant H, et al. *Neospora caninum* and *Ehrlichia canis* co-infection in a dog with meningoencephalitis. *Vet Clin Pathol.* 2018;47:289–293.

Dubey JP. Neosporosis in dogs. *CAB Rev.* 2013;8:055.

REFERENCES

1. Bjerkas I, Mohn SF, Presthus J. Unidentified cyst-forming sporozoon causing encephalomyelitis and myositis in dogs. *Z Parasitenkd.* 1984;70:271–274.
2. Dubey JP, Lappin MR. Toxoplasmosis and neosporosis. In: Greene CE (ed). *Infectious Diseases of the Dog and Cat.* 4th ed. Elsevier Saunders: St. Louis, MO.

3. Dubey JP, Carpenter JL, Speer CA, et al. Newly recognized fatal protozoan disease of dogs. *J Am Vet Med Assoc*. 1988;192:1269.
4. Silva RC, Machado GP. Canine neosporosis: perspectives on pathogenesis and management. *Vet Med (Auckl)*. 2016;7:59–70.
5. Cavalcante GT, Monteiro RM, Soares RM, et al. Shedding of *Neospora caninum* oocysts by dogs fed different tissues from naturally infected cattle. *Vet Parasitol*. 2011;179:220–223.
6. Perrucci S, Gavazza A, Rocchigiani G, et al. *Neospora caninum* oocyst shedding in a naturally infected dog from Italy. *Vet Parasitol Reg Stud Reports*. 2017;8:10–12.
7. Klein C, Barua S, Liccioli S, et al. *Neospora caninum* DNA in coyote fecal samples collected in an urban environment. *J Wildl Dis*. 2019;55:196–199.
8. Sedlák K, Bartova E, Machacova T. Seroprevalence of *Neospora caninum* in cats from the Czech republic. *Acta Parasitol*. 2014;59:359–361.
9. Lima DCV, Magalhães FJR, Andrade MR, et al. Anti-*Neospora caninum* antibodies in feral cats on the Island of Fernando de Noronha, Brazil. *Acta Parasitol*. 2018;63:645–646.
10. McAllister MM, Jolley WR, Wills RA, et al. Oral inoculation of cats with tissue cysts of *Neospora caninum*. *Am J Vet Res*. 1998;59:441–444.
11. Pusterla N, Conrad PA, Packham AE, et al. Endogenous transplacental transmission of *Neospora hughesi* in naturally infected horses. *J Parasitol*. 2011;97:281–285.
12. Walsh CP, Duncan RB, Zajac AM, et al. *Neospora hughesi*: experimental infections in mice, gerbils, and dogs. *Vet Parasitol*. 2000;92:119–128.
13. Dubey JP, Hemphill A, Calero-Bernal R, et al. *Neosporosis in Animals*. Boca Raton, FL; CRC Press.
14. Taques IIGG, Barbosa TR, Martini AC, et al. Molecular assessment of the transplacental transmission of *Toxoplasma gondii, Neospora caninum, Brucella canis* and *Ehrlichia canis* in dogs. *Comp Immunol Microbiol Infect Dis*. 2016;49:47–50.
15. McCann CM, McAllister MM, Gondim LF, et al. *Neospora caninum* in cattle: experimental infection with oocysts can result in exogenous transplacental infection, but not endogenous transplacental infection in the subsequent pregnancy. *Int J Parasitol*. 2007;37:1631–1639.
16. Williams DJ, Hartley CS, Bjorkman C, et al. Endogenous and exogenous transplacental transmission of *Neospora caninum*—how the route of transmission impacts on epidemiology and control of disease. *Parasitology*. 2009;136:1895–1900.
17. Reichel MP, Ellis JT, Dubey JP. Neosporosis and hammondiosis in dogs. *J Small Anim Pract*. 2007;48:308–312.
18. de Barros LD, Miura AC, Minutti AF, et al. *Neospora caninum* in birds: a review. *Parasitol Int*. 2018;67:397–402.
19. Oliveira S, Aizawa J, Soares HS, et al. Experimental *Neospora caninum* infection in chickens (*Gallus gallus domesticus*) with oocysts and tachyzoites of two recent isolates reveals resistance to infection. *Int J Parasitol*. 2018;48:117–123.
20. Furuta PI, Mineo TW, Carrasco AO, et al. *Neospora caninum* infection in birds: experimental infections in chicken and embryonated eggs. *Parasitology*. 2007;134:1931–1939.
21. Bandini LA, Neto AF, Pena HF, et al. Experimental infection of dogs (*Canis familiaris*) with sporulated oocysts of *Neospora caninum*. *Vet Parasitol*. 2011;176:151–156.
22. McGarry JW, Stockton CM, Williams DJ, et al. Protracted shedding of oocysts of *Neospora caninum* by a naturally infected foxhound. *J Parasitol*. 2003;89:628–630.
23. Gondim LF, McAllister MM, Gao L. Effects of host maturity and prior exposure history on the production of *Neospora caninum* oocysts by dogs. *Vet Parasitol*. 2005;134:33–39.
24. Antony A, Williamson NB. Prevalence of antibodies to *Neospora caninum* in dogs of rural or urban origin in central New Zealand. *N Z Vet J*. 2003;51:232–237.
25. Basso W, Venturini L, Venturini MC, et al. Prevalence of *Neospora caninum* infection in dogs from beef-cattle farms, dairy farms, and from urban areas of Argentina. *J Parasitol*. 2001;87:906–907.
26. Sicupira PM, de Magalhaes VC, Galvao Gda S, et al. Factors associated with infection by *Neospora caninum* in dogs in Brazil. *Vet Parasitol*. 2012;185:305–308.
27. Bruhn FR, Figueiredo VC, Andrade Gda S, et al. Occurrence of anti–*Neospora caninum* antibodies in dogs in rural areas in Minas Gerais, Brazil. *Rev Bras Parasitol Vet*. 2012;21:161–164.
28. Dijkstra T, Barkema HW, Hesselink JW, et al. Point source exposure of cattle to *Neospora caninum* consistent with periods of common housing and feeding and related to the introduction of a dog. *Vet Parasitol*. 2002;105:89–98.
29. Sloan S, Šlapeta J, Jabbar A, et al. High seroprevalance of *Neospora caninum* in dogs in Victoria, Australia, compared to 20 years ago. *Parasit Vectors*. 2017;10(1):503.
30. Barber JS, Trees AJ. Clinical aspects of 27 cases of neosporosis in dogs. *Vet Rec*. 1996;139:439–443.
31. Garosi L, Dawson A, Couturier J, et al. Necrotizing cerebellitis and cerebellar atrophy caused by *Neospora caninum* infection: magnetic resonance imaging and clinicopathologic findings in seven dogs. *J Vet Intern Med*. 2010;24:571–578.
32. Heckeroth AR, Tenter AM. Immunoanalysis of three litters born to a Doberman bitch infected with *Neospora caninum*. *Parasitol Res*. 2007;100:837–846.
33. Ordeix L, Lloret A, Fondevila D, et al. Cutaneous neosporosis during treatment of pemphigus foliaceus in a dog. *J Am Anim Hosp Assoc*. 2002;38:415–419.
34. Galgut BI, Janardhan KS, Grondin TM, et al. Detection of *Neospora caninum* tachyzoites in cerebrospinal fluid of a dog following prednisone and cyclosporine therapy. *Vet Clin Pathol*. 2010;39:386–390.
35. Fry DR, McSporran KD, Ellis JT, et al. Protozoal hepatitis associated with immunosuppressive therapy in a dog. *J Vet Intern Med*. 2009;23:366–368.
36. Aroch I, Baneth G, Salant H, et al. *Neospora caninum* and *Ehrlichia canis* co-infection in a dog with meningoencephalitis. *Vet Clin Pathol*. 2018;47:289–293.
37. Cuddon P, Lin DS, Bowman DD, et al. *Neospora caninum* infection in English Springer Spaniel littermates. Diagnostic evaluation and organism isolation. *J Vet Intern Med*. 1992;6:325–332.
38. Ishigaki K, Noya M, Kagawa Y, et al. Detection of *Neospora caninum*–specific DNA from cerebrospinal fluid by polymerase chain reaction in a dog with confirmed neosporosis. *J Vet Med Sci*. 2012;74:1051–1055.
39. Hay WH, Shell LG, Lindsay DS, et al. Diagnosis and treatment of *Neospora caninum* infection in a dog. *J Am Vet Med Assoc*. 1990;197:87–89.
40. Barber JS, Payne-Johnson CE, Trees AJ. Distribution of *Neospora caninum* within the central nervous system and other tissues of six dogs with clinical neosporosis. *J Small Anim Pract*. 1996;37:568–574.
41. Mayhew PD, Bush WW, Glass EN. Trigeminal neuropathy in dogs: a retrospective study of 29 cases (1991-2000). *J Am Anim Hosp Assoc*. 2002;38:262–270.
42. Dubey JP, Koestner A, Piper RC. Repeated transplacental transmission of *Neospora caninum* in dogs. *J Am Vet Med Assoc*. 1990;197:857–860.
43. Pumarola M, Anor S, Ramis AJ, et al. *Neospora caninum* infection in a Neapolitan mastiff dog from Spain. *Vet Parasitol*. 1996;64:315–317.
44. Meseck EK, Njaa BL, Haley NJ, et al. Use of a multiplex polymerase chain reaction to rapidly differentiate *Neospora caninum* from *Toxoplasma gondii* in an adult dog with necrotizing myocarditis and myocardial infarct. *J Vet Diagn Invest*. 2005;17:565–568.
45. Gaitero L, Anor S, Montoliu P, et al. Detection of *Neospora caninum* tachyzoites in canine cerebrospinal fluid. *J Vet Intern Med*. 2006;20:410–414.
46. Lorenzo V, Pumarola M, Siso S. Neosporosis with cerebellar involvement in an adult dog. *J Small Anim Pract*. 2002;43:76–79.
47. Holmberg TA, Vernau W, Melli AC, et al. *Neospora caninum* associated with septic peritonitis in an adult dog. *Vet Clin Pathol*. 2006;35:235–238.
48. Curtis B, Harris A, Ullal T, et al. Disseminated *Neospora caninum* infection in a dog with severe colitis. *J Vet Diagn Invest*. 2020;32:923–927.
49. Decôme M, Martin E, Bau-Gaudreault L, et al. Systemic disseminated *Neospora caninum* infection with cutaneous lesions as the initial clinical presentation in a dog. *Can Vet J*. 2019;60:1177–1181.
50. Peters M, Wagner F, Schares G. Canine neosporosis: clinical and pathological findings and first isolation of *Neospora caninum* in Germany. *Parasitol Res*. 2000;86:1–7.

51. Ruehlmann D, Podell M, Oglesbee M, et al. Canine neosporosis: a case report and literature review. *J Am Anim Hosp Assoc.* 1995;31:174–183.
52. Boyd SP, Barr PA, Brooks HW, et al. Neosporosis in a young dog presenting with dermatitis and neuromuscular signs. *J Small Anim Pract.* 2005;46:85–88.
53. Poli A, Mancianti F, Carli MA, et al. *Neospora caninum* infection in a Bernese cattle dog from Italy. *Vet Parasitol.* 1998;78:79–85.
54. McInnes LM, Irwin P, Palmer DG, et al. In vitro isolation and characterisation of the first canine *Neospora caninum* isolate in Australia. *Vet Parasitol.* 2006;137:355–363.
55. Perl S, Harrus S, Satuchne C, et al. Cutaneous neosporosis in a dog in Israel. *Vet Parasitol.* 1998;79:257–261.
56. Greig B, Rossow KD, Collins JE, et al. *Neospora caninum* pneumonia in an adult dog. *J Am Vet Med Assoc.* 1995;206:1000–1001.
57. Yakhchali M, Bahrami M, Asri-Rezaei S, et al. The enzymes and electrolytes profiles in sera of Iranian stray dogs naturally infected with *Neospora caninum*. *Ann Parasitol.* 2017;63:63–68.
58. Jones BS, Harcourt-Brown T. Comparison of serum creatine kinase and aspartate aminotransferase activity in dogs with *Neospora* meningoencephalitis and noninfectious meningoencephalitis. *J Vet Intern Med.* 2022;36:141–145.
59. Silva DA, Lobato J, Mineo TW, et al. Evaluation of serological tests for the diagnosis of *Neospora caninum* infection in dogs: optimization of cut off titers and inhibition studies of cross-reactivity with *Toxoplasma gondii*. *Vet Parasitol.* 2007;143:234–244.
60. Gondim LF, Lindsay DS, McAllister MM. Canine and bovine *Neospora caninum* control sera examined for cross-reactivity using *Neospora caninum* and *Neospora hughesi* indirect fluorescent antibody tests. *J Parasitol.* 2009;95:86–88.
61. Ghalmi F, China B, Kaidi R, et al. Detection of *Neospora caninum* in dog organs using real time PCR systems. *Vet Parasitol.* 2008;155:161–167.
62. Langoni H, Matteucci G, Medici B, et al. Detection and molecular analysis of *Toxoplasma gondii* and *Neospora caninum* from dogs with neurological disorders. *Rev Soc Bras Med Trop.* 2012;45:365–368.
63. Schatzberg SJ, Haley NJ, Barr SC, et al. Use of a multiplex polymerase chain reaction assay in the antemortem diagnosis of toxoplasmosis and neosporosis in the central nervous system of cats and dogs. *Am J Vet Res.* 2003;64:1507–1513.
64. Dubey JP, Vianna MC, Kwok OC, et al. Neosporosis in Beagle dogs: clinical signs, diagnosis, treatment, isolation and genetic characterization of *Neospora caninum*. *Vet Parasitol.* 2007;149:158–166.
65. Crookshanks JL, Taylor SM, Haines DM, Shelton GD. Treatment of canine pediatric *Neospora caninum* myositis following immunohistochemical identification of tachyzoites in muscle biopsies. *Can Vet J.* 2007;48:506–508.
66. Gottstein B, Eperon S, Dai WJ, et al. Efficacy of toltrazuril and ponazuril against experimental *Neospora caninum* infection in mice. *Parasitol Res.* 2001;87:43–48.
67. Swinger RL, Schmidt KA Jr, Dubielzig RR. Keratoconjunctivitis associated with *Toxoplasma gondii* in a dog. *Vet Ophthalmol.* 2009;12:56–60.
68. Tranas J, Heinzen RA, Weiss LM, et al. Serological evidence of human infection with the protozoan *Neospora caninum*. *Clin Diagn Lab Immunol.* 1999;6:765–767.
69. Oshiro LM, Motta-Castro AR, Freitas SZ, et al. *Neospora caninum* and *Toxoplasma gondii* serodiagnosis in human immunodeficiency virus carriers. *Rev Soc Bras Med Trop.* 2015;48(5):568–572.
70. Petersen E, Lebech M, Jensen L, et al. *Neospora caninum* infection and repeated abortions in humans. *Emerg Infect Dis.* 1999;5:278–280.
71. Calero-Bernal R, Horcajo P, Hernández M, et al. Absence of *Neospora caninum* DNA in human clinical samples, Spain. *Emerg Infect Dis.* 2019;25:1226–1227.
72. Dubey JP, Hartley WJ, Lindsay DS, et al. Fatal congenital *Neospora caninum* infection in a lamb. *J Parasitol.* 1990;76:127–130.

95

Sarcocystosis

Jitender P. Dubey, Jane E. Sykes

KEY POINTS

- Cause: Protozoan parasites belonging to order Apicomplexa, family Sarcocystidae. There are more than 200 named species of *Sarcocystis.*[1] Disease in dogs and cats results from infection with *Sarcocystis neurona* or *S. neurona*-like organisms, *Sarcocystis felis*, *Sarcocystis canis*, and *Sarcocystis caninum.*
- First Described: The encysted stage of the parasite (sarcocyst: in Greek, sarkos = flesh, kystis = bladder) was first found in the muscle of a house mouse in 1843,[2] but its life cycle remained unknown until 1970. Natural sarcocyst infection was reported in dogs in 1966[3] and in cats in 1986.[4]
- Affected Hosts: Most warm-blooded animals, humans, and some cold-blooded animals.
- Intermediate and Definitive Hosts: These vary with each *Sarcocystis* species.
- Geographic Distribution: Worldwide. Some species may be confined to geographic locations defined by the distribution of definitive or intermediate hosts. For example, *S. neurona* is confined to the Americas, dependent on the geographic location of its definitive host, the opossum (*Didelphis* spp.).
- Route of Transmission: Definitive hosts become infected by ingestion of muscles of an infected intermediate host. Intermediate hosts are infected by ingestion of food or water that has been contaminated with sporocysts.
- Major Clinical Signs: These depend on the *Sarcocystis* species and the specific intermediate hosts infected, but include fever, lethargy, neurologic signs (*S. neurona*), muscle pain, weakness (myositis due to sarcocysts), and icterus as a result of hepatitis (*S. canis, S. caninum*).
- Differential Diagnosis: Toxoplasmosis, neosporosis, hepatozoonosis, rabies, CDV infection, infectious canine hepatitis, West Nile virus infection, canine monocytic ehrlichiosis, RMSF, deep mycoses, migrating ascarid infections, neuronal storage diseases, granulomatous or eosinophilic meningoencephalitis, immune-mediated neuromuscular diseases, primary or metastatic neoplasia.
- Human Health Significance: Humans can be definitive and intermediate hosts for certain species of *Sarcocystis.* However, *Sarcocystis* species of dogs and cats do not infect humans.

ETIOLOGY AND EPIDEMIOLOGY

Sarcocystis spp. are obligatory intracellular protozoal pathogens that resemble *Toxoplasma* and *Neospora*. The epidemiology of *Sarcocystis* spp. is dependent on the various hosts involved in the organism's complex life cycle, which includes an asexual phase that culminates in the form of schizonts then sarcocysts in tissues of intermediate hosts, and a sexual cycle with formation of oocysts containing sporocysts in the small intestine of a definitive host (Fig. 95.1). Although infections occur worldwide, the distribution of the intermediate host involved affects the geographic distribution of some *Sarcocystis* spp.

Dogs and cats are definitive hosts for more than 40 species of *Sarcocystis.*[1] The life cycles of these *Sarcocystis* species are largely unknown. When dogs and cats act as definitive hosts, infection appears to be subclinical. In contrast, when dogs and cats act as intermediate hosts, infections can be clinical or subclinical. Sarcocysts have been found in the skeletal muscles or myocardium of dogs and cats worldwide, including dogs from India[3] and Kenya,[5] cats from Chile, and dogs and cats from the United States.[6] These animals typically died or were euthanized for other conditions, such as neoplasia, and sarcocysts were detected as an incidental finding.

Clinical infections can involve the CNS, muscles, liver, and less often the skin and respiratory tract, depending on the *Sarcocystis* species involved. Disease is rare, but has been described in dogs and cats as a result of infection with *Sarcocystis canis*, *Sarcocystis neurona*-like organisms, and *Sarcocystis caninum* (Table 95.1). Lower numbers of sarcocysts of another species, *Sarcocystis svanai*, were detected in the muscles of a dog from Colorado that had severe myositis and larger numbers of *S. caninum* sarcocysts, as well as in a dog from Finland with necrotizing myositis and *S. caninum* co-infection.[7] Dogs and cats with severe *Sarcocystis* infections frequently have underlying immunosuppression, due to young age,[8,9] concurrent CDV infection,[9,10] or immunosuppressive drug treatment.[11] Affected adult dogs often reside in rural areas and many have had a history of ingestion of wildlife feces, carrion, or prey.

Sarcocystis neurona is the principal parasite associated with equine protozoal encephalomyelitis. The Virginia opossum (*Didelphis virginiana*) is its definitive host in North America (see Fig. 95.1). The opossum's range includes the eastern half of the United States, the Pacific Coast states, and Mexico, with lesser population numbers in the northern states. Several other animal species, including dogs, cats, rodents, primates, marine mammals, birds, and horses, act as intermediate or aberrant hosts. Animals that ingest oocysts from opossums and serve as intermediate hosts are the nine-banded armadillo (*Dasypus novemcinctus*), striped skunk (*Mephitis mephitis*), raccoon (*Procyon lotor*), sea otter (*Enhydra lutris*), and domestic cats.[12–16] These animals develop muscle sarcocysts and are capable of infecting new opossums that ingest their carrion. Sarcocysts have been identified in the skeletal and cardiac muscles of free-ranging wild felids.[17,18] Horses are incidental or aberrant dead-end hosts because they develop encephalomyelitis with lesions only within the CNS; muscle sarcocysts have not been confirmed. Fatal encephalomyelitis with an organism that resembles *S. neurona* has also been described in Canadian lynx (*Lynx*

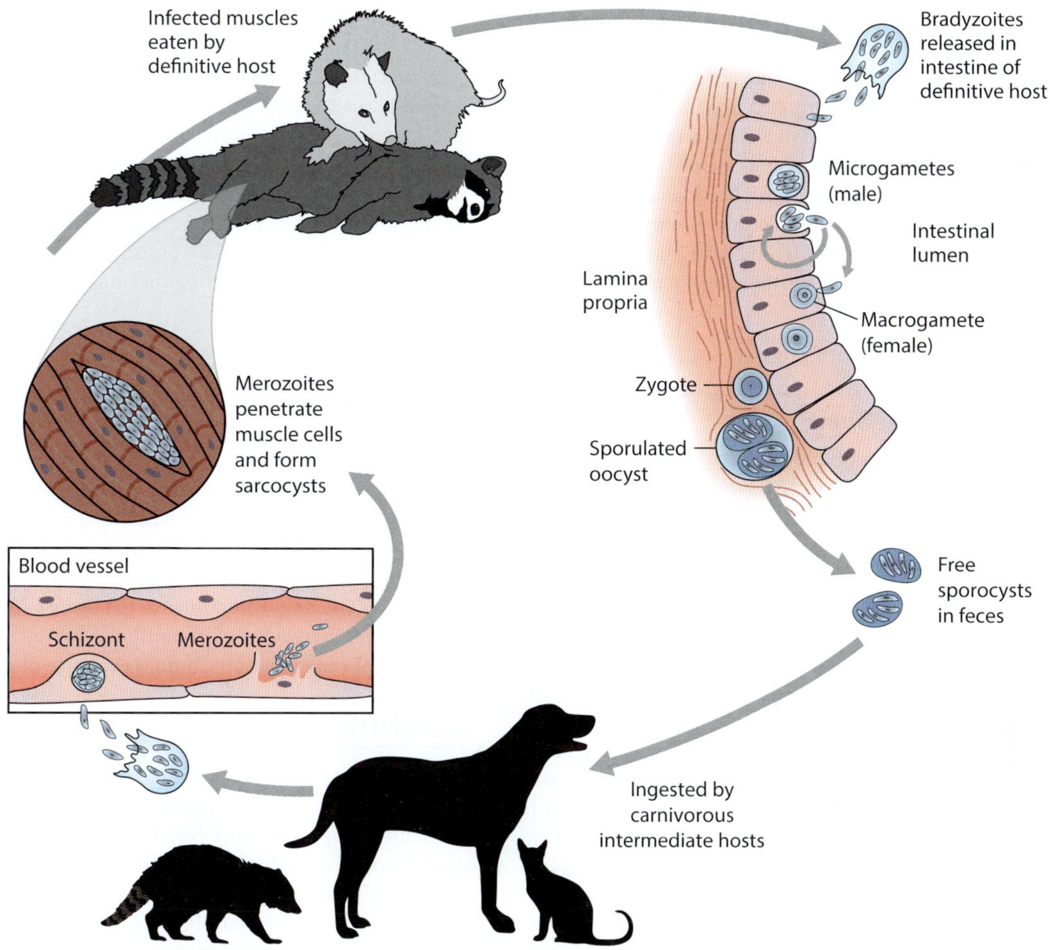

Fig. 95.1 Life cycle of *Sarcocystis*. After ingestion of infected muscles of intermediate host containing the *sarcocyst* stage, bradyzoites enclosed in the sarcocyst are released in the gut lumen and penetrate enterocytes, and transform into male and female gamonts. After fertilization, *oocysts* are formed in the lamina propria of small intestine. Oocysts sporulate *in situ* and sporulated oocysts contain two *sporocysts*, each with four sporozoites. Sporulated oocysts, but more often, sporocysts are excreted in feces. Because oocysts are trapped in the lamina propria, they are released at irregular intervals, even several months after initial infection. The intermediate host becomes infected by ingesting food or water contaminated with sporocysts. The replicative cycle in intermediate hosts varies depending on the *Sarcocystis* species involved. In general, sporozoites released from sporocysts penetrate the intestine and form *schizonts*, often in endothelial cells. After one or more replicative cycles, the organisms encyst in the muscle as sarcocysts, where they wait to be ingested by a carnivore.

TABLE 95.1 *Sarcocystis* Species that Cause Disease in Dogs and Cats and Associated Clinical Syndromes

Sarcocystis Species	Affected Host Species	Clinical Manifestations
Sarcocystis canis	Dogs	Hepatitis, meningoencephalomyelitis, pneumonia, dermatitis
Sarcocystis neurona or *S. neurona*-like	Dogs, cats	Meningoencephalomyelitis, chorioretinitis, myositis
Sarcocystis caninum/ *Sarcocystis svanai*	Dogs	Hepatitis, myositis

canadensis), raccoons, striped skunks, American mink (*Mustela vison*), Pacific harbor seals (*Phoca vitulina*), and nonhuman primates such as the rhesus monkey (*Macaca mulatta*) and lemurs (*Eulemur macaco*, *Lemur catta*). An atypical disseminated infection was described in a white-nosed coati (*Nasua narica molaris*) that had been housed for over 10 years at the Philadelphia Zoo, United States.[19] Experimentally and naturally, domestic cats have been shown to be intermediate hosts of *S. neurona*, although results have varied with individual isolates.[20] Cats experimentally fed sporocysts shed by opossums develop schizonts in their tissues and sarcocysts in their muscles, and infected cats develop high antibody titers (e.g., 1:4,000).[21,22] Opossums excrete *S. neurona* sporocysts after they are fed tissues from cats that contain sarcocysts.[14,21] There are rare reports of severe *S. neurona* or *S. neurona*-like infections in dogs and cats from the eastern, central, and southern United States, usually with CNS signs associated with the schizont stage.[23–28] Serum antibodies to *S. neurona* were detected in 13% of 310 farm cats from Ohio,[29] 9% of 232 cats from Virginia,[30] 5% of 209 cats from Pennsylvania,[30] and 5% of 196 domestic cats from Michigan whose sera were submitted for *Toxoplasma gondii* antibody testing.[31]

Sarcocystis canis has been associated with hepatic, pulmonary, cutaneous, and/or CNS infections in puppies less than 10 months of age.[8–10] Reported cases have been from Maryland, Kansas, and Colorado (United States), and one dog from Costa Rica. *Sarcocystis canis* has also been reported as a cause of hepatitis in a California sea lion and a Steller sea lion from Alaska, a striped dolphin from Spain, a Hawaiian monk seal, polar bears, a chinchilla, a horse, and a black bear.[32] Genetic characterization of the organism has been based on DNA extracted from the liver of wildlife species with hepatitis.[32] The definitive host of *S. canis* is unknown.

Sarcocystis caninum has been identified as a cause of systemic illness and myositis/necrotizing myopathy in domestic dogs from Canada, Finland, and the United States.[7,11,33,34] *Sarcocystis caninum* sarcocysts also were identified in the muscle tissue from 2 of 37 dogs on sale for dog meat consumption at a market in southwestern China.[35] The life cycle of this organism is also unknown.

CLINICAL FEATURES

Pathogenesis and Clinical Signs

After ingestion of infected muscles of intermediate host containing the sarcocyst stage, bradyzoites enclosed in the sarcocyst are released in the gut lumen and penetrate enterocytes, and transform into male and female gamonts. After fertilization, oocysts are formed in the lamina propria of small intestine. Oocysts sporulate *in situ* and sporulated oocysts contain two sporocysts, each with four sporozoites. Sporulated oocysts, but more often, sporocysts are excreted in feces. Because oocysts are trapped in the lamina propria, they are released at irregular intervals even several months after initial infection. The intermediate host becomes infected by ingesting food or water contaminated with sporocysts. The replicative cycle in intermediate hosts varies depending on the *Sarcocystis* species involved. In general, sporozoites released from sporocysts penetrate the intestine and form schizonts, often in endothelial cells. After one or more replicative cycles, the organisms encyst in the muscle as sarcocysts, where they wait to be ingested by a carnivore.

Sarcocystis canis

Sarcocystis canis can cause hepatitis, meningoencephalitis, and pneumonia in dogs, with most reports involving puppies.[8–10] Clinical signs have been complicated by comorbidities such as CDV and *Blastomyces* spp. infection, but include fever, lethargy, vomiting, diarrhea, cough, abdominal effusion, dehydration, obtundation, ataxia, abnormal placing reactions, circling, nystagmus, and seizures.[8–10] The life cycle of *S. canis* is unknown. Organisms that are morphologically similar to *S. canis* have also been found in noncanid carnivores and marine mammals,[36–38] although application of molecular methods is needed to confirm these are truly *S. canis*. In these intermediate hosts, only schizonts are present, and they are primarily confined to the liver. Recently, molecular methods were used to identify infection with an *S. canis*-like organism as well as *Sarcocystis arctosi* in a grizzly bear with fatal hepatic sarcocystosis.[39]

Sarcocystis neurona

Most dogs and cats with *S. neurona* infections have had neurologic signs secondary to meningoencephalomyelitis.[25–27,40] One dog with pelvic limb paresis was treated with glucocorticoids, and after temporary remission of signs, the dog developed progressive tetraparesis with recumbency and hyperesthesia.[27] On retrospective examination, dogs with neurologic sarcocystosis originally attributed to *S. canis* were found to be infected with *S. neurona*, and organisms were found in extraneural tissues of some dogs.[40] One dog had chorioretinitis in addition to meningoencephalitis.[26] *Sarcocystis neurona* infection was also described in a dog with myositis and muscle atrophy.[41] Sarcocysts were found in many skeletal muscles. PCR testing confirmed *S. neurona* in the muscle tissue, although the dog had received immunosuppressive therapy for its clinical illness, and whether the cysts were a cause of the disease or effect of therapy was uncertain.

Sarcocystis neurona–associated meningoencephalomyelitis was described in a 13-week-old Burmese kitten from California with progressive lethargy, vocalization, and hemiparesis.[28] Another 12-week-old kitten from Illinois developed progressive neurologic signs with ataxia 3 days after castration.[23] A third report described a 5-month-old domestic shorthair from Indiana with fever, dull mentation, spinal pain, muscle fasciculations, ataxia, postural reaction deficits, hyperesthesia, and anisocoria.[24] An *S. neurona*-like organism was detected in the brain tissue using molecular analysis.

Sarcocystis caninum

Dogs infected with *S. caninum* have had a biphasic illness characterized by variable fever, lethargy, anorexia, ptyalism, diarrhea, dehydration, icterus, thrombocytopenia, hyperbilirubinemia, and increased serum liver enzyme activities, followed by development of generalized muscle stiffness, muscle atrophy and weakness, muscle pain, delayed placing reactions, decreased segmental reflexes, and increased CK activity.[11] The latter phase resembles a systemic immune-mediated neuromuscular disease. The dog from Finland that was co-infected with *S. caninum* and *S. svanai* had signs of nonambulatory tetraparesis, and decreased to absent placing reactions, but no evidence of muscle pain.[7]

DIAGNOSIS

A diagnosis of sarcocystosis should be considered in young (<1 year) or immunosuppressed dogs and cats with systemic signs of illness, especially involving the liver, CNS, or muscle. Diagnosis most often relies on detection of protozoal organisms in tissues using light microscopy and/or PCR assays. Diagnosis of intestinal infections is dependent on microscopic examination following centrifugal zinc sulfate fecal flotation.

Laboratory Abnormalities

Complete Blood Count, Serum Biochemistry Panel, and Urinalysis

There are no specific hematologic or biochemical abnormalities that suggest sarcocystosis. When laboratory findings have been reported, the CBC has been normal or there has been evidence of mild nonregenerative anemia, neutrophilia with a left shift and toxic change, monocytosis or monocytopenia, lymphopenia, or mild to moderate eosinophilia (up to 6,300 cells/μL).[7,8,11,25,33,34] Some affected dogs and cats have had thrombocytopenia. On the serum chemistry panel, abnormalities have included hypoalbuminemia, moderate to severe elevations in the activity of serum ALT (655–3,436 U/L), mild to moderate elevations in the activity of serum ALP (312–2,203 U/L), mild to moderate hyperbilirubinemia, and/or increased CK activity (623–13,206 U/L).[8,11,33,34] One dog with *S. caninum/S. svanai* myopathy had only increased activity of serum AST (459 U/L) and CK (5,018 U/L).[7] The urinalysis may be normal or show bilirubinuria.

Cerebrospinal Fluid Analysis

Findings on CSF analysis in dogs and cats with sarcocystosis have been reported rarely. One dog with neuromuscular disease due to *S. caninum* had a mild increase in CSF protein concentration (62 mg/dL).[11] A dog with encephalomyelitis secondary to infection with *T. gondii* and *S. neurona* had lymphocytic pleocytosis (70 cells/μL) and a moderate increase in CSF protein concentration (260 mg/dL).[25] A dog seen at the author's institution with *Sarcocystis* meningoencephalitis was initially diagnosed with eosinophilic meningoencephalitis because the CSF had a total nucleated cell count of 117 cells/uL with 23% eosinophils, 34%

small mononuclear cells, 40% large mononuclear cells, and 3% neutrophils, with 54 mg/dL protein.[42] In contrast, a cat with *S. neurona* encephalomyelitis had neutrophilic pleocytosis with both intracellular and extracellular merozoites.[24] Intracellular merozoites were also described in the CSF of a dog infected with *S. neurona*.[26]

Diagnostic Imaging

Reports of diagnostic imaging findings in dogs and cats with clinical sarcocystosis have been limited. Findings on thoracic radiography in two dogs were normal.[8,11] Hepatomegaly has been described on abdominal radiography and ultrasound examination in dogs with hepatitis.[8,34] Abdominal lymphadenomegaly and mild peritoneal effusion also have been described on abdominal ultrasound examination.[8,34] MRI of the thoracolumbar spine of a dog that was co-infected with *S. neurona* and *T. gondii* revealed focal spinal cord enlargement at T4 to T6 and L2 to L4, with asymmetric intramedullary parenchymal T2 hyperintensity with associated contrast enhancement in these regions.[25] A dog with suspected *S. canis* meningoencephalitis at the author's institution had multifocal T2- and FLAIR-hyperintense, contrast-enhancing regions throughout the cerebrum, thalamus, midbrain, and brainstem with meningeal enhancement (Fig. 95.2). Evidence of mandibular lymph node reactivity was also present.

Electrodiagnostic Testing

Electrodiagnostic findings were described in one dog from the United States with *S. caninum* myositis[11] and the dog from Finland with *S. caninum/S. svanai* myopathy.[7] Electromyography (EMG) in the first case showed spontaneous activity with increased insertional activity and fibrillation potentials in a generalized distribution. There was marked decrease in motor nerve conduction velocity, and compound motor unit amplitudes were decreased with dispersion. In the dog from Finland, EMG evaluation revealed no changes in insertional activity and no spontaneous activity. Motor nerve conduction velocity was normal and compound motor unit amplitudes showed temporal dispersion with no decrement following repetitive nerve stimulation.[7]

Microbiologic Tests (Table 95.2)

Cytologic Examination

Cytological diagnosis of *Sarcocystis* infections has been reported in a cat and a dog with *S. neurona* encephalomyelitis. *Sarcocystis* merozoites were observed intracellularly and extracellularly in the CSF, and measure 2–4 µm × 4–6 µm (Fig. 95.3).[24,26]

Fecal Flotation

Fecal flotation with sugar or zinc sulfate solutions can be used to detect the sporocysts of *Sarcocystis* in feces. However, clinically affected dogs do not typically excrete oocysts. *Sarcocystis* is excreted in feces fully sporulated, often as free sporocysts when examined (Fig. 95.4). It is not possible to differentiate the species based on sporocyst size or appearance using light microscopy. Free sporocysts are small and not very dense, so they lie at a different plane of focus than other parasites.

Serology

Serologic assays for diagnosis of *Sarcocystis* infections in dogs and cats are not available commercially. Diagnosis of *S. neurona* infection in horses has involved immunoblot testing for specific antibodies to *S. neurona* in CSF, but this is not commercially available for dogs and cats due to the need for feline- and canine-specific antibody conjugates. Infected dogs and cats most often have negative antibody titers to *Toxoplasma* and *Neospora*. Nevertheless, positive antibody titers have been described,[11,33] possibly as a result of previous exposure to these pathogens.

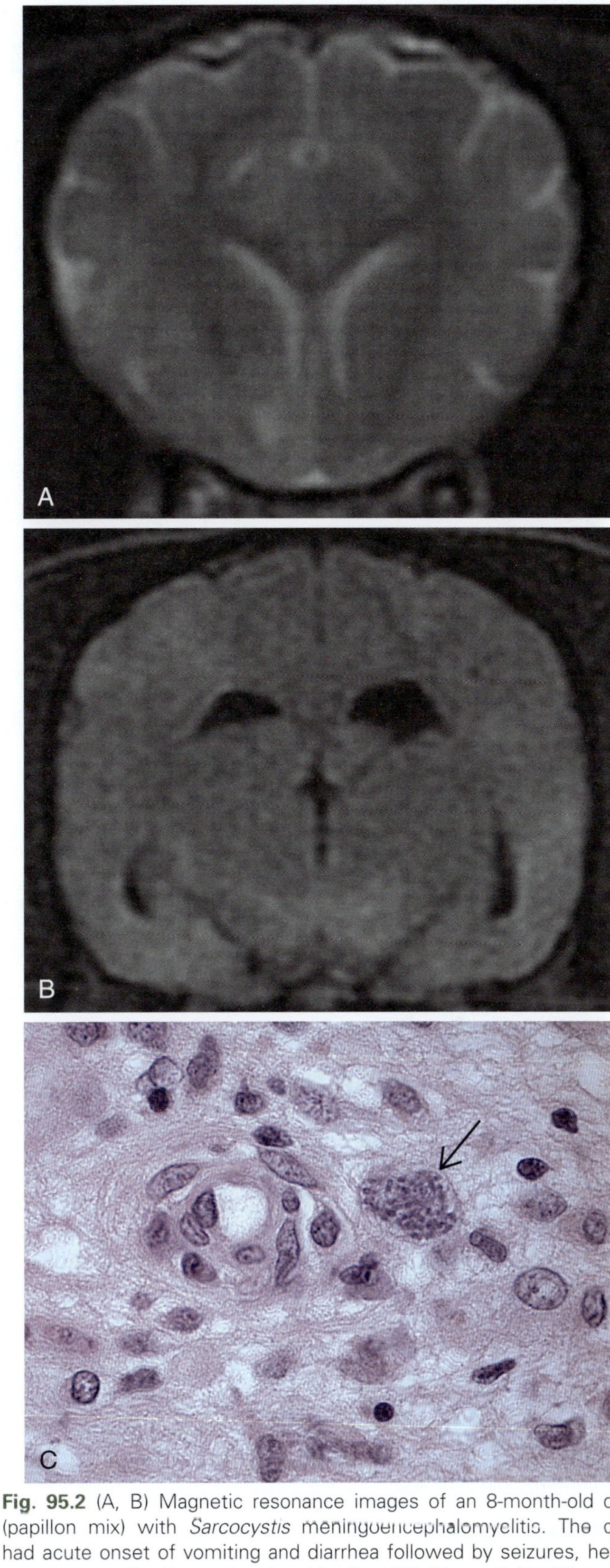

Fig. 95.2 (A, B) Magnetic resonance images of an 8-month-old dog (papillon mix) with *Sarcocystis* meningoencephalomyelitis. The dog had acute onset of vomiting and diarrhea followed by seizures, head-pressing, vocalization, and pacing. Multifocal T2 (A) and FLAIR (B) hyperintense, contrast-enhancing regions were apparent throughout the cerebrum, thalamus, midbrain, and brainstem with meningeal enhancement. At necropsy, abundant intralesional *Sarcocystis* spp. cysts were found throughout the brain parenchyma (C, *arrow*). (Courtesy University of California, Davis Diagnostic Imaging, Neurology/Neurosurgery, and Anatomic Pathology Services.)

TABLE 95.2 Diagnostic Assays Available for Sarcocystosis in Dogs and Cats

Assay	Specimen Type	Target	Performance
Fecal flotation	Feces	*Sarcocystis* sporocysts	Dogs with clinical sarcocystosis typically do not excrete oocysts, so this is not used for diagnosis.
Cytologic examination	CSF, tissue aspirates	*Sarcocystis* merozoites	Insensitive. Confirms active infection. Organisms resemble *Toxoplasma gondii* or *Neospora* tachyzoites.
Histopathology	Muscle biopsies, multiple tissues collected at necropsy	*Sarcocystis* sarcocysts, schizonts, merozoites	If organisms are detected in the presence of inflammation and necrosis, clinical sarcocystosis is likely. Immunohistochemistry can aid in the differentiation of *Sarcocystis* from *Toxoplasma* and *Neospora.*
PCR assay	Muscle biopsies, body fluids (especially CSF), tissues collected at necropsy	*Sarcocystis* DNA	Assay performance may vary between laboratories. Because positive PCR results can occur in healthy animals, they must be interpreted in light of clinical signs and other findings in the specimens tested. May not readily distinguish between *Sarcocystis* species.

CSF, cerebrospinal fluid; *PCR,* polymerase chain reaction.

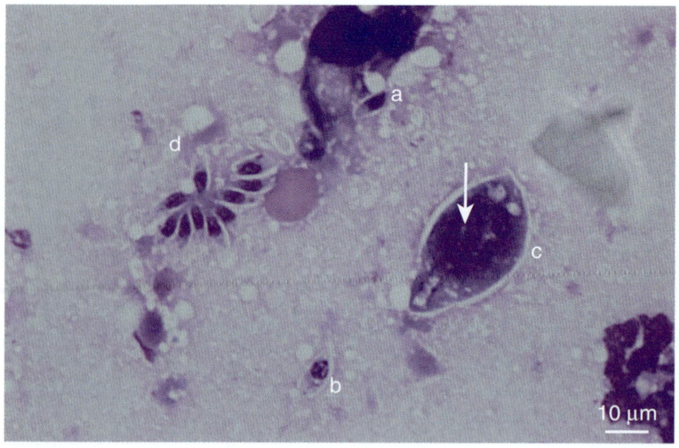

Fig. 95.3 *Sarcocystis* spp. merozoites and schizonts in varying stages of development; depicted are a merozoite *(a)*, a merozoite transitioning to a schizont *(b)*, an immature schizont with a large undivided nucleus *(arrow) (c)*, and a mature schizont with merozoites attached to a residual body *(d)*. Note erythrocyte for size comparison.

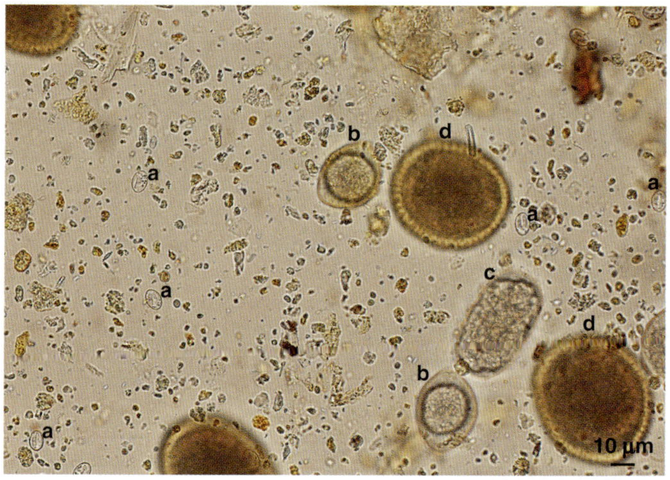

Fig. 95.4 Fecal flotation showing several *Sarcocystis* sporulated sporocysts *(a)*, *Cystoisospora felis* oocysts *(b)*, *Ancylostoma* egg *(c)*, and *Toxocara* egg *(d)*. Note that *Sarcocystis* is excreted sporulated, whereas *C. felis* is excreted unsporulated.

Molecular Diagnosis Using Nucleic Acid–Based Testing

Real-time PCR assays are commercially available for detection of *S. neurona* in horses and could be used on the CSF or aspirates of affected tissues from dogs and cats suspected to have *S. neurona* infections, although the clinical sensitivity of these assays in dogs and cats is unknown. Broad-spectrum *Sarcocystis* PCR assays that amplify 18S and ITS-1 gene sequences have been used on a research basis for diagnosis.[11,24,27,34,40,41] Sequence analysis of PCR products has limited ability to distinguish among *Sarcocystis* species, and typically species identification is based on sequence analysis of the ITS-1 gene combined with phenotypic characteristics of the organisms using light and transmission electron microscopy (e.g., sarcocyst ultrastructure, lack of rhoptries in *S. canis*). As is the case for *Neospora* and *Toxoplasma*, PCR results must always be interpreted in light of clinicopathologic findings, because *Sarcocystis* DNA can be detected in tissues from healthy dogs and cats.

Pathologic Findings

Gross lesions at necropsy may be absent, or findings such as hepatomegaly, muscle atrophy, or spinal cord swelling and discoloration may be present.[8] Histopathologic abnormalities in dogs and cats with clinical *Sarcocystis* infections of the CNS have typically included granulomatous or pyogranulomatous necrotizing meningoencephalomyelitis with intralesional merozoites and schizonts of varying stages of development (see Fig. 95.3).[26–28,40] Schizonts and merozoites have been reported within neurons and other neuropil cells. The schizonts range in size from 3 to 25 µm × 5–20 µm and contain up to 40 merozoites. The merozoites measure 1–2 × 2–5 µm and form rosettes that may surround a residual body. Perivascular cuffing with mixed mononuclear inflammatory cells (lymphocytes, plasma cells, and histiocytes) and gliosis is commonly reported in the gray and white matter. Lesions have been in the cerebral cortex, caudate nucleus, cerebellum, brainstem, and spinal cord.[23,27,28] One dog with *S. neurona* infection had chorioretinitis in addition to meningoencephalitis, with retinal necrosis and detachment, and merozoites and schizonts in all layers of the retina.[26] There was also significant involvement of skeletal muscle of the tongue. Dogs with *Sarcocystis* hepatitis have had often widespread hepatic necrosis and hepatic vasculitis with infiltrates of eosinophils, neutrophils, lymphocytes, and plasma cells.[8,10,40] In one dog, many hepatocytes were reported to contain merozoites, sometimes forming rosettes.[8] Pulmonary *Sarcocystis* infections in dogs have been characterized by necrotizing bronchiolitis and schizonts within endothelial cells, epithelial cells, or macrophages, with concurrent evidence of co-infections with organisms such as CDV.[9] The presence of multinucleated giant cells has

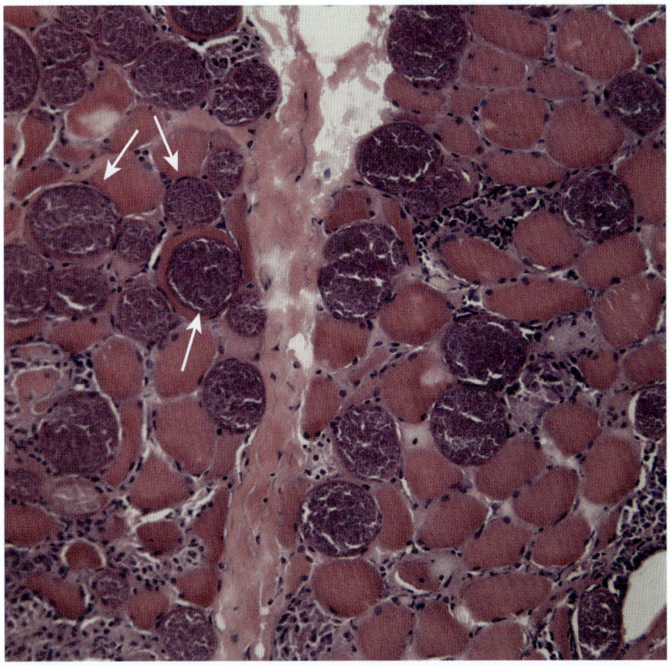

Fig. 95.5 Hematoxylin and eosin–stained cryosection of a biopsy from the deep digital flexor muscle of an 11-year-old male neutered golden retriever with myositis showing numerous myofibers containing large and encapsulated parasite cysts that were confirmed to be *Sarcocystis* spp. (200× magnification). (Reprinted from Sykes JE, Dubey JP, Lindsay LL, et al. Severe myositis associated with *Sarcocystis* spp. infection in 2 dogs. *J Vet Intern Med.* 2011;25:1277–1283.)

been reported in a variety of tissues from multiple dogs and cats with *Sarcocystis* infections.[25,26,33,40] Dogs with *S. caninum* myositis have necrotizing myositis with mixed mononuclear cell to pyogranulomatous inflammation and intracellular sarcocysts, which measure up to 1200 μm long and 25 to 75 μm wide (Fig. 95.5).[7,11] The sarcocysts have a thin wall and contain metrocytes peripherally and differentiating bradyzoites centrally. The single dog with myositis thought to be secondary to *S. neurona* infection had necrotizing, pyogranulomatous myositis with intralesional cysts that were smaller (40–100 μm × 15–40 μm) than those described for *S. caninum*. The cysts contained many circularly arranged metrocytes.[41]

IHC can be used to increase sensitivity for detection of parasitic stages and can help distinguish between *Sarcocystis* infection and infection with *Toxoplasma* and *Neospora*. Tissues from affected dogs and cats have not reacted to *Toxoplasma* and *Neospora* antisera, but had positive reactions to *Sarcocystis cruzi* or *S. neurona* antisera.[9,10,23,27,28,33,41] However, *S. canis* does not appear to react with *S. neurona* antisera.[8]

TREATMENT AND PROGNOSIS

Intestinal Infections

Sarcocystis species do not cause clinically relevant intestinal tract lesions in dogs and cats, so treatment of intestinal infections is not necessary.

Extraintestinal Infections

There are few reports of antiprotozoal treatment of dogs and cats with clinical *Sarcocystis* infections because most affected dogs and cats have been diagnosed with sarcocystosis at necropsy. Clinical signs worsened after glucocorticoid therapy in some animals, suggesting that immunosuppression may allow for proliferation of the parasite.

TABLE 95.3 Antimicrobials Used To Treat Sarcocystosis in Dogs and Cats

Drug	Dose (mg/kg)	Route	Interval (hours)	Duration (days)
Clindamycin	10–12	PO	q8h	At least 4 weeks
Trimethoprim-sulfa	15	PO	q12h	At least 4 weeks
Pyrimethamine	1	PO	q24h	At least 4 weeks
Ponazuril	20	PO	q24h	Not determined

Effective treatment of horses has involved the use of ponazuril. Other anticoccidial drugs such as clindamycin, tetracyclines, or antifolate inhibitors might also be considered, especially if parenteral therapy is considered (Table 95.3). A cat with encephalomyelitis thought to be caused by *S. neurona* was treated with ponazuril followed by a combination of clindamycin, pyrimethamine, and trimethoprim sulfonamide, and recovered with the only residual neurologic abnormality being delayed placing reaction in the right thoracic limb.[24] Treatment of a dog infected with *S. caninum* with decoquinate led to resolution of signs of myositis,[11] and two others appeared to respond clinically to treatment with clindamycin.[33,34]

IMMUNITY AND VACCINATION

Immunity to *Sarcocystis* is cell-mediated. No vaccines exist for prevention of disease in dogs and cats.

PREVENTION

Sarcocystis infections can be prevented by cooking all meat fed to animals, prevention of hunting behavior, keeping cats indoors, or feeding only commercially processed diets. Prevention of roaming and coprophagy may reduce the chance that dogs act as intermediate hosts.

PUBLIC HEALTH ASPECTS

Humans can be definitive and intermediate hosts for certain species of *Sarcocystis*. However, *Sarcocystis* species of dogs and cats do not infect humans. The primary public health significance of sarcocystosis is that it can resemble rabies, and a number of dogs and cats with *Sarcocystis* infections were euthanized because of a suspicion for rabies virus infection. The potential for zoonotic transmission in China through consumption of infected dog meat was raised in one study where sarcocysts of *S. caninum* were found in 2 of 37 dogs on sale for dog meat consumption at a market in southwestern China.[35]

SUGGESTED READINGS

Bisby TM, Holman PJ, Pitoc GA, et al. *Sarcocystis* sp. encephalomyelitis in a cat. *Vet Clin Pathol.* 2010;39:105–112.

Dubey JP, Sykes JE, Shelton GD, et al. *Sarcocystis caninum* and *Sarcocystis svanai* n. spp. (Apicomplexa: Sarcocystidae) associated with severe myositis and hepatitis in the domestic dog (*Canis familiaris*). *J Eukaryot Microbiol.* 2015;62:307–317.

Hagner K, Jokinen TS, Lavikainen A, et al. Acute fulminant necrotizing myopathy in a dog caused by co-infection with ultrastructural *Sarcocystis caninum* and *Sarcocystis svanai*-like apicomplexan protozoa. *Vet Parasitol.* 2018;252:153–156.

REFERENCES

1. Dubey JP, Calero-Bernal R, Rosenthal BM, et al. *Sarcocystosis of Animals and Humans.* 2 ed. Boca Raton, FL: CRC Press; 2016.
2. Miescher F. Über eigenthümliche Schläuche in den Muskeln einer Hausmaus. *Bericht der Verhandlungen der Naturforschenden Gesellschaft.* 1843;5:198–202.
3. Sahasrabudhe VK, Shah HL. The occurrence of *Sarcocystis* sp. in the dog. *J Protozool.* 1966;13:531.
4. Kirkpatrick CE, Dubey JP, Goldschmidt MH, et al. *Sarcocystis* sp. in muscles of domestic cats. *Vet Pathol.* 1986;23:88–90.
5. Bwangamoi O, Ngatia TA, Richardson JD. *Sarcocystis*-like organisms in musculature of a domestic dog (*Canis familiaris*) and wild dogs (*Lycaon pictus*) in Kenya. *Vet Parasitol.* 1993;49:201–205.
6. Hill JE, Chapman WL Jr , Prestwood AK. Intramuscular *Sarcocystis* sp. in two cats and a dog. *J Parasitol.* 1988;74:724–727.
7. Hagner K, Jokinen TS, Lavikainen A, et al. Acute fulminant necrotizing myopathy in a dog caused by co-infection with ultrastructural *Sarcocystis caninum* and *Sarcocystis svanai*-like apicomplexan protozoa. *Vet Parasitol.* 2018;252:153–156.
8. Allison R, Williams P, Lansdowne J, et al. Fatal hepatic sarcocystosis in a puppy with eosinophilia and eosinophilic peritoneal effusion. *Vet Clin Pathol.* 2006;35:353–357.
9. Berrocal A, Lopez A. Pulmonary sarcocystosis in a puppy with canine distemper in Costa Rica. *J Vet Diagn Invest.* 2003;15:292–294.
10. Trasti SL, Dubey JP, Webb DM, et al. Fatal visceral and neural sarcocystosis in dogs. *J Comp Pathol.* 1999;121:179–184.
11. Sykes JE, Dubey JP, Lindsay LL, et al. Severe myositis associated with *Sarcocystis* spp. infection in 2 dogs. *J Vet Intern Med.* 2011;25:1277–1283.
12. Cheadle MA, Tanhauser SM, Dame JB, et al. The nine-banded armadillo (*Dasypus novemcinctus*) is an intermediate host for *Sarcocystis neurona. Int J Parasitol.* 2001;31:330–335.
13. Cheadle MA, Yowell CA, Sellon DC, et al. The striped skunk (*Mephitis mephitis*) is an intermediate host for *Sarcocystis neurona. Int J Parasitol.* 2001;31:843–849.
14. Turay HO, Barr BC, Caldwell A, et al. *Sarcocystis neurona* reacting antibodies in Missouri feral domestic cats (*Felis domesticus*) and their role as an intermediate host. *Parasitol Res.* 2002;88:38–43.
15. Dubey JP, Saville WJ, Stanek JF, et al. *Sarcocystis neurona* infections in raccoons (*Procyon lotor*): evidence for natural infection with sarcocysts, transmission of infection to opossums (*Didelphis virginiana*), and experimental induction of neurologic disease in raccoons. *Vet Parasitol.* 2001;100:117–129.
16. Dubey JR, Rosypal AC, Rosenthal BM, et al. *Sarcocystis neurona* infections in sea otter (*Enhydra lutris*): evidence for natural infections with sarcocysts and transmission of infection to opossums (*Didelphis virginiana*). *J Parasitol.* 2001;87:1387–1393.
17. Canon-Franco WA, Lopez-Orozco N, Christoff AU, et al. Molecular and morphologic characterization of *Sarcocystis felis* (Apicomplexa: Sarcocystidae) in South American wild felids from Brazil. *Vet Parasitol.* 2016;217:15–20.
18. Anderson AJ, Greiner EC, Atkinson CT, et al. Sarcocysts in the Florida bobcat (*Felis rufus floridanus*). *J Wildl Dis.* 1992;28:116–120.
19. Dubey JP, Trupkiewicz JG, Verma SK, et al. Atypical fatal sarcocystosis associated with *Sarcocystis neurona* in a White-nosed coati (*Nasua narica molaris*). *Vet Parasitol.* 2017;247:80–84.
20. Butcher M, Lakritz J, Halaney A, et al. Experimental inoculation of domestic cats (*Felis domesticus*) with *Sarcocystis neurona* or *S. neurona*-like merozoites. *Vet Parasitol.* 2002;107:1–14.
21. Dubey JP, Saville WJ, Lindsay DS, et al. Completion of the life cycle of *Sarcocystis neurona. J Parasitol.* 2000;86:1276–1280.
22. Dubey JP, Lindsay DS, Saville WJ. Serologic responses of cats against experimental *Sarcocystis neurona* infections. *Vet Parasitol.* 2002;107:265–269.
23. Dubey JP, Benson J, Larson MA. Clinical *Sarcocystis neurona* encephalomyelitis in a domestic cat following routine surgery. *Vet Parasitol.* 2003;112:261–267.
24. Bisby TM, Holman PJ, Pitoc GA, et al. *Sarcocystis* sp. encephalomyelitis in a cat. *Vet Clin Pathol.* 2010;39:105–112.
25. Gerhold R, Newman SJ, Grunenwald CM, et al. Acute onset of encephalomyelitis with atypical lesions associated with dual infection of *Sarcocystis neurona* and *Toxoplasma gondii* in a dog. *Vet Parasitol.* 2014;205:697–701.
26. Dubey JP, Black SS, Verma SK, et al. *Sarcocystis neurona* schizonts-associated encephalitis, chorioretinitis, and myositis in a two-month-old dog simulating toxoplasmosis, and presence of mature sarcocysts in muscles. *Vet Parasitol.* 2014;202:194–200.
27. Cooley AJ, Barr B, Rejmanek D. *Sarcocystis neurona* encephalitis in a dog. *Vet Pathol.* 2007;44:956–961.
28. Dubey JP, Higgins RJ, Barr BC, et al. *Sarcocystis*-associated meningoencephalomyelitis in a cat. *J Vet Diagn Invest.* 1994;6:118–120.
29. Stanek JF, Stich RW, Dubey JP, et al. Epidemiology of *Sarcocystis neurona* infections in domestic cats (*Felis domesticus*) and its association with equine protozoal myeloencephalitis (EPM) case farms and feral cats from a mobile spay and neuter clinic. *Vet Parasitol.* 2003;117:239–249.
30. Hsu V, Grant DC, Dubey JP, et al. Prevalence of antibodies to *Sarcocystis neurona* in cats from Virginia and Pennsylvania. *J Parasitol.* 2010;96:800–801.
31. Rossano MG, Murphy AJ, Vrable RA, et al. Cross-sectional study of serum antibodies against *Sarcocystis neurona* in cats tested for antibodies against *Toxoplasma gondii. J Am Vet Med Assoc.* 2002;221:511–514.
32. Welsh T, Burek-Huntington K, Savage K, et al. *Sarcocystis canis* associated hepatitis in a Steller sea lion (*Eumetopias jubatus*) from Alaska. *J Wildl Dis.* 2014;50:405–408.
33. Chapman J, Mense M, Dubey JP. Clinical muscular sarcocystosis in a dog. *J Parasitol.* 2005;91:187–190.
34. Dubey JP, Sykes JE, Shelton GD, et al. *Sarcocystis caninum* and *Sarcocystis svanai* n. spp. (Apicomplexa: Sarcocystidae) associated with severe myositis and hepatitis in the domestic dog (*Canis familiaris*). *J Eukaryot Microbiol.* 2015;62:307–317.
35. Ye Y, Liang Y, Hu J, et al. First isolation of *Sarcocystis caninum* sarcocysts from two domestic dogs (*Canis familiaris*) from China. *Parasitol Res.* 2018;117:3613–3618.
36. Davies JL, Haldorson GJ, Bradway DS, et al. Fatal hepatic sarcocystosis in a captive black bear (*Ursus americanus*) associated with *Sarcocystis canis*-like infection. *J Vet Diagn Invest.* 2011;23:379–383.
37. Yantis D, Moeller R, Braun R, et al. Hepatitis associated with a *Sarcocystis canis*-like protozoan in a Hawaiian monk seal (*Monachus schauinslandi*). *J Parasitol.* 2003;89:1258–1260.
38. Dubey JP, Zarnke R, Thomas NJ, et al. *Toxoplasma gondii, Neospora caninum, Sarcocystis neurona*, and *Sarcocystis canis*-like infections in marine mammals. *Vet Parasitol.* 2003;116:275–296.
39. Britton AP, Bidulka J, Scouras A, et al. Fatal hepatic sarcocystosis in a free-ranging grizzly bear cub associated with *Sarcocystis canis*-like infection. *J Vet Diagn Invest.* 2019;31:303–306.
40. Dubey JP, Chapman JL, Rosenthal BM, et al. Clinical *Sarcocystis neurona, Sarcocystis canis, Toxoplasma gondii*, and *Neospora caninum* infections in dogs. *Vet Parasitol.* 2006;137:36–49.
41. Vashisht K, Lichtensteiger CA, Miller LA, et al. Naturally occurring *Sarcocystis neurona*-like infection in a dog with myositis. *Vet Parasitol.* 2005;133:19–25.
42. Sykes JE. Davis: University of California; 2017 (Unpublished observations).

96

Leishmaniosis

Gad Baneth, Christine Petersen, Laia Solano-Gallego, Jane E. Sykes

KEY POINTS

- First Described: The cause of visceral leishmaniasis was first described in India in 1903 (separately by William Leishman and Charles Donovan).[1]
- Causes: Canine and feline leishmaniosis is caused by *Leishmania infantum* (synonymous with *Leishmania chagasi*) (class Kinetoplasta, family Trypanosomatidae). Other species such as *Leishmania braziliensis* cause localized cutaneous lesions in South America (American tegumentary leishmaniosis).
- Affected Hosts: Dogs and less commonly cats; also humans, rodents, wild canids, horses, and marsupial species.
- Geographic Distribution: Primarily southern Europe and the Middle East, Asia, northern Africa, Central and South America; also some parts of the United States. Travel-related disease may occur in nonendemic regions worldwide.
- Mode of Transmission: *Phlebotomus* and *Lutzomyia* spp. sand flies. Transmission through blood transfusion as well as vertical transmission can occur.
- Major Clinical Signs: Weight loss, inappetence, scaling and/or ulcerative non-pruritic cutaneous lesions, onychogryphosis, keratoconjunctivitis, uveitis, lymphadenomegaly, hepatosplenomegaly, pallor, lameness, signs of renal failure.
- Differential Diagnoses: Differential diagnoses in dogs with systemic disease include canine monocytic ehrlichiosis, babesiosis, histoplasmosis, brucellosis, hemic neoplasia, other metastatic neoplasms, and primary autoimmune diseases such as systemic lupus erythematosus. Differential diagnoses for cutaneous lesions in dogs include demodectic mange, pyoderma, *Malassezia* dermatitis, cutaneous vasculitis, and pemphigus foliaceus. Differential diagnoses for cutaneous lesions in cats include cutaneous neoplasia, cutaneous vasculitis, herpesviral dermatitis, and dermatophytosis. The primary differential for American tegumentary leishmaniosis is sporotrichosis.
- Human Health Significance: Human infections are primarily transmitted by sand flies, and are caused by a large number of different *Leishmania* species. Dogs are considered the major reservoir for *L. infantum* infections. Precautions should be taken when handling potentially infected tissue and blood specimens.

INTRODUCTION

The leishmaniases are a group of infectious diseases that affect humans and domestic and wild animals worldwide and are caused by members of the genus *Leishmania*. Leishmaniosis is the preferred term for the disease in animals.[2] The infection is transmitted by sand flies of the genus *Phlebotomus* in the Old World (Europe, Asia, and Africa), and *Lutzomyia* in the New World (South, Central, and North America). Reservoir hosts vary within different geographic areas and can include domestic or wild animals. Leishmaniosis caused by *Leishmania infantum* (synonymous with *Leishmania chagasi*)[3] is a frequent cause of clinical illness in dogs in some regions but is less common in cats.[4] Dogs are the major reservoir for canine and human *L. infantum* infection in an area that stretches from Portugal to China and across South, Central, and parts of North America (Fig. 96.1). As reservoir hosts, dogs can infect feeding sand flies and remain subclinical carriers for extended periods. Canine leishmaniosis is sometimes found in nonendemic countries because of international tourists and immigrants who bring infected pets or because of dog importation. Leishmaniosis due to *L. infantum* has been reported among soldiers returning from Afghanistan.[5,6] Similarly, pet dogs belonging to military personnel and other individuals from *Leishmania*-endemic regions are transported back to the United States. Subclinical dogs can remain healthy for months to years after being introduced or reintroduced to the United States.

This chapter presents a global overview of leishmaniosis, followed by two recognized geographic forms of emerging disease in animals in the New World. The last section is devoted to leishmaniosis in cats.

OVERVIEW OF LEISHMANIOSIS WORLDWIDE

Leishmaniosis is caused by diphasic protozoans of the genus *Leishmania* in the class Kinetoplasta and family Trypanosomatidae. The genus *Leishmania* is divided into the subgenera *Leishmania* and *Viannia* based on differences in the location of parasite development within the sand fly. Organisms of the *Viannia* subgenus (e.g., *Leishmania braziliensis*) replicate in the sand fly hindgut (see Canine American Tegumentary Leishmaniosis, later), in contrast to the midgut replication characteristic of other *Leishmania* species. Several different species are recognized within the *Leishmania* and *Viannia* subgenera, and classification is primarily based on DNA sequence comparisons, electrophoresis migration patterns of isoenzymes (zymodemes), and reactivity to monoclonal antibodies and to membrane-shed antigens.

Phlebotomine sand flies of the genus *Phlebotomus* in the Old World (Europe, Asia, and Africa) and *Lutzomyia* in the New World (the Americas) are the natural vectors of leishmaniosis. Sand flies are small insects with a body length that seldom exceed 3 mm.[7] The biting activity of sand flies is crepuscular (at twilight) and nocturnal. In the Mediterranean and Asia, sand flies are primarily active in the warm months, from spring to late fall. In Latin America, some sand fly species are active throughout the year. Sand flies do not move long distances, and studies have shown that they are seldom dispersed more than 1 km away from their breeding sites. Many species of sand fly exist, but only some of them act as *Leishmania* vectors. Different vector species may be found in distinct geographic regions and ecologic niches. Some sand fly species exclusively transmit only one *Leishmania*

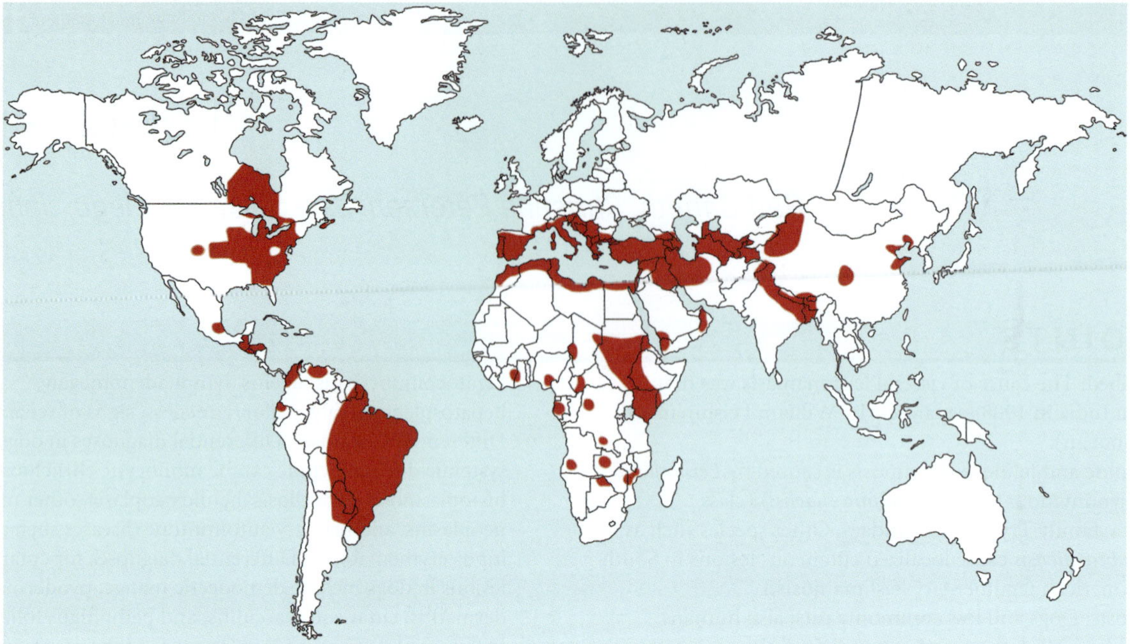

Fig. 96.1 The global distribution of visceral leishmaniosis in humans and dogs.

species, whereas others are vectors for multiple species. The capacity of different sand fly species to act as vectors appears to be related to the ability of promastigotes to specifically bind to ligands in the sand fly gut. When they do not bind to the sand fly gut, the parasites that initially replicated in the gut lumen are excreted with the sand fly feces and presumably do not reach the critical mass needed to infect a host during a second blood meal.[8]

In vertebrate hosts, *Leishmania* is found in macrophages in its nonflagellate form, the amastigote (Fig. 96.2). Amastigotes are ovoid or round, 2.5 to 5 μm long and 1.5 to 2 μm wide. In addition to a basophilic-staining nucleus, a rod-shaped, darker-staining kinetoplast is visible with Wright or Giemsa stain (Fig. 96.3). Amastigotes multiply by binary fission, and then subsequently rupture out of the macrophage to infect new cells. Sand flies can ingest amastigotes when they become engorged with blood from an infected host. In the sand fly gut, amastigotes are released from host cells; transform into the extracellular, flagellated procyclic promastigote (Fig. 96.4); and replicate. In an appropriate vector, there is sufficient replication and regulated molecular changes in the parasite's cell surface and the parasite detaches from the midgut epithelium. This results in anterior migration of infectious metacyclic promastigotes into the foregut and mouthparts of the vector. Promastigotes are injected with saliva into the skin of a vertebrate host when the female sand fly feeds again. After inoculation into the host, the promastigotes lose their flagella and transform back into amastigotes (see Fig. 96.2).

About 30 different *Leishmania* species are found in various parts of the Old World and New World. Of these, about 20 cause a wide spectrum of clinical illnesses in humans.[9] Most *Leishmania* spp. that infect humans are zoonotic, and only a few are strictly anthroponotic (i.e., transmitted directly from human to human via sand flies). Human leishmaniasis is endemic in 88 countries—66 countries in the Old World and 22 in the New World—and affects the world's poorest populations living mainly in rural and suburban areas.[10] Approximately 12 million humans are infected with leishmaniasis, and some 350 million humans are at risk of acquiring the disease, with a yearly incidence of 1 to 1.5 million new cases of cutaneous

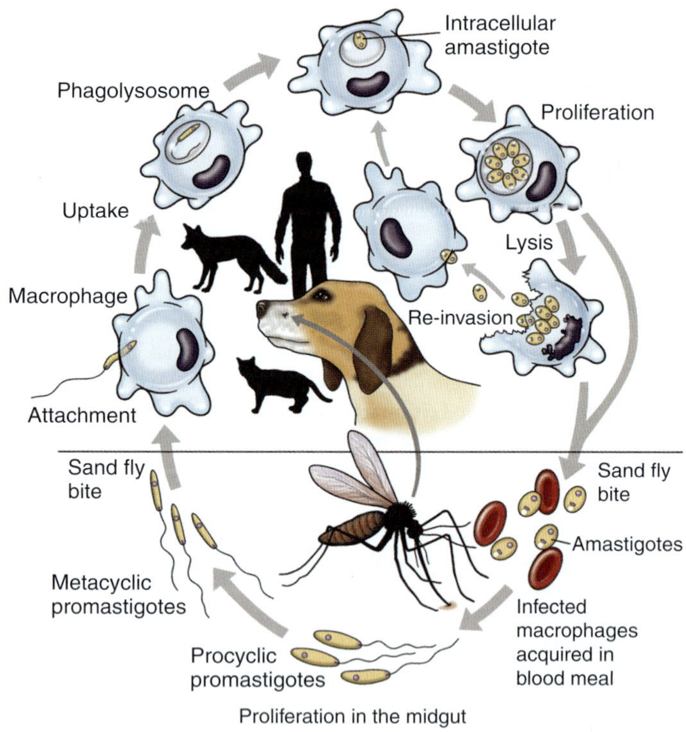

Fig. 96.2 The life cycle of *Leishmania infantum*. Dogs, cats, and humans become infected when they are bitten by a sand fly. Promastigotes are inoculated into the dermis and penetrate macrophages. Within the macrophage, they transform into amastigotes and replicate within a phagolysosome. The macrophage ruptures and new macrophages are infected. If the host fails to control the infection in the skin, amastigotes disseminate via regional lymphatics and the blood to infect the entire reticuloendothelial system. Amastigotes that are ingested by a female sand fly during feeding convert back into promastigotes, and replication of promastigotes within the sand fly completes the life cycle.

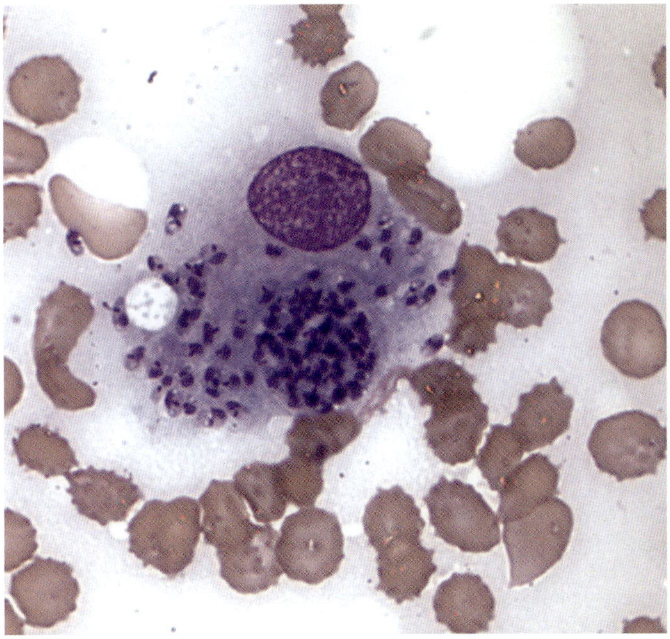

Fig. 96.3 Bone marrow aspirate cytology findings in a dog with leishmaniosis due to *L. infantum*. Numerous *Leishmania* amastigotes can be seen within the cytoplasm of a histiocyte as well as extracellularly. (Courtesy Dr. Sheri Ross, University of California Veterinary Medical Center, San Diego, CA, USA)

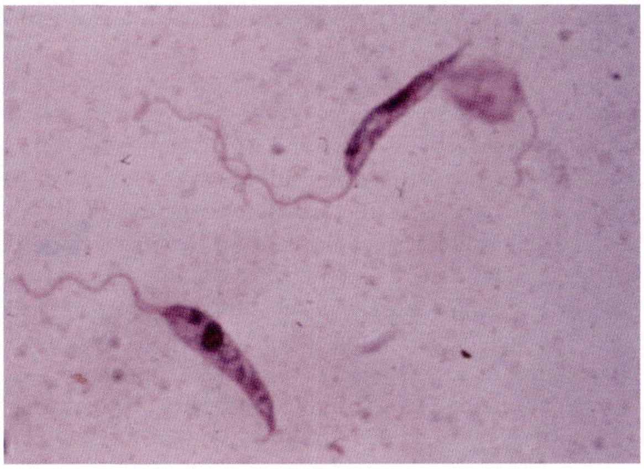

Fig. 96.4 *Leishmania* promastigotes grown in culture. Note round nuclei and rod-shaped kinetoplast (May-Grunwald-Giemsa stain, ×1000).

disease and 500,000 new cases of the potentially fatal visceral form.[11,12] Disease caused by the various *Leishmania* spp. in humans is divided into three forms according to clinical features: cutaneous leishmaniasis (CL), mucocutaneous leishmaniasis, and visceral leishmaniasis (VL). Some species cause more than one form. Anthroponotic VL caused by *Leishmania donovani* is responsible for a large part of the fatalities due to the visceral disease in humans and is present in East Africa, Bangladesh, India, and Nepal.[10] Humans are the reservoir hosts for *L. donovani*, and animals do not appear to play a significant role in the anthroponotic epidemiology of infection,[13] although dog ownership has been associated with human leishmaniasis in Ethiopia.[14] The main reservoir hosts for *Leishmania* spp. causing CL and mucocutaneous leishmaniasis in humans are rodents and other wild animal species.[15]

CANINE LEISHMANIOSIS

EPIDEMIOLOGY

Domestic dogs are the main reservoirs for human leishmaniasis caused by *L. infantum* in the Mediterranean basin, Middle East, and South America. The low genetic variability of *L. infantum*, as compared with other species of *Leishmania*, is consistent with its more contemporary importation to the New World, it is thought to have been introduced by infected dogs from Europe that arrived with early settlers to the Americas.[16] Other species of *Leishmania* that infect dogs in different geographic regions include *L. donovani*, *Leishmania tropica*, *Leishmania major*, *L. braziliensis*, *Leishmania mexicana*, *Leishmania peruviana*, *Leishmania panamensis*,[17] and *Leishmania amazonensis*.[18]

Seroprevalence studies from Spain, France, Italy, and Portugal estimate that 2.5 million dogs in these countries are infected with *L. infantum*, and infection is spreading north in Europe, reaching the foothills of the Alps,[19] Pyrenees,[20] and northwestern Spain.[21] The number of infected dogs in South America is in the millions, with high infection rates in some areas of Brazil and Venezuela.[22] In regions with a high infection rate among dogs, the incidence of clinical VL in the general human population has generally been low. In contrast, the rates of human exposure to *Leishmania* (as determined by the prevalence of specific antibodies or positive leishmanin skin test results) can be high.[22–25] This suggests that either subclinical infection or protective immunity exists in humans. Clinically healthy human blood donors from southern France[26] and the Balearic Islands[27,28] also have a high rate of infection.[29]

Canine leishmaniosis caused by *L. infantum* is an important cause of zoonotic disease in many endemic countries and areas, including Spain, Portugal, southern France, Italy, Malta, Greece, Turkey, Israel, Egypt, Tunisia, Algeria, Morocco, Iraq, Iran, the former Asian republics of the Soviet Union, Pakistan, China, Brazil, Argentina, Uruguay, Paraguay, and Venezuela.[30–34] Leishmaniosis may also be transmitted in southern Germany.[35] Sporadic cases of canine leishmaniosis occur as a result of importation or transport of infected dogs to countries where sand fly transmission of *Leishmania* does not occur, such as the Netherlands, the United Kingdom,[36] and Sweden.[37] Because many dogs in endemic areas harbor subclinical infections, infection rates are often estimated not only by the presence of clinical signs compatible with the disease but also by serologic test results, demonstration of specific CMI responses against *Leishmania*, and the presence of parasite DNA in tissues as determined using PCR assays. Canine infection rates approach 70% to 90%, as shown by PCR and serology in highly endemic foci, such as the Balearic Islands of Spain,[38] the Marseille area in France,[39] throughout Greece,[40] and the Naples area in Italy.[41] This is a much higher prevalence of infection than that associated with disease or determined by serology alone. It is thought that most or all dogs in these areas are infected at some point during their lives.[38,41] A low proportion of dogs succumb to the infection and develop disease, whereas the majority of dogs are resistant and harbor the pathogen subclinically.[17,42] In other areas, infection is not as highly prevalent, possibly because of less favorable environmental conditions for transmission and vectors.[22,43] The age distribution of clinical disease has two peaks, one in young dogs (2 to 4 years old) and another in older dogs (more than 7 years old)[44] Several dog breeds, including boxers, cocker spaniels, Rottweilers and German shepherds, are apparently more susceptible to disease.[44–46] Other breeds that arose and evolved in endemic areas, such as the Ibizan hound from the Balearic Islands, only develop mild forms of disease such as papular dermatitis and possess protective cellular immunity.[47,48]

In Europe and South America, sensitive xenodiagnostic studies, involving feeding of vector sand flies on dogs, have demonstrated that dogs with or without clinical illness and with serum antibody titers to *Leishmania* are a source of infection for a high proportion of feeding sand flies.[49] The percentage of infected sand flies increased with the presence and severity of clinical signs, high anti-*Leishmania* antibody levels, and decrease in CD4+ T-cell counts.[50–53] These findings corroborate that clinical disease and high anti-*Leishmania* antibody levels are positively correlated with high parasite burdens.[54,55] Risk of sand fly-borne transmission is reduced as parasite loads decline after treatment.[56–58]

Although *L. infantum* is transmitted most frequently through the bites of sand flies, other modes of transmission are possible. *In utero* transmission has been documented in clinical reports[59] and under experimental[60] and natural conditions as well as in humans.[61,62] Venereal transmission of leishmaniosis from infected males to healthy bitches can occur.[63] Transmission by hematophagous arthropods other than sand flies has been investigated but not proven to have epidemiologic significance. *Rhipicephalus sanguineus* ticks acquire *Leishmania* organisms in their gut after feeding on infected dogs[64]; however, the tick's competence as a vector has not been confirmed.[65] Fleas have been proposed as alternative vectors of *Leishmania* transmission, but proof of transmission is still lacking.[66,67] Transmission by blood transfusion has been reported[68,69] and is of special concern in areas where blood donors are subclinical carriers of infection.[70,71] Direct dog-to-dog transmission has been suspected in areas where sand fly vectors are apparently absent.[72] Modalities of transmission other than by sand flies require further investigation to define their relative importance in the natural history and epidemiology of leishmaniosis.[42]

Infection of dogs occurs mostly in periurban or rural areas; however, canine and human infections have been reported in urban areas and pose a threat to the well-being of dogs, cats, and humans.[73,74] The potential importance of reservoir hosts other than domestic dogs in the epidemiology of *L. infantum* infection is less well known.[49] *Leishmania infantum* infection has been reported in many domestic animals from the Old and New Worlds.[49] A high prevalence of infection based on positive serum antibody titers and PCR results has been reported in domestic cats in some areas of Europe[75] and Brazil.[76] Clinical disease occurs in cats.[77–80] Infections have also been reported infrequently in horses in Europe,[81,82] and South America[83] and cellular immunity tests in horses have shown that exposure is more frequent than clinical disease.[84,85] Serologic responses of pigs to *L. infantum* have been described in Brazil.[86] Infection has been reported in a wide range of wild carnivores and rodents in the Old World, including a seal.[49,87] In the New World, infection has been detected in crab-eating foxes (*Cerdocyon thous*) and in a range of other carnivores and rodents, including bats.[49] A high prevalence of infection exists in populations of foxes in Europe and South America.[49,87] Clinical disease has been reported in wild canids.[88,89] The majority of reports in other domestic or wild mammals describe subclinical infections.

Transmission of *Leishmania* to feeding sand flies has been confirmed from humans, black rats, domestic cats, hares,[90] crab-eating foxes, and opossums. These hosts, therefore, have the potential to act as primary or secondary reservoirs.[49,87] However, infected crab-eating foxes in Brazil exhibited low rates of transmission to the sand fly *Lutzomyia longipalpis.* Similar results were found in humans, who were not considered to be important as reservoirs of leishmaniosis in Brazil.[49,91]

Although leishmaniosis is infrequently reported in humans and domestic animals in North America, the disease has become established in dogs, predominantly hunting hounds. No autochthonous (local, non-travel-related) human cases have been reported in association with these dogs. The first report of autochthonous leishmaniosis in dogs in the United States was in a hunting hound in 1980.[92] An outbreak in 1999 among foxhounds in a New York kennel revealed a puzzling epizootiologic situation suggesting endemic transmission.[93,94] Organisms isolated from infected dogs were typed biochemically as *L. infantum* zymodeme MON-1, the most common zymodeme found in the Mediterranean region, suggesting an origin from Europe and not South America. Subsequent to the New York kennel investigation, the CDC screened sera from 13,000 foxhounds from across North America. Positive animals were found in 28 states and 2 Canadian provinces.[72] Positive serum antibody reactivity to *L. infantum* was identified in foxhounds from 69 kennels. Organisms isolated from 45 hounds across multiple states and provinces were again identified as *L. infantum* MON-1 (Fig. 96.5).[72] Leishmaniosis became enzootic in North American hunting hounds via vertical transmission.[95,96] North American dogs with leishmaniosis have the same clinical abnormalities as dogs from endemic areas.[97] Leishmaniosis can also be diagnosed in North America in any dog breed originating from endemic areas following importation and breeding of one or more infected dogs. Breeds include Corsicas, Neapolitan Mastiffs, Spinones, Cane Corso, and potentially other breeds.[98]

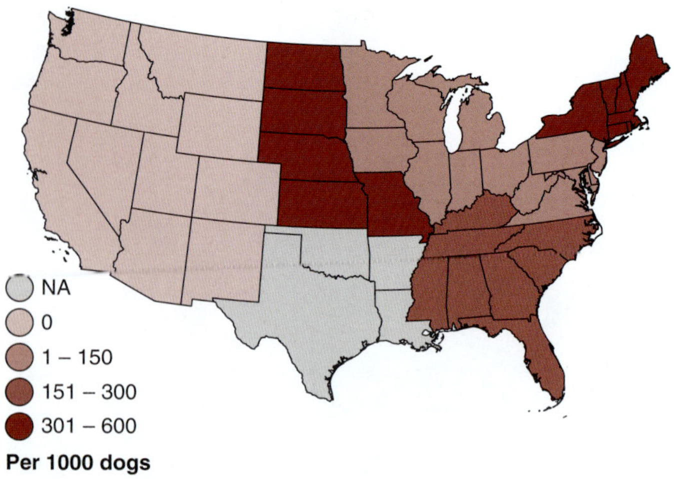

Fig. 96.5 Geographic distribution of leishmaniosis in dog kennels in North America in 2015 as determined using real-time PCR. *NA*, no specimens from these states were tested. (From Toepp AJ, Schaut RG, Scott BD, et al. *Leishmania* incidence and prevalence in U.S. hunting hounds maintained via vertical transmission. *Vet Parasitol Reg Stud Reports.* 2017;10:75–81.)

Transplacental transmission can affect almost all pups born to a subclinically infected dam, and can lead to a full spectrum of clinical outcomes over multiple years.[99] Vertical transmission of *Leishmania* spp. occurs globally in both endemic and nonendemic countries, and in humans as well as dogs, hamsters, and other rodents.[62] Blood-to-blood contact due to fighting,[100] or other direct contact could also potentially lead to transmission, but factors for direct transmission in the environment are poorly understood. Because the most common Mediterranean *L. infantum* strain (MON-1) has been identified in North America, the possibility of a suitable North American vector has been a concern for the persistence and potential spread of infection. The most prevalent sand fly in United States, found in 21 states as of 2012, is *Lutzomyia shannoni.*[101] *Lutzomyia shannoni* develops heavy parasite burdens when experimentally fed on dogs infected with *L. infantum*[102]; however, the vector competence of *Lu. shannoni* for the natural transmission of the parasite to dogs has not been established. *Lutzomyia longipalpis* is found as far north as Mexico, and *Lu. longipalpis* was able to transmit *L. infantum* from infected North American foxhounds to hamsters.[103] Because the presence and the role of sand flies as the primary vector of leishmaniosis have not been determined in North America, biologic transmission by other insects has also been investigated and rejected.[104] Evidence for transvaginal transfer of infection during parturition or spread through milk is lacking.[105] Some researchers have suggested the possibility of venereal transmission[59,76,106]; however, further investigation is needed. Leishmaniosis has been reported in Canada[72]; however, the Canadian food inspection agency lists it as one of the "non-reportable list B" diseases.

Other *Leishmania* Species

Leishmania tropica occurs in the Old World and is a rare cause of infection in dogs. *Leishmania tropica* is an important agent of CL in humans in some parts of the Middle East and Africa. It also caused VL in American soldiers returning from the Persian Gulf after the 1991 Operation Desert Storm[107] and has been described in patients from India.[108] It has been sporadically found in dogs with cutaneous lesions from Tunisia, Morocco, and Israel,[109,110] and was described in a dog from Morocco with visceral involvement and no dermal abnormalities,[111] as well as a dog from Iran.[112] *Leishmania major* infection has been associated with cutaneous disease in dogs in the Middle East.[113,114]

CLINICAL FEATURES

Pathogenesis and Clinical Signs

Infection of the vertebrate host starts when *Leishmania* promastigotes are injected along with sand fly saliva into the vertebrate host's dermis. These promastigotes are phagocytized by localized immune phagocytes including dermal macrophages and Langerhans cells. Surviving intracellular parasites shift to the aflagellar amastigote phase and multiply within parasitophorous vacuoles that have the characteristics of phagolysosomes. Upon phagocyte rupture, freed amastigotes penetrate additional host cells and disseminate primarily via lymphatic circulation from the local bite site to the draining lymph node and further to hemolymphatic organs including the spleen, bone marrow, liver, and remote dermal areas. This establishes systemic infection.

Not every dog naturally or experimentally infected with *Leishmania* develops disease.[115] The ability to mount a productive, robust, proinflammatory immune response at the time of infection and thereafter appears to be the most important factor in determining whether dogs develop generalized infection or remain healthy and whether infection will progress from a subclinical to a clinical state.[105] Infection initially is subclinical but can progress into clinical disease unless parasite replication is controlled. Dogs that are able to control infection, restricting parasite burden and remaining subclinical for long periods or life, are considered *clinically resistant.* Infected animals predisposed to disease either genetically, or due to secondary factors including comorbid infection(s), poor nutrition or other immunosuppressive disease or treatments, are considered *susceptible.* These same factors, if they occur later in life, can also lead to loss of immune control and progression of disease.[17] This occurs in human patients with HIV and *Leishmania* co-infection, as well as cats infected with FeLV or FIV.[4,116]

The innate, or pattern-based early immune response is the first line of defense encountered by *Leishmania* parasites when entering a host. One of many mechanisms by which *Leishmania* parasites evade innate immune defenses involves the ability of promastigotes to survive within macrophage phagolysosomes by producing surface glycolipids such as lipophosphoglycans that may inhibit phagosome maturation.[117]

A protective immune response to all *Leishmania* species, as an intracellular pathogen, is dependent upon a Th1 response including IL-12 production by dendritic cells and macrophages, efficient antigen presentation, and subsequent IFN-γ production from T cells.[118,119] Innate immune system–based clearance of *Leishmania* requires intracellular killing via production of oxygen radicals within the phagolysosomes of infected cells. Critical innate responses are mediated through detection of parasite surface molecules, or PAMPs, detected by pattern recognition receptors, including TLRs, NOD-like receptors, and others. TLRs appear to play an important role.[120] Generally speaking, TLR2 upregulation appears to be associated with disease, while TLR4 downregulation appears to be associated with disease progression in dogs.[121,122] There is limited information regarding the role of other TLRs such as TLR3 and TLR9, which recognize nucleic acids in canine leishmaniosis.[120,123] Surface PAMPs are key components in many current *Leishmania* vaccines as antigens, adjuvants, or both. This response is enhanced by IFN-γ stimulation of phagocytes by NK cells early after *Leishmania* infection and by IFN-γ from CD4+ T cells at later stages of infection,[124] also indicated by IL-17 expression by infected dogs.[123] Therefore, the initial understanding of a dichotomous immune response (Th1/Th2) has been expanded to include additional types of T-cell immunity including Th17, T-regulatory responses, and others.[125] Although protective immunity for leishmaniosis is still described as Th1, this response is likely to also contain elements of a Th17 response and be dampened by a regulatory response, leading to a mixed overall cytokine profile. Shorter-term robust Th1 responses are believed to control *Leishmania* infection, but alone in chronic settings or when combined with hyperinflammatory Th17 responses, inflammation is harmful and is likely to drive T cells to shift to IL-10–based regulatory immune responses.[125,126] Regulatory immunity leads to T-cell exhaustion, predominance of regulatory B-cell responses, hyperproduction of immunoglobulins, expansion of parasite burden, and clinical disease.[125,127] A strong DTH response with the leishmanin intradermal skin test indicative of a CMI response to *Leishmania* infection is found in resistant dogs that have been exposed to the parasite, and is absent in severely ill dogs.[47] While elements of cytokine production that provide protective immunity against *Leishmania* spp. are thought to be understood (high IFN-γ, low IL-10, and low IL-4),[126] development of protective immunity through vaccination has been more challenging.[119] Vaccination as immunotherapy for canine leishmaniosis has had conflicting results.[125,128] These studies demonstrated successful stimulation of a balanced Th1 response from canine cells following exposure to a TLR agonist, but inclusion of a TLR4 agonist within a subunit vaccine formulation was not successful in halting disease progression.[129,130] Perhaps more importantly, healthy yet infected dogs progressing to clinical leishmaniosis already have T-cell exhaustion,[127] which can interfere with the response to vaccines or immunotherapeutics.[125] When exposed to vaccine antigens and mitogen, CD4+ T cells from dogs with clinical leishmaniosis had significantly reduced proliferation and IFN-γ production when compared with those from healthy dogs. At its heart, leishmaniosis is an opportunistic infection which manifests clinically when there is immune compromise. Therefore, consideration of an animal's immune status before starting any immunomodulatory therapy, including vaccination, is important.

Susceptibility and resistance to canine leishmaniosis appear to have a genetic basis. Studies on polymorphisms of the *Slc11c1* (*Solute carrier family 11 member a1*) canine gene (formerly *NRAMP1*), which encodes an iron transporter protein involved in the control of intraphagosomal replication of parasites and macrophage activation, implied that susceptible dogs have polymorphism and mutations in this gene.[131–133] Similar mutations have also been described in humans.[134] A DLA class II DLA-DRB1 genotype, which is a dog MHC II allele, was linked to the risk of susceptibility to leishmaniosis in an endemic area in Brazil.[135] A similar HLA DQ/DR allele was identified to lead to human susceptibility to leishmaniasis in a multicentric study of patients in both India and Brazil.[136] Genome-wide analysis has demonstrated that multiple loci are responsible for the progression of *Leishmania* infection to clinical disease. Genetic biomarkers of susceptibility to infection and disease in canines is extensively reviewed elsewhere.[137]

Canine leishmaniosis is a chronic disease, and clinical signs may develop 3 months to 7 years or more after infection. T-cell regions in the lymphoid organs become depleted, and antibody-producing B-cell regions proliferate. The proliferation of B cells, plasma cells, histiocytes, and macrophages results in generalized lymphadenomegaly, splenomegaly, and hyperglobulinemia. As with other chronic persistent intracellular infections, the immunoglobulin response is usually excessive, not necessarily targeted at parasite antigens, not protective, and often detrimental. Autoantibodies in dogs with clinical leishmaniosis[138,139] are thought to be associated with the development of pathologic phenomena such as ITP.[140,141] Serum anti-histone antibodies have been associated with glomerulonephritis, and antigen-antibody depositions were frequent in dogs with leishmaniosis.[142,143] Impaired T-cell regulation with exuberant regulatory B-cell activity leads to large amounts of circulating immune complexes (CICs).[144] Deposition of CICs in the walls of blood vessels may cause vasculitis, polyarthritis, uveitis, and glomerulonephritis, the latter being the main cause of death. Immune complexes that activate the complement cascade also induce vasculitis and renal damage.[142] This important pathologic mechanism is responsible for tissue necrosis and accounts for dermal, visceral, and ocular lesions. Systemic vasculitis may lead to visceral and cutaneous necrosis and rarely nervous system involvement.[145–147] CICs may also include cryoglobulins. These may precipitate in the blood vessels of the extremities when exposed to cold and cause ischemic necrosis.

Canine leishmaniosis is most often associated with various skin lesions, which can be generalized rather than local because *L. infantum* disseminates systemically.[148] In addition, microscopic lesions and intralesional amastigotes are detected in normal-appearing skin from sick dogs as well as in clinically apparent dermal lesions.[149] Extracellular matrix assessment in the skin of sick dogs demonstrated a decrease in collagen type I and an increase in collagen type III fibers proportional to the severity of the skin lesion and tissue destruction.[150] Dermatologic abnormalities may occur in the apparent absence of other signs, but any animal with dermal manifestations is likely to have visceral involvement, because dissemination occurs before generalized skin lesions develop. Cutaneous lesions are present in 56% to 90% of dogs with clinical leishmaniosis.[151–153] Several dermatologic entities have been described, which are rarely associated with pruritus:[152,154,155] (1) desquamative dermatitis with alopecia, which can be generalized or localized to the face, ears, and limbs (Fig. 96.6A); (2) ulcerative dermatitis over bony prominences, and in mucocutaneous junctions, paws, and the ear pinnae (Fig. 96.6B); (3) focal or multifocal nodular dermatitis; (4) mucocutaneous proliferative dermatitis (Fig. 96.7); (5) papular dermatitis (Fig. 96.8); (6) abnormally long or brittle nails (onychogryphosis); (7) pustular dermatitis; (8) nasal and digital hyperkeratosis; and (9) multifocal alopecia.

Dogs with leishmaniosis may show hemorrhagic diatheses, manifested primarily as epistaxis, and less commonly as hematuria and hemorrhagic diarrhea. Epistaxis appears to be the result of multiple abnormalities of primary and secondary hemostasis, such as thrombocytopathy, hyperglobulinemia-induced serum hyperviscosity, and lymphoplasmacytic or granulomatous rhinitis with or without nasal mucosal ulceration.[156–158] Anemia usually develops as a sequela to inflammatory disease or CKD, but may be aggravated by blood loss.

Lymphadenomegaly of multiple superficial lymph nodes frequently develops[159] with lymph nodes enlarging to two to six times their normal size, occasionally mimicking lymphoma. Splenomegaly is also common.

Approximately 16% to 80.5% of dogs have ocular lesions, including conjunctivitis, blepharitis, keratoconjunctivitis, and anterior or posterior uveitis, glaucoma, panuveitis, and panophthalmitis (Fig. 96.9).[151,153,160–162] In keratoconjunctivitis sicca, inflammatory infiltrates located around the lacrimal ducts cause secretory retention and a decrease in tear production.[163] Less frequently, nictitating membrane or iris granulomas may be identified. In the majority of cases, ocular signs are bilateral, while unilateral ocular lesions are associated with an early diagnosis of the disease.

Weight loss and muscle atrophy are the most common signs of visceral involvement (Fig. 96.10). Some dogs lose weight despite a ravenous appetite. Muscle weakness is associated with mononuclear myositis, neutrophilic vasculitis, and IgG immune complexes in muscle tissues in conjunction with serum anti-myofiber antibodies.[164,165] Progressive CKD may be accompanied by anorexia, obtundation, polyuria, polydipsia, and vomiting. Transient diarrhea may occur. Kidney disease may be the only abnormality apparent; dogs with CKD in endemic areas should be tested for *Leishmania* infection.

In cases of overt disease, decreased physical activity is obvious and related to somnolence, decreased endurance, and locomotion disturbances. Locomotion disturbances may be caused by neuralgia, erosive and nonerosive polyarthritis, polymyositis, footpad clefts, interdigital

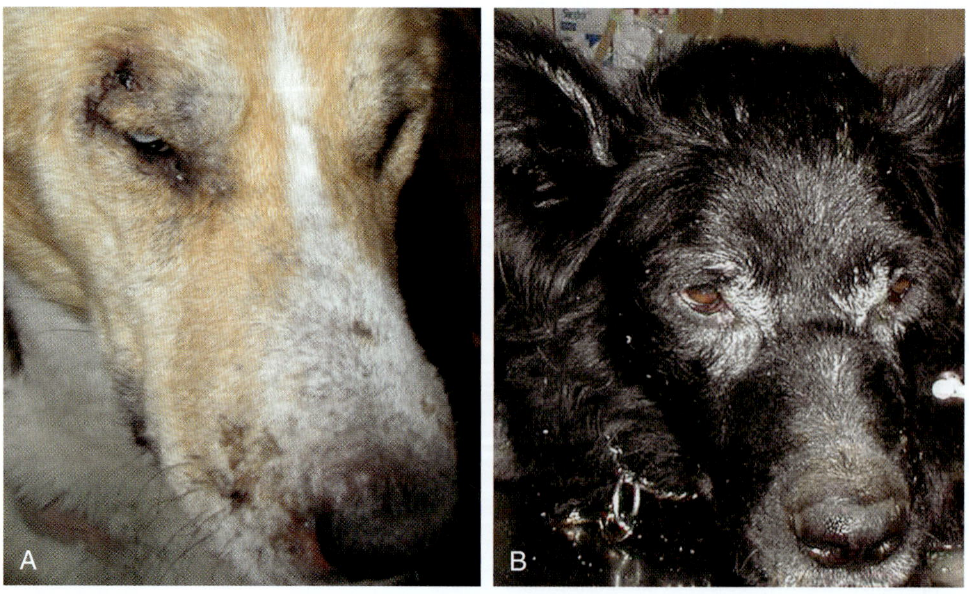

Fig. 96.6 Alopecic cutaneous lesions in dogs with leishmaniosis. (A) Periocular alopecia and crusting in an 8-year-old male neutered husky mix with leishmaniosis. The dog was evaluated in northern California and had a history of travel to Spain. Lesions were also present on the muzzle and the pinnae. (B) Typical exfoliative facial dermatitis with alopecia of the tips of the pinnae. (B, Courtesy Dr. Gad Baneth, Koret University, Israel.)

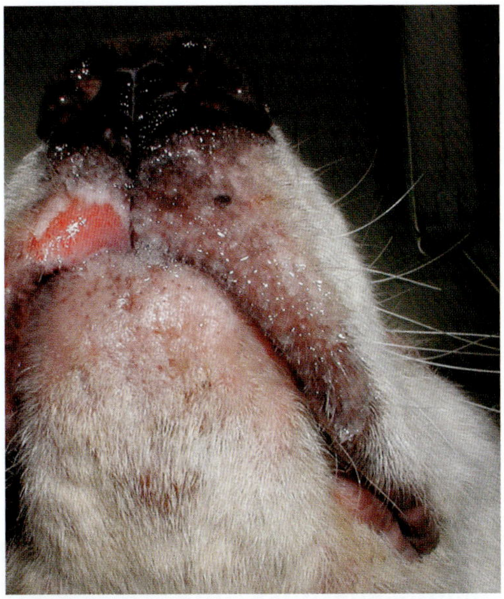

Fig. 96.7 Mucocutaneous ulceration in a dog with leishmaniosis.

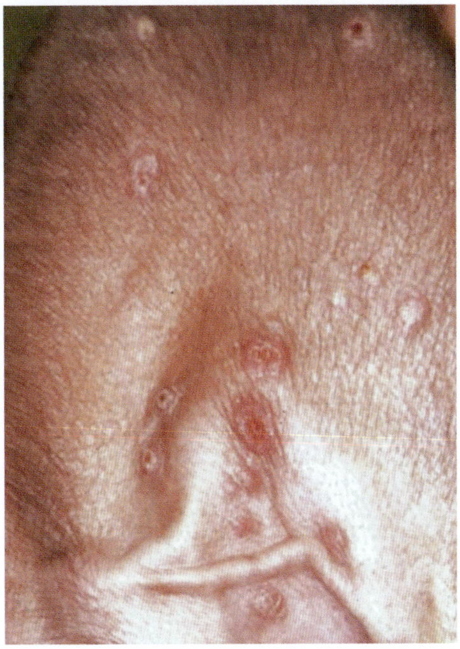

Fig. 96.8 Multiple papules due to *Leishmania infantum* in the ear of a dog with papular dermatitis. (Courtesy Dr. Laura Ordeix, Barcelona, Spain.)

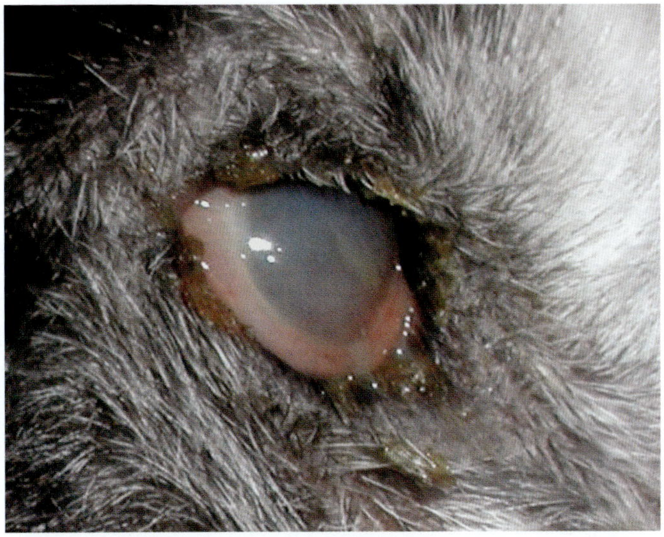

Fig. 96.9 Conjunctivitis and uveitis in a dog with leishmaniosis.

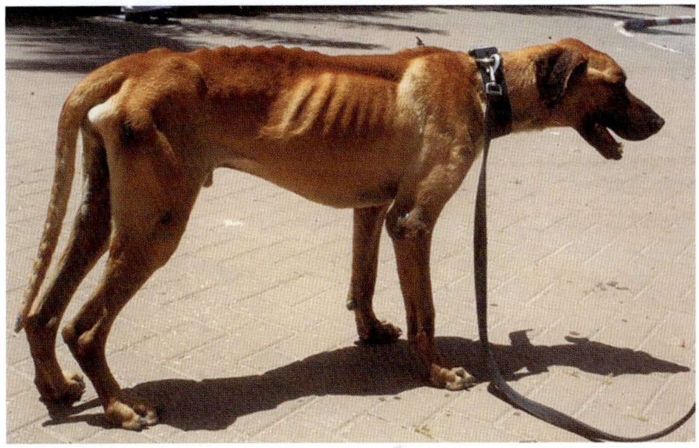

Fig. 96.10 Dog with advanced leishmaniosis. Cachexia, muscle atrophy, and generalized scaling are present.

ulcers, osteoarticular and osteolytic lesions, or proliferative periostitis.[166,167] Both CNS and peripheral nervous system can be affected.

Small and large intestinal disease such as colitis and duodenitis can occur.[168] The clinical picture may be complicated by conditions such as demodicosis, pyoderma, and pneumonia. Co-infections with other endemic infections such as *Anaplasma, Ehrlichia, Babesia, Bartonella, Dirofilaria, Hepatozoon, Rickettsia*, and *Trypanosoma* can exacerbate clinical signs and/or clinicopathologic abnormalities.[169] Case-control studies have associated clinical leishmaniosis with co-infections with *Ehrlichia canis*[170,171] and other pathogens such as *Rickettsia* and *Anaplasma* spp.[169] Co-infections may induce progression from subclinical to clinical leishmaniosis in dogs.[172] Other less common manifestations may include pericardial tamponade,[173] masticatory myositis,[165] pancreatitis,[174] meningitis,[175] and pemphigus.[176] Thrombosis can occur secondary to nephrotic syndrome.[177,178] Signs secondary to DIC may occur.[179] Cardiac and pulmonary alterations associated with leishmaniosis have been sporadically described in dogs.[180–183]

Physical Examination Findings

Canine leishmaniosis may be subclinical, a self-limiting disease, or the classical non–self-limiting and severe illness.[17] Canine leishmaniosis due to *L. infantum* is often classified as visceral disease in compliance with the classification of the disease caused by this pathogen in humans; however, dogs usually have both visceral and cutaneous involvement. Canine leishmaniosis is essentially a chronic systemic disease that may involve any organ, tissue, and biological fluid and is manifested by a plethora of clinical signs and physical examination findings.[17] The main historic and physical examination findings in typical cases are skin lesions, local or generalized lymphadenomegaly, thin body condition, exercise intolerance, inappetence, lethargy, splenomegaly, polyuria and polydipsia, ocular lesions, epistaxis, onychogryphosis, lameness, vomiting, and diarrhea (Table 96.1).[17,42,151,152] Rectal temperature may fluctuate but is usually normal. In some cases, ocular abnormalities are the only signs.[161] For this reason, it is important to perform a thorough ophthalmologic examination in dogs with suspected leishmaniosis. Epistaxis and cough are other clinical signs that may be present in isolation or with other clinical signs (Fig. 96.11).[157,158]

TABLE 96.1 Clinical Findings in Dogs with Leishmaniosis[151–153,161]

Findings	Percentage of Dogs
Clinical and Historic Findings	
Decreased endurance	67.5
Weight loss	64
Somnolence	60
Increased fluid intake	40
Anorexia	32.5
Diarrhea	30
Vomiting	26
Polyphagia	15
Epistaxis	6–15
Melena	12.5
Sneezing	10
Coughing	6
Fainting	6
Physical Examination Abnormalities	
Lymphadenomegaly	62–90
Skin involvement	81–89
Cachexia	10–48
Abnormal locomotion	37.5
Hyperthermia	4–36
Ocular disease	16–81
Palpable spleen	10–53
Abnormal nails	20–31
Rhinitis	10
Pneumonia	2.5
Icterus	2.5

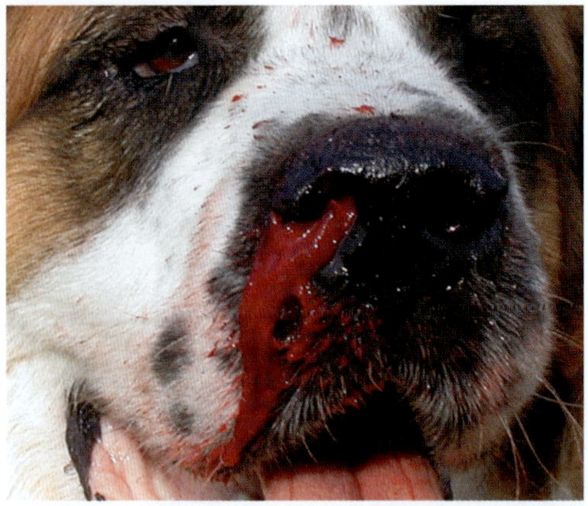

Fig. 96.11 Epistaxis in a St. Bernard with leishmaniosis and no dermal lesions.

TABLE 96.2 Clinicopathologic Abnormalities in Dogs with Leishmaniosis[151–153]

Abnormality	Percentage of Dogs
Hyperproteinemia	63.3–72.8
Hyperglobulinemia (gamma and/or beta)	76–100
Hypoalbuminemia	68–94
Decreased albumin/globulin ratio	76
Azotemia	16–45
Increased serum ALP activity	16–51
Increased serum ALT activity	16–61
Proteinuria	71.5–85
Anemia	60–73.4
Leukocytosis	24
Leukopenia	22
Thrombocytopenia	29.3–50
Detectable antinuclear antibodies	31–53
Positive Coombs' test	21–84

ALP, alkaline phosphatase; *ALT*, alanine aminotransferase

DIAGNOSIS

The diagnosis of canine leishmaniosis is complex due to its variable clinical manifestations and laboratory findings. Vaccination efforts to prevent leishmaniosis have increased the complexity of diagnosis, as serologic tests may not distinguish between naturally infected and vaccinated dogs. Prevaccination screening tests are not sufficiently sensitive to detect subclinically infected dogs, resulting in the potential for vaccination of infected animals, which then remain infectious to sand flies.[184] Diagnosis is usually performed to confirm disease in a dog with signs compatible with leishmaniosis as well as to monitor response to treatment. However, detection of infection may also be pursued for clinically healthy dogs in endemic regions such as blood donors, breeding dogs, candidates for vaccination, dogs suspected to have progression of disease, dogs travelling from endemic to nonendemic countries, and to evaluate immune responses to vaccination.[17,184,185] The diagnostic procedures used, and the approach to interpretation of test results, will vary accordingly.[17]

Accurate diagnosis requires an integrated approach consisting of clinicopathologic tests and specific diagnostic assays.[17] Specific assays include microscopic demonstration of parasites in cytologic preparations or histopathologic specimens, serology, culture, or nucleic acid detection.

Laboratory Abnormalities

A summary of clinicopathologic findings in dogs with leishmaniosis from three large case series[151–153] is shown in Table 96.2.

Complete Blood Count

Mild to moderate nonregenerative anemia and lymphopenia are frequently found on the CBC. Mild leukocytosis, leukopenia, and pancytopenia are inconsistent findings.[158,186] Serum hyperviscosity, thrombocytopathy,[158] secondary ITP,[141] impaired secondary hemostasis, and fibrinolysis[156] may also be detected. Parasites are rarely detected in peripheral blood smears.

Serum Chemistry Profile

The most consistent serum biochemistry findings are serum hyperproteinemia with hyperglobulinemia and hypoalbuminemia, which results in a decreased albumin/globulin ratio. Serum globulin concentration ranges from mild to severe (up to 8 g/dL). Leishmaniosis should be suspected in dogs from endemic regions that have polyclonal beta and gamma hyperglobulinemia with no apparent cause. Dogs with leishmaniosis may have increases in the concentration of serum acute-phase proteins such as CRP and ferritin and decreases in negative acute phase proteins such as albumin and paraoxonase 1 (PON1).[187,188] Mild increases of liver enzyme activities are frequent; however, grossly elevated liver enzyme activities, severe azotemia, or both are found in only a minority of dogs.[186] However, glomerulonephritis eventually

TABLE 96.3 Diagnostic Assays Available for Leishmaniosis in Dogs and Cats

Assay	Specimen Type	Target	Performance
Cytologic examination	Aspirates of lymph nodes, spleen, impression smears of skin lesions, bone marrow aspirates, rarely blood smears or buffy coat preparations	*Leishmania* amastigotes within mononuclear phagocytes	In the absence of experience, organisms may be confused with fungi such as *Histoplasma* or *Sporothrix*. Organisms may be few in number and in some cases are absent.
Antibody serology (IFA, immunochromatographic, or ELISA)	Serum	Antibodies to *Leishmania* spp. antigens	Most infected dogs with clinical disease test positive (sensitivity > 90%), but positive test results occur in healthy animals, so results must be interpreted in light of clinical signs. Sensitivity may be lower in cats. False positives can occur in dogs exposed to *Trypanosoma* spp. (IFA) and dogs vaccinated with the *Leishmania* vaccine.
Nucleic acid–based detection assays	Conjunctival swabs, aspirates of affected tissues, lymphoid organs, bone marrow, whole blood, skin biopsies	*L. infantum* DNA	May be useful in dogs with suggestive lesions in which organisms cannot be found cytologically. Sensitivity and specificity depends on assay design. Quantitative PCR may be useful for evaluation of treatment efficacy.
Histopathology	Biopsy specimens from affected tissues (e.g., skin lesions)	*Leishmania* amastigotes	Use of immunohistochemistry is needed to increase sensitivity and be used to confirm the presence of *Leishmania* spp. in tissues
Leishmania culture	Aspirates or biopsies of affected tissues	*Leishmania* spp.	Sensitive and specific but requires special techniques and expertise that are not widely available

develops with progressive pathologic renal dysfunction. Azotemia has been reported in 16% to 38% of dogs. Renal biomarkers, such as the serum symmetric dimethylarginine (SDMA), may also be useful to assess the extent of renal damage.[189,190] Test results for antinuclear antibodies can be positive, especially if co-infections are present.[139]

Urinalysis

Dogs with leishmaniosis may have proteinuria or isosthenuria secondary to glomerular and tubulointerstitial renal function impairment, respectively. Cylindruria may be detected in some dogs. The urinary protein/creatinine ratio and enzymuria have been proposed as tests to assess the extent of renal damage.[191–193]

Examination of Other Body Fluids

Lymphocytic and neutrophilic inflammation is observed with *Leishmania* amastigotes in the synovial fluid in dogs with both erosive and nonerosive polyarthritis.[166] Dogs with neurologic signs have most commonly a lymphocytic pleocytosis.[194] A reduction in semen quality of dogs with leishmaniosis has been reported with poor progressive motility and large score of total sperm defects and detached normal heads. Semen quality is partially reverted after long-term treatment.[195]

Bone Marrow Examination

Bone marrow cytologic alterations described in canine leishmaniosis include erythrophagocytosis, erythroid hypoplasia and dysplasia, eosinophilic hypoplasia, granulocytic hyperplasia, and increased numbers of lymphocytes and plasma cells.[196,197] Amastigotes may also be visible.

Diagnostic Imaging

Abdominal radiography or ultrasonography in dogs with leishmaniosis may reveal abdominal lymphadenomegaly, splenomegaly, and hepatomegaly. Radiographic lesions of long bones in dogs with bone involvement consist of soft periosteal proliferation, increased or decreased intramedullary opacity, and/or cortical and medullary destruction.[153,166] Lesions tend to be bilateral and symmetric. Joint radiographs in dogs with signs of arthritis may reveal erosive changes, or arthritis may be nonerosive.

Microbiologic Tests (Table 96.3)

Organism Identification by Microscopy and Culture

Diagnosis can be based on cytologic or histologic identification of amastigotes, either in macrophages or free in routinely stained smears. Organisms are often found in lymph nodes, splenic aspirates, skin touch impressions, bone marrow, or other tissues and body fluids.[193] The specificity of these methods is virtually 100%, but depending on the time spent searching for parasites, the maximum sensitivity is around 80% in dogs with clinical signs of the disease and lower in subclinically infected seropositive dogs. Cytologic studies may reveal few or no demonstrable parasites in dogs with overt clinical signs of disease.

Serologic Diagnosis

Various serologic methods have been used to detect serum anti-*Leishmania* antibodies. These include IFA testing, ELISA, immunochromatography with rapid POC devices, direct agglutination assays, and Western blotting. In general, most of these methods have good sensitivities and specificities for the diagnosis of clinical leishmaniosis. However, sensitivity and specificity greatly depend on the antigens employed. Whole-parasite extracts are sensitive for the detection of subclinical or clinical infections but provide a somewhat lower specificity.[198] On the other hand, assays that include recombinant protein antigens are very specific but may lack sensitivity for the detection of clinically healthy infected dogs, depending on the antigen employed.[199] The recombinant proteins reported to be highly sensitive for detection of infection in dogs are K39, K26, KMP11, SMT,[200,201] cysteine proteinase,[202] A2,[203] and the chimeric protein Q.[204] Another study demonstrated the high sensitivity and specificity of a ribosomal protein extract.[205]

Negative test results may reflect delayed seroconversion in some animals, which may take several months to occur. However, many dogs with clinical signs seroconvert after a long incubation period. Importantly, in endemic areas, positive serologic test results do not imply that disease is

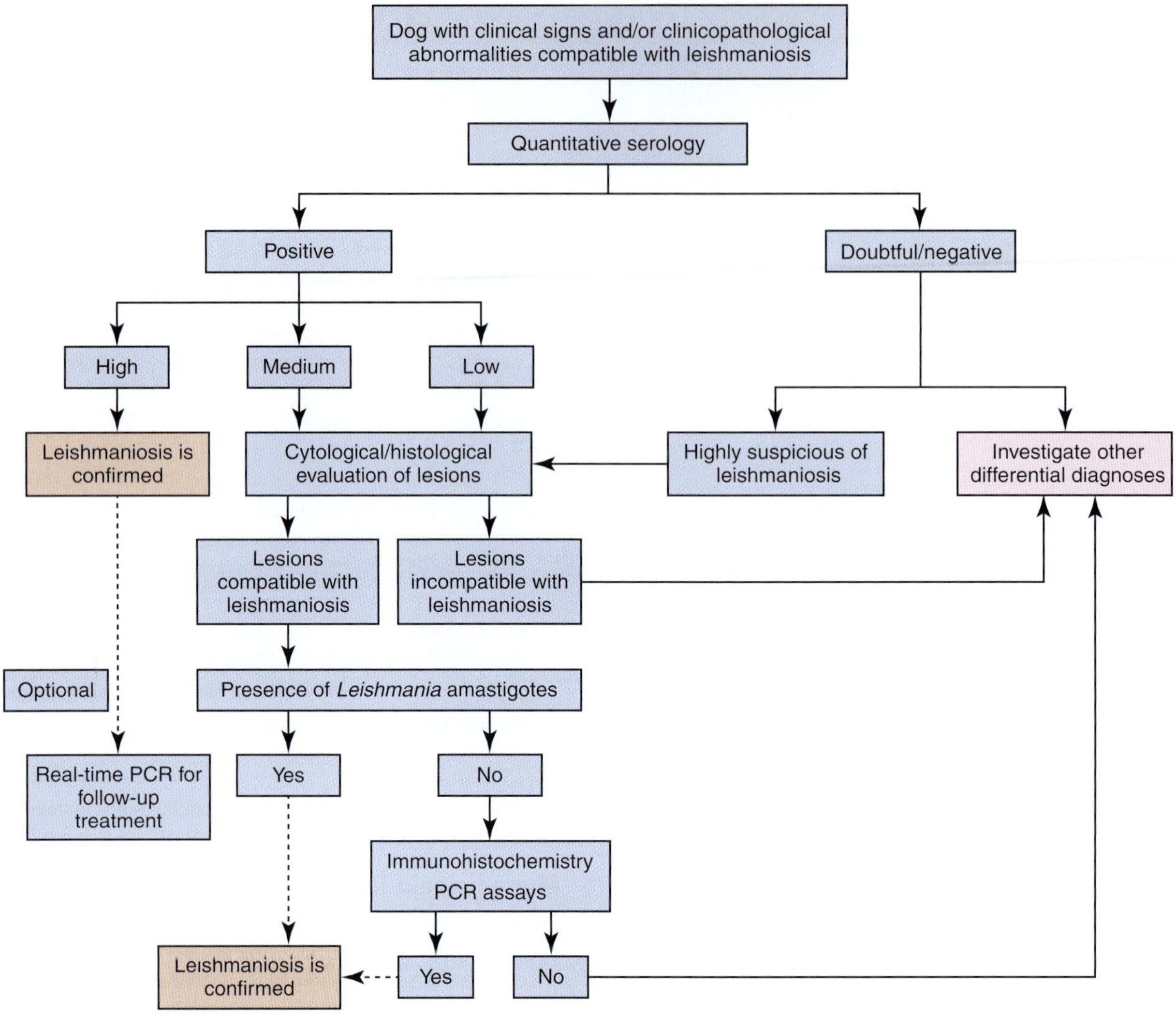

Fig. 96.12 Approach to diagnosis of leishmaniosis in dogs with compatible clinical signs and/or clinicopathologic abnormalities and no history of recent vaccination against leishmaniosis.

due to *Leishmania* spp. infection, because subclinical infections are widespread. Thus, for diagnosis of disease (leishmaniosis), results must be interpreted in conjunction with clinical findings and the results of cytologic and histopathologic evaluation of affected tissues. A diagnostic algorithm summarizing the use of antibody titers for leishmaniosis is shown in Fig. 96.12. High antibody levels are associated with high tissue parasite loads and disease.[54,55] Anti-*Leishmania* antibodies are rarely undetectable in infected dogs with clinical signs of leishmaniosis. Therefore, a high positive antibody titer strongly supports the diagnosis and is conclusive of leishmaniosis in dogs with compatible clinical signs or clinicopathologic abnormalities.[17] In cases with low antibody titers and compatible clinical signs, the use of additional detection methods is recommended to exclude or confirm the disease because a low positive titer result may be detected in dogs that are subclinical carriers (see Fig. 96.12).[17]

Serologic tests also may detect antibodies that form secondary to vaccination. This may not allow "differentiation between infected and vaccinated animals" (DIVA). Serologic cross-reactivity with other pathogens is possible with some tests, especially those based on whole-parasite antigen. Cross-reactions are less likely to occur when using recombinant peptides or extracts[199,202] or ribosomal protein extracts.[205] Cross-reactivity has been reported with other species of *Leishmania*[198,199] and *Trypanosoma*.[206] Cross-reactivity is less likely to occur to *Babesia canis* and *E. canis* antigens.[207]

Molecular Diagnosis Using Nucleic Acid–Dased Testing

PCR demonstration of *Leishmania* DNA in tissues of infected animals is sensitive. It is routinely used for diagnostic purposes, research studies, and screening for canine blood donors.[208,209] The small subunit rRNA gene, the internal transcribed spacer of the ribosomal operon, and high-copy sequences of kinetoplast DNA (kDNA) have been used as targets. The kDNA assays are considered the most sensitive due to the high copy number of this target[210] and, therefore, are the most commonly employed diagnostic assays. In contrast, rRNA assays are frequently used for speciation but are less sensitive. PCR can be performed on DNA extracted from tissues, blood, body fluids, or even histopathologic specimens.[211,212] PCR on bone marrow, lymph node, spleen, or skin is most sensitive and specific for the diagnosis of leishmaniosis.[213,214] PCR on whole blood, buffy coat, and urine is less sensitive than the aforementioned tissues.[214,215] Conjunctival swab specimens can be collected noninvasively and PCR on these specimens is accurate for diagnosis of seropositive dogs with clinical leishmaniosis.[216–218] The clinical performance of molecular assays on other noninvasively collected specimens such as oral swabs,[219] hair,[220,221] and cerumen[222] is under investigation. PCR on cytologic stained samples from the bone marrow[223] and cutaneous lesions[224] is sensitive and specific for the diagnosis of *Leishmania* infection in dogs. Isothermal assays that have the potential to be used as sensitive and specific POC tests have also been developed and require further clinical validation.[225]

Culture

The diagnosis may also be established by the culture of parasites from tissues in Novy-MacNeal-Nicolle medium or Schneider's *Drosophila* medium, but this can take weeks and is typically only performed in the research setting.

Pathologic Findings

Severely affected animals are usually cachectic and suffer from muscle atrophy. The skin and hemolymphatic organs are primarily affected. Generalized lymphadenomegaly and splenomegaly are usually present. Hepatomegaly may be present, but it is less common. Small, light-colored focal nodular granulomas may develop in various organs, including the skin and the kidneys. Mucosal ulcerations in the nasal cavity, stomach, intestine, and colon are occasionally observed. Petechiae and ecchymoses on mucosal and serosal membranes are present in some cases. Osteolytic or proliferative periosteal lesions may be found in various parts of the skeleton.[166]

Most affected tissues exhibit an inflammatory reaction associated with macrophages in the presence or apparent absence of amastigotes. Amastigote numbers may vary from very few organisms within macrophages to large numbers in rarer events. Lymphoplasmacytic inflammation is also common. Classical histopathologic lesions have been described mainly in organs with abundant mononuclear-phagocytic system cells such as the spleen, lymph nodes, bone marrow, liver, GI tract,[226] and skin. Similar inflammatory patterns may be observed in other tissues such as the eyes[160] and nasal cavity.[158] Reactive lymphoid hyperplasia is found in lymphoid organs including the lymph nodes and spleen in association with monocytic hyperplasia in the spleen and bone marrow[227–229] and variable numbers of amastigotes.

The most common cutaneous findings are periadnexal nodular to diffuse pyogranulomatous or granulomatous dermatitis, together with orthokeratotic to parakeratotic hyperkeratosis, acanthosis, crusting, and ulceration. Other histopathologic patterns, such as subcorneal pustular dermatitis, lichenoid dermatitis, vasculitis, and panniculitis, have also been described.[17,149,154,167]

Renal lesions include glomerulonephritis, tubulointerstitial nephritis, and rarely amyloidosis.[230,231,232] Membranoproliferative glomerulonephritis is more frequently associated with CKD. Mesangioproliferative lesions and minimal-change glomerulonephritis have been detected in kidney tissue from infected dogs without clinicopathologic evidence of renal disease.[233]

In the liver, mild changes have been observed with the presence of individual or clustered macrophages, mostly within the sinusoids.[234] Moderate changes, the most common finding, are characterized by mononuclear infiltration in the portal space and hepatic parenchyma.[234,235] Hepatic granulomas and collagenogenesis (intralobular fibrosis) have been reported.[235,236] More severe hepatic pathology is characterized by marked lymphoplasmacytic portal hepatitis with occasional infiltration to the parenchyma and portal fibrosis.[234]

Histopathologic changes in the eyes are observed, in order of frequency, in the conjunctiva and limbus, ciliary body, iris, cornea, sclera and iridocorneal angle, choroid, and optic nerve sheath, with different inflammatory patterns and variable numbers of amastigotes.[160]

Pathologic changes in muscle are characterized by scattered to diffuse mononuclear myositis, myonecrosis, and endomysial fibrosis.[164]

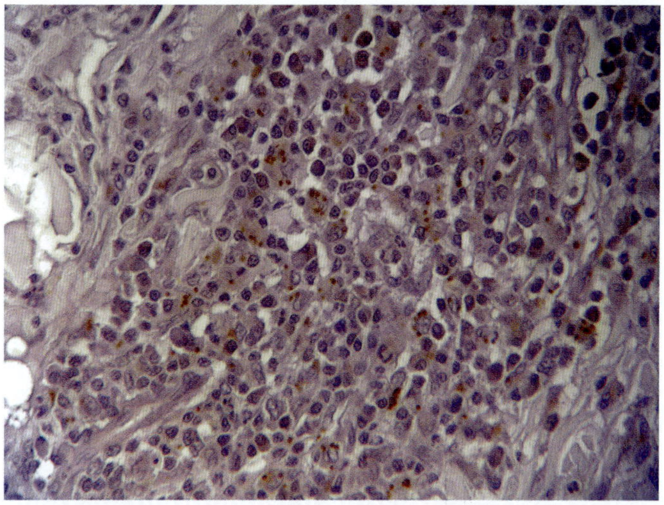

Fig. 96.13 Diffuse histiocytic dermal infiltrate with *Leishmania* amastigotes within the cytoplasm of macrophages from a dog with leishmaniosis; organisms revealed by immunohistochemical staining. *Leishmania* amastigotes are brown (×400). (Courtesy Univet, Barcelona, Spain.)

In the CNS, inflammatory cell infiltration including lymphocytes, macrophages, plasma cells, and some neutrophils was reported in the choroid plexi, subventricular zone, and leptomeninges as well as around parenchymal blood vessels in dogs with high anti-*Leishmania* antibody titers and clinical leishmaniosis with or without neurologic signs.[237] Cerebral blood vessel walls presented positive labeling against anti-*Leishmania* antibody in a histopathologic study, suggesting the deposition of circulating parasite antigens in the CNS.[237]

No gross lesions are normally detected in the external or internal genital organs of canine males and bitches.[106,238] However, a high frequency of microscopic inflammatory lesions and presence of amastigotes have been observed mainly in the epididymis, glans penis, prepuce, and testis.[106] In contrast, the only change in bitches was a mild to moderate vulvar dermatitis with no changes in other genital organs.[238]

Identification of amastigotes in formalin-fixed, paraffin-embedded sections of canine skin or visceral tissues may be facilitated by immunohistochemical methods such as immunoperoxidase staining (Fig. 96.13).[239,240]

TREATMENT AND PROGNOSIS

Canine leishmaniosis is more resistant to therapy than human leishmaniosis, and only rarely are all *Leishmania* organisms eliminated with available drugs.[241,242] Relapses necessitating retreatment are the rule rather than the exception, although dogs frequently become cured of the clinical disease. For a summary of the main drug dosages and adverse effects, see Table 96.4.[243] Follow-up and monitoring of clinical and laboratory parameters of treated dogs and healthy infected dogs are essential for adequate management.[17,184] A summary of the approach to monitoring sick and clinically healthy dogs is shown in Table 96.5.

For decades, pentavalent antimonials have been the primary drug for treatment of canine and human leishmaniosis. These selectively inhibit the protozoal enzymes required for glycolytic and fatty acid oxidation. Meglumine antimoniate (see Chapter 12) is the main antimonial used for treatment of dogs. It is administered at 75 to 100 mg/kg/day SC for 4 to 8 weeks and may cause cutaneous cellulitis or abscesses at the injection site and be potentially nephrotoxic.[56,57,243–246] The selection for *L. infantum* strains that are resistant to pentavalent antimonials has been reported in France, Spain, and Italy and is a veterinary and public health concern.[247–249]

TABLE 96.4 Antimicrobial Therapy for Canine Leishmaniosis

Drug	Dose (mg/kg)	Route	Interval (Hours)	Duration (Weeks)	Adverse Effects
Meglumine antimoniate[a]	75–100	SC	24	4–8	Local pain, pancreatitis, panniculitis, potential nephrotoxicity
Allopurinol	10	PO	12	At least 6–12 months. Some dogs need life-long treatment.	Xanthinuria, urolithiasis, renal mineralization
Miltefosine[b]	2	PO	24	4	Anorexia, vomiting, diarrhea

[a]Some studies suggest combined therapy with a 4- to 8-week course of meglumine antimoniate in combination with allopurinol. This is followed by allopurinol for at least 6–12 months and is currently considered the most effective treatment of *L. infantum* infections.
[b]Can be combined with allopurinol as an alternative to the meglumine antimoniate. In such cases, treatment with allopurinol is continued for at least 6–12 months after miltefosine discontinuation.

TABLE 96.5 Treatment Monitoring for Dogs Infected with *Leishmania infantum*[184]

Parameters	Frequency for Sick Treated Dogs	Frequency for Clinically Healthy Infected Dogs
History and physical examination; CBC, biochemical profile ± serum electrophoresis	After the first month of treatment and then every 3–4 months during the first year.	Every 3–6 months
Complete urinalysis ± UPCR and abdominal ultrasound	Every 6–12 months in dogs fully recovered clinically with treatment	
Quantitative serology[a]	Not before 6 months after initial treatment and every 3–6 months	
Real-time PCR (optional)	At the same time as serology	

[a]Some dogs have a significant decrease in antibody levels (i.e., more than three two-fold dilutions difference between samples) associated with clinical improvement within 6–12 months of therapy. A marked increase in antibody levels (i.e., more than three two-fold dilutions difference between samples) should be interpreted as a marker of relapse, especially in dogs following the discontinuation of treatment.
CBC, complete blood count; *UPCR,* urine protein to creatinine ratio.

Allopurinol is an indispensable part of the treatment of canine leishmaniosis, frequently used in combination with other drugs. It is a hypoxanthine compound that is metabolized by *Leishmania* spp. to produce an analogue of inosine. The analogue is incorporated into leishmanial RNA, causing faulty protein translation and inhibition of parasite multiplication. It is administered orally, has few adverse effects, and is readily available, even in the United States and countries where meglumine antimoniate is not marketed.[250,251] A dose of 10 mg/kg, q12h, PO often results in remarkable clinical improvement within 4 weeks and reduction of parasites to undetectable numbers. However, relapses may occur once therapy has been discontinued or while still on treatment due to selection for allopurinol resistance.[252] Even after conscientious administration of the drug for 6 months, complete recovery is rare,[253] and deterioration of kidney function may continue during allopurinol therapy despite resolution of dermal lesions and general improvement in the clinical condition. Use of allopurinol causes hyperxanthinuria, which may occasionally produce urolithiasis. Combined treatment with meglumine antimoniate and allopurinol is considered as the most effective therapy and constitutes the most frequently used protocol against the disease.[17,185] The combination is administered for 4 to 8 weeks, followed by continuation with allopurinol alone usually for at least 12 months.[254]

Miltefosine (see Chapter 12) is an alkylphospholipid with a direct toxic effect on *Leishmania* parasites that is effective for the treatment of human VL and has been introduced for use in veterinary medicine.[255,256] It is administered to dogs at 2 mg/kg/day PO for 4 weeks and is an alternative to meglumine antimoniate when combined with long-term allopurinol therapy.[243,257,258] In North America, miltefosine can be purchased from Profounda Pharmaceuticals (Orlando, FL, USA).

Additional drugs that are not recommended as first-line therapy for canine leishmaniosis because of the adverse effects associated with treatment include pentamidine, amphotericin B (AMB), and aminosidine.[259,260] Other drugs that have been evaluated for antileishmanial efficacy in dogs include ketoconazole, metronidazole and spiramycin, and marbofloxacin.[185] In a trial comparing the efficacy of conventional treatment with meglumine antimoniate and allopurinol against use of metronidazole and spiramycin, treated dogs showed some clinical improvement without a parasitologic cure, similar to control dogs.[261]

Additional treatment with immune system modulators for the prevention of disease progression is reviewed elsewhere[262] and includes dietary supplementation of nucleotides and active hexose as an adjunctive therapy.[263,264]

If dogs are seriously ill, and especially if they are in severe renal failure, it may be necessary to restore fluid and acid-base balances before antileishmanial drugs are administered. The prognosis of leishmaniosis depends on the severity of injury to the dog's systems at the time of diagnosis and the dog's individual response and rate of deterioration. In dogs that have not reached a progressive state of renal failure, treatment frequently significantly improves dermal and visceral signs of the disease. Immune responses were monitored in dogs before and after treatment and have indicated that in some cases, parasite-specific CMI that is absent before therapy is regained after drug administration but may deteriorate again during a clinical relapse.[260,265]

TABLE 96.6 Clinical Staging of Canine Leishmaniosis[184]

Clinical Stages (Antibody Levels[a])	Clinical Signs	Laboratory Abnormalities	Treatment and Prognosis
Stage I: mild disease (negative to low positive)	Mild localized peripheral lymphadenomegaly or papular dermatitis	Usually none Renal profile results within reference limits[b]	No treatment or treatment with a single drug or two combined drugs (allopurinol, meglumine antimoniate, or miltefosine)[c] Prognosis: good
Stage II: moderate disease (low to high positive)	Stage I signs *plus* diffuse or symmetric cutaneous lesions such as exfoliative dermatitis, onychogryphosis, ulcerations (planum nasale, footpads, bony prominences, mucocutaneous junctions), anorexia, weight loss, fever, and epistaxis, among others	Mild nonregenerative anemia, hypergammaglobulinemia, hypoalbuminemia Substage: a) No abnormalities in renal profile: no proteinuria b) Creatinine < 1.4 mg/dL; UPCR = 0.5–1	Allopurinol + meglumine antimoniate or miltefosine Prognosis: good to guarded
Stage III: severe disease (medium to high positive)	Stage I or II signs *plus* immune-complex lesions such as vasculitis, arthritis, uveitis, and glomerulonephritis.	Signs of stage II *and* CKD IRIS stage I with UPCR > 1 or stage II (creatinine 1.4–2 mg/dL)	Treatment: allopurinol + meglumine antimoniate or miltefosine Follow IRIS guidelines for CKD Prognosis: guarded to poor
Stage IV: very severe disease (medium to high positive)	Signs up through stage III *plus* pulmonary thromboembolism, or nephrotic syndrome and end-stage renal disease	Stage II signs *plus* CKD IRIS stage III (creatinine 2–5 mg/dL) and stage IV (creatinine > 5 mg/dL)[d] Nephrotic syndrome: marked proteinuria UPCR > 5	Specific treatment should be instituted based on individual case considerations. Follow IRIS guidelines for CKD Prognosis: poor

[a]Dogs with negative to medium-positive antibody levels should be confirmed as infected with other diagnostic techniques such as cytology, histology (preferably with immunohistochemistry), or PCR. High antibody titers in a sick dog, which was not previously vaccinated, with compatible signs and/or laboratory abnormalities are conclusive of a diagnosis of leishmaniosis and are defined as a three- to four-fold increase above the reference cutoff level in a well-established laboratory.

[b]Reference interval: creatinine < 1.4 mg/dL; UPCR < 0.5.

[c]Dogs in stage I (mild disease) are likely to require less prolonged treatment with one or two combined drugs (allopurinol, domperidone, meglumine antimoniate, or miltefosine) or alternatively monitoring with no treatment. There is limited information on dogs in this stage and, therefore, treatment options remain to be defined.

[d]IRIS (2022) http://www.iris-kidney.com/guidelines/index.html Accessed 4/9/2022.

CKD, chronic kidney disease; *IRIS*, International Renal Interest Society; *UPCR*, urine protein to creatinine ratio.

Staging

A clinical staging system for canine leishmaniosis divides the disease into four clinical stages from mild to very severe disease based on clinical signs, clinical laboratory abnormalities, and level of serum anti-*Leishmania* antibodies.[184] This system is helpful for decisions on the therapy most suitable for each patient and for consideration of a prognosis (Table 96.6). The clinical stage may change if the clinical health of the dog deteriorates or improves.

PREVENTION

Efforts to control leishmaniosis in the canine populations in some endemic countries are controversial and generally have not been considered to be successful.[50,266–269] Culling sick and seropositive dogs is obviously unacceptable to the owners, but it is also ineffective in controlling spread of the disease because subclinically infected dogs, and possibly wild canids are additional sources of parasite transmission. Furthermore, available methods for testing do not identify all infected dogs, and a population of young susceptible puppies can replace the culled animals.[43,268] Spraying for sand fly vectors and eradicating their presumptive breeding places has limited effectiveness in preventing spread of the disease. No prophylactic drug has yet been shown to be effective against infection, and medical treatment of infected dogs with antileishmanial drugs is ineffective in eliminating the parasite.

Sand fly bites can be reduced by keeping dogs indoors during the sand fly season from dusk to dawn, avoiding microhabitats favorable to sand flies in the location where the dog spends time, and using environmental insecticides and topical insecticides.[270] Topical insecticides for protecting dogs against sand fly bites include solutions, spot-on tubes, sprays, and collars. A spot-on containing imidacloprid and permethrin is recommended for dogs every 3 to 4 weeks for repelling sand flies.[271–273] Deltamethrin-impregnated collars (see Chapter 13) can protect dogs for about 8 months from more than 90% of bites from *Phlebotomus perniciosus*, the primary vector of *L. infantum* in France, Italy, and Spain; and *Lu. longipalpis*, a major South American vector.[274–276] A controlled study on the effect of using collars on dogs in a focus of VL in Iran indicated that the seroconversion rate after 1 year in dogs and children was significantly lower in intervention villages than in control villages.[277] Topical insecticide protection is valuable for dogs in endemic regions during transmission seasons and for dogs traveling to these areas. Use of collars or spot-on formulations on client-owned infected dogs treated medically and living in infected areas is warranted.

Commercial vaccines to protect dogs against canine leishmaniosis are available and widely used in Brazil and Europe. Vaccination decreases the occurrence of clinical disease, however, may not be as successful in preventing infection.[184,243,278] Domperidone is a dopamine D2 receptor agonist reported to act by the stimulation of prolactin secretion which acts as a pro-inflammatory cytokine. It is also used as a prophylactic treatment in dogs in some European countries.[279] An integrated control approach that combines vaccination with the application of topical insecticides could reduce the burden of infection in dog populations in endemic countries.[243] There is no licensed vaccine against leishmaniosis for veterinary use in the United States. Euthanasia has been promoted to prevent leishmaniosis from becoming established in North America in settings where large numbers of dogs are infected in kennel situations.

PUBLIC HEALTH CONSIDERATIONS

VL is a serious human disease that may be fatal if untreated. Malnutrition predisposes to progression of infection.[10,280,281] Traditionally, VL primarily affected young children and infants, but now it is also often a complication in adults infected with HIV or those receiving cytostatic or immunosuppressive drugs.[116,282]

Transmission of *L. infantum* from dogs to humans via sand flies is the primary route of infection. Several studies have investigated the association between canine and human leishmaniosis in the same region.[185] Increased prevalence of infection in the dog population is associated with increased incidence of human leishmaniosis.[283] Poor socioeconomic conditions are risk factors for the association between canine and human infections,[282] and dog density and infected dog ownership are risk factors for infantile human leishmaniosis.[32,284,285] The link between dog and human infections probably differs from one region and lifestyle to another and could depend on multiple factors including human nutrition, time spent outdoors, the density of dogs, and the behavior of sand fly vectors. In southern Europe, where human disease is often sporadic and the ratio between clinically affected humans and infected dogs is low, ownership of dogs is usually not perceived as being associated with an increased risk to humans. Despite this, studies from Europe have established linkage between human and canine infection at the population level.[284] Effective control of canine leishmaniosis could lead to a decrease in human leishmaniosis in endemic regions. Control measures of canine leishmaniosis include vaccines, topical insecticides, and environmental control of sand flies.[286]

Transmission by direct contact between dogs and humans is speculated to be rare, if it occurs at all. Transmission of *L. infantum* through blood products has been reported in dogs that received blood transfusions from infected canine donors and in humans.[69] Studies in Spain have documented transmission among IV drug users as a result of shared needle use.[287] Therefore, direct contact with contaminated hypodermic needles or with open wounds or exudates from dogs with leishmaniosis should be avoided.

Direct blood-to-blood transmission would likely pose a far smaller risk to humans than transmission by insects such as sand flies. However, as sand flies are able to transmit *L. infantum* from infected to susceptible dogs in North America, zoonotic vector transmission might be possible.[103,288]

Infected pets may remain disease carriers despite treatment. In areas where sand fly vectors are found, this poses a concern to owners, veterinarians, and local public health and environmental agencies. Before deciding on the fate of an infected pet, owners should be consulted and educated about the disease, its zoonotic nature, the prognosis for their dog, what should be expected from therapy, and safety precautions that should be taken. A clear, official policy based on relevant research and a calculated estimation of the risk to the community is desirable.

CANINE AMERICAN TEGUMENTARY LEISHMANIOSIS

American cutaneous (tegumentary) leishmaniosis (ATL) is caused by multiple *Leishmania* species that belong to the subgenus *Viannia*. These include *L. braziliensis*, *L. mexicana* and *L. peruviana*. The condition affects dogs and humans in Latin America; infection in dogs has been reported from Brazil, Argentina, Bolivia, Peru, Ecuador, Colombia, Venezuela, and Panama. *Leishmania braziliensis* is the most widespread *Leishmania* species causing ATL in South America.[289–291] Outbreaks of ATL have been associated with jungle deforestation.[292]

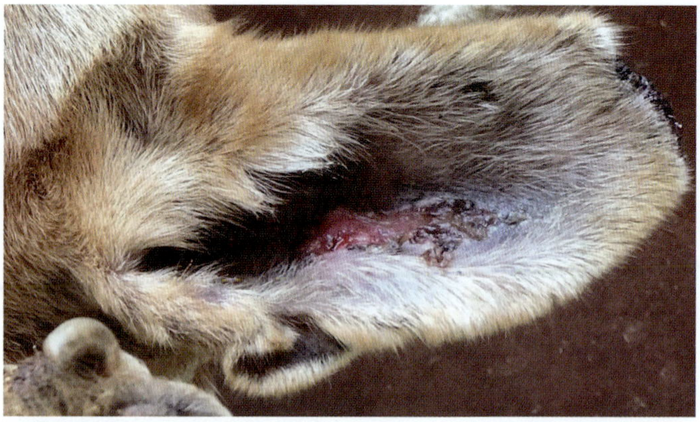

Fig. 96.14 Pinnal ulceration in a dog infected with *Leishmania braziliensis* from the northeast of Brazil.

The clinical signs of disease in dogs include single, double, or less commonly multiple chronic ulcerative lesions on the ears, scrotum, muzzle, face, or other areas of the skin, mucocutaneous erosive lesions in the mouth and nasal mucosa, and lymphadenomegaly (Fig. 96.14).[293–297] Anemia, hypoalbuminemia, and hyperglobulinemia are common clinicopathologic findings.[296] Sporotrichosis is an important differential diagnosis (see Chapter 84).[296] Diagnosis can be confirmed by microscopic detection of parasites, by serologic tests, or nucleic acid–based assays (see Table 96.3). On histopathology, a granulomatous inflammatory infiltrate is observed in the dermis, frequently without detectable parasites or in the presence of low numbers of amastigotes; however, a high percentage of dermal lesions are positive for parasites by culture.[298] It is more difficult to detect the organism in samples from hemolymphatic tissues or normal skin.[295,298] Co-infection with *L. braziliensis* and *L. infantum* has been reported in regions where both infections are endemic and poses a diagnostic challenge.[299,300] Sick dogs with ATL commonly have low levels of anti-*Leishmania* antibodies as compared to dogs with clinical visceral disease due to *L. infantum*. To add to the diagnostic challenges, several species of *Trypanosoma* are endemic in South America,[301] which can be associated with serologic cross-reactivity.[295] Reliable species-specific diagnostic assays that employ quantitative and/or recombinant antigen serologic tests,[302,303] discriminatory nucleic acid–based assays,[304] or culture are required for accurate diagnosis. The majority of infected dogs respond to systemic antimonial therapy, but they remain infected after therapy and commonly have clinical relapses.[136] Intralesional antimonial therapy has been reported to be beneficial in providing clinical improvement and limiting disease relapse.[305] Limited information is available about treatment of ATL and, therefore, the most adequate therapeutic protocol remains unclear. Numerous wildlife species including opossums and rodents can be infected with agents of ATL. Although dogs can be infected, their role as a reservoir host for human ATL is controversial.[291,306,307]

FELINE LEISHMANIOSIS

Laia Solano-Gallego and Gad Baneth

ETIOLOGY AND EPIDEMIOLOGY

Leishmania infection in a domestic cat was first described in 1912 in Algeria from the bone marrow of a 4-month-old kitten living in the same house where a dog and a child were affected by leishmaniosis.[308] Since then, clinical disease and subclinical infections have been reported sporadically in the following regions and countries where canine leishmaniosis is endemic: southern Europe, North Africa, the Middle East, and Central and South America. Clinical leishmaniosis in domestic cats has been reported to involve *L. infantum* in Europe, the Middle East, and Brazil,[80,309,310] *L. mexicana* in Texas[311] and Venezuela, and *L. braziliensis*[312] and *L. amazonensis*[313] in Brazil.

Serologic and PCR surveys of cat populations in canine leishmaniosis–endemic regions in southern Europe[75,221,314,315] and the Middle East[175] indicate that feline infection is more widespread than clinical disease. Epidemiologic studies have described seroprevalence rates ranging from 0.9% to 28%.[75,314,316,317] PCR studies on blood samples have shown rates of infection from 0.43% to 30%.[75,314,315,318,319] The true role of the cat as a reservoir of *L. infantum* infection remains unclear. Transmission of *L. infantum* to sand flies (*P. perniciosus*) from a chronically infected cat under experimental conditions has been reported.[320]

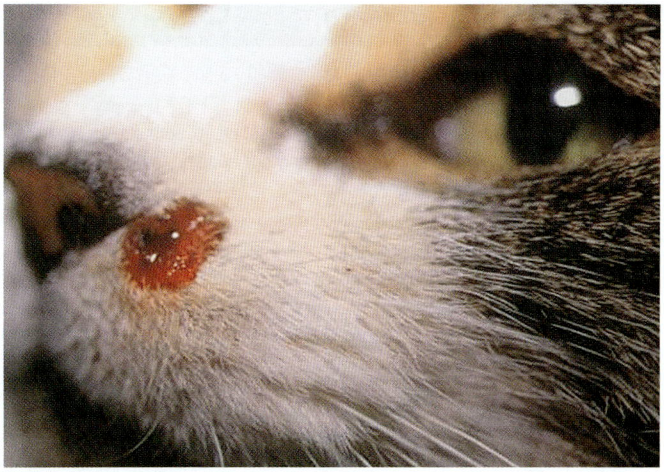

Fig. 96.15 Cutaneous ulcer in cat with leishmaniosis. (Courtesy Prof. Maria Grazia Pennisi, University of Messina, Messina, Italy.)

CLINICAL FINDINGS

The most frequently described lesions in feline leishmaniosis caused by *L. infantum* are ulcerous crusting and nodular dermatitis, alopecia, and scaling predominantly affecting the face and ears (Fig. 96.15).[77–80] Visceral forms of disease with spleen, liver, bone marrow, lymph node, uvea, and kidney involvement have been less commonly described and are thought to be associated with immunosuppression caused by FeLV and FIV infections or other concomitant diseases.[4,77,309,321–323] One cat had visceral involvement that included hepatosplenomegaly, icterus, lymphoplasmocytic gastroenteritis with abundant *Leishmania* parasites, and membranous glomerulonephritis.[77] A second cat from which *L. infantum* MON-1 zymodeme was cultured had disseminated crusty cutaneous lesions and amastigotes in the bone marrow.[309] Another cat with disseminated disease had uveitis as a predominant finding.[321] A case of pancytopenia in a cat has been reported with amastigotes in blood smears, bone marrow, spleen, and lymph nodes.[324] As with dogs, hyperproteineimia with hypergammaglobulinemia is a common finding in feline leishmaniosis.[78,79,321,325] The serum antibody titers to *Leishmania* antigen ranged from low to high levels.[77,80,309] Diagnosis was made in the majority of cases by serologic, cytologic, histologic, or PCR methods.

Reports of feline leishmaniosis in the New World have primarily described cutaneous infections with species that cause CL in humans. Nodules on the pinnae of a cat from southern Texas caused by *L. mexicana* were described in one report.[326] Thirty months after surgical removal of the affected pinna, the cat developed more diffuse lesions on the muzzle and the nasal mucosa. No visceral involvement was found on necropsy.[311] Similar lesions were described in eight cats from Texas involving the ear pinnae, or less commonly the muzzle and periorbital skin.[327] Solitary or multiple ulcerative nodular lesions due to *L. mexicana* infection, located on the nose, ears, tail, and lower limbs were diagnosed in cats from Venezuela.[328,329] Infection with a *Leishmania* (*Viannia*) species in a cat from Brazil was detected in a proliferative interdigital lesion.[330] *Leishmania braziliensis* was also isolated from cutaneous lesions from two cats in Brazil.[312,313] Experimentally, cats were susceptible to a generally self-limiting infection with a human isolate of this organism.[331] PCR has been used to confirm the presence of *Leishmania* DNA in spleen and lymph nodes of affected cats in Brazil.[332]

CASE EXAMPLE

Signalment

"Fausto," an 8-year-old male neutered husky mix from northern California, United States.

History

Fausto was referred to the University of California, Davis VMTH, for evaluation of suspected autoimmune disease. The dog had a 6-month history of progressive skin lesions that began as crusting and ulceration around the elbow and stifle joints. This was followed by development of similar lesions above both eyes, and on the dog's ears and dorsal muzzle. Three months after the skin lesions appeared, Fausto became stiff, lethargic, and was reluctant to walk. He also appeared to be lame. At that time, Fausto was taken to another veterinary clinic where an injection of triamcinolone acetonide (Vetalog®) was administered, and he was prescribed NSAID (carprofen) and trimethoprim-sulfamethoxazole. There was no improvement in the clinical signs with this treatment. The day before he was brought to the VMTH, the owner had taken Fausto to a local emergency clinic because he was reluctant to move. Blood work and arthrocentesis (left and right tarsal joints) were performed. The blood work showed a mild normocytic, normochromic nonregenerative anemia (HCT 31%); mild hypoalbuminemia (2.4 g/dL); and moderate hyperglobulinemia (7.7 g/dL). Cytologic examination of the synovial fluid analysis revealed large numbers of nondegenerate neutrophils, which was considered consistent with immune-mediated polyarthritis. Cephalexin and carprofen were prescribed and the dog was referred for further evaluation.

The owner had not noticed any coughing, sneezing, vomiting, diarrhea, or changes in thirst or urination. Fausto was fed 3 cups of a commercial dry chicken and rice-based dog food once a day, and his appetite remained good. He was fully vaccinated for rabies, CDV, CAdV, and CPV. The dog did not receive heartworm prophylaxis medication but was treated with fipronil once a month for flea control. There was one other healthy dog in the household. The owner and his dogs had moved to California from Barcelona, Spain, a few weeks around the time that the skin lesions appeared. In Spain, Fausto had worn a collar to prevent insect bites.

Continued

CASE EXAMPLE—cont'd

Physical Examination

Body weight: 34.4 kg.

General: Quiet, alert, and responsive, but reluctant to ambulate. T = 102.7°F (39.3°C), HR = 132 beats/minute, panting but eupneic, mucous membranes moist and pink.

Integument: Multiple focal regions of crusting, erythema, hyperpigmentation, thickening, and sometimes ulceration were present over the elbows and stifles, prepuce, ventral aspect of the mandible, above both eyes, and on both pinnae. Moderate pruritus was present.

Eyes, ears, nose, and throat: Apart from the skin lesions, only moderate periodontal disease was present. A fundoscopic examination showed no significant abnormalities.

Musculoskeletal: BCS 5/9. The dog was able to walk but had a shifting lameness. Pain was detected on extension of the joints but there was no palpable effusion present.

Cardiovascular: No murmurs or arrhythmias were auscultated. Femoral pulses were strong and synchronous.

Respiratory: No significant abnormalities detected.

Abdominal palpation: Splenomegaly was present.

Lymph nodes: Superficial cervical and popliteal lymph nodes were all enlarged (approximately 3 cm in diameter).

Laboratory Findings

CBC: HCT 32.4% (40%–55%), MCV 62.7 fL (65–75 fL), MCHC 35.2 g/dL (33–36 g/dL), reticulocyte count 54,500 cells/μL, WBC 9,300 cells/μL (6,000–13,000 cells/μL), neutrophils 7,533 cells/μL (3,000–10,500 cells/μL), lymphocytes 930 cells/μL (1,000–4,000 cells/μL), monocytes 651 cells/μL (150–1,200 cells/μL), eosinophils 186 cells/μL (0–1,500 cells/μL), platelets 338,000 platelets/μL (150,000–400,000 platelets/μL).

Serum chemistry profile: Sodium 140 mmol/L (145–154 mmol/L), potassium 4.4 mmol/L (4.1–5.3 mmol/L), chloride 107 mmol/L (105–116 mmol/L), bicarbonate 15 mmol/L (16–26 mmol/L), phosphorus 3.8 mg/dL (3.0–6.2 mg/dL), calcium 10.4 mg/dL (9.9–11.4 mg/dl), BUN 16 mg/dL (8–31 mg/dL), creatinine 0.9 mg/dL (0.3–1.2 mg/dL), glucose 109 mg/dL (70–118 mg/dL), total protein 10.7 g/dL (5.4–7.4 g/dL), albumin 2.1 g/dL (2.9–4.2 g/dL), globulin 8.6 g/dL (2.3–4.4 g/dL), ALT 12 U/L (19–67 U/L), AST 39 U/L (21–54 U/L), ALP 43 U/L (15–127 U/L), GGT 3 U/L (0–6 U/L), cholesterol 191 mg/dL (135–345 mg/dL), total bilirubin 0.1 mg/dL (0–0.4 mg/dL).

Serum protein electrophoresis: There was a marked increase in gamma-globulin with mild hypoalbuminemia. The gammopathy was polyclonal.

Urinalysis (cystocentesis): SpG 1.037; pH 7.0, 4+ protein (SSA), 1+ bilirubin, 1+ hemoprotein, no glucose or ketones, rare WBC/HPF, 1–3 RBC/HPF, rare hyaline casts, few lipid droplets.

Urine protein to creatinine ratio: 2.99 (normal, < 0.5).

Microbiologic Testing

IFA serology for antibodies for *Ehrlichia* spp., *Anaplasma* spp., *Rickettsia* spp., *Bartonella clarridgeiae*, *Bartonella vinsonii* subsp. *berkhoffii*, and *Bartonella henselae*: Negative.

Western immunoblot for antibodies to *Borrelia burgdorferi*: Negative.

Knott's and ELISA antigen test for *Dirofilaria immitis* infection: Negative.

Aerobic bacterial, anaerobic bacterial, and *Mycoplasma* culture of synovial fluid: Negative.

Aspiration cytology (right and left superficial cervical and popliteal lymph nodes): A heterogeneous population of lymphocytes was present, which consisted primarily of small mature lymphocytes and slightly increased numbers of intermediate-sized lymphocytes and lymphoblasts. Large numbers of plasma cells were noted, and a few macrophages were scattered throughout the specimen. Rare nondegenerate neutrophils and eosinophils were seen.

Bone marrow aspiration cytology: Many unit particles were present in a monolayer background of hemic cells and lipid vacuoles. Unit particles were normocellular and a small amount of storage iron was noted. Normal numbers of megakaryocytes were noted. The myeloid to erythroid ratio was mildly increased and both series were synchronous and complete. Increased numbers of plasma cells were noted throughout the sample with few small lymphocytes noted. Macrophages occasionally contained intracytoplasmic organisms consistent with *Leishmania* spp. amastigotes. Interpretation: mild erythroid hypoplasia, *Leishmania* spp., and mild plasma cell hyperplasia.

Skin biopsy (performed while the dog was sedated for bone marrow aspiration): There was a thick band of inflammatory cells that extended from the superficial to the mid-dermis. The inflammatory infiltrate comprised dense sheets of large foamy macrophages admixed with smaller numbers of lymphocytes and plasma cells and few neutrophils. Many of the large macrophages contained multiple, round to oval, intracytoplasmic basophilic organisms that were 1 to 2 μm in diameter. The epidermis was hyperplastic and hyperkeratotic and was covered by exudate admixed with keratin, degenerate neutrophils, and cellular debris.

Diagnosis

Canine leishmaniosis.

Treatment and Outcome

Fausto was initially treated with a combination of allopurinol (10 mg/kg, PO, q8h), ketoconazole (9 mg/kg, PO, q12h), cephalexin (30 mg/kg, PO, q12h for 4 weeks, for secondary bacterial pyoderma) and carprofen (4.4 mg/kg, PO, q24h). At a recheck examination 2 weeks later, the dog's owner reported that 1 or 2 days after treatment was started, Fausto became intensely pruritic. Fausto's appetite also decreased and he developed increased thirst and urination, but the lameness resolved. Physical examination showed severe crusting and ulceration of the face, with an associated foul odor. This extended from the dorsal nasal planum to the temporal and supra-ocular regions, as well as the inner aspect and tips of the pinnae, and had an associated foul odor. The lesions on the limbs were static or slightly improved from the last visit. A CBC was unchanged and a serum chemistry profile showed more severe hyperglobulinemia (9.3 g/dL) and hypoalbuminemia (1.9 g/dL). A drug reaction was suspected and the cephalexin was replaced with clavulanic acid-amoxicillin. Over the next month, the skin lesions improved (see Fig. 96.6A). The owner subsequently obtained meglumine antimoniate from Spain and treatment was changed to allopurinol (10 mg/kg, PO, q12h) and meglumine antimoniate (88 mg/kg, SC, q24h for 1 month). However, 6 days after treatment with meglumine commenced, the dog developed prolapsed third eyelids and was unable to catch treats when they were thrown to him. Physical examination showed healing skin lesions with evidence of hair regrowth, prolapsed third eyelids, risus sardonicus, and erect ears. A presumptive diagnosis of localized tetanus was made. A serum chemistry panel showed an albumin of 2.5 g/dL and a globulin of 6.4 g/dL, and the urine protein to creatinine ratio was 0.2. Fausto was treated with metronidazole (10 mg/kg, PO, q8h for 14 days) and tetanus antitoxin (20,000 U in 250 mL saline over 1 hour, IV, once). Clinical signs of tetanus had almost resolved 11 days later when the owner was contacted by telephone. The dog was subsequently lost to follow-up.

Comments

This case is an interesting example of travel-related canine leishmaniosis that was ultimately complicated by what appeared to be a cutaneous drug reaction to cephalexin and then localized tetanus. The diagnosis of leishmaniosis was suspected based on the clinical signs together with the travel history from southern Europe. The bone marrow aspirate and skin biopsies were obtained simultaneously for the sole purpose of cytologic diagnosis of leishmaniosis; impression smears of the skin lesions failed to yield organisms and the lymph node aspirates were also negative. The owner returned to Spain with his dog in order to obtain the meglumine antimoniate, which could not be obtained in the United States. The development of tetanus possibly may have followed use of contaminated needles by the owner for subcutaneous injection of the meglumine.

(Case example provided by Jane Sykes, University of California-Davis Veterinary Medical Teaching Hospital)

TREATMENT AND PROGNOSIS

Published information on the treatment of feline leishmaniosis is limited and controlled data on efficacy and safety is lacking. Allopurinol is the most frequently used drug, and meglumine antimoniate has also been used alone or in combination with allopurinol.[4,325] Successful treatment of cats with clinical improvement was achieved in the majority of cases with 5 to 10 mg/kg allopurinol, given twice daily.[78,79,321] Cats with disseminated forms of infection require longer allopurinol treatment of at least 6 months in comparison to the shorter course reported beneficial for cats with only cutaneous lesi ons.[78,79,321]

Prevention of feline leishmaniosis is available by using topical insecticides with activity against sand flies which are specifically licensed for cats including collars.[333] Caution must be exercised, as canine products, especially those with pyrethroids, are frequently toxic to felines. Commercial vaccines against leishmaniosis are currently not available for cats.

SUGGESTED READINGS

Solano-Gallego L, Cardoso L, Pennisi MG, et al. Diagnostic challenges in the era of canine *Leishmania infantum* vaccines. *Trends Parasitol.* 2017;33:706–717.

Miro G, Petersen C, Cardoso L, et al. Novel areas for prevention and control of canine leishmaniosis. *Trends Parasitol.* 2017;33:718–730.

Curtin JM, Aronson NE. Leishmaniasis in the United States: emerging issues in a region of low endemicity. *Microorganisms.* 2021;9:578.

REFERENCES

1. Dutta AK. Pursuit of medical knowledge: Charles Donovan (1863-1951) on kala-azar in India. *J Med Biogr.* 2008;16:72–76.
2. World Association for the Advancement of Veterinary Parasitology. Standardised nomenclature in animal parasitic diseases. https://www.waavp.org/documents/snopad-guidelines/#.X88CbUJKjOR.
3. Mauricio IL, Howard MK, Stothard JR, et al. Genomic diversity in the *Leishmania donovani* complex. *Parasitology.* 1999;119(Pt 3):237–246.
4. Pennisi MG, Cardoso L, Baneth G, et al. LeishVet update and recommendations on feline leishmaniosis. *Parasit Vectors.* 2015;8:302.
5. Halsey ES, Bryce LM, Wortmann GW, et al. Visceral leishmaniasis in a soldier returning from Operation Enduring Freedom. *Mil Med.* 2004;169:699–701.
6. Myles O, Wortmann GW, Cummings JF, et al. Visceral leishmaniasis: clinical observations in US army soldiers deployed to Afghanistan or Iraq, 2002-2004. *Arch Intern Med.* 2007;167:1899–1901.
7. Killick-Kendrick R. The biology and control of phlebotomine sand flies. *Clin Dermatol.* 1999;17:279–289.
8. Volf P, Hostomska J, Rohousova I. Molecular crosstalks in *Leishmania*-sandfly-host relationships. *Parasite.* 2008;15:237–243.
9. Ashford RW. The leishmaniases as emerging and reemerging zoonoses. *Int J Parasitol.* 2000;30:1269–1281.
10. Alvar J, Yactayo S, Bern C. Leishmaniasis and poverty. *Trends Parasitol.* 2006;22:552–557.
11. Desjeux P. Leishmaniasis. Public health aspects and control. *Clin Dermatol.* 1996;14:417–423.
12. Desjeux P. The increase in risk factors for leishmaniasis worldwide. *Trans R Soc Trop Med Hyg.* 2001;95:239–243.
13. Hassan MM, Osman OF, El-Raba'a FM, et al. Role of the domestic dog as a reservoir host of *Leishmania donovani* in eastern Sudan. *Parasit Vectors.* 2009;2:26.
14. Bashaye S, Nombela N, Argaw D, et al. Risk factors for visceral leishmaniasis in a new epidemic site in Amhara Region, Ethiopia. *Am J Trop Med Hyg.* 2009;81:34–39.
15. Tabbabi A. Review of leishmaniasis in the Middle East and North Africa. *Afr Health Sci.* 2019;19:1329–1337.
16. Tuon FF, Neto VA, Amato VS. *Leishmania*: origin, evolution and future since the Precambrian. *FEMS Immunol Med Microbiol.* 2008;54:158–166.
17. Solano-Gallego L, Koutinas A, Miro G, et al. Directions for the diagnosis, clinical staging, treatment and prevention of canine leishmaniosis. *Vet Parasitol.* 2009;165:1–18.
18. Tolezano JE, Uliana SR, Taniguchi HH, et al. The first records of *Leishmania (Leishmania) amazonensis* in dogs (*Canis familiaris*) diagnosed clinically as having canine visceral leishmaniasis from Aracatuba County, Sao Paulo State, Brazil. *Vet Parasitol.* 2007;149:280–284.
19. Maroli M, Rossi L, Baldelli R, et al. The northward spread of leishmaniasis in Italy: evidence from retrospective and ongoing studies on the canine reservoir and phlebotomine vectors. *Trop Med Int Health.* 2008;13:256–264.
20. Dereure J, Vanwambeke SO, Male P, et al. The potential effects of global warming on changes in canine leishmaniasis in a focus outside the classical area of the disease in southern France. *Vector Borne Zoonotic Dis.* 2009;9:687–694.
21. Amusategui I, Sainz A, Aguirre E, et al. Seroprevalence of *Leishmania infantum* in northwestern Spain, an area traditionally considered free of leishmaniasis. *Ann N Y Acad Sci.* 2004;1026:154–157.
22. Moreira Jr ED, Mendes de Souza VM, Sreenivasan M, et al. Assessment of an optimized dog-culling program in the dynamics of canine *Leishmania* transmission. *Vet Parasitol.* 2004;122:245–252.
23. Adini I, Ephros M, Chen J, et al. Asymptomatic visceral leishmaniasis, northern Israel. *Emerg Infect Dis.* 2003;9:397–398.
24. Moral L, Rubio EM, Moya M. A leishmanin skin test survey in the human population of l'Alacanti region (Spain): implications for the epidemiology of *Leishmania infantum* infection in southern Europe. *Trans R Soc Trop Med Hyg.* 2002;96:129–132.
25. Werneck GL, Rodrigues L, Santos MV, et al. The burden of *Leishmania chagasi* infection during an urban outbreak of visceral leishmaniasis in Brazil. *Acta Trop.* 2002;83:13–18.
26. le Fichoux Y, Quaranta JF, Aufeuvre JP, et al. Occurrence of *Leishmania infantum* parasitemia in asymptomatic blood donors living in an area of endemicity in southern France. *J Clin Microbiol.* 1999;37:1953–1957.
27. Riera C, Fisa R, Lopez-Chejade P, et al. Asymptomatic infection by *Leishmania infantum* in blood donors from the Balearic Islands (Spain). *Transfusion.* 2008;48:1383–1389.
28. Riera C, Fisa R, Udina M, et al. Detection of *Leishmania infantum* cryptic infection in asymptomatic blood donors living in an endemic area (Eivissa, Balearic Islands, Spain) by different diagnostic methods. *Trans R Soc Trop Med Hyg.* 2004;98:102–110.
29. Jimenez-Marco T, Fisa R, Girona-Llobera E, et al. Transfusion-transmitted leishmaniasis: a practical review. *Transfusion.* 2016;56(suppl 1):S45–51.
30. Baneth G, Dank G, Keren-Kornblatt E, et al. Emergence of visceral leishmaniasis in central Israel. *Am J Trop Med Hyg.* 1998;59:722–725.
31. Maroli M, Krasnonos L, Gafurov I. Epidemiological and entomological survey in a focus of visceral leishmaniasis in Pap district (Fergana Valley) of Namangan region, Uzbekistan. *Acta Trop.* 2001;80:223–228.
32. Gavgani AS, Mohite H, Edrissian GH, et al. Domestic dog ownership in Iran is a risk factor for human infection with *Leishmania infantum. Am J Trop Med Hyg.* 2002;67:511–515.
33. Rab MA, Frame IA, Evans DA. The role of dogs in the epidemiology of human visceral leishmaniasis in northern Pakistan. *Trans R Soc Trop Med Hyg.* 1995;89:612–615.
34. Trotz-Williams LA, Trees AJ. Systematic review of the distribution of the major vector-borne parasitic infections in dogs and cats in Europe. *Vet Rec.* 2003;152:97–105.
35. Koehler K, Stechele M, Hetzel U, et al. Cutaneous leishmaniosis in a horse in southern Germany caused by *Leishmania infantum. Vet Parasitol.* 2002;109:9–17.
36. Shaw SE, Langton DA, Hillman TJ. Canine leishmaniosis in the United Kingdom: a zoonotic disease waiting for a vector? *Vet Parasitol.* 2009;163:281–285.
37. Teske E, van Knapen F, Beijer EG, et al. Risk of infection with *Leishmania* spp. in the canine population in the Netherlands. *Acta Vet Scand.* 2002;43:195–201.

38. Solano-Gallego L, Morell P, Arboix M, et al. Prevalence of *Leishmania infantum* infection in dogs living in an area of canine leishmaniasis endemicity using PCR on several tissues and serology. *J Clin Microbiol.* 2001;39:560–563.
39. Berrahal F, Mary C, Roze M, et al. Canine leishmaniasis: identification of asymptomatic carriers by polymerase chain reaction and immunoblotting. *Am J Trop Med Hyg.* 1996;55:273–277.
40. Leontides LS, Saridomichelakis MN, Billinis C, et al. A cross-sectional study of *Leishmania* spp. infection in clinically healthy dogs with polymerase chain reaction and serology in Greece. *Vet Parasitol.* 2002;109:19–27.
41. Oliva G, Scalone A, Foglia Manzillo V, et al. Incidence and time course of *Leishmania infantum* infections examined by parasitological, serologic, and nested-PCR techniques in a cohort of naive dogs exposed to three consecutive transmission seasons. *J Clin Microbiol.* 2006;44:1318–1322.
42. Baneth G, Koutinas AF, Solano-Gallego L, et al. Canine leishmaniosis - new concepts and insights on an expanding zoonosis: part one. *Trends Parasitol.* 2008;24:324–330.
43. Zaffaroni E, Rubaudo L, Lanfranchi P, et al. Epidemiological patterns of canine leishmaniasis [correction of leishmaniosis] in Western Liguria (Italy). *Vet Parasitol.* 1999;81:11–19.
44. Miranda S, Roura X, Picado A, et al. Characterization of sex, age, and breed for a population of canine leishmaniosis diseased dogs. *Res Vet Sci.* 2008;85:35–38.
45. Franca-Silva JC, da Costa RT, Siqueira AM, et al. Epidemiology of canine visceral leishmaniosis in the endemic area of Montes Claros Municipality, Minas Gerais State, Brazil. *Vet Parasitol.* 2003;111:161–173.
46. Sideris V, Papadopoulou G, Dotsika E, et al. Asymptomatic canine leishmaniasis in Greater Athens area, Greece. *Eur J Epidemiol.* 1999;15:271–276.
47. Solano-Gallego L, Llull J, Ramos G, et al. The Ibizian hound presents a predominantly cellular immune response against natural *Leishmania* infection. *Vet Parasitol.* 2000;90:37–45.
48. Burnham AC, Ordeix L, Alcover MM, et al. Exploring the relationship between susceptibility to canine leishmaniosis and anti-*Phlebotomus perniciosus* saliva antibodies in Ibizan hounds and dogs of other breeds in Mallorca, Spain. *Parasit Vectors.* 2020;13;129.
49. Quinnell RJ, Courtenay O. Transmission, reservoir hosts and control of zoonotic visceral leishmaniasis. *Parasitology.* 2009;136:1915–1934.
50. Courtenay O, Quinnell RJ, Garcez LM, et al. Infectiousness in a cohort of Brazilian dogs: why culling fails to control visceral leishmaniasis in areas of high transmission. *J Infect Dis.* 2002;186:1314–1320.
51. da Costa-Val AP, Cavalcanti RR, de Figueiredo Gontijo N, et al. Canine visceral leishmaniasis: relationships between clinical status, humoral immune response, haematology and *Lutzomyia (Lutzomyia) longipalpis* infectivity. *Vet J.* 2007;174:636–643.
52. Guarga JL, Moreno J, Lucientes J, et al. Canine leishmaniasis transmission: higher infectivity amongst naturally infected dogs to sand flies is associated with lower proportions of T helper cells. *Res Vet Sci.* 2000;69:249–253.
53. Michalsky EM, Rocha MF, da Rocha Lima AC, et al. Infectivity of seropositive dogs, showing different clinical forms of leishmaniasis, to *Lutzomyia longipalpis* phlebotomine sand flies. *Vet Parasitol.* 2007;147:67–76.
54. Manna L, Reale S, Vitale F, et al. Evidence for a relationship between *Leishmania* load and clinical manifestations. *Res Vet Sci.* 2009;87:76–78.
55. Reis AB, Teixeira-Carvalho A, Vale AM, et al. Isotype patterns of immunoglobulins: hallmarks for clinical status and tissue parasite density in Brazilian dogs naturally infected by *Leishmania (Leishmania) chagasi. Vet Immunol Immunopathol.* 2006;112:102–116.
56. Ikeda-Garcia FA, Lopes RS, Marques FJ, et al. Clinical and parasitological evaluation of dogs naturally infected by *Leishmania (Leishmania) chagasi* submitted to treatment with meglumine antimoniate. *Vet Parasitol.* 2007;143:254–259.
57. Ribeiro RR, Moura EP, Pimentel VM, et al. Reduced tissue parasitic load and infectivity to sand flies in dogs naturally infected by *Leishmania (Leishmania) chagasi* following treatment with a liposome formulation of meglumine antimoniate. *Antimicrob Agents Chemother.* 2008;52:2564–2572.
58. Miro G, Galvez R, Fraile C, et al. Infectivity to *Phlebotomus perniciosus* of dogs naturally parasitized with *Leishmania infantum* after different treatments. *Parasit Vectors.* 2011;4:52.
59. da Silva SM, Ribeiro VM, Ribeiro RR, et al. First report of vertical transmission of *Leishmania (Leishmania) infantum* in a naturally infected bitch from Brazil. *Vet Parasitol.* 2009;166:159–162.
60. Rosypal AC, Lindsay DS. Non-sand fly transmission of a North American isolate of *Leishmania infantum* in experimentally infected BALB/c mice. *J Parasitol.* 2005;91:1113–1115.
61. Diaz-Espineira MM, Slappendel RJ. A case of autochthonous canine leishmaniasis in The Netherlands. *Vet Q.* 1997;19:69–71.
62. Grinnage-Pulley T, Scott B, Petersen CA. A mother's gift: congenital transmission of *Trypanosoma* and *Leishmania* species. *PLoS Pathog.* 2016;12:e1005302.
63. Silva FL, Oliveira RG, Silva TM, et al. Venereal transmission of canine visceral leishmaniasis. *Vet Parasitol.* 2009;160:55–59.
64. Coutinho MT, Bueno LL, Sterzik A, et al. Participation of *Rhipicephalus sanguineus* (Acari: Ixodidae) in the epidemiology of canine visceral leishmaniasis. *Vet Parasitol.* 2005;128:149–155.
65. Dantas-Torres F. Ticks as vectors of *Leishmania* parasites. *Trends Parasitol.* 2011;27:155–159.
66. Coutinho MT, Linardi PM. Can fleas from dogs infected with canine visceral leishmaniasis transfer the infection to other mammals? *Vet Parasitol.* 2007;147:320–325.
67. Ferreira MG, Fattori KR, Souza F, et al. Potential role for dog fleas in the cycle of *Leishmania* spp. *Vet Parasitol.* 2009;165:150–154.
68. Giger U, Oakley DA, Owens SD, et al. *Leishmania donovani* transmission by packed RBC transfusion to anemic dogs in the United States. *Transfusion.* 2002;42:381–383.
69. Owens SD, Oakley DA, Marryott K, et al. Transmission of visceral leishmaniasis through blood transfusions from infected English foxhounds to anemic dogs. *J Am Vet Med Assoc.* 2001;219:1076–1083.
70. de Freitas E, Melo MN, da Costa-Val AP, et al. Transmission of *Leishmania infantum* via blood transfusion in dogs: potential for infection and importance of clinical factors. *Vet Parasitol.* 2006;137:159–167.
71. Tabar MD, Roura X, Francino O, et al. Detection of *Leishmania infantum* by real-time PCR in a canine blood bank. *J Small Anim Pract.* 2008;49:325–328.
72. Duprey ZH, Steurer FJ, Rooney JA, et al. Canine visceral leishmaniasis, United States and Canada, 2000-2003. *Emerg Infect Dis.* 2006;12:440–446.
73. Cunha S, Freire M, Eulalio C, et al. Visceral leishmaniasis in a new ecological niche near a major metropolitan area of Brazil. *Trans R Soc Trop Med Hyg.* 1995;89:155–158.
74. Moreno J, Alvar J. Canine leishmaniasis: epidemiological risk and the experimental model. *Trends Parasitol.* 2002;18:399–405.
75. Martin-Sanchez J, Acedo C, Munoz-Perez M, et al. Infection by *Leishmania infantum* in cats: epidemiological study in Spain. *Vet Parasitol.* 2007;145:267–273.
76. da Silva AV, de Souza Candido CD, de Pita Pereira D, et al. The first record of American visceral leishmaniasis in domestic cats from Rio de Janeiro, Brazil. *Acta Trop.* 2008;105:92–94.
77. Hervas J, Chacon MDLF, Sanchez-Isarria MA, et al. Two cases of feline visceral and cutaneous leishmaniosis in Spain. *J Feline Med Surg.* 1999;1:101–105.
78. Pennisi MG, Venza M, Reale S, et al. Case report of leishmaniasis in four cats. *Vet Res Commun.* 2004;28(suppl 1):363–366.
79. Rufenacht S, Sager H, Muller N, et al. Two cases of feline leishmaniosis in Switzerland. *Vet Rec.* 2005;156:542–545.
80. Poli A, Abramo F, Barsotti P, et al. Feline leishmaniosis due to *Leishmania infantum* in Italy. *Vet Parasitol.* 2002;106:181–191.
81. Rolao N, Martins MJ, Joao A, et al. Equine infection with *Leishmania* in Portugal. *Parasite.* 2005;12:183–186.
82. Solano-Gallego L, Fernandez-Bellon H, Serra R, et al. Cutaneous leishmaniosis in three horses in Spain. *Equine Vet J.* 2003;35:320–323.
83. Limeira CH, Alves CJ, Azevedo SS, et al. Clinical aspects and diagnosis of leishmaniasis in equids: a systematic review and meta-analysis. *Rev Bras Parasitol Vet.* 2019;28:574–581.
84. Fernandez-Bellon H, Solano-Gallego L, Bardagi M, et al. Immune response to *Leishmania infantum* in healthy horses in Spain. *Vet Parasitol.* 2006;135:181–185.

85. Mhadhbi M, Sassi A. Infection of the equine population by *Leishmania* parasites. *Equine Vet J.* 2020;52:28–33.
86. Moraes-Silva E, Antunes FR, Rodrigues MS, et al. Domestic swine in a visceral leishmaniasis endemic area produce antibodies against multiple *Leishmania infantum* antigens but apparently resist to *L. infantum* infection. *Acta Trop.* 2006;98:176–182.
87. Millan J, Ferroglio E, Solano-Gallego L. Role of wildlife in the epidemiology of *Leishmania infantum* infection in Europe. *Parasitol Res.* 2014;113:2005–2014.
88. Beck A, Beck R, Kusak J, et al. A case of visceral leishmaniosis in a gray wolf (*Canis lupus*) from Croatia. *J Wildl Dis.* 2008;44:451–456.
89. Luppi MM, Malta MC, Silva TM, et al. Visceral leishmaniasis in captive wild canids in Brazil. *Vet Parasitol.* 2008;155:146–151.
90. Molina R, Jimenez MI, Cruz I, et al. The hare (*Lepus granatensis*) as potential sylvatic reservoir of *Leishmania infantum* in Spain. *Vet Parasitol.* 2012;190:268–271.
91. Courtenay O, Quinnell RJ, Garcez LM, et al. Low infectiousness of a wildlife host of *Leishmania infantum*: the crab-eating fox is not important for transmission. *Parasitology.* 2002;125:407–414.
92. Anderson DC, Buckner RG, Glenn BL, et al. Endemic canine leishmaniasis. *Vet Pathol.* 1980;17:94–96.
93. Enserink M. Infectious diseases. Has leishmaniasis become endemic in the U.S.? *Science.* 2000;290:1881–1883.
94. Gaskin AA, Schantz P, Jackson J, et al. Visceral leishmaniasis in a New York foxhound kennel. *J Vet Intern Med.* 2002;16:34–44.
95. Toepp AJ, Schaut RG, Scott BD, et al. *Leishmania* incidence and prevalence in U.S. hunting hounds maintained via vertical transmission. *Vet Parasitol Reg Stud Reports.* 2017;10:75–81.
96. Toepp AJ, Bennett C, Scott B, et al. Maternal *Leishmania infantum* infection status has significant impact on leishmaniasis in offspring. *PLoS Negl Trop Dis.* 2019;13:e0007058.
97. Gibson-Corley KN, Hostetter JM, Hostetter SJ, et al. Disseminated *Leishmania infantum* infection in two sibling foxhounds due to possible vertical transmission. *Can Vet J.* 2008;49:1005–1008.
98. Petersen CA, Barr SC. Canine leishmaniasis in North America: emerging or newly recognized?. *Vet Clin North Am Small Anim Pract.* 2009;39:1065–1074. vi.
99. Vida B, Toepp A, Schaut RG, et al. Immunologic progression of canine leishmaniosis following vertical transmission in United States dogs. *Vet Immunol Immunopathol.* 2016;169:34–38.
100. Naucke TJ, Amelung S, Lorentz S. First report of transmission of canine leishmaniosis through bite wounds from a naturally infected dog in Germany. *Parasit Vectors.* 2016;9:256.
101. Curtin JM, Aronson NE. Leishmaniasis in the United States: emerging issues in a region of low endemicity. *Microorganisms.* 2021;9:578.
102. Travi BL, Ferro C, Cadena H, et al. Canine visceral leishmaniasis: dog infectivity to sand flies from non-endemic areas. *Res Vet Sci.* 2002;72: 83–86.
103. Schaut RG, Robles-Murguia M, Juelsgaard R, et al. Vectorborne transmission of *Leishmania infantum* from hounds, United States. *Emerg Infect Dis.* 2015;21:2209–2212.
104. Dantas-Torres F. Do any insects other than phlebotomine sandflies (Diptera: Psychodidae) transmit *Leishmania infantum* (Kinetoplastida: Trypanosomatidae) from dog to dog? *Vet Parasitol.* 2006;136:379–380.
105. Boggiatto PM, Gibson-Corley KN, Metz K, et al. Transplacental transmission of *Leishmania infantum* as a means for continued disease incidence in North America. *PLoS Negl Trop Dis.* 2011;5:e1019.
106. Diniz SA, Melo MS, Borges AM, et al. Genital lesions associated with visceral leishmaniasis and shedding of *Leishmania* sp. in the semen of naturally infected dogs. *Vet Pathol.* 2005;42:650–658.
107. Magill AJ, Grogl M, Gasser Jr RA, et al. Visceral infection caused by *Leishmania tropica* in veterans of Operation Desert Storm. *N Engl J Med.* 1993;328:1383–1387.
108. Sacks DL, Kenney RT, Kreutzer RD, et al. Indian kala-azar caused by *Leishmania tropica*. *Lancet.* 1995;345:959–961.
109. Dereure J, Rioux JA, Gallego M, et al. *Leishmania tropica* in Morocco: infection in dogs. *Trans R Soc Trop Med Hyg.* 1991;85:595.
110. Baneth G, Zivotofsky D, Nachum-Biala Y, et al. Mucocutaneous *Leishmania tropica* infection in a dog from a human cutaneous leishmaniasis focus. *Parasit Vectors.* 2014;7:118.
111. Guessous-Idrissi N, Chiheb S, Hamdani A, et al. Cutaneous leishmaniasis: an emerging epidemic focus of *Leishmania tropica* in north Morocco. *Trans R Soc Trop Med Hyg.* 1997;91:660–663.
112. Mohebali M, Hajjaran H, Hamzavi Y, et al. Epidemiological aspects of canine visceral leishmaniosis in the Islamic Republic of Iran. *Vet Parasitol.* 2005;129:243–251.
113. Baneth G, Yasur-Landau D, Gilad M, et al. Canine leishmaniosis caused by *Leishmania major* and *Leishmania tropica*: comparative findings and serology. *Parasit Vectors.* 2017;10:113.
114. Morsy TA, Schnur LF, Feinsod FM, et al. Natural infections of *Leishmania major* in domestic dogs from Alexandria, Egypt. *Am J Trop Med Hyg.* 1987;37:49–52.
115. Killick-Kendrick R, Killick-Kendrick M, Pinelli E, et al. A laboratory model of canine leishmaniasis: the inoculation of dogs with *Leishmania infantum* promastigotes from midguts of experimentally infected phlebotomine sandflies. *Parasite.* 1994;1:311–318.
116. Alvar J, Aparicio P, Aseffa A, et al. The relationship between leishmaniasis and AIDS: the second 10 years. *Clin Microbiol Rev.* 2008;21:334–359.
117. Sacks D, Sher A. Evasion of innate immunity by parasitic protozoa. *Nat Immunol.* 2002;3:1041–1047.
118. Kaye PM, Aebischer T. Visceral leishmaniasis: immunology and prospects for a vaccine. *Clin Microbiol Infect.* 2011;17:1462–1470.
119. Engwerda CR, Matlashewski G. Development of *Leishmania* vaccines in the era of visceral leishmaniasis elimination. *Trans R Soc Trop Med Hyg.* 2015;109:423–424.
120. Hosein S, Blake DP, Solano-Gallego L. Insights on adaptive and innate immunity in canine leishmaniosis. *Parasitology.* 2017;144:95–115.
121. Montserrat-Sangra S, Alborch L, Ordeix L, et al. TLR-2 and TLR-4 transcriptions in unstimulated blood from dogs with leishmaniosis due to *Leishmania infantum* at the time of diagnosis and during follow-up treatment. *Vet Parasitol.* 2016;228:172–179.
122. Ordeix L, Montserrat-Sangra S, Martinez-Orellana P, et al. Toll-like receptors 2, 4 and 7, interferon-gamma and interleukin 10, and programmed death ligand 1 transcripts in skin from dogs of different clinical stages of leishmaniosis. *Parasit Vectors.* 2019;12:575.
123. Hosein S, Rodriguez-Cortes A, Blake DP, et al. Transcription of Toll-like receptors 2, 3, 4 and 9, FoxP3 and Th17 *Leishmania infantum* infection. *PLoS One.* 2015;10:e0140325.
124. Prajeeth CK, Haeberlein S, Sebald H, et al. *Leishmania*-infected macrophages are targets of NK cell-derived cytokines but not of NK cell cytotoxicity. *Infect Immun.* 2011;79:2699–2708.
125. Schaut RG, Grinnage-Pulley TL, Esch KJ, et al. Recovery of antigen-specific T cell responses from dogs infected with *Leishmania (L.) infantum* by use of vaccine associated TLR-agonist adjuvant. *Vaccine.* 2016;34:5225–5234.
126. Nylen S, Sacks D. Interleukin-10 and the pathogenesis of human visceral leishmaniasis. *Trends Immunol.* 2007;28:378–384.
127. Esch KJ, Juelsgaard R, Martinez PA, et al. Programmed death 1-mediated T cell exhaustion during visceral leishmaniasis impairs phagocyte function. *J Immunol.* 2013;191:5542–5550.
128. Trigo J, Abbehusen M, Netto EM, et al. Treatment of canine visceral leishmaniasis by the vaccine Leish-111f+MPL-SE. *Vaccine.* 2010;28:3333–3340.
129. Gradoni L, Foglia Manzillo V, Pagano A, et al. Failure of a multi-subunit recombinant leishmanial vaccine (MML) to protect dogs from *Leishmania infantum* infection and to prevent disease progression in infected animals. *Vaccine.* 2005;23:5245–5251.
130. Moreno J, Nieto J, Masina S, et al. Immunization with H1, HASPB1 and MML *Leishmania* proteins in a vaccine trial against experimental canine leishmaniasis. *Vaccine.* 2007;25:5290–5300.
131. Altet L, Francino O, Solano-Gallego L, et al. Mapping and sequencing of the canine NRAMP1 gene and identification of mutations in leishmaniasis-susceptible dogs. *Infect Immun.* 2002;70:2763–2771.

132. Sanchez-Robert E, Altet L, Sanchez A, et al. Polymorphism of Slc11a1 (Nramp1) gene and canine leishmaniasis in a case-control study. *J Hered.* 2005;96:755–758.
133. Sanchez-Robert E, Altet L, Utzet-Sadurni M, et al. Slc11a1 (formerly Nramp1) and susceptibility to canine visceral leishmaniasis. *Vet Res.* 2008;39:36.
134. Mohamed HS, Ibrahim ME, Miller EN, et al. SLC11A1 (formerly NRAMP1) and susceptibility to visceral leishmaniasis in The Sudan. *Eur J Hum Genet.* 2004;12:66–74.
135. Quinnell RJ, Kennedy LJ, Barnes A, et al. Susceptibility to visceral leishmaniasis in the domestic dog is associated with MHC class II polymorphism. *Immunogenetics.* 2003;55:23–28.
136. Leish GENC, Wellcome Trust Case Control C, Fakiola M, et al. Common variants in the HLA-DRB1-HLA-DQA1 HLA class II region are associated with susceptibility to visceral leishmaniasis. *Nat Genet.* 2013;45:208–213.
137. Maia C, Campino L. Biomarkers associated with *Leishmania infantum* exposure, infection, and disease in dogs. *Front Cell Infect Microbiol.* 2018;8:302.
138. Lucena R, Ginel PJ. Immunoglobulin isotype distribution of antinuclear antibodies in dogs with leishmaniasis. *Res Vet Sci.* 1998;65:205–207.
139. Smith BE, Tompkins MB, Breitschwerdt EB. Antinuclear antibodies can be detected in dog sera reactive to *Bartonella vinsonii* subsp. *berkhoffii, Ehrlichia canis*, or *Leishmania infantum* antigens. *J Vet Intern Med.* 2004;18:47–51.
140. Cortese L, Sica M, Piantedosi D, et al. Secondary immune-mediated thrombocytopenia in dogs naturally infected by *Leishmania infantum*. *Vet Rec.* 2009;164:778–782.
141. Terrazzano G, Cortese L, Piantedosi D, et al. Presence of anti-platelet IgM and IgG antibodies in dogs naturally infected by *Leishmania infantum*. *Vet Immunol Immunopathol.* 2006;110:331–337.
142. Esch KJ, Schaut RG, Lamb IM, et al. Activation of autophagy and nucleotide-binding domain leucine-rich repeat-containing-like receptor family, pyrin domain-containing 3 inflammasome during *Leishmania infantum*-associated glomerulonephritis. *Am J Pathol.* 2015;185:2105–2117.
143. Ginel PJ, Camacho S, Lucena R. Anti-histone antibodies in dogs with leishmaniasis and glomerulonephritis. *Res Vet Sci.* 2008;85:510–514.
144. Lopez R, Lucena R, Novales M, et al. Circulating immune complexes and renal function in canine leishmaniasis. *Zentralbl Veterinarmed B.* 1996;43:469–474.
145. Font A, Mascort J, Altimira J, et al. Acute paraplegia associated with vasculitis in a dog with leishmaniasis. *J Small Anim Pract.* 2004;45:199–201.
146. Pumarola M, Brevik L, Badiola J, et al. Canine leishmaniasis associated with systemic vasculitis in two dogs. *J Comp Pathol.* 1991;105:279–286.
147. Torrent E, Leiva M, Segales J, et al. Myocarditis and generalised vasculitis associated with leishmaniosis in a dog. *J Small Anim Pract.* 2005;46:549–552.
148. Prats N, Ferrer L. A possible mechanism in the pathogenesis of cutaneous lesions in canine leishmaniasis. *Vet Rec.* 1995;137:103–104.
149. Solano-Gallego L, Fernandez-Bellon H, Morell P, et al. Histological and immunohistochemical study of clinically normal skin of *Leishmania infantum*-infected dogs. *J Comp Pathol.* 2004;130:7–12.
150. Giunchetti RC, Mayrink W, Genaro O, et al. Relationship between canine visceral leishmaniosis and the *Leishmania (Leishmania) chagasi* burden in dermal inflammatory foci. *J Comp Pathol.* 2006;135:100–107.
151. Ciaramella P, Oliva G, Luna RD, et al. A retrospective clinical study of canine leishmaniasis in 150 dogs naturally infected by *Leishmania infantum*. *Vet Rec.* 1997;141:539–543.
152. Koutinas AF, Polizopoulou ZS, Saridomichelakis MN, et al. Clinical consideration on canine leishmaniasis in Greece: a retrospective study of 158 cases (1989–1996). *J Am Anim Hosp Assoc.* 1999;35:376–383.
153. Slappendel RJ. Canine leishmaniasis. A review based on 95 cases in The Netherlands. *Vet Q.* 1988;10:1–16.
154. Koutinas AF, Scott DW, Kontos V, et al. Skin lesions in canine leishmaniasis (kala-azar): a clinical and histopathological study of 22 spontaneous cases in Greece. *Vet Dermatol.* 1992;3:121–130.
155. Saridomichelakis MN, Koutinas AF. Cutaneous involvement in canine leishmaniosis due to *Leishmania infantum* (syn. *L. chagasi*). *Vet Dermatol.* 2014;25:61–71. e22.
156. Ciaramella P, Pelagalli A, Cortese L, et al. Altered platelet aggregation and coagulation disorders related to clinical findings in 30 dogs naturally infected by *Leishmania infantum*. *Vet J.* 2005;169:465–467.
157. Juttner C, Rodriguez Sanchez M, Rollan Landeras E, et al. Evaluation of the potential causes of epistaxis in dogs with natural visceral leishmaniasis. *Vet Rec.* 2001;149:176–179.
158. Petanides TA, Koutinas AF, Mylonakis ME, et al. Factors associated with the occurrence of epistaxis in natural canine leishmaniasis (*Leishmania infantum*). *J Vet Intern Med.* 2008;22:866–872.
159. Lima WG, Michalick MS, de Melo MN, et al. Canine visceral leishmaniasis: a histopathological study of lymph nodes. *Acta Trop.* 2004;92:43–53.
160. Pena MT, Naranjo C, Klauss G, et al. Histopathological features of ocular leishmaniosis in the dog. *J Comp Pathol.* 2008;138:32–39.
161. Pena MT, Roura X, Davidson MG. Ocular and periocular manifestations of leishmaniasis in dogs: 105 cases (1993-1998). *Vet Ophthalmol.* 2000;3:35–41.
162. Garcia-Alonso M, Blanco A, Reina D, et al. Immunopathology of the uveitis in canine leishmaniasis. *Parasite Immunol.* 1996;18:617–623.
163. Naranjo C, Fondevila D, Leiva M, et al. Characterization of lacrimal gland lesions and possible pathogenic mechanisms of keratoconjunctivitis sicca in dogs with leishmaniosis. *Vet Parasitol.* 2005;133:37–47.
164. Paciello O, Oliva G, Gradoni L, et al. Canine inflammatory myopathy associated with *Leishmania infantum* infection. *Neuromuscul Disord.* 2009;19:124–130.
165. Vamvakidis CD, Koutinas AF, Kanakoudis G, et al. Masticatory and skeletal muscle myositis in canine leishmaniasis (*Leishmania infantum*). *Vet Rec.* 2000;146:698–703.
166. Agut A, Corzo N, Murciano J, et al. Clinical and radiographic study of bone and joint lesions in 26 dogs with leishmaniasis. *Vet Rec.* 2003;153:648–652.
167. Blavier A, Keroack S, Denerolle P, et al. Atypical forms of canine leishmaniosis. *Vet J.* 2001;162:108–120.
168. Casanova MI, Martín S, Marco A, et al. Detection of *Leishmania* spp. infection by immunohistochemistry in archived biopsy samples from dogs with colitis in an area endemic for leishmaniosis. *J Comp Pathol.* 2019;167:12–17.
169. Baxarias M, Alvarez-Fernandez A, Martinez-Orellana P, et al. Does co-infection with vector-borne pathogens play a role in clinical canine leishmaniosis? *Parasit Vectors.* 2018;11:135.
170. Attipa C, Solano-Gallego L, Papasouliotis K, et al. Association between canine leishmaniosis and *Ehrlichia canis* co-infection: a prospective case-control study. *Parasit Vectors.* 2018;11:184.
171. Attipa C, Solano-Gallego L, Leutenegger CM, et al. Associations between clinical canine leishmaniosis and multiple vector-borne co-infections: a case-control serological study. *BMC Vet Res.* 2019;15:331.
172. Toepp AJ, Monteiro GRG, Coutinho JFV, et al. Comorbid infections induce progression of visceral leishmaniasis. *Parasit Vectors.* 2019;12:54.
173. Font A, Durall N, Domingo M, et al. Cardiac tamponade in a dog with visceral leishmaniasis. *J Am Anim Hosp Assoc.* 1993;29.
174. Carrasco L, de Lara FC, Martin E, et al. Acute haemorrhagic pancreatitis associated with canine visceral leishmaniasis. *Vet Rec.* 1997;141:519–521.
175. Vinuelas J, Garcia-Alonso M, Ferrando L, et al. Meningeal leishmaniosis induced by *Leishmania infantum* in naturally infected dogs. *Vet Parasitol.* 2001;101:23–27.
176. Ginel PJ, Mozos E, Fernandez A, et al. Canine pemphigus foliaceus associated with leishmaniasis. *Vet Rec.* 1993;133:526–527.
177. Fondevila D, Vilafranca M, Ferrer L. Epidermal immunocompetence in canine leishmaniasis. *Vet Immunol Immunopathol.* 1997;56:319–327.
178. Font A, Closa JM, Molina A, et al. Thrombosis and nephrotic syndrome in a dog with visceral leishmaniasis. *J Small Anim Pract.* 1993;34:466–470.
179. Font A, Gines C, Closa JM, et al. Visceral leishmaniasis and disseminated intravascular coagulation in a dog. *J Am Vet Med Assoc.* 1994;204:1043–1044.

180. Alves GB, Pinho FA, Silva SM, et al. Cardiac and pulmonary alterations in symptomatic and asymptomatic dogs infected naturally with *Leishmania (Leishmania) chagasi*. *Braz J Med Biol Res.* 2010;43:310–315.
181. Sebastian-Marcos P, Santarelli G, Gomez S, et al. Canine leishmaniasis associated with pericardial effusion in a 4-year-old dog. *J Vet Cardiol.* 2019;23:32–37.
182. Rosa FA, Leite JH, Braga ET, et al. Cardiac lesions in 30 dogs naturally infected with *Leishmania infantum chagasi*. *Vet Pathol.* 2014;51:603–606.
183. Silvestrini P, Piviani M, Alberola J, et al. Serum cardiac troponin I concentrations in dogs with leishmaniasis: correlation with age and clinicopathologic abnormalities. *Vet Clin Pathol.* 2012;41:568–574.
184. Solano-Gallego L, Cardoso L, Pennisi MG, et al. Diagnostic challenges in the era of canine *Leishmania infantum* vaccines. *Trends Parasitol.* 2017;33:706–717.
185. Miro G, Cardoso L, Pennisi MG, et al. Canine leishmaniosis: new concepts and insights on an expanding zoonosis: part two. *Trends Parasitol.* 2008;24:371–377.
186. Melendez-Lazo A, Ordeix L, Planellas M, et al. Clinicopathological findings in sick dogs naturally infected with *Leishmania infantum*: Comparison of five different clinical classification systems. *Res Vet Sci.* 2018;117:18–27.
187. Martinez-Subiela S, Tecles F, Eckersall PD, et al. Serum concentrations of acute phase proteins in dogs with leishmaniasis. *Vet Rec.* 2002;150:241–244.
188. Ceron JJ, Pardo-Marin L, Caldin M, et al. Use of acute phase proteins for the clinical assessment and management of canine leishmaniosis: general recommendations. *BMC Vet Res.* 2018;14:196.
189. Giapitzoglou S, Saridomichelakis MN, Leontides LS, et al. Evaluation of serum symmetric dimethylarginine as a biomarker of kidney disease in canine leishmaniosis due to *Leishmania infantum*. *Vet Parasitol.* 2020;277:109015.
190. Torrent E, Planellas M, Ordeix L, et al. Serum symmetric dimethylarginine as an early marker of excretory dysfunction in canine leishmaniosis (*L. infantum*) induced nephropathy. *Vet Med Int.* 2018;2018:7517359.
191. Palacio J, Liste F, Gascon M. Urinary protein/creatinine ratio in the evaluation of renal failure in canine leishmaniasis. *Vet Rec.* 1995;137:567–568.
192. Palacio J, Liste F, Gascon M. Enzymuria as an index of renal damage in canine leishmaniasis. *Vet Rec.* 1997;140:477–480.
193. Paltrinieri S, Gradoni L, Roura X, et al. Laboratory tests for diagnosing and monitoring canine leishmaniasis. *Vet Clin Pathol.* 2016;45:552–578.
194. Lima VM, Goncalves ME, Ikeda FA, et al. Anti-*Leishmania* antibodies in cerebrospinal fluid from dogs with visceral leishmaniasis. *Braz J Med Biol Res.* 2003;36:485–489.
195. Assis VP, Ribeiro VM, Rachid MA, et al. Dogs with *Leishmania chagasi* infection have semen abnormalities that partially revert during 150 days of allopurinol and amphotericin B therapy. *Anim Reprod Sci.* 2010;117:183–186.
196. Foglia Manzillo V, Restucci B, Pagano A, et al. Pathological changes in the bone marrow of dogs with leishmaniosis. *Vet Rec.* 2006;158:690–694.
197. Tropia de Abreu R, Carvalho MG, Carneiro CM, et al. Influence of clinical status and parasite load on erythropoiesis and leucopoiesis in dogs naturally infected with *Leishmania (Leishmania) chagasi*. *PLoS One.* 2011;6:e18873.
198. Ferreira Ede C, de Lana M, Carneiro M, et al. Comparison of serological assays for the diagnosis of canine visceral leishmaniasis in animals presenting different clinical manifestations. *Vet Parasitol.* 2007;146:235–241.
199. Porrozzi R, Santos da Costa MV, Teva A, et al. Comparative evaluation of enzyme-linked immunosorbent assays based on crude and recombinant leishmanial antigens for serodiagnosis of symptomatic and asymptomatic *Leishmania infantum* visceral infections in dogs. *Clin Vaccine Immunol.* 2007;14:544–548.
200. Goto Y, Howard RF, Bhatia A, et al. Distinct antigen recognition pattern during zoonotic visceral leishmaniasis in humans and dogs. *Vet Parasitol.* 2009;160:215–220.
201. Todoli F, Perez-Filgueira M, Galindo I, et al. Seroreactivity against raw insect-derived recombinant KMPII, TRYP, and LACK *Leishmania infantum* proteins in infected dogs. *Vet Parasitol.* 2009;164:154–161.
202. Pinheiro PH, Pinheiro AN, Ferreira JH, et al. A recombinant cysteine proteinase from *Leishmania (Leishmania) chagasi* as an antigen for delayed-type hypersensitivity assays and serodiagnosis of canine visceral leishmaniasis. *Vet Parasitol.* 2009;162:32–39.
203. Carvalho FA, Charest H, Tavares CA, et al. Diagnosis of American visceral leishmaniasis in humans and dogs using the recombinant *Leishmania donovani* A2 antigen. *Diagn Microbiol Infect Dis.* 2002;43:289–295.
204. Soto M, Requena JM, Quijada L, et al. Multicomponent chimeric antigen for serodiagnosis of canine visceral leishmaniasis. *J Clin Microbiol.* 1998;36:58–63.
205. Coelho EA, Ramirez L, Costa MA, et al. Specific serodiagnosis of canine visceral leishmaniasis using *Leishmania* species ribosomal protein extracts. *Clin Vaccine Immunol.* 2009;16:1774–1780.
206. Barbosa-De-Deus R, Dos Mares-Guia ML, Nunes AZ, et al. *Leishmania major*-like antigen for specific and sensitive serodiagnosis of human and canine visceral leishmaniasis. *Clin Diagn Lab Immunol.* 2002;9:1361–1366.
207. Oliveira TM, Furuta PI, de Carvalho D, et al. A study of cross-reactivity in serum samples from dogs positive for *Leishmania* sp., *Babesia canis* and *Ehrlichia canis* in enzyme-linked immunosorbent assay and indirect fluorescent antibody test. *Rev Bras Parasitol Vet.* 2008;17:7–11.
208. Ashford DA, Bozza M, Freire M, et al. Comparison of the polymerase chain reaction and serology for the detection of canine visceral leishmaniasis. *Am J Trop Med Hyg.* 1995;53:251–255.
209. Mathis A, Deplazes P. PCR and in vitro cultivation for detection of *Leishmania* spp. in diagnostic samples from humans and dogs. *J Clin Microbiol.* 1995;33:1145–1149.
210. Lachaud L, Marchergui-Hammami S, Chabbert E, et al. Comparison of six PCR methods using peripheral blood for detection of canine visceral leishmaniasis. *J Clin Microbiol.* 2002;40:210–215.
211. Ikonomopoulos J, Kokotas S, Gazouli M, et al. Molecular diagnosis of leishmaniosis in dogs. Comparative application of traditional diagnostic methods and the proposed assay on clinical samples. *Vet Parasitol.* 2003;113:99–113.
212. Roura X, Fondevila D, Sanchez A, et al. Detection of *Leishmania* infection in paraffin-embedded skin biopsies of dogs using polymerase chain reaction. *J Vet Diagn Invest.* 1999;11:385–387.
213. Maia C, Ramada J, Cristovao JM, et al. Diagnosis of canine leishmaniasis: conventional and molecular techniques using different tissues. *Vet J.* 2009;179:142–144.
214. Manna L, Reale S, Vitale F, et al. Real-time PCR assay in *Leishmania*-infected dogs treated with meglumine antimoniate and allopurinol. *Vet J.* 2008;177:279–282.
215. Solano-Gallego L, Rodriguez-Cortes A, Trotta M, et al. Detection of *Leishmania infantum* DNA by fret-based real-time PCR in urine from dogs with natural clinical leishmaniosis. *Vet Parasitol.* 2007;147:315–319.
216. Strauss-Ayali D, Jaffe CL, Burshtain O, et al. Polymerase chain reaction using noninvasively obtained samples, for the detection of *Leishmania infantum* DNA in dogs. *J Infect Dis.* 2004;189:1729–1733.
217. Leite RS, Mendes VC, Ferreira AL, et al. The use of conjunctival swab samples for PCR screening for visceral leishmaniasis in vaccinated dogs. *Rev Bras Parasitol Vet.* 2011;20:36–41.
218. Ferreira Sde A, Ituassu LT, de Melo MN, et al. Evaluation of the conjunctival swab for canine visceral leishmaniasis diagnosis by PCR-hybridization in Minas Gerais State, Brazil. *Vet Parasitol.* 2008;152:257–263.
219. Aschar M, de Oliveira ET, Laurenti MD, et al. Value of the oral swab for the molecular diagnosis of dogs in different stages of infection with *Leishmania infantum*. *Vet Parasitol.* 2016;225:108–113.
220. Belinchon-Lorenzo S, Iniesta V, Parejo JC, et al. Detection of *Leishmania infantum* kinetoplast minicircle DNA by real time PCR in hair of dogs with leishmaniosis. *Vet Parasitol.* 2013;192:43–50.
221. de Sousa Goncalves R, Franke CR, Magalhaes-Junior JT, et al. Association between *Leishmania infantum* DNA in the hair of dogs and their infectiousness to *Lutzomyia longipalpis*. *Vet Parasitol.* 2016;232:43–47.
222. Belinchon-Lorenzo S, Parejo JC, Iniesta V, et al. First detection of *Leishmania* kDNA in canine cerumen samples by qPCR. *Vet Parasitol.* 2016;228:65–68.

223. Santos TR, Carreira VS, Ferrari HF, et al. Comparison of PCR with stained slides of bone marrow and lymph nodes aspirates with suspect diagnosis for leishmaniasis. *Acta Trop.* 2014;140:137–140.
224. Lima T, Martinez-Sogues L, Montserrat-Sangra S, et al. Diagnostic performance of a qPCR for *Leishmania* on stained cytological specimens and on filter paper impressions obtained from cutaneous lesions suggestive of canine leishmaniosis. *Vet Dermatol.* 2019;30:318–e389.
225. Castellanos-Gonzalez A, Saldarriaga OA, Tartaglino L, et al. A novel molecular test to diagnose canine visceral leishmaniasis at the point of care. *Am J Trop Med Hyg.* 2015;93:970–975.
226. Adamama-Moraitou KK, Rallis TS, Koytinas AF, et al. Asymptomatic colitis in naturally infected dogs with *Leishmania infantum*: a prospective study. *Am J Trop Med Hyg.* 2007;76:53–57.
227. Barrouin-Melo SM, Larangeira DF, Santos SO, et al. A standardized cytological and immunochemical method for the analysis of fine-needle spleen aspirates: assessment of leukocyte population changes in canine visceral leishmaniosis. *Vet Immunol Immunopathol.* 2006;111:251–261.
228. Giunchetti RC, Martins-Filho OA, Carneiro CM, et al. Histopathology, parasite density and cell phenotypes of the popliteal lymph node in canine visceral leishmaniasis. *Vet Immunol Immunopathol.* 2008;121:23–33.
229. Mylonakis ME, Papaioannou N, Saridomichelakis MN, et al. Cytologic patterns of lymphadenopathy in dogs infected with *Leishmania infantum*. *Vet Clin Pathol.* 2005;34:243–247.
230. Costa FA, Goto H, Saldanha LC, et al. Histopathologic patterns of nephropathy in naturally acquired canine visceral leishmaniasis. *Vet Pathol.* 2003;40:677–684.
231. Nieto CG, Navarrete I, Habela MA, et al. Pathological changes in kidneys of dogs with natural *Leishmania* infection. *Vet Parasitol.* 1992;45:33–47.
232. Zatelli A, Borgarelli M, Santilli R, et al. Glomerular lesions in dogs infected with *Leishmania* organisms. *Am J Vet Res.* 2003;64:558–561.
233. Plevraki K, Koutinas AF, Kaldrymidou H, et al. Effects of allopurinol treatment on the progression of chronic nephritis in canine leishmaniosis (*Leishmania infantum*). *J Vet Intern Med.* 2006;20:228–233.
234. Rallis T, Day MJ, Saridomichelakis MN, et al. Chronic hepatitis associated with canine leishmaniosis (*Leishmania infantum*): a clinicopathological study of 26 cases. *J Comp Pathol.* 2005;132:145–152.
235. Melo FA, Moura EP, Ribeiro RR, et al. Hepatic extracellular matrix alterations in dogs naturally infected with *Leishmania (Leishmania) chagasi*. *Int J Exp Pathol.* 2009;90:538–548.
236. Melo F, Amaral M, Oliveira P, et al. Diffuse intralobular liver fibrosis in dogs naturally infected with *Leishmania (Leishmania) chagasi*. *Am J Trop Med Hyg.* 2008;79:198–204.
237. Melo GD, Marcondes M, Vasconcelos RO, et al. Leukocyte entry into the CNS of *Leishmania chagasi* naturally infected dogs. *Vet Parasitol.* 2009;162:248–256.
238. Silva FL, Rodrigues AA, Rego IO, et al. Genital lesions and distribution of amastigotes in bitches naturally infected with *Leishmania chagasi*. *Vet Parasitol.* 2008;151:86–90.
239. Bourdoiseau G, Marchal T, Magnol JP. Immunohistochemical detection of *Leishmania infantum* in formalin-fixed, paraffin-embedded sections of canine skin and lymph nodes. *J Vet Diagn Invest.* 1997;9:439–440.
240. Ferrer L, Rabanal RM, Domingo M, et al. Identification of *Leishmania donovani* amastigotes in canine tissues by immunoperoxidase staining. *Res Vet Sci.* 1988;44:194–196.
241. Baneth G, Shaw SE. Chemotherapy of canine leishmaniosis. *Vet Parasitol.* 2002;106:315–324.
242. Noli C, Auxilia ST. Treatment of canine Old World visceral leishmaniasis: a systematic review. *Vet Dermatol.* 2005;16:213–232.
243. Miro G, Petersen C, Cardoso L, et al. Novel areas for prevention and control of canine leishmaniosis. *Trends Parasitol.* 2017;33:718–730.
244. Slappendel RJ, Teske E. The effect of intravenous or subcutaneous administration of meglumine antimonate (Glucantime) in dogs with leishmaniasis. A randomized clinical trial. *Vet Q.* 1997;19:10–13.
245. Tassi P, Ormas P, Madonna M, et al. Pharmacokinetics of N-methylglucamine antimoniate after intravenous, intramuscular and subcutaneous administration in the dog. *Res Vet Sci.* 1994;56:144–150.
246. Valladares JE, Alberola J, Esteban M, et al. Disposition of antimony after the administration of N-methylglucamine antimoniate to dogs. *Vet Rec.* 1996;138:181–183.
247. Carrio J, Portus M. In vitro susceptibility to pentavalent antimony in *Leishmania infantum* strains is not modified during in vitro or in vivo passages but is modified after host treatment with meglumine antimoniate. *BMC Pharmacol.* 2002;2:11.
248. Carrio J, Riera C, Gallego M, et al. In vitro activity of pentavalent antimony derivatives on promastigotes and intracellular amastigotes of *Leishmania infantum* strains from humans and dogs in Spain. *Acta Trop.* 2001;79:179–183.
249. Gradoni L, Gramiccia M, Scalone A. Visceral leishmaniasis treatment, Italy. *Emerg Infect Dis.* 2003;9:1617–1620.
250. Cavaliero T, Arnold P, Mathis A, et al. Clinical, serologic, and parasitologic follow-up after long-term allopurinol therapy of dogs naturally infected with *Leishmania infantum*. *J Vet Intern Med.* 1999;13:330–334.
251. Koutinas AF, Saridomichelakis MN, Mylonakis ME, et al. A randomised, blinded, placebo-controlled clinical trial with allopurinol in canine leishmaniosis. *Vet Parasitol.* 2001;98:247–261.
252. Yasur-Landau D, Jaffe CL, David L, et al. Allopurinol resistance in *Leishmania infantum* from dogs with disease relapse. *PLoS Negl Trop Dis.* 2016;10:e0004341.
253. Lester SJ, Kenyon JE. Use of allopurinol to treat visceral leishmaniosis in a dog. *J Am Vet Med Assoc.* 1996;209:615–617.
254. Solano-Gallego L, Di Filippo L, Ordeix L, et al. Early reduction of *Leishmania infantum*-specific antibodies and blood parasitemia during treatment in dogs with moderate or severe disease. *Parasit Vectors.* 2016;9:235.
255. Manna L, Gravino AE, Picillo E, et al. *Leishmania* DNA quantification by real-time PCR in naturally infected dogs treated with miltefosine. *Ann N Y Acad Sci.* 2008;1149:358–360.
256. Mateo M, Maynard L, Vischer C, et al. Comparative study on the short term efficacy and adverse effects of miltefosine and meglumine antimoniate in dogs with natural leishmaniosis. *Parasitol Res.* 2009;105:155–162.
257. Manna L, Reale S, Picillo E, et al. Interferon-gamma (INF-gamma), IL4 expression levels and *Leishmania* DNA load as prognostic markers for monitoring response to treatment of leishmaniotic dogs with miltefosine and allopurinol. *Cytokine.* 2008;44:288–292.
258. Miro G, Oliva G, Cruz I, et al. Multicentric, controlled clinical study to evaluate effectiveness and safety of miltefosine and allopurinol for canine leishmaniosis. *Vet Dermatol.* 2009;20:397–404.
259. Poli A, Sozzi S, Guidi G, et al. Comparison of aminosidine (paromomycin) and sodium stibogluconate for treatment of canine leishmaniasis. *Vet Parasitol.* 1997;71:263–271.
260. Rhalem A, Sahibi H, Lasri S, et al. Analysis of immune responses in dogs with canine visceral leishmaniasis before, and after, drug treatment. *Vet Immunol Immunopathol.* 1999;71:69–76.
261. Pennisi MG, De Majo M, Masucci M, et al. Efficacy of the treatment of dogs with leishmaniosis with a combination of metronidazole and spiramycin. *Vet Rec.* 2005;156:346–349.
262. Baxarias M, Martinez-Orellana P, Baneth G, et al. Immunotherapy in clinical canine leishmaniosis: a comparative update. *Res Vet Sci.* 2019;125:218–226.
263. Toepp A, Larson M, Wilson G, et al. Randomized, controlled, double-blinded field trial to assess *Leishmania* vaccine effectiveness as immunotherapy for canine leishmaniosis. *Vaccine.* 2018;36:6433–6441.
264. Segarra S, Miro G, Montoya A, et al. Prevention of disease progression in *Leishmania infantum*-infected dogs with dietary nucleotides and active hexose correlated compound. *Parasit Vectors.* 2018;11:103.
265. Martinez-Orellana P, Mari-Martorell D, Montserrat-Sangra S, et al. *Leishmania infantum*-specific IFN-gamma production in stimulated blood from dogs with clinical leishmaniosis at diagnosis and during treatment. *Vet Parasitol.* 2017;248:39–47.
266. Ashford DA, David JR, Freire M, et al. Studies on control of visceral leishmaniasis: impact of dog control on canine and human visceral leishmaniasis in Jacobina, Bahia, Brazil. *Am J Trop Med Hyg.* 1998;59:53–57.

267. Dietze R, Barros GB, Teixeira L, et al. Effect of eliminating seropositive canines on the transmission of visceral leishmaniasis in Brazil. *Clin Infect Dis.* 1997;25:1240–1242.
268. Nunes CM, Lima VM, Paula HB, et al. Dog culling and replacement in an area endemic for visceral leishmaniasis in Brazil. *Vet Parasitol.* 2008;153:19–23.
269. Palatnik-de-Sousa CB, dos Santos WR, Franca-Silva JC, et al. Impact of canine control on the epidemiology of canine and human visceral leishmaniasis in Brazil. *Am J Trop Med Hyg.* 2001;65:510–517.
270. Alexander B, Maroli M. Control of phlebotomine sandflies. *Med Vet Entomol.* 2003;17:1–18.
271. Mencke N, Volf P, Volfova V, et al. Repellent efficacy of a combination containing imidacloprid and permethrin against sand flies (*Phlebotomus papatasi*) in dogs. *Parasitol Res.* 2003;90(suppl 3):S108–111.
272. Otranto D, Paradies P, Lia RP, et al. Efficacy of a combination of 10% imidacloprid/50% permethrin for the prevention of leishmaniasis in kennelled dogs in an endemic area. *Vet Parasitol.* 2007;144:270–278.
273. Podaliri Vulpiani M, Iannetti L, Di Mattia T, et al. *Leishmania infantum* in a Central Italy dog shelter: retrospective study of serologic reactivity during a 4-year period in a confined dog population subjected to preventive and therapeutic treatment. *Vet Parasitol.* 2009;160:190–197.
274. David JR, Stamm LM, Bezerra HS, et al. Deltamethrin-impregnated dog collars have a potent anti-feeding and insecticidal effect on *Lutzomyia longipalpis* and *Lutzomyia migonei*. *Mem Inst Oswaldo Cruz.* 2001;96:839–847.
275. Foglia Manzillo V, Piantedosi D, Cortese L. Detection of *Leishmania infantum* in canine peripheral blood. *Vet Rec.* 2005;156:151–152.
276. Killick-Kendrick R, Killick-Kendrick M, Focheux C, et al. Protection of dogs from bites of phlebotomine sandflies by deltamethrin collars for control of canine leishmaniasis. *Med Vet Entomol.* 1997;11:105–111.
277. Gavgani AS, Hodjati MH, Mohite H, et al. Effect of insecticide-impregnated dog collars on incidence of zoonotic visceral leishmaniasis in Iranian children: a matched-cluster randomised trial. *Lancet.* 2002;360:374–379.
278. Dantas-Torres F, Nogueira FDS, Menz I, et al. Vaccination against canine leishmaniasis in Brazil. *Int J Parasitol.* 2020;50:171–176.
279. Sabate D, Llinas J, Homedes J, et al. A single-centre, open-label, controlled, randomized clinical trial to assess the preventive efficacy of a domperidone-based treatment programme against clinical canine leishmaniasis in a high prevalence area. *Prev Vet Med.* 2014;115:56–63.
280. Anstead GM, Chandrasekar B, Zhao W, et al. Malnutrition alters the innate immune response and increases early visceralization following *Leishmania donovani* infection. *Infect Immun.* 2001;69:4709–4718.
281. Badaro R, Jones TC, Lorenco R, et al. A prospective study of visceral leishmaniasis in an endemic area of Brazil. *J Infect Dis.* 1986;154:639–649.
282. World Health Organization. Leishmaniasis: Key Facts. 2021. https://www.who.int/news-room/fact-sheets/detail/leishmaniasis
283. Margonari C, Freitas CR, Ribeiro RC, et al. Epidemiology of visceral leishmaniasis through spatial analysis, in Belo Horizonte municipality, state of Minas Gerais, Brazil. *Mem Inst Oswaldo Cruz.* 2006;101:31–38.
284. Acedo Sanchez C, Martin Sanchez J, Velez Bernal ID, et al. Leishmaniasis eco-epidemiology in the Alpujarra region (Granada Province, southern Spain). *Int J Parasitol.* 1996;26:303–310.
285. Papadopoulou C, Kostoula A, Dimitriou D, et al. Human and canine leishmaniasis in asymptomatic and symptomatic population in Northwestern Greece. *J Infect.* 2005;50:53–60.
286. Otranto D, Dantas-Torres F. The prevention of canine leishmaniasis and its impact on public health. *Trends Parasitol.* 2013;29:339–345.
287. Cruz I, Morales MA, Noguer I, et al. *Leishmania* in discarded syringes from intravenous drug users. *Lancet.* 2002;359:1124–1125.
288. Agut A, Corzo N, Murciano J, et al. Clinical and radiographic study of bone and joint lesions in 26 dogs with leishmaniasis. *Vet Rec.* 2003;153:648–652.
289. Dantas-Torres F. Canine leishmaniosis in South America. *Parasit Vectors.* 2009;2(suppl 1):S1.
290. Madeira Md Mde F, Uchoa CM, Leal CA, et al. *Leishmania (Viannia) braziliensis* in naturally infected dogs. *Rev Soc Bras Med Trop.* 2003;36:551–555.
291. Reithinger R, Davies CR. Is the domestic dog (*Canis familiaris*) a reservoir host of American cutaneous leishmaniasis? A critical review of the current evidence. *Am J Trop Med Hyg.* 1999;61:530–541.
292. Padilla AM, Marco JD, Diosque P, et al. Canine infection and the possible role of dogs in the transmission of American tegumentary leishmaniosis in Salta, Argentina. *Vet Parasitol.* 2002;110:1–10.
293. Carvalho FS, Wenceslau AA, Albuquerque GR, et al. *Leishmania (Viannia) braziliensis* in dogs in Brazil: epidemiology, co-infection, and clinical aspects. *Genet Mol Res.* 2015;14:12062–12073.
294. Lago J, Silva JA, Borja L, et al. Clinical and histopathologic features of canine tegumentary leishmaniasis and the molecular characterization of *Leishmania braziliensis* in dogs. *PLoS Negl Trop Dis.* 2019;13:e0007532.
295. Castro EA, Thomaz-Soccol V, Augur C, et al. *Leishmania (Viannia) braziliensis*: epidemiology of canine cutaneous leishmaniasis in the State of Parana (Brazil). *Exp Parasitol.* 2007;117:13–21.
296. dos Santos IB, Schubach TM, Leme LR, et al. Sporotrichosis: the main differential diagnosis with tegumentary leishmaniosis in dogs from Rio de Janeiro, Brazil. *Vet Parasitol.* 2007;143:1–6.
297. Pirmez C, Coutinho SG, Marzochi MC, et al. Canine American cutaneous leishmaniasis: a clinical and immunological study in dogs naturally infected with *Leishmania braziliensis braziliensis* in an endemic area of Rio de Janeiro, Brazil. *Am J Trop Med Hyg.* 1988;38:52–58.
298. Madeira Mde F, Schubach Ade O, Schubach TM, et al. Is *Leishmania (Viannia) braziliensis* preferentially restricted to the cutaneous lesions of naturally infected dogs? *Parasitol Res.* 2005;97:73–76.
299. de Fatima Madeira M, de OSA, Schubach TM, et al. Post mortem parasitological evaluation of dogs seroreactive for *Leishmania* from Rio de Janeiro, Brazil. *Vet Parasitol.* 2006;138:366–370.
300. Madeira MF, Schubach A, Schubach TM, et al. Mixed infection with *Leishmania (Viannia) braziliensis* and *Leishmania (Leishmania) chagasi* in a naturally infected dog from Rio de Janeiro, Brazil. *Trans R Soc Trop Med Hyg.* 2006;100:442–445.
301. Madeira MF, Sousa MA, Barros JH, et al. *Trypanosoma caninum* n. sp. (Protozoa: Kinetoplastida) isolated from intact skin of a domestic dog (*Canis familiaris*) captured in Rio de Janeiro, Brazil. *Parasitology.* 2009;136:411–423.
302. Andrade RA, Silva Araujo MS, Reis AB, et al. Advances in flow cytometric serology for canine visceral leishmaniasis: diagnostic applications when distinct clinical forms, vaccination and other canine pathogens become a challenge. *Vet Immunol Immunopathol.* 2009;128:79–86.
303. Santiago Mde A, Ribeiro FC, Mouta-Confort E, et al. Differentiation between canine cutaneous and visceral leishmaniasis by the detection of immunoglobulin G specific for *Leishmania (Viannia) braziliensis* and *Leishmania (Leishmania) chagasi* antigens using flow cytometry. *Vet Parasitol.* 2008;154:341–346.
304. de Andrade HM, Reis AB, dos Santos SL, et al. Use of PCR-RFLP to identify *Leishmania* species in naturally-infected dogs. *Vet Parasitol.* 2006;140:231–238.
305. Barbosa Santos EG, Marzochi MC, Conceicao NF, et al. N-methylglucamine antimonate (SbV+): intralesional canine tegumentary leishmaniasis therapy. *Parasite.* 1998;5:175–180.
306. Dantas-Torres F. The role of dogs as reservoirs of *Leishmania* parasites, with emphasis on *Leishmania (Leishmania) infantum* and *Leishmania (Viannia) braziliensis*. *Vet Parasitol.* 2007;149:139–146.
307. Dantas-Torres F. Dogs as reservoirs for *Leishmania braziliensis*. *Emerg Infect Dis.* 2011;17:326–327, author reply 327.
308. Sergent E, Sergent E, Lombard J, et al. La leishmaniose à Alger. Infection simultanée d'un enfant, d'un chien et d'un chat dans la même habitation. *Bull Soc Pathol Exot.* 1912;5:93–98.
309. Ozon C, Marty P, Pratlong F, et al. Disseminated feline leishmaniosis due to *Leishmania infantum* in Southern France. *Vet Parasitol.* 1998;75:273–277.
310. Savani ES, de Oliveira Camargo MC, de Carvalho MR, et al. The first record in the Americas of an autochthonous case of *Leishmania (Leishma-*

nia) infantum chagasi in a domestic cat (*Felix catus*) from Cotia County, Sao Paulo State, Brazil. *Vet Parasitol.* 2004;120:229–233.

311. Barnes JC, Stanley O, Craig TM. Diffuse cutaneous leishmaniasis in a cat. *J Am Vet Med Assoc.* 1993;202:416–418.
312. Schubach TM, Figueiredo FB, Pereira SA, et al. American cutaneous leishmaniasis in two cats from Rio de Janeiro, Brazil: first report of natural infection with *Leishmania (Viannia) braziliensis. Trans R Soc Trop Med Hyg.* 2004;98:165–167.
313. de Souza AI, Barros EM, Ishikawa E, et al. Feline leishmaniasis due to *Leishmania (Leishmania) amazonensis* in Mato Grosso do Sul State, Brazil. *Vet Parasitol.* 2005;128:41–45.
314. Ayllon T, Tesouro MA, Amusategui I, et al. Serologic and molecular evaluation of *Leishmania infantum* in cats from Central Spain. *Ann N Y Acad Sci.* 2008;1149:361–364.
315. Maia C, Gomes J, Cristovao J, et al. Feline *Leishmania* infection in a canine leishmaniasis endemic region, Portugal. *Vet Parasitol.* 2010;174:336–340.
316. Portús M, Gàllego M, Riera C, et al. Wild and domestic mammals in the life cycle of *Leishmania infantum* in Southwest Europe. A literature review and studies performed in Catalonia (Spain). *Rev Iber Parasitol.* 2002;62:72–76.
317. Solano-Gallego L, Rodriguez-Cortes A, Iniesta L, et al. Cross-sectional serosurvey of feline leishmaniasis in ecoregions around the Northwestern Mediterranean. *Am J Trop Med Hyg.* 2007;76:676–680.
318. Maia C, Nunes M, Campino L. Importance of cats in zoonotic leishmaniasis in Portugal. *Vector Borne Zoonotic Dis.* 2008;8:555–559.
319. Tabar MD, Altet L, Francino O, et al. Vector-borne infections in cats: molecular study in Barcelona area (Spain). *Vet Parasitol.* 2008;151:332–336.
320. Maroli M, Pennisi MG, Di Muccio T, et al. Infection of sandflies by a cat naturally infected with *Leishmania infantum. Vet Parasitol.* 2007;145:357–360.
321. Leiva M, Lloret A, Pena T, et al. Therapy of ocular and visceral leishmaniasis in a cat. *Vet Ophthalmol.* 2005;8:71–75.
322. Grevot A, Jaussaud Hugues P, Marty P, et al. Leishmaniosis due to *Leishmania infantum* in a FIV and FelV positive cat with a squamous cell carcinoma diagnosed with histological, serological and isoenzymatic methods. *Parasite.* 2005;12:271–275.
323. Akhtardanesh B, Moeini E, Sharifi I, et al. *Leishmania* infection in cats positive for immunodeficiency virus and feline leukemia virus in an endemic region of Iran. *Vet Parasitol Reg Stud Reports.* 2020;20:100387.
324. Marcos R, Santos M, Malhao F, et al. Pancytopenia in a cat with visceral leishmaniasis. *Vet Clin Pathol.* 2009;38:201–205.
325. Fernandez-Gallego A, Feo Bernabe L, Dalmau A, et al. Feline leishmaniosis: diagnosis, treatment and outcome in 16 cats. *J Feline Med Surg.* 2020;22:993–1007.
326. Craig TM, Barton CL, Mercer SH, et al. Dermal leishmaniasis in a Texas cat. *Am J Trop Med Hyg.* 1986;35:1100–1102.
327. Trainor KE, Porter BF, Logan KS, et al. Eight cases of feline cutaneous leishmaniasis in Texas. *Vet Pathol.* 2010;47:1076–1081.
328. Rivas AK, Alcover M, Martinez-Orellana P, et al. Clinical and diagnostic aspects of feline cutaneous leishmaniosis in Venezuela. *Parasit Vectors.* 2018;11:141.
329. Paniz Mondolfi AE, Colmenares Garmendia A, Mendoza Perez Y, et al. Autochthonous cutaneous leishmaniasis in urban domestic animals (*Felis catus / Canis lupus familiaris*) from central-western Venezuela. *Acta Trop.* 2019;191:252–260.
330. Passos VM, Lasmar EB, Gontijo CM, et al. Natural infection of a domestic cat (*Felis domesticus*) with *Leishmania* (*Viannia*) in the metropolitan region of Belo Horizonte, State of Minas Gerais, Brazil. *Mem Inst Oswaldo Cruz.* 1996;91:19–20.
331. Simoes-Mattos L, Mattos MR, Teixeira MJ, et al. The susceptibility of domestic cats (*Felis catus*) to experimental infection with *Leishmania braziliensis. Vet Parasitol.* 2005;127:199–208.
332. Coelho WM, Richini-Pereira VB, Langoni H, et al. Molecular detection of *Leishmania* sp. in cats (*Felis catus*) from Andradina Municipality, Sao Paulo State, Brazil. *Vet Parasitol.* 2011;176:281–282.
333. Brianti E, Falsone L, Napoli E, et al. Prevention of feline leishmaniosis with an imidacloprid 10%/flumethrin 4.5% polymer matrix collar. *Parasit Vectors.* 2017;10:334.

97

Babesiosis

Adam J. Birkenheuer

KEY POINTS

- First Described: Early descriptions of intraerythrocytic parasites in dogs with signs of babesiosis were made in Africa in 1893.[1] The first documented case of canine babesiosis in the United States was in 1934.[2]
- Cause: *Babesia canis, Babesia rossi, Babesia vogeli, Babesia gibsoni, Babesia conradae, Babesia vulpes, Babesia negevi* sp. nov. (dogs); *Babesia felis, B. canis, B. gibsoni, Babesia cati, Babesia lengau* (cats); several other unnamed *Babesia* species (dogs and cats) (phylum Apicomplexa).
- Affected Hosts: Domestic dogs and cats.
- Geographic Distribution: Worldwide, but different *Babesia* species vary in their geographic distribution.
- Mode of Transmission: A variety of tick vector species; fighting or biting interactions; vertical (perinatal) transmission; blood transfusion.
- Major Clinical Signs: Lethargy, pallor, splenomegaly. Many infected dogs show no overt clinical signs. Dogs with severe babesiosis (*B. rossi*) may show neurologic signs, anuria, tachypnea, and poor perfusion parameters.
- Differential Diagnoses: IMHA and/or ITP, other causes of hemolysis such as oxidative toxins or microangiopathic hemolysis (e.g., with splenic hemangiosarcoma). Other causes of protein-losing nephropathy (borreliosis, immune-mediated, amyloidosis, etc.). Canine monocytic ehrlichiosis, RMSF, bacterial endocarditis, and hemoplasmosis should also be considered.
- Human Health Significance: *Babesia* species that infect dogs and cats are not known to infect humans.

ETIOLOGY AND EPIDEMIOLOGY

Babesia spp. are intraerythrocytic protozoan parasites of the phylum Apicomplexa. Babesiosis is the disease caused by infection with organisms from the genus *Babesia.* Babesiosis is classically characterized by hemolytic anemia, thrombocytopenia, fever, and splenomegaly and can be a severe, life-threatening illness. *Babesia* infections can also be subclinical. Altogether, more than 100 species of *Babesia* have been described, and with the advent of molecular techniques such as PCR assays, new species and genotypes are identified each year. Historically, species have been named and identified based on the vertebrate host and the size of the parasite (large or small *Babesia* species). Large *Babesia* spp. are 3 to 7 µm in length, whereas small *Babesia* spp. are 1 to 3 µm in length. However, molecular phylogenetic analyses are critical for accurate identification and classification of *Babesia* spp. In most parts of the world, tick vectors are the most important means of transmission of *Babesia* species. For some *Babesia* species, such as *Babesia gibsoni* in North America and Europe, direct transmission between dogs, through fighting (and exchange of blood), or vertical (transplacental) transmission, is believed to be the most common route of transmission when competent tick vectors are absent.[3–5]

When ticks are involved in transmission, sporozoites are released from the tick salivary glands as the tick feeds and they enter the bloodstream of the vertebrate host (Fig. 97.1). They then attach to, and are endocytosed by, erythrocytes. Within the erythrocytes, they undergo asexual reproduction (merogony), and the daughter cells infect new erythrocytes. A naïve tick then ingests infected erythrocytes. It is unclear whether transformation from merozoite to gametocyte begins in the vertebrate host or in the tick. In the tick midgut, the sexual phase of reproduction occurs when the gametocytes fuse to form a zygote. The zygote invades epithelial cells of the tick gut. The resultant forms, known as ookinetes, leave the epithelial cell and invade either the salivary gland or the ovary, where they participate in transstadial or transovarial transmission, respectively. Prior to transmission, another asexual form of reproduction occurs in the salivary gland, sporogony.

Canine Babesiosis

Canine babesiosis is a disease of worldwide importance. Initially, two species of *Babesia* were recognized in dogs (*Babesia canis* and *B. gibsoni*); however, now at least nine genetically distinct canine piroplasms have been described.[6] Periodically, infections with piroplasmid species from other hosts have been documented using molecular assays.[7,8] Formal changes in eukaryotic nomenclature, including *Babesia* sp., should be proposed through the International Commission on Zoological Nomenclature (ICZN: http://www.iczn.org/). Unfortunately, there have not been formal proposals through the ICZN for the majority of *Babesia* spp. which has led to confusion when navigating the primary literature where many species are referred to using different nomenclature.

Babesia species that infect dogs vary in their geographic distribution; however, due to movement of infected animals, movement of tick vectors, and increased recognition due to improved diagnostic techniques, geographic range of many *Babesia* spp. is expanding. As new organisms are recognized, it has become more important for the clinician to understand the differences in diagnosis, prognosis, and treatment for infection with each organism.

Large *Babesia* Species

Large *Babesia* species are recognized throughout the world. The first description of a large canine *Babesia* species was by Piana in 1895 and is generally accepted to describe *B. canis.*[9] Likewise, *Babesia rossi* was first described in 1910 and 1912 by Nutall, and *Babesia vogeli* was described by Reichenow in 1935 and 1937.[10–13] In 1989, Uilenberg proposed that these organisms were all subspecies of a single species and proposed the names *B. canis canis*, *B. canis rossi*, and *B. canis vogeli.*[14] Since none

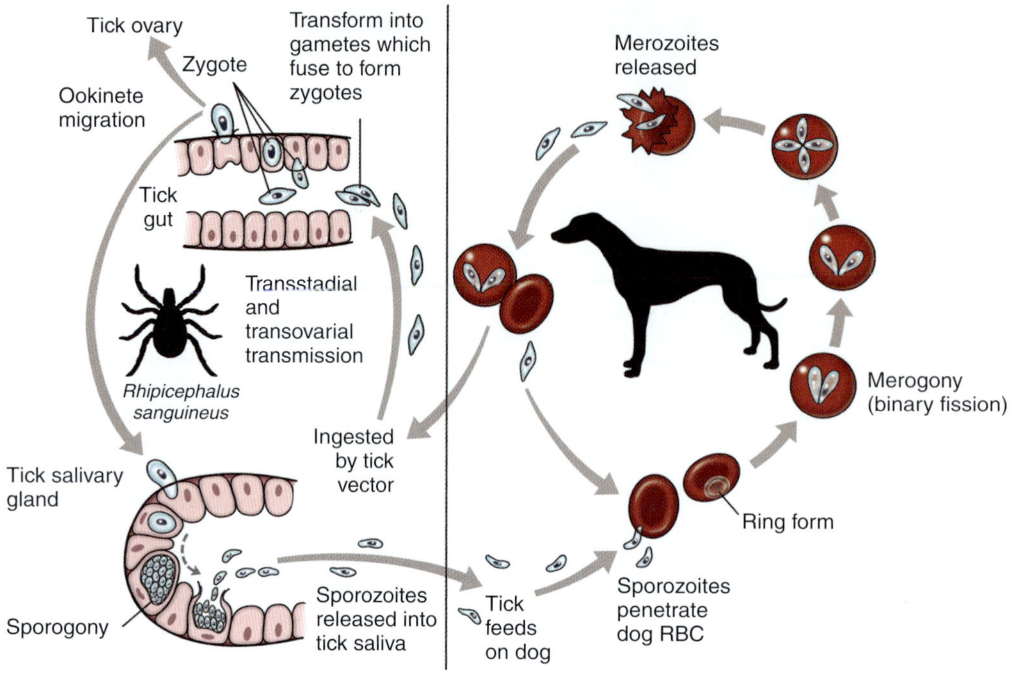

Fig. 97.1 Life cycle of *Babesia canis.*

of these descriptions or proposals have met the standards of the ICZN, the original proposed nomenclature is now used: *B. canis*, *B. rossi*, and *B. vogeli*. Genetically unique large canine *Babesia* spp. that have been more recently described will be referred to as: *Babesia* sp. (followed by author and year of original description).

Babesia vogeli is the most common large *Babesia* species in the United States and transmitted by the brown dog tick *(Rhipicephalus sanguineus)*.[15] Infection is most commonly diagnosed in warm, humid regions of the world, and while transmission may be seasonal in some regions, disease manifestation can occur throughout the year. *Babesia vogeli* can be found in Africa, Asia, Australia, Europe, and the Americas (Fig. 97.2A).[15] The reported seroprevalence of *B. vogeli* in dogs has ranged from 3.8% to 59%.[16] The prevalence of seroreactivity is higher in adult dogs than in dogs younger than 1 year.[17] Greyhounds appear to have a higher rate of exposure and infection than other breeds. There is no definitive evidence that greyhounds are more susceptible to *B. vogeli* infection than other breeds, and it is this author's opinion that the higher rates of infection are secondary to increased risks such as exposure to infected ticks and direct dog-to-dog transmission (perinatal/transplacental and bites). In an antibody serosurvey of dogs in Florida, 46% of 393 greyhounds were seroreactive.[16] The prevalence of seroreactive dogs within these kennels ranged from 17% to 100%; the lower prevalence was noted in kennels with more intensive tick control. None of 50 non-greyhound, individually housed adult pet dogs within the same geographic area were seroreactive, which implicated environment and breed susceptibility as possible risk factors in endemic areas.[16] Transplacental transmission of *B. vogeli* infections is strongly suspected but has not yet been definitively documented.[18]

Babesia canis is the most commonly detected *Babesia* sp. in Europe, but is occasionally detected in dogs that have been imported from or traveled to Europe (Fig. 97.2B). *Babesia canis* is transmitted by the ornate cow tick, *Dermacentor reticulatus*.[15,19] The incidence of infection is highest in the fall and spring. Higher prevalence rates are most commonly found in rural or suburban areas that are adjacent to prairies or woodlands that provide suitable habitat for *D. reticulatus*.[20] *Babesia canis* infection has been commonly diagnosed in France. However, infections are being reported more frequently from other European countries such as Croatia, Poland, Germany, and the United Kingdom, likely due in part to changes in the distribution of *D. reticulatus*.[21,22] Outbreaks of disease due to *B. canis* infection in Polish sled dogs share many similarities with those due to *B. vogeli* infection in North American greyhounds.[23]

Babesia rossi is transmitted by the yellow dog tick, *Haemaphysalis elliptica* (syn. *Haemaphysalis leachi*).[24] Black-backed jackals are natural hosts for *B. rossi*.[25] Reports of autochthonous *B. rossi* infection have been limited to Africa, with the vast majority of reports coming from South Africa, where more than 10% of the dogs evaluated in some veterinary hospitals may be affected.[26,27] A 2021 study of vector-borne pathogens in 209 owned or stray dogs in Malawi identified *B. rossi* as the most prevalent vector-borne pathogen, infecting 23% of dogs as determined using PCR.[28] The incidence of infection is highest during the summer months. Breed predispositions for infection have not been well studied, but the traditional fighting breeds (American pit bull terriers [APBT], Staffordshire bull terriers, and bull terriers) are more likely to die when they are diagnosed with severe babesiosis.[29] Recent surveys have suggested a decline in the number of cases of babesiosis treated in South African hospitals since 2011 with a sharp decline in 2015. This decline coincides with the introduction of isoxazoline use in South Africa and has been postulated as a possible cause for some of the decline.[30]

Unnamed Large *Babesia* Species. At least two genetically unique large *Babesia* spp. that have not been formally named have been described in dogs. One is a large *Babesia* sp. (Birkenheuer, 2004) that has been isolated from dogs in North America.[31] The majority of these dogs had been splenectomized or were undergoing chemotherapy for cancer. Infected dogs have been identified throughout the southeastern and south central United States.[31–33] Another large *Babesia* sp. (Holm, 2006) was reported in a dog from the United Kingdom that never traveled outside of that country.[34] The dog died as a result of infection. There have not been any further reports of this infection in dogs or other vertebrate species. The natural vertebrate host(s) for either species has yet to be identified.

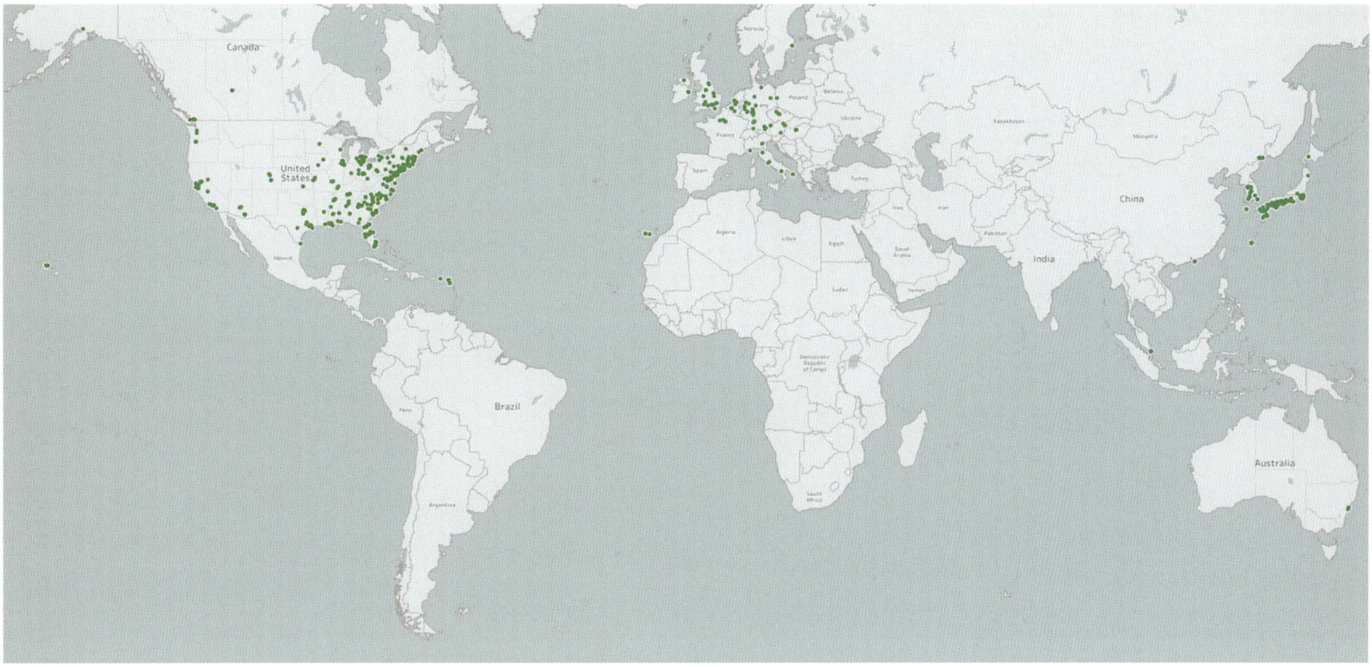

A

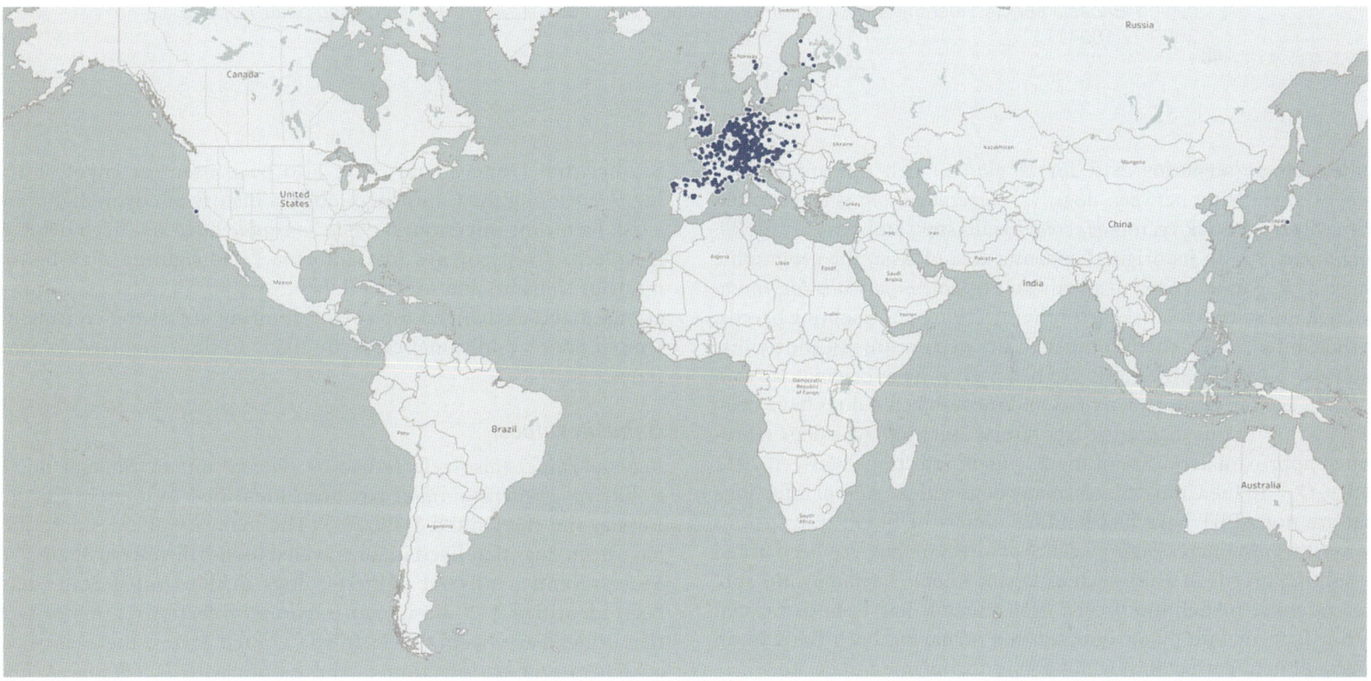

B

Fig. 97.2 Locations of positive test results for species-specific *Babesia* polymerase chain reaction assays performed by IDEXX Laboratories. Each dot represents a postal code from which one or more positive samples were submitted. (A) *Babesia vogeli*. (B) *Babesia canis*.

Continued

Babesia gibsoni

Infections with *B. gibsoni* occur throughout the world, and the insidious nature of this infection has allowed the inadvertent transport of infected dogs from Asia to other regions. *Babesia gibsoni* can be found in Africa, Asia, Australia, North and South America, and Europe (Fig. 97.2C); in a 2020 study, globally it accounted for almost 50% of positive *Babesia* PCR test results in specimens submitted to IDEXX Laboratories; this was followed by *B. canis* (35%) and *B. vogeli* (15%).[15,35] Antarctica is the only continent from which *B. gibsoni* infections have not yet been reported. *Babesia gibsoni* is the most commonly recognized *Babesia* sp. in the United States and Asia. Depending on the availability of suitable vectors, two distinct

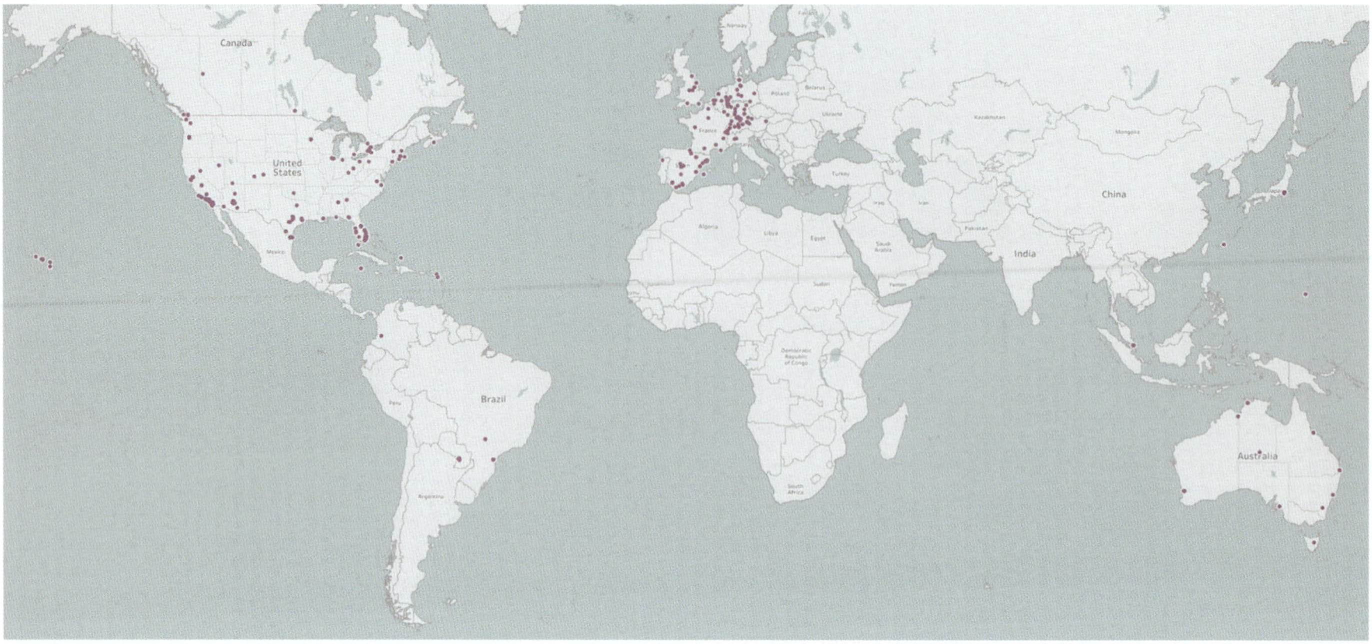

C

Fig. 97.2, cont'd (C) *Babesia gibsoni*. (From Birkenheuer AJ, Buch J, Beall MJ, et al. Global distribution of canine *Babesia* species identified by a commercial diagnostic laboratory. *Vet Parasitol Reg Stud Reports*. 2020;22:100471.)

epidemiologic scenarios exist for *B. gibsoni*: tick transmission or direct transmission between dogs.[36,37] *Babesia gibsoni* is transmitted primarily by the tick vectors *Haemaphysalis* spp., and possibly by *Rh. sanguineus*.[38–47] In its original endemic area of Asia, the geographic range of *B. gibsoni* correlates with that of *Haemaphysalis bispinosa*, and tick infestation is a risk factor for infection in nonfighting breeds. In the United States where competent tick vectors are not widely distributed, *B. gibsoni* infections are believed to have originated from dogs engaged in fighting activities and most infected dogs have been APBT.[37,48,49] In one diagnostic laboratory, "pit bull" type dogs represented approximately 75% of the *B. gibsoni* infections between 2012 and 2017.[50] In the United States, many dogs with *B. gibsoni* infections that are not APBT have had fighting contact or blood transfusions from APBT. An increased prevalence of infection has also been noted in fighting breeds in areas such as Japan, where *Haemaphysalis* spp. are endemic. In fighting breeds, transmission has been associated with a fight or bite by an infected dog or having been born to an infected bitch. Perinatal transmission is documented to occur.[3–5]

Babesia conradae

Babesia conradae (previously referred to as "the California isolate" and the "western piroplasm", which has been historically misidentified as *B. gibsoni*) was originally detected in dogs from southern California, and more recently has been reported in dogs from southcentral USA (Oklahoma).[51–53] Tick vectors have not been identified. Transmission studies that attempted to prove vector competence for *Rh. sanguineus* and *Dermacentor variabilis* were unsuccessful or inconclusive.[54] The author has identified *Rh. sanguineus* as well as soft-bodied ticks, *Ornithodoros coriaceus*, on *B. conradae*–infected dogs.[55] A high prevalence (>50%) of *B. conradae* infection has been noted in greyhound mixed-breed dogs used to hunt coyotes in California, and infected greyhounds in the southcentral United States have also been used for coyote hunting.[53,56] Among the Californian dogs, a history of coyote fights was a risk factor for infection. *Babesia conradae* DNA has been detected in spleens from coyotes in California,[57], so fighting may be one mode of transmission for this *Babesia* species. Because greyhounds are used and exchanged for coyote-hunting across the continental United States, additional cases are likely to be recognized in other states.[57]

Babesia vulpes

Babesia vulpes (also referred to as *Babesia annae*, *Babesia microti*–like or *Theileria annae*) has been identified in dogs in Europe, Russia, and the United States.[58–60] The majority of cases described have been dogs that lived in, or traveled to, northwestern Spain.[61–65] More recently, infected domestic dogs in the United States have been identified.[66–68] Similar to *B. gibsoni* infections, a majority of these dogs have been APBT. In the United States, there has been a high rate of co-infection of these dogs with *B. gibsoni*. A high percentage of European and North American foxes are infected with a genetically identical parasite and they are believed to be the natural reservoir host.[69–72] A 2019 study found a high prevalence of *B. vulpes* infections in domestic dogs.[73] A tick vector has not been definitively identified, but in Spain an association between *Ixodes hexagonus* infestation and *B. microti*–like infection has been observed.[74] *Ixodes hexagonus* is not endemic in North America, so it is not likely to be the universal vector.

Babesia negevi sp. nov.

Babesia negevi sp. nov. is a novel intermediate-sized piroplasm that was detected in five dogs with signs of babesiosis from Israel and described in 2020.[75] The organism is named after the Negev desert in southern Israel, where the first infected dog was found.

Feline Babesiosis

Feline babesiosis has not been studied as extensively as canine babesiosis, but as with canine babesiosis, there has been increased recognition of the number of species that can infect cats in recent years.[76] Several small *Babesia* species have been identified in cats, which include *Babesia felis* sensu stricto, *Babesia cati, Babesia leo,* and a novel small *Babesia* species.[77–79] *Babesia felis* is a highly pathogenic *Babesia* species that infects domestic cats in southern Africa and the Sudan.[77] Infection of domestic cats has primarily been identified along the coast of South Africa.[80,81] Affected cats are usually younger than 3 years, and there is no recognized breed or sex predilection. *Babesia cati* is less pathogenic and found primarily in India. *Babesia leo* has been detected in lions (*Panthera leo*) in Kruger National Park, as well as a single domestic cat in a molecular survey.[82] A small piroplasm was visualized in blood smears from feral cats in Rio de Janeiro, Brazil, but no molecular data were available to confirm the identity of these organisms.[83] *Babesia gibsoni* was detected in 4% of 115 apparently healthy cats in the Caribbean; *B. vogeli* was detected in 13% of cats, and mixed infections with *B. vogeli* and *B. gibsoni* were detected in 3% of cats.[84]

Large *Babesia* species also appear to infect cats. *Babesia lengau*, originally described in cheetahs, was detected in two domestic cats from South Africa with cerebral and hemolytic disease.[85] DNA sequences, most similar to those of *B. vogeli* and *B. vulpes*, have been amplified from the blood of three cats with retroviral infections from Spain and Portugal, but no organisms were visualized.[86–90] *Babesia canis presentii* was identified in two cats in Israel.[89] Possible other novel *Babesia* species have been proposed that infect cats, such as *Babesia panickeri* sp. nov. (described in a 3-month-old cat from India with severe anemia and thrombocytopenia)[91] and *Babesia hongkongensis* (described in cats from Asia).[79] Another *B. canis*–like parasite has been identified in a naturally infected cat from Poland.[92] Feline babesiosis has not been well documented in the United States.

CLINICAL FEATURES

Pathogenesis and Clinical Signs

Canine Babesiosis

The pathogenicity of *Babesia* organisms is determined primarily by the species and strain involved. Host factors, such as the age of the host and the immunologic response generated against the parasite or vector tick, are also important. Although most often subclinically infected, dogs infected with "avirulent" species such as *B. vogeli* may have severe clinical disease. Similarly, dogs infected with "virulent" species such as *B. rossi* may be subclinically infected without overt clinical or laboratory findings. However, features that should raise clinical suspicion for babesiosis include fever, thrombocytopenia, hemolytic anemia, and splenomegaly. Dogs often have nonspecific signs such as lethargy, anorexia, and weakness (Box 97.1). Occasionally, owners note jaundice, mucosal pallor, or discoloration of the urine caused by bilirubinuria or hemoglobinuria. Azotemia and proteinuria have been identified with increased frequency in dogs with *Babesia* infections.[61,93–96] Dogs infected with *B. vogeli* may have fever of unknown origin only without overt hematologic abnormalities.[97] Co-infections with other tick- or bloodborne pathogens may also influence the clinical signs of disease.

Parasite antigens are incorporated on the erythrocyte surface and induce host-opsonizing antibodies, which in turn leads to removal of infected erythrocytes by the mononuclear phagocyte system. Soluble parasite antigens can also adhere to the surface of noninfected erythrocytes and platelets. This may lead to their opsonization by antibodies, with or without complement, and account for hemolytic anemia and thrombocytopenia that is often not correlated with the level of parasitemia. Parasitemia and anemia are more severe in splenectomized dogs, and splenectomy may precipitate disease in dogs with chronic subclinical infections. Mechanisms other than immune-mediated destruction that contribute to erythrocyte damage include increased erythrocyte osmotic fragility, direct injury of erythrocytes by *Babesia* parasites, accumulation of cyclic nucleotides, and oxidative injury.[98–102] Lipid peroxidation increases erythrocyte rigidity and slows the passage of erythrocytes through capillary beds. Soluble parasite proteases activate the kallikrein system and induce fibrinogen-like protein formation. These proteins make erythrocytes more "sticky," and they sludge in capillary beds, which contributes to anemia and many of the other potential clinical signs. The most severe sludging occurs in the CNS and muscles.

Thrombocytopenia may result from immune-mediated destruction of platelets or consumption coagulopathy. Despite severely decreased platelet counts, bleeding is rarely observed in dogs infected with most *Babesia* strains, and other abnormal coagulation test results are uncommon (with the exceptions of *B. conradae* and also *B. rossi* infections). Dogs with *B. conradae* infection have experienced life-threatening hemorrhage, the pathogenesis of which requires further study.[57]

Other possible complications include membranoproliferative glomerulonephritis, which may have an immune-mediated pathogenesis.[93,94,103] Renal failure occurs in up to 40% of dogs infected with *B. vulpes*, and the presence of renal failure has been associated with increased mortality.[61,63,65,104,105] Nonregenerative anemia, azotemia, and proteinuria with high UPCRs were found in these dogs. Renal disease and proteinuria have been identified in dogs with *B. gibsoni* infections.[93,94]

BOX 97.1 Clinical Findings in Dogs with Babesiosis

Common signs

Anorexia
Lethargy
Weakness
Pyrexia
Weight loss

Uncommon/atypical signs (primarily *B. rossi*)

Ascites
Edema
Constipation
Diarrhea
Ulcerative stomatitis
Hemorrhage
Congested mucous membranes
Polycythemia
Ocular and nasal discharge
Respiratory distress
Masticatory myositis
Temporomandibular joint pain
Spinal pain
Central nervous system signs (seizures, ataxia, paresis)

Hyperacute signs (primarily *B. rossi*)

Hypothermia
Shock
Coma
Disseminated intravascular coagulation
Metabolic acidosis
Death

Acute signs

Hemolytic anemia
Icterus
Splenomegaly
Lymphadenopathy
Vomiting

Chronic signs

Intermittent pyrexia
Partial anorexia
Loss of body condition
Lymphadenomegaly
Splenomegaly
No signs

Severe Babesiosis. Virulent *B. canis* and especially *B. rossi* strains may induce a profound systemic inflammatory response, which can result in a severe sepsis-like syndrome with multiple organ dysfunction (see Chapter 123). The majority of dogs infected with *B. rossi* have uncomplicated babesiosis and can be treated as outpatients. However, up to 31% of the dogs examined at a university clinic required hospitalization, and 10% of hospitalized dogs did not survive.[29] Severe clinical illness in dogs infected with *B. rossi* results from hypotension, AKI, neurologic complications, DIC, hepatopathy, and ARDS. Tissue hypoxia results from anemia, shock, vascular stasis, excessive endogenous production of carbon monoxide, parasitic damage to hemoglobin, and decreased ability of hemoglobin to off-load oxygen.[99,106] Lactic acid generation from tissue hypoxia can result in severe metabolic acidosis.[107]

"Red biliary syndrome" is a paradoxical phenomenon of severe intravascular hemolysis (manifested as hemoglobinemia and hemoglobinuria) in combination with hemoconcentration (high reference range or elevated hematocrit).[106] The hemoconcentration is thought to occur when plasma shifts from the vascular to the extravascular compartment as a result of increased capillary permeability, with a resultant decrease in blood volume. Hemoconcentration has been associated with cerebral babesiosis, DIC, AKI, and ARDS.

Neurologic complications result from sludging of parasitized erythrocytes in CNS capillary beds, with congestion and macroscopic and microscopic hemorrhages. Severe hypoglycemia can also result in neurologic signs. Other complications of severe babesiosis include pancreatitis, rhabdomyolysis, ocular involvement, upper respiratory signs, cardiac arrhythmias, necrosis of the extremities, and fluid accumulation. Pulmonary, CNS, and renal complications are associated with a higher rate of mortality. Persistent lactate concentrations above 40 mg/dL are a poor prognostic indicator for survival.[108] In a study of 240 babesiosis cases from central Europe, serum creatinine concentrations above 5 mg/dL and albumin concentrations less than 2.2 g/dL were negative prognostic indicators. When AKI was present, 34% of dogs died, and 40% of dogs with pancreatitis died.[109]

Feline Babesiosis

Cats with babesiosis from southern Africa generally show lethargy, anorexia, weakness, an unkempt haircoat, and/or diarrhea.[81] Fever and icterus are less common. Anemia can be severe and is the underlying reason for the clinical signs. The disease is chronic, and signs may not be apparent until a later stage of illness. Cats usually adapt to the anemia and may have only mild clinical signs until they are stressed by handling. Complications of hemolytic anemia include hepatopathy, pulmonary edema, renal failure, CNS signs, and concurrent infections.

Physical Examination Findings

Physical examination abnormalities in most dogs with babesiosis consist of mucosal pallor, lethargy, splenomegaly, and bounding pulses. Fever is not consistently identified because it often waxes and wanes. Tachycardia and tachypnea may be present in severely anemic dogs. Mucosal hemorrhages and/or epistaxis may be present in dogs with *B. conradae* infections (Fig. 97.3), and excessive bleeding from venipuncture sites may be noted.

Dogs with severe babesiosis may show CNS signs such as incoordination, pelvic limb paresis, muscle tremors, nystagmus, anisocoria, intermittent loss of consciousness, seizures, stupor, coma, aggression, or vocalization.[106] Dogs with red biliary syndrome may have congested mucous membranes or icterus. Other clinical abnormalities in dogs with severe babesiosis include tachypnea, increased lung sounds, and cardiac arrhythmias.

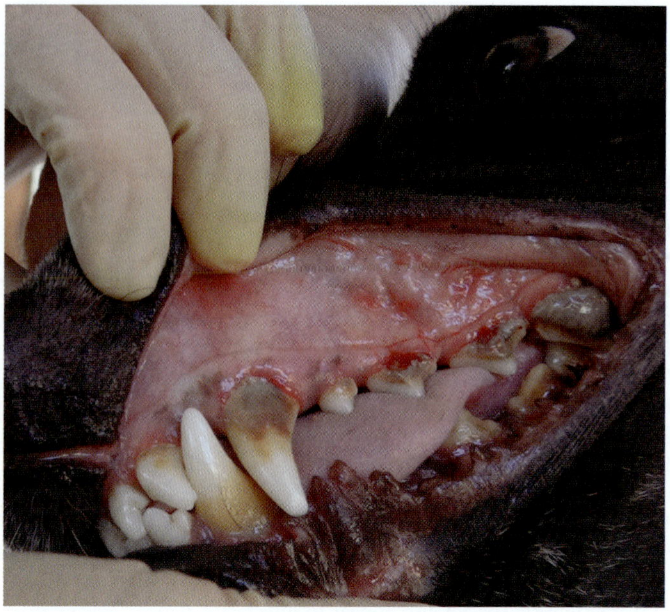

Fig. 97.3 Greyhound infected with *Babesia conradae.* Mucosal hemorrhages are apparent. These resolved after treatment with atovaquone and azithromycin. (Courtesy Dr. Jane E. Sykes, University of California, Davis.)

Affected cats may be lethargic, pale, tachycardic, and tachypneic, and in some cases, icteric.

DIAGNOSIS

Laboratory Abnormalities

Complete Blood Count

In dogs with babesiosis, the primary hematologic abnormalities are anemia and thrombocytopenia. Thrombocytopenia is the most common abnormality and is often present, even when anemia is absent. A mild, normocytic, normochromic anemia is generally noted in the first few days after infection, which becomes macrocytic, hypochromic, and regenerative as the disease progresses. Uncommonly with *B. rossi* infections, a relative polycythemia may be noted.[106] Leukocyte abnormalities are inconsistently observed but may include leukocytosis (with or without a left shift), leukopenia, neutrophilia, neutropenia, lymphocytosis, and/or eosinophilia.[56,110,111] Leukopenia or a low-normal leukocyte count due to relative neutropenia has been frequently observed in dogs from Europe with *B. canis* infections and dogs from the United States with *B. conradae* infections.[56,111] Autoagglutination, positive direct antiglobulin (Coombs') tests, and spherocytosis may also be present.[112] Some infected dogs have no hematologic abnormalities.

In cats, anemia associated with *B. felis* infection is typically macrocytic, hypochromic, and regenerative.[113] Thrombocytopenia is an inconsistent finding.

Serum Chemistry Profile

There are no pathognomonic biochemical findings in dogs with babesiosis, and serum biochemical profiles may have no abnormal findings. Common findings in North American dogs include hyperglobulinemia (which may be present in the absence of other laboratory abnormalities), mildly increased liver enzyme activities, and, less commonly, hyperbilirubinemia. A study of dual infections with *B. canis* and *Ehrlichia canis* showed that the prevalence of hyperglobulinemia was higher in dogs with dual infections than in dogs with a single infection

TABLE 97.1 Diagnostic Assays Available for Babesiosis in Dogs and Cats

Assay	Specimen Type	Target	Performance
Cell culture	Whole blood	*Babesia* spp.	Not widely offered or utilized for routine diagnostic purposes. Requires several weeks' incubation.
Cytology	Whole blood, buffy-coat smears (the area just below the buffy coat), tissue aspirates	*Babesia* spp.	Rapid and specific (i.e., when merozoites are identified by experienced cytologists, the sample is likely to be infected with *Babesia* spp.; however, *Babesia* spp. cannot be accurately differentiated based on morphology alone). Less sensitive than PCR.
Immunofluorescent antibody serology	Serum	Antibodies to *Babesia* spp.	Acute and convalescent serology may be required for diagnosis of acute infection, because initial results may be negative in dogs with acute disease and positive results may reflect previous exposure rather than active infection. Cross-reactivity can occur between *Babesia* spp. Some dogs do not develop detectable antibody titers despite chronic infection.
PCR	Whole blood, splenic aspirates	*Babesia spp.* DNA	Confirms active infection. Sensitivity and specificity varies depending on assay design and specimen type. Both false-positive and false-negative results are possible; PCR results must be interpreted in light of the clinical signs. Serial sampling (i.e., two or more tests on specimens obtained 2–4 weeks apart) will increase sensitivity, especially in chronically infected animals.

caused by either organism.[114] Hyperbilirubinemia is a more consistent finding during acute disease caused by *B. canis* and *B. rossi* but not by *B. gibsoni* or *B. conradae*.[56,110] Dogs with severe *B. rossi* infections may have hemoglobinemia, moderately increased liver enzyme activities, increased BUN and serum creatinine concentrations, hypoalbuminemia, hypoglycemia, and metabolic acidosis. Some dogs develop kidney injury with or without proteinuria and hypoalbuminemia.[61,94]

Cats infected with *B. felis* typically have elevated serum ALT activity and total bilirubin concentrations. Serum protein values are usually within reference limits, but hyperglobulinemia can occur. Renal parameters are unaffected.[113]

Urinalysis

Urinalysis abnormalities in dogs with babesiosis are variable but include bilirubinuria, hemoglobinuria, proteinuria, and, in rare cases, granular casts. Some dogs have pigmenturia consisting most commonly of bilirubin, and occasionally hemoglobin. Dogs with secondary glomerular nephritis have proteinuria and may have isosthenuria.

Coagulation Testing

The most consistent hemostatic abnormality in complicated and uncomplicated babesiosis is thrombocytopenia. DIC has been reported, but it is extremely rare. Dogs with *B. conradae* infection appear to have altered platelet function tests.[57]

Microbiologic Testing

There are three basic methods available for specific diagnosis of *Babesia* infections: microscopic identification, serologic testing, and nucleic acid–based testing (Table 97.1). The true clinical sensitivity and specificity of most of the available tests is unknown, but all modalities can have either false-positive or false-negative results. Therefore, there is no "perfect" test for *Babesia* infection, and in many cases, multiple diagnostic tests are indicated.

Cytologic Diagnosis

Light microscopic examination is highly specific for the identification of *Babesia* organisms, but because of its limit of detection (0.001% parasitemia), it has relatively poor sensitivity and is not suitable as a sole screening test. Several species/genotypes are virtually indistinguishable by light microscopy, making accurate identification to the species level impossible. However, when cytologic detection is used in combination with the history, signalment, physical examination, clinicopathologic data, and geographic location, the clinician may be able to predict the most likely species present.

Babesia canis, B. vogeli and *B. rossi* are large, pyriform organisms and usually exist singly or in pairs (Fig. 97.4A). Smaller single intracellular organisms are likely to be *B. gibsoni, B. conradae* or *B. vulpes* (Fig. 97.4B and C). However, when the parasites are rapidly replicating, the classic intraerythrocytic forms may not predominate and some more atypical irregular, amoeboid parasite forms with a wide range of sizes can be detected. During these phases of infection, some small *Babesia* spp. exhibit large forms and some large *Babesia* spp. exhibit small forms. In chronic infection, the level of parasitemia is often low, especially in dogs infected with large *Babesia* sp., and thorough examination of thin blood smears is necessary. Evaluation of stained slides requires experience and a significant time commitment on the part of the laboratory technician. For large *Babesia* spp. infections, blood collected from the peripheral capillary beds of the ear tip or nailbed may yield higher numbers of parasitized cells.[115] Rarely, phagocytized organisms and erythrocyte fragments are seen in neutrophils. Methods that concentrate and stain buffy-coat specimens may improve the sensitivity of parasite detection.[116,117]

Serologic Diagnosis

Because *Babesia* parasites are difficult to detect, especially in chronic carriers, immunodiagnostics may be used to screen for exposure. IFA assays are used most commonly to detect antibodies to *Babesia* species. Laboratory methods differ, and each laboratory should be consulted for cutoff antibody titers. As a general guideline, titers ≥ 1:64 on a single specimen are supportive of exposure. Serologic assays for *B. rossi, B. conradae,* and *B. vulpes* are not widely available at the time of writing.

Titers to multiple *Babesia* species must be measured if antibody testing is performed in geographic areas where more than one species of *Babesia* exists. Serologic cross-reactivity among *Babesia* spp. makes parasite identification by PCR necessary to definitively identify a given species. When titers against multiple species are performed, the highest titer is not always the infecting species. There are also many documented instances in which parasites or parasite DNA have been detected but anti-*Babesia* antibodies could not be detected. Very young dogs or dogs tested early in the disease course may have negative antibody test results, so convalescent serology is required in some cases. Antibodies were not detected in 36% of dogs with *B. canis* parasitemia in one study.[17] ELISAs that target several

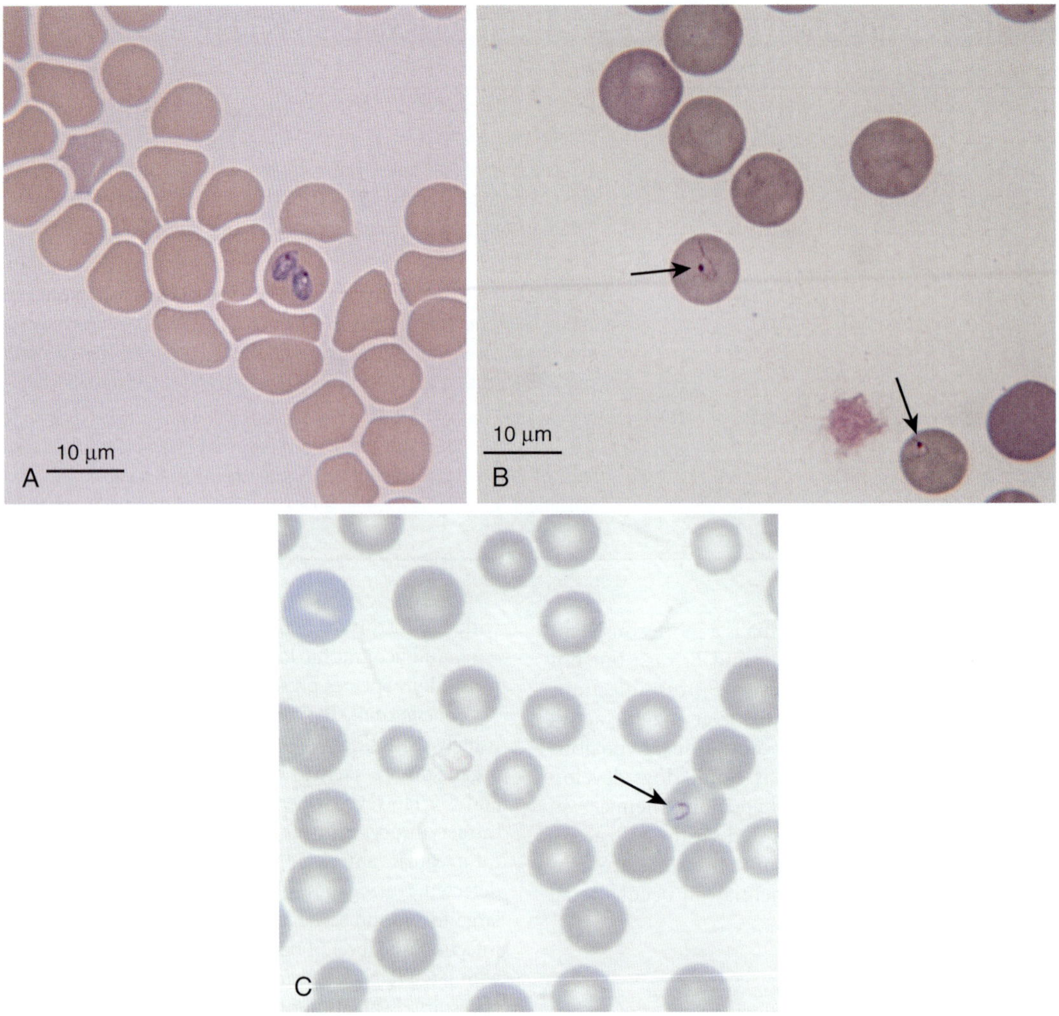

Fig. 97.4 Blood smears from dogs with babesiosis. (A) Large unnamed *Babesia* piroplasm originally identified in dogs in North Carolina. A pair of large, piriform-shape merozoites are present within an erythrocyte. (B) Individual merozoites of *Babesia gibsoni* in erythrocytes *(arrows)*. (C) *Babesia conradae* merozoite within an erythrocyte *(arrow)*. Polychromasia and anisocytosis are also present. Wright stain, 1000×.

different antigens have been developed for use in antibody or antigen detection tests and offer promise for serodiagnosis of canine babesiosis in the future. However, there are currently no commercially available ELISA assays for the detection of anti-*Babesia* antibodies in the United States.

Molecular Diagnosis Using Nucleic Acid–Based Testing

Nucleic acid amplification tests (NAATs) such as PCR assays are the most specific means of detecting infection with *Babesia* and are essential for accurate species identification. Some assays have a lower limit of detection that is more than 1300-fold more sensitive than the level (0.001% parasitized erythrocytes) of light microscopy.[118] A 2018 study found PCR to be five times more sensitive than microscopy for the identification of infection.[119] Many different NAATs have been published for the identification and differentiation of *Babesia* infections, and several commercial diagnostic laboratories offer real-time PCR assays for detection of *Babesia* infection. Species identification can then be accomplished by DNA sequencing or by the use of species-specific assays. NAATs that are designed to detect multiple *Babesia* spp. (i.e., a broad-range *Babesia* PCR) are recommended for initial screening. A well-designed species-specific assay will only detect one species; the potential downside is that a negative test may lead clinicians to falsely conclude that the patient is not infected with *Babesia* because the wrong species was targeted for testing. In addition, broad-range PCR assays have been helpful for identification of novel *Babesia* species.

Pathologic Findings

The most striking pathologic findings occur in dogs that die from severe babesiosis (usually associated with *B. rossi*). These include staining of tissues with hemoglobin or bilirubin, hepatosplenomegaly, lymphadenomegaly, and kidneys that are a dark-reddish color. Edema and hemorrhage, which may indicate vascular injury and poor tissue oxygenation in severely affected dogs, are often most severe in the lungs. Nonparasitized cells often line the endothelial surface with parasitized cells sludged in the lumen. Pathologic changes in the brain of these dogs include congestion, macroscopic and microscopic hemorrhages, sequestration of parasitized erythrocytes in capillary beds, and pavementing of parasitized cells against the endothelium. Cardiac histologic changes include hemorrhage, necrosis, inflammatory infiltrates, and fibrosis. Microthrombi

TABLE 97.2 Selected Antibabesial Compounds Used in Dogs and Cats

Generic Name[a]	Dose (mg/kg)	Route	Interval (Hours)	Duration (Days)	ORGANISM: *Babesia canis, Babesia vogeli, Babesia conradae,* large *Babesia* spp.	*Babesia gibsoni*	*Babesia conradae*	*Babesia felis*
Imidocarb dipropionate[b]	5–6.6	IM	Once	Repeat in 14	+++	+	+	—
	7.5	IM	Once	NA				
Diminazene aceturate	3.5–5	IM	Once[c]	NA	+++	++	?	+
Azithromycin[d] *and* atovaquone[d]	10 13.3	PO PO	24 8	10 10	+++	+++	+++	?
Clindamycin[e] *and* doxycycline *and* metronidazole	25 5 15	PO PO PO	12 12 12	90 90 90	+	++	?	?
Primaquine phosphate	0.5	PO	24	1–3	?	—	?	+++
	1 mg per cat[f]	IM	36	6	—	—	?	+++

[a]For specific information on each drug, see Chapter 12.
[b]For combination therapy, a dose of 3.5 mg/kg diminazene has been followed by a dose of 6.0 mg/kg imidocarb.
[c]Not available in the United States, except by compassionate use. For large *Babesia spp.*, this dose is sufficient; for *B. gibsoni*, repeat dose in 24 hours. Total dosages of 7 mg/kg or higher are associated with an increased risk of neural and parasympathomimetic toxicity.
[d]These two drugs should be used in combination. Atovaquone must be given with a fatty meal to facilitate absorption. The suspension causes minimal gastrointestinal adverse effects.
[e]Anecdotal evidence for activity against *B. vogeli*. Not effective in clearing the infection. Not recommended as sole therapy because of the potential to develop resistance. Further documentation needed to establish efficacy of this combination (see text).
[f]Note that 1 mg/kg is a lethal dose.
+++, very good; ++, good; +, fair to poor; —, not effective; *?*, unknown.

of many tissues may be evident in animals exhibiting signs of DIC. Impression smears of the spleen may substantiate the diagnosis of babesiosis at necropsy. Nonspecific findings in dogs with all forms of babesiosis include erythroid hyperplasia in the bone marrow, extramedullary hematopoiesis of the liver and spleen, mononuclear phagocyte system hyperplasia, and centrilobular necrosis of the liver. Vasculitis has been observed in *B. conradae* infections and is associated with hepatitis and lymphadenitis with multifocal deposits of IgM in inflamed arteries and renal glomeruli.[103] In chronic canine babesiosis and feline babesiosis, the only gross finding may be splenomegaly.

TREATMENT AND PROGNOSIS

Antiprotozoal Treatment

Dogs

Dogs generally show clinical improvement within 24 to 72 hours of treatment with antibabesial drugs, but some animals take as long as 7 days to respond (Table 97.2).

Imidocarb dipropionate can eliminate *B. canis*, *B. vogeli*, and *B. rossi* infections, but has shown variable efficacy for eliminating infections with large *Babesia* sp.[33] Imidocarb also eliminates infection with *B. canis* in ticks that engorge on treated animals for up to 4 weeks after treatment, and prevents infection for up to 6 weeks after a single injection.[120] A single dose of 7.5 mg/kg or a single dose of 6 mg/kg given the day after a dose of diminazene (3.5 mg/kg) also clears infection.[121] In areas where reinfection is likely, some practitioners use a lower dose, 2 mg/kg, SC, once. This approach is an attempt to induce a state of premunition. Premunition is the immunity of existing infection in which chronic subclinically affected carriers may be resistant to reinfection or at least have reduced morbidity with new infections. In contrast, animals that have been cleared of infection are more susceptible to reinfection with recurrent clinical disease. The risk of this approach is that clinical babesiosis may relapse in some chronic carriers. Therefore, this approach is not recommended for the treatment of canine babesiosis in many parts of the United States, where vector transmission and risk for reinfection are thought to be low. Imidocarb does not clear *B. gibsoni* infections, but reduces morbidity and mortality. Therefore, this is a reasonable alternative treatment for *B. gibsoni* infection if the owner cannot immediately afford more effective treatments. The same may be true for *B. conradae* infections. Pretreatment with atropine (0.025 mg/kg, SC, 30 minutes before injection) reduces the adverse effects of imidocarb (see Chapter 12).

Other related aromatic diamidines include diminazene aceturate, phenamidine isethionate, and pentamidine isethionate (see Chapter 12). Although these are not available for treatment of dogs in the United States, the first two of these drugs have been used in many other countries and are highly active against large *Babesia* sp. They do not clear *B. gibsoni* infections, but can reduce morbidity and mortality.

Atovaquone and azithromycin combination therapy is recommended for the treatment of *B. gibsoni* and *B. conradae* infections (see Table 97.2).[55,122,123] Anecdotally this author has seen clinical remissions in dogs infected with *B. vogeli* or the large *Babesia* sp. (Birkenheuer, 2004). Atovaquone and azithromycin are given for 10 days. Atovaquone must be administered with a high-fat meal to maximize drug absorption. There are also two commercially available formulations of atovaquone: a single-drug liquid suspension that is very well tolerated, and a combination tablet product (atovaquone and proguanil hydrochloride). Although the combination product is less expensive, it causes severe vomiting in some patients. Because drug absorption is critical and selection for resistance to atovaquone can occur, this author recommends *only* use of the single-drug suspension. The treatment appeared to sterilize *B. gibsoni* infections or reduce the parasitemia below detectable limits in approximately 80% of dogs in a randomized double-blind placebo-controlled trial.[122] However, in another study, this combination only eliminated *B. gibsoni* infection (or reduced parasitemia below detectable limits of PCR assay), in two of seven dogs.[124] It also did not clear experimental infection with two Australian isolates of *B. gibsoni*.[125] When atovaquone is used alone to treat *B. gibsoni* infection, recrudescence of infection develops more than 30 days after treatment.[125] Drug resistance has been identified *in vitro*, so atovaquone should always be used in combination with other drugs. Mutations in the genes that encode the putative molecular target of atovaquone have been identified in *B. gibsoni* isolates from dogs that failed to clear infection after atovaquone treatment.[50,124,126,127]

In this author's experience, dogs that fail to clear *B. gibsoni* infections after initial treatment with atovaquone and azithromycin are infected with organisms with mutations in the cytochrome B gene and will not clear their infection after a follow-up treatment with the same drugs, although clinical disease may resolve. Dogs that have been splenectomized before treatment do not always appear to clear infections with treatment.[128] Likewise, immunosuppressive therapy may reduce the ability of antibabesial treatment to clear dogs of *B. gibsoni* infection. The recommended follow-up after treatment with atovaquone and azithromycin is a minimum of two PCR tests approximately 60 and 90 days after completing treatment. Earlier testing can result in false-negative or false-positive results due to decreased circulating parasitemia or detection of dead or replication-deficient organisms.[123] A trial comparing imidocarb, atovaquone and azithromycin, and buparvaquone and azithromycin was performed in dogs with *B. vulpes* infections. None of these treatments consistently cleared the infections. The combination therapies were superior to imidocarb for reducing clinical signs and parasitemias. Atovaquone and azithromycin reduced infections below the limit of detection of the PCR test in the highest proportion of cases (approximately 50%).[129]

An alternative treatment strategy can be used to treat *B. gibsoni* infections that fail to respond to atovaquone and azithromycin.[130] This regimen involves a combination of clindamycin, metronidazole, and doxycycline for a minimum of 3 months (see Table 97.2). In an uncontrolled study, three of four experimentally infected dogs had negative PCR assay results after treatment, whereas one dog remained persistently infected and experienced clinical relapses during treatment.[130] Clearance of the infection as determined by PCR was not detected until 30 and 72 days after completing a 90-day treatment course in two dogs. The PCR test result became negative in the third dog 12 days into treatment. Three of the dogs were initially treated with three doses of diminazene aceturate. In two other studies, naturally infected dogs that had clinical relapse after or during atovaquone and azithromycin treatment had clinical recoveries after treatment with the clindamycin, metronidazole, and doxycycline combination.[124,131] The small number of cases reported and the high degree of variability in the PCR results after treatment make the efficacy of this combination uncertain. However, as with the atovaquone-azithromycin combination, PCR testing 60 and 90 days after completing therapy is recommended.

Aggressive supportive care and monotherapy with clindamycin (25 mg/kg, PO, q12h for 7 to 21 days) has been recommended if specific antibabesial drugs are not available.[132] At this dosage, clinical abnormalities resolve even if organism clearance does not occur. This author *does not* routinely recommend this practice for *B. gibsoni*–infected dogs due to concerns about the selection for macrolide resistance that could potentially interfere with subsequent atovaquone and azithromycin treatment.

Doxycycline has some activity against *Babesia* spp., but there are no controlled studies evaluating efficacy. It is this author's experience that many dogs with babesiosis have a mild reduction in morbidity with doxycycline monotherapy. This frequently leads clinicians to suspect a rickettsial or bacterial infection. Doxycycline (5 mg/kg, PO, q12h) therapy can be instituted while awaiting specific antiprotozoal drugs.

Other treatments that have been used to treat *B. canis* infections are quinuronium sulfate and 1% trypan blue solution. Trypan blue does not clear infections and results in bluish discoloration of tissues and plasma. Tafenoquine, an 8-aminoquinoline, is an anti-malarial drug and has also been shown to have activity against *Babesia gibsoni* infections in experimentally-infected dogs through oxidative damage to parasites.[133]

Cats

Treatment of feline babesiosis has not been as critically evaluated, but most antibabesial drugs appear ineffective. Primaquine phosphate, an antimalarial compound, administered orally or as an intramuscular injection, is currently the drug of choice (see Table 97.2). However, the effective dose, 0.5 mg/kg, is very close to the lethal dose (1 mg/kg). In experimental studies, rifampin and trimethoprim-sulfadiazine were not as effective as primaquine.[134]

Supportive Care

Other supportive care measures that may be required to treat animals with babesiosis are packed red blood cell transfusions and IV crystalloid fluid therapy. The administration of the plasma component of whole blood is unnecessary in the majority of dogs with babesiosis and can place the patient at risk of volume overload and transfusion reaction or the transmission of other infectious agents. If rehydration is required, crystalloid replacement solutions are preferable. Whether glucocorticoids are indicated to counteract the immune-mediated complications of babesiosis is controversial. This author does not recommend the use of glucocorticoids to treat dogs infected with *B. gibsoni* or *B. vogeli*. In one study, 21% of 134 dogs with *B. rossi* infection had hemolytic anemias that did not respond to antibabesial therapy alone.[106] This seems less common with *B. vogeli* or *B. gibsoni* infections because these often respond completely to antibabesial treatment alone. In most dogs that require glucocorticoids, the glucocorticoid dosage can be tapered and discontinued within a 2- to 3-week period. Continued glucocorticoid therapy may predispose the animals to other infections and has the potential to induce babesial relapse.

IMMUNITY AND VACCINATION

The duration of protective immunity against *Babesia* spp. infection is limited. Antibody titers may gradually decline between 3 and 5 months after infection.[120] Recovered dogs are protected against homologous infection within 5 to 8 months after infection.[120] Cross-protection between strains does not occur, and seropositivity does not guarantee protection against heterologous challenge.

A vaccine produced from cell culture–derived exoantigens of *B. canis* is available in Europe.[135] An efficacy of 70% to 100% has been reported, with the disease occasionally seen in the vaccinates generally being mild. Other field studies have been less impressive. Vaccination does not prevent infection but appears to block initiation of many of the pathologic processes involved in disease pathogenesis.[136,137] Vaccines may limit parasitemia and reduce development of anemia and splenomegaly. A bivalent vaccine derived from soluble parasite antigens from *B. canis* and *B. rossi* (Nobivac Piro, MSD Animal Health South Africa) reduces clinical signs after challenge with both species.[138] Differences in strain antigenicity limit the usefulness of the commercial vaccine in other areas. *Babesia canis* vaccines do not cross-protect against other *Babesia* species.

PREVENTION

Treatment of babesiosis is expensive and may be ineffective, so prevention is of paramount importance. Preventive measures alone may be sufficient to control *B. vogeli* outbreaks in kennels in the southeastern United States. The primary means of prevention is tick control (see Chapters 13 and 109). Early tick identification and removal is important because it likely takes a minimum of 2 to 3 days of feeding for transmission of the parasite to occur. Dogs should be tested, treated if necessary, and quarantined before being introduced into a colony. Several tick-control products (isoxazoline class, fipronil/permethrin, and imidacloprid/flumethrin) have reduced the experimental and natural transmission of *B. canis* and *B. rossi* infections.[139–149] Similar studies have not yet been performed/published for other canine *Babesia* spp. Prevention of aggressive interactions with other dogs (especially fighting breeds such as APBT) may also prevent infection. All prospective canine blood donors should be tested for babesiosis with serology and PCR assays, and animals positive by either or both methods should not be used for blood donation.

Splenectomy of at-risk breeds or exposed/infected dogs should be avoided if possible. If a nonemergent splenectomy must be performed, treatment should be considered before the procedure. Ideally treatment would be completed 60 days prior to the procedure.

PUBLIC HEALTH ASPECTS

Canine and feline *Babesia* spp. do not appear to pose a zoonotic risk to immunocompetent humans. Their risks to immunocompromised individuals are unknown, but as with many infectious diseases, people who are undergoing chemotherapy, are immunocompromised, or have been splenectomized should exercise special caution when handling blood samples from dogs. Babesiosis is a rare tick-borne zoonosis of people in Europe and in the United States, and isolated uncharacterized *Babesia* infections have been reported in Africa and Mexico.[150,151] The majority of infections are mild or asymptomatic; however, some result in severe illness and death. Splenectomized people or those older than 55 years are especially at risk.[151] No *Babesia* species has been identified that is host specific for people. Sylvan cycles with wild animal reservoirs occur in nature. People serve as accidental hosts for *Babesia* of animals when they are bitten by infected ticks. Transmission through blood transfusion has also been described. *Babesia microti* is the primary parasite that infects people in the northeast and upper Midwest of the United States. The vector tick is *Ixodes scapularis*, which can co-transmit *Anaplasma phagocytophilum* and *Borrelia burgdorferi*. The hemolytic disease with flu-like symptoms is usually mild and self-limiting or easily treated with atovaquone and azithromycin. Both asymptomatic infections and clinical babesiosis with severe anemia have been reported in people in California and Washington and is caused by the more recently described parasite *Babesia duncani*.[151]

Babesia divergens causes a severe form of human babesiosis in Europe, which usually occurs in people who have had a splenectomy and is often fatal. Babesiosis was also identified in splenectomized people from Italy and Austria with a new strain (EU1) that was more closely related to *Babesia odocoilei*.[152] Identical isolates of *Babesia* have been found in *Ixodes ricinus* ticks from Slovenia, suggesting a more widespread distribution of this organism in Europe.

CASE EXAMPLE

Signalment

"Dora," a 4-year-old female spayed American Staffordshire terrier from North Carolina.

History

Dora was evaluated for a 3- to 4-day history of anorexia and lethargy. Before referral, an ELISA that detects heartworm antigen and antibodies to *E. canis* or *B. burgdorferi* antigens was performed and the results were negative. The dog had mild anemia (HCT 28.4%) and moderate thrombocytopenia (59,000 platelets/μL) on an automated hematology analyzer. Amoxicillin-clavulanic acid, doxycycline, and famotidine were prescribed. The patient began showing signs of increased energy and appetite as well as an increase in the HCT (38%) and platelet count (147,000 platelets/μL) after 4 weeks of treatment. However, because the values did not return to within reference range, the case was referred.

Physical Examination

Body weight: 24.2 kg.

General: Bright, alert, responsive, hydrated. T = 101.6°C (38.7°F), HR = 100 beats/minute, RR = 24 breaths/minute, mucous membranes pink, CRT < 2 seconds. Physical examination was otherwise unremarkable.

Selected Laboratory Findings

	Pretreatment	Posttreatment	Reference Range
PCV (%)	41	52	39–58
Platelet count (×10³/μL)	80	361	190–468
TP (g/dL)	6.3	6.5	5.2–7.3
Albumin (g/dL)	2.7	3.8	3–3.9
Globulin (g/dL)	3.5	2.7	1.7–3.8
Albumin/globulin ratio	0.78	1.38	0.9–1.8
Visualization of *Babesia* on microscopic examination of blood smear	Negative	Negative	
Babesia canis IFA	1:256	ND	
Ehrlichia canis IFA	<1:16	ND	
Bartonella vinsonii IFA	<1:16	ND	
Bartonella henselae IFA	<1:16	ND	
Rickettsia rickettsii IFA	1:64	ND	
SNAP 4Dx ELISA	Negative for all agents	ND	
Babesia spp. PCR	Positive (*B. gibsoni*)	Negative	

Continued

CASE EXAMPLE—cont'd

Diagnosis

Babesia gibsoni infection.

Treatment

Atovaquone and azithromycin.

Comments

Dogs with babesiosis often have a positive clinical response to doxycycline, which leads clinicians to suspect rickettsial infection. Although fever is considered a classic sign of babesiosis, most dogs are afebrile during initial examination, and waxing and waning fever is often documented with serial rectal temperatures. Thrombocytopenia is often a more prominent hematologic finding than anemia and may be the only finding in some cases. Babesiosis may be associated with changes in both albumin and globulin concentrations. Hypoalbuminemia can be secondary to proteinuria (not documented in this case). Globulins are often increased, although they may not be above the high end of the reference range. Organisms are frequently not observed on routine examination of stained blood smears, and PCR assays are required to document infection. Panels that detect antibodies to tick-borne pathogens typically either do not include *Babesia* spp. at all or only detect antibodies against *B. canis*. Serologic cross reactivity among species can occur, leading to inappropriate diagnosis and treatment recommendations. The positive titer to *Rickettsia* spp. was interesting, but in this geographic location, approximately 20% to 25% of healthy dogs are seropositive to *Rickettsia* spp., so its significance was unclear. Although acute-phase serology for *B. gibsoni* was not done, a convalescent titer to *B. gibsoni* at a follow up examination was 1:64.

SUGGESTED READINGS

Birkenheuer AJ, Correa MT, Levy MG, et al. Geographic distribution of babesiosis among dogs in the United States and association with dog bites: 150 cases (2000-2003). *J Am Vet Med Assoc*. 2005:227 942–947.

Di Cicco MF, Downey ME, Beeler E, et al. Re-emergence of *Babesia conradae* and effective treatment of infected dogs with atovaquone and azithromycin. *Vet Parasitol*. 2012;187:23–27.

Jefferies R, Ryan UM, Jardine J, et al. *Babesia gibsoni*: detection during experimental infections and after combined atovaquone and azithromycin therapy. *Exp Parasitol*. 2007;117:115–123.

REFERENCES

1. Hutcheon D. Diseases amongst dogs. Malignant jaundice or bilious fever of the dog. *Agric J Cape Good Hope*. 1893;6:2.
2. Eaton P. *Piroplasma canis* in Florida. *J Parasitol*. 1934;20:2.
3. Abu M, Hara I, Naito I, Sibauchi T. *Babesia* infections in puppies: probably due to transplacental transmission. *J Vet Med B Infect Dis Vet Public Health*. 1973;609:4.
4. Fukumoto S, Suzuki H, Igarashi I, et al. Fatal experimental transplacental *Babesia gibsoni* infections in dogs. *Int J Parasitol*. 2005;35:1031–1035.
5. Itoh N, Itoh S. A case of canine babesiosis possibly developed by transplacental infection. *J Jpn Vet Med Assoc*. 1990;43:2.
6. Schreeg ME, Marr HS, Tarigo JL, et al. Mitochondrial genome sequences and structures aid in the resolution of Piroplasmida phylogeny. *PLoS One*. 2016;11:e0165702.
7. Hornok S, Horvath G, Takacs N, et al. Molecular identification of badger-associated *Babesia* sp. DNA in dogs: updated phylogeny of piroplasms infecting Caniformia. *Parasit Vectors*. 2018;11:235.
8. Rosa CT, Pazzi P, Nagel S, et al. Theileriosis in six dogs in South Africa and its potential clinical significance. *J South African Vet Assoc*. 2014;85:1114.
9. Piana GP, Galli-Valerio B. Su di Un'inezione del cane con parassiti endoglobulari nel sangue. *Il Moderno Zooiatro*. 1895;6:6.
10. Reichenow E. Uebertragungsweise und Entwicklung der Piroplasmen. *Zbl Bakt I Orig*. 1935;135:11.
11. Reichenow E. Ueber die Entwicklung von *Theileria parva*, dem Erreger des Kustenfiebers der Rinder, in *Rhipicephalus appendiculatus*. *Zbl Bakt I Orig*. 1937;140:4.
12. Nuttall GHF. On Hematozoa occuring in wild animals in Africa. *Piroplasma rossi* n. sp. and *Haemogregarina canis adusti* n. sp. found in the jackal. 2. *Spirochaeta bovis caffris* n. sp. found in the buffalo. *Parasitology*. 1910;3:8.
13. Nuttall GHF. Note on *Rossiella rossi* (Nuttall, 1910) occuring in the jackal in British East Africa. *Parasitology*. 1912;5:4.
14. Uilenberg G, Franssen FF, Perie NM, et al. Three groups of *Babesia canis* distinguished and a proposal for nomenclature. *Vet Q*. 1989;11:33–40.
15. Buch J, Braff J, Leutenegger C, et al. The occurence and speciation of *Babesia* spp. infections by PCR in a global canine population. In: *Proceedings of the 2018 ACVIM Forum*; Seattle, WA.
16. Taboada J, Harvey JW, Levy MG, et al. Seroprevalence of babesiosis in greyhounds in Florida. *J Am Vet Med Assoc*. 1992;200:47–50.
17. Bobade PA, Oduye OO, Aghomo HO. Prevalence of antibodies against *Babesia canis* in dogs in an endemic area. *Rev Elev Med Vet Pays Trop*. 1989;42:211–217.
18. Harvey JW, Taboada J, Lewis JC. Babesiosis in a litter of pups. *J Am Vet Med Assoc*. 1988;192:1751–1752.
19. Cassini R, Zanutto S, Frangipane di Regalbono A, et al. Canine piroplasmosis in Italy: epidemiological aspects in vertebrate and invertebrate hosts. *Vet Parasitol*. 2009;165:30–35.
20. Bourdoiseau G. Canine babesiosis in France. *Vet Parasitol*. 2006;138:118–125.
21. Wright I. Babesiosis in Essex, UK: monitoring and learning lessons from a novel disease outbreak. *Parasit Vectors*. 2018;11:132.
22. Zygner W, Gorski P, Wedrychowicz H. New localities of *Dermacentor reticulatus* tick (vector of *Babesia canis canis*) in central and eastern Poland. *Polish J Vet Sci*. 2009;12:549–555.
23. Welc-Faleciak R, Rodo A, Sinski E, et al. *Babesia canis* and other tick-borne infections in dogs in Central Poland. *Vet Parasitol*. 2009;166:191–198.
24. Apanaskevich DA, Horak IG, Camicas JL. Redescription of *Haemaphysalis (Rhipistoma) elliptica* (Koch, 1844), an old taxon of the *Haemaphysalis (Rhipistoma) leachi* group from east and southern Africa, and of *Haemaphysalis (Rhipistoma) leachi* (Audouin, 1826) (Ixodida, Ixodidae). *Onderstepoort J Vet Res*. 2007;74:181–208.
25. Penzhorn BL, Vorster I, Harrison-White RF, et al. Black-backed jackals (*Canis mesomelas*) are natural hosts of *Babesia rossi*, the virulent causative agent of canine babesiosis in sub-Saharan Africa. *Parasit Vectors*. 2017;10:124.
26. Collett MG. Survey of canine babesiosis in South Africa. *J South Afr Vet Assoc*. 2000;71:180–186.
27. Shakespeare AS. The incidence of canine babesiosis amongst sick dogs presented to the Onderstepoort Veterinary Academic Hospital. *J South Afr Vet Assoc*. 1995;66:247–250.
28. Chatanga E, Kainga H, Razemba T, et al. Molecular detection and characterization of tick-borne hemoparasites and Anaplasmataceae in dogs in major cities of Malawi. *Parasitol Res*. 2021;120:267–276.
29. Reyers F, Leisewitz AL, Lobetti RG, et al. Canine babesiosis in South Africa: more than one disease. Does this serve as a model for falciparum malaria? *Ann Trop Med Parasitol*. 1998;92:503–511.
30. Lavan R, Tunceli K, de Swardt H, et al. Canine babesiosis treatment rates in South African veterinary clinics between 2011 and 2016. *Parasit Vectors*. 2018;11:386.
31. Birkenheuer AJ, Neel J, Ruslander D, et al. Detection and molecular characterization of a novel large *Babesia* species in a dog. *Vet Parasitol*. 2004;124:151–160.

32. Holman PJ, Backlund BB, Wilcox AL, et al. Detection of a large unnamed *Babesia* piroplasm originally identified in dogs in North Carolina in a dog with no history of travel to that state. *J Am Vet Med Assoc.* 2009;235:851–854.
33. Sikorski LE, Birkenheuer AJ, Holowaychuk MK, et al. Babesiosis caused by a large *Babesia* species in 7 immunocompromised dogs. *J Vet Intern Med.* 2010;24:127–131.
34. Holm LP, Kerr MG, Trees AJ, et al. Fatal babesiosis in an untravelled British dog. *Vet Rec.* 2006;159:179–180.
35. Birkenheuer AJ, Buch J, Beall MJ, et al. Global distribution of canine *Babesia* species identified by a commercial diagnostic laboratory. *Vet Parasitol Reg Studies Reports.* 2020;22:100471.
36. Konishi K, Sakata Y, Miyazaki N, et al. Epidemiological survey of *Babesia gibsoni* infection in dogs in Japan by enzyme-linked immunosorbent assay using *B. gibsoni* thrombospondin-related adhesive protein antigen. *Vet Parasitol.* 2008;155:204–208.
37. Matsuu A, Kawabe A, Koshida Y, et al. Incidence of canine *Babesia gibsoni* infection and subclinical infection among Tosa dogs in Aomori Prefecture, Japan. *J Vet Med Sci.* 2004;66:893–897.
38. Higuchi S, Fujimori M, Hoshi F, et al. Development of *Babesia gibsoni* in the salivary glands of the larval tick, *Rhipicephalus sanguineus. J Vet Med Sci.* 1995;57:117–119.
39. Higuchi S, Hoshina H, Hoshi F, et al. Development of *Babesia gibsoni* in the salivary glands of the tick, *Haemaphysalis longicornis. Kitasato Arch Exp Med.* 1993;65(Suppl):147–151.
40. Higuchi S, Izumitani M, Hoshi H, et al. Development of *Babesia gibsoni* in the midgut of larval tick, *Rhipicephalus sanguineus. J Vet Med Sci.* 1999;61:689–691.
41. Higuchi S, Konno H, Hoshi F, et al. Observations of *Babesia gibsoni* in the ovary of the tick, *Haemaphysalis longicornis. Kitasato Arch Exp Med.* 1993;65(Suppl):153–158.
42. Higuchi S, Kuroda H, Hoshi H, et al. Development of *Babesia gibsoni* in the midgut of the nymphal stage of the tick, *Rhipicephalus sanguineus. J Vet Med Sci.* 1999;61:697–699.
43. Higuchi S, Oya H, Hoshi F, et al. Observations of *Babesia gibsoni* in midgut epithelial cells of the tick, *Haemaphysalis longicornis. Kitasato Arch Exp Med.* 1992;65:143–147.
44. Higuchi S, Simomura S, Yoshida H, et al. Development of *Babesia gibsoni* in the hemolymph of the vector tick, *Haemaphysalis longicornis. J Vet Med Sci.* 1991;53:491–493.
45. Higuchi S, Simomura S, Yoshida H, et al. Development of *Babesia gibsoni* in the gut epithelium of the tick, *Haemaphysalis longicornis. J Vet Med Sci.* 1991;53:129–131.
46. Jongejan F, Su BL, Yang HJ, et al. Molecular evidence for the transovarial passage of *Babesia gibsoni* in *Haemaphysalis hystricis* (Acari: Ixodidae) ticks from Taiwan: a novel vector for canine babesiosis. *Parasit Vectors.* 2018;11:134.
47. Swaminath CSaS HE. The arthropod vector of *Babesia gibsoni. Ind Jour Med Res.* 1937;25:5.
48. Birkenheuer AJ, Correa MT, Levy MG, et al. Geographic distribution of babesiosis among dogs in the United States and association with dog bites: 150 cases (2000-2003). *J Am Vet Med Assoc.* 2005;227: 942–947.
49. Wang C, Ahluwalia SK, Li Y, et al. Frequency and therapy monitoring of canine *Babesia* spp. infection by high-resolution melting curve quantitative FRET-PCR. *Vet Parasitol.* 2010;168:11–18.
50. Birkenheuer AJ, Marr HS, Wilson JM, et al. *Babesia gibsoni* cytochrome b mutations in canine blood samples submitted to a US veterinary diagnostic laboratory. *J Vet Intern Med.* 2018;32:1965–1969.
51. Kjemtrup AM, Conrad PA. A review of the small canine piroplasms from California: *Babesia conradae* in the literature. *Vet Parasitol.* 2006;138:112–117.
52. Kjemtrup AM, Wainwright K, Miller M, et al. *Babesia conradae*, sp. nov., a small canine *Babesia* identified in California. *Vet Parasitol.* 2006;138:103–111.
53. Stayton E, Lineberry M, Thomas J, et al. Energence of Babesia conradae infection in coyote-hunting greyhounds in Oklahoma, USA. *J Vet Intern Med.* 2021;14:402.
54. Yamane I, Gardner IA, Telford III SR, Elward T, Hair JA, Conrad PA. Vector competence of *Rhipicephalus sanguineus* and *Dermacentor variabilis* for American isolates of *Babesia gibsoni. Exp Appl Acarol.* 1993;17:7.
55. Di Cicco MF, Downey ME, Beeler E, et al. Re-emergence of *Babesia conradae* and effective treatment of infected dogs with atovaquone and azithromycin. *Vet Parasitol.* 2012;187:23–27.
56. Dear JD, Owens SD, Lindsay LL, et al. *Babesia conradae* infection in coyote hunting dogs infected with multiple blood-borne pathogens. *J Vet Intern Med.* 2018;32:1609–1617.
57. Sykes JE. 2021. Unpublished observations.
58. Baneth G, Cardoso L, Brilhante-Simoes P, et al. Establishment of *Babesia vulpes* n. sp. (Apicomplexa: Babesiidae), a piroplasmid species pathogenic for domestic dogs. *Parasit Vectors.* 2019;12:129.
59. Miro G, Checa R, Paparini A, et al. *Theileria annae* (syn. *Babesia microti*-like) infection in dogs in NW Spain detected using direct and indirect diagnostic techniques: clinical report of 75 cases. *Parasit Vectors.* 2015;8:217.
60. Radyuk E, Karan L. A case of *Babesia vulpes* infection in a dog in Russia. *Vet Parasitol Reg Stud Reports.* 2020;22:100467.
61. Camacho AT, Guitian EJ, Pallas E, et al. Azotemia and mortality among *Babesia microti*-like infected dogs. *J Vet Intern Med.* 2004;18:141–146.
62. Camacho AT, Guitian FJ, Pallas E, et al. Serum protein response and renal failure in canine *Babesia annae* infection. *Vet Res.* 2005;36:713–722.
63. Camacho AT, Pallas E, Gestal JJ, et al. Natural infection by a *Babesia microti*-like piroplasm in a splenectomised dog. *Vet Rec.* 2002;150:381–382.
64. Camacho AT, Pallas E, Gestal JJ, et al. Infection of dogs in north-west Spain with a *Babesia microti*-like agent. *Vet Rec.* 2001;149:552–555.
65. Garcia AT. Piroplasma infection in dogs in northern Spain. *Vet Parasitol.* 2006;138:97–102.
66. Yeagley TJ, Reichard MV, Hempstead JE, et al. Detection of *Babesia gibsoni* and the canine small *Babesia* 'Spanish isolate' in blood samples obtained from dogs confiscated from dogfighting operations. *J Am Vet Med Assoc.* 2009;235:535–539.
67. Qurollo BA, Archer NR, Schreeg ME, et al. Improved molecular detection of *Babesia* infections in animals using a novel quantitative real-time PCR diagnostic assay targeting mitochondrial DNA. *Parasit Vectors.* 2017;10:128.
68. Barash NR, Thomas B, Birkenheuer AJ, et al. Prevalence of Babesia spp. and clinical characteristics of Babesia vulpes infections in North American dogs. *J Vet Intern Med.* 2019;33:2075–2081.
69. Birkenheuer AJ, Horney B, Bailey M, et al. *Babesia microti*-like infections are prevalent in North American foxes. *Vet Parasitol.* 2010;172:179–182.
70. Criado-Fornelio A, Martinez-Marcos A, Buling-Sarana A, et al. Molecular studies on *Babesia, Theileria* and *Hepatozoon* in southern Europe. Part I. Epizootiological aspects. *Vet Parasitol.* 2003;113:189–201.
71. Cardoso L, Cortes HC, Reis A, et al. Prevalence of *Babesia microti*-like infection in red foxes (*Vulpes vulpes*) from Portugal. *Vet Parasitol.* 2013;196:90–95.
72. Farkas R, Takacs N, Hornyak A, et al. First report on *Babesia* cf. *microti* infection of red foxes (*Vulpes vulpes*) from Hungary. *Parasit Vectors.* 2015;8:55.
73. Checa R, Fidalgo LE, Montoya A, et al. The role of healthy dog carriers of *Babesia microti*-like piroplasms. *Parasit Vectors.* 2019;12:127.
74. Camacho AT, Pallas E, Gestal JJ, et al. *Ixodes hexagonus* is the main candidate as vector of *Theileria annae* in northwest Spain. *Vet Parasitol.* 2003;112:157–163.
75. Baneth G, Nachum-Biala Y, Birkenheuer AJ, et al. A new piroplasmid species infecting dogs: morphological and molecular characterization and pathogeny of *Babesia negevi* n. sp. *Parasit Vectors.* 2020;13:130.
76. Penzhorn BL, Oosthuizen MC. *Babesia* species of domestic cats: molecular characterization has opened Pandora's Box. *Front Vet Sci.* 2020;7:134.
77. Penzhorn BL, Schoeman T, Jacobson LS. Feline babesiosis in South Africa: a review. 1026:183–186.
78. Bosman AM, Penzhorn BL, Brayton KA, et al. A novel *Babesia* sp. associated with clinical signs of babesiosis in domestic cats in South Africa. *Parasit Vectors.* 2019;12:138.
79. Wang J, Wang X, Sun H, et al. Molecular evidence of piroplasm infection in companion animals in Hunan Province, China. *BMC Vet Res.* 2020;16:297.

80. Penzhorn BL, Stylianides E, Coetzee MA, et al. A focus of feline babesiosis at Kaapschehoop on the Mpumalanga escarpment. *J South Afr Vet Assoc.* 1999;70:60.
81. Jacobson LS, Schoeman T, Lobetti RG. A survey of feline babesiosis in South Africa. *J South Afr Vet Assoc.* 2000;71:222–228.
82. Bosman AM, Venter EH, Penzhorn BL. Occurrence of *Babesia felis* and *Babesia leo* in various wild felid species and domestic cats in Southern Africa, based on reverse line blot analysis. *Vet Parasitol.* 2007;144:33–38.
83. Mendes-de-Almeida F, Faria MC, Branco AS, et al. Sanitary conditions of a colony of urban feral cats (*Felis catus* Linnaeus, 1758) in a zoological garden of Rio de Janeiro, Brazil. *Rev Instit Med Trop Sao Paulo.* 2004;46:269–274.
84. Kelly PJ, Koster L, Li J, et al. Survey of vector-borne agents in feral cats and first report of *Babesia gibsoni* in cats on St Kitts, West Indies. *BMC Vet Res.* 2017;13:331.
85. Bosman AM, Oosthuizen MC, Venter EH, et al. *Babesia lengau* associated with cerebral and haemolytic babesiosis in two domestic cats. *Parasit Vectors.* 2013;6:128.
86. Andre MR, Baccarim Denardi NC, Marques de Sousa KC, et al. Arthropod-borne pathogens circulating in free-roaming domestic cats in a zoo environment in Brazil. *Ticks Tick-borne Dis.* 2014;5:545–551.
87. Andre MR, Herrera HM, Fernandes Sde J, et al. Tick-borne agents in domesticated and stray cats from the city of Campo Grande, state of Mato Grosso do Sul, midwestern Brazil. *Ticks Tick-borne Dis.* 2015;6:779–786.
88. Malheiros J, Costa MM, do Amaral RB, et al. Identification of vector-borne pathogens in dogs and cats from Southern Brazil. *Ticks Tick-Borne Dis.* 2016;7:893–900.
89. Baneth G, Kenny MJ, Tasker S, et al. Infection with a proposed new subspecies of *Babesia canis, Babesia canis* subsp. *presentii*, in domestic cats. *J Clin Microbiol.* 2004;42:99–105.
90. Georges K, Ezeokoli CD, Newaj-Fyzul A, et al. The application of PCR and reverse line blot hybridization to detect arthropod-borne hemopathogens of dogs and cats in Trinidad. *Ann New York Acad Sci.* 2008;1149:196–199.
91. Panicker VP, Sreedharannair AK, Narayanan A, et al. Molecular identification of a novel species, *Babesia panickeri* sp. *nov.*, from a naturally infected domestic cat of India and its comparison with canine *Babesia* isolates. *Acta Parasitol.* 2020;65:913–918.
92. Adaszek L, Ukaszewska J, Winiarczyk S, et al. The first case of feline babesiosis in Poland. *Zycie Weterynaryjne.* 2008;83:3.
93. Slade DJ, Lees GE, Berridge BR, et al. Resolution of a proteinuric nephropathy associated with *Babesia gibsoni* infection in a dog. *J Am Anim Hosp Assoc.* 2011;47:e138–144.
94. Ullal T, Birkenheuer A, Vaden S. Azotemia and proteinuria in dogs infected with *Babesia gibsoni. J Am Anim Hosp Assoc.* 2018;54:156–160.
95. Defauw P, Daminet S, Leisewitz AL, et al. Renal azotemia and associated clinical and laboratory findings in dogs with *Babesia rossi* infection. *Vet Parasitol.* 2018;260:22–29.
96. Kules J, Bilic P, Beer Ljubic B, et al. Glomerular and tubular kidney damage markers in canine babesiosis caused by *Babesia canis. Ticks Tick-Borne Dis.* 2018;9:1508–1517.
97. Birkenheuer AJ. 2021. Unpublished observations.
98. Hossain MA, Yamato O, Yamasaki M, et al. Serum from dogs infected with *Babesia gibsoni* inhibits maturation of reticulocytes and erythrocyte 5'-nucleotidase activity in vitro. *J Vet Med Sci.* 2003;65:1281–1286.
99. Lobetti RG, Reyers F. Met-haemoglobinuria in naturally occurring *Babesia canis* infection. *J South Afr Vet Assoc.* 1996;67:88–90.
100. Makinde MO, Bobade PA. Osmotic fragility of erythrocytes in clinically normal dogs and dogs infected with parasites. *Res Vet Sci.* 1994;57:343–348.
101. Murase T, Ueda T, Yamato O, et al. Oxidative damage and enhanced erythrophagocytosis in canine erythrocytes infected with *Babesia gibsoni. J Vet Med Sci.* 1996;58:259–261.
102. Otsuka Y, Yamasaki M, Yamato O, et al. Increased generation of superoxide in erythrocytes infected with *Babesia gibsoni. J Vet Med Sci.* 2001;63:1077–1081.
103. Wozniak EJ, Barr BC, Thomford JW, et al. Clinical, anatomic, and immunopathologic characterization of *Babesia gibsoni* infection in the domestic dog (*Canis familiaris*). *J Parasitol.* 1997;83:692–699.
104. Zahler M, Rinder H, Schein E, et al. Detection of a new pathogenic *Babesia microti*-like species in dogs. *Vet Parasitol.* 2000;89:241–248.
105. Guitian FJ, Camacho AT, Telford SR 3rd. Case-control study of canine infection by a newly recognised *Babesia microti*-like piroplasm. *Prev Vet Med.* 2003;61:137–145.
106. Jacobson LS, Clark IA. The pathophysiology of canine babesiosis: new approaches to an old puzzle. *J South Afr Vet Assoc.* 1994;65:134–145.
107. Leisewitz AL, Jacobson LS, de Morais HS, et al. The mixed acid-base disturbances of severe canine babesiosis. *J Vet Intern Med.* 2001;15:445–452.
108. Nel M, Lobetti RG, Keller N, et al. Prognostic value of blood lactate, blood glucose, and hematocrit in canine babesiosis. *J Vet Intern Med.* 2004;18:471–476.
109. Strobl A, Kunzel F, Tichy A, et al. Complications and risk factors regarding the outcomes of canine babesiosis in Central Europe - a retrospective analysis of 240 cases. *Acta Vet Hung.* 2020;68:160–168.
110. Irwin PJ, Hutchinson GW. Clinical and pathological findings of *Babesia* infection in dogs. *Aust Vet J.* 1991;68:204–209.
111. Zygner W, Gojska O, Rapacka G, et al. Hematological changes during the course of canine babesiosis caused by large *Babesia* in domestic dogs in Warsaw (Poland). *Vet Parasitol.* 2007;145:146–151.
112. Farwell GE, LeGrand EK, Cobb CC. Clinical observations on *Babesia gibsoni* and *Babesia canis* infections in dogs. *J Am Vet Med Assoc.* 1982;180:507–511.
113. Schoeman T, Lobetti RG, Jacobson LS, et al. Feline babesiosis: signalment, clinical pathology and concurrent infections. *J South Afr Vet Assoc.* 2001;72:4–11.
114. Matthewman LA, Kelly PJ, Bobade PA, et al. Infections with *Babesia canis* and *Ehrlichia canis* in dogs in Zimbabwe. *Vet Rec.* 1993;133:344–346.
115. Bohm M, Leisewitz AL, Thompson PN, et al. Capillary and venous *Babesia canis rossi* parasitaemias and their association with outcome of infection and circulatory compromise. *Vet Parasitol.* 2006;141:18–29.
116. Mattia AR, Waldron MA, Sierra LS. Use of the Quantitative Buffy Coat system for detection of parasitemia in patients with babesiosis. *J Clin Microbiol.* 1993;31:2816–2818.
117. Comazzi S, Paltrinieri S, Manfredi MT, et al. Diagnosis of canine babesiosis by Percoll gradient separation of parasitized erythrocytes. *J Vet Diagn Invest.* 1999;11:102–104.
118. Birkenheuer AJ, Levy MG, Breitschwerdt EB. Development and evaluation of a seminested PCR for detection and differentiation of *Babesia gibsoni* (Asian genotype) and *B. canis* DNA in canine blood samples. *J Clin Microbiol.* 2003;41:4172–4177.
119. Happi AN, Toepp AJ, Ugwu CA, et al. Detection and identification of blood-borne infections in dogs in Nigeria using light microscopy and the polymerase chain reaction. *Vet Parasitol Reg Stud Reports.* 2018;11:55–60.
120. Vercammen F, De Deken R, Maes L. Duration of protective immunity in experimental canine babesiosis after homologous and heterologous challenge. *Vet Parasitol.* 1997;68:51–55.
121. Penzhorn BL, Lewis BD, de Waal DT, et al. Sterilisation of *Babesia canis* infections by imidocarb alone or in combination with diminazene. *J South Afr Vet Assoc.* 1995;66:157–159.
122. Birkenheuer AJ, Levy MG, Breitschwerdt EB. Efficacy of combined atovaquone and azithromycin for therapy of chronic *Babesia gibsoni* (Asian genotype) infections in dogs. *J Vet Intern Med.* 2004;18:494–498.
123. Kirk SK, Levy JK, Crawford PC. Efficacy of azithromycin and compounded atovaquone for treatment of *Babesia gibsoni* in dogs. *J Vet Intern Med.* 2017;31:1108–1112.
124. Sakuma M, Setoguchi A, Endo Y. Possible emergence of drug-resistant variants of *Babesia gibsoni* in clinical cases treated with atovaquone and azithromycin. *J Vet Intern Med.* 2009;23:493–498.
125. Jefferies R, Ryan UM, Jardine J, et al. *Babesia gibsoni*: detection during experimental infections and after combined atovaquone and azithromycin therapy. *Exp Parasitol.* 2007;117:115–123.
126. Matsuu A, Miyamoto K, Ikadai H, et al. Short report: cloning of the *Babesia gibsoni* cytochrome B gene and isolation of three single nucleotide

polymorphisms from parasites present after atovaquone treatment. *Am J Trop Med Hyg*. 2006;74:593–597.
127. Sakuma M, Fukuda K, Takayama K, et al. Molecular epidemiological survey of the *Babesia gibsoni* cytochrome b gene in western Japan. *J Vet Med Sci*. 2012;74:1341–1344.
128. Stegeman JR, Birkenheuer AJ, Kruger JM, et al. Transfusion-associated *Babesia gibsoni* infection in a dog. *J Am Vet Med Assoc*. 2003;222:959–963.
129. Checa R, Montoya A, Ortega N, et al. Efficacy, safety and tolerance of imidocarb dipropionate versus atovaquone or buparvaquone plus azithromycin used to treat sick dogs naturally infected with the *Babesia microti*-like piroplasm. *Parasit Vectors*. 2017;10:145.
130. Suzuki K, Wakabayashi H, Takahashi M, et al. A possible treatment strategy and clinical factors to estimate the treatment response in *Babesia gibsoni* infection. *J Vet Med Sci*. 2007;69:563–568.
131. Almendros A, Burchell R, Wierenga J. An alternative combination therapy with metronidazole, clindamycin and doxycycline for *Babesia gibsoni* (Asian genotype) in dogs in Hong Kong. *J Vet Med Sci*. 2020;82:1334–1340.
132. Wulansari R, Wijaya A, Ano H, et al. Clindamycin in the treatment of *Babesia gibsoni* infections in dogs. *J Am Anim Hosp Assoc*. 2003;39:558–562.
133. Liu M, Ji S, Kondoh D, et al. Tafenoquine is a promising drug candidate for the treatment of babesiosis. *Antimicrob Agents Chemother*. 2021;65. e0020421.
134. Penzhorn BL, Lewis BD, Lopez-Rebollar LM, et al. Screening of five drugs for efficacy against *Babesia felis* in experimentally infected cats. *J South Afr Vet Assoc*. 2000;71:53–57.
135. Moreau Y, Vidor E, Bissuel G, et al. Vaccination against canine babesiosis: an overview of field observations. *Trans Royal Soc Trop Med Hyg*. 1989;83(Suppl):95–96.
136. Schetters T. Vaccination against canine babesiosis. *Trends Parasitol*. 2005;21:179–184.
137. Schetters TH, Kleuskens J, Scholtes N, et al. Strain variation limits protective activity of vaccines based on soluble *Babesia canis* antigens. *Parasite Immunol*. 1995;17:215–218.
138. Schetters TP, Kleuskens J, Carcy B, et al. Vaccination against large *Babesia* species from dogs. *Parassitologia*. 2007;49(suppl 1):13–17.
139. Beugnet F, Halos L, Larsen D, et al. The ability of an oral formulation of afoxolaner to block the transmission of *Babesia canis* by *Dermacentor reticulatus* ticks to dogs. *Parasit Vectors*. 2014;7:283.
140. Geurden T, Six R, Becskei C, et al. Evaluation of the efficacy of sarolaner (Simparica®) in the prevention of babesiosis in dogs. *Parasit Vectors*. 2017;10:415.
141. Taenzler J, Liebenberg J, Roepke RK, et al. Prevention of transmission of *Babesia canis* by *Dermacentor reticulatus* ticks to dogs treated orally with fluralaner chewable tablets (Bravecto). *Parasit Vectors*. 2015;8:305.
142. Taenzler J, Liebenberg J, Roepke RK, et al. Prevention of transmission of *Babesia canis* by *Dermacentor reticulatus* ticks to dogs after topical administration of fluralaner spot-on solution. *Parasit Vectors*. 2016;9:234.
143. Jongejan F, Fourie JJ, Chester ST, et al. The prevention of transmission of *Babesia canis* canis by *Dermacentor reticulatus* ticks to dogs using a novel combination of fipronil, amitraz and (S)-methoprene. *Vet Parasitol*. 2011;179:343–350.
144. Jongejan F, de Vos C, Fourie JJ, et al. A novel combination of fipronil and permethrin (Frontline Tri-Act®/Frontect®) reduces risk of transmission of *Babesia canis* by *Dermacentor reticulatus* and of *Ehrlichia canis* by *Rhipicephalus sanguineus* ticks to dogs. *Parasit Vectors*. 2015;8:602.
145. Fourie JJ, de Vos C, Crafford D, et al. A study on the long-term efficacy of Seresto® collars in preventing *Babesia canis* (Piana & Galli-Valerio, 1895) transmission to dogs by infected *Dermacentor reticulatus* (Fabricius, 1794) ticks. *Parasit Vectors*. 2019;12:139.
146. Fourie JJ, Stanneck D, Jongejan F. Prevention of transmission of *Babesia canis* by *Dermacentor reticulatus* ticks to dogs treated with an imidacloprid/flumethrin collar. *Vet Parasitol*. 2013;192:273–278.
147. Navarro C, Reymond N, Fourie J, et al. Prevention of *Babesia canis* in dogs: efficacy of a fixed combination of permethrin and fipronil (Effitix®) using an experimental transmission blocking model with infected *Dermacentor reticulatus* ticks. *Parasit Vectors*. 2015;8:32.
148. Last RD, Hill JM, Matjila PT, et al. A field trial evaluation of the prophylactic efficacy of amitraz-impregnated collars against canine babesiosis (*Babesia canis rossi*) in South Africa. *J South African Vet Assoc*. 2007;78:63–65.
149. Cavalleri D, Murphy M, Seewald W, et al. Two randomized, controlled studies to assess the efficacy and safety of lotilaner (Credelio) in preventing *Dermacentor reticulatus* transmission of *Babesia canis* to dogs. *Parasit Vectors*. 2017;10:520.
150. Kjemtrup AM, Conrad PA. Human babesiosis: an emerging tick-borne disease. *Int J Parasitol*. 2000;30:1323–1337.
151. Krause PJ. Human babesiosis. *Int J Parasitol*. 2019;49:165–174.
152. Herwaldt BL, de Bruyn G, Pieniazek NJ, et al. *Babesia divergens*-like infection, Washington State. *Emerg Infect Dis*. 2004;10:622–629.

98

Cytauxzoonosis

Leah A. Cohn, Adam J. Birkenheuer

KEY POINTS

- First Described: Cytauxzoonosis was first recognized in domestic cats from Missouri during the mid-1970s.[1]
- Cause: *Cytauxzoon felis* is a hematoprotozoal pathogen of domestic and wild felids.
- Affected Hosts: Only felids are infected with *C. felis.* Domestic cats often develop a severe disease but occasionally only a mild, brief or unapparent illness. The bobcat reservoir host is believed to typically demonstrate mild illness but can die as a result of infection. Other felids (e.g., cougars, tigers, and lions) can also become infected.
- Arthropod Vectors: *Amblyomma americanum* (lone star tick) is the primary vector for pathogen transmission, although *Dermacentor variabilis* (American dog ticks) may also be competent vectors.
- Geographic Distribution: In the United States, cytauxzoonosis is identified in the midwest, south-central, south-eastern, and the mid-Atlantic states; the geographic range has expanded with the expanded range of *A. americanum* ticks. Cytauxzoonosis is also reported in South America (especially Brazil). Other species of *Cytauxzoon* cause infection in felidae in Eurasia.
- Route of Transmission: *Cytauxzoon felis* is transmitted by the feeding of vector ticks.
- Major Clinical Signs: Cytauxzoonosis is a rapidly progressive febrile illness characterized by anorexia, lethargy or depressed mentation, elevation of the third eyelid, vocalization, increased respiratory effort, icterus, pallor, lymphadenomegaly, splenomegaly or hepatomegaly, and sometimes seizures.
- Differential Diagnosis: Tularemia is an important differential for outdoor cats. Depending on clinical signs present, other differentials include hemotropic mycoplasmosis, cholangiohepatitis, histoplasmosis, sepsis, primary IMHA, oxidative toxicities, toxoplasmosis, and FIP.
- Human Health Significance: None.

ETIOLOGIC AGENT AND EPIDEMIOLOGY

Feline cytauxzoonosis, an emerging infectious disease with an expanding geographic distribution, is caused by the vector-borne hematoprotozoan parasite *Cytauxzoon felis*. A member of the order Piroplasmida, the organism is part of the family Theileriidae. Like other Theileriidae, *C. felis* exists in two distinct nonerythrocytic (schizont) and erythrocytic (piroplasm) forms within the mammalian host.

Although *C. felis* is the species most relevant to the health of domestic cats in the United States, it is only one of several species of the genus *Cytauxzoon*.[2] Outside the United States, cytauxzoonosis has been described in cats in South America (especially Brazil).[3–5] Other species of *Cytauxzoon* cause infection in felidae in Europe and Asia.[6–11] A morphologically indistinguishable intraerythrocytic parasite, *Cytauxzoon manul*, has been identified in Pallas's cats (*Otocolobus manul*) imported from Mongolia.[12] Sequence analysis of the 18S rRNA gene confirms that the organism is related to, but distinct from, *C. felis.*[9] When injected into domestic cats, *C. manul* produced erythroparasitemia, but no disease, and was unable to prevent virulent disease when those cats were subsequently infected with *C. felis.*[13] Similar but distinct pathogens have been detected in both wild and domestic cats in Eurasia (e.g., Spain, Portugal, Italy, France, Germany, Switzerland, Russia, Iran, and China) (Fig. 98.1).[7,8,10,11,14–21] *Cytauxzoon europaeus* is the proposed name for a species identified in domestic cats and wild felis in Europe, with rare novel species detected in European wildcats (*Felis sylvestris sylvestris*) from Romania (*Cytauxzoon otrantorum and Cytauxzoon banethi*).[11,21] *Cytauxzoon* parasites identified in domestic cats in South America may or may not be genetically identical to the *C. felis* found in the United States.[22–25] Infection with *C. felis* or very closely related protozoa occurs in a wide variety of non-domesticated felid species, including both wild and captive (i.e., non-native) large cats.[26–33] In the United States, the presumed reservoir host for *C. felis* is the bobcat (*Lynx rufus rufus*). In bobcats, infection is believed to commonly result in brief illness followed by persistent subclinical erythroparasitemia, but unknown numbers of wild cats may die of infection in endemic areas.[32,34–37] Experimental transmission studies to many nonfelid species, including immunodeficient mice, have failed.[38]

Cytauxzoonosis can occur in cats of any age and either sex, with no identified breed predilections. Immune suppression is not necessary for cats to become infected, and there is no evidence that infection is more likely in retrovirus-infected cats than in noninfected cats. Outdoor cats are more likely to become infected because of increased exposure to tick vectors. Infections occur during the warm months with a peak incidence during the spring, and a second smaller peak in the early autumn.[39] In retrospective studies, infection has rarely been identified from November through March.[37,39,40]

For many years after its original description in Missouri during the mid-1970s,[1] feline cytauxzoonosis was recognized only in the south-central United States. With expansion of the range of the primary vector tick, *Amblyomma americanum*,[41] the geographic range has expanded subsequently, with infections now reported in cats throughout the south-central, south-eastern, and mid-Atlantic regions.[42–47] Although not yet demonstrated in domestic cats, *C. felis* infection has been demonstrated in bobcats living as far north as Pennsylvania[48] and North Dakota.[45] Although it is possible that infections outside the south-central United States were simply missed in years past, the relative ease of recognition of the parasite on examination of blood smears or by finding organisms in tissues following necropsy makes

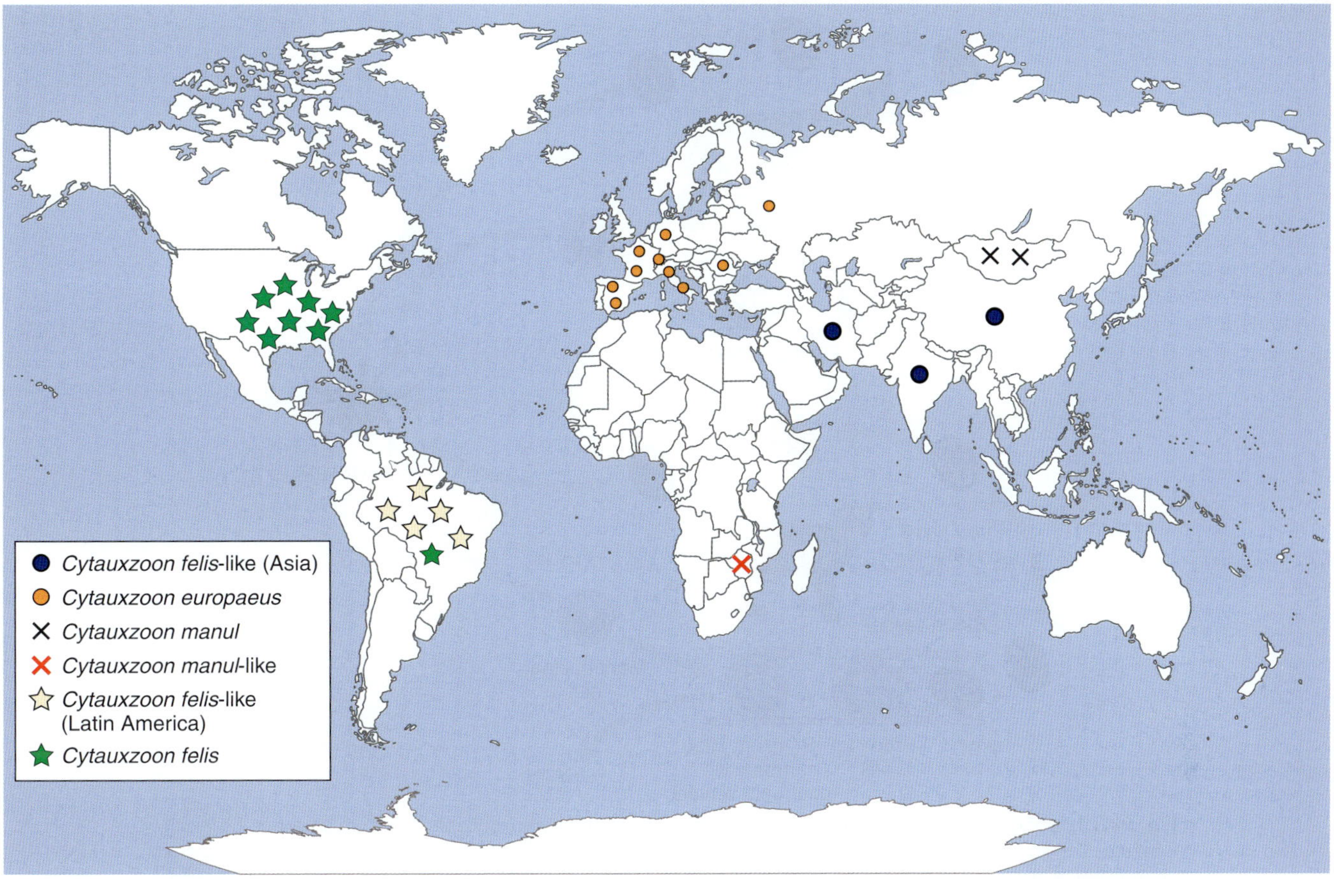

Fig. 98.1 Map of global reports of *Cytauxzoon felis* and related organisms in domestic and wild felids. Species with proposed names *Cytauxzoon banethi* and *Cytauxzoon otrantoreum* have been identified in European wildcats from Romania (see text, not marked).

this possibility seem unlikely. Instead, the parasite likely now occurs throughout a wider geographic region. The geographic range of reported *C. felis* infections in domestic cats in North America appears to overlap with the ranges inhabited by both bobcats and *Amblyomma americanum* (Fig. 98.2).[45] Ecological niche models using the distribution of tick vectors and the reservoir hosts predict a broader possible distribution of infection than models based on recognized cases in domestic cats.[37] Because the primary reservoir host for the pathogen in the United States is the bobcat, infected domestic cats are typically from rural or suburban rather than urban areas. Cats living close to wooded areas or less intensely managed land are more likely to become infected.[39] It is common for multiple cats in a neighborhood, or even a household, to become infected within a single season, likely reflecting the presence of infected carriers in the area.

There are few studies of incidence or prevalence in domestic cats. Prevalence studies focus on healthy carrier cats, but because infection is often rapidly fatal, prevalence (i.e., infections at any one time) cannot be used to estimate disease incidence (i.e., infections over a period of time). Interestingly, disease may be more virulent in some geographic regions than others, thus leading to a lower prevalence in those areas even if disease incidence is high.[49] In a study of 902 healthy cats, 18 of 60 blood samples (30%) from a single clinic in Arkansas were positive using PCR.[44,49] The clinic was in an area that was suspected to harbor a less virulent strain of the pathogen. The overall prevalence in that same study for cats tested in Arkansas (15.5%) and Missouri (12.9%) was higher than that in Oklahoma (3.4%).[44] Anecdotally, Oklahoma strains may be more virulent with few cats surviving infection despite aggressive treatment.[50] In another study

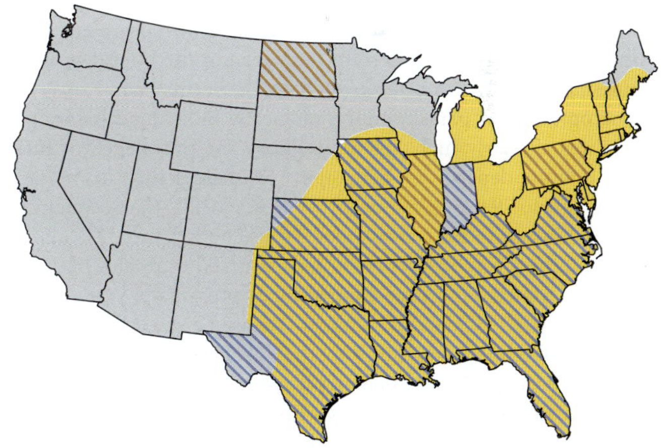

Fig. 98.2 Geographic distribution of *Cytauxzoon felis* infections in the United States. Shaded areas show confirmed cases in domestic cats (blue stripes) or bobcats only (black stripes; ND, IL and PA). The yellow region (with and without overlying stripes) represents the distribution of *Amblyomma americanum* ticks.

involving cats from northern Oklahoma, where disease is recognized only rarely, the prevalence of infection was less than 1%.[51] Few of the healthy cats that were part of TNR programs in North Carolina, Florida, and Tennessee were infected, with prevalence of 0 to 1.3%.[52] Among healthy cats considered at high risk due to outdoor exposure in endemic regions of Arkansas and Georgia, 27/89 (30.3%) of cats were PCR-positive.[53] The authors of this chapter are aware of several

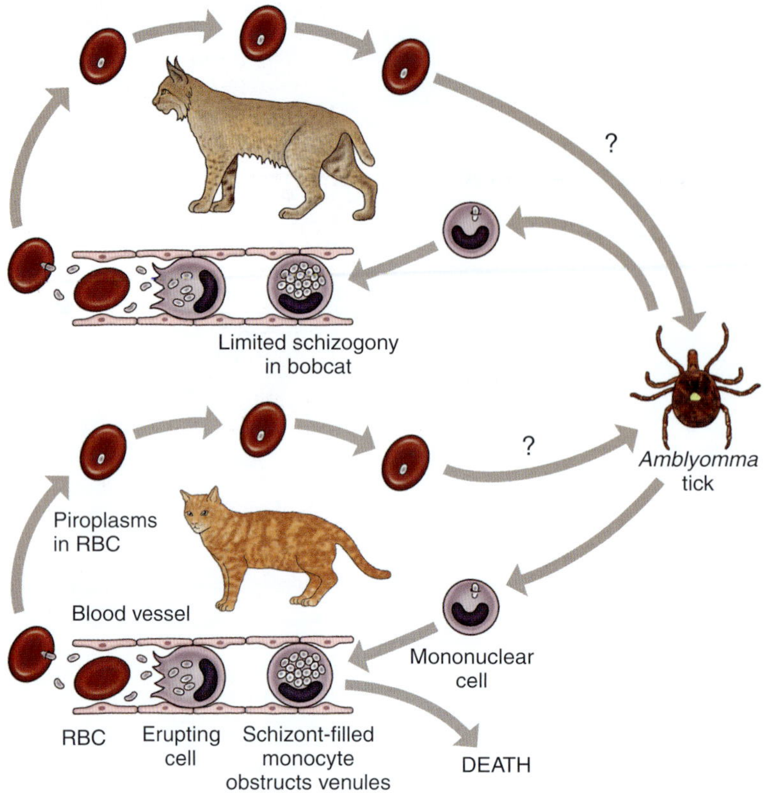

Fig. 98.3 Life cycle of *Cytauxzoon felis*. The parasite is maintained in bobcats *(top)* which are subclinically infected. The sexual cycle of the organism occurs in *Amblyomma americanum* hard ticks, which then transmit sporozoites to domestic cats. Sporozoites invade mononuclear cells, where they undergo schizogony. Schizont-filled monocytes obstruct capillaries and cause multiorgan failure and death. In cats that survive the schizogony phase, the organism infects erythrocytes and forms piroplasms. The importance of domestic cats as a reservoir for infection of ticks is uncertain. The schizogony phase in the bobcat is usually relatively mild and brief.

colonies of cats in Missouri and North Carolina with prevalence rates of up to 72%, nearly equivalent to rates seen in the bobcat reservoir in endemic areas. The prevalence of infection in cats from Brazil with a hematoprotozoan parasite morphologically indistinguishable from *C. felis* was similarly high, up to 48.5%.[24] The prevalence of infection in bobcats depends on geography; estimates range from 7% in Pennsylvania to 79% in Missouri.[45,48,54,55] In Florida, the prevalence of subclinical infection for transplanted Texas cougars was 39% and for Florida panthers was 35%.[56] There are fewer still estimates of disease incidence. Cytauxzoonosis accounted for approximately 1% of feline submissions to the Oklahoma Animal Disease Diagnostic Laboratory and 1.5% of feline admissions to the Oklahoma State University VMTH between 1995 and 2006 and between 1998 and 2006, respectively.[39] Personal communications with the authors of this chapter suggest that veterinarians in enzootic “hot spots” see as many as 5 cases of cytauxzoonosis a week during the peak season, with many more veterinarians in endemic areas reporting that they see 5–10 cases per summer.

Infection of domestic cats with *C. felis* in a natural setting requires a tick vector; ill and naïve cats can be co-housed without disease transmission.[57] Although perinatal transmission is important for other hematoprotozoal infections, there is little evidence that this is the case for *C. felis*.[58] Similarly, tick ingestion does not seem to be an important route of infection.[59] Experimentally, infection can be transmitted through inoculation of schizont-laden tissues or transfusion of blood collected during the acute illness.[34,57,60] Transfusion of blood from recovered cats, which contains only erythrocytes with piroplasms rather than mononuclear-associated schizonts, does transmit the piroplasm stage of infection but does not result in schizogony or clinical illness in the recipient.[34,61]

A variety of ticks feed on both domestic and wild felids, and *C. felis* has been recovered from *Dermacentor variabilis* and *A. americanum* ticks.[62] Although vector competence and transstadial transmission (nymphs to adults) have been demonstrated for both, *A. americanum* appears to be the primary natural vector.[41,61,63] Although neither *D. variabilis* nor *A. americanum* is found in Brazil, naturally occurring infection with *Cytauxzoon* spp. occur there.[3,5,23,25] Presumably, *Amblyomma cajennense* or another ixodid tick is the responsible vector.[64] There are no published studies investigating transovarial transmission in ticks.

When bobcats become infected with *C. felis*, there is limited schizogenous replication associated with a typically mild to moderate acute clinical illness, although fatal infection of bobcats has been described.[32,34,35] On recovery from illness, bobcats remain infected with piroplasms in their erythrocytes. Ticks become infected when they ingest piroplasms contained in erythrocytes of persistently infected carriers. These ticks then transmit sporozoites to the next felid host on which it feeds (Fig. 98.3). If the tick feeds on another bobcat, the sylvan cycle is repeated. If the tick feeds on a domestic cat, infection often results in massive schizogenous replication and profound illness.

For years, domestic cats were deemed terminal hosts because most died from cytauxzoonosis. Felids that recover from acute infection can apparently harbor piroplasms for months or even years without serious consequences.[24,49,52,53,65–68] Additionally, domestic cats that harbor piroplasms without any history of clinical illness are occasionally identified.[25,44,49,52] In an experimental setting, domestic cats can transmit infection via the tick vector.[41,69,70] Although these studies demonstrate reservoir competence, more extensive studies are necessary to establish the actual reservoir capacity of domestic cats in a natural setting. The existence of domestic cat colonies with high prevalence rates of *C. felis* infections combined with extensive exposure to competent tick vectors suggests that both the reservoir and vector capacities are likely to be high in select populations.[44,53] If so, movement of domestic carrier cats (with their owners) might help account for the expansion in the endemic geographic region for this pathogen.[26,44]

CLINICAL FEATURES

Pathogenesis and Clinical Signs

Much of what we believe to occur in the life cycle of *C. felis* is inferred from what is known about related protozoan parasites. The sexual phase of reproduction occurs in the tick gut. Ookinetes leave the gut, enter the body cavity, and migrate to the salivary glands, where they replicate as infective sporozoites. After these sporozoites enter the host during tick feeding, they penetrate and develop, primarily within mononuclear phagocytes. They are visible first as indistinct vesicular structures within the cytoplasm of infected cells and later as large, distinct, nucleated schizonts that actively undergo division by schizogony and binary fission. Multiplication of schizonts within host cells is observed ultrastructurally to be true schizogony, without host cell division. Fission of the schizont within the mononuclear cells results in the formation of merozoites.[71] The phagocytes line the lumens of vessels within almost every organ and become huge and numerous, often occluding the vessel similar to a thrombus (Fig. 98.4). The host cell probably ruptures, releasing the merozoites into the blood or tissue fluid. Merozoites appear in macrophages 1 to 3 days before they are observed in erythrocytes. These organisms then invade uninfected erythrocytes and produce late-stage parasitemias that are detected on examination of blood smears (Fig. 98.5). Piroplasms (merozoites) reproduce through asexual binary fission only in erythrocytes.

The phase of asexual schizogenous reproduction, within the host's mononuclear phagocytic cells, is responsible for the pathologic processes resulting in clinical illness. It is unclear whether only sporozoites can enter macrophages and initiate schizogony or if early schizonts can spread from macrophage to macrophage. Regardless, infection results in massive numbers of schizont-distended mononuclear cells within the vascular lumen of the interstitium of most organs. This may be especially severe in the lungs, liver, spleen, and other lymphoid tissues.[57,72] DIC, presumably activated by vascular endothelial disruption, has been a complication based on laboratory findings in naturally infected cats.[73,74] Vascular obstruction, anoxia, and release of damaging substances secondary to cell death and rupture may all contribute to multiple organ failure. The presence of piroplasms is sometimes associated with hemolysis during the later stages of the acute illness, but piroplasms are not likely a major contributor to disease.

Less virulent strains of *C. felis* might result in a more limited schizogony with less associated pathology in domestic cats. The theoretical existence of less virulent strains is supported by a regional occurrence of survivors at a greater than expected rate.[49] Using noncoding regions of rRNA known as internal transcribed spacer (ITS) regions, variability in strains of *C. felis* from naturally infected cats in Georgia and Arkansas was demonstrated.[27] Despite initial findings suggesting an association between survivability and the particular strain of *C. felis,* a subsequent study found that ITS region-sequence type could not be used to discriminate between strain pathogenicity and disease survival.[53]

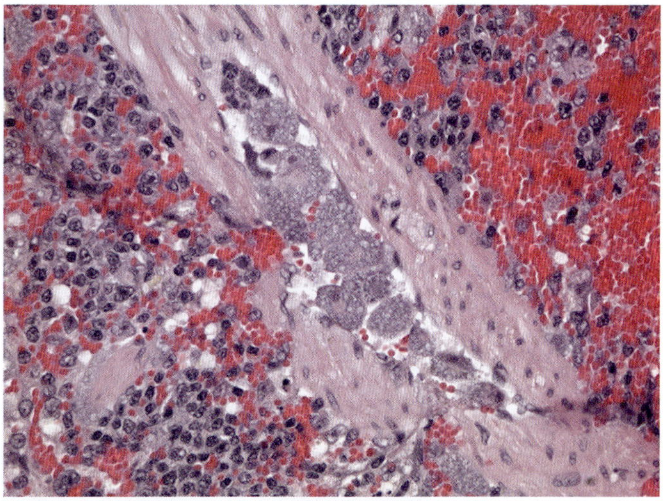

Fig. 98.4 Histologic image from the spleen of a cat that died of cytauxzoonosis demonstrates many readily recognizable schizont-laden mononuclear phagocytic cells occluding the vascular lumen (hematoxylin and eosin stain, ×100). Histologic disease diagnosis is generally straightforward. (Courtesy of Dr. Linda Berent.)

Although historic findings are nonspecific, an acute onset of anorexia, lethargy, and fever in cats given outdoor exposure within an endemic region (especially during spring, summer, or early autumn) should raise immediate suspicions for cytauxzoonosis. The onset of clinical disease occurs from 1 to 3 weeks after tick-transmitted infection.[41,61] Initial clinical signs are vague and typically include anorexia and lethargy. Within hours to days, illness becomes more severe and owners may notice increased vocalization, weakness, icterus, dark yellow urine color, respiratory distress, obtunded mentation, or even seizures.[42] Cats may become comatose shortly before death.

Physical Examination Findings

Physical examination findings are nonspecific. The most consistent alteration on physical examination is pyrexia (often marked: 39.4°C to 41.6°C [103°F to 107°F]), but hypothermia occurs in moribund animals. Higher rectal temperatures have not been associated with a poorer prognosis,[75] and in the author's experience, cats with a rapid drop in temperature after treatment is begun are less likely to survive. Mucous membranes may be icteric and/or pale. Evidence of dehydration and delayed CRT or mucosal pallor may be observed. Tachypnea and tachycardia are typical, with or without overt respiratory distress. Arrhythmia may also be identified.[76] Pleural effusion can lead to shallow breaths with inspiratory effort and paradoxical breathing. Lung sounds may be harsh due to interstitial pneumonia, or may be diminished ventrally due to effusion. Mild to moderate lymphadenomegaly, splenomegaly, and hepatomegaly are often detected. Sometimes, cats are hyperesthetic during muscle palpation and vocalize when handled. Cats may demonstrate ataxia, seizures, or become comatose shortly before death. Elevation of the third eyelid is common. The entire disease course is usually rapid, and many cats succumb within days.[42,77,78]

DIAGNOSIS

Laboratory Abnormalities

Complete Blood Count

A CBC with blood smear examination is the single most useful diagnostic test for cytauxzoonosis. Pancytopenia is often recognized in cats with cytauxzoonosis. A bone marrow crowded with schizont-laden

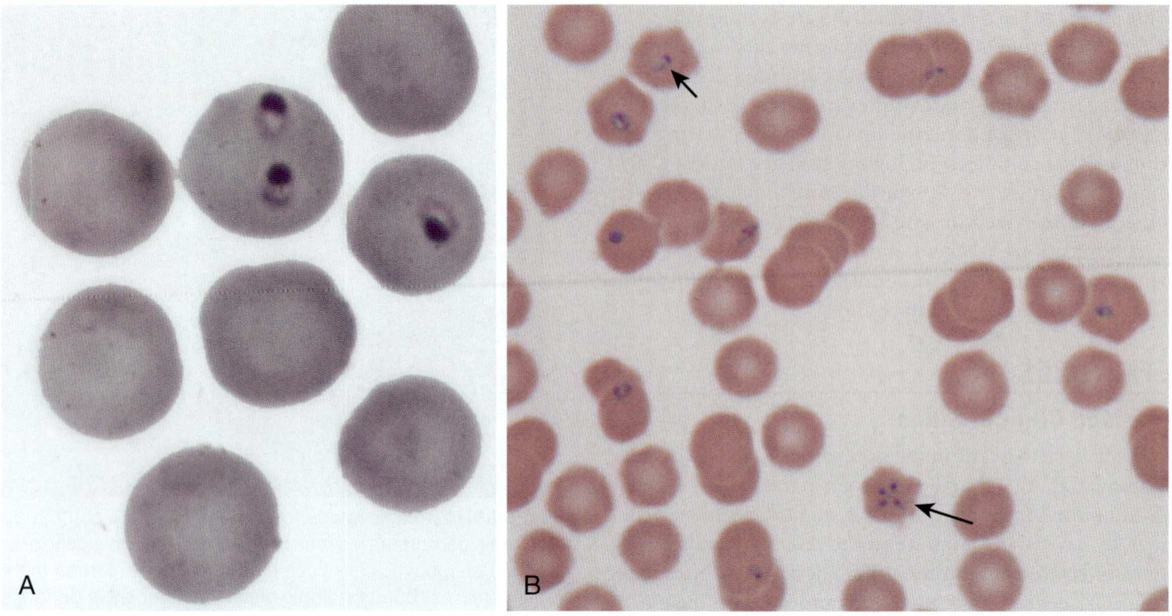

Fig. 98.5 Peripheral blood smears from cats with cytauxzoonosis that show erythrocytes infected with characteristic, signet ring-shaped *Cytauxzoon* piroplasms (Wright-Giemsa, ×1000). (A) The large, clearly evident nuclear area allows the organisms to be differentiated from hemotropic *Mycoplasma* organisms (Wright-Giemsa). (B) Multiple erythrocytes show signet ring-shaped piroplasms *(short arrow)*; a single erythrocyte contains a tetrad form *(long arrow)*. (Courtesy of Dr. Marlyn Whitney, University of Missouri—Veterinary Medical Diagnostic Laboratory.)

macrophages may lead to neutropenia, but neutrophilia resulting from an inflammatory response to infection may be identified alternatively. Leukopenia may be associated with a worsened prognosis.[75] Hemolytic anemia develops after the onset of signs and tends to be most severe as piroplasms become more numerous. Interestingly, severity of anemia has not been associated with a worse prognosis.[75] Because of the acute nature of the illness, anemia is usually normocytic, normochromic, and nonregenerative until disease recovery. Although anemia develops as piroplasms become apparent, these RBC parasites persist in low numbers for years in recovered cats without causing anemia.[42,49,66] Moderate to marked thrombocytopenia is believed to be related to consumptive processes, including the common complication of DIC. Coagulation times (e.g., activated partial prothrombin time, one-stage prothrombin time) are often prolonged as a component of DIC.[73,74,79]

Diagnosis of cytauxzoonosis can be accomplished by identification of erythroparasitemia or schizont-laden mononuclear cells on peripheral blood smears in cats with compatible history and physical examination findings. A thin, well-made blood smear can be stained with either Diff-Quik or Wright stain for identification of piroplasms. Blood smears should be scanned at low power (100×) on the outer edges as schizont-laden mononuclear cells can occasionally be seen at the feathered edge of peripheral blood smears (Fig. 98.6). Identification of even one such cell can confirm the diagnosis. Because these distended cells become lodged in the small blood vessels, they are more commonly identified on examination of tissue aspirates than peripheral blood smears. Aspirates from the spleen seem to be most useful for identification of these cells.[80] Next, the slide should be evaluated at high power (500–1000×) for piroplasms. The piroplasms of *C. felis* in erythrocytes are most often shaped as 1- to 1.5-μm signet rings, but "safety pin" and tetrad forms are also observed, or rarely chains of organisms resembling cocci (see Fig. 98.5B). Similar erythroparasites are identified in cats infected with *Babesia felis* and *C. manul*, but those pathogens have not been identified in the United States. *Mycoplasma haemofelis* might be mistaken for *C. felis* piroplasms (see Chapter 58). In addition to the

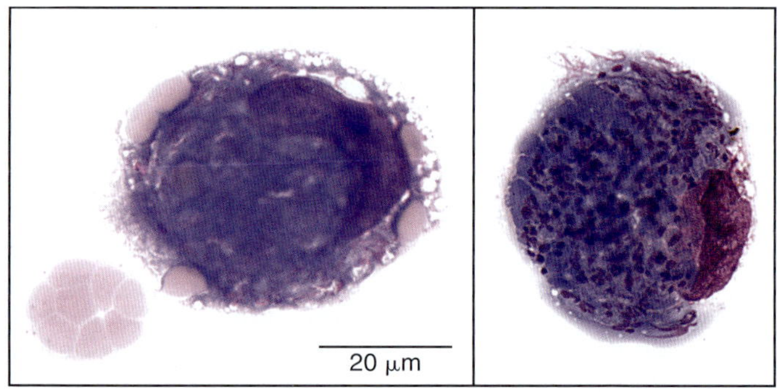

Fig. 98.6 Schizont-containing mononuclear cells on the feathered edge (cells shown from two different microscopic fields) of a Wright-Giemsa–stained peripheral blood smear from an acutely ill cat with cytauxzoonosis. (Courtesy of Dr. Marlyn Whitney, University of Missouri—Veterinary Medical Diagnostic Laboratory.)

smaller size of *M. haemofelis* (typically 0.3 to 0.8 μm), its epicellular location, frequent occurrence in pairs or short chains, and associated regenerative anemia help distinguish it from *C. felis.* Stain precipitate found overlying erythrocytes can easily be mistaken for piroplasms, but precipitate can usually be found unassociated with cells as well as overlying cells. Nuclear remnants known as Howell-Jolly bodies can likewise be mistaken for *C. felis* piroplasms.

Identification of *C. felis* piroplasms is not a sensitive method of disease diagnosis. The feathered edge of the stained blood smear must be carefully evaluated because erythroparasite burden is often low at the onset of infection. Even more importantly, piroplasms are not present in all infected cats, particularly early in the disease course. Piroplasms may be absent in up to 50% of cases at the time of initial illness, and in the author's experience there may be a several-day delay between initial clinical signs and the appearance of piroplasms on peripheral blood smear.[81]

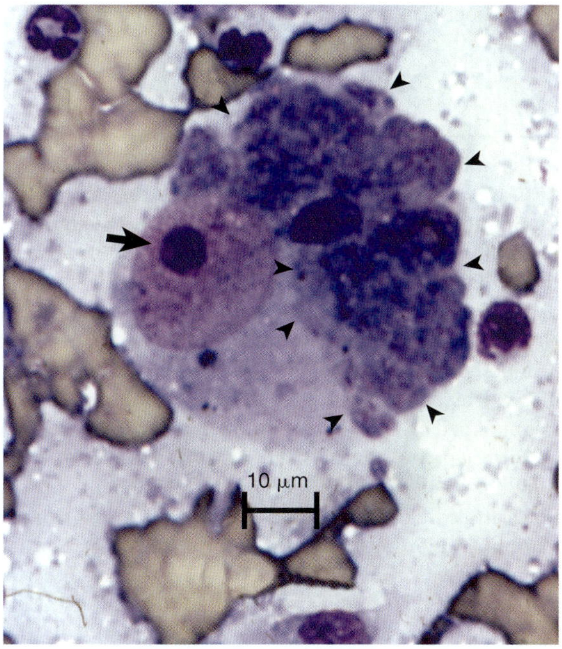

Fig. 98.7 Impression smear from a feline liver showing a macrophage that contains a developing *Cytauxzoon* schizont. The early schizont *(outlined by arrowheads)* appears as a lobulated basophilic area within the cytoplasm of the host cell. A large, prominent nucleolus is present in the host cell nucleus *(arrow)* (Wright-Giemsa, ×165).

Serum Chemistry Profile and Urinalysis

Aside from identification of protozoal pathogens on blood smear, there are no specific abnormalities on routine clinicopathologic testing. Hyperbilirubinemia is very common but rarely exceeds 5 mg/dL; more severe hyperbilirubinemia may be associated with a worsened prognosis.[75] Increased bilirubin occurs both as a result of intrahepatic infiltration of schizont-loaded macrophages as well as hemolysis.[75] Prerenal azotemia, hyperglycemia, and electrolyte and acid-base disturbances are documented in many infected cats. Other clinical chemistry changes are variable and less specific but include low serum concentrations of albumin, cholesterol, and potassium and high serum ALT activity.[42,75,77] Bilirubinuria is common, but hemoglobinuria is not observed because hemolysis is largely extravascular.[42]

Diagnostic Imaging

Imaging techniques do not contribute directly to the diagnosis of *C. felis* infection. Splenomegaly and hepatomegaly are commonly identified due to vascular occlusion by schizont-laden mononuclear cells. Pulmonary schizogeny can lead to interstitial pneumonia and edema; depending on severity, either an interstitial to alveolar lung pattern may be seen on thoracic radiographs.[5,82] Pleural effusion, and less often peritoneal effusion, are also identified in some cats.[42]

Microbiologic Tests

Cytologic Diagnosis

Fine-needle aspirates obtained antemortem or tissue imprints obtained at necropsy from parasitized tissues such as lymph node, spleen, or liver will often yield samples containing schizont-laden macrophages (Fig. 98.7).[80] Tissue biopsy is rarely employed for the diagnosis of cytauxzoonosis, but infection is easily confirmed at necropsy through microscopic identification of such schizont-laden cells.

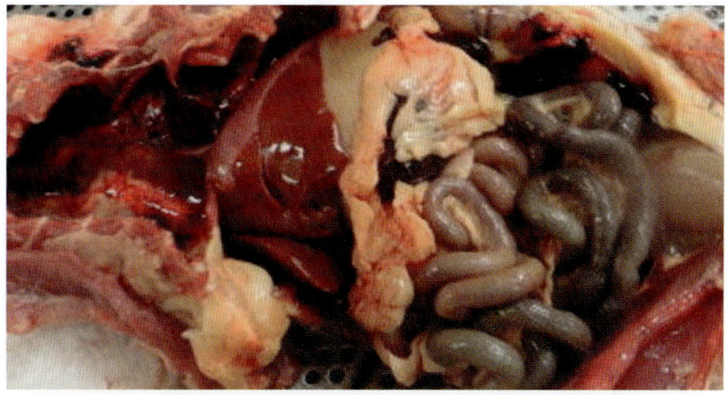

Fig. 98.8 Gross lesions in a cat naturally infected with *Cytauxzoon felis*. There is splenomegaly and an enlarged liver with rounded edges.

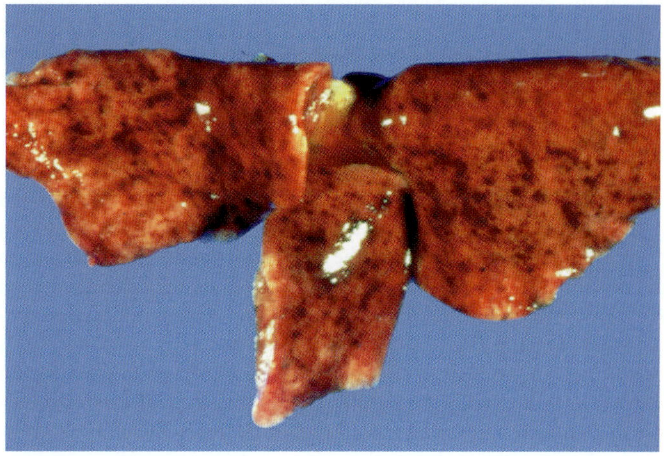

Fig. 98.9 Petechial and ecchymotic hemorrhages throughout the lungs of a cat that died from cytauxzoonosis. (Courtesy of Oklahoma State University Veterinary Pathobiology Teaching Set, Stillwater, OK.)

Molecular and Serologic Diagnosis

Diagnosis using PCR on blood is sensitive, with positive results possible many days prior to blood smear identification of pathogen.[83] Mitochondrial gene-based PCR testing was found to be even more sensitive than traditional 18S rRNA gene testing.[83] Even very early in disease, commercial PCR tests can be used to confirm the presence of *C. felis* DNA. Although test turnaround time is rapid, delays associated with sample submission are important considering the brief clinical course of illness. An important caveat to PCR testing is that PCR results may remain positive in recovered cats, meaning the test is specific for infection but not disease. Serologic testing for antibody to *C. felis* can be used in a research setting to document previous infection, but at the time of writing it is clinically impractical because infected cats may die before antibodies appear in circulation. To date, *C. felis* cannot be grown in culture.

Pathologic Findings

Experimental studies of *C. felis* infection have provided an extensive description of pathologic findings associated with acute illness.[72] Enlargement and mottling of the spleen and liver are common (Fig. 98.8), as is mild to moderate lymphadenomegaly. Interstitial pneumonia, pulmonary edema, and congestion with petechial hemorrhages on the lung surface are typical (Fig. 98.9). Petechial and ecchymotic hemorrhage may be detected in a variety of tissues. Venous distention can be appreciated grossly.

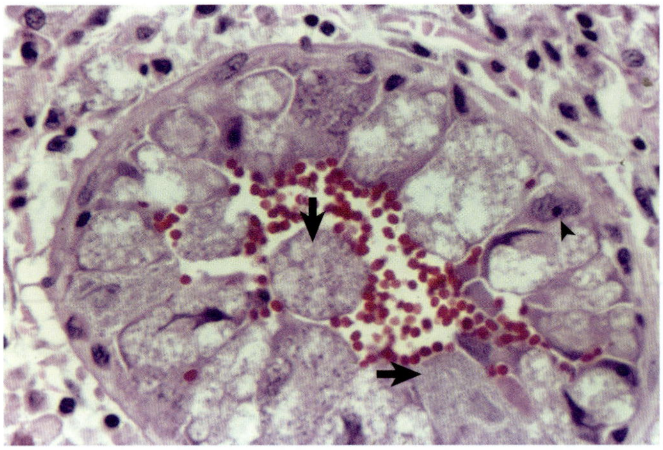

Fig. 98.10 Section of the lung from a cat with cytauxzoonosis. Schizont-containing macrophages completely line the endothelial surface and nearly occlude the lumen of a large vessel. The enlarged nucleoli of host cell nuclei are visible in some cells *(arrowhead).* Developing organisms can be seen as a faint granular appearance to the cytoplasm of some of the cells *(arrows)* (hematoxylin and eosin stain, ×66).

Histopathologic examination of tissues readily demonstrates the tissue stage of *C. felis* infection. Schizonts occur within the cytoplasm of mononuclear phagocytes in the tissues themselves, or attached to the endothelium or within the vasculature in essentially all organs (Fig. 98.10). Spleen, liver, lung, bone marrow, and lymph nodes are especially heavily parasitized. Partial or complete occlusion of blood vessels by infected mononuclear cells results in marked venous congestion of tissues. In a retrospective study of cats that died of cytauxzoonosis, all demonstrated vascular occlusion of the brain by schizont-laden macrophages with resultant edema, microgliosis, astrogliosis, microhemorrhage, and necrosis.[84] Similarly, a retrospective study of pulmonary lesions in cats that died with acute cytauxzoonosis found that vascular occlusion by parasitized macrophages was severe and consistent.[82] Other histopathologic findings in the lungs were more varied, but included interstitial pneumonia and hemorrhage. Spleen and lymph node should be used for tissue impression films, which should be stained with Wright or Giemsa stain. In situ hybridization or immunohistochemical methods can be used for specific identification of organisms within tissues.[85]

TREATMENT

Atovaquone and azithromycin combination therapy and supportive treatments are considered the standard of care for cats with cytauxzoonosis. Supportive care is indicated for ill cats although there are no studies demonstrating the utility of any specific supportive measure.[42] Crystalloid fluids are used to correct dehydration, preserve vascular volume, and maintain tissue perfusion but must be used with caution when pleural effusion or pulmonary edema are identified. Transfusion of whole blood or packed red blood cells is indicated for the treatment of anemia with associated tachypnea or tachycardia. Cytauxzoonosis is often accompanied by DIC,[73,79] so prophylactic heparinization administered to effect or by using a fixed heparin dose (Table 98.1) may prove useful in management of infected cats. Placement of nasogastric or esophageal feeding tubes can allow both nutritional support and ease in administration of oral medications (Fig. 98.11). Placement of feeding tubes early is important since most cats (even survivors) tend to develop more severe illness in the first 24 to 72 hours of hospitalization. Stressful events such as pilling or syringing medications can result in clinical decompensation and death. Although vomiting is not a common disease manifestation, maropitant may be used for cats with nausea. Because the pathogen can infect ocular vessels, identification and treatment of uveitis should be part of supportive care.[86] NSAIDs such as meloxicam have been used to provide analgesia and reduce fever. Some veterinarians treat ill cats with low-dose prednisolone. The potential benefit of NSAIDs or glucocorticoids has not been evaluated. While analgesia is important for humane reasons, in our experience, fever reduction does not correspond to improved survival. A variety of antimicrobial drugs (e.g., ampicillin, enrofloxacin, and doxycycline) have been used in infected cats alone or in combination.[77,79,87] Used alone, none of these drugs has demonstrated efficacy against protozoal agents such as *C. felis*. A combination of antimicrobials including doxycycline, metronidazole, and enrofloxacin[88] has been effective in treating dogs with *Babesia gibsoni* infection. In a small study of cats with experimentally induced cytauxzoonosis, a combination of doxycycline-metronidazole-pradofloxacin was not beneficial.[89]

TABLE 98.1 Treatment for Cytauxzoonosis

Drug[a]	Dose[b]	Route	Interval	Duration (Days)
Heparin (unfractionated)	100–200 U/kg	SC	8 hours	As needed[c]
Atropine	0.04 mg/kg	IV, IM, SC	24 hours	1[d]
Glycopyrrolate	0.005–0.01 mg/kg	IV, IM, SC	24 hours	1[d]
Imidocarb dipropionate	3.5–5.0 mg/kg	IM	14 days	14
Diminazene aceturate[e]	2 mg/kg	IM	7 days	7
Atovaquone[f]	15 mg/kg	PO	8 hours	10
and				
Azithromycin	10 mg/kg	PO	24 hours	10

[a]See Chapter 12 for specific information on each drug. Adjunctive isotonic fluid therapy is extremely important for this disease. See text.
[b]Dose per administration at specified interval.
[c]This dosage range is used until a cat's clinical signs have stabilized and hematologic abnormalities have improved. In lieu of this fixed dose, the therapeutic goal is prolongation of the baseline activated partial thromboplastin time by twofold. A variable dose would be administered at the 8-hour interval to achieve this effect.
[d]Given once, 15 minutes before injection of imidocarb or diminazene.
[e]Note that a higher dose than listed here (4 mg/kg q24h for 5 days) was not recommended due to lack of efficacy and adverse events in a 2014 study.[90]
[f]Thick, viscous liquid can be difficult to accurately dose; allow liquid to settle in syringe to confirm volume prior to administration.
IM, intramuscular; *IV*, intravenous; *PO*, oral; *SC*, subcutaneous.

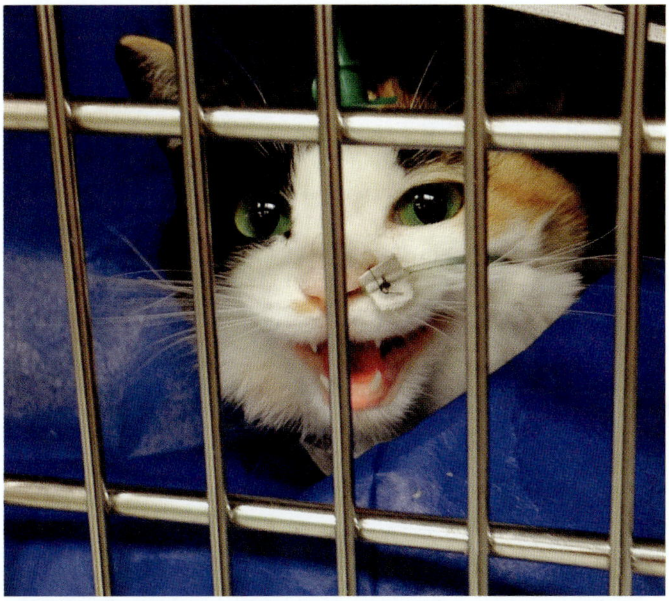

Fig. 98.11 Nasoesophageal feeding tube in a cat with cytauxzoonosis. (Courtesy of Dr. Adam Birkenheuer.)

Treatment with a combination of atovaquone (15 mg/kg, PO, q8h) and azithromycin (10 mg/kg, PO, q24h) for 10 days was associated with a 60% survival rate in a randomized, prospective clinical trial; this was significantly different from the 26% survival rate with imidocarb dipropionate (Imizol, Merck Animal Health, Madison, NJ, USA).[75] Before publication of that study, imidocarb dipropionate was widely used for the treatment of cytauxzoonosis at a variety of different dose regimens (e.g., two doses at 2 mg/kg, IM, 7 days apart, two doses at 5 mg/kg, IM, 7 days apart, two doses of 5 mg/kg, 4 days apart) with little evidence of efficacy. There was also mention in a retrospective report on cats with *C. felis* infection that imidocarb lacked efficacy for treatment of experimentally induced cytauxzoonosis.[49] If used, pretreatment with atropine or glycopyrrolate may minimize the potential adverse cholinergic effects of imidocarb. Another aromatic diamidine, diminazene aceturate, has been used to treat cytauxzoonosis. In a retrospective study, five of six cats treated with diminazene plus aggressive supportive care survived.[79] Unfortunately, diminazene is not approved for use or available in the United States. Diminazene and imidocarb are also not effective in clearing piroplasms from healthy cats with chronic *C. felis* infection.[67,68,75,90] The antiprotozoal hydroxynaphthoquinolone agents, parvaquone and buparvaquone, are the treatment of choice for *Theileria* infection of African cattle. Despite the close relationship of *C. felis* to *Theileria* spp., these drugs were ineffective for treatment of cytauxzoonosis.[78] Although treatment with atovaquone and azithromycin is currently the standard of care, improved treatments are needed as this treatment is expensive, difficult to administer, and many cats die despite treatment. At the time of writing, the authors are conducting a prospective trial on the use of the antimalarial compounds artemether and lumefantrine (Coartem, Novartis, East Hanover, NJ, USA), for the treatment of cytauxzoonosis based on preliminary success in experimentally infected cats.

It is unclear whether treatment should be administered to healthy cats with persistent erythroparasitemia. In the few cats followed for months or years, clinical disease has not developed after recovery from initial infection. However, the possibility exists that these cats may experience hemolysis or some other immune-mediated sequelae from chronic infection at a future date. Of additional importance, it is possible that these carrier cats may serve to infect naïve ticks, which could then be a source of infection for other felids.[41,63,70] The combination of atovaquone and azithromycin was unable to uniformly cure infection, but many treated cats had negative PCR results after treatment.[67,75] Recommended dosages for these drugs are listed in Table 98.1.

PROGNOSIS

Although cytauxzoonosis was once described as a uniformly fatal infection, there are now many reports of surviving cats. In many cases, cats survived clinical cytauxzoonosis with aggressive supportive care that might or might not have included specific antiprotozoal therapy.[75,78,79,87] However, healthy carriers have also been identified with no known history of clinical illness, suggesting a limited schizogenous replication as is typical for the bobcat reservoir host.[27,44,49,51,52,66,90] Survivors might be explained by differences in the dose of inoculum or route of exposure, differences in the individual cat's immune response to pathogen, or pathogen strain variation. As mentioned previously, survival with or without antecedent clinical illness is often linked to certain geographic regions suggesting strain variation.[49]

Genetic differences in the pathogen have been identified that may account for response to treatment with atovaquone.[53,91] Atovaquone is presumed to work by disrupting electron transport in the parasite mitochondria via targeting protozoal cytochrome b (cytb). A recent pharmacogenomics study identified a *C. felis* cytb genotype associated with increased survival in cats treated with atovaquone and azithromycin but not in cats treated with imidiocarb.[91] Further, a quantitative real-time PCR assay that is coupled with high-resolution melt analysis of amplified DNA has been developed that detects the *C. felis* cytb genotype associated with improved survival.[92] Such testing could provide valuable prognostic information to help owners make difficult decisions regarding treatment of sick cats. A mutation in cytb has been detected in a cat that remained persistently parasitemic despite repeated treatments with atovaquone and azithromycin.[93]

IMMUNITY AND VACCINATION

Little is known about immunity to cytauxzoonosis. In addition to possible strain differences or varied dose inoculum, individual immune responses may also impact outcome. This is especially true in experimental settings where all cats are similarly exposed to the same *C. felis* strain, yet some develop only minimal illness. Cats that are experimentally inoculated with blood that contains piroplasms form antibodies, but these antibodies do not protect from illness after inoculation of schizonts.[34,36,78] On the other hand, experimental attempts to reinfect a small number of cats that have survived illness (and therefore survived the schizont stage of infection) do not result in recurrent illness, suggesting immunologic protection from disease.[77,79] Despite the failure to induce a second illness through experimental infection, a second illness due to reinfection 7 years after the first illness has been documented in at least one domestic cat.[94] Reinfection of bobcats in the wild with multiple strains of *C. felis*, as based on ITS1 and ITS2 genotypes, has been documented.[65]

There is no available vaccine for cytauxzoonosis. Although the growth of *C. felis* has not been sustained in culture, a report from 1978 describes a cat that was protected from infection after subcutaneous inoculation with a Vero culture that had been inoculated with splenic cells from a cat dying of cytauxzoonosis. It is unclear whether the Vero cells were truly infected or if they were co-cultured, resulting in an attenuated live or even killed vaccine.[95] Recently, genomic bioinformatic methods have been used to identify potential antigen vaccine candidates; however, initial attempts at vaccination did not result in protection from experimental infection.[96,97]

Few studies have been published that describe the immune response to *C. felis*. Clearly, infection of mononuclear cells will directly impact the immune response. A small study of naturally infected cats identified increased expression of CD18, a key integrin for leukocyte adhesion to endothelium.[98] This same study found significantly increased serum TNF-α in cats that died of cytauxzoonosis when compared with healthy cats, but no statistically significant difference between survivors and non-survivors.[98] Lung tissues from cats that died of the disease stained positively for TNF-α, and many demonstrated increased staining (compared to uninfected cats) for IL-1β and IL-6.[99] Not surprisingly, these findings support the idea that cytauxzoonosis is an inflammatory disease, as is the case for other piroplasmoses.[100]

PREVENTION

For now, prevention is focused on prevention of tick bites. Indoor confinement of cats in endemic areas reduces the risk of tick bites. In a recent experimental controlled trial, ticks failed to attach and feed on cats wearing an imidacloprid 10%/flumethrin 4.5% impregnated collar and were protected from experimental tick-transmitted infection.[70] While this collar helps kill ticks on contact, other paraciticides approved for use in cats (i.e., fipronil, fluralaner) require tick feeding. The time required between tick attachment and transmission of *C. felis* can be less than 48 hours.[59] Rapid killing after tick feeding might be effective in prevention of pathogen transmission, as has been documented for topical selamectin plus sarolaner.[101] However, a number of cats reportedly treated with fipronil on a regular basis were nonetheless diagnosed with cytauxzoonosis.[75] Prophylactic chemotherapy is used to prevent malaria in humans in endemic regions. The role that prophylaxis may have in prevention of feline cytauxzoonosis remains to be determined. See Chapters 13 and 109 for more extensive information on tick control.

PUBLIC HEALTH ASPECTS

Infection with *C. felis* has only been recognized in felidae. Therefore, there are no recognized public health consequences of infection.

CASE EXAMPLE

Signalment and History

"Ginger," a 2-year-old female spayed domestic longhaired cat that lived near Springfield, Missouri, was evaluated for a 1-day history of anorexia and lethargy in April of the year. The cat was an indoor/outdoor cat with no known history of tick exposure. There were no other cats in the household.

Physical Examination

On examination, the cat's rectal temperature was 105.6°F (40.9°C), with HR of 200 beats/minute and RR of 28 breaths/minute. The spleen was prominent on abdominal palpation and the nictitans was elevated (Fig. 98.12), but examination was otherwise unremarkable.

Laboratory Findings

Blood was obtained for a CBC and retrovirus testing. The cat tested negative for FeLV antigen and FIV antibody. The cat had a mild, nonregenerative anemia (PCV 27%) and leukopenia (4,200 cells/μL, reference range 5,500–19,500 cells/μL).

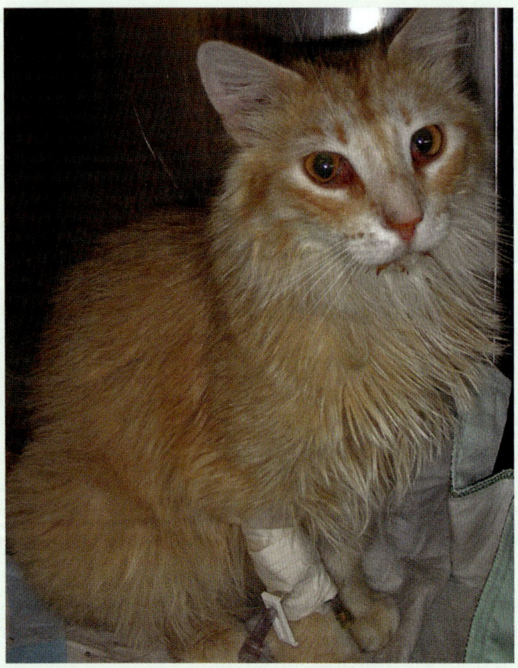

Fig. 98.12 Cat with cytauxzoonosis. There is elevation and hyperemia of the nictitating membranes.

Although the platelet count was low, platelet clumps were present. Plasma in the spun hematocrit tube was icteric. No parasites were observed on microscopic slide review.

Because of a high degree of suspicion for cytauxzoonosis, a fine-needle aspirate was obtained from the spleen. Multiple markedly enlarged mononuclear cells containing numerous merozoites were observed.

Diagnosis

Cytauxzoonosis.

Treatment and Outcome

A nasoesophageal tube was placed to facilitate administration of atovaquone suspension (15 mg/kg, PO, q8h) and azithromycin (10 mg/kg, PO, q24h). A cephalic vein catheter was placed and IV crystalloid fluids administered at a maintenance rate. Heparin (200 units/kg, SC, q8h) and buprenorphine (0.01 mg/kg, SC, q8h) were administered.

The following day, the cat's PCV was 20% and icterus was evident on physical examination. Additionally, many piroplasms were visible on cytologic analysis of a smear of peripheral blood. A serum chemistry profile confirmed hyperbilirubinemia and a mild increase in the activity of serum ALT but was otherwise unremarkable.

By day 3, the PCV was 12%, and both RR and HR were increased. The cat was administered a single unit of whole blood, after which the PCV increased to 19%. Nutritional support was administered via the nasoesophageal tube, but otherwise treatment remained unchanged.

On day 5, the PCV dropped to 11%, which necessitated another whole blood transfusion. The cat remained tachypneic after transfusion. Thoracic radiographs revealed pleural effusion and a marked diffuse interstitial lung pattern. The cat was treated with supplemental oxygen, and 25 mL of a clear, yellow, modified transudate was removed using thoracocentesis.

By day 7, the cat no longer required supplemental oxygen to maintain respiratory function, and the anemia was regenerative. The cat was discharged from the hospital on day 8 with continued administration of atovaquone and azithromycin at home, but all other treatments were discontinued.

On recheck examination 1 week later, the cat was seemingly normal to the owners, and no abnormalities were detected on physical examination. The PCV was 29%, platelet and WBC counts had normalized, and a single piroplasm was observed on careful review of the entire feathered edge of the blood smear. The cat's owners were advised to keep the cat entirely indoors and to use an ectoparasiticide regularly to minimize any risk that the cat could serve as a reservoir for infection of ticks. The cat remained healthy 1 year later.

SUGGESTED READINGS

Cohn LA, Birkenheuer AJ, Brunker JD, et al. Efficacy of atovaquone and azithromycin or imidocarb dipropionate in cats with acute cytauxzoonosis. *J Vet Intern Med.* 2011;25(55).

Reichard MV, Thomas JE, Arther RG, et al. Efficacy of an imidacloprid 10%/ flumethrin 4.5% collar (Seresto®, Bayer) for preventing the transmission of *Cytauxzoon felis* to domestic cats by *Amblyomma americanum. Parasitol Res.* 2013;112(suppl 1:11).

Sherrill MK, Cohn LA. Cytauxzoonosis: diagnosis and treatment of an emerging disease. *J Feline Med Surg.* 2015;17:940.

REFERENCES

1. Wagner JE. A fatal cytauxzoonosis-like disease in cats. *J Am Vet Med Assoc.* 1976;168:585–588.
2. Criado-Fornelio A, Gonzalez-del-Rio MA, Buling-Sarana A, et al. The "expanding universe" of piroplasms. *Vet Parasitol.* 2004;119:337–345.
3. Mendes-de-Almeida F, Faria MC, Branco AS, et al. Sanitary conditions of a colony of urban feral cats (*Felis catus* Linnaeus, 1758) in a zoological garden of Rio de Janeiro, Brazil. *Rev Inst Med Trop Sao Paulo.* 2004;46:269–274.
4. Andre MR, Baccarim Denardi NC, Marques de Sousa KC, et al. Arthropod-borne pathogens circulating in free-roaming domestic cats in a zoo environment in Brazil. *Ticks Tick Borne Dis.* 2014;5:545–551.
5. Meier HT, Moore LE. Feline cytauxzoonosis: a case report and literature review. *J Am Anim Hosp Assoc.* 2000;36:493–496.
6. Carli E, Trotta M, Chinelli R, et al. *Cytauxzoon* sp. infection in the first endemic focus described in domestic cats in Europe. *Vet Parasitol.* 2012;183:343–352.
7. Gallusova M, Jirsova D, Mihalca AD, et al. *Cytauxzoon* infections in wild felids from Carpathian-Danubian-Pontic space: further evidence for a different *Cytauxzoon* species in European felids. *J Parasitol.* 2016;102:377–380.
8. Veronesi F, Ravagnan S, Cerquetella M, et al. First detection of *Cytauxzoon* spp. infection in European wildcats (*Felis silvestris silvestris*) of Italy. *Ticks Tick Borne Dis.* 2016;7:853–858.
9. Reichard MV, Van Den Bussche RA, Meinkoth JH, et al. A new species of *Cytauxzoon* from Pallas' cats caught in Mongolia and comments on the systematics and taxonomy of piroplasmids. *J Parasitol.* 2005;91:420–426.
10. Naidenko SV, Erofeeva MN, Sorokin PA, et al. The first case of *Cytauxzoon* spp. in Russia: the parasite conquers Eurasia. *Animals (Basel).* 2022; 12:593.
11. Willi B, Meli ML, Cafarelli C, et al. *Cytauxzoon europaeus* infections in domestic cats in Switzerland and in European wildcats in France: a tale that started more than two decades ago, *Parasit Vectors.* 2022;15:19.
12. Ketz-Riley CJ, Reichard MV, Van den Bussche RA, et al. An intraerythrocytic small piroplasm in wild-caught Pallas's cats (*Otocolobus manul*) from Mongolia. *J Wildl Dis.* 2003;39:424–430.
13. Joyner PH, Reichard MV, Meinkoth JH, et al. Experimental infection of domestic cats (*Felis domesticus*) with *Cytauxzoon manul* from Pallas' cats (*Otocolobus manul*). *Vet Parasitol.* 2007;146:302–306.
14. Zou FC, Li Z, Yang JF, et al. *Cytauxzoon felis* infection in domestic cats, Yunnan Province, China, 2016. *Emerg Infect Dis.* 2019;25:353–354.
15. Alho AM, Silva J, Fonseca MJ, et al. First report of *Cytauxzoon* sp. infection in a domestic cat from Portugal. *Parasit Vectors.* 2016;9:220.
16. Millan J, Candela MG, Palomares F, et al. Disease threats to the endangered Iberian lynx (*Lynx pardinus*). *Vet J.* 2009;182:114–124.
17. Millan J, Naranjo V, Rodriguez A, et al. Prevalence of infection and 18S rRNA gene sequences of *Cytauxzoon* species in Iberian lynx (*Lynx pardinus*) in Spain. *Parasitology.* 2007;134:995–1001.
18. Zaeemi M, Razmi GR, Khoshnegah J. The first detection of *Cytauxzoon felis* in a wild cat (*Felis silvestris*) in Iran. *Comp Clin Pathol.* 2015;24:181–184.
19. Panait LC, Stock G, Globokar M, et al. First report of *Cytauxzoon* sp. infection in Germany: organism description and molecular confirmation in a domestic cat. *Parasitol Res.* 2020; July;17:1–7.
20. Moghaddam MR, Zaeemi M, Razmi GR. Preliminary study of *Cytauxzoon felis* infection in outdoor cats in Mashhad, Iran. *Parasitol Res.* 2020;119:4177–4183.
21. Panait LC, Milhallca AD, Modry D, et al. Three new species of *Cytauxzoon* in European wild felids, *Vet Parasitol.* 2021;290:109344.
22. Andre MR, Herrera HM, Fernandes S de J, et al. Tick-borne agents in domesticated and stray cats from the city of Campo Grande, state of Mato Grosso do Sul, midwestern Brazil. *Ticks Tick Borne Dis.* 2015;6:779–786.
23. Maia LM, Cerqueira Ade M, de Barros Macieira D, et al. *Cytauxzoon felis* and *'Candidatus Mycoplasma haemominutum'* coinfection in a Brazilian domestic cat (*Felis catus*). *Rev Bras Parasitol Vet.* 2013;22:289–291.
24. Mendes-de-Almeida F, Labarthe N, Guerrero J, et al. Follow-up of the health conditions of an urban colony of free-roaming cats (*Felis catus* Linnaeus, 1758) in the city of Rio de Janeiro, Brazil. *Vet Parasitol.* 2007;147:9–15.
25. Soares CO. Cytauxzoonose felina é diagnosticada e isolada pela primeira vez na América Latina. *Revista Clín Vet.* 2001;32:56–58.
26. Andre MR, Adania CH, Machado RZ, et al. Molecular detection of *Cytauxzoon* spp. in asymptomatic Brazilian wild captive felids. *J Wildl Dis.* 2009;45:234–237.
27. Brown HM, Berghaus RD, Latimer KS, et al. Genetic variability of *Cytauxzoon felis* from 88 infected domestic cats in Arkansas and Georgia. *J Vet Diagn Invest.* 2009;21:59–63.
28. Butt MT, Bowman D, Barr MC, et al. Iatrogenic transmission of *Cytauxzoon felis* from a Florida panther (*Felix concolor coryi*) to a domestic cat. *J Wildl Dis.* 1991;27:342–347.
29. Harvey JW, Dunbar MR, Norton TM, et al. Laboratory findings in acute *Cytauxzoon felis* infection in cougars (*Puma concolor couguar*) in Florida. *J Zoo Wildl Med.* 2007;38:285–291.
30. Jakob W, Wesemeier HH. A fatal infection in a Bengal tiger resembling cytauxzoonosis in domestic cats. *J Comp Pathol.* 1996;114:439–444.
31. Cerreta AJ, Yang TS, Ramsay EC, et al. Detection of vector-borne infections in lions and tigers at two zoos in Tennessee and Oklahoma, USA. *J Zoo Wildl Med.* 2022;53:50–59.
32. Blouin EF, Kocan AA, Kocan KM, et al. Evidence of a limited schizogonous cycle for *Cytauxzoon felis* in bobcats following exposure to infected ticks. *J Wildl Dis.* 1987;23:499–501.
33. Lewis KM, Cohn LA, Downey ME, et al. Evaluation of *Cytauxzoon felis* infection status in captive-born wild felids housed in an area endemic for the pathogen. *J Am Vet Med Assoc.* 2012;241:1088–1092.
34. Glenn BL, Kocan AA, Blouin EF. Cytauxzoonosis in bobcats. *J Am Vet Med Assoc.* 1983;183:1155–1158.
35. Nietfeld JC, Pollock C. Fatal cytauxzoonosis in a free-ranging bobcat (*Lynx rufus*). *J Wildl Dis.* 2002;38:607–610.
36. Cowell RL, Fox JC, Panciera RJ, et al. Detection of anticytauxzoon antibodies in cats infected with a *Cytauxzoon* organism from bobcats. *Vet Parasitol.* 1988;28:43–52.
37. Mueller EK, Baum KA, Papes M, et al. Potential ecological distribution of *Cytauxzoon felis* in domestic cats in Oklahoma, Missouri, and Arkansas. *Vet Parasitol.* 2013;192:104–110.
38. Kier AB, Wightman SR, Wagner JE. Interspecies transmission of *Cytauxzoon felis. Am J Vet Res.* 1982;43:102–105.
39. Reichard MV, Baum KA, Cadenhead SC, et al. Temporal occurrence and environmental risk factors associated with cytauxzoonosis in domestic cats. *Vet Parasitol.* 2008;152:314–320.
40. Birkenheuer AJ, Cohn LA, Levy MG, et al. Atovaquone and azithromycin for the treatment of *Cytauxzoon felis* (abstr.). *J Vet Intern Med.* 2008;22:703.
41. Reichard MV, Meinkoth JH, Edwards AC, et al. Transmission of *Cytauxzoon felis* to a domestic cat by *Amblyomma americanum. Vet Parasitol.* 2009;161.110–115.
42. Sherrill MK, Cohn LA. Cytauxzoonosis: diagnosis and treatment of an emerging disease. *J Feline Med Surg.* 2015;17:940–948.
43. Birkenheuer AJ, Le JA, Valenzisi AM, et al. *Cytauxzoon felis* infection in cats in the mid-Atlantic states: 34 cases (1998-2004). *J Am Vet Med Assoc.* 2006;228:568–571.
44. Rizzi TE, Reichard MV, Cohn LA, et al. Prevalence of *Cytauxzoon felis* infection in healthy cats from enzootic areas in Arkansas, Missouri, and Oklahoma. *Parasit Vectors.* 2015;8:13.

45. Shock BC, Murphy SM, Patton LL, et al. Distribution and prevalence of *Cytauxzoon felis* in bobcats (*Lynx rufus*), the natural reservoir, and other wild felids in thirteen states. *Vet Parasitol.* 2011;175:325–330.
46. Jackson CB, Fisher T. Fatal cytauxzoonosis in a Kentucky cat (*Felis domesticus*). *Vet Parasitol.* 2006;139:192–195.
47. MacNeill AL, Barger AM, Skowronski MC, et al. Identification of *Cytauxzoon felis* infection in domestic cats from southern Illinois. *J Feline Med Surg.* 2015;17:1069–1072.
48. Birkenheuer AJ, Marr HS, Warren C, et al. *Cytauxzoon felis* infections are present in bobcats (*Lynx rufus*) in a region where cytauxzoonosis is not recognized in domestic cats. *Vet Parasitol.* 2008;153:126–130.
49. Meinkoth J, Kocan AA, Whitworth L, et al. Cats surviving natural infection with *Cytauxzoon felis*: 18 cases (1997-1998). *J Vet Intern Med.* 2000;14:521–525.
50. Cohn LA, Nafe L. Personal communication. 2020.
51. Nagamori Y, Slovak JE, Reichard MV. Prevalence of *Cytauxzoon felis* infection in healthy free-roaming cats in north-central Oklahoma and central Iowa. *J Fel Med Surg Open Rep.* 2016;2:2055116916655174.
52. Haber MD, Tucker MD, Marr HS, et al. The detection of *Cytauxzoon felis* in apparently healthy free-roaming cats in the USA. *Vet Parasitol.* 2007;146:316–320.
53. Brown HM, Lockhart JM, Latimer KS, et al. Identification and genetic characterization of *Cytauxzoon felis* in asymptomatic domestic cats and bobcats. *Vet Parasitol.* 2010;172:311–316.
54. Glenn BL, Stair EL. Cytauxzoonosis in domestic cats: report of two cases in Oklahoma, with a review and discussion of the disease. *J Am Vet Med Assoc.* 1984;184:822–825.
55. Kocan AA, Blouin EF, Glenn BL. Hematologic and serum chemical values for free-ranging bobcats, *Felis rufus* (Schreber), with reference to animals with natural infections of *Cytauxzoon felis* Kier, 1979. *J Wildl Dis.* 1985;21:190–192.
56. Rotstein DS, Taylor SK, Harvey JW, et al. Hematologic effects of cytauxzoonosis in Florida panthers and Texas cougars in Florida. *J Wildl Dis.* 1999;35:613–617.
57. Wagner JE, Ferris DH, Kier AB, et al. Experimentally induced cytauxzoonosis-like disease in domestic cats. *Vet Parasitol.* 1980;6:305–311.
58. Lewis KM, Cohn LA, Birkenheuer AJ. Lack of evidence for perinatal transmission of *Cytauxzoon felis* in domestic cats. *Vet Parasitol.* 2012;188:172–174.
59. Thomas JE, Ohmes CM, Payton ME, et al. Minimum transmission time of *Cytauxzoon felis* by *Amblyomma americanum* to domestic cats in relation to duration of infestation, and investigation of ingestion of infected ticks as a potential route of transmission. *J Feline Med Surg.* 2018;20:67–72.
60. Kier AB, Wagner JE, Morehouse LG. Experimental transmission of *Cytauxzoon felis* from bobcats (*Lynx rufus*) to domestic cats (*Felis domesticus*). *Am J Vet Res.* 1982;43:97–101.
61. Blouin EF, Kocan AA, Glenn BL, et al. Transmission of *Cytauxzoon felis* Kier, 1979 from bobcats, *Felis rufus* (Schreber), to domestic cats by *Dermacentor variabilis* (Say). *J Wildl Dis.* 1984;20:241–242.
62. Bondy PJ Jr, Cohn LA, Tyler JW, et al. Polymerase chain reaction detection of *Cytauxzoon felis* from field-collected ticks and sequence analysis of the small subunit and internal transcribed spacer 1 region of the ribosomal RNA gene. *J Parasitol.* 2005;91:458–461.
63. Reichard MV, Edwards AC, Meinkoth JH, et al. Confirmation of *Amblyomma americanum* (Acari: Ixodidae) as a vector for *Cytauxzoon felis* (Piroplasmorida: Theileriidae) to domestic cats. *J Med Entomol.* 2010;47:890–896.
64. Peixoto PV, Soares CO, Scofield A, et al. Fatal cytauxzoonosis in captive-reared lions in Brazil. *Vet Parasitol.* 2007;145:383–387.
65. Zieman EA, Nielsen CK, Jimenez FA. Chronic *Cytauxzoon felis* infections in wild-caught bobcats (*Lynx rufus*). *Vet Parasitol.* 2018;252:67–69.
66. Brown HM, Latimer KS, Erikson LE, et al. Detection of persistent *Cytauxzoon felis* infection by polymerase chain reaction in three asymptomatic domestic cats. *J Vet Diagn Invest.* 2008;20:485–488.
67. Cohn LA, Birkenheuer AJ, Ratcliff E. Comparison of two drug protocols for clearance of *Cytauxzoon felis* infections (abstr). *J Vet Intern Med.* 2008;22:704.
68. Lewis KM, Cohn LA, Marr HS, et al. Diminazene diaceturate for treatment of chronic *Cytauxzoon felis* parasitemia in naturally infected cats. *J Vet Intern Med.* 2012;26:1490–1493.
69. Kocan AA, Kocan KM, Blouin EF, et al. A redescription of schizogony of *Cytauxzoon felis* in the domestic cat. *Ann N Y Acad Sci.* 1992;653:161–167.
70. Reichard MV, Thomas JE, Arther RG, et al. Efficacy of an imidacloprid 10 % / flumethrin 4.5 % collar (Seresto®, Bayer) for preventing the transmission of *Cytauxzoon felis* to domestic cats by *Amblyomma americanum. Parasitol Res.* 2013;112(suppl 1):11–20.
71. Simpson CF, Harvey JW, Lawman MJ, et al. Ultrastructure of schizonts in the liver of cats with experimentally induced cytauxzoonosis. *Am J Vet Res.* 1985;46:384–390.
72. Kier AB, Wagner JE, Kinden DA. The pathology of experimental cytauxzoonosis. *J Comp Pathol.* 1987;97:415–432.
73. Conner BJ, Hanel RM, Brooks MB, et al. Coagulation abnormalities in 5 cats with naturally occurring cytauxzoonosis. *J Vet Emerg Crit Care.* 2015;25:538–545.
74. Garner MM, Lung NP, Citino S, et al. Fatal cytauxzoonosis in a captive-reared white tiger (*Panthera tigris*). *Vet Pathol.* 1996;33:82–86.
75. Cohn LA, Birkenheuer AJ, Brunker JD, et al. Efficacy of atovaquone and azithromycin or imidocarb dipropionate in cats with acute cytauxzoonosis. *J Vet Intern Med.* 2011;25:55–60.
76. Jeong HW, Borgarelli M. Trifascicular block in a cat infected with *Cytauxzoon felis. J Vet Cardiol.* 2021;35:121–123.
77. Hoover JP, Walker DB, Hedges JD. Cytauxzoonosis in cats: eight cases (1985-1992). *J Am Vet Med Assoc.* 1994;205:455–460.
78. Motzel SL, Wagner JE. Treatment of experimentally induced cytauxzoonosis in cats with parvaquone and buparvaquone. *Vet Parasitol.* 1990;35:131–138.
79. Greene CE, Latimer K, Hopper E, et al. Administration of diminazene aceturate or imidocarb dipropionate for treatment of cytauxzoonosis in cats. *J Am Vet Med Assoc.* 1999;215:497–500. 482.
80. Sleznikow CR, Granick J, Cohn LA, et al. Evaluation of various sample sources for the cytologic diagnosis of *Cytauxzoon felis. J Vet Intern Med.* 2022;36:126–132.
81. Ferris DH. A progress report on the status of a new disease of American cats: cytauxzoonosis. *Comp Immunol Microbiol Infect Dis.* 1979;1: 269–276.
82. Snider TA, Confer AW, Payton ME. Pulmonary histopathology of *Cytauxzoon felis* infections in the cat. *Vet Pathol.* 2010;47:698–702.
83. Schreeg ME, Marr HS, Griffith EH, et al. PCR amplification of a multi-copy mitochondrial gene (cox3) improves detection of *Cytauxzoon felis* infection as compared to a ribosomal gene (18S). *Vet Parasitol.* 2016;225:123–130.
84. Clarke LL, Rissi DR. Neuropathology of natural *Cytauxzoon felis* infection in domestic cats. *Vet Pathol.* 2015;52:1167–1171.
85. Susta L, Torres-Velez F, Zhang J, et al. An in situ hybridization and immunohistochemical study of cytauxzoonosis in domestic cats. *Vet Pathol.* 2009;46:1197–1204.
86. Meekins J, Cino-Ozuna AG. Histologic identification of intraocular *Cytauxzoon felis* in three cats. *J Fel Med Surg Open Rep.* 2018;4:2055116918813242.
87. Walker DB, Cowell RL. Survival of a domestic cat with naturally acquired cytauxzoonosis. *J Am Vet Med Assoc.* 1995;206:1363–1365.
88. Lin MY, Huang HP. Use of a doxycycline-enrofloxacin-metronidazole combination with/without diminazene diaceturate to treat naturally occurring canine babesiosis caused by *Babesia gibsoni. Acta Vet Scand.* 2010;52:27.
89. Cohn LA, Birkenheuer AJ. Personal communication. 2020.
90. Lewis KM, Cohn LA, Marr HS, et al. Failure of efficacy and adverse events associated with dose-intense diminazene diaceturate treatment of chronic *Cytauxzoon felis* infection in five cats. *J Feline Med Surg.* 2014;16:157–163.
91. Schreeg ME, Marr HS, Tarigo J, et al. Pharmacogenomics of *Cytauxzoon felis* cytochrome b: implications for atovaquone and azithromycin therapy in domestic cats with cytauxzoonosis. *J Clin Microbiol.* 2013;51:3066–3069.

92. Schreeg ME, Marr HS, Tarigo JL, et al. Rapid high-resolution melt analysis of *Cytauxzoon felis* cytochrome b to aid in the prognosis of cytauxzoonosis. *J Clin Microbiol.* 2015;53:2517–2524.
93. Hartley AN, Marr HS, Birkenheuer AJ, et al. *Cytauxzoon felis* cytochrome b gene mutation associated with atovaquone and azithromycin treatment. *J Vet Intern Med.* 2020;34:2432–2437.
94. Cohn LA, Shaw D, Shoemake C, et al. Second illness due to subsequent *Cytauxzoon felis* infection in a domestic cat. *J Fel Med Surg Open Rep.* 2020;6:2055116920908963.
95. Shindel N, Dardiri AH, Ferris DH. An indirect fluorescent antibody test for the detection of *Cytauxzoon*-like organisms in experimentally infected cats. *Can J Comp Med.* 1978;42:460–465.
96. Tarigo JL, Scholl EH, Bird DMcK, et al. A novel candidate vaccine for cytauxzoonosis inferred from comparative apicomplexan genomics. *PLoS One.* 2013;8:e71233.
97. Schreeg ME, Marr HS, Tarigo J, et al. Identification of *Cytauxzoon felis* antigens via protein microarray and assessment of expression library immunization against cytauxzoonosis. *Clin Proteomics.* 2018;15(1):44.
98. Frontera-Acevedo K, Balsone NM, Dugan MA, et al. Systemic immune responses in *Cytauxzoon felis*-infected domestic cats. *Am J Vet Res.* 2013;74:901–909.
99. Frontera-Acevedo K, Sakamoto K. Local pulmonary immune responses in domestic cats naturally infected with *Cytauxzoon felis. Vet Immunol Immunopathol.* 2015;163:1–7.
100. Ahmed JS. The role of cytokines in immunity and immunopathogenesis of piroplasmoses. *Parasitol Res.* 2002;88:S48–S50.
101. Reichard MV, Rugg JJ, Thomas JE, et al. Efficacy of a topical formulation of selamectin plus sarolaner against induced infestations of *Amblyomma americanum* on cats and prevention of *Cytauxzoon felis* transmission. *Vet Parasitol.* 2019;270(suppl 1):S31–S37.

99

Hepatozoonosis

Nancy Vincent-Johnson, Gad Baneth, Kelly E. Allen

KEY POINTS

- Cause: Hepatozoonosis is an arthropod-borne infection caused by apicomplexan protozoa from the family Hepatozoidae in the suborder Adeleorina. Based on DNA analysis of the gene encoding for 18S rRNA and morphologic features, parasites in the genus *Hepatozoon* are most closely related to other apicomplexan parasites such as *Plasmodium* spp. and piroplasms. The genus was named *Hepatozoon* because merogonic development of the type strain *Hepatozoon muris* was observed in rat livers. However, the liver is not necessarily a major target tissue for other *Hepatozoon* spp. More than 300 *Hepatozoon* species have been described in amphibians, reptiles, birds, marsupials, and mammals Of these, more than 120 species infect snakes, and approximately 50 infect mammals. *Hepatozoon canis* and *Hepatozoon americanum* infect wild and domestic canids. *Hepatozoon* spp. infecting cats include *Hepatozoon felis*, *Hepatozoon silvestris*, and organisms closely related or identical to *H. canis* and *H. americanum.*
- First Described: *Hepatozoon canis* was first reported in dogs in 1905 in India, and has long been known to infect dogs in many regions of the world, including Asia, Africa, southern Europe, the Middle East, and more recently in North and South America and Australia. The first reports of *H. americanum* infection were from the Gulf Coast of Texas, United States, in 1978. In 1997, *H. americanum* was identified as a separate species, distinct from *H. canis.*[1,2] *Hepatozoon* sp. infection in cats was first reported in India in 1908, and infections in felids have since been documented in numerous countries.[3]
- Affected Hosts: *Hepatozoon canis*: domestic dogs, and some wild canids including foxes, jackals, African wild dogs, and coyotes. *Hepatozoon americanum*: domestic dogs, coyotes, and possibly other mammals. *Hepatozoon felis* and *H. silvestris*: domestic and wild felids; other *Hepatozoon* species infecting cats have also been reported, including *H. canis.*
- Geographic Distribution: *Hepatozoon canis* is found in canids in numerous countries in all inhabited continents. In the United States, *H. canis* has been reported in dogs from southeastern states including Alabama, Georgia, Louisiana, Mississippi, Oklahoma, New Jersey, and Virginia. *Hepatozoon americanum* infections occur primarily in the south-eastern and south-central United States. *Hepatozoon canis* and *H. americanum* co-infections in domestic dogs in North America have been reported in Alabama, Mississippi, and Louisiana. *Hepatozoon* sp. infections in domestic cats have been reported from many countries including Brazil, France, India, Israel, Nigeria, Portugal, Italy, Thailand, South Africa, Spain, and the United States.
- Route of Transmission: *Hepatozoon canis* is transmitted by ingestion of infected *Rhipicephalus sanguineus* ticks, and possibly other tick species (*Amblyomma ovale, Rhipicephalus turanicus, Rhipicephalus* (*Boophilus*) *microplus, Haemaphysalis longicornis*, and *Haemaphysalis flava*). Transplacental transmission *of H. canis* is also documented. *Hepatozoon americanum* is transmitted by ingestion of infected *Amblyomma maculatum*, and by ingestion of paratenic vertebrate hosts. The route of infection for *Hepatozoon* spp. infecting cats has not been elucidated, but may involve ingestion of infected arthropod and paratenic host tissues, and possibly transplacental transmission.
- Major Clinical Signs: *Hepatozoon canis* infections in dogs vary greatly in severity from inapparent to severe and life-threatening infection, although dogs are most often subclinically or mildly affected. A compromised immune status tends to lead to more severe disease. In patients with overt disease, clinical signs including fever, anemia, lethargy, and anorexia may be observed. *Hepatozoon americanum* causes American canine hepatozoonosis (ACH), which is associated with fever, lethargy, bilateral mucopurulent ocular discharge, pain and reluctance to move, altered gait, and muscle atrophy. The majority of cats reported with *Hepatozoon* sp. are subclinically infected.
- Differential Diagnoses: Anemia is the most common hematologic abnormality in dogs with *H. canis* infection. Therefore, other conditions causing anemia, including other vector-borne diseases, are differentials. For ACH, differential diagnoses include sterile or infectious meningitis, bacterial discospondylitis, Lyme borreliosis, canine monocytic or granulocytic ehrlichiosis, anaplasmosis, toxoplasmosis, sarcocystosis, bacteremia, and systemic immune-mediated diseases such as systemic lupus erythematosus. Cats infected with *Hepatozoon* spp. should be tested for immunosuppressive diseases including FIV and FeLV infection, and also for hemotropic mycoplasmosis.
- Human Health Significance: Canine and feline *Hepatozoon* species are not known to infect humans.

HEPATOZOON CANIS INFECTION

ETIOLOGIC AGENT AND EPIDEMIOLOGY

Hepatozoon canis was first identified in India in 1905, and has long been known to infect dogs in many regions of the Old World, including Asia, Africa, southern and central Europe, and the Middle East.[4,5] More recently, it has been identified in the New World, both in North and South America and Australia.[1,6–10] The complete genome of *H. canis*, which provides information that may be used for diagnostic test development, has been published.[11]

The main definitive host of *H. canis* is the brown dog tick, *Rhipicephalus sanguineus.*[9] However, in Brazil, *Amblyomma ovale* has been suggested as a vector, and *Rhipicephalus turanicus* collected from a naturally infected fox in southern Italy was also identified as a vector of *H. canis*.[13] *Rhipicephalus microplus* and *Haemaphysalis* spp. have been reported to harbor *H. canis* oocysts in Brazil and Japan, respectively, and are therefore considered suspected vectors.

The brown dog tick, which serves as the primary definitive host of *H. canis,* is found worldwide, and all three stages feed on dogs. Life stages of *H. canis* or morphologically indistinguishable *Hepatozoon* spp. have been reported in numerous carnivore species around the world, but the host range of *H. canis* in mammalian carnivores other than the domestic dog has not been clarified. *Hepatozoon canis* or *Hepatozoon* spp. that morphologically resemble *H. canis* have been reported in several wild canine species, from domestic and wild felids, and from other carnivores, including the wolf (*Canis lupus*), the red fox (*Vulpes vulpes*), crab-eating fox (*Cerdocyon thous*), black-backed jackal (*Canis mesomelas*), golden jackal (*Canis aureus*), African wild dog (*Lycaon pictus*), coyote (*Canis latrans*), raccoon (*Procyon lotor*), maned wolf (*Chrysocyon brachyurus*), hyena (*Crocuta crocuta*), palm civet (*Paradoxurus hermaphroditus*), white eared opposums (*Didelphis albiventris*), cheetah (*Acinonyx jubatus*), tiger (*Panthera tigris*), leopard (*Panthera pardus*), lion (*Panthera leo*), bobcat (*Lynx rufus*), Pallas's cat (*Felis manul*), ocelot (*Leopardus pardalis*), little spotted cat (*Leopardus tigrinus*), leopard cat, Iriomote wildcat (*Felis iriomotensis*), Tsushima leopard cat (*Felis bengalensis euptilura*), and flat-headed cat (*Prionailurus planiceps*).[5,14–19]

The geographic distribution of *H. canis* infections is tied closely to the distribution of *Rh. sanguineus*, the most widely distributed tick species in the world. This tick, which is now considered as a species complex and not just one species, is found in warm and temperate regions, but is adaptable to different environmental conditions. *Hepatozoon canis* is transmitted transstadially from the larva to the nymph stage, and also from the nymph to the adult stage in *Rh. sanguineus*.[20] Transovarial transmission through the tick's ovary and eggs could not be demonstrated under experimental conditions. *Rhipicephalus sanguineus* ticks can be infected experimentally through percutaneous injection of blood gamonts, allowing researchers to study the disease in ticks.[21] *Hepatozoon canis* infections are prevalent in regions with tropical, subtropical, and temperate climates. Infections have been reported in domestic dogs from all inhabited continents and numerous countries, including Greece, Italy, France, Spain, Portugal, Croatia, Albania, Romania, Poland, Ukraine, Czech Republic, Slovakia, and Bulgaria in Europe; Israel, Egypt, and Turkey in the Middle East; South Africa, Sudan, and Nigeria in Africa; India, Sri Lanka, Singapore, Malaysia, the Philippines, Thailand, and Japan in Asia; and Brazil, Argentina, and Venezuela in South America; Costa Rica and Mexico in Central America; and from Australia. *Hepatozoon canis* was also found in dogs from the Caribbean island of Grenada and the Cape Verde Islands. *Hepatozoon canis* is present in the south-eastern United States in some areas where *H. americanum* is enzootic, and co-infections with *H. americanum* and *H. canis* in dogs have been detected (Fig. 99.1).[6,7] *Hepatozoon canis* was also reported in ticks in Eastern Canada.[22] In addition, *H. canis* infections in Sweden[23] and in dogs imported into nonendemic areas have been reported in several countries, including Germany, The Netherlands, and the United Kingdom.[24]

Genetic variability exists among *H. canis* isolates.[25] Sequence identity in 18S rDNA fragments amplified from dogs ranges from 97% to 100%, whereas the diversity among dogs infected with *H. americanum* is higher, with identity that ranges from 92.7% to 99.6%.[6] Phylogenetic analyses of partial sequences of the 18S rDNA from *Hepatozoon* isolates from dogs in Japan and Brazil indicated that these isolates had a 99% identity with *H. canis* sequenced from Israel and were more distant to *H. americanum*.

Differences in the sensitivity and specificity of diagnostic techniques likely influence the observed prevalence rates among different regions. A study of 349 dogs from Turkey found that 10.6% had positive test results using blood smear evaluation for gamonts, 25.8% by PCR and 36.8% were seropositive by IFA testing. Circulating *H. canis* gamonts were detected by blood smear evaluation in 39% of dogs surveyed in rural areas of Rio de Janeiro, Brazil; 19.6% of dogs in nine

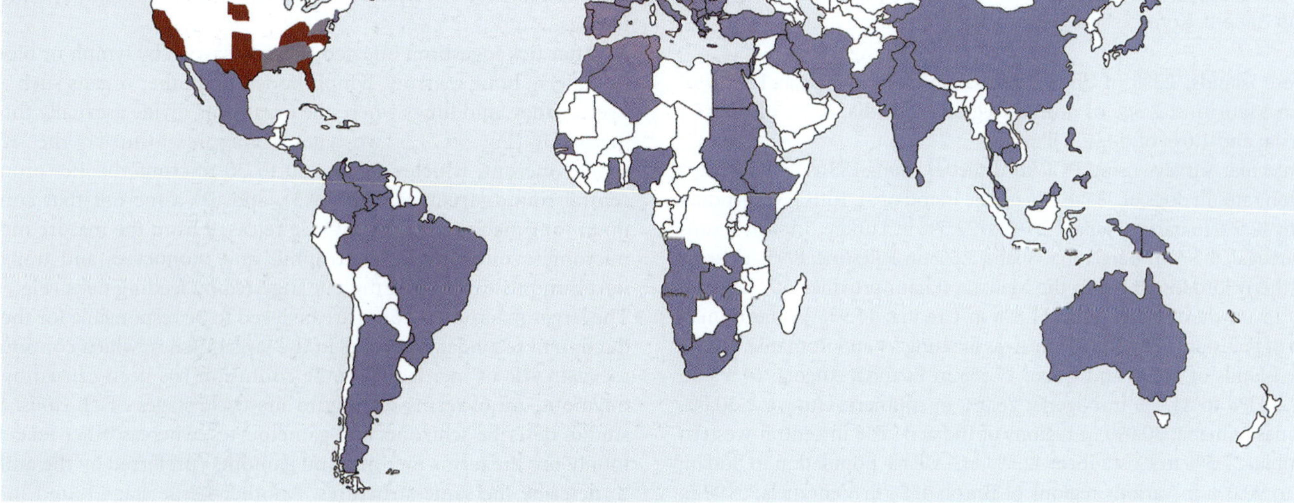

Fig. 99.1 Geographic distribution of reported *Hepatozoon canis (blue)* and *Hepatozoon americanum (red)* infections. Both species *(purple)* exist in the United States.

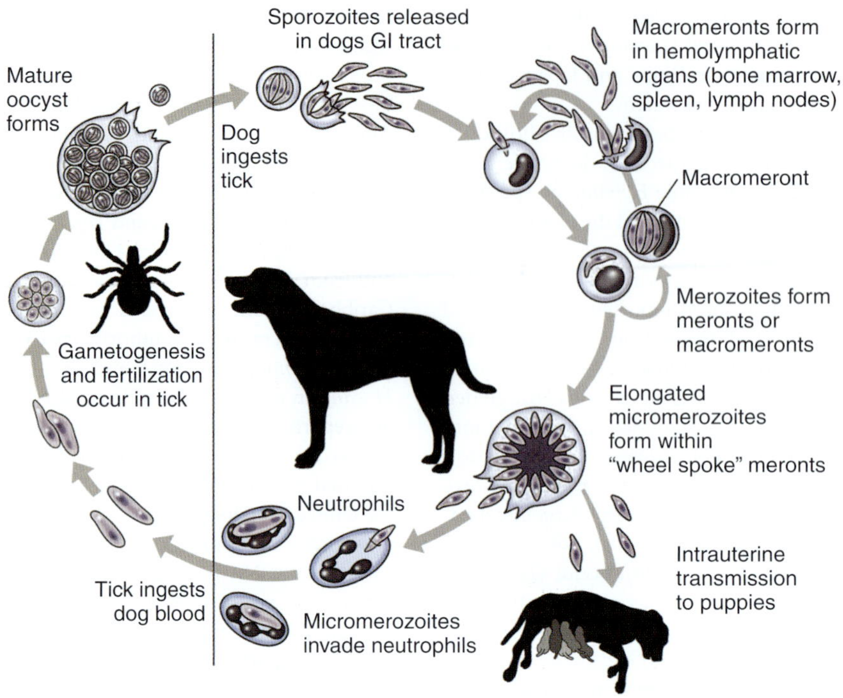

Fig. 99.2 Life cycle of *Hepatozoon canis*.

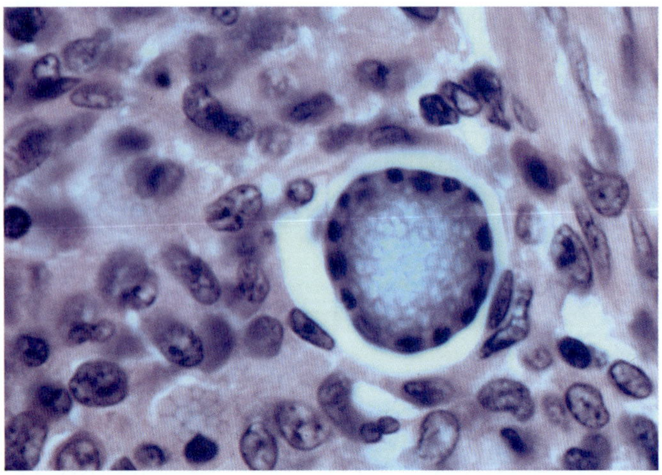

Fig. 99.3 *Hepatozoon canis* meront in splenic tissue of a dog from Israel demonstrating the typical "wheel-spoke" pattern. (Courtesy of Dr. Gad Baneth, Koret School of Veterinary Medicine, Israel.)

Japanese islands; 22% of dogs surveyed in Zaria, Nigeria; 12.5% of dogs in Mauritius; 2.3% of dogs in regions of India; 1.2% of dogs in Malaysia; and 1.0% of dogs in Turkey.

Molecular surveys using PCR to detect *H. canis* 18S rDNA revealed infection rates in dogs of 2% to 6% on the island of St. Kitts, West Indies; 2.5% to 42.9% in parts of Japan; 2.7% to 22.3% in Turkey; 3.1% in southern Portugal; 3.3% in Barcelona, Spain; 5.5% in Palestine; 8.9% in areas of northern Jordan; 10.1% in the Mahasarakham province of Thailand; 10.9% in northern Cambodia; 11.8% in Croatia; 11.9% in the Punjab region of Pakistan; 1.9% to 15% in areas of Hungary and Romania; 16.2% on the islands of Malta and Gozo; 17.5% in Luanda, Angola; 19.3% in Haiti; 20.3% to 41.4% in Nigeria; 26.0% in southern Hungary; 30.0% in Kumasi, Ghana; 30.0% in regions of India; 31.8% in central-western Colombia; 37.5% in Costa Rica; 42.3% in a village population in Sudan; 8.6% to 90.0% in various regions of Brazil; 45% in Venezuela; 51% in Rivas, Nicaragua; and 35.9% to 64% in the Cape Verde Islands.

Serologic studies using IFA revealed that 65.2% of dogs diagnosed with canine monocytic ehrlichiosis (CME) in Thessaloniki, Greece; 36.8% of dogs surveyed for *Hepatozoon* spp. infection around the Aegean coast of Turkey; 33% of the dogs surveyed in Israel; and 4.2% in the Yamaguchi region in Japan had been exposed to *H. canis*. The high seroprevalence rates suggest that most dogs infected with *H. canis* experience subclinical infection. Among dogs surveyed for *H. canis* antibodies in Israel, 3% of the 33% dogs with positive serum antibody titers had detectable blood gamonts, and only 1% had severe clinical signs.

Most dogs are thought to become infected with *H. canis* when they groom ticks from their haircoats or feeding on prey infested with parasitized ticks. An adult *Rh. sanguineus* tick might acquire *H. canis* as a larva or nymph feeding on a parasitemic dog, and then after molting, attach and feed on a new host, not necessarily a dog.[20] Ticks may also acquire infection during feeding at the adult stage as shown experimentally for *A. ovale* in Brazil. Both male and female adult *Rh. sanguineus* can harbor *Hepatozoon* oocysts and are potentially infective to dogs.

After tick ingestion, infected cells are carried by lymph or blood to the spleen, bone marrow, lymph nodes, and other organs such as the liver, kidney, and lungs where the organisms divide asexually through merogony (Fig. 99.2).[9] Two types of meronts form: (1) the "wheel-spoke" meront, which contains 20 to 30 micromerozoites around a central round structure (Fig. 99.3), and (2) a meront that contains up to four macromerozoites. Once released from the mature meront, micromerozoites invade neutrophils and monocytes and transform into gamonts, which can then be ingested by feeding ticks (Fig. 99.4). The larger macromerozoites are believed to be responsible for the production of secondary meronts in the target tissues, which continue the asexual cycle of merogony. Some confusion has been caused by synonymous use of terms relating to life-cycle stages of *H. canis*. Some studies describe schizonts and gametocytes, whereas other texts commonly use the terms meronts and gamonts (preferred by the authors) to describe the same structures. Another tissue stage found in dogs with *H. canis* but not *H. americanum* infections is a small monozoic

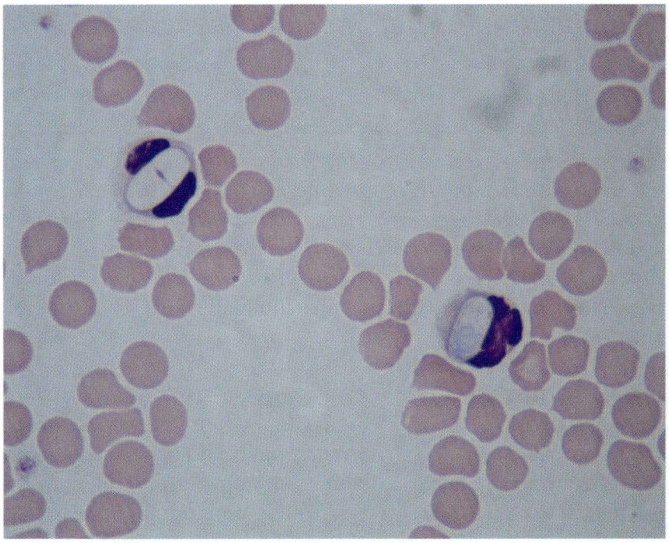

Fig. 99.4 Two *Hepatozoon canis* gamonts in neutrophils on a blood smear. The gamonts of *Hepatozoon americanum* are nearly identical in appearance to those of *H. canis,* although they are rarely seen. 1000× magnification. (Courtesy of Dr. Gad Baneth, Koret School of Veterinary Medicine, Israel.)

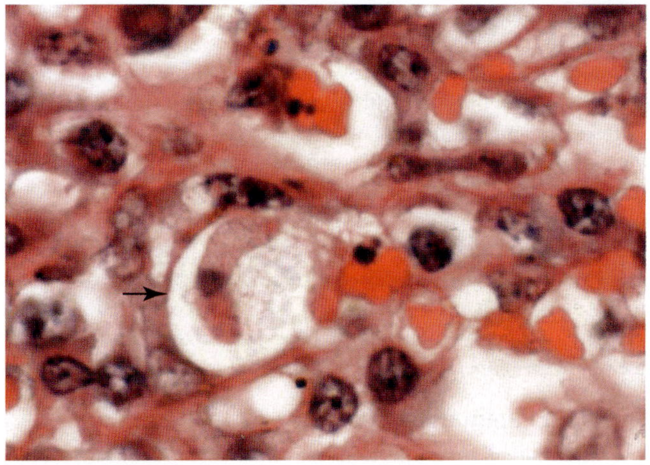

Fig. 99.5 A monozoic tissue cyst of *Hepatozoon canis (arrow)* in the splenic tissue of a naturally infected dog (hematoxylin and eosin stain, 500× magnification).

cyst (containing a single parasite) that resembles the cystozoite form in lizards and snakes affected by other *Hepatozoon* species in which transmission by predation has been shown (Fig. 99.5).[26] The predation route of transmission has not yet been proven to occur for *H. canis* and the role of these cysts in the life cycle of *H. canis* has not been clarified.

Ticks become infected when they ingest leukocytes that contain gamonts while feeding on a parasitemic dog. Morphologically indistinguishable male and female *H. canis* gamonts are released from the dog leukocytes within the tick gut, associate with one another, and differentiate in the process of gametogenesis to form distinct gametes. After fertilization, the zygote divides, and sporogony occurs with the formation of oocysts that are released into the tick's hemocoel. The oocysts are large, spherical forms consisting of a membrane that envelops hundreds of sporocysts in which the infective sporozoites are found. Sporozoites do not migrate to the feeding parts or salivary gland of the tick; therefore, the tick must be ingested to infect the dog.

The entire life cycle of *H. canis* (both tick and dog components) can be completed within 81 days. In an experimental transmission study, adult-stage *Rh. sanguineus* ticks were infective by ingestion to dogs 53 days after the ticks fed as nymphs on a naturally infected dog. Meronts were first detected in the experimentally infected dog's bone marrow 13 days postinoculation, and gamonts appeared in the blood in 28 days, thereby completing the life cycle.[9]

As for other apicomplexan parasites, such as *Toxoplasma gondii* and *Neospora caninum* (see Chapters 93 and 94), vertical transmission through the uterus from dam to its offspring has also been demonstrated for *H. canis*. Naturally infected pregnant dogs were allowed to give birth in a tick-free environment. Meronts were found in the spleen of a pup that died 16 days after birth, and blood gamonts were detectable as early as 21 days in other pups.[27]

Another likely mode of transmission that has not yet been demonstrated for *H. canis* infections is predation on another intermediate or transport host. Experimentally, infection could not be established through parenteral inoculation of tissues or blood from infected dogs but it could from inoculation of emulsified tick tissues. In an area of south-eastern Brazil with high *H. canis* prevalence, a survey study documented characteristic monozoic cysts of *Hepatozoon* spp. in many collected rodents, but molecular analysis revealed that the organism was distinct from *H. canis*. However, *H. americanum* may be transmitted by dog predation on wild rodents and rabbits harboring the tissue cyst stages of this parasite, and some other species of *Hepatozoon* that infect snakes, lizards, and frogs have also been shown to be transmitted through predation and ingestion of tissue cysts found in intermediate host tissues.[26]

No gender or breed predilection for disease caused by *H. canis* has been noted. Disease has been reported in all age groups, from pups younger than three months of age to geriatric dogs. In a case series of dogs from Greece, the female-to-male ratio was 1.2:1, and the mean age was 4.2 years. Dogs with disease caused by *H. canis* are more likely to be from a rural community as compared with an urban setting, which may reflect a higher tick exposure rate. In a study of dogs from Brazil, the presence of *Rh. sanguineus* ticks on dogs in the household was associated with at least one *H. canis*–infected dog per household.

Most dogs with disease due to *H. canis* are examined during the warmer months of the year when tick vectors are more abundant. In a case-control study of 100 dogs *H. canis* infections from Israel, 77% were admitted during the warm period of May through November. A follow-up study on the periodic appearance of *H. canis* gamonts in the blood of dogs in Japan indicated that the peak parasitemia was from spring to autumn. However, disease due to *H. canis* is also diagnosed during the colder months, when transmission by vector ticks is less likely, as a result of chronic persistent infection.

CLINICAL FEATURES

Pathogenesis and Clinical Signs

Most dogs infected with *H. canis* have a low level of parasitemia, with less than 5% of circulating leukocytes infected with gamonts. These dogs have a limited inflammatory reaction. About 15% of parasitemic dogs have a high level of parasitemia (>800 gamonts/μL).[23] The degree of parasitemia correlates with the severity of clinical signs; the sickest dogs may have parasitemia that approaches 100% of infected circulating leukocytes.[25] These dogs may develop hepatitis, glomerulonephritis, or pneumonitis in addition to severe anemia, fever, and cachexia.[26]

When a dog ingests the vector tick or tick parts, *H. canis* sporozoites are released in the intestine and penetrate the gut wall. The sporozoites invade mononuclear cells and disseminate hematogenously or via the lymph to hemolymphatic target organs that include the bone marrow, spleen, and lymph nodes and to other internal organs such as the liver, kidney, and lungs. Respectively, hepatitis, glomerulonephritis, and pneumonitis may develop. Meronts, in which asexually dividing merozoites develop, are formed in the dog's tissues in the process of merogony.

Conditions that weaken the immune responses increase the susceptibility to new infection with *H. canis* or allow existing infections to reactivate. Co-infections with other pathogens such as *Ehrlichia canis, Babesia* spp., *Anaplasma* spp., *Leishmania infantum*, CPV, or CDV can influence establishment of a new *H. canis* infection as well as progression or reactivation of an existing infection. In a litter of Dalmatians that were diagnosed with *H. canis* parasitemia, pups that developed parvoviral enteritis demonstrated a significantly higher level of parasitemia than did their littermates that did not become ill. In addition, treatment of experimentally infected dogs with an immunosuppressive dose of prednisolone was followed by the appearance of parasitemia.[21]

Physical Examination Findings

Dogs with mild *H. canis* infections may have pale mucous membranes and lethargy. Dogs with high parasitemia often exhibit fever, lethargy, and severe weight loss or cachexia, even if they maintain a good appetite. Splenomegaly and lymphadenomegaly may be detected. Dogs often have physical examination abnormalities that relate to the presence of co-infections or other comorbidities.

A variety of clinical abnormalities are associated with infection, which range in severity from an incidental hematologic finding in an apparently healthy dog to a debilitating and life-threatening illness. A low level of *H. canis* parasitemia with gamonts in less than 5% of neutrophils is the most common finding. This is usually associated with subclinical to mild disease. A high-level parasitemia that can approach 100% of infected neutrophils with leukocytosis is usually associated with severe disease. High parasitemia rates are frequently found in association with marked neutrophilic leukocytosis, as high as 150,000 cells/μL of blood.[25,26] The mechanism leading to this leukocytosis has not been elucidated.

In a case-control study of 100 dogs with disease caused by *H. canis*, dogs were categorized into low and high parasitemia groups. Of these, 85% had a low parasitemia level and 15% had a high number of circulating parasites. Dogs with low parasitemia were more anemic and had lower platelet counts than did the control dogs with other disease conditions. However, dogs with high circulating parasite numbers suffered mainly from fever, lethargy, weight loss, anemia, and hyperglobulinemia. A study of canine hepatozoonosis from Turkey also found an association between the severity of clinical signs and the level of parasitemia. Dogs with severe disease had higher parasitemia levels than dogs showing moderate or mild clinical signs.[26]

High numbers of circulating *H. canis* gamonts (e.g., 50,000 to 100,000 gamonts/μL of blood) signify significant tissue parasitism. Tissue meronts produce the numerous merozoites that eventually invade leukocytes. The load of blood and tissue parasites present in dogs with high-level parasitemia demands nutrients and exerts tissue injury. This subgroup of affected dogs typically exhibit weight loss with cachexia and profound lethargy. A study of 185 dogs from Thailand found a significant positive correlation between the number of gamonts in *H. canis* infected dogs and the plasma protein level.[30]

Concurrent infections involving *H. canis* and other canine pathogens are common. Some co-infecting organisms, including *E. canis* (see Chapter 44) and *Babesia vogeli* (see Chapter 97), are also transmitted by *Rh. sanguineus*, and are likely to be found in dogs with tick infestations in areas where these diseases are endemic in the dog population. Other pathogens reported to be involved in concurrent infections include CPV, CDV, *Anaplasma phagocytophilum, Anaplasma platys, T. gondii*, and *L. infantum*. Young puppies with hepatozoonosis and other concurrent infections may develop more severe disease. Co-infections may influence the susceptibility to establishing a new infection or the progression of an existing one. In the case of concurrent infection, clinical signs attributed to *H. canis* infection must be interpreted cautiously.

DIAGNOSIS

The pathogenesis, vector capacity, tissue tropism, and clinical signs associated with *H. canis* infection differ from those of *H. americanum* infection (see later discussion). *Hepatozoon canis* is found primarily in hemolymphatic tissues, whereas *H. americanum* infects mainly muscular tissues, causing myositis and lameness.[1,2,10] The principal differences between these two infections are summarized in Table 99.1.

Laboratory Abnormalities

Complete Blood Count

The most common laboratory finding in *H. canis* infection is anemia, which is usually normocytic, normochromic, and occasionally regenerative. Platelets are decreased about one third of the time, but this may be due to concurrent infection with *E. canis* or other disease. The white blood cell count is typically normal in cases with low parasitemia but is elevated in dogs with high parasitemia. Some dogs have neutrophil counts of 50,000 to 150,000/μL with close to 100% of these cells containing gamonts.[31]

Serum Chemistry Profile

Common serum chemistry findings in *H. canis* infection include hyperproteinemia, hyperglobulinemia, and hypoalbuminemia. The hyperglobulinemia is due to a polyclonal gammopathy. Increases in the activities of ALP and CK are usually present.

Urinalysis

Urinalysis findings are not known to be affected by *H. canis*, but because some dogs have evidence of glomerulonephritis, proteinuria may be possible.

Diagnostic Imaging

In *H. canis* infection, radiographic bone lesions are rare. Periostitis has been described in reports from Japan, India, and Italy, and in an experimental infection in Israel.

Microbiologic Tests

Diagnostic assays currently available for hepatozoonosis in dogs are described in Table 99.2.

Cytologic and Morphologic Diagnosis

In most dogs with *H. canis* infections, gamonts are found on blood smear examination in 0.5% to 5% of neutrophils and monocytes. Parasitemia may approach 100% in heavy infections. Gamonts may also be identified in dogs that are apparently healthy.

Microscopic detection of *H. canis* gamonts in Giemsa- or Diff-Quik-stained blood smears is the most common method for diagnosis. The gamonts are ellipsoidal and measure approximately 11 μm × 4 μm (Fig. 99.6) and are found in the cytoplasm of neutrophils and rarely in monocytes. Gamonts are enveloped in a thick membrane (Fig. 99.7) and are often situated in the center of the neutrophil and compress its lobulated nucleus toward the cell membrane. Examination of buffy-coat smears is more sensitive than routine blood smears for detection of the organism; however, nucleic acid amplification tests (see later discussion) are even more sensitive and specific.

Hepatozoon canis meronts can be detected in cytologic preparations made from aspirates or touch impressions of hemolymphatic tissues. With cytologic examination, meronts are round to oval and approximately 30 μm in diameter. Immature meronts appear as

TABLE 99.1 Comparison Between *Hepatozoon canis* Infection, American Canine Hepatozoonosis, and Feline Hepatozoonosis

	Hepatozoon canis Infection	American Canine Hepatozoonosis	Feline Hepatozoonosis
First described	India, 1905	Texas Gulf Coast, 1978	India, 1908
Etiologic agent	*Hepatozoon canis*	*Hepatozoon americanum*	*Hepatozoon felis, Hepatozoon silvestris, Hepatozoon canis*
Primary vector	*Rhipicephalus sanguineus* (brown dog tick), *Rhipicephalus turanicus, Ambylomma ovale*	*Amblyomma maculatum* (Gulf Coast tick)	Unknown
Route of transmission	Ingestion of tick (not a tick bite)	Ingestion of tick (not a tick bite)	Probably ingestion of tick or other hematophageous vector
Additional routes of transmission	Transplacental from dam to puppy	Ingestion of cystozoites in transport hosts; transplacental is likely	Possibly transplacental
Affected mammalian hosts	Dogs, foxes, jackals, other carnivores	Dogs, coyotes, possibly bobcats, ocelots, and other wildlife	Domestic cats, wild felids
Geographic distribution	Africa, Middle East, Asia, southern Europe, Central and South America, United States, Australia	Primarily southern and south-eastern United States	India, Africa, Israel, Brazil, Spain, France, Italy, Cyprus, Turkey, Thailand, United States
Severity of disease	Subclinical to mild; occasionally severe, especially if immunosuppressed	Usually severe, even in absence of immunosuppression	Typically subclinical unless immunosuppressed
Principal target organs	Spleen, bone marrow, lymph node	Skeletal muscle, myocardium	Myocardium, skeletal muscle, lungs, bone marrow
Major clinical signs	Lethargy, fever, weight loss	Fever, pain, lameness, ocular discharge	Nonspecific
Common laboratory abnormalities	Anemia; extreme leukocytosis is rare but may occur with high parasitemia	Marked leukocytosis (20,000–200,000 cells/μL), anemia, elevated ALP activity, low glucose concentration	Elevated CK activity
Radiographic lesions	Nonspecific; rare periostitis	Common; periosteal bone proliferation	Not reported
Histopathology findings	Hepatitis, splenitis, glomerulonephritis, pneumonitis associated with *H. canis* meronts No muscle lesions	Myositis, onion-skin cysts, pyogranulomas, and meronts in skeletal muscle	Meronts in myocardium and skeletal muscle
Unique morphologic features	"Wheel-spoked" meronts, small monozoic splenic tissue cysts	Large onion-skin cysts in muscle	
Blood smear findings	Gamonts common; parasitemia of 1%–5% is typical; rarely see parasitemia of 5%–100%	Rarely observed gamonts; parasitemia is usually < 0.1%	Parasitemia is rare; when present usually < 1% of neutrophils
Human health significance	None known	None known	None known

ALP, alkaline phosphatase; *CK*, creatine kinase.

TABLE 99.2 Diagnostic Assays Currently Available for Hepatozoonosis in Dogs

Assay	Specimen Type	Target	Performance
Cytologic examination	Whole blood smears	*Hepatozoon* spp. gamonts in leukocytes	False negatives are common because of low circulating numbers of gamonts, especially in clinical *Hepatozoon americanum* infections.
Antibody serology (ELISA or immunofluorescent antibody)	Serum	Antibodies to *Hepatozoon canis*	Positive test results indicate exposure but do not indicate the presence of the organism in circulating leukocytes and do not correlate with clinical disease.
Real-time PCR assays	Whole blood	*H. americanum* or *H. canis* DNA	Sensitivity and specificity may vary depending on assay design, but in general PCR assays are more sensitive than cytology. False-negative results may occur when organism levels are very low, such as early in disease or in very chronic infections.
Histopathology	Muscle biopsy specimens	*H. americanum* cysts, meronts, and pyogranulomas	Reliable method in both acute and chronic cases of *H. americanum* infection, but requires anesthesia.

ELISA, enzyme-linked immunosorbent assay; *PCR*, polymerase chain reaction.

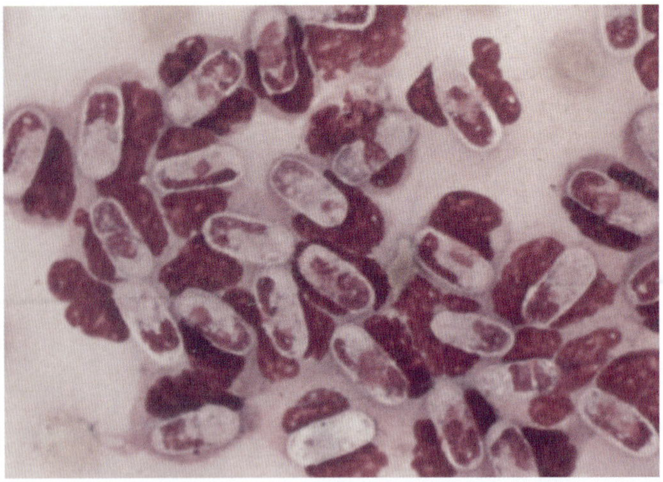

Fig. 99.6 Feathered edge of a blood smear from a dog with leukocytosis and a high *Hepatozoon canis* parasitemia. Close to 100% of the neutrophils are parasitized with gamonts (Giemsa stain, 1000× magnification).

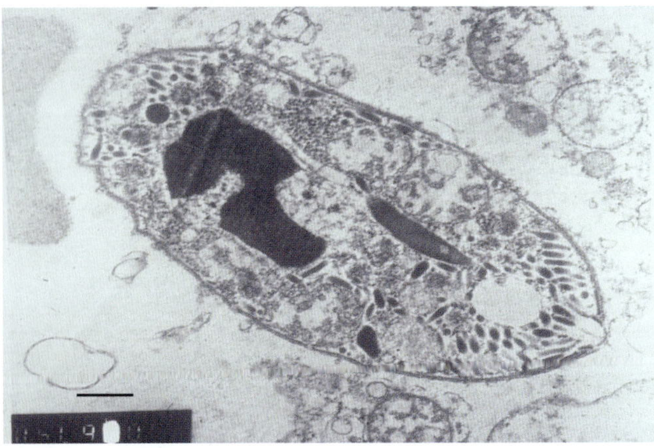

Fig. 99.7 A transmission electron microscopic image of *Hepatozoon canis* gamont from the blood of a naturally infected dog. Note the conoid at the anterior end of the parasite. A three-layer membrane envelopes the gamont (bar = 1 μm).

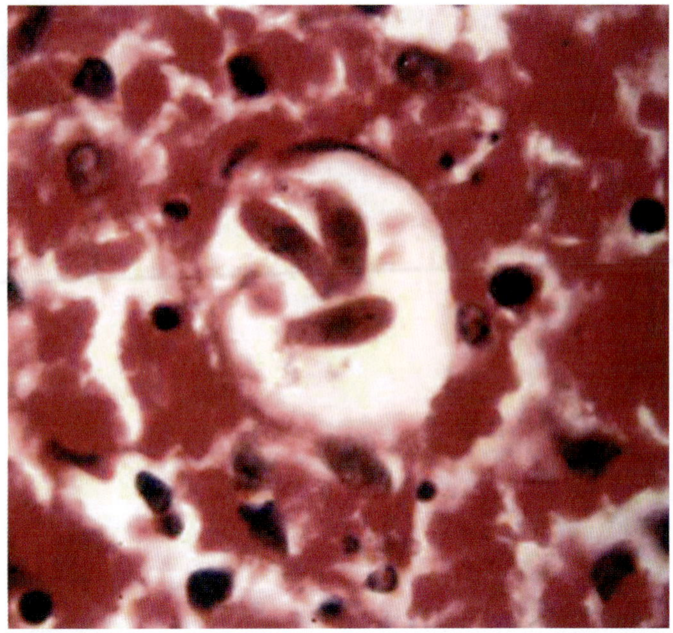

Fig. 99.8 *Hepatozoon canis* meront containing three macromerozoites in splenic tissue.

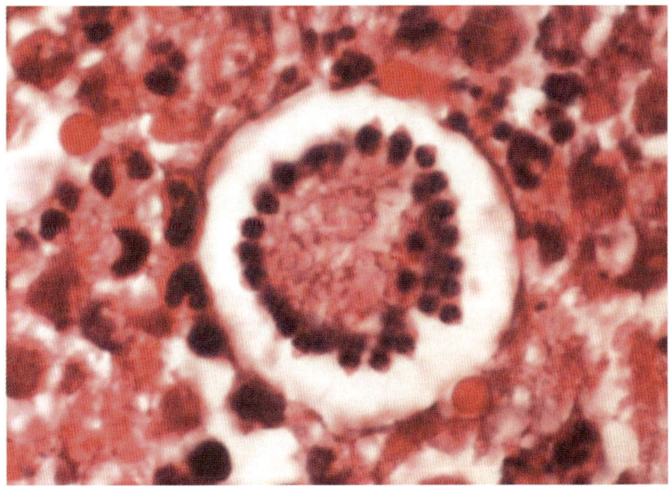

Fig. 99.9 *Hepatozoon canis* meront containing micromerozoites forming a "wheel-spoke" shape in splenic tissue (hematoxylin and eosin stain, 400× magnification).

round opacities filled with globular foam-like material. As the meront matures, basophilic-staining chromatin material forms as either two to four larger macromerozoites (Fig. 99.8) or more than 20 micromerozoites (Fig. 99.9). The micromerozoites align in a circle close to the meront wall around a central opaque core.

Hepatozoon canis can also be identified in ticks. Mature oocysts can be seen even without magnification as small white globular forms in wet preparations of the hemocoel. The observation of oocysts is verified and differentiated from the tick's organs and salivary glands by microscopy of hemocoel smears as unstained wet preparations or as Giemsa-stained specimens (Fig. 99.10). The oocysts are enveloped in a fragile membrane and contain hundreds of smaller oval sporocysts. Free sporocysts are often scattered outside the oocyst, and infective sporozoites are packed as elongated slender forms within the sporocysts.

Serologic Diagnosis

Both IFA and ELISA assays for *H. canis* antibodies have been developed. Positive serologic test results indicate exposure but do not prove active infection or correlate with clinical disease. Thus, serologic testing is mostly of use for epidemiologic studies. Both IgM and IgG antibodies were detectable in the sera of experimentally infected dogs as early as 16 and 22 days postinoculation, respectively, peaked at 7 to 9 weeks, and persisted for more than 7 months.

Molecular Diagnosis Using Nucleic Acid–Based Testing

PCR assays for the detection of *Hepatozoon* DNA have been mostly based on amplification of fragments of the *18S rRNA* gene.[6,7,32] Some of the PCR assays originally developed to detect piroplasms such as *Babesia* spp. also amplify *Hepatozoon* DNA; however, the amplified products are of different size, and their identities can be further verified by sequencing. Studies that compared the detection of *Hepatozoon* by blood smear microscopy and endpoint PCR from the same blood samples indicated that PCR was considerably more sensitive. In one study, smears were positive in 2.6% of cases versus 11.4% by PCR, in another 10.6% versus 25.8%, and in a third, 11.3% versus 53.3%, respectively. Quantitative (real-time) PCR assays for *Hepatozoon* are very sensitive and specific and have the potential to provide an estimate

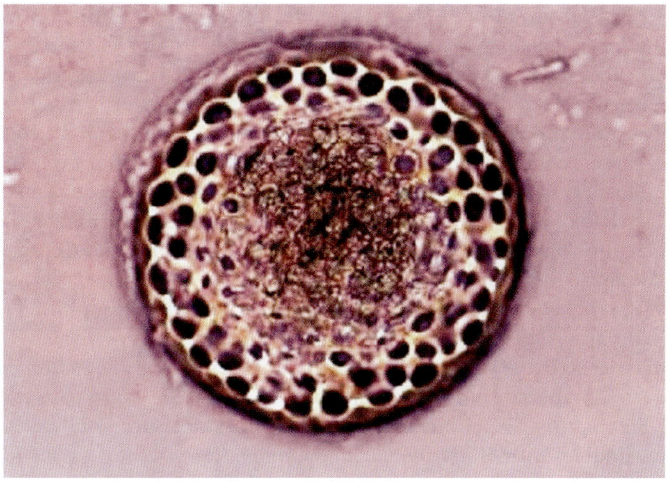

Fig. 99.10 Unstained *Hepatozoon canis* oocyst containing numerous sporocysts from the hemocoel of an adult-stage *Rhipicephalus sanguineus* tick (200× magnification).

of the parasite load in submitted specimens.[7] A loop-mediated isothermal amplfication technique for the detection of *H. canis* infection at POC has been developed.[33]

Pathologic Findings

Gross Pathologic Findings

Pathologic descriptions of infected dogs range from reports on infrequent tissue meronts termed as incidental findings to severe and occasionally fatal multiorgan involvement. A considerable variation is found in the spectrum of lesions and the number of parasitic life forms. The major macroscopic lesions found in dogs with heavy infections include splenomegaly and hepatomegaly, with a diffuse pattern of small white necrotic foci 1 to 2 mm in diameter. Necrotic foci may be larger and nodular in appearance and are also found in other tissues including the pancreas and on the pleura. Pneumonia may be evident, and lymph nodes are typically enlarged.

Histopathologic Findings

Histopathologic findings include a varying number of developing or mature meronts in tissues. "Wheel-spoke" meronts are approximately 30 μm in diameter (see Fig. 99.9). Meronts can be found in small numbers as an incidental finding in dogs from enzootic areas.

Meronts can be associated with a mild to severe inflammatory response. Focal splenic necrosis is associated with *H. canis* merogony in red and white pulp regions, with white pulp necrosis located primarily in lymphoid follicles. Hepatitis with Kupffer cell hyperplasia and mononuclear and neutrophil infiltration is associated with developing meronts in the liver. The presence of *H. canis* in the lung is associated with interstitial pneumonia and thickening of alveolar septa with inflammatory cell infiltrates. Renal lesions include glomerulonephritis and interstitial nephritis with multifocal necrosis. Mild to extensive parasitism with meronts and developing gamonts in the lymph nodes and bone marrow may also be evident.

TREATMENT AND PROGNOSIS

The current treatment protocol for *H. canis* infection is imidocarb dipropionate at 5 to 6 mg/kg, SC or IM, every 14 days, until gamonts are no longer present in blood smears. It has been recommended that all dogs, even those with only mild disease, be treated because parasitemia may increase over time. One or two injections may suffice; however, the elimination of gamonts in heavy infections using imidocarb dipropionate may require treatment for 8 weeks or longer. Doxycycline at 10 mg/kg/day, PO, for 21 days is frequently used in combination with imidocarb dipropionate to treat potential or identified rickettsial vector-borne co-infections.

Despite the clinical improvement or clearance of the parasite in the blood by microscopic methods, PCR methods may still detect the organism during follow-up evaluation after treatment. Successful treatment with the combination of toltrazuril at 10 mg/kg/day PO for 5 days followed by 5 mg/kg/day for additional 10 days, and trimethoprim-sulfonamide at 15 mg/kg PO q12h for 30 days was described in one dog. Addition of toltrazuril or clindamycin does not seem to provide any additional benefit to imidocarb therapy.

Despite lack of a parasitologic cure, clinical cure is achieved in many dogs. The rate of survival of treated dogs with a low *H. canis* parasitemia is generally good and is frequently dependent on the prognosis of any concurrent disease, if present. The prognosis for dogs with a high parasitemia is guarded. Only 7 of 15 dogs (47%) with a high parasitemia survived 2 months despite specific treatment.

IMMUNITY AND VACCINATION

Infection with *H. canis* elicits a distinct humoral immune response during the early stages of the disease.[34] No information is available on the cellular response to infection; however, because *H. canis* is an intracellular parasite, CMI probably plays a major role in the immune mechanism mounted by the host.

Current treatments do not cure infection, so dogs remain susceptible to relapse of disease, especially if immunosuppressed. In experimental *H. canis* infection, treatment with an immunosuppressive dose of glucocorticoids was followed by the appearance of parasitemia. Vaccines for *H. canis* infection are not available.

PREVENTION

Hepatozoon spp. have not been shown to be transmitted through blood transfusion, and the parasite needs to pass through the tick in which the sporozoites, the infective stage of the parasite, are produced in order to complete its life cycle. However, there is no knowledge whether tissue stages that may be infectious may circulate in dogs' blood, and therefore it seems logical that dogs infected with *Hepatozoon* species be avoided as blood donor dogs.

Prevention of *H. canis* infection should consist of an effective control of vector ticks on dogs and in the environment using external parasiticides. Dogs must be prevented from ingesting ticks while grooming or scavenging. Until the certainty that *H. canis* infection may be transmitted by ingestion of infected tissues is reached, dogs in endemic areas should be prevented from eating raw or prey meat.[5]

PUBLIC HEALTH ASPECTS

The spectrum of natural hosts for *H. canis* and *H. americanum* is not currently known. There is only one report of infection with a *Hepatozoon* spp. in a person from the Philippines. This patient was anemic and icteric, and gamonts were detected in the blood. However, no parasites were found in liver and bone marrow biopsies. The danger of direct transmission from dogs to humans is apparently low. *H. canis* is transmitted by tick ingestion rather than a tick bite, and tick ingestion is an unlikely route of transmission for humans.

Although the zoonotic importance of *Hepatozoon* spp. is not known, and it is unlikely to be a significant pathogen in immunocompetent people, caution should be used when handling infected dogs infested with ticks or when removing ticks from dogs as there is a possibility that known human pathogens may also be present.

HEPATOZOON AMERICANUM INFECTION

ETIOLOGY AND EPIDEMIOLOGY

Hepatozoon americanum, the cause of American canine hepatozoonosis (ACH), was first described in 1978 in a Texas coyote. Reports of infections in domestic dogs in Texas and additional southern states occurred over the next two decades, but the parasite was mistaken for *H. canis* due to the similar morphology of the intraleukocytic gamont stage.[1,2] However, based on several criteria including demonstrated tick definitive host, clinical manifestations in infected dogs, and genetic and antigenic differences from *H. canis, H. americanum* was recognized as a novel species infecting canids in North America in 1997.[1,10]

ACH is an emerging disease that is spreading north and east from where it was originally detected, which may be due to the geographic expansion of the tick definitive host, *Amblyomma maculatum,* the Gulf Coast tick.[10,35] The geographic distribution of ACH aligns closely with the range of the Gulf Coast tick. Although this tick is endemic in the states that surround the Gulf of Mexico, its range is expanding and it has been found in arid regions of Arizona and as far north as Kansas, Illinois, Kentucky and the Mid-Atlantic states of Virginia, Maryland, and Delaware.[35–37]

Hepatozoon americanum infection is predominantly diagnosed in south-central and south-eastern states, but occasional cases have been identified in diverse locations across the United States, including California, Nebraska, Vermont, Virginia, and Washington. Because infection may be chronic, ACH is occasionally diagnosed in dogs with a history of travel to and from endemic areas.[7] Although initially thought only to be present in North America, recent molecular data suggest that *H. americanum* or a genetically close species infects canids in Brazil.[38] There are isolated reports of DNA of a *Hepatozoon felis*–like organism detected in a dog from southern California and a *H. americanum*–like organism in an immunocompromised cat in Oklahoma, but the clinical significance and epidemiology of these infections are unknown.[37]

Significant variation in 18S rDNA sequences of *Hepatozoon* spp. that infect dogs in the United States has been identified, indicating that the species infecting dogs in North America may be more diverse than previously recognized.[6] As research using molecular diagnostics and genetic sequencing continues, it is possible that additional species will be identified.

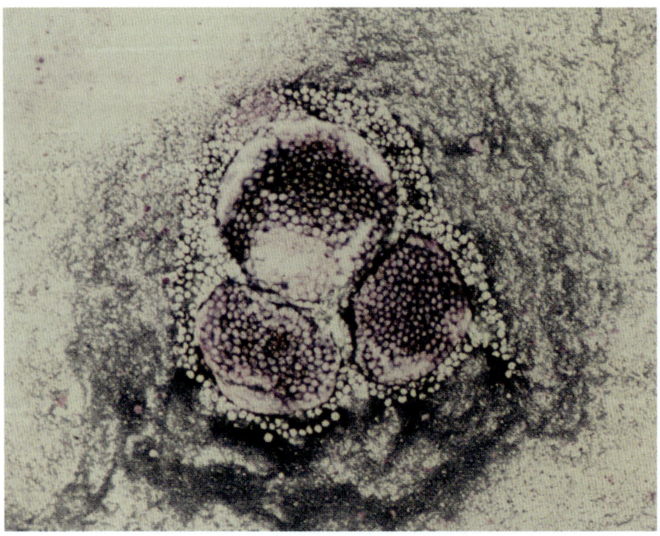

Fig. 99.11 *Hepatozoon americanum* oocysts from the hemocoel of an *Amblyomma maculatum* tick. Hundreds of small, round sporocysts are present within each oocyst. Each sporocyst contains 10 to 26 infective sporozoites.

The true prevalence of *H. americanum* infection is not entirely clear. In 2007, a collaborative molecular survey study using real-time PCR on whole blood detected *H. americanum* in 27.2% of 614 dogs with signs suggestive of hepatozoonosis from 28 states in North America, predominantly in the southeast. Accurate estimates of the prevalence of *H. americanum* infection are difficult due to the lack of available serologic tests and the insensitivity of molecular methods to detect *H. americanum* DNA in infected dogs that have no detectable parasitemia. Infections have also been reported in dogs from Alabama, Georgia, Louisiana, Mississippi, Oklahoma, New Jersey, and Virginia; a few dogs have had mixed infections with *H. americanum* and *H. canis.*[6,8,32]

Because dogs or other vertebrates serve as intermediate hosts, a vector is needed to complete the sexual phase of the life cycle of *Hepatozoon* species. In the case of *H. americanum,* the vector is the Gulf Coast tick, *A. maculatum.* Experimentally the disease has not successfully been transmitted with *Amblyomma americanum, Dermacentor variabilis,* or *Rh. sanguineus* ticks. As it feeds on an infected dog, the larval or nymphal Gulf Coast tick ingests circulating blood macrophages that contain gamonts. Within the tick's gut, the gamonts are freed from the cells and undergo further development before fertilization occurs. The resulting zygote divides through sporogony and develops into an oocyst within the hemocoel of the tick (Fig. 99.11). Oocysts mature while the tick molts to the nymphal or adult stage. Each mature oocyst contains hundreds of sporocysts, with each sporocyst containing 10 to 26 infective sporozoites.[2]

Once a dog ingests an infected tick, whether through grooming or preying on a tick-infested animal, exposure of the parasite to bile in the dog's GI tract results in release of sporozoites, which penetrate the intestinal epithelial wall and are transported to target organs and tissues, likely within mononuclear cells. In *H. americanum* infections, infected cells preferentially travel to skeletal muscle where each organism develops within its monocytic host cell, which becomes lodged between myocytes (Fig. 99.12). Concentric layers of mucopolysaccharide are

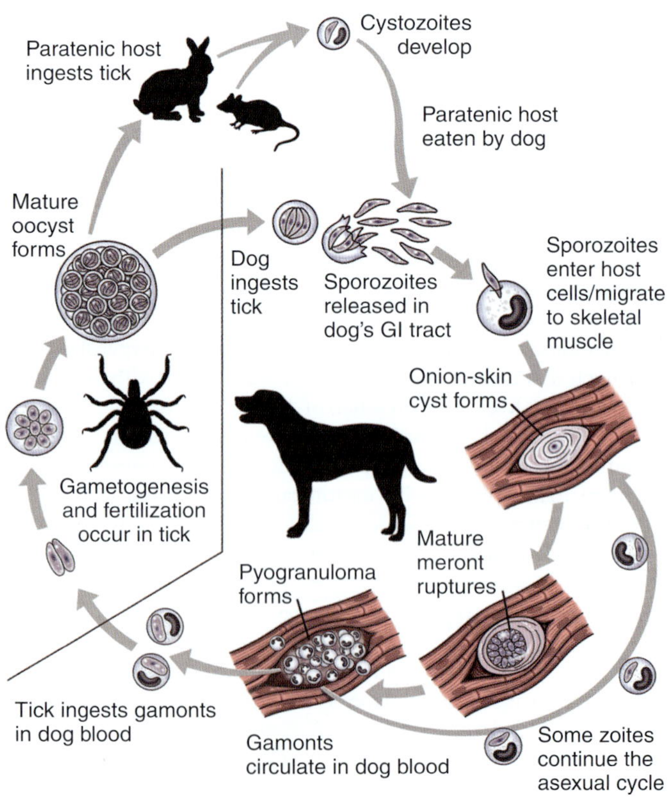

Fig. 99.12 Life cycle of *Hepatozoon americanum.*

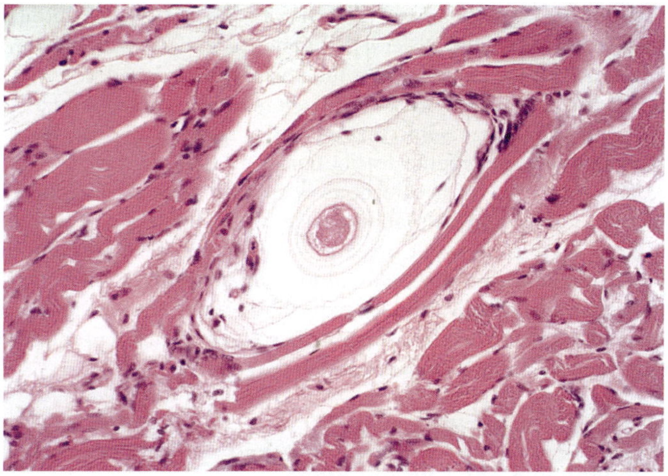

Fig. 99.13 "Onion-skin cyst" of *Hepatozoon americanum.* Concentric layers of mucopolysaccharide material produced by the host cell protect the developing organism from the host's immune system (hematoxylin and eosin stain, 400x magnification).

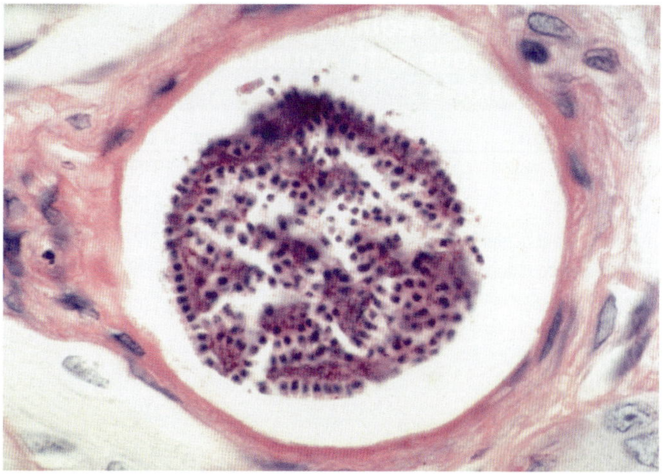

Fig. 99.14 A mature *Hepatozoon americanum* meront just before release of merozoites. Note the lack of inflammation surrounding the cystic structure (hematoxylin and eosin stain, 1200× magnification).

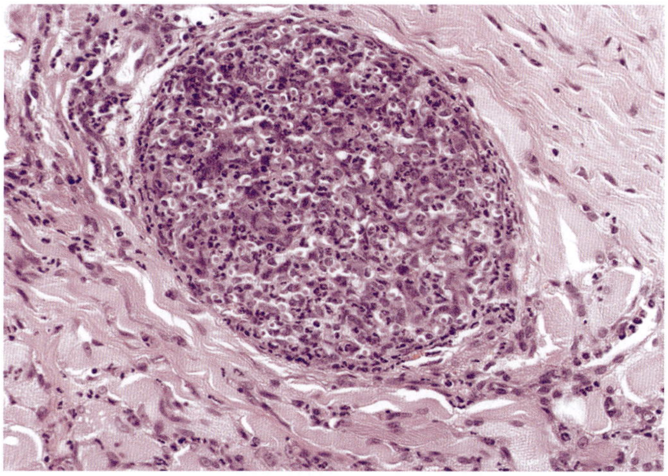

Fig. 99.15 Pyogranuloma associated with the invasion of zoites released from a meront in skeletal muscle of a dog infected with *Hepatozoon americanum.* Zoites displace the nucleus in several of the inflammatory cells.

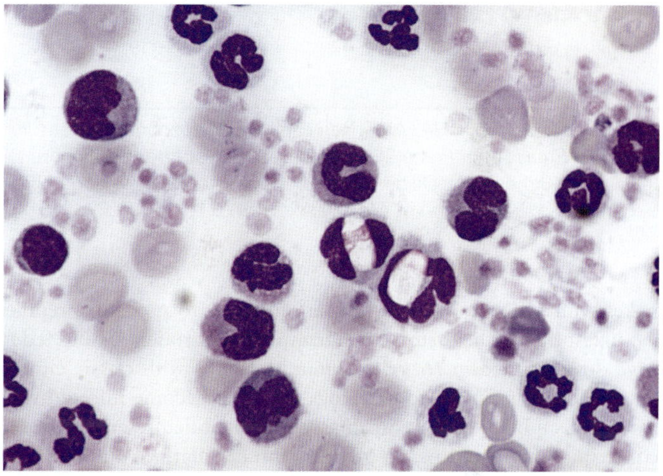

Fig. 99.16 Gamonts of *Hepatozoon americanum* in circulating neutrophils appear identical to *Hepatozoon canis* gamonts. (Giemsa stain, 1200× magnification).

laid down by the host cell to form a large "onion-skin cyst," which may protect the organism from the host immune response (Fig. 99.13). Merogony occurs within the cyst, and on maturation of the meront, the cyst ruptures and merozoites are released (Fig. 99.14). This elicits a severe inflammatory response, with recruitment of neutrophils and macrophages to the area. A pyogranuloma develops in the space where the cyst existed (Fig. 99.15). Many macrophages become infected with a single zoite. Angiogenesis within the pyogranuloma results in a highly vascular structure from which the infected cells can reenter circulation. Two morphologic forms of organism have been observed in macrophages within the pyogranulomas or peripheral blood: circulating merozoites continue the asexual cycle by redistributing to tissues to initiate repeated asexual cycles, while gamonts in peripheral blood macrophages are ingested by feeding ticks, thus completing the life cycle (Fig. 99.16).[2]

Some of the onion-skin cysts within muscle lie dormant for varying lengths of time; their activation is responsible for the waxing and waning nature of ACH as well as relapse of clinical signs that can occur months after perceived clinical cure. Cysts have been found in muscle biopsies taken from dogs for up to 5 years after the initial infection, and an experimentally infected dog remained infective to ticks for over 5 years.[2] In experimental infections, completion of the life cycle from ingestion of infected ticks to development of circulating gamonts can occur in as few as 32 days.[39] In the nymphal tick, approximately 40 days are needed for the organism to develop into mature oocysts that are present in the hemocoel of newly molted adults. Larval *A. maculatum* can also acquire *H. americanum* when they feed from infected dogs, and then support the parasite's development through the molting period. Experimental infections have been produced in both dogs and coyotes by feeding them infected *A. maculatum* ticks.[2]

Other modes of transmission also occur in hepatozoonosis. Transplacental transmission from dam to puppies has been documented for *H. canis* infections and may occur in *H. americanum* infections, although not experimentally demonstrated. Carnivory may play an important role in *H. americanum* transmission in enzootic areas, as has been demonstrated for *Hepatozoon* spp. infecting snakes, lizards, and frogs.[26] Experimentally, cotton rats, mice, and rabbits fed *H. americanum* oocysts developed inflammatory lesions that contain cystozoites (one to two merozoites within small tissue cysts). Gamonts or meronts did not develop, and illness was not documented. Morphologically, cystozoites were similar to tissue stages observed in

TABLE 99.3 Frequency of Clinical Signs in 22 Dogs with American Canine Hepatozoonosis

Clinical Sign	Number of Dogs (%)
Fever	19 (86)
Weight loss	18 (82)
Mucopurulent ocular discharge	17 (77)
Low tear production	8 (36)
Muscle atrophy	14 (64)
Pain	
All types	14 (64)
Joints	2 (9)
Lumbar	4 (18)
Cervical	5 (19)
Generalized	3 (14)
Stiffness	12 (55)
Generalized weakness	9 (41)
Pelvic limb paresis and ataxia	5 (19)
Inability to rise	5 (19)
Anorexia	5 (19)

From Vincent-Johnson NA. American canine hepatozoonosis. *Vet Clin North Am Small Anim Pract.* 2003;33:905–920. Data from Macintire DK, Vincent-Johnson N, Dillon AR, et al. Hepatozoonosis in dogs: 22 cases (1989-1994). *J Am Vet Med Assoc.* 1997;210:916–922.

snakes with hepatozoonosis which are infective to predatory reptiles that ingest them. The cystozoite-laden rabbit and rodent tissues fed to naïve dogs resulted in *H. americanum* infections with classic clinical signs. Thus, it is suspected that dogs may also become infected with this organism by predation on an as-yet unidentified reservoir host in nature. In support of this, an investigation of a natural outbreak in a pack of hunting beagles revealed that clinical signs of ACH developed 4 to 6 weeks after some of the dogs were allowed to consume a wild rabbit carcass, whereas dogs not allowed to consume the rabbit did not develop clinical signs.[26] Larval and nymphal stages of *A. maculatum* may feed on a variety of vertebrate hosts including coyotes, but preferentially feed on ground-dwelling birds and small mammals, lending credence to the supposition that noncanid reservoir hosts may serve as a source of infection to feeding ticks and predatory dogs.[2,10,40]

However, surveys of wildlife in ACH-endemic areas have detected *Hepatozoon* spp. that are related but not identical to *H. americanum* in small rodents and rabbits.[26] Bobcats, fox, ocelots, and raccoons are also documented wildlife hosts of *Hepatozoon* spp. in North America.[2,32,41]

Coyotes have long been recognized as harboring *H. americanum* in endemic areas. In a 2013 study, nearly 80% of coyotes sampled from six total locations in Oklahoma and Texas were infected with *Hepatozoon* spp. by histologic and/or molecular methods.[42] Dogs may be an aberrant, rather than natural, host of *H. americanum* due to the severity of disease that develops. Adult coyotes are reported to tolerate *H. americanum* infection better than domestic dogs, and may represent a reservoir host.[2,43] However, the severity of disease in coyotes may be influenced by age and/or infective dose. Coyote puppies developed higher-level parasitemia, more numerous parasite-induced muscle lesions, and more commonly experienced bony changes after oral administration of 50–100 oocysts than did adult coyotes in the same experiments.[44]

Although a noncanid reservoir species has not been identified, the diversity of wildlife species that could potentially serve as reservoir hosts and the persistence of the organism in infected tick populations may explain why *H. americanum* infection is recognized as an emerging disease that is infecting increasing numbers of dogs, as well as expanding its geographic distribution in the United States.[10,35,37]

The occurrence of hepatozoonosis appears to be seasonal in the warmer months or in early fall when dogs are most likely to be exposed to ticks. There is no sex or breed predilection for ACH, but hunting dogs, rural dogs, and dogs allowed to roam are most at risk.[26] Once infected, dogs typically exhibit waxing and waning clinical signs that occur throughout the year as repeated cycles of asexual reproduction and pyogranulomatous inflammation take place.[1,2,10]

CLINICAL FEATURES

Pathogenesis and Clinical Signs

In contrast to *H. canis*–infected dogs, most dogs with *H. americanum* infection exhibit moderate to severe clinical signs even in the absence of concurrent disease or immunosuppression.[1,41] Clinical signs of *H. americanum* infection are associated with the strong inflammatory response that occurs when meronts rupture, leukocytes are recruited, and pyogranulomas form in skeletal muscle. The earliest lesions occur 3 weeks after infection.[39] As the organisms multiply, the infection disseminates, which results in more severe inflammation that waxes and wanes over time. The inflammation causes fever and myositis, which is associated with locomotor abnormalities and hyperesthesia (Table 99.3).[10] The clinical signs can mimic those of meningitis or discospondylitis.[1,41]

Many affected dogs also develop bone lesions that are evident radiographically and resemble lesions seen in hypertrophic osteopathy, except they are proximal rather than distal in distribution (Fig. 99.17). It is unknown whether the bone lesions result from nearby localized muscle inflammation or from humoral factors.[2,10]

Dogs infected with *H. americanum* usually have bilateral mucopurulent ocular discharge that may be caused by pyogranulomatous inflammation of the extraocular muscles or of the lacrimal gland (Fig. 99.18). Return of ocular discharge is frequently the first clinical sign indicative of a relapse following treatment.[2,10,41]

Dogs with ACH frequently maintain a fairly normal appetite; however, weight loss, cachexia, and muscle atrophy occur over time, likely as a result of the increased caloric demands associated with a prolonged inflammatory state.[2,10] There may be a history of polyuria and polydipsia that is due to glomerulonephritis or amyloidosis, which can occur secondary to long-standing inflammation in chronic infections. Nephrotic syndrome and thromboembolic complications may ensue. Less common clinical signs include diarrhea, mucosal pallor, cough, abnormal lung sounds, and lymphadenomegaly.[1,41]

Physical Examination Findings

With *H. americanum* infection, fever (up to 105.6°F or 40.9°C) that does not resolve with antibiotic therapy is common, although because of the waxing and waning nature of the disease, body temperature may be normal at any given time.[45] Many dogs are treated for a fever of unknown origin before it is evident that abatement of clinical signs is not in response to antibiotic therapy, but attributable rather to the cyclic nature of ACH.[1,10]

Because of the myositis, dogs are typically evaluated for gait abnormalities, which range from lameness or stiffness to recumbency and an inability or unwillingness to rise. Pain from myositis is common and may appear as cervical, back, joint, or generalized pain. The stiffness and reluctance to move cause many dogs to assume a "master's voice"

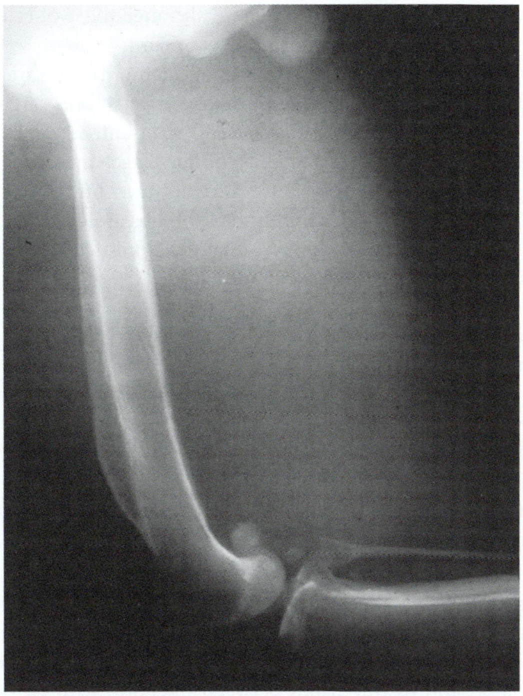

Fig. 99.17 Radiograph of the pelvic limb of a dog with *Hepatozoon americanum* infection. There is smooth periosteal proliferation on the cranial aspect of the femur. (From Vincent-Johnson NA. American canine hepatozoonosis. *Vet Clin North Am Small Anim Pract.* 2003;33:905–920.)

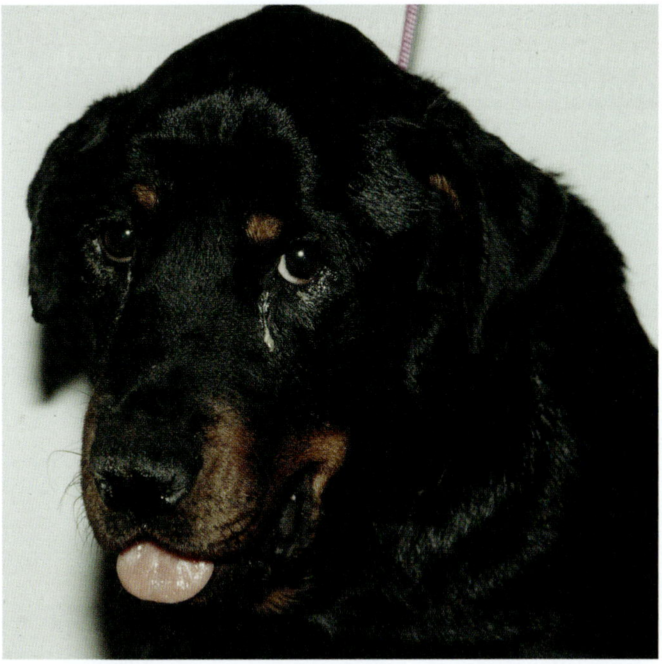

Fig. 99.18 Rottweiler with *Hepatozoon americanum* infection. Note the hunched appearance, muscle atrophy, and mucopurulent ocular discharge.

stance. Hyperesthesia, stiffness, neck guarding, and fever can easily be mistaken for meningitis or discospondylitis, but sensory deficiencies and analysis of CSF are usually unremarkable, indicating that nervous system involvement is unlikely. Generalized polymyopathy may be detected using electromyography.[1,45] Lethargy is common, and cachexia and generalized muscle atrophy may be apparent. Mucopurulent ocular discharge is often present; approximately one third of dogs with matted eyes have decreased tear production on a Schirmer tear test.[41,43] Other ocular lesions seen in ACH patients on occasion include focal retinal scars or hyper-reflectivity, increased retinal pigmentation, papilledema, and uveitis with active inflammatory fundic lesions. Mucosal pallor and lymphadenomegaly may also be present.[43]

DIAGNOSIS

A high degree of suspicion based on consistent clinical signs, radiographic findings, and laboratory abnormalities is key to the diagnosis of *H. americanum* infection. Diagnosis is most often confirmed by histopathologic findings of muscle biopsy or positive PCR assays on blood.[10,41,46]

Laboratory Abnormalities

Complete Blood Count

The most consistent laboratory abnormality in *H. americanum* infection is leukocytosis, which is often, but not necessarily, extreme (Table 99.4). White cell counts are typically 20,000 to 200,000 cells/μL, with reported means of 76,807 and 85,700 cells/μL.[1,41,43] The leukocytosis is due to a mature neutrophilia, although sometimes there is a mild to moderate left shift. A mild normocytic, normochromic nonregenerative anemia is typical. Platelets are usually normal to increased, sometimes with thrombocytosis up to 916,000 platelets/μL. When thrombocytopenia is evident, concurrent tick-borne diseases such as ehrlichiosis, RMSF, and babesiosis should be considered.[1,41,43]

Serum Chemistry Profile

In *H. americanum* infection, a mild increase in the activity of serum ALP is typical, possibly due to periosteal new bone formation. Serum glucose concentration is often decreased (40 to 60 mg/dL) and occasionally as low as 5 mg/dL. This is not a true hypoglycemia, but rather a laboratory artifact due to utilization of glucose in the specimen by the high number of white blood cells. Blood glucose values are typically in reference range if sodium fluoride is used as the anticoagulant to block glucose metabolism by leukocytes. Hypoalbuminemia is common and may be due to chronic inflammation, decreased protein intake, or renal loss from secondary glomerulonephritis or amyloidosis. Chronic inflammation causes increased production of acute-phase proteins and macroglobulins, resulting in downregulation of albumin synthesis. Hyperglobulinemia is relatively uncommon. Except in dogs with significant renal damage, serum urea nitrogen concentration is often low. The combination of increased activity of serum ALP and low glucose, serum urea nitrogen, and albumin concentrations may mislead the clinician to suspect liver disease. Serum bile acid concentrations are normal or only slightly elevated. Surprisingly, the activity of serum CK is consistently within the normal range even though *H. americanum* infection causes severe myositis.[1,41,43]

Urinalysis

Urinalysis may be normal but in patients with chronic *H. americanum* infection, proteinuria of varying degrees is a frequent finding due to the occurrence of secondary glomerular disease, protein-losing nephropathy, or amyloidosis. These dogs have decreased concentrating ability, resulting in isosthenuria and an elevated protein-creatinine ratio.[41,43]

Diagnostic Imaging

Plain Radiography

Many dogs with *H. americanum* infection show radiographic abnormalities of the skeletal system; therefore, radiographs of the pelvis or long bones can be useful to support a clinical diagnosis of ACH.[10,43,46] Young dogs are more likely to show bone lesions than older dogs. In experimental infections, bone lesions are recognizable histologically

TABLE 99.4 **Frequency of Laboratory and Radiographic Findings in 22 Dogs with American Canine Hepatozoonosis**

Finding	Number of Dogs (%)
Moderate to marked leukocytosis[a]	22 (100)
Mature neutrophilia	15 (68)
Mild left shift	7 (31)
Elevated ALP activity	22 (100)
Hypoglycemia	20 (91)
Hypoalbuminemia	19 (86)
Periosteal proliferation on radiography	18 (82)
Anemia (nonregenerative)	14 (64)
Hypocalcemia	14 (64)
Normal platelet count	11 (50)
Thrombocytosis	9 (41)
Hyperphosphatemia	7 (32)
Low BUN concentration	7 (32)
Hyperglobulinemia	4 (11)
Hypercalcemia	2 (9)
Elevated CK activity	1 (5)

[a]Minimum white cell count was 27,800 cells/μL.

ALP, alkaline phosphatase; BUN, blood urea nitrogen; *CK,* creatine kinase.

From Vincent-Johnson NA. American canine hepatozoonosis. *Vet Clin North Am Small Anim Pract.* 2003;33:905–920. Data from Macintire DK, Vincent-Johnson N, Dillon AR, et al. Hepatozoonosis in dogs: 22 cases (1989-1994). *J Am Vet Med Assoc.* 1997;210:916–922.

within 5 weeks postexposure.[2] Disseminated, symmetric periosteal new bone formation occurs most frequently and most markedly on the diaphysis of long bones, but occurs to a lesser degree on flat and irregular bones.[2,10,46] The radiographic appearance can vary from subtle irregular periosteal exostoses to thick parallel pseudocortices. Morphologically resembling hypertrophic osteopathy, the bone lesions of *H. americanum* infection typically affect the more proximal bones while sparing the distal ones.[10,41]

Sonographic Findings

Abdominal ultrasound examination of dogs with *H. americanum* infection is generally unremarkable, although dogs with secondary glomerulonephritis, interstitial nephritis, or amyloidosis may have renal hyperechogenicity and abnormalities in kidney size according to the chronicity of the condition. Ultrasound findings in the skeletal muscle have not been described in the literature, although subtle disruption in the normally well-organized muscle echotexture may be expected due to the presence of onion-skin cysts, pyogranulomas, and myositis.

Microbiologic Testing

Diagnostic assays currently available for hepatozoonosis in dogs are described in Table 99.2. Blood smears from dogs suspected to have ACH can be stained and examined for rare gamonts in circulating leukocytes. PCR assays on whole blood are more sensitive.[7]

Cytologic Diagnosis

The gamont of *H. americanum* appears as a light blue to clear oblong structure containing a faintly staining nucleus within the cytoplasm of circulating monocytes stained with Diff-Quik or Giemsa. The gamonts look nearly identical to those of *H. canis,* although those of *H. americanum* are slightly smaller, measuring 8.8 × 3.9 μm.[41,43]

In dogs with *H. americanum* infection, gamonts are rarely found on peripheral blood smears. When present, infected cells rarely exceed 0.1% of the circulating leukocytes; several thousand cells may have to be examined before an infected cell is found. The chance that gamonts are detected can be increased by examination of buffy-coat smears. Neither bone marrow nor lymph node aspirates are of much value in making a definitive diagnosis of *H. americanum* infection; organisms are not usually seen in these specimens.[10,41,43]

Serologic Diagnosis

An ELISA assay for detection of antibodies to *H. americanum* sporozoites was developed at Oklahoma State University for research purposes, but the assay is not available commercially to veterinary practitioners.[10]

Molecular Diagnosis Using Nucleic Acid–Based Testing

A quantitative, real-time PCR assay that detects *Hepatozoon* spp. is available commercially to veterinary practitioners through the Auburn University Molecular Diagnostics Laboratory and various veterinary diagnostic laboratories. The assay performed at Auburn University detects as few as seven genomic copies of *Hepatozoon* spp. per milliliter of blood and distinguishes between infection with *H. canis* and *H. americanum.* Although highly sensitive and specific and useful for detection of early infections (from around 42 days PI), false negatives can occur early in the course of infection or in chronic disease where the numbers of circulating gamonts are extremely low or absent. Muscle biopsy should be performed in dogs suspected to have *H. americanum* infection but that have negative PCR assay results.[7]

Pathologic Findings

Gross Pathologic Findings

In dogs with *H. americanum* infection, muscle atrophy and cachexia are consistent findings on gross necropsy examination. Pyogranulomas may appear as multiple 1- to 2-mm–diameter white-tan foci.[43] These are scattered diffusely throughout skeletal and cardiac muscle but may also be observed in other tissues. Roughening and thickening of bone surfaces are often present. Less common findings include lymphadenomegaly, congestion of the gastric mucosa, splenic coagulative necrosis, and pulmonary congestion.[1,43]

Histopathologic Findings

Muscle biopsy has long been considered the most reliable method for diagnosis of *H. americanum* infections. Muscle specimens (approximately 2 cm × 2 cm) can be obtained from the biceps femoris or semitendinosus muscles under general anesthesia.[10,41] Submission of multiple specimens increases diagnostic sensitivity, especially for low-level infections. Muscle lesions consist of large onion-skin cysts, pyogranulomas, and myositis. The cysts are round to oval and have mean cross-section dimensions of 186 × 150 μm.[1] At the center of the cyst is a host cell nucleus and protozoan, but depending on the plane of the cut surface, these may or may not be visible. Surrounding the center of the cyst are concentric layers of mucopolysaccharide. Occasionally meronts in various stages of development are observed within these cystic structures. The highly vascular pyogranulomas are packed with neutrophils and macrophages, many of which contain a single zoite. Myositis is characterized by muscle necrosis and atrophy with infiltration of neutrophils, macrophages, and occasional lymphocytes between muscle fibers.[47]

Although consistently identified in skeletal and cardiac muscle, *H. americanum* cysts, meronts, and pyogranulomas can sporadically

TABLE 99.5 Antimicrobial Drugs Indicated for Treatment of American Canine Hepatozoonosis

Drug	Dose[a] (mg/kg)	Route	Interval (Hours)	Duration (Days)
TCP combination:				
Trimethoprim-sulfonamide *and*	15	PO	12	14
clindamycin *and*	10	PO	8	14
pyrimethamine *and*	0.25	PO	24	14
decoquinate[b]	10–20	PO	12	730
Ponazuril regimen:				
Ponazuril *and*	10	PO	12	28
decoquinate[b]	10–20	PO	12	730

[a]Dose per administration at specified interval.
[b]Use the decoquinate 6% (27.2 g/lb) powder, Deccox (Alpharma Inc., Fort Lee, NJ). One teaspoonful is equivalent to approximately 180 mg decoquinate. Administer at a rate of 1 teaspoon per 10 kg of body weight and feed q12h mixed into moist dog food.
TCP, trimethoprim-sulfadiazine, clindamycin, and pyrimethamine; *PO*, oral.

be found in adipose tissue, intestinal smooth muscle, pancreas, liver, lymph node, spleen, skin, salivary gland, lung, and kidney.[43] The wheel-spoked meront typical of *H. canis* infection is not identified in dogs infected with *H. americanum*. Renal damage is common and manifests as focal pyogranulomatous inflammation with mild glomerulonephritis, lymphoplasmacytic interstitial nephritis, mesangioproliferative glomerulonephritis, or occasionally amyloidosis. Amyloid deposits have also been found in the spleen, lymph nodes, small intestines, and liver of affected dogs. Various organs can show vascular changes, which include fibrinoid degeneration of vessel walls, mineralization and proliferation of the vascular intima, and pyogranulomatous vasculitis.[1,2,41]

TREATMENT AND PROGNOSIS

Most dogs will die within 1 year after infection without treatment.[1,2,10,41,43] No treatment effectively eliminates the tissue stages of *H. americanum*, but remission of clinical signs can be achieved using either a combination of trimethoprim-sulfa, clindamycin, and pyrimethamine (TCP) or ponazuril (Table 99.5).[48] Response to therapy is usually dramatic, with resolution of clinical abnormalities within a week of initiating therapy. Either of these protocols must be followed by long-term administration of decoquinate in order to prevent relapse.[41,48] Without the addition of decoquinate, relapse occurs in most dogs 2 to 6 months following treatment.[41] Although these dogs generally respond well to another round of combination therapy, subsequent relapses occur more frequently, and eventually disease may become refractory to treatment.[43,49]

Persistent infections and multiple relapses lead to complications such as glomerulonephropathy, amyloidosis, vasculitis, and cachexia, which carry a guarded to poor prognosis. Decoquinate, a livestock anticoccidial agent, apparently breaks the asexual recycling of infection by arresting the development of the merozoites after their release from meronts through disruption of electron transport in the parasite's mitochondrial cytochrome system. Two years of daily decoquinate therapy is recommended.[48,49]

Alternatively, a PCR assay can be performed every 3 to 6 months, and when the results of PCR testing becomes negative, treatment can be discontinued. However, with this approach, some dogs have required treatment for longer than 2 years because of persistent positive test results. Mild relapses can occur even during treatment with decoquinate. If clinical signs are severe, another course of TCP combination therapy or ponazuril is indicated. Long-term administration of decoquinate very often results in extended survival times and excellent quality of life with a good prognosis. During the initial few days of treatment with either antiprotozoal regimen, administration of an NSAID at standard dosages can provide relief from fever and pain.[48,49]

IMMUNITY AND VACCINATION

Current treatments do not cure *H. americanum* infections, so dogs remain susceptible to relapse of disease, especially if immunosuppressed.[1,41,43] Vaccines for *H. americanum* infections are not available.

PREVENTION

Since *H. americanum* is transmitted by ingestion of ticks, the administration of topical or oral acaricides to dogs, use of environmental acaricides, and immediate removal of ticks from dogs are the most important means of prevention.[1,10,41,43] Because the organism can also be transmitted through ingestion of cystozoites in muscle from other animals, dogs should not be allowed to roam, scavenge, or engage in predatory behavior. Dogs should not be fed uncooked or undercooked game meat.[26,41]

PUBLIC HEALTH ASPECTS

See Public Health Aspects under the *H. canis* section for the discussion on this subject.

HEPATOZOON SPP. INFECTIONS IN DOMESTIC CATS

ETIOLOGIC AGENT AND EPIDEMIOLOGY

Feline hepatozoonosis occurs primarily in areas where canine hepatozoonosis exists. It has been reported in a number of countries, including India, South Africa, Nigeria, Brazil, Israel, Italy, Japan, Spain, France, Portugal, Turkey, Austria, Cyprus, Cape Verde, and Thailand.[50] In the United States, there is one report of hepatozoonosis in a domestic cat from Hawaii and an immunocompromised cat from Oklahoma. The main species of *Hepatozoon* infecting cats is *H. felis*, which primarily targets striated muscle tissues and the myocardium.[3] Another species, *Hepatozoon silvestris*, was described in Bosnia and Herzegovina in five European wild cats (*Felis silvestris silvestris*) based on molecular and morphologic characteristics.[51] The organism is found in the heart, spleen, and skeletal muscle, and is only 96% genetically similar to *H. felis* and its tissue meronts differ from those of *H. felis* in size, number, and orientation. In this same survey study, *H. felis* was also identified for the first time in wild felids in Europe.[51] Another study identified *H. felis*, *H. silvestris*, and *H. canis* infections in domestic cats in Italy.[52] Another case of a fatal infection with *H. silvestris* in a domestic cat was reported from Switzerland.[53]

A survey of blood specimens from stray cats in Bangkok, Thailand, showed that 32.3% were positive by PCR for a *Hepatozoon* sp. most closely related to *H. canis,* whereas only 0.7% of the cats had gamonts observed on blood smears. In Israel, *Hepatozoon* DNA was amplified from the blood of 36% of 152 cats, and infected cats were more likely to have access to the outdoors.[3] The vast majority of cats were infected with *H. felis*, although two cats were infected with *H. canis*. Most infections were subclinical. A survey study of 644 client-owned and stray cats in Spain documented *H. felis* infection in 1.4% of cats and *H. canis* infection in one cat.[54] Another survey from Cyprus documented that 38% of the surveyed cats were positive for *H. felis* and there was significant association for co-infection with *L. infantum* and "*Candidatus* Mycoplasma haemominutum."[55]

The vectors that transmit *Hepatozoon* spp. to domestic cats are also unknown. However, based on *Hepatozoon* spp. infecting other vertebrates, transmission of feline *Hepatozoon* spp. may be via the ingestion of an arthropod definitive host and vertebrate paratenic host tissues, and possibly transplacental transmission.[3]

CLINICAL FEATURES

Pathogenesis and Clinical Signs

Cats with hepatozoonosis are commonly immunosuppressed because of infection with FIV or FeLV. Alternatively, they may be co-infected with other vector- or blood-borne pathogens such as hemotropic mycoplasmas and/or *L. infantum*.[55,56] FIV or FeLV was detected in four of six cats with hepatozoonosis from Israel and in two cats from France.

Hepatozoonosis in cats is associated with infection of muscle tissues. *Hepatozoon* meronts have been identified in the myocardium and skeletal muscles of domestic and wild felids. Elevated activities of serum CK were found in the majority of cats with hepatozoonosis in a retrospective study, and in three cats reported from a rural area in Brazil.

A variety of clinical signs have been described in infected cats. In a parasitemic cat from Israel, weakness, hypersalivation, lingual mucosal ulceration, and lymphadenomegaly were observed. Two parasitemic cats from France that also had positive test results for FeLV had lethargy, anorexia, anemia, and thrombocytopenia. A cat from Hawaii had weight loss, ulcerative glossitis, pyrexia, progressive anemia, serous ocular discharge, and icterus. The cat also had cytologic evidence of liver infection consistent with hepatozoonosis. A cat from Cyprus had multiple ulcerated skin nodules associated with *L. infantum* infection, in addition to co-infection with *H. felis* and "*Candidatus* M. haemominutum."[55]

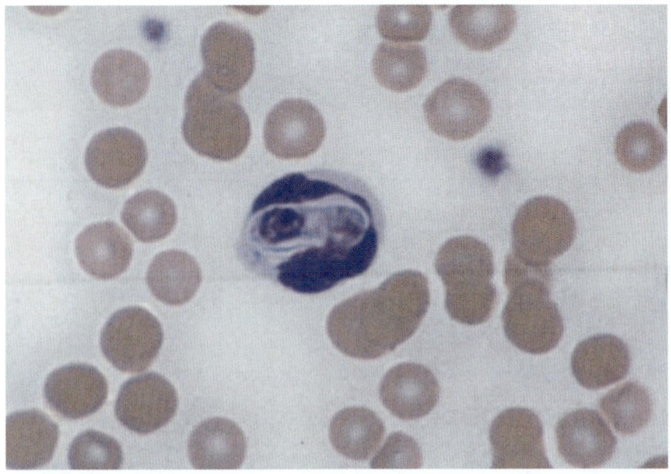

Fig. 99.19 *Hepatozoon* sp. gamont in the cytoplasm of a neutrophil from a domestic cat. The blood smear was stained with Giemsa (500× magnification).

DIAGNOSIS

The diagnosis of feline hepatozoonosis is usually performed by detection of gamonts in stained blood smears. Gamonts are located in the cytoplasm of neutrophils, have an ellipsoidal shape, and possess a round or pleomorphic nucleus (Fig. 99.19). The level of parasitemia is frequently low with less than 1% of the neutrophils containing gamonts. Application of PCR assays can be used to confirm infection.

TREATMENT AND PROGNOSIS

No controlled studies that evaluate treatment outcomes for cats infected with *Hepatozoon* spp. are documented. In rare case reports, feline hepatozoonosis has been treated with doxycycline, 5 mg/kg, PO, with no clear benefit or oxytetracycline at 50 mg/kg, PO, q12h with a single dose of primaquine (2 mg/kg, PO) with a successful outcome. A cat from Austria infected with *H. felis* was treated successfully with imidocarb dipropionate at 6 mg/kg repeated after 14 days and doxycycline 5 mg/kg twice daily for 4 weeks.[57]

CASE EXAMPLE

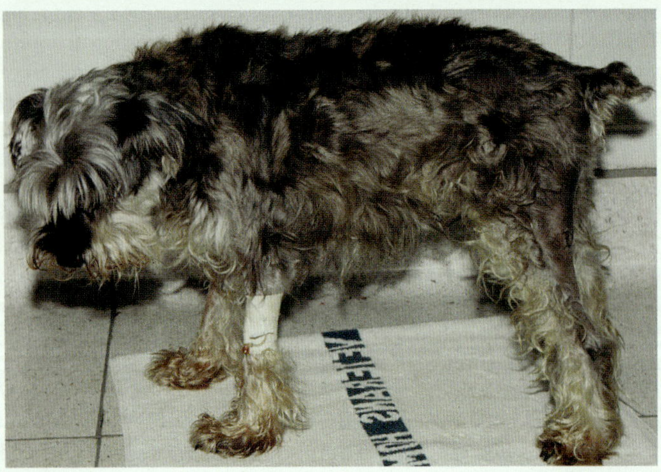

Fig. 99.20 "Pepper," a 1.5-year-old male miniature schnauzer with *Hepatozoon americanum* infection.

Signalment

"Pepper," a 1.5-year-old male miniature schnauzer from Opelika, AL (Fig. 99.20).

History

Pepper was seen for a 1-month duration of illness characterized by intermittent fever (104.0°F to 105.0°F [40.0°C to 40.6°C]), lethargy, and ocular discharge. The dog's owner reported that Pepper had also been stiff and reluctant to move. Despite a fairly good appetite, he had lost weight and muscle mass. The fever and other clinical signs had been nonresponsive to antibiotics, which included enrofloxacin and doxycycline, prescribed at the onset of illness. Pepper was a house dog but spent time outdoors in a rural environment. No vomiting, coughing, or sneezing had been reported, but he had had mild diarrhea at the onset of illness that resolved after a week. He had also had a mild increase in thirst and urination. He was fed a high-quality commercial dry dog food, received monthly heartworm preventive, and was current on all vaccinations, including CDV, hepatitis, CPV, and rabies vaccines. He had not traveled outside of the local area. The owner mentioned that she had another dog that died about 1 year earlier after exhibiting similar clinical signs, but a diagnosis was not made.

Current medications: Aspirin 11 mg/kg, PO, q12h for pain.

Continued

CASE EXAMPLE—cont'd

Physical Examination

Body weight: 7.6 kg.

General: Quiet, slightly lethargic, but responsive. Reluctant to walk or stand; appeared painful. T = 103.8°F (39.9°C), HR = 96 beats/minute, RR = 32 breaths/minute, mucous membranes pink, CRT = 1.5 seconds.

Integument: The skin and haircoat appeared normal with no evidence of ectoparasites.

Eyes, ears, nose, and mouth: A moderate amount of mucopurulent ocular discharge was present bilaterally. No other abnormalities were identified.

Musculoskeletal: BCS was 3/9 with moderate generalized muscle atrophy. The dog exhibited hyperesthesia during palpation of trunk, head, neck, and limb muscles. The dog's gait was very stiff and slow.

All other systems: Apart from abdominal splinting on palpation of the abdomen, no clinically significant abnormalities were present.

Ophthalmic Examination

Pupillary light reflex (direct and consensual): Normal.

Conjunctiva: Injected bilaterally, mucopurulent discharge bilaterally.

Cornea and lens: Normal.

Schirmer tear test: Right eye = 18 mm; left eye = 16 mm (normal > 15 mm).

Fluorescein stain: Negative.

Tonometry: Normal.

Fundoscopic examination: A small grayish, slightly raised focal lesion was identified in the right fundus.

Laboratory Findings

CBC: PCV 38.7% (37%–55%), MCV 68.7 fL (60–77 fL), MCHC 35.4 g/dL (32–36 g/dL), WBC 39,200 cells/μL (6,000–17,000 cells/μL), neutrophils 35,672 cells/μL (3,000–11,400 cells/μL), lymphocytes 1,176 cells/μL (1,000–4,000 cells/μL), monocytes 1,952 cells/μL (150–1,200 cells/μL), eosinophils 0 (100–750 cells/μL), platelets 607,000 platelets/μL (200,000–400,000 platelets/μL).

The clinical pathologist's blood smear review showed no evidence of microorganisms.

Serum chemistry profile: BUN 8 mg/dL (10–25 mg/dL), creatinine 0.6 mg/dL (0.3–1.0 mg/dL), ALP 142 U/L (19–50 U/L), ALT 37 U/L (17–66 U/L), CK 148 U/L (92–357 U/L), total bilirubin 0.3 mg/dL (0.1–0.3 mg/dL), glucose 52 mg/dL (80–100 mg/dL), sodium 153 mmol/L (146–160 mmol/L), potassium 4.7 mmol/L (3.5–5.9 mmol/L), chloride 118 mmol/L (108–125 mmol/L), calcium 10.3 mg/dL (9.5–11.8 mg/dL), phosphorus 3.9 mg/dL (3.3–5.8 mg/dL), total protein 6.4 g/dL (5.1–7.3 g/dL), albumin 2.7 g/dL (2.6–3.5 g/dL), globulin 3.7 g/dL (3.6–5.0 g/dL), total CO_2 21.8 mmol/L (13.9–31.5 mmol/L).

Urinalysis: SpG 1.035; pH 8.0, protein 1+, bilirubin negative, hemoprotein negative, glucose negative, 0 WBC/HPF, 0 RBC/HPF, no crystals, moderate lipid droplets.

Imaging Findings

Pelvic radiographs: Bilateral smooth periosteal bone formation was present on the ilium and femurs.

Abdominal ultrasound examination: No abnormalities were detected.

Bone Marrow Aspirate

The bone marrow smears were highly cellular with many particles. Megakaryocytes were adequate. In a 500-cell count, the M:E ratio was 1.7 (reference range 1.3–2.1) with normal maturation sequences in both red and white series. Multiple smears examined showed no evidence of microorganisms.

Muscle Biopsy

Histopathology showed infiltration of neutrophils and monocytes between muscle fibers. There were rare onion-skin cysts and one focal pyogranuloma. Many of the monocytes and neutrophils within the granuloma contained a single zoite. Findings were consistent with *H. americanum* infection.

Cytology Findings

Although negative at the initial evaluation, blood smears and buffy-coat smears performed a few days later showed oblong "jellybean" inclusions in the cytoplasm of < 0.1% of the leukocytes. These were characteristic of *Hepatozoon* gamonts.

Diagnosis

ACH (*H. americanum* infection).

Treatment

Triple combination therapy consisting of (1) pyrimethamine 0.25 mg/kg, PO, q24h for 14 days; (2) sulfadiazine/trimethoprim 15 mg/kg, PO, q12h for 14 days; and (3) clindamycin 10 mg/kg, PO, q8h for 14 days. This was associated with resolution of fever within 24 hours. According to his owner, Pepper was back to normal within 7 days. After the 14-day course of triple combination therapy was completed, Pepper was started on decoquinate 15 mg/kg, PO, q12h with food. At day 74, the owners ran out of decoquinate and Pepper missed 2 days of treatment before a refill was obtained. Eight days later, the owners called to say that Pepper was doing poorly, could not get up, and his eyes were matted shut with a yellow-green discharge. Physical exam and CBC findings were similar to initial findings. Another 14-day course of triple combination therapy with pyrimethamine, sulfadiazine/trimethoprim, and clindamycin was prescribed. Once again, Pepper's clinical signs resolved within a few days. Pepper has continued on the decoquinate twice daily with no further breaks in doses and no more relapses.

Comments

ACH was suspected in this dog because of the geographic location in an endemic area of the south-eastern United States, a waxing and waning fever, muscle pain, ocular discharge, leukocytosis, and other laboratory findings. As initially occurred in this case, organisms often cannot be seen on blood smear or buffy-coat exam. Muscle biopsy has been considered the most reliable way to diagnose infection, although PCR is also a very sensitive and specific diagnostic tool. This case illustrates the typical relapsing nature of the disease and the need for continuous long-term decoquinate therapy. After missing only a few doses of decoquinate, this dog suffered a relapse days later. He made a quick recovery with a second round of triple combination therapy. Effective treatment requires daily decoquinate therapy with no breaks for at least 2 years or until PCR of whole blood becomes negative.

SUGGESTED READINGS

Cardoso L, Cortes HC, Eyal O, et al. Molecular and histopathological detection of *Hepatozoon canis* in red foxes (*Vulpes vulpes*) from Portugal. *Parasit Vectors*. 2014;24(7):113.

Baneth G, Mathew JS, Shkap V, et al. Canine hepatozoonosis: two disease syndromes caused by separate *Hepatozoon* spp. *Trends Parasitol.* 2003;19(1):27–31.

Ewing SA, Panciera RJ. American canine hepatozoonosis. *Clin Microbiol Rev.* 2003;16(4):688–697.

Potter TM, Macintire DK. *Hepatozoon americanum*: an emerging disease in the south-central/southeastern United States. *J Vet Emerg Crit Care (San Antonio)*. 2010;20(1):70–76.

Vincent-Johnson NA. American canine hepatozoonosis. *Vet Clin North Am Small Anim Pract*. 2003;33:905–920.

REFERENCES

1. Vincent-Johnson NA, Macintire DK, Lindsay DS, et al. A new *Hepatozoon* species from dogs: description of the causative agent of canine hepatozoonosis in North America. *J Parasitol.* 1997;83:1165–1172.
2. Ewing SA, Panciera RJ. American canine hepatozoonosis. *Clin Microbiol Rev.* 2003;16:688–697.
3. Baneth G, Sheiner A, Eyal O, et al. Redescription of *Hepatozoon felis* (Apicomplexa: Hepatozoidae) based on phylogenetic analysis, tissue and blood form morphology, and possible transplacental transmission. *Parasit Vectors.* 2013;6:102.
4. Miterpakova M, Komjati-Nagyova M, Hurnikova Z, et al. Retrospective molecular study on canine hepatozoonosis in Slovakia - Does infection risk for dogs really exist? *Ticks Tick Borne Dis.* 2017;8:567–573.
5. Baneth G. Perspectives on canine and feline hepatozoonosis. *Vet Parasitol.* 2011;181:3–11.
6. Allen KE, Li Y, Kaltenboeck B, et al. Diversity of *Hepatozoon* species in naturally infected dogs in the southern United States. *Vet Parasitol.* 2008;154:220–225.
7. Li Y, Wang C, Allen KE, et al. Diagnosis of canine *Hepatozoon* spp. infection by quantitative PCR. *Vet Parasitol.* 2008;157:50–58.
8. Little L, Baneth G. Cutaneous *Hepatozoon canis* infection in a dog from New Jersey. *J Vet Diagn Invest.* 2011;23:585–588.
9. Greay TL, Barbosa AD, Rees RL, et al. An Australian dog diagnosed with an exotic tick-borne infection: should Australia still be considered free from *Hepatozoon canis*? *Int J Parasitol.* 2018;48:805–815.
10. Potter TM, Macintire DK. *Hepatozoon americanum*: an emerging disease in the south-central/southeastern United States. *J Vet Emerg Crit Care (San Antonio).* 2010;20:70–76.
11. Leveille AN, Baneth G, Barta JR. Next generation sequencing from *Hepatozoon canis* (Apicomplexa: Coccidia: Adeleorina): Complete apicoplast genome and multiple mitochondrion-associated sequences. *Int J Parasitol.* 2019;49:375–387.
12. Baneth G, Samish M, Shkap V. Life cycle of *Hepatozoon canis* (Apicomplexa: Adeleorina: Hepatozoidae) in the tick *Rhipicephalus sanguineus* and domestic dog (*Canis familiaris*). *J Parasitol.* 2007;93:283–299.
13. Giannelli A, Lia RP, Annoscia G, et al. *Rhipicephalus turanicus*, a new vector of *Hepatozoon canis*. *Parasitology.* 2017;144:730–737.
14. Criado-Fornelio A, Martin-Perez T, Verdu-Exposito C, et al. Molecular epidemiology of parasitic protozoa and *Ehrlichia canis* in wildlife in Madrid (central Spain). *Parasitol Res.* 2018;117:2291–2298.
15. Hodzic A, Georges I, Postl M, et al. Molecular survey of tick-borne pathogens reveals a high prevalence and low genetic variability of *Hepatozoon canis* in free-ranging grey wolves (*Canis lupus*) in Germany. *Ticks Tick Borne Dis.* 2020;11:101389.
16. Iatta R, Natale A, Ravagnan S, et al. Zoonotic and vector-borne pathogens in tigers from a wildlife safari park, Italy. *Int J Parasitol Parasites Wildl.* 2020;12:1–7.
17. Hodžić A, Georges I, Postl M, et al. Molecular survey of tick-borne pathogens reveals a high prevalence and low genetic variability of *Hepatozoon canis* in free-ranging grey wolves (*Canis lupus*) in Germany. *Ticks Tick Borne Dis.* 2020;11:101389.
18. Arrais RC, Paula RC, Martins TF, et al. Survey of ticks and tick-borne agents in maned wolves (*Chrysocyon brachyurus*) from a natural landscape in Brazil. *Ticks Tick Borne Dis.* 2021;12:101639.
19. da Silva MRL, Fornazari F, Demoner LC, et al. *Didelphis albiventris* naturally infected with *Hepatozoon canis* in southeastern Brazil. *Ticks Tick Borne Dis.* 2017;8:878–881.
20. Giannelli A, Ramos RA, Di Paola G, et al. Transstadial transmission of *Hepatozoon canis* from larvae to nymphs of *Rhipicephalus sanguineus*. *Vet Parasitol.* 2013;196:1–5.
21. Baneth G, Samish M, Alekseev E, et al. Transmission of *Hepatozoon canis* to dogs by naturally-fed or percutaneously-injected *Rhipicephalus sanguineus* ticks. *J Parasitol.* 2001;87:606–611.
22. Scott JD, Pesapane RR. Detection of *Anaplasma phagocytophilum, Babesia odocoilei, Babesia* sp., *Borrelia burgdorferi* Sensu Lato, and *Hepatozoon canis* in *Ixodes scapularis* ticks collected in Eastern Canada. *Pathogens.* 2021;10:1265.
23. Lilliehook I, Tvedten HW, Pettersson HK, et al. *Hepatozoon canis* infection causing a strong monocytosis with intra-monocytic gamonts and leading to erroneous leukocyte determinations. *Vet Clin Pathol.* 2019;48:435–440.
24. Attipa C, Maguire D, Solano-Gallego L, et al. *Hepatozoon canis* in three imported dogs: a new tickborne disease reaching the United Kingdom. *Vet Rec.* 2018;183:716.
25. Modry D, Beck R, Hrazdilova K, et al. A review of methods for detection of *Hepatozoon* infection in carnivores and arthropod vectors. *Vector Borne Zoonotic Dis.* 2017;17:66–72.
26. Johnson EM, Panciera RJ, Allen KE, et al. Alternate pathway of infection with *Hepatozoon americanum* and the epidemiologic importance of predation. *J Vet Intern Med.* 2009;23:1315–1318.
27. Murata T, Inoue M, Tateyama S, et al. Vertical transmission of *Hepatozoon canis* in dogs. *J Vet Med Sci.* 1993;55:867–868.
28. Baneth G, Harmelin A, Presentey BZ. *Hepatozoon canis* infection in two dogs. *J Am Vet Med Assoc.* 1995;206:1891–1894.
29. Baneth G, Weigler B. Retrospective case-control study of hepatozoonosis in dogs in Israel. *J Vet Intern Med.* 1997;11:365–370.
30. Hangsawek A, Chutasripanich S, Kammaled P, et al. Relationship between the number of *Hepatozoon canis* gamonts and hematobiochemical values in dogs. *Trop Biomed.* 2020;37:421–432.
31. Chhabra S, Uppal SK, Singla LD. Retrospective study of clinical and hematological aspects associated with dogs naturally infected by *Hepatozoon canis* in Ludhiana, Punjab, India. *Asian Pac J Trop Biomed.* 2013;3:483–486.
32. Allen KE, Yabsley MJ, Johnson EM, et al. Novel *Hepatozoon* in vertebrates from the southern United States. *J Parasitol.* 2011;97:648–653.
33. Singh MD, Singh H, Singh NK, et al. Development of loop-mediated isothermal amplification (LAMP) assay for detection of *Hepatozoon canis* infection in dogs. *Ticks Tick Borne Dis.* 2019;10:371–376.
34. Gonen L, Strauss-Ayali D, Shkap V, et al. An enzyme-linked immunosorbent assay for antibodies to *Hepatozoon canis*. *Vet Parasitol.* 2004;122:131–139.
35. Paddock CD, Goddard J. The evolving medical and veterinary importance of the Gulf Coast tick (Acari: Ixodidae). *J Med Entomol.* 2015;52:230–252.
36. Phillips VC, Zieman EA, Kim CH, et al. Documentation of the expansion of the gulf coast tick (*Amblyomma maculatum*) and *Rickettsia parkeri*: first report in Illinois. *J Parasitol.* 2020;106:9–13.
37. Sonenshine DE. Range expansion of tick disease vectors in North America: implications for spread of tick-borne disease. *Int J Environ Res Public Health.* 2018;15.
38. Gomes LA, Moraes PH, do Nascimento LC, et al. Molecular analysis reveals the diversity of *Hepatozoon* species naturally infecting domestic dogs in a northern region of Brazil. *Ticks Tick Borne Dis.* 2016;7:1061–1066.
39. Panciera RJ, Ewing SA, Mathew JS, et al. Canine hepatozoonosis: comparison of lesions and parasites in skeletal muscle of dogs experimentally or naturally infected with *Hepatozoon americanum*. *Vet Parasitol.* 1999;82:261–272.
40. Little SE, Allen KE, Johnson EM, et al. New developments in canine hepatozoonosis in North America: a review. *Parasit Vectors.* 2009;2(suppl 1):S5.
41. Baneth G, Vincent-Johnson NA. Hepatozoonosis. In: Shaw S, ed. *Arthropod-Borne Infectious Diseases of the Dog and Cat.* Boca Raton, FL: CRC Press; 2016:109–124.
42. Starkey LA, Panciera RJ, Paras K, et al. Genetic diversity of *Hepatozoon* spp. in coyotes from the south-central United States. *J Parasitol.* 2013;99:375–378.
43. Vincent-Johnson NA. American canine hepatozoonosis. *Vet Clin North Am Small Anim Pract.* 2003;33:905–920.
44. Garrett JJ, Kocan AA, Reichard MV, et al. Experimental infection of adult and juvenile coyotes with domestic dog and wild coyote isolates of *Hepatozoon americanum* (Apicomplexa: Adeleorina). *J Wildl Dis.* 2005;41:588–592.
45. Macintire DK, Vincent-Johnson N, Dillon AR, et al. Hepatozoonosis in dogs: 22 cases (1989-1994). *J Am Vet Med Assoc.* 1997;210:916–922.

46. Bowman D, ed. *Georgis' Parasitology for Veterinarians.* St Louis, MO: Elsevier Saunders; 2014:109–110.
47. Cummings CA, Panciera RJ, Kocan KM, et al. Characterization of stages of *Hepatozoon americanum* and of parasitized canine host cells. *Vet Pathol.* 2005;42:788–796.
48. Companion Animal Parasite Council. Current Advice on Parasite Control. Vector-borne Diseases: American hepatozoonosis. 2013. Available at: https://capcvet.org/guidelines/american-canine-hepatozoonosis/
49. Macintire DK, Vincent-Johnson NA, Kane CW, et al. Treatment of dogs infected with *Hepatozoon americanum*: 53 cases (1989-1998). *J Am Vet Med Assoc.* 2001;218:77–82.
50. Pereira C, Maia JP, Marcos R, et al. Molecular detection of *Hepatozoon felis* in cats from Maio Island, Republic of Cape Verde and global distribution of feline hepatozoonosis. *Parasit Vectors.* 2019;12:294.
51. Hodzic A, Alic A, Prasovic S, et al. *Hepatozoon silvestris* sp. nov.: morphological and molecular characterization of a new species of *Hepatozoon* (Adeleorina: Hepatozoidae) from the European wild cat (*Felis silvestris silvestris*). *Parasitology.* 2017;144:650–661.
52. Giannelli A, Latrofa MS, Nachum-Biala Y, et al. Three different *Hepatozoon* species in domestic cats from southern Italy. *Ticks Tick Borne Dis.* 2017;8:721–724.
53. Kegler K, Nufer U, Alic A, et al. Fatal infection with emerging apicomplexan parasite *Hepatozoon silvestris* in a domestic cat. *Parasit Vectors.* 2018;11:428.
54. Diaz-Reganon D, Villaescusa A, Ayllon T, et al. Molecular detection of *Hepatozoon* spp. and *Cytauxzoon* sp. in domestic and stray cats from Madrid, Spain. *Parasit Vectors.* 2017;10:112.
55. Attipa C, Papasouliotis K, Solano-Gallego L, et al. Prevalence study and risk factor analysis of selected bacterial, protozoal and viral, including vector-borne, pathogens in cats from Cyprus. *Parasit Vectors.* 2017;10:130.
56. Attipa C, Neofytou K, Yiapanis C, et al. Follow-up monitoring in a cat with leishmaniosis and coinfections with *Hepatozoon felis* and '*Candidatus* Mycoplasma haemominutum. *JFMS Open Rep.* 2017;3: 2055116917740454.
57. Basso W, Gorner D, Globokar M, et al. First autochthonous case of clinical *Hepatozoon felis* infection in a domestic cat in Central Europe. *Parasitol Int.* 2019;72:101945.

100

Trypanosomiasis

Sarah A. Hamer, Ashley B. Saunders, Karen F. Snowden, Jane E. Sykes

KEY POINTS

American Trypanosomiasis (Chagas disease)

- First Described: Chagas disease (American trypanosomiasis) was first described in humans in 1909 by Dr. Carlos Chagas.[1] The first canine Chagas disease cases in the United States were diagnosed in the early 1970s in Texas.[2]
- Cause: *Trypanosoma cruzi,* a protozoan parasite (order Kinetoplastida, family Trypanosomatidae).
- Affected Hosts: Dogs, cats, humans, horses, nonhuman primates, and other domestic and wild mammalian species.
- Geographic Distribution: Endemic across the Americas including South and Central America, Mexico, and the southern United States.
- Mode of Transmission: Contact with infected feces from, or ingestion of, triatomine (kissing bug) vectors, primarily *Triatoma* species. Transmission through blood transfusion and vertical transmission can occur.
- Major Clinical Signs: Infected dogs may be subclinically infected. Clinical disease manifests as lethargy, inappetence, mucosal pallor, lymphadenopathy, splenomegaly, arrhythmias, heart failure, or sudden death. Neurologic signs such as pelvic limb ataxia and exaggerated spinal reflexes may also occur.
- Differential Diagnoses: The differential diagnoses for suspected Chagas myocarditis include dilated cardiomyopathy, parvoviral myocarditis in puppies, canine monocytic ehrlichiosis, babesiosis, and leishmaniosis. The primary differential diagnoses for suspected Chagas meningoencephalitis in puppies are CDV infection and neosporosis, but other infectious and inflammatory causes of meningoencephalitis should also be considered.
- Human Health Significance: Chagas disease is a neglected tropical disease with as many as 8 million humans infected. Infected animals may be sentinels for human disease risk when there are infected triatomine vectors in the environment. Direct transmission from infected dog to human has not been shown. Transmission to humans has the potential to occur after needlestick injuries; caution is advised when handling tissues or clinical specimens from dogs with suspected trypanosomiasis.

African Trypanosomiasis

- First Described: Reports of African trypanosomiasis date back to Egyptian times. Trypanosomes were identified as the cause in 1895, when they were detected in cattle by a Scottish microbiologist, David Bruce (after whom *Brucella* was named).[3]
- Cause: *Trypanosoma brucei rhodesiense, Trypanosoma congolense, Trypanosoma evansi* (protozoan parasites, family Trypanosomatidae).
- Affected Hosts: Dogs and a variety of other mammalian host species. Humans are infected with *Trypanosoma brucei gambiense* and *T. brucei rhodesiense.*
- Geographic Distribution: Central Africa *(T. brucei, T. congolense)*; *T. evansi* is found in Africa as well as in Asia, Latin America, and the Canary Islands in Spain.
- Mode of Transmission: A bite from the tsetse fly *(T. brucei* or *T. congolense)* or mechanical transmission by hematophagous flies *(T. evansi)*.
- Major Clinical Signs: Lethargy, inappetence, weight loss, pallor, peripheral edema, ascites, hematemesis, hemorrhagic diarrhea, uveitis, corneal edema, neurologic signs due to meningoencephalitis.
- Differential Diagnoses: These include canine monocytic ehrlichiosis, babesiosis, leishmaniosis, and systemic immune-mediated diseases. CDV infection and neosporosis are important differential diagnoses in dogs with meningoencephalitis.
- Human Health Significance: Although most *Trypanosoma* species that cause African trypanosomiasis in dogs do not infect humans, *T. brucei rhodesiense* does, so caution is advised when handling tissues or clinical specimens from dogs or cats with suspected trypanosomiasis.

Trypanosomes, which cause trypanosomiasis, are hemoflagellate protozoans of the order Kinetoplastida and family Trypanosomatidae. The disease has been divided into American and African forms of disease because of the biologic differences in the two forms of infection (e.g., stercorarian versus salivarian transmission), different parasite species, and their tendency to exist in separate geographic regions. However, infections with African-type trypanosomes have been identified as indigenous foci in South America. These latter infections are mentioned under Epidemiology in the section on American trypanosomiasis because of their geographic location; however, the biology and treatment of these diseases are covered in more detail under the heading of African Trypanosomiasis.

AMERICAN TRYPANOSOMIASIS

ETIOLOGY AND EPIDEMIOLOGY

Chagas disease, or American trypanosomiasis, is caused by the flagellated protozoan *Trypanosoma cruzi,* and exists in several morphologic forms. In the mammalian host, the extracellular spindle-shaped trypomastigote or blood form is 15 to 20 μm long, with a central vesicular nucleus. A single, free flagellum originates from a basal body near the large posterior subterminal kinetoplast and an undulating membrane passes along the body to project anteriorly (Fig. 100.1). The second mammalian form is an oval intracellular amastigote approximately 1.5 to 4.0 μm in diameter

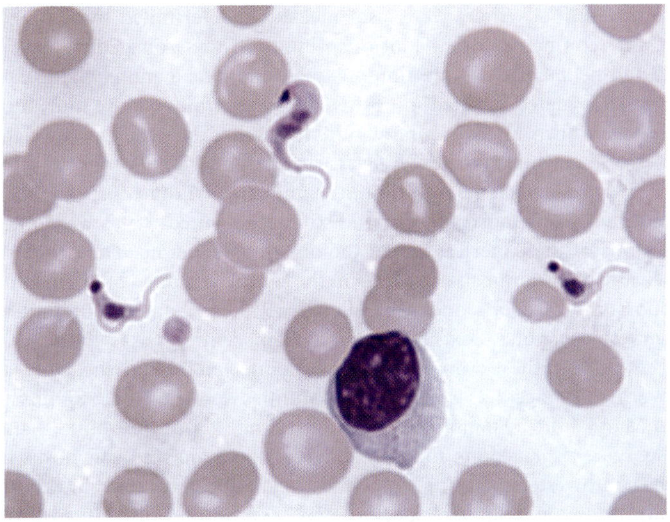

Fig. 100.1 Trypomastigotes of *Trypanosoma cruzi* in a blood smear of a dog. Wright-Giemsa stain, 100× oil magnification. (From Barr SC. Canine Chagas' disease [American trypanosomiasis] in North America. *Vet Clin North Am.* 2009;39:1055–1064.)

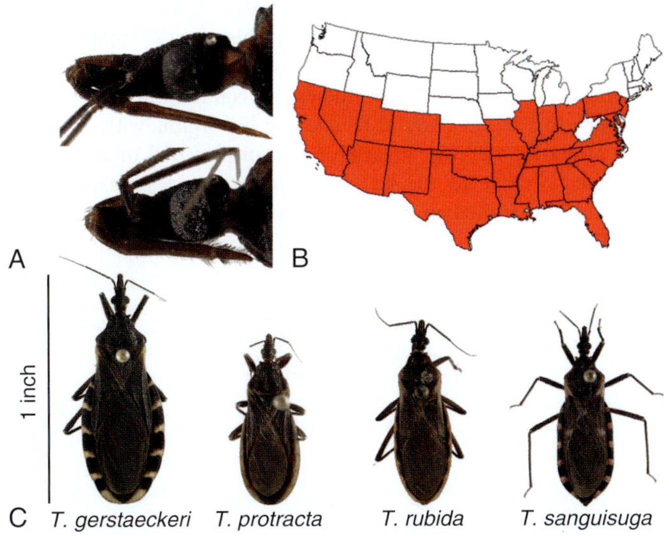

Fig. 100.2 (A) Side view of head and mouthparts of triatomine bugs. (B) Triatomine bug distribution in the United States. (C) Dorsal view of various *Triatoma* species.

that contains a large, round nucleus and rod-like kinetoplast similar to that of *Leishmania*. Epimastigotes, the third morphologic form, are found in the triatomine insect vector (Hemiptera: Reduviidae), commonly known as the *conenose bug* or *kissing bug*. This flagellated and somewhat pleomorphic form (15 to 20 µm) has a kinetoplast situated adjacent to the nucleus with a short undulating membrane and a single anterior flagellum. Six genotypes of *T. cruzi* have been identified (TcI through TcVI, also known as *discrete typing units* or *DTUs*), plus a bat-associated genotype (TcBat), which appear to differ in their vector preferences and the extent to which they cause disease.[4] Triatomine vectors are established across the southern half of the United States, with 11 species reported.[5] *Trypanosoma cruzi*–infected bugs have been reported from the majority of southern US states (Fig. 100.2).[6]

Stercorarian transmission occurs when the infected bug defecates on or near the host during or shortly after feeding and the fecal material containing trypomastigotes is subsequently rubbed into the bite wound, skin abrasions, or mucosal tissue (Fig. 100.3). Oral ingestion of infected insects will cause infection in opossums, raccoons, and wood rats and is a probable route of infection in dogs.[7–9] Other less common sources of infection in humans and possibly in dogs include blood transfusion, congenital transmission, or ingestion of meat or milk from infected lactating animals.[10] Trypomastigotes usually enter macrophages and myocytes, either locally or systemically, after hematogenous spread. Once they are intracellular, trypomastigotes transform into amastigotes, which multiply by binary fission (see Fig. 100.3). These amastigotes transform into trypomastigotes before rupture of and release from the cell. Rapid intracellular multiplication cycles ensure a rapid rise in parasitemia before effective immunity develops. The bug vector becomes infected by ingesting circulating trypomastigotes that transform to epimastigotes and multiply by binary fission. Transformation of the epimastigotes back into trypomastigotes occurs in the vector's hindgut before the trypomastigotes are passed in the feces.

Trypanosoma cruzi infection has been documented in a wide variety of dogs including 48 breeds in a medical records review in Texas.[11] Sporting and working breed groups may have lifestyle factors that increase the dogs' exposure to infected triatomine vectors, such as confinement in outdoor kennels. However, no evidence for a breed predilection for the pathogen was found in studies across diverse ecoregions in Tennessee or Texas.[12,13] Although cross-reactivity with *Leishmania* spp. is a concern in *T. cruzi* serologic surveys, histopathologic or parasitologic confirmation of *T. cruzi*

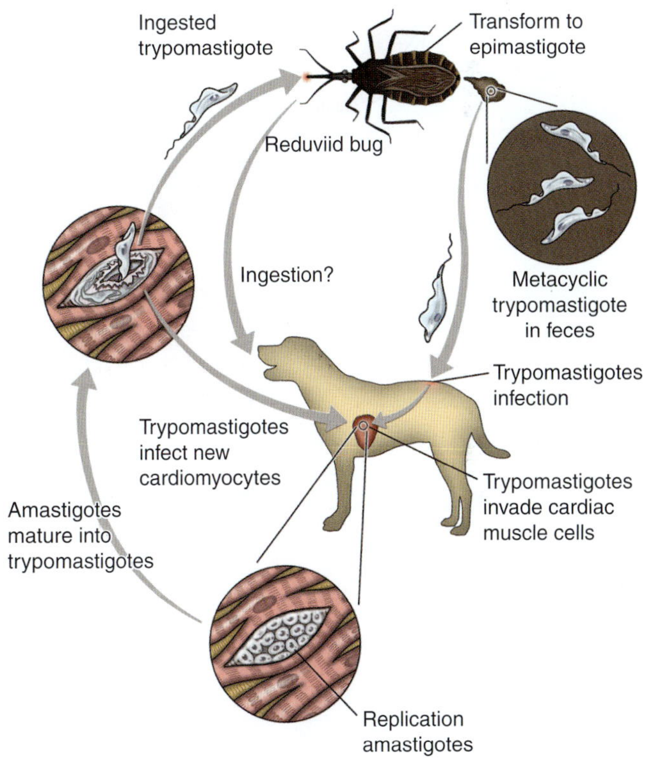

Fig. 100.3 Life cycle of *Trypanosoma cruzi*. Dogs are infected when a triatome (reduviid bug) defecates at its bite site, and possibly when dogs ingest infected triatomes. Other routes of transmission may also predominate in the United States (see text). Trypomastigotes infect cardiomyocytes (as well as other tissues) and form amastigotes, which replicate locally, leading to myocarditis.

infection has been reported in dogs from at least five states, providing further evidence of active and widespread canine Chagas disease transmission in the southern United States (Fig. 100.4).[11,14–20] An incidence of 30.7 *T. cruzi* infections per 100 dogs per year was documented in a 2021 longitudinal study of dogs across 10 kennels in Texas over a 12-month period.[21] A study of 284 shelter cats from southern Louisiana found a seroprevalence of 7.3% and blood samples from 24.6% of cats were PCR positive.[22]

As in humans, transplacental transmission in dogs may contribute to the prevalence of Chagas disease in this species. Transplacental and transmammary transmission was documented in experimentally infected dogs in very early studies.[19,23] Natural infection in eight pups born to a Walker hound female dog in Virginia with a positive serum antibody titer was suggestive of transplacental or transmammary infection due to the lack of vector presence or exposure to infected wild mammalian tissues.[14] Data from canine field studies in Argentina showed that 10% of offspring born to dams with positive serum antibody titers were also infected as determined by serologic testing compared with 4% of offspring born to seronegative dams.[24] Experimental *T. cruzi* infection of a male and female mongrel dog pair that later mated resulted in positive *T. cruzi* serology in all four pups that were born; after weaning all pups had weakness, progressive weight loss, and chronic diarrhea with cardiac dilation evident on necropsy.[25]

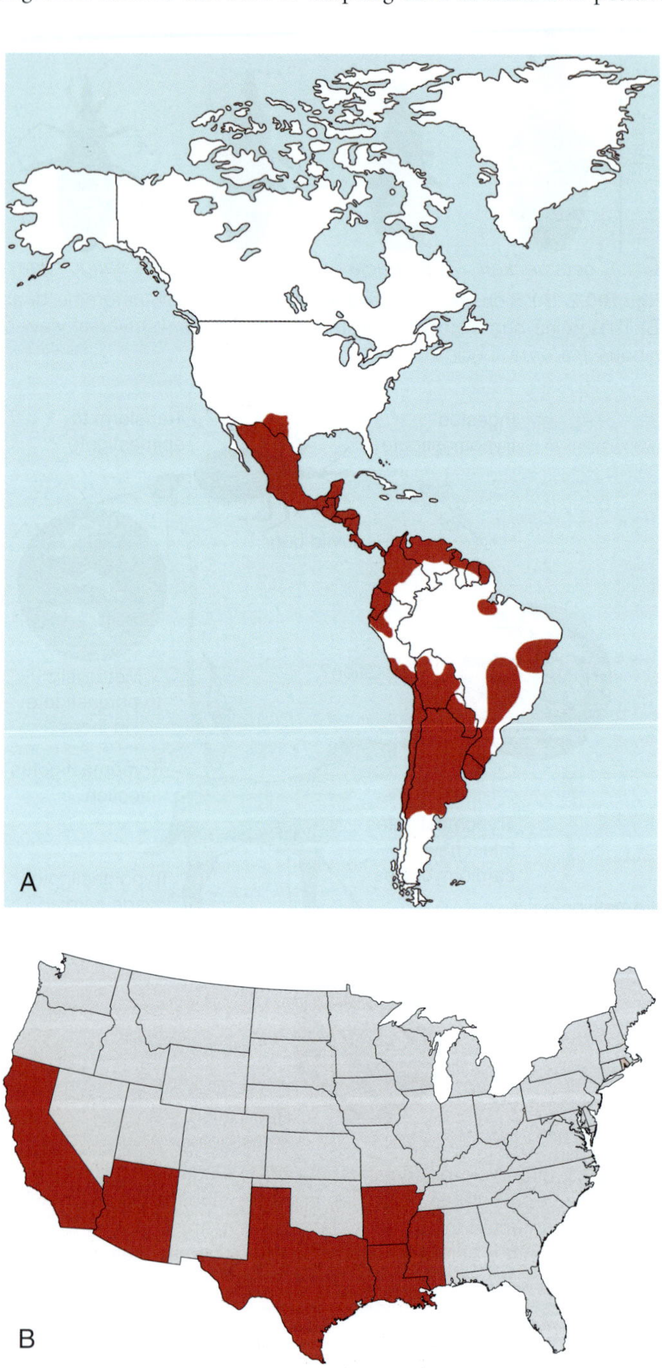

Fig. 100.4 (A) Approximate distribution of Chagas disease in humans in the Americas, showing states where autochthonous human transmission has occurred in the United States. (From Lynn MK, Bossak BH, Sandifer PA, et al. Contemporary autochthonous human Chagas disease in the USA. 2020;205:105361.) (B) States within the United States where Chagas disease is most prevalent in dogs. Occasional cases have been reported in other southern states and as far north as Virginia and Missouri.

Trypanosoma cruzi infection in mammalian wildlife hosts has been reported from most areas of the southern United States and other regions of the Americas where the disease is endemic. The principal sylvatic reservoir hosts of *T. cruzi* in the southern United States include opossums, raccoons, and armadillos.[18,26–31] Recent analysis of hunter-harvested coyotes, fox, and bobcats from central Texas found that 12%–14% of these animals had *T. cruzi*–infected heart tissue, whereas over 70% of raccoons from the same counties were infected.[32] Similarly, in Maryland,[33] Oklahoma,[34] North Carolina,[28] South Carolina,[35] and Georgia,[35–38] raccoons and opossums are the main reservoir hosts. In the southwestern states, *T. cruzi* infection has been detected in various rat, mouse, and squirrel species.[30,38,39] Triatomines distributed from the western half of Texas to California are frequently found in the nests of wood rats. Consequently, a significant percentage of wood rats in field surveys have been found to be infected with *T. cruzi* and probably serve as reservoirs in those regions.[18,40,41] Because experimental inoculation of *T. cruzi* isolates from opossums and armadillos into dogs produces a disease similar to that described in naturally acquired cases of acute and chronic canine trypanosomiasis, dogs in natural settings are likely infected with the same parasite strains as those sylvatic hosts.[42–44] Across several biomedical research facilities in the southern United States, nonhuman primates have seroconverted presumably from exposure to vectors in outdoor cages, leading to Chagas cardiomyopathy and diminishing the value of the infected animals as biomedical models.[45] Chagas disease was diagnosed in a horse in Texas with neurologic signs of ataxia and pelvic limb weakness. Amastigotes were found in the thoracic spinal cord; this constituted the first report of clinical *T. cruzi* infection in an equid.[46]

CLINICAL FEATURES

Pathogenesis, Clinical Signs and Physical Examination Findings

The host-parasite interactions in *T. cruzi* infections are complex, and it is likely that both parasite and host response contribute to the progressive cardiac damage.[47] In experimental canine infections, the intensity of inflammatory infiltrate and fibrosis in the heart varied based on the strain of the parasite in both acute and chronic phases of infection.[43,47,48] In medical literature reporting pathologic changes in acute Chagas disease in humans, a microangiopathy has been described, and an ischemic vascular component to the cardiac destruction has been suggested.[47]

The mechanism by which progressive cardiac damage occurs may be linked in part to host immune responses to the parasite. In experimentally infected beagles, high levels of the anti-inflammatory cytokine IL-10 were consistently detected in animals that showed less severe cardiac pathology during chronic infection.[49] The role of various antiparasite immunoglobulin subclasses in contributing to cardiac damage is unclear. In one study, an elevated IgG1 isotype was reported in dogs with an increased cardiac index and myocarditis.[50] Conversely, in another study, low IgG1 levels correlated with cardiomegaly in chronically infected dogs.[49]

In a review of Chagas-associated human pathology, it was hypothesized that a balance of cell-mediated immune response and inflammatory response was maintained in the indeterminate phase of infection.[47] The progressive cardiac damage and inflammation in chronic disease was attributed to mediation by cytotoxic CD8+ T cells, although the mechanism of cell-mediated myocardial damage was not clearly elucidated. An autoimmune component in cardiac damage has been proposed, especially because there is a lack of correlation between intracellular amastigote numbers and the degree of chronic myocarditis with fibrosis.

Dogs

The course of *T. cruzi* infection in dogs appears to follow the cardiac disease pattern in humans, with an acute phase, followed by an "indeterminate" or latent phase with normal clinical presentation, and a chronic phase of cardiac damage.[14,31,43,48,51,52]

Acute disease in young dogs is often sudden in onset, with signs of myocarditis, cardiac arrhythmias and heart failure, or sudden collapse and death of a previously normal young dog. Acute myocarditis results from cell damage and inflammation as trypomastigotes rupture from cardiomyocytes. Lethargy, fever, inappetence, generalized lymphadenopathy, slow capillary refill time with pale mucous membranes, and, in some cases, splenomegaly and hepatomegaly are the main signs in puppies. A weak pulse with deficits, tachyarrhythmia, and terminal hypothermia and respiratory distress are common. In some dogs over 6 months of age, parasitemia develops more slowly and clinical signs are often much less severe or not apparent at all. Sudden death, presumably from cardiac muscle failure or to malignant arrhythmias, may also occur. In adult dogs, these acute manifestations are sometimes less severe, with only transient mental depression and parasitemia.[53] The reason for variation in intensity of illness with age is unclear; however, it may relate to inherent age-related host immunity.

In one retrospective study of dogs with confirmed *T. cruzi* infections in Texas, 50.5% of the infected dogs were less than 1 year of age.[11] In that study, 42% died acutely (n = 86 dogs) and the diagnosis of Chagas disease was determined using histopathology after necropsy.[10]

In addition to cardiac manifestations, dogs may exhibit other signs of acute disease. Generalized lymphadenomegaly, anorexia, and diarrhea are common during acute illness and may precede cardiac manifestations. Although less common than signs referable to cardiac abnormalities, neurologic signs referable to meningoencephalomyelitis as a direct result of parasitic invasion of the neurologic system may also occur. Weakness, paresis, pelvic limb ataxia, and upper motor neuron (hyperreflexive) spinal reflexes have rarely been described in naturally and experimentally infected dogs.[43,54]

Survivors of acute myocarditis become aparasitemic and without overt clinical signs in the "indeterminate" or "latent" phase. Parasitemia becomes cytologically undetectable at about 30 days PI, although it can still be demonstrated by blood culture. During the long subclinical period between acute and chronic disease in the dog, ECG readings may be within reference limits, except for intermittent occurrence of ventricular arrhythmias, which can be exacerbated by exercise or excitement.[55] Sudden death during this phase can occur and is thought to be caused by fatal cardiac arrhythmias.

Although not all dogs exhibit signs of chronic disease, many develop chronic myocarditis with cardiac dilatation over a variable length of time. In experimental studies of young dogs, the onset of chronic disease was documented over an 8- to 36-month period postinoculation.[43,44] In the chronic phase, cardiac dilatation occurs, ECG abnormalities become more prevalent, and clinical signs referable to right-sided and/or bilateral cardiac failure occur. ECG abnormalities detected in naturally infected dogs in the chronic phase have included supraventricular and ventricular arrhythmias and atrioventricular block.[56,57] In experimentally infected dogs with chronic infection, clinical signs included pulse deficits, ascites, pleural effusion, hepatomegaly, and jugular venous congestion.[41] In two retrospective studies of naturally infected dogs, the most common clinical history and physical examination abnormalities included exercise intolerance, lethargy, anorexia, ascites, respiratory difficulties (tachypnea and cough), bradycardia, heart murmurs, and hepatomegaly.[11,58] Chronic *T. cruzi*–induced myocardial disease in dogs is difficult to distinguish from chronic dilative cardiomyopathy of noninfectious origin, and misdiagnosis may occur until serologic evaluation for exposure or histologic detection of parasites is available.[14,42,52]

In chronic infections, electrical conduction disturbances along with variable cardiomegaly can sometimes be overlooked. In a Texas study reviewing case records, 21.3% of dogs had electrical conduction disturbances, and a number of animals were being evaluated for pacemaker implantation.[11] A variety of electrical conduction abnormalities have been reported.[44,53] Parasite-associated damage to parasympathetic innervation in the heart and subsequent conduction disturbances are probably responsible for the cardiac arrhythmias. In experimental infections in both rats and dogs, a reduction in autonomic neurons has been documented, along with a variable intensity of inflammatory changes in histopathologic studies.[59,60] Trypanosomiasis should be considered in any dog with signs of myocarditis, cardiomyopathy, or electrical conduction disturbance in the heart. There is little information available on survival times of dogs. In a review of 11 dogs identified with chronic *T. cruzi* infection, survival times ranged from 0 to 60 months.[58]

Humans with Chagas disease can also develop severe megaesophagus or megacolon due to parasympathetic denervation,[61] but these syndromes have not been described in dogs. Morphometry of the myenteric esophagus was not altered in dogs with experimentally induced chronic *T. cruzi* infection.[62]

The most common physical examination findings in puppies with Chagas disease are lethargy, generalized lymphadenomegaly, splenomegaly, pallor, and arrhythmias. Generalized subcutaneous edema has also been reported.[63] Dogs with chronic Chagas disease may show signs of right- and/or left-sided congestive heart failure, with tachypnea, ascites, or jugular pulses. Cardiac murmurs and arrhythmias may be detected during auscultation of the heart.

Cats

Field studies in Mexico and South America (Brazil and Argentina) have documented significant levels of serum antibody reactivity to *T. cruzi* in cats and have implicated this species as a potential reservoir in the domestic transmission cycle.[64–66] Unfortunately, data on the clinical course of disease in cats are lacking in the published literature. A total of 42% of seropositive cats from shelters in Texas had evidence of myocardial inflammation and fibrosis.[67] In Louisiana, 7.3% of 234 cats were seropositive for *T. cruzi*, with 24.6% testing PCR-positive.[22] Serologic testing for *T. cruzi* antibodies in cats is not generally available in commercial diagnostic laboratories, complicating detection of infection in this host species. In the authors' experience, cats with unknown clinical disease in households with seropositive dogs and positive triatomine vectors can test positive for the presence of anti-*T. cruzi* antibodies using unvalidated assays.

DIAGNOSIS

The key to diagnosis of Chagas disease is a high degree of clinical suspicion. Chagas disease should be considered in any dog with signs of myocarditis or cardiomyopathy, particularly if it lives or has lived at any time—even years before evaluation—in an endemic region. Diagnosis of dogs in regions without endemic triatomines (e.g., the northern United States) may reflect travel histories.[68] The odds of

TABLE 100.1 Diagnostic Assays Currently Available for Trypanosomiasis in Dogs and Cats

Assay	Specimen Type	Target	Indications and Limitations
Cytologic examination	Aspirates of lymph nodes, spleen, bone marrow, blood smears, or buffy-coat preparations	*Trypanosoma* trypomastigotes or, less commonly, amastigotes	Organisms may be few in number and in chronic trypanosomiasis are often not found.
Trypanosoma culture	Blood or buffy-coat preparations, bone marrow	*Trypanosoma* spp.	Requires special techniques, laboratory biosafety containment, and expertise that are not widely available. Sensitivity may be low in chronic infections.
Antibody serology (indirect fluorescent antibody or ELISA)	Serum	Antibodies to *Trypanosoma* spp.	Most infected dogs test positive, although acutely infected dogs may test negative. Not all infected dogs will develop disease, so results must be interpreted in light of clinical signs. False positives can occur in dogs exposed to *Leishmania* or those vaccinated with *Leishmania* vaccines.
PCR assay	Whole blood, buffy coats, splenic or lymph node aspirates, CSF	*Trypanosoma* DNA	Negative results may occur in infected animals because duration of parasitemia is short. May be useful in dogs with suggestive clinical signs in which organisms cannot be found cytologically. Sensitivity and specificity depend on assay design. Limited availability.

CSF, cerebrospinal fluid; *ELISA,* enzyme-linked immunosorbent assay; *PCR,* polymerase chain reaction.

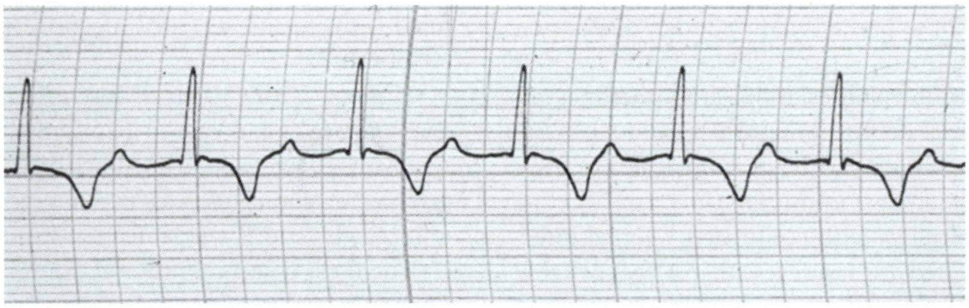

Fig. 100.5 Electrocardiogram showing second-degree heart block and depressed QRS complexes often present in dogs with acute Chagas' disease. (From Barr SC. Canine Chagas' disease [American trypanosomiasis] in North America. *Vet Clin North Am.* 2009;39:1055–1064.)

being infected with *T. cruzi* are higher in dogs with an infected littermate or housemate.[69] Diagnostic assays for trypanosomiasis are described in Table 100.1.

Laboratory Abnormalities

Complete Blood Count

Hematologic abnormalities are of little specific diagnostic value for Chagas disease. During the acute phase of infection, the CBC of some dogs may reveal anemia, leukocytosis due to a neutrophilia, eosinophilia, monocytosis, and lymphocytosis.[70–72] Thrombocytopenia, leukopenia, and/or lymphopenia have also been documented.[73] Dogs in the chronic phase of infection may have no hematologic abnormalities.

Serum Biochemical Tests

Serum ALT activity, AST activity, and creatinine and urea nitrogen concentrations can be elevated in dogs with *T. cruzi* infection, especially those that are at risk of death from severe acute myocarditis. Rarely, moderate to severe hypoalbuminemia with or without hyperglobulinemia occurs in acutely affected dogs.[63,73] Elevation in serum troponin I levels has been reported as a nonspecific indicator of myocardial damage.[56,57,69,74]

Electrocardiography

The ECG of dogs with Chagas myocarditis may show any combination of arrhythmias or conduction disturbances including sinus tachycardia, decreased R-wave amplitude, axis shifts, supraventricular and ventricular arrhythmias, and conduction abnormalities including atrioventricular block and right bundle branch block (Fig. 100.5). Ventricular arrhythmias alone or in combination with other ECG abnormalities are most often detected in seropositive dogs.[69] The damage to the myocardium and conduction system from parasites, inflammation, and fibrosis provide a substrate for the ECG abnormalities (for instance, damage to the ventricular myocardium resulting in ventricular arrhythmias).

Diagnostic Imaging

Thoracic radiography is of value in the diagnosis of cardiomegaly and congestive heart failure (pleural effusion, pulmonary edema) (Fig. 100.6).[58,75] Echocardiographic abnormalities are variable depending on the location of myocardial damage and can include enlargement of all four heart chambers and reduced ventricular systolic function (Fig. 100.7).[57,58]

Microbiologic Tests

Cytologic Examination

During acute disease, trypomastigotes may be detected on stained blood smear examination (see Fig. 100.1). In experimental infections in puppies, parasites could be detected in circulation as early as 3 days postinoculation, and parasitemia peaked about day 17, approximately at the time that clinical signs of acute myocarditis and lymphadenomegaly appeared.[53] In those animals, parasitemia persisted for up to 30 days. However, in chronic infections, parasitemia is often so low that

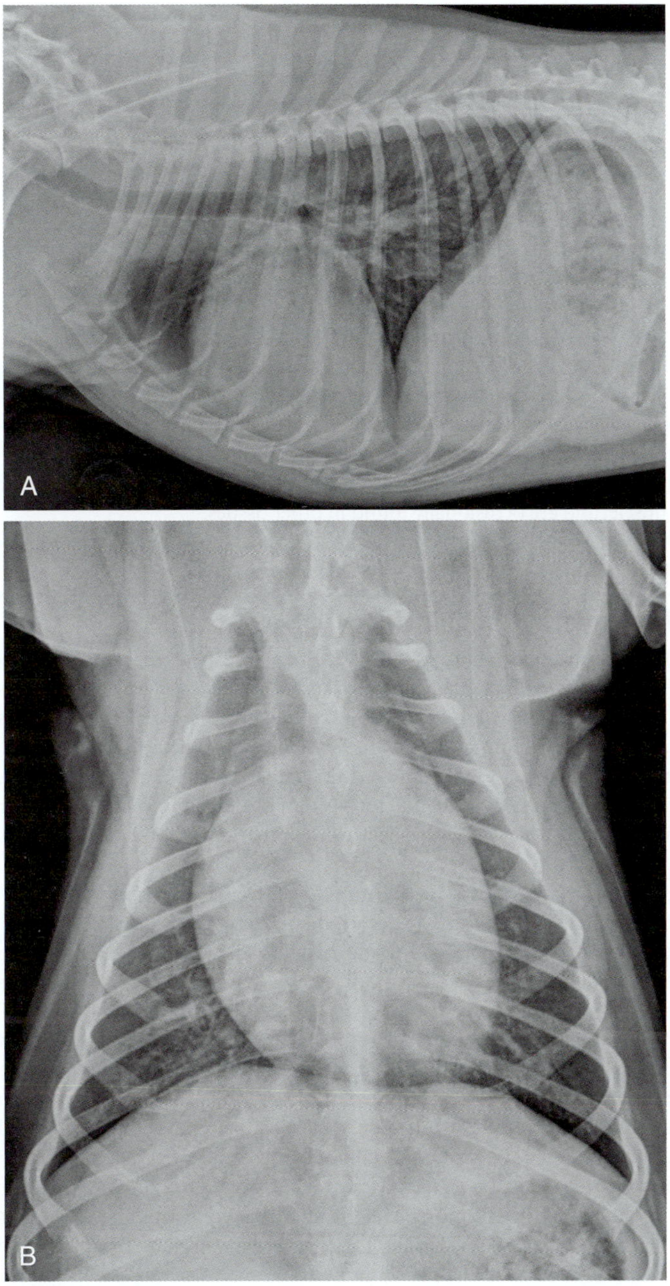

Fig. 100.6 Lateral (A) and dorsoventral (B) thoracic radiographic images of a dog with trypanosomiasis and mild generalized cardiomegaly. The pulmonary veins are mildly larger than the corresponding artery, and a slight interstitial pattern was present throughout the lungs.

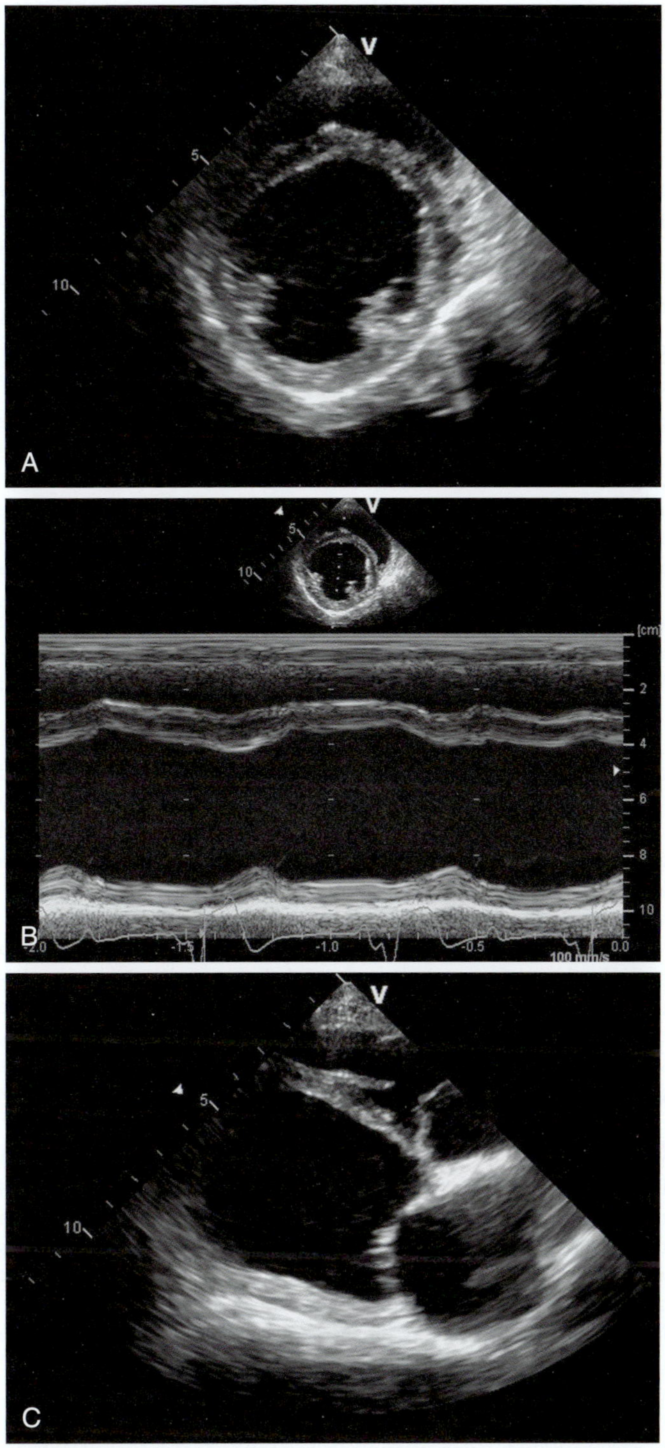

Fig. 100.7 Two-dimensional (A) and M-mode (B) transthoracic echocardiogram images obtained in a right parasternal short axis view and long axis view (C) documenting significant left ventricular enlargement and mild right ventricular enlargement.

organisms may be difficult to identify during routine examination of Wright-stained blood films. To concentrate parasites and increase the sensitivity of detection, a thick-film buffy coat smear can be stained with Wright or Giemsa stain and examined microscopically, or a buffy coat specimen may be examined as a wet preparation for trypomastigote movement.[75] Stained lymph node aspirates or impression smears may contain amastigotes, even when parasitemias are very low.[75] The larger the volume of the blood specimen collected, the greater the likelihood that organisms will be detected. Trypomastigotes may also be found on cytologic examination of lymph node aspirates and in abdominal effusions. Amastigotes were described in the lymph node of one affected dog that were cytologically indistinguishable from those of *Leishmania*.[63]

Parasite Culture and Xenodiagnosis

Culture of trypanosomes is a specialized procedure that is not routinely available in veterinary diagnostic laboratories. *Trypanosoma cruzi* can be cultured from blood in liver infusion tryptose (LIT) growth medium or other media; however, 2 to 20 weeks may be needed for the results to become positive for epimastigotes.[14,43] In one naturally infected dog, parasite cultures were established using lymph node aspirates inoculated into serum-supplemented Dulbecco's modified Eagle's medium and maintained at room temperature to yield replication of the flagellated epimastigote stage of parasite.[63]

Xenodiagnosis involves feeding colony-reared, parasite-negative triatomine vectors on suspected infected hosts and subsequently testing the vectors in order to diagnose infection in the host, and is thought to measure infectiousness of a host to vectors. These methods are used primarily in a research setting and have limited application in making a clinical diagnosis. Although specificity of bug feeding is high, the sensitivity may be low. Results of one study were only an 11% detection rate in bugs fed serially on experimentally infected dogs.[76]

Serologic Diagnosis

Serologic testing for *T. cruzi*–specific serum antibodies is the predominant diagnostic tool for detection of canine *T. cruzi* infections. A positive result, in association with clinical signs, is considered supportive for the diagnosis of *T. cruzi* infection in dogs. Due to variation in sensitivities and specificities among assays, two different serologic assays should be used to confirm a positive titer, especially in regions of low prevalence, although very few veterinary diagnostic laboratories currently offer assays for diagnosis of canine *T. cruzi* infection. In experimental infections, antibodies are usually first detected by 3 weeks PI, at the time when parasitemia is declining, and positive titers persist for the life of the animal.[27] Many apparently healthy dogs are diagnosed as positive for *T. cruzi* based on serology findings, and the prognosis is currently unknown.[13]

Antibody detection methods used by commercial diagnostic laboratories include IFA and ELISA tests. However, there may be confusion due to significant cross-reactivity and cross-infection with the closely related parasite *Leishmania*.[77,78] Depending on the clinical history and geographic location of the animal, positive serum antibody test results for *T. cruzi* should be confirmed by additional testing for antibodies to *Leishmania* to determine which organism yields the higher titer.[79]

Several immunochromatographic POC "dipstick" tests have also been developed for use in humans and show promise in canine epidemiologic research[13,80–82] but are not currently approved for canine diagnosis in the United States. These test kits have potential as rapid, simple screening tools in a clinic setting that can be used in conjunction with additional confirmatory tests.

Molecular Diagnosis Using Nucleic Acid–Based Testing

PCR testing can be used to detect DNA of *T. cruzi* in various clinical specimens including specimens that can be acquired antemortem (blood, lymph node aspirates, or ascites fluid) as well as cardiac and other organ tissues acquired at necropsy. PCR assays can be highly specific for *T. cruzi* but can have variable and sometimes low sensitivity for diagnosis of chronic infections unless multiple specimens are tested.[83] In a clinical setting, the utility of PCR may be limited in animals that are in the indeterminate state of infection when the parasite is not circulating in the blood. PCR may be useful to confirm infection when organisms are not seen on blood smears. In a research study using experimentally infected dogs, parasite DNA was easily detected in the acute phase of infection in 12 animals, but the sensitivity of the test decreased during the chronic phase of infection depending on the strain of parasite.[84] Currently, PCR assays for *T. cruzi* are not widely available from veterinary diagnostic laboratories on a commercial basis, but have been used for diagnosis of canine Chagas disease.[63,85]

Pathologic Findings

Gross Pathologic Findings

Gross pathologic findings in dogs with Chagas disease include generalized lymphadenopathy, evidence of congestive heart failure (ascites, pleural effusion, or congestion of viscera), and biventricular cardiac enlargement with thinning of the ventricular wall. Subendocardial and subepicardial hemorrhages, as well as multiple yellow to white myocardial spots and streaks may be observed.[16,60,74]

Histopathologic Findings

Histopathologic findings in acute Chagas disease include a severe diffuse granulomatous myocarditis with myocardial necrosis, often with large numbers of parasitic pseudocysts containing intracellular amastigotes, and minimal fibrosis (Fig. 100.8). Typically, the heart is the primary organ with significant lesions, but amastigotes can be identified in lymph nodes and other organs including liver, spleen, and brain.[63,74] IHC does not distinguish *Leishmania* from *Trypanosoma* amastigotes because of serologic cross-reactivity.[63] In chronically infected dogs, multifocal coalescing areas of lymphoplasmacytic inflammation and mild necrosis with extensive loss of myocardial fibers and severe interstitial fibrosis occur.[47,53] A progressive, destructive process occurs in the heart, including damage to uninfected cardiomyocytes, which has been described in infected humans.[50] In chronic infections, organisms may uncommonly be evident in cardiac muscle, and are occasionally found in other tissues.[86]

TREATMENT

Antiprotozoal Treatment

Therapeutic options for treating *T. cruzi* infections in dogs are limited. The drugs available for treatment of Chagas disease in humans include benznidazole and nifurtimox; however, neither of these drugs is available for animal use in the United States. In the United States, benznidazole was FDA-approved for pediatric use in 2017; otherwise these drugs are only available for human use through the CDC, under an investigational drug-use license. The marketing of nifurtimox has been discontinued in many countries.

In humans, these drugs are primarily effective in the acute phase of infection, and significant toxic adverse effects[87] and drug resistance[88] have been reported for both. Some early success was reported in treating experimental and natural cases of canine trypanosomiasis with nifurtimox, but severe adverse effects limited its use.[89] In one study, benznidazole was shown to induce cure in acute (63%) and to a lesser extent in chronic (39%) experimental infections in dogs.[90] However in a more recent study, benznidazole resulted in a temporary, short-term reduction in parasite load but did not prevent myocardial damage in an infected canine model.[91] The efficacy of chemotherapy in clearing *T. cruzi* infection appears dependent on an adequately functioning immune system.[92,93]

Numerous medications have been evaluated as therapeutic agents for Chagas disease with high adverse effect profiles or disappointing results in clinical trials, particularly in chronic disease.[94] Medications

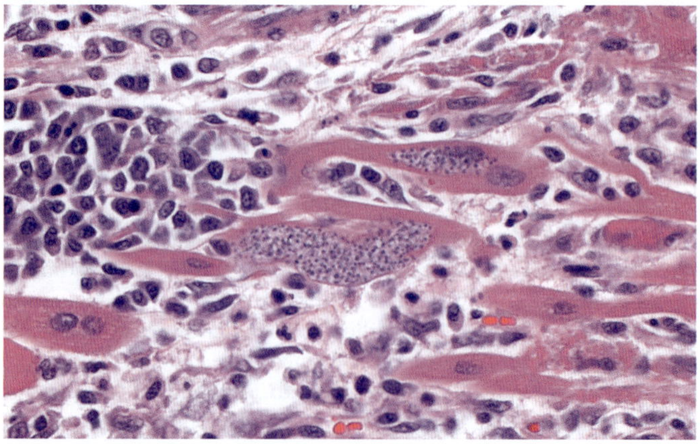

Fig. 100.8 *Trypanosoma cruzi* amastigotes in a pseudocyst within the cardiac muscle of a dog. Inflammatory cells are present as well (hematoxylin and eosin stain, ×1000).

including gossypol, allopurinol, and multiple triazole class of drugs (albaconazole, ketoconazole, itraconazole, posaconazole) have been investigated for treatment, but drug efficacies for some are less than convincing.[95–100] In some experimental models, the drug may be effective in suppressing parasite proliferation and death in infected humans or dogs; but treatment failure occurs and cure is not achieved.[93,97,99] Current research is exploring alternatives including combinations of medications and sequential therapies.[100] In a study of 105 dogs with *T. cruzi* infection, treatment with a combination of itraconazole and amiodarone for 12 months resulted in survival times that were on average 7 months longer than those of the 16 dogs in a control group.[85]

Because there is no available effective parasiticide, clinically affected animals should be managed using appropriate supportive therapy. Diuretics and positive inotropes/inodilators may be indicated in dogs with reduced ventricular systolic function that have developed congestive heart failure. Cardiac arrhythmias may require specific antiarrhythmic therapy for tachyarrhythmias and pacemaker implantation for bradyarrhythmias.[101]

PROGNOSIS

The prognosis for dogs that develop Chagas disease is often poor because of the lack of effective treatments. Dogs diagnosed at an older age (mean of 9 years) survive longer (30 to 60 months) than dogs diagnosed at a younger age (mean of 4.5 years), which survive only up to 5 months post diagnosis.[59] In a study of 44 client-owned dogs evaluated at Texas A&M University, identification of right ventricular enlargement was strongly associated with decreased time to death in a multivariable model.[57]

IMMUNITY AND VACCINATION

No vaccine is available for Chagas disease in dogs. Protective immunity was not documented in experimentally infected dogs that received five repeated infections over a 3-year period. Over time, dogs developed diminishing parasitemias and increased antibody titer results, with a progressive myocarditis similar to control animals.[102]

PREVENTION

Chagas disease prevention is centered on vector control. Implementing integrated pest management methods to reduce encounters between dogs and infected vectors will likely have the greatest effect. These measures could include housing dogs indoors at night in areas with doors and screens to exclude bugs, limiting the use of yard lights to reduce attraction of insects, and optimizing pesticide regimens. There are no pesticides in the United States specifically labeled for control of triatomine bugs. However, residual spray formulations of synthetic pyrethroids, such as deltamethrin, have proven to be very effective at killing the triatomine vectors in Latin America[103] and are available in the United States. Applications of fipronil on the coats of dogs do not appear to prevent infections in dogs or reduce the feeding of vectors,[104] but deltamethrin-treated collars do reduce feeding by *Triatoma infestans*.[105,106] Isoxazolines (fluralaner and afoxolaner) were also shown to induce triatome mortality when given as a single oral dose to dogs that were then exposed to triatomes 2, 7, 21, 34, and 51 days after treatment,[107] and in another study, fluralaner was shown to significantly reduce infestations with pyrethroid-resistant triatomes when compared with placebo.[108]

Kennels and surrounding structures (chicken houses, wood piles) in endemic areas can be sprayed monthly with a residual insecticide. Dog housing and surrounding habitats should be upgraded to remove vector nesting sites. Woody debris and other habitat that may serve as refuge for triatomine vectors or wildlife hosts (wood rats, raccoons, opossums, armadillos) should be removed from the immediate vicinity of dog kennels. Serologic testing of breeding females is advised in areas where *T. cruzi* is endemic, so the risk of transplacental and transmammary transmission can be considered. Dog-to-dog transmission, through exposure to infected blood while fighting or during rough play, has not been documented but may be possible if the infected dog is parasitemic. Although *T. cruzi* organisms were detected in the urine and saliva of dogs after experimental administration of an extremely high infective dose, transfer of parasites through these body fluids has not been documented in natural settings.[109] Limiting exposure to potentially infectious tissues of wild mammalian reservoirs may reduce disease transmission in dogs. Finally, *T. cruzi* antibody screening of canine blood donors residing in endemic areas should be considered to reduce potential blood transfusion transmission.

In the United States, it is not known if dogs with seropositive test results are significant parasite reservoirs in the vector-borne transmission cycle. The importance of dogs as reservoir hosts has been well documented throughout South America and appears to be influenced by parasite strain, infectious dose, and host health attributes such as nutritional status.[103,110,111]

PUBLIC HEALTH ASPECTS

American trypanosomiasis is a major human health problem in South and Central America and Mexico.[112,113] It is primarily a problem in impoverished regions where humans live in rural areas. Dogs are considered a reservoir for human infection in these regions because they maintain high levels of parasitemia and are a preferred host for triatomine insects. Cats may also act as a reservoir for human infection in South America.[114] Fewer than one third of infected humans ultimately develop Chagas disease.[61] More information about triatome bug species that may transmit *T. cruzi* to dogs and humans in South America and the importance of dogs as reservoirs and sentinels has become available in recent years with application of serologic and molecular methods as part of a One Health approach. Seroprevalences that exceed 30% and PCR prevalences that reach 57% have been reported in dogs in South America.[115–118]

The human health burden of Chagas disease in the United States is largely unknown, but it is estimated that over 235,000 people in the United States are infected, the majority of whom are immigrants from Chagas-endemic areas of Central or South America or Mexico.[119] At the time of writing, the CDC indicates that it is a reportable disease in humans in six states (Arkansas, Arizona, Louisiana, Mississippi, Tennessee, and Texas). Reports of cases associated with transmission by blood transfusion continue to rise.[120–122] Autochthonous cases in humans in the United States are rare, but increasingly recognized especially in Texas.[123,124] The generally higher standards of housing in the United States relative to other endemic regions may limit the degree to which vectors from colonize human dwellings. It is likely that many human cases of Chagas disease in the United States may be overlooked because of a low level of suspicion.

Although the risk of a human acquiring infection directly from an infected dog is extremely low, the presence of an infected dog often signals a landscape where infected triatomines occur, and so there is a human health risk due to the presence of infected vectors. The severity and difficulty of treating disease in humans makes this disease of considerable public health significance. Veterinarians should be careful when handling blood samples from infected dogs and warn laboratory staff of the potential infectivity of the samples. Accidental needle-stick injuries when administering therapy to or collecting specimens from infected dogs should be reported immediately to healthcare providers.

TRYPANOSOMA CANINUM INFECTION

Trypanosoma caninum has only been identified in dogs primarily from Brazil, many of which have been apparently healthy.[125–128] The pathogenicity of this organism requires further study. Importantly, infection with *T. caninum* leads to false-positive serologic test results for *Leishmania*, which can confound control methods that rely on culling of dogs that are seropositive for *Leishmania* (see Chapter 96).

AFRICAN TRYPANOSOMIASIS

African trypanosomiasis is caused by *Trypanosoma brucei* and *Trypanosoma congolense*. These organisms are transmitted by tsetse flies (*Glossina* species), which are only found in Africa. *Trypanosoma brucei* includes three subspecies: *Trypanosoma brucei, T. brucei gambiense,* and *T. brucei rhodesiense,* which are indistinguishable morphologically and are referred to as "*T. brucei* complex" organisms. *Trypanosoma evansi* also belongs to this group (see later). The epidemiology, host range, and clinical features of disease caused by these *T. brucei* complex organisms differ. *Trypanosoma brucei gambiense* and *T. brucei rhodesiense* cause "sleeping sickness" in humans from Africa (West African and East African trypanosomiasis, respectively) (Fig. 100.9). A variety of animal reservoirs of *T. brucei rhodesiense* have been established, and although naturally occurring infections of domestic animals and wildlife hosts with *T. brucei gambiense* have been identified, the relative importance of animals as reservoir hosts for this pathogen has been less clear.[129] Naturally occurring, clinical and subclinical infections of domestic dogs with *T. brucei rhodesiense*, and more recently with *T. brucei gambiense*, have been reported.[129–132] *Trypanosoma brucei* and *T. congolense* cause trypanosomiasis in a variety of domestic animal species ("nagana") but do not infect humans. Dogs are especially susceptible to *T. congolense* infection, and evidence of co-infections with *T. congolense* and *T. brucei rhodesiense* or *T. brucei* was identified using molecular methods in indigenous hunting dogs from eastern Zambia.[130] Three groups of *T. congolense* have been identified—savannah (East and West Africa), forest, and kilifi—which vary in pathogenicity, with savannah being the most pathogenic and kilifi causing mostly subclinical infections in cattle.[133] There are several reports of travel-related infections with *T. congolense* in dogs,[134–138] sometimes in association with a long period of latency.[136] Both savannah-type and forest-type infections have been identified.[132,134,135] African dogs may exhibit a degree of "trypanotolerance," whereas dogs imported into Africa may be more susceptible to infection and disease.[139]

African trypanosomes exist only as a trypomastigote in the blood of the mammalian host; in contrast to Chagas disease, there is no amastigote phase. Epimastigotes develop in the salivary glands of the tsetse fly, and the organism is transmitted in saliva when it feeds on the mammalian host. Transmission to the mammalian host results in hemolymphatic spread of the organism over weeks to months with signs that relate to proliferation of mononuclear phagocytes and increased vascular permeability. *Trypanosoma brucei* complex organisms are well known for their ability to evade the host immune response through extensive variation of their outer surface glycoproteins (known as *variant antigen types,* or *VATs*). The hemolymphatic phase may be followed by the development of meningoencephalitis in some animals. In humans, meningoencephalitis is most apparent with *T. brucei gambiense* infections and results in tremors and progressive daytime somnolescence (hence the term "sleeping sickness"). Pancarditis with arrhythmias and congestive heart failure is a more typical outcome of *T. brucei rhodesiense* infection in humans.

The clinical signs of canine African trypanosomiasis include persistent fever, lethargy, anorexia, weight loss, pallor, mucopurulent oculonasal

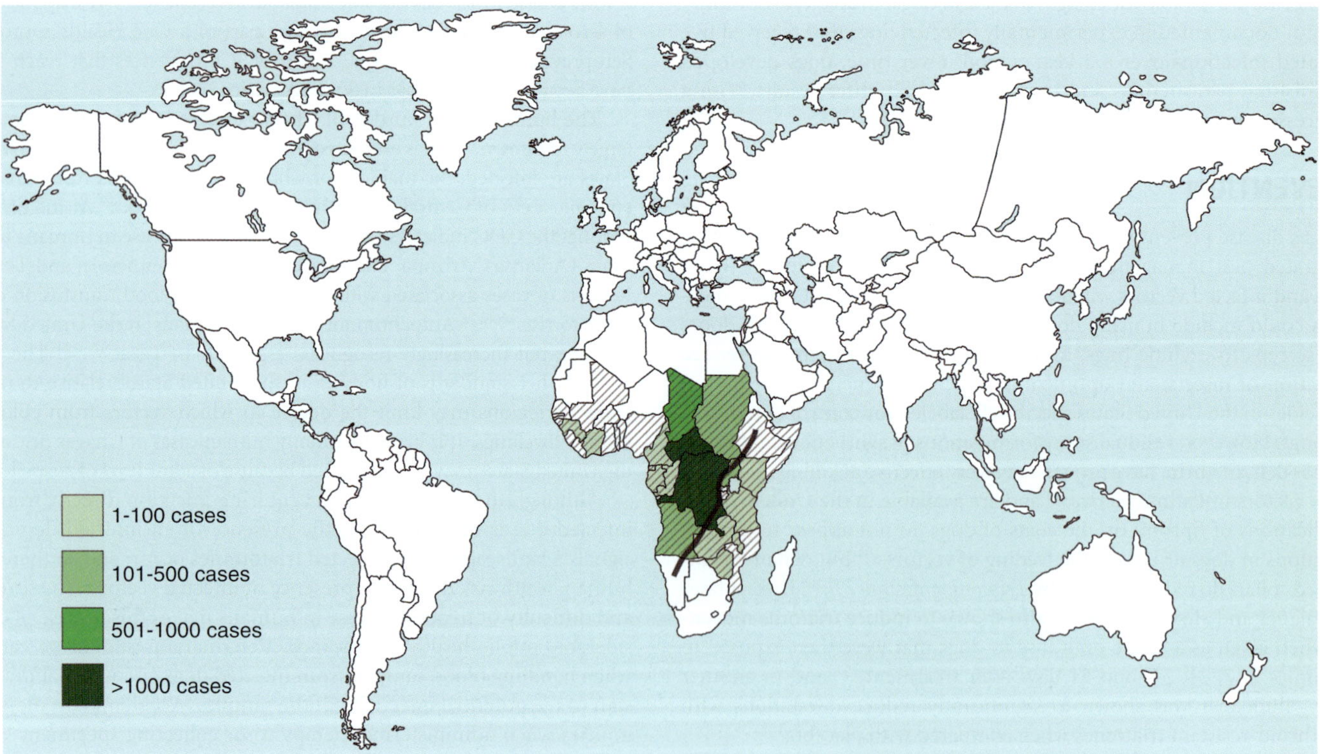

Fig. 100.9 Map showing geographic distribution of human African trypanosomiasis *(green countries)* and the number of cases reported in natives in the year 2009. *Trypanosoma brucei gambiense* is found in western Africa and *Trypanosoma brucei rhodesiense* is found in eastern Africa. The line divides the geographic distribution of the two forms of disease. *Trypanosoma brucei brucei,* which also infects dogs, occurs throughout both regions. The *hashed lines* indicate the countries in which tsetse flies are found. (Modified from Brun R, Blum J. Human African trypanosomiasis. *Inf Dis Clin North Am.* 2012;26:261–273.)

discharge, lymphadenopathy, hepatosplenomegaly, variable peripheral edema, abdominal distention due to ascites, petechial hemorrhages, signs of pancarditis, and ocular signs such as unilateral or bilateral uveitis, corneal edema, and/or keratitis (which can mimic "blue eye" due to canine adenovirus-1). In a study of indigenous hunting dogs from eastern Zambia that used a LAMP assay to detect trypanosomes in blood, bilateral corneal opacity was associated with infection (Fig. 100.10); affected dogs were infected with *T. brucei* (one dog), *T. brucei rhodesiense* (two dogs), or both *T. congolense* and *T. brucei rhodesiense* (one dog).[130] Clinical signs that include lymphadenomegaly and blindness associated with bilateral keratitis have also been described in dogs from Nigeria infected with *T. brucei gambiense.*[132] Hemorrhagic vomiting and diarrhea can occur in dogs infected with *T. congolense.*[137,140] Neurologic signs (seizures, tremors, opisthotonos, and hyperreflexia) due to meningoencephalitis have also been described in dogs infected with *T. congolense.*[137,140] In one dog, seizures were associated with severe hypoglycemia.[134]

Laboratory abnormalities in dogs with African trypanosomiasis have been most well described for *T. congolense* infections. The most common findings are regenerative or nonregenerative anemia, leukocytosis or leukopenia, and thrombocytopenia.[134–137,140] Serum biochemistry findings include increased serum liver enzyme activities, azotemia, hypoglycemia, hyperglobulinemia, and hypoalbuminemia,[134–137] but one dog had no significant abnormal serum biochemistry findings.[138] Severe and refractory hypoglycemia in another dog was thought to be secondary to massive consumption of glucose by replicating trypanosomes.[134]

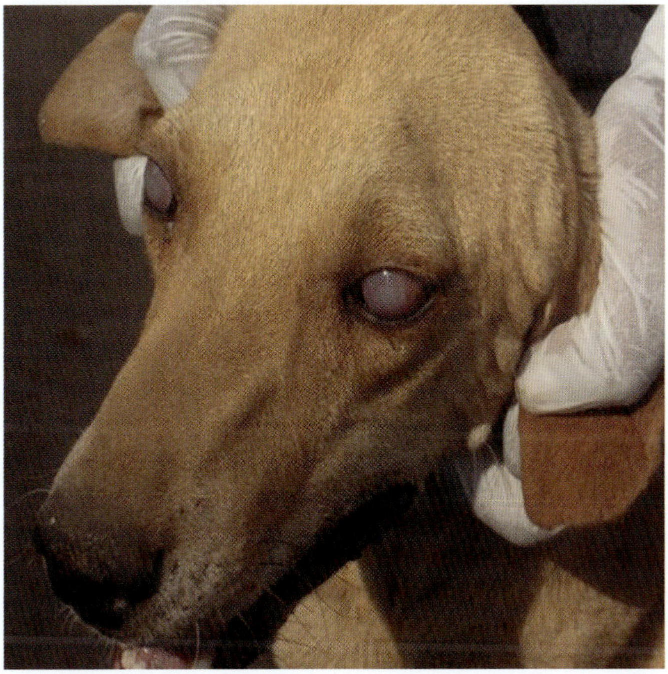

Fig. 100.10 Bilateral corneal opacities/keratitis in an indigenous dog from eastern Zambia with canine African trypanosomiasis. (From Lisulo M, Sugimoto C, Kajino K, et al. Determination of the prevalence of African trypanosome species in indigenous dogs of Mambwe district, eastern Zambia, by loop-mediated isothermal amplification. *Parasit Vectors.* 2014;7:19.)

The primary means of diagnosis is cytologic detection of the organism in aspirates, body fluids, or blood smears. Identification of the infecting species requires PCR and sequencing. The treatment of choice for dogs is diminazene aceturate, but this may not always be effective or available. Treatment of the hemolymphatic disease in humans is with pentamidine isethionate *(gambiense)* or suramin *(rhodesiense)*, whereas disease of the CNS is treated with the arsenical melarsoprol, but these drugs can have significant adverse effects. Pentamidine was used with apparent success to treat dogs with African trypanosomiasis (Table 100.2).[134,141] Prevention is through the use of insect repellants and indoor housing. Isometamidium (Trypamidium, Boehringer Ingelheim) is also used every 2 months (1 mg/kg, IM) as chemoprophylaxis for military dogs in sub-Saharan Africa, especially French working dogs in the Côte d'Ivoire,[135] although disease was reported in one dog despite use of this drug in addition to deltamethrin collars. Complete eradication of *T. congolense* forest type was reported in a dog seen in Austria following treatment with IM isometamidium chloride; before that, clinical improvement with imidocarb and miltefosine treatment was described.[142]

TRYPANOSOMA EVANSI INFECTION

Trypanosoma evansi causes surra (= "rotten") and is endemic in large parts of Asia, Africa, Latin America, and the Canary Islands of Spain. It causes disease in a variety of mammalian host species that include horses, cattle, dogs, and cats, but not humans. *Trypanosoma evansi* is very closely related to *T. brucei* and may have derived from *T. brucei* as a result of partial or complete loss of kinetoplast DNA, which stops it from developing within the insect vector. Instead, the organism is transmitted mechanically by biting flies. Ingestion of infected meat may also lead to infection. Because populations of biting flies are greatest during the rainy season, a seasonal incidence of disease has been observed in dogs.[143] Travel-related disease has been described.[144,145] The disease has an acute course; clinical signs and laboratory abnormalities resemble those of African trypanosomiasis, with lethargy, fever, anorexia, weight loss, pallor, lymphadenomegaly, hepatosplenomegaly, vomiting, arrhythmias, conjunctivitis, uveitis, corneal edema, and peripheral edema, as well as leukopenia, thrombocytopenia, and anemia on the CBC.[143–149] Hyperglobulinemia, hypoalbuminemia and proteinuria have also been reported.[17,24] Some dogs develop neurologic signs late in the course of disease due to nonsuppurative meningoencephalitis.[144] Definitive diagnosis of infection is based on cytologic examination of blood smears and/or PCR assay. A variety of antiprotozoal

TABLE 100.2 Antimicrobials Used To Treat African Trypanosomiasis in Dogs[a]

Drug	Dose (mg/kg)	Route	Interval	Duration (days)
Diminazene aceturate	3–5[b]	Deep IM	Give once or repeat 72 to 96 hours later	NA
Pentamidine isethionate	8 mg/kg on day 1, then 4 mg/kg	IM or IV infusion over 2 to 3 hours	24	10
Suramin	10–20	IV infusion over 3 minutes	Repeat every 7 days	2 months

[a]The availability of these drugs is limited and varies with country. None are readily available in the United States. The optimal dosing protocols, safety, and efficacy for these drugs for treatment of African trypanosomiasis are not well understood in dogs. Neither pentamidine nor suramin penetrate the blood-brain barrier well and so may not be effective for CNS infections. Pre-treatment with antihistamines or nonsteroidal anti-inflammatory drugs may be used to reduce adverse reactions that follow administration.

[b]Diminazene was used successfully to treat *Trypanosoma evansi* infection in cats at 3.5 mg/kg IM daily for 7 days without adverse effects in one study.

CASE EXAMPLE

Signalment

"Duke," a 5-year-old male beagle mix dog from south Texas.

History

Duke's owner reported a 7-day history of inappetence, lethargy, and decreased exercise tolerance. Two months earlier, the dog had been diagnosed with dirofilariasis and was treated with melarsomine dihydrochloride using a split protocol. He had not traveled out of his local area. He was up to date on vaccinations, which included vaccines for distemper, hepatitis, parvovirus, and rabies.

Current medications: Monthly oral ivermectin/pyrantel heartworm preventative.

Physical Examination

Body weight: 19.9 kg.

General: Lethargic. T = 101.7°F (38.7°C), HR = 142 beats/minute, RR = 48 breaths/minute, mucous membranes pink, CRT = 1 second.

Integument, eyes, ears, nose, and throat: Full, shiny haircoat. No evidence of ectoparasites was detected. No other significant abnormalities were noted.

Musculoskeletal: BCS was 6/9.

Cardiovascular: An irregular rhythm and a grade 3/6 systolic left apical murmur were detected on thoracic auscultation. Strong femoral pulses were palpated bilaterally.

Respiratory: Mild tachypnea was identified with normal breath sounds and normal respiratory effort.

GI, genitourinary, and lymph nodes: No abnormalities were detected.

Laboratory Findings

CBC: PCV 48.3% (31%–56%), MCV 66.4 fL (60–77 fL), MCHC 35 g/dL (32–36 g/dL), WBC 13,100 cells/μL (6,000–17,000 cells/μL), neutrophils 8,777 cells/μL (3,000–11,500 cells/μL), lymphocytes 2,096 cells/μL (1,000–4,800 cells/μL), monocytes 1,179 cells/μL (150–1,250 cells/μL), platelets 238,000 platelets/μL (200,000–500,000 platelets/μL).

Serum chemistry profile: Sodium 144 mmol/L (139–147 mmol/L), potassium 3.9 mmol/L (3.3–4.6 mmol/L), chloride 118 mmol/L (107–118 mmol/L), bicarbonate 22 mmol/L (20–28 mmol/L), phosphorus 3.6 mg/dL (2.9–6.2 mg/dL), calcium 9.8 mg/dL (9.3–11.8 mg/dL), BUN 19 mg/dL (5–29 mg/dL), creatinine 1.27 mg/dL (0.3–2.0 mg/dL), glucose 108 mg/dL (60–135 mg/dL), total protein 5.5 g/dL (5.7–7.8 g/dL), albumin 2.6 g/dL (2.4–3.6 g/dL), globulin 2.9 g/dL (1.7–3.8 g/dL), ALT 136 U/L (10–130 U/L), ALP 103 U/L (21–147 U/L), GGT 11 U/L (0–25 U/L), cholesterol 199 mg/dL (120–247 mg/dL), total bilirubin 0.2 mg/dL (0–0.8 mg/dL), magnesium 2.1 mg/dL (1.7–2.1 mg/dL).

Urinalysis: SpG 1.012; pH 7.5, trace protein (SSA), no bilirubin, no glucose, no WBC/HPF, 0–1 RBC/HPF.

Heartworm antigen test: Negative.

Cardiac troponin I: 0.69 ng/mL (<0.2 ng/mL).

Chagas indirect fluorescent antibody titer: Positive at 1:160.

Imaging Findings

Thoracic radiographs: The cardiac silhouette was mildly, generally enlarged. The pulmonary veins were mildly larger than the corresponding artery. A mild pulmonary interstitial pattern was present.

Echocardiogram: The left ventricular internal dimensions were enlarged, and systolic function was reduced (fractional shortening 16.1%, area shortening 26.9%; normal is >25% and >50%, respectively). Moderate mitral regurgitation was documented, and the left atrium was enlarged. The right ventricle was mildly dilated. Pulmonic and aortic velocities were within normal limits. No heartworms were visualized.

Additional Testing

Electrocardiogram: Sinus rhythm with frequent, multiform ventricular premature complexes. Sinus beats conduct with a long PR interval (0.16 seconds) consistent with first-degree atrioventricular block.

Blood pressure: Systolic blood pressure was 115 mmHg.

Diagnosis

American trypanosomiasis (Chagas disease).

Treatment

Medication to address cardiac enlargement, dysfunction, and arrhythmias included pimobendan (0.25 mg/kg, PO, q12h), enalapril (0.5 mg/kg, PO, q12h), and sotalol (1 mg/kg, PO, q12h). This was associated with improvement in clinical signs within 1 week of starting treatment.

Comments

This dog was diagnosed with trypanosomiasis based on an index of suspicion in the presence of ventricular enlargement and dysfunction in combination with multiform ventricular arrhythmias. Infection by *Leishmania* could also have caused the positive serologic test result, but this was considered unlikely based on the geographic location and clinical signs. Antiprotozoal drugs were not used to treat this dog because they do not appear to alter outcome in chronic Chagas disease and they are not available. The dog did very well clinically while being managed with cardiac medications including antiarrhythmics along with routine evaluation. After 2.5 years, ventricular arrhythmias increased in severity and were more difficult to control with antiarrhythmic therapy. He died suddenly at home 5 days after reevaluation.

treatments have been used, especially with diminazene aceturate or suramin, although diminazene aceturate is considered less effective against *T. evansi* than against *T. congolense* infection, and some affected dogs have died or had relapse of parasitemia despite treatment.[144,148,149] In one study that involved an outbreak of infection with a high mortality rate in 38 dogs on a farm in rural Brazil, clinical improvement was reported for 15 of 18 dogs treated with diminazene aceturate (3.5 mg/kg, IM, once).[149]

SUGGESTED READINGS

Vitt JP, Saunders AB, O'Brien MT, et al. Diagnostic features of acute Chagas myocarditis with sudden death in a family of Boxer dogs. *J Vet Intern Med.* 2016;30:1210–1215.

Deschamps JY, Desquesnes M, Dorso L, et al. Refractory hypoglycaemia in a dog infected with *Trypanosoma congolense*. *Parasite.* 2016;23:1.

Lisulo M, Sugimoto C, Kajino K, et al. Determination of the prevalence of African trypanosome species in indigenous dogs of Mambwe district, eastern Zambia, by loop-mediated isothermal amplification. *Parasit Vectors.* 2014;7:19.

REFERENCES

1. Chagas C. Nova tripanosomiase humana. Estudos sobre a morfologia e o ciclo evolutivo do *Schizotrypanum cruzi* n. gen., n. sp., agente etiologico de nova entradade morbida do homen. *Mem Inst Oswaldo Cruz.* 1909;1:1–9.
2. Williams GD, Adams LG, Yaeger RG, et al. Naturally occurring trypanosomiasis (Chagas disease) in dogs. *J Am Vet Med Assoc.* 1977;171:171–177.
3. Steverding D. The history of African trypanosomiasis. *Parasit Vectors.* 2008;1:3.
4. Zingales B, Miles MA, Campbell DA, et al. The revised *Trypanosoma cruzi* subspecific nomenclature: rationale, epidemiological relevance and research applications. *Infect Genet Evol.* 2012;12:240–253.
5. Bern C, Kjos S, Yabsley MJ, Montgomery SP. *Trypanosoma cruzi* and Chagas disease in the United States. *Clin Microbiol Rev.* 2001;24:655–681.
6. Curtis-Robles R, Hamer S, Lane S, et al. Bionomics and spatial distribution of Triatomine vectors of *Trypanosoma cruzi* in Texas and other southern states, USA. *Am J Trop Med Hyg.* 2018;98:113–121.

7. Montenegro VM, Jimenez M, Dias K, et al. Chagas disease in dogs from endemic areas of Costa Rica. *Mem Inst Oswaldo Cruz.* 2002;97:491–494.
8. Roellig DM, Ellis AE, Yabsley MJ. Oral transmission of *Trypanosoma cruzi* with opposing evidence for the theory of carnivory. *J Parasitol.* 2009;95:360–364.
9. Ryckman RE, Folkes DL, Olsen LE, et al. Epizootiology of *Trypanosoma cruzi* in southwestern north America. V. Host parasite specificity between *Trypanosoma cruzi* and *Triatominae* (Kinetoplastida: Trypanosomidae) (Hemiptera: Triatominae). *J Med Entomol.* 1965;2:87–108.
10. Tanowitz HB, Kirchhoff LV, Simon D, et al. Chagas disease. *Clin Microbiol Rev.* 1992;5:400–419.
11. Kjos SA, Snowden KF, Craig TM, et al. Distribution and characterization of canine Chagas disease in Texas. *Vet Parasitol.* 2008;152:249–256.
12. Rowland ME, Maloney J, Cohen S, et al. Factors associated with *Trypanosoma cruzi* exposure among domestic canines in Tennessee. *J Parasitol.* 2010;96:547–551.
13. Tenney TD, Curtis-Robles R, Snowden KF, et al. Shelter dogs as sentinels for *Trypanosoma cruzi* transmission across Texas. *Emerg Infect Dis.* 2014;20:1323–1326.
14. Barr SC, van Beek O, Carlisle-Nowak MS, et al. *Trypanosoma cruzi* infection in Walker hounds from Virginia. *Am J Vet Res.* 1995;56:1037–1044.
15. Bradley KK, Bergman DK, Woods JP, et al. Prevalence of American trypanosomiasis (Chagas disease) among dogs in Oklahoma. *J Am Vet Med Assoc.* 2000;217:1853–1857.
16. Snider TG, Yaeger RG, Dellucky J. Myocarditis caused by *Trypanosoma cruzi* in a native Louisiana dog. *J Am Vet Med Assoc.* 1992;177:247–249.
17. Nieto PD, Boughton R, Dorn PL, et al. Comparison of two immunochromatographic assays and the indirect immunoflourscence antibody test for diagnosis of *Trypanosoma cruzi* infection in dogs in south central Louisiana. *Vet Parasitol.* 2009;165:241–247.
18. Burkholder JE, Allison TC, Kelly VP. *Trypanosoma cruzi* (Chagas) (Protozoa: Kinetoplastida) in invertebrate, reservoir, and human hosts of the lower Rio Grande valley of Texas. *J Parasitol.* 1980;66:305–311.
19. Mazza S. Frecuencia e importancia de la infeccion natural de perros y gatos por *S. cruzi* y cuestion de la herencia del mismo en los primeros animales. *Novena Reunion de la Sociedad Argentina de Patologia Regional.* 1936;1:412–417.
20. Elmayan A, Tu W, Duhon B, et al. High prevalence of *Trypanosoma cruzi* infection in shelter dogs from southern Louisiana, USA. *Parasit Vectors.* 2019;12:322.
21. Busselman RE, Meyers AC, Zecca IB, et al. High incidence of *Trypanosoma cruzi* infections in dogs directly detected through longitudinal tracking at 10 multi-dog kennels, Texas, USA. *PLoS Negl Trop Dis.* 2021;15: e0009935.
22. Dumonteil E, Desale H, Tu W, et al. Shelter cats host infections with multiple *Trypanosoma cruzi* discrete typing units in southern Louisiana. *Vet Res.* 2021;52:53.
23. Souza Campos E. Transmisao intrauterina do *Trypanosoma cruzi* na infeccao experimental do cao. *Ann Fac Med Sao Paulo.* 1928;3:2–7.
24. Castanera MB, Lauricella MA, Chuit R, et al. Evaluation of dogs as sentinels of the transmission of *Trypanosoma cruzi* in a rural area of northwestern Argentina. *Ann Trop Med Parasitol.* 1998;92:671–683.
25. Rodríguez-Morales O, Ballinas-Verdugo MA, Alejandre-Aguilar R, et al. *Trypanosoma cruzi* connatal transmission in dogs with Chagas disease: experimental case report. *Vector Borne Zoonotic Dis.* 2011;11:1365–1370.
26. Barr SC, Brown C, Dennis VA, et al. The lesions and prevalence of *Trypanosoma cruzi* in opossums and armadillos from southern Louisiana. *J Parasitol.* 1991;77:624–627.
27. Barr SC, Dennis VA, Klei TR. Biological characterization of *Trypanosoma cruzi* isolated from Louisiana mammals, abstract no 66. In: *Proc Am Soc Trop Med Hyg.* 1986.
28. Karsten V, Davis C, Kuhn R. *Trypanosoma cruzi* in wild raccoons and opossums in North Carolina. *J Parasitol.* 1992;78:547–549.
29. McKeveer S, Gorman GW, Norman L. Occurrence of a *Trypanosoma cruzi*-like organisms in some mammals from southwestern Georgia and Northwestern Florida. *J Parasitol.* 1958;44:583–587.
30. Navin TR, Roberto RR, Juranek DD, et al. Human and sylvatic *Trypanosoma cruzi* infections in California. *Am J Public Health.* 1985;75:366–369.
31. Yaeger RG. The prevalence of *Trypanosoma cruzi* infection in armadillos collected at a site near New Orleans, Louisiana. *Am J Trop Med Hyg.* 1988;38:323–326.
32. Curtis-Robles R, Lewis BC, Hamer SA. High *Trypanosoma cruzi* infection prevalence associated with minimal cardiac pathology among wild carnivores in central Texas. *Int J Parasitol Parasites Wild.* 2016;5:117–123.
33. Walton BC, Bauman PM, Diamond LS, et al. The isolation and identification of *Trypanosoma cruzi* from raccoons in Maryland. *Am J Trop Med Hyg.* 1958;7:603–610.
34. John DT, Hoppe KL. *Trypanosoma cruzi* from wild raccoons in Oklahoma. *Am J Vet Res.* 1986;47:1056–1059.
35. Yabsley MJ, Noblet GP. Seroprevalence of *Trypanosoma cruzi* in raccoons from South Carolina and Georgia. *J Wildl Dis.* 2002;38:75–83.
36. Pietrzak SM, Pung OJ. Trypanosomiasis in raccoons from Georgia. *J Wildl Dis.* 1998;34:132–136.
37. Pung OJ, Banks CW, Jones DN, et al. *Trypanosoma cruzi* in wild raccoons, opossums, and triatomine bugs in southeast Georgia, USA. *J Parasitol.* 1995;81:324–326.
38. Wood SF. Additional observations on *Trypanosoma cruzi* Chagas, from Arizona in insects, rodents, and experimentally infected animals. *Am J Trop Med Hyg.* 1949;29:43–55.
39. Wood SF, Wood FD. Observations on vectors of Chagas disease in the United States: III. New Mexico. *Am J Trop Med Hyg.* 1961;10:155–165.
40. Pippin WF. The biology and vector capability of *Triatoma sanguisuga texana* (Usinger) and *Triatoma gerstaeckeri* (Stal) compared with *Rhodnius prolixus* (Stal) (Hemiptera: Triatominae). *J Med Entomol.* 1970;7:30–45.
41. Wood SF. *Trypanosoma cruzi*: new foci of enzootic Chagas disease in California. *Exp Parasitol.* 1975;38:153–160.
42. Barr SC, Dennis VA, Klei TR. Serologic and blood culture survey of *Trypanosoma cruzi* for infection in four canine populations of southern Louisiana. *Am J Vet Res.* 1991;52:570–573.
43. Barr SC, Gossett KA, Klei TR. Clinical, clinicopathologic, and parasitologic observations of trypanosomiasis in dogs infected with North American *Trypanosoma cruzi* isolates. *Am J Vet Res.* 1991;52: 954–960.
44. Barr SC, Holmes RA, Klei TR. Electrocardiographic and echocardiographic features of trypanosomiasis in dogs inoculated with North American *Trypanosoma cruzi* isolates. *Am J Vet Res.* 1992;53:521–527.
45. Dorn PL, Daigle ME, Combe CL, Tate AH, et al. Low prevalence of Chagas parasite infection in a nonhuman primate colony in Louisiana. *J Am Assoc Lab Anim Sci.* 2012;51:443–447.
46. Bryan LK, Hamer SA, Shaw S, et al. Chagas disease in a Texan horse with neurologic deficits. *Vet Parasitol.* 2016;216:13–17.
47. Andrade ZA. Immunopathology of Chagas disease. *Mem Inst Oswaldo Cruz.* 1999;94(suppl 1):71–80.
48. Guedes PMM, Veloso VM, Afonso LCC, et al. Development of chronic cardiomyopathy in canine Chagas disease correlates with high INF-γ, TNF-α and low IL-10 production during the acute infection phase. *Vet Immunol Immunopathol.* 2009;130:43–52.
49. Guedes PMM, Veloso VM, Gollob KJ, et al. IgG isotype profile is correlated with cardiomegaly in Beagle dogs infected with distinct *Trypanosoma cruzi* strains. *Vet Immunol Immunopathol.* 2008;124:163–168.
50. Cruz-Chan J, Bolio-Gonzalez M, Colin-Flores R, et al. Immunopathology of natural infection with *Trypanosoma cruzi* in dogs. *Vet Parasitol.* 2009;162:151–155.
51. Barr SC, Schmidt SP, Brown CC, et al. Pathologic features of dogs inoculated with North American *Trypanosoma cruzi* isolates. *Am J Vet Res.* 1991;52:2033–2039.
52. Barr SC, Simpson RM, Schmidt SP, et al. Chronic dilatative myocarditis caused by *Trypanosoma cruzi* in two dogs. *J Am Vet Med Assoc.* 1989;195:1237–1241.
53. Barr SC. Canine Chagas disease (American trypanosomiasis) in North America. *Vet Clin Small Anim.* 2009;39:1055–1064.
54. Berger SL, Palmer RH, Hodges CC, et al. Neurologic manifestations of trypanosomiasis in a dog. *J Am Vet Med Assoc.* 1991;198:132–134.

55. Barr SC. Canine American trypanosomiasis. *Compend Contin Educ Pract Vet.* 1991;13:745–755.
56. Meyers AC, Ellis MM, Purnell JC, et al. Selected cardiac abnormalities in *Trypanosoma cruzi* serologically positive, discordant, and negative working dogs along the Texas-Mexico border. *BMC Vet Res.* 2020;16:101.
57. Matthews DJ, Saunders AB, Meyers AC, et al. Cardiac diagnostic test results and outcomes in 44 dogs naturally infected with Trypanosoma cruzi. *J Vet Intern Med.* 2021;35:1800–1809.
58. Meurs KM, Anthony MA, Slater M, et al. Chronic *Trypanosoma cruzi* infection in dogs: 11 cases (1987-1996). *J Am Vet Med Assoc.* 1998;213:497–500.
59. Guedes PMM, Veloso VM, Talvani A, et al. Increased type 1 chemokine expression in experimental Chagas disease correlates with cardiac pathology in Beagle dogs. *Vet Immunol Immunopathol.* 2010;138:106–113.
60. Machado CR, Caliari MV, de Lana M, et al. Heart autonomic innervation during the acute phase of experimental American trypanosomiasis in the dog. *Am J Trop Med Hyg.* 1998;59:492–496.
61. Kirchhoff LV. *Trypanosoma* species (American Trypanosomiasis, Chagas disease): biology of trypanosomes. In: Mandell GL, Bennett JE, Dolin R, eds. *Principles and Practice of Infectious Diseases.* 7th ed. Philadelphia, PA: Elsevier; 2009:3481–3488.
62. Machado EM, Camilo Júnior DJ, Pinheiro SW, et al. Morphometry of submucous and myenteric esophagic plexus of dogs experimentally reinfected with *Trypanosoma cruzi. Mem Inst Oswaldo Cruz.* 2001;96:545–548.
63. Nabity MB, Barnhart K, Logan KS, et al. An atypical case of *Trypanosoma cruzi* infection in a young English Mastiff. *Vet Parasitol.* 2006;140:356–361.
64. Gürtler RE, Cecere MC, Lauricella MA, et al. Domestic dogs and cats as sources of *Trypanosoma cruzi* infection in rural northwestern Argentina. *Parasitology.* 2007;134(Pt 1):69–82.
65. Mott KE, Mota EA, Sherlock I, et al. *Trypanosoma cruzi* infection in dogs and cats and household seroreactivity to *T. cruzi* in a rural community in northeast Brazil. *Am J Trop Med Hyg.* 1978;27:1123–1127.
66. Jimenez-Corello M, Acosta-Viana KY, Guzman-Marin E, et al. Epidemiologic survey of *Trypanosoma cruzi* infection in domestic owned cats from the tropical southeast of Mexico. *Zoonoses Public Health.* 2012;59(suppl 2):102–109.
67. Zecca IB, Hodo CL, Slack S, et al. Prevalence of *Trypanosoma cruzi* infection and associated histologic findings in domestic cats (*Felis catus*). *Vet Parasitol.* 2019;278:109014.
68. Meyers AC, Purnell JC, Ellis MM, et al. Nationwide exposure of U.S. working dogs to the Chagas disease parasite, *Trypanosoma cruzi. Am J Trop Med Hyg.* 2020;102:1078–1085.
69. Meyers AC, Hamer SA, Matthews DM, et al. Risk factors and select cardiac characteristics associated with *Trypanosoma cruzi* infection in naturally infected dogs presenting to a teaching hospital in Texas. *J Vet Intern Med.* 2019;33:1695–1706.
70. Guedes PM, Veloso VM, Mineo TW, et al. Hematological alterations during experimental canine infection by *Trypanosoma cruzi. Rev Bras Parasitol Vet.* 2012;21:151–156.
71. Quijano-Hernandez IA, Castro-Barcena A, Aparicio-Burgos E, et al. Evaluation of clinical and immunopathological features of different infective doses of *Trypanosoma cruzi* in dogs during the acute phase. *Scientific World Journal.* 2012;2012. Article ID 635169.
72. Jaimes-Dueñez J, Jiménez-Leaño AP, Esteban-Mendoza M, et al. Epidemiological and clinical characteristics of *Trypanosoma cruzi* infection in dogs (*Canis lupus familiaris*) from a Chagas disease-endemic urban area in Colombia. *Prev Vet Med.* 2020;182:105093.
73. Patel JM, Rosypal AC, Zimmerman KL, et al. Isolation, mouse pathogenicity, and genotyping of *Trypanosoma cruzi* from an English Cocker Spaniel from Virginia, USA. *Vet Parasitol.* 2012;187:394–398.
74. Vitt JP, Saunders AB, O'Brien MT, et al. Diagnostic features of acute Chagas myocarditis with sudden death in a family of Boxer dogs. *J Vet Intern Med.* 2016;30:1210–1215.
75. Russell KE, Barnhart KF, Fryer JS, et al. Buffy coat smear from a puppy. *Vet Clin Pathol.* 2002;31:9–12.
76. Araujo FM, Bahia MT, Magalhaes NM, et al. Follow-up of experimental chronic Chagas disease in dogs: use of polymerase chain reaction (PCR) compared with parasitological and serological methods. *Acta Trop.* 2002;81:21–31.
77. Grosjean NL, Vrable RA, Murphy AJ, et al. Seroprevalence of antibodies against *Leishmania* spp. among dogs in the United States. *J Am Vet Med Assoc.* 2003;222:603–606.
78. Troncarelli MZ, Camargo KB, Machado JG, et al. *Leishmania* spp. and/or *Trypanosoma cruzi* diagnosis in dogs from endemic and nonendemic areas for canine visceral leishmaniasis. *Vet Parasitol.* 2009;164:118–123.
79. Duprey ZH, Steurer FJ, Rooney JA, et al. Canine visceral leishmaniasis, United States and Canada, 2000-2003. *Emerg Infect Dis.* 2006;12:440–446.
80. Cardinal MV, Reithinger R, Gurtler RE. Use of an immunochromatographic dipstick test for rapid detection of *Trypanosoma cruzi* in sera from animal reservoir hosts. *J Clin Microbiol.* 2006;44:3005–3007.
81. Nieto PD, Boughton R, Dorn PL, et al. Comparison of two immunochromatographic assays and the indirect immunofluorescence antibody test for diagnosis of *Trypanosoma cruzi* infection in dogs in south central Louisiana. *Vet Parasitol.* 2009;165:241–247.
82. Barbabosa-Pliego A, Díaz-Albiter HM, Ochoa-García L, et al. *Trypanosoma cruzi* circulating in the southern region of the State of Mexico (Zumpahuacan) are pathogenic: a dog model. *Am J Trop Med Hyg.* 2009;81:390–395.
83. Araujo FM, Bahia MT, Magalhaes NM, et al. Follow-up of experimental chronic Chagas disease in dogs: use of polymerase chain reaction (PCR) compared with parasitological and serological methods. *Acta Trop.* 2002;81:21–31.
84. Veloso VM, Guedes PMM, Andrade IM, et al. *Trypanosoma cruzi*: blood parasitism kinetics and their correlation with heart parasitism intensity during long-term infection of beagle dogs. *Mem Inst Oswaldo Cruz.* 2008;103:528–534.
85. Madigan R, Majoy S, Ritter K, et al. Investigation of a combination of amiodarone and itraconazole for treatment of American trypanosomiasis (Chagas disease) in dogs. *J Am Vet Med Assoc.* 2019;255:317–329.
86. Andrade ZA, Andrade SG, Sadigursky M, et al. The indeterminate phase of Chagas disease: ultrastructural characterization of cardiac changes in the canine model. *Am J Trop Med Hyg.* 1997;57:328–336.
87. Rodriques Coura J, de Castro SL. A critical review on Chagas disease chemotherapy. *Mem Inst Oswaldo Cruz.* 2002;97:3–24.
88. Wilkinson SR, Taylor MC, Horn D, et al. A mechanism for cross-resistance to nifurtimox and benznidazole in trypanosomes. *Proc Natl Acad Sci USA.* 2008;105:5022–5027.
89. Haberkorn A, Gonnert R. Animal experimental investigations into the activity of nifurtimox against *Trypanosoma cruzi. Arzneimittelforschung.* 1972;22:1570–1582.
90. Guedes PMM, Veloso VM, Tafuri WL, et al. The dog as model for chemotherapy of the Chagas disease. *Acta Trop.* 2002;84:9–17.
91. Santos FM, et al. Chagas cardiomyopathy: the potential effect of benznidazole treatment on diastolic dysfunction and cardiac damage in dogs chronically infected with *Trypanosoma cruzi. Acta Trop.* 2016;161:44–54.
92. Caldas IS, Talbani A, Caldas S, et al. Benznidazole therapy during acute phase of Chagas disease reduces parasite load but does not prevent chronic cardiac lesions. *Parasitol Res.* 2008;103:413–421.
93. Santos FM, Lima WG, Gravel AS, et al. Cardiomyopathy prognosis after benznidazole treatment in chronic canine Chagas disease. *J Antimicrob Chemother.* 2012;67:1987–1995.
94. Rassi Jr A, Neto MJA, Rassi A. Chronic Chagas cardiomyopathy: a review of the main pathogenic mechanisms and the efficacy of aetiological treatment following the BENznidazole Evaluation for Interrupting Trypanosomiasis (BENEFIT) trial. *Mem Inst Oswaldo Cruz.* 2017;112:224–235.
95. Gallerano RH, Marr JJ, Sosa RR. Therapeutic efficacy of allopurinol in patients with chronic Chagas disease. *Am J Trop Med Hyg.* 1990;43:159–166.
96. Guedes PMM, Urbina JA, de Lana M, et al. Activity of a new triaole derivative albaconazole against *Trypanosoma* (*Schizotrypanum*) *cruzi* in dog hosts. *Antimicrob Agents Chemother.* 2004;48:4286–4292.

97. Marr JJ, Docampo R. Chemotherapy for Chagas disease: a perspective of current therapy and considerations for future research. *Rev Infect Dis.* 1986;8:884–903.
98. Rovai LE, Aoki A, Gerez de Burgos NM, et al. Effect of gossypol on trypomastigotes and amastigotes of *Trypanosoma cruzi*. *J Protozool.* 1990;37:280–286.
99. Molina I, Gomez J, Salvador F, et al. Randomized trial of posaconazole and benznidazole for chronic Chagas disease. *N Engl J Med.* 2014;370:1899–1908.
100. Cunha ELA, Torchelsen FKVDS, Cunha LM, et al. Benznidazole, itraconazole and their combination in the treatment of acute experimental Chagas disease in dogs. *Exp Parasitol.* 2019;204:107711.
101. Saunders AB, Gordon SG, Rector MH, et al. Bradyarrhythmias and pacemaker therapy in dogs with Chagas disease. *J Vet Intern Med.* 2013;27:890–894.
102. Machado EM, Fernandes AJ, Murta SM, et al. A study of experimental reinfection by *Trypanosoma cruzi* in dogs. *Am J Trop Med Hyg.* 2001;65:958–965.
103. Rojas de Arias A, Lehane MJ, Schofield CJ, et al. Comparative evaluation of pyrethroid insecticide formulations against *Triatoma infestans* (Klug): residual efficacy on four substrates. *Mem Inst Oswaldo Cruz.* 2003;98:975–980.
104. Gurtler RE, Ceballos LA, Stariolo R, et al. Effects of topical application of fipronil spot-on on dogs against the Chagas disease vector *Triatoma infestans*. *Trans R Soc Trop Med Hyg.* 2009;103:98–304.
105. Reithinger R, Ceballos L, Stariolo R, et al. Chagas disease control: deltamethrin-treated collars reduce *Triatoma infestans* feeding success on dogs. *Trans R Soc Trop Med Hyg.* 2005;99:502–508.
106. Reithinger R, Ceballos L, Stariolo R, et al. Extinction of experimental *Triatoma infestans* populations following continuous exposure to dogs wearing deltamethrin-treated collars. *Am J Trop Med Hyg.* 2006;74:766–771.
107. Loza A, Talaga A, Herbas G, et al. Systemic insecticide treatment of the canine reservoir of *Trypanosoma cruzi* induces high level of lethality in *Triatoma infestans*, a principal vector of Chagas disease. *Parasit Vectors.* 2017;10:344.
108. Laiño MA, Cardinal MV, Gaspe MS, et al. Control of pyrethroid-resistant populations of *Triatoma infestans*, the main vector of *Trypanosoma cruzi*, by treating dogs with fluralaner in the Argentine Chaco. *Med Vet Entomol.* 2021;Dec 6. Online ahead of print.
109. Marsden PD, Hagstrom JW. Experimental *Trypanosoma cruzi* infection in beagle puppies. The effect of variations in the dose and source of infecting trypanosomes and the route of inoculation on the course of the infection. *Trans R Soc Trop Med Hyg.* 1968;62:816–824.
110. Gürtler RE, Cecere MC, Lauricella MA, et al. Domestic dogs and cats as sources of *Trypanosoma cruzi* infection in rural northwestern Argentina. *Parasitology.* 2007;134(Pt 1):69–82.
111. Petersen RM, Gurtler RE, Cecere MC, et al. Association between nutritional indicators and infectivity of dogs seroreactive for *Trypanosoma cruzi* in a rural area of northwestern Argentina. *Parasitol Res.* 2001;87:208–214.
112. Espinosa R, Carrasco HA, Belandria F, et al. Life expectancy analysis in patients with Chagas disease: prognosis after one decade (1973-1983). *Int J Cardiol.* 1985;8:45–56.
113. Estrada-Franco JG, Bhatia V, Diaz-Albiter H, et al. Human *Trypanosoma cruzi* infection and seropositivity in dogs, Mexico. *Emerg Infect Dis.* 2006;12:624–630.
114. Cardinal MV, Lauricella MA, Ceballos LA, et al. Molecular epidemiology of domestic and sylvatic *Trypanosoma cruzi* infection in rural northwestern Argentina. *Int J Parasitol.* 2008;38:1533–1543.
115. Toscano de Araújo-Neto VT, Honorato NRM, de Oliveira Santana R, et al. *Trypanosoma cruzi* circulating among dogs and triatomines in the endemic countryside of the State of Rio Grande do Norte, Brazil. *Acta Trop.* 2019;200:105067.
116. Costa TF, Rocha AVVO, Miranda LM, et al. Seroprevalence and detection of *Trypanosoma cruzi* in dogs living in a non-endemic area for Chagas disease in the legal Amazon region, Brazil. *Vet Parasitol Reg Stud Reports.* 2021;26:100648.
117. Santos F, Magalhães-Junior JT, de Oliveira Carneiro I, et al. Eco-epidemiology of vectorial *Trypanosoma cruzi* transmission in a region of northeast Brazil. *Acta Trop.* 2022;225:106184.
118. Opazo A, Bacigalupo A, Urrutia S, et al. Detection of *Trypanosoma cruzi* infection by PCR in *Canis lupus familiaris* and their ectoparasites in Chile. *Med Vet Entomol.* 2021;Oct 30. Online ahead of print.
119. Manne-Goehler J, Umeh CA, Montgomery SP, et al. E estimating the burden of Chagas disease in the United States. *PLoS Negl Trop Dis.* 2016;10(11):e0005033.
120. Kirchhoff LV. American trypanosomiasis (Chagas disease)—a tropical disease now in the United States. *N Engl J Med.* 1993;329:639–644.
121. Schmunis GA. *Trypanosoma cruzi*, the etiologic agent of Chagas disease: status in the blood supply in endemic and nonendemic countries. *Transfusion.* 1991;31:547–557.
122. Garcia MN, Woc-Colburn L, Rossmann SN, et al. *Trypanosoma cruzi* screening in Texas blood donors, 2008-2012. *Epidemiol Infect.* 2016;144:1010–1013.
123. Garcia MN, Aguilar D, Gochakov R, et al. Case report: evidence of autochthonous Chagas disease in southeastern Texas. *Am J Trop Med Hyg.* 2015;92:325–330.
124. Lynn MK, Bossak BH, Sandifer PA, et al. Contemporary autochthonous human Chagas disease in the USA. *Acta Trop.* 2020;205:105361.
125. De S, Pinto AG, Schubach TMP, Figueiredo FB, et al. Isolation of *Trypanosoma caninum* in domestic dogs in Rio de Janeiro, Brazil. *Parasitology.* 2010;137:1653–1660.
126. Madeira MF, Almeida ABPF, Barros JHS, et al. *Trypanosoma caninum*, a new parasite described in dogs in Brazil: aspects of natural infection. *J Parasitol.* 2014;100:231–234.
127. Makino H, Moreira J, Bezerra KS, et al. Clinical-dermatological, histological abnormalities and prevalence of *Trypanosoma caninum* and *Leishmania infantum* in dogs from Midwest region of Brazil. *Rev Bras Parasitol Vet.* 2020;29:e016319.
128. de Oliveira Tda S, Barros JH, Perez TD, et al. Report of new cases of *Trypanosoma caninum* in Brazil. *Rev Soc Bras Med Trop.* 2015;48:347–349.
129. Vourchakbe J, Tiofack ZAA, Kante TS, et al. Molecular identification of *Trypanosoma brucei gambiense* in naturally infected pigs, dogs and small ruminants confirms domestic animals as potential reservoirs for sleeping sickness in Chad. *Parasite.* 2020;27:63.
130. Lisulo M, Sugimoto C, Kajino K, et al. Determination of the prevalence of African trypanosome species in indigenous dogs of Mambwe district, eastern Zambia, by loop-mediated isothermal amplification. *Parasit Vectors.* 2014;7:19.
131. Matete GO. Occurrence, clinical manifestation and the epidemiological implications of naturally occurring canine trypanosomosis in western Kenya. *Onderstepoort J Vet Res.* 2003;70:317–323.
132. Umeakuana PU, Gibson W, Ezeokonkwo RC, et al. Identification of *Trypanosoma brucei gambiense* in naturally infected dogs in Nigeria. *Parasit Vectors.* 2019;12:420.
133. Fogue PS, Njiokou F, Simo G. Genetic structure of *Trypanosoma congolense* "forest type" circulating in domestic animals and tsetse flies in the South-West region of Cameroon. *Parasite.* 2017;24:51.
134. Deschamps JY, Desquesnes M, Dorso L, et al. Refractory hypoglycaemia in a dog infected with *Trypanosoma congolense*. *Parasite.* 2016;23:1.
135. Calvet F, Medkour H, Mediannikov O, et al. An African canine trypanosomosis case import: is there a possibility of creating a secondary focus of *Trypanosoma congolense* infection in France? *Pathogens.* 2020;9:709.
136. Gow AG, Simpson JW, Picozzi K. First report of canine African trypanosomosis in the UK. *J Small Anim Pract.* 2007;48:658–661.
137. Harrus S, Harmelin A, Presenty B, et al. *Trypanosoma congolense* infection in two dogs. *J Small Anim Pract.* 1995;36:83–86.
138. Museux K, Boulouha L, Majani S, et al. African *Trypanosoma* infection in a dog in France. *Vet Rec.* 2011;168:590.
139. Horchner F, Zillmann U, Metzner M, et al. West African dogs as a model for research on trypanotolerance. *Trop Med Parasitol.* 1985;36:257–258.
140. Ezeokonkwo RC, Ezeh IO, Onunkwo JI, et al. Comparative haematological study of single and mixed infections of mongrel dogs with

Trypanosoma congolense and *Trypanosoma brucei brucei*. *Vet Parasitol.* 2010;173:48–54.
141. 't Hooft EM. Canine African trypanosoma. *J Small Anim Pract.* 2008;49:487.
142. Leschnik M, Silbermayr K, Guija A, et al. Diagnosis and successful treatment of an Austrian dog infected with *Trypanosoma congolense* forest type. *Tierarztl Prax Ausg K Kleintiere Heimtiere.* 2021;49:142–147.
143. Singh B, Kalra IS, Gupta MP, et al. *Trypanosoma evansi* infection in dogs: seasonal prevalence and chemotherapy. *Vet Parasitol.* 1993;50:137–141.
144. Defontis M, Richartz J, Engelmann N, et al. Canine *Trypanosoma evansi* infection introduced into Germany. *Vet Clin Pathol.* 2012;41:369–374.
145. Hellebrekers LJ, Slappendel RJ. Trypanosomiasis in a dog imported in The Netherlands. *Vet Q.* 1982;4:182–186.
146. Aquino LP, Machado RZ, Alessi AC, et al. Clinical, parasitological and immunological aspects of experimental infection with *Trypanosoma evansi* in dogs. *Mem Inst Oswaldo Cruz.* 1999;94:255–260.
147. Bui KL, Duong DH, Bui DTA, et al. A case of *Trypanosoma evansi* in a German Shepherd dog in Vietnam. *Parasitol Int.* 2021;80:102198.
148. Dangolla A, Wijesundara DLR, Blair D, et al. Canine trypanosomosis in Sri Lanka: an emerging problem reported from three distinct geographic locations. *Parasitol Int.* 2020;77:102129.
149. Echeverria JT, Soares RL, Crepaldi BA, et al. Clinical and therapeutic aspects of an outbreak of canine trypanosomiasis. *Rev Bras Parasitol Vet.* 2019;28:320–324.

Giardiasis

Valeria Scorza, Michael R. Lappin

KEY POINTS

- Cause: *Giardia duodenalis* (multiple genetic assemblages); a flagellate protozoan (phylum Sarcomastigophora).
- First Described: Trophozoites that were likely *Giardia* spp. were first described in 1681 by Antonie van Leeuwenhoek and the genus was established in the early 1900s. Infections of dogs and cats were first described in the 1960s.[1,2]
- Affected Host Species: Dogs and cats are the definitive hosts for several different *Giardia* assemblages and pass either trophozoites (diarrhea) or cysts (diarrhea or normal stool) in feces.
- Intermediate Hosts: Although there are no intermediate hosts, there are multiple potential transport hosts that may carry *Giardia* spp. cysts and indirectly infect dogs or cats.
- Route of transmission: Fecal-oral.
- Geographic Distribution: Worldwide.
- Major Clinical Signs: Most dogs and cats harbor subclinical infections. Acute watery diarrhea that can contain mucus can occur. Steatorrhea can be observed. Chronic or intermittent diarrhea and weight loss may be noted in animals with concurrent infections or immunocompromise.
- Differential Diagnoses: All causes of small bowel diarrhea including *Cystoisospora* spp., *Cryptosporidium* spp., bacterial infections such as salmonellosis, nematode infections, dietary intolerance, exocrine pancreatic insufficiency, and inflammatory bowel disease.
- Human Health Significance: *Giardia duodenalis* assemblages that infect dogs (assemblages C and D) or cats (assemblage F) are usually not associated with clinical disease in humans but can be detected in the feces of immunocompromised people.[3] Human assemblages A and B can be found in feces of dogs and cats when animals share human environmental features (such as contaminated water). However, it is unlikely that new human infections with *G. duodenalis* assemblage A or B infections are acquired from the feces of dogs or cats.

ETIOLOGIC AGENT AND EPIDEMIOLOGY

Enteric protozoa covered in this book are limited to four protozoan genera: *Giardia*, *Tritrichomonas*, and *Entamoeba* in the phylum Sarcomastigophora (having flagella or pseudopodia); and *Balantidium* in the phylum Ciliophora (having cilia). For perspective, salient characteristics of these organisms and the diseases they may cause are presented in Table 101.1. A detailed coverage of laboratory methods for diagnosis of enteric protozoal infections is presented in Chapter 5, and more information on treatment can be found in Chapter 12.

Giardia duodenalis is a protozoan parasite with worldwide distribution that infects a variety of mammals. Several other species of *Giardia* exist that infect other hosts (Table 101.2). Molecular characterization studies report that *G. duodenalis* is a species complex comprising eight assemblages (A to H). Some of the assemblages have been detected in animals and humans, but some others are species-specific. Dogs usually harbor the species-specific C-D assemblages, and cats usually harbor the cat-specific assemblage F (Table 101.3 and Fig. 101.1). Assemblages A and B have been reported in humans and other mammals including cats and dogs (Table 101.3).[4-8] Many studies have evaluated the prevalence of *Giardia* spp. infection and different assemblages in dogs and cats worldwide, and prevalences vary widely depending on the test used and the population studied (Tables 101.4, 101.5, 101.6, and 101.7). A meta-analysis showed that *Giardia* spp. estimated pooled prevalence rates of 15.2% and 12% for dogs and cats, respectively.[9]

Giardia spp. occur in two forms, the trophozoite and the cyst form. The trophozoite (15 μm long and 8 μm wide) is the active, motile form that is found in the intestinal tract (Figs. 101.2 and 101.3). The trophozoites can be identified under light microscopy by the "smiling-face" appearance, which is formed by the two nuclei in the anterior third forming the eyes, the axonemes passing longitudinally between the nuclei forming the nose, and the median bodies located transversely in the posterior third forming the mouth; four pairs of flagella complete the shape.[10] Trophozoites are susceptible to inactivation by many environmental conditions, and are usually not responsible for spread among animals.

The cyst (12 μm long and 7 μm wide) form is the resistant stage that is mainly responsible for transmission. The cyst contains two incompletely separated but formed trophozoites, their axonemes, fragments of the ventral discs, and as many as four nuclei (Fig. 101.4). *Giardia* spp. are transmitted by the direct ingestion of fecal cysts or by indirect ingestion of contaminated water, food, transport hosts, infected prey species, or fomites (Fig. 101.5). Many infected hosts excrete fecal cysts for months, but infections may also be self-limited in 27 to 35 days in dogs and cats.

CLINICAL FEATURES

Pathogenesis And Clinical Signs

Although the pathogenesis of *Giardia* infection is not completely understood, it is suggested that is multifactorial with a combination of intestinal malabsorption and hypersecretion as the primary mechanisms associated with the development of diarrhea. *Giardia* colonize the lumen and epithelial surface but do not invade deeper mucosal layers. *Giardia* infection causes disruption of tight junctions and cytoskeleton proteins resulting in increased intestinal permeability and decreased transepithelial resistance.[11] The host-parasite interaction leads to the upregulation of genes involved in the apoptotic cascade and in the formation of reactive oxygen species.[12] The induction of

TABLE 101.1 Comparison of Some Enteric Protozoa in Dogs and Cats

Organism	Stage	Average Size (μm)	Natural Hosts	Organ Parasitized	Pathogenic Mechanisms	Clinical Signs
Giardia[a]	Tr Cy	15 × 10 × 3 10 × 8	D, C, H, other mammals	Small intestine	Damage to glycocalyx and microvilli on intestinal epithelium; inhibition of some digestive enzymes; host elicits inflammatory response	None to chronic diarrhea, continuous or intermittent, malabsorption
Entamoeba histolytica	Tr Cy	25 (diam) 12 (diam)	D, C, H, NHP	Large intestine	Invades colonic wall, producing ulcers; may spread to extraintestinal sites	None to diarrhea; dysentery
Balantidium coli	Tr Cy	60 × 35 50 (diam)	D, P, H, NHP	Large intestine	Invades colonic wall, producing ulcers, dissemination (rare)	None to diarrhea; dysentery
Pentatrichomonas hominis	Tr	8 × 5, five flagella	D, C, H, other mammals	Large intestine	Probably none; considered harmless commensal but may be opportunistic pathogen	None to diarrhea
Tritrichomonas blagburni	Tr	8 × 5, three flagella	D, C, Ca, P	Genitalia (cattle) Intestine, nasal (swine) Large intestine (cat)	Epithelial adherent, elaboration of cytotoxins and enzymes; host elicits inflammatory response	Large bowel diarrhea in cats; infertility and fetal loss in cattle

[a]Some *Giardia* species can be microscopically indistinguishable.
C, cat; *Ca*, cattle; *Cy*, cyst; *D*, dog; *H*, human; *NHP*, nonhuman primate; *P*, pig; *Tr*, trophozoite.

TABLE 101.2 *Giardia* Species and Their Corresponding Hosts[91]

Giardia Species	Host
Giardia agilis	Amphibians
Giardia ardae	Birds
Giardia microti	Muskrats and voles
Giardia muris	Rodents
Giardia psittaci	Birds
Giardia varani	Lizards
Giardia duodenalis	Mammals

TABLE 101.3 Host Distribution and Taxonomy of the Eight Currently Recognized Assemblages within *Giardia duodenalis* Species Complex[5]

Assemblage	Proposed Species Name	Main Host
A	*Giardia duodenalis*	Humans and other mammals
B	*Giardia enterica*	Humans and other mammals
C	*Giardia canis*	Domestic and wild canids
D	*Giardia canis*	Domestic and wild canids
E	*Giardia bovis*	Hoofed animals
F	*Giardia cati*	Cats
G	*Giardia simondi*	Rodents
H	None proposed	Pinnipeds

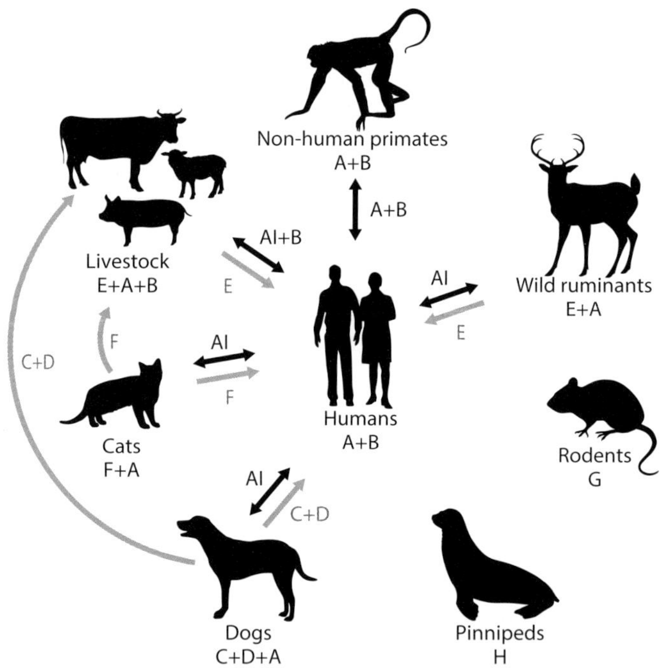

Fig. 101.1 Assemblages and transmission cycles of giardiasis. Most human infections are anthroponotic, and involve sub-assemblages AI, AII, BIII, and BIV. Sub-assemblage AI has zoonotic potential, and involves livestock, wild ruminants, nonhuman primates, cats, and dogs. Occasional reports of transmission of assemblages C, E, and F have been reported, likely originating from the animals predominantly infected by these assemblages. (Modified from Caccio, et al. *Infect Genetics Evol.* 2018: 66; 335-345.)

apoptosis increases GI permeability, allowing luminal antigens to activate host immune–dependent pathologic pathways.[12] Parasite proteins cause cellular damage affecting the intestinal permeability and cells of the adaptive immune system. *Giardia* infection stimulates chloride secretion and results in a diffuse loss of brush border microvillus length, which causes epithelial maldigestion and malabsorption of glucose, sodium, and water and reduced disaccharidase activity.[12]

The reason as to why *Giardia* can cause clinical signs in some individuals and not in others is not completely elucidated. Parasite strains, host nutritional status, the composition of intestinal microbiota, co-infection with other enteric pathogens, and immunological response are important factors that influence disease manifestations.[11] It is unknown if the different assemblages vary

TABLE 101.4 Prevalence of *Giardia* Infection in Dogs[a]

Location	Number Examined	Method	Prevalence (%)
Albania	602	Fecal antigen	35.5
Argentina	106	Microscopy	14.5
Bulgaria	294	Fecal antigen	30.3
Brazil	166	Microscopy	31.3
Brazil	97	Microscopy	19.6
Brazil	49	Microscopy	8.2
Canada	118	Fecal antigen/ microscopy	64
Canada	619	Microscopy	8.1
Canada	70	Microscopy	7.1
Canada	1216	Fecal antigen	7.2
Canada	102	Fecal antigen	7
Cambodia	94	PCR	10.6
Chile	452	Microscopy	2.2
China	205	PCR	11
China	315	PCR	3.2
China	318	Fecal antigen	16.0
China	197	PCR	15.2
China	485	PCR	26.2
China	940	PCR	14.3
Czech Republic	458	Microscopy	2.5
Czech Republic	458	Serum	36.5
France	116	Microcopy	25
Jamaica	225	Microscopy	2.7
Jamaica	225	PCR	
Germany	1281	Microscopy	2.3
Germany	100	Fecal antigen	13
Germany	341	Fecal antigen	11.4
Germany	376	Microscopy	10
Germany	376	Fecal antigen	30.6
Hungary	187	Fecal antigen	58.5
Hungary	115	Fecal antigen	37.4
India	101	PCR	20
Iran	147	Microscopy	0.68
Iran	210	Microscopy	0.95
Ireland	627	Microscopy	6.02
Italy	105	Fecal antigen	19
Italy	183	Fecal antigen	55.2
Italy	143	PCR	30
Italy	127	PCR	20.5
Italy	655	Microscopy	26.3
Italy	139	Fecal antigen	2.9
Japan	2365	Microcopy	58.8
Japan	906	Microscopy	0.9
Japan	573	Fecal antigen	25.7
Japan	1105	Microscopy	12.4
Macedonia	136	Fecal antigen	33.1
Poland	148	PCR	2.0
Poland	128	Fecal antigen	21.1
Romania	183	Fecal antigen	36.1
Scotland	101	Microscopy	13.9
Serbia	167	Microscopy	14.4
Serbia	134	Fecal antigen	65.7
Spain	1161	Microscopy	7
Spain	505	Microscopy	6.1
Spain	194	Microscopy/PCR	33
Spain	604	Microscopy	16.4
Spain	348	Microscopy/direct FA	36.5
Spain	55	Microscopy/direct FA/PCR	29
Taiwan	118	PCR	9.3
Thailand	500	Microscopy	2.8
The Netherlands	152	Fecal antigen	15.2
United Kingdom	275	Microscopy	14.5
United States	1,199,293	Microscopy	4.0
United States	5959	Fecal antigen	7.5
United States	16,114	Fecal antigen	15.6
United States	49	Direct FA	26.5
United States	120	PCR	15
United States	672	Direct FA	196

[a]Data from references 17,33,41,62,93,94,106,110,116–124,126–165,170,173,207.

in their disease-producing properties and induce a respective range of severity of clinical signs in cats and dogs. A higher prevalence of symptomatic giardiasis is observed in human infants, especially in those with pre-existing nutritional deficits, due to an immature adaptive immune system.[11] In HIV/AIDS patients, *Giardia* is not a common opportunistic pathogen, suggesting that not all forms of immunosuppression predispose to severe disease.[11] Recent findings suggest that some protozoa parasites can colonize the human gut for long periods without provoking symptoms, challenging their definition as a "pathogen" or "commensal."[13] *Giardia* and intestinal microbiota may produce persistent dysbiosis that could potentially predispose to GI disorders post infection to people with giardiasis.[13] *Giardia* colonization may cause a metabolic shift among the intestinal microbial community, and as a consequence the altered microbiota could contribute the clinical signs during the infection.[14] In dogs, the composition of the fecal bacterial microbiome was significantly different in clinically ill and subclinical *Giardia* infections.[15]

Although many cats and dogs that excrete *Giardia* do not show clinical signs of disease, *Giardia* can cause illness in other animals. Younger, immunosuppressed animals and those living in crowded environments are at the highest risk of showing clinical disease.[9,16-20] Shelter dogs showed a higher prevalence of protozoa l infections and a lower prevalence of helminth infections when compared with hunting dogs.[21] The

TABLE 101.5 Prevalence of *Giardia* in Cats[a]

Location	Number Examined	Method	Prevalence (%)
Albania	58	Fecal antigen	29.3
Australia	40	Microscopy	5
Australia	40	PCR	80
Austria	298	Fecal antigen/ microscopy	12.4
Brazil	131	Microscopy	6.1
Canada	41	Microscopy	2.4
Canada	153	Microscopy	7.2
Canada	283	Microscopy	9.9
Canada	251	Fecal antigen	6.4
Chile	230	Microscopy	19.1
China	102	Microscopy	9.8
China	160	PCR	13.1
Czech Republic	135	Microscopy	1
Czech Republic	135	Serum	57
Egypt	113	Microscopy	2
Finland	402	Fecal antigen	3.2
Germany	3167	Microscopy	10
Germany	584	Fecal antigen	6.8
Germany	145	Microscopy	6.2
Germany	145	Fecal antigen	17.9
Iran	140	Microscopy	15
Ireland	289	Microscopy	1.8
Italy	48	Fecal antigen	4
Italy	463	Microscopy/ fecal antigen	11.1
Jamaica	225	PCR	19.6
Japan	942	Microscopy	1.5
Poland	33	Fecal antigen	15.1
Spain	144	Microscopy	4.2
Spain	65	Microscopy/PCR	9.2
Spain	34	Microscopy/direct FA/PCR	5.9
Thailand	300	Microscopy	0.3
The Netherlands	305	Microscopy	1
The Netherlands	60	Fecal antigen	13.6
United Kingdom	1355	Microscopy	6
United Kingdom	48	Fecal antigen	15
United States (CO)	206	Microscopy	2.4
United States (MS)	250	Direct FA	13.6
United States (NY)	263	Microscopy	7.3
United States (PA)	335	Microscopy	10.1
United States	344	Direct FA	9.8
United States	4978	Fecal antigen	10.8

[a]Data from references 41,43,71,93,106,115,120,121,125,128,130,138, 139,149,153,155,157,158,162,166–169,171,172,174–185.

TABLE 101.6 *Giardia* Assemblages Identified in Dogs Worldwide[a]

Country	Total Number of Isolates	Assemblages (Number of Isolates) A	B	C	D	Others[b] (Number of Isolates)
Albania	17			5	12	
Australia	11			10	1	
Australia	9	1	2	4	2	
Brazil	27			7	20	
Brazil	7	7				
Brazil	10	5 (AI)	3 (BIV)	2		
Brazil	6	3 (AII)		2	1	
Brazil	16				D 2	D+AI (4), D+BIII (3), D+C (3), D+BIV (3), D+E (1)
Bulgaria	13			4	9	
Cambodia	10		2 (BIII)	4		C+D (4)
Canada	8			3	5	
Canada	73		1	31	51	
China	27	25 (AI)		2		
China	23	5			18	
China	10		6		4	
China	108	23	1	26	58	
China	80			28	33	19 mixed infections (C+D)
Croatia	16			6	10	
Croatia	96	3	10	18	21	C+D (18), B+D (11), C+B (7) and other mixed infections
Germany	55	33		5	2	A+C (15)
Germany	92			33	50	C+D (8), A+D (1)
Germany	123	11	3	32	47	Multiple combinations (30)
Germany	6	2		1	2	A+B (1)
Germany	103	2		42	55	E (2), F (2)
Hungary	15			5	9	C+D (1)
India	7	5	2			
Italy	17	2		11	1	A+C (2), C+D (1)
Italy	20	6		1	12	A+D (1)
Italy	14			8	6	
Italy	42	AII (2)		17	23	
Jamaica	44	A				
Japan	4				4	
Japan	24	14		1	6	A+D (3)
Macedonia	14			7	7	
Mexico	5	4				A+B (1)
Mexico	11	7				A4 (=probably C or D) (4)

TABLE 101.6 *Giardia* Assemblages Identified in Dogs Worldwide[a]—cont'd

Country	Total Number of Isolates	Assemblages (Number of Isolates)				Others[b] (Number of Isolates)
		A	B	C	D	
Poland	22		1	18	2	C+D (1)
Portugal	31	21		2	2	A+C (2), A+D (4)
Romania	39			8	29	C+D (1), E(1)
Romania	16			8	8	
Serbia	14			8	6	
Spain	63	3	7 BIII 15 BIV	1	7	30 mixed infections
Spain	19	7AII	1BIII 7BIV	3C	1D	
Spain	35	5	8	2	13	AII+B (4), A+D (1), A+B+D (1)
Spain	3			3		
Taiwan	11			7	4	
Thailand	13	5		1	3	A+B (3), A+D (1)
Trinidad and Tobago	26			4	21	E (1)
United States	15			15		
United States	148	41	61	22	24	83% (multiple infections)
United States	183	4AI		29	124	C+D (25), AII+C (1)
Vietnam	8			8		

[a]Data from references 41,93–97,99,101–103,106,107,109,110,115,118, 119,124,126,128,129,134,143,149,154–156,170,176,186–201,207,208.
[b]Most represent mixed infections with different assemblage types.

primary clinical signs of giardiasis include acute or chronic diarrhea and weight loss. Acute diarrhea occurs frequently in very young animals; in older cats and dogs the diarrhea can be acute, intermittent, or chronic. The diarrhea is usually mucoid, pale, and soft and has a strong odor; steatorrhea may be present as well. The organism is not usually enteroinvasive, and so blood is uncommon. Most infected cats and dogs are afebrile and do not vomit. Co-infection with other parasites is common. *Giardia/Cryptosporidium* and *Giardia/Tritrichomonas blagburni* co-infections may often be found in association with diarrhea.[22,23]

DIAGNOSIS

A variety of different *Giardia* detection tests have been evaluated for use in cats and dogs. Despite the improved specificity, there is no one test that can be performed on a single fecal specimen that has 100% sensitivity. Even more problematic is the lack of an assay with high etiologic predictive value for clinical giardiasis due to the high prevalence of infection in clinically healthy animals.

Laboratory Abnormalities

Giardia spp. infection alone is rarely associated with CBC or serum biochemical panel abnormalities.

TABLE 101.7 *Giardia* Assemblages Identified in Cats Worldwide[a]

Country	No. of Isolates	A	B	C	D	F	Others
Australia	18	6	2	2	7		E (1)
Austria	14	4				10	
Brazil	19	8				11	
Canada	13	12	1				
China	10	8				1	A+C (1)
China	18	2	6	2	1	7	
Colombia	3					3	
Germany	53	13	2	1	3	28	
Germany	17	2			1	14	
Italy	10	10					
Italy	3					3	
Japan	3					3	
Japan	44	6	1			33	A+F 4
Poland	5	1				4	
Poland	6	2	2		2		
Portugal	2	1				1	
Romania	8				8		
Spain	2	1				1	
Spain	2					2	
United States	17	6				11	
United States	8					8	
United States	17	16			1		

[a]Data from references 41,93,101,119,125,128,140,149,155,164,167, 183,187,190,191,193,196,202–207.

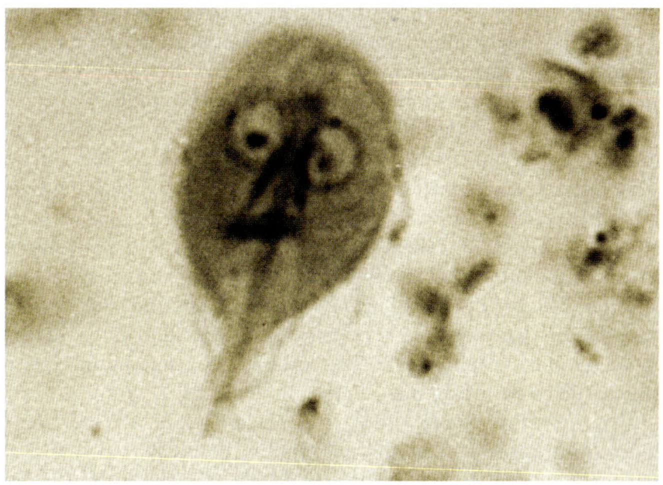

Fig. 101.2 *Giardia* trophozoite in a fecal smear stained to enhance the characteristic organelles (iron hematoxylin, ×2000.)

Diagnostic Imaging

Abdominal radiographic abnormalities are uncommon and nonspecific and, when present, are suggestive of diffuse enteritis.

Microbiologic Tests

Diagnosis Using Fecal Examination

Giardia is one of the most commonly misidentified parasites.[24] Pseudoparasites or yeasts are easily mistaken for *Giardia*, and cysts

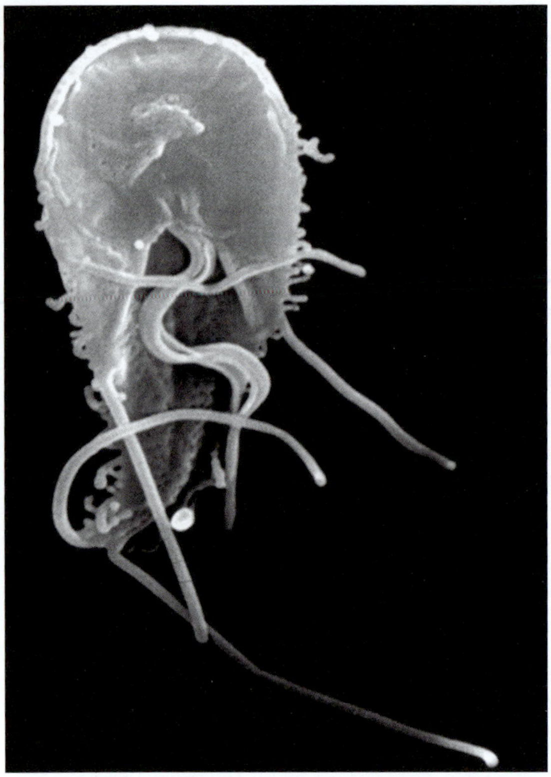

Fig. 101.3 Electron micrograph of a *Giardia* trophozoite. (Courtesy of Bayer Animal Health. In: Tangtrongsup S, Scorza V. Update on the diagnosis and management of *Giardia* spp. infections in dogs and cats. *Top Comp Anim Med.* 2010;25:155-162.)

can deteriorate in fecal flotation solutions, leading to false positive and false negative results, respectively.[24]

Direct Smear. *Giardia* trophozoites can be observed in direct smears of unstained fecal specimens using light microscopy. Trophozoites are rarely found in formed feces, refrigerated specimens, or specimens that are examined several hours after collection.[25] Although *Giardia* trophozoites can be confused with tritrichomonads that are similar in size, the latter may be differentiated by the presence of an undulating membrane, a rolling form of motility, the lack of a concave surface, and a single nucleus.[26] Further testing with *Giardia* antigen tests or fecal culture or PCR for *T. blagburni* can be used for differentiation. Once *Giardia* is detected, further cytologic examination should be performed on a fresh specimen. Although they also inactivate the parasites, the application of Lugol's solution, methylene blue, or acid-methyl green to the wet mount helps in the visualization of the internal structures of the trophozoites.[26] Examination of fresh feces on 3 different days detected 40% of the *Giardia*-infected dogs.[27]

Concentration Techniques. If trophozoites are not seen on a direct smear, examination for cysts should be performed.[24] If fecal specimens cannot be examined immediately, storage at 4°C for several days is acceptable, but specimens should not be frozen. *Giardia* cysts are best detected by Sheather's sugar centrifugation and the zinc sulfate centrifugation technique ($ZnSO_4$) (see Fig. 101.4, *B*).[26] If the feces contain much fat, formalin-ethyl acetate sedimentation is the best technique for cyst detection. The zinc sulfate centrifugation technique has also been superior to passive fecal flotation for detection of helminths and *Giardia* cysts. Flotation methods detected only 6.5% to 14.7% of samples with *Giardia* cysts, as compared to those found to contain cysts using $ZnSO_4$.[28,29] The zinc sulfate centrifugation technique recovered seven times more *Giardia* cysts than sodium nitrate when used in a commercial flotation device (StatSpin Ovatube, Iris

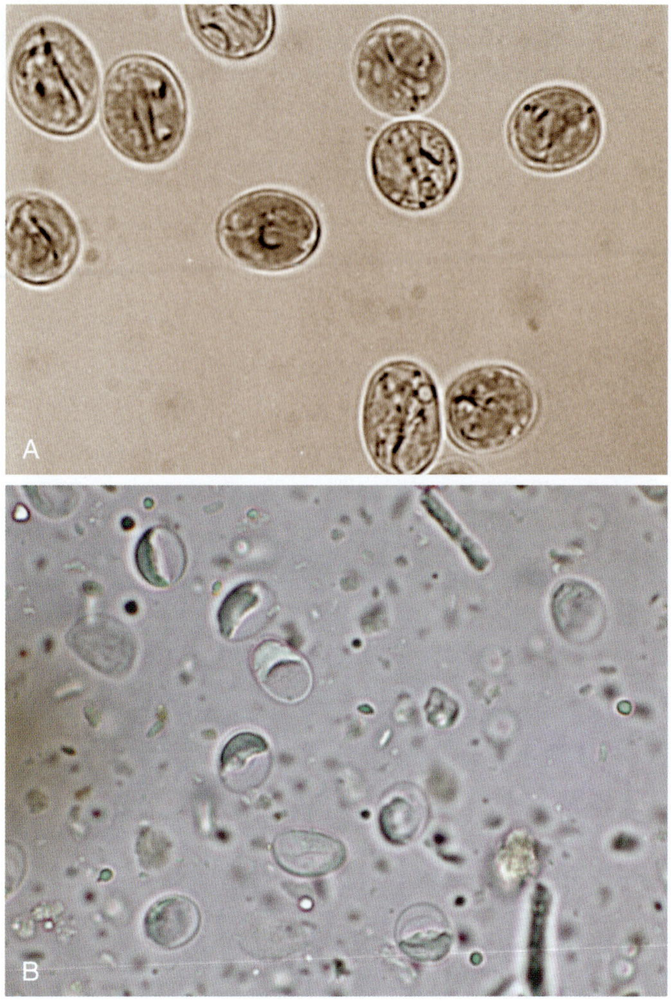

Fig. 101.4 *Giardia* cysts concentrated from the feces of a cat by the zinc sulfate centrifugal flotation technique. (A) Cyst wall, nuclei, axonemes, and median bodies are apparent in several of the cysts (iodine, ×1100). (B) Unstained with numerous cysts showing concavity (×1100).

Sample Processing, Inc., Westwood, MA, USA).[30] Barium sulfate, several proprietary antidiarrheals, and enemas administered before the collection of the feces may interfere with the detection of the cysts.[25] Because of the intermittent pattern of excretion, it is recommended that if fecal flotation alone is to be used, at least three specimens be examined over a period of about 1 week before ruling out the presence of *Giardia*.[24,25,27]Additionally, in general, dogs and cats often are not excreting large numbers of *Giardia* cysts. Another factor to consider is the type of laboratory to submit the specimen to for the diagnosis of *Giardia* infection via fecal centrifugation flotation. In one study, the frequency of *Giardia* detection was significantly lower when performed at a commercial laboratory than when it was performed at a university laboratory.[31]

Immunochemical Detection with Fluorescent Microscopy. A monoclonal antibody–based direct FA assay (Merifluor Cryptosporidium/*Giardia*, Meridian Diagnostics, Cincinnati, OH) is used to detect *Giardia* spp. cysts and *Cryptosporidium* spp. oocysts in feces. The assay has been evaluated for detection of *Giardia* infections of dogs and cats in multiple studies.[32,33] Because the assay gives both immunologic confirmation (fluorescence) and morphologic evaluation (size and shape), it is usually considered a reference standard in test comparison studies.[34] This FA assay was more sensitive and specific than zinc sulfate flotation but comparable to other antigen-detection techniques when used on refrigerated feline fecal

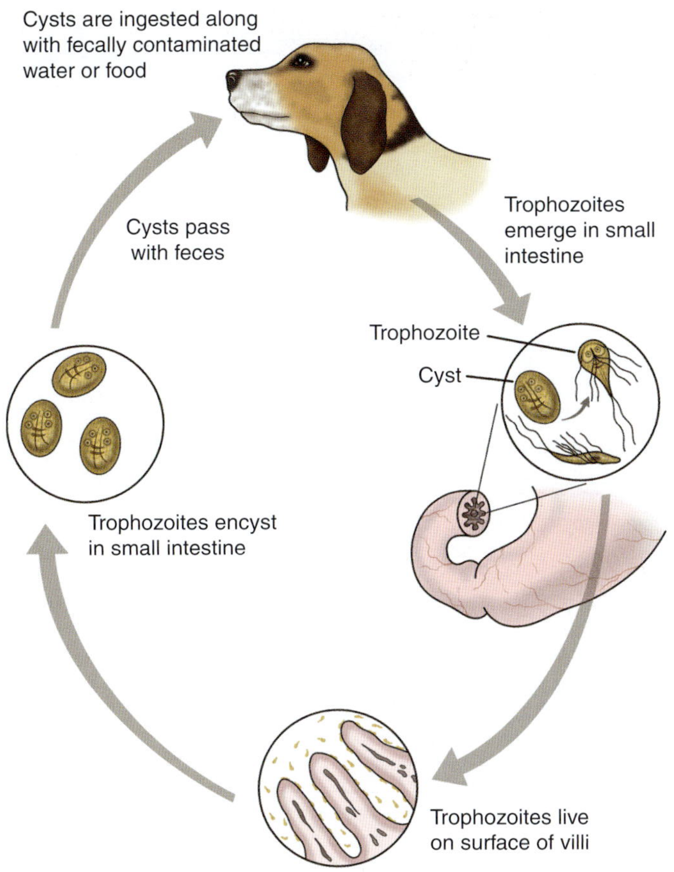

Fig. 101.5 Life cycle of *Giardia duodenalis.*

specimens and in fecal specimens from shelter dogs.[26,35] In addition, it detects *Cryptosporidium* spp., which can be found as co-pathogens. A fluorescence microscope is needed to read the FA slides, therefore this assay is usually only performed in diagnostic laboratories. Specimens can be stored at 4°C for several days but should not be frozen.

Fecal Antigen Assays

There are several POC ELISA-based kits available for the detection of *Giardia* spp. antigen in human feces, and one kit is licensed for use with dog and cat feces (SNAP *Giardia*, IDEXX Laboratories, Portland, ME). Results vary depending on the test kits used, and inconsistent results have been reported with some *Giardia* antigen tests when compared to other non–ELISA-based techniques.[9,36-42] In cats, the ELISA-based kit licensed for use with canine or feline feces had similar sensitivity and specificity when compared to $ZnSO_4$ flotation, and when the results of the two techniques were combined, the overall sensitivity was 97.8%.[43] In dogs, using the direct FA as the gold standard test, at a prevalence rate of 10%, the *Giardia* antigen assay was estimated to have a positive predictive value (PPV) and negative predictive value (NPV) of 51.0% and 97.0%, respectively, which were similar to those for $ZnSO_4$ flotation.[34]

In a study using Bayesian statistical approach, the IDEXX POC kit (SNAP *Giardia*) showed a sensitivity of 88.9% and a specificity of 95.8% with PPV and NPV of 89.6% and 95.4%, respectively, when used on dog specimens.[44] A study compared the results of $ZnSO_4$ flotation and the SNAP *Giardia* antigen test (IDEXX Laboratories Inc., Netherlands) in dog fecal specimens with the results of two additional POC ELISA-based tests: Single Antigen Rapid *Giardia* Ag and the Triple Antigen Rapid CPV-CCV-*Giardia* Ag (BioNote).[45] At a high prevalence rate in the dog population, the specificities and PPV of both tests were 100%. However, the sensitivities were 48% and 83% for the single and triple test, respectively, and the NPV was 55% and 80% for the single and triple test, respectively.[45] At lower prevalence rates, both tests showed high PPVs (100%) and the NPVs were higher with the Triple (96% to 99%) than the Single (88% to 96%) Rapid test.[45] The direct FA assay, $ZnSO_4$ flotation, SNAP *Giardia* test, ProSpecT *Giardia* EZ Microplate assay, and PCR were evaluated in fecal specimens from 136 young dogs.[42] Comparisons among the tests were done using FA as a gold standard and also using Bayesian analysis.[42] *Giardia* was detected in 41% of the specimens by FA, and $ZnSO_4$ flotation was positive in 37% of specimens with a relative sensitivity and specificity of 86% and 98%, respectively. The SNAP *Giardia* test was positive in 40% of the specimens, with a relative sensitivity and specificity of 91% and 96%, respectively. The ProSpecT test was positive in 51% of the specimens, with a relative sensitivity and specificity of 100% and 83%, respectively. The PCR was positive in 55% of the specimens, with a relative sensitivity and specificity of 58% and 56%, respectively. When the Bayesian approach was performed, the conclusions remained the same although sensitivity and specificity changed.[42] The ProSpecT was the most sensitive test, but it is not designed for dogs and is more expensive than the other tests. In another study, specimens from 573 dogs were tested by centrifugation sedimentation flotation coproscopical analysis, direct FA, the SNAP *Giardia* test, and a qPCR assay.[46] Bayesian analysis was used to evaluate test performance characteristics.[46] All tests were highly specific. The highest specificity was with the SNAP *Giardia* (99.6%) and the lowest was with qPCR (85.6%).[46] The qPCR assay had the highest sensitivity (97.0%) and centrifugation sedimentation flotation had the lowest sensitivity (48.2%). Direct FA was more sensitive than SNAP *Giardia*, but slightly less specific.[46]

Another study compared the performance of the VetScan Canine *Giardia* Rapid Test (Abaxis), Anigen Rapid CPV-CCV-*Giardia* Antigen Test (BioNote), SNAP *Giardia* Test (IDEXX), and Witness *Giardia* Test (Zoetis), ova parasite examination and the ProSpecT Microtiter Plate ELISA to FA as the gold standard.[47] The sensitivities of the SNAP, Anigen, Witness, VetScan, ova and parasite examination, and ProSpecT assays were 87.1%, 80.2%, 73.3%, 70.0%, 81.2%, and 94.1%, respectively.[47] The specificities were 93.4%, 80.3%, 71.1%, 85.5%, 93.4%, and 97.4%, respectively.[47] Although information is limited regarding detection of *Giardia* assemblages C, D, or F, in one study of four assemblage C isolates and 13 assemblage D isolates, all were positive by the SNAP *Giardia* antigen assay.[47]

The CAPC recommends that fecal antigen tests be used as an addition to fecal flotation only during the evaluation of dogs and cats with diarrhea, and not with clinically healthy pets or to follow therapy, because the clinical and zoonotic impact of an antigen result-positive, cyst presence result-negative healthy pet is unknown.[48] It is also unknown as to how long *Giardia* antigen assay results remain positive after resolution of diarrhea. Therefore, if a veterinarian chooses to assess the success of the treatment for giardiasis in cats and dogs, only fecal flotation is recommended for follow-up evaluation.

Molecular Diagnosis Using Nucleic Acid–Based Testing

Many veterinary diagnostic laboratories offer PCR diarrhea panels that include *G. duodenalis* for the detection of common enteric pathogens. However, if genotyping is desired, other PCR assays may be required.[49] At the time of writing, one diagnostic laboratory has begun to offer a PCR panel that detects nucleic acid from 20 different parasites, and differentiates zoonotic assemblages of *Giardia* (A and B) from other assemblages of *Giardia* (assemblage non-specific assay) (KeyScreen GI Parasite PCR, Antech Diagnostics, USA). A 2019 article reported that the sensitivity and specificity of a real-time PCR assay for *G. duodenalis* that was incorporated as a component of a diarrhea panel was 95.1% and 92.1%, respectively, when compared with a reference real-time PCR assay.[50] However, *Giardia* PCR assay results can also be falsely negative because of the presence of PCR inhibitors in feces. In one study, false negative results were obtained in 41% (11/27) specimens using a real-time PCR assay in comparison with direct FA or fecal flotation.[31] Therefore, PCR should not be used as the sole means of confirming *G. duodenalis* infection. The authors recommend to test initially with $ZnSO_4$ centrifugal flotation and then follow with an antigen test.

Pathologic Findings

Gross Pathologic Findings

Giardia spp. infection may cause mild intestinal thickening, and it is not enteroinvasive, so blood is generally not present within the intestinal lumen unless co-infections are recognized. Animals with chronic clinical signs of disease may be emaciated.

Histopathologic Findings

In clinically affected animals with *Giardia* infection, a diffuse loss of brush border microvillus length may be noted on histopathology of the small intestine. Increased numbers of intraepithelial lymphocytes and mast cell hyperplasia may also be present. However, diarrhea has been associated with giardiasis in dogs, cats, and people with normal intestinal biopsy results.

TREATMENT AND PROGNOSIS

Effective and approved drugs to treat giardiasis in humans include 5-nitroimidazoles and benzimidazoles derivatives, quinacrine, furazolidone, paromomycin, and nitazoxanide.[51] In veterinary medicine, many drugs can reduce the parasite burden and speed resolution of clinical signs (Table 101.8). Metronidazole has been widely used for the treatment of giardiasis in naturally and experimentally infected cats and dogs, even though controlled studies are lacking.[52,53] Central nervous system toxicity had been associated with the administration of metronidazole in some dogs and kittens but this is usually avoided by staying below 50 mg/kg total daily dose and only using the drug for days rather than weeks.[52,54] The CAPC suggests a maximum dose of 25 mg/kg, PO, q12h for 5 days.[48] Treatment for longer than 7 days should never exceed 30 mg/kg per day. Metronidazole hydrochloride is the United States Pharmacopeia (USP) formulation in tablets, which causes cats to salivate, while the benzoate form that is available in some countries is less likely to cause this problem.[55] When metronidazole benzoate was administered to cats with subclinical giardiasis, cyst excretion ceased over the time period of the study, and signs of toxicity did not develop. Use of drugs in the nitroimidazole class may also add the benefit of correcting bacterial overgrowth, which may also contribute to diarrhea. However, one study demonstrated that dogs with acute diarrhea continue to have dysbiosis and altered metabolic profiles after treatment with metronidazole for 28 days.[56] Other nitroimidazoles including ipronidazole, ronidazole, and tinidazole had been used for the treatment of giardiasis in a small number of animals. Ipronidazole added to water was effective for the treatment of giardiasis in two dogs.[57] The administration of a single dose of secnidazole at 30 mg/kg eliminated diarrhea and *Giardia* cyst excretion in 11 naturally infected cats; however, one cat showed elevation of liver enzymes.[58] This drug is not available in most countries except as a compounded formulation.[58]

Nitazoxanide was approved by FDA for the treatment of *Cryptosporidium* and *Giardia* infections in humans, it has also been used to treat some cats and dogs infected with cryptosporidiosis and giardiasis.[59] A salicylanide derivative of nitrothiazole, nitazoxanide is effective against a broad spectrum of parasites and bacteria.[60] Diarrhea resolved in some infected cats and dogs after the administration of nitazoxanide at 25 mg/kg, PO, q12h for at least 5 days.[23] Nonetheless, nitazoxanide is a GI irritant and often causes vomiting and it is not effective in the absence of an appropriate immune response.

One study of dogs that were naturally infected with *Giardia* involved administration of nitazoxanide at different dosages (37.5, 75, and 150 mg/kg) on days 0 and 14.[61] In the same study, another group of dogs

TABLE 101.8 Treatment for Giardiasis and Other Enteric Protozoal Infections

Drug	Species	Dose	Route	Interval (Hours)	Duration (Days)
Drontal Plus[a] tablets	D	25 mg/kg feb 5 mg/kg praz 5 mg/kg pyr base	PO	24	3
	C	56.5 mg/kg feb 11.3 mg/kg praz 11.3 mg/kg pyr	PO	24	5
Drontal Plus Taste tabs[a]	D	25 mg/kg feb 5 mg/kg praz 5 mg/kg pyr base	PO	24	3
Fenbendazole	B	50 mg/kg	PO	24	5
Metronidazole	B	25 mg/kg	PO	12	5–7
Ipronidazole	D	126 mg/L[b]	PO	Ad libitum	7
Tinidazole	D	44 mg/kg	PO	24	6
	C	30 mg/kg	PO	24	7–10
Nitazoxanide	B	100 mg/animal	PO	12	3–4
Quinacrine	D	9 mg/kg	PO	24	6
	D	6.6 mg/kg	PO	12	5
Furazolidone[c]	C	4 mg/kg	PO	12	7–10

[a]Elanco. See manufacturer's label for dosing recommendations based on tablet size. Some dosages noted here are based on studies where combination products were used off-label.
[b]In drinking water and given ad libitum.
[c]In suspension, 200 mg/day maximum. Has been used in children and has the ability to inhibit cyst formation. Not available in some countries. maximum recommended dosages are used for treatment of enteric protozoal infections. Neurotoxicity has been observed at levels of hydrochloride salt at ≥ 60 mg/kg per day. To facilitate the dosage to smaller animals, the 250- or 500-mg tablets may be ground, or smaller tablet size (50 to 100 mg) may be used. This may be placed in a palatable base. For cats, metronidazole benzoate formulations (62% metronidazole base) are better tolerated orally than hydrochloride formulations, but dosage needed would be 1.6 times listed.
B, both dog and cat; *C*, cat; *D*, dog; *feb*, febantel; *PO*, oral; *praz*, praziquantel; *pyr*, pyrantel.

were treated PO with a combination of pyrantel, praziquantel, and febantel for 3 consecutive days; another group of dogs were untreated control dogs.[61] Although *Giardia* excretion reduced in all treatment groups, fecal consistency did not improve. However, this study lacked an uninfected control group and some of the dogs were co-infected with other parasites.

Fenbendazole has been evaluated for the treatment of giardiasis in a number of studies of dogs and cats.[10,62-64] Fenbendazole also has activity against other parasites that have the potential to be co-pathogens. The CAPC recommends a dose of fenbendazole of 50 mg/kg, q24h, for 5 days for cats and dogs, or a combination of this dosage of fenbendazole and metronidazole (25 mg/kg, q12h, for 5 days). However, when fenbendazole was administered to cats concurrently infected with *Giardia* and *Cryptosporidium parvum*, *Giardia* cyst excretion ceased in only four of eight cats.[63] When fenbendazole was administered to naturally infected shelter dogs, the percent persistence of cyst counts per gram of feces were 84% and 78% when feces were rechecked 9 and 16 days, respectively, after treatment.[64] Fenbendazole (50 mg/kg, PO, q4h for 10 days), bathing and moving dogs into disinfected kennels while disinfecting their original kennels with a quaternary ammonium solution, and then raising the temperature in the room for 24 hours to promote drying of *Giardia* cysts, eliminated *Giardia* excretion in 34 dogs.[65]

In cats, fenbendazole was safe when administered to healthy, adult, nonpregnant cats at a dosage five times higher than the approved dosage.[66] Other benzimidazoles used in some studies of giardiasis are albendazole, oxfendazole, and febantel. Albendazole has been effective in dogs; however, because of bone marrow suppression, it is not recommended.[66,67] Oxfendazole used in conjunction with other control measures led to resolution of diarrhea and cyst excretion in one study of kenneled dogs with giardiasis.[68]

A combination of febantel, pyrantel, and praziquantel (FPP) (Drontal Plus Tablets, Bayer, Shawnee Mission, KS), using a variety of dosage protocols, has had variable results in the treatment of giardiasis in dogs and cats.[40,69-75] Two different formulations of the drug exist (see Table 101.8), and dose differences may be responsible for some of the discrepancies between results of efficacy studies. In one report of seven healthy *Giardia*-infected dogs, organisms were not detected again in 3 days after 3 consecutive days of treatment with FPP.[69] However, 6 days after the last treatment, some dogs began to excrete organisms again, probably from reinfection.[69] The efficacy of the treatment of dogs naturally infected with *Giardia* spp. for 5 consecutive days with the European formulation was not significantly better than treatment for 3 consecutive days.[74] Another study implied that when FPP was used to treat dogs with giardiasis, bathing the animal and changing its environment after treatment may be more important for preventing reinfection than duration of treatment.[40,48]

When FPP was administered at the empiric dosage of two "small dog" tablets per cat, PO, for 5 days, to six cats, a significant decrease in cyst excretion was observed in the treated group in comparison to the untreated control group.[75] In addition, four of the six treated cats had evidence of infection after administration of two immunosuppressive doses of repositol glucocorticoids.[75]

Azithromycin (10 mg/kg PO q24h for 5 days) was used for the treatment of an 8-month-old dog that had persistent diarrhea after being treated with fenbendazole and metronidazole for giardiasis.[76] After treatment the diarrhea stopped, and no adverse reactions were observed. *Giardia* cysts and DNA were not detected after examination of fecal smears and PCR of fecal samples on days 2, 4, and 6 after therapy.[76] However, azithromycin has failed to lessen *Giardia* attachment or growth *in vivo*, and so use of this drug for treatment of giardiasis in animals needs additional study.[77]

Other drugs used historically to treat giardiasis in dogs or cats included quinacrine, furazolidone, and paromomycin; however, controlled efficacy studies are lacking.[23,59,61,78]

Auranofin is a gold-containing drug that was approved by the FDA in 1985 for the treatment of rheumatoid arthritis, and it could be a promising new agent for the treatment of giardiasis. Auranofin showed anti-*Giardia* activity *in vivo* and *in vitro* at a low concentration and was effective against multiple metronidazole-resistant strains *in vitro*.[79] Auranofin inhibits the activity of a protozoal enzyme that contributes to normal protein function and that combats oxidative damage. Auranofin has activity against both the *Giardia* cyst and the trophozoite stages. It has been administered to shelter dogs with diarrhea due to *Giardia* infections alone and *Giardia* and *Cryptosporidium* co-infections.[80] No adverse effects have been observed in these dogs using a dose of 0.3 mg/kg and upwards to a maximum dose of 6 mg/day, q24h for 5 days, and dogs ceased excreting cysts and had normal stools after 5 to 10 days of treatment.[80]

Although controlled studies in dogs and cats are generally lacking, other adjunctive therapies, including fiber, silymarin, and probiotics, have been administered to some dogs or cats with giardiasis on the basis of work with other species. Although all dogs who received metronidazole, with or without silymarin, stopped excreting *Giardia* cysts, the addition of silymarin appeared to help to compensate for weight loss and increased the levels of serum total proteins and albumin when compared to dogs administered metronidazole alone.[81] Dietary fiber reduced *Giardia* infection rates in a gerbil model and controlled studies assessing the benefit in dogs are ongoing.[82] While the probiotic *Enterococcus faecium* SF68 enhanced *Giardia* immune responses in mice, positive effects on cyst excretion, fecal antigen excretion, fecal IgA concentrations, or leukocyte phagocytic activity were not recognized in samples from adult dogs with chronic subclinical infections.[83] Further work is required before these adjunctive therapies can be routinely recommended.

Common questions about treatment of *Giardia* spp. infection in dogs and cats include which drug to start with and whether dual therapy is required for treatment success. Dual therapy with fenbendazole and metronidazole has been suggested for the treatment of giardiasis in dogs and cats by some veterinarians and the combination was shown to be synergistic in a recent study in mice.[84] However, while metronidazole has adverse effects on the GI microbiome and the benzimidazole drugs fenbendazole and febantel do not, monotherapy with a benzimidazole first may be prudent with dual therapy only used in resistant cases.[56,85]

Because *Giardia* infection may be difficult to eliminate in dogs and cats, the primary goal is to resolve diarrhea. The treatment protocol used may need to be varied according to each individual patient. Additionally, control measures should be instituted to attempt to avoid reinfection. Resistance to metronidazole, nitazoxanide, albendazole, furazolidone, and quinacrine has been described in humans.[51] In dogs and cats with persistent diarrhea and detection of *Giardia* in feces after appropriate treatment, an extensive work-up should be undertaken to evaluate for other underlying disorders that may perpetuate clinical disease such as co-infections with other parasites (*Cryptosporidium* spp., *T. blagburni*), inflammatory bowel disease, bacterial overgrowth, and exocrine pancreatic insufficiency.

Although immunization has been used in the past, both the canine and feline *Giardia* vaccines previously licensed for use in dogs or cats in the United States have been discontinued.[86] However, *Giardia* vaccines are commercially available in Latin American countries for prevention of clinical illness and reduction of parasite excretion.[87] An oral vaccine with the complete repertoire of variant-specific surface protein (VSP) antigens hindered establishment of infection by trophozoites or cysts, in experimental and domestic animals (gerbils, dogs, and cats).[88] The administration of this vaccine also decreased clinical signs and reduced contamination of the environment with cysts.[88]

PREVENTION

In controlled environments (cattery or kennel situation), four main approaches should be employed to control *Giardia*: (1) decontamination of the environment, (2) antiprotozoal treatment, (3) cleaning of cysts from coats, and (4) preventing reintroduction of infection.[89]

Animals should be treated (preferably with fenbendazole or the FPP combination) before moving them into catteries or kennels. Cages or runs should be steam or chemically cleaned after all fecal material has been removed before disinfection. Five percent sodium hypochlorite (1:30 dilution) and quaternary ammonium–containing disinfectants inactivate *Giardia* cysts.[90] Quaternary ammonium compounds lose activity in the presence of organic matter, which makes it impossible to decontaminate environmental areas such as soil and grass. The kennel should be allowed to dry thoroughly after cleaning (cysts are extremely susceptible to drying) and preferably left dry and empty for several days. Animals should be bathed with a general pet shampoo to remove fecal material from their coats, rinsed, and then bathed with quaternary ammonium compounds.[40] Quaternary ammonium compounds can irritate skin and mucous membranes with repeated or prolonged exposure but appear to produce no adverse effects when applied for 3 to 5 minutes followed by thorough rinsing. The coat is allowed to dry thoroughly before returning the animal to the clean area. Animals should then be treated again, preferably with a different compound than the one initially used, once back in the clean facility. Theoretically, the only way *Giardia* can be reintroduced into a clean area is by an infected animal or by fomite transmission. Fomite transmission can be avoided by donning shoe covers before entering the facility or cleaning boots with a quaternary ammonium compound footbath. Fecal specimens should be periodically checked using $ZnSO_4$ centrifugal fecal flotation in order to determine whether the process has been effective.

PUBLIC HEALTH ASPECTS

Giardia is the most common parasite infecting humans worldwide; it is estimated that it causes approximately 280 million cases of human illness per year.[12] The majority of infections are acquired by drinking water or swallowing contaminated water while swimming in natural bodies of water or swimming pools.[12,91,92] Most dogs harbor dog-specific assemblages. However, potential zoonotic assemblages A and B have also been reported (see Table 101.6).[93-103] Assemblages A and B are subtyped into four sub-assemblages (AI-IV and BI-IV).[99,104] Human isolates mostly belonged to AI, AII, BIII, and BIV whereas isolates from animals belonged to AI, AIII, AIV, BI, and BII.[105] Nevertheless, assemblage AII has also been described in a small number of dogs worldwide. Additionally, sub-assemblages BIII and BIV were observed in 27% and 73% of dogs and 56% and 44% of humans, respectively.[4,7,93,104,106] Numerous isolates from *G. duodenalis* from animals and humans have been genetically characterized.[106-108] However, few studies have genetically compared *Giardia* isolates from animals and humans sharing the same household.[102,104,110,111] In India, assemblage A or B was found in humans and dogs living in the same household. In Brazil, a child and a dog in the same household were both harboring sub-assemblage BIV. Only a few studies have reported cat- and dog-specific assemblages in humans, but these findings were based on the detection of *Giardia* DNA and not on viable protozoa.[112,113] The fact that similar genotypes are dispersed in different hosts and that humans and pets in the same household share the same genotypes is not certain evidence of zoonotic transmission. Assemblage BIV was detected in humans, dogs, and vegetables showing a connection in the transmission dynamics of *G. duodenalis* in Southern Brazil.[98] More molecular epidemiologic studies on giardiasis in humans, animals, and the environment are needed to completely clarify the occurrence of zoonotic transmission.[4,98]

Several studies have reported an association between dogs attending dog parks and the presence of enteropathogens.[31,114] However, off leash activity showed a positive association with the transmission of *Giardia* infections, rather than attending the park alone.[115] *Giardia duodenalis* was detected in 3.8% and 9% of the dogs attending dog parks in Colorado and in California, respectively. In Colorado, dogs visiting dog parks were more likely than the control dogs to be positive for *Giardia* feces.[31,114] The *Giardia* isolates from both studies typed as dog-specific assemblages C and D.[31,114] The benefits of attending dog parks outnumber the disadvantages for both owners and dogs, therefore owners are advised to be responsible in ensuring proper disposal of dog feces, minimizing environmental contamination.

CASE EXAMPLE

Signalment

"Giada," a 3-month-old female papillon from Fort Collins, Colorado.

History

Giada was brought to a referral veterinary clinic with a history of intermittent diarrhea, weight loss, and lethargy.

Physical Examination

The dog was dehydrated and lethargic. Rectal examination revealed feces that were soft and contained traces of blood.

Laboratory Findings

The initial hemogram showed mild non-regenerative anemia.

Imaging Findings

Thoracic radiographs: Possible interstitial pneumonia and mild distention of the cervical esophagus were identified.

Fecal examination

$ZnSO_4$ centrifugal fecal flotation: Positive for *Giardia* spp. cysts.

Diagnosis

Giardiasis and possible pneumonia.

Treatment

The dog was treated wiith IV fluids (0.45% NaCl and 2.5% dextrose), sucralfate, famotidine, and cefazolin. The next day the dog improved and so was discharged with instructions to administer metronidazole (25 mg/kg, PO, q12h for 7 days) for the *G. duodenalis* infection, amoxicillin-clavulanate (21 mg/kg, PO, q12h for 7 days) for suspected interstitial pneumonia, sucralfate for the hemorrhagic diarrhea, and a vitamin supplement. After 10 days, the diarrhea was still present and grossly appeared to contain blood and mucus. The dog was active but hardly eating and drinking; metronidazole was administered for another week. After 2 weeks of metronidazole administration, the dog was still positive for *Giardia* spp. on fecal flotation and *Strongyloides* larvae were also detected. After administration of metronidazole for another 5 days, fenbendazole (50 mg/kg PO q24h) for 5 days was added to the dog's food. Thoracic radiographs at that time showed that the pneumonia was resolving. The next fecal flotation was still positive for *G. duodenalis* and so fenbendazole was prescribed for an additional 14 days. The referring veterinarian also added psyllium to the food and recommended cleaning the environment with a quaternary ammonium compound. Two weeks later the fecal flotation remained positive for *G. duodenalis* cysts and so the dose of metronidazole was increased to 35 mg/kg, PO q12h for 5 days while continuing the fenbendazole. A CBC and a chemistry panel were performed in order to assess for evidence of underlying immunodeficiency. Abnormalities noted included a lymphocytosis (5311/μL; N = 690–4500/μL) and hypoproteinemia (total protein 4.7 g/dL: RR, 5–7.4 g/dL). Treatment with amoxicillin-clavulanate (for an additional 14 days), metronidazole (for an additional 5 days), and fenbendazole (for an additional 14 days) was continued. In the meantime, the consistency of the feces was still soft. Continued treatment with fenbendazole for 90 days was begun. However, the stool consistency remained soft and the next fecal flotation remained positive for *G. duodenalis.* At that time one of the authors (MRL) was consulted and it was recommended that the dog be evaluated for *Cryptosporidium* spp. co-infection. An FA confirmed that the dog was co-infected with *G. duodenalis* and *Cryptosporidium* spp. and tylosin was administered (11 mg/kg, PO, q12h for 28 days). By day 9 of treatment, stools were normal, and the dog was negative for both parasites by FA. The medication was discontinued and a week later the dog appeared to be healthy.

CASE EXAMPLE—cont'd

Comments

In general, giardiasis is more common in young, shelter and immunosuppressed animals. The dog described here was young and had evidence of pneumonia as well as the diarrhea which may have suggested the presence of an underlying immunodeficiency. Diarrheic dogs had a higher prevalence of co-infection with enteric pathogens whereas the non-diarrhea dogs had only single infections. Certain combinations of co-pathogens tend to arise, possibly associated with common factors that promote environmental survival, similar patterns of transmission, and/or host immunodeficiency factors. For example, co-infections with *G. duodenalis* and *Cryptosporidium* (dogs and cats) or *T. blagburni* (cats) have been commonly observed. Additionally, the pathogenic mechanisms and transmission routes of *G. duodenalis* and *Cryptosporidium* are similar.

SUGGESTED READINGS

Bowman DD, Lucio-Forster A. Cryptosporidiosis and giardiasis in dogs and cats: veterinary and public health importance. *Exp Parasitol.* 2010;124:121–127.

da Rocha Gizzi AB, Tostes Oliveira S, Leutenegger CM, et al. Presence of infectious agents and co-infections in diarrheic dogs determined with a real-time polymerase chain reaction-based panel. *BMC Vet Res.* 2014;10:23.

Mizhquiri Barbecho J, Bowman DD, Liotta JL. Comparative performance of reference laboratory tests and in-clinic tests for *Giardia* in canine feces. *Parasit Vectors.* 2018;11:444.

Cacciò SM, Lalle M, Svärd SG. Host specificity in the *Giardia duodenalis* species complex. *Infect Genetics Evol.* 2018;66:335–345.

REFERENCES

1. Wolfe MS. Giardiasis. *Clin Microbiol Rev.* 1992;5:93–100.
2. Bemrick WJ. Observations on dogs infected with *Giardia. J Parasitol.* 1963;49:1031–1032.
3. Bowman DD, Lucio-Forster A. Cryptosporidiosis and giardiasis in dogs and cats: veterinary and public health importance. *Exp Parasitol.* 2010;124:121–127.
4. Ballweber LR, Xiao L, Bowman DD, et al. Giardiasis in dogs and cats: update on epidemiology and public health significance. *Trends Parasitol.* 2010;26:180–189.
5. Cacciò SM, Lalle M, Svärd SG. Host specificity in the *Giardia duodenalis* species complex. *Infect Genetics Evol.* 2018;66:335–345.
6. Lebbad M, Mattsson JG, Christensson B, et al. From mouse to moose: multilocus genotyping of *Giardia* isolates from various animal species. *Vet Parasitol.* 2010;168:231–239.
7. Xiao L, Fayer R. Molecular characterization of species and genotypes of *Cryptosporidium* and *Giardia* and assessment of zoonotic transmission. *Int J Parasitol.* 2008;38:1239–1255.
8. Ryan U, Zahedi A. Molecular epidemiology of giardiasis from a veterinary perspective. *Adv Parasitol.* 2019;106:209–254.
9. Bouzid M, Halai K, Jeffreys D, et al. The prevalence of *Giardia* infection in dogs and cats, a systematic review and meta-analysis of prevalence studies from stool samples. *Vet Parasitol.* 2015;207:181–202.
10. Barr SC, Bowman DD. Giardiasis in dogs and cats. *Compend Contin Educ Pract Vet.* 1994;16:603–611.
11. Certad G, Viscogliosi E, Chabé M, et al. Pathogenic mechanisms of *Cryptosporidium* and *Giardia. Trends Parasitol.* 2017;33:561–576.
12. Buret AG. Pathophysiology of enteric infections with *Giardia duodenalis. Parasite.* 2008;15:261–265.
13. Beatty JK, Akierman SV, Motta JP, et al. *Giardia duodenalis* induces pathogenic dysbiosis of human intestinal microbiota biofilms. *Int J Parasitol.* 2017;47:311–326.
14. Fink MY, Singer SM. The intersection of immune responses, microbiota and pathogenesis in giardiasis. *Trends Parasitol.* 2017;33:901–913.
15. Slapeta J, Dowd SE, Alanazi AD, et al. Differences in the faecal microbiome of non-diarrhoeic clinically healthy dogs and cats associated with *Giardia duodenalis* infection: impact of hookworms and coccidia. *Int J Parasitol.* 2015;45:585–594.
16. Epe C, Rehkter G, Schnieder T, et al. *Giardia* in symptomatic dogs and cats in Europe: results of a European study. *Vet Parasitol.* 2010;173:32–38.
17. Huber F, Bomfim TCB, Gomes RS. Comparison between natural infection by *Cryptosporidium* sp., *Giardia* sp. in dogs in two living situations in the West Zone of the municipality of Rio de Janeiro. *Vet Parasitol.* 2005;130:69–72.
18. Kirkpatrick CE. Feline giardiasis: a review. *J Small Anim Pract.* 1986;27:69–80.
19. Kirkpatrick CE, Farrell JP. Feline giardiasis: observations on natural and induced infections. *Am J Vet Res.* 1984;45:2182–2188.
20. Paris JK, Wills S, Balzer HJ, et al. Enteropathogen co-infection in UK cats with diarrhoea. *BMC Vet Res.* 2014;12:13.
21. Ortuño A, Scorza V, Castellà J, et al. Prevalence of intestinal parasites in shelter and hunting dogs in Catalonia, Northeastern Spain. *Vet J.* 2014;199:465–467.
22. Gookin JL, Stebbins ME, Hunt E, et al. Prevalence of and risk factors for feline *Tritrichomonas foetus* and *Giardia* infection. *J Clin Microbiol.* 2004;42:2707–2710.
23. Scorza AV. Diagnosis and Treatment of *Cryptosporidium* and Giardiasis in cats and dogs. PhD Dissertation. Department of Clinical Sciences, Colorado State University. Fort Collins, CO; 2007.
24. Dryden MW, Payne PA, Smith V. Accurate diagnosis of *Giardia* spp. and proper fecal examination procedures. *Vet Ther.* 2006;7:4–14.
25. Leib MS, Dalton MN, King SE, et al. Endoscopic aspiration of intestinal contents in dogs and cats: 394 cases. *J Vet Intern Med.* 1999;13:191–193.
26. Lappin MR, Calpin J. Laboratory diagnosis of protozoal diseases. In: Saunders W, ed. *Infectious Diseases of the Dog and Cat.* 2nd ed. Philadelphia: Elsevier; 1998:437–441.
27. Zimmer JF, Burrington DB. Comparison of four protocols for the treatment of canine giardiasis. *J Am Anim Hosp Assoc.* 1986;22:168–172.
28. Gates MC, Nolan TJ. Endoparasite prevalence and recurrence across different age groups of dogs and cats. *Vet Parasitol.* 2009;166:153–158.
29. Zajac AM, Johnson J, King SE. Evaluation of the importance of centrifugation as a component of zinc sulfate fecal flotation examinations. *J Am Anim Hosp Assoc.* 2002;38:221–224.
30. Medeiros KL, Lucio-Forster A, Bowman DD. Evaluation of parasite egg and cyst recovery using devices designed for centrifugal or stationary flotation. *J Am Anim Hosp Assoc.* 2018;54:36–45.
31. Hascall KL, Kass PH, Saksen J, et al. Prevalence of enteropathogens in dogs attending 3 regional dog parks in northern California. *J Vet Intern Med.* 2016;30:1838–1845.
32. Lappin MR, Jensen WA, Taton-Allen G. Comparison of $ZnSO_4$ centrifugation, a fecal antigen assay, and an immunofluorescent antibody assay for diagnosis of giardiasis in cats. *Proceedings of the 20th ACVIM Forum.* 2002.
33. Solarczyk P, Majewska A. A survey of the prevalence and genotypes of *Giardia duodenalis* infecting household and sheltered dogs. *Parsitol Res.* 2010;106:1015–1019.
34. Rishniw M, Liotta J, Bellosa M, et al. Comparison of 4 *Giardia* diagnostic tests in diagnosis of naturally acquired canine chronic subclinical giardiasis. *J Vet Intern Med.* 2010;24:293–297.
35. Sokolow SH, Rand C, Marks SL, et al. Epidemiological evaluation of diarrhea dogs in an animal shelter. *Am J Vet Res.* 2005;66:1018–1024.

36. Bachman D, Scorza AV, Brewer M, et al. Evaluation of chromatographic immunoassays for the diagnosis of *Giardia* spp. and *Cryptosporidium* spp. of cats and dogs. *Proceedings of the 25th ACVIM Forum*. 2007.
37. Barr SC, Bowman DD, Erb HN. Evaluation of two test procedures for diagnosis of giardiasis in dogs. *Am J Vet Res*. 1992;53:2028–2031.
38. Cirak VY, Bauer C. Comparison of conventional coproscopical methods and commercial coproantigen ELISA kits for the detection of *Giardia* and *Cryptosporidium* infections in dogs and cats. *Berl Munch Tierarztl Wochenschr*. 2004;117:410–413.
39. Clark M, Scorza AV, Lappin MR. A commercially available *Giardia* spp. antigen assay detects the assemblages isolated from dogs. *Proceedings of the 26th ACVIM Forum*. 2008.
40. Payne PA, Ridley RK, Dryden MW. Efficacy of a combination febantel-praziquantel-pyrantel product, with or without vaccination with a commercial *Giardia* vaccine, for treatment of dogs with naturally occurring giardiasis. *J Am Vet Med Assoc*. 2002;220:330–333.
41. Sommer MF, Rupp P, Pietsch M, et al. *Giardia* in a selected population of dogs and cats in Germany: diagnostics, coinfections and assemblages. *Vet Parasitol*. 2018;249:49–56.
42. Uehlinger FD, Naqvi SA, Greenwood SJ, et al. Comparison of five diagnostic tests for *Giardia duodenalis* in fecal samples from young dogs. *Vet Parasitol*. 2017;244:91–96.
43. Mekaru SR, Marks SL, Felley AJ, et al. Comparison of direct immunofluorescence, immunoassays, and fecal flotation for detection of *Cryptosporidium* spp. and *Giardia* spp. in naturally exposed cats in 4 Northern California animal shelters. *J Vet Intern Med*. 2007;21:959–965.
44. Papini R, Carreras G, Marangi M, et al. Use of a commercial enzyme-linked immunosorbent assay for rapid detection of *Giardia duodenalis* in dog stools in the environment: a Bayesian evaluation. *J Vet Diagn Invest*. 2013;25:418–422.
45. Costa M, Clarke C, Mitchell S, et al. Diagnostic accuracy of two point-of-care kits for the diagnosis of *Giardia* species infection in dogs. *J Small Anim Pract*. 2016;57:318–322.
46. Uiterwijk M, Nijsse R, Kooyman FNJ, et al. Comparing four diagnostic tests for *Giardia duodenalis* in dogs using latent class analysis *Parasit Vectors*. 11:439.
47. Mizhquiri Barbecho J, Bowman DD, Liotta JL. Comparative performance of reference laboratory tests and in-clinic test for *Giardia* in canine feces. *Parasit Vectors*. 2018;11:444.
48. Companion Animal Parasitic Council. *Giardia*. Available at: https://capcvet.org/guidelines/giardia/.
49. Cacciò SM, Ryan U. Molecular epidemiology of giardiasis. *Mol Biochem Parasitol*. 2008;160:75–80.
50. Meggiolaro MN, Roeber F, Kobylski, et al. Comparison of multiplexed-tandem real-time PCR panel with reference real-time PCR molecular diagnostic assays for detection of *Giardia intestinalis* and *Tritrichomonas foetus* in cats. *Vet Parasitol*. 2019;266:12–17.
51. Lalle M, Hanevik K. Treatment-refractory giardiasis: challenges and solutions. *Infect Drug Resist*. 2018;11:1921–1933.
52. Dow SW, LeCouteur RA, Poss ML, et al. Central nervous system toxicosis associated with metronidazole treatment of dogs: five cases (1984–1987). *J Am Vet Med Assoc*. 1989;195:365–368.
53. Groman R. Metronidazole. *Compend Contin Educ Pract Vet*. 2000;22:1104–1107.
54. Caylor KB, Cassimatis MK. Metronidazole neurotoxicosis in two cats. *J Am Hosp Assoc*. 2001;37:258–262.
55. Scorza AV, Lappin MR. Metronidazole for the treatment of feline giardiasis. *J Feline Med Surg*. 2004;6:157–160.
56. Chaitman J, Ziese AL, Pilla R, et al. Fecal microbial and metabolic profiles in dogs with acute diarrhea receiving either fecal microbiota transplantation or oral metronidazole. *Front Vet Sci*. 2020;7:192.
57. Abbitt B, Huey RL, Eugster AK, et al. Treatment of giardiasis in adult greyhounds, using ipronidazole-medicated water. *J Am Vet Med Assoc*. 1986;188:67–69.
58. Da Silva AS, Castro VS, Tonin AA, et al. Secnidazole for the treatment of giardiasis in naturally infected cats. *Parasitol Int*. 2011;60:429–432.
59. Lappin MR, Spindel M, Riggenbach L. Infectious agent prevalence rates in dogs with diarrhea and response to administration of fenbendazole or nitazoxanide. Proceedings of the 25th ACVIM Forum. 2008.
60. Smith HV, Corcoran GD. New drugs and treatment for cryptosporidiosis. *Curr Opin Infect Dis*. 2004;17:667–674.
61. Moron-Soto M, Gutierrez L, Sumano H, et al. Efficacy of nitazoxanide to treat natural *Giardia* infections in dogs. *Parasit Vectors*. 2017;10:52.
62. Barr SC, Bowman DD, Heller RL. Efficacy of fenbendazole against giardiasis in dogs. *Am J Vet Res*. 1994;55:988–990.
63. Keith CL, Radecki SV, Lappin MR. Evaluation of fenbendazole for treatment of *Giardia* infection in cats concurrently infected with *Cryptosporidium parvum*. *Am J Vet Res*. 2003;64:1027–1029.
64. Miró G, Mateo M, Montoya A, et al. Survey of intestinal parasites in stray dogs in the Madrid area and comparison of the efficacy of three anthelmintics in naturally infected dogs. *Parasitol Res*. 2007;100:317–320.
65. Saleh MN, Gilley AD, Byrnes MK, et al. Development and evaluation of a protocol for control of *Giardia duodenalis* in a colony of group-housed dogs at a veterinary medical college. *J Am Vet Med Assoc*. 2016;249:644–649.
66. Schwartz RD, Donogue AR, Baggs RB, et al. Evaluation of the safety of fenbendazole in cats. *J Am Vet Res*. 2000;61:330–332.
67. Barr SC, Bowman DD, Heller RL, et al. Efficacy of albendazole against *Giardia* sp. in dogs and cats. *Proc Am Assoc Vet Parasitol*. 1993;83:56.
68. Villeneuve V, Beugnet F, Bourdoiseau G. Efficacy of oxfendazole for the treatment of giardiosis in dogs. Experiments in dog breeding kennels. *Parasite*. 2000;7:221–226.
69. Bowman DD, Liotta JL, Ulrich M, et al. Treatment of naturally occurring, asymptomatic *Giardia* sp. in dogs with Drontal Plus flavour tablets. *Parasitol Res*. 2009;105(suppl 1):S125–S134.
70. Barr SC, Bowman DD, Frongillo MF, et al. Efficacy of a drug combination of praziquantel, pyrantel pamoate, and febantel against giardiasis in dogs. *Am J Vet Res*. 1998;59:1134–1136.
71. Barutzki D, Schaper R. Endoparasites in dogs and cats in Germany 1999-2002. *Parasitol Res*. 2003;90(suppl 3):S148–S150.
72. Bowman DD, Charles S, Heine J, et al. Efficacy of Drontal Plus flavour 950mg praziquantel, 144 mg pyrantel amboate, 150 mg febantel per tablet) against *Giardia* sp. in naturally infected dogs. *International Giardia and Cryptosporidium Conference*. Mexico: Morelia, Michoacan; 2007.
73. Giangaspero A, Traldi G, Paoletti B, et al. Efficacy of pyrantel embonate, febantel and praziquantel against *Giardia* species in naturally infected adult dogs. *Vet Rec*. 2002;150:184–186.
74. Montoya A, Dado D, Mateo M, et al. Efficacy of Drontal Flavour Plus (50 mg praziquantel, 144 mg pyrantel embonate, 150 mg febantel pr tablet) against *Giardia* sp. in naturally infected dogs. *Parasitol Res*. 2008;103:1141–1144.
75. Scorza AV, Radecki SV, Lappin MR. Efficacy of a combination of febantel, pyrantel, and praziquantel for the treatment of kittens experimentally infected with *Giardia* species. *J Feline Med Surg*. 2006;8:7–13.
76. Zygner W, Jaros D, Gójska-Zygner O, et al. Azithromycin in the treatment of a dog infected with *Giardia intestinalis*. *Pol J Vet Sci*. 2008;11:231–234.
77. Katelaris PH, Naeem A, Farthing MJ. Activity of metronidazole, azithromycin and three benzimidazoles on *Giardia lamblia* growth and attachment to a human intestinal cell line. *Aliment Pharmacol Ther*. 1994;8:187–192.
78. Lappin MR, Clark M, Scorza AV. Treatment of healthy *Giardia* spp. positive dogs with fenbendazole or nitazoxanide. *Proceedings of the 26th ACVIM Forum*. 2008.
79. Debnath A, Ndao M, Reed SL. Reprofiled drug targets ancient protozoans: drug discovery for parasitic diarrheal diseases. *Gut Microb*. 2013;4:66–71.
80. Zoafin. Available at: https://zoafin.com.
81. Chon SK, Kim NS. Evaluation of silymarin in the treatment of asymptomatic *Giardia* infections in dogs. *Parasitol Res*. 2005;97:445–451.
82. Leitch GJ, Visvesvara GS, Wahlquist SP, et al. Dietary fiber and giardiasis: dietary fiber reduces rate of intestinal infection by *Giardia lamblia* in the gerbil. *Am J Trop Med Hyg*. 1989;41:512–520.
83. Benyacoub J, Pérez PF, Rochat F, et al. *Enterococcus faecium* SF68 enhances the immune response to *Giardia intestinalis* in mice. *J Nutr*. 2005;135:1171–1176.
84. Bezagio RC, Colli CM, Romera LI, et al. Synergistic effects of fenbendazole and metronidazole against *Giardia muris* in Swiss mice naturally infected. *Parasitol Res*. 2017;116:939–944.

85. Fujishiro MA, Lidbury JA, Pilla R, et al. Evaluation of the effects of anthelmintic administration on the fecal microbiome of healthy dogs with and without subclinical *Giardia* spp. and *Cryptosporidium canis* infections. *PLoS One*. 2020;15:e0228145.
86. Olson ME, Hannigan CJ, Gaviller PF, Fulton LA. The use of a *Giardia* vaccine as an immunotherapeutic agent in dogs. *Can Vet J*. 2001;42:865–868.
87. Molina Díaz VM. Pharmacological treatment of giardiasis. In: Rodriguez-Morales AJ, ed. *Current Topics in Giardiasis*. [Internet]. London: IntechOpen; 2017:176.
88. Serradell MC, Saura A, Rupil LL, et al. Vaccination of domestic animals with a novel oral vaccine prevents *Giardia* infections, alleviates signs of giardiasis and reduces transmission to humans. *NPJ Vaccines*. 2016;1:16018.
89. Kirkpatrick CE, Laczak JP. Giardiasis in a cattery. *J Am Vet Med Assoc*. 1985;187:161–162.
90. Zimmer JF, Miller JJ, Lindmark DG. Evaluation of the efficacy of selected commercial disinfectants in inactivating *Giardia muris* cysts. *J Am Anim Hosp Assoc*. 1988;24:379–385.
91. Feng Y, Xiao L. Zoonotic potential and molecular epidemiology of *Giardia* species and giardiasis. *Clin Microbiol Rev*. 2011;24:110–140.
92. Hoque ME, Hope VT, Scragg R, Kjellström T. Children at risk of giardiasis in Auckland: a case-control analysis. *Epidemiol Infect*. 2003;131:655–662.
93. Gil H, Cano L, de Lucio A, et al. Detection and molecular diversity of *Giardia duodenalis* and *Cryptosporidium* spp. in sheltered dogs and cats in Northern Spain. *Infect Genet Evol*. 2017;50:62–69.
94. Li W, Liu C, Yu Y, et al. Molecular characterization of *Giardia duodenalis* isolates from police and farm dogs in China. *Exp Parasitol*. 2013;135:223–226.
95. Quadros RM, Weiss PH, Marques SM, et al. Potential cross-contamination of similar *Giardia duodenalis* assemblage in children and pet dogs in southern Brazil as determined by PCR-RFLP. *Rev Inst Med Trop Sao Paulo*. 2016;22:58–66.
96. Rehbein S, Klotz C, Ignatius R, et al. *Giardia duodenalis* in small animals and their owners in Germany: a pilot study. *Zoonoses Public Health*. 2019;66:117–124.
97. Berrilli F, Di Cave D, De Liberato C, et al. Genotype characterisation of *Giardia duodenalis* isolates from domestic and farm animals by SSU-rRNA gene sequencing. *Vet Parasitol*. 2004;122:193–199.
98. Colli CM, Bezagio RC, Nishi L, et al. Identical assemblage of *Giardia duodenalis* in humans, animals and vegetables in an urban area in southern Brazil indicates a relationship among them. *PLoS One*. 2015;11:3.
99. Lalle M, Pozio E, Capelli G, et al. Genetic heterogeneity at the beta-giardin locus among human and animal isolates of *Giardia duodenalis* and identification of potentially zoonotic subgenotypes. *Int J Parasitol*. 2005;35:207–213.
100. Marangi M, Berrilli F, Otranto D, et al. Genotyping of *Giardia duodenalis* among children and dogs in a closed socially deprived community from Italy. *Zoonoses Public Health*. 2010;57:e54–e58.
101. Souza SL, Gennari SM, Richtzenhain LJ, et al. Molecular identification of *Giardia duodenalis* isolates from humans, dogs, cats and cattle from the state of Sao Paulo, Brazil, by sequence analysis of fragments of glutamate dehydrogenase (gdh) coding gene. *Vet Parasitol*. 2007;149:258–264.
102. Inpankaew T, Traub R, Thompson RCA, et al. Canine parasitic zoonoses in Bangkok temples. *Southeast Asian J Trop Med Public Health*. 2007;38:247–255.
103. Volotao AC, Costa-Macedo LM, Haddad FS, et al. Genotyping of *Giardia duodenalis* from human and animal samples from Brazil using beta-giardin gene: a phylogenetic analysis. *Acta Trop*. 2007;102:10–19.
104. Sprong H, Caccio SM, van der Giessen JW, et al. Identification of zoonotic genotypes of *Giardia duodenalis*. *PLoS Negl Trop Dis*. 2009;3:e558.
105. Monis PT, Thompson RCA. *Cryptosporidium* and *Giardia*—zoonoses: fact or fiction? *Infect Gen Evol*. 2003;3:233–244.
106. Lee MF, Cadogan P, Eytle S, et al. Molecular epidemiology and multilocus sequence analysis of potentially zoonotic *Giardia* spp. from humans and dogs in Jamaica. *Parasitol Res*. 2017;116:409–414.
107. Covacin C, Aucoin DP, Elliot A, et al. Genotypic characterization of *Giardia* from domestic dogs in the USA. *Vet Parasitol*. 2011;177:28–32.
108. Himsworth CG, Skinner S, Chaban B, et al. Short report: multiple zoonotic pathogens identified in canine feces collected from a remote Canadian indigenous community. *Am J Trop Med Hyg*. 2010;83:338–341.
109. Leonhard S, Pfister K, Beelitz P, et al. The molecular characterisation of *Giardia* from dogs in southern Germany. *Vet Parasitol*. 2007;150:33–38.
110. Traub RJ, Monis PT, Robertson I, et al. Epidemiological and molecular evidence supports the zoonotic transmission of *Giardia* among humans and dogs living in the same community. *Parasitology*. 2004;128:253–262.
111. Traub RJ, Robertson ID, Irwin P, et al. Humans, dogs and parasitic zoonoses—unraveling the relationships in a remote endemic community in northeast India using molecular tools. *Parasitol Res*. 2003;90:S156–S157.
112. Gelanew T, Lalle M, Hailu A, et al. Molecular characterization of human isolates of *Giardia duodenalis* from Ethiopia. *Acta Trop*. 2007;102:92–99.
113. Štrkolcová G, Maďar M, Hinney B, et al. Dog's genotype of *Giardia duodenalis* in human: first evidence in Europe. *Acta Parasitol*. 2015;60:796–799.
114. Wang A, Ruch-Gallie R, Scorza V, et al. Prevalence of *Giardia* and *Cryptosporidium* species in dog park attending dogs compared to non-dog park attending dogs in one region of Colorado. *Vet Parasitol*. 2012;23:335–340.
115. Procter TD, Pearl DL, Finley RL, et al. A cross-sectional study examining *Campylobacter* and other zoonotic enteric pathogens in dogs that frequent dog parks in three cities in south-western Ontario and risk factors for shedding of *Campylobacter* spp. *Zoonoses Public Health*. 2014;61:208–218.
116. Shukullari E, Hamel D, Rapti D, et al. Parasites and vector-borne diseases in client-owned dogs in Albania. Intestinal and pulmonary endoparasite infections. *Parasitol Res*. 2015;114:4579–4590.
117. Taranto NJ, Pasamonte L, Marinconz R, et al. Zoonotic parasitosis transmitted by dogs in the Chaco Saltenio, Argentina. *Medicina (B Aires)*. 2000;60:270–272.
118. Fava NM, Soares RM, Scalia LAM, et al. Molecular typing of canine *Giardia duodenalis* isolates from Minas Gerais, Brazil. *Exp Parasitol*. 2016;161:1–5.
119. McDowall RM, Peregrine AS, Leonard EK, et al. Evaluation of the zoonotic potential of *Giardia duodenalis* in fecal samples from dogs and cats in Ontario. *Can Vet J*. 2011;52:1329–1333.
120. Joffe D, Van Niekerk D, Gagne F, et al. The prevalence of intestinal parasites in dogs and cats in Calgary, Alberta. *Can Vet J*. 2011;52:1323–1328.
121. Shukla R, Giraldo P, Kraliz A, et al. *Cryptosporidium* spp. and other zoonotic enteric parasites in a sample of domestic dogs and cats in the Niagara region of Ontario. *Can Vet J*. 2006;47:1179–1184.
122. Jacobs SR, Forrester CPR, Yang J. A survey of the prevalence of *Giardia* in dogs presented to Canadian veterinary practices. *Can Vet J*. 2001;42:45–46.
123. Lefebvre SL, Waltner-Toews D, Peregrine AS, et al. Prevalence of zoonotic agents in dogs visiting hospitalized people in Ontario: implications for infection control. *J Hosp Infect*. 2006;62:458–466.
124. Inpankaew T, Schär F, Odermatt P, et al. Low risk for transmission of zoonotic *Giardia duodenalis* from dogs to humans in rural Cambodia. *Parasites Vectors*. 2014;7:412.
125. Zheng G, Hu W, Liu Y, et al. Occurrence and molecular identification of *Giardia duodenalis* from stray cats in Guangzhou, Southern China. *Korean J Parasitol*. 2015;53:119–124.
126. Gu YF, Wang K, Liu DY. Molecular detection of *Giardia lamblia* and *Cryptosporidium* species in pet dogs. *Chinese J Parasitol Parasitic Dis*. 2015;33:362–367.
127. Yang D, Zhang Q, Zhang L, et al. Prevalence and risk factors of *Giardia* doudenalis in dogs from China. *Int J Environ Health Res*. 2015;25:207–213.
128. Xu H, Jin Y, Wu W, et al. Genotypes of *Cryptosporidium* spp., *Enterocytozoon bieneusi* and *Giardia duodenalis* in dogs and cats in Shanghai, China. *Parasites Vectors*. 2016;9:121.
129. Qi M, Dong H, Wang R, et al. Infection rate and genetic diversity of *Giardia duodenalis* in pet and stray dogs in Henan Province, China. *Parasitol International*. 2016;65:159–162.
130. Svobodovà V, Konvalinova J, Svodobodova M. Coprological and serological findings in dogs and cats with giardiosis and cryptosporidiosis. *Acta Vet Brno*. 1994;63:257–262.
131. Osman M, Bories J, El Safadi D, et al. Prevalence and genetic diversity of the intestinal parasites *Blastocystis* sp. and *Cryptosporidium* spp. in

household dogs in France and evaluation of zoonotic transmission risk. *Vet Parasitol*. 2015;30:167–170.
132. Epe C, Coati N, Schnieder T. Results of parasitological examinations of faecal samples from horses, ruminants, pigs, dogs, cats, hedgehogs and rabbits between 1998 and 2002. *Dtsch Tierarztl Wochenschr*. 2004;111:243–247.
133. Becker AC, Rohen M, Epe C, et al. Prevalence of endoparasites in stray and fostered dogs and cats in Northern Germany. *Parasitol Res*. 2012;111:849–857.
134. Szenasi Z, Marton S, Kucsera I, et al. Preliminary investigation of prevalence and genotype distribution of *Giardia intestinalis* in dogs in Hungary. *Parasitol Res*. 2007;101:145–152.
135. Capári B, Hamel D, Visser M, et al. Parasitic infections of domestic cats, *Felis catus*, in western Hungary. *Vet Parasitol*. 2013;192:33–42.
136. Shoorijeh S, Sadjjadi SM, Asheri A, et al. *Giardia* spp. and *Sarcocystis* spp. status in pet dogs of Shiraz, southern part of Iran. *Trop Biomed*. 2008;25:154–159.
137. Gharekhani J. Study on gastrointestinal zoonotic parasites in pet dogs in Western Iran. *Turkiye Parazitol Derg*. 2014;38:172–176.
138. Biancardi P, Papini R, Giuliani G, et al. Prevalence of *Giardia* antigen in stool samples from dogs and cats. *Revue Med Vet*. 2004;155:417–421.
139. Garcia-Campos A, Power C, O'Shaughnessy J, et al. One-year parasitological screening of stray dogs and cats in County Dublin, Ireland. *Parasitology*. 2019; 146:746–752.
140. Papini R, Gorini G, Spaziani A, et al. Survey on giardiosis in shelter dog population. *Vet Parasitol*. 2005;128:333–339.
141. Papini R, Marangi M, Mancianti F, et al. Occurrence and cyst burden of *Giardia duodenalis* in dog faecal deposits from urban green areas: implications for environmental contamination and related risks. *Prev Vet Med*. 2009;95:158–162.
142. Scaramozzino P, Cave DD, Berrilli F, et al. A study of the prevalence and genotypes of *Giardia duodenalis* infecting kenneled dogs. *Vet J*. 2009;182:231–234.
143. Pipia AP, Varcasia A, Tamponi C, et al. Canine giardiosis in Sardinia Island, Italy: prevalence, molecular characterization, and risk factors. *J Infect Dev Ctries*. 2014;14:655–660.
144. Spada E, Proverbio D, Della Pepa A, et al. Prevalence of faecal-borne parasites in colony stray cats in northern Italy. *J Fel Med Surg*. 2013;15:672–677.
145. Itoh N, Kanai K, Tominaga H, et al. *Giardia* and other intestinal parasites in dogs from veterinary clinics in Japan. *Parasitol Res*. 2011;109:253–256.
146. Yamamoto N, Kon M, Saito T, et al. Prevalence of intestinal canine and feline parasites in Saitama Prefecture, Japan. *Kansenshogaku Zasshi*. 2009;83:223–228.
147. Itoh N, Kanai K, Kimura Y, et al. Prevalence of intestinal parasites in breeding kennel dogs in Japan. *Parasitol Res*. 2015;114:1221–1224.
148. Itoh N, Kanai K, Hori Y, et al. Prevalence of *Giardia intestinalis* and other zoonotic intestinal parasites in private household dogs of the Hachinohe area in Aomori prefecture, Japan in 1997, 2002 and 2007. *J Vet Sci*. 2009;10:305–308.
149. Piekarska J, Bajzert J, Gorczykowski M, et al. Molecular identification of *Giardia duodenalis* isolates from domestic dogs and cats in Wroclaw, Poland. *Ann Agric Environ Med*. 2016;23:410–415.
150. Simpson JW, Burnie AG, Miles RS, et al. Prevalence of *Giardia* and *Cryptosporidium* infection in dogs in Edinburgh. *Vet Rec*. 1988;123:445.
151. Nikolic A, Dimitrijevic S, Djurkovic-Djakovic O, et al. Giardiasis in dogs and kittens in the Belgrade Area. *Acta Vet*. 2002;52:43–48.
152. Gracenea M, Goméz MS, Torres J. Prevalence of internal parasites in shelter dogs and cats in the metropolitan area of Barcelona (Spain). *Acta Parasitol*. 2009;54:73–77.
153. Dado D, Montoya A, Blanco MA, et al. Prevalence and genotypes of *Giardia duodenalis* from dogs in Spain: possible zoonotic transmission and public health importance. *Parasitol Res*. 2012;111:2419–2422.
154. Adell-Aledon M, Koster PC, de Lucio A, et al. Occurrence and molecular epidemiology of *Giardia duodenalis* infection in dog populations in eastern Spain. *BMC Vet Res*. 2018;14:26.
155. de Lucio A, Bailo B, Aguilera M, et al. No molecular epidemiological evidence supporting household transmission of zoonotic *Giardia duodenalis* and *Cryptosporidium* spp. from pet dogs and cats in the province of Alava, Northern Spain. *Acta Trop*. 2017;170:48–56.
156. Tseng YC, Ho GD, Chen TTW, et al. Prevalence and genotype of *Giardia duodenalis* from faecal samples of stray dogs in Hualien city of eastern Taiwan. *Trop Biomed*. 2014;31:305–311.
157. Rojekittikhun W, Chaisiri K, Mahittikorn A, et al. Gastrointestinal parasites of dogs and cats in a refuge in Nakhon Nayok, Thailand. *Southeast Asian J Trop Med Public Health*. 2014;45:31–39.
158. Overgaauw PA, van Zutphen L, Hoek D, et al. Zoonotic parasites in fecal samples and fur from dogs and cats in The Netherlands. *Vet Parasitol*. 2009;163:115–122.
159. Sykes TJ, Fox MT. Patterns of infection with *Giardia* in dogs in London. *Trans R Soc Trop Med Hyg*. 1989;83:239–240.
160. Little SE, Johnson EM, Levis D, et al. Prevalence of intestinal parasites in pet dogs in the United States. *Vet Parasitol*. 2009;166:144–152.
161. Zislin A, Goldstein M, Hustead D. Prevalence of *Giardia* in companion animal populations in the USA. In: Olson B, Olson M, Wallis P, eds. *Giardia. The Cosmopolitan Parasite*. New York: CABI Publishing; 2002:87–90.
162. Carlin EP, Bowman DD, Scarlett JM, et al. Prevalence of *Giardia* in symptomatic dogs and cats throughout the United States as determined by the IDEXX SNAP *Giardia* test. *Vet Ther*. 2006;7:199–206.
163. Jafri HS, Reedy T, Moorhead AR, et al. Detection of pathogenic protozoa in fecal specimens from urban dwelling dogs. *Proceedings of the 42nd Annual Meeting of the American Society of Tropical Medicine and Hygiene*. 1993.
164. Munoz J, Mayer G. *Toxoplasma gondii* and *Giardia duodenalis* infections in domestic dogs in New York City public parks. *Vet J*. 2016;211: 97–99.
165. Johansen KM, Castro NS, Lancaster KE, et al. Characterization of *Giardia lamblia* genotypes in dogs from Tucson, Arizona using SSU-rRNA and β-giardin sequences. *Parasitol Res*. 2014;113:387–390.
166. Knaus M, Rapti D, Shukullari E, et al. Characterisation of ecto- and endoparasites in domestic cats from Tirana, Albania. *Parasitol Res*. 2014;113:3361–3371.
167. Hinney H, Ederer C, Stengl C. Enteric protozoa of cats and their zoonotic potential—a field study from Austria. *Parasitol Res*. 2015;114:2003–2006.
168. McGlade TR, Robertson ID, Elliot AD, et al. High prevalence of *Giardia* detected in cats by PCR. *Vet Parasitol*. 2003;110:197–205.
169. Barrientos Serra CM, Antunes Uchoa CM, Alonso Coimbra R. Parasitological study with fecal samples of stray and domiciliated cats (*Felis catus domesticus*) from the metropolitan area of Rio de Janeiro, Brazil. *Rev Soc Bras Med Trop*. 2003;36:331–334.
170. David ÉB, Guimarães S, de Oliveira AP, et al. Molecular characterization of intestinal protozoa in two poor communities in the state of São Paulo, Brazil. Parasites Vectors 2016;8:103.
171. Hoopes JH, Polley L, Wagner B, et al. A retrospective investigation of feline gastrointestinal parasites in western Canada. *Can Vet J*. 2013;54:359–362.
172. López JD, Abarca K, Paredes P, et al. Intestinal parasites in dogs and cats with gastrointestinal symptoms in Santiago, Chile. *Rev Med Chile*. 2006;134:193–200.
173. Luzio A, Belmar P, Troncoso I, et al. Parasites importance in dog feces collected in parks and public squares of the city of Los Angeles, Bio-Bio, Chile. *Rev Chilena Infectol*. 2015;32:403–407.
174. Khalafalla RE. A survey study on gastrointestinal parasites of stray cats in northern region of Nile delta, Egypt. *PLoS One*. 2011;6:e20283.
175. Näreaho A, Puomio J, Saarinen K, et al. Feline intestinal parasites in Finland: prevalence, risk factors and anthelmintic treatment practices. *J Fel Med Surg*. 2012;14:378–383.
176. Beck R, Sprong H, Pozio E, et al. Genotyping *Giardia duodenalis* isolates from dogs: lessons from a multilocus sequence typing study. *Vector Borne Zoonotic Dis*. 2012;12:206–213.
177. Khademvatan S, Abdizadeh R, Rahim F, et al. Stray cats gastrointestinal parasites and its association with public health in Ahvaz city, South Western of Iran. *Jundishapur J Microbiol*. 2014;7:11079.
178. Zanzani SA, Di Cerbo AR, Gazzonis AL, et al. Canine fecal contamination in a metropolitan area (Milan, north-western Italy): prevalence of intestinal parasites and evaluation of health risks. *Scientific World Journal*. 2014;2014:132361.
179. Itoh N, Ikegami H, Takagi MJ. Prevalence of intestinal parasites in private-household cats in Japan. *J Feline Med Surg*. 2012;6:436–439.

180. Robben SR, le Nobel WE, Döpfer D, et al. Infections with helminths and/or protozoa in cats in animal shelters in The Netherlands. *Tijdschr Diergeneeskd*. 2004;129:2–6.
181. Tzannes S, Batchelor DJ, Graham PA, et al. Prevalence of *Cryptosporidium, Giardia* and *Isospora* species infections in pet cats with clinical signs of gastrointestinal disease. *J Feline Med Surg*. 2008;10:1–8.
182. Hill SL, Cheney JM, Taton-Allen GF, et al. Prevalence of enteric zoonotic organisms in cats. *J Am Vet Med Assoc*. 2000;216:687–692.
183. Vasilopulos RJ, Rickard LG, Mackin AJ, et al. Genotypic analysis of *Giardia duodenalis* in domestic cats. *J Vet Intern Med*. 2007;21:352–355.
184. Spain CV, Scarlett JM, Wade SE, et al. Prevalence of enteric zoonotic agents in cats less than 1 year old in central New York State. *J Vet Intern Med*. 2001;15:33–38.
185. Gates MC, Nolan TJ. Comparison of passive fecal flotation run by veterinary students to zinc-sulfate centrifugation flotation run in a diagnostic parasitology laboratory. *J Parasitol*. 2009;195:1213–1214.
186. Monis PT, Andrews RH, Mayrhofer G, et al. Novel lineages of *Giardia intestinalis* identified by genetic analysis of organisms isolated from dogs in Australia. *Parasitology*. 1998;11:7–19.
187. Read CM, Monis PT, Thompson RC. Discrimination of all genotypes of *Giardia duodenalis* at the glutamate dehydrogenase locus using PCR-RFLP. *Infect Genet Evol*. 2004;4:125–130.
188. Li J, Zhang P, Wang P, et al. Genotype identification and prevalence of *Giardia duodenalis* in pet dogs of Guangzhou, Southern China. *Vet Parasitol*. 2012;188:368–371.
189. Barutzki D, Thompson RC, Wielinga C, et al. Observations of *Giardia* infections in dogs from veterinary clinics in Germany. *Parasitol Res*. 2007;101:153–156.
190. Pallant L, Barutzki D, Schaper R, et al. The epidemiology of infections with *Giardia* species and genotypes in well cared for dogs and cats in Germany. *Parasit Vectors*. 2015;8:2.
191. Ravagnan S, Minazzato E, Coppellotti O, et al. Comparison of two target genes for detection and genotyping of *Giardia duodenalis* in mammals. *3rd International Giardia and Cryptosporidium Conference*. Italy: Orvieto; 2009.
192. Abe N, Kimata I, Iseki M. Identification of genotypes of *Giardia intestinalis* isolates from dogs in Japan by direct sequencing of the PCR amplified glutamate dehydrogenase gene. *J Vet Med Sci*. 2003;65:29–33.
193. Itagaki T, Kinoshita S, Aoki M, et al. Genotyping of *Giardia intestinalis* from domestic and wild animals in Japan using glutamete dehydrogenase gene sequencing. *Vet Parasitol*. 2005;133:283–287.
194. Eligio-Garcia L, Cortes-Campos A, Jimenez-Cardoso E. Genotype of *Giardia intestinalis* isolates from children and dogs and its relationship to host origin. *Parasitol Res*. 2005;97:1–6.
195. Sousa MC. Predominance of zoonotic *Giardia* assemblage A in dogs in Portugal. *3rd International Giardia and Cryptosporidium Conference*. Italy: Orvieto; 2009.
196. Gyorke A, Zsuzsa K, Mirabela Oana D, et al. *Giardia duodenalis* genotypes in domestic and wild animals from Romania identified by PCR-RFLP targeting the gdh gene. *Vet Parasitol*. 2016;217:71–75.
197. Dado D, Montoya A, Blanco MA, et al. Prevalence and genotypes of *Giardia duodenalis* from dogs in Spain: possible zoonotic transmission and public health importance. *Parasitol Res*. 2012;111:2419–2422.
198. Mark-Carew MP, Adesiyun AA, Basu A, et al. Characterization of *Giardia duodenalis* infections in dogs in Trinidad and Tobago. *Vet Parasitol*. 2013;1:199–202.
199. Sulaiman IM, Fayer R, Bern C, et al. Triosephosphate isomerase gene characterization and potential zoonotic transmission of *Giardia duodenalis*. *Emerg Infect Dis*. 2003;9:1444–1452.
200. Nguyen LP, Phungb CD, Thompson RCA. Prevalence and characterization of *Giardia* and *Cryptosporidium* in human and domestic animals in a rural area of Vietnam. *3rd International Giardia and Cryptosporidium Conference*. Italy: Orvieto; 2009.
201. Scorza AV, Ballweber LR, Tangtrongsup S, et al. Comparisons of mammalian *Giardia duodenalis* assemblages based on the beta-giardin, glutamate dehydrogenase and triose phosphate isomerase genes. *Vet Parasitol*. 2012;189:182–188.
202. Santín M, Trout JM, Vecino JA, et al. *Cryptosporidium, Giardia* and *Enterocytozoon bieneusi* in cats from Bogota (Colombia) and genotyping of isolates. *Vet Parasitol*. 2006;141:334–339.
203. Iijima Y, Itoh N, Ito Y, et al. Multilocus genotyping of *Giardia duodenalis* isolates from household cats and pet shop kittens. *Vet Parasitol*. 2018;259:44–48.
204. Jaros D, Zygner W, Jaros S, et al. Detection of *Giardia intestinalis* assemblages A, B and D in domestic cats from Warsaw, Poland. *Pol J Microbiol*. 2011;60:259–263.
205. Ferreira FS, Pereira-Baltasar P, Parreira R, et al. Intestinal parasites in dogs and cats from the district of Évora, Portugal. *Vet Parasitol*. 2011;179:242–245.
206. Fayer R, Santín M, Trout JM, et al. Detection of *Cryptosporidium felis* and *Giardia duodenalis* assemblage F in a cat colony. *Vet Parasitol*. 2006;140:44–53.
207. Sommer MF, Beck R, Ionita M, et al. Multilocus sequence typing of canine *Giardia duodenalis* from South Eastern European countries. *Parasitol Res*. 2015;114:2165–2174.
208. Lalle M, Jimenez-Cardosa E, Cacciò SM, et al. Genotyping of *Giardia duodenalis* from humans and dogs from Mexico using a beta-giardin nested polymerase chain reaction assay. *J Parasitol*. 2005;91:203–205.

102

Trichomonosis

M. Katherine Tolbert

KEY POINTS

- Cause: *Tritrichomonas blagburni* (also known as *Tritrichomonas foetus*); flagellate protozoan (phylum Sarcomastigophora, order Trichomonadida, class Parabasalia).
- First Described: Trophozoites that were likely to be *T. foetus* have been recognized in cat feces for many years, but *T. blagburni* was not definitely recognized as the primary cause of trichomonal diarrhea until 2003 (Levy).[1]
- Affected Host Species: Cats. Clinical signs of disease are most common in purebred or young cats that are housed or originate from high-density housing environments.
- Geographic Distribution: Although infections have not been documented in all countries, *T. blagburni* infection of cats is thought to have a worldwide distribution.
- Primary Mode of Transmission: Fecal-oral. There are no proven intermediate hosts, but *T. blagburni* can survive outside the host for several hours as well as survive transit through slugs, and so transport hosts are possible.
- Major Clinical Signs: Subclinical infections are common in high-risk cats. Continuous or intermittent large bowel diarrhea is most common in young, purebred cats. Swelling of the anus and fecal incontinence can occur.
- Differential Diagnoses: All causes of large bowel diarrhea, including *Cystoisospora* spp., food responsive disease, and inflammatory bowel disease. If motile trophozoites are noted on wet mount examination of feces, infections with *Giardia* spp. and *Pentatrichomonas hominis* are differential diagnoses.
- Human Health Significance: There are no known significant human health risks associated with *T. blagburni* infections of cats. However, two case reports of immunocompromised humans with *T. foetus* infections thought to be cattle or swine genotype suggest a zoonotic potential of trichomonads. Thus, cat feces should always be handled as if the possibility of zoonosis exists.

ETIOLOGIC AGENT AND EPIDEMIOLOGY

Members of the order Trichomonadida are flagellates that reproduce by binary fission and do not form true cysts (Fig. 102.1).[2,3] The trophozoite of *Tritrichomonas blagburni* is 10 to 26 μm long and 3 to 5 μm wide, spindle-to-pear shaped, and has three anterior flagella and a posteriorly directed flagellum (Fig. 102.2). A rigid, rod-shaped axostyle bisects the trichomonad and protrudes from the posterior end. In vertebrates, trichomonads are parasites of microaerophilic environments including the GI system, the reproductive system, and the upper portions of the respiratory tract. *Tritrichomonas blagburni* infects the reproductive tract of both cows and bulls and can cause abortion and other reproductive abnormalities. The organism resides as a commensal or parasite within the GI system of the cat and can be associated with diarrhea. Genetic characterization of bovine and feline *Tritrichomonas* spp. isolates has been performed, and minor differences exist.[4–6] Feline isolates of *T. blagburni* remained in the reproductive tract of heifers but did not cause the same pathologic changes as a bovine isolate in one study.[7] Similarly, a bovine isolate of *T. blagburni* did not cause diarrhea in cats as successfully as feline isolates.[8] Although a proposed name change has not been adopted by the American College of Veterinary Parasitologists, this lack of host specificity has led investigators to propose that the feline trichomonad is an entirely different species and should be renamed *Tritrichomonas blagburni*.[9] However, experimental infection of cats with the feline isolate also does not reliably reproduce disease.

Tritrichomonas blagburni is presumed to be transmitted by the direct fecal-oral route. The organism can survive for short periods of time in contaminated water, urine, feces, and cat litter,[10,11] although they do not persist under clean, dry, and aerobic conditions. Shared food bowls and litter boxes and mutual grooming likely contribute to transmission from one cat to another. In one study, the organism was shown to survive 30 minutes on dry cat food, several hours in moist cat food, and hours to days in cat feces.[10] The organism also survived transit through the GI tract of two types of slugs, which are known to eat cat feces.[12]

Cats that harbor *T. blagburni* infection have now been documented in multiple countries.[13–28] Cats in crowded environments and purebred catteries are commonly colonized; the organism is uncommon in feral cats. In one of the first large prevalence studies in the United States, 31% of 117 cats owned by 89 different breeders at an international cat show were colonized.[29] In the United Kingdom, 16 (14.4%) of 111 diarrhea specimens were positive for *T. blagburni* by PCR assay.[18] *Tritrichomonas blagburni*-associated diarrhea is most common in kittens and young cats, but adult cats can also be affected.[18,29] Catteries with a recent history of refractory diarrhea, adult cats with *Cystoisospora* spp. infections, and cats living in a facility with a small number of square feet per cat were more likely to be infected with *T. blagburni* in some studies.[18,29] Other co-infections, such as those with *Giardia* spp. and *Cryptosporidium* spp., may also increase the potential for disease.[30] Proximity of a cattery to agricultural species (pigs, cattle, horses), feeding of raw meat, type of water source, outdoor contact, or history of travel have not been identified as significant risk factors for *T. blagburni* infection in cats.

T. blagburni infection has only been identified in two dogs; these dogs were concurrently infected with *Giardia* or *Pentatrichomonas hominis*, respectively.[31,32] Thus, dogs are not considered to be natural hosts for *T. blagburni*.

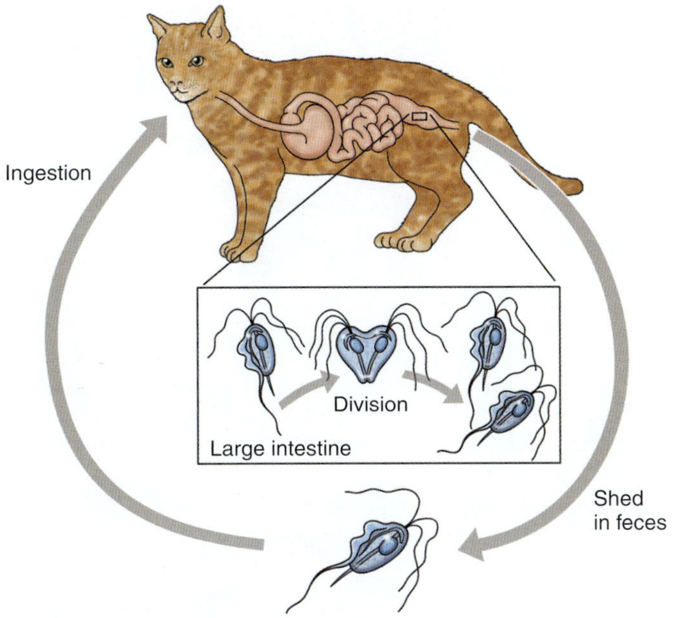

Fig. 102.1 Life cycle of *Tritrichomonas blagburni*. The organism has a direct life cycle, and the parasite replicates by binary fission.

CLINICAL FEATURES

Pathogenesis and Clinical Signs

Tritrichomonas blagburni is an obligate parasite, which like other trichomonads, resides in a nonsterile environment because it lacks many of its own metabolic pathways and, therefore, relies on the host and resident microorganisms for provision of nutrients. In experimentally infected cats, the location of *T. blagburni* is restricted to the terminal ileum, cecum, and colon where bacterial density is the highest.[33,34] Fluctuations in the colonic microflora or genetic and environmental factors may be necessary to produce the clinical signs in association with *T. blagburni* infection. The organism can persist in cats without diarrhea, and diarrhea can worsen without a change in the number of organisms present, suggesting that the underlying mechanisms that lead to diarrhea are multifactorial.[33] Other pathogenic factors associated with *T. blagburni* include adherence to host epithelium and elaboration of cytotoxins and proteolytic enzymes.[35–40] The organism adheres to the intestinal epithelium and incites a lymphoplasmacytic and neutrophilic inflammatory response.[34] An increased number of *T. blagburni* organisms and increased severity of diarrhea were associated with co-infection with *Cryptosporidium* spp. in one study.[33] However, co-infections are not always present in *T. blagburni*–associated diarrhea. There is little information available as to whether immunosuppression predisposes to chronic infection with *T. blagburni*. Administration of prednisolone did not change the fecal consistency or the frequency of positive results on direct fecal exams in one study.[33]

The clinical signs of trichomonosis are variable and range from subclinical infection to chronic intractable diarrhea. The signs often are intermittent and can resolve with antimicrobial drug treatment, only to recur after treatment is discontinued. The diarrhea is most commonly waxing and waning and large bowel in origin; characterized by increased frequency of defecation and passage of semi-formed to liquid, often foul-smelling feces, sometimes with fresh blood and mucus. When the diarrhea is severe, the anus may become edematous and fecal incontinence may develop (Fig. 102.3). Although diarrhea may persist, most affected cats maintain a good appetite and body condition score. Less frequently, but especially with poor care or housing conditions or co-infections, infected cats can have other clinical signs such as vomiting, dysrexia, abdominal pain, depression, and weight loss.[30]

Tritrichomonas blagburni was detected in the uterine contents of a cat with endometritis and pyometra.[41] However, the organism was not associated with infection or disease of the reproductive tract in a separate study of cats with *T. blagburni* infection that were housed in catteries.[42] The organism has also been identified in the nose of a young cat with chronic rhinitis.[43]

Physical Examination Findings

Cats solely infected with *T. blagburni* are generally in good body condition. Cats with co-infections or comorbidities may have poor body condition, abdominal pain, or depression.

DIAGNOSIS

Laboratory Abnormalities

Tritrichomonas blagburni infections are only rarely associated with systemic laboratory abnormalities. However, if the diarrhea is severe, decreases in potassium, sodium, and chloride concentrations may be present as a result of GI losses. Evaluation for co-infections and comorbidities in cats with more severe clinical signs or laboratory abnormalities is recommended. Further diagnostic evaluation of infected cats may include CBC; serum biochemical analysis; urinalysis; tests for viral infections such as FeLV, feline panleukopenia virus, and FIV; fecal flotation; *Giardia*-specific antigen testing; fecal direct FA for *Cryptosporidium*; molecular genetic testing for other feline enteric pathogens; and colonic mucosal biopsies. Commercial assays that detect fecal *Giardia*-specific antigen do not cross-react with antigens of *T. blagburni*.

Diagnostic Imaging

Abdominal radiographic or ultrasonographic abnormalities associated with *T. blagburni* infection are uncommon, nonspecific, and, when present, suggestive of diffuse colitis.

Microbiologic Tests

Trichomonads cannot be detected with fecal flotation methods. A direct wet mount cytology using fresh, unrefrigerated feces should be performed for all cats with large bowel or mixed diarrhea to evaluate for the presence of *T. blagburni* trophozoites (Table 102.1), using the technique described for *Giardia* (see Chapter 101). *Tritrichomonas blagburni* is similar in size to *Giardia* but can be differentiated by the presence of an undulating membrane, pear shape, a rapid forward motion, the lack of a concave surface, and a single nucleus. The trophozoite and its undulating membrane may also be identified on fecal smears stained with Diff-Quik stain using the high-dry (40-50× objective) or oil immersion microscopy. The sensitivity of direct cytology using specimens from naturally infected cats was only 14% in one study.[33] The sensitivity can be improved by analyzing multiple fresh fecal smears and by obtaining the fecal specimen from the proximal colon through fecal collection loop or colonic flush. Video clips that demonstrate how to perform the colonic flush technique and of the classic motility of the parasite can be found online (https://cvm.ncsu.edu/research/labs/clinical-sciences/tfoetus/#tabsPnl1-tab-1). *Tritrichomonas blagburni* is difficult to distinguish from *P. hominis*; however, infection with *T. blagburni* is more common, and *P. hominis* is generally easily eliminated with a short course of metronidazole.

If *T. blagburni* infection is still suspected after the initial work-up, culture can be performed using a commercially available culture system (InPouch TF, BioMed Diagnostics, White City, OR, USA). In this

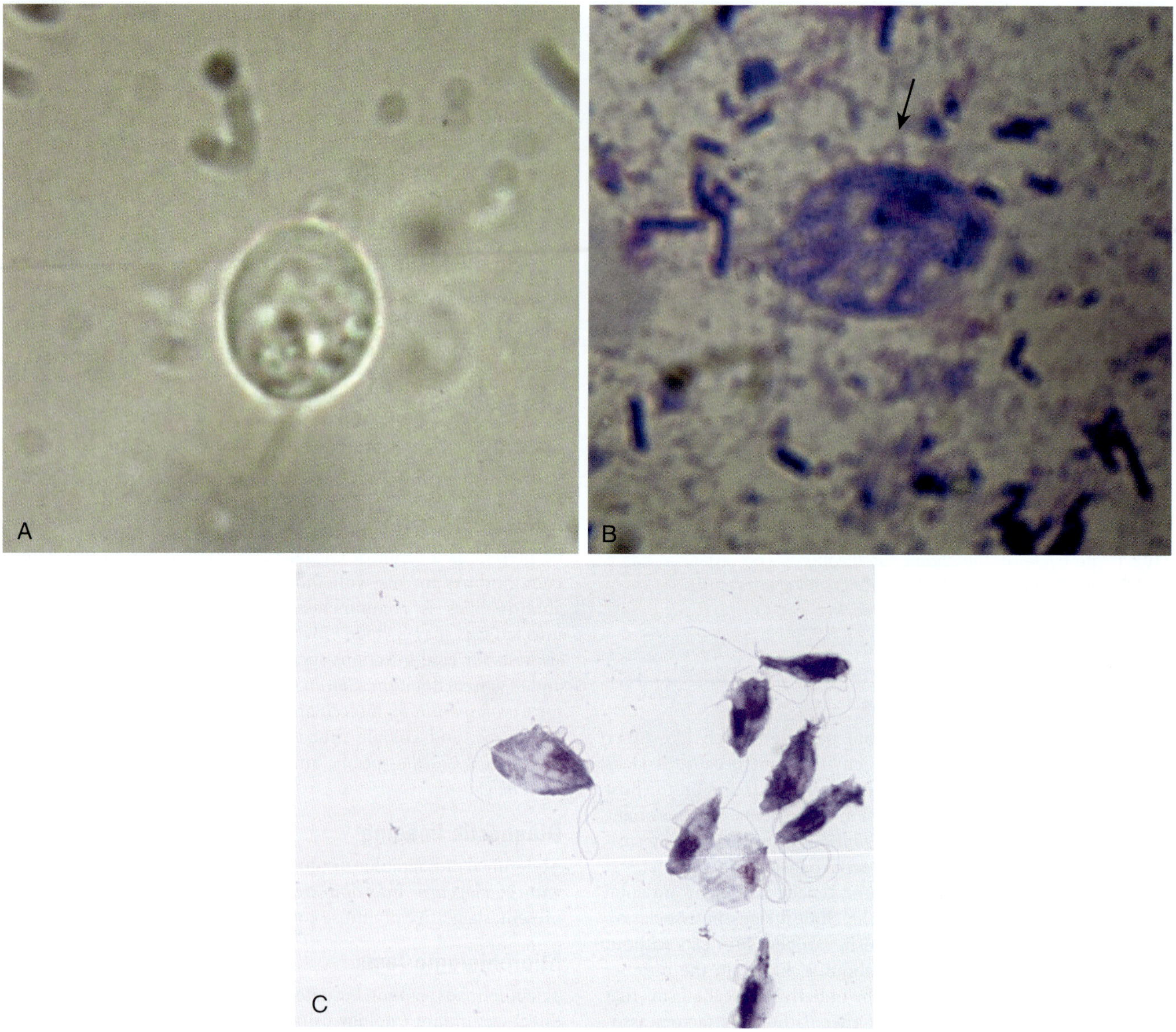

Fig. 102.2 (A) *Tritrichomonas blagburni* trophozoite seen on a saline wet mount of a fecal specimen. The organism can be recognized by its progressive forward, rolling motility. (B) Diff-Quik stain. The undulating membrane can be clearly visualized coursing along the lateral aspect of the trophozoite *(arrow)*. (C) Diff-Quik stain of a sample taken from an InPouch fecal culture. Several trichomonads can be observed. The undulating membrane, axostyle, and flagella can all be seen.

system, a tiny amount of fresh feces (~50 mg), obtained by the methods described above, is inoculated into the culture pouch. Inoculation with more feces than this can overwhelm the antibacterial agents in the culture pouch and bacteria will overgrow leading to a false-negative result. Shipment of fecal specimens to external laboratories is not recommended as the culture requires viable organisms and trichomonads often die in transit. If a fecal specimen must be transported to the clinic or diagnostic laboratory, removal of adherent litter and dilution with saline (3 mL 0.9% saline per 2 g of feces) is recommended to extend trichomonad survival.[16] The specimen should be evaluated within 6 hours of collection to preserve diagnostic sensitivity.[11] The culture pouch is incubated in an upright position in the clinic at room temperature, or preferably in a 37°C incubator, and examined daily by microscopy for evidence of protozoal growth. Positive results can occur within hours when incubated at 37°C or after several days (up to 12) when incubated at room temperature. The medium used does not support the growth of *Giardia* spp. and positive test results generally suggest infection by *T. blagburni*.[35] Rarely, *P. hominis* can be cultivated with the InPouch system.[44] Thus, positive results should be confirmed with microscopic visualization of the trichomonad (see Fig 102.2) (*P. hominis* has 5 anterior flagella) or by PCR. PCR assays are considered to be the gold standard method to diagnose *T. blagburni* infection. These assays are recommended for assessment of fecal specimens that were found negative by microscopy and fecal culture and to confirm that microscopically observed or cultivated organisms are *T. blagburni*.[31] Specimens obtained from non-diarrheic or dry stools are not suitable for use in testing for *T. blagburni* and rarely yield positive test results even if infection is present. Several PCR-based assays that are specific for *T. blagburni* and that do not amplify *Giardia* or *P. hominis* DNA are commercially available.[45] Thus, a positive PCR result from a reputable lab should be interpreted as positive for the infection. PCR can detect both viable and non-viable organisms and has a very good analytical sensitivity. The assay can detect as little as 10 *T. blagburni* organisms per 100 mg fecal specimen. However, PCR assays are

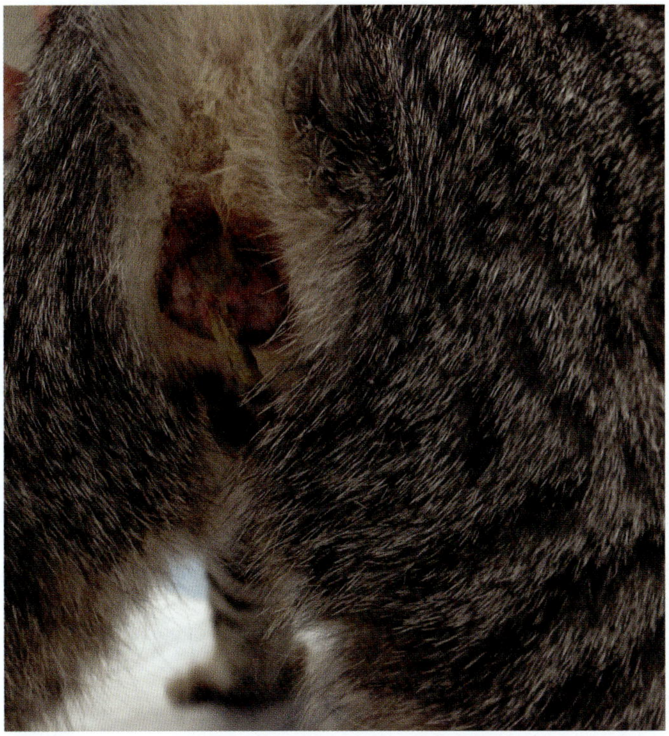

Fig. 102.3 Anal swelling and evidence of fecal incontinence in a kitten with suspected *Tritrichomonas blagburni* infection.

TABLE 102.1 Diagnostic Assays Available for Trichomonosis in Dogs or Cats

Assay	Specimen Type	Target	Performance
Cytologic examination	Feces	*Tritrichomonas* trophozoites	False negatives are common and occur when specimen size is small or low numbers of organisms are present, or because of intermittent shedding. The sensitivity of this method is < 20%.
Culture (InPouch test)	Feces	*T. blagburni*	May take days for the organism to grow. The sensitivity of this method is approximately 55%. False negatives can occur if feces are dried out, because of intermittent shedding or recent treatment with antiprotozoal drugs, or if the pouch is overgrown by intestinal bacteria.
PCR assays	Feces	*T. blagburni* DNA	The sensitivity and specificity of assays vary depending on assay design. Well-designed assays have the highest sensitivity of all diagnostic test methods, but false negatives can occur if specimen size is small or as a result of PCR inhibitors in feces.

TABLE 102.2 Drugs Commonly Used for Treatment of *Tritrichomonas blagburni* Infection in Cats

Drug	Dose	Route	Interval (Hours)	Minimum Duration (Days)
Ronidazole	30 mg/kg	PO	24	14
Tinidazole	30 mg/kg	PO	24	14

not 100% sensitive. In cases with a high index of suspicion for infection, repeat testing is recommended. For all microbiologic testing, the feces should be diarrheic, devoid of litter, and the cat should not have received antimicrobials (e.g., metronidazole, fenbendazole) within the 1–2 weeks before testing. Co-infections with organisms such as *Giardia* spp. in cats infected with *T. blagburni* are common; therefore, a positive result with any diagnostic test for *T. blagburni* does not preclude the possibility of a co-infection.

Pathologic Findings

Gross Pathologic Findings

Gross pathologic findings associated with *T. blagburni* infection in cats are nonspecific and associated primarily with the colon and terminal ileum. The colon may be normal or appear mildly thickened with or without hyperemia.

Histopathologic Findings

Lesions associated with *T. blagburni* infection in cats are most prominent in the colon but can also be identified in the terminal ileum and cecum. The organisms are noted in most experimentally infected cats, but not in all sections.[34] Thus, if colonoscopy is performed, multiple specimens should be collected for histopathologic evaluation. The organisms are usually close to the mucosal surface and are associated with mild to severe lymphoplasmacytic and neutrophilic infiltrates; crypt epithelial cell hypertrophy, hyperplasia, and increased mitotic activity; loss of goblet cells; crypt microabscesses; and attenuation of the superficial colonic mucosa.[34] In some cats, *T. blagburni* may be detected in the lumen of colonic crypts and, less commonly, can invade the lamina propria. However, trichomonads are fragile and often difficult to preserve in intestinal biopsy specimens. It is advisable to indicate that *T. blagburni* is a diagnostic consideration when submitting specimens, as a minimum of six tissue sections should be examined to achieve at least 95% confidence that trichomonads will be identified.[34] *In situ* hybridization techniques have been used to identify *T. blagburni* and *P. hominis* in biopsy specimens.[46,47]

TREATMENT AND PROGNOSIS

The treatment of choice for *T. blagburni* infections is the nitroimidazole drug ronidazole (Table 102.2). Before ronidazole was discovered as an effective treatment, multiple other treatment regimens had been attempted in cats with *T. blagburni* infections with generally poor responses.[16,48] In some cases, temporary improvement was noted with a variety of drugs, but relapse was invariable. Some of the apparent clinical improvement may have been due to secondary effects of drugs on the intestinal bacterial flora, although treatment may also prolong trophozoite shedding.

A number of drugs have also been tested *in vitro* to determine *T. blagburni* susceptibility patterns.[49,50] Ronidazole has been the most effective drug used clinically to date and is currently recommended at a dose of 30 mg/kg, PO, q24h for 14 days.[51] Clinical signs can relapse after administration of ronidazole, but generally resolve again after the treatment regimen is repeated. The pharmacokinetics have been determined for ronidazole in cats.[52,53] Higher doses of ronidazole and twice-daily dose regimens can result in neurologic signs such as ataxia and seizures.[54] This likely relates to the high oral bioavailability and slow elimination of the drug by cats.[52] Even with lower doses and once-daily regimens, cats should be monitored closely. To date, all reported cases of ronidazole-related neurotoxicity have been reversible, but irreversible neurotoxicity can occur in some cats. Signs of neurotoxicity may be easier to observe if the treated cat is engaged each day in a playful activity (e.g., chasing a laser pointer) that requires coordination and agility. If signs of toxicity are observed, owners should be advised to discontinue treatment with ronidazole. Continuing treatment after signs of toxicity are observed could result in life-threatening complications. If treatment must be discontinued because of neurotoxicity, the cat should be retested for *T. blagburni* infection. Many of these cats have received sufficient ronidazole, by the time toxicity ensues, to have cleared the infection.

Not all cats treated with high doses of ronidazole develop toxicity. In one study, a dose of 50 mg/kg, PO, q12h was used in research cats with no reported adverse effects.[55] Ronidazole is not approved by the US FDA for use in companion animals and is banned for use in food animals because of its teratogenic potential in humans. Accordingly, due diligence is required to protect humans from exposure to ronidazole, and veterinarians are advised to prescribe the drug only in cases of confirmed *T. blagburni* infection after obtaining the owner's informed consent. Ronidazole should not be used to treat pregnant or lactating queens or very young kittens. Likewise, caution is recommended with pregnant clients. Ronidazole should be obtained from a reputable compounding pharmacy and not pigeon supply warehouses because the latter may provide poor-quality preparations. Compounded chemical grade ronidazole is available from several online pharmacies. Compounding into gelatin capsules rather than liquid is recommended to avoid stability and taste concerns. A delayed-release (guar gum) formulation offers promise for targeted delivery of ronidazole to the colon and reduced likelihood of systemic adverse effects in cats.[53]

Some strains of *T. blagburni* are resistant to ronidazole.[56] Based on previous studies, approximately 60% of cats that are treated with ronidazole will have improvement or resolution of clinical signs.[57] Poor compounding can be another reason for failure of treatment in some situations. Other reasons for ronidazole failure include insufficient dose or duration of therapy, compliance failure, or re-infection from another cat in the household who may be asymptomatic. Other cats in the household/cattery should also be tested for *T. blagburni*. Ronidazole also has activity against *Giardia*.[58] However, to lessen the potential for selection of resistant strains, ronidazole should be reserved for use for *T. blagburni* infections, because multiple other drugs are effective for treatment of giardiasis.

Tinidazole, administered at 30 mg/kg for 14 days, suppressed *T. blagburni* shedding to undetectable levels in two of four cats during a 33-week period post-treatment.[49] However, this drug is currently considered inferior to ronidazole because infection was not eliminated in all cats. Veterinarians should be cautious in embracing the success of other antimicrobial drugs for treatment of *T. blagburni* infection because many drugs merely suppress detection of the organisms rather than eradicate them. Investigation into other treatments for feline trichomonosis including novel probiotics and protease inhibitors are ongoing. If owners elect not to treat for *T. blagburni* infection, the diarrhea will eventually spontaneously resolve in most cats (88%); however, this can take as long as 2 years.[16] Unfortunately, 55% of these cats remain infected based on positive PCR results for *T. blagburni* and, therefore, may be sources of infection for other cats. Owners of only one cat may find this outcome satisfactory if the cat remains healthy in other respects. However, in a cattery environment, subclinical carriers may perpetuate the infection.

IMMUNITY AND VACCINATION

Immunity to reinfection by *T. blagburni* does not occur in the short term after recovery. However, although intestinal infection can be prolonged, the development of effective immune responses as kittens mature can be followed by resolution of clinical disease. Vaccines for prevention of *T. blagburni* infection in cats are not currently available.

PREVENTION

Kittens in crowded environments are more susceptible to infection due to stress or immunologic immaturity. Thus, minimizing stress and reduction of population-dense housing conditions will likely reduce the chances of exposure to *T. blagburni*. Protocols for eliminating infections or lessening signs of *T. blagburni* infection in catteries involve testing, isolation or removal of cats that test positive, and retesting. Treatment with ronidazole does not guarantee cure even if repeated PCR assays are negative, and relapse of infection (or re-infection) can occur months after discontinuation of treatment. For this reason, re-introduction of treated cats to a cattery is not recommended.

PUBLIC HEALTH ASPECTS

Only two case reports of immunosuppressed humans infected with *T. foetus* have been reported.[59,60] The parasite was isolated from a bronchoalveolar lavage specimen in a patient with *Pneumocystis* pneumonia and from the bile of a patient with acquired agammaglobulinemia. The authors did not rule out the possibility of a human host-adapted strain of *T. blagburni*. However, because of the apparent poor host specificity of *T. blagburni* and the close contact between cats and humans, zoonotic transmission should be considered and infected kittens with diarrhea should be handled with care. In addition, the possible presence of other zoonotic pathogens should always be considered in cats with diarrhea.

CASE EXAMPLE

Signalment

"Belle," a 14-week-old intact female pixie-bob cat from Seattle, WA, United States.

History

Belle was considered a pet quality pixie-bob and so was sold into a private home at 14 weeks of age. The cattery had three queens and one tom and had bred at least six litters over the previous 2 years. No significant health problems were reported to the adoptive owner, and the cattery was retrovirus free. Belle appeared healthy the day the adoption was completed and was also pronounced healthy by the new attending veterinarian. The breeder had administered one dose of a vaccine for prevention of FHV-1, FCV, and FPV and a dose of pyrantel pamoate at 7 and 10 weeks of age. The veterinarian administered an attenuated live FVRCP vaccine subcutaneously, gave one dose of pyrantel pamoate, discharged Belle with selamectin to be applied monthly, and scheduled a re-check at 16 weeks of age for rabies vaccination. Belle was taken to her new home by car for 4 hours and then housed in her private room while attempting to socialize to the two black Labrador retrievers living at the new home. The kitten was not allowed to see the dogs the first 2 days, but the dogs were allowed to sniff under the door of the room Belle was housed in and occasionally

CASE EXAMPLE—cont'd

barked. On day 3, Belle began having diarrhea that the owner reported to be "pea soup" consistency, with white strands and fresh blood. Tenesmus was also noted.

Physical Examination

Body weight: 2.1 kg.

General: Quiet, alert, and responsive. Ambulatory on all four limbs. Body weight was 2.1 kg and BCS was 4/9. T = 101.3°F (38.5°C), HR = 180 beats/minute, RR = 24 breaths/minute, mucous membranes pink, CRT = 1 second. The only abnormality detected on physical examination was that the cat postured to defecate, and passed a small volume of diarrhea with streaks of blood and mucus when the caudal abdomen was palpated. Intestinal palpation was unremarkable.

Microbiologic Testing

Fecal wet mount examination: Motile flagellates noted with morphology and motility consistent with that of *T. blagburni*.

In-house *Giardia* ELISA assay (SNAP Giardia, IDEXX Laboratories): Negative.

Zinc sulfate centrifugal fecal flotation: Negative.

Tritrichomonas blagburni PCR: Positive.

Diagnosis

Tritrichomonas blagburni infection.

Treatment

Ronidazole at 30 mg/kg, PO, daily for 14 days was prescribed. The stool normalized 3 days later, and ultimately, Belle learned to tolerate Labrador retrievers. She was clinically healthy at the visit 2 weeks later for rabies vaccination. The breeder was informed of the findings, and it was recommended that the breeder discuss management of this agent in the cattery with a veterinarian.

Comments

The findings were characteristic of a stress-activated *T. blagburni* infection associated with moving to the new home and first contact with dogs. Many cats in catteries maintain subclinical infections that may be followed by clinical signs of large bowel diarrhea when the infected cats are subjected to stress. While *T. blagburni* can be amplified by PCR assay or grown from feces of dogs, it is unlikely that healthy adult dogs will become clinically ill, and so no tests or treatments were performed on the family dogs.

SUGGESTED READINGS

Gookin JL. An owners guide to diagnosis and treatment of cats infected with *Tritrichomonas foetus* infection. https://cvm.ncsu.edu/wp-content/uploads/2016/05/ownersguide-to-feline-t-foetus.pdf.

Rosado TW, Specht A, Marks SL. Neurotoxicosis in 4 cats receiving ronidazole. *J Vet Intern Med.* 2007;21:328–331.

REFERENCES

1. Levy MG, Gookin JL, Poore M, et al. *Tritrichomonas foetus* and not *Pentatrichomonas hominis* is the etiologic agent of feline trichomonal diarrhea. *J Parasitol.* 2003;89:99–104.
2. Scorza V, Lappin MR. Gastrointestinal protozoal infections. In: August J, ed. *Consultations in Feline Internal Medicine*, 6th ed., Saunders/Elsevier, 2006, pp. 200.
3. Payne PA, Artzer M. The biology and control of *Giardia* spp. and *Tritrichomonas foetus*. *Vet Clin North Am Small Anim Pract.* 2009;39:993–1007.
4. Reinmann K, Muller N, Kuhnert P, et al. *Tritrichomonas foetus* isolates from cats and cattle show minor genetic differences in unrelated loci ITS-2 and EF-1alpha. *Vet Parasitol.* 2012;185:138–144.
5. Slapeta J, Craig S, McDonell D, et al. *Tritrichomonas foetus* from domestic cats and cattle are genetically distinct. *Exp Parasitol.* 2010;126:209–213.
6. Sun Z, Stack C, Slapeta J. Sequence differences in the diagnostic region of the cysteine protease 8 gene of *Tritrichomonas foetus* parasites of cats and cattle. *Vet Parasitol.* 2012;186:445–449.
7. Stockdale H, Rodning S, Givens M, et al. Experimental infection of cattle with a feline isolate of *Tritrichomonas foetus*. *J Parasitol.* 2007;93:1429–1434.
8. Stockdale HD, Dillon AR, Newton JC, et al. Experimental infection of cats (*Felis catus*) with *Tritrichomonas foetus* isolated from cattle. *Vet Parasitol.* 2008;154:156–161.
9. Walden HS, Dykstra C, Dillon A, et al. A new species of *Tritrichomonas* (Sarcomastigophora: Trichomonida) from the domestic cat (*Felis catus*). *Parasitol Res.* 2013;112:2227–2235.
10. Rosypal AC, Ripley A, Stockdale Walden HD, et al. Survival of a feline isolate of *Tritrichomonas foetus* in water, cat urine, cat food and cat litter. *Vet Parasitol.* 2012;185:279–281.
11. Hale S, Norris JM, Slapeta J. Prolonged resilience of *Tritrichomonas foetus* in cat faeces at ambient temperature. *Vet Parasitol.* 2009;166:60–65.
12. Van der Saag M, McDonell D, Slapeta J. Cat genotype *Tritrichomonas foetus* survives passage through the alimentary tract of two common slug species. *Vet Parasitol.* 2011;177:262–266.
13. Bell ET, Gowan RA, Lingard AE, et al. Naturally occurring *Tritrichomonas foetus* infections in Australian cats: 38 cases. *J Feline Med Surg.* 2010;12:889–898.
14. Bissett SA, Gowan RA, O'Brien CR, et al. Feline diarrhoea associated with *Tritrichomonas* cf. *foetus* and *Giardia* co-infection in an Australian cattery. *Aust Vet J.* 2008;86:440–443.
15. Doi J, Hirota J, Morita A, et al. Intestinal *Tritrichomonas suis* (=*T. foetus*) infection in Japanese cats. *J Vet Med Sci.* 2012;74:413–417.
16. Foster DM, Gookin JL, Poore MF, et al. Outcome of cats with diarrhea and *Tritrichomonas foetus* infection. *J Am Vet Med Assoc.* 2004;225:888–892.
17. Frey CF, Schild M, Hemphill A, et al. Intestinal *Tritrichomonas foetus* infection in cats in Switzerland detected by in vitro cultivation and PCR. *Parasitol Res.* 2009;104:783–788.
18. Gunn-Moore DA, McCann TM, Reed N, et al. Prevalence of *Tritrichomonas foetus* infection in cats with diarrhoea in the UK. *J Feline Med Surg.* 2007;9:214–218.
19. Holliday M, Deni D, Gunn-Moore DA. *Tritrichomonas foetus* infection in cats with diarrhoea in a rescue colony in Italy. *J Feline Med Surg.* 2009;11:131–134.
20. Stockdale HD, Givens MD, Dykstra CC, et al. *Tritrichomonas foetus* infections in surveyed pet cats. *Vet Parasitol.* 2009;160:13–17.
21. Tysnes K, Gjerde B, Nodtvedt A, et al. A cross-sectional study of *Tritrichomonas foetus* infection among healthy cats at shows in Norway. *Acta Vet Scand.* 2011;53:39.
22. Xenoulis PG, Saridomichelakis MN, Read SA, et al. Detection of *Tritrichomonas foetus* in cats in Greece. *J Feline Med Surg.* 2010;12:831–833.
23. Kim YA, Kim HY, Cho SH, et al. PCR detection and molecular characterization of *Pentatrichomonas hominis* from feces of dogs with diarrhea in the Republic of Korea. *Korean J Parasitol.* 2010;48:9–13.
24. Kingsbury DD, Marks SL, Cave NJ, et al. Identification of *Tritrichomonas foetus* and *Giardia* spp. infection in pedigree show cats in New Zealand. *N Z Vet J.* 2010;58:6–10.
25. Kuehner KA, Marks SL, Kass PH, et al. *Tritrichomonas foetus* infection in purebred cats in Germany: prevalence of clinical signs and the role of co-infection with other enteroparasites. *J Feline Med Surg.* 2011;13:251–258.
26. Mardell EJ, Sparkes AH. Chronic diarrhoea associated with *Tritrichomonas foetus* infection in a British cat. *Vet Rec.* 2006;158:765–766.
27. Miro G, Hernandez L, Montoya A, et al. First description of naturally acquired *Tritrichomonas foetus* infection in a Persian cattery in Spain. *Parasitol Res.* 2011;109:1151–1154.
28. Queen EV, Marks SL, Farver TB. Prevalence of selected bacterial and parasitic agents in feces from diarrheic and healthy control cats from Northern California. *J Vet Intern Med.* 2012;26:54–60.

29. Gookin JL, Stebbins ME, Hunt E, et al. Prevalence of and risk factors for feline *Tritrichomonas foetus* and *Giardia* infection. *J Clin Microbiol.* 2004;42:2707–2710.
30. Xenoulis PG, Lopinski DJ, Read SA, et al. Intestinal *Tritrichomonas foetus* infection in cats: a retrospective study of 104 cases. *J Feline Med Surg.* 2013;15:1098–1103.
31. Gookin JL, Birkenheuer AJ, St John V, et al. Molecular characterization of trichomonads from feces of dogs with diarrhea. *J Parasitol.* 2005;91:939–943.
32. Tolbert MK, Leutenegger CM, Lobetti R, et al. Species identification of trichomonads and associated coinfections in dogs with diarrhea and suspected trichomonosis. *Vet Parasitol.* 2012;187:319–322.
33. Gookin JL, Levy MG, Law JM, et al. Experimental infection of cats with *Tritrichomonas foetus. Am J Vet Res.* 2001;62:1690–1697.
34. Yaeger MJ, Gookin JL. Histologic features associated with *Tritrichomonas foetus*-induced colitis in domestic cats. *Vet Pathol.* 2005;42:797–804.
35. Gould EN, Corbeil LB, Kania SA, et al. Evaluation of surface antigen TF1.17 in feline *Tritrichomonas foetus* isolates. *Vet Parasitol.* 2017;244:144–153.
36. Gould EN, Giannone R, Kania SA, et al. Cysteine protease 30 (CP30) contributes to adhesion and cytopathogenicity in feline *Tritrichomonas foetus. Vet Parasitol.* 2017;244:114–122.
37. Tolbert MK, Brand MD, Gould EN. In vitro effects of cysteine protease inhibitors on *Trichomonas foetus*-induced cytopathic changes in porcine intestinal epithelial cells. *Am J Vet Res.* 2016;77:890–897.
38. Tolbert MK, Gookin JL. Mechanisms of *Tritrichomonas foetus* pathogenicity in cats with insights from venereal trichomonosis. *J Vet Intern Med.* 2016;30:516–526.
39. Tolbert MK, Stauffer SH, Brand MD, et al. Cysteine protease activity of feline *Tritrichomonas foetus* promotes adhesion-dependent cytotoxicity to intestinal epithelial cells. *Infect Immun.* 2014;82:2851–2859.
40. Tolbert MK, Stauffer SH, Gookin JL. Feline *Tritrichomonas foetus* adhere to intestinal epithelium by receptor-ligand-dependent mechanisms. *Vet Parasitol.* 2013;192:75–82.
41. Dahlgren SS, Gjerde B, Pettersen HY. First record of natural *Tritrichomonas foetus* infection of the feline uterus. *J Small Anim Pract.* 2007;48:654–657.
42. Gray SG, Hunter SA, Stone MR, et al. Assessment of reproductive tract disease in cats at risk for *Tritrichomonas foetus* infection. *Am J Vet Res.* 2010;71:76–81.
43. Pazzini L, Mugnaini L, Mancianti F, et al. *Tritrichomonas foetus* and *Mycoplasma felis* coinfection in the upper respiratory tract of a cat with chronic purulent nasal discharge. *Vet Clin Pathol.* 2018;47:294–296.
44. Ceplecha V, Svoboda M, Cepicka I, et al. InPouch TF-Feline medium is not specific for *Tritrichomonas foetus. Vet Parasitol.* 2013;196:503–505.
45. Gookin JL, Stauffer SH, Levy MG. Identification of *Pentatrichomonas hominis* in feline fecal samples by polymerase chain reaction assay. *Vet Parasitol.* 2007;145:11–15.
46. Mostegl MM, Wetscher A, Richter B, et al. Detection of *Tritrichomonas foetus* and *Pentatrichomonas hominis* in intestinal tissue specimens of cats by chromogenic in situ hybridization. *Vet Parasitol.* 2012;183:209–214.
47. Gookin JL, Stone MR, Yaeger MJ, et al. Fluorescence in situ hybridization for identification of *Tritrichomonas foetus* in formalin-fixed and paraffin-embedded histological specimens of intestinal trichomoniasis. *Vet Parasitol.* 2010;172:139–143.
48. Gookin JL, Breitschwerdt EB, Levy MG, et al. Diarrhea associated with trichomonosis in cats. *J Am Vet Med Assoc.* 1999;215:1450–1454.
49. Gookin JL, Stauffer SH, Coccaro MR, et al. Efficacy of tinidazole for treatment of cats experimentally infected with *Tritrichomonas foetus. Am J Vet Res.* 2007;68:1085–1088.
50. Kather EJ, Marks SL, Kass PH. Determination of the in vitro susceptibility of feline *Tritrichomonas foetus* to 5 antimicrobial agents. *J Vet Intern Med.* 2007;21:966–970.
51. Gookin JL, Copple CN, Papich MG, et al. Efficacy of ronidazole for treatment of feline *Tritrichomonas foetus* infection. *J Vet Intern Med.* 2006;20:536–543.
52. LeVine DN, Papich MG, Gookin JL, et al. Ronidazole pharmacokinetics after intravenous and oral immediate-release capsule administration in healthy cats. *J Feline Med Surg.* 2011;13:244–250.
53. Papich MG, Levine DN, Gookin JL, et al. Ronidazole pharmacokinetics in cats following delivery of a delayed-release guar gum formulation. *J Vet Pharmacol Ther.* 2013;36:399–407.
54. Rosado TW, Specht A, Marks SL. Neurotoxicosis in 4 cats receiving ronidazole. *J Vet Intern Med.* 2007;21:328–331.
55. Lim S, Park SI, Ahn KS, et al. Efficacy of ronidazole for treatment of cats experimentally infected with a Korean isolate of *Tritrichomonas foetus. Korean J Parasitol.* 2012;50:161–164.
56. Gookin JL, Stauffer SH, Dybas D, et al. Documentation of in vivo and in vitro aerobic resistance of feline *Tritrichomonas foetus* isolates to ronidazole. *J Vet Intern Med.* 2010;24:1003–1007.
57. Gookin JL, Hanrahan K, Levy MG. The conundrum of feline trichomonosis. *J Feline Med Surg.* 2017;19:261–274.
58. Fiechter R, Deplazes P, Schnyder M. Control of *Giardia* infections with ronidazole and intensive hygiene management in a dog kennel. *Vet Parasitol.* 2012;187:93–98.
59. Suzuki J, Kobayashi S, Osuka H, et al. Characterization of a human isolate of *Tritrichomonas foetus* (cattle/swine genotype) infected by a zoonotic opportunistic infection. *J Vet Med Sci.* 2016;78:633–640.
60. Duboucher C, Caby S, Dufernez F, et al. Molecular identification of *Tritrichomonas foetus*-like organisms as coinfecting agents of human *Pneumocystis* pneumonia. *J Clin Microbiol.* 2006;44:1165–1168.

103

Cryptosporidiosis and Cyclosporiasis

Valeria Scorza, Michael R. Lappin

KEY POINTS

Cryptosporidiosis

- First Described: The genus *Cryptosporidium* was first described in 1910 by Tyzzer, who in 1912 also described *Cryptosporidium parvum* in the small intestine of mice.[1]
- Cause: *Cryptosporidium* is a ubiquitous coccidian genus in the phylum Apicomplexa, suborder Eimeriorina, family Cryptosporidiidae, which inhabits the epithelium of the respiratory and digestive systems of reptiles, birds, and mammals. Based on extensive biological and molecular data, *Cryptosporidium* has been recently transferred from the Coccidia, to a new subclass, Cryptogregaria, with gregarine parasites.[2]
- Affected Hosts: Mammals, birds, and reptiles.
- Intermediate Hosts: Although there are no intermediate hosts, there are multiple potential transport hosts that may carry *Cryptosporidium* spp. oocysts and indirectly infect dogs or cats.
- Geographic Distribution: Worldwide.
- Route of Transmission: Direct contact with infected humans and animals, drinking contaminated water during recreational activities, or by eating or drinking contaminated food.
- Major Clinical Signs: *Cryptosporidium* spp. have been detected in dogs and cats with and without GI signs of disease. Clinical signs include diarrhea, usually small bowel characterized by high volume, low-frequency stools, and significant weight loss.
- Differential Diagnoses: Dietary, nematode parasitic, viral, and bacterial diarrhea.
- Human Health Significance: *Cryptosporidium parvum* was the cause of numerous waterborne outbreaks. The majority of the infections in humans are caused by *Cryptosporidium hominis* and *C. parvum*. However, *Cryptosporidium canis* and *Cryptosporidium felis* DNA has also been amplified from the feces of people, and so the potential for zoonotic transmission exists (see Public Health Aspects).

Cyclosporiasis

- Causes: *Cyclospora* (phylum Apicomplexa, suborder Eimeriorina, family Eimeriidae) was first described in 1993.[3]
- Affected Hosts: Although *Cyclospora cayetanensis* oocysts have also been identified in animals, currently *C. cayetanensis* is the only species known to infect humans.
- Geographic Distribution: *Cyclospora* infections have been described worldwide. In many non-industrialized countries, infections are endemic. Sporadic reports associated with outbreaks occur in industrialized countries.
- Primary Mode of Transmission: Ingestion of contaminated food and water.
- Major Clinical Signs: Clinical illness, if any, in dogs and cats is uncertain, because definitive oocysts have been documented only in human feces. Infected humans can develop anorexia, nausea, watery diarrhea, flatulence, fatigue, abdominal cramping, low-grade fever, fatigue, and weight loss after *C. cayetanensis* infection; the most severe symptoms develop in children and in humans with HIV/AIDS.
- Differential Diagnoses. Dietary, nematode parasitic, viral, and bacterial diarrhea.
- Human Health Significance: *Cyclospora cayetanensis* seems to be the only species detected in humans, and they seem to be its specific host. However, contact with animals was considered a risk factor for human infection in many studies worldwide.

CRYPTOSPORIDIOSIS

ETIOLOGY AND EPIDEMIOLOGY

The majority of *Cryptosporidium* spp. are host-adapted and have a narrow spectrum of natural hosts (Tables 103.1, 103.2, and 103.3). Most studies report that dogs and cats are infected with the host-specific *Cryptosporidium canis* and *Cryptosporidium felis*, respectively. *Cryptosporidium muris* and *Cryptosporidium ubiquitum* have also been detected in the feces of naturally infected dogs.[4-6] More recently, the DNA of *Cryptosporidium hominis* was detected in the feces of a dog in Spain.[7] *Cryptosporidium parvum*, *C. muris*, *Cryptosporidium ryanae*, and a novel genotype related to *Cryptosporidium* rat genotype III were detected in a small number of cats.[8-12]

Prevalence rates of *Cryptosporidium* spp. in cats and dogs vary worldwide depending on the test used and the population studied (Tables 103.4 and 103.5). Infection occurs after oocysts are ingested directly (coprophagia or grooming) and indirectly (ingesting the oocysts in contaminated food or water, or after ingesting infected prey species). After ingestion, oocysts excyst in the GI tract, releasing infective sporozoites, which become enclosed as trophozoites within parasitophorous vacuoles of the microvillous surface of enterocytes (Figs. 103.1 and 103.2).[13] The trophozoites proliferate asexually by merogony to produce, sequentially, two types of meronts. Type I meronts leave the parasitophorous vacuoles to invade other epithelial cells where they develop into more type I meronts or type II meronts. Type I meronts are capable of recycling indefinitely and type II meronts produce sexual reproductive stages. The zygotes formed by sexual reproduction form either thick-walled or thin-walled oocysts, each containing four sporozoites. Approximately 20% of the oocysts produced in the gut are "thin-walled" oocysts that fail to form an oocyst wall. Instead, a series of membranes surround the developing sporozoites. Thus, *C. parvum* appears to have two autoinfective cycles: by continuous recycling of type I meronts, and by sporozoites released from ruptured thin-walled

TABLE 103.1 *Cryptosporidium* Species and Host Range

Host	Tier 1 Species	Tier 2 Species	Tier 3 Species
Humans	*Cryptosporidium hominis, Cryptosporidium parvum*	*Cryptosporidium meleagridis, Cryptosporidium felis, Cryptosporidium canis, Cryptosporidium ubiquitum, Cryptosporidium cuniculus, Cryptosporidium viatorum,* chipmunk genotype I, *Cryptosporidium muris*	*Cryptosporidium andersoni, Cryptosporidium suis, Cryptosporidium bovis,* horse genotype, *Cryptosporidium xiaoi,* skunk genotype, mink genotype, *Cryptosporidium erinacei, Cryptosporidium fayeri, Cryptosporidium scrofarum, Cryptosporidium tyzzeri*
Cats	*C. felis*	*C. muris*	*C. parvum, Cryptosporidium ryanae,* rat genotype III
Dogs	*C. canis*	*C. parvum, C. muris*	*C. scrofarum, C. ubiquitum, C. hominis*
Cattle	*C. parvum, C. bovis*	*Cryptosporidium ryanae, C. andersoni*	*Cryptosporidium occultus, C. xiaoi, C. ubiquitum*
Sheep and goats	*C. xiaoi, C. ubiquitum*	*C. parvum*	*C. andersoni*
Pigs	*C. suis, C. scrofarum*	*C. muris*	
Camels	*C. andersoni, C. muris*	*C. parvum*	
Horses and donkeys	Horse genotype, *C. parvum, C. hominis*	*C. andersoni*	*C. muris, C. tyzzeri, C. felis*(?), *C. proliferans*
Rabbits	*C. cuniculus*	-	-
House mouse	*C. tyzzeri, C. muris*	*C. parvum*	-

Tier 1 species: *Cryptosporidium* spp. that are responsible for over 90% of infections in the specified host.
Tier 2 species: *Cryptosporidium* spp. that have been each reported in at least five cases.
Tier 3 species: *Cryptosporidium* spp. for which detection has been each reported in fewer than five cases.
From Feng Y, Ryan UM, Xiao L. Genetic diversity and population structure of *Cryptosporidium. Trends Parasitol.* 2018;34:997–1011.

TABLE 103.2 *Cryptosporidium* Species/ Genotypes Identified in Cats Following Genetic Typing

Cryptosporidium Species/ Genotypes (No. of Isolates Examined)	Country
Cryptosporidium felis (16), *Cryptosporidium muris* (1), *Cryptosporidium ryanae* (1), *Cryptosporidium* rat genotype III (5)	Australia[12,67,145]
Cryptosporidium parvum (1), *C. felis* (3)	Brazil[146]
C. felis (6)	China (Shanghai)[16]
C. felis (1), *C. parvum* (1)	China (Heilongjiang province)[6]
C. felis (5), *Cryptosporidium muris* (1)	Colombia[10]
C. felis (3), *C. muris* (1)	Czech Republic[9,147,148]
C. parvum (1)	Germany[149]
C. felis (4)	Greece[150]
C. felis (8)	Japan[151]
C. felis (1)	Portugal[152]
C. felis (2)	Spain[7,153]
C. felis (2)	Thailand[154]
C. felis (32)	United States[11,155]

oocysts.[13] The thick-walled oocysts are passed in the feces and into the environment.

Cryptosporidium spp. oocysts are sporulated when passed in feces, so they are immediately infectious. *Cryptosporidium felis* oocysts are excreted in the feces 3 to 6 days after infection. The number of oocysts excreted by cats as estimated by quantitative PCR ranges from 175 to 1.1×10^5 oocysts/g of feces with a median of 3.5×10^3 oocysts/g.[12] *Cryptosporidium felis* and *C. canis* oocysts are similar in size; *C. felis* oocysts are 5 μm × 4.5 μm and *C. canis* oocysts are 4.95 μm × 4.71 μm.[14,15]

TABLE 103.3 *Cryptosporidium* Species/ Genotypes Identified in Dogs Following Genetic Typing

Cryptosporidium Species/ Genotypes (No. of Isolates Examined)	Country
Cryptosporidium canis (4)	Australia[156]
C. canis (14), *Cryptosporidium parvum* (2)	Brazil[146,157,158]
C. canis (4)	Canada[159]
C. canis (39)	China (Shanghai)[16]
C. canis (29)	China (Henan province)[17]
C. canis (5), *Cryptosporidium ubiquitum* (1)	China (Heilongjiang province)[6]
Cryptosporidium parvum (1), *Cryptosporidium meleagridis* (1)	Czech Republic[148]
C. parvum (5)	Egypt[20]
C. parvum (1)	Germany[149]
C. canis (2), *Cryptosporidium scrofarum* (1)	Greece[150]
C. parvum (7), *C. canis* (1)	Italy[160]
C. canis (15)	Japan[161-163]
C. canis (7), *Cryptosporidium hominis* (1)	Spain[7,153]
C. canis (2)	Thailand[155]
C. canis (7), *C. parvum* (1)	United States[15,74,155,164]

Risk factors for excretion of *Cryptosporidium* oocysts are living in crowded environments (shelters, pet shops), living in the same household of a cat excreting *Cryptosporidium* oocyts and *Giardia* cysts, contact with livestock, and drinking untreated water.[16-22]

Specific pathogen–free cats developed chronic infection after being inoculated with *C. parvum* but these cats showed minimal clinical signs of disease, even after the administration of glucocorticoids.[23]

TABLE 103.4 Prevalence of *Cryptosporidium* spp. in Dogs

No. Examined	Location	Test (% Prevalence)
2193	Argentina	Microscopy (2.2)[165]
195	Australia	Microscopy (7.1)[166]
450	Brazil	Microscopy (8.8), PCR (9.5)[157]
128	Brazil	Microscopy (22.6), PCR (4.6)[146]
166	Brazil	Microscopy (2.4)[167]
70	Canada	ELISA (7.4)[168]
140	Canada	Microscopy/direct FA (9.2)[159]
458	Czech Republic	Microscopy (4.6)[70]
485	China (Shanghai)	PCR (8)[16]
770	China (Henan province)	PCR (3.8)[17]
267	China (Heilongjiang province)	PCR (2.2)[6]
25	Egypt	Microscopy (12)[169]
50	Egypt	Microscopy (34), PCR (24)[20]
57	Finland	Microscopy (0)[170]
29	France	Microscopy (44.8)[171]
116	France	Microscopy (2.6)[172]
81	Germany	PCR (1.2)[149]
879	Greece	Microcopy/IFA (5.9)[150]
210	Iran	Microscopy (3.8)[173]
140	Iran	Microscopy (2.1), PCR (2.1)[22]
240	Italy	PCR (3.3)[160]
213	Japan	Microscopy (1.4)[46]
140	Japan	PCR (9.3)[161]
77	Japan	PCR (3.9)[174]
906	Japan	Microscopy (0.9)[175]
257	Korea	Microscopy (9.7)[176]
290	Norway	Microscopy/direct FA (5-22)[177]
101	Scotland	Microscopy (0)[178]
100	Scotland	Microscopy (1)[179]
81	Spain	Microscopy (7.4)[180]
505	Spain	Microscopy (6.3)[181]
55	Spain	Microscopy/direct FA (5.5)[153]
194	Spain	PCR (4.1)[7]
111	Thailand (farm dogs)	PCR (0)[155]
95	Thailand (temple dogs)	PCR (2)[154]
109	Thailand (Chiang Mai)	IFA (12.8), PCR (20)[182]
152	The Netherlands	Microscopy (8.7)[183]
4225	United Kingdom	Microscopy (0.6)[184]
130	United States (Colorado)	Microscopy (3.8)[185]
200	United States (California)	Microscopy (2)[186]
300	United States (California)	Microscopy/PCR (5.3)[187]
49	United States (Georgia)	Microscopy (10.2)[188]
100	United States (Kentucky)	Microscopy (17)[189]
84	United States (South Dakota)	PCR (4.7)[190]
390	Zambia	Microscopy (5.9)[19]

TABLE 103.5 Prevalence of *Cryptosporidium* spp. in Cats

No. Examined	Location	Test (% Prevalence)
418	Australia	Microscopy (0)[191]
40	Australia	PCR (10)[191]
162	Australia	Microscopy (1.2)[67]
345	Western Australia	PCR (9.9)[12]
298	Austria	Microscopy (1.7)[192]
49	Brazil	Microscopy (22.4), PCR (8.2)[146]
41	Canada	ELISA (7.3)[168]
653	Canada	Microscopy/direct FA (2.3)[193]
160	China (Shanghai)	PCR (3.8)[16]
52	China (Heilongjiang province)	PCR (3.8)[6]
135	Czech Republic	Serology (57)[70]
16	Egypt	Microscopy (6.2)[169]
10	France	Microscopy (0)[171]
19	Germany	PCR (0.52)[149]
264	Greece	Microscopy/IFA (6.8)[150]
60	Iraq	Microscopy (9.6), PCR (20)[194]
13	Japan	Microscopy (38.5)[14]
507	Japan	Microscopy (3.9)[46]
608	Japan	Microscopy (3.8)[36]
1079	Japan	Microscopy (2.8)[175]
55	Japan	PCR (12.7)[174]
357	Japan	PCR (2)[151]
329	Japan	PCR (0.3)[151]
57	Scotland	Microscopy (12.3)[195]
235	Scotland	Microscopy (8.1)[196]
50	Spain	Microscopy (4)[181]
65	Spain	PCR (4.6)[7]
34	Spain	Microscopy, direct FA (8.8)[153]
60	The Netherlands	Microscopy (4.6)[183]
80	Thailand	PCR (2.6)[155]
145	United Kingdom	Microscopy, direct FA (17.2)[197]
180	United States	Microscopy, direct FA (3.3)[155]

Continued

TABLE 103.5 Prevalence of *Cryptosporidium* spp. in Cats—cont'd

No. Examined	Location	Test (% Prevalence)
344	United States (California)	Microscopy, direct FA (4.7)[64]
206	United States (Colorado)	Microscopy/ELISA (5.4)[39]
263	United States (New York)	Microscopy (3.8)[38]
173	United States (North Carolina)	Microscopy, direct FA (6.5)[198]
250	United States (Mississippi)	Microscopy, direct FA (12), PCR (4.8)[18]

Cryptosporidium parvum infection (of bovine origin) developed in inoculated dogs and cats.[24] Dogs experimentally infected with *C. muris* oocysts rarely developed infections.[25] However, when *C. muris* was administered to three kittens, a large number of oocysts were excreted for extended periods.[14] In another study, puppies and kittens experimentally inoculated with *C. parvum* excreted oocysts after a prepatent period of 2 to 14 and 2 to 11 days, respectively.[26] Patent periods lasted 3 to 33 days in puppies and 2 to 25 days in kittens. None of the infected animals showed clinical illness.[26] In a 2018 study, immunocompetent dogs, immunocompromised dogs, and mice were experimentally infected with *C. canis* oocysts.[27] *Cryptosporidium canis* was not infective for immunocompetent dogs or mice with severe immunodeficiency syndrome, and immunosuppressed dogs started excreting oocysts on day 3 PI with levels peaking on days 10 and 17 PI.[27] In the same study, only the immunocompromised dogs showed lethargy and diarrhea around day 8 PI.[27]

CLINICAL FEATURES

Pathogenesis and Clinical Signs

There is little information regarding the pathogenesis of *C. felis* or *C. canis* in cats and dogs. Most evidence is from research done in humans, mice, and cattle after infection with *C. parvum*. *Cryptosporidium* spp. cause diarrhea by intestinal malabsorption of electrolytes and nutrients with hypersecretion of chloride and water.[28] The pathologic changes are caused by both the parasite factors and the host immune response against the organism. *Cryptosporidium* causes damage by attaching to host cells, penetrating the epithelium, altering the cytoskeleton, inducing apoptosis, and secreting virulence factors.[29] After infection, *Cryptosporidium* sporozoites attach to the intestinal epithelium between the cell membrane and the cell cytoplasm; this extracytoplasmic location may explain their resistance to chemotherapy.[30] Different proteins are involved in adhesion, binding, invasion, and attachment of the epithelial cells.[31] *Cryptosporidium* is intracellular but can be considered "minimally invasive," because it does not penetrate into deeper mucosal layers. However, in immunosuppressed individuals infection can spread to the epithelial cells of the biliary tract, pancreatic duct, stomach, esophagus, and respiratory tract.[29] It was suggested that *Cryptosporidium* parasites regulate gene expression of the host cells by modulating apoptosis, inhibiting the process at the trophozoite stage, and promoting it at the sporozoite and merozoite stages.[32] Cellular damage is also caused by loss of barrier function, increased rates of cell death, and the release of several enzymes and hemolysins.[29] Some protozoan parasites carry small double-stranded RNA (dsRNA) viruses, which might influence the virulence of the parasites that carry them.[29] *Cryptosporidium parvum* carries the virus *Cryptosporidium parvum* virus 1 (CSpV1) (genus *Cryspovirus*, family *Partitiviridae*) and is considered to be associated with fecundity and virulence.[33]

Regarding the host immune response, recognition of *Cryptosporidium* by receptors activates the immune response leading to induction of the expression of proinflammatory cytokines and chemokines. IFN-γ is an important cytokine secreted early in infection by natural killer (NK) cells, macrophages, and dendritic cells, which are thought to play a major role in arranging the innate and adaptive immune responses.[34] In addition, the intestinal microbiota is essential in maintaining intestinal homeostasis. A study that compared the gut microbiota of *C. parvum*–infected mice and controls reported that the parasite causes slight but significant alteration of the native intestinal microbiome.[35] The severity of cryptosporidiosis is highly dependent on the host immune response. The prevalence is usually higher in young individuals due to their immature immune system; however, not all forms of immune suppression lead to increased severity of cryptosporidiosis. Individuals with T cell immunodeficiency disorders are particularly at risk. In contrast, immune deficiencies that affect B cell function have not been associated with increased severity of cryptosporidiosis.[29]

Cryptosporidium spp. have been detected in dogs and cats with and without GI signs of disease. Host immunity is likely important in the development of infection and clinical illness following exposure to cryptosporidia, although the association with risk factors has been confusing. Because of the isolation of cryptosporidia from clinically healthy animals, finding the organism in an animal with clinical illness must always be viewed with caution as an indication of a direct role of the parasite. Clinical signs include diarrhea, usually small bowel characterized by high volume, low-frequency stools, and significant weight loss (Fig. 103.3). Fresh blood, tenesmus, and discomfort can be reported in some chronic cases.[14,36-39] Vomiting is uncommon in cats with cryptosporidiosis unless concurrent abnormalities exist. Most of the published cases with diarrhea and *Cryptosporidium* spp. infection have been immunosuppressed, had preexisting disease of the intestines, co-infections, or chronic diarrhea.[40-44] In cats with co-infections, it was difficult to determine if *Cryptosporidium* spp. were the primary cause of the observed clinical signs. *Cystoisospora* spp., *Toxocara cati*, coronavirus, *Giardia*, *Tritrichomonas blagburni*, and *Campylobacter* have been documented as co-pathogens in cats with *Cryptosporidium* spp. in feces and diarrhea.[43,45-49] However, co-infection with other parasites also has been reported in healthy cats with *Cryptosporidium* spp. infections.[45] Non-infectious diseases associated with cryptosporidiosis in cats are lymphoma and inflammatory bowel disease.[40,50]

Cryptosporidium was detected in puppies with diarrhea that had co-infections with CPV, CDV, and parasites, as well as dogs with lymphoma.[51-53] Intestinal malabsorption was reported in an adult dog with cryptosporidiosis.[54] *Cryptosporidium muris* infection was identified in the stomach of a dog that had a chronic history of vomiting and profuse diarrhea that was observed during physical examination.[55] The histopathologic findings of stomach biopsy revealed gastritis associated with cryptosporidia and bacteria compatible with *Helicobacter* spp. The dog was treated empirically for gastric helicobacteriosis with metronidazole and omeprazole and had clinical improvement during a 6-week follow-up period.

Physical Examination Findings

Most dogs or cats colonized with *Cryptosporidium* spp. have a normal physical examination. On abdominal palpation, small intestines may feel slightly thickened. Because some dogs or cats with *Cryptosporidium* spp. infection and diarrhea have had underlying

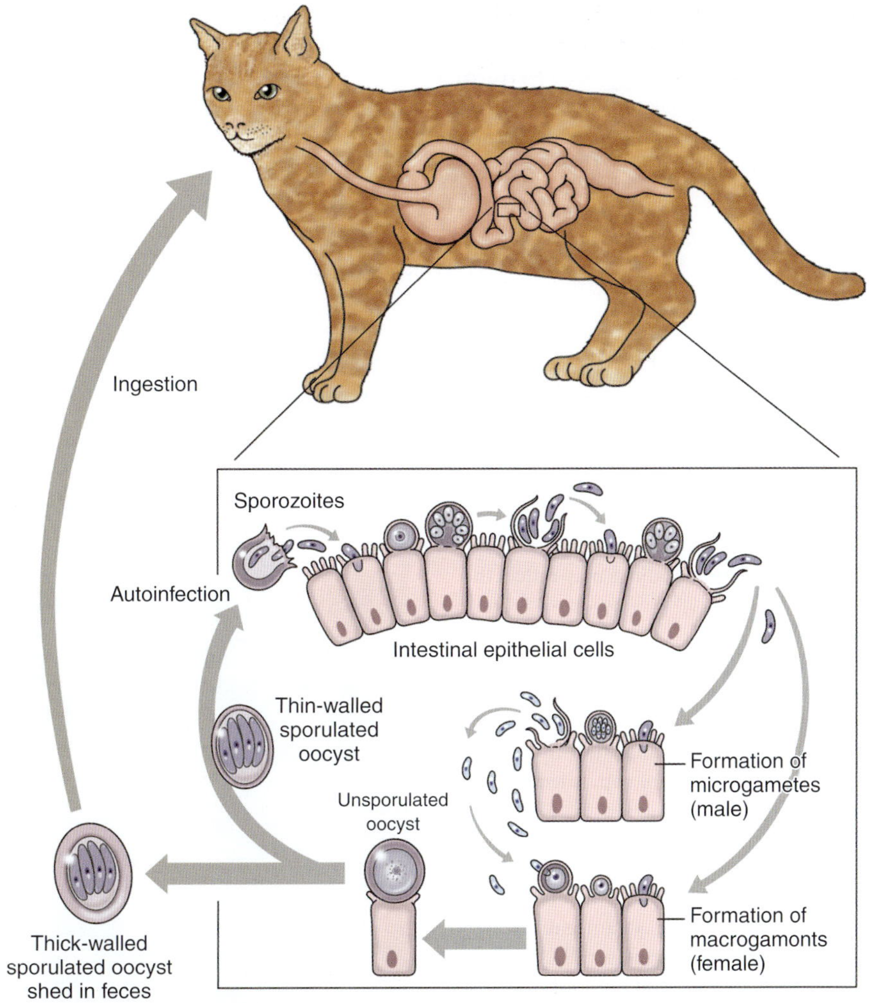

Fig. 103.1 Life cycle of *Cryptosporidium* spp.

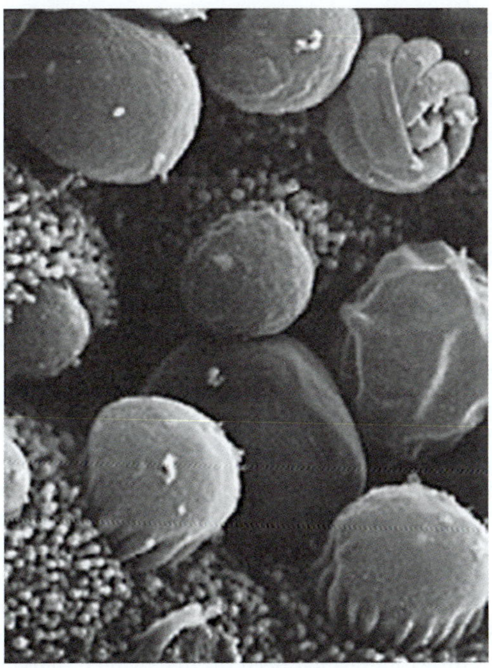

Fig. 103.2 Scanning electron microscopic image of various stages of *Cryptosporidium* on the epithelial cell microvillous surface of the cloaca of a young chicken (×5000). (Courtesy Sandy L. White, Lilly Research Labs, Greenfield, IN. From Current WL. 1988. The biology of *Cryptosporidium*. *ASM News* 54:605-612, with permission.)

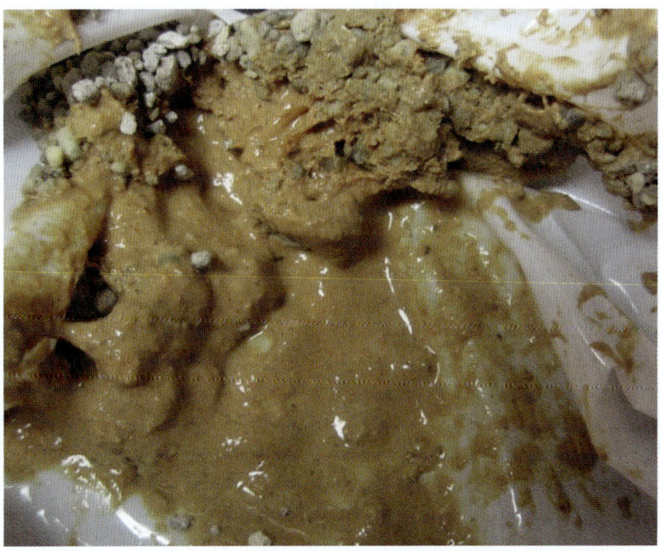

Fig. 103.3 Diarrhea induced by *Cryptosporidium* spp. and *Giardia* spp. co-infection. The image is from the case example at the end of this chapter.

TABLE 103.6 Diagnostic Assays Available for Cryptosporidiosis in Dogs or Cats

Assay	Specimen Type	Target	Performance
Cytologic examination	Feces	*Cryptosporidium* oocysts	Modified acid-fast staining has an approximately 70% sensitivity and so false negatives are common. However, the technique is more sensitive than fecal flotation.
$ZnSO_4$ centrifugal fecal flotation	Feces	*Cryptosporidium* oocysts	The small size of the oocysts and small numbers shed by dogs and cats makes this an inadequate screening procedure. The sensitivity is unknown but may be as low as 10%.
Direct FA assay	Feces	*Cryptosporidium* oocysts	Direct FA assays are available that detect both *Cryptosporidium* spp. oocysts and *Giardia* cysts. Morphology as well as fluorescence can be evaluated and so this assay is considered by most to be the gold standard. The assay appears to detect *C. felis* and *C. canis*. The sensitivity of the assay is > 70% but false negatives can occur because oocysts numbers fluctuate.
PCR assays	Feces	*Cryptosporidium* DNA	The sensitivity and specificity of assays may vary depending on assay design. Well-designed assays have the highest sensitivity of all diagnostic test methods, but false negatives can occur if low numbers of oocysts are shed, the specimen size is small, or as a result of PCR inhibitors in feces. Use of PCR as a screening assay will result in detection of many subclinical infections.

diseases or co-infections, physical examination findings may reflect the presence of these conditions.

DIAGNOSIS

The etiologic predictive value of all assays for *Cryptosporidium* spp. is low since there is a relatively high prevalence of infection in healthy dogs and cats. Diagnostic tests for *Cryptosporidium* spp. infection are summarized in Table 103.6.

Microbiologic Testing

Fecal Microscopic Examination

Cryptosporidium oocyst shedding can be sporadic, so a negative assay result does not exclude the infection. Cats and dogs generally shed relatively few oocysts. Naturally infected cats with and without diarrhea shed approximately 1817 oocysts/g of feces and 191 oocysts/g of feces, respectively.[46] In comparison, infected calves, less than 21 days old, shed a mean of 90,867 oocysts/g of feces.[56]

Concentration techniques. The threshold of detection of *Cryptosporidium* oocysts was 10^6 oocysts/g of feces using unconcentrated fecal smears.[57] Oocyst concentration procedures such as Sheather's sucrose flotation, zinc sulfate flotation, and saturated sodium chlorine methods are needed to increase the test sensitivity.[58] The consistency of the feces also affects the detection rate. For 100% test sensitivity in formed fecal specimens, 50,000 oocysts/g of feces were needed for positive results with FA examination, whereas 500,000 oocysts/g of feces were needed for acid-fast stain detection.[59] However, cats and dogs generally only shed 10^3 oocysts/g of feces, and even concentration procedures are considered insensitive for detecting infection.

Nonspecific direct oocyst staining techniques. Because oocysts are slightly smaller compared with erythrocytes, and because they are transparent, unstained preparations using conventional light microscopy make accurate identification difficult (Fig. 103.4). The stains more commonly used are safranin-methylene blue stain, Kinyoun, modified Ziehl-Neelsen (MZN), and dimethyl sulfoxide carbol fuchsin (Fig. 103.5). The average detection limit using MZN stain after concentration of human feces was 5×10^5 oocysts/g.[59] However, since cats and dogs shed only low numbers of oocysts, this technique may not be very sensitive in those species.

Immunostaining methods. Direct FA detection procedures, using monoclonal antibody reagents, can be more sensitive and specific than acid-fast or other staining methods. In one study using

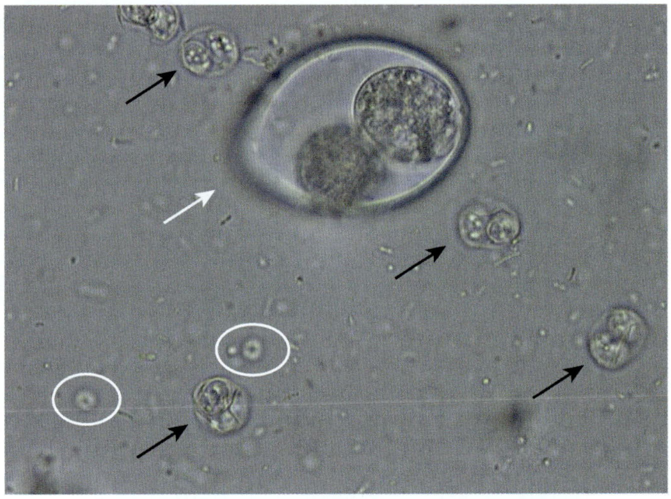

Fig. 103.4 Fecal flotation from a cat that was co-infected with *Toxoplasma gondii, Cystoisospora felis*, and *Cryptosporidium felis*. The image is magnified approximately 2000×. The *black arrows* are sporulated *T. gondii* oocysts; the *white arrow* shows *Cystoisospora felis*; the *white circles* surround *Cryptosporidium felis* oocysts.

human feces, the average detection limit using MZN was 5×10^5 oocysts/g of feces and the threshold of detection using direct FA was 5×10^4 oocysts/g of feces.[59] The disadvantage compared to other staining procedures, is that direct FA has a higher cost and requires a fluorescent microscope.

A commercially available direct FA test kit (Merifluor *Cryptosporidium/Giardia*, Meridian Bioscience, Inc., Cincinnati, OH), which simultaneously detects *Giardia* cysts and *Cryptosporidium* oocysts, has been evaluated for use in dogs and cats. In one study, this assay had a lower sensitivity than MZN staining when a single fecal specimen from a cat was tested.[60] However, the sensitivity of direct FA was the same as that of MZN when 2 to 4 consecutively collected specimens were tested. In this study, oocyst fluorescence intensity varied from an intense apple-green to a weak green fluorescence. This direct FA test has been titrated using *C. parvum* oocysts in human feces, and the variation in oocyst fluorescence may be due to antigenic diversity within *Cryptosporidium* spp. or to infection with more than one *Cryptosporidium* species.[60] Unfortunately, the

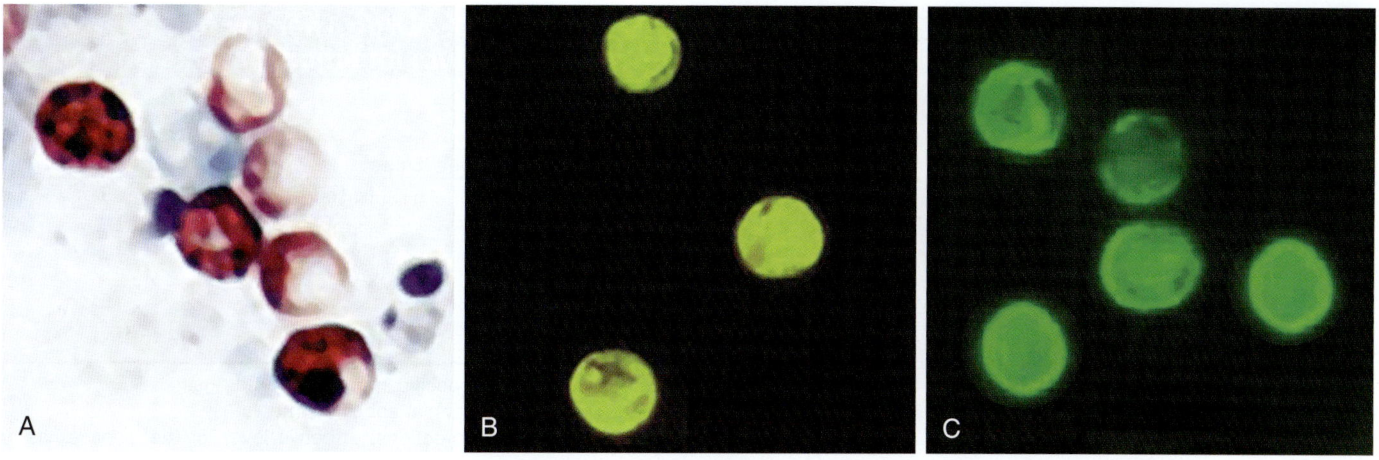

Fig. 103.5 *Cryptosporidium* is detected by demonstration of organisms in fecal specimens. This can be done using immunoassays for antigen, by microscopic detection of the organisms, or by nucleic acid amplification. Because the organisms are similar in size and shape to erythrocytes and yeasts that are normally found in feces, differential stains are required to identify the organism. These can include modified acid-fast stains (A), which stain oocysts red because they retain carbol fuchsin after decolorizing with alcohol; fluorescent stains, such as auramine-rhodamine (B), or immunofluorescent antibody stains (C) (green organisms). (From the Centers for Disease Control and Prevention).

Cryptosporidium species infecting the cats in that study were not determined. However, when the same feline specimens were tested with a polyclonal antibody, a higher sensitivity was achieved, indicating that antigenic differences exist among *C. parvum* of humans and species infecting cats.[60]

The direct FA method had a sensitivity threshold of around 10^4 to 10^5 oocysts/g of feces when used with *C. parvum*–spiked feline feces.[23]

Fecal Antigen ELISA-Based Assays

A number of different ELISA-based tests are available for detection of *C. parvum* antigen in feces. The available assays were titrated for use with human feces; therefore, sensitivity and specificity of each assay for use with dog or cat feces is unknown. The sensitivity of three fecal ELISAs and direct FA tests were compared to MZN staining.[61] Using specimens collected on day 1 of the study, the sensitivity of the three ELISA methods were 89%, 80%, and 15%. The sensitivity of these assays increased when specimens from two consecutive days were examined.[60] In another study, a comparison was made between the sensitivity of a fecal ELISA kit and carbol fuchsin stain in the detection of *Cryptosporidium* in canine and feline specimens.[62] Of 270 dog specimens, 26 (9.5%) had positive test results for *Cryptosporidium* by microscopy and 8 (3.0%) specimens had positive test results with the fecal ELISA.[62] In the same study, none of 100 cats had positive results for *Cryptosporidium* using microscopy, but 22 of 100 cats had positive results using fecal ELISA. Since observation of organisms using microscopy is considered the reference standard, it is unknown whether the ELISA results of this study were falsely positive.[38,39,62] In general, in humans, ELISA methods have had lower specificity (90.3% to 100%) when compared to direct FA.[63] When human-based ELISA test kits were applied to cat specimens, specificities were high (> 99%), but sensitivities ranged from 72.7% to 91.2% compared to direct FA.[64] Two lateral-flow POC devices for detection of *C. parvum* in human feces were insensitive for the detection of *Cryptosporidium* spp. in feline feces.[65] This may relate to antigenic differences between *C. felis* and *C. parvum*.

Molecular Diagnosis Using Nucleic Acid–Based Testing

Some studies report increased sensitivity of PCR when compared to microscopy and immunological-based techniques in clinical specimens from humans.[57,66-68] PCR has been used to amplify *Cryptosporidium* spp. DNA in feline feces, and was more sensitive than IFA.[23,57,67] A variety of PCR assays are available for detection of *Cryptosporidium* spp. DNA in feline and canine feces, including quantitative PCR panels that also detect other common GI pathogens. A positive test result does not prove that *Cryptosporidium* cause illness, because subclinical infections are common. Therefore, PCR is not considered valuable as a first-choice test for diagnosis of cryptosporidiosis in dogs or cats with diarrhea. In addition, nucleic acid–based assays are not recommended for diagnosis of *Cryptosporidium* spp. infection in clinically healthy dogs or cats (see also Public Health Aspects, later).

Serologic Diagnosis

Detection of serum antibodies has been used in a limited number of prevalence studies.[69-71] In experimentally infected cats, *C. parvum*–specific IgG was detected 4 weeks post inoculation.[71] When the results of this ELISA were compared with the presence of oocysts in feces by zinc sulfate flotation and acid-fast staining, the sensitivity, specificity, positive predictive value, and negative predictive value were 50%, 85.5%, 7.7% and 98.6%, respectively.[72] In the same study, 26 of 170 cats (15.3%) had seropositive results for *C. parvum* IgG, but only 4 of 170 cats (2%) had oocysts in feces.[72] Many cats with acute infection and diarrhea are likely to be seronegative, and it is feasible that *Cryptosporidium* IgG titers will persist for months or years as the organism is difficult to eliminate.[72] Thus, the presence of *C. parvum*–specific IgG in cat serum suggests prior infection but does not correlate highly with oocyst excretion. *Cryptosporidium* spp. infections often persist at low levels for years in some animals and so it is possible that antibody test results do not correlate to presence of oocysts in studies because of false-negative test results in fecal assays. In dogs, antibodies to *Cryptosporidium* were detected by indirect FA in 16 of 20 (80%) blood samples in one study suggesting that exposure to the

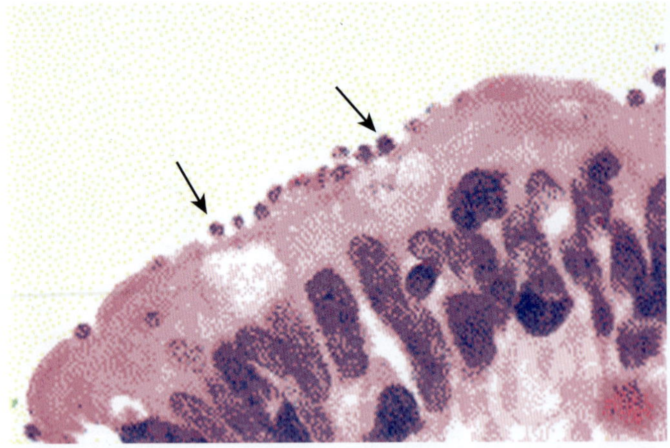

Fig. 103.6 *Cryptosporidium (arrows)* in intestine from an infected human is characteristically located at the microvillous border (hematoxylin and eosin stain). (From Petri WA. Therapy of intestinal protozoa. *Trends Parasitol.* 2003;19:523-526.)

TABLE 103.7 Drug Therapy for *Cryptosporidium* Infections in Cats and Dogs

Drug[a]	Species	Dose[b]	Route	Interval (Hours)	Minimum Duration (Days)
Azithromycin[c]	D	5–10 mg/kg	PO	12	5–7
	C	7–15 mg/kg	PO	12	5–7
Nitazoxanide	B	25 mg/animal	PO	12	5
Paromomycin[d]	B	125–165 mg/kg	PO	12–24	5
Tylosin	B	10–15 mg/kg	PO	8-12	21

[a]See Chapter 10 for specific information on drugs.
[b]Dose per administration at specified interval.
[c]Dose for systemic infections; effective level for the disease has not been established.
[d]Can be nephrotoxic and of uncertain efficacy. Never use where bloody diarrhea is observed, because the drug may be absorbed systemically.
B, both dog and cat; *C*, cat; *D*, dog

organism may be common.[71] There is no information available concerning the use of *C. canis* or *C. felis* as the antigen source in different antibody assays as previous studies used either *C. parvum* or unknown *Cryptosporidium* spp.

Intestinal Biopsy

Intestinal biopsy is costly, time-consuming, and lacks sensitivity for diagnosis of cryptosporidiosis. Specimens may be fixed in Bouin's or formalin solutions within hours after being collected. Giemsa and routine H&E stains are effective in highlighting organisms (Fig. 103.6). In naturally infected cats, loss of microvilli, degeneration of host epithelial cells, and atrophy of the villi in heavy infections, which may predispose to malabsorption or other GI dysfunction, have been documented.[40,41,73] Moderate small intestinal lymphocytic infiltrates were detected in one cat infected with *Cryptosporidium* spp. with no evidence of concurrent infection.[40] Histological findings in infected dogs included severe crypt damage with hyperplasia, dilation, marked villous atrophy, and loss of glands from the mucosa; the lamina propria has been infiltrated with lymphocytes, plasma cells, and neutrophils.[27] In dogs that were experimentally infected with *C. canis* and treated with dexamethasone acetate (6 mg/day 5 days PI), histopathologic changes consisted of epithelial metaplasia and dilation and damage to the integrity of the intestinal mucosal epithelial cells with widespread cilial atrophy.[27] Using scanning electron microscopy, *C. canis* in various developmental stages was found adherent to the surface of the duodenum and jejunum.[27] No parasites were found in the ileum, cecum, or stomach[27]; however, in one report involving an infected puppy, *C. canis* was most predominantly found within the stomach.[74]

TREATMENT AND PROGNOSIS

Treatment options for cryptosporidiosis remain limited. Many compounds with potential anti-*Cryptosporidium* activity have been evaluated in people, cattle, and mice and none consistently controlled clinical signs of disease or eliminated infection. One of the reasons proposed for lack of drug activity appears to be the unique location of the parasite in the parasitophorous vacuole, which separates it from the epithelial cell cytoplasm.[75] Because of this, supportive care and restoration of host immune response remains the mainstay of treatment in human patients.[75]

There are only a few published reports of treatment for cryptosporidiosis in cats and dogs. As a result, treatment suggestions described here are anecdotal (Table 103.7). Furthermore, some clinical responses to treatment may be due to drug activity on co-pathogens in naturally exposed cats since the presence of cryptosporidia can be an incidental finding. Therefore, only drugs with known anti-cryptosporidial activity are listed in Table 103.7. Clindamycin hydrochloride (25 mg/kg PO q24h) was administered to a cat with chronic cryptosporidiosis and lymphocytic duodenitis.[40] After 60 days of therapy there was no further improvement in stool consistency and oocysts were still detected. Tylosin was then administered (11 mg/kg PO q12h for 28 days) and stools were normal within a week of initiating therapy; *Cryptosporidium* spp. oocysts were no longer detected over a period of 6 months, intestinal inflammatory lesions resolved, and the cat remained apparently healthy for a follow-up time of 2 years after treatment. Other cats with presumed cryptosporidiosis were treated with tylosin (10 to 15 mg/kg PO q12h for 21 days), and diarrhea had resolved in about 50% of animals.[76] These observations are uncontrolled, and the signs in affected cats may have resolved spontaneously. Because tylosin has only questionable antiprotozoal effect, it is possible that its anti-inflammatory or antibacterial effects played a role in the beneficial clinical responses. Neither clindamycin nor tylosin are generally recommended as therapy for cryptosporidiosis.

Azithromycin has been evaluated in animal models of infection and in some humans with cryptosporidiosis with encouraging preliminary results.[77-80] Administration of azithromycin to dairy cows infected with *Cryptosporidium* reduced oocyst shedding and improved clinical signs of diarrhea.[77] Azithromycin is well tolerated by cats and has been administered at 10 mg/kg PO q24h for a minimum of 10 days for treatment of cryptosporidiosis with variable response.[80] The optimal duration of therapy is unknown but frequently several weeks of therapy is required for diarrhea to resolve.

Elimination of *Giardia* using drugs such as fenbendazole may have the potential to resolve *Cryptosporidium* spp. infections. Administration of ivermectin to mice co-infected with *Giardia* spp. and *Cryptosporidium* spp. decreased excretion of both parasites even though the drug has no known activity against *Cryptosporidium*.[81]

Paromomycin is an aminoglycoside antibiotic that is poorly absorbed across the gut epithelium but can be absorbed in small quantities by the apical membrane surrounding the extracytoplasmic parasite.[79,82] Studies of immunocompromised humans concluded that paromomycin alone was only partially effective for the treatment of cryptosporidiosis.[82-85] However, when paromomycin was used in combination with azithromycin, infection was cleared.[82] When paromomycin was administered to some naturally and experimentally *Cryptosporidium*-infected cats, oocyst excretion decreased to below the detectable limits of the assays used.[72,86] Paromomycin should never be administered to animals with bloody diarrhea because it can be absorbed systemically resulting in renal toxicity and ototoxicity. When cats infected with *Tritrichomonas* were treated with paromomycin, 4 out of 32 cats developed acute renal failure and three of the four cats became deaf.[84]

Nitazoxanide is the only drug approved by the US FDA for the treatment of diarrhea caused by *Cryptosporidium* in humans.[87] Nitazoxanide, a salicylanide derivative of nitrothiazole, has activity against a broad spectrum of parasites and bacteria.[88] The anti-*Cryptosporidium* activity of nitazoxanide have been proven *in vitro*, in some animal models, and in human clinical trials.[87] Nitazoxanide does not seem to be beneficial in the treatment of cryptosporidiosis in malnourished children and the immunocompromised.[34] Nitazoxanide has been used to treat some cats and dogs infected with cryptosporidiosis and giardiasis.[89] Diarrhea has resolved in some dogs and cats following administration of nitazoxanide at 25 mg/kg PO q12h for at least 5 days.[76] Nonetheless, nitazoxanide is a GI irritant, often causes vomiting, and is not effective in the absence of an appropriate immune response.

Auranofin, a gold-containing drug that was approved by the FDA in 1985 for the treatment of rheumatoid arthritis, has shown promise for the treatment of protozoal and gram-positive bacterial infections.[90] Auranofin's *in vitro* activity against *C. parvum* was similar to nitazoxanide.[90] It has been administered to shelter dogs with diarrhea due to *Giardia* infection or *Giardia* and *Cryptosporidium* co-infection (0.3 mg/kg to a maximum dose of 6 mg/d q24h for 5 days) without adverse effects.[91] Stool specimens tested negative and were formed after 5 to 10 days of treatment.

In humans, combination therapy (azithromycin and paromomycin; azithromycin, paromomycin, and nitazoxanide) has been used to reduce oocyst excretion and improve clinical signs in some individuals.[92,93]

The optimal duration of therapy for feline and canine cryptosporidiosis is uncertain, and clinical signs in some animals treated with the dosing regimens described in this chapter (Table 103.7) may improve but may not resolve by the end of the suggested treatment period. In these animals, continued treatment may be indicated if gradual improvement is noted. Animals co-infected with *Cryptosporidium* spp. and *Giardia* spp. appear to be more difficult to treat than animals infected with either organism alone.[76]

Molecular-based immunotherapy against *Cryptosporidium* and the effects of probiotic bacteria have been studied, but neither of the two protocols eradicated the parasite.[78] The use of highly active antiretroviral therapy in humans with AIDS has significantly reduced the severity of cryptosporidiosis, probably due to the recovery of the host immune responses and also due to a direct effect of protease inhibitors of host cell invasion and parasite development.[75,94,95]

Parenteral fluid replacement is indicated if dehydration is severe. Antibiotic therapy for secondary bacterial infection may be necessary. Oral rehydration solutions that contain glutamine may be helpful since absorptive-cell surface epithelium is lost and development of glutamine-dependent epithelium prevails.[96]

PREVENTION

Cryptosporidium spp. oocysts are resistant to most frequently used disinfectants, such as commercial bleach (5.25% sodium hypochlorite, see Chapter 14). Routine chlorination of drinking water does not affect oocyst viability.[97] Because filtration of this small organism is difficult, the organism can enter treated municipal water supplies. Formol saline (10% solution) and ammonia (5% solution) destroyed oocyst viability, but the required contact time was 18 hours. Concentrated ammonia solutions (50%) inactivate *Cryptosporidium* oocysts after 30 minutes.[98] Formaldehyde and hydrogen peroxide also have activity against oocysts.[99] Moist heat (steam or pasteurization [over 55°C]), freezing and thawing, or thorough drying are more practical means of disinfection. Swimming pools can be disinfected by using high chlorine concentrations for long periods (3 mg/L of water for 53 hours or 8 mg/L for 20 hours).[100] Housing dogs and cats indoors and feeding processed foods also may reduce the potential for infection since *Cryptosporidium* DNA was amplified from some raw meat diets.[101] Exceptional sanitation and use of boiling water for the cleaning of water and food bowls should decrease the possibility of contamination within crowded environments. When a human is infected with cryptosporidiosis, it is advisable to exclude that individual from work place, school, or other institutional setting until 48 hours after the last diarrhea episode.[102] This last preventive measure might be prudent for infected cats or dogs.

PUBLIC HEALTH ASPECTS

Humans become infected when they consume contaminated food and water, as well as contaminated water during recreational activities. Person-to-person or animal-to-person spread can also occur. Cryptosporidiosis in humans is generally caused by *C. hominis* and *C. parvum*.[34] Infection may be subclinical or lead to fever, severe abdominal pain, nausea, decreased appetite, weight loss, vomiting, and voluminous watery diarrhea. In developed countries, disease has occurred in association with swimming in contaminated water (such as swimming pools where fecal accidents have occurred), day-care center transmission, and less often as a result of food-borne spread.[75]

Cryptosporidium parvum is one of the few *Cryptosporidium* species with a broad host range and high genetic heterogeneity; genotyping has revealed nearly 20 subtype families, some of which are adapted to humans and some adapted to animals.[4] *Cryptosporidium hominis* is largely a human-specific *Cryptosporidium* species. However, it had been occasionally detected in cattle, sheep and goats, rodents, and dogs.[4,7]

In 2021, the AVMA reported that in 2020, there were 83.7 million dogs and 60 million cats; 45% of households owned at least one dog and 26% of households owned cats. (see also Chapter 75, Bite and Scratch Wound Infections). *Cryptosporidium felis* and *C. canis* are occasionally found in feces from humans.[97,103,104] *Cryptosporidium canis* and *C. felis* have been reported mainly in children in studies in developing countries, and these species account for 3.3% and 4.4%, respectively, of the overall *Cryptosporidium* cases.[34,105] In England, contact with dogs and cats was not a risk factor for cryptosporidiosis.[106] Furthermore, the prevalence of fecal oocyst excretion by dogs and cats owned by humans with cryptosporidiosis was no higher than that by dogs and cats owned by noninfected humans within the same studied population.[107] However, a study reported a possible case of zoonotic transmission of *C. felis* from a cat to a human living in the same household.[104] A weak statistical association was found between pediatric cryptosporidiosis and contact with dogs and cats in Guinea-Bissau and Indonesia.[108-110] In another report, *C. canis* was detected in a dog and two children in the same environment.[111] However, even when *C. canis* or *C. felis* oocysts have been reported in the same household in humans and pets, it is difficult to establish the direction, or a common source, of the infection.[92] The cross-species transmission of *Cryptosporidium* spp. among dogs or cats and their owners has been a long-standing controversy. A report from 2021 used new typing tools to identify several subtype families within both *C. canis* and *C. felis*.[112] Five subfamilies have been detected within both *C. felis* and *C. canis*; two of these subtype families in each of *C. felis* and *C. canis* have been detected in humans and cats and in humans and dogs, respectively. The use of these subtyping tools will be useful in elucidating the importance of zoonotic transmission of *Cryptosporidium* spp. from cats and dogs.

In immunocompromised individuals, such as those with AIDS and malnourished children, diarrhea can become chronic and life-threatening.[34] Life-threatening disseminated infections involve the respiratory tract, gall bladder, liver, and pancreas in addition to the GI tract. Currently, there is no effective treatment for cryptosporidiosis. Nitazoxanide, the only FDA-approved drug to treat cryptosporidiosis, does not improve clinical signs in AIDS patients and malnourished children.[34] The most beneficial treatment for these individuals has been reversal of underlying immunosuppression with highly active anti-retroviral therapy (HAART).

Since there is no effective treatment for cryptosporidiosis, prevention and risk reduction are the most important interventions, particularly for those that are immunosuppressed. Immunosuppressed individuals should be advised on prevention measures. Rigorous hand washing after handling animals, potential contact with human feces (changing diapers), and contact with soil before eating and before food preparation can reduce the risk of diarrhea in HIV-infected humans.[96] Immunosuppressed individuals also should avoid contact with animal feces, especially those of stray pets or pets less than 6 months of age. Gloves should be worn when cleaning areas that could be contaminated with pet feces. Humans with AIDS should also avoid direct exposure to calves and lambs. They should not drink water directly from lakes, canals, or rivers[96,113,114] and they should avoid accidental swallowing of water during recreational activities like swimming in public pools.[115]

The creation of dog parks has generated concerns regarding transmission of infectious agents among veterinarians, dog owners, and public health authorities. In one study, dogs attending dog parks were more likely to be positive for *Giardia* or *Cryptosporidium* than non–dog park-attending dogs. However, the only *Cryptosporidium* isolate in that study was typed as *C. canis*, which is of low risk for zoonotic transmission.[116] Since the benefits of attending dog parks outnumber the disadvantages for both owners and dogs, owners are advised to responsibly dispose of dog feces, minimizing environmental contamination of the parks.

CYCLOSPORIASIS

ETIOLOGY AND EPIDEMIOLOGY

Cyclospora cayetanensis (subclass Coccidia, phylum Apicomplexa) infects humans and animals in warm or tropical climates worldwide. *Cyclospora* are small (8 to 10 μm) obligate intracellular coccidian parasites that infect the mucosal epithelium of the intestine or bile duct of a variety of vertebrate hosts. *Cyclospora* was first identified in 1977 in Papua New Guinea as a human pathogen. The name "cyanobacterium-like bodies" was initially suggested for the organism because of its similarity to members of the blue-green algae.[117] Later the parasite was isolated from human feces and the oocysts were induced to sporulate, yielding two sporocysts that each contained two sporozoites. The parasite was considered a coccidian and named *C. cayetanensis*.[117-119] *Cyclospora cayetanensis* is closely related to *Eimeria* spp.[120] Like *Cryptosporidium*, *Cyclospora* are transmitted via the fecal-oral route by exposure to contaminated water, food, or soil.

Although the life cycle of *Cyclospora* spp. is not fully characterized, it appears to be monoxenous, requiring a single human host to complete the entire life cycle. Oocysts are passed in a noninfective form and must survive long enough to sporulate and to be ingested by a susceptible host. Depending on climate factors, oocysts may require days to weeks to sporulate and can persist and maintain infectivity for long periods in the environment even when exposed to harsh conditions.[120] Oocysts are spherical with a diameter of 7.7 to 9.9 μm. The minimum infectious dose is unknown, but it is likely that it is very low, ranging between 10 and 100 oocysts.[121]

After ingestion, sporulated oocysts excyst in the small bowel and enter epithelial cells. Asexual replication occurs in the small bowel with extruded merozoites penetrating new epithelial cells. Sexual reproduction occurs in the small-bowel epithelium and culminates with the passage of unsporulated oocysts in the feces.[122]

Outbreaks of cyclosporiasis in humans living in endemic areas usually occur during the warm and rainy season. In the United States and Canada, food-borne outbreaks related to eating contaminated raspberries also occurred during the warm rainy season.[123,124] The role that animals may play in the transmission of cyclosporiasis is controversial. Experiments conducted on nine strains of mice, rats, sand rats, chickens, ducks, rabbits, gerbils, hamsters, ferrets, pigs, dogs, and three types of monkeys have been unsuccessful in establishing an animal model for study of this parasite.[125] However, oocysts morphologically similar to *C. cayetanensis* have been detected in feces from dogs, chickens, ducks, and primates.[121] The organisms have been confirmed as *Cyclospora* only in primates. Oocysts that resembled *Cyclospora* were observed in feces from two dogs in Sao Paulo, Brazil and in one dog in Egypt.[126,127] However, another study of 140 stray dogs in the same area in Sao Paulo, Brazil, did not report evidence of such oocysts in feces.[128] The DNA of *C. cayetanensis* was amplified by PCR from feces from one chicken, two dogs, and one monkey.[129] In Mexico, oocysts morphologically and biologically similar to *C. cayetanensis* were detected in poultry feces, but not in cat feces.[130]

CLINICAL SIGNS

Clinical illness, if any, in dogs and cats is uncertain, because definitive oocysts have been documented only in human feces. Infected humans can develop anorexia, nausea, watery diarrhea, flatulence, fatigue, abdominal cramping, low-grade fever, fatigue, and weight loss after *C. cayetanensis* infection; the most severe symptoms develop in children and in humans with HIV/AIDS.[120] Asymptomatic infections are more common in endemic areas.[120] Biliary disease has also been reported in some patients with cyclosporiasis, and co-infections with *Cryptosporidium*, and other intestinal pathogens have also been described.[120]

DIAGNOSIS

Cyclospora oocysts can be identified by phase-contrast microscopy or bright-field microscopy (Table 103.8). The oocysts are spherical, refractile bodies with a central morula (Fig. 103.7A). Because the organisms are passed unsporulated in fresh feces, they can be confused with fecal yeasts. If fecal specimens are stored at 23° to 30°C for 7 to 15 days, the oocysts will sporulate and contain two sporocysts. The oocysts can also be stained with MZN acid-fast stain (Fig. 103.7B), and thus can be confused with *Cryptosporidium* and *Cystoisospora*. Some oocysts can have variable staining, with some being dark red, pale pink, or unstained.[120] Better results have been observed when the slides were heated by microwave treatment or heated to 85°C for 5 minutes in a water bath during staining (Fig. 103.7C).[120] PCR assays have been used for outbreak investigations or research; they are more sensitive than microscopy.[131-137] However, one PCR assay designed to detect *C. cayetanensis* as part of a multiplex panel was positive on a stool specimen from a dog with diarrhea in Korea; when the DNA was sequenced, the organism was identified as *Cystoisospora ohioensis*.[138] Of interest, the panel, which was reported to detect 23 enteric pathogens that were predominantly canine

TABLE 103.8 **Comparison of Some Coccidial Oocysts Features and Transmission Potential**

	Cyclospora	*Cryptosporidium*	*Cystoisospora*	*Toxoplasma*
Definitive Host	Humans, possibly animals	Humans, dogs, cats, other animals	Humans, dogs, cats, other animals	Cats
Intestinal Biopsy Findings				
Intracellular stages	T, S, M	T, S, M, G	T, S, M, G	T, S, M, G
Intracellular location	Deep seated	Intramembranous, extracytoplasmic	Deep seated	Deep seated
Size in tissue (μm)	4–16	2–5	3–15	3–15
Fecal Analysis				
Oocyst size (μm)	8–10	4–6	10–19 × 20–30 Varies with species	12 × 10
Sporulated Oocyst Features				
Number of sporocysts	2	0	2	2
Number of sporozoites per sporocyst	2	4 per oocyst (naked)	4	4
Acid-fast staining	Variable	Yes	Yes	Yes
Ultraviolet autofluorescence, 365-nm filter	Blue-green circles	None	Yes	None
Auramine fluorescence	Weak	Bright	Variable	Variable
Infectivity in fresh feces (already sporulated)	No	Yes	No	No
Zoonotic transmission	Unknown	Many animals	None, host-specific	Cats
Host-to-like-host transmission	Unknown	Yes	Yes	Yes, uncommon via oocyst

G, gametocyte; *M*, merozoite; *S*, schizont; *T*, trophozoite.

Modified from Pohjola S. Survey of cryptosporidiosis in feces of normal healthy dogs. *Nord Vet Med*. 1984;36:189–190; and Sun T, Ilardi CF, Asnis D, et al. Light and electron microscopic identification of *Cyclospora* species in the small intestine: evidence of the presence of asexual life cycle in human host. *Am J Clin Pathol*. 1996;105:216-220.

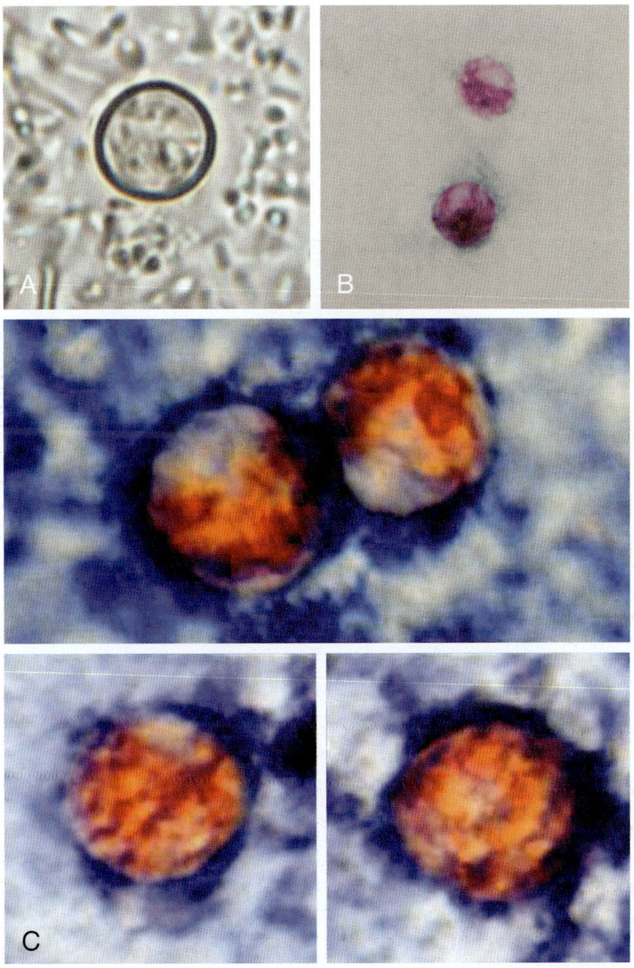

Fig. 103.7 *Cyclospora* oocysts visualized using different staining methods. (A) Wet mount. (B) Variable staining with modified acid-fast stain. (C) Uniform staining with modified safranin stain. Modification consists of heating in a microwave during staining to improve stain penetration. (From DPDx Image Library, Centers for Disease Control and Prevention, Atlanta, GA. In Bennett JE, Dolin R, Blaser MJ, eds. *Mandell, Douglas and Bennett's Principles and Practice of Infectious Diseases*. Philadelphia, PA; Elsevier: 3184-3191.)

(e.g., CDV) but sometimes human pathogens (*Lawsonia intracellularis*), did not include *Cystoisospora* spp. This underscores the importance of careful analysis of the components of "diarrhea panels" and the potential meaning of a positive or negative result for each pathogen included in the panel.

TREATMENT

The drug of choice for treatment of humans with cyclosporiasis is trimethoprim-sulfonamide, which generally leads to resolution of diarrhea after 3 to 7 days.[136,139] Ciprofloxacin was reported as an alternative for patients who are allergic to sulfonamides, but anecdotal treatment failure with this drug has also been reported.[140,141] Nitazoxanide was also effective in the treatment of cyclosporiasis in patients with sulfonamide hypersensitivity.[142,143] If a dog or cat is diagnosed with clinical cyclosporiasis, or is clinically healthy but poses a potential risk for human infection, routine dosages of trimethoprim-sulfonamide can be administered (see Chapter 10).

PUBLIC HEALTH ASPECTS

Cyclospora cayetanensis seems to be the only species detected in humans, and they seem to be its specific host. However, contact with animals was considered a risk factor for human infection in many studies worldwide.[144] Amplification of *C. cayetanensis* DNA from feces of two dogs by PCR assay increases the evidence that dogs can be exposed. However, it is unknown whether the dogs had natural infection or were just passing oocysts in feces after eating feces of another natural host. Direct human-to-human or animal-to-human transmission is unlikely, because the oocysts need a considerable amount of time to sporulate outside the host.[144] Humans tend to acquire their infection from consuming contaminated water or unwashed produce. To prevent infection, health education including personal hygiene, changing eating habits, proper sanitary infrastructures, and safe drinking water are needed. As with other coccidians, sodium hypochlorite is not an effective disinfectant for *Cyclospora* spp. oocysts. See Public Health Aspects, under *Cryptosporidia* previously, for further information on decontamination.

CASE EXAMPLE

Signalment

This case report describes the clinical management of two cats suspected to have diarrhea from *Cryptosporidium* spp. and *Giardia* spp. co-infection diagnosed by FA. Cat 1 (1-year-old, domestic longhair, male, neutered) and cat 2 (3.5-month-old, domestic longhair, male, neutered) lived in the same home in north-central Colorado.

History

The source of the cats was unknown. Both cats had been administered several conventional treatments (drugs and doses unavailable) but the diarrhea did not resolve.

Physical Examination Findings

Physical examinations were normal in both cats. Because of the dual infection and chronic diarrhea, the cats were evaluated for evidence of immunodeficiency by performing a CBC, serum biochemical panel, urinalysis, and CD4+ and CD8+ cell counts.

Laboratory Findings

The only abnormalities detected were mild neutrophilia (12,500/μL; N = 2000–12,000/μL) and a slight increase in serum ALP activity (75 IU/L; N = 7–65 IU/L) in cat 1.

Diagnosis

Prior to treatment, three fecal specimens per cat were collected (pretreatment) for evaluation for *Cryptosporidium* spp. DNA in feces by PCR, *Cryptosporidium* spp. oocysts, and *Giardia* spp. cysts by FA, and trophozoites of *Giardia* spp. and *Tritrichomonas blagburni* by wet mount examination. Specimens were then collected daily during the treatment period (intra-treatment), and then three times per week during the week after treatment (post-treatment).

Treatment

Azithromycin was administered at a dose of 10 mg/kg PO q24h for 14 days. Diarrhea did not resolve in either cat, both cats remained positive for *Cryptosporidium* DNA by PCR, and for *Giardia* spp. cysts by FA. Paromomycin was then administered at 500 mg/cat PO q24h for 5 days. After treatment, the consistency of the feces of both cats was normal and both cats were negative for *Giardia* spp. cysts by FA testing, but both cats remained positive for *Cryptosporidium* spp. DNA by PCR. In an attempt to resolve *Cryptosporidium* spp. oocyst excretion, paromomycin was administered again 1 month later. After administration of paromomycin, follow-up fecal tests were performed over 4 weeks (seven specimens) and 1 week (two specimens) for the first and second treatment periods, respectively. After treating the cats with both azithromycin and paromomycin, both cats became negative for *Giardia* spp. and *Cryptosporidium* spp. by FA but remained PCR positive for *Cryptosporidium* spp. DNA in feces. Although parasitologic clearance was not achieved, fecal consistency improved. Approximately 4 years after the administration of the last treatment, the owner reported that cats 1 and 2 were healthy and they did not have any other episodes of diarrhea.

Comments

Animals with co-infections may be more difficult to treat successfully than animals infected with either organism alone. It is possible that no drug will be generally effective for the treatment of these infections. Some treatments can help improve the clinical signs but infection may be unlikely to clear. In general, cats and dogs harbor the host-specific *Cryptosporidium* and *G. duodenalis* genotypes; currently there is no information if different assemblages might have different drug susceptibilities. Consequently, the drug and protocol should be varied according to each individual patient. In chronic cases, the possibility of underlying disorders should also be considered. Additionally, infection with *G. duodenalis* and *Cryptosporidium* does not appear to cause permanent immunity and so re-infections are likely to occur.

SUGGESTED READINGS

Lee S, Kim J, Cheon DS, et al. Identification of *Cystoisospora ohioensis* in a diarrheal dog in Korea. *Korean J Parasitol*. 2018;56:371–374.

Ortega YR, Sanchez R. Update on *Cyclospora cayetanensis*, a food-borne and waterborne parasite. *Clin Microbiol Rev*. 2010;23:218–234.

Ryan U, Zahedi A, Paparini A. *Cryptosporidium* in humans and animals: a one health approach to prophylaxis. *Parasite Immunol*. 2016;38(9):535–547.

Santin M, Trout JM. Companion animals. In: Ortega-Pierres G, Cacciò S, Fayer R, et al., eds. *Giardia and Cryptosporidium: From Molecules to Disease*. CAB International; 2008:437–449.

Xiao L, Feng Y. Zoonotic cryptosporidiosis. *FEMS Immunol Med Microbiol*. 2008;52:309–323.

REFERENCES

1. Tyzzer EE. *Cryptosporidium parvum (sp. nov.)*, a coccidium found in the small intestine of the common mouse. *Arch Protistenkunde*. 1912;26:394–412.
2. Ryan U, Paparini A, Monis P, et al. It's official - *Cryptosporidium* is a gregarine: what are the implications for the water industry? *Water Res*. 2016;105:305–313.

3. Ortega YR, Sterling CR, Gilman RH, et al. *Cyclospora* species—a new protozoan pathogen of humans. *N Engl J Med.* 1993;328:1308–1312.
4. Feng Y, Ryan UM, Xiao L. Genetic diversity and population structure of *Cryptosporidium. Trends Parasitol.* 2018;34:997–1011.
5. Lupo PJ, Langer-Curry RC, Robinson M, et al. *Cryptosporidium muris* in a Texas canine population. In: Ortega-Pierres G, Cacciò S, Fayer R, et al., eds. *Giardia and Cryptosporidium: From Molecules to Disease.* CAB International; 2008:437–449.
6. Li W, Li Y, Song M, et al. Prevalence and genetic characteristics of *Cryptosporidium, Enterocytozoon bieneusi* and *Giardia duodenalis* in cats and dogs in Heilongjiang province, China. *Vet Parasitol.* 2015;208:125–134.
7. Gil H, Cano L, de Lucio A, et al. Detection and molecular diversity of *Giardia duodenalis* and *Cryptosporidium* spp. in sheltered dogs and cats in Northern Spain. *Infect Genet Evol.* 2017;50:62–69.
8. Santin M, Trout JM. Companion animals. In: Ortega-Pierres G, Cacciò S, Fayer R, et al., eds. *Giardia and Cryptosporidium: From Molecules to Disease.* CAB International; 2008:437–449.
9. Pavlasek I, Ryan U. The first finding of a natural infection of *Cryptosporidium muris* in a cat. *Vet Parasitol.* 2007;144:349–352.
10. Santín M, Trout JM, Vecino JA, et al. *Cryptosporidium, Giardia* and *Enterocytozoon bieneusi* in cats from Bogota (Colombia) and genotyping of isolates. *Vet Parasitol.* 2006;141:334–339.
11. Fayer R, Santín M, Trout JM, et al. Detection of *Cryptosporidium felis* and *Giardia duodenalis* assemblage F in a cat colony. *Vet Parasitol.* 2006;140:44–53.
12. Yang R, Ying JL, Monis P, et al. Molecular characterisation of *Cryptosporidium* and *Giardia* in cats (*Felis catus*) in western Australia. *Exp Parasitol.* 2015;155:13–18.
13. Fayer R, Ungar BL. *Cryptosporidium* spp. and cryptosporidiosis. *Microbiol Rev.* 1986;50:458–483.
14. Iseki M. *Cryptosporidium felis* sp. n. (Protozoa: Eimeriorina) from the domestic cat. *Jpn J Parasitol.* 1979;28:285–307.
15. Fayer R, Trout JM, Xiao L, et al. *Cryptosporidium canis* sp. n. from domestic dogs. *J Parasitol.* 2001;87:1415–1422.
16. Xu H, Jin Y, Wu W, et al. Genotypes of *Cryptosporidium* spp., *Enterocytozoon bieneusi* and *Giardia duodenalis* in dogs and cats in Shanghai, China. *Parasit Vectors.* 2016;9:121.
17. Jian F, Qi M, He X, et al. Occurrence and molecular characterization of *Cryptosporidium* in dogs in Henan province, China. *BMC Vet Res.* 2014;10:26.
18. Ballweber LR, Panuska C, Huston CL, et al. Prevalence of and risk factors associated with shedding of *Cryptosporidium felis* in domestic cats of Mississippi and Alabama. *Vet Parasitol.* 2009;160:306–310.
19. Mugala L, Siwila J, Saasa N, et al. Prevalence of *Cryptosporidium* spp. oocysts in dogs in Lusaka district of Zambia. *Vet World.* 2018;11:585–589.
20. Gharieb RMA, Merwad AMA, Saleh AA, et al. Molecular screening and genotyping of *Cryptosporidium* species in household dogs and in-contact children in Egypt: risk factor analysis and zoonotic importance. *Vector Borne Zoonotic Dis.* 2018;18:424–432.
21. Moreira ADS, Baptista CT, Brasil CL, et al. Risk factors and infection due to *Cryptosporidium* spp. in dogs and cats in southern Rio Grande do Sul. *Rev Bras Parasitol Vet.* 2018;27:113–118.
22. Ranjbar R, Mirhendi H, Izadi M, et al. Molecular identification of *Cryptosporidium* spp. in Iranian dogs using seminested PCR: a first report. *Vector Borne Zoonotic Dis.* 2018;18:96–100.
23. Scorza AV, Brewer MM, Lappin MR. Polymerase chain reaction for the detection of *Cryptosporidium* spp. in cat feces. *J Parasitol.* 2003;89:423–426.
24. Darabus G, Olariu R. The homologous and interspecies transmission of *Cryptosporidium parvum* and *Cryptosporidium meleagridis. Pol J Vet Sci.* 2003;6:225–228.
25. Aydin Y, Ozkul IA. Infectivity of *Cryptosporidium muris* directly isolated from the murine stomach for various laboratory animals. *Vet Parasitol.* 1996;66:257–262.
26. Augustin-Bichl G, Boch J, Henkel G. Cryptosporidial infections in dogs and cats. *Berl Munch Tierarztl Wochenschr.* 1984;97:179–181.
27. Cui Z, Dong H, Wang R, et al. A canine model of experimental infection with *Cryptosporidium canis. Exp Parasitol.* 2018;195:19–23.
28. Huang DB, White AC. An updated review on *Cryptosporidium* and *Giardia. Gastroenterol Clin North Am.* 2006;35:291–314.
29. Certad G, Viscogliosi E, Chabe M, et al. Pathogenic mechanisms of *Cryptosporidium* and *Giardia. Trends Parasitol.* 2017;33:561–576.
30. Deng M, Rutherford MS, Abrahamsen MS. Host intestinal epithelial response to *Cryptosporidium parvum. Adv Drug Deliv Rev.* 2004;56:869–884.
31. Bouzid M, Hunter PR, Chalmers RM, et al. *Cryptosporidium* pathogenicity and virulence. *Clin Microbiol Rev.* 2013;26:115–134.
32. Mele R, Gomez Morales MA, Tosini F, et al. *Cryptosporidium parvum* at different developmental stages modulates host cell apoptosis in vitro. *Infect Immun.* 2004;72:6061–6067.
33. Jenkins MC, Higgins J, Abrahante JE, et al. Fecundity of *Cryptosporidium parvum* is correlated with intracellular levels of the viral symbiont CPV. *Int J Parasitol.* 2008;38:1051–1055.
34. Ryan U, Zahedi A, Paparini A. *Cryptosporidium* in humans and animals: a one health approach to prophylaxis. *Parasite Immunol.* 2016;38:535–547.
35. Ras R, Huynh K, Desoky E, et al. Perturbation of the intestinal microbiota of mice infected with *Cryptosporidium parvum. Int J Parasitol.* 2015;45:567–573.
36. Arai H, Fukuda Y, Hara T, et al. Prevalence of *Cryptosporidium* infection among domestic cats in the Tokyo metropolitan district. *Jpn J Med Biol.* 1990;43:7–14.
37. Asahi H, Koyama T, Arai H, et al. Biological nature of *Cryptosporidium* spp. isolated from a cat. *Parasitol Res.* 1991;77:237–240.
38. Spain CV, Scarlett JM, Wade SE, et al. Prevalence of enteric zoonotic agents in cats less than 1 year old in central New York state. *J Vet Intern Med.* 2001;15:33–38.
39. Hill SL, Cheney JM, Taton-Allen GF, et al. Prevalence of enteric zoonotic organisms in cats. *J Am Vet Med Assoc.* 2000;216:687–692.
40. Lappin MR, Dowers K, Edsell D, et al. Cryptosporidiosis and inflammatory bowel disease in a cat. *Feline Pract.* 1997;25:10–13.
41. Goodwin MA, Barsanti JA. Intractable diarrhea associated with intestinal cryptosporidiosis in a domestic cat also infected with feline leukemia virus. *J Am Anim Hosp Assoc.* 1990;26:365–368.
42. Brizee-Buxton BL, Crystal MA. Coincident enteric cryptosporidiosis [correspondence]. *J Am Anim Hosp Assoc.* 1994;30:307.
43. Gookin JL, Levy MG, Law JM, et al. Experimental infection of cats with *Tritrichomonas foetus. Am J Vet Res.* 2001;62:1690–1697.
44. Fitzgerald L, Bennett M, Ng J, et al. Morphological and molecular characterisation of a mixed *Cryptosporidium muris/Cryptosporidium felis* infection in a cat. *Vet Parasitol.* 2011;175:160–164.
45. Bennet M, Baxby D, Blundell N, et al. Cryptosporidiosis in the domestic cat. *Vet Rec.* 1985;116:73–74.
46. Uga S, Matsumura T, Ishibashi K, et al. Cryptosporidiosis in dogs and cats in Hyogo Prefecture, Japan. *Jap J Parasitol.* 1989;38:139–143.
47. Keith CL, Radecki SV, Lappin MR. Evaluation of fenbendazole for treatment of *Giardia* infection in cats concurrently infected with *Cryptosporidium parvum. Am J Vet Res.* 2003;64:1027–1029.
48. Perez Trot G, Asanovic J, Petetta L. Resolucion de un caso complejo de diarrhea en una gata. *Rev Med Vet.* 2002;84:73–74.
49. Paris JK, Wills S, Balzer HJ, et al. Enteropathogen co-infection in UK cats with diarrhoea. *BMC Vet Res.* 2014;10:13.
50. Lent SF, Burkhardt JE, Bolka D. Coincident enteric cryptosporidiosis and lymphosarcoma in a cat with diarrhea. *J Am Anim Hosp Assoc.* 1993;29:492–496.
51. Wilson RB, Holscher MA, Lyle SJ. Cryptosporidiosis in a pup. *J Am Vet Med Assoc.* 1983;183:1005–1006.
52. Aydin Y, Guvenc T, Beyaz L, et al. Intestinal cryptosporidiosis associated with distemper in a dog [abstract]. *Ankara Univ Vet Fak Derg.* 2004;51:233–235.
53. Denholm KM, Haitjema H, Gwynne BJ, et al. Concurrent *Cryptosporidium* and parvovirus infections in a puppy. *Aust Vet J.* 2001;79:98–101.
54. Greene CE, Jacobs GJ, Prickett D. Intestinal malabsorption and cryptosporidiosis in an adult dog. *J Am Vet Med Assoc.* 1990;197:365–369.
55. Ellis AE, Brown CA, Miller DL. Diagnostic exercise: chronic vomiting in a dog. *Vet Pathol.* 2010;47:991–993.

56. Nydam DV, Wade SE, Schaaf SL, et al. Number of *Cryptosporidium parvum* oocysts or *Giardia* spp. cysts shed by dairy calves after natural infection. *Am J Vet Res.* 2001;62:1612–1615.
57. Webster KA, Smith HV, Giles M, et al. Detection of *Cryptosporidium parvum* oocysts in feces: comparison of conventional coproscopical methods and the polymerase chain reaction. *Vet Parasitol.* 1996;61:5–13.
58. Kar S, Gawlowska S, Daugschies A, et al. Quantitative comparison of different purification and detection methods for *Cryptosporidium parvum* oocysts. *Vet Parasitol.* 2011;177:366–370.
59. Weber R, Bryan RT, Bishop HS, et al. Threshold of detection of *Cryptosporidium* oocysts in human stool specimens: evidence for low sensitivity of current diagnostic methods. *J Clin Microbiol.* 1991;29:1323–1327.
60. Marks SL, Hanson TE, Melli AC. Comparison of direct immunofluorescence modified acid fast staining, and enzyme immunoassay techniques for detection of *Cryptosporidium* spp. in naturally exposed kittens. *J Am Vet Med Assoc.* 2004;225:1549–1553.
61. Sabshin SJ, Levy JK, Tupler T, et al. Enteropathogens identified in cats entering a Florida animal shelter with normal feces or diarrhea. *J Am Vet Med Assoc.* 2012;241:331–337.
62. Cirak VY, Bauer C. Comparison of conventional coproscopical methods and commercially coproantigen ELISA kits for the detection of *Giardia* and *Cryptosporidium* infections in dogs and cats. *Berl Munch Tierarztl Wochenschr.* 2004;117:410–413.
63. Petry F. Laboratory diagnosis of *Cryptosporidium parvum* infection. *Contrib Microbiol.* 2000;6:33–49.
64. Mekaru SR, Marks SL, Felley AJ, et al. Comparison of direct immunofluorescence, immunoassays, and fecal flotation for detection of *Cryptosporidium* spp. and *Giardia* spp. in naturally exposed cats in 4 Northern California animal shelters. *J Vet Intern Med.* 2007;21:959–965.
65. Bachman D, Scorza AV, Brewer M, et al. Evaluation of chromatographic immunoassays for the diagnosis of *Giardia* spp. and *Cryptosporidium* spp. of cats and dogs. *Proceedings of the 25th ACVIM Forum.* 2007.
66. da Silva AJ, Bornay-Llinares FJ, Moura INS, et al. Fast and reliable extraction of protozoan parasite DNA from fecal specimens. *Mol Diagn.* 1999;4:57–64.
67. Sargent KD, Morgan UM, Elliot A, et al. Morphological and genetic characterization of *Cryptosporidium* oocysts from domestic cats. *Vet Parasitol.* 1998;77:221–227.
68. Rochelle PA, De Leon R, Stewart MH, et al. Comparison of primers and optimization of PCR conditions for detection of *Cryptosporidium parvum* and *Giardia lamblia* in water. *Appl Environ Microbiol.* 1997;63:106–114.
69. McReynolds CA, Lappin MR, Ungar B, et al. Regional seroprevalence of *Cryptosporidium parvum*-specific IgG of cats in the United States. *Vet Parasitol.* 1999;80:187–195.
70. Svobodovà V, Konvalinova J, Svobodobodova M. Coprological and serological findings in dogs and cats with giardiosis and cryptosporidiosis. *Acta Vet Brno.* 1994;63:257–262.
71. Tzipori S, Campbell I. Prevalence of *Cryptosporidium* antibodies in 10 animal species. *J Clin Microbiol.* 1981;14:455–456.
72. McReynolds C, McReynolds LM, Brewer MM, et al. *Cryptosporidium parvum* serum antibodies responses and oocyst shedding in experimentally inoculated cats. Masters Thesis. Colorado State University; 2001.
73. Poonacha KB, Pippin C. Intestinal cryptosporidiosis in a cat. *Vet Pathol.* 1982;19:708–710.
74. Miller DL, Liggett A, Radi ZA, et al. Gastrointestinal cryptosporidiosis in a puppy. *Vet Parasitol.* 2003;115:199–204.
75. White AC Jr. Cryptosporidiosis (*Cryptosporidium* species). In: Bennett JE, Dolin R, Blaser MJ, eds. *Mandell, Douglas and Bennett's Principles and Practice of Infectious Diseases.* Philadelphia, PA: Elsevier; 2015:3173–3183.
76. Scorza AV. Co-infection of *Cryptosporidium* and *Giardia* in Naturally Infected Cats. Diagnosis and Treatment of Cryptosporidiosis and Giardiasis in Cats and Dogs in the United States. PhD Thesis. Colorado State University; 2007.
77. Elitok B, Elitok OM, Pulat H. Efficacy of azithromycin dihydrate in treatment of cryptosporidiosis in naturally infected dairy calves. *J Vet Intern Med.* 2005;19:590–593.
78. Gargala G. Drug treatment and novel drug target against *Cryptosporidium. Parasite.* 2008;15:275–281.
79. Rossignol JF. Drug treatment and novel drug targets against *Giardia* and *Cryptosporidium.* In: Ortega-Pierres G, Cacciò S, Fayer R, et al., eds. *Giardia and Cryptosporidium: From Molecules to Disease.* Wallingford, Oxfordshire, UK: CAB International; 2009.
80. Scorza AV, Lappin MR. An update in three important protozoan parasitic infections in cats: cryptosporidiosis, *Giardiasis*, and tritrichomoniasis. *Vet Med (Auckl).* 2006:18–32.
81. Youssef MY, Essa MM, Sadaka HA, et al. Effect of ivermectin on combined intestinal protozoal infection (giardiasis and cryptosporidiosis). *J Egypt Soc Parasitol.* 1996;26:543–553.
82. Wallace MR, Nguyen MT, Newton JAJ. Use of paromomycin for the treatment of cryptosporidiosis in patients with AIDS. *Clin Infect Dis.* 1993;17:1070–1073.
83. Bissuel F, Cotte L, Raodonirina M, et al. Paromomycin: an effective treatment for cryptosporidial disease in patients with AIDS. *Clin Infect Dis.* 1994;18:447–449.
84. Gookin JL, Riviere JE, Gilger BC, et al. Acute renal failure in four cats treated with paromomycin. *J Am Vet Med Assoc.* 1999;215:1821–1823.
85. Hewitt RG, Yiannoutsos CT, Higgs ES, et al. Paromomycin: no more effective than placebo for treatment of cryptosporidiosis in patients with advanced human immunodeficiency virus infection. *Clin Infect Dis.* 2000;31:1084–1092.
86. Barr SC, Jamrosz GJ, Hornbuckle WE, et al. Use of paromomycin for treatment of cryptosporidiosis in a cat. *J Am Vet Med Assoc.* 1994;205:1742–1743.
87. Hemphill A, Mueller J, Esposito M. Nitazoxanide, a broad-spectrum thiazolide anti-infective agent for the treatment of gastrointestinal infections. *Expert Opin Pharmacother.* 2006;7:953–964.
88. Smith HV, Corcoran GD. New drugs and treatment for cryptosporidiosis. *Curr Opin Infect Dis.* 2004;17:667–674.
89. Lappin MR, Spindel M, Riggenbach L. Infectious agent prevalence rates in dogs with diarrhea and response to administration of fenbendazole or nitazoxanide. *Proceedings of the 25th ACVIM Forum.* 2008.
90. Debnath A, Ndao M, Reed SL. Reprofiled drug targets ancient protozoans: drug discovery for parasitic diarrheal diseases. *Gut Microb.* 2013;4:66–71.
91. Zoafin (1 mg Auranofin). Available at: www.zoafin.com.
92. Giacometti A, Burzacchini F, Cirioni O, et al. Efficacy of treatment with paromomycin, azithromycin, and nitazoxanide in a patient with disseminated cryptosporidiosis. *Euro J Clin Microbiol Infect Dis.* 1999;18:885–889.
93. Smith NH, Cron S, Valdez LM, et al. Combination drug therapy for cryptosporidiosis in AIDS. *J Infect Dis.* 1998;178:900–903.
94. Farthing MJG. Clinical aspects of human cryptosporidiosis. *Contrib Microbiol.* 2000;50:74–76.
95. Caccio SM, Chalmers RM. Human cryptosporidiosis in Europe. *Clin Microbiol Infect.* 2016;22:471–480.
96. Kaplan JE, Benson C, Holmes KK, et al. Guidelines for prevention and treatment of opportunistic infections in HIV-infected adults and adolescents; recommendations from CDC, the National Institutes of Health, and the HIV Medicine Association of the Infectious Diseases Society of America. *Morb Mortal Wkly Rep.* 2009;58:1–198.
97. Xiao L. Molecular epidemiology of cryptosporidiosis: an update. *Exp Parasitol.* 2010;124:80–89.
98. Sundermann CA, Lindsay DS, Blagburn BL. Evaluation of disinfectants for ability to kill avian *Cryptosporidium* oocysts. *Companion Anim Pract.* 1987;1:36–39.
99. Castro-Hermida JA, Pors I, Mendez-Hermida F, et al. Evaluation of two commercial disinfectants on the viability and infectivity of *Cryptosporidium parvum* oocysts. *Vet J.* 2006;171:340–345.
100. Juranek DD. Cryptosporidiosis: sources of infection and guidelines for prevention. *Clin Infect Dis.* 1995;21(suppl 1):S57–S61.
101. Strohmeyer RA, Morley PS, Hyatt DR, et al. Evaluation of bacterial and protozoal contamination of commercially available raw meat diets for dogs. *J Am Vet Med Assoc.* 2006;228:537–542.
102. Chalmers RM, Davies AP. Minireview: clinical cryptosporidiosis. *Exp Parasitol.* 2010;124:138–146.
103. Bowman DD, Lucio-Forster A. Cryptosporidiosis and giardiasis in dogs and cats: veterinary and public health importance. *Exp Parasitol.* 2010;124:121–127.

104. Beser J, Toresson L, Eitrem R, et al. Possible zoonotic transmission of *Cryptosporidium felis* in a household. *Infect Ecol Epidemiol.* 2015;5:28463.
105. Pedraza-Diaz S, Amar C, Iversen AM, et al. Unusual *Cryptosporidium* species recovered from human faeces: first description of *Cryptosporidium felis* and *Cryptosporidium* "dog type" from patients in England. *J Med Microbiol.* 2001;50:293–296.
106. Goh S, Reacher M, Casemore DP, et al. Sporadic cryptosporidiosis, north Cumbria, England, 1996-2000. *Emerg Infect Dis.* 2004;10:1007–1015.
107. Smith RP, Chalmers RM, Elwin K, et al. Investigation of the role of companion animals in the zoonotic transmission of cryptosporidiosis. *Zoonoses Public Health.* 2009;56:24–33.
108. Katsumata T, Hosea D, Ranuh IG, et al. Short report: possible *Cryptosporidium muris* infection in humans. *Am J Trop Med Hyg.* 2000;62:70–72.
109. Molbak K, Aaby P, Hojlyng N, et al. Risk factors for *Cryptosporidium* diarrhea in early childhood: a case-control study from Guinea-Bissau, West Africa. *Am J Epidemiol.* 1994;139:734–740.
110. Robinson RA, Pugh RN. Dogs, zoonoses and immunosuppression. *J R Soc Promot Health.* 2002;122:95–98.
111. Xiao L, Cama VA, Cabrera L, et al. Possible transmission of *Cryptosporidium canis* among children and a dog in a household. *J Clin Microbiol.* 2007;45:2014–2016.
112. Ryan U, Zahedi A, Feng Y, et al. An update on zoonotic Cryptosporidium species and genotypes in humans. *Animals (Basel).* 2021;11:3307.
113. Ng J, Yang R, Whiffin V, et al. Identification of zoonotic *Cryptosporidium* and *Giardia* genotypes infecting animals in Sydney's water catchments. *Exp Parasitol.* 2011;128:138–144.
114. Schets FM, van Wijnen JH, Schijven JF, et al. Monitoring of waterborne pathogens in surface waters in Amsterdam, The Netherlands, and the potential health risk associated with exposure to *Cryptosporidium* and *Giardia* in these waters. *Appl Environ Microbiol.* 2008;74:2069–2078.
115. Centers for Disease Control and Prevention. Parasites - *Cryptosporidium* (also known as "Crypto"). Available at: https://www.cdc.gov/parasites/crypto/prevention-control.html.
116. Wang A, Ruch-Gallie R, Scorza V, et al. Prevalence of *Giardia* and *Cryptosporidium* species in dog park attending dogs compared to non-dog park attending dogs in one region of Colorado. *Vet Parasitol.* 2012;184:335–340.
117. Long EG, White EH, Carmichael WW, et al. Morphologic and staining characteristics of a cyanobacterium-like organism associated with diarrhea. *J Infect Dis.* 1991;164:199–202.
118. Soave R. *Cyclospora*: an overview. *Clin Infect Dis.* 1996;23:429–435. quiz 436-427.
119. Ortega YR, Gilman RH, Sterling CR. A new coccidian parasite (Apicomplexa: Eimeriidae) from humans. *J Parasitol.* 1994;80:625–629.
120. Ortega YR, Sanchez R. Update on *Cyclospora cayetanensis*, a food-borne and waterborne parasite. *Clin Microbiol Rev.* 2010;23:218–234.
121. Sterling CR, Ortega YR. *Cyclospora*: an enigma worth unraveling. *Emerg Infect Dis.* 1999;5:48–53.
122. Ortega YR, Nagle R, Gilman RH, et al. Pathologic and clinical findings in patients with cyclosporiasis and a description of intracellular parasite life-cycle stages. *J Infect Dis.* 1997;176:1584–1589.
123. Herwaldt BL. *Cyclospora cayetanensis*: a review, focusing on the outbreaks of cyclosporiasis in the 1990. *Clin Infect Dis.* 2000;31:1040–1057.
124. Shields JM, Olson BH. *Cyclospora cayetanensis*: a review of an emerging parasitic coccidian. *Int J Parasitol.* 2003;33:371–391.
125. Eberhard ML, Ortega YR, Hanes DE, et al. Attempts to establish experimental *Cyclospora cayetanensis* infection in laboratory animals. *J Parasitol.* 2000;86:577–582.
126. Yai LE, Bauab AR, Hirschfeld MP, et al. The first two cases of *Cyclospora* in dogs, Sao Paulo, Brazil. *Rev Inst Med Trop Sao Paulo.* 1997;39:177–179.
127. Awadallah MA, Salem LM. Zoonotic enteric parasites transmitted from dogs in Egypt with special concern to *Toxocara canis* infection. *Vet World.* 2015;8:946–957.
128. Carollo MC, Amato N, Braz VLM, et al. Detection of *Cyclospora* sp. oocysts in the feces of stray dogs in greater Sao Paulo (Sao Paulo state, Brazil). *Rev Soc Bras Med Trop.* 2001;34:597–598.
129. Chacín-Bonilla L. Importance of the different species and genotypes of *Cryptosporidium* in public health. *Invest Clin.* 2002;43:67–69.
130. Garcia-Lopez HL, Rodriguez-Tovar LE, Medina-De la Garza CE. Identification of *Cyclospora* in poultry. *Emerg Infect Dis.* 1996;2:356–357.
131. Hussein EM. Molecular identification of *Cyclospora* spp. using multiplex PCR from diarrheic children compared to other conventional methods. *J Egypt Soc Parasitol.* 2007;37:585–598.
132. Hussein EM, El-Moamly AA, Dawoud HA, et al. Real-time PCR and flow cytometry in detection of *Cyclospora* oocysts in fecal samples of symptomatic and asymptomatic pediatrics patients. *J Egypt Soc Parasitol.* 2007;37:151–170.
133. Lalonde LF, Gajadhar AA. Highly sensitive and specific PCR assay for reliable detection of *Cyclospora cayetanensis* oocysts. *Appl Environ Microbiol.* 2008;74:4354–4358.
134. Mundaca CC, Torres-Slimming PA, Araujo-Castillo RA, et al. Use of PCR to improve diagnostic yield in an outbreak of cyclosporiasis in Lima, Peru. *Trans R Soc Trop Med Hyg.* 2008;102:712–717.
135. Relman DA, Schmidt TM, Gajadhar A, et al. Molecular phylogenetic analysis of *Cyclospora*, the human intestinal pathogen, suggests that it is closely related to *Eimeria* species. *J Infect Dis.* 1996;173:440–445.
136. Madico G, Gilman RH, Miranda E, et al. Treatment of *Cyclospora* infections with co-trimoxazole. *Lancet.* 1993;342:122–123.
137. Taniuchi M, Verweij JJ, Sethabutr O, et al. Multiplex polymerase chain reaction method to detect *Cyclospora, Cystoisospora*, and microsporidia in stool samples. *Diag Microbiol Infect Dis.* 2011;71:386–390.
138. Lee S, Kim J, Cheon DS, et al. Identification of *Cystoisospora ohioensis* in a diarrheal dog in Korea. *Korean J Parasitol.* 2018;56:371–374.
139. Hoge CW, Shlim DR, Ghimire M, et al. Placebo-controlled trial of co-trimoxazole for *Cyclospora* infections among travellers and foreign residents in Nepal. *Lancet.* 1995;345:691–693.
140. Maratim AC, Kamar KK, Ngindu A, et al. Safranin staining of *Cyclospora cayetanensis* oocysts not requiring microwave heating. *Br J Biomed Sci.* 2002;59:114–115.
141. Zimmer SM, Schuetz AN, Franco-Paredes C. Efficacy of nitazoxanide for cyclosporiasis in patients with sulfa allergy. *Clin Infect Dis.* 2007;44:466–467.
142. Diaz E, Mondragon J, Ramirez E, et al. Epidemiology and control of intestinal parasites with nitazoxanide in children in Mexico. *Am J Trop Med Hyg.* 2003;68:384–385.
143. Mansfield LS, Gajadhar AA. *Cyclospora cayetanensis*, a food- and water-borne coccidian parasite. *Vet Parasitol.* 2004;126:73–90.
144. Chacin-Bonilla L. Epidemiology of *Cyclospora cayetanensis*: a review focusing in endemic areas. *Acta Trop.* 2010;115:181–193.
145. Morgan UM, Deplazes P, Forbes DA, et al. Sequence and PCR-RFLP analysis of the internal transcribed spacers of the rDNA repeat unit in isolates of *Cryptosporidium* from different hosts. *Parasitology.* 1999;118(Pt 1):49–58.
146. Alves MEM, Martins FDC, Braunig P, et al. Molecular detection of *Cryptosporidium* spp. and the occurrence of intestinal parasites in fecal samples of naturally infected dogs and cats. *Parasitol Res.* 2018;117:3033–3038.
147. Ryan U, Xiao L, Read C, et al. Identification of novel *Cryptosporidium* genotypes from the Czech Republic. *Appl Environ Microbiol.* 2003;69:4302–4307.
148. Hajdusek O, Ditrich O, Slapeta J. Molecular identification of *Cryptosporidium* spp. in animals and human hosts from the Czech Republic. *Vet Parasitol.* 2004;122:183–192.
149. Sotiriadou I, Pantchev N, Gassmann D, et al. Molecular identification of *Giardia* and *Cryptosporidium* from dogs and cats. *Parasite.* 2013;20:8.
150. Kostopoulou D, Claerebout E, Arvanitis D, et al. Abundance, zoonotic potential and risk factors of intestinal parasitism amongst dog and cat populations: the scenario of Crete, Greece. *Parasit Vectors.* 2017;10:43.
151. Ito Y, Itoh N, Iijima Y, et al. Molecular prevalence of *Cryptosporidium* species among household cats and pet shop kittens in Japan. *JFMS Open Rep.* 2017;3:2055116917730719.
152. Alves M, Matos O, Fonseca IP, et al. Multilocus genotyping of *Cryptosporidium* isolates from human HIV-infected and animal hosts. *J Eukaryot Microbiol.* 2001;(suppl):17S–18S.
153. de Lucio A, Bailo B, Aguilera M, et al. No molecular epidemiological evidence supporting household transmission of zoonotic *Giardia duode-*

nalis and *Cryptosporidium* spp. from pet dogs and cats in the province of Alava, Northern Spain. *Acta Trop.* 2017;170:48–56.
154. Koompapong K, Mori H, Thammasonthijarern N, et al. Molecular identification of *Cryptosporidium* spp. in seagulls, pigeons, dogs, and cats in Thailand. *Parasite.* 2014;21:52.
155. Scorza AV, Burnett R, Lappin MR. Genotyping of *Cryptosporidium* spp. isolates from dogs and cats in the United States [abstract]. *Proceedings of the 2nd International Giardia and Cryptosporidium Conference.* 2007.
156. Palmer CS, Traub RJ, Robertson ID, et al. Determining the zoonotic significance of *Giardia* and *Cryptosporidium* in Australian dogs and cats. *Vet Parasitol.* 2008;154:142–147.
157. Lallo MA, Fernandez-Bondan E. Prevalence of *Cryptosporidium* sp. in institutionalized dogs in the city of Sao Paulo. *Rev Saude Publica.* 2006;40:120–125.
158. David ÉB, Guimarães S, de Oliveira AP, et al. Molecular characterization of intestinal protozoa in two poor communities in the state of São Paulo, Brazil. *Parasit Vectors.* 2015;8:103.
159. Uehlinger FD, Greenwood SJ, M.C JT, et al. Zoonotic potential of *Giardia duodenalis* and *Cryptosporidium* spp. and prevalence of intestinal parasites in young dogs from different populations on Prince Edward Island, Canada. *Vet Parasitol.* 2013;196:509–514.
160. Giangaspero A, Iorio R, Paoletti B, et al. Molecular evidence for *Cryptosporidium* infection in dogs in Central Italy. *Parasitol Res.* 2006;99:297–299.
161. Abe N, Sawano Y, Yamada K, et al. *Cryptosporidium* infection in dogs in Osaka, Japan. *Vet Parasitol.* 2002;108:185–193.
162. Abe N, Kimata I, Iseki M. Identification of genotypes of *Cryptosporidium parvum* isolates from a patient and a dog in Japan. *J Vet Med Sci.* 2002;64:165–168.
163. Satoh M, Matsubara-Nihei Y, Sasaki T, et al. Characterization of *Cryptosporidium canis* isolated in Japan. *Parasitol Res.* 2006;99:746–748.
164. Xiao L, Morgan UM, Limor J, et al. Genetic diversity within *Cryptosporidium parvum* and related *Cryptosporidium* species. *Appl Environ Microbiol.* 1999;65:3386–3391.
165. Fontanarrosa MF, Vezzani D, Basabe J, et al. An epidemiological study of gastrointestinal parasites of dogs from Southern Greater Buenos Aires (Argentina): age, gender, breed, mixed infections, and seasonal and spatial patterns. *Vet Parasitol.* 2006;136:283–295.
166. Johnson J, Gasser RB. Copro-parasitological survey of dogs in southern Victoria. *Aust Vet Pract.* 1993;23:127–131.
167. Huber F, Bomfim TCB, Gomes RS. Comparison between natural infections by *Cryptosporidium* sp., *Giardia* sp. in dogs in two living situations in the West Zone of the municipality of Rio de Janeiro. *Vet Parasitol.* 2006;130:69–72.
168. Shukla R, Giraldo P, Kraliz A, et al. *Cryptosporidium* spp. and other zoonotic enteric parasites in a sample of domestic dogs and cats in the Niagara region of Ontario. *Can Vet J.* 2006;47:1179–1184.
169. El-Hohary AH, Abdel-Latif AM. Zoonotic importance of cryptosporidiosis among some animals at Gharbia Province in Egypt. *Indian J Anim Sci.* 1998;68:305–307.
170. Pohjola S. Survey of cryptosporidiosis in feces of normal healthy dogs. *Nord Vet Med.* 1984;36:189–190.
171. Chermette R, Blondel S. Cryptosporidiose des carnivores domestiques, resultants preliminaries in France. *Bull Soc Franc Parasitol.* 1989;7:31–36.
172. Osman M, Bories J, El Safadi D, et al. Prevalence and genetic diversity of the intestinal parasites *Blastocystis* sp. and *Cryptosporidium* spp. in household dogs in France and evaluation of zoonotic transmission risk. *Vet Parasitol.* 2015;30:167–170.
173. Gharekhani J. Study on gastrointestinal zoonotic parasites in pet dogs in Western Iran. *Turkiye Parazitol Derg.* 2014;38:172–176.
174. Yoshiuchi R, Matsubayashi M, Kimata I, et al. Survey and molecular characterization of *Cryptosporidium* and *Giardia* spp. in owned companion animal, dogs and cats, in Japan. *Vet Parasitol.* 2010;174:313–316.
175. Yamamoto N, Kon M, Saito T, et al. Prevalence of intestinal canine and feline parasites in Saitama Prefecture, Japan. *Kansenshogaku Zasshi.* 2009;83:223–228.
176. Kim J, Wee SH, Lee CG. Detection of *Cryptosporidium* oocysts in canine fecal samples by immunofluorescence assay. *Korean J Parasitol.* 1998;36:147–149.
177. Hamnes IS, Gjerde BK, Robertson LJ. A longitudinal study on the occurrence of *Cryptosporidium* and *Giardia* in dogs during their first year of life. *Acta Vet Scand.* 2007;49:22.
178. Simpson JW, Burnie AG, Miles RS, et al. Prevalence of *Giardia* and *Cryptosporidium* infection in dogs in Edinburgh. *Vet Rec.* 1988;123:445.
179. Grimason AM, Smith HV, Parker JFW, et al. Occurrence of *Giardia* sp. cysts and *Cryptosporidium* sp. oocysts in feces from public parks in the west of Scotland. *Epidemiol Infect.* 1993;110:641–645.
180. Causape AC, Quilez J, Sanchez-Acedo C, et al. Prevalence of intestinal parasites, including *Cryptosporidium parvum*, in dogs in Zaragoza city, Spain. *Vet Parasitol.* 1996;67:161–167.
181. Gracenea M, Goméz MS, Torres J. Prevalence of internal parasites in shelter dogs and cats in the metropolitan area of Barcelona (Spain). *Acta Parasitol.* 2009;54:73–77.
182. Tangtrongsup S, Scorza AV, Reif JF, et al. Prevalence and multilocus genotyping analysis of *Cryptosporidium* and *Giardia* isolates from dogs in Chiang Mai, Thailand. *Vet Sci.* 2017;4:26.
183. Overgaauw PA, van Zutphen L, Hoek D, et al. Zoonotic parasites in fecal samples and Fur from dogs and cats in The Netherlands. *Vet Parasitol.* 2009;163:115–122.
184. Batchelor DJ, Tzannes S, Graham PA, et al. Detection of endoparasites with zoonotic potential in dogs with gastrointestinal disease in the UK. *Transbound Emerg Dis.* 2008;55:99–104.
185. Hackett T, Lappin MR. Prevalence of enteric pathogens in dogs of north-central Colorado. *J Am Anim Hosp Assoc.* 2003;39:52–56.
186. El-Ahraf A, Tacal JV, Sobin M, et al. Prevalence of cryptosporidiosis in dogs and human beings in San Bernardino County, California, USA. *J Am Vet Med Assoc.* 1991;198:631–634.
187. Hascall KL, Kass PH, Saksen J, et al. Prevalence of enteropathogens in dogs attending 3 regional dog parks in northern California. *J Vet Intern Med.* 2016;30:1838–1845.
188. Jafri H, Moorhead AR, Reedy T, et al. Detection of pathogenic protozoa in fecal specimens from urban dwelling dogs. *Am J Trop Med Hyg.* 1993;49:269–275.
189. Juett BW, Otero RB, Bishop WH. *Cryptosporidium* in the domestic dog population of central Kentucky. *Trans Ky Acad Sci.* 1996;57:18–21.
190. Scorza AV, Lappin MR. Prevalence of selected zoonotic and vector-borne agents in dogs and cats on the Pine Ridge reservation. *Vet Sci.* 2017;4:43.
191. McGlade TR, Robertson ID, Elliot AD, et al. Gastrointestinal parasites of domestic cats in Perth, Western Australia. *Vet Parasitol.* 2003;117:251–262.
192. Hinney H, Ederer C, Stengl C. Enteric protozoa of cats and their zoonotic potential—a field study from Austria. *Parasitol Res.* 2015;114:2003–2006.
193. Hoopes JH, Polley L, Wagner B, et al. A retrospective investigation of feline gastrointestinal parasites in western Canada. *Can Vet J.* 2013;54:359–362.
194. Ahmed ZK, Abbas AK. Prevalence of *Cryptosporidium* in domestic and stray cats in Baghdad, Iraq. *Onl J Vet Res.* 2018;22:715–720.
195. Nash AS, Mtambo MMA, Gibbs HA. *Cryptosporidium* infection in farm cats in the Glasgow area. *Vet Rec.* 1993;133:576–577.
196. Mtambo MMA, Nash AS, Blewett DA, et al. *Cryptosporidium* infection in cats: prevalence of infection in domestic and feral cats in the Glasgow area. *Vet Rec.* 1991;129:502–504.
197. Scorza V, Willmott A, Gunn-Moore D, et al. *Cryptosporidium felis* in faeces from cats in the UK. *Vet Rec.* 2014;174:609.
198. Nutter FB, Dubey JP, Levine JF, et al. Seroprevalence of antibodies against *Bartonella henselae* and *Toxoplasma gondii* and fecal shedding of *Cryptosporidium* spp., *Giardia* spp., and *Toxocara cati* in feral and pet domestic cats. *J Am Vet Med Assoc.* 2004;225:1394–1398.

Cystoisosporiasis and Other Enteric Coccidioses

Michael R. Lappin, Jitender P. Dubey

KEY POINTS

- First Described: Coccidian parasites were first described in dogs and cats in the 1800s; the organisms were placed in the genus *Isospora* spp. in 1906.[1] Once it was discovered that the parasites have an extraintestinal phase, the genus was transferred to *Cystoisospora*.
- Cause: *Cystoisospora* spp., protozoan coccidian parasites (phylum Apicomplexa).
- Mode of Transmission: Fecal-oral; ingestion of intermediate/paratenic hosts.
- Affected Host Species: Dogs and cats are the definitive host of different *Cystoisospora* spp. The sexual phase of the organism is completed in the small intestine, which culminates in the passage of oocysts in feces.
- Intermediate Hosts: Most vertebrates can serve as intermediate/paratenic hosts (whereby the parasite encysts but does not multiply); invertebrates can serve as transport hosts by carrying *Cystoisospora* spp. oocysts.
- Geographic Distribution: Worldwide.
- Major Clinical Signs: Most dogs and cats harbor subclinical infections. Watery diarrhea that can contain blood occasionally occurs in puppies and kittens.
- Differential Diagnoses: These include other protozoal infections (e.g., *Giardia, Tritrichomonas blagburni*), enteropathogenic bacterial infections (e.g., *Clostridium perfringens, Campylobacter* spp.), and nematode infestations.
- Human Health Significance: *Cystoisospora* spp. of dogs and cats do not infect humans.

CYSTOISOSPORIASIS

ETIOLOGIC AGENT AND EPIDEMIOLOGY

Cystoisospora spp. are protozoan coccidian parasites that have been recognized for years as potential pathogens in dogs and cats.[2-5] The sexual phase of reproduction occurs in the intestines of dogs and cats and culminates in the passage of oocysts in feces (Table 104.1). Cats are the definitive hosts for *Cystoisospora felis* and *Cystoisospora rivolta*. *Cystoisospora canis, Cystoisospora ohioensis, Cystoisospora neorivolta*, and *Cystoisospora burrowsi* are described in dogs.[2] There is some overlap in the size of oocysts among *C. ohioensis, C. neorivolta*, and *C. burrowsi*. While *C. ohioensis* is distinct from the other species based on the location of intestinal endogenous stages, *C. neorivolta* and *C. burrowsi* currently cannot be distinguished and so it is proposed that these agents be referred to as *C. ohioensis*-like organisms.[6]

Cystoisospora spp. are host specific and have worldwide distribution.[4] Infections are very common, particularly in young animals. In the United States, the Companion Animal Parasite Council reports that prevalence rates for *Cystoisospora* spp. infection in dogs and cats vary from 3% to more than 30%.[7] In a study of more than one million fecal specimens from dogs in the United States, 4.4% contained *Cystoisospora* spp. oocysts.[8] Another study of 2586 fecal specimens from cats submitted to the veterinary parasitology laboratory at Oklahoma State University over a 12-year period noted that "*Cystoisospora* spp. oocysts was the most common parasite stage (9.4%)[9]; in fecal specimens from dogs it was the second most common parasite stage (5%) after *Ancylostoma* eggs (8.2%)."[10] In a study of 1355 cats in the United Kingdom, *C. felis* oocysts were detected in 3%.[11] Gender and breed do not usually influence *Cystoisospora* spp. excretion rates, but young animals are usually more likely to be excreting oocysts than adults. For example, in one Austrian study, 8.7% of dogs less than 2 years of age were infected; 78% of the positive specimens were in puppies less than 4 months of age.[12] In the study from the United Kingdom, *C. felis* was found in the feces of 9% of cats less than 6 months of age.[11]

CLINICAL FEATURES

Pathogenesis and Clinical Signs

Infection by *Cystoisospora* spp. in dogs or cats is initiated by ingestion of sporulated oocysts in the environment or by ingestion of tissues of other infected vertebrate or transport hosts (Fig. 104.1).[12,13] Infection can also occur if the dog or cat ingests sporulated oocysts carried mechanically by flies, cockroaches, or dung beetles.[14] The enteroepithelial phase occurs in the small intestine of infected animals and culminates in the passage of unsporulated oocysts in feces. The prepatent period (time between infection and appearance of oocysts in the feces) and patent period (time that the organism can be detected in the body) vary slightly by the species. In one study of dogs experimentally infected with *C. canis*, the mean prepatent period was 9.8 days (range, 9 to 11 days, n = 22 dogs), the patent period was 8.9 days (range, 7 to 18 days, n = 20 dogs), and all of the puppies developed diarrhea.[13] In contrast, the prepatent period for *C. ohioensis* in one study was 6 to 7 days, and diarrhea was variable.[12] The number of oocysts excreted by infected animals can vary dramatically.[12,13] Depending on the environmental conditions, sporulation can occur in as little as 12 hours.

Cystoisospora can invade extraintestinal tissues of cats, dogs, and other animals and can encyst (at a stage known as the *tissue cyst*) but does not multiply in this location or cause tissue damage. However, dogs or cats can become infected by eating tissues of these infected animals (*paratenic hosts*). In addition, invertebrates (such as cockroaches) can mechanically transport oocysts in the environment.

Clinical disease is most common in young, debilitated, and immunocompromised animals. All the different *Cystoisospora* spp. replicate in the small intestine, but the regions with the heaviest infection vary by species. The presence of co-infections may increase potential for clinical illness associated with *Cystoisospora* spp.[15] Fecal microbiome differences were detected between cats with and without *Cystoisospora* spp. oocysts in feces; whether this finding is associated with development of clinical disease will need to be assessed further.[16]

TABLE 104.1 *Cystoisospora* spp. Oocyst Characteristics After Detection by Centrifugal Fecal Flotation

	Oocyst Dimensions
Cats	
Cystoisospora felis	30 × 40 μm
Cystoisospora rivolta	20 × 25 μm
Dogs	
Cystoisospora canis	30 × 38 μm
Cystoisospora ohioensis and *C. ohioensis*-like	19 × 23 μm

Cystoisospora spp. infections are generally only associated with disease in puppies and kittens. However, adult animals treated with immune-suppressive drugs may also have activated cystoisosporiasis and resultant disease.[17] Clinically ill puppies and kittens can show signs of vomiting, abdominal discomfort, inappetence, and watery diarrhea that sometimes contains blood. Depending on the age of the animal and the parasite burden, severe dehydration and death can occur. Puppies and kittens with subclinical infection can repeat shedding and clinical signs of disease during periods of stress.

DIAGNOSIS

When illness from cystoisosporiasis occurs, diarrhea is most common and so proving the presence of the agent in feces is the most important part of the diagnostic plan. However, because *Cystoisospora* spp. can be

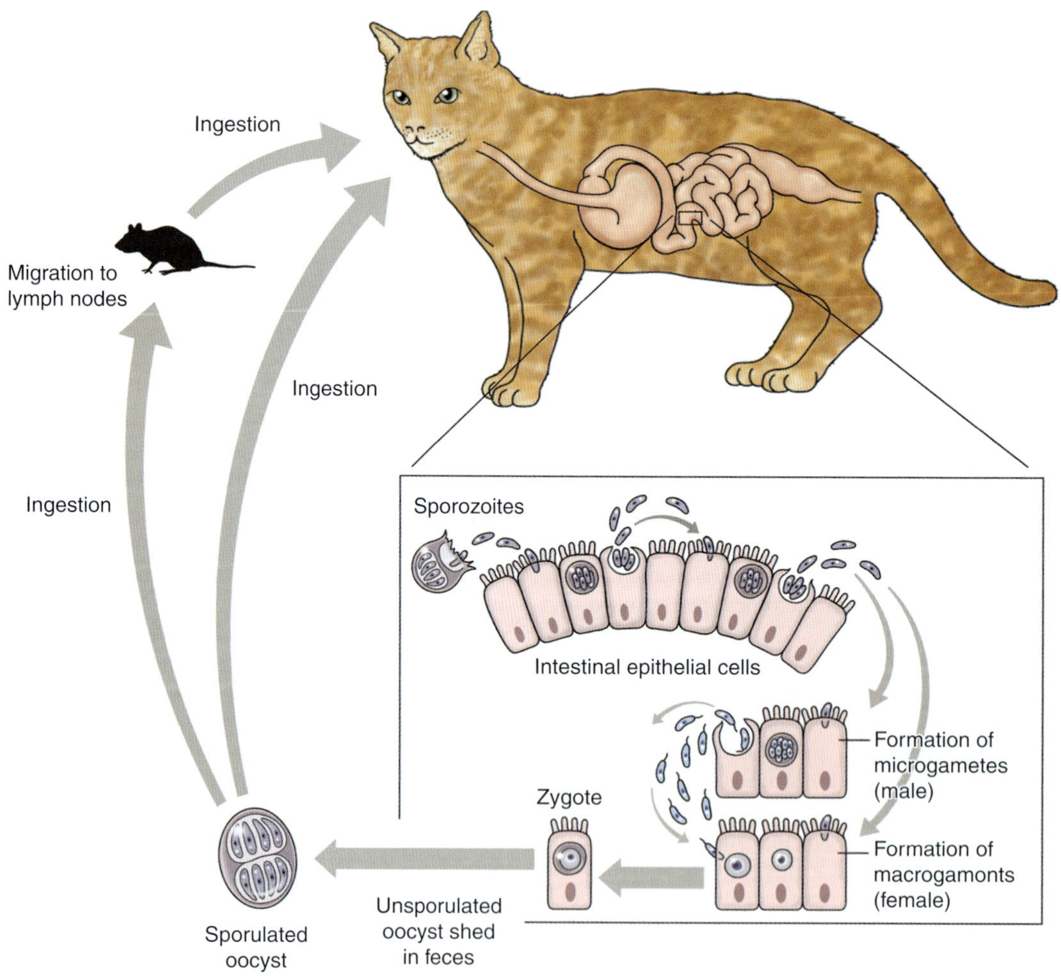

Fig. 104.1 Life cycle of *Cystoisospora* spp. The host species (in this case, cats) can be infected by ingestion of sporulated oocysts or ingestion of prey that have organisms encysted in their mesenteric lymph nodes. Oocysts shed in the feces can sporulate in as little as 12 hours under optimal environmental conditions.

detected in the feces of normal animals, a positive test result does not prove the agent is the cause of the clinical abnormalities.

Laboratory Abnormalities

Cystoisospora spp. infections only rarely lead to systemic laboratory abnormalities. In theory, regenerative anemia could develop from blood loss in puppies or kittens with heavy parasite loads. Other CBC abnormalities are uncommon. Decreases in serum total protein, albumin, and globulin concentrations can occur concurrently with blood loss. If diarrhea is severe, potassium, sodium, and chloride concentrations may decrease as a result of GI losses.

Diagnostic Imaging

Abdominal radiographic abnormalities in puppies and kittens with cystoisosporiasis are uncommon and nonspecific and, when present, are suggestive of diffuse enteritis.

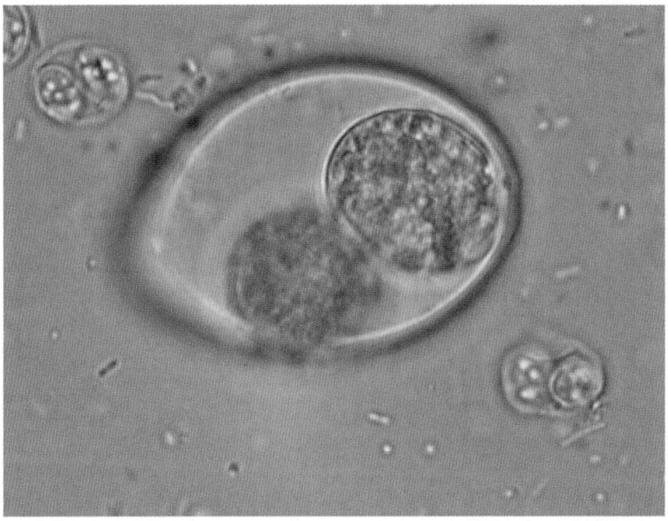

Fig. 104.2 Oocysts of *Cystoisospora felis* from a kitten with diarrhea (1000× magnification). (From Lappin MR. Update on the diagnosis and management of *Cystoisospora* spp. infections in dogs and cats. *Top Companion Anim Med.* 2010;25:133-135.)

Microbiologic Testing

The definitive diagnosis of coccidiosis can be made by demonstrating oocysts in fecal specimens from affected animals. *Cystoisospora* spp. oocysts are large and often numerous and so are generally easy to identify on microscopic examination of feces after centrifugal fecal flotation (Fig. 104.2). However, as discussed, animals with normal stool can pass *Cystoisospora* spp. oocysts, and so positive test results do not prove a disease association. False-negative fecal flotation results are uncommon in clinically infected animals, but occasionally clinical signs precede oocyst shedding, and so a second fecal flotation may be needed to prove infection in some cases.

Molecular diagnostic assays can be used to amplify the DNA of *Cystoisospora* spp. in feces. The detection of parasite DNA in feces will be used more in the future as a diagnostic test for cystoisosporiasis.[18-20] However, careful assay design is important in order to ensure that the DNA of related organisms is not amplified[20]; laboratories should be able to provide evidence that the assay is specific for detection of *Cystoisospora* spp. DNA. In one small study of experimentally inoculated kittens, fecal PCR results were positive in several specimens that were negative for oocysts after fecal flotation.[21]

Pathologic Findings

Clinically affected puppies and kittens may be emaciated. Other parasites such as roundworms or hookworms may be noted. The small intestines of clinically ill puppies and kittens may be hyperemic, edematous, or thickened. Microscopic lesions observed in some infected animals include villous atrophy, sloughing of villi in the intestinal lumen, dilation of lacteals, and hyperplasia of lymph nodes in Peyer's patches.

TREATMENT AND PROGNOSIS

Coccidiosis is generally self-limited, and clinical signs in most puppies and kittens resolve without therapy. However, treatment can hasten resolution of clinical disease and may lessen environmental contamination and the potential for infecting other, in-contact animals, particularly if the coccidiocidal drugs (see Chapter 12) ponazuril or toltrazuril are used (Table 104.2).[22-25]

In the United States, ponazuril is licensed for the treatment of *Sarcocytis neurona* infection in horses and has been used most frequently in this country for the treatment of canine or feline

TABLE 104.2 Drugs Used for the Treatment of *Cystoisospora* spp. Infections[a]

Drug	Species	Dose	Route	Interval and Duration
Amprolium	C D	60–100 mg total 300–400 mg total	PO	q24h for 5 days
Furazolidone	C, D	8–20 mg/kg	PO	q12-24h for 5 days
Ponazuril	C, D	50 mg/kg	PO	q24h for 3 days
Toltrazuril[b]	C, D	9 mg/kg	PO	Once
Sulfadimethoxine	C, D	50–60 mg/kg	PO	q24h for 5 to 20 days
Trimethoprim sulfonamide	C, D	15–30 mg/kg	PO	q12–24h for 5 days
Amprolium-sulfadimethoxine	D	150 mg amprolium and 25 mg/kg sulfadimethoxine	PO	q24h for 14 days

[a]Sulfadimethoxine is the only approved drug for the treatment of coccidiosis in the United States. Sulfonamides or trimethoprim-sulfonamide combinations can cause macrocytic anemia, keratoconjunctivitis sicca, type III hypersensitivity reactions (primarily Doberman pinschers), and acute hepatic necrosis. See also Chapter 10.

[b]In Europe, toltrazuril has been available in combination with emodepside (Procox Oral Suspension for Dogs, Bayer Animal Health) for treatment of cystoisosporiasis and roundworm infections in puppies over 2 weeks of age. The suspension contains 18 mg/mL of toltrazuril.

C, cats; *D,* dogs.

cystoisosporiasis. Several treatment protocols have been recommended over the years. In one study, the optimal protocol was to administer 50 mg/kg, PO, daily for 3 days.[23] In Europe, toltrazuril has been available in combination with the anthelmintic emodepside (Procox Oral Suspension for Dogs, Bayer Animal Health) for treatment of cystoisosporiasis and roundworm infections in puppies over 2 weeks of age (see Chapter 12 for additional information). The only approved treatment for coccidiosis in the United States is sulfadimethoxine. Other drug regimens have been used with some success, and these include trimethoprim-sulfa (30 to 60 mg/kg of trimethoprim daily for 6 days in animals >4 kg; or 15 to 30 mg/kg trimethoprim daily for 6 days in animals <4 kg) and a variety of protocols using amprolium alone or in combination with sulfadimethoxine. Amprolium can cause anorexia, diarrhea, lethargy, and CNS disease due to induction of thiamine deficiency. However, these other drugs have only static effects and so are inferior to ponazuril or toltrazuril.

Use of prebiotics (food ingredients that stimulate the growth or activity of beneficial bacteria), or probiotics and/or dietary manipulation may speed up resolution of diarrhea, but controlled data are lacking.[16]

Most *Cystoisospora* spp.–infected dogs and cats survive infection, and so the prognosis is considered good to excellent.

IMMUNITY AND VACCINATION

Dogs previously infected with *C. canis* and challenged with *C. canis* did not show any signs of illness.[26] In contrast, dogs previously infected with *C. ohioensis* excreted *C. canis* oocysts and some developed diarrhea. These results suggested some immunity to repeat infection by the homologous species. However, the duration of immunity is likely not permanent because repeated excretion, clinical signs, and infection can occur. While *Cystoisospora* spp. infestation can be prolonged, immune responses usually block the development of clinical disease as puppies and kittens grow older. Vaccines for *Cystoisospora* spp. that infect dogs and cats are not currently available.

PREVENTION

Cystoisospora spp. oocysts are resistant to environmental conditions and disinfectants. The key to control is to provide good sanitation, including prompt removal of feces before oocyst sporulation. Steam cleaning can be used to destroy oocysts that contaminate surfaces, provided the water is hot enough (> 70°C) when it reaches contaminated surfaces. Treatment of dams and queens with anticoccidials before parturition can lessen the occurrence of coccidiosis in young animals. In environments with heavy infections, treatment of all in-contact animals, particularly puppies and kittens, could be considered. Ponazuril administered to all at-risk puppies and kittens on intake to shelters may aid in the control of coccidiosis.

PUBLIC HEALTH ASPECTS

Cystoisospora spp. of dogs and cats do not infect people. However, some infected animals are co-infected with other parasites with potential for zoonotic transfer to people, such as *Cryptosporidium* spp. and *Giardia* spp. Thus, a complete diagnostic workup should be completed for animals with diarrhea.

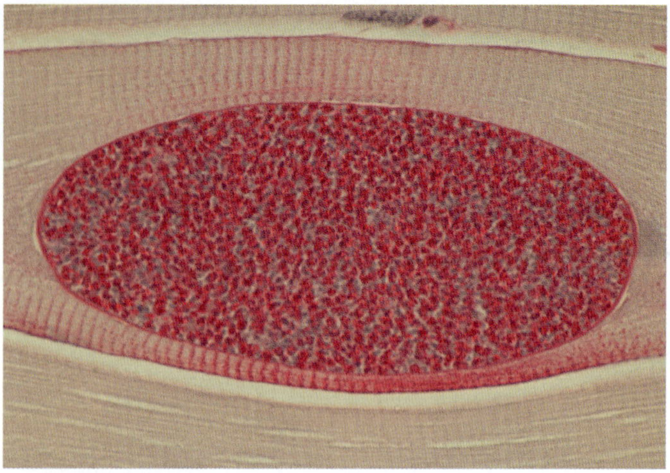

Fig. 104.3 *Hammondia hammondii* tissue cyst in skeletal muscle of a mouse. Note the thin cyst wall enclosing hundreds of PAS-positive bradyzoites (PAS stain, ×750).

OTHER ENTERIC COCCIDIOSES

Other enteric coccidia that infect the intestines of dogs and cats include *Hammondia*, *Besnoitia*, a variety of intestinal *Sarcocystis* species (see Chapter 95), *Toxoplasma gondii* (see Chapter 93), and *Neospora caninum* (see Chapter 94).

Hammondia species, unlike *Isospora* species, have obligatory two-host life cycles. Domestic cats and the European wildcat (*Felis sylvestris*) are the definitive hosts of *H. hammondii*; goats and rodents are natural intermediate hosts, but a number of other warm-blooded animals have been infected as intermediate hosts experimentally. *Hammondia hammondii* does not invade extraintestinal tissues of the cat, and cats are infected only by eating tissue cysts. Intermediate hosts become infected when they ingest sporulated oocysts, which resemble those of *T. gondii*. Sporozoites excyst in the intestinal lumen, invade the intestinal wall, and multiply as tachyzoites in the intestines, mesenteric lymph nodes, and other tissues. The parasite then encysts principally in muscles (Fig. 104.3).

The life cycle of *Hammondia heydorni* is not fully known but appears similar to that of *H. hammondii*. Dogs and other canids are definitive hosts; cattle, sheep, goats, deer, and a variety of other herbivores are intermediate hosts. In dogs, the oocyst of *H. heydorni* resembles that of *N. caninum* (Fig. 104.4).

Hammondia spp. are largely thought to be nonpathogenic in dogs and cats. However, there have been some reports that have suggested an association between *H. heydorni* infection in dogs and diarrhea (see also Fig. 104.4).[27-29] In addition, *H. heydorni* or a closely related *Hammondia* species was associated with cholangiohepatitis in an 11-year-old Jack Russell terrier mix from a horse farm in Wisconsin, USA.[30] Another dog with intrahepatic biliary coccidiosis was also reported from the United States, although the organism could not be identified to the species level.[31]

Cats are the definitive host for several *Besnoitia* species, including *Besnoitia darlingi* (intermediate hosts: opossums and possibly lizards), *Besnoitia wallacei* (rodents), *Besnoitia oryctofelisi* (rabbits), and *Besnoitia neotomofelis* (woodrats). The life cycle is similar to *T. gondii*; schizonts may be found not only in intestinal tissues but also in extraintestinal organs. The oocysts are difficult to distinguish from those of *T. gondii*. *Besnoitia* spp. infections are considered nonpathogenic in cats.

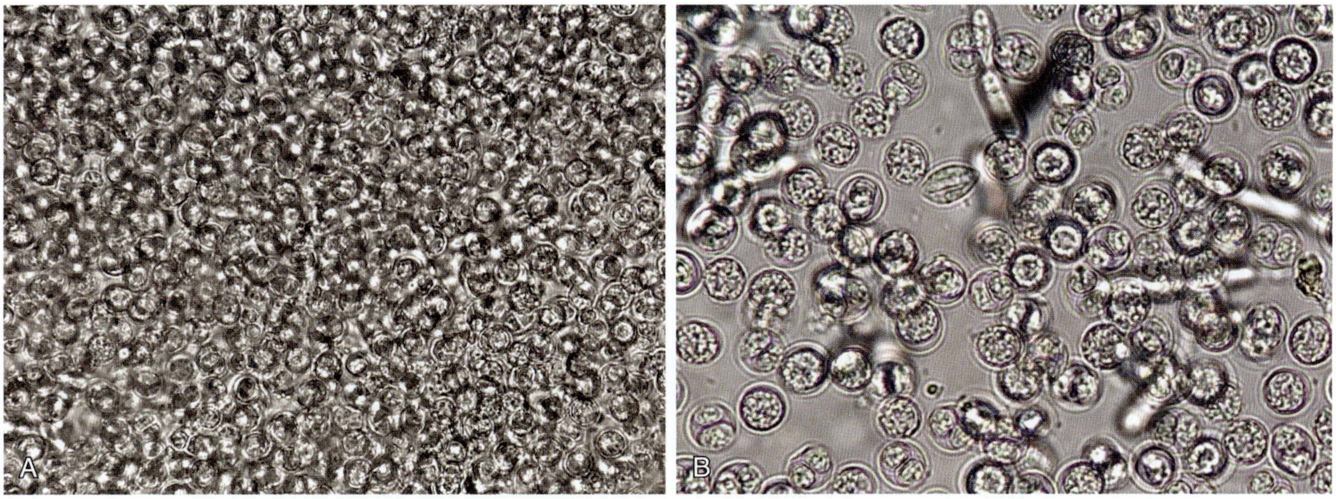

Fig. 104.4 Massive numbers of both sporulated and unsporulated *Hammondii heydorni* oocysts in a fecal flotation from a 7-year-old Great Dane with acute vomiting, diarrhea, and weight loss. The oocysts were initially thought to be *Neospora caninum*, but were later identified as *H. heydorni* using molecular methods. (Courtesy Dr. Lauren Camp, Veterinary Parasitology Service, University of California, Davis.)

CASE EXAMPLE

Signalment

"No-name," an 8-week-old, intact male, domestic shorthair cat from a pet store in Fort Collins, CO.

History

No-name was housed in a pet store. The kitten appeared small for his age and weighed 25% less than the littermates also housed at the pet store. Although he was eating well, he was thin. Small bowel diarrhea was the other historical complaint, and stool character varied from soft to watery with occasional flecks of what appeared to be fresh blood but no mucus. The source of the kitten was not disclosed. His first vaccine (an attenuated live vaccine for prevention of FHV-1, FCV, and FPV infections) had been administered subcutaneously 2 weeks previously. He had been fed a commercial processed food followed by a bland diet with no improvement noted in body weight or diarrhea. The other littermates were normal according to the pet store owner. The kitten was administered pyrantel pamoate once on entry to the pet store; no other treatments had been administered.

Physical Examination

Quiet, alert, and responsive. Ambulatory on all four limbs. Body weight was 1.1 kg and body condition score was 3/9. T = 101.3°F (38.5°C), HR = 180 beats/min, RR = 24 breaths/min, mucous membranes pink, CRT = 1 s. The cat's haircoat was dull but there was no evidence of ectoparasites. Abdominal palpation revealed mild diffuse thickening of the small intestinal loops. No other significant abnormalities were detected.

Results of Microbiologic Testing

FeLV antigen ELISA assay: Negative.

FIV antibody ELISA assay: Negative.

Fecal wet mount examination: No motile flagellates were noted.

Fecal flotation: Oocysts that were morphologically consistent with *C. felis* were noted.

Diagnosis

Cystoisospora felis infection.

Treatment

Ponazuril at 20 mg/kg PO q24h for 2 days; the littermates were treated as well. A commercially available intestinal diet was administered until the stool normalized 5 days later.

Comments

The findings were characteristic of *Cystoisospora* spp. infection. Although the littermates were clinically normal, ponazuril was administered to try to lessen oocysts shedding into the pet store environment and lessen the potential for reinfection.

SUGGESTED READINGS

Dubey JP, Lindsay DS. Coccidiosis in dogs-100 years of progress. *Vet Parasitol.* 2019;266:34–55.

Dubey JP, ed. *Coccidiosis in Livestock, Poultry, Companion Animals, and Humans.* Boca Raton, London, New York: CRC Press, Taylor and Frances; 2020:381.

Irvine KL, Walker JM, Friedrichs KR. Sarcocystid organisms found in bile from a dog with acute hepatitis: a case report and review of intestinal and hepatobiliary Sarcocystidae infections in dogs and cats. *Vet Clin Pathol.* 2016;45:57–65.

REFERENCES

1. Lühe M. *Die im Blute schmarotzenden Protozoen und ihre nächsten Verwandten.* Leipzig, Germany: Verlag; 1906.
2. Dubey JP. The evolution of the knowledge of cat and dog coccidia. *Parasitology.* 2009;136:1469–1475.
3. Dubey JP. A review of *Cystoisospora felis* and *C. rivolta*-induced coccidiosis in cats. *Vet Parasitol.* 2018;263:34–48.
4. Dubey JP, Lindsay DS. Coccidiosis in dogs: 100 years of progress. *Vet Parasitol.* 2019;266:34–55.

5. Lappin MR. Update on the diagnosis and management of *Cystoisospora* spp. infections in dogs and cats. *Top Companion Anim Med.* 2010;25:133–135.
6. Dubey JP. Re-evaluation of merogony of a *Cystoisospora ohioensis*-like coccidian and its distinction from gametogony in the intestine of a naturally infected dog. *Parasitology*. 2019;146:740–745.
7. Companion Animal Parasite Council. http://www.capcvet.org.
8. Little SE, Johnson EM, Lewis D, et al. Prevalence of intestinal parasites in pet dogs in the United States. *Vet Parasitol.* 2009;166:144–152.
9. Nagamori Y, Payton ME, Looper E, et al. Retrospective survey of parasitism identified in feces of client-owned cats in North America from 2007 through 2018. *Vet Parasitol.* 2020;277:109008.
10. Nagamori Y, Payton ME, Looper E, et al. Retrospective survey of endoparasitism identified in feces of client-owned dogs in North America from 2007 through 2018. *Vet Parasitol.* 2020;282:109137.
11. Tzannes S, Batchelor DJ, Graham PA, et al. Prevalence of *Cryptosporidium, Giardia* and *Isospora* species infections in pet cats with clinical signs of gastrointestinal disease. *J Feline Med Surg.* 2008;10:1–8.
12. Buehl IE, Prosl H, Mundt HC, et al. Canine isosporosis - epidemiology of field and experimental infections. *J Vet Med B Infect Dis Vet Public Health.* 2006;53:482–487.
13. Mitchell SM, Zajac AM, Charles S, et al. *Cystoisospora canis* Nemeseri, 1959 (syn. *Isospora canis*), infections in dogs: clinical signs, pathogenesis, and reproducible clinical disease in beagle dogs fed oocysts. *J Parasitol.* 2007;93:345–352.
14. Saitoh Y, Itagaki H. Dung beetles, *Onthophagus* spp., as potential transport hosts of feline coccidia. *Nihon Juigaku Zasshi.* 1990;52:293–297.
15. Duijvestijn M, Mughini-Gras L, Schuurman N, et al. Enteropathogen infections in canine puppies: (co-)occurrence, clinical relevance and risk factors. *Vet Microbiol.* 2016;195:115–122.
16. Slapeta J, Dowd SE, Alanazi AD, et al. Differences in the faecal microbiome of non-diarrhoeic clinically healthy dogs and cats associated with *Giardia duodenalis* infection: impact of hookworms and coccidia. *Int J Parasitol.* 2015;45:585–594.
17. Cervone M, Gavazza A, Zbriger A, et al. Intestinal parasite infections in dogs affected by multicentric lymphoma and undergoing chemotherapy. *Comp Immunol Microbiol Infect Dis.* 2019;63:81–86.
18. Cama VA, Mathison BA. Infections by intestinal coccidia and *Giardia duodenalis. Clin Lab Med.* 2015;35:423–444.
19. He P, Li J, Gong P, et al. *Cystoisospora* spp. from dogs in China and phylogenetic analysis of its 18S and ITS1 gene. *Vet Parasitol.* 2012;190:254–258.
20. Lee S, Kim J, Cheon DS, et al. Identification of *Cystoisospora ohioensis* in a diarrheal dog in Korea. *Korean J Parasitol.* 2018;56:371–374.
21. Scorza AV, Tyrrell P, Wennogle S, et al. Experimental infection of cats with *Cystoisospora felis. J Vet Intern Med.* 2021;35:269–272.
22. Daugschies A, Mundt HC, Letkova V. Toltrazuril treatment of cystoisosporosis in dogs under experimental and field conditions. *Parasitol Res.* 2000;86:797–799.
23. Litster AL, Nichols J, Hall K, et al. Use of ponazuril paste to treat coccidiosis in shelter-housed cats and dogs. *Vet Parasitol.* 2014;202:319–325.
24. Lloyd S, Smith J. Activity of toltrazuril and diclazuril against *Isospora* species in kittens and puppies. *Vet Rec.* 2001;148:509–511.
25. Petry G, Kruedewagen E, Kampkoetter A, et al. Efficacy of emodepside/toltrazuril suspension (Procox® oral suspension for dogs) against mixed experimental *Isospora felis/Isospora rivolta* infection in cats. *Parasitol Res.* 2011;109(suppl 1):S29–S36.
26. Houk AE, O'Connor T, Pena HF, et al. Experimentally induced clinical *Cystoisospora canis* coccidiosis in dogs with prior natural patent *Cystoisospora ohioensis*-like or *C. canis* infections. *J Parasitol.* 2013;99:892–895.
27. Abel J, Schares G, Orzeszko K, et al. *Hammondia* isolated from dogs and foxes are genetically distinct. *Parasitology*. 2006;132:187–192.
28. Schares G, Pantchev N, Barutzki D, et al. Oocysts of *Neospora caninum, Hammondia heydorni, Toxoplasma gondii* and *Hammondia hammondi* in faeces collected from dogs in Germany. *Int J Parasitol.* 2005;35:1525–1537.
29. Steffl M, Nautscher N. Detection of *Hammondia heydorni*-like oocysts in feces of a dog with recurrent diarrhea. *Tierarztl Prax Ausg K Kleintiere Heimtiere.* 2019;47:189–192.
30. Irvine KL, Walker JM, Friedrichs KR. Sarcocystid organisms found in bile from a dog with acute hepatitis: a case report and review of intestinal and hepatobiliary Sarcocystidae infections in dogs and cats. *Vet Clin Pathol.* 2016;45:57–65.
31. Lipscomb TP, Dubey JP, Pletcher JM, et al. Intrahepatic biliary coccidiosis in a dog. *Vet Pathol.* 1989;26:343–345.

105

Emerging and Miscellaneous Protozoal Diseases

Mary Marcondes, Marc Kent, Elizabeth W. Howerth, Jane E. Sykes

KEY POINTS

Rangeliosis

- Cause: *Rangelia vitalii*, a protozoan parasite of the phylum Apicomplexa, class Aconoidasida, order Piroplasmida; phylogenetically close to the family Babesiidae.
- First Described: 1908, in dogs from Brazil (Carini, 1908).[1]
- Affected Hosts: Domestic dogs and wild canids (the crab-eating fox *Cerdocyon thous*, and the pampas fox *Lycalopex gymnocercus*).
- Geographic Distribution: South America, especially in the south and south-east of Brazil, Argentina, and Uruguay.
- Mode of Transmission: *Amblyomma aureolatum* ticks.
- Major Clinical Signs: Lethargy, inappetence, weakness, weight loss, fever, pallor, jaundice, splenomegaly, lymphadenomegaly, pelvic limb edema, and hemorrhagic disorders including persistent hemorrhage from the tips and external surface of the pinnae, nose (epistaxis), oral cavity (including hematemesis), venipuncture sites, and GI tract (hemorrhagic diarrhea).
- Differential Diagnosis: Other tick-borne diseases (e.g., canine babesiosis and canine monocytic ehrlichiosis), leptospirosis, leishmaniosis, immune-mediated disorders.
- Human Health Significance: There is no evidence that *R. vitalii* can infect humans.

Amebiasis and Balantidiasis

- Cause: Nonenteric (free-living) amebiasis in dogs is caused by organisms belonging to the genera *Acanthamoeba* and *Balamuthia.* Amebic keratitis caused by *Acanthamoeba* spp. has rarely been reported in companion animals. GI amebiasis in dogs is rare and caused by *Entamoeba histolytica.* Balantidiasis is also rare and caused by *Balantioides coli* (formerly *Balantidium coli*)
- Affected Hosts: Domestic dogs.
- Geographic Distribution: Worldwide.
- Mode of Transmission: Unclear, but inhalation (systemic disease) or ingestion (systemic or GI disease) from environmental sources are suspected.
- Major Clinical Signs: The major clinical signs of canine systemic amebiasis are lethargy, inappetence, weakness, weight loss, fever, and a variety of neurologic signs. Rare cases of localized amebic keratitis have been described in dogs with chronic keratoconjunctivitis sicca treated with topical immunosuppressive drugs. GI amebiasis may be characterized by signs of large bowel diarrhea and inappetence.
- Differential Diagnosis: Systemic amebiasis must be differentiated from other viral, bacterial, protozoal, and fungal pathogens that cause chronic progressive CNS signs; and noninfectious diseases of the CNS (see Chapter 129). Differential diagnoses for amebic keratitis include squamous cell carcinoma, leishmaniosis, and toxoplasmosis. GI amebiasis and balantidiasis must be differentiated from other subacute and chronic infectious and inflammatory causes of large bowel diarrhea.
- Human Health Significance: GI ameba and *Balantioides* can cause mild to severe diarrhea in humans, and systemic ameba can cause life-threatening disease. However, there is no strong evidence for a role of companion animals in zoonotic transmission.

RANGELIOSIS

Mary Marcondes

ETIOLOGIC AGENT AND EPIDEMIOLOGY

Rangeliosis is a severe tick-borne hemorrhagic disease of dogs caused by *Rangelia vitalii,* a protozoan parasite of the phylum Apicomplexa, class Aconoidasida, order Piroplasmida; phylogenetically close to the family Babesiidae.[2,3] *Rangelia vitalii* infection has been reported only in domestic and wild canids.[4-14] The taxonomy of *R. vitalii* is not completely understood.[15] Molecular phylogenetic analyses of *R. vitalii,* based on fragments of the 18S rRNA and heat shock protein 70 (*hsp70*) genes, demonstrated that *R. vitalii* forms a new branch of piroplasms, which is located in the *Babesia* spp. *sensu stricto* clade.[2,3,16] Analysis of 18S rRNA gene sequences shared the highest degree of sequence identity (95%) with *Babesia* spp., and 92% to 94% sequence identity with *Babesia canis* and *Babesia gibsoni,* while DNA sequences of the *hsp70* gene shared the highest degree of sequence identity (87%) with *Babesia bigemina* and only 82% to 86% sequence identity with *B. canis* and *B. gibsoni.*[3] However, further analysis is needed for a clearly defined phylogenetic classification of *R. vitalii.*[3,17] What is known about life cycle and host cell tropisms of *R. vitalii* also differ from those of organisms in the *Babesia* spp. *sensu stricto* clade.

The first reference in the literature to rangeliosis in dogs was by Antônio Carini in 1908.[1] Two years later, in 1910, the Brazilian protozoologist Bruno Rangel Pestana published two articles describing a disease that affected dogs in several parts of the country that was known as "nambiuvú," (which means "bleeding ears" in the indigenous language Tupi-Guarani), "bleeding plague," or "yellow fever of dogs."[18,19] According to Pestana, the disease was possibly caused by a novel piroplasm, which he named *Piroplasma vitalii* in honor of the Brazilian scientist Vital Brazil.[19] Despite the similarities with other piroplasms, namely *Piroplasma canis* (a former synonym of *Babesia canis*), its status as a new species relied on its additional intracellular presence within endothelial cells, which has never been reported for any other canine piroplasm. In 1914, Carini and Maciel studied this same disease and reached similar conclusions to those described by Rangel. The authors stated that a tick was probably the source of the infection and, as a tribute to Rangel Pestana, proposed that a new genus of protozoan was created, designated *Rangelia*. From that time, the etiologic agent became known as *Rangelia vitalii* and the disease was called rangeliosis.[20]

Over the years, clinical signs of rangeliosis characterized by ear margin bleeding, epistaxis, anemia, jaundice, and a history of tick exposure were erroneously associated with numerous diseases, including visceral leishmaniosis, babesiosis, ehrlichiosis, hepatozoonosis, and toxoplasmosis,[5,21] or were described using various names throughout Brazil.[22,23] Veterinarians did not consider *R. vitalii* in their differential diagnosis as most were unfamiliar with this pathogen, and almost no information about it was published between 1948[24] and 2003,[23] after which more studies and clinical cases were reported.[4,6,17,25-27] Canine rangeliosis is now recognized as a reemerging disease in Brazil.[22]

At the time of writing, canine rangeliosis has been reported only in dogs from South America, especially in the south and south-east of Brazil,[2,4,6,7,17,22,23] Argentina,[16,28] Uruguay,[29] and Paraguay.[30] Among the three piroplasmids recognized to infect dogs in South America (*Babesia vogeli, B. gibsoni,* and *R. vitalii*), *R. vitalii* is the only one that has not been found outside South America.[12] In the southern part of Brazil the disease has been identified not only in rural areas, but also in the outskirts of cities, where dogs have direct access to forest and mountain areas, and where tick species that infest dogs are present.[5]

Although *Amblyomma aureolatum* (commonly known as the yellow dog tick) and *Rhipicephalus sanguineus* (brown dog tick) are the ixodid ticks that have been found on dogs infected with *R. vitalii*,[3,5,22] vector competence for *R. vitalii* has only been confirmed for *A. aureolatum*, which transstadially transmits the agent from nymph to adult.[31,32] *Rangelia vitalii* DNA has also been detected in *Amblyomma sculptum* ticks that were found on crab-eating foxes (*Cerdocyon thous*) in endemic areas.[33] The distribution of *A. aureolatum* includes southeastern and southern Brazil, northeastern Argentina, and Uruguay; this reflects the distribution of rangeliosis (Fig. 105.1).[29,34] In an experimental study of dogs exposed to infected ticks, clinical signs appeared after the engorged females had dropped off the dogs, around 14 to 19 days post infestation. Since the period of engorgement of *A. aureolatum* ranges from 9 to 15 days, female ticks found on dogs with signs of rangeliosis are not necessarily those that transmitted the agent to the dog. This explains the fact that some dogs have no ticks at the time they develop clinical signs.[31]

Rangelia vitalii has been described infecting two species of wild canids—the crab-eating fox (*C. thous*) and the pampas fox (*Lycalopex gymnocercus*); these are possible natural reservoirs of the parasite in Brazil.[9,10,12-14] Although the first confirmed *R. vitalii* infection in crab-eating foxes was reported in six subclinically infected animals, disease was reproduced in a domestic dog inoculated with blood and bone marrow from one of those foxes, suggesting a higher pathogenicity of the parasite in domestic dogs than in *C. thous*.[12] However, severe rangeliosis was also documented in a captive crab-eating fox in Brazil, indicating that disease can also occur in this species.[35]

There is limited information about the seasonality of canine rangeliosis. Although the disease is described throughout the year, the highest number of cases appear to occur in the summer, when ticks are more abundant.[5] *Rangelia vitalii* affects mainly young dogs, although adult dogs may also be affected, especially those in rural areas. Hunting dogs may be predisposed due to increased exposure.

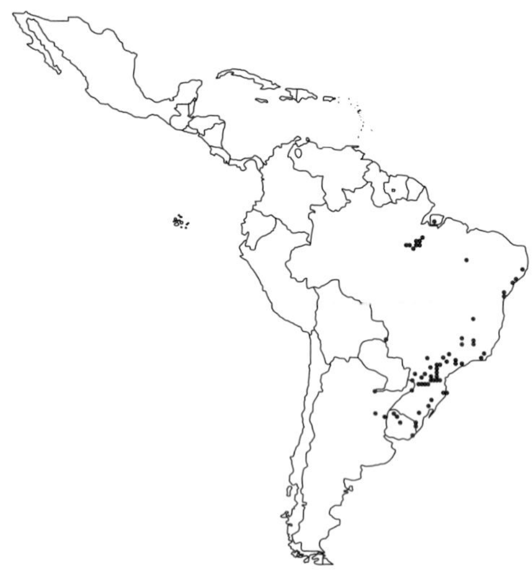

Fig. 105.1 Geographic distribution of *Amblyomma aureolatum* (and canine rangeliosis). (Modified from Guglielmone AA, Estrada-Pena A, Mangold AJ. *Amblyomma aureolatum* (Pallas, 1772) and *Amblyomma ovale* Koch, 1844 (Acari: Ixodidae): hosts, distribution and 16S rDNA sequences. *Veterinary Parasitology.* 113;2003:273-288.)

CLINICAL FEATURES

Pathogenesis and Clinical Signs

There is little information on the pathogenesis of *R. vitalii* infection. Spontaneously occurring disease may have a clinical course of a few days to up to 3 months. In early reports, the disease was classified as an acute or icteric form, a subacute or hemorrhagic form, and a mild and benign chronic form.[18-20] However, overlap of these clinical forms can occur.[5,23] Experimental studies showed that the clinical course can range from 3 days (acute form) to 8 to 15 days (subacute form) or up to 18 to 25 days (chronic form).[5] Infected dogs often have nonspecific clinical signs such as lethargy, anorexia, chronic weight loss, and intermittent fever. Mucosal pallor, jaundice, generalized lymphadenomegaly, and splenomegaly are usually noted. Pelvic limb edema may occur. Hemorrhagic disorders, such as petechiae and ecchymoses of mucosal membranes, persistent bleeding from the tips and external surface of the pinnae, planum nasale, venipuncture sites, GI tract (including hematemesis and hemorrhagic diarrhea), and epistaxis are commonly observed.[4-6,8,17,22] The pathogenesis of the hemorrhagic disorders is still unclear.[17] Consumptive coagulopathy related to DIC secondary to endothelial damage caused by the intracellular replication of this organism may be one mechanism. The observation of microthrombi in the lumina of small blood vessels supports this possibility.[5,17] Another possible cause of bleeding is thrombocytopenia related to other mechanisms such as immune-mediated destruction.[6,17,36] Additionally, thrombocytopenia may be related to possible altered enzymatic activity of the purinergic system.[37] Trauma inflicted by hematophagous flies feeding on the tips of the ears, and the vigorous scratching and head shaking to alleviate the pain and irritation of these areas, may also contribute to auricular hemorrhage.[17]

The infection in dogs consists of an intraerythrocytic and an extraerythrocytic phase that occurs in endothelial cells of internal

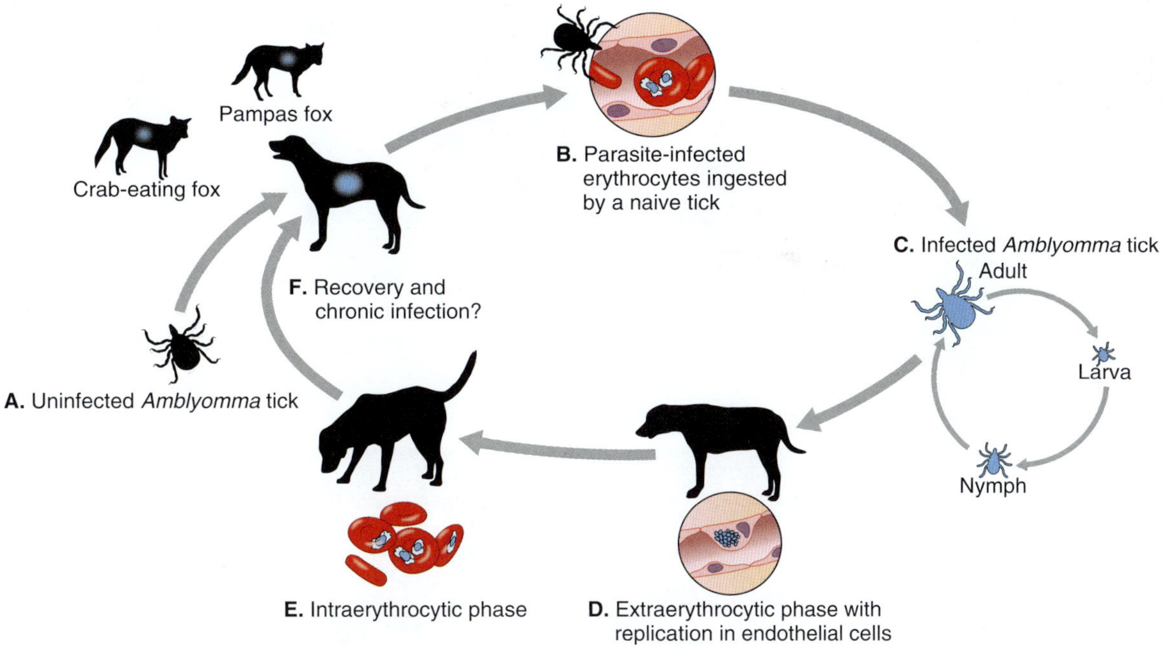

Fig. 105.2 Possible life cycle of *Rangelia vitalii.* (A) Uninfected ticks feed on infected dogs and possible wild canids (acting as reservoir hosts) and (B) ingest parasite-infected blood cells. (C) Transovarial transmission of *R. vitalii* occurs in female ticks. Inoculation of domestic dogs with *R. vitalii* during tick feeding leads to disease (D and E). Two phases of replication occur in the canid host, an extraerythrocytic phase that involves infection of endothelial cells (D), and an intraerythrocytic phase that involves infection of erythrocytes (E). Surviving dogs may remain subclinically infected and serve as reservoirs for infection of new ticks.

organs (tissue phase) (Fig. 105.2).[17,22] Although some authors state that the intraerythrocytic form of the parasite is mostly observed during the acute stage of the disease,[18-20] the tissue phase appears to occur before the intraerythrocytic stage.[31] Thrombocytopenia precedes detection of the parasites in a blood smear, leading to the belief that infection of the vascular endothelium is pre-erythrocytic, and that thrombocytopenia could be the result of platelet consumption in vascular lesions caused by the protozoan exiting the vascular endothelium.[31] The severe anemia may reflect IMHA, leading to prehepatic jaundice.[4,6,22,23] Evidence for an immune-mediated process includes the presence of regenerative anemia, spherocytosis, erythrophagocytosis in the blood, spleen and lymph nodes, and a favorable response to corticosteroids during treatment;[4,6,22,23] however, the Coombs test has not been evaluated in affected dogs. The presence of hemosiderophages in the bone marrow is also consistent with an excessive erythrocyte breakdown.[17]

Physical Examination Findings

Physical examination abnormalities in most dogs with rangeliosis include lethargy, weakness, dehydration, intermittent fever, mucosal pallor, jaundice, generalized peripheral lymphadenomegaly, splenomegaly on abdominal palpation, pelvic limb edema and hemorrhagic disorders that most often occur as persistent bleeding from the tips and external surface of the pinnae and planum nasale (Fig. 105.3), and epistaxis and excessive bleeding from venipuncture sites. Petechiae and ecchymoses of mucosal surfaces can also be observed.[4-6,8,17,22] The severe bilateral pinnal hemorrhage is a characteristic (but not pathognomonic) clinical sign.[22] The outer surface of the ears or planum nasale may show extensive hemorrhagic crusting.[4-6,17]

DIAGNOSIS

A presumptive diagnosis of rangeliosis is based on history, typical clinical signs, and hematological changes. Ticks may have detached from the dog by the time the animal is examined.[17] Definitive diagnosis requires detection of parasites in peripheral blood smears or in tissues, through histopathological evaluation,[3,4,6,17,26] or molecular diagnostics.[3,15,28] Differential diagnoses include babesiosis, leptospirosis, monocytic ehrlichiosis, and leishmaniosis.[5,17,33,34]

Laboratory Abnormalities

Complete Blood Count

CBC findings in canine rangeliosis include severe regenerative anemia and mild to severe thrombocytopenia.[4,6,8,22,23,31] In experimental infections, *R. vitalii* reduced platelet aggregation.[37] A normocytic, normochromic anemia is usually observed in the first days of infection, which becomes macrocytic and hypochromic as the disease progresses. Reticulocytosis, anisocytosis, polychromasia, metarubricytosis, and Howell-Jolly bodies are common findings on blood smears. Spherocytosis, microscopic agglutination of RBCs, and erythrophagocytosis are also noted.[4-6,23,25] The plasma can be icteric and, in some cases, macroscopic erythrocyte agglutination can be seen in the blood collection tube.[4,23] Leukocyte abnormalities are inconsistent but may include leukocytosis, neutrophilia, lymphocytosis, monocytosis, or neutropenia.[4,6,8,23,25,31]

Serum Chemistry Profile and Urinalysis

Increased activities of ALT, AST, and CK are reported in experimental infections with *R. vitalii.*[38] An increase in serum bilirubin concentration due to extravascular hemolysis may also occur.[39] In experimentally

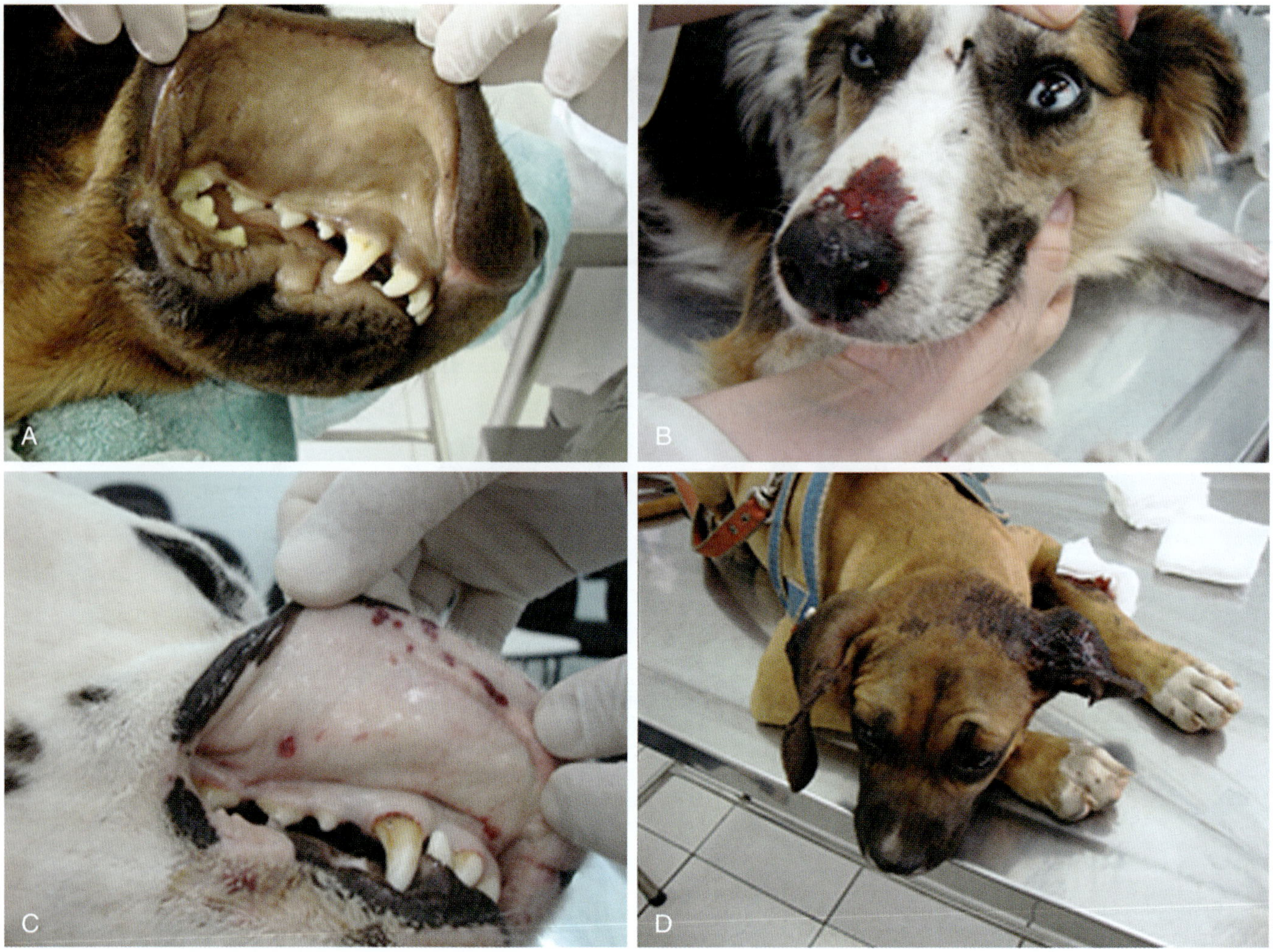

Fig. 105.3 Physical examination findings in dogs with rangeliosis. (A) Yellow discoloration of the oral mucosa (jaundice); (B) hyphema and epistaxis; (C) petechiae and ecchymoses scattered throughout the oral mucosa, and mucosal pallor (anemia); (D) severe bleeding on the outer surface of the right pinna and on a venipuncture site on the right forelimb. (From França, RT et al. Canine rangeliosis due to *Rangelia vitalii*: from first report in Brazil in 1910 to current day – a report. *Ticks and Tick-borne Diseases*. 2014;5:466–474. Elsevier. Figure 4). *Continued*

infected dogs, total protein, albumin, alpha-2 globulin, and beta-2 globulin concentrations decreased, while there was an increase in alpha-1 globulin and gamma-globulin levels.[40] Urinalysis may reveal bilirubinuria and hemoglobinuria.[39]

Microbiologic Tests

Rangeliosis can be diagnosed by microscopic identification of the parasite and/or molecular diagnostic assays. To date, there are no serologic tests for detection of antibodies to *R. vitalii.*

Cytologic Diagnosis

Examination of peripheral blood smears for *R. vitalii* is insensitive, because in many cases the number of circulating parasites is low.[41] The parasite can be found free in plasma or inside erythrocytes, neutrophils, and monocytes (Fig. 105.4). The probability of finding the parasite is higher when blood is collected during an episode of high fever in the acute stage of the disease.[5,18-20] Parasitized erythrocytes tend to be found on the feathered edge of blood smears.[22] Depending on the study, parasites were seen in blood smears in 11% to 71% of cases.[4,6] Within cells, *R. vitalii* is a round, oval, or teardrop-shaped organism found singly or in pairs.[22] The zoites of *R. vitalii* are 3 μm long and 2 μm wide (nucleus 1 μm long and 0.8 μm wide).[42] In blood smears stained with Giemsa, intraerythrocytic merozoites have a pale basophilic cytoplasm and an eccentric magenta nucleus.[3]

Diagnosis Using Nucleic Acid–Based Assays

A quantitative PCR assay to detect and quantify a fragment of the 18S rRNA gene of *R. vitalii* in canine blood samples has been validated,[15] but there are no commercial veterinary diagnostic laboratories performing PCR analysis for *R. vitalii.*

Pathologic Findings

Necropsy findings commonly observed in dogs with rangeliosis include diffuse pallor or jaundice, splenomegaly, hepatomegaly, generalized enlargement of peripheral and visceral lymph nodes, and enlarged tonsils. Diffuse subcutaneous edema of the pelvic limbs and multiple petechiae and ecchymoses are observed on the serosa of many organs and the mucous membranes. There may be pulmonary and cardiac hemorrhage. Lungs are edematous, heavy, and fail to collapse. The stomach and intestines can be filled with blood. Mild to moderate hydrothorax, hydropericardium, and ascites can also be noted.[4,17,22,23]

Microscopic findings include the presence of zoites in endothelial cells of blood capillaries in many organs; the zoites are located inside intracytoplasmic membrane-bound parasitophorous vacuoles.[4,17,22,23]

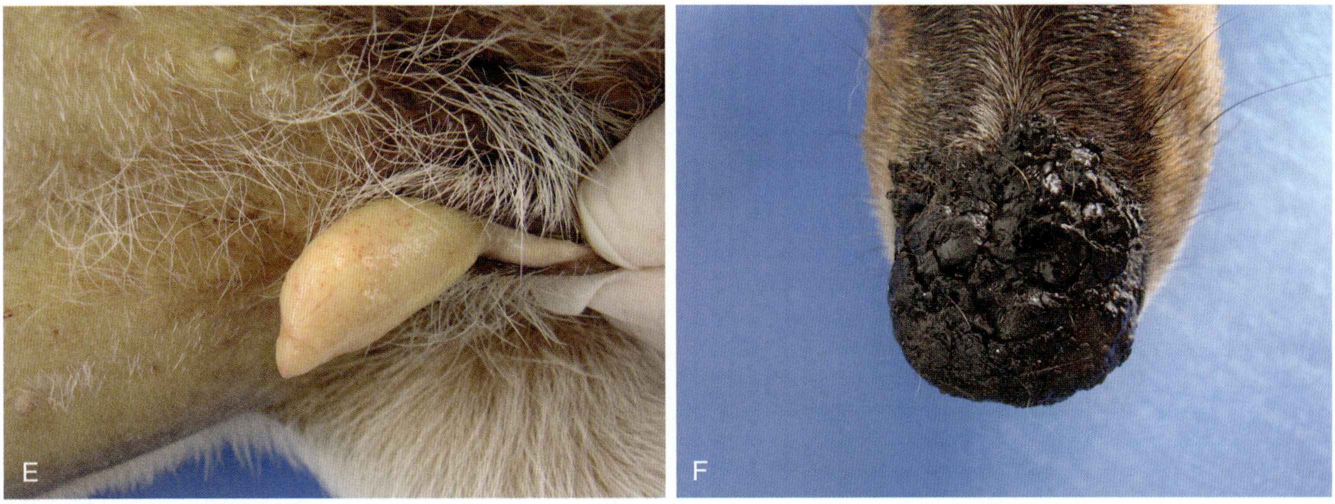

Fig. 105.3 cont'd. (Courtesy of Rafael Fighera, UFSM, Santa Maria, Brazil.)

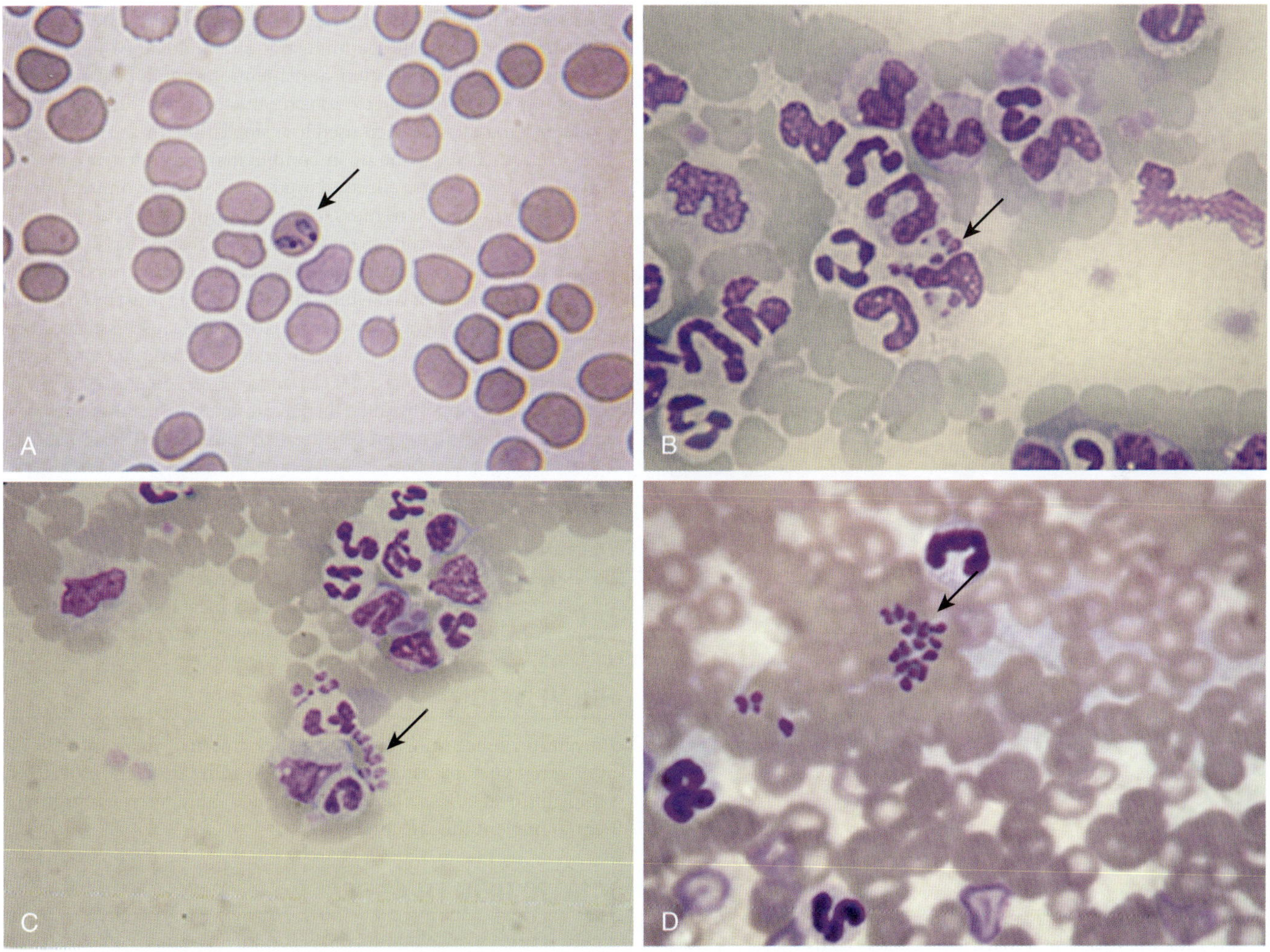

Fig. 105.4 Blood smear from a dog with rangeliosis showing intraerythrocytic *R. vitalii* piroplasms (arrows). (A), inside leukocytes (B), and (C and D) free in the plasma. (From França, RT et al. Canine rangeliosis due to *Rangelia vitalii*: from first report in Brazil in1910 to current day – a report. *Ticks Tick Borne Dis.* 2014;5:466-474. Elsevier. Figure 1.)

The organisms are round or oval, homogeneous and basophilic with H&E, and are found most often in peripheral lymph nodes, liver, tonsils, bone marrow, kidneys, lungs, adrenal medulla, and choroid plexus (Fig. 105.5).[4,17,22,23] The cytoplasm of the parasites is pale with a prominent basophilic and eccentrically located nucleus.[17] Parasitized endothelial cells can be markedly distended by organisms.[17]

Tissues often show a mononuclear inflammatory infiltrate, predominantly plasmacytic, of variable severity.[4,17,22] Reactive hyperplasia of the lymph nodes with prominent secondary follicles, multinucleated giant cells, and erythrophagocytosis within medullary sinuses are often observed (Fig. 105.5).[4,17] Follicular hyperplasia of the splenic white pulp is observed in many cases.[17] There is also increased cellularity of the red

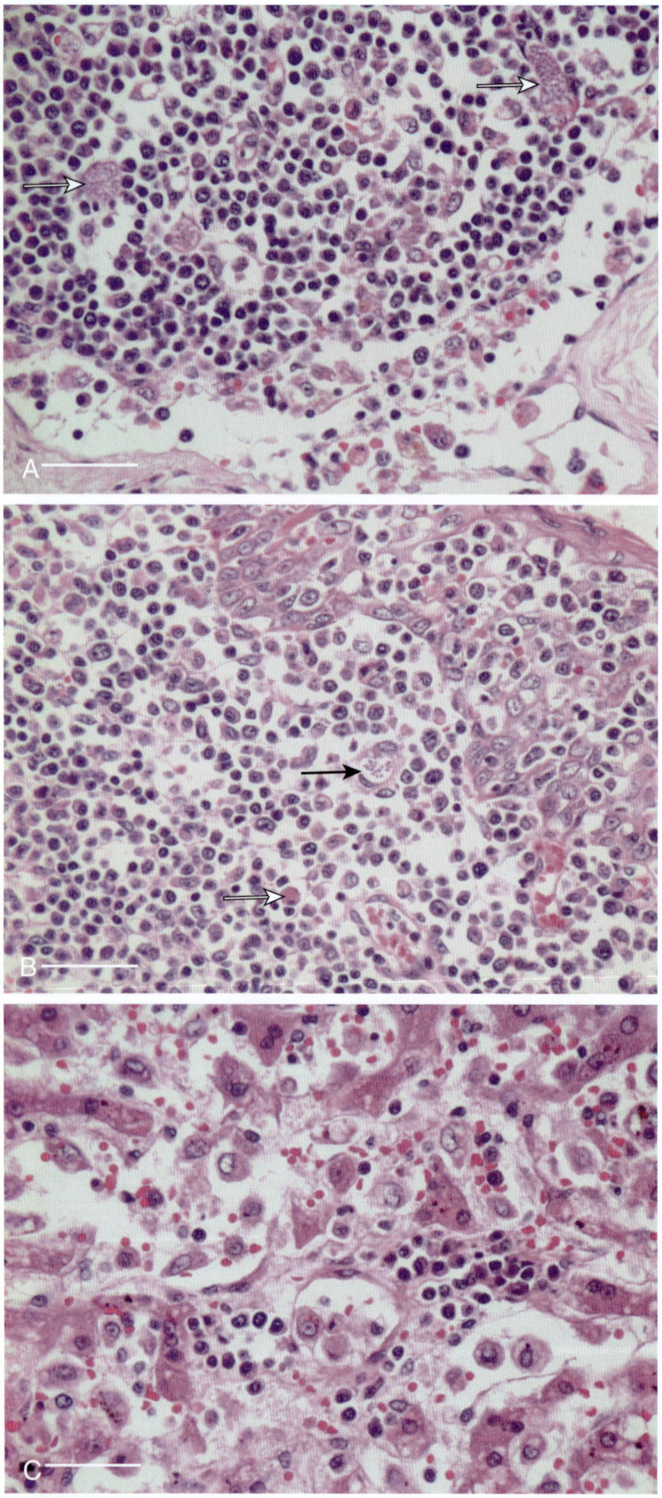

Fig. 105.5 Histopathologic findings in canine rangeliosis. There are multiple zoites of *R. vitalii* within capillary endothelial cells *(arrows)*. (A) Lymph node showing plasmacytic hyperplasia within the medullary cords with sinus histiocytosis. (B) In the tonsil, there is lymphoid and marked plasmacytic hyperplasia; a Mott cell is present in the center of the image *(black arrow)*. (C) Lymphoplasmacytic hepatitis with marked Kupffer cell hyperplasia (hematoxylin and eosin stain, bar = 100 μm). (Courtesy of Rafael Fighera, UFSM, Santa Maria, Brazil.)

pulp, due to proliferation of plasma cells and extramedullary hematopoiesis.[4] In the liver, there may be periportal inflammation, or less often, inflammation surrounding central veins, extramedullary hematopoiesis, and Kupffer cell hyperplasia (Fig. 105.5). There may also be centrilobular or midzonal necrosis, microthrombi, and evidence of biliary stasis.[4,17]

Renal changes include cortical and occasionally medullary interstitial inflammation, evidence of acute tubular necrosis, and accumulation of hemosiderin in tubular epithelial cells.[4,17,22] Mononuclear cell infiltrates surround glomeruli, and *R. vitalii* may be seen in capillary endothelial cells. Hyperplasia of all cell lines may be observed in the marrow. Hemosiderin-laden macrophages can be seen.[17]

Other changes may include myocarditis; pulmonary edema and interstitial inflammation with lymphocytes, plasma cells, and macrophages; and meningitis.[4,17,23]

TREATMENT AND PROGNOSIS

Drugs used for treatment of rangeliosis have included diminazene aceturate, imidocarb dipropionate, doxycycline, and trypan blue (Table 105.1).[5,25,28,42,43] Diminazene aceturate (3.5 mg/kg IM, once) was used successfully to treat dogs with experimental infection with *R. vitalii*.[25,42] Blood smears were negative for *R. vitalii* within 24 hours, and 9 days after treatment, all dogs were PCR negative for the parasite.[25] Nevertheless, diamizene aceturate has a low therapeutic index and neurotoxicosis has been reported.[6,17,44] The toxicity of the drug is cumulative and usually dose-related, but individual variation in susceptibility and idiosyncratic reactions can occur. Repeat administration should be avoided for at least 2 weeks after the first injection, and attention should be paid to the animal's body weight to avoid overdosing and toxicosis.[44] Imidocarb dipropionate (5 mg/kg) has been used as a single dose or as two doses given at 2-week intervals, alone or in combination with doxycycline.[6,17,28,29] Anticholinergic adverse effects of imidocarb, such as vomiting, diarrhea, salivation, and muscle tremors, can be controlled with atropine (0.005 mg/kg SC).[44] Doxycycline (5 mg/kg q12h for 28 days) has been used with apparent success.[5,6,17] Trypan blue was used in the first reported cases of the disease; however, it is no longer used. The drug must be administered IV and, in case of perivascular extravasation, can cause tissue necrosis.[5,43]

Glucocorticoids have been used to address the immune-mediated consequences of the disease (i.e., IMHA and ITP) in some cases.[5,6,17,42] Blood transfusion and supportive fluid therapy are necessary in those cases in which anemia is severe.[5,17] If not properly treated, rangeliosis is usually fatal.[22]

IMMUNITY AND VACCINATION

Dogs that recover spontaneously or are treated for rangeliosis may develop immunity against a new infection by *R. vitalli*, but parasite persistence for months in the face of subclinical infection has also been documented.[17] Vaccines for *R. vitalii* infection are not available.

PREVENTION

Prevention relies on avoidance of tick-infested areas and the use of appropriate ectoparasite preventives. Routine inspection of dogs and rapid removal of ticks after outdoor activities, such as hunting, can help to prevent the infection.

PUBLIC HEALTH ASPECTS

There is no evidence that *R. vitalii* can infect humans.

NONENTERIC (FREE-LIVING) AMEBIASIS

Marc Kent, Elizabeth W. Howerth

INTRODUCTION

Amebas that belong to the genera *Acanthamoeba, Balamuthia*, and *Naegleria* are free-living, amphizoic, and opportunistic protozoa that are ubiquitous in nature. Infections with these amebae are rarely reported in

TABLE 105.1 Antimicrobials Used in the Treatment of Rangeliosis

Drug	Dose (mg/kg)	Route	Interval (Hours)	Duration
Diminazene aceturate	3.5	IM	Once	NA
Imidocarb dipropionate	5	IM	Once	Repeat in 14 days
Doxycycline	5	PO, IV	12 hours	28 days
Trypan blue	10	IV	Once	NA

IM, intramuscular; NA, not applicable; PO, oral.

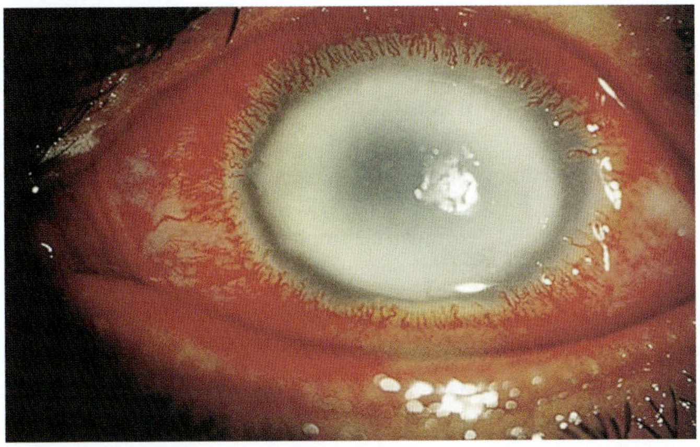

Fig. 105.6 *Acanthamoeba* keratitis with characteristic corneal ring infiltrate in a human patient. The disease can be sight-threatening and lead to corneal perforation. (From Garg P, Rao GN. Corneal ulcer: diagnosis and management. *J Comm Eye Health.* 1999;12:21.)

humans and companion animals. Infections often are disseminated, with frequent involvement of the CNS; the respiratory system and kidneys may also be involved. Localized corneal infections with *Acanthamoeba* occur in humans, most often associated with contact lens or corneal trauma, as well as following LASIK procedures (Fig. 105.6). *Acanthamoeba* spp. keratitis has also rarely been reported in dogs and cats. In humans, CNS infections with *Acanthamoeba* spp. and *Balamuthia mandrillaris* are referred to as *granulomatous amebic encephalitis* (GAE), whereas infections with *Naegleria* are referred to as *primary amebic meningoencephalitis* (PAM) in an effort to denote restriction of the infection to the CNS. Systemic infections with *Acanthamoeba* spp. and *B. mandrillaris* have only been described in dogs and not cats, and PAM has not been reported in companion animals.

ETIOLOGIC AGENT AND EPIDEMIOLOGY

Acanthamoebae are ubiquitous free-living amebae found in a multitude of water sources including fresh and salt water, as well as soil, dust, and sewage.[45-51] The classification of the genus *Acanthamoeba* and separation from the closely related genera have had a confusing history that is becoming resolved only with the use of molecular techniques.[52] Acanthamoebae are classified as distinct genera based on morphologic differences in the trophozoite shape and cyst wall structure, nutritional requirements, and serologic responses by infected hosts.

Acanthamoeba spp. have been divided into three morphologic groups (I, II, and III) based on trophozoite and cyst size and structure. Although this morphologic classification is used, genetic comparisons have suggested the need for additional taxonomic reevaluation. Twenty different genotypes (T1 to T20) exist based on rRNA sequencing.[53] The majority of infections in human beings (those not in association with ocular keratitis) involve the T4 genotype.[51,54] Too few cases have been reported in dogs to identify a common genotype. The T4 genotype has been documented in dogs with and without disease.[55-59] Interestingly, the T1 genotype also has been documented in affected dogs.[60,61] All the pathogenic ameba are known to harbor obligate intracellular prokaryotes including bacteria, chlamydiae, and viruses. The role of these endosymbionts in the production of disease or transport of these organisms is uncertain.

The life cycle of *Acanthamoeba* involves two stages: one, a dormant free-living cyst in the environment, and the other, a vegetative trophozoite form capable of parasitizing and feeding in host tissues. The vegetative replicating trophozoite has two distinct phagotrophic niches: (1) feeding on bacteria in aquatic habitats and (2) acting as opportunists of host cells in the body. The cyst phase is often able to resist adverse environmental conditions, including desiccation and possibly host immune responses. Cysts can survive exposure to temperatures between −20°C and +42°C and a pH of 3.9 to 9.75.[62]

In the environment, *Acanthamoeba* species are omnipresent and abundant. They have been isolated from all fresh-water sources and vegetation. In the atmosphere, they are carried on pollutants, and their concentrations have been used as potential monitors of air quality. After ingestion, they may be inhabitants of the GI tracts of many animals and human beings and can be found in their feces.[63]

Several *Acanthamoeba* species are pathogenic for animals and human beings. They can subclinically colonize superficial epithelial surfaces but can also produce ocular surface infections and may disseminate in immunocompromised individuals. Disseminated infections usually involve the CNS. *Parachlamydia acanthamoebae,* a chlamydial endosymbiont of *Acanthamoeba* spp., has been associated with pneumonia in human beings.[64] *Parachlamydia acanthamoebae* has also been detected in topical ocular specimens from human beings[65,66] and cats[67,68] with conjunctivitis with or without keratitis. The prevalence of infection was similar in cats with or without corneal disease, indicating that clinically healthy cats may harbor this organism.[69] Cats in this latter study also had an equal prevalence of infection whether they were kept indoors or outdoors. Furthermore, they harbored *P. acanthamoebae* without *Acanthamoeba* spp. being detected.[69]

Three related amebae, *B. mandrillaris, Naegleria fowleri,* and *Sappinia pedata,* also cause meningoencephalitis or encephalitis in human beings and nonhuman primates (also known as "brain-eating ameba").[70] Of these organisms, disseminated infection with *B. mandrillaris* has been reported in several dogs with granulomatous meningoencephalitis,[71-74] one with concurrent granulomatous nephritis[72] and another with concurrent pneumonitis.[73] One dog had a history of exposure to stagnant water.[74] Systemic infections with *Acanthamoeba* spp. develop in immunocompromised human beings; however, those caused by *N. fowleri* and *B. mandrillaris* spp. can affect immunocompetent humans. Infection with *N. fowleri* is acquired through swimming in contaminated waters, with the infection spreading through the olfactory neuroepithelium to the CNS, and reports typically involve children. In contrast, infections with *Acanthamoeba* and *B. mandrillaris* are subacute infections that may also follow hematogenous spread of organisms from pulmonary or cutaneous sites to the CNS. Most human infections with *B. mandrillaris* in the United States have come from California, followed by Texas and Arizona.

In dogs, epizootics of acanthamebiasis have been observed in greyhounds.[75] Affected greyhounds ranged from 4 to 13 months of age. During outbreaks, organisms are thought to be acquired from a common environmental source rather than from other animals. However, most reported cases of acanthamebiasis involve a single dog. Young dogs appear to be most susceptible. Affected breeds reported include two German shepherd dogs, one 6 months old and one 4 years old;[76,77] a 1-year-old Labrador-type dog;[60] an immunosuppressed Akita;[78] an immunosuppressed 10-month-old boxer;[61] and a 22-month-old Spanish water dog.[58] While most are disseminated infections, *Acanthamoeba* infection with genotype T4 was reported in the prostate of a 10-year-old mixed breed dog.[56] *Balamuthia* spp. infections have been reported in a golden retriever (Melbourne, Australia), Australian blue heeler (Melbourne, Australia), great Dane (northern California, USA), and Siberian husky dog (Oklahoma, USA).[71-74]

The source of infection and the incubation period in dogs are unknown. Immunosuppression is likely involved in the development of most infections. In one dog infected with *Acanthamoeba castellanii,* T cell function was abnormal based on lymphocyte blastogenesis in response to various mitogens, consistent with immunosuppression or T cell–mediated immunodeficiency.[78] Although immunocompetency is often not evaluated, affected dogs often have been treated with immunosuppressive drugs when infection was diagnosed.[61] In other cases, infection has occurred in dogs obtained from shelters.[60,77] Concurrent acanthamebiasis and distemper in affected dogs further supports the role of an incompetent immune system in the pathogenesis of the infection.[79]

Acanthamoeba infection is rare in cats. Despite this, strains consistent with *A. castellanii* genotype T4 were isolated from 10 of 64 cats with clinical signs of keratoconjunctivitis.[80]

CLINICAL FEATURES

Pathogenesis, Clinical Signs, and Physical Examination Findings

The pathogenesis of nonenteric amebiasis in dogs is unknown. In humans, routes of infection may include inhalation of organisms from water while swimming or from contaminated air. The organisms can replicate in the upper or lower respiratory tract after inhalation, or may replicate in skin or other tissues after penetrating injuries and then spread to the CNS by hematogenous means. Alternatively, infection of the cornea and nasal passage might lead to a spread to the nervous system via optic and olfactory nerves, respectively. In one dog with acanthamebiasis, distribution of the brain lesions suggested penetration of the cribriform plate.[77] Experimentally, *Balamuthia* has been shown to infect the brain via the olfactory nerves in immunodeficient mice,[81] and this may be a likely route for natural infection.

Acanthamoeba sp. infection was identified in two dogs from Florida with preexisting chronic keratoconjunctivitis sicca treated with topical immunosuppressive drugs that developed localized granulomatous keratitis, which was evident on ocular examination as fleshy mass lesions.[82] Clinical manifestations of systemic canine acanthamebiasis often include mild ocular and nasal discharge, anorexia, lethargy, and fever.[60,74,78] In many dogs, acute onset of respiratory distress and neurologic dysfunction are present.[61] Neurologic signs include incoordination, head tilt, stumbling, dysmetria, and seizures. Severely affected dogs are tetraplegic and in lateral recumbency. Cough and dyspnea may be observed together with neurological signs, or respiratory signs may develop a few days after the onset of neurological signs. In one dog, progressive neurologic signs developed as a result of meningoencephalitis, as well as the syndrome of inappropriate antidiuretic hormone secretion (SIADH).[77]

A dog with disseminated balamuthiasis developed lethargy, anorexia, diarrhea, and hematuria followed by neurologic dysfunction, including intermittent seizures, rotary nystagmus, recumbency, and coma.[72] Another dog had an 8-month history of generalized seizures that had been controlled with phenobarbital.[73] Two months before referral, the dog had been evaluated for deafness, a left-sided head tilt, and circling. A diagnosis of CNS lymphoma was suspected based on CSF analysis, which revealed a lymphocytic pleocytosis with atypical lymphocytes. The dog was treated with glucocorticoid and lomustine therapy. Four weeks later, the dog was evaluated for respiratory distress and hypotension and was euthanized.[73] In one dog with no previous history of illness, acute signs of left-sided central vestibular dysfunction developed. Balamuthiasis localized to the cerebellum was observed at necropsy.[74] Acute onset of seizures was reported in another dog that had right cerebral frontal cortex involvement at necropsy.[71]

DIAGNOSIS

Laboratory Abnormalities

Laboratory abnormalities in animals with systemic amebiasis are nonspecific. The CBC often reveals a neutrophilic leukocytosis. In some animals, leukopenia is observed. Leukopenia in greyhounds is a result of marked lymphopenia and in other breeds is caused by a reduction in all types of blood leukocytes.[76,78] Similar laboratory findings have been documented in dogs with *B. mandrillaris* infection. On the serum biochemistry panel, increased serum liver enzyme activities and renal azotemia may be observed if kidney and liver involvement is present. Azotemia may also reflect dehydration.

Cerebrospinal Fluid Analysis

In dogs with neurological signs, CSF may have a pleocytosis and elevated protein concentration. The degree of pleocytosis has ranged from 234 nucleated cells/μL to 2,925 nucleated cells/μL and has been characterized by a mixture of nondegenerative neutrophils and large mononuclear cells and lymphocytes.[74,77] Protein concentration may be greater than 1 g/dL.[77]

Diagnostic Imaging

Plain Radiography

In one dog with pulmonary infection, thoracic radiographs disclosed a diffuse bronchial to interstitial pattern.[61]

Sonographic Findings

Nonspecific changes are observed on abdominal ultrasound examination which likely reflect infection involving organs such as the liver and kidney. In a dog with *Acanthamoeba* infection localized to the prostate, multiple cysts in the prostate were identified.[56]

Advanced Imaging

Too few cases with neurological signs have undergone advanced imaging using CT or MRI examinations to characterize lesions. In one dog, CT disclosed a ring-enhancing lesion in the cerebellum.[74] In another dog, MRI disclosed a heterogenous mass that was ring-enhancing following contrast administration.[79]

Microbiologic Tests

Cytological Diagnosis

Antemortem diagnosis of amebic infection is rare; the diagnosis necessitates the identification of trophozoites or cysts. Organisms are rarely observed in CSF. Despite the lack of clinical reports that document evidence of infection in specimens obtained from the respiratory tract, it may be possible to make a diagnosis using BAL or lung biopsy in animals with respiratory disease.

Molecular Diagnosis Using Nucleic Acid–Based Testing

Because these amebae are difficult to distinguish morphologically, PCR testing offers the most specific and reliable means of species identification.[57,58,70,83,84] PCR-based assays have been used frequently on isolates in culture as well as from necropsy specimens. Demonstration of *Acanthamoeba* and *Balamuthia* have been documented in archived, formalin-fixed, and paraffin-embedded specimens using molecular techniques.[84]

Cell Culture

Acanthamoeba spp. can be easily cultured on non-nutrient agar plates coated with bacteria such as *Escherichia coli* or *Enterobacter aerogenes*.[51]

Amebae demonstrate a preference for nonencapsulated and nonpigmented bacteria as the mucoid capsules of the bacteria inhibit phagocytosis by the ameba and bacterial pigments may be toxic.[51] Early in the cultivation process, plaque-like clearings in the bacterial lawn may be observed; once the bacteria have been consumed, amebae encyst.[51] Cysts remain viable for prolonged periods of time, especially if the agar plate is sealed to prevent drying and kept at a reduced temperature.[51] Isolation of the parasitic amebae is possible using fresh frozen (−70°C) tissue that has been stored for up 2 months.[60] Cultivation using bacteria-free medium is also possible.

Pathologic Findings

Gross Pathologic Findings

A definitive diagnosis of systemic amebiasis is almost always made at necropsy. In dogs with acanthamebiasis, lung and brain lesions have been observed grossly in almost all reports, but small nodules that range in color from white to reddish-brown may be observed in the kidney and liver.[60,61] Lung lesions vary from light-tan to deep-red, raised, semisolid nodules distributed uniformly throughout all lobes.[61,76,78] The nodules have a tendency to coalesce, and intralesional cavitations have been noted. Brain lesions may be large, multifocal, and visible on the meningeal surfaces of the cerebrum and cerebellum and vary from red to tannish-brown as a result of recent hemorrhage or necrosis.

Histopathologic Findings

Microscopically, multifocal necrotizing and often hemorrhagic meningoencephalitis and pneumonia with purulent, pyogranulomatous, or granulomatous inflammation and intralesional amebic trophozoites and cyst forms, sometimes in macrophages, are seen (Figs. 105.7 and 105.8). In brain lesions, sometimes the amebae are best visualized in perivascular and subarachnoid spaces, because in the neural parenchyma they are often masked by the presence of infiltrating inflammatory cells. Similar necrotizing and purulent to granulomatous foci containing amebae may be seen in other tissues, including kidney, heart, liver, adrenal, lymph node, and pancreas.[60,61,76-78] Histopathology of biopsy specimens obtained from the two dogs with localized amebic keratitis revealed chronic granulomatous superficial keratitis with intralesional trophozoites and cysts.[82] Histologic and direct fluorescent antibody methods can be used to demonstrate and identify the organism in tissues. Free-living pathogenic amebae are difficult to differentiate microscopically from certain mammalian cells, especially macrophages.[85] The diagnostic feature of *Acanthamoeba* in histologic sections, which should help differentiate them from macrophages, is the eccentric nucleus with a large centrally located nucleolus (*targetoid karyosome*) and vacuolated cytoplasm. Gomori's methenamine silver and PAS stains can be used to help demonstrate the organism, but they only stain the cyst wall. Trophozoites are 15 to 50 μm in diameter, and cysts are 15 to 25 μm, depending on species.[51] The cysts have an outer wrinkled cyst wall and a variably shaped, PAS-positive inner wall. Direct fluorescent antibody staining is specific and reliable on deparaffinized sections of formalin-fixed tissue and, with specific conjugates, can be used to distinguish among the various species of *Acanthamoeba*. Nucleic acid–based assays have been used to document infection and for strain genotyping.[60,61,72,82]

In dogs with *B. mandrillaris* infection, grossly visible granulomas have been present in the kidneys, lung, and brain (Figs. 105.9 and 105.10).[15,16] In one dog, the kidneys had marked interstitial edema and necrosis with perivascular granulomatous inflammation (Fig. 105.11), and the brain had fibrinoid necrosis of vessels with marked perivascular pyogranulomatous inflammation mixed with fibrin and malacia surrounding the affected vessels. Trophozoite and fewer cyst forms were admixed with the perivascular infiltrates. Trophozoites are 15 to 45 μm in diameter and round to oval, with short cytoplasmic pseudopodia (Fig. 105.12) and a centrally located nucleus with one or

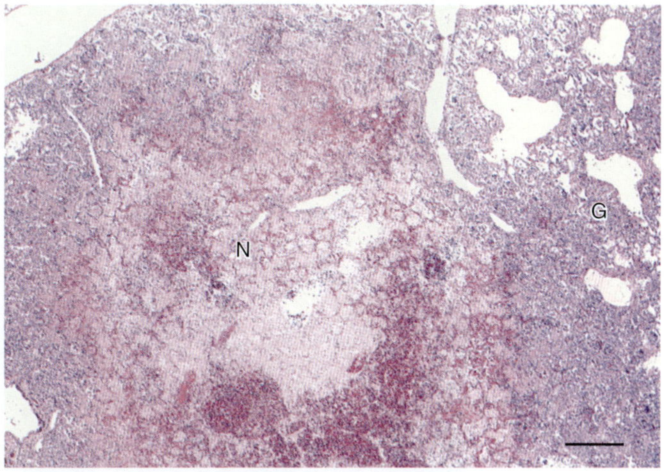

Fig. 105.7 Lung from a greyhound with acanthamebic pneumonia characterized by necrosis and hemorrhage (*N*) surrounded by pyogranulomatous inflammation (*G*) (hematoxylin and eosin stain, bar = 0.3 mm).

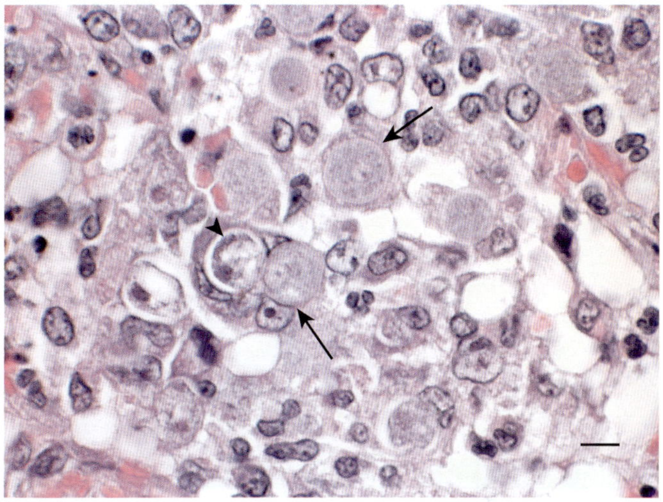

Fig. 105.8 Lung from a greyhound with acanthamebic pneumonia. *Acanthamoeba* trophozoites (*arrows*) and developing cysts (*arrowhead* shows mature cyst) are present in pyogranulomatous inflammation in an alveolus (hematoxylin and eosin stain, bar = 30 μm).

two nucleoli. Cysts are 15 to 20 μm in diameter and surrounded by a double wall with an outer undulating wall and a thick round inner wall (Fig. 105.13). In a second dog, there was embolic pneumonia with small numbers of neutrophils and macrophages and large numbers of amebic trophozoites and fewer cysts, whereas the brain had chronic multifocal nonsuppurative meningoencephalitis in which amebic forms outnumbered inflammatory cells. Immunohistochemistry, fluorescent antibody staining, and PCR have been used on paraffin-embedded tissue for diagnosis.

TREATMENT AND PROGNOSIS

Information on treatment of topical and systemic amebic infections in animals is lacking, and most infections are diagnosed at necropsy. Amebic keratitis was reported in one dog when topical tacrolimus for keratoconjunctivitis sicca was switched to topical 2% cyclosporine, and in another dog following topic treatment with 0.02% chlorhexidine digluconate and 0.02% polyhexamethylene biguanide.[82]

No therapeutic regimen for systemic acanthamebiasis in humans has been well established, and drug susceptibility has been inconsistent. Only a small number of humans have survived CNS involvement

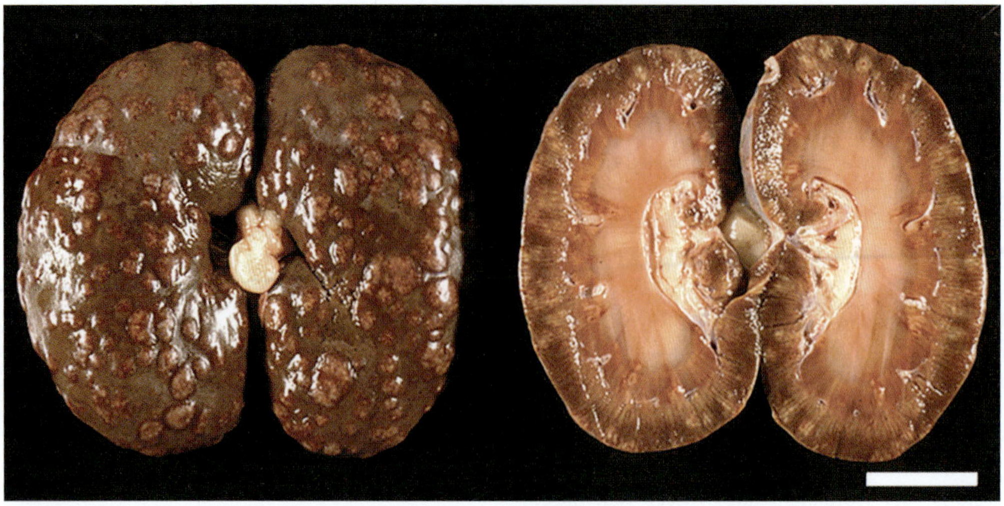

Fig. 105.9 Kidney from a dog with numerous granulomatous lesions throughout the cortex as a result of disseminated *Balamuthia mandrillaris* infection (bar = 2 cm). (From Foreman O, Sykes J, Ball L, et al. Disseminated infection with *Balamuthia mandrillaris* in a dog. *Vet Pathol.* 2004;41:506-510.)

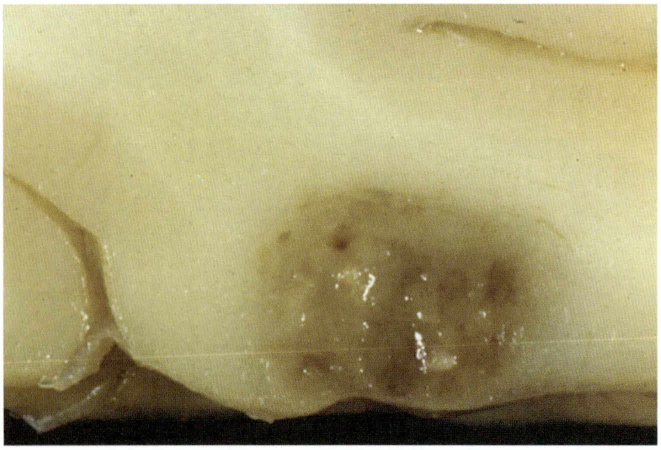

Fig. 105.10 Focal necrotizing lesion in right occipital lobe of cerebral cortex of a dog with *Balamuthia mandrillaris* infection. (From Foreman O, Sykes J, Ball L, et al. Disseminated infection with *Balamuthia mandrillaris* in a dog. *Vet Pathol.* 2004;41:506-510.)

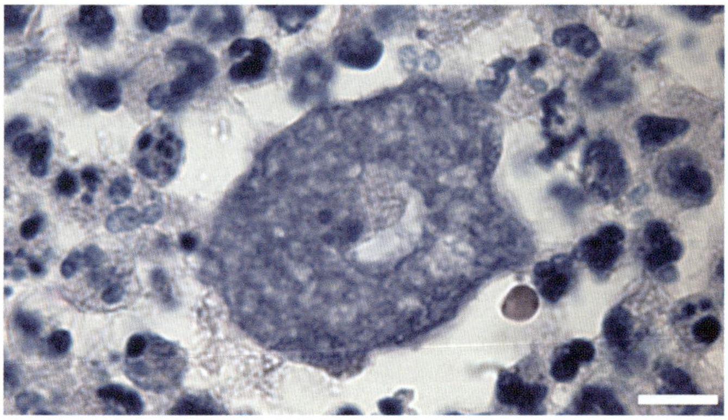

Fig. 105.12 Trophozoite of *Balamuthia mandrillaris* in the brain of a dog showing vacuolated cytoplasm (bar = 10 μm). (Courtesy Oded Foreman, Davis, CA.)

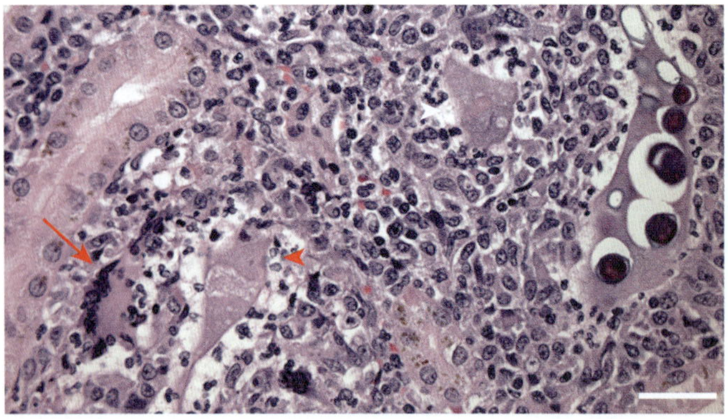

Fig. 105.11 Histopathology of the kidney from a dog with *Balamuthia mandrillaris* infection. Small cluster of organism cysts on right and trophozoite stages (*arrowhead*) are accompanied by mononuclear infiltration and multinucleated giant cell (*arrow*; hematoxylin and eosin stain, bar = 33 μm). (From Foreman O, Sykes J, Ball L, et al. Disseminated infection with *Balamuthia mandrillaris* in a dog. *Vet Pathol.* 2004;41:506-510.)

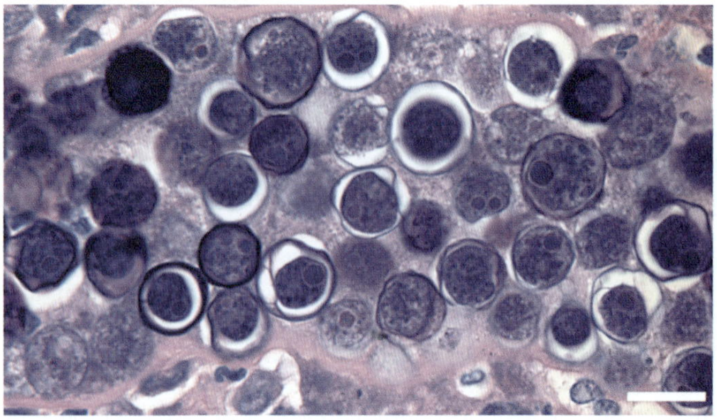

Fig. 105.13 Dog kidney containing cystic stages of *Balamuthia mandrillaris* infection. Note outer undulating membrane and prominent karyosomes (Giemsa stain, bar = 15 μm). (From Foreman O, Sykes J, Ball L, et al. Disseminated infection with *Balamuthia mandrillaris* in a dog. *Vet Pathol.* 2004;41:506-510.)

worldwide. Drugs active against *Acanthamoeba* and some other amebae *in vitro* include polyene antifungals (amphotericin B); azoles (ketoconazole, fluconazole, and voriconazole); trimethoprim-sulfamethoxazole; and flucytosine.[47,50,86,87] Multidrug therapy is most often employed.[47,50,86-88] Of the azole drugs, voriconazole may be considered a first-line treatment for *Acanthamoeba* infection and is often used in multidrug regimens in humans.[86]

In addition to traditional antimicrobials such as voriconazole, the use of a statin drug with voriconazole may be effective.[89] This combination may cause cell death through apoptosis rather than necrosis and consequently provoke less of an inflammatory reaction which may lessen the morbidity associated with CNS inflammation.[89] Of note, voriconazole appears less effective against *B. mandrillaris.*[90,92] Instead, other medications including amlodipine, loperamide, and prochlorperazine have shown *in vitro* activity against *B. mandrillaris.*[92] Given the time it takes for identification and susceptibility testing, several combinations of medication have shown *in vitro* activity against both *Acanthamoeba* and *B. mandrillaris*. These combinations include prochlorperazine plus loperamide; prochlorperazine plus apomorphine; and procyclidine plus loperamide.[87] Such combinations may be used along with traditional antimicrobials (i.e., azole and trimethoprim-sulfamethoxazole). Despite the knowledge of *in vitro* susceptibility, it is unknown whether or not such medications would be effective in veterinary patients. Most drugs used for treatment are amebistatic with few being amebicidal, therefore successful treatment likely necessitates months or years of therapy.[47]

Early detection seems crucial to successful treatment in humans. In humans surviving infection, early diagnosis of cutaneous infection may enable implementation of treatment before dissemination occurs. In humans, skin lesions often precede CNS infections by weeks to months.[47] To date, successful therapy in dogs has not been described due to advanced disease at presentation, with dissemination to the CNS.

PREVENTION

As these ameba species are ubiquitous in the environment, prevention is difficult. It is likely that dogs are exposed to low numbers of *Acanthamoeba* organisms throughout their lifetimes. Because these amebae are free-living, infection prevention may involve avoiding access to contaminated water especially in animals with a compromised immune system.

PUBLIC HEALTH ASPECTS

Human infections are believed to originate from exposure to free-living amebae in the environment such as soils and water sources. Transmission from an infected animal to another is unlikely. However, the dog is sentinel for human infection because of common environmental exposure. Strains infecting dogs have been genotypically identical to those infecting humans.

GASTROINTESTINAL AMEBIASIS AND BALANTIDIASIS

Jane E. Sykes

Ameba species that belong to the genus *Entamoeba* and the ciliate protozoan *Balantioides coli* (formerly *Balantidium coli*) (da Silva et al, 2021) can infect the colon of dogs and cats.[92] Balantidiasis has been reported very rarely in dogs but not cats. Dogs with balantidiasis showed signs of large bowel diarrhea with hematochezia and tenesmus, although co-infections with *Trichuris* have been reported.[93,94] Cysts and occasionally trophozoites can be seen in fecal flotations, as well as in colonic biopsy specimens using histopathology (Fig. 105.14).

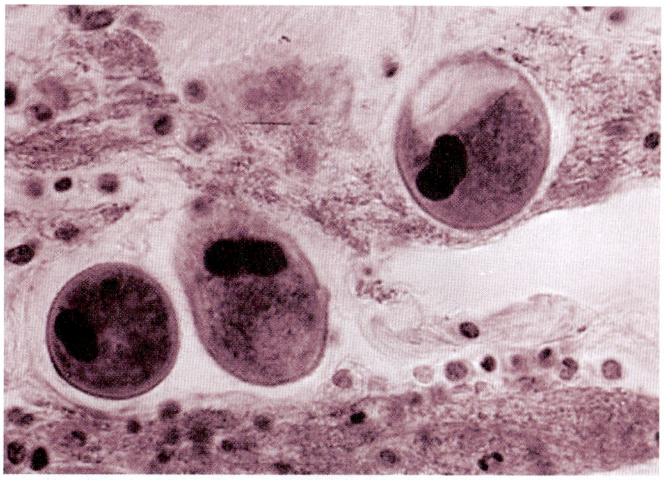

Fig. 105.14 *Balantioides coli* trophozoites in a section from the wall of a human colon. Note the prominent parasite macronuclei and the surrounding inflammatory response (hematoxylin and eosin stain, ×250).

There are several species in the genus *Entamoeba*, but only *Entamoeba histolytica* is recognized as a pathogen; in humans, *Entamoeba dispar* is considered a commensal and the pathogenic potential of *Entamoeba moshkovskii* is unclear. *Entamoeba histolytica* infection occurs worldwide and is an important cause of disease in humans and nonhuman primates. The life cycle of the organism as it relates to human infections is shown in Figure 105.15. Infection has also been described in both dogs and cats. A high prevalence of infection in dogs in Malaysia with *E. histolytica*, *E. moshkovskii* and *E. dispar* was documented in one study using PCR.[95] Most *Entamoeba* infections are subclinical, but large bowel diarrhea and anorexia can also occur.[96,97] Diagnosis is based on the finding of trophozoites in feces (Fig. 105.16) or in colonic biopsies using histopathology (Fig. 105.17). Dogs and cats may acquire infection from humans in the household, so the owners of pets diagnosed with *E. histolytica* infection should be referred to their physician for medical advice.

BLASTOCYSTOSIS

Jane E. Sykes

Blastocystis spp. are waterborne protozoal organisms that inhabit the intestinal tracts of humans and a wide variety of vertebrate animals. Analysis of the small subunit (SSU) rRNA gene suggests that they belong to the stramenopiles, a diverse group of protists that include the brown algae and diatoms; however, analysis of other portions of the genome indicates that they are related to *E. histolytica*. Analysis of the SSU rRNA gene also has identified 28 different subtypes (ST1 to ST32)[98]; ST1 to ST4 are the most frequently found in humans.

The significance of *Blastocystis* spp. lies in the fact that it is the most prevalent protozoa found in human fecal specimens worldwide, but its role in GI disease remains controversial because they are found widely as commensals. In humans, they have been incriminated as contributing to acute or chronic diarrhea, flatulence, irritable bowel syndrome, refractory ulcerative colitis, and colorectal cancer.[99] However, a large metagenomic study found no clear association between infection and disease among organisms worldwide, instead finding a higher prevalence of infection in healthy individuals.[100]

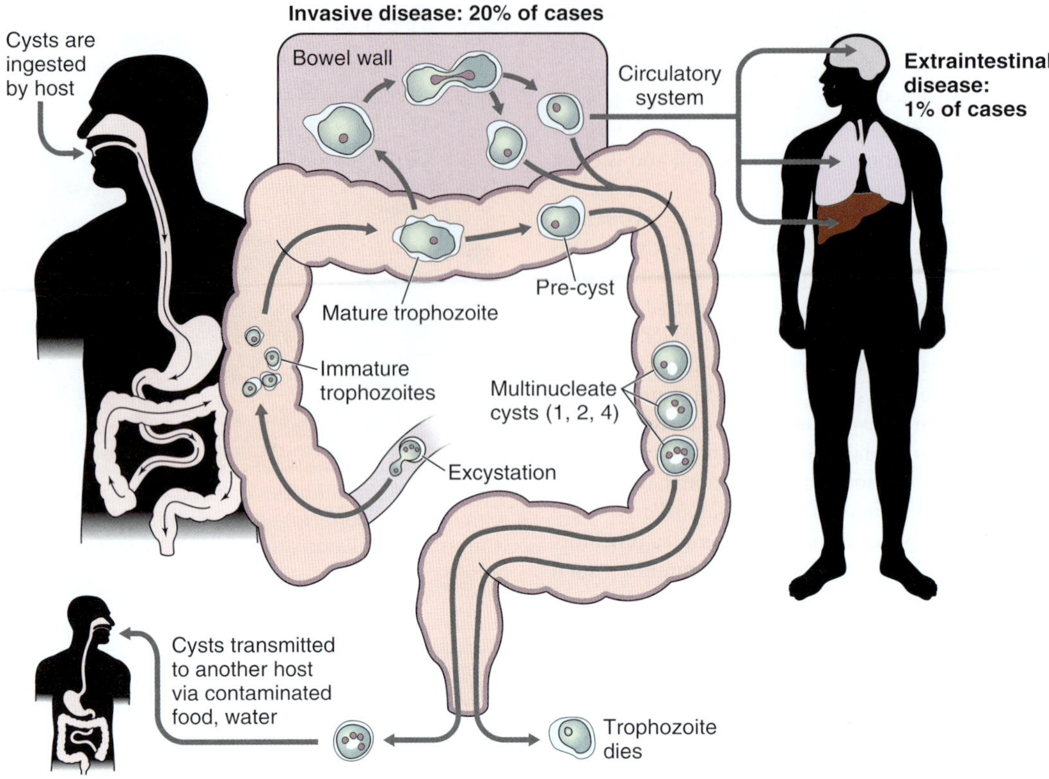

Fig. 105.15 Life cycle of *Entamoeba histolytica.* Infection is normally initiated by the ingestion of fecally contaminated food or water that contains cysts. Excystation occurs in the bowel lumen, where motile and potentially invasive trophozoites form. In most infections, trophozoites aggregate in the intestinal mucin layer and form new cysts, which results in self-limited and asymptomatic infection. In some cases, however, adherence to and lysis of colonic epithelium leads to invasion of the colon by trophozoites. Extraintestinal spread to the peritoneum, liver, and other sites may follow.

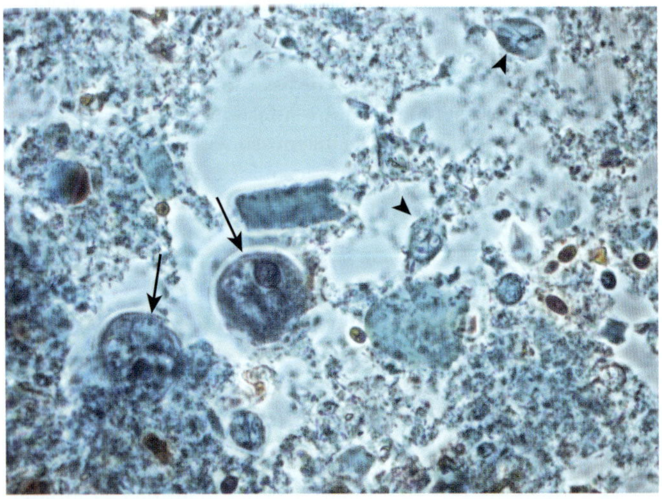

Fig. 105.16 Fecal smear from a woman who had recently traveled to India and developed severe diarrhea. Trophozoites of *Entamoeba histolytica (arrows)* and *Giardia (arrowheads)* are present. Trichrome stain. (Courtesy Dr. Patricia Conrad.)

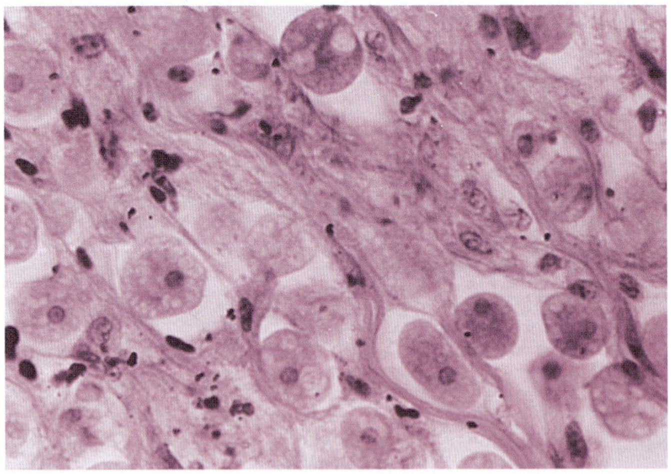

Fig. 105.17 Numerous *Entamoeba histolytica* trophozoites in a section from the wall of a human colon. Each organism contains a single, darkly stained nucleus; in some of the trophozoites, pale vacuoles are apparent (hematoxylin and eosin stain, ×540).

The life cycle is believed to involve ingestion of a cyst form, with excystation in the large intestine. The cyst then transforms into a vacuolar form which then encysts and is excreted. Risk factors in humans for infection have included immunocompromise, travel to and residence within developing countries, and exposure to contaminated food and water. Several investigators have examined subtypes of *Blastocystis* spp. in companion animals because of interest in the possibility of zoonotic transmission.[101,102] Cysts can be identified in wet mounts as irregular structures (2–25 μm in diameter) with barely discernable organelles, an outer rim of cytoplasm, and a central vacuole (Fig. 105.18A). They can be stained with Lugol's iodine, Wright, or trichrome stains (Fig. 105.18B). The internal structures are more discernable using electron microscopy (Fig. 105.18C). PCR-based assays have also been developed for their detection. Identification of *Blastocystis* spp. organisms in canine and feline fecal specimens should be considered an incidental finding.

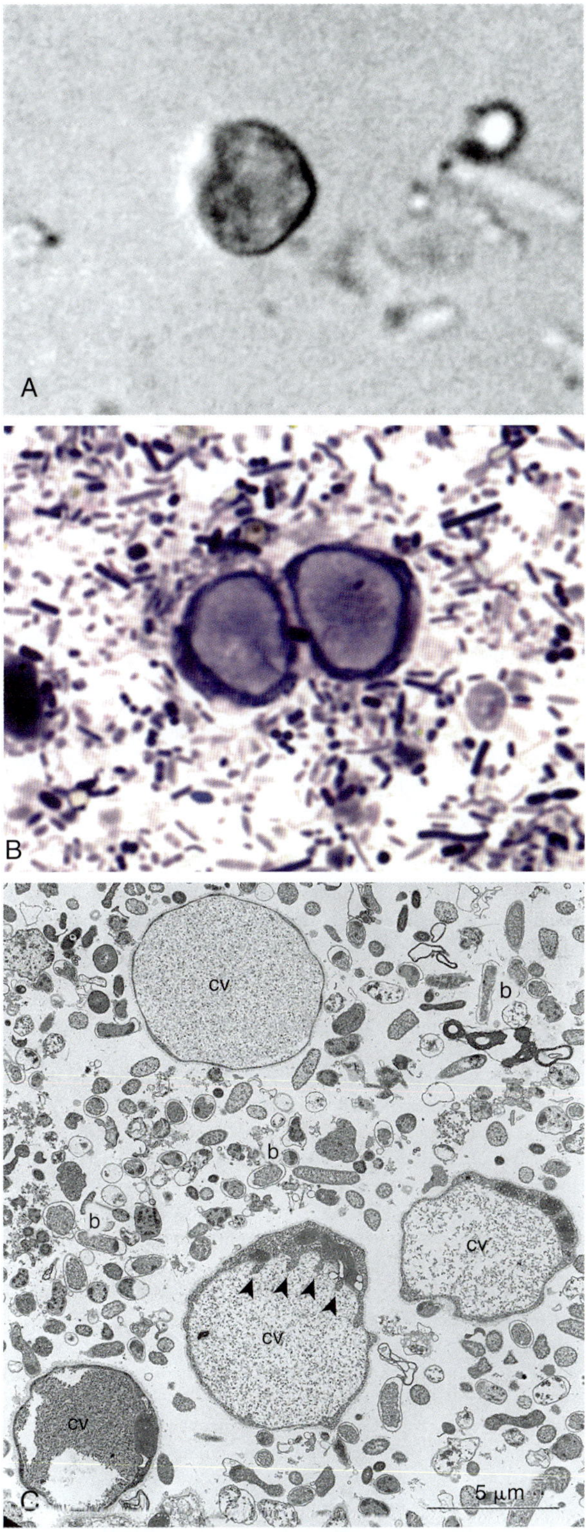

Fig. 105.18 *Blastocystis* sp. in canine fecal material. (A) Unstained wet mount (×1000). (B) Diff-Quik stain (×1000). (C) Transmission electron micrograph showing cell morphology. Variability is noted in the central vacuolar (*cv*) contents. One cell shows projections of the cytoplasm (*arrowheads*) into the central vacuole. Numerous bacteria (*b*) are present in the culture. (A and C, Courtesy Deborah Stenzel, Queensland University of Technology, Brisbane, Australia.)

CASE EXAMPLE

Signalment

"Luna", 10-month-old female German shepherd dog from Porto Alegre, RS, Brazil.

History

Luna's owner reported a 6-day history of lethargy and progressive inappetence. Two days before evaluation the owner noted diarrhea containing fresh blood, and bleeding from the tips of Luna's ears. Luna lived on a hobby farm with frequent exposure to ticks, and her owner had removed some engorged ticks from Luna before taking her to the clinic. She had never traveled out of her local area, and was up to date on vaccinations.

Physical Examination Findings

Luna was weak and quiet, and estimated to be 10% dehydrated. T = 104.5°F (40.3°C), with icteric mucous membranes. There was no evidence of ectoparasites. Peripheral lymphadenomegaly was present. Abdominal palpation revealed splenomegaly and a fluid-filled intestinal tract. Bloody diarrhea was present on the thermometer. There was extensive hemorrhagic crusting on the outer surface of the pinnae, and excessive bleeding from a venipuncture site was noted.

Laboratory Findings

CBC: HCT 20% (40–55%), MCV 80 fL (65–75 fL), MCHC 32.5 g/dL (33–36 g/dL), WBC 11,900 cells/μL (6000–13,000 cells/μL), neutrophils 6188 cells/μL (3000–10,500 cells/μL), lymphocytes 3808 cells/μL (1000–4000 cells/μL), monocytes 1904 cells/μL (150–1200 cells/μL), platelets 58,000 platelets/μL (150,000–400,000 platelets/μL). Blood smear evaluation revealed intraerythrocytic merozoites consistent with *Rangelia vitalii*.

Diagnosis: Rangeliosis

Treatment

Diminazene aceturate (3.5 mg/kg IM, single dose), immunosuppressive doses of glucocorticoids for 1 week and supportive treatment.

Comments

Rangeliosis was suspected in this case because of the geographic location (southern Brazil), clinical signs (especially bleeding from the tips of the pinnae), and history of tick exposure. Although examination of peripheral blood smears is not a sensitive diagnostic procedure, the diagnosis was confirmed in this case based on cytological examination. The probability of finding the parasite is higher when blood is collected during an episode of high fever, as was present in this case. After 36 hours Luna showed clinical improvement, and made a full recovery in 3 weeks.

SUGGESTED READINGS

Franca RT, Da Silva AS, Loretti AP, et al. Canine rangeliosis due to *Rangelia vitalii*: from first report in Brazil in 1910 to current day - a review. *Ticks Tick Borne Dis.* 2014;5:466–474.

Foreman O, Sykes J, Ball L, et al. Disseminated infection with *Balamuthia mandrillaris* in a dog. *Vet Pathol.* 2004;41:506–510.

Gompf SG, Garcia C. Lethal encounters: the evolving spectrum of amoebic meningoencephalitis. *ID Cases.* 2019;15:e00524.

REFERENCES

1. Carini A. Notícias sobre zoonoses observadas no Brasil. *Rev Méd São Paulo.* 1908;22:459–462.
2. Lemos TD, Cerqueira Ade M, Toma HK, et al. Detection and molecular characterization of piroplasms species from naturally infected dogs in southeast Brazil. *Rev Bras Parasitol Vet.* 2012;21:137–142.

3. Soares JF, Girotto A, Brandao PE, et al. Detection and molecular characterization of a canine piroplasm from Brazil. *Vet Parasitol.* 2011;180:203–208.
4. Fighera RA, Souza TM, Kommers GG, et al. Pathogenesis, clinical, hematological, and pathological aspects of *Rangelia vitalii* infection in 35 dogs (1985-2009). *Pesq Vet Bras.* 2010;30:974–987.
5. Loretti AP, Barros SS. Parasitismo por *Rangelia vitalli* em cães ("nambiuvú", "peste de sangue") - uma revisão crítica sobre o assunto. *Arq Inst Biol.* 2004;71:101–131.
6. França RT, Paim FC, Silva AS, et al. *Rangelia vitalii* in dogs in southern Brazil. *Comp Clin Pathol.* 2010;19:383–387.
7. Gottlieb J, André MR, Soares JF, et al. *Rangelia vitalii, Babesia* spp. and *Ehrlichia* spp. in dogs in Passo Fundo, state of Rio Grande do Sul, Brazil. *Rev Bras Parasitol Vet.* 2016;25:172–178.
8. Lemos TD, Toma HK, Assad RQ, et al. Clinical and hematological evaluation of *Rangelia vitalii*-naturally infected dogs in southeastern Brazil. *Rev Bras Parasitol Vet.* 2017;2:307–313.
9. de Quadros RM, Soares JF, Xavier JS, et al. Natural infection of the wild canid *Lycalopex gymnocercus* by the protozoan *Rangelia vitalii*, the agent of canine rangeliosis. *J Wildl Dis.* 2015;51:787–789.
10. Silva MRLD, Mattoso CRS, Costa A, et al. *Rangelia vitalii* and *Hepatozoon canis* coinfection in pampas fox *Lycalopex gymnocercus* from Santa Catarina State, Brazil. *Rev Bras Parasitol Vet.* 2018;27:377–383.
11. Silveira JA, D'Elia ML, de Oliveira Avelar I, et al. *Rangelia vitalii* in a free-ranging maned wolf (*Chrysocyon brachyurus*) and co-infections. *Int J Parasitol Parasites Wildl.* 2016;5:280–285.
12. Soares JF, Dall'Agnol B, Costa FB, et al. Natural infection of the wild canid, *Cerdocyon thous*, with the piroplasmid *Rangelia vitalii* in Brazil. *Vet Parasitol.* 2014;202:156–163.
13. Fredo G, Bianchi MV, De Andrade CP, et al. Natural infection of wild canids (*Cerdocyon thous* and *Lycalopex gymnocercus*) with the intraendothelial piroplasm *Rangelia vitalii* in southern Brazil. *J Wildl Dis.* 2015;51:880–884.
14. de Souza VK, Dall'Agnol B, Souza UA, et al. Detection of *Rangelia vitalii* (Piroplasmida: Babesiidae) in asymptomatic free-ranging wild canids from the Pampa biome, Brazil. *Parasitol Res.* 2019;118:1337–1342.
15. Paim FC, dos Santos AP, do Nascimento NC, et al. Development of a quantitative PCR for the detection of *Rangelia vitalii. Vet Parasitol.* 2016;217:113–117.
16. Eiras DF, Craviotto MB, Baneth G, et al. First report of *Rangelia vitalii* infection (canine rangeliosis) in Argentina. *Parasitol Int.* 2014;63:729–734.
17. Loretti AP, Barros SS. Hemorrhagic disease in dogs infected with an unclassified intraendothelial piroplasm in southern Brazil. *Vet Parasitol.* 2005;134:193–213.
18. Pestana BR. O nambyuvú (nota preliminar). *Rev Soc Cientif São Paulo.* 1910;5:14–17.
19. Pestana BR. O nambyuvú. *Rev Med São Paulo.* 1910;22:423–426.
20. Carini A, Maciel J. Sobre a molestia dos cães, chamada nambiuvú, e o seu parasita (*Rangelia vitalii*). *Ann Paul Med Cir.* 1914;3:65–71.
21. Pocai EA, Frozza L, Headley SA, et al. Leishmaniose visceral (calazar): cinco casos em cães de Santa Maria, Rio Grande do Sul, Brasil. *Cienc Rural.* 1998;28:501–505.
22. Franca RT, Da Silva AS, Loretti AP, et al. Canine rangeliosis due to *Rangelia vitalii*: from first report in Brazil in 1910 to current day - a review. *Ticks Tick Borne Dis.* 2014;5:466–474.
23. Kruaspenhar C, Fighera RA, Graça DL. Anemia hemolítica em cães associada a protozoários. *Rev Cient Med Vet Peq Anim Anim Estimação – MEDVEP.* 2003;1:273–281.
24. Carini A. Sobre o ciclo de desenvolvimento exoeritrocítico de um piroplasma de cão. *Arq Biol.* 1948;285:49–52.
25. Franca RT, Da Silva AS, Costa MM, et al. Hematologic and bone marrow changes in dogs experimentally infected with *Rangelia vitalii. Vet Clin Pathol.* 2013;42:31–39.
26. Paim CB, Paim FC, Da Silva AS, et al. Thrombocytopenia and platelet activity in dogs experimentally infected with *Rangelia vitalii. Vet Parasitol.* 2012;185:131–137.
27. Silva BRD, Ferreira MFK, Maffezzolli G, et al. Detection molecular of *Rangelia vitalii* in dogs from Parana State, Southern Brazil. *Rev Bras Parasitol Vet.* 2019;28:310–313.
28. Borras P, Salvador F, Rinaldi V, et al. Use of molecular tools for the diagnosis of rangeliosis by *Rangelia vitalii* in Argentina: a case report. *Vet Parasitol Reg Stud Reports.* 2020;21:100426.
29. Soares JF, Carvalho L, Maya L, et al. Molecular detection of *Rangelia vitalii* in domestic dogs from Uruguay. *Vet Parasitol.* 2015;210:98–101.
30. Inácio EL, Pérez-Macchi S, Alabi A, et al. Prevalence and molecular characterization of piroplasmids in domestic dogs from Paraguay. *Ticks Tick Borne Dis.* 2019;10:321–327.
31. Soares JF. *História Natural da Rangeliose.* São Paulo: Faculdade de Medicina Veterinária e Zootecnia, Universidade de São Paulo; 2014. Thesis.
32. Soares JF, Costa FB, Girotto-Soares A, et al. Evaluation of the vector competence of six ixodid tick species for *Rangelia vitalii* (Apicomplexa, Piroplasmorida), the agent of canine rangeliosis. *Ticks Tick Borne Dis.* 2018;9:1221–1234.
33. Campos SDE, Toma HK, Machado CSC, et al. Novel record of a tick *Amblyomma sculptum* with detection of piroplasm *Rangelia vitalii* DNA. *Vet Parasitol Reg Stud Reports.* 2018;13:228–229.
34. Guglielmone AA, Estrada-Pena A, Mangold AJ, et al. *Amblyomma aureolatum* (Pallas, 1772) and *Amblyomma ovale* Koch, 1844 (Acari: Ixodidae): hosts, distribution and 16S rDNA sequences. *Vet Parasitol.* 2003;113:273–288.
35. Copat B, Bastiani PV, Castellarin Jaconi F, et al. Presentation of hemolytic and hemorrhagic rangeliosis in *Cerdocyon thous. Ticks Tick Borne Dis.* 2019;10:690–693.
36. França RT, Pillat MM, da Silva CB, et al. Surface immunoglobulins of erythrocytes and platelets in dogs naturally infected by *Rangelia vitalii. Microb Pathog.* 2018;121:245–251.
37. Paim CB, Da Silva AS, Paim FC, et al. Activities of ectonucleotidases and adenosine deaminase in platelets of dogs experimentally infected with *Rangelia vitalii. Exp Parasitol.* 2012;131:252–257.
38. Costa MM, Franca RT, Da Silva AS, et al. *Rangelia vitalii*: changes in the enzymes ALT, CK and AST during the acute phase of experimental infection in dogs. *Rev Bras Parasitol Vet.* 2012;21:243–248.
39. Fighera RA. Rangeliose. *Acta Sci Vet.* 2007;35:261–263.
40. Paim FC, Da Silva AS, Paim CB, et al. Serum proteinogram, acute phase proteins and immunoglobulins in dogs experimentally infected with *Rangelia vitalii. Vet Parasitol.* 2013;192:137–142.
41. Da Silva AS, Martins DB, Soares JF, et al. Canine rangeliosis: the need for differential diagnosis. *Parasitol Res.* 2013;112:1329–1332.
42. Da Silva AS, Franca RT, Costa MM, et al. Experimental infection with *Rangelia vitalii* in dogs: acute phase, parasitemia, biological cycle, clinical-pathological aspects and treatment. *Exp Parasitol.* 2011;128:347–352.
43. Carini A, Maciel JJ. Contribuição ao tratamento do nanbyuvú pelo trypamblau. *Rev Vet Zoot.* 1914;1:63–64.
44. Irwin P. Babesiosis and cytauxzoonosis. In: Day MJ, ed. *Arthropod-borne Infectious Diseases of the Dog and Cat.* 2nd ed. Abingdon: CRC Press; 2016:77–95.
45. Martinez AJ, Visvesvara GS. Free-living, amphizoic and opportunistic amebas. *Brain Pathol.* 1997;7:583–598.
46. Schuster FL, Visvesvara GS. Free-living amoebae as opportunistic and non-opportunistic pathogens of humans and animals. *Int J Parasitol.* 2004;34:1001–1027.
47. Schuster FL, Visvesvara GS. Opportunistic amoebae: challenges in prophylaxis and treatment. *Drug Resist Updat.* 2004;7:41–51.
48. Siddiqui R, Khan NA. Biology and pathogenesis of *Acanthamoeba. Parasit Vectors.* 2012;5:6.
49. Trabelsi H, Dendana F, Sellami A, et al. Pathogenic free-living amoebae: epidemiology and clinical review. *Pathologie-biologie.* 2012;60:399–405.
50. Visvesvara GS. Amebic meningoencephalitides and keratitis: challenges in diagnosis and treatment. *Curr Opin Infect Dis.* 2010;23:590–594.
51. Visvesvara GS, Moura H, Schuster FL. Pathogenic and opportunistic free-living amoebae: *Acanthamoeba* spp., *Balamuthia mandrillaris, Naegleria fowleri*, and *Sappinia diploidea. FEMS Immunol Med Microbiol.* 2007;50:1–26.

52. Vodkin MH, Howe DK, Visvesvara GS, et al. Identification of *Acanthamoeba* at the generic and specific levels using the polymerase chain reaction. *J Protozool.* 1992;39:378–385.
53. Fuerst PA, Booton GC, Crary M. Phylogenetic analysis and the evolution of the 18S rRNA gene typing system of *Acanthamoeba. J Euk Microbiol.* 2015;62:69–84.
54. Booton GC, Visvesvara GS, Byers TJ, et al. Identification and distribution of *Acanthamoeba* species genotypes associated with nonkeratitis infections. *J Clin Microbiol.* 2005;43:1689–1693.
55. Carlesso AM, Mentz MB, da Machado ML, et al. Characterization of isolates of *Acanthamoeba* from the nasal mucosa and cutaneous lesions of dogs. *Curr Microbiol.* 2014;68:702–707.
56. Lorenzo-Morales J, Valladares M, Sancho J, et al. First report of a case of prostatitis due to *Acanthamoeba* in a dog. *Acta Protozool.* 2013;52:325.
57. Valladares M, Reyes-Batlle M, Martin-Navarro CM, et al. Molecular characterization of *Acanthamoeba* strains isolated from domestic dogs in Tenerife, Canary Islands, Spain. *Arch Microbiol.* 2015;197:639–643.
58. Valladares M, Reyes-Batlle M, Mora-Peces I, et al. A multisystemic *Acanthamoeba* infection in a dog in Tenerife, Canary Islands, Spain. *Vet Parasitol.* 2014;205:707–711.
59. Karakus M, Aykur M, Ozbel Y, et al. Molecular detection and genotyping of *Acanthamoeba* spp. among stray dogs using conjunctival swab sampling. *Acta Trop.* 2016;164:23–26.
60. Dubey JP, Benson JE, Blakeley KT, et al. Disseminated *Acanthamoeba* sp. infection in a dog. *Vet Parasitol.* 2005;128:183–187.
61. Kent M, Platt SR, Rech RR, et al. Multisystemic infection with an *Acanthamoeba* sp in a dog. *J Am Vet Med Assoc.* 2011;238:1476–1481.
62. Greene CE, Howerth EW, Kent M. Nonenteric amebiasis: Acanthamebiasis, hartmannelliasis, and balamuthiasis. In: Greene CE, ed. *Infectious Diseases of the Dog and Cat.* 4th ed. St. Louis, MO: Elsevier/Saunders; 2012:1354.
63. Gonzalez P, Carbonell E, Urios V, et al. Coprology of *Panthera tigris altaica* and *Felis bengalensis euptilurus* from the Russian Far East. *J Parasitol.* 2007;93:948–950.
64. Greub G. *Parachlamydia acanthamoebae*, an emerging agent of pneumonia. *Clin Microbiol Infect.* 2009;15:18–28.
65. Fritsche TR, Gautom RK, Seyedirashti S, et al. Occurrence of bacterial endosymbionts in *Acanthamoeba* spp. isolated from corneal and environmental specimens and contact lenses. *J Clin Microbiol.* 1993;31:1122–1126.
66. Fritsche TR, Horn M, Wagner M, et al. Phylogenetic diversity among geographically dispersed Chlamydiales endosymbionts recovered from clinical and environmental isolates of *Acanthamoeba* spp. *Appl Environ Microbiol.* 2000;66:2613–2619.
67. von Bomhard W, Polkinghorne A, Lu ZH, et al. Detection of novel chlamydiae in cats with ocular disease. *Am J Vet Res.* 2003;64:1421–1428.
68. von Bomhard W, Pospischil A, Richter M, et al. Amoebic infections in cats with ocular disease. *Vet Rec.* 2002;150:556.
69. Richter M, Matheis F, Gonczi E, et al. *Parachlamydia acanthamoebae* in domestic cats with and without corneal disease. *Vet Ophthalmol.* 2010;13:235–237.
70. Marciano-Cabral F. Free-living amoebae as agents of human infection. *J Infect Dis.* 2009;199:1104–1106.
71. Chien RC, Telford CR, Roy S, et al. Canine amoebic meningoencephalitis due to *Balamuthia mandrillaris. Vet Parasitol Reg Stud Reports.* 2018;13:156–159.
72. Foreman O, Sykes J, Ball L, et al. Disseminated infection with *Balamuthia mandrillaris* in a dog. *Vet Pathol.* 2004;41:506–510.
73. Finnin PJ, Visvesvara GS, Campbell BE, et al. Multifocal *Balamuthia mandrillaris* infection in a dog in Australia. *Parasitol Res.* 2007,100. 423–426.
74. Hodge PJ, Kelers K, Gasser RB, et al. Another case of canine amoebic meningoencephalitis—the challenges of reaching a rapid diagnosis. *Parasitol Res.* 2011;108:1069–1073.
75. Bauer RW, Harrison LR, Watson CW, et al. Isolation of *Acanthamoeba* sp. from a greyhound with pneumonia and granulomatous amebic encephalitis. *J Vet Diagn Invest.* 1993;5:386–391.
76. Ayers KM, Billups LH, Garner FM. Acanthamoebiasis in a dog. *Vet Pathol.* 1972;9:221–226.
77. Brofman PJ, Knostman KA, DiBartola SP. Granulomatous amebic meningoencephalitis causing the syndrome of inappropriate secretion of antidiuretic hormone in a dog. *J Vet Intern Med.* 2003;17:230–234.
78. Pearce JR, Powell HS, Chandler FW, et al. Amebic meningoencephalitis caused by *Acanthamoeba castellani* in a dog. *J Am Vet Med Assoc.* 1985;187:951–952.
79. Reed LT, Miller MA, Visvesvara GS, et al. Diagnostic exercise. Cerebral mass in a puppy with respiratory distress and progressive neurologic signs. *Vet Pathol.* 2010;47:1116–1119.
80. Ithoi I, Mahmud R, Abdul Basher MH, et al. *Acanthamoeba* genotype T4 detected in naturally-infected feline corneas found to be in homology with those causing human keratitis. *Trop Biomed.* 2013;30:131–140.
81. Kiderlen AF, Laube U. *Balamuthia mandrillaris*, an opportunistic agent of granulomatous amebic encephalitis, infects the brain via the olfactory nerve pathway. *Parasitol Res.* 2004;94:49–52.
82. Beckwith-Cohen B, Gasper DJ, Bentley E, et al. Protozoal infections of the cornea and conjunctiva in dogs associated with chronic ocular surface disease and topical immunosuppression. *Vet Ophthalmol.* 2016;19:206–213.
83. Qvarnstrom Y, Nerad TA, Visvesvara GS. Characterization of a new pathogenic *Acanthamoeba* species, *A. byersi* n. sp., isolated from a human with fatal amoebic encephalitis. *J Euk Microbiol.* 2013;60:626–633.
84. Yagi S, Schuster FL, Visvesvara GS. Demonstration of *Balamuthia* and *Acanthamoeba* mitochondrial DNA in sectioned archival brain and other tissues by the polymerase chain reaction. *Parasitol Res.* 2008;102:211–217.
85. Culbertson CG. The pathogenicity of soil amebas. *Annu Rev Microbiol.* 1971;25:231–254.
86. Cabello-Vilchez AM, Martin-Navarro CM, Lopez-Arencibia A, et al. Voriconazole as a first-line treatment against potentially pathogenic *Acanthamoeba* strains from Peru. *Parasitol Res.* 2014;113:755–759.
87. Kulsoom H, Baig AM, Siddiqui R, et al. Combined drug therapy in the management of granulomatous amoebic encephalitis due to *Acanthamoeba* spp., and *Balamuthia mandrillaris. Exp Parasitol.* 2014;145(suppl):S115–120.
88. Maritschnegg P, Sovinz P, Lackner H, et al. Granulomatous amebic encephalitis in a child with acute lymphoblastic leukemia successfully treated with multimodal antimicrobial therapy and hyperbaric oxygen. *J Clin Microbiol.* 2011;49:446–448.
89. Martin-Navarro CM, Lopez-Arencibia A, Sifaoui I, et al. Statins and voriconazole induce programmed cell death in *Acanthamoeba castellanii. Antimicrob Agents Chemother.* 2015;59:2817–2824.
90. Schuster FL, Guglielmo BJ, Visvesvara GS. In-vitro activity of miltefosine and voriconazole on clinical isolates of free-living amebas: *Balamuthia mandrillaris, Acanthamoeba* spp., and *Naegleria fowleri. J Euk Microbiol.* 2006;53:121–126.
91. Kalsoom H, Baig AM, Khan NA, et al. Laboratory testing of clinically approved drugs against *Balamuthia mandrillaris. World J Microbiol Biotechnol.* 2014;30:2337–2342.
92. da Silva RKM, Dib LV, Amendoeira MR, et al. Balantidiasis in humans: a systematic review and meta-analysis. *Acta Trop.* 2021;223:106069.
93. Bailey WS, Williams AG. *Balantidium* infection in the dog. *J Am Vet Med Assoc.* 1949;114:238.
94. Ewing SA, Bull RW. Severe chronic canine diarrhea associated with *Balantidium-Trichuris* infection. *J Am Vet Med Assoc.* 1966;149:519–520.
95. Ngui R, Hassan NA, Nordin NMS, et al. Copro-molecular study of *Entamoeba* infection among the indigenous community in Malaysia: a first report on the species-specific prevalence of *Entamoeba* in dogs. *Acta Trop.* 2020;204:105334.
96. Wittnich C. *Entamoeba histolytica* infection in a German shepherd dog. *Can Vet J.* 1976;17:259–263.
97. Shimada A, Muraki Y, Awakura T, et al. Necrotic colitis associated with *Entamoeba histolytica* infection in a cat. *J Comp Pathol.* 1992;106:195–199.
98. Higuera A, Herrera G, Jimenez P, et al. Identification of multiple *Blastocystis* subtypes in domestic animals from Colombia using amplicon-based next generation sequencing. *Front Vet Sci.* 2021;8:732129.

99. Suh KN, Kozarsky P, Keystone JS. *Cyclospora cayetanensis, Cystoisospora (Isospora) belli, Sarcocystis* species, *Balantidium coli*, and *Blastocystis* species. In: Bennett JE, Dolin R, Blaser MJ, eds. *Mandell, Douglas and Bennett's Principles and Practice of Infectious Diseases*. Philadelphia, PA: Elsevier Saunders; 2015:3184–3191.
100. Beghini F, Pasolli E, Truong TD, et al. Large-scale comparative metagenomics of *Blastocystis*, a common member of the human gut microbiome. *ISME J*. 2017;11:2848–2863.
101. Gazzonis AL, Marangi M, Zanzani SA, et al. Molecular epidemiology of *Blastocystis* sp. in dogs housed in Italian rescue shelters. *Parasitol Res*. 2019;118:3011–3017.
102. Paulos S, Koster PC, de Lucio A, et al. Occurrence and subtype distribution of *Blastocystis* sp. in humans, dogs and cats sharing household in northern Spain and assessment of zoonotic transmission risk. *Zoonoses Public Health*. 2018;65:993–1002.

SECTION 5

Metazoan Parasites and Parasitic Diseases

Susan E. Little

Metazoan parasites include some of the most common and medically important pathogens of dogs and cats. In the absence of careful, consistent control strategies, both external parasites (e.g., fleas, ticks, mites; Chapters 106–110) and internal parasites (e.g., intestinal helminths, heartworm; Chapters 111–118) can quickly become established in companion animals, leading to poor body condition, disease, and, in severe cases, death. Fortunately, well cared for pets maintained on preventives are unlikely to develop clinical disease due to parasites; however, because many dogs and most cats are not routinely treated, the conditions caused by these preventable infections and infestations remain familiar to those in general practice. In addition, less commonly encountered parasites of dogs and cats, including gastrointestinal nematodes like *Physaloptera* or *Strongyloides stercoralis*, lungworms, and trematodes (Chapter 116–118) occasionally infect and cause clinical signs in pets. Diagnosis of a parasitic infection or infestation is readily achieved by identifying the organisms directly; examining skin scrapes, blood, or feces by microscopy; or detecting antigen using widely available commercial tests (Chapter 5).

The goal of Section 5 is to convey the relevant features of epidemiology and natural history that lead to the presence of each of the most common types of parasites in dogs and cats and to explain some key strategies for effective diagnosis, treatment, and prevention. These organisms can also create a zoonotic risk, so public health issues associated with parasites are discussed in each chapter. A related risk not always fully appreciated in clinical practice is the damage parasites can cause to the human-animal bond; because most pet owners find metazoan parasites unpleasant or repulsive, effective control strategies are critically important in fostering and maintaining a close relationship between pets and their owners. Ideally, pets would be protected from parasites through careful management to limit infection risk and routine use of preventives. However, because these organisms are almost ubiquitous, and because many pets do not receive veterinary care, eliminating infection risk is all but impossible. Thus, although prevention is the preferred strategy, a second goal of Section 5 is to provide an overview of the best treatments currently available to clear parasites from pets when they occur and to limit, to the extent possible, the pathology caused by these infections and infestations. Parasite treatment is also covered comprehensively in Chapters 12 and 13.

106

Fleas and Lice

Susan E. Little

KEY POINTS

Fleas

- First Described: Familiar since antiquity, fleas (*Pulex irritans, Tunga penetrans*) were first described in the 10th edition of *Systema Naturae* published by Linnaeus in 1758. *Ctenocephalides canis* was first described by Curtis in 1826, *Ctenocephalides felis* by Bouché in 1835, *Echidnophaga gallinacea* by Westwood in 1875, and *Pulex simulans* by Baker in 1895.
- Cause: *Ctenocephalides felis* (cat flea) most common on dogs and cats worldwide; also *Ctenocephalides canis* (dog flea), *Echidnophaga gallinacea* (sticktight flea), *Pulex* spp. (human flea), *Xenopsylla cheopis* (rat flea) (family Pulicidae, order Siphonaptera); *Tunga penetrans* (chigoe flea, jigger) (family Hectopsyllidae (formerly Tungidae), order Siphonaptera).
- Affected Hosts: Dogs, cats, other domestic animals, and peridomestic wildlife.
- Geographic Distribution: Most fleas of companion animals (*Ctenocephalides* spp., *Pulex* spp., *E. gallinacea*) are found worldwide, sparing high altitude and arid regions; *T. penetrans* is native to the Caribbean, Central America, and South America, and has been introduced to and established in sub-Saharan Africa, especially East Africa, and India.
- Primary Mode of Transmission: Infestations are most often acquired through direct contact with emerging fleas from pupae in the environment. Fleas are persistent or permanent ectoparasites of the host; although considered a secondary infestation route, a few fleas may occasionally move directly from an infested animal to another animal in close, prolonged proximity.
- Major Clinical Signs: Pruritus; anemia; flea allergy dermatitis consisting of tail head or abdominal alopecia, seborrhea, pyotraumatic dermatitis, and secondary infections (dogs); or miliary dermatitis especially around the neck (cats). Pruritus may be the primary clinical sign or, in some flea-infested animals, absent. Direct evidence of flea infestation (fleas, flea frass) is absent in the majority of dogs and cats with flea allergy dermatitis. Fleas also serve as vectors for common pathogens, including *Bartonella* spp. and *Dipylidium caninum*.
- Differential Diagnoses: Atopic dermatitis; dermatophytosis, bacterial pyoderma, *Malassezia* dermatitis, mite infestations (*Cheyletiella* spp., *Demodex* spp., *Notoedres cati, Otodectes cynotis, Sarcoptes scabiei, Lynxacarus radovskyi*), lice infestation, mosquito allergy, cutaneous adverse food reactions, autoimmune disease.
- Human Health Significance: Humans, especially those sharing a home with infested pets, are at risk of experiencing flea bites, particularly on the feet, ankles, and lower legs. The bites occur when adult fleas emerge from pupae and feed on humans instead of pets. Children less than 10 years of age are particularly likely to develop a localized allergic reaction to the bites.

Lice (pediculosis)

- First Described: *Trichodectes canis* was first described in 1778 by De Geer. *Linognathus setosus* was described in 1816 by von Olfers, and *Heterodoxus spiniger* by Enderlein in 1909. *Felicola subrostratus* was first described in 1838 by Burmeister as *Trichodectes subrostratus* and moved to a newly erected genus, *Felicola*, by Ewing in 1929.
- Cause: Dogs: *Trichodectes canis, Linognathus setosus, Heterodoxus spiniger*; cats: *Felicola subrostratus* (family T*richodectidae* [*T. canis, F. subrostratus*], *Boopiidae* [*H. spiniger*], and *Linognathidae* [*L. setosus*], order Psocodea, clade Phthiraptera.
- Affected Hosts: Dogs and closely related wild canids (coyotes, wolves) are infested with *T. canis* and *L. setosus. Heterodoxus spiniger* evolved on dingo hosts but is now found on domestic dogs and other wild canids (jackals, coyotes, wolves, foxes), and occasionally on cats, primarily in warmer areas of the world. Domestic cats are hosts for *F. subrostratus.*
- Geographic Distribution: Lice are found on dogs and cats worldwide although prevalence and species composition vary by geography and climate. Lice are more common in free-roaming populations and in dogs and cats not regularly treated with ectoparasiticides. Some species (e.g., *T. canis*) are more common in colder areas, while others (*H. spiniger*) predominate in warmer regions.
- Primary Mode of Transmission: Infestations are acquired through direct contact between animals, including from dam to nursing young in the neonatal period. Lice may also be spread through fomites (e.g., brushes, bedding). All stages of the louse life cycle are found on the host.
- Major Clinical Signs: Pruritus; alopecia; anemia (*L. setosus*); presence of eggs (nits) adherent to and different stages of lice grasping the hair shaft.
- Differential Diagnoses: Flea allergy dermatitis; atopic dermatitis; dermatophytosis, bacterial pyoderma, *Malassezia* dermatitis, mite infestations (*Cheyletiella* spp., *Demodex* spp., *Notoedres cati, Otodectes cynotis, Sarcoptes scabiei, Lynxacarus radovskyi*), mosquito allergy, cutaneous adverse food reactions, autoimmune disease.
- Human Health Significance: None. Lice are host-specific parasites, and people acquire lice from other people, not from pets or from an environment with pets.

FLEAS: *CTENOCEPHALIDES* SPP.

ETIOLOGY AND EPIDEMIOLOGY

Despite decades of safe, effective control products, the cat flea (*Ctenocephalides felis*) remains the most important ectoparasite of dogs and cats and infestations are commonly seen even in well-cared-for pets.[1] Dogs are sometimes also infested with *Ctenocephalides canis*, the dog flea, and subspecies of *C. felis* have been described, but *Ctenocephalides felis felis* predominates on both dogs and cats in most regions worldwide and will be the focus of this chapter.[2,3] Adult *C. felis*, like all fleas, are obligatory blood feeders in the order

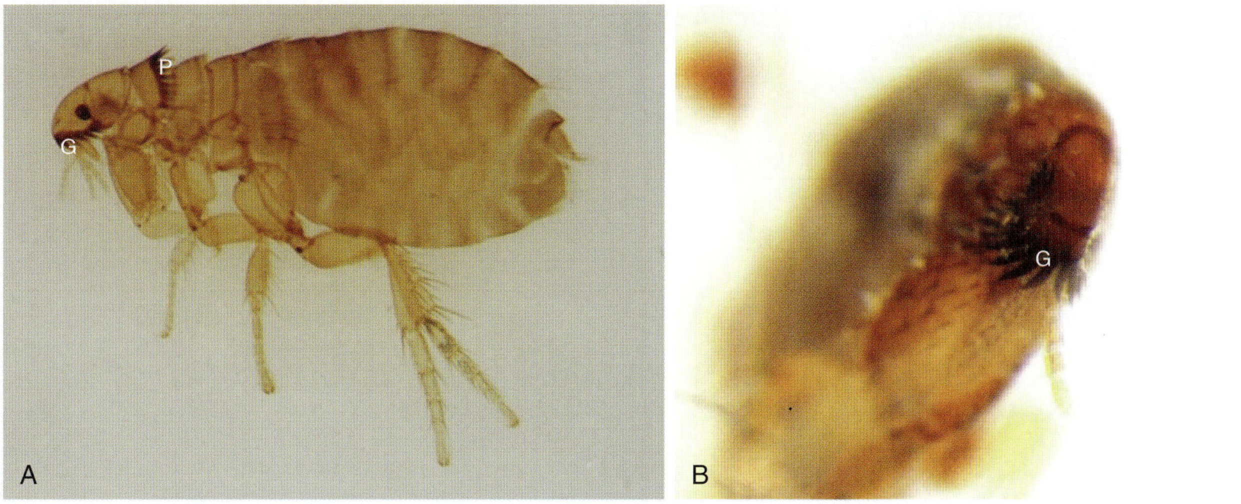

Fig. 106.1 Adult female *Ctenocephalides felis,* lateral view and en face showing genal *(G)* and pronotal *(P)* comb. (From the National Center for Veterinary Parasitology.)

Siphonaptera. They are small (1–2 mm), laterally compressed, and reddish-brown in color. Both a genal ctenidium (comb) on the anteroventral aspect of the head and a pronotal ctenidium on the first thoracic segment are present (Fig. 106.1). Although morphologically very similar, *C. felis* can be distinguished from *C. canis* by the relative length of the first genal spine, shape of the head, and number of tibial teeth.[4,5] Fleas live in the haircoat of infested animals, rarely leaving once they have located a host, and both males and females feed on capillary blood.[6,7] Fleas begin feeding almost immediately after acquiring a host, with 25% of fleas engorged after 5 minutes and all fed in the first hour.[8]

Mating occurs within 8 to 24 hours of initial infestation and most females are mated by 34 hours. Egg production can be initiated as soon as 24 to 36 hours after the first blood meal and peaks 4 to 9 days after infestation, with each female producing 40 to 50 eggs per day during peak reproduction. If not removed by host grooming, 85% of females and 58% of males will survive on the host at least 50 days, and a few continue to persist for more than 100 days.[2,6,9] However, host grooming is a major source of flea mortality, with approximately 4% to 18% of fleas removed each day. Accordingly, the longevity of fleas on the host averages 7.8 days.[10] Flea-allergic cats remove a higher number of fleas than nonallergic cats; egg production is also reduced in female fleas fed on allergic cats.[11]

Eggs begin to fall from the host once dry (~2–8 hours after oviposition occurs), accumulating in the carpet, soil, or other substrate where the pet spends most of its time. The first instar larvae hatch and molt to second and third instars in the environment, feeding on flea feces that has also fallen from the haircoat. Flea eggs are also a major source of nutrition for maturing larvae, with some estimates suggesting that each larva may consume more than 20 eggs as it develops.[12,13] Larvae usually develop near where eggs are deposited, with most migrating < 15 cm; larvae are susceptible to desiccation and negatively phototactic, burrowing to the base of carpet or below sandy soil to develop. Mortality of immature stages is high; a majority do not develop to adult fleas.[2] Once fully mature, third instar larvae develop a pupal case to which debris often adheres (Fig. 106.2) and begin the process of metamorphosis to the adult flea. Adults emerge from the pupal case upon sensing host cues such as warmth or mechanical pressure. Females usually emerge before males. Newly emerged adults immediately seek a host and begin to feed and mate.[2] The timing of the life cycle is variable but can be completed in 3 to 8 weeks. Development from egg to adult fleas is faster in warmer

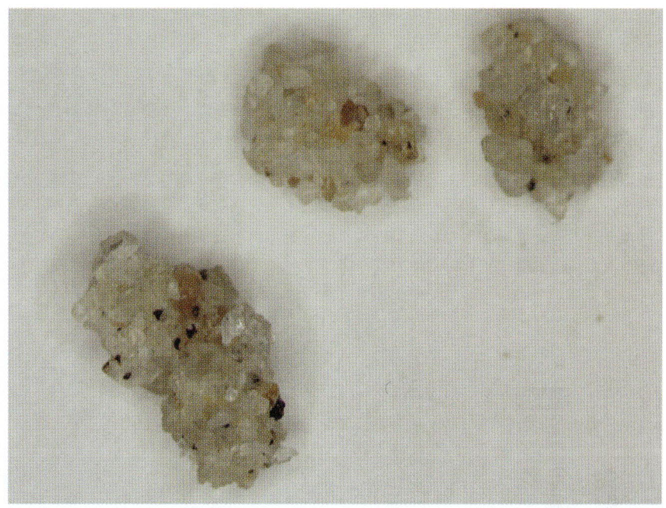

Fig. 106.2 Pupae of *Ctenocephalides felis.* Note the debris adherent to the pupal case. (From the National Center for Veterinary Parasitology.)

months (20 to 24 days) than in the winter (36 to 50 days); if protected in the environment under soil, vegetation, or leaf litter, pupae can survive frosts and some adults may emerge > 5 months after egg production.[14,15] In warmer areas, larvae can also survive outdoors year-round.[15,16] Several excellent comprehensive reviews of biology and life history of cat fleas are available.[1–3,6,15]

In most surveys, *C. felis* is the most common ectoparasite collected from free-roaming and pet dogs and cats. In warmer areas, prevalence of infestation in free-roaming animals exceeds 50% and, for some populations, approaches 100% (Tables 106.1 and 106.2); in temperate areas, 9.2%–25.6% of pet cats and 4.4%–16.3% of pet dogs seen at veterinary practices have evidence of flea infestation.[17–20] Prevalence of infestation is usually higher in cats than in dogs in the same region, and although seasonal patterns are evident and infestations peak in summer and early fall, fleas can be found throughout the year.[18,20–22] Risk factors for infestation in pet dogs and cats include outdoor access, failure to administer any flea control product, and multipet households.[18,20,23,24] In areas where *C. felis* occurs, flea allergy dermatitis (FAD) is often the most common allergic dermatologic disease of dogs and cats seen.[25–27]

TABLE 106.1 Representative Surveys Reporting Prevalence of Fleas and Lice on Free-Roaming and Pet Dogs[a]

Geographic Location	Parasite	Species	Prevalence (%)	Lifestyle
Malawi	Fleas	*Ctenocephalides* sp.	98.0	F
	Lice	*Trichodectes canis*	25	
Ethiopia	Fleas	*Ctenocephalides felis*	95	F
	Licc	*Pulcx irritans*	20.5	
		Echidnophaga gallinacea	9	
		Xenopsylla cheopis	0.5	
		Heterodoxus spiniger	5	
		Linognathus setosus	1.5	
		Tr. canis	0.5	
Thailand	Fleas	*C. felis*	86.2	F
	Lice	*E. gallinacea*	1.	
		H. spiniger	7.4	
Korea	Fleas	*C. canis*	6.8	F
	Lice	*Tr. canis*	1.0	
Malawi	Fleas	*Ctenocephalides* sp.	35.0	P
	Lice	*Tr. canis*	10	
Brazil	Fleas	*C. felis*	64.4	P
	Lice	*Rhopalopsyllus lutzi*	4.0	
		Tunga penetrans	2.0	
		Tr. canis	7.9	
Nigeria	Fleas	*C. canis*	32.1	P
	Lice	*P. irritans*	6.6	
		T. penetrans	0.5	
		Tr. canis	10.6	
Iran	Fleas	*C. canis*	25.2	P
	Lice	*P. irritans*	4.2	
		Tr. canis	5.6	
		L. setosus	2.8	
Chile	Fleas	*C. felis*	19.1	P
		C. canis	26.0	
		P. irritans	14.5	
		E. gallinacea	1.5	
Italy	Fleas	*C. felis*	16.3	P
		C. canis	1.5	
United Kingdom (England, Scotland)	Fleas	*C. felis*	13.0	P
		C. canis	0.5	
		Spilopsyllus cuniculi	0.3	
		Archaeopsylla erinacei	0.2	
		Ceratophyllus spp.	0.3	
Albania	Fleas	*C. canis*	4.8	P
	Lice	*C. felis*	3.0	
		P. irritans	0.2	
		Tr. canis	0.2	
United States	Fleas	Flea infestation (not specified)	4.4	P

[a]Data from references 17, 19, 20, 30, 83, 93, 131–136.
F, free-roaming; *P*, pet.

Ctenocephalides felis is also commonly identified on peridomestic wildlife including opossums, foxes, coyotes, raccoons, bobcats, mustelids, and hedgehogs.[6,15] Historically, *C. canis* was identified more widely; predominance of *C. canis* persists in a few regions, including at higher altitudes.[5,18,28] Where *C. canis* is found, both *C. canis* and

TABLE 106.2 Representative Surveys Reporting Prevalence of Fleas and Lice on Free-Roaming and Pet Cats[a]

Geographic Location	Parasite	Species	Estimated Prevalence (%)	Lifestyle
United States (Florida)	Fleas	*Ctenocephalides felis*	92.5	F
		Pulex simulans	4.5	
		Echidnophaga gallinacea	5.5	
United States (Oklahoma, Kansas)	Fleas	*C. felis*	71.6%	F
	Lice	*Pulex* spp.	69.6	
		Felicola	2.0	
		subrostratus	1.0	
Ethiopia	Fleas	*C. felis*	61.7	F
		Pulex irritans	1.5	
		Xenopsylla cheopis	0.7	
Brazil	Fleas	*C. felis*	60.0	F
	Lice	*F. subrostratus*	5.4	
Israel	Fleas	*C. felis*	54.7	F
	Lice	*F. subrostratus*	14.4	
Mexico	Fleas	*C. felis*	53	F
		C. canis	18	
		P. irritans	7	
		E. gallinacea	1	
Malaysia	Fleas	*C. felis*	41.8	F
	Lice	*F. subrostratus*	7.7	
		Heterodoxus spiniger	0.4	
Greece	Fleas	*C. felis*	24.3	F
	Lice	*F. subrostratus*	0.6	
Hungary	Fleas	*C. felis*	70.7	P
	Lice	*C. canis*	3.7	
		P. irritans	2.4	
		F. subrostratus	1.2	
Albania	Fleas	*C. felis*	51.2	P
	Lice	*C. canis*	2.0	
		F. subrostratus	8.3	
United Kingdom (England, Scotland)	Fleas	*C. felis*	25.6	P
		C. canis	0.4	
		S. cuniculi	1.1	
		Archaeopsylla erinacei	0.3	
		Ctenocephalides spp.	0.4	
Europe (Austria, Belgium, France, Hungary, Italy, Romania, and Spain)	Fleas	*C. felis*	15.5	P
	Lice	*F. subrostratus*	0.9	
United States	Fleas	Flea infestation (not specified)	9.2	P

[a]Data from references 17–19, 21, 31, 49, 116, 132, 137–141.
F, free-roaming; *P*, pet.

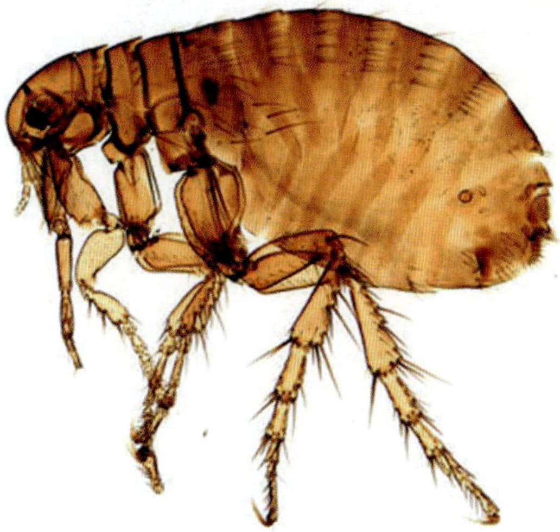

Fig. 106.3 *Pulex irritans*, the human flea, and the morphologically similar *Pulex simulans*, can be distinguished from *Ctenocephalides* spp. by the absence of genal and pronotal combs. (From the National Center for Veterinary Parasitology.)

C. felis may be recovered from dogs, while primarily *C. felis* (and some other flea genera, see below) is identified on cats.[29] In some areas, low humidity and temperatures reduce flea populations dramatically and *Ctenocephalides* spp. are rarely found. Other fleas are occasionally found on pets. Brief summaries of *Echidnophaga gallinacea*, the sticktight flea, and *Tunga penetrans*, the chigoe flea, are provided at the end of this section. Other species sometimes reported from pets or free-roaming dogs and cats but considered of minimal clinical significance include *Pulex* spp. (Fig. 106.3), *Xenopsylla cheopis*, *Cediopsylla simplex*, *Leptopsylla segnis*, *Nosopsyllus fasciatus*, and *Rhopalopsyllus lutzi*.[17,21,30,31] Representative surveys documenting the prevalence of different flea species on dogs and cats are summarized in Tables 106.1 and 106.2.

PATHOGENESIS

Adult male and female fleas feed on blood. Female *C. felis* consume 13.6 μL daily, more than 15 times their body weight, with much of it excreted incompletely digested as flea frass and available as a nutrient source to larvae in the environment.[32] Intense infestations lead to blood loss and severe, iron deficiency anemia, particularly in young kittens, puppies, and small-breed dogs; fatalities can occur.[2,3,15] Feeding fleas also inject saliva that contains histamine-like compounds and other proteins which induce localized dermal inflammation at the bite site. Histologically, a perivascular eosinophilic dermal infiltrate develops; endothelial swelling, edema, and vesicles are evident.[27]

In animals with FAD, compounds in flea saliva induce type I (immediate), type IV (delayed), and cutaneous basophil hypersensitivity reactions; up to 30% of dogs only experience a delayed reaction.[15,27] Histologic changes are nonspecific and include edema and perivascular infiltration of eosinophils.[33] In dogs, basophils may be present, peaking 4 to 18 hours after exposure.[34,35] Flea-allergic dogs also have a higher number of mast cells before flea exposure, greater eosinophil infiltration after exposure, and a higher number of IgE+ cells after exposure than nonallergic dogs.[36] Cats with FAD demonstrate antigen-induced wheal formation and infiltration of lymphocytes and mast cells in response to flea antigen.[37]

Fleas are also important disease vectors, and infested pets are at risk of infection with *Bartonella* spp. (see Chapter 70), flea-borne *Rickettsia* spp. (see Chapter 46), *Acanthocheilonema reconditum* (see Chapter 111), and *Dipylidium caninum* (see Chapter 115). *Dipylidium caninum* was detected in 2.2% and 5.2% of individual *C. felis* collected from cats and dogs, respectively; 3.1% of *C. canis* from dogs were infected.[29] Distinct canine and feline genotypes of *D. caninum* have been identified by molecular comparison of proglottids shed by dogs and cats. When cysticercoids were present in fleas collected from animals, almost all *C. felis* (>95%) and all (100%) *C. canis* and *Pulex irritans* from dogs harbored *D. caninum* canine genotype. Similarly, when infected, almost all *C. felis* (>95%) recovered from cats carried the *D. caninum* feline genotype.[38,39]

CLINICAL FEATURES

Fleas are a major cause of pruritus and allergic dermatitis. In warmer areas with high humidity, fleas can be responsible for most dermatology issues seen in primary practice. All flea bites induce some local inflammation; true FAD, or an exaggerated response to antigen in flea saliva, develops in a subset of infested animals dependent on the frequency of flea exposure and degree of hypersensitivity in a given patient.[40] Intermittent flea exposure, as occurs with irregular use of flea control, is thought to promote development of FAD.[15,27] In an animal model, both intermittently and continuously exposed dogs developed FAD although erythema developed earlier and persisted longer with intermittent exposure.[41] In dogs with simple pruritus associated with flea infestation, fleas or flea frass can often be identified at physical examination (see Diagnosis). Skin lesions vary from mild irritation to pyotraumatic dermatitis. In contrast, direct evidence of flea infestation is lacking in the majority of dogs with FAD.

No breed or sex predisposition is seen with FAD. Although age can be affected, most dogs that develop FAD are between 2 and 5 years old. Atopy may also be present, and mixed signs of atopic dermatitis and FAD are common.[27,42] In some patients, addressing the flea infestation can support resolution of other allergies.[27] Classic lesions include erythema and alopecia in the lumbosacral area and base of the tail that extend down the pelvic limbs (Fig. 106.4); in canine FAD patients, the abdomen or caudomedial aspects of the pelvic limbs may also be affected. Excoriations, crusts, lichenification, or hyperpigmentation develop over time. Many nonallergic cats tolerate flea infestations well and remain subclinically infected. Cats with FAD are more likely to be pruritic, groom excessively, and often develop miliary dermatitis on the neck and head as well as alopecia at the base of the tail, in a stripe along the dorsum, on the face, and on the legs. Eosinophilic granuloma complex can develop—indolent ulcers are present in a majority of flea-allergic cats.[27,43] In temperate areas, lesions often resolve in winter months and recur in summer and early fall.[15,27,42]

Kittens, puppies, and small-breed dogs with flea anemia are usually covered with hundreds of fleas when examined. Entire litters may be affected and the diagnosis is readily confirmed by evaluating PCV. The history often includes outdoor exposure; housing in a shed, barn, or other open structure; and lack of flea control in the dam.[15] Flea-infested animals can also develop secondary bacterial or fungal dermatitis (see Chapters 79 and 119), flea-transmitted bacterial infections (see Chapters 46, 70, and 73), or present with *A. reconditum* microfilaremia (see Chapter 111) or *D. caninum* proglottids in the feces (see Chapter 115).

DIAGNOSIS

Direct Microscopic Examination

Although many animals with pruritus due to FAD do not present with direct evidence of fleas, infestation can be confirmed in some pets by identifying adult fleas or flea frass ("flea dirt"). Close examination of the haircoat and skin is required; recovery of fleas is facilitated by use of a fine-toothed comb (32 teeth/inch) and by systematic examination of the top of head, dorsal neck and midline, left and right lateral

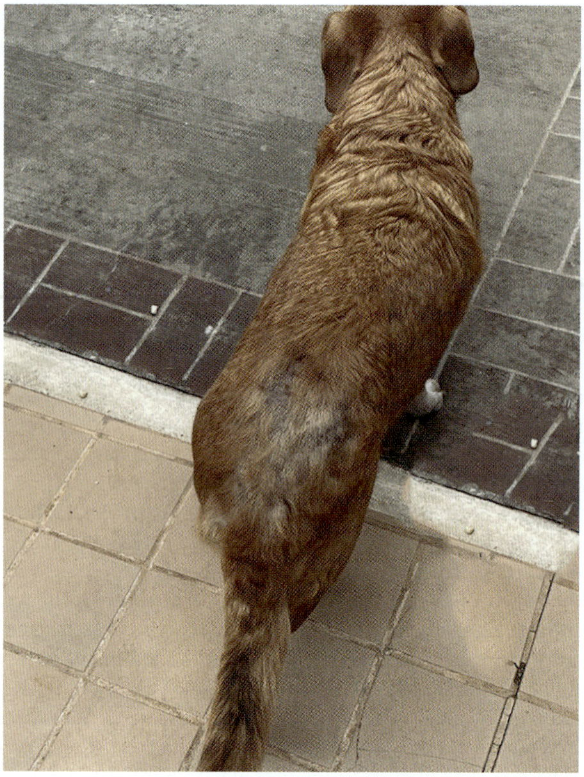

Fig. 106.4 A 5-year-old mixed breed dog with lumbosacral alopecia, excoriations, and pruritus consistent with flea allergy dermatitis.

thorax, ventral neck, and ventral midline. On cats, most fleas are found on the head and neck and the lowest number are on the tail and legs.[44] Adult fleas are approximately 3- to 4-mm long and can be adhered to clear tape and examined with a microscope. *Ctenocephalides* spp. have both a genal and pronotal comb and rounded head (see Fig. 106.1). If specific identification is desired, fleas should be placed in 70% ethanol and submitted to a parasitology laboratory. Flea frass is often present on infested pets even when adult fleas are not identified. This dark, granular or coiled material can be confirmed to be the dried blood of flea feces by placing on a white paper towel and wetting slightly to reveal the dark-red color. Glistening white eggs approximately 0.5-mm long are occasionally found on pets with an active infestation.[3,15,45]

Serology

Flea-specific IgE can be measured in serum samples although levels do not necessarily predict severity of clinical disease due to FAD. In dogs continuously exposed to fleas, IgE concentrations correspond to clinical signs of FAD, but in dogs intermittently exposed, significant IgE titers may not develop even in patients for which FAD is confirmed.[41,46]

Laboratory Abnormalities

Anemia or eosinophilia can develop in animals heavily infested with or allergic to fleas, respectively. However, these changes are less likely to be seen in dogs. In an evaluation of a canine model for FAD, blood values remained normal despite clinical, serologic, and intradermal confirmation of flea allergy.[4] In contrast, in an animal model of feline FAD, cats developed eosinophilia, and a multiyear study documented FAD in 20.5% of cats with eosinophilia.[47,48] Cats also may be more prone to anemia from fleas. In a survey of urban cats submitted to a spay/neuter program in Brazil, 12.7% of cats were anemic, most anemic cats (78.4%) were infested with fleas, and there was a significant association between anemia and flea infestation.[49]

Flea allergy can be evaluated by intradermal or blood IgE tests although a treatment trial with a highly effective flea control product is more commonly used to confirm a diagnosis in practice.[46] At least 3 months of flea control is recommended prior to intradermal skin testing for other possible allergens.[46,50] A majority of dogs with FAD have both immediate and delayed positive skin test reactions to flea antigen; approximately 30% have only mild, delayed reactions. Some normal dogs also react.[27]

Gross Pathologic Findings

Flea feeding activity on dogs results in pruritic, erythematous wheals and papules which are often crusted. Erythema is variable, and moist, pyotraumatic dermatitis or acral lick granulomas may be present.[3,15] Dogs with acute FAD develop erythematous macules, papules, which are often crusted, and self-induced alopecia due to the persistent chewing induced by the intense pruritus. Lesion pattern (lumbosacral region, base of tail, caudolateral pelvic limbs) is distinct. When FAD is chronic and untreated, lichenification and hyperpigmentation occur due to chronic pruritus.[3,15,46] Cats infested with fleas may appear normal or show evidence of mild dermal reactions and pinpoint lesions where fleas have fed. Cats with FAD also develop erythematous wheals, crusted papules, and dorsal or lumbosacral alopecia as well as miliary dermatitis on the neck and head; erythema is absent and the abdomen is usually spared.[3,15,48] Kittens and puppies with flea anemia present with pale mucous membranes.[3,15]

TREATMENT AND PROGNOSIS

Elimination of mild to moderate flea infestations can be achieved by consistently treating pets with highly effective flea adulticides; in certain situations, severe infestations may warrant also treating the environment to reduce the burden of fleas likely to emerge and speed resolution of a home infestation. When almost all adult fleas on the pet are rapidly killed, and when insecticidal efficacy of pet-administered compounds persists for several weeks, ensuring new fleas acquired from the environment will also be killed, treating the pet alone is adequate. Environmental treatment becomes important when efficacy of persistent products wanes. Numerous field studies demonstrate that pet treatment alone controls home flea infestations as long as highly effective products are consistently administered.[50–65] Several studies conducted in the same region (west central Florida, United States) over the past 25 years provide incontrovertible evidence that pet-only treatments reduce or eliminate active, severe home infestations in challenging environments although efficacy of specific compounds may have shifted over time (Table 106.3).[50–58] Resistance to some older insecticides has been described in fleas although laboratory confirmation can be difficult. When using current flea control products, lack of efficacy is more likely due to issues with administration, compliance, and continued emergence of fleas from the environment.[66]

Flea control products are discussed in detail in Chapter 13. Compounds with activity against adult fleas include fipronil, indoxacarb, isoxazolines (e.g., afoxolaner, fluralaner, lotilaner, sarolaner), neonicotinoids (e.g., dinotefuran, imidacloprid, nitenpyram), pyrethrins, pyrethroids (e.g., deltamethin, permethrin), selamectin, and spinosyns (e.g., spinetoram, spinosad). Significant adulticidal activity persists for as short as 1 day to as long as 8 months depending on the compound and formulation. Care must be taken to ensure that all pets in the household are treated; untreated pets provide a reservoir supporting continued infestation. Similarly, free-roaming dogs or cats or peridomestic wildlife can increase flea populations around the home, allowing reintroductions to occur. Insect growth regulators (e.g., methoprene, pyriproxyfen) and insect development inhibitors (e.g., lufenuron) provide added

TABLE 106.3 **Studies of Flea Control Efficacy in Naturally Infested Homes**[a]

Year Field Work Conducted	Treatment Evaluated, Administered Monthly	Reduction in Flea Count, 28-30 days (%)	Reduction in Flea Count, 54-60 days (%)	Reduction in Flea Count, 84-90 days (%)
1997	Fipronil, D, C	97.0	96.7	98.8
	Imidacloprid, D, C	97.4	100	99.1
2010	Dinotefuran / pyriproxyfen / permethrin, D	83.6	95.2	NR
	Fipronil/s-methoprene, D	88.7	95.5	NR
2013	Indoxacarb, D, C	95.0	99.1	NR
	Fipronil/(s)-methoprene, D, C	49.5	54.8	NR
2014	Afoxolaner, D	99.9	100	100
2015	Fluralaner[b], D	100	100	100
	Afoxolaner, D	99.9	99.9	100
2016	Sarolaner, D	99.7	99.9	NR
	Spinosad, D	84.6	92.0	NR
2017	Fluralaner[b], C	98.5	99.2	100
	Selamectin, C	77.8	91.0	91.3
	Fluralaner[b], D	100	100	100
	Sarolaner, D	99.9	100	100
2018	Lotilaner, D	99.6	100	NR
	Spinosad, D	98.0	100	NR
2019	Sarolaner / selamectin, C	98.5	100	100
	Flurlaner[b], C	99.5	99.9	100

[a]Data from references 49, 51-58.
[b]Administered once, per label repeat every 12 weeks.
C, cat; *D*, dog; *NR*, not reported.

support to flea control efforts by limiting development of immature fleas in the environment. Some flea adulticides also reduce production or development of eggs or larvae.[1,15] Essential oils and other plant-derived flea products have poor or unknown efficacy.[1] Several essential oils have documented toxicity and should not be applied to pets.[67–69]

Kittens and puppies with flea anemia can be treated with fast-acting, mild insecticides, and combed to remove fleas. Depending on severity, management of anemia may require supportive care, iron supplementation, or blood transfusion to allow recovery; fatalities are reported.[3] Management of FAD in both dogs and cats requires consistent administration of highly effective flea control products to all animals in the household. The identification of bacteria using skin cytology sometimes supports prescription of antimicrobials to manage secondary infections associated with FAD. If pruritus is intense, a short course of oral glucocorticoids may be helpful. When effective, persistent insecticides are used, environmental treatment is not usually necessary; skin lesions and pruritus associated with FAD are significantly reduced by flea treatment alone.[54–65] Environmental cleaning to remove immature stages can be helpful for reducing the overall flea population, allowing more rapid eradication of the infestation. When owners consistently administer effective flea control to all pets in the home, dramatic reduction or elimination of flea populations is readily achieved.

IMMUNITY

Cats and dogs do not acquire natural immunity to flea infestations, and development of a vaccine for fleas, and for arthropods in general, is challenging.[1,15,70] One study showed a modest reduction (32%–46%) in flea egg hatching success following vaccination with recombinant antigens, suggesting immunity may be able to reduce flea populations over time.[71] Immunotherapy that combines antigens from flea saliva and T-cell suppression proteins reduced FAD in cats but is not commercially available.[1,48]

PREVENTION

Preventing flea infestations on pets involves consistent use of flea control products; when flea control is not administered, active infestations lead to environmental burdens of immature fleas, including pupae, which provide a source of infestation for several months. The CAPC recommends all pets be routinely treated throughout the year. All pets in the home that can support cat fleas (i.e., dogs, cats, rabbits, ferrets) should be treated to eliminate reservoirs. Keeping cats indoors and limiting roaming in dogs reduces acquisition of new fleas from contaminated outdoor areas. Exclusion of wildlife and free-roaming dogs and cats from the area immediately surrounding the home further decreases the likelihood of introduction of fleas. Routine use of insect development inhibitors or insect growth regulators, vacuuming areas where pets spend the majority of their time, and frequent cleaning of pet bedding limits accumulation of immature stages in the environment. Premise infestations can be avoided at shared animal facilities (e.g., boarding kennels, dog day care, veterinary practices) by requiring evidence of flea control or treating animals at intake to eliminate fleas.[2,3,15]

PUBLIC HEALTH ASPECTS

Cat fleas readily feed on people that share a home environment with infested pets or come in contact with areas where adults are emerging from pupae. Feeding by *C. felis* induces pruritus and erythematous edematous papules on the lower legs of people; bites are often clustered and vesiculobullous lesions may be present.[72] Lesions are moderately or intensely pruritic and often excoriated.[73] In sensitized individuals, particularly children, papular urticaria may develop as a delayed hypersensitivity reaction.[72] Antihistamines and 1% hydrocortisone cream are helpful for symptomatic relief, but eradicating the infestation is key to preventing future bites.[73]

Treatment of all pets in the home that can serve as a source of *C. felis* (e.g., dogs, cats, rabbits, ferrets) with safe, label-approved, persistent insecticides is critical to control flea populations and protect public health. In all but the most extreme situations, pets should not be removed from a home with fleas as treated pets will attract fleas that will then be killed; removing pets drives newly emerging fleas in the environment to feed on the humans that remain. When homes are heavily infested, environmental cleaning (thorough vacuuming and immediate removal and disposal of vacuum bags) followed by environmental application of insect growth regulators or compounds to desiccate flea larvae can reduce the immature stages that constitute the majority of the flea population. Environmental efforts should focus on pet resting areas where immature flea stages are most likely to accumulate.[2,3,15]

Fleas also transmit potentially zoonotic infections.[74] Cats are the reservoir for *Bartonella henselae*, the causative agent of cat scratch disease, and *C. felis* is the primary arthropod vector maintaining feline infection (see Chapter 70). Fleas that feed on bacteremic cats will shed *B. henselae* in their frass; the organisms are transmitted to the cat's teeth or claws during normal grooming behavior and humans become infected when bitten or scratched.[75] Treating cats for fleas prevents *B. henselae* transmission.[76,77] Similarly, fleas shed *Rickettsia typhi* and *Rickettsia felis* in their feces (see Chapter 46) that can be transmitted to humans when inoculated into flea bite wounds or mucous membranes.[78] Although *R. typhi* is historically associated with *X. cheopis*, a rat flea, a cycle involving *C. felis*, opossums, domestic animals, and human disease has been described in the United States.[79] Plague is also associated with infestation with *X. cheopis* and other rodent fleas; *C. felis* is considered a poor vector for *Yersinia pestis* (see Chapter 73). Cats can become infected with *Y. pestis* from rodents while hunting. Flea control and keeping cats indoors to prevent hunting are recommended for prevention.[74] *Dipylidium caninum* can be transmitted to humans, usually young children, by accidental ingestion of fleas containing cysticercoids (see Chapter 115). Infections are usually asymptomatic or associated with mild anal pruritus.[80]

FLEAS: *ECHIDNOPHAGA GALLINACEA*

Commonly known as the sticktight flea or the stickfast flea, *Echidnophaga gallinacea* is a semi-permanent, sedentary ectoparasite; fertilized adult females attach to the host with serrated laciniae, feeding for prolonged periods of time. Preferred sites include the skin of the comb, wattle, and around the eye of chickens; many other domestic and peridomestic birds are also infested although the extensive host list leads some to suggest that mammals may be a more common host than birds.[81] Eggs are deposited by females while still attached to the host and develop in the environment. While not common on pets, *E. gallinacea* is occasionally found on dogs in rural areas worldwide (see Table 106.1), often in association with domestic poultry, and attaches to less haired areas around the eyes, margins of the pinna, between the toes, on the scrotum, and the perianal region.[82,83] Surveys in Georgia and Florida, United States, documented that 3.7%–6.9% of fleas removed from dogs were *E. gallinacea*.[84,85] Stickfast fleas account for as many as 16.6% of fleas from dogs in Western Australia although they were not recovered on dogs or cats in the rest of the country.[86,87] Attached *E. gallinacea* can be removed by securely grasping with forceps and applying rearward traction. Sticktight fleas are smaller than *C. felis* and *C. canis*, lack pronotal and genal combs, and have a sharply angular head (Fig. 106.5).[5]

Ulcerative lesions develop at *E. gallinacea* attachment sites due to laceration by flea mouthparts and secondary infections; hypersensitivity reactions are also described. Female fleas remain attached for as long as 19 days. A related species in Australia, *Echidnophaga myremecobii*, can transmit the myxamotosis agent to rabbits although European rabbit fleas (*Spilopsyllus cuniculi*) are more important vectors.[5] Treatment of infested pets is achieved by physical removal of attached fleas and use of insecticides. Flea control products are not label-approved for *E. gallinacea*, but standard options (e.g., fipronil, isoxazolines, neonicotinoids, spinosad) would be expected to be effective. Dead fleas may remain attached to the host after treatment. Sticktight fleas occasionally attach to humans in contact with areas frequented by domestic poultry, wild birds, or other hosts.[88–90]

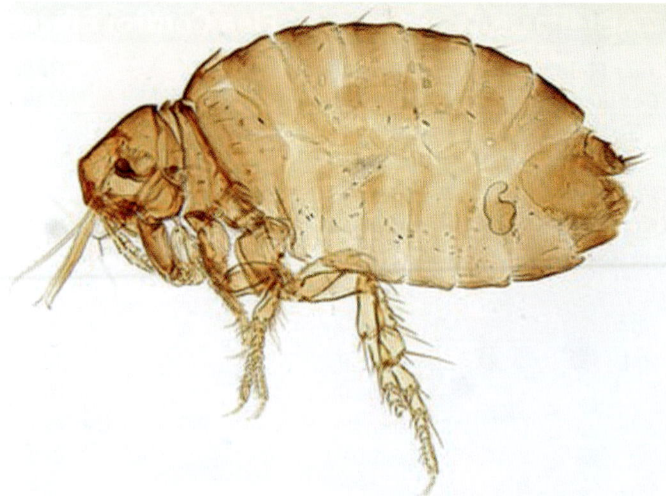

Fig. 106.5 The sticktight flea, *Echidnophaga gallinacea*, is usually found attached to hosts and has a distinct angular head; combs are absent.

FLEAS: *TUNGA PENETRANS*

The chigoe, jigger, or sand flea, *T. penetrans* is a very small (~1 mm) burrowing flea with an angled head similar to *E. gallinacea*. Fertilized females invade host skin and increase dramatically in size, resulting in formation of a nodule approximately 4–10 mm in diameter. The female genital aperture protrudes through an opening in the skin to allow eggs to be deposited in sandy soil in the environment for development. Originally native to South America, *T. penetrans* is now found throughout many tropical regions, including Latin America, the Caribbean, sub-Saharan Africa, and southern India.[5] Cases have been associated with translocation of infested dogs to other areas of the world.[91]

Dogs, cats, and humans in resource-limited areas are commonly infested although people in affected regions are more aware of human tungiasis than animal infestations.[92] Dogs are considered an important animal host; pigs and cats are also frequently infested.[93–95] In two communities in northeastern Brazil, *T. penetrans* was found in 52.1% and 54.4% of people, 30.9% and 67.1% of dogs, and 32.4% and 49.6% of cats surveyed.[96] Prevalence is high throughout the year, with one study showing 62.1% of dogs infested in August and 82.2% in November; sex and age were not associated with infestation risk.[97] In dogs, most lesions (89.1%) develop on the toe pads; other affected areas include the nipples, abdomen, testicles, elbows, and nose pad (Fig. 106.6). Lesions are often painful and erythematous. Hyperkeratosis, deep fissures, onychogryphosis, and lameness can develop, leading to progressive debilitation. Lesions commonly cluster and higher numbers are seen in younger dogs.[98]

Treatment of dogs with imidacloprid/permethrin insecticides reduced canine infestations and may help decrease distribution of eggs in the environment, thereby preventing human infestations.[99] Prevalence of human tungiasis is reportedly higher in homes with infested dogs or cats, and early recognition and treatment of infestations in dogs has been recommended as an important public health measure.[94,98] Frequent inspection of dog paws in endemic areas allows lesions to be recognized early and treatment instituted.[98] Repellents and protective clothing (i.e., shoes) are recommended for people to prevent skin penetration.[100,101] In people with only a few lesions, surgical extraction of the fleas can be used for treatment.[102]

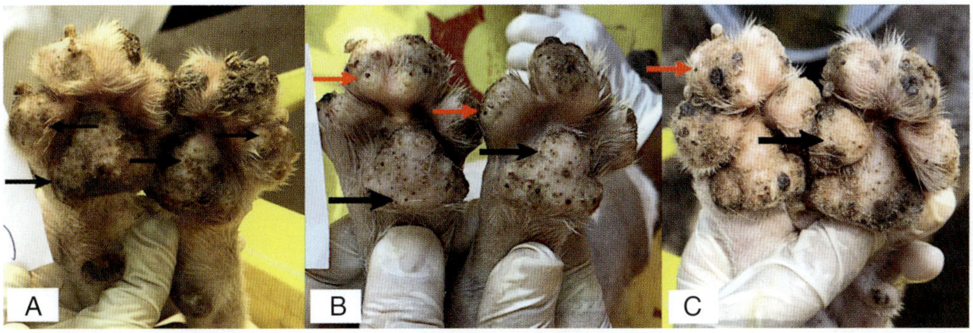

Fig. 106.6 *Tunga penetrans* lesions on a dog's paws. Multiple active *Tunga penetrans* flea lesions on a dog's paws in varying stages of development (examples shown with black and red arrows). Each panel shows evolution of lesions on days 0 (A), 7 (B) and 21 (C). (From dos Santos KC, Chiummo RM, Heckeroth AR, et al. Efficacy of oral fluralaner (Bravecto) against *Tunga penetrans* in dogs: A negative control, randomized field study in an endemic community in Brazil. *PLoS Negl Trop Dis.* 2022;16:e0010251)

LICE

ETIOLOGY AND EPIDEMIOLOGY

Lice infestations in dogs and cats may be caused by chewing lice (*Trichodectes canis* and *Heterodoxus spiniger* in dogs, *Felicola subrostratus* in cats) or blood-sucking lice (*Linognathus setosus* in dogs). Historically, chewing lice, also referred to as "biting lice," were grouped together in an order or suborder referred to as "mallophaga" but subsequent analysis has shown that the taxa are not monophyletic. Both *T. canis* and *F. subrostratus* are in the suborder Ischnocera, family Trichodectidae, while *H. spiniger* is in the suborder Amblycera, family Boopiidae. A single species of blood-sucking lice, *L. setosus* (suborder Anoplura), is also found on dogs in some regions. Chewing lice have prominent mandibles and feed on skin scales, hair, and tissue fluids; *H. spiniger* is an exception in that it primarily feeds on blood released by chewing activity.[103,104] As a blood-sucking louse, *L. setosus* mouthparts are adapted to pierce skin and imbibe blood directly from capillary beds.[27,103]

The life cycle of lice occurs entirely on the host. Females cement the eggs to hair shafts. First-stage nymphs hatch from the eggs in approximately 1 to 2 weeks depending on the species by dislodging the operculum on the anterior end of the egg. The nymphs then molt through two subsequent nymphal stages before developing in to adults. The entire life cycle can be completed in 3 to 4 weeks. Infestations are more commonly identified in young, aged, or debilitated animals. Infestations of *L. setosus* and *F. subrostratus* are more common in long-haired breeds and in cats that do not self-groom.[105] Reported predilection sites for *T. canis* include the head, neck, tail, and perianal region; in wolves, *T. canis* is most commonly found in the dorsal hindquarters and the inguinal region.[103,106] *Linognathus setosus* is more commonly found on the back, ears, and neck, especially below the collar.[103,107] Both *H. spiniger* and *F. subrostratus* may be found anywhere on the host.[103]

In most surveys, lice are recovered less commonly than fleas from dogs and cats. Prevalence of lice in domestic dogs ranges from 1% to 10% depending on lifestyle of the population considered and geographic location (see Table 106.1). Similarly, surveys reveal *F. subrostratus* infestations on less than 1% of pet cats to as many as 14% of free-roaming cats (see Table 106.2). However, although under-reported, lice infestations of pets may be common in colder climates, perhaps due in part to reduced use of routine insecticides for flea control.[108,109] In Finland and Sweden, *L. setosus* predominates on dogs and is most common in the winter months.[109] In other regions, *T. canis* is the most common species found on dogs.[110] *Trichodectes canis* infestations are also frequently identified in coyotes and wolves in colder regions of North America, with per animal infestation intensity ranging from 14 to an estimated 80,000.[106,111,112] *Heterodoxus spiniger* is more common in warmer or tropical climates and, although reported, is considered rare in North America.[113]

PATHOGENESIS

Lice are active on hosts, feeding on skin or blood and causing irritation. Common chewing lice (*T. canis, F. subrostratus*) abrade host skin with mandibles and then feed on skin cells, broken hairs, or tissue fluids. Although also chewing lice, *H. spiniger* are facultative hematophages that scrape the host skin until it bleeds and then ingest the blood. Blood-sucking lice (*L. setosus*) insert stylets through the skin to puncture a capillary, secrete saliva with anticoagulants, and imbibe blood.[103] Regardless of the method, lice feeding induces pruritus, increasing host grooming activity. Alopecia and skin damage from host scratching results in excoriations and secondary bacterial infections. If blood loss is severe, anemia may develop, particularly in malnourished young animals with multiple parasitic infections and infestations.[27] Lice also transmit pathogens to dogs. Although fleas (*C. felis*) are considered epidemiologically more important, chewing lice (*T. canis*) can serve as an intermediate host for *D. caninum* (see Chapter 115) and *H. spiniger* can be an intermediate host for *A. reconditum* (see Chapter 111).[103,114]

CLINICAL FEATURES

Animals with lice present with moderate to intense pruritus. History usually reveals an absence of insecticide use. On long-haired animals, eggs are often evident but the motile nymphs and adults cluster at the base of the hair shaft near the skin surface; parting the hair to allow closer examination is necessary. The hair is often matted and may have a fetid odor. Lice are more commonly seen in animals that have not received regular veterinary care, are housed in conditions of poor sanitation, and have frequent contact with other animals. Young animals with intense *L. setosus* infestations may be anemic, lethargic, and debilitated. Adult *L. setosus* tend to move more slowly and are readily collected for examination; adult *T. canis* and *F. subrostratus* move quickly through the haircoat, making collection more difficult.[27,103]

DIAGNOSIS

Direct Microscopic Examination

Lice are dorsoventrally flattened and can be collected for examination by combing or by adhering to clear tape; collecting nits is facilitated by clipping hair. Unlike with fleas, lice are invariably present on infested animals although close inspection may be needed to recover specimens for microscopic examination.[27] Chewing lice (*T. canis, H. spiniger*) have a head that is broader than the thorax (Fig. 106.7); antennae of *T. canis* project posteriorly and maxillary palps are absent, whereas *H. spiniger* antennae are within lateral grooves and distinct maxillary palps bearing post-palpal processes are evident.[103] In canine blood-sucking lice (*L.*

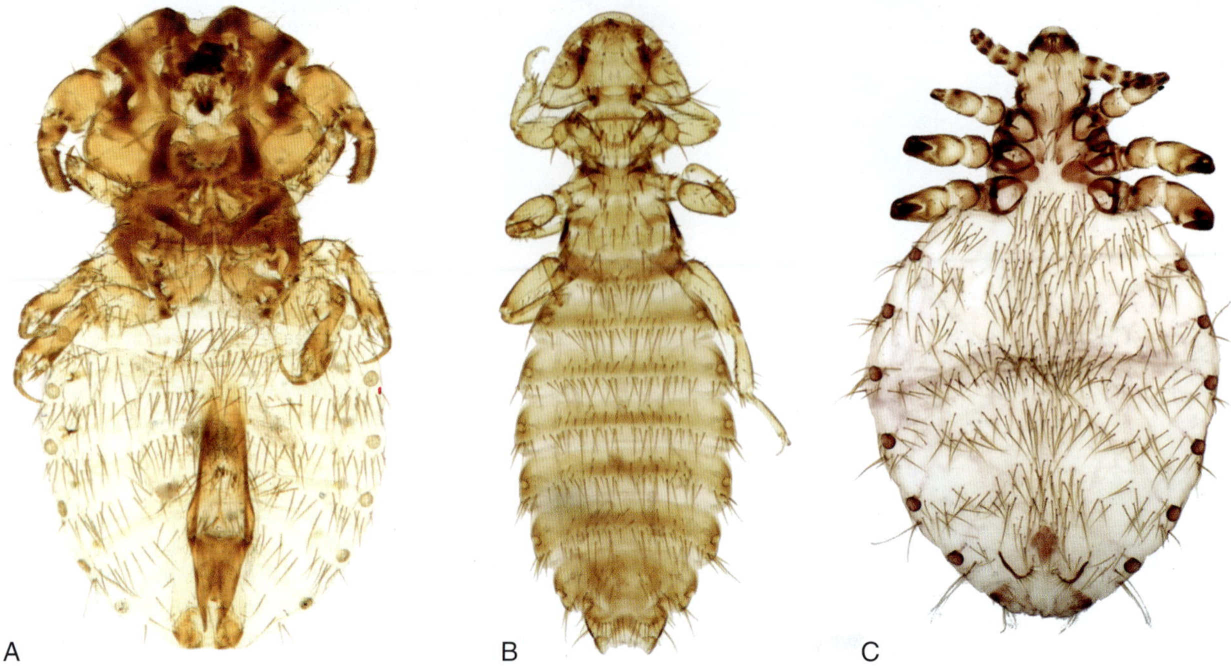

Fig. 106.7 Lice of domestic dogs. (A) *Trichodectes canis*, (B) *Heterodoxus spiniger*, (C) *Linognathus setosus*. (Photographs by Lorenza Beati and Lance A. Durden. In: Mullen GR, Durden LA. *Medical and Veterinary Entomology*. 3rd edition. Academic Press; 2019:79–106.)

setosus), the head is narrower than the thorax and the segmented antennae project laterally or anteriorly. Blood-sucking lice are larger than chewing lice and if fed may be dark red. *Felicola subrostratus* resembles *T. canis* but has a triangular rather than rounded head (Fig. 106.8). In most regions, *F. subrostratus* is the only feline louse present, although *H. spiniger* has been rarely reported from cats in tropical areas.[115,116]

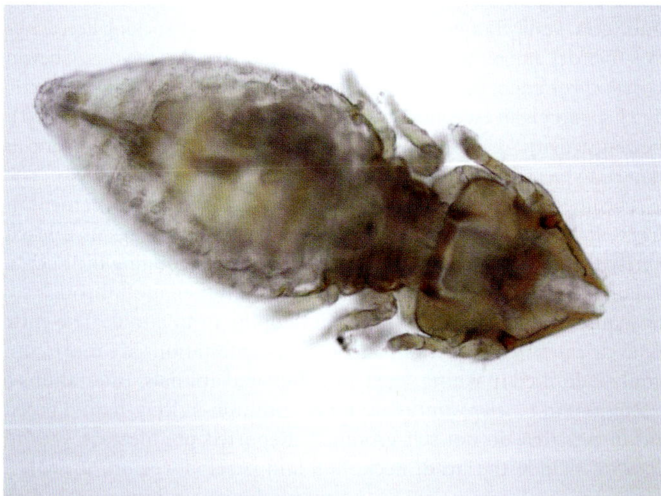

Fig. 106.8 Adult *Felicola subrostratus* from a cat. This chewing louse feeds on superficial tissue debris. (From the National Center for Veterinary Parasitology.)

Laboratory Abnormalities

Heavy infestations of puppies with *L. setosus* and *H. spiniger*, both of which feed on blood, may lead to anemia.[27,103]

Gross Pathologic Findings

Damage to the hair coat including broken hairs due to self-trauma caused by host scratching or chewing is often present. Alopecia and self-excoriations may be evident. When infestations are chronic, papules, crusts, and secondary dermatitis may develop; skin discoloration can occur, but deep pyoderma is rare. Lesions can resemble FAD in dogs or miliary dermatitis in cats.[27]

TREATMENT AND PROGNOSIS

Although not all are label-approved for this purpose in all regions, lice infestations are readily treated with insecticides commonly used in dogs and cats for flea control including dinotefuran, fipronil, imidacloprid, and selamectin.[117–122] In dogs, high-concentration permethrin can be used.[107,123] Fluralaner is effective at eliminating blood-sucking lice (*L. setosus*) from dogs, and a selamectin/sarolaner combination product is label-approved for the treatment of biting lice (*F. subrostratus*) in cats in Europe.[124] Bathing with a neem-seed extract has also been shown to be effective.[125] Traditional treatments using lime sulfur, pyrethroid, organophosphate, or carbamate dips, or the off-label use of high-dose large animal macrocyclic lactone products, are no longer necessary or recommended to eliminate lice infestations.

When a large number of nits are evident or the fur matted, the hair should be clipped to reduce the infestation; bathing may also be indicated to address dermatitis and secondary infections. In severely anemic animals, supportive care, including blood transfusions, should be considered. Off-host survival of lice is limited, but washing bedding and grooming tools in hot water can be helpful to reduce their role as fomites.[27,126,127] In a multi-animal home or facility, all contact animals of the same species should be treated. When infestations are intense, multiple treatments, and, depending on the product used, more frequent application may be indicated. The prognosis is excellent; although lice are very contagious between dogs or between cats, insecticide treatment readily eliminates the infestations.[27,45]

IMMUNITY

Lice infestations are more common in young, debilitated animals, suggesting immune restriction plays a role in limiting infestations.[27] *Trichodectes canis* prevalence in dogs decreases with increasing age.[128]

PREVENTION

Lice infestations can be prevented by routine use of insecticides as is recommended for flea control. In areas where flea control is commonly used, lice are rare in well-cared-for pets and usually only encountered by veterinarians who work with shelter, rescue, or free-roaming animals. In colder climates where flea control may not be as widely practiced, lice infestations may be seen in pets, particularly in dogs that attend dog day care or those allowed to roam; avoiding direct contact with other dogs and cats, especially those not on control products, and with wildlife hosts, limits risk of infestations. Shelters and multi-animal facilities should routinely treat all new animals, especially young puppies and kittens, with insecticides during quarantine to avoid introducing lice into the larger population. When lice are diagnosed in a pet, infestation of all pets of that species in the home should be assumed, regardless of findings on clinical examination, and all same-species contacts treated.[126,127]

PUBLIC HEALTH ASPECTS

Lice from pets are not zoonotic, and pets play no role in the maintenance or transmission of human lice. Humans, particularly children, are commonly infested with head lice (*Pediculus capitis*) worldwide; body lice (*Pediculus humanus*) are less common and primarily seen when conditions of poverty, war, or homelessness prevail. Transmission occurs following direct contact with an infested person, or, less commonly, through shared fomites (e.g., hairbrushes, clothing).[129] Pubic lice (*Phthirus pubis*) usually infest the groin and perianal region, but infestations are also described from facial hair, eyelashes, eyebrows, and, occasionally, the scalp.[130] People acquire pubic lice through direct, intimate contact with other infested individuals; humans are the only host.

CASE EXAMPLE

Signalment

"Grover," a 4-week-old intact male domestic shorthair cat from northern California.

History

Grover is an orphan kitten that was rescued with no known medical history. He was brought to the University of California-Davis, VMTH, with signs of an upper respiratory tract infection.

Physical Examination

Body weight: 268 g.

General: Dull, rectal temperature too low to read, R = 30, HR = 130 beats/minute, BCS 2/9, CRT = 2 seconds, pale/white mucous membranes, 8%–10% dehydrated, sternally recumbent for most of the examination but ambulatory.

Integument: Full haircoat with large numbers of fleas and flea frass over the entire body.

Eyes, ears, nose, and throat: Eyes crusted closed with dry discharge. Moderate to severe mucopurulent ocular discharge OU and nasal discharge. Mild ceruminous debris in both ears.

Cardiovascular: Regular cardiac rhythm with no murmurs auscultated.

Respiratory: Normal breath sounds.

All other systems: No clinically significant abnormalities noted.

Laboratory Findings

PCV: 11%, blood glucose 283 mg/dL.

Venous blood gas: pH 7.267, pCO_2 47.9 mmHg, pO_2 40.8 mmHg, bicarbonate 21.1 mmol/L, CO_2 total 22.6 mmol/L, base deficit –4.7 mmol/L, sodium 149 mEq/L, potassium 3.8 mEq/L, ionized calcium 1.44 mmol/L, chloride 117 mEq/L, glucose 150 mg/dL, lactate 0.8 mol/L, creatinine 0.2 mg/dL, anion gap 14.5 mmol/L.

Diagnosis

Anemia likely secondary to severe flea infestation, feline URTD (conjunctivitis neonatorum).

Treatment

Nitenpyram (5.7 mg PO); doxycycline (5 mg/kg, PO, q12h); famciclovir (90 mg/kg, PO, q12h), topical ofloxacin (1 drop OU, q12h), IV lactated Ringer's solution. Grover was also given a transfusion with 6 mL packed RBCs (Fig. 106.9A) after which his PCV was 22% and total protein was 6 g/dL. After 5 hours in the intensive care unit, Grover's mentation improved significantly and he began to eat. He was discharged the following day. At a recheck 2 months later, he was bright and alert and weighed 1.8 kg; mucous membranes were pink and CRT was < 2 seconds. Ocular examination was normal (Fig. 106.9B). There were no fleas or flea frass noted on examination of the haircoat. An FeLV antigen and FIV antibody test was negative.

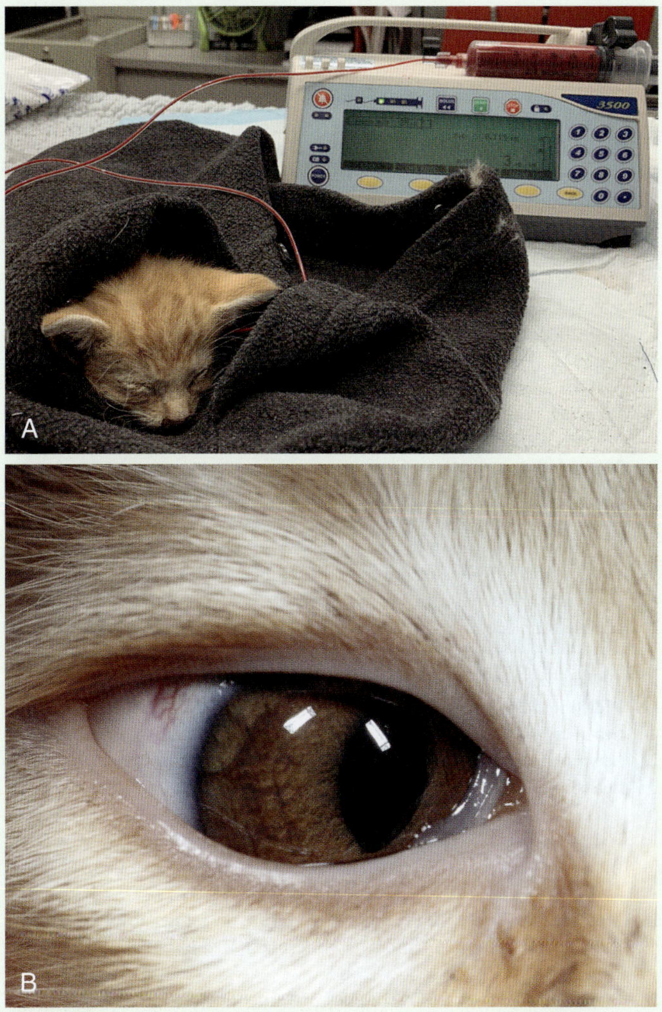

Fig. 106.9 (A) A 1-month-old intact male domestic shorthair kitten receiving a packed red blood cell transfusion to treat anemia secondary to flea infestation. The kitten's eyelids are glued together by crusty exudate secondary to feline upper respiratory tract disease. (B) A recheck examination 2 months later after treatment with antimicrobials and oral famciclovir showed only mild serous ocular discharge and no clinical evidence of anemia. (Courtesy of University of California Davis Veterinary Medical Teaching Hospital.)

Continued

CASE EXAMPLE—cont'd

Comments

Although the cause of this kitten's anemia was not proven to be flea infestation, this seemed most likely based on the large numbers of fleas present and the kitten's small size. Other differentials that were considered were retrovirus infection or hemoplasmosis; however, typically the incubation periods for these diseases are longer than 4 weeks and hemoplasmosis is rare in kittens. Antimicrobial therapy for the upper respiratory tract infection was clearly indicated based on the presence of mucopurulent ocular discharges and systemic illness. Differentials for the upper respiratory tract disease included FHV-1, FCV, *Bordetella bronchiseptica*, or *Chlamydia felis* infection; multiple pathogens may be present in some cases. FHV-1 has most often been associated with conjunctivitis neonatorum, hence the decision to treat with famciclovir. Treatment with antimicrobials and famciclovir was continued for 3 weeks, and the owner was instructed to continue regular flea prevention year-round.

SUGGESTED READINGS

Blagburn BL, Dryden MW. Biology, treatment, and control of flea and tick infestations. *Vet Clin North Am Small Anim Pract*. 2009;39:1173–1200.

Durden LA. Lice (Phthiraptera). In: Mullen G, Durden L, eds. *Medical and Veterinary Entomology*. 3rd ed. Academic Press; 2019:79–106.

Rust MK. Recent advancements in the control of cat fleas. *Insects*. 2020;11:668.

REFERENCES

1. Rust MK. Recent advancements in the control of cat fleas. *Insects*. 2020;11:668.
2. Rust MK, Dryden MW. The biology, ecology, and management of the cat flea. *Annu Rev Entomol*. 1997;42:451–473.
3. Dryden MW, Rust MK. The cat flea: biology, ecology and control. *Vet Parasitol*. 1994;52:1–19.
4. Fox I. *Fleas of eastern United States*. Ames: Iowa State College Press; 1940:191.
5. Durden LA, Hinkle NC. Fleas (Siphonaptera). In: Mullen G, Durden L, eds. *Medical and Veterinary Entomology*. 3rd ed. Academic Press; 2019:145–168.
6. Rust MK. The biology and ecology of cat fleas and advancements in their pest management: a review. *Insects*. 2017;8:118.
7. Franc M, Bouhsira E, Beugnet F. Direct transmission of the cat flea (*Ctenocephalides felis*) between cats exhibiting social behaviour. *Parasite*. 2013;20:49.
8. Cadiergues MC, Hourcq P, Cantaloube B, Franc M. First bloodmeal of *Ctenocephalides felis felis* (Siphonaptera: Pulicidae) on cats: time to initiation and duration of feeding. *J Med Entomol*. 2000;37:634–636.
9. Dryden MW. Host association, on host longevity and egg production of *Ctenocephalides felis felis*. *Vet Parasitol*. 1989;34:117–122.
10. Hinkle NC, Koehler PC, Patterson RS. Host grooming efficiency for regulation of cat flea (Siphonaptera: Pulicidae) populations. *J Med Entomol*. 1998;35:266–269.
11. McDonald BJ, Foil CS, Foil LD. An investigation on the influence of feline flea allergy on the fecundity of the cat flea. *Vet Dermatol*. 1998;9:75–79.
12. Lawrence W, Foil LD. The effects of flea egg consumption on larval cat flea (Siphonaptera: Pulicidae) development. *J Vector Ecol*. 2000;25:98–101.
13. Hsu MH, Hsu YC, Wu WJ. Consumption of flea faeces and eggs by larvae of the cat flea, *Ctenocephalides felis*. *Med Vet Entomol*. 2002;16:445–447.
14. Metzger ME, Rust MK. Effect of temperature on cat flea (Siphonaptera: Pulicidae) development and overwintering. *J Med Entomol*. 1997;34:173–178.
15. Blagburn BL, Dryden MW. Biology, treatment, and control of flea and tick infestations. *Vet Clin North Am Small Anim Pract*. 2009;39:1173–1200.
16. Kern WH, Richman DL, Koehler PG, Brenner RJ. Outdoor survival and development of immature cat fleas (Siphonaptera: Pulicidae) in Florida. *J Med Entomol*. 1999;36:207–211.
17. Abdullah S, Helps C, Tasker S, et al. Pathogens in fleas collected from cats and dogs: distribution and prevalence in the UK. *Parasit Vectors*. 2019;12:71.
18. Beugnet F, Bourdeau P, Chalvet-Monfray K, et al. Parasites of domestic owned cats in Europe: co-infestations and risk factors. *Parasit Vectors*. 2014;7:291.
19. Lund EM, Armstrong PJ, Kirk CA, et al. Health status and population characteristics of dogs and cats examined at private veterinary practices in the United States. *J Am Vet Med Assoc*. 1999;214:1336–1341.
20. Rinaldi L, Spera G, Musella V, et al. A survey of fleas on dogs in southern Italy. *Vet Parasitol*. 2007;148:375–378.
21. Thomas JE, Staubus L, Goolsby JL, Reichard MV. Ectoparasites of free-roaming domestic cats in the central United States. *Vet Parasitol*. 2016;228:17–22.
22. Beck W, Boch K, Mackesen H, et al. Qualitative and quantitative observations on the flea population dynamics of dogs and cats in several areas of Germany. *Vet Parasitol*. 2006;137:130–136.
23. Bond R, Riddle A, Mottram L, et al. Survey of flea infestation in dogs and cats in the United Kingdom during 2005. *Vet Rec*. 2007;160:503–506.
24. Farkas R, Gyurkovszky M, Solymosi N, Beugnet F. Prevalence of flea infestation in dogs and cats in Hungary combined with a survey of owner awareness. *Med Vet Entomol*. 2009;23:187–194.
25. White SD, Ihrke PJ. Allergy disease. In: Pratt PW, ed. *Feline Medicine*. Santa Barbara, CA: American Veterinary Publications; 1983:577–580.
26. Stopler R. Flea allergy dermatitis in dogs diagnosed by intradermal skin test. *Res Vet Sci*. 1994;57:21–27.
27. Miller WH, Griffin CE, Campbell KL. Parasitic skin disease. In: *Muller and Kirk's Small Animal Dermatology*. 7th ed. Elsevier Mosby; 2012: 284–342.
28. Franc M, Choquart P, Cadiergues MC. Species of fleas found on dogs in France. *Rev Med Vet*. 1998;149:135–140.
29. Beugnet F, Labuschagne M, Fourie J, et al. Occurrence of *Dipylidium caninum* in fleas from client-owned cats and dogs in Europe using a new PCR detection assay. *Vet Parasitol*. 2014;205:300–306.
30. Rodrigues DF, Daemon E, Rodrigues AF. Characterization of ectoparasites on dogs in the nucleus of urban expansion of Juiz de Fora, Minas Gerais, Brazil. *Rev Bras Parasitol Vet*. 2008;17:185–188.
31. Knaus M, Rapti D, Shukullari E, et al. Characterisation of ecto- and endoparasites in domestic cats from Tirana, Albania. *Parasitol Res*. 2014;113:3361–3371.
32. Dryden M, Gaafar S. Blood consumption by the cat flea, *Ctenocephalides felis felis* (Siphonaptera: Pulicidae). *J Med Entomol*. 1991;28:394–400.
33. Kwochka KW, Bevier DE. Flea dermatitis. In: Nesbitt GE, ed. *Contemporary Issues in Small Animal Practice. Dermatology*. Vol. 9. New York: Churchill Livingstone; 1987:pp21–55.
34. Halliwell RE, Schemmer KR. The role of basophils in the immunopathogenesis of hypersensitivity to fleas (*Ctenocephalides felis*) in dogs. *Vet Immunol Immunopathol*. 1987;15:203–213.
35. Halliwell RE, Preston JF, Nesbitt JG. Aspects of the immunopathogenesis of flea allergy dermatitis in dogs. *Vet Immunol Immunopathol*. 1987;17:483–494.
36. Wuersch K, Brachelente C, Doherr M, et al. Immune dysregulation in flea allergy dermatitis: a model for the immunopathogenesis of allergic dermatitis. *Vet Immunol Immunopathol*. 2006;110:311–323.
37. Jin J, Ding Z, Meng F, et al. An immunotherapeutic treatment against flea allergy dermatitis in cats by co-immunization of DNA and protein vaccines. *Vaccine*. 2010;28:1997–2004.

38. Labuschagne M, Beugnet F, Rehbein S, et al. Analysis of *Dipylidium caninum* tapeworms from dogs and cats, or their respective fleas - Part 1. Molecular characterization of *Dipylidium caninum*: genetic analysis supporting two distinct species adapted to dogs and cats. *Parasite.* 2018;25:30.
39. Beugnet F, Labuschagne M, Vos C, et al. Analysis of *Dipylidium caninum* tapeworms from dogs and cats, or their respective fleas - Part 2. Distinct canine and feline host association with two different *Dipylidium caninum* genotypes. *Parasite.* 2018;25:31.
40. Dryden MW, Blakemore JC. A review of flea allergy dermatitis in the dog and cat. *Companion Anim Prac.* 1989;19:10–17.
41. Wilkerson MJ, Bagladi-Swanson M, Wheeler DW, et al. The immunopathogenesis of flea allergy dermatitis in dogs, an experimental study. *Vet Immunol Immunopathol.* 2004;99:179–192.
42. Kramer F, Mencke N. *Flea Biology and Control.* Berlin: Springer-Verlag; 2001.
43. Colombini S, Hodgin EC, Foil CS, et al. Induction of feline flea allergy dermatitis and the incidence and histopathological characteristics of concurrent indolent lip ulcers. *Vet Dermatol.* 2001;12:155–161.
44. Hsu MH, Hsu TC, Wu WJ. Distribution of cat fleas (Siphonaptera: Pulicidae) on the cat. *J Med Entomol.* 2002;39:685–688.
45. Greiner E. Arthropods. In: Zajac A, Conboy G, eds. *Veterinary Clinical Parasitology*. 8th ed. Wiley-Blackwell; 2012:217–303.
46. Hensel P, Santoro D, Favrot C, et al. Canine atopic dermatitis: detailed guidelines for diagnosis and allergen identification. *BMC Vet Res.* 2015;11:196.
47. Center SA, Randolph JF, Erb HN, Reiter S. Eosinophilia in the cat: a retrospective study of 312 cases (1975 to 1986). *J Am Anim Hosp Assoc.* 1990;26:349–358.
48. Jin J, Ding Z, Meng F, et al. An immunotherapeutic treatment against flea allergy dermatitis in cats by co-immunization of DNA and protein vaccines. *Vaccine.* 2010;28:1997–2004.
49. Mendes-de-Almeida F, Crissiuma AL, Gershony LC, et al. Characterization of ectoparasites in an urban cat (*Felis catus* Linnaeus, 1758) population of Rio de Janeiro, Brazil. *Parasitol Res.* 2011;108:1431–1435.
50. Dryden MW, Payne PA, Smith V, et al. Evaluation of indoxacarb and fipronil (s)-methoprene topical spot-on formulations to control flea populations in naturally infested dogs and cats in private residences in Tampa FL, USA. *Parasit Vectors.* 2013;6:366.
51. Dryden MW, Denenberg TM, Bunch S. Control of fleas on naturally infested dogs and cats and in private residences with topical spot applications of fipronil or imidacloprid. *Vet Parasitol.* 2000;93:69–75.
52. Dryden MW, Payne PA, Vicki S, et al. Efficacy of dinotefuran-pyriproxyfen, dinotefuran-pyriproxyfen-permethrin and fipronil-(S)-methoprene topical spot-on formulations to control flea populations in naturally infested pets and private residences in Tampa, FL. *Vet Parasitol.* 2011;182:281–286.
53. Dryden MW, Smith V, Chwala M, et al. Evaluation of afoxolaner chewables to control flea populations in naturally infested dogs in private residences in Tampa FL, USA. *Parasit Vectors.* 2015;8:286.
54. Dryden MW, Canfield MS, Kalosy K, et al. Evaluation of fluralaner and afoxolaner treatments to control flea populations, reduce pruritus and minimize dermatologic lesions in naturally infested dogs in private residences in west central Florida USA. *Parasit Vectors.* 2016;9:365.
55. Dryden MW, Canfield MS, Niedfeldt E, et al. Evaluation of sarolaner and spinosad oral treatments to eliminate fleas, reduce dermatologic lesions and minimize pruritus in naturally infested dogs in west Central Florida, USA. *Parasit Vectors.* 2017;10:389.
56. Dryden MW, Canfield MS, Bocon C, et al. In-home assessment of either topical fluralaner or topical selamectin for flea control in naturally infested cats in West Central Florida, USA. *Parasit Vectors.* 2018;11:422.
57. Dryden MW, Canfield MS, Herrin BH, et al. In-home assessment of flea control and dermatologic lesions in dogs provided by lotilaner (Credelio®) and spinosad (Comfortis®) in west central Florida. *Vet Parasitol X.* 2019;1:100009.
58. Dryden MW, Herrin BH, Canfield MS, et al. Evaluation of a topical sarolaner-selamectin combination to control flea populations on naturally infested cats in private residences in West Central Florida. *Vet Parasitol.* 2020;283:109172.
59. Fisara P, Sargent RM, Shipstone M, et al. An open, self-controlled study on the efficacy of topical indoxacarb for eliminating fleas and clinical signs of flea-allergy dermatitis in client-owned dogs in Queensland, Australia. *Vet Dermatol.* 2014;25:195-e49.
60. Fisara P, Shipstone M, von Berky A, von Berky J. A small-scale open-label study of the treatment of canine flea allergy dermatitis with fluralaner. *Vet Dermatol.* 2015;26:417–420, e97-8.
61. Crosaz O, Chapelle E, Cochet-Faivre N, et al. Open field study on the efficacy of oral fluralaner for long-term control of flea allergy dermatitis in client-owned dogs in Ile-de-France region. *Parasit Vectors.* 2016;9:174.
62. Karadzovska D, Chappell K, Coble S, et al. A randomized, controlled field study to assess the efficacy and safety of lotilaner flavored chewable tablets (Credelio™) in eliminating fleas in client-owned dogs in the USA. *Parasit Vectors.* 2017;10:528.
63. Briand A, Cochet-Faivre N, Prélaud P, et al. Open field study on the efficacy of fluralaner topical solution for long-term control of flea bite allergy dermatitis in client owned cats in Ile-de-France region. *BMC Vet Res.* 2019;15:337.
64. Becskei C, Fias D, Mahabir SP, Farkas R. Efficacy of a novel oral chewable tablet containing sarolaner, moxidectin and pyrantel (Simparica Trio™) against natural flea and tick infestations on dogs presented as veterinary patients in Europe. *Parasit Vectors.* 2020;13:72.
65. Kryda K, Mahabir SP, Inskeep T, Rugg J. Safety and efficacy of a novel oral chewable combination tablet containing sarolaner, moxidectin and pyrantel (Simparica Trio™) against natural flea infestations in client-owned dogs in the USA. *Parasit Vectors.* 2020;13:98.
66. Coles TB, Dryden MW. Insecticide/acaricide resistance in fleas and ticks infesting dogs and cats. *Parasit Vectors.* 2014;7:8.
67. Villar D, Knight MJ. Toxicity of melaleuca oil and related essential oils applied topically on dogs and cats. *Vet Hum Toxicol.* 1994;36:139–142.
68. Bischo K, Guale F. Australian tea tree (*Melaleuca alternifolia*) oil poisoning in three purebred cats. *J Vet Diag Investig.* 1998;10:208–210.
69. Genovese AG, McLean MK, Khan SA. Adverse reactions from essential oil-containing natural flea products exempted from Environmental Protection Agency regulations in dogs and cats. *J Vet Emerg Crit Care.* 2012;22:470–475.
70. Nesbit AJ, Huntly JF. Progress and opportunities in the development of vaccines against mites, fleas and myiasis-causing flies of veterinary importance. *Parasite Immunol.* 2006;28:165–172.
71. Contreras M, Villar M, Artigas-Jerónimo S, et al. A reverse vaccinology approach to the identification and characterization of *Ctenocephalides felis* candidate protective antigens for the control of cat flea infestations. *Parasites Vectors.* 2018;11:43.
72. Peres G, Tacito Yugar LB, Haddad Junior V. Breakfast, lunch, and dinner sign: a hallmark of flea and bedbug bites. *An Bras Dermatol.* 2018;93:759–760.
73. Rensch GP, Elston DM. What's eating you? Cat flea (*Ctenocephalides felis*) revisited. *Cutis.* 2019;104:182–183.
74. McElroy KM, Blagburn BL, Breitschwerdt EB, et al. Flea-associated zoonotic diseases of cats in the USA: bartonellosis, flea-borne rickettsioses, and plague. *Trends Parasitol.* 2010;26:197–204.
75. Chomel BB, Kasten RW, Floyd-Hawkins K, et al. Experimental transmission of *Bartonella henselae* by the cat flea. *J Clin Microbiol.* 1996;34:1952–1956.
76. Bradbury CA, Lappin MR. Evaluation of topical application of 10% imidacloprid-1% moxidectin to prevent *Bartonella henselae* transmission from cat fleas. *J Am Vet Med Assoc.* 2010;236:869–873.
77. Lappin MR, Davis WL, Hawley JR, et al. A flea and tick collar containing 10% imidacloprid and 4.5% flumethrin prevents flea transmission of *Bartonella henselae* in cats. *Parasit Vectors.* 2013;6:26.
78. Blanton LS, Walker DH. Flea-borne rickettsioses and rickettsiae. *Am J Trop Med Hyg.* 2017;96:53–56.
79. Adjemian J, Parks S, McElroy K, et al. Murine typhus in Austin, Texas, USA, 2008. *Emerg Infect Dis.* 2010;16:412–417.
80. Hogan CA, Schwenk H. *Dipylidium caninum* infection. *N Engl J Med.* 2019;380:e39.
81. Boughton RK, Atwell JW, Schoech SJ. An introduced generalist parasite, the sticktight flea (*Echidnophaga gallinacea*), and its pathology in the threatened Florida scrub-jay (*Aphelocoma coerulescens*). *J Parasitol.* 2006;92:941–948.

82. Kalkofen UP, Greenberg J. *Echidnophaga gallinacea* infestation in dogs. *J Am Vet Med Assoc.* 1974;165:447–448.
83. Abarca K, Garate D, Lopez J, et al. Flea and tick species from dogs in urban and rural areas in four districts in Chile. *Arch Med Vet.* 2016;48:247–253.
84. Beard CB, Butler JF, Hall DW. Prevalence and biology of endosymbionts of fleas (Siphonaptera: Pulicidae) from dogs and cats in Alachua County, Florida. *J Med Entomol.* 1990;27:1050–1061.
85. Durden LA, Judy TN, Martin JE, et al. Fleas parasitizing domestic dogs in Georgia, USA: species composition and seasonal abundance. *Vet Parasitol.* 2005;130:157–162.
86. Slapeta J, King J, McDonell D, et al. The cat flea (*Ctenocephalides f. felis*) is the dominant flea on domestic dogs and cats in Australian veterinary practices. *Vet Parasitol.* 2011;180:383–388.
87. Schloderer D, Owen H, Clark P, et al. *Rickettsia felis* in fleas, Western Australia. *Emerg Infect Dis.* 2006;12:841–843.
88. Elston DM. What's eating you? *Echidnophaga gallinacea* (the sticktight flea). *Cutis.* 2001;68:250.
89. Carlson JC, Fox MS. A sticktight flea removed from the cheek of a two-year-old boy from Los Angeles. *Dermatol Online J.* 2009;15:4.
90. Kapoor R, Elston DM. What's eating you? The sticktight flea (*Echidnophaga gallinacea*). *Cutis.* 2012;89:157–158.
91. Loft KE, Nissen MH. *Tunga penetrans* in a young dog imported to Denmark from Brazil; a case report. *Vet Dermatol.* 2009;20:300–303.
92. Mutebi F, Krücken J, von Samson-Himmelstjerna G, et al. Animal and human tungiasis-related knowledge and treatment practices among animal keeping households in Bugiri District, south-eastern Uganda. *Acta Trop.* 2018;177:81–88.
93. Ugbomoiko US, Ariza L, Heukelbach J. Pigs are the most important animal reservoir for *Tunga penetrans* (jigger flea) in rural Nigeria. *Trop Doct.* 2008;38:226–227.
94. Pilger D, Schwalfenberg S, Heukelbach J, et al. Investigations on the biology, epidemiology, pathology, and control of *Tunga penetrans* in Brazil: VII. The importance of animal reservoirs for human infestation. *Parasitol Res.* 2008;102:875–880.
95. Mutebi F, Krucken J, Feldmeier H, et al. Pigs have been identified as the most important animal reservoirs of *T. penetrans* in sub-Saharan Africa. *BMC Vet Res.* 2017;13:206.
96. Heukelbach J. Revision on tungiasis: treatment options and prevention. *Expert Rev Anti Infect Ther.* 2006;4:151–157.
97. Harvey TV, Heukelbach J, Assunção MS, et al. Seasonal variation and persistence of tungiasis infestation in dogs in an endemic community, Bahia State (Brazil): longitudinal study. *Parasitol Res.* 2019;118:1711–1718.
98. Harvey TV, Dos Santos Freire Z, Dos Santos KC, et al. Clinical and macroscopic morphological features of canine tungiasis. *Parasitol Res.* 2021;120:807–818.
99. Klimpel S, Mehlhorn H, Heukelbach J, et al. Field trial of the efficacy of a combination of imidacloprid and permethrin against *Tunga penetrans* (sand flea, jigger flea) in dogs in Brazil. *Parasitol Res.* 2005;97(suppl 1):S113–S119.
100. de Carvalho RW, de Almeida AB, Barbosa-Silva SC, et al. The patterns of tungiasis in Araruama township, state of Rio de Janeiro, Brazil. *Mem Inst Oswaldo Cruz.* 2003;98:31–36.
101. Feldmeier H, Kehr JD, Heukelbach J. A plant-based repellent protects against *Tunga penetrans* infestation and sand flea disease. *Acta Trop.* 2006;99:126–136.
102. Heukelbach J, Costa AM, Wilcke T, et al. The animal reservoir of *Tunga penetrans* in severely affected communities of north-east Brazil. *Med Vet Entomol.* 2004;18:329–335.
103. Durden LA. Lice (Phthiraptera). In: Mullen G, Durden L, eds. *Medical and Veterinary Entomology*. 3rd ed. Academic Press; 2019:79–106.
104. Koungoulos L, Contos P. Global expansion of the Australian biting louse *Heterodoxus spiniger* facilitated by human transport of dog (*Canis familiaris*), and implications for prehistoric cultural interaction in Australasia. *Environ Arch.* 2021;26:3,281–294.
105. Wall R, Shearer D. Lice (Phthiraptera). In: *Veterinary Ectoparasites: Biology, Pathology, and Control.* 2nd ed. Oxford: Blackwell Science; 1998:162–178.
106. Woldstad TM, Dullen KN, Hundertmark KJ, Beckmen KB. Restricted evaluation of *Trichodectes canis* (Phthiraptera: Trichodectidae) detection methods in Alaska gray wolves. *Int J Parasitol Parasites Wildl.* 2014;3:239–241.
107. Gunnarsson L, Christensson D, Palmér E. Clinical efficacy of selamectin in the treatment of naturally acquired infection of sucking lice (*Linognathus setosus*) in dogs. *J Am Anim Hosp Assoc.* 2005;41:388–394.
108. Hanssen I, Mencke N, Asskildt H, et al. Field study on the insecticidal efficacy of Advantage against natural infestations of dogs with lice. *Parasitol Res.* 1999;85:347–348.
109. Kohler-Aanesen H, Saari S, Armstrong R, et al. Efficacy of fluralaner (Bravecto™ chewable tablets) for the treatment of naturally acquired *Linognathus setosus* infestations on dogs. *Parasit Vectors.* 2017;10:426.
110. Pollmeier M, Pengo G, Jeannin P, Soll M. Evaluation of the efficacy of fipronil formulations in the treatment and control of biting lice, *Trichodectes canis* (De Geer, 1778) on dogs. *Vet Parasitol.* 2002;107:127–136.
111. Foreyt WJ, Long GG, Gates NL. *Trichodectes canis*: severe pediculosis in coyotes. *Vet Med Small Anim Clin.* 1978;73:503–505.
112. Schwartz CC, Stephenson R, Wilson N. *Trichodectes canis* on the gray wolf and coyote on Kenai Peninsula, Alaska. *J Wildl Dis.* 1983;19:372–373.
113. Baak-Baak C, Garcia-Rejon J, Tzuc-Dzul J, et al. Four species of under-reported parasitic arthropods in Mexico and their potential role as vectors of pathogens. *J Parasitol.* 2020;106:835–842.
114. Nelson G. *Dipetalonema reconditum* (Grassi, 1889) from the dog with a note on its development in the flea, *Ctenocephalides felis* and the louse, *Heterodoxus spiniger*. *J Helminthol.* 1962;36:297–308.
115. Norhidayu S, Mohd Zain SN, Jeffery J, Lewis JW. The dog louse *Heterodoxus spiniger* from stray cats in Penang, Malaysia. *Trop Biomed.* 2012;29:301–303.
116. Mohd Zain SN, Sahimin N, Pal P, Lewis JW. Macroparasite communities in stray cat populations from urban cities in Peninsular Malaysia. *Vet Parasitol.* 2013;196:469–477.
117. Cooper PR, Penaliggon J. Use of fipronil to eliminate recurrent infestation by *Trichodectes canis* in a pack of bloodhounds. *Vet Rec.* 1996;139:95.
118. Pollmeier M, Pengo G, Jeannin P, Soll M. Evaluation of the efficacy of fipronil formulations in the treatment and control of biting lice, *Trichodectes canis* (De Geer, 1778) on dogs. *Vet Parasitol.* 2002;107:127–136.
119. Pollmeier M, Pengo G, Longo M, Jeannin P. Effective treatment and control of biting lice, *Felicola subrostratus* (Nitzsch in Burmeister, 1838), on cats using fipronil formulations. *Vet Parasitol.* 2004;121:157–165.
120. Hanssen I, Mencke N, Asskildt H, et al. Field study on the insecticidal efficacy of Advantage against natural infestations of dogs with lice. *Parasitol Res.* 1999;85:347–348.
121. Shanks DJ, Gautier P, McTier TL, et al. Efficacy of selamectin against biting lice on dogs and cats. *Vet Rec.* 2003;152:234–237.
122. Gunnarsson L, Christensson D, Palmér E. Clinical efficacy of selamectin in the treatment of naturally acquired infection of sucking lice (*Linognathus setosus*) in dogs. *J Am Anim Hosp Assoc.* 2005;41:388–394.
123. Endris RG, Reuter VE, Nelson J, Nelson JA. Efficacy of a topical spot-on containing 65% permethrin against the dog louse, *Trichodectes canis* (Mallophaga:Trichodectidae). *Vet Ther.* 2001;2:135–139.
124. Kohler-Aanesen H, Saari S, Armstrong R, et al. Efficacy of fluralaner (Bravecto™ chewable tablets) for the treatment of naturally acquired *Linognathus setosus* infestations on dogs. *Parasit Vectors.* 2017;10:426.
125. Mehlhorn H, Walldorf V, Abdel-Ghaffar F, et al. Biting and bloodsucking lice of dogs: treatment by means of a neem seed extract (MiteStop®, Wash Away Dog). *Parasitol Res.* 2012;110:769–773.
126. Prior IC, Stich WR. Canine arthropods: class insect — recommendations from the Companion Animal Parasite Council. *Today's Vet Pract.* 2014;6:51–55.
127. Starkey LA, Stewart J. Feline arthropods — recommendations from the Companion Animal Parasite Council. *Today's Vet Pract.* 2015;1:59–64.
128. Ugbomoiko US, Ariza L, Heukelbach J. Parasites of importance for human health in Nigerian dogs: high prevalence and limited knowledge of pet owners. *BMC Vet Res.* 2008;4:49.

129. Veracz A, Raoult D. Biology and genetics of human head and body lice. *Trends Parasitol.* 2012;28:563–571.
130. Veraldi S, Pontini P, Nazzaro G. *Phthirus pubis* infestation of the scalp: a case report and review of the literature. *Korean J Parasitol.* 2018;56:487–489.
131. Alvåsen K, Johansson SM, Höglund J, et al. A field survey on parasites and antibodies against selected pathogens in owned dogs in Lilongwe, Malawi. *J S Afr Vet Assoc.* 2016;87:e1–6.
132. Kumsa B, Abiy Y, Abunna F. Ectoparasites infesting dogs and cats in Bishoftu, central Oromia, Ethiopia. *Vet Parasitol Reg Stud Reports.* 2019;15:100263.
133. Changbunjong T, Buddhirongawatr R, Suwanpakdee S, et al. A survey of ectoparasitic arthropods on domestic animals in Tak Province, Thailand. *Southeast Asian J Trop Med Public Health.* 2009;40:435–442.
134. Chee JH, Kwon JK, Cho HS, et al. A survey of ectoparasite infestations in stray dogs of Gwang-ju City, Republic of Korea. *Korean J Parasitol.* 2008;46:23–27.
135. Jamshidi S, Maazi N, Ranjbar-Bahadori S, et al. A survey of ectoparasite infestation in dogs in Tehran, Iran. *Rev Bras Parasitol Vet.* 2012;21:326–329.
136. Shukullari E, Rapti D, Visser M, et al. Parasites and vector-borne diseases in client-owned dogs in Albania: infestation with arthropod ectoparasites. *Parasitol Res.* 2017;116:399–407.
137. Akucewich LH, Philman K, Clark A, et al. Prevalence of ectoparasites in a population of feral cats from north central Florida during the summer. *Vet Parasitol.* 2002;109:129–139.
138. Salant H, Mumcuoglu KY, Baneth G. Ectoparasites in urban stray cats in Jerusalem, Israel: differences in infestation patterns of fleas, ticks and permanent ectoparasites. *Med Vet Entomol.* 2014;28:314–318.
139. Cantó GJ, Guerrero RI, Olvera-Ramírez AM, et al. Prevalence of fleas and gastrointestinal parasites in free-roaming cats in central Mexico. *PLoS One.* 2013;8:e60744.
140. Lefkaditis MA, Sossidou AV, Panorias AH, et al. Urban stray cats infested by ectoparasites with zoonotic potential in Greece. *Parasitol Res.* 2015;114:3931–3934.
141. Capári B, Hamel D, Visser M, et al. Parasitic infections of domestic cats, *Felis catus*, in western Hungary. *Vet Parasitol.* 2013;192:33–42.

107 Mosquitoes and Other Blood-Feeding Flies

Meriam N. Saleh

KEY POINTS

- First Described: Aristotle gave true flies their name "Diptera" (two-winged) in the fourth century BC. In Aristotle's *History of Animals* (335 BC), he accurately observed "the diptera have the sting in the front" and "no insect with only two wings has a sting in the rear." The earliest Diptera appeared in the Triassic period ca. 240 million years ago.[1]
- Causes: A variety of blood-feeding flies feed on dogs and cats in North America, including members of the families Culicidae (e.g., mosquitoes), Simuliidae (e.g., black flies), Psychodidae (e.g., sand flies), and Muscidae (e.g., stable flies).
- Affected Hosts: Blood-feeding flies feed on a wide variety of reptiles, birds, and mammals, including dogs and cats.
- Geographic Distribution: Mosquitoes, black flies, and muscid flies are found on every continent except Antarctica. Sand flies can be found throughout tropical and subtropical Europe, Asia, Africa, and in parts of the Americas.
- Primary Mode of Transmission: Fly bites occur upon contact with environments where blood-feeding flies are present. The specific environment of risk varies with each particular fly species.
- Major Clinical Signs: Blood-feeding flies cause skin lesions leading to irritation, erythema, pruritus, inflammation, hypersensitivity reactions, and anemia. In addition, blood-feeding flies transmit numerous pathogens as biologic (e.g., *Dirofilaria immitis*) or mechanical (e.g., anthrax) vectors.
- Differential Diagnoses: Skin lesions from other ectoparasites including ticks, mites, fleas, and lice; other cutaneous hypersensitivities (e.g., atopic dermatitis); eosinophilic plaque; autoimmune disorders; photoinduced dermatitis (e.g., solar dermatitis, photosensitive dermatitis).
- Human Health Significance: Many species of blood-feeding flies readily feed on humans.

ETIOLOGY AND EPIDEMIOLOGY

True flies (Diptera) are among the most varied order of insects. Approximately 158,000 species have been described with great diversity in their biology and life histories.[2] Historically the order was divided into three major suborders: Nematocera containing mosquitoes, black flies, sand flies, and gnats; Brachycera containing horse flies and deer flies; and Cyclorrhapha containing the house flies, flesh flies, tsetse flies, and keds. However, major taxonomic revision has led to most current studies classifying the true flies into five infraorders: Culicomorpha (mosquitoes and black flies), Psychodomorpha (sand flies), Brachycera (horse flies, deer flies, and house flies), Bibionomorpha (gnats), and Tipulomorpha (crane flies).[2,3] This chapter focuses on families that contain blood-feeding Diptera known to feed on dogs and cats: Culicidae and Simuliidae of the infraorder Culicomorpha, Psychodidae of Psychodomorpha, and Muscidae of Brachycera.

Like other insects, the body of adult Diptera are divided into three parts: the head, thorax, and abdomen. The head contains the eyes, antennae, and specialized mouthparts that vary greatly among species. Variation in antennae structure and number, along with mouthpart morphology, play an important role in taxonomy and species distinction. Blood-feeding Diptera have specialized mouthparts made for piercing or biting the skin to imbibe blood meals.[4,5] Hematophagous flies first appeared in the Jurassic period,[6,7] and only a minority of known Diptera (approximately 11,000 species) have evolved to feed on blood.[8] Most Diptera have two wings (one pair) as adults, although there are some species of wingless adults. True flies have modified structures called halteres rather than hind wings; these club-shaped organs are used for balance and are present even in the wingless Diptera.[8] Wing venation is also important for identification and classification of different species. The abdomen consists of 11 or fewer segments, with the posterior segments modified for copulation or ovipositing.

All Diptera have a complex life cycle and undergo complete metamorphosis with egg, larval, pupal, and adult stages. The larval stages are commonly referred to as maggots, while the pupal stage usually involves development within a cocoon.[8] In most blood-feeding species, only the female imbibes blood from the host. However, there are some examples where both sexes take blood meals (e.g., stable flies). Feeding behavior is a major component of a blood-feeding fly's ability to serve as a vector for a pathogen, and differences in host preference or feeding patterns directly influence vector potential. Table 107.1 provides examples of different pathogens that can be transmitted to dogs or cats by members of each family.

Culicidae (Mosquitoes)

Adult mosquitoes are delicate flies (Fig. 107.1) with long segmented antennae and an extended proboscis containing a bundle of stylets used in feeding. Mosquitoes persist and thrive in a variety of environments. They feed on dogs, cats, people, and many other animals worldwide; mosquitoes also transmit a wide variety of human and veterinary disease agents. Important genera that readily feed on and transmit pathogens to dogs and cats include *Aedes, Anopheles, Culex,* and *Psorophora*.[9,10]

The mosquito life cycle is depicted in Fig. 107.2. Mosquitoes oviposit in aquatic environments or in dry areas that flood seasonally, with some species being able to utilize moist soil.[11] A small body of water (e.g., a backyard puddle) can provide a suitable habitat for a large number of eggs. In some species, eggs remain dormant in dry

TABLE 107.1 Blood-Feeding Diptera of Dogs and Cats and Associated Pathogens

Family	Common Name	Important Genera	Examples of Pathogens Transmitted	Affected Species
Culicidae	Mosquito	*Aedes, Anopheles, Culex,* and *Psorophora*	*Dirofilaria immitis*	Dogs and Cats
Simuliidae	Black fly	*Simulium*	*Onchocerca lupi*	Dogs and Cats
Psychodidae	Sand fly	*Phlebotomus* (Old World) *Lutzomyia* (New World)	*Leishmania* spp.	Dogs and Cats
Muscidae	Stable fly	*Stomoxys*	*Coxiella burnetti* *Trypanosoma evansi* (mechanical)	Dogs

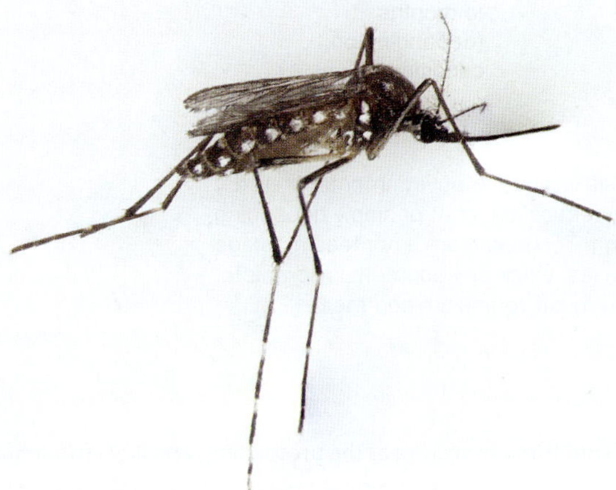

Fig. 107.1 Female mosquito (*Aedes aegypti*). Note the delicate appearance and long proboscis.

conditions for months, hatching only after an area is inundated by floods or heavy rain. Several abiotic factors, particularly temperature and moisture, play a role in determining when eggs will hatch or when pupae become adults.[11,12] After hatching, mosquito larvae molt four times within an approximately 2-week period before pupating. The pupae may persist from 2 days to a week depending on the species (Fig. 107.2).

Only the female mosquito takes a blood meal, which is required for oviposition, while the males feed on plant nectar.[13] In some species the female undergoes autogeny (production of eggs without a blood meal), but most only do so for an initial clutch.[11] The female mosquito takes blood meals every few days and rests and develops eggs between feedings.[14,15] After oviposition the female seeks a new host. Repeated feeding on new hosts contributes greatly to pathogen transmission.

Mosquitoes utilize complex behaviors that support the location of a host and subsequently a blood meal. Chemical cues such as the detection of carbon dioxide, lactic acid, and acetone from the skin, sweat, and breath may be used.[16,17] Mosquito mouthparts have evolved to efficiently pierce skin and obtain a blood meal.[13] Mosquito saliva contains anticoagulants that are injected into the wound during feeding;[13] if not interrupted, feeding is usually concluded within 3 to 4 minutes.[18] Abdominal stretch receptors alert the nervous system when adequate blood has been consumed and feeding stops.[15]

Simuliidae (Black flies)

Black flies are among the smallest of the blood-feeding Diptera, measuring 1 to 6 mm in length. Black flies have stout bodies with short segmented antennae and they vary in color from black or gray to a yellow-brown. Sometimes referred to as the humpback fly because of the shape visible in profile behind their head (Fig. 107.3), black flies are a major pest of poultry and livestock, and livestock deaths from hypersensitivity reactions, anemia, or toxin from fly saliva have been reported.[14] Black flies also readily feed on dogs and cats and can cause pruritic bloody lesions.[14] In areas where black flies are common, reports often describe dogs plagued by swarms during the summer months.[19,20] Black flies are also considered a putative vector of *Onchocerca lupi* in dogs and cats in the United States.[21,22]

Like mosquitoes, black flies also use water to complete their life cycle (Fig. 107.4). Female black flies deposit eggs in clear, running water in natural areas.[23] Larval and pupal stages are adapted to an aquatic environment, and only the females imbibe a blood meal while the males feed on plant nectar, similar to mosquitoes.[23] Black flies are notorious for their aggressive feeding and markedly large swarms involving huge numbers of flies; asphyxiation of livestock has reportedly occurred following inhalation due to the extreme abundance of black flies at certain times of the year.[24,25] Females oviposit on the water's surface or on partially submerged objects.[14] Species differ in seasonality and annual fecundity. In areas of North America with mild climates, some species are multivoltine (produce multiple broods annually) and can complete seven or more generations per year.[23] The eggs of multivoltine species hatch in a few days, but eggs of univoltine species (one brood of eggs per year) will not hatch until the following year. In some species of black flies, females can reproduce without taking a blood meal; for these species the mouthparts lack teeth and cannot cut the host's skin.[23]

Black flies feed during the day, and their activity is highly seasonal in temperate areas, with more feeding occurring during the spring and summer.[8] Several host attractants have been identified, including carbon dioxide, host shape, size, and color.[16] The black fly has short mouthparts consisting of serrated stylets that cut into host skin.[8] Stylets enter the host's skin and anchor the mouthparts; blood then begins to pool at the feeding site and is imbibed from the pool.[23] The saliva contains anticoagulants and local anesthetic to enhance vasodilation.[26] Black flies are persistent feeders and often do not leave a host until completing their blood meal, which can require as long as 3 to 6 minutes; this behavior renders them poor mechanical vectors as they do not take multiple interrupted feedings.[23]

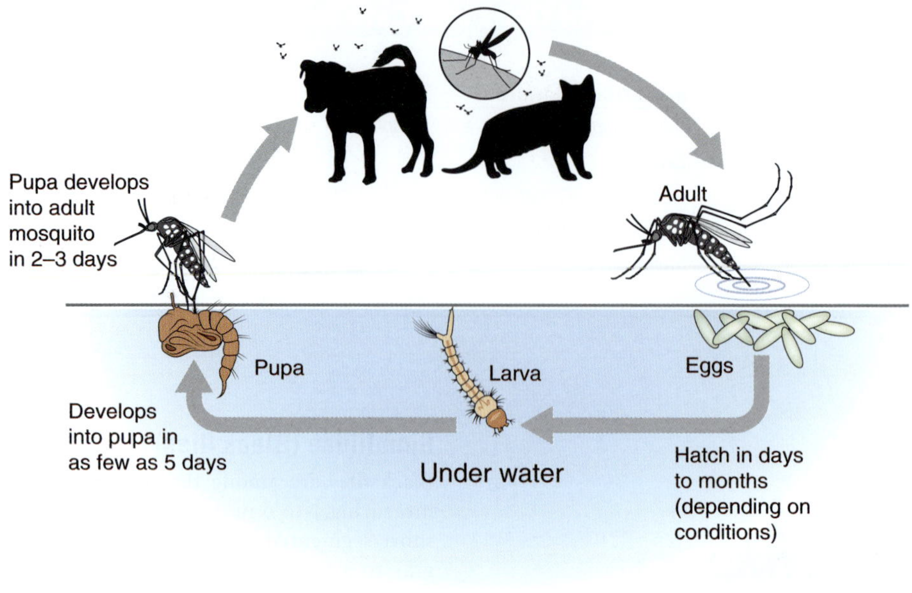

Fig. 107.2 Mosquito life cycle. Female mosquitoes oviposit in aquatic environments or in dry areas that flood seasonally. Eggs are deposited either in clusters called a raft or singly depending on species. Larvae hatch and molt four times before pupating. The pupae are a nonfeeding stage and can persist from 2 days to a week depending on the species. Once development is complete, adults emerge and rest on the water surface to dry and then fly off to find a blood meal.

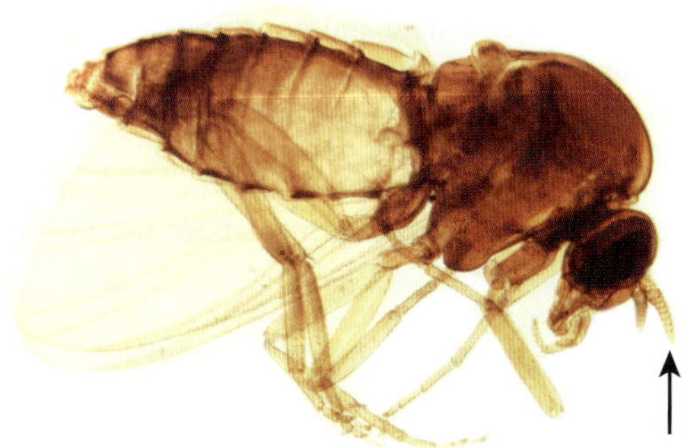

Fig. 107.3 Black fly (*Simulium* sp.). Note the hump behind the head and the short segmented antennae. (Courtesy of Dr. Brian Herrin, Kansas State University.)

Psychodidae (Sand flies)

Sand flies of veterinary importance are in the subfamily Phlebotomine. These small fuzzy-appearing flies have long legs and antennae (Fig. 107.5) and are readily distinguished from other Diptera by wings held above the body forming a vertical "V" shape.[27] The adults are weak fliers and are mainly active at night. Sand flies can typically be found near breeding and resting sites such as tree hollows, plant leaves, cracks and crevices between rocks or other masonry, and other dark humid sites that offer shelter.[28] The sand fly life cycle is depicted in Figure 107.6. Breeding and ovipositing occur in humid and terrestrial areas.[28] Sand flies are vectors of the protozoan parasite *Leishmania* spp. (see Chapter 96).

Only female sand flies feed on blood. As is the case with Culicidae and Simuliidae, some sand fly species are autogenous, but females of these species need to imbibe blood meals for successful oviposition. Blood feeding generally occurs on exposed skin such as ears, nose, lips, and feet.[28] The sand fly has tiny mouthparts (less than 0.6 mm) and mandibles with teeth that cut like scissors, creating a small pool of blood from which to imbibe (similar to black flies).[27] Less is known about the host-seeking behavior and cues of sand flies compared to mosquitoes.[29]

Muscidae (Stable Flies)

Most Muscidae adults do not imbibe blood, but one subfamily, the Stomoxyinae, contains several blood-feeding species.[30] The stable fly, *Stomoxys calcitrans*, is a filth fly and a blood feeder of medical and veterinary importance. Stable flies closely resemble the common house fly (*Musca domestica*), but the mouthparts differ (Fig. 107.7A). Stable fly mouthparts bear a nonretractable, long, sharp proboscis for piercing the host skin and imbibing blood (Fig. 107.7B). Unlike many other blood-feeding flies, both males and females imbibe blood. As a filth fly, stable fly eggs are laid in decaying organic material such as damp hay, lawn clippings, or animal manure. The complete life cycle is illustrated in Figure 107.8. The adults mate in the air and do not spend significant time on the host.

Stable flies are usually active and attacking hosts on warm days and often stop seeking hosts and blood meals during cold weather.[14] Livestock are the primary hosts, but stable flies will often feed on people and dogs, so much so that in some areas they are commonly referred to as the dog fly or kennel fly, as dogs are often repeatedly bitten.[30] Stable flies are a common cause of allergic fly bite dermatitis in

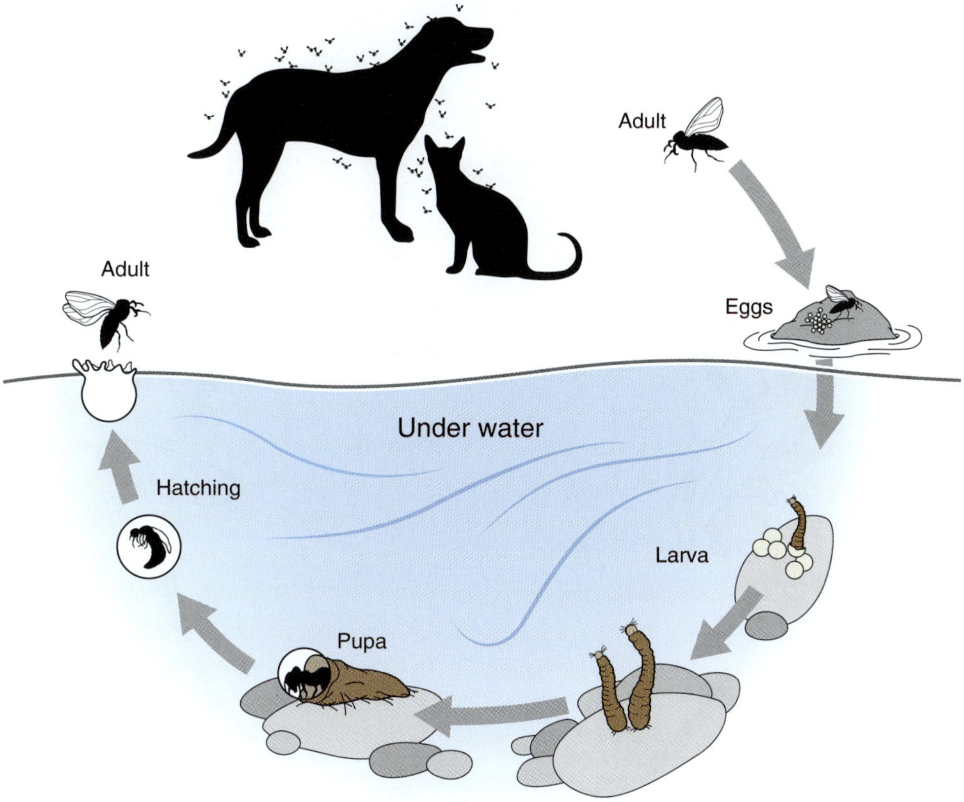

Fig. 107.4 Black fly life cycle. Female black flies oviposit after taking a blood meal, depositing their eggs in clear running water. The larval stages are adapted to an aquatic lifestyle and anchor themselves to rocks, vegetation, or other debris and feed on organic matter in the current. After passing through several instars (4–9 depending on the species), the larvae spin cocoons and pupate underwater. Pupae are attached to the substrate via a silken thread. Adults emerge from the pupae underwater and are carried to the surface in a bubble of air. The mature adult then searches for a blood meal.

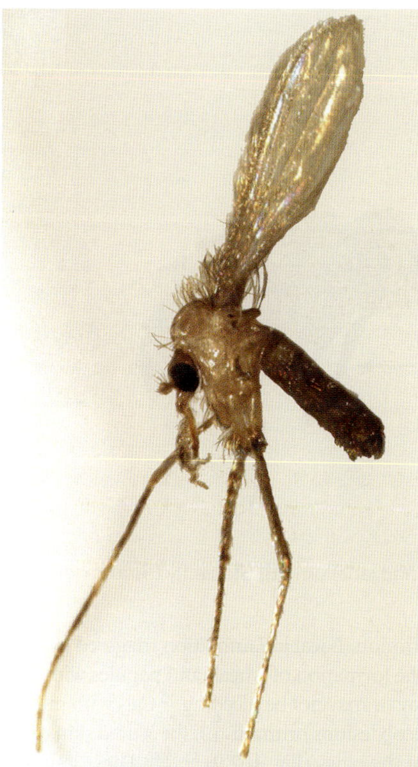

Fig. 107.5 Old World sand fly (*Phlebotomus perniciosus*). Note the long legs relative to the body and the fuzzy appearance. (Courtesy of Dr Emilie Bouhsira, National Veterinary School of Toulouse, France.)

dogs, particularly in dogs housed in outdoor kennels where they cannot readily escape the flies.[31] Mechanical transmission of *Trypanasoma evansi* and *Coxiella* spp. by *Stomoxys* spp. has been documented.[32]

CLINICAL FEATURES

Pathogenesis and Clinical Signs

Blood feeding by flies causes a wide range of effects, from no reaction by the host, to general annoyance, the appearance of pruritic bloody spots at the feeding site, and the potential for pathogen transmission. Fly feeding injuries often result in mechanical damage to the host skin and immediately underlying tissues. A wound can form at the feeding site causing further irritation, erythema, dermatitis, papular eruptions, and, in some cases, hypersensitivity reactions.[33] Stable flies can cause necrotic dermatitis on the ear tips of dogs as well as exudative dermatitis.[34] Hypersensitivity reactions to mosquito feeding are particularly common in some cats resulting in eosinophilic dermatitis that can lead to nodules, scaling, and alopecia.[33,35]

Excessive blood feeding by flies can result in significant blood loss and subsequent anemia. Mosquitoes can ingest up to three times their body weight when taking a blood meal,[36] and heavy swarms have caused the death of cattle and horses,[37,38] therefore exsanguination of smaller mammals is also possible, although rare. The saliva of a biting fly contains anticoagulants, toxins, and other secretions that aid in blood flow at the wound site and allow the fly to continue to successfully feed.[30] For example, sand flies inject a particularly powerful vasodilation peptide into the feeding site which results in a pool of blood for feeding.[39] Salivary components also stimulate an immune

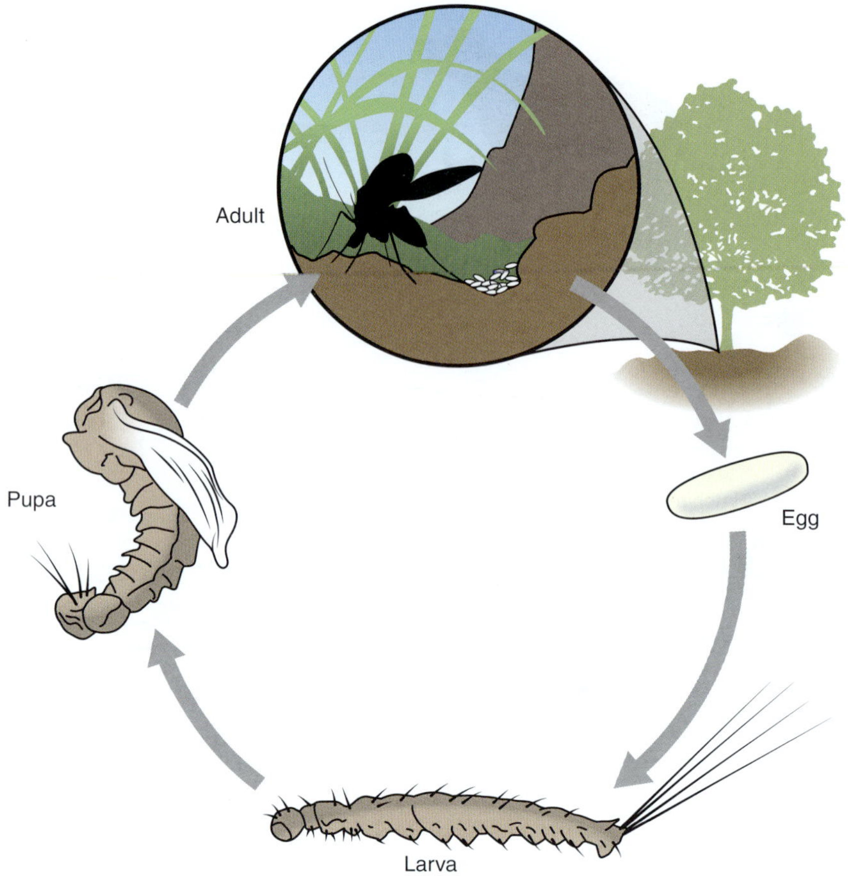

Fig. 107.6 Sand fly life cycle. Female sand flies oviposit after a blood meal and deposit eggs in cracks and crevices between rocks or other masonry, tree hollows, or other dark humid areas that offer shelter. Sand flies progress from egg, to larva going through four instars before pupating and the emergence of adults. Unlike mosquitoes and black flies, the immature sand fly stages are not aquatic.

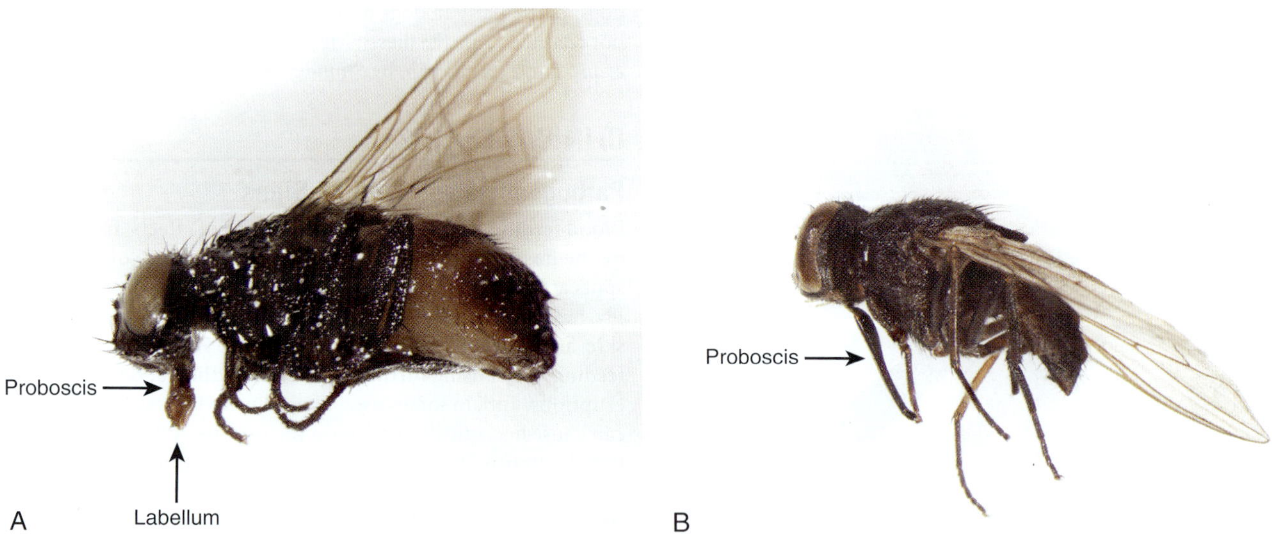

Fig. 107.7 (A) House fly (*Musca domestica*) with retractable proboscis and labellum. (B) Stable fly (*Stomoxys calcitrans*) with long, pointed proboscis.

response that often results in local inflammation. In some instances, individual dogs or cats may become hypersensitive, developing more severe reactions as they encounter more flies.

Physical Examination Findings

Blood feeding by flies is often painful, although reactions vary greatly among individual animals. Inflammatory reactions and pruritus at the bite site are common. Local inflammation triggered by blood-feeding flies may result in the formation of wheals and papules with a central puncture wound that may or may not be bleeding.[40] Cats with mosquito bite hypersensitivity develop lesions primarily on the haired skin of the nose, pinnae, and margins of the paws (Fig. 107.9).[33,35,40] These lesions initially appear as erythematous papules that, over time, become crusts, erosions, areas of alopecia, or ulcers and may be either hyper- or hypopigmented.

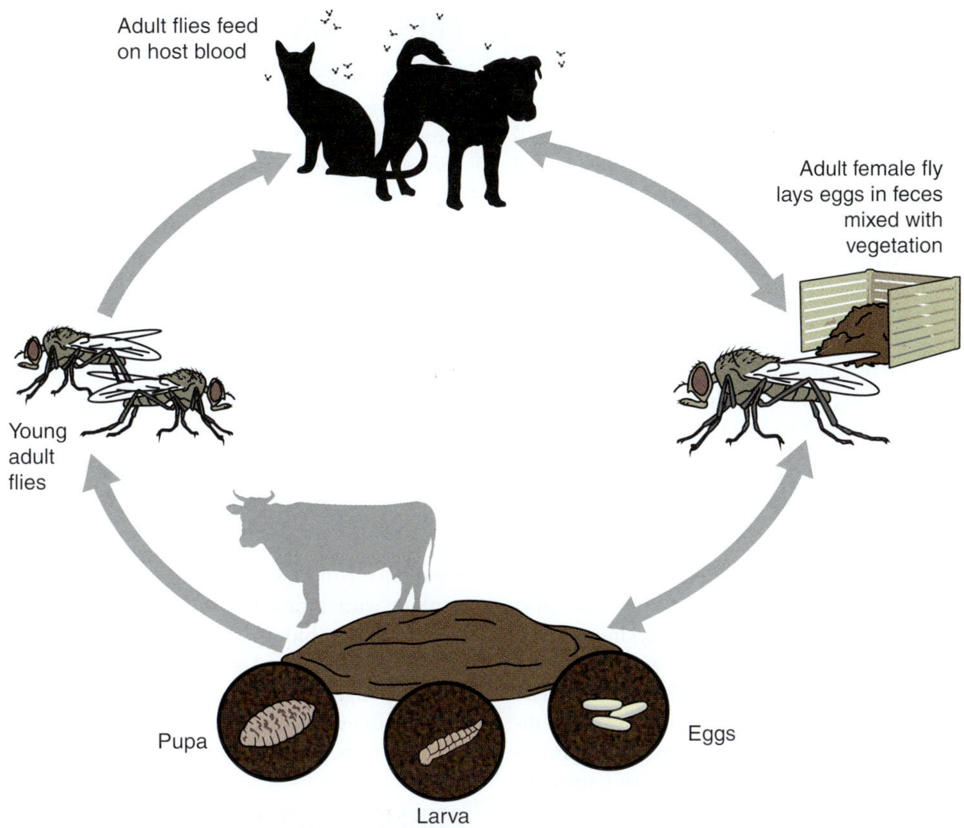

Fig. 107.8 Stable fly life cycle. Stable flies deposit eggs in moist, decaying organic matter such as feces. The adult female deposits multiple clutches of eggs, with each clutch requiring a separate blood meal. Eggs hatch into the first instar larvae, which feed and mature through three instars. The third instar larvae pupate in the organic material and adult stable flies can fly within an hour of emerging.

DIAGNOSIS

Definitive diagnosis can be achieved by identifying flies directly; however, observing flies feeding on pets is unlikely. Because flies are usually not present on examination, a detailed history—including attention to the season and awareness of arthropods commonly active in a given habitat and geographic region—is necessary to help identify the cause of the skin lesions. The identification of a specific vector-borne disease or pathogen transmitted by the biting fly also would indicate a previous fly bite. Differential diagnoses for blood-feeding flies include other arthropod bite wounds such as those induced by ticks, mites, fleas, lice, and bed bugs as well as a number of different skin conditions. Reactions to food and environmental antigens, head and neck excoriations, photoinduced dermatitis, and autoimmune conditions can result in similar lesions.

Biting flies that readily feed on dogs or cats can be differentiated from other ectoparasites morphologically. Diptera bodies are differentiated into head, thorax, and abdomen. The head contains the eyes, antennae, and specialized mouthparts adapted for blood feeding that can vary greatly among species; the thorax bears six legs and a pair of wings; and the abdomen contains the reproductive organs.[4,5]

Morphologic keys are available to identify all stages of biting flies.[41-43] If the adult fly is available and the specimen is not damaged, an identification can be made by a trained parasitologist or medical entomologist using morphologic keys.[14,30,44]

LABORATORY ABNORMALITIES

Most bloodwork findings on animals with fly bites are unremarkable. When massive blood loss from feeding has occurred, anemia can be present.

Pathologic Findings

Histopathologic Findings

Early fly bite lesions may include a central area of epidermal necrosis surrounded by edema and dermal hemorrhage; in some cases, a hemorrhagic crust covers the necrotic area. Mixed mononuclear, neutrophilic, and eosinophilic inflammatory infiltrates may be present, along with intraepidermal eosinophils, sometimes contained within eosinophilic pustules.[44] The histologic findings of feline mosquito bite hypersensitivity include extensive superficial and deep perivascular and interstitial eosinophilic and mixed dermatitis. Focal areas of degranulated eosinophils with eosinophilic folliculitis and furunculosis may also be present.[44]

TREATMENT AND PROGNOSIS

Animals with hypersensitivity or other dermatologic reactions to blood-feeding flies should be treated as their clinical signs dictate. Feline mosquito bite hypersensitivity can be addressed by keeping the cat housed indoors and administering immunomodulatory drugs such as glucocorticoids and antihistamines until lesions resolve.[45] In the case of feline mosquito bite hypersensitivity, as long as mosquitoes are kept from biting, the reaction can be contained and the prognosis for recovery is good, but the reappearance of mosquitoes and subsequent bites will lead to continued hypersensitivity reactions.[45] As for all blood-feeding flies, preventing contact with flies is crucial for a good prognosis. Repellents containing permethrin can be helpful in limiting bites from mosquitoes, sand flies, and *Stomoxys* on dogs but cannot be used safely on cats.[46] Some studies have documented reduced transmission of heartworm to dogs when a mosquito repellent is used; this approach should always be combined with consistent use of heartworm preventive (see Chapter 111).[47] Dogs and cats that are routinely pestered by blood-feeding flies, particularly by persistent and aggressive feeders such as black flies or *Stomoxys* spp., should be kept indoors to limit contact with the offending flies.

IMMUNITY AND VACCINATION

The immune response to a biting fly is largely directed against salivary proteins. The saliva of blood-feeding flies contains numerous enzymes to assist in blood meal acquisition and minimize the host immune response, including kinases that destroy bradykinin, which is responsible for mediating pain and itch in the host, as well as other histamine-binding proteins.[48] Fly feeding activity induces both a Th1 and Th2 response in the host. The Th1 respsonse is stimulated by salivary components that do not function as antigens because of their low molecular weight, but instead bind to collagen and other skin proteins of the host, acting as haptens.[48] Repeated exposure to these haptens can induce delayed hypersensitvity reactions.

Mosquito saliva has been shown to elicit an immune response that leads to Type 1 and Type 4 hypersensitivity reactions as well as IgE-mediated reactions and antibody-independent T-cell reactions.[49] Mast cells also play a key role in the hypersensitivity reactions caused by exposure to mosquito saliva. The adaptive immune response to biting fly saliva can also impact pathogen transmission. Immunity to sand fly saliva can lead to strong protection against *Leishmania* spp. infection by limiting parasite proliferation.[50] Numerous salivary proteins from different sand fly species have been evaluated as potential candidates for vaccines against leishmaniosis.[51] A phase I clinical trial in humans showed that a mosquito vaccine appeared to be safe and incited an immune response when adjuvanted.[52] However, at the time of writing no commercially available vaccine exists for mosquitoes, sand flies, or any other biting flies for any species.

PREVENTION

Keeping pets indoors and limiting contact between the pets and blood-feeding flies are particularly helpful in preventing fly bites. However, some biting flies, especially certain endophilic mosquito species, will readily enter the home or other buildings.[15] Ensuring that windows and doors are properly screened will help prevent access by mosquitoes. In addition, removing any potential breeding sites, such as standing water for mosquitoes or decaying vegetation associated with compost piles for *Stomoxys* spp., can limit populations of biting flies in the environment.[53,54]

In dogs, some topical pyrethroids have efficacy as mosquito, sand fly, and stable fly repellents and can reduce the feeding activity of these biting flies.[55-58] In areas where vector transmission of pathogens is common, permethrin or deltamethrin repellents are used to protect pets from fly feeding and can reduce transmission risks.[59] Pyrethroid repellents have also been shown to prevent sand flies from transmitting *Leishmania* spp. to dogs in endemic areas.[57,60] An effective prevention strategy combines the use of safe, effective repellents with lifestyle management (habitat avoidance) to limit the contact with blood-feeding flies, and barriers to prevent mosquitoes and other blood-feeding flies from gaining entry into the home. Isoxazoline insecticides will kill mosquitoes and sand flies after feeding; although their use does not prevent feeding altogether, killing the flies does reduce the overall population and limit transmission to the next host.[61,62]

PUBLIC HEALTH ASPECTS

Mosquitoes and other biting flies also are of significant human health importance. People often develop localized reactions from arthropod feeding as well as hypersensitivity resulting in erythema, pruritus, and edema.[63] Biting flies also transmit a number of pathogens to people. Recommended protection methods include habitat modifications to reduce fly populations, avoiding areas with actively feeding flies, wearing protective clothing, and using repellents containing permethrin or N, N-diethyl-meta-toluamide (DEET). No DEET-containing products are labeled for veterinary use and DEET should not be used in pets as seizures may result, especially in cats.[14] In leishmaniosis-endemic regions, dogs can serve as a reservoir host; sand fly control on dogs has been shown to limit transmission risk to people (see Chapter 96).

CASE EXAMPLE

Signalment

"Tom," a 3-year-old male neutered domestic shorthair from Glen Ellen, California, USA.

History:

Tom was evaluated in June for multiple skin nodules and ulcerations on his nasal planum and pinnae that first appeared in April (2 months previously). He had a similar problem last spring that began as a few small nodules on his nose and ears. His owner reported that the nodules increase in number and eventually ulcerate if untreated. The lesions were nonpruritic. Last spring, he was treated with a glucocorticoid injection, ivermectin IM, and possibly antimicrobials. The lesions resolved completely until this episode. Tom is an indoor/outdoor cat that lives on a half-acre of land with a dog, goats, and chickens. None of the other animals have skin conditions.

Current Medications:

Topical monthly flea prevention (owner unaware of name).

Other Medical History:

Previous medical problems included transient pyrexia of unknown origin a year previously, and a migrating plant awn in the inguinal fat pad a month previously that was removed surgically. At that time the skin lesions were present. He was treated with cefovecin sodium SC, but there was no change in the skin lesions after the injection.

Physical Examination

Body weight: 6.2 kg

General: Bright, alert, hydrated, responsive. Mucous membranes pink, HR 190, RR 50, temperature 100°F (37.8°C)

CASE EXAMPLE—cont'd

Integument: There was focal alopecia, crusting, and ulceration on the bridge of the nose and multiple crusted nodules on both pinnae (see Fig. 107.9A and B). A thickened area of skin was present in the inguinal fat pad where surgery had been performed a month previously. No ectoparasites were evident.

Eyes, ears, nose, and throat: Mild gingivitis was present.

No other clinically significant findings were found on physical examination.

Cytology Findings

Cytology of a skin scraping revealed increased numbers of neutrophils and cocci.

Serology

A feline heartworm antibody test was negative.

Diagnosis:

Suspected mosquito bite hypersensitivity.

Treatment

Tom was treated with a tapering course of prednisolone (1 mg/kg q12h PO for 5 days, then q24h for 5 days, then 0.5 mg/kg q24h for 5 days then q48h for 5 days). He was also treated with clavulanic acid-amoxicillin (10 mg/kg q12h PO). Monthly treatment with topical selamectin was commenced. The lesions resolved completely.

Comments

A presumptive diagnosis of mosquito bite hypersensitivity was made in this cat based on the seasonality of disease, the cat's lifestyle and geographic location, and the suggestive appearance and distribution of lesions. The owner was offered a biopsy but declined. Other diagnostic tests that could be considered in this case are retrovirus testing as well as a heartworm antigen test (see Chapter 111).

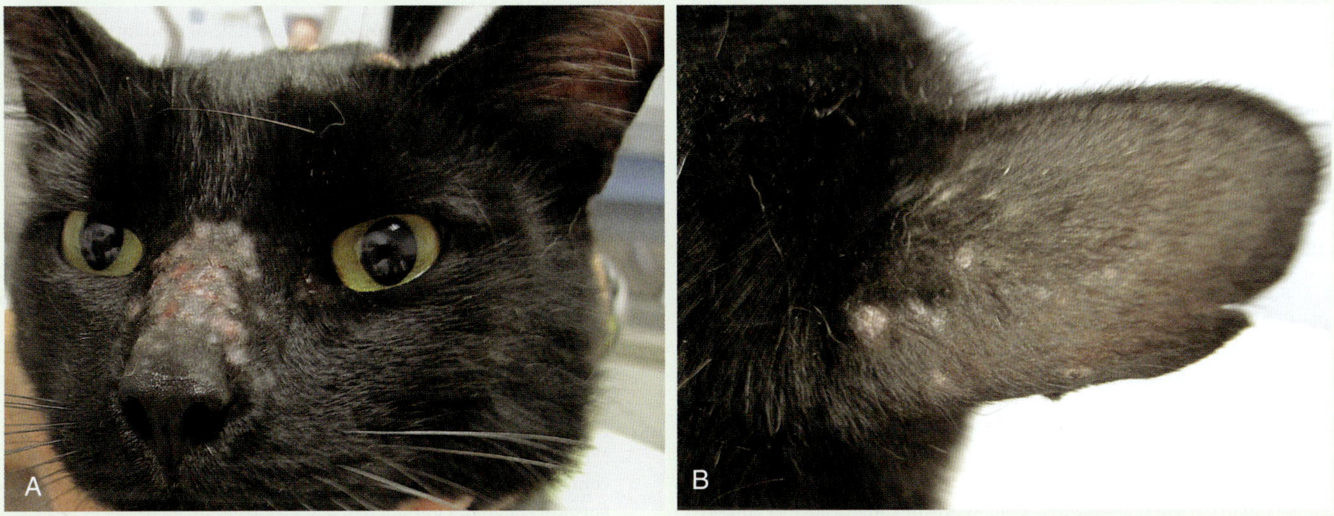

Fig. 107.9 Suspected mosquito bite hypersensitivity dermatitis lesions on (A) the bridge of the nose and (B) the pinna of a 3-year-old male neutered domestic shorthair. (Courtesy of University of California-Davis Veterinary Dermatology Service.)

SUGGESTED READINGS

Mullen GR, Durden LA. *Medical and Veterinary Entomology*. San Diego: Elsevier Science & Technology; 2018.

Day MJ. In: *Arthropod-Borne Infectious Diseases of the Dog and Cat*. 2nd ed. CRC Press; 2016.

Russell RC, Domenico O, Wall R. *The Encyclopedia of Medical and Veterinary Entomology*. Wallingford, Oxfordshire, UK: CABI; 2013.

REFERENCES

1. Krzeminski W, Krzeminska E, Papier F. *Grauvogelia arzvilleriana* sp. n. - the oldest Diptera species (Lower/Middle Triassic of France). *Acta Zoologica Cracovensia*. 1994;37:95–99.
2. Wiegmann BM, Richards S. Genomes of diptera. *Curr Opin Insect Sci*. 2018;25:116–124.
3. Wiegmann BM, Yeates DK. Phylogeny of diptera. In: Kirk-Spriggs AH, Sinclair BJ, eds. *Manual of Afrotropical Diptera. Volume 1. Introductory Chapters and Keys to Diptera Families Suricata*. SANBI Graphics & Editing; 2017:253–266.
4. Grimaldi DA, Engel MS. *Evolution of the Insects*. Cambridge: Cambridge University Press; 2005:468–547.
5. Hall RD, Gerhardt RR. Flies (Diptera). In: Mullen G, Durden L, eds. *Medical and Veterinary Entomology*. San Diego: Academic Press; 2002:127–145.
6. Kalugina NS. New mesozoic Simuliidae and Leptoconopidae and the origin of blood-sucking in the lower Diptera. *Paleontol Zh*. 1991;1:81–84.
7. Lukashevich ED, Mostovski MB. Hematophagous insects in the fossil record. *J Paleontol*. 2003;37:48–56.
8. Crosskey RW. Introduction to the diptera. In: Lane RP, Crosskey RW, eds. *Medical Insects and Arachnids*. Dordrecht: Springer; 1993:51–77.
9. Ledesma N, Harrington LC. Mosquito vectors of dog heartworm in the United States: vector status and factors influencing transmission efficiency. *Top Companion Anim Med*. 2011;26:178–185.
10. Lok JB, Walker ED, Scoles GA. Filariasis. In: Eldridge BF, Edman JD, eds. *Medical Entomology*. Boston: Kluwer Academic Publishers; 2000:299–375.
11. Becker N, Boase C, Dahl C, et al. *Mosquitoes and Their Control*. Berlin: Springer; 2010:9–24.
12. Brust RA, Costello RA. Mosquitoes of Manitoba. II. The effect of storage temperature and relative humidity on hatching of eggs of *Aedes vexans* and *Aedes abserratus* (Diptera: Culicidae). *Can Ent*. 1969;101:1285–1291.
13. Clements AN. In: *The Biology of Mosquitoes, Vol. 1; Development, Nutrition and Reproduction*. London: Chapman and Hall; 1992.
14. Bowman DD. *Georgis' Parasitology for Veterinarians*. 11th ed. St. Louis, MO: Elsevier Saunders; 2021:10–89.
15. Reiskind MH, Little SE. Biology, ecology, and vector role of mosquitoes. In: Beugnet F, ed. *Guide to Vector Borne Disease of Pets*. Lyon, France: Merial; 2013:4.
16. Sutcliffe JF, McIver SB. Fine structure of tarsal sensilla of male and female *Simulium vittatum* (Diptera: Simuliidae). *J Morphol*. 1987;192:13–26.

17. Bowen MF. The sensory physiology of host seeking behavior in mosquitoes. *Ann Rev Entomol.* 1991;36:139–158.
18. Gillett JD. Natural selection and feeding speed in a blood-sucking insect. *Proc R Soc Lond B Biol Sci.* 1967;167(1008):316–329.
19. Wendt K. How you can protect your dog from black fly bites. WIVB, May 26, 2017. Available at: www.wivb.com/news/local-news/how-you-can-protect-your-dog-from-black-fly-bites/1045741826.
20. Hughes V. Black flies: are they biting your dog? FOX 28 Spokane, July 11, 2017. Available at: fox28spokane.com/black-flies-are-they-biting-your-dog/.
21. Hassan HK, Bolcen S, Kubofcik J, et al. Isolation of *Onchocerca lupi* in dogs and black flies, California, USA. *Emerg Infect Dis.* 2015;21:789–796.
22. Verocai GG, Conboy G, Lejeune M, et al. *Onchocerca lupi* nematodes in dogs exported from the United States into Canada. *Emerg Infect Dis.* 2016;22:1477–1479.
23. Adler PH, McCreadie JW. Black flies (Simuliidae). In: Mullen G, Durden L, eds. *Medical and Veterinary Entomology.* 2nd ed. San Diego, CA: Elsevier; 2009:183–200.
24. Knapp FW. Arthropod pests of horses. In: Williams RE, Hall RD, Broce AB, Scholl PJ, eds. *Livestock Entomology.* New York: John Wiley & Sons; 1985:297–313.
25. Wright RE. Arthropod pests of beef cattle on pasture and range land. In: Williams RE, Hall RD, Broce AB, Scholl PJ, eds. *Livestock Entomology.* New York: John Wiley & Sons; 1985:191–206.
26. Cupp EW, Cupp MS. Black fly (Diptera:Simuliidae) salivary secretions: importance in vector competence and disease. *J Med Entomol.* 1997;34: 87–94.
27. Lane RP. Sandflies (*Phlebotominae*). In: Lane RP, Crosskey RW, eds. *Medical Insects and Arachnids.* Dordrecht: Springer; 1993:78–119.
28. Rutledge LC, Gupta RK. 2009. Mothflies and sandflies. In: Mullen G, Durden L, eds. *Medical and Veterinary Entomology.* 2nd ed. San Diego, CA: Elsevier; 2009:153–168.
29. Pardo RH, Santamaría E, Cabrera OL. Entering and exiting behavior of the phlebotomine sand fly *Lutzomyia longiflocosa* (Diptera: Psychodidae) in rural houses of the sub-Andean region of Colombia. *Mem Inst Oswaldo Cruz.* 2017;112:19–30.
30. Crosskey RW. Stable-flies and horn-flies (bloodsucking Muscidae). In: Lane RP, Crosskey RW, eds. *Medical Insects and Arachnids.* Dordrecht: Springer; 1993:389–402.
31. Fankhauser B, Irwin JP, Stone ML, et al. Repellent and insecticidal efficacy of a new combination of fipronil and permethrin against stable flies (*Stomoxys calcitrans*). *Parasit Vectors.* 2015;8:61.
32. Baldacchino F, Muenworn V, Desquesnes M, et al. Transmission of pathogens by *Stomoxys* flies (Diptera, Muscidae): a review. *Parasite.* 2013;20:26.
33. Medleau L, Hnilica KA. Hypersensitivity disorders. In: *Small Animal Dermatology: A Color Atlas and Therapeutic Guide.* 2nd ed. St. Louis, MO: Elsevier; 2006:159–188.
34. Yeruham I, Braverman Y. Skin lesions in dogs, horses and calves caused by the stable fly *Stomoxys calcitrans* (Diptera: Muscidae). *Rev Elev Med Vet Pays Trop.* 1995;48:347–349.
35. Clare AC, Medleau L. Case management workshop (mosquito bite hypersensitivity in a cat). *Vet Med.* 1997;92:728.
36. Nayar K, Sauerman DM. The effects of nutrition on survival and fecundity in Florida mosquitoes: part 3. Utilization of blood and sugar for fecundity. *J Med Entomol.* 1975;12:220–225.
37. Bishopp FC. Mosquitoes kill livestock. *Science.* 1933;77:115–116.
38. Abbitt B, Abbitt LG. Fatal exsanguination of cattle attributed to an attack of salt marsh mosquitoes (*Aedes sollicitans*). *J Am Vet Med Assoc.* 1981;179:1397–1400.
39. Ribeiro JC, Modi GB, Tesh RB. Salivary apyrase activity of some Old World phlebotomine sand flies. *Insect Biochem.* 1989;19:409–412.
40. Hargis AM, Myers S. The integument. In: Zachary JF, ed. *Pathologic Basis of Veterinary Disease.* 6th ed. St. Louis, MO: Saunders/Elsevier; 2017:1009–1146.
41. Oldroyd H. *The Natural History of Flies.* London: Weidenfeld and Nicolson; 1964.
42. Cole FR. *The Flies of Western North America.* Berkeley: University of California Press; 1969.
43. McAlpine JF, Peterson BV, Shewell GE, et al. *Manual of Nearctic Diptera, Volumes 1—2.* Quebec: Canadian Govt. Publishing Centre; 1987.
44. Zajac AM, Conboy GA, Little SE, Reichard MV. *Veterinary Clinical Parasitology.* 9th ed. Hoboken, NJ: Wiley-Blackwell; 2021:322–345.
45. Mason KV, Evans AF. Mosquito bite-caused eosinophilic dermatitis in cats. *J Am Vet Med Assoc.* 1991;198:2086–2088.
46. Martin A, Campbell A. Permethrin toxicity in cats. *Vet Rec.* 2000;147:639.
47. McCall JW, Varloud M, Hodgkins E, et al. Shifting the paradigm in *Dirofilaria immitis* prevention: blocking transmission from mosquitoes to dogs using repellents/insecticides and macrocyclic lactone prevention as part of a multimodal approach. *Parasit Vectors.* 2017;10(suppl 2):525.
48. Tizard IR. *Veterinary Immunology.* St. Louis, MO: Saunders/Elsevier; 2013:312–327.
49. Boulanger N. Arthropod saliva and its role in pathogen transmission: insect saliva. In: Boulanger N, ed. *Skin and Arthropod Vectors.* Academic Press; 2018:83–119.
50. Kamhawi S, Jesus G, Valenzuela JG, et al. Role of sand fly saliva on *Leishmania* infection and the potential of vector salivary proteins as vaccines. In: Boulanger N, ed. *Skin and Arthropod Vectors.* Academic Press; 2018:83–119.
51. Gomes R, Oliveira F. The immune response to sand fly salivary proteins and its influence on *Leishmania* immunity. *Front Immunol.* 2012;3:110.
52. Manning JE, Oliveira F, Coutinho-Abreu IV, et al. Safety and immunogenicity of a mosquito saliva peptide-based vaccine: a randomised, placebo-controlled, double-blind, phase 1 trial. *Lancet.* 2020;395:1998–2007.
53. Axtell RC. *Fly Control in Confined Livestock and Poultry Production.* Ciba-Geigy, Technical Monograph; 1986.
54. Richards SL, Ghosh SK, Zeichner BC, et al. Impact of source reduction on the spatial distribution of larvae and pupae of *Aedes albopictus* (Diptera: Culicidae) in suburban neighborhoods of a Piedmont community in North Carolina. *J Med Entomol.* 2008;45:617–628.
55. Mencke N, Volf P, Volfova V, et al. Repellent efficacy of a combination containing imidacloprid and permethrin against sand flies (*Phlebotomus papatasi*) in dogs. *Parasitol Res.* 2003;90:S108.
56. Fourie L. The efficacy of a topically applied combination of imidacloprid and permethrin against *Stomoxys calcitrans* on dogs. *Int J Appl Res Vet Med.* 2006;4:29.
57. Otranto D, Paradies P, Lia RP, et al. Efficacy of a combination of 10% imidacloprid/50% permethrin for the prevention of leishmaniasis in kennelled dogs in an endemic area. *Vet Parasitol.* 2007;144:270–278.
58. Fankhauser B, Irwin JP, Stone ML, et al. Repellent and insecticidal efficacy of a new combination of fipronil and permethrin against stable flies (*Stomoxys calcitrans*). *Parasit Vectors.* 2015;8:61.
59. Solano-Gallego L, Koutinas A, Miro G, et al. Directions for the diagnosis, clinical staging, treatment and prevention of canine leishmaniosis. *Vet Parasitol.* 2009;165:1–18.
60. Otranto D, Dantas-Torres F. Canine and feline vector-borne diseases in Italy: current situation and perspectives. *Parasit Vectors.* 2010;3:2.
61. Queiroga TBD, Ferreira HRP, dos Santos WV, et al. Fluralaner (Bravecto®) induces long-term mortality of *Lutzomyia longipalpis* after a blood meal in treated dogs. *Parasites Vectors.* 2020;13:609.
62. Liebenberg J, Fourie J, Lebon W, et al. Assessment of the insecticidal activity of afoxolaner against *Aedes aegypti* in dogs treated with NexGard®. *Parasite.* 2017;24:39.
63. Foster WA, Walker ED. Mosquitoes (Culicidae). In: Mullen G, Durden LA, eds. *Medical and Veterinary Entomology.* 2nd ed. San Diego, CA: Elsevier; 2009:207–274.

108

Myiasis

Jane E. Sykes, Lindsay Merkel, Susan E. Little

KEY POINTS

- First Described: Myiasis in humans and animals has been recognized for centuries. The most well-accepted description of myiasis was reported in 1965 by Fritz Zumpt, a German entomologist.[1] Infestations with *Cuterebra* spp. in cats in the United States were first described in the late 1800s.[2]
- Cause: A variety of fly species that obligately or facultatively infest the skin of vertebrates. The most common species that infest dogs and cats belong to the order Diptera; families Oestridae (bot flies or warble flies), Calliphoridae (blow flies), Sarcophagidae (flesh flies), and Muscidae (house flies). Examples include *Cuterebra* spp., *Hypoderma* spp., *Dermatobia hominis,* and *Oestrus* spp. (Oestridae); *Cochliomyia hominivorax*, *Lucilia* spp., and *Chrysomya* spp. (Calliphoridae); *Sarcophaga* spp. and *Wohlfahrtia* spp. (Sarcophagidae); and *Musca domestica* (Muscidae).
- Affected Hosts: Dogs, cats, and a large number of other vertebrate host species, especially livestock and wildlife species.
- Geographic Distribution: Worldwide, although the geographic distribution of individual fly species varies.
- Route of Transmission: For *Cuterebra* spp., eggs or larvae that are normally deposited around rodent or lagomorph burrows contaminate the skin and migrate into tissues. For most other fly species, eggs or larvae are deposited directly on to the vertebrate host. This may be where wounds or skin maceration are present, around body orifices (e.g., nasal cavity, perianal region), or on intact skin of weak or debilitated animals that are unable to groom.
- Major Clinical Signs: Cutaneous ulceration, which may have a putrid odor; subcutaneous masses ("warbles"), which may be pruritic or have evidence of larval movement; upper respiratory signs (e.g., sneezing, nasal discharge, stertorous respiration); neurologic signs (e.g., seizures, paralysis); ophthalmologic signs (impaired vision, uveitis, corneal edema, ocular discharge, distortion of the globe).
- Differential Diagnoses: Depend on parasite location and include a variety of other infectious diseases and neoplasia of the skin, ocular tissues, upper respiratory tract, and CNS; and migrating foreign bodies (e.g., plant awns). Aberrant CNS migration by *Cuterebra* spp. has been identified as a cause of feline ischemic encephalopathy in some regions.
- Human Health Significance: Humans can be infested by some of the same Diptera species that infest dogs and cats; myiasis is more often seen in impoverished people living in unhygienic conditions, travelers returning from tropical jungles, and children. Infestations are not directly transmitted from dogs and cats to humans. Blow fly larvae, especially *Lucilia sericata*, are also used as a recognized treatment in humans for debridement of necrotic wounds.

INTRODUCTION

Myiasis is defined as the infestation of live human and vertebrate animals with dipterous larvae, which, at least for a certain period, feed on the host's dead or living tissue, liquid body-substances, or ingested food. Myiasis has been divided into *obligatory myiasis*, where a living host is required for fly development, and *facultative myiasis*, where flies that normally use carrion or decaying organic matter for development occasionally infest macerated tissue or wounds of living hosts. *Pseudomyiasis* is when maggots are found in the intestinal or urogenital tract as passersby; they have accidentally been swallowed or migrated into these areas without actually feeding on tissues.

Myiasis may also be defined based on the anatomic region infested: cutaneous, auricular, ophthalmic, neurologic, urogenital, GI, and nasopharyngeal. Cutaneous myiasis includes *furuncular (subcutaneous) myiasis*, *traumatic (superficial cutaneous) myiasis*, and *creeping obligatory myiasis.* Creeping obligatory myiasis is when dipteran larvae create burrows in the skin and is usually caused by *Gasterophilus* spp. To date, this has not been reported in dogs or cats.

Ophthalmic myiasis has been divided into three types depending on the location of affected ocular tissues: *ophthalmomyiasis externa* (orbital or external ocular tissues), *ophthalmomyiasis interna posterior* (posterior portion of the globe), and *ophthalmomyiasis interna anterior* (anterior chamber).

A large number of fly species have been implicated in myiasis, which can be broadly grouped into the families Oestridae (bot flies or warble flies), Calliphoridae (blow flies), Sarcophagidae (flesh flies), and Muscidae (house flies). Often the exact species of Diptera involved is not identified in clinical cases. However, examples of species that have been identified in dogs and cats are listed in Table 108.1.

CUTEREBRA SPP. INFESTATIONS (CUTEREBRIASIS/CUTEREBROSIS)

ETIOLOGIC AGENT AND EPIDEMIOLOGY

Cuterebra spp. (family Oestridae) are large, bee-like flies (bot flies) that normally deposit their eggs in or around rodent (depending on

TABLE 108.1 Examples of Fly Species Implicated in Obligatory or Facultative Myiasis in Dogs and Cats

Species	Common Name	Normal Hosts	Geographic Distribution	Site of Egg/Larval Deposition	Comments
Oestridae (bot flies, warble flies)					
Cuterebra spp.	Rodent bot fly, rabbit bot fly	Rodents, rabbits	North America (especially northeastern United States and southeastern Canada), northern Central America	E	Large larvae capable of causing significant respiratory, ocular, CNS, or cutaneous lesions
Dermatobia hominis	Human bot fly Torsalo American warble fly	Humans	Tropical and subtropical Central and South America	H	Large flies that resemble bumblebees. Important cause of furuncular myiasis in impoverished humans. Eggs may be vectored to tissues by mosquitos or muscoid flies
Hypoderma spp.	Heel fly Gad fly Warble fly	Cattle, deer	Northern hemisphere, 25–60 degree latitude; especially North Africa, India	H	Rare. Primarily lays eggs on cattle. Can cause furuncular, CNS, and ocular myiasis in humans
Oestrus spp.	Nasal bot Sheep bot fly	Sheep and to a lesser extent deer, goats	Worldwide	H	Normally deposits first-stage larvae in nostrils of sheep, sporadically affects the nasal cavity of humans and dogs
Calliphoridae (blow flies)					
Cochliomyia hominivorax	New World screw-worm fly	Warm-blooded animals including humans	Southern North America, Central and South America; largely eradicated from North America	H	Adults lay hundreds of eggs in exposed host flesh; wound disturbance causes maggots to invade more deeply
Chrysomya spp., especially *Chrysomya bezziana*	Old World blow fly Old World screw-worm fly (*Ch. bezziana*)	Warm-blooded animals especially livestock	Tropical Africa, southeast Asia, Middle East, India, Papua New Guinea	H	*Ch. bezziana* adults lay 150–200 eggs in wounds and mucous membranes; larvae feed on living (rather than necrotic) tissue of animals, sometimes causing permanent tissue damage. Importation into nonendemic regions has been a concern
Cordylobia spp., especially *Cordylobia anthropophaga* ("human eater")	Tumbu fly, mango fly	Warm-blooded animals, especially dogs and rodents	Subtropics of Africa	E	Larvae penetrate host skin and cause furuncles
Lucilia spp., especially *Lucilia sericata*	Common green bottle fly Sheep blow fly (United Kingdom, Australia)	Sheep, other warm-blooded animals	Temperate and tropical regions worldwide	H	Eggs laid in carrion and sometimes wounds or macerated skin of living hosts. Maggots have been used for wound debridement therapy
Sarcophagidae (flesh flies)					
Sarcophaga spp., e.g., *Sarcophaga haemorrhoidalis*	Flesh fly Red-tailed flesh fly	Carrion	Worldwide	H	Usually lay eggs on carrion but can cause wound myiasis in debilitated hosts; aural, nasal, and gastrointestinal (rectal) myiasis have been described in humans
Wohlfahrtia spp., e.g., *Wohlfahrtia magnifica*	Spotted flesh fly	Primarily livestock and horses	Tropical and subtropical regions worldwide	H	Most species lay eggs on carrion but can cause wound myiasis; *W. magnifica* is obligatory parasite; cases of aural, nasal, genital, and oral myiasis have been described
Muscidae (house flies)					
Musca domestica	House fly	Decomposing organic matter in the environment	Worldwide	H	Rare cause of wound myiasis in debilitated hosts

E, environment; *H*, host.

the *Cuterebra* species, various squirrels, chipmunks, woodrats, house mice) (subgenus *Cuterebra*) and lagomorph burrows (subgenus *Trypoderma*). They are the most common cause of furuncular myiasis in North America. Approximately 34 different species have been identified in North America, with approximately 12 species in the subgenus *Cuterebra* and 22 in the subgenus *Trypoderma*.[3] Adult flies, which live only a few weeks, lay 5 to 15 eggs per site (one to several thousand per lifetime) on vegetation during the summer months, and in response to heat from vertebrate hosts and optimal environmental conditions, eggs hatch and release first-stage larvae, which are 2 to 4 mm long (Fig. 108.1A). The sticky larvae then adhere to the fur of their target hosts and penetrate the host body by entering natural orifices. Often this is the upper respiratory tract, especially the nasopharyngeal or tracheal mucosa. Larvae then migrate through pleural and peritoneal tissues to a subcutaneous location. After about a week, the larva molts to the second instar, penetrates the epidermis, and creates a small air pore ("warble pore") by which it uses to breathe and excrete waste. The second-stage instar is gray to white and about 5 to 10 mm long. After another week, development to a third-stage larva occurs, then the larva enlarges the pore, emerges, drops to the ground, burrows into detritus and soil, and pupates. At the pre-pupal stage, third-stage larvae may be 2 to 4 cm long, are dark, thick, have two black mouth hooks, and are covered in cuticular spines (platelets) (Fig. 108.1B). The spines of *Cuterebra* species that prefer rodents have been described as flattened and plate-like, occasionally somewhat conical, usually bifid to many pointed in the anterior and posterior bands of spines on most segments. In contrast, species that prefer lagomorphs have conical, single-pointed spines, especially in the anterior and posterior bands on most segments.[4] Precise species determination is not possible based on larval morphology and requires molecular assays or pupation in the laboratory environment; unfortunately, larvae recovered from aberrant hosts often will fail to pupate to adults. The total time for larval maturation, from infection to exit from the warble, ranges from 3 to 8 weeks. The time required for the adult fly to emerge from the pupal case may be a month to several years.

Dogs, cats, humans, and a variety of other wildlife species such as raccoons and skunks are accidental or atypical hosts, developing more severe clinical disease than rabbits and rodents, sometimes with aberrant larval migration to sites such as the CNS and upper respiratory tract. It has been suggested that most infestations in dogs and cats involve *Cuterebra* spp. with a preference for lagomorph burrows.[5] Most affected dogs and cats documented in the literature have been from the midwestern and northeastern states of the United States, where only six different species of *Cuterebra* exist (Table 108.2). However, many cases have also been reported from eastern Canada,[6,7] along with isolated cases from other states of the United States (e.g., Georgia, Louisiana, Florida, Kansas, Texas), where other species of *Cuterebra* are present, potentially with slightly different host species as well as target site predilections. For example, in a case report of ophthalmomyiasis externa in an 8-week old Scottish terrier puppy, it was

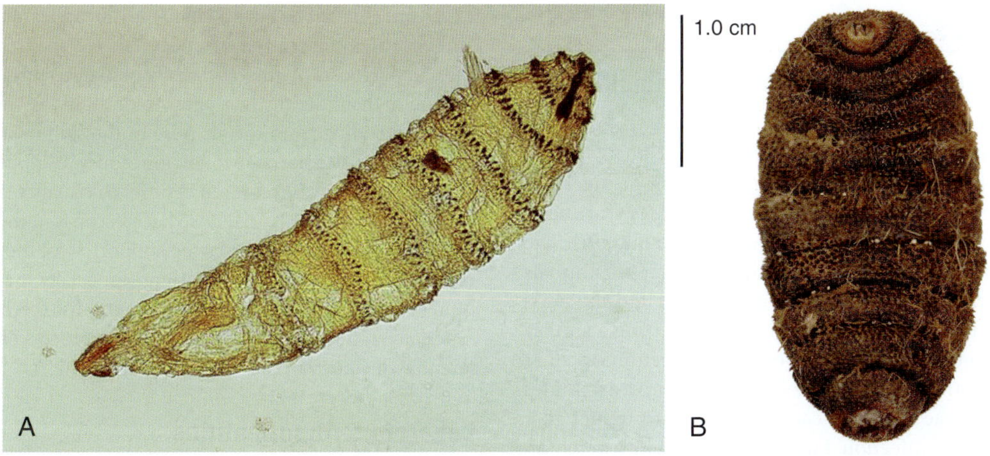

Fig. 108.1 *Cuterebra* spp. larvae. (A) First-stage larva. Note the rows of anterior hooklets that can anchor the feeding larva to the dermis. (B) Third-stage larva. (A, From Diaz JH. Myiasis and tungiasis. In: Bennett JE, Dolin R, Blaser MJ, eds. *Mandell, Douglas, and Bennett's Principles and Practice of Infectious Diseases.* Philadelphia, PA: Elsevier; 2020:3492–3496. B, Modified from Lara-Lagunes N, Jaume-Schinkel S, Ibáñez-Bernal S. An incidental case of gastric pseudomyiasis in *Canis latrans* (Carnivora: Canidae) by a rabbit bot fly *Cuterebra* sp. (Diptera: Oestridae). *Rev Mex de Bioversidad.* 2017;88:410–414.)

TABLE 108.2 *Cuterebra* Species of the Northeastern United States

Subgenus	Order of Preferred Host	Species	Common Name	Preferred Host
Cuterebra	Rodentia	*Cuterebra emasculator*	Tree squirrel bot fly	Squirrels, chipmunks
		Cuterebra fontinella	Mouse bot fly	White footed mouse (*Peromyscus leucopus*)
		Cuterebra americana[a]	Woodrat bot fly	Eastern woodrat (*Neotoma floridana*)
Trypoderma	Lagomorpha	*Cuterebra abdominalis*	Rabbit bot fly	Cottontail rabbit (*Sylvilagus floridanus*)
		Cuterebra buccata		
		Cuterebra cuniculi[b]		

[a]Found primarily in southeastern states as far south as Florida.
[b]Found primarily in southeastern coastal regions (Florida and southern Georgia); other species can be found throughout the east.

suggested that *Cuterebra jellisoni* might be involved, a species in the region that typically targets the head of rabbits, especially periocular tissues.[8] Although unpublished in the peer-reviewed literature, cases are common in Colorado (Jane Sykes, personal communication),[9,10] and occasional cases occur in the western United States (author's personal observations).[11,12]

Infestations are usually recognized in late summer to early fall; 90% of 42 cases (20 dogs and 22 cats) in one study that included cases from Michigan (United States) and Ontario (Canada) were seen in July and August, and the remainder in September.[6] A similar temporal pattern of infection has been noted in cats with CNS cuterebriasis.[13,14] The mean body weight of affected dogs in the series from Michigan and Ontario was 4.1 kg, and 80% of dogs were ≤ 4.5 kg; only one dog weighed > 9.1 kg. Eight of the dogs were Yorkshire terriers, and this breed was significantly overrepresented. A Yorkshire terrier with cerebral cuterebriasis confirmed molecularly to be *C. abdominalis* was also described from Texas.[15] However, anecdotally, small-breed white-coated dogs such as West Highland white terriers are most often affected in Colorado. Mean age of the dogs was 55.7 months (range, 8–110 months) and that of the cats was 17.8 months (range, 1–97 months); median age of 11 cats with CNS cuterebriasis was 2 years.[14] No sex predisposition has been noted. Both indoor-only, indoor/outdoor, and exclusively outdoor animals were affected; however, free roaming increases risk for infection. Although only one larva is usually identified, occasionally multiple larvae are removed; the presence of multiple larvae has most often been reported in kittens,[6] which also have the potential to be infected by larvae transferred from the fur of a queen.

CLINICAL FEATURES

Pathogenesis, Clinical Signs, and Physical Examination Findings

Furuncular myiasis in dogs and cats may occur when *Cuterebra* spp. larvae penetrate wounds or migrate following inhalation or ingestion to a subcutaneous location, forming subcutaneous masses (furuncles or "warbles") with a 2 to 4 mm air pore with well-defined margins. The exact route of migration to subcutaneous tissues in domestic animals is unknown, but evidence of migration through muscle and the peritoneal cavity has been identified in some animals, suggesting a similar pattern of migration to that in rabbits or rodents.[6] Secretion of collagenase, proteases, and other digestive enzymes by the larva facilitates migration. Migrating larvae may also carry bacteria into tissues that leads to secondary bacterial infection. Furuncles are usually located on the head, neck, or trunk. The pore may ooze serosanguinous fluid such that the hair covering the furuncle becomes matted. Occasionally, the larva may also be observed to intermittently extrude from the pore.

Aberrant migration of larvae can involve the nasal cavity, pharynx, trachea, eye, and CNS. Occasionally, animals exhibit systemic signs in association with infection, such as inappetence or lethargy. Fever may also be present, possibly resulting from secondary bacterial infection or toxins excreted by the migrating larva. DIC, sepsis, and anuric renal failure secondary to acute tubular necrosis have been documented in dogs, but not cats.[6] Animals with infection of the upper respiratory tract or pharynx typically show signs that include epistaxis, sneezing, stertor, nasal discharge, gagging, cough, or inspiratory stridor and dyspnea with tracheal involvement.[6,12,16] Occasionally a larva is sneezed out of the nasal cavity, coughed or vomited out, or extrudes from the nares. Other physical examination findings include decreased nasal airflow, and swelling of the soft palate or pharynx. Ocular cuterebriasis is associated with ocular discharge, corneal edema, periocular swelling or masses, chemosis, blepharospasm, uveitis, and sometimes blindness.[17,18] A larva may be observed in periocular masses (ophthalmomyiasis externa) or within the anterior or posterior chambers (ophthalmomyiasis interna).[17] Involvement of the anterior chamber appears to incite more inflammation than involvement of the posterior chamber. CNS migration (cerebrospinal cuterebriasis) is most often reported in cats, but also has been described in a small number of dogs.[19–21] Based on the frequent finding of *Cuterebra* spp. in the olfactory bulbs or peduncles and cribriform plate at necropsy, it is suspected that larvae gain access to the brain from the nasal cavity.[14] The neurologic signs that follow depend on the path of larval migration. Acute onset of seizures (documented in approximately 25% of cats), head tilt, nystagmus, circling, falling to one side, central blindness, evidence of cranial nerve dysfunction, head pressing, obtundation, ataxia, abnormal placing reactions, pelvic limb weakness, behavioral changes, thermoregulatory disturbances, vomiting, and vocalization have been described.[11,13,14,21–23] Signs are often lateralizing (and in one study, left lateralizing),[14] typically progress rapidly and end in death due to ischemic necrosis and inflammation; rarely, recovery with or without residual neurologic signs occurs. Rarely larvae are found within the spinal canal.[24] Respiratory signs (especially sneezing) often precede CNS signs, most often by 1 to 2 weeks, but occasionally 4 to 10 weeks.[4] CNS cuterebriasis has been suggested as the cause of feline ischemic encephalopathy, based on a similar geographic distribution and seasonality as well as findings on CNS histopathology[11]; it has also been suggested as a possible cause of feline idiopathic vestibular disease.[14,23]

DIAGNOSIS

Cuterebra spp. larvae have a characteristic appearance as described above, and because other causes of myiasis in North America are rare, in most cases, a diagnosis of cuterebriasis is made presumptively, without confirmation of their identity by a parasitologist. If a larva is not visualized in the eye or extruding from the air pore in the skin or upper respiratory tract, diagnosis can also be made following biopsy. Clipping the hair over cutaneous furuncles may be required in order to visualize the pore. Cerebrospinal cuterebriasis is usually diagnosed at necropsy, although findings on MRI examination of the brain may be supportive of the diagnosis. In endemic regions, a history of respiratory signs (especially sneezing) before the onset of neurologic signs should raise suspicion for cerebrospinal cuterebriasis, especially in the summer or early fall. Cryptococcosis is an important differential diagnosis in cats with this history.

Laboratory Abnormalities

Complete Blood Count, Serum Chemistry Profile, Urinalysis, and Clotting Function

Findings on routine blood work and urinalysis in dogs and cats with cuterebriasis are nonspecific and may be normal. Neutrophilic leukocytosis, eosinophilia, thrombocytopenia, increased serum liver enzyme activity, azotemia, hypoalbuminemia, and hyperglobulinemia have been described in some animals.[6,14] In the study of dogs and cats from Michigan and Ontario, proteinuria was documented in all 13 animals that had urinalysis performed; urine protein-to-creatinine ratios (UPCRs) that were performed in six dogs were consistent with the magnitude expected with glomerular proteinuria (3.2 to 16). Some animals have granular casts in the urine.[6] Clotting function is usually normal, but evidence of DIC may be present in infestations that are complicated by SIRS or sepsis.

Cerebrospinal Fluid Analysis

The CSF in dogs and cats with cerebrospinal cuterebriasis may have evidence of hemorrhage and pleocytosis, in some cases with a predominance of eosinophils.[14,19,23] Total protein concentration may be moderately to markedly increased.[19,21] Given that some animals have had evidence of increased intracranial pressure, collection of CSF may carry some risk for brain herniation; however, this has not been reported in the literature.

Diagnostic Imaging

Plain radiography of affected tissues can reveal soft tissue submucosal or subcutaneous masses, sometimes with evidence of chitinous larval fragments, which appear as radiodensities.[6] Brain MRI of dogs and cats with cerebrospinal cuterebriasis can reveal single tubular lesions (tracts) that course through the brain parenchyma; these have been described as hyperintense with a hypointense rim on T2-weighted images, and hypointense on T1-weighted images, relative to normal gray matter. In one case report, the hypointense rim enhanced strongly with gadolinium on T1-weighted images, and T2-weighted and FLAIR sequences revealed evidence of edema surrounding the tract (hyperintense signal).[19] Brain lesions extended from the cribriform plate, suggesting entry through the nasal cavity. One cat had evidence of subtentorial and transforaminal brain herniation, with intraparenchymal T2-hyperintense, T1-contrast-enhancing meandering tracts that correlated with eosinophilic tract lesions on histopathology.[23] Few descriptions exist of the larvae themselves, but blooming artifacts have been described on T2* (T2-star) sequences in humans with CNS myiasis that have the potential to be caused by larval materials rather than hemorrhage (Fig. 108.2).[25]

Rhinoscopy and tracheoscopy in animals with respiratory involvement allow direct visualization of warbles or larvae and in some cases, endoscopic removal of larvae (Fig. 108.3). Larvae may be observed to intermittently extrude from a warble.[12]

Parasitologic Tests

Serologic Diagnosis and Molecular Diagnosis Using Nucleic Acid–Based Testing

No serologic tests are commercially available for diagnosis of cuterebriasis in dogs and cats. However, development of an ELISA assay that detects IgG antibodies to *Cuterebra* spp. antigen was reported which showed some promise for aiding diagnosis when larvae could not be visualized, especially in the case of cerebrospinal cuterebriasis.[24] Unfortunately, for unclear reasons, some cats with large larvae remained seronegative, and no further developments on this assay have been reported at the time of writing. PCR-based assays have been used to differentiate fly species causing myiasis in livestock (including *Cuterebra* spp.)[26,27] and humans,[3] but

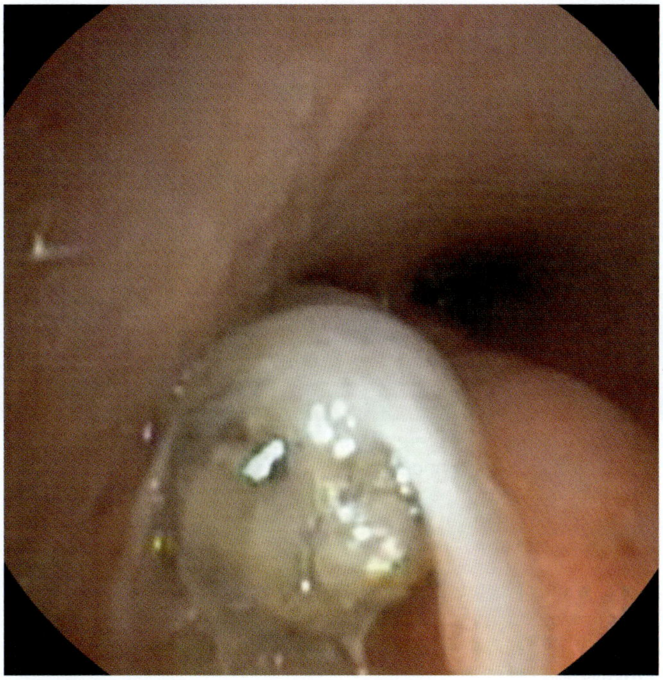

Fig. 108.3 Endoscopic image of the trachea of a 6-year-old intact female wire-haired dachshund that was seen for lethargy, cough, apparent odynophagia, intermittent fever, and inappetence. On one instance hemoptysis was observed. A *Cuterebra* sp. larva was visualized on the left ventrolateral trachea. The larva was removed using suction. A large erosion remained on the tracheal mucosa. Recovery was uneventful.

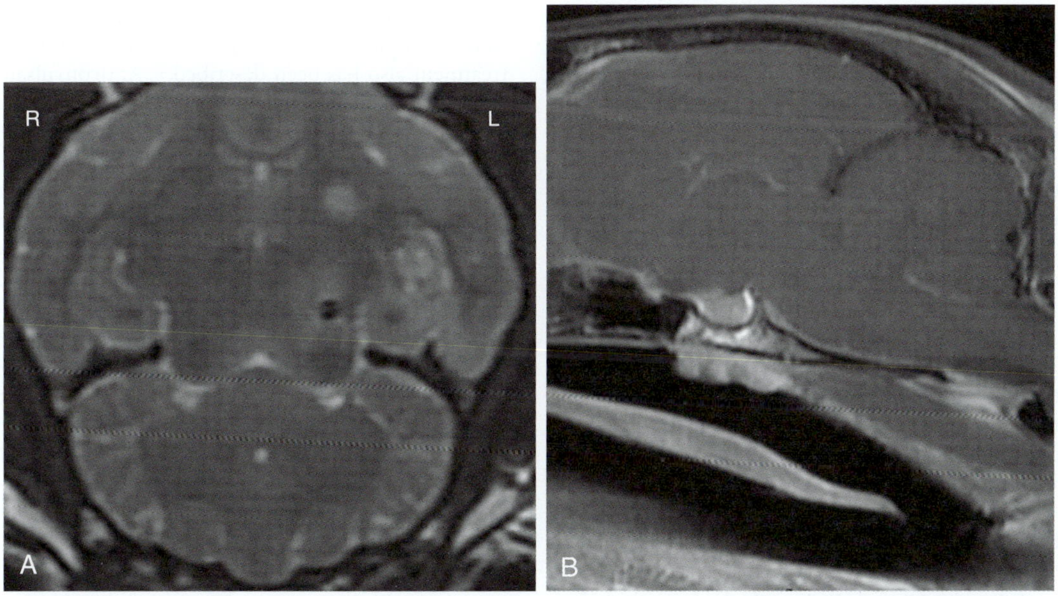

Fig. 108.2 MRI images from a 1-year-old intact female domestic shorthair cat with presumptive cerebrospinal cuterebriasis. (A) Multiple T2-weighted hyperintense lesions are present throughout the cerebral parenchyma. (B) T1-weighted post-contrast image showing markedly contrast-enhancing lesion in the nasopharynx suspected to be the site of a furuncle.

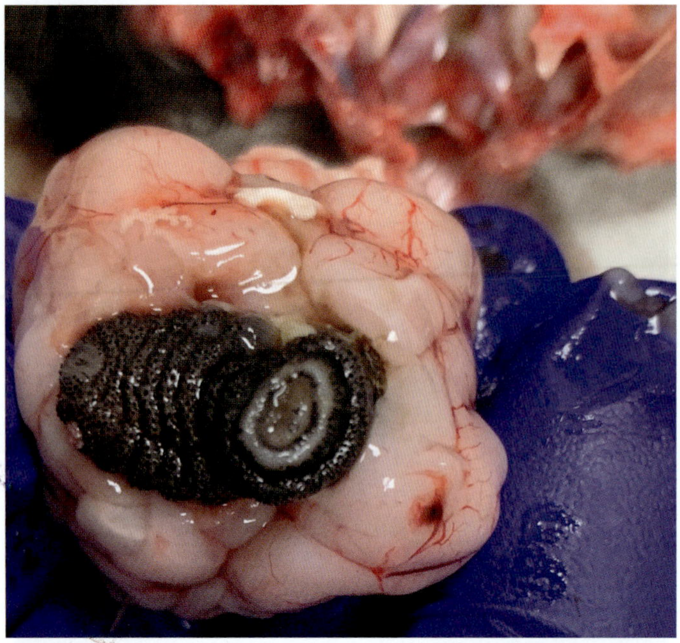

Fig. 108.4 Migrating *Cuterebra* spp. larva in the brain of a kitten from Minnesota, USA, with neurologic signs. The larva was discovered following submission of the head for rabies testing. (Courtesy of Dr. Lindsay Merkel, University of Minnesota College of Veterinary Medicine.)

these have only recently been applied for identification of larvae recovered from companion animals.[15] However the dearth of accurately identified specimens for reference purposes makes molecular confirmation difficult in many cases.[3,24]

Pathologic Findings

Gross pathology of the brain in dogs and cats with CNS involvement can reveal focal or multifocal areas of yellow discoloration (malacia) and hemorrhage, often within the olfactory bulbs or peduncles, with a single intralesional larva (Fig. 108.4).[13] Histopathology may reveal a larva within the brain parenchyma accompanied by neutrophilic and or eosinophilic meningoencephalitis. However, larvae are not found in many cases.[14]

Parasitic migratory tracts have most often been identified in or near the caudate nucleus and thalamus in cats, and have been characterized by spongy degeneration, cerebral infarction, and hemorrhage; cerebrocortical necrosis; astrogliosis; and focal granulomatous encephalitis surrounding a larva.[13,19,21] Larvae have also been found at necropsy in association with the optic nerve, cribriform plate, or ventral cranial cavity.[13] It has been suggested that a larval toxin may induce some of the pathology found within the brain that resembles that described for feline ischemic encephalopathy.

TREATMENT AND PROGNOSIS

Treatment of furuncular cuterebriasis or infestations that involve the respiratory tract or eye involves removal of the larva using forceps as well as broad-spectrum antimicrobial therapy for secondary bacterial infection. It has been recommended not to squeeze or disrupt the larva during removal as release of antigens has the potential to trigger an anaphylactic reaction, and residual fragments may lead to a foreign body reaction and abscessation. However, this is anecdotal and in practice, gentle compression of the base of a cutaneous furuncle to extrude the larva rarely has adverse consequences. The area should be debrided as much as possible, lavaged with copious amounts of saline, and allowed to heal by granulation. In human medicine, asphyxiation of the larvae by covering the air pore with petrolatum jelly or other fatty substances has been advocated to trigger spontaneous extrusion of the larva, rather than removing it surgically. Such treatments have not been documented in the veterinary literature. A short (72-hour) course of NSAIDs may help to reduce pruritus following extraction of cutaneous larvae, and for cases that involve the nasopharynx or trachea, a tapering course of glucocorticoids should be administered if there is severe swelling that obstructs respiration. Where multiple larvae are identified, administration of ivermectin should be considered (e.g., 100 to 400 μg/kg, PO, once). Application of topical fluralaner or oral sarolaner was used to successfully treat furuncular myiasis caused by *Dermatobia hominis* in cats and dogs, respectively.[28,29] Larvae located within the respiratory tract may be removed using endoscopic guidance.[16,30] Descriptions exist of surgical approaches to remove larvae of various stages from the tracheal submucosa[12,16] and in cases of ophthalmomyiasis interna by keratotomy or vitrectomy techniques.[12,17,31,32] IV fluid therapy and other supportive care measures may be required for debilitated animals. Angiotensin-converting enzyme inhibitors and low-dose aspirin have been used to treat animals with secondary protein-losing nephropathy.[19]

The optimal treatment for suspected cerebrospinal cuterebriasis is not known. Ivermectin has been the most commonly reported antiparasitic treatment, with doses that range from 20 to 400 μg/kg SC or PO; in some cases, more than one treatment was given at intervals ranging from q24h, q48h, and 14 days.[14,19,23] Ivermectin normally does not penetrate the blood-brain barrier; its use has been based on the assumption that barrier disruption occurs secondary to larval migration and inflammation and evidence of efficacy for treatment of other cerebrospinal myiases.[19] Death of larvae may trigger a type I hypersensitivity reaction, and so pretreatment with diphenhydramine (4 mg/kg IM) 1 to 2 hours before ivermectin (400 μg/kg, SC, q24h for 3 treatments) and dexamethasone (0.1 mg/kg IV) has been used in some cases.[14,19] It may be necessary to continue treatment with tapering anti-inflammatory doses of glucocorticoids to reduce brain edema and inflammation. Mannitol may also be indicated if increased intracranial pressure is suspected. Surgical removal of a migrating larva by craniotomy was attempted in one dog, but the larva was not identified, and instead biopsy was performed.[19] This dog ultimately recovered following treatment with an escalating dose of ivermectin (20 μg/kg on day 1, 25 μg/kg on day 2, and 30 μg/kg on day 3) and methylprednisolone sodium succinate (30 mg/kg IV q24h). Recovery without ivermectin treatment also has been described.[21] Anticonvulsants such as phenobarbital have been used to manage seizures acutely, and were required for long-term management of residual cluster seizures in one otherwise recovered dog.[19] An overall mortality rate of 17% was reported among 42 dogs and cats with cuterebriasis from North America.[6] Only 1 of 22 cats died, and this was as a result of suspected septic peritonitis secondary to larval migration through the peritoneal cavity. In contrast, 6 of 20 dogs died; all weighed ≤ 4.5 kg and had SIRS, DIC, or both.

PREVENTION

Keeping cats indoors, limiting roaming of pets, and maintaining yards to reduce long grass and rodent/lagomorph habitats can help reduce infection. It is possible that the use of heartworm prophylaxis and flea control, including systemic insecticides (e.g., isoxazolines), may also reduce the risk of infection, but this has not been evaluated experimentally.[6]

PUBLIC HEALTH ASPECTS

Human cases of cuterebriasis have been reported in North America, including cases of ophthalmomyiasis, respiratory infections, and cuterebrid cutaneous furunculosis.[33] Most cases occur in the northeastern

United States, with humans encountering eggs or larvae when they engage in outdoor activities. The rabbit bot fly species *Cuterebra buccata* has been identified as the cause of a small number of human myiasis cases in the United States; however, as with dogs and cats, the species is rarely identified.[3] Furuncles are most commonly identified in lesions of the scalp, face, and neck down to the upper torso. Cutaneous and respiratory infestation with *C. buccata* was described in a 74-year-old man from Connecticut who reported doing yard work, including mowing his lawn, without a shirt.[3] Similar lesions occur with *Dermatobia hominis* infestations (New World or human bot fly), which occurs in the Caribbean, Central America, and South America. Although theoretically animals could bring first-stage *Cuterebra* spp. larvae adherent to their coats into close proximity with humans, human disease is extremely rare and no human case has been linked to contact with companion animals.

WOUND MYIASIS (MAGGOT INFESTATION)

ETIOLOGIC AGENTS AND EPIDEMIOLOGY

In North America, most maggots found associated with skin wounds are facultative parasites that feed on decaying, necrotic tissue and include members of the Calliphoridae (blow flies), Sarcophagidae (flesh flies), and, rarely, Muscidae (house flies). In other regions of the world, a few species are obligatory parasites that feed on healthy tissue. Examples of obligatory myiasis flies include the primary New World screwworm fly, *Cochliomyia hominivorax*; the Old World screwworm fly, *Chrysomya bezziana*; the tumbu fly, *Cordylobia anthropophaga;* and the spotted flesh fly, *Wohlfahrtia magnifica*. The latter two species are non–bot fly agents of furuncular myiasis not present in the Americas.[34]

Diptera associated with wound myiasis have a similar life cycle. Females deposit eggs or larvae on the edge of a wound or, for some species, on a moist mucous membrane. For obligatory myiasis flies, a wound as small as a tick bite may be adequate. In some patients, no primary trauma is identified.[34] Larvae feed on necrotic tissue and decaying organic material (e.g., feces, vegetation) adherent to the skin or, in the case of primary screwworm larvae and other obligatory myiasis flies, healthy tissue. After 3 to 10 days on the host, fully developed larvae drop to the environment and pupate in the soil. Environmental development, activity of adult flies, and fecundity are species, temperature, and humidity dependent. Some species thrive in more tropical areas, whereas others are found seasonally in temperate regions. At lower temperatures, flies may remain in the pupal stage for several months.[34]

Adult New World screwworm flies are two to three times larger than house flies, metallic blue to blue-black, and have three stripes along the dorsal surface; the center stripe of *Co. hominivorax* is shorter than the outer ones, and in *Cochliomyia macellaria* all stripes appear to be of the same length.[35] Larvae of *Co. hominivorax* grow as long as 17 mm and can be identified by the presence of pigmented tracheal trunks. Tissue destruction by feeding *Co. hominivorax* may attract other blow flies resulting in a mixed population of maggots. The primary screwworm can only survive in areas with mild (warm) temperatures and adequate humidity, and, although historically found in the southern United States, has been eradicated from North America and most of Central America.[36] Populations remain in southern Panama, South America, and in some Caribbean islands with occasional re-introductions into North America reported.[37,38] Adult female *Co. hominivorax* only mate once; large-scale release of sterile male flies allowed initial eradication and continues to be employed when re-introductions occur.[36,38] The Old World screwworm fly, *Ch. bezziana*, is found in tropical areas in Southeast Asia, Africa, the Middle East, and some Pacific islands. Adults are metallic green or blue. Larvae have pigmented tracheal trunks, but the pattern differs from that of *Co. hominivorax*.[35] Other *Chrysomya* spp. (*Chrysomya rufifacies*, *Chrysomya putoria*) primarily develop in carcasses but are also involved in some cases of facultative myiasis.[34] *Cordylobia anthropophaga* is unusual in that larvae hatch from eggs deposited in the environment and then directly penetrate the skin to develop in furuncles prior to emerging to pupate in the environment, similar to bot flies.[34]

Like *Chrysomya* spp., *Lucilia* spp., *Calliphora* spp., and *Phormia* spp. are referred to as bottle flies due to the dramatic metallic green or blue color of the adults. *Lucilia sericata*, the common green bottle fly, is found worldwide and thrives in warm humid areas although it can also survive in drier regions. Although associated with sheep, *L. sericata* will also deposit eggs on necrotic tissue on dogs and cats, resulting in fly strike.[39] Other *Lucilia* spp. (e.g., *Lucilia* [*Phaenicia*] *eximia*), *Calliphora* spp. (e.g., *Calliphora vicina*), and *Phormia* spp. (e.g., *Phormia regina*) can also be involved.[40–43]

Adult flesh flies (Sarcophagidae: *Sarcophaga* spp., *Wohlfahrtia* spp.) are large, greyish flies approximately twice as large as house flies and can be recognized by the distinct checkerboard pattern (*Sarcophaga* spp.) or rows of oval black spots (*Wohlfahrtia* spp.) on the abdomen.[34] Female *Sarcophaga* spp. deposit fully formed larvae (or, for some species, hatching eggs) onto decaying flesh; development to mature larvae can proceed in as little as 3 to 4 days. Several *Sarcophaga* spp. (*Sarcophaga pernix* [= *haemorrhoidalis*], *Sarcophaga argyrostoma*, *Sarcophaga tibialis*) have been reported in cases of facultative myiasis in dogs and cats.[43] Larvae of *W. magnifica* are obligatory parasites that infest wounds or natural body orifices (nares, ears, eyes, genitals) of mammals and birds in southern Europe, Asia, and the Middle East. As with *Sarcophaga* spp., female *Wohlfahrtia* spp. deposit formed larvae. Canine infestations are often associated with livestock, especially small ruminants, but infestations in shelter dogs have also been reported.[44–46] *Wohlfahrtia* spp. in North America (*Wohlfahrtia vigil*, *Wohlfahrtia opaca*) normally infest wildlife (fox, rabbits) and have been historically reported in dogs and cats but are presently considered rare causes of furuncular myiasis in the region.[47,48] House flies (*Musca domestica*) occasionally lay eggs in decaying tissues but are not a common cause of wound myiasis.

Wound myiasis disproportionally affects animals in poor condition that are kept outside.[49] Feral cats, and dogs and cats that experience trauma and are not presented for treatment, are at increased risk; ages vary and intact males are overrepresented.[50–53] Fight-related wounds are considered particularly high risk.[53] Other identified risk factors include paresis and obesity.[41,43] An association with exposure to livestock is evident in many case reports, and cases of myiasis are more likely in months with warm, humid weather when fly activity is highest.[45,49]

CLINICAL FEATURES

Pathogenesis, Clinical Signs, and Physical Examination Findings

Facultative myiasis flies are attracted to dogs and cats by the presence of adherent blood, feces, or decaying tissue. Obligatory species seek out pets kept outdoors regardless of overall condition, although debilitated animals may be more susceptible. Female flies deposit eggs or larvae directly onto animals, selecting warm, moist regions such as wounds, which may be as minor as arthropod feeding lesions, or mucous membranes. Predisposing, traumatic conditions that attract female flies include wounds that develop following a fight, fall, or vehicular collision; untreated surgical incisions; abrasions from a collar; dermatitis associated with infection, which may be secondary to fecal and urine contamination of skin or matted fur; ectoparasite infestation; or decubitus ulcers secondary to prolonged immobility.[39]

Dogs and cats infested with maggots are malodorous and often debilitated. Stabilizing the patient may be necessary prior to instituting therapy. The extent of the infestation may be obscured by the hair-coat, particularly in long-haired or dense-coated animals, or by other material adherent to the wound. Careful inspection, including clipping the hair, is usually necessary to adequately assess overall condition; sedation with analgesia may be required to allow full examination of affected areas. A complete history that includes questions about recent injuries, pre-existing conditions, housing conditions, and, for potentially introduced species of myiasis flies, travel, can be helpful in formulating an effective treatment plan.

DIAGNOSIS

In animals with wound myiasis, maggots are usually grossly apparent on ulcerated skin lesions. To confirm the etiology, a representative sample of larvae should be removed with forceps, placed in 70% ethanol, and submitted to a diagnostic laboratory.[54] Mixed infestations commonly occur, including with primary screwworm fly; submitting several larvae (20–30) collected from different areas is recommended. Third-stage larvae are more readily identified; when possible, larger larvae should be selected for submission. In cases of furuncular myiasis, larvae are removed from subcutaneous cysts for identification as described for cuterebriasis.

Laboratory Abnormalities

Complete Blood Count, Serum Chemistry Profile, Urinalysis, and Clotting Function

Findings on routine blood work and urinalysis in dogs and cats with wound myiasis may be normal or, if abnormal, associated with either the infestation or the underlying condition. Dogs infested with *W. magnifica* had neutrophilic leukocytosis, but all other parameters were normal.[45] Some case reports of wound myiasis describe increased serum hepatic enzyme activities, increased CK concentration, and hypergammaglobulinemia, as well as mild anemia, decreased serum albumin concentration, and decreased serum albumin-to-globulin ratio.[55–54] Evidence of dehydration due to fluid loss may be present in dogs and cats with advanced wound myiasis lesions.

Parasitologic Tests

Larval identification is made by examining the spiracles, cuticular spines, and, for *Co. hominivorax*, tracheal trunks.[54] If primary screwworm flies are suspected, representative specimens should be placed in 70% ethanol and submitted to a diagnostic parasitologist for confirmation of identification. In many areas of the world, including North America, primary screwworm flies must be promptly reported to regulatory agencies.[38,58] The identity of larvae in ethanol can also be evaluated using molecular assays; formalin distorts some morphologic features and reduces utility for subsequent molecular assays. Morphologic identification of larvae of some fly species can be challenging, and appropriate keys should be used by a trained, boarded entomologist or veterinary parasitologist. Many larvae cannot be identified to species based on morphology alone, and molecular data are not available for all species. In these cases, partnering with a specialist to collect live larvae and rear them to adults can allow identification.

Pathologic Findings

Wound myiasis is usually present in ulcerated, necrotic tissue. Invasion of major organs or sepsis following secondary infections may occur.[59] Because wound myiasis is grossly apparent, histopathology is not usually pursued. Examination of otic discharge and preputial lavage fluid from dogs with *W. magnifica* infestations revealed bacterial cocci, neutrophils, and epithelial cells; *Staphylococcus aureus* and coagulase-negative staphylococci were isolated.[45]

TREATMENT AND PROGNOSIS

Treatment of wound myiasis involves a combination of insecticidal and manual removal of fly larvae followed by wound management. The hair should be clipped to visualize the extent of the infestation. Systemic insecticides useful for treatment of wound myiasis include nitenpyram, spinosad, sarolaner, afoxolaner, milbemycin oxime, and other macrocyclic lactones. Nitenpyram administered twice, 6 hours apart, to dogs infested with *Co. hominivorax* resulted in expulsion of 86% of larvae by 6 hours and 94% by 18 hours; all larvae were killed as well as expelled.[60,61] Administration of spinosad to dogs infested with *Co. hominivorax* resulted in expulsion of most (70%) larvae by 6 hours after treatment although not all larvae were killed; sarolaner expelled fewer larvae than spinosad but all (100%) larvae in sarolaner-treated dogs were dead 24 hours after treatment.[62,63] A combination spinosad/milbemycin treatment killed all larvae by 7 hours post-treatment. In groups receiving afoxolaner or spinosad, all larvae were killed within 24 hours.[61] Other approved isoxazolines (fluralaner, lotilaner) are also considered effective.[64] Historically, topical organophosphates or pyrethroids were applied to wounds, but their use has largely been supplanted by systemic insecticides.[65] Any remaining larvae in the wound after insecticide treatment should be manually removed. Larvae can be removed from affected tissues with forceps and the tissue lavaged and cleaned with chlorhexidine and povidone-iodine.[54]

Insecticide treatment and manual removal of larvae alone are not adequate for resolving cases of wound myiasis; careful wound management, treatment of underlying conditions, and change in owner care practices are also necessary. Once larvae are removed, necrotic tissue should be debrided and other issues caused by larvae or responsible for initial wounds appropriately addressed (e.g., skin resection, complete excision to allow primary closure, enucleation, amputation). Pain management (e.g., meloxicam, 0.2 mg/kg q24h until resolved) and both systemic and topical antibiotic therapy should be provided as indicated; continuing antibiotics for at least 2 weeks past clinical resolution is recommended.[54,62,63] Larvae involved in furuncular myiasis (e.g., *W. magnifica, Co. anthropophaga*) can be removed with forceps and the skin lesion managed as described for cuterebriasis.[34] Prognosis is dependent on the extent of the lesions at presentation, the body systems affected, any underlying conditions, and the ability of the owner to provide appropriate housing and follow-up care. Uncomplicated cases or those in which co-morbidities can be readily addressed are likely to recover, even when infestations are severe.

PREVENTION

Keeping dogs and cats indoors and protected from flies, particularly when debilitated or if skin wounds are present, largely eliminates risk of myiasis. Outdoor pets should be routinely bathed, groomed to remove mats, and kept in clean, dry areas free of fecal debris or other decomposing material (e.g., garbage, compost) that will attract flies; screening kennels if possible is strongly encouraged.[54] Postsurgical discharge instructions should advise owners to house pets indoors and protected from flies until wounds are completely healed, particularly during warmer months. Pets with skin lesions, including pyotraumatic or atopic dermatitis, or those infested with mites, lice, ticks, or fleas, are at increased risk. Addressing other health issues, such as incontinence or malodorous dermatitis or otitis externa, that might lead some owners to house animals outdoors or in structures unprotected from flies (e.g., sheds, barns) supports prevention. Risk is higher for older,

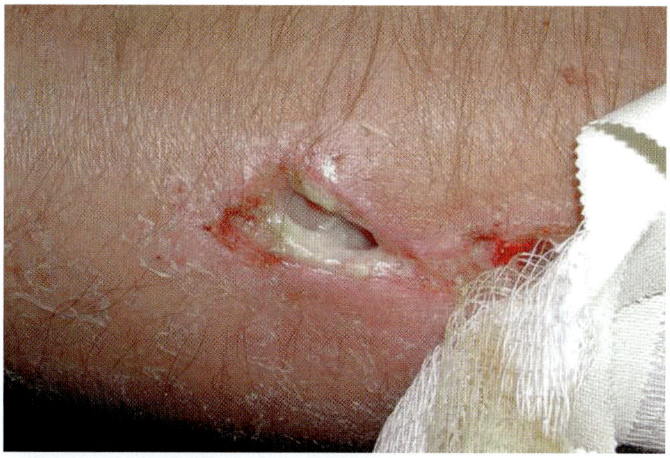

Fig. 108.5 Forearm exit site wound of a third-stage (instar) New World screwworm fly larva, *Cochliomyia hominivorax*. (From Seppänen M, Virolainen-Julkunen A, Kakko I, et al. Myiasis during adventure sports race. *Emerg Infect Dis.* 2004;10:137–139.)

debilitated dogs that may develop decubital ulcers and for intact dogs and cats allowed to roam and thus prone to trauma or fight wounds. Accordingly, neutering indirectly reduces risk.[53] Routine use of macrocyclic lactones for heartworm prevention and insecticides for flea control, including systemic isoxazolines, would be expected to limit wound myiasis, but this has not been evaluated experimentally.

PUBLIC HEALTH ASPECTS

In areas where the flies are endemic, primary screwworm fly larvae (*Co. hominivorax*, *Ch. bezziana*) feed on human as well as animal tissues (Fig. 108.5). Myiasis caused by both species can result in extensive tissue destruction, including bone loss; in severe cases and without treatment, fatalities occur.[66–68] A systematic review of 291 cases revealed that human infestation with *Ch. bezziana* usually occurs in concert with poor hygiene, low socioeconomic status, advanced age, substance abuse, or the presence of underlying diseases including infections, age-related diseases, and noninfectious chronic diseases.[67] Similar factors have been identified in analysis of human cases of *Co. hominivorax*, with infestations more common in warmer months and associated with poor hygiene, psychiatric disorders, substance abuse, and co-infestation with lice or scabies; older men are overrepresented.[68,69] In Africa, humans acquire *Co. anthropophaga* larvae from the environment, developing furuncular myiasis on the arms, abdomen, and lower back; other species of *Cordylobia* described from humans include the Lund's fly, *Cordylobia rodhaini*.[70]

Facultative wound myiasis readily develops on humans and is usually associated with lack of access to housing, neglect, and the presence of comorbidities, including substance abuse and peripheral vascular disease. Cases of wound myiasis in the United States are more common in older men (average age 60 years, male-to-female ratio 5.5:1).[59] *Lucilia sericata* is the most common species, but other blow flies and flesh flies have been described in people. A majority of patients are homeless and present with larvae from late spring through early fall.[59] In Brisbane, Australia, where *Lucilia cuprina* was the most commonly identified species, cases similarly occurred during warm weather and disproportionately affected elderly, ill, and debilitated patients.[71] do not contribute to the risk of facultative wound myiasis in humans. Dogs are considered a reservoir of *Co. anthropophaga* in Africa, and translocation of infested pets is a potential source for re-introduction and geographic spread of primary screwworm flies, but dogs and cats are not epidemiologically important in the life cycle of any other obligatory or facultative myiasis flies.[34,38]

ACCIDENTAL MYIASIS (PSEUDOMYIASIS)

Accidental myiasis refers to the presence of larvae (maggots) in feces or vomit of animals following ingestion of fly eggs or larvae in food, carrion, or garbage.[54] Common species include any of the blow fly or bottle fly larvae that invade carcasses (*Lucilia* spp., *Calliphora* spp., *Phormia* spp.) or muscid flies whose larvae develop in decomposing food materials (e.g., *Musca* spp., *Muscina* spp.). *Sarcophaga* spp. have also been detected in feces following ingestion in carrion.[34] The larvae are present due to dietary indiscretion, not because of ongoing development in the GI tract. Since the pet is not infected, treatment is not indicated.[54] Accidental myiasis would be expected to be more commonly seen in free-roaming pets that are likely to encounter and ingest decomposing carcasses or rotting food with fly larvae. Confirmation of pseudomyiasis can be achieved by confining the pet for 2–3 days and feeding only fresh, commercial food; larvae will no longer be evident in the feces.

Pseudomyiasis can also occur when larvae are found in feces submitted for parasite examination because specimens are collected from the environment rather than per rectum. Female flies oviposit on uncovered feces in the environment almost immediately after it is deposited, and larvae rapidly develop but are not of diagnostic significance.[72] When confirmation of the absence of larvae is desired, a fresh fecal specimen can be collected and examined.

In humans, accidental myiasis is commonly associated with *Piophila casei*, the cheese skipper, following ingestion of cured or smoked meats and cheese on which the flies have fed.[34,73] The condition has also been reported in children and adults that ingest *Drosophila* spp. on produce, meat with *Sarcophaga* spp., and in a child fed overripe bananas with *Muscina stabulans*.[34,74,75]

CASE EXAMPLE

Signalment

"Prim," a 1-year-old intact female domestic shorthair from Minneapolis, MN, United States.

History

Prim was evaluated by the University of Minnesota Small Animal Emergency Service on July 6 for acute onset of ataxia and possible loss of vision. The owner noted that she was disinterested in food, she appeared to be walking very cautiously with a low stance, her pupils were enlarged, and she was not responsive to voice or other stimuli.

Current Medications

None.

Other Medical History

Prim was an indoor cat that was allowed outdoors but only with supervision. She was up to date on core vaccinations, including rabies.

Physical Examination

Body weight: 3.5 kg.

Continued

CASE EXAMPLE—cont'd

General: Bright, alert, and responsive. T = 102.6°F (39.2°C), HR = 160 beats/minute, RR = 80 breaths/minute, mucous membranes pink and moist, CRT < 2 seconds.

All other body systems: No clinically significant findings.

Neurologic examination: Decreased withdrawal reflex for the left pelvic limb and absent withdrawal reflex for the right thoracic limb. Menace response was normal OS but not OD. All other aspects of the neurologic examination were unremarkable.

Laboratory Findings

CBC: HCT 35.3% (29.5%–47%), MCV 40.5 fL (37.4–50.4 fL), MCHC 34.7 g/dL (32.1–39.7 g/dL), WBC 13,280 cells/μL (1,830–16,270 cells/μL), neutrophils 11,820 cells/μL (1,200–13,200 cells/μL), eosinophils 400 cells/μL (0–1,900 cells/μL), basophils 0 cells/μL (0–300 cells/μL), lymphocytes 660 cells/μL (200–9,400 cells/μL), monocytes 400 cells/μL (0–800 cells/μL), platelets clumped but adequate. Rare reactive lymphocytes.

Serum chemistry profile: Sodium 145 mmol/L (147–158 mmol/L), potassium 4.2 mmol/L (3.9–5.3 mmol/L), chloride 111 mmol/L (113–123 mmol/L), bicarbonate 14.2 mmol/L (12–20 mmol/L), phosphorus 4.1 mg/dL (3.3–7.8 mg/dL), calcium 9.9 mg/dL (8.3–10.9 mg/dL), BUN 13 mg/dL (12–39 mg/dL), creatinine 1.0 mg/dL (0.5–2.1 mg/dL), glucose 209 mg/dL (74–143 mg/dL), total protein 7.0 g/dL (5.9–8.2 g/dL), albumin 3.8 g/dL (2.4–4.1 g/dL), globulin 3.2 g/dL (2.5–5.3 g/dL), ALT 70 U/L (16–127 U/L), AST 84 U/L (14–42 U/L), ALP 32 U/L (2–88 U/L), creatine kinase 3285 U/L (54–744 U/L), GGT < 3 U/L (0–3 U/L), cholesterol 118 mg/dL (56–226 mg/dL), total bilirubin 0.2 mg/dL (0–0.3 mg/dL), magnesium 1.9 mg/dL (1.6–2.4 mg/dL).

Urinalysis: not available.

Imaging Findings

MRI: Multiple T2-, T2 FLAIR-hyperintense and poorly-defined lesions were identified throughout the cerebral parenchyma: specifically, within the left frontal lobe, left thalamus, left midbrain, and left hippocampus (see Fig. 108.2A). With the exception of mild contrast enhancement associated with the left hippocampal lesion, these lesions were not contrast-enhancing. However, there was mild left pachymeningeal enhancement that extended from the forebrain to the occipital lobe. Associated with the lesions within the hippocampus and left midbrain is ill-defined T2-hypointensity, T1- and isointensity with a susceptibility artifact on the T2* (T2-star)-weighted image, compatible with acute hemorrhage. Within the dorsal aspect of the left cerebellar hemisphere is similar patchy T2-hyperintensity with minimal patchy contrast enhancement. The caudal fossa is slightly crowded and the cerebellar vermis is mildly flattened and displaced caudally without overt herniation.

Extra-calvarial structures: Originating from the dorsal aspect of the mid nasopharyngeal wall was a broad-based, 0.5 × 1 cm, T1-, T2-isointense (to gray matter) and markedly contrast-enhancing structure (see Fig. 108.2B). Both medial retropharyngeal lymph nodes were moderately generally enlarged and markedly heterogenously contrast-enhancing.

Conclusions: multifocal intra-axial lesions affecting the forebrain, midbrain, and cerebellum with mild pachymeningeal enhancement. Broad-based structure within the dorsal aspect of the nasopharynx of uncertain etiology but could be related to the intracranial lesions if this is parasitic. Crowding of the caudal fossa is likely secondary to increased intracranial pressure. Medial retropharyngeal lymphadenopathy that is likely reactive is present.

CSF Analysis

Total protein, 41 mg/dL; RBC, 163 cells/μL; total nucleated cells, 9 cells/μL. Total nucleated cells comprised 70% neutrophils, 7% small mononuclear cells, 19% large mononuclear cells, and 4% eosinophils. The neutrophils were largely non-degenerate although occasional hyper-segmented and rare degenerate forms were identified. The large mononuclear cells were often vacuolated. No infectious agents were noted.

Diagnosis: Minimal mixed (neutrophilic and eosinophilic) pleocytosis.

Serologic Tests

FeLV/FIV serology (IDEXX SNAP, IDEXX Laboratories, ME, USA): Negative for FeLV antigen and FIV antibody.

Toxoplasma gondii IgG/IgM: Negative.

Diagnosis

Presumptive cerebrospinal cuterebriasis.

Treatment

Ivermectin (300 μg/kg PO, two doses, 48 hours apart), prednisolone (0.7 mg/kg PO q12h), clindamycin (20 mg/kg q12h for 7 days.)

Comments

Although not confirmed, a diagnosis of CNS cuterebriasis seemed likely in this cat based on the geographic location, time of year, left lateralizing CNS signs, MRI findings (including the structure in the nasopharyngeal wall, which may have represented a furuncle), and negative *T. gondii* titers. Upon recovery from the MRI, two partial seizures were observed, 12 hours apart, that involved the face. Following treatment, Prim made a full recovery although the seizures continued and were managed with zonisamide (7 mg/kg, PO, q12h). Three years later, at the time of writing, she is still alive and otherwise apparently healthy.

SUGGESTED READINGS

Francesconi F, Lupi O. Myiasis. *Clin Microbiol Rev.* 2012;25(1):79–105.

Stafford KC, Ridge GE, Molaei G, et al. Rabbit bot fly furuncular, tracheopulmonary, and human bot fly infestations in Connecticut (Oestridae: Cuterebrinae). *J Med Entomol.* 2021;58:114–120.

Thomas JE, Reichard MV. Managing maggots and bots in dogs and cats. *Veterinary Team Brief.* 2018;5:33–37.

Tieber LM, Axlund TW, Simpson ST, et al. Survival of a suspected case of central nervous system cuterebrosis in a dog: clinical and magnetic resonance imaging findings. *J Am Anim Hosp Assoc.* 2006;42:238–242.

REFERENCES

1. Zumpt FKE. *Myiasis in Man and Animals in the Old World: A Textbook for Physicians, Veterinarians and Zoologists.* London, UK: Butterworths; 1965.
2. Pezzi M, Bonacci T, Leis M, et al. Myiasis in domestic cats: a global review. *Parasit Vectors.* 2019;12:372.
3. Stafford KC, Ridge GE, Molaei G, et al. Rabbit bot fly furuncular, tracheopulmonary, and human bot fly infestations in Connecticut (Oestridae: Cuterebrinae). *J Med Entomol.* 2021;58:114–120.
4. Bowman A. Cuterebra species. American Association of Veterinary Parasitologists; 2014. Available at: https://www.aavp.org/wiki/arthropods/insects/cuteribridae/cuterebra-species/.

5. Slansky F. Feline cuterebrosis caused by a lagomorph-infesting *Cuterebra* spp. larva. *J Parasitol.* 2007;93:959–961.
6. Rutland BE, Byl KM, Hydeskov HB, et al. Systemic manifestations of *Cuterebra* infection in dogs and cats: 42 cases (2000-2014). *J Am Vet Med Assoc.* 2017;251:1432–1438.
7. Bau-Gaudreault L, Overvelde S, Martin D. What is your diagnosis? Subcutaneous temporal mass from a cat. *Vet Clin Pathol.* 2018;47:324–325.
8. Crumley WR, Rankin AJ, Dryden MW. Ophthalmomyiasis externa in a puppy due to *Cuterebra* infestation. *J Am Anim Hosp Assoc.* 2011;47:e150–155.
9. Pikes Peak Veterinary Clinic. Cuterebras get under your pets' skin!; 2010. Available at: https://pikespeakvet.com/cuterebras-get-under-your-pets-skin/.
10. Wheeler SR. Beware of outdoor hazards for pets. Denver Post; 2009. Available at: https://www.denverpost.com/2009/08/28/beware-of-outdoor-hazards-for-pets/.
11. Rissi DR, Howerth EW. Pathology in practice. Ischemic encephalopathy caused by aberrant migration of a *Cuterebra* larva. *J Am Vet Med Assoc.* 2013;243:493–495.
12. Bordelon JT, Newcomb BT, Rochat MC. Surgical removal of a *Cuterebra* larva from the cervical trachea of a cat. *J Am Anim Hosp Assoc.* 2009;45:52–54.
13. Williams KJ, Summers BA, de Lahunta A. Cerebrospinal cuterebriasis in cats and its association with feline ischemic encephalopathy. *Vet Pathol.* 1998;35:330–343.
14. Glass EN, Cornetta AM, deLahunta A, et al. Clinical and clinicopathologic features in 11 cats with *Cuterebra* larvae myiasis of the central nervous system. *J Vet Intern Med.* 1998;12:365–368.
15. Park JY, Sobotyk C, Edwards EE, et al. Fatal cerebral cuterebrosis in a dog. Vet Parasitol Reg Stud Reports. 2021;26:100636.
16. Dvorak LD, Bay JD, Crouch DT, et al. Successful treatment of intratracheal cuterebrosis in two cats. *J Am Anim Hosp Assoc.* 2000;36:304–308.
17. Stiles J, Rankin A. Ophthalmomyiasis interna anterior in a cat: surgical resolution. *Vet Ophthalmol.* 2006;9:165–168.
18. Wyman M, Starkey R, Weisbrode S, et al. Ophthalmomyiasis (interna posterior) of the posterior segment and central nervous system myiasis: *Cuterebra* spp. in a cat. *Vet Ophthalmol.* 2005;8:77–80.
19. Thawley VJ, Suran JN, Boller EM. Presumptive central nervous system cuterebriasis and concurrent protein-losing nephropathy in a dog. *J Vet Emerg Crit Care.* 2013;23:335–339.
20. Sartin EA, Hendrix CM, Dillehay DL, et al. Cerebral cuterebrosis in a dog. *J Am Vet Med Assoc.* 1986;189:1338–1339.
21. Tieber LM, Axlund TW, Simpson ST, et al. Survival of a suspected case of central nervous system cuterebrosis in a dog: clinical and magnetic resonance imaging findings. *J Am Anim Hosp Assoc.* 2006;42:238–242.
22. McKenzie BE, Lyles DI, Clinkscales JA. Intracerebral migration of *Cuterebra* larva in a kitten. *J Am Vet Med Assoc.* 1978;172:173–175.
23. James FM, Poma R. Neurological manifestations of feline cuterebriasis. *Can Vet J.* 2010;51:213–215.
24. Davis LL, Puozzo A, Vitalo DC, et al. Enzyme-linked immunosorbent assay using a crude antigen extract to measure *Cuterebra*-specific immunoglobulin G in sera of cats with systemic infections. *J Vet Diagn Invest.* 2013;25:395–401.
25. Marco de Lucas E, Diez C, Gutierrez A, et al. wUnusual MRI findings in a patient with history of frontal fracture and skin infestation by fly larvae, as a possible sign of intracerebral myiasis. *Clin Neurol Neurosurg.* 2008;110:725–728.
26. Otranto D, Traversa D, Tarsitano E, et al. Molecular differentiation of *Hypoderma bovis* and *Hypoderma lineatum* (Diptera, Oestridae) by polymerase chain reaction-restriction fragment length polymorphism (PCR-RFLP). *Vet Parasitol.* 2003;112:197–201.
27. Noel S, Tessier N, Angers B, et al. Molecular identification of two species of myiasis-causing *Cuterebra* by multiplex PCR and RFLP. *Med Vet Entomol.* 2004;18:161–166.
28. Andriotti PA, Souza CP. Oliveita PC, et al. Effectiveness of sarolaner in the clinical management of furuncular myiasis in dogs naturally infested with *Dermatobia hominis*. Parasit Vectors. 2021;14:401.
29. Campos DR, Pereira de Assis RC, de Oliveira Chaves JK, et al. Furuncular myiasis caused by *Dermatobia hominis* in five cats and efficacy of topical fluralaner for its treatment. *Vet Dermatol.* 2021;32:438–e117.
30. Yates JL, Stroup ST. Case report: endoscopic removal of a nasal *Cuterebra* larva from a puppy. *Compend Contin Educ Vet.* 2011;33:E1–E4. quiz E5.
31. Harris BP, Miller PE, Bloss JR, et al. Ophthalmomyiasis interna anterior associated with *Cuterebra* spp. in a cat. *J Am Vet Med Assoc.* 2000;216:352–355. 345.
32. Edelmann ML, Lucio-Forster A, Kern TJ, et al. Ophthalmomyiasis interna anterior in a dog: keratotomy and extraction of a *Cuterebra* sp. larva. *Vet Ophthalmol.* 2014;17:448–453.
33. Diaz JH. Myiasis and tungiasis. In: Bennett JE, Dolin R, Blaser MJ, eds. *Mandell, Douglas, and Bennett's Principles and Practice of Infectious Diseases.* Philadelphia, PA: Elsevier; 2020:3492–3496.
34. Scholl PJ, Colwell DD, Cepeda-Palacios R. Myiasis (Muscoidea, Oestroidea). In: Mullen, Durden, eds. *Medical and Veterinary Entomology.* 3rd ed. Academic Press; 2019:383–419.
35. Animal Health Australia. *Old World Screw-Worm Fly: A Diagnostic Manual.* 3rd ed. Canberra: Animal Health Australia; 2017. Available at: https://www.animalhealthaustralia.com.au/wp-content/uploads/SWF-Manual_Full_digital.pdf.
36. Krafsur ES, Whitten CJ, Novy JE. Screwworm eradication in North and Central America. *Parasitol Today.* 1987;3(5):131–137.
37. Welch JB. *Cochliomyia hominivorax* (New World screwworm) datasheet. CABI Invasive Species Compendium; 2016.
38. Skoda SR, Phillips PL, Welch JB. Screwworm (Diptera: Calliphoridae) in the United States: response to and elimination of the 2016-2017 outbreak in Florida. *J Med Entomol.* 2018;55:777–786.
39. Pezzi M, Scapoli C, Chicca M, et al. Cutaneous myiasis in cats and dogs: cases, predisposing conditions and risk factors. *Vet Med Sci.* 2021;7:378-384.
40. Azeredo-Espin AM, Madeira NG. Primary myiasis in dog caused by *Phaenicia eximia* (Diptera: Calliphoridae) and preliminary mitochondrial DNA analysis of the species in Brazil. *J Med Entomol.* 1996;33:839–843.
41. Rodríguez JM, Pérez M. Cutaneous myiasis in three obese cats. *Vet Q.* 1996;18:102–103.
42. Pekmezci D, Pekmezci GZ, Açıcı M, et al. A case of auricular, anal and umbilical myiasis caused by the larvae of *Phormia regina* (Meigen) (Diptera: Calliphoridae) in neonatal kittens. *Turkiye Parazitol Derg.* 2014;38:71–75.
43. Pezzi M, Bonacci T, Leis M, et al. Myiasis in domestic cats: a global review. *Parasit Vectors.* 2019;12(1):372.
44. Gaglio G, Brianti E, Abbene S, Giannetto S. Genital myiasis by *Wohlfahrtia magnifica* (Diptera, Sarcophagidae) in Sicily (Italy). *Parasitol Res.* 2011;109:1471–1474.
45. Orfanou DC, Papadopoulos E, Cripps PJ, et al. Myiasis in a dog shelter in Greece: epidemiological and clinical features and therapeutic considerations. *Vet Parasitol.* 2011;181:374–378.
46. Raele DA, Galante D, Pugliese N, Cafiero MA. Traumatic cutaneous myiasis by *Wohlfahrtia magnifica* in a stray dog in Italy. *J Small Anim Pract.* 2017;58:539.
47. Kingscote AA. Myiasis in man and animals due to infection with the larvae of *Wohlfahrtia vigil* (Walker). *Report Ontario Vet College.* 1935;14:51–69.
48. James MT, Gassner FX. The immature stages of the fox maggot, *Wohlfahrtia opaca.* *J Parasitol.* 1947;33:241–244.
49. Farkas R, Hall MJ, Bouzagou AK, et al. Traumatic myiasis in dogs caused by *Wohlfahrtia magnifica* and its importance in the epidemiology of wohlfahrtiosis of livestock. *Med Vet Entomol.* 2009;23(suppl 1):80–85.
50. de Souza CP, Verocai GG, Ramadinha RH. Myiasis caused by the New World screwworm fly *Cochliomyia hominivorax* (Diptera: Calliphoridae) in cats from Brazil: report of five cases. *J Feline Med Surg.* 2010;12:166–168.
51. Pezzi M, Whitmore D, Chicca M, et al. Traumatic myiasis caused by an association of *Sarcophaga tibialis* (Diptera: Sarcophagidae) and *Lucilia sericata* (Diptera: Calliphoridae) in a domestic cat in Italy. *Korean J Parasitol.* 2015;53:471–475.
52. Pezzi M, Whitmore D, Bonacci T, et al. Facultative myiasis of domestic cats by *Sarcophaga argyrostoma* (Diptera: Sarcophagidae), *Calliphora vicina* and *Lucilia sericata* (Diptera: Calliphoridae) in northern Italy. *Parasitol Res.* 2017;116:2869–2872.
53. Han HS, Toh PY, Yoong HB, et al. Canine and feline cutaneous screwworm myiasis in Malaysia: clinical aspects in 76 cases. *Vet Dermatol.* 2018;29. 442-e148.

54. Thomas JE, Reichard MV. Managing maggots and bots in dogs and cats. *Veterinary Team Brief.* 2018;5:33–37.
55. Muñoz-García CI, Lorenzo-Burgunder D, Gumi-Castillo G, et al. Canine myiasis by *Lucilia eximia* in North America. *Trop Biomed.* 2016;33:494–499.
56. Muñoz AAF, Caceres AFB, León JCP. First report of myiasis in dogs caused by *Cochliomyia hominivorax* (Coquerel 1858) in Colombia. *Vet Parasitol Reg Stud Reports.* 2020;19:100356.
57. Choi J, Kim H, Na J, et al. Cutaneous myiasis associated with tick infestations in a dog. *J Vet Clin.* 2015;32:473–475.
58. Garris G. Veterinarian averts screwworm outbreak. *J Am Vet Med Assoc.* 1998;212:159.
59. Sherman RA. Wound myiasis in urban and suburban United States. *Arch Intern Med.* 2000;160:2004–2014.
60. Correia TR, Scott FB, Verocai GG, et al. Larvicidal efficacy of nitenpyram on the treatment of myiasis caused by *Cochliomyia hominivorax* (Diptera: Calliphoridae) in dogs. *Vet Parasitol.* 2010;173:169–172.
61. Han HS, Chen C, Schievano C, Noli C. The comparative efficacy of afoxolaner, spinosad, milbemycin, spinosad plus milbemycin, and nitenpyram for the treatment of canine cutaneous myiasis. *Vet Dermatol.* 2018;29:312-e109.
62. Oliveira PC, Moraes PA, Scott FB, et al. Efficacy of spinosad on the treatment of myiasis caused by *Cochliomyia hominivorax* (Diptera: Calliphoridae) in dogs. *Vet Parasitol.* 2018;258:53–56.
63. Oliveira PC, Almeida GPS, Cardoso JD, et al. Efficacy of sarolaner on the treatment of myiasis caused by *Cochliomyia hominivorax* (Diptera: Calliphoridae) in dogs. *Vet Parasitol.* 2019;276:108966.
64. Hnilica KA, Patterson AP. *Small Animal Dermatology: A Color Atlas and Therapeutic Guide.* 4th ed. St. Louis, MO: Elsevier; 2017:132–172.
65. Mcnae JC, Lewis SJ. Retrospective study of Old World screwworm fly (*Chrysomya bezziana*) myiasis in 59 dogs in Hong Kong over a one year period. *Aust Vet J.* 2004;82(4):211–214.
66. Oliva A, Ramos NL, Bosio L. Fatal scalp myiasis: autopsy finding of *Cochliomyia hominivorax* (Diptera: Calliphoridae) in the brain cavity. *Can Soc Forensic Sci J.* 2007;40:183.
67. Zhou X, Kambalame DM, Zhou S, et al. Human *Chrysomya bezziana* myiasis: a systematic review. *PLoS Negl Trop Dis.* 2019;13:e0007391.
68. Ruiz-Zapata JD, Figueroa-Gutiérrez LM, Mesa-Franco JA, Moreno-Gutierrez PA. Umbilical myiasis by *Cochliomyia hominivorax* in an infant in Colombia. *Front Med.* 2020;6:292.
69. Batista-da-Silva JA, Moya-Borja GE, Queiroz MM. Factors of susceptibility of human myiasis caused by the New World screw-worm, *Cochliomyia hominivorax* in São Gonçalo, Rio de Janeiro, Brazil. *J Insect Sci.* 2011;11:14.
70. Lachish T, Marhoom E, Mumcuoglu KY, et al. Myiasis in travelers. *J Travel Med.* 2015;22:232–236.
71. Lukin LG. Human cutaneous myiasis in Brisbane: a prospective study. *(Med J Aust).* 1989;150:237–240.
72. Zajac A, Conboy G. Fecal examination for the diagnosis of parasitism. In: *Veterinary Clinical Parasitology.* 8th ed. Wiley-Blackwell; 2012:3–169.
73. Peckenscneider LE, Pokorny C, Hellwig CA. Intestinal infestation with maggots of the cheese fly (*Piophila casei*). *J Am Med Assoc.* 1952;149:262–263.
74. Centers for Disease Control. Intestinal myiasis: Washington. *Morb Mortal Wkly Rep.* 1985;34:141–142.
75. Ly P, Aizenberg A, Martin T, et al. Intestinal myiasis caused by *Sarcophaga* spp. in Cusco, Peru: a case report and review of the literature. *Case Rep Infect Dis.* 2018;3685439.

109

Ticks

Jennifer E. Thomas, Mason V. Reichard

KEY POINTS

- First Described: The earliest written records of ticks date to ancient Greek literature. Homer mentioned ticks in his poem Odyssey (800 BC) as did Aristotle in the *History of Animals* (335 BC). *Rhipicephalus sanguineus* adults and nymphs were recovered from a mummified dog dating to Roman Egypt.[1] Occurrence of ticks in the fossil record indicate the parasites originated during the Cretaceous period (65–146 mya).[2]
- Causes: Ticks that infest dogs and cats belong to two taxonomic families, the Ixodidae or hard ticks, and the Argasidae or soft ticks. The most common ticks found on dogs and cats in North America are hard ticks and include *Amblyomma americanum* (lone star tick), *Amblyomma maculatum* (Gulf Coast tick), *Dermacentor andersoni* (Rocky Mountain wood tick), *Dermacentor occidentalis* (Pacific Coast tick), *Dermacentor variabilis* (American dog tick), *Haemaphysalis longicornis* (longhorn tick), *Ixodes pacificus* (western black-legged tick), *Ixodes scapularis* (deer tick; black-legged tick), and *Rhipicephalus sanguineus* (brown dog tick; kennel tick). The soft tick most commonly encountered in dogs and cats is *Otobius megnini* (spinose ear tick). However, other soft ticks including *Ornithodoros* spp. can also infest dogs and cats.
- Affected Hosts: All dogs and cats are susceptible to tick infestation.
- Geographic Distribution: Worldwide with the highest abundances in tropical and temperate climates.
- Primary Mode of Transmission: Contact with environments contaminated with ticks. Intrastadial transfer of ticks from one infested animal to another.
- Major Clinical Signs: Painful bite, erythema, pruritus, inflammation, swelling, ulceration, hypersensitivity reactions, otitis externa, paralysis, and anemia. Ticks are vectors of several pathogens capable of resulting in severe disease with variable clinical signs in dogs and cats.
- Differential Diagnoses: Other ectoparasites including mites, fleas, lice, and bed bugs. For tick paralysis, key differential diagnoses include botulism, polyradiculoneuritis, acute peripheral neuropathies, snakebite, and hypokalemia.
- Human Health Significance: Several species of ticks (e.g., *A. americanum* and *I. scapularis*) readily bite and feed on humans. Pets that are not maintained on tick control can transport ticks indoors increasing the risk of exposure to humans. Owners removing embedded ticks from infested pets with improper technique or without protection risk infections with tick-borne pathogens.

ETIOLOGY

Ticks (Acari: Ixodida) are obligate parasites that feed on the blood of vertebrates. There are about 900 extant species of ticks known.[3] These species are divided into three families: Ixodidae (hard ticks; ca. 700 species), Argasidae (soft ticks; ca. 200 species), and Nuttalliellidae (one species, *Nuttalliella namaqua*). *Nuttalliella namaqua* occurs only in southern Africa and exhibits biology related to both hard and soft ticks as well as traits specific to itself. This tick primarily infests lizards[4] and has not been reported from dogs or cats.

Numerous species of ticks feed on dogs and cats throughout the world (Table 109.1).[5] The focus of this chapter will be ticks in North America[6] but the chapter will also mention important ticks from other parts of the world. The ticks most commonly recovered from dogs and cats include *Amblyomma americanum, Amblyomma maculatum, Dermacentor andersoni, Dermacentor occidentalis, Dermacentor variabilis, Haemaphysalis longicornis, Ixodes pacificus, Ixodes scapularis, Rhipicephalus sanguineus,* and *Otobius megnini* (Tables 109.1 and 109.2; Figs. 109.1 and 109.2).[5,7,8] Ticks are highly specialized arachnids with three distinct regions to their bodies[9]: the gnathostoma (or capitulum), idiosoma (body), and segmented appendages (legs). The gnathostoma contains the mouthparts (e.g., palps, chelicerae, hypostome, basis capituli). The idiosoma is the largest part of a tick and contains the internal organs. Legs connect to the anterior half of the idiosoma through coxae. The tarsus of the first pairs of legs contains Haller's organ. Haller's organ is a sensory structure used to locate hosts by detecting odors, temperature, humidity, and possibly other external stimuli.[9] Ticks also contain chemoreceptors in their palps that help them sense their environment.[9,10]

Hard and soft ticks differ in several key characteristics. The most conspicuous difference is that hard ticks possess a scutum. The scutum is a sclerotized plate that covers nearly the entire dorsal surface of males and the anterior half of females and immature stages (larvae and nymphs). Soft ticks lack a scutum and have a cuticle covered in mammillae. When examining hard ticks from the dorsal aspect, mouthparts project anteriorly. The mouthparts do not project beyond the anterior margin of the body in adult soft ticks and can be visualized only from the ventrum.

EPIDEMIOLOGY

There are four developmental stages in the life cycle of ticks: eggs, larvae, nymphs, and adults. There is little variation on this basic developmental plan for hard ticks in that each motile, feeding stage (i.e., larvae, nymphs, and adults) feeds once on a host. Soft ticks are more variable having more than one nymphal stage and feeding multiple times as adults; the number of nymphal stages is not consistent across species.

Hard ticks are categorized as one-, two-, or three-host ticks. Three-host ticks are the most common and comprise the majority of ticks that infest dogs and cats. Three-host ticks are defined by each feeding

TABLE 109.1 Ticks that Commonly Infest Dogs and Cats

Continent	Tick	Common Name
Africa	*Haemaphysalis elliptica*	African yellow dog tick
	Haemaphysalis leachi	Yellow dog tick, African dog tick
	Ixodes spp.	Various depending on species
	Otobius megnini	Spinose ear tick
	Rhipicephalus gertrudae	–
	Rhipicephalus sanguineus	Brown dog tick, kennel tick
Antarctica	None that infest dogs and cats	
Asia	*Haemaphysalis longicornis*	Asian longhorn tick, bush tick
	Rhipicephalus haemaphysaloides	–
	Rhipicephalus sanguineus	Brown dog tick, kennel tick
Australia	*Amblyomma triguttatum*	Kangaroo tick
	Haemaphysalis bancrofti	Wallaby tick
	Haemaphysalis longicornis	Asian longhorn tick, bush tick
	Ixodes cornuatus	Southern paralysis tick, Tasmanian paralysis tick
	Ixodes holocyclus	Eastern paralysis tick
	Ixodes tasmani	Tasmanian possum tick
	Rhipicephalus sanguineus	Brown dog tick, kennel tick
Europe	*Dermacentor reticulatus*	Meadow tick, marsh tick, ornate cow tick
	Haemaphysalis concinna	Bush tick, relict tick
	Haemaphysalis punctata	Red sheep tick
	Ixodes ricinus	Sheep tick, castor bean tick
	Ixodes canisuga	Dog tick, fox tick
	Ixodes hexagonus	Hedgehog tick
	Rhipicephalus sanguineus	Brown dog tick, kennel tick
North America	*Amblyomma americanum*	Lone star tick
	Amblyomma maculatum	Gulf coast tick
	Dermacentor variabilis	American dog tick
	Haemaphysalis longicornis	Asian longhorn tick, bush tick
	Ixodes pacificus	Western black-legged tick
	Ixodes scapularis	Black-legged tick, deer tick
	Otobius megnini	Spinose ear tick
	Rhipicephalus sanguineus	Brown dog tick, kennel tick
South America	*Amblyomma aureolatum*	Yellow dog tick
	Amblyomma ovale	–
	Amblyomma triste	–
	Rhipicephalus sanguineus	Brown dog tick, kennel tick

stage taking a blood meal from a host, falling off that host, molting to the next stage, and then finding another host. For the common three-host ticks of dogs and cats, adult ticks feed and mate on the third host after which replete (fully fed) females drop off the host and lay eggs in the environment. Larvae hatch from the eggs and the cycle is repeated. For two-host ticks, fed larvae are retained on the first host, molt to the nymphal stage, feed, and then drop off and molt to adults. Adults find the second host where they feed and mate. Larvae, nymphs, and adults of one-host ticks all feed on the same individual host animal without spending time in the environment (off the host), between stages.

In general, soft ticks utilize a multitude of hosts in their life cycle. In addition to having multiple nymphal stages, soft ticks display biology that distinguish them from hard ticks. Soft ticks visit their vertebrate hosts only to take a blood meal and they feed quickly (15 to 30 minutes). In some instances, soft ticks may not take a blood meal before molting to the next life stage. Soft tick females lay several clutches of eggs from a single blood meal and may take multiple blood meals at various stages. In comparison, hard ticks attach and feed on their hosts from days to just over a week depending on species and life cycle stage, only take one blood meal per motile stage, and females deposit one clutch of eggs from their single blood meal.

Ticks persist in two environments: on hosts and off hosts. Ticks infest a wide variety of vertebrates including amphibians, reptiles, birds, and mammals. Host predilection is the host preferred by a tick species. Host range is the variety of hosts that a tick species can utilize for a blood meal. Different stages of ticks and tick species often have different host predilections and ranges (see Table 109.2). Relatively few tick species feed on dogs and cats[11-14] with the majority parasitizing wildlife species.[6,15] Understanding the preferred host and the host range of ticks is critical to understanding population dynamics of ticks, tick-borne diseases, and the risks to pets and humans.

Dogs are significant hosts for ticks throughout the world.[16] Examination of dogs seen at veterinary hospitals in 339 US cities across 40 states from 2002 to 2004 demonstrated that ticks were observed during 42,090 of 8,088,288 dog visits.[17] That is, the prevalence of dog visits in which ticks were found was 0.52% (95% CI, 0.51–0.53%). The highest prevalence of dogs with ticks were in Oklahoma (2.5%; 2.3–2.7%), Arkansas (2.4%; 2.1–2.7%), Connecticut (1.4%; 1.2–1.6%), West Virginia (1.3%; 1.1–1.6%), and Rhode Island (1.2%; 1.0–1.5%). States with the lowest prevalence of ticks on dogs included Michigan (0.03%; 0.02–0.06%), Utah (0.04%; 0.03–0.06%), Nevada (0.05%; 0.04–0.07%), Colorado (0.1%; 0.09–0.1%), and Washington (0.2%; 0.1–0.2%). The highest prevalence of ticks on dogs were observed late spring into summer during April, May, June, and July. The lowest prevalence was during winter in November, December, January, and February. Factors that increased the risk for infestation were age of 6 months to 1 year (OR [95% CI] = 1.54 [1.47–1.62]), male sex (OR [95% CI] = 1.08 [1.06–1.10]) and being sexually intact (OR [95% CI] = 1.46 [1.43–1.49]).[17] These factors likely indicate time before client compliance with ectoparasite preventive regimens and a tendency of intact animals to roam, increasing contact with environments harboring ticks. Similarly, dogs less than 1 year of age from Mexicali, Mexico were found to be 2.8 times more likely to be infested with *Rh. sanguineus* when compared with dogs over one year of age.[18] A comparison of the prevalence of ticks among dog breeds demonstrated that toy-breed dogs were least likely to be infested.[17] It is likely that the lower prevalence of ticks on toy-breed dogs is reflective of the dog's lifestyle and being less exposed to environments with ticks than toy-breed dogs being less susceptible to infestation with ticks.

Less information is known about ticks on cats, and primary literature reports of cats naturally infested with ticks are limited to a

TABLE 109.2 **Common Ticks of Dogs and Cats in North America—Preferred Hosts, Geographic Distribution, and Examples of Pathogens Transmitted to Dogs and Cats**

Tick	Common Name	Preferred Hosts	Geographic Distribution	Examples of Pathogens Transmitted (Chapter Number)
Amblyomma americanum	Lone star tick	Larvae: Medium-sized and larger mammals including dogs, cats, deer, cattle, other domestic and wild animals Nymphs: Medium-sized and larger mammals including dogs, cats, deer, cattle, other domestic and wild animals Adults: Large mammals including dogs, cats, cattle, deer, other domestic and wild animals	Southeastern and southcentral US north to southern Michigan. Atlantic Coast of US from Florida to southern Maine	*Cytauxzoon felis* (98) *Ehrlichia chaffeensis* (44) *Ehrlichia ewingii* (44) *Francisella tularensis* (74)
Amblyomma maculatum	Gulf Coast tick	Larvae: Small mammals and ground-dwelling birds Nymphs: Small mammals, ground-dwelling birds, and larger mammals Adults: Medium- and large-sized mammals including dogs	Gulf Coast states of US inland to southern Kansas. North along the Atlantic Coast to Virginia	*Hepatozoon americanum* (99)
Dermacentor andersoni	Rocky Mountain wood tick	Larvae: Rodents Nymphs: Rodents Adults: Medium- to large-sized mammals	Rocky Mountain states and provinces of US and Canada from elevation of 4000 to 15,000 feet (1219 to 4572 m)	*Rickettsia rickettsii* (46) *Francisella tularensis* (74)
Dermacentor occidentalis	Pacific Coast tick	Larvae: Small rodents Nymphs: Small rodents Adults: Larger mammals including dogs and cats	Pacific Coast of US	*Francisella tularensis* (74) *Rickettsia rickettsii* (46)
Dermacentor variabilis	American dog tick	Larvae: Small rodents Nymphs: Small- and medium-sized mammals Adults: Medium-sized mammals	Prairie states and provinces of US and Canada east of the Rocky Mountains to the Atlantic Coast. California coast of US to southern Oregon	*Cytauxzoon felis* (98) *Francisella tularensis* (74) *Rickettsia rickettsii* (46)
Ixodes pacificus	Western black-legged tick	Larvae: Lizards, birds, and small mammals Nymphs: Birds, small mammals, and lizards Adults: Large and medium-sized mammals	Pacific Coast of US	*Anaplasma phagocytophilum* (45) *Borrelia/Borreliella* (*incertae sedis*) *burgdorferi* (69)
Ixodes scapularis	Deer tick; black-legged tick	Larvae: Rodents, birds, and reptiles Nymphs: Rodents, birds, reptiles, dogs, and cats Adults: Medium- and large-sized mammals including dogs and cats	Southcentral and southeastern US north along the Atlantic Coast into the northeastern US and Canada. Upper Midwest of US	*Anaplasma phagocytophilum* (45) *Borrelia/Borreliella burgdorferi* (69)
Otobius megnini	Spinose ear tick	Larvae: Medium- and large-sized mammals Nymphs: Medium- and large-sized mammals Adults: None, adults are free living	Southern Canada through the US. Also found in Central America, South America, Africa, and India. In the US, most common in arid regions of the west	None known
Rhipicephalus sanguineus sensu lato	Brown dog tick; kennel tick	Larvae: Dogs Nymphs: Dogs Adults: Dogs	Cosmopolitan throughout the world	*Anaplasma platys* (suspected) (45) *Babesia canis* (97) *Babesia gibsoni* (not confirmed in North America) (97) *Ehrlichia canis* (44) *Hepatozoon canis* (not confirmed in North America) (99) *Rickettsia rickettsii* (46)

handful.[6,19-26] The importance of ticks infesting cats is often overlooked possibly due to the misperception that cats are not suitable hosts and are fastidious groomers. A survey of ectoparasites on feral cats in Florida[20] only recovered a few adults of *A. americanum*, *D. variabilis*, *I. scapularis*, and *Rh. sanguineus*. A comparable survey of free-roaming cats in Oklahoma[25] also demonstrated adults of *A. americanum*, *D. variabilis*, *I. scapularis*, and *Rh. sanguineus* on 18.7% (15.9–21.9%) of the cats examined. However, larvae and nymphs comprised 54.7% of

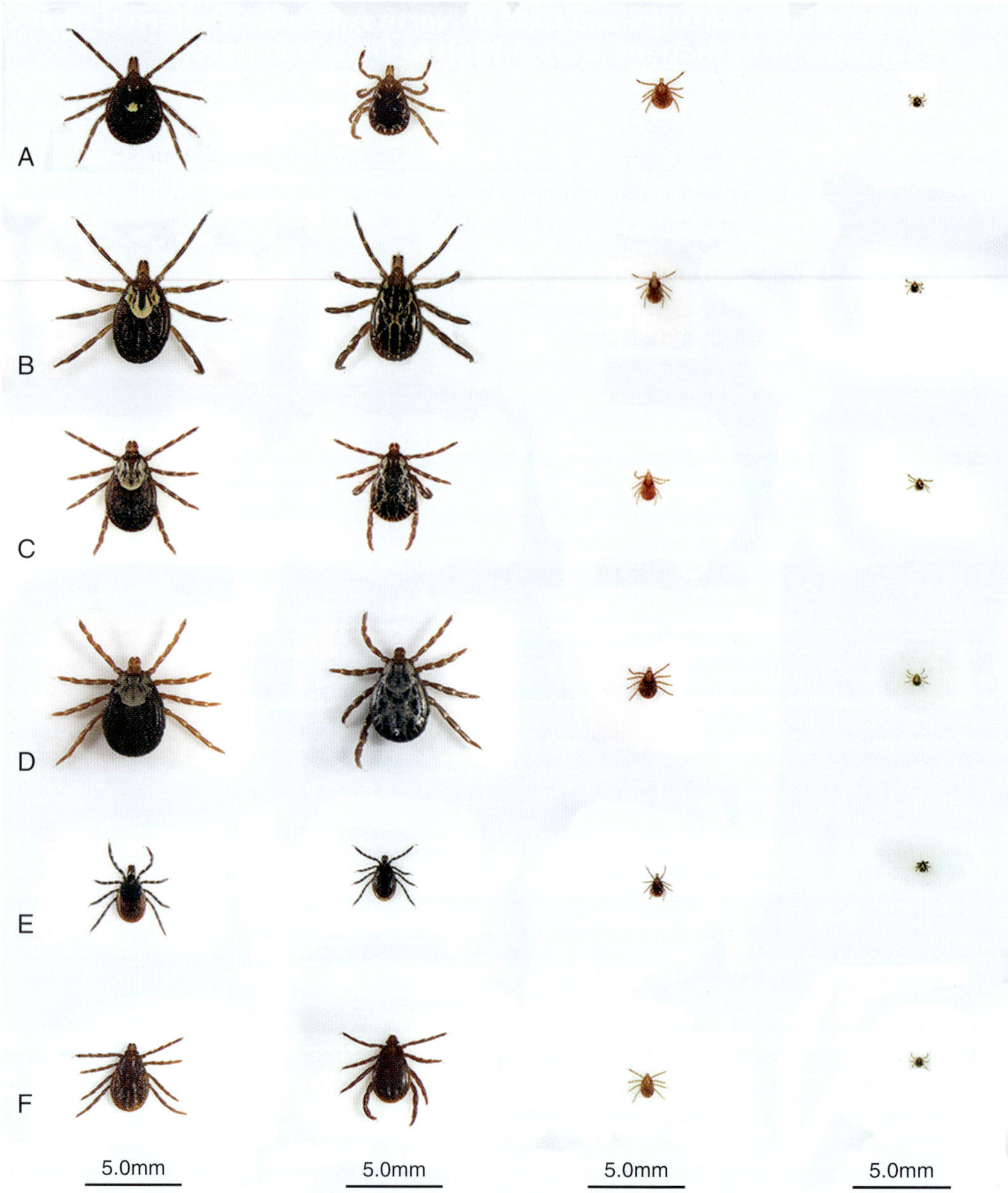

Fig. 109.1 Size and morphological comparisons of life stages of unengorged (A) *Amblyomma americanum*, (B) *Amblyomma maculatum*, (C) *Dermacentor variabilis*, (D) *Dermacentor andersoni*, (E) *Ixodes scapularis*, and (F) *Rhipicephalus sanguineus*. Scale bar is 5.0 mm, magnification is 1.25×. (Courtesy of the National Center for Veterinary Parasitology.)

the ticks (mostly *A. americanum*) recovered from infested cats. Ticks were found infesting cats in all months surveyed.[25]

Three-host hard ticks are intermittent parasites and spend 95% of their lifespan in the external environment.[27] In general, soft ticks spend even more time in the external environment and only visit hosts briefly to feed. *Otobius megnini* is an exception. This is a soft tick whose larvae and two nymphal stages are parasitic in the ear canal of dogs, cats, and other animals.[28] Adult *O. megnini* are free living and do not feed.

Hard ticks thrive in habitats rich with vertebrate hosts, like mammals, lizards, and ground-dwelling birds. The preferred habitats for most wildlife ticks are brushy, wooded, or weedy areas, especially moist woodlands and vegetated areas at the edge of forests, along animal and hiking trails and in overgrown weedy or grassy fields. One hard tick, *Rh. sanguineus*, is more likely to be found in or around homes or kennels with dogs. Soft ticks are generally found in animal burrows, dens, caves, or dilapidated human dwellings such as huts, cabins, or sheds. In addition, soft ticks readily thrive in hot and dry conditions. Dogs and cats become infested with ticks through contact with contaminated environments. Pets may also become infested with ticks through intrastadial (same life stage) transfer from one infested animal to a naïve one (e.g., an adult tick transfers from one dog in the household to another pet).[29]

In the external environment, tick survival is dependent upon a multitude of factors including climate, vegetation, host availability, photoperiod, and human activities.[30] Ticks that are off hosts are most susceptible to arid conditions and temperature extremes.[27] Mortality of ticks in the external environment results from freezing in winter, dehydration during arid summers, overheating during summer, drowning in floodwater, and exhaustion of energy resources because they fail to find a host.[31] Nonetheless, ticks are well adapted to survive off hosts and live longer than any other arthropod without food or water.[27] Ticks can become active at temperatures not thought to be conducive to tick activity and they can occur in locations considered atypical by most pet owners presenting

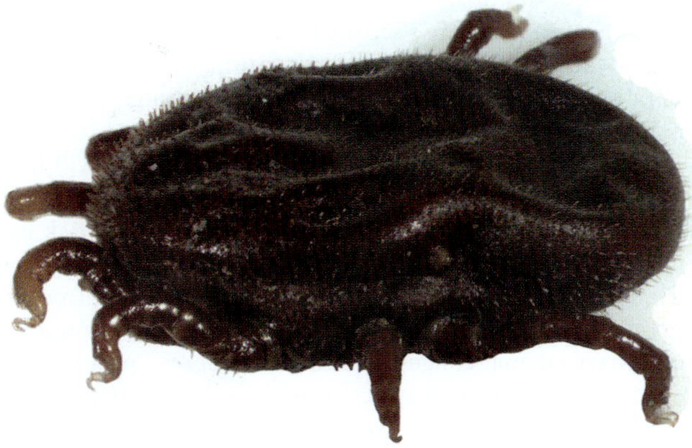

Fig. 109.2 Nymph of *Otobius megnini* recovered from an infested dog. Note spiny protuberances (mamillae) covering the body. Magnification 2.4×.

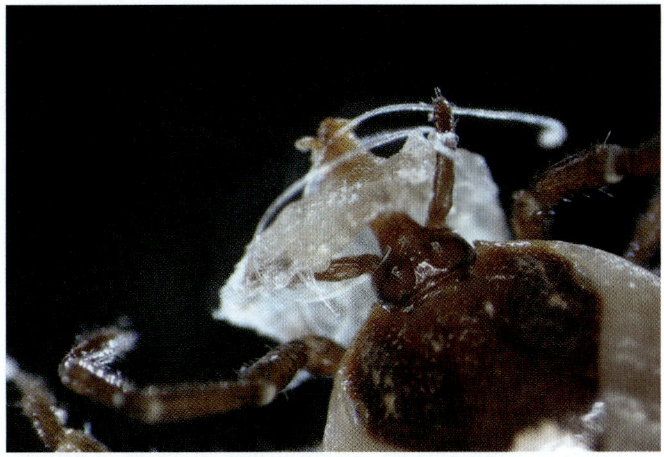

Fig. 109.3 Partially engorged *Amblyomma americanum* female with cement cone surrounding hypostome.

unforeseen risks to pets. For example, the threshold temperature in which *I. scapularis* adults quest is 4°C (32°F).[32] *Rhipicephalus sanguineus* is adapted to completing its life cycle indoors but can also survive outdoors in mild climates if hosts and environmental refuges are available.[33] With the ability to survive and reproduce indoors, as well as the ability to transmit *Rickettsia rickettsii* (causative agent of Rocky Mountain spotted fever), *Rh. sanguineus* presents a significant public health concern.[34]

Current thinking suggests that human development and population growth, movement of wild and domestic animals, and climate change will all have an impact on tick distribution and abundances.[35,36] What that impact will be has yet to be determined. Within recent history, we have seen an expansion of the ranges of *A. americanum*, *A. maculatum*, *D. variabilis*, and *I. scapularis*. *Amblyomma americanum*, historically found in the southeastern and southcentral United States, has expanded rapidly in the northeast and Midwest.[37] *Amblyomma maculatum* was historically found within a couple hundred miles of the Gulf of Mexico. Over the last two decades, the geographic range of *A. maculatum* has expanded northward along the Atlantic coast to Maryland as well as north into mid-western states including Arkansas, Oklahoma, Kansas, and southwestern Tennessee. *Dermacentor variabilis*, historically found in prairie states and provinces east of the Rocky Mountains, has moved westward and northward in Canada.[38] and is now commonly found infesting dogs and cats in Rocky Mountain states.[44] Finally, *Ixodes scapularis* (historically found in the southcentral, southeastern, northeastern, and upper Midwest) has expanded into Canada.[40] The distribution of *I. scapularis* in the United States has also shifted. Since 1998 the number of counties in the United States reporting *I. scapularis* has increased by 44.7%.[31] Moreover, the greatest increase in the number of counties reporting *I. scapularis* occurred in the northeastern states and upper Midwest. It has been suggested that the historic foci of *I. scapularis* populations in New England states and upper Midwest are converging in the Ohio River Valley.[31] *Haemaphysalis longicornis* was initially found in the United States on sheep in New Jersey in late 2017[41] and has since been found in at least 17 states throughout the eastern and southcentral United States.

CLINICAL FEATURES

Pathogenesis

Insertion of mouthparts and feeding activities may result in mechanical injury, irritation, inflammation, hypersensitivity reactions, transmission of pathogens, and toxicosis (see tick paralysis). A tick bite lesion is created upon insertion of the tick's chelicerae and hypostome into the host's skin.[42] Once a tick finds a suitable location, insertion of the mouthparts occurs in four phases: surface coursing, superficial attachment, cheliceral insertion, and hypostomal envelopment.[43] Ticks may remain attached at one location or they may remove their mouthparts and reattach at a different site. Insertion of chelicerae and the hypostome are not adequate holdfast organs to support the extended duration needed for ixodid ticks to feed. Most ixodid ticks secrete cement proteins[44] for extended attachment. Tick cement is a latex-like substance secreted by the tick within 5 to 30 minutes of attachment.[42] The cement hardens quickly forming a gasket between the tick's mouthparts (Fig. 109.3) and the host's epidermis, securing the attachment. Soft ticks do not produce cement[42] and feed rapidly by inserting their mouth parts deeply into their hosts.

Insertion of a tick's mouthparts damages capillaries and small blood vessels creating pools of extravasated blood that is ingested. While on hosts, ticks are in a gorging state[27] and must modulate the host's defenses in order to successfully feed. A variety of bioactive proteins and lipids are produced to combat host hemostasis, tissue repair at the feeding site, and development of an anti-tick response. Over 3500 putative salivary proteins have been identified from a variety of tick species.[45] These substances include anticoagulants, antiplatelet aggregators, vasodilators, anti-inflammatories, and immunomodulators that allow ticks to feed successfully to repletion.[46] Ticks are important vectors of pathogens and transmit a greater variety of disease agents (Table 109.2) than any other arthropod vector group.[16] Transfer of pathogens from ticks to hosts most commonly occurs through the passage of contaminated saliva during feeding.[47] However, tick-borne pathogens may also be transferred to hosts through regurgitation, coxal fluid, tick feces,[48] and ingestion of infected ticks as seen with *Hepatozoon americanum* and *Hepatozoon canis* (see Chapter 99).[49]

Galactose-alpha-1,3-galactose Hypersensitivity Reactions

In humans, an association has been made between bites of certain tick species and subsequent development of delayed (3 to 8 hours) anaphylactic reactions to red meat. In 2009, it was reported that bites from *A. americanum* induced a delayed anaphylaxis to red meat in humans due to IgE antibodies against galactose-alpha-1,3-galactose (alpha-gal) in the US.[50,51] Alpha-gal is a carbohydrate naturally produced in all mammals besides humans, great apes, and new-world monkeys. It is a carbohydrate moiety of post-translational modification of proteins for proper protein folding and stability as well as intracellular movement of proteins. The mechanism by which this antibody response develops has yet to be determined. Possibilities include, but are not limited to: the presence of alpha-gal in ticks to which hosts are exposed; host antibody development against a non-alpha-gal carbohydrate or protein which is cross-reactive with alpha-gal; and host exposure to alpha-gal ingested from a previous blood meal, including from the blood meal of the previous motile life stage. This phenomenon has also been demonstrated in Europe (*Ixodes ricinus*), Australia (*Ixodes holocyclus*), Asia (tick species not identified), and Central America (*Amblyomma cajennense* suspected).[52] Food allergy as a result of anti-alpha-gal antibodies is not likely to develop in dogs and cats as these species naturally produce alpha-gal. Production of anti-alpha-gal antibodies would represent a catastrophic autoimmune disorder, unlikely to be overlooked.

Tick Paralysis

Tick paralysis results from the inoculation of toxins present in tick saliva into hosts. Dogs, cats, and numerous other animals are susceptible to these toxins.[53–55] Tick paralysis in animals and humans occurs worldwide.[56] Most tick bites do not result in paralysis and the condition is rare in North America. Approximately 70 species of hard and soft ticks have been implicated in, or suspected to cause, paralysis in hosts.[57] Most cases of tick paralysis in dogs, cats, and humans in North America are due to infestation with *D. andersoni* or *D. variabilis*.[57] However, all of the ticks common on dogs and cats in North America are capable of causing tick paralysis.[54–57] Other medically important ticks that cause paralysis are *I. holocyclus* (eastern paralysis tick) and *Ixodes cornuatus* (southern paralysis tick) in Australia[58,59] and *Ixodes rubicundus* and *Rhipicephalus evertis* in Africa.[60] A third *Ixodes* species in Australia, *Ixodes hirsti*, has been reported as a cause of paralysis in cats.[59] The onset of paralysis coincides with rapid engorgement of female ticks regardless of the species.[57] Feeding of male ticks does not result in paralysis likely as a result of lower levels of saliva injected during feeding compared to females.[61] Large numbers of larvae or nymphs are believed to cause toxicosis. For *Dermacentor* species, rapid engorgement of females occurs after mating with a male after about 5 days of attachment and feeding. In cases of tick paralysis in humans, ticks are commonly found attached to the scalp, behind the ear, the neck, and the groin.[56] In veterinary medicine, it is commonly believed that ticks attached to the head, base of the skull, or along the spine are most likely to result in paralysis. The ability of *D. andersoni* adults to cause paralysis is a heritable trait and virulent strains of ticks can be selected.[60]

Paralysis due to *I. holocyclus* results from a temperature-dependent inhibition of acetylcholine release from the neuromuscular junction.[62] Muscle paralysis can be experimentally induced by inhibiting the dependence of transmitter release on extracellular calcium.[58] Direct cardiotoxicity and GI signs (vomiting and regurgitation), with aspiration pneumonia, have also been identified in dogs. The exact mechanism of paralysis caused by *D. andersoni* is not known and is thought to be distinct from that of *I. holocyclus*.[57] Feeding *D. andersoni* females are known to affect neurons of the efferent pathway but not the afferent; the neuromuscular junction of peripheral nerves is targeted through inhibition of acetylcholine release from the synapse, suggesting a presynaptic target.[63]

Clinical Signs

Tick bites are painful and irritating. They incite local inflammatory reactions and pruritus. The attachment of a few ticks is well tolerated by most dog and cat hosts. However, severe infestations can lead to anemia[64] and possibly death by exsanguination. It is important to remember that tick burden is relative to patient size and concurrent morbidities. A female tick will ingest between 0.5 and 1.5 mL of blood from the host, depending on tick species.[65] Hypersensitivity reactions to tick attachment and feeding may result in focal areas of necrosis and ulceration; erythematous macules or nodules that may or may not be pruritic and ulcerated; and pruritic pododermatitis.[66] Ticks that feed in or around the ears (e.g., *O. megnini*) may cause secondary otitis externa[67] and pruritic or painful ear disease (head tilt, altered pinnal carriage). Cases of tick paralysis present as acute, symmetric, ascending paresis/paralysis. The longer the inciting tick(s) remains attached, the higher the likelihood that ascending neuromuscular paralysis will lead to respiratory failure and death. Unilateral facial paralysis and anisocoria have been noted in dogs and cats presenting with tick paralysis due to *I. holocyclus*.[53] Additional signs include cough; gagging; hypersalivation; inappetence; urinary incontinence due to sphincter incompetence; and dyspnea and increased breath sounds due to pulmonary edema, congestive heart failure, or aspiration pneumonia.[68,69] Hypothermia may occur in moribund animals. Physical examination findings can be confounded if a tick-borne disease is also present. Sudden death may also occur.

Physical Examination Findings

Physical examination findings of dogs and cats infested with ticks are highly variable. Cases with only a few ticks attached will be subclinical. Infestation by only a few ticks or by immature ticks can be easily missed during physical examination.[25] Ticks can be found attached anywhere on a dog or cat requiring close inspection of the entire surface of a pet, as well as mucous membranes. If tick infestation is severe enough to lead to anemia, expected findings may include dull mentation, generalized weakness, pale mucous membranes, tachycardia, tachypnea, and poor peripheral pulses.[64]

Cutaneous lesions include erythematous macules, papules, or nodules around the site of tick attachment (Fig. 109.4). These lesions may be up to 2 cm in diameter. Surface ulceration/erosion and crusting will develop after tick detachment and may be subtle. Self-induced trauma may make the lesions more dramatic. After a tick detaches or is removed, acute feeding lesions of 1 to 2 mm deep and 1 to 3 mm wide remain (Fig. 109.5). Tick bite lesions typically heal in about 3 weeks but may be complicated by secondary infection. Granuloma formation at the bite site has been described in humans and domestic animals, and may persist for months to years.[70,71]

Dogs and cats with tick paralysis have generalized lower motor neuron signs (including ataxia, lateral recumbency, decreased withdrawal reflexes) and may also have signs related to the respiratory and GI tract described earlier. Respiratory signs may predominate in cats.[68]

DIAGNOSIS

Diagnosis is achieved by identifying ticks recovered from infested pets during physical examination. The burden of ticks on pets can range from a few that are subclinical to severe infestation that results in anemia requiring a blood transfusion.[64] Thorough examination of infested animals is often necessary to locate immature stages of ticks that are easily missed because of their small size.[25] Utilization of a flea comb can help recover ticks but combing is not efficient for recovering small, attached, unengorged (i.e., flat) ticks aligned close to the surface of the pet's skin. By examining dogs during peak activity times of *A. americanum*, *D. variabilis*, *I. scapularis*, and *Rh. sanguineus* activity, predilection sites have been described for each species.[72] Adult *A. americanum* were evenly distributed on dogs including the perianal region and between the pelvic limbs. However, 43% of *A. americanum* adults were recovered from the ears, head, and neck of infested dogs. The majority (80%) of adult *D. variabilis* were also recovered from the ears, head, and neck of infested dogs. Adult *I. scapularis* were most commonly recovered from anterior body regions of infested dogs. Adult *Rh. sanguineus* were retrieved from all body regions of dogs with

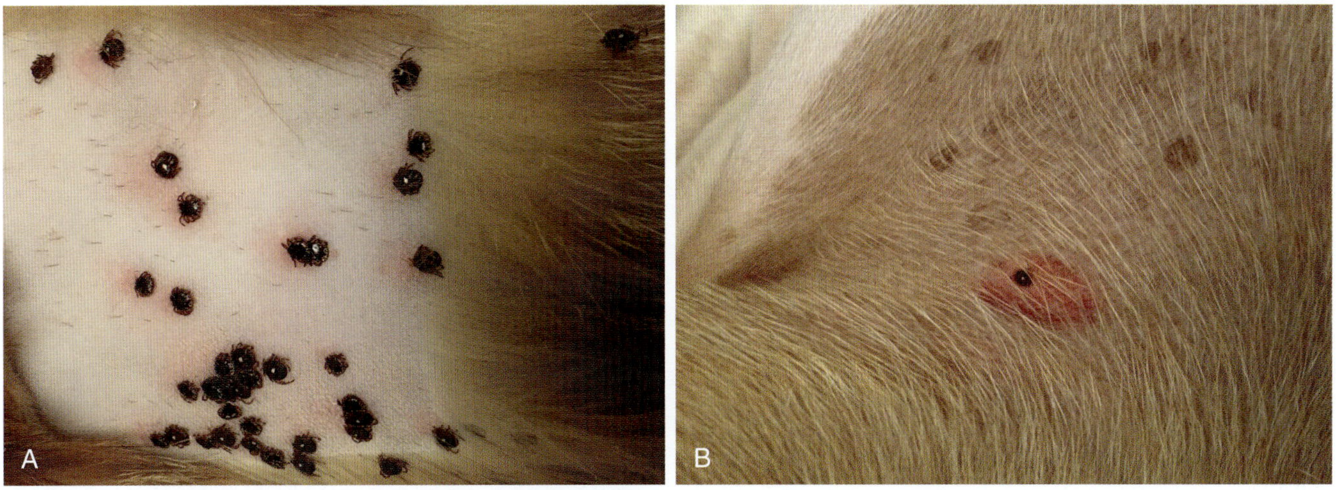

Fig. 109.4 Erythema associated with attached ticks. (A) Poorly defined erythematous macules around feeding *Amblyomma americanum* adults on an artificially infested cat. (B) Markedly erythematous, semi-fluctuant epidermal swelling around an attached female *A. americanum* in the axilla of a 5-year-old dog.

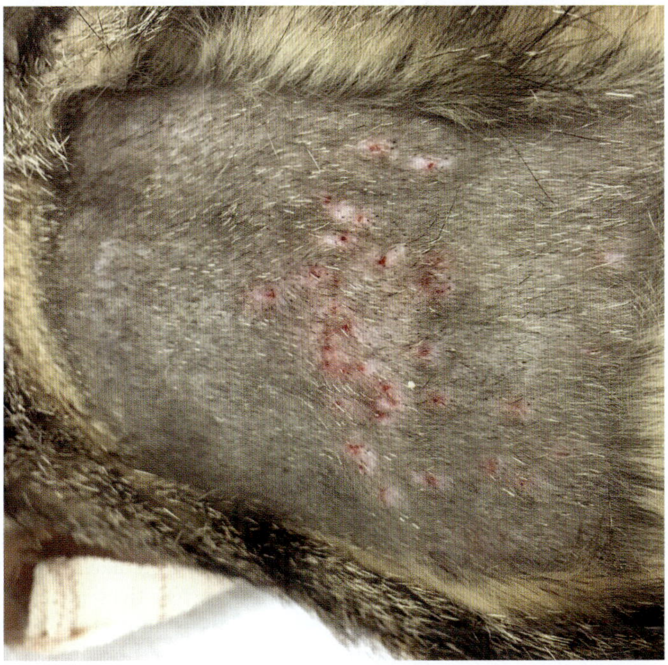

Fig. 109.5 Erythematous papules with central hemorrhagic crusts remaining after a large number of *Amblyomma americanum* adults were removed. Tick frass (feces) can still be observed around feeding sites. Hair clipped for improved visualization of lesions.

the head, neck, and back being most commonly infested.[72] Larvae and nymphs of *Rh. sanguineus* were evenly distributed on infested dogs with the fewest on the dorsum. Predilection sites of ears, head, interdigital spaces, back, inguinal region, and axilla were also reported for *Rh. sanguineus*.[33]

Differential diagnoses for acariasis includes infestation with other parasites such as mites, fleas (especially *Echidnophaga gallinacea*, the sticktight flea), lice, and bed bugs. Ticks are arachnids that can be easily differentiated from other ectoparasites.[13,73] Arachnids do not have wings, have four pairs of legs in the adult stage, and undivided bodies. Insects (e.g., fleas and lice) have bodies divided into three regions (head, thorax, and abdomen), six pair of legs, and mouthparts outside the head capsule. Mites (see Chapter 110) are also arachnids but can be easily distinguished from ticks. Ticks are larger than mites, and have a leathery cuticle and spiracles near the coxa of the fourth pair of legs.[6]

Ticks are identified based on the morphology of key anatomical structures. Dichotomous keys are available for identification of adults,[74,75] nymphs,[75–78] and larvae.[75,78–81] However, dichotomous keys are problematic in that they are often limited to specific taxa, life stage, or geographic location. Identification of immature ticks to species can be challenging and is not practical in a clinical setting. Common adult hard ticks (see Fig. 109.1) and *O. megnini* (see Fig. 109.2) can be readily identified in clinic with the aid of a magnifying lens or dissecting microscope. Websites are available[82,83] to assist in gross identification of common adult ticks found on pets and humans.

Amblyomma americanum is a medium-sized, reddish-brown bodied, ornate tick with long mouthparts and festoons.[84] The female *A. americanum* is distinguished by a white spot (hence the name "lone star" tick) on the posterior margin of the scutum. Male *A. americanum* are readily identified having white spots on the festoons. *Amblyomma maculatum* is a medium- to large-sized, reddish-brown bodied, ornate tick with long mouthparts and festoons.[85] This tick is distinguished from other ticks based on its large size and diffuse pattern of white on the scutum of both males and females.

Dermacentor andersoni, *D. occidentalis*, and *D. variabilis* are morphologically similar. They are medium- to large-sized, reddish-brown bodied, ornate ticks with short mouthparts, a square basis capitulum, and festoons. A primary difference among these ticks is the geographic locales where they are most abundant. *Dermacentor andersoni*, the Rocky Mountain wood tick, is found in the Rocky Mountains in western North America.[86] *Dermacentor occidentalis*, the Pacific Coast tick has a range restricted to far western North America.[87] *Dermacentor variabilis*, the American dog tick, is widely distributed in North America east of the Rocky Mountains and some areas along the Pacific Coast (see Fig. 46.1 for maps). The coloration and patterns of adult *Dermacentor* spp. look most similar to those of *A. maculatum* and the ticks may be confused for each other in areas where their distributions overlap. Nonetheless, *Dermacentor* spp. are readily differentiated from *A. maculatum* due to their short mouthparts.

Haemaphysalis longicornis is an inornate, reddish-brown, medium-sized tick with rectangular basis capitulum, short mouth parts, and lateral projection of the second palpal segment.[88] Morphologically, *H. longicornis* is most similar to and easily mistaken for *Rh. sanguineus*. However, upon close inspection under magnification, one can easily identify the flared second palpal segment of *H. longicornis* as compared to the flared basis capitulum of *Rh. sanguineus* (see following text).

Ixodes pacificus and *I. scapularis* are morphologically similar ticks. *Ixodes pacificus*, the western black-legged tick, is found along the west coast of the United States.[31] *Ixodes scapularis*, the black-legged tick or deer tick, is widely distributed in eastern North America with dense populations in the northeast and upper Midwest (see Fig. 45.2).[31] As their common names suggest, the legs of these adult ticks are black as is their scutum. They have long mouthparts and an anal groove located anterior to the anus; this is also true for other ticks that belong to the *Ixodes persulcatus* complex.

Rhipicephalus sanguineus, the brown dog tick or kennel tick, is found throughout the world.[33] *Rhipicephalus sanguineus* is a brown tick that is inornate and has a flared basis capitulum and short mouthparts.

Otobius megnini, the spinose ear tick, is the soft tick that is most commonly encountered in dogs and cats.[7] This tick has no scutum and only larvae and nymphs of *O. megnini* are parasitic, infesting the ears of their hosts.[28] Larvae of *O. megnini* resemble tiny shriveled grapes[7] and nymphs are covered in spines, conveying its common name. *Otobius megnini* is most commonly found in arid areas of western North America.[7,89]

Tick paralysis is diagnosed when acute onset of ascending paralysis is accompanied by tick infestation. Inciting tick(s) may be difficult to locate on the affected animals necessitating a complete and thorough search of the pet. Ticks may be attached in areas not typically considered including deep within the ears, in the mouth (both mucosa and transverse palatine ridges of the hard palate), preputial sheath, vulvar folds, and perianal folds. Clinical laboratory tests are not available outside of research labs to aid the veterinary practitioner in diagnosing tick paralysis nor infestation with ticks. Diagnosis is confirmed by resolution of clinical signs following tick removal. Clinical scoring systems have been developed to classify neurologic and respiratory signs in canine[69,90] and feline[68,91] tick paralysis patients for prognostication purposes and to monitor recovery.

Laboratory Abnormalities

Responses of cats and dogs to infestation with ticks are non-specific and variable. Most cases of infestation in which only a few ticks are attached are unremarkable. Laboratory abnormalities range from no abnormalities to eosinophilia, hypoproteinemia, and non-regenerative or regenerative anemia. No significant difference in CBC findings were detected in dogs repeatedly infested with >50 adult *Rh. sanguineus* versus non-infested dogs.[92] Two dogs severely infested with nymphal and adult *Rh. sanguineus* (i.e., thousands of ticks) were described with severe regenerative anemia, hypoproteinemia, and leukocytosis.[64]

Pathologic Findings

Histologic lesions of tick bites include congestion, edema, and sometimes focal hemorrhage (Fig. 109.6). Inflammation consists of perivascular to diffuse accumulations of neutrophils, eosinophils, and basophils.[93] After about 24 hours of infestation with *A. americanum*, there is mild, focal epidermal necrosis with a minimal increase in dermal cellular infiltrates. The tick bite lesion extends through the epidermis into the dermis. By 48 hours post infestation, the predominant patterns include a moderate perivascular neutrophilic dermatitis with extension into the dermis and subcutis, and a moderate diffuse neutrophilic panniculitis. Coagulated collagen degeneration is observed by 48 hours. By 96 hours post infestation, a focally severe neutrophilic dermatitis and panniculitis is observed, with focal areas of necrosis and fibrin deposition extending through the subcutis into the muscle band of the deep subcutis. The most intense cellular infiltration into the dermis and epidermis is by 96 hours post infestation. Mast cells and mononuclear leukocytes are also present.[94]

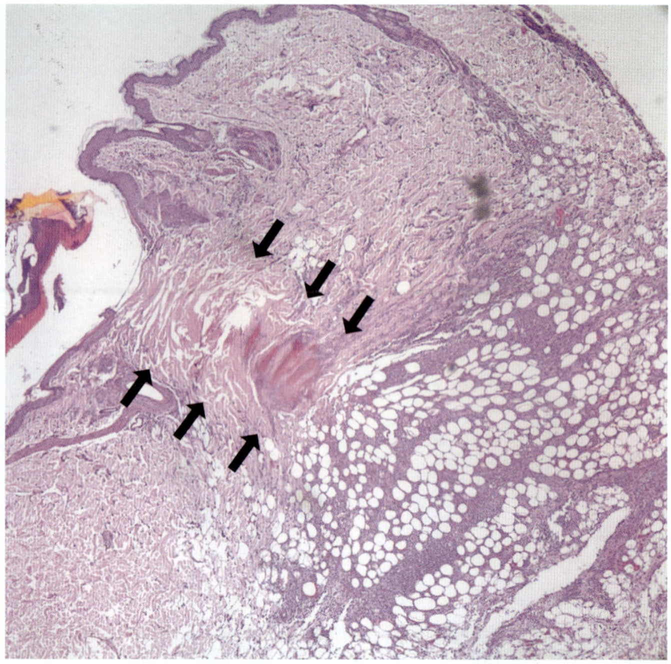

Fig. 109.6 Histologic section showing lesion created from a tick bite on a domestic cat with focally severe, perivascular neutrophilic dermatitis and panninculitis associated with tick feeding. Focal areas of necrosis and fibrin deposition extend through the deep subcutis. Coagulated collagen degeneration is present in the dermis, prominently in the central feeding lesion. Feeding lesion, which extends into the deep dermis, denoted by arrows (hematoxylin and eosin stain).

TREATMENT AND PROGNOSIS

All attached ticks should be removed from infested pets as quickly as possible to minimize pathogenesis and reduce the likelihood of pathogen transmission. For pets with only a few ticks attached, manual removal of ticks with gloved hands is indicated. Ticks are easily removed using fine-tipped tweezers. The tick should be grasped as close to the surface of the skin as possible and pulled perpendicular to the skin with steady, even pressure. Jerking or twisting should be avoided as this will increase the likelihood of breaking off the tick's mouthparts. If mouthparts do break off, they should be removed from the skin with fine-tipped tweezers. Ticks should not be squeezed or crushed as this may cause the tick to regurgitate gut contents or stimulate salivary gland secretion. After ticks are removed, the lesion should be cleaned to reduce risk of secondary bacterial infection, using dilute chlorhexidine or iodine, rubbing alcohol, or soap and water.

Other popularized remedies suggesting that attached ticks be removed by some method of burning (e.g., lit match or cigarette), suffocation (e.g., painting with fingernail polish, petrolatum jelly, oils), or chemical irritation (e.g., alcohol, oils, perfume, diatomaceous earth) do not work, are ill-advised, and could increase the risk of pathogen transmission to hosts.

Live, motile ticks can be secured by placing them in a sealed plastic bag or adhering between two layers of tape. Secured ticks should be disposed of in the trash. Ticks are also killed by long-term submersion in alcohol or freezing at −20°C for a minimum of 24 hours. Ticks can be tested for specific pathogens at various commercial laboratories. Testing ticks for the presence or absence of pathogens should not be used as a proxy for the clinical assessment of a patient. It is impossible to tell if a pathogen was transmitted from a tick to a host by testing the tick after it has been removed from the host. Tick pathogen screens are, by nature, not comprehensive for all pathogens the tick may carry.

Pets heavily infested with ticks can be treated with an approved acaricide (Table 109.3 and Chapter 13). Depending on the level of infestation and the amount of injury that results, severely infested animals may require treatment for secondary skin infections, topical or systemic glucocorticoid therapy, fluid therapy, and/or blood transfusion.[64] Historically, it was recommended to bath severely infested pets with warm water and an acaricide-containing shampoo, sometimes daily until all ticks were removed.[64] However, the majority of acaricide-containing shampoos and dips available in the US market contain pyrethrins, pyrethroids, and their synergists. As of 2021, amitraz dip for dogs is not currently being manufactured in the United States. Clinicians should weigh the risks of dermal irritation of exposing broken and damaged skin to these compounds, along with potential risks of increased dermal absorption of these compounds in highly infested animals. Similar clinical judgment should be used when considering topical sprays. Common topical acaricidal sprays in the US market may contain a variety of active ingredients, including: pyrethrins, pyrethroids, fipronil, etofenprox, and tetrachlorvinphos (see Table 109.3). Acaricidal powders are generally avoided in small animal medicine due to risk of respiratory irritation, eye irritation, and exposure to veterinary staff and clients. A clinician may elect to use an effective systemic acaricide for the patient, and determine if the addition of an EPA-approved topical product is necessary.

Routine treatment and control of ticks on dogs and cats is accomplished through regular and continuous use of approved acaricides (see Table 109.3). Year-round use of acaricides on dog and cats is warranted because pets are host to several tick species that have varying degrees of activity throughout the year, ticks can be active in colder months of the year, common ticks that infest dogs and cats are expanding in distribution, and because *Rh. sanguineus* can infest homes and kennels and be active indoors throughout the year. All animals in close association with an infested animal should be treated and maintained on an approved acaricide.

In the United States, ectoparasiticides are regulated by the Environmental Protection Agency (EPA) or the FDA. As a general rule, if a product is applied topically to an animal to treat ectoparasites, and the compound is not absorbed systemically, it likely falls under the jurisdiction of the EPA. If a product is administered orally, by injection, or if it is applied topically for systemic absorption, it likely falls under the jurisdiction of the FDA. This distinction is important for practitioners to recognize, because there is no legal extra-label use of products regulated by the EPA. Label directions must be followed regarding species treated, product concentration, product dosage, individuals allowed to administer application, and re-treatment interval. Because products regulated by the FDA are approved animal drugs, extra-label use may be allowed under the Animal Medicinal Drug Use and Clarification Act (AMDUCA).

Acaricides currently approved for use in cats and dogs are formulated for topical ("spot on" products, collars, sprays) or oral administration (see Table 109.3). Care must be taken to use acaricides only on or in the host species for which they are approved. Dog products should not be administered to cats, and vice versa. In areas where ticks are abundant and there is increased risk of infestation to pets, practitioners can combine tick treatment and control products, alternating and overlapping application of products yet keeping within label directions. Acaricide resistance has been documented in various locations throughout the world, predominately in livestock.[95] The continued use and in some cases misuse of acaricides would be expected to select for ticks that are drug-resistant. Resistance of *A. americanum* to benzene hexachloride (BHC)/cyclodienes; *D. variabilis* to BHC/cyclodienes and

TABLE 109-3 Examples of Ectoparasiticides Approved for Dogs and Cats in the United States.[a]

ORAL PRODUCTS

Product	Source	Insecticide	IGR	Acaracide (Other)	Species Label	Earliest Age; Weight	Label: Flea vs Tick
AcuGuard (VCA Label)	Vethical	Spinosad	No	No	C, D	14 weeks; C: 4.1 lbs D: 5 lbs	F
Advantus soft chew	Elanco	Imidacloprid	No	No	D	10 weeks	F
Bravecto Chews for Dogs	Merck Animal Health	Fluralaner	No	Fluralaner	D	8 weeks; > 4.4 lbs	F&T
Bravecto 1-Month Chews for Dogs	Merck Animal Health	Fluralaner	No	Fluralaner	D	8 weeks; > 4.4 lbs	F&T
Capstar	PetIQ Inc.	Nitenpyram	No	No	C, D	4 weeks; 2 lbs	F
Comfortis chewable tablets	Elanco	Spinosad	No	No	C, D	14 weeks; C: 4.1 lbs D: 5 lbs	F
Credelio chewable tablets	Elanco	Lotilaner	No	Lotilaner	D	8 weeks; 4.4 lbs	F&T
Credelio CAT chewable tablets	Elanco	Lotilaner	No	Lotilaner	C	8 weeks; 2 lbs	F&T
NexGard chewables	Boehringer Ingelheim	Afoxolaner	No	Afoxolaner	D	8 weeks; 4 lbs	F&T
Simparica chewables	Zoetis	Sarolaner	No	Sarolaner	D	6 months; 2.8 lbs	F&T
Simparica Trio chewables	Zoetis	Sarolaner	No	Sarolaner, (moxidectin)	D	8 weeks; 2.8 lbs	F&T

Continued

TABLE 109.3 Examples of Ectoparasiticides Approved for Dogs and Cats in the United States.[a]—cont'd

TOPICAL PRODUCTS							
Product	**Source**	**Insecticide**	**IGR**	**Acaracide (Other)**	**Species Label**	**Earliest Age; Weight**	**Label: Flea vs Tick**
Activyl for Cats & Kittens	Merck Animal Health	Indoxacarb	No	No	C	8 weeks, > 2 lbs	F
Activyl for Dogs & Puppies	Merck Animal Health	Indoxacarb	No	No	D	8 weeks, 4 lbs	F
Activyl Tick Plus for Dogs & Puppies	Merck Animal Health	Indoxacarb; Permethrin	No	Permethrin	D	8 weeks, 4 lbs	F&T
Adams Plus Flea & Tick Spot On for Cats	Farnam	Etofenprox	(s)-methoprene	Etofenprox	C	12 weeks, 5 lbs	F&T
Adams Plus Flea & Tick Prevention Spot On for Dogs	Farnam	Etofenprox	(s)-methoprene, pyriproxyfen	(MGK 264; PBO)	D	12 weeks, 5 lbs	F&T
Advantage II for Cats	Elanco	Imidacloprid	Pyriproxyfen	No	C	8 weeks	F
Advantage II for Dogs	Elanco	Imidacloprid	Pyriproxyfen	No	D	8 weeks	F
Advantage Multi for Cats	Elanco	Imidacloprid	No	(moxidectin)	C	9 weeks; > 2 lbs	F
Advantage Multi for Dogs	Elanco	Imidacloprid	No	(moxidectin)	D	7 weeks; > 3 lbs	F
Advecta Plus Flea Protection for Cats	PetIQ	Imidacloprid	Pyriproxyfen	No	C	8 weeks, 5 lbs	F
Advecta Ultra Flea & Tick Protection for Dogs	PetIQ	Imidacloprid; Permethrin	Pyriproxyfen	Permethrin	D	7 weeks, 4 lbs	F&T
Banfield label (see First Shield)							
Bio Spot Active Care Flea & Tick Spot On for Cats	Farnam	Etofenprox	(s)-methoprene	Etofenprox	C	12 weeks, 5 lbs	F&T
Bio Spot Active Care Flea & Tick Spot On for Dogs	Farnam	Etofenprox	Pyriproxyfen, (s)-methoprene	Etofenprox; (MGK 264; PBO)	D	12 weeks	F&T
Bravecto Plus Topical Solution for Cats	Merck Animal Health	Fluralaner	No	Fluralaner; (moxidectin)	C	6 months, 2.6 lb	F&T
Bravecto Topical Solution for Cats	Merck Animal Health	Fluralaner	No	Fluralaner	C	6 months, 2.6 lb	F&T
Bravecto Topical Solution for Dogs	Merck Animal Health	Fluralaner	No	Fluralaner	D	6 months; 4.4 lbs	
Catego for Cats	Ceva	Fipronil; Dinotefuran	Pryiproxyfen	Fipronil	C	> 8 weeks, > 1.5 lbs	F&T
Cheristin for Cats	Elanco	Spinetoram	No	No	C	8 weeks; 1.8 lbs	F
Certifect	*Merial*	*Fipronil*	*(s)-methoprene*	*Amitraz*	*D*	*8 weeks*	*F&T*
Effipro Plus Topical Solution for Cats	Virbac	Fipronil	Pyriproxyfen	Fipronil	C	8 weeks, 1.5 lbs	F&T
Effipro Plus Topical Solution for Dogs	Virbac	Fipronil	Pyriproxyfen	Fipronil	D	8 weeks, 5 lbs	F&T
Effitix Plus Topical Solution for Dogs	Virbac	Fipronil; Permethrin	Pyriproxyfen	Fipronil; Permethrin	D	8 weeks, 5 lbs	F&T
First Shield for Cats & Kittens (Banfield label)	Schuyler	Dinotefuran	Pyriproxyfen	No	C	8 weeks	F
First Shield for Dogs & Puppies (Banfield label)	Schuyler	Dinotefuran	Pyriproxyfen	No	D	8 weeks	F

TABLE 109.3 Examples of Ectoparasiticides Approved for Dogs and Cats in the United States.[a]—cont'd

TOPICAL PRODUCTS							
Product	**Source**	**Insecticide**	**IGR**	**Acaracide (Other)**	**Species Label**	**Earliest Age; Weight**	**Label: Flea vs Tick**
First Shield Trio (Banfield label)	Schuyler	Dinotefuran	Pyriproxyfen	Permethrin	D	7 weeks	F&T
Frontline Gold for Cats	Boehringer Ingelheim	Fipronil	Pyriproxyfen, (s)-methoprene	Fipronil	C	8 weeks; 3 lbs	F&T
Frontline Gold for Dogs	Boehringer Ingelheim	Fipronil	Pyriproxyfen, (s)-methoprene	Fipronil	D	8 weeks; 5 lbs	F&T
Frontline Plus for Cats	Boehringer Ingelheim	Fipronil	(s)-methoprene	Fipronil	C	8 weeks; > 1.5 lbs	F&T
Frontline Plus for Dogs	Boehringer Ingelheim	Fipronil	(s)-methoprene	Fipronil	D	8 weeks; 5 lbs	F&T
Frontline Shield for Dogs	Boehringer Ingelheim	Fipronil; Permethrin	Pyriproxyfen	Fipronil; Permethrin	D	9 weeks; 5 lbs	F&T
Hartz InControl Advanced Flea & Tick Cat Drops	Hartz	Etofenprox	(s)-methoprene	Etofenprox	C	12 weeks	F&T
Hartz UltraGuard Flea & Tick Powder	Hartz	Tetrachlorvinphos	No	Tetrachlorvinphos	C, D	12 weeks	F&T
Hartz UltraGuard Topical Flea & Tick Prevention for Cats & Kittens	Hartz	Etofenprox	No	Etofenprox	C	12 weeks	F&T
Hartz UltraGuard DualAction Topical Flea & Tick Prevention for Dogs & Puppies	Hartz	Etofenprox	Pyriproxyfen	Etofenprox; (MGK 264; PBO)	D	12 weeks, 5 lbs	F&T
Hartz UltraGuard Plus Topical Flea & Tick Prevention for Cats & Kittens	Hartz	Etofenprox	(s)-methoprene	Etofenprox	C	12 weeks, 5 lbs	F&T
Hartz UltraGuard Plus Topical Flea & Tick Prevention for Dogs & Puppies	Hartz	Etofenprox	Pyriproxyfen; (s)-methoprene	Etofenprox; (MGK264; PBO)	D	12 weeks	F&T
Hartz UltraGuard Pro Topical Flea & Tick Treatment for Cats & Kittens	Hartz	Etofenprox	(s)-methoprene	Etofenprox	C	12 weeks, 5 lbs	F&T
Hartz UltraGuard Pro Topical Flea & Tick Treatment for Dogs & Puppies	Hartz	Etofenprox	Pyriproxyfen	Etofenprox; (PBO)	D	12 weeks, > 5 lbs	F&T
Hartz UltraGuard Pro Triple Action Flea & Tick Drops for Dogs & Puppies	Hartz	Etofenprox	Pyriproxyfen; (s)-methoprene	Etofenprox; (MGK 264; PBO)	D	12 weeks, 5 lbs	F&T
Imoxi Topical Solution for Cats	Vetoquinol	Imidacloprid	No	No; (moxidectin)	C	9 weeks, 2 lbs	F
Imoxi Topical Solution for Dogs	Vetoquinol	Imidacloprid	No	No; (moxidectin)	D	7 weeks, 3 lbs	F
K9 Advantix II	Elanco	Imidacloprid; Permethrin	Pyriproxyfen	Permethrin	D	7 weeks	F&T
Parastar for Dogs	Elanco	Fipronil	No	Fipronil	D	8 weeks	F&T
Parastar Plus for Dogs	Elanco	Fipronil; Cyphenothrin	No	Fipronil; Cyphenothrin	D	12 weeks	F&T

Continued

TABLE 109.3 **Examples of Ectoparasiticides Approved for Dogs and Cats in the United States.[a]—cont'd**

TOPICAL PRODUCTS							
Product	**Source**	**Insecticide**	**IGR**	**Acaracide (Other)**	**Species Label**	**Earliest Age; Weight**	**Label: Flea vs Tick**
PetAction Plus for Cats	PetIQ	Fipronil	(s)-methoprene	Fipronil	C	8 weeks, > 1.5 lbs	F&T
PetAction Plus for Dogs	PetIQ	Fipronil	(s)-methoprene	Fipronil	D	8 weeks, 5 lbs	F&T
PetArmor Flea & Tick Treatment for Cats	PetIQ	Fipronil	No	Fipronil	C	8 weeks, 1.5 lbs	F&T
PetArmor Flea & Tick Treatment for Dogs	PetIQ	Fipronil	No	Fipronil	D	8 weeks, 5 lbs	F&T
PetArmor Max for Dogs	PetIQ	Imidacloprid; Permethrin	Pyriproxyfen	Permethrin	D	7 weeks, 4 lbs	F&T
PetArmor Plus Flea & Tick Protection for Cats	PetIQ	Fipronil	(s)-methoprene	Fipronil	C	8 weeks, > 1.5 lbs	F&T
PetArmor Plus Flea & Tick Protection for Dogs	PetIQ	Fipronil	(s)-methoprene	Fipronil	D	8 weeks, 5 lbs	F&T
Revolution for Cats	Zoetis	Selamectin	No	No	C	8 weeks	F
Revolution for Dogs	Zoetis	Selamectin	No	Selamectin	D	6 weeks	F&T
Revolution for Puppies & Kittens	Zoetis	Selamectin	No	(Selamectin-dogs)	C, D	C: 8 weeks; ≤ 5 lbs D: 6 weeks; ≤ 5 lbs	F (cat) F&T (dog)
Revolution Plus for Cats	Zoetis	Fluralaner; Selamectin	No	Fluralaner	C	8 weeks; 2.8 lbs	F&T
Senergy Topical Parasiticide for Dogs and Cats	Virbac	Selamectin	No	(Selamectin-dogs)	C, D	C: 8 weeks D: 6 weeks	F&T
Sergeant's Evolve Flea & Tick Squeeze-On for Dogs	PetIQ	Etofenprox	Pyriproxyfen	Etofenprox	D	12 weeks, 11 lbs	F&T
Sergeant's Flea & Tick Squeeze-On for Dogs	PetIQ	Permethrin	(s)-methoprene	Permethrin	D	12 weeks, 7 lbs	F&T
Sergeant's Gold Squeeze-On for Cats & Kittens	PetIQ	Etofenprox	Pyriproxyfen	Etofenprox	C	> 12 weeks	F&T
Sergeant's Guardian Topical Prevention for Dogs	PetIQ	Permethrin	No	Permethrin	D	6 months, 7 lbs	F&T
Sergeant's Silver Squeeze-On for Cats & Kittens	PetIQ	Etofenprox	No	Etofenprox	C	> 12 weeks	F&T
SimpleGuard for Cats and Kittens (VCA label)	Vethical	Dinotefuran	Pyriproxyfen	No	C	8 weeks, < 9 lbs	F
SimpleGuard for Cats (VCA label)	Vethical	Dinotefuran	Pyriproxyfen	No	C	≥ 9 lbs	F
SimpleGuard 3 (VCA label)	Vethical	Dinotefuran	Pyriproxyfen	Permethrin	D	7 weeks; > 2.5 lbs	F&T
VCA label (see SimpleGuard)							
Vectra for Cats & Kittens	Ceva	Dinotefuran	Pyriproxyfen	No	C	8 weeks, 2 lbs	F
Vectra for Cats	Ceva	Dinotefuran	Pyriproxyfen	No	C	8 weeks	F
Vectra for Dogs & Puppies	Ceva	Dinotefuran	Pyriproxyfen	No	D	8 weeks; 2.5 lbs	F
Vectra 3D	Ceva	Dinotefuran	Pyriproxyfen	Permethrin	D	7 weeks; 3.3 lbs	F&T

TABLE 109.3 **Examples of Ectoparasiticides Approved for Dogs and Cats in the United States.[a]—cont'd**

COLLARS

Product	Source	Insecticide	IGR	Acaracide (Other)	Species Label	Earliest Age; Weight	Label: Flea vs Tick
Activyl Protector Band for Dogs	Merck Animal Health	Deltamethrin	No	Deltamethrin	D	12 weeks	F&T
Adams Flea & Tick Collar for Dogs & Puppies	Farnam	Deltamethrin	No	Deltamethrin	D	12 weeks	F&T
Adams Flea & Tick Collar Plus for Dogs & Puppies	Farnam	Deltamethrin	Pyriproxyfen	Deltamethrin	D	12 weeks	F&T
Adams Flea & Tick Control Collar for Dogs & Puppies	Farnam	Tetrachlorvinphos	(s)-methoprene	Tetrachlorvinphos	D	12 weeks	F&T
Adams Plus Flea & Tick Collar for Cats	Farnam	Tetrachlorvinphos	(s)-methoprene	Tetrachlorvinphos	C, D	12 weeks	F&T
Bio Spot Active Care Flea & Tick Collar for Cats	Farnam	Tetrachlorvinphos	(s)-methoprene	Tetrachlorvinphos	C	12 weeks	F&T
Bio Spot Active Care Flea & Tick Collar for Dogs and Puppies	Farnam	Tetrachlorvinphos	(s)-methoprene	Tetrachlorvinphos	D	6 weeks	F&T
Hartz InControl Flea & Tick Collar for Dogs and Puppies	Hartz	Deltamethrin	(s)-methoprene	Deltamethrin	D	12 weeks	F&T
Hartz UltraGuard Flea & Tick Collar	Hartz	Tetrachlorvinphos	No	Tetrachlorvinphos	C, D	12 weeks	F&T
Hartz UltraGuard Plus Flea & Tick Collar for Dogs	Hartz	Tetrachlorvinphos	(s)-methoprene	Tetrachlorvinphos	D	12 weeks	F&T
Hartz UltraGuard Pro Flea & Tick Collar	Hartz	Tetrachlorvinphos	(s)-methoprene	Tetrachlorvinphos	C, D	12 weeks	F&T
Hartz UltraGuard ProMax Flea & Tick Collar for Dogs	Hartz	Deltamethrin	(s)-methoprene	Deltamethrin	D	12 weeks	F&T
PetArmor Flea and Tick Collar for Dogs	PetIQ	Deltamethrin	No	Deltamethrin	D	12 weeks	F&T
PetArmor Plus Flea and Tick Collar for Dogs	PetIQ	Deltamethrin	Pyriproxyfen	Deltamethrin	D	12 weeks	F&T
Preventic Tick Collar for Dogs	Virbac	No	No	Amitraz	D	12 weeks	T
Sentry Flea & Tick Collar for Dogs	PetIQ	Deltamethrin	No	Deltamethrin	D	12 weeks	F&T

Continued

TABLE 109.3 **Examples of Ectoparasiticides Approved for Dogs and Cats in the United States.[a]—cont'd**

COLLARS

Product	Source	Insecticide	IGR	Acaracide (Other)	Species Label	Earliest Age; Weight	Label: Flea vs Tick
Sentry Dual Action Flea & Tick Collar for Dogs & Puppies	PetIQ	Deltamethrin	No	Deltamethrin	D	12 weeks	F&T
Seresto for Cats	Elanco	Imidacloprid; Flumethrin	No	Flumethrin	C	10 weeks	F&T
Seresto for Dogs	Elanco	Imidacloprid; Flumethrin	No	Flumethrin	D	7 weeks	F&T

SPRAYS

Product	Source	Insecticide	IGR	Acaracide (Other)	Species Label	Earliest Age; Weight	Label: Flea vs Tick
Adams Flea & Tick Spray	Farnam	Etofenprox	(s)-methoprene	Etofenprox; (PBO)	C, D	C: 12 weeks D: 10 weeks	F&T
Bio Spot Active Care Flea & Tick Spray	Farnam	Etofenprox	(s)-methoprene	Etofenprox; (PBO)	C, D	C: 12 weeks D: 10 weeks	F&T
Frontline Spray Treatment for Cats and Dogs	Boehringer Ingelheim	Fipronil	No	Fipronil	C, D	8 weeks	F&T
Hartz UltraGuard Plus Flea & Tick Spray	Hartz	Tetrachlorvinphos	(s)-methoprene	Tetrachlorvinphos	C, D	12 weeks	F&T
PetArmor FastAct Flea and Tick Spray for Dogs and Cats	PetIQ	Pyrethrins	Pyriproxyfen	Pyrethrins; (MGK264, PBO)	C, D	12 weeks	F&T
Sentry Pro Flea & Tick Spray Dog & Cat	PetIQ	Pyrethrins	Pyriproxyfen	Pyrethrins; (MGK 264; PBO)	C, D	12 weeks	F&T
Sergeant's Gold Flea & Tick Spray	PetIQ	Pyrethrins	Pyriproxyfen	Pyrethrins; (MGK 264; PBO)	C, D	12 weeks	F&T

[a]Product names which appear in italics are no longer being manufactured, though EPA estimates that they will remain available for sale through 2020 or later, and in households for use. Note: The EPA no longer permits the manufacturing of propoxur-containing flea and tick collars in the US. In 2020, the EPA determined that tetrachlorvinphos in powder for use on companion animals or kennels poses unacceptable risks, but remains acceptable for on-pet use according to revised residential exposure and risk assessments in collar and spray formulations.

C, cat; *D*, dog; *F*, flea; *F&T*, flea and tick; *IGR*, insect growth regulator; *T*, tick. MGK 264 (n-octyl bicycloheptene dicarboximide) and PBO (piperonyl butoxide) are pyrethrin/pyrethroid synergists.

DDT; and *Rh. sanguineus* to amitraz, BHC/cyclodienes, and organophosphates has been reported.[96] *Rhipicephalus sanguineus* removed from dogs in Florida and Texas were resistant to permethrin and tolerant to fipronil.[97] *Rhipicephalus sanguineus* from dogs in Yucatan, Mexico were resistant to amitraz and cypermethrin,[98] and ivermectin.[99]

IMMUNITY AND VACCINATION

Both innate and acquired immune defenses are involved in the response of hosts to tick attachment and feeding. Tick feeding induces a complex array of host immune responses involving antigen-presenting cells, T cells, B cells, antibodies, cytokines, complement, basophils, mast cells, eosinophils, and a number of other bioactive molecules.[100] Hosts show varying degrees of susceptibility to ticks. Some hosts can develop resistance to ticks after repeated infestations. Dogs are less likely to acquire resistance to the host-adapted *Rh. sanguineus*[101] but do develop a cutaneous,[102] immediate[92] hypersensitivity reaction induced by the tick's attachment and feeding.

In naïve hosts, local reactions to tick bites are inflammatory with a predominance of neutrophils; in contrast, in sensitized hosts, rapid and more intense reactions occur locally and cutaneous lesions present at a greater distance from the site of attachment with basophils, eosinophils, and neutrophils present in the epidermis and dermis.[93] Cutaneous basophil hypersensitivity, a form of delayed-type hypersensitivity (DTH), plays an important role in immunity to ticks.[93] Acquired resistance to ticks manifests in reduced engorgement weight, increased duration of feeding, decreased numbers of eggs, reduced viability of eggs, inhibition of moulting, and death of engorged ticks.[100]

Ticks counteract innate and acquired host defenses by producing a complex array of pharmacologically active proteins differentially expressed over the course of tick feeding.[100] Distinct differences occur in the composition of secreted proteins for different tick species.[103] Molecules produced in the salivary glands of ticks function for vasodilation, platelet aggregation inhibition, anticoagulation, fibrinolysis, complement inhibition, immunosuppression, immunomodulation, chemokine binding, delayed wound healing, and angiogenesis.[46]

No commercial vaccine exists for use in dogs and cats to prevent ticks from attaching and feeding. A tick vaccine was developed and commercialized in the early 1990s for control of *Rhipicephalus* (*Boophilus*) *microplus* (a one-host tick) on cattle in several Latin American countries and in Australia.[104] The vaccine contained recombinant *Rh.* (*Boophilus*) *microplus* gut antigens and showed efficacy by reducing the number of engorged female ticks, their weight, and reproductive capacity.[104] Despite demonstrated efficacy when combined with strategic acaricide application and integrated tick management, the vaccine experienced a number of difficulties in commercialization.[104] Tick vaccines still offer promise for reducing tick burdens on animals while concurrently reducing dependence on acaricides. Current research efforts in tick vaccine development target the unique physiology of ticks and their dependence on a parasitic lifestyle, modern molecular biology techniques, and bioinformatics.[105]

PREVENTION

Veterinarians and pet owners should not rely solely on the application of approved acaricides to pets to prevent infestation. No compound is 100% effective all of the time. Combining a tick treatment and control plan for pets with other control strategies to formulate an integrated tick management (ITM)[106] program provides the most comprehensive and successful approach to prevent infestation with ticks. The goal of an ITM program is to reduce the risk of tick infestation on pets. This is accomplished by:

1. Maintaining all pets in a household on approved acaricides for the entire year. Thoroughly checking pets each day for ticks and removing any ticks as quickly as possible.
2. Modifying the habitat where pets reside to become less suitable to ticks while off hosts. This includes keeping the yard mowed, removing leaf litter, and trimming bushes and trees that are overgrown to let in more sunlight.
3. Excluding other animals from the backyard where pets spend their time. This includes adding secure fencing and, moving bird feeders, water baths, and woodpiles. Keep pets in managed areas to reduce the risk that they come in contact with ticks.
4. Applying approved environmental acaricides that target off host ticks to the perimeter of a yard where natural wooded areas come in contact with the lawn. Optimal results are obtained using a trained and licensed pesticide applicator.
5. Using targeted acaricide treatment of wildlife species that are key reservoirs of ticks and tick-borne pathogens. Several devices exist that target white-tailed deer[102-104] and small rodents[110] (Tick Control Tubes, Thermacell, MA, USA) to deliver acaricides safely to wildlife and reduce the size of tick populations.

Arguably, the biggest obstacle that veterinarians face when implementing an effective tick prevention program is owner compliance. Analysis of 559 dog owners at 24 veterinary hospitals across the United States demonstrated that the average owner believed their pet needed only 10.5 months of flea and tick prevention despite their veterinarian's recommendation of 12 months.[111] Moreover, only 62% of the 559 dog owners remembered their veterinarian's recommendation of 12 months of flea and tick prevention.[111] Common causes of tick product failure include product not applied at correct frequency, product not applied to all pets in a household, product improperly applied by owner, insufficient dosing rate by owner, unrealistic expectations of owner (no compound is 100% effective all of the time), and overwhelming numbers of ticks in the environment.

PUBLIC HEALTH ASPECTS

As for pets, tick bites in humans are painful and annoying. Humans throughout the world are exposed to ticks[112] and ticks are often found on people in the United States[113] and Canada.[114,115] Most cases of tick infestation on humans are due to ixodid ticks; however, cases of argasid tick bites of humans are also reported.[112,116] Based on specimens submitted to the US National Tick Collection, 44 species of ticks (33 ixodid and 11 argasid) were recovered from infested humans. The predominant tick species on humans was variable and predictable based on geographic location in the United States.[113] All motile stages of *A. americanum* were common in the southern United States and Atlantic coastal states. Adults of *D. variabilis* and all stages of *I. scapularis* were common on people in the eastern and northern United States. In Rocky Mountain and western states, *D. andersoni* was most common whereas in far western states, adult *I. pacificus* were most commonly recovered from humans.[113] Tick paralysis in humans occurs worldwide.[56,117,118] In North America, the majority of human tick paralysis cases are in the Pacific northwest of the United States and adjacent areas of southwestern Canada.[119] However, occurrence is rare.[56] Children 2 to 5 years old are at highest risk.[120]

Humans exposed to natural areas with wildlife present are at increased risk of exposure to ticks and tick-borne diseases.[116] Outdoor activities related to contact with wood (e.g., sitting on logs, gathering wood, sitting against trees, walking, stirring and sitting on leaf litter, just sitting on leaf litter) resulted in greater acquisition of *I. pacificus* nymphs.[121] Coming in contact with wild and domestic animals infested with ticks increases the risk of tick bites to humans.[116] Maintaining pets on year-round tick prevention under the direction of a veterinarian will minimize the potential for animals to bring ticks into the home. Perhaps the biggest impact ticks have on humans globally is as pathogen vectors.[116,122] Ticks are second only to mosquitoes in this respect,[16] and they will continue to play a significant role in emerging zoonotic diseases.[123–125]

CASE EXAMPLE

Signalment

"Amos," a 2-year-old mastiff mix male dog from north-central Oklahoma.

History

The mastiff mix was reported to be roaming for 5 to 7 days and a municipality's Department of Animal Welfare was notified for pick-up. The dog was given the name "Amos" and examined by a veterinarian. After 4 days for stray hold (according to city animal welfare protocol), Amos was presented to a local animal shelter for castration and vaccination. Amos was adopted after 10 days at the shelter. There was no history of known medication.

Physical Examination

Body weight: 31 kg (68 lb).

General: Quiet, alert, responsive. Body condition score 2/9. Euhydrated. T = 101.6°C (38.7°F). P = 100 beats/min, R = 24 breaths/min, mucous membranes pink, CRT <2 s.

Integument, eyes, ears, nose, and throat: Dermatological abnormalities were limited to the sites of ectoparasite attachment. An asymmetric pattern of attached ticks was present over the patient's dorsum and convex surfaces of the pinnae (Fig. 109.7). Nodular swellings underlay each attachment point. The ticks were at various stages of rapid engorgement. Mild small, loose scale was present throughout the coat. Neither alopecia nor hypotrichosis were seen. No adult fleas were observed with flea comb exam. The interdigital webbing was normal. Ocular mucopurulent discharge was noted OU with mild hyperemia of the conjunctiva. There was mild ectropion OU. Corneas were clear. A Schirmer tear test was normal. Otoscopic examination revealed moderate brown, waxy exudate adherent to non-erythematous, non-edematous canal walls AU. Tympanic membranes intact AU. Nasal orifices free of discharge. Oral exam had no abnormalities noted.

Musculoskeletal: Ambulation was assessed by allowing the patient to roam in a small enclosure as Amos was not accustomed to walking on a leash. All joints palpated had normal range of motion with no swelling noted. There was no evidence of pain, and weight bearing was equal on all four limbs. Pain score was assessed to be 1/5.

Cardiovascular, respiratory, gastrointestinal, and genitourinary: No murmurs or arrhythmias were ausculted. All lung fields were clear on auscultation. No cough was elicited on tracheal palpation. Abdominal palpation was unremarkable. A smooth enlarged spleen was noted. Unilateral cryptorchidism was noted with the right testicle retained in the abdomen. Rectal examination was unremarkable.

Lymph nodes: Within normal limits.

Neurologic examination: Patient interacts appropriately with surroundings. No neurologic abnormalities were detected during an abbreviated neurologic examination.

Laboratory Findings

CBC: HCT 39% (36%–60%), MCV 68 fL (58–79 fL), MCHC 35 g/dL (30–38 g/dL), WBC 17,500 cells/μL (4000–15,500 cells/μL), neutrophils 9450 cells/μL (2060–10,600 cells/μL), lymphocytes 4375 cells/μL (690–4500 cells/μL), monocytes 1225 cells/μL (0–840 cells/μL), eosinophils 2450 cells/μL (0–1200 cells/μL), basophils 0 cells/μL (0–150 cells/μL), platelet 244,000 cells/μL (170,000–400,000 cells/μL).

Serum chemistry profile: Albumin 2.8 g/dL (2.7–4.4 g/dL), globulin 4.6 g/dL (1.6–3.6 g/dL), AST 37 IU/L (15–66 IU/L), ALT 71 IU/L (12–118 IU/L), ALP 73 IU/L (5–131 IU/L), GGT 2 IU/L (1–12 IU/L), total bilirubin 0.1 mg/dL (0.1–0.3 mg/dL), BUN 15 mg/dL (6–31 mg/dL), creatinine 0.8 mg/dL (0.5–1.6 mg/dL), phosphorus 4.3 mg/dL (2.5–6.0 mg/dL), glucose 96 mg/dL (70–138 mg/dL), calcium 10.1 mg/dL (8.9–11.4 mg/dL), magnesium 1.7 mEq/L (1.5–2.5 mEq/L), sodium 144 mEq/L (139–154 mEq/L), potassium 4.2 mEq/L (3.6–5.5 mEq/L), chloride 105 mEq/L (102–120 mEq/L), cholesterol 183 mEq/L (92–324 mEq/L), triglyceride 76 mg/dL (29–291 mg/dL), amylase 726 IU/L (290–1125 IU/L), precision PSL 42 U/L (24–140 U/L), CPK 138 IU/L (59–895 IU/L).

Urinalysis: Not performed

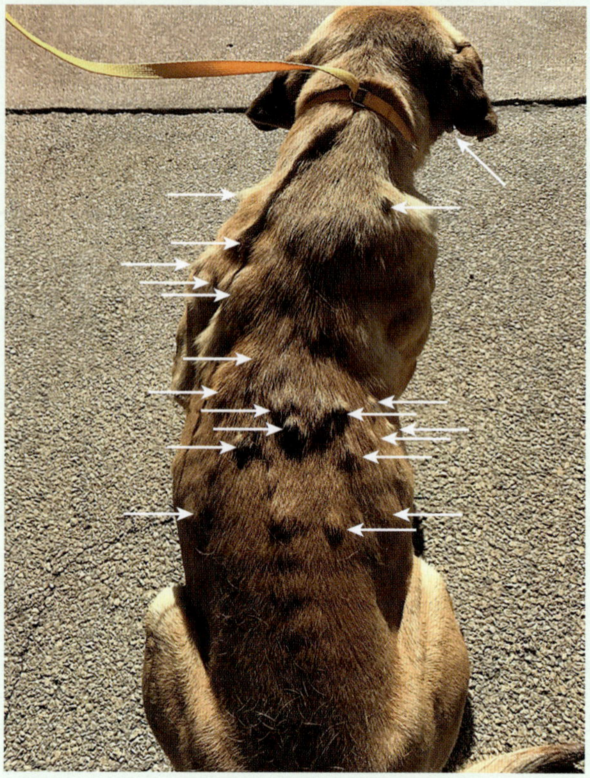

Fig. 109.7 Adult male intact mastiff mix infested with *Amblyomma maculatum* and *Dermacentor variabilis*. Engorged female ticks were first observed as "lumps" in the haircoat *(arrows)*. (Photo and case information courtesy of Dr. Katrina Meinkoth, Oklahoma State University.)

Parasitological Testing

Gross parasites identified as *Amblyomma maculatum* (Gulf Coast ticks) and *Dermacentor variabilis* (American dog ticks).

Fecal flotation (sugar with centrifugation) demonstrated moderate numbers of *Ancylostoma caninum* (hookworm) eggs.

SNAP 4Dx Plus test (IDEXX Laboratories): Negative for *Borreliella burgdorferi* antibodies; negative for antibodies to *Anaplasma* spp.; negative for antibodies to *Ehrlichia canis, E. ewingii*; negative for *Dirofilaria immitis* antigen.

Diagnosis

Infestation with ticks, infection with hookworms; malnutrition.

Treatment

Amos was treated with 8.80% imidacloprid + 44.00% permethrin + 0.44% pyriproxyfen (Advantix II, Bayer) for ticks and 272 μg ivermectin + 227 mg pyrantel pamoate (Heartgard Plus, Boehringer Ingelheim) for hookworms. He was vaccinated for canine distemper, canine adenovirus type 2, canine parainfluenza, canine parvovirus type 2, *Bordetella bronchiseptica*, and rabies. Amos received a balanced, commercially available dry dog food to improve his nutritional status and elevate his body condition score.

CASE EXAMPLE—cont'd

Comments

This was a typical case of a stray dog seen at an animal shelter in the south-central United States. Amos was malnourished and moderately infested with ticks. Upon further examination, he was also found to be infected with hookworms. The moderate eosinophilia and mild monocytosis was consistent with parasitic infestation and infection. The extent of eosinophilia caused by the ticks versus hookworms was not known. The likelihood that a parasite will generate an eosinophilia is proportional to the degree of tissue contact. Prolonged injection of tick saliva, migration of juvenile *A. caninum*, and feeding of adult *A. caninum* in the small intestines would all produce an eosinophilia. It is possible that infection with vector-borne pathogens was too recent for an antibody response to have developed. The presence of fully engorged female *A. maculatum* and *D. variabilis* suggested that infestation had been present for at least 7 to 10 days, which is the average amount of time required for female ticks to attach, breed, engorge fully, and detach. Both *A. maculatum* and *D. variabilis* are capable of transmitting pathogens to dogs (see Table 109.1). Due to the substantial and year-round activity of various tick species in the central United States and the potential for tick-borne pathogen transmission, the necessity of continuous administration of acaricides and control of other parasites was discussed with Amos' new owners.

SUGGESTED READINGS

Blagburn BL, Dryden MW. Biology, treatment, and control of flea and tick infestations. *Vet Clin North Am Small Anim Pract*. 2009;39:1173–1200.

Dantas-Torres F. Biology and ecology of the brown dog tick, *Rhipicephalus sanguineus*. *Parasites & Vectors*. 2010;3:26.

Saleh, MN, Allen KE, Lineberry MW, et al. Ticks infesting dogs and cats in North America: biology, geographic distribution, and pathogen transmission. *Vet Parasitol*. 2021;294:109392.

REFERENCES

1. Huchet JB, Callou C, Lichtenberg R, Dunand F. The dog mummy, the ticks and the louse fly: archaeological report of severe ectoparasitosis in Ancient Egypt. *Int J Paleopathol*. 2013;3:165–175.
2. De La Fuente J. The fossil record and the origin of ticks (Acari: Parasitiformes: Ixodida). *Exp Appl Acarol*. 2003;29:331–344.
3. Guglielmone A, Robbins R, Apanaskevich D, et al. The Argasidae, Ixodidae and Nuttalliellidae (Acari: Ixodida) of the world: a list of valid species names. *Zootaxa*. 2010:1–28.
4. Mans BJ, de Klerk DG, Pienaar R, Latif AA. The host preferences of *Nuttalliella namaqua* (Ixodoidea: Nuttalliellidae): a generalist approach to surviving multiple host-switches. *Exp Appl Acarol*. 2014;62:233–240.
5. Saleh MN, Allen KE, Lineberry MW, et al. Ticks infesting dogs and cats in North America: biology, geographic distribution, and pathogen transmission. *Vet Parasitol*. 2021;294:109392.
6. Bishopp FC, Trembley HL. Distribution and hosts of certain North American ticks. *J Parasitol*. 1945;81:1–54.
7. Blagburn BL, Dryden MW. Biology, treatment, and control of flea and tick infestations. *Vet Clin North Am Small Anim Pract*. 2009;39:1173–1200 (viii).
8. Dryden MW, Payne PA. Biology and control of ticks infesting dogs and cats in North America. *Vet Ther*. 2004;5:139–154.
9. Sonenshine DE, Roe RM. *Biology of Ticks*. 2nd ed. New York: Oxford University Press; 2013.
10. Carr AL, Roe M. Acarine attractants: chemoreception, bioassay, chemistry and control. *Pest Biochem Physiol*. 2016;131:60–79.
11. Bowman DD. *Georgis' Parasitology for Veterinarians*. 11th ed. St. Louis, MO: Elsevier; 2020.
12. Soulsby EJL. *Helminths, Arthropods, & Protozoa of Domesticated Animals*. 6th ed. Baltimore: Baltimore: Williams and Wilkins Co.; 1968.
13. Zajac AM, Conboy GA, Little SE, et al. *Veterinary Clinical Parasitology*. 9th ed. Hoboken, NJ: John Wiley & Sons; 2021.
14. Mullen GR, Durden LA. *Medical and Veterinary Entomology*. 3rd ed. Cambridge, MA: Academic Press; 2019.
15. Anderson JF, Magnarelli LA. Biology of ticks. *Infect Dis Clin North Am*. 2008;22:195–215.
16. Jongejan F, Uilenberg G. The global importance of ticks. *Parasitol*. 2004;129:S3–S14.
17. Raghavan M, Glickman N, Moore G, et al. Prevalence of and risk factors for canine tick infestation in the United States, 2002-2004. *Vector Borne Zoonotic Dis*. 2007;7:65–75.
18. Tinoco-Gracia L, Quiroz-Romero H, Quintero-Martinez MT, et al. Prevalence of *Rhipicephalus sanguineus* ticks on dogs in a region on the Mexico-USA border. *Vet Rec*. 2009;164:59–61.
19. Adolph C. *Prevalence, Disease Implications, and Diagnostic Assays for Parasites and Vector-Borne Infections of Cats in Northeastern Oklahoma*. Stillwater, OK: M.S. Thesis, Oklahoma State University; 2013.
20. Akucewich LH, Philman K, Clark A, et al. Prevalence of ectoparasites in a population of feral cats from north central Florida during the summer. *Vet Parasitol*. 2002;109:129–139.
21. Anderson JF, Magnarelli LA. Vertebrate host relationships and distribution of ixodid ticks (Acari, Ixodidae) in Connecticut, USA. *J Med Entomol*. 1980;17:314–323.
22. Burroughs JE, Thomasson JA, Marsella R, et al. Ticks associated with domestic dogs and cats in Florida, USA. *Exp Appl Acarol*. 2016;69:87–95.
23. Curran KL, Fish D. Increased risk of Lyme-disease for cat owners. *N Engl J Med*. 1989;320:183.
24. Magnarelli LA, Anderson JF, Levine HR, Levy SA. Tick parasitism and antibodies to *Borrelia burgdorferi* in cats. *J Am Vet Med Assoc*. 1990;197:63–66.
25. Thomas JE, Staubus L, Goolsby JL, Reichard MV. Ectoparasites of free-roaming domestic cats in the central United States. *Vet Parasitol*. 2016;228:17–22.
26. Saleh, MN, Sundstrom KD, Duncan KT, et al. Show us your ticks: a survey of ticks infesting dogs and cats across the USA. *Parasit Vectors*. 2019;12:595.
27. Needham GR, Teel PD. Off-host physiological ecology of ixodid ticks. *Annu Rev Entomol*. 1991;36:659–681.
28. Parish HE. Recent studies on life history and habits of the ear tick. *J Econ Entomol*. 1949;42:416–419.
29. Little SE, Hostetler J, Kocan KM. Movement of *Rhipicephalus sanguineus* adults between co-housed dogs during active feeding. *Vet Parasitol*. 2007;150:139–145.
30. Randolph SE. Epidemiological consequences of the ecological physiology of ticks. In: Simpson SJ, Casas J, eds. *Advances in Insect Physiology, Vol 37: Physiology of Human and Animal Disease Vectors*. San Diego: Elsevier Academic Press Inc; 2009:297–329.
31. Eisen RJ, Eisen L, Beard CB. County-scale distribution of *Ixodes scapularis* and *Ixodes pacificus* (Acari: Ixodidae) in the Continental United States. *J Med Entomol*. 2016;53:349–386.
32. Duffy DC, Campbell SR. Ambient air-temperature as a predictor of activity of adult *Ixodes scapularis* (Acari, Ixodidae). *J Med Entomol*. 1994;31:178–180.
33. Dantas-Torres F. Biology and ecology of the brown dog tick, *Rhipicephalus sanguineus*. *Parasite Vectors*. 2010;3:26.
34. Nicholson WL, Paddock CD, Demma L, et al. Rocky Mountain spotted in fever in Arizona: documentation of heavy environmental infestations of *Rhipicephalus sanguineus* at an endemic site. *Ann N Y Acad Sci*. 2006;1078:338–341.
35. Dantas-Torres F. Climate change, biodiversity, ticks and tick-borne diseases: the butterfly effect. *Int J Parasitol Parasites Wildl*. 2015;4:452–461.
36. Sonenshine DE. Range expansion of tick disease vectors in North America: implications for spread of tick-borne disease. *Int J Environ Res Public Health*. 2018;15:478.
37. Monzon JD, Atkinson EG, Henn BM, Benach JL. Population and evolutionary genomics of *Amblyomma americanum*, an expanding arthropod disease vector. *Genome Biol Evol*. 2016;8:1351–1360.

38. Dergousoff SJ, Galloway TD, Lindsay LR, et al. Range expansion of *Dermacentor variabilis* and *Dermacentor andersoni* (Acari: Ixodidae) near their northern distributional limits. *J Med Entomol.* 2013;50:510–520.
39. Duncan KT, Saleh MN, Sundstrom KD, Little SE. *Dermacentor variabilis* is the predominant *Dermacentor* spp. (Acari: Ixodidae) feeding on dogs and cats throughout the United States. *J Med Entomol.* 2021;58:1241–1247.
40. Ogden NH, Lindsay LR, Morshed M, et al. The emergence of Lyme disease in Canada. *Can Med Assoc J.* 2009;180:1221–1224.
41. Rainey T, Occi JL, Robbins RG, Egizi A. Discovery of *Haemaphysalis longicornis* (Ixodida: Ixodidae) parasitizing a sheep in New Jersey, United States. *J Med Entomol.* 2018;55:757–759.
42. Kemp D, Stone B, Binnington K. Tick attachment and feeding: role of the mouthparts, feeding apparatus, salivary gland secretions, and the host response. In: Obenchain FD, Galun R, eds. *Physiology of Ticks.* Elmsford, NY: Pergamon Press Inc.; 2012:119–167.
43. Richter D, Matuschka FR, Spielman A, Mahadevan L. How ticks get under your skin: insertion mechanics of the feeding apparatus of *Ixodes ricinus* ticks. *Proc R Soc B-Biol Sci.* 2013;280:6.
44. Moorhouse DE. Morphogenesis of the attachment cement of some ixodid ticks. In: Daniel M and Rosicky B, eds. *Proceedings of the 3rd International Congress of Acarology.* 1971.
45. Francischetti IMB, Sa-Nunes A, Mans BJ, et al. The role of saliva in tick feeding. *Front Biosci.* 2009;14:2051–2088.
46. Kazimirova M, Stibraniova I. Tick salivary compounds: their role in modulation of host defences and pathogen transmission. *Front Cell Infect Microbiol.* 2013;3:19.
47. Liu XY, Bonnet SI. Hard tick factors implicated in pathogen transmission. *PLoS Negl Trop Dis.* 2014;8:8.
48. Sonenshine DE, Mather TN. *Ecological Dynamics of Tick-Borne Zoonoses.* New York, NY: Oxford University Press; 1994.
49. Allen KE, Johnson EM, Little SE. *Hepatozoon* spp. infections in the United States. *Vet Clin North Am Small Anim Pract.* 2011;41:1221–1238.
50. Commins SP, James HR, Kelly LA, et al. The relevance of tick bites to the production of IgE antibodies to the mammalian oligosaccharide galactose-alpha-1,3-galactose. *J Allergy Clin Immunol.* 2011;127:1286–1293.
51. Steinke JW, Platts-Mills TAE, Commins SP. The alpha-gal story: lessons learned from connecting the dots. *J Allergy Clin Immunol.* 2015;135:589–596.
52. van Nunen S. Tick-induced allergies: mammalian meat allergy, tick anaphylaxis and their significance. *Asia Pac Allergy.* 2015;5:3–16.
53. Holland CT. Asymmetrical focal neurological deficits in dogs and cats with naturally occurring tick paralysis (*Ixodes holocyclus*): 27 cases (1999-2006). *Aust Vet J.* 2008;86:377–384.
54. Otranto D, Dantas-Torres F, Tarallo VD, et al. Apparent tick paralysis by *Rhipicephalus sanguineus* (Acari: Ixodidae) in dogs. *Vet Parasitol.* 2012;188:325–329.
55. Anderson WI, Waters RH. Tick paralysis in a cat. *Mod Vet Pract.* 1985;66:1006.
56. Edlow JA, McGillicuddy DC. Tick paralysis. *Infect Dis Clin North Am.* 2008;22:397–413.
57. Mans J, Gothe R, Neitz AWH. Biochemical perspectives on paralysis and other forms of toxicoses caused by ticks. *Parasitol.* 2004;129: S95–S111.
58. Chand KK, Lee KM, Lavidis NA, et al. Tick holocyclotoxins trigger host paralysis by presynaptic inhibition. *Sci Rep.* 2016;6:29446.
59. Barker D, Barker SC. Survey of cases of tick-paralysis and the presence of the eastern paralysis tick, *Ixodes holocyclus*, and the southern paralysis tick, *Ixodes cornuatus*, in the Greater Melbourne Area. *Aust Vet J.* 2020;98:2–10.
60. Masina S, Broady KW. Tick paralysis: development of a vaccine. *Int J Parasitol.* 1999;29:535–541.
61. Lysyk TJ. Tick paralysis caused by *Dermacentor andersoni* (Acari: Ixodidae) is a heritable trait. *J Med Entomol.* 2010;47:210–214.
62. Cooper BJ, Spence I. Temperature dependent inhibition of evoked acetylcholine release in tick paralysis. *Nature.* 1976;263:693–695.
63. Gothe R, Neitz AWH. Tick paralyses: pathogenesis and etiology. In: Harris KF, ed. *Advances in Disease Vector Research.* New York, NY: Springer New York; 1991:177–204.
64. Herndon A, Little S. Complications of severe tick infestation. *NAVC Clinician's Brief.* 2015:19–21.
65. Koch HG, Sauer JR. Quantity of blood ingested by 4 species of hard ticks (Acari: Ixodidae) fed on domestic dogs. *Ann Entomol Soc Am.* 1984;77:142–146.
66. Miller WH, Griffin CE, Campbell KL, eds. *Muller & Kirk's Small Animal Dermatology.* 7th ed. St. Louis, MO: Elsevier/Mosby; 2013.
67. Roth L. Pathologic changes in otitis externa. *Vet Clin North Am Small Anim Pract.* 1988;18:755–764.
68. Leister E, Morton J, Atwell R, et al. Clinical presentations, treatments and risk factors for mortality in cats with tick paralysis caused by *Ixodes holocyclus*: 2077 cases (2008-2016). *J Feline Med Surg.* 2018;20:465–478.
69. Westwood MN, Emery DL, Dhand NK. Clinical presentation and treatment of tick paralysis in dogs and cats in Sydney (2001-2010). *Aust Vet J.* 2013;91:491–498.
70. Gashaw B, Mersha CK. Pathology of tick bite lesions in naturally infested skin and hides of ruminants: a review. *Acta Parasitologica Globalis.* 2013;4:59–63.
71. Demain JG. Papular urticaria and things that bite in the night. *Curr Allergy Asthma Rep.* 2003;3:291–303.
72. Koch HG. Seasonal incidence and attachment sites of ticks (Acari, Ixodidae) on domestic dogs in southeastern Oklahoma and northwestern Arkansas, USA. *J Med Entomol.* 1982;19:293–298.
73. Mathison BA, Pritt BS. Laboratory identification of arthropod ectoparasites. *Clin Microbiol Rev.* 2014;27:48–67.
74. Keirans JE, Litwak TR. Pictoral key to the adults of hard ticks, family Ixodidae (Ixodida, Ixodoidea), east of the Mississippi River. *J Med Entomol.* 1989;26:435–448.
75. Robbins RG, Keirans JE. *Systematics and Ecology of the Subgenus Ixodiopsis (Acari: Ixodidae: Ixodes).* Lanham, MD: Entomological Society of America; 1992:159.
76. Keirans JE, Durden LA. Illustrated key to nymphs of the tick genus *Amblyomma* (Acari : Ixodidae) found in the United States. *J Med Entomol.* 1998;35:489–495.
77. Durden LA, Keirans JE. *Nymphs of the Genus Ixodes (Acari: Ixodidae) of the United States: Taxonomy, Identification Key, Distribution, Hosts, and Medical/Veterinary Importance.* Lanham, MD: Entomological Society of America; 1996:95.
78. Dubie TR, Grantham R, Coburn L, Noden BH. Pictorial key for identification of immature stages of common ixodid ticks found in pastures in Oklahoma. *Southwest Entomol.* 2017;42:1–14.
79. Clifford CM, Anastos G, Van der Borght-Elbl A. *The Larval Ixodid Ticks of the Eastern United States (Acarina-Ixodidae).* College Park, MD: Entomological Society of America; 1961.
80. Kleinjan JE, Lane RS. Larval keys to the genera of Ixodidae (Acari) and species of Ixodes (Latreille) ticks established in California. *Pan-Pacific Entomol.* 2008;84:121–142.
81. Webb JP Jr, Bennett SG, Challet GL. The larval ticks of the genus *Ixodes* Latreille (Acari: Ixodidae) of California. *Bulletin Soc Vector Ecol.* 1990;15:73–124.
82. Centers for Disease Control and Prevention (CDC). Tick ID. Available at: https://www.cdc.gov/ticks/tickbornediseases/tickID.html.
83. The University of Rhode Island. TickEncounter. Available at: http://www.tickencounter.org/tick_identification.
84. Childs JE, Paddock CD. The ascendancy of *Amblyomma americanum* as a vector of pathogens affecting humans in the United States. *Annu Rev Entomol.* 2003;48:307–337.
85. Paddock CD, Goddard J. The evolving medical and veterinary importance of the Gulf coast tick (Acari: Ixodidae). *J Med Entomol.* 2015;52:230–252.
86. James AM, Freier JE, Keirans JE, et al. Distribution, seasonality, and hosts of the Rocky Mountain wood tick in the United States. *J Med Entomol.* 2006;43:17–24.
87. Padgett KA, Bonilla D, Eremeeva ME, et al. The eco-epidemiology of pacific coast tick fever in California. *PLoS Negl Trop Dis.* 2016;10:17.
88. Egizi AM, Robbins RG, Beati L, et al. A pictorial key to differentiate the recently detected exotic *Haemaphysalis longicornis* Neumann, 1901

(Acari, Ixodidae) from native congeners in North America. *ZooKeys.* 2019;18:117–128.

89. Rich GB. The ear tick, *Otobius megnini* (Duges), (Acarina: Argasidae), and its record in British Columbia. *Can J Comp Med Vet Sci.* 1957;21: 415–418.
90. Atwell RB, Campbell FE, Evans EA. Prospective survey of tick paralysis in dogs. *Aust Vet J.* 2001;79:412–418.
91. Schull DN, Litster AL, Atwell RB. Tick toxicity in cats caused by *Ixodes* species in Australia: a review of published literature. *J Feline Med Surg.* 2007;9:487–493.
92. Szabo MPJ, Aoki VL, Sanches FPS, et al. Antibody and blood leukocyte response in *Rhipicephalus sanguineus* (Latreille, 1806) tick-infested dogs and Guinea pigs. *Vet Parasitol.* 2003;115:49–59.
93. Zachary JF, McGavin MD. *Pathologic Basis of Veterinary Disease.* Elsevier Health Sciences; 2016.
94. Szabo MPJ, Bechara GH. Sequential histopathology at the *Rhipicephalus sanguineus* tick feeding site on dogs and Guinea pigs. *Exp Appl Acarol.* 1999;23:915–928.
95. Food and Agriculture Organization. *Guidelines: Resistance Management and Integrated Parasite Control in Ruminants.* Rome; 2004.
96. Coles TB, Dryden MW. Insecticide/acaricide resistance in fleas and ticks infesting dogs and cats. *Parasit Vectors.* 2014;7:10.
97. Eiden AL, Kaufman PE, Oi FM, et al. Detection of permethrin resistance and fipronil tolerance in *Rhipicephalus sanguineus* (Acari: Ixodidae) in the United States. *J Med Entomol.* 2015;52:429–436.
98. Rodriguez-Vivas RI, Ojeda-Chi MM, Trinidad-Martinez I, Bolio-Gonzalez ME. First report of amitraz and cypermethrin resistance in *Rhipicephalus sanguineus* sensu lato infesting dogs in Mexico. *Med Vet Entomol.* 2017;31:72–77.
99. Rodriguez-Vivas RI, Ojeda-Chi MM, Trinidad-Martinez I, Pérez de León AA. First documentation of ivermectin resistance in *Rhipicephalus sanguineus* sensu lato (Acari: Ixodidae). *Vet Parasitol.* 2017;233:9–13.
100. Brossard M, Wikel SK. In: Bowman AS, Nuttall PA, eds. *Ticks: Biology, Disease and Control.* Cambridge, UK: Cambridge University Press; 2008.
101. Szabo MPJ, Mukai LS, Rosa PCS, Bechara GH. Differences in the acquired resistance of dogs, hamsters, and guineapigs to repeated infestations with adult ticks *Rhipicephalus sanguineus* (Acari: Ixodidae). *Braz J Vet Res Anim Sci.* 1995;32:43–50.
102. Szabo MPJ, Morelli J, Bechara GH. Cutaneous hypersensitivity induced in dogs and Guinea-pigs by extracts of the tick *Rhipicephalus sanguineus* (Acari:Ixodidae). *Exp Appl Acarol.* 1995;19:723–730.
103. Steen NA, Barker SC, Alewood PF. Proteins in the saliva of the Ixodida (ticks): pharmacological features and biological significance. *Toxicon.* 2006;47:1–20.
104. de la Fuente J, Almazan C, Canales M, et al. A ten-year review of commercial vaccine performance for control of tick infestations on cattle. *Anim Health Res Rev.* 2007;8:23–28.
105. de la Fuente J, Kopacek P, Lew-Tabor A, Maritz-Olivier C. Strategies for new and improved vaccines against ticks and tick-borne diseases. *Parasite Immunol.* 2016;38:754–769.
106. Stafford KC. *Tick Management Handbook: An Integrated Guide for Homeowners, Pest Control Operators, and Public Health Officials for the Prevention of Tick-Associated Disease.* New Haven, Conn: Connecticut Agricultural Experiment Station; 2007.
107. Carroll JF, Allen PC, Hill DE, et al. Control of *Ixodes scapularis* and *Amblyomma americanum* through use of the '4-poster' treatment device on deer in Maryland. *Exp Appl Acarol.* 2002;28:289–296.
108. Harmon JR, Hickling GJ, Scott MC, Jones CJ. Evaluation of 4-poster acaricide applicators to manage tick populations associated with disease risk in a Tennessee retirement community. *J Vector Ecol.* 2011;36:404–410.
109. Pound JM, Miller JA, George JE, Lemeilleur CA. The '4-poster' passive topical treatment device to apply acaricide for controlling ticks (Acari : Ixodidae) feeding on white-tailed deer. *J Med Entomol.* 2000;37: 588–594.
110. Deblinger RD, Rimmer DW. Efficacy of permethrin-based acaricide to reduce the abundance of *Ixodes dammini* (Acari, Ixodidae). *J Med Entomol.* 1991;28:708–711.
111. Lavan RP, Tunceli K, Zhang DM, et al. Assessment of dog owner adherence to veterinarians' flea and tick prevention recommendations in the United States using a cross-sectional survey. *Parasite Vectors.* 2017;10:7.
112. Parola P, Raoult D. Ticks and tickborne bacterial diseases in humans: an emerging infectious threat. *Clin Infect Dis.* 2001;33:897–928.
113. Merten HA, Durden LA. A state-by-state survey of ticks recorded from humans in the United States. *J Vector Ecol.* 2000;25:102–113.
114. Lindquist EE, Galloway T, Artsob H, et al. *A Handbook to the Ticks of Canada.* Biological Survey of Canada. 2016:326.
115. Nelder MP, Russell C, Lindsay LR, et al. Population-based passive tick surveillance and detection of expanding foci of blacklegged ticks *Ixodes scapularis* and the Lyme disease agent *Borrelia burgdorferi* in Ontario, Canada. *PLoS One.* 2014;9.
116. Dantas-Torres F, Chomel BB, Otranto D. Ticks and tick-borne diseases: a One Health perspective. *Trends Parasitol.* 2012;28:437–446.
117. Diaz JH. A 60-year meta-analysis of tick paralysis in the United States: a predictable, preventable, and often misdiagnosed poisoning. *J Med Toxicol.* 2010;6:15–21.
118. Felz MW, Swift TR, Hobbs W. Tick paralysis in the United States: a photographic review. *Arch Neurol.* 2000;57:1071–1072.
119. Greenstein P. Tick paralysis. *Med Clin N Am.* 2002;86:441–446.
120. Schmitt N, Bowmer EJ, Gregson JD. Tick paralysis in British Columbia. *Can Med Assoc J.* 1969;100:417–421.
121. Lane RS, Steinlein DB, Mun J. Human behaviors elevating exposure to *Ixodes pacificus* (Acari: Ixodidae) nymphs and their associated bacterial zoonotic agents in a hardwood forest. *J Med Entomol.* 2004;41:239–248.
122. Brites-Neto J, Duarte KMR, Martins TF. Tick-borne infections in human and animal population worldwide. *Vet World.* 2015;8:301–315.
123. Patz JA, Olson SH, Uejio CK, Gibbs HK. Disease emergence from global climate and land use change. *Vet World.* 2008;92:1473–1491.
124. Han BA, Kramer AM, Drake JM. Global patterns of zoonotic disease in mammals. *Trends Parasitol.* 2016;32:565–577.
125. Jones KE, Patel NG, Levy MA, et al. Global trends in emerging infectious diseases. *Nature.* 2008;451.

110

Mites

Susan E. Little, Roberto Cortinas

KEY POINTS

***Cheyletiella* spp. ('Walking Dandruff')**

- First Described: *Cheyletiella parasitovorax* was first described from the fur of rabbits by Megnin in 1878 as the genus "*Cheyletus.*" In 1885, Canestrini erected the genus *Cheyletiella.* Robert Smiley described *Cheyletiella yasguri* as a primary infestation on dogs in 1965, and *Cheyletiella blakei* as a new species from cats in 1970.
- Cause: *Cheyletiella yasguri, Cheyletiella blakei* (family Cheyletidae, order Actinedida).
- Affected Hosts: Dogs *(C. yasguri)*, cats *(C. blakei).*
- Geographic Distribution: Worldwide.
- Primary Mode of Transmission: Direct contact with infested animals or with mites in the environment.
- Major Clinical Signs: Mild to moderate dermatitis, excessive scaling, and alopecia usually along the dorsal aspect of the head, neck, and back. Pruritus may be the primary presenting complaint or, in subclinical carriers of mites, absent.
- Differential Diagnoses: Flea allergy dermatitis, other mite infestations *(Demodex* spp., *Notoedres cati, Otodectes cynotis, Sarcoptes scabiei)*, lice, mosquito allergy, dermatophytosis, bacterial pyoderma, *Malassezia* dermatitis, atopic dermatitis, cutaneous adverse food reactions, autoimmune disease.
- Human Health Significance: Humans, especially those in frequent contact with infested animals through shared households or animal care teams, are very susceptible to infestation with *Cheyletiella* spp. and may develop pruritus and a papular, erythematous dermatitis, particularly on regions of the body in direct contact while holding infested animals, such as the forearms or abdomen.

***Demodex* spp. (Hair Follicle Mites, Red Mange, Demodicosis, Demodectic Mange)**

- First Described: *Demodex canis* was first described by Leydig in 1859. *Demodex cati* was first described by Megnin in 1877 as *Demodex folliculorum* var. *cati*, and then later as *D. cati* by Hirst in 1919. In 1997, Hillier and Desch described *Demodex injai*, and in 1999, *Demodex gatoi* was described from a cat in Louisiana, United States, by Desch and Stewart. Morphologic variants (e.g., "*Demodex cornei*") have occasionally been described but later synonymized with existing species. Skin lesions and otitis externa caused by unnamed *Demodex* spp. have also been reported.
- Cause: *Demodex canis, Demodex injai, Demodex cati, Demodex gatoi, Demodex* sp. (family Demodicidae, suborder Prostigmata, order Trombidiformes).
- Affected Hosts: Dogs (*D. canis, D. injai*); cats (*D. cati, D. gatoi, Demodex* sp.).
- Geographic Distribution: Worldwide, with *D. canis* and *D. cati* reported more commonly and in a wider distribution than the other species.
- Primary Mode of Transmission: Most *Demodex* species are thought to be transferred from dam to offspring early in the neonatal period upon close contact during nursing. Some species (e.g., *D. gatoi*) are contagious and can be transmitted via direct contact among co-housed young or adult animals.
- Major Clinical Signs: Localized demodicosis: focal regions of mild to moderate alopecia and hyperkeratosis, often on the face and usually not pruritic. Generalized demodicosis (juvenile or adult onset): moderate to severe alopecia, erythema, and alopecia with folliculitis and furunculosis; pustules and crusts are often present and secondary pyoderma, which may be pruritic, can lead to sepsis. Lesions develop anywhere on the body, including periorbital, pedal, or associated with otitis externa.
- Differential Diagnoses: Flea allergy dermatitis, other mite infestations (*N. cati, O. cynotis, S. scabiei*), lice, mosquito allergy, dermatophytosis, bacterial pyoderma (often present with demodicosis), *Malassezia* dermatitis, atopic dermatitis, cutaneous adverse food reactions, autoimmune disease.
- Human Health Significance: None known. *Demodex* spp. of dogs and cats are not transmitted to humans.

***Sarcoptes scabiei* (Itch Mite, Scabies, Sarcoptic Mange)**

- First Described: *Sarcoptes scabiei* was first described in 1689 by Bonomo and Cestoni, and is widely considered to be the first known human disease with a confirmed microscopic etiology (Arlian and Morgan, 2017). Mites infesting different hosts are generally regarded as somewhat host-specific varieties of the larger *S. scabiei* species group.
- Cause: *Sarcoptes scabiei* var. *canis* (family Sarcoptidae, order Sarcoptiformes).
- Affected Hosts: Dogs, wild canids, especially coyotes, wolves, and red fox (*Vulpes vulpes*); rarely cats.
- Geographic Distribution: Worldwide.
- Primary Mode of Transmission: Highly contagious through direct contact with infested animals.
- Major Clinical Signs: Intense pruritus, hyperkeratosis, alopecia, self-excoriations. If chronic, weight loss and decreased body condition. Lesions are often most pronounced on the margins of pinnae, lateral elbows, and lateral tarsi. If immunocompromised, profound hyperkeratosis may develop in a condition referred to as "crusted scabies."
- Differential Diagnoses: Flea allergy dermatitis, other mite infestations (*Demodex* spp., *O. cynotis*), lice, mosquito allergy, dermatophytosis, bacterial pyoderma, *Malassezia* dermatitis, atopic dermatitis, cutaneous adverse food reactions, autoimmune disease.
- Human Health Significance: Humans, especially those in frequent contact with infested animals through shared households or animal care teams, are very susceptible to infestation with *S. scabiei* var. *canis* from dogs and may develop pruritus and a papular, erythematous dermatitis, particularly on regions of the body in direct contact while holding infested animals, such as the forearms or abdomen. However, outbreaks of human scabies that occur in

shared housing (e.g., nursing homes, prisons, dormitories) are caused by *Sarcoptes scabiei* var. *hominis* and are of human origin.

Notoedres cati **(Feline Head and Neck Mange)**

- First Described: *Notoedres cati* was first described as a small feline *Sarcoptes* sp. by Hering in 1838, and then as a distinct genus and species by Railliet in 1893.
- Cause: *Notoedres cati* (family Sarcoptidae, order Sarcoptiformes).
- Affected Hosts: Cats, wild felids.
- Geographic Distribution: Worldwide.
- Primary Mode of Transmission: Highly contagious through direct contact with infested animals.
- Major Clinical Signs: Intense pruritus, alopecia, and hyperkeratotic crusts, particularly on the pinnae, head, and feet, often presenting with self-excoriation which can be severe.
- Differential Diagnoses: Flea allergy dermatitis, other mite infestations (*Demodex* spp., *O. cynotis*), lice, mosquito allergy, dermatophytosis, bacterial pyoderma, *Malassezia* dermatitis, atopic dermatitis, cutaneous adverse food reactions, autoimmune disease.
- Human Health Significance: Humans, especially those in frequent contact with infested cats through shared households or animal care teams, are very susceptible to infestation with *N. cati* and may develop pruritus and a papular, erythematous dermatitis, particularly on regions of the body in direct contact while holding infested animals, such as the forearms or abdomen.

Otodectes cynotis **(Ear Mites)**

- First Described: Ear mites were originally described as *Sarcoptes cynotis* by Hering in 1838 and reclassified as *Otodectes cynotis* by Neveu-Lemaire in 1938.
- Cause: *Otodectes cynotis* (family Psoroptidae, order Sarcoptiformes).
- Affected Hosts: Cats, dogs.
- Geographic Distribution: Worldwide.
- Primary Mode of Transmission: Direct contact with infested animals; transfer particularly common during neonatal period.
- Major Clinical Signs: Otitis externa characterized by otic pruritus, excessive dark cerumen, head shaking, and, in some cases, bloody discharge; mites usually confined to ear canal.
- Differential Diagnoses: Other otic mite infestations (*Demodex* spp.), mosquito allergy, dermatophytosis, otitis externa caused by bacteria or *Malassezia*, atopic dermatitis, cutaneous adverse food reactions, autoimmune disease.
- Human Health Significance: Although rare, there are a few isolated anecdotal case reports of human infestation with *O. cynotis*.

INTRODUCTION

The term "mites" refers to a large, diverse group of arthropods in the class Arachnida, subclass Acari, and include free-living, commensal, and parasitic species. Closely related to ticks, parasitic mites can cause considerable disease in infested hosts. Knowledge of their preferred hosts, location, collection strategies, and identifying features can assist in diagnosis and selection of effective treatment and control strategies. Most parasitic mites are difficult to observe without a light microscope. As obligate parasites, most common mites remain on the host for the entirety of their life cycle and are transmitted among animals by direct contact; because of this, large populations can develop on susceptible animals. Chiggers (trombiculid mites) are a notable exception and are acquired as larvae from the environment.

CHEYLETIELLA SPP.

ETIOLOGY AND EPIDEMIOLOGY

Cheyletiella spp. are prostigmatid mites that infest the fur and skin of cats, dogs, and rabbits worldwide. The genus is easily recognizable by its distinct, large palpal claws (Fig. 110.1). Identifying *Cheyletiella* to the species level can be challenging. Individual species are not host-specific but have strong host associations, with *Cheyletiella yasguri* most commonly associated with dogs, *Cheyletiella blakei* with cats, and *Cheyletiella parasitovorax* with rabbits. All three species have been reported in human *Cheyletiella* infestations.[1–3]

The mites are intimate ectoparasites, spending their entire life cycle on the host. They have six developmental stages: egg, prelarva, larva, a first and second nymphal stage, and adult.[4] All motile stages are parasitic. Adult females deposit single, elliptical eggs that range in size 190–260 μm by 110–140 μm.[1,5] Eggs are wrapped in finely woven threads attached to the hair shaft approximately 2–3 mm above the base.[5]

The prelarva and larva develop within the egg. The prelarva is a legless, inactive, nonfeeding stage. The larva hatches from the egg and molts through the first (protonymph) and second (deutonymph) nymphal stages before developing in to adults. Adult *Cheyletiella* spp. are yellowish and large, barely visible to the unaided eye. Adult females measure approximately 500 × 315 μm and males measure approximately 350 × 225 μm.[1,5] All parasitic stages have large palpal claws that lie lateral to the mouthparts (gnathostoma) and feather-like appendages (empodia) at the distal extremities of the legs (tarsi) (see Fig. 110.1). The life cycle varies in duration from 21 to 35 days.[3,6–10]

Cheyletiella spp. mites live in the hair of the host and travel to the epidermis to feed on the keratin layer.[4] The mites do not burrow in the epidermis.[3,9] Instead, they pierce the epidermis with their chelicerae to feed on tissue fluids.[3,5] Regardless of humidity or temperature, immature stages and males die within 48 hours of leaving the host, whereas females may be hardier and can live off the host for 10 days if kept in cool conditions.[5]

Transmission of mites is by direct and indirect contact; mites may also be acquired from the environment. Humans are transiently infested and human-mediated transfer among animals is possible. Infestations are contagious among young animals and can spread quickly in multiple-animal situations, such as kennels and catteries. The introduction of a new cat or dog, even if apparently healthy, is a risk factor for infestation of other animals in the household.[11,12] Transmission is likely on fomites, such as brushes and collars. "Phoresy," whereby *Cheyletiella* spp. mites attach themselves to other arthropods for the purpose of travel, has been suggested, including *C. blakei* and *C. parasitovorax* with fleas, and *C. yasguri* with the dog louse fly, *Hippobosca longipennis*.[13-16]

PATHOGENESIS

The feeding of mites on the keratin layer of the epidermis results in a subacute, nonsuppurative dermatitis with slight hyperkeratosis and vacuolization of epidermal cells. Varying degrees of superficial perivascular dermatitis may be observed with nonspecific inflammatory cell infiltrate.[5,12,17] Occasionally, lymphoplasmacytic dermatitis develops. Eosinophils vary from few to many. Mite segments may be present in hyperkeratotic stratum corneum.[10,12]

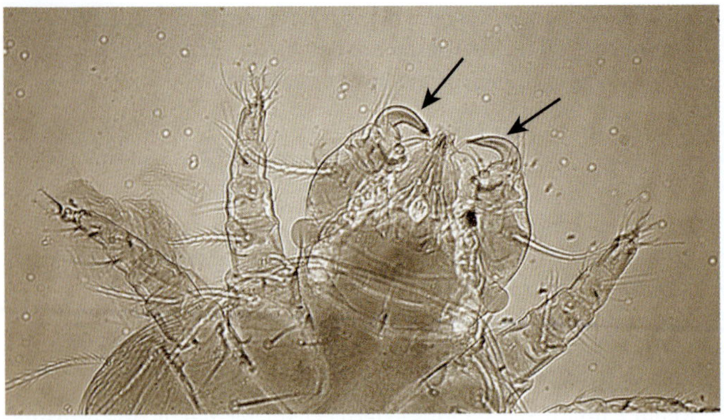

Fig. 110.1 Adult *Cheyletiella* sp., causative agent of "walking dandruff" on dogs, cats, and rabbits, are usually found in superficial hyperkeratotic flakes shed from infested animals. The large palpal claws *(arrows)* confirm the identification. (Courtesy of National Center for Veterinary Parasitology.)

CLINICAL FEATURES

Clinical signs associated with *Cheyletiella* sp. infestation include scaling, crusting, and dermatitis; infestations may not cause clinical signs in some individuals. Skin scaling, characterized by powdery, meal-like scurf or dandruff, is usually observed on the dorsum, particularly in the sacral region.[5,6,18] Scaling may not be obvious in animals that aggressively groom; self-trauma commonly occurs. In severe cases, scaling and mites may be present over most of the body surface. Pruritus can vary from absent to severe.[6,18] The intensity of clinical signs may not be proportionate to the mite density and is thought to be related to a hypersensitivity reaction.[9,12] Infestations on young dogs may be more severe, with older dogs more likely to be subclinical carriers.[3,5]

DIAGNOSIS

Direct Microscopic Examination

Diagnosis of cheyletiellosis is performed by directly visualizing the mites or by microscopic examination of material collected from the infested animal. Evidence of mites moving among debris, often with adherent scales, has given cheyletiellosis the common name of "walking dandruff." Combing is a recommended diagnostic technique but fails to confirm mites in 15% of infested dogs and 58% of cats.[9,19–21] To examine by combing, the haircoat on the back, especially over the sacral area, is parted and a flea comb or brush used to collect scurf; scales and other material are placed on dark paper and examined for movement among the debris. Material can also be transferred to a microscope slide with a few drops of mineral oil, a coverslip applied, and examined microscopically.[19] Other collection methods include using clear tape to examine scurf, superficial skin scrapes, and hair plucks to evaluate for eggs; clipping the hair in long-haired animals may facilitate examination.[22] A modified vacuum technique with in-line filters has been described and was demonstrated to be more efficient than tape preparations, skin scraping, or hair plucking but is not widely available.[9] Fecal flotation may also demonstrate mites and their eggs, particularly in cats that frequently groom.[8]

Regardless of the method employed, finding mites may be difficult.[8,12,21] The number of mites present may be highly variable and low, particularly if the animal is over-grooming or if the area being sampled is small.[8,9,12,21] Combing in combination with other diagnostic tests may yield better results.[9,23] In some cases in which mites are not demonstrated but there is considerable suspicion, empiric treatment may be warranted; in these circumstances, other animals in the household should also be treated.[23]

Comparatively speaking, *Cheyletiella* spp. are one of the larger mites encountered. Adults are yellowish, have a waist-like appearance (more pronounced in females), and very large palps that end with prehensile claws, giving the appearance of an extra pair of legs. An M-shaped peritreme can be observed in the gnathostome, just posterior to the chelicerae. The legs terminate with comb-like appendages (empodia). In addition to the number and arrangement of setae, the shape of the sensory organs (solenidia) on genu I of the legs has been used to identify *Cheyletiella* to species—the organs on *C. yasguri* are heart-shaped, those on *C. blakei* are conical, and *C. parasitovorax* has spherical organs.[4] However, there is much variation in solenidia shape in immature stages, and variation can even sometimes be observed on an individual adult.[4]

Serology

Serologic assays have not been developed to detect *Cheyletiella* spp. antibodies. In one study, protein electrophoresis was used to assess infested dogs, but gammopathy was not demonstrated.[12] Immunologic cross-reactions between *Cheyletiella* spp. and the dust mites *Dermatophagoides farinae* and *Dermatophagoides pteronyssinus* have been documented, a phenomenon also observed with other parasitic mites.[12]

Laboratory Abnormalities

CBCs and chemistry panels from infested animals are generally unremarkable. In one study, mild peripheral eosinophilia was observed in 2 of 23 infested dogs that resolved after treatment.[12]

Gross Pathologic Findings

Scaling, crusting, and dermatitis are commonly seen in animals with cheyletiellosis, although subclinical infestations also occur. Lesions are most evident on the back, particularly over the sacral region. Desquamation results in bran-like exfoliative debris in affected areas. In an uncomplicated case, very little dermatitis or pruritus is observed and alopecia is mild or absent. However, papular, crusting eruptions, scabies-like lesions, alopecia, and severe pruritus can develop due to hypersensitivity reactions.[10,12,24]

TREATMENT AND PROGNOSIS

No products are FDA label-approved for use against *Cheyletiella* mites, but several efficacious off-label treatments have been described. Treatments reported to be effective include transdermal selamectin applied for 3 consecutive months to cats, or every 2 weeks to dogs for four treatments;[8,23] two treatments of transdermal moxidectin (applied in combination with imidacloprid) administered 4 weeks apart also cleared *Cheyletiella* sp. infestations in a group of dogs.[25] Sarolaner was reported to be effective in treating cheyletiellosis in four dogs; other systemic isoxazolines are also expected to be effective.[26] Milbemycin oxime was also effective in treating dogs (2 mg/kg, PO, q7d for 3 to 9 weeks).[12] Although effective when given PO or SC, high-dose, off-label large animal preparations of ivermectin or other macrocyclic lactones are not recommended due to safety concerns; if used, treatment must be continued weekly for as long as 6 to 8 weeks.[19–21]

Topical fipronil has been used with success to treat canine cheyletiellosis using a 0.25% spray, and a 10% (w/v) spot-on was effective for cats.[27,28] Other topical therapies include lime sulfur dips and pyrethroid sprays and shampoos.[22] Amitraz topically at 250 ppm has been used to treat canine cheyletiellosis but is contraindicated in cats and is not considered the treatment of choice for dogs and canine amitraz products are not available in many areas.[19,29] An alternative topical treatment for cats and dogs is 3-weekly baths with 1.0% selenium sulfide shampoo.[22]

Regardless of the treatment used, continuing to treat for a sufficient period of time is of particular importance. The treatment period may be adjusted to address the severity of infestation, number of animals involved, the product being used, housing conditions, and the possibility of environmental contamination.[20] Because the mites are not highly host-specific and some animals remain subclinical, all animals in a household or facility should be treated simultaneously. Reinfestation from off-host females and eggs is considered possible; accordingly, the environment should be cleaned and treated with products that have acaricidal activity. Bedding and grooming tools should be discarded, washed using hot temperatures, or treated with an acaricide. Diagnostic procedures should be repeated to ensure treatment success, but due to the difficulty of isolating mites and the hardiness of eggs to treatment, therapy should continue for at least 2 to 4 weeks after signs have resolved regardless of the results of examination for mites.[19] Hypersensitivity reactions and accompanying pruritus may be alleviated if miticidal treatment is accompanied by a short course of anti-inflammatory glucocorticoid treatment if not contraindicated. Treatment of cheyletiellosis usually has a good prognosis when all animals can be treated and reinfestation prevented.

IMMUNITY

Studies investigating the immune response during cheyletiellosis have not been reported. Observations that young animals appear predisposed to infestation and that infestations can be self-limiting suggests that immunity develops.[1,3] Severe cases are in all probability the result of hypersensitivity reactions.[12]

PREVENTION

Prevention of cheyletiellosis entails that there is no direct or indirect transmission of the mite. When new pets are introduced to a household, they should be checked for mites and treated. Previously used grooming tools and other fomites should be avoided. Routine use of products effective against *Cheyletiella* spp. (e.g., transdermal macrocyclic lactones, oral or transdermal isoxazolines) would also be expected to limit infestations. Anecdotal observations have been made that in warmer areas where year-round flea control is practiced, the prevalence of *Cheyletiella* spp. mites has substantially decreased.[30]

PUBLIC HEALTH ASPECTS

Pet owners, animal care teams, and others who are in frequent contact with infested animals are susceptible to developing dermatitis associated with *Cheyletiella* spp. Approximately 20%–40% of owners of infested animals are affected.[1–4,7–9,18] Small, pruritic, erythematous papules are most frequently observed on areas of the body that are in contact while holding infested animals, such as the arms, abdomen, or legs.[2,3,7] The lesions develop into vesicles or pustules, and eventually demonstrate central necrosis.[3] Arthralgia and peripheral eosinophilia have been reported in some affected individuals.[31] In some cases, the first indication that a pet is infested may be the owners' dermatitis if the pet is apparently healthy. Mites are rarely recovered from people and do not reproduce on humans; treatment of all animals in the household prevents further lesions from developing.[8]

DEMODEX SPP.

ETIOLOGY AND EPIDEMIOLOGY

Demodex spp. are prostigmatid mites that live primarily in the pilosebaceous unit or the stratum corneum of mammals; mites occasionally venture to the surface and can be transferred between hosts of the same species by direct contact. At present, two species infest dogs and three are reported from cats although additional variants have been described.[32] *Demodex* spp. mites have elongated bodies (Fig. 110.2) that consist of a cranial gnathosoma where the mouthparts are located, a podosoma bearing short, stubby legs, and a caudal opisthosoma; an anus is absent. *Demodex canis* and *Demodex cati* are considered normal commensal fauna ubiquitous on dogs and cats, respectively, live in the hair follicles and sebaceous glands, and are transmitted early in

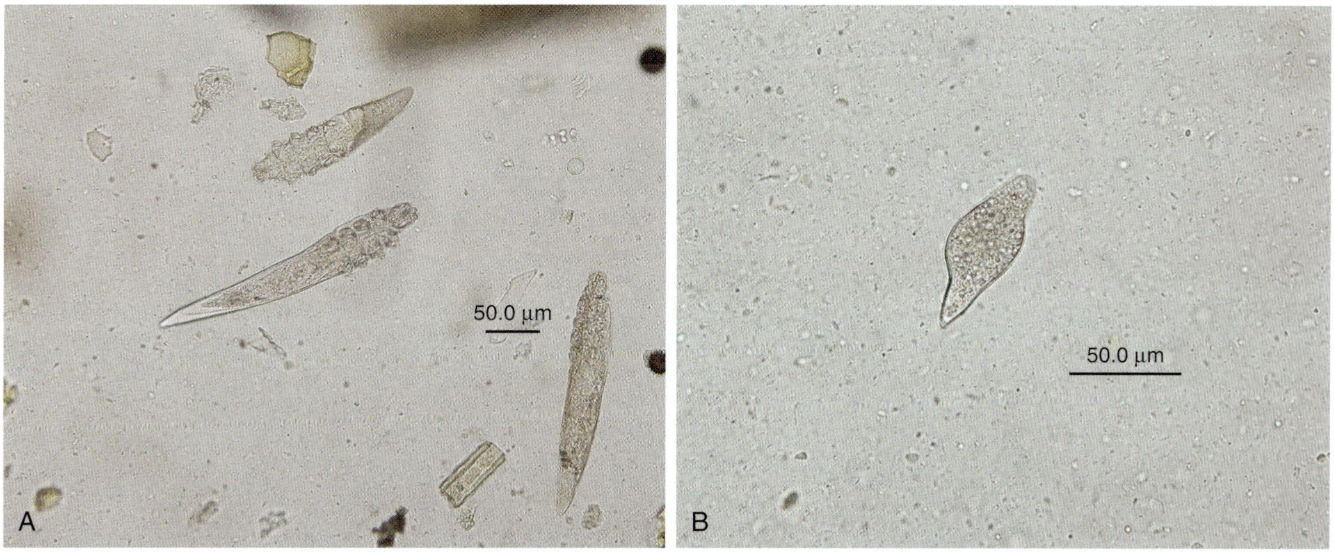

Fig. 110.2 Elongated adults (A) and spindle-shaped egg (B) of *Demodex canis* are readily found on skin scrapes from dogs with generalized demodicosis. (Courtesy of Megan Lineberry, National Center for Veterinary Parasitology.)

life by direct contact from dams to nursing neonates.[33,34] Dogs may also harbor *Demodex injai*, which has a long, thin opisthosoma and is associated with hyperplasia of sebaceous glands and excess sebum production.[32] Cats can be infested with a shorter, unnamed *Demodex* sp., or with *Demodex gatoi*, which is very short and stubby; both primarily infest the stratum corneum.[30]

Demodex spp. females deposit eggs in the infested hair follicles. Larvae hatch from eggs, feed, and molt, developing through two nymphal stages before becoming adults. Comprehensive life history studies on *Demodex* spp. of pets are lacking, but the life cycle is thought to be completed in 14 to 21 days. Females are diploid and males haploid. Infestations with *D. canis* and *D. cati* are considered universal and treatment of contact animals is not required to effectively address cases. In contrast, *D. gatoi* can be transferred between individual cats, and thus this mite should be considered contagious and managed accordingly.[30,32]

PATHOGENESIS

Most *Demodex* spp. mites are commensal organisms, and populations are kept in check by the host immune system; contagious feline *D. gatoi* infestations that spread in multi-cat facilities are the exception.[32] Immune restriction occasionally fails in young, otherwise healthy dogs, and in adult, immunocompromised dogs or cats, allowing mite populations to increase dramatically and leading to clinical disease. In dogs, localized demodicosis and juvenile-onset generalized demodicosis are thought to develop following temporary alterations in CMI; the tendency to develop the condition has a genetic basis.[32] Although the pathogenesis is not fully understood, specific DLA haplotypes have been associated with juvenile-onset generalized demodicosis in some predisposed breeds.[35]

Risk factors associated with juvenile-onset (<1.5 years old) generalized demodicosis in dogs include coccidiosis, hookworm infection, pyoderma, short haircoat, and pit bull-type breed.[36] Although any breed of dog may be affected, including mixed breeds, increased risk of disease has been reported for the American Staffordshire terrier, Staffordshire bull terrier, Chinese shar-pei, French bulldog, English bulldog, pit bull-type dog, boxer, Argentinian mastiff, and Sealyham terrier.[35–37]

Immunocompromising conditions and the use of immunosuppressive therapies are thought to be responsible for adult-onset (>4 years old) canine demodicosis, and for feline demodicosis caused by *D. cati*.[32,33] Conditions associated with adult-onset canine demodicosis include hyperadrenocorticism, hypothyroidism, leishmaniosis, and other vector-borne infections (babesiosis, ehrlichiosis). A history of neoplasia or atopic dermatitis has also been associated with generalized demodicosis but may be related to chemotherapy or glucocorticoid treatment.[32] Wire-haired fox terriers and other terrier breeds are more often reported with disease due to *D. injai* infestation and associated hyperplastic sebaceous glands; affected dogs are older (average age of 8 years) and often have a history of allergy, endocrine disease, neoplasia, or immunosuppression.[38–40]

Predisposing conditions for feline demodicosis caused by *D. cati* include FIV or FeLV infection, hyperadrenocorticism, systemic lupus erythematosus, diabetes mellitus, and xanthoma.[32,33] Localized *D. cati*–associated feline demodicosis has been described with squamous cell carcinoma.[41] Clear breed predispositions have not been identified for feline demodicosis although some consider the condition more common in Siamese and Burmese cats.[30] Infestations with *D. gatoi* can result in pruritis although not all infested cats develop clinical signs.[42] Clusters of feline *D. gatoi* infestations have been reported in multi-cat households involving several breeds and all ages of cats.[42]

CLINICAL FEATURES

Dogs

Dogs with localized demodicosis due to *D. canis* typically exhibit few (1 to 4), small (≤2.5 cm diameter), nonpruritic areas of alopecia and scaling. When localized, the condition is of only minor cosmetic concern. In contrast, dogs with generalized demodicosis can have moderate to severe disseminated skin lesions, deep pyoderma, and systemic illness.[10,32] Juvenile-onset generalized demodicosis develops in dogs less than 1.5 years of age and is considered due to an underlying genetic defect, whereas adult-onset (>4 years of age) is thought to be associated with immunocompromising disease state or administration of immunosuppressive drugs.[43] Mite proliferation in the hair follicles and sebaceous glands leads to large focal or multifocal areas of alopecia, comedone formation, and erythema, with lesions often coalescing over time. Severe pododemodicosis may develop and, when present on at least two feet, is considered indicative of generalized demodicosis even if feet are the only area affected. Follicular hyperpigmentation can be evident. In dogs with mild to moderate demodicosis due to *D. canis* infection but without secondary bacterial infection, pruritus is usually absent. As disease progresses and secondary bacterial or fungal infections establish, associated pruritus may become evident. Over time, deep, pustular pyoderma can develop with draining tracts, lymphadenomegaly, fever, and lethargy; in the absent of treatment, fatality from sepsis can occur.[32] Dogs with demodicosis due to *D. injai* also present with alopecia and an erythematous dermatitis as well as characteristic excessive sebum production dorsally and hyperplastic sebaceous glands.[39]

Cats

Cats with demodicosis due to *D. cati* infection develop localized or generalized areas of alopecia, scale, crusting, and erythema; pruritus is variable and pyoderma is rare.[30] Lesions most commonly appear first on the face and can be associated with otitis externa either as the primary focus of the infestation or as part of a generalized demodicosis.[44] Mite proliferation can also be localized to carcinoma *in situ* lesions. In cats with clinical signs due to *D. gatoi*, pruritus is often the primary owner complaint and other clinical signs (e.g., alopecia) associated with excessive grooming secondary to intense pruritus are often found on the abdomen and thorax. Hypersensitivity appears to develop in some cats infested with *D. gatoi*, while others remain subclinically infected.[32,33,42,44] Due to the contagious nature of *D. gatoi* infestations, many animals in a cattery or multi-cat household may harbor mites or experience clinical disease.[42,45,46]

DIAGNOSIS

Direct Microscopic Examination

Demodex spp. mites are readily recovered from dogs with localized or generalized demodectic mange. Although considered normal fauna, when present together with characteristic pathology and in high enough numbers to readily detect using light microscopic examination of skin scrapings, treatment is indicated. To collect material for microscopic examination, a scalpel blade with a small amount of mineral oil is used to scrape affected areas of skin in the direction of hair growth; application of lateral pressure to a skin fold while scraping increases the recovery of mites. Scrapes should be collected from multiple affected areas, when present. Primary lesions with pustules or alopecia are more likely to have mites than ulcerated areas. Collected material is transferred to microscope slides, coverslips applied, and examined for mites. When infestations are active, eggs may be numerous and all stages of mites (larvae, nymphs, adults) present; mites are often active in fresh mineral oil preparations.[32]

Other methods useful to examine for mites include clear tape preparations from patients with seborrheic dermatitis; direct examination of purulent material expressed from pustules or draining tracts in dogs with deep pyoderma; and trichograms or hair plucks, which may be preferred for collecting specimens from areas of the face and feet that are difficult to scrape. If using trichograms, many (50–100) plucked hairs should be collected, transferred to a microscope slide with mineral oil, and applied to a coverslip to facilitate examination. When lymphadenomegaly is present, mites may be identified in lymph node aspirates. Otic swabs allow identification of *Demodex* sp. mites associated with otitis externa. Mites ingested by dogs that chew affected skin can also be found on fecal flotation; however, this method alone is not considered a sensitive means of diagnosis.[32,34] In general, recovery of *Demodex* sp. mites is more challenging in cats, and especially from cats infested with *D. gatoi*, which is superficial and may elicit hypersensitivity leading to excessive grooming.[44] Cats that are active groomers reduce mite populations on the skin and may only have mites detected in feces.[46]

To allow mites to be easily visualized, the microscope lighting should be adjusted to optimize contrast by closing the condenser. *Demodex* spp. mites are readily identified by their characteristic shape (Fig. 110.2A); measurements that allow identification of different species are provided in Table 110.1. Eggs are spindle-shaped (Fig. 110.2B) and often recovered on fecal flotation or skin scraping at initial diagnosis before treatment is instituted.[34] The number and stage of mites present in skin scrapings can be used to monitor progress during treatment. As lesions resolve, mite populations will be reduced; only a small number of adults may be found, eggs are rare if present at all, and many mites are dead.[10]

Serology

Serologic assays to confirm demodicosis are not available. Common *Demodex* spp. mites (e.g., *D. canis, D. cati*) are considered part of normal flora and infestations universal.

Laboratory Abnormalities

Dogs with generalized demodicosis and deep pyoderma may have anemia of inflammatory disease or an inflammatory leukogram; an elevated concentration of C-reactive protein and haptoglobin, reduced butyrylcholinesterase activity, and reduced paraoxonase-1 activity that normalize with treatment.[47] Cats may have normal hemograms or changes associated with co-morbidities.[33]

TREATMENT AND PROGNOSIS

Dogs

Localized demodicosis usually resolves without treatment within 2 months.[32] If topical treatment is desired, benzoyl peroxide shampoo or gel or rotenone ointment can be used.[32,43] Progression to generalized demodicosis is considered rare and prognosis is excellent. Prescribing transdermal moxidectin and imidacloprid for heartworm, intestinal parasite, and flea control, or an isoxazoline for flea and tick control, would be expected to protect against progression although this approach has not been evaluated experimentally. Dogs with only demodectic otitis externa or pododermatits benefit from acaricidal treatment even though mites and lesions are localized.[32,43]

Dogs with juvenile-onset generalized demodicosis can usually be treated with acaricides and, if indicated, antibiotics for secondary bacterial pyoderma. Underlying conditions are not considered common; further diagnostic testing is not considered necessary and the prognosis for recovery is good.[32] In contrast, adult-onset generalized demodicosis is a more serious condition and successful treatment requires long-term commitment; although most dogs recover with treatment, lifelong therapy may be required in some patients to restrict mite proliferation, particularly if the underlying condition cannot be identified and addressed. Without treatment, fatalities can result, and relapse following treatment is common, particularly when therapy is terminated early.[32]

Successful treatment of adult-onset generalized demodicosis involves a thorough diagnostic evaluation to identify and address any underlying conditions, management of pyoderma when present, and acaricidal treatment of mites. Although recurrence with estrus is considered anecdotal, intact females should be spayed once the skin has healed to allow surgery to both limit recurrence and breeding of susceptible animals. Topical antimicrobial shampoos (e.g., benzoyl peroxide, chlorhexidine) are adequate to manage secondary bacterial infections in most cases; occasionally the severity of pyoderma and risk of sepsis necessitates use of systemic antibiotics. Symptomatic relief may result from acaricidal therapy alone, but recurrence is likely if underlying conditions are not identified and addressed. Continued regular monitoring of the overall health of dogs with adult-onset generalized demodicosis is recommended as underlying conditions not evident at initial presentation may become apparent over time.[10,32,43]

Widely available miticidal treatments include systemic isoxazolines and macrocyclic lactones; all are off-label in the United States. Systemic isoxazolines (afoxolaner, fluralaner, lotilaner, sarolaner) approved in dogs for flea and tick control are effective against generalized demodicosis when administered according to label directions,

TABLE 110.1 Morphology and Preferred Location of *Demodex* spp. Mites from Dogs and Cats

Species	Host	Length (µm)	Approximate Ratio Opisthosoma: Total Length (%)	Description	Preferred Location
Demodex canis	D	150–250	50–60	Long tail	Hair follicles and sebaceous glands
Demodex injai	D	270–390	60–70	Long, thin, sharply tapered tail	Hair follicles and sebaceous glands
Demodex cati	C	180–220	60–70	Long, slender, 5:1 length-to-width ratio of opisthosoma	Hair follicles and sebaceous glands
Demodex gatoi	C	90–110	40–50	Stubby, 2:1 length-to-width ratio of opisthosoma	Stratum corneum
Demodex sp.	C	140–175	50–60	Shorter, rounder than *D. cati*, 2:1 length-to-width ratio of opisthosoma	Stratum corneum

C, cat; *D*, dog.

every 4 to 12 weeks depending on product used.[32,48–57] Most (afoxolaner, fluralaner, lotilaner) are available for use in dogs > 8 weeks of age and all should be used with caution in dogs with a history of seizures. Transdermal moxidectin/imidacloprid administered weekly is effective against demodicosis and labeled for this purpose in Europe; use of weekly transdermal moxidectin/imidacloprid is recommended only for mild to moderate cases.[32,58,59] Milbemycin oxime (1 to 2 mg/kg/day PO) is also safe and effective although cost of daily use may be prohibitive.[56,60] Reports evaluating efficacy of milbemycin oxime/afoxolaner combination products are not yet available.[32] Response to treatment should be monitored with monthly skin scrapes and miticidal therapy continued for at least 8 weeks past first negative skin scrape.[32]

Historically, large animal formulations of macrocyclic lactones or amitraz rinses were used to treat generalized demodicosis. Daily, high-dose, off-label use of large animal formulations of ivermectin (0.3 to 0.6 mg/kg/day PO) or moxidectin (0.2 to 0.5 mg/kg/day), or weekly administration of doramectin (0.6 mg/kg/week PO or SC) is effective. However, neurologic toxicity may occur and these approaches are no longer necessary or recommended as the first-choice therapy.[56] Amitraz is a well-established treatment for generalized demodicosis and FDA label-approved for use at 0.025% concentration every 2 weeks; efficacy improves when amitraz is used off-label weekly and at higher concentrations (0.05%) although toxicity risk also increases.[32,59] Long-haired animals should be clipped prior to applying the dip. Sale of the approved canine formulation of amitraz (Mitaban, Zoetis, USA) was discontinued in the United States in 2018.

Although management is involved and the treatment course may be long and expensive, most dogs with generalized demodicosis can recover and euthanasia is no longer a common consideration. The prognosis for recovery from generalized demodicosis is better in young dogs (<1.5 years) than in older dogs. Spontaneous resolution from generalized demodicosis has been reported in younger dogs although the incidence is unknown and likely varies with breed and underlying condition.[32,43,59] Spontaneous resolution is not thought to occur in older dogs; without treatment, the condition can be fatal.

Cats

Demodicosis in cats may be treated with topical dips, systemic macrocyclic lactones, or systemic isoxazolines. Weekly lime sulfur dips (2%) have long been a mainstay of feline demodicosis treatment; weekly amitraz rinses (0.0125%) have also been used.[32] However, feline patients often do not tolerate both approaches well, and when several individual cats in a multi-cat household are affected, application of topical, body-wide rinses weekly can be challenging. Weekly administration of transdermal moxidectin/imidacloprid is also effective and more easily achieved.[32,60] Fluralaner and sarolaner are also effective for treatment of feline demodicosis[61–63]; other isoxazolines approved for cats (i.e., lotilaner) may also be effective. Combination macrocyclic lactone/isoxazoline products (e.g., moxidectin/fluralaner, selamectin/sarolaner) are available for cats; inclusion of both drug classes in treatment likely supports efficacy.

IMMUNITY

An underlying immune deficit is considered responsible for development of localized and generalized demodicosis; addressing stress caused by poor nutrition or presence of other infections improves patient health and supports treatment of demodicosis. A comparison of pit bull terrier-type dogs with juvenile-onset generalized demodicosis with healthy age- and breed-matched controls revealed significantly higher serum concentrations of IL-2, IL-18, and monocyte chemoattractant protein-1 in dogs with generalized demodicosis, a finding interpreted to reflect an appropriate immune response.[64]

The beneficial effects of immunostimulants in demodicosis treatment are not clear, and most studies evaluating potential adjunctive therapies are small.[32] Inactivated *Parapoxvirus ovis* administered subcutaneously together with amitraz dips decreased time to remission (85 days) when compared with amitraz dips alone (104 days).[65] Insufficient evidence is available to support use of vitamin E, muramyl dipeptide, or herbal and homeopathic products in treatment of demodicosis.[43]

PREVENTION

Judicious breeding can limit the number of litters that develop demodicosis.[10] The American Academy of Veterinary Dermatology and the consensus guidelines from the World Association for Veterinary Dermatology have consistently recommended neutering all dogs with generalized demodicosis and state that both dogs with demodicosis and their parents should not be used for breeding.[32] Although more research is needed, administering fluralaner 10 days before breeding reduced the number of puppies that developed disease.[66] Monthly administration of moxidectin/imidacloprid may prevent relapse in dogs with generalized demodectic mange.[67] Administering isoxazolines reduces but does not eliminate populations of *Demodex* sp. mites from treated dogs.[68] Routine administration of isoxazolines would also be expected to support remission for dogs with generalized demodicosis. Quarantine and prophylactic treatment of newly acquired cats should limit introduction of *D. gatoi* into a facility.

Underlying conditions should be identified and addressed whenever possible. Improving nutrition, identifying and eliminating intestinal parasites, and reducing environmental stress in stray or rescued dogs supports recovery. Co-morbidities and other inciting causes are not always identified, but one review of 41 cases of adult-onset demodicosis identified exogenous glucocorticoid use in allergy patients (24%), hyperadrenocorticism (19%), chemotherapy (15%), and hypothyroidism (12%) as common potential underlying problems.[69] Relapse after treatment occurs in 10% to 45% of canine patients due to stress (including during estrus, pregnancy, or lactation), as well as when systemic diseases are not well controlled.[10,43] Avoiding immunosuppressive drugs (e.g., glucocorticoids, oclacitinib maleate, cyclosporine) in patients with a history of generalized demodicosis is also recommended to reduce incidence of relapse.[43]

PUBLIC HEALTH ASPECTS

Canine and feline demodicosis are not zoonotic. Humans develop disease due to overgrowth of *Demodex* spp. mites that only infest humans (*Demodex folliculorum* and *Demodex brevis*) and that are normal commensals of hair follicles and sebaceous glands. Lesions most commonly appear on the face and include acne, rosacea, pityriasis folliculorum, and blepharitis. A meta-analysis found that prevalence and density of *Demodex* spp. mites were significantly higher in patients with rosacea than in controls.[70,71]

SARCOPTES SCABIEI VAR. *CANIS*

ETIOLOGY AND EPIDEMIOLOGY

Sarcoptes scabiei var. *canis* is a burrowing mite in the order Sarcoptiformes, family Sarcoptidae. Sarcoptid mites have a distinctly rounded morphology with short legs that scarcely project beyond the body margin. The anterior pretarsi of *S. scabiei* consist of long, unsegmented pedicels, also referred to as stalks, that terminate in caruncles (suckers); females have these structures on the first and second pairs of legs, and males have them on the first, second, and fourth pair of legs.[34] The dorsum has numerous transverse ridges and triangular scales or spines and the anus is located at the posterior edge of the body. The *S. scabiei* species complex is found worldwide and has been reported from more than 100 species of mammals.[72,73] However, infestations are generally regarded as caused by host-adapted strains or "varieties" of the same core species, with host varieties spread more readily among species to which each has adapted. *Sarcoptes scabiei* var. *canis* is the strain reported from domestic dogs and wild canids. Although *S. scabiei* var. *canis* will transfer to and cause dermatitis on other hosts, including humans, these infestations are generally considered self-limiting.[22,72] Sarcoptic mange is rare in cats but occasionally reported.[22,74] Mites from cats suspected to be *S. scabiei* may be *Notoedres cati* (see below) and should be submitted to a parasitologist with appropriate diagnostic expertise for accurate diagnosis.

Sarcoptic mange has been described from domestic dogs and wild canids worldwide. Sex and breed predilections have not been reported, but younger dogs are overrepresented in case series.[75,76] Mites are found in 1% or fewer of dogs in surveys and are not recovered from many infested, clinically affected dogs even when pruritus is severe.[77–79] Accordingly, the true prevalence of *S. scabiei* var. *canis* is not known. In areas where infestations are common in dogs, antibodies may be present in a majority of animals tested. One survey in Nigeria found antibodies to *S. scabiei* in 67% of dogs.[78] A survey that utilized a remote camera in Texas, United States, found lesions consistent with sarcoptic mange in 72% of coyotes.[73] Sarcoptic mange is considered a major mortality factor for red fox in the southeastern United States, and mites are more readily recovered from wild canids or domestic dogs with crusted scabies.[10,80]

After mating, fertilized female mites burrow into the stratum corneum, creating horizontal tunnels. The mites feed on fluids leaking from damaged tissues. While in tunnels, females oviposit 2 to 3 eggs per day over a lifespan of 2 months. The eggs hatch in 3 to 5 days. The larvae then crawl out onto the skin surface and make shallow superficial burrows termed "molting pockets" wherein they feed and molt. After 2 to 3 days, larvae molt to the nymphal stage and after 3 to 4 days, nymphs undergo two subsequent molts to the adult stage. Males make their way to the skin surface where they seek immature females. Mating may take place on the skin surface or in molting pockets depending on the location of the immature female. Immature and adult mites are transmitted by direct contact to other hosts and *S. scabiei* is considered highly contagious; all dogs with known contact with an infested dog should be treated. Infestation following indirect contact via fomites (e.g., clippers, bedding) has also been reported although off-host survival is limited. The entire life cycle usually takes 17 to 21 days to complete, but generation times as short as 10 days have been described.[22]

PATHOGENESIS

The burrowing activity of the fertilized female and its destructive feeding behavior, as well as the deposition of eggs, molted cuticles, and mite feces within the upper layers of the epidermis, lead to varying levels of dermatitis characterized by intense pruritus, alopecia, and hyperkeratotic lesions. Pruritus is observed early after infestation and may be evident as early as 1 week prior to development of lesions. A hypersensitivity reaction to mite antigens, including mite feces, contributes to the pruritus. Mites also release immunomodulating substances that shift immune responses, including upregulation of IL-20 which may promote hyperkeratosis.[72,81] Initial lesions consist of erythematous maculopapular eruptions with alopecia and often first appear in areas where hair is sparse. Predilection sites include the ears, particularly the margins of the pinnae, periocular region, face, lateral elbows, and lateral hocks. As infestation spreads, the ventral thorax and ventral abdomen may be affected and lesions can eventually cover the majority of the body. Extensive alopecia and generalized lymphadenomegaly may be evident.[3,76] When untreated, fatalities can result.

Biopsy of affected areas reveals acanthosis, spongiosis, hyperkeratosis, and prominent rete ridge formation; intracorneal pustules may be present.[82] Biopsy lesions contain mixed cellular infiltrates comprising mononuclear cells, neutrophils, plasma cells, and mast cells.[83] Direct evidence of infestation (e.g., mites, eggs, mite feces) confirms infestation but may not be consistently evident. In chronic infestations, lichenification and hyperpigmentation may be apparent and associated with self-excoriation. Secondary bacterial infections are common and may be promoted by mite-mediated inhibition of host complement.[84,85] In some individuals, crusted scabies develops with profound hyperkeratosis and an enormous number of mites present. In humans, patients with crusted scabies develop a more pronounced IgE response than patients with routine scabies.[86]

CLINICAL FEATURES

Intense pruritus is the most common clinical sign reported in dogs with sarcoptic mange. In some case series, pruritus is reported in only 56% to 74% of cases although severe hypersensitivity reactions responsible for pruritus may limit mite populations, precluding confirmation of infestation and inclusion in case series reports.[76,87] Other common signs include alopecia (43%), crusts (41%–78%), lesions on the pinnae (41%), and scaling (24%–44%).[76,87] In one study evaluating treatment of naturally infested dogs, pruritus, alopecia, and crusts or scales were reported in virtually all cases.[88] Lesions may occur anywhere but are most pronounced on the margins of the pinnae, lateral elbows, and lateral tarsi.[3,10] However, sarcoptic mange should be considered in any dog with a history of pruritus. Young or immunocompromised animals may develop "crusted scabies" characterized by marked, profound hyperkeratosis associated with extremely large numbers of mites; patients with crusted scabies are usually not pruritic. This condition is common in red fox in the southeastern United States and has been reported in young, malnourished dogs, dogs co-infected with *Leishmania* sp., and, rarely, in cats.[80,89,90]

DIAGNOSIS

Direct Microscopic Examination

Although mites are not recovered from approximately 50% of canine patients, sarcoptic mange can be confirmed directly by identifying *S. scabiei* mites using microscopic examination of multiple skin scrapes from the margin of affected areas. To perform skin scrapes, a small amount of mineral oil is applied to a scalpel blade used to gently abrade affected areas; the scurf thus collected is transferred to a microscope slide, a coverslip applied, and the material examined for characteristic mites. Females are 300–400 μm long and males are ~250 μm long. Pretarsi on the first two pairs of legs have long, unsegmented pedicels each bearing a caruncle; males also have these structures on the fourth pair of legs. Numerous transverse ridges and triangular scales are present on the dorsum and the anus is located at the posterior edge of the body (Fig. 110.3). Because skin scraping is relatively insensitive for confirming a diagnosis of sarcoptic mange, multiple areas should be examined and failure to detect mites should not be used to eliminate *S. scabiei* var. *canis* as a potential etiology.[10,22]

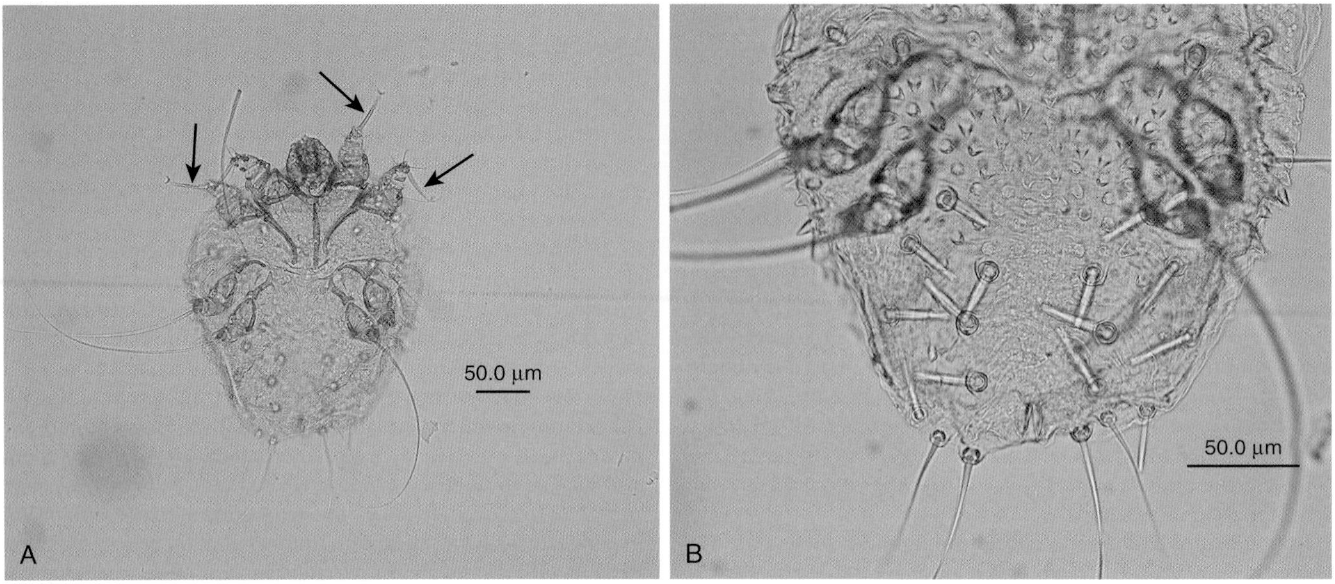

Fig. 110.3 Adult *Sarcoptes scabiei* var. *canis* showing unjointed pedicles bearing suckers *(arrows)* on first and second pairs of legs (A). Magnified view of dorsum with characteristic spines (B). Mites of *S. scabiei* var. *canis* are often present in low numbers making them difficult to find on some infested dogs, even when pruritus is intense. (Courtesy of Megan Lineberry, National Center for Veterinary Parasitology.)

Serology

Although not widely available, ELISAs have been developed to support the diagnosis of *S. scabiei* in dogs. In field evaluations using microscopic detection of mites as the comparator, ELISA has had 84%–96% sensitivity and 90% specificity.[78,91] Antibodies are not detected until 4 weeks after infestation. Specificity can be compromised by cross-reactivity with antibodies to common dust mites (*Dermatophagoides* spp.) and false positives have been reported in dogs with documented atopy associated with dust mites.[92,93] Values on serum chemistry profiles are usually unchanged.[94]

Laboratory Abnormalities

Blood values in dogs with sarcoptic mange are largely unremarkable. Hemoglobin and hematocrit concentrations decrease with infestation, and neutrophil counts increase, but in the absence of sepsis secondary to pyoderma, all remain within normal limits. Eosinophilia is reported in some individual dogs but is not consistently evident.[94]

Gross Pathologic Findings

Dogs with sarcoptic mange develop erythematous, follicular, papular dermatitis that is initially focal but spreads to become multifocal and then generalized. Alopecia, hyperkeratosis, and self-excoriations are common, and abundant crusts are often noted. In the absence of treatment, secondary pyoderma commonly develops. Mites are not easily recovered particularly early in the course of disease; a high index of suspicion and response to treatment can support a clinical diagnosis.[10,22]

TREATMENT AND PROGNOSIS

Transdermal moxidectin and selamectin are FDA label-approved for treatment of sarcoptic mange in dogs. In some countries, amitraz dips or oral milbemycin oxime may also be approved.[95] Isoxazolines (e.g., afoxolaner, fluralaner, lotilaner, sarolaner) have been shown to be effective; multiple doses may be necessary depending on the product used.[87,88,95–97] Fipronil is label-approved to aid in the control of sarcoptic mange and may help limit infestations but is not recommended as a stand-alone treatment. Older therapies, including high-dose, off-label macrocyclic lactones intended for use in large animals or phosmet dips are no longer recommended due to safety concerns and the wide availability of safer, label-approved choices. Most dogs with sarcoptic mange respond well to treatment. Pruritus is relieved within a few days of instituting effective acaricidal therapy, and lesions resolve so long as treatment course is completed and immunocompromise, malnutrition, or other co-morbidities can be addressed.

IMMUNITY

Both field and experimental data indicate that dogs develop immunity to *S. scabiei* var. *canis*. The preponderance of young dogs in case series of clinical sarcoptic mange has been interpreted as older dogs becoming less susceptible to infestation, presumably due to prior exposure.[76] In experimental infestation trials, seven of eight dogs developed immunity to *S. scabiei* var. *canis*; although reinfested, immune dogs self-cleared mites within 1 to 2 months of reinfestation and some dogs eliminated reinfestation in 3 to 4 weeks.[83] Biopsy specimens from immune dogs documented that monocytes and neutrophils predominated in challenge infestations and appeared more rapidly in sensitized dogs than in naïve dogs undergoing a primary infestation; immune dogs also had a more rapid antibody response that decreased as mite populations decreased.[83]

PREVENTION

Vaccines for *S. scabiei* are not available. Prevention requires avoiding direct contact with dogs or wild canids that are likely to harbor mites, limiting roaming, and routine use of control products effective against *S. scabiei*.[10] Dogs diagnosed with sarcoptic mange should be confined and all shared animal facilities (e.g., dog parks, groomers, boarding kennels, dog day care) avoided until treatment is completed and lesions are fully resolved. All dogs in the same household or that have had direct contact with an infested dog should be presumed infested and treated simultaneously, including dogs that are not showing evidence of clinical disease; subclinical carriers of mites contribute to perpetuating infestations.[98] Routine use of products effective against *S. scabiei* (e.g., transdermal macrocyclic lactones, oral or transdermal isoxazolines) would also be expected to limit infestations.

PUBLIC HEALTH ASPECTS

Sarcoptes scabiei var. *hominis* is a human parasite that affects approximately 200 to 300 million people worldwide each year and infests as many as 10% of children in developing countries.[99] Scabies is recognized as a neglected tropical disease by the WHO, and cases appear to be increasing in developed countries.[100,101] Patients with primary scabies due to *S. scabiei* var. *hominis*, the variety responsible for direct human-to-human transmission, develop an erythematous, papular rash characterized by intense pruritus; serpiginous burrows where mites have tunneled are often apparent. Lesions associated with *S. scabiei* var. *hominis* most commonly appear in the interdigital region, wrists, elbows, knees, abdomen, and groin, and mites are transmitted between humans by prolonged, intimate contact. Institutional outbreaks are frequently reported in nursing homes, dormitories, and prisons; transmission among family members is also common but *S. scabiei* var. *hominis* is not known to infest pets.[98,101] People are most often treated with topical permethrin or oral ivermectin.[99]

While zoonotic, cases of *S. scabiei* var. *canis* infestation are only a concern in individuals that have direct contact with infested dogs or wild canids. The rash usually develops within 1 to 4 days after contact with an infested dog. Mites are rarely present and history is key to reaching a diagnosis.[102] Although intensely pruritic, once acquired by a person, *S. scabiei* var. *canis* mites do not transfer to other humans. Preventing dermatitis associated with zoonotic infestations requires use of appropriate preventives in dogs to avoid development of infestations, prompt diagnosis and treatment of infested dogs, and careful handling of dogs with skin conditions consistent with mange or known to harbor mites.[98] Dogs or red fox with crusted scabies harbor a huge number of mites and thus present an elevated zoonotic risk. Zoonotic infestations may be managed symptomatically with topical hydrocortisone creams or, if severe, treated systemically.[3,98]

NOTOEDRES CATI

ETIOLOGY AND EPIDEMIOLOGY

Notoedres cati is a burrowing sarcoptid mite (order Sarcoptiformes, family Sarcoptidae) of domestic cats and wild felids. Infestations with *N. cati* have been reported in at least 18 different host species, including rabbits, and, rarely, dogs.[103,104] The parasite is most commonly described from domestic cats and bobcats (*Lynx rufus*). Although the rounded appearance and pretarsi (long, unjointed pedicels ending in caruncles) are morphologically similar to *S. scabiei*, *N. cati* is smaller (150–225 μm) than *S. scabiei*, lacks dorsal spines, and the anus is dorsal rather than terminal (Fig. 110.4).[34] Other species of *Notoedres* infest rodents, procyonids, and bats.[103]

The life cycle of *N. cati* is similar to that of *S. scabiei*, with larvae, nymphs, and adults burrowing in the host skin, and requires approximately 2 weeks. Females deposit eggs in burrows in the skin of the face, ears, and, occasionally, legs of the host. Mites are transferred between cats by direct contact. Cats infested with *N. cati* are reported worldwide albeit less commonly than dogs with *S. scabiei* var. *canis*. In North America, reports are more common in the southern United States and Mexico.[30,103]

A survey of feline parasites in pet cats from several countries in Europe identified *N. cati* in only 3 of 1,519 cats but infestations are

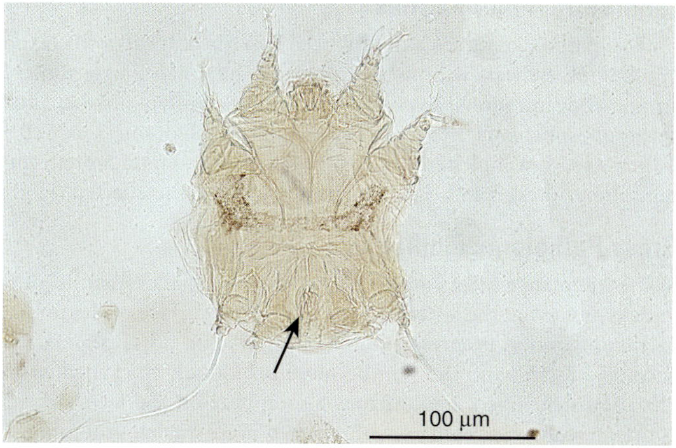

Fig. 110.4 Adult *Notoedres cati* showing dorsal anus *(arrow)* that distinguishes it from *Sarcoptes scabiei.* (Courtesy of National Center for Veterinary Parasitology.)

considered more common in some countries, including Greece (where prevalence in stray cats in a survey was 2.4%) and Brazil.[105–107] Local epizootics have also been reported and long-haired cats are predisposed.[105,108] Infestations with *N. cati* are highly contagious and may be seen as entire litters affected, in multi-cat facilities, and in free-ranging felid populations.[10,108–110]

PATHOGENESIS

Similar to *S. scabiei*, *N. cati* activity elicits inflammation. Mites burrowing in the stratum corneum lead to an erythematous, papular dermatitis that progresses to thickened skin covered with crusts. Alopecia and intense pruritus are common, and secondary infections occur, particularly with self-excoriation.[10]

CLINICAL FEATURES

Notoedric mange is characterized by intense pruritus and development of hyperkeratotic crusts and alopecia on the dorsal pinnae. Hypersensitivity contributes to pruritus and leads to intense grooming which can result in secondary excoriations. In chronically infested cats with advanced disease, anorexia, weight loss, and poor condition may be evident.[10]

DIAGNOSIS

Direct Microscopic Examination

Mites are present in high numbers and are readily recovered in skin scrapings from affected areas. Although rare, *S. scabiei* has been reported in cats; feline sarcoptiform mites must be carefully examined to distinguish *N. cati* from those of *S. scabiei*. Use of clear tape to collect material for microscopic examination from affected areas may be less stressful for feline patients and appears to be of equal diagnostic sensitivity for *N. cati*.[107] Like other mites (e.g., *Demodex* sp., *Lynxacarus* sp.), *N. cati* is occasionally detected on fecal flotation of infested cats due to ingestion during grooming.[111] Fecal PCR has been developed for survey of wild felid populations but is not commercially available for testing domestic cats.[112]

Serology

Serologic assays to detect antibodies to *N. cati* have not been described, and *S. scabiei* ELISA is not validated for use in cats with notoedric mange.

Laboratory Abnormalities

Clinical pathology values have not been described in cats with *N. cati* infestations. Bobcats with notoedric mange have had low serum creatinine concentrations, hypoglycemia, and electrolyte abnormalities (hyperphosphatemia, hypernatremia, and hyperchloremia), as well as decreased serum cholesterol, albumin, globulin, and total protein concentrations, presumably due to protein loss across the affected skin.[113]

Gross Pathologic Findings

Notoedric mange most commonly presents as facial dermatitis, often initially involving the anterior edge and dorsal surface of the pinnae. As the infestation progresses, the head, neck, and dorsal thorax may become affected, and the skin becomes profoundly thickened, wrinkled, and lichenified. Lesions may also appear on the feet, tail, and perineum following contact with affected areas during grooming. In chronic infestations, most of the body surface can be affected, peripheral lymphadopathy develops, and fatality may occur.[10]

TREATMENT AND PROGNOSIS

Although FDA label-approved options to treat *N. cati* are not available, treatment is similar to that recommended for *S. scabiei*, with transdermal eprinomectin, moxidectin, or selamectin recommended; combination products in which both active ingredients have efficacy against mites (e.g., eprinomectin/fipronil, selamectin/sarolaner, moxidectin/fluralaner) are likely of even greater efficacy.[114–116] Isoxazolines approved for cats (i.e., fluralaner, lotilaner, sarolaner) would also be considered effective. High-dose off-label cattle preparations of macrocyclic lactones have been used historically but are not recommended due to safety concerns; repeating the treatment at 14-day or monthly intervals may be necessary to remove mites that hatch from eggs which remain after treatment and eliminate the infestation. If a dip is preferred, a 2% to 3% warm lime sulfur solution can be applied topically and allowed to dry on the skin every 7 days for at least 6 weeks and until lesions resolve.[10] Because some cats may be subclinical carriers, all cats in the household should be treated for *N. cati* infestation regardless of clinical appearance. Cats with notoedric mange respond well to treatment so long as all cats in the household can be treated, re-exposure is prevented, and treatment can be repeated, if necessary, until infestations completely resolve.[10]

IMMUNITY

The extent to which cats develop immunity to *N. cati* has not been investigated. The occurrence of epizootics in wild felid populations that stabilize over time suggests that, although notoedric mange can be responsible for population declines, immunity may develop similar to what has been described for *S. scabiei* in some wild canid populations.[103]

PREVENTION

Vaccines are not available for prevention of *N. cati* infections. Prevention involves keeping cats indoors, avoiding contact with other cats likely to be infested, and, for multi-cat households, treating new arrivals during initial quarantine to prevent introduction. Although not evaluated experimentally, routine use of control products effective against mites, including macrocyclic lactones and isoxazolines, would also be expected to prevent infestation.[30,117] Cats with notoedric mange should be isolated until cleared of the infestation. All littermates or adult cats in the same household should be treated regardless of clinical appearance as subclinical infestations may be present in some cats, creating a reservoir for future infestations.[10]

PUBLIC HEALTH ASPECTS

People in direct contact with infested cats often develop self-limiting dermatitis characterized by intense pruritus and an erythematous papular rash; lesions are common on areas in contact with infested cats including the hands, wrists, forearms, and abdomen.[108,118] As with pruritus due to zoonotic *S. scabiei* varieties, *N. cati* mites create a transient infestation in humans and are not transmitted to other humans.[10]

OTODECTES CYNOTIS

ETIOLOGY AND EPIDEMIOLOGY

Otodectes cynotis (order Sarcoptiformes, family Psoroptidae) is the common ear mite of domestic cats, dogs, and ferrets; infestations have been reported in many other mammals.[30] Although most commonly reported from domestic and free-roaming cats, *O. cynotis* is well recognized as a parasite of ferrets and dogs. Adults of *O. cynotis* are approximately the same size (300–450 µm) as *S. scabiei*; at 350–450 µm, females may be grossly visible to the unaided eye. The pretarsi consist of a caruncle (sucker) attached to a very short pedicel (stalk) on the first two pairs of legs of the female and all four pairs of legs on the male; males also have distinct copulatory structures on the ventral surface.[34] *Otodectes cynotis* is the only member of the genus.

Completion of the life cycle of *O. cynotis* requires approximately 3 weeks, with larvae, nymphs, and adults developing in the ear canal and feeding on superficial epidermal debris; under warmer conditions, the life cycle is completed more rapidly.[30] Females adhere eggs to the epidermal surface of the ear canal; larvae hatch from eggs in approximately 4 days and then develop through two nymphal stages (protonymph, deutonymph) to the adults. Motile stages largely remain in the ceruminous exudate and cellular material that accumulates in infested ears, occasionally venturing to the surface. Mites are transferred between animals by direct contact, including from dams to nursing young, and off-host survival is limited. However, experimentally mites can survive for 5 to 17 days off host depending on temperature and relative humidity.[119,120] Cats and, less commonly, dogs, infested with *O. cynotis* are reported worldwide; ear mites are also very common in ferrets and both wild and farmed foxes.

The prevalence of *O. cynotis* infestation in cats ranges from 0.9% of pet cats in the United Kingdom to 37% of free-roaming cats in the United States (Florida) (Table 110.2).[120–122] Failure to microscopically examine otic exudate from every cat underestimates prevalence and may explain some of the variation seen.[121,122] In a multi-institutional survey of 1,519 cats in seven different countries in Europe, *O. cynotis* was present in 17.4% of pet cats and was more commonly recovered from cats than any other ectoparasite, including fleas (15.5%).[106] Although infestations are frequently found in kittens and in cats with outdoor access, age-related differences in prevalence have not been clearly established in all feline populations and ear mite infestations also occur in adult cats.[22,123–125] Prevalence in dogs has ranged from 2.8% (Albania) to 6% (Brazil); age, sex, and breed have not been associated with risk of infestation in dogs.[126,127] *Otodectes cynotis* is also commonly identified in pet ferrets and wild canids.[128–131] In wild canid populations, *O. cynotis* infestations tend to be focused in certain geographic areas. For example, 4% of Arctic foxes across Iceland were infested, but all were from a single county where the prevalence of infestation was 38%.[132]

PATHOGENESIS

Infestation with *O. cynotis* is an important inciting cause of otitis externa in cats and, less commonly, dogs. Ear mites do not burrow

TABLE 110.2 Prevalence of *Otodectes cynotis* in Pet and Free-Roaming Cats and Dogs

Location	Host	Lifestyle	Prevalence	Reference
Europe (Austria, Belgium, France, Hungary, Italy, Romania, and Spain)	Cat	Pet	17.4%	106
Greece (Thessaloniki area)	Cat	Pet kittens (0 – 6 months), first exam	14%	125
Greece (northern)	Cat	Pet cats, clinically normal	25.5%	123
United States	Cat	Pet	7.4%	155
Japan	Cat	Pet	9.4%	124
United Kingdom (England, Wales)	Cat	Pet and rescue cats	0.9%	122
Greece (Thessaloniki area)	Cat	Free roaming	15.8%	105
Spain (Murcia)	Cat	Free-roaming	30%	156
Spain (central)	Cat	Free-roaming	10.6%	157
United States (Oklahoma, Arkansas)	Cat	Free-roaming	19.3%	158
United States (Florida)	Cat	Free-roaming	37%	121
Albania	Dog	Pet	2.8%	126
Albania	Dog	Pet	6.7%	159
Brazil	Dog	Pet	6.0%	127
Iran (Ahvaz)	Dog	Pet	4.8%	160
Korea (Gwang-Ju City)	Dog	Free-roaming	22.3%	161
Mexico (Yucatán)	Dog	Free-roaming	3.5%	162

but instead feed on superficial epithelial cells and associated exudate; occasionally tissue fluid is imbibed.[10] The inflammatory response leads to erythema of the ear canal and development of dark brown, granular, ceruminous exudate. As mite populations expand, miliary dermatitis may develop on adjacent areas of the head and, less commonly, on the feet or tail following transfer during grooming.[3] Some estimate that as many as 85% of feline otitis externa cases and 50% of canine otitis externa cases are caused by ear mites.[133] In a survey of free-roaming cats in northern Italy, 55% had evidence of otitis externa with *O. cynotis* found in a majority (53.3%) of affected cats.[134] When treatment is delayed, secondary bacterial and fungal infections can develop.[135] In some infested pets, diffuse hypersensitivity resembling flea allergy dermatitis and associated with ectopic mites has been described.[10] The chronic ceruminous gland hyperplasia resulting from untreated *O. cynotis* infestations has been associated with development of ceruminous gland tumors.[131]

CLINICAL FEATURES

Ear mite infestations lead to a wide variety of clinical presentations. Some infested animals appear normal, whereas others develop intense otic pruritus accompanied by head shaking and frequent, persistent scratching of the ears. Acne-like lesions on the face have been described.[123] Affected ears may contain copious amounts of dark, granular discharge described as resembling coffee grounds. In severe cases, self-excoriation leads to traumatic injury of the skin, bleeding, development of aural hematomas, and secondary infections. Purulent otitis externa may develop. Dermatitis may also be seen, particularly when mites are present outside the ear canals; common sites for ectopic mites and associated alopecia and pruritus include the neck, back, feet, and tail.[10,30] However, some animals will have large numbers of mites with minimal discharge or pruritus evident. In cats, there is not a clear correlation between the number of mites and the severity of lesions that develop, or the amount of otic discharge and the relative degree of pruritus. Dogs are usually pruritic with only minimal discharge evident.[10]

DIAGNOSIS

Direct Microscopic Examination

Ear mites can be visualized directly during otoscopic examination or by microscopic examination of exudate collected on a swab; mineral oil aids in collection of material for examination and transfer to a microscope slide. Direct microscopic examination of material collected from the ear canal is key to reaching an accurate diagnosis. In one study, otoscopic examination alone failed to identify *O. cynotis* in 39% of infested cats, including eight cats with an ear canal that appeared normal and had only mild ceruminous exudate.[121] Another study showed that otoscopic examination identified only 67% of infestations and that sensitivity was increased by use of curettage to collect the cerumen.[136] Flushing the external ear canal with a small amount of mineral oil further enhances recovery and increases prevalence of infestation when used for surveys of clinically normal pet cats but is likely impractical in a clinical setting.[123] Immature and adult *O. cynotis* are motile when collected and are readily identified by their large size (200–450 μm), characteristic rounded appearance, and presence in the ear canal (Fig. 110.5). The other mite occasionally found associated with otitis externa is *Demodex* spp., which has a distinct elongated morphology. Males and deutonymphs (pre-females) of *O. cynotis* are often found in copulation; eggs are commonly seen within females or in collected exudate.[34] Ectopic *O. cynotis* may occasionally be recovered on skin scrape of the neck or tail.[10]

Serology

Serologic tests for ear mites are not available. Cross-reactions with dust mites can occur on intradermal skin tests similar to that seen with *S. scabiei* and *Cheyletiella* spp.[137]

Laboratory Abnormalities

Blood values in cats and dogs with *O. cynotis* infestations are largely unremarkable. Significant changes on CBCs, including eosinophilia, have not been demonstrated.[138]

Gross Pathologic Findings

Classically, *O. cynotis* induces erythematous hyperplasia and hyperkeratosis in the ear canal epithelium. Pronounced hyperplasia of the sebaceous and ceruminous glands is commonly seen together with dilated blood vessels and increased numbers of macrophages

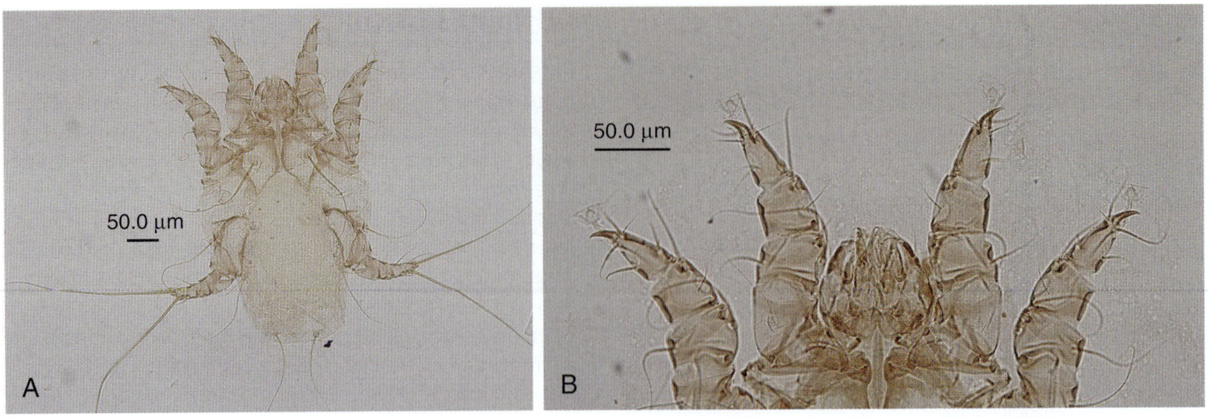

Fig. 110.5 (A) Adult *Otodectes cynotis*. (B) Magnified view showing suckers at the end of short pedicels on the first and second pair of legs. (Courtesy of Megan Lineberry, National Center for Veterinary Parasitology.)

and mast cells.[10,30] Copious dark, ceruminous otic discharge often packs the ear canal and must be removed to allow complete examination. However, many cats and dogs confirmed to be infested as documented by the presence of mites on ear swabs do not develop significant pathology and otoscopic examination is unremarkable.[121]

TREATMENT AND PROGNOSIS

Otodectes cynotis is readily treated with macrocyclic lactones, including otic preparations of ivermectin or milbemycin oxime developed for treating ear mites, or transdermal, systemic formulations of eprinomectin, moxidectin, or selamectin with broad-spectrum efficacy against many internal and external parasites.[22,139,140] Otic preparations may lead to more rapid clearance of mites.[141] Systemic isoxazolines (afoxolaner, fluralaner, lotilaner, sarolaner) are also effective against ear mites and may be given alone or in combination with macrocyclic lactones to further support efficacy.[142–148] In one study, a single administration of a label-approved formulation of fluralaner plus moxidectin eliminated ear mites from treated cats.[147] Historically, ear mites have been treated with otic preparations of pyrethrin, rotenone, fipronil, or lindane, or by using high-dose large animal preparations of macrocyclic lactones off-label; toxicities have been reported and these strategies are no longer recommended.[149] Mineral oil alone is effective although repeated treatments are needed, an overly aggressive approach can exacerbate otitis, and an oily residue is left on the cats.[30,150]

Otic cytology should be evaluated prior to cleaning; when present, secondary bacterial or fungal infections should also be treated. If debris is present, ear canals can be gently cleaned with ceruminolytics to provide symptomatic relief to the patient and to remove mites, taking care not to irritate the epidermal lining.[150] When otic acaricides are to be used, cleaning should occur before application. Eliminating ectopic mites with systemic macrocyclic lactones or isoxazolines should resolve traumatic alopecia associated with excessive grooming due to pruritus from a diffuse hypersensitivity reaction. If pruritus is severe, symptomatic care may be indicated while infestations resolve. All dogs and cats in contact with the patient should also be treated with acaricides; subclinical infestations are common, and these animals may serve as reservoirs to perpetuate the cycle of infestation. When the primary patient and any direct contacts (e.g., other cats or dogs in the household) can be treated, and any secondary infections addressed, animals routinely recover.[10]

IMMUNITY

The negative association between age and intensity of *O. cynotis* infestation suggests immunity may develop, and this reaction could limit mite populations in older animals.[123,151] However, ear mites are still present in many adult cats and dogs, and reinfestation following treatment has been described.[137]

PREVENTION

Preventing *O. cynotis* infestation can be achieved by avoiding contact with other cats and dogs likely to be infested, including keeping cats indoors and preventing roaming in dogs. Young animals are particularly susceptible to acquiring infestations from dams in the neonatal period due to prolonged, intimate contact while nursing; treating breeding females before or during pregnancy, prior to parturition, would be expected to eliminate mites and reduce risk of transmission to kittens and puppies. In addition, routine use of products known to have efficacy against *O. cynotis*, including macrocyclic lactones and isoxazolines used to control heartworm, intestinal parasites, fleas, and ticks, would also limit infestations with ear mites.[142–148] A combination fipronil, S-methoprene, eprinomectin, and praziquantel product has been shown to protect cats from *O. cynotis* infestation.[152]

PUBLIC HEALTH ASPECTS

Although a few isolated cases of human infestation or dermatitis associated with *O. cynotis* in pets have been reported, transmission from pets to people appears quite rare.[153,154] Ear mites pose minimal, if any, zoonotic risk.

PNEUMONYSSOIDES CANINUM (NASAL MITE)

Nasal mites (*Pneumonyssoides caninum*, also *Pneumonyssus caninum*) are an uncommon finding in pet dogs in most of the world. The large (1.0–1.5 mm) mites live in paranasal sinuses and nasal cavity, and transmission occurs with direct or indirect contact between dogs. Nasal mites appear more common in Scandinavia, with prevalence estimated to be 7% in Norway and 23% in Sweden.[163,164] One survey in Uppsala, Sweden documented *P. caninum* in 20% of dogs surveyed; infestations were more common in older (>3 years) and large-breed dogs, and dolichocephalic breeds may be more commonly infested.[165] Cases have also been described in North America and the United Kingdom, but the true prevalence is not known.[166–169]

Clinical signs vary from nasal irritation, nasal discharge, sneezing, nasal pruritus, and stertorous breathing, to epistaxis, hyposmia, and head shaking.[169] Diagnosis can be made by visualizing mites with rhinoscopy or by retrograde saline nasal flush.[163] Nasal biopsy may reveal an eosinophilic inflammatory response, and transient peripheral eosinophilia has been described.[169,170] Selamectin applied every 2 weeks for three treatments is effective and clinical signs resolve within a few days of initial treatment.[169,171] Milbemycin oxime (1 mg/kg, PO, q10d × 3 doses) is also effective.[163] All dogs in the home should be treated. Nasal mites are not known to be zoonotic.

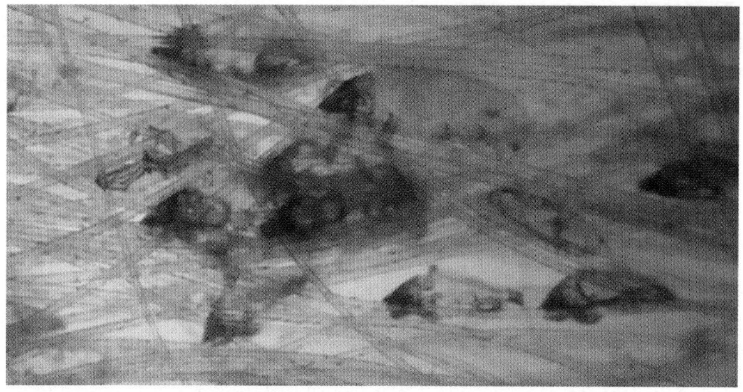

Fig. 110.6 Adult *Lynxacarus radovsky* in hairs collected from an infested cat. (Courtesy of National Center for Veterinary Parasitology.)

LYNXACARUS RADOVSKYI (FUR MITE, HAIR CLASPING MITE)

The fur mite, *Lynxacarus radovskyi*, is laterally compressed and primarily found infesting cats in tropical areas. Mites attach eggs to the hairs of cats. Larvae, nymphs, and adults clasp the hairs with the anterior end oriented toward the hair shaft (Fig. 110.6). The complete life cycle has not been described, but off-host survival is considered limited.[30] Mite populations are higher on the caudal area of the body, including the base of the tail, tail tip, and perianal region.[172,173] *Lynxacarus radovskyi* may be found on more than 70% of pet cats in Malaysia and free-roaming cats in the Caribbean.[172,173] Many infested cats are subclinically infested, with pruritus, presumably due to a hypersensitivity reaction, only occasionally observed.[174]

Infested cats develop a dry, dull hair coat, alopecia, and, occasionally, pruritus; the stippled appearance to the fur is often described as "peppered." Excessive grooming leads to alopecia that is most pronounced in the perianal region, caudolateral hind legs, base of tail, and abdomen.[173] An association between fur mite infestation and feline eosinophilic granuloma complex has been suggested.[175] Diagnosis can be made by identifying mites grasping hairs plucked from affected areas. Clear tape applied to the fur also recovers mites and identifies more infested animals.[172] Effective treatments include moxidectin/imidacloprid or selamectin applied every 2 weeks, fluralaner once, or sarolaner.[173,173,176,177] All cats in the home should be treated. Humans in contact with infested cats may develop a papular rash that resolves with treatment of the pet.[178]

TROMBICULID MITES (CHIGGERS, RED BUGS, BERRY BUGS, HARVEST MITES, SCRUB ITCH OR GRASS ITCH MITES)

ETIOLOGY AND EPIDEMIOLOGY

Chiggers (family Trombiculidae, order Trombidiformes) are minute, larval mites that cause chigger dermatitis (trombiculosis). They are found in many tropical and temperate terrestrial habitats. Although usually parasites of wildlife, trombiculids occasionally found on dogs and cats include *Eutrombicula* spp. (North, Central, and South America), *Neotrombicula* spp. and *Ericotrombidium* spp. (Europe), and *Leptotrombidium* spp. (Asia, Australia).[179–186] Over 1,200 species of trombiculid mites have been identified, but many only as larvae. More than 50 species have been recorded infesting humans and approximately 20 are recognized as capable of causing animal and human disease. Specific identification is often not pursued, and the full diversity of species involved is likely under-recognized.[183] *Eutrombicula alfredugessi* is the most common and widespread chigger in the Western Hemisphere and is found from Canada to Argentina and the Caribbean.[187] In the United States, *E. alfreddugesi* is more common east of the Rocky Mountains, *Eutrombicula splendens* is found in the eastern United States, and *Eutrombicula lipovskyi* is encountered in the southern United States from Arkansas, Oklahoma and Kansas to Alabama and Tennessee.[187] *Walchia americana*, a mite in the family Walchiidae and in the same superfamily as the trombiculids (Trombiculoidea), is found in the southwest and eastern United States, and commonly infests squirrels and other rodents although larvae can infest cats.[180] *Neotrombicula autumnalis*, the harvest mite, is the most common chigger in Europe, found throughout the continent and the British Isles.[187] *Neotrombicula inopinata* is found in England, Spain and France, and portions of central and Eastern Europe, from Germany and Poland to Ukraine and the Northern Caucasus region of Russia.[188] A related trombidioid mite of foxes, *Straelensia cynotis* (family Leeuwenhoekiidae), parasitizes dogs in Portugal, Spain, France, Italy, and Israel.[189–193] *Leptotrombidium* spp., the vectors for scrub typhus, are found in Southeast Asia, the southwestern Pacific Islands, and northern Australia.[194]

The life history of trombiculid mites encompasses the egg, prelarva, larva, prenymph, nymph, tritonymph, and adult stages. The female adult oviposits on the ground and larvae hatch and begin to search for new hosts in 12 days. The larvae, which are obligate parasites, have little host specificity and will feed on a wide variety of terrestrial vertebrates, including domestic animals and humans. Larvae feed for 1 to 5 days, but generally, most will complete feeding by the second day. Engorged larvae then drop to the ground where they molt into the prenymph stage. Following another molt, nymphs prey on invertebrates and, following two more molts, become adults. Nymphal and adult stages are either predatory on invertebrates or scavengers; they are usually found in soil. The adults are typically bright red or yellow, and about 1 mm in length. Covered in plumose setae, adults appear to be covered in velvet and are sometimes referred to as red velvet or true velvet mites.

Pets become infested when they encounter larval stages in the environment, often in brushy areas frequented by wildlife. In temperate regions, larvae usually begin to appear in the mid-summer and their populations peak in the late summer and early fall, and in tropical and subtropical areas, larval populations may be host-seeking throughout the year.[187,195,196] The harvest mite, *N. autumnalis*, is active on warm, sunny days[187] and *E. alfreddugesi* larvae are most active at dawn and late afternoon–early evening, with low levels of activity during the midday and night.[197]

CLINICAL FEATURES

Larvae are round, 0.2 to 0.5 mm long, often orange or red in color, and have six legs. The mouthparts (gnathostoma) include the chelicerae, or cutting plates, that are used for piercing and holding onto the host. Attached larvae eject saliva into the epidermis through a buccal aperture. The saliva digests host tissue and aids in formation of a stylostome, or feeding tube, through which the larva can imbibe fluid. After feeding, or if dislodged by the host, the larva falls to the ground and the stylostome is left behind, resulting in persistent, intense pruritus; chiggers do not burrow.[187] Irritation reactions appear to become more severe with repeated feeding episodes, likely due to a hypersensitivity reaction. In cats, the ears are most frequently infested, but clusters of orange-red trombiculid larvae may be visible on margins of pinnae, periorbital region, ventrum, or interdigital skin; alopecia is often evident, and associated lesions are dry and crusted. Papules, measuring 0.1 to 0.3 cm, may be observed with mild wheals, crusting, and yellow exudate. Involvement of the feet may present with swollen paws and cracked claws.[180] Pruritus was the most common clinical sign although a majority (57%) of infested cats in one study did not have clinical signs.[198] Neurologic signs have been reported in dogs heavily infested with *Neotrombicula* spp.[199,200]

In contrast, larvae of *S. cynotis* infest hair follicles of dogs and cause a nonpruritic nodular dermatitis on the dorsal head and trunk; when severe, nodules may be painful and dogs lethargic and anorexic. Infestations with *S. cynotis* are associated with contact with fox dens where the nymph and adult mites live and have been reported in dogs and, occasionally, cats, in Spain, Portugal, France, and Israel.[189–191,193,201] Histologically, the cysts comprise large, dilated hair follicles containing a larva; the follicular epithelium is hyperplastic and infiltrates of plasma cells and mast cells are evident.[190] Inflammatory infiltrates are usually mild and eosinophils are rarely observed.

DIAGNOSIS

When there is an abundant and recent infestation, clumps of reddish- to orange-colored larvae can be observed on the skin. Diagnosis of chiggers can be made by close inspection of lesions, gently scraping mites from affected areas or collecting with clear tape, or, in the case of *S. cynotis*, examining biopsy specimens of the nodular dermatitis.

TREATMENT AND PREVENTION

Treatments for trombiculid mites reported to be effective in cats include transdermal selamectin or fipronil.[202–205] Dogs have been treated successfully with topical fipronil, permethrin-pyriproxyfen, and permethrin-fipronil combinations.[202,206,207] *Straelensia cynotis* infestations do not consistently respond to systemic treatment with ivermectin.[190,191] Treatment failures may relate to the mite's endofollicular location. Topical or systemic antibiotics may be indicated to treat secondary infections, and glucocorticoids would provide relief. Anecdotally, isoxazolines may also have good efficacy, eliminating chiggers on dogs within 6–8 hours.[200]

Modifying chigger habitat so as to make it inhospitable for mite survival can reduce the likelihood of exposure. Routinely mowing grassy areas, clearing brush, and raking leaves can decrease chigger exposure. Reinfestation in cats (and dogs and humans, as well) is very likely after treatment if there are no changes in lifestyle.[198] Avoidance of sites where chiggers are active, especially during the times of the year when larvae are active, is useful in minimizing chigger exposure. Limiting activity in those areas to the midday hours during chigger season may also minimize exposure as the larvae are less likely to be seeking hosts during the warmest and driest part of the day.

PUBLIC HEALTH ASPECTS

Although humans are considered accidental hosts, about 20 mite species are considered medically relevant because their bites can elicit dermatitis and hypersensitivity reactions, as well as being vector pathogens.[194] In addition, scrub typhus (tsutsugamushi disease), caused by the bacterium *Orientia tsutsugamushi*, is transmitted by chiggers of *Leptotrombidium* spp. in far eastern Russia, the Korean Peninsula, Japan, South east Asia, India, and northern coastal Australia.[194] Larvae are efficient vectors because the bacterium is transovarially transmitted.

In humans, chigger bites usually occur on the lower limbs. Small (1–2 mm) papules appear approximately 3 to 24 hours post-exposure, which can develop into pustules. Intense pruritus begins to subside after 1 week and accompanying skin lesions may last 3 weeks.

People are advised to prevent mite exposure by avoiding known and suspected chigger areas, wearing protective clothing, and using repellents. Although direct contact with host-seeking larvae on vegetation is the likeliest route of transmission, there are two suspected cases of animal-to-human transmission in the literature.[208,209]

CASE EXAMPLE

Signalment

"Ginger," a 5-year-old female spayed domestic shorthair cat from Muscogee, Oklahoma, United States.

History

Ginger was evaluated in July for alopecia and mild to moderate pruritus on the head, pinnae, and shoulder. Her owner reported excessive grooming over the past month when the lesions first appeared; this included pawing at the ears, scratching, and occasionally chewing the affected area on the shoulder. Ginger was an indoor-only cat that had been housed in a long-term, limited access private shelter. Ginger joined the shelter population in April (3 months ago) following the death of a previous owner. The owner's impression was that Ginger was removing her own hair with the excessive grooming, perhaps due to stress, but she had not observed any difficult interactions with other cats in the facility. The current owner managed the shelter and had not noted pruritus or similar skin lesions in any of the other 14 cats in residence.

Current Medications: Topical monthly flea control (imidacloprid).

Other Medical History: No medical problems or skin lesions were noted at intake. Ginger was negative for feline retroviruses and feline heartworm antigen. *Giardia* sp. cysts were present on fecal flotation in April; 3 days of fenbendazole (50 mg/kg) was administered to avoid introducing *Giardia* sp. into the shelter population. For the past 3 weeks, the owner had fed Ginger a commercial hydrolyzed protein dry kibble diet; pruritus and skin lesions persisted.

Physical Examination

Body weight: 6.4 kg; BCS 6/9.

General: Bright, alert, hydrated, responsive. Mucous membranes pink, HR = 170 beats/minute, RR = 50 breaths/minute, T = 100.8°F (38.2°C).

Continued

CASE EXAMPLE—cont'd

Integument: Alopecia, scaling, and broken hairs were evident on the dorsal neck, right shoulder and right lateral thorax (Fig. 110.7). Alopecia and scaling were present on the dorsal surface of the head and the external pinnae; excoriations were noted on the left pinna. Flea frass, fleas, or other grossly apparent ectoparasites were not recovered by combing. Fluorescence was not noted with ultraviolet illumination of affected areas; culture of plucked hairs in dermatophyte test medium did not reveal color change or fungal growth.

Eyes, ears, nose, and throat: Mild amount of light tan cerumen in both ears. No other clinically significant findings were found on physical examination.

Skin Cytology and Skin Biopsy Findings

Mites were not evident on multiple ($n = 6$) skin scrapings collected from affected areas. Cytologic examinations of skin scrapings revealed no significant findings. Skin biopsy revealed mild hyperkeratosis and mild to moderate perivascular dermatitis.

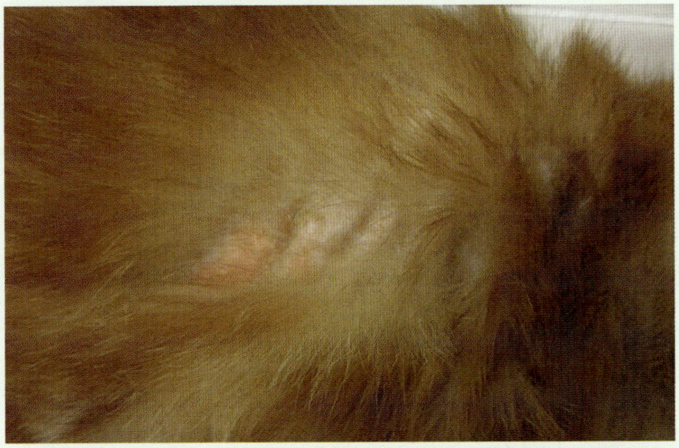

Fig. 110.7 Alopecia, mild erythema, and mild to moderate scaling on the dorsal neck, shoulder, and lateral thorax of a cat with demodicosis.

Fecal Flotation Findings

Demodex gatoi mites, with characteristic stubby appearance and each approximately 90–110 μm long, were recovered on centrifugal fecal flotation using 33% zinc sulfate (Fig. 110.8).[45]

Diagnosis

Demodex gatoi infestation.

Treatment

Ginger was treated with transdermal moxidectin/imidacloprid administered weekly for three consecutive treatments and monthly thereafter. Clavulanic acid-amoxicillin (10 mg/kg, q12h, PO) was also administered; antibiotics were discontinued after 7 days. The pruritus and associated lesions began to resolve in the first week of treatment. Mites were detected on fecal flotation 7 days after treatment but not at 14 days or 21 days. At 1-month follow-up examination, the skin appeared normal.

Comments

Mites are not consistently recovered in skin scrapings from cats with demodicosis, including those with *D. gatoi* infestation. Examination of material collected with tape strips may be more successful for confirmation of diagnosis.[42] However, because the pruritus associated with demodicosis causes cats to groom excessively, mites are ingested and frequently identified on fecal flotation.[46] Fecal examination should be requested for cats seen for pruritus. Skin biopsy was not necessary in this case and could have been avoided if fecal flotation had been performed initially. Although this cat was treated with transdermal moxidectin, isoxazolines (lotilaner, fluralaner, sarolaner) are available for cats, and sometimes in combination with macrocyclic lactones (selamectin, moxidectin) and would also be expected to be effective. Unlike most other *Demodex* spp., *D. gatoi* causes contagious pruritus and when co-housed, multiple cats are often infested.[42] Ginger should be isolated until treatment has been completed and other in-contact cats closely evaluated for skin lesions. Prophylactic treatment of all cats in the facility with selamectin/sarolaner or moxidectin/fluralaner may be warranted.

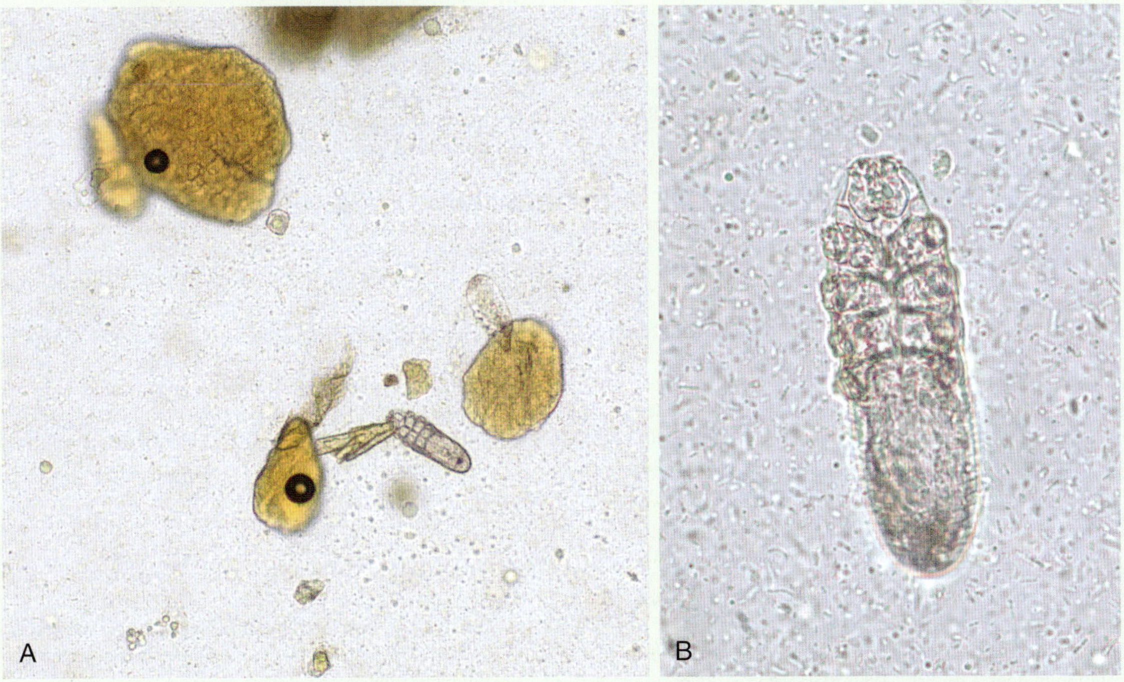

Fig. 110.8 *Demodex gatoi* mites recovered on fecal flotation as viewed with 10× (A) and 40× (B) objectives (100× and 400× magnification, respectively).

SUGGESTED READINGS

Arlian LG, Morgan MS. A review of *Sarcoptes scabiei*: past, present and future. *Parasit Vectors*. 2017;10:297.

Curtis CF. Current trends in the treatment of *Sarcoptes, Cheyletiella* and *Otodectes* mite infestations in dogs and cats. *Vet Dermatol*. 2004;15:108–114.

Mueller RS, Rosenkrantz W, Bensignor E, et al. Diagnosis and treatment of demodicosis in dogs and cats: clinical consensus guidelines of the World Association for Veterinary Dermatology. *Vet Dermatol*. 2020;31:5–27.

Yang C, Huang HP. Evidence-based veterinary dermatology: a review of published studies of treatments for *Otodectes cynotis* (ear mite) infestation in cats. *Vet Dermatol*. 2016;27:221–e56.

REFERENCES

1. Ayalew L, Vaillancourt M. Observations on an outbreak of infestation of dogs with *Cheyletiella yasguri* and its public health implications. *Can Vet J*. 1976;17:184–191.
2. Cohen SR. *Cheyletiella* dermatitis. A mite infestation of rabbit, cat, dog, and man. *Arch Dermatol*. 1980;116:435–437.
3. Scott DW, Horn RT. Zoonotic dermatoses of dogs and cats. *Vet Clin North Am Small Anim Pract*. 1987;17:117–144.
4. Bronswijk JE, De Kreek EJ. *Cheyletiella* (Acari: Cheyletiellidae) of dog, cat and domesticated rabbit, a review. *J Med Entomol*. 1976;13:315–327.
5. Foxx TS, Ewing SA. Morphologic features, behavior, and life history of *Cheyletiella yasguri*. *Am J Vet Res*. 1969;30:269–285.
6. Humphreys M. *Cheyletiella parasitivorax* infestation of the dog. *Vet Rec*. 1958;70:442.
7. Kunkle GA, Miller WH. *Cheyletiella* infestation in humans. *Arch Dermatol*. 1980;116:1345.
8. Chailleux N, Paradis M. Efficacy of selamectin in the treatment of naturally acquired cheyletiellosis in cats. *Can Vet J*. 2002;43:767–770.
9. Saevik BK, Bredal W, Ulstein TL. *Cheyletiella* infestation in the dog: observations on diagnostic methods and clinical signs. *J Small Anim Pract*. 2004;45:495–500.
10. Miller WH, Griffin CE, Campbell KL. Parasitic skin disease. In: *Muller and Kirk's Small Animal Dermatology*. 7th ed. Elsevier Mosby; 2012:284–342.
11. Wagner R, Stallmeister N. *Cheyletiella* dermatitis in humans, dogs and cats. *Br J Dermatol*. 2000;143:1110–1112.
12. White SD, Rosychuk RA, Fieseler KV. Clinicopathologic findings, sensitivity to house dust mites and efficacy of milbemycin oxime treatment of dogs with *Cheyletiella* sp. infestation. *Vet Dermatol*. 2001;12:13–18.
13. Rothschild M. *Cheyletiella parasitivorax* (Megnin)(Acar., Cheyletidae) feeding upon the rabbit flea (*Spilopsyllus cuniculi* (Dale)). *Entomol Mon Mag*. 1969;105:216.
14. Rak H. *Cheyletiella parasitovorax* (Megnin) Acaridae, Cheyletidae from cat flea (*Ctenocephaldes felis felis*) (Bouche) in Iran. *Entomol Mon Mag*. 1972;108:62.
15. Guzman RF. *Cheyletiella blakei* (Acari: Cheyletiellidae) hyperparasitic on the cat flea *Ctenocephalides felis felis* (Siphonaptera: Pulicidae) in New Zealand. *N Z Entomol*. 1982;7:322–323.
16. Vercammen-Grandjean P, Rak H. *Cheyletiella yasguri* Smiley, 1965, un parasite de canides aux etats-unis et hyperparasite d'hippoboscide en Iran (Acarina: Cheyletidae). *Ann Parasitol Hum Comp*. 1968;43:405–412.
17. Schaffer MH, Baker NF, Kennedy PC. 1958. Parasitism by *Cheyletiella parasitivorax*; a case report of the infestation in a female dog and its litter. *Cornell Vet*. 1958;48:440–447.
18. Thomsett LR. Mite infestations of man contracted from dogs and cats. *Br Med J*. 1968;3:93–95.
19. Ghubash R. Parasitic miticidal therapy. *Clin Tech Small Anim Pract*. 2006;21:135–144.
20. Paradis M, Villeneuve A. Efficacy of ivermectin against *Cheyletiella yasguri* infestation in dogs. *Can Vet J*. 1988;29:633–635.
21. Paradis M, Scott D, Villeneuve A. Efficacy of ivermectin against *Cheyletiella blakei* infestation in cats. *J Am Anim Hosp Assoc*. 1990;26:125–128.
22. Curtis CF. Current trends in the treatment of *Sarcoptes, Cheyletiella* and *Otodectes* mite infestations in dogs and cats. *Vet Dermatol*. 2004;15:108–114.
23. Mueller RS, Bettenay SV. Efficacy of selamectin in the treatment of canine cheyletiellosis. *Vet Rec*. 2002;151:773.
24. Ottenschot TR, Gil D. Cheyletiellosis in long-haired cats. *Tijdschr Diergeneeskd*. 1978;103:1104–1108.
25. Loft KE, Willesen JL. Efficacy of imidacloprid 10 % / moxidectin 2.5% spot-on in the treatment of cheyletiellosis in dogs. *Vet Rec*. 2007;160:528–529.
26. Falconi ID, Billi M, Cornegliani L. Use of sarolaner therapy in dogs with *Cheyletiella* sp. infestation: a case series. Summa. *Animali da Compagnia*. 2018;35:61–64.
27. Chadwick AJ. Use of a 0.25% fipronil pump spray formulation to treat canine cheyletiellosis. *J Small Anim Pract*. 2007;38:261–262.
28. Scarampella F, Pollmeier M, Visser M, et al. Efficacy of fipronil in the treatment of feline cheyletiellosis. *Vet Parasitol*. 2005;129:333–339.
29. Folz SD, Kakuk TJ, Henke CL, et al. Clinical evaluation of amitraz for treatment of canine scabies. *Mod Vet Pract*. 1984;65:597–600.
30. Bowman DD, Hendrix CM, Lindsay DS, Barr SC. *The Arthropods. In: Bowman et al., eds*. Feline Clinical Parasitology. Iowa State University Press; 2001:355–445.
31. Dobrosavljevic DD, Popovic ND, Radovanovic SS. Systemic manifestations of *Cheyletiella* infestation in man. *Int J Dermatol*. 2007;46:397–399.
32. Mueller RS, Rosenkrantz W, Bensignor E, et al. Diagnosis and treatment of demodicosis in dogs and cats: clinical consensus guidelines of the World Association for Veterinary Dermatology. *Vet Dermatol*. 2020;31:5–27.
33. Löwenstein C, Beck W, Bessmann K, Mueller RS. Feline demodicosis caused by concurrent infestation with *Demodex cati* and an unnamed species of mite. *Vet Rec*. 2005;157:290–292.
34. Greiner E. Arthropods. In: Zajac A, Conboy G, eds. *Veterinary Clinical Parasitology*. 8th ed. Wiley-Blackwell; 2012:217–303.
35. It V, Barrientos L, Lopez Gappa J, et al. Association of canine juvenile generalized demodicosis with the dog leukocyte antigen system. *Tissue Antigens*. 2010;76:67–70.
36. Plant JD, Lund EM, Yang M. A case-control study of the risk factors for canine juvenile-onset generalized demodicosis in the USA. *Vet Dermatol*. 2011;22:95–99.
37. Bowden DG, Outerbridge CA, Kissel MB, et al. Canine demodicosis: a retrospective study of a veterinary hospital population in California, USA (2000–2016). *Vet Dermatol*. 2018;29:19–e10.
38. Robson DC, Burton GG, Bassett R, et al. Eight cases of demodicosis caused by a long-bodied *Demodex* species (1997–2002). *Aust Vet Pract*. 2003;33:64–72.
39. Ordeix L, Bardagí M, Scarampella F, et al. *Demodex injai* infestation and dorsal greasy skin and hair in eight wirehaired fox terrier dogs. *Vet Dermatol*. 2009;20:267–272.
40. Sgarbossa RS, Sechi GV, Pacheco BD, et al. The epidemiological and clinical aspects of *Demodex injai* demodicosis in dogs: a report of eight cases. *Semina: Ciências Agrárias, Londrina*. 2017;38:3387–3394.
41. Guaguere E, Olivry T, Delverdier-Poujade A, et al. *Demodex cati* infestation in association with feline cutaneous squamous cell carcinoma in situ: a report of five cases. *Vet Dermatol*. 1999;10:61–67.
42. Saari SA, Juuti KH, Palojärvi JH, et al. *Demodex gatoi*-associated contagious pruritic dermatosis in cats: a report from six households in Finland. *Acta Vet Scand*. 2009;51:40.
43. Koch SN. Updates on the management of canine demodicosis. *Today's Vet Pract*. 2017;7:77–85.
44. Beale K. Feline demodicosis: a consideration in the itchy or overgrooming cat. *J Feline Med Surg*. 2012;14:209–213.
45. Desch CE Jr, Stewart TB. *Demodex gatoi*: new species of hair follicle mite (Acari: Demodecidae) from the domestic cat (Carnivora: Felidae). *J Med Entomol*. 1999;36:167–170.

46. Silbermayr K, Joachim A, Litschauer B, et al. The first case of *Demodex gatoi* in Austria, detected with fecal flotation. *Parasitol Res.* 2013;112:2805–2810.
47. Martínez-Subiela S, Bernal LJ, Tvarijonaviciute A, et al. Canine demodicosis: the relationship between response to treatment of generalised disease and markers for inflammation and oxidative status. *Vet Dermatol.* 2014;25(72–6):e23–e24.
48. Fourie JJ, Liebenberg JE, Horak IG, et al. Efficacy of orally administered fluralaner (Bravecto™) or topically applied imidacloprid/moxidectin (Advocate®) against generalized demodicosis in dogs. *Parasit Vectors.* 2015;8:187.
49. Six RH, Becskei C, Mazaleski MM, et al. Efficacy of sarolaner, a novel oral isoxazoline, against two common mite infestations in dogs: *Demodex* spp. and *Otodectes cynotis. Vet Parasitol.* 2016;222:62–66.
50. Beugnet F, Halos L, Larsen D, de Vos C. Efficacy of oral afoxolaner for the treatment of canine generalised demodicosis. *Parasite.* 2016;23:14.
51. Snyder DE, Wiseman S, Liebenberg JE. Efficacy of lotilaner (Credelio™), a novel oral isoxazoline against naturally occurring mange mite infestations in dogs caused by *Demodex* spp. *Parasit Vectors.* 2017;10:532.
52. Becskei C, Cuppens O, Mahabir SP. Efficacy and safety of sarolaner against generalized demodicosis in dogs in European countries: a non-inferiority study. *Vet Dermatol.* 2018;29: 203-e72.
53. Duangkaew L, Larsuprom L, Anukkul P, et al. A field trial in Thailand of the efficacy of oral fluralaner for the treatment of dogs with generalized demodicosis. *Vet Dermatol.* 2018;29: 208-e74.
54. Lebon W, Beccati M, Bourdeau P, et al. Efficacy of two formulations of afoxolaner (NexGard® and NexGard Spectra®) for the treatment of generalised demodicosis in dogs, in veterinary dermatology referral centers in Europe. *Parasit Vectors.* 2018;11:506.
55. Fourie JJ, Meyer L, Thomas E. Efficacy of topically administered fluralaner or imidacloprid/moxidectin on dogs with generalised demodicosis. *Parasit Vectors.* 2019;12:59.
56. Perego R, Spada E, Foppa C, Proverbio D. Critically appraised topic for the most effective and safe treatment for canine generalised demodicosis. *BMC Vet Res.* 2019;15:17.
57. Petersen I, Chiummo R, Zschiesche E, et al. A European field assessment of the efficacy of fluralaner (Bravecto®) chewable and spot-on formulations for treatment of dogs with generalized demodicosis. *Parasit Vectors.* 2020;13:304.
58. Mueller RS, Meyer D, Bensignor E, Sauter-Louis C. Treatment of canine generalized demodicosis with a 'spot-on' formulation containing 10% moxidectin and 2.5% imidacloprid (Advocate, Bayer Healthcare). *Vet Dermatol.* 2009;20:441–446.
59. Mueller RS. An update on the therapy of canine demodicosis. *Compend Contin Educ Vet.* 2012;34:E1–E4.
60. Short J, Gram D. Successful treatment of *Demodex gatoi* with 10% imidacloprid/1% moxidectin. *J Am Anim Hosp Assoc.* 2016;52:68–72.
61. Matricoti I, Maina E. The use of oral fluralaner for the treatment of feline generalised demodicosis: a case report. *J Small Anim Pract.* 2017;58:476–479.
62. Duangkaew L, Hoffman H. Efficacy of oral fluralaner for the treatment of *Demodex gatoi* in two shelter cats. *Vet Dermatol.* 2018;29:262.
63. Simpson AC. Successful treatment of otodemodicosis due to Demodex cati with sarolaner/selamectin topical solution in a cat. *JFMS Open Rep.* 2021:7: 2055116920984386.
64. Souza CP, Schissler JR, Contreras ET, et al. Evaluation of immunological parameters in pit bull terrier-type dogs with juvenile onset generalized demodicosis and age-matched healthy pit bull terrier-type dogs. *Vet Dermatol.* 2018;29:482-e162.
65. Pekmezci D, Pekmezci GZ, Guzel M, et al. Efficacy of amitraz plus inactivated parapoxvirus ovis in the treatment of canine generalised demodicosis. *Vet Rec.* 2014;174:556.
66. Mueller RS, Shipstone MA. Update on the diagnosis and treatment of canine demodicosis (workshop report). In: Torres SMF, Roudebush P, eds. *Advances in Veterinary Dermatology.* Vol. 8. Wiley Online Books; 2017:206–207. Available at: https://onlinelibrary.wiley.com/doi/book/10.1002/9781119278368.
67. Colombo S, Leone F, Vercelli A, Cornegliani L. Monthly application of 10 % moxidectin and 2.5 % imidacloprid spot-on to prevent relapses in generalised demodicosis: a pilot study. *Vet Rec.* 2012;171:272.
68. Djuric M, Milcic Matic N, Davitkov D, et al. Efficacy of oral fluralaner for the treatment of canine generalized demodicosis: a molecular-level confirmation. *Parasit Vectors.* 2019;12:270.
69. Charach MG. Demodicosis: new treatment, common misdiagnosis. *Can Vet J.* 2018;59:545–547.
70. Chang YS, Huang YC. Role of *Demodex* mite infestation in rosacea: a systematic review and meta–analysis. *J Am Acad Dermatol.* 2017;77:441–447,e6.
71. Foley R, Kelly P, Gatault S, Powell F. *Demodex*: a skin resident in man and his best friend. *J Eur Acad Dermatol Venereol.* 2021;35:62–72.
72. Arlian LG, Morgan MS. A review of *Sarcoptes scabiei*: past, present and future. *Parasit Vectors.* 2017;10:297.
73. Brewster K, Henke SE, Hilton C, et al. Use of remote cameras to monitor the potential prevalence of sarcoptic mange in southern Texas, USA. *J Wildl Dis.* 2017;53:377–381.
74. Hardy JI, Sinclair G, Fox MT, Loeffler A. Feline sarcoptic mange in the UK: a case report. *Vet Rec.* 2012;171:351.
75. Curtis C, Paradis M. Sarcoptic mange, cheyletiellosis and trombiculosis. In: Foster AP, Foil CS, eds. *BSAVA Manual of Small Animal Dermatology.* Gloucester: British Small Animal Veterinary Association; 2003:146–149.
76. Feather L, Gough K, Flynn RJ, Elsheikha HM. A retrospective investigation into risk factors of sarcoptic mange in dogs. *Parasitol Res.* 2010;107:279–283.
77. Arlian LG. Biology, host relations, and epidemiology of *Sarcoptes scabiei. Annu Rev Entomol.* 1989;34:139–161.
78. Nwufoh OC, Sadiq AN, Emikpe BO. The seroprevalence of *Sarcoptes scabiei* var. *canis* and its associated risk factors in dogs in Ibadan, Southwest Nigeria. *J Immunoassay Immunochem.* 2019;40:473–484.
79. Nagamori Y, Payton ME, Looper E, et al. Retrospective survey of endoparasitism identified in feces of client-owned dogs in North America from 2007 through 2018. *Vet Parasitol.* 2020;282:109137.
80. Little SE, Davidson WR, Howerth EW, et al. Diseases diagnosed in red foxes from the southeastern United States. *J Wildl Dis.* 1998;34:620–624.
81. Morgan MS, Arlian LG, Markey MP. *Sarcoptes scabiei* mites modulate gene expression in human skin equivalents. *PLoS One.* 2013;8:e71143.
82. Morris DO, Dunstan RW. A histomorphological study of sarcoptic acariasis in the dog: 19 cases. *J Am Anim Hosp Assoc.* 1996;32:119–124.
83. Arlian LG, Morgan MS, Rapp CM, Vyszenski-Moher DL. The development of protective immunity in canine scabies. *Vet Parasitol.* 1996;62:133–142.
84. Mika A, Reynolds SL, Pickering D, et al. Complement inhibitors from scabies mites promote streptococcal growth - a novel mechanism in infected epidermis? *PLoS Negl Trop Dis.* 2012;6:e1563.
85. Swe PM, Fischer K. A scabies mite serpin interferes with complement-mediated neutrophil functions and promotes staphylococcal growth. *PLoS Negl Trop Dis.* 2014;8:e2928.
86. Arlian LG, Morgan MS, Estes SA, et al. Circulating IgE in patients with ordinary and crusted scabies. *J Med Entomol.* 2004;41:74–77.
87. Taenzler J, Liebenberg J, Roepke RK, et al. Efficacy of fluralaner administered either orally or topically for the treatment of naturally acquired *Sarcoptes scabiei* var. *canis* infestation in dogs. *Parasit Vectors.* 2016;9:392.
88. Chiummo R, Petersen I, Plehn C, et al. Efficacy of orally and topically administered fluralaner for treatment of client-owned dogs with sarcoptic mange under field conditions. *Parasit Vectors.* 2020;13:524.
89. Kaltsogianni F, Farmaki R, Koutinas AF. Norwegian or crusted sarcoptic mange in two leishmanial dogs. *J Am Anim Hosp Assoc.* 2017;53:326–330.
90. Malik R, McKellar Stewart K, et al. Crusted scabies (sarcoptic mange) in four cats due to *Sarcoptes scabiei* infestation. *J Feline Med Surg.* 2006;8:327–339.
91. Lower KS, Medleau LM, Hnilica K, Bigler B. Evaluation of an enzyme-linked immunosorbent assay (ELISA) for the serological diagnosis of sarcoptic mange in dogs. *Vet Dermatol.* 2001;12:315–320.

92. Arlian LG, Morgan MS. Serum antibody to *Sarcoptes scabiei* and house dust mite prior to and during infestation with *S. scabiei*. *Vet Parasitol.* 2000;90:315–326.
93. Schumann RJ, Morgan MS, Glass R, Arlian LG. Characterization of house dust mite and scabies mite allergens by use of canine serum antibodies. *Am J Vet Res.* 2001;62:1344–1348.
94. Arlian LG, Morgan MS, Rapp CM, Vyszenski-Moher DL. Some effects of sarcoptic mange on dogs. *J Parasitol.* 1995;81:698–702.
95. Becskei C, De Bock F, Illambas J, et al. Efficacy and safety of a novel oral isoxazoline, sarolaner for the treatment of sarcoptic mange in dogs. *Vet Parasitol.* 2016;222:56–61.
96. Beugnet F, de Vos C, Liebenberg J, et al. Efficacy of afoxolaner in a clinical field study in dogs naturally infested with *Sarcoptes scabiei*. *Parasite.* 2016;23:26.
97. Romero-Núñez C, Bautista-Gómez LG, Sheinberg G, et al. Efficacy of afoxolaner plus milbemycin oxime and afoxolaner alone as treatment for sarcoptic mange in naturally infested dogs. *Can J Vet Res.* 2020;84:212–216.
98. Day MJ. Pet-related infections. *Am Fam Physician.* 2016;94:794–802.
99. Leung AKC, Lam JM, Leong KF. Scabies: a neglected global disease. *Curr Pediatr Rev.* 2020;16:33–42.
100. Amato E, Dansie LS, Grøneng GM, et al. Increase of scabies infestations, Norway, 2006 to 2018. *Euro Surveill.* 2019;24:190020.
101. Thomas C, Coates SJ, Engelman D, et al. Ectoparasites: scabies. *J Am Acad Dermatol.* 2020;82:533–548.
102. Burroughs RF, Elston DM. What's eating you? Canine scabies. *Cutis.* 2003;72:107–109.
103. Foley J, Serieys LE, Stephenson N, et al. A synthetic review of *Notoedres* spp. mites and mange. *Parasitology.* 2016;143:1847–1861.
104. Leone F. Canine notoedric mange: a case report. *Vet Dermatol.* 2007;18:127–129.
105. Lefkaditis MA, Sossidou AV, Panorias AH, et al. Urban stray cats infested by ectoparasites with zoonotic potential in Greece. *Parasitol Res.* 2015;114:3931–3934.
106. Beugnet F, Bourdeau P, Chalvet-Monfray K, et al. Parasites of domestic owned cats in Europe: co-infestations and risk factors. *Parasit Vectors.* 2014;7:291.
107. Sampaio KO, de Oliveira LM, Burmann PM, et al. Acetate tape impression test for diagnosis of notoedric mange in cats. *J Feline Med Surg.* 2017;19:702–705.
108. Foley RH. A notoedric mange epizootic in an island's cat population. *Feline Prac.* 1991;19:8–10.
109. Pence DB, Matthews FD 3rd, Windberg LA. Notoedric mange in the bobcat, *Felis rufus*, from south Texas. *J Wildl Dis.* 1982;18:47–50.
110. Klein Serieys LE, Foley J, Owens S, et al. Serum chemistry, hematologic and post-mortem findings in bobcats (*Lynx rufus*) with notoedric mange. *J Parasitol.* 2013;99:989–996.
111. Wyrosdick HM, Chapman A, Martinez J, Schaefer JJ. Parasite prevalence survey in shelter cats in Citrus County, Florida. *Vet Parasitol Reg Stud Reports.* 2017;10:20–24.
112. Stephenson N, Clifford D, Worth SJ, et al. Development and validation of a fecal PCR assay for *Notoedres cati* and application to notoedric mange cases in bobcats (*Lynx rufus*) in Northern California, USA. *J Wildl Dis.* 2013;49:303–311.
113. Serieys LE, Foley J, Owens S, et al. Serum chemistry, hematologic, and post-mortem findings in free-ranging bobcats (*Lynx rufus*) with notoedric mange. *J Parasitol.* 2013;99:989–996.
114. Knaus M, Capári B, Visser M. Therapeutic efficacy of Broadline against notoedric mange in cats. *Parasitol Res.* 2014;113:4303–4306.
115. Itoh N, Muraoka N, Aoki M, Itagaki T. Treatment of *Notoedres cati* infestation in cats with selamectin. *Vet Rec.* 2004;154:409.
116. Hellmann K, Petry G, Capari B, et al. Treatment of naturally *Notoedres cati*-infested cats with a combination of imidacloprid 10 % / moxidectin 1 % spot-on (Advocate® / Advantage® multi, Bayer). *Parasitol Res.* 2013;112(suppl 1):57–66.
117. Dryden MW, Payne P. Preventing parasites in cats. *Vet Ther.* 2005;6:260–267.
118. Sivajothi S, Sudhakara Reddy B, et al. *Notoedres cati* in cats and its management. *J Parasit Dis.* 2015;39:303–305.
119. Otranto D, Milillo P, Mesto P, et al. *Otodectes cynotis* (Acari: Psoroptidae): examination of survival off-the-host under natural and laboratory conditions. *Exp Appl Acarol.* 2004;32:171–179.
120. Yang C, Huang HP. Evidence-based veterinary dermatology: a review of published studies of treatments for *Otodectes cynotis* (ear mite) infestation in cats. *Vet Dermatol.* 2016;27:221–e56.
121. Akucewich LH, Philman K, Clark A, et al. Prevalence of ectoparasites in a population of feral cats from north central Florida during the summer. *Vet Parasitol.* 2002;109:129–139.
122. Tyler S, Swales N, Foster AP, et al. Otoscopy and aural cytological findings in a population of rescue cats and cases in a referral small animal hospital in England and Wales. *J Feline Med Surg.* 2020;22:161–167.
123. Sotiraki ST, Koutinas AF, Leontides LS, et al. Factors affecting the frequency of ear canal and face infestation by *Otodectes cynotis* in the cat. *Vet Parasitol.* 2001;96:309–315.
124. Itoh N, Itoh S. Prevalence of *Otodectes cynotis* infestation in household cats. *J Japan Vet Med Assoc.* 2002;55:155–158.
125. Lefkaditis MA, Koukeri SE, Mihalca AD. Prevalence and intensity of *Otodectes cynotis* in kittens from Thessaloniki area, Greece. *Vet Parasitol.* 2009;163:374–375.
126. Shukullari E, Rapti D, Visser M, et al. Parasites and vector-borne diseases in client-owned dogs in Albania: infestation with arthropod ectoparasites. *Parasitol Res.* 2017;116:399–407.
127. Souza CP, Ramadinha RR, Scott FB, Pereira MJS. Factors associated with the prevalence of *Otodectes cynotis* in an ambulatory population of dogs. *Pesqui Vet Bras.* 2008;28:375–378.
128. Le Sueur C, Bour S, Schaper R. Efficacy and safety of the combination imidacloprid 10 % / moxidectin 1.0 % spot-on in the treatment of ear mite infection (*Otodectes cynotis*) in ferrets. *Parasitol Res.* 2011;109(suppl 1):S149–S156.
129. Briceño C, González-Acuña D, Jiménez JE, et al. Ear mites, *Otodectes cynotis*, on wild foxes (*Pseudalopex* spp.) in Chile. *J Wildl Dis.* 2020;56:105–112.
130. Perrucci S, Verin R, Mancianti F, Poli A. Sarcoptic mange and other ectoparasitic infections in a red fox (*Vulpes vulpes*) population from central Italy. *Parasite Epidemiol Control.* 2016;1:66–71.
131. Moriarty ME, Vickers TW, Clifford DL, et al. Ear mite removal in the Santa Catalina Island Fox (*Urocyon littoralis catalinae*): controlling risk factors for cancer development. *PLoS One.* 2015;10:e0144271.
132. Gunnarsson E, Hersteinsson P, Adalsteinsson S. Prevalence and geographical distribution of the ear canker mite (*Otodectes cynotis*) among arctic foxes (*Alopex lagopus*) in Iceland. *J Wildl Dis.* 1991;27:105–109.
133. Wall R, Shearer D, eds. *Veterinary Ectoparasites: Biology, Pathology and Control.* 2nd ed. Oxford, London: USA Blackwell Sciences, Iowa State University; 2001:262.
134. Perego R, Proverbio D, Bagnagatti De Giorgi G, et al. Prevalence of otitis externa in stray cats in northern Italy. *J Feline Med Surg.* 2014;16:483–490.
135. Roy J, Bédard C, Moreau M. Treatment of feline otitis externa due to *Otodectes cynotis* and complicated by secondary bacterial and fungal infections with Oridermyl auricular ointment. *Can Vet J.* 2011;52:277–282.
136. Combarros D, Boncea AM, Brément T, et al. Comparison of three methods for the diagnosis of otoacariasis due to *Otodectes cynotis* in dogs and cats. *Vet Dermatol.* 2019;30:334-e96.
137. Saridomichelakis MN, Koutinas AF, Gioulekas D, et al. *Sensitization to Dust Mites in Cats with Otodectes Cynotis Infestation.* University of Thessaly Institutional Repository; 1999. Available at: https://ir.lib.uth.gr/xmlui/handle/11615/32878.
138. Powell MB, Weisbroth SH, Roth L, Wilhelmsen C. Reaginic hypersensitivity in *Otodectes cynotis* infestation of cats and mode of mite feeding. *Am J Vet Res.* 1980;41:877–882.
139. Six RH, Clemence RG, Thomas CA, et al. Efficacy and safety of selamectin against *Sarcoptes scabiei* on dogs and *Otodectes cynotis* on dogs and cats presented as veterinary patients. *Vet Parasitol.* 2000;91:291–309.
140. Arther RG, Davis WL, Jacobsen JA, et al. Clinical evaluation of the safety and efficacy of 10% imidacloprid + 2.5% moxidectin topical solution for the treatment of ear mite (*Otodectes cynotis*) infestations in dogs. *Vet Parasitol.* 2015;210:64–68.

141. Nunn-Brooks L, Michael R, Ravitz LB, et al. Efficacy of a single dose of an otic ivermectin preparation or selamectin for the treatment of *Otodectes cynotis* infestation in naturally infected cats. *J Feline Med Surg.* 2011;13:622–624.
142. Six RH, Becskei C, Mazaleski MM, et al. Efficacy of sarolaner, a novel oral isoxazoline, against two common mite infestations in dogs: *Demodex* spp. and *Otodectes cynotis. Vet Parasitol.* 2016;222:62–66.
143. Carithers D, Crawford J, de Vos C, et al. Assessment of afoxolaner efficacy against *Otodectes cynotis* infestations of dogs. *Parasit Vectors.* 2016;9:635.
144. Becskei C, Reinemeyer C, King VL, et al. Efficacy of a new spot-on formulation of selamectin plus sarolaner in the treatment of *Otodectes cynotis* in cats. *Vet Parasitol.* 2017;238(suppl 1):S27–S30.
145. Machado MA, Campos DR, Lopes NL, et al. Efficacy of afoxolaner in the treatment of otodectic mange in naturally infested cats. *Vet Parasitol.* 2018;256:29–31.
146. Taenzler J, de Vos C, Roepke RK, et al. Efficacy of fluralaner against *Otodectes cynotis* infestations in dogs and cats. *Parasit Vectors.* 2017;10:30.
147. Taenzler J, de Vos C, Roepke RKA, Heckeroth AR. Efficacy of fluralaner plus moxidectin against *Otodectes cynotis* infestations in cats. *Parasit Vectors.* 2018;11:595.
148. Bosco A, Leone F, Vascone R, et al. Efficacy of fluralaner spot-on solution for the treatment of *Ctenocephalides felis* and *Otodectes cynotis* mixed infestation in naturally infested cats. *BMC Vet Res.* 2019;15:28.
149. Meekins JM, Guess SC, Rankin AJ. Retinopathy associated with ivermectin toxicosis in five cats. *J Am Vet Med Assoc.* 2015;246:1238–1241.
150. Nuttall T, Cole LK. Ear cleaning: the UK and US perspective. *Vet Dermatol.* 2004;15:127–136.
151. Weisbroth SH, Powell MB, Roth L, Scher S. Immunopathology of naturally occurring otodectic otoacariasis in the domestic cat. *JAVMA.* 1974;165:1088–1093.
152. Beugnet F, Bouhsira E, Halos L, Franc M. Preventive efficacy of a topical combination of fipronil--(S)-methoprene--eprinomectin--praziquantel against ear mite (*Otodectes cynotis*) infestation of cats through a natural infestation model. *Parasite.* 2014;21:40.
153. Van de Heyning J, Thienpont D. Otitis externa in man caused by the mite *Otodectes cynotis. Laryngoscope.* 1977;87:1938–1941.
154. Herwick RP. Lesions caused by canine ear mites. *Arch Dermatol.* 1978;114:130.
155. Lund EM, Armstrong PJ, Kirk CA, et al. Health status and population characteristics of dogs and cats examined at private veterinary practices in the United States. *J Am Vet Med Assoc.* 1999;214:1336–1341.
156. Fanelli A, Doménech G, Alonso F, et al. *Otodectes cynotis* in urban and peri-urban semi-arid areas: a widespread parasite in the cat population. *J Parasit Dis.* 2020;44:481–485.
157. Montoya A, García M, Gálvez R, et al. Implications of zoonotic and vector-borne parasites to free-roaming cats in central Spain. *Vet Parasitol.* 2018;251:125–130.
158. Thomas JE, Staubus L, Goolsby JL, Reichard MV. Ectoparasites of free-roaming domestic cats in the central United States. *Vet Parasitol.* 2016;228:17–22.
159. Xhaxhiu D, Kusi I, Rapti D, et al. Ectoparasites of dogs and cats in Albania. *Parasitol Res.* 2009;105:1577–1587.
160. Mosallanejad B, Alborzi A, Katvandi N. A survey on ectoparasite infestations in companion dogs of Ahvaz District, southwest of Iran. *J Arthropod Borne Dis.* 2012;6:70–78.
161. Chee JH, Kwon JK, Cho HS, et al. A survey of ectoparasite infestations in stray dogs of Gwang-ju City, Republic of Korea. *Korean J Parasitol.* 2008;46:23–27.
162. Rodriguez-Vivas RI, Ortega-Pacheco A, Rosado-Aguilar JA, Bolio GM. Factors affecting the prevalence of mange mite infestations in stray dogs of Yucatán, Mexico. *Vet Parasitol.* 2003;115:61–65.
163. Bredal W, Vollset I. Use of milbemycin oxime in the treatment of dogs with nasal mite (*Pneumonyssoides caninum*) infection. *J Small Anim Pract.* 1998;39:126–130.
164. Rehbinder C, Christensson D, Bornstein S, et al. Undersnrkning av ett obduktionsmaterial - *Pneumonyssus caninum* - ett kvalster i huvudets luftvagar hos hund. *Svensk Ver.* 1994;46:489–495.
165. Gunnarsson LK, Zakrisson G, Egenvall A, et al. Prevalence of *Pneumonyssoides caninum* infection in dogs in Sweden. *J Am Anim Hosp Assoc.* 2001;37:331–337.
166. Brandt RW. *Pneumonyssus caninum* (nasal mite) in four Golden Retrievers. *Can Vet J.* 1988;29:741.
167. McClelland RB, McClelland FE Jr. *Pneumonyssus caninum* in a dog in Western New York. *Cornell Vet.* 1952;42:337–338.
168. Blagburn BL, Didier PJ, Todd KS. *Pneumonyssoides caninum* in a dog. Veterinary Medicine. *Small Animal Clinician.* 1982;77:768–769.
169. Wills SJ, Arrese M, Torrance A, et al. *Pneumonyssoides* species infestation in two Pekingese dogs in the UK. *J Small Anim Pract.* 2008;49:107–109.
170. Gunnarsson L, Zakrisson G, Lilliehook I, et al. Experimental infection of dogs with the nasal mite *Pneumonyssoides caninum. Vet Parasitol.* 1998;77:179–186.
171. Gunnarsson L, Zakrisson G, Christensson D, Uggla A. Efficacy of selamectin in the treatment of nasal mite (*Pneumonyssoides caninum*) infection in dogs. *J Am Anim Hosp Assoc.* 2004;40:400–404.
172. Ketzis JK, Dundas J, Shell LG. *Lynxacarus radovskyi* mites in feral cats: a study of diagnostic methods, preferential body locations, co-infestations and prevalence. *Vet Dermatol.* 2016;27:425-e108.
173. Han HS, Chua HL, Nellinathan G. Self-induced, noninflammatory alopecia associated with infestation with *Lynxacarus radovskyi*: a series of 11 cats. *Vet Dermatol.* 2019;30:356-e103.
174. Han HS. A survey of the prevalence of *Lynxacarus radovskyi* in cats in Malaysia. *Vet Dermatol.* 2015;26:68.
175. da Rocha CM, Farias PCG, Gorza L, et al. Association between infestation by *Lynxacarus radovskyi* (Acari: Lystrophoridae) and the occurrence of feline eosinophilic granuloma complex. *J Parasit Dis.* 2019;43:726–729.
176. Han HS, Noli C, Cena T. Efficacy and duration of action of oral fluralaner and spot-on moxidectin/imidacloprid in cats infested with *Lynxacarus radovskyi. Vet Dermatol.* 2016;27:474-e127.
177. Campos DR, Chaves JKO, Assis RCP, et al. Efficacy of oral sarolaner against *Lynxacarus radovskyi* in naturally infested cats. *Vet Dermatol.* 2020;31:355-e92.
178. Foley RH. Parasitic mites of dogs and cats. *Comp Cont Ed Pract Vet.* 1991;13:783–800.
179. Hardison JL. A case of *Eutrombicula alfreddugesi* (chiggers) in a cat. *Vet Med Small Anim Clin.* 1977;72:47.
180. Lowenstine LJ, Carpenter JL, OConnor BM. Trombiculosis in a cat. *J Am Vet Med Assoc.* 1979;175:289-2.
181. Heyne H, Ueckermann EA, Coetzee L. First report of a parasitic mite, *Leptotrombidium* (Hypotrombidium) *subquadratum* (Lawerence) (Acari: Trombiculidae: Trombiculinae), from dogs and children in the Bloemfontein area, South Africa. *J S Afr Vet Assoc.* 2001;72:105–106.
182. Giannoulopoulos GD, Desilla LJ, Desilla ES, et al. First report of *Neotrombicula autumnalis* infestation in a cat and a dog from Corfu (Greece) and in a cat from Limassol (Cyprus). *Vector Borne Zoonotic Dis.* 2012;12:1065–1067.
183. Stekolnikov AA, Waap H, Gomes J, Antunes T. Chigger mites of the genus *Ericotrombidium* (Acariformes: Trombiculidae) attacking pets in Europe. *Vet Parasitol.* 2016;221:60–63.
184. Areso Apesteguía M, Areso Portell JB, Halaihel Kassab N, Gracia Salinas MJ. Severe trombiculiasis in hunting dogs infested with *Neotrombicula inopinata* (Acari: Trombiculidae). *J Med Entomol.* 2019;56:1389–1394.
185. Ramilo DW, Costa P, Stekolnikov AA, et al. First report of *Ericotrombidium ibericense* in domestic dogs. *Acta Parasitol.* 2021;66:253–258.
186. Cousandier G, Bassini-Silva R, Huang-Bastos M, et al. First record of *Eutrombicula tinami* (Oudemans, 1910) (Trombidiformes: Trombiculidae) parasitizing a cat in Brazil. *Parasitol Res.* 2021;120:337–339.
187. Mullen GR, O'Connor BM. Mites. In: Mullen G, Durden L, eds. *Medical and Veterinary Entomology.* 3rd ed. Academic Press; 2018:533–602.
188. Stekolnikov AA, Santibáñez P, Palomar AM, et al. *Neotrombicula inopinata* (Acari: Trombiculidae)–a possible causative agent of trombiculiasis in Europe. *Parasit Vectors.* 2014;7:1–9.
189. Le Net JL, Fain A, George C, et al. Straelensiosis in dogs: a newly described nodular dermatitis induced by *Straelensia cynotis. Vet Rec.* 2002;150:205–209.

190. Seixas F, Travassos PJ, Pinto ML, et al. Dermatitis in a dog induced by *Straelensia cynotis*: a case report and review of the literature. *Vet Dermatol.* 2006;17:81–84.
191. Ramírez GA, Altimira J, García B, et al. Clinical, histopathological and epidemiological study of canine straelensiosis in the Iberian Peninsula (2003-2007). *Vet Dermatol.* 2009;20:35–41.
192. Vercelli A, Cornegliani L. First report of *Straelensia cynotis* in a dog in Italy: dermatological lesions, diagnostic approach and treatment of an unusual ectoparasitosis. *Veterinaria (Cremona).* 2011;25:33–38.
193. Kaufmann R, Bourdeau P, Waldman L, et al. Straelensiosis in two cats and ten dogs from Israel. *J Small Anim Pract.* 2015;56:723–727.
194. Santibáñez P, Palomar AM, Portillo A, et al. The role of chiggers as human pathogens. In: *An Overview of Tropical Diseases.* Intech Open Limited; 2015:173–202.
195. Schöler A, Maier WA, Kampen H. Multiple environmental factor analysis in habitats of the harvest mite *Neotrombicula autumnalis* (Acari: Trombiculidae) suggests extraordinarily high euryoecious biology. *Exp Appl Acarol.* 2006;39:41–62.
196. McGarry JW, Hansen R, Greene S. Canine trombiculosis and seasonal canine illness. *Vet Rec.* 2012;171:406.
197. Clopton RE, Gold RE. Distribution and seasonal and diurnal activity patterns of *Eutrombicula alfreddugesi* (Acari: Trombiculidae) in a forest edge ecosystem. *J Med Entomol.* 1993;30:47–53.
198. Leone F, Di Bella A, Vercelli A, Cornegliani L. Feline trombiculosis: a retrospective study in 72 cats. *Vet Dermatol.* 2013;24:535-e126.
199. Prosl H, Rabitsch A, Brabenetz J. Trombiculid mite--*Neotrombicula autumnalis* (Shaw 1790)--in veterinary medicine. Nervous systems in dogs following massive infestation. *Tierarztl Prax.* 1985;13:57–64.
200. Santibáñez P, Gallo E, Palomar AM, Portillo A, et al. Trombiculiasis in a dog with severe neurologic disorders, Spain. *Emerg Infect Dis.* 2020;26:819–820.
201. Font A. Straelensiosis in a dog in Spain. *Vet Dermatol.* 2007;18:67–68.
202. Nuttall TJ, French AT, Cheetham HC, Proctor FJ. Treatment of *Trombicula autumnalis* infestation in dogs and cats with a 0.25 per cent fipronil pump spray. *J Small Anim Pract.* 1998;39:237–239.
203. Leone F, Albanese F. Efficacy of selamectin spot-on formulation against *Neotrombicula autumnalis* in eight cats. *Vet Dermatol.* 2004;15(suppl 1). 49-10.
204. Fisher MA, Shanks DJ. A review of the off-label use of selamectin (Stronghold/Revolution) in dogs and cats. *Acta Vet Scand.* 2008;50:46.
205. Cadiergues MC, Navarro C, Castilla-Castaño E, et al. Treatment of *Neotrombicula* species infestation in cats using a 10% (w/v) fipronil topical spot-on formulation: a pilot study. *J Feline Med Surg.* 2018;20:587–590.
206. Smal D, Jasmin P, Mercier P. Treatment of *Neotrombicula autumnalis* dermatitis in dogs using two topical permethrin-pyriproxyfen combinations. *J Small Anim Pract.* 2004;45:98–103.
207. Lecru LA, Combarros D, Castilla-Castaño E, et al. Treatment of harvest mite infestation in dogs using a permethrin 54.5% and fipronil 6.1% (Effitix®) topical spot-on formulation. *Vet Sci.* 2019;6:100.
208. Guarneri F, Pugliese A, Giudice E, et al. Trombiculiasis: clinical contribution. *Eur J Dermatol.* 2005;15:495–496.
209. Parcell BJ, Sharpe S, Jones B, Alexander CL. Conjunctivitis induced by a red bodied mite, *Neotrombicula autumnalis*. *Parasite.* 2013;20:25.

Heartworm and Related Nematodes

C. Thomas Nelson

KEY POINTS

- First Described: Heartworm was first described in dogs in Italy in 1626[1] and in the United States in 1847.[2]
- Cause: *Dirofilaria immitis,* belonging to the superfamily Filarioidea and family Onchocercidae. A related nematode, *Dirofilaria repens,* is found in southern and central Europe, Africa, and Asia but is not currently endemic in North America.
- Affected Hosts: Although canids (domestic dogs, coyotes, foxes, wolves, and other wild canids) are the definitive hosts for heartworms, the parasite has been found in more than 30 species of animals, including domestic cats and wild felids, bears, ferrets, seals, sea lions, and humans.
- Intermediate Hosts: There are multiple mosquito vectors in every region of the United States. More than 70 species of mosquitoes have been shown to be capable of transmitting heartworms; 25 species have been proven to be significant vectors.
- Geographic Distribution: Heartworm is endemic in North, Central, and South America; the Caribbean Islands; the coastal regions of Africa, southern Europe, and Asia; Japan; Indonesia; and Australia.
- Route of Transmission: Female mosquitoes feeding on a microfilaremic canine host ingest microfilariae. The ingested microfilariae undergo a transformation and two molts over a 2- to 4-week period to become infective third-stage larvae (L_3). The L_3 are then deposited on a dog's skin in a droplet of hemolymph by a feeding female mosquito. The L_3 enter through the bite wound into the subcutaneous tissue.
- Major Clinical Signs: Signs of heartworm disease can range from a cough and exercise intolerance to dyspnea, abnormal heart and lung sounds, hepatomegaly, syncope, ascites, and death.
- Differential Diagnoses: These include primary pulmonary diseases (pneumonia, chronic bronchitis, allergic lung disease), pulmonary thromboembolism, pulmonary hypertension, and right-sided heart failure.
- Human Health Significance: *Dirofilaria immitis* is of public health concern even though the number of reports of infection in humans is relatively small. The most common clinical syndrome reported in human infections is the formation of a pulmonary nodule or nodules within the lung parenchyma.

CANINE HEARTWORM DISEASE

ETIOLOGIC AGENT AND EPIDEMIOLOGY

Heartworm disease is caused by the parasitic filarial nematode *Dirofilaria immitis,* belonging to the superfamily Filarioidea and family Onchocercidae. Nine filarial nematode species infect dogs worldwide, and three have been diagnosed in the United States: *D. immitis, Dirofilaria repens,* and *Acanthocheilonema reconditum* (formerly *Dipetalonema reconditum*). Only *D. immitis* and *A. reconditum* are considered endemic, but conditions exist for *D. repens* to become established. Heartworm was first described in dogs in Italy in 1626[1] and in the United States in 1847.[2] Although canids (domestic dogs, coyotes, foxes, wolves, and other wild canids) are the definitive hosts for heartworms, the parasite has been found in more than 30 species of animals, including domestic cats and wild felids, bears, ferrets, seals, sea lions, and humans. There has even been one confirmed case in a bird.[3] Information specific to the cat is presented in the second part of this chapter.

Heartworms are endemic in North, Central, and South America; the Caribbean Islands; the coastal regions of Africa, southern Europe, and Asia; Japan; Indonesia; and Australia.[4,5] In the United States, heartworm has progressed from being a parasitic disease primarily in the southeast to being diagnosed in all 50 states (Fig. 111.1). Alaska is the only state in which transmission has not been documented; however, there are mosquito vectors and climatic conditions present in regions of central Alaska to support the transmission of heartworms for brief periods.[6] The yearly incidence of identified cases of canine heartworm infection continues to rise despite the availability of many chemoprophylactic drugs. The increased incidence has been prominent in the western half of the United States over the past 30 years. Two factors are likely responsible: (1) heartworm-infected dogs have been relocated to western regions as humans have moved from endemic areas, thus establishing a reservoir of infection, and (2) mosquito habitats have been created as a result of irrigation of newly developed areas and the subsequent influx of suitable vector mosquitoes. A sylvatic cycle has developed in the coyote population, as the rate of heartworm infection is over 90% in many western areas.[7] The prevalence of infection elsewhere in the United States varies by region with over 90% of unprotected dogs along the Gulf Coast, lower Atlantic Coast, and Mississippi River valley being infected.[8] The severity of clinical illness also varies by region. The worm biomass in an infected dog is typically higher in dogs coming from the high-prevalence areas just listed. However, there are isolated pockets of infection with high prevalence and severity of infection throughout the United States.

The natural cycle and transmission of heartworms requires a reservoir of infection, a competent mosquito vector, and favorable climatic conditions. Unprotected domestic and feral dogs as well as wild canids serve as the reservoir hosts. Relocation of heartworm-infected dogs and expansion of the territories of microfilaremic wild canids into other areas continue to precipitate the spread of heartworms.

There are multiple mosquito vectors in every region of the United States.[9] More than 70 species of mosquitoes have been shown to be capable of transmitting heartworms; 25 species have been proven to be significant vectors. Importation of new mosquito species into an area, environmental changes created by humans, and natural climatic conditions can affect heartworm transmission. *Aedes albopictus* (Asian tiger mosquito), originally introduced into southeast Texas in 1985, has increased the exposure rate of dogs in many regions of the United States.[10] This mosquito can now be found in 35 states primarily in the Southeast, the Midwest, and the Atlantic seaboard as far north as New Jersey, southern New York, and Pennsylvania.[11] This large urban-dwelling mosquito can reproduce in small water-containing vessels such as flower pots. It voraciously feeds throughout the day, not just at dusk and dawn. The female lives for 3 months and is capable of overwintering. *Aedes albopictus* was introduced into Italy in 1990 and has spread over much of southern Europe, becoming a major vector of *D. immitis* and *D. repens*. *Aedes sierrensis* (western tree-hole mosquito) has had its geographic range extended in the western United States as a result of the continuing development of previously semiarid areas by the installation of irrigation systems and the planting of trees in new urban home sites.

Laboratory studies have determined that a minimum temperature of 57°F is necessary for the development of heartworm larvae to the infective third-stage larva (L_3).[12] This has led to the common practice of seasonal, rather than year-round, heartworm prevention in states north of the 37th parallel. Unfortunately, the heat island effect (Fig. 111.2) in urban areas can create microenvironments that are capable of supporting heartworm larva development even during winter months in northern states.[13] Furthermore, *Culex* spp. mosquitoes are competent vectors that are frequently found indoors. Therefore, transmission can continue even during cooler months in large indoor kennels. These factors along with the northward spread of *A. albopictus* have prompted the American Heartworm Society (AHS) to recommend year-round administration of heartworm preventive to dogs and cats in the continental United States and Hawaii.[14]

A knowledge of the heartworm life cycle is important for development and implementation of prevention and treatment strategies (Fig. 111.3). The life cycle of *D. immitis* is 7 to 9 months (210 to 270 days). Female mosquitoes feeding on a microfilaremic canine host ingest microfilariae. The ingested microfilariae then undergo a transformation into first-stage larvae (L_1) after entering a mosquito.[15] The L_1 will undergo two molts over the next 2 to 4 weeks, depending on the average ambient temperature, at which time they become infective L_3. The L_3 are then deposited on the dog's skin in a droplet of hemolymph by a feeding female mosquito (Fig. 111.3A). The L_3 enter through the bite wound into the subcutaneous tissue, where most L_3 molt to fourth-stage larvae (L_4) within a couple of days. The L_4 migrates in the subcutaneous tissue and muscle toward the thorax, and from approximately 50 to 70 days after initial infection L_4 undergo a final molt to juvenile worms. These juvenile worms subsequently penetrate the muscle tissue and eventually enter the circulation. Historically, the juvenile worm has been referred to as a fifth-stage larva (L_5). Because this stage does not undergo another molt, it should not be considered a larval stage. It is an immature or juvenile worm that matures into an adult over the next several months. After entering a peripheral vein, the blood then carries immature worms to and through the heart and into the

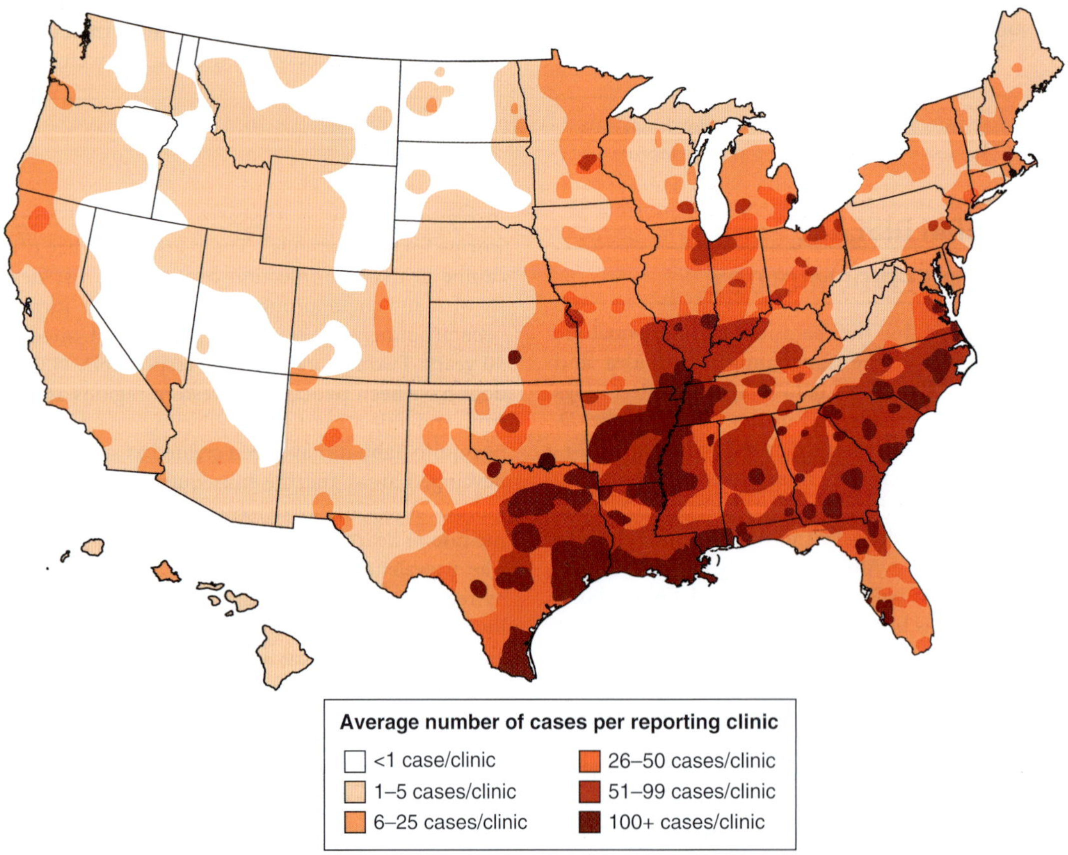

Fig. 111.1 Heartworm incidence in the United States, 2019. The severity of heartworm incidence as shown in this map is based on the average number of cases per reporting clinic. Some remote regions of the United States lack veterinary clinics; therefore, we have no reported cases from these areas. (Courtesy The American Heartworm Society.)

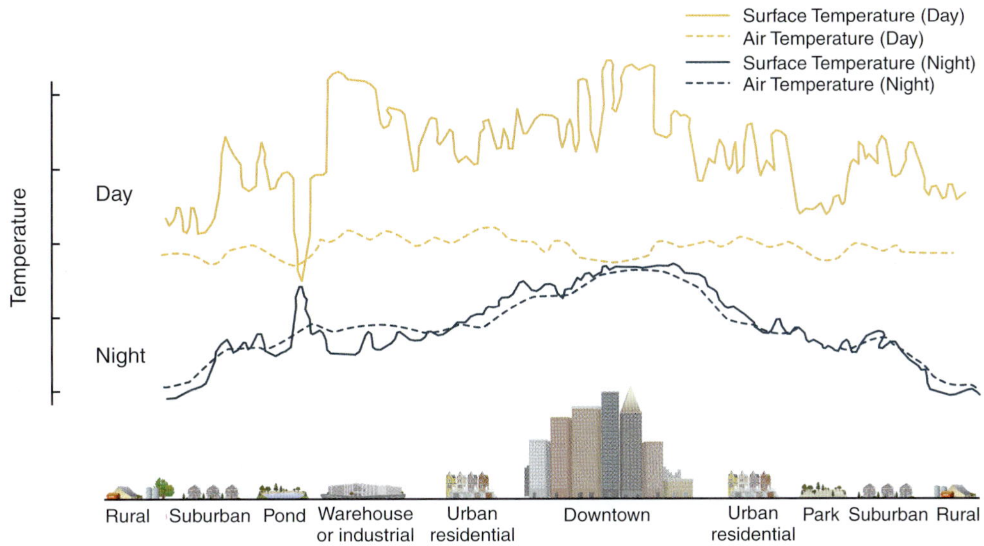

Fig. 111.2 The heat island effect in urban environments keeps urban temperatures relatively high compared to suburban and rural areas.

pulmonary arteries, arriving as early as 70 days PI.[16] By 120 days PI, virtually all juvenile worms have entered the pulmonary vasculature. Final maturation to adult worms and mating occurs in the pulmonary vessels. Microfilariae are then produced, typically around 180 to 210 days (but up to 270 days) PI, completing the life cycle. Mature adult males range from 15 to 18 cm in length and females from 25 to 30 cm with a life expectancy of 5 to 7 years.[17]

CLINICAL FEATURES

Pathogenesis and Clinical Signs

Heartworm infections primarily cause damage to the pulmonary arteries and lungs. Juvenile worms entering the pulmonary vasculature 3 months PI initiate an eosinophilia and eosinophilic pneumonitis.[18] Mature worms cause endothelial damage to pulmonary vessels, villous proliferation, and neutrophilic infiltrates in the vessel walls (Fig. 111.3B). Heartworms harbor the rickettsial endosymbiont *Wolbachia pipientis* that produces *Wolbachia* surface proteins (WSPs). These WSPs activate IL-8 transcription and stimulate chemokinesis in canine neutrophils.[19] In dogs infected with *D. immitis*, neutrophils accumulate in the pulmonary arterial walls and may help incite the pulmonary vasculature changes that develop. WSPs can be detected using IHC in glomerular capillaries from heartworm-infected dogs (Fig. 111.4) which suggests that glomerulonephropathy associated with heartworm disease may be the direct result of *D. immitis* that harbor *Wolbachia*.[20] The WSP also stimulates IL-10 and prostaglandin E_2 responses and IFN-γ production and IgG1 antibody responses in humans infected with *Onchocerca volvulus*, another filarial nematode that harbors *Wolbachia*.[21]

The severity of disease can be affected by the number of worms and the duration of the infection; but of equal importance, if not greater, is the activity level of the dog. Dogs in which 50 worms were surgically implanted and that were exercise-restricted took longer to develop clinical disease, and developed less pulmonary vascular resistance, than dogs infected with 14 heartworms that were allowed moderate activity.[22] This is also evident in naturally infected dogs in which there is no correlation between the number of heartworms and pulmonary vascular resistance, indicating that the individual host-parasite interaction plays an important role in the severity of disease.[22] Results of a subsequent study included similar findings in dogs being treated with melarsomine.[23] Whereas live heartworms can cause endarteritis and muscular hypertrophy of arteriole walls, primarily of the caudal pulmonary arteries, the pathologic changes seen in clinical disease are primarily the result of the effects of dying heartworms. As worms die from either natural causes or as a result of administration of adulticidal drugs, they decompose. Small worm fragments lodge in the distal pulmonary arteriole and capillary beds in the caudal lung lobes, blocking blood flow. These worm fragments, along with the inflammation that they elicit and platelet aggregation, result in pulmonary thromboembolism. During periods of increased activity or exercise, the increased blood flow to these blocked vessels can cause fragile capillaries to rupture with resultant pulmonary hemorrhage and subsequent fibrosis.[24] This fibrosis, along with the release of vasoactive substances by heartworms, leads to increased pulmonary vascular resistance and subsequent pulmonary hypertension.[25] The sequelae to these pulmonary vascular events is cor pulmonale and potential right-sided heart failure.

Ectopic lesions, due to aberrant migration of worms into the eye, CNS, abdominal cavity, and systemic circulation, can occur.[15] "Caval syndrome," which occurs in a small percentage of cases, results from heartworms located in the posterior vena cava and right atrium causing interference with tricuspid valve function (see Fig. 111.3C). Luminal obstruction, which can result in a peracute hemolytic crisis from traumatic injury to erythrocytes, contributes to the development of overt right-sided heart failure. "Caval syndrome" is usually associated with excessively large worm burdens in the right ventricle and atrium and may result from a combination of cardiac insufficiency and increased pulmonary vascular resistance, which allows the heartworms in the pulmonary artery to move back into the right heart. Glomerulonephropathy may also occur as a result of antigen-antibody complexes leading to proteinuria, and anemia, hemoglobinemia, and hemoglobinuria are often present (Table 111.1).

Many dogs infected with heartworms have no clinical signs, because dogs can tolerate live heartworms very well, especially if they are not very active. Factors that can affect the onset of clinical signs are the number of worms present in relationship to the size of the dog; the duration of infection; the individual host response to the parasite; and, most importantly, the activity level of the dog. Clinical signs usually develop gradually, with a mild cough being the most common sign noticed. This will be followed by exercise intolerance and an unthrifty appearance. Clinical signs associated with more advanced disease can

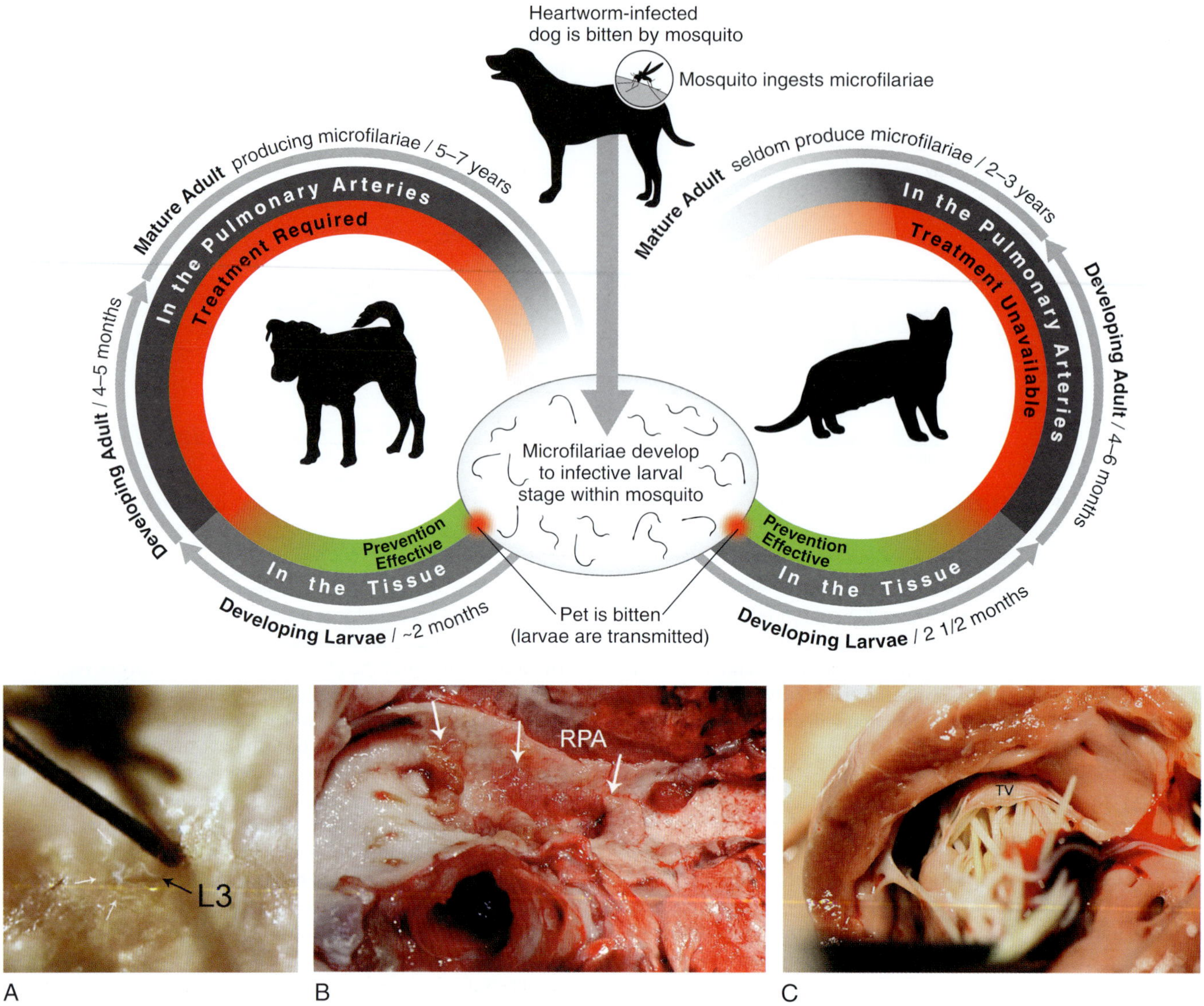

Fig. 111.3 Life cycle of heartworm infection. Microfilaria are ingested by the mosquito. After undergoing transformation to first-stage larvae (L_1), they undergo two molts over a period that can span 10 to 28 days, depending on ambient temperature. During this transformation, they first enter the malpighian tubules, then the body cavity, finally migrating toward the head and into the labium. (A) During feeding, the third-stage larvae (L_3) are deposited in a droplet of hemolymph (*white arrows*) on the animal's skin surface and migrate into subcutaneous tissue. In dogs, they molt into fourth-stage larvae (L_4) within 3 to 4 days post-infection (PI), and migrate in the subcutaneous tissue and muscle moving toward the thorax. L_4 molt into juvenile worms (sexually immature adult stage) within 50 to 70 days PI. Juvenile worms enter the venous circulation within the muscle tissue and between 70 and 120 days PI have migrated to the heart and pulmonary vasculature. The juvenile worm grows to a sexually mature adult during the range of 120 to 210 days PI, and female worms release increasing levels of antigen. *In dogs*, pulmonary vascular changes include blunting of the arteries, intraluminal thrombi and pulmonary hypertension (B). Adult worms usually reside in the pulmonary arteries and in severe infections, in the right side of the heart including the cranial and caudal vena cava (arrows indicate right pulmonary artery [RPA]). (C) A heart from a dog with caval syndrome as viewed from the right ventricle toward the tricuspid valve (*TV*). A mass of heartworms completely occludes the valve preventing it from closing. Right atrial, ventricular, and pulmonary artery enlargement are apparent. *In cats*, 90% to 95% of infections do not go past the juvenile stage, and 50% of cats have negative antibody titer results by 8 months. Dying immature worms produce heartworm-associated respiratory disease (HARD) syndrome consisting of occlusive hypertrophy of pulmonary arterioles, peribronchial infiltrates, and alveolar inflammatory infiltrates and consolidation. (A, Courtesy Boehringer Ingleheim; B, Photographic images courtesy of Stephen Jones, DVM.)

also develop acutely as a result of the natural death and disintegration of a heartworm that leads to sudden pulmonary thromboembolism. As the disease progresses and pulmonary pathology worsens, signs associated with right-sided heart involvement such as abnormal heart sounds and ascites appear.[15] Dogs that have experienced pulmonary thromboembolism from dead worms may be febrile and have hemoptysis. Those with caval syndrome present with acute, often profound, lethargy and weakness. Four classes of heartworm disease have been described with associated clinical signs (see Table 111.1). Classification of disease based on clinical severity has been used to determine treatment strategies and prognosis. However, although class 3 patients are statistically at a greater risk for severe complications and death after treatment, class 1 and 2 patients can experience the same levels of complications.[14] Dogs with caval syndrome (class 4) are severely ill and require surgery to survive.

Physical Examination Findings

Physical examination findings in dogs with heartworm disease may be normal in mild or early infections. Dogs may exhibit a thin body condition, tachypnea, dyspnea, a right-sided heart murmur from tricuspid insufficiency, cardiac gallop, and jugular distension with pulsation. Auscultation of lung fields could reveal pulmonary crackles primarily in the caudal lung lobes. Dogs with caval syndrome are severely lethargic, have pale mucous membranes and delayed capillary refill time, weak peripheral pulses, and often have dark urine due to hemoglobinuria.

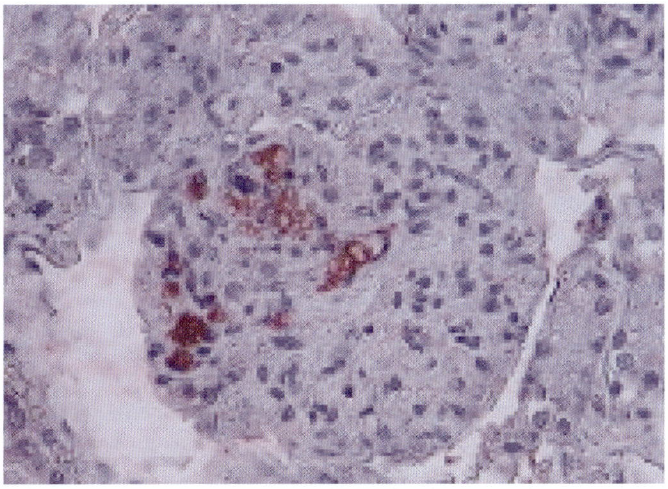

Fig. 111.4 Immunohistochemical staining for *Wolbachia* surface protein in a dog with natural *Dirofilaria immitis* infection showing a positive reaction in a renal glomerulus (×40). (From Kramer LH, Tamarozzi F, Morchon R, et al. Immune response to and tissue localization of the *Wolbachia* surface protein (WSP) in dogs with natural heartworm (*Dirofilaria immitis*) infection. *Vet Immunol Immunopathol.* 2005;106:303–308, with permission.)

TABLE 111.1 Classification of Canine Heartworm Disease Based on Clinical Severity

Severity	Class	Clinical Signs
Early infection	Class 1	No signs
Mild disease	Class 1	Cough
Moderate disease	Class 2	Cough, exercise intolerance, abnormal lung sounds
Severe disease	Class 3	Cough, exercise intolerance, dyspnea, abnormal heart and lung sounds, hepatomegaly, syncope, ascites, hemoptysis and death
Caval syndrome	Class 4	Sudden onset of severe lethargy and weakness accompanied by hemoglobinemia and hemoglobinuria

DIAGNOSIS

The diagnosis of heartworm disease is primarily done using serum immunoassays, but other testing modalities are useful in determining the severity of disease present.

Laboratory Abnormalities

Abnormal clinical laboratory results occur but are not uniquely diagnostic for heartworm infection. Hemogram abnormalities may include eosinophilia, basophilia, neutrophilia, nonregenerative anemia, and thrombocytopenia. Elevated liver enzyme activities,

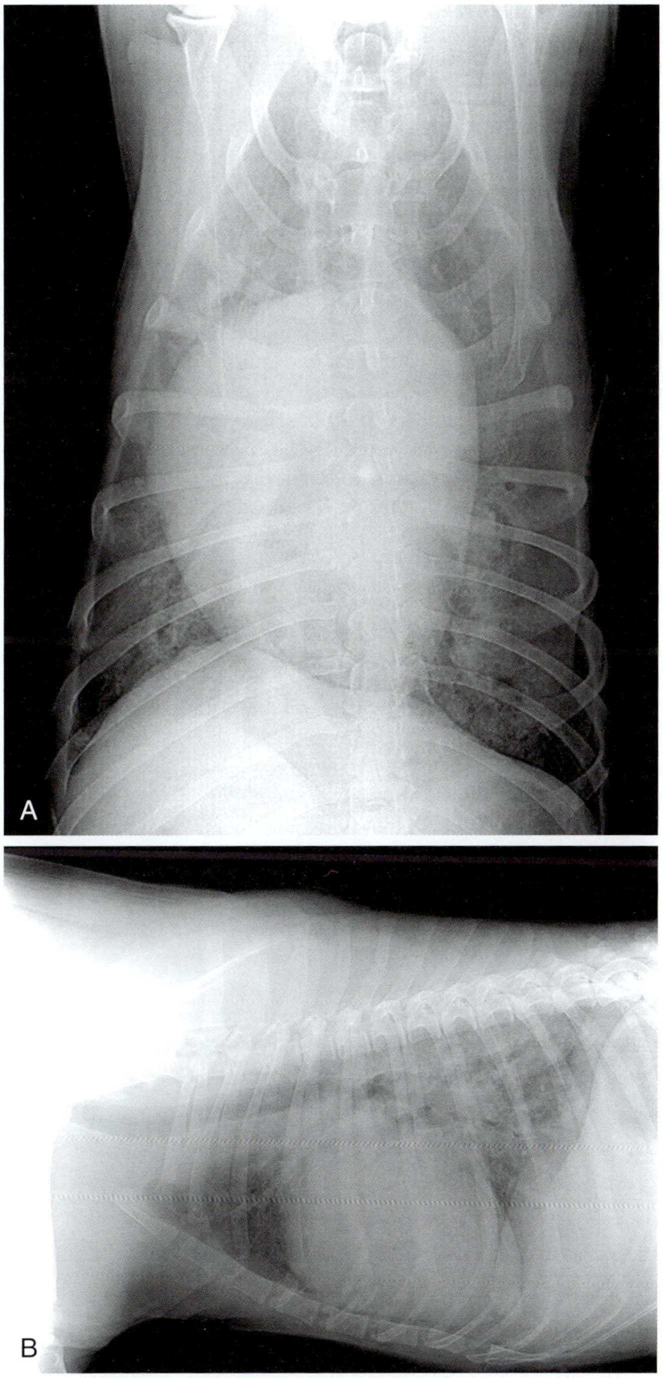

Fig. 111.5 (A) Ventrodorsal and (B) lateral thoracic radiographs of a dog with class 3 heartworm infection.

azotemia, and hyperbilirubinemia may be noted in results of serum chemistries, and proteinuria may be detected on urinalysis.

Diagnostic Imaging

Plain Radiography

Radiography is an effective way of evaluating the severity of cardiopulmonary disease, and before the availability of serologic testing, it was the method used to diagnose occult (nonmicrofilaremic) heartworm disease. The heart silhouette appears as a reversed "D" and caudal lobar pulmonary arteries are enlarged, tortuous, and often truncated. These vascular changes are accompanied by varying degrees of pulmonary parenchymal disease (Fig. 111.5).[26]

Parasitologic Tests

The AHS recommends annual screening using both a microfilariae and an antigen test for all dogs over 7 months of age; and testing is indicated 6 months after starting prophylaxis in dogs over 8 weeks of age; before starting prophylaxis in dogs over 7 months of age; and on days 0, 180, and 360 when there has been noncompliance or a change in prophylactic treatment product.

Detection of Microfilaria

Microfilaria can be identified microscopically by direct examination of a drop of anticoagulated blood, with concentration techniques using a Millipore filter, or centrifugation using the modified Knott's procedure (see Chapter 5). Microfilariae may not be detected in as many as 20% of heartworm-infected dogs. These "occult" infections may occur as a result of single-sex infections, host immune responses suppressing reproduction, and if the dog has been on a heartworm preventive.[15] For various reasons, microfilariae may be present in dogs with negative blood antigen result. It is possible for puppies to acquire microfilariae *in utero* when the bitch has a high microfilaria count. Because microfilariae can survive in the dog's bloodstream for over 2 years, dogs treated with an adulticide or dogs whose infection has cleared naturally can have microfilariae and have negative antigen test results. Heartworm microfilariae must be differentiated from those of *A. reconditum* (Fig. 111.6 and Table 111.2).

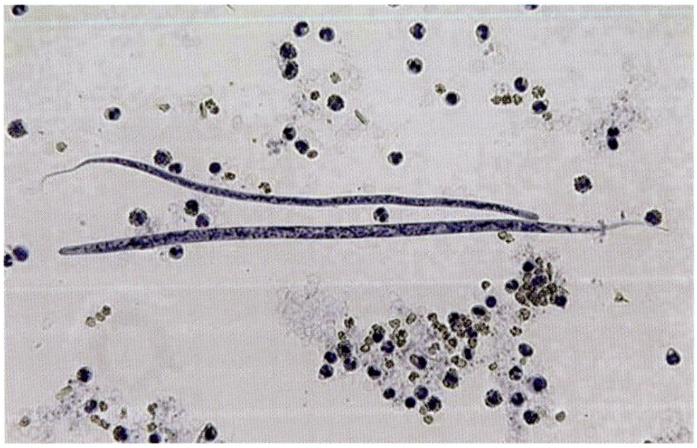

Fig. 111.6 *Acanthocheilonema reconditum* (top) and *Dirofilaria immitis* (bottom). (Courtesy Byron Blagburn, Auburn University, Auburn, AL.)

Serologic Testing

Antigen detection, which, together with microfilaria testing is the recommended method for diagnostic screening in dogs, is accomplished by using one of several commercially available antigen tests kits. These are available as POC tests or well-based tests that are used by reference laboratories to process large numbers of specimens. These tests detect a glycoprotein secreted mainly by adult female heartworms and are the most sensitive diagnostic method currently available.

Commercially available antigen test systems are based on enzyme immunoassay methods that have been adapted to laboratory or POC kits. The sensitivity (95% to 100%) and specificity (100%) of these test systems are excellent in infections when three or more female worms are present. Most POC test kit systems have low sensitivity in dogs with fewer than three female worms. In dogs with one female worm, the sensitivity ranged from 65% to 85%, and with two female worms, it ranged from 85% to 95%.[27] However, when comparing the presence or absence of female worms at necropsy, the sensitivity of one in-clinic instrument-based agglutination immunoassay test system ranged between 50% and 72% compared with 92% and 99.6% for a kit-based enzyme immunoassay.[28] False-positive results are rare, and, therefore, it is better to accept rather than reject a positive test result. However, it is prudent to repeat a test when positive results are found for dogs residing in hypoendemic areas, and in animals that receive heartworm preventive. Confirmation of the positive test result can be obtained if circulating microfilaria are identified, or if another positive result is generated using a different type of antigen test. An animal with clinical signs of heartworm disease that has a negative test result should also be retested. The amount of antigen present in the circulation can be quantitated and does have a relationship to the number of female worms, but this is not an accurate determination of the total worm burden. Male and immature female worms could be present but not producing detectable antigen. Likewise, shortly after the death of a female worm, large amounts of antigen are released into the circulation, giving the appearance of a heavy worm burden in quantitative test results.[14]

False-negative test results occur most commonly when infections are light, female worms are still immature, only male worms are present, and/or the test kit instructions have not been followed. There are also documented cases of antigen blocking, presumably from antigen-antibody complexes, interfering with antigen testing, resulting in false-negative test results. Laboratory studies have shown that heating the sample test-tube to 104°C for 10 minutes degrades the complexes, which releases antigen, yielding more accurate results.[29,30] The routine

TABLE 111.2 Comparison of Microfilariae of *Acanthocheilonema reconditum* and *Dirofilaria immitis*

	Number in Blood	Motion	Shape	Length (Modified Knott Test)
A. reconditum	Usually few	Progressive	Curved body Blunt head Curved or "button-hook" tail	250–288 μm
D. immitis	Usually many	Stationary	Straight body and tail Tapered head	307–322 μm

TABLE 111.3 Treatment for Canine Heartworm Disease

Drug[a]	Dose	Route	Interval	Duration (Days)
Melarsomine	2.5 mg/kg[b]	Deep IM	Once; repeat in 4 weeks followed by third dose 24 hours later	3 doses
Macrocyclic lactones[c]	Varies	PO, topical	30 days	Indefinite[c]
Doxycycline	10 mg/kg; 5 mg/kg in cases of severe gastrointestinal signs	PO	q12h	28
Prednisolone	0.5 mg/kg	PO	q12h	7[d]

[a]See Chapter 13 for specific information on each anti-infective drug.
[b]This drug has a low margin of safety: three times the single dose indicated (7.5 mg/kg) can result in severe pulmonary inflammation, edema, and death. Dose calculations must be very accurate and given over the extended period specified.
[c]Ivermectin, milbemycin, moxidectin, selamectin: See manufacturers' dosage recommendations.
[d]Dosage is reduced to 0.5 mg/kg every 24 hours for the next 7 days and 0.5 mg/kg every other day for 1 to 2 weeks thereafter.

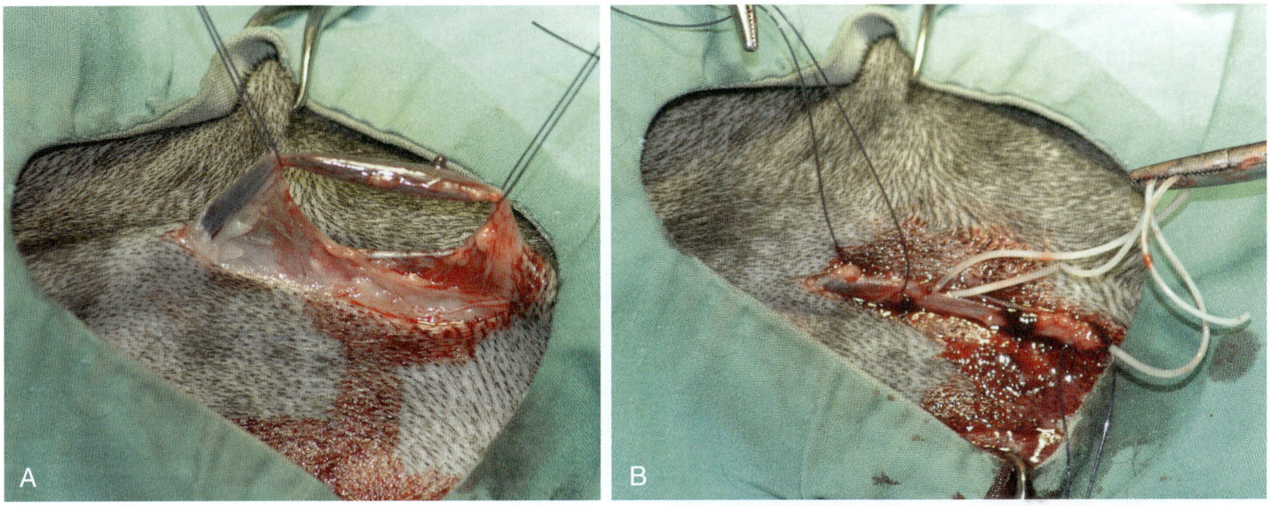

Fig. 111.7 Surgical removal of *Dirofilaria immitis* from a dog with caval syndrome. (A) Isolation of the right jugular vein. (B) Extraction of worms. (Courtesy of C. Thomas Nelson.)

heating of all blood samples is not recommended at this time as this is contrary to the label instructions for these tests and could interfere with the results of combination tests that include an antibody test for detection of other infectious agents. Due to this, and other mentioned considerations, heartworm test results should only be recorded as positive or no antigen detected (NAD) and should not be written as "negative." Antigen test results should be interpreted carefully, taking other relevant clinical information into consideration.

Antigen may be detected as early as 5 months PI and consistently by 7 months PI. Antigenemia may be delayed until 9 months PI in some infected dogs that receive preventives. Microfilaria can be detected microscopically 6 months PI, by examining fresh blood, or with concentration techniques. Screening dogs for the presence of microfilaria is complementary to antigen testing, because it adds sensitivity without compromising specificity,[31] confirms the infection and alerts the veterinarian of a potential adverse reaction that may occur after administration of microfilaricidal doses of macrocyclic lactones. Because of the prepatent period, dogs should not be tested with either microfilariae or antigen tests until they are at least 7 months old.[14]

Molecular diagnostic methods are occasionally used in research for diagnosis of heartworm infection. A multiplex PCR assay has been developed that can detect and discriminate *D. immitis* from *D. repens*.[32]

TREATMENT

Successful management and treatment of heartworm disease requires a thorough understanding of the life cycle of *D. immitis,* the host-parasite relationship, and the susceptibility of the various life stages to microfilaricidal and adulticidal drugs. The goals of any heartworm treatment are to improve the clinical condition of the animal and to eliminate all adult heartworms and developmental stages with minimal post-treatment complications. Before initiation of therapy, a thorough physical examination, clinical laboratory testing, and thoracic radiographs should be performed. Clinical or laboratory problems of concern should be controlled or stabilized before the dog receives adulticidal therapy. This may involve the administration of glucocorticoids to reduce pulmonary inflammation as well as angiotensin-converting enzyme inhibitors to improve cardiac function. In severe cases of right-sided heart failure, abdominal drainage may be necessary to remove ascitic fluid to initially reduce diaphragmatic pressure followed by maintenance therapy with furosemide and sildenafil (see Table 111.3 for doses of drugs used to treat canine heartworm disease).

Caval syndrome is an often fatal manifestation of heartworm disease in dogs that have a high worm burden that obstructs blood flow. Severe pulmonary arteriolar hypertension and decreased cardiac output occur. Heartworms can be surgically extracted via a right jugular venotomy and introduction of alligator forceps, a flexible snare, or brush (Fig. 111.7).[33] The use of a C-arm imaging device is useful but not imperative. This procedure is done as an emergency measure that is reserved for dogs with this syndrome. Medical management of heartworm disease is used in all other patients as discussed in the following sections.

Melarsomine

Melarsomine is an arsenic-based drug and is the only adulticidal drug approved by the FDA for heartworm treatment in the United States. It is administered by deep intramuscular injection into the epaxial lumbar muscles. The two-dose protocol recommended on the package insert for treating class 1 and 2 heartworm infections (see Table 111.1) kills 90% of adult worms present. The "alternate" or three-dose protocol recommended for treating class 3 heartworm infections kills 98% of the adult worms. Approximately 50% of adult worms are killed by the first dose, and most of the remaining worms are killed by the second and third injection administered 4 to 8 weeks later. The three-dose protocol is recommended by the AHS as the adulticidal treatment of choice because of its increased safety margin and efficacy.

Macrocyclic Lactones

The heartworm preventive products belonging to the macrocyclic lactones contain ivermectin, milbemycin, moxidectin, or selamectin.

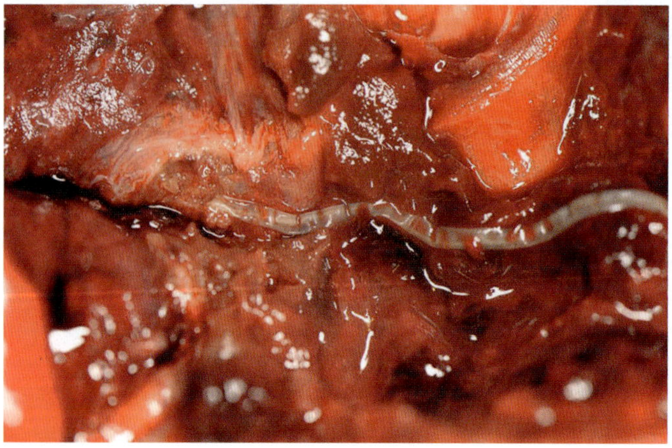

Fig. 111.8 Heartworm cuticle after 3 years of ivermectin preventive administration. (Courtesy of Stephen Jones, DVM.)

In the past, long-term administration of heartworm preventives has been advocated to prevent reinfection while waiting for existing adult heartworms to die. This approach is not recommended because it can take 2 to 3 years to completely clear the infection, during which time pulmonary and cardiovascular abnormalities can progress (Fig. 111.8). There is also the chance of selection for resistant strains of *D. immitis*.

Doxycycline

Because the metabolites (WSP) of *Wolbachia* contribute to the disease process, doxycycline has been the subject of several studies in heartworm treatment, and is now being used in the treatment of several human filarial diseases. Results of two studies were compared: heartworm test–positive dogs treated with ivermectin and doxycycline before melarsomine injections versus those with melarsomine alone had fewer gross pulmonary pathologic changes associated with the death of the heartworms.[34,35] In one study, there was a 78% reduction in heartworm numbers using ivermectin and doxycycline only after 36 weeks of therapy.[34] Other studies have shown similar results.[36] Histopathologic changes in the lung tissue included an intense inflammatory reaction and positive staining for WSP in the dogs treated with melarsomine. The inflammation was significantly reduced and staining for WSP was virtually absent in dogs receiving doxycycline-ivermectin-melarsomine combination therapy (Fig. 111.9).[37] Doxycycline administered at 10 mg/kg q12h for 4 weeks eliminates the presence of *Wolbachia* DNA. The dose can be reduced to 5 mg/kg q12h if GI adverse effects occur. In one study, 40% of heartworm-infected dogs receiving doxycycline developed elevated serum liver enzyme activities. This does not appear to be clinically significant in dogs with normal liver function. The elevated activities are transient and they typically return to pretreatment values without intervention.[38] Microfilariae from dogs treated with doxycycline developed into L_3 after ingestion by mosquitoes, but those L_3 did not develop into adult worms when inoculated into a new canid host. This impaired maturation of L_3 would result in decreased transmission and reduces the potential for selection of resistant strains of *D. immitis*.[39,40]

Macrocyclic Lactones/Doxycycline Combinations

Select macrocyclic lactones (ivermectin and moxidectin) coupled with doxycycline individually suppress embryogenesis and weaken adult heartworms. Administration of doxycycline in combination with ivermectin provided more rapid adulticidal activity than

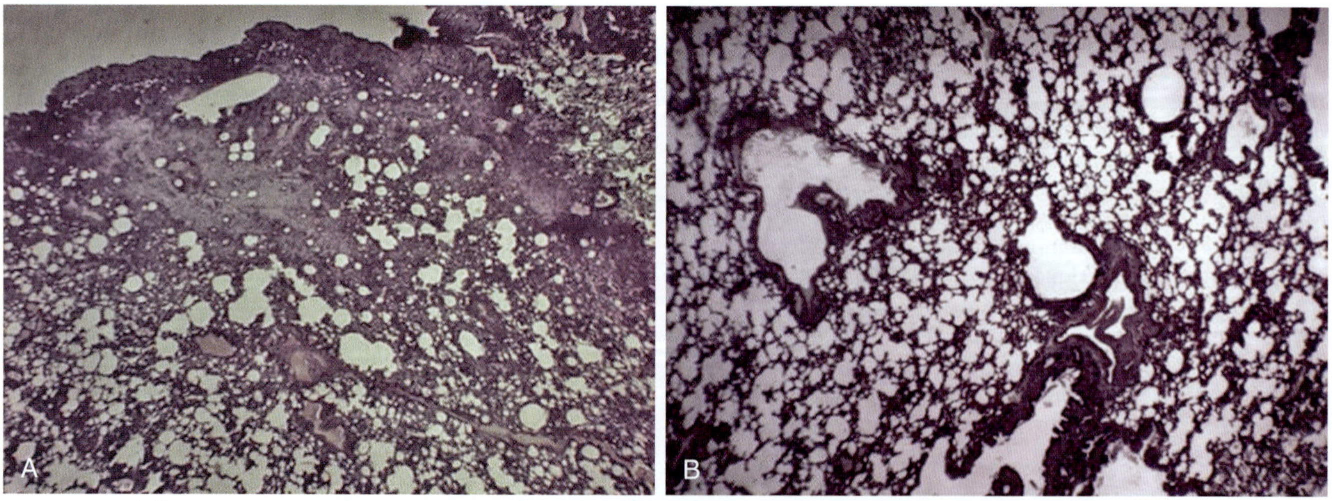

Fig. 111.9 Histopathologic appearance of the lung tissue from dogs experimentally infected with heartworms. (A) Treatment with melarsomine only. (B) Combined treatment with ivermectin, doxycycline, and melarsomine. (Courtesy Laura Kramer, University of Parma Veterinary School, Parma, Italy.)

ivermectin alone, and reduced *Wolbachia* burden to a greater extent than doxycycline alone.[41] Topical moxidectin in combination with doxycycline had 95.9% efficacy in killing adult worms after 10 months of treatment.[42] In cases where arsenic therapy is not possible or is contraindicated, the use of a monthly heartworm preventive containing ivermectin or topical moxidectin along with doxycycline at 10 mg/kg q12h for a 4-week period might be considered. This protocol is not recommended by the AHS as a standard first-line treatment but instead as a salvage procedure. The safety and long-term effects of these protocols have not been evaluated. An antigen test should be performed every 6 months and the dog not considered cleared until two consecutive negative heartworm antigen tests have been obtained. Heat treatment of samples from dogs being treated with only preventive and doxycycline prior to antigen testing is necessary because false-negative antigen tests are common in such patients.[43] If a dog treated this way is still antigen positive after 1 year, doxycycline therapy should be repeated. Exercise should be rigidly restricted for the duration of the treatment process.

Prednisone

Thromboembolism is an unavoidable sequela of any heartworm treatment protocol. Emboli primarily consist of worm fragments with associated perivascular inflammation; grossly visible clots are not usually present. The treatment of choice to help reduce the inflammatory response is prednisone. The dosage is 0.5 mg/kg q12h for the first week, 0.5 mg/kg q24h for the second week, and 0.5 mg/kg q48h for 1 to 2 weeks. Aspirin had been advocated in years past, but has been shown to be contraindicated in heartworm treatments because it leads to greater pulmonary vascular extravasation of blood. Prednisone reduces parenchymal and arterial wall damage resulting in less reparative fibrosis. Arterial elasticity is better preserved, which leads to reduced pulmonary vascular resistance, and subsequently fewer right-sided heart complications.[44] In dogs experimentally infected with heartworms, efficacy of therapy with melarsomine and prednisone was the same as that in dogs treated only with melarsomine, in either two- or three-dose protocols.[45]

AHS-Recommended Treatment Protocol

The treatment protocol outlined in Table 111.4 is designed to eliminate *Wolbachia* organisms and allows time for clearance of *Wolbachia*-associated metabolites such as WSP. Pretreatment with a macrocyclic lactone heartworm preventive and doxycycline halts embryogenesis and makes the adult worms unthrifty and smaller. This is followed by the three-dose melarsomine protocol, which provides a 99% kill rate of adult worms. Results of a retrospective study of naturally infected dogs treated with the AHS protocol compared with an identical protocol with the exception of doxycycline showed a decrease in overall post-treatment complications and mortality with the AHS protocol.[46] A second study that compared cardiopulmonary biomarkers between a classic melarsomine two-injection protocol and the AHS approach showed higher levels of D-dimer in the melarsomine treatment group.[47]

PROGNOSIS

Most heartworm infections can be cleared successfully, but there is usually residual damage to the pulmonary vasculature and parenchyma. The extent of the damage depends on the number of worms, activity level of the dog before and after treatment, and the host-parasite relationship. Strict exercise restriction during and after treatment along with utilizing the AHS treatment protocol provides the best opportunity to minimize permanent lung damage.[46]

TABLE 111.4 Example of Treatment Protocols for Canine Heartworm Disease

Day	Treatment
0	Dog diagnosed and verified as heartworm positive
	If the dog has clinical signs, attempt to stabilize the dog with angiotensin-converting enzyme inhibitor and furosemide. If dog is severely ascitic, also perform abdominal drainage.
	Administer heartworm preventive. (If microfilariae are present, pretreat with antihistamine and glucocorticosteroid if not already on prednisone.) Apply topical mosquito repellant approved for use in dogs
	Begin exercise restriction. The more pronounced the clinical signs, the stricter the exercise restriction.
1–7	Prednisone: 0.5 mg/kg PO q12h (only if clinical signs are present)
1–28	Doxycycline: 10 mg/kg PO for 4 weeks
8–14	Prednisone: 0.5 mg/kg PO q24h
15–28	Prednisone: 0.5 mg/kg PO q48h
30	Administer heartworm preventive Apply topical mosquito repellant approved for use in dogs
60	Administer heartworm preventive Apply topical mosquito repellant approved for use in dogs
61	Melarsomine: 2.5 mg/kg IM
61–67	Prednisone: 0.5 mg/kg PO q12h; further decrease activity level; cage rest in severe cases
68–74	Prednisone: 0.5 mg/kg PO q24h
75–88	Prednisone: 0.5 mg/kg PO q48h
90	Administer heartworm preventive and second melarsomine injection 2.5 mg/kg IM
91	Administer heartworm preventive and third melarsomine injection 2.5 mg/kg IM
91–97	Prednisone: 0.5 mg/kg PO q12h
98–104	Prednisone: 0.5 mg/kg PO q24h
105–118	Prednisone: 0.5 mg/kg PO q48h; continue exercise restriction for 6–8 weeks after last melarsomine injection
120	Test for microfilaria and if positive treat with a microfilaricide and retest in 4 weeks. Continue a year-round heartworm prevention program as described in prevention section.
365	Antigen test 9 months after last melarsomine injection. If still positive, re-treat with doxycycline followed by two doses of melarsomine 24 hours apart.

IMMUNITY AND VACCINATION

Attempts to produce a vaccine, while successful, have not been commercially marketed as vaccine efficacy was less than the current preventives on the market.

PREVENTION

Dirofilaria immitis infection can be prevented with commercially available macrocyclic lactone heartworm preventives (see Table 13.2), which should be recommended no later than 8 weeks of age. These products vary in their claims of efficacy against other internal and external parasites and are offered as orally administered flavored or chewable tablets (ivermectin, milbemycin oxime, and moxidectin), as topically applied liquids (moxidectin and selamectin), or as a slow-release formulation of subcutaneously injected drug (moxidectin). The oral and topical forms are administered once monthly, and the injectable product licensed in the United States is available in a 6-month and 12-month formulation.[14] The macrocyclic lactones are formulated to kill the tissue stages (L_3 and L_4) of *D. immitis.* The final molt from L_4 to juvenile worm can occur as early as 50 days PI, so it is imperative that the product be given at a 30-day interval, because late L_4 stages have reduced susceptibility.[48] These preparations also help to control other internal and external parasites.[49]

There have been increased reports of lack of efficacy (LOE) according to the Center for Veterinary Medicine of the FDA.[50] Evidence of LOE is defined by the FDA as having positive heartworm test results in the face of consistent heartworm preventive use. Unless the injectable form is given, it is very difficult to assess client compliance with regard to product administration. Other reasons for LOE are possible. Underdosing may occur in animals that have gained weight. Dosing intervals may be prolonged beyond efficacy, because doses may be inadvertently skipped or animals may fail to retain a dose because they spit out or vomit tablets shortly after administration. There is also the possibility of biological variation in how an individual animal metabolizes a drug or whether or not a strain of *D. immitis* has developed drug resistance.

In experimental studies that have evaluated these products against apparently resistant strains of *D. immitis*, dogs being given preventives developed adult worms.[51,52] Therefore, the drugs generally cannot be assumed to be 100% effective and clients should be so informed. Furthermore, genetic variations associated with decreased susceptibility to macrocyclic lactones occur among *D. immitis* isolates, indicating resistant strains exist.[53,54] Because drug resistance is selected for and does not randomly develop, it is imperative that any dog suspected of harboring a more tolerant or resistant strain be treated immediately with an adulticidal protocol that incorporates doxycycline and melarsomine. Doxycycline will eliminate *Wolbachia* and reduce the potential for transmission of the resistant strain. A three-injection melarsomine treatment protocol will eliminate 98% of the total worm burden. With this protocol, usually 100% of the male worms needed for sexual reproduction will be eliminated, thus impairing microfilaria production. This approach, along with the extensive refugia of wild-type genes, may limit resistance from becoming widespread.

Addition of topical products that repel and kill mosquitoes will also enhance the efficacy of the macrocyclic lactones. Use of a topical dinotefuran-permethrin-pyriproxyfen product in conjunction with a macrocyclic lactone heartworm preventive was able to prevent experimental heartworm infection by a known resistant strain.[55] Reduction of exposure to mosquitoes through standard environmental control of mosquitoes and their breeding environments, and when possible, reducing outdoor exposure during key mosquito feeding periods is also recommended.

Diethylcarbamazine citrate is an older medication that is no longer marketed in the United States but is still available for heartworm prevention in other parts of the world. Its effect is at the molt between L_3 and L_4 and, therefore, it must be given every day to be effective.

PUBLIC HEALTH ASPECTS

Dirofilaria immitis is of public health concern, even though the number of reports of infection in humans is relatively small. However, there is no serologic test to detect infection, so invasive procedures that involve biopsy of lesions is usually necessary.[56] The most common clinical syndrome reported in human infections is the formation of a pulmonary nodule or nodules within the lung parenchyma.[57,58] This lesion appears on radiographs as circular density and has been described as a "coin lesion." These lesions resemble those of pulmonary adenocarcinomas and often are not diagnosed until after a person has undergone a thoracotomy for the removal of a lung lobe. Histopathologic findings are granulomatous inflammation surrounding the remnants of an immature heartworm. Granulomatous lesions have also been recorded in the eye, skin, testicle, and other tissues.[58] Infected dogs or blood with microfilaria do not present a direct risk of infection to humans because the parasite can only be transmitted by mosquitoes. Prevention is best accomplished through mosquito-abatement programs and by using mosquito repellents, wearing protective clothing, and remaining indoors during mosquito feeding periods. See Chapter 13 for further information on insect control measures.

FELINE HEARTWORM DISEASE

ETIOLOGY AND EPIDEMIOLOGY

Heartworm disease was first discovered in cats in Brazil in 1921[59] and in the United States in 1922.[60] Its geographic distribution mirrors that of canine heartworm infections, as long as there is a competent mosquito vector present that will feed on both dogs and cats.[61] The means of transmission and life cycle are identical in the cat and dog until the juvenile heartworm (also referred to as an immature adult or fifth stage) reaches the pulmonary arteries (see Fig. 111.3). Most juvenile worms in dogs mature to adults over 3 to 4 months, after which they mate and produce microfilariae. However, in the cat, most of the juvenile worms die 3 to 4 months PI, resulting in an abbreviated infection.[62] In a small percentage of cats, a few worms mature to be adults and live for 2 to 4 years.[63] Microfilaria will be produced and may be found 8 months PI in 20% of mature worm infections. They will be removed from the circulation by the cat's immune response within 2 months and not found again.[62]

CLINICAL FEATURES

Pathogenesis and Clinical Signs

There are three stages of heartworm disease in cats. The first stage begins shortly after the arrival of the juvenile worms in the caudal pulmonary arteries 75 days PI. There is an acute vascular and parenchymal inflammatory response to the presence and subsequent death of most of these immature worms approximately 90 days PI. Light and electron microscopic lesions can be detected in the lungs of experimentally infected cats as early as 42 days PI.[64] Vascular disease can be found in the caudal lung lobes by day 75 PI, followed by interstitial and alveolar disease by day 90 PI.[65,66] The vascular lesions are described as severe muscular hypertrophy of the medium- and small-sized arteries. These same types of lesions are found in cats that have positive results for anti-heartworm antibodies but have no adult heartworms at necropsy.[66] Therefore, cats do not have to have fully mature adult worms to have pulmonary disease.

A study of experimentally infected cats compared the pulmonary pathologic changes between cats receiving heartworm prevention, cats with abbreviated juvenile worm infections, and cats with adult heartworms. Vascular lesions were found in both cats that had mature heartworms and cats with abbreviated infections (Fig. 111.10). The lesions in the bronchioles and alveoli of the abbreviated juvenile worm were almost identical to those found in cats with adult worm infections (Figs. 111.11 and 111.12).[68] Thus, pulmonary disease occurs in cats as a result of juvenile worm infections even if they do not progress to the mature adult worm stage. Because heartworm disease in the cat is primarily a pulmonary disease, the term "heartworm-associated respiratory disease" (HARD) has been adopted to describe heartworm infections in cats.[68,69]

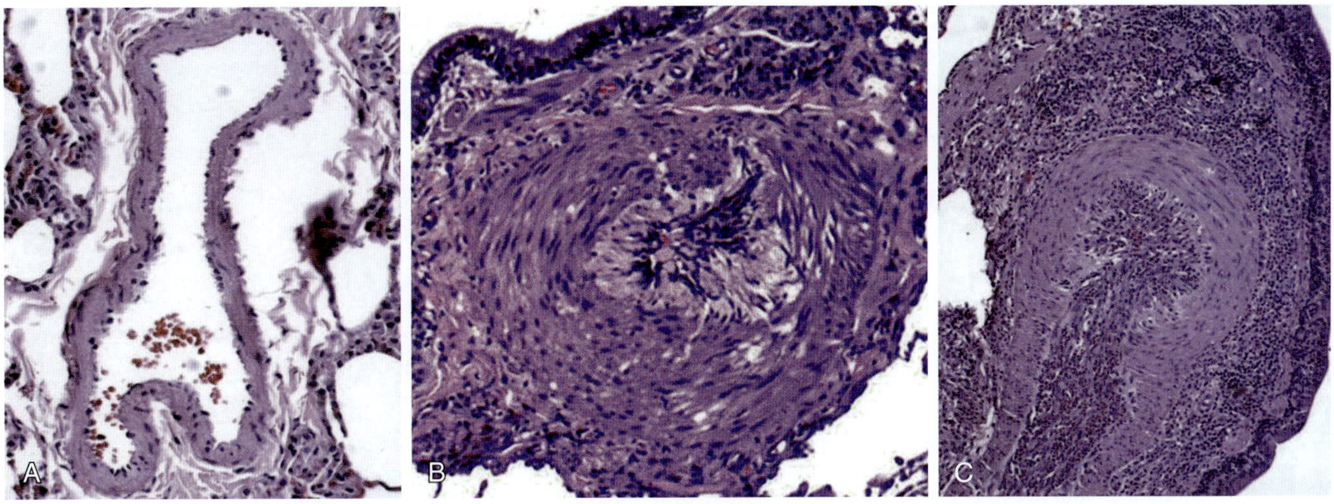

Fig. 111.10 Histopathologic view of arterioles from heartworm-challenged cats. (A) Cat receiving monthly heartworm preventive. (B) Cat with abbreviated juvenile worm infection. (C) Adult heartworm infection (hematoxylin and eosin stain, ×40). (Courtesy Drs. Ray Dillon and Byron Blagburn, Auburn University, Auburn, AL.)

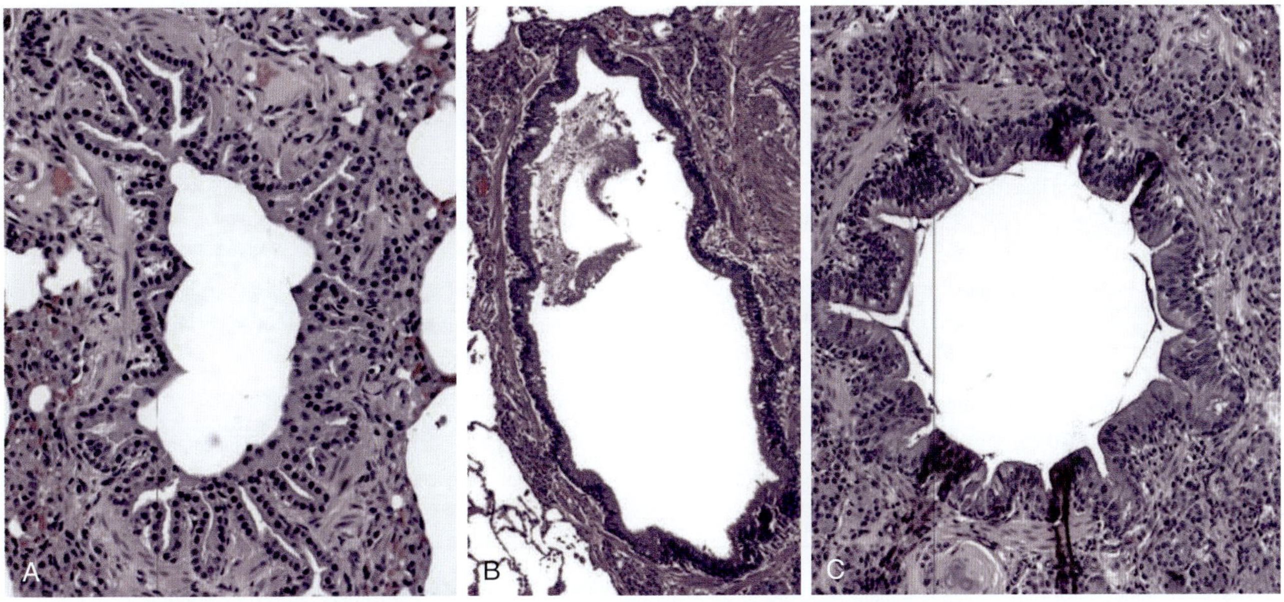

Fig. 111.11 Histopathologic view of bronchioles from heartworm-challenged cats. (A) Cat receiving monthly heartworm preventive. (B) Cat with abbreviated juvenile worm infection. (C) Adult heartworm infection (hematoxylin and eosin stain, ×20). (Courtesy Drs. Ray Dillon and Byron Blagburn, Auburn University, Auburn, AL.)

Adult heartworms have the ability to suppress the activity of the pulmonary intravascular macrophage, the main component of the cat's reticuloendothelial system.[70,71] Therefore, if the juvenile worm matures to the adult worm, suppression of the host immune response occurs and there may be some resolution of clinical signs. However, when heartworms die, this downregulation of the immune system ceases and the degenerating parasite causes an intense inflammatory reaction and thromboembolism, which can lead to a catastrophic acute lung injury and sudden death. Sudden death has been reported to occur in 10% to 20% of cats with mature adult heartworm infections.[63,72] If the cat survives this insult, there is hyperplasia of type II alveolar cells, which replace the normal type I cell, and may cause permanent pulmonary dysfunction.[24,71] This can lead to chronic respiratory disease, the third manifestation of heartworm disease in cats.

Arterial intimal proliferation of the pulmonary arteries, resembling the characteristic heartworm arteritis found in dogs, can occur in cats. These lesions are localized and ordinarily fail to cause sufficient obstruction to produce clinically significant pulmonary hypertension in cats. Consequently, right ventricular hypertrophy and right heart failure are less common in cats than in dogs. Ectopic migration of worms, however, appears more common in cats.

Proteinuria occurs as a consistent complication in experimentally infected cats.[73] Naturally infected cats also have a greater prevalence of proteinuria (90% versus 35%) than do age- and gender-matched control cats.[73] The mechanism for the proteinuria is presumed to be renal in origin; however, further investigation is needed to determine its cause and significance.

The most common clinical signs observed in cats are cough or dyspnea (64%) and intermittent vomiting unrelated to eating (38%); 28% of infected cats are clinically healthy.[72] The large proportion of subclinically affected cats is probably a result of the sedentary lifestyle of many cats, because exercise is a major factor in precipitating

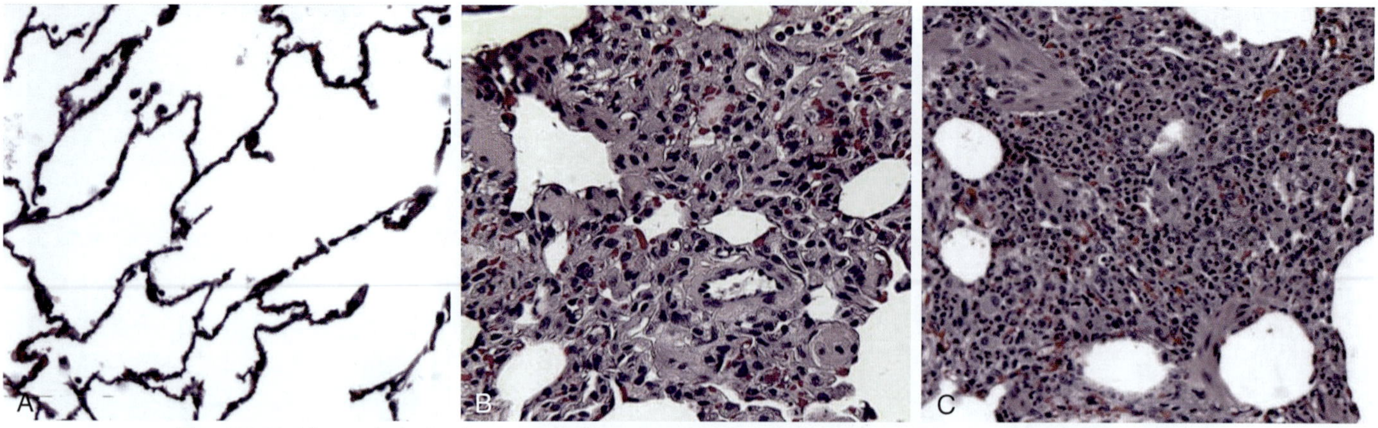

Fig. 111.12 Histopathologic view of pulmonary alveoli from heartworm-challenged cats. (A) Cat receiving monthly heartworm preventive. (B) Cat with abbreviated juvenile worm infection. (C) Adult heartworm infection (hematoxylin and eosin stain, ×20). (Courtesy Drs. Ray Dillon and Byron Blagburn, Auburn University, Auburn, AL.)

TABLE 111.5 Comparison of Diagnostic Tests for Feline Heartworm Disease[a]

Test	Brief Description	Result	Interpretation	Limitations
Antibody test	Detects antibodies produced by the cat in response to presence of heartworm larvae, immature adults, or adult worms. May detect infections as early as 8 weeks post-transmission by the mosquito	Negative	Does not rule out heartworms	Antibodies confirm infection with heartworm larvae, immature adults, or mature adults. Studies have shown significant false-negative results
		Positive	Indicates a current or recent infection; 50% or more cats will have pulmonary arterial disease	
Antigen test	Detects antigen produced by the adult female heartworm or from the dying male (>5) or female heartworms	Negative	Does not rule out heartworms	Immature or male-only worm infections are rarely detected. Does not detect larvae or immature worm infections
		Positive	Confirms presence of heartworms	
Thoracic radiography	Detects vascular enlargement (inflammation caused by immature worms and, later, hypertrophy), pulmonary parenchymal inflammation, and edema (the latter only in ARDS-like reaction)	Normal	Lower index of suspicion	Radiographic signs subjective and affected by clinical interpretation
		Signs consistent with FHWD	Enlarged arteries greatly increases index of suspicion	
Echocardiography	Detects echogenic walls of the immature or mature heartworm residing in the lumen of the pulmonary arterial tree, if within the visual window of the ultrasound	No worms seen	No change to index of suspicion	Ultrasonographer experience with heartworm detection appears to influence accuracy rate
		Worms seen	Confirms presence of heartworms in the structure	

[a]Courtesy of the American Heartworm Society.
Note: In cats, a combination of test results is usually required to determine the likelihood of heartworm disease. While antigen tests are highly specific for detecting adult heartworm antigen, they will not detect infections with only live male worms.
ARDS, acute respiratory distress syndrome; *FHWD*, feline heartworm disease.

cardiopulmonary manifestations of heartworm disease in dogs. Ascites, hydrothorax, chylothorax, pneumothorax, ataxia, seizures, and syncope have been reported in cats, but are uncommon. A peracute syndrome consisting of some combination of signs including respiratory distress, ataxia, collapse, seizures, hemoptysis, or sometimes sudden death may arise without warning.

DIAGNOSIS

Diagnosis of heartworm disease in cats can be challenging because there is no test that can reliably detect all stages of disease (Table 111.5). Running multiple tests increases the chances of making a diagnosis. It is difficult to make a diagnosis using a single method unless there is a positive antigen test result or a worm is found on ultrasound. Additional testing must be considered if results do not support clinical suspicion. In a study of 22 heartworm-infected cats, where thoracic radiography, echocardiography, and antigen and antibody testing were performed, pulmonary enlargement was detected using radiography in 64%; worms were visualized by echocardiography in 64%; 55% had antigen-positive results; and 82% had antibody-positive results.[74] In a multicenter study of 215 cats when clinical signs were correlated to serologic and radiographic findings, 44% of cats with coughing or dyspnea and intermittent vomiting unrelated to eating had positive antibody test results.[75] This was twice the positive antibody result rate for clinically healthy cats in the same geographic area. Of cats with radiographic signs consistent with heartworm disease, 58% had positive antibody test results.[76]

Diagnostic Imaging

Radiology

A bronchointerstitial lung pattern (Fig. 111.13A) can also be found in cats with heartworm disease but is not specific. The most common radiographic

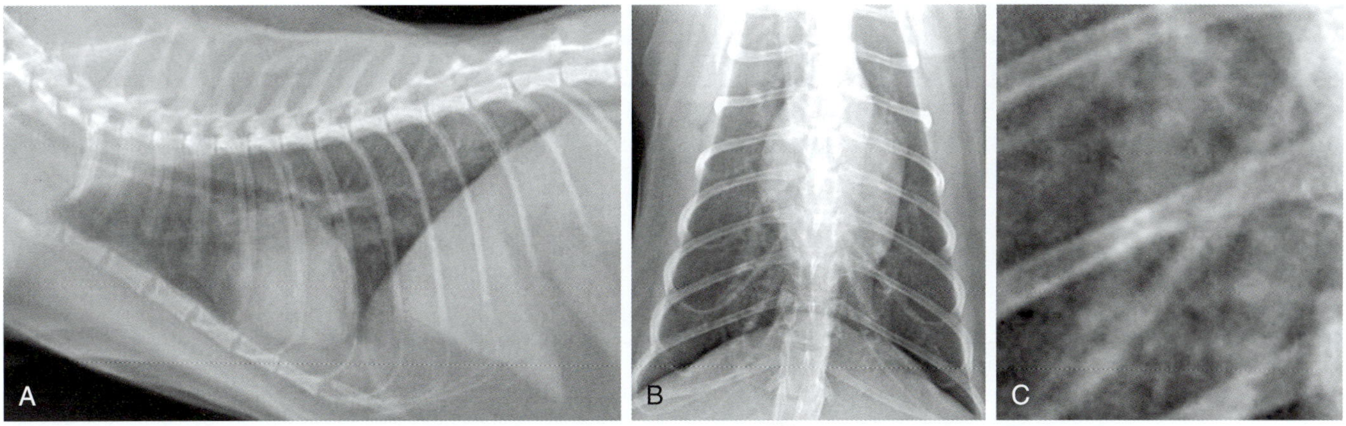

Fig. 111.13 Thoracic radiographs from a cat with heartworm infection and bronchointerstitial lung pattern. (A) Lateral view. (B) Dorsoventral view. (C) Closer view of enlarged right caudal lobar pulmonary artery.

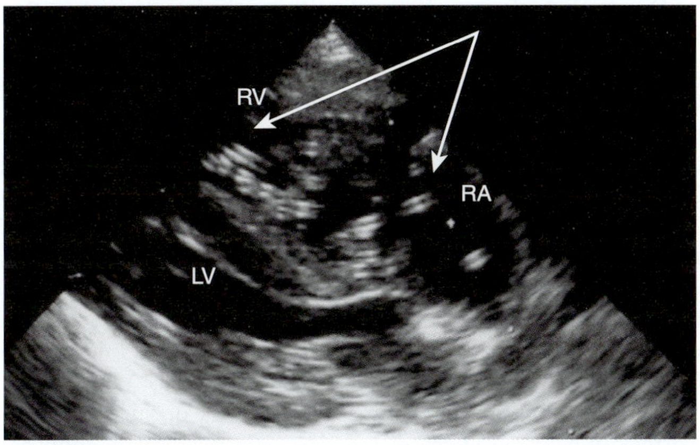

Fig. 111.14 Echocardiogram of a heartworm-infected cat. Arrows point to heartworm signatures. *LV,* left ventricle; *RA,* right atrium; *RV,* right ventricle. (Courtesy Dr. Clarke Atkins, North Carolina State University, Raleigh, NC.)

abnormality is an enlargement of what appears to be the right caudal lobar pulmonary artery, which is best seen in a ventrodorsal view (Fig. 111.13B and C). This apparent enlargement is a result of inflammatory infiltrates surrounding the vessel and producing a radiographic shadow. Cats with these lesions may be misdiagnosed as having allergic bronchitis or asthma, and if treated with glucocorticoids, the radiographic signs improve, further supporting the misdiagnosis. Other less commonly seen findings are hyperinflation of the lungs with flattening of the diaphragm, focal parenchymal radiodensities, consolidated lung lobes, pleural effusion, and pneumothorax. The use of radiography does have limitations, as found in one study where only 6 of 10 cats with heartworm antigen-positive test results had radiographic signs consistent with heartworm disease.[76]

Echocardiography

Ultrasound examination can detect adult heartworm infections, but the caudal pulmonary arteries must be examined up to the bifurcation within the lung fields, because this is where most adult heartworms are found. The cuticle of the adult heartworm is strongly echogenic and produces short, segmented, parallel lines ("heartworm signatures") where the imaging plane crosses the worm (Fig. 111.14). Heartworm signatures on echocardiography have been described as "equal signs" (=). Because the imaging beam may cross the worm multiple times, quantification of the number of worms is difficult. Reports cite echocardiography as detecting heartworms in 68% of naturally infected cats[77] and 88% of experimentally infected cats.[78]

Microfilarial Detection

Microfilaremia in the cat is rare for multiple reasons. More than 90% of infections in cats are abbreviated and do not reach the adult stage. When adult worms are present, the infections are frequently single sex, and if microfilariae are produced, their presence is transient because the cat's immune response will eliminate them from circulation.

Serologic Testing

Antigen Detection

Both antigen and antibody testing are available for cats, but a thorough understanding of their limitations is essential for interpretation of results. Antigen tests are considered the gold standard for diagnosis of heartworm disease in dogs. Because the available antigen tests detect a glycoprotein primarily produced by the uterus of the mature female worm, these tests will not detect early or male-only worm infections as readily. The most common form of heartworm disease in cats results from the death of juvenile worms at 3 to 4 months PI and will not be detected by an antigen test. If mature adult heartworms do develop, most cats have only one or two adult worms. Single-sex infections are common, and these are frequently male-only infections. Multiple studies have reported the sensitivity of antigen test in mature heartworm infections to be 50% to 86%.[79–81] Antigen-antibody complexes, as described earlier in this chapter for dogs, also occur in cats further decreasing sensitivity.[82] Blocked antigen is particularly common early in feline infection, and multiple testing modalities may be needed to reach a diagnosis.[83] Blocked antigen was identified in 5.3% of shelter and free-roaming cats in the southern United States and a majority (77%) were also antibody positive.[84] As a result, a negative antigen test result cannot be used to rule out heartworm infections in cats.

Antibody Detection

Tests that measure serum antibody detect infection with late L_4, juvenile and adult worm infections. They have been reported to be 93% to 100% sensitive in experimental models[85,86] but are less sensitive in naturally infected cats. A retrospective study involving 50 cats with heartworms had a 14% false-negative antibody test result rate.[72] Results of a necropsy study of shelter cats in Texas revealed 50% false-negative antibody test results.[80] In a similar necropsy study of shelter cats in Florida, 11% to 68% had false-negative test results using eight different antibody test methods.[81] In this study, 21 of 31 cats with heartworms had negative test results on at least one of six antibody methods that were evaluated. A number of the assays described in these references are no longer available. Clearly however, a negative antibody test result cannot be used to

TABLE 111.6 **Treatment for Feline Heartworm Disease**

Drug[a]	Dose	Route	Interval	Duration (Days)
Macrocyclic lactones[b]	Varies	PO	30 days	Indefinite[b]
Doxycycline[c]	5 mg/kg	PO	q12h	28
Prednisolone				
Anti-inflammatory	1–2 mg/kg	PO	q12h	7[d]
Shock, pulmonary	50–100 mg/cat	IV	q24h	prn
Dexamethasone (shock, pulmonary)	1–2 mg/kg	IM, IV	q24h	prn
Aminophylline (respiratory distress)	6.6 mg/kg	IV	q24h	prn

[a]See Chapter 13 for specific information on antiparasitics.
[b]Eprinomectin, ivermectin, milbemycin, moxidectin, selamectin; see manufacturers' dosage recommendations.
[c]Give as suspension or else round up and use whole tablets, or use monohydrate salt. Damaged or cracked tablets in the esophagus can cause esophagitis and esophageal strictures.
[d]Dosage is reduced to 0.5 mg/kg q12h for the next 7 days and 0.5 mg/kg q48h for 1 to 2 weeks thereafter.

rule out heartworm infection in cats, and more sensitive and specific assays are badly needed for diagnosis of heartworm infection in cats.

TREATMENT AND PROGNOSIS

Table 111.6 summarizes the drug dosages used to treat cats with heartworm disease. Cats with clinical or radiographic signs of heartworm disease should be treated with daily anti-inflammatory doses of glucocorticoids (prednisolone 1 to 2 mg/kg PO). This dosage should be reduced on a weekly basis, over a 3- to 4-week period. If clinical signs recur or persist, then alternate-day glucocorticoid therapy is given at the lowest dose effective for control of clinical signs. Radiographic evaluation and serologic testing are repeated periodically to monitor the course of the disease. Infected cats can be started on a once-monthly heartworm preventive, because cats are rarely microfilaremic, and even when microfilaria are present, their numbers are low, so reactions do not occur.

Cats with acute respiratory distress should be given oxygen and "shock doses" of glucocorticoids (dexamethasone sodium phosphate, 1 to 2 mg/kg, IM or IV; or prednisolone sodium succinate, 50 to 100 mg/cat, IV) and bronchodilators (such as theophylline or terbutaline). Supportive therapy (IV fluids and external thermal regulation) is maintained until the cat's clinical condition is stabilized.

Results of retrospective studies are that between 10% to 20% of cats with adult heartworm infections will die within 4 years.[63] If cats are diagnosed with adult heartworms by antigen test or echocardiography, their owners must be made aware of this risk and instructed to seek prompt medical attention at any sign of respiratory distress, because timely treatment is critical. It may be prudent to send home dexamethasone sodium phosphate (10 mg), with instruction to administer it IM in case of a respiratory emergency, to initiate treatment. This is not in lieu of, but before, seeking emergency veterinary care.

There is no form of adulticidal therapy proven to improve the survival rate of heartworm-infected cats. Theoretically, the use of antileukotrienes might help because cytokines contribute to the disease process. IL-8 is produced in response to *Wolbachia*, an intracellular rickettsial endosymbiont found in all stages of heartworms and IL-4 can be found in the secretions recovered by bronchoalveolar lavage from heartworm-infected cats. There is anecdotal evidence that antileukotrienes such as montelukast (2 mg, PO, q24h) may be beneficial in thwarting a respiratory crisis in heartworm-infected cats.[87]

Doxycycline therapy is another theoretical treatment option. Elimination of *Wolbachia* reduces the pathologic changes associated with worm death in dogs.[34,35] Doxycycline is now being used to treat some filarial nematode infections in humans.[88,89] Although this form of therapy in cats is unproven, considering the 20% chance of a heartworm-related death in cats with adult worms, its use could be considered in cases where the owner wants to pursue all options. The recommended protocol would be to administer doxycycline 5 mg/kg q12h for 1 month with once-monthly administration of a macrocyclic lactone heartworm preventive. If doxycycline hyclate is used, a suspension is preferred to prevent esophagitis and potential esophageal strictures. If tablets are used, follow with a minimum of 6 mL of water.

Although not shown to improve outcomes or survival, heartworms can be surgically extracted via a right jugular venotomy and introduction of a flexible snare or brush that is guided into the pulmonary artery using a C-arm imaging device. During removal, care must be taken to keep the worms intact, because partial or complete traumatic transection of a worm may result in acute circulatory collapse and death.[90]

PREVENTION

All cats in endemic areas, whether residing indoors or outdoors, should receive heartworm preventives. Indoor cats are at similar risk of exposure as outdoor cats. There are many commercially available products on the market labeled for cats that are safe and virtually 100% effective (see Chapter 13). Ivermectin is available as a chewable treat, milbemycin as a flavored tablet, and selamectin, eprinomectin, and moxidectin as topical applications. All products have activity against *D. immitis* as well as a variety of other internal and external parasites.[69] Of 400 animal sheltering agencies in the southeastern United States, only 23% performed heartworm testing and 31% provided preventive medication for cats for cats.[91] Expense and the perception that the risk of feline infection in the region was low were reasons for these low prevalences. Further financial support and education are required concerning this disease in cats.

PUBLIC HEALTH ASPECTS

See Canine Heartworm Infection.

CASE EXAMPLE

Signalment

"Possum," a 2-year-old female spayed blue heeler from Roanoke, AL.

History

Possum's owner reported that Possum had shown signs of lethargy, cough, and inappetence for several days. When abdominal distention was noted and she vomited a few times, Possum was taken to her regular veterinarian where a rectal temperature of 105°F and harsh lung sounds were documented. A presumptive diagnosis of pneumonia was made, as well as possible intestinal obstruction, as the dog had a history of chewing and swallowing foreign objects. Possum was discharged with a course of antibiotics and instructions to return the following day for abdominal radiographs if vomiting continued. That evening the abdominal distention became more pronounced and labored respirations developed, so Possum was taken to a 24-hour facility where she was admitted to the critical care unit. Possum was up to date on core vaccines and was given monthly ivermectin-based heartworm preventive. Upon further questioning, the owner admitted to missing an occasional dose and that the preventive had not been started until the dog was 6 months old.

Current Medications

Ivermectin 136 μg/pyrantel 114 mg PO q30d for monthly heartworm prevention and intestinal parasite control.

Physical Examination

Body weight: 15 kg.

General: Quiet, alert and responsive. Ambulatory on all four limbs. Temperature = 102.1°F (38.9°C), HR = 132 beats/minute, respiratory rate = 148 breaths/minute, mucous membranes pale pink, CRT = 2 seconds.

Integument: No clinically significant abnormalities.

Eyes, ears, nose, and throat: No significant abnormalities.

Musculoskeletal: BCS of 5/9; no clinically significant abnormalities.

Cardiovascular: Grade 3/6 systolic murmur loudest at sternum.

Respiratory: Breath sounds harsh with labored breathing.

GI and genitourinary: Abdomen distended and firm but not painful. Urinary tract appears normal.

Lymph nodes: Within normal limits.

Laboratory Findings

CBC: HCT 42.8% (37%–55%), MCV 74.3 fL (60–77 fL), MCHC 33.6 g/dL (30–37.5 g/dL), WBC 23,680 cells/μL (5,500–16,900 cells/μL), neutrophils 20,550 cells/μL (2,000–12,000 cells/μL), lymphocytes 900 cells/μL (500–4,900 cells/μL), monocytes 1,900 cells/μL (300–2,000 cells/μL), platelets 264,000 platelets/μL (175,000-500,000 platelets/μL).

Serum chemistry profile: Sodium 147 mmol/L (144–160 mmol/L), potassium 4.0 mmol/L (3.5–5.8 mmol/L), chloride 111 mmol/L (109–122 mmol/L), BUN 22 mg/dL (7–27 mg/dL), creatinine 1.0 mg/dL (0.5–1.8 mg/dL), glucose 101 mg/dL (74–143 mg/dL), total protein 7.9 g/dL (5.2–8.2 g/dL), albumin 3.2 g/dL (3.0–4.4 g/dL), globulin 4.7 g/dL (1.8–3.9 g/dL), ALT 49 U/L (10–100 U/L), ALP 76 U/L (23–212 U/L).

Imaging Findings

Thoracic radiographs: Enlarged reversed D cardiac silhouette with large, tortuous caudal lobar arteries and areas of consolidation consistent with heartworm disease. Evidence of pulmonary embolism of the left caudal lobar artery was identified (Fig. 111.15).

Abdominal radiographs: No evidence of GI foreign body obstruction. Loss of abdominal detail suggesting ascites (Fig. 111.16).

Abdominal ultrasound: Hepatic congestion, distended caudal vena cava, and free abdominal fluid. Abdominocentesis was performed and yielded serosanguineous fluid.

Fluid analysis: Color – serosanguineous; total solids 2.8 g/dL, few mesothelial cells and RBCs noted on microscopic review, no bacteria. Consistent with a modified transudate.

Fecal examination: No parasite ova seen.

Heartworm test: Antigen strong positive, no microfilariae on Knott's test.

Diagnosis

Class 3 heartworm disease.

Treatment

Possum was placed on flow-by oxygen and 450 mL of serosanguineous fluid was removed from the abdominal cavity to relieve severe abdominal distension, which was considered to be impacting respiration. The dog was also started on prednisone 10 mg

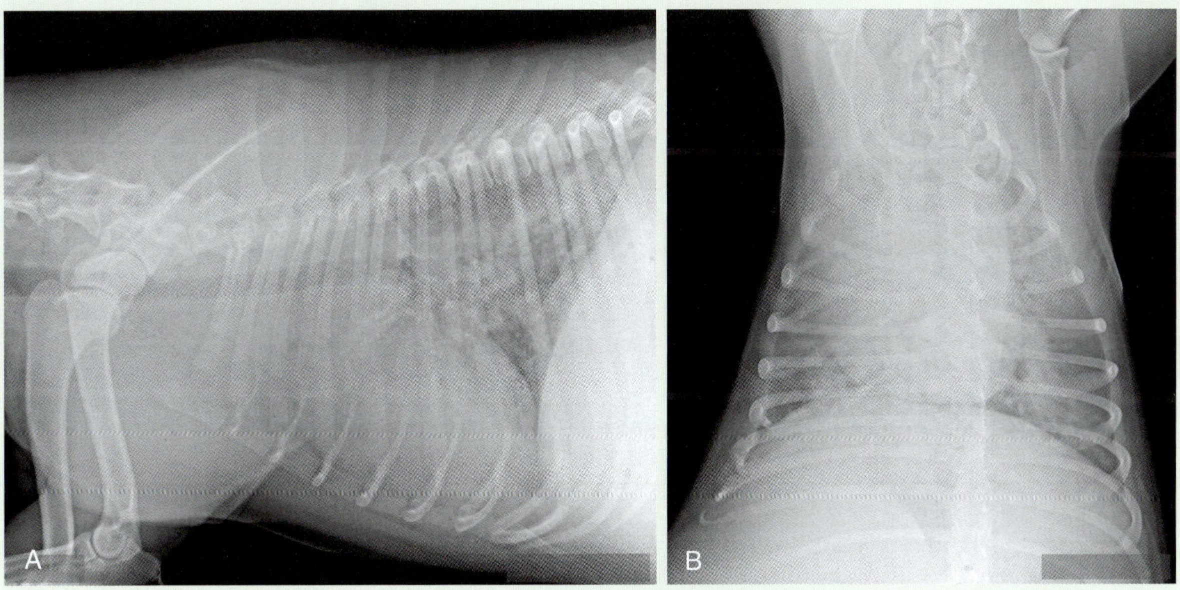

Fig. 111.15 Lateral (A) and ventrodorsal (B) radiographs of the thorax of a 2-year-old female spayed blue heeler with heartworm disease before treatment (day 0). Enlarged reversed D cardiac silhouette is evident with large, tortuous caudal lobar arteries and areas of consolidation consistent with heartworm disease.

Continued

CASE EXAMPLE—cont'd

q24h for 2 weeks then reduced to 10 mg q48h, doxycycline 150 mg q12h for 30 days, enalapril 5 mg q12h, and furosemide 12.5 mg. Possum responded favorably to therapy and was weaned off oxygen within 24 hours and released from the hospital the following day with instructions for strict exercise restriction for the duration of treatment.

Possum returned for a recheck examination 2 weeks later. Her appetite had returned, her lung sounds were greatly improved and the heart murmur was no longer noted. Radiographs showed significant improvement, and the dog was scheduled to start melarsomine therapy in 6 weeks.

Possum continued to do well clinically although significant abnormalities persisted on thoracic radiography (Fig. 111.17A). The first melarsomine injection was given on day 62. The dose of prednisone was increased to 10 mg q24h for 2 weeks, then the dosage interval was reduced to q48h. The furosemide dosage interval was decreased to q48h. The owners were reminded of the importance of exercise restriction. The second and third melarsomine injections were given on days 97 and 98. Again, the prednisone dosage interval was increased to q24h for 2 weeks then reduced to q48h. Possum returned on day 128 for a recheck. No abnormalities were detected on physical examination, and the furosemide, enalapril, and prednisone doses were reduced by 50%. On day 160, thoracic radiographs revealed reduction in the size of the right heart and pulmonary arteries (Fig. 111.17B). The owner perceived that Possum had a normal appetite and activity level. The enalapril, furosemide, and prednisone were discontinued and Possum was allowed to resume normal activity. Follow-up radiographs taken 7 years later revealed persistent cardiac, vascular and pulmonary parenchymal changes that resulted from worm death (Fig. 111.17C).

Comments

This dog was not treated with preventives until 6 months of age. When preventive treatment was initiated, she was not tested 6 months later and was likely infected during the first few months of life. By starting a dog in a highly endemic region on preventives after 6 months of age (i.e., after infection), a "slow kill" form of heartworm treatment was essentially implemented, which is not recommended. Death of worms lead to pulmonary thromboembolism and right-sided heart failure at an early age, and was likely exacerbated by the fact that she was a very active dog. Puppies should be started on heartworm preventives no later than 8 weeks of age, and if started after 8 weeks of age, they should be tested 6 months later.

Possum was treated with the protocol described in this chapter. Although the heartworm infection was cleared and the dog survived, the radiographs taken 7 years later revealed how permanent damage to cardiopulmonary structures can occur.

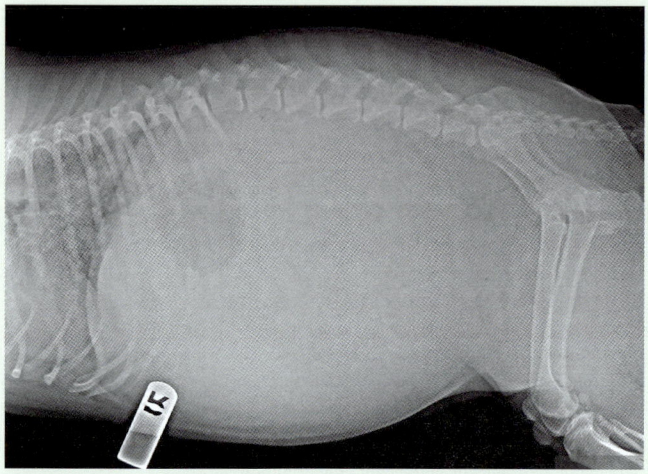

Fig. 111.16 Lateral radiograph of the abdomen of a 2-year-old female spayed blue heeler with heartworm disease before treatment showing marked abdominal distention and evidence of ascites.

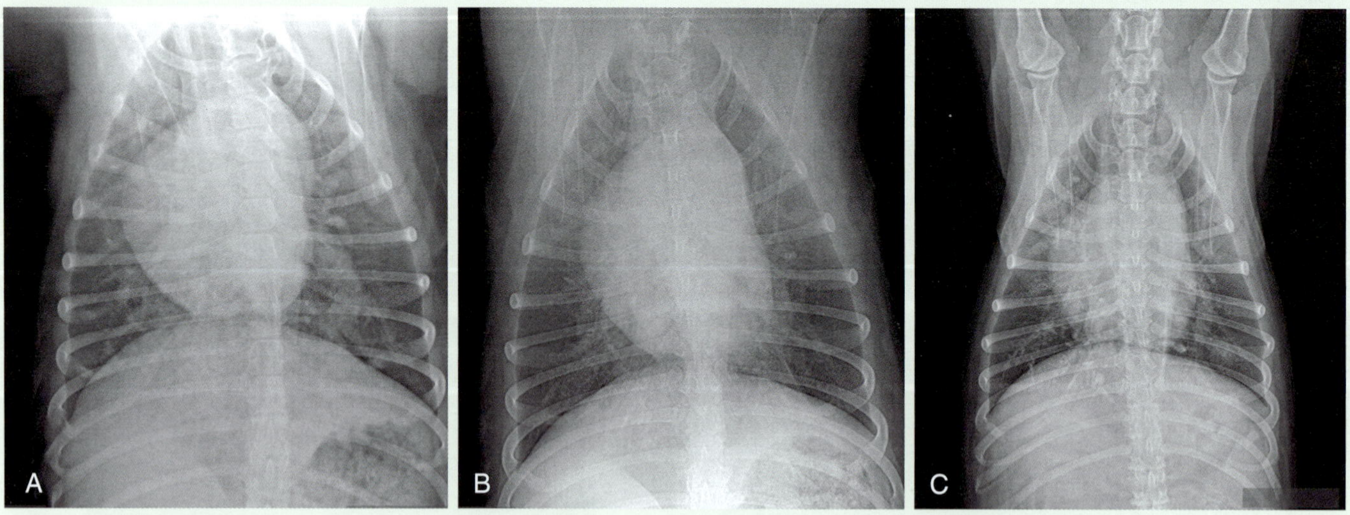

Fig. 111.17 Ventrodorsal radiographs of the thorax of the same dog in 110-15 after 62 days (A), 160 days (B) and 7 years (C) of treatment as described in the case report. There is progressive radiographic improvement but even at 7 years after treatment, persistent abnormalities remain.

SUGGESTED READINGS

Nelson CT, McCall JW, Jones S, et al. *Current Canine Guidelines for the Prevention, Diagnosis, and Management of Heartworm (Dirofilaria immitis) Infection in Dogs*. American Heartworm Society; 2020. Available at: https://d3ft8sckhnqim2.cloudfront.net/images/pdf/AHS_Canine_Guidelines_11_13_20.pdf?1605556516.

Jones S, Graham W, von Simson C, et al. *Current Feline Guidelines for the Prevention, Diagnosis, and Management of Heartworm (Dirofilaria immitis) Infection in Cats*. American Heartworm Society; 2020. Available at: https://d3ft8sckhnqim2.cloudfront.net/images/pdf/2020_AHS_Feline_Guidelines_11_12.pdf?1605556516.

REFERENCES

1. Birago F. *Trattato Cinegenetico, Ouero Della Caccia del Sig. Francesco Bitago, Signor di Metono, & di Siciano*. Milan, Italy: G. B. Bidelli; 1626:58–60.
2. Osborne TC. Worms found in the heart and blood vessels of a dog; symptoms of hydrophobia. *Western J Med Surg*. 1847;8:491–492.
3. Sano Y, Aoki M, Takahashi H, et al. The first record of *Dirofilaria immitis* infection in a Humboldt penguin, *Spheniscus humboldti*. *J Parasitol*. 2005;91:1235–1237.
4. Roncalli RA. Tracing the history of heartworm: a 400 year perspective. In: Seward RL, ed. *Recent Advances in Heartworm Disease: Symposium '98*. Batavia, IL: American Heartworm Society; 1998:1–14.
5. Vezzani D, Carbajo AE, Fontanarrosa MF, et al. Epidemiology of canine heartworm in its southern distribution in South America: risk factors, inter-annual trend and spatial patterns. *Vet Parasitol*. 2011;176:240–249.
6. Terrell SP, Courtney CH. Heartworm in Alaska: prevalence in domestic dogs and wild canids. In: Seward RL, ed. *Recent Advances in Heartworm Disease: Symposium '98*. Batavia, IL: American Heartworm Society; 1998:83–86.
7. Sacks BN. Increasing prevalence of canine heartworms in coyotes from California. *J Wildl Dis*. 1998;34:386–389.
8. McTier TL, McCall JW, Dzimianski MT, et al. Epidemiology of heartworm infection in beagles naturally exposed to infection in three southeastern states, pp 47-57. In: Soll MD, ed. *Proceedings of the Heartworm Symposium '92*. Batavia, IL: American Heartworm Society; 1992:47–57.
9. Scoles GA. Vectors of canine heartworm in the United States: a review of the literature including new data from Indiana, Florida and Louisiana. In: Seward RL, ed. *Recent Advances in Heartworm Disease: Symposium '98*. Batavia, IL: American Heartworm Society; 1998:21–36.
10. Scoles GA, Dickson SL. New foci of canine heartworm associated with introductions of new vector species. In: Sol MD, Knight DH, eds. *Proceedings of the Heartworm Symposium '95*. Batavia, IL: American Heartworm Society; 1995:27–35.
11. Rochlin I, Ninivaggi DV, Hutchinson ML, Farajollahi A. Climate change and range expansion of the Asian tiger mosquito (*Aedes albopictus*) in northeastern USA: implications for public health practitioners. *PLoS One*. 2013;8(4):e60874.
12. Lok JB, Knight DH. Laboratory verification of a seasonal heartworm transmission model. In: Seward RL, ed. *Recent Advances in Heartworm Disease: Symposium '98*. Batavia, IL: American Heartworm Society; 1998:15–20.
13. Nelson CT. Evaluation of temperature variation in microclimes in multiple locales in the United States and its effect on accuracy of models for prediction of mosquito survival and heartworm transmission. In: *Heartworm Disease: The Science, the Practice, the Future. Proceedings of the American Heartworm Society Triennial Symposium*. 2016.
14. Nelson CT, McCall JW, Jones S, et al. *Current Canine Guidelines for the Prevention, Diagnosis, and Management of Heartworm (Dirofilaria immitis) Infection in Dogs*. American Heartworm Society; 2020. https://d3ft8sckhnqim2.cloudfront.net/images/pdf/AHS_Canine_Guidelines_11_13_20.pdf?1605556516.
15. Bowman DD. Dirofilaria. In: Bowman DD, Lynn RC, Eberhard ML, Alcarez A, eds. *Georgi's Parasitology for Veterinarians*. 8th ed. St Louis, MO: Saunders; 2003:216–222.
16. Kotani K, Powers KG. Developmental stages of *Dirofilaria immitis* in the dog. *Am J Vet Res*. 1982;43:2199–2206.
17. Rawlings CA. *Heartworm Disease in Dogs and Cats*. Philadelphia: WB Saunders; 1986:329.
18. Calvert CA, Losonsky JM. Occult heartworm-disease associated allergic pneumonitis. *J Am Vet Med Assoc*. 1985;186:1097.
19. Bazzochi C, Genchi C, Paltrinieri S, et al. Immunological role of the endosymbionts of *Dirofilaria immitis*: the *Wolbachia* surface protein activates canine neutrophils with production of IL-8. *Vet Parasitol*. 2003;117:77–83.
20. Kramer LH, Tamarozzi F, Morchon R, et al. Immune response to and tissue localization of the *Wolbachia* surface protein (WSP) in dogs with natural heartworm (*Dirofilaria immitis*) infection. *Vet Immunol Immunopathol*. 2005;106:303–308.
21. Brattig NW, Bazzocchi C, Kirshing CJ, et al. The major surface protein of *Wolbachia* endosymbionts in filarial nematodes elicits immune responses through TLR2 and TLR 4. *J Immunol*. 2004;173:437–445.
22. Dillon AR, Brawner W, Hanrahan L. Influence of number of parasites and exercise on the severity of heartworm disease in dogs. In: Sol MD, Knight DH, eds. *Proceedings of the Heartworm Symposium '95*. Batavia, IL: American Heartworm Society; 1995 :113.
23. Fukami N, Hagio M, Okano S, et al. Influence of exercise on recovery of dogs following heartworm adulticide treatment with melarsomine. In: Seward RL, ed. *Recent Advances in Heartworm Disease: Symposium '98*. Batavia, IL: American Heartworm Society; 1998:225–227.
24. Dillon AR, Warner AE, Molina RM. Pulmonary parenchymal changes in dogs and cats after experimental transplantation of dead *Dirofilaria immitis*. In: Sol MD, Knight DH, eds. *Proceedings of the Heartworm Symposium '95*. Batavia, IL: American Heartworm Society; 1995:97–101.
25. Kitoh KA, Oka A, Kitagawa H, et al. Relaxing and contracting activities of heartworm extract on isolated canine abdominal aorta. *J Parasitol*. 2001;87:522–526.
26. Losonsky JM, Thrall DE, Lewis RE. Thoracic radiographic abnormalities in 200 dogs with heartworm infestation. *Vet Radiol*. 1983;24:124.
27. McCall JW, Supakorndej N, Donoghue AR, et al. Evaluation of the performance of canine heartworm antigen test kits licensed for use by veterinarians and canine heartworm test kits conducted by diagnostic laboratories. In: Seward RL, Knight DH, eds. *Recent Advances in Heartworm Disease: Symposium '01*. Batavia, IL: American Heartworm Society; 2001:91–104.
28. Lee ACY, Bowman DD, Lucio-Forster A, et al. Evaluation of a new in-clinic method for the detection of canine heartworm antigen. *Vet Parasitol*. 2011;77:387–391.
29. Little SE, Munzing C, Heise SR, et al. Pre-treatment with heat facilitates detection of antigen of *Dirofilaria immitis* in canine samples. *Vet Parasitol*. 2014;203:250–252.
30. Velasquez L, Blagburn BL, Duncan-Decoq R, et al. Increased prevalence of *Dirofilaria immitis* antigen in canine samples after heat treatment. *Vet Parasitol*. 2014;206:67–70.
31. Lane JN, Litster A, Little SE, et al. Optimizing heartworm diagnosis in dogs using multiple test combinations. *Parasit Vectors*. 2021;14:224.
32. Gioia G, Lecova L, Genchi M, et al. Highly sensitive multiplex PCR for simultaneous detection and discrimination of *Dirofilaria immitis* and *Dirofilaira repens* in canine peripheral blood. *Vet Parasitol*. 2010;172:160–163.
33. Bove CM, Gordon SG, Saunders AB, et al. Outcome of minimally invasive surgical treatment of heartworm caval syndrome in dogs: 42 cases (1999-2007). *J Am Vet Med Assoc*. 2010;236:187–192.
34. McCall JW, Genchi C, Kramer L, et al. Heartworm and *Wolbachia:* therapeutic implications. *Vet Parasitol*. 2008;158:204–214.
35. Kramer L, Grandi G, Passeri B, et al. Evaluation of lung pathology in *Dirofilaria immitis*-experimentally infected dogs treated with doxycycline or a combination of doxycycline and ivermectin before administration of melarsomine dihydrochloride. *Vet Parasitol*. 2011;176:357–360.
36. Grandi G, Quintavalla C, Mavropoulou A, et al. A combination of doxycycline and ivermectin is adulticidal in dogs with naturally acquired heartworm disease *(Dirofilaria immitis)*. *Vet Parasitol*. 2010;169:347–351.
37. Kramer L, Grandi G, Leoni L, et al. *Wolbachia* and its influence on the pathology and immunology of *Dirofilaria immitis*. *Vet Parasitol*. 2008;158:191–195.

38. Savadelis MD, Coleman AE, Rapoport GS, et al. Clinical assessment of heartworm-infected beagles treated with a combination of imidacloprid/moxidectin and doxycycline, or untreated. *J Vet Intern Med.* 2020;34:1734–1745.
39. McCall JW, Kramer L, Genchi C, et al. Effects of doxycycline on heartworm embryogenesis, transmission, circulating microfilaria, and adult worms in microfilaremic dogs. *Vet Parasitol.* 2014;206:5–13.
40. McCall JW, Jun JJ, Bandi C. *Wolbachia* and the antifilarial properties of tetracycline. An untold story. *Ital J Zool.* 1999;66:7–10.
41. Bazzocchi C, Mortarina M, Grandi G, et al. Combined ivermectin and doxycycline treatment has microfilaricidal and adulticidal activity against *Dirofilaria immitis* in experimentally infected dogs. *Int J Parasitol.* 2008;38:1401–1410.
42. Savadelia MD, Ohmes CM, Hostetler JA, et al. Assessment of parasitological findings in heartworm-infected beagles treated with Advantage Multi® for dogs (10% imidacloprid+2.5% moxidectin) and doxycycline. *Parasites Vectors.* 2017;10:245.
43. Drake J, Gruntmeir J, Merritt H, et al. False negative antigen tests in dogs infected with heartworm and placed on macrocyclic lactone preventives. *Parasites Vectors.* 2015;8:68.
44. Atwell R, Tarish JH. The effect of oral low-dose prednisolone on the extent of pulmonary pathology associated with dead *Dirofilaria immitis* in a canine lung model. In: Soll MD, Knight DH, eds. *Proceedings of the Heartworm Symposium '95.* Batavia, IL: American Heartworm Society; 1995.
45. Dzimianski M. The effect of prednisone on the efficacy of melarsomine dihydrochloride against adult *Dirofilaria immitis* in experimentally infected beagles. In: *Proceedings of the 13th Triennial State of the Heartworm Symposium.* 2010.
46. Nelson CT, Myrick ES, Nelson TA. Clinical benefits of incorporating doxycycline into a canine heartworm treatment protocol. *Parasites Vectors.* 2017;10(suppl 2):515.
47. Carretón E, Morchón R, Simón F, et al. Evaluation of cardiopulmonary biomarkers during classic adulticide treatment versus the American Heartworm Society recommended treatment protocol in dogs infected with *Dirofilaria immitis. Vet Parasitol.* 2014;206:55–59.
48. Paul AJ, Todd KS, Sundberg JP, et al. Efficacy of ivermectin against *Dirofilaria immitis* larvae in dogs 30 and 45 days after induced infection. *Am J Vet Res.* 1986;47:883–884.
49. Gates MC, Nolan TJ. Efficacy of heartworm preventatives against ascarids and hookworms in client-owned dogs: a retrospective case control study. *J Vet Pharmacol Ther.* 2010;34:116–119.
50. Hampshire V. Evaluation of efficacy of heartworm preventives products in the USA. *Vet Parasitol.* 2005;133:191–196.
51. Blagburn BL, Dillon AR, Arther RG, et al. Comparative efficacy of four commercially available heartworm preventive products against the MP3 laboratory strain of *Dirofilaria immitis. Vet Parasitol.* 2011;176: 189–194.
52. Snyder DE, Wiseman S, Cruthers LR, et al. Ivermectin and milbemycin oxime in experimental adult heartworm *(Dirofilaria immitis)* infection of dogs. *J Vet Intern Med.* 2011;25:61–64.
53. Bourguinat C, Keller K, Prichard RK, et al. Genetic polymorphisms in *Dirofilaria immitis. Vet Parasitol.* 2011;176:368–373.
54. Bourguinat C, Keller K, Blagburn B, et al. Correlation between loss of efficacy of macrocyclic lactone heartworm anthelmintics and P-glycoprotein genotype. *Vet Parasitol.* 2011;176:374–381.
55. McCall JW, Hodgkins E, Varloud M, et al. Blocking of the transmission of *Dirofilaria immitis* L3 (JYD-34 ML resistant strain) from infected mosquitoes to dogs and prevention of infection in dogs treated topically with dinotefuran-permethrin-pyriproxyfen and orally with milbemycin oxime alone or in combination. San Antonio, TX: *Proceedings of the American Association of Veterinary Parasitiologists 61st Annual Meeting.* 2016.
56. Lee ACY, Montgomery SP, Theis JH, et al. Public health issues concerning the widespread distribution of canine heartworm disease. *Trends Parasitol.* 2010;26:168–173.
57. Beskin CA, Colvin SH, Beaver PC. Pulmonary dirofilariasis cause of pulmonary nodular disease. *J Am Med Assoc.* 1996;198:197–199.
58. Theis JH. Public health aspects of dirofilariasis in the United States. *Vet Parasitol.* 2005;133:157–180.
59. Travassous LP. Notas helminthologicas. *Brazil Med.* 1921;35:67.
60. Riley WA. *Dirofilaria immitis* in the heart of a cat. *J Parasitol.* 1922;9:48.
61. Venco L, Genchi M, Genchi C, et al. Can heartworm prevalence in dogs be used as a provisional data for assessing the prevalence of the infection in cats? *Vet Parasitol.* 2011;176:300–303.
62. McCall JW, Dzimianski MT, McTier TL, et al. Biology of experimental heartworm infection in cats. In: Soll MD, ed. *Proceedings of the Heartworm Symposium '92.* Batavia, IL: American Heartworm Society; 1992:77–79.
63. Genchi C, Venco L, Ferrari N, et al. Feline heartworm (*Dirofilaria immitis*) infection: a statistical elaboration of the duration of the infection and life expectancy in asymptomatic cats. *Vet Parasitol.* 2008;158:177–182.
64. Maia FCL, McCall JW, Silva VA, et al. Structural and ultrastructural changes in the lungs of cats *Felis catus* (Linnaeus, 1758) experimentally infected with *D. immitis* (Leidy, 1856). *Vet Parasitol.* 2011;176:304–312.
65. Donahoe JMR, Kneller SK, Lewis RE. Hematological and radiographic changes in cats after inoculation with infective larvae of *D. immitis. J Am Vet Med Assoc.* 1976;168:413–417.
66. Holmes RA, Clark JN, Casey HW, et al. Histopathologic and radiographic studies of the development of heartworm pulmonary vascular disease in experimentally infected cats. In: Soll MD, ed. *Proceedings of the Heartworm Symposium '92.* Batavia, IL: American Heartworm Society; 1992:81–89.
67. Brown LE, Carter TD, Levy JK, et al. Pulmonary arterial disease in cats seropositive for *Dirofilaria immitis* but lacking adult heartworms in the heart and lungs. *Am J Vet Res.* 2005;66:1544–1549.
68. Dillon AR, Tillson DM, Wooldridge A, et al. Effect of pre-cardiac and adult stages of *Dirofilaria immitis* in pulmonary disease in cats: CBC, bronchial lavage cytology, serology, radiographs, CT images, bronchial reactivity, an histopathology. *Vet Parasitol.* 2014;206:24–37.
69. Jones S, Graham W, von Simson C, et al. *Current Feline Guidelines for the Prevention, Diagnosis, and Management of Heartworm (Dirofilaria immitis) Infection in Cats.* American Heartworm Society; 2020. Available at: https://d3ft8sckhnqim2.cloudfront.net/images/pdf/2020_AHS_Feline_Guidelines_11_12.pdf?1605556516.
70. Dillon AR, Warner A, Hudson J, et al. Role of PIM in inflammatory lung disease of cats and dogs. *J Vet Intern Med.* 1996;10:162.
71. Dillon AR, Warner AE, Brawner W, et al. Activity of pulmonary intravascular macrophages in cats and dogs with and without adult *Dirofilaria immitis. Vet Parasitol.* 2008;158:171–176.
72. Atkins CE, DeFrancesco TC, Coats JR, et al. Heartworm infection in cats: 50 cases (1985-1997). *J Am Vet Med Assoc.* 2000;217:355–358.
73. Atkins CE, Vaden SL, Arther RG, et al. Renal effects of *Dirofilaria immitis* in experimentally and naturally infected cats. *Vet Parasitol.* 2011;176:317–323.
74. DeFrancesco TC, Atkins CE, Mille MW, et al. Use of echocardiography for the diagnosis of heartworm disease in cats: 43 cases (1985–1997). *J Am Vet Med Assoc.* 2001;218:66–69.
75. Dillon AR, Brawner WR, Robertson-Plough CK, et al. Feline heartworm disease: correlations of clinical signs, serology, and other diagnostics: results of a multicenter study. *Vet Ther.* 2000;1:176–182.
76. Brawner WR, Dillon AR, Robertson-Plough CK, et al. Radiographic diagnosis of feline heartworm disease and correlation to other clinical criteria: results of a multicenter clinical case study. *Vet Ther.* 2000;1:81–87.
77. Defrancesco TC, Atkins CE. The utility of echocardiography in the diagnosis of feline heartworm disease: a review of published reports. In: Seward RL, ed. *Recent Advances in Heartworm Disease: Symposium '98.* Batavia, IL: American Heartworm Society; 1998:103–105.
78. Atkins CE, Arther RG, Ciszewski DK, et al. Echocardiographic quantification of *Dirofilaria immitis* in experimentally-infected cats. *Vet Parasitol.* 2008;158:164–170.
79. McCall JW, Guerrero J, Supakorndej P, et al. Evaluation of the accuracy of heartworm antigen and antibody test for cats. In: Seward RL, ed. *Recent Advances in Heartworm Disease: Symposium '98.* Batavia, IL: American Heartworm Society; 1998:127–134.
80. Nelson CT, Self TS. Incidence of *Dirofilaria immitis* in shelter cats in southeast Texas. In: Seward RL, ed. *Recent Advances in Heartworm Disease: Symposium '98.* Batavia, IL: American Heartworm Society; 1998:63–66.

81. Snyder PS, Levy JK, Salute ME, et al. Performance of serologic tests used to detect heartworm infection in cats. *J Am Vet Med Assoc*. 2000;216: 693–700.
82. Little SE, Raymond MR, Thoams JE, et al. Heat treatment prior to testing allows detection of antigen of *Dirofilaria immitis* in feline serum. *Parasites Vectors*. 2014;7:1.
83. Hays KM, Rodriguez JY, Little SE, et al. Heartworm prevalence in dogs versus cats: multiple diagnostic modalities provide new insights. *Vet Parasitol*. 2020;4:100027.
84. Gruntmeir JM, Adolph CB, Thomas JE, et al. Increased detection of *Dirofilaria immitis* antigen in cats after heat pretreatment of samples. *J Feline Med Surg*. 2017;19:1013–1016.
85. Bestul KJ, McCall JW, Nonglak S, et al. Evaluation of the Assure/FH Antibody Assay for the detection of feline heartworm infection. In: Seward RL, ed. *Recent Advances in Heartworm Disease: Symposium '98*. Batavia, IL: American Heartworm Society; 1998:179–186.
86. Donoghue AR, Mondesire RR, Porter JP. Detection of antibodies to *Dirofilaria immitis* in the cat using a highly specific recombinant antigen. In: *Proceedings of the North American Veterinary Conference*. 1997.
87. Richards J. *Heartworm-Associated Respiratory Disease in Cats*. Miami, FL: Roundtable discussion, AAFP Winter Meeting; 2007.
88. Hoerauf A, Mand S, Adjei O, et al. Depletion of *Wolbachia* in *Onchocerca volvulus* by doxycycline and microfilaridermia after ivermectin treatment. *Lancet*. 2001;357:1415–1416.
89. Taylor MJ, Bandi C, Hoerauf AM, Lazdins J. *Wolbachia* bacteria of filarial nematodes: a target for control? *Parasitol Today*. 2000;16:179–180.
90. Venco L, Borgarelli M, Ferrari E, et al. Surgical removal of heartworms from naturally-infected cats. In: Seward RL, ed. *Recent Advances in Heartworm Disease: Symposium '98*. Batavia, IL: American Heartworm Society; 1998:241–246.
91. Dunn KF, Levy JK, Colby KN, et al. Diagnostic, treatment, and prevention protocols for feline heartworm infection in animal sheltering agencies. *Vet Parasitol*. 2011;176:342–349.

112

Ascarids

Michael J. Yabsley, Sarah G.H. Sapp

KEY POINTS

- First Described: *Toxocara canis* and *Toxocara cati* have been recognized since the late 1700s. *Toxascaris leonina* was first described in 1902. *Baylisascaris procyonis* was first described in raccoons (*Procyon lotor*) in Poland in 1951, and first reported in dogs in 1988 (Michigan, United States).
- Cause: Ascarids (order Ascaridida) are large robust nematodes that primarily infect the small intestine of their definitive hosts. The anterior end of this group of nematodes has three prominent lips and males lack copulatory bursa. Representatives of this group include important pathogens of several domestic animals, wildlife species, and humans. This chapter will focus on the four primary ascarid species that infect dogs and cats: *Toxocara canis* and *Toxascaris leonina* in dogs, *Toxocara cati* and *T. leonina* in cats, and *Baylisascaris procyonis* (raccoon roundworm), which rarely occurs in dogs.
- Affected Hosts: Domestic dogs and wild canids can become infected with *T. canis* and *T. leonina,* whereas domestic cats and wild felids are the hosts of *T. cati* and *T. leonina*. Although the raccoon is the primary host of *B. procyonis*, domestic dogs can develop patent infections.
- Paratenic Hosts: An intermediate host is not required for ascarids, but many species utilize paratenic hosts. Rodents are the primary paratenic host species, although birds can also become infected with *Toxocara* spp. and *B. procyonis*.
- Geographic Distribution: *Toxocara canis, T. cati*, and *T. leonina* have cosmopolitan distributions. *Baylisascaris procyonis* is native to many regions of the United States and Canada but has been introduced to parts of Asia and Europe through translocation of raccoons.
- Route of Transmission: *Toxocara canis* can be transmitted to canids by ingestion of embryonated eggs or paratenic hosts or by transplacental or transmammary routes. *Toxocara cati* can be transmitted to felids by ingestion of embryonated eggs or paratenic hosts and through the transmammary route. *Toxascaris leonina* is transmitted to canids or felids by ingestion of embryonated eggs or paratenic hosts. *Baylisascaris procyonis* is transmitted to canids by ingestion of embryonated eggs or paratenic hosts.
- Major Clinical Signs: Young dogs and cats are more likely to develop signs which may include unthriftiness, lethargy, abdominal tenderness, rough haircoat, poor body condition and potbellied appearance, cough, and mucoid diarrhea. Adult animals are less likely to develop signs, as are those animals with low parasite burdens.
- Differential Diagnoses: Parasitic ova of other GI helminths must be differentiated from ascarid eggs. In dogs and cats, other large parasitic helminths or pseudoparasites (e.g., *Physaloptera* spp., free-living planarian *Bipalium,* horsehair worms/nematomorpha) may be passed in feces or vomitus and must be differentiated from ascarids.
- Human Health Significance: *Toxocara* spp. and *B. procyonis* are zoonotic. Infections are acquired by ingestion of embryonated eggs in the environment.

TOXOCARA CANIS

ETIOLOGIC AGENT

The common dog roundworm *Toxocara canis* is one of three ascarids that occur in the small intestine of domestic dogs. The other two ascarids are *Toxascaris leonina* and *Baylisascaris procyonis* (raccoon roundworm); the latter rarely occurs in dogs. *Toxocara canis* is transmitted to dogs by ingestion of embryonated eggs or paratenic hosts, or by transplacental or transmammary routes (see Transmission, later in this section). Infection is of zoonotic importance because of the potential for *T. canis* to cause ocular larva migrans (OLM) and visceral larva migrans (VLM) in humans.

Toxocara canis can most readily be distinguished from *T. leonina* by the presence of cervical alae in *T. leonina* which are absent or inconspicuous in *T. canis* (Table 112.1; Fig. 112.1). In addition, the eggs of these two species are easily distinguished based on morphology but not size (see Table 112.1; Fig. 112.2). Eggs of *T. canis* are pitted, whereas *T. leonina* are smooth with an undulating, prominent vitelline membrane on the inner boundary of the shell (which is not apparent in *T. canis*). Therefore, if there is any doubt to identity of adult worms, female worms can be teased open and egg morphology examined. Eggs of *T. canis* are most similar to those of *B. procyonis*; eggs of the latter tend to be smaller in diameter with a zygote that usually does not fill the shell, and possess a darker coat that is less distinctly pitted (see Fig. 112.2).[1] Another species, *Toxocara tanuki*, has been described from the raccoon dog (*Nyctereutes procyonoides*) in South Korea and Japan, but it has not been reported in domestic dogs.[2] Morphologically, *T. tanuki* is similar to *T. canis* (similar width of cervical alae and egg size) but the two can be distinguished based on spicule length (*T. tanuki* spicules are longer than those of *T. canis* and *T. cati*) and by sequence analysis of several gene targets.

EPIDEMIOLOGY

Toxocara canis is ubiquitous in canine populations worldwide and the prevalence varies among regions.[3–14] In the United States, prevalence varies considerably among studies in different regions or among different populations of dogs (e.g., owned dogs with low risk of infection

TABLE 112.1 Morphologic Characteristics of the Four Primary Ascarid Species Found in Domestic Dogs and Cats

	Toxocara canis	*Toxocara cati*	*Toxascaris leonina*	*Baylisascaris procyonis*
Authority	Werner 1782	Schrank 1788	Von Linstow 1902	Stefanski and Zarnowski 1951
Historical Synonyms	*Ascaris marginata* *Belascaris marginata*	*Ascaris teres* *Ascaris cati* *Ascaris felis* *Belascaris mystax* *Belascaris cati* *Toxocara mystax*	*Ascaris leptoptera* *Ascaris leonina*	*Ascaris columnaris* *Ascaris procyonis*
Adult size				
Female	6.5–10 cm	4–10 cm	6–10 cm	5–33 cm
Male	4–6 cm	3–7 cm	3–7 cm	4–11 cm
Cervical alae	Somewhat inconspicuous	Very prominent, arrow shaped	Prominent, spear shaped	Inconspicuous
Maximal L_3 size				
Length	400–500 μm	400–450 μm	650–750 μm	1,400–1,800 μm
Diameter	18–20 μm	15–16 μm	32–43 μm	60–75 μm
Average egg size	75 × 65 μm	75 × 65 μm	65 × 80 μm	70 × 60 μm
Egg morphology	Yellow to amber, round to slightly pear-shaped, pitted surface, zygote usually fills shell	Very similar to *T. canis,* pits may be smaller	Translucent to pale yellow, slightly ellipsoid, smooth surface	Amber, slightly ellipsoid, granular, irregularly pitted surface
Definitive hosts	Mostly dogs, infrequently cats	Cats only	Both dogs and cats	Raccoons, dogs
Zoonotic	Yes; common	Yes; relative frequency not known	Unlikely	Yes; rare

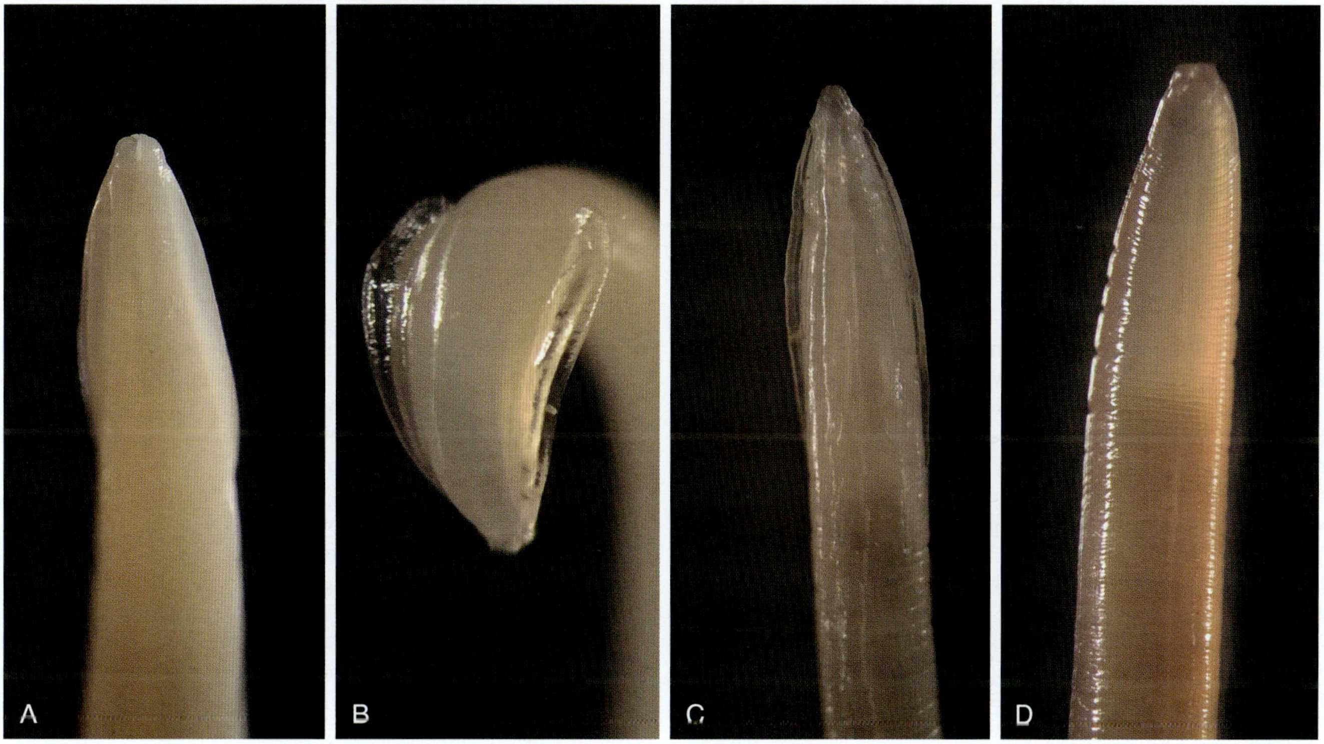

Fig. 112.1 Anterior end of four ascarid species found in domestic dogs and cats: (A) *Toxocara canis,* (B) *Toxocara cati,* (C) *Toxascaris leonina,* and (D) *Baylisascaris procyonis.*

versus stray/shelter dogs). However, even in areas where infection is believed to be infrequent, prevalence can change. For example, using a long-term dataset (capcvet.org), the prevalence of *T. canis* in dogs in Colorado was shown to have increased nearly 36% between 2013 and 2017.[15] Although lower in prevalence, *T. leonina* is considered widespread in canid populations.

Age resistance to *T. canis* is well documented but not absolute. Puppies spontaneously lose many adult worms after 6–8 weeks and patent infections are less likely to develop in dogs older than 6 months following ingestion of eggs.[16] In subsequent exposures, larvae are more likely to undergo somatic migration than to successfully complete the tracheal migration necessary for development. However, patent

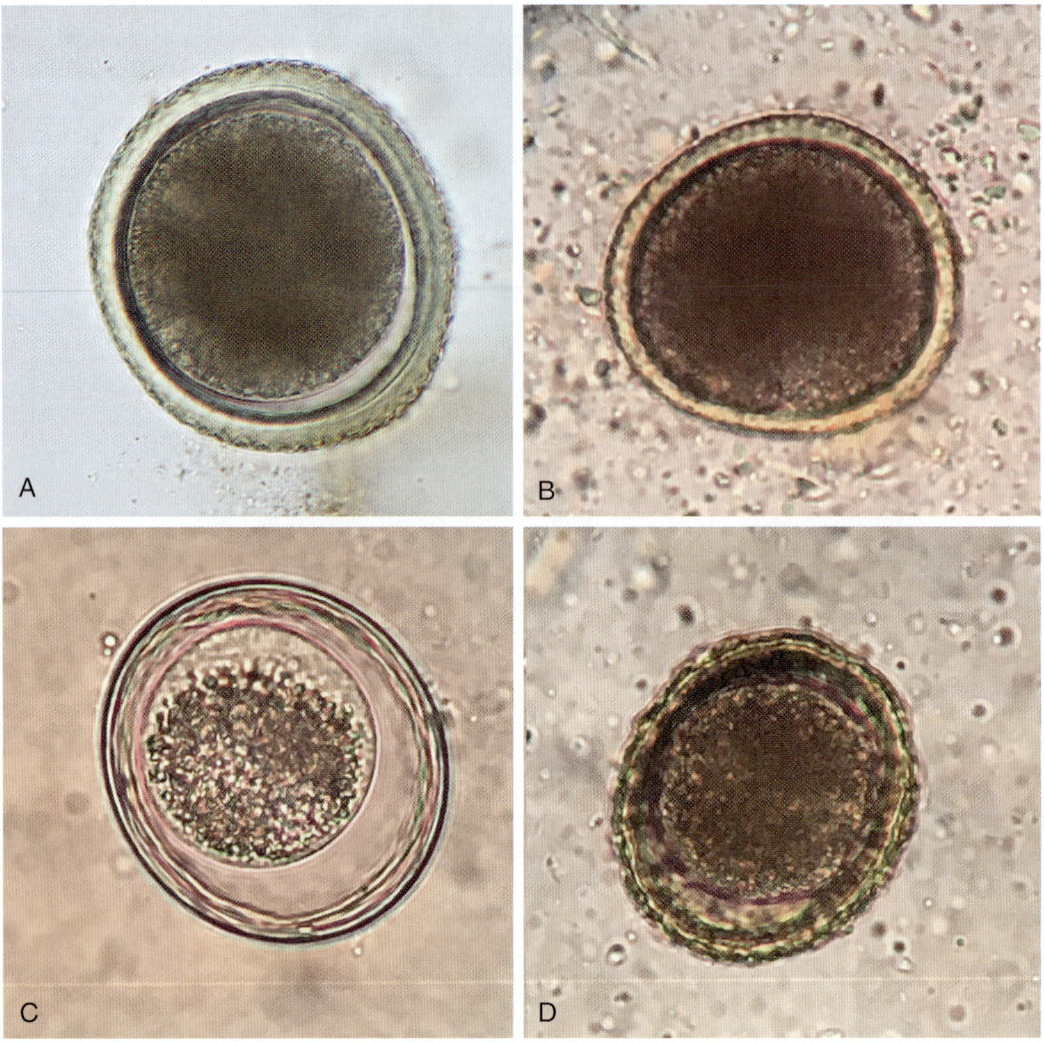

Fig. 112.2 Eggs of four ascarid species found in domestic dogs and cats: (A) *Toxocara canis*, (B) *Toxocara cati*, (C) *Toxascaris leonina*, and (D) *Baylisascaris procyonis*.

infections are still capable of developing in adult dogs and are detected occasionally; these dogs, even with low worm burdens, are sufficient to provide substantial environmental contamination; transmission.[17,18] Male dogs are somewhat more frequently infected than female dogs, although it is not clear if this is due to biological or epidemiologic factors,[19–21] and the opposite has also been noted.[22] Among owned dogs, prevalence is generally greater in dogs used for hunting or pastoral purposes than in companion dogs.[20,23–25]

Similar to most ascarids, large numbers of eggs are passed by infected dogs. Each female worm can release thousands of eggs, so a single puppy could excrete 10,000 to more than 100,000 eggs per gram of feces (EPG).[26–28] Eggs passed by dogs are unembryonated and require at least 2–4 weeks under ideal conditions to become infectious. Larval development ceases below 10°C and most larvae die if frozen (–15°C).[29] Once embryonated, eggs retain infectivity for a considerable period of time, up to 14 months in experimental settings, and are generally resistant to freezing.[30,31]

Seasonality has been noted for identification of *T. canis* in dogs in the United States.[32–34] Evaluation of more than 39 million fecal float test results at national service laboratories from 2012 to 2018 compiled by the CAPC (capcvet.org) revealed monthly prevalence of detection was consistent among years but highest (2.4%–2.7%) in the winter (December–January) and lowest (1.2%–1.5%) in the summer (May–June).[35] Similar seasonality was noted for whipworms, but the opposite seasonality was noted for hookworms, indicating that year-round control of intestinal parasites is important. On Prince Edward Island, Canada, the highest prevalence of *T. canis* infections in dogs occurred in the autumn (September–December) and winter (December–March).[22]

Numerous studies have shown that *T. canis* eggs may adhere to the haircoat of dogs and possibly present a risk, if a small one, for transmission to humans or other animals with direct contact to pet dogs.[36–39] In one study, 100% of stray puppies and over half of stray adult dogs had *Toxocara* spp. eggs adhering to perianal hair. Puppies also had a significantly higher mean concentration of eggs on hair (1,499 EPG) versus adult dogs (mean 42 EPG).[40] Among owned dogs, 8.8% were positive for *Toxocara* spp. eggs on hair on the head, neck, back, and/or perianal areas. Concentrations were very low compared to stray dogs (mean 4.4 EPG).[41] Despite the frequency of contamination, the risk of transmission is negligible unless these adherent eggs are embryonated. Eggs are capable of developing on hair in a laboratory environment, although dogs would likely groom away this fecal contamination before embryonation could occur.[42] While most studies have recovered predominately nonviable or unembryonated eggs, some dogs acquire embryonated eggs on fur from contaminated environments.[36] Appropriate hand hygiene after contact with dog fur should be observed to reduce risk of zoonotic transmission, particularly for dog groomers and individuals caring for stray dogs, especially young puppies.

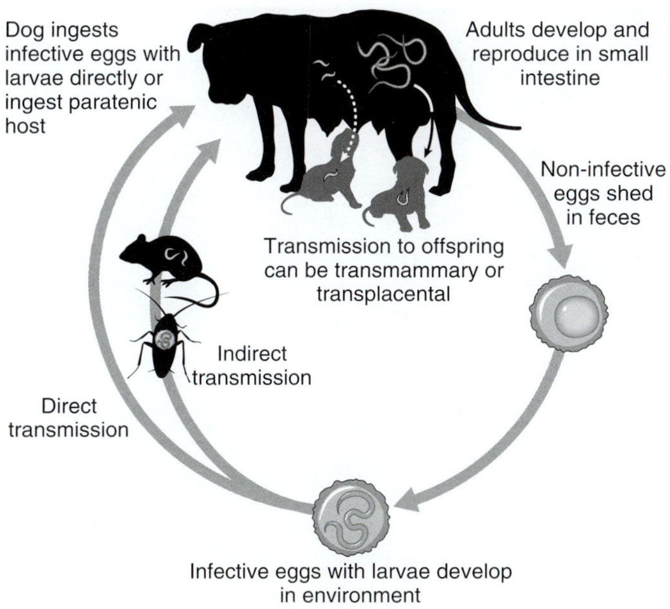

Fig. 112.3 Life cycle and transmission routes of *Toxocara canis.*

There is growing interest in the canine and public health risks associated with contamination of the environment with *T. canis* eggs. Numerous studies have shown that soil and/or dog feces in dog parks, city parks, children's playgrounds, etc. can contain *Toxocara* spp. eggs.[43–46] In a 2020 study from the United States, 9% of 3,006 fecal specimens from dogs that were using off-leash parks were positive for at least one intestinal nematode, 17 of which were ascarids.[47] Overall, intestinal parasites were detected in over 20% of dogs and at 85% of dog parks across the study areas.

CLINICAL FEATURES

Pathogenesis

Toxocara canis is transmitted to canid hosts by numerous routes including the ingestion of embryonated eggs from the environment or ingestion of paratenic hosts (Fig. 112.3). However, transplacental, and to a lesser extent transmammary, routes of transmission are very common, which is why nearly all puppies are born infected or become infected early in life. The migration of larvae in the canine host is complex and influenced by age, route of infection, and host immunity.

Transmission by Egg Ingestion

When eggs with infectious third-stage larvae (L_3) are ingested by young dogs, the eggs hatch in the duodenum and the L_3 penetrate the small intestinal wall to enter circulation. Within approximately 24 hours, circulating larvae are transported to the liver via the portal vein where they exit via the vena cava and are carried to the lungs. Larvae exit the circulation through the alveoli, then are coughed up and swallowed, reentering the GI tract in what is referred to as *hepatotracheal migration.* Once in the stomach, the L_3 molt to L_4; another molt to the L_5 (subadult) stage occurs in the small intestine. It takes approximately 1 to 2 weeks for this migration to be completed. Completion of maturation and patency typically occurs after 4 to 6 weeks, tending towards longer periods in older experimentally inoculated animals.[17,19] Some larvae do not complete the hepatotracheal migration; instead they reenter circulation after exiting the lungs. These larvae then undergo somatic migration and cause VLM. When larvae become trapped in capillaries during migration, they become encapsulated in granulomas produced by host immune mechanisms and arrest at the L_3 stage.

An interesting observation regarding infection via ingestion of eggs is the effect of dose on infection success. Ascarid-naïve puppies inoculated with 10 to 1,000 eggs developed intestinal infections, but no infections were detected in those inoculated with 10,000 eggs, suggesting this resistance is not a result of pre-existing immunity.[48] Similar results have been observed with 3-week-old puppies inoculated with 3,000 eggs.[49]

Transmission by Paratenic Host Ingestion

When a susceptible paratenic host, such as a rodent or bird, ingests infectious eggs, the larvae hatch in the GI tract and enter the circulation. Larvae in paratenic hosts do not undergo hepatotracheal migration, but instead undergo somatic migration and accumulate in the liver, lung, kidney, skeletal muscle, and nervous tissues.[50] Invasion of the CNS by larvae is referred to as neural larva migrans (NLM), and these migrating larvae may produce neurologic disease which can be fatal. Larvae can also invade the eye (OLM) and cause vision damage or blindness. Larvae can remain viable in tissues of paratenic hosts for months to years.[50–54] Experimentally, cockroaches and earthworms can ingest eggs and serve as paratenic hosts.[53–56] Reviews of the ecology and impacts of *Toxocara* spp. infections in paratenic hosts have been published.[50,54]

These larvae, regardless of location in the paratenic host, are infectious to the canine definitive host or other paratenic hosts.[57] When a dog ingests larvae in paratenic host tissues, tracheal migration may not always occur, presumably because larvae have developed sufficiently during migration within the paratenic host.[58] In experimental inoculations of dogs with *T. canis* larvae within mouse tissues, infection develops, in some instances, without breaching the GI tract as few to no larvae are recovered from sites other than the GI wall/lumen.[49,58] When development proceeds without tracheal migration, prepatent periods (PPPs) tend to be short (as early as 33 days in one experimental infection study).[57]

Transplacental and Transmammary Transmission

The majority of, if not all, infections of very young puppies with *T. canis* are acquired through the transplacental (intrauterine, prenatal) route. Infection of the dam either during gestation or prior to conception can result in vertical transmission. Hypobiotic larvae in tissues of the dam can become reactivated during gestation, but it is unknown how long these larvae can persist. The mechanism by which hypobiotic larvae become activated is also not understood, although it is likely mediated by complex hormonal changes (e.g., estradiol, progestin, prolactin) and immunosuppression that occur during pregnancy.[59] The timing of infection of a dam during gestation can impact transplacental transmission, with more frequent transmission occurring when dams become infected later in gestation.[60] For example, inoculation at 35 days post-conception did not result in transmission, whereas five of six pups from a dam inoculated at 56 days post-conception had larvae within their tissues.[60] In another study, larvae were first noted in a single fetus in a dam infected 43 days post-conception, and the infection of dams after 47 days post-conception resulted in the presence of larvae within fetuses.[61]

In puppies born to experimentally inoculated pregnant dams, L_3 were present in the heart and lungs of the puppies at parturition. Larvae had migrated to the GI tract within 3 days and molted to the L_4 stage with in ~1 week. In these puppies, mature *T. canis* were detected as early as 3 weeks post-parturition.[49,61]

Larvae that fail to establish infection in the intestine in young puppies may be passed in the feces. Dams may become reinfected postpartum by swallowing these expelled larvae during grooming of pups.[62] Also, adult worms are frequently expelled in large numbers by older puppies, especially around 9 to 10 weeks or age.

Lactogenic (transmammary) transmission can also occur, but this is considered a minor route of infection in dogs compared with the transplacental route.[63] As with larvae acquired through ingestion of paratenic hosts, the ingested L_3 do not undergo hepatotracheal migration.

Transplacental transmission has also been demonstrated in paratenic hosts. Experimental infections in mice revealed the presence of larvae in the placenta and fetal tissues after inoculation at mid-gestation. This process is generally thought to be prolactin-mediated.[59,64]

Clinical Signs and Physical Examination Abnormalities

Clinical signs of *T. canis* infestation are most severe and most likely to occur in young puppies. Most adult dogs with intestinal *T. canis* infections are subclinically infected. Heavy burdens can cause unthriftiness, abdominal tenderness, poor body condition, lethargy, vomiting, diarrhea, and cough. Puppies will often present with a "potbellied" appearance. Extremely high worm burdens can cause intestinal obstructions or intussusception. Larval migration though the lungs creates hemorrhage, but respiratory distress is not usually evident unless infections are particularly intense. In rare cases, very young puppies may die acutely due to the migration of large numbers of prenatally acquired larvae out of the lungs after birth. In some cases, puppies vomit developing mature worms when worm burdens are high.

Rarely, migrating larvae may become encapsulated in granulomas and, if numbers of larvae are high, cause morbidity or mortality.[65,66] A few unusual cases of retinitis attributed to ocular toxocariasis in puppies have been reported. In one case, four puppies developed retinopathy leading to blindness, and *T. canis* larvae were recovered from the eye of the one puppy that was necropsied. These puppies had been fed raw pork liver, which may have contained a large number of encysted larvae.[67]

Toxocara canis is capable of causing VLM in cats following experimental inoculation. Cats inoculated with *T. canis* eggs developed granulomatous lesions in the liver, lungs, and kidneys accompanied with peripheral eosinophilia, but clinical signs were mild to absent.[68] However, a naturally infected cat that was evaluated for pyrexia and eosinophilic pulmonary endarteritis had disseminated lesions containing *T. canis* larvae, suggesting that migrating *T. canis* larvae are capable of causing disease in cats in the field.[69]

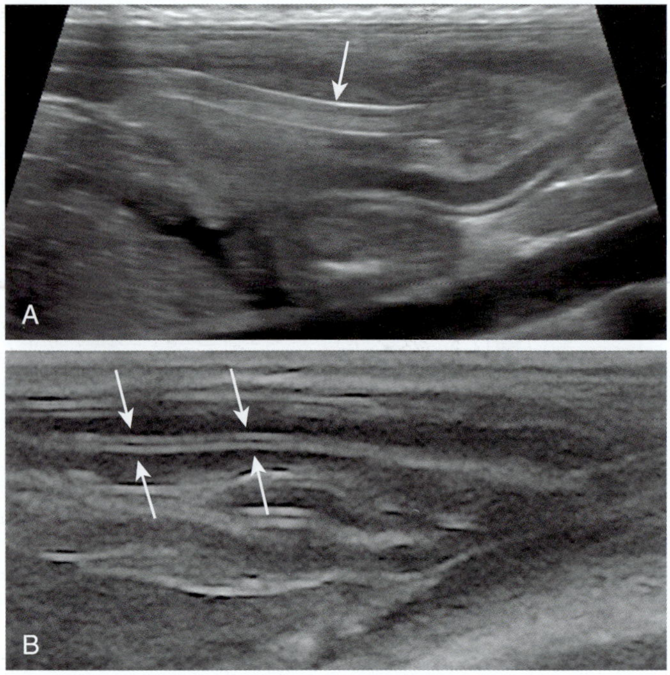

Fig. 112.4 (A) Abdominal ultrasound of a 9-week-old golden retriever puppy. Within a loop of jejunum, an ascarid is recognized as long thin parallel hyperechoic lines *(arrow)*. (B) Ultrasound of a 15-day-old dachshund puppy showing an intraluminal ascarid *(arrows)*. (A, Courtesy of K. Gendron DACVR, The University of Georgia, USA. B, Courtesy of A. Corda, University of Sassari, Italy.)

DIAGNOSIS

Laboratory Abnormalities and Diagnostic Imaging

Laboratory abnormalities in dogs with *T. canis* infections are nonspecific; peripheral eosinophilia may be present, and increased serum liver enzyme activities have been documented as a result of hepatic migration.[58] Radiographs may reveal diffuse mixed pulmonary opacities as a result of larval migration. Ascarids may be visible as linear foreign objects within the GI tract following barium administration; they may also be seen on ultrasound examination as two non-shadowing parallel hyperechoic lines ("train tracks") on longitudinal section and ring-shaped hyperechoic structures on transverse section (Fig. 112.4). In one study from Sardinia, Italy, ascarids were visible in the intestinal tract of newborn puppies using ultrasonography on days 10, 15, 20, and 25 after birth, even before eggs were visible on zinc sulfate fecal flotation.[70]

Microbiologic Tests

Diagnosis Using Fecal Examination

All dogs should be tested for ascarid infections by fecal flotation with centrifugation (see Chapter 5), although all puppies should be assumed infected and thus dewormed. Recently, a commercial test that detects antigens shed by developing and adult ascarids has become available.[71] Puppies should be tested more frequently than adult dogs; testing at least four times a year for puppies and at least 1 to 2 times a year for adults is recommended.

Ascarid eggs float in most salt- and sugar-based flotation solutions (e.g., $ZnSO_4$ SpG 1.18; sugar SpG 1.25). Although ascarids produce large numbers of eggs, increased sensitivity is gained from using centrifugation of fecal floats. This is especially important because not all parasites in dogs may produce large numbers of ova. *Toxocara* spp. eggs must be differentiated from those of *T. leonina* and *B. procyonis* (see Table 112.1; Fig. 112.2; see also section on Etiology, earlier). Coprophagy is an important consideration when examining fecal floats, especially if the dog has access to cat feces, as eggs of *T. canis* and *T. cati* are morphologically similar. If a dog tests positive for *Toxocara* spp. eggs but the history suggests a patent infection is unlikely (e.g., owner compliance regarding monthly preventive use is not in question or dog has had recent treatment), additional fecal specimens should be evaluated after the dog has been leash-confined to prevent coprophagy.

An ELISA that detects antigens produced by immature and adult ascarids is available (IDEXX Laboratories, Inc., Westbrook, ME, USA).[72] Because this test can detect antigens released by immature worms, detection of infection can occur before patency. Experimentally, the ELISA detected *T. canis* coproantigen 31 to 38 days PI.[71] Single-sex infections can also be detected. However, the assay does not differentiate between the ascarid species, so microscopic examination of feces is still recommended (e.g., patent infections with either *T. canis* or *B. procyonis* can result in a positive ELISA result).[73] As noted earlier, coprophagy may confuse interpretation of coproantigen test results; if a dog is coproantigen negative but fecal float positive, one should consider coprophagy. Several studies have noted that a high number of canine fecal specimens with *Toxocara* spp. eggs actually harbor *T. cati* eggs.[74,75] Additionally, older dogs are more likely to have discordant results (antigen negative, fecal egg positive).[72] Retesting of specimens after prevention of coprophagy should be recommended.

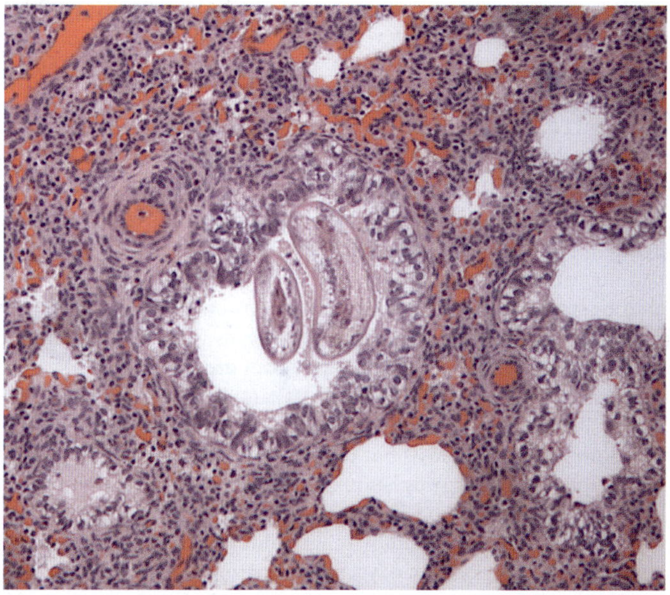

Fig. 112.5 Histopathology image showing severe, diffuse, acute, eosinophilic interstitial pneumonia with intralesional migrating ascarid larvae in a 36-hour-old great Pyrenees puppy that died acutely together with three other puppies. Severe perivascular eosinophilic hepatitis was also present, consistent with hepatopulmonary migration of larvae that were most likely obtained by transplacental infection, given the young age of the puppy. The puppy also had spina bifida and an associated acute suppurative meningitis. (Courtesy Jane E. Sykes, University of California-Davis.)

Sometimes adult worms will be detected in the vomitus of dogs. Ascarids can be differentiated from *Physaloptera* spp. by their large size and the three prominent lips on the anterior end. In contrast, *Physaloptera* spp. are smaller, are frequently more coiled, and have a triangle-shaped anterior end that often has a swelling of the cuticle (cervical collar); male *Physaloptera* spp. have large caudal alae (see Chapter 116).

Pathologic Findings

Gross pathologic findings in puppies that die as a result of large numbers of migrating ascarids include pulmonary congestion and hemorrhages, as well as hepatic congestion (which may be secondary to shock). On histopathology, eosinophilic enteritis, hepatitis, and interstitial pneumonia may be identified with intralesional ascarid larvae (Fig. 112.5).

TREATMENT AND PREVENTION

Treatment for *T. canis* is necessary for several reasons: (1) treatment of clinically ill dogs, (2) to prevent contamination of the environment with environmentally resistant eggs, (3) to prevent transmission from the dam to puppies, and (4) to reduce the risk of human disease. All dogs should be on a monthly product with efficacy against *T. canis* to limit reinfections. Also, limiting the ability of dogs to ingest possible paratenic hosts will minimize infection risk. Another final consideration for prevention of infection in dogs is to avoid raw diets; raw animal tissues (e.g., liver) can be a source of infection if tissues include *Toxocara* spp. larvae, as has been noted in humans.

Currently, numerous anthelmintics are approved for the treatment of *T. canis* including fenbendazole, milbemycin oxime, moxidectin, and pyrantel pamoate. In addition, pyrantel in combination with ivermectin, pyrantel in combination with ivermectin and praziquantel, and febantel in combination with pyrantel and praziquantel are approved for treatment of *T. canis* infections (see https://capcvet.org/parasite-product-applications/). All are effective when administered at the label-approved dose; repeated treatment may be necessary to eliminate all stages.

To prevent excretion of eggs into the environment, all pups should be routinely treated at 2, 4, 6, and 8 weeks of age and then placed on a monthly preventive with activity against *T. canis*. Nursing dams should be treated for ascarids on the same schedule as the puppies. If possible, pregnant dams should be treated during pregnancy to prevent vertical transmission to the pups. Daily fenbendazole (50 mg/kg, PO, q24h), selamectin (6–12 mg/kg applied topically), and monthly topical moxidectin/imidacloprid have been shown to prevent infection from dam to pups when administered late in pregnancy.[76–78]

PUBLIC HEALTH ASPECTS

VLM in humans can likely occur with both *T. canis* and *T. cati* infections, although most cases are thought to be associated with *T. canis* infection. Most cases are reported in children due to geophagia/pica. Signs and symptoms are generally nonspecific and variable depending on which tissues larvae migrate through, which can complicate diagnosis. Common manifestations of acute infection include fever, cough, abdominal pain, eosinophilia, and sometimes respiratory signs; diagnosis is confirmed with case history and serologic testing (typically, a *T. canis* excretory-secretory ELISA to detect specific IgG).[79] *Toxocara canis* larvae rarely invade the brain, but there are a few documented cases of cerebral toxocariasis.[80] Children should be encouraged to practice hand hygiene and be prevented from engaging in geophagia to prevent exposure to *T. canis* eggs.

OLM causes diffuse unilateral subacute retinitis (DUSN) involving unilateral vision loss and strabismus, again more in children than adults (Fig. 112.6). Symptoms can wax and wane, or it may be an incidental finding on routine ocular examination. Granuloma formation may be misdiagnosed as retinoblastoma and result in unnecessary enucleation, so awareness of ocular toxocariasis is critical for physicians.[81] Unlike VLM, OLM is thought to be associated with exposure to a low number of eggs, which would not generate a sufficient immune response to prevent larvae from invading the eye.[82] Furthermore, this low degree of immunologic activation complicates diagnosis as antibody levels may be minimal to undetectable.[83]

Antibodies to *Toxocara* spp. have been detected in people throughout the world, but seroprevalence varies regionally and with socioeconomic development.[84] In the United States, three large nationally representative surveys revealed that 5.1% to 13.9% of individuals were seropositive, with the greatest prevalence among lower socioeconomic strata.[85–88] The presence of antibodies in otherwise asymptomatic individuals is sometimes referred to as *covert toxocariasis*. Multiple epidemiologic studies have found statistical associations between covert toxocariasis and other health conditions such as urticaria, allergies, diminished lung capacity, occult seizures, and cognitive delay in children, although the role of *Toxocara* as the causative agent is not always clear.[89]

TOXOCARA CATI

ETIOLOGIC AGENT

The cat roundworm, *T. cati*, is the most common ascarid detected in domestic cats. Unlike *T. leonina*, the other ascarid likely to be found in domestic cats, adult *T. cati* have very prominent, broad, "arrow-shaped" cervical alae which are less prominent and more spear-shaped in *T. leonina* (see Table 112.1; Fig. 112.1). In addition, the eggs

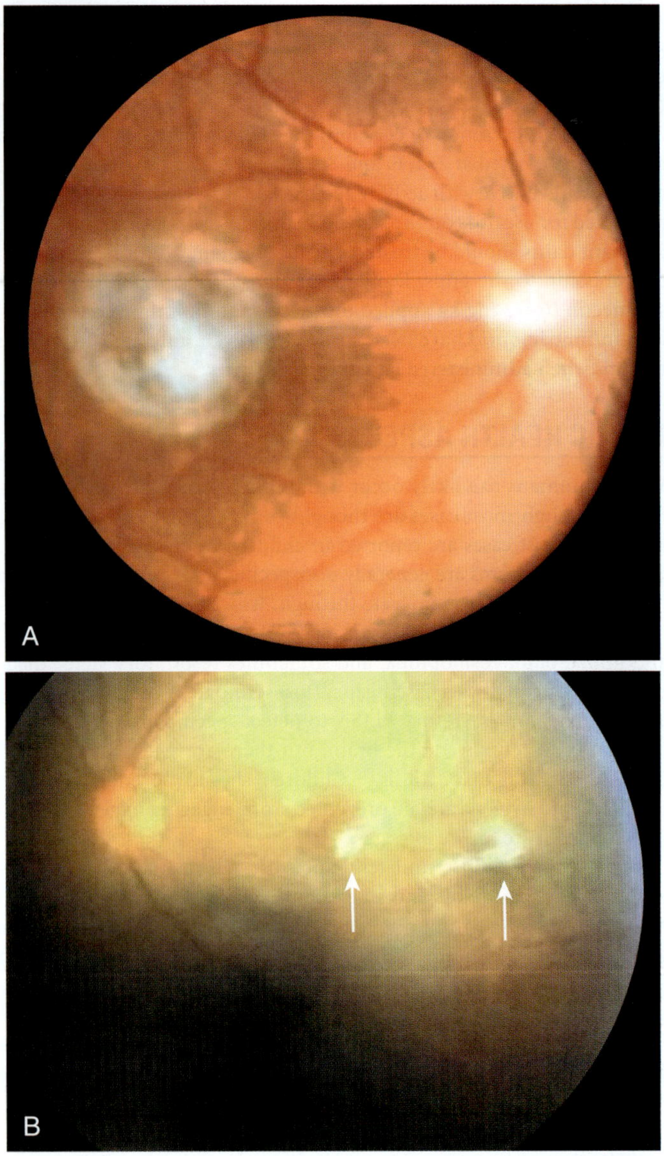

Fig. 112.6 Fundoscopic lesions in humans with ocular toxocariasis (ocular larva migrans). (A) Peripheral retinal and vitreous lesion with a localized mass of whitish tissue ("snow bank") involving the retina and peripheral vitreous. There is also a fibrocellular band that runs from the peripheral lesion toward the optic nerve or posterior retina. (B) White retinal lesions *(arrows)* caused by the migration of *Toxocara cati*. (A, From Rubinsky-Elefant G, Hirata CE, Yamamoto JH, et al. Human toxocariasis: diagnosis, worldwide seroprevalences and clinical expression of the systemic and ocular forms. *Ann Trop Med Parasitol.* 2010;104:3–23. B, From ZibaeiM, Sadijadi SM, Jahadi-Hosseini SH. Toxocara cati larvae in the eye of a child: a case report. *Asian Pacific J Trop Biomed.* 2014;4:S53–S55.)

of these two species are easily distinguished based on morphology, but not size (see Table 112.1; Fig. 112.2). Eggs of *T. cati* are pitted, whereas *T. leonina* are smooth, and *T. leonina* eggs contain prominent vitelline membranes which are absent in *T. cati*. Therefore, if there is any doubt to identity of adult worms, female worms can be teased open and egg morphology examined. In a geographically limited area of Asia, a third ascarid (*Toxocara malayasiensis*) has been reported from domestic cats. Morphologically, *T. malayasiensis* lacks the prominent broad cervical alae of *T. cati* (thus is morphologically most similar to *T. canis*).

EPIDEMIOLOGY

Toxocara cati is widespread in felid populations worldwide, although the prevalence varies among regions.[5–9,11–13,90] Its prevalence tends to be highest in shelter/unowned cats or cats without veterinary care; prevalence in these groups is often > 20%. This high prevalence in free-roaming cats likely explains the frequently detected contamination of outdoor spaces (e.g., parks, children's playgrounds).[46,91,92] In many of these environmental studies, more *T. cati* eggs were detected than *T. canis* eggs. Similar to *T. canis* in dogs, *T. cati* prevalence varies seasonally in cats (highest prevalence in winter) and in the environment.[34,91]

The PPP can be as early as 21 days if infections develop from ingestion of paratenic hosts but can take approximately 38 to 55 days if infections follow egg ingestion. As for *T. canis*, large numbers of eggs can be passed in the feces of infected cats, although egg numbers are more variable and generally range from 200 to 23,000 EPG. Eggs require about 3 weeks in an oxygenated environment to become infective. No development occurs below 10°C.[29]

Dogs may develop VLM following ingestion of *T. cati* eggs, with larvae recovered from the skeletal muscle and lung tissue, but patent intestinal infections have never been successfully established in dogs.[93]

Toxocara cati has been reported in cats worldwide. It has also been reported in wild felids.[94] Prevalence varies greatly based on location and host factors.[5–9,11–13,90] Young cats (<1 year) are more commonly infected than older cats.[14,16,95,96] Stray cats have a much greater prevalence of *T. cati* infection versus owned cats, and among owned cats, those with outdoor access are at increased risk of infection.[97–100] Cats receiving more than three anthelmintic treatments per year had a significantly reduced prevalence compared with those receiving fewer, although prevalence was still 10.4% in this group.[97]

Toxocara cati is frequently detected in soil specimens, particularly in urban areas. For example, in Poland, *T. cati* was more prevalent in soil in urban regions than *T. canis*, presumably due to the presence of feral cats.[101] However, the majority of surveys do not distinguish between the *Toxocara* species, so data on individual *Toxocara* species and environmental contamination is limited.[102]

CLINICAL FEATURES

Pathogenesis, Clinical Signs, and Physical Examination Findings

Similar to *T. canis* infection in dogs, transmission of *T. cati* to cats can occur after ingestion of either infectious eggs or paratenic host tissues containing larvae (Fig. 112.7). Transmammary transmission from dam to offspring occurs but is less important than the other two routes. Currently there is no evidence to suggest that prenatal or transplacental transmission occurs in cats even though it is a major transmission route for *T. canis* in dogs.[93,103,104]

Transmission by Egg Ingestion

As with *T. canis* infections, ingestion of *T. cati* eggs is followed by hepatotracheal migration. During the first 5 to 10 days after infection, the larvae migrate through the liver and lungs; some of the larvae migrate up the trachea, where they are swallowed. Other larvae migrate to muscle tissues. Those that return to the stomach enter the stomach wall and begin to grow from about 0.3–0.4 mm in length to approximately 1.0 mm, at which point they molt to the L_4 stage and enter the intestinal lumen.[93] L_4 stages proceed to develop to adults after passage into the lumen.

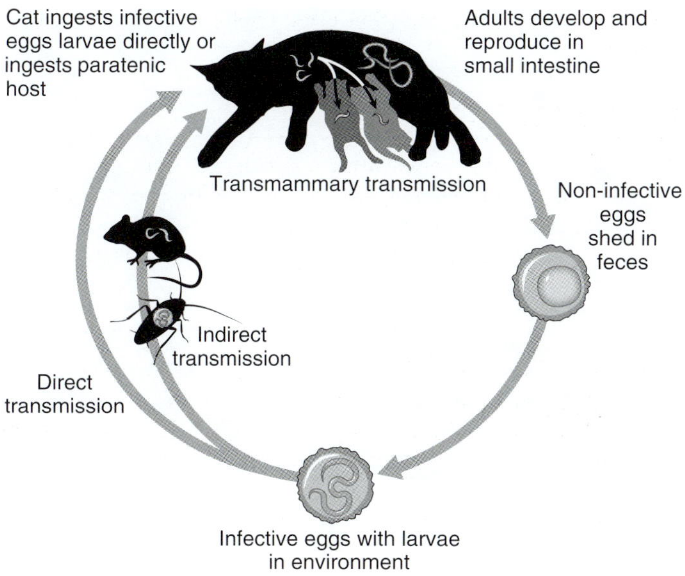

Fig. 112.7 Life cycle and transmission routes of *Toxocara cati*.

Transmission by Paratenic Host Ingestion

Predation of paratenic hosts such as rodents, birds, and some invertebrates (earthworms, beetles) is likely the most important transmission route for *T. cati* infections. When vertebrate hosts ingest eggs, the larvae migrate through the liver, lungs, skeletal muscle, and other tissues where they can remain infectious for several months.[54,105] In general, fewer *T. cati* larvae migrate to the CNS or eyes compared with *T. canis*; however, should they migrate into these tissues, they can cause clinical disease.[106–108] In a mouse model, *T. cati* appeared to have a preference for the cerebellum, whereas *T. canis* localized primarily in the cerebrum.[109] These differences may explain observed behavioral differences in neurologic manifestations between *T. canis*– and *T. cati*–induced neurotoxocariasis.[110] Although most work on paratenic hosts revolves around understanding transmission to cats, disease due to larval migrans can be important for vulnerable or endangered species (e.g., North Island brown kiwi (*Apteryx mantelli*)).[111] Reviews of the ecology and impacts of *T. cati* infections on paratenic hosts have been published.[50,54] Within paratenic hosts, larval width differentiates *T. cati* (maximum 18 μm) from *T. canis* (generally ≥ 18 μm). Several PCR assays have also been developed for detection and distinction of ascarid larvae in tissues and other specimens.[112,113] When larvae in paratenic host tissues are ingested by cats, they generally do not undergo hepatotracheal migration, although a few larvae may be recovered from the lungs or liver.

Transmammary Transmission

Transmammary transmission is most likely to occur following acute infection during pregnancy or soon after birth, after which the larvae migrate to mammary glands and infect nursing kittens. However, transmammary transmission also has been documented from chronically infected queens. Larvae are abundant in mammary glands and appear in milk throughout lactation.[95] Larvae acquired by kittens via this route do not undergo hepatotracheal migration.

Larva migrans can follow egg ingestion in cats. When large numbers of eggs are ingested, early migration of larvae in lungs can produce focal hemorrhages, pulmonary arterial lesions, and inflammation, resulting in dyspnea and cough. Complete vessel occlusion can occur as a result of arterial wall hyperplasia.[114,115] In cats that were experimentally infected with 6,000 eggs, treatment with a commercial preventive (topical moxidectin/imidacloprid) prior to inoculation did not prevent larval migration through the lungs, although it did ameliorate

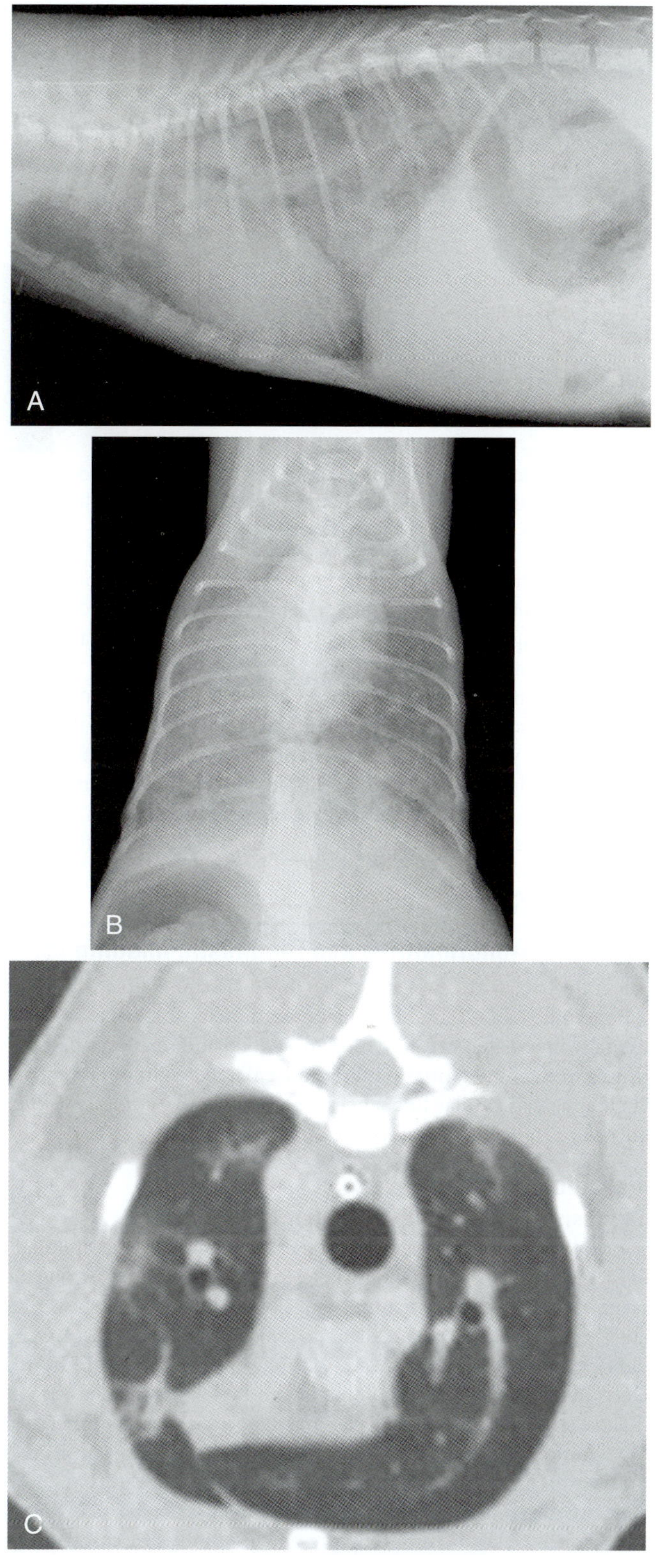

Fig. 112.8 (A) Lateral and (B) ventrodorsal radiograph showing evidence of diffuse pneumonia secondary to ascarid migration in a kitten. (C) Computed tomography scan of a cat 11 days after experimental inoculation with 3,000 *Toxocara cati* eggs. Patchy pulmonary densities are present throughout the lung parenchyma. (A,B Courtesy University of California-Davis Diagnostic Imaging Service. C, From Dillon AR, Tillson DM, Hathcock J, et al. Lung histopathology, radiography, high-resolution computed tomography, and bronchio-alveolar lavage cytology are altered by *Toxocara cati* infection in cats and is independent of development of adult intestinal parasites. *Vet Parasitol.* 2013;193:413–426.)

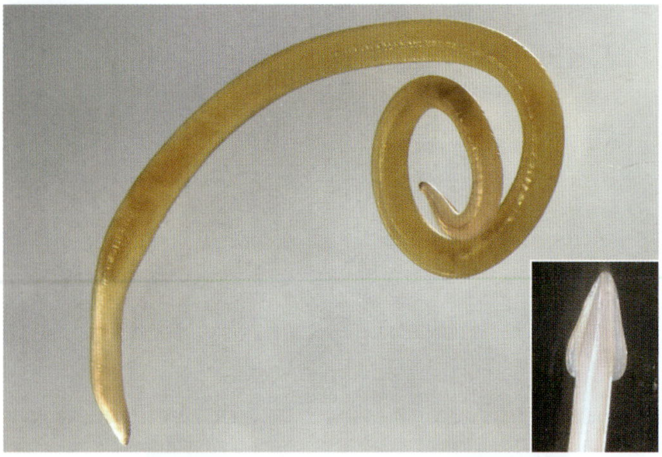

Fig. 112.9 *Toxocara cati* found in vomitus of 4-year-old spayed female domestic shorthair cat from Edmond, Oklahoma, United States (see Case Example). *Inset*: magnified view of anterior end.

pathologic changes to some degree and prevented maturation in the intestine.[116] Therefore *T. cati* larva migrans should be considered as a differential diagnosis in cases of acute and chronic lung disease in cats even if a preventive is being utilized.

Intestinal infections with mature *T. cati* are nearly always subclinical. Occasionally worms may migrate in a retrograde manner to the stomach and incite vomiting (see Case Example). Unthriftiness may occur in heavy infections in young kittens or older cats with other underlying health conditions. Heavily infected kittens may present with a potbellied appearance, poor haircoat, vomiting, anorexia, and weakness.

DIAGNOSIS

Laboratory Abnormalities and Diagnostic Imaging

Cats infected with *T. cati* may have peripheral eosinophilia. Radiographic and CT findings due to pulmonary migration in experimentally inoculated cats have been described and include a patchy to diffuse bronchointerstitial pattern and enlarged pulmonary arteries, which appeared similar to changes associated with *Dirofilaria immitis* and *Aelurostrongylus abstrusus* infection (Fig. 112.8).[116]

Microbiologic Tests

Diagnosis Using Fecal Examination

As for dogs, cats should be tested for ascarid infections by fecal flotation with centrifugation. Kittens should be tested at least four times during their first year and then one to two times annually as adults. Cats can be infected with *T. cati* and/or *T. leonina* but, as described earlier, their eggs are readily differentiated (see Table 112.1; Fig. 112.2). A commercial ELISA that detects antigens produced by immature and adult ascarids has become available and can be used to detect *T. cati* antigens in fecal specimens.[71]

Migration of *T. cati* adults into the stomach can cause vomiting, so adult worms are commonly detected in the vomitus of cats (Fig. 112.9). These worms must be differentiated from *Physaloptera* spp. nematodes which are also commonly present in vomitus of cats. Ascarids are larger and have three prominent lips, whereas *Physaloptera* are smaller and have a triangle-shaped anterior end that often has a swelling of the cuticle (see Chapter 116). Nonparasitic free-living planarians (*Bipalium*) can also be found in the vomitus of cats and are identified by their large triangle-shaped anterior end.

Pathologic Findings

Kittens that were experimentally inoculated with larvated *T. cati* eggs had multifocal depressed lesions on the surface of their lungs at necropsy. Histopathologic findings included pulmonary artery intimal

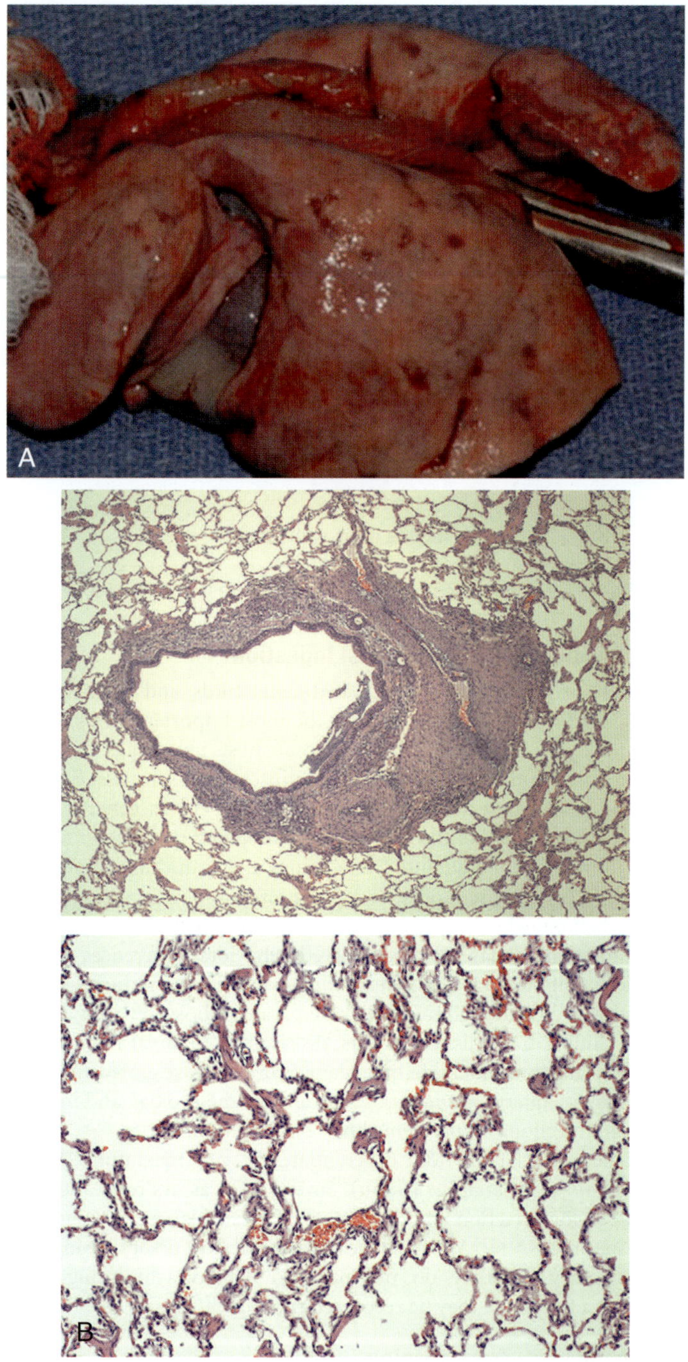

Fig. 112.10 (A) Lungs of a cat that was experimentally inoculated with *Toxocara cati* eggs following hepatotracheal migration. There are multifocal depressions on the lung surface. (B) Histopathology showing arterial smooth muscle and intimal hypertrophy in association with bronchi *(top)* and alveolar interstitium *(bottom)*. (From Dillon AR, Tillson DM, Hathcock J, et al. Lung histopathology, radiography, high-resolution computed tomography, and bronchio-alveolar lavage cytology are altered by *Toxocara cati* infection in cats and is independent of development of adult intestinal parasites. *Vet Parasitol.* 2013;193:413–426.)

and smooth muscle hyperplasia that was associated with bronchial inflammation as well as inflammatory infiltrates within the alveolar interstitium (Fig. 112.10).

TREATMENT

There are numerous commercially available products for the treatment of ascarids in cats and many of these products, when used regularly, limit reinfection (e.g., fenbendazole, milbemycin oxime, eprinomectin, moxidectin, selamectin, emodepside, pyrantel pamoate, and combinations thereof; see Chapter 13). An interactive quick product reference guide that lists all of the currently approved drugs for treatment of *T. cati* and other parasites can be found on the CAPC website (https://capcvet.org/parasite-product-applications/). Treatment of larva migrans in the cat may also be needed, especially since disease can be associated with migration through the lung and other tissues. Topical emodepside/praziquantel (Profender; Elanco) is approved for the treatment of larvae, and efficacy was 98.5% when used to treat kittens 5 days after inoculation with *T. cati*. However, oral milbemycin oxime/praziquantel was not efficacious.[117]

Vertical transmission may be prevented by treatment of pregnant queens before parturition. Application of topical emodepside/praziquantel 5–6 days before parturition in experimentally inoculated queens resulted in negative fecal egg counts in both the queen and litter, where untreated queens and their kittens were coproscopically positive.[118] When queens were inoculated with eggs daily from 50 to 60 days after conception, then treated with the same topical medication, treatment was 98.7% efficacious in preventing vertical transmission to kittens.[119]

PUBLIC HEALTH ASPECTS

Most reports of human toxocariasis (VLM or OLM) are presumed to be due to *T. canis*, but a few reports of confirmed *T. cati* larva migrans have been detected by biopsy.[120,121] Additional cases of *T. cati* larva migrans likely exist given the global distribution of the parasite, but current serologic diagnostic techniques cannot distinguish between the two species.[83,122] A high antibody titer to *T. cati* antigen but a low titer to *T. canis* antigen may be suggestive of *T. cati* infection.

Rarely, adult *T. cati* are recovered from vomit or feces of humans, typically children. Given the lack of seroconversion and consistent clinical signs, and the low likelihood that *T. cati* could mature in the human intestine, these cases may have been the result of children consuming adult *T. cati* possibly passed by pet cats.[123,124]

TOXASCARIS LEONINA

ETIOLOGIC AGENT AND EPIDEMIOLOGY

Toxascaris leonina can be found in both wild and domestic canids and felids, although in most locations, the prevalence in domestic animals is lower compared with *Toxocara* spp.[3,96] As noted earlier, the anterior end of the worm and egg morphology can be used to differentiate *T. leonina* from *Toxocara* spp. (see Table 112.1; Figs. 112.1 and 112.2).

Worldwide, *T. leonina* is a common parasite of many wild felids and canids. Wild felid hosts include nearly all extant species across subfamilies Pantherinae (e.g., lions, tigers, ocelots) and Felinae (e.g., bobcats, wildcats, pumas, leopards). Within Canidae, infection has been reported in foxes, wolves, jackals, and coyotes, among others. Molecular studies have suggested that *T. leonina* is a species complex consisting of three phylogenetically distinct clades; a canid clade (domestic dogs, wolf), a felid clade (cheetah, lynx, tigers), and parasites from foxes. However, additional work is needed to determine if the canid and felid parasites are genetic variants or separate species.[125,126] Interestingly, *T. leonina* was recently molecularly confirmed in an ~17,000-year-old coprolite from a cougar (*Puma concolor*) from Argentina.[127]

Younger dogs are more likely to be infected; however, prevalence does not drop off as sharply with age as it does for *Toxocara* spp.[128,129] Patent infections have been detected in weaning-age puppies, presumably from contamination of the whelping environment by the dam.[130] The rapid development of *T. leonina* eggs relative to *Toxocara* spp. necessitates rigorous sanitation of facilities to prevent reinfections after treatment. Because of the wide host range and persistence of eggs, *T. leonina* infection is common among captive wildlife species that do not receive regular preventives.[131]

Unlike *Toxocara* spp., *T. leonina* does not undergo liver-lung-tracheal migration in the host and completes development solely within the GI tract. After ingestion of larvated eggs or tissues from infected paratenic hosts, larvae penetrate into the intestinal mucosa and emerge into the lumen after 3 to 4 weeks of development as either L_4 stage or small adults. The PPPs range from 45 to 80 days (average, ~50 days).[132,133] Eggs of *T. leonina* reach infectivity more rapidly than those of *Toxocara* spp. or *Baylisascaris* spp., capable of becoming embryonated as soon as 4 days to 1 week under ideal conditions. Also, *T. leonina* eggs can develop at low temperatures (6°C–8°C).[134] Vertical transmission of *T. leonina* does not occur due to lack of somatic migration.[132]

Although *T. leonina* infects both dogs and cats, some studies suggest there may be some host-adapted strains. Cats inoculated with eggs of *T. leonina* derived from a dog did not develop patent infections; either no larvae were recovered or arrested L_3 were found months after inoculation. However, cats were successfully infected when fed mice infected with canine-strain larvae.[132,133] Some dogs inoculated with "feline-strain" eggs became infected, whereas others did not develop patent infections.[133] In addition, morphologic variation (esophageal length differences) has been noted among canine- and feline-derived isolates.[133,135]

Occasionally, larvae persist in the intestinal wall or lumen as L_4 stage in developmental arrest. In a cat experimentally co-infected with *T. leonina* and *T. cati*, the PPP of *T. leonina* was prolonged to 22 weeks, and at necropsy 1 year after inoculation, many immature L_4 and few adult *T. leonina* were found, suggesting that competition may occur.[133]

In paratenic hosts, *T. leonina* undergoes somatic migration; the majority of larvae become encapsulated in the mesentery and intestinal wall. A smaller proportion are recovered from other organs (liver, lung, skeletal muscle).[133,136] Migration to the brain has not been observed.[136] Some evidence suggests that host-adapted strains (i.e., canine and feline isolates) may have differential growth characteristics in the paratenic host.[133]

Overall, *T. leonina* infection is associated with few or no clinical signs. Very heavy infections may cause unthriftiness and GI distress.

DIAGNOSIS, TREATMENT AND PREVENTION

See sections earlier on *Toxocara* spp. infections.

PUBLIC HEALTH ASPECTS

There are no confirmed cases of *T. leonina* larva migrans in humans. One unusual report of infection with adult worms exists in which nematodes were purportedly extracted from a subcutaneous abscess[137]; however, this could represent a misidentification with other large nematodes that would be more likely to cause such signs (e.g., *Eustrongylides, Dirofilaria, Onchocerca*). *Toxascaris leonina* can cause VLM in paratenic hosts, so it is possible that some human VLM cases that are assumed to be *Toxocara* spp. infections may be due to *T. leonina* infection. However, there appears to be little or no serologic cross-reaction between these genera based on the excretory-secretory antigen fractions commonly used for diagnosis of *Toxocara* spp. VLM in humans.[138,139]

BAYLISASCARIS PROCYONIS

ETIOLOGIC AGENT AND EPIDEMIOLOGY

Baylisascaris procyonis, a common zoonotic ascarid of raccoons (*Procyon lotor*), is widespread in North America. Domestic dogs can serve as alternative definitive hosts and excrete eggs into the

TABLE 112.2 **Published Reports of *Baylisacaris procyonis* Infections in Dogs (Patent Infections and Larva Migrans)**

Number Of Dogs	Age	Natural/ Experimental	Route	Signs/Outcome	Diagnosis	Source
1	10 months	Natural	Likely larvated egg[a]	Encephalomyelitis; acute onset ataxia, deterioration, euthanized within 48 hours.	Histopathology	178
2	5–6 months	Natural	Unknown	Patent intestinal infection in one dog which passed 3 adults; 2 adult females passed by other dog which did not reach patency	Fecal flotation, recovery of worms after treatment	150
2	NS	Natural	Unknown	Patent intestinal infection; 7 male and 19 females from both dogs recovered.	Fecal flotation, necropsy	1
1	12 weeks	Natural	Likely larvated egg[a]	Progressive weakness, ataxia, imbalance deteriorating to severe CNS disease within 24 hours; euthanized.	Histopathology	179
1	NS	Natural	Unknown	Vomiting, anorexia, eosinophilia (peripheral and CSF), sublumbar lymphadenopathy, progressive neurologic deterioration, euthanized within 24 hours.	MRI and histopathology	180
7	NS	Experimental	Larvae[a]	Patent intestinal infection in 4/7 dogs after 42–80 days.	Fecal flotation, necropsy	146
7	NS	Experimental	Larvated eggs	Unthriftiness and abdominal tenderness followed by severe CNS signs within 10 days in 2 dogs fed 100,000 and 200,000 eggs, dead at 14 days. Ataxia and incoordination in one dog fed 10,000 eggs by day 19.	Necropsy	151
4	10 months	Experimental	Larvae[b]	Patent intestinal infection in 3/4 dogs	Fecal flotation; recovery of worms after treatment followed by necropsy	141
12	6 months	Experimental	Larvae or larvated eggs	Patent intestinal infection in 2/6 dogs inoculated with larvae (low dose group)	Fecal flotation and fecal antigen ELISA (IDEXX Laboratories)	72

[a]Had access to a cage that had previously housed a raccoon suggesting ingestion of larvated eggs as the likely route of exposure; however, only one of three puppies in the litter became ill.
[b]Larvae in tissues of infected laboratory mice.
CNS, central nervous system; *CSF,* cer ebrospinal fluid; *ELISA,* enzyme-linked immunosorbent assay; *NS,* not specified.

environment or can act as paratenic hosts and develop clinical disease due to larva migration.[73,140] Morphologically, adults resemble *T. canis* and differ from *T. leonina* by the presence of inconspicuous cervical alae (see Table 112.1; Fig. 112.1). The males of *B. procyonis* can be differentiated from those of *T. canis* by the presence of a roughened anal patch. Eggs of *B. procyonis* can be differentiated from those of *T. leonina* by their smooth egg shells and polar filaments (see Fig. 112.2). As noted previously, *T. canis* and *B. procyonis* eggs can be difficult to distinguish, but the latter tend to be darker amber and are more ellipsoid.

Although there are numerous other *Baylisascaris* spp. in North America (e.g., *B. columnaris* in skunks, *B. transfuga* in bears), none have been reported from domestic dogs. However, diagnosis of infection in dogs is generally by fecal examination and the eggs of most *Baylisascaris* spp. cannot be reliably distinguished based on morphology.[141]

Sporadic patent infections have been reported in the United States and Canada and a 2017 report of reference laboratory data described *Baylisascaris* spp. eggs in 504/9,486,672 (0.005%) fecal specimens.[140,142] Prevalence was also low in a study on Prince Edward Island, Canada (7/242 dogs; 0.36%).[143] However, prevalence in stray dogs or dogs not receiving regular veterinary care is likely higher. Also, unreported infections may be detected during POC fecal examinations or as a result of misidentification of eggs as *Toxocara* spp. eggs. In the United States, prevalence in dogs was lower in the southern and central regions, which corresponds with the known prevalence and distribution of the parasite in raccoons.[142] Most of these positive dogs were large breeds in the sporting and working groups (AKC breed classifications). These dogs may be more likely to be kept outdoors unsupervised where they have access to raccoon feces and/or infected paratenic hosts, such as rodents. Like the eggs of other ascarids, *B. procyonis* eggs are extremely hardy and are resistant to low and freezing temperatures, desiccation, and disinfectants.[144,145] Only temperatures > 60°C will destroy eggs[145] although bleach removes their mammilated outer layer, making them easier to remove from surfaces.

CLINICAL FEATURES

Pathogenesis, Clinical Signs, and Physical Examination Findings

The life cycle of *B. procyonis* is similar to that of other ascarids. Like raccoons, dogs can develop patent infections (i.e., act as definitive hosts) but unlike raccoons, some infected dogs, particularly puppies, can develop VLM. Definitive hosts are infected when they ingest embryonated eggs or tissues of infected paratenic hosts. Depending on the route of infection, the PPP for dogs can range from 42 to 48 days after ingestion of paratenic hosts to ~60 days after infection with eggs, although data are limited.[146,147] Some PPPs may be longer.[73] It is unknown if *B. procyonis* larvae undergo hepatotracheal migration in the definitive host after egg ingestion as reported for *Toxocara* infections, although this has been reported for *Baylisascaris laevis* in rodents.[148] Eggs excreted in feces require 2 to 3 weeks under ideal conditions to embryonate.

When eggs are ingested by paratenic hosts (including dogs), they hatch and larvae exit the GI tract and migrate through tissues. After an initial liver-lung migration, larvae migrate throughout the somatic tissues of the host, including the CNS and eyes, causing NLM and OLM, respectively. As with *Toxocara* spp., VLM can also produce disease if significant numbers of larvae are present. The paratenic host range is remarkably broad and encompasses over 150 species of mammals and birds.[140]

Some evidence exists for vertical transmission of *Baylisascaris* spp. in definitive and paratenic hosts. *Baylisascaris procyonis* eggs have been detected in the feces of puppies as young as 2 months of age[140,142] and *Baylisascaris* sp. larvae were detected in a neonatal lamb with neurologic disease suggesting infection via the transplacental or transmammary route.[149] Additionally, *B. transfuga* (a parasite of bears) was found in the cerebrum of two newborn sibling moose calves with neurologic disease who were born to a dam shot for aggressive behavior.[150]

Migration of larvae in susceptible paratenic hosts can lead to VLM, NLM, and/or OLM; these can be severe or fatal. When larvae hatch from eggs, they are ~300 μm in length but within 10–15 days grow to ~1,500–1,800 μm. Histologically, these larvae are ~60–80 μm in diameter and have distinct lateral alae visible in cross-section. In contrast, larvae of *Toxocara* spp. and *T. leonina* are significantly shorter and have smaller diameters (see Table 112.1). The larger size of *Baylisascaris* spp. larvae compared with *Toxocara* spp. larvae and the growth of larvae during migration leads to more significant inflammation and tissue damage.

In raccoons, intestinal infections with *B. procyonis* are nearly always subclinical and the same is likely true for dogs when they act as definitive hosts. Very high worm burdens could theoretically cause signs that are similar to heavy *T. canis* infections. However, because dogs are not the normal definitive host for *B. procyonis*, such high worm burdens may not develop. In the few case reports that exist, burdens ranged from only 2 to 13 worms.[1,151] Also, not all dogs experimentally exposed to *B. procyonis* develop infections, which is further indication that they are not an ideal host for the parasite (Table 112.2).[73,146,147]

Cerebral baylisascariasis in paratenic hosts can result in behavioral changes, agitation, ataxia, lethargy, and confusion that deteriorates into paralysis, seizures, coma, and death. Eosinophilic meningitis or encephalomyelitis with moderate to high peripheral eosinophilia are common outcomes of CNS infection. Although ocular manifestations are poorly studied in animals, *Baylisascaris*-associated OLM in humans is often associated with DUSN which can lead to diminished vision or blindness.[140] Although most natural paratenic hosts are rodents or birds, there have been cases in numerous species of lagomorphs, and carnivores, as well as domestic animals (e.g., sheep, chickens) and captive exotics (e.g., primates, prosimians, marsupials, flying fox, parrots).[140]

Several cases of larva migrans in puppies have been reported (see Table 112.2). Puppies generally showed neurologic signs, and larvae morphologically consistent with *B. procyonis* were found in association with inflammatory lesions. However, not all puppies develop disease; there have been several instances of puppies (<2 months) passing eggs in feces which were presumed to be early patent infections.[140,142] NLM has also been experimentally induced in adult dogs inoculated with high doses of *B. procyonis* eggs (see Table 112.2). Two dogs given > 100,000 embryonated eggs developed clinical signs by 2–3 days PI, including lethargy, pale mucosa, anorexia, ataxia, and reduced activity (which was likely due to VLM). By 10 days PI, their condition deteriorated and severe neurologic signs (inability to stand or right self, extensor rigidity, repetitive limb movements) developed and both dogs died by 14 days PI. Both dogs had large, ulcerated, hemorrhagic foci in the pyloric stomach presumably due to larvae migration out of the GI tract.[152] Two additional dogs were given 10,000 eggs and although one remained clinically normal, the other developed ataxia and incoordination by 19 days PI. However, this dog never developed signs as severe as the other two dogs given a higher dose. Some behavioral changes and agitation were noted in a dog inoculated with 50,000 eggs, but no neurologic disease developed. No major histologic lesions were noted in the dogs receiving 10,000 to 50,000 eggs.[152] In another study, a single dog given 5,000 eggs orally did not develop any clinical disease and no larvae were recovered from tissues.[153]

DIAGNOSIS

Centrifugal fecal flotation to recover eggs is the primary method for diagnosis of patent *Baylisascaris* spp. infections in dogs. Given their morphologic similarities, care should be taken to distinguish *Baylisascaris* spp. eggs from those of *T. canis* (see Fig. 112.2). Coprophagy has the potential to contribute to diagnostic confusion in domestic dogs. For example, oocysts of *Eimieria* spp., common raccoon parasites, were detected in 15% of canine fecal specimens positive for *Baylisascaris* spp. eggs.[142] The finding of embryonated *Baylisascaris* spp. eggs or *Eimeria* spp. oocysts indicates that coprophagy has occurred.

PCR-based protocols can be used to confirm the presence of *Baylisascaris* spp. eggs in fecal specimens.[154] Also, a commercial coproantigen ELISA (IDEXX Laboratories Inc., Westbrook, ME), developed for the detection of more common roundworm genera (*Toxocara, Toxascaris*), can also detect antigen shed from *B. procyonis* in the intestine.[73]

A diagnosis of *B. procyonis* larva migrans cannot be confirmed antemortem as serologic tests are not available for dogs. A history of exposure to raccoon feces can suggest a risk. Larvae recovered from tissues by artificial digestion or in histologic sections can be identified morphologically and/or with molecular tools. It is possible that *B. procyonis* NLM in dogs is under-recognized given these diagnostic challenges and the variable nature of disease progression and clinical signs.

TREATMENT AND PREVENTION

There are no anthelmintics approved for the treatment of *B. procyonis* in dogs. However, anthelmintics labeled for treatment of *T. canis* appear effective for the elimination of intestinal *B. procyonis* infections. Single doses of pyrantel (20 mg/kg) and moxidectin (1 mg/kg) were efficacious in experimentally infected raccoons.[155] Three daily doses of fenbendazole (50 mg/kg) and flubendazole (22 mg/kg) were also effective.[155] High-burden infections may require re-treatment to eliminate all worms. For example, in a study of *B. procyonis*–infected dogs, a single oral dose of milbemycin oxime was effective for dogs infected with 25 worms; but in two dogs with more than 25 nematodes, infection was not eliminated using this protocol.[142]

Treatment of *Baylisascaris* spp. larva migrans in dogs has not been investigated. In some recent human cases, early intervention with anthelmintics (typically albendazole, use of which should be avoided in dogs and cats) and glucocorticoids to control inflammation resulted in favorable clinical outcomes with full or nearly full recoveries.[156,157]

Use of monthly products labeled for prevention of other ascarids should control *B. procyonis* infection. Prevention of coprophagy is important for two reasons: it prevents exposure and the subsequent development of a patent infection and/or larva migrans and also prevents passive excretion of *B. procyonis* eggs by dogs into a domestic environment.

Preventing contact with captive raccoons and any structures/substrates that may be contaminated is also important. Raccoons should not be kept as pets, and any raccoons in captivity should be routinely examined for *B. procyonis* infection and treated if necessary.

PUBLIC HEALTH ASPECTS

Over 50 human cerebral and ocular baylisascariasis cases have been reported. Case fatality rates for NLM are ~40%; however, treatment is more successful now given improved diagnostic tests as well as increased awareness.[140,157] However, NLM survivors are still frequently left with permanent sequelae, and OLM can cause permanent vision defects.[140] While human infections are rare, the potentially severe consequences warrant awareness and prevention efforts. Some infections may occur covertly as with toxocariasis; however, the implications of seropositivity in asymptomatic individuals are not well understood.[158]

Although prevalence is very low in dogs, infected dogs may represent a greater risk for human and other companion animal exposure due to their indiscriminate defecation habits (versus raccoons that utilize defined latrine sites). No human cases have been linked to contact with infected dogs, but veterinarians should provide information to clients about the risks of *B. procyonis* infection and prevention strategies, especially in areas where raccoons are ubiquitous and the parasite occurs at a high prevalence.

OTHER ASCARIDS

TOXOCARA MALAYASIENSIS INFECTION

A relatively recently described species, *Toxocara malayasiensis*, has been detected in domestic cats in Southeast Asia. *Toxocara malayasiensis* shares many morphologic characteristics with *T. canis* but can be differentiated based on appearance of cervical alae in transverse section (curved versus straight in *T. canis*), shorter spicule length, and lip morphology.[159] Molecular analysis also supports the validity of this species.[160]

Little is known about the distribution and epidemiology of *T. malayasiensis* in cats. Worms collected from domestic cats in China and Malaysia were confirmed to be *T. malayasiensis* using nucleic acid–based methods.[161] In stray cats from Malaysia, the prevalence of *T. malayasiensis* infection was higher than that of *T. cati* infection.[162] This emphasizes the need for further investigation into potential cryptic *Toxocara* species globally.

LAGOCHILASCARIS SPP. INFECTION

The genus *Lagochilascaris* includes zoonotic ascarids of domestic and wild felids from Mexico south to Argentina. This genus is distinguished from other Ascarididae based on unique lip and anterior end morphology; involutions in each lip create a "hare-lipped" appearance (for which the genus is named), and the lips are of equal width to or wider than the cuticular collar. The two primary species that infect domestic cats are *Lagochilascaris minor* and *Lagochilascaris major*. The females of both species are 18 to 22 mm long, while males are 17 to 20 mm.[163] The lips of *L. major* protrude over the collar more compared with *L. minor*. Eggs of both species are similarly sized, ~60 μm wide and generally spherical, with a prominently pitted surface, but the species differ in the number of pits on the surface of the eggs (*L. minor* 15 to 25; *L. major* 33 to 45).

The life cycle of *L. minor* has been elucidated in experimental infections.[164] The adult nematodes form tumor-like masses and fistulous lesions in the larynx, pharynx, tongue, and palate, and occasionally in the esophagus and stomach of cats, although this is not always observed (especially in wild felids, presumably the "natural" host). Clinical signs became apparent within 10 days of inoculation, including dyspnea, poor body condition, decreased vocalization, decreased activity, and frequent sneezing.[164] One study observed mild to moderate neurologic impairment in some experimentally infected cats, such as imbalance, mild ataxia, and torticollis, although other cats appeared normal in behavior.[165]

Infections became patent ~2 weeks PI and eggs were excreted in feces.[164] Some lesions contained adults at variable stages, larvae, and embryonated eggs, suggesting that autoinfection may occur.[164,165] *Lagochilascaris* spp. are believed to be obligatory heteroxenous (requiring at least two host species to complete their life cycle) as no cats inoculated with eggs of *L. minor* became infected, but all mice inoculated with eggs developed VLM.[164] It is possible that young cats could become infected through egg ingestion, but this has not been evaluated. Natural infections of *L. minor* in domestic cats are variable in presentation, ranging from benign subcutaneous nodules around the head and neck to large, fistulated abscesses in the upper respiratory tract.[166–169] Both young (<1 year) and adult cats are susceptible.

The life cycle of *L. major* has not been demonstrated experimentally, but is presumably similar; reports of natural infections in cats exist and resemble those of *L. minor*. The adults of *L. major* may cause fistulated, purulent pharyngeal abscesses that result in cough, dyspnea, and difficulty swallowing.[163] Abscesses may contain 50 or more adult worms.

In humans, larvae migrate to subcutaneous sites of the head, neck, throat and particularly the submandibular area, where large nodules may develop. If these form in proximity to the eyes, severe, persistent ocular disease may result.[170] At least one human case has been associated with fatal NLM.[171] More than 60 cases have been reported in Mexico, Trinidad, Suriname, Venezuela, Colombia, Bolivia, Brazil, and Argentina.[172] The transmission route to humans is unknown, although in some communities it may be due to the practice of eating wild intermediate hosts such as capybara, agouti, and opossums.[165,173] One suspected *L. major* larva migrans case has been reported from a dog and involved a purulent abscess.[174]

Treatment in humans and felids typically involves surgical excision of the nodules, followed by lavage of the area and anthelmintic therapy to remove any remaining larvae. Levamisole and ivermectin appear to be the drugs of choice; diethylcarbamazine and benzimidazoles appear to lack efficacy in some human cases and experimental infections.[175–177] Prolonged or multiple rounds of anthelmintic therapy may be required to prevent recrudescence via autoinfection.[170] Antibiotic treatment may be necessary if secondary bacterial infection of subcutaneous abscesses has occurred.

CASE EXAMPLE

Signalment

"Chloe," a 4-year-old female spayed domestic shorthair cat from Edmond, Oklahoma, United States.

History

Chloe was evaluated in April for a recent episode of acute vomiting. Her owners reported finding motile nematodes in the vomitus; one was brought for examination (see Fig. 112.9). Chloe was an indoor/outdoor cat that lived in a wooded subdivision. She was current on vaccinations and wore a flumethrin/imidacloprid collar for flea and tick control. Her owners denied that she hunted often but reported occasionally finding dead, eviscerated mice and birds around their home.

Current medications: No treatments other than the flumethrin/imidacloprid collar. Owners reported applying a new collar each March.

Other medical history: Previous medical problems included flea infestation and ear mites as a kitten, both of which resolved with treatment. Owners declined earlier recommendations for comprehensive monthly internal parasite control (selamectin), opting instead to only protect Chloe from fleas and ticks.

Physical Examination

Body weight: 3.7 kg; BCS: 4/9.

General: Bright, alert, hydrated, responsive. Mucous membranes pink, HR = 180 beats/minute, RR = 40 beats/minute, T = 101.2°F (38.4°C).

GI and genitourinary: Normal palpation. No abdominal mass, pain, or other abnormalities detected.

Integument: Normal haircoat. No ectoparasites were evident.

Eyes, ears, nose, and throat; musculoskeletal; respiratory; cardiovascular; lymph nodes: No clinically significant findings were noted.

Fecal flotation, fecal antigen test, and parasite identification results: Numerous eggs of *T. cati* were present on examination of zinc sulfate centrifugal fecal flotation, and fecal specimen was positive for antigen of *Toxocara* spp. (FecalDx®, IDEXX Laboratories, Inc.). The adult nematode (see Fig. 112.9) was morphologically identified as a female *T. cati* ascarid.

Serology

A feline heartworm antibody test and antigen test were negative.

Diagnosis

Toxocara cati infection.

Treatment

Chloe was treated with a single transdermal dose of emodepside/praziquantel. Topical moxidectin/fluralaner administered every 8 weeks was commenced and the owners were advised to discontinue the flumethrin/imidacloprid collar. No further incidents of vomiting were reported.

Comments

A definitive diagnosis of *T. cati* infection was made based on identification of adult worms in vomitus, eggs on fecal flotation, and antigen detected in feces. Although normally present in the small intestine, ascarids often migrate in a retrograde manner to the stomach, irritate the gastric mucosa, and are expelled through vomiting. The distinct arrowhead-shaped anterior end allows adults of *T. cati* to be distinguished from those of *Physaloptera* spp., another nematode found in cat vomit us that requires a different treatment (see Chapter 116). Treatment with emodepside/praziquantel was recommended to address potential co-infection with *Taenia* sp. tapeworms which are difficult to detect on fecal examination and commonly found together with ascarid infections in cats with access to prey species.[178] Treating only with moxidectin/fluralaner every 2 months would eliminate the *T. cati* infection and address the need for ongoing flea and tick control but would not provide efficacy against tapeworms.

SUGGESTED READINGS

Bowman DD. Toxocara and toxocariasis. *Adv Parasitol.* 2020;109:2–883.

Kazacos KR. *Baylisascaris Larva Migrans - Circular 1412.* U.S. Geological Survey. 2016. Available at: https://pubs.usgs.gov/circ/1412/cir1412.pdf.

Centers for Disease Control and Prevention. *Toxocariasis.* 2020. Available at: https://www.cdc.gov/parasites/toxocariasis/.

Lee AC, Schantz PM, Kazacos KR, et al. Epidemiologic and zoonotic aspects of ascarid infections in dogs and cats. *Trends Parasitol.* 2010;26:155–161.

REFERENCES

1. Averbeck G, Vanek J, Stromberg B, et al. Differentiation of *Baylisascaris* species, *Toxocara canis*, and *Toxascaris leonina* infections in dogs. *Compend Contin Educ Vet.* 1995;29:475–478.
2. Alexander U, Lim CW, Kim B, et al. Morphological and molecular characterization of *Toxocara tanuki* (Nematoda: Ascaridae) from Korean raccoon dog, *Nyctereutes procyonoides koreensis. Korean J Parasitol.* 2018;56:567–575.
3. Rostami A, Riahi SM, Hofmann A, et al. Global prevalence of *Toxocara* infection in dogs. *Adv Parasitol.* 2020;109:561–583.
4. Jenkins DJ. *Toxocara canis* in Australia. *Adv Parasitol.* 2020;109:873–878.
5. Ketzis JK, Lucio-Forster A. *Toxocara canis* and *Toxocara cati* in domestic dogs and cats in the United States, Mexico, Central America and the Caribbean: a review. *Adv Parasitol.* 2020;109:655–714.
6. Dantas-Torres F. *Toxocara* prevalence in dogs and cats in Brazil. *Adv Parasitol 2020.* 2020;109:715–741.
7. López-Osorio S, Penagos-Tabares F, Chaparro-Gutiérrez JJ. Prevalence of *Toxocara* spp. in dogs and cats in South America (excluding Brazil). *Adv Parasitol.* 2020;109:743–778.
8. Overgaauw P, Nijsse R. Prevalence of patent *Toxocara* spp. infections in dogs and cats in Europe from 1994 to 2019. *Adv Parasitol.* 2020;109:779–800.
9. Lukashev AN, Ruzina MN, Akhmadishina LV. *Toxocara* prevalence in dogs, cats and the environment in Russia. *Adv Parasitol.* 2020;109:801–817.
10. Lejeune M, Gnani Charitha V, Mathivathani C, et al. Canine toxocariosis: its prevalence, incidence and occurrence in the Indian subcontinent. *Adv Parasitol.* 2020;109:819–842.
11. Zheng WB, Zou Y, Liu GH, et al. Epidemiology of *Toxocara* spp. in dogs and cats in mainland China, 2000–2019. *Adv Parasitol.* 2020;109:843–860.
12. Chidumayo NN. Prevalence of *Toxocara* in dogs and cats in Africa. *Adv Parasitol.* 2020;109:861–871.
13. Jenkins EJ. *Toxocara* spp. in dogs and cats in Canada. *Adv Parasitol.* 2020;109:641–653.
14. Martínez-Barbabosa I, Vázquez Tsuji O, Romero Cabello R, et al. The prevalence of *Toxocara cati* in domestic cats in Mexico City. *Vet Parasitol.* 2003;114:43–49.
15. Drake J, Parrish R. Dog importation and changes in canine intestinal nematode prevalence in Colorado, USA, 2013-2017. *Parasit Vectors.* 2020;13:404.
16. Barutzki D, Schaper R. Age-dependant prevalence of endoparasites in young dogs and cats up to one year of age. *Parasitol Res.* 2013;112:119–131.
17. Fahrion AS, Staebler S, Deplazes P. Patent *Toxocara canis* infections in previously exposed and in helminth-free dogs after infection with low numbers of embryonated eggs. *Vet Parasitol.* 2008;152:108–115.
18. Sager H, Moret CS, Grimm F, et al. Coprological study on intestinal helminths in Swiss dogs: temporal aspects of anthelminthic treatment. *Parasitol Res.* 2006;98:333–338.

19. Overgaauw PA. Prevalence of intestinal nematodes of dogs and cats in The Netherlands. *Vet Q.* 1997;19:14–17.
20. Papazahariadou M, Founta A, Papadopoulos E, et al. Gastrointestinal parasites of shepherd and hunting dogs in the Serres Prefecture, Northern Greece. *Vet Parasitol.* 2007;148:170–173.
21. Zanzani SA, Gazzonis AL, Scarpa P, et al. Intestinal parasites of owned dogs and cats from metropolitan and micropolitan areas: prevalence, zoonotic risks, and pet owner awareness in northern Italy. *Biomed Res Int.* 2014:696508.
22. Morandi B, Greenwood SJ, Conboy GA, et al. Endoparasites in dogs and cats diagnosed at the veterinary teaching hospital (VTH) of the University of Prince Edward Island between 2000 and 2017. A large-scale retrospective study. *Prev Vet Med.* 2020;175:104878.
23. Habluetzel A, Traldi G, Ruggieri S, et al. An estimation of *Toxocara canis* prevalence in dogs, environmental egg contamination and risk of human infection in the Marche region of Italy. *Vet Parasitol.* 2003;113:243–252.
24. Mircean V, Dumitrache M, Mircean M, et al. Prevalence and risk factors associated with endoparasitic infection in dogs from Transylvania (Romania): a retrospective study. *Vet Parasitol.* 2017;243:157–161.
25. Ortuño A, Scorza V, Castellà J, et al. Prevalence of intestinal parasites in shelter and hunting dogs in Catalonia, Northeastern Spain. *Vet J.* 2014;199:465–467.
26. Barriga OO. A critical look at the importance, prevalence and control of toxocariasis and the possibilities of immunological control. *Vet Parasitol.* 1988;29:195–234.
27. Fisher MA, Jacobs DE, Hutchinson MJ, et al. Studies on the control of *Toxocara canis* in breeding kennels. *Vet Parasitol.* 1994;55:87–92.
28. Overgaauw PAM, van Knapen F. Veterinary and public health aspects of *Toxocara* spp. *Vet Parasitol.* 2013;193:398–403.
29. Overgaauw PAM. Aspects of *Toxocara* epidemiology: toxocarosis in dogs and cats. *Crit Rev Microbiol.* 1997b;23:233–251.
30. Fan CK, Lin YH, Du WY, et al. Infectivity and pathogenicity of 14-month-cultured embryonated eggs of *Toxocara canis* in mice. *Vet Parasitol.* 2003;113:145–155.
31. O'Lorcain P. The effects of freezing on the viability of *Toxocara canis* and *T. cati* embryonated eggs. *J Helminthol.* 1995;69:169–171.
32. Lightner L, Christensen BM, Beran GW. Epidemiologic findings on canine and feline intestinal nematode infections from records of the Iowa State University Veterinary Clinic. *J Am Vet Med Assoc.* 1978;172:564–567.
33. Kirkpatrick CE. Epizootiology of endoparasitic infections in pet dogs and cats presented to a veterinary teaching hospital. *Vet Parasitol.* 1988;30:113–124.
34. Nolan TJ, Smith G. Time series analysis of the prevalence of endoparasitic infections in cats and dogs presented to a veterinary teaching hospital. *Vet Parasitol.* 1995;59:87–96.
35. Drake J, Carey T. Seasonality and changing prevalence of common canine gastrointestinal nematodes in the USA. *Parasit Vectors.* 2019;12:430.
36. Aydenizöz-Özkayhan M, Yağci BB, Erat S. The investigation of *Toxocara canis* eggs in coats of different dog breeds as a potential transmission route in human toxocariasis. *Vet Parasitol.* 2008;152:94–100.
37. Öge H, Öge S, Özbakiş G, et al. Comparison of *Toxocara* eggs in hair and faecal samples from owned dogs and cats collected in Ankara, Turkey. *Vet Parasitol.* 2014;206:227–231.
38. Maurelli MP, Santaniello A, Fioretti A, et al. The presence of *Toxocara* eggs on dog's fur as potential zoonotic risk in animal-assisted interventions: a systematic review. *Animals (Basel).* 2019;9:827.
39. Sasannejad N, Khoshnegah J, Bakhshani A, et al. Survey of *Toxocara* eggs on dog hair as a potential transmission route in human toxocariasis in Northeastern Iran. *Iran J Parasitol.* 2020;15:248–252.
40. Roddie G, Holland C, Stafford P, et al. Contamination of dog hair with eggs of *Toxocara canis. Vet Parasitol.* 2008;82:293–296.
41. Keegan JD, Holland CV. Contamination of the hair of owned dogs with the eggs of *Toxocara* spp. *Vet Parasitol.* 2010;173:161–164.
42. Keegan JD, Holland CV. A comparison of *Toxocara canis* embryonation under controlled conditions in soil and hair. *J Helminthol.* 2012;87:78–84.
43. Eisen AKA, Demoliner M, Oliveira KG, et al. Soil contamination of a public park by human and canine mastadenovirus, as well as hookworms and *Toxocara* spp. eggs. *Rev Inst Med Trop Sao Paulo.* 2019;61:60.
44. Savadelis MD, Evans CC, Mabry KH, et al. Canine gastrointestinal nematode transmission potential in municipal dog parks in the southeast United States. *Vet Parasitol Reg Stud Reports.* 2019;18:100324.
45. Duncan KT, Koons NR, Litherland MA, et al. Prevalence of intestinal parasites in fecal samples and estimation of parasite contamination from dog parks in central Oklahoma. *Vet Parasitol Reg Stud Reports.* 2020;19:100362.
46. Tyungu DL, McCormick D, Lau CL, et al. *Toxocara* species environmental contamination of public spaces in New York City. *PLoS Negl Trop Dis.* 2020;14:e0008249.
47. Stafford K, Kollasch TM, Duncan KT, et al. Detection of gastrointestinal parasitism at recreational canine sites in the USA: the DOGPARCS study. *Parasit Vectors.* 2020;13:275.
48. Dubey JP. Patent *Toxocara canis* infection in ascarid-naive dogs. *J Parasitol.* 1978;64:1021–1023.
49. Sprent JFA. Observations on the development of *Toxocara canis* (Werner 1782) in the dog. *Parasitol.* 1958;48:184–209.
50. Strube C, Heuer L, Janecek E. *Toxocara* spp. infections in paratenic hosts. *Vet Parasitol.* 2013;193:375–389.
51. Beaver PC. The nature of visceral larva migrans. *J Parasitol.* 1969;55:3–12.
52. Lescano SZ, Queiroz ML, Chieffi PP. Larval recovery of *Toxocara canis* in organs and tissues of experimentally infected *Rattus norvegicus. Mem Inst Oswaldo Cruz.* 2004;99:627–628.
53. Pahari TK, Sasmal NK. Experimental infection of Japanese quail with *Toxocara canis* larvae through earthworms. *Vet Parasitol.* 1991;39:337–340.
54. Wu T, Bowman DD. Visceral larval migrans of *Toxocara canis* and *Toxocara cati* in non-canid and non-felid hosts. *Adv Parasitol.* 2020;109:63–88.
55. Okoshi S, Usui M. Experimental studies on *Toxascaris leonina*. VI. Experimental infection of mice, chickens and earthworms with *Toxascaris leonina, Toxocara canis* and *Toxocara cati. Japanese J Vet Sci.* 1968;30:151–166.
56. Sasmal NK, Pahari TK, Laha R. Experimental infection of the cockroach *Periplaneta americana* with *Toxocara canis* and the establishment of patent infections in pups. *J Helminthol.* 2008;82:97–100.
57. Pahari TK, Sasmal NK. Infection of Japanese quail with *Toxocara canis* larvae and establishment of patent infection in pups. *Vet Parasitol.* 1990;35:357–364.
58. Schnieder T, Laabs EM, Welz C. Larval development of *Toxocara canis* in dogs. *Vet Parasitol.* 2011;175:193–206.
59. Jin Z, Akao N, Ohta N. Prolactin evokes lactational transmission of larvae in mice infected with *Toxocara canis. Parasitol Int.* 2008;57:495–498.
60. Scothorn M, Koutz F, Groves H. Prenatal *Toxocara canis* infection in pups. *J Am Vet Med Assoc.* 1965;146:45–48.
61. Koutz F, Groves H, Scothorn M. The prenatal migration of *Toxocara canis* larvae and their relationship to infection in pregnant bitches and in pups. *Am J Vet Res.* 1966;27:789–795.
62. Sprent JFA. Post-parturient infection of the bitch with *Toxocara canis. J Parasitol.* 1961;47.
63. Burke TM, Roberson EL. Prenatal and lactational transmission of *Toxocara canis* and *Ancylostoma caninum*: experimental infection of the bitch at midpregnancy and at parturition. *Int J Parasitol.* 1985;15:485–490.
64. Lee K, Min H, Soh C. Transplacental migration of *Toxocara canis* larvae in experimentally infected mice. *J Parasitol Vector Biol.* 1976;62:460–465.
65. Buckle KN, Hardcastle MR, Scott I, et al. *Toxocara canis* larval migration causing verminous pneumonia in fading puppies from 2 Scottish terrier litters. *Vet Pathol.* 2019;56:903–906.
66. Miller AD. Pathology of larvae and adults in dogs and cats. *Adv Parasitol.* 2020;109:537–544.
67. Johnson B, Kirkpatrick C, Whiteley H, et al. Retinitis and intraocular larval migration in a group of border collies. *J Am Anim Hosp Assoc.* 1989;25:623–629.
68. Parsons JC, Bowman DD, Grieve R. Pathological and haematological responses of cats experimentally infected with *Toxocara canis* larvae. *Int J Parasitol.* 1989;19:479–488.

69. Parsons JC, Bowman DD, Gillette DM, et al. Disseminated granulomatous disease in a cat caused by larvae of *Toxocara canis*. *J Comp Pathol*. 1988;99:343–346.
70. Corda A, Tamponi C, Meloni R, et al. Ultrasonography for early diagnosis of *Toxocara canis* infection in puppies. *Parasitol Res*. 2019;118:873–880.
71. Elsemore DA, Geng J, Cote J, et al. Enzyme-linked immunosorbent assays for coproantigen detection of *Ancylostoma caninum* and *Toxocara canis* in dogs and *Toxocara cati* in cats. *J Vet Diagn Investig*. 2017;29:645–653.
72. Elsemore DA. Antigen detection: Insights into *Toxocara* and other ascarid infections in dogs and cats. *Adv Parasitol*. 2020;109:545–559.
73. Sapp SGH, Elsemore DA, Hanna R, et al. Experimental comparison of *Baylisascaris procyonis* definitive host competence between domestic dogs and raccoons (*Procyon lotor*). *Parasitology*. 2020:1–8.
74. Fahrion AS, Schnyder M, Wichert B, et al. *Toxocara* eggs shed by dogs and cats and their molecular and morphometric species-specific identification: is the finding of *T. cati* eggs shed by dogs of epidemiological relevance? *Vet Parasitol*. 2011;177:186–189.
75. Nijsse R, Mughini-Gras L, Wagenaar JA, et al. Coprophagy in dogs interferes in the diagnosis of parasitic infections by faecal examination. *Vet Parasitol*. 2014;204:304–309.
76. Burke TM, Roberson EL. Fenbendazole treatment of pregnant bitches to reduce prenatal and lactogenic infections of *Toxocara canis* and *Ancylostoma caninum* in pups. *J Am Vet Med Assoc*. 1983;183:987–990.
77. Krämer F, Hammerstein R, Stoye M, et al. Investigations into the prevention of prenatal and lactogenic *Toxocara canis* infections in puppies by application of moxidectin to the pregnant dog. *J Vet Med B Infect Dis Vet Public Health*. 2006;53:218–223.
78. Payne-Johnson M, Maitland TP, Sherington J, et al. Efficacy of selamectin administered topically to pregnant and lactating female dogs in the treatment and prevention of adult roundworm (*Toxocara canis*) infections and flea (*Ctenocephalides felis felis*) infestations in the dams and their pups. *Vet Parasitol*. 2000;91:347–358.
79. Woodhall DM, Fiore AE. Toxocariasis: a review for pediatricians. *J Pediatric Infect Dis Soc*. 2013;3:154–159.
80. Chun CS, Kazacos KR, Glaser C, et al. Global neurologic deficits with *Baylisascaris* encephalitis in a previously healthy teenager. *Pediatr Infect Dis J*. 2009;28:925–927.
81. Cortez RT, Ramirez G, Collet L, et al. Ocular parasitic diseases: a review on toxocariasis and diffuse unilateral subacute neuroretinitis. *J Pediatr Ophthalmol Strabismus*. 2010;48:204–212.
82. Pawlowski Z. Toxocariasis in humans: clinical expression and treatment dilemma. *J Helminthol*. 2001;75:299–305.
83. Fillaux J, Magnaval JF. Laboratory diagnosis of human toxocariasis. *Vet Parasitol*. 2013;193:327–336.
84. Bowman DD. *Toxocara* and toxocariasis. *Adv Parasitol*. 2020;109:2–883.
85. Won KY, Kruszon-Moran D, Schantz PM, et al. National seroprevalence and risk factors for zoonotic *Toxocara* spp. infection. *Am J Trop Med Hyg*. 2008;79:552–557.
86. Farmer A, Beltran T, Choi YS. Prevalence of *Toxocara* species infection in the US: results from the National Health and Nutrition Examination Survey, 2011-2014. *PLoS Negl Trop Dis*. 2017;11:e0005818.
87. Liu EW, Chastain HM, Shin SH, et al. Seroprevalence of antibodies to *Toxocara* species in the United States and associated risk factors, 2011–2014. *Clin Infect Dis*. 2018;66:206–212.
88. Bradbury RS, Hobbs CV. *Toxocara* seroprevalence in the USA and its impact for individuals and society. *Adv Parasitol*. 2020;109:317–339.
89. Hotez PJ, Wilkins PP. Toxocariasis: America's most common neglected infection of poverty and a helminthiasis of global importance? *PLoS Negl Trop Dis*. 2009;3:1–4.
90. Rostami A, Sepidarkish M, Ma G, et al. Global prevalence of *Toxocara* infection in cats. *Adv Parasitol*. 2020;109:615–639.
91. Mizgajska-Wiktor H, Jarosz W, Fogt-Wyrwas R, et al. Distribution and dynamics of soil contamination with *Toxocara canis* and *Toxocara cati* eggs in Poland and prevention measures proposed after 20 years of study. *Vet Parasitol*. 2017;234:1–9.
92. Choobineh M, Mikaeili F, Sadjjadi SM, et al. Molecular characterization of *Toxocara* spp. eggs isolated from public parks and playgrounds in Shiraz, Iran. *J Helminthol*. 2019;93:306–312.
93. Sprent JFA. The life history and development of *Toxocara cati* (Schrank 1788) in the domestic cat. *Parasitology*. 1956;46:54–78.
94. Vega RM, González Prous C, Krivokapich S, et al. Toxocariasis in Carnivora from Argentinean Patagonia: species molecular identification, hosts, and geographical distribution. *Int J Parasitol Parasites Wildl*. 2018;7:106–110.
95. Hoggard KR, Jarriel DM, Bevelock TJ, et al. Prevalence survey of gastrointestinal and respiratory parasites of shelter cats in northeastern Georgia, USA. *Vet Parasitol Reg Stud Reports*. 2019;16:100270.
96. Nagamori Y, Payton ME, Looper E, et al. Retrospective survey of endoparasitism identified in feces of client-owned dogs in North America from 2007 through 2018. *Vet Parasitol*. 2020;282:109137.
97. Beugnet F, Bourdeau P, Chalvet-Monfray K, et al. Parasites of domestic owned cats in Europe: co-infestations and risk factors. *Parasit Vectors*. 2014;7:291.
98. Nijsse R, Ploeger HW, Wagenaar JA, et al. Prevalence and risk factors for patent *Toxocara* infections in cats and cat owners' attitude towards deworming. *Parasitol Res*. 2016;115:4519–4525.
99. Nagamori Y, Payton ME, Duncan-Decocq R, et al. Fecal survey of parasites in free-roaming cats in northcentral Oklahoma, United States. *Vet Parasitol Reg Stud Reports*. 2020;14:50–53.
100. Chalkowski K, Wilson AE, Lepczyk CA, Zohdy S. Who let the cats out? A global meta-analysis on risk of parasitic infection in indoor versus outdoor domestic cats (*Felis catus*). *Biol Lett*. 2019;15:20180840.
101. Mizgajska-Wiktor H, Jarosz W. A comparison of soil contamination with *Toxocara canis* and *Toxocara cati* eggs in rural and urban areas of Wielko-Polska district in 2000-2005. *Wiad Parazytol*. 2007;53:219–225.
102. Nijsse R, Overgaauw P, Ploeger H, et al. Sources of environmental contamination with *Toxocara* spp.: an omnipresent parasite. *Adv Parasitol*. 2020;109:585–614.
103. Coati N, Schnieder T, Epe C. Vertical transmission of *Toxocara cati*. Schrank 1788 (Anisakidae) in the cat. *Parasitol Res*. 2004;92:142–146.
104. Swerczek T, Neilsen S, Hemboldt C. Transmammary passage of *Toxocara cati* in the cat. *Am J Vet Res*. 1971;32:89–92.
105. Taira K, Saitoh Y, Kapel CMO. *Toxocara cati* larvae persist and retain high infectivity in muscles of experimentally infected chickens. *Vet Parasitol*. 2011;180:287–291.
106. Prociv P. *Toxocara pteropodis, T. canis,* and *T. cati* infections in Guinea pigs. *Trop Biomed*. 1986;3:97–106.
107. Havasiová-Reiterová K, Tomasovicová O, Dubinský P. Effect of various doses of infective *Toxocara canis* and *Toxocara cati* eggs on the humoral response and distribution of larvae in mice. *Parasitol Res*. 1995;81:13–17.
108. Akao N, Takayanagi TH, Suzuki R, et al. Ocular larva migrans caused by *Toxocara cati* in Mongolian gerbils and a comparison of ophthalmologic findings with those produced by *T. canis*. *J Parasitol*. 2000;86:1133–1135.
109. Janecek E, Beineke A, Schnieder T, et al. Neurotoxocarosis: marked preference of *Toxocara canis* for the cerebrum and *T. cati* for the cerebellum in the paratenic model host mouse. *Parasit Vectors*. 2014;7:194.
110. Janecek E, Waindok P, Bankstahl M, et al. Abnormal neurobehaviour and impaired memory function as a consequence of *Toxocara canis*- as well as *Toxocara cati*-induced neurotoxocarosis. *PLoS Negl Trop Dis*. 2017;11:e0005594.
111. French AF, Castillo-Alcala F, Gedye KR, et al. Nematode larva migrans caused by *Toxocara cati* in the North Island brown kiwi (*Apteryx mantelli*). *Int J Parasitol Parasites Wildl*. 2020;11:221–228.
112. Durant JF, Irenge LM, Fogt-Wyrwas R, et al. Duplex quantitative real-time PCR assay for the detection and discrimination of the eggs of *Toxocara canis* and *Toxocara cati* (Nematoda, Ascaridoidea) in soil and fecal samples. *Parasit Vectors*. 2012;5:288.
113. Wang Z, Shibata M, Nguyen YTH, et al. Development of nested multiplex polymerase chain reaction (PCR) assay for the detection of *Toxocara canis, Toxocara cati* and *Ascaris suum* contamination in meat and organ meats. *Parasitol Int*. 2018;67:622–626.
114. Swerczek TW, Nielsen SW, Helmboldt CF. Ascariasis causing pulmonary arterial hyperplasia in cats. *Res Vet Sci*. 1970;11:103–104.
115. Weatherley AJ, Hamilton JM. Possible role of histamine in the genesis of pulmonary arterial disease in cats infected with *Toxocara cati*. *Vet Rec*. 1984;114:347–349.

116. Dillon AR, Tillson DM, Hathcock J, et al. Lung histopathology, radiography, high-resolution computed tomography, and bronchio-alveolar lavage cytology are altered by *Toxocara cati* infection in cats and is independent of development of adult intestinal parasites. *Vet Parasitol.* 2013;193:413–426.
117. Wolken S, Böhm C, Schaper R, et al. Treatment of third-stage larvae of *Toxocara cati* with milbemycin oxime plus praziquantel tablets and emodepside plus praziquantel spot-on formulation in experimentally infected cats. *Parasitol Res.* 2012;111:2123–2127.
118. Wolken S, Schaper R, Mencke N, et al. Treatment and prevention of vertical transmission of *Toxocara cati* in cats with an emodepside/praziquantel spot-on formulation. *Parasitol Res.* 2009;105:S75–S81.
119. Böhm C, Petry G, Schaper R, et al. Prevention of lactogenic *Toxocara cati* infections in kittens by application of an emodepside/praziquantel spot-on (Profender) to the pregnant queen. *Parasitol Res.* 2015;114:S175–S184.
120. Fisher M. *Toxocara cati:* an underestimated zoonotic agent. *Trends Parasitol.* 2003;19:167–170.
121. Shimokawa H, Nakashima T, Akagi K, et al. Visceral larva migrans by *Toxocara cati. Fukuoka Igaku Zasshi.* 1982;73:64–69.
122. Poulsen CS, Skov S, Yoshida A, et al. Differential serodiagnostics of *Toxocara canis* and *T. cati* - is it possible? *Parasite Immunol.* 2015;37:204–207.
123. Eberhard ML, Alfano E. Adult *Toxocara cati* infections in U.S. children: report of four cases. *Am J Trop Med Hyg.* 1998;59:404–406.
124. Wiseman RA, Lovel TW. Human infection with adult *Toxocara cati. Br Med J.* 1969;3:454–455.
125. Fogt-Wyrwas R, Dabert M, Jarosz W, et al. Molecular data reveal cryptic speciation and host specificity in *Toxascaris leonina* (Nematoda: Ascarididae). *Vet Parasitol.* 2019;266:80–83.
126. Jin YC, Li XY, Liu JH, et al. Comparative analysis of mitochondrial DNA datasets indicates that *Toxascaris leonina* represents a species complex. *Parasit Vectors.* 2019;12:194.
127. Petrigh RS, Martínez JG, Mondini M, et al. Ancient parasitic DNA reveals *Toxascaris leonina* presence in final pleistocene of South America. *Parasitology.* 2019;146:1284–1288.
128. Okoshi S, Usui M. Experimental studies on *Toxascaris leonina*. I. Incidence of *T. leonina* among dogs and cats in Japan. *Japanese J Vet Sci.* 1967;29:185–194.
129. Schantz PM, Biagi F. Coexistence of *Toxocara* and *Toxascaris* in dogs in Mexico city. *J Parasitol.* 1968;54:185–186.
130. Fisher MA, Murphy MG, Siedek EM. Epidemiology of *Toxascaris leonina* infection post-weaning within a colony of dogs. *J Helminthol.* 2002;76:27–29.
131. Abdel-Rasoul K, Fowler M. An epidemiologic approach to the control of ascariasis in zoo carnivores. Erkrankungen der Zootiere Verhandlungsbericht des XXII. *Int Symp uber die Erkrankungen der Zootiere.* 1980:273–277.
132. Okoshi S, Usui M. Experimental studies on *Toxascaris leonina*. V. Experimental infection of dogs and cats with eggs of canine, feline and Felidae strains. *Japanese J Vet Sci.* 1968;30:81–91.
133. Sprent J. The life history and development of *Toxascaris leonina* (von Linstow 1902) in the dog and cat. *Parasitology.* 1959;49:330–371.
134. Okoshi S, Usui M. Experimental studies on *Toxascaris leonina*. IV. Development of eggs of three ascarids, *T. leonina, Toxocara canis*, and *Toxocara cati*, in dogs and cats. *Japanese J Vet Sci.* 1968;30:29–38.
135. Okoshi S, Usui M. Experimental studies on *Toxascaris leonina*. III. Morphology of worms and eggs obtained from various animals. *Japanese J Vet Sci.* 1967;29:329–336.
136. Matoff K, Komanderev S. Comparative studies on the migration of the larvae of *Toxascaris leonina* and *Toxascaris transfuga*. *Zeitschrift für Parasitenkd.* 1965;25:538–555.
137. Grinberg AI. Rare cases of *Toxascaris leonina* and *Toxocara mystax* in man. *Meditsinskaya Parazitol i Parazit Bolezn.* 1961;30:626.
138. Cuéllar C, Fenoy S, Guillén JL. Cross-reactions of sera from *Toxascaris leonina* and *Ascaris suum* infected mice with *Toxocara canis, Toxascaris leonina* and *Ascaris suum* antigens. *Int J Parasitol.* 1995;25:731–739.
139. Hogarth-Scott R. Visceral larva migrans-an immunofluorescent examination of rabbit and human sera for antibodies to the ES antigens of the second stage larvae of *Toxocara canis, Toxocara cati* and *Toxascaris leonina* (Nematoda). *Immunology.* 1966;10:217.
140. Kazacos KR. *Baylisascaris Larva Migrans - Circular 1412.* U.S. Geological Survey. 2016. Available at: https://pubs.usgs.gov/circ/1412/cir1412.pdf.
141. Sapp SGH, Gupta P, Martin MK, et al. Beyond the raccoon roundworm: the natural history of non-raccoon *Baylisascaris* species in the New World. *Int J Parasitol Parasites Wildl.* 2017;6:85–99.
142. Yabsley MJ, Sapp SGH. Prevalence of *Baylisascaris* in domestic dog coprological examinations in the United States, 2013–2016. *Vet Parasitol Reg Stud Reports.* 2017;9:65–69.
143. Conboy G, Stewart TA, Taylor A. *Baylisascaris procyonis* infection in raccoons and dogs on Prince Edward Island, Canada. *Proceed Am Assoc Vet Parasitol.* 2010;55:56.
144. Ogdee JL, Henke SE, Wester DB, et al. Permeability and viability of *Baylisascaris procyonis* eggs in southern Texas soils. *J Parasitol.* 2016;102:608–612.
145. Shafir SC, Sorvillo FJ, Sorvillo T, et al. Viability of *Baylisascaris procyonis* eggs. *Emerg Infect Dis.* 2011;17:1293–1295.
146. Bowman DD, Ulrich MA, Gregory DE, et al. Treatment of *Baylisascaris procyonis* infections in dogs with milbemycin oxime. *Vet Parasitol.* 2005;129:285–290.
147. Miyashita M. Prevalence of *Baylisascaris procyonis* in raccoons in Japan and experimental infections of the worm to laboratory animals. *J Urban Living Heal Assoc.* 1993;37:137–151.
148. Babero BB. Studies on the larval morphology of *Ascaris laevis* Leidy, 1856. *Am Midl Nat.* 1960;64:349–361.
149. Anderson BC. Congenital *Baylisascaris* sp. larval migrans in a newborn lamb. *J Parasitol.* 1999;85:128–129.
150. Hoberg EP, Burek-Huntington K, Beckmen K, et al. Transuterine infection by *Baylisascaris transfuga*: neurological migration and fatal debilitation in sibling moose calves (*Alces alces gigas*) from Alaska. *Int J Parasitol Parasites Wildl.* 2018;7:280–288.
151. Greve JH, O'Brien SE. Adult *Baylisascaris* infections in two dogs. *Companion Anim Pract.* 1989;19:41–53.
152. Snyder DE. The Prevalence, Cross-Transmissibility to Domestic Animals and the Adult Structure of *Baylisascaris procyonis* from Illinois Raccoons (*Procyon lotor*) 1983. University of Illinois at Urbana-Champaign.
153. Dubey JP. *Baylisascaris procyonis* and eimerian infections in raccoons. *J Am Vet Med Assoc.* 1982;181:1292–1294.
154. Dangoudoubiyam S, Vemulapalli R, Kazacos KR. PCR assays for detection of *Baylisascaris procyonis* eggs and larvae. *J Parasitol.* 2009;95:571–577.
155. Bauer C, Gey A. Efficacy of six anthelmintics against luminal stages of *Baylisascaris procyonis* in naturally infected raccoons (*Procyon lotor*). *Vet Parasitol.* 1995;60:155–159.
156. Peters JM, Madhavan VL, Kazacos KR, et al. Good outcome with early empiric treatment of neural larva migrans due to *Baylisascaris procyonis*. *Pediatrics.* 2012;129:806–811.
157. Sircar AD, Abanyie F, Blumberg D, et al. Raccoon roundworm infection associated with central nervous system disease and ocular disease - six states, 2013-2015. *Morb Mortal Wkly Rep.* 2016;65:930–933.
158. Sapp SGH, Rascoe LN, Wilkins PP, et al. *Baylisascaris procyonis* roundworm seroprevalence among wildlife rehabilitators, United States and Canada, 2012-2015. *Emerg Infect Dis.* 2016;22:2012–2015.
159. Gibbons L, Jacobs D, Sani R. *Toxocara malaysiensis* n. sp. (Nematoda: Ascaridoidea) from the domestic cat (*Felis catus* Linnaeus, 1758). *J Parasitol.* 2001;87:660–665.
160. Zhu XQ, Jacobs DE, Chilton NB, et al. Molecular characterization of a *Toxocara* variant from cats in Kuala Lumpur, Malaysia. *Parasitology.* 1998;117:155–164.
161. Li MW, Zhu XQ, Gasser RB, et al. The occurrence of *Toxocara malaysiensis* in cats in China, confirmed by sequence-based analyses of ribosomal DNA. *Parasitol Res.* 2006;99:554–557.
162. Zain MSN, Sahimin N, Pal P, et al. Macroparasite communities in stray cat populations from urban cities in Peninsular Malaysia. *Vet Parasitol.* 2013;196:469–477.
163. Amato JFR, Grisi L, Pimentel Neto M. Two cases of fistulated abcesses caused by *Lagochilascaris major* in the domestic cat. *Mem Inst Oswaldo Cruz.* 1990;85:471–473.
164. Volcan GS, Medrano CE, Payares G. Experimental heteroxenous cycle of *Lagochilascaris minor* Leiper, 1909 (Nematoda: Ascarididae) in white mice and in cats. *Mem Inst Oswaldo Cruz.* 1992;87:525–532.

165. Paçô JM, Campos DMB, De Oliveira JA. Wild rodents as experimental intermediate hosts of *Lagochilascaris minor* Leiper, 1909. *Mem Inst Oswaldo Cruz.* 1999;94:441–449.
166. Castro O, Venzal JM, Félix ML. Two new records of helminth parasites of domestic cat from Uruguay: *Alaria alata* (Goeze, 1782) (Digenea, Diplostomidae) and *Lagochilascaris major* Leiper, 1910 (Nematoda, Ascarididae). *Vet Parasitol.* 2009;160:344–347.
167. Dos Reis RA, Cristiane R, Mangoni F, et al. *Lagochilascaris minor* (Nematoda, Ascarididae) em gato doméstico: relato de caso. *Veterinária em Foco.* 2014;9:2011.
168. Faccio L, Oliveira CB, Denardin CA, et al. Case report: feline infection by *Lagochilascaris* sp. in the state of Rio Grande do Sul, Brazil. *Vet Parasitol.* 2013;196:541–543.
169. Sakamoto T, Cabrera PA. Subcutaneous infection of *Lagochilascaris minor* in domestic cats from Uruguay. *Vet Parasitol.* 2002;108:145–152.
170. Aquino RTR, Magliari MER, Vital Filho J, et al. Lagochilascariasis leading to severe involvement of ocular globes, ears and meninges. *Rev Inst Med Trop Sao Paulo.* 2008;50:355–358.
171. Rosemberg S, Lopes MBS, Masuda Z, et al. Fatal encephalopathy due to *Lagochilascaris minor* infection. *Am J Trop Med Hyg.* 1986;35:575–578.
172. Martinez-Hernandez F, Prado-Calleros HM, Ramirez-Hinojosa, et al. An unexpected case of lagochilascariasis: interdisciplinary management and use of 12S and 18S rDNA analysis. *Am J Med Sci.* 2020;359:235–241.
173. Moncada LI, Alvarez CA, Castellanos C, et al. *Lagochilascaris minor* in a patient from the Colombian Amazon: a case report. *Rev Inst Med Trop Sao Paulo.* 1998;40:387–389.
174. Craig TM, O'Quinn BO, Robinson RM, et al. Parasitic nematode (*Lagochilascaris major*) associated with a purulent draining tract in a dog. *J Am Vet Med Assoc.* 1982;181:69–70.
175. Barbosa CAL, Campos DMB, Oliveira JA. Assessment of ivermectin therapeutic efficacy on third-stage larvae of *Lagochilascaris minor* in mice experimentally infected. *Rev Inst Med Trop Sao Paulo.* 1998;40:137–144.
176. Botero D, Little MD. Two cases of human *Lagochilascaris* infection in Colombia. *Am J Trop Med Hyg.* 1984;33:381–386.
177. Oostburg BFJ. Thiabendazole therapy of *Lagochilascaris minor* infection in Surinam. *Am J Trop Med Hyg.* 1971;20:580–583.
178. Little S, Adolph C, Downie K, et al. High prevalence of covert infection with gastrointestinal helminths in cats. *J Am Anim Hosp Assoc.* 2015;51:359–364.

113

Hookworms

Dwight D. Bowman, Araceli Lucio-Forster, Alice C.Y. Lee

KEY POINTS

- First Described: The canine hookworm, now known as *Ancylostoma caninum*, was first described by Ercolani in a veterinary textbook in Italy in 1859, and in 1911, the species was moved to the genus *Ancylostoma*.[1] *Ancylostoma tubaeforme* was first described by Zeder in 1800 as a hookworm of the cat; it was later considered the same as the dog hookworm until 1962 when Burrows showed it was a distinct species.[2] *Ancylostoma braziliense* was described as a new species by de Faria in 1910 from specimens collected from dogs and cats in Brazil. It was then synonymized with *Ancylostoma ceylanicum* until 1951 when Biocca showed they were distinct species.[3] *Ancylostoma ceylanicum* was first described by Looss in 1911[1] based on specimens from a civet and then in three people in India.[4] *Uncinaria stenocephala* was initially named *Dochmoides stenocephala* in France in 1884 by Railliet and then later transferred to the genus *Uncinaria*.
- Cause: Five members of the hookworm family Ancylostomatidae: *Ancylostoma caninum* (canine ancylostomiasis), *Ancylostoma tubaeforme* (feline ancylostomiasis), *Ancylostoma braziliense* (the creeping eruption hookworm of people), *Uncinaria stenocephala* (canine uncinariasis), and in tropical areas of Australasia, *Ancylostoma ceylanicum* (causing ancylostomiasis in dogs, cats, and humans).
- Affected Hosts: *Ancylostoma caninum* is a parasite of dogs and other canids; *A. tubaeforme* is a parasite of the domestic cat and other felids; *A. braziliense* is a parasite of canids and felids; adults of *A. ceylanicum* can be found in canids, felids, and people; and *U. stenocephala* is found in dogs, foxes, and other canids. There are no intermediate hosts; however, all these hookworms can utilize some invertebrates and mammals as paratenic hosts.
- Geographic Distribution: *Ancylostoma caninum* and *A. tubaeforme* have a cosmopolitan distribution. *Ancylostoma braziliense* tends to be restricted to the southeastern United States and the coastal areas of the Atlantic, through the Caribbean, the eastern coastal areas of Mexico, Central and South America, southeast Asia, and the northern coast of Australia. *Ancylostoma ceylanicum* occurs in India, Taiwan, central Thailand, Malaysia, Indonesia, Borneo, and likely New Guinea; it is also in Surinam in South America. *Uncinaria stenocephala* is found in the northern United States and Canada, as well as the EU, Africa, and it has been reported from Australia.
- Primary Mode of Transmission: Hookworms infect their final hosts through either oral or percutaneous routes. *Ancylostoma caninum* is the only species capable of infecting offspring through transmammary transmission. Relative to transmission into their carnivorous final hosts, all four species of *Ancylostoma* persist in the tissues of murine paratenic hosts for extended periods, with the exception being *A. ceylanicum* where a very small percentage of larvae (<1%) survive in mice one month PI. It has been reported that the larvae of *U. stenocephala* can also persist in the tissues of mice after either oral or percutaneous infection; however, others consider *U. stenocephala* to have strictly a direct life cycle.
- Major Clinical Signs: When present in sufficient numbers, hookworms can cause anemia, leading to pale mucous membranes, tachycardia, and lethargy. Inappetence, emaciation or failure to gain weight, and poor haircoat are often evident. During acute infections, feces can contain blood and mucus. Dark, tarry feces may be produced when there is significant blood loss into the intestinal lumen.
- Differential Diagnoses: Other parasitisms (e.g., fleas, ticks, coccidia, *Babesia* spp.), bacterial or viral enteritis (e.g., parvovirus, feline panleukopenia virus, *Salmonella*, enterohemorrhagic *Escherichia coli*), IMHA, hemotropic *Mycoplasma* infections, FeLV or FIV infections, portosystemic shunt, hereditary hemophilia, toxicity (e.g., rodenticide, NSAID, garlic, onion), and neoplasia.
- Human Health Significance: *Ancylostoma braziliense* and, to a lesser extent, *A. caninum* cause cutaneous larva migrans in humans ("creeping eruption"). *Ancylostoma caninum* can mature to the adult stage in the human intestine on rare occasions, eliciting an eosinophilic enteritis.

ETIOLOGY AND EPIDEMIOLOGY

Hookworm infections in cats and dogs are caused by species of nematodes in the genera *Ancylostoma* and *Uncinaria*. The species of *Ancylostoma* infecting companion animals in the Americas include: *Ancylostoma caninum* in dogs, *Ancylostoma tubaeforme* in cats, and *Ancylostoma braziliense* in both hosts. *Uncinaria stenocephala* infects dogs and other canids, and although the nematode has been previously reported in cats, infections in feline hosts are rare. In companion animals, these parasites are important because of the anemia they induce as they feed from the mucosa of the small intestine. The major differences in the pathology induced in their hosts are related to: (1) the modes of infection utilized by each species, and (2) the amount of blood loss induced by individual worms within the intestinal tract, which varies with the species of hookworm involved. Aside from the exotic *Ancylostoma ceylanicum* that routinely develops to the adult stage in humans, the zoonotic importance of canine and feline hookworms stems from the ability of the larvae to penetrate skin and produce cutaneous lesions in humans.

The general life cycle of hookworms requires that the feces from an infected host be deposited at a site where it will be mixed with porous soil that remains moist; in this manner, the eggs will be protected from being overly heated, frozen, or dried. Then, in about a week, larvae develop within the egg, hatch as first-stage larvae, feed and grow, molt twice, and become non-feeding infective third-stage larvae. The larvae of *A. caninum* develop optimally at 25°C to 30°C, taking only 3 days to become infective at 30°C compared to 22 days if maintained at 15°C.[5] *Ancylostoma tubaeforme* and *U. stenocephala* develop optimally at 20°C.[5,6] Fecal cultures harboring both *A. caninum* and *U. stenocephala* eggs, if held at 15°C, will produce only *U. stenocephala* larvae 8 days after the cultures are initiated; the eggs and larvae of *U. stenocephala* are tolerant to cold and can survive temperatures near freezing, for days to weeks, while the same conditions will kill *A. caninum* eggs and larvae in a few days.[5] There have been no similar studies on the development of *A. braziliense*, but its presence only in warmer climes would suggest that it develops most successfully at warmer temperatures and may not develop in soils of colder climates.

Infective-stage hookworm larvae that develop in the soil can enter their final canine or feline hosts in three different ways. One means of infection is to penetrate the skin, be carried to the lungs via the circulatory system, and then enter the intestine after migrating up the trachea and being swallowed. Second, they can be ingested as free larvae from the soil or on contaminated plants or fomites. Third, they can be ingested as infective-stage larvae in the tissues of prey paratenic hosts. All four species of *Ancylostoma* persist in tissues of rodent paratenic hosts for extended periods, with the exception of *A. ceylanicum* where a small percentage of larvae (< 1%) survive in mice a month PI.[7–9] Additional work with *A. caninum* has shown that it will persist in the tissues of cockroaches, rodents, cats, sheep, and goats.[10] Chickens appear refractory to *A. caninum* larval infection with < 1% of the inoculum being recovered from muscle after 2 months,[11] and no larvae were recovered from chickens 20 days after infection with *A. tubaeforme*.[7] *Uncinaria stenocephala* can also persist in the tissues of mice after oral or percutaneous infection[12]; however, others consider *U. stenocephala* to have strictly a direct life cycle.[13] *Ancylostoma caninum* of dogs is the only species discussed herein that infects neonates through transmammary transmission (Fig. 113.1).[14] In this case, larvae that have been sequestered in the tissues of the dam will enter the mammary gland and make their way into the milk after the female begins lactation. Thus, very young pups can be infected with a large number of *A. caninum* relative to their body size, which can lead to severe and even fatal anemia. The pre-patent and patent periods for *A. caninum*, *A. tubaeforme*, *A. braziliense*, and *U. stenocephala*, respectively, are: 15–26, 18–28, 14–16, and 15–17 days before eggs are produced; and about 6, 18–24, 4–8, and 6–12 months of egg excretion.[15–18]

Ancylostoma caninum and *A. tubaeforme* have a cosmopolitan geographic distribution. *Uncinaria stenocephala*, the most cold tolerant of the species,[19] is found in the northern United States and Canada, as well as in the EU, Africa, and has been reported from Australia.[20] The CAPC prevalence maps for the United States show the results for over 10 million dog fecal examinations; in 2021, about 2.9% contained hookworm eggs. The CAPC maps for cats, representing almost 1.8 million fecal specimens, show that 0.8% contained hookworm eggs. Much higher infection rates were reported in animals not receiving routine veterinary care or endoparasitic treatments, and those having access to prey and contaminated environments.[21–23] The areas with the highest prevalence rates were in the southeastern and southcentral states, and the areas with the lowest rates of infection were the southwestern states. *Ancylostoma braziliense,* based on reported cases of "creeping eruption" in humans and surveys of dogs and cats in the United States, is located mainly in the southeastern and southcentral states bordering the shores of the Atlantic and the Gulf of Mexico.[24–26] Globally, cutaneous larva migrans (CLM) occurs in warmer climates, is endemic in many countries in the developing world, and has increasingly been a problem in southern Europe. The disease has been a problem among travelers returning to North America from the Caribbean[27]; a study that included over 17,000 travelers consulting specialized travel or tropical medicine clinics on six continents after holidays identified the disease in 2%–3% of patients.[28] Sites of exposure, in decreasing order of frequency, were the Caribbean, Southeast Asia, Central America and South America, and the northern coast of Australia.[15,29] (see Public Health Significance). *Ancylostoma ceylanicum* occurs in India, Taiwan, central Thailand, Malaysia, Indonesia, Borneo, and likely New Guinea; it is also in Surinam in South America.[15,29]

CLINICAL FEATURES

Pathogenesis

The disease produced by adult hookworms is anemia. In 1992, Dr. Jay Georgi, who for years studied blood loss from hookworm infection and haemonchosis, described the blood lost due to *A. caninum* as follows: "The amount of blood removed is directly proportional to the weight of adult hookworms in the small intestine and amounts to a daily loss of about 30 μL of erythrocytes per mg of worm. An adult female *A. caninum* weighs 2.0 to 2.6 mg and a male, about 0.8 mg. Therefore, a population of only 50 females and 25 males would exact a toll of about 4 mL of erythrocytes each day, a substantial drain on the hemopoietic resources of any puppy. The imposition of such a burden during the nursing period could prove fatal. To make matters worse, peak blood loss is experienced even before eggs appear in the feces. This not only renders diagnosis difficult but constitutes a sudden hemorrhagic shock that very young puppies are ill-equipped to compensate. The other species of *Ancylostoma* remove less blood than *A. caninum*, and *U. stenocephala* least of all."[30–32]

It has also been estimated that amount of blood lost in dogs per worm is 10–200 μL for *A. caninum*, 14 μL for *A. ceylanicum*, 1 μL for *A. braziliense*, and 0.3 μL for *U. stenocephala*.[31] Thus, *A. caninum* causes far greater blood loss than the other species. In the case of puppies, not only do they have a markedly lower total blood volume than adults but also they do not receive large amounts of iron in the milk from the dam, limiting their ability to regenerate red blood cells. By the end of the third week postpartum, a heavily infected pup can lose 25% of its circulating erythrocyte volume; this can be fatal.[33]

The same number of worms will cause as much blood loss in an adult dog as they do in puppies, however, a well-nourished adult dog can compensate for the blood loss. "Compensated" and "decompensated" hookworm disease has been described.[30] In compensated disease, well-maintained dogs will have no signs other than fecal egg excretion or reductions in erythrocyte parameters. In decompensated hookworm disease, animals that are malnourished or emaciated may require supportive protein and iron supplements along with treatment for intestinal hookworms.

Hookworms secrete a family of anticoagulative proteins into the host blood that prevents fibrin clot formation and also enhances the dissolution of formed clots. They act by several mechanisms, including inhibition of platelet aggregation and clotting factor activity (Xa, VIIa/tissue factor complex), as well as degradation of fibrinogen into nonfunctional components.[34,35] Consequently, hemorrhage can continue from hookworm-abandoned feeding sites within the intestine until hemostasis is re-established (Fig. 113.2). This intestinal hemorrhage, in combination with that lost through direct feeding by the worms, contributes to anemia and hypoproteinemia in heavily infected animals.

Dogs and cats infected with hookworm species other than *A. caninum* can have large numbers of worms without significant clinical signs, because these other species are not passed directly from the mother to offspring, they cause less blood loss per worm, and they are less pathogenic. However, all hookworm infections cause blood loss, and signs are commensurate with the number of worms present. Thus, a high egg count in adult animals indicates a larger number of adult female worms, and greater blood loss than an animal with low egg counts, in most cases. Though anemia is uncommon with *U. stenocephala* and *A. braziliense* infections, hypoproteinemia may still develop as a result of villous atrophy with associated malabsorption and protein loss.[36] Additionally, intestinal mucosal thickening can be observed when *U. stenocephala* worm numbers reach 1,000 or more.[36]

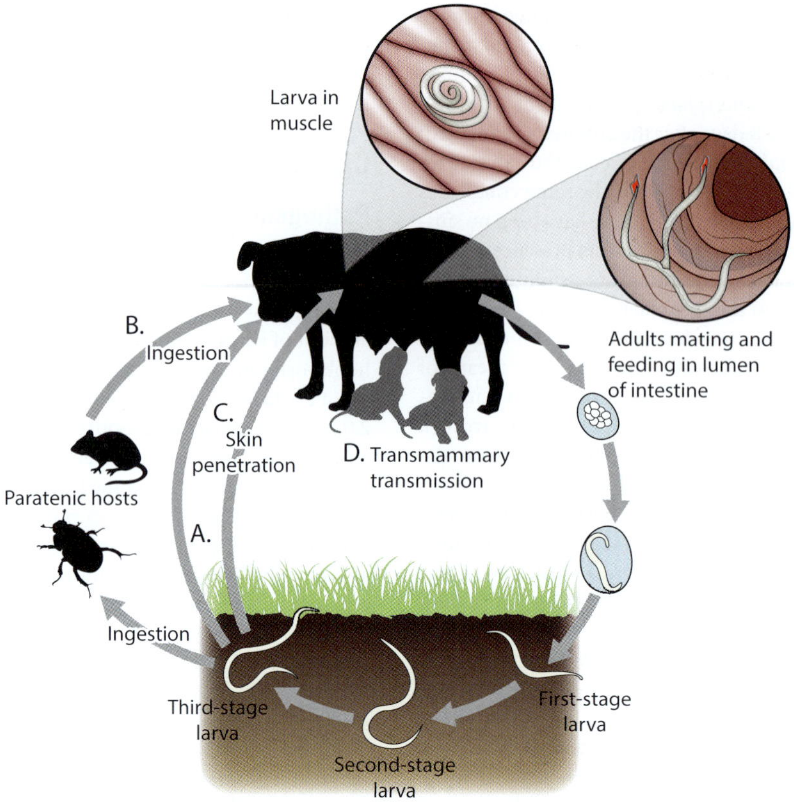

Fig. 113.1 Life cycle of *Ancylostoma caninum*, the most common hookworm in dogs in the United States. The nematode can infect dogs in the same manner as the other hookworms of cats and dogs (i.e., ingestion of free larvae from the environment, ingestion of larvae in prey tissues, and through skin penetration), but it is the only hookworm species in these hosts that is capable of transmammary transmission through the reactivation of hypobiotic larvae from the tissues of the dam.

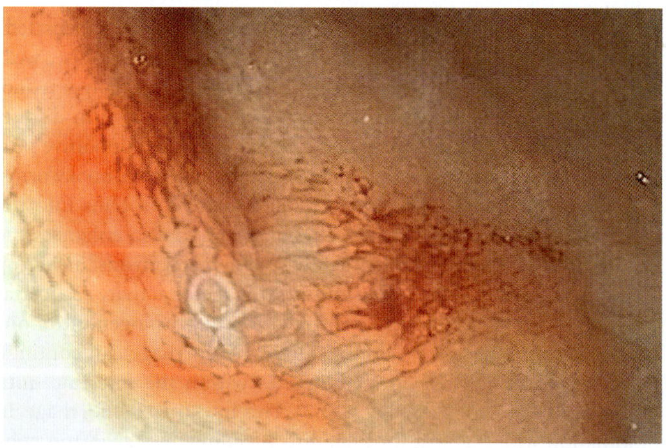

Fig. 113.2 Endoscopic evidence of hemorrhage associated with an immature worm feeding in the small intestine of a dog experimentally infected with *Ancylostoma caninum* (11 days post-infection).

Clinical Signs and Physical Examination Findings

Peracute clinical disease is seen in neonatal pups infected by *A. caninum* through transmammary transmission. Pups often appear healthy in the first week of life, then rapidly deteriorate and die at 2–3 weeks of age. Acute disease affects older pups and kittens, and even adult animals exposed to overwhelming numbers of infectious larvae. Clinical signs include diarrhea with melena and/or mucus, mucosal pallor, lethargy, inappetence, emaciation or failure to gain weight, and poor haircoat. Tachycardia, tachypnea, and weak pulses may be present on physical examination in severely anemic and hypoproteinemic animals. In peracute—and sometimes acute—hookworm disease, clinical signs may occur before eggs appear in the feces, so an accurate diagnosis relies on a good history and physical examination findings. Animals with chronic, compensated hookworm infections are subclinically infected, though decreases in hematologic parameters such as erythrocyte count and hemoglobin concentration may be evident.

Uncinaria stenocephala infection is most commonly associated with dermatitis, though *Ancylostoma* spp. are also capable. These cutaneous manifestations typically occur in kenneled greyhounds.[37] There is typically dermatitis with keratitis of the paw pads, but associated lesions can also often be observed on the ventral thorax and abdomen as well as the limbs. Thickened intestinal loops may also be palpable on physical examination in heavy infections of *U. stenocephala*.

DIAGNOSIS

Fecal Analysis

Fecal Flotation

Patent hookworm infections may be diagnosed by recovery of eggs from fresh or refrigerated fecal specimens examined by routine fecal centrifugal flotation; stationary (noncentrifuged) flotations will recover a markedly lower percentage of hookworm eggs from any given fecal specimens. Hookworm eggs are thin-shelled, smooth and oval, containing an embryo in a morula (generally 4–8 cells) stage.

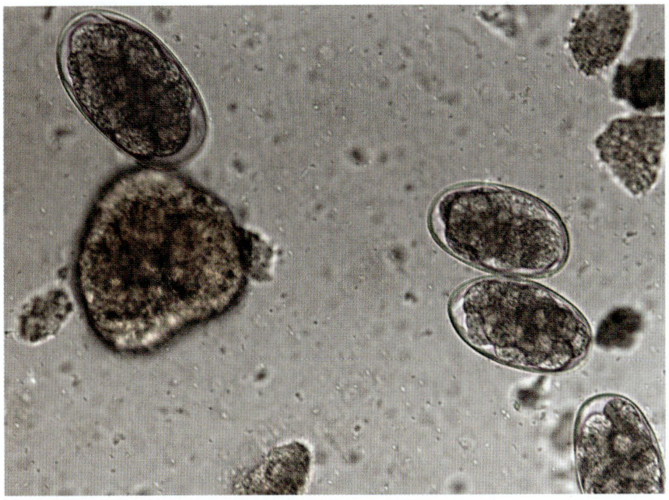

Fig. 113.3 A single egg of *Uncinaria stenocephala (top left corner)* and three eggs of *Ancylostoma caninum* recovered by centrifugal flotation of a fecal specimen from a naturally infected dog.

Careful measurement of length and width, and consideration of the host species, can aid identification of the species of hookworm involved. The eggs of *A. caninum* and *A. tubaeforme* are similarly sized, but can be distinguished based upon the host specificity of the parasite. Dogs and cats can both be infected with *A. braziliense*, but the smaller egg of this species allows it to be distinguished from the dog- and cat-specific hookworms. *Uncinaria stenocephala* eggs are larger than any of the *Ancylostoma* spp. (Fig. 113.3). The egg measurements (length by width) of the four hookworm species in micrometers are: 48–57 × 34–39 µm for *A. braziliense*, 58–66 × 38–42 µm for *A. tubaeforme*, 58–76 × 36–41 µm for *A. caninum*, and 71–92 × 35–58 µm for *U. stenocephala*.[38,39] Mixed infections are possible. In the case of *U. stenocephala*, the major confounder in fecal examinations is the presence of strongyle or trichostrongyle eggs in the feces of a dog that has ingested either prey or the feces of ruminants, equids, or other animals.

Fecal Antigen Detection

Coproantigen detection of hookworms via a fecal ELISA is commercially available (IDEXX Laboratories, Inc., Westbrook, ME, USA). This test can detect a protein excreted by *Ancylostoma* spp. and *U. stenocephala* worms in the intestine of cats and dogs, but cannot differentiate species. This test detects both patent and nonpatent infections, i.e., young and adult nematodes of either sex in the intestine.[40] It is recommended that coproantigen testing be paired with fecal centrifugal flotation tests to optimize detection of concurrent infections and to provide information on egg excretion (and hence environmental contamination).

Adult Nematode Morphology

Adult worms recovered from the feces or during necropsy may be identified to species level by examination of the buccal capsule and the teeth present on its anterior margin. *Ancylostoma* species can be differentiated by the number of teeth present: one large tooth on either side of the midline in *A. braziliense*, and three lateral teeth on either side for *A. caninum* and *A. tubaeforme*. *Uncinaria stenocephala*, on the other hand, is armed with a cutting plate on each side rather than teeth (Fig. 113.4). Although adult *A. caninum* resemble *A. tubaeforme*, they can be differentiated based on the length of the spicules of the males. However, cats and dogs are refractory to infections with *A. caninum* and *A. tubaeforme*, respectively, so such efforts for differentiation are seldom warranted.

Molecular Identification

Molecular identification of hookworm eggs, larvae, or adults to the species level is possible by performing PCR amplification-sequencing. In early 2022, a real-time PCR assay was released in North America that detects the DNA of *Ancylostoma* spp. and *U. stenocephala* as part of a panel designed to detect the DNA of 20 different parasites (KeyScreen GI Parasite PCR, Antech, CA, USA). The assay also detects a genetic marker for benzimidazole (fenbendazole) resistance in *A. caninum* (see Treatment, below). Additional peer-reviewed studies are required to assess the performance of this panel.

Laboratory Abnormalities

In animals with hookworm infections, the CBC may reveal acute normocytic, normochromic anemia progressing to microcytic, hypochromic anemia. Eosinophilia may also be observed. Hypoalbuminemia is present in severe cases, and increased BUN concentration may be evident as a result of intestinal bleeding.

Diagnostic Imaging

Although not practical or economical as a primary means of diagnosing hookworm infection, intestinal hookworms in both dogs and cats can be detected using conventional flexible endoscopy (see Fig. 113.2).[41] Capsule endoscopy is another option in dogs.[42]

Pathologic Findings

Grossly, translucent, white, or red-colored nematodes up to 2 cm long are found attached to the intestinal mucosa in hookworm infections. Pinpoint red lesions are visible in the mucosa at sites where hookworms previously fed. The contents of the intestinal lumen are dark red in color due to waste produced by the hookworms and ongoing hemorrhage. In severely anemic animals, extreme pallor of the intestines, liver, and other internal organs is observed. Serous effusion may be found in the abdominal and thoracic cavities as a consequence of hypoproteinemia. Intestinal thickening may be apparent in animals heavily infected with *U. stenocephala*.

TREATMENT AND PROGNOSIS

Products approved for *A. caninum* treatment in dogs include fenbendazole, milbemycin, moxidectin, pyrantel, and a pyrantel/febantel/praziquantel combination. All of these, aside from milbemycin, are also labeled for treatment of *U. stenocephala* infections. The ivermectin-based heartworm preventives that contain a pyrantel component also are labeled for the treatment of *A. braziliense* infections. Approved products for the treatment of *A. tubaeforme* infection in cats include emodepside, ivermectin, milbemycin, moxidectin, pyrantel, and selamectin; in cats, the ivermectin dose used for heartworm prophylaxis is also approved for treatment of *A. braziliense* infections.

The prognosis for recovery from acute and chronic hookworm disease is good to excellent after effective anthelmintic treatment. Unfortunately, in recent years, veterinarians have observed an increase in the number of cases where *A. caninum* infections have not been successfully cleared by treatment with multiple doses or even multiple classes of anthelmintics approved for this purpose. Initially the "larval leak" phenomenon was suspected to be largely responsible (see Prevention, below), but subsequently, emergence of anthelmintic resistance has been documented in *A. caninum* in the United States. Resistance of *A. caninum* to pyrantel was first reported in pet dogs in Australia in 2007.[43] In the United States, resistance was first suspected in pet greyhounds that failed to stop excreting hookworm eggs despite aggressive treatment with a combination of topical moxidectin, oral

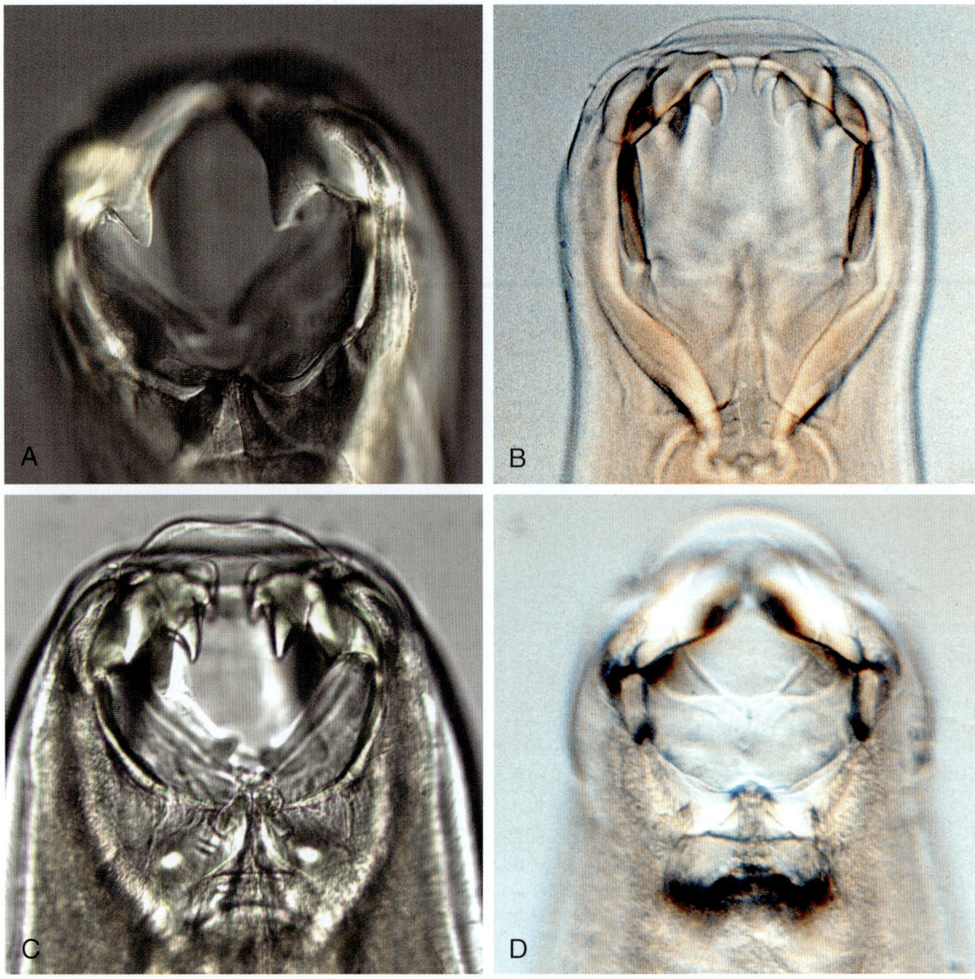

Fig. 113.4 Dorsoventral view of the buccal cavity of adult worms: (A) *Ancylostoma braziliense*, (B) *Ancylostoma caninum*, (C) *Ancylostoma tubaeforme*, and (D) *Uncinaria stenocephala*.

pyrantel, and oral febantel. However, uncertainty about client compliance limited full interpretation.[44] Subsequent work with hookworm isolates from pet greyhounds and pet dogs of other breeds confirmed infection with multidrug resistant *A. caninum* through poor reduction in fecal egg counts and elevated resistance ratios.[45,46] The problem appears to have initially developed in greyhound kennels, and although resistance is also described from other breeds, greyhounds are overrepresented in reports of *A. caninum* resistance.[47] Initial data indicate that canine hookworms resistant to pyrantel, benzimidazoles, and macrocyclic lactones can be cleared with emodepside treatment.[48] An oral product containing emodepside is available for dogs in Europe (but not in the United States) and is effective for treating *A. caninum* infections.[49] A topical feline emodepside product is available in the United States and appears effective against multidrug resistant hookworm infections when administered to dogs orally. However, due to toxicity concerns, the topical feline formulation should only be administered orally to dogs by a veterinarian and care must be taken to avoid severe reactions in heartworm-infected dogs.[50] The geographic distribution of multidrug resistant hookworm populations in the United States has not been fully defined but appears widespread. It is strongly recommended that veterinarians follow up with suspected resistant cases post-treatment to confirm that egg excretion has ceased. If egg clearance cannot be accomplished, owners must be careful to promptly dispose of feces to prevent larval development that may lead to reinfection of the dog or infection risk for humans. Emodepside treatment under the close supervision of a veterinarian may also be considered.[50]

The prognosis for recovery from peracute hookworm disease due to *A. caninum* is guarded to poor, even when effective treatment is instituted. Whole blood transfusion and other colloid therapy are often necessary for supportive care and to allow time for worms to be killed by anthelmintics. Supplemental oxygen may be required. Additional ongoing support in the form of iron supplementation and a high-protein diet is warranted.

IMMUNITY AND VACCINATION

Greyhounds appear to develop immunity to infections with *U. stenocephala*.[51] A vaccine for hookworms was previously available that utilized irradiated larvae, similar to the commercial vaccine for the bovine lungworm, *Dictyocaulus viviparus*.[52] Thus, dogs do develop immunity to hookworm infections, but it does not appear to be sterile immunity. Also, work has shown that when dogs receive less than adequate nutrition, their immunity wanes and they can be reinfected with hookworms.[53]

PREVENTION

With current heartworm prevention products that are effective against hookworm infections, along with the other excellent anthelmintics labeled for treatment of hookworms, there is every reason to believe that hookworm infections can be controlled through routine prevention. Dogs and cats receiving broad-spectrum heartworm prevention should in most instances remain relatively hookworm-free (caveat: dormant larvae present in the tissues are not removed until they reactivate, migrate to the intestines, and are killed when the next dose of anthelmintic is administered). If they are not receiving such prevention, cats and dogs should have two to four fecal examinations each year to insure that any worms detected at that time are removed through proper treatment. Some intact females, especially rescue dogs, may have large numbers of sequestered larvae in their tissues that can reactivate and infect nursing pups, and there is currently no approved means of preventing transmammary infection in these dogs. Thus, veterinarians need to remain aware that post-natal hookworm infections are likely to occur and can prove fatal to pups. For all puppies, the recommendation is to deworm with pyrantel every 2 weeks beginning at 2 weeks of age until they can be transitioned to a monthly heartworm preventive product with activity against hookworms. For a dam with a history of *A. caninum*-related peracute disease in a previous litter, decreased transmission to subsequent litters can be achieved by the off-label use of one of the following: daily fenbendazole (50 mg/kg, PO, given from the 40th day of gestation to the 14th day postpartum; this regimen can be costly), ivermectin (0.5 mg/kg, SC, given 4–9 days before parturition and then again 10 days later), transdermal moxidectin (4–4.6 mg/kg given on the 56th day of gestation), or injectable moxidectin (1 mg/kg, SC, on the 55th day of gestation).[54]

Some dogs persistently excrete eggs in spite of treatment. Even when treatment successfully removes the population of worms in the intestine, sequestered larvae in the dog's tissues—the same ones that awaken to infect pups—constantly reactivate to repopulate the intestine and mature to egg-producing adults.[55–57] This "larval leak" phenomenon was a common occurrence before monthly control products became available. Some dogs on monthly preventives, especially those coming from heavily contaminated environments, continue to shed eggs despite many months of repeated hookworm treatments. In these dogs, the goal should be to use the monthly preventives to remove any worms reactivated since the last dose in order to maintain low populations of feeding worms in the intestine, and preclude disease in the animal as well as egg excretion into the environment.

PUBLIC HEALTH ASPECTS

The hookworms of dogs and cats in the United States can all penetrate the skin of mammals. At the same time, the vast majority of reports of creeping eruption from hookworms occur in areas where the species *A. braziliense* is found. *Ancylostoma braziliense* is also the species for which larvae have been recovered from human skin and identified using molecular methods.[58] Migrating larvae cause pruritic, serpiginous tracks in the skin that can persist for weeks if not treated (Fig. 113.5).

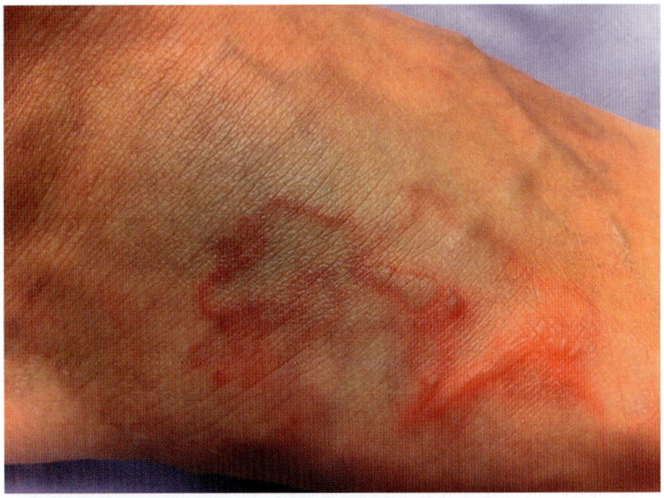

Fig. 113.5 Serpiginous tracts secondary to cutaneous larva migrans. (Reprinted from Kinkaid L, Klowak M, Klowak S, et al. Management of imported cutaneous larva migrans: A case series and mini-review. *Travel Med Infect Dis.* 2015;13:382–387.)

An often overlooked aspect of canine and feline hookworm infections is that these parasites utilize mammalian paratenic hosts as part of their life cycles. All four of these hookworms persist for long periods in the tissues of rodents, and a hookworm larva was identified in a muscle biopsy from a person 3 months after diagnosis of CLM.[59] *Ancylostoma caninum* larvae can persist in the muscles of sheep after percutaneous infection.[10] Thus, it seems likely that in patients with CLM, larvae will migrate into the musculature where they will begin a long-term residence.

Among the hookworm species found in the United States, only *A. caninum* is known to develop to the adult stage in humans. The worms have been found in the intestine and cause eosinophilic enteritis with abdominal pain as the main symptom.[21]

CASE EXAMPLE

Signalment

"Tonka," a 13-week-old intact male basset hound from Ithaca, NY, USA.

History

Tonka's owner reported a 24-hour history of lethargy and inappetence, with one episode of a small amount of bile being vomited. Tonka had had diarrhea with intermittently black and tarry feces since he was acquired from a local breeder 1 week ago. He had been eating, drinking, and urinating normally up until the previous day. According to the owner, Tonka had been vaccinated by the breeder at 8 and 12 weeks of age with a "9-way" vaccine, and had also been dewormed. He was not on any current medications.

Physical Examination Findings

Body weight: 7.6 kg.

General: Quiet, alert, and responsive. Temperature = 100.5°F (38.1°C), HR = 188 beats/minute, RR = 24 breaths/minute, pale mucous membranes, CRT < 2 seconds.

Integument: Normal haircoat. No petechiation and no evidence of ectoparasites.

Eyes, ears, nose, and throat: Mild waxy debris within both ear canals. No other abnormalities noted.

Cardiovascular: Sinus tachycardia. Femoral pulses strong and synchronous. No murmurs were detected on auscultation. Mucous membranes were pale and tacky.

GI and genitourinary: The abdomen was large and distended, with fluid-filled intestinal loops. No pain was elicited upon palpation. No other abnormalities noted.

Musculoskeletal, respiratory, lymph nodes: No clinically significant abnormalities noted.

Laboratory Findings

Rapid assessment tests: PCV 17%, TP 5.1 g/dL, BUN 15–26 mg/dL.

Coagulation panels: PT and aPTT within normal limits.

Parvovirus fecal antigen ELISA test: Negative.

Blood smear: Normal RBC morphology with no spherocytes observed. WBCs (lymphocytes, neutrophils, eosinophils) were subjectively increased. Approximately 15 platelets/HPF were observed.

Continued

CASE EXAMPLE—cont'd

Fecal Examination Results

Fecal flotation: *Ancylostoma caninum* eggs, >100 per 10× field.

Diagnosis

Anemia due to ancylostomiasis.

Treatment

Tonka was given an IV bolus of 20 mL/kg of Plasmalyte for cardiovascular support, followed by 175 mL of packed RBCs. Anthelmintic treatment was initiated with fenbendazole (50 mg/kg, PO, q24h for 3 days). Famotidine (0.5 mg/kg, q12h) and sucralfate (0.5 g slurry, q8h) for 5 days were also prescribed for gastroprotection.

Comments

This puppy was evaluated by a veterinary emergency service. It was unclear from the history provided by the owners what drug and protocol the breeder used for deworming. Based on the severity of the clinical signs, the large numbers of eggs in the feces, and the large numbers of *A. caninum* worms passed in the feces a day after the initiation of anthelmintic treatment (Fig. 113.6), it seemed likely that whatever parasite protocol the breeder utilized was insufficient for hookworm control. Adherence to the recommendation for deworming every 2 weeks starting at 2 weeks of age until puppies can be placed on a broad-spectrum heartworm preventive should prevent this condition.

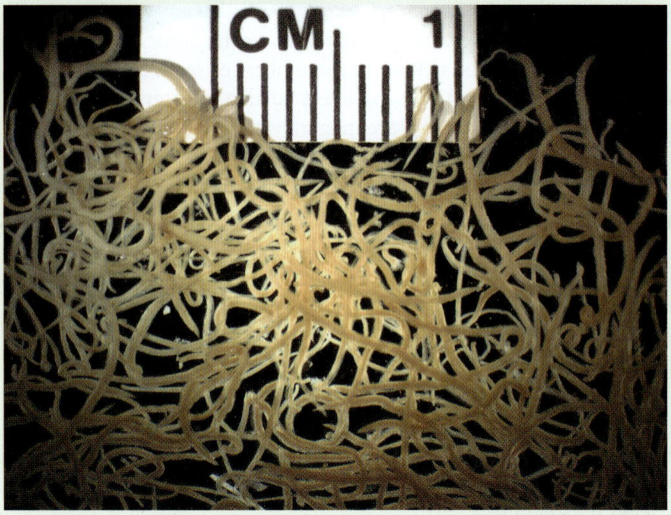

Fig. 113.6 *Ancylostoma caninum* worms recovered from the feces of the 13-week-old intact male basset hound pup with severe anemia described in the case example. Hookworms were passed after treatment with fenbendazole.

SUGGESTED READINGS

Bowman DD, Montgomery SP, Zajac AM, et al. Hookworms of dogs and cats as agents of cutaneous larva migrans. *Trends Par.* 2010;26:162–167.

Le Joncour A, Lacour SA, Lecso G, et al. Case report. Molecular characterization of *Ancylostoma braziliense* larvae in a patient with hookworm-related cutaneous larva migrans. *AJTMH.* 2012;86:843–845.

Lucio-Forster A, Liotta JL, Yaros JP, et al. Morphological differentiation of eggs of *Ancylostoma caninum, Ancylostoma tubaeforme*, and *Ancylostoma braziliense* from dogs and cats in the United States. *J Parasit.* 2012;98:1041–1044.

REFERENCES

1. Looss A. The anatomy and life history of *Agchylostoma duodenale* Dub. A monograph. *Records of the School of Medicine Cairo.* 1911:613.
2. Burrows RB. Comparative morphology of *Ancylostoma tubaeforme* and *Ancylostoma caninum. J Parasit.* 1962;48:715–718.
3. Biocca E. On *Ancylostoma braziliense* (de Faria 1910) and its morphological differentiation from *A ceylanicum* (Looss, 1911). *J Helminthol.* 1951;25:1–10.
4. Lane C. *Agchylostoma ceylanicum*, a new human parasite. *The Indian Medical Gazette.* 1913:217–218.
5. Hill RL Jr, Roberson EL. Temperature-induced separation of larvae of *Uncinaria stenocephala* from a mixed fecal culture containing *Ancylostoma caninum. J Parasitol.* 1985;71:390–391.
6. Okoshi S, Murata Y. Experimental studies on ancylostomiasis in cats. III. Egg culture of *Ancylostoma tubaeforme* Zeder, 1800 and *Ancylostoma caninum* Ercolani, 1859. *Jpn J Vet Sci.* 1967;29:174–177.
7. Okoshi S, Murata Y. Experimental studies on ancylostomiasis in cats. VII. Experimental infection and visceral migration of larvae of *Ancylostoma tubaeforme* and *A. caninum* in mice and chickens. *Jpn J Vet Sci.* 1968;30:97–107.
8. Norris DE. The migratory behavior of the infective-stage larvae of *Ancylostoma braziliense* and *Ancylostoma tubaeforme* in rodent paratenic hosts. *J Parasitol.* 1971;57:989–1009.
9. Fukutome S. The migratory behaviour and development of *Ancylostoma braziliense* and *Ancylostoma ceylanicum* in the mouse. *Jpn J Parasit.* 1975;24:49–54.
10. Jeschke BU, Stoye M. Untersuchungen iiber die galaktogene Transmission dritter Larven von *Ancylostoma caninum* Ercolani 1859 (Ancylostomidae) bei paratenischen Wirten. *Zbl. Vet. Med. B.* 1978;25:623–640.
11. Mittra S, Sasmal NK. Experimental infection of pups with *Ancylostoma caninum* larvae from an abnormal host, the chicken. *J Helminthol.* 1985;59:303–306.
12. Mihatsch D. *Zum Verhalten der Larven von Uncinaria stenocephala Railliet 1884 (Ancylostomidae) in der Maus.* Hannover, Germany: Thesis, Tierarztliche Hochschule; 1984:47.
13. Reperant LA, Hegglin D, Fischer C, et al. Influence of urbanization on the epidemiology of intestinal helminths of the red fox (*Vulpes vulpes*) in Geneva Switzerland. *Par Res.* 2007;101:605–611.
14. Stone WM, Girardeau M. Transmammary passage of *Ancylostoma caninum* larvae in dogs. *J Parasitol.* 1968;54:426–429.
15. Bowman DD, Hendrix CM, Lindsay DS, Barr SC. *Feline Clinical Parasitology.* Iowa State University Press; 2002:469.
16. Anderson RC. *Nematode Parasites of Vertebrates, their Development and Transmission.* 2nd ed. CABI Press; 2000:650.
17. Gibbs HC. Studies on the life cycle and developmental morphology of *Dochmoides stenocephala* (Railliet 1884) (Ancylostomidae Nematoda). *Can J Zool.* 1996;39:325-348.
18. Okoshi S, Murata Y. Experimental studies on ancylostomiasis in cats. IV. Experimental infection of *Ancylostoma tubaeforme* and *A. caninum* to cat. *Jpn J Vet Sci.* 1967;29:251–258.
19. Balasingam E. Comparative studies on the effects of temperature on free-living stages of *Placoconus lotoris, Dochmoides stenocephala* and *Ancylostoma caninum. Can J Zool.* 1964;42:907–918.
20. Levine ND. *Nematode Parasites of Domestic Animals and Man.* 2nd ed. Minneapolis, MN: Burgess Publishing Co; 1980:477.
21. Little SE, Johnson EM, Lewis D, et al. Prevalence of intestinal parasites in pet dogs in the United States. *Vet Parasitol.* 2009;166:144–152.
22. Companion Animal Parasite Council. https://capcvet.org/maps/#/2021/all-year/hookworm/dog/united-states Last accessed May 24, 2022.
23. Companion Animal Parasite Council. https://capcvet.org/maps/#/2021/all-year/hookworm/cat/united-states Last accessed May 24, 2022.
24. Bowman DD, Montgomery SP, Zajac AM, et al. Hookworms of dogs and cats as agents of cutaneous larva migrans. *Trends Par.* 2010;26:162–167.
25. Liotta JL, Koompapong KN, Yaros JP, et al. Prevalence of *Ancylostoma braziliense* in cats in three northern counties of Florida, United States. *J Parasitol.* 2012;95:1032–1033.

26. Liotta JL, Youn HJ, Aksel S, et al. Prevalence of *Ancylostoma braziliense* in dogs from Alachua and Marion counties, Florida, United States. *J Parasitol.* 2012;98:1039–1040.
27. Kinkaid L, Klowak M, Klowak S, et al. Management of imported cutaneous larva migrans: a case series and mini-review. *Travel Med Infect Dis.* 2015;13:382–387.
28. Freedman DO, Weld LH, Kozarsky PE, et al. Spectrum of disease and relation to place of exposure among ill returned travelers. *N Engl J Med.* 2006;354:119–130.
29. Traub RJ, Hobbs RP, Adams PJ, et al. A case of mistaken identity – reappraisal of the species of canid and felid hookworms (*Ancylostoma*) present in Australia and India. *Parasitol.* 2007;134:113–119.
30. Georgi JR, Georgi ME. *Canine Clinical Parasitology*. Philadelphia, PA: Lea and Febiger; 1992:227.
31. Georgi JR. Estimation of erythrocyte loss in hookworm infection by whole-body ^{59}Fe counting. *J Parasitol.* 1968;54:417.
32. Georgi JR, Le Jambre LF, Ractliffe LH. *Ancylostoma caninum* burden in relationship to erythrocyte loss in dogs. *J Parasitol.* 1969;55:1205.
33. Kelly JD. *Canine Parasitology*. Sydney, Australia: University of Sydney, Post-Graduate Foundation in Veterinary Science; 1977.
34. Hotez PJ, Cerami A. Secretion of a proteolytic anticoagulant by *Ancylostoma* hookworms. *J Exp Med.* 1983;157:1594–1603.
35. Stanssens P, Bergum P, Gansemans Y, et al. Anticoagulant repertoire of the hookworm *Ancylostoma caninum*. *Proc Natl Acad Sci USA.* 1996;93:2149–2154.
36. Uzai FA, Plattner BL, Hostetter JM. Alimentary system. In: Maxie MG, ed. *Jubb, Kennedy, and Palmer's Pathology of Domestic Animals*. 6th ed. Vol. 2. St Louis, MO: Elsevier Saunders; 2016:1–257.
37. Chu S, Myers SL, Wagner B, et al. Hookworm dermatitis due to *Uncinaria stenocephala* in a dog from Saskatchewan. *Can Vet J.* 2015;54:743–747.
38. Lucio-Forster A, Liotta JL, Yaros JP, et al. Morphological differentiation of eggs of *Ancylostoma caninum, Ancylostoma tubaeforme*, and *Ancylostoma braziliense* from dogs and cats in the United States. *J Parasit.* 2012;98:1041–1044.
39. Zajac AM, Conboy GA. *Veterinary Clinical Parasitology*. Hoboken, NJ: Wiley-Blackwell; 2011.
40. Elsemore DA, Geng J, Cote J, et al. Enzyme-linked immunosorbent assays for coproantigen detection of *Ancylostoma caninum* and *Toxocara canis* in dogs and *Toxocara cati* in cats. *J Vet Diagn Invest.* 2017;29:645–653.
41. Liotta JL, Lee ACY, Aksel S, et al. Obtaining an isolate of *Ancylostoma braziliense* from dogs without the need for necropsy. *J Parasitol.* 2012;98:1034–1036.
42. Lee ACY, Epe C, Simpson KW, Bowman DD. Utility of capsule endoscopy for evaluating anthelmintic efficacy in fully conscious dogs. *Int J Parasitol.* 2011;41:1377–1383.
43. Kopp SR, Coleman GT, McCarthy JS, Kotze AC. Application of in vitro anthelmintic sensitivity assays to canine parasitology: detecting resistance to pyrantel in *Ancylostoma caninum*. *Vet Parasitol.* 2008;152: 284–293.
44. Hess LB, Millward LM, Rudinsky A, et al. Combination anthelmintic treatment for persistent *Ancylostoma caninum* ova shedding in greyhounds. *J Am Anim Hosp Assoc.* 2019;55:160–166.
45. Kitchen S, Ratnappan R, Han S, et al. Isolation and characterization of a naturally occurring multidrug-resistant strain of the canine hookworm, *Ancylostoma caninum*. *Int J Parasitol.* 2019;49:397–406.
46. Jimenez Castro PD, Howell SB, Schaefer JJ, et al. Multiple drug resistance in the canine hookworm *Ancylostoma caninum*: an emerging threat? *Parasit Vectors.* 2019;12:576.
47. Jimenez Castro PD, Venkatesan A, Redman E, et al. Multiple drug resistance in hookworms infecting greyhound dogs in the USA. *Int J Parasitol Drugs Drug Resist.* 2021;17:107–117.
48. Jimenez Castro PD, Mansour A, Charles S, et al. Efficacy evaluation of anthelmintic products against an infection with the canine hookworm (*Ancylostoma caninum*) isolate Worthy 4.1F3P in dogs. *Int J Parasitol Drugs Drug Resist.* 2020;13:22–27.
49. Schimmel A, Altreuther G, Schroeder I, et al. Efficacy of emodepside plus praziquantel tablets (Profender tablets for dogs) against mature and immature adult *Ancylostoma caninum* and *Uncinaria stenocephala* infections in dogs. *Parasitol Res.* 2009;105(suppl 1):S9–S16.
50. Jimenez Castro PD, Kaplan RM. Persistent or suspected-resistant hookworm infections. *Clinician's Brief.* 2020;8:61–68.
51. Jacobs DE. The epidemiology of hookworm infections of dogs in the UK. *Vet Annual.* 1978;18:220–224.
52. Miller TA. Vaccination against the canine hookworm diseases. *Adv Parasitol.* 1971;9:153–183.
53. Foster AO, Cort WW. The effect of diet on hookworm infestation in dogs. *Science.* 1931;73:681–683.
54. Bowman DD. *Georgis' Parasitology for Veterinarians*. St Louis, MO: Elsevier Saunders; 2014.
55. Little MD. Dormant *Ancylostoma caninum* larvae in muscle as a source of subsequent patent infection in the dog. In: *Proceedings of the Fifty-Third Annual Meeting of the American Society of Parasitology*. 1978.
56. Schad GA. Experimentally induced arrested development of parasite larvae of hookworms. *Proc 3rd Int Congr Parasitol.* 1974;2:772.
57. Schad GA, Page MR. *Ancylostoma canium*: adult worm removal, corticosteroid treatment, and resumed development of arrested larvae in dogs. *Exp Parasitol.* 1982;54:303.
58. Le Joncour A, Lacour SA, Lecso G, et al. Case report. Molecular characterization of *Ancylostoma braziliense* larvae in a patient with hookworm-related cutaneous larva migrans. *AJTMH.* 2012;86:843–845.
59. Little MD, Halsey NA, Cline BL, Katz SP. *Ancylostoma* larva in a muscle fiber of man following cutaneous larva migrans. *Am J Trop Med Hyg.* 1983;32:1285–1288.

114

Whipworms

David A. Elsemore, Jennifer K. Ketzis

KEY POINTS

- First Described: *Trichuris vulpis* was first described in 1789 by von Frölich, who isolated it from a dog in Europe. *Trichuris serrata* and *Trichuris campanula*, described in 1879 and 1888, respectively, were first isolated from cats in Brazil by von Linstow.[1,2] It has been proposed that these are the same species and should be renamed *Trichuris felis*.[3]
- Cause: *Trichuris vulpis*, which occurs in dogs, and *Trichuris felis* (*Trichuris serrata* and *Trichuris campanula*), which occurs in cats, are commonly referred to as whipworms (family Trichuridae).
- Affected Hosts: *Trichuris vulpis* infects dogs and wild canids. *Trichuris felis* infects domestic cats and wild felids.
- Geographic Distribution: The distribution of *T. vulpis* is worldwide, although prevalence is reportedly lower in extremely cold and extremely hot arid climatic zones.[1] *Trichuris felis* is considered a more exotic infection except in tropical and subtropical zones with infection being common in South America and the Caribbean. Less frequent reports of infection have come from the USA, Australia, and Europe.
- Route of Transmission: Dogs and cats become infected with whipworms by ingestion of eggs with infective first-stage larvae.
- Major Clinical Signs: In general, *T. vulpis* infections are of low pathogenicity. However, infections can be associated with intermittent diarrhea and, with heavy infections, chronic and/or severe diarrhea, dehydration, lethargy, anorexia, and anemia. Little is known regarding feline disease. Theoretically, cats could have similar clinical signs as dogs, although there are no published case studies suggesting infection results in clinical signs.
- Differential Diagnoses: The clinical signs are representative of many large bowel disorders (gastroenteritis, dietary indiscretion, gastrointestinal foreign body, inflammatory bowel disease, and other nematode infections). In some cases, infection can be associated with pseudo-hypoadrenocorticism. Presence of *Trichuris* eggs does not necessarily indicate that whipworms are the cause of the clinical signs, given the general low pathogenicity of infection.
- Human Health Significance: *Trichuris vulpis* has been proposed as a zoonotic pathogen. While there have been a few reported human infections, genetic sequencing to confirm the *Trichuris* sp. has been limited. There are no reports of *T. felis* infecting humans.

ETIOLOGIC AGENT AND EPIDEMIOLOGY

Dogs

Trichuris spp. belong to the superfamily Trichinelloidea and the family Trichuridae. While the name of this genus can be translated as "hair-tail," it is actually the anterior portion (forming up to ¾ of the body) that is filamentous and the posterior portion that is thick, resulting in the typical whip-like appearance.[4] *Trichuris vulpis* adults range from 4.5 to 7.5 cm in length (Fig. 114.1).[5] They have a stichosome esophagus and a bacillary band in the esophageal region. The male adults have a single spicule and a coiled posterior while the females have a straight uterus and straight posterior.[6] The eggs range from 70 to 90 μm long by 30 to 50 μm wide, are lemon shaped with symmetrical bipolar plugs, and contain a single cell in fresh feces (Fig. 114.2).[5,7,8]

Several experimental infections have been conducted to determine the life cycle of *T. vulpis* (Fig. 114.3).[7,9–11] Infection occurs via ingestion of an egg with an infective first-stage larva. On arrival in the small intestine, the plugs are digested and the larvae are released primarily in the duodenum and upper portion of the jejunum with some delayed until the upper portion of the ileum.[9,11] The larvae enter the mucosa via the crypts of Lieberkühn where they remain tightly coiled for 6 to 15 days.[9,11] Some minor destruction of the host tissue cells surrounding the larvae can occur. By 15 days PI, the larvae enter the lumen and travel to the cecum or colon where they enter the mucosa, molt three times, and then mature to adults. As the larvae molt from an immature stage (which are not whip-shaped and more uniform in diameter) to an adult, the anterior end remains in the epithelium and the posterior end begins to protrude into the lumen. The final adult worm lives with the anterior esophagus in a "tunnel" in the mucosa, formed by the destruction of the lateral membranes while the apical and basal surfaces remain intact.[12] The embedded portion of the adult worm is normally limited to the superficial tunica propria although some individual nematodes penetrate more deeply into lymph follicles resulting in focal coagulative necrosis surrounding the region.[7,9–11]

In low-burden infections, *T. vulpis* can be found crowded together in the cecum. However, in heavier infections, the worms also can be found in the colon and, rarely, near the rectum. The prepatent period is long (70 to 112 days) with the single-cell eggs excreted in the feces.[7,9–11,13] Adult worms can live for several months to over a year with female worms having the capability of excreting 1000 to 5000 eggs per day, with potentially fewer eggs per female with high burden infections.[7,9,13,14] While the impact of crowding has not been well studied in dogs, *Trichuris* spp. in other hosts have been shown to decrease in size and fecundity with higher burden infections.[15–18] Also, egg excretion can vary significantly on a daily basis. The eggs require <2 weeks to 1.5 months to develop to the infective stage, depending on the soil temperature and moisture level (e.g., 1.5 months at 20°C, 1 month at 25 to 30°C).[7,19,20] Infective eggs contain a first-stage larvae and have a slightly rounder appearance. At cool temperatures (e.g., 4°C), development can be delayed but resumes when temperatures increase, while long periods of freezing temperatures and direct sunlight can destroy eggs. Though generally considered relatively hardy, *Trichuris* eggs do not survive desiccation and heat as well as ascarid eggs do.[7,10,11,19–21]

Given the susceptibility of eggs to freezing temperatures and arid conditions, it is not surprising that prevalence of infections in dogs is lower in hot arid regions and regions with long cold winters. While

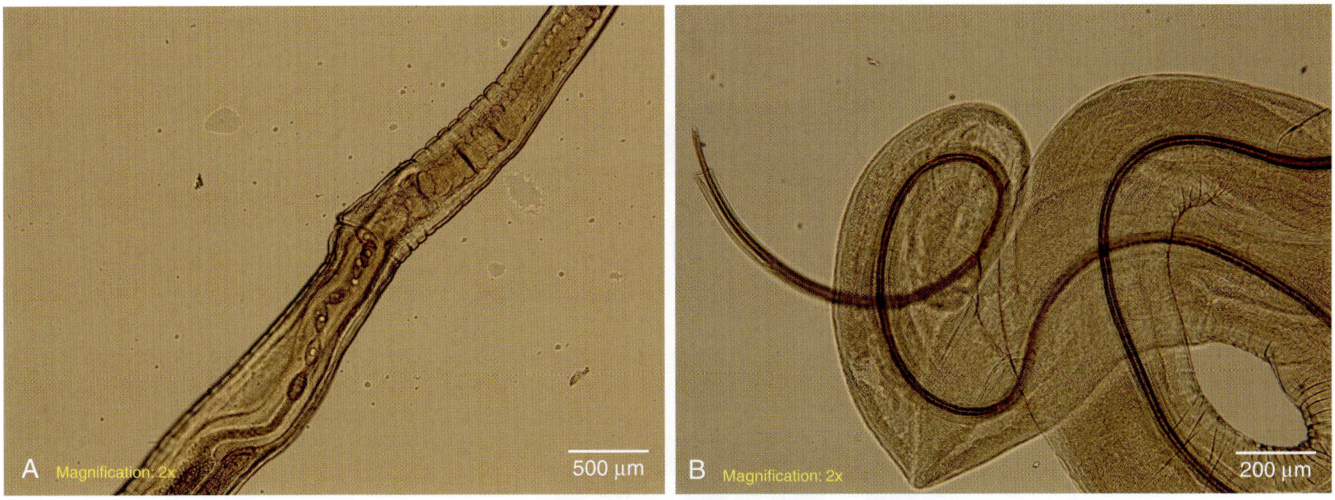

Fig. 114.1 Features of adult *Trichuris vulpis* nematodes. (A) Female vulva. (B) Male spicule. (Courtesy of Dr. Jinming Geng, IDEXX Laboratories, Inc. Copyright © 2017, IDEXX Laboratories, Inc. All rights reserved. Used with permission.)

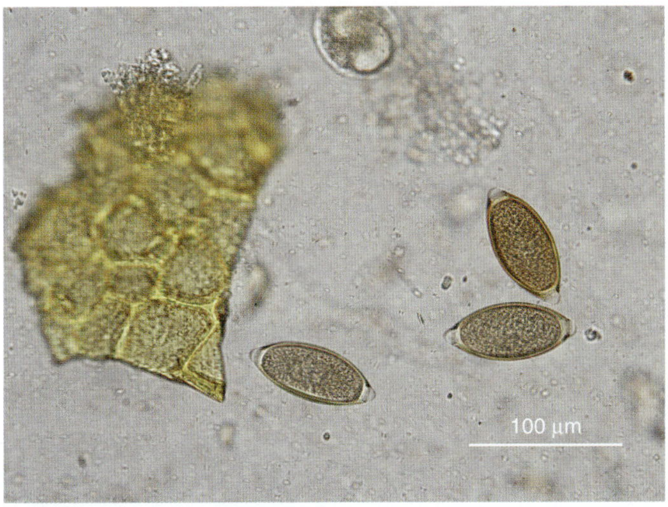

Fig. 114.2 *Trichuris vulpis* eggs in a fresh fecal specimen, examined using centrifugation with Sheather's sugar flotation solution; eggs range in size from 70 to 90 µm by 30 to 50 µm. (Courtesy of Dr. Kathryn Duncan, National Center for Veterinary Parasitology, Oklahoma State University.)

challenging to compare prevalence studies due to differences in the diagnostic methods used and source of dogs, it appears that prevalence in well-cared-for pet dogs is decreased in many regions, likely attributable to regular anthelmintic treatment. Data from CAPC indicate that prevalence in pet dogs is <1% in the United States (vs. 8 to 81% in the US in the 1930s to 1950s) and <0.5% in Canada.[7,21] Other United States–based studies have found prevalence to range from <1% to 10%.[22,23] In Australia, a study from 1975 showed a prevalence of 60.6% in shelter dogs, whereas a study from 2004–2005 found only 3.1% to be infected, with <1% of owned dogs infected.[24] In Europe, more contemporary studies have also indicated that prevalence is generally low among owned dogs (0.1 to <4%) although it is higher in regions of Greece, Hungary, and Italy (9.6 to 23.3%).[4,25,26] Higher prevalences (14 to >50%) have been documented in dogs from rural areas, kennels, shelters, and stray dogs as well as other regions of the world, which is likely reflective of parasite control and dog ownership practices.[27–32]

In addition to occurring worldwide in domestic dogs, *T. vulpis* has been documented in red foxes (*Vulpes vulpes*), coyotes (*Canis latrans*), and wolves (*Canis lupus*) in the United States, Europe, Asia, and Africa with prevalences ranging from 0.5 to 33%, and an indication that in the Netherlands, it might be increasing in prevalence.[33–39] These canids could serve as a source of environmental contamination and hence domestic dog infection.

Cats

Much less is known about the whipworm species that infect cats and their epidemiology when compared with dog whipworm species. While two separate species, *Trichuris serrata* and *Trichuris campanula*, were described, it has been proposed that they are one species and should be renamed *Trichuris felis*.[3] In the original descriptions, the presence of a vulva appendage in *T. serrata* and differences in the size of the adults, spicule, and eggs were used as differing characteristics.[1,2] *Trichuris serrata* adult females range from 14.7 to 49.5 mm in length; males from 12.8 to 40 mm; and their eggs are 54 to 60 µm long by 35 to 40 µm wide. *Trichuris campanula* adult females range from 22.5 to 31.5 mm in length; males from 21.5 to 36 mm; and their eggs are 63 to 72 µm long by 34 to 39 µm wide.[40–43] Given that adult worm size can vary based on infection intensity and variation in egg size has been demonstrated with other *Trichuris* spp., size is an unreliable characteristic for species differentiation.[15,16] Twenty-two females (with the vulva appendage and classified as *T. serrata*) and 12 males harvested from 12 cats and eggs from the feces of nine of these cats were measured and shown to overlap with the measurements for *T. serrata* and *T. campanula*, supporting the theory that there is just one species.[43] While the 18S rRNA gene of these "*T. serrata*" were sequenced, at the time of writing, sequences are not available from *Trichuris* spp. from cats that lack the vulva appendage.[44] Therefore it remains to be determined if cats host two *Trichuris* species or one. Given the lack of information on the separate species, these are, herein, referred to as *T. felis* (Figs. 114.4–114.6).

Based on one experimental study, the prepatent period of *T. felis* is believed to range from 62 to 91 days.[42] The life cycle is the same as that of *T. vulpis*. However, since it has not been as extensively studied as *T. vulpis*, less is known about the timeframe for each stage of development. Less also is known about the factors that influence egg development, although they are likely similar to *T. vulpis* and other *Trichuris* species.

Trichuris felis are generally present in low prevalence in much of the world with most reported infections occurring in the Caribbean and South America.[3] In a study from Argentina, 16% of cats were infected.[45] On St. Kitts, 71% of feral cats and 22% of owned cats were

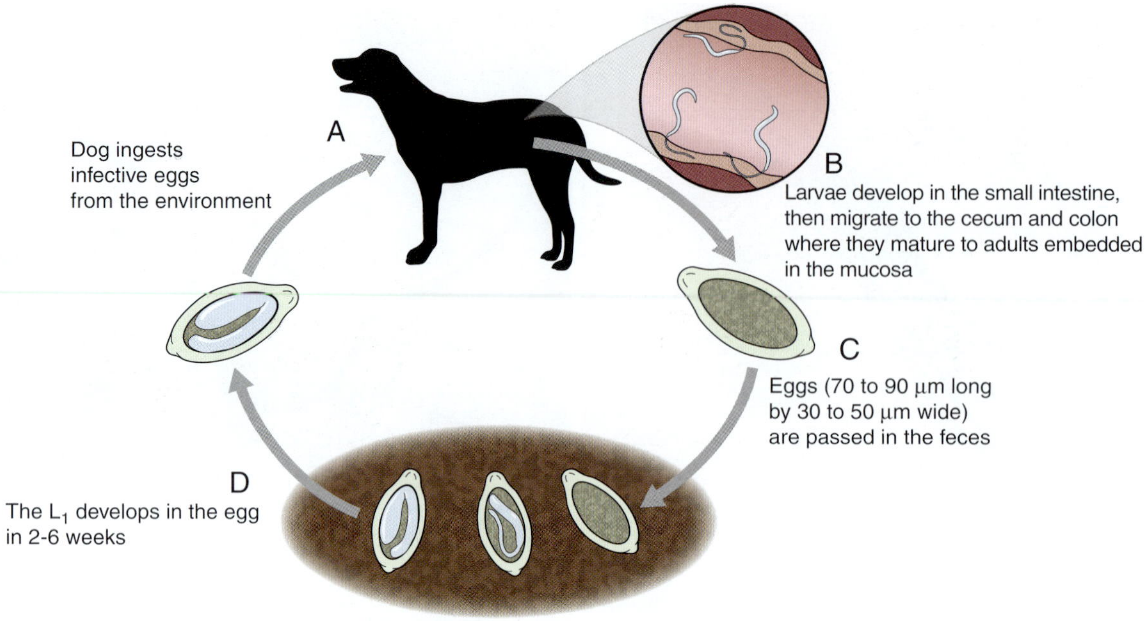

Fig. 114.3 Life cycle of *Trichuris vulpis*.

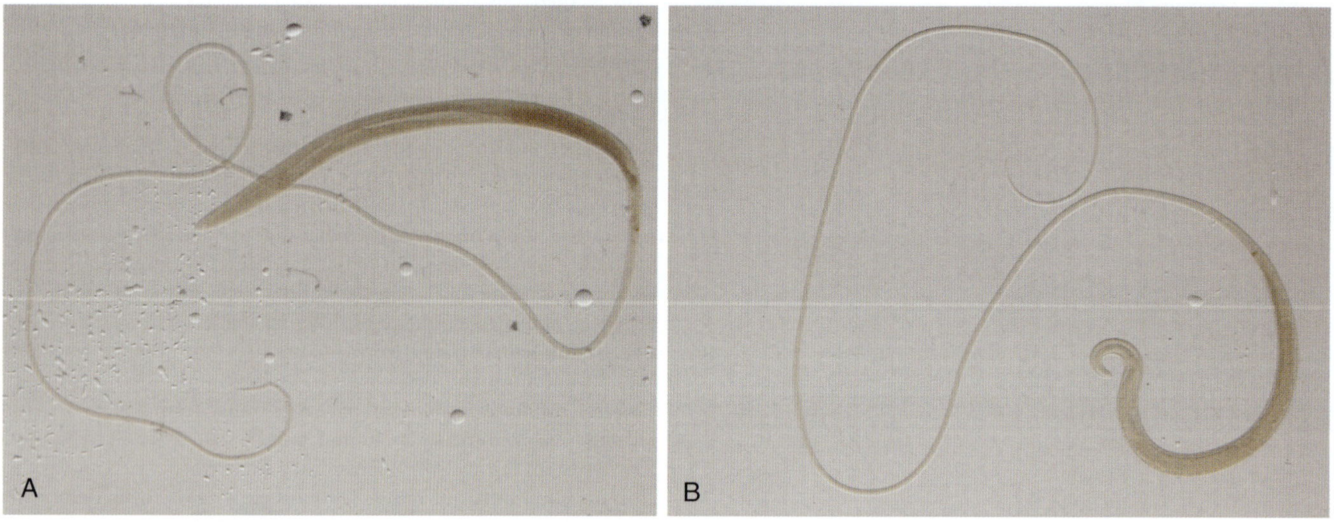

Fig. 114.4 Adult *Trichuris felis* worms. (A) Female; length ranges from 14.7 to 49.5 mm. (B) Male; length ranges from 12.8 to 40.0 mm. (Courtesy of Jennifer K. Ketzis, Ross University School of Veterinary Medicine, St. Kitts, West Indies.)

positive.[46,47] In a 1975 study from Australia, 1.5% of cats were infected, although infections have not been reported in more recent studies.[24,48] In the United States there have been infrequent reports of infection in cats from the Midwest, Southeast, and Northeast. A study from 2003 reported a prevalence of 0.03% in owned cats.[3,42,49] A 2015 study of a shelter in Miami, Florida, however, found 25 (38%) of 65 cats to be infected, suggesting that prevalence can be higher among certain regional populations.[50] In Europe, most prevalence studies have not detected *Trichuris* sp. in cats.[51,52] However, two studies from Italy (one with owned and the other stray cats) and a study from Serbia (owned cats) found 0.9 to 2.9% to be infected; these infections were referred to as *T. vulpis*.[26,53] Based on a small study in Nigeria where 5.8% of cats were positive, feline *Trichuris* sp. infection also occurs in Africa.[54]

Trichuris felis infections have been reported in two oncillas (*Leopardus tigrinus*, 1851 in Brazil and 1963 in Venezuela) and from ocelots (*Leopardus pardalis*, 1937 in Trinidad; *Oncifelis geoffroyi*, 2005 in Argentina).[3,40,55]

CLINICAL FEATURES

Pathogenesis and Clinical Signs

During the prepatent stage of infection, the embedding of larvae in the mucosa of the small intestine can cause mechanical damage resulting in localized inflammation, mucosal hyperemia, and hemorrhage.[7,9–11,56] Immature and adult worms in the cecum (and colon in heavy infections) also cause mechanical damage to the mucosa due to the penetration and movement of the embedded anterior end and mouth stylet. Hemorrhage and inflammatory cell infiltration of the mucosa and submucosa are localized around worms.[7,9–11,56] *Trichuris* spp. release cytolytic and hemolytic enzymes, believed to enable them to consume tissue fluids that contribute to the localized reactions.[9,11,56] *Trichuris* also consume blood (at a low level compared to hookworms) and mucosal epithelium.[57]

In many cases, *T. vulpis* infection is of low pathogenicity and there are no or limited clinical signs. The most common clinical sign is

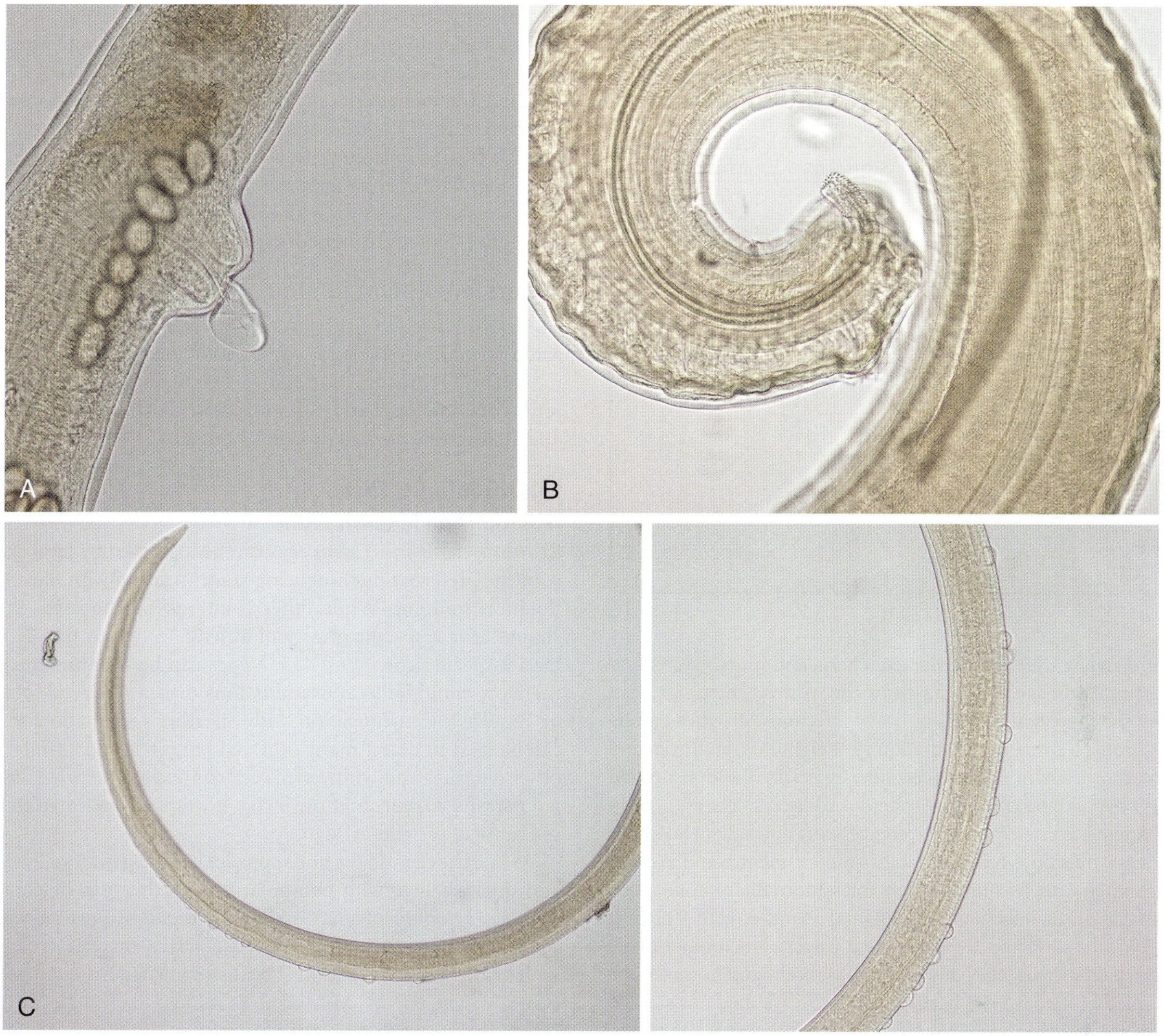

Fig. 114.5 Features of adult *Trichuris felis* nematodes. (A) Female vulva appendage. (B) Male spicule. (C) Bacillary band. (Courtesy of Jennifer K. Ketzis, Ross University School of Veterinary Medicine, St. Kitts, West Indies.)

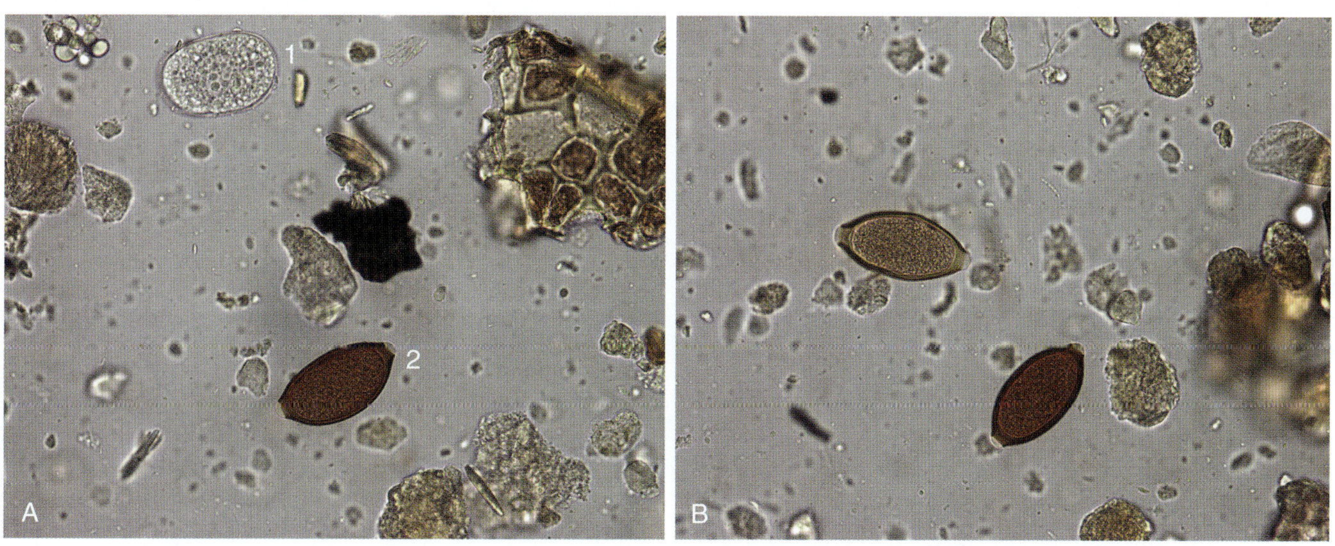

Fig. 114.6 *Trichuris felis* eggs in a fresh fecal specimen, examined using centrifugation with Sheather's sugar flotation solution; eggs range in size from 54 to 72 μm by 34 to 40 μm. (A) Comparison of *Ancylostoma tubaeforme* (1) to *Trichuris felis* (2). (B) Variation in color of eggs. (Courtesy of Jennifer K. Ketzis, Ross University School of Veterinary Medicine, St. Kitts, West Indies.)

BOX 114.1 Clinical Signs and Physical Examination Results in Dogs with *Trichuris*-associated Pseudo-hypoadrenocorticism

Clinical Sign	Number of Dogs with Sign/Total Examined
Diarrhea	20/20
Dehydration	20/20 (2 mild, remainder moderate to severe)
Vomiting	8/20
Lethargy, weakness, and/or depression	11/13
Anorexia or inappetence	5/13
Weight loss	3/13
Polydipsia and polyuria	3/13
Episodes of collapse/acute collapse	2/13
Trembling/muscle twitching	2/13
Hypothermia	3/7
Pale mucus membranes	2/7
Bradycardia	1/7
Abdominal pain	1/7

intermittent diarrhea with variable hematochezia and mucus secondary to the mechanical damage being caused by the worms. These signs can begin during the prepatent period. In heavy infections, diarrhea can be severe and chronic leading to dehydration.[5,8] Weight loss, anorexia, and lethargy also can occur in severe infections, especially those associated with pseudo-hypoadrenocorticism (pseudo-Addison's disease) (Box 114.1).[58–64] Anemia is listed in many references as a clinical sign; however, few experimental infections have been able to induce anemia, and in other hosts (e.g., children with *Trichuris trichiura* infestation) there has not been a strong association of infection with anemia.[65] Studies with *Trichuris muris* and *Trichuris suis* have demonstrated a parasite-microbiota interaction which could increase the pathology and clinical signs; however, the changes in microbiota have not been consistent.[66–68] While not studied with *T. vulpis*, this variable interaction with the microbiota has the potential to explain the occurrence of pseudo-hypoadrenocorticism.

No clinical signs have been associated with *T. felis* infections in cats. This apparent lack of clinical disease has been attributed to most infections being low intensity (1 to 10 adult worms).[3] However, cats can harbor >100 adult worms, so more studies are required to ascertain whether infections in cats can be associated with signs of disease.[43,45]

Physical Examination Findings

Most dogs have no abnormal findings on physical examination except in high-intensity infections.[5,8] Infections with a large number of whipworms may result in chronic or severe diarrhea, with dehydration, lethargy, weight loss, pale mucus membranes, and even hypothermia noted on physical examination. Dehydration may be severe and can lead to acute collapse, bradycardia, and weak pulses.[58–64] Rectal examination may indicate the presence of diarrheic feces with blood flecks and mucus. Rectal prolapse has not been associated with *T. vulpis* infection in dogs as it has in humans and pigs.

No abnormal physical examination findings have been reported in cats with *T. felis* infections.

DIAGNOSIS

The most common method used to identify *T. vulpis* and *T. felis* infection is fecal examination for the identification of eggs. A commercial fecal antigen test (IDEXX Laboratories, Inc., Westbrook, ME USA) became available in 2015 but is not in a POC format. Adult *T. vulpis* worms can be seen at necropsy, and the stichosome esophagus and bacillary bands can be used for identification in histology. Because of the long prepatent period, clinical signs can appear before eggs can be detected in the feces. Intermittent shedding can also lead to failure to detect infection on a single fecal flotation. In these situations, failure to treat dogs with chronic diarrhea can result in the somewhat unfortunate occasional diagnosis with colonoscopy, a significantly more costly procedure than assessment of response to treatment (Fig. 114.7).

Laboratory Abnormalities

In cases of pseudo-hypoadrenocorticism, hyponatremia, metabolic acidosis, and hyperkalemia are present. An adrenocorticotropic hormone (ACTH) stimulation test can be used to rule out true hypoadrenocorticism. Basal and poststimulation cortisol levels will be normal and aldosterone normal or high (Table 114.1).[58–64]

Microbiologic Tests

Isolation and Identification

Trichuris vulpis and *T. felis* eggs can be identified by fecal examination with the preferred method being centrifugation with Sheather's sugar flotation solution. While other solutions can be used, the solution should have a specific gravity of at least 1.2, given that *T. vulpis* eggs have a specific gravity of 1.15.[66] Eggs can be intermittently shed and therefore multiple fecal examinations over a one-week period might be required. Centrifugation with Sheather's sugar flotation solution can be used to detect many other GI parasites, and co-infections with other parasites and whipworms are common. The presence of intestinal parasite co-infection can make it more complicated to determine the cause of the clinical signs.

While the eggs of *Trichuris* spp. are distinct (oval, yellowish-brown, and thick-shelled, with two polar plugs), they can be confused with *Eucoleus aerophilus* (syn. *Capillaria aerophila*), *Eucoleus boehmi*, and *Aoncotheca putorii* (Table 114.2). Also, if fecal material is contaminated with urine, *Trichuris* eggs must be distinguished from *Pearsonema plica* (*Capillaria plica*).[69–71] Misdiagnosis is more likely to occur with *T. felis* infections, due to the similarity in size with *Eucoleus* spp. eggs. Because of this, some cases of *T. felis* diagnosed in the United States may have represented *Eucoleus* infections and vice versa.[3,71] However, in regions where *T. felis* is uncommon, it is reasonable to presumptively identify eggs with bipolar plugs as *Eucoleus* eggs, provided there is no travel history. Bipolar plugged eggs also may be found in cat feces following consumption of rodents or other wildlife harboring infection with *Trichuris* spp. or *Capillaria* spp.[69] Confining the pet to prevent additional predation or coprophagy and repeating fecal flotation 2 to 3 days later should facilitate differentiation of these pseudoinfections.

Molecular Diagnosis Using Nucleic Acid–Based Testing

Specific PCR assays have been used to detect nucleic acid of *Trichuris* spp. in feces. However, this approach is not used for clinical specimens, is not effective for eggs (unless eggs are first crushed to release nucleic acid), and sequencing is required to differentiate the species.[72–74]

Fecal Antigen Testing

A fecal antigen test (IDEXX Laboratories, Inc., Westbrook, ME, USA) became available in 2015 and was offered at some commercial veterinary diagnostic laboratories. This test has been validated for detection of *T. vulpis* and *T. felis* antigen and can detect infections not identifiable on fecal examination including single-sex infections (male or female) and prepatent infections. Antigen tests also have been demonstrated to differentiate between true infection and eggs in feces from coprophagy.[50,75,76]

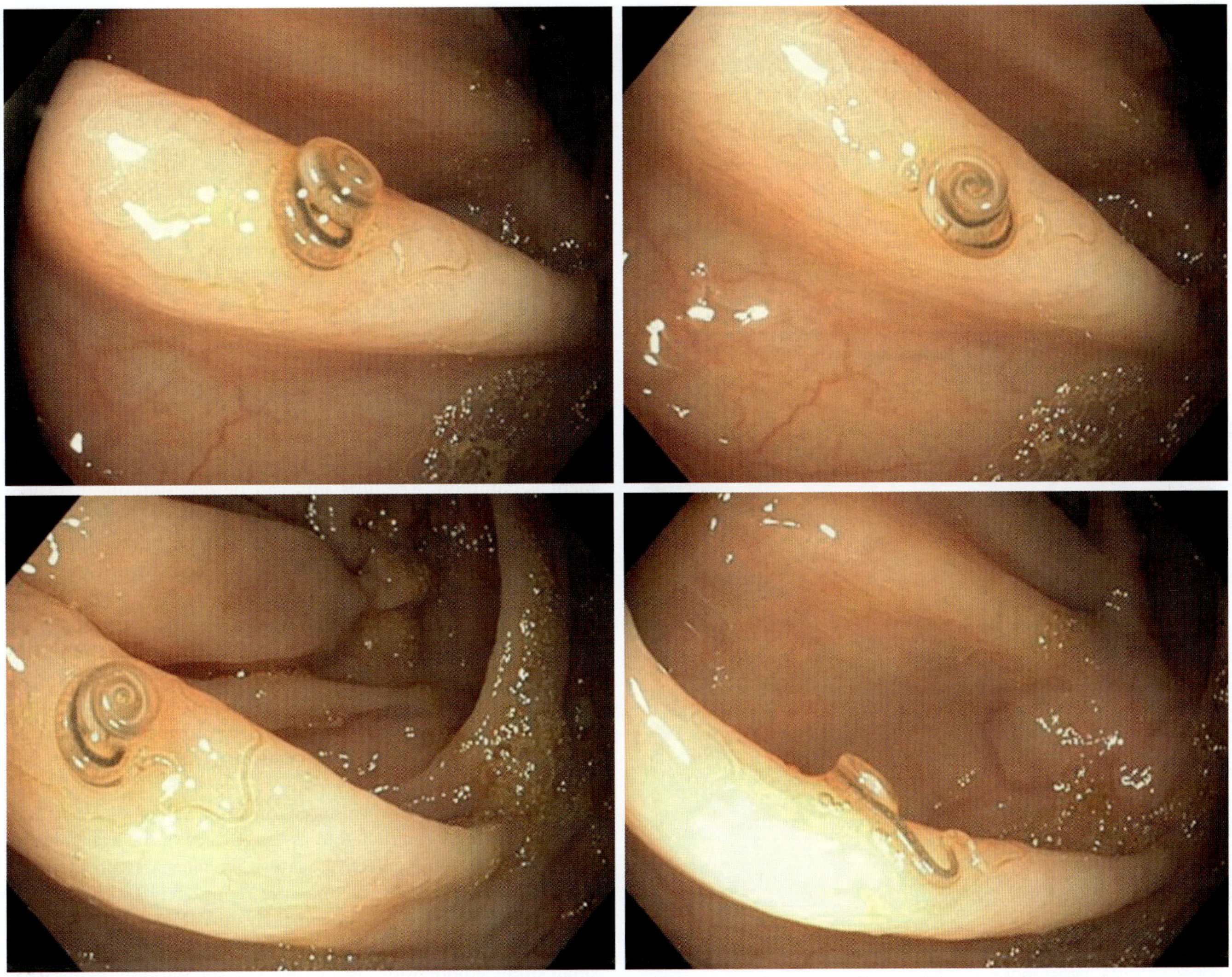

Fig. 114.7 Image obtained at the level of the ileocecal valve using colonoscopy from a 50-year-old woman infested with *Trichuris trichiura*. She was referred for a 20-pound weight loss over 2 months and had immigrated to New York, USA from Bangladesh 15 years previously. (From Sunkara T, Sharma SR, Ofosu A. *Trichuris trichiura*—an unwelcome surprise during colonoscopy. *Am J Trop Med Hyg*. 2018;99:555–556.)

TABLE 114.1 **Summary of Clinical Chemistry Findings in Reported *Trichuris*-Associated Pseudo-hypoadrenocorticism**

	2013[64] (1 case)	2011[62] (1 case)	2011[63] (1 case)	2002[61] (2 cases)	1994[60] (5 cases[b])	1990[59] (3 cases)	1985[58] (7 cases)
Sodium mmol/L (reference range)	123 (141–156)	113 (139–154)	132 (140–155)	119; 119 (144.6–156.1)	113-149 (146–156)	107-128 (137–150)	101-134 (140–155)
Potassium mmol/L (reference range)	6.4 (4–5.6)	6.5 (3.5–5.5)	5.7 (3.8–5.2)	7.7; 9.0 (4.2–5.1)	4.9–7.3 (3.6–5.5)	7.0–7.6 (3.5–4.8)	4.9–9.6 (3.8–5.3)
Na:K ratio (reference range)	19.2 (>27)	17 (NR)	23 (27–40)	15.4; 13.2 (NR)	14.8–26.7 (27–38)	14–17 (>26)	14–26 (27–40)
Cortisol[a]	Normal	Normal	Normal	Normal	2 elevated; 3 normal	NR	Mixed results[c]
Aldosterone	NR	NR	NR	High	High 3 dogs	NR	NR

[a]Cortisol: basal and response to ACTH stimulation.
[b]There were five dogs with one dog having two episodes (e.g., six cases); only the first episode for this dog is reported here. In addition, for one dog, Na, K, and the Na:K ratio were not reported although the dog's records indicated that it was hyponatremic and hyperkalemic.
[c]Results were mixed: one dog normal; one low with a normal response; four elevated (3 to >10 times normal) of which two had a normal response and two did not; one not tested.
NR, not reported or not determined.

TABLE 114.2 Egg Size, Plug, and Shell Wall Comparison for *Trichuris, Eucoleus,* and *Aonchotheca*[70,71]

	Trichuris vulpis	*Trichuris felis*	*Eucoleus aerophilus (Capillaria aerophilia)*	*Eucoleus boehmi*	*Aonchotheca putorii*
Length (μm)	70–90	54–72	58–85	50–60	56–72
Width (μm)	30–50	34–40	25–40	30–35	23–32
Bipolar plugs	Symmetrical Ringed	Symmetrical	Asymmetrical	Asymmetrical	Asymmetrical
Shell wall	Smooth	Smooth	Striated Anastomosing ridges	Pitted	Sides parallel Anastomosing ridges

Note: The symmetry of the bipolar plugs listed is the most common form; however, those that are typically symmetrical can occasionally be asymmetrical and vice versa.

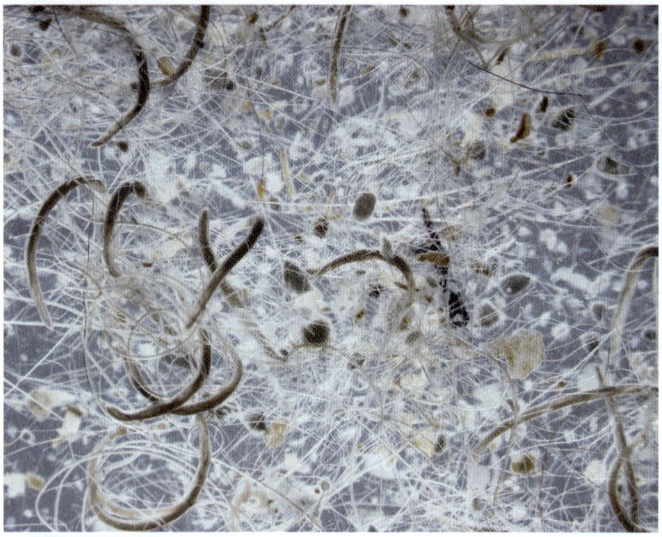

Fig. 114.8 "Medusa's head" appearance of large numbers of *T. felis*. (Courtesy of Jennifer K. Ketzis, Ross University School of Veterinary Medicine, St. Kitts, West Indies.)

Pathologic Findings

Adult *Trichuris* spp. can be seen grossly at necropsy with either only the posterior end visible in the lumen or whole worms with the classic whip shape in the lumen of the cecum and colon. In heavy infections, if the adult whipworms have released from the mucosa, they will be tangled together forming a "Medusa's head" (Fig. 114.8). Occasionally, the worms contain a reddish or pinkish fluid due to blood consumption. In histopathologic sections, the stichosome esophagus and the bacillary band(s) are key characteristics for differentiation from other nematodes.

Histologic changes that can be observed include pyknotic nuclei in cells of the lamina propria, coagulative necrosis, hyperemia, and lymphocytic invasion. Immediately after infection, hyperemia in the duodenal and jejunal mucosa and desquamation of the epithelium can be seen. Larvae in the lamina muscularis of the duodenum and jejunum are surrounded with clusters of eosinophils. Larvae and adults in the cecum and colon are associated with diffuse lymphohistiocytic infiltration of the submucosa and mucosa. Mucoid dystrophy and vascular hyperemia also are present.[56,77]

TREATMENT AND PROGNOSIS

Several anthelmintics are approved for the treatment of *T. vulpis* (Table 114.3). Repeat treatments (e.g., 3 monthly treatments) are usually recommended since few anthelmintics have efficacy against the immature stages and reinfection from a contaminated environment is common. *Trichuris* spp. can be dose-limiting parasites for some anthelmintics and the best treatment and control are achieved with consistent use of monthly broad-spectrum anthelmintics. When infection is associated with pseudo-hypoadrenocorticism, complete recovery is possible with prompt treatment for the infection and supportive therapy for the dehydration. As with all cases of severe dehydration and electrolyte imbalance, slow correction of the serum sodium concentration is required to prevent CNS disorders and death. Hypokalemia can develop in these pseudo-hypoadrenocorticism–associated cases if mineralocorticoids for hypoadrenocorticism are administered; however, the hypokalemia will resolve when steroid administration is stopped.[60]

No anthelmintics are registered for the treatment of *T. felis* and few studies have been conducted to assess efficacy of the available anthelmintics. Compounds effective against *T. vulpis* are considered likely effective against *T. felis*. In one case report, fenbendazole (Panacur 10% oral suspension, Merck Animal Health) at 50 mg/kg administered for 5 days was effective at treating a cat infected with *T. felis*.[78] In a small study, emodepside (Profender Topical Solution, Elanco) at 3 to 15 mg/kg also was effective.[79]

IMMUNITY AND VACCINATION

Dogs and cats do not develop strong immunity and are susceptible to reinfection. Self-curing and some resistance to reinfection has been noted in a few dogs that were experimentally infected. However, dogs and cats of all ages, regardless of previous exposure, have been identified with *Trichuris* spp. infestations. Therefore, any immunity that develops appears to be of a limited nature. Vaccination is not available.

PREVENTION

Given the hardiness of whipworm eggs, the key to prevention is removal of feces from the environment. This recommendation applies to gardens, yards, public parks, and other locations where dogs and cats roam. Once soil contamination has occurred, removing eggs is not feasible. In kennels and shelters, thorough cleaning is important. Regular fecal examinations using centrifugation and antigen testing, especially in adult dogs and cats (in areas where feline infections are prevalent), with prompt treatment of all positive animals, can assist in decreasing environmental contamination. Given the long prepatent period and the lower efficacy of treatments against immature stages, multiple treatments may be required. Alternatively, use of treatments

TABLE 114.3 Treatments for *Trichuris vulpis* Infections

Active Compound Product[a] (Additional Compounds in the Product)	Dose[b] (mg/kg)	Route	Interval/Duration
Emodepside Procox Oral Suspension (toltrazuril)[c] Profender Tablet (praziquantel)[c]	0.45, 1	PO	Once
Febantel Drontal Plus (pyrantel pamoate, praziquantel)	25	PO	Once[d]
Fenbendazole Panacur	50	PO	24h/3 days[d]
Milbemycin oxime Interceptor Interceptor Plus (praziquantel) Sentinel (lufenuron) Sentinel Spectrum (lufenuron, praziquantel) Trifexis (spinosad) Nexgard Spectra (afoxolaner)	0.5	PO	Once[e]
Moxidectin Advantage Multi (imidacloprid) (Advocate in Europe)	2.5	Topical	Once[e]
Oxantel embonate Dolpac (praziquantel, pyrantel embonate)[c]	20	PO	Once

[a]Products listed were available as of December 2020 and registered with the U.S. Food and Drug Administration unless otherwise indicated. Generics (e.g., products with the same active compound, same combination of actives, and same indication but different brand names) are not listed. Instead, only the original registered product is listed.
[b]All doses have activity against adults only, except the higher dose of emodepside, which also has activity against L_4 and immature adults
[c]These products were not available in the USA as of December 2020 but were available in Europe and registered with the European Medical Agency.
[d]Three monthly administrations are recommended.
[e]Monthly use is approved (for heartworm prevention), which can be used to treat and control *T. vulpis* infection.

with efficacy against immature stages of whipworms or the use of monthly broad-spectrum anthelmintics with efficacy against whipworms can be used to control and prevent infections.

For *T. felis*, given the lack of information regarding the optimal conditions for egg development, it is unclear if the prevalence of this parasite could increase outside the Caribbean and South America. It is possible that the distribution of this parasite could extend with global climate change and translocation of cats. Given increased travel of pet cats with owners, measures should be implemented to prevent transport of *T. felis* to nonendemic locations. Treatment should be administered before departure from endemic areas with follow-up fecal examinations and treatment as needed upon arrival in nonendemic areas.

PUBLIC HEALTH ASPECTS

There have been no reports of *T. felis* infecting humans. Zoonotic transmission of *T. vulpis* has been proposed with reports of *T. vulpis* completing its development in humans. Reported incidence has ranged from <0.2% to >7% with infections primarily in children.[80,81] These infections have been asymptomatic or caused clinical signs ranging from abdominal upset, diarrhea, nausea, vomiting, and eosinophilia. Humans have their own species of *Trichuris*, *T. trichiura*, which can be misidentified as *T. vulpis*; disease caused by *T. trichiura* primarily occurs in children living in poverty in the tropics and subtropics. Adult worms (excreted post treatment) can be distinguished based on spicule length and cloaca of the males and the vagina and uterus of the females, with *T. trichiura* convoluted and *T. vulpis* straight.[16] Traditionally, however, egg size has been used to distinguish *T. vulpis* from *T. trichiura* infections in humans. *Trichuris trichiura* eggs (50–56 μm by 21–26 μm) are normally half the size of *T. vulpis* (72–90 μm by 32–40 μm); however, a small percentage of *T. trichiura* eggs overlap in size with *T. vulpis*. Therefore, when egg size is used to determine the species infecting people, misidentification can occur.[16,78,80] *Trichuris vulpis* has rarely been reported to cause visceral larva migrans in people[82]; however, none of these reports have been confirmed and the evidence more strongly suggests that these were not *T. vulpis* infections, particularly since there is no evidence of larval migration with *T. vulpis*.

CASE EXAMPLE

Signalment

"Rusty," an 8-year-old female spayed boxer mix from Tennessee, USA.

History

The owner reported that Rusty had a history of weight loss, lethargy, and anorexia. The last recorded body weight (4 years previously) was 34 kg. Vaccinations were not current and the dog was not on any medications, including heartworm preventive.

Physical Examination

Ambulatory on all four limbs. Body weight: 23.4 kg. Temperature = 99.5°F (37.5°C).

Faint/muffled heart sounds, strong pulses, and slightly increased respiratory noise. No significant abnormalities were noted in examination of the eyes, ears, nose, and throat. Mucous membranes pink and tacky; decreased skin turgor. Lymph nodes were normal. Abdominal palpation was unremarkable. No evidence

Continued

CASE EXAMPLE—cont'd

of ectoparasites. After hospitalization, Rusty had an episode of voluminous diarrhea, which was liquid in consistency and without obvious blood or mucus.

Laboratory Findings

CBC: WBC 35,820 cells/μL (6000–17,000 cells/μL), neutrophils 32,550 cells/μL (3000–12,000 cells/μL), HCT 60% (37–55%); all other parameters were within the normal range.

Serum chemistry profile: BUN 118 mg/dL (7–25 mg/dL), creatinine 2.5 mg/dL (0.3–1.4 mg/dL), phosphorus 11.3 mg/dL (2.9–6.6 mg/dL), glucose 267 mg/dL (60–110 mg/dL), potassium 6.4 mmol/L (3.7–5.8 mmol/L), sodium 109 mmol/L (138–160 mmol/L); all other parameters were within the normal range.

ACTH stimulation test (cosyntropin, 125 mg, IV) with samples taken at times 0 (<1.0 μg/dL; normal range 1.0–5.0 μg/dL) and 1 hour (6.1 μg/dL; normal range 8–17 μg/dL).

Imaging Findings

Thoracic radiographs revealed decreased cardiac size, clear lung fields, and no pleural effusion or masses.

Microbiologic Testing

Fecal flotation revealed large numbers of hookworm and whipworm eggs.

Diagnosis

Pseudo-hypoadrenocorticism secondary to whipworm and hookworm infestation. The initial differential diagnoses were hypoadrenocorticism (Addison's disease), whipworm infestation, neoplasia, and renal failure.

Treatment

After initial examination, Rusty was hospitalized for IV fluid administration; dexamethasone sodium phosphate was also administered (4 mg, once, IV). On the following day, when the fecal and ACTH stimulation results became available, IV fluids were continued and the following medications were started: sucralfate 1 g PO q12h and fenbendazole PO q24h for 3 days.

Comments

Rusty's condition rapidly improved and he began eating and drinking by the evening after the first dose of fenbendazole. Stools were firm within 2 days of instituting treatment and electrolyte and renal values were normal when retested 3 days after treatment commenced. The fenbendazole treatment was repeated 3 weeks and 3 months later.

Case example provided courtesy of Dr. Gary Del Gaudio.

SUGGESTED READINGS

Hurst RJ, Else KJ. *Trichuris muris* research revisited: a journey through time. *Parasitol.* 2013;140:1325–1339.

Traversa D. Are we paying too much attention to cardio-pulmonary nematodes and neglecting old-fashioned worms like *Trichuris vulpis*? *Parasit Vectors.* 2011;4:32.

Venco L, Valenti V, Genchi M, Grandi G. A dog with pseudo-Addison disease associated with *Trichuris vulpis* infection. *J Parasitol Res.* 2011:682039.

REFERENCES

1. von Linstow OFB. Helminthologisches. *Arch Naturgesch.* 1889;54:235–246.
2. von Linstow OFB. Helminthologische Untersuchungen. *Jh Ver Vaterl Naturk Wurttemb.* 1879;35:313–342.
3. Bowman DD, Hendrix CM, Lindsay DS, Barr SC. *Trichuris felis*. In: Bowman DD, ed. *Feline Clinical Parasitology*. Ames, IA: Iowa State University Press; 2002:348–350.
4. Hansen TVA. Drug treatment of *Trichuris spp.* infections – an attempt to explain porr drug efficacy of benzimidazoles. Thesis (PhD). Faculty of Health and Medical Sciences. University of Copenhagen; 2014:19–23.
5. Hendrix CM, Blagburn BL, Lindsay DS. Whipworms and intestinal threadworms. *Vet Clin North Am Small Anim Pract.* 1987;17:1355–1375.
6. Lanfredi RM, De Souza W, Gomes DC. Comparative study of four species of *Trichuris* Roederer, 1761 (Nematoda, Trichurinae) by scanning electron microscopy. *Mem Inst Oswaldo Cruz, Rio de Janeiro.* 1995;90:489–496.
7. Rubin R. Studies on the common whipworm of the dog, *Trichuris vulpis*. *Cornell Vet.* 1954;44:36–49.
8. Dryden MW, Gaafar SM. Whipworm infection in small animals. *Companion Anim Practice.* 1988;2:17–22.
9. Miller MJ. Studies on the life history of *Trichocephalus vulpis*, the whipworm of dogs. *Can J Res Section D Zoological Sci.* 1947;25:1–11.
10. Opitz HM. *Untersuchungen über die Entwicklung des Peitschenwurmes des Hundes Trichuris vulpis (Froelich 1789). Inaugural Dissertation.* Berlin, Germany: Freie University; 1963:41.
11. Kirkova Z. Studies on the life cycle of *Trichuris vulpis*. *Bulgarina J Vet Med.* 2003;6:35–42.
12. Tilney LG, Connelly PS, Guild GM, et al. Adaptation of a nematode parasite to living within the mammalian epithelium. *J Exp Zool Comp Exp Biol.* 2005;303:927–945.
13. Miller MJ. Quantitative studies on *Trichocephalus vulpis* infections in dogs. *Amer J Hygiene Section D Helminthol.* 1941;33:58–70.
14. Miller MJ. The egg-count index of *Trichocephalus vulpis* infections in dogs. *Proc Soc Exp Biol Med.* 1939;42:301–303.
15. Michael E, Bundy DAP. Density dependence in establishment, growth and worm fecundity in intestinal helminthiasis: the population biology of *Trichuris muris* (Nematoda) infection in CBA/Ca mice. *Parasitol.* 1989;98:451–458.
16. Yoshikawa H, Yamada M, Matsumoto Y, Yoshida Y. Variations in egg size of *Trichuris trichiura*. *Parasitol Res.* 1989;75:649–654.
17. Churcher TS, Filipe JAN, Basáñez M-G. Density dependence and the control of helminth parasites. *J Anim Ecology.* 2006;75:1313–1320.
18. Walker M, Hall A, Anderson RM, Basáñez M-G. Density-dependent effects on the weight of female *Ascaris lumbricoides* infections of humans and its impact on patterns of egg production. *Parasit Vectors.* 2009;2:11–28.
19. Spindler LA. A study of the temperature and moisture requirements in the development of the eggs of the dog Trichurid (*Trichuris vulpis*). *J Parasitol.* 1929;16:41–46.
20. Miller MJ. Studies on embryonation and hatching of the eggs of the dog whipworm, *Trichocephalus vulpis*. *Proc Soc Exp Biol Med.* 1939;42:303–305.
21. Companion Animal Parasite Council. Parasite Prevalence Maps. Whipworm, 2021. Available at: https://capcvet.org/maps/#/2021/all-year/whipworm/dog/united-states
22. Blagurn BL. Prevalence of canine and feline parasites in the United States. Bayer Zoonosis Symposium. *Suppl Comp Cont Ed Pract Vet.* 2001;23:5–10.
23. Gates MC, Nolan TJ. Endoparasite prevalence and recurrence across different age groups of dogs and cats. *Vet Parasitol.* 2009;166:153–158.
24. Palmer CS, Andrew Thompson RC, Traub RJ, et al. National study of the gastrointestinal parasites of dogs and cats in Australia. *Vet Parasitol.* 2008;151:181–190.
25. Barutzki D, Schaper R. Results of parasitological examinations of faecal samples from cats and dogs in Germany between 2003 and 2010. *Parasitol Res.* 2011;109:S45–S60.
26. Ilić T, Kulišić Z, Antić N, et al. Prevalence of zoonotic intestinal helminths in pet dogs and cats in the Belgrade area. *J Applied An Res.* 2017;45:204–208.

27. Dubná S, Langrová I, Nápravník J, et al. The prevalence of intestinal parasites in dogs from Prague, rural areas, and shelters of the Czech Republic. *Vet Parasitol.* 2007;145:120–128.
28. Martínez-Carrasco C, Berriatua E, Garijo M, et al. Epidemiological study of non-systemic parasitism in dogs in southeast Mediterranean Spain assessed by coprological and post-mortem examination. *Zoonoses Public Health.* 2007;54:195–203.
29. Neves D, Lobo L, Simões PB, Cardoso L. Frequency of intestinal parasites in pet dogs from an urban area (Greater Oporto, northern Portugal). *Vet Parasitol.* 2014;200:295–298.
30. Zanzani SA, Gazzonis AL, Scarpa P, et al. Intestinal parasites of owned dogs and cats from metropolitan and micropolitan areas: prevalence, zoonotic risks, and pet owner awareness in northern Italy. *BioMed Res Int.* 2014;2014:696508.
31. Johnson SA, Gakuya DW, Mbuthia PG, et al. Prevalence of gastrointestinal helminths and management practices for dogs in the Greater Accra region of Ghana. *Heliyon.* 2015;1(1):e00023.
32. Rehbein S, Kaulfuß K, Visser M, et al. Parasitenbefall von schaf-hütehunden in Mitteldeutschland [Parasites of sheep herding dogs in central Germany]. *Berl Münch Tierärztl Wochenschr.* 2016;129:56–64.
33. Craig HL, Craig PS. Helminth parasites of wolves (*Canis lupus*): a species list and an analysis of published prevalence studies in Nearctic and Palaearctic populations. *J Helminthol.* 2005;79:95–103.
34. Saeed I, Maddox-Hyttel C, Monrad J, Kapel CM. Helminths of red foxes (*Vulpes vulpes*) in Denmark. *Vet Parasitol.* 2006;139:168–179.
35. Franssen F, Nijsse R, Mulder J, et al. Increase in number of helminth species from Dutch red foxes over a 35-year period. *Parasit Vectors.* 2014;7:166.
36. Lahmar S, Boufana B, Boubaker SB, Landolsi F. Intestinal helminths of golden jackals and red foxes from Tunisia. *Vet Parasitol.* 2014;204:297–303.
37. Otranto D, Cantacessi C, Dantas-Torres F, et al. The role of wild canids and felids in spreading parasites to dogs and cats in Europe. Part II: helminths and arthropods. *Vet Parasitol.* 2015;213:24–37.
38. Figueiredo A, Oliveira L, Madeira de Carvalho L, et al. Parasite species of the endangered Iberian wolf (*Canis lupus signatus*) and a sympatric widespread carnivore. *Int J Parasitol Parasites Wildl.* 2016;5:164–167.
39. Redman WK, Bryant JE, Ahmad G. Gastrointestinal helminths of coyotes (*Canis latrans*) from Southeast Nebraska and Shenandoah area of Iowa. *Vet World.* 2016;9:970–975.
40. Cameron TWM. Studies on the endoparasitic fauna of Trinidad mammals. V. Further parasites from the Ocelot. *Can J Res.* 1937;15:24–27.
41. Ng BK, Kelly JD. Isolation of *Trichuris campanula* von Listow 1889 from Australian cats. *Aus Vet J.* 1975;51:450–451.
42. Hass DK, Meisels LS. *Trichuris campanula* infection in a domestic cat from Miami, Florida. *Am J Vet Res.* 1978 Sep;39(9):1553–1555.
43. Ketzis J. *Trichuris* spp. infecting domestic cats on St. Kitts: identification based on size or vulvar structure? *SpringerPlus.* 2015;4(1):115. (Note: error in this article regarding the bacillary band of *T. campanula*; while omitted from the original description, all *Trichuris* have a band).
44. Ketzis JK, Verma A, Burgess G. Molecular characterization of *Trichuris serrata. Parasitol Res.* 2015;114:1993–1995.
45. Santa Cruz AM, Lombardero OJ. Parasitological results of 50 necropsies of cats in Corrientes City, Argentina. *Vet Argent.* 1987;4:735–739.
46. Krecek RC, Moura L, Lucas H, Kelly P. Parasites of stray cats (*Felis domesticus* L., 1758) on St. Kitts, West Indies. *Vet Parasitol.* 2010;172:147–149.
47. Ketzis JK, Shell L, Chinault S, et al. The prevalence of *Trichuris* spp. infection in indoor and outdoor cats on St. Kitts. *J Infect Dev Ctries.* 2015;9:111–113.
48. Ng BK, Kelly JD. Anthropozoonotic helminthiases in Australasia: Part 3: studies on the prevalence and public health implications of helminth parasites of dogs and cats in urban environments. *Int J Zoonoses.* 1975;2:76–91.
49. De Santis AC, Raghavan M, Caldanaro RJ, et al. Estimated prevalence of nematode parasitism among pet cats in the United States. *J Am Vet Med Assoc.* 2006;228:885–892.
50. Geng J, Elsemore D, Ketzis J, Oudin N. Diagnosis of feline whipworm infection in southern Florida. In: *Proceedings of the American Association of Veterinary Parasitologists 60th Annual Meeting, 59th Livestock Insect Workers' Conference, 13th International Symposium on Ectoparasites of Pets.* 2015.
51. Coati N, Hellmann K, Mencke N, Epe C. Recent investigation on the prevalence of gastrointestinal nematodes in cats from France and Germany. *Parasitol Res.* 2003;90:S146–S147.
52. Beugnet F, Bourdeau P, Chalvet-Monfray K, et al. Parasites of domestic owned cats in Europe: co-infestations and risk factors. *Parasit Vectors.* 2014;7:291.
53. Spada E, Proverbio D, Della Pepa A, et al. Prevalence of faecal-borne parasites in colony stray cats in northern Italy. *J Feline Med Surg.* 2013;15:672–677.
54. Umeche N, Ima AE. Intestinal helminthic infections of cats in Calabar, Nigeria. *Folia Parasitol.* 1988;35:165–168.
55. Beldomenico PM, Kinsella JM, Uhart MM, et al. Helminths of Geoffroy's cat, *Oncifelis geoffroyi* (Carnivora, Felidae) from the Monte desert, central Argentina. *Acta Parasitol.* 2005;50:263–266.
56. Kirkova Z, Dinev I. Morphological changes in the intestine of dogs, experimentally infected with *Trichuris vulpis. Bulgarina J Vet Med.* 2005;8:239–243.
57. Burrows RB, Lillis WG. The whipworm as a blood sucker. *J Parasitol.* 1964;50:675–680.
58. DiBartola SP, Johnson SE, Davenport DJ, et al. Clinicopathologic findings resembling hypoadrenocorticism in dogs with primary gastrointestinal disease. *J Am Vet Med Assoc.* 1985;187:60–63.
59. Malik R, Hunt GB, Hinchliffe JM, Church DB. Severe whipworm infection in the dog. *J Small Anim Pract.* 1990;31:185–188.
60. Graves TK, Schall WD, Refsal K, Nachreiner RF. Basal and ACTH-stimulated plasma aldosterone concentrations are normal or increased in dogs with trichuriasis-associated pseudohypoadrenocorticism. *J Vet Intern Med.* 1994;8:287–289.
61. Ruckstuhl N, Hoerauf A, Tomsa K, Reusch C. Pseudohypoadrenocorticism in two Siberian huskies with gastrointestinal parasitoses. *Schweiz Arch Tierheilkd.* 2002;144:75–81.
62. Peterson ME. Q&A: pseudo-Addison's disease in a dog with whipworms. *Insights into Veterinary Endocrinology.* 2011. Available at: https://endocrine-vet.blogspot.com//2011/05/q-pseudo-addisons-disease-in-dog-with.html
63. Venco L, Valenti V, Genchi M, Grandi G. A dog with pseudo-Addison disease associated with *Trichuris vulpis* infection. *J Parasitol Res.* 2011:682039.
64. Cooper R. Whipworm in a dog: could it be more? *Clinician's Brief.* 2013:81–83.
65. Kirkova Z, Petkov P, Goundasheva D. Clinical and haematological studies in dogs, experimentally infected with *Trichuris vulpis. Bulgarina J Vet Med.* 2005;8:141–148.
66. Leung JM, Graham AL, Knowles SCL. Parasite-microbiota interactions with the vertebrate gut: synthesis through an ecological lens. *Front Microbiol.* 2018;9:843.
67. Peachey LE, Jenkins TP, Cantacessi C. This gut ain't big enough for both of us. Or is it? Helminth-microbiota interactions in veterinary species. *Trends Parasitol.* 2017;33:619–632.
68. Li RW, Wu S, Li W, et al. Alterations in the porcine colon microbiota induced by the gastrointestinal nematode *Trichuris suis. Infect Immun.* 2012;80:2150–2157.
69. Di Cesare A, Castagna G, Meloni S, et al. Mixed trichuroid infestation in a dog from Italy. *Parasit Vectors.* 2012;5:128.
70. Traversa D, Di Cesare A, Lia RP, et al. New insights into morphological and biological features of *Capillaria aerophila* (Trichocephalida, Trichuridae). *Parasitol Res.* 2011;109:S97–S104.
71. Traversa D, Di Cesare A, Conboy G. Canine and feline cardiopulmonary parasitic nematodes in Europe: emerging and underestimated. *Parasit Vectors.* 2010;3:62.
72. Guardone L, Deplazes P, Macchioni F, et al. Ribosomal and mitochondrial DNA analysis of Trichuridae nematodes of carnivores and small mammals. *Vet Parasitol.* 2013;197:364–369.
73. Callejón R, Nadler S, De Rojas M, et al. Molecular characterization and phylogeny of whipworm nematodes inferred from DNA sequences of cox1 mtDNA and 18S rDNA. *Parasitol Res.* 2013;112:3933–3949.

74. Demeler J, Ramünke S, Wolken S, et al. Discrimination of gastrointestinal nematode eggs from crude fecal egg preparations by inhibitor-resistant conventional and real-time PCR. *PLoS One*. 2013;8:e61285.
75. Elsemore DA, Geng J, Flynn L, et al. Enzyme-linked immunosorbent assay for coproantigen detection of *Trichuris vulpis* in dogs. *J Vet Diagn Invest*. 2014;26:404–411.
76. Geng J, Elsemore D, Ketzis JK. ELISA Detection of *Trichuris serrata* Coproantigen in cats. In: *Proceedings of the American Association of Veterinary Parasitologists 59th Annual Meeting*. 2014.
77. Fernandes M, Saliba AM. Estudo histológico e histoquímico das lesões produzidas por *Trichuris vulpis* (Fröelich, 1789) no ceco de cães. *Rev Fac Med vet Zootec Univ. S. Paulo*. 1974;11:59–68.
78. Gattenuo T, Ketzis J, Shell L. Fenbendazole treatment for *Mammomonogamus* species infection of a domestic cat on St Kitts, West Indies. *J Feline Med Surg*. 2014;16:864–866.
79. Pérez Tort G, Fernanda Iglesias M, Prieto O, et al. Field evaluation of the efficacy of the emodepside/praziquantel spot on solution for the control of *Trichuris campanula* in naturally infected domestic cats. In: *Proceedings of the World Small Animal Veterinary Association/FECAVA World Congress*. 2008.
80. Areekul P, Putaporntip C, Pattanawong U, et al. *Trichuris vulpis* and *T. trichiura* infections among schoolchildren of a rural community in northwestern Thailand: the possible role of dogs in disease transmission. *Asian Biomed*. 2010;4:49–60.
81. Kenney M, Eveland LK. Infection of man with *Trichuris vulpis*, the whipworm of dogs. *Am J Clin Pathol*. 1978;69:199.
82. Coulter JB, Jewsbury JM, Beesley WN, Bailey W. Visceral larva migrans and *Trichuris vulpis*. *Arch Dis Child*. 1981;56:406.

Tapeworms

Christopher B. Adolph, Andrew S. Peregrine

KEY POINTS

Dipylidium caninum

- First Described: *Dipylidium caninum* has been known to infect pets since ancient times. Linnaeus named this parasite *Taenia cania* in 1758; Leuckart created the genus *Dipylidium* in 1863.
- Cause: *Dipylidium caninum* (order Cyclophyllidea).
- Geographic Distribution: Worldwide.
- Affected Hosts: Dogs and cats, as well as other canids and felids, serve as definitive hosts for adult *D. caninum.*
- Primary Mode of Transmission: Infected definitive hosts intermittently shed segments that contain egg packets which break down in the environment. When a suitable arthropod intermediate host (e.g., *Ctenocephalides felis felis* [flea], *Trichodectes canis* [biting louse]) ingests the eggs, a metacestode stage (a cysticercoid) develops within the arthropod. Final hosts become infected and develop patent intestinal infections upon ingestion of an infected intermediate host.
- Major Clinical Signs: Heavy infections in dogs and cats may cause constipation and diarrhea. However, the most common clinical situation arises when an owner discovers segments in the hair coat, bedding, or recently passed feces, of a healthy animal.
- Differential Diagnoses: Other GI parasites, dietary indiscretion, pancreatitis, intestinal bacterial overgrowth, IBD, GI neoplasia, exocrine pancreatic insufficiency, hepatobiliary disease, GI foreign body, and intestinal perforation. When segments are present, these need to be differentiated from other tapeworms that shed segments.
- Human Health Significance: *Dipylidium caninum* occasionally infects people that accidentally ingest infected fleas.

Taenia spp.

- First Described: *Taenia* was first described by Linnaeus in 1758.
- Cause: Multiple cyclophyllidean species that belong to the family Taeniidae. The family contains two generally accepted genera: *Taenia* and *Echinococcus.*
- Geographic Distribution: Essentially worldwide. However, the importance of different *Taenia* species varies depending on the geographic region.
- Affected Hosts: *Taenia pisiformis, Taenia crassiceps, Taenia hydatigena, Taenia ovis, Taenia serialis,* and *Taenia multiceps* all infect dogs as the definitive host. The predominant *Taenia* species infecting cats globally is *Taenia taeniaeformis.*
- Primary Mode of Transmission: Infected dogs and cats intermittently pass egg-laden segments into the environment. Eggs are then consumed by a suitable mammalian intermediate host (e.g., rabbit, sheep, mice, rats) resulting in the formation of the metacestode, larval, tapeworm in that host's tissues; the type of metacestode varies with the *Taenia* spp. involved. Dogs and cats develop patent intestinal infections after consuming an infected intermediate host.
- Major Clinical Signs: Intestinal infections with *Taenia* spp. in dogs and cats have long been thought to be well tolerated with no associated clinical signs. When clinical signs occur, they are relatively non-specific and may include vomiting and diarrhea. Rarely, cats require an enterotomy to relieve a cestode impaction.
- Differential Diagnoses: Differentials include other GI parasites, dietary indiscretion, pancreatitis, intestinal bacterial overgrowth, IBD, GI neoplasia, exocrine pancreatic insufficiency, hepatobiliary disease, GI foreign body, and intestinal perforation. When segments are present, these need to be differentiated microscopically from segments of other tapeworms.
- Human Health Significance: In general, zoonotic *Taenia* spp. are limited to species that utilize cattle and pigs as intermediate hosts (e.g., *T. saginata*, *T. solium*); dogs and cats are not involved in the life cycles. However, adult *T. taeniaeformis* have been recovered from the intestinal tract of humans. Humans may also occasionally be infected with the metacestode stage of *T. multiceps* or *T. serialis*, which utilize dogs as a definitive host. When eggs are accidentally ingested by humans, they hatch in the GI tract; oncospheres are released and circulate in the bloodstream until they lodge in organs where coenuri develop. For *T. multiceps*, coenuri may be found in the brain and eyes, while those of *T. serialis* are found in subcutaneous tissue.

Echinococcus spp.

- First Described: *Echinococcus granulosus* s.l. was first described by Batsch in 1786, and *Echinococcus multilocularis* was first described by Leuckart in 1863.
- Causes: *Echinococcus granulosus* sensu lato (s.l.) and *Echinococcus multilocularis* (family Taeniidae).
- Geographic Distribution: *Echinococcus granulosus* s.l. comprises multiple genotypes/species that differ in their geographic distribution due to differences in host specificity. The genotype most important for human disease is *E. granulosus* sensu stricto (s.s.), which is primarily associated with sheep and found worldwide. *Echinococcus multilocularis* occurs throughout much of the northern hemisphere (Europe, Asia, and North America).
- Affected Hosts: Adult stages of both cestodes are a few millimeters in length and occur in the small intestine of carnivores. Definitive hosts for *E. granulosus* s.l. are primarily dogs and, to a lesser extent, wild canids, which excrete infective eggs into the environment in feces. *Echinococcus multilocularis* occurs primarily in a wildlife cycle with wild canids (arctic/red fox, coyote, raccoon dog, wolf) as definitive hosts. Dogs, and to a lesser extent cats, may also be definitive hosts. Dogs occasionally may also be accidental hosts that develop metacestodes.
- Primary Mode of Transmission: Ingestion of *E. granulosus* s.l. eggs by intermediate hosts (e.g., sheep, cattle, goats, pigs, horses)

and accidental hosts (e.g., people) results in the development of a hydatid cyst within the liver, lungs, or other internal organs. The resultant disease is termed *cystic echinococcosis* (CE). After ingestion of *E. multilocularis* eggs by rodents, the typical intermediate host, the metacestode stage develops most commonly within the liver, behaves like an invasive tumor, and produces *alveolar echinococcosis* (AE). Ingestion of eggs by accidental hosts (e.g., people, dogs) also results in AE. Thus, dogs can be both definitive and accidental hosts for *E. multilocularis.* Dogs, cats, and wild canids develop intestinal infections following ingestion of metacestode-infected rodents.

- Major Clinical Signs: Intestinal infections are rarely clinical. AE in dogs is typically associated with hepatic injury; clinical signs include abdominal pain and/or distension, lethargy, anorexia, and vomiting.
- Differential Diagnoses: Both cats and dogs excrete eggs morphologically identical to those of *Taenia* spp. and require DNA analysis to determine the genus/species. Differential diagnoses for hepatic AE in dogs include tumors, abscesses, and cysts (sterile, congenital).
- Human Health Significance: Most species of *E. granulosus* s.l. can infect people. However, globally, most human cases of CE are due to *E. granulosus* s.s. (sheep strain). This strain occurs in both domestic and wildlife cycles. However, the domestic cycle is of particular zoonotic significance as human infections are typically associated with ingestion of eggs in the feces of dogs. The resultant hydatid cysts are usually large, fluid-filled structures that behave like a space-occupying lesion. While often clinically silent, they may cause CE, a potentially severe disease of the liver, lungs, bone, brain, or other organs. While *E. multilocularis* occurs in wild and domestic life cycles, most human infections are associated with ingestion of eggs in the feces of dogs. In humans, AE is typically associated with development of the metacestode stage in the liver and has a high case fatality rate when left untreated; the metacestode behaves like an invasive tumor and often metastasizes to other organs. The clinical incubation period is 5 to 15 years. Both AE and, to a lesser extent, CE, have high pathogenic potential and are considered two of the most important helminthic zoonoses. In a veterinary environment, infection risk in people when handling dogs and cats can essentially be eliminated by strict attention to hand hygiene.

Mesocestoides spp.

- First Described: Valliant described *Mesocestoides ambiguous* in 1863.
- Causes: Cestodes that belong to the *Mesocestoides* genus. Questions remain as to how to define the species because the life cycle has not been fully defined for any species.
- Geographic Distribution: Worldwide.
- Affected Hosts: Dogs, cats, and raccoons are definitive hosts for *Mesocestoides* spp.; there are a variety of intermediate hosts (e.g., mammals, amphibians, birds, reptiles). Peritoneal larval cestodiasis occasionally occurs in dogs or cats following ingestion of an infected intermediate host.
- Primary Mode of Transmission: Definitive hosts become infected by ingesting intermediate hosts that contain the second metacestode stage, a tetrathyridium, located in the peritoneal cavity. The first intermediate stage is thought to be a cysticercoid that develops from an oncosphere in a coprophagic insect, but this has yet to be proven. Tetrathyridia develop into adult tapeworms in the intestinal tract of the definitive host. Subsequently, sections of the strobila, or body, are excreted in feces, rather than individual segments like *D. caninum* or *Taenia* spp. Segments contain eggs that vary in maturity. Peritoneal larval cestodiasis occurs when dogs and cats ingest an infected intermediate host and larval parasites migrate through the intestinal wall and multiply as the tetrathyridial stage within the peritoneal cavity by asexually dividing or budding.
- Major Clinical Signs: Dogs and cats infected with *Mesocestoides* spp. typically have subclinical intestinal infections. Dogs with peritoneal larval cestodiasis may show abdominal distention with or without systemic signs of anorexia, weight loss, vomiting, diarrhea, lethargy, ascites, and tachypnea. Clinical signs in one cat from Sicily, Italy included anorexia, moderate abdominal swelling, cough, and dyspnea.
- Differential Diagnoses: *Mesocestoides* spp. segments are significantly smaller than those of more common cestodes (i.e., *D. caninum* and *Taenia* spp.) and may be confused with those of *Echinococcus* spp. Differentials for peritoneal larval cestodiasis include other causes of ascites, such as right-sided heart failure, neoplasia, pancreatitis, GI foreign body, and intestinal perforation.
- Human Health Significance: Rarely, humans can become infected with adult *Mesocestoides* spp. by ingestion of undercooked organs (e.g., raw snake liver, chicken viscera) containing tetrathyridia leading to abdominal pain and passage of segments in the stool. Infected dogs and cats are not a direct zoonotic risk to people.

Diphyllobothrium spp.

- First Described: Linnaeus, 1758.
- Causes: Cestodes of the *Diphyllobothrium* genus (family Diphyllobothriidae). Globally, *Diphyllobothrium latum* (*Dibothriocephalus latus*) is the most important species.
- Geographic Distribution: *Diphyllobothrium latum* has a circumboreal distribution involving Alaska, the Great Lakes region of the USA/Canada, northern Europe, Russia, and parts of Asia and South America.
- Affected Hosts: Adult tapeworms occur in the small intestine of dogs, cats, people, pigs, foxes, mink, and other fish-eating animals.
- Primary Mode of Transmission: Ingestion of the plerocercoid stage in raw or undercooked freshwater fish.
- Major Clinical Signs: Infections in both dogs and cats are typically subclinical.
- Differential Diagnoses: Segments of *D. latum* within feces are typically larger in size than those of *Spirometra* spp., *Taenia* spp., and *D. caninum.* Unlike *Taenia* spp. and *D. caninum*, segments of *D. latum* and *Spirometra* spp. have a medial uterine pore.
- Human Health Significance: Humans acquire *D. latum* infection by ingestion of raw or undercooked fish; infections are most commonly asymptomatic. Dogs and cats infected with *D. latum* are not a direct risk to human health.

Spirometra spp.

- First Described: Rudolphi first described *Spirometra erinaceieuropaei* (syn. *Diphyllobothrium erinaceieuropaei*) in 1819. In 1882, Mason described *Spirometra mansoni.* In 1935, Mueller described *Spirometra mansonoides.*
- Causes: *Spirometra* spp. (family Diphyllobothriidae); a cestode closely related to *Diphyllobothrium* spp.
- Geographic Distribution: *Spirometra erinaceieuropaei* occurs in Asia, Australia, and Europe. *Spirometra mansonoides* occurs in North and South America. *Spirometra mansoni* is predominantly found in Asia.
- Affected Hosts: Adult *Spirometra* spp. occur in the small intestine of dogs, cats, wild felids, wild canids, raccoons, and other carnivores. Proliferative sparganosis (proliferation of plerocercoids) occasionally occurs in the abdominal or thoracic cavity, or connective tissue, of dogs and cats.
- Primary Mode of Transmission: Infected definitive hosts shed eggs in feces that hatch in water to release a coracidium. When ingested

by freshwater copepods (e.g., *Cyclops* spp.), the coracidium develops into a procercoid. Following ingestion of infected copepods by a second intermediate host (e.g., amphibians, reptiles, birds, mammals), the procercoid develops into a plerocercoid (or spargana). Definitive hosts become infected following ingestion of muscle or connective tissue of second intermediate hosts or paratenic hosts containing a plerocercoid. The plerocercoid then attaches to the intestinal wall and develops into an adult tapeworm. Proliferative sparganosis occurs following ingestion of water containing copepods infected with procercoids, or plerocercoids in second intermediate hosts or paratenic hosts.

- Major Clinical Signs: Dogs and cats infected with adult *Spirometra* spp. often have subclinical infections. However, enteritis, diarrhea, weight loss, and vomiting have been associated with infection, particularly in cats. Occasionally, the only evidence of infection is the presentation of chains of segments by owners to a veterinarian. Clinical signs associated with proliferative sparganosis depend on the location of the plerocercoids.
- Differential Diagnoses (Intestinal Infections): Other GI parasites, dietary indiscretion, pancreatitis, intestinal bacterial overgrowth, IBD, GI neoplasia, exocrine pancreatic insufficiency, hepatobiliary disease, and GI foreign body.
- Human Health Significance: *Spirometra* spp. cause sparganosis in people. This occurs when the plerocercoid stage (spargana) is transferred to humans following ingestion of raw or undercooked meat (e.g., frog) or when copepods infected with the procercoid larval stage are consumed by drinking untreated water. This condition is rare, and usually presents as a subcutaneous nodule containing a plerocercoid. However, in some cases, proliferative sparganosis involving the CNS or other organs has been reported.

INTRODUCTION

Cestodes are flatworms that are divided into two orders of veterinary significance, Cyclophyllidea and Diphyllobothriidea (formerly Pseudophyllidea).[1] The Cyclophyllidea comprise *Dipylidium caninum, Echinococcus* spp., *Mesocestoides* spp., and *Taenia* spp. The Diphyllobothriidea, or primitive tapeworms, contain *Diphyllobothrium* spp. and *Spirometra* spp.. Definitions that are related to cestode infections are shown in Box 115.1.

DIPYLIDIUM CANINUM

ETIOLOGY AND EPIDEMIOLOGY

Dipylidium caninum is the only *Dipylidium* species of veterinary importance and commonly infects dogs, cats, and other canids and felids. Molecular characterization of *D. caninum* isolates obtained from infected fleas and proglottids of both dogs and cats has demonstrated the existence of two distinct genotypes, suggesting the possibility of two separate species within *D. caninum*. Extensive evaluation of infected fleas from the United States and Europe as well as adult tapeworms from South Africa, France, and China has demonstrated that the two genotypes (dog and cat) generally appear to be species specific around the world.[2] The success of this tapeworm can partially be attributed to the global distribution of flea intermediate hosts. However, multiple additional factors are involved including societal attitudes toward dogs and cats as pets, ability and willingness to institute proper flea control, and the low sensitivity of current detection methods. Thus, *D. caninum* has been documented in North America,[3] South America (e.g., Brazil),[4] Europe,[5] the Middle East (e.g., Iran),[6] Russia,[7] Asia (e.g., China),[8] and Africa (e.g., Nigeria).[9]

Dogs and cats become infected when they ingest arthropod intermediate hosts that include fleas (*Ctenocephalides felis, Ctenocephalides canis,* and *Pulex irritans*) and chewing lice (*Trichodectes canis*) (Fig. 115.1).[3] Dogs and cats pass gravid segments intermittently in feces. Pre-adult stages of the intermediate host (e.g., flea larvae) ingest eggs of the cestode once the segment breaks down in the environment. As the intermediate host develops to adulthood, the oncosphere (tapeworm embryo) develops to the metacestode stage, a cysticercoid, within the intermediate host. Dogs and cats become infected when infected arthropods are ingested. The cysticercoid then develops to an adult tapeworm within the lumen of the small intestine and attaches to the small intestine wall via muscular suckers on the scolex and small hooks on the rostellum. The body of the tapeworm (strobila) elongates and the most mature (gravid) segments on the distal end detach and are passed in feces. Gravid segments may be shed by dogs and cats as soon as 2 to 3 weeks after being infected with cysticercoids.[10,11]

Proglottids do not have an opening for eggs to escape and each segment is packed with eggs. The oncospheres are contained within

BOX 115.1 Definitions Used in Reference to Cestodes

Alveolar echinococcosis	Disease due to the metacestode stage of *E. multilocularis*
Brood capsule	Fluid-filled bladder found within hydatid cyst that contains multiple protoscolices
Calcareous corpuscle	Ovoid mineral structures, 2–30 μm in size, found in all tapeworms
Cestode	Tapeworm; a parasitic flatworm of the class Cestoda
Cystic echinococcosis	Disease due to the metacestode stage of *E. granulosus* s.l.
Hydatid cyst	Metacestode stage of *E. granulosus* s.l.
Intermediate host	Animal species in which development of the metacestode stage occurs
Metacestode	Immature stage that occurs in the intermediate host
Oncosphere	Immature stage that hatches from egg
Patent infection	Shedding of eggs in feces or presence of proglottids in feces or perianal region
Prepatent period	Time from ingestion of metacestode stage to development of adult parasites and shedding of eggs or proglottids in feces
Protoscolices	Juvenile scolices (plural of scolex) formed from germinal layer of a metacestode
Scolex	Adult tapeworm holdfast organ that attaches to the host intestinal wall
Strobila	Chain of individual adult tapeworm segments that progressively mature as the tapeworm elongates

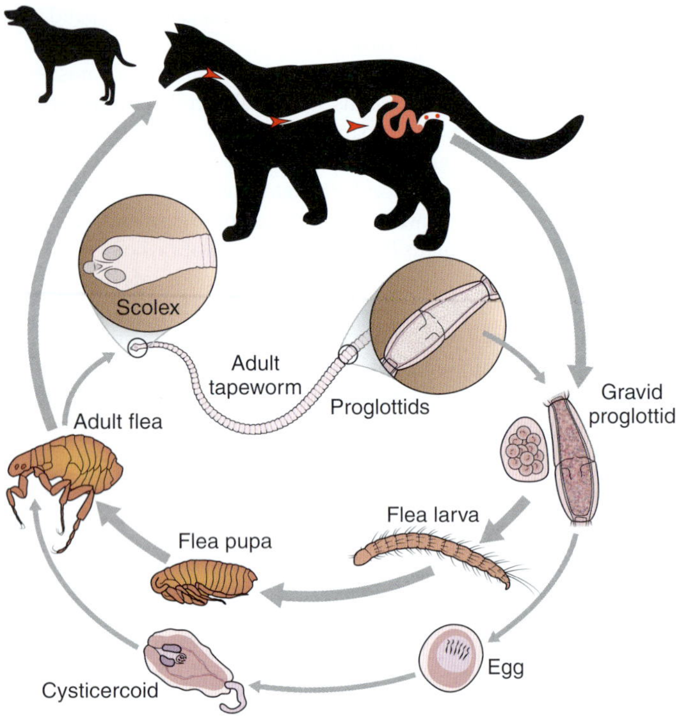

Fig. 115.1 Life cycle of *Dipylidium caninum*.

a packet and each packet may contain 25 to 30 oncospheres (Fig. 115.2A).[3] Evidence of the longevity of *D. caninum* is unclear; estimates vary widely, from as short as 3 months to 3 years.[12]

Previous surveys in New Jersey and Wisconsin, USA, reported *D. caninum* prevalences of 10.4% and 13.0% in cats, respectively. The same two surveys also reported prevalences for dogs of 0.4% and 4.0%, respectively.[13,14] In the New Jersey survey, 318 feral cats were examined by both fecal flotation and necropsy; 33 were infected with *D. caninum* at necropsy (10.4%); none tested positive by zinc sulfate fecal flotation. In a more recent survey in Oklahoma, USA, 40 of 116 (34.5%) cats were positive for *D. caninum* at necropsy; however, 0 of 40 of these infections were detected utilizing two different flotation methods (passive and centrifugal).[15] These data indicate that prevalence determinations based solely on fecal examination underestimate the true prevalence of infection. This finding is consistent with the biological characteristic of proglottids passing singly in feces without release of eggs in the intestinal tract.[16]

CLINICAL FEATURES

Pathogenesis and Clinical Signs

Adult *D. caninum* cause little pathology and are well tolerated by the host. Dogs and cats with tapeworm proglottids visible on the perineal area, or detected in freshly passed feces, have been observed to drag their anus on the ground. However, such behavior can also happen in the absence of infection.[11] Occasionally, cats infected with *D. caninum* have developed convulsions and seizures.[10] More commonly,

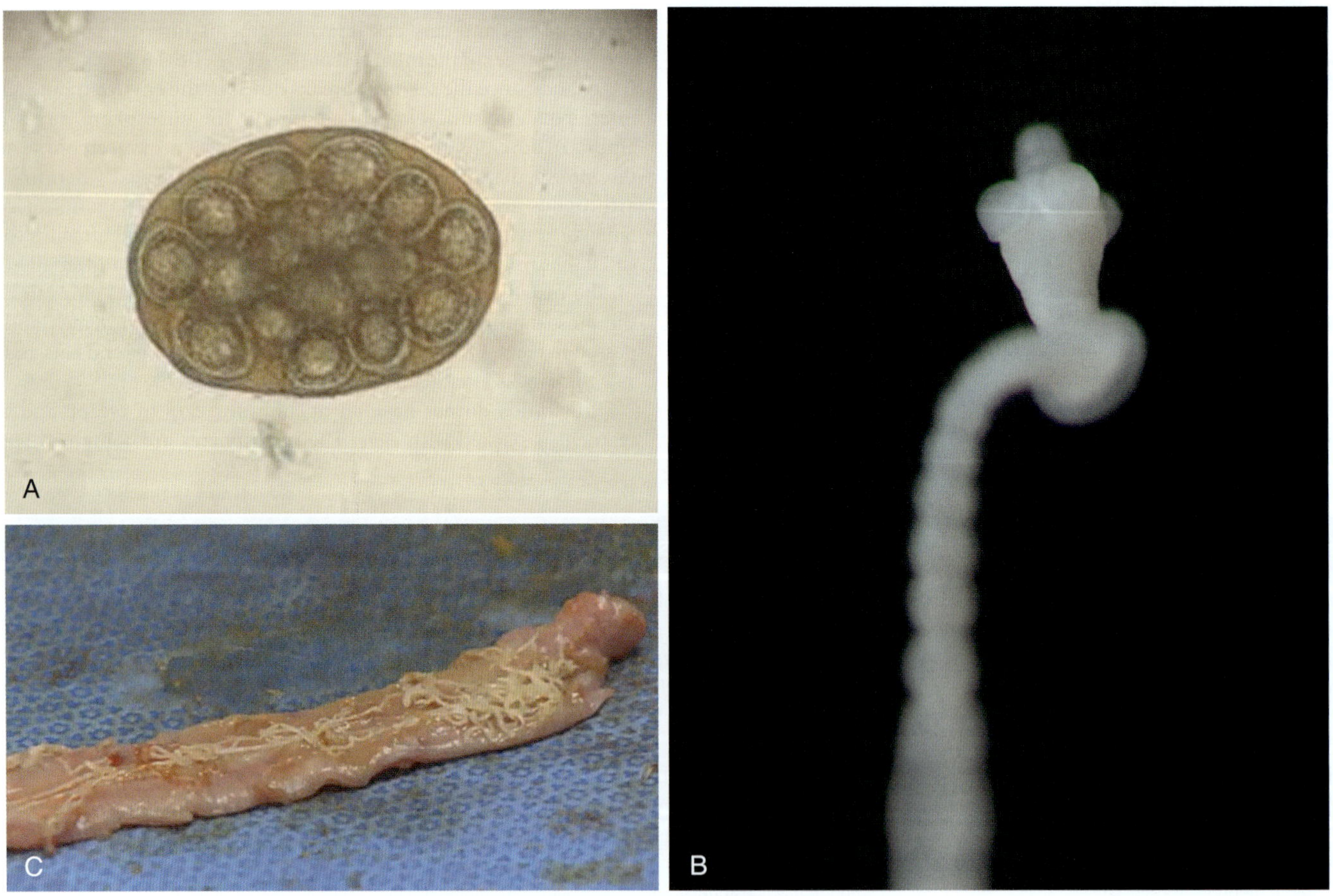

Fig. 115.2 Morphologic features of *Dipylidium caninum*. (A) Egg packet from a proglottid. Eggs containing a hexacanth embryo are visible inside the egg packet. (B) Scolex. The rostellum is retractable and armed with small hooks and four suckers. (C) Strobila in the small intestine of a cat. (B, courtesy of Megan Lineberry, National Center for Veterinary Parasitology, Oklahoma State University). *Continued*

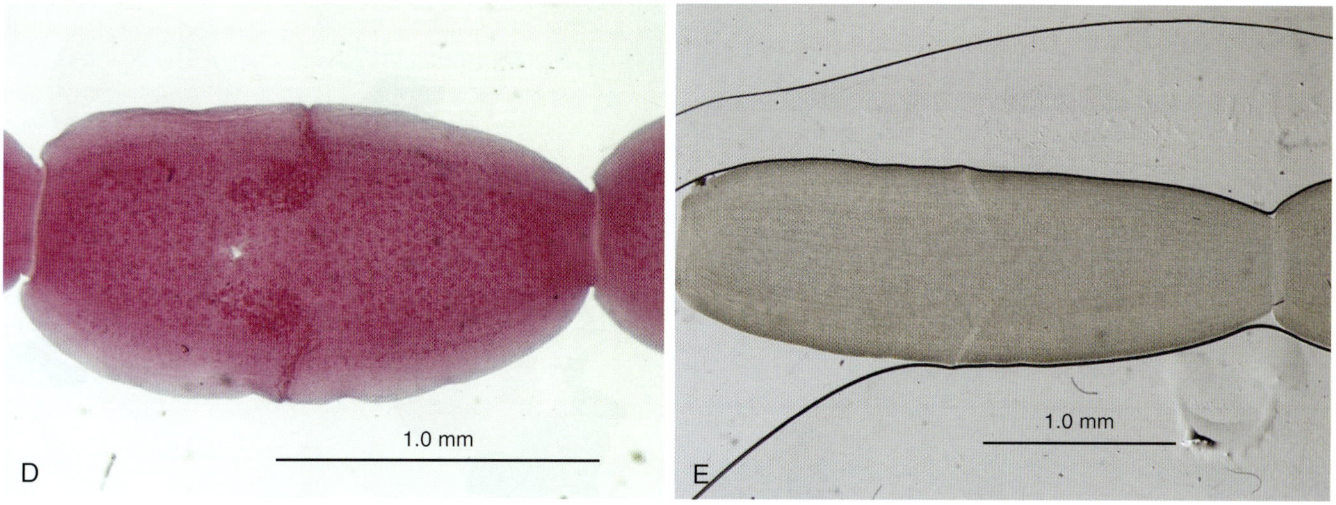

Fig. 115.2 cont'd (D) Stained and (E) unstained segment showing bilateral genital pores. (D, E courtesy of Megan Lineberry, National Center for Veterinary Parasitology, Oklahoma State University.)

young animals with clinical signs exhibit an unthrifty, potbellied appearance.[17]

In a 2015 survey in Oklahoma, cats infected with *D. caninum* had gross intestinal lesions, including distension of the small intestine, mural thickening, hemorrhage, and ulceration in association with the presence of tapeworms. Because of this, it appears that the current understanding of pathology associated with intestinal tapeworm infections requires more study.[15]

Most clients have strong emotional reactions to detecting a proglottid in their pet's feces or on the pet's perianal region and will often contact their veterinarian for assistance. Differentiating proglottids of *D. caninum* from other cestodes will allow the clinician to appropriately treat the current infection, because certain tapeworms require higher dosages of anticestodal medications and for longer periods of time, and to address the risk of reinfection.

DIAGNOSIS

Adult *D. caninum* tapeworms may be detected at necropsy and are usually 15 to 30 cm in length (Fig. 115.2C).[10] The scolex has a retractable rostellum with 30 to 150 small thorn-like hooks arranged in circles and four muscular suckers (Fig. 115.2B). Gravid segments are 10 to 12 mm in length, narrowed at both ends, and contain two genital pores. The common name, "cucumber seed" tapeworm, is based on the appearance of the gravid segment (Fig. 115.2D and E).[3] Diagnosis of *D. caninum* antemortem typically relies on detection of the characteristic proglottid on the host or in the feces, as well as detection of the characteristic egg packet on fecal flotation. However, egg packets can be difficult to float and astute veterinary team members are more likely to detect proglottids on gross examination than egg packets on flotation.[15] Occasionally, the egg packet may be disrupted during specimen preparation and individual eggs observed in feces. Generally, high specific gravity solutions (e.g., Sheather's sucrose solution, SpG 1.27) have a higher probability of floating heavier helminth eggs than lower specific gravity solutions.[18]

Tapeworm proglottids should be definitively identified prior to initiating anticestodal therapy. Environmental structures may be confused for proglottids, and determining the genus of the tapeworm and addressing risk factors is important to prevent reinfection. Rehydrating suspected proglottids in water or saline for 10 to 30 minutes prior to microscopic examination often aids identification of the bilateral genital pores characteristic of *D. caninum* (see Fig. 115.2D and E). Eggs can be observed by adding a drop of saline and crushing the proglottid between two glass slides. Occasionally, proglottids are sterile and one may only observe calcareous corpuscles (ovoid mineral concentrations that contain calcium carbonite) that vary in size from 2 to 30 μm.[19] However, these are typical of all cestodes. Regardless of the detection method (flotation or proglottid preparation), egg packets are 120 to 200 μm long and contain 25 to 30 individual ova. Each egg measures 35 to 60 μm and contains a hexacanth embryo (see Fig. 115.2A).[20] Copro-antigen and PCR detection methods are not yet commercially available for detection of *D. caninum* infections but would be expected to dramatically improve diagnosis. These strategies have been used on a research basis to detect *D. caninum* in fleas and to differentiate *D. caninum* from other cestode species.[21,22]

TREATMENT AND PROGNOSIS

Effective treatment of *D. caninum* infections requires both treatment for tapeworms and for the flea intermediate host. To avoid reinfection, every dog and cat on the premise must be treated for fleas. Treatment with appropriate anticestodal medication at both the time of the initial diagnosis and at conclusion of environmental flea elimination (2 to 4 months is a reasonable expectation with proper flea control of all pets) will eliminate all current and newly acquired tapeworms.

Praziquantel is available as both oral and injectable formulations for both dogs and cats. Dogs and cats are dosed at 5 mg/kg PO or 5.7 mg/kg when administered either SC or IM (Table 115.1). These dosages eliminate 100% of the adult and immature stages.[23] Praziquantel (12 mg/kg) is also available as a topical formulation in combination with emodepside or eprinomectin, and as a standalone formulation (8 mg/kg) for cats. Epsiprantel is an oral medication with efficacy against adult stages of *D. caninum* and is dosed at 5.5 mg/kg in dogs and 2.75 mg/kg in cats.[11] Nitroscanate is approved for use in dogs in some countries. A dosage of 25 mg/kg eliminated natural infections with *D. caninum*.[24] However, nitroscanate is approved in Canada for treatment of *D. caninum* infections in dogs at a dosage of 50 mg/kg. Nitazoxanide has been given to dogs and cats infected with *D. caninum* and was 100% effective at a single dosage of 100 mg/kg.[25] Over the last few years, there have been reports of *D. caninum* infections in dogs in the USA that could not be eliminated despite effective flea control and therapeutic dosages of either praziquantel or epsiprantel.

TABLE 115.1 Recommended Drugs for Treating *Dipylidium caninum* Infections in Dogs and Cats

Drug	Species	Dose (mg/kg)	Route	Interval
Praziquantel	B	5.0	PO	Once
	B	5.7	IM/SC	Once
	C	8.0	TD	Once
Epsiprantel	D	5.5	PO	Once
	C	2.75	PO	Once
Nitroscanate	D	50	PO	Once
Nitazoxanide	B	100	PO	Once

B, both dog and cat; *C*, cat; *D*, dog; *TD*, transdermal.

Cases were resolved following treatment with either nitroscanate or a compounded pyrantel/praziquantel/oxantel formulation.[26]

PREVENTION

With proper flea control and use of an effective anticestodal medication, *D. caninum* infections should be eliminated and the risk of reinfection minimized.

PUBLIC HEALTH ASPECTS

Dipylidium caninum can infect people. Young children are at greatest risk due to their propensity to sample their environment orally leading to ingestion of flea intermediate hosts.[27] Human infections have been reported worldwide. A recent publication described 349 human cases of dipylidiasis, distributed among 24 countries; more than 100 cases were reported in Italy, followed by the USA (86 cases), Japan (81 cases), China (30 cases), Chile (18 cases), Poland (6 cases), India (5 cases), and Mexico, Brazil, Canada, Sri Lanka, and Uruguay (each had 2). Individual cases were reported in other countries. More than two-thirds of the cases were in small children.[28] Most humans with dipylidiasis are asymptomatic; however, anal pruritus, diarrhea, or mild abdominal pain may occur. Flea control in pets should eliminate environmental infestations and minimize the risk of human infection.

TAENIA SPP. INFECTIONS

ETIOLOGY AND EPIDEMIOLOGY

The *Taenia* genus belongs to the cyclophyllidean group of tapeworms and has multiple species that utilize dogs, and one that utilizes cats, as definitive hosts. Like *D. caninum*, definitive hosts are infected by ingestion of the metacestode (immature or larval) stage within the tissues of an intermediate host (Fig. 115.3). *Taenia* species typically form one of three different kinds of metacestode: a cysticercus, strobilocercus, or coenurus (Table 115.2). A cysticercus is composed of a single bladder within which is a single immature parasite with a protoscolex. A strobilocercus also consists of a single bladder that contains a single immature parasite; however, unlike a cysticercus, the strobilocercus contains a protoscolex with a long segmented body. Thus, elongation and segmentation has begun in the intermediate host. A coenurus is composed of a single bladder, within which are many protoscolices; each protoscolex has the potential to develop into a mature tapeworm. Dogs are infected with *Taenia pisiformis* when the cysticercus is consumed in the viscera of rabbits or rodents (see Table 115.2). For *Taenia*

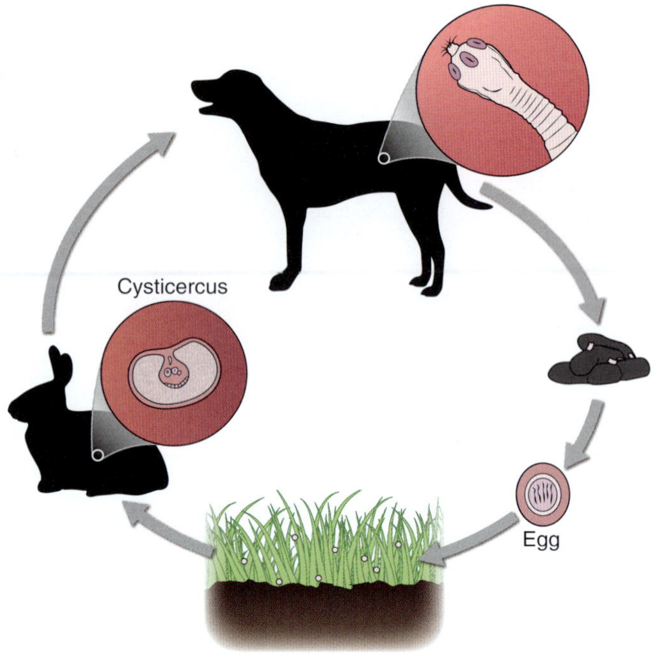

Fig. 115.3 Life cycle of *Taenia pisiformis.*

crassiceps, dogs are infected when the cysticercus is consumed in the viscera of rodents. Dogs are infected with *Taenia hydatigena* when the cysticercus is consumed in the viscera of ruminants, horses, and pigs. *Taenia ovis* infects dogs when the cysticercus is ingested in the muscle of sheep or goats (see Table 115.2). The metacestode stage of *Taenia multiceps* is a coenurus and infects dogs following consumption of the brain or spine of sheep or cattle. The metacestode of *Taenia serialis* is also a coenurus and infects dogs following consumption of connective tissue of rabbits or rodents. Cats are infected with *T. taeniaeformis* by ingesting rodents containing a strobilocercus, typically within the liver (see Table 115.2).[3]

Once the metacestode stage is consumed by a dog or cat, it develops into an adult tapeworm in the lumen of the small intestine. Gravid tapeworm segments containing eggs detach and are excreted in feces. *Taenia pisiformis* reaches patency in approximately 56 days, *T. crassiceps* in 27 to 31 days, *T. hydatigena* in 51 days, *T. ovis* in 42 to 63 days, *T. multiceps* in 30 days, *T. serialis* in 1 to 2 months, and *T. taeniaeformis* in 40 days.[11,29] If a suitable intermediate host ingests the eggs, which are immediately infective in fresh feces, the oncosphere hatches, penetrates the intestinal wall, and migrates to the preferred organ. Here the embryo grows, cavitates, and forms the metacestode stage that is infective to the definitive host.[11]

Necropsy surveys indicate that *Taenia* spp. infections are common in dogs and cats; prevalences in North America have been reported between 25.0% and 29.7% for dogs (*T. pisiformis*), and between 25.9 and 33.0% in cats (*T. taeniaeformis*).[13–15] In Iran, 90 dogs were necropsied; *T. hydatigena* was recovered in 43%, *T. multiceps* in 11%, and *T. ovis* in 3%.[6] In Albania, 111 dogs were necropsied; *T. hydatigena* was recovered in 2.7%.[30]

When fecal flotation is utilized as the sole detection method, the observed prevalence of infection is typically much lower than that observed by necropsy.[13,15,31] However, the sensitivity of fecal flotation depends on the flotation method used. For example, in a 2015 study from Oklahoma, 30/116 (25.9%) cats were detected as infected with *T. taeniaeformis* by necropsy. Fecal flotation was performed on all the cats utilizing two flotation methods: passive flotation with $NaNO_3$ and centrifugal flotation with Sheather's sucrose solution.

TABLE 115.2 *Taenia* Species that Infect Dogs and Cats

Species	Definitive Host	Prepatent Period (Days)	Intermediate Host	INFECTIVE METACESTODE Type	Location
Taenia pisiformis	Dog, wild canids	56	Rabbit, rodents	Cysticercus	Abdominal cavity, liver
Taenia crassiceps	Dog, wild canids	27–31	Rodents	Cysticercus	Abdominal or thoracic cavity
Taenia hydatigena	Dog, wild canids	51	Ruminants, horses, pigs	Cysticercus	Abdominal cavity, liver
Taenia ovis	Dog, wild canids	42–63	Sheep, goat	Cysticercus	Muscle
Taenia multiceps	Dog, wild canids	30	Sheep, cattle	Coenurus	Brain, spinal cord
Taenia serialis	Dog, wild canids	30–60	Rabbit, rodents	Coenurus	Connective tissue
Taenia taeniaeformis	Cat, wild felids	40	Rodents	Strobilocercus	Liver

Centrifugal flotation detected 8/30 infected cats (26.7%); passive flotation detected only 3/30 infected cats (10.0%).[15] In fecal flotations, *Taenia* species eggs are morphologically indistinguishable from one another and from *Echinococcus* spp.; a diagnosis to species level requires identification of adults procured at necropsy or the use of molecular techniques. For example, a recent study in Turkey demonstrated that 27 of 100 dogs were positive for taeniid eggs by centrifugal flotation and sedimentation. *Echinococcus granulosus*-specific PCR products were obtained in 14/27 (51.9%) taeniid specimens. Since additional PCR analysis was not conducted, the remaining 13/27 positive taeniid specimens can be presumed to be other *Echinococcus* or *Taenia* spp.[32]

CLINICAL FEATURES

Pathogenesis and Clinical Signs

The current dogma is that *Taenia* spp. infections in dogs and cats are generally not associated with clinical signs. As for dipylidiasis, some infected animals will exhibit scooting behavior associated with anal pruritus, but other conditions such as impacted anal glands will lead to the same behavior. Several case reports describe cats with *Taenia* sp. impactions.[33,34]

Dogs and cats are rarely infected with the metacestode stages of *Taenia* spp. However, disseminated abdominal, thoracic, or subcutaneous cysticercosis due to *T. crassiceps* has been reported in dogs;[35–37] a compromised immune system may have played a role in the pathogenesis. Occasional cases of feline cerebral coenurosis due to *T. serialis* have been described in Australia and North America. In all cases the diagnosis was made at necropsy following morphological identification of cerebral coenuri (i.e., fluid-filled cysts containing characteristic protosolices). *Taenia serialis* normally utilizes a dog as the definitive host and a lagomorph or rodent as the intermediate host. The rare cat that develops cerebral coenurosis presumably is infected by ingesting eggs passed by an infected dog; the larvae then aberrantly migrate to the cat's cerebrum.[38] Neurocysticercosis due to *T. crassiceps* has been rarely described in cats.[39]

DIAGNOSIS

When fully intact *Taenia* spp. are grossly identified, characteristic features include a scolex with four suckers and a non-retractable rostellum armed with two rows of hooks (Fig. 115.4A). Depending on the maturity of the specimen, the length of the tapeworm can range from tens to hundreds of centimeters. The segments are rectangular with alternating unilateral genital pores (Fig. 115.4B and C). Typical taeniid eggs are usually observed in gravid segments (Fig. 115.4D). Morphologic identification is based on the number and size of rostellar hooks and the morphology of mature segments.[40] It is recommended that fresh (in saline) specimens be submitted to a reference laboratory for speciation efforts; fixation in formalin may preclude proper identification.

Diagnosis of *Taenia* spp. infection in dogs and cats is most commonly based on detection of segments on the haircoat or skin of the host or in freshly passed feces, as well as detection of eggs by fecal flotation. As for *D. caninum*, both methods are very insensitive;[15,31] segments are excreted intermittently and eggs are only present in feces if the segment is damaged in the GI tract or during preparation of the fecal specimen for examination. However, segments should be examined when present as identification informs advice on prevention of reinfection. A single lateral genital pore may be observed (see Fig. 115.4B) which differentiates *Taenia* spp. from *D. caninum*. Furthermore, segments can be differentiated from those of *Echinococcus* spp. as *Taenia* spp. segments are more rectangular and much larger (Fig. 115.5). As with other tapeworms, the presence of calcareous corpuscles allows one to distinguish between a cestode segment and a pseudoparasite (e.g., small foreign body).[41] Molecular techniques allow identification of adult parasites or segments to the species level.[42]

Eggs may be identified in segments or free in feces. They have a thick shell wall with radial striations, are brown, and 25 to 40 μm in diameter. *Taenia* spp. eggs are morphologically indistinguishable from those of *Echinococcus* spp. (Fig. 115.4D).

Two methods for characterization of taeniid eggs in fecal specimens have been developed: PCR and copro-antigen detection by ELISA. In a study from Iran, 450 canine fecal specimens were evaluated; taeniid eggs were observed in 25 specimens (5.6%) by microscopic examination using formalin-ethyl acetate sedimentation. Use of a multiplex PCR assay identified *E. granulosus* in 2/25 (8.0%), *Taenia* spp. in 17/25 (68.0 %), and co-infection with *E. granulosus* and *Taenia* spp. in 6/25 (24.0%) of the positive specimens. *Echinococcus multilocularis* DNA was not detected in any of the specimens.[42] Multiplex PCR has also been utilized to distinguish individual *Taenia* spp.; an Australian study identified *T. ovis, T. hydatigena, T. serialis,* and *T. pisiformis* in the feces of red foxes (*Vulpes vulpes*) and wild dogs.[43] Detection of parasite antigen in feces is another promising area of focus for detection of *Taenia* spp. and *Echinococcus* spp. However, while these tests typically have high sensitivity, they are generally genus specific. Even so, this approach offers several advantages, namely: antigen can be detected in feces weeks before patency, the levels of antigen in feces are independent of egg production, copro-antigen is stable in feces for days at a range of temperatures and for several months in formalin-fixed feces, and copro-antigen levels drop rapidly, in 1 to 5 days, following successful treatment.[44]

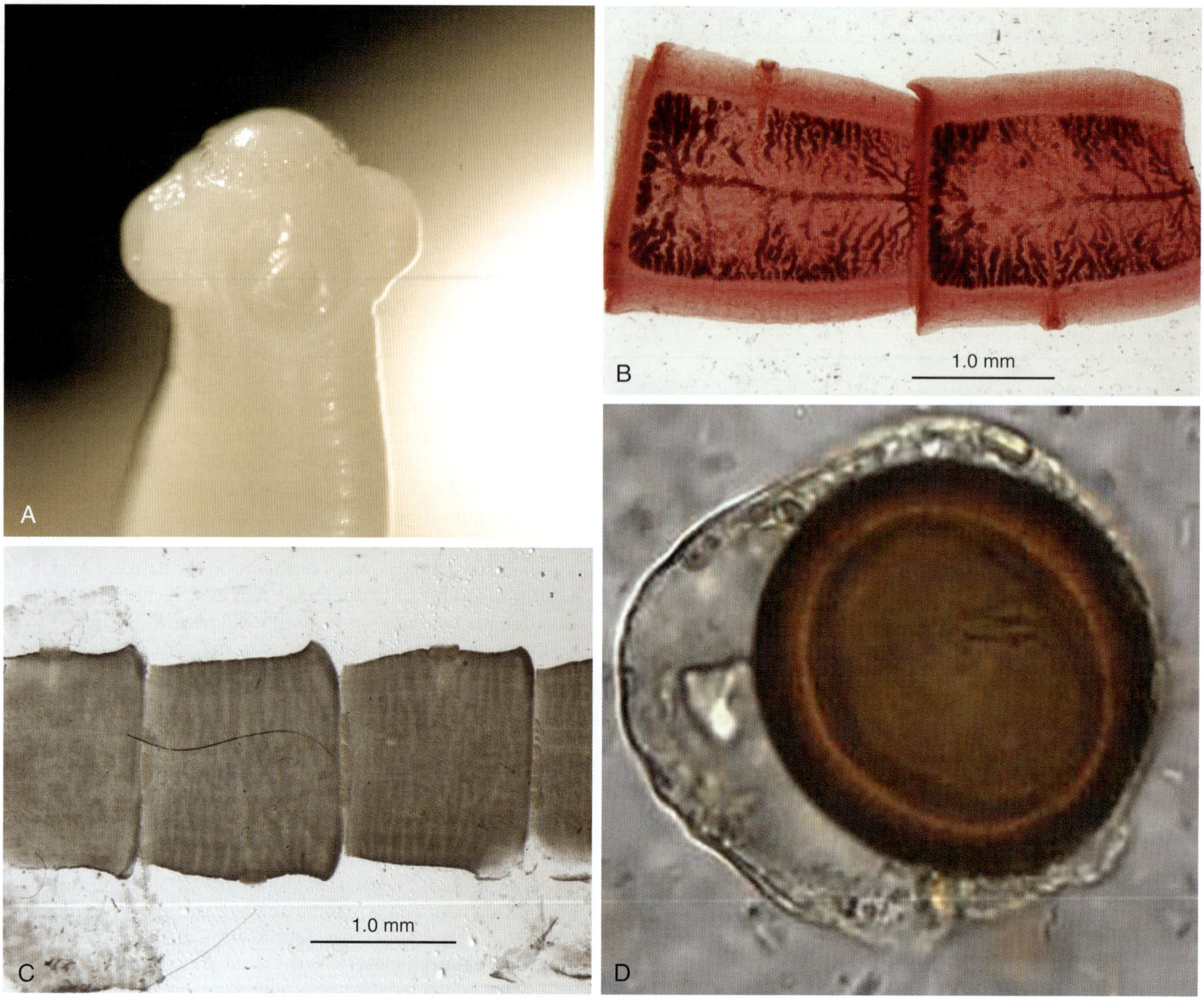

Fig. 115.4 Morphologic features of *Taenia* sp. (A) Scolex. Note the non-retractable rostellum armed with rows of hooks and four suckers. (B) Stained and (C) unstained segment showing alternating unilateral genital pore. (D) Egg. Note the thick shell wall and two of the six hooks visible in the embryo. (A, B, and C courtesy of Megan Lineberry, National Center for Veterinary Parasitology, Oklahoma State University.)

TREATMENT AND PROGNOSIS

Praziquantel or epsiprantel are effective for treatment of *Taenia* spp. infections using the same dosages as used for *D. caninum* (Table 115.3).[23] In the USA, fenbendazole is approved at 50 mg/kg q24h for 3 consecutive days for *T. pisiformis* in dogs; in the UK, the same drug dosage is approved for use in dogs and cats for *Taenia* spp.. Nitroscanate is approved in some countries for use in dogs; a dosage of 50 mg/kg was 98% effective against *T. hydatigena*, *T. ovis*, and *T. pisiformis*.[24] Nitazoxanide has been used to treat dogs and cats infected with *T. pisiformis* and *T. taeniaeformis*, respectively. The drug was 100% effective against both cestodes at a single dose of 100 mg/kg.[25]

PREVENTION

Prevention of *Taenia* spp. infections is essentially limited to minimizing the risk of ingestion of infected intermediate hosts, which requires confinement. Ideally, the *Taenia* species infecting a dog or cat should be identified as this will allow one to determine the most likely source of infection. Pets can then be administered an effective anticestodal medication periodically based on risk factors for exposure. Depending on the *Taenia* spp. involved, *Taenia* spp. that infect dogs and cats have PPPs of 27 to 63 days (see Table 115.2). If limiting predation of intermediate hosts is not possible, anticestodal medication could be considered every 6 to 12 weeks; preventive treatment at intervals slightly greater than the PPP typically provides adequate control because not all intermediate hosts are infected with the metacestode.

PUBLIC HEALTH ASPECTS

Occasionally, the metacestode stages of *T. crassiceps*, *T. multiceps*, *T. serialis*, and *T. taeniaeformis* have been described in people. However, overall, the risk of zoonotic infection by these *Taenia* spp. is very low and often associated with immunosuppression;[45] infections are likely

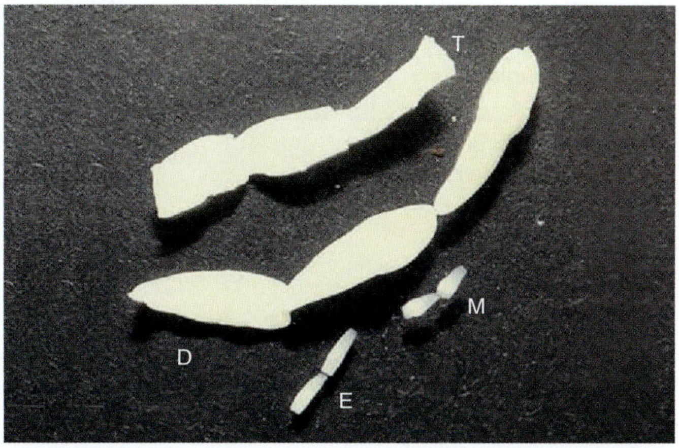

Fig. 115.5 Mature tapeworm segments passed in the feces may be observed by owners and presented for identification. *Taenia* segments *(T)* are square to rectangular in shape, *Dipylidium* segments *(D)* are more barrel shaped, and *Mesocestoides (M)* has club-shaped segments. Both *Mesocestoides* and *Echinococcus (E)* segments are small and are often overlooked. Identification can be confirmed by examining eggs from the segments. (From *Veterinary Clinical Parasitology*, 8th edition, page 77, Fig 1.97; used with permission from John Wiley and Sons License number 4530290914537.)[20]

TABLE 115.3 Recommended Drugs for Treatment of *Taenia* spp. in Dogs and Cats

Drug	Species	Indication	Dosage (mg/kg)[d]	Route
Praziquantel	B	*T. pisiformis*[a,b], *T. multiceps*[b], *T. hydatigena*[b], *T. ovis*[b] *T. taeniaeformis*[a]	5.0	PO
	B	*T. pisiformis*[a] *T. taeniaeformis*[a]	5.7	IM/SC
Epsiprantel	C	*Taenia* spp.[b]	8.0	TD
	D	*T. pisiformis*[a]	5.5	PO
	C	*T. taeniaeformis*[a]	2.75	PO
Fenbendazole	D	*T. pisiformis*[a]	50	PO
	B	*Taenia* spp.[b]	50	PO
Nitroscanate	D	*Taenia* spp.[c]	50	PO
Nitazoxanide	D	*T. pisiformis*	100	PO
	C	*T. taeniaeformis*	100	PO

[a]USA; [b]United Kingdom; [c]Canada.
[d]All doses are for one time administration, with the exception of fenbendazole, which is given q24h for 3 days.
B, both dog and cat; *C*, cat; *D*, dog; *TD*, transdermal.

acquired via ingestion of eggs in the feces of dogs or cats. Dogs and cats are not involved in the life cycle of *T. saginata* (beef tapeworm) and *T. solium* (pork tapeworm).

ECHINOCOCCUS SPP. INFECTIONS (ECHINOCOCCOSIS)

ETIOLOGY AND EPIDEMIOLOGY

All species in the genus *Echinococcus* have a predator-prey, indirect life cycle that commonly involves wildlife. However, some occur in significant domestic life cycles. The adult tapeworms of all species are only a few millimeters in length and reside within the small intestine of carnivores, especially canids. Intermediate hosts range from livestock to rodents. Most species are infective for people. However, globally, the two most important species are *E. granulosus* sensu lato (s.l.) and *Echinococcus multilocularis*.

Echinococcus granulosus sensu lato Infections

Echinococcus granulosus s.l. occurs in animals and people and is found worldwide, except for Greenland and Iceland which are considered free of the parasite.[46] This etiologic agent is composed of multiple genotypes/species that differ in host specificity, morphology, geographical distribution, and human pathogenicity (Table 115.4).[47–49] Dogs are the definitive host for most genotypes/species. However, wild canids can also be definitive hosts for some. Following ingestion of eggs, the intermediate stage, a hydatid cyst, develops within internal organs of intermediate hosts (primarily ruminants, horses, pigs) and accidental hosts (people and other mammals). The resultant disease is termed cystic echinococcosis (CE). Furthermore, while most species/strains of *E. granulosus* s.l. have been associated with CE in people, the majority of human cases are due to *E. granulosus* sensu stricto (s.s.) (sheep strain) (dangerous dog tapeworm, dwarf dog tapeworm).[48,50] This genotype is therefore the primary focus of the rest of this section.

Dogs are the primary definitive host for *E. granulosus* s.s. However, wild canids such as foxes, coyotes, and dingoes may also serve as definitive hosts. Domestic herbivores and omnivores (e.g., sheep, cattle, buffalo, goat, camel, pig) are the predominant intermediate hosts. Furthermore, while sheep are the primary intermediate host in many regions, reindeer constitute the primary intermediate host in parts of northern Europe and northern Russia; camels are the main reservoir in parts of the Middle East.[51]

Adult tapeworms develop within the small intestine of definitive hosts and live for approximately 6 months. Once segments are fully mature, they usually disintegrate within the intestine to release eggs that are shed in feces and are immediately infective. Both intermediate hosts and accidental hosts, including people, are infected by ingestion of eggs. Subsequently, oncospheres hatch from eggs within the small intestine, penetrate blood vessels, and travel primarily to the liver where they develop into hydatid cysts, the metacestode stage. Hydatid cysts are composed of an outer acellular laminated layer and an inner germinal layer. Weeks to months following infection, the germinal layer may generate brood capsules, 0.25 to 1.5 mm in diameter, that each contain up to approximately 40 protoscolices. Brood capsule walls may subsequently rupture. Thus, hydatid cysts occur either as a single, fluid-filled, cyst or one large cyst containing multiple smaller cysts; hydatid fluid is composed of protoscolices, calcareous corpuscles, and potentially brood capsules that collectively are referred to as "hydatid sand". Cysts may take 6 to 12 months to mature and, depending on the host species, age of the animal, and organ involved, may vary in diameter from 1 mm to 20 cm. In intermediate hosts and people, the liver and lungs are the primary organs involved. Less commonly, cysts develop in body cavities, the CNS, eye, kidney, muscle, or spleen. Cysts may remain viable for lengthy periods (Fig. 115.6). The life cycle is completed when fertile hydatid cysts are eaten by dogs and wild canids. In dogs, the PPP is 34 to 58 days.[52,53]

Although *E. granulosus* s.s. occurs in wildlife species, it is the domestic life cycle that is of particular zoonotic concern. Thus, CE in people is especially common in parts of Africa, Asia, Australia, Europe, the Middle East, and South America where the following condition(s) occur that facilitate establishment of the domestic cycle: (1) large sheep and dog populations, (2) dogs that have access to dead livestock or offal, (3) cestocide treatment of dogs is lacking, (4) communities have a low socioeconomic status. Prevalences of hydatid cyst detection in sheep in excess of 40% have been demonstrated in parts of China,

TABLE 115.4 **Species, Strains, and Genotypes of *Echinococcus granulosus* sensu lato**

Species/Strain/Genotype	Distribution	Definitive Host	Intermediate Host	Occurrence of Cystic Echinococcosis in People
Echinococcus granulosus s.s. sheep (and buffalo) strains G1-G3	Worldwide	Dog Wild canids	Sheep, cattle, buffalo, goat, camel, yak	Yes
Echinococcus equinus horse strain G4	Africa, Europe, Middle East, USA	Dog	Horse, donkey, zebra	Not reported
Echinococcus ortleppi cattle strain G5	Africa, Asia, Central & South America, Europe	Dog	Cattle, buffalo, goat, sheep	Yes
Echinococcus canadensis cluster				
Camel strain G6	Africa, Asia, South America	Dog	Camel, cattle, goat, sheep	Yes
Pig strain G7	Worldwide focally	Dog	Pig, wild boar, (cattle)	Yes
Cervid strains G8, G10	Eurasia, North America	Dog Wild canids	Moose, reindeer, wapiti	Yes
Echinococcus felidis lion strain	Africa	Lion	Warthog	Not reported

After Thompson (2008),[50] Deplazes et al (2016),[53] and Romig T, Deplazes P, Jenkins D, et al. Chapter Five – Ecology and life cycle patterns of *Echinococcus* species. *Adv Parasitol.* 2017;95:213–314.

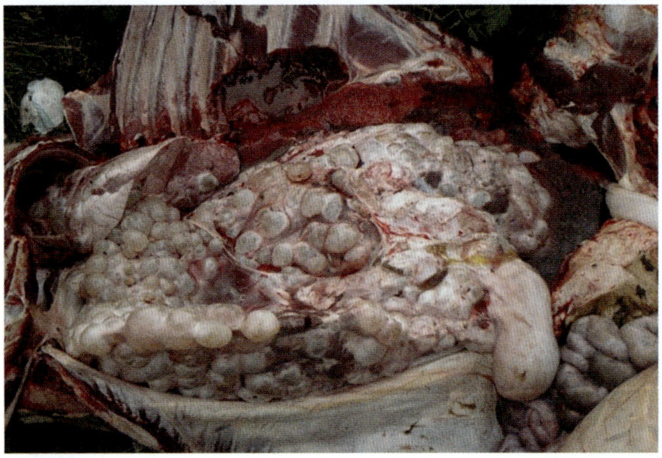

Fig. 115.6 Large burden of hydatid cysts throughout the abdomen of a cow in Kosovo. (Courtesy of Dr. Naim Zeqiri and Dr. Arsim Ademi, Kosovo.)

Ethiopia, Iran, Italy, and Kyrgystan.[51] While few studies have evaluated the prevalence of *E. granuosus* s.l. in dogs in many of these regions, in some areas of Italy the prevalence of hydatid cysts in sheep has been 23.5% to 27.9%; in the same areas, 24.6% of dogs were copro-antigen-positive for *E. granulosus* s.l.; significant levels of CE have been identified in people in the same region.[54]

Human infections only occur following ingestion of eggs, which primarily occur in feces or an environment contaminated with feces, or on the skin and coat, of dogs. Unfortunately, little information is available on the typical prevalence of infection in dogs in endemic areas. *Echinococcus granulosus* s.l. infection prevalences of 3.8% were reported for farm dogs in Lithuania[55] and 10.6% for farm dogs in Wales.[56]

In moist environments, eggs can remain viable for weeks to months. However, the duration of viability is greatly reduced in low humidity. At temperatures of 75 to 100°C, eggs are destroyed within minutes; at −80°C this takes approximately 48 hours. Commonly used chemical disinfectants do not destroy eggs.[53]

While cats are not definitive hosts for *E. granulosus* s.l., a few cases of CE have been reported in cats. CE due to *E. granulosus* s.s. (genotype 1) has been described in cats from Russia and Uruguay;[57,58] and CE due to *E. granulosus* s.l. was reported in a cat in Turkey.[59] One of the cats was co-infected with FIV;[58] the other two cats were not tested for retrovirus infection.

Echinococcus multilocularis (Dwarf Fox Tapeworm)

Echinococcus multilocularis is a zoonotic tapeworm that occurs throughout the northern hemisphere, primarily in a wildlife-associated life cycle. Across its distribution, only minor genetic variation has been observed.[60] In North America, *E. multilocularis* has historically been considered to occur in two distinct geographic regions: the Northern Tundra Zone that extends from the west coast of Alaska to parts of the Canadian arctic,[61] and the North Central Region that includes the southern parts of three Canadian provinces (Alberta, Saskatchewan, Manitoba) and 13 midwestern US states (North Dakota, South Dakota, Iowa, Minnesota, Montana, Wyoming, Nebraska, Illinois, Wisconsin, Indiana, Ohio, Missouri, Michigan).[61–63] However, the geographical range has been expanding into parts of British Columbia and Ontario, Canada.[64,65] In Europe, the parasite has historically occurred in Austria, France, Germany, and Switzerland. However, over the last two decades the distribution of the parasite has extended into western, northern, and eastern parts of Europe, involving a total of 21 countries; those with the highest prevalence of infection in definitive hosts (>10%) include the Czech Republic, Estonia, France, Germany, Latvia, Liechtenstein, Lithuania, Poland, Slovakia, and Switzerland. European countries currently free of *E. multilocularis* in wild canids are Finland, Ireland, the United Kingdom, and mainland Norway.[66,67] The parasite also occurs throughout much of the Middle East (e.g., Turkey, Iran) and Asia (e.g., Russia, China, Japan).[68,69]

Adult *E. multilocularis* reside within the distal small intestine of definitive hosts, which are primarily wild canids. In Europe, the red fox is the primary definitive host. In North America, coyotes, wolves, and arctic foxes also harbor adult parasites and may play a significant role in the epidemiology. Domestic dogs may also be definitive hosts. Dogs also can play an important role in the epidemiology in parts of Alaska and Asia (e.g., China).[53,70] Domestic cats and wild felids occasionally develop intestinal infections but are of minor importance in the epidemiology due to the short duration, and low levels, of fecal egg excretion.[71]

Like *E. granulosus* s.l. eggs, eggs of *E. multilocularis* are morphologically indistinguishable from eggs of *Taenia* spp. and are immediately infective for intermediate and accidental hosts. Intermediate hosts for *E. multilocularis* are primarily wild rodents.[72] Accidental hosts include humans, non-human primates, pigs, horses, and dogs. Both intermediate and accidental hosts become infected by ingestion of eggs (Fig. 115.7). Subsequently, an oncosphere hatches from the egg, typically travels to the liver via the hepatic portal circulation, and develops into

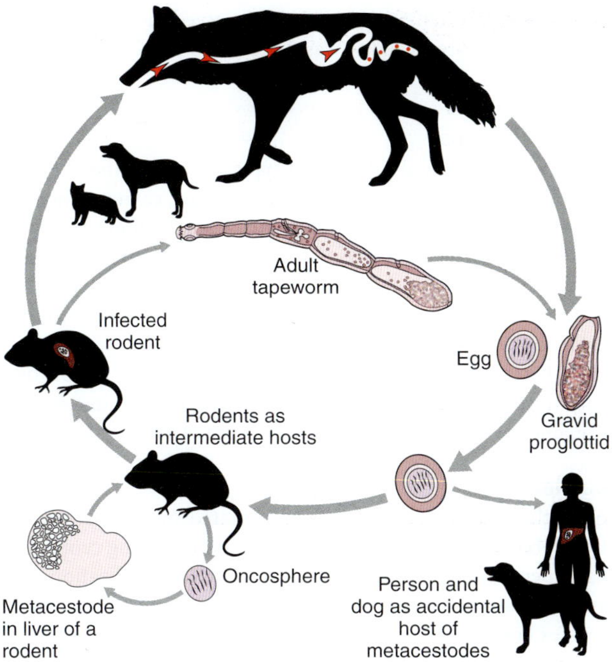

Fig. 115.7 Life cycle of *Echinococcus multilocularis*.

the metacestode. This stage comprises numerous small vesicles that vary in size from <1 mm to 3 cm in diameter; the wall is composed of an outer laminated layer and an inner germinal epithelium from which multiple protoscolices may develop. In intermediate hosts that are highly susceptible to infection, protoscolices develop in 2 to 4 months. In less susceptible hosts, the rate of development is slower or the number of protoscolices that develop is reduced or absent. Unlike hydatid cysts caused by *E. granulosus* s.l., the metacestode of *E. multilocularis* undergoes exogenous budding. During this process, the metacestode buds smaller portions of its cystic-like structure that invade neighboring tissue and may spread to distant organs, mimicking an invasive tumor.[46] By the time clinical signs develop, there is usually substantive involvement of the liver. The resultant disease, alveolar echinococcosis (AE), is usually associated with extensive hepatic damage and occasionally spreads to other locations (e.g., lungs, brain, bone). The life cycle is completed when an infected intermediate host is ingested by a definitive host; development of adult tapeworms takes approximately 4 to 5 weeks.[71] Thereafter, egg excretion usually lasts a few weeks. However, some parasites persist for up to 12 months. In experimental work, the duration and level of egg excretion in cats has been substantively less than in dogs.[73,74]

Across Europe, pooled prevalence estimates of infection in red foxes range from <1% to >50%.[67] Furthermore, within endemic areas the focal prevalence of infection in red foxes shows regional variability.[75,76] High prevalences have been observed in fox populations that have established in multiple European cities over the last two decades. For example, in Geneva, Stuttgart, and Zurich in Switzerland, the prevalence of infection in red foxes ranges from 17% to 44%.[77] This, in turn, has been associated with the establishment of urban parasite life cycles. For example, fecal analysis of 660 randomly selected, privately owned dogs in a densely populated part of eastern Switzerland demonstrated an *E. multilocularis* prevalence of 0.3%; in the same area, 0.4% of 263 cats were infected.[78] Among dogs in endemic European countries, a pooled estimate for the prevalence of intestinal infections was 0.3%.[67] However, among dogs that roam freely and have access to rodents, a prevalence as high as 8.1% has been described.[79]

Infected dogs, particularly in urban environments, constitute a significant risk for human infection. For example, in central Europe, 4% to 19% of environmental contamination with *E. multilocularis* eggs is associated with domestic dogs. The contribution of cats is considered insignificant (<0.3%).[80] Within North America, there are very few reports of intestinal infections in dogs or cats in either the USA or Canada. Historically, prevalences of infection up to 12% have been observed in some dog populations on St. Lawrence Island, Alaska.[81] However, outside Alaska, intestinal infections in dogs appear to have been evaluated only three times; using molecular methods, *E. multilocularis* was identified in feces of 1/218 (0.5%) dogs in Alberta[63] and 0/477 (0%) dogs in Ontario[82]; an intestinal infection has recently been described in a dog in Missouri.[83] Similarly, only five cats have been reported with intestinal infections (three in Saskatchewan;[84] two in North Dakota).[85] Under central European summer conditions, with adequate moisture, eggs of *E. multilocularis* survive in the environment for 2 to 3 months. Under cooler conditions and at −20°C, eggs may remain viable for months. However, as with *E. granulosus* s.l., eggs are susceptible to desiccation. Temperatures in excess of 70°C inactivate eggs. At −80°C, infectivity is lost after 48 hours.[53]

Alveolar Echinococcosis in Dogs

Since the late 1980s, cases of AE, primarily involving the liver, have been described in domestic dogs in Switzerland, Germany, France, and Belgium.[72,86] These cases are thought to occur either as a result of ingestion of large numbers of infective eggs (e.g., in the feces of foxes) or by autoinfection in association with the presence of adult *E. multilocularis* in the small intestine.[87,88] Of the cases seen in Switzerland, the median age at diagnosis is 3.1 years (range = 1.1–10.7 years), with no significant breed predilection.[88]

Prior to 2009, AE had not been diagnosed in a dog in North America. However, in 2009, hepatic AE was diagnosed in a 3-year-old dog that had lived permanently in British Columbia,[64] a Canadian province previously considered free of *E. multilocularis*. Subsequently, examination of wild canids in the area where the dog resided indicated that 11/33 (33%) were infected with *E. multilocularis*.[89] Between 2009 and 2020, at least 25 dogs have been described with AE in Canada: in British Columbia, Alberta, Saskatchewan, Manitoba, and southern Ontario.[19,65,69,90,91] Furthermore, the Ontario dogs were generally from an area where the prevalence of *E. multilocularis* in wild canids is >30%.[92] In 2020, AE was described in an 8-year-old Labrador retriever that was acquired as a puppy from Mississippi and brought to Virginia,[93] which is the first case reported in the United States.

CLINICAL FEATURES

Pathogenesis and Clinical Signs

Echinococcus granulosus s.l. Infection

Dogs (definitive host). Parasites are typically found in the proximal small intestine, deeply embedded within crypts and attached to the mucosa via the scolex. This usually results in minimal damage, even when substantive parasite burdens are present (similar to Fig. 115.8); minor damage to the epithelium and mild cellular infiltration of the mucosa may be observed. Thus, intestinal infections are typically subclinical, even when large numbers of parasites are present. When parasite burdens are heavy, segments of *Echinococcus* spp. are occasionally found on the perianal region or in feces; they are white and 0.5 to 3.0 mm long.

Cats (accidental hosts). In all three cats described in the literature, large numbers (>150) of fluid-filled, transparent-white, hydatid cysts,

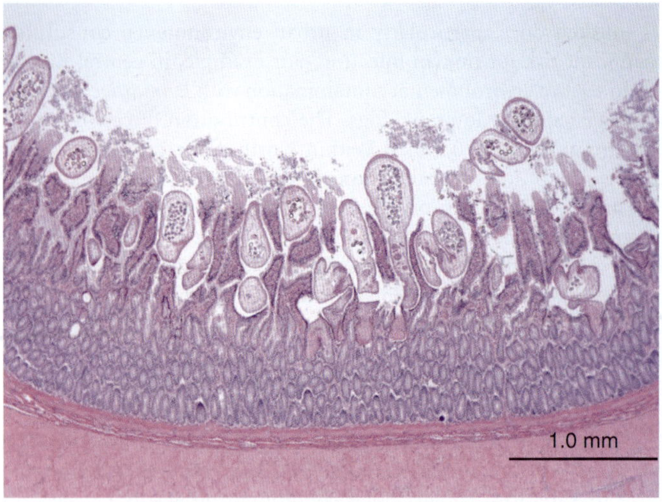

Fig. 115.8 Histopathology of the small intestine of a coyote (*Canis latrans*) infected with *Echinococcus multilocularis*. Multiple cross and longitudinal sections of *E. multilocularis* are present between villi. Note the presence of eggs within segments. There is no associated tissue response or inflammation. (Courtesy of Dr. Jamie L. Rothenburger, Faculty of Veterinary Medicine, University of Calgary, and Canadian Wildlife Health Cooperative.)

0.1 to 5.0 cm in diameter, were found free in the abdomen and attached to serosal surfaces. In one cat, multiple cysts were also present within hepatic parenchyma.[57–59] However, despite substantive cyst burdens, minimal pathology was described. Signs were primarily associated with a progressive space-occupying lesion within the abdomen; all cats had a history of progressive abdominal enlargement. Additional clinical signs included anorexia, dull mentation, polydipsia, dyspnea, and constipation.[57–59] One of the three cats was co-infected with FIV;[58] immunosuppression has been associated with an increased risk of AE in people.[94]

Echinococcus multilocularis Infection

Dogs and cats (definitive hosts). Adult parasites are found attached to the small intestinal mucosa via the scolex, typically deep within intestinal crypts (see Fig. 115.8). Intestinal burdens in dogs are much greater than in cats.[71] However, even when large numbers of parasites are present, lesions are minimal and infections are rarely clinical.

Dogs (accidental hosts). Cases of AE in dogs are typically associated with lesions in the liver; usually, there is significant involvement by the time a diagnosis is made, with lesions up to 10 to 15 cm in diameter. Furthermore, because of the ability of the metacestode to metastasize, secondary lesions may be found elsewhere in the body, both within and outside the abdomen.[95] Dogs with AE usually have signs of abdominal distention, lethargy, anorexia, and vomiting.[87,88] Other, less common, signs include abdominal pain, diarrhea, weight loss, polypnea, fever, and polyphagia.

DIAGNOSIS

Laboratory Abnormalities

Complete Blood Count, Serum Chemistry Profile, and Urinalysis

In dogs and cats with *Echinococcus* spp. intestinal infections, the CBC, serum biochemical tests, and urinalysis are typically unremarkable. In a European study on 11 dogs with AE, the most common serum chemistry abnormalities were hypoalbuminemia (10/11), hyperproteinemia (9/11), increased serum amylase (7/11), and hyperglobulinemia (3/11). Increased liver enzyme activities were only observed in 2/11 dogs. The most significant CBC abnormality was a decreased PCV (3/11).[96]

Diagnostic Imaging

Sonographic Findings

In dogs with AE, abdominal ultrasound typically reveals the presence of one or more large, heterogeneous, poorly limited, cavitated hepatic masses, with or without wall mineralization. Usually, there is a thick hyperechoic outer surface, an irregular inner surface, and a centrally located cavity filled with echogenic fluid.[88,96] Non-cavitated ultrasound patterns are thought to represent early infiltration prior to central liquefaction or cavity formation. A lack of vascularity of masses is evident.[96] Extension to neighboring organs is observed in approximately one-third of cases. Free abdominal fluid is present in a similar proportion and is generally attributed to rupture of cystic structures.[88]

Advanced Imaging

CT of dogs with AE usually reveals cystic to cavitated, or granular, masses within liver lobes; cavitated masses have a hypoattenuating center and a distinct hyperattenuating wall (Fig. 115.9).[96,97] Mineralization may be observed in walls of cavitated masses. The absence of enhancement within masses has been observed and is a characteristic CT feature of AE in people.[98] Progressive mineralization over time is considered a sign of chronic disease and of dystrophic tissue metaplasia because of medical therapy.[99] A lack of vascularity of masses is evident.[96]

Microbiologic Tests

Cytologic Diagnosis

In many dogs, ultrasound-guided fine-needle aspirates of intralesional or peritoneal fluid generates specimens with cytologic morphology consistent with AE, namely, calcareous corpuscles and folded membranous structures (Fig. 115.10).[19] While the former may be associated with any cestode, the folded membranes have only been described in AE cases.

Isolation and Identification

In heavy parasite burdens, a presumptive diagnosis of intestinal infection may be made if segments are found in feces or on the perianal region. However, *Echinococcus* spp. segments are much smaller than those of *Taenia* spp. and *Dipylidium caninum* (see Fig. 115.5) and usually disintegrate before being passed in feces. Eggs of *Echinococcus* spp. may be found in feces using flotation methods. However, this is insensitive and the eggs are indistinguishable from *Taenia* spp. eggs (see *Taenia* earlier in this chapter).[20,53] Eggs of both species are immediately infective for people and appropriate biosecurity practices must be followed when handling intestinal contents and feces.

At necropsy, adult parasites are most likely to be found by: (1) stereoscopic examination of the small intestine, (2) intestinal scraping, and (3) examination of small intestine wash fluid using the sedimentation and counting technique (SCT).[100] The latter method has the highest sensitivity. *Echinococcus granulosus* s.l. are generally located within the proximal small intestine. Adult parasites are 1 to 7 mm in length with a scolex containing two rows of hooks and four suckers. Typically, three (two to six) segments are present. The genital pore is located approximately equidistant from either end of the segment. *Echinococcus multilocularis* are generally located within the distal small intestine.[101] Adult parasites are 2 to 4 mm in length with a scolex containing two rows of hooks and four suckers. Typically, five (two to six) segments are present. The genital pore is located within the anterior half of the segment.

The sensitivity of necropsy examination for diagnosis of intestinal echinococcosis is high (>97%). However, when low parasite burdens are present (<6 parasites), false-negative results may occur, particularly

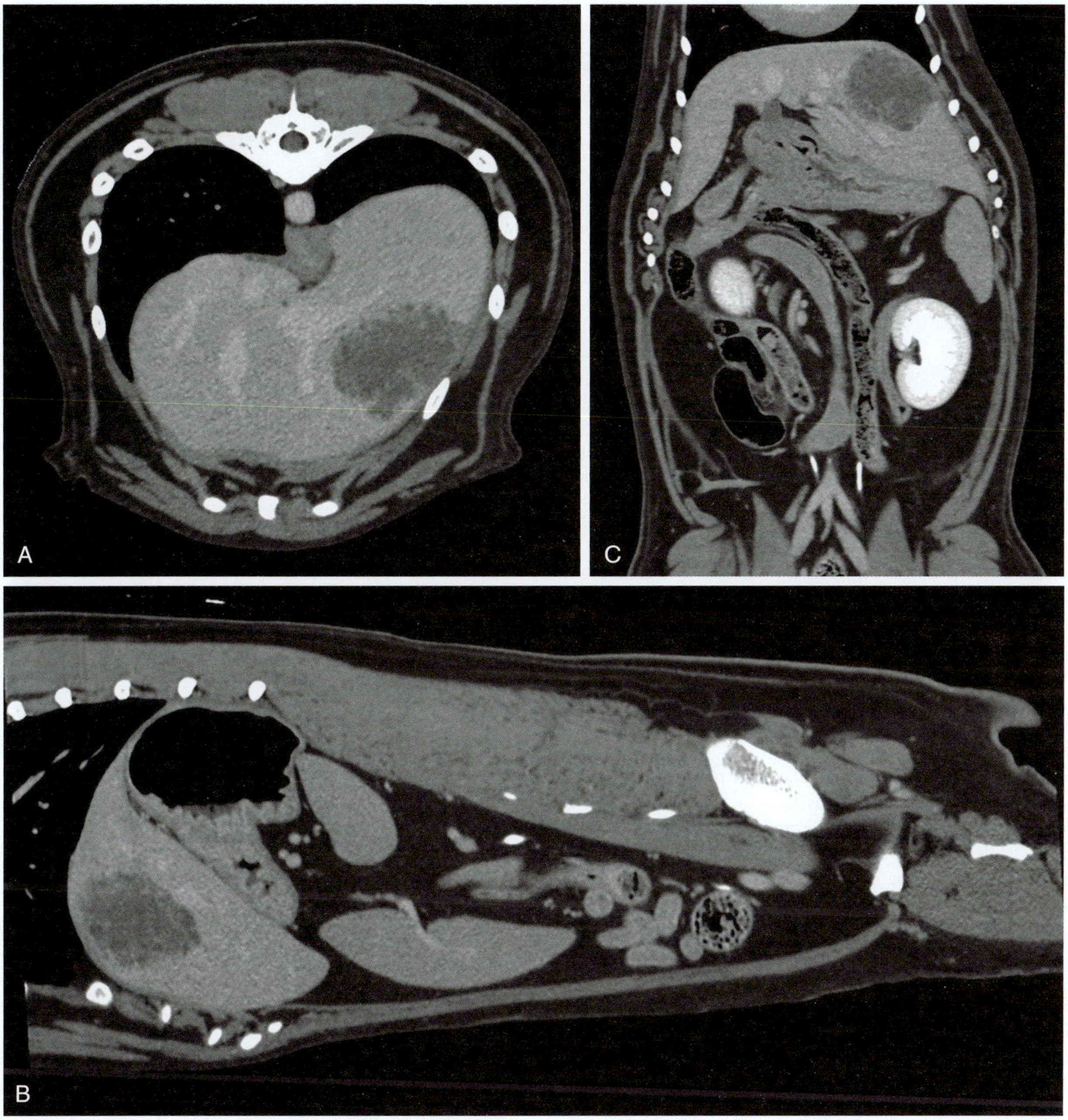

Fig. 115.9 Computed tomography images of a dog with hepatic alveolar echinococcosis. (A) Transverse. (B) Sagittal. (C) Dorsal. (Courtesy of Dr. Taizha Ciasca, Dr. Chris Warren-Smoth, and VetCT.)

if SCT is not performed.[102] Confirmation of the parasite species recovered can be carried out by DNA analysis.[103]

Serologic Diagnosis (Fecal Antigen Detection)

Multiple copro-antigen-detection ELISAs have been developed for examining fecal specimens from dogs for *Echinococcus* spp. but are generally genus specific. Sensitivities of these tests range from 60% to 92%; specificities range from 70% to 96%. Copro-antigen ELISA sensitivity is influenced by parasite burden.[53,102] Cross-reactions are generally associated with infection with *T. hydatigena* but likely also occur with other *Taenia* spp.. Thus, when used on dogs or cats, copro-antigen ELISA-positive results should ideally be confirmed with nucleic acid–based testing.[53]

Serology

Most dogs with AE develop antibodies to an *E. multilocularis*-specific antigen.[88,104] At the time of writing, this diagnostic tool is only available at the Universities of Bern and Zurich, Switzerland. Due to abortive infections, some dogs will seroconvert but not develop AE.[105,106]

Molecular Diagnosis Using Nucleic Acid–Based Testing

Multiple PCR-based assays have been described for detection of *E. granulosus* s.l.[102] and *E. multilocularis*, some of which require isolation of eggs. While most assays have high specificity, sensitivity has been variable; some methods have low sensitivity, presumably due to PCR inhibitors in feces or intermittent shedding of eggs. One *E. multilocularis* PCR assay had an overall sensitivity of 88%; in animals with more than 100 parasites, sensitivity was 95.7%; specificity was at least 99.9%. This assay was selected for use in national surveillance programs of wild canids in Europe and has been used to detect infection in fecal specimens from dogs and cats.[107]

Multiple *Echinococcus* species-specific assays also have been developed for use on tissue specimens. For example, DNA sequence data for

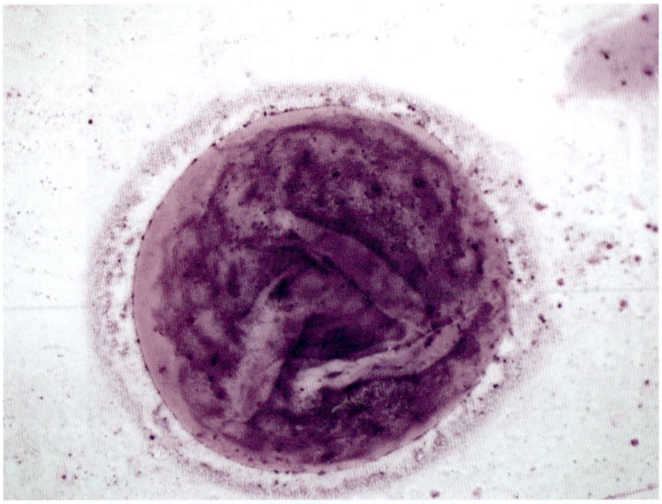

Fig. 115.10 Sediment smear of an aspirate from an abdominal mass in a dog with alveolar echinococcosis showing folded membrane structure. Wright stain, 200× magnification.

PCR-generated fragments of the mitochondrial *12S rRNA* gene[108] and restriction fragment length polymorphism analysis of the *12S rRNA* gene and *NADH dehydrogenase 1* gene[109] can be used to confirm the presence of *E. multilocularis*. Similar methods are available for detection and identification of *E. granulosus* s.l.[48,102]

Pathologic Findings

Gross Pathologic Findings

In dogs with hepatic AE, multiple nodular firm pale-tan masses are typically present that can be readily mistaken for neoplasia, or sometimes abscesses, without histologic examination (Fig. 115.11A). Furthermore, while the liver is the most common organ affected, extension(s) into neighboring organs such as the omentum, peritoneum, and diaphragm may occur.[88] Exogenous budding of the metacestode has also been associated with lesions in the lungs, spleen, vertebral bodies, brain, and prostate of dogs.[87,97]

Histopathologic Findings

Histological examination of tissue biopsies is extremely helpful for diagnosis of AE as morphology is characteristic for *E. multilocularis*;[64,72] hepatic architecture is replaced by multi-loculated coalescing cystic structures surrounded by fibrosis.[88] Lining individual cysts is an eosinophilic hyaline membrane ("laminated layer") that stains with PAS (Fig. 115.11B and C). The inner lining of the hyaline membrane is typically composed of a germinal epithelial layer and a basophilic matrix that contains occasional calcareous corpuscles. Intraluminal protoscolices are sometimes observed. A prominent chronic eosinophilic and granulomatous inflammation is also usually present. The combination of histopathology and a positive *E. multilocularis* species-specific PCR assay is the gold standard for diagnosis of AE.[88,109]

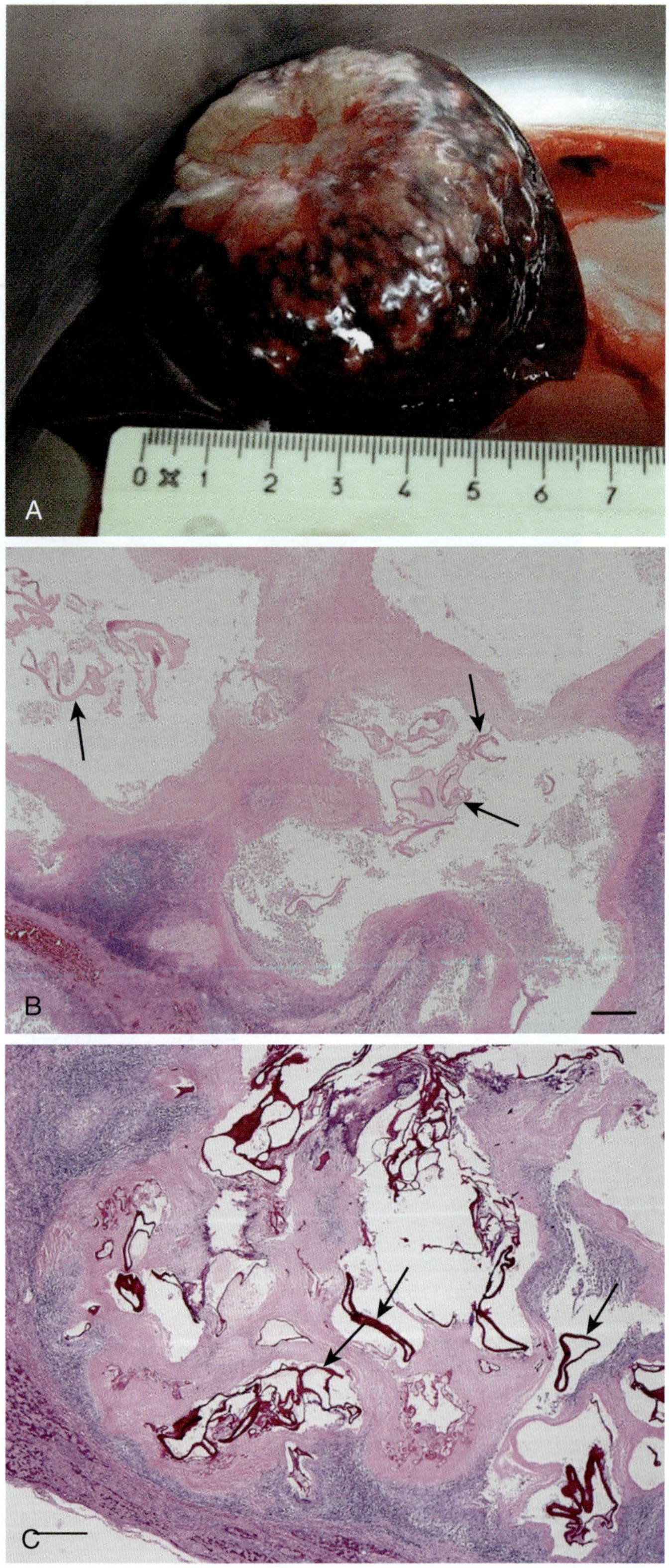

Fig. 115.11 Gross (A) and histopathology (B and C) images of a resected liver lobe from a dog with hepatic alveolar echinococcosis. (B) Degenerating cysts in the liver are lined by a hyaline membrane ("laminated layer"; *arrows*). Hematoxylin and eosin stain, bar = 50 μm. (C) PAS stain demonstrating PAS-positive hyaline membranes *(arrows)* surrounded by eosinophilic granulomatous inflammation and necrosis. Bar = 250 μm. (A, courtesy of Dr. Michelle Oblak. B and C courtesy of Dr. Britta Knight, Ontario Veterinary College, University of Guelph.)

TREATMENT AND PROGNOSIS

E. granulosus s.l. and *E. multilocularis* Intestinal Infections

Praziquantel is most commonly used and typically recommended as a single treatment as it kills both adult and immature parasites in the intestine (see Table 115.5).[110] However, two treatments 24 hours apart

TABLE 115.5 Recommended Drugs for Treating *Echinococcus* spp. Infections in Dogs and Cats

Parasite/Drug (Indication)	Species	Dosage (mg/kg)	Route
E. granulosus s.l.			
Praziquantel (intestinal infection)	D	5.0 5.7	PO IM
Epsiprantel (intestinal infection)	D	5.5	PO
E. multilocularis			
Praziquantel[a] (intestinal infection)	B B C	5.0 5.7 8.0	PO IM TD
Epsiprantel[a,b] (intestinal infection)	B	5.5	PO
Albendazole[c] (alveolar echinococcosis)	D	10	PO

[a]In order to ensure adequate dosing, retreat 24 hours after the first treatment.
[b]At least one repeat treatment is required as the efficacy is less than praziquantel; in contrast to praziquantel, which kills adult and immature *E. multilocularis*, epsiprantel only kills adult parasites. Epsiprantel is not approved for treatment of *E. multilocularis* in the USA. However, the drug has been used in Finland for this purpose.
[c]Administer q24h for life.
B, both dog and cat; *C*, cat; *D*, dog; *TD*, transdermal.
From Domingo M, Boue F, Conraths F, et al. Assessment of the risk of echinococcosis introduction into the UK, Ireland, Sweden, Malta and Finland as a consequence of abandoning national rules. *The EFSA Journal*. 2006;441:1–54.

are recommended for *E. multilocularis* infections to ensure adequate dosing. Epsiprantel may also be used but efficacy is typically less than that of praziquantel.[111] Neither praziquantel nor epsiprantel are ovicidal, and infective eggs may be shed in feces for up to 3 days following treatment. As a result, when treating infected dogs and cats, animals should be maintained in an environment that is easy to clean, feces should be safely disposed of for 3 days following treatment, animals should be washed entirely after treatment using a shampoo to remove eggs from the coat, and people should ideally wear mouth protection (e.g., surgical mask or cloth face covering), gloves, and protective clothing.[3]

Alveolar Echinococcosis

The metacestode of *E. multilocularis* in the abdomen of dogs does not constitute a direct risk to human health. However, some dogs with hepatic AE may also have patent intestinal infections[112] and therefore may constitute a zoonotic risk. Thus, as soon as a presumptive diagnosis of hepatic AE is made, dogs should be treated with praziquantel to eliminate intestinal infection;[110] treatment should be repeated 24 hours later. Praziquantel has little efficacy against the metacestode.

Once a definitive diagnosis of AE is made, treatment should be initiated with albendazole at 10 mg/kg PO q24h for life.[96] In some dogs, albendazole can cause bone marrow toxicity leading to aplastic anemia.[113] Therefore dogs receiving albendazole should be monitored weekly for 1 month, then every 3 to 4 months thereafter, with a CBC. This treatment regimen is recommended whether or not surgical excision is pursued. As in people, surgery is only recommended if complete removal of the metacestode can be achieved.[88] Dogs with any type of intervention (albendazole, surgery, or both) live significantly longer than those that have no intervention.[88] At present, there is no evidence that debulking surgery (cytoreduction) followed by treatment with albendazole results in a superior outcome compared to treatment with albendazole alone.[88]

Historically, it has been assumed that medical management of dogs with AE is associated with short-term survival. However, four of six dogs managed with only daily albendazole were in remission 0.5, 0.5, 2.6, and 9.5 years after the initial diagnosis.[88]

IMMUNITY AND VACCINATION

A recombinant vaccine (EG95) for *E. granulosus* s.l. has been developed for use in sheep and cattle intermediate hosts which results in a substantive reduction (>95%) in hydatid cyst burdens. As such, this vaccine is approved for use in a number of countries (e.g., Argentina, China)[53,114,115] and constitutes a useful tool in *E. granulosus* s.l. control programs. A similar vaccine is currently being developed for AE in people.[68] Although vaccines are not available for dogs, they have been considered desirable, and vaccine trials in dogs have yielded promising results.[115]

PREVENTION

E. granulosus s.l. Infections

In some countries with high prevalence of infection in dogs and high incidence of CE in people, control programs have been implemented (e.g., Argentina, Chile, Cyprus, New Zealand, Uruguay) that include: (1) strict regulation of animal slaughter and disposal of offal, (2) control of dog populations, (3) treatment of all dogs every 6 weeks with a cestocide, and (4) education of the public about transmission of *E. granulosus* s.l. and the importance of cooking raw offal or freezing it at −18°C for a minimum of 3 days prior to feeding it to dogs.[3,116,117] Such programs are costly and take >10 years before the prevalence of infection in dogs and intermediate hosts declines to low levels. Incorporation of (EG95) vaccination of both intermediate and definitive hosts into these control programs will likely have a more rapid and sustainable impact on the prevalence of infection in different hosts.[53,115]

E. multilocularis Infections

In areas endemic for *E. multilocularis*, administration of praziquantel at 5.0 mg/kg PO every 4 weeks is recommended for dogs with access to rodents.[88] In such areas, a risk assessment should be carried out on a regular basis to determine if such preventive treatment is necessary. Since AE in dogs may be associated with autoinfection, such a protocol may also reduce the risk of AE in dogs.

In order to reduce the risk of importation of *E. multilocularis* into countries free of this parasite, some countries require dogs from endemic areas to be treated with a cestocide at the time of entry, for example, Finland, Iceland, Ireland, mainland Norway, Malta, and the United Kingdom.[118,119]

PUBLIC HEALTH ASPECTS

People only become infected with *E. granulosus* s.l. and *E. multilocularis* by ingestion of eggs. Thus, in a veterinary environment, this will typically only occur by contamination of hands. Since the eggs of both parasites are immediately infective in fresh feces of dogs or cats, strict attention to hand hygiene whenever handling feces, materials contaminated by feces, or a potentially infected animal will effectively eliminate the risk of infection. When performing a necropsy on a dog potentially infected with *Echinococcus* spp., masks, gloves, and protective clothing should be used if the intestine is opened.

Cystic Echinococcosis

While many genotypes/species of *E. granulosus* s.l. infect people, >88% of human infections that have been typed are *E. granulosus* s.s. genotype G1,[48] indicating that sheep are the intermediate hosts. Many infections in people remain clinically inapparent for lengthy periods, even when large hydatid cyst(s) are present.[120] Disease ranges from mild to fatal and is associated with the space-occupying nature of cysts that usually occur in the liver and lungs and, less commonly, in the bone, CNS, or spleen. Liver involvement is typically associated with abdominal pain. With lung involvement, patients may present with chest pain, cough, dyspnea, and hemoptysis.[121] Diagnosis is based on detection of cysts by imaging (ultrasound, CT, MRI) combined with *Echinococcus* spp. serology.[120] Surgical excision is the preferred management as this is the only approach likely to result in cure.[122] When surgery is not an option, prolonged treatment with albendazole or mebendazole is carried out which, while usually not curative, reduces the cyst size and the associated clinical signs.[122]

Alveolar Echinococcosis

Only approximately 1% to 10% of people that are exposed to eggs of *E. multilocularis* and seroconvert develop disease.[68,98] When infections are not eliminated, the clinical incubation period is 5 to 15 years. People usually present with symptoms associated with hepatic neoplasia, such as epigastric pain, fatigue, jaundice, and weight loss.[122,123] Disease has been reported in all ages, but is most commonly diagnosed in people aged 50 to 55 years.[124,125] AE is usually diagnosed by imaging (ultrasound, CT, MRI) followed by *Echinococcus* spp. serology. However, imaging is usually suggestive of a neoplasm; suspicion of AE typically only occurs after histological examination of a biopsy.[120]

AE in people often presents in an advanced stage[124] and mortality rates are typically much greater than CE. When left untreated, AE has a chronic course that lasts weeks to years. Surgical excision of the entire lesion, followed by treatment with a benzimidazole (albendazole or mebendazole), is the only intervention that can result in cure, but is an option for only approximately one-third of cases. For individuals with non-resectable lesions, long-term treatment with a benzimidazole is recommended.[68] Since this treatment is parasitostatic rather than parasitocidal, regular imaging (e.g., PET scan) is required to determine the duration of therapy; in some individuals, life-long treatment may be required.[123] Data from Europe indicate that the 10-year survival rate in untreated individuals is 6% to 25%. However, this increases to 80% to 89% in people on long-term benzimidazole treatment.[126]

In a recent systematic review and meta-analysis of the literature, risk factors associated with AE in people included dog-related factors (e.g., playing with dogs, dog ownership), gender (being female), vocational factors (e.g., being a farmer, handling foxes), sociocultural factors (e.g., low income), and human habits (e.g., chewing grass). However, these potential risk factors likely vary in importance in different endemic areas of the world.[127] For example, strong associations between AE in people and dogs have been observed in parts of Alaska and China.[81,128] If exposure of people to *E. multilocularis* eggs is a concern, serological testing for up to 12 months following exposure is recommended.[129–131]

In North America, despite the large geographic distribution of *E. multilocularis* in wildlife, only a small number of cases of autochthonous alveolar echinococcosis in people had been described before 2013—one from Manitoba in 1937,[132] and one from Minnesota in 1977.[133] This low number of cases led some to conclude that the genetic variants of *E. multilocularis* occurring in North America are of lower infectivity or pathogenicity for people than those in Europe.[134] However, since 2013, reports of disease in humans associated with a European-type strain began to emerge, including seventeen cases from Alberta, one from Saskatechewan, and one from Vermont, USA.[135,136] The case from Vermont was a 36-year-old woman who owned a dog and had grown up fox-hunting in Maryland; she had traveled extensively throughout the USA, Costa Rica, Rome/Naples, and Montreal, but not to regions in Europe or Canada where the majority of European haplotype strain cases have been described.

MESOCESTOIDES SPP. INFECTION

ETIOLOGY AND EPIDEMIOLOGY

There is still much to learn about *Mesocestoides* spp., including the number of species and the identity of the first intermediate hosts.[137,138] At present, there are no accepted specific criteria that can be used to define a species, so numerous species appear in the literature. In 1932, Witenberg recognized one species, *Mesocestoides lineatus* in dogs, foxes, jackals, and cats, and synonymized or discounted 24 described species.[17,139] In 1980, Loos-Frank created the name *Mesocestoides leptothylacus* for the species commonly found in foxes in Europe.[140] In 1991, Etges proposed the name *Mesocestoides vogae* to replace the species *Mesocestoides corti* first described by Hoeppi in 1925, utilizing specimens collected from a mouse in Colorado, USA.[141] The most common European species are *M. vogae*, *M. leptothylacus*, and *M. lineatus*. However, some authors believe the name of the latter is taxonomically incorrect; the first descriptions were based on specimens that were not available for future authors to compare and none of the descriptions matched the original description. Therefore it has been proposed that all descriptions under the name *M. lineatus* be revised.[140]

Mesocestoides spp. occasionally infect dogs and cats, and essentially have a worldwide distribution. In Europe, the adult stage of *Mesocestoides* spp. occurs mainly in foxes, with a prevalence in some areas of up to 70%.[142] The prevalence in dogs and cats is considerably less. For example, the prevalence of *Mesocestoides* spp. in feral cats in Denmark at necropsy was 3.0%.[143] The prevalence of *Mesocestoides* spp. in owned cats in central Italy was 1.2% by fecal flotation.[144] In Iran, *M. lineatus* was reported in 19% of stray dogs at necropsy.[145] In Russia, *M. lineatus* was found in 1.7% to 23.5% of dogs at necropsy.[146] *Mesocestoides* spp. have also been reported in North and South America.[147,148] In North American dogs and cats, both fecal examination and necropsy studies have revealed a low prevalence (0%–1%); infections are more commonly detected in the southeastern and western United States.[14,15,148,149]

Adult *Mesocestoides* spp. develop in the intestine of dogs and cats following ingestion of the infective metacestode stage (tetrathyridium) within the abdominal cavity of various intermediate hosts, which include over 200 species of reptiles, amphibians, mammals, and birds (Fig. 115.12).[150] However, strangely, despite this breadth of information, the first stage and first intermediate host for *Mesocestoides* spp. remain a mystery. It is currently believed that a cysticercoid stage occurs in an arthropod such as an ant, and that this precedes

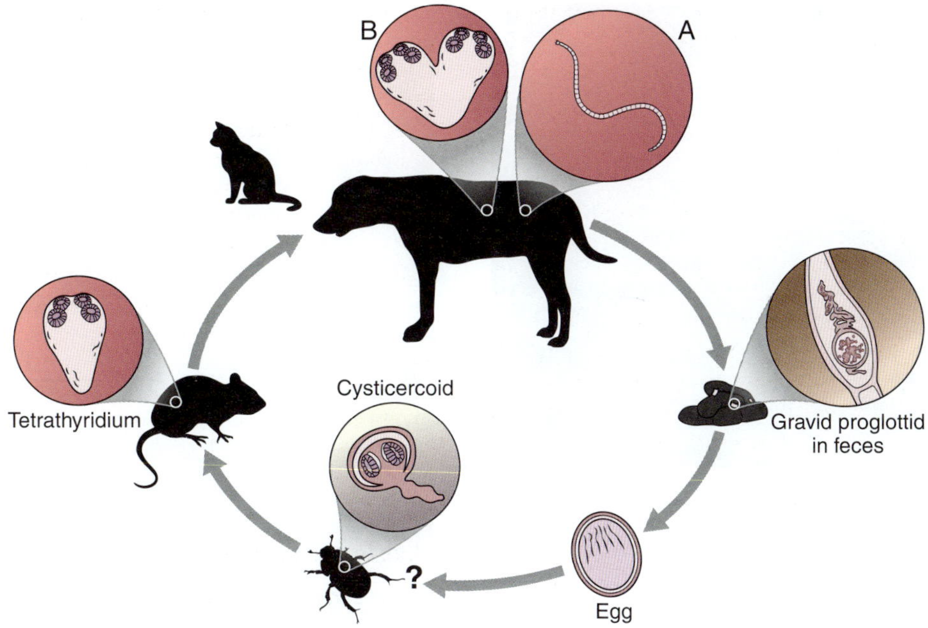

Fig. 115.12 Life cycle of *Mesocestoides* sp. A, within the intestine. B, peritoneal infection.

the tetrathyridial stage. However, experimental infections have yet to confirm this.[137,151] One study examined thousands of soil-inhabiting invertebrates from areas heavily contaminated with *Mesocestoides* spp. gravid segments shed by experimentally infected foxes, but cysticercoids were not found.[137]

Once infected with *Mesocestoides* spp., gravid segments may be detected in the feces of dogs and cats 20 to 30 days later.[11] Peritoneal tetrathyridial infection in dogs and cats may follow ingestion of a first-stage larva in the still-unidentified first intermediate host or a tetrathyridium in a second intermediate host.[152] In *M. vogae* (syn. *M. corti*), both the tetrathyridium and adult tapeworm can undergo asexual reproduction.[153] Thus, this species can repopulate the intestinal tract without further exposure if not eliminated by anthelmintic treatment.[154] Chronic glucocorticoid treatment may be a risk factor for peritoneal disease in dogs; Welsh Corgis appeared to be overrepresented in a study of 60 dogs from the United States, comprising 10% of the affected dogs.[155]

CLINICAL FEATURES

Pathogenesis and Clinical Signs

Intestinal infection appears to be subclinical in dogs and cats. Most reported cases of peritoneal infections have been dogs from North America. Of 60 dogs in the United States with peritoneal infections, most (50) were from California, with three cases from Oregon, and single cases from Washington, Arizona, Florida, and Oklahoma.[155] Single cases have also been reported in dogs from New Mexico and Washington state, and British Columbia, Canada.[138,156,157] Additional affected dogs have been reported in other countries (e.g., Germany, Japan).[142,158] Disease is associated with asexual division or budding of the parasite and development of large numbers in the peritoneal cavity; viable tetrathyridial or non-viable acephalic metacestodes may be produced. Infected dogs and cats may appear clinically normal, especially if infected with relatively few metacestodes; subclinical infections may be an incidental finding during abdominal surgery. Clinically affected dogs may have abdominal distension secondary to ascites, anorexia, weight loss, vomiting, diarrhea, and tachypnea.[155] Some affected cats have abdominal pain and vomiting.[152,159,160]

DIAGNOSIS

Laboratory Abnormalities

In dogs with peritoneal larval cestodiasis, leukocytosis, eosinophilia, and thrombocytopenia have been demonstrated on CBC. Serum chemistry analysis may show azotemia, hyperphosphatemia, hyponatremia, panhypoproteinemia, and hyperbilirubinemia.[142,158]

Diagnostic Imaging

Abdominal radiographs typically show a general loss of detail secondary to ascites. Abdominal ultrasound may reveal round, thin-walled, anechoic cysts. Some may contain a 1-mm to 5-mm rounded structure compatible with a tetrathyridium.[142,158,159] Large quantities of hyperechoic free peritoneal fluid is often present that is highly suggestive of the disease (Fig. 115.13).

Microbiologic Tests

Diagnosis Using Fecal Examination

Diagnosis of intestinal infections is by detection of segments in feces (Fig. 115.14A and B) or, rarely, detection of eggs via fecal flotation (Fig. 115.14C). Gravid segments are 3 to 4 mm in size and club shaped; they are similar in size to segments of *Echinococcus* spp. but smaller than those of *Taenia* spp. and *D. caninum* (see Fig. 115.5). For definitive identification, segments should be flattened between two glass slides after adding water or saline to the segment; the genital pore is positioned mid-ventrally. Furthermore, *Mesocestoides* spp. possess a thick-walled parauterine organ in mature segments where eggs accumulate; this is rarely found in other cyclophyllideans.[11,161] Segments can also be disrupted to release eggs (if present). As for other cestodes, calcareous corpuscles also may be seen.[41]

Although fecal flotation is insensitive (as for other cestode infections), *Mesocestoides* eggs are unique; they are 30 to 40 μm in diameter and possess a thin, clear, smooth shell wall. Hooks of the hexacanth embryo can help distinguish the egg from a pseudoparasite.[3]

Cytologic Diagnosis

Peritoneal larval cestodiasis is diagnosed by detection of either tetrathyridia or calcareous corpuscles in abdominal fluid; abdominal

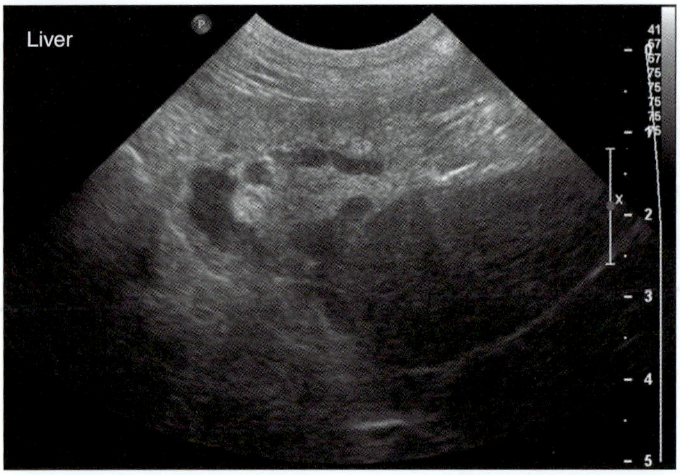

Fig. 115.13 Abdominal ultrasound image of a 4-year-old male neutered beagle mix with peritoneal larval cestodiasis. Clinical signs were chronic weight loss in the face of polyphagia. (Courtesy University of California-Davis Veterinary Diagnostic Imaging Service.)

fluid is collected via centesis or during an exploratory laparotomy.[153] Grossly, free fragments of white, flocculated material that vary in size from less than 1 mm to 5 mm may be seen in abdominal fluid that appears clear to serosanguinous (Fig. 115.15). Microscopically, tetrathyridia of *Mesocestoides* spp. have four suckers, calcareous corpuscles, and the absence of hooks or a rostellum (Fig. 115.16).[142,158,159]

Molecular Diagnosis Using Nucleic Acid–Based Testing

Molecular methods can be used to definitively identify acephalic metacestodes.[138] PCR-DNA analysis targeting the mitochondrial (mt) *12S rRNA* gene and mt cytochrome *c* oxidase subunit 1 gene has been used to identify *M. vogae* (syn. *M. corti*),[158] as well as the mt *12S rRNA* gene of *M. lineatus*.[142]

TREATMENT AND PROGNOSIS

A single dose of praziquantel (5 mg/kg PO or 5.7 mg/kg SC or IM) can eliminate intestinal *Mesocestoides* spp. infections in dogs and cats (Table 115.6).[11,162] However, dogs with peritoneal infections require long-term use of high dosages of fenbendazole (100 mg/kg q12h for 28 days) along with peritoneal lavage following laparotomy to remove tetrathyridia (see Table 115.6).[138] One case report concluded that praziquantel was more effective than fenbendazole at treating canine peritoneal cestodiasis; however, this was only in one dog that had previously been treated with fenbendazole. In this case, praziquantel was dosed at 5.0 mg/kg and repeated 15 days later.[163] Long-term follow-up is indicated as some dogs will experience recurrence of clinical disease even after 28 days of high dosages of fenbendazole.[155] Dogs that fail fenbendazole treatment or have adverse effects of high-dose fenbendazole (typically gastrointestinal or neurologic signs in the editor's experience) after peritoneal lavage may respond to 8 mg/kg praziquantel q24h for 2 weeks (Sykes JE, personal observations).

In the 60 dogs from California, Oregon, Washington, Arizona, Florida, and Oklahoma, dogs received one, two, or three of the following treatment options: surgery/lavage, fenbendazole at any dosage, or fenbendazole at 100 mg/kg for >28 days (termed high dose). Overall, survival was 72.3% at 6 months and 60.5% at 1 year. Both clinical severity at the time of diagnosis and treatment regimen significantly influenced the treatment outcome; dogs treated with high-dose fenbendazole, or both peritoneal lavage/surgery and any dosage

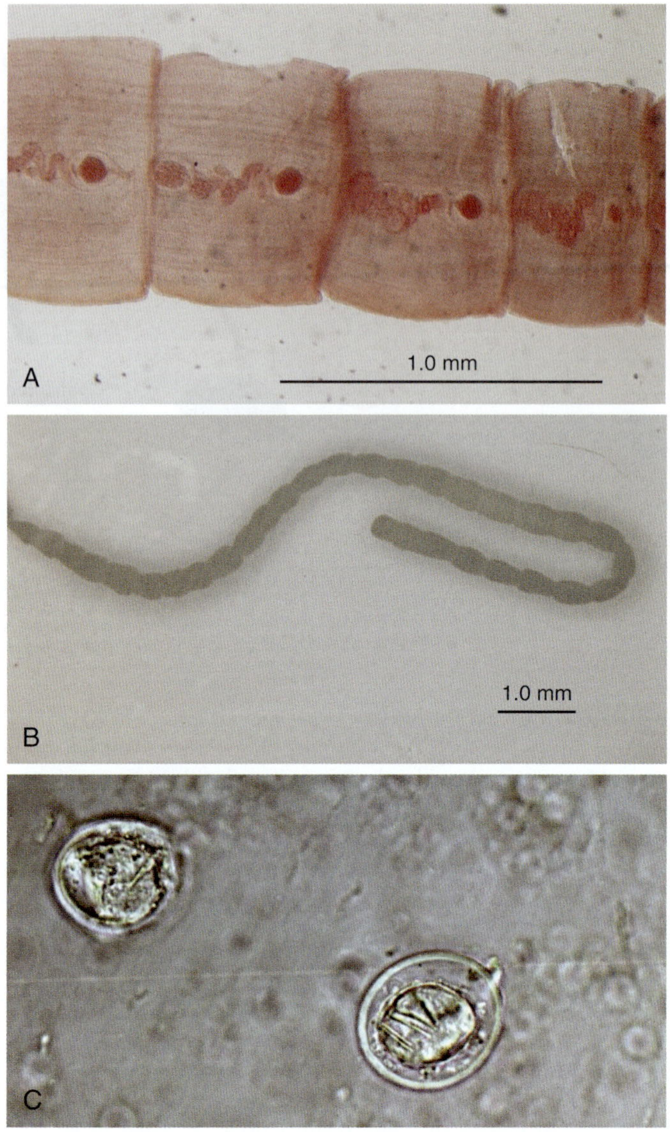

Fig. 115.14 Features of *Mesocestoides* sp. cestodes. (A) Mature segments. Note eggs contained within the medially located parauterine organ. (B) Strobila (body). (C) Egg. Note the hooks visible in the embryo. (A and B, courtesy of Megan Lineberry, Oklahoma State University. C, courtesy of National Center for Veterinary Parasitology, Oklahoma State University.)

of fenbendazole, had less than one-fifth the risk of dying compared to dogs that were not treated in this manner.[155] If there is a history of chronic treatment with glucocorticoids or other immunosuppressive medications, these should be tapered and discontinued if possible.

When parasites are present in pockets or cysts, ultrasound guidance may be needed to locate and drain these areas when lavage is impractical (e.g., invasion of tissue by parasites, substantive fibrous adhesions); surgery may be required to remove parasites and affected tissues.[155] Dogs that remain persistently infected should be treated with fenbendazole at 50 to 100 mg/kg daily for life (if tolerated).[155] Nitazoxanide (100 mg/kg) was found to be 100% effective against adult *M. lineatus* infections in cats.[25]

PREVENTION

The only preventive measure available is minimizing the risk of consumption of intermediate hosts by dogs and cats. Since the tetrathyridium stage (the stage infective to dogs and cats) has been reported in

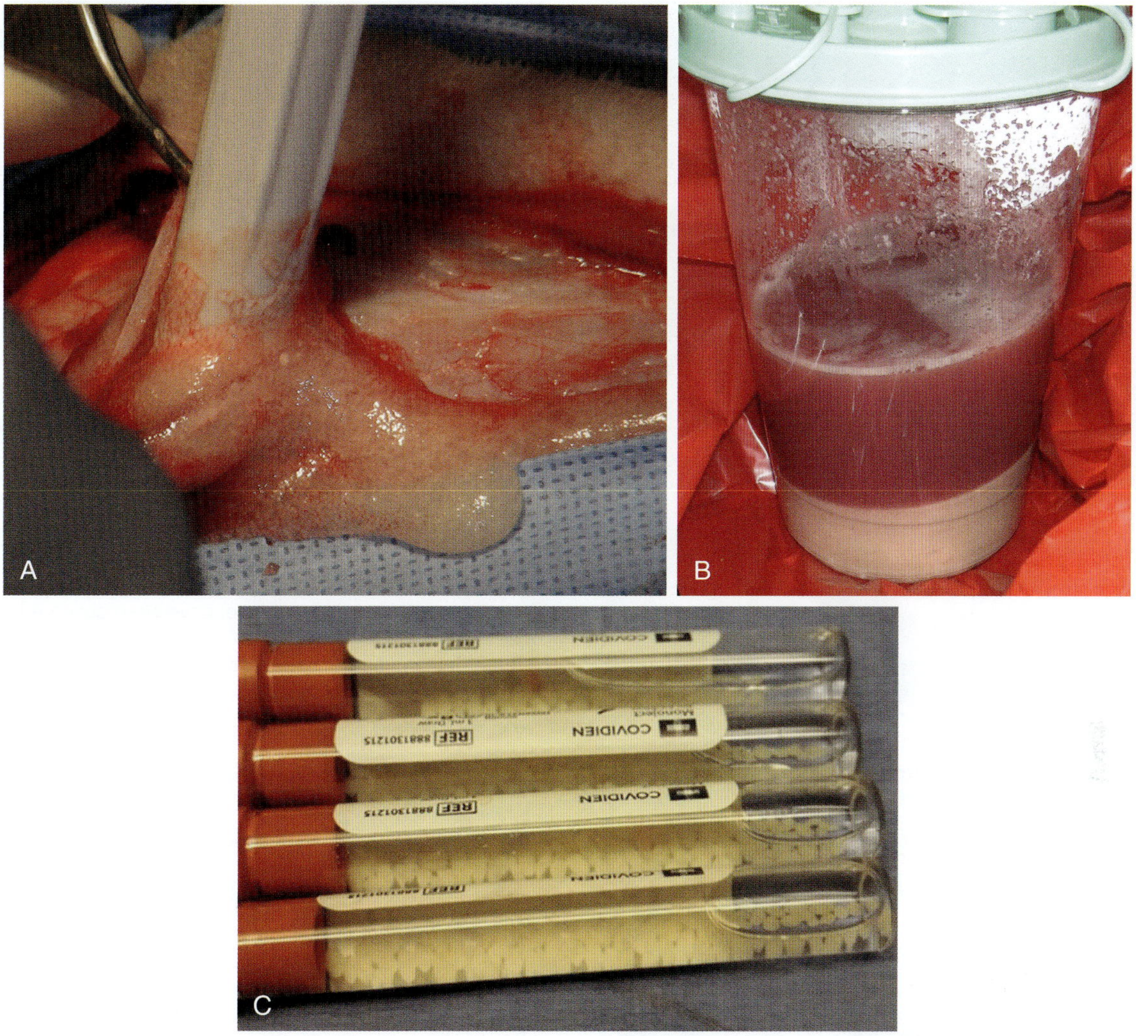

Fig. 115.15 (A) Peritoneal fluid containing *Mesocestoides* sp. tetrathyridia oozing from an initial laparotomy incision in the dog in Fig. 115.13. (B) Suction canister after surgery that contained serosanguineous fluid and what was estimated to be 11,500,000 tetrathyridia. (C) *Mesocestoides* sp. tetrathyridia lavaged from the peritoneal cavity of a 1.5-year-old German shepherd. (A and B, courtesy of Dr. Jane E. Sykes, University of California-Davis. C, courtesy of Dr. Joe Dubois, Mountain View Animal Clinic, Poteau, Oklahoma and Dr. Mason Reichard, National Center for Veterinary Parasitology, Oklahoma State University.)

over 200 species of reptiles, amphibians, mammals, and birds, the best recommendation is to limit unsupervised roaming outdoors.[150]

PUBLIC HEALTH ASPECTS

Humans have very rarely been reported to develop intestinal adult *Mesocestoides* spp. infections, but infected dogs and cats are not a direct risk to humans. The first report of a human infection was in Texas, USA (1942), where a girl was diagnosed with an *M. lineatus* infection.[164] Other cases include a 19-month-old boy from Louisiana diagnosed with an *M. variabilis* infection; the proposed origin of infection was food-borne.[165] Six other human cases of *M. lineatus* or *Mesocestoides* spp. have been reported in the USA in Texas, Missouri, New Jersey, Ohio, Mississippi, and California.[166] In Japan, a 35-year-old man was diagnosed with *M. lineatus* infection and thought most likely to have acquired the infection by eating raw snake liver.[167] These infections all appeared to be well tolerated and were diagnosed by finding segments in the feces. Treatment with praziquantel is typically effective. In addition, niclosamide and paromomycin sulfate have been used.[166,167]

DIPHYLLOBOTHRIUM SPP. INFECTION

ETIOLOGY AND EPIDEMIOLOGY

The *Diphyllobothrium* genus contains approximately 50 species of which 14 have been reported in humans.[168] All occur as adult parasites within the intestinal tract of fish-eating mammals and birds. Globally, *Diphyllobothrium latum* (*Dibothriocephalus latus*)[169] is the most important species. Regionally important species include *Diphyllobothrium dendriticum* (Russia, Argentina, Chile) and *Diphyllobothrium nihonkaiense* (Pacific Coast of Asia and North America).[168,170]

Diphyllobothrium latum (the fish tapeworm, broad tapeworm) infects both dogs and cats; other definitive hosts include humans, bears, foxes, pigs, mink, and seals. The parasite occurs in North America (Alaska and the Great Lakes region of Canada and the USA), northern Europe (Estonia, Finland, Hungary, Lithuania, Poland, Sweden and sub-Alpine lakes in France, Italy, Switzerland), and Russia. However, cases have also been reported in South America (Argentina, Brazil, Chile, Peru) and occasionally in parts of Asia (Japan, Korea, Philippines, Taiwan).[171–173]

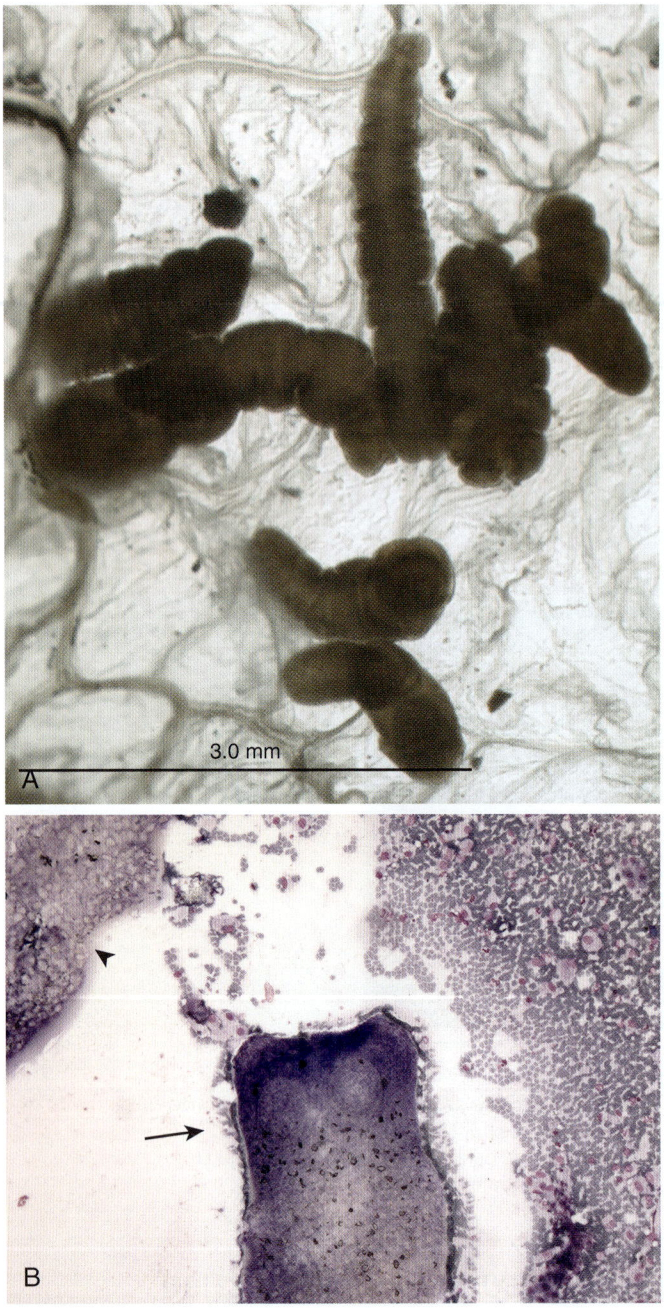

Fig. 115.16 (A) Light microscopic appearance of unstained tetrathyridia of *Mesocestoides* sp. in a specimen from the abdomen of a cat. Note the lack of hooks or a rostellum and the presence of suckers and an elongated body. (B) Romanowsky-stained cytospin specimen of peritoneal fluid from an adult mixed-breed dog with *Mesocestoides* sp. peritonitis. Note the tetrathyridium *(arrow)* and calcareous corpuscles *(arrowhead)*. (A, courtesy of Dr. Mason Reichard, Oklahoma State University. B, courtesy Dr. William Vernau, University of California-Davis Veterinary Clinical Pathology Service.)

TABLE 115.6 Recommended Drugs for Treating *Mesocestoides* spp. Infections in Dogs and Cats

Drug (Indication)	Species	Dosage (mg/kg)[a]	Route
Praziquantel (intestinal infection)	B	5.0 5.7	PO IM/SC
Nitazoxanide (intestinal infection)	C	100	PO
Fenbendazole (peritoneal larval cestodiasis)[b,c]	D	100	PO
Praziquantel (peritoneal larval cestodiasis)	D	5–8	PO

[a]Doses are for one time administration with the exception of fenbendazole, which should be given q12h for 28 days; and praziquantel (peritoneal larval cestodiasis), which should be given twice, 15 days apart, or q24h for 14 days (based on limited anecdotal evidence).
[b]Combine with peritoneal lavage and debridement to remove as many tetrathyridia as possible.
[c]Long-term follow-up is necessary. Neurologic signs and GI signs (twitching, vomiting, inappetence) have been observed using such high doses.
B, both dog and cat; *C*, cat; *D*, dog.

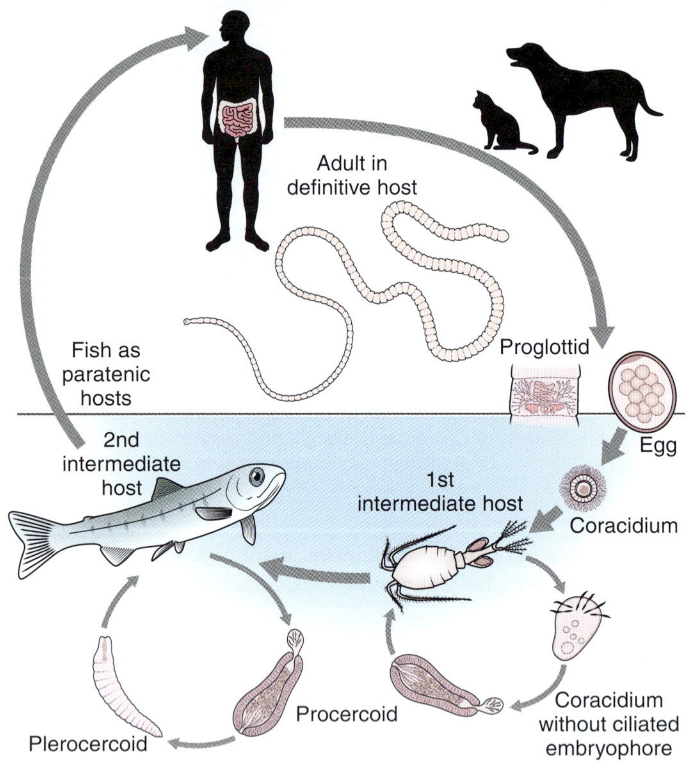

Fig. 115.17 Life cycle of *Diphyllobothrium latum.*

Diphyllobothrium latum has a three-host life cycle (Fig. 115.17). Adult parasites occur within the small intestine of dogs, cats, people, and other definitive hosts. Each parasite releases up to 1,000,000 eggs per day in to the intestinal contents via a single uterine pore that is present in each segment.[174] Eggs are then shed into the environment in feces. In fresh water, a ciliated coracidium hatches from the egg[174] and is ingested by the first intermediate host, aquatic copepods (*Cyclops* and *Diaptomus* species).[175] The coracidium matures into a procercoid within the body cavity of the copepod. When ingested by the second intermediate host, fresh water fish, the procercoid invades the peritoneal cavity, internal organs, or muscles and matures to a 1- to 3-cm long pleroceroid that resembles a small tapeworm. Plerocercoids can survive for extended periods in these locations.[176] If a fish infected with a plerocercoid is ingested by another fish, the plerocercoid can transfer to the new fish, that is, fish may be paratenic hosts. Dogs, cats, and other definitive hosts develop intestinal infections after consuming fish infected with a plerocercoid. In dogs and cats, the prepatent period is 5 to 6 weeks.[11]

Fish intermediate hosts for *D. latum* are primarily non-salmonids.[172] Plerocercoids are most commonly found in perch, pike, burbot (Europe), and walleye (North America).[177] Prevalence of infection in these species is highly variable. However, in Lake Geneva, France/Switzerland, the prevalence of plerocercoids in perch in 2003–2005 was 4% to 10%.[178] By contrast, in Lake Como, Italy, the prevalence of infection from 2013 to 2014 in perch and pike was 25.4% and 84.2%, respectively.[179]

Little information is available on the prevalence of *D. latum* in dogs and cats. In North America, most infections are diagnosed in dogs.[3] In Europe, *D. latum* infections are generally rare. Thus, in dog populations examined in both Finland and Switzerland, *D. latum* infections were detected in 0.4% of dogs.[180,181] By contrast, in parts of Russia, up to 90% of cats have been shown to be infected.[182,183]

One of the most important components of the epidemiology of *D. latum* is contamination of freshwater environments by untreated human sewage, although dogs can also be an important source of environmental contamination.[184,185]

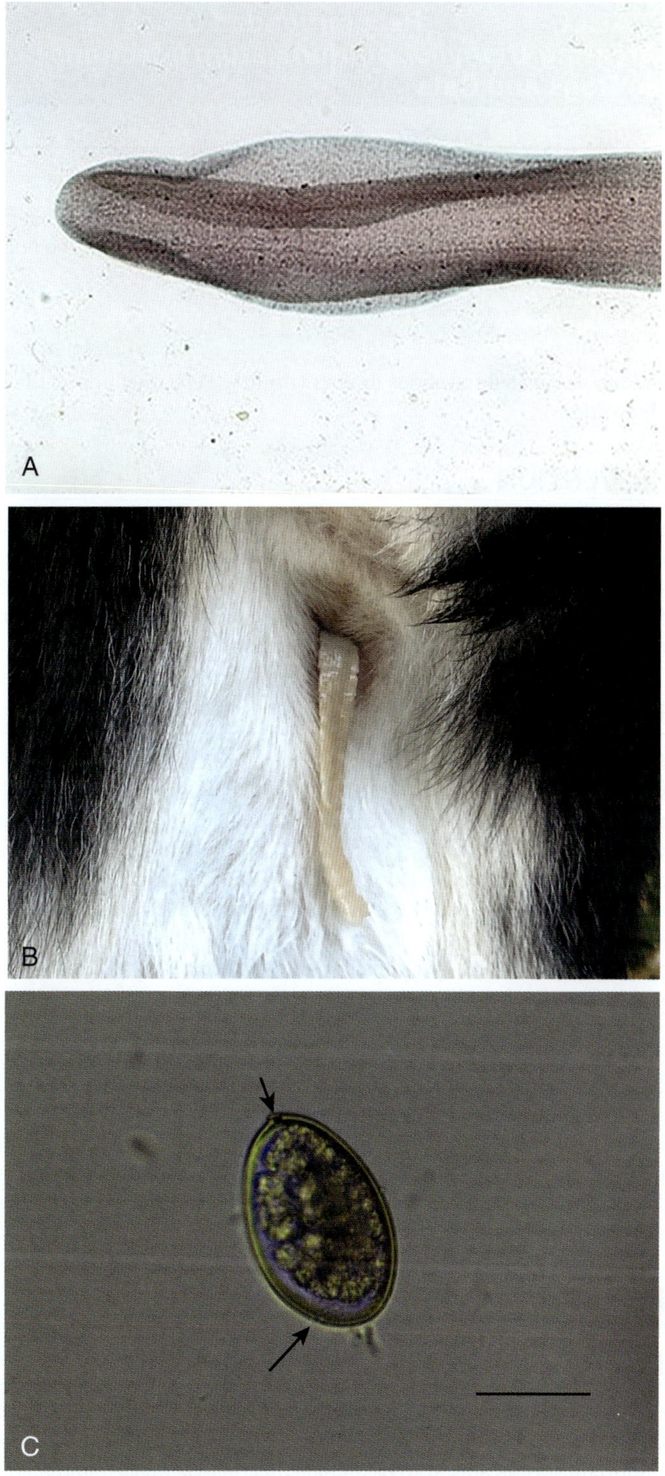

Fig. 115.18 Morphologic features of *Diphyllobothrium* sp. Anterior end (A) and chain (B) of *Diphyllobothrium* segments (proglottids) protruding from the anus of a 6-month old shepherd mix dog. (C) Egg. Note the operculum *(long arrow)* and pore in shell wall *(short arrow)*. Bar = 30 μm. (A, courtesy of National Center for Veterinary Parasitology, Oklahoma State University. B, courtesy of Dr. Marissa Bessell, Aspen Springs Animal Hospital, Bowmanville, Ontario.)

CLINICAL FEATURES

Pathogenesis and Clinical Signs

Intestinal infections in both dogs and cats are usually subclinical. While anemia has been associated with *D. latum* intestinal infections in people, this phenomenon has not been described in naturally infected dogs or cats. Experimental *D. latum* infections in dogs have been associated with decreased red cell numbers and decreased total hemoglobin levels.[186] The possibility of infection is generally only considered after owners report the presence of chains of segments (typically empty of eggs) in feces.[3]

DIAGNOSIS

Laboratory Abnormalities

Laboratory abnormalities are generally unremarkable in dogs and cats with *D. latum* infections.

Microbiologic Tests

Isolation and Identification

Adult *D. latum* are found in the small intestine and measure 1 to 12 m in length. As with other pseudophyllidean tapeworms, the scolex lacks hooks and suckers. Instead, it contains two shallow longitudinal grooves (bothria). The strobila contains up to 3000 segments. Anterior segments are broader than long (width = 12–20 mm); posterior segments are approximately square shaped (Fig. 115.18). Segments have a number of characteristic features that include a medioventral uterine pore and a centrally located, rosette-shaped uterus. Unlike the more common tapeworms of dogs and cats (i.e., *Taenia* spp. and *D. caninum*), segments of *D. latum* continuously release eggs until the uterine contents are exhausted. Thus, terminal segments are typically not gravid, that is, do not contain eggs. Furthermore, they usually detach in chains, not individually.

Eggs of *D. latum* are oval, light brown, have an operculum at one pole, and measure 58 to 76 μm × 40 to 51 μm. They resemble eggs produced by *Spirometra* spp. and digenetic trematodes. However, a pore is often visible in the shell wall at the pole opposite the operculum in association with a small amount of material that protrudes from it (Fig. 115.18C). Eggs may be recovered by fecal flotation but are most readily detected using sedimentation.[20,176] Precise identification of different *Diphyllobothrium* species is most reliably achieved by PCR sequencing.[187]

TREATMENT AND PROGNOSIS

Praziquantel has been reported to be efficacious for treatment of *D. latum* infections in dogs and cats, but increased dosages are required beyond label recommendations (Table 115.7). Some authors have reported efficacy in dogs at 7.5 mg/kg, PO, either singly or for 2 consecutive days.[11,188] However, both the authors of this chapter and others have observed infections in dogs that have not been eliminated by these dosage regimens. A single dose of 35 mg/kg eliminated *D. latum* from infected cats[189]

TABLE 115.7 Recommended Drugs for Treating *Diphyllobothrium latum* Infections in Dogs and Cats

Drug	Species	Dose (mg/kg)	Route
Praziquantel	D	7.5[a]	PO
	C	35	PO

[a]Some authors recommend a second treatment, 24 hours after the first. In some dogs, a higher dose (35 mg/kg) is required.
C, cat; *D*, dog.

and has eliminated infections in dogs (Andrew Peregrine, unpublished observations).

PREVENTION

Diphyllobothrium latum infections in dogs and cats are acquired by ingestion of raw or undercooked fish. However, freezing fish for over 48 hours at −18°C, or cooking fish (core temperature ≥ 50°C) for ≥ 5 minutes, will eliminate infection risk.[178] Preventing animals from roaming freely or scavenging dead fish will also prevent infection.[190]

PUBLIC HEALTH ASPECTS

Diphyllobothrium latum infection is an important fish-borne zoonosis,[172] but dogs and cats infected with *D. latum* are not a direct risk to humans. Worldwide, approximately 20 million people are infected with *Diphyllobothrium* spp., of which *D. latum* and *D. nihonkaiense* are the most common.[172,178] As with dogs and cats, human infections are acquired by ingestion of raw or undercooked fish that contains plerocercoids. Smoking or marinating fish typically does not kill the plerocercoid.[191] Increased consumption of carpaccio, ceviche, sushi, sashimi, and other dishes made from raw fish has been associated with increased risk of *D. latum* infection in people.[172,184] Intestinal infections in people are typically clinically silent. However, some individuals experience poorly defined symptoms that may include mild abdominal discomfort, nausea, diarrhea, constipation, and weakness. Occasionally, heavy, prolonged *D. latum* infections may result in a megaloblastic anemia due to absorption of vitamin B_{12} by tapeworms.[192] Infections are readily eliminated by treatment with praziquantel or niclosamide.[178]

SPIROMETRA SPP. INFECTION

ETIOLOGY AND EPIDEMIOLOGY

Spirometra spp. are diphyllobothridean tapeworms and infect wild and domestic carnivores, including cats and occasionally dogs. The most important species appear to be *Spirometra erinaceieuropaei/Spirometra erinacei* (Asia, Australia, Europe), *Spirometra mansonoides* (North and South America), and *Spirometra mansoni* (Asia). Adult parasites are found in the small intestine of cats, dogs, and wild carnivores.[193] In the USA, infection is most common in cats in the Gulf Coast and southeastern states, with additional reports from Hawaii, New Jersey, New York, and Pennsylvania.[194] In stray cat populations from Syracuse, New York and New Jersey, the prevalence was 3% and 1%, respectively.[13,195] *Spirometra* sp. was detected in 7.9% of shelter cats in Florida.[196] Typically, higher prevalences have been detected in the Gulf Coast states of southeastern United States (e.g., Florida) where aquatic ecosystems support the life cycle of *Spirometra* spp. In a necropsy study

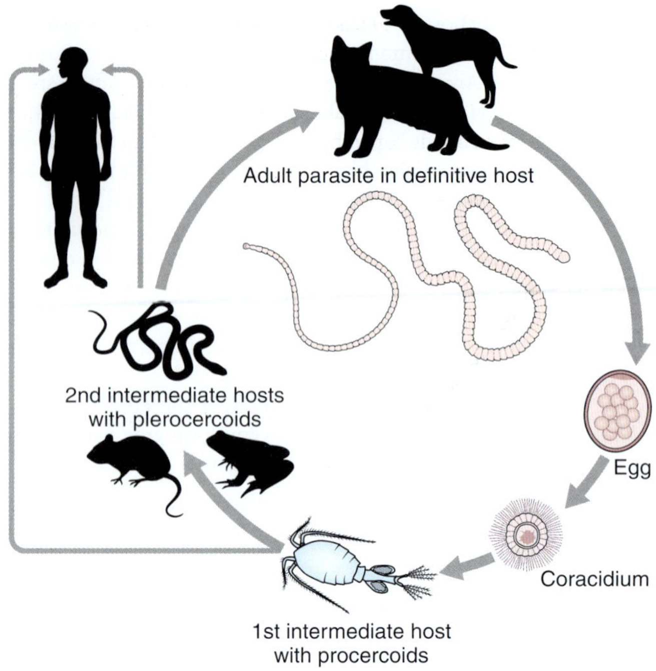

Fig. 115.19 Life cycle of *Spirometra* sp.

in Brazil, 4.1% of cats were infected with *S. mansonoides*.[4] In northern Portugal, 0.3% of dogs living on farms were positive for *Spirometra* sp. using fecal flotation and sedimentation.[197] In Iran, *Spirometra* spp. were found in 7.4% of dogs and 33.3% of cats at necropsy.[198] In Japan, 1.7% of owned cats were infected with *S. erinacei* as determined using fecal sedimentation.[199] In China, 40.5% of cats and 27.5% of dogs from 23 villages had eggs of *S. mansoni* detected in feces using the Kato-Katz technique.[200] In Malaysia, 9.2% of stray cats and 3.5% of stray dogs were positive for *Spirometra* sp. by fecal sedimentation.[201] In Thailand, 4.0% of cats and 0.6% of dogs from an animal refuge were infected with *S. mansoni* by fecal sedimentation.[202]

Like *Diphyllobothrium* spp., *Spirometra* spp. differ from the more common cyclophyllidean tapeworms in several aspects of their life cycle (Fig. 115.19). Firstly, they shed individual eggs into the intestinal tract through a mid-ventral uterine pore of individual segments, rather than detach an egg-laden segment from the strobila. Secondly, the egg is operculated, hatches once it reaches water, and releases a ciliated coracidium that is free-swimming. The coracidium is then ingested by the first intermediate host, a copepod (e.g., *Cyclops* spp.) and matures into a procercoid. Thereafter, infected copepods are consumed accidentally by the second intermediate host (i.e., amphibians, reptiles, birds, rodents) while drinking water. In the second intermediate host, the procercoid develops into a plerocercoid, also referred to as a *spargana*, in the muscle or connective tissue. The plerocercoid stage is highly paratenic, meaning it can remain in this stage through a series of paratenic hosts. For example, if a tadpole is infected with plerocercoids and is consumed by a water snake, the plerocercoids will migrate through the snake's tissues but remain as plerocercoids in this new paratenic host. The parasite will survive this way until an infected paratenic host is ultimately consumed by a carnivore definitive host (e.g., cat or dog). This increases the odds that *Spirometra* spp. cestodes find their way into a definitive host. When an infected second intermediate host, or paratenic host, is consumed by a definitive host, the plerocercoid attaches to the small intestine wall and develops into an adult tapeworm. The prepatent period is 10 to 60 days in dogs and cats.

Furthermore, infection can persist up to 3.5 years in cats.[194,195,203] The duration of infection in dogs is unclear.

When plerocercoids are ingested by accidental hosts (e.g., rodents, pigs, humans), they may penetrate the intestinal wall and invade serous cavities, connective tissue, or internal organs (proliferative sparganosis). Such infections occasionally also occur in dogs, cats, and other definitive hosts.[195,204–206]

CLINICAL FEATURES

Pathogenesis and Clinical Signs

Infection with adult *Spirometra* spp. appears to be well tolerated by cats and dogs; however, vomiting, diarrhea, and weight loss have been reported.[13,195] The mechanism underlying disease has not been fully elucidated. Selective uptake of vitamin B_{12} by the adult and plerocercoid stage has been demonstrated,[207] but the significance of this phenomenon in cats and dogs is unknown. Clinical signs usually resolve quickly following treatment.

In sparganosis, spargana proliferate in abdominal and thoracic cavities, affecting the stomach, lungs, liver, and spleen, as well as in subcutaneous tissues. This is associated with chronic inflammation and fibrosis. Proliferative sparganosis is rare, but has been reported in dogs from Australia,[205] and cats and dogs from the USA.[204,206] Probable exposure routes include ingestion of copepods infected with procercoids in contaminated drinking water, and ingestion of plerocercoids in second intermediate or paratenic hosts.[3] Clinical signs vary depending on the tissue involved and disease can range from mild to severe. In Gainesville, Florida, USA, a 6-year-old cat was evaluated for abdominal pain; physical examination revealed a palpable abdominal mass. Proliferative sparganosis was diagnosed at necropsy; the liver and spleen and wall of the cat's stomach contained numerous spargana.[204] Two cats from southern Georgia were described that had subcutaneous cystlike masses.[208] In Tampa, Florida, a 21-month-old border collie was evaluated for progressive right thoracic limb lameness and subcutaneous edema. The subcutaneous tissue and intermuscular fascia contained multiple cavities filled with spargana. Septic pleuritis and peritonitis were detected later in the course of the disease. At necropsy, multiple spargana were found in the pleural and peritoneal cavities.[206] In Australia, five dogs have been reported with sparganosis; spargana were detected free in the abdominal cavity, in association with chronic fibrinous peritonitis or inflammation of the serosal surface of the GI tract or liver. Signs in three dogs included a palpable abdominal mass (n = 1) and abdominal distension (n = 2); in the remaining two dogs, sparganosis was an incidental finding at surgery (n = 2).[205] Another dog from southeastern Australia was evaluated for pneumothorax secondary to pulmonary involvement; exploratory thoracotomy revealed numerous white nodules throughout the pleura and pulmonary parenchyma (Fig. 115.20).[209]

DIAGNOSIS

Laboratory Abnormalities and Diagnostic Imaging

In animals with proliferative sparganosis, laboratory abnormalities and diagnostic imaging findings depend on the location of affected tissues. For example, pneumothorax was evident in one dog on plain thoracic radiographs, together with irregular soft-tissue opacities in the region of the distal eighth and ninth ribs (Fig. 115.20A).

Microbiologic Tests

Diagnosis Using Fecal Examination

Short (usually < 5 cm) chains of mature segments may be recovered from feces or vomit. Occasionally, longer chains are recovered (Fig. 115.21A and B). These segments can be identified as diphyllobothridean tapeworms by the presence of a medial uterine pore and operculated eggs within segments.[3,194]

Eggs can be recovered by flotation. However, lower SpG flotation solutions may be inadequate to float the heavy eggs; the diagnostic sensitivity of flotation methods using $ZnSO_4$ (specific gravity 1.18) or $NaNO_3$ (specific gravity 1.18) is significantly less than sucrose (specific gravity 1.27) for recovery of *Spirometra* spp. eggs.[194,210] Fecal sedimentation can also be used to recover *Spirometra* spp. eggs.[20] *Spirometra* spp. eggs are yellow-brown and 60 to 75 μm × 35 to 37 μm, have an operculum at one end, and are narrowed at both ends (Fig. 115.21C). They may be mistaken for the similar, but more rounded, eggs of *Diphyllobothrium* spp.[3,20] Geographic location can suggest the species involved. In the Americas, while *D. latum* is most common in the Great Lakes region of North America, *S. mansonoides* is most common in the southeastern USA and parts of South America.[17,194] Eggs of *Spirometra* spp. can also be mistaken for trematode eggs. Both *Spirometra* spp. and *Paragonimus* spp. produce eggs that are unembryonated when shed, but *Spirometra* spp. eggs are smaller than those of *Paragonimus kellicotti* (lung fluke; North America; eggs 75–118 μm × 42–67 μm) and other *Paragonimus* species around the world (e.g., *Paragonimus westermani*, the Japanese lung fluke, and *Paragonimus heterotremus* in Asia). The liver fluke of cats (*Platynosomum concinnum*), found in the southeastern USA and the Caribbean, produces smaller operculated eggs that contain a miracidium (see Chapter 118).[11,20,194]

Recovery of plerocercoids from tissue is necessary for diagnosis of sparganosis. Additionally, molecular identification can be performed by isolating DNA from segments of the tapeworm. PCR assays have been utilized to identify *S. erinacei*[209,211] and *S. mansonoides*.[212] In dogs, inflammatory tissue cysts may be filled with both intact and degenerate white spargana surrounded by red, cloudy, thick fluid.[206] Microscopic findings include large numbers of spargana surrounded by large numbers of pyogranulomatous inflammatory cells in variably sized cystic spaces and reactive fibrocollagenous stroma. Larval parenchyma is strongly PAS positive.[208] The absence of scolices and suckers helps differentiate plerocercoid larvae from those of cyclophyllidean tapeworms (*Mesocestoides*, *Echinococcus* spp.).

TREATMENT AND PROGNOSIS

There is no approved treatment for infection with *Spirometra* spp. in dogs or cats. Treating animals infected with adult parasites requires higher dosages of praziquantel than is required for *Taenia* spp. or *D. caninum*; a protocol of 25 mg/kg of praziquantel (PO or SC) for 2 consecutive days is effective (Table 115.8).[194] Treatment of proliferative sparganosis in dogs utilizing combination therapy with praziquantel (50 mg/kg SC once a week for 3 weeks) and fenbendazole (100 mg/kg PO q12h for 28 days), along with abdominal lavage to remove as many plerocercoids as possible, may be attempted, but prognosis is guarded.[206] There is also a report of a dog surviving proliferative sparganosis utilizing a protocol of alternating 3-week courses of mebendazole (20 mg/kg PO q24h for 21 days) and praziquantel (5 mg/kg PO q24h for 21 days) for 3 months.[205] The effect of substituting other benzimidazoles for mebendazole is unknown.[3]

PREVENTION

While reinfection in endemic areas is likely, the only preventive measure is to limit access to intermediate host species.[194] Therefore limiting a dog's or cat's access to amphibians, birds, reptiles, and small mammals that are potential intermediate hosts should aid in preventing *Spirometra* spp. infections.

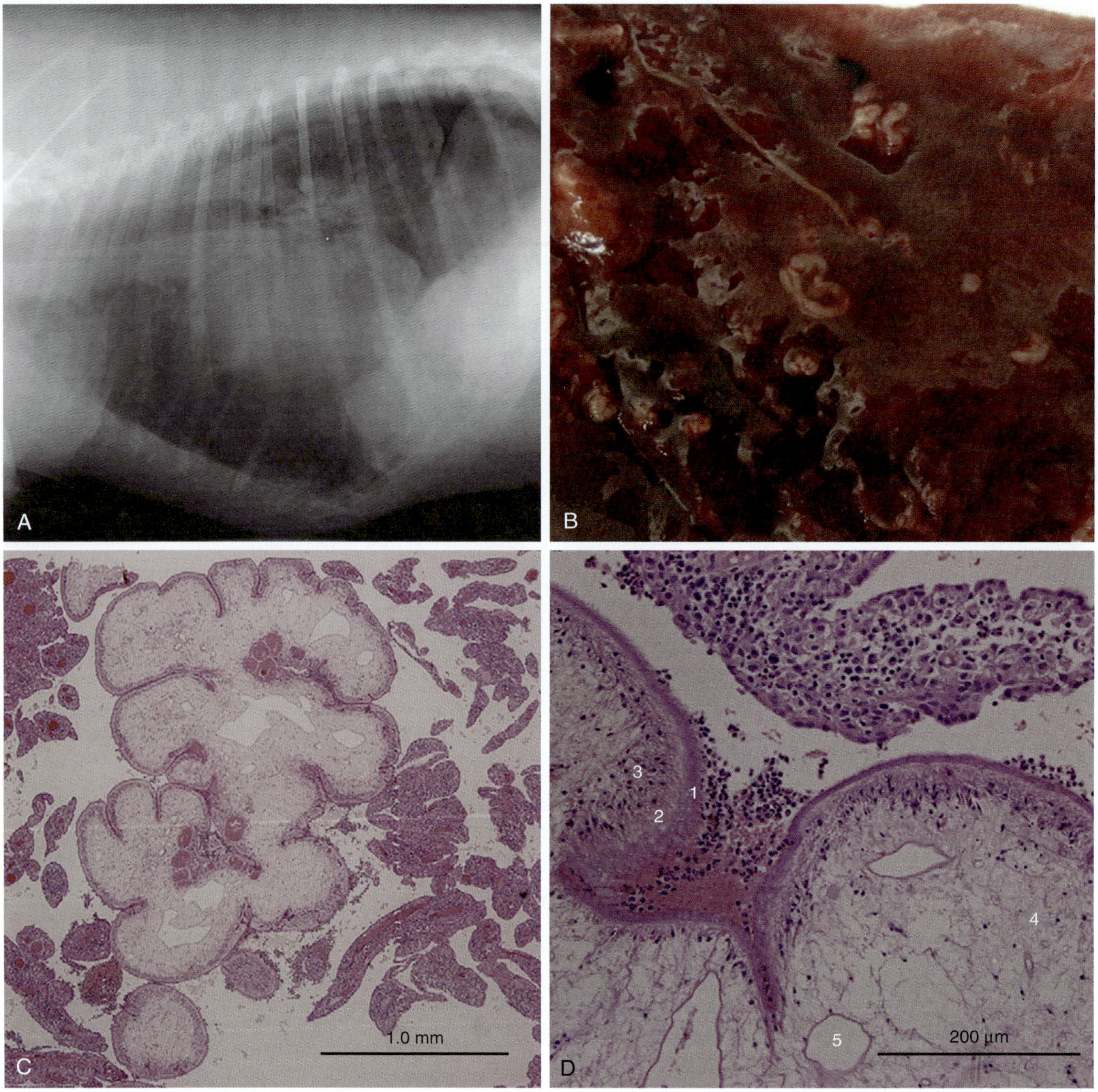

Fig. 115.20 Clinical images from a 12-year-old female spayed Labrador retriever from southeastern Australia with pulmonary sparganosis due to *Spirometra erinacei.* (A) Left lateral thoracic radiograph. There is evidence of pneumothorax, and soft-tissue opacities are present adjacent to the pleural surface of the diaphragm. (B) Pleural surface of the diaphragm with *Spirometra* plerocercoids. (C) Histological section of a plerocercoid and surrounding thickened omentum. (D) Histological section of omentum and plerocercoids showing the parasite's tegument *(1)*, subtegumental muscles *(2)*, perikaryon *(3)*, parenchyma *(4)*, and osmoregulatory canals *(5)*. There is neutrophilic inflammation around the parasite. (Reprinted from Simpson C, Jabbar A, Mansfield CS, et al. Molecular diagnosis of sparganosis associated with pneumothorax in a dog. *Mol Cell Probes.* 2012;26:60–62.)

PUBLIC HEALTH ASPECTS

Sparganosis of humans is caused by the plerocercoid stage of various tapeworms within the *Spirometra* genus. Humans can be infected by several routes including drinking water containing copepods infected with procercoids, ingesting the flesh of second intermediate hosts infected with plerocercoids (e.g., snakes, frogs), and via direct migration into a wound or across a mucous membrane from infected flesh (e.g., applying the incised body of a freshly caught frog to an open wound or injured eye as a traditional poultice).[11,203,213] Human sparganosis is a food-borne disease, therefore the risk of a human developing sparganosis directly from an infected dog or cat is minimal. Epidemiological data suggest

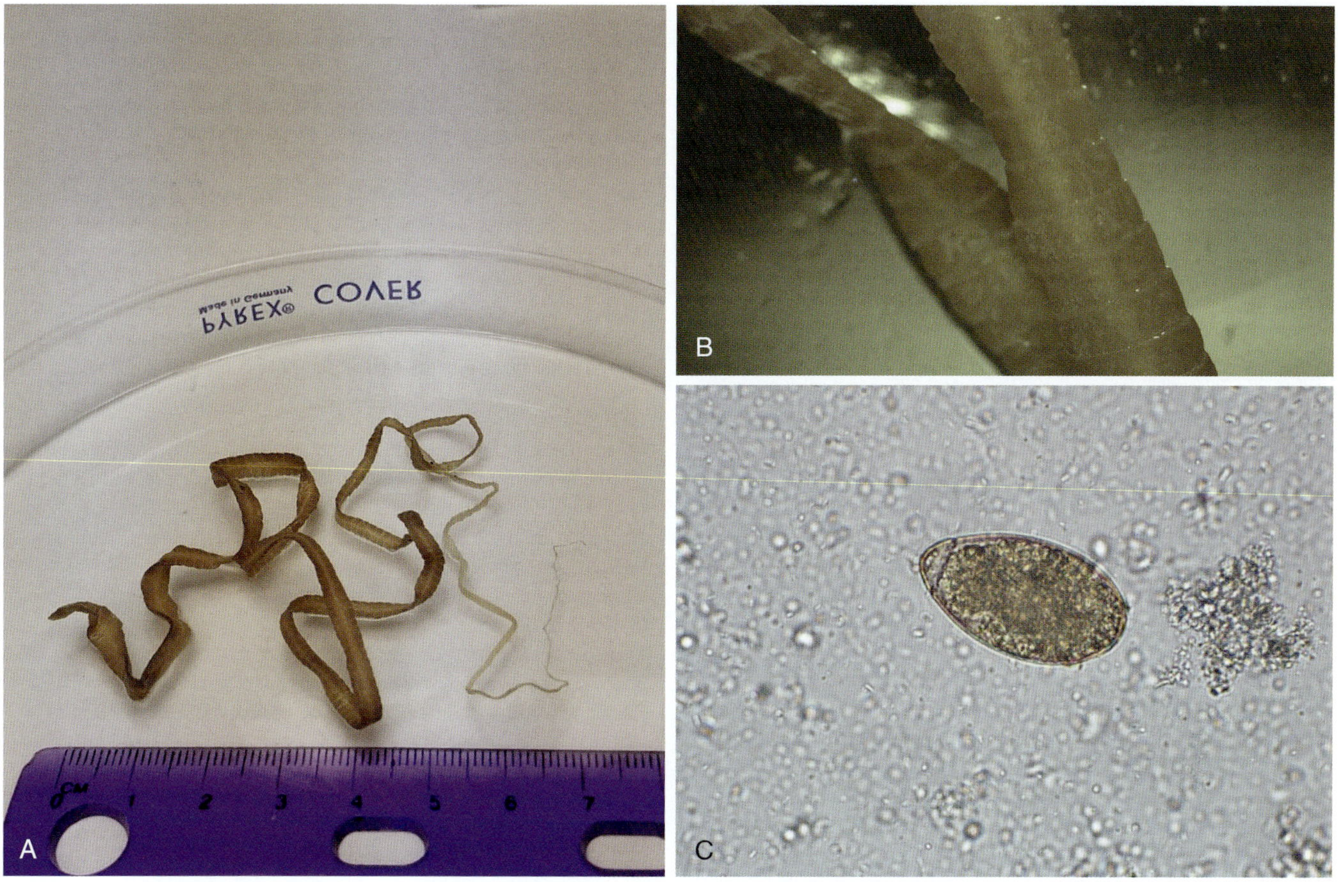

Fig. 115.21 Morphologic features of *Spirometra* sp. cestodes. (A) Formalin-fixed *Spirometra* sp. specimen of segments from a domestic cat. Note the small proximal segments relative to the larger distal (mature) segments with centrally located genital pores. (B) Strobila. Note the medial genital pores giving the appearance of a zipper. (C) Operculated egg from a fecal flotation of a cat. Unlike cyclophyllidean tapeworms, *Spirometra* spp. eggs resemble trematode eggs. (A, courtesy of Dr. Lindsay Starkey and B,C courtesy of Jamie Butler, Auburn University.)

TABLE 115.8 Recommended Drugs for Treating *Spirometra* spp. Infections in Dogs and Cats[a]

Indication/Drug	Species	Dosage (mg/kg)	Route	Interval	Days
Adult infection:					
Praziquantel	B	7.5	PO/SC	Daily	2
	B	25[b]	PO/SC	Daily	2
Proliferative sparganosis[c]:					
Praziquantel	D	50	SC	Weekly	21[d]
Fenbendazole	D	100	PO	BID	28[d]
Praziquantel	D	5.0	PO	Daily	21[e]
Mebendazole	D	20	PO	Daily	21[e]

[a]No anthelmintics are labeled for elimination of adult *Spirometra* spp.
[b]Preferred dosage.[103]
[c]Guarded prognosis.
[d]At the same time.
[e]Alternating 3-week protocol for 3 months (based on one case).
B, both dog and cat; *D*, dog.

that the most common cause of human sparganosis is consumption of raw freshwater frogs or snakes.[203] Human sparganosis most often presents as subcutaneous nodules containing a plerocercoid; scrotal and breast nodules are also described, and surgical removal is indicated.[214,215] Occasionally, the plerocercoid develops in the lungs, peritoneal cavity, eyes, or CNS. Cerebral sparganosis is of particular concern as it may be associated with neurological signs and even death.[194] Such infections have primarily been described in eastern and southeastern Asia.

CASE EXAMPLE

Signalment

"Zoe," a 5-year-old female, spayed, shar-pei/beagle mix that lived in southern Ontario, Canada.

History

Zoe was evaluated at a Veterinary Emergency and Referral Hospital in southern Ontario with a history of urinary incontinence for the previous 18 months. She was able to urinate and postured normally during micturition. There was no history of polyuria, polydipsia, or stranguria. Bloodwork and urinalysis performed 12 months earlier by the referring veterinarian were unremarkable, but at this visit a CBC revealed non-regenerative anemia (HCT 34% [RR, 38–57%], MCHC 32.1 [RR: 32.6-39.2 g/L]). On urinalysis, SpG was 1.026; some calcium oxalate crystals were noted. The urine protein:creatinine ratio was unremarkable and aerobic bacterial urine culture was negative. An abdominal ultrasound examination revealed no abnormalities of the urinary tract. However, a poorly defined, 5 × 3 cm mass was detected within the left liver lobe adjacent to the diaphragm. Due to the location of the lesion, fine-needle aspirates were not possible. Thoracic radiographs were unremarkable. An abdominal CT scan revealed a 4.5-cm diameter, rounded mass lesion in the left cranioventral and lateral aspect of the hepatic parenchyma in close proximity to the diaphragm. The mass was suspected to involve the left medial and left lateral lobes (see Fig. 115.9). After contrast administration, small septations were evident in the lesion creating a subtle honeycomb appearance. The periportal, gastric, splenic, and pancreaticoduodenal lymph nodes were mildly enlarged. No other abnormalities were detected.

Zoe was started on phenylpropanolamine for suspected sphincter mechanism incontinence. However, the incontinence appeared to worsen. The phenylpropanolamine dose was increased, but without improvement. Zoe had a history of aggression and was known to bite dogs and people. As a result, limited physical examinations had been performed; sedation was required for any procedure. Two months after being seen at the referral hospital, Zoe was evaluated at Ontario Veterinary College. At that time the owner reported she had been eating and drinking normally; no vomiting or diarrhea had been noted. She was still incontinent despite daily treatment with phenylpropanolamine.

Physical Examination Findings

The dog was bright, alert, and responsive. Body weight was 19.8 kg. After sedation (15 μg/kg dexmedetomidine IM and 0.4 mg/kg butorphanol IM), pulse was 48/minute, respiration rate was 28/minute, temperature was 99.3°F (37.4°C). No heart murmurs, arrhythmias, or abnormal breath sounds were auscultated. No masses or organomegaly were detected on abdominal palpation. No abnormalities of the genitourinary tract were detected. All other parameters were unremarkable.

Laboratory Findings

A PCV and total protein by refractometry were unremarkable.

Imaging Findings

Abdominal ultrasound examination revealed an 8 × 8 × 6 cm mass in the left liver, close to the diaphragm, with echogenic material in the center.

The initial differential diagnosis for the hepatic mass was hepatic neoplasia (hepatocellular carcinoma, adenoma, hemangiosarcoma, lymphoma, other) or a benign liver mass (nodular regeneration, granuloma, hematoma). In order to obtain a biopsy specimen, exploratory laparotomy was performed. A 7 × 6 × 4 cm mass was identified within the left medial liver lobe that was white/brown and slightly nodular (see Fig. 115.11A). The affected lobe was removed using a thoracoabdominal stapler; two circumferential ligatures were placed on remaining hilar vessels. The remainder of the liver and other abdominal organs were grossly unremarkable.

Pathologic Findings

On cut section, the resected mass was soft, white, and irregular, and contained multiple small (1 to 5 mm) cavities. On histopathology, effacing and replacing 80% to 90% of the hepatic parenchyma was a well-demarcated, partially encapsulated, expansile nodule composed of coalescing cystic spaces. These spaces were surrounded by abundant, variably mature, fibrovascular tissue and mixed inflammatory cells. Cystic spaces were lined by a variably folded eosinophilic, homogeneous, laminated (hyaline) membrane and an inner, variably intact, germinal epithelial layer. Cysts contained eosinophilic necrotic debris and mixed inflammatory cells. Rare small calcareous corpuscles were observed. However, no protoscolices were seen in the sections (see Fig. 115.11B). The same tissue sections stained positive with PAS stain.

Microbiologic Testing

Fresh frozen liver tissue was submitted for PCR testing. A PCR product was generated using primers specific for *E. multilocularis.*[109] The sequence generated was 100% identical (344/344 bp) to reference sequence of *E. multilocularis.*

Diagnosis

Hepatic alveolar echinococcosis (AE).

Treatment

Zoe was treated with praziquantel (5 mg/kg PO), to eliminate a potential intestinal infection. When the results of nucleic acid testing became available, treatment with albendazole (10 mg/kg PO q24h) for life was commenced.

Comments

Because this mass was located at the liver hilus, it was possible that a small amount of affected liver tissue remained after surgery. Treatment with albendazole was therefore particularly important. Since albendazole can occasionally cause bone marrow suppression in dogs, a CBC was recommended every week for the first month, monthly for the first 3 months, then every 3 months thereafter. A repeat abdominal ultrasound/CT scan was recommended every 6 to 12 months to monitor for recurrent disease. The diagnosis of AE in this case was an incidental finding and not likely associated with the urinary incontinence, which remained unresolved.

SUGGESTED READINGS

1. Corsini M, Geissbuhler U, Howard J, et al. Clinical presentation, diagnosis, therapy, and outcome of alveolar echinococcosis in dogs. *Vet Rec.* 2015;177:569.
2. Deplazes P, van Knapen F, Schweiger A, et al. Role of pet dogs and cats in the transmission of helminthic zoonoses in Europe, with a focus on echinococcosis and toxocarosis. *Vet Parasitol.* 2011;182:41–53.
3. Polish LB, Pritt B, Barth TFE, et al. First European haplotype of *Echinococcus multilocularis* identified in the United States: an emerging disease? *Clin Infect Dis.* 2021;72:1117–1123.
4. Wen H, Vuitton L, Tuxun T, et al. Echinococcosis: advances in the 21st century. *Clin Microbiol Rev.* 2019;32:e00075. 18.
5. Chai J-Y, Murrell KD, Lymbery AJ. Fish-borne parasitic zoonoses: status and issues. *Int J Parasitol.* 2005;35:1233–1254.
6. Scholz T, Garcia HH, Kuchta R, et al. Update on the human broad tapeworm (Genus *Diphyllobothrium*), including clinical relevance. *Clin Microbiol Rev.* 2009;22:146–160.

REFERENCES

1. Kutcha R, Scholz T, Bravec J, et al. Suppression of the tapeworm order Pseudophyllidea (Platyhelminthes: Eucestoda) and the proposal of two new orders, Bothriocephalidea and Diphyllobothriidea. *Int J Parasitol.* 2008;38:49–55.
2. Labuschange M, Beugnet F, Rehbein S, et al. Analysis of *Dipylidium caninum* tapeworms from dogs and cats, or their respective fleas. Part 1. Molecular characterization of *Dipylidium caninum*: genetic analysis supporting two distinct species adapted to dogs and cats. *Parasite.* 2018;25:30.

3. Conboy G. Cestodes of dogs and cats in North America. *Vet Clin Small Anim*. 2009;39:1075–1090.
4. Dantas-Torres F, Otranto D. Dogs, cats, parasites, and humans in Brazil: opening the black box. *Parasit Vectors*. 2014;56:1–56.
5. Beugnet F, Meyer L, Fouire J, et al. Preventive efficacy of NexGard Spectra® against *Dipylidium caninum* infection in dogs using a natural flea (*Ctenocephalides felis*) infection model. *Parasite*. 2017;24:16.
6. Emampour S, Borji H, Nagibi A. An epidemiological survey on intestinal helminths of stray dogs in Mashhad, North-east of Iran. *J Parasit Dis*. 2015;39:266–271.
7. Moskvina T, Ermolenka A. Helminth infections in domestic dogs from Russia. *Vet World*. 2016;9:1248–1258.
8. Dai R, Li Z, Li F, et al. Severe infection of adult dogs with helminths in Hunan Province, China poses significant public health concerns. *Vet Parasitol*. 2009;160:348–350.
9. Umar Y. Intestinal helminthoses in dogs in Kaduna Metropolis, Kaduna State, Nigeria. *Iran J Parasitol*. 2009;4:34–39.
10. Boreham R, Boreham P. *Dipylidium caninum*: life cycle, epizootiology, and control. *Compend Cont Educ Vet*. 1990;12:667–676.
11. Bowman DD. *Georgis' Parasitology for Veterinarians*. 10th edition. St. Louis, MO: Elsevier Saunders; 2014:477.
12. Hinaidy HK. Beitrag zur Biologie des *Dipylidium caninum*. 2. Mitteilung. *J Vet Med B*. 1991;38:329–336.
13. Lillis W. Helminth survey of dogs and cats in New Jersey. *J Parasitol*. 1967;53:1082–1084.
14. Amin O. Helminth and arthropod parasites of same domestic animals in Wisconsin. *Wisc Acad Sci Arts Letters*. 1980;68:106–110.
15. Little S, Adolph C, Downie K, et al. High prevalence of covert infection with gastrointestinal helminths in cats. *J Am Anim Hosp Assoc*. 2015;51:359–363.
16. Griffiths H. Helminths. In: *A Handbook of Veterinary Parasitology of Domestic Animals in North America*. Minneapolis, MN: University of Minnesota Press; 1978:119.
17. Bowman DD, Hendrix CM, Lindsay DS, et al. *Dipylidium caninum* (Linnaeus, 1758) Leuckart, 1863. In: *Feline Clinical Parasitology*. Ames, IA: Iowa State University Press; 2002:205–211.
18. Dryden MW, Payne PA, Ridley R, et al. Comparison of common fecal flotation techniques for the recovery of parasitic eggs and oocysts. *Vet Ther*. 2005;6:15–28.
19. Oscos-Snowball A, Tan E, Peregrine A, et al. What is your diagnosis? Fluid aspirated from an abdominal mass in a dog. *Vet Clin Pathol*. 2015;44:167–168.
20. Zajac A, Conboy G. *Veterinary Clinical Parasitology*. 8th edition. Wiley-Blackwell; 2012:354.
21. Beugnet F, Labuschagne M, Fourie J, et al. Occurrence of *Dipylidium caninum* in fleas from client-owned cats and dogs in Europe using a new PCR detection assay. *Vet Parasitol*. 2014;205:300–306.
22. Zhu G, Li L, Ohiolei JA, et al. A multiplex PCR assay for simultaneous detection of *Taenia hydatigena, T. multiceps, T. pisiformis* and *Dipylidium caninum* infections. *BMC Infect Dis*. 2019;19:854.
23. Thomas H, Gonnert R. The efficacy of praziquantel against cestodes in cats, dogs, and sheep. *Res Vet Sci*. 1978;24:20–25.
24. Boray J, Strong M, Allison J, et al. Nitroscanate, a new broad spectrum anthelmintic against nematodes and cestodes of dogs and cats. *Aust Vet J*. 1979;55:45–53.
25. Euzeby J, Prom Tep S, Rossignol J. Study of the anthelmintic properties of nitazoxanide in dog, cat, and sheep. *Rev Med Vet*. 1980;131:687–696.
26. Jesudoss Chelladurai J, Kifleyohannes T, Scott J, et al. Praziquantel resistance in the zoonotic cestode *Dipylidium caninum*. *Am J Trop Med Hyg*. 2018;99.1201–1205.
27. Taylor T, Zitzmann M. *Dipylidium caninum* in a 4-month old male. *Clin Lab Sci*. 2011;24:212–214.
28. Peng J, Xi Z, Ruo Dan L, et al. A human case of zoonotic dog tapeworm, *Dipylidium caninum* (Eucestoda: Dilepiidae), in China. *Korean J Parasitol*. 2017;55:61–64.
29. Miyaji S, Oku Y, Rausch R, et al. Growth of Japanese isolate of *Taenia crassiceps* in intermediate and definitive hosts. *Parasitol Res*. 1990;76:351–354.
30. Xhaxhiu D, Kusi I, Rapti D, et al. Principal intestinal parasites of dogs in Tirana, Albania. *Parasitol Res*. 2011;108:341–353.
31. Adolph C, Barnett S, Beall M, et al. Diagnostic strategies to reveal covert infections with intestinal helminths in dogs. *Vet Parasitol*. 2017;247:108–112.
32. Oge H, Oge S, Bahadir G, et al. Coprodiagnosis of *Echinococcus granulosus* infection in dogs from Ankara, Turkey. *Vet Parasitol*. 2017;242:44–46.
33. Wilcox R, Bowman D, Barr S, et al. Intestinal obstruction caused by *Taenia taeniaeformis* infection in a cat. *J Am Anim Hosp Assoc*. 2009;45:93–96.
34. Adolph C, Nutt G. Dysuria in a cat: could it be more? *Clin Brief*. 2015;13:24–27.
35. Hoberg E, Ebinger W, Render J. Fatal cysticercosis by *Taenia crassiceps* (Cyclophyllidea: Taeniidae) in a presumed immunocompromised canine host. *J Parasitol*. 1999;85:1174–1178.
36. Chemette R, Bussieras J, Mialot M, et al. Subcutaneous *Taenia crassiceps* cysticercosis in a dog. *J Am Vet Med Assoc*. 1993;203:263–265.
37. Nolte A, Strube C, Raue K, et al. Subcutaneous *Taenia crassiceps*-cysticercosis in a dog with Cushing's syndrome. *Tierarzliche Paraxis Kleintiere*. 2016;1:53–58.
38. Jull P, Browne E, Schonier, et al. Cerebral coenurosis in a cat caused by *Taenia serialis*: neurological, magnetic resonance imaging and pathological features. *J Feline Med Surg*. 2012;14:646–649.
39. Wünschmann A, Garlie V, Averbeck G, et al. Cerebral cysticercosis by *Taenia crassiceps* in a domestic cat. *J Vet Diagn Invest*. 2003;15:484–488.
40. Loos-Frank B. An up-date of Vester's (1969) 'Taxonomic revision of the genus *Taenia Linnaeus*' (Cestoda) in table format. *Syst Parasitol*. 2000;45:155–183.
41. Chalar C, Salome M, Sanorale-Pose M, et al. A high resolution analysis of the structure and chemical composition of the calcareous corpuscles from *Mesocestoides corti*. *Micron*. 2013;44:185–192.
42. Kohansal M, Nourian A, Hanilo A, et al. Molecular detection of *Taenia* spp. in dogs' feces in Zanjan Province, Northwest of Iran. *Vet World*. 2017;10:445–449.
43. Jenkins D, Urwin N, Williams T, et al. Red foxes (*Vulpes vulpis*) and wild dogs (dingoes (*Canis lupus dingo*) and dingo/domestic dog hybrids) as sylvatic hosts for Australian *Taenia hydatigena* and *Taenia ovis*. *Int J Parasitol Parasites Wildl*. 2014;3:75–80.
44. Allen J, Craig P. Coproantigens in taeniasis and echinococcosis. *Parasitol Int*. 2006;55:S75–S80.
45. Hoberg E. *Taenia* tapeworms: their true biology, evolution, and socioeconomic significance. *Microbes Infect*. 2002;4:859–866.
46. Eckert J, Deplazes P. Biological, epidemiological and clinical aspects of echinococcosis, a zoonosis of increasing concern. *Clin Microbiol Rev*. 2004;17:107–135.
47. McManus DP, Thompson RC. Molecular epidemiology of cystic echinococcosis. *Parasitology*. 2003;127:S37–S51.
48. Alvarez Rojas CA, Romig T, Lightowlers MW. *Echinococcus granulosus sensu lato* genotypes infecting humans – review of current knowledge. *Int J Parasitol*. 2014;44:9–18.
49. Lymbery AJ, Jenkins EJ, Schurer JM, et al. *Echinococcus canadensis, E. borealis*, and *E. intermedius*. What's in a name? *Trends Parasitol*. 2015;31:23–29.
50. Thompson RCA. The taxonomy, phylogeny and transmission of *Echinococcus*. *Exp Parasitol*. 2008;119:439–446.
51. Cardona GA, Carmena D. A review of the global prevalence, molecular epidemiology and economics of cystic echinococcosis in production animals. *Vet Parasitol*. 2013;192:10–32.
52. Thompson RCA, Kumaratilake LM, Ecker J. Observations on *Echinococcus granulosus* of cattle origin in Switzerland. *Int J Parasitol*. 1984;14:283–291.
53. Deplazes P, Eckert J, Mathis A, et al. Genus *Echinococcus*. In: *Parasitology in Veterinary Medicine*. The Netherlands: Wageningen Academic Publishers; 2016:653.
54. Garippa G, Manfredi MT. Cystic echinococcosis in Europe and in Italy. *Vet Res Commun*. 2009;33(Suppl 1):S35–S39.
55. Bružinskaite R, Šarkunas M, Torgerson PR, et al. Echinococcosis in pigs and intestinal infection with *Echinococcus* spp. in dogs in southwestern Lithuania. *Vet Parasitol*. 2009;160:237–241.
56. Mastin A, Brouwer A, Fox M, et al. Spatial and temporal investigation of *Echinococcus granulosus* coproantigen prevalence in farm dogs in South Powys, Wales. *Vet Parasitol*. 2011;178:100–107.

57. Konyaev SV, Yanagida T, Ivanov MV, et al. The first report on cystic echinococcosis in a cat caused by *Echinococcus granulosus* sensu stricto (G1). *J Helminthol.* 2012;86:391–394.
58. Armua-Fernandez MT, Castro OF, Crampet A, et al. First case of peritoneal cystic echinococcosis in a domestic cat caused by *Echinococcus granulosus* sensu stricto (genotype 1) associated to feline immunodeficiency virus infection. *Parasitol Int.* 2014;63:300–302.
59. Burgu A, Vural SA, Sarimehmetoglu O. Cystic echinococcosis in a stray cat. *Vet Rec.* 2004;155:711–712.
60. Nakao M, Xiao N, Okamoto M, et al. Geographic pattern of genetic variation in the fox tapeworm *Echinococcus multilocularis. Parasitol Int.* 2009;58:384–389.
61. Eckert J, Conraths FJ, Tackmann K. Echinococcosis: an emerging or re-emerging zoonosis? *Int J Parasitol.* 2000;30:1283–1294.
62. Kazacos KR. Cystic and alveolar hydatid disease caused by *Echinococcus* species in the contiguous United States. *Suppl Compend Contin Educ Pract Vet.* 2003;25:16–20.
63. Massolo A, Liccioli S, Budke C, et al. *Echinococcus multilocularis* in North America: the great unknown. *Parasite.* 2014;21:73.
64. Peregrine AS, Jenkins EJ, Barnes B, et al. Alveolar hydatid disease (*Echinococcus multilocularis*) in the liver of a Canadian dog in British Columbia, a newly endemic region. *Can Vet J.* 2012;53:870–874.
65. Skelding A, Brooks A, Stalker M, et al. Hepatic alveolar hydatid disease (*Echinococcus multilocularis*) in a boxer dog from southern Ontario. *Can Vet J.* 2014;55:551–553.
66. Davidson RK, Romig T, Jenkins E, et al. The impact of globalisation on the distribution of *Echinococcus multilocularis. Trends Parasitol.* 2012;28:239–247.
67. Oksanen A, Siles-Lucas M, Karamon J, et al. The geographical distribution and prevalence of *Echinococcus multilocularis* in animals in the European Union and adjacent countries: a systematic review and meta-analysis. *Parasites Vectors.* 2016;9:519.
68. Gottstein B, Stojkovic M, Vuitton DA, et al. Threat of alveolar echinococcosis to public health – a challenge for Europe. *Trends Parasitol.* 2015;31:407–412.
69. Deplazes P, Rinaldi L, Alvarez Rojas CA, et al. Global distribution of alveolar and cystic echinococcosis. *Adv Parasitol.* 2017;95:315–493.
70. Stehr-Green JK, Stehr-Green PA, Schantz PM, et al. Risk factors for infection with *Echinococcus multilocularis* in Alaska. *Am J Trop Med Hyg.* 1988;38:380–385.
71. Deplazes P, van Knapen F, Schweiger A, et al. Role of pet dogs and cats in the transmission of helminthic zoonoses in Europe, with a focus on echinococcosis and toxocarosis. *Vet Parasitol.* 2011;182:41–53.
72. Deplazes P, Eckert J. Veterinary aspects of alveolar echinococcosis – a zoonosis of public health significance. *Vet Parasitol.* 2001;98:65–87.
73. Kapel CMO, Togerson PR, Thompson RCA, et al. Reproductive potential of *Echinococcus multilocularis* in experimentally infected foxes, dogs, raccoon dogs and cats. *Int J Parasitol.* 2006;36:79–86.
74. Thompson RCA, Kapel CMO, Hobbs RP, et al. Comparative development of *Echinococcus multilocularis* in its definitive hosts. *Parasitology.* 2006;132:709–716.
75. König A, Romig T, Thoma D, et al. Drastic increase in the prevalence of *Echinococcus multilocularis* in foxes (*Vulpes vulpes*) in southern Bavaria, Germany. *Eur J Wildl Res.* 2005;51:277–282.
76. Tanner F, Hegglin D, Thoma R, et al. *Echinococcus multilocularis* in Grisons: distribution in foxes and presence of potential intermediate hosts. *Schweiz Arch Tierheilkd.* 2006;148:501–510.
77. Deplazes P, Hegglin D, Gloor S, et al. Wilderness in the city: the urbanization of *Echinococcus multilocularis. Trends Parasitol.* 2004;20:77–84.
78. Deplazes P, Alther P, Tanner I, et al. *Echinococcus multilocularis* coproantigen detection by enzlyme-linked immunosorbent assay in fox, dog, and cat populations. *J Parasitol.* 1999;85:115–121.
79. Svobodová V, Lenská B. Echinococcosis in dogs in the Czech Republic. *Acta Vet Brno.* 2002;71:347–350.
80. Hegglin D, Deplazes P. Control of *Echinococcus multilocularis*: strategies, feasibility and cost-benefit analyses. *Int J Parasitol.* 2013;43:327–337.
81. Schantz PM, Chai J, Craig PS, et al. Epidemiology and control of hydatid disease. In: Thompson RCA, Lymbery AJ, eds. *Echinococcus and Hydatid Disease.* England, UK: CAB International; 1995:233–331.
82. Kotwa JD, Greer T, Jardine CM, et al. Evaluation of the prevalence of *Echinococcus multilocularis* in dogs that visit off-leash dog parks in southern Ontario, Canada. *Zoonoses Public Health.* 2021;68:533–537.
83. Kuroki K, Morishima Y, Neil J, et al. Intestinal echinococcosis in a dog from Missouri. *J Am Vet Med Assoc.* 2020;256:1041–1046.
84. Wobeser G. The occurrence of *Echinococcus multilocularis* (Leukart, 1863) in cats near Saskatoon, Saskatchewan. *Can Vet J.* 1971;12:65–67.
85. Leiby PD, Kritsky DC. *Echinococcus multilocularis*: a possible domestic life cycle in central North America and its public health implications. *J Parasitol.* 1972;58:1213–1215.
86. Carmena D, Cardona GA. Canine echinococcosis: global epidemiology and genotypic diversity. *Acta Trop.* 2013;128:441–460.
87. Weiss A, Bauer C, Kohler K. Canine alveolar echinococcosis: morphology and inflammatory response. *J Comp Pathol.* 2010;143:233–238.
88. Corsini M, Geissbuhler U, Howard J, et al. Clinical presentation, diagnosis, therapy, and outcome of alveolar echinococcosis in dogs. *Vet Rec.* 2015;177:569.
89. Gesy K, Hill JE, Schwantje H, et al. Establishment of a European-type strain of *Echinococcus multilocularis* in Canadian wildlife. *Parasitology.* 2013;140:1133–1137.
90. Pinard C, Cuq B, Gibson T, et al. Alveolar echinococcosis in an Ontario dog resembling a hepatic abscess. *Can Vet J.* 2019;60:1099–1103.
91. Schurer JM, Tsybina P, Gesy KM, et al. Molecular evidence for local acquisition of human alveolar echinococcosis in Saskatchewan, Canada. *J Infect Dis.* 2021;223:1015–1018.
92. Kotwa JD, Isaksson M, Jardine CM, et al. *Echinococcus multilocularis* infection, Southern Ontario, Canada. *Emerg Infect Dis.* 2019;25:265–272.
93. Zajac A, Fairman D, McGee E, et al. Alveolar echinococcosis in a dog in the eastern United States. *J Vet Diagn Invest.* 2020;32:742–746.
94. Vuitton DA, Demonmerot F, Knapp J, et al. Clinical epidemiology of human AE in Europe. *Vet Parasitol.* 2015;213:110–120.
95. Gendron K, Goepfert C, Linon E, et al. Pulmonary *Echinococcus multilocularis* metastasis in a dog. *Can Vet J.* 2015;56:267–271.
96. Scharf G, Deplazes P, Kaser-Hotz B, et al. Radiographic, ultrasonographic, and computed tomographic appearance of alveolar echinococcosis in dogs. *Vet Radiol Ultrasound.* 2004;45:411–418.
97. Geigy CA, Kuhn K, Rutten M, et al. Unusual presentation of alveolar echinococcosis as prostatic and paraprostatic cysts in a dog. *BMC Vet Res.* 2013;9:159.
98. Reuter S, Nussle K, Kolokythas O, et al. Alveolar liver echinococcosis: a comparative study of three imaging techniques. *Infection.* 2001;29:119–125.
99. Czermak BV, Unsinn KM, Gotwald T, et al. *Echinococcus multilocularis* revisited. *Am J Roentgenol.* 2001;176:1207–1212.
100. Deplazes P, Eckert J. Diagnosis of the *Echinococcus multilocularis* infection in final hosts. *Appl Parasitol.* 1996;37:245–252.
101. Taylor MA, Coop RL, Wall RL. Echinococcus. In: *Veterinary Parasitology.* 4th edition. Wiley Blackwell:612-614.
102. Craig P, Mastin A, van Kesteren F, et al. *Echinococcus granulosus*: epidemiology and state-of-the-art of diagnostics in animals. *Vet Parasitol.* 2015;213:132–148.
103. Sobrino R, Gonzales LM, Vicente J, et al. *Echinococcus granulosus* (Cestoda, Taeniidae) in the Iberian wolf. *Parasitol Res.* 2006;99:753–756.
104. Staebler S, Grimm F, Glaus T, et al. Serological diagnosis of canine alveolar echinococcosis. *Vet Parasitol.* 2006;141:243–250.
105. Rausch RL, Wilson JF, Schantz PM, et al. Spontaneous death of *Echinococcus multilocularis*: cases diagnosed serologically (by Em2 ELISA) and clinical significance. *Am J Trop Med Hyg.* 1987;36:576–585.
106. Gottstein B, Wang J, Blagosklonov O, et al. *Echinococcus* metacestode: in search of viability markers. *Parasite.* 2014;21:63.
107. Isaksson M, Hagström Ä, Armua-Fernandez MT, et al. A semi-automated magnetic capture probe based DNA extraction and real-time PCR method applied in the Swedish surveillance of *Echinococcus multilocularis* in red fox (*Vulpes vulpes*) faecal samples. *Parasites Vectors.* 2014;7:583.
108. Dinkel A, von Nickisch-Rosenegk M, Bilger B, et al. Detection of *Echinococcus multilocularis* in the definitive host: coprodiagnosis by PCR as an alternative to necropsy. *J Clin Microbiol.* 1998;36:1871–1876.
109. Trachsel D, Deplazes P, Mathis A. Identification of taeniid eggs in the faeces from carnivores based on multiplex PCR using targets in mitochondrial DNA. *Parasitology.* 2007;134:911–920.

110. Panel on Animal Health and Welfare. *Echinococcus multilocularis* infection in animals. *EFSA J.* 2015;13:4373.
111. Thompson RC, Reynoldson JA, Manger BR. *In vitro* and *in vivo* efficacy of epsiprantel against *Echinococcus granulosus*. *Res Vet Sci.* 1991;51:332–334.
112. Deplazes P, Arnold P, Kaser-Holtz B, et al. Concurrent infections of the liver and intestine with *Echinococcus multilocularis* in dogs. *Arch Int Hidatid.* 1997;31:202–203.
113. Plumb DC. Albendazole. In: *Plumb's Veterinary Drug Handbook*. 8th edition. Wisconsin: Wiley Blackwell Publishing Co.; 2015:25–27.
114. Gauci C, Heath D, Chow C, et al. Hydatid disease; vaccinology and development of the EG95 recombinant vaccine. *Expert Rev Vaccines.* 2005;4:103–112.
115. Wen H, Vuitton L, Tuxun T, et al. Echinococcosis: advances in the 21st century. *Clin Microbiol Rev.* 2019;32:e00075–18.
116. Cabrera PA, Lloyd S, Haran G, et al. Control of *Echinococcus granulosus* in Uruguay: evaluation of different treatment intervals for dogs. *Vet Parasitol.* 2002;103:333–340.
117. Soriano SV, Pierangeli NB, Roccia I, et al. A wide diversity of zoonotic intestinal parasites infects urban and rural dogs in Neuquén, Patagonia, Argentina. *Vet Parasitol.* 2010;167:81–85.
118. Torgerson PR, Craig PS. Risk assessment of importation of dogs infected with *Echinococcus multilocularis* into the UK. *Vet Rec.* 2009;165:366–368.
119. Davidson RK, Robertson LJ. European pet travel: misleading information from veterinarians and government agencies. *Zoonoses Public Health.* 2012;59:575–583.
120. King CH. Cestodes (tapeworms). In: Mandell GL, Bennett JE, Dolin R, eds. *Principles and Practice of Infectious Diseases*. Philadelphia, PA: Saunders; 2005:3290–3293.
121. Arinc S, Kosif A, Ertugrul M, et al. Evaluation of pulmonary hydatid cyst cases. *Int J Surg.* 2009;7:192–195.
122. WHO. Guidelines for treatment of cystic and alveolar echinococcosis in humans. WHO Informal Working Group on Echinococcosis. *Bull World Health Organ.* 1996;74:231–242.
123. Craig P. Echinococcus multilocularis. *Curr Opin Infect Dis.* 2003;16:437–444.
124. Kern P, Bardonnet K, Renner E, et al. European echinococcosis registry: human alveolar echinococcosis, Europe, 1982–2000. *Emerg Infect Dis.* 2003;9:343–349.
125. Schweiger A, Ammann RW, Candinas D, et al. Human alveolar echinococcosis after fox population increase, Switzerland. *Emerg Infect Dis.* 2007;13:878–882.
126. Kadry Z, Renner EC, Bachmann LM, et al. Evaluation of treatment and long-term follow-up in patients with hepatic alveolar echinococcosis. *Br J Surg.* 2005;92:1110–1116.
127. Conraths FJ, Probst C, Possenti A, et al. Potential risk factors associated with human alveolar echinococcosis: systematic review and meta-analysis. *PLoS Negl Trop Dis.* 2017;11:e0005801.
128. Vuitton DA, Zhou H, Bresson-Hadni S, et al. Epidemiology of alveolar echinococcosis with particular reference to China and Europe. *Parasitology.* 2003;127:S87–S107.
129. Gottstein B, Jacquier P, Bresson-Hadni S, et al. Improved primary diagnosis of alveolar echinococcosis in humans by an enzyme-linked immunosorbent assay using the Em2plus antigen. *J Clin Microbiol.* 1993;31:373–376.
130. Müller NE, Frei S, Nuñez B, et al. Improved serodiagnosis of alveolar echinococcosis of humans using an *in vitro*-produced *Echinococcus multilocularis* antigen. *Parasitology.* 2007;134:879–888.
131. Trotz-Williams L, Mercer N, Walters J, et al. Public health investigation of suspected exposure to *Echinococcus multilocularis* in southwestern Ontario. *Zoonoses Public Health.* 2017;64:460–467.
132. James E, Boyd W. *Echinococcus alveolaris* (with the report of a case). *Can Med Assoc J.* 1937;36:354–356.
133. Gamble WG, Segal M, Schantz PM, et al. Alveolar hydatid disease in Minnesota. First human case acquired in the contiguous United States. *J Am Med Assoc.* 1979;241:904–907.
134. Jenkins EJ, Peregrine AS, Hill JE, et al. Detection of European strain of *Echinococcus multilocularis* in North America. *Emerg Infect Dis.* 2012;18:1010–1012.
135. Polish LB, Pritt B, Barth TFE, et al. First European haplotype of *Echinococcus multilocularis* identified in the United States: an emerging disease? *Clin Infect Dis.* 2021;72:1117–1123.
136. Houston S, Belga S, Buttenschoen K, et al. Epidemiological and clinical characteristics of alveolar echinococcosis: an emerging infectious disease in Alberta, Canada. *Am J Trop Med Hyg.* 2021;104:1863–1869.
137. Loos-Frank B. One or two intermediate hosts in the life cycle of *Mesocestoides* (cyclophyllidea, mesocestoididae)? *Parasitol Res.* 1991;77:726–728.
138. Crosbie P, Boyce W, Platzer E, et al. Diagnostic procedures and treatment of eleven dogs with peritoneal infections caused by *Mesocestoides* spp. *J Am Vet Med Assoc.* 1998;213:1578–1583.
139. Witenberg G. Studies on the cestode genus *Mesocestoides*. *Arch Zool Ital.* 1932;20:467–509.
140. Loos-Frank B. The common vole, *Microtus arvalis* pall. as intermediate host of *Mesocestoides* (Cestoda) in Germany. *Z Parasitenkd.* 1980;63:129–136.
141. Etges F. The proliferative tetrathyridium of *Mesocestoides vogae* sp. n. (Cestoda). *J Helminthol Wash.* 1991;58:181–185.
142. Wirtherle N, Wiemann A, Ottenjann M, et al. First case of canine peritoneal larval cestodosis caused by *Mesocestoides lineatus* in Germany. *Parasitol Int.* 2007;56:317–320.
143. Takeuchi-Storm N, Mejer H, Al-Sabi M, et al. Gastrointestinal parasites of cats in Denmark assessed by necropsy and concentration McMaster technique. *Vet Parasitol.* 2015;214:327–332.
144. Riggio F, Mannella R, Ariti G, et al. Intestinal and lung parasites in owned dogs and cats from central Italy. *Vet Parasitol.* 2013;193:78–84.
145. Adinezadeh A, Kia E, Mohebali M, et al. Endoparasites of stray dogs in Mashad, Khorasan Razavi Provence, Northeast Iran with special reference to zoonotic parasites. *Iran J Parasitol.* 2013;8:459–466.
146. Moskvina T, Ermolenko A. Helminth infections in domestic dogs from Russia. *Vet World.* 2016;9:1248–1258.
147. Loennberg E. Cestoden. In: Hamburger Malhaenische Sammelreise, 10 pages. (Cited in Witenberg, 1932). Studies on the cestode genus *Mesocestoides*. *Arch Zool Ital.* 1896;20:467–509.
148. Blagburn B, Lindsay D, Vaughan J, et al. Prevalence of canine parasites based on fecal flotation. *Compend Contin Educ Vet.* 1996;18:483–510.
149. Jordan H, Mullins S, Stebbins M. Endoparasitism in dogs: 21,583 cases (1981–1990). *J Am Vet Med Assoc.* 1993;203:547–549.
150. Rausch R. Family Mesocestoididae. In: Khalil L, Jones A, Bray R, eds. *Keys to the Cestode Parasites of Vertebrates*. CAB International; 1994:309–314.
151. Padgett K, Boyce W. Ants as the first intermediate hosts of *Mesocestoides* on San Miguel Island, USA. *J Helminthol.* 2005;79:67–73.
152. Eleni C, Scaramozzino P, Busi M, et al. Proliferative peritoneal and pleural cestodiasis in a cat caused by metacestodes of *Mesocestoides* sp. Anatomohistopathological findings and genetic identification. *Parasite.* 2007;14:71–76.
153. Conn D. The rarity of asexual reproduction among *Mesocestoides* tetrathyridia (Cestoda). *J Parasitol.* 1990;76:453–455.
154. Eckert L, von Brand T, Voge M. Asexual multiplication of *Mesocestoides corti* (Cestoda) in the intestines of dogs and skunks. *J Parasitol.* 1969;55:241–249.
155. Boyce W, Shender L, Schultz L, et al. Survival analysis of dogs diagnosed with canine peritoneal larval cestodiasis (*Mesocestoides* spp.). *Vet Parasitol.* 2011;180:256–261.
156. Barsanti J, Jones B, Bailey W, et al. Diagnosis and treatment of peritonitis caused by a larval cestode *Mesocestoides* spp. in a dog. *Cornell Vet.* 1979;69:45–53.
157. Parker M. An unusual cause of abdominal distention in a dog. *Vet Medicine.* 2002;97:189–195.
158. Kashiide T, Matsumoto J, Yamaya Y, et al. Case report; first confirmed case of canine peritoneal larval cestodiasis caused by *Mesocestoides vogae* (syn. *M. corti*) in Japan. *Vet Parasitol.* 2014;201:154–157.
159. Venco L, Kramer L, Pagliaro L, et al. Ultrasonographic features of peritoneal cestodiasis caused by *Mesocestoides* sp. in a dog and cat. *Vet Radiol Ultrasound.* 2005;46:417–422.
160. Lanteri G, di Caro G, Capucchio M, et al. *Mesocestoides* and multivisceral tetrathyridiosis in a European cat. *Veterinarni Medicina.* 2017;62:356–362.
161. Hrckova G, Miterpakova M, O'Connor A, et al. Molecular and morphological circumscription of *Mesocestoides* tapeworms from red foxes (*Vulpes vulpes*) in central Europe. *Parasitology.* 2011;138:638–647.
162. Tamura Y, Ohta H, Kashiide T, et al. Case Report: Protein-losing enteropathy caused by *Mesocestoides vogae* (syn. *M. corti*) in a dog. *Vet Parasitol.* 2014;205:412–415.

163. Papini R, Matteini A, Bandinelli P, et al. Effectiveness of praziquantel for treatment of peritoneal larval cestodiasis in dogs: a case report. *Vet Parasitol.* 2010;170:158–161.
164. Chandler A. First case of human infection with *Mesocestoides. Science.* 1942;96:112.
165. Fuentes M, Galan-Puchades M, Malone J. Short report: a new case report of human *Mesocestoides* infection in the United States. *Am J Trop Med Hyg.* 2003;68:566–567.
166. Gleason N, Kornblum Walzer P. *Mesocestoides* (Cestoda) in a child in New Jersey treated with niclosamide (Yomesan®). *Am Trop Med Hyg.* 1973;22:757–760.
167. Ohtomo H, Hioki A, Ito A, et al. 13th human case of the infection with *Mesocestoides lineatus* in Japan treated with paromomycin sulfate. *Jpn J Antibiot.* 1983;36:152–157.
168. Kuchta R, Brabec J, Kubácková P, et al. Tapeworm *Diphyllobothrium dendriticum* (Cestoda) – neglected or emerging human parasite? *PLoS Negl Trop Dis.* 2013;7:e2535.
169. Waeschenbach A, Brabec J, Scholz T, et al. The catholic taste of broad tapeworms – multiple routes to human infection. *Int J Parasitol.* 2017;47:831–843.
170. Kuchta R, Oros M, Ferguson J, et al. *Diphyllobothrium nihonkaiense* tapeworm larvae in salmon from North America. *Emerg Infect Dis.* 2017;23:351–353.
171. Dick TA, Nelson PA, Choudhury A. Diphyllobothriasis: update on human cases, foci, patterns and sources of human infections and future considerations. *Southeast Asian J Trop Med Public Health.* 2001;32(Suppl 2):59–76.
172. Chai J-Y, Murrell KD, Lymbery AJ. Fish-borne parasitic zoonoses: status and issues. *Int J Parasitol.* 2005;35:1233–1254.
173. Rivero MR, Motta CE, Salas MM, et al. *Diphyllobothrium* sp. in *Canis familiaris* from the subtropical area of Argentina (Puerto Iguazú, Misiones). *Rev Argent Microbiol.* 2015;47:196–200.
174. von Bonsdorff B. *Diphyllobothriasis in Man.* New York, NY: Academic Press; 1977:189.
175. Eguchi S. *Diphyllobothrium latum* (Linnaeus, 1758). *Proc Med Parasitol Jpn.* 1973;5:127–144.
176. Deplazes P, Eckert J, Mathis A, et al. Genus *Diphyllobothrium.* In: *Parasitology in Veterinary Medicine.* The Netherlands: Wageningen Academic Publishers; 2016:208–210.
177. Andersen K, Gibson DI. A key to three species of larval *Diphyllobothrium* Cobbold, 1858 (Cestoda: Pseudophyllidea) occurring in European and North American freshwater fishes. *Syst Parasitol.* 1989;13:3–9.
178. Scholz T, Garcia HH, Kuchta R, et al. Update on the human broad tapeworm (Genus *Diphyllobothrium*), including clinical relevance. *Clin Microbiol Rev.* 2009;22:146–160.
179. Gustinelli A, Menconi V, Prearo M, et al. Prevalence of *Diphyllobothrium latum* (Cestoda: Diphyllobothriidae) plerocercoids in fish species from four Italian Lakes and risk for the consumers. *Int J Food Microbiol.* 2016;235:109–112.
180. Pullola T, Vierimaa J, Saari S, et al. Canine intestinal helminths in Finland: prevalence, risk factors and endoparasite control practices. *Vet Parasitol.* 2006;140:321–326.
181. Sager H, Moret CS, Grimm F, et al. Coprological study on intestinal helminths in Swiss dogs: temporal aspects of anthelmintic treatment. *Parasitol Res.* 2006;98:333–338.
182. Shamarina AG, Kazantseva NA, Zavgorodnyaya NF, et al. The role of waterbodies in the spread of human diphyllobothriasis and opisthorchiasis in the Perm region. *Biol Resu vodo sapad Urala.* 1980:145–147.
183. Bowman DD, Hendrix CM, Lindsay DS, et al. *Diphyllobothrium latum* (Linnaeus, 1758) Cobbold, 1858. In: *Feline Clinical Parasitology.* Ames, IA: Iowa State University Press; 2002:185–189.
184. Dupouy-Camet J, Peduzzi R. Current situation of human diphyllobothriasis in Europe. *Euro Surveill.* 2004;9:31–35.
185. Torres P, Cuevas C, Tang M, et al. Introduced and native fishes as infection foci of *Diphyllobothrium* spp. in humans and dogs from two localities at Lake Panguipulli in Southern Chile. *Comp Parasitol.* 2004;70:111–117.
186. Wardle RA, Gotschall MJ, Horder LJ. The influence of *Diphyllobothrium latum* infestation upon dogs. *Trans Roy Soc Can.* 1937;31:59–69.
187. Wicht B, Yanagida T, Scholz T, et al. Multiplex PCR for differential identification of broad tapeworms (*Cestoda: Diphyllobothrium*) infecting humans. *J Clin Microbiol.* 2010;48:3111–3116.
188. Kirkpatrick CE, Knochenhauer AW, Jacobson SI. Use of praziquantel for treatment of *Diphyllobothrium* sp. infection in a dog. *J Am Vet Med Assoc.* 1987;190:557–558.
189. Sakamoto T. The anthelmintic efficacy of Droncit on adult tapeworms of *Hydatigera taeniaeformis, Mesocestoides corti, Echinococcus multilocularis, Diphyllobothrium erinacei,* and *D. latum. Vet Med Rev.* 1977;1:64–74.
190. Hendrix CM, Blagburn BL. Common gastrointestinal parasites. *Vet Clin North Am.* 1983;13:627–646.
191. Beldsoe GE, Oria MP. Potential hazards in cold-smoked fish: parasites. *J Food Sci.* 2001;66:1100–1103.
192. Hochberg NS, Bhadelia N. Infections associated with exotic cuisine: the dangers of delicacies. *Microbiol Spectrum.* 2015;3:10.1128/microbiolspec.IOL5-0010-2015.
193. Hendrix C. Helminth infections of the feline small and large intestines: diagnosis and treatment. *Vet Med.* 1995;90:456–472.
194. Little S, Ambrose D. *Spirometra* infection in cats and dogs. *Compend Contin Educ Vet.* 2000;22:299–305.
195. Mueller J, Strano A. *Sparganum proliferum,* a *Sparganum* infected with a virus? *J Parasitol.* 1974;60:15–19.
196. Wyrosdick H, Chapman A, Martinez J, et al. Parasite prevalence survey in shelter cats in Citrus County, Florida. *Vet Parasitol.* 2017;10:20–24.
197. Cardoso A, Figueiredo C, Conceicao M. The occurrence of zoonotic parasites in rural dog populations from northern Portugal. *J Helminthol.* 2014;88:203–209.
198. Vafae Eslahi A, Kiam E, Mobedi I, et al. Road killed carnivores illustrate the status of zoonotic helminthes in Caspian Sea littoral of Iran. *Iran J Parasitol.* 2017;12:230–235.
199. Itoh N, Ikegami H, Takagi M, et al. Prevalence of intestinal parasites in private-household cats in Japan. *J Feline Med Surg.* 2012;14:436–439.
200. Hong Q, Feng J, Liu H, et al. Prevalence of *Spirometra mansoni* in dogs, cats, and frogs and its medical relevance in Guangzhou, China. *Int J Infect Dis.* 2016;53:41–45.
201. Tun S, Ithoi I, Mahmud R, et al. Detection of helminth eggs and identification of hookworm species in stray cats, dogs, and soil from Klang Valley, Malaysia. *PLoS ONE.* 2015;10:e0142231.
202. Rojekittikhun W, Chaisiri K, Mahittkorn A, et al. Gastrointestinal parasites of dogs and cats in a refuge in Naknon Nayok, Thailand. *Southeast Asian J Trop Med Public Health.* 2014;45:31–39.
203. Liu Q, Li M, Wang Z, et al. Review: Human sparganosis, a neglected food-borne zoonosis. *Lancet Infect Dis.* 2015;15:1226–1235.
204. Buergelt C, Greiner E, Senior D. Proliferative sparganosis in a cat. *J Parasitol.* 1984;70:121–125.
205. Beveridge I, Friend S, Jeanathan N, et al. Proliferative sparganosis in Australian cattle dogs. *Aust Vet J.* 1998;76:757–759.
206. Drake D, Carreno A, Blagburn B, et al. Proliferative sparganosis in a dog. *J Am Vet Med Assoc.* 2008;233:1756–1760.
207. Marchiondo A, Weinstein P, Muller J. Significance of the distribution of ^{57}Co-vitamin B_{12} in *Spirometra mansonoides* (Cestoidea) during growth and differentiation in mammalian intermediate and definitive hosts. *Int J Parasitol.* 1989;19:119–124.
208. Woldemeskel M. Subcutaneous sparganosis, a zoonotic cestodiasis, in two cats. *J Vet Diagn Invest.* 2014;26:316–319.
209. Simpson C, Jabbar A, Mansfield CS, et al. Molecular diagnosis of sparganosis associated with pneumothorax in a dog. *Mol Cell Probes.* 2012;26:60–62.
210. Kirkpatrick C. *Spirometra* sp. in a domestic cat in Pennsylvania. *J Am Vet Med Assoc.* 1983;183:111–112.
211. Ugarte C, Thomas D, Gasser R, et al. *Spirometra erinacei/S. erinaceieuropaei* in a feral cat in Manawatu with chronic intermittent diarrhea. *N Z Vet J.* 2005;53:347–351.
212. Lee S, Huh S, Phares C. Genetic comparison between *Spirometra erinacei* and *S. mansonoides* using PCR-RFLP analysis. *Korean J Parasitol.* 1997;35:277–282.
213. Roberts L, Janovy J. Tapeworms. In: *Foundations of Parasitology.* 5th edition. Dubuque, IA: Wm C. Brown Publishers; 1996:325–353.
214. Chung S, Park K, Lee Y. Breast sparganosis: mammographic and ultrasound features. *J Clin Ultrasound.* 1995;23:447–451.
215. Ishida Y, Naitoh Y, Nishida M, et al. A case of *Sparganosis mansoni* with a painless mass in the inguinal region and the scrotum. *Hinyokika Kiyo.* 1996;42:983–985.

116

Miscellaneous Nematode Infections

Jennifer K. Ketzis, Susan E. Little, Judit M. Wulcan

KEY POINTS

Physaloptera spp. Infection

- First Described: *Physaloptera praeputialis* was first isolated from a domestic cat and described in 1889 (von Linstow). *Physaloptera rara* was first isolated from a domestic dog in North America and described in 1918 (Hall and Wigdor).
- Cause: *Physaloptera praeputialis* and *Physaloptera rara.*
- Affected Hosts: Domestic and wild dogs and cats.
- Geographic Distribution: Worldwide (*P. praeputialis*), North America (*P. rara*).
- Route of Transmission: Ingestion of intermediate insect or paratenic hosts.
- Major Clinical Signs: May cause chronic intermittent vomiting. Infections often are subclinical.
- Differential Diagnosis: Any GI or systemic cause of chronic vomiting (e.g., idiopathic gastritis, gastric foreign body, gastric neoplasia, food intolerance/allergy, chronic pancreatitis). Eggs must be differentiated from those of *Spirocerca lupi.* Vomited nematodes must be differentiated from *Toxocara canis*, *Toxocara cati*, and *Toxascaris leonina.*
- Human Health Significance: *Physaloptera* spp. of dogs and cats are not considered a zoonosis.

Spirocerca lupi Infection

- First Described: Karl Asmund Rudolphi (Swedish parasitologist and "father" of helminthology), 1809.
- Cause: *Spirocerca lupi* (esophageal worm), superfamily Spiruroidea, order Spirurida.
- Affected Hosts: Domestic dogs, wild canids, and other carnivores; rarely cats.
- Geographic Distribution: Worldwide but primarily in tropical and subtropical regions with the highest prevalence in the southern United States, Brazil, the Caribbean, South Africa, and the Middle East.
- Route of Transmission: Dogs become infected after ingestion of the intermediate host (coprophagous beetles in the family Scarabaeidae, order Coleoptera) or paratenic hosts (e.g., birds, frogs, lizards and other reptiles, rodents) containing a third-stage larva.
- Major Clinical Signs: Vomiting or regurgitation, odynophagia, ptyalism, respiratory difficulty, cough, weight loss, and fever.
- Differential Diagnoses: Differentials for regurgitation include esophageal foreign bodies, esophageal strictures, esophageal neoplasia or granulomas of other origin, and megaesophagus. Differentials for vomiting include any GI or systemic cause of chronic vomiting (e.g., idiopathic gastritis, gastric foreign body, gastric neoplasia, food intolerance/allergy, chronic pancreatitis). Eggs must be differentiated from *Physaloptera* spp.
- Human Health Significance: *Spirocerca lupi* infection is not considered a zoonosis.

Strongyloides spp. Infection

- First Described: Larval stages of *Strongyloides stercoralis* were first isolated from human feces in 1876; the first identification of natural infection in a dog was in 1914. In cats, *Strongyloides planiceps* was isolated by Leiper from a rusty tiger cat (*Felis planiceps*) in 1927. *Strongyloides felis* was first isolated from cats in India in 1925. While *Strongyloides tumefaciens* was first noted in cats in the USA in 1929, it was not described or named until 1941.
- Cause: *Strongyloides* are commonly referred to as threadworms and belong to the family Strongyloididae in the order Rhabditida.
- Affected Hosts: *Strongyloides stercoralis* occurs in dogs, cats, non-human primates, and people. *Strongyloides felis* and *S. tumefaciens* have been described in domestic and wild cats; *S. planiceps* in domestic and wild cats, dogs, and wild carnivores.
- Geographic Distribution: Worldwide.
- Route of Transmission: Oral, percutaneous, and, less frequently, transmammary infections occur in dogs. Oral and percutaneous transmission occur in cats.
- Major Clinical Signs: Subclinical infections are common. Cough and other signs of bronchial involvement can occur in the early stage of infection in dogs. Severe enteritis with profuse diarrhea can occur in the later stage of infection. Skin papules are sometimes seen when larvae enter the dog percutaneously. In cats, clinical signs are rare, but diarrhea has been reported in some infections.
- Differential Diagnoses: The clinical signs are nonspecific and must be differentiated from other causes of diarrhea, for example, dietary, infectious, inflammatory, toxic, or extraintestinal causes of diarrhea. In puppies, *S. stercoralis* must be differentiated from other parasites that have larval lung migration stages (e.g., *Toxocara canis, Ancylostoma caninum*), cause diarrhea, and are able to enter the animal percutaneously (e.g., *Ancylostoma caninum, Uncinaria stenocephala*). In cats and dogs, recovered larvae must be distinguished from lungworm; hookworm larvae.
- Human Health Significance: *Strongyloides stercoralis* can be transmitted from dogs to people and from people to dogs. Zoonotic transmission of cat *Strongyloides* has not been studied; there have been no reports of *Strongyloides* being transmitted from cats to people.

Mammomonogamus spp. Infection

- First Described: *Mammomonogamus ierei* (synonym *Syngamus ierei*) was first described by Buckley in 1934, who isolated it from a domestic cat in Trinidad. *Mammomonogamus auris* (synonym *Syngamus auris*) was first described by Faust and Tank in 1934, who isolated it from the middle ear of several cats in China.
- Cause: *Mammomonogamus ierei* and *Mammomonogamus auris*, which occur in cats, are commonly referred to as gapeworms. These nematodes belong to the family Syngamidae.

- Affected Hosts: *Mammomonogamus ierei* and *M. auris* infect domestic cats.
- Geographic Distribution: The distribution of *Mammomonogamus* is disparate, with *M. ierei* reported in the Caribbean and *M. auris* found in Asia.
- Route of Transmission: Unknown. Given the life cycle of other parasites in this family, it is likely that paratenic hosts are involved.
- Major Clinical Signs: Subclinical infections are common. However, infections can be associated with inflammation of the nasopharynx resulting in a mucoid nasal discharge, coughing, sneezing episodes, and weight loss with *M. ierei*. Head shaking has been seen in a cat with *M. auris* infection.
- Differential Diagnoses: Other infections that cause nasal discharge and sneezing (e.g., viral infections, *Eucoleus aerophilus*, *Cuterebra* spp.). In the case of *M. auris*, *Otodectes cynotis* also can result in head shaking. The dark cerumen associated with *O. cynotis* infection does not occur with *M. auris* infection. Eggs of *M. ierei* and *M. auris* can be seen in a fecal flotation.
- Human Health Significance: There are no reports of *M. ierei* and *M. auris* infecting humans and neither are believed to be zoonotic.

Dioctophyme renale Infection

- First Described: *Dioctophyme renale* was first described by the German zoologist Johann Goeze in 1782; earlier reports of giant kidney worms date back to the late 1500s.
- Cause: *Dioctophyme renale*, the giant kidney worm, is the largest parasitic nematode of domestic animals (family Dioctophymidae in the order Ascaridida).
- Affected Hosts: Most cases of *D. renale* in domestic animals are reported in dogs, with infections occasionally seen in cats and other host species, including humans. Fish-eating vertebrates, especially mink and other mustelids, are the natural definitive host.
- Geographic Distribution: *Dioctophyme renale* has a sporadic, worldwide distribution although reports of infection are rare in Africa and Asia. The parasite is widespread in the Americas and has been reported from dogs and other hosts from Canada to Brazil.
- Route of Transmission: Eggs are shed in the urine of infected definitive hosts. First-stage larvae develop inside the eggs and hatch following ingestion by aquatic oligochaete annelid intermediate hosts found in the detritus of ponds and streams. Third-stage larvae develop within the tissues of the annelids and may be passed to paratenic hosts, such as fish and frogs, when they ingest the intermediate hosts. Dogs and other final hosts are infected upon ingestion of annelids, or, more commonly, by ingesting third-stage larvae in fish paratenic hosts.
- Major Clinical Signs: Most infections are subclinical. Some dogs have hematuria, renal pain, renal enlargement, abdominal pain, and abdominal effusion. Development of worms in subcutaneous fat has also been reported.
- Differential Diagnoses: Other causes of cystitis; renal neoplasia; or a retroperitoneal, abdominal, or subcutaneous mass. Abdominal *D. renale* infection in cats can resemble FIP. Eggs of *D. renale* are not always present in urine sediment and thus diagnosis may sometimes be made by ultrasound or exploratory laparotomy.
- Human Health Significance: Although rare, zoonotic infections with *D. renale* have been reported and are associated with ingestion of larvae in undercooked fish or frogs.

Dracunculus insignis Infection

- First Described: *Dracunculus* spp. have been described since antiquity. *Dracunculus medinensis* was described by Linnaeus in 1758, and *Dracunculus insignis* by Leidy in 1858.
- Cause: *Dracunculus insignis*, a subcutaneous worm of raccoons and other carnivores that also infects dogs, is a spirurid nematode closely related to the human Guinea worm, *Dracunculus medinensis*.
- Affected Hosts: Most cases of *D. insignis* infection in domestic animals are reported in dogs, although ferrets are also susceptible; a limited number of cases have been described in cats. Wild carnivores, especially raccoons, are most commonly infected and considered the natural definitive host of this parasite in North America. Although primarily a human parasite, *D. medinensis* also readily infects dogs in endemic areas.
- Geographic Distribution: *Dracunculus insignis* has only been reported from Canada and the United States. Due to concerted eradication efforts, *D. medinensis* is currently limited to three countries in Africa. Other *Dracunculus* spp. have been reported from mammals, snakes, and turtles in the Western Hemisphere and from snakes in Europe, Africa, Asia, and Australia.
- Route of Transmission: Gravid female *Dracunculus* spp. migrate to the extremities of the definitive host and form subcutaneous cysts. The presence of the nematode induces the formation of blisters; when immersed in water, the uterus of the nematode ruptures, releasing hundreds of thousands of larvae into the water. The motile larvae are ingested by copepod intermediate hosts. After third-stage larvae develop, copepods are ingested by definitive hosts drinking water; the nematodes then migrate to subcutaneous locations, mature, mate, and eventually form new cysts to continue the life cycle. Alternatively, infected copepods may be ingested by aquatic vertebrates which can then serve as paratenic hosts.
- Major Clinical Signs: Dogs with *D. insignis* present with fluctuant subcutaneous swellings, usually on a distal extremity or, less commonly, the thorax. Lesions are often pruritic and painful. The skin may appear ulcerated or bear a patent opening; when the affected limb is immersed in water, an adult nematode may emerge.
- Differential Diagnoses: Other, more common causes of subcutaneous masses include lipoma, reactive lymph nodes, neoplasia, or other dermal parasites (e.g., *Cuterebra*, *Dirofilaria repens*). However, the distinct location on a distal extremity and, when present, the appearance of a patent ulcer through which a nematode emerges, considerably narrows potential diagnoses. Specimen collection using fine-needle aspiration often leads to recovery of *D. insignis* larvae. Long female nematodes may be encountered during surgical exploration of the cystic lesion.
- Human Health Significance: Human infection is most commonly by *D. medinensis*. Recent reports of *D. medinensis* in domestic dogs have created challenges in the final stages of eradication efforts for the human Guinea worm.

Ocular Nematodes

- First Described: *Onchocerca lupi* was first described in a feral wolf in Russia. *Thelazia callipaeda* was first described by Ralliet and Henry in 1910 and *Thelazia californiensis* by Price in 1930.
- Cause: *Onchocerca lupi* and *Thelazia* spp. Aberrant migration has also resulted in other species of nematodes reported from the eye, including *Dirofilaria* spp., *Dracunculus* spp., and *Toxocara* spp.
- Affected Hosts: *Onchocerca lupi* is primarily a parasite of domestic dogs although feline onchocerciasis has been reported. *Thelazia callipaeda* and *T. californiensis* are described from dogs and cats with occasional reports from wildlife definitive hosts. Other *Thelazia* spp. infect the eyes of large animals.
- Geographic Distribution: Ocular nematodes occur sporadically around the world, with *O. lupi* reported from northern Asia, southern and central Europe, and the southwestern United States; *T. callipaeda* from Asia and, more recently, Europe; and *T. californiensis* from western North America.

- Route of Transmission: The life cycle of *O. lupi* is not fully understood, but other *Onchocerca* spp. are transmitted between definitive hosts by arthropod intermediate hosts, including black flies (*Simulium* spp.) and biting midges (*Culicoides* spp.). *Thelazia* spp. are transmitted by muscid flies feeding around the eyes.
- Major Clinical Signs: Ocular lesions due to *O. lupi* and *Thelazia* spp. may be mild to severe although many animals appear largely subclinical. In the acute phase of *O. lupi* infection, general ocular discomfort is seen with excessive lacrimation and photophobia. In chronic infections, nodules develop on the sclera, conjunctiva, and eyelids. Infection with *Thelazia* spp. may be associated with chronic conjunctivitis but nodules are not present.
- Differential Diagnoses: Many infectious, inflammatory, and traumatic conditions can cause ocular irritation and conjunctivitis. However, once nematodes are visualized coiled in inflammatory tissue on the conjunctiva (*O. lupi*) or free under the eyelids or nictitating membrane (*Thelazia* spp.), the diagnostic list of differentials is short. Other nematodes that occasionally migrate aberrantly to the eyes include *Angiostrongylus vasorum, Dirofilaria* spp., *Dracunculs insignis, Toxocara* spp., and *Trichinella spiralis* (eyelid).
- Human Health Significance: Human infection with both *O. lupi* and *Thelazia* spp. occasionally occurs resulting in ocular irritation, excessive lacrimation, and the presence of intraocular nematodes.

INTRODUCTION

This chapter reviews clinically relevant aspects of several nematode parasites of dogs and cats that are occasionally encountered in veterinary practice. Some affect the GI system, including *Physaloptera*, a stomach worm associated with chronic vomiting, and *Strongyloides stercoralis. Strongyloides stercoralis* is a nematode that alternates between a free-living and parasitic lifestyle and that, when parasitizing the small intestine, can induce severe diarrhea, particularly in puppies. Other nematodes in this chapter may cause esophageal (*Spirocerca lupi*), otic or nasopharyngeal (*Mammomonogamus* spp.), dermal (*Dracunculus insignis*), renal (*Dioctophyme renale*), or ocular (*Onchocerca lupi, Thelazia* spp.) pathology.

PHYSALOPTERA SPP. INFECTION

ETIOLOGY AND EPIDEMIOLOGY

Physaloptera is a genus of spirurid nematodes belonging to the family Physalopteridae in the order Spirurida. Numerous species have been reported in a variety of vertebrate hosts worldwide, but only two species, *Physaloptera praeputialis* and *Physaloptera rara*, are regularly reported in dogs and cats. *Physaloptera praeputialis*, first described in 1889 (von Linstow), occurs worldwide and is considered primarily a parasite of cats, although it infects a variety of other mammals including domestic dogs, foxes, and wild felids.[1–5] *Physaloptera rara,* first described in 1918 (Hall and Wigdor), occurs in North America and is considered primarily a parasite of coyotes but also is found in domestic dogs and cats, raccoons, and other wild animals.[1,2,6–8]

Adult nematodes are between 2 and 6 cm long, white or pink, and have a cephalic collar and triangular, toothed pseudolabia. The males are slightly shorter than the females and have pedunculated caudal papillae and alae, joined anterior to the anus (Fig. 116.1).[3,6,9] *Physaloptera praeputialis* can be differentiated from *P. rara* by a cuticular sheath that covers the posterior end.[2] The eggs of the two species are indistinguishable and are small (49 to 59 μm x 30 to 34 μm), oval, thick-shelled, and contain fully formed larvae in fresh feces (Fig. 116.2).[2,10,11]

The life cycle of *Physaloptera* spp. includes intermediate insect hosts from the orders Coleoptera, Orthoptera, and Blattodea (beetles, crickets, and roaches) and paratenic hosts (snakes, lizards, frogs, hedgehogs). The complete diversity of insect and paratenic hosts is unknown. Cats and dogs become infected via the consumption of intermediate or paratenic hosts or feces from these hosts containing third-stage larvae (L_3). Adult *Physaloptera* spp. and larvae reside mainly in the stomach with some also found in the cranial duodenum, usually with their anterior end attached to the mucosa.[9,12] Larvae are not known to migrate. The prepatent period ranges from as few as 35 days to 156 days, with most infections requiring at least 60 days to reach patency. This wide variation in the prepatent period is potentially due to the source of infection (intermediate or paratenic

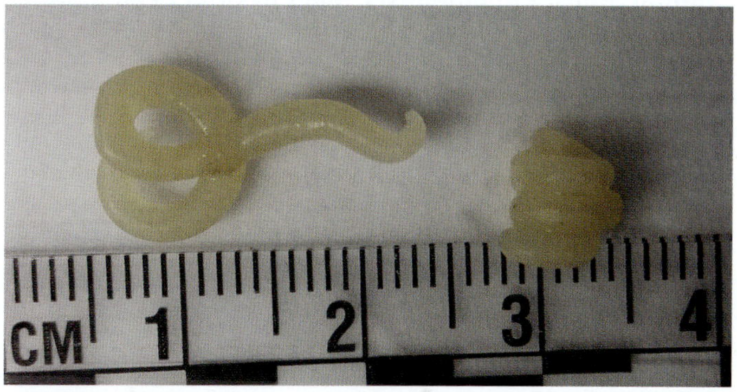

Fig. 116.1 *Physaloptera sp.* adults; adults range from 2 to 6 cm long. (Courtesy J. Ketzis.)

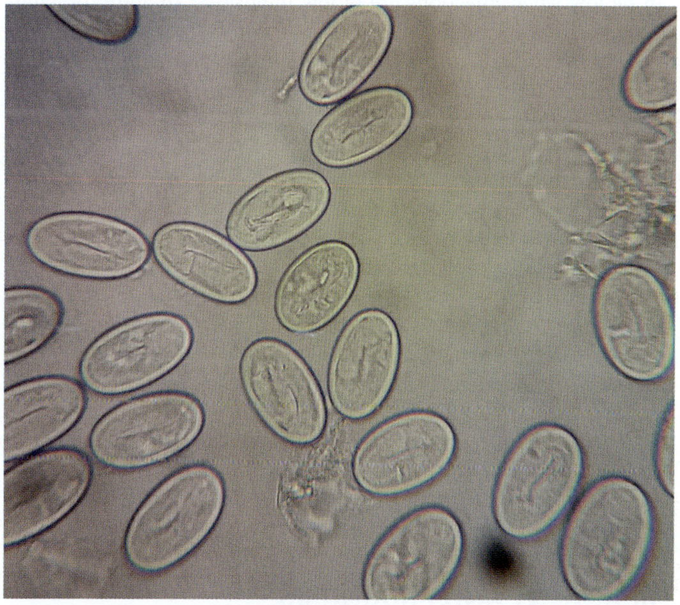

Fig. 116.2 *Physaloptera sp.* eggs isolated from a female adult; eggs are larvated in fresh feces and are approximately 49 to 59 μm x 30 to 34 μm. (Courtesy J. Ketzis.)

host).[2,3,6,12] In cats and dogs, most infections consist of only a few adult worms (1 to 8), although much higher numbers have been found in feral cats (25 to 30).[13,14]

Physaloptera spp. occur worldwide with most reports of infections in cats and dogs from North and South America, Australia, and Asia. There have only been a few reports of *Physaloptera* spp. in Europe and Africa in domestic dogs and cats.[2,15] In domestic dogs and cats, prevalence is typically below 5% with most studies in dogs showing a prevalence of <2% and cats with the higher prevalence.[10,15–24] This contrasts with some older studies from the 1940s to the mid-1980s where prevalence in cats was found to be from 20% to 40% and differs from wildlife species where it can be over 50%.[6,25,5,26,27]

Given the issues with diagnosis using many common fecal flotation solutions with lower specific gravity (e.g., <1.3), the prevalence of *Physaloptera* spp. in domestic dogs and cats could be underestimated. At the same time, prevalence could be decreasing with more widespread use of regular monthly heartworm preventives. Conversely, the high prevalence in wildlife species could potentially pose a concern where these animals frequent urban areas, which could increase exposure of domestic dogs and cats.

CLINICAL FEATURES

Clinical Signs, Pathogenesis, and Physical Examination Findings

Physaloptera spp. attach to the gastric or duodenal mucosa and feed on blood and tissue. Adult and immature *Physaloptera* can induce a catarrhal gastritis which may manifest as chronic, intermittent vomiting. Diarrhea, anorexia, and weight loss also can occur, although many infections are subclinical.[13,18,28] Differentials for *Physaloptera* spp. are broad and can include any GI or systemic cause of chronic vomiting (e.g., idiopathic gastritis, gastric foreign body, gastric neoplasia, food intolerance/allergy, chronic pancreatitis).[29]

DIAGNOSIS

Physaloptera eggs are particularly heavy compared to other common nematode eggs and occur intermittently in feces; overall egg numbers can be low when infections are of low intensity.[30] In addition, clinical signs can be induced by larval stages before eggs are present in the feces. Therefore fecal diagnosis is insensitive. When eggs are present, flotation methods with solutions of specific gravity >1.3 can be used; however, many standard flotation solutions are <1.3 SpG.[31,32] Direct smear can overcome the heavy egg issue but also lacks sensitivity due to the limited quantity of feces examined.[18,31–33] When eggs are seen, they must be differentiated from those of *Spirocerca lupi*.

Frequently, a diagnosis is made when dogs or cats vomit nematodes or following gastroscopy.[13,28] When nematodes are vomited, they must be differentiated from *Toxocara canis*, *Toxocara cati*, and *Toxascaris leonina*. Although adult worms are readily visible using gastroscopy, immature stages, which also induce clinical signs, might be more challenging to see. Peripheral eosinophilia has been reported in a minority of cases.[13,28]

On gross necropsy examination the gastric wall may be normal or thickened, with mucosal petechiae or ecchymoses. Histologically, a diffuse lymphoplasmacytic gastritis is most commonly reported, sometimes with concurrent mucosal congestion, catarrhal gastritis, and histiocytic or eosinophilic infiltrates.[13,14]

TREATMENT AND PROGNOSIS

No anthelmintics are registered for the treatment of *Physaloptera* spp. infections in cats and dogs. Pyrantel pamoate (20 mg/kg PO repeated at 2 week intervals for a total of 2 to 3 administrations) is recommended, and with this treatment, prognosis is good.[33] Treatment with lower and single doses of pyrantel pamoate has shown limited efficacy; pyrantel pamoate (5 to 20 mg/kg PO) did not clear infections in cats.[34,35] In a single case report of infection in a dog, 5 mg/kg administered twice at a 2-week interval was effective; however, in a study of 10 dogs in which adult worms were removed via endoscopy prior to treatment, 15 mg/kg administered twice at 2- to 3-week intervals did not result in resolution of clinical signs in two dogs.[13,18] Other anthelmintics that have been used include ivermectin (200 µg/kg SC) in two dogs and two cats, fenbendazole (50 mg/kg, PO q24h for three days) in a single dog after manual removal of worms by endoscopy, and levamisole (8 mg/kg SC) in two cats.[13,28] The dose of ivermectin used was significantly higher than that in heartworm preventives and should not be used in sensitive breeds.

Endoscopic removal of adult nematodes can be effective. However, not all adult nematodes may be seen and larval stages can remain, requiring a follow-up anthelmintic treatment.[13,33]

IMMUNITY, VACCINATION, AND PREVENTION

There are no published data suggesting that dogs and cats develop immunity to reinfection and there are no vaccines to prevent infection. The primary means of prevention is to limit access to intermediate and paratenic hosts. No studies on the efficacy of monthly heartworm preventives (e.g., macrocyclic lactones) in preventing the establishment of *Physaloptera* spp. have been performed; however, data with ivermectin suggest that monthly heartworm preventives could limit infections.[28,33]

PUBLIC HEALTH ASPECTS

Physaloptera spp. of dogs and cats are not considered zoonotic.

SPIROCERCA LUPI INFECTION (SPIROCERCOSIS)

ETIOLOGIC AGENT AND EPIDEMIOLOGY

Spirocerca lupi, first described by Rudolphi in 1809, belongs to the superfamily Spiruroidea in the order Spirurida.[36] *Spirocerca lupi* infects domestic and wild canids with some other mammals such as raccoons occasionally serving as a final host.[37–40] Adult *S. lupi* reside in nodules in the esophagus, are pink to red in color, and range in size from 3 to 7 cm, with the males being smaller than the females.[41–43] The eggs released by the female worms enter the lumen of the esophagus and are passed in the

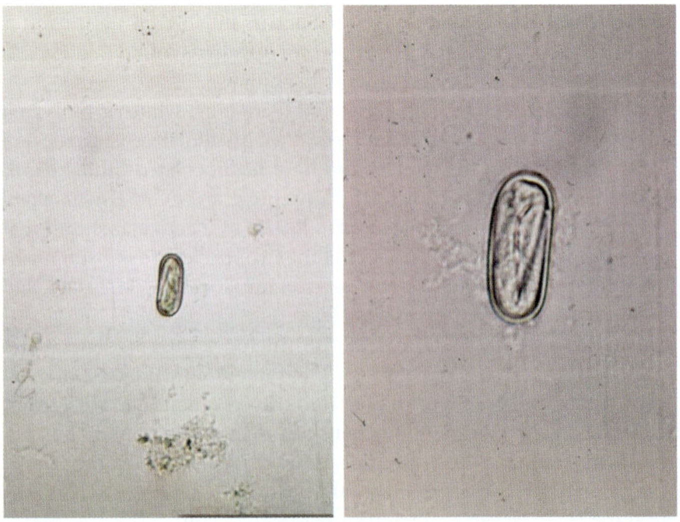

Fig. 116.3 *Spirocerca lupi* egg; eggs are larvated in fresh feces and are approximately 20 to 37 µm x 11 to 18 µm. (Courtesy of National Center for Veterinary Parasitology, Oklahoma State University.)

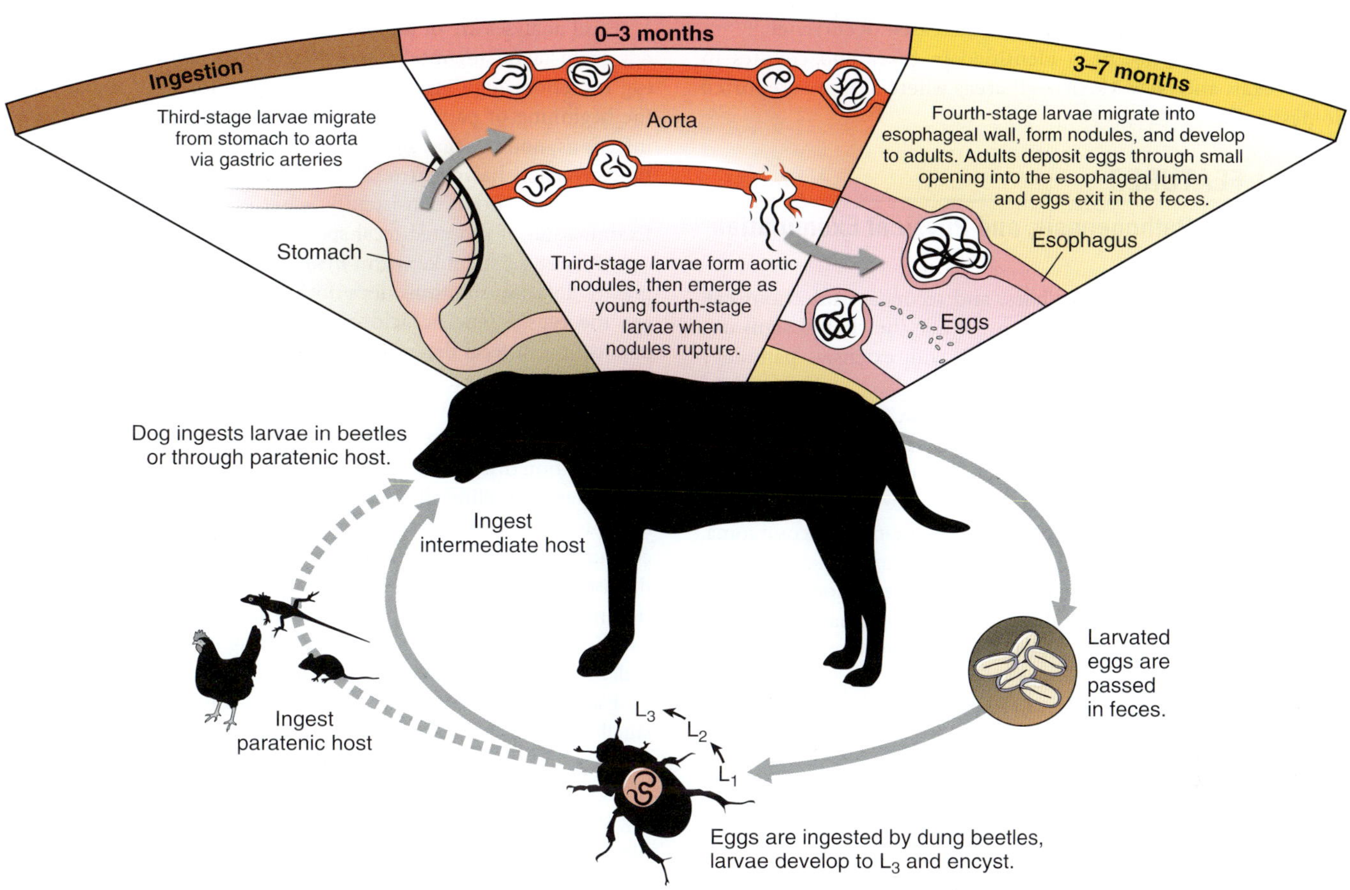

Fig. 116.4 Life cycle of *Spirocerca lupi.*

feces. Eggs recovered from fresh feces contain a first-stage larva (L_1) and are thick-shelled, elongated with parallel sides, and range in size from 20 to 37 µm x 11 to 18 µm (Fig. 116.3).[41,43,44] Coprophagous beetles from the family Scarabaeidae, order Coleoptera consume the eggs whereby the larva is released, develops to the third stage, and encysts. Dogs become infected when they ingest beetles with third-stage larvae (L_3) or by consuming paratenic hosts such as birds, frogs, lizards and other reptiles, and rodents (Fig. 116.4).[41,45–47] Once consumed, the L_3 are released in the stomach of the dog and proceed to penetrate the stomach mucosa and migrate toward the thoracic aorta via the gastric and celiac arteries. This migration typically requires 3 weeks. Once in the wall of the thoracic artery, the nematode develops to an immature adult stage in approximately 3 months, after which it migrates to the esophagus where further development to the adult stage occurs. During development from a larva to a mature adult, a tissue reaction develops in the esophageal wall, resulting in the esophageal nodule in which the adult nematode lives (Fig. 116.5). These nodules initially consist of granulation-like tissue, which later gradually is replaced by proliferating fibroblasts. They are often incorrectly referred to as granulomas.[41,43,45] The prepatent period is 3 to 6 months.[41,43]

Most reports of *S. lupi* infection in dogs are from the southern United States (Alabama, Mississippi, Oklahoma, Texas), South and Central America (Brazil, Mexico), the Caribbean, the Middle East, and South Africa with infrequent reports in Europe.[41,42,45,48–51] In general, occurrence in domestic dogs is <1% although in some areas, particularly in stray dogs, it can be as high as 40%.[22,25,52–54] The density of intermediate and paratenic hosts influences differences in occurrence in rural and urban areas and prevalence can be underestimated if less-sensitive diagnostic methods are used and overestimated if based solely on stray dogs.[45,49] Older dogs, working and sporting dogs, and large-breed dogs are at risk of infection.[49,55]

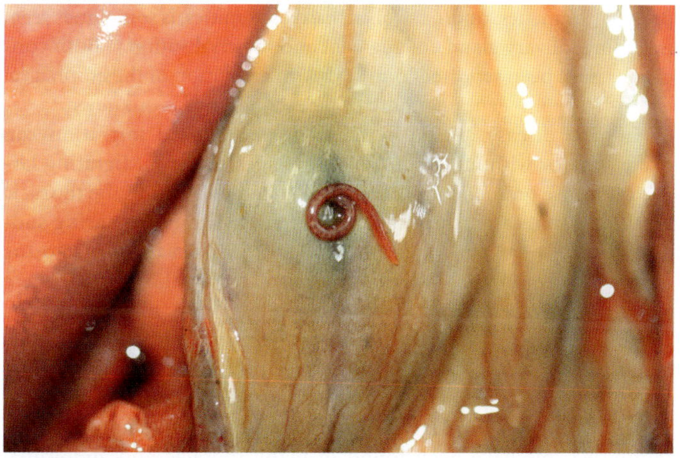

Fig. 116.5 *Spirocerca lupi* adult and esophageal nodule; adults range from 3 to 7 cm long. (Courtesy of Ross University School of Veterinary Medicine.)

Incidence has decreased in some locations and in Italy it is referred to as an "old-fashioned" parasite due to its lack of occurrence.[40] Reasons cited for decreasing prevalence are use of insecticides killing the intermediate host, changes in dog diets, and use of monthly heartworm preventives.[41,45] In endemic areas where macrocyclic lactones are used as a preventive, there is some concern that anthelmintic resistance development could occur. While no resistance has been documented, it does require investigation.[49]

In locations where *S. lupi* currently is rare in domestic dogs, there are concerns that migration of wild animal hosts, urbanization of foxes and raccoons, and the movement of domestic dogs could pose a risk of reintroduction or increased occurrence.[40,56,57] In the USA, *S. lupi* has been identified in foxes and coyotes in Florida, Texas, and New Mexico, all areas where *S. lupi* is reported in domestic dogs.[27,39]

CLINICAL FEATURES

Clinical Signs, Pathogenesis, and Physical Examination Findings

Larval migration, esophageal nodules, and secondary infections can cause clinical signs in *S. lupi* infections. While the clinical signs can be severe, many infections are subclinical, with extensive pathology occurring prior to diagnosis.

The esophageal nodules may be single or few, <1 to several cm in diameter, and are typically located just a few centimeters cranial to the caudal esophageal sphincter.[45,49,58–61] The nodules may undergo malignant transformation and approximately 20% of affected dogs are diagnosed with either esophageal fibrosarcoma, osteosarcoma, or undifferentiated sarcoma.[45,49,59] These tumors may metastasize to lungs and other organs.[62,63] Small benign esophageal nodules can be subclinical, whereas larger nodules can disrupt normal swallowing, causing clinical signs such as regurgitation/vomiting, odynophagia, and weight loss.[45,49,59–61] Respiratory signs such as cough or dyspnea are not uncommon and may be secondary to physical compression by esophageal nodules or complications associated with migration or malignant transformation.[49,59,60,64] Fever may be present on physical examination.

A frequent but typically subclinical concurrent finding is a caudal thoracic spondylitis, which is seen in approximately 30% of cases. The pathogenesis of this periosteal bone reaction is not known, but is so rarely seen without *S. lupi* lesions that the combination of a caudal esophageal mass and caudal thoracic spondylitis by some is considered pathognomonic.[59–61] Concurrent hypertrophic osteopathy, which may present as lameness and/or swollen, hard extremities, is sometimes seen, including salivary gland enlargement and hypersalivation.[59] Both conditions have been reported to resolve with resolution of the esophageal lesion. The pathogenesis of both of these conditions is unknown.[65–67]

Clinical disease caused by aberrant or standard migration can occur with or without concurrent esophageal lesions. Migrating larvae can cause permanent intimal scars and aneurysms in the thoracic aorta. In some cases, the weakened aorta may rupture, causing sudden death.[41,52,68,69] In other cases, migration from the aorta to the esophagus causes mediastinitis, pleuritis, or pyothorax.[59,64] There also have been reports of thromboembolic disease, likely caused by turbulent blood flow through aortic aneurysms, presenting as peracute paresis/paralysis of pelvic limbs; and painful, cold, dysfunctional lower extremities with absent or weak femoral pulses.[70,71] Aberrant migration of larvae is not uncommon and nodules containing worms have been found in many thoracic and abdominal organs.[60] There are several reports of aberrant migration through the spinal cord presenting as acute-onset paresis or paralysis of one or both pelvic limbs. Apart from neurological deficits associated with spinal lesions, physical examination findings in these cases included pain along the spine.[72–75]

DIAGNOSIS

A diagnosis of canine spirocercosis heavily relies on diagnostic imaging and esophageal endoscopy. Clinical pathological findings are variable and unspecific. Findings compatible with inflammation such as inflammatory leukograms (typically characterized by neutrophilia and/or monocytosis), evidence of an acute phase reaction (e.g., increased serum CRP concentration), and non-regenerative anemia are sometimes, but not always, seen.[45,76]

Fecal analyses are of limited sensitivity for several reasons: pathology from larval migration and nodule formation can occur before egg excretion; high egg production occurs for only a short time at the beginning of patency; and few or no eggs are shed in single-sex infections, nodules that lack opercula, and late in infection if neoplastic conversion has occurred.[41,43–45,77] Regardless of the fecal analysis method used, none consistently achieves >70% sensitivity.[44,48,60,77] Examination of repeated fecal specimens improves detection, but by only 8 to 28%.[60] Unlike with *Physaloptera* spp., use of higher specific gravity flotation solutions does not improve sensitivity and can damage the eggs.[44] Nucleic acid–based detection methods have limited application in fecal diagnosis but could enable diagnosis using tissue specimens and have the potential to increase detection during early infection.[77]

Where infections are endemic, a tentative diagnosis can be made on identification of a soft-tissue mass in the caudal esophagus. The esophageal masses in clinically affected patients can be large enough to be seen on thoracic radiographs.[45] Radiographs also can be used to detect concurrent thoracic spondylitis, hypertrophic osteopathy, and other disease complications. Sensitivity of radiographs for nodule detection may be improved with administration of liquid barium sulfate in subclinically infected dogs where screening is considered desirable in order to prevent malignant transformation in hyperendemic regions.[48]

Esophageal endoscopy is useful for confirmation or detection of smaller lesions but requires general anesthesia and can only detect nodules and adult nematodes that are protruding into the lumen of the esophagus.[48,78] Computed tomography, in addition to detecting small esophageal nodules, can be used to detect extraesophageal nodules, aortic lesions, and potential metastasis in cases of neoplastic transformation.[45]

Endoscopic-guided biopsy has high specificity but low sensitivity for diagnosis of malignant transformation; instead, diagnosis is often made after surgical excision or on necropsy. In sections of nodules collected at necropsy, nematodes, eggs, or migratory tracts can be seen in most nonneoplastic nodules, but in only a minority of neoplastic nodules.[59]

The diagnosis of intraspinal *S. lupi* infection is extraordinarily challenging as esophageal nodules and patent infections are not always present. Nonspecific changes can be seen on CT or MRI. CSF analysis regularly shows marked pleocytosis with variable proportions of neutrophils and eosinophils; however, definitive diagnosis usually is made by direct visualization of nematodes during surgery or at necropsy.[72] There is one case report, however, where nematode eggs were visualized directly in CSF.[79]

TREATMENT AND PROGNOSIS

There are no registered anthelmintics for the treatment of *S. lupi*. In dogs without neoplastic nodules, treatment with doramectin, milbemycin oxime, and moxidectin halts egg excretion, resolves clinical signs (if present) within weeks, and results in disappearance of esophageal nodules in 95 to > 500 days (Table 116.1). These macrocyclic lactones must be used with caution in certain dog breeds. There have been mixed reports of ivermectin efficacy (0.4 mg/kg, SC, six doses at 2-week intervals; 0.6 mg/kg, SC, two doses at 2-week intervals).[49,80] Levamisole does not appear to be effective.[40] Prognosis, with treatment, is typically good for cases without malignant transformation.[45,59,81] This requires early detection, even in subclinically infected dogs, which can be challenging due to the limitations of routine fecal diagnostic methods.

Surgical treatment is required for dogs with neoplastic transformation. Partial esophagectomies may be successful, but median survival time after surgery is usually short (3 to 9 months), with metastatic disease reported as the most common cause of death.[63,82,83] More

TABLE 116.1 **Extra-label Treatments with Reported Activity Against Adult *Spirocerca lupi***

Doramectin SC	Moxidectin Topical	Milbemycin Oxime Oral
0.2 mg/kg, 3 doses at 2-week intervals	2.5 to 6.25 mg/kg weekly for 19 weeks	0.5 to 1 mg/kg, 2 doses 1 week apart, third dose 2 weeks later
0.4 mg/kg, 6 doses at 2-week intervals		Initial treatment followed by monthly administration for 6 months or more
0.5 mg/kg, 2 doses 2 weeks apart		
0.8 mg/kg, 2 doses 1 week apart		
Additional treatments can be required; SC can be followed by 0.5 mg/kg PO q24h for 42–126 days		

See references 49, 82, 205–210.

recently, transendoscopic esophageal mass ablation has been described as a method for removing nodules.[82,84,85] Removal of nodules is often combined with chemotherapy (doxorubicin or carboplatin as monotherapies or combined), but neither the use nor the type of drug has been demonstrated to increase survival time.[82] Esophageal resections have been attempted but are typically not successful, as patients often die within the immediate postoperative period.[63]

IMMUNITY, VACCINATION, AND PREVENTION

There is no indication that dogs develop immunity to reinfection and there is no vaccine available. Prevention should focus on limiting a dog's access to the intermediate and paratenic hosts. Removal of vomit and feces from the environment can decrease dung beetle access to the eggs.

Moxidectin 2.5%/imidacloprid 10% (Advocate for dogs in Europe and Advantage Multi in the USA; previously Bayer, now Elanco) applied monthly is approved in Europe as a preventive for *S. lupi* infection. Natural exposure studies have shown a preventive fraction of 94.7%.[86] Other macrocyclic lactones are active against immature stages, reducing establishment of *S. lupi* adults and the size of nodules. Milbemycin oxime (minimum 0.5 mg/kg, monthly for up to six treatments) decreased aortic lesions, establishment in the thoracic aorta, and establishment of adults; efficacy for prevention of adult infections ranged from 92.3% to 100% in experimental and natural infections.[87-89] Doramectin and ivermectin (0.2 mg/kg every 3 months) have been used as preventives in endemic areas, although the efficacy of these regimens have not been evaluated.[49]

PUBLIC HEALTH ASPECTS

Spirocerca lupi has not been identified as a zoonosis.

STRONGYLOIDES SPP. (STRONGYLOIDIASIS)

ETIOLOGIC AGENT AND EPIDEMIOLOGY

Strongyloides stercoralis (family Strongyloididae, order Rhabditida) has a unique life cycle; adult females reside in the host and reproduce via parthenogenesis (asexual reproduction), and free-living adult females and males reproduce sexually. In dogs, females reside in the small intestine and can be identified by their filariform esophagus, which is approximately one third of the length of their body. Larvated eggs and, more commonly, first-stage rhabditiform larvae (L_1) with straight tails can be recovered in host feces. These larvae can develop to L_3 (homogonic cycle), or, depending on environmental conditions, free-living adult rhabditiform female and male nematodes (heterogonic cycle) that produce offspring that develop into infective L_3. The environmental cycle can take as few as 2 days (homogonic cycle) and as long as 7 days (heterogonic cycle).[90-95] Infective L_3 primarily enter the host percutaneously. Oral infection can occur, although this more typically results in penetration of the oral mucosa by L_3.[96,97] The migration route varies with strain and species; pulmonary migration is common but not required.[98] Some larvae can arrest but the majority reach the small intestine within 4 to 6 days. The female then develops in the mucosal epithelium and lays eggs in small intestinal crypts. The prepatent period ranges from 5 to 21 days. *Strongyloides stercoralis* females range from slightly < 2 mm to 3.5 mm; mean egg dimensions are 42 to 58 μm x 30 to 34 μm; and L_1 recovered in feces are approximately 180 to 380 μm long with most 250 to 300 μm long.[90,91,93,97]

Although less common, transmammary infection is possible if the infection in the mother occurs in late gestation or early lactation.[99,100] Autoinfection is rare but can occur with the L_1 hatching from the egg and molting into an L_3 while in the host.[101,102] Hyperinfection, used to refer to high levels of autoinfection and migrating larvae, also can occur. In humans, "disseminated infection" refers to the migration of larvae beyond the GI tract, peritoneum, and lungs. This term is not directly applicable to dogs since the normal migratory route can be extrapulmonary.

The life cycle of *Strongyloides* in cats has not been as extensively studied but likely is similar to that in dogs with a few important exceptions. Female *Strongyloides* spp. worms in cats also can inhabit the colon and neither transmammary, autoinfection nor hyperinfection have been confirmed.[93-95] Also, with *Strongyloides planiceps,* embryonated eggs almost as large as *Ancylostoma* eggs are found in the feces instead of L_1.[93]

While *S. stercoralis* is the species found in dogs, the species infecting cats is much less clear. *Strongyloides planiceps*, first isolated in 1927 and described in 1943, has only been reported in cats and some wildlife species in Malaya and Japan.[93,103] *Strongyloides felis*, described in 1925, has been reported in India and Australia.[91,95] *Strongyloides tumefaciens*, the last to be described (1941) and the only species in which the parasitic female resides in the large intestine, has been reported in North and South America.[94,104-106] Reports of *S. stercoralis* in cats have been infrequent although it has been proposed that *S. felis* and *S. tumefaciens* are strains or subspecies of *S. stercoralis*; this has been supported by work with dog and human strains.[91,107-111] Nematodes in tissue that were thought to be *S. tumefaciens* based on lesion location and pathology were recently subjected to PCR-sequencing and determined to be *S. stercoralis*, supporting the theory of strains or subspecies.[112] However, given the difference in morphology that exists, *S. planiceps* is likely a distinct species. Hence, in the rest of this chapter, infections in cats are referred to as *Strongyloides* spp. unless the information is specific to *S. planiceps*.

In both cats and dogs, *Strongyloides* spp. occur worldwide, although prevalence is typically low; most studies report a prevalence of <5% in dogs (range, 0 to 50%).[113-124] The higher prevalence is reported more in tropical and subtropical regions. In cats, prevalence is typically 0 to 4% but up to 46% has been seen in some population s.[24,95,125-128] *Strongyloides* infections in dogs and cats are likely underreported, given that release of eggs and L_1 can be intermittent and routine fecal diagnostic methods lack sensitivity for *Strongyloides* spp. detection.

CLINICAL FEATURES

Clinical Signs, Pathogenesis, and Physical Examination Findings

Most *Strongyloides* spp. infections in dogs and cats are subclinical. Dogs with heavy infections can have chronic intermittent diarrhea and weight loss or stunted growth. Feces is typically of watery, mucoid consistency and can contain blood. Severe infections may be fatal.[114,115,121,123] In some cases, GI signs are preceded by respiratory signs and hemorrhagic pododermatitis. These signs may be caused by pulmonary migration and percutaneous infection, respectively.[129,130] As in humans, *Strongyloides* infection of dogs with immunosuppressive conditions (e.g., glucocorticoid therapy) can result in accelerated autoinfection or hyperinfection that is associated with exacerbated GI and pulmonary signs.[101,102,130,131] Less is known about clinical signs of infection in cats. However, infections have been associated with chronic diarrhea, weight loss, and death.[94,104,105]

DIAGNOSIS

Strongyloides infection is challenging to diagnose using conventional fecal analysis techniques due to a low parasite load and irregular larval output. Use of serial specimen collection and the Baermann test can increase sensitivity.[132] When L_1 are recovered (Fig. 116.6), *Strongyloides* spp. larvae can be differentiated from *Ancylostoma* spp. larvae by their shorter buccal capsule and a prominent genital primordium. If filariform L_3 are seen, these can be distinguished by their truncated notched tail and long esophagus. If eggs are seen, they are larvated in fresh feces and are smaller than *Ancylostoma* spp. eggs.

There are no commercially available serological or PCR assays for detection of *Strongyloides* spp. in dogs or cats. PCR methods have had variable sensitivity when used to detect *Strongyloides* spp. in humans. IFA tests and ELISA have good sensitivity but are of limited availability.[119]

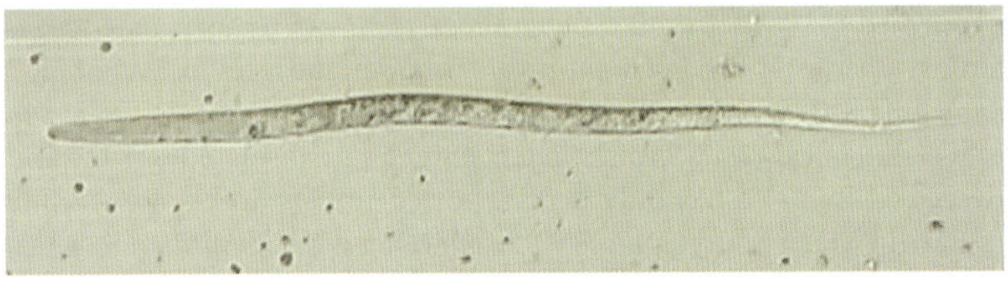

Fig. 116.6 *Strongyloides* larva from a Baermann examination; first-stage rhabditiform larvae range from 180 to 380 μm in length. (Courtesy of Ross University School of Veterinary Medicine.)

CBC and serum chemistry results in clinically affected animals are nonspecific and may include stress leukograms, mild anemia, hypoproteinemia, and increased serum CRP.[121] While eosinophilia is typically associated with many parasitic infections, it is not consistently seen with *Strongyloides* spp. infections.[121,133]

On necropsy, parasitic females are typically located in the duodenal mucosa. The nematodes are small and may easily be overlooked on gross examination, but can be found on microscopic examination of duodenal scrapings or on histopathological sections. Pathological findings in clinically affected dogs range from none to mild to marked lymphoplasmacytic enteritis and may, in addition to the duodenum, affect the proximal jejunum, or occasionally the whole intestinal tract.[114,121,129] *Strongyloides* spp. also can be found in the anterior portion of the small intestine in cats.[95] However, in cats, parasitic female adult nematodes also can be found within nodules in the colonic submucosa (Figs. 116.7 and 116.8).[94,105,112]

TREATMENT AND PROGNOSIS

No anthelmintics are registered for the treatment of *Strongyloides* in dogs and cats, and effective doses are higher than those required for most other GI nematode infections. In dogs, ivermectin (0.2 mg/kg PO), fenbendazole (50 mg/kg PO for 3 to 5 days), and albendazole (100 mg/kg PO twice daily for 3 days) have been used.[134-136] In the treatment of hyperinfections, ivermectin (0.2 mg/kg PO) administered every 4 days with a total of three or four administrations and fenbendazole (50 mg/kg PO) for 7 to 14 days have been used.[136] Due to toxicity concerns, extra-label use of high-dose ivermectin or albendazole is not recommended in dogs or cats. Less is known about effective treatments in cats although ivermectin (0.2 mg/kg PO) and thiabendazole (25 mg/kg PO q12h for 2 days) have been suggested. Fenbendazole (20 mg/kg PO for 3 days), pyrantel emboate (12.5 mg/kg PO), and pyrantel pamoate (25 mg/kg PO) were not effective in cats.[137]

With treatment, dogs fully recover from non-hyperinfections. The prognosis for dogs with hyperinfections is poor. In cats, very little work on treatment has been performed and prognosis is difficult to assess. Most cats are subclinically infected.

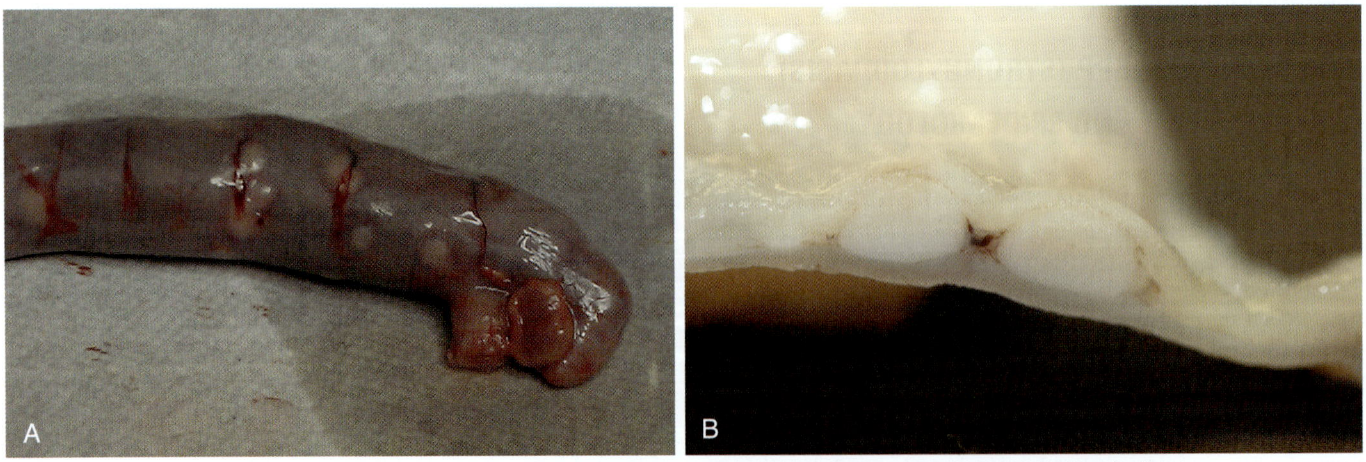

Fig. 116.7 *Strongyloides*-associated colonic nodules in the proximal colon of a cat. (A) Multifocal slightly raised, off-white nodules randomly distributed in the colonic wall. (B) Cut surface of colonic nodules. (Courtesy of Jennifer Ketzis and Dr. Lewis Bogdanovic, Ross University School of Veterinary Medicine.)

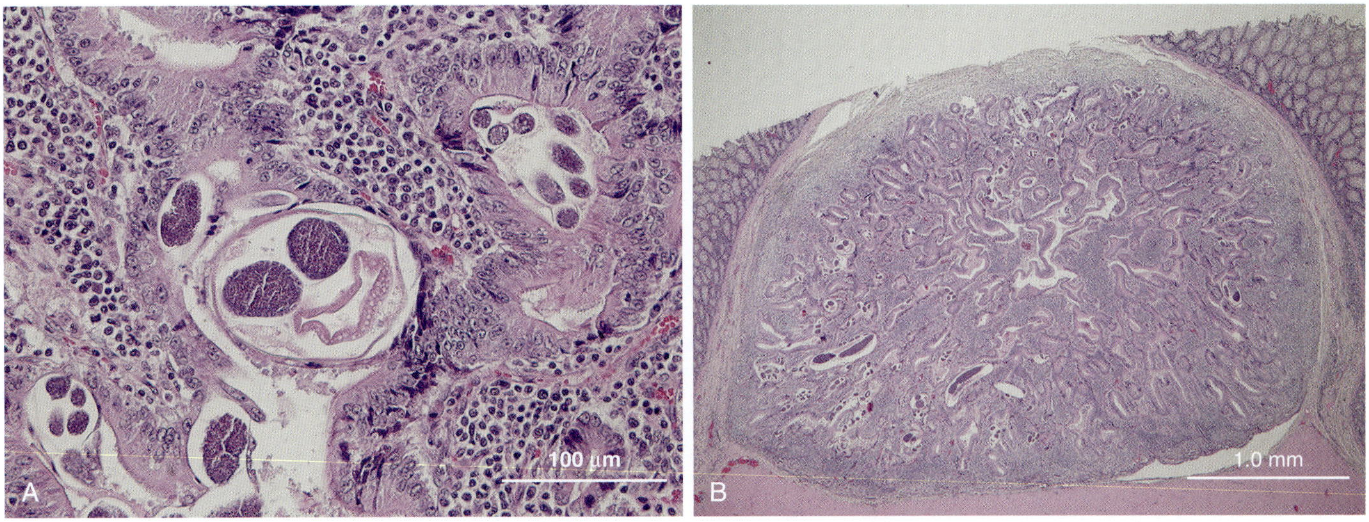

Fig. 116.8 Histopathology showing *Strongyloides*-associated colonic nodules in the proximal colon of a cat. (A) A submucosal, encapsulated collection of colonic crypts containing cross-sections of adult and larval *Strongyloides* surrounded by lymphocytes and plasma cells. (B) Adult nematodes have morphological characteristics typical of *Strongyloides* spp., i.e., platymyarian musculature, an intestine composed of uninucleate cells, and paired reproductive structures. (Hematoxylin and eosin stain). (Courtesy of Dr. Lewis Bogdanovic, Ross University School of Veterinary Medicine.)

IMMUNITY AND PREVENTION

Dogs develop limited immunity to reinfection with *S. stercoralis*. Infections can be chronic with female worms living for months or longer. Immunosuppression can result in recrudescence of larval shedding, higher autoinfection, and extensive dissemination of the larvae, which can be fatal.[101,130,133,138] Development of immunity has not been studied in cats. Prevention is primarily through hygiene, especially in kennel situations.

PUBLIC HEALTH ASPECTS

Strongyloides stercoralis is zoonotic. DNA and RNA sequencing have shown that people and dogs share some strains of *S. stercoralis*, while others are host specific, therefore people potentially serve as a source of infection for dogs and vice versa.[107-111]

Even if zoonotic infections are strain-specific, *S. stercoralis* must be considered a serious zoonosis. Between 30 and 100 million people are estimated to be infected with *S. stercoralis* worldwide. In the USA, community-based studies suggest a prevalence of 2.7%[139]; IgG seroprevalences of 12 to 77% have been reported in certain immigrant groups in North America from southeast Asia, Somalia, and Sudan. Hyperinfection, while rare, can be fatal and people with asymptomatic infections can develop hyperinfection when glucocorticoids are administered.

There have been no reports of cat *Strongyloides* spp. infecting people, and the role of cat infections in providing a reservoir for human or dog infections is unknown.

MAMMOMONOGAMUS SPP. INFECTIONS

ETIOLOGIC AGENT AND EPIDEMIOLOGY

Mammomonogamus spp. (family Syngamidae) typically reside in the upper respiratory tract. While five species have been described in either domestic or wild cats, three of the species, *Mammomonogamus dispar*, *Mammomonogamus felis*, and *Mammomonogamus mcgaughei*, have only been seen once or twice and are likely conspecific with other *Mammomonogamus* spp.[140] The remaining two species, *Mammomonogamus ierei* and *Mammomonogamus auris*, infect domestic cats and have been associated with upper respiratory signs and head shaking, respectively.[141,142] Both *M. ierei* and *M. auris* were first described in 1934; *M. ierei* was isolated from a domestic cat in Trinidad[143] and *M. auris* from the middle ear of several cats in China.[144] There have been reports of *Mammomonogamus* spp. infections in wild felids, but the species involved are unclear. *Mammomonogamus laryngeus*, a species found in ruminants, is morphologically similar to *M. ierei* and the two species have overlapping distribution. While it has been suggested that they might be synonyms, genetic sequence information does not support this theory.[140]

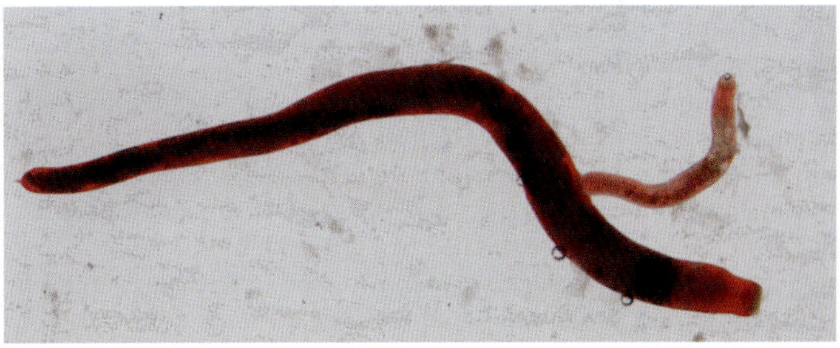

Fig. 116.9 *Mammomonogamus ierei* adult female and male; females range from 13.8 to 23.8 mm long and the males range from 3 to 6.9 mm long. (Courtesy of J. Ketzis.)

Mammomonogamus spp. are thick-bodied nematodes with large buccal capsules. They are characterized by the "Y" shape formed by male and female adult worms attached in permanent copulation (Fig. 116.9). The males are less than half the length of the females. Adult *M. ierei* reside in the nares and nasopharynx and are red to reddish-brown, and *M. auris* adults reside in the middle ear and are orange to red.[140,143,144] Both are considered haematophagous. Location in the host is the main differentiating feature for the two species. Sizes of the male and female worms are similar: *M. ierei* females are 13.8 to 23.8 mm long and the males are 3 to 6.9 mm long; *M. auris* females are 13.7 to 30 mm long and males are 3.3 to 8.1 mm long.[140,143-145]

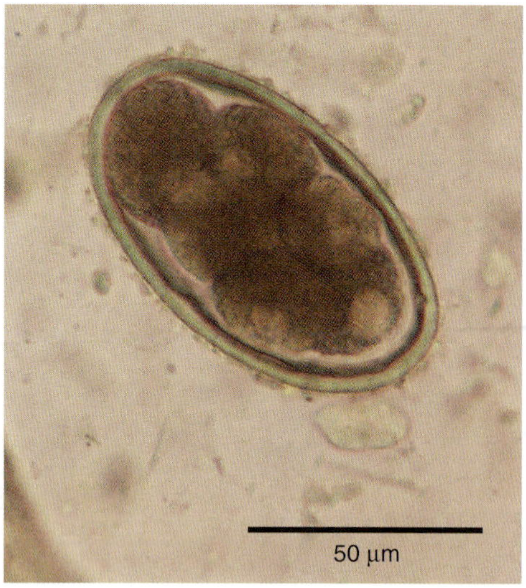

Fig. 116.10 *Mammomonogamus ierei* egg in a Sheather's sugar flotation; eggs are 78 to 100 μm long x 46 to 58 μm wide. (Courtesy of J. Ketzis.)

The eggs of both species can be found in feces or sputum with the eggs of *M. ierei* also found in nasal discharge. The eggs are oval with a clear, slightly thick shell and are 78 to 100 μm long x 46 to 58 μm wide (Fig. 116.10).[143-145] In fresh fecal material, the eggs are in the four- to eight-celled morula stage.[143,144]

The complete life cycle of the various *Mammomonogamus* species has yet to be determined. Neither oral infection nor percutaneous infection has been successful in limited studies, as is the case for other *Mammomonogamus* species.[143,146] It has been hypothesized that paratenic hosts are involved. The migratory path of the larvae to their respective predilection sites is not known. For *M. ierei*, eggs are likely coughed up and swallowed while those of *M. auris* are believed to pass down the Eustachian tubes into the pharynx where they are swallowed.[143,144] Larvae develop to the third stage in the egg before hatching and there are no data on differentiating the eggs or L_3 of the two species. The prepatent period is unknown but is potentially as short as a few days and as long as 2 weeks or more.[147-150]

All confirmed reports of *M. ierei* infection have come from the Caribbean islands. *Mammomonogamus auris* occurs in Asia with reports from China, Japan, Sri Lanka, and islands in the northwest Pacific Ocean.[140,142,144,145,151] There have been sporadic reports from other locations with the species not identified.[140,152] There are few recent studies on prevalence of infection in cats in endemic areas. A 2015 study from St. Kitts of 41 owned cats (indoor/outdoor and indoor only) found 2% to be infected and a 2010 study from the same location with 100 feral cats found 45% to be infected.[153,154] In less recent studies in the Caribbean, prevalence ranged from 32.5% to 47%.[142,141] In the case of *M. auris*, a 1934 study in China found 11 (23%) of 48 cats to be infected, and 5.6% (7 of 124 cats) were found to be infected in a 1982 study from Japan.[144,145] Little is known about infection intensity; one to four pairs of worms are most often seen although 27 pairs of *M. ierei* were described in one cat and six pairs of *M. auris* in another cat.[141,143,144]

CLINICAL FEATURES

Clinical Signs, Pathogenesis, and Physical Examination Findings

Most cats are subclinically infected. Clinical signs have included mucoid nasal discharge, cough, sneezing episodes, upper respiratory tract congestion, open mouth breathing, and weight loss with *M. ierei*.[141,153,155] Head shaking has been seen in a cat with *M. auris* infection.[142] Inflammation and hemorrhage of the nasopharyngeal mucosa have been observed in infections with both species.[141,143,144] In cats with *M. auris* infection, the tympanic membrane appears unaffected.[144]

DIAGNOSIS

Mammomonogamus spp. infections can be confirmed via fecal or sputum flotation. While simple flotation, direct smear, and sedimentation have been used, flotation with centrifugation and Sheather's sugar flotation solution (1.27 to 1.3 SpG) appears to be the most sensitive method.[140,154] On otoscopic examination, *M. auris* adults can be visible and on occasion *M. ierei* can be expelled during a sneeze. Both species can be recovered at necropsy, with *M. ierei* firmly attached to the mucosa.[141,143]

TREATMENT AND PROGNOSIS

In a single case report, fenbendazole (50 mg/kg PO q24h for 5 days) was effective for the treatment of an *M. ierei* infection.[155] Selamectin and a combination of thiabendazole, dexamethasone, and neomycin were used to treat an *M. auris* infection.[142] Thiabendazole, mebendazole, and ivermectin have been used with apparent success to treat *Mammomonogamus* spp. in other hosts, which suggests that both benzimidazoles and macrocyclic lactones could be effective.[147] Physical removal of nematodes from the ear also is possible and on occasion, cats eliminate the nematodes with forceful sneezing. With treatment or physical removal of the worms, cats fully recover.[141,142,152,155]

IMMUNITY, VACCINATION, AND PREVENTION

Cats are not known to develop immunity to *Mammomonogamus* spp. infection and there is no vaccine. Given that the route of infection is unknown, control/prevention measures are unclear. However, since infection is likely through paratenic hosts, preventing cats from hunting should decrease infection in endemic areas.

PUBLIC HEALTH ASPECTS

Neither *M. ierei* nor *M. auris* has been identified as zoonotic. Reports of *Mammomonogamus* spp. infecting people are extremely rare (approximately 100 cases in the literature), almost always associated with residence in or travel to the Caribbean or Brazil, and largely attributed to *M. laryngeus*. In humans, infections involve the trachea and are followed by violent coughing until the worms are expelled.[148] Molecular studies of *Mammomonogamus* spp. found in people are required to confirm that the species involved is the same as that infecting ruminants.

DIOCTOPHYME RENALE INFECTION (DIOCTOPHYMATOSIS, DIOCTOPHYMIASIS)

ETIOLOGY AND EPIDEMIOLOGY

Dioctophyme renale (also referred to as *Dioctophyma renale*, especially in the human literature), the giant kidney worm, is the largest nematode of domestic animals. The parasite has a sporadic, worldwide distribution although reports of infection are rare in Africa and Asia. It is widespread in the Americas and has been reported from dogs and other hosts from Canada to Brazil. Adults are usually dark red and thick, often measuring 1 cm or more in diameter; immature worms may be creamy white and smaller. Females are larger than males, and may measure as long as 50 to 100 cm. *Dioctophyme renale* is found in a variety of fish-eating mammals; mink and other mustelids are considered definitive hosts. Adult nematodes do not become as large when in mink. In domestic animals, infection with *D. renale* is most commonly reported in dogs and, occasionally, cats, but has also been described in pigs, cattle, and horses.[156,157] Whether the name of the genus was *Dioctophyme* or *Dipctophyma* was contentious for over 2 centuries, but was resolved as "*Dioctophyme*" in 1989 (International Commission on Zoological Nomenclature).

Eggs are passed in the urine of an infected host and are long-lived in the environment. First-stage larvae develop within eggs, a process dependent on temperature; larvae may develop in as early as 30 days at 25 to 30°C or as late as 7 months at lower temperatures.[158] Aquatic oligochaete annelids commonly referred to as mud worms (e.g., *Lumbriculus variegatus*) serve as intermediate hosts. The annelids ingest the eggs; the larvae then hatch, penetrate the tissues, and develop through successive molts to third-stage larvae. These larvae are immediately infective to mink and dog definitive hosts if annelids are ingested. However, more commonly, a fish or frog bridges the ecologic gap by ingesting the annelid and serving as a paratenic host.[158]

Mink, dogs, and, rarely, cats become infected when they ingest infective larvae in the tissues of paratenic hosts, most commonly freshwater fish. Larvae emerge from paratenic host tissues, penetrate the wall of the duodenum, and migrate directly to the kidney. Based on anatomical proximity to the duodenum, the right kidney is most frequently infected. Adult worms develop over several months, with infections becoming patent in 4 to 6 months or as long as 2 years.[158] Adult worms also can remain in the abdominal cavity.

Infection of dogs with *D. renale* is largely sporadic and few epidemiologic studies have been undertaken. Dogs with *D. renale* infection in Manitoba were co-infected with *Metorchis conjunctus* and clinically normal when examined, but at necropsy had extensive destruction of the right kidney and, occasionally, hypertrophied left kidneys.[159] In Brazil, dogs with *D. renale* infection were more likely to be female, fed fish or fish offal by their owners, known to eat frogs, and reported to drink water from a river known to harbor infected annelids.[159] Some authors do not consider dogs to be definitive hosts because few worms are usually present in infected dogs and infections are often not patent. However, eggs recovered from dogs have been shown to be fertile and develop larvae, and thus dogs are thought to contribute to transmission of the parasite in some environments.[160]

CLINICAL FEATURES

Clinical Signs, Pathogenesis, and Physical Examination Findings

A majority of renal infections are unilateral, involving only the right kidney, and subclinical; when both kidneys are involved, disease is more severe. When clinical signs are present, hematuria, polyuria, and pyuria are most commonly reported. Renal pain or generalized abdominal pain may be present. Some dogs are reluctant to move and anorexia, ascites, weight loss, and polydipsia may be present. When renal damage is severe, dogs can develop uremia, with associated lethargy, anorexia, and seizures. Adhesions and peritonitis may develop when *D. renale* is present in the abdominal cavity.[156,161]

Adult worms in the renal pelvis cause compression atrophy resulting in hemorrhagic, suppurative pyelitis. Over time, the renal tubules atrophy and fibrose, the pelvis dilates, and the entire parenchyma is lost resulting in a renal capsule that contains only large, coiled *D. renale* and hemorrhagic exudate. Adult worms in the abdominal cavity can result in adhesions and a serosanguinous exudate. Entrapment of a liver lobe with subsequent rupture and hemoperitoneum has been reported. A minority of dogs have both renal and abdominal *D. renale* nematodes.[157]

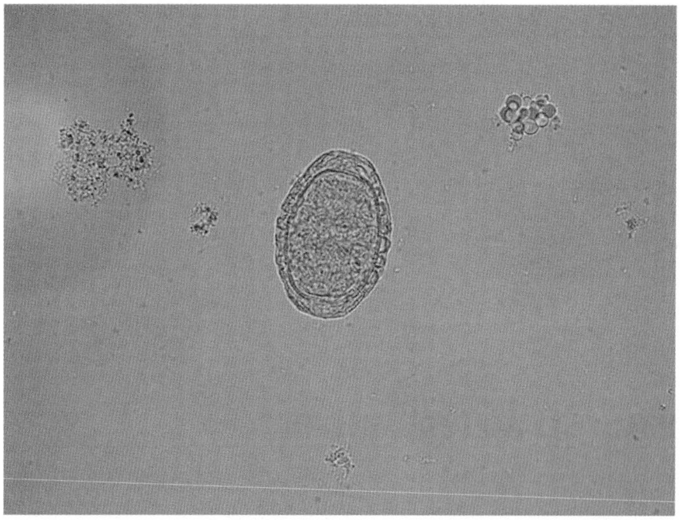

Fig. 116.11 Egg of *Dioctophyme renale* in urine sediment; eggs are 60 to 80 μm x 40 to 47 μm, oval, and have a dramatically corrugated surface. (Courtesy of National Center for Veterinary Parasitology, Oklahoma State University.)

DIAGNOSIS

Classical diagnosis of *D. renale* infection relies on detection of the characteristic eggs in urine sediment. Eggs are not detected in all infected patients; many dogs with a single nematode in the renal pelvis, and all dogs with nematodes only in the abdominal cavity, will not be excreting eggs in urine. When present, the eggs of *D. renale* have a distinct appearance; they are oval, 60 to 80 μm x 40 to 47 μm, often yellowish to brown in color, and have bipolar plugs and a dramatically pitted, rough outer coat (Fig. 116.11). A serum ELISA has been developed for research use but is not available commercially.[160]

Infection with *D. renale* may also be suspected radiographically when a distended right kidney is evident, but ultrasonography is preferred for confirmation. The large adults of *D. renale* will appear as ring-like structures with hyperechoic walls and a hypoechoic core that, when viewed laterally, are arrayed as bands in the renal pelvis of the right kidney.[162] Because confusion with normal structures can occur, ultrasound should be interpreted with care when attempting to identify *D. renale* in the abdominal cavity. When nematodes are present in the renal pelvis, compressive atrophy of the parenchyma is often evident; in advanced cases, nothing remains of the affected kidney except a capsule containing the adult worms and hemorrhagic exudate.

Entire adult nematodes are also occasionally found free or encysted in the abdominal cavity during routine surgical procedures such as ovariohysterectomy. They can also be found encapsulated during exploration of cystic lesions in tissues such as mammary glands, subcutaneous fat in the inguinal region, or mesenteric lymph nodes.[156,163] Adult worms have also been found in the urinary bladder, uterus, ovary, and urethra. The nematodes are usually dark red and very large; females are 30 to 100 cm x 1 cm and males are 15 to 45 cm x 0.5 cm. Histologic examination of affected tissues with encapsulated nematodes may reveal cross-sections of the distinct eggs, which appear as birefringent double-walled circular structures with regular radial striations.[164]

TREATMENT AND PROGNOSIS

Nephrectomy is recommended for animals with only one affected kidney as complete atrophy of the renal parenchyma is usually present; most dogs recover well.[165] Less commonly, in patients with both kidneys affected, nephrotomy may be attempted to remove the parasites and allow recovery of renal function but the prognosis is more guarded; careful evaluation of remaining renal structure and function should guide surgical decisions. Exploratory laparotomy to remove any nematodes free in the abdominal cavity is also recommended. Ectopic worms in subcutaneous fat or mammary tissue can also be removed surgically; when lesions are not complicated, the prognosis for recovery is excellent.

IMMUNITY AND PREVENTION

Prevention strategies focus on not feeding raw fish or fish offal to dogs or cats and keeping pets confined to prevent ingestion of frogs or other potential paratenic hosts. Infection may also occur by direct ingestion of the aquatic oligochaete annelid intermediate hosts in water, but this route is considered less common. Immunity to infection has not been described.

PUBLIC HEALTH ASPECTS

Human infection with *D. renale* is extremely rare (approximately 40 cases in the literature) but has been reported following ingestion of undercooked fish or frogs, as well as contaminated unfiltered and unboiled water.[164,166,167] Most cases have been from China.[168] Occasionally, nematodes develop in the kidneys or retroperitoneal space but in most cases developing larvae become encapsulated in subcutaneous nodules.

DRACUNCULUS INSIGNIS INFECTION (DRACUNCULOSIS)

ETIOLOGY AND EPIDEMIOLOGY

Dracunculus insignis is a spirurid nematode closely related to the human Guinea worm, *Dracunculus medinensis*.[169] *Dracunculus insignis* causes subcutaneous infections in raccoons and other carnivores, including domestic dogs. *Dracunculus* spp. have been described since antiquity. *Dracunculus medinensis* was described by the Swedish botanist Linnaeus in 1758, and *D. insignis* by Leidy (Pennsylvania, USA) in 1858.[158] Traditional treatments in people involved slowly winding the female nematodes around a stick over a period of several days.

Adult female *Dracunculus* spp. are long and thin and usually found coiled in subcutaneous cysts. Most reports of *D. insignis* include female nematodes 20 to 30 cm in length although longer specimens have been described; males die in subcutaneous tissues before the mature cysts form and are rarely encountered in clinical cases. *Dracunculus insignis* infections only occur in North America (especially in the southeast); wild carnivores, especially raccoons, are most commonly infected and considered the natural definitive host. Most cases of *D. insignis* infection in domestic animals are reported in dogs, although ferrets are also susceptible; a limited number of cases have been described in cats.[170-174] Because males are necessary to confirm species identification, although assumed *D. insignis*, most of these are now considered to be reports of *Dracunculus* sp. infection. Although primarily a human parasite, *D. medinensis* also infects dogs in Africa.[174,175]

Larvae are deposited directly into water from ulcerative cutaneous lesions on the limbs of the definitive hosts and ingested by cyclopoid copepod intermediate hosts, which are small crustaceans found widely in freshwater and saltwater habitats. First-stage larvae molt to third-stage in 3 to 4 weeks at temperatures of 24°C; at lower temperatures, development in the copepod is delayed or does not occur.[176,177] Infected copepods may be ingested directly by definitive hosts when they drink water, or by paratenic hosts, notably frogs, with definitive hosts ultimately infected through predation. Male and female *Dracunculus* spp. become sexually mature in approximately 2 to 3 months and mate in the subcutaneous tissues of the thorax or inguinal region; in experimental studies, fertilized females are identified as early as 4 months PI. Males die in the subcutaneous tissue after mating, while females migrate to the extremities, form cysts, become gravid, and release larvae into water. After larvae are expelled the females senesce and calcify.[158]

The identification of *D. insignis* infections in wildlife species follows a seasonal pattern. Historically, the highest prevalence of mature females in subcutaneous cysts was reported in the spring and early summer; these infections result from ingestion of copepods or paratenic hosts the previous year as mature females take as long as 10 to 12 months to develop in the definitive host.[178] A 2018 review of infections in North American dogs and cats showed that dogs could be diagnosed with dracunculosis in every month of the year, but 72% of infected dogs were seen in December to May, with the highest number of cases in March.[174] Although less common, *D. insignis* infections in cats were also seen between November and April. Cases were widespread throughout eastern North America. The average age at initial examination was 5.3 years, although patients ranged from 7 months to 15 years of age; no sex predilection was observed.[174]

CLINICAL FEATURES

Clinical Signs, Pathogenesis, and Physical Examination Findings

Most dogs infected with *D. insignis* are evaluated for non-painful skin nodules or subcutaneous swellings that are usually located on the extremities. Other common locations include the thoracic and abdominal wall, although nodules have been reported from a variety of locations including the head.[174] The skin overlying the nodule may be ulcerated or bear a patent opening; when the affected limb is immersed in water, an adult nematode may emerge.[179] Localized hair loss is often seen. Occasionally lesions are pruritic.

Nodule formation and ulceration are thought to be due to the inflammatory response to the adult female nematode. Ulcer formation is necessary to allow release of the larvae from the uterus into water to continue the life cycle. Most infected dogs have a single nodule containing only one adult female nematode, but multiple nodules and multiple nematodes have been reported. In one particularly severe case, more than 100 nematodes were removed from a dog over the course of a year.[180]

DIAGNOSIS

When characteristic nematodes are encountered in subcutaneous cysts on a leg, diagnosis is straightforward. Fine-needle aspirate of the subcutaneous cyst usually yields serosanguineous fluid containing numerous *Dracunculus* spp. larvae with a distinctly long, thin tail and measuring 600 to 800 μm (Fig. 116.12). Females can be removed by careful dissection (see Treatment); intact nematodes should be submitted to a diagnostic veterinary parasitologist for confirmation of their identity. This is particularly important when adults suspected to be *Dracunculus* spp. are recovered from unusual locations such as the eye or scrotum. Specimens can be submitted immediately in saline; alternatively, placing nematodes in 70% ethanol preserves key

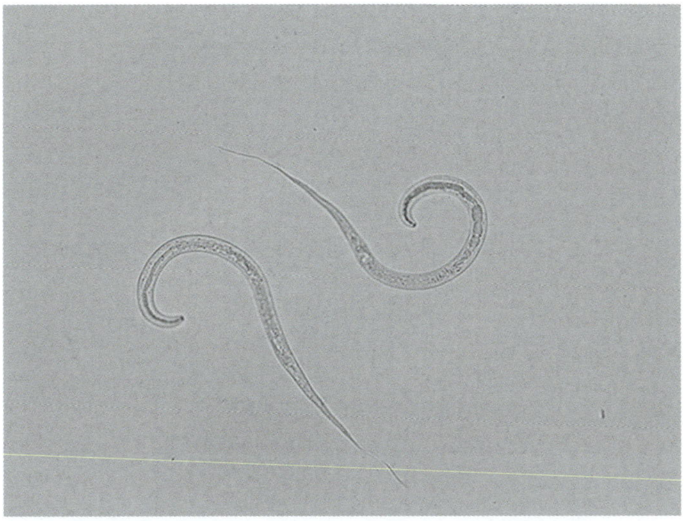

Fig. 116.12 Larvae of *Dracunculus insignis.* Often present on fine-needle aspirate from a cyst containing adult female worms; the larvae are approximately 600 to 800 μm long and have a long, thin tapering tail. (Courtesy of National Center for Veterinary Parasitology, Oklahoma State University.)

morphologic features while also allowing subsequent evaluation of key nucleic acid sequences. Formalin is not recommended. Definitive morphologic confirmation of the species requires recovery of males which are usually not available.[175]

TREATMENT AND PROGNOSIS

Treatment of *D. insignis* in dogs with uncomplicated skin lesions usually involves careful surgical exploration of subcutaneous cysts and removal of any nematodes present followed by routine wound management. Care should be taken not to cut or break the nematodes during removal. Anthelmintic protocols to prevent or treat infection have not been reported. Some dogs that develop lesions are reported by their owners to be current on heartworm preventives, and experimental treatment trials in ferrets using ivermectin, albendazole, or diethylcarbamazine were not rewarding.[174,181] Despite the lack of data, follow-up treatment with macrocyclic lactones, including ivermectin at 0.2 mg/kg administered parenterally and repeated in 2 weeks, or transdermal 2.5% moxidectin/10% imidacloprid at the label-approved dose, is often recommended to attempt to eliminate developing, immature larvae that have not yet formed subcutaneous cysts. Prognosis is good in uncomplicated cases that involve a single nematode in the skin. When nematodes have migrated aberrantly, such as to the eye, scrotum, or other locations, or when numerous cysts are present, surgical removal is still recommended but prognosis may be more guarded.

IMMUNITY AND PREVENTION

Limiting *D. insignis* infection in dogs requires complete avoidance of ingestion of copepod intermediate hosts in natural bodies of water or predation on potential paratenic hosts. Dogs should be prevented from roaming, particularly in areas where raccoons or other definitive hosts known to be infected with *D. insignis* are also present.

PUBLIC HEALTH ASPECTS

Human infections with *D. insignis* have not been reported despite the fact that non-human primates are susceptible to experimental infection.[182] *Dracunculus medinensis*, also known as the Guinea worm or Medina worm, is currently limited in distribution to three countries in Africa; historically this parasite was much more widespread in Africa, southwestern Asia, and to a lesser extent, northeastern South America and the West Indies. Infection follows ingestion of water contaminated with infected copepods, with transmission occurring when people stand in water when filling water containers. Extensive eradication efforts have dramatically reduced both the number and geographic distribution of *D. medinensis* cases in people in Africa.[183] Canine infections with *D. medinensis*, while low in number and restricted geographically, continue to be monitored.

OCULAR NEMATODE INFECTIONS

ETIOLOGY AND EPIDEMIOLOGY

Ocular nematodes reported from small animals include *Onchocerca lupi* in dogs, and *Thelazia* spp. in dogs and, less commonly, cats. Aberrant migration has also resulted in other species of nematodes reported from the eye, including *Dirofilaria* spp., *Dracunculus* spp., and *Toxocara* spp. *Onchocerca lupi* was first described in a feral wolf in Russia,[184] and causes onchocerciasis in dogs in northern Asia, southern and central Europe, and the southwestern United States. *Thelazia callipaeda* was first described by Ralliet and Henry (France) in 1910; infections occur in Asia, and more recently in Europe. *Thelazia californiensis* was first described by Price in 1930 and causes infections in dogs in western North America.

Onchocerca lupi infections are most commonly reported in domestic dogs although occasionally the parasite has been described in captive wild canids, domestic cats, and people.[185,186] Prevalence of infection is highest in adult dogs over 3 years of age, likely due to the very long development time of the nematodes, and particularly common in dogs kept outside.[187] German shepherds are overrepresented in case series.[188,189] In a survey in Greece and Portugal, 8.4% of adult dogs were infected.[190] Many infected dogs are subclinically infected. Knowledge of the epidemiology of *O. lupi* infections is hindered by lack of a full understanding of the vectors and intermediate hosts. In California, *Simulium tribulatum* was identified as a putative vector when PCR surveys revealed 2.8% harbored DNA of *O. lupi.*[191] Adults of *O. lupi* are found in conjunctival nodules and produce microfilaria which are distributed in the skin. Blood-feeding fly vectors ingest these microfilaria which then develop to third-stage larvae and are transmitted to the next host by subsequent feeding.[158]

Thelazia callipaeda and *T. californiensis* are described from dogs and cats with occasional reports from wildlife definitive hosts. Other *Thelazia* spp. infect the eyes of large animals.[158]Adults of *Thelazia* spp. are found in the conjunctiva, under the nictitating membrane, or in the lacrimal glands of definitive hosts. Larvae are shed in lachrymal secretions and are ingested by muscid flies feeding around the eyes. In Europe, *T. callipaeda* vectors are *Phortica* and *Amiota* spp., and drosophilid fruit flies. Prevalence in dogs can reach up to 40 to 60% in highly endemic areas.[192,193] In North America, *T. californiensis* is thought to be transmitted by latrine flies (*Fannia* spp.) although fruit flies may also be involved. Third-stage larvae develop in the flies in approximately 2 weeks, migrate to the mouthparts, and are deposited directly into the eyes of the next host when the fly again feeds.[158]

CLINICAL FEATURES

Clinical Signs, Pathogenesis, and Physical Examination Findings

Onchocerca lupi infections result in the development of episcleral and subconjunctival nodules. In acute infections, dogs have conjunctivitis with episcleral and conjunctival hyperemia and periorbital swelling

(Fig. 116.13A). As infections become chronic, mature nematodes are found within granulomatous nodules in the sclera, conjunctiva, orbital fascia, or eyelid. Exophthalmos and protrusion of the nictitating membrane may be present, along with edema, ocular discharge, lacrimation, and photophobia. Nematodes or nematode fragments are present in excised nodules. Occasionally, mild dermatitis develops in response to microfilaria in the skin.[187,194]

The presence of larval and adult *Thelazia* sp. results in lacrimation, ocular discharge, epiphora, conjunctivitis, keratitis, and, when trauma is severe or prolonged, corneal ulcers. Conjunctivitis appears more severe when gravid females are present. *Thelazia* sp. adults have a serrated cuticle that causes damage to the corneal epithelium; the resultant ocular discharge is both characteristic of the disease seen and important to continuing the life cycle by attracting secretophagous fly intermediate hosts. Nematodes are readily observed and collected during ocular examination (Fig. 116.14).[192,195]

DIAGNOSIS

Ocular onchocerciasis can be confirmed when nematodes are found within excised orbital nodules (Fig. 116.13B). Examination of saline digest of skin snips reveals microfilaria; preferred locations where *O. lupi* microfilaria concentrate include the head, ears, and intrascapular region.[190] Microfilaria are not present in blood and heartworm antigen tests do not appear to cross-react with antigen of *O. lupi*.

Thelazia spp. infections are diagnosed directly by observation of nematodes in the conjunctival sac (Fig. 116.14). Often several nematodes are present, necessitating thorough examination to allow complete removal. Once removed, nematodes can be submitted to a specialist for confirmation of identity by morphology, including the presence of distinct transverse striations on the cuticle.[192] Specimens should be submitted in 70% ethanol or 0.9% saline to preserve nucleic acid for amplification.

TREATMENT AND PROGNOSIS

Treatment of ocular *O. lupi* in dogs involves surgical removal of the nodules and the nematodes followed by anthelmintics to eliminate any remaining nematodes, reducing the recurrence of nodules after surgery (Fig. 116.13C).[187] Melarsomine (two injections 24 hours apart) and macrocyclic lactones are recommended.[188] However, some dogs infected with *O. lupi* were reportedly current on heartworm prevention and thus it is not clear if all macrocyclic lactone–based heartworm preventives protect dogs from infection. With appropriate surgery and postsurgical care, most dogs recover from ocular onchocerciasis.[187,188] One dog that appeared refractory to treatment appeared to benefit from addition of doxycycline for nematode-associated *Wolbachia* spp. infection (5–10 mg/kg PO q12h) as well as topical demecarium bromide (1 drop q12h in affected eye), which induces miosis and may have some activity against *Onchocerca* spp. (Fig. 116.13).

Macrocyclic lactones (extra-label) are effective for treatment of *Thelazia* spp., including application of label-approved doses of transdermal moxidectin/imidacloprid or oral milbemycin oxime.[196,197] Worms can also be manually extracted using forceps after application of topical proparacaine (Fig. 116.14). Prognosis for recovery is excellent, and treatment with sustained-release injectable moxidectin also provides protection.[198]

IMMUNITY AND PREVENTION

Preventing infection with *O. lupi* and *Thelazia* spp. requires protecting dogs and cats from the fly intermediate hosts. Keeping animals inside

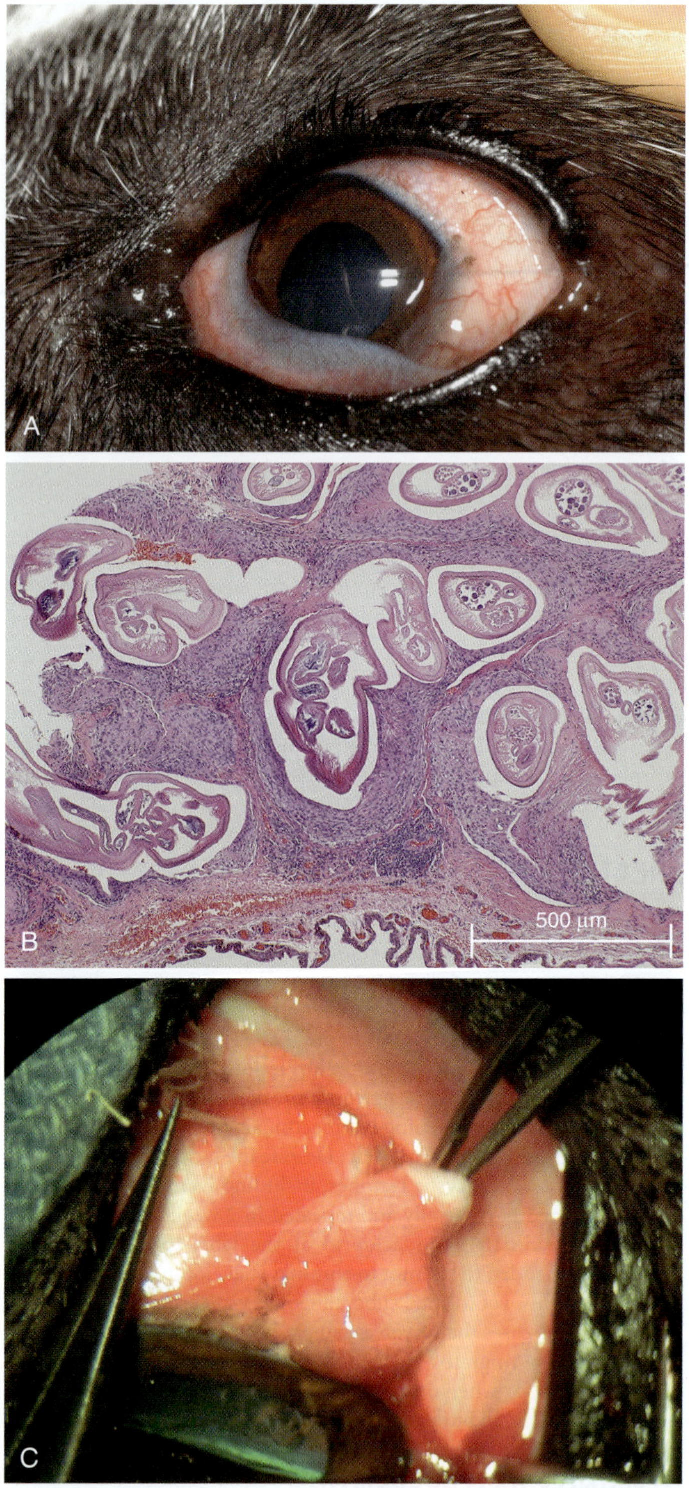

Fig. 116.13 Onchocerciasis in a 7-year-old female spayed Australian cattle dog mix. The signs began about 1 year after the dog moved from New Mexico and Arizona to northern California. (A) The initial problem was marked scleral swelling. (B) Histopathology of nodule biopsy showing *Onchocerca lupi* within granulomas (hematoxylin and eosin stain). (C) Treatment with surgical extraction and medical therapy with ivermectin and melarsomine was not immediately successful; ongoing treatment with monthly ivermectin, topical demecarium bromide and prednisone acetate, and oral doxycycline ultimately resolved the infection. (A, courtesy of University of California-Davis Veterinary Ophthalmology Service; B,C courtesy of Dr. Patricia Smith)

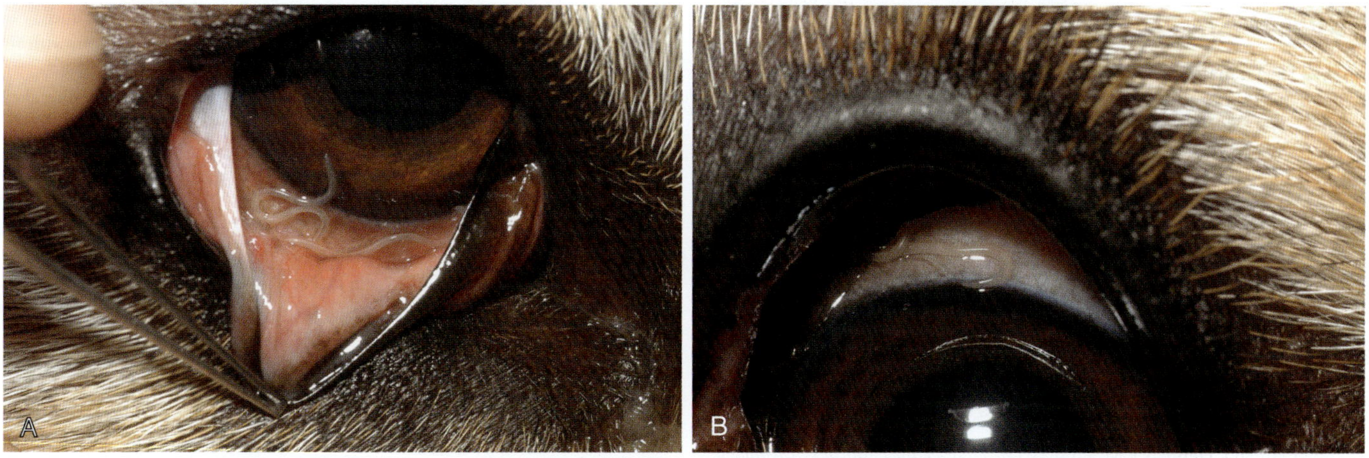

Fig. 116.14 *Thelazia californiensis* in a 1-year-old male intact malamute mix from Colfax in northern California. The dog was evaluated for a positive heartworm antigen test and the nematode was an incidental finding. A total of 15 worms were manually extracted from the conjunctival sac using forceps following application of topical proparacaine. (Courtesy of University of California-Davis Veterinary Ophthalmology Service.)

behind screens should reduce the risk of infection. Pyrethroid repellents in the form of topical, liquid permethrin spot-on products or deltamethrin collars are available for dogs and would also be expected to provide some protection from infection. A study in France showed that transdermal 2.5% moxidectin/10% imidacloprid protected dogs from *Thelazia callipaeda* infection;[199] a similar strategy may also be effective for treating *O. lupi* infections early, before development of clinical signs.

PUBLIC HEALTH ASPECTS

Human infection with both *O. lupi* and *Thelazia* spp. occasionally occurs, resulting in ocular irritation, excessive lacrimation, and the presence of intraocular nematodes.[200-202] Patients with *O. lupi* infections in most areas of the world develop conjunctival hyperemia and subconjunctival nodules containing nematodes; diagnosis is usually made upon histopathologic examination of excised tissues. In the United States, human patients are more commonly reported to have subdermal, spinal, and orbital nodules. In addition to removal of affected tissues and nematodes, treatment involves a combination of anthelmintics and antibiotics together with glucocorticoids to reduce inflammation.[203,204] Patients with *Thelazia* spp. infections generally report ocular discomfort and a foreign body sensation; nematodes are identified directly upon ophthalmologic examination and removed with forceps.[191] Prevention of zoonotic infection with *O. lupi* and *Thelazia* spp. requires avoiding contact with the respective fly vectors.

CASE EXAMPLE

Signalment

"Pirro," an adult male neutered mixed breed dog from St. Kitts, West Indies.

History

Pirro was seen for lethargy, anorexia, and regurgitation (approximately once daily), which were of a few days' duration. Pirro was adopted from an animal neglect situation 10 months before initial examination. At that time he was treated with Drontal Plus (praziquantel/pyrantel pamoate/febantel), and shortly thereafter he was vaccinated and started on monthly heartworm preventives (ivermectin/pyrantel pamoate). Shortly after adoption, a firm, indolent, 2 × 2 cm prominence was noted over the left third metatarsal.

Physical Examination

The dog was in adequate body condition (BCS 3/5). Apart from mild pyrexia, and an approximately 4 × 4 cm firm, indolent swelling over the left dorsal metatarsals, physical examination findings were within normal limits.

Laboratory Findings

There was moderate hypoalbuminemia (1.3 g/dL, reference interval 2.5–4.4 g/dL) and mild hyperglobulinemia (6.3 g/dL, reference interval 2.3–5.2 g/dL). All other CBC and serum biochemical parameters were within normal limits.

Fecal flotation and sedimentation: No parasite oocysts, ova, or larvae were seen.

Imaging Findings

Thoracic radiographs: A soft-tissue opacity, compatible with an esophageal mass was seen in the caudal thorax.

Left distal pelvic limb radiographs: Palisades of periosteal new bones were seen on the dorsal surface of the left metatarsal bones, consistent with hypertrophic osteopathy.

Esophagoscopy: A large (9 × 6 × 6 cm) intraluminal mass with superficial hemorrhage was partly obliterating the caudal esophageal lumen.

Pathologic Findings

Endoscopic biopsies: Histopathology revealed necrotic debris admixed with pieces of plant material.

Surgical biopsy (via gastrotomy): Osteosarcoma.

Diagnosis

Distal esophageal osteosarcoma.

Treatment

The dog was initially treated with ivermectin for presumed *S. lupi* infection. A lack of clinical response and the biopsy diagnosis of osteosarcoma led to a decision of humane euthanasia.

Necropsy Findings

The antemortem diagnoses of caudal esophageal osteosarcoma and hypertrophic osteopathy was confirmed at necropsy. No adult or larval stages of *S. lupi* were found.

Comments

In this case, an underlying previous spirocercosis was presumed based on the finding of an esophageal osteosarcoma in an endemic region.

Case example provided courtesy of Ross University School of Veterinary Medicine.

SUGGESTED READINGS

Campbell KL, Graham JC. *Physaloptera* infection in dogs and cats. *Compend Cont Educ Pract Vet.* 1999;21(4):299–314.

Mylonakis ME, Rallis T, Koutinas AF. Canine spirocercosis. *Compend Contin Educ Vet.* 2008;30(2):111–116.

Stancampiano L, Morandi F, Usai F, Benazzi C, Pietra M. An unusual case of fatal *Strongyloides stercoralis* hyperinfection. *Veterinaria.* 2011;25(4):39.

Červená B, Hrazdilová K, Vallo P, et al. *Mammomonogamus* nematodes in felid carnivores: a minireview and the first molecular characterization. *Parasitol.* 2018;21:1–10.

REFERENCES

1. Morgan BB. The *Physaloptera* (Nematoda) of carnivores. *Trans Wisc Acad Sci Arts Lett.* 1944;36:375–388.
2. Bowman DD, Hendrix CM, Lindsay DS, et al. *Feline Clinical Parasitology.* John Wiley & Sons; 2008.
3. Rausch RL, Maser C, Hoberg EP. Gastrointestinal helminths of the cougar, *Felis concolor* L., in northeastern Oregon. *J Wildl Dis.* 1983;19:14–19.
4. Olsen JL. Life history of *Physaloptera rara* Hall and Wigdor, 1918 (Nematoda: Physalopteroidia) of canids and felids in definitive, intermediate, and paratenic hosts. *Rev Iber Parasitol.* 1980;40(4):489–525.
5. Napoli E, Anile S, Arrabito C, et al. Survey on parasitic infections in wildcat (*Felis silvestris silvestris* Schreber, 1777) by scat collection. *Parasitol Res.* 2016;115:255–261.
6. Petri LH. Life cycle of *Physaloptera rara* Hall and Wigdor (Nematoda : Spiruroidea) with the cockroach, *Blatella germánica*, serving as the intermediate host. *Trans Kans Acad Sci.* 1918;1950(53):331–337.
7. Kresta AE, Henke SE, Pence DB. Gastrointestinal helminths in raccoons in Texas. *J Wildl Dis.* 2009;45:1–13.
8. Pence DB, Tewes ME, Laack LL. Helminths of the ocelot from southern Texas. *J Wildl Dis.* 2003;39:683–689.
9. Ackert JE. *Physaloptera felidis* n.sp., a nematode of the cat. *Trans Am Microsc Soc.* 1936;55:250–254.
10. Tongson MS, San Pablo FG. A study on the prevalence of gastrointestinal worms of cats in metropolitan Manila. *Philipp J Vet Med.* 1979;18:1–15.
11. Zajac AM, Conboy GA. *Veterinary Clinical Parasitology.* John Wiley & Sons; 2012.
12. Widmer EA. Development of third-stage *Physaloptera* larvae from *Crotalus viridis rafinesque*, 1818 in cats with notes on pathology of the larvae in the reptile. (Nematoda, Spiruroidea). *J Wildl Dis.* 1970;6:89–93.
13. Theisen SK, LeGrange SN, Johnson SE, et al. *Physaloptera* infection in 18 dogs with intermittent vomiting. *J Am Anim Hosp Assoc.* 1998;34:74–78.
14. Naem S, Abbass Farshid A, Tanhai Marand V. Pathological findings on natural infection with *Physaloptera praeputialis* in cats. *Vet Arh.* 2006;76(4):315–321. Available at: https://hrcak.srce.hr/file/8247.
15. Guardone L, Magi M, Prati MC, et al. Cardiorespiratory and gastrointestinal parasites of dogs in north-west Italy. *Helminthologia.* 2016;53:8.
16. Adolph CB. Prevalence, disease implications, and diagnostic assays for parasites and vector-borne infections of cats in northeastern Oklahoma. Master of Science, Center for Veterinary Health Sciences, Oklahoma State University, Stillwater, OK, USA; 2013.
17. Abu-Madi MA, Behnke JM, Prabhaker KS, et al. Intestinal helminths of feral cat populations from urban and suburban districts of Qatar. *Vet Parasitol.* 2010;168:284–292.
18. Clark JA. *Physaloptera* stomach worms associated with chronic vomition in a dog in Western Canada. *Can Vet J.* 1990;31:840.
19. Kazacos KR. Gastrointestinal helminths in dogs from a humane shelter in Indiana. *J Am Vet Med Assoc.* 1978;173:995–997.
20. Craig TM, Zarate Ramos JJ, Guzman Garcia MA, et al. Gastritis verminosa por *Physaloptera praeputialis* en el gato. *Veterinaria.* 1991;22:185–190.
21. Ash LR. Helminth parasites of dogs and cats in Hawaii. *J Parasitol.* 1962;48:63–65.
22. Cantó GJ, García MP, García A, et al. The prevalence and abundance of helminth parasites in stray dogs from the city of Queretaro in central Mexico. *J Helminthol.* 2011;85:263–269.
23. Borji H, Razmi G, Ahmadi A, et al. A survey on endoparasites and ectoparasites of stray cats from Mashhad (Iran) and association with risk factors. *J Parasit Dis.* 2011;35:202–206.
24. Adams PJ, Elliot AD, Algar D, et al. Gastrointestinal parasites of feral cats from Christmas Island. *Aust Vet J.* 2008;86:60–63.
25. Barton MA, McEwan DR. Spirurid nematodes in dogs and cats from central Australia. *Aust Vet J.* 1993;70:270.
26. Ubelaker JE, Griffin BS, Konicke GM, et al. Helminth parasites from the Kit fox, *Vulpes macrotis* (Carnivora: Canidae), from New Mexico. *Comp Parasitol.* 2014;81:100–104.
27. Foster GW, Main MB, Kinsella JM, et al. Parasitic helminths and arthropods of coyotes (*Canis latrans*) from Florida, U.S.A. *Comp Parasitol.* 2003;70:162–166.
28. Gustafson BW. Ivermectin in the treatment of *Physaloptera preputialis* in two cats. *J Am Anim Hosp Assoc.* 1995;31:416–418.
29. Batchelor DJ, Devauchelle P, Elliott J, et al. Mechanisms, causes, investigation and management of vomiting disorders in cats: a literature review. *J Feline Med Surg.* 2013;15:237–265.
30. David ED, Lindquist WD. Determination of the specific gravity of certain helminth eggs using sucrose density gradient centrifugation. *J Parasitol.* 1982;68:916–919.
31. Kazacos KR. How do you detect *Physaloptera* species eggs. *Vet Med.* 2010;105:472–473.
32. Ehrenford FA. Diagnosis of *Physaloptera* in dogs by stool examination. *J Parasitol.* 1954. Available at: https://www.cabdirect.org/cabdirect/abstract/19540801446.
33. Companion Animal Parasite Council. *Physaloptera* spp. 2016 Available at: https://capcvet.org/guidelines/physaloptera-spp/.
34. Gennari SM, Kasai N, Nishi SM, et al. Anthelmintic efficacy of three doses of an association of pyrantel pamoate plus, oxantel pamoate and praziquantel in naturally infected cats. *Braz J Vet Res Anim Sci.* 1997;34:284–287.
35. Santen DR, Chastain CB, Schmidt DA. Efficacy of pyrantel pamoate against *Physaloptera* in a cat. *J Am Anim Hosp Assoc.* 1993;29:53–55.
36. Chitwood BG. The status of *Spirocerca sanguinola* (Rudolphi, 1819) Seurat. *J Parasitol.* 1913;1934:20.
37. Popiołek M, Szczęsna-Staśkiewicz J, Bartoszewicz M, et al. Helminth parasites of an introduced invasive carnivore species, the raccoon (*Procyon lotor* L.), from the Warta Mouth National Park (Poland). *J Parasitol.* 2011;97:357–360.
38. Morrison EE, Gier HT. Parasitic infection of *Filaroides osleri, Capillaria aerophila* and *Spirocera lupi* in coyotes from the Southwestern United States. *J Wildl Dis.* 1979;15:557–559.
39. Ubelaker JE, Griffin BS, Duszynski DW, et al. Distribution records for helminths of the red fox *Vulpes vulpes* from New Mexico. *Southwest Nat.* 2013;58:111–112.
40. Giannelli A, Baldassarre V, Ramos RAN, et al. *Spirocerca lupi* infection in a dog from southern Italy: an "old fashioned" disease? *Parasitol Res.* 2014;113:2391–2394.
41. Bailey WS. *Spirocerca lupi*: a continuing inquiry. *J Parasitol.* 1972;58:3–22.
42. Mylonakis ME, Rallis T, Koutinas AF. Canine spirocercosis. *Compend Contin Educ Vet.* 2008;30:111–116.
43. Sen K, Anantaraman M. Some observations on the development of *Spirocerca lupi* in its intermediate and definitive hosts. *J Helminthol.* 1971;45:123–131.
44. Christie J, Schwan EV, Bodenstein LL, et al. The sensitivity of direct faecal examination, direct faecal flotation, modified centrifugal faecal flotation and centrifugal sedimentation/flotation in the diagnosis of canine spirocercosis. *J S Afr Vet Assoc.* 2011;82:71–75.
45. van der Merwe LL, Kirberger RM, Clift S, et al. *Spirocerca lupi* infection in the dog: a review. *Vet J.* 2008;176:294–309.
46. Anantaraman M, Sen K. Experimental spirocercosis in dogs with larvae from a paratenic host, *Calotes versicolor*, the common garden lizard in Madras. *J Parasitol.* 1966;52:911–912.
47. Gottlieb Y, Markovics A, Klement E, et al. Characterization of *Onthophagus sellatus* as the major intermediate host of the dog esophageal worm *Spirocerca lupi* in Israel. *Vet Parasitol.* 2011;180:378–382.

48. Fisher MM, Morgan JP, Krecek RC, et al. Radiography for the diagnosis of spirocercosis in apparently healthy dogs, St. Kitts, West Indies. *Vet Parasitol.* 2009;160:337–339.
49. Aroch I, Markovics A, Mazaki-Tovi M, et al. Spirocercosis in dogs in Israel: a retrospective case-control study (2004-2009). *Vet Parasitol.* 2015;211:234–240.
50. Wright I, Stafford K, Coles G. The prevalence of intestinal nematodes in cats and dogs from Lancashire, north-west England. *J Small Anim Pract.* 2016;57:393–395.
51. Lobetti R. Follow-up survey of the prevalence, diagnosis, clinical manifestations and treatment of *Spirocerca lupi* in South Africa. *J S Afr Vet Assoc.* 2014;85:e1–e7.
52. Chikweto A, Bhaiyat MI, Tiwari KP, et al. Spirocercosis in owned and stray dogs in Grenada. *Vet Parasitol.* 2012;190:613–616.
53. Oryan A, Sadjjadi SM, Mehrabani D, et al. Spirocercosis and its complications in stray dogs in Shiraz, southern Iran. *Vet Med.* 2008;53:617–624.
54. Shubhagata D, Alim MA, Hassan MM, et al. Spirocercosis in stray dogs of Chittagong metropolitan area of Bangladesh: an epidemiological and pathological investigation. *Vet World.* 2011;4:485–491.
55. Mylonakis ME, Koutinas AF, Liapi MV, et al. A comparison of the prevalence of *Spirocerca lupi* in three groups of dogs with different life and hunting styles. *J Helminthol.* 2001;75:359–361.
56. Al-Sabi MNS, Hansen MS, Chriél M, et al. Genetically distinct isolates of *Spirocerca* sp. from a naturally infected red fox (*Vulpes vulpes*) from Denmark. *Vet Parasitol.* 2014;205:389–396.
57. Psáder R, Balogh M, Pápa K, et al. Occurrence of *Spirocerca lupi* infection in Hungarian dogs referred for gastroscopy. *Parasitol Res.* 2017;116:99–108.
58. Avner A, Herrtage ME. Computed tomographic features of spirocercosis with putative benign oesophageal nodules in dogs. *Isr J Vet Med.* 2013;68:87–93.
59. Dvir E, Kirberger RM, Malleczek D. Radiographic and computed tomographic changes and clinical presentation of spirocercosis in the dog. *Vet Radiol Ultrasound.* 2001;42:119–129.
60. Mazaki-Tovi M, Baneth G, Aroch I, et al. Canine spirocercosis: clinical, diagnostic, pathologic, and epidemiologic characteristics. *Vet Parasitol.* 2002;107:235–250.
61. Mylonakis ME, Rallis T, Koutinas AF, et al. Clinical signs and clinicopathologic abnormalities in dogs with clinical spirocercosis: 39 cases (1996-2004). *J Am Vet Med Assoc.* 2006;228:1063–1067.
62. Dvir E, Clift SJ, Williams MC. Proposed histological progression of the *Spirocerca lupi*-induced oesophageal lesion in dogs. *Vet Parasitol.* 2010;168:71–77.
63. Ranen E, Lavy E, Aizenberg I, et al. Spirocercosis-associated esophageal sarcomas in dogs. A retrospective study of 17 cases (1997-2003). *Vet Parasitol.* 2004;119:209–221.
64. Klainbart S, Mazaki-Tovi M, Auerbach N, et al. Spirocercosis-associated pyothorax in dogs. *Vet J.* 2007;173:209–214.
65. Schroeder H, Berry WL. Salivary gland necrosis in dogs: a retrospective study of 19 cases. *J Small Anim Pract.* 1998;39:121–125.
66. van der Merwe LL, Christie J, Clift SJ, et al. Salivary gland enlargement and sialorrhoea in dogs with spirocercosis: a retrospective and prospective study of 298 cases. *J S Afr Vet Assoc.* 2012;83:920.
67. Craig LE, Dittmer KE, Thompson KG. Bones and joints. In: Maxie MG, ed. *Jubb, Kennedy and Palmer's Pathology of Domestic Animals Volume 1.* 6th ed. St. Louis, MO: Elsevier; 2016:16–163.
68. Elias F, Barros RM, Santos-Junior HL, et al. Pathological alterations in dogs resulting from parasitism by *Spirocerca lupi. Acta Scientiae Veterinariae.* 2016:44(Suppl 1):145.
69. Joubert KE, McReynolds MJ, Strydom F. Acute aortic rupture in a dog with spirocercosis following the administration of medetomidine. *J S Afr Vet Assoc.* 2005;76:159–162.
70. Gal A, Kleinbart S, Aizenberg Z, et al. Aortic thromboembolism associated with *Spirocerca lupi* infection. *Vet Parasitol.* 2005;130:331–335.
71. Kirberger RM, Zambelli A. Imaging diagnosis-aortic thromboembolism associated with spirocercosis in a dog. *Vet Radiol Ultrasound.* 2007;48:418–420.
72. Chai O, Yas E, Brenner O, et al. Clinical characteristics of *Spirocerca lupi* migration in the spinal cord. *Vet Parasitol.* 2018;253:16–21.
73. Chai O, Shelef I, Brenner O, et al. Magnetic resonance imaging findings of spinal intramedullary spirocercosis. *Vet Radiol Ultrasound.* 2008;49:456–459.
74. Du Plessis CJ, Keller N, Millward IR. Aberrant extradural spinal migration of *Spirocerca lupi*: four dogs. *J Small Anim Pract.* 2007;48:275–278.
75. Dvir E, Perl S, Loeb E, et al. Spinal intramedullary aberrant *Spirocerca lupi* migration in 3 dogs. *J Vet Intern Med.* 2007;21:860–864.
76. Nivy R, Caldin M, Lavy E, et al. Serum acute phase protein concentrations in dogs with spirocercosis and their association with esophageal neoplasia - a prospective cohort study. *Vet Parasitol.* 2014;203:153–159.
77. Traversa D, Avolio S, Modrý D, et al. Copromicroscopic and molecular assays for the detection of cancer-causing parasitic nematode. *Spirocerca lupi. Vet Parasitol.* 2008;157:108–116.
78. Markovics A, Medinski B. Improved diagnosis of low intensity *Spirocerca lupi* infection by the sugar flotation method. *J Vet Diagn Invest.* 1996;8:400–401.
79. Klainbart S, Chai O, Vaturi R, et al. Nematode eggs observed in cytology of cerebrospinal fluid diagnostic for intramedullary *Spirocerca lupi* spinal cord migration. *Vet Clin Pathol.* 2018;47:138–141.
80. Mylonakis ME, Rallis TS, Koutinas AF, et al. A comparison between ethanol-induced chemical ablation and ivermectin plus prednizolone in the treatment of symptomatic esophageal spirocercosis in the dog: a prospective study on 14 natural cases. *Vet Parasitol.* 2004;120:131–138.
81. Lavy E, Aroch I, Bark H, et al. Evaluation of doramectin for the treatment of experimental canine spirocercosis. *Vet Parasitol.* 2002;109:65–73.
82. Pazzi P, Kavkovsky A, Shipov A, et al. *Spirocerca lupi* induced oesophageal neoplasia: predictors of surgical outcome. *Vet Parasitol.* 2018;250:71–77.
83. Ranen E, Dank G, Lavy E, et al. Oesophageal sarcomas in dogs: histological and clinical evaluation. *Vet J.* 2008;178:78–84.
84. Yas E, Kelmer G, Shipov A, et al. Successful transendoscopic oesophageal mass ablation in two dogs with *Spirocerca lupi* associated oesophageal sarcoma. *J Small Anim Pract.* 2013;54:495–498.
85. Shipov A, Kelmer G, Lavy E, et al. Long-term outcome of transendoscopic oesophageal mass ablation in dogs with *Spirocerca lupi*-associated oesophageal sarcoma. *Vet Rec.* 2015;177:365.
86. Le Sueur C, Bour S, Schaper R. Efficacy of a combination of imidacloprid 10%/moxidectin 2.5% spot-on (Advocate® for dogs) in the prevention of canine spirocercosis (*Spirocerca lupi*). *Parasitol Res.* 2010;107:1463–1469.
87. Kok DJ, Schenker R, Archer NJ, et al. The efficacy of milbemycin oxime against pre-adult *Spirocerca lupi* in experimentally infected dogs. *Vet Parasitol.* 2011;177:111–118.
88. Kok DJ, Williams EJ, Schenker R, et al. The use of milbemycin oxime in a prophylactic anthelmintic programme to protect puppies, raised in an endemic area, against infection with *Spirocerca lupi. Vet Parasitol.* 2010;174:277–284.
89. Beugnet F, Crafford D, de Vos C, et al. Evaluation of the efficacy of monthly oral administration of afoxolaner plus milbemycin oxime (NexGard Spectra®, Merial) in the prevention of adult *Spirocerca lupi* establishment in experimentally infected dogs. *Vet Parasitol.* 2016;226:150–161.
90. Grove DI. Human strongyloidiasis. *Adv Parasitol.* 1996;38:251–309.
91. Chandler AC. The species of *Strongyloides* (Nematoda). *Parasitology.* 1925;17:426–433.
92. Genta RM. *Strongyloides stercoralis* infection in animals. In: Grove DI, ed. *Strongyloidiasis: A Major Roundworm Infection of Man.* Taylor & Francis; 1989:251–269.
93. Rogers WP. A new species of *Strongyloides* from the cat. *J Helminthol.* 1939;17:229–238.
94. Price EW, Dikmans G, U.S. Bureau of Animal Industry. Adenomatous tumors in the large intestine of cats caused by *Strongyloides tumefaciens* n. sp. *Proc Helminthol Soc Wash.* 1941;8:41–44.
95. Speare R, Tinsley DJ. *Strongyloides felis*: an "old" worm rediscovered in Australian cats. *Aust Vet Pract.* 1986;16:10–18.
96. Galliard H. Recherches sur l'infestation expérimentale a *Strongyloides stercoralis* au Tonkin (2e note). *Ann Parasitol Hum Comp.* 1951;26:67–84.
97. Galliard H. Recherches sur l'infestation expérimentale a *Strongyloides stercoralis* au Tonkin (3e note). *Ann Parasitol Hum Comp.* 1951;26:201–227.

98. Mansfield LS, Alavi A, Wortman JA, et al. Gamma camera scintigraphy for direct visualization of larval migration in *Strongyloides stercoralis*-infected dogs. *Am J Trop Med Hyg.* 1995;52:236–240.
99. Mansfield LS, Schad GA. Lack of transmammary transmission of *Strongyloides stercoralis* from a previously hyperinfected bitch to her pups. *J Helminthol Soc Wash.* 1995;62:80–83.
100. Shoop WL, Michael BF, Eary CH, et al. Transmammary transmission of *Strongyloides stercoralis* in dogs. *J Parasitol.* 2002;88:536–539.
101. Genta RM, Schad GA, Hellman ME. *Strongyloides stercoralis*: parasitological, immunological and pathological observations in immunosuppressed dogs. *Trans R Soc Trop Med Hyg.* 1986;80:34–41.
102. Grove DI, Heenan PJ, Northern C. Persistent and disseminated infections with *Strongyloides stercoralis* in immunosuppressed dogs. *Int J Parasitol.* 1983;13:483–490.
103. Fukase T, Chinone S, Itagaki H. *Strongyloides planiceps* (Nematoda; Strongyloididae) in some wild carnivores. *Nihon Juigaku Zasshi.* 1985;47:627–632.
104. Malone JB, Butterfield AB, Williams JC, et al. *Strongyloides tumefaciens* in cats. *J Am Vet Med Assoc.* 1977;171:278–280.
105. Moura MAO, Jorge EM, Gomes do Nascimento KK et al. Colonic epithelial nodular hyperplasia associated with strongyloidiasis in cats in the Amazon region, Pará State, Brazil. Ciência Rural. 2017;47. Available at: http://www.scielo.br/scielo.php?script=sci_abstract&pid=S0103-84782017000100502&lng=pt&nrm=iso&tlng=en.
106. Lindsay DS, Blagburn BL, Stuart BB, et al. *Strongyloides tumefaciens* infection in a cat. *Comp An Pract.* 1987;1:12–13.
107. Hasegawa H, Sato H, Fujita S, et al. Molecular identification of the causative agent of human strongyloidiasis acquired in Tanzania: dispersal and diversity of *Strongyloides* spp. and their hosts. *Parasitol Int.* 2010;59:407–413.
108. Barratt JLN, Lane M, Talundzic E, et al. A global genotyping survey of *Strongyloides stercoralis and Strongyloides fuelleborni* using deep amplicon sequencing. PLoS Negl Trop Dis. 2019 13:e0007609.
109. Schär F, Guo L, Streit A, et al. *Strongyloides stercoralis* genotypes in humans in Cambodia. *Parasitol Int.* 2014;63:533–536.
110. Streit A, Jaleta T, Forrer A, et al. Different *Strongyloides stercoralis* populations in humans and dogs in rural Cambodia. In: *Proceedings of the 13th International Congress of Parasitology*. 2014.
111. Jaleta TG, Zhou S, Bemm FM, et al. Different but overlapping populations of *Strongyloides stercoralis* in dogs and humans: dogs as a possible source for zoonotic strongyloidiasis. *PLoS Negl Trop Dis.* 2017;11. e0005752.
112. Wulcan JM, Dennis MM, Ketzis JK, et al. *Strongyloides* spp. in cats: a review of the literature and the first report of zoonotic *Strongyloides stercoralis* in colonic epithelial nodular hyperplasia in cats. *Parasit Vectors.* 2019;12:349.
113. Asano K, Suzuki K, Matsumoto T, et al. Prevalence of dogs with intestinal parasites in Tochigi, Japan in 1979, 1991 and 2002. *Vet Parasitol.* 2004;120:243–248.
114. Dillard KJ, Saari SA, Anttila M. *Strongyloides stercoralis* infection in a Finnish kennel. *Acta Vet Scand.* 2007;49:37.
115. Eydal M, Skirnisson K. *Strongyloides stercoralis* found in imported dogs, household dogs and kennel dogs in Iceland. *Icel Agric Sci.* 2016;29:39–51.
116. Gates MC, Nolan TJ. Endoparasite prevalence and recurrence across different age groups of dogs and cats. *Vet Parasitol.* 2009;166:153–158.
117. Gaunt MC, Carr AP. A survey of intestinal parasites in dogs from Saskatoon, Saskatchewan. *Can Vet J.* 2011;52:497–500.
118. Itoh N, Kanai K, Hori Y, et al. Prevalence of *Giardia intestinalis* and other zoonotic intestinal parasites in private household dogs of the Hachinohe area in Aomori prefecture, Japan in 1997, 2002 and 2007. *J Vet Sci.* 2009;10:305–308.
119. Júnior AF, Gonçalves-Pires MRF, Silva DAO, et al. Parasitological and serological diagnosis of *Strongyloides stercoralis* in domesticated dogs from southeastern Brazil. *Vet Parasitol.* 2006;136:137–145.
120. Palmer CS, Thompson RCA, Traub RJ, et al. National study of the gastrointestinal parasites of dogs and cats in Australia. *Vet Parasitol.* 2008;151:181–190.
121. Paradies P, Iarussi F, Sasanelli M, et al. Occurrence of strongyloidiasis in privately owned and sheltered dogs: clinical presentation and treatment outcome. *Parasit Vectors.* 2017;10:345.
122. Paulos D, Addis M, Fromsa A, et al. Prevalence of gastrointestinal helminthes among dogs and owners perception about zoonotic dog parasites in Hawassa Town, Ethiopia. *J Public Health Epidemiol.* 2012;4:205–209.
123. Riggio F, Mannella R, Ariti G, et al. Intestinal and lung parasites in owned dogs and cats from central Italy. *Vet Parasitol.* 2013;193:78–84.
124. Robinson RD, Thompson DL, Lindo JF. A survey of intestinal helminths of well-cared-for dogs in Jamaica, and their potential public health significance. *J Helminthol.* 1989;63:32–38.
125. Mircean V, Titilincu A, Vasile C. Prevalence of endoparasites in household cat (*Felis catus*) populations from Transylvania (Romania) and association with risk factors. *Vet Parasitol.* 2010;171:163–166.
126. Mohd Zain SN, Sahimin N, Pal P, et al. Macroparasite communities in stray cat populations from urban cities in Peninsular Malaysia. *Vet Parasitol.* 2013;196:469–477.
127. Speare R, Tinsley DJ. Survey of cats for *Strongyloides felis. Aust Vet J.* 1987;64:191–192.
128. Takeuchi-Storm N, Mejer H, Al-Sabi MNS, et al. Gastrointestinal parasites of cats in Denmark assessed by necropsy and concentration McMaster technique. *Vet Parasitol.* 2015;214:327–332.
129. Malone JB, Breitschwerdt EB, Little MD, et al. *Strongyloides stercoralis*-like infection in a dog. *J Am Vet Med Assoc.* 1980;176:130–133.
130. Cervone M, Giannelli A, Otranto D, et al. *Strongyloides stercoralis* hyper-infection in an immunosuppressed dog from France. *Revue Vétérinaire Clinique.* 2016;51:55–59.
131. Schad GA, Hellman ME, Muncey DW. *Strongyloides stercoralis*: hyper-infection in immunosuppressed dogs. *Exp Parasitol.* 1984;57:287–296.
132. Ericsson CD, Steffen R, Siddiqui AA, et al. Diagnosis of *Strongyloides stercoralis* infection. *Clin Infect Dis.* 2001;33:1040–1047.
133. Stancampiano L, Morandi F, Usai F, et al. Un caso atipico di iperinfestazione mortale sostenuta da *Strongyloides stercoralis* nel cane. *Veterinaria.* 2011;25:39.
134. Grove DI, Lumsden J, Northern C. Efficacy of albendazole against *Strongyloides ratti* and *S. stercoralis in vitro*, in mice, and in normal and immunosuppressed dogs. *J Antimicrob Chemother.* 1988;21:75–84.
135. Itoh N, Kanai K, Hori Y, et al. Fenbendazole treatment of dogs with naturally acquired *Strongyloides stercoralis* infection. *Vet Rec.* 2009;164:559–560.
136. Nolan TJ. Canine strongyloidiasis. In: Bowman DD, ed. *Companion and Exotic Animal Parasitology.* International Veterinary Information Service; 2001.
137. Mansfield LS, Niamatali S, Bhopale V, et al. *Strongyloides stercoralis*: maintenance of exceedingly chronic infections. *Am J Trop Med Hyg.* 1996;55:617–624.
138. Genta RM. *Strongyloides stercoralis*: loss of ability to disseminate after repeated passage in laboratory beagles. *Trans R Soc Trop Med Hyg.* 1989;83:539–541.
139. Schär F, Trostdorf U, Giardina F, et al. *Strongyloides stercoralis*: global distribution and risk factors. *PLoS Negl Trop Dis.* 2013;7: e2288.
140. Červená B, Hrazdilová K, Vallo P, et al. *Mammomonogamus* nematodes in felid carnivores: a minireview and the first molecular characterization. *Parasitol.* 2018;21:1–10.
141. Cuadrado R, Maldonado-Moll JF, Segarra J. Gapeworm infection of domestic cats in Puerto Rico. *J Am Vet Med Assoc.* 1980;176:996–997.
142. Tudor EG, Lee ACY, Armato DG, Bowman DD. *Mammomonogamus auris* infection in the middle ear of a domestic cat in Saipan, Northern Mariana Islands, USA. *J Feline Med Surg.* 2008;10:501–504.
143. Buckley JJC. On *Syngamus ierei* sp. *nov.* from domestic cats, with some observations on its life-cycle. *J Helminthol.* 1934;12:89–98.
144. Faust EC, Tang C-C. A new species of *Syngamus (S. auris)* from the middle ear of the cat in Foochow, China. *Parasitol.* 1934;26:455–459.
145. Sugiyama E, Kano R, Kage N, Hayashi S. A new record of *Mammomonogamus auris* from the middle ear of the domestic cats in Japan. *Japanese J Parasitol.* 1982;31:471–476.

146. Euzeby J, Graber M, Gevrey J, Mejia A. Recent findings concerning *Mammonmonogamus* infection in America and the West Indies. *Bull Acad Vet France*. 50:267–273.
147. Bowman DD, Hendrix CM, Lindsay DS, Barr SC. The Nematodes. In: Bowman DD, ed. *Feline Clinical Parasitology*. Ames, IA: Iowa State University Press; 2002:148–150.
148. Gardiner CH, Schantz PM. *Mammomonogamus* infection in a human. Report of a case. *Am J Trop Med Hyg*. 1983;32:995–997.
149. Leers WD, Sarin MK, Arthurs K. Syngamosis, an unusual cause of asthma: the first reported case in Canada. *Can Med Assoc J*. 1985;132:269–270.
150. Nosanchuk JS, Wade SE, Landolf M. Case report and description of parasite in *Mammomonogamus laryngeus* (human syngamosis) infection. *J Clin Microbiol*. 1995;33:998–1000.
151. Seneviratne P. *Syngamus mcgaughei* sp. nov. in domestic cats in Ceylon. *Ceylon Vet J*. 1954;2:55–60.
152. Lindquist DW, Austin ER. Exotic parasitism in a Siamese cat. *Feline Pract*. 1981;11:9–10.
153. Ketzis JK, Shell L, Chinault S, et al. The prevalence of *Trichuris* spp. infection in indoor and outdoor cats on St. Kitts. *J Infect Dev Ctries*. 2015;9:111–113.
154. Krecek RC, Moura L, Lucas H, Kelly P. Parasites of stray cats (*Felis domesticus* L., 1758) on St. Kitts, West Indies. *Vet Parasitol*. 2010;172:147–149.
155. Gattenuo T, Ketzis J, Shell L. Fenbendazole treatment for *Mammomonogamus* species infection of a domestic cat on St. Kitts, West Indies. *J Feline Med Surg*. 2014;16:864–866.
156. Verocai GG, Measures LN, Azevedo FD, et al. *Dioctophyme renale* (Goeze, 1782) in the abdominal cavity of a domestic cat from Brazil. *Vet Parasitol*. 2009;161:342–334.
157. Cianciolo RE, Mohr FC. Urinary system. In: Maxie MG, ed. *Jubb, Kennedy, and Palmer's Pathology of Domestic Animals*. 6th ed. St. Louis, MO: Elsevier; 2016:449.
158. Anderson RC. *Nematode Parasites of Vertebrates. Their Development and Transmission*. 2nd ed. Wallingford, Oxon (UK): CABI Publishing; 2000:650.
159. McLeod JA. *Dioctophyma renale* infections in Manitoba. *Can J Zool*. 1967;45:505–508.
160. Pedrassani D, Nascimento AA, André MR, Machado RZ. *Dioctophyme renale*: prevalence and risk factors of parasitism in dogs of São Cristóvão district, Três Barras County, Santa Catarina State, Brazil. *Rev Bras Parasitol Vet*. 2017;26:39–46.
161. Nakagawa TL, Bracarense AP, dos Reis AC, et al. Giant kidney worm (*Dioctophyma renale*) infections in dogs from Northern Paraná. *Brazil. Vet Parasitol*. 2007;145:366–370.
162. Rahal SC, Mamprim MJ, Oliveira HS, et al. Ultrasonographic, computed tomographic, and operative findings in dogs infested with giant kidney worms (*Dioctophyme renale*). *J Am Vet Med Assoc*. 2014;244:555–558.
163. Mattos-Junior DG, Pinheiro J. *Dioctophyma renale* in subcutaneous tissues of the inguinal region of a dog. *Arq Bras Med Vet Zootec*. 1994;46:301–302.
164. Fernando SS. The giant kidney worm (*Dioctophyma renale*) infection in man in Australia. *Am J Surg Pathol*. 1983;7:281–284.
165. Ferreira VL, Medeiros FP, July JR, Raso TF. *Dioctophyma renale* in a dog: clinical diagnosis and surgical treatment. *Vet Parasitol*. 2010;168:151–155.
166. Sun T, Turnbull A, Lieberman PH, Sternberg SS. Giant kidney worm (*Dioctophyma renale*) infection mimicking retroperitoneal neoplasm. *Am J Surg Pathol*. 1986;10:508–512.
167. Ignjatovic I, Stojkovic I, Kutlesic C, Tasic S. Infestation of the human kidney with. *Dioctophyma renale*. *Urol Int*. 2003;70:70–73.
168. Yang F, Zhang W, Gong B, et al. A human case of *Dioctophyma renale* (giant kidney worm) accompanied by renal cancer and a retrospective study of dioctophymiasis. *Parasite*. 2019;26:22.
169. Muller R. *Dracunculus* and dracunculiasis. *Adv Parasitol*. 1971;9:73–151.
170. Dikmans G. Another case of Guinea worm, *Dracunculus* sp., infestation in a dog in the United States. *Proc Helm Soc Wash*. 1948;15:39–40.
171. Ewing SA, Hibbs CM. *Dracunculus insignis* (Leidy, 1858) in dogs and wild carnivores in the Great Plains. *Am Nat*. 1966;76:515–519.
172. Eberhard ML, Ruiz-Tiben E, Wallace SV. *Dracunculus insignis*: experimental infection in the ferret. *Mustela putorius Furo*. *J Helminthol*. 1988;62:265–270.
173. Lucio-Forster A, Eberhard ML, Cama VA, et al. First report of *Dracunculus insignis* in two naturally infected cats from the northeastern USA. *J Fel Med Surg*. 2014;16:194–197.
174. Williams BM, Cleveland CA, Verocai GG, et al. *Dracunculus* infections in domestic dogs and cats in North America: an under-recognized parasite? *Vet Parasitol Reg Stud Reports*. 2018;13:148–155.
175. Cleveland CA, Garretta KB, Cozadb RA, et al. The wild world of Guinea worms: a review of the genus *Dracunculus* in wildlife. *IJP: Parasites and Wildlife*. 2018;7:289–300.
176. Fedchenko AP. Concerning the structure and reproduction of the Guinea worm (*Filaria medinensis* L.). *Am J Trop Med Hyg*. 1871;20:511–523.
177. Crichton VFJ, Beverley-Burton M. Migration, growth, and morphogenesis of *Dracunculus insignis* (Nematoda: Dracunculoidea). *Can J Zool*. 1975;63:105–113.
178. Crichton VFJ, Beverley-Burton M. Observations on the seasonal prevalence, pathology, and transmission of *Dracunculus insignis* in the raccoon in Ontario. *J Wildl Dis*. 1977;13:273–280.
179. Panciera DL, Stockham SL. *Dracunculus insignis* in a dog. *J Am Vet Med Assoc*. 1988;192:76–78.
180. Beyer TA, Pinckney RD, Cooley AJ. Massive *Dracunculus insignis* infection in a dog. *J Am Vet Med Assoc*. 1999;214:366–368.
181. Eberhard ML, Brandt FH, Ruiz-Tiben E, Hightower A. Chemoprophylactic drug trials for treatment of dracunculiasis using the *Dracunculus insignis*-ferret model. *J Helminthol*. 1990;64:79–86.
182. Beverley-Burton M, Crichton VFJ. Attempted experimental cross infections with mammalian Guinea worms, *Dracunculus* spp. (Nematoda: Dracunculoidea). *Am J Trop Med Hyg*. 1976;25:704–708.
183. Molyneux D, Sankara DP. Guinea worm eradication: progress and challenges—should we beware of the dog? *PLoS Neglected Trop Dis*. 2017;11. e0005495.
184. Rodonaja TE. A new species of nematode, *Onchocerca lupi* n. sp. from *Canis lupus cubanensis*. *Soobshchenyia Akad Nauk Gruzinskoy USSR*. 1967;45:715–719.
185. Labelle AL, Daniels JB, Dix M, Labelle P. *Onchocerca lupi* causing ocular disease in two cats. *Vet Ophthalmol Suppl*. 2011;1:105–110.
186. Labelle AL, Maddox CW, Daniels JB, et al. Canine ocular onchocercosis in the United States is associated with. *Onchocerca lupi*. *Vet Parasitol*. 2013;193(1–3):297–301.
187. Otranto D, Giannelli A, Scotty Trumble N, et al. Clinical case presentation and a review of the literature of canine onchocercosis by *Onchocerca lupi* in the United States. *Parasit Vectors*. 2015;8:89.
188. Komnenou A, Eberhard ML, Kaldrymidou E, et al. Subconjunctival filariasis due to *Onchocerca* sp. in dogs: report of 23 cases in Greece. *Vet Ophthal*. 2002;5:119–126.
189. Komnenou A, Egyed Z, Sréter T, et al. Canine onchocercosis in Greece: report of further 20 cases and molecular characterization of the parasite and its *Wolbachia* endosymbiont. *Vet Parasitol*. 2003;118:151–155.
190. Otranto D, Dantas-Torres F, Giannelli A, et al. Zoonotic *Onchocerca lupi* in dogs from Greece and Portugal. *Emerg Infect Dis*. 2013;19:2000–2003.
191. Hassan HK, Bolcen S, Kubofcik J, et al. Isolation of *Onchocerca lupi* in dogs and black flies, California, USA. *Emerg Infect Dis*. 2015;21(5):789–796.
192. Otranto D, Lia RP, Traversa D, Giannetto S. *Thelazia callipaeda* (Spirurida, Thelaziidae) of carnivores and humans: morphological study by light and scanning electron microscopy. *Parasitologia*. 2003;45(3–4):125–133.
193. Miró G, Montoya A, Hernández L, et al. *Thelazia callipaeda*: infection in dogs: a new parasite for Spain. *Parasit Vectors*. 2011;4:148.
194. Zarfoss MK, Dubielzig RR, Eberhard ML, Schmidt KS. Canine ocular onchocerciasis in the United States: two new cases and a review of the literature. *Vet Ophthalmol*. 2005;8(1):51–57.
195. Otranto D, Traversa D. *Thelazia* eyeworm: an original endo- and ecto-parasitic nematode. *Trends Parasitol*. 2005;21(1):1–4.
196. Bianciardi P, Otranto D. Treatment of dog thelaziosis caused by *Thelazia callipaeda* (Spirurida, Thelaziidae) using a topical formulation of imidacloprid 10% and moxidectin 2.5%. *Vet Parasitol*. 2005;129:89–93.

197. Motta B, Schnyder M, Basano FS, et al. Therapeutic efficacy of milbemycin oxime/praziquantel oral formulation (Milbemax®) against *Thelazia callipaeda* in naturally infested dogs and cats. *Parasit Vectors.* 2012;5:85.
198. Rossi L, Rigano C, Tomio E, et al. Use of sustained-release moxidectin to prevent eyeworm (*Thelazia callipaeda*) infection in dogs. *Vet Rec.* 2007;161(24):820–821.
199. Lechat C, Siméon N, Pennant O, et al. Comparative evaluation of the prophylactic activity of a slow-release insecticide collar and a moxidectin spot-on formulation against *Thelazia callipaeda* infection in naturally exposed dogs in France. *Parasit Vectors.* 2015;8:93.
200. Biswas A, Yassin MH. An unexpected cause of eye irritation: a case of zoonotic ocular onchocerciasis. *Case Rep Infect Dis.* 2013;2013:504749.
201. Eberhard ML, Ostovar GA, Chundu K, et al. Zoonotic *Onchocerca lupi* infection in a 22-month-old child in Arizona: first report in the United States and a review of the literature. *Am J Trop Med Hyg.* 2013;88(3):601–605.
202. Otranto D, Dutto M. Human thelaziasis, Europe. *Emerg Infect Dis.* 2008;14(4):647–649.
203. Grácio AJ, Richter J, Komnenou AT, Grácio MA. Onchocerciasis caused by *Onchocerca lupi*: an emerging zoonotic infection. Systematic review. *Parasitol Res.* 2015;114(7):2401–2413.
204. Cantey PT, Weeks J, Edwards M, et al. The emergence of zoonotic *Onchocerca lupi* infection in the United States–a case-series. *Clin Infect Dis.* 2016;62(6):778–783.
205. Berry WL. *Spirocerca lupi* esophageal granulomas in 7 dogs: resolution after treatment with doramectin. *J Vet Intern Med.* 2000;14:609–612.
206. Lobetti R. Successful resolution of oesophageal spirocercosis in 20 dogs following daily treatment with oral doramectin. *Vet J.* 2012;193:277–278.
207. Austin CM, Kok DJ, Crafford D, et al. The efficacy of a topically applied imidacloprid 10% / moxidectin 2.5% formulation (Advocate®, Advantage® Multi, Bayer) against immature and adult *Spirocerca lupi* worms in experimentally infected dogs. *Parasitol Res.* 2013;112(suppl 1):91–108.
208. Okanishi H, Matsumoto J, Aoki H, et al. Successful resolution of esophageal granulomas in a dog infected with. *Spirocerca lupi. J Vet Med Sci.* 2013;75:1629–1632.
209. Kelly PJ, Fisher M, Lucas H, et al. Treatment of esophageal spirocercosis with milbemycin oxime. *Vet Parasitol.* 2008;156:358–360.
210. Zorzella MM, Jark PC, Legatti E, et al. Diagnóstico endoscópico e parasitológico e avaliação do tratamento com milbemicina oxima em um caso de *Spirocerca lupi* em cão. *Vet Zootec.* 2011:553–557.

117

Nematode Infections of the Respiratory Tract

Gary A. Conboy, Jane E. Sykes

KEY POINTS

Aelurostrongylus abstrusus Infection (Aelurostrongylosis)

- First Described: First recovered from a cat in 1890, the cat lungworm was described and named as *Strongylus abstrusus* by Railliet in France in 1898 and renamed *Aelurostrongylus abstrusus* by Cameron in 1927.
- Causes: *Aelurostrongylus abstrusus* (cat lungworm). Nematode in the superfamily Metastrongyloidea, family Angiostrongylidae.
- Affected Hosts: Adult worms occur in the terminal bronchioles and alveolar ducts in the lungs of cats and some wild felids.
- Intermediate Hosts: Terrestrial gastropods (slugs and land snails) serve as intermediate hosts. Various amphibians, birds, reptiles, and rodents can serve as paratenic hosts.
- Geographic Distribution: Endemic throughout the world and reported from all continents except Antarctica.
- Route of Transmission: Cats may acquire infection by the ingestion of infective third-stage larvae in the tissues of the terrestrial gastropod intermediate hosts (slugs, land snails); however, transmission probably more commonly occurs by the ingestion of infected paratenic hosts (amphibians, birds, reptiles, rodents). Infection may also occur through ingestion of infective third-stage larvae released into the environment by infected gastropods.
- Major Clinical Signs: Cough, nasal discharge, tachypnea, and dyspnea. Weight loss and emaciation may occur in some cases. Infections can be fatal.
- Differential Diagnoses: Allergic respiratory disease, bacterial or viral pneumonia or infection with lungfluke (*Paragonimus kellicotti*), other metastrongyloids (*Oslerus rostratus, Troglostrongylus* spp.), or the capillarid nematode *Eucoleus aerophilus.*
- Human Health Significance: There are no reports of zoonotic infection; *A. abstrusus* is not considered a human health concern.

Crenosoma vulpis Infection (Crenosomosis)

- First Described: Recovered by Dujardin from a specimen bottle in a natural history museum in Paris in 1844, the fox lungworm was described and named as *Liorhynchus vulpis* and renamed *Crenosoma vulpis* by Railliet in 1915.
- Cause: *Crenosoma vulpis* (fox lungworm); nematode in the superfamily Metastrongyloidea, family Crenosomatidae.
- Affected Hosts: Adult worms occur in the bronchi, bronchioles, and trachea of dogs, wild canids, bears, badgers, and martens.
- Intermediate Hosts: Terrestrial gastropods (slugs and land snails).
- Geographic Distribution: Endemic in the northeastern quarter of North America as well parts of Europe and Asia.
- Route of Transmission: Dogs acquire infection by ingestion of infective third-stage larvae in the tissues of the terrestrial gastropod intermediate hosts (slugs, land snails). Infection may also occur through ingestion of infective third-stage larvae released into the environment by infected gastropods.
- Major Clinical Signs: Chronic productive cough, gagging.
- Differential Diagnoses: Airway collapse, chronic bronchitis, airway neoplasia, eosinophilic bronchopneumopathy, or other infectious respiratory diseases that can cause cough. Parasitic infections on the differential diagnosis list when examining fecal specimens include lung fluke (*Paragonimus kellicotti*), other metastrongyloids (*Angiostrongylus vasorum, Filaroides hirthi, Filaroides milksi, Oslerus osleri*), the capillarid nematode *Eucoleus aerophilus*, or intestinal threadworm (*Strongyloides stercoralis*).
- Human Health Significance: There are no reports of zoonotic infection; presently *C. vulpis* is not considered a human health concern.

Filaroides spp. Infection (Filaroidiosis)

- First Described: *Filaroides milksi* was first recovered and described from a dog in New York by Whitlock in 1956. *Filaroides hirthi* was first detected by Hirth and Hottendorf in research beagles in New York in 1973 and described and named by Georgi and Anderson in 1975.
- Causes: *Filaroides hirthi* and *Filaroides milksi* are nematodes in the superfamily Metastrongyloidea, family Filaroididae. These species are similar in morphology so there is some debate as to whether they may be the same species.
- Affected Hosts: *Filaroides hirthi* infection has only been reported in dogs. Subclinical infections have been reported in laboratory colony research beagles. Prevalence within research colonies may be high. Infrequent cases with severe clinical disease have been reported in client-owned dogs. These are usually associated with concurrent immunosuppression or some underlying disease process. *Filaroides milksi* has been reported from dogs and skunks.
- Intermediate Hosts: None—both species have a direct life cycle; L_1 are the infective stage.
- Geographic Distribution: *Filaroides hirthi* has been reported from the USA, Canada, Europe, Australia, Israel, and Japan. *Filaroides milksi* has been reported from the USA.
- Route of Transmission: Dogs acquire *F. hirthi* infection by ingestion of L_1 larvae in sputum, feces, or vomitus. The life cycle of *F. milksi* is unknown.
- Major Clinical Signs: Adult worms of both species occur in bronchioles and embedded in the lung parenchyma. Most *F. hirthi* infections are likely subclinical. With immunosuppression or the presence of another underlying disease or stress condition, a potentially fatal hyperinfection with signs of dyspnea, cough, cyanosis, and obtundation may occur.
- Differential Diagnoses: Other severe pulmonary conditions including CDV infection, bacterial bronchopneumonia (e.g., bordetellosis, *Streptococcus equi* subsp. *zooepidemicus*), toxoplasmosis, fungal pneumonia, heartworm disease, left-sided congestive heart failure, pulmonary thromboembolism, idiopathic eosinophilic pulmonary diseases, and infection with other metastrongyloid, capillarid, or trematode lungworms.

- Human Health Significance: There are no reports of zoonotic infection; neither *Filaroides* species is considered a human health concern.

Oslerus osleri Infection (Oslerosis)

- First Described: First recovered from dogs in Montreal, Canada by Sir William Osler in 1877, *Oslerus osleri* was described and named by Cobbold in 1879.
- Cause: *Oslerus osleri* is a nematode in the superfamily Metastrongyloidea, family Filaroididae.
- Affected Hosts: Wild and domestic canids.
- Intermediate Hosts: None—the life cycle is direct; L_1 are the infective stage.
- Geographic Distribution: Reported from all continents except Antarctica.
- Route of Transmission: Dogs acquire infection by the ingestion of infective L_1 in sputum or vomitus.
- Major Clinical Signs: Adult worms occur in nodules clustered at the bifurcation of the trachea. Signs include a non-productive hacking cough which may be paroxysmal, wheezing and in severe cases dyspnea, cyanosis, bronchospasm, and emaciation may occur. Infection can be fatal.
- Differential Diagnoses and Human Health Significance: See *Filaroides* spp. infection.

Angiostrongylus vasorum Infection (Angiostrongylosis)

- First Described: *Angiostrongylus vasorum* was first described in 1853 in a dog from southern France.
- Causes: *Angiostrongylus vasorum* (French heartworm), is a nematode in the superfamily Metastrongyloidea, family Angiostrongylidae.
- Affected Hosts: Domestic and wild canids, especially domestic dogs and red foxes.
- Intermediate Hosts: Terrestrial gastropods (slugs and land snails) are the primary intermediate hosts. Frogs can also serve as intermediate hosts. Both frogs and chickens can be paratenic hosts.
- Geographic Distribution: Infection is endemic throughout most of Europe, parts of Africa, and South America, and in North America it is restricted to the Canadian provinces of Newfoundland-Labrador and most recently in Nova Scotia.
- Route of Transmission: Dogs acquire infection by the ingestion of infective L_3 in the tissues of terrestrial gastropod intermediate hosts (slugs, land snails), or infected paratenic hosts (such as frogs or chickens). Infection may also occur through ingestion of infective L_3 released into the environment by infected gastropods. The importance of paratenic hosts or environmental contamination in transmission is unclear.
- Major Clinical Signs: Cough, gagging, dyspnea, tachypnea, exercise intolerance, evidence of bleeding disorders, neurological signs, uveitis, anorexia. Infections can be fatal.
- Differential Diagnoses: These include heartworm disease, other infectious causes of tracheitis and bronchopneumonia including other lungworms (metastrongyloids, *Eucoleus aerophilus*, *Paragonimus kellicotti*), systemic neoplasia, anticoagulant rodenticide toxicity, pulmonary thromboembolism, pulmonic stenosis, cardiomyopathy, and a variety of infectious and inflammatory disorders of the CNS and eye (rabies, CDV infection, toxoplasmosis, neosporosis, cryptococcosis, other CNS-migrating parasitic diseases such as *Baylisascaris procyonis* migration and cerebrospinal myiasis).
- Human Health Significance: *Angiostrongylus vasorum* does not infect humans.

Eucoleus aerophilus and Eucoleus boehmi Infection (Eucoleosis/Capillariosis)

- First Described: First recovered from a wolf in 1839 by Creplin (*Eucoleus aerophilus*) and from the frontal sinuses of a wolf (*Eucoleus boehmi*) in 1953 by Supperer.
- Cause: *Eucoleus aerophilus* (previously *Capillaria aerophila*) and *Eucoleus boehmi* (previously *Capillaria boehmi*) are nematodes in the superfamily Trichinelloidea, family Trichuridae, subfamily Capillariinae that parasitize the trachea, bronchi, and bronchioles (*E. aerophilus*) and nasal cavity and frontal sinuses (*E. boehmi*).
- Affected Hosts: *Eucoleus aerophilus*: Dogs, cats, wild carnivores (e.g., mustelids, foxes), occasionally people. *Eucoleus boehmi*: Dogs and various wild canids.
- Intermediate Hosts: The life cycle is unclear. Direct (i.e., without an intermediate host) or indirect involving earthworms have been proposed for both *Eucoleus* species.
- Geographic Distribution: Endemic throughout the world.
- Route of Transmission: Whether definitive hosts acquire infection by the ingestion of larvated eggs (fecal-oral) or earthworm intermediate hosts is unknown.
- Major Clinical Signs: Most infections are subclinical. Non-productive cough, nasal discharge, sneezing, tachypnea, and dyspnea may occur with heavy infections. Secondary bacterial bronchopneumonia may occur and may exacerbate clinical signs.
- Differential Diagnoses: These include allergic respiratory disease, bacterial, fungal, or viral pneumonia or infection with lungfluke (*Paragonimus kellicotti*), or other metastrongyloids (*Angiostrongylus vasorum, Crenosoma vulpis, Filaroides hirthi, Oslerus osleri* in dogs; *Aelurostrongylus abstrusus, Oslerus rostratus, Troglostrongylus* spp. in cats). In dogs, the bipolar-plugged eggs may also be mistaken for those of *Trichuris vulpis.*
- Human Health Significance: Very rare (< 20) cases of human infection by *E. aerophilus* exist in the literature.

OVERVIEW OF METASTRONGYLOID INFECTIONS OF THE RESPIRATORY TRACT

Metastrongyloids ("lungworms") are a varied group of nematode parasites of mammals. As the common name suggests, most species occur in the lungs; however, a few species occur in the pulmonary artery, veins, or frontal sinuses of the host. The life cycles for the majority of metastrongyloids are indirect, most often involving terrestrial gastropods as intermediate hosts; however, direct life cycles occur in a few species.[1] Although the significance remains unclear, recent studies have indicated that spontaneous shedding of infective third-stage larvae (L_3) into the environment by infected gastropods is widespread within the metastrongyloids and that these L_3 survive outside the host for several weeks to up to 4 months.[2] Therefore animals have the potential to acquire infections through ingestion or licking of grass and other plant sources. In North America, *Aelurostongylus abstrusus* occurs in the lungs of cats and *Angiostrongylus vasorum* in the pulmonary arteries and *Crenosoma vulpis, Filaroides hirthi, Filaroides milksi*, and *Oslerus osleri* in the lungs of dogs.[3] First-stage larvae (L_1) are passed in the feces of infected dogs or cats for each of these species. Typical of the metastrongyloids, fecal larval excretion patterns may be sporadic.[4] Due to sporadic larval excretion and difficulty in recovery and identification of nematode larvae, diagnosis of metastrongyloid infection in dogs and cats tends to be challenging. An additional and perhaps the most significant impediment to diagnosis is a failure to consider metastrongyloid infection as a differential diagnosis in dogs and cats with signs of respiratory disease.

AELUROSTRONGYLUS ABSTRUSUS INFECTION (AELUROSTRONGYLOSIS)

ETIOLOGIC AGENT AND EPIDEMIOLOGY

Aelurostrongylus abstrusus adult worms are 4 to 10 mm in length.[5] The bursa in males is greatly reduced, and the vulva in females is near the anus just anterior to the tail.[6] Mature females produce undifferentiated eggs which develop in the lung tissue and hatch L_1.

Aelurostrongylus abstrusus infects cats and wild felids (Amur cat, cheetah, Eurasian lynx, leopard, lion, ocelot, tiger) and has a worldwide distribution.[7–9] In North America, infection has been reported in the eastern USA (Alabama, Connecticut, Florida, Georgia, Maryland, Massachusetts, New Jersey, New York, North Carolina, Pennsylvania, South Carolina, Tennessee, Virginia) and in the western coastal states (California, Oregon, Washington) as well as in Hawaii and Puerto Rico.[10–14] In Canada, infection has been reported in Ontario and diagnosis based on fecal examination has occurred in British Columbia, Newfoundland-Labrador, New Brunswick, and Nova Scotia (author's unpublished observations).[15] In other global regions, infection has been reported in Africa (Kenya, South Africa), Asia, Australia, Europe (Albania, Bulgaria, Denmark, England, France, Germany, Greece, Hungary, Italy, Netherlands, Poland, Portugal, Romania, Scotland, Serbia, Spain, Switzerland, Turkey), the Middle East (Iran, Israel), and South America (Argentina, Brazil).[16–30] Infection in cats has been reported with increasing frequency in Europe in the last decade.[31] There have also been reports of *A. abstrusus* infection in dogs based solely on detection of L_1 on fecal examination.[10] These may be spurious diagnoses due to coprophagy. Attempts to experimentally infect dogs with *A. abstrusus* have been unsuccessful indicating dogs are probably not a susceptible host.[5]

The prevalence of infection varies within endemic regions. Fecal flotation surveys, which likely underestimate prevalence, indicated *A. abstrusus* infection rates in North America in cats as low as 0.1 to 1.1% in Pennsylvania, Connecticut, and New Jersey to 6.2% in upstate New York.[10–12,32] Although it may reflect a regional difference, a much higher prevalence (18.5%) was found in a fecal survey of cats in Alabama which utilized the more sensitive Baermann technique.[33] Various surveys have found prevalence values that range from 0.5 to 50% in Europe and 14 to 39.2% in Australia.[31] Infection appears to be more common in younger cats (3 months to 3 years), cats with access to outdoors, and in those living in rural environments.[17,27,34–38]

CLINICAL FEATURES

Pathogenesis

The life cycle of *A. abstrusus* is indirect involving terrestrial gastropods as intermediate hosts (Fig. 117.1). L_1 are passed in the feces of infected felids; slugs and land snails become infected while feeding on cat excrement. L_3 develop in tissues of the gastropod in about 3 to 4 weeks.[1] Cats acquire infection by ingestion of L_3 contained in the gastropod or in a wide range of paratenic hosts (amphibians, reptiles, birds, small rodents).[1] Recent studies have indicated that infected gastropods spontaneously excrete L_3 into the environment; this may be an additional exposure route for cats or paratenic host species by direct ingestion of L_3 through ingestion of plant material.[2] The PPP is about 5 to 6 weeks; infected cats may excrete L_1 in feces for about 2 to 7 months (peak excretion 10 to 17 weeks PI).[14,39,40] A prolonged period of larval excretion (1 to 2 years) occurs in some cats.[39,40] L_1 may survive for 5 months in moist soil.[14] In cats that have been re-exposed, there is a delayed onset of patency, a reduced excretion level, and a more erratic larval excretion pattern than that typical of a first exposure.[39,40] Cats may excrete large numbers of L_1 in the feces with counts as high as 144,800 larvae per gram of feces.[36]

Heavy infections can result in severe, potentially fatal, interstitial bronchopneumonia. Severe clinical disease occurred 6 weeks PI in experimentally infected kittens fed 800 L_3.[41] Chronic catarrhal

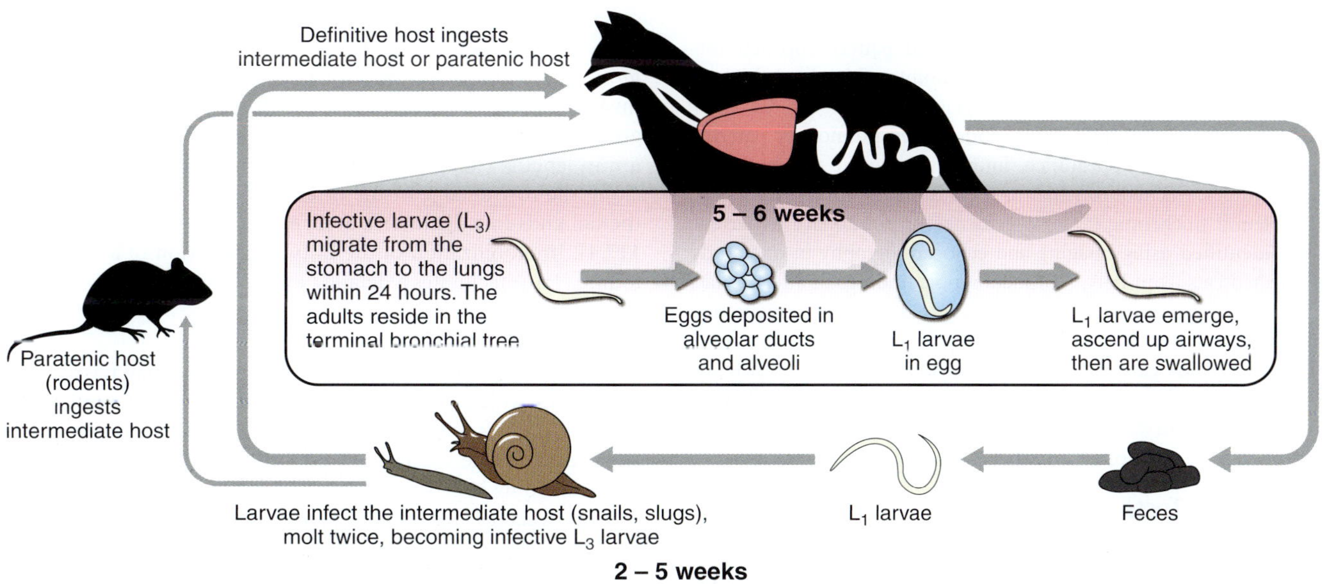

Fig. 117.1 Life cycle of *Aelurostrongylus abstrusus.*

eosinophilic bronchiolitis occurs in response to the presence of adult worms, eggs, and larvae. A necropsy survey of anesthetic-associated deaths in cats in New York found 9% were infected with *A. abstrusus*.[42] The infections were subclinical at the time of anesthesia and it was speculated that death may have occurred due to hypoxia and systemic hypotension secondary to lungworm infection resulting in cardiovascular collapse and arrest. Pneumothorax and pyothorax secondary to *A. abstrusus* infection has been reported in a kitten. Migrating L_3 may have become contaminated with *Salmonella typhimurium* in the lumen of the intestine and carried it to the lungs.[43] Although rare, there have been several reports of invasion of the large intestine by L_1 of *A. abstrusus*; in one of these cases, hyperinfection was considered the cause of death.[44,45]

Clinical Signs and Physical Examination Abnormalities

Most infections are subclinical and self-limiting.[14,21,39] Heavily infected cats show signs of cough, wheezing, dyspnea, and may suffer from anorexia and emaciation. Most cats are afebrile. Usually, cough can be elicited on tracheal palpation. Increased vesicular lung sounds may be noted on auscultation. Enlarged mandibular lymph nodes, nasal discharge, and increased respiratory rate (> 50/min) may be noted.[46]

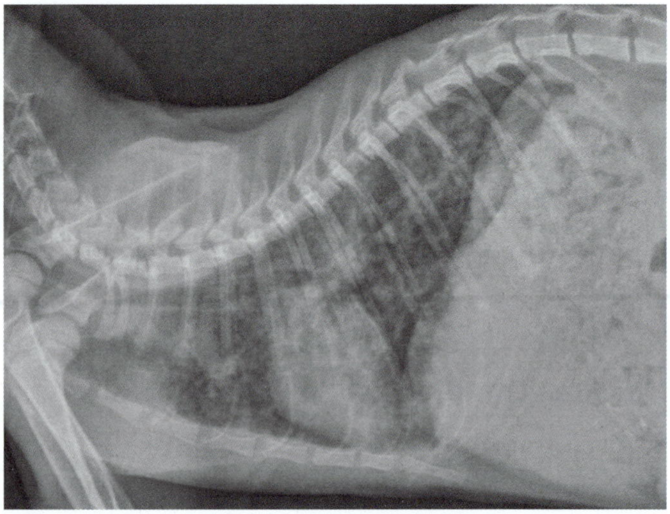

Fig. 117.2 Lateral thoracic radiograph showing a severe, diffuse, bronchointerstitial pattern with peribronchial cuffing in a 6-month-old intact female Himalayan cat with *Aelurostrongylus abstrusus* infection. (Courtesy of University of California-Davis Diagnostic Imaging Service.)

DIAGNOSIS

Definitive diagnosis of *A. abstrusus* infection is achieved by the detection of L_1 in the feces or mucus of infected cats. The L_1 can be specifically identified based on size and morphology. Larvae can be detected in feces by both direct smear and flotation; however, the method of choice is the Baermann technique (see Chapter 5). In general, larval excretion in the feces of animals infected with metastrongyloids tends to be sporadic.[4] In *A. abstrusus* infections, the fecal larval excretion pattern becomes sporadic typically after 10 to 17 weeks of infection.[14] As a consequence, false-negative fecal examination results can occur. Examination of multiple fecal specimens increases detection sensitivity; most recommendations suggest the evaluation of three fecal specimens before discounting the possibility of metastrongyloid infection.[4]

Laboratory Abnormalities

In many cases, no abnormalities are detected. The CBC may show a peripheral eosinophilia.[47]

Diagnostic Imaging

Radiographic changes usually involve a mixed pattern (bronchointerstitital and alveolar), or may show bronchointerstitial, bronchial, or diffuse unstructured interstitial patterns (Fig. 117.2).[31,38,48,49] CT findings have also been described and include mixed pulmonary patterns with a "ground glass" appearance, interstitial-alveolar patterns, pulmonary nodules, tracheobronchial or mediastinal lymphadenomegaly, and subpleural thickening.[49–51] No evidence of pulmonary hypertension was identified using imaging and echocardiography in one study of 14 infected cats from Italy.[49] Bronchoscopic findings in affected cats include airway hyperemia and stenosis, increased bronchial mucus, airway collapse, and bronchiectasis (Fig. 117.3). In a small study that compared findings in 24 cats with aelurostrongylosis to 12 cats with feline idiopathic bronchial disease, bronchiectasis was only found in cats with aelurostrongylosis; airway hyperemia, epithelial irregularities, and bronchial stenosis were more often found in cats with bronchial disease.[52]

Microbiologic Tests

Diagnosis Using Fecal Examination

Although insensitive, examination of a direct fecal smear for L_1 is the simplest, least expensive, and quickest diagnostic test. A small speck of feces is mixed in a single drop of saline or water on a slide, coverslipped, and examined microscopically for L_1. In one study, direct smears identified larvae in 3 of 12 *A. abstrusus*-infected cats.[21] This test will only detect cats that excrete high numbers of larvae in the feces.

Centrifugal fecal flotation using zinc sulfate ($ZnSO_4$), sodium chloride, or sugar has been used to detect L_1. Flotation is less sensitive than the Baermann method and larval morphology may be damaged by the high specific gravity flotation media; this can complicate identification. Detection sensitivity of centrifugal flotation using $ZnSO_4$ was reported to be superior to that of sugar but both were inferior to the Baermann technique.[53]

The Baermann technique is the most sensitive method for detection of most species of nematode larvae.[4] Larval detection by this method requires that the L_1 are vigorous and motile. Only fresh fecal specimens should be evaluated. In cats this usually means restricting the use of a clean litterbox to one cat and collecting the next available specimen. Feces that cannot be submitted within several hours of collection should be refrigerated. False-positive results can occur if specimens are incubated at room temperature for about a day before collection due to the presence of newly hatched *Ancylostoma tubaeforme* eggs. Additionally, specimens collected from grass or soil can be invaded by free-living nematodes if left for prolonged periods on the ground before collection.[4] *Aelurostrongylus abstrusus* L_1 are 360–400 μm in length. There is a cephalic button (symmetrical indentations along the rostral edge of the head) present at the anterior end and the tail ends in a distinctive S-shaped kink with a dorsal spine (Fig. 117.4). Immobilization of the L_1 by the addition of a drop of dilute iodine (1:10) facilitates a detailed examination of the morphology.[4]

Cytologic Diagnosis

Analysis of respiratory lavage specimens in cats may reveal increased cell counts with mixed neutrophilic and eosinophilic inflammation, as found in cats with idiopathic bronchial disease. However, bronchoalveolar lavage specimens were normal in 21% of 24 cats in one study, and only 33% of specimens had evidence of eosinophilic inflammation.[52] Larvae may also be recovered from transtracheal wash or bronchoalveolar lavage specimens. In one study, larvae were found in bronchoalveolar lavage specimens from 5 (21%) of 24 cats with aelurostrongylosis (Fig. 117.5).

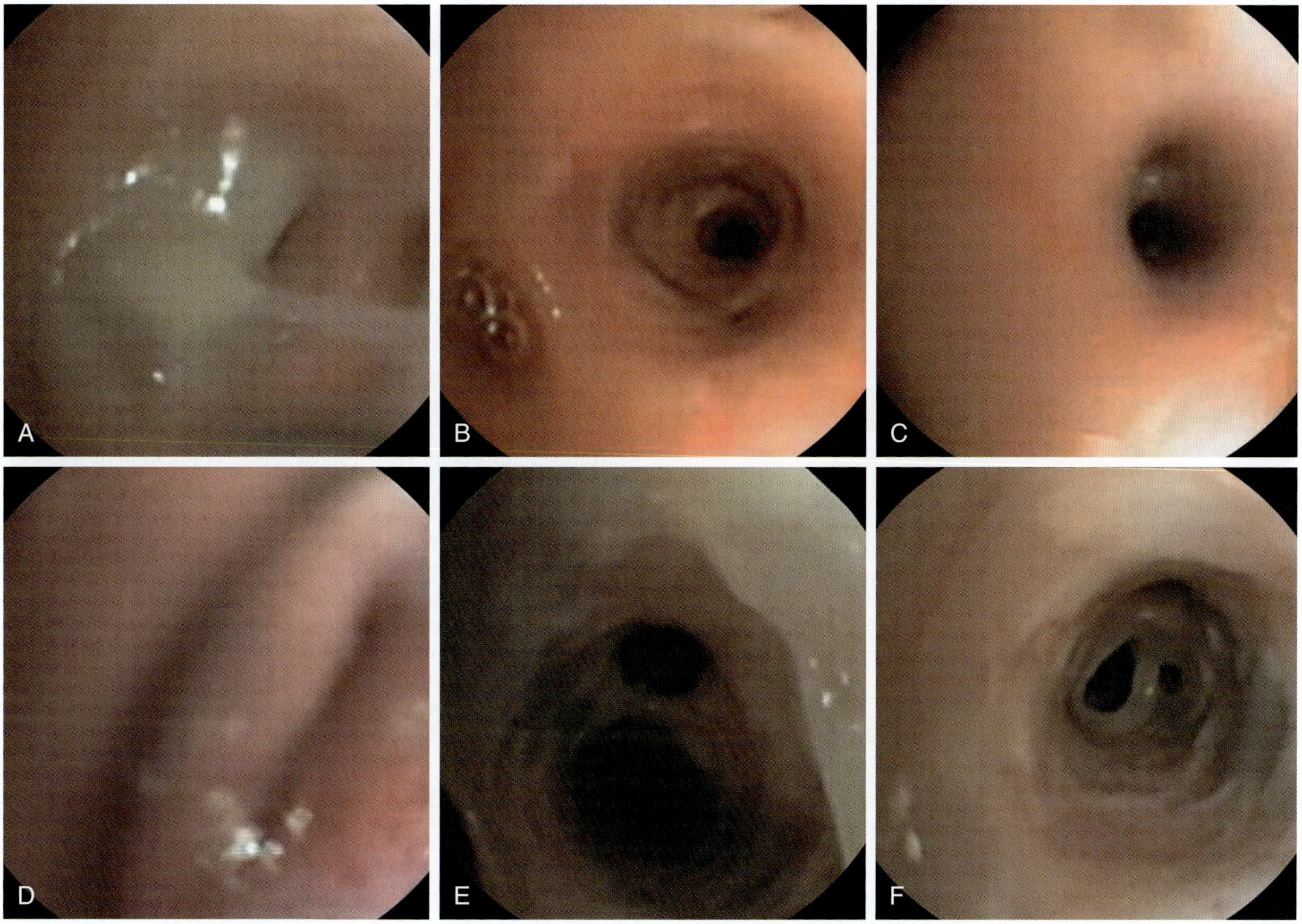

Fig. 117.3 Bronchoscopic findings in cats with aelurostrongylosis. (A) Mucus plug and bronchial obstruction; (B, C) hyperemia and stenosis; (D) bronchial collapse; (E, F) bronchiectasis and mucus accumulation. (From Crisi PE, Johnson LR, Di Cesare A, et al. Evaluation of bronchoscopy and bronchoalveolar lavage findings in cats with *Aelurostrongylus abstrusus* in comparison to cats with feline bronchial disease. *Front Vet Sci.* 2019;6:337.)

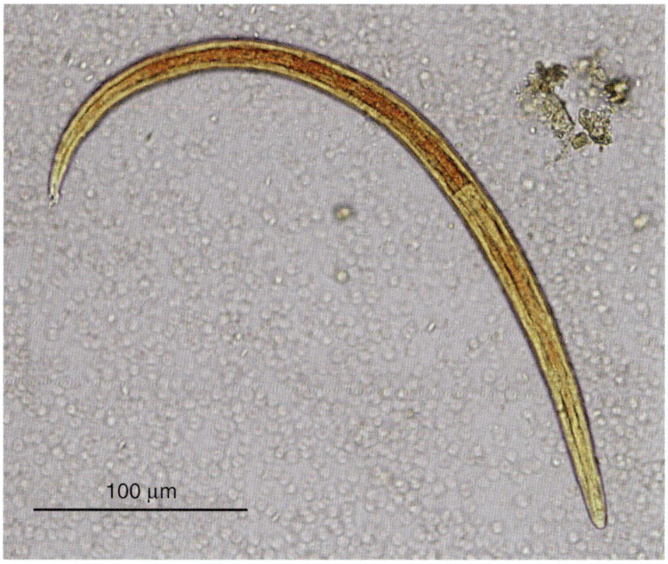

Fig. 117.4 First-stage larva of *Aelurostrongylus abstrusus* recovered on Baermann examination of a fecal specimen from a domestic cat.

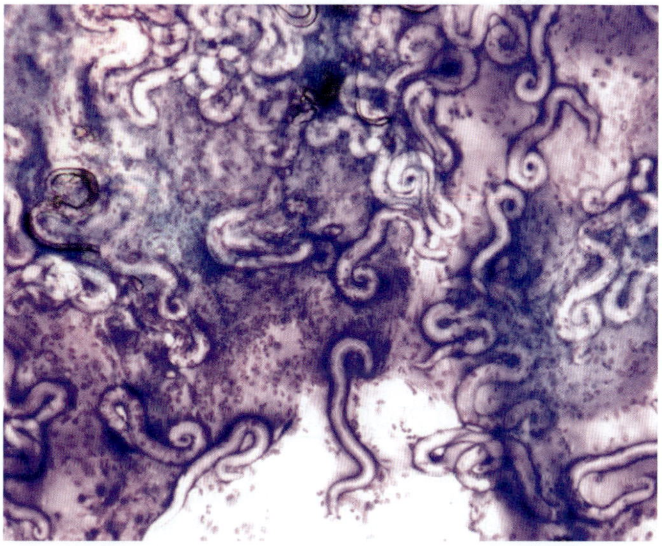

Fig. 117.5 Larvae of *Aelurostrongylus abstrusus* in a bronchoalveolar lavage specimen. Diff-Quik stain (40× magnification). (From Crisi PE, Johnson LR, Di Cesare A, et al. Evaluation of bronchoscopy and bronchoalveolar lavage findings in cats with *Aelurostrongylus abstrusus* in comparison to cats with feline bronchial disease. *Front Vet Sci.* 2019;6:337.)

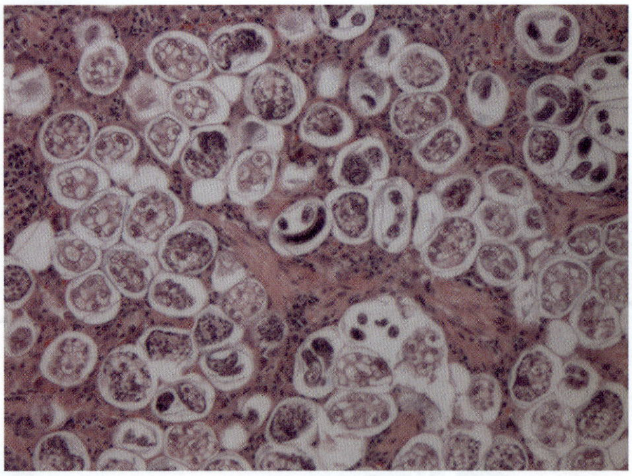

Fig. 117.6 Histopathology image of *Aelurostrongylus abstrusus* in the lung of a 15-year-old female spayed domestic shorthair with diabetes mellitus and fragile skin syndrome. Pyogranulomatous nephritis with intralesional coronavirus antigen (consistent with FIP), intestinal ascariasis, multiple biliary cystadenomas, and *A. abstrusus* infection were incidental findings at necropsy. This is also another example of a smiley-face pathogen image (see Fig. 58.2). (Courtesy of Dr. Jane Sykes, University of California-Davis Veterinary Medical Teaching Hospital.)

Molecular Diagnosis Using Nucleic Acid–Based Testing

A PCR assay for *A. abstrusus* infection used on Baermann sediment, feces, and pharyngeal swabs has been developed and shows promise; it had a reported specificity of 100% and sensitivity of 96.6%.[53–55]

Pathologic Findings

Yellow, firm protruding nodules (1–10 mm in diameter) may be apparent throughout the lungs on necropsy examination of cats with aelurostrongylosis. Histologically, a granulomatous (eosinophils, neutrophils, monocytes, and multinucleated giant cells) response occurs around adult worms, eggs, and larvae (Fig. 117.6). The uterus of adult female worms contain only undifferentiated eggs and undifferentiated eggs may be visible in the lung parenchyma. In most metastrongyloid species infecting companion animals, adult females produce fully formed L_1; only in the Angiostrongylidae (including *A. abstrusus* and *Angiostrongylus chabaudi* in wild felids) are undifferentiated eggs produced.[1] Although domestic cats are susceptible to infection with *Angiostrongylus* spp., infections are very rare and the few infections reported have been non-patent.[56] Therefore the detection of undifferentiated metastrongyloid eggs in the lung parenchyma of cats in histologic sections is nearly pathognomonic for *A. abstrusus* infection. There is hypertrophy and hyperplasia of smooth muscle in the walls of bronchioles and alveolar ducts.[21,31] Identification of *A. abstrusus* nematodes may be an incidental finding on necropsy of cats with other disorders.

TREATMENT AND PROGNOSIS

Emodepside, eprinomectin, fenbendazole, moxidectin, and selamectin have been used to treat cats with aelurostrongylosis. Based on fecal larval counts, emodepside (3 mg/kg, in combination with praziquantel) had an efficacy of 99% when used in a single topical application and 100% with two bi-weekly applications.[57,58] In an efficacy study based on total worm counts at necropsy, a single application of 3 mg/kg emodepside had an efficacy of 73%; with two doses 14 days apart, the efficacy rose to 99%.[59]

Based on fecal larval counts, an efficacy of 90% was reported for a single topical application of eprinomectin (with fipronil and praziquantel) at 0.5 mg/kg in naturally infected cats.[60] Efficacies of 91.6 to 98.9% with a single application and 99.9% after two treatments of eprinomectin (0.5 mg/kg) was reported in cats infected with *A. abstrusus*.[61]

Fenbendazole (50 mg/kg PO q24h for 3 days) greatly reduced but did not eliminate larval excretion in *A. abstrusus*-infected cats.[57,62] Extension of treatment duration appears to increase effectiveness. Dosages of 20 mg/kg for 5 days, 25 mg/kg for 5 days, and 50 mg/kg for 15 days have all been reported as effective treatments.[63–65] The efficacy of a single topical application of moxidectin (in combination with imidacloprid) at 1 mg/kg was 100% based on fecal larval counts.[66] Efficacy of topical moxidectin based on necropsy worm counts was reduced to 88% for a single application; administering two to three monthly applications resulted in an efficacy of 99 to 100% when used as either a treatment or preventive.[67] A single topical application of selamectin (6 mg/kg) resulted in cessation of fecal larval excretion in one of three naturally infected cats.[63] Administration of two selamectin treatments 23 days apart resulted in clinical improvement and negative post-treatment fecal examinations in 9 of 10 naturally infected cats.[68]

With timely diagnosis and treatment, prognosis is good. Case reports of fatal infections often involve prolonged periods of time from the onset of clinical disease to diagnosis. To what degree a delay in diagnosis contributes to a fatal outcome is unknown. Some airway changes, such as bronchiectasis, may be irreversible and predispose cats to chronic bronchial disease.

IMMUNITY AND VACCINATION

Infection in most cats is mild and self-limiting. Re-exposed cats have a delayed onset of patency and tend to shed lower numbers of larvae than that occurring with naïve exposures.[39,40] Cats likely develop some degree of immunity through previous exposure. No vaccines are currently available.

PREVENTION

Curtailing access of cats to the outdoors limits exposure to terrestrial gastropods and paratenic hosts. Topical eprinomectin and moxidectin have potential for use as monthly preventive treatments.[61,67] Most of the anthelmintics with activity against *A. abstrusus* are approved for monthly use to prevent infection with a range of different parasites. To what degree cats receiving monthly treatments with these anthelmintics are protected from developing clinical aelurostrongylosis is unknown.

PUBLIC HEALTH ASPECTS

There are no reports of zoonotic infection with *A. abstrusus*, and currently *A. abstrusus* is not considered to have any public health significance.

METASTRONGYLOIDS OF WILD FELIDS

Reports from Europe have indicated a growing recognition that domestic cats acquire infection with metastrongyloids (*Angiostrongylus chabaudi, Oslerus rostratus, Troglostrongylus brevior, Troglostrongylus subcrenatus*) that naturally occur in wild felids.[56,69] Previously, domestic cats infected with these wild felid lungworms were likely misdiagnosed as having *A. abstrusus* infections. In North America, *O. rostratus* and *Troglostrongylus wilsoni* have been reported from lynx and bobcats in the USA (Alabama, Arkansas, Georgia, North Carolina, Texas, Virginia, West Virginia) and Canada (Alberta, Nova Scotia, Ontario).[70–75] To date, there have been no reports of domestic cat infection with either of these wild felid metastrongyloids in North America.

CRENOSOMA VULPIS INFECTION (CRENOSOMOSIS)

ETIOLOGIC AGENT AND EPIDEMIOLOGY

Adult *Crenosoma vulpis* nematodes are 4 to 15 mm in length and are characterized by a distinctive anterior-end morphology; there are 18 to 26 ringlike folds in the cuticle.[3] Males possess a copulatory bursa, and female worms produce thin-shelled larvated eggs which hatch shortly after being laid.

The definitive hosts of *C. vulpis* are primarily wild and domestic canids. The natural definitive host is the red fox (*Vulpes vulpes*). Infection has also been reported in such wildlife as the arctic fox (*Alopex lagopus*), gray fox (*Urocyon cinereoargenteus*), coyote (*Canis latrans*), raccoon-dog (*Nyctereutes procyonoides*), and wolf (*Canis lupus*) and non-canid hosts such as the badger (*Meles meles*), black bear (*Ursus americanus*), and martens (*Martes* spp.).[1] Wildlife, particularly red fox, serve as reservoir hosts of infection for dogs.

In North America, *C. vulpis* is mainly restricted to the northeast. Endemic infection in dogs or wild canids has been reported in Canada (New Brunswick, Newfoundland-Labrador, Nova Scotia, Ontario, Prince Edward Island, Quebec) and the USA (Illinois, Massachusetts, New York).[76–82] The sole report of infection outside this region was in an arctic fox on St. Lawrence Island, Alaska.[83] Endemic infections have been reported throughout most of Europe.[30] Infection in a dog based on fecal examination was reported in South Korea.[84] Prevalence of infection in the red fox in North America ranges from 21 to 87% and is particularly high in the Atlantic Canadian provinces.[78,79,82]

Dogs acquire *C. vulpis* infection by ingestion of infective L_3 in the tissues of the terrestrial gastropod intermediate hosts.[1] Multiple slug and land snail species appear to be suitable intermediate hosts; however, gastropod species involved in natural infections are unknown.[3] Infected gastropods release L_3 in mucus trails and feces; shed L_3 may survive for periods of weeks to months free in the environment. Therefore the potential exists that dogs may also acquire infection when they ingest L_3 during consumption of grass and other vegetation.[2] The prevalence of infection in dogs is unknown for most regions. A necropsy survey of humane society dogs on Prince Edward Island, Canada, found 3.2% were infected with *C. vulpis*.[76] Crenosomosis is a frequent cause of chronic canine respiratory disease in Atlantic Canada with *C. vulpis* infection detected in 21% of the dogs with chronic cough.[85] There are no age, breed, or sex predispositions. Ages of infected dogs have ranged from 3 months to 16 years. In North America, the majority of the diagnoses occur from November to May.[85]

CLINICAL FEATURES

Upon ingestion, L_3 penetrate the duodenal wall, enter the liver, and travel to the heart and lungs via the hepatic portal circulation. The L_3 break through the pulmonary capillaries into the alveolar airspace and migrate to the bronchioles and bronchi to mature to the adult stage. In cases of heavy infection, adult worms may also be found in the trachea. The PPP is 18 to 21 days and the adult worm lifespan is about 10 months.[1] The magnitude of the exposure dose necessary to cause clinical disease and the prodromal period are unknown. The consequences of repeated exposure are also unknown. Infection results in eosinophilic bronchitis; signs consist solely of chronic, usually productive cough which may be accompanied by gagging.[86,87] The gagging may be so pronounced that the owner may perceive that the dog has esophageal obstruction. Affected dogs are otherwise usually bright, alert, and responsive with normal temperature and appetite. Mild hyperpnea may be detected. In most cases, a cough response is easily elicited through tracheal palpation.[86,87]

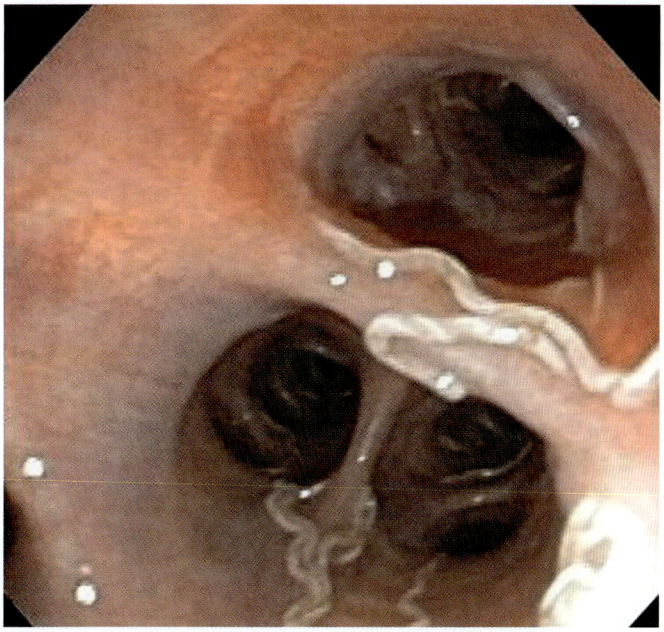

Fig. 117.7 Bronchoscopy image showing *Crenosoma vulpis* in the airways of a 6-year-old female spayed golden retriever-poodle mix with a 1-month history of cough, lethargy, and inappetence. (Courtesy of Dr. Michelle Miller and Dr. Lynelle Johnson, University of California-Davis Small Animal Internal Medicine Service.)

DIAGNOSIS

Laboratory Abnormalities

Bloodwork results in dogs with crenosomosis are generally unremarkable. Eosinophilia, basophilia, and mild monocytosis may be detected on CBC.[87]

Diagnostic Imaging

Thoracic radiographs in affected dogs may reveal an interstitial to bronchointerstitial pattern; focal alveolar patterns have also been described.[86,87] Findings on thoracic CT include diffuse bronchial wall thickening, parenchymal consolidation, multifocal peribronchial "ground glass" attenuation, parenchymal bands, and cylindrical bronchiectasis.[88] Airway mucus and hyperemia, irregular bronchial wall thickening, nodules, and adult worms may be visualized on bronchoscopy (Fig. 117.7).[89–91] Occasionally, adult worms may be identified using bronchoscopy when Baermann fecal examination is negative.[89]

Microbiologic Tests

Definitive diagnosis of crenosomosis is best achieved by detection and identification of L_1 in feces or sputum of infected dogs. Fecal flotation lacks detection sensitivity for *C. vulpis* L_1. In specimens where L_1 are present, the morphology may be too severely affected by osmotic damage to allow larval identification. Centrifugal fecal flotation using zinc sulfate as the flotation media has been reported to detect *C. vulpis* larvae in about 10% of infected dogs.[85] The fecal examination method of choice is the Baermann technique (see Chapter 5).[3] As for aelurostrongylosis, the intermittent shedding pattern typical of metastrongyloids limits sensitivity. In order to minimize the chance of a false-negative result, submission of feces from 3 consecutive days is recommended.[3,4]

Recovered larvae should be killed by addition of a drop of dilute (1:10) iodine prior to examination on microscopy. Larvae are identified based on size (264 to 340 μm in length) and morphology (cephalic button, long esophagus, tail ends in a simple point lacking kinks and spines but showing a slight deflection) (Fig. 117.8).[4] A false-positive diagnosis of crenosomosis can occur as a result of larvae excreted passively as a result of coprophagia or predation. Additionally, fecal specimens collected from grass or soil hours to days after deposit may be invaded by free-living nematodes, which may be confused with *C. vulpis*. Finally, if fresh feces are not examined, hookworm eggs in fecal specimens may hatch and release larvae, which can also be confused with metastrongyloids.[4]

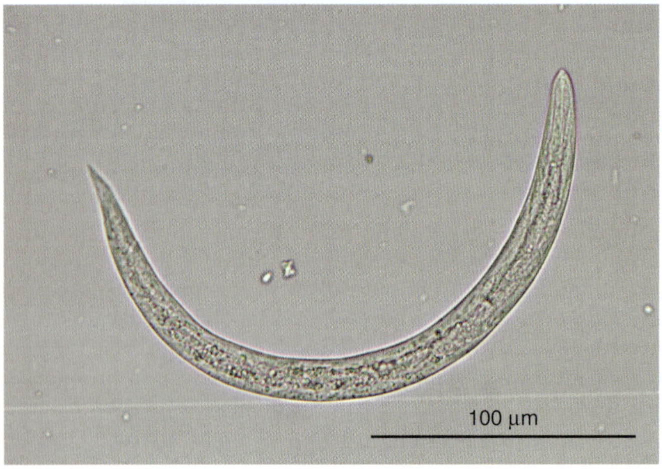

Fig. 117.8 First-stage larva of *Crenosoma vulpis* recovered on Baermann examination of a canine fecal specimen.

Cytologic Diagnosis

Analysis of respiratory lavage specimens in dogs with crenosomosis may reveal increased cell counts with mixed neutrophilic and eosinophilic inflammation. In one study of 10 affected dogs, bronchial lavage specimens revealed a predominance of eosinophils in seven dogs, eosinophils and neutrophils in two dogs, and neutrophils in one dog; larvae were identified in specimens from five dogs.[87]

Pathologic Findings

Since there have been no reports of fatal infection, details on gross and histologic lesions in dogs are limited. Slightly depressed red to purple discolored areas of consolidation in the mid to ventral portions of the lung lobes have been reported. On histopathology, multifocal histiocytic, eosinophilic bronchopneumonia may be present with complete blockage by inflammatory cells, nematodes, and debris occurring in bronchioles and in some cases, bronchi (Fig. 117.9).[92]

TREATMENT AND PROGNOSIS

Fenbendazole, milbemycin oxime, and moxidectin have been used to treat dogs infected with *C. vulpis*. Fenbendazole (50 mg/kg, PO, q24h for 3 to 10 days) has been used widely with resolution of clinical signs and cessation of larval excretion.[86,93] Milbemycin oxime (0.5 mg/kg, PO, single dose) had an efficacy of 99% in the treatment of experimentally infected dogs.[85,92] A single topical application of moxidectin (2.5 mg/kg) was similarly effective.[94]

The prognosis is excellent. In most dogs, full recovery occurs within 7 to 10 days of anthelmintic treatment. In some dogs, cough worsens in the first 48 hours after treatment. This is invariably followed by marked improvement and a full recovery.

IMMUNITY AND VACCINATION

As for cats with *A. abstrusus* infections, the onset of fecal larval shedding is delayed and the number of larvae shed is greatly reduced in dogs that have been re-infected with *C. vulpis* (author's unpublished observations). This likely reflects the induction of some degree of immunity from exposure. No vaccines are available.

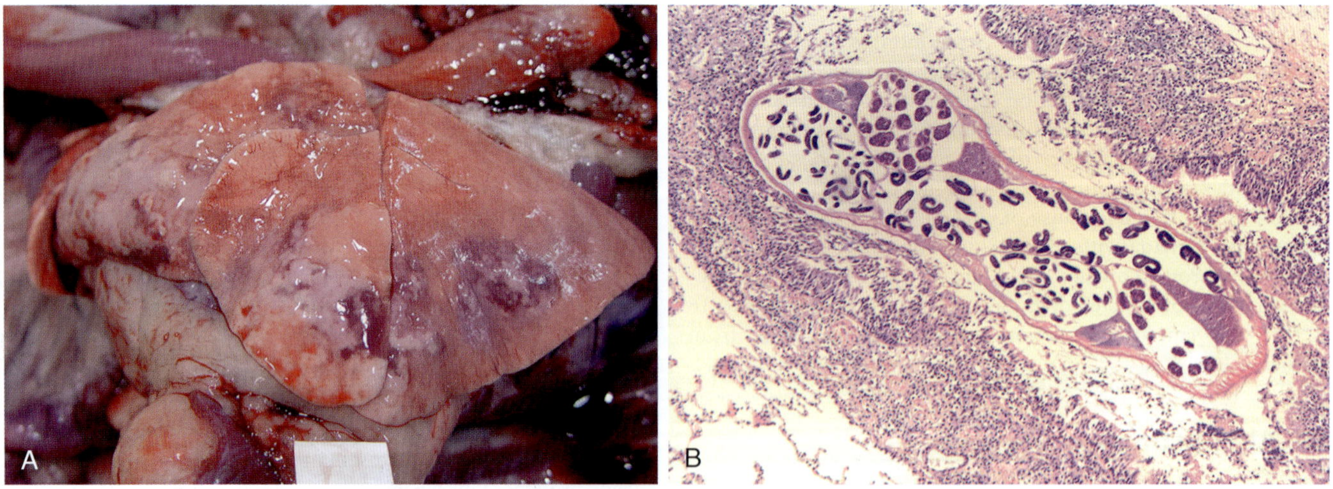

Fig. 117.9 Gross (A) and histopathologic (B) lesions in dogs 49 days after experimental infection with *Crenosoma vulpis*. Slightly depressed areas of consolidation are present, especially in the mid to ventral regions of the lung lobes. On histopathology, there is multifocal histiocytic, eosinophilic bronchopneumonia with obstruction of bronchi and bronchioles by inflammatory cells and nematodes (here shown in cross-section). (Reprinted from Conboy G, Bourque A, Miller L, et al. Efficacy of Milbemax (milbemycin oxime + praziquantel) in the treatment of dogs experimentally infected with *Crenosoma vulpis*. *Vet Parasitol.* 2013;198:319–324.)

PREVENTION

Dogs placed on monthly milbemycin oxime or topical moxidectin for heartworm prevention or other reasons are unlikely to develop clinical disease due to *C. vulpis* infection.

PUBLIC HEALTH ASPECTS

Crenosoma vulpis is not considered to have any public health significance.

FILAROIDES SPP. INFECTION (FILAROIDOSIS)

ETIOLOGIC AGENT AND EPIDEMIOLOGY

Filaroides milksi was first found in 1956 as an incidental finding at necropsy in the bronchioles and coiled in nests in the lung parenchyma of a 10-year-old Boston terrier.[95] Adult worms were 3.4 to 10.9 mm in length. *Filaroides hirthi* was first reported, also as an incidental finding at necropsy, in the bronchioles and lung parenchyma of beagles from a purpose-bred research colony in 1975.[96,97] Adult worms were 2.3 to 13 mm in length. The morphology of both species is similar, with the vulva in the female located near the anus just anterior to the termination of the tail and the male tail lacking a well-developed bursa.[6] The two species are differentiated based on subtle differences in worm size and male spicule morphology and length.[98] Whether the two are different species or the same has been the subject of some debate.[98–100] There are few reports of *F. milksi* infection in dogs. Diagnosis based solely on histopathology has been reported in dogs in Australia, Canada, and the USA.[101–103] However, differentiation between *F. hirthi* and *F. milksi* is not possible based on histopathology and therefore these may have been *F. hirthi*.[100] Since the original description of *F. milksi* infection in 1956, there is only one other report of its diagnosis in a dog based on recovery and identification of adult male worms from a dog in Michigan.[104] There have been several reports of *F. milksi* infection in skunks.[99,105]

Filaroides hirthi infection has been reported in laboratory research dogs from Australia, Germany, Great Britain, Israel, Japan, and the USA, with a prevalence of infection in colonies as high as 78%.[96,106–111] However, most likely as a result of heightened awareness and control efforts, there have been no reports of infection in laboratory research beagle colonies since 1996. Diagnosis has been relatively rare in non-research colony dogs. Infected client-owned dogs have been reported from the USA (Alabama, Georgia, New York, Pennsylvania, Texas, Washington), Europe (France, England, Ireland, Spain), and Australia.[112–122] Most case reports involve young (< 3 years of age) toy breed dogs (Chihuahua, toy poodle, West Highland white terrier, Yorkshire terrier).

The life cycle of *F. milksi* is unknown. Transmission of *F. hirthi* occurs by ingestion of infective L_1 usually through coprophagy of fresh fecal material or in sputum, saliva, or vomitus. In research beagle colonies, this is thought to occur from mother to pup by 4 to 5 weeks of age through exposure to feces from infected dams.[123] The PPP is 35 days.[124] Infections appear to be long lived and may persist due to re-exposure to infective L_1 through autoinfection.[125]

CLINICAL FEATURES

Adult worms of both species occur in bronchioles and embedded in the lung parenchyma. Most infections of *F. hirthi* in dogs are probably subclinical. Clinical signs are usually associated with immunosuppression or comorbid diseases. Glucocorticoid therapy, concurrent demodectic mange, CDV infection, severe trauma, and neoplasia have all been associated with clinical disease.[108,109,112-114,116,117] Presumably, through autoinfection such dogs develop massive hyperinfections with life-threatening granulomatous pneumonia; larvae have also been found in mesenteric lymph nodes, the intestinal wall, and the liver. Most often, affected dogs develop a non-productive cough that progresses to dyspnea, tachypnea, cyanosis, and sometimes death. Dogs may become emaciated.

DIAGNOSIS

Laboratory Abnormalities

Eosinophilia may be detected on bloodwork. Other bloodwork abnormalities may be detected depending on the presence of co-existing diseases.

Diagnostic Imaging

Radiographic changes are non-specific. Radiographs may show an interstitial pattern with linear and nodular infiltrates involving all lung lobes.[113,117,119,126] Bronchoscopy can be done to rule out the possibility of *Oslerus osleri* infection. The absence of nodules at the bifurcation of the trachea in a dog in which L_1 are detected suggests *Filaroides* spp. infection.

Diagnosis Using Fecal Examination

Complicating the diagnosis of *Filaroides* spp. infection is the lack of a reliable fecal examination method. For reasons poorly understood, the L_1 of *Filaroides* spp. excreted in feces of infected dogs lack vigor to the point of being moribund and are therefore not reliably recovered by the Baermann method.[124] Zinc sulfate centrifugal flotation has greater detection sensitivity than the Baermann method but is still insensitive. Osmotic damage due to the high specific gravity flotation media may obscure the larval morphology preventing accurate identification. Larvae can be detected using fecal sedimentation, but this is time-consuming and laborious to perform.

Larval detection is best achieved through examination of sputum, saliva, or respiratory lavage specimens. This is the method of choice; larvated eggs and L_1 may be detected. The eggs are thin walled and measure about 38 × 80 μm; L_1 are 240 to 290 μm in length and have a bluntly rounded head (i.e., lack a cephalic button) and the tail has a kink (Fig. 117.10).[124] The L_1 of *Filaroides* spp.

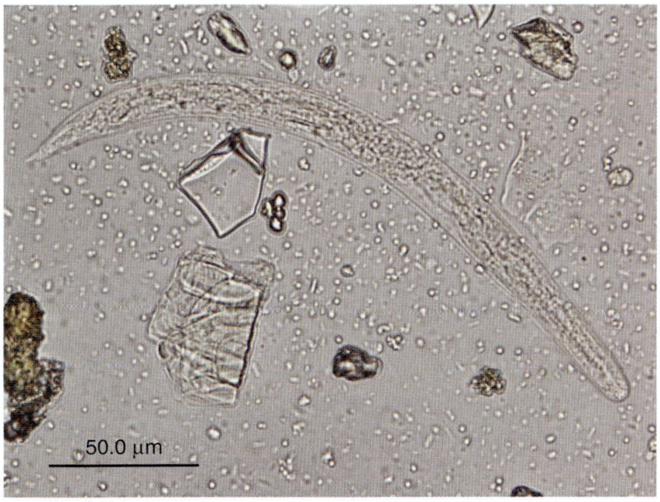

Fig. 117.10 First-stage larva of *Filaroides hirthi* recovered on a fecal sedimentation examination of a canine sample. Note the head lacks a cephalic button and the tail ends in a kink.

and *Oslerus osleri* are difficult to differentiate due to similarities in size and morphology.

Pathologic Findings

Grossly, the lungs of dogs infected with *Filaroides* spp. are firm and red. A large number of thin (35 to 102 μm wide) adult worms may be observed extruding from the cut surface of the lung tissue. Histopathology reveals granulomatous verminous pneumonia with adult worms in bronchioles and nested in the lung parenchyma. In some cases, only eggs and larvae are observed. Hepatic granulomas surrounding worms have also been also observed.[108,109,112,113,115-117,124] In massive infections, larvae may be found in mesenteric lymph nodes, liver, the intestinal wall, and the lungs.[108]

TREATMENT AND PROGNOSIS

There is no anthelmintic approved for use in the treatment of *Filaroides* spp. infection in dogs. Albendazole, fenbendazole, and ivermectin have been used to treat dogs infected with *F. hirthi*.[3] Albendazole and high-dose ivermectin are not approved for use in dogs and, due to safety concerns, are not recommended. Fenbendazole (50 mg/kg PO q24h) for 14 to 21 days has been used to successfully treat several dogs with clinical disease signs due to *F. hirthi* infection.[114,117,121] One dog was successfully treated with fenbendazole at 100 mg/kg PO q24h for 7 days.[122] Depending on the nature of the predisposing disease condition, prognosis may be guarded to poor. Infections in immunocompromised dogs may be overwhelming and fatal despite treatment.

IMMUNITY, VACCINATION, AND PREVENTION

Routine use of anthelmintics should prevent *Filaroides* spp. infections in research dogs.

PUBLIC HEALTH ASPECTS

Neither *Filaroides* spp. is considered to have any public health significance.

OSLERUS OSLERI INFECTION (OSLEROSIS)

ETIOLOGIC AGENT AND EPIDEMIOLOGY

Oslerus osleri infects the trachea and bronchi of dogs and various wild canids (coyotes, dingos, wolves).[1] Adult worms are 6.5 to 13.5 mm long; males lack a well-developed bursa and the vulva and anus in females occurs at the termination of the tail.[6,127] Adult worms reside within wart-like nodules that are attached to the surface of the lumen in the trachea and bronchi clustered at the bifurcation.[127,128] Nodules range in size from 1 to 14 mm and can become confluent if present in large numbers.[129–135] Nodules from naturally infected coyotes contained 1 to > 100 worms per nodule.[136]

Oslerus osleri has a worldwide distribution. In North America, infection has been reported in wild and domestic canids in the USA (Alabama, Arizona, California, Colorado, Connecticut, Georgia, Illinois, Iowa, Hawaii, Kansas, Massachusetts, Michigan, Minnesota, Montana, Nebraska, New Mexico, New York, North Carolina, Ohio, Oklahoma, Pennsylvania, Rhode Island, South Dakota, Texas, Utah, Washington, Wyoming), Canada (Alberta, British Columbia, Manitoba, Ontario, Quebec, Saskatchewan, Nova Scotia), and Mexico.[13,137–148] Other endemic regions of the world include Australia, parts of Europe, Japan, New Zealand, and South Africa.[127–129,131,133–135,149–153] Infection can be common in wild canids, particularly in coyotes and Australian dingos, with a prevalence as high as 52%.[148] However, wild canids do not appear to serve as an infection reservoir for dogs; dogs exposed to infective larvae recovered from coyotes failed to become infected.[146] Infection in dogs appears to be relatively infrequent.[13] However, *O. osleri* infection was found to be the cause of 18% of the cases of chronic respiratory disease in dogs in a retrospective survey from the 1980s in England.[149]

The *O. oslerus* life cycle is direct with the L_1 as the infective stage. Female worms partially protrude through pores in the nodule to deposit thin-shelled larvated eggs (90 × 60 μm) into the lumen of the trachea and bronchi. The eggs hatch releasing the L_1 while in the process of being coughed up to either pass to the outside in the saliva or be swallowed and pass in the feces.[1] As for *F. hirthi*, larvae recovered from the feces tend to be sluggish and are often found to be dead and degenerating. Transmission in wild canids is thought to occur at the time of weaning from dam to puppy by regurgitative feeding.[150] Transmission in domestic dogs is likely also from dam to puppy but occurs more through exposure to L_1 in saliva when the dam cleans puppies by licking.[148] Infection may also follow ingestion of larvae in contaminating fecal matter but this is likely of lesser importance.[128,150] The PPP is about 70 to 126 days.[150,154] Consistent with exposure at an early age, infections are more common in younger dogs (6 months to 2 years of age).[148,149,155]

CLINICAL FEATURES

After ingestion, L_1 penetrate through the wall of the duodenum and travel to the heart via the lymphatics or hepatic portal circulation; they then travel to the lungs via the pulmonary artery. Immature worms arrive in the trachea about 34 days after exposure and by 70 days PI, nodules that contain adult worms become apparent.[150] In heavily infected dogs, nodules may be so large and numerous that they may obstruct 50% to almost the entire lumen of the trachea and bronchi.[130–132,149,152] Infection results in a chronic, non-productive cough which may become worse with exercise and is readily elicited on tracheal palpation. In some cases, wheezing, dyspnea, and cyanosis occur.[148] Severely affected dogs will show weight loss, emaciation, collapse, and even death.[156] Pneumothorax secondary to bronchial rupture was reported in one dog.[130] Subclinical infections occur in some dogs.

DIAGNOSIS

Laboratory Abnormalities

Bloodwork findings are mild and non-specific; a peripheral eosinophilia may be detected.

Diagnostic Imaging

Tracheal nodules or narrowing of the tracheal lumen secondary to a mural soft-tissue mass are occasionally visible using thoracic radiography.[131,132,134,135,149,155,157,158] Definitive diagnosis of *O. osleri* infection occurs by detection of the nodules by bronchoscopy (Fig. 117.11) along with the identification of nematode larvae with consistent morphology from respiratory specimens or feces. The absence of nodules at the bifurcation of the trachea in a dog excreting such larvae indicates *Filaroides* spp. infection.

Microbiologic Tests

The same fecal examination challenges that exist for *Filaroides* spp. exist for *O. osleri*. The diagnostic test of choice is examination of respiratory lavage specimens for larvated eggs and L_1. The eggs are thin walled and measure about 60 × 90 μm; L_1 have a bluntly rounded head

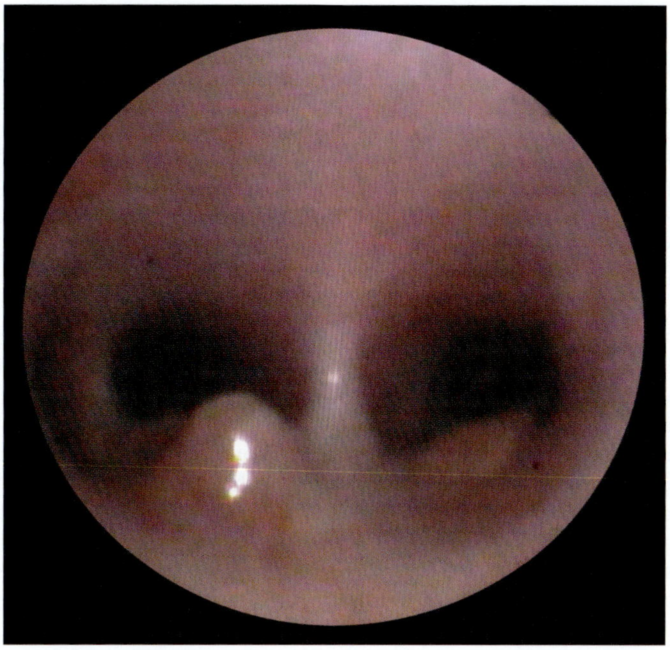

Fig. 117.11 Bronchoscopy image showing tracheal nodules associated with *Oslerus osleri* infection in a 1-year-old intact female toy poodle with a 6-month history of cough and gagging. (Courtesy of University of California-Davis Small Animal Internal Medicine Service.)

(i.e., lack a cephalic button) and a kinked tail.[150] Larvae recovered from mucus are 232 to 266 µm in length; those recovered from feces measure 326 to 378 µm (Fig. 117.12A).[128,151] The L_1 of *F. hirthi*, *F. milksi*, and *O. osleri* are similar in size and morphology.[4]

Pathologic Findings

Grossly, nodules are readily seen attached to the epithelial surface of the lumen in the trachea and bronchi clustered at the bifurcation. Individual nodules may be as large as 12 mm in diameter and contain adult worms coiled inside. Portions of female worms may be seen extruding out from the surface of the nodule. The presence of coiled adult worms in the nodule with the females containing a uterus with developing larvated eggs can be confirmed on histopathology, either following endoscopic biopsy of tracheal nodules or at necropsy (Fig. 117.12B).[128]

TREATMENT AND PROGNOSIS

There are no anthelmintics approved for use in the treatment of dogs infected with *O. osleri*. Variable results using a number of older anthelmintics (diethylcarbamazine, thiacetarsemide, thiabendazole, levamisole, oxfendazole) have been cited in the literature.[133,155,157,159–162] Currently, fenbendazole and high-dose ivermectin are treatment options. Fenbendazole (50 mg/kg PO q24h) for 7 to 14 days was reported to be effective in 19 of 20 dogs with clinical *O. osleri* infections.[149] The one remaining dog required a second 14-day course of treatment and although it showed marked clinical improvement, it still had evidence of a few tracheal nodules and a small number of larvae present on post-treatment examination. Fenbendazole at the same dose for approximately 1 month was reportedly effective in another dog with severe tracheal involvement.[158] Ivermectin (0.4 mg/kg, SC, repeated every 3 weeks for 4 treatments) was reported to be effective in the treatment of four dogs resulting in a clinical cure and resolution of tracheobronchial nodules.[163] This dose of ivermectin is not safe to administer to collies, collie-type breeds, and other dogs with a mutation in the multidrug resistance gene (*mdr1*). Marked clinical improvement was reported

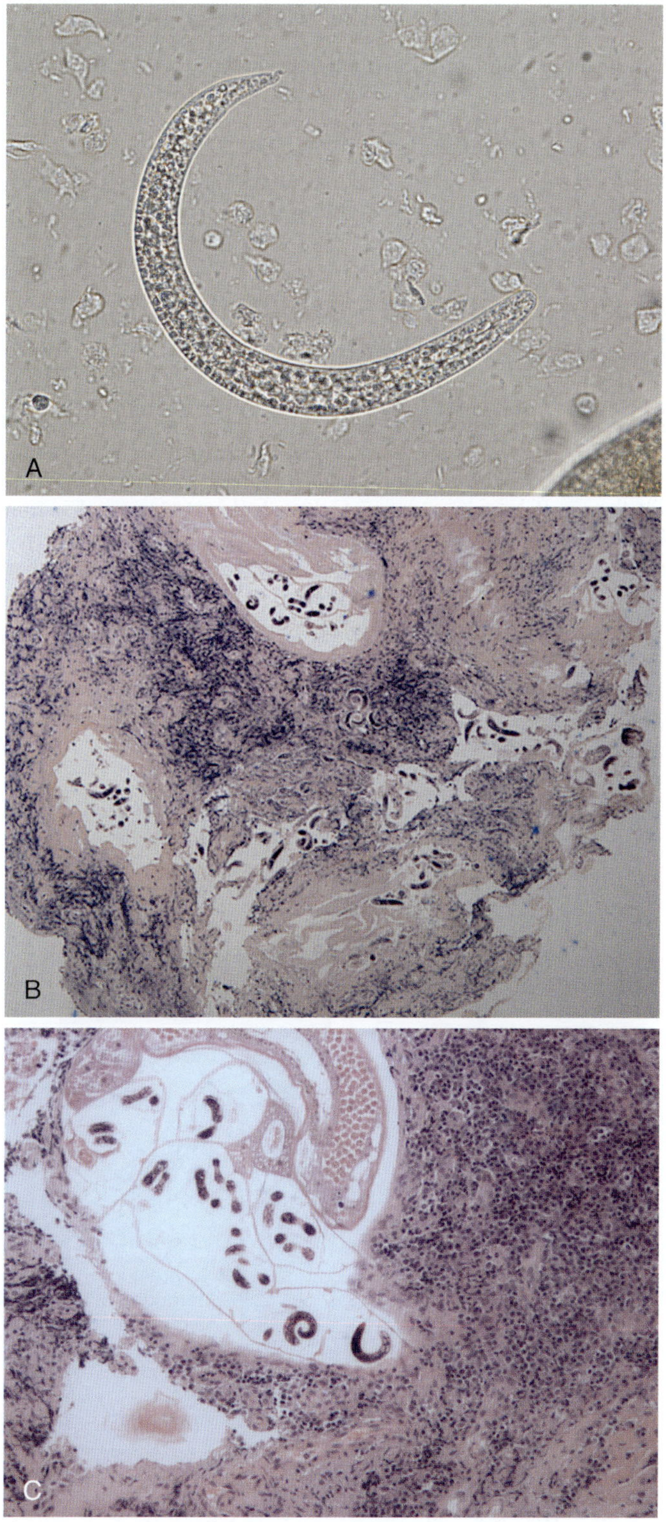

Fig. 117.12 (A) First-stage larvae of *Oslerus osleri* recovered from an impression smear of a nodule removed from the surface of the tracheal lumen of a coyote from Prince Edward Island, Canada. Note the lack of a cephalic button and the tail ends in a kink. (B, C) Histopathology of biopsies collected from nodules observed using bronchoscopy (the same dog as described in Fig. 117.11). Hematoxylin and eosin stain.

in a dog given a single oral dose of ivermectin (0.4 mg/kg); however, nodules persisted after treatment.[133] In general, prognosis for recovery following appropriate treatment is good to excellent.

IMMUNITY, VACCINATION, AND PREVENTION

Routine use of anthelmintics should prevent *Oslerus* spp. infections.

PUBLIC HEALTH ASPECTS

There are no reports of zoonotic infection with *O. osleri* and it is not considered to have any public health significance.

ANGIOSTRONGLYUS VASORUM INFECTIONS (ANGIOSTRONGYLOSIS)

ETIOLOGY AND EPIDEMIOLOGY

Angiostrongylus vasorum (French heartworm) is a nematode in the superfamily Metastrongyloidea, family Angiostrongylidae. *Angiostrongylus vasorum* was first described in 1853 in a dog from southern France.[164] The life cycle is indirect with a wide variety of gastropods (slugs and land snails) as well as the frog as intermediate hosts, and both frogs and chickens reported as paratenic hosts (Figure 117.13). Although the precise role it may play in natural infection is unknown, the possibility of exposure through direct ingestion of L_3 has been suggested. Recent studies have shown a portion of the infective L_3 contained in the tissues of infected gastropods are shed into the environment where they can survive outside of a host for several weeks to several months.[2] This suggests that dogs might become infected through licking or eating grass and other plant materials.[2] Somewhat limited in geographic distribution, *A. vasorum* has shown a remarkable capability for expansion over the past 40 years with endemic foci currently occurring in southwestern France, the United Kingdom (espeically southwestern England and Wales), Ireland, Denmark; sporadic cases from other parts of Scandinavia (Finland, Sweden), the Netherlands, Austria, Switzerland, Italy, Hungary, Spain, Greece, Turkey, Argentina, Brazil, Colombia, Uganda, and Canada. *Angiostrongylus vasorum* is a significant pathogen of dogs, causing life-threatening cardiopulmonary and neurological disease. Various species of foxes, particularly the red fox, are considered to be the natural definitive host, but infections can also occur in other wild canids including the wolf (*Canis lupus*), coyote (*Canis latrans*), and jackal (*Canis aureus*). Disease is occasionally recognized in non-endemic regions following importation of infected dogs, including a dog imported into the United States (Michigan) from Ireland,[165] a dog imported into Canada (Alberta) from Cornwall, England, and another imported into Australia (Perth, Western Australia) from southern England.[166,167] Autochthonous cases in domestic dogs have not been reported from the United States, but infection based on histopathology was recognized in 2014 in a red fox from West Virginia;[168] and a focus of infection has been identified in domestic dogs, red foxes, and subsequently coyotes in Newfoundland, Canada.[169] Recently, infection in coyotes has been reported from the Canadian province of Nova Scotia, indicating the parasite has spread

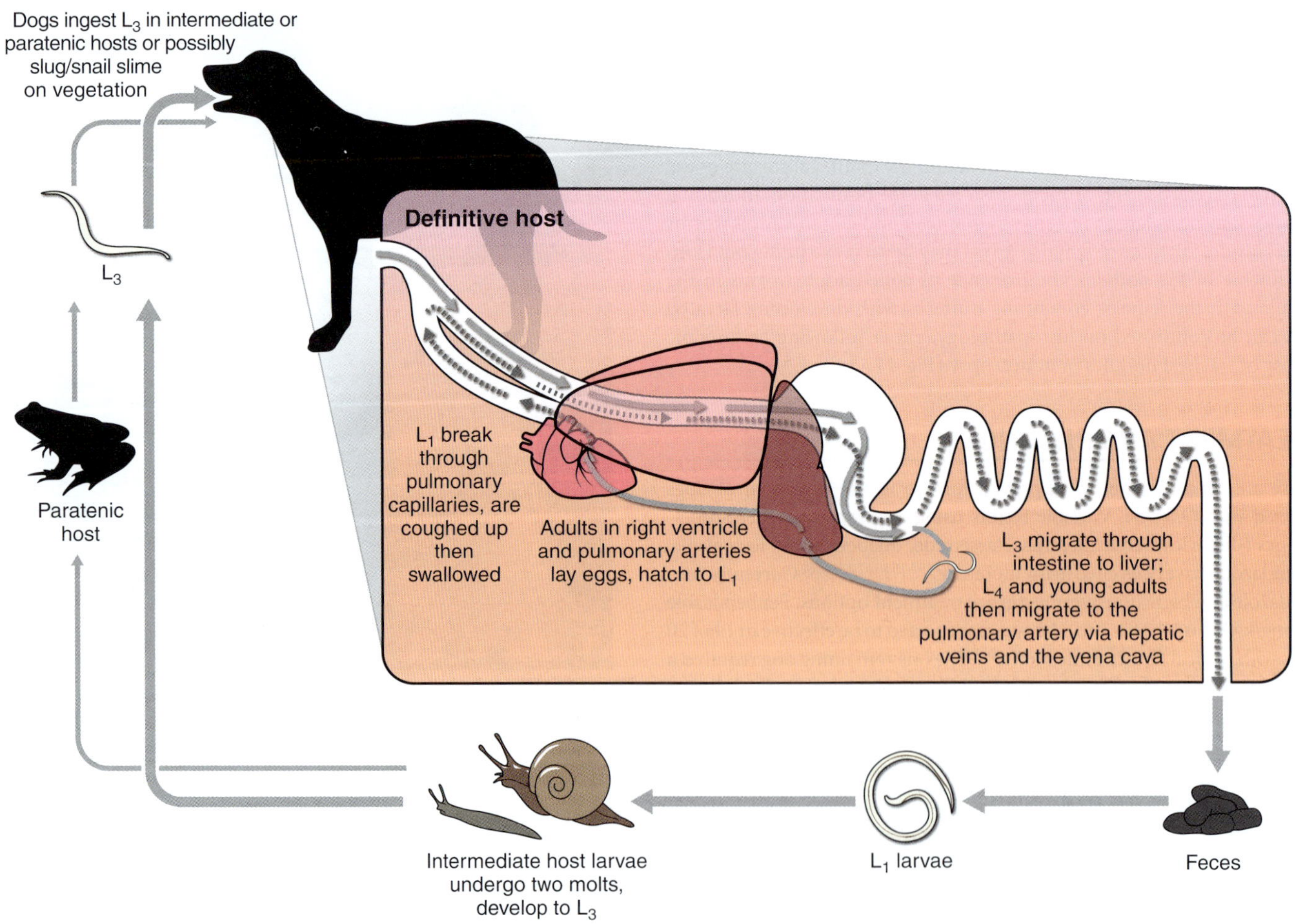

Fig. 117.13 Life cycle of *Angiostrongylus vasorum*.

from the island of Newfoundland to the mainland. The ongoing expansion of the geographic range of this parasite has raised concern about its impact following introduction into nonendemic regions as a result of climate change and the movement of foxes and gastropods (international movement of gastropods as a result of horticulture industry activities is significant).[170] Computer modelling has predicted that there is a high likelihood that the parasite will become established in much of North America, becoming endemic throughout the eastern half of the continent and in the states and provinces on the west coast.[171]

In endemic regions, the overall prevalence of infection in domestic dogs has ranged from 0.3 to 9.8%, and depends on factors such as the coprological method used to detect L_1 and the dog population studied (e.g., stray vs. owned dogs). In contrast, the prevalence of infection in foxes has ranged from 5 to 56%.[172] Increased awareness of the parasite and improved diagnostic testing has likely contributed to disease emergence as well.[173] Although infections with *A. vasorum* have been reported from South America (primarily Brazil, but also Argentina and Colombia),[174] molecular studies suggest that isolates from Europe and South America may be genetically distinct.[175]

There is no clear breed predisposition for angiostrongylosis. In the United Kingdom, purebred dogs, especially Cavalier King Charles spaniels, Staffordshire bull terriers, and beagles have been overrepresented.[172,176] Studies from other countries have shown no breed predisposition; in Newfoundland, Canada, hunting dogs were at greatest risk.[171,172] The median age of dogs in one case series was 10 months,[176] and in another survey of 160 dogs, over 50% of affected dogs were ≤ 1 year of age.[177] However, dogs from 3 months to 14 years of age have been affected. No breed predilection has been identified. In Canada, the majority of the cases are diagnosed from October to March with a similar winter-spring pattern (December to May) reported in Denmark.[176]

CLINICAL FEATURES

Adult nematodes live within the pulmonary arteries and right ventricle where they deposit undifferentiated eggs. The eggs lodge in capillaries in the lungs where they become larvated and hatch. The L_1 break through the pulmonary capillaries into the airways, are coughed up, swallowed, and passed in the feces. L_1 are ingested by the snail, slug, or frog intermediate host and mature into L_3 over about 10 to 16 days when conditions are optimal.[172] Domestic dogs acquire infection by ingesting intermediate or paratenic hosts; although the epidemiological significance remains unknown, infection may also be acquired by consumption of vegetation contaminated with L_3 released from gastropods in feces and mucus.[2,178] Frogs and chickens can act as paratenic hosts after ingestion of slugs or snails.[179] The L_3 are then released into the intestinal tract and migrate to the mesenteric lymph nodes, where they develop into L_4. L_4 migrate via the portal vasculature and liver to the lung by 9 to 10 days PI. The PPP is 38 to 57 days, but can range from 28 to 108 days (see Figure 117.13).[172]

Clinical signs of infection in domestic dogs can range from subclinical to life threatening, with varying organ involvement; the disease has been referred to as "the great pretender"[180] because of the varying manifestations of illness. Respiratory signs are the most common manifestations of infection. The granulomatous response to the developing eggs and movement of L_1 through the capillary wall into the alveolar airspace results in fibrosis which eventually can affect large areas of the lungs.[181] This in turn is responsible for signs of productive or non-productive cough, dyspnea, tachypnea, syncope, exercise intolerance, and sometimes ascites. Increased lung sounds and a right-sided heart murmur secondary to tricuspid regurgitation may be detected on thoracic auscultation. Dogs may develop a coagulopathy that results in hemorrhage. Hemorrhage may lead to anemia with evidence of mucosal pallor on physical examination. Signs of hemorrhage include scleral ecchymoses, hyphema, retinal hemorrhage, epistaxis, hemoptysis, melena, gingival bleeding, excessive post-surgical bleeding, subcutaneous hematomas, or thoracic or abdominal cavity hemorrhage. The pathogenesis of the coagulopathy is poorly understood, but chronic DIC has been suggested to play a role.[182–184] Neurologic signs in dogs with *A. vasorum* infection are usually secondary to CNS hemorrhage, and include seizures, ataxia, nystagmus, blindness, tremors, paralysis, and coma. Rarely CNS signs have been reported to occur as a result of aberrant migration of L_1.[167,185] The acute onset of neurological signs may be the only evidence of infection.[186] Other reported signs include vomiting, diarrhea, abdominal pain, lumbar pain, inappetence, and weight loss. Sudden death may occur secondary to abdominal, cerebral, or thoracic hemorrhage or the rupture of a major blood vessel due to worm migrations.[184,187] Aberrant migration of L_1 has also been identified to the skin, myocardium, kidney, spleen, adrenal gland, thyroid gland, diaphragm, and pancreas.[172,177]

Rarely, visualization of aberrant migrating larvae in the anterior chamber has been reported on ocular examination, sometimes with accompanying signs of blepharospasm, epiphora, uveitis, episcleral congestion, hyphema, and corneal edema.[188]

DIAGNOSIS

Laboratory Abnormalities

Complete Blood Count, Serum Chemistry Profile, and Urinalysis

Findings on bloodwork are non-specific and include non-regenerative or regenerative anemia, leukocytosis due to a neutrophilia, bandemia, lymphopenia, mild to moderate eosinophilia (up to 2800 cells/μL in one study) and/or mild basophilia, and mild to moderate thrombocytopenia. Findings on serum chemistry profile are variable and include hyperglobulinemia, hypercalcemia, azotemia, and increased activity of serum ALP. Hypercalcemia has been reported secondary to granulomatous inflammation.[185,189] Urinalysis is often unremarkable, but proteinuria has been reported.[190]

Clotting Function

In dogs with evidence of a coagulopathy secondary to *A. vasorum* infection, coagulation test results are variable. In one study of 30 affected dogs, 18 dogs had signs of bleeding on physical examination.[183] Of these 18 dogs, 17 had thromboelastography results consistent with hypocoagulation. A total of 22 of 25 dogs had increased D-dimer concentrations, and fibrinogen concentrations were significantly lower in dogs with evidence of hemorrhage compared with those that did not. Although coagulation times (PT and APTT) were abnormal in some dogs, these were not associated with clinically evident hemorrhage.

Cytologic Analysis of Body Fluids

Analysis of the CSF in dogs with neurological signs may show no abnormalities or a mixed pleocytosis, variable degrees of hemorrhage, and increased protein concentration. Eosinophilic pleocytosis and L_1 were reported in the CSF of a dog with CNS signs secondary to aberrant larval migration.[185]

Bronchoalveolar lavage specimens have increased cellularity with a predominance of neutrophils; eosinophils may also be present. In one study, L_1 were found in 7 of 10 specimens.[176]

Diagnostic Imaging

Plain Radiography

Findings on thoracic radiography include interstitial, bronchial, and/or alveolar lung patterns with a patchy, peripheral distribution; mild pleural effusion; pneumothorax; subcutaneous emphysema; and a widened cranial mediastinum. Right ventricular enlargement may be evident as well as truncated pulmonary arteries, but these findings are more common with dirofilariasis (see Chapter 111).[190]

Advanced Imaging

MRI of the brain and spinal cord of dogs with *A. vasorum* infection and neurological signs may reveal evidence of intramedullary and intraparenchymal hemorrhage, including ill-defined T1-isointense, T2-hyperintense lesions and areas of signal void that are consistent with infarction on T2-weighted image gradient echo sequences.[186,191] In cases where CNS signs have been secondary to aberrant larval migration, evidence of focal meningitis has been described, with meningeal thickening and hyperintensity in T2-weighted images.[185]

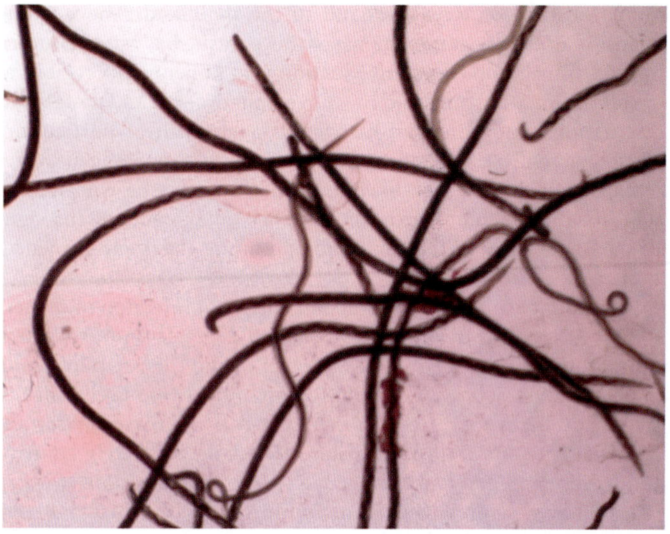

Fig. 117.14 Adult *Angiostrongylus vasorum* recovered from the pulmonary artery of a red fox from Newfoundland, Canada. Note the intestine filled with ingested blood entwined with the lighter-colored reproductive tract giving the worms a "barber's pole" appearance.

Sonographic Findings

Echocardiography can reveal evidence of pulmonary hypertension with concentric and eccentric right ventricular hypertrophy, right atrial dilation, tricuspid valve regurgitation, pulmonic valve insufficiency, and a bulging interatrial septum. In one dog, a ruptured chordae tendineae was evident as a systolic flail of the anterior leaflet of the tricuspid valve, which represented the first report of tricuspid valve chordae tendineae rupture in any dog.[192] Abdominal ultrasonography may reveal ascites and distended hepatic veins in dogs with right-sided congestive heart failure.

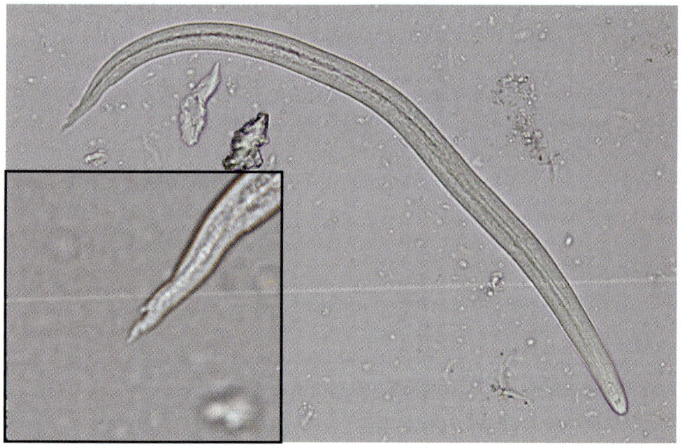

Fig. 117.15 First-stage larva (L_1) of *Angiostrongylus vasorum* recovered from the feces of a dog using the Baermann technique. Note the cephalic button and the kinked tail with a dorsal spine (see insert of tail).

Parasitological Tests

Adult worms may be identified at necropsy. They are approximately one-tenth the size of adult *D. immitis*; males are 14 to 18 mm long, with visible bursa, bursal rays, and spicules and females are 18 to 25 mm long and have the "barber's pole" appearance that has been described for *Haemonchus* spp. (Fig. 117.14).[172] L_1, the form shed in the feces, can be detected using the Baermann technique on feces and respiratory lavage specimens and are occasionally detected in the CSF or eye. They are 340 to 399 μm long, have an anterior cephalic button, and their tail ends with a marked kink with a dorsal spine (Fig. 117.15). In contrast, *Crenosoma vulpis* larvae have a straight tail and *Oslerus* spp. and *Filaroides* spp. larvae have a kinked tail but lack the dorsal spine. Because the larvae are highly motile, accurate identification requires the immobilization of the L_1 in order to examine them in detail. This can be achieved by the application of a drop of diluted Lugol's iodine (1:10) to the edge of the coverslip. Zinc sulfate fecal flotation may also reveal larvae, but is only 60% sensitive compared with the Baermann technique. Because the Baermann technique is time-consuming, a direct smear, which may detect L_1 in about half of the infections, can be used in order to rapidly assess for larvae initially. If the direct smear is negative, a Baermann examination should be done. Regardless of the method used, false-negative results can occur as a result of intermittent excretion of larvae in the feces. Examination of multiple (at least three) fecal specimens collected over a 7- to 10-day period or daily for 3 consecutive days can increase sensitivity. With the availability of tests for circulating antigen and PCR assays, which can be used in combination with fecal examination, the requirement for serial fecal examinations may be reduced.

Serologic Diagnosis

Sensitive and specific ELISA assays have been developed for detection of circulating antigens and antibodies to *A. vasorum* and can detect infection before 7 weeks PI, the period of patency. These assays have been made available by some university diagnostic laboratories. A rapid (15-minute) POC antigen-detection assay is also available in Europe (Angio Detect, IDEXX Laboratories). When applied to 214 dogs with suspected or confirmed disease, the sensitivity of this assay compared with the Baermann assay was 97.1% and specificity was 98.9%; there was no evidence of cross-reactivity with other common nematode parasites, including *Dirofilaria immitis*.[193] However, in one study of experimentally inoculated dogs, the Baermann assay became positive at 8 weeks, laboratory ELISA antigen assay at 11 weeks, and the POC assay at 14 weeks after inoculation, so the sensitivity of the POC assay may be low early in the course of infection.[194] Antibody testing has the potential to be positive with subclinical infection or in recovered dogs, so may lack predictive value.

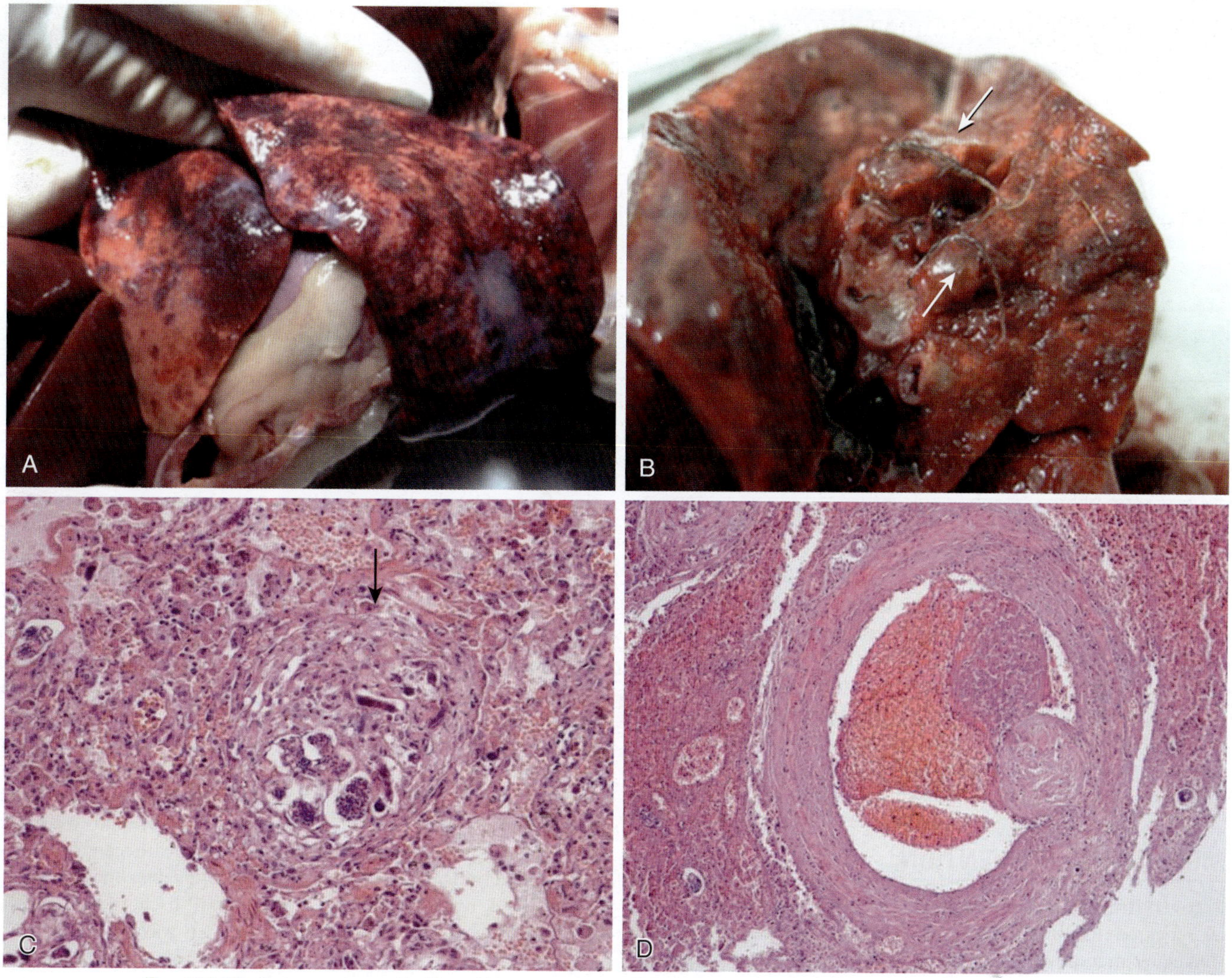

Fig. 117.16 Gross necropsy (A, B) and histopathologic (C, D) findings in a dog with *Angiostrongylus vasorum* infection. Findings at necropsy include mottled and congested lungs, multifocal pleural fibrosis, evidence of systemic petechial or ecchymotic hemorrhages, and adult worms in the pulmonary arteries. Histopathology of the lungs in dogs infected with *A. vasorum* reveals multifocal granuloma (C) that is accompanied by hemorrhage and arterial thrombosis (D). (A and B, from Di Cesare et al. Elusive *Angiostrongylus vasorum* infections. *Parasites Vectors.* 2015;8:438. C and D, from Rinaldi L, Cortese L, Meomartino L, et al. *Angiostrongylus vasorum:* epidemiological, clinical and histopathological insights. *BMC Vet Res.* 2014;10:236.)

The POC assay has been used to look for evidence of other angiostrongylid infections in domestic cats in Europe that were either positive or negative (50 cats each) for metastrongyloid nematodes on Baermann examination, none of which were positive. Cross-reactivity occurs with antigens of *Gurltia paralysans*, a related metastrongyloid nematode found in domestic and wild felids in South America.[195] *Gurltia paralysans* has a tropism for veins of the subarachnoid space, and causes chronic eosinophilic meningomyelitis and progressive paraparesis in cats (gurltiosis).

The POC assay has also been used to monitor resolution of infection with treatment,[196] but can also remain positive up to 7 weeks after treatment, possibly due to slow elimination of antigens from dying worms.[194]

Molecular Diagnosis Using Nucleic Acid–Based Testing

Nucleic acid–based assays have been developed to detect *A. vasorum* DNA. These have been used to identify the parasite in gastropod intermediate hosts, as well as to detect infection in respiratory lavage specimens. In one study, use of a real-time PCR assay for *A. vasorum* on bronchoalveolar lavage specimens was more sensitive than Baermann analysis or detection of circulating antigen using the IDEXX POC assay.[197]

Pathologic Findings

Gross findings at necropsy include mottled and congested lungs, multifocal pleural fibrosis, evidence of systemic petechial or ecchymotic hemorrhages, and adult worms in the pulmonary arteries (Fig. 117.16A and B). Histopathology of the lungs in dogs infected with *A. vasorum* reveals multifocal granulomas in the periphery of the lungs that is accompanied by hemorrhage, arterial thrombosis, periarteritis, and with chronicity, fibrosis (Fig. 117.16C and D). Detection of undifferentiated metastrongyloid eggs together with L_1 in histologic sections of the lungs is considered pathognomonic for *A. vasorum* infection in the dog.

TABLE 117.1 **Differential Features of Eggs of *Trichuris vulpis, Eucoleus aerophilus,* and *Eucoleus boehmi***

Nematode Species	Length (μm)	Width (μm)	Morphological Features	Plugs	Shell
Trichuris vulpis	72–94	31–42	Lemon-shaped, brownish	Symmetrical presence of rings	Thick, smooth wall
Eucoleus aerophilus	60–65	25–40	Barrel-shaped, zygote fills egg	Asymmetrical, no rings	Striated outer shell with a network of anastomosing ridges and bridges
Eucoleus boehmi	50–60	30–35	Barrel-shaped, clear to gold, space between the embryo and wall	Asymmetrical, no rings	Tiny pits on wall surface

Modified from Di Cesare A, Castagna G, Meloni S, et al. Mixed trichuroid infestation in a dog from Italy. *Parasit Vectors.* 2012;5:128.

TREATMENT AND PROGNOSIS

Treatment of *A. vasorum* infections has most often involved the use of fenbendazole (20–50 mg/kg PO for 5 to 21 days or 20–25 mg/kg PO for 20 days), topical moxidectin/imidocloprid (minimum 2.5 mg/kg moxidectin and up to 6.25 mg/kg; minimum 10 mg/kg imidacloprid and up to 25 mg/kg; one or two monthly treatments), or milbemycin oxime (0.5 mg/kg PO once weekly for 4 weeks).[190] Use of the latter two protocols represents licensed use in Europe. In addition, supportive care measures are often needed depending on clinical signs present, such as intravenous fluids, blood products, supplemental oxygen, anticonvulsants, treatment for congestive heart failure (diuretics, angiotensin-converting enzyme inhibitors), and sildenafil.

IMMUNITY AND PREVENTION

On recovery from infection, dogs are not immune and can experience repeated infections. Repeated infection also has been documented experimentally.[190] No vaccine is available. Prevention relies on minimizing access to slugs and snails as well as regular treatment with prophylactic anthelmintics. Licensed prophylactic treatments in Europe are topical moxidectin/ivermectin or oral milbemycin oxime in combination products. A single dose of a moxidectin (24 μg/kg) in combination with sarolaner (1.2 mg/kg) and pyrantel (5 mg/kg) (Simparica Trio, Zoetis) had a 95% efficacy in prevention of development of immature adults in dogs experimentally infected with *A. vasorum*; doses of 3 mg/kg and 12 mg/kg had efficacies of 7.2% and 54.5%, respectively.[198] Milbemycin oxime (0.75 to 1.0 mg/kg, PO) in combination with spinosad had an efficacy of 98.8% when administered 30 days after exposure to *A. vasorum*.[199]

PUBLIC HEALTH ASPECTS

Angiostrongylus vasorum does not infect humans.

NON-METASTRONGYLOID NEMATODE INFECTIONS OF THE RESPIRATORY TRACT

EUCOLEUS AEROPHILUS AND *EUCOLEUS BOEHMI* INFECTION (EUCOLEOSIS/CAPILLARIASIS)

Eucoleus aerophilus and *Eucoleus boehmi* (previously *Capillaria* spp.; the species name *Capillaria aerophila* was revised to *Eucoleus aerophilus*) are trichuroid nematodes with a worldwide distribution that infect the lower and upper respiratory tract, respectively. Infection with *E. aerophilus* occurs in dogs, cats, and various wild animals; *E. boehmi* infection only occurs in dogs and wild canids. Adult worms are embedded in the mucosal epithelium—*E. aerophilus* in the trachea, bronchi, and bronchioles; and *E. boehmi* in the turbinates of the nasal cavity. The life cycle of both nematode species is incompletely described although earthworms have been proposed as a possible intermediate host for *E. boehmi*.[200] Adults mate and produce bipolar-plugged eggs that are coughed up, swallowed, and passed unembryonated in the feces. Most infections appear to be subclinical, but animals infected with *E. aerophilus* may show episodes of non-productive cough, gagging, retching, tachypnea, and dyspnea. Secondary bacterial infections may lead to bronchopneumonia and a productive cough, and death can result from heavy infections.[201] Dogs infected with *E. boehmi* may show signs of sneezing, reverse sneezing, and/or nasal discharge. In addition, aberrant migration of *E. boehmi* to the CNS was reported in a dog from Texas that was evaluated for seizures and a possible meningioma based on findings on MRI.[202]

Thoracic radiographs in dogs and cats infected with *E. aerophilus* may show tracheal narrowing and mixed pulmonary patterns if secondary bacterial infection occurs. The nematodes can be visualized and retrieved for identification of adults and eggs using tracheobronchoscopy (*E. aerophilus*) or rhinoscopy (*E. boehmi*). Identification of eggs on centrifugal fecal flotation can also be used for diagnosis.[3,203] The eggs have bipolar plugs, similar to those of whipworms. Because the eggs of these nematodes may be misidentified as *Trichuris* spp., the true prevalence of *Eucoleus* spp. infections in dogs may be underestimated. Capillarid eggs can be differentiated from those of *Trichuris* spp. based on their morphologic appearance (Table 117.1). The eggs of *T. vulpis* are larger (72–90 × 32–40 μm) with a smooth shell wall surface, the plugs are symmetrical on the longitudinal midline (in most eggs), and the plugs have a series of "threaded" lines making them appear as if they were "screwed" into the shell wall (Fig. 117.17A). In contrast, capillarid (*Eucoleus* spp.) eggs are smaller, the plugs are asymmetrical on the longitudinal midline (in most eggs), the plugs lack "threaded" lines, and there is a surface shell wall pattern unique to each species (Fig. 117.17B). Eggs of *E. aerophilus* are 58–79 × 29–40 μm in size and the shell wall surface has a net-like pattern of interconnected ridges (Fig. 117.18A and B). Eggs of *E. boehmi* are 54–60 × 30–35 μm in size and the shell wall surface is covered with small pits (Fig. 117.18C and D).[3,4] In addition, a PCR assay that detects the mitochondrial *cox1* gene of

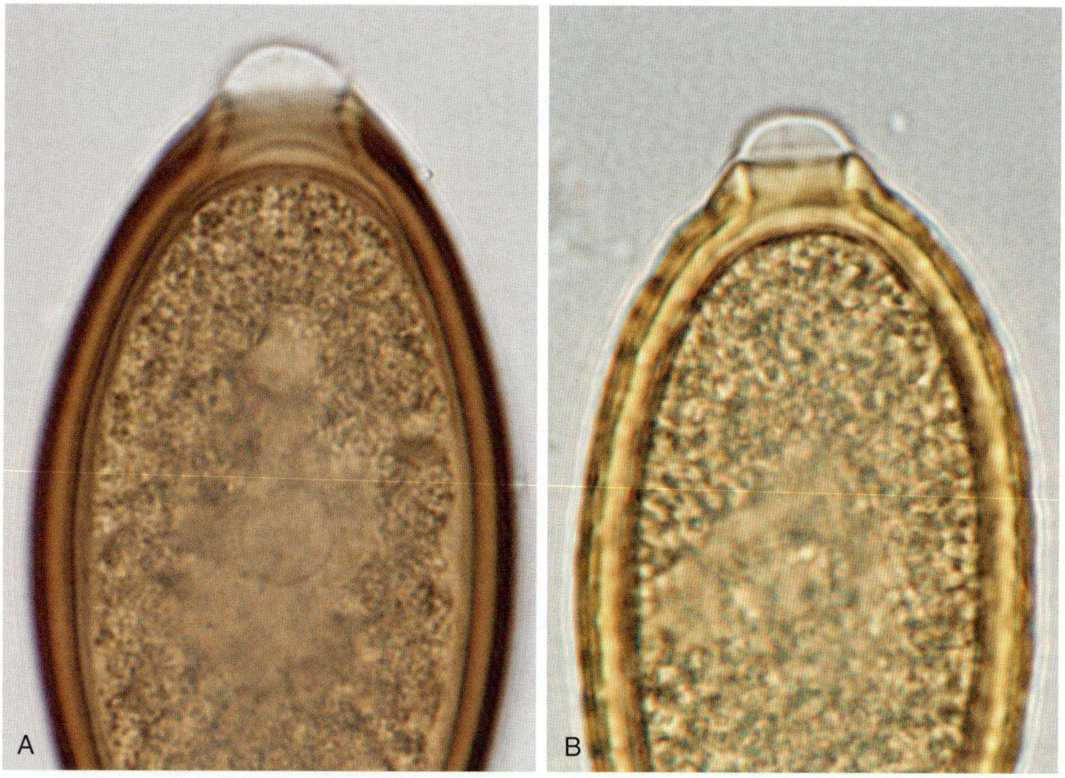

Fig. 117.17 Comparison of the morphology of trichuroid (*Trichuris* spp.) and capillarid (*Eucoleus* spp.) bipolar plugs. (A) Plug of a *Trichuris vulpis* egg from the feces of a dog. Note the "threaded lines" giving the appearance as if the plug has been "screwed" into the shell wall. (B) Plug of a *Eucoleus aerophilus* egg from the feces of a dog. Capillarid egg plugs of *Eucoleus* spp. lack the threaded lines.

nematodes in the subfamily Capillariinae has been used to identify *Eucoleus* spp. in stool specimens and differentiate them from *T. vulpis*.[203]

There are currently no anthelmintics approved for use in the treatment of dogs and cats infected with *E. aerophilus* or dogs infected with *E. boehmi*. Eprinomectin, fenbendazole, and moxidectin have been used to successfully treat cats infected with *E. aerophilus*. A single topical application of eprinomectin (0.5 mg/kg) in combination with fipronil, (S)-methoprene, and praziquantel had an efficacy of 82.4% in cats naturally infected with *E. aerophilus*. In a case report involving a single animal, fenbendazole (50 mg/kg, PO, q24h for 14 days) was reported as an effective treatment in a cat; clinical signs resolved after treatment; however, a second 14-day course was required due to a return of egg excretion.[204] Efficacies (based on fecal egg counts) of 99.8 to 100% were reported with topical moxidectin (1.0 mg/kg) combined with imidicloprid in cats infected with *E. aerophilus*.[205,206] Fenbendazole and milbemycin oxime have been used to successfully treat dogs infected with *E. aerophilus*. Treatment with fenbendazole (50 mg/kg, PO, q24h for 14 days) resulted in a clinical cure and the cessation of fecal egg shedding in a dog with Addison's disease also infected with *E. aerophilus*.[207] Negative fecal examination results occurred after the first treatment of eight dogs infected with *E. aerophilus* in a 6-month field study on monthly use of milbemycin oxime (0.5–1.0 mg/kg) combined with afoxolaner.[208] Fenbendazole, ivermectin, and moxidectin have been used successfully to treat dogs infected with *E. boehmi*. Fenbendazole at several dosages (50 mg/kg, PO, q24h for 14 days or 110 mg/kg q12h for 14 days), ivermectin (0.2 mg/kg, PO, once), and milbemycin oxime (2 mg/kg, PO, once) have been reported to be effective in the treatment of dogs infected with *E. boehmi*.[202,209–211] In several field studies using topical moxidectin (2.5–6.25 mg/kg) in combination with imidacloprid to treat dogs naturally infected with *E. boehmi*, reported efficacies based on fecal egg counts were 99 to 99.7% with a single application and 100% after two applications.[203] A short course of glucocorticoids may be indicated for animals with severe respiratory difficulty to reduce tracheitis or bronchitis (e.g., prednisolone sodium succinate, dexamethasone sodium phosphate). There have been several reports of treatment failures with multiple anthelmintics (fenbendazole, milbemycin oxime, and moxidectin) in dogs infected with *E. aerophilus* and *E. boehmi*.[212,213] Whether failure to respond adequately to treatment reflects reinfection from the environment or is due to some other factor remains unknown. In some cases, further treatments are required, as well as efforts to clean the environment and limit coprophagy by dogs. Post-treatment fecal surveillance to monitor anthelmintic effectiveness is extremely important in the management of cases of capillarid infections in both dogs and cats. Rare (< 20) cases of human infection by *E. aerophilus* have been reported in the literature.[214]

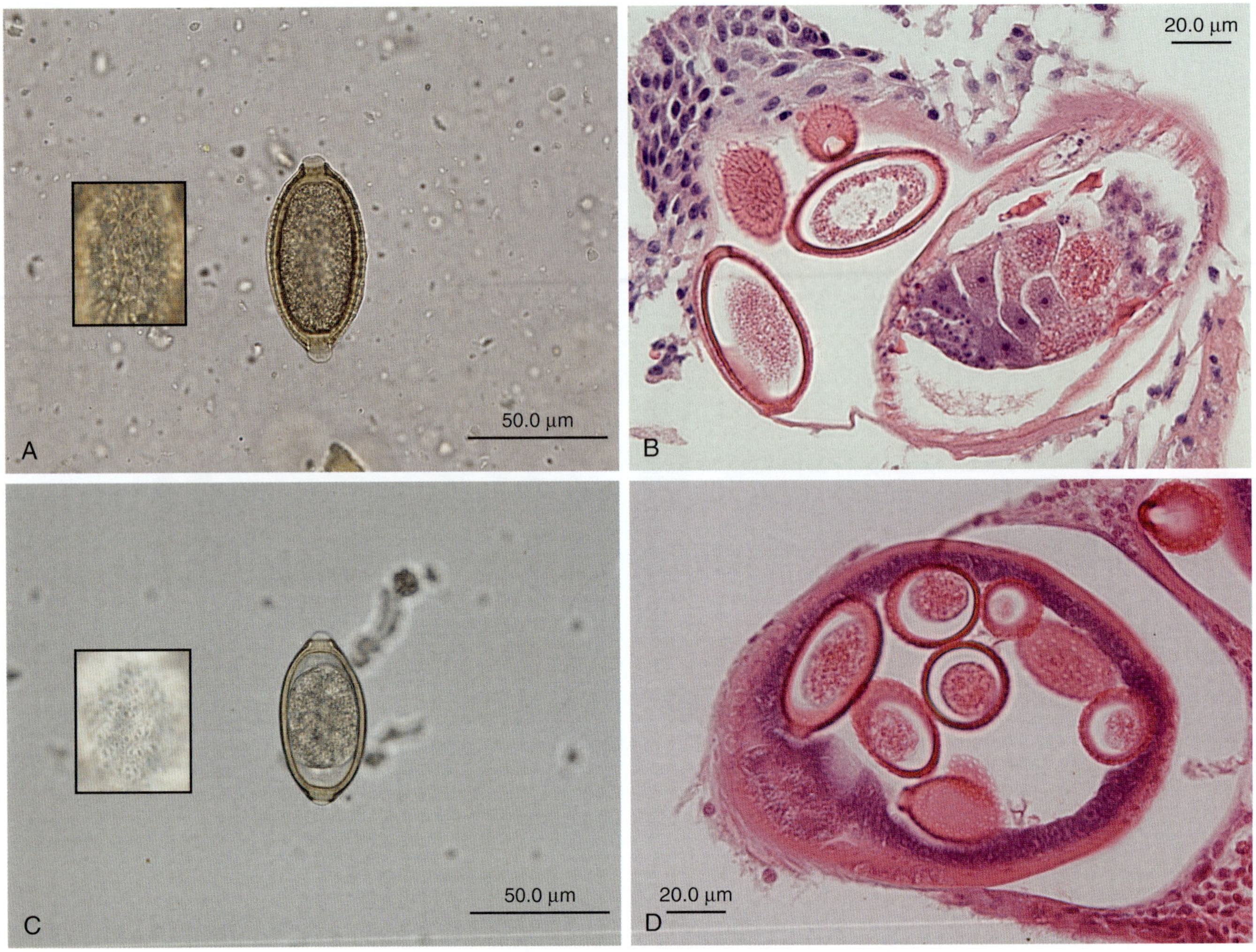

Fig. 117.18 Comparative features of *Eucoleus aerophilus* and *Eucoleus boehmi* eggs. (A) *Eucoleus aerophilus* egg recovered from the feces of a cat. Inserted is a high-magnification view of the shell wall surface showing the net-like pattern of interconnecting ridges. (B) Histologic section of an adult female *E. aerophilus* in the bronchi of a red fox. Plugs and the net-like ridges on the surface are visible in several of the eggs. Hematoxylin and eosin stain. (C) *Eucoleus boehmi* egg recovered from the feces of a dog. Inserted is a high-magnification view of the shell wall showing the small pits on the surface. (D) Histologic section of an adult female *E. boehmi* in the nasal turbinates of a red fox. Plugs and the pitted shell wall surface are visible in several of the eggs. Hematoxylin and eosin stain.

CASE EXAMPLE

Signalment

"Sass," a 1-year-old intact female toy poodle from West Sacramento in northern California.

History

Sass was evaluated at the University of California-Davis VMTH for a 6-month history of chronic intermittent cough and gagging that began 1 month after she was acquired. Episodes of clinical signs were sometimes associated with inappetence and lethargy and persisted for several weeks at a time; at least 8 episodes were reported. The cough was not associated with eating, drinking, or exercise. Diagnostics performed at several other veterinary clinics over the course of illness included thoracic and abdominal radiographs, CBC, chemistry profile, pancreatic lipase immunoreactivity, and a direct fecal smear and flotation, all of which had been negative. Sass had also been treated with clavulanic acid-amoxicillin and doxycycline with mild clinical improvement.

Current Medications

None

Other Medical History

There was no other known medical history. Sass was an indoor/outdoor dog and was current on routine vaccinations. The owner reported feeding a homemade chicken- and rice-based diet with some potato and dry dog food added.

Physical Examination

Body weight: 2.5 kg

Sass was quiet, alert, and responsive; had pale pink mucous membranes, HR 140 beats/min, RR 30 breaths/min, T = 102°F, and BCS 5/9. A cough was easily elicited on tracheal palpation. No other clinically significant abnormalities were identified on physical examination.

Centrifugal zinc sulfate fecal flotation and Baermann examination: Negative for parasites.

CASE EXAMPLE—cont'd

Imaging Findings

Tracheal fluoroscopy: There was no evidence of tracheal collapse when a cough was elicited. However, dynamic narrowing of the mainstem bronchi was noted that was suggestive of bronchiectasis.

Bronchoscopy: Four soft-tissue nodules were identified at the level of the carina (see Fig. 117.11). The remainder of the respiratory tract was within normal limits.

Cytology Findings

Bronchoalveolar lavage: Total nucleated cell count 1940 cells/μL with 9% neutrophils, 4% lymphocytes, 16% macrophages, 65% eosinophils, and 6% mast cells. The cytofuge specimen was highly cellular with moderate accumulations of mucinous material in a clear background. Large numbers of eosinophils were admixed with macrophages, some of which contained foamy cytoplasmic vacuoles.

Impression smear of nodule biopsy: There were numerous parasite larvae either free or within eggs in a moderately cellular background.

Histopathology of Nodule Biopsy (see Fig. 117.12B)

Sections are composed of nodules of extensively inflamed fibrous connective tissue that contains numerous tangential and cross sections of nematode parasites. The nodules are variably covered by a pseudostratified columnar ciliated-to-low cuboidal epithelium. The nematodes have a pseudocoelomic body cavity and an intestine. Consistent with metastrongyloids, the cuticle is smooth, the intestine is composed of a few multinucleate cells with short microvilli, and the uterus of female worms contain developing L_1. There are a few free larvae within the inflammatory nodules. Many of the nematodes are surrounded by a dense fibrous capsule. Inflammatory cells include numerous lymphocytes, plasma cells, and histiocytes that extensively expand the submucosal fibrovascular connective tissue separating collagen bundles.

Diagnosis

Oslerus osleri infection.

Treatment

Fenbendazole, 50 mg/kg PO q12h for 14 days and butorphanol (0.05 mg/kg PO up to q8h) for cough. Larvae were not detected on zinc sulfate centrifugal flotation and simple sedimentation fecal examinations performed 2 weeks later and the dog had improved clinically. The owner was informed that a second bronchoscopy to re-evaluate the nodules was advisable and additional treatment may be required. However, 2 days later she was brought to the emergency room when her owners found her vomiting and obtunded in their back yard. She was found to be in hypovolemic shock and was diagnosed with hemoabdomen. The owners elected euthanasia based on the guarded prognosis and financial concerns.

Comments

This dog was diagnosed with *O. osleri* infection based on the presence of nodules that contained parasitic larvae that had morphology supportive of that diagnosis. Larvae were not detected in the feces both before and after treatment by any of the methods employed (Baermann, flotation, sedimentation). Baermann examination has poor detection sensitivity due to the moribund state of *O. osleri* L_1 excreted in the feces; the primary use of the Baermann test in this case was to screen for possible infection with *A. vasorum* or *C. vulpis*. Although zinc sulfate centrifugal flotation has greater detection sensitivity than the Baermann examination, it also has a low sensitivity. The most reliable fecal examination method for detecting *O. osleri* L_1 is fecal sedimentation. Due to the considerable time and effort necessary to perform the fecal sedimentation test, it is useful to attempt to detect the larvae first by zinc sulfate centrifugal flotation. Larvae were also not detected by fecal sedimentation and this was likely due to the erratic shedding pattern typical of metastrongyloids. Had the *O. osleri* infection diagnosis not been made by the detection of nodules and larvae on bronchoscopy, further fecal specimens would have been requested before ruling out lungworm infection. The cause of the hemoabdomen was unknown, but the dog was reported to roam freely outdoors and had access to rodenticide, so anticoagulant rodenticide toxicity was considered most likely in light of the signalment and history.

SUGGESTED READINGS

1. Crisi PE, Johnson LR, Di Cesare A, et al. Evaluation of bronchoscopy and bronchoalveolar lavage findings in cats with *Aelurostrongylus abstrusus* in comparison to cats with feline bronchial disease. *Front Vet Sci.* 2019;6:337.
2. Helm JR, Morgan ER, Jackson MW, et al. Canine angiostrongylosis: an emerging disease in Europe. *J Vet Emerg Crit Care (San Antonio).* 2010;20:98–109.

REFERENCES

1. Anderson RC. *Nematode Parasites of Vertebrates: Their Development and Transmission.* 2nd ed. Wallingford, UK: CAB Publishing; 2000:151–191.
2. Conboy G, Guselle N, Schaper R. Spontaneous shedding of metastrongyloid third-stage larvae by experimentally infected *Limax maximus. Parasitol Res.* 2017;116:S41–S54.
3. Conboy G. Helminth parasites of the canine and feline respiratory tracts. *Vet Clin North Am Small Anim.* 2009;39:1109–1126.
4. Zajac AM, Conboy GA., Little SE, Reiuchard MV. Fecal examination for the diagnosis of parasitism. In: *Veterinary Clinical Parasitology.* 9th ed. Ames, IA: Wiley-Blackwell; 2021:1–95.
5. Hobmaier M, Hobmaier A. Mammalian phase of the lungworm *Aelurostrongylus abstrusus* in the cat. *J Am Vet Med Assoc.* 1935;87:191–198.
6. Anderson RC. No. 5 Keys to genera of the superfamily Metastrongyloidea. In: Anderson RC, Chabaud AG, Willmott S, eds. *CIH Keys to the Nematode Parasites of Verterbrates* UK: CAB; 1978:1–40.
7. Bowmann DD, Hendrix CM, Lindsay DS, et al. Metastrongyloidea. In: *Feline Clinical Parasitology.* Ames: Iowa State University Press; 2002:267–271.
8. Di Cesare A, Laiacona F, Iorio R, et al. *Aelrostrongylus abstrusus* in wild felids of South Africa. *Parasitol Res.* 2016;115:3731–3735.
9. Patton S, Rabinowitz AR. Parasites of wild felidae in Thailand: a coprological survey. *J Wildl Dis.* 1994;30:472–475.
10. Lillis WG. Helminth survey of dogs and cats in New Jersey. *J Parasitol.* 1967;53:1082–1084.
11. Nolan T, Smith G. Time series analysis of the prevalence of endoparasitic infections in cats and dogs presented to a veterinary teaching hospital. *Vet Parasitol.* 1995;59:87–96.
12. Rembiesa C, Richardson DJ. Helminth parasites of the house cat, *Felis catus*, in Connecticut, USA. *Comp Parasitol.* 2003;70:115–119.
13. Becklund WW. Revised checklist of internal and external parasites of domestic animals in the United States and possessions and in Canada. *Am J Vet Res.* 1964;25:1380–1416.
14. Scott DW. Current knowledge of aelurostrongylosis in the cat. *Cornell Vet.* 1973;63:483–500.
15. Kennedy MJ. Superfamily Metastrongyloidea. In: *Synopsis of the Parasites of Domesticated Mammals of Canada.* Edmonton: Alberta Agriculture Animal Health; 1986:17.
16. Barutzki D, Schaper R. Occurrence and regional distribution of *Aelurostrongylus abstrusus* in cats in Germany. *Parasitol Res.* 2013;112:855–861.
17. Beugenet F, Bourdeau P, Chalvet-Monfray K, et al. Parasites of domestic owned cats in Europe: co-infestations and risk factors. *Parasites Vectors.* 2014;7:291.
18. Burgu A, Sarimehmetoglu O. *Aelurostrongylus abstrusus* infection in two cats. *Vet Rec.* 2004;154:602–604.
19. Coman BJ, Jones EH, Driesen MA. Helminth parasites and arthropods of feral cats. *Aust Vet J.* 1981;57:324–327.

20. Diakou A, Di Cesare A, Barros LA, et al. Occurrence of *Aelurostrongylus abstrusus* and *Troglostrongylus brevior* in domestic cats in Greece. *Parasites Vectors.* 2015;8:590.
21. Dubey JP, Bevereley JKA, Crane WAJ. Lung changes and *Aelurostrongylus abstrusus* infestation in English cats. *Vet Rec.* 1968;83:191–194.
22. Gathumbi PK, Waruiru RM, Buoro I. A case of feline *Aelurostrongylus abstrusus* infection in Kenya. *Bull Anim Hlth Prod Africa.* 1991;39:361–363.
23. Gavrilovic P, Jovanovic M. Fatal aelurostrongylosis in a kitten in Serbia. *Acta Parasitol.* 2017;62:488–491.
24. Gerichter CB. Studies on the nematodes parasitic in the lungs of felidae in Palestine. *Parasitol.* 1949;39:251–262.
25. Headley SA. *Aelurostrongylus abstrusus* induced pneumonia and epidemiological findings of 38 cases (1987–1996). *Semina Ciencias Agrarias Londrina.* 2005;26:373–380.
26. Kamenov Y, Radev V, Zlateva N. On diagnosis and clinic of angiostrongylosis of cats. *Exp Path Parasitol.* 1999;2:51–54.
27. Mircean V, Titlincu A, Vasile C. Prevalence of endoparasites in household cat (*Felis catus*) populations from Transylvania (Romania) and associated risk factors. *Vet Parasitol.* 2010;171:163–166.
28. Taubert A, Pantchev N, Vrhovec MG, et al. Lungworm infections (*Angiostrongylus vasorum, Crenosoma vulpis, Aelurostrongylus abstrsus*) in dogs and cats in Germany and Denmark in 2003-2007. *Vet Parasitol.* 2009;159:175–180.
29. Thiengo SC, Fernandez MA, Torres JL, et al. First record of a nematode Metastrongyloidea (*Aelurostrongylus abstrusus* larvae) in *Achatina (Lissachatina) fulica* (Mollusca, Achatinidae) in Brazil. *J Invert Path.* 2008;98:34–39.
30. Traversa D, Di Cesare A, Conboy G. Canine and feline cardiopulmonary parasitic nematodes in Europe: emerging and underestimated. *Parasit Vectors.* 2010;3:62.
31. Elsheikha HM, Schnyder M, Traversa D, et al. Updates on feline aleurostrongylosis and research priorities for the next decade. *Parasit Vectors.* 2016;9:389.
32. Lucio-Forster A, Bowman DD. Prevalence of fecal-borne parasites detected by centrifugal flotation in feline samples from two shelters in upstate New York. *J Feline Med Surg.* 2011;13:300–303.
33. Willard MD, Roberts RE, Allison N, et al. Diagnosis of *Aelurostrongylus abstrusus* and *Dirofilaria immitis* infections in cats from a humane shelter. *J Am Vet Med Assoc.* 1988;192:913–916.
34. Iorio R, Traversa D. New epidemiological and molecular insights into feline lungworm infection. *Ann NY Acad Sci.* 2008;1149:174–176.
35. Traversa D, Lia RP, Iorio R, et al. Diagnosis and risk factors of *Aelurostrongylus abstrusus* (Nematoda, Strongylida) infection in cats from Italy. *Vet Parasitol.* 2008;153:182–186.
36. Genchi M, Ferrari N, Fonti P, et al. Relation between *Aelurostrongylus abstrusus* larvae excretion, respiratory and radiographic signs in naturally infected cats. *Vet Parasitol.* 2014;206:182–187.
37. Hamilton JM. *Aelurostrongylus abstrusus* infestation of cat. *Vet Rec.* 1963;75:417–422.
38. Losonsky JM, Smith FG, Lewis RE. Radiographic findings of *Aelurostrongylus abstrusus* infection in cats. *J Am Anim Hosp Assoc.* 1978;14:348–355.
39. Hamilton JM. Studies on re-infestation of the cat with *Aelurostrongylus abstrusus. J Comp Path.* 1968;78:69–72.
40. Ribeiro VM, Lima WS. Larval production in cats infected and re-infected with *Aelurostrongylus abstrusus* (Nematoda: Protostrongylidae). *Rev de Med Vet.* 2001;152:815–829.
41. Hamilton JM. The number of *Aelurostrongylus abstrusus* larvae required to produce pulmonary disease in the cat. *J Comp Path.* 1967;77:343–346.
42. Gerdin JA, Slater MR, Makolinski KV, et al. Post-mortem findings in 54 cases of anesthetic associated death in cats from two spay-neuter programs in New York State. *J Feline Med Surg.* 2011;13:959–966.
43. Barrs VR, Swinney GR, Martin P, et al. Concurrent *Aelurostrongylus abstrusus* infection and salmonellosis in a kitten. *Austral Vet J.* 1999;77:229–232.
44. Ellis AE, Brown CA, Yabsley MJ. *Aelurostrongylus abstrusus* larvae in the colon of two cats. *J Vet Diagn Invest.* 2010;22:652–655.
45. Philbey AW, Krause S, Jefferies R. Verminous pneumonia and enteritis due to hyperinfection with *Aelurostrongylus abstrusus* in a kitten. *J Comp Path.* 2014;150:357–360.
46. Hansen AP, Skarbye LK, Vinther LM, et al. Occurrence and clinical significance of *Aelurostrongylus abstrusus* and other endoparasites in Danish cats. *Vet Parasitol.* 2017;234:31–39.
47. Center SA, Randolph JF, Erb HN, Reiter S. Eosinophilia in the cat: a retrospective study of 312 cases (1975 to 1986). *J Amer Anim Hosp Assoc.* 1990;26:349–358.
48. Mahaffrey MB. Radiographic-pathologic findings in experimental *Aelurostrongylus abstrusus* infection in cats. *J Am Vet Rad Soc.* 1979;20:81.
49. Lacava G, Zini E, Marchesotti F, et al. Computed tomography, radiology and echocardiography in cats naturally infected with. *Aelurostrongylus abstrusus. J Fel Med Surg.* 2017;19:446–453.
50. Dennler M, Bass DA, Gutierrez-Crespo B, et al. Thoracic computed tomography, angiographic computed tomography, and pathology findings in six cats experimentally infected with *Aelurostrongylus abstrusus. Vet Radiol Ultrasound.* 2013;54:459–469.
51. Payo-Puente P, Diez A, Gonzalo-Orden, et al. Computed tomography in cats infected by *Aelurostrongylus abstrusus*: 2 clinic cases. *Intern J Appl Res Vet Med.* 2005;3:339–343.
52. Crisi PE, Johnson LR, Di Cesare A, et al. Evaluation of bronchoscopy and bronchoalveolar lavage findings in cats with *Aelurostrongylus abstrusus* in comparison to cats with feline bronchial disease. *Front Vet Sci.* 2019;6:337.
53. Traversa D, Di Cesare A, Milillo P, et al. *Aelurostrongylus abstrusus* in a feline colony from central Italy: clinical features, diagnostic procedures and molecular characterization. *Parasitol Res.* 2008;103:1191–1196.
54. Traversa D, Guglielmini C. Feline aelurostrongylosis and canine angiostrongylosis: a challenging diagnosis for two emerging verminous pneumonia infections. *Vet Parasitol.* 2008;157:163–174.
55. Traversa D, Ioria R, Otranto D. Diagnostic and clinical implications of a nested PCR specific for ribosomal DNA of the feline lungworm *Aelurostrongylus abstrusus* (Nematoda, Strongylida). *J Clin Microbiol.* 2008;46:1811–1817.
56. Di Cesare A, Morelli S, Colombo M, et al. Is angiostrongylosis a realistic threat for domestic cats? *Frontiers Vet Sci.* 2020;7:195.
57. Traversa D, Milillo P, Di Cesare A, et al. Efficacy and safety of emodepside 2.1%/praziquantel 8.6% spot-on formulation in the treatment of feline aelurostrongylosis. *Parasitol Res.* 2009;105:S83–S89.
58. Crisi PE, Di Cesare A, Traversa D, et al. Controlled field study evaluating the clinical efficacy of a topical formulation containing emodepside and praziquantel in the treatment of natural cat aelurostrongylosis. *Vet Rec.* 2020;187:e34.
59. Bohm C, Wolken S, Schynder M, et al. Efficacy of emodepside/praziquantel spot-on (Profender) against adult *Aelurostrongylus abstrusus* in experimentally infected cats. *Parasitol Res.* 2015;114(Suppl 1):S155–S164.
60. Gianelli A, Brianti E, Varcasia A, et al. Efficacy of Broadline spot-on against *Aelurostrongylus abstrusus* and *Troglostrongylus brevior* lungworms in naturally infected cats in Italy. *Vet Parasitol.* 2015;209:273–277.
61. Knaus M, Chester ST, Rosentel J, et al. Efficacy of a novel topical combination of fipronil, (S)-methoprene, eprinomectin and praziquantel against larval and adult stages of the cat lungworm, *Aelurostrongylus abstrusus. Vet Parasitol.* 2014;202:64–68.
62. Roberson EL, Burke TM. Evaluation of granulated fenbendazole (22.2%) against induced and naturally occurring helminth infections in cats. *Am J Vet Res.* 1980;41:1499–1502.
63. Grandi G, Calvi LE, Venco L, et al. *Aelurostrongylus abstrusus* (cat lungworm) infection in five cats from Italy. *Vet Parasitol.* 2005;134:177–182.
64. Hamilton JM, Weatherley A, Chapman AJ. Treatment of lungworm disease in the cat with fenbendazole. *Vet Rec.* 1984;114:40–41.
65. Miller BH, Roudebush P, Ward HG. Pleural effusion as a sequela to aelurostrongylosis in a cat. *J Am Vet Med Assoc.* 1984;185:556–557.
66. Traversa D, Di Cesare A, Milillo P, et al. Efficacy and safety of imidacloprid 10%/moxidectin 1% spot-on formulation in the treatment of feline aelurostrongylosis. *Parasitol Res.* 2009;105:S55–S62.
67. Heuer L, Petry G, Pollmeier M, et al. Efficacy of imidacloprid 10%/moxidectin 1% spot-on formulation (Advocate®) in the prevention and treatment of feline aelurostrongylosis. *Parasit Vectors.* 2020;13:65.
68. Iannino F, Iannetti L, Paganico D, et al. Evaluation of the efficacy of selamectin spot-on in cats infested with *Aelurostrongylus abstrusus* (Strongylida, Filaroididae) in a central Italy cat shelter. *Vet Parasitol.* 2013;197:258–262.

69. Brianti E, Gaglio G, Gianetto S, et al. *Troglostrongylus brevior* and *Troglostrongylus subcrenatus* (Strongylida: Crenosomatidae) as agents of broncho-pulmonary infestation in domestic cats. *Parasit Vectors.* 2012;5:178.
70. Daoust PY, McBurney SR, Godson DL, et al. Canine distemper virus-associated encephalitis in free-living lynx (*Lynx canadensis*) and bobcats (*Lynx rufus*) of eastern Canada. *J Wildl Dis.* 2009;45:611–624.
71. Reichard MV, Caudell DL, Kocan AA. Survey of helminth lung parasites of bobcats (*Lynx rufus*) from Alabama, Kansas, New Mexico, Oklahoma, and Virginia, USA. *Comp Parasitol.* 2004;71:88–90.
72. Sarmiento L, Stough HD. *Troglostrongylus wilsoni* (Stough, 1953) n. comb. (Nematoda: Metastrongylidae) from the lungs of the bobcat, *Lynx rufus. J Parasitol.* 1956;42:45–48.
73. Smith JD, Addison EM, Joachim DG, Smith LM. Helminth parasites of Canada lynx (*Felis canadensis*) from northern Ontario. *Can J Zool.* 1986;64:358–364.
74. Van Zyll de Jong CG. Parasites of the Canada lynx, *Felis (Lynx) canadensis* (Kerr). *Can J Zool.* 1966;44:499–509.
75. Watson TG, Nettles VF, Davidson WB. Endoparasites and selected infectious agents in bobcats (*Felis rufus*) from West Virginia and Georgia. *J Wildl Dis.* 1981;17:547–554.
76. Bihr T, Conboy GA. Lungworm (*Crenosoma vulpis*) infection in dogs on Prince Edward Island. *Can Vet J.* 1999;40:555–559.
77. Craig RE, Anderson RC. The genus *Crenosoma* (Nematoda: Metastongyloidea) in New World mammals. *Can J Zool.* 1972;50:1555–1561.
78. Goble FC, Cook AH. Notes on the lungs and frontal sinuses of New York fur-bearers. *J Parasitol.* 1942;28:451–455.
79. Jeffery RA, Lankester MW, McGrath MJ, et al. *Angiostrongylus vasorum* and *Crenosoma vulpis* in red fox (*Vulpes vulpes*) in Newfoundland, Canada. *Can J Zool.* 2004;82:66–74.
80. Nelson TA, Gregory DG, Burroughs C, et al. Prevalence of lungworms in Illinois coyotes. *Trans IL State Acad Sci.* 2007;100:89–95.
81. Rankin JS. Helminth parasites of birds and mammals in western Massachusetts. *Am Midld Nat.* 1946;35:756–768.
82. Smith HJ. Parasites of red foxes in New Brunswick and Nova Scotia. *J Wildl Dis.* 1978;14:366–370.
83. Rausch RL, Fay FH, Willamson FSL. The ecology of *Echinococcus multilocularis* (Cestoda: Taeniidae) on St. Lawrence Island, Alaska. II. - Helminth populations in the definitive host. *Annals Parasitol Hum Comp.* 1990;65:131–140.
84. Choi S, Sim C, Kim HC, et al. Natural infection of *Crenosoma vulpis* (nematode: Crenosomatidae) in an urban Korean dog. *Korean J Vet Res.* 2014;54:127–129.
85. Conboy G. Natural infections of *Crenosoma vulpis* and *Angiostrongylus vasorum* in dogs in Atlantic Canada and their treatment with milbemycin oxime. *Vet Rec.* 2004;155:16–18.
86. Shaw DH, Conboy GA, Hogan PM, et al. Eosinophilic bronchitis caused by *Crenosoma vulpis* infection in dogs. *Can Vet J.* 1996;37:361–363.
87. Unterer S, Deplazes P, Arnold P, et al. Spontaneous *Crenosoma vulpis* infection in 10 dogs: laboratory, radiographic and endoscopic findings. *Schweiz Arch Tierheilkd.* 2002;144:174–179.
88. Mortier JR, Fina CJ, Edery E, et al. Computed tomographic findings in three dogs naturally infected with *Crenosoma vulpis. Vet Radiol Ultrasound.* 2018;59:27–31.
89. Caron Y, Merveille AC, Losson B, Billen F. *Crenosoma vulpis* infection in two young dogs in Belgium. *Vet Rec Case Reports.* 2014;2:e000098-e000098.
90. Husnik R, Sloboda M, Kovarikova S, Koudela B. Infection with *Crenosoma vulpis* lungworm in a dog in the Czech Republic. *Helminthologia.* 2010;48:56–58.
91. Matos B, Colella V, Alho AM, et al. *Crenosoma vulpis* infection in a four-month old puppy. *Helminthologia.* 2016;53:276–280.
92. Conboy G, Bourque A, Miller L, et al. Efficacy of Milbemax (milbemycin oxime + praziquantel) in the treatment of dogs experimentally infected with *Crenosoma vulpis. Vet Parasitol.* 2013;198:319–324.
93. Petersen EN, Barr SC, Gould WJ, et al. Use of fenbendazole for treatment of *Crenosoma vulpis* infection in a dog. *J Am Vet Med Assoc.* 1993;202:1483–1484.
94. Conboy G, Hare J, Charles S, et al. Efficacy of a single topical application of Advantage Multi (= Advocate) topical solution (10% imidacloprid + 2.5% moxidectin) in the treatment of dogs experimentally infected with *Crenosoma vulpis. Parasitol Res.* 2009;105:S49–S54.
95. Whitlock JH. A description of a new dog lungworm, *Filaroides milksi* n sp (Nematoda, Metastrongyloidea). *Wien Tierarztl Monat.* 1956;43:730–738.
96. Hirth RS, Hottendorf GH. Lesions produced by a new lungworm in beagle dogs. *Vet Pathol.* 1973;10:385–407.
97. Georgi JR, Anderson RC. *Filaroides hirthi* sp. n. (Nematoda: Metastrongyloidea) from the lung of the dog. *J Parasitol.* 1975;61:337–339.
98. Georgi JR. Differential characters of *Filaroides milksi* Whitlock, 1956 and *Filaroides hirthi* Georgi and Anderson, 1975. *Proc Helminthol Soc Wash.* 1979;46:142–145.
99. Pence DB. Notes on two species of *Filaroides* (Nematoda: Metastrongyloidea) from carnivores in Texas. *Proc Helminthol Soc Wash.* 1978;45:103–110.
100. Webster WA. *Andersonstrongylus milksi* (Whitlock, 1956) n. comb. (Metastrongyloidea: Angiostrongylidae) with a discussion of related species in North American canids and mustelids. *Proc Helminthol Soc Wash.* 1981;48:154–158.
101. Mills JHL, Nielsen SW. Canine *Filaroides osleri* and *Filaroides milksi* infection. *J Am Vet Med Assoc.* 1966;149:56–63.
102. Greenway JA, Stockdale PHG. A case tentatively diagnosed as *Filaroides milksi* in a dog. *Can Vet J.* 1970;11:203–204.
103. Robinson WF, Dunsmore JD, Paterson AJ. A species of lungworm in a dog in western Australia. *Aust Vet J.* 1978;54:361–362.
104. Corwin RM, Legendre AM, Dade AW. Lungworm (*Filaroides milksi*) infection in a dog. *J Am Vet Med Assoc.* 1974;165:180–181.
105. Levine ND, Ivens V, Reilly JR, Simon J. *Filaroides milksi* (Nematoda: Filaroididae) in the lungs of a striped skunk, *Mephitis mephitis. J Parasitol.* 1965;51:628–630.
106. Erb HN, Georgi JR. Control of *Filaroides hirthi* in commercially reared beagle dogs. *Lab Anim Sci.* 1982;32:394–396.
107. Beveridge I, Dunsmore JD, Harrigan KE, et al. *Filaroides hirthi* in dogs. *Aust Vet J.* 1983;60:59.
108. Genta RM, Schad GA. *Filaroides hirthi*: hyperinfective lungworm infection in immunosuppressed dogs. *Vet Pathol.* 1984;21:349–354.
109. Spencer A, Rushton B, Munro H. *Filaroides hirthi* in a British bred beagle dog. *Vet Rec.* 1985;117:8–10.
110. Waner T, Pirak M, Nyska A. Lungworm (*Filaroides hirthi*) infestation in a batch of beagle dogs: a case report and review of the literature. *Isr J Vet Med.* 1991;46:106–109.
111. Bauer C, Bahnemann R. Control of *Filaroides hirthi* infections in beagle dogs by ivermectin. *Vet Parasitol.* 1996;65:269–273.
112. Craig TM, Brown TW, Shefstad DK, et al. Fatal *Filaroides hirthi* infection in a dog. *J Am Vet Med Assoc.* 1978;172:1096–1098.
113. August JR, Powers RD, Bailey WS, et al. *Filaroides hirthi* in a dog: fatal hyperinfection suggestive of autoinfection. *J Am Vet Med Assoc.* 1980;176:331–334.
114. Rubash JM. *Filaroides hirthi* infection in a dog. *J Am Vet Med Assoc.* 1986;189:213.
115. Andreasen CB, Carmichael P. What is your diagnosis? *Vet Clin Path.* 1992;21:77–78.
116. Valentine BA, Georgi ME. *Filaroides hirthi* hyperinfection associated with adrenal cortical carcinoma in a dog. *J Comp Path.* 1987;97:21–225.
117. Pinckney RD, Studer AD, Genta RM. *Filaroides hirthi* infection in two related dogs. *J Am Vet Med Assoc.* 1988;193:1287–1288.
118. Bourdeau P, Ehm JP. Cas original de Filaroidose due a *Filaroides* sp. chez le chien. *Rev de Med Vet.* 1992;168:315–321.
119. Torgerson PR, McCarthy G, Donnelly WJC. *Filaroides hirthi* verminous pneumonia in a west Highland white terrier bred in Ireland. *J Small Anim Pract.* 1997;38:217–219.
120. Carrasco L, Hervais J, Gomez-Villamandos, et al. Massive *Filaroides hirthi* infestation associated with canine distemper in a puppy. *Vet Rec.* 1997;140:72–73.
121. Caro-Vadillo A, Martinez-Merlo E, Garcia-Real I, et al. Verminous pneumonia due to *Filaroides hirthi* in a Scottish terrier in Spain. *Vet Rec.* 2005;157:586–589.

122. Crawford P. What is your diagnosis? *J Small Anim Pract.* 2000;41(95):133–134.
123. Georgi JR, Georgi ME, Fahnestock GR, et al. Transmission and control of *Filaroides hirthi* lungworm infection in dogs. *Am J Vet Res.* 1979;40:829–831.
124. Georgi JR, Fahnestock GR, Bohm MFK, et al. The migration and development of *Filaroides hirthi* larvae in dogs. *Parasitology* 1979;79:39–47.
125. Georgi JR, Georgi ME, Cleveland DJ. Patency and transmission of *Filaroides hirthi* infection. *Parasitology.* 1977;75:251–257.
126. Rendano VT, Georgi JR, Fahnestock GR, et al. *Filaroides hirthi* lungworm infection in dogs: its radiographic appearance. *J Am Radiol Soc.* 1979;20:2–9.
127. Mills JHL. Filaroidiasis in the dog: a review. *J Small Anim Pract.* 1967;8:37–43.
128. Urquhart GM, Jarrett FH, O'Sullivan JG. Canine tracheo-bronchitis due to infection with *Filaroides osleri. Vet Rec.* 1954;66:143–145.
129. Keep JM. *Filaroides osleri* infestation in conjunction with a generalized infection in a greyhound. *Aust Vet J.* 1951;27:43–45.
130. Burrows CF, O'Brien JA, Biery DN. Pneumothorax due to *Filaroides osleri* infestation in the dog. *J Small Anim Pract.* 1972;3:613–618.
131. Barr SC, Lavelle RB, Harrigan KE, et al. *Oslerus (Filaroides) osleri* in a dog. *Aust Vet J.* 1986;63:334–337.
132. Lappin MR, Prestwood AK. *Oslerus osleri*: clinical case, attempted transmission, and epidemiology. *J Am Anim Hosp Assoc.* 1988;24:153–158.
133. Levitan DM, Matz ME, Findlen CS, et al. Treatment of *Oslerus osleri* infestation in a dog: case report and literature review. *J Am Anim Hosp Assoc.* 1996;32:435–438.
134. Bredal W, Gjerde B, Heiene R, et al. First verified case of *Oslerus osleri* infection in a dog from Norway. *Norsk Vet.* 1997;109:573–578.
135. Metcalfe SS. *Filaroides oslerus* in a dog. *Aust Vet Practit.* 1997;27:65–67.
136. Polley L. Quantitative observations on populations of the lungworm *Oslerus osleri* (Cobbold, 1889) in coyotes (*Canis latrans* Say). *Can J Zool.* 1986;64:2384–2386.
137. Erickson AB. Helminths of Minnesota canidae in relation to food habits and a host and key list of the species reported from North America. *Am Midl Nat.* 1944;32:358–372.
138. Holmes JC, Podesta R. The helminths of wolves and coyotes from the forested regions of Alberta. *Can J Zool.* 1968;46:1193–1204.
139. Thornton JE, Bell RR, Reardon MJ. Internal parasites of coyotes in southern Texas. *J Wildl Dis.* 1974;10:232–236.
140. Byman D, Van Ballenberghe V, Schlotthauer JC, et al. Parasites of wolves, *Canis lupus* L., in northeastern Minnesota, as indicated by analysis of fecal samples. *Can J Zool.* 1977;55:376–380.
141. Conder GA, Loveless RM. Parasites of the coyote (*Canis latrans*) in central Utah. *J Wildl Dis.* 1978;14:247–249.
142. Morrison EE, Gier HT. Lungworms in coyotes on the Great Plains. *J Wildl Dis.* 1978;14:314–316.
143. Seesee FM, Sterner MC, Worley DE. Helminths of the coyote (*Canis latrans* Say) in Montana. *J Wildl Dis.* 1983;19:54–55.
144. Pence DB, Windberg LA. Population dynamics across selected habitat variables of the helminth community in coyotes, *Canis latrans*, from south Texas. *J Parasitol.* 1984;70:735–746.
145. Carlson BL, Nielsen SW. Prevalence of *Oslerus osleri* (Cobbold, 1879) in coyotes (*Canis latrans* Say) from Connecticut. *J Wildl Dis.* 1985;21:64–65.
146. Foreyt WJ, Foreyt KM. Attempted transmission of *Oslerus (Oslerus) osleri* (=*Filaroides osleri*) from coyotes to domestic dogs and coyotes. *J Parasitol.* 1981;67:284–286.
147. Power J, Weather-Bee M, Boudreau M, et al. Diversity and ecology of pulmonary metastrongyloidosis in Coyotes (*Canis latrans*) of Nova Scotia, Canada. *Comp Parasitol.* 2015;82:85–93.
148. Yao C, O'Toole D, Driscoll M, et al. *Filaroides osleri* (*Oslerus osleri*): two case reports and a review of canid infections in North America. *Vet Parasitol.* 2011;179:123–129.
149. Brownlie SE. A retrospective study of diagnosis in 109 cases of canine lower respiratory disease. *J Small Anim Pract.* 1990;31:371–376.
150. Dunsmore JD, Spratt DM. The life history of *Filaroides osleri* in wild and domestic canids in Australia. *Vet Parasitol.* 1979;5:275–286.
151. Dorrington JE. Studies on *Filaroides osleri* infestation in dogs. *Onderstepoort J Vet Res.* 1968;35:225–286.
152. Jones BR, Clark WT, Collins GH, et al. *Filaroides osleri* in a dog. *New Zealand Vet J.* 1977;25:103–104.
153. Kotani T, Horie M, Yamaguchi S, et al. Lungworm, *Filaroides osleri*, infection in a dog in Japan. *J Vet Med Sci.* 1995;57:573–576.
154. Polley L, Creighton SR. Experimental direct transmission of the lungworm *Filaroides osleri* in dogs. *Vet Rec.* 1977;100:136–137.
155. Darke PGG. Use of levamisole in the treatment of parasitic tracheobronchitis in the dog. *Vet Rec.* 1976;99:293–294.
156. Clayton HM, Lindsay FEF. *Filaroides osleri* infection in a dog. *J Small Anim Pract.* 1979;20:773–782.
157. Bennett D, Beresford-Jones WP. Treatment of *Filaroides osleri* infestation in a 16-month-old male Yorkshire terrier with thiabendazole. *Vet Rec.* 1973;93:226–227.
158. Reagan JK, Aronsohn MG. Acute onset of dyspnea associated with *Oslerus osleri* infection in a dog. *J Vet Emerg Crit Care.* 2012;22:267–272.
159. Dietrich LE. Treatment of canine lungworm infection with thiacetarsamide. *J Am Vet Med Assoc.* 1962;140:572–573.
160. Hill BL, McChesney AE. Thiabendazole treatment of a dog with *Filaroides osleri. J Am Anim Hosp Assoc.* 1976;12:487–489.
161. Randolph JF, Rendano VT. Treatment of *Filaroides osleri* infestation in a dog with thiabendazole and levamisole. *J Am Anim Hosp Assoc.* 1984;20:795–798.
162. Kelly PJ, Mason PR. Successful treatment of *Filaroides osleri* infection with oxfenbendazole. *Vet Rec.* 1985;116:445–446.
163. Outerbridge CA, Taylor SM. *Oslerus osleri* tracheobronchitis: treatment with ivermectin in 4 dogs. *Can Vet J.* 1998;39:238–240.
164. Serres E. Entozoaires trouvés dans l'oreille droite, le ventricule correspondant et l'artère pulmonaire d'un chien. *J Vet Midi.* 1854;7:70.
165. Williams JF, Lindemann B, Padgett GA, et al. Angiostrongylosis in a greyhound. *J Am Vet Med Assoc.* 1985;186:1101–1103.
166. Tebb AI, Johnson VS, Irwin PJ. *Angiostrongylus vasorum* (French heartworm) in a dog imported into Australia. *Aust Vet J.* 2007;85:23–28.
167. Perry AW, Hertling R, Kennedy MJ. Angiostrongylosis with disseminated larval infection associated with signs of ocular and nervous disease in an imported dog. *Can Vet J.* 1991;32:430–431.
168. Kistler WM, Brown JD, Allison AB, et al. First report of *Angiostrongylus vasorum* and Hepatozoon from a red fox (Vulpes vulpes) from West Virginia, USA. *Vet Parasitol.* 2014;200:216–220.
169. Conboy G. Natural infections of *Crenosoma vulpis* and *Angiostrongylus vasorum* in dogs in Atlantic Canada and their treatment with milbemycin oxime. *Vet Rec.* 2004;155:16–18.
170. Taylor CS, Garcia Gato R, Learmount J, et al. Increased prevalence and geographic spread of the cardiopulmonary nematode *Angiostrongylus vasorum* in fox populations in Great Britain. *Parasitology* 2015;142:1190–1195.
171. Conboy GA. Canine angiostrongylosis: the French heartworm: an emerging threat in North America. *Vet Parasitol.* 2011;176:382–389.
172. Elsheikha HM, Holmes SA, Wright I, et al. Recent advances in the epidemiology, clinical and diagnostic features, and control of canine cardio-pulmonary angiostrongylosis. *Vet Res.* 2014;45:92.
173. Olivieri E, Zanzani SA, Gazzonis AL, et al. *Angiostrongylus vasorum* infection in dogs from a cardiopulmonary dirofilariosis endemic area of Northwestern Italy: a case study and a retrospective data analysis. *BMC Vet Res.* 2017;13:165.
174. Penagos-Tabares F, Lange MK, Chaparro-Gutierrez JJ, et al. *Angiostrongylus vasorum* and *Aelurostrongylus abstrusus*: neglected and underestimated parasites in South America. *Parasit Vectors.* 2018;11:208.
175. Jefferies R, Shaw SE, Viney ME, et al. *Angiostrongylus vasorum* from South America and Europe represent distinct lineages. *Parasitology* 2009;136:107–115.
176. Chapman PS, Boag AK, Guitian J, et al. *Angiostrongylus vasorum* infection in 23 dogs (1999-2002). *J Small Anim Pract.* 2004;45:435–440.
177. Koch J, Willesen JL. Canine pulmonary angiostrongylosis: an update. *Vet J.* 2009;179:348–359.
178. Morgan ER, Shaw SE, Brennan SF, et al. *Angiostrongylus vasorum*: a real heartbreaker. *Trends Parasitol.* 2005;21:49–51.
179. Bolt G, Monrad J, Frandsen F, et al. The common frog (*Rana temporaria*) as a potential paratenic and intermediate host for *Angiostrongylus vasorum. Parasitol Res.* 1993;79:428–430.

180. Corda A, Carta S, Varcasia A, et al. Pulmonary arterial response to *Angiostrongylus vasorum* in naturally infected dogs: echocardiographic findings in two cases. *Parasit Vectors.* 2019;12:286.
181. Bourque AC, Conboy G, Miller LM, et al. Pathological findings in dogs naturally infected with *Angiostrongylus vasorum* in Newfoundland and Labrador, Canada. *J Vet Diagn Invest.* 2008;20:11–20.
182. Glaus T, Sigrist N, Hofer-Inteeworn N, et al. Unexplained bleeding as primary clinical complaint in dogs infected with *Angiostrongylus vasorum. Schweiz Arch Tierheilkd.* 2016;158:701–709.
183. Adamantos S, Waters S, Boag A. Coagulation status in dogs with naturally occurring *Angiostrongylus vasorum* infection. *J Small Anim Pract.* 2015;56:485–490.
184. Cury MC, Lima WS, Guimaraes MP, et al. Hematological and coagulation profiles in dogs experimentally infected with *Angiostrongylus vasorum* (Baillet, 1866). *Vet Parasitol.* 2002;104:139–149.
185. Negrin A, Cherubini GB, Steeves E. *Angiostrongylus vasorum* causing meningitis and detection of parasite larvae in the cerebrospinal fluid of a pug dog. *J Small Anim Pract.* 2008;49:468–471.
186. Gredal H, Willesen JL, Jensen HE, et al. Acute neurological signs as the predominant clinical manifestation in four dogs with *Angiostrongylus vasorum* infections in Denmark. *Acta Vet Scand.* 2011;53:43.
187. Oliveira-Junior SD, Barcante JM, Barcante TA, et al. Ectopic location of adult worms and first-stage larvae of *Angiostrongylus vasorum* in an infected dog. *Vet Parasitol.* 2004;121:293–296.
188. Colella V, Lia RP, Premont J, et al. *Angiostrongylus vasorum* in the eye: new case reports and a review of the literature. *Parasit Vectors.* 2016;9:161.
189. Boag AK, Murphy KF, Connolly DJ. Hypercalcaemia associated with *Angiostrongylus vasorum* in three dogs. *J Small Anim Pract.* 2005;46:79–84.
190. Helm JR, Morgan ER, Jackson MW, et al. Canine angiostrongylosis: an emerging disease in Europe. *J Vet Emerg Crit Care (San Antonio).* 2010;20:98–109.
191. Alcoverro E, Bersan E, Sanchez-Masian D, et al. Eosinophilic cerebrospinal fluid pleocytosis associated with neural *Angiostrongylus vasorum* infection in a dog. *Vet Clin Pathol.* 2019;48:78–82.
192. Szatmari V. Spontaneous tricuspid valve chordal rupture in a dog with severe, irreversible pulmonary hypertension caused by *Angiostrongylus vasorum* infection. *BMC Vet Res.* 2020;16:311.
193. Liu J, Schnyder M, Willesen JL, et al. Performance of the Angio Detect in-clinic test kit for detection of *Angiostrongylus vasorum* infection in dog samples from Europe. *Vet Parasitol Reg Stud Reports.* 2017;7:45–47.
194. Schnyder M, Stebler K, Naucke TJ, et al. Evaluation of a rapid device for serological in-clinic diagnosis of canine angiostrongylosis. *Parasit Vectors.* 2014;7:72.
195. Deak G, Gherman CM, Ionica AM, et al. Use of a commercial serologic test for *Angiostrongylus vasorum* for the detection of *A. chabaudi* in wildcats and *A. daskalovi* in badgers. *Vet Parasitol.* 2017;233:107–110.
196. Bird LE, Bilbrough G, Fitzgerald R, et al. Determining resolution of *Angiostrongylus vasorum* in dogs following anthelmintic treatment with an imidacloprid 10 per cent/moxidectin 2.5 per cent spot-on. *Vet Rec Open.* 2018;5:e000215.
197. Canonne AM, Billen F, Losson B, et al. Angiostrongylosis in dogs with negative fecal and in-clinic rapid serological tests: 7 Cases (2013-2017). *J Vet Intern Med.* 2018;32:951–955.
198. Becskei C, Thys M, Doherty P, et al. Efficacy of orally administered combination of moxidectin, sarolaner and pyrantel (Simparica Trio) for the prevention of experimental *Angiostrongylus vasorum* infection in dogs. *Parasit Vectors.* 2020;13:64.
199. Bohm C, Schnyder M, Thamsborg SM, et al. Assessment of the combination of spinosad and milbemycin oxime in preventing the development of canine *Angiostrongylus vasorum* infections. *Vet Parasitol.* 2014;199:272–277.
200. Radman N, Venturini L, Denegri G. Comprobación experimental de la presencia en Argentina de *Capillaria aerophila* Creplin, 1839 (Nematoda-Capillaridae). *Rev Ibérica Parasitol.* 1986;46:267–272.
201. Di Cesare A, Castagna G, Otranto D, et al. Molecular detection of *Capillaria aerophila*, an agent of canine and feline pulmonary capillariosis. *J Clin Microbiol.* 2012;50:1958–1963.
202. Clark AC, Lopez FR, Levine JM, et al. Intracranial migration of *Eucoleus (Capillaria) boehmi* in a dog. *J Small Anim Pract.* 2013;54:99–103.
203. Veronesi F, Morganti G, Di Cesare A, et al. A pilot trial evaluating the efficacy of a 10% imidacloprid/2.5% moxidectin spot-on formulation in the treatment of natural nasal capillariosis in dogs. *Vet Parasitol.* 2014;200:133–138.
204. Elhamiani Khatat S, Rosenberg D, Benchekroun G, et al. Lungworm *Eucoleus aerophilus* (*Capillaria aerophila*) infection in a feline immunodeficiency virus-positive cat in France. *J Feline Med Surg Open Rep.* 2016;2. 2055116916651649.
205. Di Cesare A, Veronesi F, Capelli G, et al. Evaluation of the efficacy and safety of an imidacloprid 10% / moxidectin 1% spot-on formulation (Advocate®, Advantage®Multi) in cats naturally infected with *Capillaria aerophila. Parasitol Res.* 2017;116:55–64.
206. Traversa D, Di Cesare A, Di Giulio E, et al. Efficacy and safety of imidacloprid 10%/moxidectin 1% spot-on formulation in the treatment of feline infection by *Capillaria aerophila. Parasitol Res.* 2012;111:1793–1798.
207. Burgess H, Ruotsalo K, Peregrine AS, et al. *Eucoleus aerophilus* respiratory infection in a dog with Addison's disease. *Can Vet J.* 2008;49:389–392.
208. Abbate JM, Napoli E, Arfuso F, et al. Six-month field efficacy and safety of the combined treatment of dogs with Frontline Tri-Act® and NexGard Spectra. *Parasit Vectors.* 2018;11:425.
209. Evinger JV, Kazacos KR, Cantwell HD. Ivermectin for treatment of nasal capillariasis in a dog. *J Am Vet Med Assoc.* 1985;186:174–175.
210. Baan M, Kidder AC, Johnson SE, et al. Rhinoscopic diagnosis of *Eucoleus boehmi* infection in a dog. *J Am Anim Hosp Assoc.* 2011; 47:60–63.
211. Conboy G, Stewart T, O'Brien S. Treatment of E. *boehmi* infection in a mixed-breed dog using milbemycin oxime. *J Am Anim Hosp Assoc.* 2013;49:204–209.
212. Morandi B, Sabetti MC, Veronesi F, et al. A case of a dog refractory to different treatments for pulmonary capillariasis. *Parasitol Res.* 2021;120:1137–1141.
213. Gillis-Germitsch N, Muller S, Gori F, et al. *Capillaria boehmi* (syn. *Eucoleus boehmi*): challenging treatment of a rarely diagnosed nasal nematode in dogs and high prevalence in Swiss foxes. *Vet Parasitol.* 2020;281:109103.
214. Lalosevic D, Lalosevic V, Klem I, et al. Pulmonary capillariasis miming bronchial carcinoma. *Am J Trop Med Hyg.* 2008;78:14–16.

118

Trematodes

Karen F. Snowden, Jennifer K. Ketzis

KEY POINTS

Heterobilharzia americana **Infection (Heterobilharziasis/Canine Schistosomiasis)**

- First Described: *Heterobilharzia americana* was first described as an adult worm recovered from a bobcat (*Lynx rufus*) in 1929, and more fully described in specimens from a raccoon (*Procyon lotor*) in 1943. The parasite was first reported in dogs in Louisiana in 1961.
- Cause: *Heterobilharzia americana* (Platyhelminthes, Trematoda, Digenea, Strigeidida, Schistosomatidoidea, Schistosomatidae).
- Affected Hosts: A variety of wildlife hosts, most commonly the raccoon (*P. lotor*). Dogs are the most frequently identified domestic animal hosts, but the parasite has also been shown to cause disease in horses and llama.
- Intermediate hosts: Freshwater snails in the lymnaeid family, with Galba (previously Fossaria or Lymnaea), *Galba humilis,* and *Pseudosuccinia columella* confirmed as intermediate hosts by experimental infection.
- Geographic Distribution: Primarily the southeastern United States, but the range appears to be expanding.
- Route of Transmission: Penetration of intact skin by the larval cercarial stage that is released from snails in fresh water.
- Major Clinical Signs: Many infections are subclinical, but the most frequent signs are chronic or recurrent diarrhea, weight loss, and sometimes hematochezia in response to adult parasites in the mesenteric veins and migrating eggs in the intestinal mucosa. Hepatic fibrosis and pancreatitis can occur due to inflammatory changes associated with hematogenously disseminated eggs in various tissues.
- Differential Diagnoses: Depending on signs, these are a wide variety of neoplastic, toxic, or infectious/inflammatory causes. In a case series review, possible differentials included cholecalciferol toxicity, ethylene glycol toxicity, lymphoma, and pancreatitis. A variety of infectious pathogens can cause enteritis and hemorrhagic diarrhea. The differential diagnosis for hypercalcemia (sometimes present) includes malignancy-associated disease, endocrinopathies, renal failure, or a variety of infectious or inflammatory diseases.
- Human Health Significance: No human infections with *H. americana* have been reported. However, it is possible that the free-swimming cercarial stage may be able to penetrate human skin causing "cercarial dermatitis" as reported from the closely related avian schistosomes found in waterfowl.

Paragonimus kellicotti **Infection (Paragonomiasis)**

- First Described: *Paragonimus kellicotti* was described as a new species by Ward in 1908 after a careful review of eggs and other parasitologic specimens from humans from different geographic localities.
- Cause: Over a dozen respiratory trematode species have been described in dogs and cats on a global basis. In the United States, *Paragonimus kellicotti* (Platyhelminthes, Trematoda, Paragonomidae) is the helminth parasite that localizes in cystic spaces in the lung parenchyma of dogs and cats.
- Affected Hosts: *Paragonimus* spp. infect domestic dogs and cats, and less frequently are reported in a variety of wildlife hosts and humans.
- Intermediate hosts: The first intermediate hosts for *Paragonimus* spp. are aquatic snails, and the second intermediate hosts are typically crabs or crayfish, depending on the parasite species. For *P. kellicotti*, reported snail intermediate hosts include *Pomatiopsis lapidaria, Pomatiopsis cincinnatiensis* or *Oncomelania nosophora*, and the crayfish hosts, *Cambarus* spp. or *Orconectes* spp.
- Geographic Distribution: Various species of *Paragonimus* are globally distributed in temperate climates, with *P. kellicotti* being the important species in North America.
- Route of Transmission: Mammalian hosts become infected by ingesting the metacercaria larval stage found in the tissues of the second intermediate host (crab or crayfish). Ingestion of infected paratenic hosts may also occur.
- Major Clinical Signs: *Paragonimus* infections may be subclinical or may be associated with signs of respiratory disease, most often intermittent or chronic cough.
- Differential Diagnoses: *Paragonimus kellicotti* is found in cystic spaces in the pulmonary parenchyma, so major differential diagnostic considerations include pulmonary abscesses, metastatic neoplasia, cavitated neoplasms, and mycotic pneumonia.
- Human Health Significance: *Paragonimus kellicotti* is a zoonotic parasite that causes respiratory disease in humans. Humans become infected through the ingestion of raw or undercooked crab or crayfish intermediate hosts, so contact with dogs or cats does not pose a direct risk to humans.

Platynosomum illiciens **Infection (Platynosomiasis)**

- First Described: *Platynosomum illiciens* (synonyms *Platynosomum concinnum* and *Platynosomum fastosum*) was isolated from civet cat by Braun in 1901 (named *Dicrocelium concinnum*) and *Felis minuta* by Kossack in 1910. Other potential synonyms are *Dicrocelium lanceolatum* var *symmetricum* and *Concinnum concinnum.*
- Cause: *Platynosomum illiciens* (previously *Platynosomum fastosum*), a liver fluke of cats, which belongs to the class Trematoda and family Dicrocoeliidae.
- Affected Hosts: Domestic cats and a variety of wild cats. *Platynosomum* spp. also have been found in other hosts (e.g., opossums, ferrets, mice, non-human primates, and birds); it is unclear if these are true or incidental hosts, or if it is *P. illiciens* or another species in these hosts.
- Intermediate and paratenic hosts: The first intermediate host of *P. illiciens* is a land snail (e.g., *Subulina octona*). Isopods (*Oniscidea* spp. and *Nagurus* spp.) are considered the primary second intermediate host. Paratenic hosts include reptiles and amphibians (e.g., *Anolis* spp., *Hemidactylus* spp., *Tropidurus* spp., *Bufo* spp.) with mice potentially serving as paratenic hosts and final hosts.

- Geographic Distribution: Tropical and subtropical regions of the world, including those in Central and South America, the Caribbean, Asia, and Africa. In North America, *P. illiciens* occurs in Florida; there are no reports of infection in cats from Europe.
- Route of Transmission: Ingestion of excysted metacercariae in paratenic hosts or encysted metacercariae in a second intermediate host.
- Major Clinical Signs: Most infections are subclinical. Clinical signs are consistent with liver disease and include anorexia, weight loss, jaundice, vomiting and diarrhea.
- Differential Diagnoses: Differentials include polycystic liver disease, biliary carcinoma, and other nonparasitic causes of liver disease. When geographic distribution overlaps or cats have traveled between endemic areas, differentials include other fluke species that infect the liver and bile ducts (e.g., *Opisthorchis felineus*).
- Human Health Significance: *Platynosomum illiciens* is not considered to be zoonotic.

Alaria spp. Infections

- First Described: The mesocercaria larval stage of *Alaria marcianae* was first described by La Rue (1917) in a garter snake and named *Cercaria marcianae.*[1] Walton (1949) proposed the scientific name *A. marcianae* based on studies in frogs.[2] The first description of *Alaria alata* was attributed to Goeze (1782). Adult *Alaria* parasites were first described in naturally infected cats (*A. marcianae*) and dogs *(Alaria canis*) in 1965.[3] Additional species have been described in dogs, cats, and a number of wildlife hosts, and several parasite species have been synonymized. Due to challenges in parasite identification, several clinical reports use only the genus name (*Alaria* sp.)
- Cause: Members of the genus *Alaria* are Diplostomatid trematode parasites that localize in the small intestine of the definitive mammalian host. Multiple species have been described in the cat and dog, especially *Alaria marcianae* (cats) and *Alaria alata* (dogs).
- Affected Hosts: Domestic dogs, domestic cats, a variety of wild canids and felids, and other small mammals serve as definitive hosts.
- First intermediate host: In the United States, planorbid snails including *Heliosoma trivola* and *Heliosoma campanulatum*; other snail species are first intermediate hosts on other continents.
- Second intermediate host: In the United States, frogs in the Ranidae family, including *Rana catesbeiana, Rana clamitans, Rana utricularia, Myla cinerea,* and *Gastrophryne carolinensis.* Other amphibian intermediate hosts have been identified for various *Alaria* spp.
- Paratenic host: A number of nonessential hosts such as rodents, frogs, garter snakes, feral swine, and domestic chickens have been described and may be important in maintaining the parasite until the life cycle is completed in the carnivore definitive host.
- Geographic Distribution: Temperate climates across North America from Canada to Louisiana, Mexico, and South America; Europe; Middle East; and Africa.
- Route of Transmission: Ingestion of an intermediate or paratenic host that contain mesocercaria.
- Major Clinical Signs: Adult *Alaria* spp. attach to the small intestinal mucosa but do not cause signs in dogs and cats. In other hosts, adult flukes may cause enteritis, and migrating larval stages may cause damage, inflammation, and hemorrhage in the lungs or other viscera.
- Differential Diagnoses: Infections are subclinical, so this is not applicable.
- Human Health Significance: *Alaria* spp. are generally considered zoonotic parasites. The migrating larval mesocercariae may cause serious clinical disease, and human fatalities have been reported. Humans become infected by ingesting raw or poorly cooked frogs or paratenic hosts, but human association with infected dogs or cats does not pose a direct transmission risk.

HETEROBILHARZIA AMERICANA INFECTION (HETEROBILHARZIASIS/CANINE SCHISTOSOMIASIS)

ETIOLOGIC AGENT AND EPIDEMIOLOGY

Heterobilharzia americana (Platyhelminthes, Trematoda, Digenea, Strigeidida, Schistosomatidoidea, Schistosomatidae) is a trematode parasite of wildlife and domestic mammals in North America, and it is the only species in this genus.[4–9] It was originally described by Price (1929) who reported an adult worm in a bobcat (*Lynx rufus*) in Florida, and was later redescribed from specimens recovered from a raccoon (*Procyon lotor*) in Texas.[4,5] The parasite was first described in dogs in Louisiana in 1961.[6] *Heterobilharzia americana* belongs to the Schistomatidae family that includes several species such as *Schistosoma mansoni, Schistosoma haematobium*, and *Schistosoma japonicum* that are of global importance as "neglected tropical disease" pathogens in humans.[10] Adult worms of the majority of these species infect the blood vessels of the host intestine, with a few species infecting the vasculature of other organs. This group of parasites are informally called "schistosomes" and the clinical infection is often referred to as "schistosomiasis."

The life cycle of the parasite is maintained in wildlife and has been reported most frequently in raccoons,[11,12] as well a variety of other mammals including nutria (*Myocastor coypus*), swamp rabbit (*Sylvilagus aquaticus*),[6] opossum (*Didelphis virginianis*),[13] beaver (*Castor canadensis*),[14] and white-tailed deer (*Odocoileus virginianus*).[15] *Heterobilharzia americana* has also been identified in various wild carnivores such as coyote (*Canis latrans*),[16] mink (*Mustela vison*),[11] and black bear (*Ursus americanus*).[12] On occasion, *H. americana* also infects horses (*Equus ferus caballus*) and zebras (*Equus burchelli boehmi*).[17,18]

Cases in dogs have been reported across the southern United States, including Louisiana, Florida, North Carolina, Kansas, Arkansas, Georgia, and Texas.[7,19–21] The identification of cases in the last decade from California, Oklahoma, Kansas, Utah, and Illinois indicates a wider geographic distribution of the parasite than is generally recognized (Sykes, unpublished observations).[21,23,24]

The life cycle of *H. americana* requires fresh water for transmission among hosts (Fig. 118.1). Long slender adult male and female worms (6 to 12 mm in length) are typically paired *in copula*, and reside in the mesenteric veins. Eggs that contain already developed miracidia are excreted from adult females in mesenteric veins. The eggs then migrate through the small intestinal tissue to the gut lumen and are passed in feces. When eggs are deposited in water, the larval miracidium hatches and infects the first intermediate host, small conical aquatic lymnaeid snails (*Galba* (previously *Fossaria* or *Lymnaea*) *cubensis, Pseudosuccinia columella, Galba humulis*).[25–28] Following asexual multiplication through two sporocyst larval stages, motile cercarial larvae are released from the snails into the water and actively penetrate the intact skin of

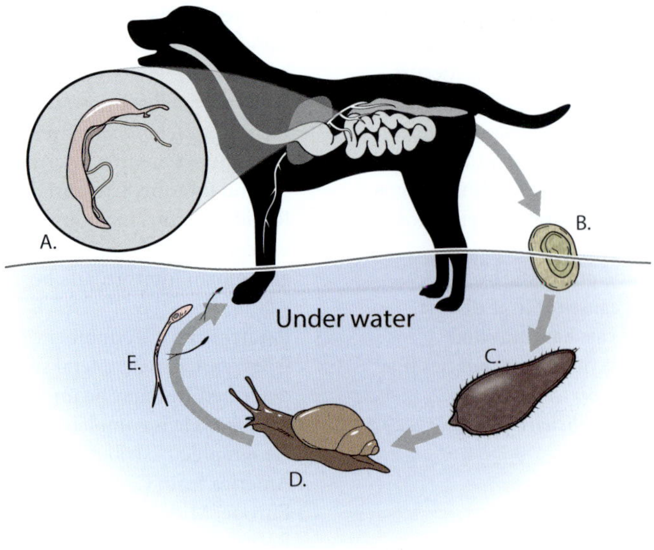

Fig. 118.1 Life cycle of *Heterobilharzia americana*. Adult trematodes in the mesenteric veins (A) produce eggs which pass through the intestinal wall and are excreted in the feces (B). When the egg contacts fresh water, a fully developed miracidium is released (C) and infects a snail first intermediate host (D). After asexual development in the snail, motile cercaria emerge and penetrate the skin of the definitive host (E) where they migrate to the mesenteric veins and, in 2–4 months, develop into adults.

mammalian hosts. The prepatent period (PPP) is estimated at 2 to 4 months based on egg excretion at 61 to 70 days and 65 to 121 days in a small number of experimentally infected dogs in two studies.[27,29] The longevity of adult *Heterobilharzia* in the mammalian definitive host has not been well studied, but closely related schistosome adult parasites live an average of 3 to 10 years and have been documented for as long as 40 years in humans.[10]

Only limited information is available on risk factors for canine schistosomiasis. In one report of 214 cases from Texas, the age range was 3 months to 17 years (median 5.5 years) with an even gender distribution.[7] All American Kennel Club breed groups were represented, with herding and sporting breeds and mixed breed dogs in the highest numbers. Affected dogs typically have an outdoor lifestyle with exposure to fresh water sources, which is consistent with the route of parasite transmission. No significant seasonality has been noted, but for 12 cases more than one dog in a household was infected, suggesting that multiple dogs were exposed to a common infected water source.

CLINICAL FEATURES

The clinical signs associated with heterobilharziasis range widely from no clinical signs to signs with a fatal outcome, and various stages of the parasite life cycle result in a spectrum of clinical problems. The presence of paired adult parasites in the mesenteric veins and migration of eggs through the intestinal wall from the serosa to the intestinal lumen typically results in signs associated with inflammatory intestinal lesions including intermittent diarrhea with or without blood and mucus, anorexia/hyporexia, weight loss of variable duration, and hematochezia.[7,8,21,30–32] Additionally, eggs may be carried by portal circulation to the liver causing chronic granulomatous inflammation and hepatic fibrosis.[7] Less frequently, eggs disseminate hematogenously to other organs including pancreas, spleen, lungs, lymph nodes, and kidneys and cause granulomatous inflammation resulting in organ-specific problems such as pancreatitis and glomerulonephritis.[7,32–34] The intensity and duration of infection impact the spectrum and severity of clinical problems.

DIAGNOSIS

Diagnosis of *H. americana* infections can be challenging because the parasite infection is under-recognized and the clinical signs are nonspecific and varied. Often infection is diagnosed at necropsy, and sometimes it is considered an incidental finding rather than the primary cause of clinical disease or fatality. In one retrospective case series of 22 dogs, the diagnosis was obtained by necropsy, histopathology, or fecal examination; in approximately one third of cases, *H. americana* infection was an incidental finding.[32] In another review of 238 cases, the diagnosis was confirmed by histopathology, egg identification on fecal examinations, or fecal PCR assays; a number of cases were positive using multiple methods.[7] In that study, infection was considered an incidental finding in 42% of dogs. In another retrospective evaluation of 60 cases from 2010 to 2019, diagnosis was made most commonly by fecal PCR alone (82%) followed by identification of eggs in feces or lesions on histopathology, and infection considered incidental in 12%.[22]

Laboratory Abnormalities

Complete Blood Count

Consistent hematologic changes in white or red blood cell counts are not seen in association with infection with this parasite although a mild anemia has been noted in a few case reports, probably secondary to chronic inflammation.[20,31,32] Anemia was reported in 18% and eosinophil count > 500/μL in 42% of dogs confirmed to be infected.[22]

Serum Chemistry Profile and Urinalysis

The most frequently reported clinical chemistry abnormalities are hyperglobulinemia and a variable, but inconsistent, hypercalcemia.[7,21,30–32,34] In one case series, more than 40% of dogs infected with *H. americana* were hypergammglobulinemic, while hypercalcemia caused by *H. americana* was identified in a minority (7%) of infected dogs and 17% were hypocalcemic.[22] Parathyroid hormone or parathyroid hormone-related protein concentrations have been within normal limits or increased.[21,30,31,34] In some patients with *H. americana* infection, renal function is compromised based on increased BUN and/or creatinine concentrations, or significant proteinuria that suggests the presence of glomerulitis.[7,21,33] Other clinical chemistry changes occasionally reported include increased serum liver enzyme activities (ALT and/or ALP) or hypoalbuminemia.[7,12,20,22,32–35]

Diagnostic Imaging

Plain Radiography

Imaging techniques may be suggestive of granulomatous inflammatory tissue changes associated with chronic *H. americana* infection. Abdominal radiography can be helpful in documenting focal mineralized lesions associated with the chronic granulomas that may be distributed in the small intestine or other tissues.[21,35,36] Hepatomegaly may also be noted.[31]

Sonographic Findings

In a few canine case reports, abdominal ultrasonography showed thickened walls of small intestinal loops or enlarged mesenteric lymph nodes and splenomegaly.[20,21,34] In one case series, 8 of 13 infected dogs had hepatic abnormalities on abdominal ultrasonography.[32] One of the often-noted lesions in chronic infections are hyperechoic foci in small intestine and sometimes kidney or liver indicating egg-associated mineralized granulomas.[21,31,36,37]

Parasitologic Tests

Diagnosis Using Fecal Examination

Detection of eggs using fecal sedimentation test is a simple but insensitive diagnostic method that can be conducted in a primary care setting.[38] Since adult female *H. americana* intermittently produce thin-shelled eggs (clear to golden, round to oval, 74–113 × 60–80 μm) that are passed in feces, the likelihood of egg detection is increased if the test is conducted on three or more fecal specimens collected on different days (Fig. 118.2A). Unlike most trematode eggs, there is no obvious operculum as a distinctive morphologic feature, but a freshly voided egg contains a developed miracidium which serves as a distinguishing characteristic. Since these larval miracidia readily hatch from eggs in fresh water, it is important to use saline (0.9% to 1.2% NaCl) rather than water in the fecal sedimentation test. In multiple case reports, trematode eggs were recovered by sedimentation, confirming active infections, and often negative tests were considered as an indicator of successful treatment.[21,31]

Although eggs can be identified on a direct fecal smear or saline wet mount, those methods have very low sensitivity and are not recommended for diagnosis.[33] In several case reports, no eggs were recovered by fecal flotation, the most widely used routine parasitologic fecal screening test.[20,21,30] These negative results are not surprising since most trematode eggs are relatively dense and are not typically recovered by flotation methods.

Cytologic Diagnosis

Heterobilharzia americana infection can be diagnosed by light microscopic examination of biopsied tissues retrieved by upper GI endoscopy, exploratory laparotomy, or FNA.[19–21,23,31–33] Diagnosis is usually inferred based on the presence of eggs or egg fragments, or characteristic multifocal granulomatous lesions in the intestine, liver, or sometimes other tissues. In 24 dogs where diagnosis of *H. americana* infection was achieved by biopsy,[7] associated disease was present in 16 dogs, whereas the parasite was considered an incidental finding in 8 dogs. Interestingly, heterobilharziasis was not considered as a differential diagnosis in 14 of those cases, and biopsies were conducted based on suspected neoplasia or other hepatic disease. The sensitivity of biopsies for diagnosis depends on the intensity and distribution of granulomas and eggs in various tissues and the size of the specimen collected.

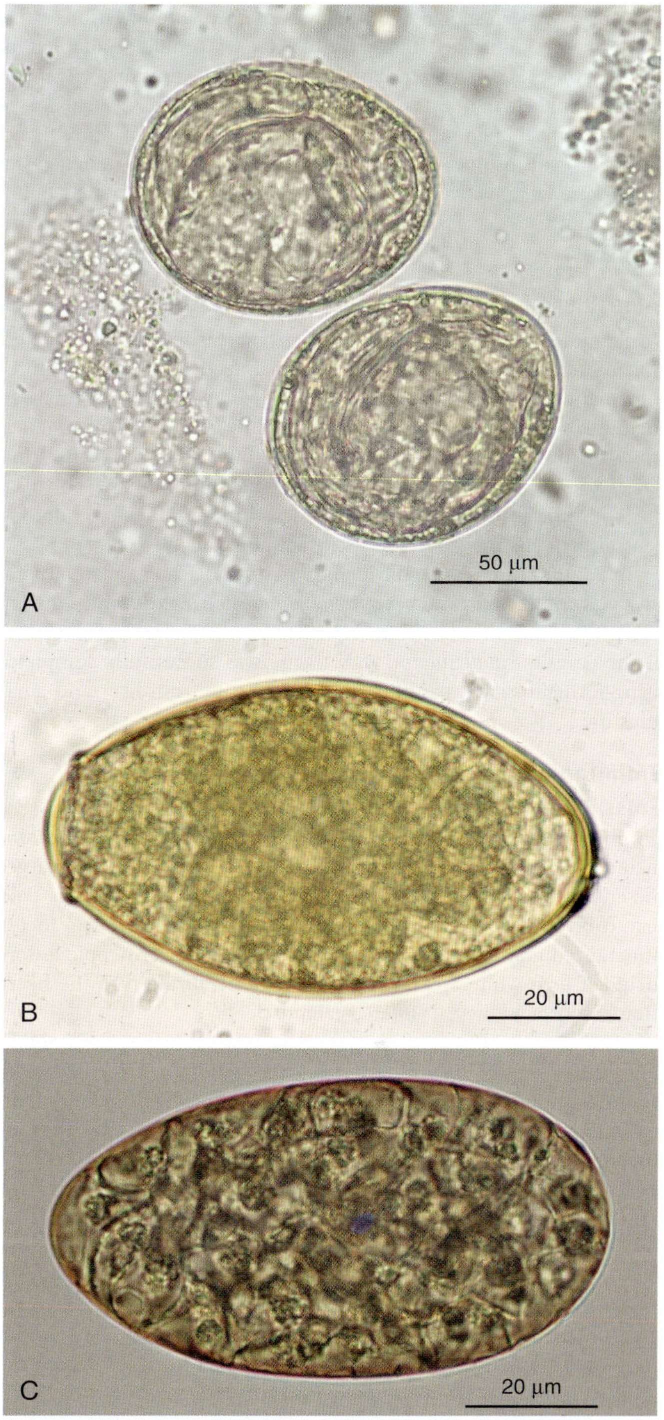

Fig. 118.2 Diagnostically important trematode eggs. (A) *Heterobilharzia americana* eggs containing developed miracidia at the time of detection on a fecal sedimentation test; bar = 50 μm. (B) *Paragonimus* sp. egg showing characteristic operculum with a lip and a small button structure on the opposite pole; bar = 25 μm. (C) *Alaria* sp. egg with an indistinct operculum and an undifferentiated embryo surrounded by yolk cells; bar = 20 μm. (A, Courtesy of Dr. Jessica Rodriguez, Zoetis Animal Health; C, Courtesy of Dr. Yoko Nagamori, Oklahoma State University, College of Veterinary Medicine.)

Serologic Diagnosis

Numerous immunologic methods for diagnosis of human schistosomiasis are described in the scientific literature. Both antigen and parasite-specific antibody detection tests are commercially available for use in individual cases or in serologic surveys in humans.[10] Since several antigens have been shown to be highly conserved among various schistosome species, it is likely that some of these tests could be adapted for veterinary use. However, a lack of demand for these tests on a large scale makes it unlikely that tests validated for use in dogs will be available in the near future. In an interesting case report, an antigen capture ELISA detecting schistosome circulating anodic antigen and designed for human use was positive in a confirmed canine case.[20] Repeated ELISA testing showed a decrease in serum antigen level following anthelmintic treatment.

Molecular Diagnosis Using Nucleic Acid–Based Testing

While molecular diagnostic methods are increasingly used for detection of schistosome parasites in human infections, there is limited information on the molecular detection of *H. americana* in animals. At the time of writing, there is one commercially available fecal *H. americana* qPCR test for dogs (Texas A&M University, Gastrointestinal Laboratory, College Station, TX). Although commonly used for diagnosis at some academic centers, a full description of the methodology, gene target, sensitivity and specificity are not available.[21]

In another case report, the identity of histologically apparent parasites was confirmed at necropsy as *H. americana.* End-point (conventional) PCR amplification and sequencing of a 487 base pair sequence of the parasite *small subunit rRNA* gene was successfully completed using formalin-fixed, paraffin-embedded tissue from liver and small intestine.[35]

Pathologic Findings

Gross Pathologic Findings

Commonly reported gross lesions in dogs infected with *H. americana* include segmental areas of thickened small intestinal walls and enlarged mesenteric lymph nodes.[34,35] Other findings sometimes include pale, firm (fibrotic) liver, or pale kidneys with or without pale, firm foci of mineralized granulomas.[34] In some case reports, macroscopic lesions included firm white areas of dystrophic mineralization in the heart, thoracic aorta, kidney, or intercostal muscle.[30,35]

Histopathologic Findings

The most notable histopathologic finding in dogs with heterobilharziasis is granulomatous inflammation associated with eggs that are disseminated in a variety of tissues. In 39 dogs that were necropsied, the most commonly affected tissues were small intestine, liver, and pancreas, with occasional egg-associated lesions in the large intestine and rectum, kidney, and lung.[7] Thin-walled, clear to golden-colored eggs or egg shell fragments are sometimes visualized microscopically in association with granulomas in various tissues (Fig. 118.3). In the small intestine, eggs are sometimes arranged in linear rows as they migrate through the intestinal wall to enter the lumen.[5,35] Sections of adult parasites may be identified in veins of the small intestine, colon, rectum, liver, lung, or pancreas. In addition to granulomas, local to focally extensive lymphoplasmacytic and sometimes eosinophilic inflammation can be present. Other reported histopathologic changes include fibrosis, hemosiderin pigment in macrophages, focal mineralization associated with granulomas, and bile duct hyperplasia. In hypercalcemic dogs, dystrophic mineralization has been noted in the gastric mucosa, cardiac tissues, and skeletal muscle.[30,34,35]

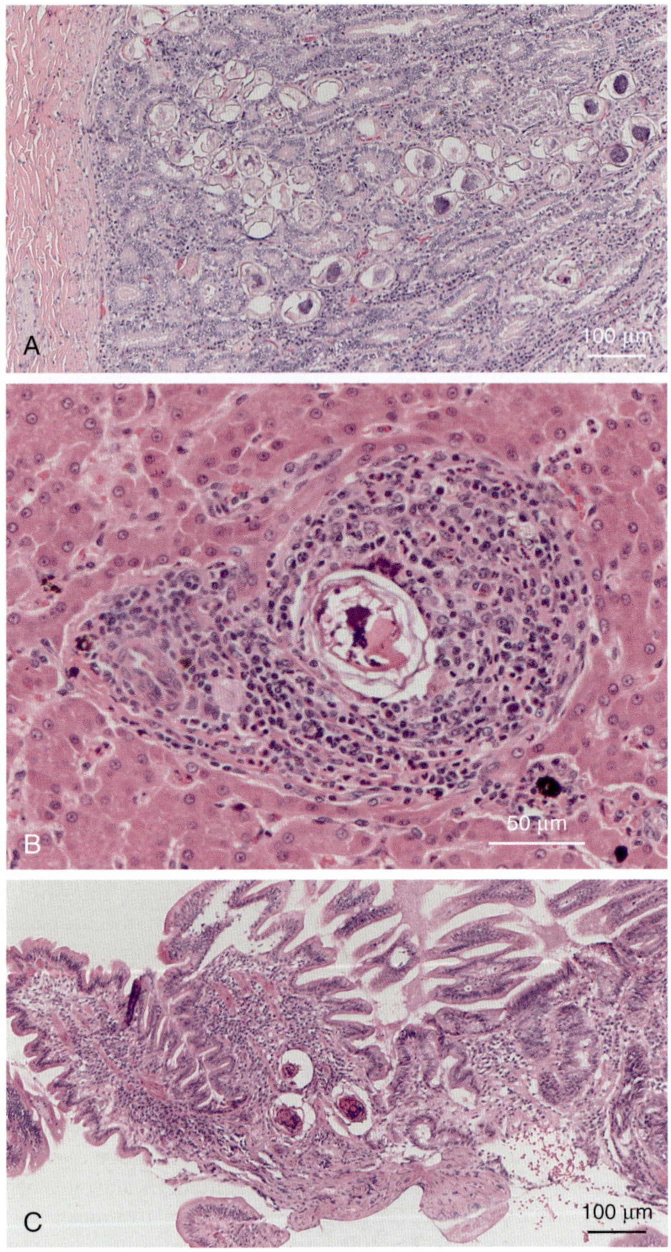

Fig. 118.3 Histologic sections (hematoxylin and eosin staining) of canine tissues with *Heterobilharzia americana* eggs and associated inflammatory changes. (A) Small intestine showing many eggs in linear rows migrating to the intestinal lumen; bar = 100 μm. (B) Liver showing eggs within a granuloma in the hepatic parenchyma; bar = 50 μm. (C) Intestinal biopsy showing eggs in the lamina propria; bar = 100 μm. (Courtesy of Dr. Carolyn Hodo, Texas A&M University, College of Veterinary Medicine.)

TREATMENT AND PROGNOSIS

No anthelmintics are label-approved for the treatment of *H. americana* infection and current extra-label recommendations are mostly anecdotal. No data from clinical trials comparing different treatment protocols have been published. Praziquantel and fenbendazole have been used individually, sequentially, or in combination in various clinical reports (Table 118.1). In several cases, praziquantel at varying doses was generally effective. The canine dose of praziquantel labeled for the control of cestodes (5 mg/kg, PO) is inadequate for treating many trematode infections. Praziquantel is the treatment of choice for human schistosome infections (40 to 60 mg/kg, PO, depending on the parasite species).[10] The most significant adverse effect of high-dose praziquantel is GI irritation and vomiting, which can be mitigated by dividing the daily dose into several treatments and administering the drug with food.

In a clinical report and in one experimentally infected dog, fenbendazole treatment was considered effective.[21,39] In other case reports, a

TABLE 118.1 Anthelmintic Treatments Used for Canine *Heterobilharzia americana* Infection as Documented in Clinical Reports

Drug(s)	Dose (mg/kg)	Frequency	Duration (Days)	No. Dogs Treated	Basis of Outcome
Praziquantel[32]	15, 20, or 25	q8h	1, 2, or 3	7	C
Praziquantel[20]	5 then increased to 30	q24h	unknown	1	C F (1 month)
Fenbendazole[39]	40	q24h	10	1	N
Fenbendazole[30]	50	q24h	10	1	F
Fenbendazole[30]	50	q24h	17	1	F
Fenbendazole + praziquantel[30]	40 25	q24h q8h	10 2	1	Treatment repeated then C
Fenbendazole + praziquantel[32]	50 15 or 20 or 25	q24h q8h	10 1, 2, or 3	3	C
Fenbendazole + praziquantel[38]	24 10	q24h q8h	7 2	1	C F (2 or 3 months)
Fenbendazole + praziquantel[7]	25 25	q12h q8h	14 1	1	Unsuccessful (F)
Fenbendazole + praziquantel[40]	24 5	q24h q8h	7 2	12	F (successful 12 dogs; 2 months) PCR (successful 8 dogs; 2 months)

C, clinical improvement; *F*, fecal egg excretion (time of testing post treatment); *N*, identification of flukes at necropsy.

combination of praziquantel and fenbendazole had varied therapeutic success using several different dosing regimens or repeated treatments.[7,21,32,33,40] In some cases, successful treatment was defined as remission of clinical signs, whereas in other cases, negative fecal sedimentation tests were used to determine therapeutic success (see Table 118.1). Both praziquantel and fenbendazole are readily available and labeled for use in dogs as treatment for infections by other helminths; concurrent extra-label use of these drugs at higher than labeled doses is currently considered the best treatment option.

IMMUNITY AND VACCINATION

No vaccines are available for canine schistosomiasis, and studies regarding protective immunity have not been reported. Reinfection has been noted in multiple clinical cases, so it is unlikely that dogs develop protective immunity.

PREVENTION

Based on the mode of transmission, the most obvious way to prevent infection is to limit dog access to surface water locations (wading or swimming in water). The lymnaeid snail intermediate hosts are typically found in shallow, stagnant fresh water such as persistent puddles and pond edges (not fast-running streams). They are small, conical snails which may not be obvious based on casual observation of the aquatic environment.[25,26] Since raccoons are common hosts, the presence of wildlife around a water source would increase the likelihood of contamination of the area with egg-containing feces, leading to establishment of the life cycle. Historically, the use of molluscicides for snail control was recommended in developing countries as part of human schistosome control programs, but no such efforts have been reported in the United States for this parasite.[41]

PUBLIC HEALTH ASPECTS

There are no reports of human infection with adult *H. americana*, and the parasite is not considered a zoonotic risk. However, it is theoretically possible that if larval cercariae have access to humans who are wading/swimming in fresh water, the parasite should be able to penetrate intact skin. The transient pruritic rash called "cercarial dermatitis" is typically attributed to skin penetration by the cercariae of avian schistosome parasites that are associated with ducks and other waterfowl that use the aquatic environment.[42] It is unknown whether *H. americana* cercariae may play a minor role in causing transient cercarial dermatitis in humans or other mammalian hosts.

PARAGONIMUS KELLICOTTI INFECTION (PARAGONOMIASIS)

ETIOLOGIC AGENT AND EPIDEMIOLOGY

On a global basis, a number of trematodes in the genus *Paragonimus* and the closely related genera *Euparagonimus* and *Pagumogonimus* infect the respiratory tract of dogs or cats (Table 118.2).[43–45] Various species have been reported in dogs and cats across the Americas, Africa, and Asia. All have indirect life cycles involving an aquatic snail first intermediate host and a second intermediate host, usually a crab or crayfish, ingested by the mammalian definitive host (Table 118.3).[46,47] Ingestion of infected paratenic hosts may also lead to infection.[48] This chapter will focus on *Paragonimus kellicotti*, which is geographically located in much of the eastern half of North America from Canada to Louisiana, and the Mississippi River basin.[49,50]

The monoecious (hermaphrodite) adult trematode occurs in the lung parenchyma of a number of mammalian hosts including dogs, cats, a variety of wildlife species (skunk, red fox, coyote, raccoon, bobcat, mink), and rarely humans.[49–51] Adults are approximately 10 × 5 mm in size, ovoid, with typical oral and ventral suckers, and are found in pairs within encapsulated cysts in the lung parenchyma with connections to bronchiole airways. Operculated eggs are shed from adult flukes, coughed up in bronchial secretions, swallowed, and passed in feces. The life cycle requires fresh water for several stages. When eggs are deposited in water, the larval miracidium stage develops and hatches from the egg and infects the first intermediate host, aquatic snails (*Pomatiopsis lapidaria, Pomatiopsis cincinnatiensis, Oncomelania*

TABLE 118.2 Taxonomic Identification, Definitive Host, Intermediate Host, and Geographic Source of Description for Various *Paragonimus* and Related Species in Naturally Infected Dogs or Cats[a]

Scientific Name	DH	IH	Geographic Source
Euparagonimus, Paragonimus africanus, P. uterobilateralis, P. westermani-like	D,C	NR	Cameroon, Democratic Republic of the Congo, Gabon, Republic of Côte d'Ivoire
P. caliensis, P. peruvianus	D	Cr: *Pseudothelphusa chilensis*	Peru
P. heterotremus	D	NR	Vietnam
P. loktsuenensis	D	NR	Japan
P. inca n. sp.	C, wild felids	Cr: *P. chilensis*	Peru
P. kellicotti	D	NR	Canada, Israel,[b] USA (incl. GA, MI)
P. kellicotti	D, C	NR	USA (incl. NJ, OH)
P. kellicotti	C	NR	Canada, USA (incl. LA, MO, OK, TN, KY, and VA)
P. kellicotti	C	S: *Pomatiopsis lapidaria, Pomatiopsis cincinnatiensis* Cr: *Cambarus bartonii, Orconectes juvenilis*	Kentucky, USA
P. miyazakii	D	NR	Japan
P. miyazakii, P. westermani	C	NR	Japan
P. mexicanus	C	S: *Aroapyrgus alleei*	Mexico
P. ohirai	D	NR	Japan
P. peruvianus n. sp./*P. mexicanus*	C	NR	Peru
P. pulmonalis	D, C	Cr: *Geothelphusa dehaani, Eriocheir japonicus*	Japan (reviews other reports in Asia)
P. uterobilateralis	D	NR	Liberia, West Africa
P. westermani	D	NR	Japan
P. westermani	D	NR	India
P. westermani	C	NR	India
Paragonimus sp.	D	Cr: *Sudanonautes africanus, S. aubryi, S. granulatus*	Cameroon
Paragonimus sp.	D	NR	South Africa
Paragonimus sp.	C	NR	North Carolina, USA

[a]Reference list associated with this table available on request to the chapter authors. For more description of reports of *Paragonimus* spp., please see Diaz JH. Paragonimiasis acquired in the United States: native and nonnative species. *Clin Microbiol Rev.* 2013;26(3):493–504.
[b]Possibly misidentified.
C, cat; *Cr*, crab/crayfish (second intermediate host); *D*, dog; *DH*, definitive host; *IH*, intermediate host; *NR*, not reported; *S*, snail (first intermediate host).

nosophora).[45,46] Following asexual replication as sporocyst and redia stages, cercarial larvae are released into water, penetrate the second intermediate crayfish host (*Cambarus* spp., *Orconectes* spp.), and develop to metacercaria.[49] The mammalian definitive host becomes infected through ingestion of an infected crayfish or paratenic host such as an infected rodent, so infection is possible in a dog or cat without direct access to crayfish and fresh water.[48] Metacercariae excyst in the duodenum, penetrate the intestinal wall into the peritoneal cavity, then migrate through the abdominal wall and diaphragm to the lungs, where they become encapsulated and mature into adults. Infections have been reported to last as long as 4 years in a dog, following a PPP of 5 to 7 weeks.[49] Human infections with the parasite have been reported to persist for several decades.[50]

Most descriptions of *P. kellicotti* infections in dogs and cats are included in the literature as case reports, and little information on risk factors is available. In a Louisiana survey of domestic cats with respiratory tract disease, 3 of 65 cats with clinical signs were infected with *P. kellicotti*, whereas 0 of 65 control cats were infected.[52] In a 5-year survey of parasitic infections in dogs and cats from New Jersey that was published in 1965, eggs of *P. kellicotti* were identified in three cats and one dog.[45] In a survey of 123 stray adult dogs from Michigan from 1964, *P. kellicotti* was identified in a single animal.[44]

CLINICAL FEATURES

In dogs or cats, *P. kellicotti* infections are often subclinical. Long-lived adult flukes localize in cystic spaces in lung parenchyma and intermittently shed eggs into the bronchial tree. Clinical disease in naturally infected dogs is characterized by a chronic or intermittent cough, which may be productive with frothy white sputum.[53,54] A mild, intermittent cough was the most frequently reported clinical sign in experimentally infected dogs.[55] Similarly, infected cats may have a mild cough.[56] In a study of 10 infected client-owned cats, the predominant reason for evaluation was cough.[57] In another feline case series, four of five infected cats were seen with a history of cough lasting from 3 days to 1 year.[58] Over time, exercise or exertion may exacerbate the cough in some animals. Infrequently, parasitic cysts may rupture causing acute pneumothorax, sometimes with sudden death.[55,59–61]

TABLE 118.3 Taxonomic Identification and Geographic Distribution of Various *Paragonimus* and Related Species in Dog or Cat Definitive Hosts (Experimentally Infected from Naturally Infected Intermediate Hosts to Confirm Life Cycles)[a]

Scientific Name	DH	IH Source, Naturally Infected	Geographic Source
Paragonimum caliensis	D	Cr: *Pseudothelphusa chilensis*	Peru
P. cheni	C	Crab	China
P. filipinus n. sp.	D	Cr: *Sundathelphusa picta*	Philippines
P. harinasutai	C	Crab	Vietnam
P. heterotremus	C, D	Cr: *Ranguna luangprabansensis*	Vietnam
P. iloktsuenensis	C, D	Crab	Korea
P. kellicotti	D	Crayfish	USA
P. kellicotti	C		USA
P. kellicotti	C	S: *Pomatiopsis cincinnatiensis, Pomatiopsis lapidria, Oncomelania nosophora* Cr: *Cambarus robustus*	Laboratory infections to identify new snail IH
P. kellicotti	C	Cr: *Orconectes propinquus*	North America
P. kellicotti	C	Crayfish	USA
P. kellicotti	C	Cr: *Orconectes propinquus*	
Paragonimus macrorchis	D	Cr: *Parathelphusa rugosa, Parathelphusa enodis*	Ceylon
P. ohirai	C, D	Cr: *R. luangprabansensis*	Vietnam
P. mexicanus	C		Peru
P. mexicanus	C	Cr: *Pseudothelphusa dilatata*	Mexico
P. mexicanus/P. peruvianus syn.	C	S: *Aroapyrgus costaricensis* Cr: *Ptychophallus tristani, Ptychophallus costaricensis*	Costa Rica
P. peruvianus	D	Cr: *P. chilensis*	Peru
P. peruvianus	C		Peru
P. proliferus	C	Cr: *Potamiscus mieni*	Vietnam
P. pseudoheterotremus	C	Cr: *Larnaudia larnaudii*	Thailand
P. siamensis	C	Cr: *Parathelphusa diagasti, Parathelphusa germaini*	Thailand
P. westermani	D	S: *Semisulcospira libertine* Cr: *Geothelphusa, Procambarus clarkii*	Japan
P. westermani	D		Korea
Pagumogonimus veocularis	C	S: *Tricula fujianensis, Erhaia jianouensis* Cr: *Sinopotamon fujianensis*	China
Pagumogonimus skrjabini	C	Cr: *Sinopotamon fujianensis*	China

[a]Reference list associated with this table available on request to the chapter authors. For more description of reports of *Paragonimus* spp., please see Diaz JH. Paragonimiasis acquired in the United States: native and nonnative species. *Clin Microbiol Rev.* 2013;26(3):493–504.
C, cat; *Cr*, crab/crayfish (second intermediate host); *D*, dog; *DH*, definitive host; *IH*, intermediate host; *S*, snail (first intermediate host).

Most animals are afebrile with an adequate appetite and normal hydration.[53,62] The most notable finding on physical examination in infected animals is abnormal lung sounds on thoracic auscultation in both dogs and cats.[53,62,63] In some cases, cough can be elicited by tracheal palpation.[54,63]

DIAGNOSIS

The diagnosis of pulmonary paragonimiasis is usually based on recognition of suggestive lesions on thoracic radiographs. Confirmation of the infection is usually based on detection of *Paragonimus* eggs in fecal specimens or respiratory secretions.

Laboratory Abnormalities

CBC and serum chemistry test results are often within normal limits in naturally and experimentally infected cats and dogs.[62–64] In a case series of 10 infected cats, leukocyte counts ranged from normal to slightly high, sometimes with a neutrophilia or an eosinophilia.[57] Serum chemistry results for total protein concentration, BUN, and serum ALT activity in those cats were within normal limits. In a single canine case report, total serum protein was elevated with a hyperglobulinemia and hypoalbuminemia.[53] Secondary pneumonia in association with *Paragonimus* infection may be associated with elevated WBC counts and neutrophilia.[59]

Diagnostic Imaging

Plain Radiography

Cystic structures containing adult parasites are radiographically detectable on thoracic radiographs in both dogs and cats.[53,59,62,65] Lesions are described as interstitial nodular opacities or as thin-walled cavitated pulmonary cystic structures, usually ranging from 2 to 5 cm in diameter. Air-filled cysts containing adult parasites may be multilocular.

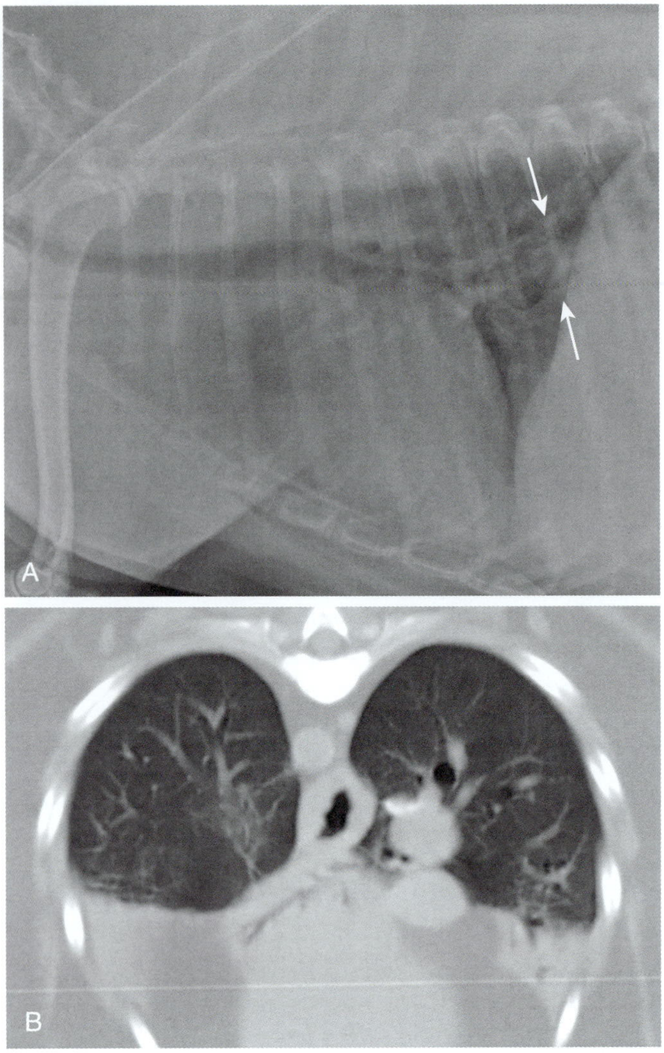

Fig. 118.4 Right lateral thoracic radiograph (A) and computed tomography (CT) scan (B) from a 10-year-old male neutered kelpie dog mix with paragonimiasis. There is a single soft tissue nodular opacity superimposed over the eighth rib in the caudodorsal thorax (arrows). On the CT scan there is a soft tissue spherical mass with a medial mineralized portion that abuts the pleural margin in the right dorsal aspect of the accessory lobe; the mass is also associated with the lobar bronchus. (Courtesy of the University of California, Davis Diagnostic Imaging Service.)

The caudal lung lobes are most frequently affected.[59] Other abnormalities include secondary pneumonia, peribronchial infiltrates, or rarely pneumothorax due to rupture of a cyst. Differential diagnoses include pulmonary abscesses, metastatic neoplasia, cavitated neoplasms, and mycotic pneumonia.[58] Findings on thoracic CT have been described in human patients and include peripheral lung nodules that are 1 to 3.5 cm in size with peripheral ground glass opacity. Sometimes linear tracks may be seen connecting nodules to the pleural surface.[66] One dog seen at the editor's institution had a solitary soft tissue spherical mass in the right dorsal aspect of the accessory lung lobe. The mass was adjacent to the pleura, associated with the bronchus and had a medial mineralized portion (Fig. 118.4A and B).

Serial thoracic images in the months following treatment reveal slowly resolving lesions; nodules may no longer be visualized, may decrease in size, or may change in appearance from cavitated to solid soft tissue opacities.[62] In experimentally infected dogs and cats, radiographic lesions were evident at 3 weeks PI.[64] Radiographic lesions resolved in dogs by 2 weeks post-treatment with praziquantel, but lesions were variably resolved by 4 weeks post-treatment in cats.

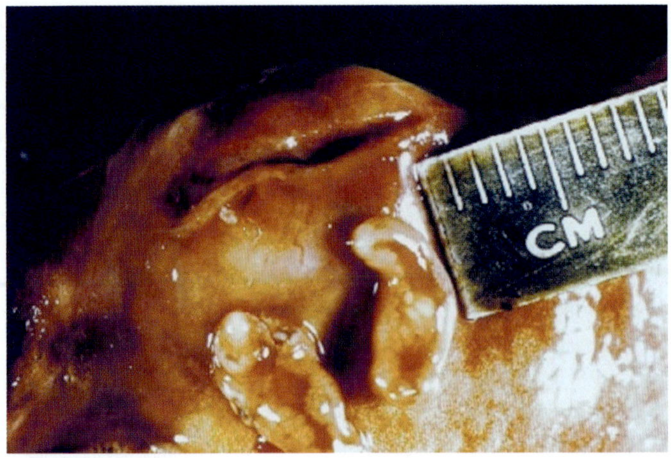

Fig. 118.5 Gross image of cat lung with an incised *Paragonimus* cyst and two adult flukes that were removed from the cyst.

Parasitologic Tests

Diagnosis Using Fecal Examination

Definitive diagnosis of *P. kellicotti* infection is made by detection of the oval, yellow-brown operculated egg (74–118 × 42–67 μm) in feces or respiratory secretions (Fig. 118.2B).[35] Eggs have a distinctive lip or ridge along the edge of the operculum, sometimes described as "flask-shaped," that is a key diagnostic feature. When evaluating fecal specimens, the eggs are dense and are difficult to detect in fecal flotation tests, so a fecal sedimentation test is the parasitologic method of choice. Eggs are excreted intermittently; a single fecal sedimentation test has a low sensitivity and multiple tests on multiple fecal specimens may increase the likelihood of egg detection.

Cytologic Diagnosis

Although adult flukes in lung parenchymal cysts are not visualized on bronchoscopy, characteristic "flask-shaped" eggs may be detected by cytologic evaluation of bronchial lavage secretions.[53]

Serologic Diagnosis and Nucleic Acid–Based Testing

No immunodiagnostic tests have been reported as diagnostic tools for detection of *P. kellicotti* infection in dogs or cats. The use of several experimental immunodiagnostic assays for *Paragonimus westermani*, *Paragonimus siamensis,* or *Paragonimus heterotremus* has been described in scientific literature to detect antibody production in experimentally infected cats.[67,68] Similarly, PCR-based assays have been used experimentally to detect *P. heterotremus* DNA in feces of experimentally infected cats, but the use of molecular tests that detect *P. kellicotti* DNA has not been reported for diagnostic purposes in dogs or cats.[69,70]

Pathologic Findings

At necropsy, subpleural cystic lesions up to several centimeters in size may be visualized as raised dark reddish-brown nodules on the lung surface, or may be located deeper in the lung parenchyma. On cut section, the nodules have a thin, dense fibrotic capsule and usually contain one or two adult flukes along with a small amount of brownish fluid (Fig. 118.5).[59] Bronchial lymph nodes may or may not be enlarged. Pulmonary areas adjacent to the parasitic nodules are usually grossly and histologically normal. Histologically, parasitic cystic structures are composed of fibrous capsular tissue with a variable collection of mixed inflammatory infiltrate cells including macrophages, plasma cells, and eosinophils surrounding the cyst wall (Fig. 118.6).[65,71] Sometimes eggs may also be visualized in the lung parenchyma or small bronchioles surrounded with a localized granulomatous inflammatory infiltrate.

TREATMENT AND PROGNOSIS

No anthelminthics are label-approved for the treatment of *Paragonimus* spp. infection in dogs or cats. However, praziquantel, fenbendazole, and albendazole have been reported to be effective in a variety of studies (Table 118.4). Multiday treatment of dogs or cats with praziquantel administered at higher than the labeled dose has been generally reported as successful.[54,64,72,73] The most significant adverse effect of high-dose praziquantel is GI irritation and vomiting, which may be mitigated by dividing the the daily dose into several treatments and administering the drug with food. The recommended treatment for human paragonimiasis is also praziquantel (25 mg/kg, q8h, for 3 days).[50]

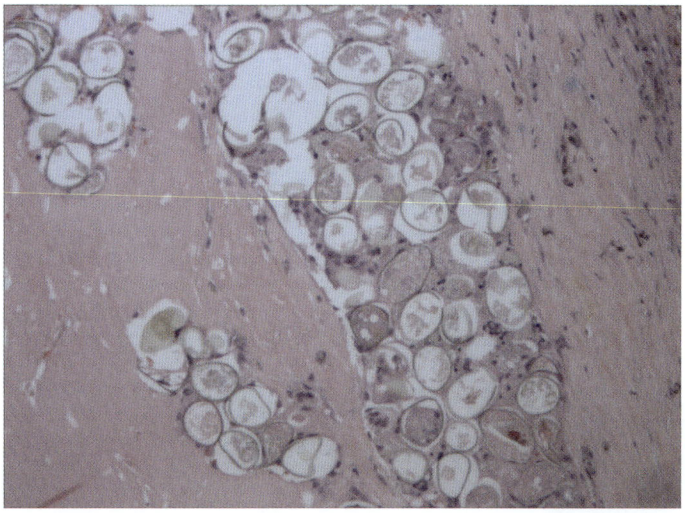

Fig. 118.6 Section of lung from a 10-year-old female spayed kelpie mix with paragonomiasis. There are multiple large coalescing cystic spaces at the edge of the lung that contain trematode eggs and are surrounded by inflammation.

Successful, multiday, high-dose fenbendazole treatment has also been reported in naturally infected cats and experimentally infected dogs.[63,74] Similarly, albendazole administered in varying doses for a prolonged period has been reported as effective in a small number of experimentally infected cats and in one naturally infected dog (see Table 118.4).[75,76] Albendazole is not label-approved for use in dogs or cats and can induce aplastic anemia, so alternative therapies are suggested.

IMMUNITY AND VACCINATION

No vaccines are available for paragonomiasis, and studies regarding protective immunity have not been reported.

PREVENTION

Prevention of paragonomiasis is focused on limiting dog and cat access to crayfish and their aquatic habitat, as well as paratenic hosts such as rodents. Since a variety of wild mammals can serve as reservoir hosts, proximity to wildlife associated with ponds or

TABLE 118.4 Anthelmintic Treatments for *Paragonimus kellicotti* Infection in Dogs or Cats as Documented in Clinical Reports

Drug(s)	Dose (mg/kg)[a]	Frequency	Duration (Days)	Host	No. Animals	Basis of Outcome
Praziquantel[55]	5	q24h	2	D	1	Unsuccessful
Praziquantel[55]	25	q8h	2	D	1	R
Praziquantel[72]	25	q8h	2	D	2	F × 6 days
Praziquantel[64]	23	q8h	3	D, C	6, 6	R, F
Praziquantel + febantel[172]	0.29 g/kg	q24h	3	C	1	Unsuccessful
Fenbendazole[74]	25	q12h	14	D[b]	4	F, N
Fenbendazole[74]	100	q24h	10	D[b]	2	F, N
Fenbendazole + prednisone[62]	28 + 0.6	q12h q12h then taper	21	C	1	F; regimen repeated
Albendazole[173]	25	q12h	10	C	2	R, F
Albendazole[75]	20	q24h	14+	C[b]	2	Unsuccessful
Albendazole[75]	50	q24h	14+	C[b]	1	F, N
Albendazole[75]	100	q24h	14+	C[b]	2	F, N
Albendazole[58]	50	q24h	11-24	C	10	Variable success
Albendazole[76]	30	q24h	12	D	1	F, N
Bithionol[174]	110	q24h	7	C	1	R, F
Bithionol acetate[175]	100	q48h	30	D	1	F
Bithionol[176]	25	q12h	4	D	1	F

[a]Unless specified otherwise.
[b]Experimental infection.
C, cat; *D*, dog; *F*, fecal egg excretion; *N*, necropsy; *R*, radiographic resolution of lung lesions.

streams increases the likelihood that the parasite life cycle will become established in a local environment.

PUBLIC HEALTH ASPECTS

Pulmonary paragonimiasis is considered a foodborne infection that affects as many as 23 million people, primarily in Asia and Africa.[51] Most of these infections are attributed to *P. westermani* or other closely related species.[51,77] A limited number of autochthonous cases of North American paragonimiasis have been described in humans caused by *P. kellicotti* infection and associated with ingestion of raw or undercooked crayfish.[51,78] Clinical disease in humans ranges from asymptomatic to serious respiratory disease, with similar clinical expression as the disease in dogs and cats. Eosinophilic meningitis has also been reported.[79]

Frequency of transmission in humans depends on dietary habits since mammalian definitive hosts, including humans, become infected by ingesting metacercaria in crab or crayfish intermediate hosts. Therefore, although *P. kellicotti* is considered a parasite with zoonotic potential, direct or indirect contact with infected pets or mammalian wildlife poses no direct risk to humans.

PLATYNOSOMUM ILLICIENS (PREVIOUSLY *FASTOSUM*) INFECTION (PLATYNOSOMIASIS)

ETIOLOGIC AGENT AND EPIDEMIOLOGY

Platynosomum illiciens (previously *fastosum*) belongs to the family Dicrocoeliidae and is synonymous with *Platynosomum concinnum* and *Platynosomum fastosum*. While most literature has used "*fastosum*" for infections in mammals and "*illiciens*" for infections in birds, molecular studies indicate these are the same with the trematode having a low host specificity. The name *P. illiciens* has been recommended rather than *P. fastosum* and so will be used from this point onwards.[80–85] Adult *P. illiciens* is found in the intrahepatic biliary ducts of the final host, domestic cats and a variety of wild cats,[86–88] and other hosts including non-human primates, opossums, birds of prey and parrots,[84] with no predilection for a specific hepatic lobe or lobule, and the gallbladder.[89] In heavy infections, adult trematodes also can be found within the pancreatic ducts, small intestine, and lungs.[87,88,90] Mature *P. illiciens* are 2.1 to 8 mm long and 0.5 to 2.5 mm wide (Fig. 118.7).[81,91,92] The location of the testes, ventral sucker, ovaries, and vitelline glands can be used to distinguish *P. illiciens* from other flukes in the biliary

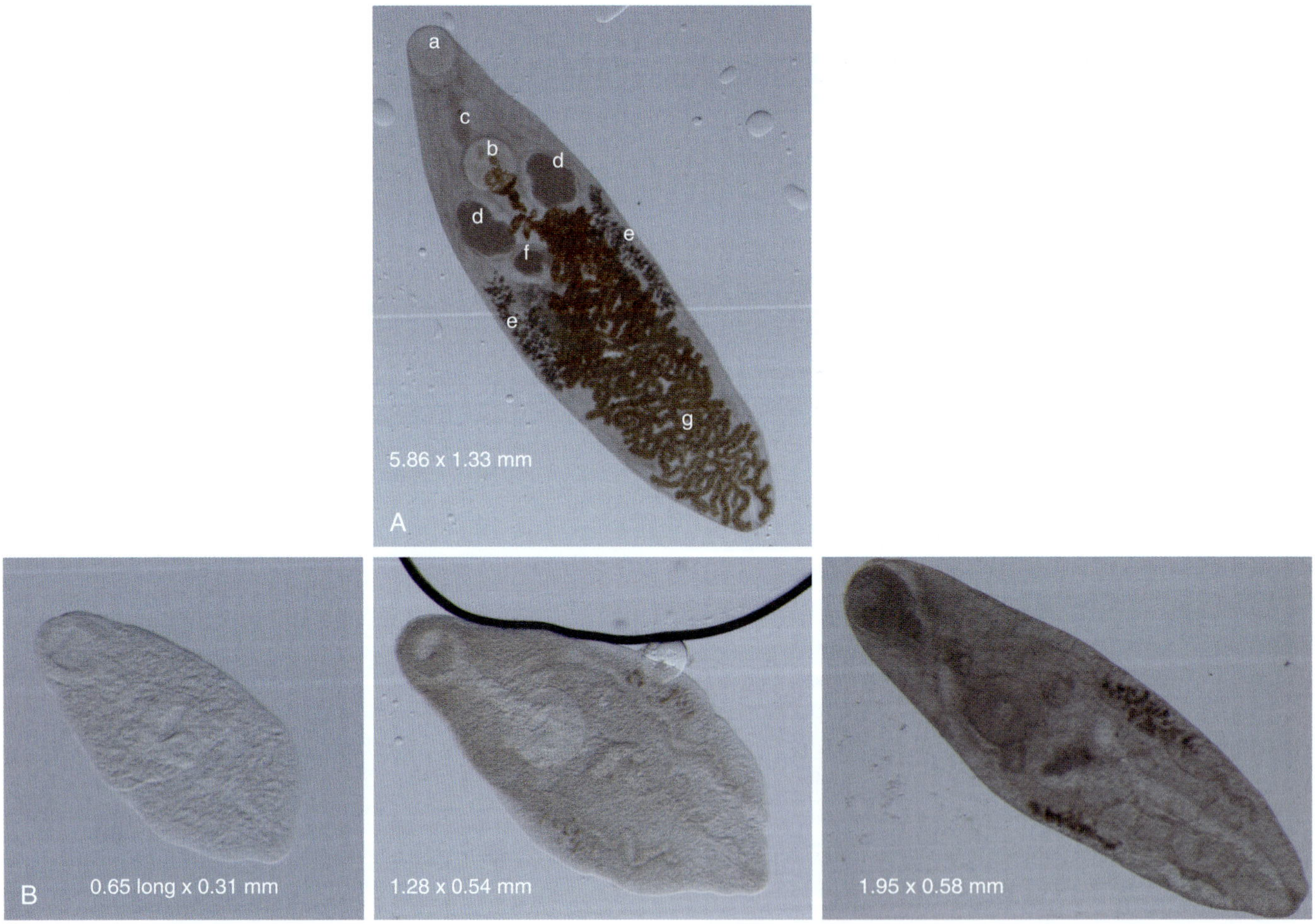

Fig. 118.7 (A) Adult *Platynosomum illiciens* and morphologic characteristics; *a,* oral sucker; *b,* ventral sucker; *c,* genital pore; *d,* two bilateral testes; *e,* two bilateral vitelline glands; *f,* ovary; *g,* oviducts. Testes are located just ventrolateral to the ventral sucker, the ovaries ventral to the testis, and the vitelline glands lateral to the testis. The genital pore is dorsal to the ventral sucker with the distance between these organs changing with maturity of the fluke. (B) With maturity, the digestive and reproductive tracts of *P. illiciens* develop and the trematode increases in size. The digestive tract forms in the first days after infection, the testis 2 to 3 weeks post infection followed by the vitelline glands, with the female genital tract and eggs forming approximately 4 to 5 weeks post infection.

TABLE 118.5 Comparison of Distinguishing Characteristics of Selected Flukes of the Biliary System or Pancreas of Cats

	DICROCOELIDAE		OPISTHORCHIDAE		
	Platynosomum illiciens	***Eurytrema procyonis***	***Amphimerus pseudofelineus***	***Clonorchis sinensis***	***Opisthorchis felineus***
Primary source of infection	Lizards, amphibians	Arthropods suspected	Freshwater fish	Freshwater fish	Freshwater fish
Geographic area of overlap	—	Texas, Florida	Central and South America	Asia	Endemic in Europe[a]
Site of infection	Bile ducts Gallbladder Rarely pancreas	Pancreatic duct	Bile ducts Gallbladder	Bile ducts Gallbladder Rarely pancreas	Bile ducts Gallbladder Rarely pancreas
Adult trematode	5–8 mm long Vitelline glands at mid-body Paired anterior testes	1.7–3.3 mm long Smaller testes and ovary	5–28 mm long Anterior and posterior sets of vitelline glands Testes posterior; one anterior to the other	10–25 mm long Branched testes Uterus between ventral sucker and the ovary	7–15 mm long Lobed testes
Egg	34–50 × 20–35 μm Indistinct operculum	45–53 × 29–36 μm	27–31 × 15 μm	28–35 × 12–19 μm Distinct operculum	22–32 × 10–22 μm
Clinical significance	Subclinical or liver cirrhosis Bile duct blockage	Subclinical or pancreatitis	See *P. illiciens*	See *P. illiciens*	See *P. illiciens* Choleliths
Other comments	Not zoonotic Praziquantel 20–40 mg/kg Daily consecutive treatment	Not zoonotic Praziquantel likely effective Raccoons are the definitive final host	Infects humans[b] Praziquantel likely effective	Infects humans[b] Praziquantel some efficacy	Infects humans[b] Praziquantel likely effective

[a]Included here for cats travelling between Europe and *P. illiciens*–endemic areas.
[b]Eggs in cat feces are not infective to people. Human infection is via consumption of the intermediate host or paratenic hosts.
See references 82, 177–183.

system in areas where more than one species is endemic (Fig. 118.7 and Table 118.5).[81]

The eggs, which are smaller than those produced by many other fluke species, are light brown, more oval than round, approximately 30 × 50 μm, and have an operculum that can be obscure (Fig. 118.8).[81,88] Damaged and immature eggs also occur in feces. Damaged eggs are shrunken and clear to pink; and immature eggs are clear, more ovoid, and smaller (16–20 × 27–30 μm).[88,92]

The life cycle of *P. illiciens* is indirect and utilizes two intermediate hosts and several paratenic hosts (Fig. 118.9).[81,93–95] Cats become infected when they ingest excysted metacercariae in a paratenic host or encysted metacercariae in the second intermediate host. Metacercariae are released in the intestine and the immature flukes travel to the common bile duct and within 3 days develop a digestive tract. In the following weeks, the fluke increases in size and the reproductive tract develops. Full maturity is reached in 8 to 12 weeks. Mature adult *P. illiciens* release 10 to 100 eggs per day which are stored within the gallbladder, released with bile into the GI tract, and excreted in feces.[81] The life span of *P. illiciens* can be > 1.5 years.[89]

Eggs are ingested by land snails (primarily *Subulina octona* but also *Eulota similaris*), the first intermediate host, resulting in the release of miracidia which move to the snails' connective tissues surrounding the respiratory tract. In the respiratory cavity, sporocysts develop resulting in cercariae. The cercariae release a glandulous fluid that helps the sporocysts exit the snail and re-enter the environment via the respiratory tract or the tunica propria, killing the snail in the process. Moisture and decreased light signal the exit of the sporocysts. A snail on average releases 7.6 sporocysts (approximately 134 cercariae) with the process from miracidium to sporocyst release requiring approximately 60 days.[81,89,91,96]

Isopods are considered the most likely second intermediate hosts.[81,89,91,96] These are tiny terrestrial crustaceans (woodlice), specifically *Oniscidea* sp. ("roly-polys") and *Nagurus* sp. (e.g., the "greenhouse woodlouse"). These consume cercariae in the environment, which then mature to metacercariae and encyst. Cats can become infected if they consume isopods, although most infections are believed to originate from the consumption of a paratenic host. In paratenic hosts the metacercariae excyst and reside in the hepatic and biliary systems. For many years, lizards, particularly *Anolis* spp. lizards (anoles), were considered an obligate paratenic host, resulting in the common name of "lizard poisoning" for platynosomiasis. Subsequent work has shown that several other lizard species (e.g. *Tropidurus* spp., *Hemidactylus* spp., *Lygosoma metallicum*), toads (*Bufo* spp.), frogs (*Eleutherodactylus* spp.), and, potentially, mice also can serve as paratenic hosts.[81,89,91,96–98] There are few studies on the prevalence and impact of metacercariae in paratenic hosts. A study from Puerto Rico found > 30% of *Anolis* spp. lizards examined to be infected (mean number of 16 metacercariae) with heavy infections (e.g., >300 metacercariae) associated with hyperplasia of the bile duct and atrophy of the gallbladder.[81]

Platynosomum illiciens can be found in cats in the Caribbean and other tropical and subtropical regions of the world, including Central and South America, southern areas of North America, Asia, and Africa.[88,90,93–95,99–102] In Australia, *P. illiciens* was found in cats in quarantine and treatment was pursued to prevent importation of the parasite.[103] In North America, *P. illiciens* occurs in Florida and Texas in the United States. It also has been found in cats outside of these regions such as in Ohio, Illinois, and Oklahoma within the United States; and Siberia, Russia. In some of these cases, the cats have originated from

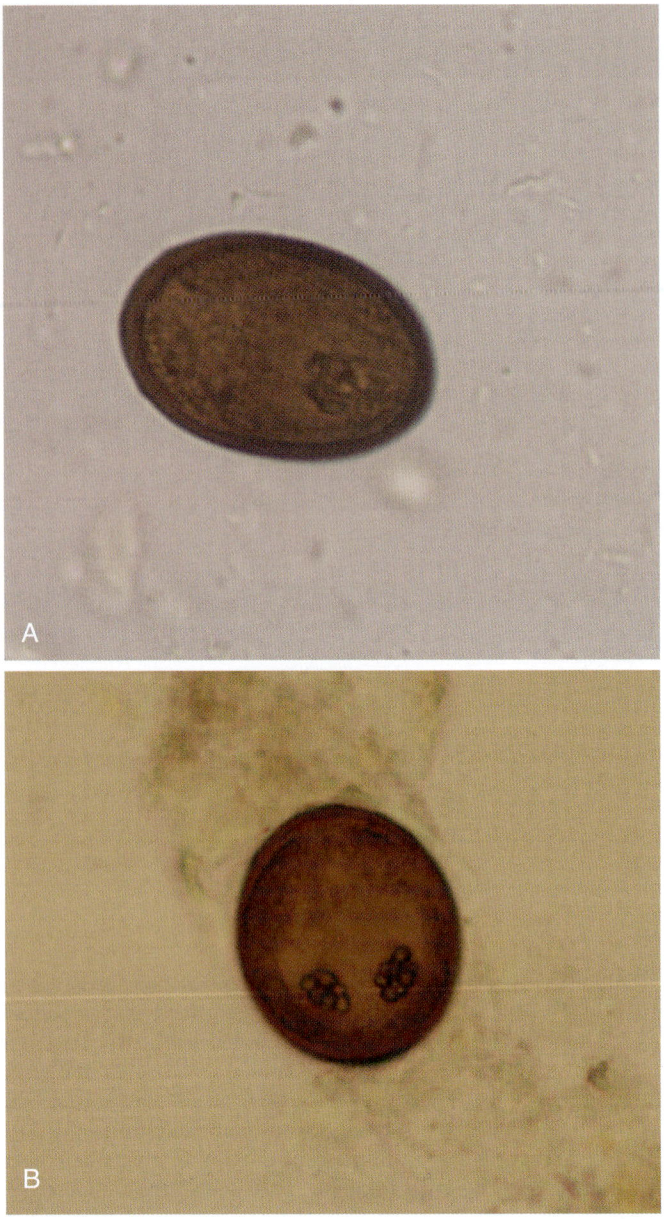

Fig. 118.8 *Platynosomum illiciens* eggs (30 × 50 μm) (A) in a fresh fecal specimen, examined using double centrifugation with Sheather's sugar flotation solution, and (B) in bile collected using percutaneous ultrasound-guided cholecystocentesis.

endemic areas.[104,105] However, travel was not demonstrated in all cases indicating that *P. illiciens* might have the potential to be present in or spread to nonendemic areas. This is supported by the presence of the trematode in non-feline hosts in areas where *P. illiciens* is not considered endemic in felids.

Within endemic areas, there are few recent studies on prevalence of infection in cats. Studies from St. Kitts in the Caribbean suggest that 22% of owned cats (indoor/outdoor and indoor only) and 81% of free-roaming cats are infected, with other Caribbean islands reporting a prevalence of <15% to >80%.[88,100,102] The prevalence in Brazil has been reported as <3% to >42%; in Yucatan, Mexico as 45%; and in different Asian countries, <1% to 73%.[1,88,106,107] Because paratenic hosts can gain access to homes, both indoor and outdoor cats are at risk for infection.[102,108]

Infection burden ranges from 1 to >4,000 flukes with average burden of 202 in St. Kitts and 110 in Yucatan; approximately one fourth of cats have high-burden infections (>125 flukes).[92,95] Older cats are more likely to be infected than younger cats, and some studies have suggested that female cats are more likely to be infected than male cats, a difference attributed to hunting behavior to feed offspring.[95,109]

While domestic and wild cats have been considered to be the definitive final host, other animals can be infected. Mice (*Mus musculus*) and birds (Australian parakeets, *Melopsittacus undulatus*) have been successfully experimentally infected with *P. illiciens* metacercariae, although the infection establishment level was lower than in cats.[89,91,96] *Platynosomum* adults also have been found in opossums (*Didelphis virginiana*), ferrets (*Grisson vittatus*), skunks (*Spilogale putorius*), North American hawks (*Buteo platypterus*), and nonhuman primates (marmosets, [*Callithrix jachhus*], orangutans [*Pongo pygmaeus*], monkeys [*Macaca* spp.]).[93,97,110–115] Molecular studies now suggest that all of these hosts contain the same species of *Platynosoumum*, indicating that the distribution is much larger then previously defined.

CLINICAL FEATURES

Most cats are subclinically infected and signs, when they do occur, are nonspecific. The presence of the flukes in the biliary system is associated with hepatic cirrhosis, cholangitis, and cholangiohepatitis. The occurrence of clinical signs are related to the parasitic load within the biliary system, level of continuous exposure to infection, chronicity of infection, and the cats' individual reaction to the parasite.[109] Increasing liver and biliary tract pathology result in general malaise, poor body condition, anorexia, weight loss, alopecia, vomiting, diarrhea, emaciation, dehydration, anemia, enlarged abdomen, hepatic encephalopathy, and progressive icterus.[89,109,116–119] On physical examination, hepatomegaly can be palpable.

While few studies have been conducted on the pathogenesis of *P. illiciens* infection, much can be extrapolated from the more studied liver flukes such as *Clonorchis* spp., *Opisthorchis* spp., *Dicrocoelium* spp., and *Fasciola hepatica*. Immature and adult flukes cause mechanical destruction of liver tissue via migration, attachment, and feeding. Localized toxic reactions and localized inflammatory reactions occur with fluke excretion/secretion products leading to eosinophilia. Fluke maturation and growth leads to bile duct dilation and adenomatous hyperplasia with duct dilation contributing to parenchymal cell damage and altered duct walls resulting in blood leakage. Younger flukes are believed to reside in the intrahepatic biliary ducts with more mature and larger flukes migrating to the extrahepatic biliary ducts.[91] As the flukes mature and their growth rate decreases, fibrotic connective tissues around the bile duct decrease bile and fluke excretion/secretion product flow into the parenchymal tissue limiting parenchymal tissue pathology.

Partial mechanical obstruction of the common bile duct or irritation of the common bile duct resulting in dyskinesia causes bile retention. Bile stagnation is believed to result in an environment conducive to secondary bacterial infections; however, little is known about secondary bacterial infection with *P. illiciens* infection.[88,97,109,110,120] With *Clonorchis* spp. infections, development of biliary calculi also has been attributed to bile stagnation and these are considered a factor in the occurrence of cholangiocarcinoma. While choleliths have not been identified in *P. illiciens* infections, cholangiocarcinomas have been noted, albeit rarely.

In experimental infections that involve a single exposure, clinical signs have not been seen during the early stages of infection. Approximately 2 months PI, lethargy, inappetence, slight weight loss, and abdominal distension have been documented with exposure to

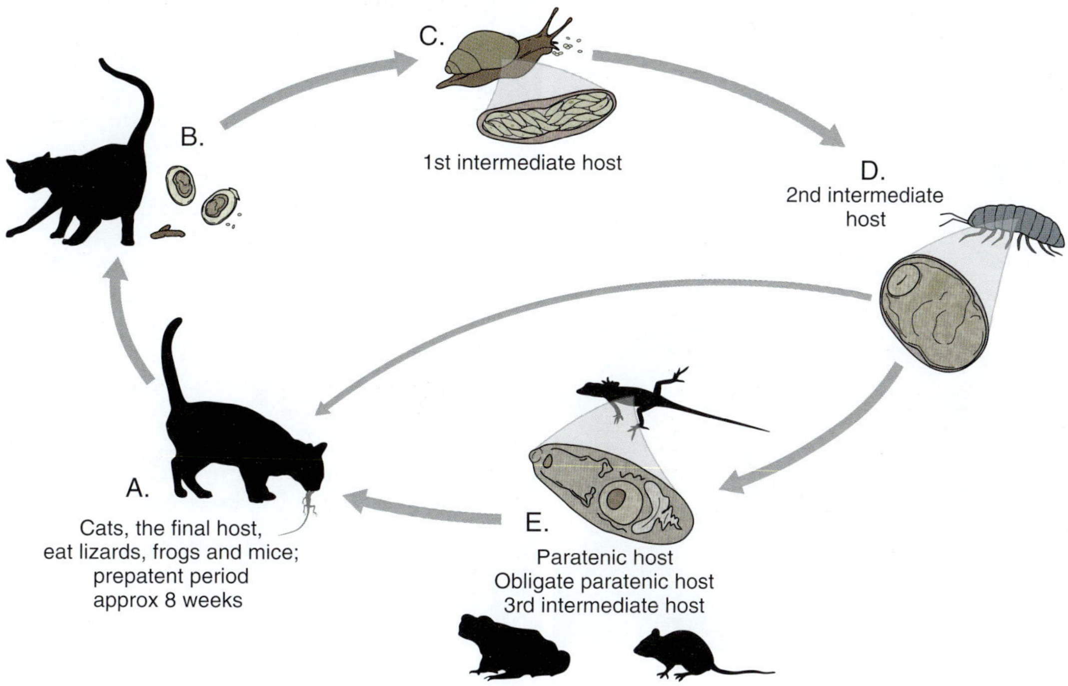

Fig. 118.9 The life cycle of *Platynosomum illiciens* includes the cat, two intermediate hosts, and frog, lizard, or rodent paratenic hosts. The adult trematode resides in the bile ducts of cats (A) with eggs released into bile and excreted in feces (B). Eggs are ingested by a snail and within approximately 2 months develop from miracidia to sporocysts containing several cercariae (C) which are released into the environment. These infect isopods (D) where they encyst as metacercariae. Paratenic hosts (usually lizards but also frogs and mice) (E) consume the isopods and are in turn consumed by the cat.

large numbers of trematodes, although most clinical signs resolved by 4 months PI with the cats remaining subclinical for up to an additional year. Less is known about progression of clinical signs during natural, continuous exposure. Natural infections of cats with > 125 flukes have been classified as high-intensity infections, with infection associated with pathology and clinical signs. Conversely, cats with > 1,000 flukes have been subclinical. It is possible that differences in pathology and clinical signs might differ between cats infected by consumption of a few paratenic hosts with a high number of metacercariae compared with those that develop more chronic infections as they consume many paratenic hosts that each harbor only a few metacercariae.

DIAGNOSIS

Fecal analysis is the recommended method for diagnosis of platynosomiasis.[88,121] However, the number of eggs recovered might not reflect the intensity of infection and negative fecal specimens can occur in heavy infections where there is partial or complete occlusion of bile ducts.[87,102,121] Bile collected using percutaneous ultrasound-guided cholecystocentesis can be used as an alternative to fecal specimen for retrieval of eggs and might be a more sensitive method.[122] Laboratory findings, abdominal ultrasound examination, and liver biopsy also can be useful for assessing the extent of liver damage but do not reveal findings specific for *P. illiciens* infection.[114,118] At necropsy, adult *P. illiciens* can be recovered from the liver and/or gallbladder and eggs can be found in bile.

Laboratory Abnormalities

Routine bloodwork can assist in determining the cause of liver disease and assessment of the extent of liver damage. The leukogram may be normal; however, an inflammatory leukogram with eosinophilia is a common finding, and occasionally a neutrophilia.[88,119] Anemia can be present in some infected cats.[119] Increased activities of serum AST and ALT can occur 4 to 5 months after infection and are indicative of cholestasis and hepatocyte damage.[88,108,110,118,119] Serum ALP activity may be normal, which is not unusual for cats even with severe or obstructive cholestastic disease.[123] Serum total bilirubin and bile acid concentrations may be increased in proportion to the severity of the infection. Serum pancreatic enzyme activities can also increase with *P. illiciens* invasion.

Diagnostic Imaging

The results of abdominal ultrasound examination are nonspecific in cats infected with *P. illiciens*, with some studies finding no significant abnormalities of the gallbladder, bile ducts, and liver of infected cats.[87,123,124] However, in endemic areas and when *P. illiciens* infection is suspected, changes in these structures would support examining multiple fecal specimens or bile for eggs. Changes that have been noted include distention of the gallbladder with a hyperechoic wall, distended and tortuous bile ducts and common bile duct, and hepatomegaly.[114,123–126] In one case study, cystic structures consistent with intrahepatic biliary duct dilatation were observed.[108] While *P. illiciens* can invade the pancreas, ultrasonographic changes to the pancreas have not been described.[126] Some relationship between intensity of infection and pathologic changes detected with ultrasound has been noted, but changes are likely also to be related to the chronicity of the infection.[109,123–125]

Parasitologic Tests

Diagnosis Using Fecal or Bile Examination

Two fecal diagnostic methods for egg recovery have been proposed as the "gold-standard" for diagnosis of platynosomiasis: traditional

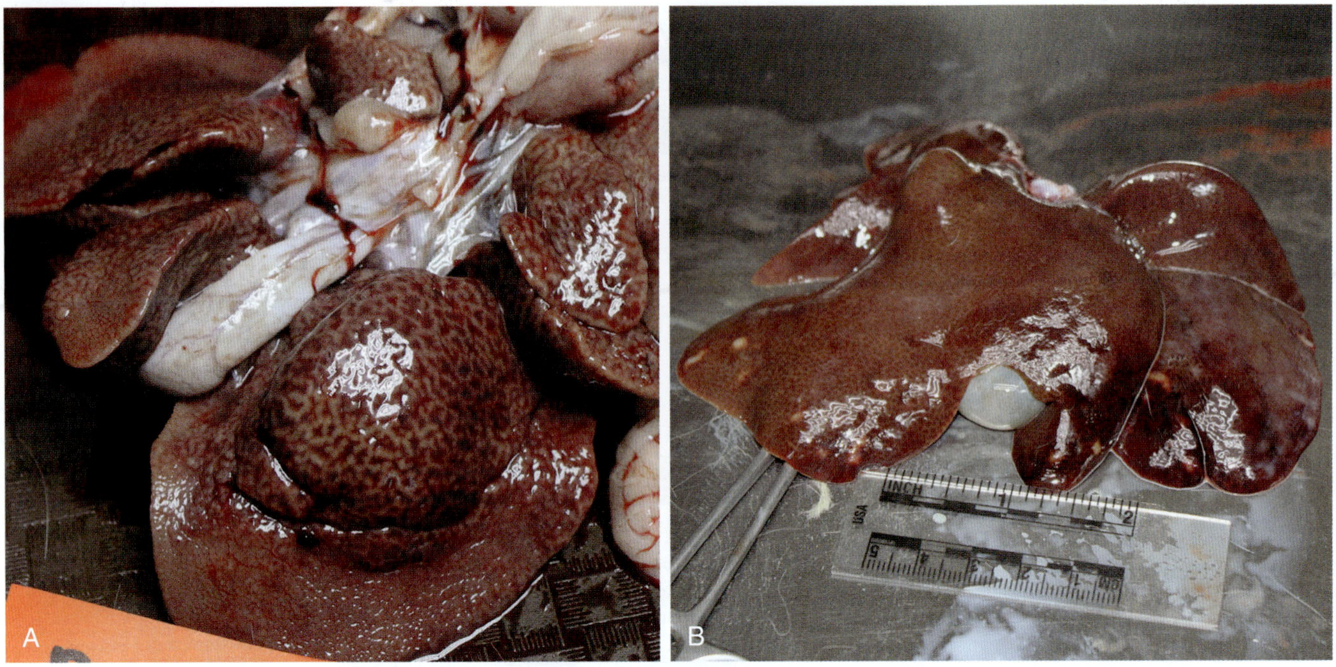

Fig. 118.10 (A) Firm liver with a focal domed mass in the right medial lobe with a prominent accentuated lobular pattern. The cat, euthanized for nonrelated reasons, had a chronic *Platynosomum illiciens* infection. (B) Mottled, discolored appearance and a diffuse reticular pattern in a *P. illiciens*–infected liver of a cat.

formalin-ether sedimentation and the more sensitive double centrifugation (500 g for 5 minutes) with Sheather's sugar flotation solution (SpG ≥ 1.27).[94,100,121,127,128] Safety issues with the use of formalin-ether solutions make this method less desirable, and centrifugation and flotation also permit identification of a greater variety of other parasites.[129] False-negative results can occur due to intermittent egg excretion in feces, biliary obstruction, and low numbers of eggs in general.[89,118,130] Multiple fecal analyses, as well as complementary diagnostics should be performed before eliminating *P. illiciens* infection as a cause of liver disease in cats.

Light microscopic examination of bile can be a more sensitive diagnostic method than fecal analysis. Use of 10 to 20 μL in a direct smear preparation is considered sufficient to identify eggs (Fig. 118.8B).[102,122,130] In severe platynosomiasis, few to no eggs may be found in feces due to biliary obstruction, but are present in bile.[118] Bile collection, via percutaneous ultrasound-guided cholecystocentesis, can be safely performed in *P. illiciens*–positive cats even in cases when severe pathology of the gallbladder is present.[122]

Pathologic Findings

At necropsy, *P. illiciens* adults can be collected from the liver and gallbladder. To recover the parasites, the liver can be cut into pieces (approximately 1 to 2 cm) and massaged and washed over a sieve. The gallbladder also can be opened and washed over a sieve to retrieve adult flukes. Bile can be collected and a direct smear viewed using a 10× objective (100× magnification) for identification of eggs, which can be more sensitive than adult trematode collection.[123]

Gross pathologic findings include icterus, hepatomegaly, an accentuated hepatic parenchymal lobular or reticular pattern, intraparenchymal parasitic cysts, biliary obstruction, a distended gallbladder, ascites (usually a transudate), and abdominal lymphadenomegaly (Fig. 118.10).[88–90,95,104,105,108,116,119,130–132] Cholangiocarcinomas and polycystic livers have been described in a few cats.[108,131,133]

Histologic findings include: atrophy and fatty infiltration of hepatocytes, hepatic and biliary duct fibrosis, hyperplasia of epithelium lining biliary tubules, and infiltration by eosinophils, lymphocytes, plasma calls, and neutrophils.[89,109,116–119,130–134] Ultimately, this is associated with increasingly severe cholangitis and nonsuppurative cholangiohepatitis. If cholangiocarcinomas develop, metastasis to other organs may follow.[130,133]

TREATMENT AND PROGNOSIS

The treatment of choice for platynosomiasis is praziquantel (20–40 mg/kg, PO, q24h for 3–10 days). This use and dose is extra-label but within tested safety limits for healthy cats. Adverse events may include GI irritation causing vomiting, diarrhea, and salivation. Praziquantel disrupts the tegument of flukes causing permeability alterations in the membrane, disintegration of the tegument, and spastic paralysis.[135–137] The antigen presentation of the trematode to the host changes, permitting it to be recognized by the host immune system; hence the host's immune system can work synergistically with the treatment to eliminate the infection.[136,137] Disintegration of the tegument and spastic paralysis results in increased release of eggs with corresponding higher fecal egg counts after treatment. In most *P. illiciens* infections, if there are no signs of liver failure, prognosis is good with praziquantel treatment. Prognosis is poor in cats with diffuse liver pathology and with clinical signs of liver failure, with euthanasia being the outcome in many case studies.[99,108,118,119] Immature flukes may be more resistant to treatment, so treatment may need to be repeated 2 to 12 weeks later.[88,137–139] Drugs found insufficient to treat *P. illiciens* infections include fenbendazole, mebendazole, levamisole, thiabendazole, diamphenethide, rafoxanide, and pyrantel pamoate.[89,103,134]

The efficacy of the praziquantel dose and dosing regimen is based on case series rather than on controlled studies. In one study, five cats infected with adult mature flukes were treated with a single dose of praziquantel at 20 mg/kg, after which they appeared to be cured.[103] The use of 10 mg/kg for 3 consecutive days resulted in reversal of clinical signs in mildly to moderately ill cats.[90] In a field study with seven cats, 20 mg/kg, q24h, for 3 days and repeated 3 months later resulted in cure, although the assessment of cure was based on single fecal egg counts following formalin-ether sedimentation.[140]

Oral administration of 20 mg/kg praziquantel can be challenging for the pet owner. Also, in high-burden infections, mass trematode death has the potential to cause acute bile duct blockage, which may worsen outcome. Alternative regimens of 20 mg/kg, IM, q24h, for 3 days or lower doses of praziquantel have been investigated with limited success.[92] In a study of six naturally infected cats with immature and adult flukes, praziquantel at 20 mg/kg, IM, for 3 days cured three cats based on fluke counts performed at necropsy 10 days after treatment. Two of the remaining cats had low-burden infections (1–2 flukes) and one cat had 40 flukes.[92] Adverse events from injection administration may include pain and/or swelling at the site of injection, vomiting, diarrhea, muscle tremors, weakness or lassitude, and anorexia. In addition, in a small study where one cat received 27 mg/kg, gross muscle pathology was noted at the injection site (paralumbar muscle) at necropsy. Histopathology revealed focal rhabdomyositis with evidence of myofiber regeneration.[92]

A dose of 5 mg/kg (the labeled dose of praziquantel, although the use is extra-label) administered twice at a 2- to 4-week interval has been proposed. In a case study, fecal egg excretion ceased after the initial dose but recommenced weeks later. After a second 5-mg dose, fecal egg count remained negative over an 8-month monitoring period.[141] In a study of six cats with natural infections (unknown fluke maturity), none of the cats were cured, based on fluke counts at necropsy, after being administered 5 mg/kg, twice, 2 weeks apart. However, egg counts and fluke burden decreased.[100] An advantage of this dose is that fewer tablets are administered and products in which praziquantel is combined with nematicides could be used, increasing the options available in a clinical setting. While this lower dose can be more convenient to administer, without further proof of efficacy it should be used with caution.

Regardless of the dose and regimen used, efficacy of treatment should be assessed, since chronic infections contribute to ongoing hepatobiliary damage. Fecal egg counts to assess efficacy should not be performed until 14 days after treatment. As a result of slow release from the bile or a few surviving adult flukes, eggs can continue to be excreted at low levels intermittently for up to 9 weeks post treatment.[103]

Other treatments administered to *P. illiciens*–infected cats with complicated infections include fluid therapy, nutritional support, antimicrobial drugs for secondary bacterial cholangiohepatitis, cholecystotomy, cholecystectomy, complete or partial liver lobectomy, or choledochoenterostomy. Prognosis is poor in these situations.[142]

IMMUNITY

Cats do not develop immunity to *P. illiciens* infection. Chronic infections and reinfection are common.

PREVENTION

Given the variety of intermediate and paratenic hosts, prevention of infection in endemic areas is challenging. Even indoor cats are at risk with paratenic hosts such as anoles able to enter homes. In endemic areas, regular examination of feces of indoor and outdoor cats is needed to identify infections and treat them before extensive biliary tract pathology develops. Administration of monthly praziquantel might be beneficial for cats at a high risk of infection, although the efficacy of the low dose of praziquantel is uncertain and the potential exists for selection for anthelmintic-resistant parasites. The selection for resistant flukes has been suspected in the case of other fluke species in other hosts, although most cases of reduced treatment efficacy have been attributed to overwhelming infections or incorrect dose.[135,137]

Reports of *P. illiciens* infection in cats outside endemic areas are a concern. While most of these cats have a history of travel from an endemic area, it is unknown if *P. illiciens* can adapt to other intermediate hosts and establish in new locations. Therefore, measures should be implemented to prevent transport of *P. illiciens* to currently nonendemic locations. Treatment should be administered before departure from endemic areas with follow-up fecal examinations and treatment as needed after arrival in nonendemic areas. Given the long PPP, need for repeated treatments to eliminate infection, the lack of sensitivity of the diagnostic methods, and the long lifespan of adult flukes, prevention of transporting infections to nonendemic areas represents a challenge.

PUBLIC HEALTH ASPECTS

Platynosomum illiciens is not considered a public health issue. There have been no reports of human infections.

ALARIA SPP. INFECTIONS

ETIOLOGIC AGENT AND EPIDEMIOLOGY

Members of the genus *Alaria* are Diplostomatid trematode parasites that localize in the small intestine of a variety of domestic and wild carnivores. Species described in domestic dogs and cats include *A. alata* (Goeze, 1782), *A. marcianae* (La Rue, 1917 and Walton, 1949); *A. canis* (La Rue & Fallis, 1936); *Alaria arisaemoides* (Augustine & Uribe, 1927); *Alaria americana* (Hall & Wigdor, 1918); *Alaria nasuae* (La Rue & Townsend, 1932); and *Alaria minnesotae* (Chandler, 1954) (Table 118.6).[1,143–147] Several *Alaria* species such as *A. canis*, *A. minnesotae*, and *A. americana* have been considered synonymous with *A. marcianae* by some authors,[148–152] while separate species identities are supported by other reports.[153] In relatively recent scientific literature, *A. marcianae* is most frequently identified in the intestinal tract of domestic cats, whereas *A. alata* is reported primarily in dogs. Due to challenges in morphologic identification of the various species in some clinical reports, the parasite is identified only to the genus level as *Alaria* sp.[154–158]

The life cycle of *Alaria* spp. is complex with multiple life stages in at least three hosts. In addition to dogs and cats, adult parasites are found in the small intestine of a variety of wild carnivores including wolves (*Canis lupus*), red fox (*Vulpes vulpes*), grey fox (*Urocyon cinereoargenteus*), mountain lion (*Felis (Puma) concolor*), striped skunk (*Mephistis mephistis*), and coyote (*C. latrans*).[147,148,152,159,160] The relative importance of these wildlife reservoirs with regard to dog or cat infections is unclear.

Alaria adults usually range in length from 1.5 to 4 mm and have an unusual two-compartment body structure. The flattened forebody contains oral and ventral suckers and a bulbous trybocytic organ, and attaches to the intestinal mucosa. The cylindrical hind body contains the reproductive organs and extends into the lumen of the small intestine.[143,148,161] Large, oval eggs with indistinct opercula (98–134 × 62–68 μm) are shed in the feces of the definitive host (Fig. 118.2C).[35] When the egg contacts fresh water, the larval miracidium develops and hatches in about 2 weeks. The motile miracidia infect planorbid snails of the genus *Helisoma* and undergo asexual replication as sporocysts. Motile cercaria are released into the water and penetrate the skin of larval amphibians (tadpoles) and transform into mesocercaria. Several frog species serve as second intermediate hosts by maintaining the larval stage in tissues as an adult.[148,159,162] Alternatively, the infected tadpole may be ingested by frogs, snakes, rodents, chickens, or other paratenic hosts.[148] The dog or cat definitive host becomes infected by ingesting an infected frog or paratenic host.

TABLE 118.6 Taxonomic Identification, Definitive and Intermediate Hosts, and Geographic Source of Various *Alaria* Species in Dogs or Cats[a]

Scientific Name	DH	IH, Naturally Infected	Geographic Source
Alaria alata	C	NR	Spain, Uruguay
A. alata	D, jackal	NR	Iran
A. alata	D	NR	Argentina, Denmark, Serbia, Sweden, Turkey
Alaria canis	D	NR	New Jersey, USA
Alaria marcianae	C	NR	New Jersey, USA
A. marcianae	C, bobcat, raccoon	S: *Helisoma trivolvis* F: *Rana catesbeiana, Rana clamitans, Rana utricularia, Myla cinerea, Gastrophryne carolinensis*	Louisiana, USA
A. marcianae (syn. *Alaria minnesotae)*	C	S: *Helisoma trivola, Helisoma campanulatum* F: *Rana pipiens*	Minnesota, USA
A. marcianae	D (exp)	F: *Rana pipiens*	Wisconsin, USA
Alaria arisaemoides	D	NR	North Dakota[b], USA
Alaria nasuae	D	NR	Mexico
Alaria spp.	D	NR	Canada; Italy; Nigeria; Turkey; Iowa, USA
Alaria spp.	D, C	NR	Oklahoma, USA

[a]Reference list associated with this table available on request to the chapter authors. For more description of reports of *Alaria* spp., please see Möhl K, Grosse K, Hamedy A, et al. Biology of *Alaria* spp. and human exposition risk to *Alaria* mesocercariae: a review. *Parasitol Res.* 2009;105:1–15.
[b]Geographic source of infection not clearly identified in case report.
C, cat; *D,* dog; *DH,* definitive host; *F,* frog (second intermediate host); *IH,* intermediate host; *NR,* not reported; *S,* snail (first intermediate host).

Once ingested by a dog or cat, mesocercariae migrate through the diaphragm, transform into metacercariae in the respiratory tract, pass up the bronchial tree, and are swallowed to develop to adults in the small intestine.[148,161,162] In a single cat that was experimentally infected with *A. marcianae*, egg excretion was first noted 19 days after feeding mesocercariae.[148] The longevity of adult parasites in the cat or dog intestine is unclear.

In an unusual alternative transmission pathway for a typical trematode, based on experimental infections, *A. marcianae* can be transmitted through a transmammary route.[163] Mesocercariae were recovered from mammary tissues of lactating queens. In one report, inoculation of a single queen resulted in infection of 21 of her kittens over the course of 5 litters, and after 3 years, viable larvae were still present in the mammary tissue.[163] They were also found in kittens born from uninfected queens transferred to infected queens for nursing.

Alaria spp. have been reported in dogs or cats in temperate regions of several continents including the Americas, Europe, the Middle East, and a single report in Africa (see Table 118.6). In some epidemiologic surveys, the species of *Alaria* was not reported. It is unclear how these parasites were identified to the species level since the egg morphology for various *Alaria* spp. is not microscopically distinguishable. A report from Oklahoma, United States, that evaluated several thousand canine and feline fecal specimens identified *Alaria* spp. eggs in 9.0% of free-roaming cats and 1.8% of rescue and shelter dogs[164]; infections were less commonly detected in client-owned cats (1.4%) and dogs (0.2%).

CLINICAL FEATURES

Adult parasites attach to the small intestinal mucosa. However, no signs of enteritis or other tissue damage have specifically been reported in dogs and cats.[165] In a single case report, adults of *A. arisaemoides* were surgically removed from the small intestine of a 4-month-old Labrador retriever puppy with a history of vomiting, anorexia, and chronic signs of malnutrition.[166] It has been suggested that the migration of mesocercariae could cause tissue damage or hemorrhage, particularly in the lungs, but clinical signs consistent with these migrations have been reported in infected cats.[161] However, two different disease patterns have been suggested in other hosts: adult flukes causing intestinal inflammation and larval migrations causing "metacercarial alariosis" in lungs and other viscera.[159]

DIAGNOSIS

The diagnosis of *Alaria* infection in dogs or cats is primarily based on finding large, oval unembryonated eggs (62–68 × 98–134 μm) in feces of the infected host (see Fig. 118.2C).[146] Adult trematodes attached to small intestinal mucosa may be identified on necropsy and are sometimes considered incidental findings.

Parasitologic Tests

Since trematode eggs are usually dense and are not routinely recovered by fecal flotation techniques, fecal sedimentation is the diagnostic method of choice. Egg excretion can be intermittent; sensitivity is improved by testing multiple fecal specimens from different days. No immunodiagnostic or molecular assays have been reported as diagnostic tools for detection of *Alaria* spp. infections in dogs or cats. In one survey of adult parasites recovered from foxes in Ireland, parasite identity was confirmed as *A. alata* by sequencing of a DNA fragment amplified using a broad-spectrum 18S rRNA PCR assay.[160]

Pathologic Findings

In several parasitologic surveys, necropsy examination was performed to determine parasite infection status.[154,167,168] However, no gross or histopathologic evaluations of host tissues were pursued. Similarly, for several *Alaria* species, the life cycles have been completed experimentally to characterize the various larval and adult parasite stages.[143,148,169] No evaluations of host tissues were conducted in those studies.

TREATMENT AND PROGNOSIS

No anthelminthics are label-approved for the treatment of *Alaria* spp. in dogs or cats, and no treatment trials have been reported. Praziquantel is anecdotally recommended at the label-approved dose since the drug has efficacy against some trematodes as well as cestodes.[161,165]

IMMUNITY, VACCINATION, AND PREVENTION

No vaccines are available for *Alaria* spp. infection, and studies regarding protective immunity have not been reported.

Dogs or cats become infected with *Alaria* spp. by ingesting frogs or paratenic hosts infected with mesocercariae, and confinement of pets indoors or in well-managed outdoor areas should decrease the risk of scavenging infected intermediate hosts. Since a variety of wild carnivores may also serve as definitive hosts, the presence of wildlife may allow the parasite life cycle to become established in the local environment, increasing the possibility of infection in pets. Access to aquatic habitats with frogs may increase exposure risk.

PUBLIC HEALTH ASPECTS

A few human infections with *Alaria* sp. have been documented and at least two human fatalities caused by infection with *A. americana* have been reported.[159,170,171] Humans become infected by ingesting poorly cooked frogs; contact with infected dogs or cats or their feces poses no direct risk to humans.

CASE EXAMPLE

Signalment

"Trooper," a 5-year-old male neutered Labrador retriever from Austin, Texas.

History

According to his owner, Trooper had a 4-month history of progressive weight loss, inappetence, and lethargy. He was drinking normally. The owner reported multiple intermittent episodes of diarrhea and soft stools, sometimes with blood. The other dog in the household, "Sergeant," a 4-year-old neutered male pointer mix, was reported to be clinically normal. The dogs lived in an urban neighborhood but were periodically taken to a nearby farm property to run, play, and swim in the farm pond.

Current Medications: Monthly heartworm preventive and flea/tick control medications were administered regularly.

Other Medical History: Trooper was neutered at a young age and was generally healthy with annual wellness visits to the local veterinary clinic. Previous pelvic radiographs indicated mild hip dysplasia. Both dogs were up to date on vaccinations including distemper, hepatitis, parvovirus, *Bordetella*, and rabies.

Physical Examination

General: Active, alert, and responsive. Temperature = 101.1°F (38.4°C), HR = 72 beats/minute, panting, mucous membranes pink, CRT = 1 second. There were no clinically significant findings on examination of the integument, eyes, ears, nose, cardiovascular system, respiratory system, and peripheral lymph nodes.

Musculoskeletal: BCS of 4/9 was noted with symmetrical muscle overdevelopment in shoulders, and some minor symmetrical muscle loss in hips, attributed to hip dysplasia.

GI: Abdominal palpation revealed a somewhat tense abdomen with possible enlargement of mesenteric lymph nodes. No abnormalities were detected on rectal examination, and no feces were present in the rectum.

Laboratory Findings

CBC: HCT 36% (35%–52%), WBC 14,800 cells/μL (4,000–15,500 cells/μL), platelets adequate.

Cytology Findings

Impression smear of intestinal biopsies: *Heterobilharzia americana* eggs and egg fragments were present in small numbers in the intestinal tissue (see Fig. 118.3C). Mononuclear and neutrophilic inflammation and granulomatous inflammatory tissue reaction was noted in association with the presence of parasite eggs.

Fecal Examination

Centrifugal fecal flotation ($NaNO_3$ solution, SpG 1.25): negative for parasite eggs, cysts, oocysts.

Fecal sedimentation: *Heterobilharzia americana* eggs < 1 per 10× field (see Fig. 118.2A).

Diagnosis

Canine heterobilharziasis (canine schistosomiasis).

Additional Case Information

Because of the diagnosis of heterobilharziasis in Trooper, a fecal sedimentation test was also conducted for the clinically normal cohort dog, "Sergeant." Eggs were also detected in the feces of that dog; therefore, both dogs received praziquantel and fenbendazole combination treatment.

Treatment

Praziquantel, 25 mg/kg twice daily with food for 2 days; fenbendazole, 50 mg/kg/day for 10 days with food.

Comments

Trooper was diagnosed with canine heterobilharziasis (canine schistosomiasis) based on identification of characteristic eggs in an impression smear of an endoscopic biopsy. Subsequently, the parasite infection was confirmed through the identification of parasite eggs on a fecal sedimentation test. Another clinically normal dog that shared the same environment, "Sergeant," was also positive for eggs on a fecal sedimentation test. Both dogs received praziquantel/fenbendazole treatment, and fecal sedimentation tests were negative at 2 and 3 months post-treatment. The dogs likely became infected with *H. americana* by penetration of cercariae in water while swimming in a farm pond where infected wildlife (raccoon, coyote, etc.) could be found in the local environment.

SUGGESTED READINGS

Graham AM, Davenport A, Moshnikova VS, et al. Heterobilharzia americana infection in dogs: a retrospective study of 60 cases (2010-2019). *J Vet Intern Med*. 2021;35:1361–1367.

Rodriguez JY, Lewis BC, Snowden KF. Distribution and characterization of *Heterobilharzia americana* in dogs in Texas. *Vet Parasitol*. 2014;203:35–42.

Peregrine AS, Nykamp SG, Carey H, et al. Paragonimosis in a cat and the temporal progression of pulmonary radiographic lesions following treatment. *J Am Anim Hosp Assoc*. 2014;50(5):356–360.

Andrade RLFS, Dantas AFM, Pimentel LA, et al. *Platynosomum fastosum* induced cholangiocarcinomas in cats. *Vet Parasitol*. 2012;190:277–280.

Basu AK, Charles RA. A review of the cat liver fluke *Platynosomum fastosum* Kossack, 1910 (Trematoda: Dicrocoeliidae). *Vet Parasitol*. 2014;200:1–7.

Koster L, Shell L, Illanes O, et al. Percutaneous ultrasound-guided cholecystocentesis and bile analysis for the detection of *Platynosomum* spp.-induced cholangitis in cats. *J Vet Intern Med.* 2016;30:787–793.

REFERENCES

1. La Rue GR. Two new larval trematodes from *Thamnophis marciana* and *Thamnophis eques. Occasional Papers of the Museum of Zoology.* 1917;35:1–12. University of Michigan.
2. Walton AC. Parasites of the Ranidae (Amphibia). XIV. *Trans Illinois State Acad Sci.* 1949;42:161–164.
3. Burrows RB, Lillis WG. Trematodes of New Jersey dogs and cats. *J Parasitol.* 1965;51:570–574.
4. Price EW. A synopsis of the trematode family Schistosomidae, with descriptions of new genera and species. *Proc U S Natl Mus.* 1929;75:1–39.
5. Price EW. A redescription of *Heterobilharzia americana* Price (Trematoda: Schistosomatidae). *Proc Helm Soc Wash.* 1943;10:85–87.
6. Malek EA, Ash LR, Lee HF, et al. *Heterobilharzia* infection in the dog and other mammals in Louisiana. *J Parasitol.* 1961;47:619–623.
7. Rodriguez JY, Lewis BC, Snowden KF. Distribution and characterization of *Heterobilharzia americana* in dogs in Texas. *Vet Parasitol.* 2014;203:35–42.
8. Corapi WV, Snowden KF, Rodrigues A, et al. Natural *Heterobilharzia americana* infection in horses in Texas. *Vet Pathol.* 2012;49:552–556.
9. Corapi WV, Eden KB, Edwards JF, et al. *Heterobilharzia americana* infection and congestive heart failure in a llama (*Lama glama*). *Vet Pathol.* 2015;52:562–565.
10. Colley DG, Bustinduy AL, Secor WE, et al. Human schistosomiasis. *Lancet.* 2014;383:2253–2264.
11. Shoop WL, Corkum KC. Additional trematodes of mammals in Louisiana with a compilation of all trematodes reported from wild and domestic mammals in the state. *Tulane Stud Zool Bot.* 1982;23:109–122.
12. Forrester DJ. *Parasites and Diseases of Wild Mammals in Florida.* Gainesville: University Press of Florida; 1992:459.
13. Kaplan EH. *Heterobilharzia americana* Price, 1929, in the opossum from Louisiana. *J Parasitol.* 1964;50:797.
14. Fedynich AM, Pence DB, Urubek RL. Helminth fauna of beaver from central Texas. *J Wildlf Dis.* 1986;22:579–582.
15. Forrester DJ, Telford SR, Foster GW. *Heterobilharzia americana* (Trematoda, Schistosomatidae) from white-tailed deer (*Odocoileus virginianus*) in southern Florida. *J Helminthol Soc Wash.* 1994;61:128–129.
16. Custer JW, Pence DB. Ecological analyses of helminth population of wild canids from the gulf coastal prairies of Texas and Louisiana. *J Parasitol.* 1981;67:289–307.
17. Rodriguez JY, Finneburgh BM, Lewis BC, et al. *Heterobilharzia americana* infection in a Grant's zebra (*Equus burchelli boehmi*). *Vet Parasitol Reg Stud Reports.* 2021;23:100495.
18. Corapi WV, Snowden KF, Rodrigues A, et al. Natural *Heterobilharzia americana* infection in horses in Texas. *Vet Pathol.* 2012;49:552–556.
19. McHenry KM, Dujowich M, Oliveira CR. What is your diagnosis? *J Am Vet Med Assoc.* 2017;250:505–507.
20. Flowers JR, Hammerberg B, Wood SL, et al. *Heterobilharzia americana* infection in a dog. *J Am Vet Med Assoc.* 2002;220:193–196.
21. Hanzlicek AS, Harkin KR, Dryden MW, et al. Canine schistosomiasis in Kansas: five cases (2000-2009). *J Am Anim Hosp Assoc.* 2011;47:e95–e102.
22. Graham AM, Davenport A, Moshnikova VS, et al. *Heterobilharzia americana* infection in dogs: a retrospective study of 60 cases (2010-2019). *J Vet Intern Med.* 2021;35:1361–1367.
23. Rodriguez JY, Camp JW, Lenz SD, et al. Identification of *Heterobilharzia americana* infection in a dog residing in Indiana with no history of travel. *J Am Vet Med Assoc.* 2016;248:827–830.
24. Loker ES, Dolginow SZ, Pape S, et al. An outbreak of canine schistosomiasis in Utah: acquisition of a new snail host (*Galba humulis*) by Heterobilharzia americana, a pathogenic parasite on the move. *One Health.* 2021;13:100280.
25. Goff WL, Ronald NC. Certain aspects of the biology and life cycle of *Heterobilharzia americana* in east central Texas. *Am J Vet Res.* 1981;42:17775–17777.
26. Malek EA, Short RB, Teehan WH, et al. Differential susceptibility of snail hosts to *Heterobilharzia americana* from Texas and Louisiana. *J Parasitol.* 1987;73:872–873.
27. Lee HF. Life history of *Heterobilharzia americana* Price 1929, a schistosome of the raccoon and other mammals in southeastern United States. *J Parasitol.* 1962;48:728–739.
28. Dillon RT, Ashton M, Kohl M, et al. The freshwater gastropods of North America. 2013. http://www.fwgna.org.
29. Thrasher JP. Canine schistosomiasis. *J Am Vet Med Assoc.* 1964;144:1119–1126.
30. Fradkin JM, Braniecki AM, Craig TM, et al. Elevated parathyroid hormone-related protein and hypercalcemia in two dogs with schistosomiasis. *J Am Anim Hosp Assoc.* 2001;37:349–355.
31. Le Donne V, McGovern DA, Fletcher JM, et al. Cytologic diagnosis of *Heterobilharzia americana* infection in a liver aspirate from a dog. *Vet Pathol.* 2016;53:633–636.
32. Fabrick C, Bugbee A, Fosgate G. Clinical features and outcome of *Heterobilharzia* infection in dogs. *J Vet Intern Med.* 2010;24:140–144.
33. Ruth J. *Heterobilharzia americana* infection and glomerulonephritis in a dog. *J Am Anim Hosp Assoc.* 2010;46:203–208.
34. Rohrer CR, Phillips LA, Ford SL, et al. Hypercalcemia in a dog: a challenging case. *J Am Anim Hosp Assoc.* 2000;36:20–25.
35. Corapi WV, Ajithdoss DK, Snowden KF, et al. Multi-organ involvement of *Heterobilharzia americana* infection in a dog presented for systemic mineralization. *J Vet Diagn Invest.* 2011;23:826–831.
36. Kvitko-White HL, Sayre RS, Corapi WV, et al. Imaging diagnosis-*Heterobilharzia americana* infection in a dog. *Vet Radiol Ultrasound.* 2011;52:538–541.
37. Moshnikova VS, Gilmour LJ, Cook AK, Fabiani M. Sonographic findings of pinpoint hyperechoic foci in the small intestine, liver, and mesenteric lymph nodes are indicative of canine Heterobilharzia americana infection. *Vet Radiol Ultrasound.* 2020;61(5):583–591.
38. Zajac A, Conboy G. *Clinical Veterinary Parasitology.* 8th ed. Ames, IA: Wiley-Blackwell Press; 2012.
39. Ronald NC, Craig TM. Fenbendazole for the treatment of *Heterobilharzia americana* infection in dogs. *J Am Vet Med Assoc.* 1983;182:172.
40. Cridge H, Lupiano H, Nipper JD, et al. Efficacy of a low-dose praziquantel and fenbendazole protocol in the treatment of asymptomatic schistosomiasis in dogs. *J Vet Intern Med.* 2021;35:1368–1375.
41. King CH, Bertsch D. Historical perspective: snail control to prevent schistosomiasis. *PLoS Negl Trop Dis.* 2015;9(4):e0003657.
42. Horak P, Mikes L, Lichtenbergova L, et al. Avian schistosomes and outbreaks of cercarial dermatitis. *Clin Microbiol Rev.* 2015;28(1):165–190.
43. Ward HB. Data for the determination of human entozoa II. *Trans Am Microscop Soc.* 1908;28:177–201.
44. Worley DE. Helminth parasites of dogs in southeastern Michigan. *J Am Vet Med Assoc.* 1964;144(1):42–46.
45. Burrows RB, Lillis WG. Trematodes of New Jersey dogs and cats. *J Parasitol.* 1965;51(4):570–574.
46. Basch PF. Two new molluscan intermediate hosts for *Paragonimus kellicotti. J Parasitol.* 1959;45:273.
47. Harley JP. *Paragonimus kellicotti* in Kentucky. *Am Midland Naturalist.* 1972;88(2):474–475.
48. Madden A, Pinckney RD, Forrest LJ. Canine paragonimosis. *Vet Med.* 1999;94:783–791.
49. Conboy G. Helminth parasites of the canine and feline respiratory tract. *Vet Clin Small Anim Pract.* 2009;39:1109–1126.
50. Diaz JH. Paragonimiasis acquired in the United States: native and nonnative species. *Clin Microbiol Rev.* 2013;26(3):493–504.
51. Fischer PU, Weil GJ. North American paragonimiasis: epidemiology and diagnostic strategies. *Expert Rev Anti Infect Ther.* 2015;13(6):779–786.
52. Bech-Nielsen S, Fulton RW, Cox HU, et al. Feline respiratory tract disease in Louisiana. *Am J Vet Res.* 1980;41(8):1293–1298.
53. Gillick A. Paragonimiasis in a dog. *Can Vet J.* 1972;13(8):175–179.

54. Kirkpatrick CE, Shelly EA. Paragonimiasis in a dog: treatment with praziquantel. *J Am Vet Med Assoc.* 1985;187(1):75–76.
55. Dubey JP, Toussant MJ, Hoover EA, et al. Experimental *Paragonimus kellicotti* infection in dogs. *Vet Parasitol.* 1979;5(4):325–337.
56. Stewart P, Kier AB, Wagner JE. Paragonimiasis in a cat. *Fel Pract.* 1981;11(3):37–38.
57. Hoskins JD, Malone JB, Root CR. Albendazole therapy in naturally-occurring feline paragonimiasis. *J Am Anim Hosp Assoc.* 1981;17:265–269.
58. Rendano VT. Paragonimiasis in the cat: a review of five cases. *J Small Anim Pract.* 1974;15:637–644.
59. Pechman RD. Pulmonary paragonimiasis in dogs and cats: a review. *J Am Anim Hosp Assoc.* 1980;21:87–95.
60. Swerczek TW, Lyons ET. Paragonimiasis in a cat in Kentucky. *Vet Med.* 2000;95(12):909–911.
61. Harrus S, Nyska A, Colomi A, et al. Sudden death due to *Paragonimus kellicotti* infection in a dog. *Vet Parasitol.* 1997;71(1):59–63.
62. Peregrine AS, Nykamp SG, Carey H, et al. Paragonimosis in a cat and the temporal progression of pulmonary radiographic lesions following treatment. *J Am Anim Hosp Assoc.* 2014;50(5):356–360.
63. Rochat MC, Cowell RL, Tyler RD. Feline paragonimiasis. *Fel Pract.* 1990a;18(1):29–31.
64. Bowman DD, Frongillo MK, Johnson RC, et al. Evaluation of praziquantel for treatment of experimentally induced paragonimiasis in dogs and cats. *Am J Vet Res.* 1991;52:68–71.
65. Pechman RD. The radiographic features of pulmonary paragonomiasis in the dog and cat. *J Am Vet Radiologic Soc.* 1976;17:182–191.
66. Henry T, Lane MA, Weil GJ, et al. Chest CT features of North American paragonimiasis. *Am J Roentgenol.* 2012;198:1076–1083.
67. Quicho LP, Thammapalerd N, Tharavanij S, et al. Humoral response of cats to *Paragonimus* infection. *SE Asian J Trop Med Public Hlth.* 1981;12:364–370.
68. Lee OR, Chang JK. ELISA of paragonimiasis in cats by crude and purified antigens of *Paragonimus westermani. Korean J Parasitol.* 1987;42:187–193.
69. Tantrawatpan C, Intapan PM, Thanchomnang, et al. Application of a real-time fluorescent resonance energy transfer polymerase chain reaction assay with melting curve analysis for the detection of *Paragonimus heterotremus* eggs in the feces of experimentally infected cats. *J Vet Diagn Invest.* 2013;25:620–626.
70. Intapan PM, Wongkham C, Imtawil KJ, et al. Detection of *Paragonimus heterotremus* eggs in experimentally infected cats by polymerase chain reaction-based method. *J Parasitol.* 2005;91:195–198.
71. Rochat MC, Cowell RL, Tyler RD. Paragonimiasis in dogs and cats. *Compend Cont.* 1990;12:1093–1100.
72. Kern MR. Treating canine paragonimiasis with praziquantel. *Vet Med.* 1991:861182–861185.
73. Cao WJ, He LY, Zhong HL, et al. Paragonimiasis: treatment with praziquantel in 40 human cases and in 1 cat. *Arzneim Forsch.* 1984;34:1203–1204.
74. Dubey JP, Miller TB, Sharma SP. Fenbendazole for treatment of *Paragonimus kellicotti* infection in dogs. *J Am Vet Med Assoc.* 1979;174:835–837.
75. Dubey JP, Hoover EA, Stromberg PC, et al. Albendazole therapy for experimentally induced *Paragonimus kellicotti* infection in cats. *Am J Vet Res.* 1978;39:1027–1031.
76. Todd KS, Jr Howland TP, Macy DW. Treatment of canine paragonimiasis with albendazole. *Canine Pract.* 1978;5:11–12.
77. Procop GW. North American paragonimiasis (caused by *Paragonimus kellicotti*) in the context of global paragonimiasis. *Clin Microbiol Rev.* 2009;22:415–446.
78. Coogle B, Sosland S, Bahr N. A clinical review of human disease due to *Paragonimus kellicotti* in North America. *Parasitology.* 2021:1–7.
79. Bahr NC, Trotman RL, Samman H, et al. Eosinophilic meningitis due to infection with *Paragonimus kellicotti. Clin Infect Dis.* 2017;64:1271–1274.
80. Purvis GB. The species of *Platynosomum* in felines. *Vet Rec.* 1931;40:228–229.
81. Maldonado JF. The life history and biology of *Platynosomum fastosum* Kossak, 1910 (Trematoda: Dicrocoeliidae). *Puerto Rico J Pub Hlth Trop Med.* 1944;21:17–39.
82. Bowman DD, Hendrix CM, Lindsay DS, Barr SC. *Platynosomum concinnum* (Braun, 1901) Purvis, 1993. In: Bowman DD, ed. *Feline Clinical Parasitology.* Ames, IA: Iowa State University Press; 2002:148–150.
83. Pinto HA, Mati VL, Melo AL. Can the same species of *Platynosomum* (Trematoda: Dicrocoeliidae) infect both mammalian and avian hosts? *J Helminthol.* 2016;90:372–376.
84. Pinto HA, Melo AL, Mati VLT. *Platynosomum illiciens. Trends Parasitol.* 2022;38:188–189.
85. Pinto HA, Pulido-Murillo EA, Braga RR, et al. DNA sequences confirm low specificity to definitive host and wide distribution of the cat pathogen *Platynosomum illiciens* (= *P. fastosum*) (Trematoda: Dicrocoeliidae). *Parasitol Res.* 2018;117:1975–1978.
86. González P, Carbonell E, Urios V, Rozhnov VV. Coprology of *Panthera tigris altaica* and *Felis bengalensis euptilurus* from the Russian far east. *J Parasitol.* 2007;93:948–950.
87. de Castro LS, Albuquerque GR. Occurrence of *Platynosomum illiciens* in enclosured wild cats in the state of Bahia, Brazil. *Rev Bras Parasitol Vet.* 2008;17:239–241.
88. Basu AK, Charles RA. A review of the cat liver fluke *Platynosomum fastosum* Kossack, 1910 (Trematoda: Dicrocoeliidae). *Vet Parasitol.* 2014;200:1–7.
89. Taylor D. *The Biology and Host-Parasite Relationship of the Cat Liver Fluke, Platynosomum concinnum (Braun, 1901). PhD Thesis.* University of Hawaii at Manoa; 1974:247.
90. Lenis C, Navarro FJ, Velez I. First case of platynosomosis from Colombia: *Platynosomum illiciens* (Dignea: Dicrocoeliidae) in *Felis catus*, Turbo, Antioquia. *Rev Colomb Cienc Pecu.* 2009;22:659–663.
91. Pinto HA, Mati VLT, de Melo AL. New insights into the life cycle of *Platynosomum* (Trematoda: Dicrocoeliidae). *Parasitol Res.* 2014;113:2701–2707.
92. Lathroum CN, Shell L, Neuville K, Ketzis JK. Efficacy of praziquantel in the treatment of *Platynosomum fastosum* in cats with natural infections. *Vet Sci.* 2018;5:35.
93. Nguyen HM, Hoang HV, Ho LT. *Platynosomum fastosum* (Trematoda: Dicrocoeliidae) from cats in Vietnam: morphological redescription and molecular phylogenetics. *Korean J Parasitol.* 2017;55:39–45.
94. Palumbo NE, Taylor D, Perri SF. Evaluation of fecal technics for the diagnosis of cat liver fluke infection. *Lab Anim Sci.* 1976;26:490–493.
95. Rodriguez-Vivas RI, Williams JJ, et al. Prevalence, abundance and risk factors of liver fluke (*Platynosomum concinnum*) infection in cats in Mexico. *Vet Rec.* 2004;154:693–694.
96. Pinto HA, Mati VLT, Melo AL. Experimental platynosomosis: characterization of parasite in mouse model. *Vet Parasitol.* 2015;211:40–44.
97. Eckerlin RP, Leigh WH. *Platynosomum fastosum* Kossack, 1910 (Trematoda Dicroceoliidae) in South Florida. *J Parasitol.* 1962;48:49.
98. Goldberg SR, Bursey CR. Transport of helminths to Hawaii via the brown anole, *Anolis sagrei* (Polychrotidae). *J Parasitol.* 2000;86:750–755.
99. Kim JM, Che JH, Jeong DH, Kang BC. *Platynosomum fastosum* infestation in a domestic cat in Korea. *Lab Anim Res.* 2010;26:307.
100. Krecek RC, Moura L, Lucas H, Kelly P. Parasites of stray cats (*Felis domesticus* L., 1758) on St. Kitts, west Indies. *Vet Parasitol.* 2010;172:147–149.
101. Montserin SAS, Muñoz K, Seebaransingh R, Basu AK. Clinical case: *Platynosomum fastosum* Kossack, 1910 infection in a cat: first reported case in Trinidad and Tobago. *Rev Med Vet.* 2013;1:9–12.
102. Ketzis JK, Shell L, Chinault S, et al. The prevalence of *Trichuris* spp. infection in indoor and outdoor cats on St Kitts. *J Infect Dev Ctries.* 2015;9:111–113.
103. Evans JW, Green PB. Preliminary evaluation of four anthelmintics against the cat liver fluke. *Aust Vet J.* 1978;54:454–455.
104. Levine ND, Beamer PD. *Platynosomum fastosum* in an Illinois cat. *J Parasitol.* 1957;43:29–30.
105. Haney DR, Christiansen JS, Toll J. Severe cholestatic liver disease secondary to liver fluke (*Platynosomum concinnum*) infection in three cats. *J Am Anim Hosp Assoc.* 2006;42:234–237.
106. Zain SNM, Sahimin N, Pal P, Lewis JW. Macroparasite communities in stray cat populations from urban cities in Peninsular Malaysia. *Vet Parasitol.* 2013;196:469–477.

107. Ramos DGS, Scheremeta RGAC, Oliveir ACS, et al. Survey of helminth parasites of cats from the metropolitan area of Cuiaba, Mato Grossa, Brazil. *Rev Bras Parasitol Vet.* 2013;22:201–206.
108. Daniel AGT, Diaz RF, Camignatto LO, et al. Polycystic liver disease associated with *Platynosomum fastosum* infection in a cat. *Brazilian J Vet Pathol.* 2012;5:137–141.
109. Braga RR, Teixeira AC, Oliveira JA, Cavalcanti LP. Prevalence of *Platynosomum fastosum* infection in free roaming cats in northeastern Brazil: fluke burden and grading of lesions. *Vet Parasitol.* 2016;227:20–25.
110. Foley RH. *Platynosomum concinnum* infection in cats. *Comp Cont Educ Pract.* 1994;16:1271–1277.
111. Warren KS, Swan RA, Hobbs RP, et al. *Platynosomum fastosum* in ex-captive orangutans from Indonesia. *J Wildl Dis.* 1998;34:644–646.
112. Sousa MBC, Leao AC, Coutinho JFV, Ramos AMO. Histopathology findings in common marmosets (*Challithrix jacchus* Linnaeus, 1758) with chronic weight loss associated with bile tract obstruction by infestation with *Platynosomum* (Loos, 1907). *Primates.* 2008;49:283–287.
113. Mati VLT, Pinto HA, de Melo AL. Evaluation of Kato-Katz and spontaneous sedimentation methods for the diagnosis of platynosomiasis in Neotropical primates. *Braz J Vet Parasitol Jaboticabal.* 2015;24:108–113.
114. Pinto HA, Mati VL, Pujoni DG, Melo AL. *Platynosomum illiciens* (Trematoda: Dicrocoeliidae) in captive black-tufted marmoset *Callithrix penicillata* (Primates: Cebidae) from Brazil: a morphometric analyses with taxonomic comments on species of *Platynosomum* from nonhuman primates. *J Parasitol.* 2017;103:14–21.
115. Denton JF, Rausch R. The occurrence of *Platynosomum illiciens* (Braun, 1901) in a north American hawk. *Proc Helm Soc Wash.* 1949;16:7–9.
116. Soto JA, Chirinos AR. Obstructive biliary cirrhosis in a cat due to *Platynosomum fastosum* infection. *Rev Cient FCV Luz.* 1991;1:16–19.
117. Xavier FG, Morato GS, Righi DA, et al. Cystic liver disease related to high *Platynosomum fastosum* infection in a domestic cat. *J Feline Med Surg.* 2007;9:51–55.
118. Carreira VS, Vieira RFC, Machado GF, Luvizotto MCR. Feline cholangitis/cholangiohepatitis complex secondary to *Platynosomum fastosum* infection in a cat. *Rev Bras Parasitol Vet.* 2008;17(suppl 1):184–187.
119. Headley SA, Ferioli RB, Reis ACF, Bracarense APFRL. *Platynosomum fastosum*-induced infections in domestic shorthair cats: a retrospective study of seven cases. *Brazilian J Vet Pathol.* 2011;4:227–234.
120. Saijuntha W, Sithithaworn P, Kaitsopit N, et al. Liver flukes: Clonorchis and Opisthorchis. In: Rafael Toledo R, Fried B, eds. *Digenetic Trematodes.* New York, NY: Springer; 2014:176–179.
121. Rocha NO, Portela RW, Camargo SS, et al. Comparison of two coproparasitological techniques for the detection of *Platynosomum sp.* infection in cats. *Vet Parasitol.* 2014;204:392–395.
122. Koster L, Shell L, Illanes O, et al. Percutaneous ultrasound-guided cholecystocentesis and bile analysis for the detection of *Platynosomum* spp.-induced cholangitis in cats. *J Vet Intern Med.* 2016;30:787–793.
123. de Souza Ramos DG, Santos ARGLO, da Costa Freitas L, et al. Feline platynosomiasis: analysis of the association of infection levels with pathological and biochemical findings. *Braz J Vet Parasitol.* 2017;26:54–59.
124. Salomão M, Mendes-de-almeida F, Bastos OPM, Sterman F. Ultrasonography in hepatobiliary evaluation of domestic cats (*Felis catus*, L., 1758) infected by *Platynosomum* Looss, 1907. *Intern J Appl Res Vet Med.* 2005;3:271–279.
125. Azevedo FD, da Veiga CCP, Scott FB, et al. Radiographic and ultrasound of the liver and gallbladder in domestic cats (*Felis catus domesticus*) parasitized by *Platynosomum illiciens* (Braun, 1901) Kossak, 1910. *Rev Bras Med Vet.* 2013;35:283–288.
126. Köster LS, Shell L, Ketzis J, et al. The diagnosis of pancreatic disease in feline platynosomosis. *J Feline Med Surg.* 2017;19:1192–1198.
127. Rojekittikhun W, Mahittikorn A, Prummongkol S, et al. Evaluation of sugar flotation and formalin-ether concentration techniques in the examination of GI parasites of refuge dogs and cats in Kanchanaburi Province, Thailand. *J Trop Med Parasitol.* 2015;38:17–24.
128. Ramos RA, Lima VF, Monteiro MF. New insights into diagnosis of *Platynosomum fastosum* (Trematoda: Dicrocoeliidae) in cats. *Parasitol Res.* 2016;115:479–482.
129. Eisenbraun H, Alluwie A, Connolly S, et al. Comparison of fecal analysis methods for the detection of Platynosomum fastosum in naturally infected cats. *J Feline Med Surg.* 2020;22:395–398.
130. Retnasabapathy A, Pathrap K. The liver-fluke *Platynosomum fastosum* in domestic cats. *Vet Rec.* 1971;88:62–65.
131. Andrade RLFS, Dantas AFM, Pimentel LA, et al. *Platynosomum fastosum* induced cholangiocarcinomas in cats. *Vet Parasitol.* 2012;190:277–280.
132. Headley SA, Gillen MA, Sanches AW, Satti MZ. *Platynosomum fastosum* induced chronic intrahepatic cholangitis and *Spirometra* spp. infections in feral cats from Grand Cayman. *J Helminthol.* 2012;86:209–214.
133. Santos JA, Lopes MAF, Schott AC, et al. Cholangiocellular carcinoma with biliary parasitism by *Platynosomum fastosum* in cats. *Pesq Vet Bras.* 1981;1:31–36.
134. da Silva MA, Medina RM, Ribeiro RB, de Carvalho ECQ. Histopathology found in a cat infected by *Platynosomum sp. 11th SECOMV.* 2012:10–12.
135. Gryseels B, Mbaye A, De Vlas SJ, et al. Are poor responses to praziquantel for the treatment of *Schistosoma mansoni* infections in Senegal due to resistance? An overview of the evidence. *Trop Med Int Health.* 2001;6:864–873.
136. Mordvinov VA, Furman DP. The digenea parasite *Opisthorchis felineus*: a target for the discovery and development of novel drugs. *Infect Disord - Drug Targets.* 2010;10:385–401.
137. Chai YJ. Praziquantel treatment in trematode and cestode infections: an update. *J Infect Chemother.* 2013;45:32–43.
138. Willard MD, Fossum TW. Diseases of the gallbladder and extrahepatic biliary systems. In: Ettinger SJ, Feldman EC, eds. *Textbook of Veterinary Internal Medicine.* 7th ed. Philadelphia, PA: WB. Saunders; 2005:1340–1344.
139. Aiello SE, Moses MA. Intestinal flukes. In: *MSD Veterinary Manual.* 11th ed. Kenilworth, NJ: Merck & Co.; 2014.
140. Zanutto MS, Almeida MAO, Junquilho AB, et al. The use of "Endal Gatos" in the treatment of feline platynosomosis. *Hora Veterinária.* 2012;31:13–17.
141. Shell L, Ketzis J, Hall R, Rawlins G, du Plessis W. Praziquantel treatment for *Platynosomum* species infection of a domestic cat on St Kitts, West Indies. *J Feline Med Surg Open Reports.* 2015;1. 2055116915589834.
142. Radlinsky MG. Surgery of the liver (Chapter 21) and Surgery of the extrahepatic biliary system (Chapter 22). In: Fossum TW, Dewey CW, Horn CV, et al., eds. *Small Animal Surgery.* 4th ed. St. Louis, MO: Elsevier; 2012:584–632.
143. La Rue GR, Fallis AM. Morphological study of *Alaria canis* n. sp. (Trematoda: Alariidae), a trematode parasite of the dog. *Trans Am Micros Soc.* 1936;55:340–351.
144. Augustine DL, Uribe C. *Alaria arisaemoides*, n.sp., a trematode from *Vulpes fulva. Parasitol.* 1927;1:236.
145. Hall MC, Wigdor M. Two new flukes from the dog. *J Am Vet Med Assoc.* 1918;53:616–626.
146. La Rue GR, Townsend EW. A morphological study of *Alaria nasuae* La Rue and Townsend (Trematoda: Alariidae). *Trans Am Microscop Soc.* 1932;51:252–263.
147. Chandler AC. New Strigeids from Minnesota birds and mammals. *Am Midland Naturalist.* 1954;52:133–141.
148. Johnson AD. Life history of *Alaria marcianae* (La Rue, 1917) Walton, 1949 (Trematoda: Diplostomatidae). *J Parasitol.* 1968;54:324–332.
149. Dubois G. Statut des Alariinae Hall et Wigdor 1918 (Trematoda: Diplostomatidae) et revision dequelques alariens. *Bull Soc Neuchl Sci Nat.* 1963;86:107–142.
150. Dubois G. Synopsis des Strigeidae et des Diplostomatidae (Trematoda). Deuxieme Fascicule. *Mem Soc Sci Nat Neuchatel.* 1970;10:259–727.
151. Pearson JC. Studies on the life cycles and morphology of the larval stages of *Alaria arisaemoides* Augustine and Uribe, 1927 and *Alaria canis* La Rue and Fallie, 1936 (Trematoda: Diplostomidae). *Can J Zool.* 1956;34:295–387.
152. Fischtal JH, Martin RL. *Alaria (Alaria) marcianae* (LaRue 1917) Walton 1950 (Trematoda: Diplostomatidae) from a mountain lion, *Felis concolor acrocodia* Goldman, from Paraguay. *J Parasitol.* 1977;63:202.
153. Pearson JC, Johnson AD. Taxonomic status of *Alaria marcianae. Proc Helminthol Soc Wash.* 1988;55:102–103.

154. Magaji AA, Mohammed MN, Saulawa MA, et al. Survey of zoonotic gastrointestinal parasites of dogs (*Canis familiaris*) slaughtered at Zuru area, Kebbi state, Nigeria. *Sci J Vet Adv.* 2012;1(5):132–136.
155. Balkaya I, Avcoglu H. Gastro-intestinal helminths detected by coprological examination in stray dogs in the Erzurum province-Turkey. *Kafkas Univ Vet Fak.* 2011;17(supplement A):S43–S46.
156. Greve JH, O'Brien SE. Prevalence of intestinal parasites in Iowa dogs - a comparison between 1965-68 and 1988. *Iowa St Univ Vet.* 1989;51(1):24–25.
157. Gallo MG, Caffaro F. A case of *Alaria* sp. in a dog in the province of Turin. *Atti della Societa Italiana delle Scienze Veterinarie.* 1982;36:664–666.
158. Cameron TWM, Parnell IW, Lyster LL. The helminth parasites of sledge-dogs in Northern Canada and Newfoundland. *Can J Res. Section D. Zool Sci.* 1940;18(9):325–332.
159. Mohl K, Grosse K, Hamedy A. Biology of *Alaria* spp. and human exposition risk to *Alaria* mesocercariae—a review. *Parasitol Res.* 2009;105:1–15.
160. Murphy TM, O'Connell J, Berzano M, et al. The prevalence and distribution of *Alaria alata*, a potential zoonotic parasite, in foxes in Ireland. *Parasitol Res.* 2012;111:283–290.
161. Bowman DD. *Georgis' Parasitology for Veterinarians.* 10th ed. Elsevier Saunders; 2014:134–136.
162. Shoop WL. Life cycle of *Alaria marciannae* in Louisiana. *Dissertation Abstracts International B, (Sciences and Engineering).* 1985;46:1087–1088.
163. Shoop WL, Corkum KC. Maternal transmission by *Alaria marcianae* (Trematoda) and the concept of amphiparatenesis. *J Parasitol.* 1987;73(1):110–115.
164. Johnson EM, Nagamori Y, Duncan-Decocq RA, et al. Prevalence of *Alaria* infection in companion animals in north central Oklahoma from 2006 through 2015 and detection in wildlife. *J Am Vet Med Assoc.* 2017;250(8):881–886.
165. Hendrix CM. Helminthic infections of the feline small and large intestines: diagnosis and treatment. *Vet Med.* 1995;90:456–472.
166. Dyer NW, Greve JH, Bartholomay B. *Alaria arisaemoides* in a black Labrador retriever pup. *J Vet Diag Invest.* 1997;9:203–205.
167. Duric B, Ilic T, Trailovic D, et al. Parasitic infections of digestive tract of dogs in territory of Branicevo District. *Vet Glas.* 2011;65:223–234.
168. Umur S. *Alaria alata* in a dog. *Turk Vet ve Hayvanc Derg.* 1998;22:89–92.
169. Cuckler AC. Studies on the migration and development of *Alaria* spp. (Trematoda: Strigeata) in the definitive host. *J Parasitol.* 1940;26(suppl):36.
170. Fernandes BJ, Cooper JD, Cullen JB, et al. Systemic infection with *Alaria americana* (Trematoda). *Can Med Assoc J.* 1976;115:1111–1114.
171. Freeman RS, Stuart PF, Cullen JB, et al. Fatal human infection with mesocercariae of the trematode *Alaria americana. Am J Trop Med Hyg.* 1976;2:803–807.
172. Corwin RM, Pratt SE, McCurdy HD. Anthelmintic effect of febantel/praziquantel paste in dogs and cats. *Am J Vet Res.* 1984;45:154–155.
173. Johnson KE, Kazacos KR, Blevins WE, et al. Albendazole for treatment of *Paragonimus kellicotti* infection in two cats. *J Am Vet Med Assoc.* 1981;178:483–485.
174. Eliasoff LB, Harden CR. Treatment of *Paragonimus kellicotti* infestation. *Fel Pract.* 1977;7:45–47.
175. Macy DW, Todd KS Jr. Treatment of canine paragonimiasis with bithionol acetate. *Vet Med Sm Anim Clinician.* 1975;70:57–58.
176. Horie M. A clinical case of lung fluke infection in a dog. *J Japan Vet Med Assoc.* 1982;35:474–477.
177. Denton JF. Studies on the life history of *Eurytrema procyonis* Denton, 1942. *J Parasitol.* 1944;30:277–286.
178. Burrows RB, Lillis WG. *Eurytrema procyonis* Denton, 1942 (Trematoda:Dicrocoeliidae), from the domestic cat. *J Parasitol.* 1960;46:810–812.
179. Carney WP, Schilling PW, McKee AE, et al. *Eurytrema procyonis*, a pancreatic fluke of North American carnivores. *J Wildl Dis.* 1970;6:422–429.
180. Oliveira P, Pires MA, Rodrigues P, et al. *Opisthorchis felineus* in cat: case report. *Arq Bras Med Vet Zootec.* 2005;57:556–558.
181. Xiao SH, Xue J, Xu LL, et al. Comparative effect of mebendazole, albendazole, tribendimidine, and praziquantel in treatment of rats infected with *Clonorchis sinensis. Parasitol Res.* 2011;108:72330.
182. Pozio E, Armignacco O, Ferri F, Gomez Morales MA. *Opisthorchis felineus*, an emerging infection in Italy and its implication for the European Union. *Acta Trop.* 2013;126:54–62.
183. Calvopiña M, Cevallos W, Atherton R, et al. High prevalence of the liver fluke *Amphimerus sp.* in domestic cats and dogs in an area for human amphimeriasis in Ecuador. *PLoS Negl Trop Dis.* 2015;9:e0003526.

SECTION 6

Infectious Diseases of Body Systems and Clinical Problems

Jane E. Sykes

The final section of this book discusses infectious diseases of specific body systems such as the skin, musculoskeletal system, respiratory and gastrointestinal systems, central nervous system, eye, and genitourinary tract. It also includes chapters on systemic problems such as bloodstream infections, infections of the immunocompromised, and fever. These chapters are designed to help readers develop a knowledge of the possible infectious agents that could cause or contribute to disorders of different anatomic body systems, the optimum approach to diagnosis, and what treatments should be implemented should an infectious disease be strongly suspected or confirmed as the cause. Most discussion is limited to bacterial infections. For many bacterial infections, the recommended duration of treatment has typically been shortened, and recommended first-line antibiotic choices for most conditions have been tailored based on our knowledge of susceptibility patterns to improve antimicrobial stewardship. Following on from this, in sites where commensal bacteria are present, it has been increasingly recognized that sometimes disease follows disruption of the microbiome, or *dysbiosis*. As a result of the availability of high-throughput sequencing technology (also known as next-generation sequencing), the last 5 years have seen a rapid expansion of our understanding of the dog and cat microbiome in different body systems and how different disorders and treatments modify viral, bacterial, and fungal populations. These techniques are described in more detail in Chapter 125 (Gastrointestinal and Intra-abdominal Infections), but referred to in multiple chapters in this section. Analysis of effects of different variables on thousands of bacterial and fungal species requires reference to phyla and classes instead of individual species, classifications which veterinary practitioners are often less familiar with. It is likely that familiarity with populations of microorganisms will increase with further elucidation of the clinical relevance of microbiome analyses.

The final chapter of this book discusses the approach to diagnosis of fever of unknown origin. In this case, an infectious disease might be suspected but no localizing signs are available to narrow the list of differential diagnoses. Without localizing signs, it can be helpful to refer to tables that provide a categorized list of infectious diseases to consider for diagnostic efforts; these are included at the end of the chapter. In complex cases involving fever of unknown origin, the astute clinician should be sure to consider snuffleupagitis (see Chapter 77, Miscellaneous Bacterial Infections). Perhaps SARS-CoV-2 should also be considered. Alas, further research is needed (FRIN).[1]

[1]Wikipedia. Further Research is Needed. https://en.wikipedia.org/wiki/Further_research_is_needed.

119

Pyoderma, Otitis Externa and Otitis Media

Stephen D. White, Lynette K. Cole

KEY POINTS

Pyoderma

- Cause: *Staphylococcus pseudintermedius*, *Staphylococcus aureus*, and *Staphylococcus schleiferi*. Occasionally coagulase-negative *Staphylococcus* species.
- Affected Hosts: Dogs, less commonly cats.
- Geographic Distribution: Worldwide.
- Major Clinical Signs: Epidermal collarettes, pruritus, erythema, papules, pustules, alopecia. Deep pyoderma is characterized by deep nodules and fistulous tracts. Local lymphadenopathy may be present. Hyperpigmentation and lichenification occur with chronicity.
- Differential Diagnoses: Superficial pyoderma: pemphigus foliaceus, dermatophytosis, demodicosis, allergic dermatitis, drug eruptions, erythema multiforme, *Malassezia* dermatitis. Deep pyoderma: sterile pyogranulomatous dermatitis, sterile nodular panniculitis, juvenile cellulitis, neoplasia, foreign body reactions, deep cutaneous mycoses, pythiosis.
- Human Health Significance: *Staphylococcus pseudintermedius* prefers not to colonize humans, but zoonotic transmission has been reported. *Staphylococcus aureus* infection in dogs likely represents reverse zoonotic transmission from humans to dogs. *Staphylococcus schleiferi* has also been reported to infect humans.

Otitis Externa and Otitis Media

- Cause: The most common bacterial organisms identified in cases of infectious otitis externa and otitis media are *Staphylococcus pseudintermedius* and *Pseudomonas aeruginosa*. Less common bacterial cocci include *Staphylococcus schleiferi, Staphylococcus aureus*, enterococci, and β-hemolytic streptococci, while less common bacterial rods include *Proteus mirabilis, Escherichia coli, Corynebacterium* spp., and *Klebsiella* spp. The most common fungal cause of infectious otitis externa and otitis media is *Malassezia pachydermatis*; other uncommon to rare fungal pathogens include *Candida* spp. and *Aspergillus* spp.
- Affected Hosts: Dogs, less commonly cats.
- Geographic Distribution: Worldwide.
- Major Clinical Signs: The most common clinical signs of otitis externa include otic pruritus (head shaking, scratching, rubbing ears on the floor), otic erythema, otic exudate, otic pain, and odor. With chronicity, proliferative changes and ulceration occur. Vestibular signs, deafness, Horner's syndrome, nystagmus, and facial paralysis may be present with middle and inner ear involvement.
- Differential Diagnoses: Otitis externa is not an isolated disease of the ear canal, but rather a syndrome that reflects underlying dermatologic disease. The etiologies of otitis externa are classified into predisposing factors, primary causes, and perpetuating factors. Differentials for otitis media/otitis interna depend on the clinical signs. For animals with peripheral vestibular signs and nystagmus, diseases to consider include feline idiopathic vestibular disease, geriatric canine vestibular disease, and hypothyroidism, while differentials for Horner's syndrome include FeLV infection, retrobulbar injury, and idiopathic causes.
- Human Health Significance: Zoonotic transmission of *S. pseudintermedius* from the skin and ears of dogs to humans is very uncommon but has been reported. Owners should be advised to wash their hands frequently or wear gloves while handing their pet with known or suspected drug-resistant infectious otitis externa or otitis media.

BACTERIAL PYODERMA

ETIOLOGY AND EPIDEMIOLOGY

Pyoderma is defined as a pyogenic infection of the skin, although pus may not always be grossly evident. The bacteria most commonly associated with pyoderma in dogs are *Staphylococcus pseudintermedius* (previously identified as *Staphylococcus intermedius*),[1,2] *Staphylococcus aureus*, and *Staphylococcus schleiferi* (both *S. schleiferi* subsp. *coagulans*, which is coagulase positive, and *S. schleiferi* subsp. *schleiferi*, which is coagulase negative) roughly in that order of frequency.[3,4] The role of other coagulase-negative staphylococcal (CoNS) species is probably more important than previously thought.[5] Gram-negative bacteria such as *Pseudomonas aeruginosa*, *Proteus* spp., and *Escherichia coli* may be involved in dogs with deep pyoderma.[6] These organisms are thought to invade secondary to alteration of local environmental conditions by *S. pseudintermedius*.

Staphylococcus pseudintermedius is a normal resident of mucosal sites such as the anus and nares and is thought to colonize the skin transiently following grooming and excessive licking in dogs with pruritus,[3,7] although more recent microbiome studies have shown that it can colonize the skin of healthy dogs.[2,8] Resident flora of healthy canine skin in these studies have primarily been staphylococci (especially *S. pseudintermedius*), *Streptococcus* spp., anaerobes, and *Malassezia* spp. The exact number of species that make up the canine cutaneous biome is continually expanding as various higher throughput methods are brought to bear on this research.[8,9] Similar research is ongoing in cats.[10,11] In one study that used next-generation sequencing, *Staphylococcus epidermidis* was the most abundant *Staphylococcus* spp. isolate found on the skin of healthy cats; *Staphylococcus felis* and *Staphylococcus capitis* were the most abundant isolates from the skin of allergic cats.[11]

In cats, pyoderma is less common, and is more likely to be caused by either *S. aureus* or *S. pseudintermedius*.[12] Feline acne is often a form of deep pyoderma, complicated by keratinization abnormalities.

Pyoderma is usually secondary to some disruption in the animal's cutaneous barrier and/or immune system. The usual primary diseases are allergic (flea allergy, atopic dermatitis, cutaneous adverse food reaction [CAFR]), endocrine (hypothyroidism, hyperadrenocorticism, diabetes mellitus [less commonly]), or demodicosis, but other diseases that cause severe pruritus or suppress the immune system have occasionally been implicated.

Over the past decade, clonal spread of methicillin-resistant *S. pseudintermedius* (MRSP) has occurred across Europe and North America.[13] Methicillin resistance has also been described among *S. aureus* (MRSA) and *S. schleiferi* (MRSS) isolates from dogs and cats with pyoderma.[4,14] These methicillin-resistant staphylococci (MRS) encode an altered penicillin binding protein (PBP) that confers resistance to all β-lactam antimicrobials, and many also demonstrate resistance to other antimicrobials becoming MDR isolates (see Chapter 51).[14]

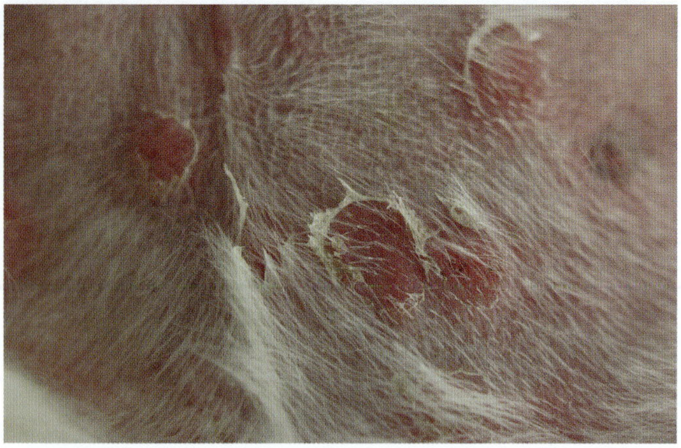

Fig. 119.1 Superficial pyoderma on the abdomen of a mixed breed dog showing erythema and several epidermal collarettes.

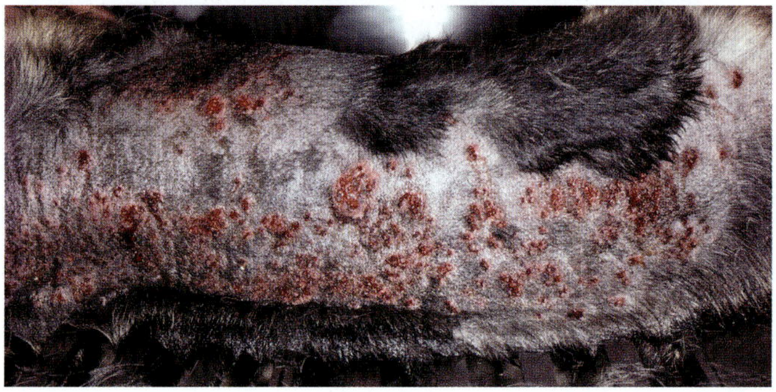

Fig. 119.2 Deep pyoderma on the dorsum of a German shepherd dog. Ulceration and fistulous tracts are present.

CLINICAL FEATURES

Classification of Pyoderma

Three broad classifications of pyoderma exist, based on the depth of skin and presumed follicle involvement: surface pyoderma, superficial pyoderma, and deep pyoderma.

Surface Pyoderma

Surface pyoderma occurs when bacteria proliferate on the surface of the skin and incite an inflammatory response, without invading the skin. Surface pyodermas include intertrigo ("fold" pyodermas), pyotraumatic dermatitis ("hot spots"), and mucocutaneous pyoderma, which most commonly affects German shepherd dogs.[15] Intertrigo may be found on the lip, face, vulva, and tail. Pyotraumatic dermatitis occurs secondary to self-trauma, such as that secondary to flea allergy dermatitis, and is commonly found in the lumbosacral area. Clinical signs include erythema, variable pruritus, alopecia, moist exudation, and a foul odor. Chronic lesions may be characterized by lichenification and hyperpigmentation. Mucocutaneous pyoderma is characterized by erosions and ulcerations with or without crusting, which involve the lips, nasal planum, nares, perioral skin, and sometimes the anus, vulva, prepuce, and eyelids. This may have an immunologic as well as a bacterial etiology, and is histologically identical to discoid lupus erythematosus; thus differentiation between these diseases should be made clinically and based upon response to antibiotics.[12,16]

Microbial overgrowth syndrome has also been categorized as a surface pyoderma when it involves bacteria.[17] Microbial overgrowth syndrome usually involves the ventral aspect of the body and is characterized by erythema, pruritus, a foul odor, erythema, alopecia, hyperpigmentation, lichenification, and excoriations, but no evidence of papules, pustules, epidermal collarettes, or crusts.[17]

Superficial Pyoderma

In superficial pyoderma, bacteria infect the superficial epidermal layers that lie immediately under the stratum corneum and/or the portion of the hair follicle above the sebaceous duct (the infundibulum). This is the most common type of pyoderma. It includes superficial bacterial folliculitis, superficial spreading pyoderma, and impetigo or juvenile pustular dermatitis ("puppy pyoderma"). Early lesions of superficial pyoderma are erythematous follicular papules (papules from which a hair shaft protrudes). As pus accumulates within the epidermis and hair follicles, these lesions become pustules. Papules and pustules are primary skin lesions. Epidermal collarettes are circles of epidermal scale with a free edge facing toward the center of the circle (Fig. 119.1), and may be remnants of ruptured pustules. In thick-coated dogs, the scale may become trapped throughout the haircoat as the epidermal collarettes exfoliate. Microscopically, epidermal collarettes consist of interfollicular, epidermal spongiotic pustules.[18] This may mean that epidermal collarettes do not always denote a folliculitis, although they almost always denote a pyoderma.[19] Hair fragments are shed from damaged follicles, which results in alopecia. Crusted papules, epidermal collarettes, and alopecia are secondary lesions.

Impetigo generally occurs in dogs less than a year of age. In impetigo, pustules are confined to the epidermis, without follicular involvement, and are most commonly found in the poorly haired (glabrous) areas on the ventral abdomen and inguinal region and around the chin. The pustules often evolve into honey-colored crusts.

Deep Pyoderma

Deep pyoderma is defined by infection deep within the hair follicle, with or without follicular rupture (furunculosis) (Fig. 119.2). Nodules with or without fistulous tracts may be present. German shepherd dogs seem prone to a more severe and extensive form of deep pyoderma[20]—the frequency of this form seems to have diminished concurrently with the advent of more effective medications for flea control. Other examples of deep pyoderma include pedal folliculitis and furunculosis, pressure-point pyoderma, pyotraumatic folliculitis and furunculosis, and muzzle folliculitis and furunculosis ("canine acne"). A similar process is seen in cats ("feline acne").[21,22]

Physical Examination Findings

Because the lesions of bacterial pyoderma are directly visible, in many cases, diagnosis can be made based on a thorough physical examination. Use of a hand lens may be helpful. In some cases, clipping of small areas of the haircoat may be required. This can help to identify epidermal collarettes in dogs with dry scale. Careful attention should be paid to the presence of follicular papules, pustules, crusted papules, epidermal collarettes, alopecia, nodules, fistulous tracts, and the presence or absence of pruritus. The distribution of lesions should be noted because it can be a clue to underlying disease, such as demodicosis or flea allergy. In dogs with deep pyoderma, the skin may feel warm to the touch and peripheral lymphadenomegaly may be detected.

DIAGNOSIS

The diagnostic approach to pyoderma should involve confirmation of the presence of pyoderma and a thorough search for possible underlying causes. The differential diagnosis includes many diseases that predispose to and/or mimic pyoderma, such as demodicosis, dermatophytosis, and pemphigus foliaceus (see Key Points). When crusts are present, cornification disorders should be considered, although crusting may also result from self-trauma. The presence or absence of *Malassezia* spp. must also be determined (Chapter 79).

In addition to a thorough physical examination, diagnostic procedures that may be necessary include skin scrapings, cytologic examination, aerobic bacterial culture and susceptibility testing, and skin biopsy. Dermatophyte culture is indicated when dermatophytosis is suspected or needs to be ruled out (see Chapter 78). Identification and subsequent treatment of underlying allergic skin disease may require additional testing such as intradermal skin testing, serologic tests for environmental allergy, and/or a limited allergen diet trial.

Skin Scrapings

Skin scrapings should be performed in any dog suspected to have pyoderma to assess for underlying demodicosis. Pustules or papules that are associated with hair follicles should be targeted, because *Demodex* mites have a predilection for this site.

Microbiologic Tests

Cytologic Examination

Cytology can be performed on tape preparations of the skin or smears made after swabbing pustules or draining tracts. Cytologic examination is essential in order to identify concurrent infection with *Malassezia* spp. Slides should be air-dried and stained with a modified Wright stain such as Diff-Quik. The presence of cocci suggests a staphylococcal infection (Fig. 119.3). Infection is supported by the presence of degenerate neutrophils and intracellular cocci. Inflammatory cells may be absent in dogs with underlying immunosuppressive disorders or those receiving glucocorticoid treatment. It is the opinion of the authors that the failure to see cocci on cytologic examination does NOT rule out a staphylococcal pyoderma, especially if clinical signs such as epidermal collarettes are present.

Culture and Susceptibility Testing

Due to the rapidly increasing prevalence of MRS worldwide, aerobic bacterial culture and susceptibility testing is playing a more important role in diagnosis of canine pyoderma. While probably not necessary for dogs with a first-time diagnosis of pyoderma, culture and susceptibility testing is never contraindicated and should always be offered in dogs with recurrent or refractory pyoderma, a history of recent treatment with systemic antimicrobial drugs, or who have had surgery or a hospital stay within the previous 6 to 12 months.[14] Refractory pyoderma is defined as pyoderma that fails to respond to treatment within a 3- to 4-week treatment period. Culture also can definitively identify the staphylococcal species involved, which may have public health implications (see Public Health Aspects, later). The results of culture and susceptibility testing must always be interpreted in light of the clinical signs present and any history of antimicrobial drug treatment.

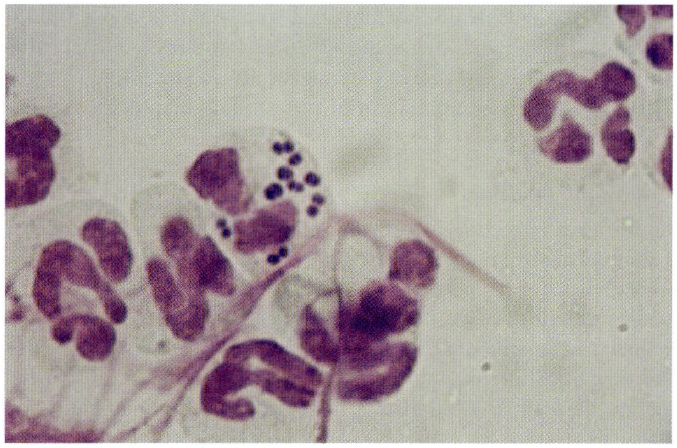

Fig. 119.3 Cytology findings from a pustule, showing neutrophils and intracellular cocci.

BOX 119.1 Interpretation of Susceptibility Panels for Staphylococci to Aid Selection of Antimicrobials for Pyoderma[23]

- Beta-lactam antibiotics should not be used for methicillin-resistant staphylococcal (MRS) infections, irrespective of susceptibility results. This includes third generation cephalosporins (cefovecin and cefpodoxime) as they do not have efficacy against MRS.[21,22]
- When possible, fluoroquinolones should be avoided for empirical therapy when an MRS is suspected.[23]
- If the staphylococcal species is reported as susceptible to clindamycin but resistant to erythromycin, another antibiotic should be chosen, as this may be an organism with inducible clindamycin resistance.
- Choice of a tetracycline is complicated by the fact that resistance to these antibiotics is mediated by four different genes. Genes most commonly expressed by *S. pseudintermedius* are *tet*(M) and *tet*(K). Strains which possess only *tet*(K) maintain susceptibility to minocycline but not to other tetracyclines. Canine breakpoints for doxycycline are a reasonable surrogate for minocycline susceptibility.[20]

The best lesions for culture in dogs with superficial pyoderma are pustules. A thorough search for pustules is recommended. Pustules can be ruptured using a sterile needle, and a swab used to obtain purulent material. If pustules cannot be detected, culture can be performed on swab specimens collected from the skin that lies beneath crusts or from under the edge of epidermal collarettes.[19] No surface antisepsis should be performed. Any hair should be clipped from the lesion using sterile scissors, and crusts should be lifted with sterile forceps. Alternatively, a sterile culturette can be rolled two to three times over the collarette. Papules can be biopsied using local anesthesia and submitted for culture. In this case, surface antisepsis with a single 70% alcohol wipe may be performed before collection of the biopsy. Culture of biopsy specimens from nodules and furuncles is best for dogs with deep pyoderma. After collection of the biopsy, the epidermis can be removed using a sterile blade and the deeper tissues submitted for macerated tissue culture.

Minimum reporting by microbiology laboratories should include complete speciation of staphylococci—regardless of tube coagulase status—and complete antibiotic susceptibility results. The pathogenic potential of any CoNS isolate obtained from a skin lesion should be interpreted in light of the clinical findings and with respect to any other pathogenic species of bacteria that may be co-isolated with it.[23] Other suggestions about interpretation of susceptibility panels are outlined in Box 119.1.

Pathologic Findings

Findings on histopathology in dogs with uncomplicated pyoderma include a neutrophilic infiltrate and abundant bacterial organisms. Folliculitis, furunculosis, or the features noted in epidermal collarettes[18] (described above) are all potential findings. Histopathologic evaluation of skin biopsy specimens allows classification of the extent and type of pyoderma and identification of other conditions such as allergic dermatitis, demodicosis, dermatophytosis, pemphigus foliaceus, neoplasia, deep mycoses, and vasculitides. Biopsy should be considered in recurrent or refractory cases, in dogs with deep pyoderma, or when the underlying cause is not apparent. Biopsies can be performed under local anesthesia using a 6-mm punch biopsy. When possible, the biopsy specimen can be halved with half submitted for culture and half for histopathology. The biopsy site should be sutured after the specimen has been collected.

Molecular Diagnosis Using Nucleic Acid–Based Testing

Molecular strain typing methods are research tools used to investigate the epidemiology and ecology of MRS. However, at this time, strain typing often has no impact on patient- or clinic-level management, even in the context of most outbreaks.[23]

TREATMENT AND PROGNOSIS

Factors to consider when treating dogs for pyoderma include the underlying disease, the severity and extent of lesions, and the local geographic prevalence of staphylococcal resistance. Veterinarians' reliance on systemic antimicrobial drug treatment has been challenged by the increasing prevalence of MDR staphylococci. Topical treatments that help to restore skin structure and function, as well as topical antimicrobial therapy, should be considered as alternatives. In dogs with mild disease, treatment aimed at the underlying disorder may be sufficient to resolve infection (see Prevention). Guidelines for the treatment of superficial bacterial pyoderma have been developed by ISCAID.[24]

Topical Treatments

Topical therapy should be used as the sole on-animal antibacterial treatment for surface and superficial infections whenever the pet and owner can be expected to be compliant.

Antibacterial shampoos may be effective alone in some dogs with surface or mild superficial pyoderma and should be used as adjunctive therapy in dogs with deep pyoderma. They aid in debridement, reduce surface bacterial numbers, and decrease pain and pruritus. Options include shampoos that contain ethyl lactate, chlorhexidine, miconazole (in combination with chlorhexidine), benzoyl peroxide, or sodium hypochlorite. Initially, they should be used at least twice weekly with a 10-minute contact time. A combination of chlorhexidine and miconazole may be particularly effective.[25] Benzoyl peroxide shampoos can be drying and so are best reserved for dogs with greasy dermatitides. Daily shampooing may be required for dogs with deep pyoderma. If available, treatment with daily whirlpool baths containing chlorhexidine may also be helpful for these dogs. Important points about shampooing are noted in Box 119.2.

Topical antimicrobial drugs and antiseptics in ointment or cream form result in high concentrations of drug at the skin surface that can overwhelm bacterial drug resistance mechanisms, and can be useful when pyoderma is limited to small areas of skin. Aside from having the potential to be messy, these drugs have minimal adverse effects and result in minimal exposure of bystander organisms (such as intestinal flora) to antimicrobial drugs. Examples of topical drugs with excellent activity against staphylococci include neomycin, gentamicin, polymyxin B, bacitracin, hydroxyl acids (such as acetic acid), novobiocin, and silver sulfadiazine. Mupirocin and fusidic acid are additional topical antimicrobial drug preparations that may also be useful for treatment of pyoderma that is restricted to small areas. While resistance to mupirocin and fusidic acid has been documented in MRSA isolates from humans,[26,27] *in vitro* evidence of resistance of *S. pseudintermedius* to these two medications is rare.[27,28] However, there is a report of subclinical nasal carriage of a mupirocin-resistant MRSA isolate in a pet dog, so some caution is warranted.[29]

BOX 119.2 Points to Optimize the Use of Shampoos for Prevention of Pyoderma

- Water temperature should be lukewarm, not hot. If the dog is bathed outside using a hose, the owner should be told to run the water first to make sure it is not hot—water in hoses in the summer can easily reach temperatures capable of causing burns.
- A hand-palm size amount of shampoo should be used, often placed in 0.5 to 1 gallon of water before it is applied to the haircoat. This reduces frustration associated with the decreased lathering tendency of medical shampoos.
- The shampoo should always be applied in the direction of the hair, not against it. Aggressive scrubbing should be avoided, as this may lead to follicular damage and even post-bathing folliculitis-furunculosis.[25]
- Sprays, mousses, wipes, and conditioners with the same or similar medications used following or in between shampoo sessions may also be useful.[26,27]
- *Diluted* sodium hypochlorite (bleach) has been used as a leave on, then rinse off after, application. Starting as a commercial 6.15% solution, a dilution of 1:32 with water was effective *in vitro* against *Staphylococcus pseudintermedius*, including methicillin-resistant strains.[28,29]

Systemic Antimicrobial Drug Therapy

When pyoderma is widespread, deep, or topical treatment is ineffective or impractical, treatment with systemic antimicrobial drugs may be required. If an antibiotic is selected for empiric treatment, it should be based on the local prevalence of resistance, and narrow-spectrum drugs that target staphylococci are preferable. Clindamycin, first-generation cephalosporins (such as cephalexin), lincomycin, and amoxicillin-clavulanic acid are reasonable first choices (Table 119.1). Other acceptable alternatives when the local regional susceptibility of *S. pseudintermedius* is known include doxycycline, trimethoprim- or ormetoprim-potentiated sulfonamides.

The use of third-generation cephalosporins for empiric therapy is controversial because their use in particular has been associated with selection for MRS in humans and they have the potential to select for resistant populations of gram-negative bacteria in the GI tract.[30] Whether this holds true for dogs and cats is unknown at present. What is known is that the percentage of MRS and MDR isolates among all species of *Staphylococcus* is increasing.[14,23,31] However, there is little evidence for a difference in outcome between MRS and methicillin-susceptible *Staphylococcus* infections in animals, and the prognosis for MRS skin infections in pets is good, depending on the underlying cause and co-morbidities.[23]

It is currently recommended that treatment be for a minimum of 4 weeks for superficial pyoderma and 8 weeks for deep pyoderma. Dogs should be re-evaluated at the end of the suggested periods while still

TABLE 119.1 Oral Antibacterial Drugs Useful for Treating Canine Pyoderma and Otitis Externa/Otitis Media[a]

Drug (Dose)	Advantages	Disadvantages	Assessment/Indication
Clindamycin (10 mg/kg q12h, or 11 mg/kg q24h or q12h)	Infrequent dosing	Only ~75% effective, development of resistance during therapy	Second-choice therapy for a once-daily drug. Can be used for staphylococcal otitis
Ormetoprim-sulfadimethoxine (27.5 mg/kg q24h)[b]	Less frequent dosing, broad spectrum, useful for MRS	Relatively expensive	Good first empiric choice, especially if need once-daily drug, useful for MRS. Rarely used for staphylococcal otitis
Cephalexin or cefadroxil (22–30 mg/kg q12h)	Less frequent dosing, broad spectrum, resistance uncommon, good tissue penetration	Cefadroxil expensive, some generics moderately expensive	Excellent first empiric choice, choice for refractory-recurrent deep pyoderma, twice-daily drug. Can be used for staphylococcal otitis
Enrofloxacin (5–20 mg/kg q24h)	Less frequent dosing, broad spectrum, rapidly absorbed, excellent tissue penetration	Expensive, cannot use in growing dogs	Excellent choice for refractory-recurrent deep pyoderma, once-daily drug. Can be used for otitis
Marbofloxacin (2.5–5 mg/kg q24h)	As for enrofloxacin	As for enrofloxacin	As for enrofloxacin
Orbifloxacin (7.5 mg/kg q24h)	As for enrofloxacin	As for enrofloxacin	As for enrofloxacin. Rarely used for otitis
Amoxicillin-clavulanate (12.5–20 mg/kg q12h)	Broad spectrum, adverse effects rare	Expensive, moisture sensitive, *in vivo* effect may not be as good as would be predicted, slow response	Reasonable first empiric choice, somewhat expensive. Can be used for staphylococcal otitis
Trimethoprim-sulfonamide (22 mg/kg q12h)	Inexpensive, less frequent dosing, broad spectrum, useful for MRS	Adverse effects: keratoconjunctivitis sicca, severe cutaneous drug reactions, hepatic necrosis	Good empiric choice, concern for adverse drug reactions, useful for MRS. Can be used for staphylococcal otitis
Cefpodoxime proxetil (5–10 mg/kg q24h)	Less frequent dosing, relatively broad spectrum, good penetration of tissues, low toxicity, can give with food	Expensive, not recommended for longer than 28-day intervals	Second choice because of expense, first choice where multiple daily dosing of medication is problematic. Can be used for staphylococcal otitis
Doxycycline (5 mg/kg q12h)	Helpful in treating MRS	Moderately expensive	Second choice due to expense. Can be used for staphylococcal otitis
Ciprofloxacin (30 mg/kg q24h)	Inexpensive, less frequent dosing	Variable absorption in dogs	Helpful in large-breed dogs due to less expense. Can be used for otitis due to *Pseudomonas* spp. and *Staphylococcus* spp.
Azithromycin (5–10 mg/kg q24h)	Often effective against MRS	Expensive, GI adverse effects; contraindicated in animals with liver disease	Long-term dosage regimen not well worked out in small animals. Not been reported for use for staphylococcal otitis

[a]For additional information on listed drugs, see Chapter 10. Treatment generally lasts for a *minimum* of 21 days for pyoderma. *Staphylococcus pseudintermedius* and *Pseudomonas aeruginosa* are the most common pathogenic bacterial organisms cultured from the external and middle ears of dogs; however, other organisms cultured from the external and middle ears may also be pathogens. Therefore, systemic antibacterial therapy should be selected based on the results of a bacterial culture and susceptibility test. Treatment for infectious otitis externa/otitis media should be continued until the otic infection has resolved.
[b]Give dose q12h on the first day.
GI, gastrointestinal; *MRS*, methicillin-resistant staphylococci.

receiving antibiotic therapy. Continued clinical signs such as pruritus in the face of resolution of the pyoderma (reduction or absence of epidermal collarettes or follicular papules) should prompt investigation of underlying diseases. For superficial pyodermas, treatment should be continued for at least 7 days beyond clinical resolution of lesions, because inflammation subsides before infection is completely resolved. For deep or recurrent superficial pyoderma, treatment should be continued for 14 days beyond clinical resolution. It is possible that in the future, shorter durations of treatment may be recommended to reduce antimicrobial selection pressure, especially when combinations of topical and systemic treatment are used together with control of the underlying cause.

Although intermittent administration of antimicrobials on a regular basis ("pulse therapy") has been used to treat some dogs with recurrent pyodermas, there is concern for induction of resistance using these protocols. This mode of therapy was initiated in the early 1980s, when the current high incidence of resistance was not present, and it may not be relevant or advisable at this time. If necessary, referral to a veterinary dermatologist is recommended.

PREVENTION

Prevention of recurring pyoderma relies on addressing the underlying cause or causes whenever possible. This may involve investigating the possibility of food allergy, flea allergy, atopic dermatitis, *Demodex* spp. infestation, hypothyroidism, or hyperadrenocorticism. This could include skin scraping, initiating or increasing flea control, frequent bathing to restore skin condition, dietary management for dogs with food allergies, management of atopic dogs, and/or breeding practices that aim to select against atopic dogs and dogs with abundant skin folds. Specific prevention of MRS infections relies on hand washing, disinfection practices, as well as judicious use of antimicrobial drugs, as outlined earlier. Previous treatment with antibiotics, previous hospitalization, and cohabitant dogs have been identified as risk factors for the development of infection with MRS.[14,32,33] There is currently not enough evidence to recommend routine decolonization of MRS carrier animals.[23]

When treatment of the underlying cause or use of topical therapy is unsuccessful in preventing recurrence of pyoderma, subcutaneous administration of autogenous bacterins or commercial bacterial antigens (such as Staphage Lysate, Delmont Laboratories, USA) may be beneficial in some dogs.[34,35] These are generally given once or twice weekly.

PUBLIC HEALTH ASPECTS

In vitro studies have shown that the majority of *S. pseudintermedius* adhere better to canine than human corneocytes.[36] However, human infection has been reported occasionally, including among veterinarians.[37,38] In these cases, pet dog contact was reported and suggested to be the source of infection. In one case, an isolate from the dog matched that isolated from the human as determined using pulsed-field gel electrophoresis.

In contrast, contact with human hospitals and children may be risk factors for acquisition of MRSA infections by dogs, as *S. aureus* infections in dogs appear to be a reverse zoonosis. MRSA isolated from animals has been shown to be human clonal in nature.[39] Colonization is generally transient in dogs and cats, so specific treatment to decolonize dogs and cats is neither necessary nor effective.[40] See the suggested reading list for a complete discussion of screening for MRSA in both dogs and humans.[23]

Although it may be carried elsewhere on the body, *S. schleiferi* subsp. *coagulans* has been isolated primarily from dogs with otitis externa and has been reported as a cause of endocarditis in an immunocompromised person, while *S. schleiferi* subsp. *schleiferi* was reported as causing a prostatic abscess and bacteremia in a man.[41,42]

Frequent and proper hand washing using soap and water and disinfectant foams or gels is the number one practice that limits spread of these infections in human hospitals. Hands should be washed before and after handling each patient. Clean clothing should be worn and doctors' coats changed regularly. Attention should be paid to regular disinfection of other fomites such as stethoscopes, cell phones, rectal thermometers, computer keyboards and mice, calculators, and bandage scissors. Disinfectant wipes that contain alcohol or accelerated hydrogen peroxide can be used to clean these surfaces.

OTITIS EXTERNA AND OTITIS MEDIA

ETIOLOGY AND EPIDEMIOLOGY

Otitis Externa

Otitis externa is defined as inflammation of the external ear canal; in some cases, the inflammation may extend onto the surface of the pinna. Etiologies of otitis externa have been divided into predisposing factors, primary causes, and perpetuating factors (Box 119.3). Successful treatment of otitis externa depends on identification, along with controlling or eliminating these factors and causes. Simply treating the complicating infection without addressing the primary cause, or eliminating the primary cause without control of the secondary infection, likely will result in treatment failure.

BOX 119.3 Etiologies of Otitis Externa

Predisposing Factors

Conformation: stenotic canals, hair in canals, pendulous pinnae
Excessive moisture: "swimmer's ear," high-humidity climate
Treatment effects: improper antibacterial use, cotton swab trauma, irritant antiseptic solutions

Primary Causes

Allergic disease: atopic dermatitis, cutaneous adverse food reaction, contact allergy
Parasites: *Otodectes cynotis, Demodex canis, Demodex cati, Otobius megnini*
Foreign bodies
Juvenile cellulitis
Keratinization disorders: primary idiopathic seborrhea
Endocrine disorders: hypothyroidism
Autoimmune diseases: pemphigus foliaceus
Masses: neoplasia, nasopharyngeal polyps

Perpetuating Factors

Progressive pathologic changes, bacterial infections, yeast infections, otitis media

Modified from August JR. *Solvay Veterinary Inc: The Complete Manual of Ear Care.* Trenton, NJ: Veterinary Learning Systems; 1986.

In a retrospective study evaluating 100 dogs with acute (37%) and chronic-recurrent (63%) otitis externa, the most common primary causes were allergic dermatitis ($n = 43$ dogs; e.g., CAFR, canine atopic dermatitis), parasites (13 dogs), and grass awns (12 dogs).[43] Most bacterial and yeast infections are perpetuating factors and therefore are secondary to the primary, underlying disease. In cats, the most common primary causes of recurrent otitis externa are *Otodectes cynotis* and nasopharyngeal polyps. Unlike dogs, underlying allergic diseases such as CAFRs and feline atopic skin syndrome are much less commonly associated with secondary infectious otitis externa. A rare painful idiopathic proliferative and necrotizing feline otitis externa (PNOE) has been reported, which may or may not involve the concave pinnae.[44,45]

In health, the external ear canal is colonized by numerous bacterial as well as yeast species. Species that can be cultured from the external ears of dogs without ear disease include CoNS, *Bacillus* spp., coagulase-positive staphylococci (e.g., *S. pseudintermedius*), *E. coli, Corynebacterium* spp., streptococci, *Micrococcus* spp., and *Malassezia* spp. However, it is uncommon to culture bacteria from healthy ears (with the exception of *Bacillus* spp., CoNS, and low numbers of coagulase-positive staphylococci). *Pseudomonas* spp. and *Proteus* spp. are rarely cultured from clinically healthy ears. Instead, these microorganisms proliferate when there is inflammation in the ear canal as a result of primary conditions. Although less common, *S. schleiferi* subsp. *schleiferi* also has been isolated from the external ear canal of dogs. More recent studies that have used next-generation sequencing to analyze the microbiota of healthy ears have shown a diverse microbial community with the most abundant species being *Cutibacterium acnes* (previously *Propionibacterium acnes*), *S. pseudintermedius*, and *Streptococcus* spp.[8]

Bacterial organisms cultured from the external ear canal in dogs with chronic otitis externa include *S. pseudintermedius, P. aeruginosa, Proteus* spp., β-streptococci, *Corynebacterium* spp., *Enterococcus* spp., and *E. coli*, with the most commonly identified cocci and rods being *S. pseudintermedius* and *P. aeruginosa*, respectively. Using next-generation sequencing, the most abundant species were *Malassezia* spp., *S. pseudintermedius*, *S. schleiferi*, and a variety of anaerobes.[8]

Knowledge of the most likely organism based on cytologic examination allows one to commence early and targeted antimicrobial therapy.

Staphylococcus schleiferi subsp. *schleiferi* has been isolated from the ears of dogs with recurrent otitis, and *S. schleiferi* subsp. *coagulans* can be found in dogs with both first-time and recurrent otitis externa. Infectious otitis externa is much less common in cats than in dogs. Organisms identified in the ear canals of cats associated with otitis externa include CoNS, *S. aureus, S. pseudintermedius,* and *Pasteurella* spp.

Otomycoses have been reported in dogs and cats, with the most common organism being *Malassezia pachydermatis*; *Candida* spp. is an uncommon fungal pathogen. *Aspergillus* spp. is a rare cause of otitis externa and otitis media in both dogs and cats.[46]

The ear mite *O. cynotis* may be responsible for most feline cases of otitis externa; dogs have a much lower prevalence of this infestation. Most animals develop a hypersensitivity reaction to the mite that results in an inflammatory reaction; however, some animals are subclinical carriers. In others, the inflammation may lead to a secondary bacterial or yeast-associated otitis externa that can eventually result in the death of the mites.

In a study of 3,707 small animal consultations from 20 general practices, the reported prevalence of otitis externa was 4.5% for dogs (of 2,322 dogs) and 1.2% for cats (of 1,043 cats).[47] Breeds that are overrepresented among dogs with otitis externa include the cocker spaniel, Jura des Alpes, and Brittany spaniel.[43] However, any breed as well as mixed-breed dogs may develop otitis externa. Among cats, the incidence of otitis externa has been reported to be highest in Himalayan and Persian cats.[48]

Otitis Media

Otitis media is defined as inflammation of the middle ear. Causes of otitis media may be divided into those that are infectious and those that are noninfectious. Infectious otitis media (bacterial, fungal) is an important perpetuating cause of recurrent otitis externa. Animals may traumatize their external ears because of discomfort caused by irritation in the middle ear. Infectious otitis media occurs as a direct extension from an existing otitis externa through a ruptured tympanic membrane. Less common routes of infection include extension through the auditory tube or the hematogenous route. The reported prevalence of infectious otitis media in dogs with acute otitis externa is 16%, whereas in dogs with chronic, recurrent otitis externa the reported prevalence is 50% to 82.5%.[49,50] Although a ruptured tympanic membrane is indicative of otitis media, the presence of an intact tympanic membrane does not rule out otitis media because the defect in the membrane may have healed.

The middle ear of dogs, like the external ear canal, has a resident microflora consisting of low numbers of yeasts and bacteria including *E. coli, Staphylococcus* spp., *Branhamella* spp., *Streptococcus* spp., *Enterococcus* spp., *Bacillus* spp., *Bordetella bronchiseptica,* and *Clostridium perfringens.* The most common organisms isolated from dogs with infectious otitis media include yeasts, *S. pseudintermedius, P. aeruginosa, Proteus* spp., β-hemolytic streptococci, *Corynebacterium* spp., and *Enterococcus* spp. The resident microflora of the feline middle ear has not been described. In cats with infectious otitis media secondary to nasopharyngeal polyps, the most common bacterial organism identified was *S. pseudintermedius.* Other bacterial organisms in the middle ears of cats with infectious otitis media include *P. aeruginosa, B. bronchiseptica, Bacteroides* spp., *Fusobacterium* spp., and *Mycoplasma* spp.

There are also noninfectious causes of otitis media (congenital palatine defects, trigeminal nerve disorders, primary secretory otitis media [PSOM], otic masses, cholesteatomas, cholesterol granulomas, sinonasal disease, parasitic nematodes, trauma, grass awns). Congenital palatine defects (i.e., secondary cleft palate, soft palate hypoplasia) have been associated with radiographic signs of middle ear disease in both dogs and cats.[51–53] Neurologic signs indicative of otitis media were identified in cats but not in dogs. Trigeminal nerve disorders due to neoplasia, neuritis, or neuropathy in dogs have been associated with a middle ear effusion. Interruption of trigeminal nerve innervation of the tensor veli palatine muscle (which opens the pharyngeal opening of the auditory tube) alters the function of the auditory tube, which could result in the middle ear effusion. PSOM has been described in the Cavalier King Charles spaniel. These dogs do not have a history of concurrent otitis externa. Clinical signs include moderate to severe pain in the head or cervical region; neck/ear scratching; neurologic signs, such as facial paralysis, nystagmus, or head tilt; and hearing loss.[54,55] An increased soft palate thickness and decreased nasopharyngeal dimension are associated with bilateral middle ear effusion in this breed. These changes may then result in auditory tube dysfunction with resultant bullae effusion.[56–58] The majority of middle ear and external ear cultures from these dogs are negative, so the role of bacteria in this disorder remains unclear.[59]

Masses can occur in the external ear canal as well as in the middle ear and can be neoplastic (benign or malignant) or nonneoplastic. Ceruminal gland neoplasia is the most common neoplastic mass of the external ear canal. In cats, these tumors are usually malignant, whereas in dogs, they are usually benign. Tumors that occur in both the ear canal and tympanic bulla are usually malignant, but biopsy is needed for confirmation. Nasopharyngeal (inflammatory) polyps are nonneoplastic masses. Although inflammatory polyps can contribute to chronic recurrent otitis externa, they originate in the auditory tube and can expand into the tympanic bulla or pharynx or both. Whereas inflammatory polyps are common in cats, especially kittens, they are relatively uncommon in dogs.[60] Feline ceruminal cystomatosis is an uncommon, nonneoplastic otic condition consisting of striking multiple blue-gray to purple papules and nodules often mistaken for melanotic or vascular tumors.[61] It is important to biopsy all masses for histopathologic identification.

Cholesteatomas are abnormal growths of the epithelium within the middle ear consisting of keratinizing stratified squamous epithelium, inflammatory cells, and ceruminous debris. These may occur congenitally or secondary to chronic otitis media. Cholesterol granulomas are granulomatous lesions containing cholesterol crystals that may also occur in the middle ear. These two entities can present similarly, but cholesteatomas typically cause more bony destruction of the tympanic bulla and more severe clinical signs and have only been reported in dogs, while cholesterol granulomas have been reported in both dogs and cats. Furthermore, in dogs, cholesteatomas and cholesterol granulomas may co-exist.[61–63]

Cats with sinonasal disease (e.g., rhinitis, neoplasia) are at increased risk of having concurrent bulla effusion and may not exhibit any clinical signs of middle ear disease.[64] *Mammomonogamus auris*, a strongylid nematode that resides in the middle ear, has been identified as the cause of head shaking in domestic cats in Asia and the Caribbean (see Chapter 116).[65,66]

Otoliths (stone-like mineral concretions of necrotic material within the bulla) of the middle ear have been reported in three dogs. The clinical significance of otoliths is unknown, as only one of the dogs reported with these had clinical signs of vestibular disease.[67] In a retrospective study, stalked bony globular structures that have been named *hyperostotic tympanic bone spicules* were identified in the middle ear; these should be considered on a differential diagnosis list for otolith-like structures identified on a CT scan but can only be differentiated from otoliths histologically.[68]

BOX 119.4 Questions for Owners Regarding Recurring Otitis Externa

When did the problem begin?
Did it begin unilaterally or bilaterally?
Is it seasonal or nonseasonal?
What are the current and previous treatment(s) used?
What has been the posttreatment outcome?
Have there been any adverse effects to medications?
Was there previous treatment with glucocorticoids?
Are there other dermatologic concerns: pruritus, alopecia, "rash"?
What are current and previous diets and treats?
What are current medications for other concurrent diseases?
What current preventive treatments are being administered (flea or tick control, heartworm prevention)?
Are there any others (human or animal) in the home with skin problems?

CLINICAL FEATURES

The most common clinical signs of otitis externa include otic pruritus (head shaking, scratching, rubbing ears on the floor), otic erythema, otic exudate, otic pain, and odor. Additional clinical signs (e.g., pedal pruritus, indicating primary underlying allergic disease) may be present and identification of these signs can help with determination of the primary cause of the otitis externa.

Usually, the only clinical signs of otitis media are those also seen with otitis externa listed above. Specific clinical signs indicative of otitis media are facial nerve paralysis and Horner's syndrome. Injury to the facial nerve, as it courses near the middle ear, produces clinical signs such as drooping of or inability to move the ear or lip, drooling of saliva, or decreased or absent palpebral reflex. In one study, 21.5% of 79 dogs and 18.8% of 16 cats had facial neuropathy (facial paresis, paralysis, hemifacial spasm, or contracture) secondary to otitis media/interna. Cocker spaniels with facial neuropathy were more likely to have otitis media/interna as the underlying cause compared to other breeds with facial neuropathy.[69] Horner's syndrome is due to injury to the sympathetic nerve fibers, which course near the middle ear, and is characterized by ptosis, miosis, enophthalmos, and protrusion of the nictitating membrane. In one study of Horner's syndrome, the underlying cause was otitis media/interna in 27% of cats and 2.7% of dogs.[70] Keratoconjunctivitis sicca may occur if the parasympathetic nerves that innervate the tear gland are injured. The parasympathetic nerve fibers course with the facial nerve, so keratitis may be aggravated by concurrent facial paralysis.

Otitis media may lead to otitis interna, which is associated with damage to the vestibular and cochlear branches of cranial nerve eight (CN VIII). Clinical signs of otitis interna include horizontal nystagmus, asymmetrical ataxia, head tilt, circling, falling, or rolling toward the affected side.

Physical Examination Findings

Obtaining a complete and thorough history from the owner is critical before a physical examination is performed. Providing the client with a dermatologic history form to complete before the appointment can facilitate this (Box 119.4).

A complete dermatologic examination as well as an otic examination should be performed. In some cases, a neurologic examination may be needed if concurrent otitis media or otitis interna is suspected. However, the most common clinical sign of otitis media is recurrent otitis externa. A head tilt, circling, and nystagmus may indicate otitis interna. Central extension of otitis media/interna into the adjacent subarachnoid space and brainstem can be a life-threatening complication.[71,72]

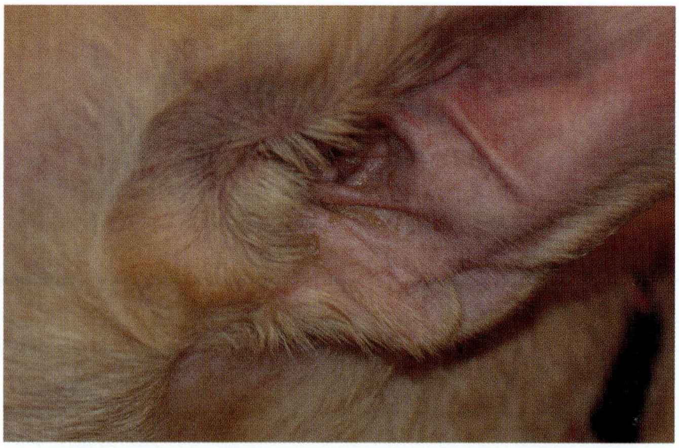

Fig. 119.4 Erythema of the inner pinna as well as erythema and mild yellow ceruminous exudate at the opening of the vertical ear canal in a dog with acute otitis externa.

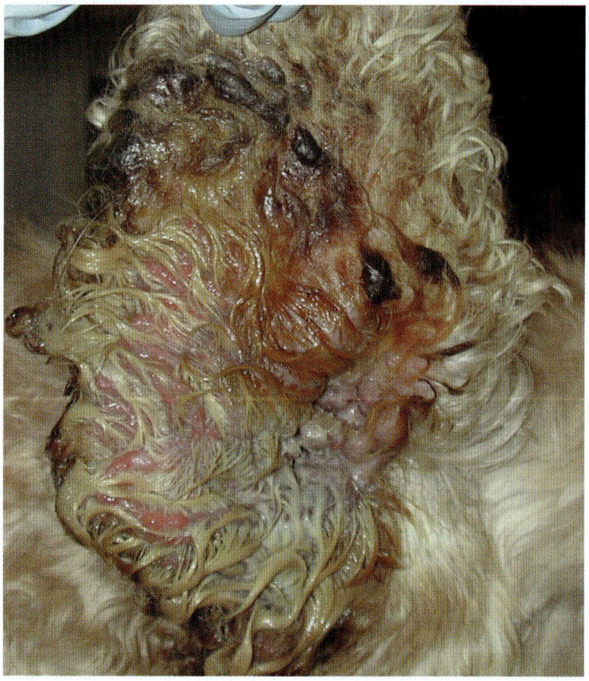

Fig. 119.5 Right ear of a dog with chronic, recurrent otitis externa, with purulent exudate and ulceration on the entire inner pinna, as well as hyperplasia and stenosis of the opening of the vertical ear canal.

The pinnae should be examined for alopecia and excoriations. The vertical and horizontal ear canals should be palpated. In acute otitis externa, clinical findings may be minimal and only include erythema and ceruminous discharge (Fig. 119.4). The tissue surrounding the external auditory meatus may be swollen, occluding the canal. In chronic or recurrent otitis externa, an increase in the otic discharge is evident, along with varying degrees of hyperplasia and canal stenosis (Fig. 119.5). Palpation of the ear canals may reveal thickened or calcified canals or elicit discomfort (Fig. 119.6).

The otic examination is performed with either a handheld or video otoscope. The purpose of the otic examination is to evaluate the vertical and horizontal ear canal for evidence of hyperplasia, stenosis, and ulceration. It is also used to evaluate the amount, consistency, and

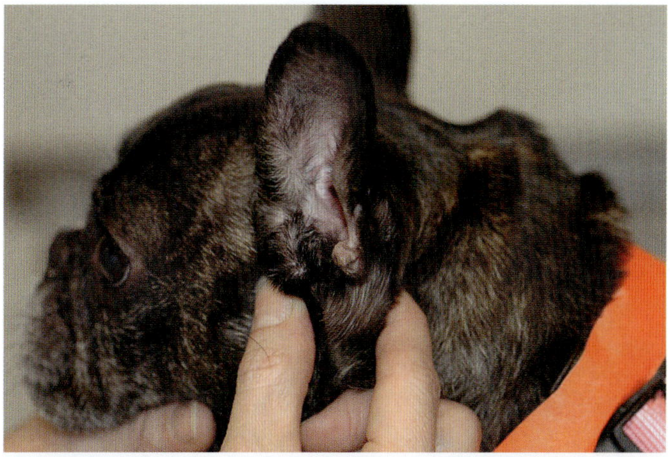

Fig. 119.6 Palpation of the vertical and horizontal ear canals is necessary to evaluate for progressive pathologic changes such as calcification.

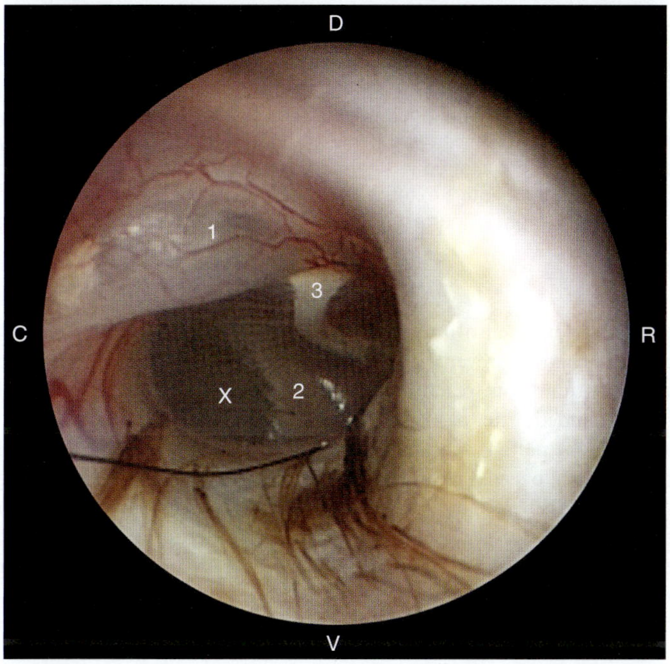

Fig. 119.7 The right tympanic membrane of the dog. The *X* depicts the proper area on the tympanic membrane for performing a myringotomy incision (caudoventral quadrant). *1*, Pars flaccida; *2*, pars tensa; *3*, stria mallearis; *C*, caudal; *D*, dorsal; *R*, rostral; *V*, ventral. (Courtesy of The Ohio State University, Columbus, OH.)

color of the otic exudate. If possible, the tympanic membrane is examined. In some instances, there is so much disease in the ear canal that otic examination is not possible. In those cases, the otic examination is delayed until after initial treatments have been implemented.

The tympanic membrane is divided into two sections, the small upper pars flaccida and the larger lower pars tensa (Fig. 119.7). When visualizing the tympanic membrane, the healthy pars tensa should be translucent and concave. Otitis media should be suspected if the pars tensa is ruptured, bulging, opaque, or cloudy. However, an intact tympanic membrane does not rule out otitis media in the dog. If the tympanic membrane is intact, it should be examined to determine if it is normal (translucent) or if the pars tensa is abnormal. A healthy pars flaccida is the pink, small, loosely attached region forming the upper

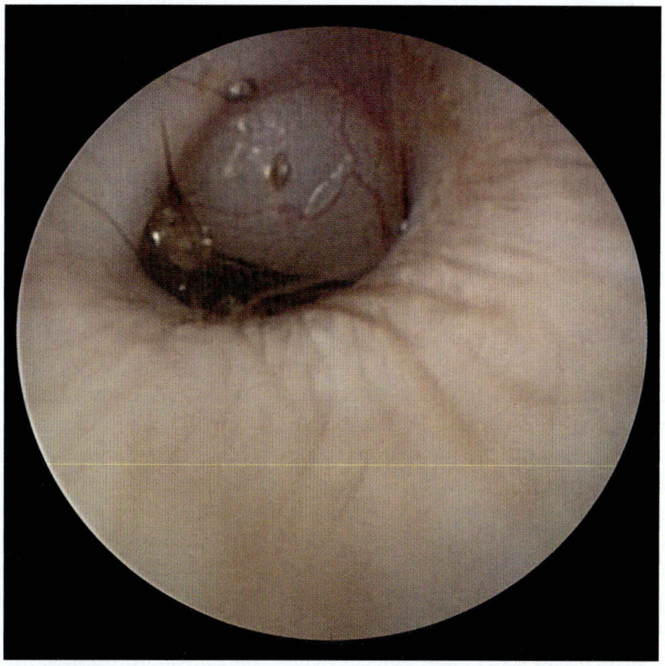

Fig. 119.8 Right ear of a Cavalier King Charles spaniel with primary secretory otitis media (PSOM). Note the large, bulging pars flaccida.

quadrant of the tympanic membrane that contains small blood vessels. On otic examination, the pars flaccida in most dogs is flat. Bulging pars flaccidas, although uncommon, may be found in the ears of clinically healthy dogs, as well as in ears of dogs with otitis. No histologic differences have been identified between flat and bulging pars flaccidas in clinically healthy dogs, so it appears unlikely that a structural difference explains a bulging pars flaccida.[73] In the Cavalier King Charles spaniel, a bulging pars flaccida is indicative of PSOM (Fig. 119.8). Unfortunately, a flat pars flaccida does not rule out PSOM.[55]

DIAGNOSIS

The diagnostic approach to otitis includes identification and management of the primary cause as well as identification and treatment of the infectious (e.g., bacteria, *Malassezia*) agent(s). In addition, predisposing factors need to be controlled or eliminated. Perpetuating factors such as otitis media and progressive pathologic changes must be diagnosed and treated. If all aspects of otitis are not identified, treated, and managed, the otitis will become recurrent and chronic. Additional diagnostics to identify predisposing factors may include, but are not limited to, a food trial, serum allergy testing, biopsy, skin scraping, or clinical laboratory evaluation (CBC, biochemical profile, thyroid testing).

Microbiologic Tests

Cytologic Examination

After the otoscopic examination, otic exudate should be collected for cytologic evaluation using a cotton swab. Specimens should be collected from each external ear canal because the organisms may differ between ears and a separate, clean otoscopic cone should be used for each ear to prevent cross-contamination. It is also important to soak otoscopic cones for 20 minutes before their use, in either 2% chlorhexidine gluconate or a dual quaternary ammonium compound (Cetylcide-II).[74] If otoscopic cones are to be stored in a solution, the optimum solution is glutaraldehyde (Cetylcide-G) (glutaraldehyde).[75]

The material obtained is rolled onto a microscope slide, which is heat fixed, then stained with a Romanowsky-type stain (Wright stain, Giemsa stain, Diff-Quik) or Gram stain. After staining, the slides should be rinsed and allowed to dry. If there is a possibility of the patient having aural mites, a second specimen should be obtained from each ear. The cotton tip should be rolled into a drop of mineral oil on a slide, a cover-slip placed on top of the slide, and examined for *Otodectes* or *Demodex* mites.

Once the slide for cytologic evaluation is dry, it should be viewed microscopically. The slide is first scanned with the low power lens (10× objective; 100× magnification) to find keratinized squamous epithelial cells or inflammatory cells, which are typically associated with infectious agents. Once these are located, they should be examined under oil immersion (100× objective; 1000× magnification). Smears should be evaluated for the number and morphology of bacteria, the number of yeast, the number and type of leukocytes, the presence of excessive cerumen, the presence of excessive keratinized squamous epithelial cells, and the presence of neoplastic cells. Ten fields under oil immersion should be evaluated, allowing estimation of the number of organisms and leukocytes in those 10 fields. For consistency, a grading system of the numbers of organisms and leukocytes counted should be developed. In one report, 2 or fewer yeast organisms per high-dry field (HDF, 40× objective, 400× magnification) in dogs and cats were within reference limits, whereas 5 or more yeast per HDF in dogs and 12 or more yeast in cats were abnormal.[76] Any rod bacteria detected cytologically should be considered abnormal. For coccoid bacteria, 5 or fewer per HDF in dogs and 4 or fewer per HDF in cats were within reference limits, whereas 25 or more per HDF in dogs and 15 or more per HDF in cats were considered of pathogenic significance. The intermediate values were considered suspect, and the decision to treat should be based on clinical signs as well as the results of cytology. Cytologic examination should be performed at the initial visit as well as at each recheck to monitor the response to therapy. Evaluation for mites should be conducted with the low power lens (10× objective; 100× magnification) with the condenser in the lowest position. Leukocytes should not be present on cytologic examination of otic specimens from healthy patients and only on occasion are identified from animals with ceruminous otitis; however, leukocytes may be abundant in purulent otic debris.

Culture and Susceptibility Testing

Bacterial culture and susceptibility testing are not needed at every visit. The purpose of performing bacterial culture and susceptibility testing is to identify the organism(s) present in the ear and to be used to guide the use of systemic (oral) antimicrobial therapy. Topical otic antimicrobial treatments may attain 100 to 1,000 times higher drug concentrations in the ear than can be attained in the plasma. This exposes the bacteria to very high concentrations of the antimicrobial agent, far exceeding the levels that may be attained with an orally administered antimicrobial agent. Therefore, susceptibility testing is not clinically useful for determining the appropriate topical otic antimicrobial agent. Some examples of indications to perform a bacterial culture are when rod-shaped bacteria are detected cytologically (to verify the organism is *P. aeruginosa*), when the patient is not responding to appropriate oral empiric therapy, or when otitis media is suspected (to identify an oral antibiotic for treatment).

Diagnostic Imaging

General anesthesia is required to perform diagnostic imaging procedures and is recommended to properly flush and clean the ears for examination of the deep canal if discomfort of the patient or occlusion of the canal have prevented adequate visualization. Anesthesia, rather than sedation, is also imperative for myringotomy because endotracheal intubation prevents any of the otic flush solutions that enter the auditory tube from reaching the nasopharynx and larynx. A general recommended order of procedure follows.

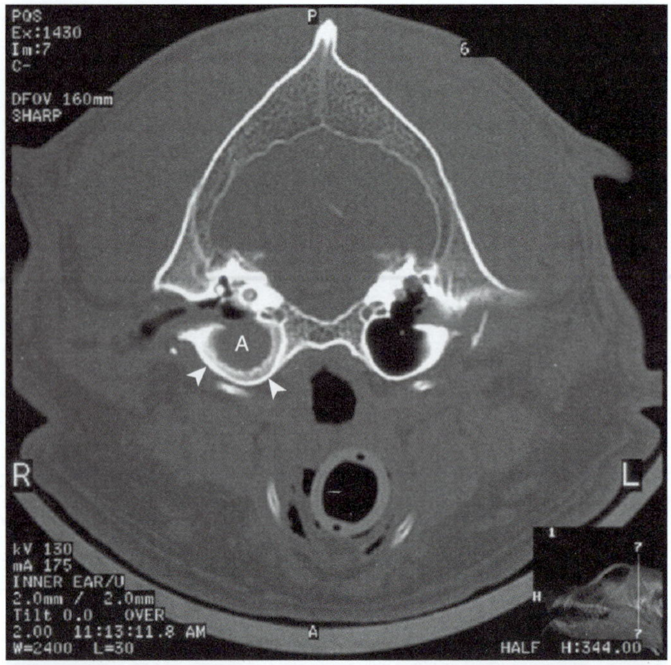

Fig. 119.9 A computed tomography scan of the tympanic bulla in a dog, which has a soft tissue density in the right bulla *(A)* with a significantly thickened wall *(arrowhead)*, a thickened right ear canal that is partially occluded, and a thickened left ear canal that is occluded. Tomographic diagnosis: Bilateral otitis externa, right-sided otitis media and bulla osteitis. *L*, left; *R*, right. (Courtesy of The Ohio State University, Columbus, OH.)

Once the patient is under anesthesia, radiographic imaging should be done first, because cleaning or flushing fluid in the ears can obscure structures that require visualization. Radiographic imaging (bulla radiographs, CT, MRI) is indicated when there is chronic otitis externa, or if neurologic signs (facial paralysis, Horner's syndrome, vestibular disturbances, deafness) are present, to determine the extent of involvement of the middle and inner ear. Radiographic changes indicative of middle ear disease include increased soft tissue opacity in the tympanic bulla, sclerosis and thickening of the tympanic bulla wall, sclerosis and bony proliferation of the petrous temporal bone, bone lysis of the bulla and petrous temporal bone, and increased soft tissue opacity within the tympanic bulla. However, normal radiographic imaging results do not rule out otitis media. With significant radiographic changes, such as sclerosis or lysis, surgical intervention (total ear canal ablation with bulla osteotomy or ventral bulla osteotomy) may be required for resolution. The most commonly used radiographic projections for examining the bullae include the dorsoventral, right and left lateral obliques, and rostroventral-caudodorsal open-mouth views. The rostroventral-caudodorsal open-mouth view is the most useful projection but the most difficult to obtain. It is valuable for comparing the thickness and opacity of the osseous bullae for asymmetry, which reflects chronic osteomyelitis. In cats, the rostro 10 degrees ventrocaudodorsal oblique view is easier to perform and as accurate as the rostroventral-caudodorsal open-mouth view.[77]

CT examination allows cross-sectional imaging of the external, middle, and internal parts of the ear and is used to better define bony structures. The overall accuracy and specificity of CT and conventional

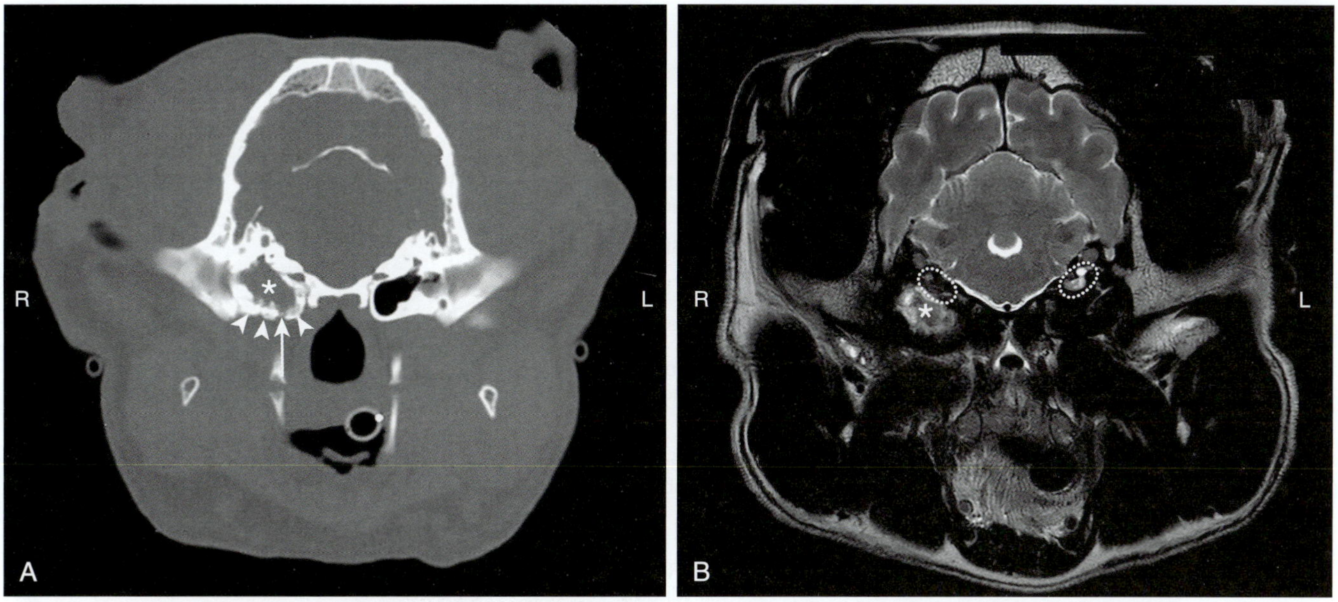

Fig. 119.10 (A) A computed tomography (CT) scan and (B) magnetic resonance imaging (MRI) scan of the tympanic bullae, inner ear, and brain in a 6-year-old male castrated French bulldog with a 2-week history of right-sided head tilt and facial paralysis. On the CT scan, there is soft tissue material completely occupying the right tympanic bulla *(asterisk)*. The right tympanic bulla is thickened, irregular *(arrowheads)*, with ill-defined areas of lysis *(arrow)*. On the MRI, the right tympanic bulla is filled with T2-weighted hyperintense material *(asterisk)*; the left bulla is unremarkable. There is lack of signal from the inner ear fluid of the right cochlea compared with the left *(dots outlining inner ear)*. Tomographic diagnosis CT scan: Right otitis media with tympanic bulla osteitis. Tomographic diagnosis MRI: Right otitis media and interna. Without the CT scan, the bulla osteitis diagnosis would have been missed while without the MRI, the diagnosis of the otitis interna would have been missed. *L*, left, *R*, right. (Courtesy of The Ohio State University, Columbus, OH.)

radiography for the diagnosis of otitis media are similar; however, CT is a more sensitive indicator of otitis media.[78,79] Both CT and conventional radiography are more accurate for predicting severity of otitis media, rather than its presence,[78] and the absence of radiographic evidence of otitis media does not rule it out. Evidence of otitis media on CT images include change in the bulla contour, presence of bony proliferation, or osteolysis of the bulla, with or without increased fluid or tissue within the bulla (Fig. 119.9). MRI and CT are complimentary modalities: MRI is superior to CT for detecting soft tissue changes, in the inner ear and brain, while CT is superior to MRI for detecting bony changes, such as in the bullae (Fig. 119.10A and B).

Ultrasound imaging of the canine tympanic bulla has been performed on healthy greyhounds[80]; cadaver dogs with gel or saline infused into their middle ears[81,82]; beagles with no evidence of middle ear disease in which saline was infused into their ear canals as well as the bulla via a myringotomy[83]; cadaver cats with lubricant infused into their ventral tympanic cavity via a needle through the bony septum[84]; Cavalier King Charles spaniels suspected of having PSOM[55]; and dogs with chronic otitis externa.[84] In dogs with chronic otitis externa, using CT results as the gold standard, a combination of conventional radiographic and ultrasonographic examinations provides a more accurate assessment of the bulla than either technique alone, but the accuracy of ultrasonographic results is operator dependent.[85] In the Cavalier King Charles spaniel, sensitivity and specificity of bulla ultrasonography is too low for accurate diagnosis of PSOM.[55] In cats, CT remains the gold standard for differentiating fluid from gas in the bulla; ultrasonography was slightly better than plain radiography.[84]

Positive-contrast ear canalography can be used to help evaluate the patency of the tympanic membrane. A 1:1 concentration of either iohexol or urografin and sterile saline is infused into the ear canals of an anesthetized dog, and pre- and postcontrast bullae radiographs are performed. The presence of the contrast medium in the bulla confirms a ruptured tympanic membrane; however, lack of contrast medium in the tympanic bulla does not rule it out. This procedure should always be the last imaging procedure, because it will obscure details of all the other methods.

Specimen Collection During Deep Ear Flushing and Cleaning

Knowledge of the anatomy of the middle ear is important to understand the relationship of the inner ear structures to the middle ear, in order to avoid damaging them during flushing or myringotomy. Possible complications of these procedures are Horner's syndrome, facial nerve paralysis, vestibular disturbances, and deafness. Owners should understand these complications and sign a consent form before the procedure.

The middle ear consists of an air-filled tympanic cavity, three auditory ossicles and their associated muscles and ligaments, and the tympanic membrane (Fig. 119.11). The round (cochlear) window is covered by a thin membrane that oscillates to dissipate the vibratory energy of the perilymph in the scala tympani (tympanic duct). The oval (vestibular) window lies above the round window adjacent to the pars flaccida. It is covered by a thin diaphragm to which the footplate of the stapes is attached. Movement of the stapes against the vestibular window is transmitted to the perilymph. When flushing the middle ear, one must be very careful to avoid damaging these windows, which in turn can damage the inner ear. The auditory tube equalizes pressure on both sides of the tympanic membrane. The tympanic cavity consists of a small epitympanic recess, a large ventral cavity, and the tympanic cavity proper. In dogs, there is an elliptical opening in the dorsal wall of the ventral cavity (the bulla septum), which

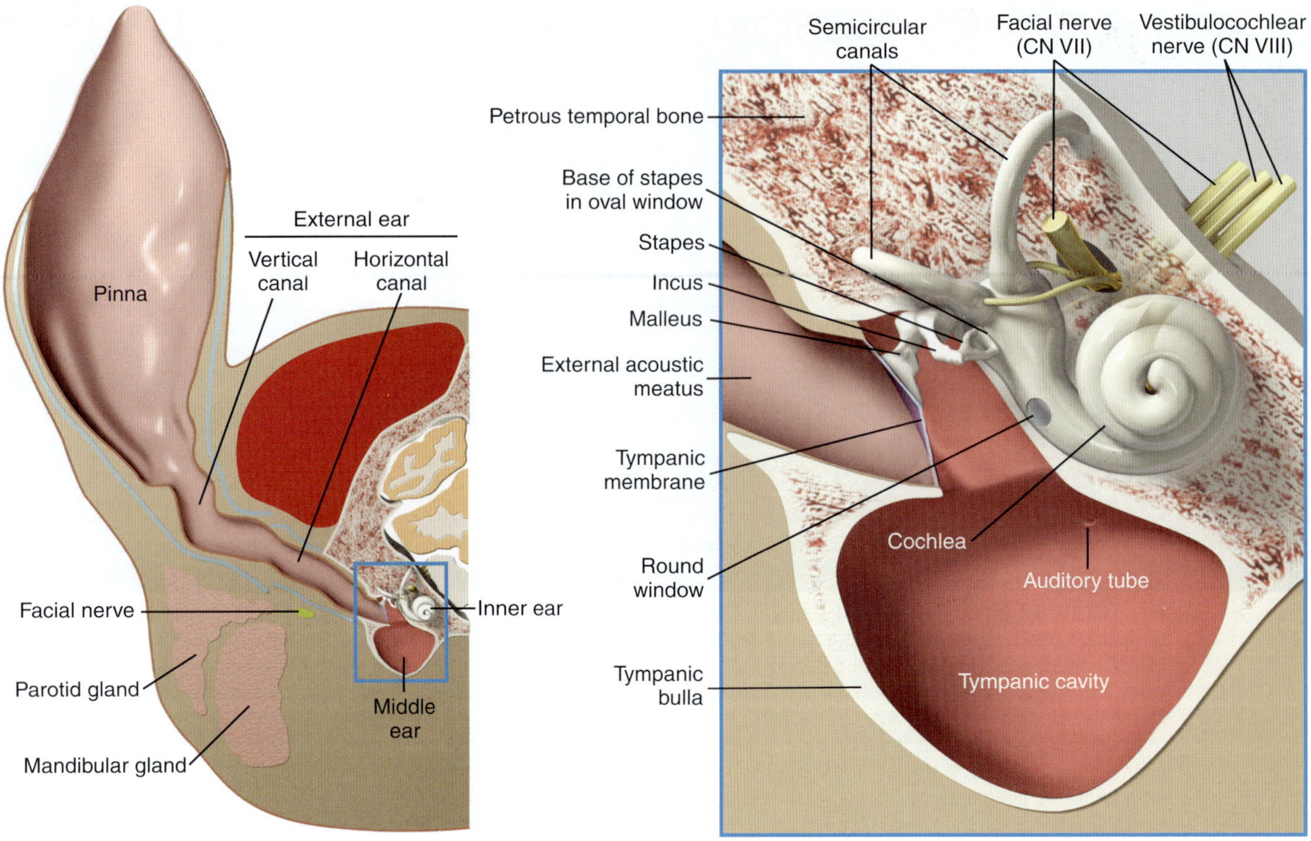

Fig. 119.11 Structures of the external, middle, and inner ear of the dog. (Courtesy of The Ohio State University, Columbus, OH.)

communicates with the tympanic cavity proper. Therefore, in dogs, both compartments of the bulla can be flushed. The middle ear cavity of cats is divided by a septum into two separate cavities. In the small dorsolateral compartment lie the auditory ossicles, the ostium of the auditory tube, and the tympanic membrane. The larger ventromedial compartment is the air-filled tympanic bulla. In order to remove exudate or a mass from the ventromedial compartment, the bony septum needs to be perforated and thus can only be accessed surgically. Rough handling of the septum may result in damage to the postganglionic sympathetic nerves, resulting in Horner's syndrome.

Deep ear flushing is best done under general anesthesia to completely clean and evaluate the ear and tympanic membrane. Indications for deep flushing are chronic, recurrent otitis externa; persistence of exudate in the external canals despite at-home cleaning; lack of response to medical management; and the presence of concurrent neurologic deficits that suggest middle or inner ear disease. First, the external ear canal is soaked for 10 minutes with a non-ototoxic ceruminolytic ear cleaner. Cerumene (Vetoquinol, Buena, NJ) is recommended, because unlike most ceruminolytic agents, it is non-ototoxic. The ear is then flushed with warm sterile isotonic saline and a bulb syringe used to remove large debris and exudate. This is followed by flushing with saline using a 12-mL syringe attached to an 8F polypropylene catheter passed through an otoscopic cone. Additional ear cleaning is performed using a video otoscope with an external flushing unit, if available.

The tympanic membrane can then be visualized. If the tympanic membrane is not intact, then the patient most likely has otitis media, and additional specimens should be obtained from the middle ear cavity. If a handheld otoscope is being used, this can be done by inserting a small sterile otoscopic cone into the horizontal ear canal and passing a sterile swab into the middle ear cavity. The first swab is used for bacterial culture and susceptibility testing. A second swab is used to collect a specimen for cytologic analysis. If a video otoscope is used, an open-end 3.5F diameter "Tomcat" catheter or 5F catheter attached to a 12-mL syringe is placed through the otoscope port. Sterile saline (1 mL) is flushed into the middle ear cavity and aspirated back for cytologic evaluation, and this process is repeated to obtain a specimen for culture. After this, the middle ear can be cleaned by flushing repeatedly with a 12-mL syringe containing 1 mL of warm sterile isotonic saline through the catheter placed in the middle ear. This procedure is repeated until the aspirated saline is clear.

Once the ear canal has been cleaned, any masses noted in the vertical ear canal, horizontal ear canal, or middle ear should be biopsied using biopsy forceps and submitted for histopathology. The biopsy should be the last procedure performed, because blood from the biopsy site may obscure visualization of more proximal structures in the ear. Foreign bodies can also be visualized and removed using forceps.

Myringotomy for Specimen Collection. If the tympanic membrane is intact but the pars tensa appears abnormal, or if otitis media was diagnosed on imaging, a myringotomy is needed to obtain diagnostic specimens and to flush the middle ear cavity. An intact tympanic membrane does not rule out otitis media. Using a handheld otoscope, the cone is inserted into the horizontal ear canal and the tympanic membrane visualized. Using a small sterile swab passed through the otoscope, a perforation is made into the caudoventral quadrant of the tympanic membrane (the pars tensa). The swab is then removed and retained for culture. A second swab is inserted into the original incision for cytologic analysis. If a video otoscope is used, one of the catheters described above for flushing is placed through the otoscope port, and used to perforate the caudoventral quadrant of the pars tensa (Fig. 119.12). Sterile saline (1 mL) is flushed into the middle ear cavity and aspirated back using a 12-mL syringe. The first specimen is used for culture and the second for cytologic evaluation. Thereafter, the middle ear is flushed as described above. Provided the ear is kept free of infection after myringotomy, the tympanic membrane should heal in 21 to 35 days.

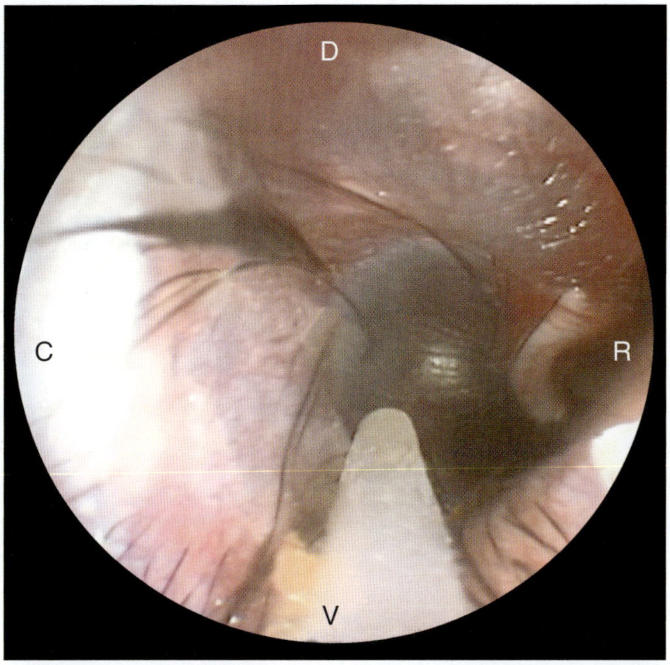

Fig. 119.12 Proper site for performing a myringotomy, right tympanic membrane. The caudoventral quadrant of the pars tensa is approached with a tomcat catheter. *C*, caudal; *D*, dorsal; *R*, rostral; *V*, ventral. (From Cole LK. Otoscopic evaluation of the ear canal. *Vet Clin North Am Small Anim Pract.* 2004;34:397–410.)

Flushing the middle ear with saline does not eliminate all bacteria from the tympanic cavity in dogs with otitis media.[86] However, when middle ear flushing was combined with at-home treatment, the otitis media resolved in 36 of 44 dogs, with a mean time to resolution of 117 days (range 30 to 360 days). At-home treatment included otic cleaners and antimicrobial agents (40 dogs treated with both topical and systemic antimicrobial agents and 4 treated with topical agents only).[87]

TREATMENT

The most common treatment for infectious otitis externa are cleaning and drying agents and combination antimicrobial/anti-inflammatory topical therapies. In severe cases, the epithelium in addition to the lumen of the vertical ear canal is infected,[50] and oral antimicrobial agents are indicated as well. The probability of successful management of the ear disease without topical therapy is low. Furthermore, when inflammation and associated ear pain is severe, a short course of systemic glucocorticoids is indicated in addition to topical therapies. For parasitic otitis externa, such as ear mites, topical or systemic therapies are used.

The goals of medical management of otitis media are to reduce inflammation and resolve infection. As for otitis externa, topical therapy is recommended and may include ear cleaning and drying agents, glucocorticoids, antibacterials, and antifungals. Systemic antibacterials and antifungals are indicated in patients with otitis media. The selection of systemic antibacterial agents should be made based on culture and susceptibility results from the middle ear. However, therapy may be initiated based on cytologic results while awaiting the culture results.

Cleansing Agents (Table 119.2)

Topical cleaning agents are divided into *ceruminolytic agents* and *cleansing and drying agents*. Ceruminolytic agents remove ceruminous and purulent exudate from the external ear canal during ear flushing. They may also be sent home with the owner if the tympanic membrane is intact. These agents work by surfactant, detergent, or effervescent activity. They are contraindicated with a ruptured tympanic membrane, because many are ototoxic, with the exception of the squalene-containing ceruminolytic Cerumene (Vetoquinol, Buena, NJ). Water-miscible preparations containing dioctyl sodium sulfosuccinate or propylene glycol are well tolerated. Oils, such as squalene or mineral oil, are effective but messy. Products containing urea peroxide are very potent and recommended for in-hospital use only.

Once the ear has been flushed with the ceruminolytic, at-home cleaning is done with a topical cleaning and drying agent in order to minimize exudate accumulation. Most products contain acids, some in combination with isopropyl alcohol, to dry the ear canal and discourage overgrowth of bacterial and yeast organisms. These products may also be used after swimming or bathing to prevent "swimmer's ear." Cleansing and drying agents are also used before topical antimicrobial agents for treatment of infectious otitis externa.

In vitro antimicrobial efficacy has been demonstrated for EpiOtic Advanced (Virbac Corporation, Fort Worth, TX), MalAcetic Otic (Dechra Veterinary Products, Overland Park, KS), and TrizCHLOR Flush (Tromethamine [Tris], EDTA, chlorhexidine 0.15%, Dechra Veterinary Products). Antimicrobial activity has been demonstrated for EpiOtic Advanced in dogs with bacterial- and yeast-related otitis externa, whereas MalAcetic Otic has benefit for dogs with yeast-related otitis externa. In some cases, use of these products for cleaning and drying alone may be sufficient to treat infection.

Application of Ear Cleaners

In some cases of otitis, the exudate in the ear canal can be kept to a minimum with routine at-home cleaning. The frequency of ear cleaner application depends on the chronicity of the otitis externa, the severity of the infection, and the amount of exudate in the ear canal. The goal is to begin treatment with the most frequent application (e.g., daily) and over time, decrease to a maintenance frequency (e.g., weekly). It is important to explain proper cleaning technique to the owner, and in some cases demonstrate the technique. The owner should fill the ear with the cleaner, gently massage the ear, let the animal shake its head, then gently wipe the opening of the vertical ear canal with a cotton ball or gauze sponge. The use of cotton-tipped applicators to clean the ear should be discouraged, because it can cause trauma to an already inflamed ear, induce ulcerations in the ear canal, or push exudate further down the ear canal. In some cases when at-home cleaning is ineffective or there is too much exudate in the ear canal, in-hospital deep ear flushing is the best option for cleaning the ear (see Deep Ear Flushing and Cleaning earlier).

Topical Glucocorticoid Therapy

Glucocorticoids are antipruritic, anti-inflammatory, and antiproliferative. During acute otitis, the ear canal becomes edematous and erythematous. As the inflammation progresses, the dermis becomes infiltrated with inflammatory cells. Apocrine glands dilate and become hyperplastic, which leads to excessive cerumen production. Glucocorticoids decrease both inflammation and sebaceous and apocrine secretions. Therefore, they decrease the pain, pruritus, stenosis, and edema associated with otitis. They are usually used in combination with other agents, but may be beneficial when used alone in treatment of allergic animals with otitis and in some animals with ceruminous otitis. To prevent iatrogenic hyperadrenocorticism, the lowest potency glucocorticoid at the lowest frequency needed to control otitis, should be used. Cort/Astrin Solution (Vedco, St. Joseph, MO) contains a low-potency topical glucocorticoid (1% hydrocortisone) in addition to a drying solution (Burrow's solution) in a water-miscible propylene glycol base. A more potent product is Synotic Otic Solution (Zoetis, Inc., Parsippany, NJ, USA), which contains 0.01% fluocinolone acetonide and 60% dimethyl sulfoxide (DMSO). DMSO is anti-inflammatory and facilitates the absorption of fluocinolone into the epidermis and dermis. This product is very effective in the management of proliferative otitis.

TABLE 119.2 **Topical Otic Ceruminolytic and Cleaning and Drying Agents**

Ceruminolytic Agents	
Name (Company)	**Ingredients**
Cerumene (Vetoquinol)	25% squalene in isopropyl myristate liquid petrolatum base
Douxo Micellar Solution (Ceva)	Phytosphingosine, nonionic surface-acting agent, polidocanol, polysaccharides, light fragrance
KlearOtic (Dechra)	22% squalene
pHnotix Ear Cleaner and Wax Remover (Vetoquinol)	Calendula, capryloyl glycine, glycerin, isopropyl alcohol, labrasol, lemon synthetic perfume, polysorbate 80, transcutol V, tromethamine, undecylenoyl glycine
Milytic Otic Ear Cleanser (VetBiotek)	Micellar solution (PEG-6 caprylic/capric glycerides, polysorbate 80, disodium EDTA, cetrimonium bromide), methyl-chloroisothiazolinone, methylisothiazolinone, fragrance, N-octadecanoylphytosphingosine
Dermoscent PYOclean Oto (Animal Dermocare)	Lipoaminoacids, honey and propolis, essential oil of red myrtle, N-acetylcysteine
Cleaning/Drying Agents	
Name (Company)	**Ingredients**
DermaPet Malacetic Otic (Dechra)	Acetic acid, boric acid, surfactants
Epi-Otic Advanced (Virbac)	Salicylic acid 0.2%, disodium EDTA, docusate sodium, PCMX, a monosaccharide complex (l-rhamnose, d-galactose, d-mannose)
Ear Cleansing Solution (Vetoquinol)	Denatured alcohol 10%, lactic acid 1.76%
Nolvasan Otic (Zoetis)	Special solvent, surfactant
Oti-Clens (Zoetis)	Purified water USP, propylene glycol, malic acid, menthol/citronella fragrance, benzoic acid, salicylic acid, simethicone
OtoCetic Solution (Vedco)	2% boric acid, 2% acetic acid, surfactants

TABLE 119.3 **Otic Topical Medications**

Medication	Use/Infectious Agents	Active Ingredients	Vehicle
Baytril Otic Emulsion (Elanco)	Chronic otitis/bacterial (rods/cocci)	Enrofloxacin 0.5%, silver sulfadiazine 1%	Emulsion
Claro Otic Solution (Elanco)	Acute otitis/bacterial (cocci)/yeast	Florfenicol, terbinafine, mometasone furoate	Solution
EasOtic (Virbac) Otic Suspension	Acute otitis/bacterial (cocci/rods), yeast	Gentamicin sulfate, miconazole nitrate, hydrocortisone aceponate	Suspension
GenOne Otic Solution (VetOne)	Acute otitis/bacterial (cocci/rods)	Gentamicin sulfate, betamethasone valerate	Solution
Miconazole 1% lotion (generics)	Acute otitis or chronic otitis/yeast	Miconazole	Lotion
Mometamax Otic Suspension (Merck Animal Health)	Acute otitis/bacterial (cocci/rods), yeast	Gentamicin sulfate, clotrimazole, mometasone furoate monohydrate	Suspension
Osurnia Otic Gel (Dechra)	Acute otitis/bacterial (cocci)/yeast	Florfenicol, terbinafine, betamethasone acetate	Gel
Otomax Ointment (Merck Animal Health)	Acute otitis/bacterial (cocci/rods), yeast	Gentamicin sulfate, clotrimazole, betamethasone valerate	Ointment
Posatex Otic Suspension (Merck Animal Health)	Chronic otitis/bacterial (cocci/rods), yeast	Orbifloxacin, posaconazole, mometasone furoate mono-hydrate	Suspension
Surolan Otic Suspension (Vetoquinol)	Chronic otitis/bacterial (cocci/rods), yeast	Polymyxin B sulfate, miconazole, prednisolone acetate	Suspension
Tresaderm Dermatologic Solution (Boehringer Ingelheim)	Acute otitis/bacterial (cocci/rods), yeast	Neomycin sulfate, thiabendazole, dexamethasone	Solution
Tritop Ointment (Zoetis)	Acute otitis/bacterial (cocci/rods) I don't think any component of Tritop is anti-yeast	Neomycin sulfate, isoflupredone acetate, tetracaine hydrochloride	Ointment

Topical Antimicrobial Therapy

Topical antimicrobial therapy is indicated in all cases of otitis externa (Table 119.3). Commercially available topical preparations usually contain various combinations of glucocorticoids, antibacterials, and/or antifungals in a vehicle base. Selection of the active ingredient of the topical product should be based on cytology results. The patient's progress while on these medications should be monitored cytologically at each re-evaluation and the topical therapy adjusted accordingly. Most topical otic treatments are administered twice daily, and the volume administered should reflect the size of the animal's ear canal, ranging from a few drops in very small dogs and cats to up to 1 mL in large-breed dogs. Topical antiseptics such as acetic acid and chlorhexidine have also been used to treat otitis externa. However, these products are usually used in addition to topical antimicrobials.

Most cases of acute bacterial otitis externa, whether due to gram-positive or gram-negative organisms (even *P. aeruginosa*), respond to aminoglycosides (e.g., neomycin, gentamicin). Antifungal agents are used in cases of acute or chronic otitis externa caused by *Malassezia* spp. or *Candida* spp. Ingredients that are active against yeast include nystatin, miconazole, ketoconazole, posaconazole, terbinafine, and clotrimazole. Furthermore, animals with acute otitis externa usually have clinical improvement after a short course of topical antimicrobial agents, such as a "triple" combination product (antibacterial, antifungal, glucocorticoid), either in an ointment vehicle (e.g., Otomax, Merck Animal Health, Madison, NJ) or solution vehicle (e.g., Tresaderm, Boehringer Ingelheim, Duluth, GA). Newer FDA-approved topical antimicrobials (e.g., Claro Otic Solution, Elanco Animal Health and Osurnia Otic gel, Dechra) which are administered in the clinic may be preferred, as the client does not have to treat the ears at home and these products are efficacious for 30 to 45 days, respectively. Unlike lanolin otic packs, these products coat the ear canal, and do not "pack" the ear and cause temporary conductive hearing loss.

Chronic or recurrent otitis externa does not respond as well to products that contain an ointment or suspension vehicle, possibly because it is difficult for an ointment or suspension to penetrate the stenotic and hyperplastic ear canals. Products containing a solution, emulsion, gel, or lotion vehicle are preferred.

Chronic infections due to *P. aeruginosa* are one of the most challenging otic diseases to treat because of *P. aeruginosa*'s high level of resistance to antimicrobial agents. Antibacterial treatments for acute otitis externa are usually not effective, and the next line of topical antimicrobial agents is needed, which includes enrofloxacin, orbifloxacin, silver sulfadiazine, and polymyxin B. Presoaking the ear canals for 15 minutes with a tromethamine EDTA (Tris-EDTA) product before application of the topical otic agent is recommended. Cell surfaces of gram-negative bacteria are damaged by exposure to EDTA, whereas tromethamine (Tris) enhances the antibacterial effect of EDTA.

None of the commercially available otic topical treatments or any extra-label otic preparations are labeled for use with a perforated tympanic membrane. However, some of these products have been used to treat otic infections in dogs with otitis media.

Ototoxicity and Topical Otic Treatments

It is the author's (LKC) opinion that the use of ointment- or suspension-based otic topical agents or otic packs in ears with a perforated tympanic membrane should be avoided. Owners should always be warned of the possibility of neurologic signs following administration of topical medications when the tympanic membrane is damaged.

Numerous compounds and classes of compounds of drugs can be ototoxic, including antibiotics (e.g., aminoglycosides), loop diuretics, antiseptics (e.g., chlorhexidine), antineoplastic agents, and miscellaneous agents (e.g., ceruminolytic agents). Toxicity may result from parenteral or topical applications. In veterinary medicine, topical otic use of aminoglycosides, chlorhexidine, and ceruminolytic agents is common. Few studies have been published evaluating ototoxicity of topically administered agents. Topical aminoglycosides and topical chlorhexidine are ototoxic in humans as well as in cats. However, treatment of healthy greyhounds with experimentally ruptured tympanic membranes with topical gentamicin sulfate[88] or topical 0.2% chlorhexidine[89] for 21 days failed to induce clinical vestibular or brainstem auditory evoked potential changes. Another study evaluated the ototoxicity of four ceruminolytic agents instilled into the middle ears of 24 dogs: these each contained dioctyl sodium sulfosuccinate; carbamide peroxide; triethanolamine; and squalene, respectively. Only the product that contained 25% squalene (Cerumene) did not cause morphologic and/or histologic changes in the majority of bulla at necropsy on day 29.[90] Results of a study determined that a Tris-EDTA and polyhexamethylene biguanide solution was not ototoxic when applied daily to dogs' ears for 21 and 14 days, with an intact and experimentally ruptured tympanic membrane, respectively.[91]

Systemic Glucocorticoid Therapy

When severe chronic changes to the ear canal exist, treatment with systemic glucocorticoids for an initial period of 2 to 3 weeks, with re-evaluation at the end of the treatment period, is recommended. Dose and frequency should be adjusted depending on the severity of the otitis. For mild otitis externa in dogs, prednisone or prednisolone (0.5 mg/kg, PO, q24h for 7 days) can be used. Dose frequency is then decreased to every other day. For more chronic changes, 1 mg/kg, q24h is used; for severe disease, 2 mg/kg, q24h, for 3 days is used, and then the dose is decreased to 1 mg/kg, q24h. Although rarely needed, prednisolone or dexamethasone can be used in cats.

Systemic Antimicrobial Therapy (see Table 119.1)

In most cases of otitis externa, topical antimicrobial treatment is sufficient. However, in severe cases, deep infection of ear tissue is present, and both topical and systemic therapy is necessary. Although every attempt should be made to treat topically, some owners are not able to administer topical medications properly, in which case systemic antimicrobial therapy may be required. Oral antibacterial selection is the same for otitis media as for otitis externa and should be based on culture and susceptibility results (see Table 119.1).

While awaiting culture results, empiric treatment for otitis may be initiated based on the cytologic results. Good empiric oral antimicrobial choices if cocci are seen include amoxicillin-clavulanic acid or cephalexin. Poor choices would be penicillin, ampicillin, and amoxicillin.

If rods are detected cytologically, *P. aeruginosa* should be suspected. Fluoroquinolones are appropriate choices, with reported susceptibilities of *P. aeruginosa* isolates from ears of 75%, 66.7%, and 46.9% for ciprofloxacin, marbofloxacin, and enrofloxacin, respectively.[92,93] However, variable absorption has been reported for ciprofloxacin in dogs, so the use of this oral antibiotic in some patients could result in treatment failure.[94]

If the bacterial culture and susceptibility data indicate intermediate susceptibility or resistance to the chosen antimicrobial agent, the oral drug should be discontinued. Another drug to which the bacteria are susceptible should be started, if one exists. As noted above, MICs are irrelevant for topical drugs because of the high concentrations reached. In the case of MDR *P. aeruginosa* or other bacteria, the only option is topical therapy alone to treat the infection.

In most cases of *M. pachydermatis* otitis externa, systemic therapy is not indicated. However, for severe yeast otitis externa, an oral antifungal agent (usually an azole or terbinafine) may be administered in addition to a topical antifungal medication (see Chapters 11 and 79).

Surgical Therapy

Animals that fail to respond to medical management of otitis media are candidates for surgical intervention. In dogs with end-stage otitis externa, the surgery of choice is total ear canal ablation with *lateral* bulla osteotomy (TECABO) and bulla curettage. This procedure removes the infected ear canal tissues as well as a portion of the ventrolateral wall of the osseous bulla to aid in complete removal of debris and epithelium within the tympanic cavity. Bacterial cultures should be obtained from the tissue (mucosa) and exudate from the tympanic bulla during this procedure. This procedure has a potential for numerous postoperative complications; however, they are usually short-lived and resolve with medical treatment. Recurrent infectious otitis media occurs in approximately 10% of dogs after TECABO. Because these recurrences rarely respond to systemic antibacterial treatment alone, a second surgical procedure (*ventral* bulla osteotomy and curettage) may be required to resolve the otitis media.[95]

Inflammatory polyps in the cat are usually treated surgically via a ventral bulla osteotomy. However, if the inflammatory polyp is in the nasopharyngeal region only, traction, plus postoperative prednisolone at anti-inflammatory dosages, is an effective alternative to surgery.[92] Inflammatory polyps in the dog are uncommon and have been successfully treated by either a ventral bulla osteotomy or TECABO.[60]

PROGNOSIS

The prognosis for infectious otitis externa is good for cases that are acute, those without progressive pathologic changes to the ear canal (stenosis, hyperplasia), those without concurrent otitis media, and those for which the underlying primary disease has been diagnosed and controlled. Chronic otitis media may occur if infection does not completely resolve. Rarely, an aural cholesteatoma (epithelial-lined cavity) will develop in the middle ear secondary to chronic otitis media. Should these complications develop, and if the ear becomes calcified, the prognosis for medical management is poor, and surgical intervention is required for resolution. Intracranial sepsis is a rare complication of bacterial otitis media/interna, but may have grave consequences if it is not diagnosed and treated promptly.[96]

CASE EXAMPLE

Signalment

"Colonel", a 3-year-old golden retriever living in the Central Valley of California.

History

The dog was evaluated for a history of pruritus for approximately 2 months. Pruritus was first noted on the ventral abdomen, but had since spread to the axilla and on the ventral neck. The dog was on flea control (afoxolaner monthly), as was the cat in the household (selamectin monthly). A plant awn had been removed from between the 3rd and 4th digits of the left pelvic limb paw 1 month previously, for which the dog received ampicillin PO for 10 days.

Physical Examination

Multiple epidermal collarettes and erythema were found on the entire ventrum and ventral neck. There was interdigital erythema, especially on the thoracic limbs.

Cytology Findings

Deep skin scraping: No evidence of *Demodex* spp.

Multiple superficial scrapings: No evidence of *Sarcoptes scabei* (in addition, treatment with afoxolaner made mite infestation unlikely).

Acetate tape preparations (inguinal, axillary and ventral neck areas): many neutrophils with numerous intracellular and extracellular cocci.

Microbiologic Findings

Aerobic bacterial culture (epidermal collarette; done because of the recent exposure to antimicrobial drugs): *Staphylococcus pseudintermedius*, resistant to ampicillin but otherwise broadly susceptible, including to cephalexin.

Diagnosis

Superficial pyoderma.

Treatment

Cephalexin (30 mg/kg, PO, q12h) for 30 days.

Outcome

At a follow-up examination 2 weeks after starting cephalexin, pruritus had reduced by approximately 30%, along with reduction in erythema and the number of epidermal collarettes. Cytologic examination of tape preparations showed fewer neutrophils and cocci than at the initial visit. Follow-up at 30 days after starting treatment continued to show lessened erythema, epidermal collarettes, neutrophils, and cocci, but the pruritus persisted. Because of concern for an underlying allergy, a hypoallergenic diet trial using a prescription diet composed of proteins to which the dog had not been previously exposed was used. The owners were instructed to stop all other foods, and switched to a topical anti-flea product (afoxolaner is flavored with soy protein). Because there was still both cytologic and clinical evidence of the pyoderma, cephalexin was continued for another 30 days. After the second month of the cephalexin, the erythema, epidermal collarettes, and pyoderma had resolved, and cytologic examination of tape preparations revealed no abnormal findings. Cephalexin was discontinued. After another month of feeding the new diet, the dog remained apparently healthy. The original diet was reinstated, and after 5 days the pruritus returned.

Comments

This dog had a dietary allergy, which led to pruritus. Mechanical trauma from pruritus led to disruption of the cutaneous barrier, with secondary *S. pseudintermedius* pyoderma. This resolved with the cephalexin, and was apparently making a 30% contribution to the pruritus. After the owners re-commenced the prescription diet, they then tried adding various proteins for a week at a time. With this approach, a beef allergy was identified. The owner was instructed to avoid beef protein-based diets in the future. The afoxolaner was recommenced.

SUGGESTED READINGS

Hillier A, Lloyd DH, Weese JS, et al. Guidelines for the diagnosis and Antimicrobial therapy of canine superficial bacterial folliculitis (antimicrobial Guidelines Working Group of the International Society for Companion Animal Infectious Diseases). *Vet Dermatol.* 2014;25:163-e143.

Morris DO, Loeffler A, Davis MF, et al. Recommendations for approaches to meticillin-resistant staphylococcal infections of small animals: diagnosis, therapeutic considerations and preventative measures: Clinical Consensus Guidelines of the World Association for Veterinary Dermatology. *Vet Dermatol.* 2017;28:304–e369.

Bajwa J. Canine otitis externa. Treatment and complications. *Can Vet J.* 2019;60:97–99.

REFERENCES

1. Sasaki T, Kikuchi K, Tanaka Y, et al. Reclassification of phenotypically identified *Staphylococcus intermedius* strains. *J Clin Microbiol.* 2007;45:2770–2778.
2. Older CE, Rodrigues Hoffmann A, Hoover K, et al. Characterization of cutaneous bacterial microbiota from superficial pyoderma forms in atopic dogs. *Pathogens.* 2020;9:638.
3. Allaker RP, Lloyd DH, Simpson AI. Occurrence of *Staphylococcus intermedius* on the hair and skin of normal dogs. *Res Vet Sci.* 1992;52:174–176.
4. Griffeth GC, Morris DO, Abraham JL, et al. Screening for skin carriage of methicillin-resistant coagulase-positive staphylococci and *Staphylococcus schleiferi* in dogs with healthy and inflamed skin. *Vet Dermatol.* 2008;19:142–149.
5. Rook KA, Brown DC, Rankin SC, et al. Case-control study of *Staphylococcus lugdunensis* infection isolates from small companion animals. *Vet Dermatol.* 2012;23:476–e490.
6. Hillier A, Alcorn JR, Cole LK, et al. Pyoderma caused by *Pseudomonas aeruginosa* infection in dogs: 20 cases. *Vet Dermatol.* 2006;17:432–439.
7. Miller WH Jr, Griffin CE, Campbell KL. Bacterial skin diseases. In: *Muller and Kirk's Small Animal Dermatology*. 7th ed. St Louis, MO: Elsevier; 2013:184–222.
8. Tang S, Prem A, Tjokrosurjo J, et al. The canine skin and ear microbiome: a comprehensive survey of pathogens implicated in canine skin and ear infections using a novel next-generation-sequencing-based assay. *Vet Microbiol.* 2020;247:108764.
9. Meason-Smith C, Diesel A, Patterson AP, et al. What is living on your dog's skin? Characterization of the canine cutaneous mycobiota and fungal dysbiosis in canine allergic dermatitis. *FEMS Microbiol Ecol.* 2015:91:fiv139.
10. Meason-Smith C, Diesel A, Patterson AP, et al. Characterization of the cutaneous mycobiota in healthy and allergic cats using next generation sequencing. *Vet Dermatol.* 2017;28:71-e17.
11. Older CE, Diesel AB, Starks JM, et al. Characterization of staphylococcal communities on healthy and allergic feline skin. *Vet Dermatol.* 2021;32:61-e10.

12. Abraham JL, Morris DO, Griffeth GC, et al. Surveillance of healthy cats and cats with inflammatory skin disease for colonization of the skin by methicillin-resistant coagulase-positive staphylococci and *Staphylococcus schleiferi* ssp. *schleiferi*. *Vet Dermatol*. 2007;18:252–259.
13. Perreten V, Kadlec K, Schwarz S, et al. Clonal spread of methicillin-resistant *Staphylococcus pseudintermedius* in Europe and North America: an international multicentre study. *J Antimicrob Chemother*. 2010;65:1145–1154.
14. Eckholm NG, Outerbridge CA, White SD, et al. Prevalence of and risk factors for isolation of meticillin-resistant *Staphylococcus* spp. from dogs with pyoderma in northern California, USA. *Vet Dermatol*. 2013;24:154–161, e134.
15. Wiemelt SP, Goldschmidt MH, Greek JS, et al. A retrospective study comparing the histopathological features and response to treatment in two canine nasal dermatoses, DLE and MCP. *Vet Dermatol*. 2004;15:341–348.
16. Gross TL, Ihrke PJ, Walder EJ, et al. Lichenoid diseases of the dermis. In: *Skin Diseases of the Dog and Cat*. 2nd ed. Ames, IA: Blackwell Science; 2008:261–263.
17. Pin D, Carlotti DN, Jasmin P, et al. Prospective study of bacterial overgrowth syndrome in eight dogs. *Vet Rec*. 2006;158:437–441.
18. Banovic F, Linder K, Olivry T. Clinical, microscopic and microbial characterization of exfoliative superficial pyoderma-associated epidermal collarettes in dogs. *Vet Dermatol*. 2017;28:107–e123.
19. White SD, Brown AE, Chapman PL, et al. Evaluation of aerobic bacteriologic culture of epidermal collarette specimens in dogs with superficial pyoderma. *J Am Vet Med Assoc*. 2005;226:904–908.
20. Rosser EJ Jr. German shepherd dog pyoderma. *Vet Clin North Am Small Anim Pract*. 2006;36:203–211 (viii).
21. Jazic E, Coyner KS, Loeffler DG, et al. An evaluation of the clinical, cytological, infectious and histopathological features of feline acne. *Vet Dermatol*. 2006;17:134–140.
22. White SD, Bourdeau P, Blumstein P, et al. Feline acne and results of treatment with mupirocin: 25 cases (1994-1996). *Vet Dermatol*. 1997;8:157–164.
23. Morris DO, Loeffler A, Davis MF, et al. Recommendations for approaches to meticillin-resistant staphylococcal infections of small animals: diagnosis, therapeutic considerations and preventative measure: Clinical Consensus Guidelines of the World Association for Veterinary Dermatology. *Vet Dermatol*. 2017;28:304–e369.
24. Hillier A, Lloyd DH, Weese JS, et al. Guidelines for the diagnosis and antimicrobial therapy of canine superficial bacterial folliculitis (Antimicrobial Guidelines Working Group of the International Society for Companion Animal Infectious Diseases). *Vet Dermatol*. 2014;25:163-e143.
25. Morris DO, Rook KA, Shofer FS, et al. Screening of *Staphylococcus aureus*, *Staphylococcus intermedius*, and *Staphylococcus schleiferi* isolates obtained from small companion animals for antimicrobial resistance: a retrospective review of 749 isolates (2003-04). *Vet Dermatol*. 2006;17:332–337.
26. Castanheira M, Watters AA, Bell JM, et al. Fusidic acid resistance rates and prevalence of resistance mechanisms among *Staphylococcus* spp. isolated in North America and Australia, 2007-2008. *Antimicrob Agents Chemother*. 2010;54:3614–3617.
27. Godbeer SM, Gold RM, Lawhon SD. Prevalence of mupirocin resistance in *Staphylococcus pseudintermedius*. *J Clin Microbiol*. 2014;52:1250–1252.
28. Clark SM, Loeffler A, Bond R. Susceptibility in vitro of canine methicillin-resistant and -susceptible staphylococcal isolates to fusidic acid, chlorhexidine and miconazole: opportunities for topical therapy of canine superficial pyoderma. *J Antimicrob Chemother*. 2015;70:2048–2052.
29. Manian FA. Asymptomatic nasal carriage of mupirocin-resistant, methicillin-resistant *Staphylococcus aureus* (MRSA) in a pet dog associated with MRSA infection in household contacts. *Clin Infect Dis*. 2003;36:e26–28.
30. Tacconelli E, De Angelis G, Cataldo MA, et al. Does antibiotic exposure increase the risk of methicillin-resistant *Staphylococcus aureus* (MRSA) isolation? A systematic review and meta-analysis. *J Antimicrob Chemother*. 2008;61:26–38.
31. Detwiler A, Bloom P, Petersen A, et al. Multi-drug and methicillin resistance of staphylococci from canine patients at a veterinary teaching hospital (2006-2011). *Vet Q*. 2013;33:60–67.
32. Hamilton E, Kruger JM, Schall W, et al. Acquisition and persistence of antimicrobial-resistant bacteria isolated from dogs and cats admitted to a veterinary teaching hospital. *J Am Vet Med Assoc*. 2013;243:990–1000.
33. Han JI, Yang CH, Park HM. Prevalence and risk factors of *Staphylococcus* spp. carriage among dogs and their owners: a cross-sectional study. *Vet J*. 2016;212:15–21.
34. Curtis CF, Lamport AI, Lloyd DH. Masked, controlled study to investigate the efficacy of a *Staphylococcus intermedius* autogenous bacterin for the control of canine idiopathic recurrent superficial pyoderma. *Vet Dermatol*. 2006;17:163–168.
35. DeBoer DJ, Moriello KA, Thomas CB, et al. Evaluation of a commercial staphylococcal bacterin for management of idiopathic recurrent superficial pyoderma in dogs. *Am J Vet Res*. 1990;51:636–639.
36. Latronico F, Moodley A, Nielsen SS, et al. Enhanced adherence of methicillin-resistant *Staphylococcus pseudintermedius* sequence type 71 to canine and human corneocytes. *Vet Res*. 2014;45:70.
37. Morris DO, Boston RC, O'Shea K, et al. The prevalence of carriage of meticillin-resistant staphylococci by veterinary dermatology practice staff and their respective pets. *Vet Dermatol*. 2010;21:400–407.
38. Stegmann R, Burnens A, Maranta CA, et al. Human infection associated with methicillin-resistant *Staphylococcus pseudintermedius* ST71. *J Antimicrob Chemother*. 2010;65:2047–2048.
39. Wipf JR, Perreten V. Methicillin-resistant *Staphylococcus aureus* isolated from dogs and cats in Switzerland. *Schweiz Arch Tierheilkd*. 2016;158:443–450.
40. Weese JS, van Duijkeren E. Methicillin-resistant *Staphylococcus aureus* and *Staphylococcus pseudintermedius* in veterinary medicine. *Vet Microbiol*. 2010;140:418–429.
41. Kumar D, Cawley JJ, Irizarry-Alvarado JM, et al. Case of *Staphylococcus schleiferi* subspecies *coagulans* endocarditis and metastatic infection in an immune compromised host. *Transpl Infect Dis*. 2007;9:336–338.
42. Merchant C, Villanueva DD, Lalani I, et al. PBP-2 Negative methicillin resistant *Staphylococcus schleiferi* bacteremia from a prostate abscess: an unusual occurrence. *Case Rep Infect Dis*. 2016;2016:8979656.
43. Saridomichelakis MN, Farmaki R, Leontides LS, et al. Aetiology of canine otitis externa: a retrospective study of 100 cases. *Vet Dermatol*. 2007;18:341–347.
44. Borio S, Massari F, Abramo F, et al. Proliferative and necrotising otitis externa in a cat without pinnal involvement: video-otoscopic features. *J Feline Med Surg*. 2013;15:353–356.
45. Mauldin EA, Ness TA, Goldschmidt MH. Proliferative and necrotizing otitis externa in four cats. *Vet Dermatol*. 2007;18:370–377.
46. Goodale EC, Outerbridge CA, White SD. *Aspergillus* otitis in small animals: a retrospective study of 17 cases. *Vet Dermatol*. 2016;27:3-e2.
47. Hill PB, Lo A, Eden CA, et al. Survey of the prevalence, diagnosis and treatment of dermatological conditions in small animals in general practice. *Vet Rec*. 2006;158:533–539.
48. Baba E, Fukata T. Incidence of otitis externa in dogs and cats in Japan. *Vet Rec*. 1981;108:393–395.
49. Spreull JSA. Treatment of otitis media in the dog. *J Small Anim Pract*. 1964;5:107–152.
50. Cole LK, Kwochka KW, Kowalski JJ, et al. Microbial flora and antimicrobial susceptibility patterns of isolated pathogens from the horizontal ear canal and middle ear in dogs with otitis media. *J Am Vet Med Assoc*. 1998;212(4):534–538.
51. Gregory SP. Middle ear disease associated with congenital palatine defects in seven dogs and one cat. *J Small Anim Pract*. 2000;41:398–401.
52. White RN, Hawkins HL, Alemi VP, et al. Soft palate hypoplasia and concurrent middle ear pathology in six dogs. *J Small Anim Pract*. 2009;50:364–372.
53. Woodbridge NT, Baines EA, Baines SJ. Otitis media in five cats associated with soft palate abnormalities. *Vet Rec*. 2012;171:124.
54. Stern-Bertholtz W, Sjostrom L, Hakanson NW. Primary secretory otitis media in the Cavalier King Charles spaniel: a review of 61 cases. *J Small Anim Pract*. 2003;44:253–256.
55. Cole LK, Samii VF, Wagner SO, et al. Diagnosis of primary secretory otitis media in the cavalier King Charles spaniel. *Vet Dermatol*. 2015;26:459–466:e106-457.
56. Hayes GM, Friend EJ, Jeffery ND. Relationship between pharyngeal conformation and otitis media with effusion in Cavalier King Charles spaniels. *Vet Rec*. 2010;167:55–58.

57. Kent M, Glass EN, de Lahunta A, et al. Prevalence of effusion in the tympanic cavity in dogs with dysfunction of the trigeminal nerve: 18 cases (2004-2013). *J Vet Intern Med.* 2013;27:1153–1158.
58. Wessmann A, Hennessey A, Goncalves R, et al. The association of middle ear effusion with trigeminal nerve mass lesions in dogs. *Vet Rec.* 2013;173:449.
59. Cole LK, Rajala-Schultz PJ, Lorch G, et al. Bacteriology and cytology of otic exudates in 41 cavalier King Charles spaniels with primary secretory otitis media. *Vet Dermatol.* 2019;30:151-e144.
60. Pratschke KM. Inflammatory polyps of the middle ear in 5 dogs. *Vet Surg.* 2003;32:292–296.
61. Sula MJ. Tumors and tumorlike lesions of dog and cat ears. *Vet Clin North Am Small Anim Pract.* 2012;42:1161–1178.
62. Ilha MR, Wisell C. Cholesterol granuloma associated with otitis media in a cat. *J Vet Diagn Invest.* 2013;25:515–518.
63. Van der Heyden S, Butaye P, Roels S. Cholesterol granuloma associated with otitis media and leptomeningitis in a cat due to a *Streptococcus canis* infection. *Can Vet J.* 2013;54:72–73.
64. Detweiler DA, Johnson LR, Kass PH, et al. Computed tomographic evidence of bulla effusion in cats with sinonasal disease: 2001-2004. *J Vet Intern Med.* 2006;20:1080–1084.
65. Sugiyama E, Kano R, Kagei N, et al. A new record of *Mammomonogamus auris* from the middle ear of the domestic cats in Japan. *Jpn J Parasitol.* 1982;31:471–478.
66. Tudor EG, Lee AC, Armato DG, et al. *Mammomonogamus auris* infection in the middle ear of a domestic cat in Saipan, Northern Mariana Islands, USA. *J Feline Med Surg.* 2008;10:501–504.
67. Ziemer LS, Schwarz T, Sullivan M. Otolithiasis in three dogs. *Vet Radiol Ultrasound.* 2003;44:28–31.
68. Parzefall B, Rieger A, Volk HA, et al. Prevalence and characterization of small tympanic bone spicules and drumstick-like hyperostotic tympanic bone spicules in the middle ear cavity of dogs. *Vet Radiol Ultrasound.* 2015;56:25–32.
69. Kern TJ, Erb HN. Facial neuropathy in dogs and cats: 95 cases (1975-1985). *J Am Vet Med Assoc.* 1987;191:1604–1609.
70. Kern TJ, Aromando MC, Erb HN. Horner's syndrome in dogs and cats: 100 cases (1975-1985). *J Am Vet Med Assoc.* 1989;195:369–373.
71. Martin-Vaquero P, da Costa RC, Daniels JB. Presumptive meningoencephalitis secondary to extension of otitis media/interna caused by *Streptococcus equi* subspecies *zooepidemicus* in a cat. *J Feline Med Surg.* 2011;13:606–609.
72. Sturges BK, Dickinson PJ, Kortz GD, et al. Clinical signs, magnetic resonance imaging features, and outcome after surgical and medical treatment of otogenic intracranial infection in 11 cats and 4 dogs. *J Vet Intern Med.* 2006;20:648–656.
73. Cole LK, Weisbrode SE, Smeak DD. Variation in gross and histopathologic appearance of the canine pars flaccida. *Vet Dermatol.* 2007;18:464–468.
74. Newton HM, Rosenkrantz WS, Muse R, et al. Evaluation of otoscope cone cleaning and disinfection procedures commonly used in veterinary medical practices: a pilot study. *Vet Dermatol.* 2006;17:147–150.
75. Kirby AL, Rosenkrantz WS, Ghubash RM, et al. Evaluation of otoscope cone disinfection techniques and contamination level in small animal private practice. *Vet Dermatol.* 2010;21:175–183.
76. Ginel PJ, Lucena R, Rodriguez JC, et al. A semiquantitative cytological evaluation of normal and pathological samples from the external ear canal of dogs and cats. *Vet Dermatol.* 2002;13:151–156.
77. Hammond GJ, Sullivan M, Weinrauch S, et al. A comparison of the rostrocaudal open mouth and rostro 10 degrees ventro-caudodorsal oblique radiographic views for imaging fluid in the feline tympanic bulla. *Vet Radiol Ultrasound.* 2005;46:205–209.
78. Rohleder JJ, Jones JC, Duncan RB, et al. Comparative performance of radiography and computed tomography in the diagnosis of middle ear disease in 31 dogs. *Vet Radiol Ultrasound.* 2006;47:45–52.
79. Love NE, Kramer RW, Spodnick GJ, et al. Radiographic and computed tomographic evaluation of otitis media in the dog. *Vet Radiol Ultrasound.* 1995;36:375–379.
80. Dickie AM, Doust R, Cromarty L, et al. Ultrasound imaging of the canine tympanic bulla. *Res Vet Sci.* 2003;75:121–126.
81. Dickie AM, Doust R, Cromarty L, et al. Comparison of ultrasonography, radiography and a single computed tomography slice for the identification of fluid within the canine tympanic bulla. *Res Vet Sci.* 2003;75: 209–216.
82. Griffiths LG, Sullivan M, O'Neill T, et al. Ultrasonography versus radiography for detection of fluid in the canine tympanic bulla. *Vet Radiol Ultrasound.* 2003;44:210–213.
83. Lee J, Eom K, Seong Y, et al. Ultrasonographic evaluation of the external ear canal and tympanic membrane in dogs. *Vet Radiol Ultrasound.* 2006;47:94–98.
84. King AM, Weinrauch SA, Doust R, et al. Comparison of ultrasonography, radiography and a single computed tomography slice for fluid identification within the feline tympanic bulla. *Vet J.* 2007;173:638–644.
85. Doust R, King A, Hammond G, et al. Assessment of middle ear disease in the dog: a comparison of diagnostic imaging modalities. *J Small Anim Pract.* 2007;48:188–192.
86. Hettlich BE, Boothe HW, Simpson RB, et al. Effect of tympanic cavity evacuation and flushing on microbial isolates during total ear canal ablation with lateral bulla osteotomy in dogs. *J Am Vet Med Assoc.* 2005;227:748–755.
87. Palmeiro BS, Morris DO, Wiemelt SP, et al. Evaluation of outcome of otitis media after lavage of the tympanic bulla and long-term antimicrobial drug treatment in dogs: 44 cases (1998-2002). *J Am Vet Med Assoc.* 2004;225:548–553.
88. Strain GM, Merchant SR, Neer TM, et al. Ototoxicity assessment of a gentamicin sulfate otic preparation in dogs. *Am J Vet Res.* 1995;56:532–538.
89. Merchant SR, Neer TM, Tedford BL, et al. Ototoxicity assessment of a chlorhexidine otic preparation in dogs. *Prog Vet Neurol.* 1993;4:72–75.
90. Mansfield PD, Steiss JE, Boosinger TR, et al. The effects of four, commercial ceruminolytic agents on the middle ear. *J Am Anim Hosp Assoc.* 1997;33:479–486.
91. Mills PC, Ahlstrom L, Wilson WJ. Ototoxicity and tolerance assessment of a TrisEDTA and polyhexamethylene biguanide ear flush formulation in dogs. *J Vet Pharmacol Ther.* 2005;28:391–397.
92. McKay L, Rose CD, Matousek JL, et al. Antimicrobial testing of selected fluoroquinolones against *Pseudomonas aeruginosa* isolated from canine otitis. *J Am Anim Hosp Assoc.* 2007;43:307–312.
93. Wildermuth BE, Griffin CE, Rosenkrantz WS, et al. Susceptibility of *Pseudomonas* isolates from the ears and skin of dogs to enrofloxacin, marbofloxacin, and ciprofloxacin. *J Am Anim Hosp Assoc.* 2007;43:337–341.
94. Papich MG. Ciprofloxacin pharmacokinetics and oral absorption of generic ciprofloxacin tablets in dogs. *Am J Vet Res.* 2012;73:1085–1091.
95. Smeak DD, Crocker CB, Birchard SJ. Treatment of recurrent otitis media that developed after total ear canal ablation and lateral bulla osteotomy in dogs: nine cases (1986-1994). *J Am Vet Med Assoc.* 1996;209:937–942.
96. Spangler EA, Dewey CW. Meningoencephalitis secondary to bacterial otitis media/interna in a dog. *J Am Anim Hosp Assoc.* 2000;36:239–243.

Abscesses and Cellulitis

Jane E. Sykes

KEY POINTS

- Abscesses and cellulitis occur in any tissue and are one of the most frequent conditions of cats.
- Anaerobes and *Pasteurella multocida* are most often isolated from abscesses when culture is performed.
- Many abscesses will heal following incision and drainage. Lavage with copious volumes of saline and surgical placement of a Penrose drain may also be indicated. For large abscesses or where there is evidence of cellulitis and systemic signs, treatment with antimicrobials for 5 to 10 days is recommended. A drug with activity against anaerobes and *Pasteurella* spp. is recommended, such as amoxicillin.
- In endemic regions, plague and tularemia should be considered as differential diagnoses for abscesses in dogs and cats with systemic illness, lymphadenomegaly, fever, and subcutaneous lesions because of their zoonotic significance. When lesions are in the inguinal region of cats, mycobacterial infections should be considered because routine surgical approaches to treatment have the potential to exacerbate disease.
- Testing for FeLV and FIV should be considered for cats with bite and fight wounds, with a follow-up test no earlier than 60 days later.

ETIOLOGY AND PATHOGENESIS

Abscesses, which are characterized by an accumulation of pus, can occur in any tissue. Subcutaneous abscesses are the most common bacterial infections of feline skin and probably the most common site of abscess formation in dogs and cats (Fig. 120.1). The following discussion focuses on feline cutaneous abscesses, although the principles of diagnosis and treatment are similar in any location. In general, abscesses are more commonly diagnosed in cats than in dogs, likely because of frequent fighting behavior and needle-like teeth and claws that facilitate inoculation of bacteria under the skin through a small wound. Feline skin is also elastic and readily seals over small contaminated puncture wounds, with accumulation of subcutaneous exudate. The size and extent of abscessation also depends on the overlying skin tension, amount of dead space, and gravitation of exudate below the point of penetration. Pus-filled cavities that form above a puncture site drain easily. Cavities that gravitate below the puncture site may repeatedly drain through the puncture site without complete resolution.

Because subcutaneous abscesses in cats usually result from bites and scratches, the most common organisms found within them are resident oral microflora (Table 120.1). Anaerobes are isolated from more than two-thirds of abscesses, and the most common facultative aerobe isolated is *Pasteurella multocida*. Chapter 75 includes a more detailed discussion of bacteria isolated from cat-bite wounds. Cats that sustain bite injuries are more likely to become infected with FIV and to a lesser extent FeLV.[1]

CLINICAL FEATURES

Clinical Signs and Physical Examination Findings

Cat-bite/fight abscesses are usually located around the limbs, head, dorsum, and base of the tail. Some cats have discernable cutaneous masses with few other signs of illness, whereas more extensive infection is associated with fever (103.6° F to 105.2° [39.7° C to 40.6°C]), anorexia, lethargy, and regional lymphadenomegaly. Pain is usually present at the site of infection, and obvious swelling or warmth may or may not be present. Mature abscesses that are at the point of rupture are usually tender with a soft, fluctuant central area. Erythema or discoloration is occasionally apparent. Drainage of purulent material occurs spontaneously or after surgical lancing. Foul-smelling, red-brown discharges occur, especially with tissue necrosis and anaerobic bacterial infection (Fig. 120.2). Systemic signs often resolve once the abscess ruptures, and the only evidence of infection may be matted hair at the site of drainage. Careful examination in the area of swelling usually reveals a small puncture wound covered by a crust. Recurrent abscesses at the same site suggest underlying osteomyelitis or neoplasia, poor surgical drainage, immunodeficiency (e.g., FeLV or FIV infection), antimicrobial resistance, or the presence of a foreign body. Abscesses associated with foreign bodies, underlying osteomyelitis, or certain fastidious organisms such as *Nocardia* or *Mycobacterium*, or fungi such as *Sporothrix schenckii* also tend to recur, persist, or spread in tissues. Abscesses in dogs and cats are often associated with noticeable regional lymphadenomegaly. Sometimes the overlying skin may become necrotic.

Additional clinical manifestations reflect possible involvement of other organs or tissues. Lameness or paralysis may be apparent with myositis, osteomyelitis, septic arthritis, or discospondylitis. Stiffness, lethargy, nuchal rigidity, or seizures can be seen with meningitis. Osteomyelitis may be manifested by chronic or recurrent draining fistulas that only temporarily respond to antibacterial drugs. Respiratory distress, dyspnea, and stridor are noted with pyothorax or abscesses that occur in the cervical region. Vestibular signs can be noted if otitis media or interna develops. Signs of bacteremia and systemic infection include malaise and fever or reflect those of another organ system of hematogenous localization.

Retrobulbar abscesses or cellulitis are associated with proptosis, decreased globe mobility, oculonasal discharge, chemosis, conjunctival congestion, protrusion of the third eyelid, pain while opening the mouth,

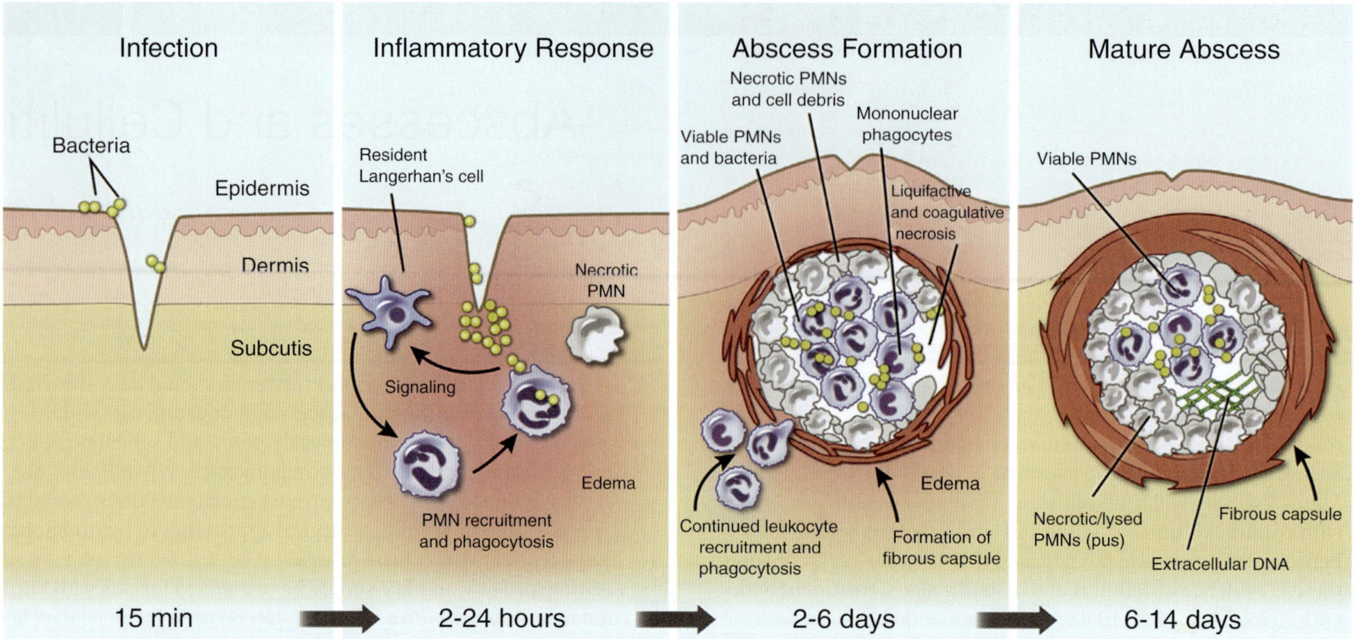

Fig. 120.1 Pathogenesis of abscess formation. (Modified from Kobayashi SD, Malachowa N, DeLeo FR. Pathogenesis of *Staphylococcus aureus* abscesses. *Am J Pathol.* 2015;185(6):1518–1527.)

TABLE 120.1 Examples of Bacteria Isolated from Feline Abscesses[a]

Genus	Species Examples
Anaerobes	
Porphyromonas spp.	*gingivalis, tectum, heparinolyticus, salivosa, melaninogenicus, corrodens, fragilis, circumdentaria,* others
Fusobacterium spp.	*nucleatum, necrophorum, russii,* others
Prevotella spp.	
Peptostreptococcus spp.	*anaerobius*
Clostridium spp.	*perfringens, novyi, sordellii, septicum, chauvoei, tetani, villosum*
Cutibacterium (formerly *Propionibacterium*) spp.	*acnes*
Bifidobacterium spp.	
Eubacterium spp.	*lentum*
Facultative Aerobes	
Pasteurella spp.	*multocida*
Actinomyces spp.	*viscosus, odontolyticus*
Nocardia spp.	
Staphylococcus spp.	
Rhodococcus	*equi*
Enterobacterales	
Streptococcus spp.	
Enterococcus spp.	
Lactobacillus spp.	

[a]See references 5, 8, 10, 11, 15–21.

periocular swelling or discomfort, lethargy, weight loss, and fever. Corneal ulcers may develop from exposure keratitis or self-trauma associated with retrobulbar pain. In some cases, swelling and discoloration may be seen caudal to the maxillary molar teeth on opening the mouth.

DIAGNOSIS

Diagnosis of abscesses and cellulitis is usually based on the history and physical examination findings. The possibility of an abscess should also be considered in cats that develop acute or subacute fever of unknown origin before extensive and invasive diagnostic tests are performed. It should be considered in cats that are acutely anorexic and/or lame, even in the absence of a subcutaneous swelling, given that formation of visible abscesses may be delayed or hidden. In endemic regions, plague and tularemia should be on the differential diagnosis list in febrile cats with subcutaneous swellings, lymphadenopathy, and fever. Although much rarer than cat-bite abscesses, they have the potential to cause life-threatening infections in exposed humans. Atypical bacteria such as *Nocardia* spp., *Mycobacterium* spp., and fungal pathogens, especially *Sporothrix* spp. and *Cryptococcus* spp., should be considered should there be a lack of response to standard treatment. Mycobacterial infections should be high on the differential diagnosis list for subcutaneous lesions that occur in the inguinal region of cats. It is critical that these be considered early because attempts to drain these abscesses surgically as if they were routine bacterial infections have the potential to spread infection further in tissues and worsen disease.

Culture of typical abscess wounds is not generally indicated because surgical debridement with or without empiric antimicrobial therapy is often effective, anaerobes are difficult to culture, and aerobic and anaerobic culture adds significant expense for owners. In addition, unless there is evidence of systemic illness, laboratory findings on bloodwork usually do not reveal abnormalities that would change treatment. Testing for retroviruses is recommended for cats with an unknown retrovirus status. Because it can take several weeks for cats

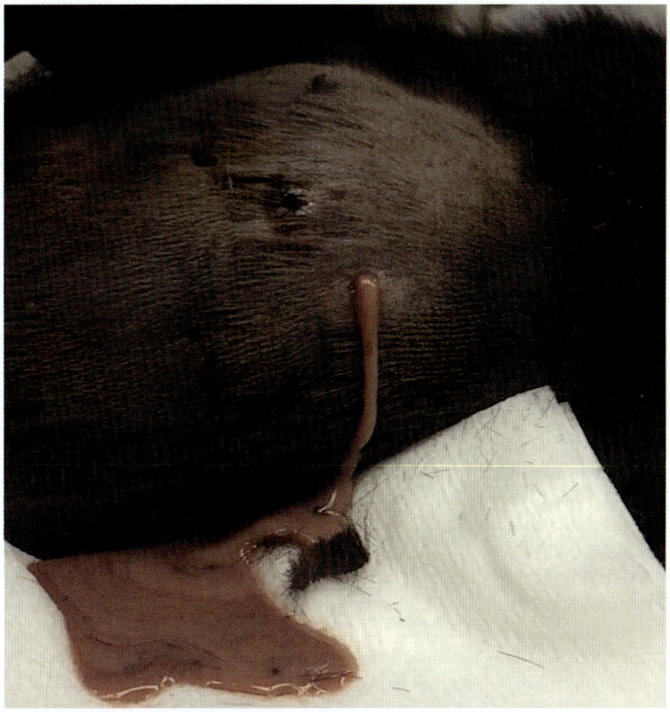

Fig. 120.2 Subcutaneous abscess in a domestic shorthair. Incision under sedation released a large amount of red-brown purulent fluid. Lavage of the abscess cavity, placement of a Penrose drain, and treatment with 5 to 7 days of oral amoxicillin with re-evaluation and removal of the drain at this time would be recommended for treatment. (Courtesy Dr. Steven Epstein, University of California, Davis Veterinary Emergency and Critical Care Service.)

to become FeLV antigen–positive or FIV antibody–positive after exposure, retesting is recommended 2 months after a cat is seen for a cat fight wound.[1]

Ultrasonography can be used to view the extent of a swelling, locate accumulations of fluid or pus in soft-tissue planes, and evaluate for foreign bodies, which are more common in dogs than in cats. Grass awns characteristically appear as double or triple spindle-shaped echogenic objects within soft tissues.[2,3] Minimally invasive ultrasound-guided retrieval of foreign material has also been helpful in avoiding standard surgical methods.[2,4] Instillation of radiographic contrast medium may be helpful in determining the extent or depth of a draining fistulous tract if a foreign body is likely, although improvements in ultrasound image quality have reduced the requirement for such procedures. Use of ultrasound guidance to inject methylene blue dye around a plant awn can facilitate identification and removal of awns during surgery.

Chronic or recurrent draining abscesses should be evaluated by radiography for underlying osteomyelitis, by cytology and culture for possible fungal or atypical bacterial infection, or by surgical exploration for the presence of a foreign body or fly larva.

TREATMENT

Abscesses vary in severity and in the extent of therapeutic intervention required. Small, localized abscesses that drain spontaneously by the time animals are examined require that the hair around the wound be clipped, and the margins of the wound be cleaned. Should abscesses not be open, incision and drainage (IAD) may be needed under sedation or general anesthesia. The abscess cavity should then be lavaged with copious amounts of normal saline (500 mL–1 L) or a dilute antiseptic such as 0.05% chlorhexidine or 0.1% povidone iodine. Consideration should be given to the use of normal saline. There is no evidence that antiseptics improve outcome; they have the potential to damage tissue, and severe nosocomial infections have been reported in association with use of antiseptic solutions that become contaminated with antiseptic-resistant bacteria such as *Pseudomonas* spp.. In one report, five cats developed *Burkholderia cepacia* complex (formerly *Pseudomonas cepacia*) skin infections and the organism was isolated from a 2% chlorhexidine scrub solution in the clinic; two cats developed sepsis and died.[5] More extensive infections that cause signs of systemic illness may require parenteral antibacterial administration, surgical drainage, or supportive care with hospitalization and intravenous fluid administration. Considerable variability in the approach to treatment of cutaneous abscesses has been observed in human medicine.[6]

Antibacterial Therapy

Antibacterial therapy has a decided but not absolute role in the management of abscesses in cats. Although mortality and complications resulting from abscesses have been reduced with the use of antibacterials, these agents should not be given indiscriminately or in the absence of other adjunctive measures. Antibacterials alone are ineffective in penetrating walled-off abscesses that require drainage. Indiscriminate antimicrobial use may also select for drug-resistant bacteria or cause drug reactions.[7]

Although antimicrobials are often routinely used in veterinary practice for cat-bite abscesses, drainage and lavage may be sufficient to resolve the abscesses in many cases. In human medicine, antimicrobials are only considered necessary when there are systemic signs of infection, comorbidities such as immunosuppressive illnesses and diabetes mellitus, or if there is extensive (> 5 cm in humans) surrounding cellulitis.[8] No difference in outcome was identified when humans with uncomplicated subcutaneous abscesses were treated with drainage with or without antimicrobials.[9] If antimicrobials are used, they should be given for a short duration (e.g., 5 to 7 days). Penicillin derivatives such as amoxicillin are antibacterials of choice for treating abscesses because they are active against *Pasteurella* spp. and anaerobes; addition of clavulanic acid is generally not necessary, adds expense, and is more likely to cause GI adverse effects (Table 120.2). Other antimicrobials likely to be effective are clindamycin and metronidazole, but these are less well tolerated by cats. Although effective against pathogens found in cat-bite abscesses,[10-12] widespread use of third-generation cephalosporins (e.g., cefovecin, cefpodoxime) and pradofloxacin has raised concerns about selection for resistant bacterial populations.[13] Cefovecin is widely used because it requires only a single injection, and one study from Australia showed that the most common reason for administration of cefovecin in cats was cat fight injuries and abscesses.[13] In another study of 4.4 million veterinary visit records from Australia, cefovecin and clavulanic acid-amoxicillin were the most common antimicrobials prescribed for dogs and cats.[14] Although convenient, because of concerns about resistance, cefovecin and pradofloxacin should only be used for treatment of cat-bite abscesses when there is a need for antibiotics and oral amoxicillin is not tolerated. In general, systemic antibacterial therapy may be beneficial in minimizing abscess formation when given immediately after bite wound contamination in order to prevent abscess formation or with diffuse cellulitis (see also Chapter 75). Antimicrobial treatment of abscesses in cats should also be considered when there are systemic signs of illness and lesions are large. Without surgical drainage, medical therapy could be continued for 7 to 10 days.

Surgery

Diffuse cellulitis or early abscesses may need to be monitored for accumulation of pus before surgical drainage is performed. Applying warm compresses daily may hasten this process. Surgical therapy usually

TABLE 120.2 Antimicrobial Drugs for Treatment of Skin and Soft Tissue Infections in Cats

Drug	Dose	Route	Interval (Hours)	Duration (Days)
Ampicillin, amoxicillin	20 mg/kg	PO, IV	12	5–7
Cefadroxil	22 mg/kg	PO	12	5–7
Cefovecin	8 mg/kg	SC	once	NA
Clindamycin	10 mg/kg	PO, IM	12	5–7
Metronidazole	10 mg/kg	PO, IV	8–12	5–7
Pradofloxacin	7.5 mg/kg	PO	24	7

involves creating drainage openings at the most ventral portion of an abscess cavity. Controversy exists as to the degree and type of surgical closure indicated. The abscess cavity can be debrided and a small portion of overlying skin removed to prevent premature closure. Placement of a Penrose drain that exits at the lowest point of incision with partial closure can also be used to maintain a drainage opening. The drain should only have a ventral exit through a new stab incision; the proximal aspect of the drain should be placed in the dorsal aspect of the wound and can be secured to the skin in this location with a mattress suture. The drain should be removed within 3 to 5 days when drainage becomes serosanguineous or decreases in volume.

Surgical drainage must be established whenever abscess formation occurs within closed cavities. Retrobulbar abscesses can be drained by passing a probe from immediately behind the last upper molar upward into the retrobulbar space. Infraorbital abscesses are usually associated with infection of the upper carnassial tooth, which must be extracted. Abscesses of the middle ear also require surgical drainage with debridement of bone because of the loculation of pus within cavities surrounded by bone. Abscesses associated with underlying osteomyelitis must be treated by surgical debridement of infected bone. Foreign bodies or material must be removed from abscess cavities before they heal.

Castration and indoor housing are recommended as a preventive measure to abscess formation because they reduce the fighting and roaming behavior of male cats.

SUGGESTED READINGS

Wong JK, Chambers LC, Elsmo EJ, et al. Cellulitis caused by the *Burkholderia cepacia* complex associated with contaminated chlorhexidine 2% scrub in five domestic cats. *J Vet Diagn Invest*. 2018;30:763–769.

Hardefeldt L, Hur B, Verspoor K, et al. Use of cefovecin in dogs and cats attending first-opinion veterinary practices in Australia. *Vet Rec*. 2020;187:e95.

Stevens DL, Bisno AL, Chambers HF, et al. Practice guidelines for the diagnosis and management of skin and soft tissue infections: 2014 update by the Infectious Diseases Society of America. *Clin Infect Dis*. 2014;59:e10–52.

REFERENCES

1. Little S, Levy J, Hartmann K, et al. 2020 AAFP feline retrovirus testing and management guidelines. *J Feline Med Surg*. 2020;22:5–30.
2. Caivano D, Birettoni F, Rishniw M, et al. Ultrasonographic findings and outcomes of dogs with suspected migrating intrathoracic grass awns: 43 cases (2010-2013). *J Am Vet Med Assoc*. 2016;248:413–421.
3. Gnudi G, Volta A, Bonazzi M, et al. Ultrasonographic features of grass awn migration in the dog. *Vet Radiol Ultrasound*. 2005;46:423–426.
4. Della Santa D, Rossi F, Carlucci F, et al. Ultrasound-guided retrieval of plant awns. *Vet Radiol Ultrasound*. 2008;49:484–486.
5. Wong JK, Chambers LC, Elsmo EJ, et al. Cellulitis caused by the *Burkholderia cepacia* complex associated with contaminated chlorhexidine 2% scrub in five domestic cats. *J Vet Diagn Invest*. 2018;30:763–769.
6. Thomas O, Ramsay A, Yiasemidou M, et al. The surgical management of cutaneous abscesses: a UK cross-sectional survey. *Ann Med Surg (Lond)*. 2020;60:654–659.
7. Hall M. Antimicrobial treatment of simple cutaneous abscesses. *J Am Vet Med Assoc*. 2010;236:620.
8. Stevens DL, Bisno AL, Chambers HF, et al. Practice guidelines for the diagnosis and management of skin and soft tissue infections: 2014 update by the Infectious Diseases Society of America. *Clin Infect Dis*. 2014;59:e10–52.
9. Lopez J, Gomez G, Rodriguez K, et al. Comparative study of drainage and antibiotics versus drainage only in the management of primary subcutaneous abscesses. *Surg Infect (Larchmt)*. 2018;19:345–351.
10. Six R, Cleaver DM, Lindeman CJ, et al. Effectiveness and safety of cefovecin sodium, an extended-spectrum injectable cephalosporin, in the treatment of cats with abscesses and infected wounds. *J Am Vet Med Assoc*. 2009;234:81–87.
11. Stegemann MR, Sherington J, Passmore C. The efficacy and safety of cefovecin in the treatment of feline abscesses and infected wounds. *J Small Anim Pract*. 2007;48:683–689.
12. Silley P, Stephan B, Greife HA, et al. Comparative activity of pradofloxacin against anaerobic bacteria isolated from dogs and cats. *J Antimicrob Chemother*. 2007;60:999–1003.
13. Hardefeldt L, Hur B, Verspoor K, et al. Use of cefovecin in dogs and cats attending first-opinion veterinary practices in Australia. *Vet Rec*. 2020;187:e95.
14. Hur BA, Hardefeldt LY, Verspoor KM, et al. Describing the antimicrobial usage patterns of companion animal veterinary practices; free text analysis of more than 4.4 million consultation records. *PLoS One*. 2020;15:e0230049.
15. Hoshuyama S, Kanoe M, Amimoto A. Isolation of obligate and facultative anaerobic bacteria from feline subcutaneous abscesses. *J Vet Med Sci*. 1996;58:273–274.
16. Jang SS, Lock A, Biberstein EL. A cat with *Corynebacterium equi* lymphadenitis clinically simulating lymphosarcoma. *Cornell Vet*. 1975;65:232–239.
17. Kanoe M, Kido M, Toda M. Obligate anaerobic bacteria found in canine and feline purulent lesions. *Br Vet J*. 1984;140:257–262.
18. Love DN, Jones RF, Bailey M. Characterization of *Fusobacterium* species isolated from soft tissue infections in cats. *J Appl Bacteriol*. 1980;48:325–331.
19. Love DN, Jones RF, Bailey M. Characterization of *Bacteroides* species isolated from soft tissue infections in cats. *J Appl Bacteriol*. 1981;50:567–575.
20. Love DN, Jones RF, Bailey M, et al. Isolation and characterisation of bacteria from abscesses in the subcutis of cats. *J Med Microbiol*. 1979;12:207–212.
21. Norris JM, Love DN. The isolation and enumeration of three feline oral *Porphyromonas* species from subcutaneous abscesses in cats. *Vet Microbiol*. 1999;65:115–122.

121

Osteomyelitis, Discospondylitis, and Infectious Arthritis

Jane E. Sykes, Amy S. Kapatkin

KEY POINTS

- Causes: The most common causes of osteomyelitis and infectious monoarthritis in dogs are *Staphylococcus* spp., but streptococci, other gram-negative bacteria, anaerobes, and fungi may be involved. *Bartonella, Nocardia,* and *Mycobacterium* can also cause osteomyelitis. *Brucella* can cause osteomyelitis and discospondylitis. Polyarthritis may be caused by a wide range of gram-positive and gram-negative bacteria; vector-borne bacterial pathogens (*Rickettsia rickettsii, Ehrlichia canis, Anaplasma phagocytophilum, Ehrlichia ewingii, Borrelia burgdorferi*); protozoa (*Leishmania*); and fungi.
- Geographic Distribution: Worldwide, although the prevalence of brucellosis and vector-borne and fungal causes varies geographically.
- Major Clinical Signs: Pain, lameness, fever, inappetence, lethargy, draining skin lesions, and soft tissue swelling may occur with osteomyelitis. Spinal pain, fever, lethargy, inappetence, and pelvic limb paresis or paralysis can occur with discospondylitis. A stiff gait, reluctance to move, lameness, fever, inappetence, lethargy, and swollen joints may occur with polyarthritis.
- Differential Diagnoses: Differential diagnoses for suspected osteomyelitis, monoarthritis, and discospondylitis include bone neoplasia, sterile foreign body reactions, and degenerative osteoarthritis. Primary immune-mediated polyarthritis is the major differential diagnosis for suspected infectious polyarthritis.
- Human Health Significance: When draining wounds are present, resistant bacteria such as methicillin-resistant *Staphylococcus* spp. associated with osteomyelitis and arthritis in dogs and cats may have the potential to colonize human patients. Discospondylitis and polyarthritis caused by *Brucella* spp. can be transmitted to humans through contact with infected urine. Because vector-borne pathogens and fungi of importance to human health can cause polyarthritis, hospital staff should take special care to avoid sharps injuries when working with animals with polyarthritis.

Infectious osteomyelitis is defined as infection of the cortical bone, periosteum, and myeloid cavity, and the associated inflammatory response. The axial and/or appendicular skeleton may be involved. *Discospondylitis* refers to inflammation of the intervertebral discs and adjacent cartilaginous endplates, and almost always results from infection by bacteria or fungi. *Infectious arthritis* refers to inflammation of the synovium, synovial fluid, and associated cartilage secondary to infectious causes.

Osteomyelitis, discospondylitis, and arthritis can result from: (1) hematogenous spread of bacteria or fungi to these sites, or (2) from direct introduction of bacteria as a result of penetrating wounds or surgery. When fungi are involved, molds such as *Aspergillus* spp. or *Paecilomyces* spp. are more likely than yeasts to cause osteomyelitis and discospondylitis (especially in genetically predisposed breeds such as German shepherds, see Chapter 86); *Candida* has rarely been associated with discospondylitis in dogs.[1] In contrast, osteomyelitis can be caused by opportunistic molds or dimorphic fungi, especially *Coccidioides* spp. or *Blastomyces* spp. Fungal arthritis is uncommon but has been associated with infection by *Coccidioides* spp., *Blastomyces* spp., and *Cryptococcus* spp.

OSTEOMYELITIS

ETIOLOGIC AGENTS AND EPIDEMIOLOGY

Bacterial osteomyelitis most often results from direct introduction of bacteria into wounds adjacent to bone. Bacteria can be introduced into the bone as a result of penetrating foreign bodies, surgical wounds (especially orthopedic surgeries with implant placement), traumatic wounds, bite wounds, or extension of soft tissue infections. In one study from Brazil, 78% of cases followed a motor vehicle accident, 17% dog bite wounds, and 5% were secondary to pododermatitis.[2] Human research shows a low incidence of osteomyelitis for elective procedures, but high (33%) reinfection rates after a *Staphylococcus* infection occurs. There are three ways that staphylococci from an implant biofilm invade bone tissue and evade inactivation: (1) formation of abscesses in the soft tissues and bone marrow; (2) glycocalyx formation on the implant; and (3) colonization of the osteocyte lacuna-canalicular network of cortical bone.[3] Veterinary orthopedic infection rates are poorly reported. Infection rates reported depend on the orthopedic procedure.[4] Tibial plateau leveling osteotomy (TPLO) surgery for cranial cruciate rupture, one of the most common orthopedic surgical procedures performed, has a postoperative implant removal rate of 2.7% to 8.5% because of confirmed implant-associated infection.[5–11] For unknown reasons, the surgical site infection (SSI) rate after TPLO appears to be higher than that after routine "clean" orthopedic surgeries that involve osteotomy (as opposed to fracture repair). In a report that was published before the TPLO procedure was described, the overall infection rate after any orthopedic surgery procedure was 3 (<1%) of 502 surgeries.[12] In contrast, radiographically detectable osteomyelitis was reported in 14 (7.3%) of 193 dogs that underwent TPLO surgery and was the single most common complication of the procedure.[6] A 1% rate of osteomyelitis was reported in a prospective study of 100 dogs undergoing stifle surgery, whereas the incision infection rate was 8%.[13] One recent review reported TPLO infection rates that ranged from 0.8% to 14.3%.[14] Total joint replacement infection rate was reported to be up to 11%.[4,15,16] Infection rate after fracture repair varies. It was 9 (8%) of 110 surgeries in one study.[17] In this study, 20% of the fractures were open. Open fractures were 4 times more likely to be contaminated with bacteria at the time of surgery than the closed fractures, and contaminated wounds were 5 times more likely to develop complications (seroma, drainage, and dehiscence) than those without contamination. Distal radius/ulna and tibial fractures were 10.5 times and 7.5 times more likely to be contaminated than femoral fractures, respectively. Animals with a normal postoperative temperature and a clean surgical wound did not develop postoperative complications.

Although gram-positive aerobes such as staphylococci and, to a lesser extent, streptococci predominate as a cause of osteomyelitis in dogs and cats, the organisms present and the bone(s) affected generally reflect the underlying type of injury that led to infection. For example, osteomyelitis that follows SSI is often caused by *Staphylococcus pseudintermedius*, a common commensal of canine skin (Table 121.1). *Staphylococcus aureus* and gram-negative bacterial infections can also cause orthopedic SSIs.[8] In contrast, anaerobes (e.g., *Bacteroides, Cutibacterium acnes, Peptostreptococcus, Clostridium, Fusobacterium, Actinomyces*) and aerobic gram-positive bacteria (staphylococci, enterococci, streptococci) or gram-negative bacteria (*Pseudomonas, Escherichia coli, Klebsiella pneumoniae, Proteus, Pasteurella*) predominate in osteomyelitis that results from bite wound infections, tooth root abscesses, or penetrating foreign bodies.[18,19] Such mixed bacterial infections are also common in dogs with digital osteomyelitis. Anaerobes were isolated from 64% of osteomyelitis cases in dogs in one study.[19]

Osteomyelitis secondary to bacteremia, also known as *hematogenous osteomyelitis*, is very rare and usually affects young to middle-aged animals.[4,20] The metaphyseal regions are often involved, sometimes with extension to the epiphyses and joints (Fig. 121.1). The pathogenesis remains obscure. It has been suggested that discontinuous endothelium in the primary spongiosa may predispose to extravasation of erythrocytes and bacteria in this region.[21] In humans, acute hematogenous osteomyelitis results from bacterial seeding secondary to transient bacteremia, which may result from conditions such as otitis media. Trauma to the bone and upregulation of bacterial virulence factors may also be important for allowing establishment of infection.[22] Sternal, pelvic, and vertebral osteomyelitis can also result from hematogenous spread of bacteria.[20] Osteomyelitis occasionally also results from hematogenous spread of fastidious bacteria such as *Brucella, Bartonella, Mycobacterium, Nocardia,* and *Nocardiopsis* spp.

CLINICAL FEATURES

Pathogenesis and Clinical Signs

The development of bacterial osteomyelitis requires the presence not only of bacteria but also of compromised bone. Bone necrosis can result from trauma (i.e., fracture), surgery, or underlying bone neoplasia. Bacteria adhere to fibronectin, a connective tissue glycoprotein, through the use of a variety of adhesins. The presence of foreign material promotes persistence of infection in the form of biofilm (Fig. 121.2). *Staphylococcus pseudintermedius, S. aureus, Pseudomonas aeruginosa,* and *E. coli* are particularly apt to form biofilms. Adherent bacteria produce a matrix of condensed exopolysaccharides known as a glycocalyx.[23] The biofilm is composed of a cluster of microorganisms and glycocalyx on an inanimate surface. Embedded in the biofilm mixture of glycocalyx, host-derived serum proteins, and cellular debris, bacteria often form into microcolonies. Within biofilm, bacteria evade opsonization and phagocytosis and are protected from the effects of antimicrobial drugs. Staphylococci can reside within osteoblasts, and when cell death occurs, they are released and can re-establish a productive infection.[23] Bacteria within biofilms intercommunicate via cytokines (quorum sensing), and this appears to assist them in their ability to evade host defense mechanisms. Bone sequestra can also become colonized by bacteria, which evade host defenses in the absence of adequate blood supply. Loose implants and fracture instability contribute to bone resorption, compromised blood supply, and persistent infection.[21] Some implant types are more apt to be colonized by bacteria.

TABLE 121.1 Bacteria Isolated from 31 Dogs with Surgical Site Infections After Tibial Plateau Leveling Operations[a]

Bacterial Classification	Species	Number of Isolates (%)	Proportion of Staphylococci Methicillin Resistant	Proportion of Staphylococci Multidrug Resistant[b]
Gram-positive aerobes (*n* = 30)	*Staphylococcus pseudintermedius*	20 (49)	4/20 (20%)	7/20 (35%)
	Staphylococcus aureus	3 (7)	2/3	1/3
	Coagulase-negative staphylococci	3 (7)	1/3	0
	Staphylococcus schleiferi subsp. *coagulans*	1 (2)	0	0
	Enterococcus spp.	3 (7)	NA	2/3
Gram-negative aerobes (*n* = 9)	Enterobacterales (*Escherichia coli, Proteus, Klebsiella pneumoniae*)	4 (10)	NA	1/2[c]
	Pseudomonas aeruginosa	3 (7)	NA	2/3
	Eugonic fermenter-4–like	1 (2)	NA	0
	Pasteurella canis	1 (2)	NA	0
Anaerobes (*n* = 2)	*Actinomyces*	1 (2)	NA	ND
	Cutibacterium acnes	1 (2)	NA	ND

Mixed infections with two or three bacterial species or strains were present in 7 (23%) of the dogs (total 41 isolates).
[a]Cases seen at the University of California-Davis Veterinary Medical Teaching Hospital.
[b]Resistant to three or more classes of antimicrobial drugs.
[c]One of two *E. coli* and the *Proteus* isolate did not undergo susceptibility testing because isolation was performed at necropsy.
NA, not applicable; *ND,* not done.

Stainless-steel plates have been associated with a higher risk of SSIs than titanium plates.[24] In one study, Slocum TPLO plates were more likely to be removed than other types of TPLO plates because of local bacterial infection and clinical signs of inflammation.[11] In another retrospective study of 104 TPLO procedures, the rate of SSI was higher among dogs treated with Synthes implants than among those with Slocum implants, but there was no significant difference in the rate of infection among the New Generation, Synthes, and Slocum implants.[25]

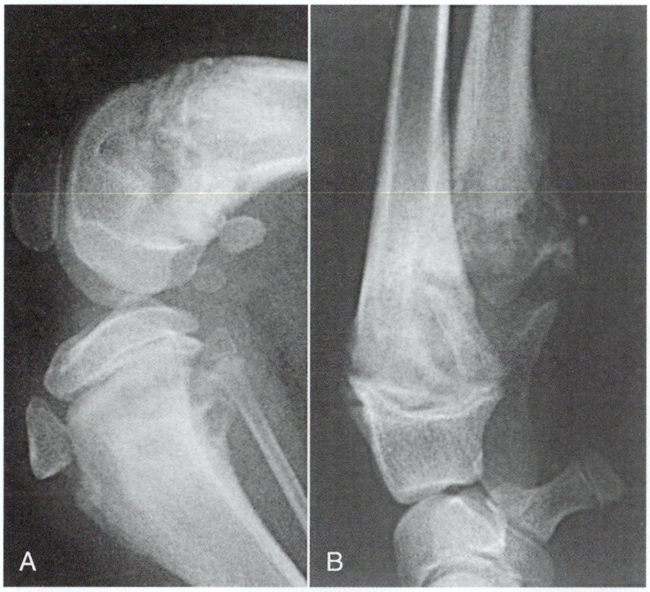

Fig. 121.1 Polyostotic metaphyseal osteomyelitis in a Border collie puppy that had persistent neutropenia. (A) Disruption of metaphyseal architecture of distal femur and proximal tibia, with irregular areas of radiolucency and sclerosis and some adjacent periosteal new bone. (B) Similar changes are evident in the distal radius and ulna. (From Ettinger SJ, Feldman EC, eds. *Textbook of Veterinary Internal Medicine*. 7th ed. St. Louis, MO: Saunders; 2010.)

Inflammatory cells recruited to the site of infection release enzymes that cause additional bone necrosis, with destruction of cancellous and cortical bone and abscessation of associated soft tissue. The end result is focal swelling, pain, draining skin lesions, and lameness. Small draining skin lesions often represent the "tip of the iceberg", with extensive bone involvement hidden beneath the skin (see Fig. 121.2). The presence of anaerobes can be associated with a foul odor or gas production. Fever, inappetence, lethargy, and leukocytosis are occasionally present in animals with acute osteomyelitis but are often absent in chronic osteomyelitis. In a 2018 study of dogs that required removal of tibial tuberosity advancement (TTA) cages to resolve SSIs, the mean time to appearance of signs related to SSI was 403 days after surgery (median: 287 days, range: 10 to 1,547 days).[26] Occasionally, infection reactivates in dogs years after surgery and implant placement. In human patients, latent periods between infection and development of osteomyelitis can last many decades.[27]

Physical Examination Findings

Physical examination findings in dogs and cats with osteomyelitis include lameness, localized pain, soft tissue swelling, muscle atrophy, and the presence of draining tracts. Fever and lethargy can also be identified in some animals.

DIAGNOSIS

In most cases, osteomyelitis is diagnosed on the basis of history, physical examination, and diagnostic imaging findings. Aerobic and anaerobic bacterial culture of affected bone or any implants present is required for definitive diagnosis.

Laboratory Abnormalities

The CBC of animals with osteomyelitis may be unremarkable or reveal mild anemia, neutrophilia with bandemia, and monocytosis. The serum biochemistry panel and urinalysis are usually unremarkable, unless bacteremia or other systemic disease is also present.

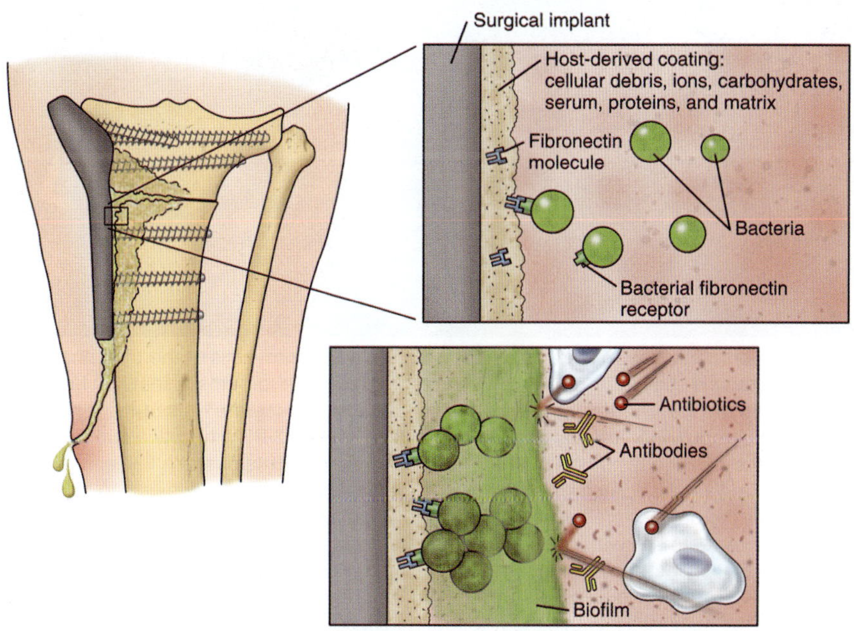

Fig. 121.2 Pathogenesis of osteomyelitis. Necrotic bone is colonized by bacteria, which adhere to fibronectin and in the presence of foreign material (in this case, an implant) can form biofilm. Biofilm consists of bacterial aggregates embedded in a matrix of exopolysaccharide (bacterial slime). The biofilm protects the bacteria from antibodies, phagocytosis, and antimicrobial drugs.

Diagnostic Imaging

Radiographic changes in dogs and cats with osteomyelitis vary considerably in extent and character. In some dogs and cats, only soft tissue swelling may be evident. Plain radiography is insensitive and can be poorly specific for diagnosis of osteomyelitis, and interpretation can vary from one board-certified radiologist to another. In one study, plain radiographic findings were interpreted as osteomyelitis by two radiologists in only five of eight dogs with experimentally induced osteomyelitis.[28] One radiologist diagnosed osteomyelitis in only three of the eight dogs, but that radiologist was less likely than the other radiologists to diagnose osteomyelitis when infection was absent.

When radiographic bony changes are evident, they consist of periosteal proliferation, which may be smooth or speculated; focal osteopenia with cortical resorption or thinning; loss of trabecular markings; lucency around implants such as cages, plates, or screws; and sequestration (Fig. 121.3). Pathologic fractures may be evident in dogs with fungal osteomyelitis. Scintigraphy with technetium-99m methylene diphosphonate, gallium-67 citrate, and indium-111-labeled leukocytes has been used in human medicine but is considered expensive and can lack specificity.[29] Bone scintigraphy has also been used for diagnosis of hematogenous arthritis in dogs with multiple site involvement.[20] Ultrasound imaging, contrast CT, MRI, and 18F-flurodeoxyglucose PET are sensitive diagnostic tools and may be useful for identification of sequestra, foreign material, and abscess formation. IV administration of ultraparamagnetic iron oxide nanoparticles during MRI, which are taken up by macrophages, has shown promise for detection of vertebral osteomyelitis and differentiation of osteomyelitis from aseptic inflammation.[4,30,31] Serum immunoassays that detect antibody responses to staphylococcal proteins, such as iron acquisition proteins and secreted toxins, have also shown utility for diagnosis and prognostication in human patients with osteomyelitis, although they can lack specificity due to previous exposure or asymptomatic colonization.[3]

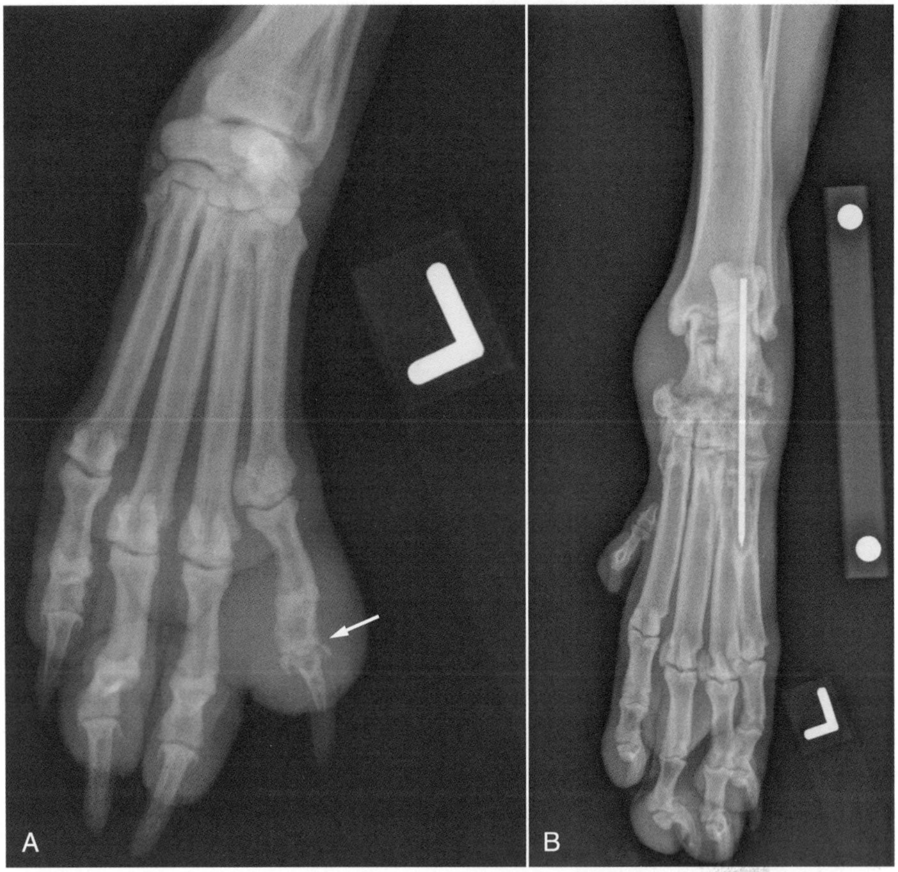

Fig. 121.3 Radiographic changes in bacterial osteomyelitis. (A) Osteomyelitis of the third phalanx of the fifth digit in a 7-year-old female spayed fox terrier with systemic lupus erythematosus that had been treated with prednisone and cyclosporine. There is severe soft tissue swelling, moderate lysis of the distal aspect of the third phalanx, and an irregular cortical margin with loss of the normal P2-P3 joint space *(arrow)*. A *Nocardia* sp. was isolated from the draining lymph node. (B) Radiographs of the left tarsus of a 5-year-old male neutered pit bull terrier with implant-associated osteomyelitis. A partial left tarsal arthrodesis had been performed a year previously after the dog suffered a traumatic injury. Draining tracts then developed in association with the screw heads, and treatment with cephalexin was unsuccessful. There is severe irregular bone lysis on both sides of the proximal intertarsal joint. A surgical pin extends from the proximal calcaneus through the tarsal joint to the level of the mid-diaphysis of the fifth metatarsal bone. There is a region of lucency that surrounds the tip of the surgical pin within the fifth metatarsal bone. The cortex of the fourth metatarsal bone adjacent to the pin is thickened with a slightly irregular periosteal reaction. The first phalanx of the first digit is incomplete (likely congenital). There is marked soft tissue swelling associated with the tarsus. A methicillin-susceptible *Staphylococcus aureus* was cultured from the implant at surgery to remove the pin. Tobramycin-impregnated calcium sulfate beads were used to fill the pin tract.

Microbiologic Tests

Isolation and Identification

Aerobic and anaerobic bacterial culture and susceptibility should be performed on aspirates of pus, bone biopsies, or removed implants from dogs and cats with osteomyelitis. Aspirates should be collected in a sterile manner from the focus of infection to avoid contamination with surface bacteria (e.g., via aspiration of lesions through healthy skin after skin antisepsis, or through collection of biopsies or implants during surgical exploration). Negative culture results may reflect an insufficient specimen size, or the presence of fastidious bacteria such as anaerobes, *Bartonella, Brucella, Nocardia,* or *Mycobacterium* spp. Sonication of implants removed from humans that had implant-associated osteomyelitis increased the sensitivity of culture from 67% to 90%.[32] Blood cultures should be performed if hematogenous osteomyelitis is suspected based on the history and clinical findings (young animal, multiple sites affected, sternal or vertebral involvement, other systemic illness, or immunosuppression).

Pathologic Findings

Pathologic findings in osteomyelitis depend on the causative agent and chronicity of infection. Inflammatory cell infiltrates may range from suppurative (acute osteomyelitis) to pyogranulomatous or lymphoplasmacytic. The neutrophilic infiltrate in dogs with acute osteomyelitis may be accompanied by the presence of fibrin, free red blood cells, and necrotic debris. There may be evidence of bone resorption with multinucleated osteoclasts and new bone and fibrous tissue formation. In some cases, intralesional bacteria or fragments of foreign material (such as plant material) are observed (Fig. 121.4).

TREATMENT AND PROGNOSIS

Treatment recommendations for focal osteomyelitis secondary to trauma, surgery, or foreign body penetration depends on the severity and chronicity of disease, the location of osteomyelitis, the presence or absence of foreign material or implant, and the extent of blood supply to the bone. In animals with fractures, early detection and treatment of osteomyelitis is critical to prevent extensive bone necrosis and nonunion. Antimicrobial drug treatment alone is usually not sufficient to resolve chronic bacterial osteomyelitis, because sequestra and biofilm are avascular and are not effectively penetrated by antimicrobial drugs. In general, treatment requires debridement, removal of sequestra and foreign material, dead space removal, copious lavage with sterile saline, rigid fracture stabilization, systemic and/or local administration of appropriate antimicrobial drugs, and grafting of bone deficits. Because implants may ultimately need to be removed to resolve infection, fractures may need stabilization through alternative means, such as external skeletal fixation or one- or two-stage implant replacement revision surgeries. Removal of the infected implant and replacing it at the time of debridement helps to prevent colonization of the lacunar canaliculi by staphylococci.[33] Maintenance of bone stabilization is considered paramount in human medicine, because unstable fractures or surgical sites are considerably more prone to infection than those that are stable.[29] It is considered better to leave an implant in place and maintain stabilization than to remove an implant early. In a study of 121 people with infection after fracture fixation, approximately 70% of the time, stable implants could be salvaged following extensive irrigation, debridement, and appropriate systemic antibiotics.[34] Systemic antimicrobial drug therapy (and often regional antibiotic therapy in the form of antimicrobial drug–impregnated beads or gel) is required while the bone heals. In some cases, foci of osteomyelitis may be removed en bloc without the need for further graft placement or stabilization (e.g., digital osteomyelitis). Resected bone should be submitted for histopathology (to confirm the presence of osteomyelitis and identify other processes such as fungal infection or neoplasia) as well as aerobic and anaerobic culture and susceptibility testing. Wounds are left open after debridement if continued debridement is needed via wet-to-dry bandaging. In severely infected cases, vacuum-assisted wound closure techniques are recommended. If all nonviable tissue has been removed, closed irrigation systems or vascularized tissue flaps may be used to manage dead space. A sterile dressing should be used to cover the wounds, with daily bandage changes until exudation resolves. If needed, autogenous cancellous bone graft placement is delayed until infection has been controlled and granulation tissue has begun to fill the wound (usually 1 to 2 weeks after initiation of antimicrobial drug treatment).[35] When graft placement or fracture stabilization is not possible because of financial concerns or uncontrollable infection, amputation may be necessary.

The choice of antimicrobial drugs should be based on the results of aerobic and anaerobic bacterial culture and susceptibility. If the animal is stable, treatment should be withheld until results are available, and medications to manage pain should be administered. If earlier antimicrobial

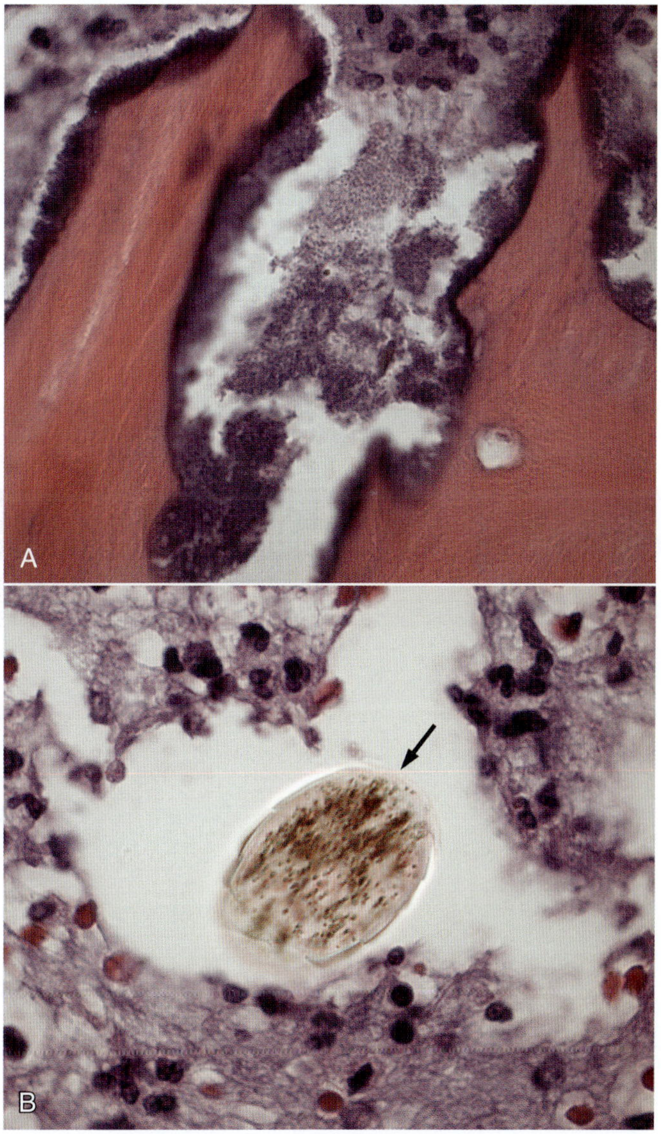

Fig. 121.4 Histopathology from the right pelvic fourth digit of a 3-year-old intact male Labrador retriever with an open articular fracture and chronic suppurative bacterial osteomyelitis. (A) Large numbers of bacteria are adhered to bone fragments (eosinophilic material) with an associated neutrophilic inflammatory response. (B) In other fields, intralesional plant material was visible *(arrow)*.

treatment is deemed necessary pending the results of culture and susceptibility, the drug chosen should be based on the history (e.g., postsurgical infection versus bite wound infection) and local prevalence data for the practice (Table 121.2). The presence of anaerobes should be assumed if anaerobic culture is not performed, or anaerobes are not isolated, especially if the underlying insult was a bite wound or a traumatic injury. Clindamycin is a reasonable initial choice for infections that could include susceptible staphylococci and/or anaerobic bacteria and was effective in experimental models of *S. aureus* osteomyelitis in dogs,[36] but a significant proportion of MRS exhibit clindamycin resistance or inducible clindamycin resistance (see Chapter 51). In a study of dogs with osteomyelitis from Brazil, nearly 60% of isolates exhibited clindamycin resistance.[2] In that study, a greater proportion of isolates (79%) were susceptible to amoxicillin-clavulanic acid. If gram-negative bacteria or MRS are suspected, the addition of an aminoglycoside may be necessary if treatment must be instituted before the results of culture and susceptibility become available. However, aminoglycosides penetrate poorly into purulent material, so adequate debridement is essential. Combinations of antibiotics are sometimes required in animals with polymicrobial infections. Systemic antibiotic treatment should be continued for at least 4 to 6 weeks. Longer periods of treatment may be required in some dogs and cats, especially if an implant is present. The duration of therapy should be considered on a case-by-case basis, depending on the underlying problem (fracture, corrective osteotomy, bite wound), the likely organisms present, and depth of infection. Antimicrobial drugs should be given parenterally in the hospital for at least the first 3 to 5 days, and for longer if possible. There is evidence that use of fluoroquinolones may delay bone healing, and so in human medicine it is recommended that the use of fluoroquinolones be avoided if possible.[29] The use of linezolid has been reported for treatment of MDR orthopedic MRSP SSIs in 4 dogs.[37] Adverse effects of vomiting, lethargy, and anorexia (2 dogs) and regenerative anemia (1 dog) were reported. Infections recurred in 2 dogs after discontinuation of treatment.

In addition to systemic treatment, antibiotic-impregnated beads or gel can be used to treat chronic osteomyelitis and septic arthritis in dogs.[38,39] Beads are prepared in the operating room by mixing an antimicrobial drug with commercially available calcium sulfate bead sets and setting through the use of a rubber mold. The beads are placed at the site of infection, where they deliver high concentrations of drug to the site (e.g., initially 500-fold that of normal serum concentrations with systemic treatment), sometimes for several weeks, without systemic adverse effects.[40] The antimicrobial drugs used are generally heat stable, hydrophilic, and have activity against MRS, such as aminoglycosides (gentamicin or tobramycin) or vancomycin. Gentamicin-impregnated beads were shown to reduce biofilm formation by methicillin-resistant *S. pseudintermedius*.[41] Other products include antibiotic-impregnated collagen, bone graft substitutes such as calcium phosphate (Fig. 121.5), and a variety of synthetic polymers such as polylactic acid, polylactide-co-glycolides, and cross-linked polydimethylsiloxane.[40] Tobramycin-impregnated calcium phosphate beads have been used successfully to treat osteomyelitis in dogs.[39] Polymers have been engineered to control the duration and concentration of antibiotic treatment at the site. Hydrogel is another medium to deliver antibiotics. The gel is aliquoted and then sterilized before use. It has to be refrigerated and mixed with the antimicrobial of choice in a hood to avoid contamination. The gel can be injected through a rubber catheter or placed in the site before wound closure. It has the advantage of being less expensive than beads but has a shorter duration of antimicrobial elution. The gel may be preferred when the infection is near a joint or a surgical approach is not being used.[38] Recently, IV administration of activated mesenchymal stem cells in conjunction with antibiotic therapy has also shown efficacy for treatment of chronic osteomyelitis.[42] Optimization of local antibiotic delivery systems in order to promote continuous delivery of appropriate concentrations of antibiotics, while avoiding colonization of the materials used, is currently the subject of extensive research.

TABLE 121.2 Suggested Initial Antimicrobial Drug Doses for Stable Animals with Bacterial Orthopedic Infections Pending Culture and Susceptibility Results

Disease	Drug	Dose (mg/kg)	Route	Interval (Hours)
Osteomyelitis or monoarthritis	Clindamycin hydrochloride, clindamycin phosphate	11–33 (dogs) 11 (cats) 10	PO PO IV,[a] IM	12 (dogs) 24 (cats) 12
	Enrofloxacin[b]	5–20 (dogs)	IV, IM, PO	24
	Gentamicin sulfate[c]	14 (dogs) 8 (cats)	IV, IM, SC	24
	Amikacin[c]	15–30 (dogs) 10–14 (cats)	IV, IM, SC	24
Discospondylitis	Ampicillin sodium	20	IV	6
	Ampicillin-sulbactam[d]	20	IV	8
	Amoxicillin–clavulanic acid	20–25	PO	12
	Cefazolin sodium	20–35	IV, IM	8
	Cephalexin	20–30	PO	6–8

[a]For IV administration, dilute 1:10 in 0.9% saline and administer over 30–60 minutes.
[b]Addition of fluoroquinolones to clindamycin or a β-lactam is indicated if gram-negative bacteria may be present and methicillin resistance among staphylococci is not prevalent in the region. In cats, other fluoroquinolones such as pradofloxacin or marbofloxacin are preferred because of the risk of retinopathy (see Chapter 10 for doses and contraindications). Use of pradofloxacin has been associated with bone marrow suppression in dogs, especially at high doses.
[c]Addition of aminoglycosides to clindamycin or a β-lactam is indicated if gram-negative bacteria and/or methicillin-resistant staphylococci may be present. See Chapter 10 for contraindications.
[d]Dose based on ampicillin component.
IM, intramuscular; *IV,* intravenous; *PO,* oral; *SC,* subcutaneous.

PREVENTION

Although not a substitute for sterile surgical technique and strict hospital infection control measures (see Chapter 15), perioperative antimicrobial drug treatment is an accepted aid for prevention of soft tissue surgical infections and osteomyelitis, especially when orthopedic implants are anticipated. Recommendations published for human medicine state that adequate prophylaxis requires: (1) antimicrobial agents with activity against organisms likely to be encountered in the surgical field; (2) timely preoperative antimicrobial drug administration (within 60 minutes of incision); (3) bactericidal concentrations of drug in the serum and tissues during the time that the wound is open; and (4) a duration of 24 hours after surgery.[43] Additional intraoperative doses should be given if the procedure lasts longer than two half-lives of the drug being administered (usually at least 2 hours). However, one study showed that administration of antibiotics longer than 60 minutes before incision was associated with a higher SSI rate than when antibiotics were administered within 60 minutes of incision, but the risk of SSI did not increase if antibiotic administration occurred after incision.[44] In practices where the prevalence of postoperative infections with MRS is low, preoperative treatment with cefazolin may be effective. Where the regional prevalence of skin colonization with MRS is high (e.g., >10%), preoperative treatment with cefazolin and an aminoglycoside such as amikacin could be used. Nevertheless, use of perioperative vancomycin in humans undergoing orthopedic procedures to prevent SSI was associated with an increased risk of SSI (OR 1.75), whereas administration of cefazolin decreased the risk of SSI (OR 0.49).[44] Whether administration of antimicrobials for multiple days postoperatively decreases the risk of infections after orthopedic procedures in dogs has been controversial, with some studies showing no significant benefit, and others showing reduction in the prevalence of SSIs. In a prospective study of 400 dogs that underwent implant surgery, dogs were randomized to receive either 5 days of postoperative antibiotics, or only perioperative antibiotics. The rate of SSI was similar between the two groups.[45] In another prospective study of 100 dogs undergoing clean orthopedic procedures that required stainless-steel plates, postoperative administration of antimicrobials (cephalexin or amoxicillin-clavulanic acid) for 7 days was associated with a lower risk of SSI (4.3%) than for dogs that did not receive postoperative antimicrobials.[46] Prophylactic treatment should never be continued for longer than 24 hours after surgery because it can select for drug-resistant bacterial infections. In human patients, antibiotic-impregnated implants have been used to prevent attachment of bacteria to their surface.[3,40,47] Silver-impregnated coatings show promise for prevention of colonization by *S. pseudintermedius*.[48] Minimization of surgery time, careful surgical technique, and use of plate types that are associated with a lower risk of postoperative infection (i.e., non–Slocum-type TPLO plates) may also prevent postsurgical osteomyelitis.[11] Metals used in implants should be of the same type (e.g., plate and screws) to minimize the chance of galvanic corrosion. Galvanic corrosion occurs when metals of different electrochemical properties are placed in close proximity in an electrolytic environment. This can predispose to implant loosening, local infection, or sarcoma formation.[49] Currently, it is considered acceptable to leave implants in place after healing unless the animal has persistent pain associated with the implant, or radiographic evidence of osteomyelitis or osteopenia is present. This is because the process of implant removal itself can be costly and may be followed by osteomyelitis or fracture. However, owners of pets with implants should be advised that although rare, possible long-term complications of implant placement include reactivation of infection in the future or development of malignancy at the implant site.

PUBLIC HEALTH ASPECTS

Dogs and cats with bacterial osteomyelitis can shed antibiotic-resistant gram-positive and gram-negative bacteria that have the potential to colonize humans and later be a source of human infection. Infections acquired after orthopedic surgeries, especially TPLOs, and joint replacements are problematic. Most dogs are infected with *S. pseudintermedius*, but a smaller percentage of dogs are infected with *S. aureus*,

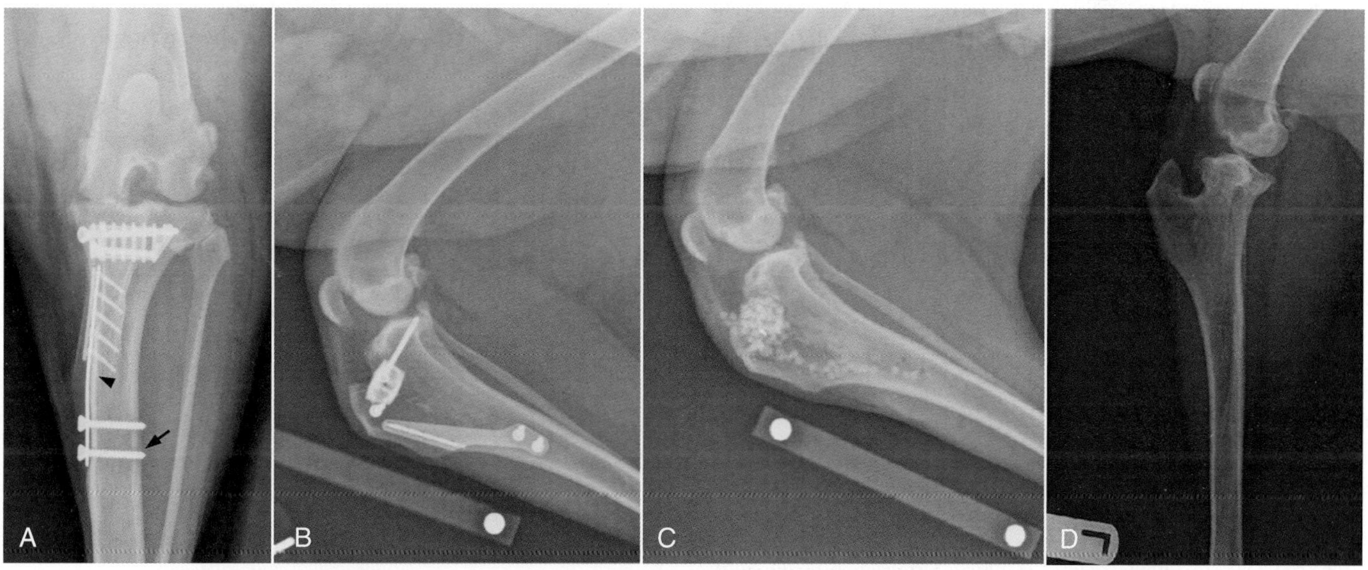

Fig. 121.5 Lateral radiographs of the left stifle from a 10-year-old female spayed greyhound–pit bull terrier mix that developed osteomyelitis at the site of a left tibial tuberosity advancement surgery (see Case Example). (A) Anteropalmar and (B) lateral radiographs of the left stifle 13 months after the surgery. The osteotomy site has filled with bone to some extent, but the site is still visible as a result of incomplete union. There was also lucency in the region of the most distal screw *(arrow)* and thinning of the cortical bone adjacent to the plate *(arrowhead)*. (C) The cage was removed by drilling around it, and calcium sulfate (Osteoset) beads were used to fill the defect. (D) Radiograph taken 13 months postoperatively showing resolution of osteomyelitis and degradation of the calcium sulfate beads. The region of cage removal never refilled with bone.

which is more likely to colonize humans (see Table 121.1). However, in some cases, the human in the household may have been the source of *S. aureus* infection. Some hospitals experience a high prevalence (>10%) of postoperative wound infections with MRS. In a case-control study that included dogs with methicillin-resistant *S. aureus* infection (cases) and dogs with methicillin-susceptible *S. aureus* infection (controls), surgical implant placement was associated with a 33-fold increased risk of methicillin-resistant *S. aureus* infection ($P = .001$).[50] Infected osteomyelitis wounds should be covered with a suitable dressing at all times, and owners should be advised to wear gloves when handling their pets (especially if the wound is infected) and to wash their hands properly afterwards. In the hospital, animals with draining orthopedic surgical wound infections due to methicillin-resistant or MDR bacteria should be handled by a limited number of individuals who wear gloves, a gown, and dedicated equipment, and signage should be posted. Hand washing should be performed after protective wear is removed, and all equipment used should be disinfected properly (see Chapter 15).

DISCOSPONDYLITIS

ETIOLOGIC AGENTS, PATHOGENESIS, AND EPIDEMIOLOGY

Discospondylitis most often follows hematogenous spread of bacteria or fungi to the cartilaginous vertebral endplates, with extension to the intervertebral discs. Bacteria or fungi are thought to lodge in the endplates because blood flow slows in this region. In most cases, the source of infection cannot be identified, but infection can originate from the urogenital tract, abscesses, skin wounds, respiratory tract infections, or the oral cavity. Occasionally, discospondylitis follows extension of infection from an adjacent site, such as following vertebral column SSIs, complications of epidural anesthesia, bite wounds, or migrating grass awns.

Risk factors for discospondylitis in dogs include male sex, older age, and breed.[1] Predisposed breeds are often large-breed dogs, such as great Danes, boxers, rottweilers, English bulldogs, German shepherd dogs, and Doberman pinschers. German shepherds and Rhodesian ridgebacks are predisposed to systemic mold infections that can target the intervertebral discs.[51] Although discospondylitis is frequently diagnosed in Labrador and golden retrievers, these dogs are popular breeds and were not found to be at risk.[1] Discospondylitis is extremely rare in cats and usually follows trauma such as cat bites, with associated meningomyelitis.[52–56] Concurrent disorders identified in dogs include genitourinary tract infections (prostatitis, orchitis, metritis, and/or UTI), pyoderma and otitis, immunosuppressive drug treatment, heartworm disease, recent vertebral column surgery, respiratory tract infection, bite wounds and other traumatic injuries, migrating foreign bodies, recent nonvertebral surgery, septic arthritis, severe intestinal parasitism, and infective endocarditis.

The incidence of discospondylitis in dogs and prevalence of different causative infectious agents vary geographically. In one study in the United States, the incidence of discospondylitis was higher in the southern states than in the northern states.[1] In 123 dogs with discospondylitis from the southern United States, the most common pathogen isolated was *Staphylococcus* (41% of 63 isolates), followed by *Streptococcus* (12%), and *E. coli* (11%).[1] Other bacteria included *Klebsiella*, *Brucella canis*, *Pseudomonas*, *Proteus*, and *Actinomyces* spp. (<10% each). When the results of *Brucella* serology and culture were combined, 13 of the dogs were diagnosed with brucellosis. Only two dogs were infected with fungal organisms, one with *Candida tropicalis* and the other with an unidentified fungal agent. Mixed infections were detected in 11 (9%) dogs. In 23 dogs with discospondylitis from the Pacific northwest of the United States, 10 of 18 isolates were staphylococci, 3 were streptococci, and 3 were *E. coli*; *Brucella* infection was not reported and a filamentous fungal species (*Phialemonium* or *Paecilomyces*) was isolated from two dogs.[57] In contrast, filamentous fungal species were isolated from nearly one third of dogs diagnosed with discospondylitis at the University of California, Davis (Table 121.3). The most common bacterial isolate was methicillin-susceptible *S. pseudintermedius*; MRS were not detected. In more than half of dogs with discospondylitis, the causative agent is not identified. Lumbar discospondylitis caused by *Actinomyces* spp. and anaerobic bacteria may occur as a result of migration of inhaled grass awns, which lodge in the retroperitoneal space. Sexually intact male dogs and dogs from the southeastern states are at increased risk for *B. canis* discospondylitis,[58] but it can occur in any region and in dogs of any sex. In a German study, 4 dogs with *B. canis* discospondylitis were described; the dogs were young (7–30 months of age) and had been imported into Germany from eastern Europe (Moldavia, Macedonia, Romania).[59] Other reported agents include *Enterobacter*, *Nocardia*, *Salmonella*, and *Erysipelothrix*.[60–64]

CLINICAL FEATURES

Pathogenesis and Clinical Signs

Clinical signs of discospondylitis include fever, lethargy, inappetence, weight loss, spinal pain, a hunched stance, lameness, reluctance to move, and/or reluctance to jump or climb stairs. The duration of signs is extremely variable, but are usually present for less than 1 month.[58] Spinal cord compression as a result of vertebral subluxation, abscess formation, disc protrusion or extrusion, and soft tissue proliferation can lead to neurologic deficits such as delayed or absent placing reactions, paresis with ataxia or paralysis, and loss of deep pain sensation. Neurologic deficits were detected in 59 (48%) of 123 dogs in one study.[1] In another study, paresis or paralysis was detected in 20 (87%) of 23 dogs and 8 of these dogs were nonambulatory.[58] The neurologic signs reflect the severity and location of discospondylitis lesions; in the latter study, the severity of neurologic signs was correlated with the number of compressive lesions and the percentage of spinal cord or cauda equina compression.[58] The majority (50% to 60%) of dogs have lesions in the thoracolumbar spine (especially the lumbosacral junction); cervical lesions are present in fewer than 20% of dogs.[1,58,65,66] Around 30% to 40% of dogs have multiple lesions. Thus, tetraparesis (which reflects the

TABLE 121.3 Infectious Agents Isolated from 31 Dogs with Culture-Positive Discospondylitis[a]

Organism Type	Infectious Agent	Number of Isolates (%)
Gram-positive aerobes (n = 15, 42%)	*Staphylococcus pseudintermedius* (methicillin-susceptible)	12 (33)
	Coagulase-negative staphylococci	2 (6)
	Streptococcus equisimilis	1 (3)
Gram-negative aerobes (n = 5, 14%)	*Klebsiella pneumoniae*	2 (6)
	Escherichia coli	2 (6)
	Brucella canis	1 (3)
Anaerobes (n = 4, 11%)	*Actinomyces* spp., *Prevotella*, *Fusobacterium*, *Porphyromonas*	4 (11)
Fungi (n = 11, 31%)	*Aspergillus* spp.	6 (17)
	Paecilomyces spp.	3 (8)
	Other molds	2 (3)

[a]Cases seen at the University of California-Davis Veterinary Medical Teaching Hospital. Based on culture of blood and/or disc material (26 dogs) or urine only (5 dogs; 3 with mold infections, 1 with *E. coli*, and 1 with *K. pneumoniae* infections).

presence of compressive cervical lesions) is less common (<5% of dogs) than pelvic limb paresis or paralysis (33% of dogs). The location of discospondylitis lesions (e.g., L7 to S1 versus C5 to C6) does not seem to affect the likelihood of cord compression.[66]

Physical Examination Findings

Dogs with discospondylitis may have fever (although it is often absent), lethargy, weakness, and pain on palpation or manipulation of the spine. Spinal pain is not consistently present. In some dogs, pain is difficult to localize or manifests as apparent abdominal pain when the abdomen is palpated, especially if upward pressure is placed on the spine. Dogs with neurologic deficits can be tetraparetic or have pelvic limb paresis or paralysis. Loss of deep pain sensation can occur in dogs with severe compression lesions. Neurologic examination may reveal delayed or absent placing reactions and exaggerated or reduced segmental reflexes. Evaluation for abnormalities that reflect the presence of concurrent disorders (such as cardiac murmurs in dogs with endocarditis or swollen joints in dogs with polyarthritis) should be carefully performed. Occasionally, discospondylitis is an incidental finding on plain radiography (performed to evaluate concurrent disease such as fever of unknown origin), and clinical signs that suggest discospondylitis are absent.

DIAGNOSIS

Diagnosis of discospondylitis is based on physical examination findings; imaging (plain radiography, CT/MRI); culture of blood, CSF, or aspirates of disc material; and serologic testing for *Brucella* spp. (antibody tests) or fungi (antigen tests). The reader is referred to Chapter 71 (Brucellosis) and Chapter 86 (Aspergillosis and Penicilliosis) for information on serologic testing for these diseases. Serologic testing for *Aspergillus* galactomannan antigen is inexpensive, and positive results (galactomannan indices > 1.5) correlate strongly with an underlying mold infection.[67] Rarely, mixed infections with bacteria and fungi occur, and bacterial contaminants can complicate interpretation of blood and disc aspirates. Thus, all dogs with discospondylitis should ideally be tested for *Aspergillus* antigen before antibiotic treatment is initiated. It is especially important to test predisposed breeds such as German shepherds and Rhodesian ridgebacks. Affected dogs should be evaluated for evidence of disease at other anatomic sites. If possible, this should consist of thoracic radiographs and abdominal ultrasound, echocardiography (for infective endocarditis), and aerobic bacterial culture of the urine.

Laboratory Abnormalities

Often the CBC and biochemistry panel are surprisingly unremarkable in dogs with discospondylitis. There may be mild to moderate neutrophilia with bandemia and/or lymphopenia on the CBC. Mild hypoalbuminemia and mild to moderate hyperglobulinemia are the most common abnormalities on the biochemistry panel. Dogs with fungal discospondylitis may be azotemic because of concurrent fungal pyelonephritis.[51] Urinalysis may show pyuria, bacteriuria, funguria, proteinuria, and/or cylindruria in dogs with concurrent UTIs. Analysis of the CSF often reveals mild to markedly increased CSF protein concentration and rarely increased total nucleated cell count.[57]

Diagnostic Imaging

Plain Radiography

Radiographic changes in dogs (and cats) with discospondylitis include narrowing or widening of the intervertebral space, irregularity or lysis of the vertebral body endplates, endplate lucency, sclerosis at the margins of bone loss, proliferative or osteolytic lesions within adjacent vertebral bones and bridging spondylosis, and, in some cases, vertebral subluxation or fracture (Fig. 121.6).[63] It has been suggested that there may be differences in the radiographic appearance of lesions in young dogs when compared with adult dogs, but more studies would help to verify this. Because multiple disc spaces are frequently affected, radiographs of the entire spine should be performed to properly assess the extent and severity of disease. Radiographic changes may lag behind clinical signs for as long as 6 weeks in dogs with discospondylitis, so radiographs should be repeated every 1 to 2 weeks if discospondylitis is suspected and plain radiographs are initially normal. Alternatively, advanced imaging with CT or MRI may reveal lesions not seen on plain radiographs. Plain radiography does not allow visualization of the degree of spinal cord compression, so advanced imaging is required to further evaluate dogs with neurologic signs. Ultrasonography may be useful for detection of retroperitoneal grass awns in dogs with localized lumbar discospondylitis on plain radiography, and can also show changes associated with discospondylitis, such as loss of reverberation artefact. Bone phase nuclear scintigraphy may also be helpful for diagnosis.

Contrast Radiography

Myelography can identify the site(s), type (vertebral subluxation or soft tissue proliferation), and extent of spinal cord compression in dogs with discospondylitis and allow planning for decompressive surgery (Fig. 121.7).[66] However, MRI is less invasive, more sensitive, and is now the preferred method for diagnosis of cord compression due to discospondylitis.

Advanced Imaging

CT and MRI may have increased sensitivity for diagnosis of discospondylitis when compared with plain radiography. MRI is the gold standard

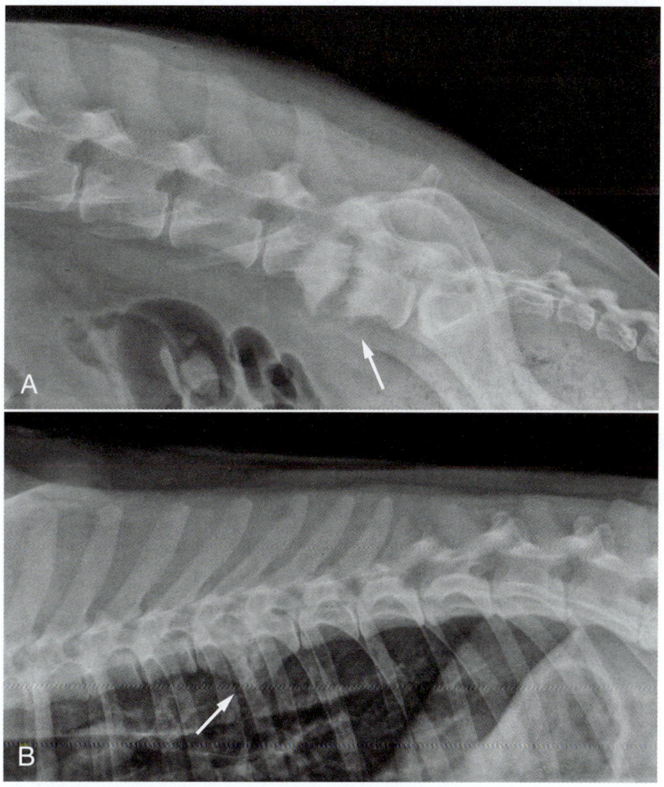

Fig. 121.6 Radiographic changes in discospondylitis. (A) Lateral radiograph of the lumbosacral region of a 3-year-old female spayed German shepherd with *Aspergillus* spp. discospondylitis. There is severe destruction of the endplates at L6-L7 *(arrow)* with sclerosis and ventral periosteal proliferation. (B) Lateral radiograph of the thoracic spine of a 1-year-old female malamute. Resolving discospondylitis is present at T8-T9 *(arrow)*. There is lysis and irregularity to the endplates of these vertebrae. There is bridging spondylosis ventrally.

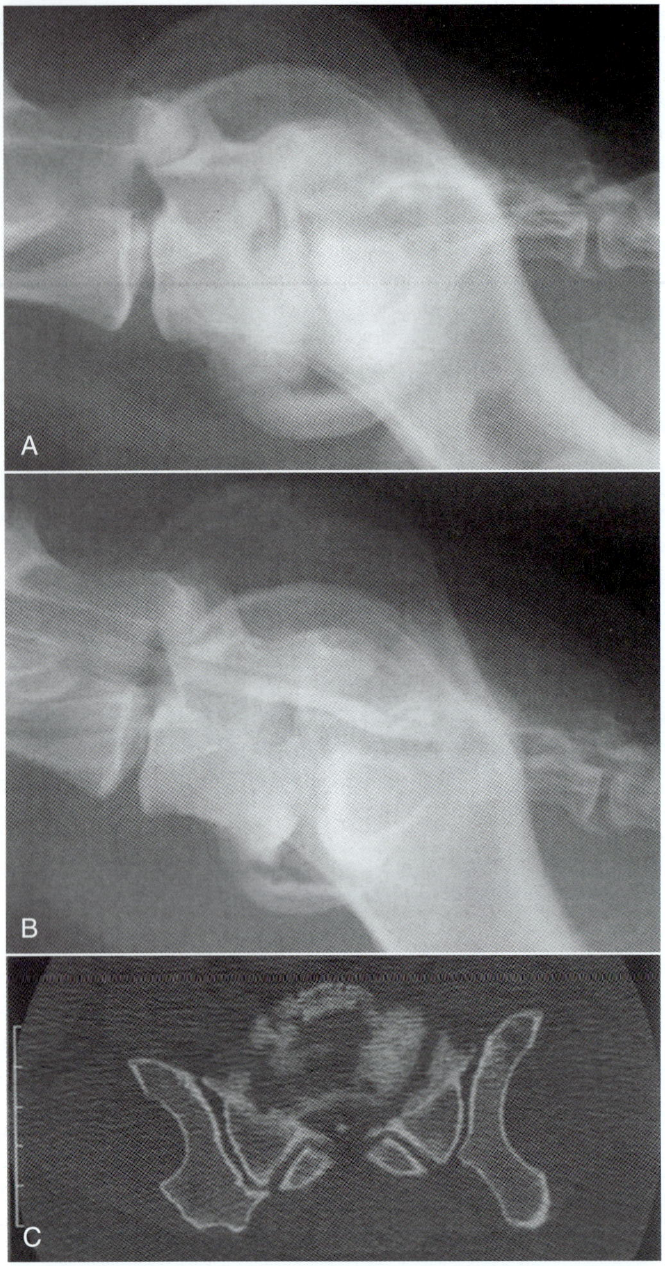

Fig. 121.7 Images from a 9-year-old intact male rottweiler with a 3-day history of difficulty standing and decreased appetite. Findings on neurologic examination included lumbosacral spinal pain, left pelvic limb paresis, and right pelvic limb paralysis. Blood and synovial fluid cultures yielded a methicillin-susceptible *Staphylococcus pseudintermedius*. Radiographic findings were consistent with chronic discospondylitis at the lumbosacral disc space and secondary compression of the spinal cord. (A) Plain lateral radiograph of the pelvis. The lumbosacral joint space is narrowed and there is significant bridging spondylitis, with endplate osteolysis. (B) Myelogram. Dorsal elevation of the conus is present at the lumbosacral junction. (C) Contrast tomography of the lumbosacral junction. There is substantial endplate osteolysis. (All images courtesy the University of California, Davis, Veterinary Neurology/Neurosurgery Service.)

for diagnosis of discospondylitis in human patients and is the method of choice for diagnosis and characterization of discospondylitis in dogs.[57,63,65,68] Affected vertebral bodies are classically hypointense on T1-weighted images (which illustrate bone lesions) and may be hypointense (most commonly), isointense, or hyperintense on T2-weighted images when compared with normal surrounding structures.[57,65] T2-weighted images highlight tissues with high water content, including the nucleus pulposus, CSF, epidural fat, and inflammatory lesions. Hyperintensity of the vertebral bodies in dogs is even more commonly observed in short tau inversion recovery (STIR) images, which suppress the signal from fat. Two adjacent vertebrae are consistently involved. Intervertebral discs are hyperintense on T2-weighted and STIR images when discospondylitis is present. Marked uniform or heterogenous contrast enhancement is usually apparent in vertebral endplates, within the disc, and in surrounding soft tissue (Fig. 121.8). Paravertebral soft tissues may also be hyperintense on T2-weighted and especially STIR images.[57] Hyperintensity of adjacent spinal cord on T2-weighted images has also been described.[63] With more chronic infection, there is loss of definition and cortical continuity and destruction of cortical margins in T1-weighted images. Distortion and narrowing of the disc space is also apparent, and subluxation and disc protrusion with associated spinal cord compression can be easily identified. The severity of spinal cord compression on MRI correlates with severity of neurologic signs, whereas this does not appear to be true for myelography.

Microbiologic Tests

Isolation and Identification

The optimal specimens for identification of the causative agent of discospondylitis are blood or fluoroscopically guided disc aspirates (or biopsies performed during decompressive surgery), because organisms isolated from these specimens are most likely to reflect those involved in disc destruction. Blood cultures are indicated in all dogs with discospondylitis (see Chapter 3 for blood culture technique and interpretation). Because anaerobes are uncommonly isolated from dogs with discospondylitis and they have predictable susceptibilities, the decision to perform anaerobic blood culture should be considered in light of any underlying disease processes and client financial constraints. Negative blood cultures occur in more than half of dogs with discospondylitis and may reflect low-level bacteremia or fungemia, the presence of fastidious or unculturable organisms such as *Brucella* or anaerobes, or recent antimicrobial drug treatment. Urine cultures may reveal the causative organism when blood cultures are negative, but not uncommonly bacterial species present in the urine differ from the organism present in affected discs. However, isolation of a mold species from the urine suggests a disseminated mycosis. Serologic testing for *Aspergillus* antigen and *Brucella* antibody should be performed in dogs with culture-negative discospondylitis. *Aspergillus* serology should also be considered for dogs that have blood culture-positive discospondylitis, especially in predisposed breeds (such as German shepherds, Rhodesian ridgebacks, vizslas) because mixed infections with fungi and bacteria can rarely occur. Dogs with *Paecilomyces* discospondylitis can have positive *Aspergillus* serum and urine antigen tests due to serologic cross-reactions between these fungi.[67]

When blood cultures are negative, disc aspirates can be obtained under anesthesia with fluoroscopic (or other advanced imaging such as CT) guidance after preparation of the skin in a sterile manner.[69] Aspiration is performed with a 22-G, 1.5- to 2.5-inch spinal needle into a syringe that contains a small amount of sterile saline. In one study, 0.3 to 0.5 mL of sterile saline was injected and immediately reaspirated,[69] but dry aspiration can also be performed into the needle. The saline in the syringe can then be used to flush the contents of the needle into a plain sterile tube, which is submitted for bacterial and fungal culture. Only 3 of 11 aspirates or biopsies were positive in one study.[1] However, in another study, positive bacterial cultures were obtained in 9 of 12 disc aspirates.[69] Other specimens that may yield growth include CSF, aspirates of cellulitis or abscesses adjacent to sites of discospondylitis, or synovial fluid. When disease is present at other sites, every effort should be made to perform culture for aerobic and anaerobic bacteria and fungi from these sites in order to identify an infectious etiology.

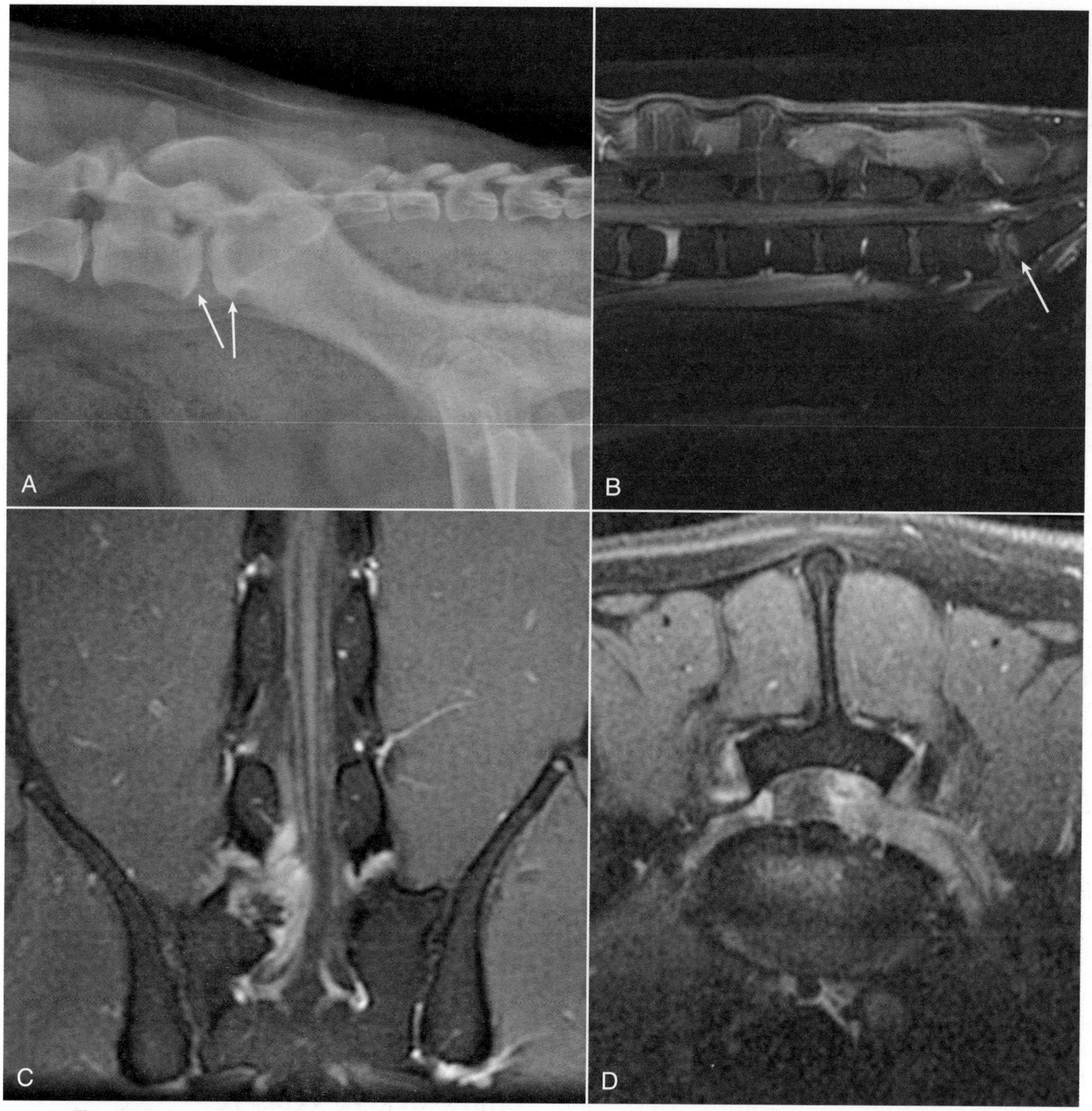

Fig. 121.8 Images from a 5-year-old intact male German shepherd dog with a history of progressive reluctance to jump over the previous 18 months. Neurologic examination revealed decreased pelvic limb placing reactions and lumbosacral pain. Blood cultures were negative. Clinical signs and radiographic lesions improved dramatically with cephalexin treatment. (A) Plain right lateral radiograph of the pelvis. The lumbosacral disc space is narrowed and there is vertebral endplate sclerosis *(arrows)*. There is also bony proliferation of the endplates at the level of the vertebral canal. (B) Sagittal T1-postcontrast magnetic resonance imaging with fat saturation, caudal lumbar and lumbosacral vertebral column. There is strong contrast enhancement in the endplates of L7 and S1 *(arrow)* on either side of the disc space. (C) Dorsal view. There is diffuse contrast enhancement of the tissues around the seventh lumbar nerve root with displacement of neural structures. (D) Transverse view. There is marked enlargement and strong uniform enhancement of the right seventh lumbar spinal nerve. The primary differential based on radiologic findings was chronic lumbosacral discospondylitis with regional soft tissue inflammation on the right, and severe neuritis of the right seventh lumbar nerve. The impingement of the right seventh lumbar nerve by contrast-enhancing material was thought to result from granulation tissue formation. (All images courtesy the University of California, Davis, Veterinary Neurology/Neurosurgery Service.)

Pathologic Findings

Gross pathologic findings in dogs with discospondylitis include the presence of pus and necrotic debris in the intervertebral disc spaces, irregularity and collapse of the disc spaces, and discoloration and friability of the vertebral endplates (Fig. 121.9). Protrusion of disc material and compression of the spinal cord may be apparent. There may also be evidence of bony callus material (ankylosing spondylosis). The nature of the inflammatory infiltrates on histopathology varies with the chronicity of the lesions and the underlying cause. For example, fungal discospondylitis may be associated with granulomatous or pyogranulomatous inflammation and intralesional fungal hyphae, whereas chronic bacterial discospondylitis lesions typically display neutrophilic

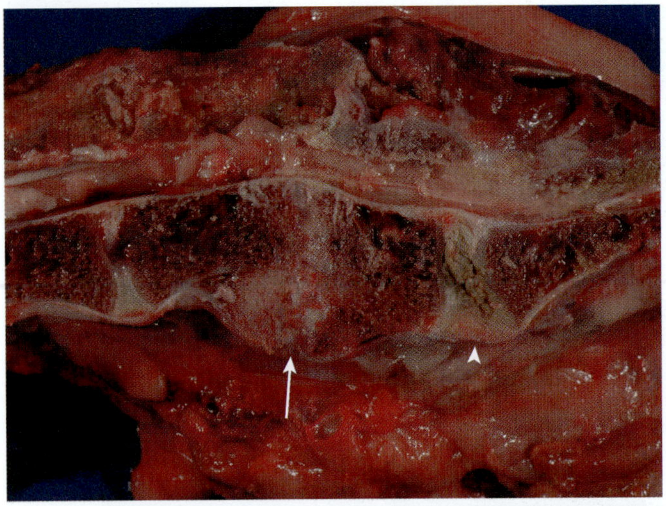

Fig. 121.9 Vertebral column of a 4-year-old female spayed German shepherd at necropsy that had multifocal discospondylitis caused by *Aspergillus* spp. The L6-L7 disc space *(arrow)* is collapsed with degenerate disc material, sclerotic endplates, and marked ventral proliferation of bone. The lumbosacral disc space *(arrowhead)* has an irregular annulus with friable, pale tan nuclear material that protrudes ventrally. (Courtesy of the University of California, Davis, Veterinary Anatomic Pathology Service.)

and lymphoplasmacytic infiltrates, with perilesional fibrosis and granulation tissue. Osteonecrosis may be present, as well as necrosis of the compressed spinal tissue.

TREATMENT AND PROGNOSIS

Treatment of discospondylitis involves prolonged antimicrobial drug treatment and strict restriction of movement for several weeks to prevent herniation of disc material or subluxation, with a gradual increase in movement once lesions have healed. It is important to stress to owners of dogs with discospondylitis that it is a serious, life-threatening condition. Analgesics such as fentanyl patches can also be administered provided they do not encourage excessive movement. NSAIDs may also be beneficial. Gabapentin may alleviate neurogenic pain and can be used with opioids and nonsteroidal drugs.[70]

The antibiotic chosen to treat discospondylitis should ideally be based on the results of culture and susceptibility. Treatment recommendations for dogs with *Brucella* discospondylitis are described in Chapter 71. Dogs with fungal discospondylitis should be treated with antifungal drugs that have activity against molds, such as voriconazole (if finances allow) or itraconazole (*not* fluconazole, which is not active against molds) with or without amphotericin B; prognosis is guarded, and lifelong treatment may be required (see Chapter 86). Dogs with culture-negative discospondylitis that have negative serum or urine *Aspergillus* galactomannan antigen tests should be treated with high doses of a drug with activity against susceptible staphylococci and *E. coli*, such as amoxicillin-clavulanic acid or cephalexin (see Table 121.2). Amoxicillin-clavulanic acid also has activity against penicillinase-producing anaerobes. However, occasionally gram-negative organisms such as *K. pneumoniae* or *P. aeruginosa*, and MRSP cause discospondylitis, and these may not respond to treatment with β-lactam drugs. Addition of a fluoroquinolone or an aminoglycoside should be considered if there is no improvement after 1 week of treatment with a β-lactam drug. Linezolid was used successfully in one case report to treat a dog with MDR MRSP discospondylitis.[71] Use of critical antimicrobials such as linezolid should be based on culture and susceptibility testing. For dogs that are systemically unwell or that have neurologic abnormalities, antimicrobials should be administered parenterally in the hospital for as long as possible (ideally at least 10 days) before changing to oral administration. Antimicrobial drugs should be administered for at least 6 to 8 weeks; in some cases, treatment may need to be extended for many months. In one study, the mean ± standard deviation for duration of antimicrobial treatment in dogs that were cured of discospondylitis was 54 ± 45 weeks; for dogs with staphylococcal infections, it was 74 ± 62 weeks.[1] Dogs with fungal discospondylitis may require lifelong treatment with antifungal drugs (see Chapter 86). Dogs should be reevaluated clinically and radiographically every 3 to 4 weeks. Improvement is characterized by resolution of bone lysis, sclerosis of bone, and vertebral fusion, although radiographic improvement can lag behind clinical improvement by 1 to 2 months, and there may be progression of osteolysis in addition to sclerosis and increased osseous proliferation within the first month.[63] It has been recommended that antimicrobial drug treatment be continued until lysis resolves completely, but whether this is truly needed is controversial. MRI may be the most sensitive imaging technique to confirm resolution of active infection, but requires general anesthesia. Imaging should also be performed 1 to 2 months after antimicrobial drugs are discontinued. If clinical deterioration occurs during treatment, additional imaging (ideally with MRI) should be offered to evaluate for development of new lesions, abscessation, subluxation, fracture, or disc protrusion.

Dogs with severe neurologic deficits (such as paralysis) may require decompressive surgery, debridement of abscesses or vertebral osteomyelitis, and stabilization of the vertebral column. Discospondylitis of L7-S1 may be a particular therapeutic challenge. Although antimicrobial therapy will produce an apparent initial cure, relapse will occur in about 25% of cases, possibly due to residual instability of the intervertebral articulation that predisposes the disc to reinfection or prevents total resolution of the original infection by interfering with neovascularization. Surgical distraction and arthrodesis of the articular facets between L7 and S1 is recommended by some clinicians in conjunction with antibacterial therapy.

Return of neurologic function can sometimes occur with antimicrobial drug treatment alone, provided deep pain is present. Decompressive surgery should be performed within 24 hours if deep pain is absent. Referral to a specialist surgeon is recommended in this situation. In one study, 9 of 27 dogs with discospondylitis received some form of decompressive surgery.[66] Physical therapy may also be beneficial in these animals.

PUBLIC HEALTH ASPECTS

The most important public health consideration in dogs with discospondylitis is the possibility of *Brucella* infection. Human disease has occurred as a result of contact with dogs with *B. canis* discospondylitis and is typically an influenza-like illness. The possibility of *B. canis* infection should be considered in all dogs with discospondylitis, and precautions such as routine hand washing, minimization of exposure to urine, and the wearing of gloves should be taken until appropriate diagnostic testing has ruled out *Brucella* as a cause.

ARTHRITIS

ETIOLOGIC AGENTS, PATHOGENESIS, AND EPIDEMIOLOGY

Infectious arthritis may be classified as *monoarthritis* or *polyarthritis*. Bacterial monoarthritis can follow orthopedic surgeries that involve the joint (such as TPLOs, arthroscopies, or joint arthrodesis), spread from soft tissue or bone infection at adjacent sites, or result from trauma or bite wound infections. Less commonly, monoarthritis follows systemic spread of bacteria to a single joint. Bacterial causes of monoarthritis are similar to those involved in osteomyelitis; the most common causes are *Staphylococcus* spp., especially *S. pseudintermedius* but also *S. aureus* and CoNS. Other reported causes are *Streptococcus canis* and *Streptococcus equi* subsp. *zooepidemicus*, *E. coli*, and *P. aeruginosa*.[72,73]

Systemic spread of bacteria to the joints more often results in polyarthritis. Infection with a variety of bacteria, protozoa, fungi, and, rarely, viruses (West Nile virus in dogs, calicivirus in cats) have been associated with polyarthritis in dogs and cats. In areas where tick-borne infections are endemic, the most common bacterial causes are *Anaplasma phagocytophilum, Ehrlichia ewingii, Ehrlichia canis, Borrelia burgdorferi,* and *Rickettsia rickettsii,* but non–vector-borne bacteria such as *S. canis, S. aureus, Erysipelothrix, Salmonella, Brucella,* and mycoplasmas can also be involved. Although its importance as a cause of polyarthritis remains unclear, *Bartonella* should also be considered. Endocarditis is frequently (if not almost always) present in dogs with polyarthritis caused by facultative aerobic gram-positive and gram-negative bacteria, and among dogs with endocarditis, *S. canis* infections are most likely to be associated with polyarthritis. Worldwide, the most important cause of protozoal polyarthritis in dogs is *Leishmania.* Fungal polyarthritis is uncommon but can result from infection by dimorphic fungi and, very rarely, molds such as *Aspergillus.* Infectious polyarthritis is an important differential diagnosis for primary (idiopathic) immune-mediated polyarthritis (IMPA) in dogs. Although infectious polyarthritis is less common than primary IMPA, failure to identify an underlying infection can have disastrous consequences when treatment with immunosuppressive drugs is initiated. In some cases, polyarthritis is a secondary immune-mediated reaction to systemic infections that are not localized in the joint (in human medicine, a condition known as "reactive arthritis").

After bacterial localization in the joint, an acute inflammatory response occurs within the joint. There is a marked synovial effusion, causing increased intra-articular pressure, ischemia, and release or activation of cartilage matrix-damaging enzymes. Cartilage damage occurs quickly and, if severe, is irreversible. Glycosaminoglycan depletion occurs within the first 5 days followed by cartilage softening and fissuring. This leads to mechanical weakening of the subchondral bone, as well as the cascade of changes within the synovial fluid and articular cartilage. After recovery from infection, persistent inactivated antigens or bacterial fragments may perpetuate the inflammatory process.

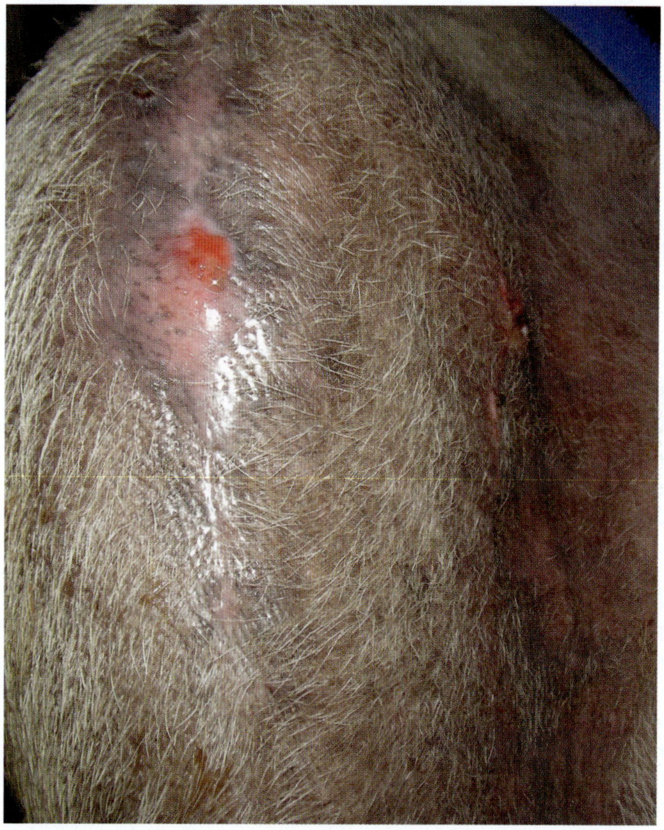

Fig. 121.10 Surgical site of a 5-year-old male neutered mastiff dog with non–weight-bearing lameness and a draining skin lesion that developed along the incision site approximately 1 month after a tibial plateau leveling operation. The right stifle was swollen and warm. Synovial fluid aspirated from the joint was red and turbid and contained 161,550 nucleated cells/μL (98% nondegenerate neutrophils) and 90,000 red blood cells/μL. Aerobic and anaerobic cultures of the fluid yielded a methicillin-resistant, multidrug-resistant *Staphylococcus pseudintermedius* that was resistant to all β-lactams, macrolides, and clindamycin, fluoroquinolones, and trimethoprim-sulfamethoxazole. The infection was treated successfully with joint exploration, lavage, and oral chloramphenicol for 8 weeks.

CLINICAL FEATURES

Clinical signs of monoarthritis may be acute or chronic in onset and include variable fever, lethargy, inappetence, lameness that involves a single limb, and a swollen joint that may be erythematous, warm to the touch, and occasionally drain purulent or blood-tinged fluid (Fig. 121.10). The draining lymph node may be enlarged and firm. Occasionally, edema of the distal limb may be apparent. The most common joints affected in one study were the stifle and elbow joints, followed by the tarsi and coxofemoral joints, and signs developed within 2 to over 8 weeks after articular or periarticular surgery.[72] In polyarthritis, multiple peripheral joints are affected, and dogs (and less commonly cats) show signs of recumbency, reluctance to move, generalized peripheral lymphadenopathy, a stiff gait, and/or shifting leg lameness; drainage of fluid is not usually apparent. Dogs with bacterial polyarthritis can also show signs of severe sepsis.

DIAGNOSIS

Diagnosis of infectious arthritis is based on the history, clinical signs, and cytology and culture of joint fluid; serologic assays for *B. canis* and fungal pathogens; and/or molecular diagnostic and/or serologic testing for vector-borne pathogens in endemic regions. Blood cultures may also allow identification of the underlying etiology in dogs with bacterial polyarthritis. As for discospondylitis, dogs with bacterial polyarthritis should ideally be evaluated for evidence of disease at other sites with thoracic radiographs, spinal radiographs (for concurrent discospondylitis) and abdominal ultrasound, echocardiography (for endocarditis), and aerobic bacterial culture of the urine. However, it should be kept in mind that bacterial isolates made from urine may represent unrelated subclinical bacteriuria.

Laboratory Abnormalities

Routine laboratory testing in animals with bacterial arthritis typically shows leukocytosis due to a neutrophilia, which can be accompanied by bandemia. The CBC may also be normal. Thrombocytopenia may be present in dogs with bacteremia or vector-borne bacterial infections and should prompt diagnostic evaluation for vector-borne infections with PCR assays and serology, or at least assessment of response to treatment with doxycycline in the absence of client funds to pursue a diagnosis. Urinalysis may be normal or show pyuria, bacteriuria, proteinuria, and/or cylindruria in dogs with concurrent aerobic bacterial UTIs.

Synovial fluid from affected joints is often yellow or blood-tinged, cloudy, increased in volume, and thin or watery in consistency (normal synovial fluid is clear and tenacious). Cytologic examination of synovial fluid reveals increased numbers of leukocytes (>5000 cells/μL), with a predominance of nondegenerate and/or degenerate neutrophils. Importantly, in the majority of dogs with septic arthritis, degenerate neutrophils are not visualized,[72,73] so the presence of only nondegenerate neutrophils does not rule out an underlying bacterial infection. Rarely, bacteria or fungal organisms are visualized extracellularly or within leukocytes. Morulae are occasionally seen within neutrophils in synovial fluid of dogs infected with *A. phagocytophilum* or *E. ewingii* (see Fig. 45.1C).

Diagnostic Imaging

When changes are apparent, radiographs of the joints in dogs and cats with infectious arthritis most often reveal soft tissue swelling and joint effusion. In severe and chronic bacterial monoarthritis, associated osteomyelitis may be present, with subchondral bone lysis, articular erosion, and periarticular new bone formation.

Microbiologic Tests

Isolation and Identification

Confirmation of bacterial arthritis requires culture of synovial fluid or of the synovium itself. Synovial fluid from dogs with neutrophilic polyarthritis should be submitted for aerobic bacterial culture and susceptibility, and anaerobic, fungal, or *Mycoplasma* culture should at least be considered if the history is suggestive. Inoculation of blood culture bottles with synovial fluids followed by subculture may increase sensitivity. Situations in which anaerobic culture may be indicated include a history of foreign body (such as plant awn) exposure or bite wounds. Although rare, the possibility of *Mycoplasma* arthritis should be considered in cats and dogs with a history of immune compromise, surgery, or bite wounds, and when treatment with β-lactam drugs fails (see Chapter 57). Dogs with fungal polyarthritis may have lesions elsewhere (e.g., chorioretinitis, pulmonary disease) that support a diagnosis of disseminated fungal disease. However, anaerobic and *Mycoplasma* culture may be insensitive (especially when there are delays in specimen transport to the laboratory); *Mycoplasma* and fungal cultures require prolonged incubation; and anaerobes, fungi, and mycoplasmas tend to have predictable susceptibilities. Broad-spectrum 16S rRNA PCR has also been used to detect and speciate bacteria in synovial fluid from dogs, but in one study, it was not more sensitive than culture and yielded more false-positive results.[74] Aerobic blood cultures may assist in identification of bacteria involved in polyarthritis.

If arthroscopy or arthrotomy is performed as part of evaluation and treatment of bacterial monoarthritis, a biopsy of the synovium could also be submitted for culture and susceptibility and may yield growth when synovial fluid culture is negative.[73] In most cases, synovial fluid culture alone is sufficient for diagnosis of bacterial arthritis.

TREATMENT AND PROGNOSIS

Treatment of infectious arthritis depends on whether one joint is involved or whether polyarthritis is present, as well as on the identity of the causative agent. Infectious monoarthritis may require surgical exploration, lavage and drainage, and treatment with appropriate antimicrobial drugs based on the results of culture and susceptibility. Monoarthritis is considered a surgical emergency, and lavage should be performed immediately after diagnosis, either via an ingress-egress approach, an arthroscope, or with open surgery. For ingress-egress lavage, large-bore (14- to 16-G) needles are inserted percutaneously into two to three fluid pockets around the joint while the animal is heavily sedated or anesthetized. Several liters of sterile saline is then administered through one portal under pressure and allowed to drain from the other portal(s). The sites of ingress and egress are switched until the fluid becomes clear. Arthroscopy can also be used. Arthrotomy may be necessary if there are large accumulations of fibrin or inspissated purulent debris that cannot be effectively flushed from the joint. If implants are present, they should be removed when healing has occurred or if stabilization has failed. If the implant is stable but the bone has not healed, lavage is performed and the implant is often left in place because bone can heal if rigidly stable despite infection. Implant exchange is the "gold standard" in human medicine to decrease the bacterial load from the biofilm.[3] Cost may be prohibitive in animals and subjectively, many of the cases in animals will heal with rigid stability and can be removed later. Usually, the implant must ultimately be removed and should be done as soon as possible after healing. Antimicrobial drugs should initially be given parenterally if possible. Treatment should continue until implants can be removed if left in place. Once implants are removed, treatment may need to be continued for another 2 to 4 weeks, depending on the severity of infection. If local antibiotic therapy is used in associated osteomyelitis lesions (i.e., impregnated beads), systemic antimicrobial drug treatment should also be used. Activated mesenchymal stem cells IV can be considered as an adjunct therapy with antibiotics.[42] The prognosis depends on the degree of cartilage and bone destruction, the degree to which progressive osteoarthritis occurs, and the joint affected. Unfortunately, evidence-based clinical studies that document long-term prognosis or prognostic indicators for infectious monoarthritis are not available. In one retrospective study, dogs that fully recovered tended to have a shorter duration of lameness before treatment (median, 11 days compared with 26 days) and lower synovial fluid cell counts (median, 54×10^9 cells/mL compared with 100×10^9 cells/mL) than dogs that never fully recovered, and had significantly lower body weights (median, 29 kg compared with 44 kg).[72]

Polyarthritis caused by vector-borne bacteria usually responds to treatment with doxycycline within 24 to 48 hours. Antimicrobials for treatment of polyarthritis caused by other bacteria should be selected based on the results of cytologic examination of synovial fluid (cocci versus rods) and culture and susceptibility of blood or synovial fluid. Because streptococci, staphylococci, and *Erysipelothrix* are usually involved, a β-lactam drug such as amoxicillin-clavulanic acid (or amoxicillin if streptococci are more likely) could be used. Because bacterial polyarthritis is frequently associated with endocarditis or discospondylitis, the duration of treatment should be based on resolution of these lesions. The reader is referred to Chapters 122 and 123 for additional information on treatment of bacteremia and sepsis.

PUBLIC HEALTH ASPECTS

Polyarthritis can be caused by organisms of public health significance, such as *Salmonella, Brucella, S. aureus*, pathogenic fungi, *Leishmania*, and vector-borne bacterial pathogens of importance to human health. This should be kept in mind when handling dogs with polyarthritis. Care should be taken to avoid needle-stick injuries during venipuncture, arthrocentesis, and aspiration of other tissues such as lymph nodes. Deep sedation or anesthesia is recommended for arthrocentesis.

CASE EXAMPLE

Signalment

"Tilly," a 10-year-old female spayed greyhound/pit bull terrier mix from Davis, CA (Fig. 121.11).

History

Tilly was brought to the University of California, Davis, VMTH Orthopedic Surgery service, for evaluation of a draining tract on her left medial proximal tibia that developed after a TTA surgery for left cranial cruciate ligament tear. The ligament tear had been diagnosed at the VMTH 15 months previously after an acute onset of lameness, and the surgery was performed 2 months after diagnosis at another veterinary hospital after there had been no improvement with conservative management (activity restriction and anti-inflammatory drugs). Immediately after the surgery, the dog was placed on a 10-day course of doxycycline. The tract was first observed 2 weeks after the doxycycline course had finished, and the owner (a veterinary student) noted that the tract subsequently healed over, then drained again. When the wound initially appeared, treatment with doxycycline was reinstituted for a month, with no improvement. A radiograph of the limb was performed at the end of the course of treatment at the VMTH. Soft tissue swelling was identified at the medial aspect of the stifle, but there was no radiographic evidence of implant infection or motion. Regional osteopenia of the left tibial tuberosity and proximal tibia was present, and there was progressive left stifle osteoarthrosis. Culture of the wound yielded very small numbers of *S. canis* and a CoNS. The wound subsequently closed over again and antibiotic treatment was not initiated, but 11 months later the tract reappeared. Since the surgery, the incision had appeared healthy. Tilly had been bearing progressively more weight on the limb, although some lameness persisted. Other treatments had included activity restriction and carprofen (2 mg/kg, PO, q12h) for pain relief. Tilly had no other significant medical history apart from multiple lipomas that had been evaluated with FNA cytology, which had not changed in size.

Physical Examination

Body weight: 37.2 kg.

General: Bright, alert, responsive. T = 101.0°F (38.3°C), HR = 80 beats/minute, panting.

Eyes, ears, nose, and throat: No abnormalities were identified apart from moderate periodontal disease.

Musculoskeletal: Left pelvic limb lameness was present, but there was intermittent right pelvic limb lameness and muscle atrophy of both pelvic limbs. There was pain on extension of both coxofemoral joints. Examination of the left pelvic limb revealed a 1-cm, open round wound on the medial aspect of the proximal left tibia, which oozed serosanguineous fluid. A positive cranial drawer sign and tibial thrust were present.

All other systems: No clinically significant abnormalities were detected.

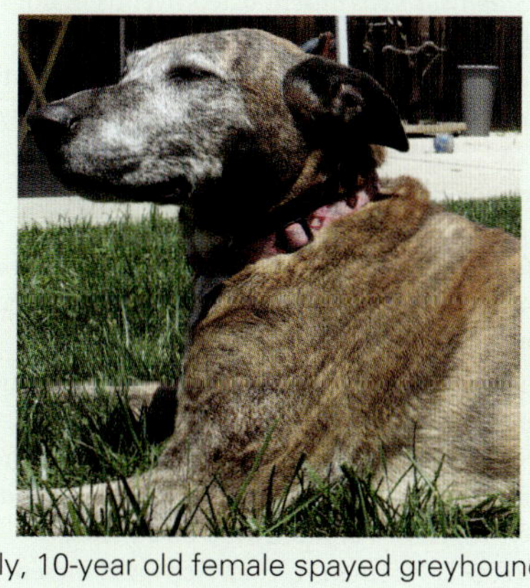

Fig. 121.11 Tilly, 10-year old female spayed greyhound–pit bull terrier mix that developed osteomyelitis at the site of a left tibial tuberosity advancement surgery.

Imaging Findings

Plain radiographs (pelvis): Bilaterally there was poor coverage of the femoral heads by the acetabulae. The femoral heads and necks were thickened and irregularly margined. There was periarticular osteophytosis of the acetabulae. Atrophy of the pelvic musculature was appreciated bilaterally although somewhat worse on the left than the right. Findings were consistent with bilateral hip dysplasia with severe degenerative change.

Plain radiographs (left stifle): The implants associated with the TTA procedure were in place and intact (see Fig. 121.5A and B). The osteotomy site had filled in with bone to some extent, although the site was still visible nearly its entire length, and bridging bone was absent at the proximal aspect of the osteotomy and around the basket implant. There was thinning of the cortical bone adjacent to the TTA plate that was associated with the tibial tuberosity and proximal tibial diaphysis, and mild lucency surrounded the medial aspect of the distal-most screw, which suggested implant-associated osteomyelitis. A gap was present between the bone plate and the tibia. Distal to the bone plates, there was smooth periosteal proliferation. The patella was displaced distally. There was moderate intracapsular soft tissue swelling of the stifle. There was also persistent, moderate periarticular osteophytosis of the distal femur and proximal tibia.

Diagnosis

TTA implant-associated osteomyelitis with incomplete union of osteotomy; severe canine hip dysplasia.

Treatment

Surgical exploration of the left stifle joint was performed. The draining tract was followed to the plate and screws. The TTA plate and screws were removed. The cage was removed by drilling around it, which left a 2-cm round defect in the tibia. During the procedure, it was discovered that a titanium plate had been used together with 316L steel screws, which led to concerns that osteomyelitis may have developed secondary to a galvanic reaction. The area was extensively flushed, and the defect was filled with calcium sulfate beads. Beads were also placed in the area previously occupied by the plate (see Fig. 121.5C). The fascia, subcutaneous tissue, and skin were closed, and a modified Robert-Jones bandage was placed. Aerobic and anaerobic bacterial cultures of the implant yielded small numbers of methicillin-susceptible *S. pseudintermedius*. The organism was resistant to ampicillin, penicillin, ticarcillin, and doxycycline. Tilly was therefore treated with amoxicillin-clavulanic acid (10 mg/kg, PO, q12h). At the time of suture removal 2 weeks later, Tilly was weight bearing on the left pelvic limb, and the draining tract had resolved. A small draining tract reappeared 2 weeks later, and a swab from the tract again grew *S. pseudintermedius* with the same antibiogram, but only from the enrichment broth. Treatment was continued for an additional month, all lesions resolved, and lameness was reduced. Several years later, the dog was doing well and there had been no recurrence of draining tracts (see Fig. 121.5D).

Comments

Diagnosis and treatment of osteomyelitis in this case was delayed because of the lag in radiographic changes and the appearance and disappearance of the draining tract. This illustrates the difficulties associated with diagnosis of osteomyelitis. Although unconfirmed, use of two different metals may have contributed to development of osteomyelitis in this dog, which required costly and difficult surgical intervention with implant removal. The defects were closed with biodegradable beads and infection resolved after 2 months of systemic antimicrobial drug treatment, based on the results of culture and susceptibility.

SUGGESTED READINGS

Aiken MJ, Hughes TK, Abercromby RH, et al. Prospective, randomized comparison of the effect of two antimicrobial regimes on surgical site infection rate in dogs undergoing orthopedic implant surgery. *Vet Surg.* 2015;44:661–667.

Ruoff CM, Kerwin SC, Taylor AR. Diagnostic imaging of discospondylitis. *Vet Clin North Am Small Anim Pract.* 2018;48:85–94.

Clements DN, Owen MR, Mosley JR, et al. Retrospective study of bacterial infective arthritis in 31 dogs. *J Small Anim Pract.* 2005;46:171–176.

Masters EA, Trombetta RP, de Mesy Bentley KL, et al. Evolving concepts in bone infection: redefining "biofilm", "acute vs. chronic osteomyelitis", "the immune proteome" and "local antibiotic therapy". *Bone Res.* 2019;7:20.

REFERENCES

1. Burkert BA, Kerwin SC, Hosgood GL, et al. Signalment and clinical features of diskospondylitis in dogs: 513 cases (1980-2001). *J Am Vet Med Assoc.* 2005;227:268–275.
2. Siqueira EG, Rahal SC, Ribeiro MG, et al. Exogenous bacterial osteomyelitis in 52 dogs: a retrospective study of etiology and in vitro antimicrobial susceptibility profile (2000-2013). *Vet Q.* 2014;34:201–204.
3. Masters EA, Trombetta RP, de Mesy Bentley KL, et al. Evolving concepts in bone infection: redefining "biofilm", "acute vs. chronic osteomyelitis", "the immune proteome" and "local antibiotic therapy". *Bone Res.* 2019;7:20.
4. Gieling F, Peters S, Erichsen C, et al. Bacterial osteomyelitis in veterinary orthopaedics: Pathophysiology, clinical presentation and advances in treatment across multiple species. *Vet J.* 2019;250:44–54.
5. Pacchiana PD, Morris E, Gillings SL, et al. Surgical and postoperative complications associated with tibial plateau leveling osteotomy in dogs with cranial cruciate ligament rupture: 397 cases (1998-2001). *J Am Vet Med Assoc.* 2003;222:184–193.
6. Priddy NH 2nd, Tomlinson JL, Dodam JR, et al. Complications with and owner assessment of the outcome of tibial plateau leveling osteotomy for treatment of cranial cruciate ligament rupture in dogs: 193 cases (1997-2001). *J Am Vet Med Assoc.* 2003;222:1726–1732.
7. Stauffer KD, Tuttle TA, Elkins AD, et al. Complications associated with 696 tibial plateau leveling osteotomies (2001-2003). *J Am Anim Hosp Assoc.* 2006;42:44–50.
8. Fitzpatrick N, Solano MA. Predictive variables for complications after TPLO with stifle inspection by arthrotomy in 1000 consecutive dogs. *Vet Surg.* 2010;39:460–474.
9. Gallagher AD, Mertens WD. Implant removal rate from infection after tibial plateau leveling osteotomy in dogs. *Vet Surg.* 2012;41:705–711.
10. Stine SL, Odum SM, Mertens WD. Protocol changes to reduce implant-associated infection rate after tibial plateau leveling osteotomy: 703 dogs, 811 TPLO (2006-2014). *Vet Surg.* 2018;47:481–489.
11. Thompson AM, Bergh MS, Wang C, et al. Tibial plateau levelling osteotomy implant removal: a retrospective analysis of 129 cases. *Vet Comp Orthop Traumatol.* 2011;24:450–456.
12. Griffiths GL, Bellenger CR. A retrospective study of osteomyelitis in dogs and cats. *Aust Vet J.* 1979;55:587–591.
13. Andrade N, Schmiedt CW, Cornell K, et al. Survey of intraoperative bacterial contamination in dogs undergoing elective orthopedic surgery. *Vet Surg.* 2016;45:214–222.
14. Bergh MS, Peirone B. Complications of tibial plateau levelling osteotomy in dogs. *Vet Comp Orthop Traumatol.* 2012;25:349–358.
15. Dyce J, Olmstead ML. Removal of infected canine cemented total hip prostheses using a femoral window technique. *Vet Surg.* 2002;31:552–560.
16. Gemmill TJ, Pink J, Renwick A, et al. Hybrid cemented/cementless total hip replacement in dogs: seventy-eight consecutive joint replacements. *Vet Surg.* 2011;40:621–630.
17. Stevenson S, Olmstead ML, Kowalski J. Bacterial culturing for prediction of postoperative complications following open fracture repair in small animals. *Vet Surg.* 1986;15:99–102.
18. Johnson KA, Lomas GR, Wood AK. Osteomyelitis in dogs and cats caused by anaerobic bacteria. *Aust Vet J.* 1984;61:57–61.
19. Muir P, Johnson KA. Anaerobic bacteria isolated from osteomyelitis in dogs and cats. *Vet Surg.* 1992;21:463–466.
20. Rabillard M, Souchu L, Niebauer GW, et al. Haematogenous osteomyelitis: clinical presentation and outcome in three dogs. *Vet Comp Orthop Traumatol.* 2011;24:146–150.
21. Johnson KA. Osteomyelitis in dogs and cats. *J Am Vet Med Assoc.* 1994;204:1882–1887.
22. Funk SS, Copley LA. Acute hematogenous osteomyelitis in children: pathogenesis, diagnosis, and treatment. *Orthop Clin North Am.* 2017;48:199–208.
23. Cook GE, Markel DC, Ren W, et al. Infection in orthopaedics. *J Orthop Trauma.* 2015;29(suppl 12):S19–S23.
24. Arens S, Schlegel U, Printzen G, et al. Influence of materials for fixation implants on local infection. An experimental study of steel versus titanium DCP in rabbits. *J Bone Joint Surg Br.* 1996;78:647–651.
25. Savicky R, Beale B, Murtaugh R, et al. Outcome following removal of TPLO implants with surgical site infection. *Vet Comp Orthop Traumatol.* 2013;26:260–265.
26. Serratore VR, Barnhart MD. Results and complications after removal of tibial tuberosity advancement cage for treatment of surgical site infections: a retrospective study. *Vet Surg.* 2018;47:768–773.
27. Gallie WE. First recurrence of osteomyelitis eighty years after infection. *J Bone Joint Surg Br.* 1951;33-B:110–111.
28. Braden TD, Tvedten HW, Mostosky UV. The sensitivity and specificity of radiology and histopathology in the diagnosis of post-traumatic osteomyelitis. *Vet Comp Orthop Traumatol.* 1989;3:98–103.
29. Berbari EF, Steckelberg JM, Osmon DR. Osteomyelitis. In: Bennett JE, Dolin R, Blaser MJ, eds. *Mandell, Douglas, and Bennett's Principles and Practice of Infectious Diseases.* Philadelphia, PA: Elsevier Saunders; 2015:1318–1327.
30. Kruskal JB. Can USPIO-enhanced spinal MR imaging help distinguish acute infectious osteomyelitis from chronic infectious and inflammatory processes? *Radiology.* 2008;248:1–3.
31. Neuwelt A, Sidhu N, Hu CA, et al. Iron-based superparamagnetic nanoparticle contrast agents for MRI of infection and inflammation. *AJR Am J Roentgenol.* 2015;204:W302–W313.
32. Puig-Verdie L, Alentorn-Geli E, Gonzalez-Cuevas A, et al. Implant sonication increases the diagnostic accuracy of infection in patients with delayed, but not early, orthopaedic implant failure. *Bone Joint Lett J.* 2013;95-B:244–249.
33. de Mesy Bentley KL, Trombetta R, Nishitani K, et al. Evidence of *Staphylococcus aureus* deformation, proliferation, and migration in canaliculi of live cortical bone in murine models of osteomyelitis. *J Bone Miner Res.* 2017;32:985–990.
34. Berkes M, Obremskey WT, Scannell B, et al. Maintenance of hardware after early postoperative infection following fracture internal fixation. *J Bone Joint Surg Am.* 2010;92:823–828.
35. Bardet JF, Hohn RB, Basinger R. Open drainage and delayed autogenous cancellous bone grafting for treatment of chronic osteomyelitis in dogs and cats. *J Am Vet Med Assoc.* 1983;183:312–317.
36. Braden TD, Johnson CA, Wakenell P, et al. Efficacy of clindamycin in the treatment of *Staphylococcus aureus* osteomyelitis in dogs. *J Am Vet Med Assoc.* 1988;192:1721–1725.
37. Chou PY, Yoon J, Hersh-Boyle R, et al. Multidrug-resistant orthopaedic surgical site infections treated with linezolid in four dogs. *VCOT Open.* 2020;3:e72–e76.
38. Cobb LH, McCabe EM, Priddy LB. Therapeutics and delivery vehicles for local treatment of osteomyelitis. *J Orthop Res.* 2020;38:2091–2103.
39. Ham K, Griffon D, Seddighi M, et al. Clinical application of tobramycin-impregnated calcium sulfate beads in six dogs (2002-2004). *J Am Anim Hosp Assoc.* 2008;44:320–326.
40. Gogia JS, Meehan JP, Di Cesare PE, et al. Local antibiotic therapy in osteomyelitis. *Semin Plast Surg.* 2009;23:100–107.
41. Morrison S, Singh A, Rousseau J, et al. Impact of polymethylmethacrylate additives on methicillin-resistant *Staphylococcus pseudintermedius* biofilm formation in vitro. *Am J Vet Res.* 2015;76:395–401.
42. Johnson V, Webb T, Norman A, et al. Activated mesenchymal stem cells interact with antibiotics and host innate immune responses to control chronic bacterial infections. *Sci Rep.* 2017;7:9575.
43. Miliani K, L'Heriteau F, Astagneau P. Non-compliance with recommendations for the practice of antibiotic prophylaxis and risk of surgical site

infection: results of a multilevel analysis from the INCISO Surveillance Network. *J Antimicrob Chemother*. 2009;64:1307–1315.
44. Hawn MT, Richman JS, Vick CC, et al. Timing of surgical antibiotic prophylaxis and the risk of surgical site infection. *JAMA Surg*. 2013;148:649–657.
45. Aiken MJ, Hughes TK, Abercromby RH, et al. Prospective, randomized comparison of the effect of two antimicrobial regimes on surgical site infection rate in dogs undergoing orthopedic implant surgery. *Vet Surg*. 2015;44:661–667.
46. Pratesi A, Moores AP, Downes C, et al. Efficacy of postoperative antimicrobial use for clean orthopedic implant surgery in dogs: a prospective randomized study in 100 consecutive cases. *Vet Surg*. 2015;44:653–660.
47. Romano CL, Tsuchiya H, Morelli I, et al. Antibacterial coating of implants: are we missing something? *Bone Joint Res*. 2019;8:199–206.
48. Azab MA, Allen MJ, Daniels JB. Evaluation of a silver-impregnated coating to inhibit colonization of orthopaedic implants by biofilm forming methicillin-resistant *Staphylococcus pseudintermedius*. *Vet Comp Orthop Traumatol*. 2016;29:347–350.
49. Serhan H, Slivka M, Albert T, et al. Is galvanic corrosion between titanium alloy and stainless steel spinal implants a clinical concern? *Spine J*. 2004;4:379–387.
50. Soares Magalhaes RJ, Loeffler A, Lindsay J, et al. Risk factors for methicillin-resistant *Staphylococcus aureus* (MRSA) infection in dogs and cats: a case-control study. *Vet Res*. 2010;41:55.
51. Schultz RM, Johnson EG, Wisner ER, et al. Clinicopathologic and diagnostic imaging characteristics of systemic aspergillosis in 30 dogs. *J Vet Intern Med*. 2008;22:851–859.
52. Aroch I, Shamir M, Harmelin A. Lumbar diskospondylitis and meningomyelitis caused by *Escherichia coli* in a cat. *Feline Pract*. 1999;27:20–22.
53. Malik RM, Latler M, Love DN. Bacterial diskospondylitis in a cat. *J Small Anim Pract*. 1990;31:404–406.
54. Norsworthy GD. Discospondylitis as a cause of posterior paresis. *Feline Pract*. 1979;9:39–40.
55. Packer RA, Coates JR, Cook CR, et al. Sublumbar abscess and diskospondylitis in a cat. *Vet Radiol Ultrasound*. 2005;46:396–399.
56. Watson E, Roberts RE. Diskospondylitis in a cat. *Vet Radiol*. 1993;34:397–398.
57. Harris JM, Chen AV, Tucker RL, et al. Clinical features and magnetic resonance imaging characteristics of diskospondylitis in dogs: 23 cases (1997-2010). *J Am Vet Med Assoc*. 2013;242:359–365.
58. Kerwin SC, Lewis DD, Hribernik TN, et al. Diskospondylitis associated with *Brucella canis* infection in dogs: 14 cases (1980-1991). *J Am Vet Med Assoc*. 1992;201:1253–1257.
59. Buhmann G, Paul F, Herbst W, et al. Canine brucellosis: insights into the epidemiologic situation in Europe. *Front Vet Sci*. 2019;6:151.
60. Golini L, Morgan JP, Glaus T, et al. Successful medical treatment of *Erysipelothrix rhusiopathiae*-induced lumbosacral diskospondylitis in a dog. *Vet Rec*. 2012;170:543.
61. Hilligas J, Van Wie E, Barr J, et al. Vertebral osteomyelitis and multiple cutaneous lesions in a dog caused by *Nocardia pseudobrasiliensis*. *J Vet Intern Med*. 2014;28:1621–1625.
62. Plessas IN, Jull P, Volk HA. A case of canine discospondylitis and epidural empyema due to *Salmonella* species. *Can Vet J*. 2013;54:595–598.
63. Ruoff CM, Kerwin SC, Taylor AR. Diagnostic imaging of discospondylitis. *Vet Clin North Am Small Anim Pract*. 2018;48:85–94.
64. Kent M, Boozer L, Glass EN, et al. Post-operative *Salmonella* surgical site infection in a dog. *Can Vet J*. 2017;58:936–940.
65. Carrera I, Sullivan M, McConnell F, et al. Magnetic resonance imaging features of discospondylitis in dogs. *Vet Radiol Ultrasound*. 2011;52:125–131.
66. Davis MJ, Dewey CW, Walker MA, et al. Contrast radiographic findings in canine bacterial discospondylitis: a multicenter, retrospective study of 27 cases. *J Am Anim Hosp Assoc*. 2000;36:81–85.
67. Garcia RS, Wheat LJ, Cook A, et al. Sensitivity and specificity of a blood and urine galactomannan antigen assay for diagnosis of systemic aspergillosis in dogs. *J Vet Intern Med*. 2012;26:911–919.
68. Gendron K, Doherr MG, Gavin P, et al. Magnetic resonance imaging characterization of vertebral endplate changes in the dog. *Vet Radiol Ultrasound*. 2012;53:50–56.
69. Fischer A, Mahaffey MB, Oliver JE. Fluoroscopically guided percutaneous disk aspiration in 10 dogs with diskospondylitis. *J Vet Intern Med*. 1997;11:284–287.
70. Moore SA. Managing neuropathic pain in dogs. *Front Vet Sci*. 2016;3:12.
71. Foster JD, Trepanier LA, Ginn JA. Use of linezolid to treat MRSP bacteremia and discospondylitis in a dog. *J Am Anim Hosp Assoc*. 2014;50:53–58.
72. Clements DN, Owen MR, Mosley JR, et al. Retrospective study of bacterial infective arthritis in 31 dogs. *J Small Anim Pract*. 2005;46:171–176.
73. Marchevsky AM, Read RA. Bacterial septic arthritis in 19 dogs. *Aust Vet J*. 1999;77:233–237.
74. Scharf VF, Lewis DD, Wellehan JF, et al. Comparison of synovial fluid culture and 16S rRNA PCR in dogs with suspected septic arthritis. *Aust Vet J*. 2015;93:204–207.

122

Cardiovascular Infections (Bacteremia, Endocarditis, Myocarditis, Infectious Pericarditis)

Steven E. Epstein, Joshua A. Stern, Jane E. Sykes

KEY POINTS

- Causes: Most common bacterial causes are staphylococci, streptococci, and *Escherichia coli.* Gram-negative bacterial etiologies predominate in cats. Culture-negative infections of the bloodstream may be caused by *Bartonella* spp. or other fastidious bacteria. Anaerobes, fungi, and mycobacteria are less commonly involved. *Rickettsia rickettsii* can cause vasculitis and myocarditis.
- Geographic Distribution: Worldwide.
- Major Clinical Signs: Highly variable. Fever, inappetence, lethargy, and tachycardia are common with sepsis. GI signs such as vomiting and diarrhea may also be present. Additional findings in infective endocarditis patients include cardiac murmurs, lameness, and neurologic signs due to thromboembolic disease. Spinal pain, paresis or paralysis may occur when discospondylitis complicates bacteremia or fungemia.
- Differential Diagnoses: Noninfectious conditions that can mimic sepsis include pancreatitis, trauma, hypoadrenocorticism, heat stroke, anaphylaxis, pulmonary thromboembolism, hemorrhage, cardiac tamponade, and some toxicities. Dogs with primary immune-mediated disorders may also show clinical signs that resemble those of chronic bacteremia and infective endocarditis. The major differential for infectious pericarditis is idiopathic or benign pericardial effusion and neoplastic disorders such as mesothelioma.
- Human Health Significance: Dogs and cats with cardiovascular infections may be infected with pathogens that have the potential to cause disease in humans, such as *Salmonella* spp., *Bartonella* spp., *Brucella* spp., and *R. rickettsii.*

ETIOLOGIC AGENTS, EPIDEMIOLOGY AND CLINICAL FEATURES

A variety of pathogens can cause infections of the cardiovascular system, including viruses, bacteria, fungi, protozoa, and parasites. This chapter focuses on bacterial infections of the cardiovascular system; information on other types of pathogens can be found in their respective chapters in this book. Bacterial infections of the cardiovascular system include bacteremia, infective endocarditis (IE), myocarditis, and infectious pericarditis. These infections are frequently associated with *sepsis,* or the host systemic inflammatory response to infection. Various terminologies are used to define the clinical manifestations associated with sepsis (see Chapter 123).

Bacteremia

Bacteremia has been defined as *uncomplicated* and *complicated bacteremia* (Table 122.1). Transient, low-level (≤10 CFU/mL) subclinical bacteremia follows a variety of procedures such as dental prophylaxis, endoscopy, GI surgery, and catheter placement. This is typically cleared rapidly (within 15 to 30 minutes) by a functional mononuclear phagocyte system. However, persistent release of large numbers of bacteria into the bloodstream can overwhelm the host immune response and culminates in clinically significant bacteremia. Overwhelming bacteremia can occur with disorders such as pyelonephritis, pyothorax, severe pyoderma, bacterial peritonitis, pyometra, pneumonia, pancreatitis, a variety of GI disorders, bite wounds, orthopedic infections, or catheter-related infections. Underlying immune system dysfunction (such as occurs with diabetes mellitus, malignancy, and neutropenia) also predisposes to clinically significant bacteremia because unhindered multiplication of bacteria occurs in the bloodstream.

The most common organisms isolated from the bloodstream of sick, bacteremic dogs are *Staphylococcus* spp., *Streptococcus* spp. (especially *Streptococcus canis*), and *Escherichia coli* (Table 122.2).[1] Less than 10% of bacteremic dogs in the authors' hospital are infected with anaerobes, but in a study of critically ill dogs and cats from Colorado, anaerobes were isolated from 31% of 39 dogs and 40% of 10 cats.[2] With the exception of bartonellosis, bacteremia is less commonly recognized in cats than in dogs, and usually results from infection with gram-negative bacterial pathogens.[1] Polymicrobial infections of the blood are common and typically occur in 10% to 20% of dogs and cats with positive blood culture results. Mixed infections with two or more different strains of a single bacterial species can also occur. Polymicrobial infections often occur when anaerobes are involved or secondary to compromise of the GI tract.

In addition to sepsis and septic shock (see Chapter 123), bacteremia may be followed by the development of IE, discospondylitis, and metastatic abscess formation in a variety of tissues. Chronic bacteremia may be associated with secondary immune-mediated disorders, especially immune-mediated polyarthritis and glomerulonephritis, and rarely IMHA. This can result in erroneous diagnosis of a primary immune-mediated disorder and inappropriate treatment with immunosuppressive drugs, sometimes with fatal outcome.

Infective Endocarditis

The reported incidence of canine IE has ranged from < 0.1% of cases evaluated by veterinary teaching hospitals to approximately 1% of cases evaluated by veterinary cardiologists.[3–6] IE is uncommonly diagnosed in cats; in one study, cats with IE represented < 0.01% of cats evaluated by a university teaching hospital.[7] Most cats were diagnosed with congestive heart failure (CHF) at the time of IE diagnosis and prognosis

TABLE 122.1 Definitions that Apply to Cardiovascular Infections in Dogs and Cats[a]

Term	Definition
Bacteremia	The presence of viable or cultivable bacteria in the bloodstream
Uncomplicated bacteremia	Positive blood culture results and the following: exclusion of endocarditis; no implants; negative follow-up cultures 2–4 days after the initial set; defervescence within 72 hours of initiation of effective treatment; and no evidence of metastatic sites of infection
Complicated bacteremia	Animals with positive blood culture results that do not meet the criteria for uncomplicated bacteremia
Fungemia	The presence of viable fungi in the bloodstream
Infective endocarditis	Infection of one or more endocardial surfaces of the heart; almost always involves a cardiac valve

[a]See Table 123.1 for definitions that apply to SIRS and sepsis.

was poor. Dogs with IE are typically middle aged to older, large-breed dogs such as German shepherd dogs, golden and Labrador retrievers, Weimaraners, mastiffs, and rottweilers. For unclear reasons, male dogs are affected approximately twice as often as females. Factors that predispose to IE are similar to those that predispose to continuous bacteremia. However, virulence factors possessed by bacteria subsequently impact whether IE develops, which explains why some bacterial species (especially gram-positive bacteria) are more likely to produce IE than others (gram-negative bacteria). Although congenital heart defects, especially subaortic stenosis (SAS), may predispose young dogs to development of IE, the vast majority of dogs with SAS never develop IE, and over 80% of dogs with IE have no identifiable underlying cardiac abnormality.[5,8] It remains unclear if the associated risk of IE in patients with SAS is related to the pathophysiology of this condition or simply an association secondary to the increased incidence of IE in large-breed dogs and a similarly increased incidence of this common, inherited heart disease in this population of large, sporting-breed dogs. Furthermore, IE is rarely diagnosed in small-breed dogs, which are predisposed to myxomatous mitral valve degeneration. The observed link between periodontal disease and IE in human subjects is less clear in dogs and cats. One study found no association between periodontal disease and IE in dogs.,[8] A 2016 investigation identified the same enterococcal pathogen from the mouth and IE lesions in 7 out of 32 dogs with IE and periodontal disease.[9] However, in 2021 this publication was retracted because of concerns about the validity of the results.[10]

The most commonly reported etiologic agents in canine IE are streptococci, staphylococci, and to a lesser extent, gram-negative rods, enterococci, and *Bartonella* spp. (Table 122.3).[4,8,11–13] Organisms that are less commonly incriminated include fungi, gram-positive rods, mycobacteria, and anaerobes. In dogs, the mitral and/or the aortic valves are most commonly affected (Fig. 122.1). The larger, septal leaflet of the mitral valve may be more commonly affected than the mural leaflet.[5] The tricuspid valve and ventricular wall are rarely involved. This distribution correlates with the degree of pressure that rests on the closed valve. Classically, vegetative lesions develop along the line of valve closure. In a case series of cats with IE, the aortic valve was affected 62% of the time while the mitral valve was affected in 38% of cats.[7]

The development of IE begins with colonization of a heart valve by bacteria, and deposition of fibrin, platelets, leukocytes, and erythrocytes. Colonization may be facilitated by changes in the valve surface as a result of turbulent blood flow, which in turn leads to the deposition of platelets, fibrin, and fibronectin; the end result is a sterile vegetation, or *nonbacterial thrombotic endocarditis.* Bacteria then adhere to this matrix, induce inflammatory cytokine and tissue factor release, and become covered with additional layers of platelets and fibrin, which promote bacterial growth to extremely high densities in an environment that is protected from the immune system. Properties of bacteria known to promote valve colonization include adhesins such as *fimA* in streptococci, and clumping factor and fibronectin-binding proteins in staphylococci,[14,15] as well as factors that cause platelet aggregation. Portions of the vegetation that results can then dislodge and embolize in a variety of different tissues, especially the kidneys, spleen, brain, joints, and muscles, with a huge spectrum of associated clinical manifestations. Thromboembolic complications are more likely to occur in dogs with mitral valve involvement than those with aortic valve IE.[5] Regardless of the valve affected, valvular dysfunction can lead to impaired cardiac output and CHF. CHF secondary to moderate to severe valvular insufficiency is a common sequela to IE in cats.[7]

As in humans, IE in dogs may be best classified on the basis of the etiologic agent involved, because the etiologic agent often determines the clinical course of disease, disease manifestations, prognosis, and the most appropriate antimicrobial drugs for treatment. For example, *Bartonella* IE is more likely to involve the aortic valve than the mitral valve; often occurs in the absence of fever; has a high prevalence of CHF when compared with IE caused by other bacterial pathogens; and is negatively correlated with survival (see Fig. 70.7). In contrast, *S. canis* IE usually involves the mitral valve and is often associated with neutrophilic polyarthritis. Dogs with gram-negative IE appear less likely to develop CHF than those with IE caused by other pathogens.[11]

The clinical signs and physical examination abnormalities that occur with IE are extremely variable and depend not only on the causative organism but also on the valve affected, the presence or absence of thromboembolic complications, and the sites and extent of thromboembolism. Common historic findings include lethargy; inappetence; locomotory problems such as lameness, shifting lameness, joint pain, reluctance to move, and inability to walk; as well as vomiting, respiratory difficulty, weight loss, and/or cough. Locomotory abnormalities can result from peripheral arterial thromboembolism, embolic or immune-mediated polyarthritis, neurologic abnormalities, and rarely, hypertrophic osteopathy. The most common initial physical examination findings in dogs with IE are fever, tachycardia, and a cardiac murmur (Table 122.4).[5] In one study of dogs with IE, fever was documented in the history or serial physical examinations of only 41 (60%) of 68 dogs with IE, and a cardiac murmur in 53 (76%) of 70 dogs with IE, so an absence of fever or a cardiac murmur does not make IE an unlikely diagnosis.[5] Although diastolic murmurs may be suggestive of IE, more than 90% of dogs with murmurs due to IE have systolic murmurs.

Infectious Myocarditis

Infectious myocarditis in dogs and cats usually results from hematogenous spread of microorganisms to the myocardium or extension of IE lesions to the myocardium. Viruses, bacteria, protozoa, or fungi may be involved. Certain organisms appear to have a particular tropism for the myocardium (Table 122.5). Infectious myocarditis is rare in cats.

Myocarditis may be subclinical or result in a variety of arrhythmias, CHF, or sudden death. Simultaneous infection of a variety of other organs is frequent for the majority of pathogens that cause myocarditis, so clinical signs of systemic infection (fever, lethargy) and other organ dysfunction are often present. In one case series of dogs with myocarditis, fever was present in 21% of dogs and a heart murmur in 19%.[16] Definitive diagnosis is often only made at necropsy.

TABLE 122.2 Organisms Cultivable Using Routine Blood Culture from Dogs and Cats with Bacteremia[1,2,11]

	Dogs	Cats
Common (>10% of isolates)	*Staphylococcus* spp., including *S. pseudintermedius*, *S. aureus*, and coagulase-negative staphylococci *Streptococcus* spp., especially *S. canis*, but also *S. bovis* complex organisms and rarely other streptococci *E. coli*	*Escherichia coli* Other Enterobacterales (*Klebsiella pneumoniae*, *Citrobacter freundii*, *Enterobacter cloacae*) Anaerobes
Uncommon (1% to 10% of isolates)	*Enterococcus* spp. *K. pneumoniae*, *Serratia* spp., *E. cloacae* *Pasteurella canis* and *Pasteurella dagmatis* *Pseudomonas aeruginosa* Anaerobes (*Clostridium perfringens*, *Prevotella* spp., *Bacteroides* spp., *Fusobacterium* spp., *Actinomyces* spp., *Peptostreptococcus* spp.)	*Salmonella* spp. Non-Enterobacterales gram-negative bacteria (*Pasteurella multocida*, *Pseudomonas aeruginosa*, *Acinetobacter baumanii*) Staphylococci Streptococci
Rare (≤1% of isolates)	*Erysipelothrix* spp. *Brucella* spp. *C. freundii* *Acinetobacter* spp. *Salmonella* spp. *Mycobacterium* spp. *Campylobacter* spp. Other nosocomial pathogens, e.g., *Ralstonia pickettii*, *Burkholderia cepacia*, *Achromobacter xylosoxidans*	*Enterococcus* spp.

TABLE 122.3 Causes of Infective Endocarditis in Dogs

Microorganism	Prevalence[11]
Streptococci (primarily *S. canis* but also *S. bovis* complex)	29%
Bartonella spp.	20%
Staphylococci (*S. pseudintermedius*, *S. aureus*, and coagulase-negative staphylococci)	15%
Gram-negative rods (most commonly *Escherichia coli*, but also *Pseudomonas aeruginosa*, *Salmonella* spp., *Citrobacter freundii*, *Klebsiella pneumoniae*, *Proteus* spp., *Pasteurella* spp., *Brucella* spp.)	15% (7% *E. coli*; < 5% other species)
Other gram-positive bacteria (*Erysipelothrix* spp., *Granulicatella adiacens*, *Actinomyces* spp., *Corynebacterium* spp., *Mycobacterium* spp.)	7% (<5% each species)
Enterococcus spp.	5%
Fungi (e.g., *Aspergillus* spp.)	<5%

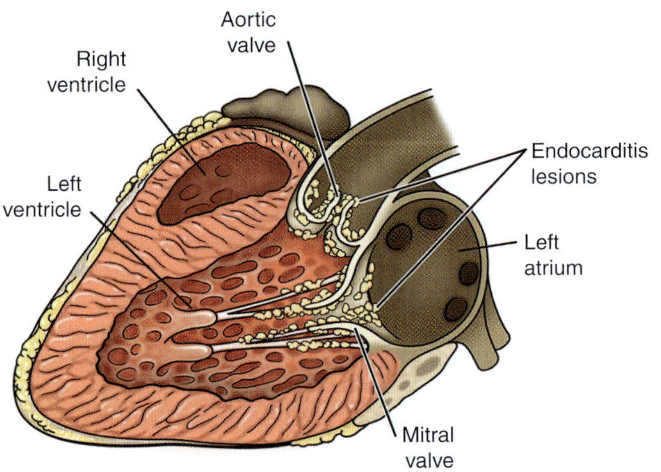

Fig. 122.1 Infective endocarditis. Vegetations are attached to the mitral and aortic valves and may be mobile or sessile.

Infectious Pericarditis

Infectious pericarditis may result from direct inoculation of organisms into the pericardium (such as occurs with penetrating wounds),[17,18] extension of infection from adjacent organs such as the pleural space or lungs, or hematogenous dissemination of viral, bacterial, protozoal, or fungal pathogens to the pericardium. Bite wounds or grass awn migration often result in mixed aerobic-anaerobic infections that involve organisms such as *Actinomyces* spp. (see Chapter 59). Infectious pericarditis as a result of hematogenous spread of pathogens is rare. Idiopathic pericardial effusion and heart base neoplasia are the most common causes of inflammatory or hemorrhagic pericardial effusion in dogs; neoplasia and hypertrophic cardiomyopathy were the most common causes of pericardial effusion in cats in one study.[19] Pathogens with particular tropism for the pericardial sac include FIP virus and *Coccidioides* spp. Pericardial effusion was also reported in association with *Leishmania* infection.[20] Pericarditis results in diastolic cardiac dysfunction with subsequent development of right-sided heart failure, which is manifested as weak pulses, tachycardia, jugular venous pulsation or distension, ascites, and pleural effusion. Muffled heart sounds may be detected on cardiac auscultation as a result of pericardial and/or pleural effusion.

DIAGNOSIS

Antemortem diagnosis of bacteremia is based on culture of bacteria from the bloodstream. Reasons to consider blood culture are shown

TABLE 122.4 Physical Examination Findings in 70 Dogs with Infective Endocarditis Seen at the University of California, Davis William R. Pritchard VMTH[a]

Physical Examination Finding	Number Affected (%)
Cardiac murmur	41 (59)
Tachycardia	34 (50)
Fever	26 (38)
Tachypnea	24 (35)
Abnormal lung sounds	24 (34)
Recumbency	21 (30)
Mental dullness	19 (27)
Neurologic signs (ataxia, decreased conscious proprioception, strabismus, nystagmus, head tilt, obtundation)	16 (23)
Swollen joints	15 (21)
Stiffness or lameness	13 (19)
Arrhythmias	14 (19)
Dehydration	11 (16)
Bounding pulses	10 (14)
Muscle atrophy	10 (14)
Thin body condition	9 (13)
Weak pulses	8 (11)
Reluctance to stand	8 (11)
Peripheral edema	7 (10)
Spinal pain	7 (10)
Abdominal pain, mucosal pallor, red mucous membranes, muscle pain, weakness, cyanosis, cool or cold limbs, oral ulceration, abdominal enlargement, hepatomegaly, icterus, uveitis, petechial or ecchymotic hemorrhages, cutaneous ulceration	6 or fewer (< 10)

[a]Cases seen at the University of California-Davis Veterinary Medical Teaching Hospital.

Modified from Sykes JE, Kittleson MD, Chomel BB, et al. Clinicopathologic findings and outcome in dogs with infective endocarditis: 71 cases (1992-2005). *J Am Vet Med Assoc.* 2006;228:1735–1747.

in Box 122.1. The diagnosis of IE is based on a set of criteria modified from the Duke criteria used for diagnosis of IE in human patients, which consider the results of blood culture and echocardiography as major criteria, and other clinical manifestations of IE as minor criteria (Table 122.6). Diagnosis of infective pericarditis relies on echocardiography and the results of cytologic examination and culture of pericardial fluid, or alternatively, histopathologic examination and culture of pericardial biopsies obtained during thoracotomy or thoracoscopy. In dogs and cats, infectious myocarditis is usually a necropsy diagnosis because myocardial biopsy is rarely performed. However, bacterial myocarditis may be suspected based on echocardiographic abnormalities, the presence of arrhythmias, increased serum cardiac troponin I, concentration and positive blood cultures or serologic testing.

Laboratory Abnormalities

Complete Blood Count

Common CBC findings in dogs and cats with bloodstream infections are mild nonregenerative anemia, neutrophilia with a left shift and neutrophil toxicity, bandemia, lymphopenia, and/or monocytosis.

TABLE 122.5 Infectious Causes of Myocarditis in Dogs and Cats

Pathogen Type	Examples	Affected Host
Viruses	West Nile virus	D
	Canine parvovirus 2	D
	Feline panleukopenia virus	C
	Pseudorabies virus	D
Bacteria	Gram-negative and gram-positive bacteria	D, C
	(e.g., extension of endocarditis)	D, C
	Bartonella spp.	D
	Borrelia burgdorferi	D
	Rickettsia spp.	
Fungi	*Blastomyces* spp.	D
	Candida albicans	D
	Cryptococcus neoformans	D
	Aspergillus spp.	D
	Paecilomyces variotii	D
	Other molds	D
Algae	*Prototheca* spp.	D
Protozoa	*Trypanosoma cruzi*	D
	Sarcocystis felis	C
	Leishmania spp.	D
	Neospora caninum	D
	Hepatozoon americanum	D
	Toxoplasma gondii	D, C

C, cats; *D*, dogs.

BOX 122.1 Reasons to Consider Blood Culture in Dogs and Cats

Fever (especially when viral infection is not likely or underlying immunosuppression or barrier disruption is present)
Unexplained peripheral edema in dogs
Evidence of thromboembolism in dogs (e.g., organ infarction, cold limbs)
Neutrophilic polyarthritis in dogs
Discospondylitis in dogs
Echocardiographic evidence of infective endocarditis or new heart murmur (dogs or cats)
Neutrophilic lymphadenitis (dogs or cats)
Severe pneumonia or pyothorax (dogs or cats)
Peritonitis (dogs or cats)
Development of leukopenia, bandemia or leukocytosis in association with immunosuppression, catheters or other devices (dogs or cats)
Thrombophlebitis in association with an indwelling catheter (dogs or cats)
Sepsis in a patient from which a culture cannot be obtained from the suspected source (e.g., pneumonia in severely hypoxemic patient, GI bacterial translocation)

Degenerative left shifts may be present, and dogs and cats with DIC may be thrombocytopenic or have evidence of schistocytosis. Rarely, bacteria may be seen within circulating leukocytes on blood smear examination.

Serum Biochemical Tests

The serum chemistry profile may show evidence of sepsis, or bacterial embolization and infarction. Abnormalities include azotemia, increased activities of liver enzymes, mild to moderate hyperbilirubinemia

TABLE 122.6 **Modified Duke Criteria Used for Diagnosis of Infective Endocarditis in Dogs and Cats**[5,28]

Major Criteria	Minor Criteria
Identification of a typical organism using blood culture	Predisposing heart condition (congenital valvular malformation)
• *Streptococcus* spp.	New or worsening heart murmur
• *Staphylococcus* spp.	Fever (≥103°F [39.4°C])
• *Escherichia coli*	Presence of vascular/embolic phenomena
Growth in all 3, or most of 4, separate blood cultures, with first and last specimens drawn at least 1 hour apart	Immunologic phenomena: nondegenerate neutrophilic polyarthritis, glomerulonephritis, immune-mediated hemolytic anemia
Two positive blood cultures for any microorganism, when blood cultures are drawn more than 12 hours apart	Microbiologic phenomena: positive blood culture not meeting major criteria, *or* serologic evidence of infection with a typical organism, *or* detection of a typical organism using a nucleic acid amplification test
Findings on echocardiogram positive for infective endocarditis	

Definite endocarditis: 2 major criteria, or histopathologic confirmation of endocarditis.
Possible endocarditis: Positive echocardiographic findings and 1 minor criteria, or 1 major and 3 minor criteria, or 5 minor criteria. In recent human guidelines, 1 major and 3 minor criteria, or 5 minor criteria, are considered sufficient evidence for diagnosis of definitive endocarditis.[24]

(usually < 5 mg/dL), and electrolyte and acid-base abnormalities (such as a high anion gap metabolic acidosis due to azotemia or lactic acidosis). Hyperglycemia may be present early in sepsis in cats while hypoglycemia may develop in either cats or dogs. Hypoglycemia may also be present as a result of decreased hepatic gluconeogenesis or upregulation of non–insulin-dependent glucose transporters. Hypoalbuminemia occurs in most dogs with IE, ranges from mild to severe, and may result from decreased hepatic production, increased vascular permeability, or as part of the inflammatory response (albumin is a negative acute-phase reactant protein). Dogs with thromboembolism to muscle tissue may have markedly increased activity of serum CK.

Urinalysis

Urinalysis findings in dogs and cats with bacteremia or IE may include proteinuria, pyuria, cylindruria, microscopic hematuria, and bacteriuria. Severe proteinuria (urine protein-to-creatinine ratio > 5) may occur as a result of glomerular damage in dogs with IE which may contribute to a hypercoagulable state.

Coagulation Profile

Dogs and cats with DIC may have prolonged aPTT and PT, increased concentrations of fibrin degradation products or D-dimers, and/or decreased concentrations of plasma fibrinogen and antithrombin. If viscoelastic testing is used, either hyper- or hypocoagulability may be documented in dogs.[21] In dogs with IE, PT is often shortened, and fibrinogen concentration is often increased.[5]

Cardiac Biomarkers

A large body of evidence has accumulated to support that cardiac biomarkers, such as the N-terminal fragment of the prohormone B-type natriuretic peptide (NT-proBNP) and cardiac troponin I, represent biochemical tests with acceptable sensitivity and specificity for the diagnosis of myocardial injury, stress, or stretch.[22,23] Serum cardiac troponin I is a useful, quantitative assessment of myocardial injury. Although not specific for endocarditis or myocarditis, one study showed that serum cardiac troponin I concentrations were significantly higher in dogs with IE (n = 29) than dogs with stage-B myxomatous mitral valve disease (n = 27) and dogs with immune-mediated disease (n = 16).[25] A cut-off value of 0.625 ng/mL had 100% specificity and 52% sensitivity for diagnosis of IE in that study. Severe myocardial injury such as myocardial infarction and myocarditis is commonly associated with significantly increased concentrations of serum cardiac biomarker molecules. However, a small percentage of dogs with myocarditis may have normal serum cardiac troponin I concentrations.[16] Ultimately, increased concentrations of cardiac biomarkers supports a diagnosis of cardiovascular infection but is not required for diagnosis.

Diagnostic Imaging

Plain Radiography

Thoracic radiographs in dogs with IE often show no detectable abnormalities. When present, abnormal findings include pulmonary infiltrates as a result of pneumonia, ARDS or CHF; generalized cardiomegaly; left atrial enlargement; pulmonary venous distension; mild pleural effusion; and occasionally, even microcardia or vascular attenuation (see Fig. 70.10). Infectious pericarditis may be associated with radiographic evidence of pleural effusion or cardiomegaly. Changes to the intervertebral disc spaces that suggest discospondylitis may also be detected in dogs with bacteremia or endocarditis (see Chapter 121).

Echocardiography

Echocardiography is indicated when IE, myocarditis, or pericarditis is suspected based on the history and physical examination findings (such as fever, arrhythmia, a new murmur, or signs of left- or right-sided CHF). It is also indicated for all dogs and cats with bacteremia, even in the absence of a cardiac murmur or arrhythmia; for dogs with neutrophilic polyarthritis; and for dogs and cats with evidence of systemic thromboembolic disease. Echocardiographic findings in IE can include valvular hyperechogenicity, thickening and irregularity, and valvular vegetations, which may be nodular, discrete, or have a shaggy or moth-eaten appearance (Fig. 122.2 and see Fig. 70.13). Large vegetations may oscillate or vibrate, and follow-up echocardiography sometimes reveals disappearance of a vegetative lesion in association with thromboembolism. Mild or severe valvular regurgitation or insufficiency may be present in association with lesions. Other echocardiographic findings include left ventricular eccentric hypertrophy, chamber dilation, mural hyperechogenicity, ruptured chordae tendineae, acquired defects in the valves or myocardium, and mild pericardial effusion. Echocardiography is a sensitive tool for diagnosis of IE (87.5% in one study of dogs with IE when necropsy was used as the gold standard),[5] but negative results do not completely rule out the possibility of IE. Echocardiography is also useful for monitoring treatment of IE (see Treatment).

Echocardiographic findings in infectious pericarditis include pericardial effusion, adhesions of the pericardium to the epicardium, and sometimes focal or diffuse pericardial thickening and hyperechogenicity (Fig. 122.3). Restrictive disease is characterized by impairment of diastole, with decreased left ventricular internal dimensions during diastole, and variation of blood flow velocity across the mitral valve with the respiratory cycle (increased with expiration and decreased with inspiration). In addition, deviation of the interventricular septum

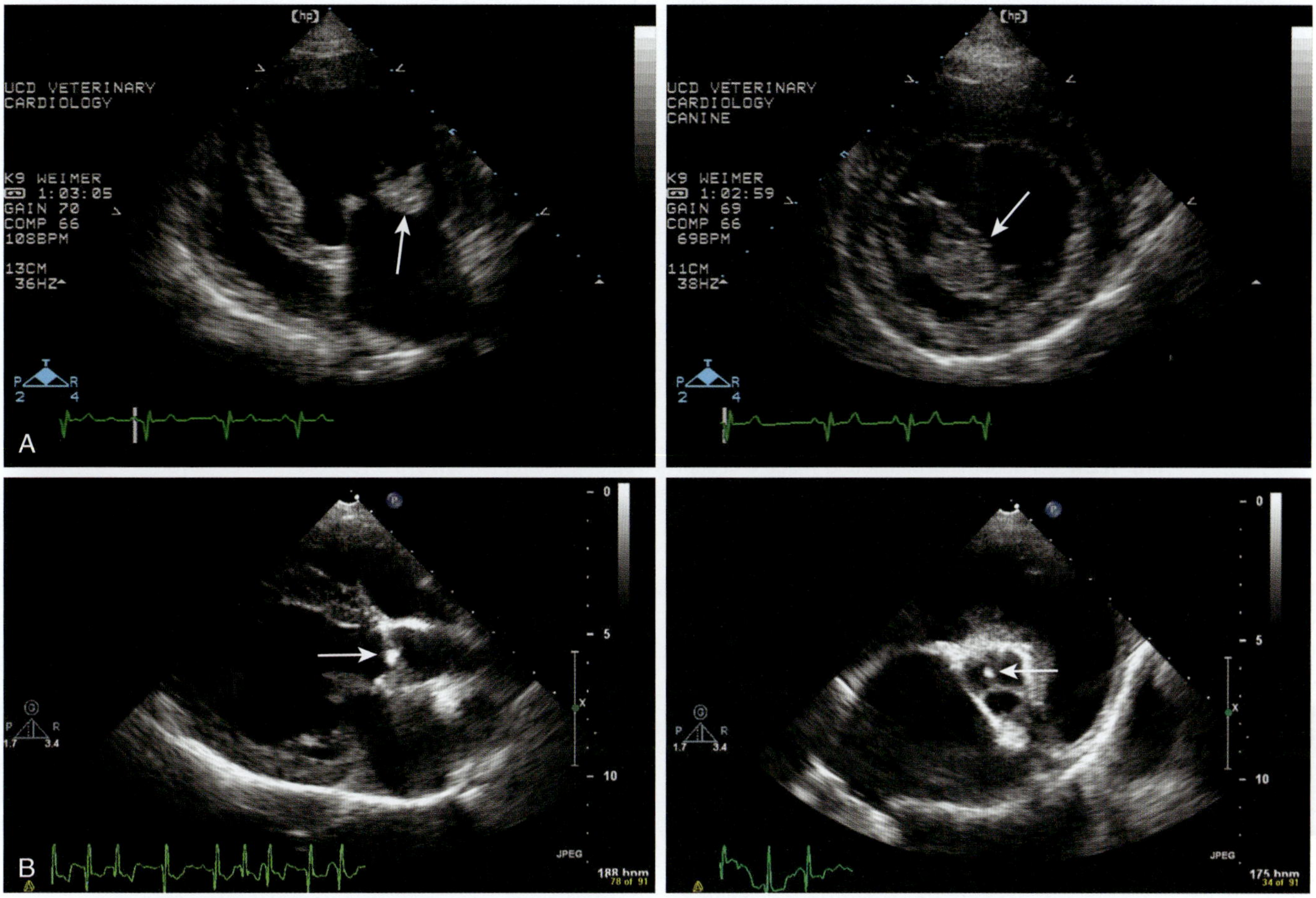

Fig. 122.2 Canine endocarditis lesions as viewed using transthoracic echocardiography. (A) Right parasternal (left) and short axis (right) views from a 7-year-old male neutered Weimaraner with *Enterococcus faecium* endocarditis that followed a perineal urethrostomy procedure. There is a large vegetative lesion attached to the anterior leaflet of the mitral valve *(arrow)*. A smaller lesion is attached to the septal leaflet. (B) Right parasternal (left) and short axis (right) views of the aortic valve from a 4-year-old intact male Doberman pinscher with aortic and mitral valve culture-negative endocarditis. A nodular, hyperechoic lesion is associated with the aortic valve *(arrow)*.

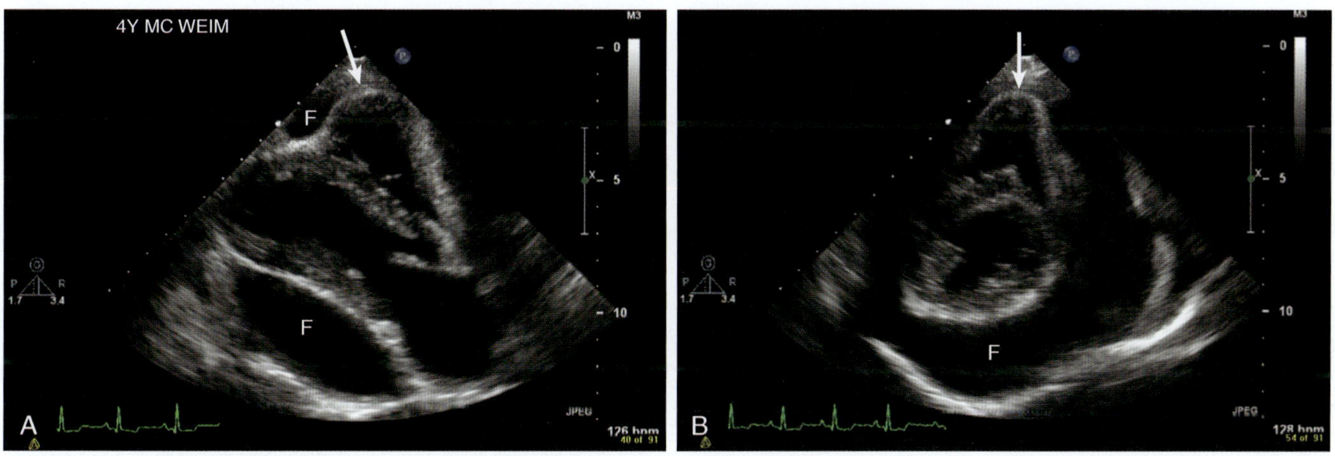

Fig. 122.3 Long axis (A) and short axis (B) echocardiography images that show pericarditis in a 4 year old male neutered Weimaraner with disseminated coccidioidomycosis. The epicardium is adhered to the pericardium *(arrow)* and a moderate quantity of anechoic pericardial fluid *(F)* can be appreciated. The cardiac chambers are distorted.

into the left ventricle can occur during inspiration and right ventricle during expiration. Echocardiographic findings in myocarditis may include a heterogeneous appearance to the ventricular myocardium, systolic dysfunction, and volume overload.[16] Regional septal or free-wall motion abnormalities may be seen in areas of more severe ischemia or infarction.

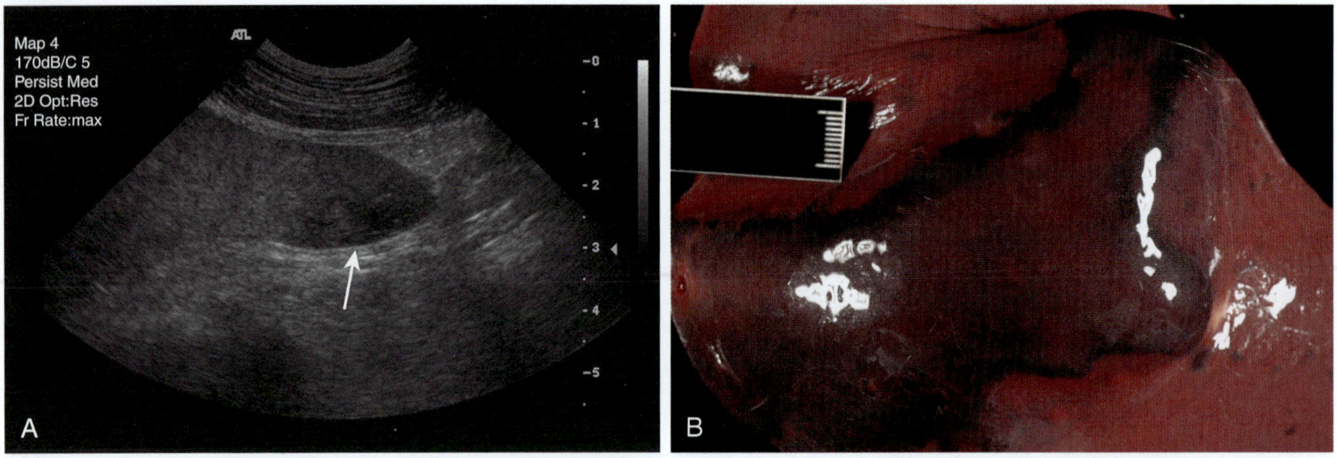

Fig. 122.4 (A) Abdominal ultrasound image that shows a splenic infarct *(arrow)* in a 6-year-old female spayed Bouvier des Flandres with *Staphylococcus aureus* infective endocarditis. (B) Splenic infarct at necropsy.

Abdominal Sonographic Findings

Sonographic abnormalities may be present in a variety of organs in dogs with IE, and may reflect underlying disease processes (such as neoplasia or bacterial peritonitis) or septic thromboembolism. Infarction and hemorrhage secondary to thromboembolic disease may result in focal cavitary or hypoechoic lesions in the spleen (Fig. 122.4) or focal hyperechoic or hypoechoic lesions in the kidney. Thrombi may be found in the iliac arteries or aorta.

Microbiologic Tests

Culture

Routine blood cultures assist in identification of infecting pathogens and permit susceptibility testing. Ideally, at least three blood cultures should be obtained from separate sites within a 24-hour period. A suggested protocol for blood cultures is outlined in Chapter 3 (Box 3.2). Although the use of separate venipuncture sites has been suggested, this is not considered essential for diagnosis of human IE; however, the use of indwelling catheters should be avoided.[24] If a catheter-related bloodstream infection is suspected, collection of paired specimens has been recommended in humans, with one specimen collected from the catheter prior to removal and the other collected from a peripheral site.[26] The skin should be prepared in the same manner used for surgery, and utmost care should be taken to avoid contamination with commensal bacteria. Because IE is generally associated with continuous bacteremia, positive results in a single bottle should be interpreted with caution. Positive results for *Bacillus* spp. or coagulase-negative staphylococci in a single bottle generally reflect contamination.

The decision to perform anaerobic blood culture should be considered in light of the animal's underlying disease process and client financial constraints. For example, anaerobic culture may not be cost effective in dogs with IE, given the rare involvement of anaerobes in this condition. Anaerobes are more likely to be present in dogs with histories that suggest involvement of plant awn foreign bodies, bite wounds, GI, or biliary tract compromise.

False-negative blood cultures may occur as a result of low-level bacteremia or fungemia, the presence of fastidious or unculturable organisms such as *Bartonella*, insufficient specimen size, or recent antimicrobial treatment. Nevertheless, blood culture is still indicated in animals with a history of antimicrobial treatment, especially if antimicrobials have only been administered for 2 to 3 days. If an animal with IE is in stable condition, discontinuation of existing antibiotic treatment for several days (ideally 7 to 10 days) could be considered before blood cultures are obtained. Specific culture and serology for *Bartonella* is also indicated in dogs and cats with IE or suspected myocarditis (see Chapter 70). This should be considered even if routine blood cultures are positive, because polymicrobial infections that include *Bartonella* spp. and other bacteria can occur.[11] Special media used to isolate *Bartonella* spp. (*Bartonella* alpha-Proteobacteria growth medium [BAPGM]) may also yield other fastidious bacteria such as *Sphingomonas* spp., the clinical significance of which requires further study.[27] Serologic testing for *Brucella* antibody and *Aspergillus* antigen could also be considered for dogs with culture-negative IE (see Chapters 71 and 86, respectively).

Attempts should also be made to isolate causative organism(s) from other sites that are suspected to be a source of infection based on the history and clinical findings. Appropriate specimens could include transtracheal or bronchoalveolar lavage specimens, urine, ascites fluid, wounds, or pleural effusion. UTIs may reflect ascending pyelonephritis or spread of bacteria from the blood into the urine. However, bacteria cultured from the urine may not always reflect those present in the bloodstream,[11] so blood cultures should always be performed even when urine cultures are positive. Isolation of the same organism from the blood as well as an additional site facilitates interpretation of the significance of a single positive blood culture and aids decisions regarding appropriate antimicrobial drug treatment.

Molecular Diagnosis Using Nucleic Acid–Based Testing

PCR assays have been used to rapidly detect bacterial DNA within whole blood and especially valvular tissue (obtained at necropsy) of animals with IE, and are especially useful for detection of fastidious bacteria such as *Bartonella* spp. within the heart valves (see Chapter 70). These assays use broad-range primers that target bacterial 16S ribosomal subunit DNA, and the identity of the organism is determined by sequence analysis of resulting PCR products.

In one prospective study that examined the performance of a conventional broad-range bacterial PCR assay on whole blood for diagnosis of the etiology of IE in 18 dogs, there was no difference in the overall sensitivity of the PCR assay and culture, but the combined use of the PCR assay and blood culture was more sensitive than the use of either assay alone.[28] This was because the PCR assay detected several fastidious organisms, which included *Bartonella vinsonii*, *Brucella*, and *Granulicatella adiacens*, but appeared less sensitive than culture for detection of less fastidious organisms such as streptococci. Studies that include larger numbers of dogs and cats, and that examine the performance of other PCR assays such as real-time PCR assays are required before broad-range bacterial PCR can be recommended for routine diagnosis of bacteremia and IE in dogs and cats, but they show promise when used in conjunction with blood cultures. Of major concern is the possibility of false positives with highly sensitive PCR assays due to detection of contaminating bacteria. Even in human medicine, evidence is considered insufficient to recommend the routine use of whole blood or serum real-time PCR assays for the diagnosis of culture-negative IE.[24]

Pathologic Findings

There are no specific pathologic findings in sepsis or bacteremia, but underlying causes such as pneumonia, pyometra, or peritonitis may be apparent. Microabscesses may be present in multiple tissues of animals with bacteremia. Isolation of the same bacterial species from multiple different tissues is supportive of a diagnosis of bacteremia. Pathologic findings in IE include valvular vegetations; avulsion or perforation of valvular structures; and gross and histopathologic evidence of infarction, widespread thrombosis, and CHF (Fig. 122.5). The inflammatory process may be chronic, with lymphoplasmacytic and histiocytic cell infiltrates and fibrosis; or acute, suppurative, and fibrinous, with or without microscopically visible intralesional bacteria (see Fig. 50.7). *Bartonella* IE is characterized by chronic inflammation and may be associated with valvular mineralization (see Fig. 70.14), whereas IE due to other microorganisms may be acute or chronic, and is rarely associated with valvular mineralization.[11] Use of tissue Gram stains and silver stains can reveal the presence of organisms within valvular vegetations. Necrotizing vasculitis may also be present in organs such as the lungs, myocardium, kidney, spleen, liver, and/or brain. Erythrophagocytosis has been described in reticuloendothelial tissues of dogs with IE due to gram-positive cocci. Membranoproliferative, membranous, or necrosuppurative glomerulonephritis may also be identified.[5]

Gross examination of the heart of animals with myocarditis may reveal focal or multifocal areas of myocardial pallor and/or friability. Histopathologic characterization of myocarditis in dogs showed that the most frequent type of inflammation present in the myocardium was lymphoplasmacytic, although granulocytic and eosinophilic inflammation may also be present.[29] The pericardium of dogs and cats with pericarditis may be thickened and discolored, and pericardial effusion may be present. Histopathology reveals acute or chronic inflammatory infiltrates, depending on the underlying cause, sometimes with intralesional bacteria or fungi.

TREATMENT AND PROGNOSIS

The mainstay of treatment of bacteremia, IE, sepsis, and bacterial myocarditis or pericarditis is early antimicrobial drug treatment. The initial choice of antimicrobial drugs should be based on knowledge of the prevalent bacterial species and their antimicrobial drug susceptibilities for each hospital and/or geographic region, as well as the likely source of infection (which provides information about the likely bacterial species involved) (Tables 122.7 and 122.8). The presence or absence of IE and/or sepsis also affects treatment recommendations. The treatment of sepsis and septic shock is covered in detail in Chapter 123.

In addition to antimicrobial drug therapy, the underlying cause of infection or chronic bacteremia should be identified and removed if possible. All catheters or devices should be removed and replaced at new sites if they are still needed. An attempt should be made to locate foreign bodies such as grass awns with imaging techniques and surgically remove them. Surgery may be required to resolve GI compromise,

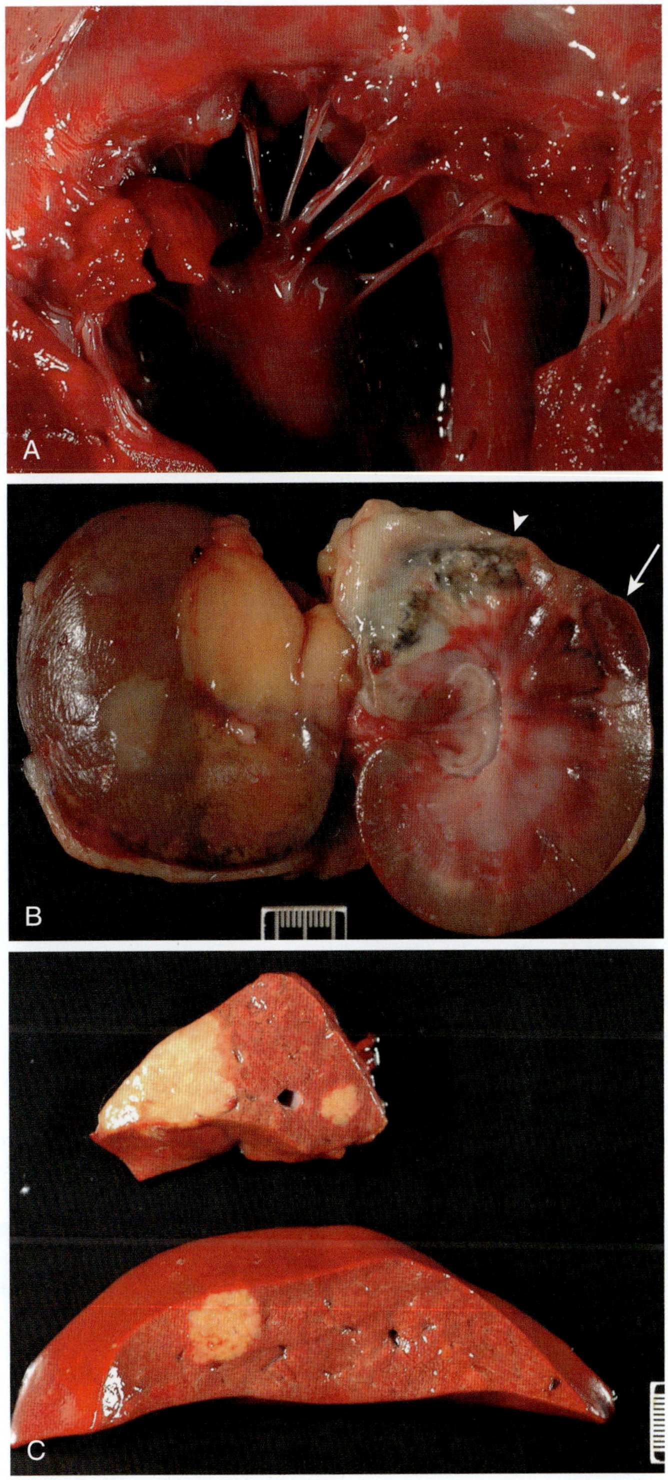

Fig.122.5 Gross pathology findings in a 12-year-old male neutered Irish water spaniel with *Enterococcus durans* infective endocarditis and widespread thromboembolic disease. (A) Mitral valve. The leaflets are thickened and nodular. (B) Left kidney. Multiple, variably sized, well-demarcated red foci with dark red rims and numerous well-demarcated tan slightly depressed foci are present. On cut surface, these foci extend to and beyond the corticomedullary junction as wedge-shaped lesions *(arrow)*. On one pole there is a 2.0 cm × 1.5 cm × 1.4 cm tan to brown-green abscess *(arrowhead)*. (C) Spleen. Several well-demarcated lesions that measured 0.3 to 0.5 cm in diameter are present. (Courtesy of the University of California, Davis, Veterinary Anatomic Pathology Service.)

TABLE 122.7 Suggested Empiric Antimicrobial Drug Choices for Intravenous Use in Dogs and Cats with Severe Sepsis or Septic Shock[a]

Antimicrobial Drug	Spectrum	Suspected Source of Infection	Comments
Ampicillin or clindamycin AND an aminoglycoside[b]	Activity against gram-negative bacteria, MRS, streptococci, enterococci, and most anaerobes.	Urinary tract, abdomen	Good first choice for most infections, except when the respiratory tract is involved. Consider use of ampicillin-sulbactam instead of ampicillin or addition of metronidazole if infection with penicillinase-producing anaerobes is possible (e.g., gastrointestinal compromise or plant foreign body, IE absent).
Ampicillin or clindamycin AND a fluoroquinolone	Active against most anaerobes, streptococci, susceptible staphylococci, and aerobic gram-negative rods. Not active against some MRS, enterococci, and MDR gram-negative bacteria.	Lung, urinary tract, abdomen, pyothorax	Consider when MDR gram-negative bacteria, enterococci or MRS are *unlikely* based on local resistance patterns and aminoglycosides are contraindicated due to toxicity or concerns related to drug penetration. Consider use of ampicillin-sulbactam instead of ampicillin or addition of metronidazole if infection with penicillinase-producing anaerobes is likely.
Meropenem	Active against aerobic gram-negative rods including *Pseudomonas*, anaerobes, streptococci. Not active against MRS and enterococci.	Abdomen, aspiration pneumonia	Use when infection with MDR gram-negative bacteria and anaerobes is likely but aminoglycosides are contraindicated due to toxicity or concerns related to drug penetration (e.g., airway involvement). Consultation with a respiratory or infectious disease veterinary specialist or veterinary pharmacologist recommended prior to use.
Vancomycin AND meropenem	MRS, streptococci, MDR aerobic gram-negative bacilli, anaerobes	Skin/soft tissue, urinary tract, abdomen	Last line for treatment of mixed infection with MDR gram-negative bacteria, MDR enterococci, anaerobes, and MRS when aminoglycosides are contraindicated due to toxicity or concerns related to inadequate drug penetration. Consultation with a respiratory or infectious disease veterinary specialist or veterinary pharmacologist recommended prior to use.

[a]Pending the results of blood culture and susceptibility testing, which should be followed by reduction in spectrum as appropriate.
[b]In human patients, amikacin is less nephrotoxic than gentamicin and may be preferable for treatment of dogs and cats with severe sepsis or septic shock.
Dosages for IV administration (normal renal function). See Chapter 10 for precautions.
Amikacin 15 mg/kg q24h (dogs)
Ampicillin sodium, 20mg/kg q6h
Ampicillin sulbactam, 20-50 mg/kg q6-8h
Clindamycin phosphate, 10 mg/kg q12h (dilute 1:10 in sterile saline and give slowly over 30 minutes)
Enrofloxacin, 15 mg/kg IV q24h (dogs)
Gentamicin sulfate, 14 mg/kg q24h (dogs), 8 mg/kg q24h (cats)
Meropenem, 12 mg/kg q8–12h
Vancomycin, 15 mg/kg q8h (dilute in sterile saline and give slowly over 30 minutes)
IE, infective endocarditis; *MDR,* multidrug resistant; *MRS,* methicillin-resistant staphylococci.

TABLE 122.8 Suggested Empiric Antimicrobial Drug Treatment for Intravenous Use in Dogs and Cats with Infective Endocarditis[b]

Antimicrobial Drug	Spectrum	Comments
Ampicillin AND gentamicin	Streptococci, *Bartonella*, MRS, enterococci, aerobic gram-negative rods	Covers all major causes of IE including most MDR gram-negative rods. Consider substitution of gentamicin with a fluoroquinolone if impairment of renal function is present.
Vancomycin AND meropenem	MRS, enterococci, gram-negative aerobes	Use only when infection with MRS is likely and aminoglycosides are contraindicated due to toxicity (e.g., refractory pyoderma, history of orthopedic surgery or antimicrobial treatment or hospitalization in the last year, contact with other animals or humans known to have MRS infections). Consultation with a respiratory or infectious disease veterinary specialist or veterinary pharmacologist recommended prior to use.

[a]Pending the results of blood culture and susceptibility testing, which should be followed by reduction in spectrum as appropriate.
IE, infective endocarditis; *MDR,* multidrug resistant; *MRS,* methicillin-resistant staphylococci.

such as occurs with foreign bodies, intestinal neoplasia, or torsion. Underlying immunosuppressive disease such as neoplasia or diabetes mellitus should be identified and treated if possible.

Infective Endocarditis

Guidelines for the treatment of IE in humans have been published and updated.[24,30] However, many factors considered for treatment of human patients do not apply to dogs and cats, and include the availability of valve replacement; penicillin allergy in some patients; the higher incidence of infections with MRS and VRE; evidence that supports use of specific antimicrobial drugs or drug combinations; and the possibility of long hospitalization times for parenteral antimicrobial drug therapy. In many human IE patients, valve replacement is also essential for resolution. Indications for cardiac surgery in humans include severe acute regurgitation or valve obstruction with refractory pulmonary edema; uncontrolled infection with enlarging vegetations; persistent fever and positive blood culture for at least 10 days after appropriate antimicrobial drug treatment is commenced, infection caused by fungi or MDR bacteria, and large vegetations (> 10 mm) in association with embolic episodes or other complications, and isolated large vegetations (> 15 mm).[24]

For dogs and cats, valve replacement is not a readily available option, so treatment must rely on antimicrobial drugs and resolution of any predisposing factors. Where the local prevalence of MDR gram-negative bacteria and MRS is low, a combination of ampicillin and an aminoglycoside is a good choice for empiric treatment of IE pending the results of culture and susceptibility. Where MDR gram-negative bacteria and MRS are locally prevalent, empiric recommendations made for human patients could be considered for dogs and cats pending the results of culture and susceptibility, provided there is a chance of treatment success in the absence of valve replacement. When severe sepsis is absent and IE follows an indolent course, it is recommended in human patients that antimicrobial treatment be withheld pending the results of culture and susceptibility, or a combination of penicillin with or without low-dose gentamicin (1 mg/kg, IV, q12h) be administered until results are available. Aminoglycosides are used at this low dose, twice daily for their synergistic activity with penicillin against enterococci and viridans streptococci, which are uncommon causes of IE in dogs. Empiric treatment protocols that have activity against drug-resistant bacteria are used in human patients pending results of culture and susceptibility when severe sepsis is present, such as vancomycin and low-dose gentamicin (no risk factors present for gram-negative bacterial infection), or vancomycin and meropenem (risk factors present for MDR Enterobacterales and *Pseudomonas* infection). However, the use of vancomycin and meropenem in dogs and cats has been controversial and may not be permitted or feasible in some geographic locations.

Recommendations for treatment of IE in dogs once the microbial etiology is known are shown in Table 122.9. Intravenous antimicrobial drugs should be continued in hospital for as long as possible (ideally at least 7 to 10 days). A switch to oral medications is not recommended for human IE patients because of poor activity when compared with IV medications.[24] However, oral antibiotic treatment has been used with success to treat some dogs with IE and may be the only viable option. At-home treatment with IV drugs through peripheral indwelling catheters may be possible for some dogs, but dog, owner, and drug factors should be considered very carefully and proper client education is critical. If oral antimicrobial drugs are used, bactericidal drugs with good oral bioavailability are preferable.

The role of antiplatelet therapy is controversial in human and veterinary patients with IE. The importance of thromboembolic disease in canine and feline IE is well documented; however, prospective studies identifying any risks or benefits of concomitant antiplatelet therapy are lacking. In the authors' hospital, the use of antiplatelet therapy such as clopidogrel is largely driven by clinician preference. Antiplatelet therapy is administered to animals considered at risk of or with clinical evidence of thromboembolic events such as those with spontaneous contrast on echocardiography, or ultrasonographic evidence of organ infarction. Given the high frequency of CHF and apparent thromboembolic events associated with IE in cats, antiplatelet therapy with clopidogrel may be warranted in this population.[7] The use of antiplatelet therapy should be carefully weighed against the risk of hemorrhage particularly in patients with concurrent thrombocytopenia or potential hypocoagulable states.

Medical treatment should be continued for at least 4 to 6 weeks, and until the underlying disease process has resolved, and valvular lesions have also resolved based on echocardiographic examinations. In the authors' experience, this treatment often extends well beyond 6 weeks before resolution of lesions is observed. Echocardiography should be

TABLE 122.9 Suggested Antimicrobial Drugs for Treatment of Major Causes of Infective Endocarditis in Dogs and Cats Once Cause Is Known

Cause	Preferred Treatment	Oral Equivalent
Methicillin-susceptible *Staphylococcus* spp.	Ampicillin IV Ampicillin-sulbactam IV (beta-lactamase producer)	Amoxicillin PO Flucloxacillin PO Clavulanic acid-amoxicillin PO
Methicillin-resistant but rifampin-susceptible *Staphylococcus* spp.	Gentamicin IV and rifampin PO OR vancomycin IV and rifampin (compromised renal function)	None
Streptococcus spp.	Benzylpenicillin IV Ampicillin IV	Amoxicillin PO
Penicillin-susceptible enterococci	Ampicillin IV	Amoxicillin PO
Penicillin-resistant enterococci	Vancomycin IV and gentamicin IV	None. Linezolid may be given orally but is bacteriostatic so may be ineffective.
Aerobic gram-negative rods	Ampicillin IV and gentamicin IV Ampicillin IV and fluoroquinolone IV Meropenem IV (or base on susceptibility)	Base on susceptibility
Bartonella spp.	Ampicillin IV and gentamicin IV Doxycycline IV and rifampin PO	Doxycycline PO and rifampin PO
Aspergillus spp.	Voriconazole or posaconazole	Voriconazole or posaconazole

repeated after 4 weeks, or earlier if there is evidence of complications (CHF, embolic disease) or inadequate treatment response. Successful resolution of IE is associated with reduction in size and consolidation of valvular vegetations. With unsuccessful treatment, lesions remain unchanged, and/or new lesions may appear on other valves.[5]

Infective Pericarditis

In addition to specific antimicrobial drug treatment, surgery may be required in dogs with infective pericarditis in order to debride the pericardium and minimize cardiac diastolic function. This carries a significant risk of mortality, and if feasible, referral to an experienced cardiac surgeon is recommended.

Prognosis

The prognosis for dogs and cats that develop IE, myocarditis, or pericarditis is guarded and depends on underlying disease processes, the severity of organ damage, and the etiologic agent or agents. In a study of dogs with IE, mortality rate due to IE was at least 40/71 (56%), and median survival time was only 54 days.[5] Factors strongly associated with negative outcome in dogs with IE were thrombocytopenia, increased serum creatinine concentration, renal complications, thromboembolic complications, and IE associated with *Bartonella* infection.

PREVENTION

Methods to prevent bloodstream infections and sepsis include limitation of the use of invasive devices and catheters unless absolutely necessary and attention to routine hygiene in the hospital to minimize nosocomial infections. Other measures include management of immunosuppressive disorders such as diabetes mellitus, minimizing use of immunosuppressive drugs such as glucocorticoids, and prompt attention to wounds or other underlying infections that have the potential to spread to the bloodstream.

The role of prophylactic antimicrobial drugs to prevent bacteremia and sepsis has been controversial. Beneficial outcomes have been reported when antimicrobials are used to prevent infection after chemotherapy. In one study, the use of a 14-day course of a trimethoprim-sulfonamide reduced morbidity and mortality in dogs with osteosarcoma or lymphoma during the first 14 days after treatment with doxorubicin.[31] In human patients a 7-day course of a fluoroquinolone during the expected neutropenic period after chemotherapy for solid tumors and lymphomas was shown to reduce the incidence of fever, probable infection, and hospitalization.[32] Prophylactic treatment with antimicrobial drugs could also be considered for animals with severe neutropenia (<500 cells/μL), although more studies are required that examine the prevalence of bacteremia in neutropenic animals and the benefits of prophylactic antimicrobial drug treatment. Finally, prophylactic antimicrobial drug treatment has been suggested for dogs and cats with congenital heart defects that undergo dental procedures, but evidence to support the need for this practice is lacking.

PUBLIC HEALTH ASPECTS

Dogs with bloodstream infections may harbor bacteria such as MRSA that have the potential to colonize humans, and so routine precautions should be taken when these dogs are handled, with special attention to hand hygiene and fomite disinfection. Dogs and cats with signs of cardiovascular infection may also be infected with important human pathogens such as *Salmonella* spp., *Bartonella* spp., *Brucella* spp., and *Rickettsia rickettsii*, so caution should be taken when handling blood from animals with cardiovascular infections and needle-stick injuries should be avoided.

CASE EXAMPLE

Signalment

"Rugby," a 12-year-old male neutered Labrador retriever from Napa, CA.

History

Rugby was seen at the University of California-Davis, VMTH emergency service for treatment of possible sepsis. One week before he was evaluated, he had been swimming in the lake in the owner's backyard and when exiting was shivering and reluctant to move. Since then, he has had a waxing and waning appetite. Over the last day, he had been unwilling to walk. He was taken to the local veterinary clinic that evening where his temperature was 104.6°F (40.3°C), he was laterally recumbent, moderately obtunded, had thoracolumbar pain, and had decreased patellar reflexes bilaterally. Blood work showed moderate leukocytosis, thrombocytopenia, hypoglycemia, hyperbilirubinemia, and a mildly elevated activity of serum ALP. Oscillometric blood pressure was normal, and hydromorphone was administered. Abdominal radiographs showed bridging spondylosis and multiple narrowed intervertebral disc spaces. Rugby was up to date on vaccinations, including for rabies.

Physical Examination

Body weight: 44 kg.

General: Obtunded, laterally recumbent, T = 104.4°F (40.2°C), HR = 120 beats/minute, RR = 20 breaths/minute, mucous membranes dark pink, CRT = 1 s.

Integument: Multiple generalized small freely moveable subcutaneous masses.

Musculoskeletal: Nonambulatory and unable to stand. BCS was 8/9.

Cardiovascular: A grade 3/6 systolic murmur with a musical quality was auscultated. Strong, symmetric femoral pulses were palpated bilaterally with frequent pulse deficits noted.

Respiratory: Increased bronchovesicular sounds were present in all fields.

Abdominal palpation: Moderate abdominal distention was noted. Palpation was difficult because of recumbency and the large size of the patient.

Neurologic evaluation: Mentation was severely obtunded with intact cranial nerves. Postural placing reactions were delayed to absent in all limbs, worse in the pelvic limbs. Segmental reflexes were intact bilaterally. Apparent pain on palpation of caudal thoracic vertebra. Neuroanatomic localization: Intracranial +/− T_3-L_3 myelopathy.

All other systems: No abnormalities detected.

Laboratory Findings

Venous blood gas: pH 7.386, pCO_2 25.6 mmHg, pO_2 35.4 mmHg, base deficit −9.0 mmol/L, bicarbonate 15.0 mmol/L, lactate 2.3 mmol/L, glucose 65 mg/dL.

CBC: HCT 43.7% (40%–55%), MCV 72.2 fL (65–75 fL), MCHC 33.4 g/dL (33–36 g/dL), WBC 40,500 cells/μL (6,000–13,000 cells/μL), neutrophils 34,020 cells/μL (3,000–10,500 cells/μL), band neutrophils 405 cells/μL, lymphocytes 1,215 cells/μL (1,000–4,000 cells/μL), monocytes 4,860 cells/μL (150–1,200 cells/μL), platelets clumped (150,000–400,000 platelets/μL).

Serum chemistry profile: Anion gap 29 mmol/L (12–20 mmol/L), sodium 152 mmol/L (143–151 mmol/L), potassium 4.2 mmol/L (3.6–4.8 mmol/L), chloride 112 mmol/L (108–116 mmol/L), bicarbonate 15 mmol/L (20–29 mmol/L), phosphorus 6.1 mg/dL (2.6–5.2 mg/dL), calcium 9.9 mg/dL (9.6–11.2 mg/dL), BUN 15 mg/dL (11–33 mg/dL), creatinine 116 mg/dL (0.8–1.5 mg/dL), glucose 60 mg/dL (86–118 mg/dL), total protein 6.4 g/dL (5.4–6.9 g/dL), albumin 3.3 g/dL (3.4–4.4 g/dL), globulin 3.1 g/dL (1.7–3.1 g/dL), ALT 63 U/L (21–72 U/L), AST 84 U/L (20–49 U/L), creatinine kinase 394 U/L (55–257 U/L), ALP 213 U/L

CASE EXAMPLE—cont'd

(14–91 U/L), cholesterol 384 mg/dL (139–353 mg/dL), total bilirubin 1.1 mg/dL (0–0.2 mg/dL), magnesium 2.1 mg/dL (1.9–2.5 mg/dL).

Urinalysis (free catch): SpG 1.022; pH 7.0, 150 mg/dL protein (SSA), 6 mg/dL bilirubin, 150 erythrocytes/μL hemoprotein, no glucose or ketones, 4–10 WBC/HPF, 3–5 RBC/HPF, no bacteria or casts seen.

Arterial blood gas (post–dextrose bolus) (FiO_2 21%): pH 7.401, pCO_2 20.8 mmHg, pO_2 78.1 mmHg, ionized calcium 1.30 mmol/L, bicarbonate 12.7 mmol/L, base deficit −11.2 mmol/L, lactate 1.9 mmol/L, glucose 157 mg/dL.

Electrocardiography

The ECG rhythm showed an underlying sinus rhythm with frequent uniform ventricular premature complexes and paroxysms of an accelerated idioventricular rhythm (120 beats/minute).

Imaging Findings

Thoracic radiographs: Diffuse bronchointerstitial pattern most pronounced caudodorsally. There was an additional wispy alveolar pattern associated with the right middle lung lobe compatible with aspiration pneumonia. The cardiovascular structures were within normal limits.

Abdominal ultrasound: The liver was diffusely hypoechoic and the spleen was mildly enlarged. The gallbladder wall was edematous. Bright mesentery surrounded the left limb of the pancreas. Throughout the small intestine, there was a segmental thickening of the submucosa layer with more subtle segmental thickening of the muscularis layer.

Echocardiography

The left and right ventricles and atria were normal in size. There was laminar flow through the pulmonary artery and aorta. There was no tricuspid, pulmonic, or aortic regurgitation. There was a pedunculated and independently oscillating vegetative lesion seen on the atrial surface of the anterior mitral valve leaflet with associated mild mitral valve regurgitation (Fig. 122.6).

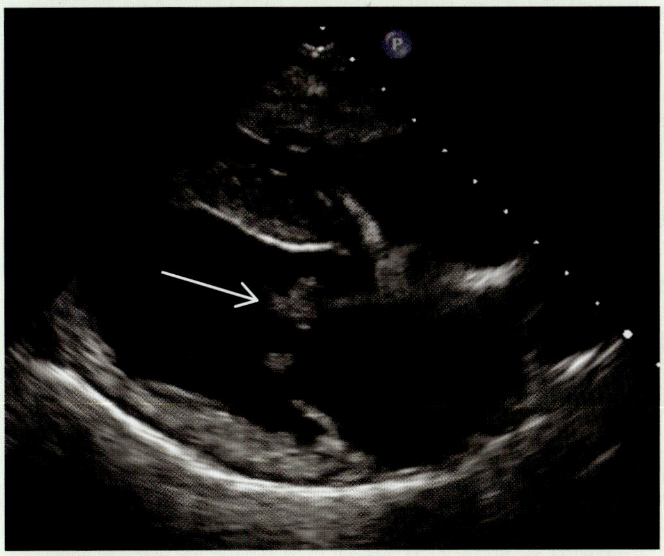

Fig. 122.6 Right parasternal view of the heart from a 12-year-old male neutered Labrador retriever with *Streptococcus dysgalactiae* endocarditis. There is a large vegetative lesion attached to the anterior leaflet of the mitral valve *(arrow)*.

Microbiologic Testing

Aerobic urine culture not performed due to concern for bleeding following cystocentesis in association with reported thrombocytopenia.

Aerobic and anaerobic blood culture (6 specimens): Large numbers of *Streptococcus dysgalactiae* from the 6 of 6 bottles. Susceptible to all antimicrobials tested.

Diagnosis

Streptococcus dysgalactiae IE with arterial thromboembolus formation.

Treatment and Outcome

Lactated Ringer's solution with 2.5% supplemental dextrose was started at a maintenance fluid rate to maintain normoglycemia and ampicillin/sulbactam constant rate infusion (CRI) was started (6 mg/kg/hour), enrofloxacin (15 mg/kg, IV, q24h), and hydromorphone (0.05 mg/kg, IV, q4h). Continuous ECG and arterial blood pressure monitoring, and urine output via urinary catheter were started. Mean arterial pressure was > 80 mmHg overnight and supplemental oxygen was provided via nasal cannulas to keep P_aO_2 > 80 mmHg. Over the next 3 days, the patient's mentation steadily improved and he was able to stand for short periods with support. However, he remained anorexic. On day 4, the arterial blood pressure tracing suddenly disappeared from continuous blood pressure monitoring; on abdominal ultrasound examination, a thrombus was detected in the caudal abdominal aorta that extended into the right external iliac artery. Multiple cortical renal infarcts were also present. A nasogastric tube was placed and a commercial liquid diet was fed starting at 25% RER to increase until full RER was reached 3 days later. Enoxaparin (0.8 mg/kg, SC, q6h) and clopidogrel (75 mg by nasogastric tube q24h) were started on day 4. On day 8, a recheck CBC showed a mild neutrophilia (23,800 cells/μL) and normalization of platelet count (304,000 platelets/μL). Biochemical analysis showed persistent hyperbilirubinemia (1.1 mg/dL) and hypoalbuminemia (1.6 g/dL). The ampicillin-sulbactam CRI was switched to intermittent dosing (50 mg/kg, IV, q8h). The dog was still not able to stand independently, but could with support. Over the following 6 days, his ambulatory status improved until he could walk with harness support. His appetite returned so he was consuming 1.25 RER voluntarily. On day 14, a focused recheck abdominal ultrasound showed diminishing clot size in the aorta and external iliac artery. He was discharged on day 15 with oral amoxicillin-clavulanate (17 mg/kg, PO, q12h) and enrofloxacin (11 mg/kg, PO, q12h) along with his anticoagulant medications until scheduled recheck in 2 weeks.

Comments

This dog had mitral valve IE with associated sepsis. Echocardiography was performed as the patient had a fever and a new-onset murmur. Broad-spectrum antibiotics were initiated based on the level of illness of the patient and multiple potential sources of infection (endocarditis and aspiration pneumonia). An antibiotic CRI of a beta-lactam was initiated in an attempt to provide 100% of time > MIC. It is likely that the arterial thrombus represented a thromboembolus based on the presence of a large oscillating valvular vegetation; portions of such lesions may break off and embolize in the periphery. The source of bacteremia and endocarditis was not apparent.

SUGGESTED READINGS

Langhorn R, Willesen JL. Cardiac troponins in dogs and cats. *J Vet Intern Med.* 2016;30:36–50.

Palerme JS, Jones AE, Ward JL, et al. Infective endocarditis in 13 cats. *J Vet Cardiol.* 2016;18:213–225.

Sykes JE, Kittleson MD, Pesavento PA, et al. Evaluation of the relationship between causative organisms and clinical characteristics of infective endocarditis in dogs: 71 cases (1992-2005). *J Am Vet Med Assoc.* 2006;228:1723–1734.

Sykes JE, Kittleson MD, Chomel BB, et al. Clinicopathologic findings and outcome in dogs with infective endocarditis: 71 cases (1992-2005). *J Am Vet Med Assoc.* 2006;228:1735–1747.

REFERENCES

1. Greiner M, Wolf G, Hartmann K. A retrospective study of the clinical presentation of 140 dogs and 39 cats with bacteraemia. *J Small Anim Pract.* 2008;49:378–383.
2. Dow SW, Curtis CR, Jones RL, et al. Bacterial culture of blood from critically ill dogs and cats: 100 cases (1985-1987). *J Am Vet Med Assoc.* 1989;195:113–117.
3. Lombard CW, Buergelt CD. Vegetative bacterial endocarditis in dogs; echocardiographic diagnosis and clinical signs. *J Small Anim Pract.* 1983;24:325–339.
4. MacDonald KA, Chomel BB, Kittleson MD, et al. A prospective study of canine infective endocarditis in northern California (1999-2001): emergence of *Bartonella* as a prevalent etiologic agent. *J Vet Intern Med.* 2004;18:56–64.
5. Sykes JE, Kittleson MD, Chomel BB, et al. Clinicopathologic findings and outcome in dogs with infective endocarditis: 71 cases (1992-2005). *J Am Vet Med Assoc.* 2006;228:1735–1747.
6. Taboada J, Palmer GH. Renal failure associated with bacterial endocarditis in the dog. *J Am Anim Hosp Assoc.* 1989;25.
7. Palerme JS, Jones AE, Ward JL, et al. Infective endocarditis in 13 cats. *J Vet Cardiol.* 2016;18:213–225.
8. Peddle GD, Drobatz KJ, Harvey CE, et al. Association of periodontal disease, oral procedures, and other clinical findings with bacterial endocarditis in dogs. *J Am Vet Med Assoc.* 2009;234:100–107.
9. Semedo-Lemsaddek T, Tavares M, Sao Braz B, et al. Enterococcal infective endocarditis following periodontal disease in dogs. *PLoS One.* 2016;11:e0146860.
10. PLoS ONE Editors. Retraction: Enterococcal infective endocarditis following periodontal disease in dogs. *PLoS One.* 2021;16:e0259200.
11. Sykes JE, Kittleson MD, Pesavento PA, et al. Evaluation of the relationship between causative organisms and clinical characteristics of infective endocarditis in dogs: 71 cases (1992-2005). *J Am Vet Med Assoc.* 2006;228:1723–1734.
12. Calvert CA. Valvular bacterial endocarditis in the dog. *J Am Vet Med Assoc.* 1982;180:1080–1084.
13. Sisson D, Thomas WP. Endocarditis of the aortic valve in the dog. *J Am Vet Med Assoc.* 1984;184:570–577.
14. Que YA, Haefliger JA, Piroth L, et al. Fibrinogen and fibronectin binding cooperate for valve infection and invasion in *Staphylococcus aureus* experimental endocarditis. *J Exp Med.* 2005;201:1627–1635.
15. Piroth L, Que YA, Widmer E, et al. The fibrinogen- and fibronectin-binding domains of *Staphylococcus aureus* fibronectin-binding protein A synergistically promote endothelial invasion and experimental endocarditis. *Infect Immun.* 2008;76:3824–3831.
16. Lakhdhir S, Viall A, Alloway E, et al. Clinical presentation, cardiovascular findings, etiology, and outcome of myocarditis in dogs: 64 cases with presumptive antemortem diagnosis (26 confirmed postmortem) and 137 cases with postmortem diagnosis only (2004-2017). *J Vet Cardiol.* 2020;30:44–56.
17. Costa A, Lahmers S, Barry SL, et al. Fungal pericarditis and endocarditis secondary to porcupine quill migration in a dog. *J Vet Cardiol.* 2014;16:283–290.
18. Sheehan NK, Kellihan HB, Yarnall B, et al. Septic pericarditis and pericardial abscess secondary to a migrating foreign body in a dog. *J Vet Cardiol.* 2019;23:122–128.
19. Davidson BJ, Paling AC, Lahmers SL, et al. Disease association and clinical assessment of feline pericardial effusion. *J Am Anim Hosp Assoc.* 2008;44:5–9.
20. Sebastian-Marcos P, Santarelli G, Gomez S, et al. Canine leishmaniasis associated with pericardial effusion in a 4-year-old dog. *J Vet Cardiol.* 2019;23:32–37.
21. Wiinberg B, Jensen AL, Johansson PI, et al. Thromboelastographic evaluation of hemostatic function in dogs with disseminated intravascular coagulation. *J Vet Intern Med.* 2008;22:357–365.
22. Langhorn R, Willesen JL. Cardiac troponins in dogs and cats. *J Vet Intern Med.* 2016;30:36–50.
23. Oyama MA, Singletary GE. The use of NT-proBNP assay in the management of canine patients with heart disease. *Vet Clin North Am Small Anim Pract.* 2010;40:545–558.
24. Gould FK, Denning DW, Elliott TS, et al. Guidelines for the diagnosis and antibiotic treatment of endocarditis in adults: a report of the Working Party of the British Society for Antimicrobial Chemotherapy. *J Antimicrob Chemother.* 2012;67:269–289.
25. Kilkenny E, Watson C, Dukes-McEwan J, et al. Evaluation of serum cardiac troponin-I concentrations for diagnosis of infective endocarditis in dogs. *J Vet Intern Med.* 2021;35:2094-2101.
26. Mermel LA, Allon M, Bouza E, et al. Clinical practice guidelines for the diagnosis and management of intravascular catheter-related infection: 2009 Update by the Infectious Diseases Society of America. *Clin Infect Dis.* 2009;49:1–45.
27. Davenport AC, Mascarelli PE, Maggi RG, et al. Phylogenetic diversity of bacteria isolated from sick dogs using the BAPGM enrichment culture platform. *J Vet Intern Med.* 2012;26:786–787 (abstr).
28. Meurs KM, Heaney AM, Atkins CE, et al. Comparison of polymerase chain reaction with bacterial 16S primers to blood culture to identify bacteremia in dogs with suspected bacterial endocarditis. *J Vet Intern Med.* 2011;25:959–962.
29. Janus I, Noszczyk-Nowak A, Nowak M, et al. Myocarditis in dogs: etiology, clinical and histopathological features (11 cases: 2007-2013). *Ir Vet J.* 2014;67:28.
30. Habib G, Hoen B, Tornos P, et al. Guidelines on the prevention, diagnosis, and treatment of infective endocarditis (new version 2009): the Task Force on the prevention, diagnosis, and treatment of infective endocarditis of the European Society of Cardiology (ESC). Endorsed by the European Society of Clinical Microbiology and Infectious Diseases (ESCMID) and the International Society of Chemotherapy (ISC) for Infection and Cancer. *Eur Heart J.* 2009;30:2369–2413.
31. Chretin JD, Rassnick KM, Shaw NA, et al. Prophylactic trimethoprim-sulfadiazine during chemotherapy in dogs with lymphoma and osteosarcoma: a double-blind, placebo-controlled study. *J Vet Intern Med.* 2007;21:141–148.
32. Cullen M, Steven N, Billingham L, et al. Antibacterial prophylaxis after chemotherapy for solid tumors and lymphomas. *N Engl J Med.* 2005;353:988–998.

123

Sepsis

Deborah Silverstein, Cynthia M. Otto

KEY POINTS

- Sepsis is the systemic inflammatory response to an infectious agent. The presence of organ function is now included in the human definitions.
- The pathophysiology of sepsis is complex and includes both a proinflammatory and anti-inflammatory response that, when exuberant, can lead to organ dysfunction and death of the host.
- Potential septic foci should be determined as soon as possible, and cultures of infected fluid or tissue obtained to help guide long-term therapy.
- Pending culture results, treatment should be aimed at the most likely etiologic agent(s) and tissue infected.
- Intensive monitoring and aggressive supportive care are of utmost importance to increase the chance for survival. The presence of multiple organ dysfunction syndrome increases the mortality rate.
- The prognosis for patients with sepsis relies on the severity and pathogenicity of the underlying infection, as well as the ability to provide appropriate and early treatment.

DEFINITIONS AND EPIDEMIOLOGY

Bacteremia is defined as live microorganisms in circulation. *Endotoxemia* refers to circulation of the LPS component of the gram-negative bacterial cell wall and may or may not be associated with the presence of live bacteria. *Sepsis* represents the clinical signs associated with a systemic inflammatory response to an infectious agent.[1] More recently, sepsis was redefined as a life-threatening organ dysfunction caused by a dysregulated host response to infection.[2] Bacteremia in dogs and cats is expected to occur in a variety of infections (e.g., peritonitis, mastitis, prostatitis, pneumonia, pulmonary abscess, pyothorax, pyometra, pyelonephritis, intra-abdominal abscess, biliary tract infections), as well as during dentistry, but is not always associated with a systemic inflammatory response.[3]

Subclinical bacteremia probably also occurs during rectal palpation, intestinal endoscopy and surgery, and when indwelling venous or arterial catheters have been placed. Normally, circulating bacteria are cleared by the mononuclear-phagocyte system; therefore, blood cultures are not always reliable in documenting bacteremia. Bacterial molecules, along with molecules from other infectious agents (e.g., fungi, virus), are referred to as "pathogen-associated molecular patterns" or PAMPs.[4] Macrophages and other cells of the innate immune system recognize these PAMPs through toll-like receptors (TLRs) and initiate a complex local inflammatory response and upregulate systemic host defenses, thus preparing the animal to combat potential spread of infection.[5]

Typical clinical signs associated with bacteremia include altered body temperature, tachycardia, tachypnea, and neutrophilia or neutropenia; these signs represent the systemic inflammatory response syndrome (SIRS) which, when initiated by an infectious agent and accompanied by organ dysfunction, is referred to as sepsis. Not all patients with bacteremia demonstrate clinical signs of sepsis.[3] Dysregulated inflammation and SIRS is characterized by a complex cytokine-mediated response and can also be initiated by endogenous danger signals (danger-associated molecular pathogens or DAMPs) from damaged cells as a result of trauma, pancreatitis, hypoxia, and other insults.[4] The host benefits if the inflammatory response remains localized and balanced by anti-inflammatory pathways; however, systemic inflammation or failure to resolve the inflammatory response can lead to high mortality.

The terminologies *SIRS* and *sepsis* were clarified in the 1990s in human medicine[1]; relevant terms and the various categories of severity are defined in Table 123.1. SIRS criteria, however, are very insensitive and nonspecific features of sepsis that were designed to identify patients eligible for clinical trials of antisepsis therapies (Tables 123.2 and 123.3). Subsequently, a human consensus conference[6] identified a more elaborate classification system (PIRO) that focuses on host factors (predisposition), infectious agent factors (infection), the host-organism interaction (response), and the consequences of systemic inflammation (organ failure) (Table 123.4). In 2016, updated definitions were introduced in an attempt to more accurately identify patients at high risk for morbidity and mortality from sepsis. These new definitions, Sepsis-3, are based on the presence of an abnormal mentation using the Glasgow coma scale, RR > 20 breaths/minute, and/or a Doppler blood pressure < 100 mmHg.[2,5] The terms SIRS and severe sepsis were eliminated. Sepsis or severe inflammatory diseases often lead to an inappropriate, dysregulated generalized systemic response that leads to a progression of severe sepsis, septic shock, and ultimately multiple organ dysfunction syndrome (MODS) (see Table 123.1).[7] This chapter will continue to refer to the terms SIRS and severe sepsis because they have been core to so many studies in the recent past that have contributed to our understanding of sepsis, and the PIRO system cannot be applied to animals. Much of our knowledge of sepsis has been derived from experimental animal models and human (and a few veterinary) clinical studies. Animal models of sepsis can be divided by the type of insult, the route of administration of the infectious agent or substance, and the endpoints of the study.[8] One of the most commonly used agents to study the physiologic response to systemic bacteria has relied on the use of endotoxin. Endotoxin (lipopolysacharride [LPS]) consists of a lipid A moiety (the toxic component) and polysaccharides (O antigens) (see Fig. 53.2). LPS is released from the outer membrane of gram-negative bacteria when they lyse and is normally confined within the gut and portal circulation. The source of endotoxin is usually a member of the Enterbacterales family (*Escherichia* spp., *Klebsiella* spp., *Enterobacter* spp., *Proteus* spp.), as well as *Pseudomonas* spp. Studies of endotoxemia are highly reproducible, but administration of endotoxin to animal models does not account for all of the factors involved in clinical conditions in which endotoxin is a component of the disease. The innate immune system has evolved to recognize and respond to LPS in tissues and fluids early in gram-negative infections.[9] A major function of the innate immune system is to recognize threats to host survival. These threats can be exogenous or pathogen-associated (PAMPs), or endogenous danger signals released from damaged or dying cells (DAMPs).[4] The pathway for recognition of endotoxin has been well defined and is the prototypical example of activation of the innate immune response. The innate immune system is also capable of recognizing gram-positive bacterial products, flagellin, bacterial or viral DNA, and fungal products via the TLR (Table 123.5).[10,11]

TABLE 123.1 Definitions of Systemic Inflammatory Response Syndrome and Sepsis[1,213]

Term	Definition
Bacteremia	Living bacterial organisms in circulating blood
Endotoxemia	Lipopolysaccharide of gram-negative bacterial cell wall circulating in blood
Systemic inflammatory response syndrome	Systemic signs of inflammation (two of the four criteria; this term has been removed from the Sepsis-3 definitions in human medicine)
Sepsis	Confirmed infection plus systemic signs of inflammation. In human medicine, this is now defined as life-threatening organ dysfunction[a] caused by a dysregulated host response to infection.
Severe sepsis	Sepsis plus sepsis-induced organ dysfunction or tissue hypoperfusion (this term has been removed in the Sepsis-3 definitions for humans)
Sepsis-induced hypotension	Systolic blood pressure (SBP) < 90 mmHg, mean arterial pressure < 70 mmHg, or a decrease in SBP of > 40 mmHg
Septic shock	Sepsis-induced hypotension despite adequate fluid resuscitation. In the Sepsis-3 definitions for humans, this is now defined as sepsis and vasopressor therapy needed to maintain mean arterial pressure ≥ 65 mmHg and lactate to ≥ 2 mmol/L despite adequate fluid resuscitation
Sepsis-induced hypoperfusion	Septic shock with an elevated lactate or oliguria

[a]As assessed by an acute change of ≥ 2 points in the sequential organ failure assessment score (components: PaO_2/FIO_2 ratio, Glasgow coma scale, mean arterial pressure, vasopressor use, serum creatinine or urine output, bilirubin, and platelet count).

The prevalence of naturally occurring sepsis in dogs and cats is unknown, even though the dog has been used for many years as a model of sepsis and endotoxemia for humans.[12] Risk factors for endotoxemia, with or without concurrent bacteremia, in dogs include canine parvovirus (CPV) enteritis, gastric dilation and volvulus, pyometra, mastitis, other gram-negative infections, and heat stroke. Endotoxemia can develop when hepatic clearance of LPS is reduced, as in hepatic insufficiency and portosystemic shunts. Obstructive biliary disease may be a risk factor because bile salts bind endotoxin in the gut. Endotoxin may also play an important role in the pathogenesis of severe acute pancreatitis in dogs.[13] In the dog, sepsis is most commonly associated with disruption of the normal mucosal barrier and movement of bacteria into the circulation or tissues. The most commonly reported causes of sepsis in dogs include peritonitis (from GI or urogenital origins) and pneumonia.[14–16] Dogs receiving chemotherapy are susceptible to developing sepsis.[17] Smaller dogs with lymphoma, after receiving doxorubicin, or vincristine are at highest risk.

Sepsis is recognized less commonly in cats. Even severely affected cats do not commonly display the classic hyperdynamic signs of sepsis (tachycardia, red mucous membranes, fever, bounding/hyperkinetic pulses), making diagnosis a challenge.[18,19] In an experimental study of low-dose endotoxin infusion, cats developed hypotension but not tachycardia.[20] Risk factors for severe sepsis in cats include pyothorax, septic peritonitis, bacteremia secondary to GI disease, pneumonia, endocarditis, pyelonephritis, osteomyelitis, pyometra, and bite wounds.[21] In cats with pyothorax, identified risk factors include indoor-outdoor environment and multicat households.[22] In cats with peritonitis, neoplasia[23] or trauma[24] are the most commonly recognized causes. Endotoxemia is likely a component of some of these

TABLE 123.2 Systemic Inflammatory Response Syndrome Criteria for Dogs, Cats, and Humans

Criteria	Cats	Dogs	Humans
Temperature	< 37.8°C, > 40.0°C	< 37.2°C, > 39.2°C	< 36.0°C, > 38.0°C
	(< 100°F, > 103.5° F)	(< 99°F, > 102.6°F)	(< 96.8°F, > 100.4°F)
Heart rate, beats/minute	< 140, > 225	> 140	> 90
Respiratory rate, breaths/minute	> 40	> 30	> 20
Leukocyte count, × 10^3/µL	< 5,000, > 19,500	< 6,000, > 19,000	< 4,000, > 12,000

TABLE 123.3 Various Proposed Canine Systemic Inflammatory Response Syndrome Criteria

Heart Rate (Beats/Min)	Respiratory Rate (Breaths/Min)	Temperature (°F)	Leukocyte Count (×10^3 Cells/µL)	Reference
160	20	100.0–103.5	4.0–12.0	209
120	20	100.4–104.0	5.0–18	210
120	20	100.6–102.6	6.0–16.0	211
160	40	100.0–103.5	4.0–12.0	106
140	30	100.0–102.5	6.0–19.0	212

infections. Sepsis is also recognized as a cause of neonatal death in puppies and kittens.

In a human study performed in a tertiary care hospital, 68% of individuals admitted to the wards or the ICU had signs of SIRS. Of those patients, 26% went on to develop sepsis, 18% developed sepsis with hypotension or hypoperfusion, and only 4% developed septic shock. Not all patients, even those who developed septic shock, had bacteremia. Pneumonia and UTIs were the most common sources of infection in patients with septic shock. Diseases associated with development of septic shock included cardiovascular disease, neoplasia, GI disease, diabetes mellitus, renal disease, respiratory disease, and pancreatitis.[25] Uncomplicated sepsis is not a negative prognostic finding if recognized early and managed appropriately; however, the prognosis worsens as an animal develops septic shock and MODS.

TABLE 123.4 PIRO System for Staging Sepsis[6]

	Present	Future
Predisposition	Concurrent illness Age, sex, species, breed	Genetic expression of inflammatory response
Insult/infection	Culture and susceptibility of infection site Disease that is controllable	Assay of microbial products (LPS, bacterial DNA)
Response	SIRS, other signs of sepsis, shock	Nonspecific markers of inflammatory response (PCT or IL-6), impaired host responsiveness (HLA-DR), or specific detection of target therapy (protein C, TNF, PAF)
Organ dysfunction	Number of organ systems with dysfunction or composite score (SOFA)	Dynamic measures of cellular response to insult—apoptosis, cytopathic hypoxia, cell stress

HLA-DR, human leukocyte antigen-DR; *IL,* interleukin; *LPS,* lipopolysaccharide; *PAF,* platelet activating factor; *PCT,* procalcitonin; *PIRO,* predisposition, infection, response, organ dysfunction; *SIRS,* systemic inflammatory response syndrome; *SOFA,* sequential organ failure assessment score; *TNF,* tumor necrosis factor.

CLINICAL FEATURES

Pathogenesis and Clinical Signs

Molecular Pathogenesis

The clinical signs of sepsis described earlier in this chapter occur as a result of expression of proinflammatory cytokines and activation of the coagulation cascade.[5] Endotoxin is released into the intestinal lumen or tissues when gram-negative bacteria lyse, as occurs with rapid bacterial replication or with bactericidal action of some antibacterials. Within the intestinal lumen, most endotoxin is bound by bile salts and contained by the mucosal barrier; the small amounts normally absorbed into the portal circulation are cleared by hepatic macrophages. Endotoxin absorbed through the lymphatic system is cleared in regional lymph nodes. Thus, endotoxin levels in the systemic circulation are usually extremely low to immeasurable. Clinical signs of endotoxemia occur only when binding and clearance mechanisms are overwhelmed. Bacteria can also translocate into the bloodstream as a result of disruption of the intestinal epithelial barrier. Bacteria and other pathogens can also gain access to the circulatory system from other mucosal surfaces, surgical or traumatic wounds, or invasive monitoring devices. The innate immune system is equipped with pattern recognition receptors that allow a response without prior exposure to the pathogen. These receptors are part of the TLR pathway.[5,10,11]

The first step in recognition of gram-negative bacteria is the binding of LPS to the acute-phase protein known as LPS-binding protein (the canine molecule has been described and cloned).[26]

TABLE 123.5 Microorganism Features That Are Recognized by Toll-like Receptors[214]

TLR	Host Ligand	Parasites	Fungi	Viruses	Bacteria	Small Molecules	Other
1, 2	HMGB1	GPI-linked proteins	Zymosan		Di- and triacyl lipopeptides Lipomannan, lipoteichoic acid	HSP 60, HSP 70, HSP 96	
3	mRNA			Double-stranded RNA			
4	HSP60, HSP 70, HSP 96, fibrinogen, fibronectin, hyaluronic acid, HMGB1, OxLDL*, beta amyloid* (*in association with TLR6)			F protein	LPS		
5					Flagellin		
2–6		GPI-linked proteins	Zymosan		Diacyl lipopeptides		
7 or 8	Single stranded RNA, microRNA, possibly mRNA			Single-stranded RNA		Imiquimod, resiquimod	
9	Self DNA			Herpesvirus DNA	CpG DNA sequences		Synthetic CpG oligoDNA
11					Uropathogenic bacteria		

CpG, regions of DNA where a cytosine (C) nucleotide occurs next to a (G) guanine nucleotide, where p represents the phosphodiester backbone, found abundantly in bacterial DNA; *GPI,* glycosylphosphatidylinositol; *HSP60,* heat shock protein 60; *LPS,* lipopolysaccharide; *mRNA,* messenger RNA; *TLR,* toll-like receptor.

This protein complexes with LPS and shuttles it to the macrophage, where the complex binds to the surface receptor, CD14, a glycosylphosphatidylinositol-anchored membrane protein that lacks a transmembrane domain. CD14 can be shed from cells, and soluble (free) CD14-endotoxin complexes can bind to endothelial cells and induce a cytokine response. Recognition of the TLR4 receptor provided the missing link between LPS binding to CD14 and the initiation of the signaling cascade.[27]

In response to the activation of the TLR4 receptor, transcription factor NF-κB (originally identified in B cells) is activated and leads to the expression of many cytokines.[28] This activation requires the recruitment and activation of a series of adapter proteins and signaling molecules. Myeloid differentiation primary response protein 88 (MyD88) is an adapter protein found on all of the TLR. TLR4 activation and MyD88 recruitment leads to the activation of the IL-1 receptor-associated kinase (IRAK) family members, and TNF receptor-associated factor-6 subsequent signaling pathways. Phosphorylated IRAK1 associates with TRAF6 and forms a complex with another signaling molecule, transforming growth factor β activated kinase (TAK1). NF-κB resides in the cytoplasm as a complex with inhibitory proteins of the inhibitors of NF-κB (I-κB) family. Eventually, TAK1 activation leads to phosphorylation of the I-κB kinase complex (IKK), releasing the transcription factor, NF-κB.[9] This also leads to activation of the NF-κB pathway.[9,10] Activation of NF-κB via phosphorylation of the inhibitory proteins (referred to as the canonical pathway of activation) can be triggered by cellular interactions with bacteria and bacterial products, viruses, parasites, and cytokines, involving activation of the TRL receptors 2, 3, 5, 6, and 9, or cytokine receptors.[28] The phosphorylation step involves three IKKs and results in proteosomal degradation of the inhibitory protein. Once released from the inhibitory I-κB, NF-κB is free to translocate to the nucleus and regulate expression of numerous genes involved in the inflammatory response. NF-κB can also be activated independent of the IKK complex by hypoxia, free radicals, and ultraviolet radiation.[28] Activation of NF-κB may be a biomarker of inflammation and serve as a therapeutic target for diseases of excessive inflammation. The wide range of genes regulated by NF-κB, however, may result in untoward systemic effects if the transcription factor is completely inhibited. Similar to endotoxin, products of gram-positive bacteria, fungi, and bacterial or viral DNA are capable of binding TLR receptors and activating the innate immune response. In SIRS, the innate immune system is activated by DAMPs such as the DNA-binding protein, high mobility group box 1 (HMGB1).[29] This highly conserved ubiquitous nuclear protein is released from cells dying from necrosis and, after acetylation or ADP ribosylation, can be actively secreted by macrophages, monocytes, and dendritic cells. HMGB1 activates TLRs 2, 4, and 9 and the receptor for advanced glycation end products. In addition, HMGB1 can enhance the response to other danger signals. Circulating HMGB1 levels persist longer than most other cytokines in acute inflammatory states, and HMGB1 may represent a therapeutic target to limit inflammation. HMGB1 induces the release of numerous cytokines from inflammatory cells, including TNF-α, IL-1 α and β, IL-1 receptor antagonist, IL-6, IL-8, and macrophage inflammatory protein-1 α and β.

The macrophage is the main cell of the innate immune system that initiates the response to PAMPs and DAMPs (Fig. 123.1). The early macrophage response to endotoxin is characterized by release of multifunctional proinflammatory cytokines, especially IL-1β and TNF-α. In dogs, TNF-α levels increase within 15 minutes of exposure to LPS, peak at 2 hours, and return to baseline levels in 4 hours. TNF-α mediates many immune and inflammatory functions, as well as further stimulating macrophages to secrete IL-1, IL-6, macrophage colony-stimulating factor, and granulocyte-macrophage colony-stimulating

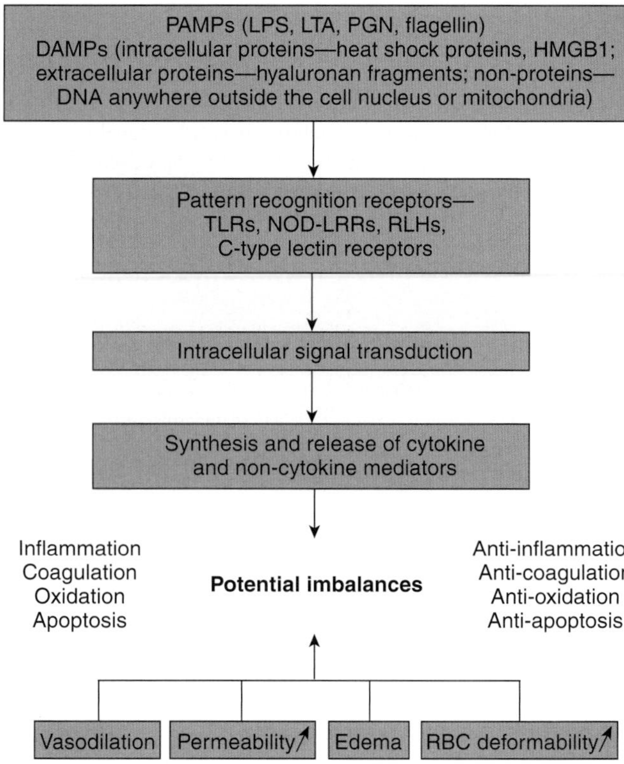

Fig. 123.1 Pathophysiology of severe septic shock. *DAMPs,* danger-associated molecular pathogens; *HMGB1,* high mobility group box 1; *LPS,* lipopolysaccharide; *LTA,* lipoteichoic acid; *NOD-LRRs,* nucleotide-binding oligomerization leucine-rich repeats; *PAMPS,* pathogen-associated molecular patterns; *PGN,* peptidoglycan; *RBC,* red blood cell; *RLHs,* retinoic acid inducible gene-like helicase; *TLRs,* toll-like receptors. (Adapted from Cinel I, Opal SM. Molecular biology of inflammation and sepsis: a primer. *Crit Care Med.* 2009;37:293–304, with permission.)

factor. IL-1 is released in similar burst fashion; it is a major co-stimulator of Th2 cells, stimulates the acute-phase response, induces fever, and has a multitude of other proinflammatory effects. Other cytokines, such as IL-6, IL-8, and IFN-α, are additional early mediators in sepsis.[30] Proinflammatory cytokines are released early and transiently in response to endotoxin, before the animal shows clinical signs. Novel therapeutics directed toward these mediators have not demonstrated significant benefit in most human clinical trials.[31] However, late mediators, such as HMGB1, may be more appropriate therapeutic targets.[21] The cytokine cascades increase the levels or activity (or both) of inflammatory phospholipid-derived mediators (prostacyclin, thromboxane, and platelet-activating factor),[32] coagulation factors, complement, reactive oxygen species, and nitric oxide (NO; which is an important molecule associated with hypotension),[33–36] endothelin-1 (a vasoconstrictor),[37] β-endorphin, histamine, serotonin, vasopressin, angiotensin II, and catecholamines. The biologic effects of these mediators include neutrophil activation, aggregation, and chemotaxis; platelet activation and aggregation; a procoagulable state; increased activity of plasma proteases; and vasodilation and potentially systemic hypotension, generalized endothelial inflammation, increased vascular permeability, and GI ulceration.[38,39] Lysosomal enzymes such as elastase and chymotrypsin deplete fibronectin and activate blood clotting, triggering DIC.

There are multiple effects of sepsis on the coagulation cascade (Fig. 123.2).[40] Sepsis promotes coagulation, inhibits anticoagulation, and impairs fibrinolysis. Early in sepsis, patients exhibit a procoagulant state which is followed by DIC.[41,42] Inflammation

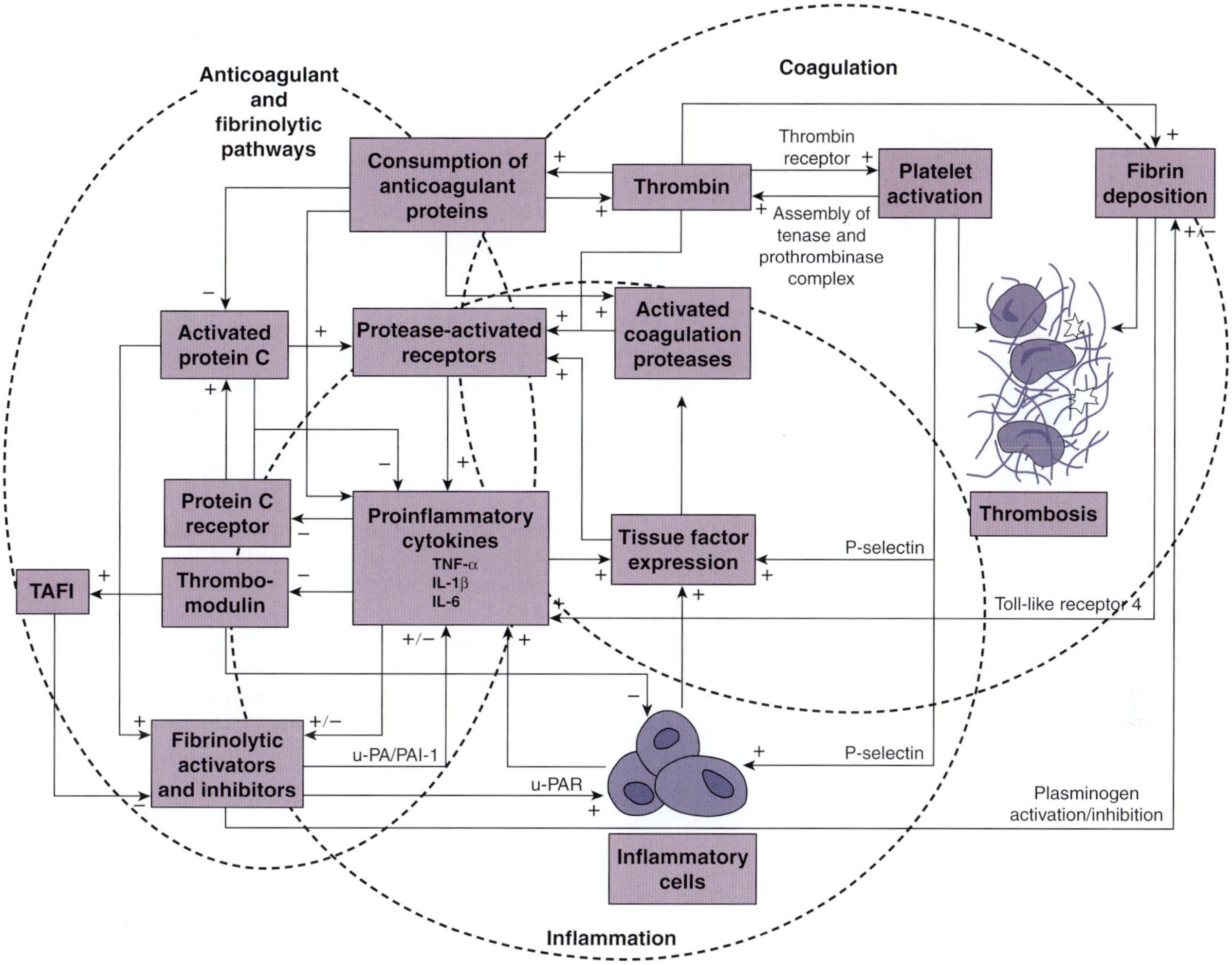

Fig. 123.2 Overview of the interrelationships between the pathways of coagulation, anticoagulation, fibrinolysis, and inflammation. +, stimulatory; –, inhibitory; *IL*, interleukin; *PAI-1*, plasminogen activator inhibitor-1; *TAFI*, thrombin activatable fibrinolysis inhibitor; *TNF*, tumor necrosis factor; *u-PA*, urinary plasminogen activator; *u-PAR*, urokinase-type plasminogen activator receptor. (From Levi M, van der Poll T. The central role of the endothelium in the crosstalk between coagulation and inflammation in sepsis. *Adv Sepsis*. 2004;3:93–101, with permission.)

leads to the exposure and induction of tissue factor, a potent procoagulant that complexes with factor VII(a) to activate factor IX and factor X and eventually lead to fibrin formation. Platelets are also activated by endotoxin, proinflammatory cytokines, and thrombin. Endothelial cell damage associated with sepsis results in the release of von Willebrand's factor and further platelet aggregation. Activation of platelets leads to release of proinflammatory mediators and consumption of platelets. Clinically, septic patients frequently have low platelet counts. The three main anticoagulant protein systems, antithrombin (AT), tissue factor pathway inhibitor (TFPI), and protein C (PC), are all deranged during sepsis. Endothelial cells are actively involved in the production/activation of TFPI and PC. TFPI is secreted by and then bound to endothelial cells and inhibits the activation of factor X by tissue factor–factor VII(a) complexes. Sepsis impairs the binding of TFPI to endothelial cells and appears to decrease its effectiveness. The other anticoagulant protein that relies on normal endothelial function is PC. Healthy endothelial cells express the surface protein thrombomodulin, which binds circulating thrombin (see Figs. 123.2 and 123.3). When thrombin is bound to thrombomodulin, it is not available for cleavage by fibrinogen, and the complex acts to cleave PC into active PC (aPC). Endothelial cells exposed to cytokines have a reduction in thrombomodulin expression; thus, less PC can be activated. In addition, aPC is consumed in the inactivation of factor Va and factor VIIIa. Septic patients and dogs have reduced PC, which may be related to survival.[43] The only clinical trial in sepsis that has shown any outcome benefit was a trial of aPC in patients with severe sepsis.[44] Unfortunately, the benefits of aPC do not seem to be generalizable to wider populations,[45] and has subsequently been withdrawn from the sepsis market. In addition, the expense and species specificity of the recombinant aPC have precluded clinical trials in dogs. A major advance that resulted from investigations of aPC was recognition of the interaction between coagulation and inflammation. aPC inhibits neutrophil-endothelial interactions, limits proinflammatory cytokine production, blocks chemotaxis of neutrophils, and protects endothelial barrier function.[45]

AT is another anticoagulant protein reported to have anti-inflammatory functions (i.e., increase prostacyclin and decrease neutrophil-endothelial cell interactions). AT is reduced in sepsis through multiple mechanisms.[40] Although AT therapy looked promising in experimental models of sepsis, no benefit of AT supplementation has been demonstrated in human clinical trials.[46]

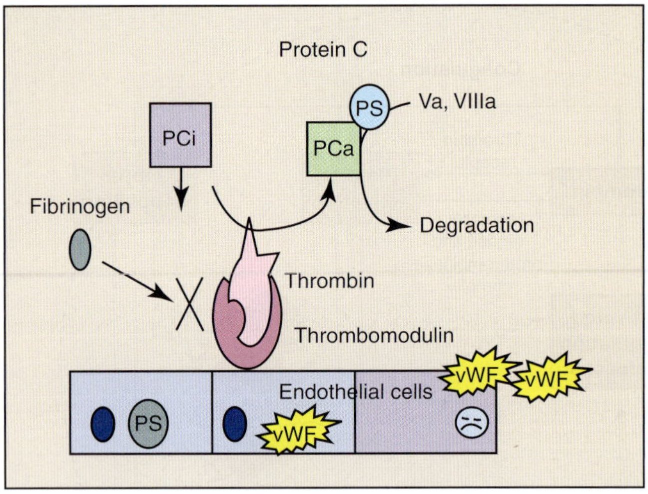

Fig. 123.3 Interaction of protein C with coagulation. The normal endothelium expresses thrombomodulin, which binds thrombin, removing it from the coagulation cascade and altering its substrate from fibrinogen to protein C *(PCi)*. Activation of protein C *(PCa)* allows it to associate with protein S *(PS)* and leads to the degradation of activated factors V and VIII. Endothelial cell injury leads to release of von Willebrand's factor *(vWF)* and decreased expression of thrombomodulin.

In addition to increased activation of procoagulants and decreased anticoagulants, fibrinolysis is also impaired during sepsis. Initially, plasmin (the main fibrinolytic protein) activation is accelerated by increased release of plasminogen activators (tissue plasminogen activator and urokinase-type plasminogen activator) from the endothelial cells. This effect is short-lived as cytokines induce the production and release of plasminogen activator inhibitor.[40] Thrombin-activatable fibrinolysis inhibitor antigen was increased in dogs with sepsis and not in other evaluated diseases.[47] Fibrin deposition results from impairment of all components of the coagulation cascade and can contribute to tissue hypoxia and development of multiple organ dysfunction.

The innate immune system includes the complement system.[48] Complement functions in neutrophil chemotaxis, drawing neutrophils to the sites of infection and inflammation, enhancing clearance of bacteria through opsonization, and causing lysis of cells (both bacterial and host). Complement is also involved in the integration between the innate and adaptive immune system and facilitates removal of apoptotic cells and immune complexes. Complement can be activated by one of three pathways, all of which converge with the activation of C3. Cleavage of C3 leads to production of the anaphylatoxin C3a and the eventual cleavage and activation of C5. C5 cleavage produces the chemotactic protein and anaphylatoxin C5a and C5b, a major component of the membrane attack complex responsible for lysing cells. The classic pathway is activated by immune complexes on cells, apoptotic cells, and some bacteria and viruses. The mannose-binding lectin pathway provides an antibody-independent mechanism to activate the complement cascade by binding bacterial mannose residues. Independent of antibody binding, endotoxin and other surface molecules on bacteria activate the alternate pathway.[48,49] In sepsis, high levels of C3a and C5a are associated with a worse prognosis. In addition to its role as a chemotactic protein, C5a activates endothelial cells, causes vasodilation, and increases vascular permeability. Like many inflammatory mediators, the effects of C5a appear to be complex. C5 can be proinflammatory or protective or even lead to immune paralysis. The response, at least in part, appears to depend on the amount of C5a, the receptor it binds, and the presence of proinflammatory or anti-inflammatory cytokines.[50] Strategies to limit C5 activation continue to be investigated.

If the systemic inflammatory state progresses, structural and metabolic changes develop in vascular endothelial cells. Endothelial adhesion molecules are upregulated, and neutrophils and platelets are sequestered in various organs. The endothelium also becomes more permeable, and plasma proteins move from the intravascular space to the interstitium, resulting in edema. In addition to the vasodilation mentioned earlier, the vascular endothelium may become unresponsive to commonly used vasopressor therapy, a condition termed *catecholamine-refractory vasodilatory shock.*

Despite normalization of macrohemodynamic indices (blood pressure, perfusion, and global tissue oxygenation), multiorgan dysfunction and failure may still develop in septic patients. Advances in the ability to study the microcirculation have found alterations in blood flow through the arterioles, capillaries, and venules. These changes have significant prognostic implications in people with severe sepsis.[51] Even though the percentage of perfused small vessels and vascular density are similar at the onset of shock in both survivors and nonsurvivors, small vessel perfusion improves with time only in survivors.[52,53] However, both survivors and nonsurvivors have similar measures of global perfusion and cardiovascular parameters after initial stabilization, demonstrating that microcirculation, not macrocirculation, is important for determining prognosis and survival. This may provide a valuable monitoring tool in veterinary patients to help guide diagnostic and therapeutic decisions and monitoring.[9]

Concurrent with inflammatory mediator upregulation, anti-inflammatory mediators are secreted to balance and limit the inflammatory response. An insufficient or inappropriate anti-inflammatory response can allow sepsis to progress.[38]

The prevailing theory has been that sepsis is a result of a *cytokine storm*, leading to uncontrolled systemic inflammation. Newer studies indicate that, for at least some patients, the hyperinflammatory state is followed by severe acute immunosuppression, caused by the apoptosis of B cells, CD4+ T cells, and follicular dendritic cells. The mechanism of immunosuppression is not known; however, release of endogenous glucocorticoids may be an important contributor.[54] Thyroid hormone production and secretion have been impaired in endotoxin-treated dogs.[55]

In summary, PAMPs act as a signal to the immune system that pathogens have invaded the host, whereas DAMPs are signals of damage to host cells (see Fig. 123.1). A localized response along with a primed or controlled systemic response is beneficial in containing and resolving the infection, whereas an uncontrolled host response leads to systemic inflammation, immunosuppression, severe sepsis, septic shock, and ultimately organ failure.

Organ Dysfunction in Sepsis

Abnormalities of the coagulation and fibrinolytic pathways play a major role in the development of organ dysfunction in septic patients. Mechanisms for derangements of the coagulation system include: (1) activation of the coagulation cascade; (2) defective physiologic anticoagulant pathways; and (3) impaired fibrinolysis. Clinically, activation of procoagulant pathways can lead to an early hypercoagulable or prothrombotic state that is difficult to diagnose but can contribute to organ dysfunction through inflammatory mediators and development of microthrombi. As sepsis progresses, coagulation disorders reflect a consumptive coagulopathy, impairment of anticoagulant mechanisms, and inhibition of fibrinolysis that is recognized clinically as DIC.[44,56–59]

Cardiovascular system. Disruption of normal cardiovascular function is common in patients with sepsis. Circulating cytokines have been implicated in leading to these derangements via three primary mechanisms: increased vascular endothelial permeability, which allows leakage of intravascular fluid into the extravascular space, leading to hypovolemia and tissue edema; impaired cardiac contractility and subsequent decrease in cardiac output; and heterogenous loss of vasomotor tone, causing maldistribution of blood flow. Although a single "myocardial depressant factor" was previously implicated as the cause of impaired cardiac performance in septic animals and humans, several circulating cytokines have been found to play a role (e.g., TNF-α, IL-1β, IL-2, and IL-6).[60,61] Additional factors might include alterations in intracellular calcium trafficking with a reduction in systolic intracellular calcium concentration and decreased myocyte contraction; downregulation of beta receptors in the heart; and myocardial "hibernation" to preserve cardiac myocytes via decrease in oxygen consumption, energy requirements, and ATP demands.[50,62]

Respiratory system. Acute respiratory distress syndrome (ARDS), a severe form of acute lung injury (ALI), is the manifestation of lung injury that may occur in human and veterinary patients with sepsis and SIRS.[63–66] ARDS and ALI are labels that describe the syndrome of SIRS- or sepsis-associated lung injury, rather than disease entities themselves. Impaired gas exchange in patients with ALI and ARDS is multifactorial and involves endothelial and epithelial injury; neutrophil-dependent lung injury; proinflammatory cytokines; abnormalities of the coagulation system; and abnormalities in the production, composition, and function of surfactant. Ultimately there is an accumulation of protein-rich fluid in the alveoli and infiltration of the alveolar interstitial space with inflammatory cells, fluid, and debris. This is typically recognized as alveolar infiltrates on thoracic radiographs. The lungs are the shock organ in cats and are especially vulnerable to injury during sepsis in this species; tachypnea was a common finding in cats with severe sepsis and, although only 11 of 29 cats in one study had an underlying respiratory cause of sepsis (pneumonia or pyothorax), 17 of 29 had clinical or radiographic signs of respiratory disease.[18] Septic cats are commonly fluid intolerant and quite susceptible to fluid overload. Veterinary definitions for the development of ARDS and ALI have been published (Box 123.1).[67]

Urinary system. Acute kidney injury (AKI) is a common sequela to sepsis in humans. A retrospective study proposed a scoring system for AKI in dogs (Box 123.2). Although there are no veterinary clinical studies that have investigated the incidence of AKI in patients with sepsis, retrospective sepsis studies and clinical impression suggest that sepsis-induced AKI is infrequent in dogs and cats, except in dogs with severe babesiosis.[18,23,68,69] Dogs with bacterial endocarditis may be another exception.[70] Sepsis-associated AKI has been historically attributed to acute tubular necrosis secondary to renal ischemia (e.g., due to afferent arteriolar vasoconstriction and/or poor cardiac output).[37,70–72] However, sepsis-associated AKI may be more complicated than a simple reduction in renal blood flow.[29,71–73] Tissue injury may be due to ischemia-reperfusion injury and/or activation of macrophages and neutrophils; alterations in NO metabolism; cytopathic hypoxia; and renal apoptosis. Reactive oxygen species may contribute to vasoconstriction directly or through depletion of endogenous vasodilators such as prostacyclin and NO. Apoptotic pathways may be activated in reaction to potentially lethal insults (e.g., TNF, ischemia, bacterial toxins).[71,72] Based on the human literature and retrospective veterinary studies, there has been debate as to the role of hydroxyethyl starch in contributing to AKI in veterinary patients.[74,75]

BOX 123.1 Veterinary Definitions for Acute Respiratory Distress Syndrome and Acute Lung Injury

ARDS: Acute respiratory distress syndrome. Acute fulminant respiratory failure leading to diffuse lung injury resulting from a variety of causes.

ALI: Acute lung injury, similar to ARDS but with less severe defects in gas exchange (classically defined as a PaO_2/FiO_2 ratio < 300 mmHg versus ARDS < 200 mmHg)

Diagnostic Criteria for Veterinary ARDS

1. Acute onset (<72 hours) of tachypnea and labored breathing at rest
2. Presence of known risk factors
3. Evidence of pulmonary capillary leak without increased pulmonary capillary pressure
4. Evidence of inefficient gas exchange
5. Evidence of diffuse pulmonary inflammation

BOX 123.2 Scoring System for Acute Kidney Injury in Dogs[216]

Stage 0	Creatinine increase < 150% from baseline
Stage 1	Creatinine increase of 150%–199% from baseline
	OR
	Creatinine increase of 26.5 µmol/L (0.3 mg/dL) from baseline
Stage 2	Creatinine increase of 200%–299% from baseline
Stage 3	Creatinine increase of ≥ 300% from baseline
	OR
	An absolute creatinine value > 354 µmol/L (4.0 mg/dL)

Neurologic dysfunction. Sepsis-associated neurologic dysfunction is poorly characterized or understood. CNS signs such as decreased alertness, stupor, coma, or seizures are common in people with septic shock. Anatomic, histopathologic, and reversible neurologic changes may be responsible for these derangements, including a direct effect from toxins of infectious organisms, a reduction in cerebral blood flow, capillary leakage, and dysfunction of the blood-brain barrier.[76,77] The incidence and pathogenesis of neurologic dysfunction in dogs and cats with sepsis remains to be determined.

Gastrointestinal and hepatic systems. GI dysfunction in septic patients often manifests as ileus, poor tolerance to enteral feedings, vomiting, diarrhea, GI ulceration, melena, and hematochezia. Subsequent disturbances often include malnutrition, fluid and electrolyte losses, and small intestinal bacterial overgrowth. An increase in GI mucosal permeability frequently occurs and may predispose the patient to bacterial translocation into the lymphatics and/or the bloodstream. Human patients in the ICU were found to have altered microbiota that were associated with inflammation, contained a loss of diversity, and were more pathogenic than healthy individuals.[78] Because of the prominent role of the liver in host defense, the derangements in liver function can contribute to both the initiation and progression of sepsis. The reticuloendothelial system of the liver acts as a first line of defense in clearing bacteria and their products; therefore, liver dysfunction leads to a spillover of these products into the systemic circulation. Possible mechanisms of increased GI epithelial permeability and hepatic dysfunction include dysregulation of blood flow, alterations in energy metabolism and mitochondrial function, oxidant stress, or direct effects of cytokines promoting apoptosis.[79–82] The liver is commonly referred to as the "shock organ" in dogs, and hepatic dysfunction can result in hypoalbuminemia, coagulopathies, hypoglycemia, icterus, mental depression, and encephalopathy. Decreased albumin levels may also result from loss into the extravascular space, a shift toward production of acute-phase proteins, and, secondary to LPS-induced downregulation of NF-κB.

Microcirculatory system. In addition to alterations in smooth muscle tone and microcirculatory perfusion, vascular endothelial cells are also commonly involved in the septic process.[83–85] This negatively influences their normal roles in antithrombosis, profibrinolysis, and inhibition of platelet and leukocyte aggregation, often resulting in DIC and further negative effects on microcirculatory perfusion. In addition, sepsis-induced alterations in vascular endothelial function and perfused capillary density may result in capillary leak syndromes and heterogenous blood flow within organs. Tissue ischemia may result from decreases in both diffusive (i.e., tissue edema) and convective (i.e., decreased perfused capillary density) oxygen delivery, possibly due to changes in the endothelial glycocalyx.[86–90] In this sense, endothelial dysfunction can be implicated as the "motor of MODS." Technology such as sidestream dark field imaging has been studied in dogs and cats and enables visualization and assessment of microcirculatory derangements during sepsis and in response to therapy.[51–53,91,92] The use of endothelial biomarkers such as endocan, syndecan-1, angiopoietin-2, and soluble vascular endothelial cadherin (sVE-cadherin) to predict the severity of sepsis and outcome is currently under investigation in human medicine.[93,94] Proteomic panels have also been used to identify differential inflammatory biomarker expression that could help to predict outcome in patients with sepsis.[95]

DIAGNOSIS

The clinical features of sepsis result from the systemic inflammatory response to microbial products. The diagnosis of sepsis is often presumptive in clinical practice, based on the accumulation of clinicopathologic and biochemical data. Although a "sepsis test" does not exist, it is possible to use the patient's clinical picture combined with a high level of suspicion to quite accurately diagnose a septic patient. However, it has been reported that 82% and 60% of bacteremic dogs and cats, respectively, were found to suffer from clinical sepsis in one retrospective study.[3] It is important to maintain a high index of suspicion for sepsis since recent studies found that 6.2% of cats and 4.2% of dogs admitted to a hospital were septic and 1.5% of cats and 1.6% of dogs developed sepsis while hospitalized.[96,97]

The diagnosis of sepsis must always begin with suspicion based on the patient's clinical signs and history. Additional diagnostics that may be indicated include imaging of the thorax and abdomen, spinal radiographs, echocardiography, diagnostic peritoneal lavage, tracheal or bronchoalveolar lavage, arthrocentesis, and CSF collection. The use of serum biomarkers is an area of intense investigation and may prove quite useful in differentiating septic and nonseptic SIRS in dogs and cats.[98,99]

Laboratory Abnormalities

Complete Blood Count

The most common hematologic abnormalities in people with sepsis include anemia, leukocytosis, thrombocytopenia, and activation of the hemostatic system.[100] Similar changes have been reported in dogs and cats.[15,18,23,101,102] A leukocytosis with bandemia and cytologic evidence of toxic neutrophils indicate ongoing and premature release of leukocytes from the bone marrow and continued inflammation.[101] Increased vascular endothelial permeability due to vasculitis, platelet sequestration in the lymphoreticular system, and DIC can all contribute to thrombocytopenia. Blood loss (e.g., GI loss secondary to poor perfusion and ulcerations), hemolysis, and/or decreased erythrocyte production may all lead to anemia (more common in septic cats than dogs). Potential causes of anemia in septic animals include premature clearance by the reticuloendothelial system with a low-grade hemolysis and increased susceptibility to oxidative damage leading to a Heinz body anemia, especially in cats.[102–105]

Serum Chemistry Profile

Biochemical profile changes in animals with sepsis are typically reflective of the underlying disease process (e.g., azotemia with pyelonephritis), but may also be due to sepsis-induced changes (e.g., cholestasis). Patients with severe sepsis and septic shock often develop derangements indicative of organ dysfunction or failure (e.g., hepatic failure, DIC). Some of the more common, nonspecific abnormalities include hyperglycemia, hypoglycemia, hypoalbuminemia, and hyperbilirubinemia.[15,18,56,106,107]

Clotting Function

DIC is common in humans and animals with sepsis.[15,42,47,108,109] Hemostatic derangements are typically characterized by hypercoagulability initially, then hypocoagulability as the disease progresses. It is often challenging to diagnose hypercoagulability clinically; therefore, this stage is often overlooked. Some potential clues might include a progressively decreasing platelet count and fibrinogen levels, low AT activity, elevated D-dimers and fibrin/fibrinogen degradation products (FDPs), the presence of schistocytes on blood smear evaluation, evidence of hypercoagulability using viscoelastic indices, or clinical evidence of abnormal clotting (e.g., catheters, anticoagulated blood samples, vascular thromboses to major organs). The later hypocoagulable state is more frequently recognized clinically and typifies the progression of a septic patient into DIC.[15,42] A statistically significant lower PC and AT activity and higher PT, PTT, D-dimer, and FDPs compared with controls have been described.[15] Dogs with naturally occurring CPV enteritis had decreased AT activity and increased maximum amplitude on the thromboelastogram, consistent with hypercoagulability.[42] Hematologic and hemostatic changes in septic animals are summarized in Table 123.6.

Biomarkers

Early detection of sepsis is desirable because mortality increases with the development of organ dysfunction, hypotension, and hyperlactatemia. Early clinical signs such as tachypnea, tachycardia, fever, and leukocytosis are nonspecific, so research investigating the use of biomarkers is ongoing. Ideal biomarkers of sepsis would be able to not only detect the presence of infection but also temporally track severity of infection and progression from sepsis to septic shock. Their ability to allow monitoring response to treatment and provide prognostic information is also desirable. Potential categories of early diagnostic biomarkers might include markers of infection (e.g., LPS, bacterial DNA), markers of cellular responsiveness (intercellular cellular adhesion molecule 1, CD11/CD18),[110] and products of inflammatory cells and humoral activation (ILs, AT, aPC).[15] Procalcitonin and neutrophil CD64 appear to be potentially useful biomarkers for human sepsis, but their application to veterinary patients is yet to be defined.[111–114] Heparin-binding protein was more predictive of septic shock in people compared with several other well-studied biomarkers.[115] Additional biomarkers that have received attention in people include IL-6, aPC, IL-8, acute-phase proteins (CRP, amyloid A, haptoglobin, fibrinogen,

TABLE 123.6 Hematologic and Hemostatic Changes in Sepsis[215]

Hematologic Parameter	Tests Available	Possible Abnormalities
WBC count	WBC count, differential	Leukocytosis or leukopenia
	Blood smear, cytologic evaluation	Toxic changes; immature neutrophils
	Bone marrow evaluation	Myeloid hyperplasia
RBC count	Hematocrit	Hemoconcentration or anemia
	Reticulocyte count	Nonregenerative anemia
	Blood smear, cytologic evaluation	Heinz bodies (cats)
	Bone marrow evaluation	Erythroid hypoplasia
Platelets	Platelet count	Thrombocytopenia
	Blood smear, cytologic evaluation	Thrombocytopenia
Hemostatic parameters	PT	Normal (early) or prolonged (late)
	PTT	Normal (early) or prolonged (late)
	Activated coagulation time	Normal (early) or prolonged (late)
	FDP	Increased
	D-dimers	Increased (late)
	Antithrombin[a]	Decreased activity
	Thromboelastography[a]	Increased coagulation index
	Protein C[a]	Decreased

[a]Less commonly performed tests; may only be available through reference laboratories.

FDP, fibrinogen degradation products; *PT*, prothrombin time; *PTT*, partial thromboplastin time; *WBC*, white blood cell; *RBC*, red blood cell.

α-1-acid glycoprotein, and ceruloplasmin), LPS, LPS-binding protein, nitrate/nitrite concentrations (byproducts of NO metabolism), soluble intercellular cellular adhesion molecule 1, AT, TFPI, CD14, CD11b/CD18, T-cell function assays, IL-12, neutrophil gelatinase-associated lipocalin, and IL-1 receptor antagonist.[116–119] Serum IL-6 has been studied in experimental models of endotoxemia or inflammation in dogs; this biomarker rises within hours, stays elevated for days when inflammation persists, and may have a prognostic role in this species.[120–123] Initial serum CRP concentration in dogs with sepsis did not correlate with survival.[124,125] However, decreasing concentrations were observed with recovery from sepsis. Monocyte chemoattractant protein-1 is increased in critically ill dogs and highest levels have been observed in those with sepsis.[126] This level of cytokine mediator in dogs appeared to increase in proportion to the severity of sepsis, similar to what has been observed in humans. aPC is decreased in septic human patients and canine models of sepsis and represents a therapeutic target that reduces mortality in limited populations with severe sepsis.[127–129] Treatment of sepsis with aPC failed to improve survival in a large randomized clinical trial,[130] the product, when it was available was quite costly and species specific; therefore, clinical use of this product was not investigated in veterinary medicine. Plasma von Willebrand factor antigen concentration, a marker of endothelial activation, was increased in dogs with sepsis compared with that in clinically healthy control dogs.[131] However, there was no significant difference between levels in surviving and nonsurviving dogs.

Microbiologic Tests

Bacterial Isolation and Identification

The identification of a septic focus and the procurement of infected tissue or fluid for culture and sensitivity testing are of paramount importance. Although this might be difficult in certain patients (e.g., those that are unstable, coagulopathic), cytology or histopathology can also be used to make a definitive diagnosis of infection.[16,18,23,132] Specimen collection is further described in Chapter 3. Faster turnaround times for canine and feline blood cultures (<24 hours) may soon be clinically available to help guide earlier therapy.[133]

Molecular Diagnosis Using Nucleic Acid–Based Testing and Metagenomic Approaches

Rapid NAAT tests are increasingly being used in human medicine for rapid identification of pathogens associated with sepsis. Such assays may detect more pathogens than culture, have a shorter turnaround time, and may still be positive in the face of empirical antimicrobial therapy.[134–136] Commercially-available diagnostic tests that use metagenomic approaches such as next-generation sequencing (NGS) are also increasingly available and in clinical use in human patients; an example is the Karius NGS test (Karius, CA, USA). At the time of writing, these assays can be expensive and their performance and value requires further study.[136]

Pathologic Findings

Because sepsis is not a specific disease, but rather a clinical entity describing the host response to systemic inflammation initiated by a pathogen, there are no specific gross or histopathologic findings that are diagnostic for sepsis. Histologic findings associated with SIRS include widespread vascular endothelial injury, neutrophil margination, edema, and microthrombosis. The focus of infection will often represent the key pathologic abnormality (e.g., CPV enteritis, pyometra, bacterial endocarditis).

Necropsy studies do not definitively reveal the cause of death in many human patients with sepsis, and there is frequently discordance between histologic findings and the degree of clinical and laboratory indices of organ dysfunction. One possible reason for this might be the occurrence of *cell stunning*, in which sepsis activates defense mechanisms that cause cellular processes to be reduced to basic housekeeping roles, but further investigation is required. Many animals develop secondary organ dysfunction that may prove life-threatening; derangements of the coagulation, cardiovascular, respiratory, renal, GI, hepatic, and microcirculatory systems are most common.

TREATMENT

The mainstay of therapy for septic patients remains source control to remove the inciting cause and provide supportive care.

Circulatory Support

Septic patients commonly suffer from circulatory collapse despite volume resuscitation; therefore, cardiovascular support is a primary objective of treatment. To maintain adequate tissue perfusion and prevent the development of MODS, aggressive fluid therapy is essential. Isotonic crystalloids, hypertonic crystalloid solutions, synthetic colloids, and blood component therapy are typically administered during fluid resuscitation and maintenance of the septic patient.[137,138] Many septic patients have increased vascular endothelial permeability and hypoalbuminemia; thus, judicious use of fluid products is recommended. Synthetic colloids may prove helpful in animals with severe decreases in colloid osmotic pressure, and colloidal blood component therapy, including human/canine albumin or plasma, may be beneficial in animals that are severely hypoalbuminemic or coagulopathic, respectively. Although not proven in small animals, the use of hydroxyethyl starch in humans with sepsis has been found to increase the risk for AKI.[139] Because large volumes of fresh frozen plasma are required for albumin replacement (e.g., 22 mL/kg of plasma to raise the albumin concentration by 0.5 g/dL),[140] fresh frozen plasma is used primarily for animals that are coagulopathic or to prevent a further decline in those with severe hypoalbuminemia.

Human and canine serum albumin are in the early stages of clinical use in veterinary medicine, and further research is ongoing. The 25% human serum albumin solution is hyperoncotic (100 mmHg) and should be used judiciously in patients with limited fluid tolerance. Anemia and thrombocytopenia may prompt the use of erythrocyte- or platelet-containing products (e.g., packed RBCs, fresh whole blood, lyophilized platelets). In contrast to the debated value of placement of a central venous catheter in humans, in veterinary patients this tool provides a way to monitor trends in central venous pressures during aggressive fluid therapy.[137] In a landmark study, the use of early goal-directed therapy, including central venous oxygen saturation, was shown to improve outcome in humans with sepsis and septic shock[141]; however, subsequent large-scale clinical trials failed to confirm a survival benefit of this approach.[142,143] Noninvasive cardiac output monitoring may prove useful in management of septic patients by providing trends in systemic vascular resistance, cardiac output, and pulmonary capillary wedge pressure.[143] This information will assist with treatment decisions regarding the use of fluids, vasopressors, and/or inotropes. Frequent monitoring of body weight and urine output via placement of an indwelling urinary catheter is also helpful in assessing total fluid balance. Various fluid types and doses can be found in Table 123.7.

Cardiovascular Support

Persistent hypotension (mean arterial pressure less than 65 mmHg or Doppler less than 90 mmHg) despite restoration of a normal intravascular volume signals the need for vasopressor and/or inotropic therapy to support oxygen delivery to the tissues and prevent organ damage.[141,144] The choice of treatment drug depends on the clinical picture combined with objective information regarding the septic patient (Table 123.8). Vasopressors such as norepinephrine, dopamine, phenylephrine, and vasopressin are typically used in patients with peripheral vasodilation. The use of dopamine has been discouraged in septic humans due to an increased risk for arrhythmias, but this has not been proven in dogs or cats.[145] Phenylephrine is a pure α-agonist, whereas norepinephrine and dopamine have a combination of both α- and β-agonist activity.[146] Vasopressin, also known as antidiuretic hormone, is a nonadrenergic vasopressor agent that aids in the regulation of free water balance in healthy animals, but serves as an important endogenous vasoconstrictor during states of hypotension.[147] Decreased vasopressin concentrations have been found in animals and humans with catecholamine-refractory shock, and exogenous vasopressin treatment works synergistically with adrenergic pressor substances, primarily norepinephrine. Therapeutic restoration of blood vasopressin levels in patients suffering from shock works primarily via the vasopressin-1 receptor to cause vasoconstriction of most capillary vessels, although the cerebral, renal, pulmonary, and mesenteric vessels are spared with low-dose therapy.[148,149] A combination of vasopressin and glucocorticoids may further increase survival.[150] Use of vasopressin in dogs and cats is limited thus far, but preliminary findings in dogs are promising.[151–153]

Hypotensive animals that are most likely to benefit from vasopressor therapy include those with clinical evidence of peripheral vasodilation, such as bright red mucous membranes, bounding pulses, and fast CRTs. However, cats rarely exhibit these signs. Invasive or noninvasive measurements of systemic vascular resistance can also guide the use of vasopressor therapy but can be difficult to measure in the clinical setting. Vasoconstricting drugs are often effective at increasing arterial blood pressure but may also result in excessive vasoconstriction to some areas, particularly the splanchnic and/or renal circulation, which may lead to GI and/or renal ischemia and dysfunction. Especially in the septic canine patient, splanchnic vasoconstriction may exacerbate the endotoxemia by compromising normal intestinal integrity and enabling bacterial translocation into the bloodstream.

Positive inotropes such as dobutamine are generally used in septic patients with evidence of impaired myocardial contractility (e.g., decreased fractional shortening on M-mode echocardiography, decreased cardiac output on invasive or noninvasive measurements of cardiac output). The β-agonist drug most commonly used for the treatment of decreased systolic function is dobutamine, although isoproterenol, epinephrine, and dopamine also have beta-adrenergic activity.[148]

TABLE 123.7 Fluid Choices for Circulatory Support

Fluid Type	Dose	Comments
Isotonic crystalloids	Dog: up to 90 mL/kg (start with 20–30 mL/kg) Cat: up to 60 mL/kg (start with 10–20 mL/kg)	Used in animals for intravascular and interstitial volume deficits. May cause edema in animals with capillary leak or a low oncotic pressure.
Synthetic colloid solutions (hydroxyethyl starches)	Dog: 5–20 mL/kg Cat: 5–10 mL/kg	Used in animals for volume replacement and oncotic support. May cause coagulopathies and increase the risk for acute kidney injury in humans.
Human albumin	2 g/kg or calculate albumin deficit (g): 10 × (desired-patient albumin) × weight (kg) × 0.3	Used for albumin and oncotic support and volume replacement. Monitor closely for reactions. One-time dose recommended.
Canine albumin	1–2 g/kg	Limited safety studies thus far. Use with caution.
Fresh frozen plasma	10–15 mL/kg as needed	Used to treat clotting factor deficiencies and provide albumin-containing oncotic support.
Frozen or cryoprecipitate-poor plasma		Used to provide albumin-containing oncotic support or for treatment of rodenticide toxicity.
Packed red blood cells	10–15 mL/kg to raise HCT by 10%–15%	Used to treat anemia.
Fresh whole blood	20–25 mL/kg	Used to treat anemia, thrombocytopenia, and clotting factor deficiencies and provide albumin-containing oncotic support.

HCT, hematocrit.

TABLE 123.8 Dosages and Receptor Activity of Vasopressor and Inotropic Drugs

Drug	Alpha Activity	Beta Activity	Dosage	Comments
Dobutamine	+	B_1 +++, B_2 ++	2–20 μg/kg/min	May cause seizures in cats
Dopamine (low dose)	0 to +	0 to +	1–4 μg/kg/min	Vasodilatory dose
Dopamine (medium dose)	+ to ++	+ to +++	5–10 μg/kg/min	Inconsistent plasma levels
Dopamine (high dose)	+++	+ to +++	10–20 μg/kg/min	Inconsistent plasma levels
Epinephrine	+++	++ to +++	0.05–1.0 μg/kg/min	Significant adverse effects
Norepinephrine	+++	+ to ++	0.05–1.0 μg/kg/min	Primarily alpha adrenergic activity
Phenylephrine	+++	0 to +	0.1–1.0 μg/kg/min	Significant vasoconstriction and potential adverse effects
Vasopressin	0	0	0.5–5 mU/kg/min	Nonadrenergic vasopressor activity via vasopressin receptors

0, zero; +, slight; ++, moderate; +++, strong.

Antimicrobial Use in Sepsis

The Surviving Sepsis Campaign Guidelines were updated in 2012, 2016, and 2021 and recommend the administration of broad-spectrum antibacterial therapy within 1 hour of diagnosis of severe sepsis or septic shock.[154,155] Timely localization of the septic focus and procurement of infected tissue or fluid for bacterial identification and determination of antibacterial susceptibility are of paramount importance in the treatment of a septic patient. However, sample collection may be impossible because of cardiopulmonary instability or the presence of a coagulopathy in some patients. Pending culture and susceptibility results, empiric antibacterial therapy should be selected based on the following factors: antibacterial properties (bactericidal versus static); the expected bacterial flora in the affected tissue; the ability of the antibacterial to penetrate the infected tissue; recent history of antibacterial use and considerations for resistance; and source of infection (whether nosocomial or community-acquired). Readers are referred to Chapters 8 and 10 for further details.

Appropriate empiric therapy is vital for success. Broad-spectrum bactericidal antimicrobial agents are typically administered to septic patients via the IV route. Adjustments are made pending availability of antibacterial susceptibility testing results. Box 123.3 contains examples of four-quadrant, empiric therapy (i.e., effective against many gram-positive and gram-negative aerobes and anaerobes). One study highlighted the importance of appropriate antibacterial selection; in five dogs in which inappropriate antibacterial drugs were empirically administered, mortality was 80%.[16] Studies have failed to show an association between appropriate antimicrobial use and mortality[156,157]; the complexity of management of septic patients warrants a prospective study to define the impact of early appropriate antimicrobial administration. Polymyxin B, an antibacterial which binds to the lipid A subunit of endotoxin molecules, has been used in the treatment of cats with experimental endotoxemia.[158] When administered IV, at a rate of 1 mg/kg over 30 minutes, polymyxin B reduced the plasma TNF activity and increased leukocyte counts with no adverse effect. Further studies in naturally affected cats will be helpful to determine its clinical efficacy. Delaying administration of antimicrobials or withholding their use in a septic patient increases the ability of the organisms to reproduce, spread, and induce a greater inflammatory response.

Gastrointestinal Protectants

The initial strategy to prevent GI complications in critically ill dogs and cats is to ensure adequate GI perfusion and employ early enteral nutrition. High-risk patients should receive pharmacologic prophylaxis for stress-related GI hemorrhage. Based on the available evidence in human medicine, it appears that proton pump inhibitors (PPIs) are superior to histamine-2 receptor antagonists (H2RAs), which are superior to sucralfate in the prevention of stress-related mucosal disease in adult critical care patients.[159–161] Drugs available include omeprazole (0.7–1.0 mg/kg, PO, q24h); pantoprazole (0.7–1.0 mg/kg, IV, q12–24h); famotidine (0.5–1.0 mg/kg, IV, q12–24h); and sucralfate (0.25–1 g/25 kg, PO, q6–8h). Lower doses of sucralfate (0.1–0.2 mg/kg) have claimed equal efficacy.[162]

BOX 123.3 Examples of Empiric, Broad-Spectrum (Four-Quadrant) Antibacterial Therapy for the Treatment of Sepsis

Ampicillin and: enrofloxacin, amikacin, gentamicin, cefoxitin, cefotaxime, or ceftazidime
Clindamycin and: enrofloxacin, amikacin, gentamicin, or ceftazidime
Imipenem or meropenem

Additional Treatment Strategies for Sepsis

There have been a number of landmark studies in human medicine regarding treatment strategies for sepsis over the past several years, some of which have subsequently been called into question. Some strategies, however, may also prove applicable to small animal medicine, although further research is needed. These highly acclaimed strategies include early goal-directed therapy to direct resuscitation treatment of relative adrenal insufficiency, tight glycemic control, neutralization of endotoxin, and physiologic anticoagulant therapy. The benefits of treatment of human patients with IV vitamin C and thiamine in combination with hydrocortisone is also being studied.[163] This has occurred in response to evidence of low vitamin C and thiamine concentrations in septic patients, and some initial evidence of positive outcomes in initial human clinical trials.

Early goal-directed therapy was initially shown to decrease mortality and severity of illness in humans with sepsis, although more recent investigations have not confirmed these earlier findings.[141,144,164] Preliminary evidence suggests a beneficial response in dogs treated with goal-directed therapy.[165] This invasive approach uses multiple criteria, including central venous oxygen saturation > 70%, central venous pressure ≥ 8–12 mmHg, mean arterial pressure ≥ 65 mmHg, urine output ≥ 0.5 mL/kg/hour, oxygen saturation ≥ 93%, and hematocrit ≥ 30%, as a rapid goal within the first 6 hours of hospitalization in humans. In an observational study,[166] 38% of canine shock patients had central venous oxygen saturation < 70% despite normalization of blood pressure, HR, and physical parameters. Although formal studies have not been performed in veterinary patients, it seems reasonable to expect that a rapid correction of hemodynamic and organ function indices would be beneficial to the animal. The use of central venous oxygen saturation monitoring in animals is limited, primarily because of the expense of the equipment required.

The hypothalamic-pituitary-adrenal axis is crucial for host response to infection. The early inflammatory response to sepsis stimulates endogenous release of cortisol, which subsequently modulates the synthesis and release of pro- and anti-inflammatory mediators to restrict inflammation of infected tissues. The cause of critical illness-related corticosteroid insufficiency (CIRCI)[167] in septic patients appears to be multifactorial, including factors such as vascular or ischemic damage, inflammation, and apoptosis within the hypothalamic-pituitary-adrenal axis; use of drugs that modify cortisol metabolism; and/or tissue resistance to glucocorticoids.[168,169] CIRCI may occur in up to 70% of people with sepsis and is correlated to hypotension and death in these patients. Preliminary research in dogs, cats, and foals suggests that a similar phenomenon also occurs with critical illness in these species.[170–174] Sepsis-induced CIRCI in humans is not easily diagnosed and a matter of considerable controversy.[45] Some recommendations suggested that a diagnosis could be made by identifying a basal cortisol less than 10 μg/dL or a change in cortisol (delta cortisol) of less than 9 μg/dL after administration of ACTH. Administration of ACTH to diagnose the syndrome is no longer recommended, rather administration of hydrocortisone is recommended in patients who have not responded to adequate fluid resuscitation and vasopressor therapy.[155] The use of physiologic doses of hydrocortisone has been found to improve 28-day mortality rates and decrease the duration of vasopressor therapy in septic humans with a poor response to ACTH testing.[175] However, one systematic review performed in 2013 found no clear benefit of glucocorticoids on mortality, although subgroup analysis of low-dose glucocorticoid use is suggestive of a beneficial drug effect on short-term mortality, particularly in more critically ill patients.[155] In contrast, a 2019 meta-analysis showed faster shock reversal, fewer vasopressor-dependent days and decreased length of ICU stay, in addition to a reduced 28-day mortality rate. In summary, although routine use of hydrocortisone in adults with sepsis is still controversial, its use is recommended in adult patients with septic shock who are poorly responsive to fluid and vasopressor therapy, as well as pediatric patients with suspected or proven adrenal insufficiency.[153,176,177] The diagnosis and treatment of CIRCI in veterinary medicine is also subject to controversy.[170] In one study, critically ill dogs with a delta cortisol ≤ 83 nmol/L were almost six times as likely to need vasopressor therapy.[174] Similar to the Surviving Sepsis Guidelines for humans,[155] the use of hydrocortisone should be limited to those veterinary patients in shock who have not responded to adequate fluid resuscitation and vasopressor treatment, until further evidence provides more specific recommendations.

Prevention of hyperglycemia in septic and critically ill patients has been the focus of much research, and glycemic control was recommended in the 2021 Surviving Sepsis Guidelines.[153,155,178–181] Although there are several etiologies for the elevated glucose in septic animals, hepatic insulin resistance appears to play a major role.[181] Hyperglycemia may serve to potentiate the proinflammatory response and cause endothelial and neutrophil dysfunction.[182,183] A decrease in morbidity and mortality, as well as the incidence of sepsis, was found when intensive insulin therapy was used to strictly regulate glucose levels (e.g., >180 mg/dL) in critically ill humans.[155,184–187] Tight glycemic control (glucose < 110 mg/dL) is associated with an increased prevalence of hypoglycemia. In a series of randomized controlled studies, tight glycemic control was either associated with no improvement or an increase in mortality and a high incidence of hypoglycemia.[155] Current recommendations from the Surviving Sepsis Guidelines are to maintain blood glucose ≤ 180 mg/dL.[155] There are few studies concerning glucose monitoring in small animals, but preliminary data show a similar trend.[188–191] Until there is more evidence of a broad benefit and institution of precise monitoring in small animals, the risk of hypoglycemia likely outweighs the benefit of tight glucose control. Critically ill small animal patients may benefit from strategies to maintain their glucose between 80 and 180 mg/dL.

Directed therapy of sepsis has attempted to follow the advances in our understanding of the cascade of inflammation.[192] The most common and potent trigger of SIRS in sepsis is bacterial endotoxin. Several strategies have been investigated to eliminate or neutralize endotoxin. The list of promising agents included glucocorticoids, anti-endotoxin antibodies, competitive inhibitors (e.g., lipid X), and natural inhibitors (e.g., bactericidal permeability increasing protein). Despite survival benefits in experimental animals, none of these agents has proven successful in human or veterinary (bactericidal permeability increasing protein) trials.[193,194] One of the proposed reasons for the failure of this strategy was that endotoxin is an early and transient mediator that initiates the cascade of events in the host immune response. Therefore, in the next wave of investigations, attention was directed toward the inflammatory cytokines and other later mediators. Similar to the experience with endotoxin inhibition, inhibition of cytokines and other individual inflammatory mediators has failed to show benefit and, in some cases, was detrimental. These circulating mediators have been demonstrated in septic veterinary patients, but there are no veterinary clinical trials investigating inhibition of these compounds. Immune paralysis has been recognized in some patients with sepsis. Immune stimulation using granulocyte colony-stimulating factor in puppies with CPV was not beneficial.[195] However, investigations in experimental animals and clinical trials are ongoing. Overall strategies targeting individual mediators of sepsis have failed.

The use of aPC therapy in humans with septic shock has received much attention over the past 10 years as it was the only directed therapy that had shown any benefit in human sepsis clinical trials. aPC inhibits factor Va and factor VIIIa and has effects on *in vitro* coagulation, fibrinolysis, and the immune system. Although initial studies showed a decrease in mortality in patients with sepsis and septic shock, subsequent trials failed to demonstrate a benefit and the drug was withdrawn from the market.[130,196] aCP was quite expensive and associated with an increased risk of serious bleeding in humans; the human formulation was known to have a short half-life and to be antigenic in dogs and, therefore, was not well studied in small animals.

Novel Drugs With Potential for Benefit in Sepsis

Nitric Oxide

NO is an important molecule in vasoregulation and the immune system.[197] In the endothelial cell, the enzyme responsible for NO production (endothelial NO synthase) is constitutively expressed. In the vascular system, NO is released at low levels and mediates vascular smooth muscle relaxation and opposes the interactions between endothelial cells and leukocytes. In the inflammatory response, macrophages are responsible for generation of large quantities (100-fold greater than the endothelial cells) of NO that are important in bactericidal activity. Excessive production of NO leads to tissue damage, particularly as a result of interactions with superoxide and the formation of the highly reactive peroxynitrite. The effects of sepsis on NO synthesis are complex. Although NO is implicated as a mediator of septic hypotension and cardiac depression (among other things), global inhibition of NO has multiple adverse effects and has failed to demonstrate a benefit in human clinical trials.[198]

Statins

Statins have been used in the treatment and prevention of atherosclerosis and lower serum lipids through the inhibition of 3-hydroxy-3-methylglutaryl coenzyme A reductase. These drugs also affect intracellular signaling, including NF-κB activation, in the inflammatory response. The anti-inflammatory effects of statins have been documented on both innate and acquired immunity, the coagulation system (promoting an anticoagulant state and enhancing the synthesis of aCP), and the vascular endothelium (improving endothelial function and normalizing NO production). Despite evidence from experimental studies and a meta-analysis of the observational studies,[199–201] two published randomized controlled trials evaluating statins in patients with ARDS[202,203] failed to demonstrate a benefit of treatment.

Toll-Like Receptor Antagonists

The attempt to intervene in the response to endotoxin has not proven beneficial in the past through anti-endotoxin antibodies, soluble CD14 (which conversely increased the inflammatory response), or through LPS-binding agents (BPI). Another target of the endotoxin pathway has been the TLR4 receptor. In a phase II clinical trial, one TLR4 antagonist did not show any more adverse events than the placebo and overall did not change mortality. In a phase III multinational study of 1,961 patients with severe sepsis, treatment with a TLR4 antagonist failed to demonstrate an effect on mortality.[204] Targeting TLR pathways continues to be an area of investigation for treatment of sepsis.[205,206]

High Mortality Group Box 1

HMGB1 is a nuclear protein that has been shown to be a late biomarker in sepsis. Serum levels of HMGB1 are measurable in mouse models of sepsis/endotoxemia within 8 hours and remain elevated for up to 32 hours.[29,207] In addition to its value as a biomarker, it appears that HMGB1 mediates part of the inflammatory response, thus making it a potential target for therapy. Antibodies to HMGB1 were protective in a mouse model of sepsis, even when they were administered 24 hours after the onset of sepsis.[207] Several agents have been shown to modify HMGB1 activity or release and these include anticoagulant agents (i.e., AT, thrombomodulin), endogenous hormones (i.e., insulin, vasoactive intestinal peptide, ghrelin), vagus nerve stimulation, green tea, the Chinese herb danshen, and ethyl pyruvate. Despite promising experimental studies, there are no clinical trials documenting the benefit of HMGB1 inhibition in patients with sepsis.[29,208,209]

Nuclear Factor-κB Inhibitors

Although NF-κB is a major transcription factor involved in the inflammatory response, it is also vital in several other pathways including the anti-inflammatory response and antiapoptotic pathways. Several compounds known to influence NF-κB signaling have failed clinical trials, (e.g., glucocorticoids, NSAIDs, antioxidants). These drugs have numerous other effects, and potentially improved specificity and selective timing of administration will still have a role in the future of sepsis therapy.[209]

Individualized Approach

One concept that arises from the PIRO scheme (see Table 123.4) is that each patient may require tailored therapy based on predisposition, age, sex, genetic background, and, in the case of veterinary patients, species and breed. Furthermore, the type and location of infection influence how a patient is treated. This approach is employed in antibacterial selection, but as additional information accumulates, it may also guide specific treatment that enhances or downregulates specific signaling pathways. Defining the host response as monitored by biomarkers is becoming more commonplace and has great potential to identify patients that could benefit from either suppression or enhancement of the host immune response depending on whether the patient was in a state of hyperinflammation or immune paralysis. The final component of PIRO is organ failure. One of the few advances in treating septic patients has come from implementing "protective ventilation" strategies in which low (6 mL/kg) tidal volume mechanical ventilation is used in patients with ARDS. Individualizing treatments and multimodal approaches are likely to be important in sepsis, given the heterogeneity in the patients and the inciting cause and the dynamic nature of response to sepsis.[209]

PROGNOSIS

Most dogs suffering from sepsis have a guarded prognosis. The published survival rate in dogs and cats with sepsis is 33% to 68%, respectively, and survival in animals with septic shock is worse.[15,168,210,211] Mortality rate increases as the number of dysfunctional organ systems increases.[7] In septic peritonitis, this survival rate does not seem to have improved over the past 20 years despite improvements in critical care management.[14] To maximize success, appropriate diagnostics as well as timely and aggressive therapeutic support are necessary. Future studies in veterinary medicine will likely focus on novel diagnostic modalities as well as superior treatment options.

CASE EXAMPLE

Signalment

"Opal," a 9-year-old, female spayed Siamese cat from Philadelphia, PA.

History

Opal's owner reported a 1 week history of fever, lethargy, and anorexia. There had been no vomiting, diarrhea, coughing, or sneezing. Two months prior to evaluation, the owner noticed that the cat was drinking and urinating more than usual for 1 week, but this resolved without treatment. Opal was an indoor-only cat with no travel history and was up to date on all vaccinations. Opal was not on flea, tick, or heartworm preventative. Opal received no medications and had no prior medical history. She ate a commercial cat food and there was no recent diet change.

Physical Examination

Body weight: 3.4 kg.

General: Quiet, alert, and responsive. Ambulatory on all four limbs. Temperature = 104.1°F (40.1°C), HR = 140 beats/minute, RR = 52 breaths/minute, mucous membranes pale and dry, CRT = 1.5 second.

Integument: A full, mildly dry haircoat was present and there was no evidence of ectoparasites.

Eyes, ears, nose, and throat: No significant abnormalities were noted. There was intermittent ptyalism and a mild amount of brown waxy debris in both ear canals.

Musculoskeletal: A BCS of 4/9 with symmetrical muscling was noted.

Continued

CASE EXAMPLE—cont'd

Cardiovascular: Weak femoral pulses were noted. No murmurs or arrhythmias were detected on thoracic auscultation.

Respiratory: An increased RR was observed and there were clear breath sounds in all lung fields on auscultation.

GI and genitourinary: The cranial abdomen was tense with abdominal splinting upon abdominal palpation. No masses were palpated, although the liver and kidneys were subjectively enlarged. A rectal examination was not performed.

Lymph nodes: All peripheral lymph nodes were < 0.5 cm.

Doppler BP: 60 mmHg (120–160 mmHg)

Laboratory Findings

CBC: HCT 31.0% (31.7%–48.0%), MCV 51.2 fL (36.7–53.7 fL), MCHC 31.1 g/dL (30.1–35.6 g/dL), WBC 13.9 × 10^3 cells/μL (4.04–18.7 × 10^3 cells/μL), neutrophils 12.9 × 10^3 cells/μL (2.3–14 × 10^3 cells/μL), band neutrophils 0.42 × 10^3 cells/μL, lymphocytes 0.56 × 10^3 cells/μL (0.8–6.1 × 10^3 cells/μL), monocytes 0 cells/μL (0–0.7 × 10^3 cells/μL), platelets 148,000 platelets/μL (175,000–500,000 platelets/μL). A clinical pathologist reviewed the slide and noted moderate toxic changes in many WBCs. Bacterial rods were noted infrequently within neutrophils (Fig. 123.4) and rarely extracellularly.

Serum chemistry profile: Sodium 149 mmol/L (146–157 mmol/L), potassium 4.0 mmol/L (3.5–4.8 mmol/L), chloride 118 mmol/L (116–126 mmol/L), bicarbonate 20 mmol/L (16–25 mmol/L), phosphorus 3.5 mg/dL (3.0–6.6 mg/dL), calcium 7.1 mg/dL (9.1–11.2 mg/dL), BUN 42 mg/dL (15–32 mg/dL), creatinine 1.6 mg/dL (1.0–2.0 mg/dL), glucose 170 mg/dL (67–168 mg/dL), total protein 4.9 g/dL (6.0–8.6 g/dL), albumin 2.0 g/dL (2.4–3.8 g/dL), globulin 2.9 g/dL (3.1–5.0 g/dL), ALT 63 U/L (33–152 U/L), AST 84 U/L (137 U/L), ALP < 20 U/L (27–87 U/L), GGT < 10.0 U/L (5–19 U/L), cholesterol 116 mg/dL (96–248 mg/dL), total bilirubin 1.5 mg/dL (0.1–0.8 mg/dL), magnesium 3.3 mg/dL (1.9–2.6 mg/dL).

Urinalysis: SpG 1.024; pH 7.0, 3+ protein (SSA), 2+ glucose, no ketones, no bilirubin, 4+ hemoprotein, 31–40 WBC/HPF, 0–5 RBC/HPF, mild epithelial cells, moderate bacterial rods.

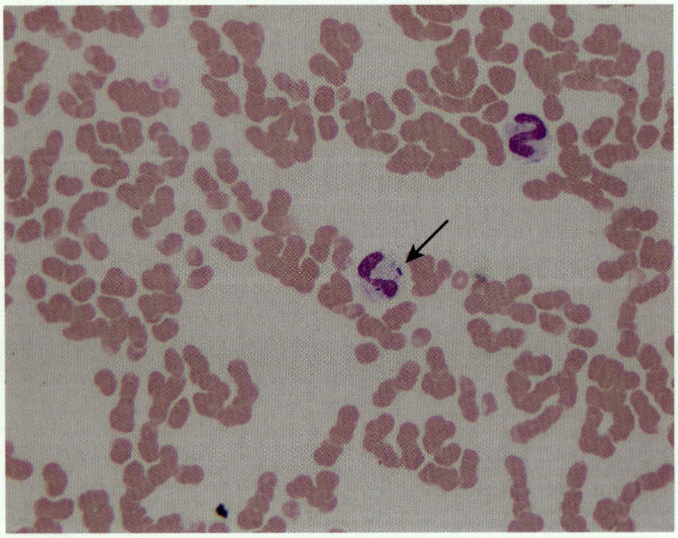

Fig. 123.4 A blood smear from the case example, Opal. Note the intracellular rod *(arrow)* that supports a diagnosis of bacteremia. Magnification 100×. (Courtesy of Dr. Dana Clarke.)

Urine culture: >100,000 CFU/mL *Escherichia coli*, susceptible to all antimicrobials tested.

Blood culture and susceptibility testing: *Escherichia coli* resistant to ampicillin with or without clavulanate or sulbactam.

SNAP FeLV/ FIV ELISA antigen/antibody (IDEXX Laboratories): Negative.

Imaging Findings

Thoracic radiographs: The cardiovascular and pulmonary structures appeared within normal limits.

Abdominal ultrasound: There was a small amount of sludge in the gallbladder. The right kidney was enlarged (47.4 mm long) with pyelectasia (3.9mm). Mild to moderate retroperitoneal effusion with perirenal steatitis and renal mineralization were present. The right ureter was dilated throughout its length (proximal: 3.5 mm in diameter; mid: 3.6 mm; distal: 4.2 mm) with a thickened wall. Within the ureter at the ureterovesicular junction there was a 2.0-mm calculus. The left kidney had decreased corticomedullary definition with hyperechoic speckling throughout the medullary cavity. Several calculi were within the renal pelvis (largest 3.9 mm in length). The left lobe of the pancreas was mildly heterogeneous with hyperechoic foci throughout, and there was a mild rim of hyperechoic surrounding fat. Very scant free peritoneal effusion was seen.

Treatment

Aggressive fluid therapy was instituted due to the hypotension. Despite 30 mL/kg of isotonic crystalloid fluids administered over 45 minutes, blood pressure only increased to 85 mmHg. Norepinephrine was administered at 0.1–0.5 μg/kg/minute as an IV infusion as needed to keep Doppler BP ≥ 100 mmHg. A vasopressin infusion was also necessary to maintain normotension (0.5–0.8 mU/kg/hour). An isotonic fluid infusion was administered at 4 mL/kg/hour. Clindamycin (10 mg/kg, IV, q12h) and ceftazidime (40 mg/kg, IV, q6h) were administered pending blood and urine culture results. Clindamycin was discontinued after 72 hours when susceptibility testing from the cultures was completed.

Opal developed clinically significant anemia and became coagulopathic based on a prolonged PT and APTT. Packed RBCs (15 mL/kg) and fresh frozen plasma were administered. Vitamin K1 was also administered (1 mg/kg, SC, q24h). Treatment with gastroprotectants, including pantoprazole (1 mg/kg, IV, q 24h) and maropitant (1 mg/kg, IV, q24h), were also started. Analgesia with methadone (0.1–0.2 mg/kg, IV, q4h) was initially used for pain control. This was later switched to a fentanyl infusion for management of continued discomfort (2–4 μg/kg/hour IV). A repeat ultrasound 1 and 2 days following initial evaluation revealed that the ureteral calculus had passed into the urinary bladder. Surgery was therefore not necessary.

Comments

This cat had several abnormalities that are common in cats with sepsis. Although this species does not get the classic hyperdynamic physical examination changes, as typically seen in dogs, the presence of an increased rectal temperature, bradycardia, and tachypnea represents a SIRS. The additional findings of pale mucous membranes, poor femoral pulse quality, hypotension, mildly increased bilirubin, toxicity and a left shift on the CBC, and the presence of bacteria in the intracellular and extracellular space upon blood smear evaluation all raise the suspicion for sepsis. Multiple organ dysfunction, as evidenced by vasoplegia and coagulopathy, is common and frequently involves additional organs such as the heart, lungs, GI tract, liver, and kidneys. The need for vasopressor therapy following fluid resuscitation indicates the cat was suffering from septic shock. Aggressive, rapid, and empiric therapy pending culture and susceptibility led to a successful outcome in this cat.

SUGGESTED READINGS

Singer M, Deutschman CS, Seymour Warren C, et al. The third international consensus definitions for sepsis and septic shock (sepsis-3). *JAMA.* 2016;315(8):801–810.

Gotts JE, Matthay MA. Sepsis: pathophysiology and clinical management. *BMJ.* 2016;353:i1585.

Peri AM, Harris PNA, Paterson DL: Culture-independent detection systems for bloodstream infection, *Clin Microbiol Infect.* 2022;28:195–201.

van der Poll T, Shankar-Hari M, Wiersinga WJ: The immunology of sepsis, *Immunity.* 2021;54:2450–2464.

REFERENCES

1. American College of Chest Physicians/Society of Critical Care Medicine Consensus Conference: definitions for sepsis and organ failure and guidelines for the use of innovative therapies in sepsis. *Crit Care Med.* 1992;20:864–874.
2. Singer M, Deutschman CS, Seymour CW, et al. The Third International Consensus Definitions for Sepsis and Septic Shock (Sepsis-3). *JAMA.* 2016;315:801–810.
3. Greiner M, Wolf G, Hartmann K. A retrospective study of the clinical presentation of 140 dogs and 39 cats with bacteraemia. *J Small Anim Pract.* 2008;49:378–383.
4. Lotze MT, Zeh HJ, Rubartelli A, et al. The grateful dead: damage-associated molecular pattern molecules and reduction/oxidation regulate immunity. *Immunol Rev.* 2007;220:60–81.
5. van der Poll T, Shankar-Hari M, Wiersinga WJ: The immunology of sepsis, *Immunity.* 2021;54:2450–2464.
6. Levy MM, Fink MP, Marshall JC, et al. 2001 SCCM/ESICM/ACCP/ATS/SIS International Sepsis Definitions Conference. *Intensive Care Med.* 2003;29:530–538.
7. Kenney EM, Rozanski EA, Rush JE, et al. Association between outcome and organ system dysfunction in dogs with sepsis: 114 cases (2003-2007). *J Am Vet Med Assoc.* 2010;236:83–87.
8. Buras JA, Holzmann B, Sitkovsky M. Animal models of sepsis: setting the stage. *Nat Rev Drug Discov.* 2005;4:854–865.
9. O'Neill LA. Immunity's early-warning system. *Sci Am.* 2005;292:24–31.
10. Akira S, Takeda K. Toll-like receptor signalling. *Nat Rev Immunol.* 2004;4:499–511.
11. Lien E, Ingalls RR. Toll-like receptors. *Crit Care Med.* 2002;30:S1–S11.
12. Natanson C. Studies using a canine model to investigate the cardiovascular abnormality of and potential therapies for septic shock. *Clin Res.* 1990;38:206–214.
13. Ruaux CG. Pathophysiology of organ failure in severe acute pancreatitis in dogs. *Compend Cont Educ Pract Vet.* 2000;22:531–542.
14. Bentley AM, Otto CM, Shofer FS. Comparison of dogs with septic peritonitis: 1988-1993 versus 1999-2003. *J Vet Emerg Crit Care.* 2007;17:391–398.
15. de Laforcade AM, Freeman LM, Shaw SP, et al. Hemostatic changes in dogs with naturally occurring sepsis. *J Vet Intern Med.* 2003;17:674–679.
16. King LG. Postoperative complications and prognostic indicators in dogs and cats with septic peritonitis: 23 cases (1989-1992). *J Am Vet Med Assoc.* 1994;204:407–414.
17. Sorenmo KU, Harwood LP, King LG, et al. Case-control study to evaluate risk factors for the development of sepsis (neutropenia and fever) in dogs receiving chemotherapy. *J Am Vet Med Assoc.* 2010;236:650–656.
18. Brady CA, Otto CM, Van Winkle TJ, et al. Severe sepsis in cats: 29 cases (1986-1998). *J Am Vet Med Assoc.* 2000;217:531–535.
19. Rothwell PM, Udwadia ZF, Lawler PG. Cortisol response to corticotropin and survival in septic shock. *Lancet.* 1991;337:582–583.
20. DeClue AE, Williams KJ, Sharp C, et al. Systemic response to low-dose endotoxin infusion in cats. *Vet Immunol Immunopathol.* 2009;132:167–174.
21. Andersson U, Wang H, Palmblad K, et al. High mobility group 1 protein (HMG-1) stimulates proinflammatory cytokine synthesis in human monocytes. *J Exp Med.* 2000;192:565–570.
22. Waddell LS, Brady CA, Drobatz KJ. Risk factors, prognostic indicators, and outcome of pyothorax in cats: 80 cases (1986-1999). *J Am Vet Med Assoc.* 2002;221:819–824.
23. Costello MF, Drobatz KJ, Aronson LR, et al. Underlying cause, pathophysiologic abnormalities, and response to treatment in cats with septic peritonitis: 51 cases (1990-2001). *J Am Vet Med Assoc.* 2004;225:897–902.
24. Parsons KJ, Owen LJ, Lee K, et al. A retrospective study of surgically treated cases of septic peritonitis in the cat (2000-2007). *J Small Anim Pract.* 2009;50:518–524.
25. Rangel-Frausto MS, Pittet D, Costigan M, et al. The natural history of the systemic inflammatory response syndrome (SIRS). A prospective study. *JAMA.* 1995;273:117–123.
26. Usui M, Hanamura N, Hayashi T, et al. Molecular cloning, expression and tissue distribution of canine lipopolysaccharide (LPS)-binding protein. *Biochim Biophys Acta.* 1998;1397:202–212.
27. Hodgson JC. Endotoxin and mammalian host responses during experimental disease. *J Comp Pathol.* 2006;135:157–175.
28. Perkins ND. Integrating cell-signalling pathways with NF-kappaB and IKK function. *Nat Rev Mol Cell Biol.* 2007;8:49–62.
29. Wang H, Ward MF, Sama AE. Novel HMGB1-inhibiting therapeutic agents for experimental sepsis. *Shock.* 2009;32:348–357.
30. Tizard IR. *Veterinary Immunology, an Introduction.* 6 ed. Philadelphia: WB Saunders; 2000.
31. Marshall JC. Such stuff as dreams are made on: mediator-directed therapy in sepsis. *Nat Rev Drug Discov.* 2003;2:391–405.
32. Tsuchiya R, Kyotani K, Scott MA, et al. Role of platelet activating factor in development of thrombocytopenia and neutropenia in dogs with endotoxemia. *Am J Vet Res.* 1999;60:216–221.
33. Doursout MF, Kilbourn RG, Hartley CJ, et al. Effects of N-methyl-L-arginine on cardiac and regional blood flow in a dog endotoxin shock model. *J Crit Care.* 2000;15:22–29.
34. Mitaka C, Hirata Y, Masaki Y, et al. S-Methylisothiourea sulfate improves renal, but not hepatic dysfunction in canine endotoxic shock model. *Intensive Care Med.* 2000;26:117–124.
35. Mitaka C, Hirata Y, Yokoyama K, et al. L-canavanine, a selective inhibitor of inducible NO synthase, increases plasma endothelin-1 concentrations in dogs with endotoxic shock. *J Crit Care.* 2001;16:17–23.
36. Preiser JC, Zhang H, Vray B, et al. Time course of inducible nitric oxide synthase activity following endotoxin administration in dogs. *Nitric Oxide.* 2001;5:208–211.
37. Mitaka C, Hirata Y, Yokoyama K, et al. Improvement of renal dysfunction in dogs with endotoxemia by a nonselective endothelin receptor antagonist. *Crit Care Med.* 1999;27:146–153.
38. McKenzie AG. Guillain-Barre syndrome may be associated with HIV infection. *Anaesthesia.* 2001;56:193–194.
39. Morresey PR. Synthesis of proinflammatory mediators in endotoxemia. *Compend Cont Educ Pract Vet.* 2001;23:829–852.
40. Schouten M, Wiersinga WJ, Levi M, et al. Inflammation, endothelium, and coagulation in sepsis. *J Leukoc Biol.* 2008;83:536–545.
41. Gando S, Nanzaki S, Sasaki S, et al. Activation of the extrinsic coagulation pathway in patients with severe sepsis and septic shock. *Crit Care Med.* 1998;26:2005–2009.
42. Otto CM, Rieser TM, Brooks MB, et al. Evidence of hypercoagulability in dogs with parvoviral enteritis. *J Am Vet Med Assoc.* 2000;217:1500–1504.
43. de Laforcade AM, Rozanski EA, Freeman LM, et al. Serial evaluation of protein C and antithrombin in dogs with sepsis. *J Vet Intern Med.* 2008;22:26–30.
44. Bernard GR, Vincent JL, Laterre PF, et al. Efficacy and safety of recombinant human activated protein C for severe sepsis. *N Engl J Med.* 2001;344:699–709.
45. Dellinger RP, Levy MM, Rhodes A, et al. Surviving sepsis campaign: international guidelines for management of severe sepsis and septic shock. *Crit Care Med.* 2012;41:580–637.
46. Afshari A, Wetterslev J, Brok J, et al. Antithrombin III for critically ill patients. *Cochrane Database Syst Rev.* 2008:CD005370.
47. Jessen LR, Wiinberg B, Kjelgaard-Hansen M, et al. Thrombin-activatable fibrinolysis inhibitor activity in healthy and diseased dogs. *Vet Clin Pathol.* 2010;39:296–301.

48. Walport MJ. Complement. First of two parts. *N Engl J Med.* 2001;344:1058–1066.
49. Flierl MA, Schreiber H, Huber-Lang MS. The role of complement, C5a and its receptors in sepsis and multiorgan dysfunction syndrome. *J Invest Surg.* 2006;19:255–265.
50. Flierl MA, Rittirsch D, Huber-Lang MS, et al. Molecular events in the cardiomyopathy of sepsis. *Mol Med.* 2008;14:327–336.
51. Trzeciak S, Dellinger RP, Parrillo JE, et al. Early microcirculatory perfusion derangements in patients with severe sepsis and septic shock: relationship to hemodynamics, oxygen transport, and survival. *Ann Emerg Med.* 2007;49(88–98):98:e81–82.
52. Trzeciak S, McCoy JV, Phillip Dellinger R, et al. Early increases in microcirculatory perfusion during protocol-directed resuscitation are associated with reduced multi-organ failure at 24 h in patients with sepsis. *Intensive Care Med.* 2008;34:2210–2217.
53. Goodnight ME, Cooper ES, Butler AL. Assessment of microcirculatory perfusion in healthy anesthetized cats undergoing ovariohysterectomy using sidestream dark field microscopy. *J Vet Emerg Crit Care.* 2015;25:349–357.
54. Hotchkiss RS, Karl IE. The pathophysiology and treatment of sepsis. *N Engl J Med.* 2003;348:138–150.
55. Panciera DL, Ritchey JW, Ward DL. Endotoxin-induced nonthyroidal illness in dogs. *Am J Vet Res.* 2003;64:229–234.
56. Moseley RH. Sepsis and cholestasis. *Clin Liver Dis.* 2004;8:83–94.
57. Estrin MA, Wehausen CE, Jessen CR, et al. Disseminated intravascular coagulation in cats. *J Vet Intern Med.* 2006;20:1334–1339.
58. Kitchens CS. Thrombocytopenia and thrombosis in disseminated intravascular coagulation (DIC). *Hematology Am Soc Hematol Educ Program.* 2009:240–246.
59. Weiss DJ, Rashid J. The sepsis-coagulant axis: a review. *J Vet Intern Med.* 1998;12:317–324.
60. Hunter JD, Doddi M. Sepsis and the heart. *Br J Anaesth.* 2010;104:3–11.
61. Zanotti-Cavazzoni SL, Hollenberg SM. Cardiac dysfunction in severe sepsis and septic shock. *Curr Opin Crit Care.* 2009;15:392–397.
62. Rudiger A, Singer M. Mechanisms of sepsis-induced cardiac dysfunction. *Crit Care Med.* 2007;35:1599–1608.
63. Fein AM, Calalang-Colucci MG. Acute lung injury and acute respiratory distress syndrome in sepsis and septic shock. *Crit Care Clin.* 2000;16:289–317.
64. Luce JM. Acute lung injury and the acute respiratory distress syndrome. *Crit Care Med.* 1998;26:369–376.
65. Parent C, King LG, Walker LM, et al. Clinical and clinicopathologic findings in dogs with acute respiratory distress syndrome: 19 cases (1985-1993). *J Am Vet Med Assoc.* 1996;208:1419–1427.
66. Ware LB. Pathophysiology of acute lung injury and the acute respiratory distress syndrome. *Semin Respir Crit Care Med.* 2006;27:337–349.
67. Wilkins PA, Otto CM, Baumgardner JE, et al. Acute lung injury and acute respiratory distress syndromes in veterinary medicine: consensus definitions: the Dorothy Russell Havemeyer Working Group on ALI and ARDS in Veterinary Medicine. *J Vet Emerg Crit Care.* 2007;17:333–339.
68. Camacho AT, Pallas E, Gestal JJ, et al. *Babesia canis* infection in a splenectomized dog. *Bull Soc Pathol Exot.* 2002;95:17–19.
69. Jacobson LS. The South African form of severe and complicated canine babesiosis: clinical advances 1994-2004. *Vet Parasitol.* 2006;138:126–139.
70. Sisson D, Thomas WP. Endocarditis of the aortic valve in the dog. *J Am Vet Med Assoc.* 1984;184:570–577.
71. Di Giantomasso D, May CN, Bellomo R. Vital organ blood flow during hyperdynamic sepsis. *Chest.* 2003;124:1053–1059.
72. Schrier RW, Wang W. Acute renal failure and sepsis. *N Engl J Med.* 2004;351:159–169.
73. Wan L, Bellomo R, Di Giantomasso D, et al. The pathogenesis of septic acute renal failure. *Curr Opin Crit Care.* 2003;9:496–502.
74. Hayes G, Benedicenti L, Mathews K. Retrospective cohort study on the incidence of acute kidney injury and death following hydroxyethyl starch (HES 10% 250/0.5/5:1) administration in dogs (2007-2010). *J Vet Emerg Crit Care.* 2016;26:35–40.
75. Yozova ID, Howard J, Adamik KN. Retrospective evaluation of the effects of administration of tetrastarch (hydroxyethyl starch 130/0.4) on plasma creatinine concentration in dogs (2010-2013): 201 dogs. *J Vet Emerg Crit Care.* 2016;26:568–577.
76. Chelazzi C, Consales G, De Gaudio AR. Sepsis associated encephalopathy. *Curr Anesth Crit Care.* 2008;19:15–21.
77. Consales G, De Gaudio AR. Sepsis associated encephalopathy. *Minerva Anesthesiol.* 2005;71:39–52.
78. Agudelo-Ochoa GM, Valdes-Duque BE, Giraldo-Giraldo NA, et al. Gut microbiota profiles in critically ill patients, potential biomarkers and risk variables for sepsis. *Gut Microb.* 2020:1–16.
79. Fink MP. Intestinal epithelial hyperpermeability: update on the pathogenesis of gut mucosal barrier dysfunction in critical illness. *Curr Opin Crit Care.* 2003;9:143–151.
80. Gimson AE. Hepatic dysfunction during bacterial sepsis. *Intensive Care Med.* 1987;13:162–166.
81. Strassburg CP. Gastrointestinal disorders of the critically ill. Shock liver. *Best Pract Res Clin Gastroenterol.* 2003;17:369–381.
82. Venkataraman R, Fink MP. Mechanisms responsible for intestinal barrier dysfunction in critical illness. In: Evans TW, Fink MP, eds. *Mechanisms of Organ Dysfunction in Critical Illness.* New York: Springer; 2002:282–300.
83. Hotchkiss RS, Karl IE. Endothelial cell apoptosis in sepsis: a case of habeas corpus? *Crit Care Med.* 2004;32:901–902.
84. Mutunga M, Fulton B, Bullock R, et al. Circulating endothelial cells in patients with septic shock. *Am J Respir Crit Care Med.* 2001;163:195–200.
85. Silverstein DC, Montealegre CD, Shofer FS, et al. The association between vascular endothelial growth factor levels and clinically evident peripheral edema in dogs with systemic inflammatory response syndrome. *J Vet Emerg Crit Care.* 2009;19:459–466.
86. Butler AL, Campbell VL. Assessment of oxygen transport and utilization in dogs with naturally occurring sepsis. *J Am Vet Med Assoc.* 2010;237:167–173.
87. Chappell D, Westphal M, Jacob M. The impact of the glycocalyx on microcirculatory oxygen distribution in critical illness. *Curr Opin Anaesthesiol.* 2009;22:155–162.
88. De Backer D, Creteur J, Preiser JC, et al. Microvascular blood flow is altered in patients with sepsis. *Am J Respir Crit Care Med.* 2002;166:98–104.
89. De Backer D, Donadello K, Favory R, et al. Link between coagulation abnormalities and microcirculatory dysfunction in critically ill patients. *Curr Opin Anaesthesiol.* 2009;22:150–154.
90. Goligorsky MS, Sun D. Glycocalyx in endotoxemia and sepsis. *Am J Pathol.* 2020;190:791–798.
91. Sakr Y, Dubois MJ, De Backer D, et al. Persistent microcirculatory alterations are associated with organ failure and death in patients with septic shock. *Crit Care Med.* 2004;32:1825–1831.
92. Seilenkamper AW, Ellis CG, Kvietys P. The microcirculation in sepsis. In: Evans TW, Fink MP, eds. *Mechanisms of Organ Dysfunction in Critical Illness.* 1 ed. New York: Springer; 2002.
93. Mihajlovic D, Brkic S, Lendak D, et al. Endothelial biomarkers in the light of new sepsis definition. *Biomark Med.* 2019;13:341–351.
94. Yu W, McNeil JB, Wickersham NE, et al.: Angiopoietin-2 outperforms other endothelial biomarkers associated with severe acute kidney injury in patients with severe sepsis and renal failure, *Crit Care.* 2021;25:48.
95. D'Onofrio V, Heylen D, Pusparum M, et al.: A prospective observational cohort study to identify inflammatory biomarkers for the diagnosis and prognosis of patients with sepsis, *J Intensive Care.* 2022;10:13.
96. Babyak JM, Sharp CR. Epidemiology of systemic inflammatory response syndrome and sepsis in cats hospitalized in a veterinary teaching hospital. *J Am Vet Med Assoc.* 2016;249:65–71.
97. Guenther-Yenke CL, Torre DM, Maranda LS, et al. Epidemiology of canine sepsis in a veterinary teaching hospital. In: *International Veterinary Emergency and Critical Care Symposium.* 2007. New Orleans, LA.
98. Goggs R, Letendre JA. Evaluation of the host cytokine response in dogs with sepsis and noninfectious systemic inflammatory response syndrome. *J Vet Emerg Crit Care.* 2019;29:593–603.
99. Kules J, Horvatic A, Guillemin N, et al. The plasma proteome and the acute phase protein response in canine pyometra. *J Proteomics.* 2020;223:103817.

100. Bone RC, Grodzin CJ, Balk RA. Sepsis: a new hypothesis for pathogenesis of the disease process. *Chest*. 1997;112:235–243.
101. Segev G, Klement E, Aroch I. Toxic neutrophils in cats: clinical and clinicopathologic features, and disease prevalence and outcome: a retrospective case control study. *J Vet Intern Med*. 2006;20:20–31.
102. Weiss DJ, Krehbiel JD, Lund JE. Studies of the pathogenesis of anemia of inflammation: mechanism of impaired erythropoiesis. *Am J Vet Res*. 1983;44:1832–1835.
103. Christopher MM. Relation of endogenous Heinz bodies to disease and anemia in cats: 120 cases (1978-1987). *J Am Vet Med Assoc*. 1989;194:1089–1095.
104. Christopher MM, White JG, Eaton JW. Erythrocyte pathology and mechanisms of Heinz body-mediated hemolysis in cats. *Vet Pathol*. 1990;27:299–310.
105. Weiss DJ, McClay CB. Studies on the pathogenesis of the erythrocyte destruction associated with the anemia of inflammatory disease. *Vet Clin Pathol*. 1988;17:90–93.
106. Sganga G, Siegel JH, Brown G, et al. Reprioritization of hepatic plasma protein release in trauma and sepsis. *Arch Surg*. 1985;120:187–199.
107. Taboada J, Meyer DJ. Cholestasis associated with extrahepatic bacterial infection in five dogs. *J Vet Intern Med*. 1989;3:216–221.
108. Aird WC. The hematologic system as a marker of organ dysfunction in sepsis. *Mayo Clin Proc*. 2003;78:869–881.
109. Levi M. The coagulant response in sepsis. *Clin Chest Med*. 2008;29:627–642 (viii).
110. Weiss DJ, Welle M, Mortiz A, et al. Evaluation of leukocyte cell surface markers in dogs with septic and nonseptic inflammatory diseases. *Am J Vet Res*. 2004;65:59–63.
111. Hochreiter M, Kohler T, Schweiger AM, et al. Procalcitonin to guide duration of antibiotic therapy in intensive care patients: a randomized prospective controlled trial. *Crit Care*. 2009;13:R83.
112. Hoffmann JJ. Neutrophil CD64: a diagnostic marker for infection and sepsis. *Clin Chem Lab Med*. 2009;47:903–916.
113. Martinez-Albarran M, Perez-Molina Jde J, Gallegos-Castorena S, et al. Procalcitonin and C-reactive protein serum levels as markers of infection in a pediatric population with febrile neutropenia and cancer. *Pediatr Hematol Oncol*. 2009;26:414–425.
114. Oh JS, Kim SU, Oh YM, et al. The usefulness of the semiquantitative procalcitonin test kit as a guideline for starting antibiotic administration. *Am J Emerg Med*. 2009;27:859–863.
115. Linder A, Christensson B, Herwald H, et al. Heparin-binding protein: an early marker of circulatory failure in sepsis. *Clin Infect Dis*. 2009;49:1044–1050.
116. Ceron JJ, Eckersall PD, Martynez-Subiela S. Acute phase proteins in dogs and cats: current knowledge and future perspectives. *Vet Clin Pathol*. 2005;34:85–99.
117. Ceron JJ, Martinez-Subiela S, Ohno K, et al. A seven-point plan for acute phase protein interpretation in companion animals. *Vet J*. 2008;177:6–7.
118. Shapiro NI, Trzeciak S, Hollander JE, et al. A prospective, multicenter derivation of a biomarker panel to assess risk of organ dysfunction, shock, and death in emergency department patients with suspected sepsis. *Crit Care Med*. 2009;37:96–104.
119. Vodovotz Y, Liu S, McCloskey C, et al. The hepatocyte as a microbial product-responsive cell. *J Endotoxin Res*. 2001;7:365–373.
120. Miyamoto T, Fujinaga T, Yamashita K, et al. Changes of serum cytokine activities and other parameters in dogs with experimentally induced endotoxic shock. *Jpn J Vet Res*. 1996;44:107–118.
121. Moeniralam HS, Bemelman WA, Romijn JA, et al. Origin of endotoxemia influences the metabolic response to endotoxin in dogs. *J Surg Res*. 1997;73:47–53.
122. Rau S, Kohn B, Richter C, et al. Plasma interleukin-6 response is predictive for severity and mortality in canine systemic inflammatory response syndrome and sepsis. *Vet Clin Pathol*. 2007;36:253–260.
123. Sakaue Y, Nezu Y, Yanagisawa S, et al. Effects of continuous low-dose infusion of lipopolysaccharide on expression of E-selectin and intercellular adhesion molecule-1 messenger RNA and neutrophil accumulation in specific organs in dogs. *Am J Vet Res*. 2005;66:1259–1266.
124. Gebhardt C, Hirschberger J, Rau S, et al. Use of C-reactive protein to predict outcome in dogs with systemic inflammatory response syndrome or sepsis. *J Vet Emerg Crit Care*. 2009;19:450–458.
125. Wiwanitkit V. C-reactive protein in sepsis. *J Vet Emerg Crit Care*. 2010;20:1.
126. Duffy AL, Olea-Popelka FJ, Eucher J, et al. Serum concentrations of monocyte chemoattractant protein-1 in healthy and critically ill dogs. *Vet Clin Pathol*. 2010;39:302–305.
127. Bernard GR. Drotrecogin alfa (activated) (recombinant human activated protein C) for the treatment of severe sepsis. *Crit Care Med*. 2003;31:S85–S93.
128. Madden RM, Ward M, Marlar RA, et al. Protein C activity levels in endotoxin-induced disseminated intravascular coagulation in a dog model. *Thromb Res*. 1989;55:297–307.
129. Shorr AF, Bernard GR, Dhainaut JF, et al. Protein C concentrations in severe sepsis: an early directional change in plasma levels predicts outcome. *Crit Care*. 2006;10:R92.
130. Ranieri VM, Thompson BT, Barie PS, et al. Drotrecogin alfa (activated) in adults with septic shock. *N Engl J Med*. 2012;366:2055–2064.
131. Rogers CL, Rozanski EA. Von Willebrand factor antigen concentration in dogs with sepsis. *J Vet Intern Med*. 2010;24:229–230.
132. Bonczynski JJ, Ludwig LL, Barton LJ, et al. Comparison of peritoneal fluid and peripheral blood pH, bicarbonate, glucose, and lactate concentration as a diagnostic tool for septic peritonitis in dogs and cats. *Vet Surg*. 2003;32:161–166.
133. Ulrich S, Gottschalk C, Straubinger RK, et al. Acceleration of the identification of sepsis-inducing bacteria in cultures of dog and cat blood. *J Small Anim Pract*. 2020;61:42–45.
134. Trung NT, Thau NS, Bang MH, et al. PCR-based Sepsis@Quick test is superior in comparison with blood culture for identification of sepsis-causative pathogens. *Sci Rep*. 2019;9:13663.
135. Mishra D, Satpathy G, Wig N, et al. Evaluation of 16S rRNA broad range PCR assay for microbial detection in serum specimens in sepsis patients. *J Infect Public Health*. 2020;13:998–1002.
136. Peri AM, Harris PNA, Paterson DL. Culture-independent detection systems for bloodstream infection. *Clin Microbiol Infect*. 2022;28:195–201.
137. Balakrishnan A, Silverstein DC. Shock fluids and fluid challenge. In: Silverstein DC, Hopper K, eds. *Small Animal Critical Care Medicine*. St. Louis: Saunders Elsevier; 2015:321–327.
138. Silverstein DC, Santoro-Beer K. Daily intravenous fluid therapy. In: Silverstein DC, Hopper K, eds. *Small Animal Critical Care Medicine*. St Louis: Saunders Elsevier; 2015:316–321.
139. Muller RB, Haase N, Lange T, et al. Acute kidney injury with hydroxyethyl starch 130/0.42 in severe sepsis. *Acta Anaesthesiol Scand*. 2015;59:329–336.
140. Mazzaferro EM, Rudloff E, Kirby R. The role of albumin replacement in the critically ill veterinary patient. *J Vet Emerg Crit Care*. 2002;12:113–124.
141. Rivers EP, Coba V, Whitmill M. Early goal-directed therapy in severe sepsis and septic shock: a contemporary review of the literature. *Curr Opin Anaesthesiol*. 2008;21:128–140.
142. Gupta RG, Hartigan SM, Kashiouris MG, et al. Early goal-directed resuscitation of patients with septic shock: current evidence and future directions. *Crit Care*. 2015;19:286.
143. Waddell LS, Brown AJ. Hemodynamic monitoring. In: Silverstein DC, Hopper K, eds. *Small Animal Critical Care Medicine*. St Louis: Saunders Elsevier; 2015:957–962.
144. Nguyen HB, Jaehne AK, Jayaprakash N, et al. Early goal-directed therapy in severe sepsis and septic shock: insights and comparisons to ProCESS, ProMISe, and ARISE. *Crit Care*. 2016;20:160.
145. De Backer D, Biston P, Devriendt J, et al. Comparison of dopamine and norepinephrine in the treatment of shock. *N Engl J Med*. 2010;362:779–789.
146. Simmons JP, Wohl JS. Catecholamines. In: Silverstein DC, Hopper K, eds. *Small Animal Critical Care Medicine*. St Louis: Saunders Elsevier; 2015:829–835.
147. Silverstein DC. Vasopressin. In: Silverstein DC, Hopper K, eds. *Small Animal Critical Care Medicine*. St Louis: Saunders Elsevier; 2015:835–840.

148. Luckner G, Dunser MW, Jochberger S, et al. Arginine vasopressin in 316 patients with advanced vasodilatory shock. *Crit Care Med.* 2005;33:2659–2666.
149. Ruggiero MS. Effects of vasopressin in septic shock. *AACN Adv Crit Care.* 2008;19:281–287.
150. Russell JA, Walley KR, Gordon AC, et al. Interaction of vasopressin infusion, corticosteroid treatment, and mortality of septic shock. *Crit Care Med.* 2009;37:811–818.
151. Guzman JA, Rosado AE, Kruse JA. Vasopressin vs norepinephrine in endotoxic shock: systemic, renal, and splanchnic hemodynamic and oxygen transport effects. *J Appl Physiol.* 2003;95:803–809.
152. Minneci PC, Deans KJ, Banks SM, et al. Differing effects of epinephrine, norepinephrine, and vasopressin on survival in a canine model of septic shock. *Am J Physiol Heart Circ Physiol.* 2004;287:H2545–H2554.
153. Silverstein DC, Waddell LS, Drobatz KJ, et al. Vasopressin therapy in dogs with dopamine-resistant hypotension and vasodilatory shock. *J Vet Emerg Crit Care.* 2007;17:399–408.
154. Dellinger RP, Levy MM, Carlet JM, et al. Surviving Sepsis Campaign: international guidelines for management of severe sepsis and septic shock. *Crit Care Med 2008.* 2008;36:296–327.
155. Evans L, Rhodes A, Alhazzani W, et al.: Surviving Sepsis Campaign: International Guidelines for Management of Sepsis and Septic Shock 2021, *Crit Care Med.* 2021;49:e1063–e1143.
156. Dickinson AE, Summers JF, Wignal J, et al. Impact of appropriate empirical antimicrobial therapy on outcome of dogs with septic peritonitis. *J Vet Emerg Crit Care.* 2015;25:152–159.
157. Keir I, Dickinson AE. The role of antimicrobials in the treatment of sepsis and critical illness-related bacterial infections: examination of the evidence. *J Vet Emerg Crit Care.* 2015;25:55–62.
158. Sharp CR, DeClue AE, Haak CE, et al. Evaluation of the anti-endotoxin effects of polymyxin B in a feline model of endotoxemia. *J Feline Med Surg.* 2010;12:278–285.
159. Metz DC. Preventing the gastrointestinal consequences of stress-related mucosal disease. *Curr Med Res Opin.* 2005;21:11–18.
160. Metz J, McGrath KM, Copperchini ML, et al. Appropriateness of transfusions of red cells, platelets and fresh frozen plasma. An audit in a tertiary care teaching hospital. *Med J Aust.* 1995;162:572–573, 576-577.
161. Stollman N, Metz DC. Pathophysiology and prophylaxis of stress ulcer in intensive care unit patients. *J Crit Care.* 2005;20:35–45.
162. Papich M. *Saunders Handbook of Veterinary Drugs.* 2 ed. St Louis: Saunders; 2002.
163. Hager DN, Hooper MH, Bernard GR, et al. The Vitamin C, Thiamine and Steroids in Sepsis (VICTAS) Protocol: a prospective, multi-center, double-blind, adaptive sample size, randomized, placebo-controlled, clinical trial. *Trials.* 2019;20:197.
164. Rivers E, Nguyen B, Havstad S, et al. Early goal-directed therapy in the treatment of severe sepsis and septic shock. *N Engl J Med.* 2001;345:1368–1377.
165. Conti-Patara A, de Araujo Caldeira J, de Mattos-Junior E, et al. Changes in tissue perfusion parameters in dogs with severe sepsis/septic shock in response to goal-directed hemodynamic optimization at admission to ICU and the relation to outcome. *J Vet Emerg Crit Care.* 2012;22:409–418.
166. Young BC, Prittie JE, Fox P, et al. Decreased central venous oxygen saturation despite normalization of heart rate and blood pressure post shock resuscitation in sick dogs. *J Vet Emerg Crit Care.* 2014;24:154–161.
167. Marik PE. Critical illness-related corticosteroid insufficiency. *Chest.* 2009;135:181–193.
168. Prigent H, Maxime V, Annane D. Clinical review: corticotherapy in sepsis. *Crit Care.* 2004;8:122–129.
169. Prigent H, Maxime V, Annane D. Science review: mechanisms of impaired adrenal function in sepsis and molecular actions of glucocorticoids. *Crit Care.* 2004;8:243–252.
170. Burkitt JM, Haskins SC, Nelson RW, et al. Relative adrenal insufficiency in dogs with sepsis. *J Vet Intern Med.* 2007;21:226–231.
171. Costello MF, Fletcher DJ, Silverstein DC, et al. Adrenal insufficiency in feline sepsis. In: *35th Critical Care Congress Society of Critical Care Medicine.* 2006. San Francisco, CA.
172. Martin LG, Groman RP. Relative adrenal insufficiency in critical illness. *J Vet Emerg Crit Care.* 2004;14:149–157.
173. Martin LG, Groman RP, Fletcher DJ, et al. Pituitary-adrenal function in dogs with acute critical illness. *J Am Vet Med Assoc.* 2008;233:87–95.
174. Prittie JE, Barton LJ, Peterson ME. Hypothalamo-pituitary-adrenal axis function in critically ill cats. In: *9th International Veterinary Emergency and Critical Care Symposium.* 2003:771. New Orleans, LA.
175. Annane D, Sebille V, Charpentier C, et al. Effect of treatment with low doses of hydrocortisone and fludrocortisone on mortality in patients with septic shock. *JAMA.* 2002;288:862–871.
176. Annane D. Adrenal insufficiency in sepsis. *Curr Pharm Des.* 2008;14:1882–1886.
177. Marik PE, Pastores SM, Annane D, et al. Recommendations for the diagnosis and management of corticosteroid insufficiency in critically ill adult patients: consensus statements from an international task force by the American College of Critical Care Medicine. *Crit Care Med.* 2008;36:1937–1949.
178. Day KM, Haub N, Betts H, et al. Hyperglycemia is associated with morbidity in critically ill children with meningococcal sepsis. *Pediatr Crit Care Med.* 2008;9:636–640.
179. Hirasawa H, Oda S, Nakamura M. Blood glucose control in patients with severe sepsis and septic shock. *World J Gastroenterol.* 2009;15:4132–4136.
180. Lewis KS, Kane-Gill SL, Bobek MB, et al. Intensive insulin therapy for critically ill patients. *Ann Pharmacother.* 2004;38:1243–1251.
181. Zenni GC, McLane MP, Law WR, et al. Hepatic insulin resistance during chronic hyperdynamic sepsis. *Circ Shock.* 1992;37:198–208.
182. Andersen SK, Gjedsted J, Christiansen C, et al. The roles of insulin and hyperglycemia in sepsis pathogenesis. *J Leukoc Biol.* 2004;75:413–421.
183. Marik PE, Raghavan M. Stress-hyperglycemia, insulin and immunomodulation in sepsis. *Intensive Care Med.* 2004;30:748–756.
184. Dronge AS, Perkal MF, Kancir S, et al. Long-term glycemic control and postoperative infectious complications. *Arch Surg.* 2006;141:375–380.
185. Gibson BR, Galiatsatos P, Rabiee A, et al. Intensive insulin therapy confers a similar survival benefit in the burn intensive care unit to the surgical intensive care unit. *Surgery.* 2009;146:922–930.
186. Mesotten D, Swinnen JV, Vanderhoydonc F, et al. Contribution of circulating lipids to the improved outcome of critical illness by glycemic control with intensive insulin therapy. *J Clin Endocrinol Metab.* 2004;89:219–226.
187. Van den Berghe G, Wilmer A, Hermans G, et al. Intensive insulin therapy in the medical ICU. *N Engl J Med.* 2006;354:449–461.
188. Chan DL, Freeman LM, Rozanski E. Prevalence of hyperglycemia in cats presented to the emergency service. *J Vet Emerg Crit Care.* 2002;12:199.
189. Ray CC, Callahan-Clark J, Beckel NF, et al. The prevalence and significance of hyperglycemia in hospitalized cats. *J Vet Emerg Crit Care.* 2009;19:347–351.
190. Syring RS, Otto CM, Drobatz KJ. Hyperglycemia in dogs and cats with head trauma: 122 cases (1997-1999). *J Am Vet Med Assoc.* 2001;218:1124–1129.
191. Torre DM, de Laforcade A, Chan DL. Incidence and clinical relevance of hyperglycemia in critically ill dogs. *J Vet Intern Med.* 2007;21:971–975.
192. Riedemann NC, Guo RF, Ward PA. Novel strategies for the treatment of sepsis. *Nat Med.* 2003;9:517–524.
193. Giroir BP, Scannon PJ, Levin M. Bactericidal/permeability-increasing protein: lessons learned from the phase III, randomized, clinical trial of rBPI21 for adjunctive treatment of children with severe meningococcemia. *Crit Care Med.* 2001;29:S130–S135.
194. Otto CM, Jackson CB, Rogell EJ, et al. Recombinant bactericidal/permeability-increasing protein (rBPI21) for treatment of parvovirus enteritis: a randomized, double-blinded, placebo-controlled trial. *J Vet Intern Med.* 2001;15:355–360.
195. Rewerts JM, McCaw DL, Cohn LA, et al. Recombinant human granulocyte colony-stimulating factor for treatment of puppies with neutropenia secondary to canine parvovirus infection. *J Am Vet Med Assoc.* 1998;213:991–992.

196. Kaziani K, Vassiliou AG, Kotanidou A, et al. Activated protein C has no effect on pulmonary capillary endothelial function in septic patients with acute respiratory distress syndrome: association of endothelial dysfunction with mortality. *Infect Dis Ther.* 2018;7:15–25.
197. Thomas DD, Ridnour LA, Isenberg JS, et al. The chemical biology of nitric oxide: implications in cellular signaling. *Free Radic Biol Med.* 2008;45:18–31.
198. Lopez A, Lorente JA, Steingrub J, et al. Multiple-center, randomized, placebo-controlled, double-blind study of the nitric oxide synthase inhibitor 546C88: effect on survival in patients with septic shock. *Crit Care Med.* 2004;32:21–30.
199. Kopterides P, Falagas ME. Statins for sepsis: a critical and updated review. *Clin Microbiol Infect.* 2009;15:325–334.
200. Terblanche M, Almog Y, Rosenson RS, et al. Statins and sepsis: multiple modifications at multiple levels. *Lancet Infect Dis.* 2007;7:358–368.
201. Tleyjeh IM, Kashour T, Hakim FA, et al. Statins for the prevention and treatment of infections: a systematic review and meta-analysis. *Arch Intern Med.* 2009;169:1658–1667.
202. McAuley DF, Laffey JG, O'Kane CM, et al. Simvastatin in the acute respiratory distress syndrome. *N Engl J Med.* 2014;371:1695–1703.
203. National Heart, Lung, and Blood Institute ARDS Clinical Trials Network, Truwit JD, Bernard GR, et al. Rosuvastatin for sepsis-associated acute respiratory distress syndrome. *N Engl J Med.* 2014;370:2191–2200.
204. Opal SM, Laterre PF, Francois B, et al. Effect of eritoran, an antagonist of MD2-TLR4, on mortality in patients with severe sepsis: the ACCESS randomized trial. *JAMA.* 2013;309:1154–1162.
205. Leon CG, Tory R, Jia J, et al. Discovery and development of toll-like receptor 4 (TLR4) antagonists: a new paradigm for treating sepsis and other diseases. *Pharm Res (N Y).* 2008;25:1751–1761.
206. Tidswell M, Tillis W, Larosa SP, et al. Phase 2 trial of eritoran tetrasodium (E5564), a toll-like receptor 4 antagonist, in patients with severe sepsis. *Crit Care Med.* 2010;38:72–83.
207. Yang H, Ochani M, Li J, et al. Reversing established sepsis with antagonists of endogenous high-mobility group box 1. *Proc Natl Acad Sci U S A.* 2004;101:296–301.
208. Cohen J. Non-antibiotic strategies for sepsis. *Clin Microbiol Infect.* 2009;15:302–307.
209. Wheeler DS, Zingarelli B, Wheeler WJ, et al. Novel pharmacologic approaches to the management of sepsis: targeting the host inflammatory response. *Recent Pat Inflamm Allergy Drug Discov.* 2009;3:96–112.
210. Greenfield CL, Walshaw R. Open peritoneal drainage for treatment of contaminated peritoneal cavity and septic peritonitis in dogs and cats: 24 cases (1980-1986). *J Am Vet Med Assoc.* 1987;191:100–105.
211. Hosgood G, Salisbury SK. Generalized peritonitis in dogs: 50 cases (1975-1986). *J Am Vet Med Assoc.* 1988;193:1448–1450.
212. Mantione N, Otto CM: Characterization of the use of antiemetic agents in dogs with parvoviral enteritis treated at a veterinary teaching hospital: 77 cases (1997-2000), *J Am Vet Med Assoc.* 2005;227:1787–1793.
213. Gotts JE, Matthay MA. Sepsis: pathophysiology and clinical management. *British Med J.* 2016;353:i1585.
214. Jimenez-Dalmaroni MJ, Gerswhin ME, Adamopoulos IE. The critical role of toll-like receptors: from microbial recognition to autoimmunity: a comprehensive review. *Autoimmun Rev.* 2016;15:1–8.
215. Boller EM, Otto CM. Sepsis and septic shock. In: Silverstein DC, Hopper K, eds. *Small Animal Critical Care Medicine.* St Louis: Elsevier; 2015:472–480.
216. Thoen ME, Kerl ME. Characterization of acute kidney injury in hospitalized dogs and evaluation of a veterinary acute kidney injury staging system. *J Vet Emerg Crit Care.* 2011;21:648–657.

124

Bacterial Respiratory Infections (Tracheobronchitis, Pneumonia, and Pyothorax)

Carol Reinero, Tekla Lee-Fowler

KEY POINTS

Bacterial Tracheobronchitis and Pneumonia

- Causes: Primary bacterial pathogens include *Bordetella bronchiseptica* and *Mycoplasma* spp. A wide variety of secondary bacterial pathogens can also be implicated including anaerobes, *Escherichia coli*, *Pasteurella* spp., *Staphylococcus* spp., and *Streptococcus* spp.
- Geographic Distribution: Worldwide.
- Mode of Transmission: Community acquired (contagious) or secondary to aspiration or impaired local or systemic immune defenses.
- Major Clinical Signs: Cough, nasal discharge, sneeze, tachypnea, respiratory distress, cyanosis, and systemic signs of illness (lethargy, anorexia, fever).
- Differential Diagnoses: Differentials for bacterial tracheobronchitis include other nonbacterial infectious airway disorders (primarily viral and parasitic), noninfectious inflammatory airway disease, and structural airway disorders; differentials for bacterial pneumonia include other infectious pneumonia (viral [especially CDV infection], fungal, parasitic, protozoal), noninfectious inflammatory pneumonia (sterile aspiration pneumonia and foreign body pneumonia), neoplasia, interstitial lung disease, cardiogenic or noncardiogenic pulmonary edema, pulmonary vascular disease, and hemorrhage.
- Human Health Significance: *Bordetella bronchiseptica* can cause disease in immunocompromised humans. While further study is needed, MDR bacteria colonizing the canine and feline respiratory tract may be able to colonize humans.

Bacterial Pyothorax

- Causes: Pyothorax is often polymicrobial. Anaerobic bacteria and mixtures of anaerobic and facultative aerobic bacteria are common in both dogs and cats. Although more often cultured from the pleural fluid of cats, *Pasteurella* is also implicated in both species.
- Geographic Distribution: Worldwide.
- Primary Mode of Transmission: Direct inoculation of the pleural cavity (e.g., migrating foreign material, bite wounds, trauma), extension of local infection (e.g., pneumonia, lung abscess, thoracic wall infection), hematogenous spread.
- Major Clinical Signs: Restrictive respiratory pattern (rapid, shallow respiration with increased inspiratory effort), obtundation, exercise intolerance, cough, lethargy, anorexia, weight loss, and fever. Cats may exhibit hypothermia, bradycardia, and hypersalivation.
- Differential Diagnoses: Other nonbacterial infections that can be associated with pleural effusion (e.g., *Aspergillus* spp.), chylothorax, hemothorax, neoplasia, FIP (cats).
- Human Health Significance: Because commensal organisms of the oral cavity and upper respiratory tract are most typically associated with pyothorax in dogs and cats, pyothorax does not have human health significance.

BACTERIAL TRACHEOBRONCHITIS AND PNEUMONIA

ETIOLOGY, EPIDEMIOLOGY, AND PATHOGENESIS

There is a continuum between the conducting airways and pulmonary parenchyma without a physical barrier separating the respiratory tract from the external environment. In healthy dogs, cultivable bacteria have been identified from the upper airways, lower airways, and thoracotomy-derived pulmonary parenchyma, with the assumption that bacteria identified in the lung were transient populations derived from the pharynx due to aspiration.[1] In cats, an analogous study with culture of lung tissue has not been performed, but healthy cats similarly have cultivable bacteria from their upper and lower airways.

Common bacterial isolates have been obtained from nasal swabs (Table 124.1) and airway lavage specimens (Table 124.2) of clinically healthy dogs and cats. In one study, bacterial isolates from the trachea in healthy dogs included *Streptococcus* spp., *Staphylococcus* spp., *Pasteurella multocida*, *Klebsiella pneumoniae*, and *Corynebacterium* spp.; when considering simultaneous positive cultures from the pharynx and trachea, in 80% of dogs, the same organism found in the trachea was identified in the pharynx.[2] These results underscore the fact that presence of bacteria cultured from the respiratory tract does not equate with infection; healthy dogs and cats have an abundance of respiratory commensal organisms. Respiratory disease may occur due to a shift in abundance of one or more commensal species to create inflammation and damage to tissue. Certain bacteria considered to be contagious may also exist as part of the respiratory microbiome, including *Bordetella bronchiseptica*, *Mycoplasma* spp., and some *Streptococcus* strains. Bacterial respiratory tract infections may also originate from primary pathogens in the environment and/or reservoir hosts such as *Nocardia* spp., *Mycobacterium* spp., or *Yersinia* spp.

Complimentary techniques to standard laboratory-based cultures have provided a wealth of information on resident complex microbial populations in the respiratory tract. Using next-generation sequencing of microbial DNA, healthy dogs have been shown to harbor a rich and diverse respiratory microbiota.[3–5] While bacterial communities from the upper and lower airways are topographically continuous, sharing

TABLE 124.1 Bacterial Species Frequently Isolated from Nasal Swabs of Healthy Dogs and Cats[a]

Dogs[122–124]	Cats[125]
Gram-positive aerobic or facultative	
Staphylococcus spp. (coagulase negative)	*Streptococcus* spp.
Streptococcus spp. (alpha and non-hemolytic)	*Staphylococcus* spp.
Corynebacterium spp.	*Corynebacterium* spp.
Bacillus spp.	*Micrococcus* spp.
Staphylococcus spp. (coagulase positive)	
Streptococcus spp. (beta-hemolytic)	
Gram-negative aerobic or facultative	
Neisseria spp.	*Pasteurella multocida*
Escherichia coli	*Escherichia coli*
Enterobacter spp.	*Pseudomonas aeruginosa*
Pasteurella multocida	*Proteus* spp.
Moraxella spp.	*Klebsiella* spp.
Proteus spp.	*Enterobacter* spp.
Pseudomonas aeruginosa	*Bordetella bronchiseptica*
Alcaligenes spp.	*Moraxella* spp.
Bordetella bronchiseptica	*Mycoplasma* spp.
Obligate anaerobes	*Clostridium* spp.

[a]Bacteria are listed in approximate order of frequency of isolation.

many bacterial species, there are distinct differences between sites suggesting each possesses unique resident communities, and lower airway populations are not solely a reflection of aspirated upper airway bacteria.[3] Healthy cats evaluated over time demonstrated a rich lower airway microbiome with dynamic respiratory bacterial populations.[6] The microbiome of the feline nasal cavity has also been examined, and was shown to display a high degree of individual variability; the most prevalent species in healthy cats and cats with URTD was *Moraxella* spp.[7] Use of DNA-based sequencing to characterize resident bacterial populations may provide insight to interpretation of microbial cultures as well as aid in an understanding of the impact of the respiratory microbiome on health and disease. Similar to GI dysbiosis in which disruption of the normally dominating species and imbalances of other minority species has been associated with a variety of local and systemic illnesses, respiratory dysbiosis has been identified in dogs and cats with inflammatory airway disease[8,9] and dogs treated with antimicrobial drugs.[5] Understanding deviations from a healthy respiratory microbiome is relevant to tracheobronchial and pulmonary bacterial infections and is a field that is still in its infancy.

Identification of bacteria solely using routine cultures is not synonymous with bacterial infection. A positive culture needs to be interpreted in light of clinical signs, evidence of concurrent suppurative inflammation ideally with intracellular bacteria, and bacterial growth conditions (e.g., heavy growth, single species). In general, the host effectively prevents bacterial respiratory infections by physical and chemical barriers and the innate and adaptive immune system. Traditionally, bacterial infection of the airways or pulmonary parenchyma has been thought to result secondary to inhalation of primary respiratory pathogens (aerosols or direct oronasal contact), macro- or microaspiration, compromised respiratory defenses, direct extension (e.g., migrating foreign body, penetrating wound, bronchoesophageal fistula), or hematogenous spread. Additional research is needed

TABLE 124.2 Bacterial Species Frequently Isolated from Tracheal and Bronchoalveolar Lavage Specimens from Healthy Dogs and Cats

Dogs[1,2]	Cats[12,126]
Staphylococcus spp. (coagulase positive and negative)	*Staphylococcus* spp.
Streptococcus spp. (alpha and non-hemolytic)	*Streptococcus* spp.
Pasteurella multocida	*Micrococcus* spp.
Klebsiella pneumoniae	*Escherichia coli*
Enterobacter aerogenes	*Pasteurella multocida*
Acinetobacter spp.	*Pseudomonas aeruginosa*
Moraxella spp.	*Klebsiella* spp.
Corynebacterium spp.	*Enterobacter* spp.
	Proteus spp.
	Haemophilus felis

to determine the role of dysbiosis in bacterial tracheobronchitis and pneumonia when co-morbid respiratory disorders alter the local microenvironment.

Bacterial tracheobronchitis and pneumonia are two separate disease syndromes that can share routes of exposure (and thus types of infecting bacteria) as well as predisposing factors of susceptibility. Both conditions can be acute or chronic and primary or secondary.

Primary bacterial tracheobronchitis in immunocompetent dogs (i.e., community-acquired CIRD complex; the reader is referred to Chapter 28 for more details) is generally self-limiting with supportive care. Primary bacterial tracheobronchitis in cats is rare, with very common upper respiratory tract infections nearly always causing nasal and ocular but not tracheobronchial pathology. Unlike in dogs where *B. bronchiseptica* is often considered a highly contagious primary pathogen, *B. bronchiseptica* can be found in healthy cats and in cats without cough (with or without upper respiratory tract infections) housed in shelters with canine outbreaks.[10,11] *Mycoplasma* species are considered normal commensals of the upper respiratory tract and have the potential to be opportunistic invaders. Attempts to isolate *Mycoplasma* spp. from the lower airway of clinically healthy cats have not been successful,[12,13] but they are typically associated with concurrent airway disease suggesting that they are most likely opportunistic invaders. Their role as a primary pathogen causing bronchitis is still unclear (see Suggested Reading list for more information).[14] (Editor's note: In 2021, a novel bacterial species belonging to the genus *Filobacterium* was reported in association with chronic neutrophilic bronchitis in cats from Europe and Australia.[15] The name *Filobacterium felis* was proposed; a related organism, *Filobacterium rodentium* (previously cilia-associated respiratory bacillus [CARB]) is considered a primary pathogen of rodents. The existence of similar organisms has been described in cats with and without respiratory disease from the United States.[16,17]

Secondary bacterial tracheobronchitis is usually associated with inflammatory or structural airway disease of the dog and cat and can be responsible for clinical disease exacerbation. Bacterial tracheobronchitis has been reported secondary to airway collapse,[18,19] chronic bronchitis, eosinophilic bronchitis/eosinophilic bronchopneumopathy, bronchiectasis, or bronchomalacia in dogs. In cats, reports of positive bacterial cultures have been linked to airway disease including asthma, chronic bronchitis, and bronchiectasis. Bacterial tracheobronchitis that is associated with bacterial species that are not "community-acquired" should prompt a search for an underlying disorder. It is reiterated

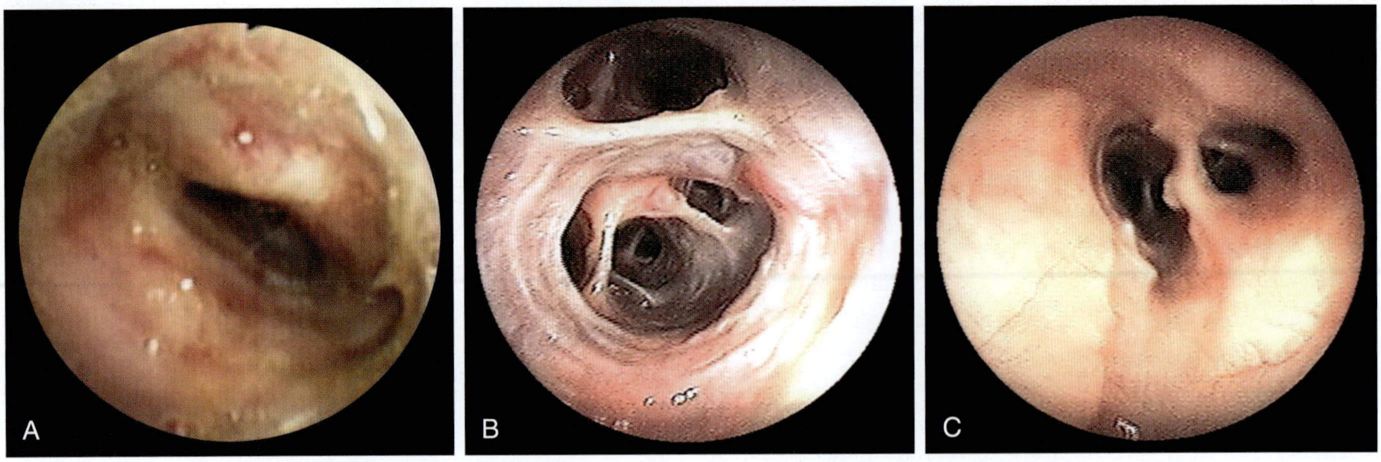

Fig. 124.1 A–C Endoscopic appearance of airway disorders that may predispose to secondary bacterial infection. (A) In tracheal collapse, the dorsal tracheal membrane sags into the lumen and the tracheal cartilages become flattened. In this case, there is accumulation of mucoid and purulent secretions associated with a positive bacterial culture. (B) Bronchiectatic airways are dilated and cavernous, failing to taper appropriately with distal progression of the endoscope. (C) The endoscopic appearance of bronchomalacia reflects a reduced and irregular airway lumen from softening of the cartilage. Note the loss of circular outlines of the airways (i.e., flattening, distortion, and narrowing) leading to airway collapse. (Courtesy of Dr. Carol Reinero, University of Missouri.)

that identifying cultivable bacteria does not necessarily imply active infection.

Dogs

Tracheal Collapse (Fig. 124.1A)

While bacteria can be frequently cultured from specimens collected from the trachea in dogs with tracheal collapse, the absence of concurrent evidence of inflammation or intracellular bacteria makes diagnosis of secondary bacterial infections unlikely in most cases.[19] The prevalence of positive bacterial cultures of dogs with tracheal collapse decreased in one study after tracheal stent placement.[20]

Chronic Bronchitis

Chronic bronchitis is classically associated with cough, mucus hypersecretion, and neutrophilic airway inflammation.[21] Chronic bronchitis is considered a sterile process that occurs secondary to airway epithelial damage and impaired mucociliary function. While dogs with chronic bronchitis have impaired mucosal defense and can theoretically be predisposed to infection, infection appears uncommon especially when quantitative, not qualitative cultures are performed.[22] Qualitative cultures using the threshold of $> 1.7 \times 10^3$ CFU/mL of BAL fluid are proposed to represent clinically relevant bacterial growth. Unlike qualitative cultures, quantitative cultures take into consideration the possibility of contamination from upper airways and/or microaspiration (subclinical aspiration of upper GI secretions) without true infection.

Eosinophilic Bronchopneumopathy

Eosinophilic bronchopneumopathy has been associated with positive BAL cultures (albeit qualitative) including growth of *Pseudomonas aeruginosa*, *K. pneumoniae*, and *Aeromonas* spp., among others.[23] As eosinophilic bronchopneumopathy can be associated with bronchiectasis, it is unclear if the aforementioned identified bacteria were a sequela to eosinophilic inflammation and/or bronchiectasis. Another study of 75 dogs with eosinophilic inflammation in BAL fluid (due to eosinophilic bronchopneumopathy, eosinophilic bronchitis, or eosinophilic pneumonia) reported bacterial growth in BAL cultures rarely; only three dogs had positive culture results (*Pasteurella* spp., *Pasteurella canis*, and mixed growth of *Escherichia coli* and *Streptococcus* spp.).[24]

Bronchiectasis (Fig. 124.1B)

Bronchiectasis may be a consequence of primary ciliary dyskinesia, chronic bronchitis, infectious pneumonia, eosinophilic bronchopneumopathy, and tracheal collapse.[24–28] Bronchiectasis can also predispose to recurrent bacterial infection because of poor clearance of mucus and exudate in the distal airways and impaired local immune responses. This in turn creates a vicious cycle of inflammation, secondary infection, and further airway damage. In one study of dogs with bronchiectasis, bacterial growth from airway lavage specimens was frequent (17/18 dogs) with a variety of bacterial species isolated as either alone (7 dogs) or as part of polymicrobial infections (10 dogs).[26] In another study, bacteria (predominantly *Streptococcus* spp., *Pasteurella* spp., enterics, and *Stenotrophomonas maltophila*) were isolated in 24/86 dogs (28%) with bronchiectasis.[27]

Bronchomalacia (Fig. 124.1C)

In bronchomalacia, weakened bronchial walls, with associated static or dynamic reduction of airway diameters results in clinical signs of cough, wheeze, and respiratory distress. In one study, intracellular bacteria were noted on cytologic examination of BAL specimens in 25/45 dogs with bronchomalacia; cultures were not performed.[29] Another study documented intra- and extracellular bacteria in 39% of specimens, with cultures yielding one isolate in 62% and two isolates in 39% of specimens.[30] The most common isolates were *B. bronchiseptica*, *Alcaligenes* spp., *Pasteurella* spp., and *Bacillus* spp. Dogs that had bronchoscopic evaluation for other causes of cough that had concurrent tracheal and bronchial collapse were less likely to have bacterial infection than dogs without evidence of airway collapse.[31]

Bacterial Pneumonia

Bacterial pneumonia generally arises due to local or systemic immune compromise and can be life-threatening. Primary bacterial pneumonia caused by *B. bronchiseptica*, virulent strains of *Streptococcus* spp., and possibly *Mycoplasma* (particularly *Mycoplasma cynos*) tends to occur most frequently in dogs under a year of age, and dogs with immune defects (overexuberant or insufficient immune responses), concurrent respiratory infections, or those in stressful or overcrowded environments.[32–34] Dogs with a variety of predisposing factors including dysphagia, regurgitation, gastroesophageal reflux, vomiting, diminished consciousness (secondary to drugs including anesthesia, or neurologic disease), and impaired airway defenses (e.g., brachycephalic airway syndrome) can develop aspiration pneumonia.[35–41] Aerodigestive disorders often go unrecognized because aspiration pneumonia can develop in the absence of GI signs.[42]

Aspiration pneumonia is not synonymous with bacterial infection, as a sterile chemical pneumonitis may occur. Commonly identified bacteria from dogs with aspiration pneumonia include *E. coli*, *Mycoplasma* spp., *Pasteurella* spp., *Staphylococcus* spp., *Klebsiella* spp., and *Enterococcus* spp.[38] Impaired airway defenses can also cause pneumonia even in the absence of aspiration, and these disorders can be congenital or acquired.[43] Direct extension of bacterial infection to the parenchyma can occur from inhaled[35] or migrating foreign bodies.[39,44,45] The most common isolates from dogs with foreign bodies include anaerobes, *Pasteurella* spp., *Streptococcus* spp., and *Actinomyces* spp.[46] Often foreign bodies are inhaled into caudodorsal principle bronchi; in other words the accessory, right, and left caudal bronchi.

Ventilator-associated pneumonia represents a type of nosocomial infection that is hospital-acquired.[39] Patients requiring mechanical ventilation have a different spectrum of bacterial isolates from airway cultures when compared with other patients with respiratory disease; these isolates are more likely to be resistant to the common antimicrobials used to treat patients with pneumonia.[47]

Cats

Chronic Bronchitis

In cats, secondary bacterial bronchitis is far less common than noninfectious inflammatory airway disease. Importantly, quantitative tracheobronchial lavage cultures in healthy cats were positive in 8 of 24 cats in one study[12] and 10 of 13 (77%) in another.[10] In the latter study, cultures yielded 100–100,000 CFU/mL, and organisms such as *Staphylococcus* spp., *Streptococcus* spp., *B. bronchiseptica*, and *P. multocida* were identified. In that same study, 42% of cats with bronchopulmonary disease (i.e., asthma and chronic bronchitis) had positive cultures, mostly yielding low numbers of bacteria.[10] Positive cultures for *Mycoplasma* species were not identified in the first study or performed in the second, but are of interest as in human asthma, mycoplasmas are postulated to contribute to induction of and exacerbation of disease. In a more recent study, *Mycoplasma* spp. were detected in BAL fluid from 6 of 17 cats with asthma/chronic bronchitis and 4 of 9 sick cats without respiratory disease, which was not a significant difference.[48] Overall, bacterial bronchitis (without involvement of the pulmonary parenchyma) in cats is rare, with 1/245 cats with necropsy-confirmed lower respiratory tract infection attributed to bronchitis alone.[49]

Bronchiectasis

Bronchiectasis in cats has been associated with inflammatory airway disease, pneumonia, and neoplasia.[50–53] Radiographic evidence of bronchiectasis was noted in 43% of cats with aspiration pneumonia, inflammatory airway disease, and bronchopneumonia in one study.[53] It has also been reported in cats with bronchial dysgenesis, presumptive primary ciliary dyskinesia, and broncholithiasis.[54–56] Bronchiectasis is rarely described in cats when compared with dogs, with too few positive cultures to reliably report common bacterial species that act as secondary invaders.[50]

Bacterial Pneumonia

Bacterial pneumonia is rare in the cat. Even when present, it may be difficult to identify as some cats may lack clinical signs, inflammatory leukograms, or classic radiographic lesions.[57] Bacteria often gain access to the respiratory tract through a hematogenous route, including from the GI tract, uterus, umbilicus, gingiva, and bite wounds.[57] Other reported routes include inhalation (aspiration or from inhaling airborne bacteria) and local extension.[53,57] Although an uncommon condition in the cat compared with the dog, approximately one third of cats treated for laryngeal paralysis with bilateral arytenoid lateralization developed aspiration pneumonia.[58] The most common underlying conditions in cats with aspiration pneumonia in another study from a tertiary referral institution were megaesophagus, esophageal stricture, esophageal dysmotility, and acute or chronic vomiting; 27% had a recent history of general anesthesia.[53] Mycoplasmas, *Pasteurella* spp., *Streptococcus* spp., and anaerobes represented the most common bacterial isolates from airway lavage specimens from cats with bronchopneumonia.[53] In contrast, mycoplasmas were not isolated from cats with aspiration pneumonia; cultures from these cats yielded aerobic gram-positive or gram-negative bacteria and/or anaerobes.

CLINICAL FEATURES

Clinical Signs and Physical Examination Findings

Dogs with primary or secondary bacterial bronchitis may show no signs, or have respiratory signs, generally cough. Contagious causes of tracheobronchitis may be associated with involvement of other parts of the respiratory tract, thus additional clinical signs referable to those sites may be noted (e.g., sneezing or nasal discharge, see Chapter 28). Dogs with secondary bacterial bronchitis may have clinical signs associated with an underlying disorder, for example, stridor or wheeze with airway collapse. Secondary infection should be suspected in stable patients with chronic tracheobronchial disorders that suddenly develop signs of disease exacerbation.

If systemic signs such as fever, lethargy, or inappetence are present, this should prompt search for pneumonia or another co-morbid respiratory condition as systemic signs are rarely seen in dogs with bacterial bronchitis. There should be a high index of suspicion for CDV infection in young dogs that develop these signs. Canine bacterial pneumonia may be associated with local signs such as nasal discharge, cough, tachypnea, adventitial lung sounds, decreased lung sounds in regions of consolidation, exercise intolerance, respiratory distress (mixed inspiratory and expiratory distress), and cyanosis; additionally, systemic signs can be seen such as fever, anorexia, lethargy, dehydration, weakness, and weight loss.[38,39,59] Some animals with pneumonia show no signs or only a few of these signs. Hemoptysis is rare but reported in dogs.[60] Other clinical signs may reflect an underlying illness, for example, vomiting or regurgitation in the case of aspiration pneumonia.[38]

As mentioned above, there is controversy about the role of *B. bronchiseptica* and *Mycoplasma* spp. in feline tracheobronchitis as these organisms can be isolated from many clinically healthy cats that lack respiratory signs (see Chapters 55 and 57).[48] Cats with secondary bronchial infection may be subclinically infected or have clinical signs (usually cough; sometimes wheeze, tachypnea, and respiratory distress) relative to their underlying inflammatory airway disease or bronchiectasis.[10,48,50] Many owners do not recognize cough in cats, confusing it with "hacking" up hairballs or retching. Cats with aspiration pneumonia may show only systemic signs of illness such as fever, lethargy, and/or inappetence. In contrast to dogs, cats with pneumonia often lack clinical respiratory signs, especially cough. In one retrospective study, cough was significantly more common in cats with bacterial pneumonia (25/26 cats, 96%) or inflammatory airway disease (30/44 cats, 68%) than in cats with aspiration pneumonia (8/33 cats, 24%). In another study of cats with fatal infectious pneumonia (of which 54% were bacterial), 36% lacked clinical signs referable to the respiratory tract.[57] Of the cats displaying respiratory signs, tachypnea or respiratory distress and nasal discharge were most common; cough was present in only 8%

of cats. Systemic signs of illness (anorexia, lethargy, and fever) were absent in 41% of these cats despite histopathologic evidence of systemic infection in 74% of cats. A high index of suspicion for pneumonia is required in cats, especially if evidence of infection exists in other organs. In a review of 21 cases of lower respiratory tract infection in cats that were not all fatal, signs were chronic cough (11), acute cough (6), respiratory distress (2), anorexia (1), and neurologic signs (1).[61]

DIAGNOSIS

The diagnosis of bacterial tracheobronchitis or pneumonia is made based on a combination of historical information (e.g., exposure to contagious pathogens, underlying co-morbid respiratory conditions or disorders predisposing to aspiration, etc.), clinical signs, radiographic findings and ideally findings on cytologic examination of respiratory specimens (suppurative inflammation with extra- or intracellular bacteria), and a positive culture. With the exception of the transtracheal wash and FNA, collection of respiratory specimens is performed under general anesthesia. A step-wise approach should be taken: functional laryngeal examination using doxapram to stimulate deep respiration, thorough oropharyngeal examination (including sweeping the tonsillar crypts for foreign material), CT imaging (if indicated), endoscopic examination of the trachea and bronchi (if indicated), collection of respiratory specimens for cytology and culture, and choanal examination (retroflexed view using an endoscope). Before anesthesia, there are a wide variety of minimally invasive respiratory diagnostics that can help define underlying or concurrent conditions and gauge severity, extent, and cause of infection (discussed below).

Laboratory Findings

Complete Blood Count, Serum Biochemical Profile, and Urinalysis

Although not specific to the respiratory system, the minimum database, including a CBC, serum biochemical profile, and urinalysis, can provide useful information regarding systemic health. Especially in the case of bacterial pneumonia, a systemic response to infection or organ dysfunction may be detected. Dogs and cats with bacterial pneumonia can have normal or abnormal leukograms.[38,39,57,59] Abnormalities include a neutrophilia with a left shift or neutropenia. Peripheral eosinophilia may be present in dogs with eosinophilic bronchopneumopathy[23,24] or cats with asthma.[62] Because bacterial pneumonia can result from hematogenous spread of bacterial infection originating elsewhere in the body, sepsis and multiple organ dysfunction can contribute to morbidity and mortality, making a serum biochemical profile and urinalysis useful to determine the extent of disease. They may also reflect an underlying disorder associated with impaired immune function (e.g., endocrinopathy).[43]

Diagnostic Tests for Pathogens Other Than Bacteria

Other infectious agents affecting the respiratory tract should be considered in the differential diagnosis (viruses such as CDV, atypical bacteria, protozoa such as *Toxoplasma gondii*, fungi, and parasites), with diagnostic tests selected based on the history (geographic location, season, length of illness, other systemic signs), minimum database (e.g., presence of thrombocytopenia), and physical examination findings. Tests may include fecal analysis (fecal flotation or Baermann analysis for parasites) or blood or urine testing (e.g., serology for antibodies to *Leptospira*, *T. gondii*; parasite or fungal antigen testing).

Assessment of Oxygenation and Ventilatory Status

Arterial blood gas analysis is useful to determine the severity of respiratory compromise as it can provide information on gas exchange and acid-base balance which can be disrupted with bacterial respiratory disease (in particular pneumonia). Hypoxemia ($PaO_2 \leq 80$ mmHg at sea level) can be detected in roughly three quarters of dogs with aspiration pneumonia that have arterial blood gases measured.[38,59] Hypocapnia or hypercapnia has also been described.[59] The alveolar-arterial (A-a) oxygen gradient can be increased; values > 15 mmHg indicate lung dysfunction.[38] Serial use of arterial blood gas measurements can help to determine what treatment to use (e.g., supplemental oxygen, mechanical ventilation) as well as provide information on response to treatment. Pulse oximetry is a simple, rapid, widely available, and noninvasive indicator of oxygen status, but is relatively insensitive and does not provide information on ventilatory or acid-base status. In patients receiving mechanical ventilation, capnography can provide information about ventilatory status.

Diagnostic Imaging

Radiography, fluoroscopy, ultrasonography, and CT have been used to image the respiratory tract. Each have distinct advantages and disadvantages.

Plain Radiography

Thoracic and possibly cervical radiography should be performed first, with a minimum of two views (lateral and ventrodorsal or dorsoventral); however, both right and left lateral views are recommended because differential aeration that results from positional atelectasis can improve or impair visualization of lesions.[39] Static airway collapse may be appreciated with standard views (Fig. 124.2), however, inspiratory and expiratory cervical and thoracic radiographs aid in diagnosis of dynamic tracheal or mainstem bronchial collapse. Thoracic radiography may demonstrate bronchial or bronchointerstitial patterns with chronic bronchitis, eosinophilic bronchitis (Fig. 124.3), or feline asthma, with hyperinflation and/or lobar atelectasis in the latter condition.[62,63] Radiographic findings in eosinophilic bronchopneumopathy

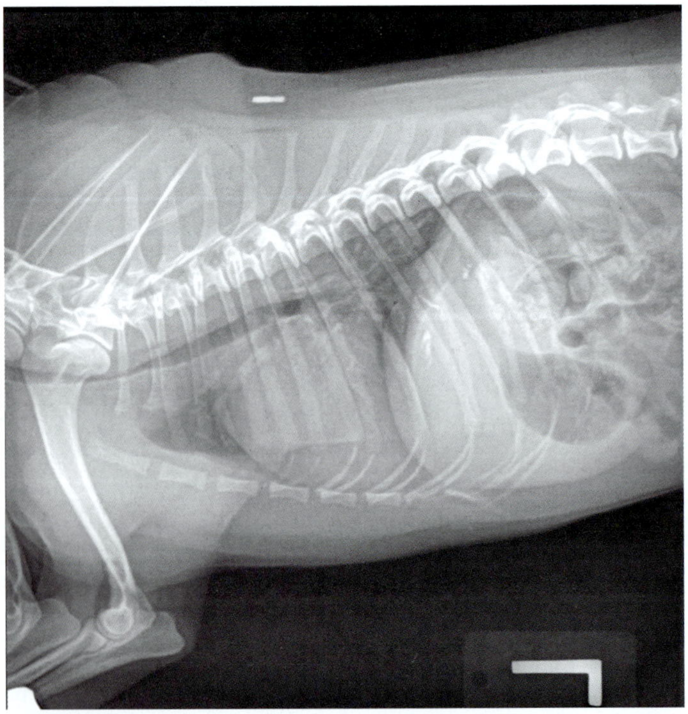

Fig. 124.2 Left lateral thoracic radiograph showing tracheal collapse in the region of the thoracic inlet. (Courtesy of Dr. Carol Reinero, University of Missouri.)

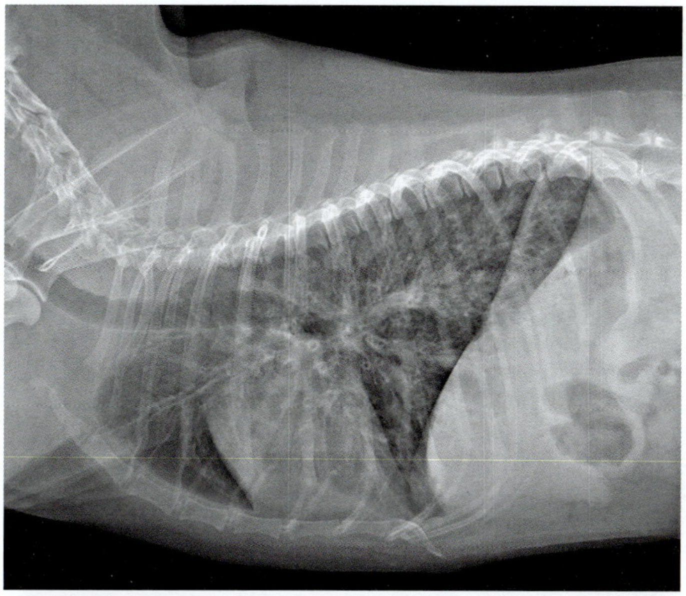

Fig. 124.3 Left lateral thoracic radiograph from a dog with eosinophilic bronchitis demonstrating a severe bronchointerstitial pattern with prominent peribronchial cuffing. (Courtesy of Dr. Carol Reinero, University of Missouri.)

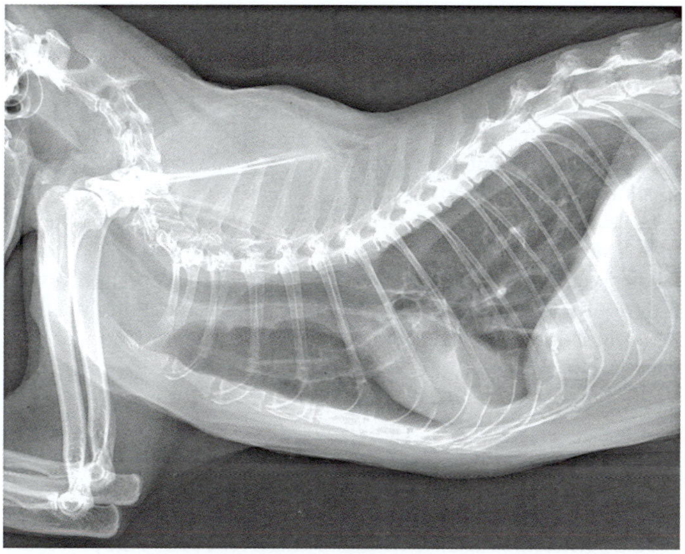

Fig. 124.4 Right lateral thoracic radiograph demonstrating bronchiectasis in a cat. There is a large poorly tapering bronchus (proximally larger in diameter than the trachea) leading to the left cranial lung lobe. (Courtesy of Dr. Carol Reinero, University of Missouri.)

in dogs include a bronchial or bronchointerstitial pattern or an alveolar pattern; bronchiectasis was seen in 26% of cases in one report[23] and 60% in another.[24]

Radiographic features of bronchiectasis include thickened airway walls with a lack of tapering as the airways track to the periphery with either a cylindrical or saccular (cystic) shape (Fig. 124.4).[26,50] Dogs with bronchomalacia generally lack radiographic evidence of bronchial collapse, but can have bronchial or bronchointerstitial patterns, poor visibility of their lobar bronchi, or have normal radiographs.[29,30] In dogs and cats with pneumonia, interstitial, alveolar, and mixed patterns are commonly seen with focal, multifocal, and diffuse distributions.[39,57] Aspiration pneumonia in dogs most commonly affects the right middle lung lobe, and plant awn pneumonia frequently involves the accessory and caudal lobes; however, any lung lobe can be affected.[38,39,45] Right middle lung lobe consolidation in cats can occur not only with aspiration pneumonia but also with bronchopneumonia and inflammatory airway disease.[53]

Videofluoroscopy

Videofluoroscopy allows visualization of the intra- and extra-thoracic trachea and mainstem bronchi during the breathing cycle and with spontaneous and induced cough. It can be helpful for diagnosis of airway collapse that is not appreciated on static plain radiographs. Videofluoroscopic swallow studies (VFSS) can also be used to determine if a swallowing disorder may be contributing to aspiration pneumonia.[42,64] Although under-recognized, there are many respiratory disorders that result from aspiration (aside from aspiration pneumonia) which affect the airways and parenchyma and can contribute to secondary bacterial infections.[35]

Ultrasonographic Examination

Thoracic ultrasonography can be used to evaluate the lungs and pleural space in cases of lung lobe consolidation, masses, pulmonary abscess, and foreign bodies.[44,45,65] A combination of transthoracic, transesophageal, and intraoperative ultrasonography helped to identify 91% of dogs with migrating grass awns in one study.[44] Lung ultrasonography was also useful for identification and monitoring of cardiogenic pulmonary edema; this is evidenced by an increase in the number of artifacts known as "B-lines" caused by increased pulmonary water.[67] Ultrasonography can also be used to guide collection of specimens by FNA. The Vet BLUE (veterinary bedside lung ultrasound exam) scan is emerging as a rapid POC examination used to screen dogs and cats with respiratory compromise, including those with lung consolidation.[67,68] A major limitation of ultrasound is the requirement for lesions to extend to the periphery as ultrasound cannot penetrate through aerated lung.

Computed Tomography

Cervical and thoracic CT can be performed to obtain further information regarding structural abnormalities and provide more accurate correlative information with histopathologic lesions. Advantages over plain radiography include increased sensitivity and ability to provide three-dimensional reconstructions to eliminate superimposition of body parts. In particular, CT is more sensitive for detection of bronchiectasis than plain radiography.[39] It can also be a useful tool for surgical planning. Paired inspiratory and expiratory scans achieved with breath holds at end inspiration and end expiration can highlight dynamic airway collapse inclusive of tracheal collapse and bronchomalacia (Fig. 124.5A and B). Peribronchial cuffing or increases in the peribronchovascular density may be seen with inflammatory airway disorders. CT changes associated with eosinophilic bronchopneumopathy include increased bronchial wall thickening, intraluminal bronchial plugging, opacity of the parenchyma (e.g., nodules and masses), and bronchiectasis.[69] Pneumonia can present with increased opacity of the lung including ground glass opacity and consolidation. In some cases, foreign bodies may be seen, such as in airways.[39,45] CT findings can also raise suspicion for some infectious diseases of the lung other than "routine" bacterial infections, such as mycobacterial, fungal, and parasitic diseases.

Tracheobronchoscopy

Endoscopic examination allows direct visualization of the trachea and bronchi which is valuable for diagnosing structural abnormalities such as tracheal collapse, bronchiectasis, and bronchomalacia (see Fig.

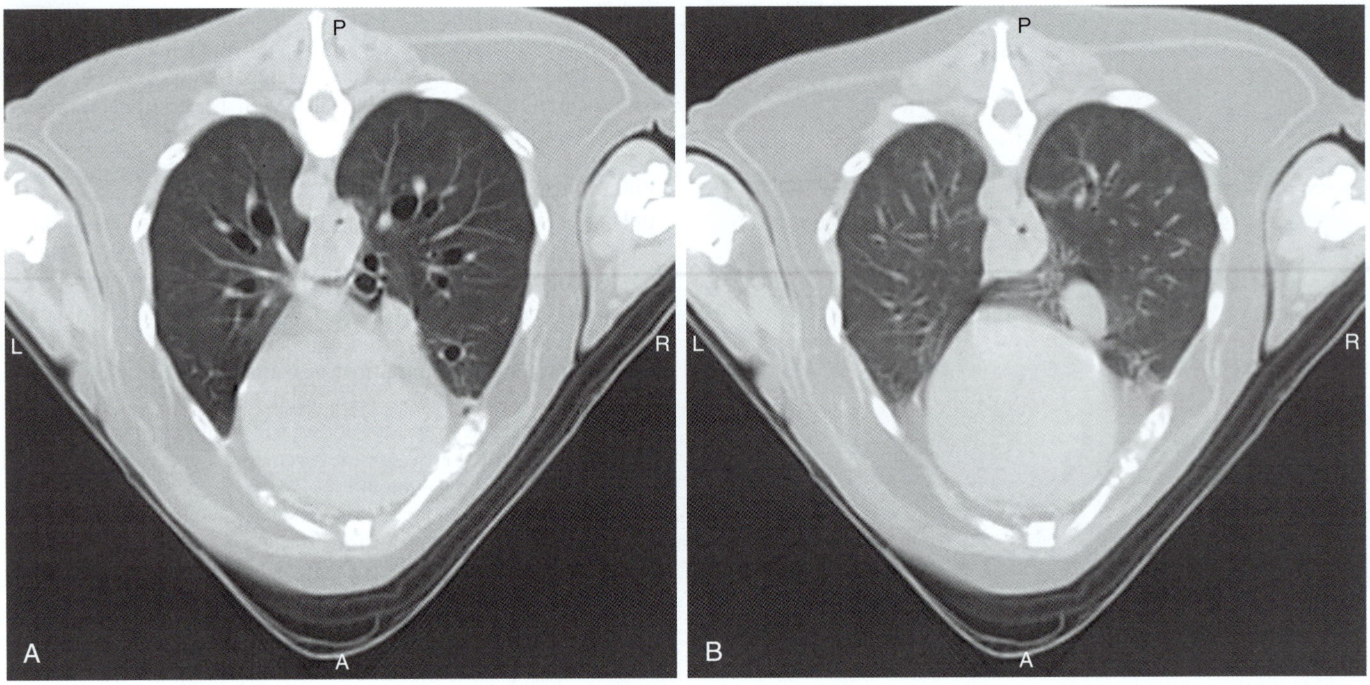

Fig. 124.5 Axial computed tomographic images at the same section from a dog with dynamic airway collapse. During inspiration (A) bronchi are round and open but collapse nearly completely during expiration (B). (Courtesy of Dr. Carol Reinero, University of Missouri.)

124.1A–C). Nonspecific changes associated with inflammatory airway disease such as thickened mucosa, hyperemia, and mucus hypersecretion may also be seen. Another use of endoscopy is to facilitate collection of specimens using brush catheters, transbronchial needles, BAL, and biopsy forceps for culture or microscopic examination from locally affected areas of the lung. Endoscopy can also be used to remove foreign bodies (e.g., grass awn) (Fig. 124.6).

Microbiologic Tests

Cytologic Diagnosis

Specimens for cytologic evaluation can be collected using FNA, transtracheal washing, endotracheal washing, BAL, bronchial brushing, or by making impression smears from tissue collected using biopsy forceps. Visible strands of exudate may then be teased onto a microscope slide, smeared, and stained. Small quantities of material can be centrifuged and smears made of the sediment. New methylene blue wet mounts and Wright-Giemsa or Gram stain of air-dried smears can be used for identification of cellular elements and bacteria. Bacterial infections are typically associated with degenerate neutrophils and intracellular bacteria; in addition, excess mucus, proteinaceous material, and activated alveolar macrophages can be present. Bacteria are demonstrable only in a fraction of washings from pneumonic animals, and their absence in cytologic specimens, especially if the patient has been placed on antibacterial therapy, does not rule out bacterial pneumonia.

Transtracheal lavage. This is well tolerated by the majority of large dogs and requires only minimal restraint of the unanesthetized patient, although some dogs require mild sedation. Endotracheal washing with anesthesia (see later discussion) is usually used for small dogs and cats. Although complications from transtracheal washing and aspiration are uncommon, the procedure is not without risk. Transtracheal washing should not be attempted in the fractious or uncooperative patient without adequate chemical and manual restraint. Contraindications include defects in hemostasis, severe pyoderma of the ventral skin of the neck, and respiratory distress. The most common complication associated with transtracheal washing is subcutaneous emphysema. Other complications include endotracheal hemorrhage, tracheal laceration, and infection at the puncture site.

Endotracheal lavage. Endotracheal lavage is recommended for small dogs and cats and requires short-acting general anesthesia. The volume of sterile nonbacteriostatic saline recommended has ranged in small animals from 3 to 10 mL per animal. Advantages of endotracheal lavage over transtracheal lavage is avoidance of tracheal injury, the need for minimal supplies, and its ease in cats and small dogs. Disadvantages are the potential for oropharyngeal contamination, a lack of airway visualization to guide specimen collection, especially when focal disease is present, and comparatively poor retrieval of fluid when compared with BAL.

Blind BAL technique. A blind BAL can be performed using short-acting general anesthesia without an endoscope.[70] This method is similar to endotracheal lavage except the red rubber catheter used is advanced through the endotracheal tube until gentle resistance is felt; this should correspond to wedging in a small airway. The catheter should be measured against the endotracheal tube before the procedure to ensure it advances well past the point of the end of the tube. The authors use 10 mL aliquots of saline in patients ≤ 3 kg, and 20 mL aliquots of saline in patients > 3 kg. If negative pressure is felt during aspiration, the catheter is slightly withdrawn, and suction reapplied until air appears in the syringe. The presence of foam in the lavage reflective of surfactant indicates a deep wash. With bacterial infection, the BAL fluid may be visibly purulent.

Bronchoscope-guided BAL. Bronchoscope-guided BAL allows collection of a specimen from an affected airway or lung lobe. In general, cytologic preparations collected using this method are superior to those obtained by transtracheal or endotracheal lavage because larger volumes of cells and proteinaceous materials are obtained from the deeper portions of the lungs. Collection of multiple specimens from different parts of the lung is recommended when disease is multifocal or diffuse, as findings may vary from one lobe to another.[39] Suppurative inflammation with or without intra- or extracellular bacteria supports a diagnosis of bacterial infection. Quantification of

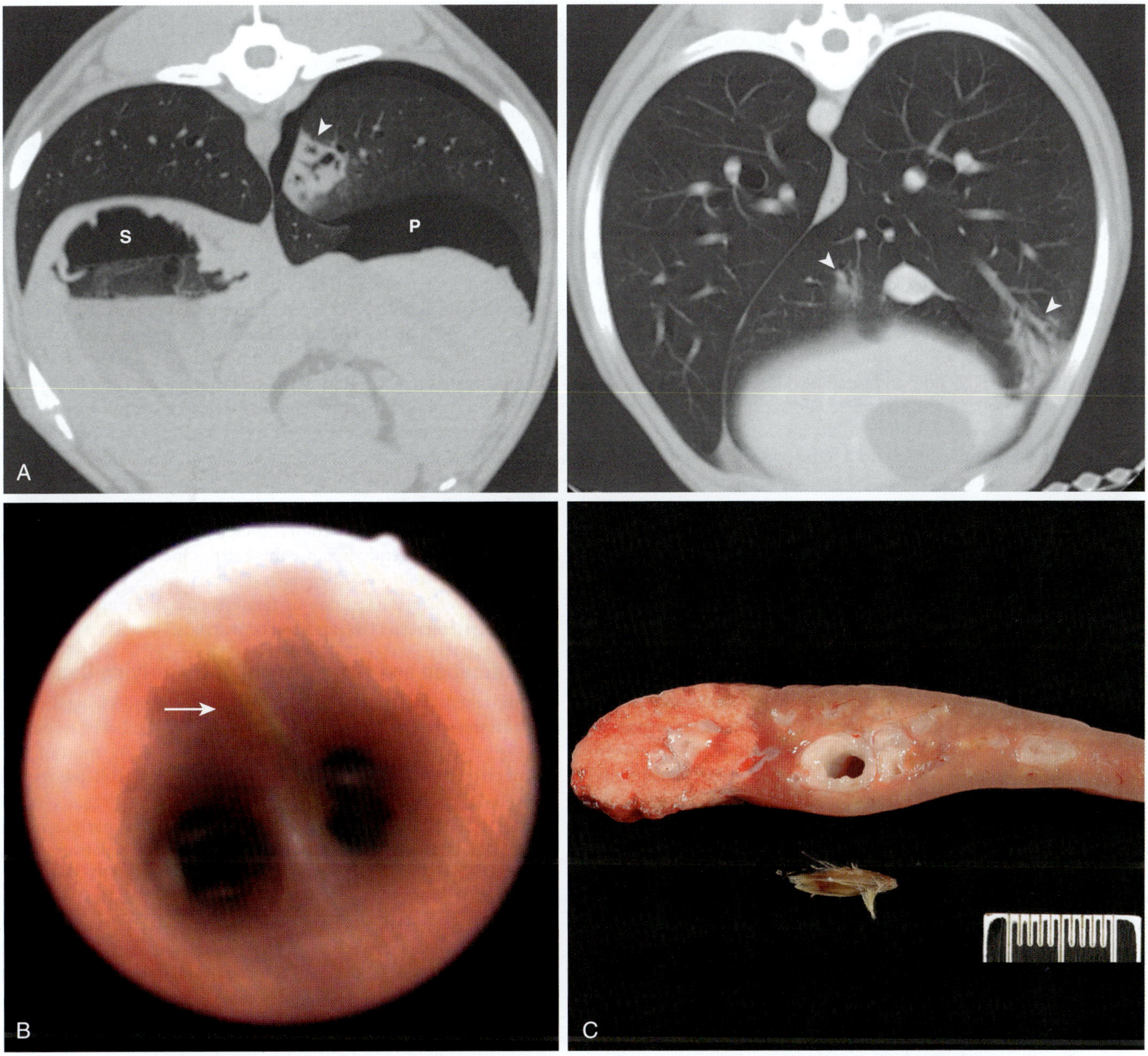

Fig. 124.6 Migrating plant awn foreign bodies. (A) Computed tomography scan images from a 1-year-old female spayed German short-haired pointer dog. A pneumothorax *(left, P)* and multifocal opacities *(arrowheads)* are present (*S*, stomach). (B) Bronchoscopic image showing a plant awn in a bronchus of a 2-year-old male neutered Belgian Malinois. (C) Portion of the right middle lung lobe of a 2-year-old female spayed Labrador retriever, which was removed during thoracotomy. A 1-cm plant awn was removed from a pocket of mucoid material within a bronchus. (C, courtesy of UC Davis Veterinary Anatomic Pathology Service.)

bacteria present is needed to distinguish lower airway contamination or transient colonization from actual infection. In addition to BAL, brush catheters can be passed through the biopsy channel of the endoscope to obtain specimens. Given the expense of a catheter system that can be used only once, the authors feel there is no advantage of using brush catheters compared with BAL for identification of bacterial infection.

Fine-needle aspiration. FNA can be performed without guidance in or with the aid of ultrasound, fluoroscopy, CT, or endoscopy to procure material for culture and cytologic examination.[71–73] Transthoracic FNA may have a higher diagnostic yield than lavage (especially tracheal washings and blind BAL) when focal lesions are present. Transbronchial needle aspiration can be performed using bronchoscopic guidance. Needles that are designed to pass through the endoscope can be used to aspirate enlarged hilar lymph nodes or discrete masses. Use of FNA (typically with a 25 or 27 gauge, 1.5″ needle and a 6-mL syringe) is less risky than use of a Tru-Cut needle, which can cause severe pulmonary hemorrhage or pneumothorax. The recommended size of the needle is 25 or 27 gauge and 1.5 inches in length but may vary depending on patient size.

Culture and Susceptibility Testing

Specimens obtained by FNA or transtracheal or BAL should be cultured for aerobic and anaerobic bacteria. Mycoplasmas can either be cultured using special media (requires laboratory notification) or

Mycoplasma-specific PCR assays can be requested. The latter is more sensitive because many *Mycoplasma* species are very fastidious or uncultivable, although the clinical significance of positive *Mycoplasma* spp. PCR results is unclear. A Gram stain can help make an early diagnosis of bacterial infection, and an acid-fast stain may be of use in dogs with suspected *Mycobacterium* spp. or *Nocardia* spp. infections. Bacterial colonization versus infection must be differentiated by use of cytology and quantitative bacterial cultures.[22] The threshold for clinically relevant bacterial growth in BAL specimens from dogs is proposed to be over 1.7×10^3 CFU/mL of BAL fluid.[22] The identification of more than two intracellular bacteria after microscopic examination of 50 oil immersion fields of a Gram-stained slide also supports the presence of bacterial infection.[22]

Dogs or cats with severe bacterial pneumonia may have substantial respiratory compromise, and invasive airway specimen collection can be risky and/or relatively contraindicated. While yet to be definitively proven, in some cases, blood cultures could represent an option to identify relevant bacteria and provide information about antimicrobial susceptibility. Further studies need to be performed to determine the utility of blood cultures in dogs and cats with bacterial pneumonia.

Pathologic Findings

Histopathologic specimens of the respiratory tract can be obtained by endoscopic biopsy (generally either masses or superficial mucosal tissue), surgical biopsy (thoracoscopy or thoracotomy), and, rarely, for consolidated and peripheral mass-like lesions, ultrasound or CT-guided biopsy. Histopathologic evaluation of masses within the upper and lower respiratory tracts can help confirm a definitive diagnosis of an underlying/predisposing cause of infection and identify intralesional bacteria. Special stains can also be applied to increase the sensitivity of organism detection. This assessment must be coupled with culture to definitively identify causative agents and determine their antimicrobial susceptibility. Although invasive, biopsy can provide complementary and additional information in complicated cases of pulmonary parenchymal disease,[51,74,75] and lung lobectomy may provide cure in cases of isolated bronchiectasis, foreign body pneumonia, and isolated lobar pneumonia unresolved by antimicrobial therapy. It also allows collection of larger specimens for culture and molecular detection methods (with improved sensitivity than techniques such as FNA or airway lavage).

TREATMENT

When designing a therapeutic plan for a patient with bacterial bronchitis or pneumonia, an investigation for all co-morbid conditions is important as secondary infections may not fully resolve or will recur if the primary disease condition is not simultaneously treated. In addition, because the presence of bacteria does not necessarily equate with infection, positive cultures must be interpreted in light of clinical signs and clinicopathologic findings. Veterinarians play an important role in promoting antimicrobial stewardship, so indiscriminate use of antibiotics should be avoided. Antibiotics should not be a first-line drug for dogs with acute cough in the absence of systemic signs where CIRD complex is suspected, as many are of viral etiology and the vast majority resolve with supportive care.[76] They are also not recommended for dogs with uncomplicated tracheal collapse or cats with cough that is likely secondary to inflammatory lower airway disease. To minimize selection for antimicrobial resistance, whenever possible, culture and susceptibility testing should be used to guide antimicrobial therapy. Additionally, certain antibiotics do not pass the blood-bronchus barrier, and while they may be useful for pneumonia, are not effective for bacterial bronchitis. Antimicrobials such as tetracyclines and fluoroquinolones are examples of drugs that cross the blood-bronchus barrier.

More aggressive antimicrobial therapy is indicated for bacterial pneumonia when compared with upper airway infections. Supportive therapies (discussed in more detail below) including systemic and airway hydration, nebulization and coupage, and supplemental oxygen are also important components of therapy, especially in severe cases. Cough suppressants are absolutely contraindicated in cases of pneumonia, as they prevent the beneficial reflex intended to clear secretions from the respiratory tract. Furosemide should be given only if critical to manage congestive heart failure as it will dry respiratory secretions and impair activity of the mucociliary apparatus. If furosemide is administered, increasing the frequency or duration of nebulization may help counterbalance this. Antihistamines are also known to dry secretions and should be avoided. There have been no studies on the use of bronchodilators in bacterial pneumonia in dogs or cats, but they may worsen ventilation:perfusion mismatch by dilating airways leading to consolidated regions of lung where gas exchange is ineffective. It is the authors' opinion that bronchodilators are most appropriately used in cats with evidence of bronchospasm (e.g., asthma). Although not routinely recommended, a trial in cats might be warranted for emergency treatment of bronchospasm and acute respiratory distress with terbutaline (0.01–0.02 mg/kg SC). Care must be taken with administration of theophylline if chloramphenicol or fluoroquinolones are being used concurrently because these drugs increase the serum theophylline concentration. Other suggested treatments without scientific evidence of efficacy in canine or feline bacterial pneumonia include N-acetylcysteine, NSAIDs, and glucocorticoids.

Identification and Management of Underlying Causes

A comprehensive discussion of the treatment for underlying disorders contributing to secondary bacterial infection of the lower respiratory tract is beyond the scope of this chapter, but brief mention of management/treatment strategies is warranted. Tracheal collapse requires a combination of weight management, avoidance of triggers of clinical signs (robust exercise, excitement, etc.), use of a harness instead of a neck collar, cough suppressants, and anxiolytics/sedatives. Canine chronic bronchitis, whether eosinophilic or neutrophilic, and feline chronic bronchitis and asthma, should be managed with avoidance of inhaled triggers (antigens such as environmental smoke; particulates such as cleaning aerosols/powders or dusty cat litter; or allergens), weight management, and glucocorticoids (oral or inhaled, tapered to the lowest effective dose). The use of bronchodilators is best reserved for asthmatic cats with episodic expiratory respiratory distress. Recurrent infections are particularly problematic in patients with bronchiectasis. If bronchiectasis is confined to a single lobe, surgical lobectomy may be curative. If bronchiectasis is generalized, recurrent infections must be managed as they arise, and low doses of glucocorticoids (0.25–0.5 mg/kg of prednisone or prednisolone in dogs and cats, respectively) may help reduce concurrent inflammation. Reduction of environmental inhaled irritants and allergens and weight management are also helpful; airway humidification may help reduce tenacious secretions. Bronchomalacia, like bronchiectasis, also requires management of underlying or co-morbid respiratory conditions and may benefit from environmental modulation, weight management, and airway humidification. If sterile inflammation is documented during a period where there is no concurrent infection, addition of low-dose glucocorticoid therapy may also be helpful. Bronchodilators have not been proven to be useful for this condition as airway smooth muscle constriction is not part of the underlying pathology.

Implementing appropriate husbandry practices and when available (based on patient risk), vaccination for causes of contagious tracheobronchitis may help reduce incidence of these diseases. As previously mentioned, identifying underlying causes of bacterial pneumonia and addressing them directly is also important in the overall management strategy and to help prevent recurrence.

Antimicrobial Drug Treatment

No single antibacterial drug is routinely effective against the wide variety of organisms causing bacterial pneumonia. Selection of an antibacterial drug based on identification of the pathogen and its antimicrobial susceptibility results in recovery of substantially more patients than when therapy is empiric.[77] Recent antimicrobial therapy that is empiric also negatively impacts susceptibility to subsequently required antimicrobials.[78] Over half (57.4%) of dogs with pneumonia previously treated empirically with antibiotics and subsequently referred for airway lavage were infected with bacteria that exhibited resistance to the empirically used antibiotic.[78] Thus, if absolutely necessary to select an antimicrobial without culture and susceptibility testing, recently administered antimicrobials should be avoided.

Morphologic characteristics of bacteria on a Gram-stained slide can aid in selection of an antibacterial drug while awaiting the results of bacterial culture and susceptibility.[22] Doxycycline has been recommended for treatment of suspected *B. bronchiseptica* or *Mycoplasma* spp. pneumonia.[76] When streptococcal pneumonia is suspected (e.g., shelter outbreak of pneumonia associated with Gram-positive cocci), a penicillin is the drug of choice.[76] Additional detail on treatment of dogs with pneumonia due to CIRD complex can be found in Chapter 28.

Because aspiration pneumonia is not always associated with bacterial infection, routine antimicrobial use is controversial. Antimicrobial treatment should ideally be delayed until secondary bacterial infection can be documented or until the animal fails to respond appropriately to other supportive therapy. When infection plays a role in aspiration pneumonia, a multiplicity of aerobic and anaerobic organisms can be involved,[38] and combination antimicrobial therapy may be required, ideally guided by results of culture and susceptibility. Cough or respiratory distress, fever, leukocytosis, and radiographic evidence of severe interstitial or alveolar patterns do not definitively prove the pneumonia is due to bacterial infection. In one study of canine aspiration pneumonia, roughly 25% of dogs had negative cultures; however, only 47 of 125 dogs in this study had airway lavage cultures and only 2 of 126 dogs had BAL instead of an upper airway wash, so focal infections may have been overlooked.[38] The consensus opinion of the Working Group of ISCAID is that in the absence of evidence of systemic sepsis, either no treatment or parenteral treatment with a beta-lactam antimicrobial may be sufficient for cases of aspiration pneumonia.[76]

Empiric antimicrobial therapy is particularly important to initiate early (within 1 to 2 hours) in dogs or cats with evidence of sepsis (see Chapter 123). A broad-spectrum parenteral antimicrobial strategy should be considered to address the possibility of gram-negative bacteria (e.g., a fluoroquinolone) and gram-positive and anaerobic bacteria (e.g., ampicillin or clindamycin) which is later adjusted based on culture and susceptibility results.[76] The reader is referred to ISCAID Working Group Guidelines (see Suggested Reading list) for detailed discussion of antimicrobial treatment options for canine and feline respiratory tract infections, including doses and other considerations.[76] Regardless of initial selection of antimicrobial, results of culture and susceptibility testing should be used to modify therapy, including de-escalation when possible.

In stable patients with documented evidence of bacterial infection of the airways or pulmonary parenchyma, oral antibiotic monotherapy that is prescribed on an outpatient basis should be sufficient. If patients are hospitalized, parenteral antimicrobial therapy is recommended regardless of disease severity; when discharged from the hospital, they can be transitioned to oral antimicrobials.[76]

Routine intratracheal or aerosol administration of antimicrobials is not recommended in pneumonia. With severe alveolar consolidation in pneumonia, airway penetration of antimicrobials is inferior to systemic administration. Inhaled aminoglycosides have been used to treat refractory *B. bronchiseptica* pneumonia in dogs, but concerns have been raised about the possibility of toxicity. Treatment of experimental dogs with inhaled gentamicin at 7, 14, and 41 mg/kg was associated with renal tubular necrosis at the highest dose, but with no evidence of respiratory tract irritation (in contrast to findings in rats in the same report).[79] Another study of dogs with naturally occurring *B. bronchiseptica* pneumonia concluded that use of an undiluted 5% solution of gentamicin in a nebulizer for 10 minutes twice daily was safe and effective.[80]

Duration of antimicrobial therapy for bacterial pneumonia has long been recommended for 3–6 or more weeks, and at least 1–2 weeks beyond clinical and radiographic resolution of signs of disease.[39] This recommendation has not been based on evidence and differs from recommendations for humans with bacterial pneumonia. In humans, meta-analyses show that in randomized controlled clinical trials of bacterial pneumonia, use of longer courses of antibiotics versus shorter courses do not lead to significant differences with respect to clinical success, bacterial eradication, adverse effects, or mortality.[81] Additionally, radiographic improvement in humans lags far behind the clinical response and offers no benefit in identifying treatment failure over physician or patient assessment of symptoms, underscoring the lack of utility of this diagnostic to guide therapy.[81–83] Until controlled peer-reviewed studies can be performed, the ISCAID Working Group consensus statement recommends reevaluation of patients with pneumonia in 10 to 14 days after initiating antimicrobial therapy.[76] One prospective study reported no difference in outcome in dogs treated for 10 days with pneumonia compared with those treated for 21 days.[84] While the best means to monitor efficacy of therapy is currently lacking, consensus opinion is that a recheck should consist of physical examination, CBC, and thoracic radiography, keeping in mind that radiographic changes may lag behind clinical improvement.

Ancillary Supportive Therapy

Maintenance of normal systemic and airway hydration is an important therapeutic objective in hospitalized patients with bacterial pneumonia. Dehydration hinders mucociliary clearance and mobilization of secretions because normal respiratory secretions are more than 90% water. Judicious use of IV fluids is recommended. Airway hydration can be directly addressed using aerosol therapy to mobilize secretions by adding water to the mucociliary blanket. A nebulizer that produces particles between 0.5 and 3.0 μm ensures that water is deposited in the lower airways. Water vaporizers or humidifiers are inadequate because the water particulate size is larger and droplets are generally deposited in the nasal cavity. For nebulization, the animal is placed in an enclosed chamber, and a bland aerosol (normal saline) is nebulized into the chamber. Physiotherapy should always be performed immediately after aerosolization to enhance secretion clearance. Methods include increased cough frequency by chest wall coupage or tracheal manipulation, mild exercise, and postural drainage. The animal should be nebulized two to six times daily for 10 to 20 minutes per treatment. Careful attention must be paid to appropriate cleaning/sterilization of the nebulizer.

Animals with severe tachypnea, respiratory distress, or moderate to marked hypoxemia (arterial oxygen tension below 80 mmHg or $SpO_2 < 94\%$ on room air) require supplemental oxygen therapy. Oxygen should be humidified to prevent drying of respiratory membranes. Oxygen can be administered in a cage, by intratracheal cannula or nasal catheter (unilateral or bilateral), or in intubated patients with or without a mechanical ventilator. Mechanical ventilation may be required when there is severe hypoxemia unresponsive to oxygen supplementation or evidence of labored respiration with inappropriate oxygenation for the degree of ventilation and with increasing $PaCO_2$ (i.e., impending respiratory muscle fatigue). High-flow oxygen therapy using high-flow nasal prongs may be an alternative approach for dogs failing traditional oxygen therapy when mechanical ventilation is not a viable option.[85]

If aspiration pneumonia is a complicating factor or has the potential to be a complicating factor, maintaining sternal recumbency with the cranial part of the body elevated, and minimizing gastric volume by small frequent feedings or use of antiemetics or prokinetics (e.g., maropitant, ondansetron, cisapride) can be considered. A pilot study in four dogs with acquired idiopathic megaesophagus indicated a potential benefit of at-home intermittent esophageal suctioning (via esophagostomy tube or per os) for prevention of aspiration pneumonia, and deserves further study as a long-term management strategy.[86] A perioperative IV CRI of metoclopramide did not affect the incidence of aspiration pneumonia in dogs undergoing arytenoid lateralization surgery.[87] If a patient with bacterial pneumonia is receiving immunosuppressants or chemotherapeutics and it can be safely done, temporary withdrawal of these drugs or a decrease in their dose may aid in resolution of pneumonia.

Surgery

Surgical intervention may be required in patients in which appropriate antimicrobial therapy has failed to fully resolve all clinical and/or radiographic lesions. For example, surgery may be indicated if, after discontinuing antimicrobial therapy, pneumonia recurs in the same lobe, which may raise suspicion for a foreign body or focal bronchiectasis. In some pulmonary abscesses, a residual nidus of infection may persist even after long-term antimicrobial therapy. Lobectomy may be curative. Additionally, histopathologic examination of lung biopsies may reveal evidence of co-morbid respiratory conditions requiring targeted therapy.

PROGNOSIS

Bacterial tracheobronchitis and bacterial bronchitis are not generally considered life-threatening, but bacterial infection can be an important contributor to clinical signs and exacerbation of co-morbid respiratory conditions. Prognosis depends on the severity of disease, response to treatment, and reversibility of pathology, if any.

Studies have shown survival to discharge rates of dogs with "community-acquired" pneumonia to be 96% and with aspiration pneumonia to be 77%–83%.[37,38,78] There was no association between survival rates and more severe evidence of disease on radiographs or duration of hospitalization in one study,[37] but multiple lobe involvement had a worse outcome than single lobe involvement in another study.[38] Prognosis for survival was not correlated with the number or types of bacteria responsible for aspiration pneumonia, the underlying cause for aspiration, or the existence of multiple underlying reasons for aspiration.[37,38] When evaluating long-term follow-up in dogs having unilateral arytenoid lateralization with postoperative aspiration pneumonia, 1-, 2-, 3-, and 4-year survival rates were 83%, 64%, 52%, and 26%, respectively, underscoring the importance of the larynx in upper airway protection.[36] Collectively, these findings demonstrate the importance of identifying and aggressively managing any underlying cause for aspiration to prevent subsequent recurrence of pneumonia and other permanent damage to the airways and pulmonary parenchyma (e.g., bronchiectasis).

PREVENTION

Contagious causes of bacterial tracheobronchitis and pneumonia can be prevented using good husbandry practices and targeted vaccination (see Chapters 17, 22, 26, and 28). For secondary bacterial infections of the respiratory tract, appropriate early identification and management of underlying disorders is critical. The risk of aspiration pneumonia can be minimized by fasting prior to anesthesia, altering feeding practices in dysphagic dogs (optimizing food/liquid consistency, low-fat diets and prokinetics to facilitate gastric emptying, upright feedings, and in some cases [e.g., megaesophagus] placement of gastric tubes with multiple frequent feedings), and use of antiemetics for animals with severe or protracted vomiting. Prophylactic antimicrobials are not recommended for animals with recurrent aspiration. Overuse or inappropriate use of antimicrobials is likely to predispose patients to infections with MDR bacteria.

PUBLIC HEALTH ASPECTS

Humans and their pets share the same environment, and close contact can lead to exposure of susceptible humans with zoonotic pathogens. A few bacterial pathogens causative of respiratory tract infection in dogs and cats are considered to have the potential to be zoonotic including *B. bronchiseptica, Streptococcus equi* subsp. *zooepidemicus, Mycobacterium tuberculosis,* and *Yersinia* spp.[88] The likelihood of infection as well as the severity of disease is higher in immunocompromised humans. Routes of transmission of zoonotic bacteria are unclear but could include inhalation of aerosols and ingestion; thus, immunocompromised individuals should minimize contact with dogs that are sneezing or coughing, and routine precautions including use of appropriate personal protective equipment and thorough hand washing are prudent for all in-contact humans. An additional concern given widespread and often indiscriminate veterinary use of antimicrobials is the MDR bacteria that may be isolated from the respiratory tract as was demonstrated in one dog with bronchopneumonia.[89]

PYOTHORAX

ETIOLOGY, EPIDEMIOLOGY, AND PATHOGENESIS

Purulent pleuritis, pyothorax, and thoracic empyema describe septic processes of the pleural cavity that are associated with exudate accumulation. The pleural cavity normally contains a small amount of transudative fluid. With bacterial infections, the resultant host inflammatory immune response leads to alterations in vascular permeability and lymphatic function leading to an effusion rich in cells and protein.

Pyothorax can result from either local or systemic disease. Local disease follows extension of infection from the thoracic wall, tracheobronchial tree, pulmonary parenchyma, or esophagus. Examples include bacterial infection from penetrating bite wounds, parapneumonic spread, migrating foreign bodies or parasites, thoracic trauma (including iatrogenic inoculation), and esophageal perforation, among others. Pyothorax that is part of a systemic disease process implies hematogenous or lymphatic spread of bacteria.

Definitive identification of the source of bacterial pleuritis is frequently not achieved.[90] Pleural infections are commonly polymicrobial in nature.[45,91–98] There is a high prevalence of obligate anaerobic bacteria as sole pathogens or in combination of facultative aerobes and other anaerobes.[95–97] The most prevalent organisms isolated from pleural exudate of the dog and cat are summarized in Table 124.3.

TABLE 124.3 Common Bacterial Species Associated with Pyothorax in Dogs and Cats[a]

Dogs	Cats
Bacteroides spp. (34)	*Pasteurella* spp. (41)
Fusobacterium spp. (34)	*Bacteroides* spp. (29)
Escherichia coli (31)	*Fusobacterium* spp. (23)
Pasteurella spp. (29)	*Clostridium* spp. (20)
Peptostreptococcus spp. (29)	*Peptostreptococcus* spp. (17)
Actinomyces spp. (28)	*Actinomyces* spp. (12)
Prevotella spp. (24)	*Porphyromonas* spp. (10)
Staphylococcus pseudintermedius (12–20)[b]	*Prevotella* spp. (8)
Streptococcus spp. (10–18)[b]	
Nocardia spp. (12)	
Corynebacterium spp. (11)	
Clostridium spp. (7)	
Klebsiella spp. (6)	
Porphyromonas spp. (6)	
Acinetobacter spp. (5)	

[a]Numbers in parentheses represent total cumulative number of isolates reported. Organisms with fewer than five isolates reported were not included.
[b]Study by Rooney and Monnet[95] did not differentiate between these two organisms; therefore, range accounts for eight isolates that could be either.
Data taken from references 92,93,95–98,107,117.

Dogs

Pyothorax in dogs most commonly occurs in young adult medium to large breeds, especially of working and sporting varieties.[92,93,95] These breeds are thought to be at risk because they are prone to grass awn inhalation during vigorous exercise. When *Actinomyces* spp. are isolated, there should be a high index of suspicion for plant material (grass awns) as the underlying cause.[99,100] Barbed awns migrate down the bronchial tree, carrying commensal microflora from the oropharyngeal cavity into the lung parenchyma. The awns may exit the visceral pleura and enter the pleural cavity where they can cause pyothorax. The relative importance of grass awns as a cause of pyothorax in dogs may be regionally variable, with only 3 of 50 dogs in a UK retrospective study being associated with plant inhalation.[93] Pyothorax may also occur in dogs due to penetrating trauma to the thoracic wall, bite wounds, or esophageal trauma. For example, the esophageal parasite *Spirocerca lupi* has also been responsible for pyothorax in dogs from damage to the esophagus at the site of granulomas and leakage of esophageal material into the thoracic cavity (see Chapter 117).[101] Pyothorax can also be a complication of thoracic drainage techniques (e.g., thoracostomy tube placement and maintenance) or thoracic surgery.[102,103] When pyothorax is a complication of indwelling thoracostomy tubes, it is typically diagnosed within 4 days of tube placement.[102]

Cats

Risk factors for pyothorax in cats include young age and being part of a multiple-cat household, but not indoor or outdoor status (i.e., free roaming does not appear to increase risk).[96] Possible overrepresentation of male cats has been documented in some studies, but this has not been a statistically significant finding. Feline pyothorax generally results from contamination of the pleural cavity with

TABLE 124.4 Characteristics of Pleural Fluid from Dogs and Cats with Pyothorax

Parameter	Reference Characteristics	Pyothorax
Physical characteristics	Color: clear, transparent	Color: variable yellow to reddish-brown, opaque, flocculent; sometimes granules can be odorous
Cells	<500/μL	>7,000/μL
Protein	<1.5 g/dL	>3 g/dL
Specific gravity	<1.017	≥1.025
Biochemistry of fluid	LDH activity and glucose concentration in reference blood range	LDH activity increased; glucose concentration decreased compared with blood[a]

[a]These changes have presently been documented in cats and humans.
LDH, lactate dehydrogenase.

oropharyngeal flora. The most common aerobic organism isolated in feline pyothorax is *Pasteurella,* although anaerobes are frequently cultured as well.[91,94,96,97] Parapneumonic spread and bite wounds are the most common routes of infection.[91,104] Previously, bite wounds were thought to be the major route of infection, especially in young, free-roaming intact male cats.[105] However, with more cats being neutered and kept indoors, pyothorax secondary to bite wounds is seen less frequently.

CLINICAL SIGNS AND PHYSICAL EXAMINATION FINDINGS

Clinical signs of pyothorax result from restrictive respiratory disease, including increased respiratory rate, shallow respirations, inspiratory respiratory distress, and orthopnea. Other signs include obtundation, exercise intolerance, cough, lethargy, anorexia, weight loss, and fever. Physical examination may reveal muffled heart sounds and decreased breath sounds in the dependent areas of the thorax. Chronic or severe infections may result in a dehydrated, debilitated, collapsed, or hypothermic patient. Approximately one half of cats with pyothorax develop sepsis.[96] In cats with pyothorax, hypersalivation and bradycardia can occur and are associated with a worse clinical outcome.[96,106]

DIAGNOSIS

The diagnosis of pyothorax in dogs and cats is usually established based on radiography and microbiologic and cytologic analyses of pleural effusion (summarized in Tables 124.3 and 124.4).

Laboratory Abnormalities

Complete Blood Count, Serum Biochemical Tests, and Urinalysis

Abnormalities on CBC are typically nonspecific including mild-to-moderate nonregenerative anemia, neutrophilic leukocytosis of varying severity with or without a left shift, and presence of toxic neutrophils.[91,93,95,96,107,108] In some patients, the CBC may be unremarkable. In cases of sepsis and concurrent DIC, thrombocytopenia may also be present. Serum biochemistry profile abnormalities may include hyponatremia, hypochloremia, hypoalbuminemia, hyperglobulinemia, azotemia, hyperglycemia or hypoglycemia, and hypocalcemia.[93–96] Hyperbilirubinemia may also be present in cats.[94,96]

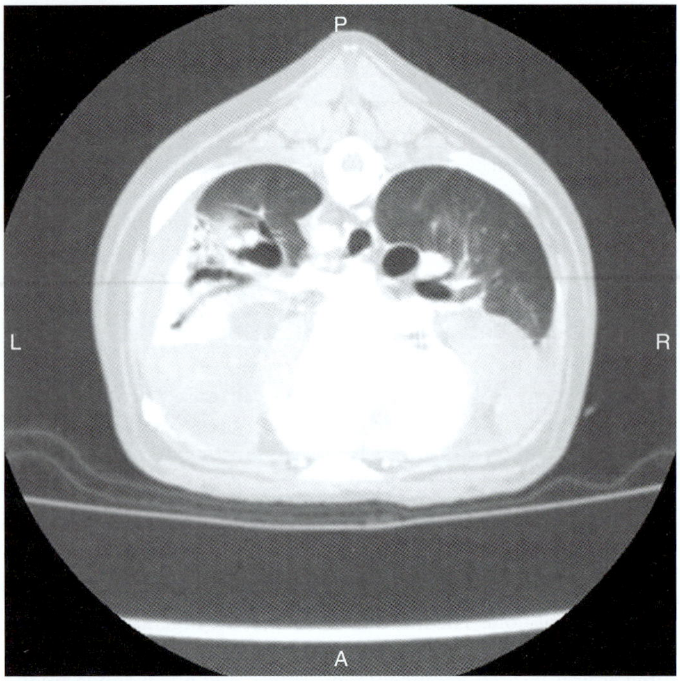

Fig. 124.7 Computed tomography image (0.625-mm thick slice during arterial phase of contrast administration) of a dog presented for increased respiratory effort and lethargy. A large volume of pleural effusion is present with a concurrent lesion in the pulmonary parenchyma of the left cranial lung lobe. (Courtesy of Dr. Tekla Lee-Fowler, Auburn University.)

Diagnostic Imaging

Thoracic Radiography

Pleural effusion is noted on thoracic radiography, particularly if this is performed prior to thoracocentesis. Bilateral effusion is most common, but unilateral effusion may be seen.[91–93,95,96,109] Thoracic radiography should be repeated after drainage of pleural effusion to evaluate for underlying etiology such as lesions in the pulmonary parenchyma, pleural space, and lymphadenomegaly.

Ultrasonographic Examination

Thoracic ultrasound (TFAST) can be used to visualize pleural effusion location and presence of fibrinous adhesions. Pleural effusion associated with pyothorax is typically echogenic. Ultrasonographic examination can also be used to further evaluate consolidated lung parenchyma, possible abscesses, intrathoracic masses, and thoracic lymph nodes. In some cases, foreign material (e.g., plant awns) may be identified.[45,110] Ultrasound can be useful to guide needles for specimen collection or thoracocentesis, particularly when loculated fluid is present.

Advanced Imaging

CT may provide more detail regarding pulmonary parenchymal lesions and correlates well with findings at surgery (Fig. 124.7).[111] CT reliably provides information on the presence and volume of pleural fluid.[111] Pleural gas may be noted, either due to procedures such as thoracocentesis or as a result of plant foreign body migration.[111] Pleural thickening, mediastinal lesions, and lymphadenomegaly can all be reliably detected.[111] Improved identification of pulmonary parenchymal lesions is also a benefit of CT over plain radiography, and lesions may be identified that are not evident at surgery.[111] For this reason, CT results can be useful to guide surgical intervention. Use of a combination of CT and bronchoscopy may be most effective for identification of migrating plant awns.[112]

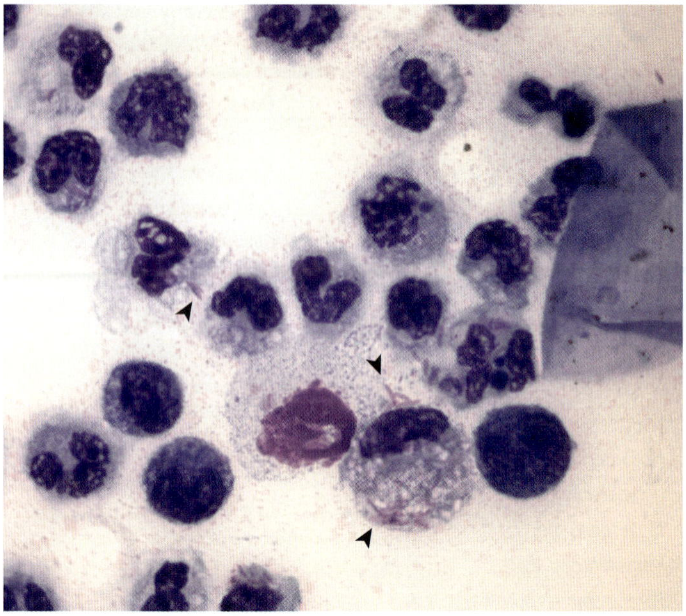

Fig. 124.8 Cytology of pleural effusion from a 3-year-old male neutered domestic shorthair cat with pyothorax. There are many neutrophils, which are variably karyolytic. Many of them contain bacterial rods, which can also be seen extracellularly *(arrowheads)*. Anaerobic bacterial culture yielded *Fusobacterium russii,* and aerobic culture was negative.

Microbiologic Tests

Cytologic Diagnosis

Grossly, pleural exudate obtained using thoracocentesis from dogs and cats with pyothorax is typically turbid and/or hemorrhagic and may contain flocculent debris. In anaerobic infections, it may also be malodorous. Sulfur granules within the effusion may be visualized with *Actinomyces* spp. or *Nocardia* spp. infections. Bacteria can often be identified microscopically, and mixed populations of bacteria may be noted; however, failure to identify bacteria does not rule out bacterial pyothorax. Infection with nonstaining bacteria such as *Mycoplasma* spp. or a history of antimicrobial therapy may mean bacteria are not visible. *Actinomyces* or *Nocardia* infection should be suspected if filamentous bacteria are seen microscopically (Fig. 124.8).

Culture and Susceptibility Testing

Specimens for aerobic and anaerobic culture should be collected before antimicrobial administration whenever possible. Pleural fluid should be placed into appropriate tubes, including anaerobic transport medium, with minimal exposure to air to optimize the chance of positive cultures. Specimens intended for anaerobic culture should not be refrigerated and should be processed with minimal delay.[90] Consideration should also be given to specific culture for *Mycoplasma* spp., and it is recommended that the laboratory be informed if there is a clinical suspicion of *Actinomyces* spp. or *Nocardia* spp. infection. Because anaerobic cultures and *Mycoplasma* spp. cultures are often low yield when transported to a commercial diagnostic laboratory from a practice environment (as opposed to immediate submission to an on-site laboratory as occurs in teaching hospital environments), aerobic bacterial culture and empiric therapy for anaerobes (which are almost always present) is a suitable alternative.

TREATMENT

Treatment of pyothorax should be prompt and aggressive. Initial goals are to relieve respiratory distress by removal of effusion from the pleural space, to provide appropriate IV fluid therapy and supportive care, and to inactivate bacteria using systemic antimicrobial drugs.

Drainage and Lavage

Drainage of pleural exudates is essential for management of pyothorax. Delayed pleural drainage leads to incomplete resolution of signs and predisposes to formation of loculated abscesses and fibrosis, which could necessitate later thoracotomy. Placement of indwelling thoracostomy tubes has been recommended as the initial treatment of choice in most cats, with 95% of cats having resolution when this is combined with appropriate concurrent antibacterial drug therapy.[91] Dogs may also benefit from indwelling tube placement and aggressive medical management. Indwelling tubes have the advantages of closed chest drainage and facilitate pleural fluid sampling to monitor therapeutic response; the tubes also allow direct instillation of isotonic lavage fluid (with or without additives) into the pleural space (see later). Disadvantages of indwelling tubes include challenges associated with maintenance of drain placement and patency and the risks of pneumothorax and infection.[102] Large-bore thoracostomy tubes have been traditionally utilized to minimize the chance of obstruction with purulent fluid. However, small-bore wire-guided thoracostomy tubes have been shown to be suitable for the management of pyothorax without any occurrences of tube obstruction.[113] When these tubes were used, thoracic lavage was incorporated into the management protocol, which may explain why obstruction did not occur. Small-bore tubes offer advantages such as patient tolerance of placement and ease of placement.

After fluid removal, radiographs should be taken to more accurately evaluate the pulmonary parenchyma, pleural space, and mediastinum for lesions that may alter treatment plans. Additionally, post-drainage radiographs can be used to assess whether drainage is complete, especially on the contralateral side. If fluid removal is incomplete, bilateral tube placement may be required. Intermittent suction every 2 to 4 hours or continuous suction can be used.[114] Use of one-way continuous suction requires close monitoring as the risk of potentially fatal complications in cases of malfunction is increased. The median duration of indwelling thoracostomy tubes for drainage has been approximately 6 to 7 days (range, a few hours to 21 days).[91–93,96]

A single-needle thoracocentesis has not been routinely advocated for management of pyothorax although one study reported complete long-term resolution of pyothorax in 15 of 16 dogs after complete drainage and 6 weeks of treatment with ampicillin and metronidazole.[107] Single drainage protocols are usually not curative if pulmonary lobar masses (associated with abscesses or consolidation) are evident by radiography after initial fluid drainage. Repeated thoracocentesis is relatively simple and inexpensive but is generally not recommended due to associated morbidity.

Thoracic lavage may be performed through indwelling thoracostomy tubes. There is controversy about the efficacy of lavage of the pleural cavity. Lavage may facilitate removal of accumulated pus and bacteria and break down clots and fibrin bands; in addition, it may dilute bacteria and other inflammatory mediators. However, prospective studies are lacking. Some retrospective studies have suggested that lavage led to decreased duration of thoracostomy tube drainage[93] and increased the likelihood of survival.[92] However, one retrospective study in cats concluded that thoracic lavage should not be routinely recommended as the benefits of lavage did not outweigh the risks.[96] Lavage has been implemented as part of a medical management protocol in some studies with apparently good success[91–93,115]; however, it is unclear how much of the beneficial outcome was directly related to lavage and not to the other medical management strategies or differences in patient populations.

Fluid volumes for lavage are generally 10 to 20 mL/kg of warmed 0.9% saline infused slowly over 5 to 10 minutes two to four times per day.[116] Respiratory pattern and effort are monitored closely during infusion, and infusion is discontinued and fluid immediately aspirated if respiratory distress occurs. The fluid volume can then be reduced for subsequent lavage. The patient can be rotated from side to side, or mild coupage can be performed followed by immediate removal of any accessible fluid. Lavage can be continued until the removed fluid is clear of pus. Cytologic improvement is exhibited by decreasing cell count, with loss of degenerative changes in neutrophils, and absence of bacteria. Repeated culture is also recommended to confirm resolution of infection. Addition of antimicrobial agents to the lavage fluid is controversial and is currently not recommended based on limited data.[76]

Antimicrobial Therapy

Systemic antimicrobial therapy is indicated for pyothorax, but it is usually insufficient without lavage or drainage of the infected pleural cavity. Initial empiric antibacterial selection should be active against a mixture of facultative and obligate anaerobic bacteria.[76,97] Penicillin or penicillin derivatives are often given because they are active against obligate anaerobes, *Pasteurella* spp., or *Actinomyces* spp. As an initial empirical choice, a combination of a fluoroquinolone (e.g., enrofloxacin or marbofloxacin) with a penicillin or clindamycin is recommended.[76] Culture and susceptibility testing should be evaluated in light of clinical condition for further adjustments to antibacterial therapy. Regardless of the anaerobic or facultative anaerobic bacteria that are cultured, the regimen should always contain drugs effective against anaerobes. Systemic antibacterial therapy should ideally be continued for at least 4 to 6 weeks.[76]

Surgery

Surgical intervention is more costly, particularly when medical management has been attempted first and failed.[117] Therefore, it is important to try to identify candidates that require surgical intervention as early in the disease course as possible.[117] Evidence of foreign material, pulmonary or mediastinal masses, radiographic evidence of fluid encapsulation, repeated blockage of drainage tubes, recurrent pneumothorax, and lack of significant improvement in fluid consistency during lavage are indications for surgical exploration and/or lobectomy.[93,95,96] Because *Actinomyces* spp. have been associated with a high likelihood of plant material,[100,118,119] isolation of these bacteria is another potential indication for surgical exploration. Although surgical exploration is expensive, one report suggested that dogs having surgical exploration and debridement followed by medical management have a better outcome after treatment than those undergoing pleural evacuation and lavage alone.[95] Thoracoscopy (or *video-assisted thoracic surgery, VATS*) is a less invasive alternative to thoracotomy.[109,120,121] In one study, conversion to open thoracotomy was only required for 2 of 14 dogs with pyothorax that underwent thoracoscopy, and only 1 dog had recurrence of pyothorax that required a second surgery 17 months later (median follow-up time: 143 days, range: 14–2,402 days).[121]

Monitoring

Radiographic monitoring is essential during treatment and follow-up of pleural infections. Serial radiographic examinations should be performed first after initial thoracocentesis, when the chest tube is removed, 10 to 14 days after starting antibacterial therapy, and at completion of therapy.[76] Additionally, radiographs can be acquired 1 to 2 weeks after discontinuing antimicrobials to monitor for subclinical recurrence of disease. If there is persistence of effusion or recurrence, repeated thoracocentesis, fluid analysis, and culture and susceptibility should be performed.

PROGNOSIS

The highest period of mortality for dogs and cats with pyothorax is within the initial 48 hours of drainage and stabilization.[93] After that time, prognosis improves. Survival to discharge of 74% and long-term survival of 63% were reported in one study,[92] whereas other studies have reported higher percentages.[93,107,117] Recurrence rates have been reported to be < 20% with most recurrences occurring within a few months of discharge [92,93,95,96,107,109,115,117]

PREVENTION

When possible, reducing exposure of dogs to areas where grass awns are prominent may assist in pyothorax prevention. Grooming dogs that are exposed to areas of abundant grass awns thoroughly and frequently may reduce the risk of related complications.[100] Housing cats indoors and in stable colonies may reduce the risk of pyothorax.

CASE EXAMPLE

Signalment

"Sam," a 5-year-old, female, intact, English pointer from the southeastern United States.

History

Sam was evaluated for a 3-day history of behavioral change and 2-day history of anorexia. Labored breathing was noted the morning of evaluation which prompted presentation on an emergent basis. The patient was up-to-date on vaccinations and routine parasite prevention. The dog lived in an outdoor kennel setting and was an active field trial dog that traveled frequently to events. There was no history of prior illness.

Physical Examination Findings

Body weight: 17.5 kg, BCS 3/9.

General: Obtunded but responsive, 5% dehydration, T = 102.4°F (39.1°C), HR = 140 beats/minute, RR = 50 breaths/minute, mucous membranes pink, CRT = 2 seconds.

Ears, eyes, nose, and throat: Mild mucoid ocular discharge bilaterally.

Respiratory: Restrictive respiratory pattern (shallow with greater effort on inspiration), decreased bronchovesicular sounds ventrally over both the right and left thorax.

Lymph nodes: Mild bilateral lymphadenomegaly of the superficial cervical lymph nodes.

No clinically significant abnormalities were noted in other systems following full physical examination.

Laboratory Findings

CBC: HCT 44.1% (38.7%–59.2%), MCV 69.6 fL (60.5–73.8 fL), MCHC 34.6 mg/dL (32–37.2 mg/dL), platelets 468,000/μL (152,000–518,000 platelets/μL), WBC 28,820 cells/μL (5,090–17,410 cells/μL), neutrophils 26,806 cells/μL (2,600–10,400 cells/μL), band neutrophils 576 cells/μL (0–300 cells/μL), lymphocytes 865 cells/μL (390–6,730 cells/μL), monocytes 576 cells/μL (160–1,160 cells/μL), eosinophils 0 cells/μL (10–2,050 cells/μL), cell morphology – slight toxic granulocytes.

Serum chemistry profile: Total protein 6.4 g/dL (5.5–7.7 g/dL), albumin 1.6 g/dL (3–4.3 g/dL), globulin 4.8 g/dL (2–4.3 g/dL), ALP 177 U/L (14–152 U/L), ALT 22 U/L (13–151 U/L), AST 29 U/L (18–55 U/L), total bilirubin 0.1 mg/dL (0–0.2 mg/dL), creatine kinase 145 U/L (53–337 U/L), BUN 9.0 mg/dL (9–34 mg/dL), creatinine 0.3 mg/dL (0.5–1.6 mg/dL), calcium 9.1 mg/dL (9.6–12 mg/dL), phosphorus 5.5 mg/dL (2.6–7.9 mg/dL), glucose 84 mg/dL (76–116 mg/dL), cholesterol 328 mg/dL (132–335 mg/dL), bicarbonate 15.2 mmol/L (14–29 mmol/L), sodium 141 mmol/L (142–151 mmol/L), potassium 3.6 mmol/L (3.6–4.9 mmol/L), chloride 104 mmol/L (105–117 mmol/L).

Imaging Findings

At the time of initial examination, a brief thoracic ultrasound was performed and confirmed the presence of pleural effusion. Thoracic radiographs revealed a moderate amount of pleural effusion characterized by retraction of the lung lobes, partial silhouetting of the cardiac outline and numerous pleural fissure lines. An alveolar pattern was also noted within the caudal aspect of the left cranial lung lobe. Interpretation: Pleural effusion. Alveolar pattern within the caudal aspect of the left cranial lung lobe was most consistent with pneumonia. An underlying presence of a foreign body could not be ruled out.

Cytologic Findings

A pleural effusion specimen was obtained for analysis using thoracocentesis.

Fluid analysis: Color: red; transparency: cloudy; nucleated cells: 124,900/μL; RBC: 370,000/μL; protein: 4.0 g/dL; specific gravity: 1.027.

Cytologic description: Predominance of neutrophils with fewer macrophages and scattered reactive mesothelial cells. Neutrophils were degenerative, and low numbers had phagocytized thin, filamentous rod bacteria and fewer small cocci. Bacteria were also seen free in the background.

Interpretation: Septic inflammation.

Microbiologic Testing

Aerobic and anaerobic culture: *Actinomyces* spp. from broth only and heavy growth of *Bacteroides capillosus.*

Diagnosis

Bacterial pyothorax.

Treatment

The patient was stabilized upon initial presentation with thoracocentesis and IV fluid therapy. Once results of the pleural fluid analysis were available, an exploratory thoracotomy was performed via median sternotomy. Effusion was suctioned from the thoracic cavity and thorough lavage was performed. The right caudal lung lobe was abnormal in appearance with an apparent mass present, and a right caudal lung lobectomy was performed. Foreign material was not visualized within the thoracic cavity. A thoracostomy tube was placed on the right side.

The patient recovered from surgery without complication. IV fluids were continued postoperatively, postoperative analgesic therapy was instituted, and empiric antimicrobial therapy was begun with ampicillin-sulbactam (30 mg/kg, IV, q8h) and clindamycin (11 mg/kg, IV, q12h). Pleural effusion was manually suctioned q4h. The thoracostomy tube was removed on day 5 post-hospitalization when very little pleural fluid production was documented, and antibiotic therapy was transitioned to clavulanic acid-amoxicillin (20 mg/kg, PO, q12h) and clindamycin (8 mg/kg, PO, q12h). Histopathology of surgically resected lung tissue revealed focal suppurative pneumonia, chronic pyogranulomatous pleuritis, and mediastinitis. Sam was discharged on day 6 of hospitalization. He continued to recover well after discharge. No evidence of recurrence was documented as of follow-up 18 months after discharge.

Comments

The growth of *Actinomyces* spp. and the mass lesion in one lung lobe in this dog suggested the possibility of plant awn migration as a cause of the pyothorax.

SUGGESTED READINGS

Dear JD. Bacterial pneumonia in dogs and cats: an update. *Vet Clin North Am Small Anim Pract.* 2020;50:447–465.

Stillion JR, Letendre JA. A clinical review of the pathophysiology, diagnosis, and treatment of pyothorax in dogs and cats. *J Vet Emerg Crit Care.* 2015;25:113–129.

Lappin MR, Blondeau J, Boothe D, et al. Antimicrobial use guidelines for treatment of respiratory tract disease in dogs and cats: Antimicrobial Guidelines Working Group of the International Society for Companion Animal Infectious Diseases. *J Vet Intern Med.* 2017;31:279–294.

REFERENCES

1. Lindsey JO, Pierce AK. An examination of the microbiologic flora of normal lung of the dog. *Am Rev Respir Dis.* 1978;117:501–505.
2. McKiernan B, Smith A, Kissil M. Bacterial isolates from the lower trachea of clinically healthy dogs. *J Am Anim Hosp Assoc.* 1984;20:139–142.
3. Ericsson AC, Personett AR, Grobman ME, et al. Composition and predicted metabolic capacity of upper and lower airway microbiota of healthy dogs in relation to the fecal microbiota. *PLoS One.* 2016;11:e0154646.
4. Fastres A, Roels E, Vangrinsven E, et al. Assessment of the lung microbiota in dogs: influence of the type of breed, living conditions and canine idiopathic pulmonary fibrosis. *BMC Microbiol.* 2020;20:84.
5. Fastres A, Taminiau B, Vangrinsven E, et al. Effect of an antimicrobial drug on lung microbiota in healthy dogs. *Heliyon.* 2019;5:e02802.
6. Vientos-Plotts AI, Ericsson AC, Rindt H, et al. Dynamic changes of the respiratory microbiota and its relationship to fecal and blood microbiota in healthy young cats. *PLoS One.* 2017;12:e0173818.
7. Dorn ES, Tress B, Suchodolski JS, et al. Bacterial microbiome in the nose of healthy cats and in cats with nasal disease. *PLoS One.* 2017;12:e0180299.
8. Ericsson AC, Personett AR, Rindt H, et al. Respiratory dysbiosis and population-wide temporal dynamics in canine chronic bronchitis and non-inflammatory respiratory disease. *PLoS One.* 2020;15. e0228085. Edinburgh, Scotland.
9. Vientos-Plotts A, Ericsson AC, Rindt H, et al. Development of respiratory dysbiosis as cats transition from healthy to asthmatic airways. In: *Proceedings of the 2016 Veterinary Comparative Respiratory Society Symposium*. Lansing, MI, USA.
10. Dye JA, McKiernan BC, Rozanski EA, et al. Bronchopulmonary disease in the cat: historical, physical, radiographic, clinicopathologic, and pulmonary functional evaluation of 24 affected and 15 healthy cats. *J Vet Intern Med.* 1996;10:385–400.
11. Foley JE, Rand C, Bannasch MJ, et al. Molecular epidemiology of feline bordetellosis in two animal shelters in California, USA. *Prev Vet Med.* 2002;54:141–156.
12. Padrid PA, Feldman BF, Funk K, et al. Cytologic, microbiologic, and biochemical analysis of bronchoalveolar lavage fluid obtained from 24 healthy cats. *Am J Vet Res.* 1991;52:1300–1307.
13. Randolph JF, Moise NS, Scarlett JM, et al. Prevalence of mycoplasmal and ureaplasmal recovery from tracheobronchial lavages and of mycoplasmal recovery from pharyngeal swab specimens in cats with or without pulmonary disease. *Am J Vet Res.* 1993;54:897–900.
14. Lee-Fowler T. Feline respiratory disease: what is the role of *Mycoplasma* species? *J Feline Med Surg.* 2014;16:563–571.
15. Načeradská M, Pekova S, Danesi P, et al. A novel Filobacterium sp. can cause chronic bronchitis in cats. *PLoS One.* 2021;16. e0251968.
16. Ramos-Vara JA, Franklin C, Miller MA. Bronchitis and bronchiolitis in a cat with cilia associated respiratory bacillus-like organisms. *Vet Pathol.* 2002;39:501–504.
17. Highland MA, Lowensteine LJ, Johnson LR, et al. CAR bacillus-like organisms in a cat with bronchiectasis. In: *Proceedings of the West Coast Veterinary Pathology Conference*. Davis, CA, USA: University of California-Davis; 2008.
18. Buback JL, Boothe HW, Hobson HP. Surgical treatment of tracheal collapse in dogs: 90 cases (1983-1993). *J Am Vet Med Assoc.* 1996;208:380–384.
19. Johnson LR, Fales WH. Clinical and microbiologic findings in dogs with bronchoscopically diagnosed tracheal collapse: 37 cases (1990-1995). *J Am Vet Med Assoc.* 2001;219:1247–1250.
20. Lesnikowski S, Weisse C, Berent A, et al. Bacterial infection before and after stent placement in dogs with tracheal collapse syndrome. *J Vet Intern Med.* 2020;34:725–733.
21. Rozanski E. Canine chronic bronchitis. *Vet Clin North Am Small Anim Pract.* 2014;44:107–116.
22. Peeters DE, McKiernan BC, Weisiger RM, et al. Quantitative bacterial cultures and cytological examination of bronchoalveolar lavage specimens in dogs. *J Vet Intern Med.* 2000;14:534–541.
23. Clercx C, Peeters D, Snaps F, et al. Eosinophilic bronchopneumopathy in dogs. *J Vet Intern Med.* 2000;14:282–291.
24. Johnson LR, Johnson EG, Hulsebosch SE, et al. Eosinophilic bronchitis, eosinophilic granuloma, and eosinophilic bronchopneumopathy in 75 dogs (2006-2016). *J Vet Intern Med.* 2019;33:2217–2226.
25. Edwards DF, Patton CS, Kennedy JR. Primary ciliary dyskinesia in the dog. *Probl Vet Med.* 1992;4:291–319.
26. Hawkins EC, Basseches J, Berry CR, et al. Demographic, clinical, and radiographic features of bronchiectasis in dogs: 316 cases (1988-2000). *J Am Vet Med Assoc.* 2003;223:1628–1635.
27. Johnson LR, Johnson EG, Vernau W, et al. Bronchoscopy, imaging, and concurrent diseases in dogs with bronchiectasis: (2003-2014). *J Vet Intern Med.* 2016;30:247–254.
28. Marolf A, Blaik M, Specht A. A retrospective study of the relationship between tracheal collapse and bronchiectasis in dogs. *Vet Radiol Ultrasound.* 2007;48:199–203.
29. Bottero E, Bellino C, De Lorenzi D, et al. Clinical evaluation and endoscopic classification of bronchomalacia in dogs. *J Vet Intern Med.* 2013;27:840–846.
30. Adamama-Moraitou KK, Pardali D, Day MJ, et al. Canine bronchomalacia: a clinicopathological study of 18 cases diagnosed by endoscopy. *Vet J.* 2012;191:261–266.
31. Johnson LR, Pollard RE. Tracheal collapse and bronchomalacia in dogs: 58 cases (7 /2001-1 /2008). *J Vet Intern Med.* 2010;24:298–305.
32. Radhakrishnan A, Drobatz KJ, Culp WT, et al. Community-acquired infectious pneumonia in puppies: 65 cases (1993-2002). *J Am Vet Med Assoc.* 2007;230:1493–1497.
33. Byun JW, Yoon SS, Woo GH, et al. An outbreak of fatal hemorrhagic pneumonia caused by *Streptococcus equi* subsp. *zooepidemicus* in shelter dogs. *J Vet Sci.* 2009;10:269–271.
34. Priestnall SL, Mitchell JA, Walker CA, et al. New and emerging pathogens in canine infectious respiratory disease. *Vet Pathol.* 2014;51:492–504.
35. Nafe LA, Grobman ME, Masseau I, et al. Aspiration-related respiratory disorders in dogs. *J Am Vet Med Assoc.* 2018;253:292–300.
36. Wilson D, Monnet E. Risk factors for the development of aspiration pneumonia after unilateral arytenoid lateralization in dogs with laryngeal paralysis: 232 cases (1987-2012). *J Am Vet Med Assoc.* 2016;248:188–194.
37. Kogan DA, Johnson LR, Sturges BK, et al. Etiology and clinical outcome in dogs with aspiration pneumonia: 88 cases (2004-2006). *J Am Vet Med Assoc.* 2008;233:1748–1755.
38. Tart KM, Babski DM, Lee JA. Potential risks, prognostic indicators, and diagnostic and treatment modalities affecting survival in dogs with presumptive aspiration pneumonia: 125 cases (2005-2008). *J Vet Emerg Crit Care.* 2010;20:319–329.
39. Dear JD. Bacterial pneumonia in dogs and cats: an update. *Vet Clin North Am Small Anim Pract.* 2020;50:447–465.
40. Maatta OLM, Laurila HP, Holopainen S, et al. Reflux aspiration in lungs of dogs with respiratory disease and in healthy West Highland white terriers. *J Vet Intern Med.* 2018;32:2074–2081.
41. Lindsay B, Cook D, Wetzel JM, et al. Brachycephalic airway syndrome: management of post-operative respiratory complications in 248 dogs. *Aust Vet J.* 2020;98:173–180.
42. Grobman ME, Masseau I, Reinero CR. Aerodigestive disorders in dogs evaluated for cough using respiratory fluoroscopy and videofluoroscopic swallow studies. *Vet J.* 2019;251:105344.

43. Dear JD. Bacterial pneumonia in dogs and cats. *Vet Clin North Am Small Anim Pract*. 2014;44:143–159.
44. Caivano D, Birettoni F, Rishniw M, et al. Ultrasonographic findings and outcomes of dogs with suspected migrating intrathoracic grass awns: 43 cases (2010-2013). *J Am Vet Med Assoc*. 2016;248:413–421.
45. Schultz RM, Zwingenberger A. Radiographic, computed tomographic, and ultrasonographic findings with migrating intrathoracic grass awns in dogs and cats. *Vet Radiol Ultrasound*. 2008;49:249–255.
46. Tenwolde AC, Johnson LR, Hunt GB, et al. The role of bronchoscopy in foreign body removal in dogs and cats: 37 cases (2000-2008). *J Vet Intern Med*. 2010;24:1063–1068.
47. Epstein SE, Mellema MS, Hopper K. Airway microbial culture and susceptibility patterns in dogs and cats with respiratory disease of varying severity. *J Vet Emerg Crit Care*. 2010;20:587–594.
48. Schulz BS, Richter P, Weber K, et al. Detection of feline *Mycoplasma* species in cats with feline asthma and chronic bronchitis. *J Feline Med Surg*. 2014;16:943–949.
49. Bart M, Guscetti F, Zurbriggen A, et al. Feline infectious pneumonia: a short literature review and a retrospective immunohistological study on the involvement of *Chlamydia* spp. and distemper virus. *Vet J*. 2000;159:220–230.
50. Norris CR, Samii VF. Clinical, radiographic, and pathologic features of bronchiectasis in cats: 12 cases (1987-1999). *J Am Vet Med Assoc*. 2000;216:530–534.
51. Norris CR, Griffey SM, Samii VF, et al. Thoracic radiography, bronchoalveolar lavage cytopathology, and pulmonary parenchymal histopathology: a comparison of diagnostic results in 11 cats. *J Am Anim Hosp Assoc*. 2002;38:337–345.
52. Ballegeer EA, Forrest LJ, Stepien RL. Radiographic appearance of bronchoalveolar carcinoma in nine cats. *Vet Radiol Ultrasound*. 2002;43:267–271.
53. Dear JD, Vernau W, Johnson EG, et al. Clinicopathologic and radiographic features in 33 cats with aspiration and 26 cats with bronchopneumonia (2007-2017). *J Vet Intern Med*. 2021;35:480–489.
54. LaRue MJ, Garlick DS, Lamb CR, et al. Bronchial dysgenesis and lobar emphysema in an adult cat. *J Am Vet Med Assoc*. 1990;197:886–888.
55. Talavera J, del Palacio MJ, Bayon A, et al. Broncholithiasis in a cat: clinical findings, long-term evolution and histopathological features. *J Feline Med Surg*. 2008;10:95–101.
56. Roperto F, Brunetti A, Saviano L, et al. Morphologic alterations in the cilia of a cat. *Vet Pathol*. 1996;33:460–462.
57. Macdonald ES, Norris CR, Berghaus RB, et al. Clinicopathologic and radiographic features and etiologic agents in cats with histologically confirmed infectious pneumonia: 39 cases (1991-2000). *J Am Vet Med Assoc*. 2003;223:1142–1150.
58. Hardie RJ, Gunby J, Bjorling DE. Arytenoid lateralization for treatment of laryngeal paralysis in 10 cats. *Vet Surg*. 2009;38:445–451.
59. Kogan DA, Johnson LR, Jandrey KE, et al. Clinical, clinicopathologic, and radiographic findings in dogs with aspiration pneumonia: 88 cases (2004-2006). *J Am Vet Med Assoc*. 2008;233:1742–1747.
60. Bailiff NL, Norris CR. Clinical signs, clinicopathological findings, etiology, and outcome associated with hemoptysis in dogs: 36 cases (1990-1999). *J Am Anim Hosp Assoc*. 2002;38:125–133.
61. Foster SF, Martin P, Allan GS, et al. Lower respiratory tract infections in cats: 21 cases (1995-2000). *J Feline Med Surg*. 2004;6:167–180.
62. Trzil JE, Reinero CR. Update on feline asthma. *Vet Clin North Am Small Anim Pract*. 2014;44:91–105.
63. Moise NS, Wiedenkeller D, Yeager AE, et al. Clinical, radiographic, and bronchial cytologic features of cats with bronchial disease: 65 cases (1980-1986). *J Am Vet Med Assoc*. 1989;194:1467–1473.
64. Harris RA, Grobman ME, Allen MJ, et al. Standardization of videofluoroscopic swallow study protocol to investigate dysphagia in dogs. *J Vet Intern Med*. 2017;31:383–393.
65. Gaschen L, Kircher P, Hoffmann G, et al. Endoscopic ultrasonography for the diagnosis of intrathoracic lesions in two dogs. *Vet Radiol Ultrasound*. 2003;44:292–299.
66. Murphy SD, Ward JL, Viall AK, et al. Utility of point-of-care lung ultrasound for monitoring cardiogenic pulmonary edema in dogs. *J Vet Intern Med*. 2021;35:68–77.
67. Boysen SR, Lisciandro GR. The use of ultrasound for dogs and cats in the emergency room: AFAST and TFAST. *Vet Clin North Am Small Anim Pract*. 2013;43:773–797.
68. Cole L, Pivetta M, Humm K. Diagnostic accuracy of a lung ultrasound protocol (Vet BLUE) for detection of pleural fluid, pneumothorax and lung pathology in dogs and cats. *J Small Anim Pract*. 2021;62:178–186.
69. Mesquita L, Lam R, Lamb CR, et al. Computed tomographic findings in 15 dogs with eosinophilic bronchopneumopathy. *Vet Radiol Ultrasound*. 2015;56:33–39.
70. Reinero CR. Bronchoalveolar lavage fluid collection using a blind technique. *NAVC Clinician's Brief*. 2010. Available at: https://www.cliniciansbrief.com/article/bronchoalveolar-lavage-fluid-collection-using-blind-technique.
71. DeBerry JD, Norris CR, Samii VF, et al. Correlation between fine-needle aspiration cytopathology and histopathology of the lung in dogs and cats. *J Am Anim Hosp Assoc*. 2002;38:327–336.
72. Tidwell AS, Johnson KL. Computed tomography-guided percutaneous biopsy in the dog and cat: description of technique and preliminary evaluation in 14 patients. *Vet Radiol Ultrasound*. 1994;35:445–446.
73. Wood EF, O'Brien RT, Young KM. Ultrasound-guided fine-needle aspiration of focal parenchymal lesions of the lung in dogs and cats. *J Vet Intern Med*. 1998;12:338–342.
74. Norris CR, Griffey SM, Samii VF, et al. Comparison of results of thoracic radiography, cytologic evaluation of bronchoalveolar lavage fluid, and histologic evaluation of lung specimens in dogs with respiratory tract disease: 16 cases (1996-2000). *J Am Vet Med Assoc*. 2001;218:1456–1461.
75. Norris CR, Griffey SM, Walsh P. Use of keyhole lung biopsy for diagnosis of interstitial lung diseases in dogs and cats: 13 cases (1998-2001). *J Am Vet Med Assoc*. 2002;221:1453–1459.
76. Lappin MR, Blondeau J, Boothe D, et al. Antimicrobial use guidelines for treatment of respiratory tract disease in dogs and cats: Antimicrobial Guidelines Working Group of the International Society for Companion Animal Infectious Diseases. *J Vet Intern Med*. 2017;31:279–294.
77. Thayer GW, Robinson S K. Bacterial bronchopneumonia in the dog: a review of 42 cases. *J Am Anim Hosp Assoc*. 1984;20:731–735.
78. Proulx A, Hume DZ, Drobatz KJ, et al. In vitro bacterial isolate susceptibility to empirically selected antimicrobials in 111 dogs with bacterial pneumonia. *J Vet Emerg Crit Care*. 2014;24:194–200.
79. Conway H, Dix KJ, McDonald JD, et al. Comparison of inhalation toxicity studies of gentamicin in rats and dogs. *Inhal Toxicol*. 2013;25:714–724.
80. Morgane Canonne A, Roels E, Menard M, et al. Clinical response to 2 protocols of aerosolized gentamicin in 46 dogs with Bordetella bronchiseptica infection. *J Vet Intern Med*. 2012-2018;2020(34):2078–2085.
81. Pinzone MR, Cacopardo B, Abbo L, et al. Duration of antimicrobial therapy in community acquired pneumonia: less is more. *Scientific World J*. 2014;2014:759138.
82. Bruns AH, Oosterheert JJ, El Moussaouri R. Routine radiographic follow-up of community-acquired pneumonia is not warranted. *J Gen Intern Med*. 2009;17:156–157.
83. El Solh AA, Aquilina AT, Gunen H, et al. Radiographic resolution of community-acquired bacterial pneumonia in the elderly. *J Am Geriatr Soc*. 2004;52:224–229.
84. Vientos-Plotts AI, Masseau I, Reinero CR. Comparison of short- versus long-course antimicrobial therapy of uncomplicated bacterial pneumonia in dogs: A double-blinded, placebo-controlled pilot study. *Animals (Basel)*. 2012;11:3096.
85. Keir I, Daly J, Haggerty J, et al. Retrospective evaluation of the effect of high flow oxygen therapy delivered by nasal cannula on PaO2 in dogs with moderate-to-severe hypoxemia. *J Vet Emerg Crit Care*. 2016;26:598–602.
86. Manning K, Birkenheuer AJ, Briley J, et al. Intermittent at-home suctioning of esophageal content for prevention of recurrent aspiration pneumonia in 4 dogs with megaesophagus. *J Vet Intern Med*. 2016;30:1715–1719.
87. Milovancev M, Townsend K, Spina J, et al. Effect of metoclopramide on the incidence of early postoperative aspiration pneumonia in dogs with acquired idiopathic laryngeal paralysis. *Vet Surg*. 2016;45:577–581.
88. Sykes JE. Bacterial bronchopneumonia and pyothorax. In: Sykes JE, ed. *Canine and Feline Infectious Diseases*. 1st ed. St. Louis, MO: Elsevier; 2013:847–858.

89. Sykes JE, Mapes S, Lindsay LL, et al. *Corynebacterium ulcerans* bronchopneumonia in a dog. *J Vet Intern Med.* 2010;24:973–976.
90. Stillion JR, Letendre JA. A clinical review of the pathophysiology, diagnosis, and treatment of pyothorax in dogs and cats. *J Vet Emerg Crit Care.* 2015;25:113–129.
91. Barrs VR, Allan GS, Martin P, et al. Feline pyothorax: a retrospective study of 27 cases in Australia. *J Fel Med Surg.* 2005;7:211–222.
92. Boothe HW, Howe LM, Boothe DM, et al. Evaluation of outcomes in dogs treated for pyothorax: 46 cases (1983-2001). *J Am Vet Med Assoc.* 2010;236:657–663.
93. Demetriou JL, Foale RD, Ladlow J, et al. Canine and feline pyothorax: a retrospective study of 50 cases in the UK and Ireland. *J Small Anim Pract.* 2002;43:388–394.
94. Ottenjann M, Lubke-Becker A, Linzmann H, et al. Pyothorax in 26 cats: clinical signs, laboratory results and therapy (2000-2007). *Berl Munch Tierarztl Wochenschr.* 2008;121:365–373.
95. Rooney MB, Monnet E. Medical and surgical treatment of pyothorax in dogs: 26 cases (1991-2001). *J Am Vet Med Assoc.* 2002;221:86–92.
96. Waddell LS, Brady CA, Drobatz KJ. Risk factors, prognostic indicators, and outcome of pyothorax in cats: 80 cases (1986-1999). *J Am Vet Med Assoc.* 2002;221:819–824.
97. Walker AL, Jang SS, Hirsh DC. Bacteria associated with pyothorax of dogs and cats: 98 cases (1989-1998). *J Am Vet Med Assoc.* 2000;216:359–363.
98. Crawford AH, Halfacree ZJ, Lee KC, et al. Clinical outcome following pneumonectomy for management of chronic pyothorax in four cats. *J Feline Med Surg.* 2011;13:762–767.
99. Doyle JL, Kuipers von Lande RG, Worth AJ. Intra-thoracic pyogranulomatous disease in four working dogs. *N Z Vet J.* 2009;57:346–351.
100. Hicks A, Golland D, Heller J, et al. Epidemiological investigation of grass seed foreign body-related disease in dogs of the Riverina District of rural Australia. *Aust Vet J.* 2016;94:67–75.
101. Klainbart S, Mazaki-Tovi M, Auerbach N, et al. Spirocercosis-associated pyothorax in dogs. *Vet J.* 2007;173:209–214.
102. Hung GC, Gaunt MC, Rubin JE, et al. Quantification and characterization of pleural fluid in healthy dogs with thoracostomy tubes. *Am J Vet Res.* 2016;77:1387–1391.
103. Meakin LB, Salonen LK, Baines SJ, et al. Prevalence, outcome and risk factors for postoperative pyothorax in 232 dogs undergoing thoracic surgery. *J Small Anim Pract.* 2013;54:313–317.
104. Barrs VR, Beatty JA. Feline pyothorax - new insights into an old problem: part 1. Aetiopathogenesis and diagnostic investigation. *Vet J.* 2009;179:163–170.
105. Jonas LD. Feline pyothorax: a retrospective study of twenty cases. *J Am Anim Hosp Assoc.* 1983:865–871.
106. Stone MS, Pook H. Lung infections and infestations. Therapeutic considerations. *Probl Vet Med.* 1992;4:279–290.
107. Johnson MS, Martin MW. Successful medical treatment of 15 dogs with pyothorax. *J Small Anim Pract.* 2007;48:12–16.
108. Robertson SA, Stoddart ME, Evans RJ, Gaskell CJ, Gibbs C. Thoracic empyema in the dog; a report of twenty-two cases. *J Small Anim Pract.* 1983;24:103–119.
109. Pelaez MJ, Jolliffe C. Thoracoscopic foreign body removal and right middle lung lobectomy to treat pyothorax in a dog. *J Small Anim Pract.* 2012;53:240–244.
110. Gnudi G, Volta A, Bonazzi M, et al. Ultrasonographic features of grass awn migration in the dog. *Vet Radiol Ultrasound.* 2005;46:423–426.
111. Swinbourne F, Baines EA, Baines SJ, et al. Computed tomographic findings in canine pyothorax and correlation with findings at exploratory thoracotomy. *J Small Anim Pract.* 2011;52:203–208.
112. Gibson EA, Balsa IM, Mayhew PD, et al. Utility of bronchoscopy combined with surgery in the treatment and outcomes of dogs with intrathoracic disease secondary to plant awn migration. *Vet Surg.* 2019;48:1309–1317.
113. Valtolina C, Adamantos S. Evaluation of small-bore wire-guided chest drains for management of pleural space disease. *J Small Anim Pract.* 2009;50:290–297.
114. Turner WD, Breznock EM. Continuous suction drainage for management of canine pyothorax-a retrospective study. *J Am Anim Hosp Assoc.* 1988;24:485–494.
115. Piek CJ, Robben JH. Pyothorax in nine dogs. *Vet Q.* 2000;22:107–111.
116. Scott JA, Macintire DK. Canine pyothorax: clinical presentation, diagnosis, and treatment. *Compend Contin Educ Pract Vet.* 2003:180–194.
117. Bach JF, Balakrishnan A. Retrospective comparison of costs between medical and surgical treatment of canine pyothorax. *Can Vet J.* 2015;56:1140–1143.
118. Brennan KE, Ihrke PJ. Grass awn migration in dogs and cats: a retrospective study of 182 cases. *J Am Vet Med Assoc.* 1983;182:1201–1204.
119. Frendin J. Pyogranulomatous pleuritis with empyema in hunting dogs. *Zentralbl Veterinarmed A.* 1997;44:167–178.
120. Kovak JR, Ludwig LL, Bergman PJ, et al. Use of thoracoscopy to determine the etiology of pleural effusion in dogs and cats: 18 cases (1998-2001). *J Am Vet Med Assoc.* 2002;221:990–994.
121. Scott J, Singh A, Monnet E, et al. Video-assisted thoracic surgery for the management of pyothorax in dogs: 14 cases. *Vet Surg.* 2017;46:722–730.
122. Bailie WE, Stowe EC, Schmitt AM. Aerobic bacterial flora of oral and nasal fluids of canines with reference to bacteria associated with bites. *J Clin Microbiol.* 1978;7:223–231.
123. Clapper WE, Meade GH. Normal flora of the nose, throat, and lower intestine of dogs. *J Bacteriol.* 1963;85:643–648.
124. Smith JE. The aerobic bacteria of the nose and tonsils of healthy dogs. *J Comp Pathol.* 1961;71:428–433.
125. Padrid PA. Do respiratory infections play a role in feline bronchial disease? In: *Proceedings of the 1996 Comparative Respiratory Society Symposium.* Orlando, FL, USA.
126. Inzana TJ, Johnson JL, Shell L, et al. Isolation and characterization of a newly identified *Haemophilus* species from cats: "*Haemophilus felis*". *J Clin Microbiol.* 1992;30:2108–2112.

125

Gastrointestinal and Intra-Abdominal Infections

Jane E. Sykes, Ingrid Balsa, William T.N. Culp, Boaz Arzi, Sina Marsilio, Stanley L. Marks

KEY POINTS

- Causes: A wide variety of gram-negative and gram-positive bacteria can infect the GI tract and peritoneal cavity, including *Escherichia coli, Enterococcus* spp., other gram-negative aerobes, *Streptococcus,* and *Staphylococcus* spp. and anaerobes. *Candida* spp. may also be involved, particularly in immunocompromised patients or patients receiving antibacterial drug therapy. Viruses, atypical bacteria (e.g., *Mycobacterium* spp.), protozoa (e.g., *Toxoplasma gondii, Giardia duodenalis, Tritrichomonas blagburni*), endemic fungi (e.g., *Histoplasma spp.*), algae (*Prototheca* spp.), and helminth parasites also cause GI disease.
- Mode of Transmission: Most GI infections result from opportunistic invasion by commensal bacteria and fungi of the GI and urogenital tracts. Other pathogens are transmitted by a variety of different routes.
- Major Clinical Signs: Signs are extremely variable depending on the site of infection, the underlying etiology, and the immunocompetence of the host, but include dysphagia, hypersalivation, inappetence, fever, vomiting, diarrhea, and abdominal pain.
- Human Health Significance: Enteric bacteria involved may be multidrug-resistant organisms that have the potential to colonize humans. In addition, certain assemblages of *Giardia duodenalis* have the potential to be zoonotic.

THE GASTROINTESTINAL MICROBIOME AND METABOLOME

Thousands of microbial species reside within the GI tract as commensal organisms. The resident gut microbiome is composed of viruses, bacteria, and eukaryotic organisms that perform a number of vital functions, including resisting colonization with pathogenic microbes by maintaining oxygen tension, competing with nutrients, and producing antibacterial substances (bacteriocins); assisting with nutrient breakdown and synthesizing essential vitamins and short-chain fatty acids; stimulating and maintaining mucosal immunity; metabolizing bile acids and drugs; and inactivating potentially carcinogenic and toxic ingested substances.[1,2] Antimicrobial administration can induce gut dysbiosis, with broad-spectrum antibiotics causing rapid and significant drops in taxonomic richness, diversity, and evenness. In addition, disruption of the gut microbiome as a result of disease, immunosuppression, or antimicrobial therapy can adversely affect the health of the GI tract and has the potential to allow organisms that are normally nonpathogenic to proliferate opportunistically and cause disease.

For decades, our understanding of the identity and quantity of the resident microflora was hampered because of a reliance on traditional culture methods. This is because the use of culture methods overestimates the species that are culturable and underestimates those that are fastidious or unculturable. The more recent advent of high-throughput molecular approaches has revolutionized our understanding of the intestinal microbiome in health and disease, especially when layered upon our existing knowledge based on culture-dependent methods. Application of next-generation sequencing (NGS) methods (also known as massive parallel sequencing) allows rapid sequencing of 1 million to 43 billion short reads (up to 1000 bp) with each run. Microbial DNA is amplified using PCR and then sequenced; several different types of sequencing methods can be used but common methods applied are 454 pyrosequencing, reversible dye terminator (Illumina) sequencing, and real-time sequencing.[3] The PCR assays used commonly target bacterial 16S rRNA genes. The internal transcribed spacer (ITS) gene has also been used as a target; across bacterial populations, the ITS gene is more variable than the 16S rRNA gene, and so ITS gene PCR methods offer improved discrimination between bacterial species (taxonomic resolution). In-depth whole metagenomic sequencing (WMS) methods capture total microbial DNA (rather than just 16S rRNA gene information) and are not subject to bias that results from preferential amplification of certain 16S rRNA gene sequences; however, they are more expensive than amplification-based methods and so amplification-based methods continue to be utilized.[2] The use of mixed methodology across studies and often small numbers of animals has led to considerable variation in microbiome composition results, but as more studies accumulate, our understanding of the canine and feline microbiome is improving. Targeted techniques such as FISH (see Chapter 6) are complementary to these studies and allow identification of bacteria or fungi within lesions in formalin-fixed tissues (Fig. 125.1).

Because microbiome analysis provides information on the identity of hundreds of bacterial species, including many previously unidentified organisms, data are usually presented by grouping bacteria into phyla, and within phyla, orders. Descriptions of microbial populations generally only refer to individual species when those species represent a significant proportion of organisms within an order. Table 125.1 provides examples of common phyla found within the GI tract, and some of the orders and species within those phyla. A phylum can contain both aerobes and anaerobes, but they tend to be primarily gram-negative or gram-positive species (e.g., organisms that belong to the Firmicutes are generally gram positive).

Terms used to describe microbiome communities include *diversity*, *richness*, *abundance*, and *evenness.* Richness is the total number of bacterial species present in a microbiome; a rich microbiome has many species present. Species diversity is a measure of the number

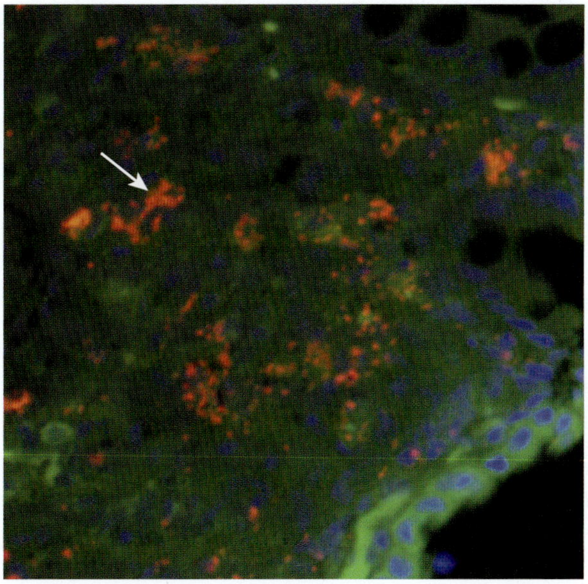

Fig. 125.1 Fluorescence in situ hybridization image using probes *E. coli*-cy3 and non-EUB 338-6FAM. *E. coli* stain red and are found abundantly in the mucosal tissue and within cells (*arrow*) in areas of inflammatory cell infiltrates. DAPI-stained nuclei (DNA) are blue. In healthy colonic tissue the bacteria are only found in superficial mucus and glandular lumens on the bowel surface (×400). (Courtesy Kenny Simpson, Cornell University, Ithaca, NY.)

of species *and* the abundance of each species. Alpha-diversity is the diversity within a particular region or sample, and beta-diversity is the diversity between two regions or samples (measured as the number of species that are unique to each region being compared). Evenness describes the distribution of abundance across a population; an even population is when all species in the population have the same abundance. Indices have been developed in order to quantify diversity (e.g., Shannon's index) and evenness (e.g., Pielou's evenness index) using mathematical equations. A *canine dysbiosis index (DI)* is a PCR-based algorithm that allows veterinarians to quantify gut dysbiosis and can be used to monitor disease progression and response to treatment.[4] A DI ≥ 2 indicates dysbiosis, a negative DI suggests normobiosis, and values in between have been considered equivocal.[5] Antimicrobial administration induces a rapid and significant drop in taxonomic richness, diversity, and evenness. In light of this phenomenon, there has been renewed vigor to study the effects of probiotics, prebiotics, and fecal microbiota transplantation (FMT) on reversing intestinal dysbiosis and optimizing the intestinal microbiome.

Several studies also have described the metabolic products generated by the canine and feline intestinal microbiota, including volatile fatty acids; amino acids such as tryptophan; lactate; ammonia; and other end products.[6,7] The chemical signature that results is reflective of the bacterial populations present, and is referred to as the GI metabolome.

INFECTIONS OF THE ORAL CAVITY

THE ORAL MICROBIOME

The resident microbial flora of the canine and feline oral cavity is composed of a wide variety of aerobic bacteria and facultative and obligate anaerobic bacteria, mycoplasmas, and yeasts, but differs significantly from that in humans. Examples of anaerobes found in canine saliva using culture include *Actinomyces, Streptococcus,* and *Granulicatella* (previously nutritionally variant streptococci), and in dental plaque, *Porphyromonas, Actinomyces,* and *Neisseria.*[8]

High-throughput sequencing methods have demonstrated the diversity of species in the bacterial and fungal biomes in the oral cavity of healthy dogs and cats and those with periodontal disease, with considerable variations from one anatomic region to another.[9] In one study, three different niches were identified in dogs—saliva, supragingival plaque, and the soft-tissue structures of the tongue and buccal mucosa.[9] The most abundant organisms were *Filofactor villosus* for supragingival plaque (5% of total DNA composition), an unclassified Pasteurellaceae for buccal mucosa (12%), *Conchiformibius* sp. for the dorsal tongue mucosa (17%), and an unclassified *Escherichia coli-Shigella* sp. for saliva (20%). Proteobacteria were the dominant group for all of the sites except supragingival plaque, where Firmicutes were dominant. Supragingival plaque also exhibited the greatest microbial diversity. *Capnocytophaga, Porphyromonas, Neisseria,* and *Fusobacterium* spp. were all observed among core microbiota. In healthy cats, the most prevalent species in swabs from the oral cavity in one study was an unidentified Pasteurellaceae (19%), followed by *Moraxella* spp. (11%). When the subgingival microbiota was examined, *Porphyromonas* spp. was most abundant, followed by *Moraxella* spp. and *Fusobacterium*.[10] In another study of cats with and without periodontal disease, the most abundant genera in healthy cats were *Enhydrobacter, Moraxella,* and *Capnocytophaga* spp.[11] Organisms that are found to a greater extent in cats with periodontal disease than healthy cats are *Filofactor* spp. and the spirochete *Treponema* spp.

Antimicrobial agents used in treating oral infections such as gingivitis and stomatitis should be chosen with the composition of the resident microflora in mind. However, clearly not all organisms that comprise the resident microflora are capable of causing disease or replicating when inoculated into tissue; bacterial virulence factors, the local tissue environment, and the host response to infection ultimately influence what bacteria are able to replicate and cause pathology. Some of the organisms are found in bite wound infections (see Chapter 75).

GINGIVITIS AND PERIODONTITIS

Inflammation and recession of the gingival margins are common findings in dogs and cats. Factors that predispose dogs and cats to periodontal disease include tooth crowding and rotation, persistent deciduous dentition, malocclusions, congenital abnormalities, trauma, soft food diets, and genetic factors.[12] Lesions are initially caused by excessive accumulation of dental plaque resulting from deposition of by-products from breakdown of food and saliva by normal resident microflora. Plaque is an organic matrix of salivary glycoproteins and polysaccharides that adheres to the tooth surface and provides sites for oral bacteria to proliferate. Resident bacteria produce a glycopolysaccharide referred to as a *glycocalyx*, which facilitates the attachment of other bacteria. This biofilm is further consolidated into a film, or plaque. Plaque accumulation results in inflammation of the gingiva. Plaque can become mineralized, resulting in calculus deposition (Fig. 125.2). The deposition of calculus facilitates additional plaque formation and periodontal inflammation.

In dogs, periodontitis is associated with proliferation of gram-positive and gram-negative anaerobic organisms that belong to the Firmicutes, Actinobacteria (such as *Actinomyces* spp.), Bacteroidetes (especially *Porphyromonas* spp. and *Fusobacterium* spp.), and Spirochaetes (e.g., *Treponema* spp.).[13,14] In humans, periodontitis has been associated with an increased population of *Porphyromonas gingivalis, Tannerella forsythia,* and *Treponema denticola* (collectively referred to as "the red complex").[15] Pups have very few *Porphyromonas* species in their dental plaque; however, bacterial numbers increase as

TABLE 125.1 Common Phyla Present in the Gastrointestinal Microbiome

Phylum	Class Examples	Order Examples	Species Examples
Firmicutes (mostly gram positive)	Clostridia	Clostridiales	*Clostridium filofactor* *Peptostreptococcus* *Eubacterium*
	Bacilli	Bacillales	*Bacillus* *Listeria* *Staphylococcus*
		Lactobacillales	*Lactobacillus* *Streptococcus* *Enterococcus*
	Erysipelotrichia	Erysipelotrichales	*Erysipelothrix*
Proteobacteria (mostly gram negative)	Gammaproteobacteria	Enterobacterales	*Escherichia* *Enterobacter* *Klebsiella* *Proteus* *Salmonella* *Yersinia*
		Pasteurellales	*Pasteurella* *Haemophilus*
	Epsilonproteobacteria	Campylobacterales	*Helicobacter* *Campylobacter*
	Betaproteobacteria	Neisseriales	*Neisseria*
Bacteroidetes (mostly gram negative)	Bacteroidia	Bacteroidales	*Bacteroides* *Prevotella* *Porphyromonas*
Fusobacteria	Fusobacteria	Fusobacteriales	*Fusobacterium*
Spirochaetes	Spirochaetia	Spirochaetales	*Treponema* *Leptospira* *Borrelia (Borreliella)*
Actinobacteria	Actinobacteria	Actinomycetales	*Actinomyces* *Nocardia* *Mycobacterium* *Corynebacterium*
		Bifidobacteriales	*Bifidobacterium*

puppies mature and inevitably periodontal disease develops. Although spirochetes such as *Treponema* spp. have been considered important pathogens in canine periodontal disease, one study found no difference in the prevalence of various *Treponema* species as detected using nucleic acid–based methods in gingival plaque from dogs with and without periodontal disease.[16]

Subgingival plaque incites an inflammatory response in the gingival tissue that can lead to chronic periodontal disease with eventual loss of teeth. Early bacterial damage occurs in the subgingival epithelial tissues with penetration of the interdental rete pegs. Many bacteria possess proteolytic enzymes that allow them to colonize and invade periodontal tissues. Periodontal pathogens destroy the integrity of the dentition and oral mucosae.

Endodontal disease and periodontitis can also develop whenever tooth damage occurs, exposing the dental pulp. Acute periapical periodontitis (i.e., periapical lesion) begins within 20 days of pulp exposure in dogs and progresses with time.[17] Fractures of teeth usually result in pulp infection before revascularization of the canal by vital tissue can occur. In advanced human root canal infections, anaerobes, corynebacteria, and streptococci predominate.[18] Although not widely practiced in veterinary medicine and human endodontics, debridement and treatment of the canal with a triple antibacterial paste (ciprofloxacin, minocycline, and metronidazole) in a resorbable matrix base early after injury may eliminate endodontal infection and promote revascularization of the pulp canal.[19]

Radiographic examination of the teeth and associated bony structures is required to determine the condition of the tooth roots and secondary bone or tooth resorption before treatment. Furthermore, endodontal involvement, neoplastic destruction of bone, and nasal and sinus passages can be evaluated to determine the extent of disease before treatment.

Treatment includes the extraction of severely affected teeth, debridement of necrotic or proliferative gingival margins, root planing with curettes, and scaling calculi from the remaining involved supragingival and subgingival dental surfaces by manual or ultrasonic means. Complete removal of all supragingival and subgingival calculus and plaque is essential in control of periodontal disease. More aggressive surgical debridement is needed for advanced periodontal disease.

Although bacterial pathogens are important in periodontitis, antimicrobial therapy alone does not eliminate progression of disease. Because proinflammatory cytokines, such as TNF-α, Il-1β, and matrix metalloproteinases have been important in the progression of periodontal disease, a variety of anti-inflammatory and immunomodulatory drugs and dietary supplements have been examined

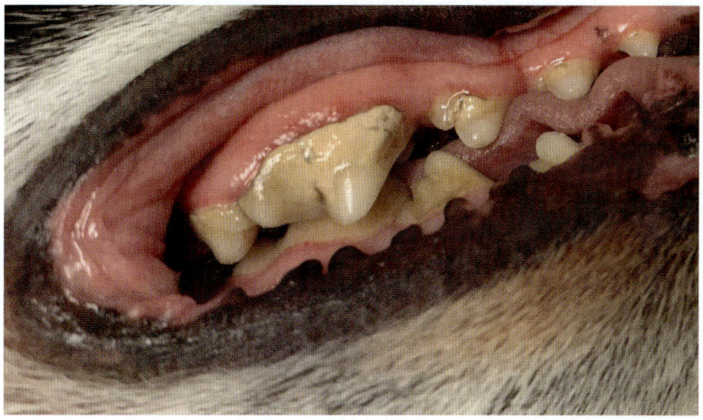

Fig. 125.2 Moderate to severe periodontal disease with accumulation of dental calculus in a 9-year-old male neutered terrier mix. (Courtesy University of California-Davis Community Medicine Service.)

as treatments.[20,21] Genetic predisposition to periodontal disease in humans may reflect differences in cytokine responses to invasion of tissues by oral cavity bacteria.[21] Oral IFN-α administered to dogs and cats with naturally occurring gingivitis reduced both periodontal bacterial counts and associated gingival inflammation.[22,23] The use of anti-inflammatory diets or supplements with omega-3 fatty acids may reduce the local gingival inflammatory response and has shown some benefit in small human clinical trials.[24] However, a prospective study in dogs showed no benefit for reduction of gingivitis, plaque, or calculus when a diet supplemented with either corn oil or fish oil was fed.[25]

Although administration of systemic antimicrobial drugs such as tetracyclines, clindamycin, metronidazole, and tinidazole have been shown to reduce gingivitis, plaque accumulation, halitosis, and alveolar bone resorption in dogs and cats,[26-28] the use and efficacy of systemic antimicrobial therapy for this purpose has been questioned as an alternative for indicated dental procedures[29] and may select for antimicrobial-resistant bacterial populations. Currently it is recommended by AAHA that the use of systemic antimicrobials in conjunction with dental procedures be considered on a case-by-case basis.[30] In most cases, antimicrobials are not required. Postoperative treatment with clindamycin or amoxicillin-clavulanic acid is indicated for at least 7 to 14 days if there is radiographic evidence of osteomyelitis.[30] Treatment for several days before surgery has been suggested for animals with Stage IV disease to facilitate tissue handling, but this may not be necessary and has the potential to select for resistant bacteria.

Perioceutics are pharmaceutical formulations that are placed into periodontal pockets to allow for sustained antimicrobial activity against periodontal pathogens. They are used as an adjunct to scaling and cleaning the dental surfaces. The perioceutics containing antimicrobials are delivered into the periodontal pocket via a blunt cannula. Once there, the biodegradable polymer gels coagulate, allowing for sustained release of the drug for up to 13 weeks. Products that contain 2% clindamycin gel or 8.5% doxycycline hyclate are available for veterinary use.[12] Their use has been recommended by AAHA when a > 5-mm cleaned pocket exists in dogs with Stage II or Stage III periodontal disease. However, one study evaluated the use of these gels in conjunction with closed root planing in dogs with periodontal pockets that ranged from 3.5 to 5.5 mm deep.[12] Use of the gels did not lead to greater improvement in periodontal disease indices over closed root planing alone.

Long-term intermittent periodontal care for dogs is highly recommended because it slows the progression of gingival recession and depth of periodontal crevices that develop in dogs not receiving dental hygiene.[31] Gingival enlargement and abscess formation are sequelae of calculus formation.[32] The type of microflora present, diet, and the animal's chewing habits may influence the formation of calculus.[33,34] Daily tooth brushing is more effective than diet for optimization of oral health in dogs; in one study it was three times as effective at controlling plaque accumulation than a dental diet or daily dental chews.[35] Tooth brushing has also been shown to be effective in cats.[36,37] The use of special diets supplemented with dental chews can reduce calculus deposition further in dogs and cats.[37] Feeding of a commercial dental food to dogs significantly reduced plaque and gingivitis by 39% and 36%, respectively, compared with daily feeding of a control dry-food diet.[38] Cats fed large kibbles with mechanical cleaning qualities had less gingivitis and calculus than cats on small kibble diets with or without daily brushing.[39]

Flushing dental surfaces once daily with 0.1% to 0.2% chlorhexidine and/or alternate-day brushing may delay accumulation of dental calculus. A commercial product formulated especially for dental purposes (Nolvadent, Zoetis) does not stain teeth blue like other chlorhexidine formulations. Daily application of chlorhexidine gel was effective in reducing recurrence of dental plaque in dogs.[40] Numerous cleansers and brushes have been developed for daily brushing of dogs' teeth, and they warrant consideration when a dog has a tendency to form calculus. Oral probiotics have been examined for their ability to prevent the growth of pathogenic bacteria or modulate mucosal immunity in the oral cavity. Oral probiotic bacteria should adhere to and colonize on dental tissue and should be part of the biofilm. They should not ferment sugars, which subsequently lowers the pH and is detrimental to dental health.[41] A split-mouth, double-blind randomized pilot study, involving eight beagle dogs with moderate experimentally induced periodontitis, documented the impact of multiple subgingival applications of pellets containing *Streptococcus sanguinis, Streptococcus salivarius,* and *Streptococcus mitis*.[42] The bone density within periodontal pockets treated with the beneficial bacteria improved significantly after 12 weeks, whereas there was a nonsignificant change in the control group that received a single root planing at baseline. In addition, there was a significant increase in the alveolar bone level at the end of the study based on repeat radiographs compared to the control group. Unfortunately, a randomized controlled clinical trial in humans with Stage III periodontitis showed no benefit of a *Lactobacillus* probiotic or azithromycin as an adjunct to scaling and root planing.[43] Also, a study that examined the effect of an oral probiotic containing *Enterococcus faecium* (Fortiflora, Purina) showed no change in the oral microbiota of dogs, which remained stable over a 7-week time period regardless of diet or administration of the probiotic.[44] More needs to be known about what organisms are capable of restoring and maintaining health when delivered in a probiotic format. The Veterinary Oral Health Council website lists products that have been shown to be effective for retarding plaque and calculus deposition in dogs and cats (vohc.org/all_accepted_products.html).

A *P. denticanis-gulae-salivosa* bacterin that was commercially available as an aid in preventing periodontal disease is no longer licensed due to concerns surrounding lack of efficacy.

Systemic Effects of Oral or Periodontal Infections

Ophthalmic manifestations can occur from dental disease because of the close proximity of the caudal maxillary teeth and the orbit. Systemic complications of periodontal disease, including cerebral and myocardial infarction, systemic hypertension, adverse pregnancy outcomes and early mortality, have been described in people.[45,46] Human patients with poorly controlled diabetes mellitus are at an increased risk of developing periodontal disease[47] and resolution of periodontal inflammation can improve metabolic control of blood glucose in diabetics.[48]

Associations between periodontal inflammation and heart (endocarditis, cardiomyopathy), liver, and kidney (CKD) disease have been reported in dogs.[49-53] These have included studies that have correlated lesions at necropsy with whole mouth periodontal scoring. In other retrospective studies, no statistical association was found between bacterial endocarditis in dogs and either dental or oral surgical procedures or oral infection.[54,55] However, detailed prospective screening and grading of oral cavity changes were not undertaken in these studies.

Bacteremia associated with dental manipulations may be subclinical or has the potential to cause sepsis or subsequently result in bacterial endocarditis or localized embolic tissue infections (see Chapter 122). In cats with periodontitis undergoing dental scaling and extraction, 36% had positive blood culture results at the time of the dental procedures.[56] Bacteria most commonly isolated were *Cutibacterium* (formerly *Propionibacterium) acnes, Pasteurella multocida,* and *Staphylococcus epidermidis.* None of the cats subsequently became ill. Similarly, blood culture results have shown subclinical bacteremia in 30% of dogs with periodontal disease undergoing periodontal treatment and tooth extraction, although a group of control dogs that were anesthetized but that did not undergo dental procedures had a similar prevalence of bacteremia.[57] It is generally recommended that dental procedures should not be performed at the same time as other surgical procedures, because the release of bacteria from the dental procedure may have the potential to establish themselves in tissue injured or devitalized by routine surgical procedures, sutures, or foreign implants. Current guidelines from AAHA recommend that intraoperative antibiotic administration be used for immunosuppressed animals or those with implants or subaortic stenosis to reduce the likelihood of bacteremia. A rational approach is to follow the recommendations for prophylactic antimicrobial use for "dirty" surgical procedures or when the implications of a surgical site infection may be devastating (see Chapter 76). In summary, the goal is to maintain therapeutic drug levels throughout the period of risk by administering the first dose IV 30 to 60 minutes before starting the procedure, with intraoperative dosing every 2 half-lives of the antimicrobial as long as the procedure is underway. Ampicillin is a rational choice for dental procedures, and it has a half-life of 20 minutes in the dog and 72 minutes in the cat, meaning intraoperative redosing is indicated every 40 and 145 minutes, respectively. Prerinsing the oral cavity with chlorhexidine solutions can also be performed just before the procedure. Drug administration should be terminated no longer than 24 hours after the dental procedure because no additional benefits are gained and additional antimicrobial exposure increases the risk of selection for resistant bacteria. Interestingly, IV administration of aqueous penicillin during ultrasonic scaling in dogs did not alter the prevalence of bacteremia before or after dental manipulation.[58] More studies are required to examine the effects of intraoperative antimicrobial administration on bacteremia in dogs undergoing dental procedures and whether prophylaxis impacts outcomes.

Because of the large numbers of bacteria in the oral cavity and especially the gingival crevices, public health considerations are important when dental procedures are performed. Face masks, ocular shields, and gloves should always be worn by humans who clean animals' teeth. In addition, biofilms that form on the inside surface of water lines of ultrasonic scalers may harbor *Legionella* species, which might produce acute pneumonia in susceptible individuals.[59]

GLOSSITIS AND STOMATITIS

Glossitis may be caused by viruses, bacteria, fungi, and protozoa. Fungi such as *Blastomyces* spp. and protozoa such as *Leishmania* spp. typically cause nodular tongue lesions.[60] Viral causes in dogs include CDV, canine calicivirus, and CPV. In cats, FCV and FHV-1 can cause lingual ulceration as well as ulceration of the buccal mucosa. *Rickettsia rickettsii* can cause lingual ulceration as a result of endothelial cell damage. Primary physical injury can occur via trauma, bite wounds, burns, caustic substances, and foreign bodies, with secondary infection with bacteria or *Candida* spp. Lesions in the mouth that disrupt the normal host barriers include those caused by eosinophilic granuloma complex and neoplasms such as squamous cell carcinoma and epitheliotropic T-cell lymphoma. Systemic disorders that may lead to lingual ulceration include uremia; autoimmune diseases such as pemphigus vulgaris, bullous pemphigoid, erythema multiforme, and systemic lupus erythematosus; and embolic disease (including septic thromboemboli). Organisms are not often found on histologic examination; however, suppuration and overlying ulceration are usually apparent. Foreign material such as hair, bone, or plant matter can be present in lingual wound infections.

The most prevalent disorders associated with gingivostomatitis in dogs and cats are canine chronic ulcerative stomatitis (CUS; also known as chronic ulcerative paradental stomatitis) and feline gingivostomatitis. Canine CUS is a chronic painful ulcerative condition of the mouth with an unclear pathogenesis.[61] Predisposed breeds include the Maltese terrier, Cavalier King Charles spaniel, greyhound, and Labrador retriever. Male neutered dogs are also overrepresented. Ulcers typically occur on the buccal mucosa opposite the dental plaque, but can also occur on the lateral margins of the tongue, the palatoglossal folds, and the mucocutaneous border of the lips (Fig. 125.3).

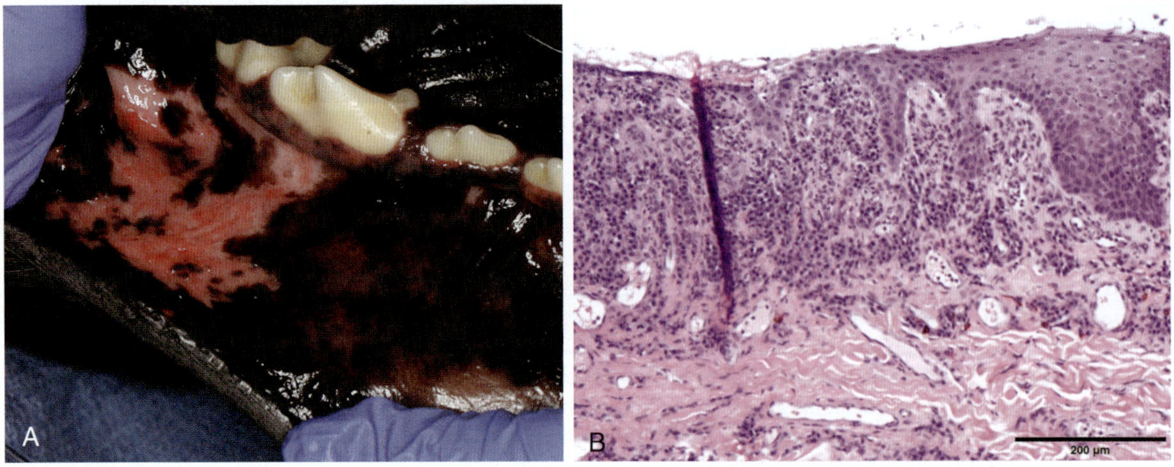

Fig. 125.3 Chronic ulcerative paradental stomatitis in a 4-year old female spayed German shepherd dog. (A) Ulcerative lesions on the buccal mucosa seen on examination of the oral cavity. (B) Histopathology findings of a biopsy from the buccal mucosa showing severe, diffuse, lymphoplasmacytic, ulcerative gingivitis. H&E stain. (Courtesy the Dentistry and Oral Surgery Service and Veterinary Anatomic Pathology Service, University of California-Davis.)

Histopathology reveals a lymphoplasmacytic infiltrate at the interface between the mucosal epithelium and the subepithelial connective tissue that is comprised of CD79+ B cells, plasma cells, CD3+ T cells, and regulatory T cells.[61,62] There has also been evidence of IL-17 expression in the lesions, a cytokine that is often associated with regulation of autoimmune diseases. Infectious agents have not been identified in association with CUS. Extraction of teeth opposite the ulcers may result in clinical improvement.[61]

Feline chronic gingivostomatitis (FCGS) is a common and painful disease of the oral cavity characterized by inflammation of the buccal and caudal oral mucosa, lateral to the palatoglossal folds. Ulcerative/erosive and proliferative phenotypes have been described (Fig. 125.4).[63] Often young adult cats are affected, and in some cats there may be minimal evidence of accompanying periodontal disease. However, most cats with FCGS often have significant generalized periodontitis and are more likely to have external inflammatory root resorptive lesions.[64] Affected cats may show evidence of dysphagia with reduced appetite, weight loss, halitosis, ptyalism, pawing at the mouth, and reduced grooming. Some of the signs may also result from esophagitis, which has been detected using endoscopy in affected cats.[65]

Although a variety of infectious agents have been associated with this disorder, direct causation has not been proven because most of the pathogens postulated to play a role commonly infect cats without causing clinical signs; these have included FeLV, FIV, FCV, FHV-1, and *Bartonella* spp.[63,66-68] The strongest associations have been made with FCV infections, although not all evidence has supported a role for this virus (see Chapter 35).[63] Disease may occur in a number of cats within a household and tends to be recurrent after the initial treatment or is unresponsive to treatment. Cessation of FCV shedding was associated with resolution of chronic gingivostomatitis in one cat.[67] Coinfections with FIV or FeLV may result in more severe lesions. In one study, cats with chronic gingivostomatitis were more likely to shed FCV and FHV-1 together than either virus alone.[68] Biopsy of affected regions reveals lymphoplasmacytic inflammation. Large numbers of B cells and both CD4+ and CD8+ T cells can be found within the lesions, as well as regulatory T cells.[69] In another study, compared with nondiseased cats, affected cats showed a significant increase in expression of IL-2, IL-4, IL-6, IL-10, IL-12 (p35 and p40), and IFN-γ.[70] The predominant bacterial species present in the oral cavity of cats with FCGS in one study with *Pasteurella multocida* subsp. *multocida*.[71] Hyperproteinemia due to a polyclonal gammopathy is often present on the serum chemistry panel, and may be moderate to severe, likely reflective of chronic antigenic stimulation.

Treatment with antibiotics that have activity against anaerobes (such as clindamycin) can result in some improvement; however, the response is temporary. Other medical treatments that have been used are topical lactoferrin and oral IFN-ω (see Chapter 9). Treatment with prednisolone may also result in some clinical improvement, but long-term treatment tends to have gradual reduction in efficacy and is not recommended because of adverse effects.[63] Although the number of cats was small, treatment with cyclosporine also seemed to be effective when compared to a placebo-treated group, and 5 of 11 cats followed for 3 or more months remained in remission.[72] If cyclosporine is used, measurement of trough concentrations is recommended on a regular basis to avoid excessive immunosuppression, and the drug should be used at the lowest possible dose that controls clinical signs. To date, the most effective treatment has been proper management of periodontal disease, and, for refractory cases, partial- or full-mouth tooth extractions. Because the outcome following extraction of all premolar and molar teeth does not appear to differ significantly from that following full-mouth extractions, premolar-molar extraction has been recommended initially, moving to full-mouth extraction 1 to 4 months later if there is insufficient reduction in clinical signs.[63,73] In cases with generalized periodontitis and stomatitis, full-mouth tooth extraction is recommended. It is estimated that approximately 20% to 30% of cats will show minimal or no improvement.

INFECTIONS OF THE ESOPHAGUS AND STOMACH

Infections of the esophageal wall in dogs and cats usually follow esophageal perforation or full-thickness ulceration secondary to foreign bodies, esophageal neoplasia, or gastroesophageal reflux during anesthesia.[74] Uncommon infectious causes of esophagitis that have been documented in dogs include *Candida* spp. esophagitis and *Pythium insidiosum* esophagitis. *Candida* spp. were isolated from two immunocompromised chow-chow puppies that were coinfected with CAdV-2 and CDV,[75] and *Pythium*-associated esophagitis was confirmed on necropsy in two dogs from rural Tennessee, USA.[76] One of the authors (SLM) has also confirmed *Pythium*-associated esophagitis in three dysphagic large-breed hunting dogs from northern California via esophageal biopsy and immunohistochemistry, and positive serum

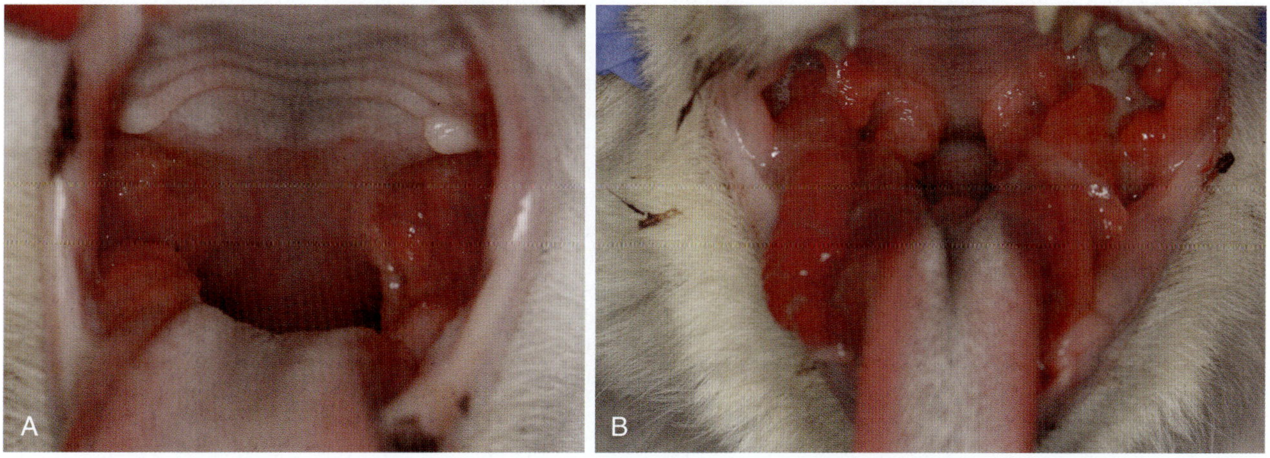

Fig. 125.4 Feline gingivostomatitis. (A) Severe proliferative form. (B) Ulceroproliferative lesions. (Courtesy University of California-Davis Dentistry and Oral Surgery Service.)

anti-*P. insidiosum* ELISA. Nevertheless, uncommon complications, esophageal abscesses, mediastinal empyema, or pyothorax may result. Migrating plant awns have been incriminated as an underlying cause in some cases.[77] Clinical signs include inappetence, ptyalism, fever, lethargy, weight loss, regurgitation, odynophagia, tachypnea, cough, and abdominal pain.[77,78] One dog developed respiratory distress secondary to tracheal collapse and bilateral laryngeal paralysis that were associated with a paratracheal abscess that had entrapped the recurrent laryngeal nerves.[79] Plain radiography may show evidence of pleural effusion or mass lesions associated with the esophagus. CT imaging and ultrasound may also be useful for visualizing esophageal abscess lesions.[77,78] Esophagoscopy findings were normal in several dogs and a cat with caudal mediastinal paraesophageal abscesses.[77,78] Treatment has generally involved open surgical drainage (lateral thoracotomy or median sternotomy) or omentalization through a diaphragmatic incision. Antimicrobials indicated for pyothorax are likely to be appropriate for paraesophageal abscesses.

Because of the acidic milieu of the stomach and the presence of pepsin, the stomach has relatively low concentrations of resident microflora relative to other portions of the GI tract, and bacterial gastritis and gastric abscesses rarely occur. *Physaloptera* spp. infection can cause gastritis, and should be considered in dogs and cats with chronic vomiting, especially those with a history of consuming insects or vertebrate prey (see Chapter 116). A higher dose and longer duration of fenbendazole in combination with pyrantel pamoate is recommended for treatment of suspected or confirmed infections. Reinfection is common in some dogs and should not be viewed as treatment failure. *Ollulanus tricuspis* nematodes are worms found in the gastric mucosa of the cat, and rarely in dogs.[80,81] The parasite has a direct life cycle and does not require an intermediate host. Clinical signs of chronic vomiting, weight loss, and anorexia are most commonly reported. Effective therapies include tetramisole at 5 mg/kg (single dose) and fenbendazole at 50 mg/kg (PO q24h for 5 days).

The reader is referred to Chapter 66 for information on gastric helicobacteriosis.

INFECTIONS OF THE INTESTINAL TRACT

THE INTESTINAL MICROBIOME

Concentrations of bacteria in the proximal small bowel are relatively low because of the influence of gastric acid and bile, but they gradually increase toward the ileocecal region. Numbers of microorganisms in the distal small bowel or the large bowel are not affected by feeding and remain relatively constant after meals. Increased numbers of resident organisms may be found in the stomach and upper small intestine, or pathogenic organisms may proliferate when normal bowel defenses are impaired. Excessive use of acid suppressants, intestinal obstruction, ileus, impaired bile acid signaling, exocrine pancreatic insufficiency, or decreased mucosal or IgA secretions can result in disruption of the normal microbiome and bacterial overgrowth in the small intestine.[82] In contrast to cats with GI illness, clinically healthy cats have much higher concentrations of bacteria in the duodenum and jejunum.[83,84]

Puppies and kittens lacking normal microflora at birth derive their microflora from exposure to their dam and littermates or from their environment by 2 to 3 weeks of life.[85] Studies performed using 16S rRNA gene PCR methods have shown that the composition of the intestinal microflora may change with age in dogs and cats, with Enterobacterales and enterococci decreasing in abundance with age in cats, and lactobacilli and enterococci decreasing in abundance with age in dogs.[86,87] Another study that used 16S rRNA gene PCR showed that the microbial diversity in dogs tended to decrease as dogs aged.[88] Changes in diet, nutritional status, and physiologic state of the host may influence the proportions of residing bacteria.[2,89] Small intestinal bacterial overgrowth (SIBO) in dogs is a condition thought to result from dysbiosis, and is most commonly associated with exocrine pancreatic insufficiency, ileus, malabsorption of nutrients, and deficiency of sIgA. The diagnosis of SIBO is a topic of debate, because it has traditionally been defined as proliferation of small intestinal bacteria to concentrations $> 10^5$/mL, which have now been identified even in healthy dogs.[90] The term "intestinal dysbiosis" is far more common in dogs, and refers to an alteration of the intestinal microbiota independent of bacterial numbers.

In general, the important phyla that make up the intestinal microbiota in dogs and cats are Fusobacteria, Bacteroidetes, and Firmicutes. Proteobacteria and Actinobacteria are the two other major taxa present. Some of the more important genera are *Fusobacterium*, *Lactobacillus*, *Streptococcus* (dogs) and *Enterococcus* (cats), *Clostridium*, *Prevotella*, and *Bacteroides*.

Use of 16S rRNA gene pyrosequencing has shown that the stomach of healthy dogs is primarily occupied by Proteobacteria (99.6%), with a predominance of *Helicobacter*. The remaining organisms belong to the Firmicutes, primarily *Lactobacillus*.[82] The duodenum and upper jejunum primarily harbor aerobes and facultative anaerobes. The main phyla of the duodenum in dogs are Firmicutes (approximately 45%), Proteobacteria (approximately 20%), and Bacteroidetes (approximately 10%).[82,91] Prevalent orders in duodenal fluid have included Clostridiales and Lactobacillales, with only low numbers of the anaerobes Fusobacteriales and Bacteroidales.[92] In the jejunal mucosa, the ratio of Firmicutes to Proteobacteria appears to change, with one study showing 47% of the microbiome to be Proteobacteria (primarily Gamma Proteobacteria) and 15% to be Firmicutes; the remaining phyla were Spirochaetes (15%), Actinobacteria (11%), Bacteroidetes (6%), and Fusobacteria (4%).[93] In jejunal fluid, Clostridiales and Lactobacillales remained prevalent, but Enterobacterales and Fusobacteriales were identified in greater concentrations than in duodenal juice.[93] In colonic contents, Proteobacteria have diminished dramatically (comprising < 2% of organisms; this includes *E. coli*) and the population is dominated by Fusobacteria, Bacteroidetes, and Firmicutes, in even distribution.[93] The same phyla are found in canine fecal specimens, although the distribution has varied among studies; in most studies, Firmicutes have comprised a significant proportion of organisms, especially clostridia.[94] The maximum numbers of microorganisms and the greatest biodiversity are found in the large intestine when compared with the small intestine.[92] A single gram of feces contains 10^{11} to 10^{12} organisms and 15,000 to 36,000 different species.[95,96] The concentration of many anaerobes is reduced in the feces during diarrhea because these organisms normally require intestinal stasis and low oxygen tension for growth.

The composition and concentration of the intestinal microflora is altered in dogs with GI disease. For example, in one study of dogs with acute diarrhea, episodes of diarrhea were associated with increased abundance of Clostridiales (especially *Clostridium perfringens*) and enterococci.[97] In dogs with inflammatory bowel disease (IBD), one study showed reduced species richness and a higher proportion of Enterobacterales;[91] another found a greater proportion of Proteobacteria and a lower abundance of Clostridia.[98] Dogs with chronic enteropathies (food-responsive, antibiotic-responsive, or immunosuppressant-responsive) are also significantly more likely to have positive dysbiosis indices when compared with healthy dogs.[5] Although treatment of dogs with immunosuppressant-responsive enteropathies (IBD) results in clinical improvement, microbial dysbiosis may persist.[99]

The effect of intestinal disease on the GI microbiome in cats has also been examined, although relatively few studies exist. In addition, studies that have examined the microbiome of healthy cats have had somewhat conflicting results, with different percentages of the major phyla (Firmicutes, Bacteroides, Actinobacteria, and Proteobacteria) varying between individuals and being influenced by age and diet.[100,101] A study that used Illumina sequencing showed that cats with chronic enteropathies (IBD and alimentary small cell lymphoma) had reduced fecal bacterial population diversity when compared with healthy cats, with an increase in Enterobacterales and Streptococcaceae and a decrease in abundance of organisms that belonged to the phyla Firmicutes and Actinobacteria (*Bifidobacterium*) and *Bacteroidetes*.[102] There were no detectable differences between cats with IBD and cats with small cell lymphoma.

The prevalence and diversity of fungal organisms in the GI tract of dogs and cats has had limited study. The most abundant phylum in both healthy dogs and dogs with acute diarrhea in one study that used pyrosequencing was Ascomycota (approximately 98%), followed by Basidiomycota (1%).[103] In both groups, the most abundant genus was *Candida*, the primary species being *Candida natalensis*. In another study that used similar methodology, Ascomycota was the most abundant phylum in dogs and the only phylum identified in cats.[104] In that study, the most abundant genus in dogs was *Nacaseomyces* and in cats were *Saccharomyces* and *Aspergillus*.

The Effect of Diet on the Microbiome

Dietary composition can impact the diversity and abundance of different bacterial species in the microbiome. In one study, feeding a raw food diet to dogs was associated with increased abundance of Proteobacteria and Fusobacteria in the fecal microbiota; in dogs fed a commercial diet, Firmicutes were more abundant.[89] It is important to consider the differences in the macronutrient composition of raw and commercial diets, because the increased fiber and carbohydrate in a commercial extruded diet can impact the microbiota significantly. A prebiotic is defined as a "nondigestible food ingredient which beneficially affects the host by selectively stimulating the growth of and/or activates the metabolism of one or a limited number of health-promoting bacteria in the intestinal tract."[105] A variety of prebiotics have been added to dog and cat diets in order to promote GI health. The most common prebiotics studied are fructans, although other prebiotics such as mannans, lactosucrose, and lactulose are also being evaluated. Short-chain fructooligosaccharides (scFOSs) are polymers of glucose that have been added to commercial diets as a source of soluble fiber. They occur naturally in plants or mammalian milk, or are synthesized from fermentation. Chicory root is one example of a naturally occurring source of scFOS. Other natural sources rich in soluble fiber are oat bran or wheat pulp. scFOSs are not digested by the mammalian small intestine, and they reach the colon intact. There they are fermented by anaerobic bacteria such as *Bifidobacterium* spp. or lactobacilli into short-chain fatty acids such as acetate, propionate, and butyrate. These anaerobic organisms proliferate and inhibit growth of other potentially pathogenic microbes such as *Clostridium* species and *E. coli*. Fructan supplementation attenuated some of the pathologic responses to experimental *Salmonella* challenge of weanling pups.[106] In general, studies evaluating the effect of dietary supplementation with scFOS have shown an increase in fecal bifidobacteria and lower fecal clostridia numbers in dogs.[94] However, these studies relied upon traditional culture methods to identify and quantify relative proportions of bacteria. When 16S rRNA gene pyrosequencing was used to assess the effect of a diet that contained beet pulp on fecal microbiota in dogs, the abundance of Clostridia increased within the Firmicutes and the abundance of the phyla Actinobacteria and Fusobacteria decreased.[107] The appearance of butyrate-producing bacterial species that may possess anti-inflammatory effects was also noted. Administration of a scFOS or pectin-based diet to cats was associated with an increase in the abundance of *Bifidobacterium* and *Lactobacillus*, respectively, when compared with a control diet.[108] In this study, genus-specific PCR assays were used to amplify bacterial DNA.

Probiotics

Probiotics are viable microorganisms that, when administered orally in adequate amounts, confer a health benefit on the host. Enterococci, lactobacilli, and bifidobacteria—normal colonic inhabitants—have often been administered after antimicrobial treatment, intestinal infections, weaning, stress, or dietary changes in an attempt to reestablish the intestinal microbiota. Many of these microorganisms become transient constituents of the enteric microflora. In humans, these bacteria have been administered in the form of yogurt, cheese, and milk products, and efforts have been made to include these in canine and feline diets. Theoretical benefits of probiotics include the production of antibacterial substances (bacteriocins) and competitive inhibition of pathogen and toxin adherence to the intestinal epithelium, reestablishment of enteric microflora after antimicrobial treatment, enhancement of host innate immunity, regulation of host immune responses, and regulation of intestinal epithelial cell functions. Synbiotics are combinations of prebiotics and probiotics.

A number of studies addressing the role of probiotics in the management of canine and feline diarrhea have been published to date, with most studies evaluating the efficacy of this therapeutic modality for the management of acute diarrhea, and results have been mixed depending on the type of probiotic and the underlying disorder being managed. The effect of probiotics in both healthy dogs and those with enteropathies have been published, with mixed results. Two studies were randomized, placebo-controlled clinical trials of dogs with food-responsive enteropathy.[109,110] In one of those studies, all of the dogs clinically improved when placed on an elimination diet. However, they showed no specific changes in the inflammatory cytokine patterns or any specific benefit of a probiotic.[109] In the second study,[110] dogs with acute diarrhea, with or without vomiting, were divided into placebo or probiotic groups. The probiotic formulation consisted of a mixture of live strains of *Lactobacillus, Bacillus*, and *Pediococcus* species. The mean time from treatment to resolution of the diarrhea was 1 day shorter in the probiotic group. Administration of *Lactobacillus kefiri* to dogs, a species found in kefir, had no impact on fecal IgA concentrations or the composition of the microbiome.[111] Several publications have described beneficial effects in prospective studies of a probiotic that contains four strains of *Lactobacillus*, three strains of *Bifidobacterium*, and *Streptococcus salivarius* subsp. *thermophilus*. Treatment of dogs with IBD with this probiotic in one randomized study appeared to have the same effect as treatment with metronidazole and prednisone, with improvement in clinical and histopathological scores.[99] In another multicenter study, dogs with IBD were randomized to receive treatment with diet and prednisone alone; or diet, prednisone, and the eight-strain probiotic.[112] There was rapid clinical remission in both groups over 60 days despite no improvement in inflammation assessed histopathologically; dogs treated with diet and prednisone alone had an increase in *Bifidobacterium* spp. using FISH on endoscopic biopsies, and those treated with the probiotic had an increase in *Lactobacillus* spp. Treatment of healthy dogs with this 8-strain probiotic preparation as a dietary supplement for 60 days resulted in a decrease in the abundance of *C. perfringens* and an increase in the abundance of *Bifidobacterium* and *Lactobacillus* spp. when compared to a control group fed the diet alone.[113] Treatment of healthy dogs and dogs with food-responsive diarrhea with a synbiotic that contained *Enterococcus faecium*, FOS, and gum arabic had no impact on fecal microbiota diversity or richness.[114] Additional studies are warranted in dogs to further assess the immunomodulatory effects of probiotics and to evaluate their safety.

There are fewer publications pertaining to probiotic use in cats, and one randomized, placebo-controlled study in 217 shelter cats administered the probiotic, *Enterococcus faecium* SF68 or placebo, showed that the percentage of cats with diarrhea ≥ 2 days was significantly lower ($P = 0.03$) in the probiotic group (7.4%) when compared with the placebo group (20.7%).[115] One study showed that a microencapsulated probiotic formulation that contained three *Lactobacillus* species—*Bifidobacterium bifidum*, *Enterococcus faecium*, and *Saccharomyces cerevisiae*—was able to modulate the fecal microbiota of healthy cats by increasing lactic acid bacterial counts.[116] A mixture of FOS and gum arabic was used for encapsulation. Treatment of laboratory-reared cats with amoxicillin-clavulanic acid for 7 days with or without *Enterococcus faecium* strain SF68 for 14 days was associated with decreased microbiome diversity in both groups, with no detectable differences between groups.[117] However, the probiotic-treated cats had improved diarrhea scores when compared with the cats treated with amoxicillin-clavulanic acid alone.

Fecal Microbiota Transplantation

FMT can be infused by various methods, including nasogastric tube, nasojejunal tube, upper tract endoscopy (esophagogastroduodenoscopy), colonoscopy, or retention enema, and has been used to treat dysbiosis associated with a wide array of disorders in humans. The therapeutic modality has recently received attention for treatment of refractory chronic enteropathies and acute diarrheas in dogs and cats. A fresh fecal specimen is collected from a healthy donor dog or cat, mixed with saline or another isotonic solution, filtered to remove particulate matter, and administered by endoscopy into the colon or enema. Repeated treatments may be given on a regular basis (such as every 3 to 5 days or even on a weekly basis). An optimum method of preparation, dose, or dosing frequency has not been established. Apparent clinical responses to treatment have occurred in animals that were refractory to traditional medical therapies.[118,119] In one report, the fecal microbiome of a recipient dog converted to that of the donor after multiple treatments, with a dramatic decrease in the abundance of Proteobacteria and increase in the abundance of Fusobacteria.[118] As in humans, randomized prospective studies are required to evaluate the efficacy of FMT to treat enteropathies in dogs and cats. Although complications associated with FMT are extremely infrequent in people, the risk of infectious hazards needs to be taken seriously, particularly in recipients who are severely immunocompromised. A recent report of infection with extended-spectrum beta-lactamase (ESBL)-producing *E. coli* in two human patients following FMT underscores the importance of comprehensive screening of donors and of the material to be transplanted.[120] Both of the ill recipients had severe underlying diseases – cirrhosis with hepatic encephalopathy in one and hematologic dysplasia treated by means of hematopoietic-cell transplantation in the other. Both patients also had concomitant and previous use of antibiotics that were broadly active against gut luminal bacteria, which may have diminished the microbiota that normally provide resistance to introduced pathogens. Both recipients developed severe infections following FMT and one of the patients died after they received FMT capsules from the same donor. It is readily apparent that FMT may carry risks that can only be identified after the fact, and improved screening of FMT donors and of the material to be transplanted should help reduce the risks of infections by known pathogens. It is highly probable that as the use of FMT is broadened in veterinary medicine and more compromised patients are treated, complications may be more frequently observed.

Bacterial Translocation

The GI tract is a known reservoir of microorganisms, which under certain circumstances can spread via the portal circulation or intestinal lymphatics to extraintestinal sites, including the mesenteric lymph nodes, liver, spleen, and pancreas, and to other organs by systemic circulation. In one study of 50 clinically healthy entire females undergoing ovariohysterectomy, a variety of aerobic and anaerobic bacterial species could be isolated using culture from the mesenteric lymph nodes of 26 dogs; in most dogs a single isolate was obtained.[121] Corresponding peripheral venous and portal venous blood cultures yielded a gram-positive coccus and a coagulase-negative *Staphylococcus* species from the peripheral blood of one of the dogs. It is highly plausible that the prevalence of bacterial translocation in healthy dogs is even higher than that documented in this study given the limitations and insensitivity of routine bacterial culture compared to molecular-based methods. In the human literature, bacterial translocation has been divided into "healthy" translocation, whereby bacteria and fragments of bacteria (DNA, LPS, peptidoglycan, flagellin) are continuously presented to the reticuloendothelial system in the liver and serve to promote host immunity. In contrast, "pathologic" bacterial translocation occurs when significant numbers of bacteria are able to cross a damaged intestinal barrier in a sustained manner and cause or contribute to disease (Fig. 125.5).

Pathologic bacterial translocation occurs with conditions of reduced mucosal perfusion; these can result from systemic hypotension, decreased peristalsis (such as with intestinal obstruction or ileus), intestinal resection, abdominal trauma, burns, abdominal radiation therapy, pancreatitis, and obstructive biliary disease. Paradoxically, antimicrobial therapy has been shown to promote bacterial translocation in mouse models.[122] Administration of glucocorticoids or NSAIDs can result in reduction in GI mucus production, a normal protective defense of the bowel against bacteria. In one study of 448 humans undergoing laparotomy in the United Kingdom, bacterial translocation was detected in 15% of patients, with the main species isolated being *E. coli*.[123] Furthermore, 41% of patients that had evidence of bacterial translocation developed septic complications, compared with only 14% of those that did not have evidence of bacterial translocation. Furthermore, gut microbes were responsible for the majority of septic events. Bacteria may translocate via transcellular or paracellular pathways; paracellular translocation of bacteria and LPS is facilitated by disruption of tight junctions. Currently the best approach to prevention of bacterial translocation is early treatment of the underlying condition, and the use of intraoperative antimicrobial drugs during contaminated procedures (see Chapter 76). A number of treatments, such as dietary modification with antioxidants, prebiotics, probiotics, and vitamin D have been suggested to reduce the impact of chronic translocation of bacteria and LPS in humans with chronic disease states by working to improve the integrity of the mucosal barrier.[124]

PATHOPHYSIOLOGIC MECHANISMS OF INFECTIOUS DIARRHEA

Enteropathogenic organisms, unlike resident and nonpathogenic transient microflora, have acquired means of overcoming the host defense mechanisms and the inhibitory properties of the normal microflora. Adherence factors (e.g., somatic pili) that permit intestinal pathogens to establish infection also allow them to attach to, multiply on, and colonize the intestinal mucosa. Some pathogenic bacteria that cause diarrhea remain on the mucosal surface and produce potent enterotoxins that disrupt fluid flux across the intestinal mucosa. Others are able to penetrate intact epithelial cells, producing inflammatory damage in the underlying mucosa. Enteric viruses damage the intestine by replicating within and destroying selected populations of epithelial cells. Often, multiple mechanisms are involved. Various mechanisms by which microorganisms produce intestinal injury are covered in relevant chapters on enteropathic viruses and bacteria in this book.

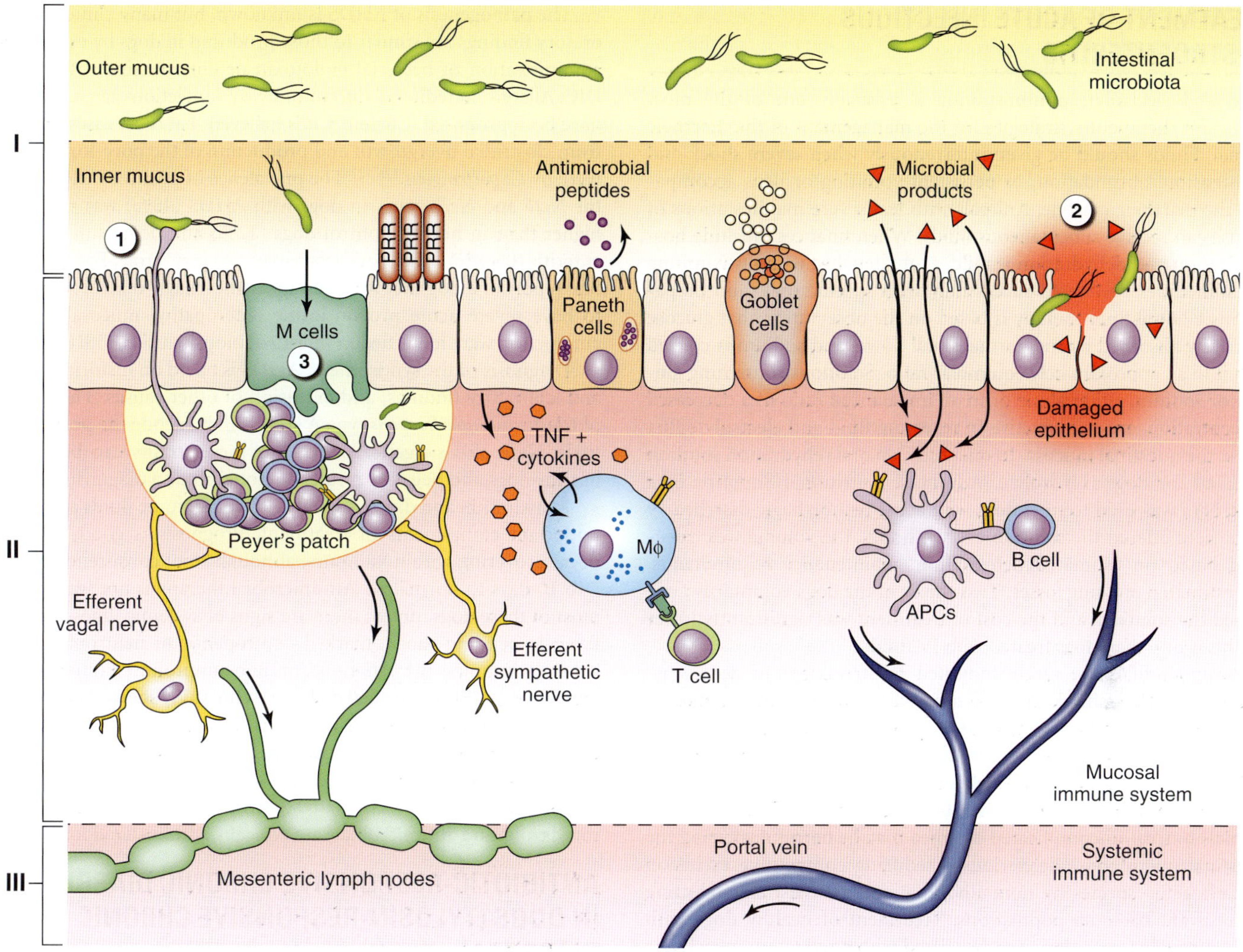

Fig 125.5 Compartments and key players involved in mediating pathological bacterial translocation (BT) and the associated host response. Three different routes *(1–3)* of BT can be separated: (1) direct sampling of luminal bacteria by dendritic cells via processes between epithelial cells, not affecting tight junction function; (2) injured/inflamed epithelium with dysfunctional epithelial barrier; and (3) M-cells overlying Peyer's patches as specialized cells providing access of microbial products to antigen-presenting cells. Moreover, three different levels of barriers (I–III) against bacterial translocation are shown: (I) lumen and secretory component (e.g., inner and outer mucus layer, antimicrobial peptides) of gut barrier; (II) mechanical epithelial barrier and the gut-associated lymphatic tissue (GALT) beneath with response elements to BT (e.g., TNF and other proinflammatory cytokines) and autonomic nervous system; (III) systemic immune system as a third barrier in case of spreading of bacteria beyond mesenteric lymph node including hematogenous (portal venous) and lymphatic (thoracic duct) route of delivery. *PRR*, pattern recognition receptors. (From Wiest R, Lawson M, Geuking M. Pathological bacterial translocation in liver cirrhosis. *J Hepatol.* 2014;60:197-209.)

DIAGNOSIS OF ACUTE INFECTIOUS GASTROENTERITIS

Diagnosis of many enteropathogenic infections is notoriously challenging because many organisms are present in both healthy and sick dogs and cats. When outbreaks of diarrhea occur, testing specimens from multiple affected and unaffected animals is recommended, because an organism is more likely to be the cause of illness when found in more than one animal and when more prevalent in diarrheic than nondiarrheic animals. Examination of fecal smears from a wet-prep may be useful when positive for *Tritrichomonas blagburni* or *Giardia* spp., but this is a highly insensitive diagnostic approach. Many veterinary diagnostic laboratories offer "GI panels" which comprise a combination of diagnostic tests for organisms that have the potential to cause diarrhea. An understanding of the limitations of each of the assays included in these panels is critical for proper interpretation. For example, some panels include culture on selective media for *Salmonella* and *Campylobacter* and ELISA assays that detect clostridial toxins; some are panels that combine fecal flotation for parasites with special stains for *Giardia* (e.g., direct FA) or *Cryptosporidium* (e.g., direct FA, acid fast stains); and others are PCR-based assays that detect clostridial toxin genes or the DNA of multiple different enteric viral, bacterial, and protozoal pathogens. It should be emphasized that the detection of bacterial DNA does not equate with infection, and that the detection of toxin genes does not equate with expression of that gene. Collection of a sufficient quantity of fresh feces is important, with the amount required depending on the assay being performed. The laboratory (or laboratory's website) should be consulted for information on the correct specimen type, quantity, and handling and transport conditions. Specific pathogen chapters in this book also include information on specimen collection and handling to optimize diagnostic yield.

TREATMENT OF ACUTE INFECTIOUS GASTROENTERITIS

Fluid and electrolyte administration is probably one of the most important therapeutic strategies for the management of the diarrheic animal. Fluids should be given intravenously when severe shock and hypotension, obtundation, or persistent vomiting or ileus accompanies the diarrheic episode. Animals with less severe manifestations of disease can receive subcutaneous fluids. When finances preclude hospitalization and dehydration is mild, acute diarrhea without vomiting can sometimes be treated successfully with specific oral fluid preparations.[125] Oral fluid therapy is based on the observation that glucose is actively absorbed by the normal small bowel and sodium is carried with it in an approximately equimolar ratio. Solutions containing glucose or sodium, either alone or in an imbalanced ratio of a decreased concentration, are not effective in reversing fluid and electrolyte flux across the intestinal mucosa. In one study, an oral rehydration solution designed for dogs (Hydrolyte, Advanced Nutritional Support, Elka Park, NY) was used to treat dogs with acute hemorrhagic diarrhea.[125] Dogs were offered the solution every 4 hours, the volume was calculated based on estimated dehydration, maintenance requirements, and estimated ongoing losses. Two-thirds of the dogs voluntarily consumed the solution, and the cost of treatment was significantly lower for this group than dogs treated with IV fluids.

Antimicrobials are rarely indicated for treatment of acute gastroenteritis. They should only be used when episodes of diarrhea or vomiting are accompanied by signs of systemic illness, including fever, severe lethargy, and impending shock, and the presence of leukopenia or leukocytosis with a marked left shift. These findings suggest sepsis secondary to translocation of microbes or their toxins. Use of antimicrobials to treat uncomplicated diarrhea may be harmful, altering the intestinal microbiome deleteriously, reducing competitive exclusion of pathogenic species by nonpathogenic commensals, and selecting for resistant bacterial populations. Treatment of healthy dogs with metronidazole for 14 days was associated with a reduction in richness of the fecal microbiome with increased abundance of Proteobacteria and decreased abundance of Fusobacteria and Bacteroidetes (assessed using 16S rRNA gene PCR-Illumina sequencing). Furthermore, disturbances in the population persisted for 4 weeks after the drug was discontinued.[6] When indicated, antibacterial therapy should be combined with supportive care measures such as dietary modification, fluid therapy, and antiemetics. In addition to complicated diarrhea with suspected bacterial translocation, antimicrobial treatment is indicated for antibiotic-responsive chronic diarrhea and granulomatous colitis. Antibiotic-responsive chronic diarrhea (ARD) and acute hemorrhagic diarrhea syndrome (AHDS) are described in the following section; information on granulomatous colitis can be found in Chapter 63.

ACUTE HEMORRHAGIC DIARRHEA SYNDROME

AHDS (previously known as hemorrhagic gastroenteritis [HGE]) is a syndrome characterized by acute onset of profuse, mucoid, bloody diarrhea, sometimes (80% of cases) with vomiting. The name of the syndrome was changed because of the frequent lack of gastric involvement. Acute hemorrhagic diarrheal syndrome associated with *Clostridium perfringens* infection has primarily been described in small-breed dogs between 2 and 4 years of age (see Chapter 64). Affected dogs are often lethargic, dehydrated, and may show evidence of abdominal pain on palpation. The syndrome is also marked by hematologic findings that include relative polycythemia, with a normal or low plasma protein concentration, and coagulation test results suggestive of DIC and occasionally, acute oliguric renal failure.

The pathogenesis of AHDS is unknown, but many clinical and laboratory findings are similar to those produced in dogs by experimental administration of bacterial endotoxin or enterotoxins with resultant DIC. Allergic, hereditary, autoimmune, and infectious causes for AHDS have been proposed. Currently it is believed that most cases may result from clostridial overgrowth and production of the pore-forming toxin NetF by *C. perfringens*.[126,127] The prevalence of positive PCR results for the *NetF* and *NetE* genes in dogs with AHDS (48%) was significantly higher than in healthy control dogs (12%) and dogs with parvovirus enteritis (0%).[128] Other pathogens may also play a role. For example, in one report of a dog that was seen for hemorrhagic diarrhea and found to have severe acute protein-losing enteropathy, mucosally invasive enterococci were identified in intestinal biopsies using FISH.[129]

Diagnosis of the syndrome of AHDS is based on historical, clinical, and laboratory findings, and exclusion of other causes. The detection of *Clostridium perfringens* type A strains that encode the pore-forming toxin NetF also suggests AHDS, but these strains can be found in healthy dogs and negative results do not exclude a diagnosis of AHDS.

Rehydration and diuresis with polyionic isotonic fluids are the most important components of treatment. Prognosis is good, with most dogs recovering within 48 hours, although stool consistency may take 7 to 10 days to normalize. Antimicrobial therapy is not warranted for most of these dogs, unless there are signs of systemic illness, including fever, impending shock, marked neutropenia, or neutrophilia with a left shift, or unless the patient is immunocompromised (chemotherapy for cancer, poorly controlled diabetes). One study showed no difference in outcome for dogs with AHDS lacking signs of sepsis when clavulanic acid-amoxicillin was used as part of treatment when compared with no antimicrobials.[130] The drugs of choice for the management of *Clostridium perfringens*-associated diarrhea include amoxicillin or metronidazole, and antimicrobials are typically administered for < 7 days.

ANTIBIOTIC-RESPONSIVE CHRONIC DIARRHEA IN DOGS (TYLOSIN-RESPONSIVE CHRONIC DIARRHEA)

Chronic or intermittent diarrhea of small intestinal character that responds to tylosin therapy has been described in dogs.[131,132] Affected dogs are usually middle-aged, large-breed dogs. The diarrhea is chronic or intermittent in nature, and typically watery, mucoid, or bloody in consistency. The frequency of defecation varies markedly depending on whether the diarrhea is associated with the small or large bowel. In addition, borborygmus and flatulence are common with a low prevalence of vomiting, weight loss, or hyporexia. Diagnostic investigation is important to rule out underlying causes for these signs and to help confirm the diagnosis of ARD (a diagnosis of exclusion). Treatment of dogs with ARD utilizing anthelmintics, antiprotozoals, anti-inflammatories, immunosuppressives, probiotics, prebiotics, other antimicrobials, pancreatic enzymes, or dietary modifications is typically unrewarding. The presence of known enteropathogenic bacteria has not been detected. The presence of an as-yet undiscovered tylosin-susceptible enteropathogen or an anti-inflammatory effect of tylosin have been speculated as possible reasons for response to treatment.[132] Tylosin causes a marked alteration in the bacterial flora of dogs, with an increase in fecal enterococci and lactobacilli, and a probiotic effect has most recently been suggested as its mechanism of action.[93,131] The recommended dose for tylosin is 5 to 10 mg/kg PO q12 to 24h for an initial period of 4 weeks.[133] If signs relapse at this stage, then a longer course of therapy may be required. Many cases require long-term or lifelong therapy to maintain remission of signs. Alternative therapeutic strategies including administration of probiotics or FMT are currently being investigated. For further information on tylosin see Chapter 10.

PANCREATITIS AND PANCREATIC ABSCESSES

Pancreatitis in dogs and cats is usually noninfectious in etiology, and secondary bacterial infection of the pancreas is rare. Nevertheless, infectious diseases should remain on the differential diagnosis list as possible etiologies when a diagnosis of suspected pancreatitis is made, especially when signs of other organ involvement exist or when response to conventional treatment is poor. In dogs, pancreatitis can be caused by *Leptospira* spp. and fungi such as *Cryptococcus neoformans*, often as part of a more widely disseminated infection. *Toxoplasma gondii* can also cause pancreatitis. *Enterococcus hirae* enteropathy was associated with ascending cholangitis and pancreatitis in a kitten.[134] Pancreatic abscesses are usually sterile and treatment requires surgical intervention and drainage.[135,136]

Use of antibacterials in dogs and cats with pancreatitis is controversial. In animals with noninfectious necrotizing pancreatitis, local intestinal damage as a result of spillage of pancreatic enzymes and decreased intestinal perfusion can cause bacterial translocation from the intestine to the diseased pancreatic tissue, with the potential for secondary bacterial infection. Bacterial infection may also occur as a result of infection that ascends the pancreatic ducts. In cats, experimental inoculation of pancreatic ducts with *E. coli* resulted in infection with concurrent pancreatitis, whereas bacteria were cleared in cats with healthy pancreatic tissue.[137] When antimicrobial therapy was started 12 hours after inoculation, infection developed in 73% of animals receiving no antibacterials and in none of the cats receiving antibacterials. In dogs with intestinal colonization by genetically labeled *E. coli*, organisms had spread to the pancreas and mesenteric lymph nodes after experimentally induced pancreatitis.[138]

If antibiotics are used, they should be capable of penetrating damaged pancreatic tissue and have activity against enteric bacteria. Parenteral administration is typically required because affected animals are usually vomiting or have evidence of nausea, and decreased GI perfusion may impair bioavailability. Drugs that reach adequate concentrations in inflamed pancreatic tissue that could be considered are clindamycin, metronidazole, a fluoroquinolone, or third-generation cephalosporins.

BACTERIAL PERITONITIS AND INTRA-ABDOMINAL ABSCESSES

ETIOLOGY AND PATHOGENESIS

Bacterial peritonitis can be classified as primary, secondary, or tertiary/recurrent secondary. Primary bacterial peritonitis, or spontaneous bacterial peritonitis, is an uncommonly reported scenario where there is no identifiable intraperitoneal source of infection or history of a peritoneal penetration.[139,140] This type of infection appears to be more common in cats than in dogs. In 56% of reported canine cases of primary bacterial peritonitis and 100% of feline cases, bacterial culture yielded only one isolate with the majority of organisms in both species being gram positive.[139] Although the pathophysiology is not entirely elucidated, the most common route of infection is believed to be hematogenous spread. Infection may also follow dissemination by the lymphatic route, or transmural migration from the GI or genitourinary (GU) tract. Because primary bacterial peritonitis is uncommon in dogs and cats, risk factors have not been identified. Primary bacterial peritonitis occurs with greater frequency in humans with impaired immune systems, alcoholic cirrhosis, nephrotic syndrome, malignancy, and acute viral hepatitis.[141-143]

Secondary bacterial peritonitis is the most common type of bacterial peritonitis. In approximately 60% of dogs and cats, it results from leakage of commensal bacteria from the GI tract due to either postsurgical wound dehiscence or rupture or perforation of the GI tract.[144,145] Rupture and perforation may occur as sequelae to gastric dilatation-volvulus, perforating ulcers, intestinal mass lesions, or a foreign body. Generalized secondary bacterial peritonitis or localized secondary peritonitis potentially with intra-abdominal abscess formation may also follow pancreatitis, penetrating abdominal wounds, ischemic intestinal injury (e.g., intussusception, foreign bodies, torsion) (Fig. 125.6), rupture of viscera (gallbladder, pyometra, urinary tract), and surgical contamination. Bile salts, along with gastric mucin, hemoglobin, and barium have the potential to enhance the severity of peritonitis. Idiopathic purulent mesenteric lymphadenitis or lymph node abscessation may be infectious or noninfectious with 50% of cases from one case series yielding positive bacterial cultures.[146]

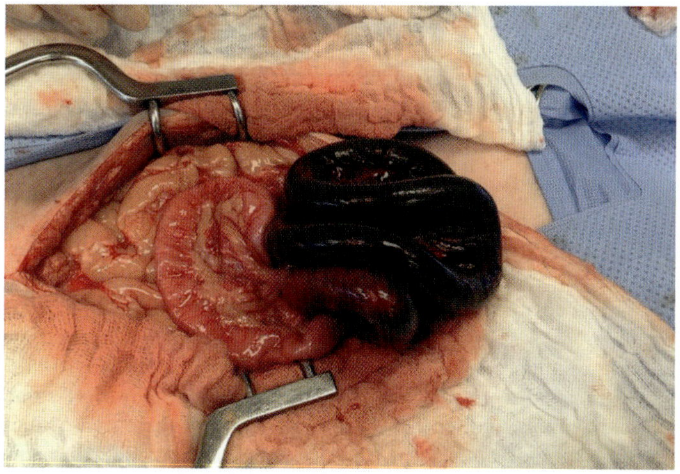

Fig. 125.6 Ischemic injury secondary to partial mesenteric torsion in a cat. Though no perforation was identified in the intestine, *E. coli*, *Enterococcus* sp., and anaerobes were cultured from a peritoneal swab.

Tertiary peritonitis may be defined as intra-abdominal infection that persists or recurs 48 hours following successful and adequate surgical source control. There is uncertainty in the human and veterinary literature how best to diagnose and treat this disease process; however, it is associated with nosocomial or resistant infections in human medicine. True tertiary peritonitis is rarely reported in the veterinary literature. However, some studies describe patients that have failed treatment for secondary septic peritonitis as having recurrent septic secondary peritonitis following a perceived successful surgical source control.[147,148] This description could fit the definition of tertiary peritonitis. Dogs that were at risk for recurrent secondary peritonitis were those that had lower serum albumin concentrations, higher PCVs, and septic peritonitis of GI origin, especially when GI foreign bodies were present.[148]

Bacterial species involved in peritonitis often reflect the normal flora of the GI tract. Secondary bacterial peritonitis is commonly polymicrobial.[149,150] Mixed aerobic-anaerobic infections, with up to four different bacterial species, occur in more than 50% of affected dogs and cats.[139,149] *Escherichia coli* is the most common isolate from both dogs and cats, followed by *Enterococcus* and *Clostridium* spp.[139,149,151] Other isolates include staphylococci, streptococci, *Pseudomonas aeruginosa* or *Acinetobacter* spp., a variety of anaerobes, gram-negative Enterobacterales (*Proteus, Citrobacter, Serratia, Klebsiella,* or *Enterobacter* spp.), *Actinomyces* spp., or, in cats, *Pasteurella multocida*.[152,153] In one study, a greater proportion of dogs with primary peritonitis had gram-positive bacterial infections than dogs with secondary peritonitis.[139] Uncommonly, *Candida albicans* can be isolated, especially if there is a history of antibiotic treatment.[154,155]

CLINICAL SIGNS AND PHYSICAL EXAMINATION FINDINGS

The most common clinical signs in dogs and cats with bacterial peritonitis are lethargy, anorexia, vomiting, and diarrhea, although clinical signs can be quite variable. Weakness and collapse can also occur in animals with septic shock. Diarrhea and vomiting may result from intestinal hypermotility or ileus or may be secondary to underlying intestinal disease.

Physical examination findings may include dull mentation, fever, dehydration, mucosal pallor, abdominal pain, thin body condition, abdominal enlargement, and a palpable fluid wave due to fluid accumulation.[139,149,156] Peritoneal fluid generally cannot be detected on physical examination until the volume reaches greater than 10 mL/kg.[157] Tachypnea or tachycardia may be present; however, some affected animals, and especially cats, show none of these signs. More than one-third of cats lack any evidence of abdominal pain.[149,156] Signs of septic shock may be present, including tachycardia, tachypnea, weak pulses, and injected mucous membranes in dogs, or hypothermia and bradycardia in cats (see Chapter 123).

DIAGNOSIS

Preoperative diagnosis of bacterial peritonitis is based on abdominal imaging findings, cytologic examination of peritoneal fluid, and aerobic and anaerobic bacterial culture of the fluid.

Laboratory Abnormalities

Complete Blood Count, Serum Chemistry Panel, and Urinalysis

Qualitative and quantitative abnormalities in leukocytes are common with septic peritonitis; however, they are generally nonspecific. Anemia of inflammatory disease is common. Depending on severity of disease, an increase or decrease in neutrophils may be present along with a regenerative or degenerative left shift.[158] Thrombocytopenia may be present in animals with septic shock and DIC.[159] Changes on the serum chemistry panel include electrolyte and acid-base abnormalities and/or hypoalbuminemia due to inflammation or third-space losses. Mild to moderate increases in serum liver enzyme activities may be detected. Hypoglycemia or hyperglycemia may be detected and hyperbilirubinemia can be present.[139,149] In patients with vomiting and diarrhea pre-renal azotemia may be present. Azotemia may be post-renal in animals with a ruptured urinary tract. Several abnormalities may be present on blood gas analysis depending on severity of disease. Increased serum lactate concentration has received the most attention in the veterinary literature.

Clotting Function

Although not indicated in all dogs with septic peritonitis, a subset of dogs and cats that develop DIC as a sequela to bacterial peritonitis may have PT or APTT prolongation, increased plasma D-dimer or fibrin degradation product concentrations, and/or decreased plasma antithrombin concentration, therefore coagulation panel evaluation may be considered in dogs with bacterial peritonitis.

Diagnostic Imaging

Imaging of the abdomen should ideally take place prior to abdominocentesis to avoid iatrogenic pneumoperitoneum and the inadvertent misdiagnosis of ruptured abdominal viscera.

Plain Radiography

Abdominal radiographs in dogs and cats with diffuse septic peritonitis may show loss of serosal detail potentially indicating free peritoneal fluid, presence of free gas, identification of foreign material, segmental dilation of bowel, or the presence of abnormal organ enlargement. Oral administration of a contrast agent may be used to better identify GI foreign bodies, ileus, or evidence of perforation. Barium should not be used as a GI contrast agent when there is concern for perforation as it can contribute to peritonitis.

Sonographic Findings

Findings on abdominal ultrasound examination include focal or diffuse hyperechogenicity of the mesentery and the presence of even small quantities of ascites. The echogenicity of the ascites will differ depending on its cellularity. Evidence of underlying disease may be present, such as an intestinal mass or foreign body. Though nonspecific, corrugation of the small intestine with or without increase in intestinal wall thickness has been associated with peritonitis. Focal bowel ischemia and associated localized peritonitis can also be detected with ultrasound. The presence of pneumoperitoneum; a dilated, air-filled stomach or bowel loops; or severe abdominal pain may interfere with complete ultrasound examination of some patients.

Advanced Imaging

Although not routinely used for the evaluation of septic peritonitis in veterinary patients, abdominal CT scans are the imaging modality of choice in humans with acute peritonitis. Its lack of routine use in veterinary medicine may be due to availability, cost, or the need for general anesthesia. In veterinary patients, a CT scan is most useful in cases of penetrating abdominal wounds secondary to trauma or focal abscessation.

Analysis of Peritoneal Fluid

Specimens for cytologic examination from animals with peritonitis may be collected by blind or ultrasound-guided abdominal paracentesis or diagnostic peritoneal lavage (DPL). With the increased availability and sensitivity of ultrasound to detect and guide collection of small quantities of undiluted intra-abdominal fluid, DPL is now uncommonly performed. Ascites fluid should be collected in a sterile EDTA tube for cytologic examination, and a sterile red top tube for aerobic and anaerobic bacterial culture and susceptibility testing.

Ascites fluid from dogs and cats with bacterial peritonitis is typically a modified transudate or exudate, although fluid from dogs with primary peritonitis may be more likely to be a modified transudate or transudate.[139] Fluid analysis from most animals with peritonitis reveals a high protein concentration and an increased erythrocyte and total nucleated cell count (usually >500 cells/μL and up to 160,000 cells/μL). There is typically a predominance of neutrophils that may have a degenerate appearance, and foreign material and/or intracellular and extracellular bacteria may be seen. The presence of intracellular bacteria is generally considered diagnostic for bacterial peritonitis. The presence of bile pigments suggests the hepatobiliary system is the origin of peritonitis.

Because absence of bacteria does not rule out bacterial peritonitis, submission of fluid for culture is essential to guide appropriate antimicrobial therapy, especially with the rise in prevalence of antimicrobial resistance.[149,160] Although it is preferable to submit specimens after therapeutic lavage at surgery, one study showed that culture results were the same regardless of whether samples were collected before or after therapeutic lavage.[161]

In addition to cytologic examination and culture of ascites fluid, other tests may be performed on the fluid to better characterize the type and source of the peritonitis. Comparing blood glucose and lactate concentrations to that of the abdominal fluid has proven to be useful to diagnose dogs with septic peritonitis. A blood-to-fluid glucose difference greater than 20 mg/dL was 100% sensitive and 100% specific for a diagnosis of bacterial peritonitis in one study of dogs and cats.[152] A peritoneal fluid lactate level greater than 2.5 mmol/L had 100% sensitivity and 91%

TABLE 125.2 Interpretation of Results of Peritoneal Fluid Analysis

Chemical Analysis	Septic Peritonitis	Uroperitoneum	Chyloperitoneum	Bile Peritonitis
Glucose (mg/dL)	< 50			
Ratio Fluid:Serum Concentration				
Glucose	< 0.05×			
Creatinine		Fluid > 2.4×		
Potassium		Fluid >1.4×		
Triglycerides			Fluid >3×	
Bilirubin				Fluid > 2×

specificity for diagnosis a septic effusion in dogs; however, this was not repeatable in cats.[162] Another report examined a variety of biomarkers as predictors of septic peritonitis in dogs.[163] Glucose, the chemokine CCL2, IL-6, IL-10, and lactate were found in significantly higher concentrations in peritoneal fluid than in serum, and serum lactate concentration was the most useful predictor. Lactate and glucose concentrations should only be used as a guide to help predict septic peritonitis in dogs that have not recently undergone an exploratory celiotomy, which has the potential to create similar perturbations based on studies in healthy research animals.[164] No single cut-off offers 100% sensitivity and specificity for distinguishing septic from nonseptic peritonitis. Measurement of fluid concentrations of creatinine, potassium, and total bilirubin and comparing these concentrations to those in serum can be helpful for identifying uroperitoneum or bile peritonitis (Table 125.2).[165]

TREATMENT

Antimicrobial Drugs

Intravenous antimicrobial drugs should be initiated as soon as a patient has been diagnosed with septic peritonitis. While waiting for culture and susceptibility test results, a knowledge of whether cocci or rods are present may be considered to help tailor antibiotic therapy. Empiric antimicrobial therapy can also be selected based on the probable source of infection, if one is suspected. However, because most infections are polymicrobial, and unculturable anaerobes may be present, initial therapy should be broad-spectrum, with activity against gram-positive and gram-negative bacteria, as well as anaerobes and aerobic bacteria. Suggested empiric antibiotic options for septic patients are outlined in Chapters 122 and 123. De-escalation of the type of antimicrobial may be considered when bacterial culture and susceptibility results are available.

Surgery

The standard treatment for secondary bacterial peritonitis is emergent exploratory laparotomy with surgical source control and proper antibiotic therapy; however, without proper surgical debridement, lavage, and drainage, it is unlikely that antimicrobial therapy alone will be successful. It is recommended that the patient is hemodynamically stable prior to anesthesia and surgical exploration. Surgical exploration for primary bacterial peritonitis may not be indicated; however, diagnosis of these conditions may require exploratory surgery.

Surgery should be performed via a standard ventral midline celiotomy from xiphoid to pubis. The entire peritoneal cavity should be explored in a systematic fashion. The source of the bacteria should be removed, in most cases, or repaired. The use of monofilament suture is generally recommended whenever possible. Placement of omentum adjacent to the surgical area (intestinal resection and anastomosis) or abscess cavity should be considered to enhance blood flow and lymphatic drainage. Copious peritoneal lavage with warm isotonic saline should be continued until the fluid returning via suction is clear (suggested 200 to 300 mL/kg). It is recommended, though not required, that a closed suction drain, such as a Jackson-Pratt drain, be placed.[166] Open peritoneal drainage is only recommended in cases of severe visceral contamination or when a planned re-exploratory surgery is required.[167] Likewise, there are reports of the use of vacuum-assisted peritoneal drainage in the veterinary literature. At this time, open drainage and vacuum-assisted drainage have not been shown to result in superior outcomes to closed suction drains and both carry significant added expense and a second anesthetic event to ultimately close the abdomen.[168] However, randomized, prospective, clinical trials regarding the need for and the optimal type of drain in patients with septic peritonitis are lacking in veterinary medicine.

Supportive Care

Patients with bacterial peritonitis often require intensive supportive care and monitoring regarding fluid replacement, cardiovascular stability, and electrolyte derangements. Additionally, transfusion, nutritional support, and analgesics are all important factors for consideration in patients with bacterial peritonitis. Use of surgically placed gastrostomy tubes for enteral nutrition is recommended and was associated with a low rate of complications.[169] Though essential for successful outcome in these patients, discussion of these topics is outside the scope of this chapter and the authors refer readers to other texts. Additionally, anesthetic protocols for patients with septic peritonitis is outside the scope of this chapter; however, a recent retrospective article on intraoperative lidocaine constant rate infusions indicated significantly greater short-term survival than in dogs that did not receive lidocaine intraoperatively.[170]

PROGNOSIS

Survival rates of 32% to 87% have been reported in dogs with secondary peritonitis.[139,151,159,166,168,170] Survival rates of 44% to 70% after surgery have been reported for cats.[139,149,156,171] In the author's experience hospitalization times vary greatly; however, most range from 3 to 10 days. When death occurs, it usually results from septic shock, DIC, lack of source control, or multiple organ dysfunction; prolonged hospitalization is often due to pancreatitis and/or ileus. Negative prognostic indicators identified in dogs with bacterial peritonitis include a diagnosis of primary as opposed to secondary peritonitis,[139] and preoperative anemia, leukocytosis, or hypoproteinemia.[172] Hypoproteinemia (<5 g/dL) and hypoalbuminemia (< 2.5 g/dL) has been correlated with an increased risk of leakage after intestinal anastomosis and resultant peritonitis;[173] however, these findings have not been consistent among studies.[174] Lower serum albumin concentration and increased PCV were risk factors for recurrent secondary peritonitis in one study, as was a GI source of peritonitis, especially foreign bodies.[148] Dogs with a foreign body were 7 times more likely to require a second surgery than those with GI sepsis occurring for reasons other than a foreign body.[148] Postoperative administration of glucocorticoids has been identified as a risk factor for death in dogs with septic peritonitis.[173] Low preoperative median serum ALT activity (56 U/L for surviving cats compared with 179 U/L for nonsurvivors) was the only positive prognostic indicator in one study of cats with peritonitis.[149] Significant differences between ALT and gamma-glutamyl transferase values were noted between survivors and nonsurvivors in dogs.[145] In another study, a high plasma lactate concentration was a negative prognostic indicator in cats with bacterial peritonitis.[156] In a retrospective study of 83 dogs with septic peritonitis, admission plasma lactate concentrations were also correlated with survival.[175] Admission plasma lactate concentrations > 4 mmol/L yielded a sensitivity of 36% and a specificity of 92% for nonsurvival. Because these prognostic factors were determined using retrospective studies with different populations and treatments, it is difficult to make firm conclusions, especially in the face of conflicting results between studies.

TABLE 125.3 Common Pathogens Encountered During Abdominal Surgical Procedures[178]

Location of Operation	Common Pathogen
Esophageal, gastroduodenal	Enteric gram-negative rods Gram-positive cocci
Colorectal	Enteric gram-negative rods Anaerobes Enterococci
Hepatobiliary	Enteric gram-negative rods Enterococci Clostridia
Genitourinary	Enteric gram-negative rods Enterococci
Penetrating trauma	Gram-negative rods Gram-positive cocci *Actinomyces/Nocardia*

Survival rates of dogs with recurrent secondary peritonitis have been reported to be 44%. One study did not identify any significant prognostic indicators for dogs with recurrent peritonitis.[147] The survival rate of cats with recurrent or tertiary bacterial peritonitis is unknown. Intestinal anastomotic and enterotomy dehiscence rates remains around 10% in the literature in dogs with and without septic peritonitis and remains an important factor to discuss with owners prior to GI surgery.[174-177]

MANAGEMENT OF SURGICAL CONTAMINATION

Surgical contamination and spillage of organ contents can often be anticipated, and a knowledge of the normal enteric flora can assist in appropriate choice of prophylactic antibiotics (Table 125.3). Spillage of intestinal contents in dogs and cats can be minimized by appropriate isolation of bowel loops and stomach with laparotomy pads and appropriate use of an assistant and suction. Although previously advocated in experimental models of septic peritonitis, intra-abdominal instillation of antimicrobials and disinfectants (e.g., povidone-iodine) is not recommend and can lead to chemical peritonitis. Sterile saline used alone (without systemic antimicrobials) to lavage the abdominal cavity as described above has been unsuccessful in consistently resulting in negative bacterial cultures, despite its diluting effect on the spilled material.[153]

CASE EXAMPLE

Signalment

"Colby," a 2-year-old male golden retriever from Davis in northern California.

History

Colby had a 3-week history of waxing and waning lethargy and inappetence that had worsened the week before examination. One week before examination at the University of California, Davis VMTH, he was examined at an emergency clinic. Abnormalities found on bloodwork were a leukocytosis (22,820 cells/μL) due to a mature neutrophilia (20,470 cells/μL); the serum chemistry panel was unremarkable. Abdominal radiographs showed decreased detail in the caudal abdomen secondary to small volume of effusion or peritonitis, and gastroenteritis was suspected. Colby was discharged with instructions to feed a bland, low-fat diet.

Physical Examination

General: Bright, alert, responsive, with adequate hydration; T: 101.5°F (38.6°C), HR: 80 beats/min with strong, symmetrical pulses. Respiration was panting, pink mucous membranes, CRT 2s, weight 29 kg, BCS 5/9. The remainder of the physical examination indicated no clinically significant abnormalities. There was mild dental calculus; the abdomen was soft and nonpainful, with no palpable masses; a rectal examination revealed some evidence of liquid stool.

Laboratory Findings

A CBC revealed a leukocytosis (21,750 cells/μL; RR, 6000–13,000 cells/μL) with 18,270/μL mature neutrophils (RR, 3000–10,500 cells/μL), and 870 bands/μL with slight toxicity. The serum biochemistry panel revealed only mild hypochloremia 107 mmol/L (108–118 mmol/L), hypocalcemia 9.5 mg/dL (9.7–11.5 mg/dL), hypoglycemia 63 mg/dL (64–123 mg/dL), hypoalbuminemia 2.9 g/dL (3.0–4.4 g/dL), and hyperglobulinemia 4.0 g/dL (1.8–3.9 g/dL). A urinalysis was unremarkable, Spec cPL® (IDEXX Laboratories) within reference range, and serum resting cortisol concentration 1.3 μg/dL.

Imaging Findings

Abdominal ultrasound: In the mid descending colon there is focal severe thickening of the colonic wall. An adjacent thick-walled, fluid and gas-filled structure, extending toward midline, is confluent with the colonic wall and gas is seen tracking through the colonic wall and into this adjacent structure. The surrounding mesentery is hyperechoic and there is a small volume of echogenic fluid surrounding the colon, adjacent small bowel, and mesentery. The remainder of the colon as well as the small intestinal tract and stomach are within normal limits. There are multiple severely enlarged, rounded, hypoechoic to heterogenous lymph nodes between the abnormal portion of the colon and the left kidney. A more caudal colic lymph node is also enlarged and hypoechoic. The spleen contains multiple small, hypoechoic nodules. The prostate is hyperechoic and large, consistent with the intact status of the patient.

Impressions: Focal colonic thickening and perforation with adjacent abscess formation; differentials include perforating foreign body, perforating neoplasia, or fungal infection. The adjacent mesentery and fluid may represent septic or sterile peritonitis. Severely abnormal adjacent lymph nodes may be reactive, but are concerning for metastatic or round cell neoplasia. Splenic nodules have a typically benign appearance, although metastatic or disseminated round cell neoplasia is not excluded.

Cytology Findings

Cytologic examination of an ultrasound-guided fine-needle aspirate of an enlarged lymph node in the caudal abdomen: A markedly expanded population of large lymphocytes is present. These cells have a small amount of deeply basophilic cytoplasm.

CASE EXAMPLE—cont'd

Nuclear chromatin is finely stippled and prominent nucleoli are observed, and there are many mitotic figures. The lymphocytes are CD79a positive, CD3 negative using immunostaining.

Diagnosis

B-cell lymphoma, high grade.

Treatment

Surgery was recommended to address the colonic perforation and associated abscess. Preoperatively, Colby was treated with intravenous fluids and parenteral ampicillin-sulbactam, enrofloxacin, maropitant, and methadone. Exploratory laparotomy was performed and the colonic mass was resected. The abdomen was lavaged and a closed suction drain was placed.

Microbiologic Testing

Sample: purulent fluid from colonic mass.

Direct smear: moderate numbers small gram-negative rods, very small numbers thin filamentous gram-negative rods, very small numbers large gram-positive rods.

Aerobic culture: very small numbers hemolytic *E. coli* (susceptible to all antimicrobials tested) and fastidious gram-negative rods. Anaerobic culture: large numbers *Bacteroides* spp./*Prevotella* spp. (β-lactamase negative), *Peptostreptococcus anaerobius* and *Fusobacterium nucleatum* (β-lactamase negative).

Diagnosis

Localized secondary septic peritonitis secondary to ruptured colonic large B-cell lymphoma.

Outcome

After the surgery, Colby was treated with L-asparaginase for lymphoma. He recovered for 5 days in hospital and was subsequently discharged. Ten days after the surgery, he continued chemotherapy with the Medical Oncology Service. Histopathology of the mass was consistent with completely excised colonic B-cell lymphoma with serosal perforation and mucosal ulceration.

Comments: In this case, spillage of colonic contents was contained by the mesentery and omentum, leading to a localized septic peritonitis. Colby recovered uneventfully from surgery with appropriate antibiotic therapy and supportive care, and experienced complete remission with chemotherapy (CHOP—cyclophosphamide, doxorubicin, vincristine, and prednisone). Three years later (at the time of writing), he remains in remission.

SUGGESTED READINGS

Hooda S, Minamoto Y, Suchodolski JS, et al. Current state of knowledge: the canine gastrointestinal microbiome. *Anim Health Res Rev*. 2012;13:78–88.

Bellows J, Berg ML, Dennis S, et al. 2019 AAHA Dental Care Guidelines for Dogs and Cats. *J Am Anim Hosp Assoc*. 2019;55:49–69.

Werner M, Suchodolski JS, Lidbury JA, et al. Diagnostic value of fecal cultures in dogs with chronic diarrhea. *J Vet Intern Med*. 2021;35:199–208.

Costello MF, Drobatz KJ, Aronson LR, et al. Underlying cause, pathophysiologic abnormalities, and response to treatment in cats with septic peritonitis: 51 cases (1990-2001). *J Am Vet Med Assoc*. 2004;225:897–902.

REFERENCES

1. Srikanth CV, McCormick BA. Interactions of the intestinal epithelium with the pathogen and the indigenous microbiota: a three-way crosstalk. *Interdiscip Perspect Infect Dis*. 2008;2008:626827.
2. Alessandri G, Argentini C, Milani C, et al. Catching a glimpse of the bacterial gut community of companion animals: a canine and feline perspective. *Microb Biotechnol*. 2020;13:1708–1732.
3. Siqueira JF Jr, Fouad AF, Rocas IN. Pyrosequencing as a tool for better understanding of human microbiomes. *J Oral Microbiol*. 2012;4.
4. AlShawaqfeh MK, Wajid B, Minamoto Y, et al. A dysbiosis index to assess microbial changes in fecal samples of dogs with chronic inflammatory enteropathy. *FEMS Microbiol Ecol*. 2017;93.
5. Werner M, Suchodolski JS, Lidbury JA, et al. Diagnostic value of fecal cultures in dogs with chronic diarrhea. *J Vet Intern Med*. 2021;35:199–208.
6. Pilla R, Gaschen FP, Barr JW, et al. Effects of metronidazole on the fecal microbiome and metabolome in healthy dogs. *J Vet Intern Med*. 2020;34:1853–1866.
7. Pilla R, Suchodolski JS. The role of the canine gut microbiome and metabolome in health and gastrointestinal disease. *Front Vet Sci*. 2019;6:498.
8. Elliott DR, Wilson M, Buckley CM, et al. Cultivable oral microbiota of domestic dogs. *J Clin Microbiol*. 2005;43:5470–5476.
9. Ruparell A, Inui T, Staunton R, et al. The canine oral microbiome: variation in bacterial populations across different niches. *BMC Microbiol*. 2020;20:42.
10. Harris S, Croft J, O'Flynn C, et al. A pyrosequencing investigation of differences in the feline subgingival microbiota in health, gingivitis and mild periodontitis. *PLoS One*. 2015;10:e0136986.
11. Rodrigues MX, Bicalho RC, Fiani N, et al. The subgingival microbial community of feline periodontitis and gingivostomatitis: characterization and comparison between diseased and healthy cats. *Sci Rep*. 2019;9:12340.
12. Martel DP, Fox PR, Lamb KE, et al. Comparison of closed root planing with versus without concurrent doxycycline hyclate or clindamycin hydrochloride gel application for the treatment of periodontal disease in dogs. *J Am Vet Med Assoc*. 2019;254:373–379.
13. Wallis C, Milella L, Colyer A, et al. Subgingival microbiota of dogs with healthy gingiva or early periodontal disease from different geographical locations. *BMC Vet Res*. 2021;17:7.
14. Ozavci V, Erbas G, Parin U, et al. Molecular detection of feline and canine periodontal pathogens. *Vet Anim Sci*. 2019;8:100069.
15. Holt SC, Ebersole JL. *Porphyromonas gingivalis, Treponema denticola*, and *Tannerella forsythia*: the "red complex", a prototype polybacterial pathogenic consortium in periodontitis. *Periodontol 2000*. 2005;38:72–122.
16. Nises J, Rosander A, Pettersson A, et al. The occurrence of *Treponema* spp. in gingival plaque from dogs with varying degree of periodontal disease. *PLoS One*. 2018;13:e0201888.
17. Kovacevic M, Tamarut T, Jonjic N, et al. The transition from pulpitis to periapical periodontitis in dogs' teeth. *Aust Endod J*. 2008;34:12–18.
18. Zahran S, Witherden E, Mannocci F, et al. Characterization of root canal microbiota in teeth diagnosed with irreversible pulpitis. *J Endod*. 2021;47:415–423.
19. Alasqah M, Khan SIR, Alfouzan K, et al. Regenerative endodontic management of an immature molar using calcium hydroxide and triple antibiotic paste: a two-year follow-up. *Case Rep Dent*. 2020;2020:9025847.
20. Aral K, Milward MR, Cooper PR. Inflammasome dysregulation in human gingival fibroblasts in response to periodontal pathogens. *Oral Dis*. 2020. Online ahead of print.
21. Kozak M, Dabrowska-Zamojcin E, Mazurek-Mochol M, et al. Cytokines and their genetic polymorphisms related to periodontal disease. *J Clin Med*. 2020;9:4045.
22. Ito A, Isogai E, Yoshioka K, et al. Ability of orally administered IFN-alpha4 to inhibit naturally occurring gingival inflammation in dogs. *J Vet Med Sci*. 2010;72:1145–1151.
23. Yamaki S, Hachimura H, Ogawa M, et al. Long-term follow-up study after administration of a canine interferon-alpha preparation for feline gingivitis. *J Vet Med Sci*. 2020;82:232–236.
24. Woelber JP, Gartner M, Breuninger L, et al. The influence of an anti-inflammatory diet on gingivitis. A randomized controlled trial. *J Clin Periodontol*. 2019;46:481–490.

25. Lourenco AL, Booij-Vrieling HE, Vossebeld CB, et al. The effect of dietary corn oil and fish oil supplementation in dogs with naturally occurring gingivitis. *J Anim Physiol Anim Nutr.* 2018;102:1382–1389.
26. Sarkiala E, Harvey C. Systemic antimicrobials in the treatment of periodontitis in dogs. *Semin Vet Med Surg Small Anim.* 1993;8:197–203.
27. Warrick JM, Inskeep GA, Yonkers TD, et al. Effect of clindamycin hydrochloride on oral malodor, plaque, calculus, and gingivitis in dogs with periodontitis. *Vet Ther.* 2000;1:5–16.
28. Norris JM, Love DN. In vitro antimicrobial susceptibilities of three *Porphyromonas* spp. and in vivo responses in the oral cavity of cats to selected antimicrobial agents. *Aust Vet J.* 2000;78:533–537.
29. Hoffman SL, Kressin DJ, Verstraete FJ. Myths and misconceptions in veterinary dentistry. *J Am Vet Med Assoc.* 2007;231:1818–1824.
30. Bellows J, Berg ML, Dennis S, et al. 2019 AAHA dental care guidelines for dogs and cats. *J Am Anim Hosp Assoc.* 2019;55:49–69.
31. Ingham KE, Gorrel C. Effect of long-term intermittent periodontal care on canine periodontal disease. *J Small Anim Pract.* 2001;42:67–70.
32. Nemec A, Pavlica Z, Stiblar-Martincic D, et al. Histological evaluation of the pulp in teeth from dogs with naturally occurring periodontal disease. *J Vet Dent.* 2007;24:212–223.
33. Logan EI. Dietary influences on periodontal health in dogs and cats. *Vet Clin North Am Small Anim Pract.* 2006;36:1385–1401 (ix).
34. Carroll MQ, Oba PM, Sieja KM, et al. Effects of novel dental chews on oral health outcomes and halitosis in adult dogs. *J Anim Sci.* 2020;98:skaa274.
35. Allan RM, Adams VJ, Johnston NW. Prospective randomised blinded clinical trial assessing effectiveness of three dental plaque control methods in dogs. *J Small Anim Pract.* 2019;60:212–217.
36. Ingham K. Effect of a dental chew on dental substrates and gingivitis in cats. *J Vet Dent.* 2003;20:136.
37. Ingham KE, Gorrel C, Bierer TL. Effect of a dental chew on dental substrates and gingivitis in cats. *J Vet Dent.* 2002;19:201–204.
38. Logan EI, Finney O, Hefferren JJ. Effects of a dental food on plaque accumulation and gingival health in dogs. *J Vet Dent.* 2002;19:15–18.
39. Vrieling HE, Theyse LF, van Winkelhoff AJ, et al. Effectiveness of feeding large kibbles with mechanical cleaning properties in cats with gingivitis. *Tijdschr Diergeneeskd.* 2005;130:136–140.
40. Hennet P. Effectiveness of a dental gel to reduce plaque in beagle dogs. *J Vet Dent.* 2002;19:11–14.
41. Meurman JH. Probiotics: do they have a role in oral medicine and dentistry? *Eur J Oral Sci.* 2005;113:188–196.
42. Nackaerts O, Jacobs R, Quirynen M, et al. Replacement therapy for periodontitis: pilot radiographic evaluation in a dog model. *J Clin Periodontol.* 2008;35:1048–1052.
43. Morales A, Contador R, Bravo J, et al. Clinical effects of probiotic or azithromycin as an adjunct to scaling and root planning in the treatment of stage III periodontitis: a pilot randomized controlled clinical trial. *BMC Oral Health.* 2021;21:12.
44. Bell SE, Nash AK, Zanghi BM, et al. An assessment of the stability of the canine oral microbiota after probiotic administration in healthy dogs over time. *Front Vet Sci.* 2020;7:616.
45. Sanz M, Marco Del Castillo A, Jepsen S, et al. Periodontitis and cardiovascular diseases: Consensus report. *J Clin Periodontol.* 2020;47:268–288.
46. Bobetsis YA, Graziani F, Gursoy M, et al. Periodontal disease and adverse pregnancy outcomes. *Periodontol 2000.* 2020;83:154–174.
47. Wu CZ, Yuan YH, Liu HH, et al. Epidemiologic relationship between periodontitis and type 2 diabetes mellitus. *BMC Oral Health.* 2020;20:204.
48. Ata-Ali F, Melo M, Cobo T, et al. Does non-surgical periodontal treatment improve glycemic control? A comprehensive review of meta-analyses. *J Int Acad Periodontol.* 2020;22:205–222.
49. DeBowes LJ, Mosier D, Logan E, et al. Association of periodontal disease and histologic lesions in multiple organs from 45 dogs. *J Vet Dent.* 1996;13:57–60.
50. Pereira Dos Santos JD, Cunha E, Nunes T, et al. Relation between periodontal disease and systemic diseases in dogs. *Res Vet Sci.* 2019;125:136–140.
51. Glickman LT, Glickman NW, Moore GE, et al. Association between chronic azotemic kidney disease and the severity of periodontal disease in dogs. *Prev Vet Med.* 2011;99:193–200.
52. Pavlica Z, Petelin M, Juntes P, et al. Periodontal disease burden and pathological changes in organs of dogs. *J Vet Dent.* 2008;25:97–105.
53. Glickman LT, Glickman NW, Moore GE, et al. Evaluation of the risk of endocarditis and other cardiovascular events on the basis of the severity of periodontal disease in dogs. *J Am Vet Med Assoc.* 2009;234:486–494.
54. Peddle GD, Drobatz KJ, Harvey CE, et al. Association of periodontal disease, oral procedures, and other clinical findings with bacterial endocarditis in dogs. *J Am Vet Med Assoc.* 2009;234:100–107.
55. Sykes JE, Kittleson MD, Chomel BB, et al. Clinicopathologic findings and outcome in dogs with infective endocarditis: 71 cases (1992-2005). *J Am Vet Med Assoc.* 2006;228:1735–1747.
56. Harari J, Gustafson S, Meinkoth K. Dental bacteremia in cats. *Feline Pract.* 1991;19:27–29.
57. Harari J, Besser TE, Gustafson SB, et al. Bacterial isolates from blood cultures of dogs undergoing dentistry. *Vet Surg.* 1993;22:27–30.
58. Black AP, Crichlow AM, Saunders JR. Bacteremia during ultrasonic teeth cleaning and extraction in the dog. *J Am Anim Hosp Assoc.* 1980;16:611–616.
59. Dahlen G. Biofilms in dental unit water lines. *Monogr Oral Sci.* 2021;29:12–18.
60. Tangalidi MK, Oikonomidis IL, Psalla D, et al. Nodular granulomatous glossitis as the sole clinical sign in canine leishmaniosis. *Vet Clin Pathol.* 2016;45:710–714.
61. Anderson JG, Peralta S, Kol A, et al. Clinical and histopathologic characterization of canine chronic ulcerative stomatitis. *Vet Pathol.* 2017;54:511–519.
62. Anderson JG, Kol A, Bizikova P, et al. Immunopathogenesis of canine chronic ulcerative stomatitis. *PLoS One.* 2020;15:e0227386.
63. Lee DB, Verstraete FJM, Arzi B. An update on feline chronic gingivostomatitis. *Vet Clin North Am Small Anim Pract.* 2020;50:973–982.
64. Farcas N, Lommer MJ, Kass PH, et al. Dental radiographic findings in cats with chronic gingivostomatitis (2002-2012). *J Am Vet Med Assoc.* 2014;244:339–345.
65. Kouki MI, Papadimitriou SA, Psalla D, et al. Chronic gingivostomatitis with esophagitis in cats. *J Vet Intern Med.* 2017;31:1673–1679.
66. Sykes JE, Westropp JL, Kasten RW, et al. Association between *Bartonella* species infection and disease in pet cats as determined using serology and culture. *J Feline Med Surg.* 2010;12:631–636.
67. Addie DD, Radford A, Yam PS, et al. Cessation of feline calicivirus shedding coincident with resolution of chronic gingivostomatitis in a cat. *J Small Anim Pract.* 2003;44:172–176.
68. Lommer MJ, Verstraete FJ. Concurrent oral shedding of feline calicivirus and feline herpesvirus 1 in cats with chronic gingivostomatitis. *Oral Microbiol Immunol.* 2003;18:131–134.
69. Vapniarsky N, Simpson DL, Arzi B, et al. Histological, immunological, and genetic analysis of feline chronic gingivostomatitis. *Front Vet Sci.* 2020;7:310.
70. Harley R, Helps CR, Harbour DA, et al. Cytokine mRNA expression in lesions in cats with chronic gingivostomatitis. *Clin Diagn Lab Immunol.* 1999;6:471–478.
71. Dolieslager SM, Riggio MP, Lennon A, et al. Identification of bacteria associated with feline chronic gingivostomatitis using culture-dependent and culture-independent methods. *Vet Microbiol.* 2011;148:93–98.
72. Lommer MJ. Efficacy of cyclosporine for chronic, refractory stomatitis in cats: a randomized, placebo-controlled, double-blinded clinical study. *J Vet Dent.* 2013;30:8–17.
73. Jennings MW, Lewis JR, Soltero-Rivera MM, et al. Effect of tooth extraction on stomatitis in cats: 95 cases (2000-2013). *J Am Vet Med Assoc.* 2015;246:654–660.
74. Adami C, Di Palma S, Gendron K, et al. Severe esophageal injuries occurring after general anesthesia in two cats: case report and literature review. *J Am Anim Hosp Assoc.* 2011;47:436–442.
75. Gabriel AL, Masuda EK, Ramos AT, et al. Canine adenovirus type-2 and canine distemper virus pulmonary co-infection in two Chow-Chow puppies with *Candida* sp. esophagitis. *Braz J Vet Pathol.* 2008;1:47–51.

76. Patton CS, Hake R, Newton J, et al. Esophagitis due to *Pythium insidiosum* infection in two dogs. *J Vet Intern Med.* 1996;10:139–142.
77. Brissot HN, Burton CA, Doyle RS, et al. Caudal mediastinal paraesophageal abscesses in 7 dogs. *Vet Surg.* 2012;41:286–291.
78. Jung J, Choi M. Nonsurgical resolution of caudal mediastinal paraesophageal abscess in a cat. *J Vet Med Sci.* 2015;77:499–502.
79. Salisbury SK, Forbes S, Blevins WE. Peritracheal abscess associated with tracheal collapse and bilateral laryngeal paralysis in a dog. *J Am Vet Med Assoc.* 1990;196:1273–1275.
80. Nagamori Y, Payton ME, Looper E, et al. Retrospective survey of parasitism identified in feces of client-owned cats in North America from 2007 through 2018. *Vet Parasitol.* 2020;277:109008.
81. Kato D, Oishi M, Ohno K, et al. The first report of the ante-mortem diagnosis of *Ollulanus tricuspis* infection in two dogs. *J Vet Med Sci.* 2015;77:1499–1502.
82. Garcia-Mazcorro JF, Suchodolski JS, Jones KR, et al. Effect of the proton pump inhibitor omeprazole on the gastrointestinal bacterial microbiota of healthy dogs. *FEMS Microbiol Ecol.* 2012;80:624–636.
83. Johnston K, Lamport A, Batt RM. An unexpected bacterial flora in the proximal small intestine of normal cats. *Vet Rec.* 1993;132:362–363.
84. Johnston KL, Lamport A, Ballevre O, et al. A comparison of endoscopic and surgical collection procedures for the analysis of the bacterial flora in duodenal fluid from cats. *Vet J.* 1999;157:85–89.
85. Ishikawa H, Baba E, Matsumoto H. Studies on bacterial flora of the alimentary tract of dogs. III. Fecal flora in clinical and experimental cases of diarrhea. *Nihon Juigaku Zasshi.* 1982;44:343–347.
86. Masuoka H, Shimada K, Kiyosue-Yasuda T, et al. Transition of the intestinal microbiota of dogs with age. *Biosci Microbiota Food Health.* 2017;36:27–31.
87. Masuoka H, Shimada K, Kiyosue-Yasuda T, et al. Transition of the intestinal microbiota of cats with age. *PLoS One.* 2017;12:e0181739.
88. Mizukami K, Uchiyama J, Igarashi H, et al. Age-related analysis of the gut microbiome in a purebred dog colony. *FEMS Microbiol Lett.* 2019;366:fnz095.
89. Schmidt M, Unterer S, Suchodolski JS, et al. The fecal microbiome and metabolome differs between dogs fed Bones and Raw Food (BARF) diets and dogs fed commercial diets. *PLoS One.* 2018;13:e0201279.
90. German AJ, Day MJ, Ruaux CG, et al. Comparison of direct and indirect tests for small intestinal bacterial overgrowth and antibiotic-responsive diarrhea in dogs. *J Vet Intern Med.* 2003;17:33–43.
91. Xenoulis PG, Palculict B, Allenspach K, et al. Molecular-phylogenetic characterization of microbial communities imbalances in the small intestine of dogs with inflammatory bowel disease. *FEMS Microbiol Ecol.* 2008;66:579–589.
92. Suchodolski JS, Camacho J, Steiner JM. Analysis of bacterial diversity in the canine duodenum, jejunum, ileum, and colon by comparative 16S rRNA gene analysis. *FEMS Microbiol Ecol.* 2008;66:567–578.
93. Suchodolski JS, Dowd SE, Westermarck E, et al. The effect of the macrolide antibiotic tylosin on microbial diversity in the canine small intestine as demonstrated by massive parallel 16S rRNA gene sequencing. *BMC Microbiol.* 2009;9:210.
94. Hooda S, Minamoto Y, Suchodolski JS, et al. Current state of knowledge: the canine gastrointestinal microbiome. *Anim Health Res Rev.* 2012;13:78–88.
95. Collins JE, Bergeland ME, Lindeman CJ, et al. *Enterococcus (Streptococcus) durans* adherence in the small intestine of a diarrheic pup. *Vet Pathol.* 1988;25:396–398.
96. Walk ST, Young VB. Emerging insights into antibiotic-associated diarrhea and *Clostridium difficile* infection through the lens of microbial ecology. *Interdiscip Perspect Infect Dis.* 2008;2008:125081.
97. Bell JA, Kopper JJ, Turnbull JA, et al. Ecological characterization of the colonic microbiota of normal and diarrheic dogs. *Interdiscip Perspect Infect Dis.* 2008;2008:149694.
98. Suchodolski JS, Xenoulis PG, Paddock CG, et al. Molecular analysis of the bacterial microbiota in duodenal biopsies from dogs with idiopathic inflammatory bowel disease. *Vet Microbiol.* 2010;142:394–400.
99. Rossi G, Pengo G, Caldin M, et al. Comparison of microbiological, histological, and immunomodulatory parameters in response to treatment with either combination therapy with prednisone and metronidazole or probiotic VSL#3 strains in dogs with idiopathic inflammatory bowel disease. *PLoS One.* 2014;9:e94699.
100. Bermingham EN, Young W, Butowski CF, et al. The fecal microbiota in the domestic cat (*Felis catus*) is influenced by interactions between age and diet; a five year longitudinal study. *Front Microbiol.* 2018;9:1231.
101. Lyu Y, Su C, Verbrugghe A, et al. Past, present, and future of gastrointestinal microbiota research in cats. *Front Microbiol.* 2020;11:1661.
102. Marsilio S, Pilla R, Sarawichitr B, et al. Characterization of the fecal microbiome in cats with inflammatory bowel disease or alimentary small cell lymphoma. *Sci Rep.* 2019;9:19208.
103. Foster ML, Dowd SE, Stephenson C, et al. Characterization of the fungal microbiome (mycobiome) in fecal samples from dogs. *Vet Med Int.* 2013;2013:658373.
104. Handl S, Dowd SE, Garcia-Mazcorro JF, et al. Massive parallel 16S rRNA gene pyrosequencing reveals highly diverse fecal bacterial and fungal communities in healthy dogs and cats. *FEMS Microbiol Ecol.* 2011;76:301–310.
105. Gibson GR, Roberfroid MB. Dietary modulation of the human colonic microbiota: introducing the concept of prebiotics. *J Nutr.* 1995;125:1401–1412.
106. Apanavicius CJ, Powell KL, Vester BM, et al. Fructan supplementation and infection affect food intake, fever, and epithelial sloughing from *Salmonella* challenge in weanling puppies. *J Nutr.* 2007;137:1923–1930.
107. Middelbos IS, Vester Boler BM, Qu A, et al. Phylogenetic characterization of fecal microbial communities of dogs fed diets with or without supplemental dietary fiber using 454 pyrosequencing. *PLoS One.* 2010;5:e9768.
108. Barry KA, Wojcicki BJ, Middelbos IS, et al. Dietary cellulose, fructooligosaccharides, and pectin modify fecal protein catabolites and microbial populations in adult cats. *J Anim Sci.* 2010;88:2978–2987.
109. Sauter SN, Benyacoub J, Allenspach K, et al. Effects of probiotic bacteria in dogs with food responsive diarrhoea treated with an elimination diet. *J Anim Physiol Anim Nutr.* 2006;90:269–277.
110. Herstad HK, Nesheim BB, L'Abee-Lund T, et al. Effects of a probiotic intervention in acute canine gastroenteritis—a controlled clinical trial. *J Small Anim Pract.* 2010;51:34–38.
111. Gaspardo A, Zannoni A, Turroni S, et al. Influence of *Lactobacillus kefiri* on intestinal microbiota and fecal IgA content of healthy dogs. *Front Vet Sci.* 2020;7:146.
112. White R, Atherly T, Guard B, et al. Randomized, controlled trial evaluating the effect of multi-strain probiotic on the mucosal microbiota in canine idiopathic inflammatory bowel disease. *Gut Microb.* 2017;8:451–466.
113. Rossi G, Pengo G, Galosi L, et al. Effects of the probiotic mixture Slab51(r) Ssivomixx(r)) as food supplement in healthy dogs: evaluation of fecal microbiota, clinical parameters and immune function. *Front Vet Sci.* 2020;7:613.
114. Pilla R, Guard BC, Steiner JM, et al. Administration of a synbiotic containing *Enterococcus faecium* does not significantly alter fecal microbiota richness or diversity in dogs with and without food-responsive chronic enteropathy. *Front Vet Sci.* 2019;6:277.
115. Bybee SN, Scorza AV, Lappin MR. Effect of the probiotic *Enterococcus faecium* SF68 on presence of diarrhea in cats and dogs housed in an animal shelter. *J Vet Intern Med.* 2011;25:856–860.
116. Rodrigues BM, Olivo PM, Osmari MP, et al. Microencapsulation of probiotic strains by lyophilization is efficient in maintaining the viability of microorganisms and modulation of fecal microbiota in cats. *Int J Microbiol.* 2020;2020:1293481.
117. Torres-Henderson C, Summers S, Suchodolski J, et al. Effect of *Enterococcus faecium* strain SF68 on gastrointestinal signs and fecal microbiome in cats administered amoxicillin-clavulanate. *Top Companion Anim Med.* 2017;32:104–108.
118. Niina A, Kibe R, Suzuki R, et al. Improvement in clinical symptoms and fecal microbiome after fecal microbiota transplantation in a dog with inflammatory bowel disease. *Vet Med (Auckl).* 2019;10:197–201.
119. Sugita K, Yanuma N, Ohno H, et al. Oral faecal microbiota transplantation for the treatment of *Clostridium difficile*-associated diarrhoea in a dog: a case report. *BMC Vet Res.* 2019;15:11.

120. DeFilipp Z, Bloom PP, Torres Soto M, et al. Drug-resistant *E. coli* bacteremia transmitted by fecal microbiota transplant. *N Engl J Med.* 2019;381:2043–2050.
121. Dahlinger J, Marks SL, Hirsh DC. Prevalence and identity of translocating bacteria in healthy dogs. *J Vet Intern Med.* 1997;11:319–322.
122. Knoop KA, McDonald KG, Kulkarni DH, et al. Antibiotics promote inflammation through the translocation of native commensal colonic bacteria. *Gut.* 2016;65:1100–1109.
123. O'Boyle CJ, MacFie J, Mitchell CJ, et al. Microbiology of bacterial translocation in humans. *Gut.* 1998;42:29–35.
124. Ghosh SS, Wang J, Yannie PJ, et al. Intestinal barrier dysfunction, LPS translocation, and disease development. *J Endocr Soc.* 2020;4:bvz039.
125. Reineke EL, Walton K, Otto CM. Evaluation of an oral electrolyte solution for treatment of mild to moderate dehydration in dogs with hemorrhagic diarrhea. *J Am Vet Med Assoc.* 2013;243:851–857.
126. Mehdizadeh Gohari I, Unterer S, Whitehead AE, et al. NetF-producing *Clostridium perfringens* and its associated diseases in dogs and foals. *J Vet Diagn Invest.* 2020;32:230–238.
127. Mehdizadeh Gohari I, Parreira VR, Nowell VJ, et al. A novel pore-forming toxin in type A *Clostridium perfringens* is associated with both fatal canine hemorrhagic gastroenteritis and fatal foal necrotizing enterocolitis. *PLoS One.* 2015;10:e0122684.
128. Sindern N, Suchodolski JS, Leutenegger CM, et al. Prevalence of *Clostridium perfringens* netE and netF toxin genes in the feces of dogs with acute hemorrhagic diarrhea syndrome. *J Vet Intern Med.* 2019;33:100–105.
129. Cartwright JA, Perez-Accino J, Timothy C, et al. Acute ulcerative enterocolitis with severe protein loss due to mucosal invasion with *Enterococcus* spp. in a dog with exocrine pancreatic insufficiency: a case report. *Front Vet Sci.* 2020;7:577642.
130. Unterer S, Strohmeyer K, Kruse BD, et al. Treatment of aseptic dogs with hemorrhagic gastroenteritis with amoxicillin/clavulanic acid: a prospective blinded study. *J Vet Intern Med.* 2011;25:973–979.
131. Kilpinen S, Rantala M, Spillmann T, et al. Oral tylosin administration is associated with an increase of faecal enterococci and lactic acid bacteria in dogs with tylosin-responsive diarrhoea. *Vet J.* 2015;205:369–374.
132. Kilpinen S, Spillmann T, Syrja P, et al. Effect of tylosin on dogs with suspected tylosin-responsive diarrhea: a placebo-controlled, randomized, double-blinded, prospective clinical trial. *Acta Vet Scand.* 2011;53:26.
133. Kilpinen S, Spillmann T, Westermarck E. Efficacy of two low-dose oral tylosin regimens in controlling the relapse of diarrhea in dogs with tylosin-responsive diarrhea: a prospective, single-blinded, two-arm parallel, clinical field trial. *Acta Vet Scand.* 2014;56:43.
134. Lapointe JM, Higgins R, Barrette N, et al. *Enterococcus hirae* enteropathy with ascending cholangitis and pancreatitis in a kitten. *Vet Pathol.* 2000;37:282–284.
135. Johnson MD, Mann FA. Treatment for pancreatic abscesses via omentalization with abdominal closure versus open peritoneal drainage in dogs: 15 cases (1994-2004). *J Am Vet Med Assoc.* 2006;228:397–402.
136. Anderson JR, Cornell KK, Parnell NK, et al. Pancreatic abscess in 36 dogs: a retrospective analysis of prognostic indicators. *J Am Anim Hosp Assoc.* 2008;44:171–179.
137. Widdison AL, Karanjia ND, Reber HA. Antimicrobial treatment of pancreatic infection in cats. *Br J Surg.* 1994;81:886–889.
138. Kazantsev GB, Hecht DW, Rao R, et al. Plasmid labeling confirms bacterial translocation in pancreatitis. *Am J Surg.* 1994;167:201–206. discussion 206-207.
139. Culp WT, Zeldis TE, Reese MS, et al. Primary bacterial peritonitis in dogs and cats: 24 cases (1990-2006). *J Am Vet Med Assoc.* 2009;234:906–913.
140. Laroche M, Harding G. Primary and secondary peritonitis: an update. *Eur J Clin Microbiol Infect Dis.* 1998;17:542–550.
141. Bernardi M. Spontaneous bacterial peritonitis: from pathophysiology to prevention. *Intern Emerg Med.* 2010;5(suppl 1):S37–S44.
142. Uncu N, Bulbul M, Yildiz N, et al. Primary peritonitis in children with nephrotic syndrome: results of a 5-year multicenter study. *Eur J Pediatr.* 2010;169:73–76.
143. Conn HO. Spontaneous bacterial peritonitis: variant syndromes. *South Med J.* 1987;80:1343–1346.
144. Hosgood G, Salisbury SK. Generalized peritonitis in dogs: 50 cases (1975-1986). *J Am Vet Med Assoc.* 1988;193:1448–1450.
145. Winkler KP, Greenfield CL. Potential prognostic indicators in diffuse peritonitis treated with open peritoneal drainage in the canine patient. *J Vet Emerg Crit Care.* 2000;10:259–265.
146. Salavati Schmitz S. Retrospective characterisation and outcome of canine idiopathic mesenteric purulent lymphadenitis and lymph node abscesses at a teaching hospital from 2005 to 2015. *J Small Anim Pract.* 2016;57:690–697.
147. Barfield DM, Tivers MS, Holahan M, et al. Retrospective evaluation of recurrent secondary septic peritonitis in dogs (2000–2011): 41 cases. *J Vet Emerg Crit Care.* 2016;26:281–287.
148. Fink O, Buysse A, Drobatz KJ, et al. Identification of risk factors for recurrent secondary septic peritonitis following initial surgical treatment of secondary septic peritonitis in dogs. *J Vet Emerg Crit Care.* 2020;30:213–220.
149. Costello MF, Drobatz KJ, Aronson LR, et al. Underlying cause, pathophysiologic abnormalities, and response to treatment in cats with septic peritonitis: 51 cases (1990-2001). *J Am Vet Med Assoc.* 2004;225:897–902.
150. Salisbury SK, Hosgood GL. Management of the patient with generalized peritonitis. *Problems Vet Med.* 1989;1:168–182.
151. Marshall H, Sinnott-Stutzman V, Ewing P, et al. Effect of peritoneal lavage on bacterial isolates in 40 dogs with confirmed septic peritonitis. *J Vet Emerg Crit Care.* 2019;29:635–642.
152. Bonczynski JJ, Ludwig LL, Barton LJ, et al. Comparison of peritoneal fluid and peripheral blood pH, bicarbonate, glucose, and lactate concentration as a diagnostic tool for septic peritonitis in dogs and cats. *Vet Surg.* 2003;32:161–166.
153. Swayne SL, Brisson B, Weese JS, et al. Evaluating the effect of intraoperative peritoneal lavage on bacterial culture in dogs with suspected septic peritonitis. *Can Vet J.* 2012;53:971–977.
154. Ong RKC, Raisis AL, Swindells KL. *Candida albicans* peritonitis in a dog. *J Vet Emerg Crit Care.* 2010;20:143–147.
155. Rogers CL, Gibson C, Mitchell SL, et al. Disseminated candidiasis secondary to fungal and bacterial peritonitis in a young dog. *J Vet Emerg Crit Care.* 2009;19:193–198.
156. Parsons KJ, Owen LJ, Lee K, et al. A retrospective study of surgically treated cases of septic peritonitis in the cat (2000-2007). *J Small Anim Pract.* 2009;50:518–524.
157. Kirby BK. Peritoneum and retroperitoneum. In: Tobias KM, Johnston SA, eds. *Veterinary Surgery: Small Animal.* Elsevier; 2012:1391–1423.
158. Hauptman JG, Walshaw R, Olivier NB. Evaluation of the sensitivity and specificity of diagnostic criteria for sepsis in dogs. *Vet Surg.* 1997;26:393–397.
159. Bentley AM, Mayhew PD, Culp WT, et al. Alterations in the hemostatic profiles of dogs with naturally occurring septic peritonitis. *J Vet Emerg Crit Care.* 2013;23:14–22.
160. Mueller MG, Ludwig LL, Barton LJ. Use of closed-suction drains to treat generalized peritonitis in dogs and cats: 40 cases (1997-1999). *J Am Vet Med Assoc.* 2001;219:789–794.
161. Kalafut SR, Schwartz P, Currao RL, et al. Comparison of initial and postlavage bacterial culture results of septic peritonitis in dogs and cats. *J Am Anim Hosp Assoc.* 2018;54:257–266.
162. Levin GM, Bonczynski JJ, Ludwig LL, et al. Lactate as a diagnostic test for septic peritoneal effusions in dogs and cats. *J Am Anim Hosp Assoc.* 2004;40:364–371.
163. Martiny P, Goggs R. Biomarker guided diagnosis of septic peritonitis in dogs. *Front Vet Sci.* 2019;6:208.
164. Szabo SD, Jermyn K, Neel J, et al. Evaluation of postceliotomy peritoneal drain fluid volume, cytology, and blood-to-peritoneal fluid lactate and glucose differences in normal dogs. *Vet Surg.* 2011;40:444–449.
165. Ludwig LL, McLoughlin MA, Graves TK, et al. Surgical treatment of bile peritonitis in 24 dogs and 2 cats: a retrospective study (1987–1994). *Vet Surg.* 1997;26:90–98.
166. Lanz OI, Ellison GW, Bellah JR, et al. Surgical treatment of septic peritonitis without abdominal drainage in 28 dogs. *J Am Anim Hosp Assoc.* 2001;37:87–92.

167. Greenfield CL, Walshaw R. Open peritoneal drainage for treatment of contaminated peritoneal cavity and septic peritonitis in dogs and cats: 24 cases (1980-1986). *J Am Vet Med Assoc.* 1987;191:100–105.
168. Buote NJ, Havig ME. The use of vacuum-assisted closure in the management of septic peritonitis in six dogs. *J Am Anim Hosp Assoc.* 2012;48:164–171.
169. Elmenhorst K, Perez Lopez P, Belch A, et al. Retrospective study of complications associated with surgically-placed gastrostomy tubes in 43 dogs with septic peritonitis. *J Small Anim Pract.* 2020;61:116–120.
170. Bellini L, Seymour CJ. Effect of intraoperative constant rate infusion of lidocaine on short-term survival of dogs with septic peritonitis: 75 cases (2007-2011). *J Am Vet Med Assoc.* 2016;248:422–429.
171. Babyak JM, Sharp CR. Epidemiology of systemic inflammatory response syndrome and sepsis in cats hospitalized in a veterinary teaching hospital. *J Am Vet Med Assoc.* 2016;249:65–71.
172. Ralphs SC, Jessen CR, Lipowitz AJ. Risk factors for leakage following intestinal anastomosis in dogs and cats: 115 cases (1991-2000). *J Am Vet Med Assoc.* 2003;223:73–77.
173. Grimes JA, Schmiedt CW, Cornell KK, et al. Identification of risk factors for septic peritonitis and failure to survive following gastrointestinal surgery in dogs. *J Am Vet Med Assoc.* 2011;238:486–494.
174. Snowdon KA, Smeak DD, Chiang S. Risk factors for dehiscence of stapled functional end-to-end intestinal anastomoses in dogs: 53 cases (2001-2012). *Vet Surg.* 2016;45:91–99.
175. Cortellini S, Seth M, Kellett-Gregory LM. Plasma lactate concentrations in septic peritonitis: a retrospective study of 83 dogs (2007-2012). *J Vet Emerg Crit Care.* 2015;25:388–395.
176. Rosenbaum JM, Coolman BR, Davidson BL, et al. The use of disposable skin staples for intestinal resection and anastomosis in 63 dogs: 2000 to 2014. *J Small Anim Pract.* 2016;57:631–636.
177. Weisman DL, Smeak DD, Birchard SJ, et al. Comparison of a continuous suture pattern with a simple interrupted pattern for enteric closure in dogs and cats: 83 cases (1991-1997). *J Am Vet Med Assoc.* 1999;214:1507–1510.
178. Cornell K. Wound healing. In: Tobias KM, Johnston SA, eds. *Veterinary Surgery: Small Animal.* Elsevier; 2012:125–139.

126

Hepatobiliary Infections

Jane E. Sykes, Sina Marsilio, Stanley L. Marks

KEY POINTS

- The liver and biliary tree contain a complex immune defense system that protects the body against bacteria that enter from the portal system, through arterial channels, or that ascend the biliary tree. Diseases that disrupt these processes can predispose to infection.
- Bacteria that most commonly cause hepatobiliary infections are *Escherichia coli*, *Enterococcus* spp., and anaerobes; less often other gram-negative aerobes, *Streptococcus* and *Staphylococcus* spp. are involved.
- Several viruses, atypical bacteria, protozoa, fungi, and helminths also can cause hepatobiliary infections in dogs and cats.
- Major clinical signs of bacterial cholangitis or cholangiohepatitis are inappetence, lethargy, fever, vomiting, diarrhea, abdominal pain, and icterus.
- Ultrasound is a relatively sensitive tool for imaging the hepatobiliary system and can be used to guide collection of specimens for cytologic examination and culture.
- Treatment includes antimicrobial drugs and supportive care for hepatobiliary disease; cholecystectomy may be required when biliary tract obstruction is severe, gall bladder mucocele is present, there is rupture of the biliary tract, or cholelithiasis.

HEPATOBILIARY INFECTIONS

Hepatobiliary infections include a variety of viral, bacterial, protozoal, or fungal infections that can spread hematogenously to the liver as part of a systemic infection; ascending infections of the biliary tree; and possibly bacterial translocation from the portal circulation (Table 126.1). The focus of this chapter is bacterial infections of the biliary tree; hepatic abscesses are considered in a separate section that follows. The main mechanism thought to be involved is ascending infections of the biliary tree, although hematogenous spread and bacterial translocation from the portal system are other proposed mechanisms.[1,2] Ascension of bacteria occurs when normal hepatic defense mechanisms are overwhelmed (Box 126.1). Those mechanisms include the mechanical barrier presented by the sphincter of Oddi, the flushing action of bile, antibacterial effects of bile salts, and local immune defenses as described in the following text (IgA, mucus, Kupffer cells). Inflammatory bowel disease, neoplasia, inflammatory liver disease, biliary obstruction, and systemic immunosuppression can all interfere with these mechanisms and predispose to infection. An understanding of normal hepatobiliary defense mechanisms can facilitate improved understanding of the pathogenesis and treatment of hepatobiliary infections.

NORMAL HEPATOBILIARY DEFENSE MECHANISMS

Kupffer Cells

Hepatic Kupffer cells comprise the largest compartment of tissue macrophages in the body, representing 80 to 90% of the total fixed macrophages and approximately 35% of the nonparenchymal liver cells.[3,4] Residing mainly within the lumen of hepatic sinusoids and adherent to endothelial cells by long cytoplasmic processes, Kupffer cells are most numerous in the periportal area (zone 1, see later) where they offer first-line defense against bacteria, endotoxin, and microbial debris delivered from the GI tract.[3] A number of other immune cells also participate in the hepatic innate immune response by patrolling sinusoids, including natural killer cells and γδ-T cells.[3]

Activation of Kupffer cells by endotoxin and other signaling molecules is mechanistic to their protective and disease-producing effects. Kupffer cells possess both Fc and C_3 receptors and phagocytize a wide variety of opsonized and nonopsonized particulates.[3] Kupffer cells express complement receptor of the Ig superfamily (CRIg), which is a receptor for C_3. This can directly bind lipoteichoic acid, a pathogen-associated molecular pattern associated with gram-positive bacteria, without the need for complement activation.[3]

Normally, hepatic Kupffer cells efficiently clear endotoxin to attenuate systemic exposure. Endotoxin extraction is enabled by LPS-binding glycoproteins on hepatocytes that facilitate transfer to high-affinity LPS receptors on Kupffer cells. Contact with LPS activates Kupffer cells directly via TLR signaling or indirectly by triggering complement activation. On exposure to endotoxin, activation of Kupffer cells initiates a multitude of signaling pathways resulting in a spectrum of inflammatory responses.[4] However, there is a degree of "endotoxin tolerance" that results from constant, low-level exposure of the liver to endotoxin.[5,6]

Because enteric bile acids bind and inactivate endotoxin, patients with extrahepatic bile duct occlusion or severe intrahepatic cholestasis with impaired enterohepatic bile acid circulation have higher risk for endotoxin translocation.[7] Dogs with induced chronic liver disease associated with intrahepatic portal hypertension and acquired portosystemic shunts develop significantly greater endotoxin concentrations in portal venous, hepatic venous, and caudal vena cava blood, compared to healthy control dogs.[8]

On activation, Kupffer cells release superoxide radicals, hydrogen peroxide, nitric oxide, hydrolytic enzymes, and eicosanoids (prostaglandins and leukotrienes) that can assist in antigen destruction. They also release a large number of immunoregulatory and inflammatory cytokines, including Il-1, Il-6, TNF-α, platelet-activating factor, transforming growth factor-β, and IFN-γ. Kupffer cells associated with zone 1 are larger, more phagocytic, and generate greater amounts of TNF-α, Il-1, prostaglandin E, and lysosomal enzymes. Less-active Kupffer cells are associated with zone 3; these exhibit greater cytotoxic activity to

TABLE 126.1 Infectious Agents Capable of Causing Liver Disease in Dogs and Cats

Organism Type	Example
Viruses	CAdV-1 FCoV (FIP) FCV
Bacteria	Gram-negative Enterobacterales, especially *Escherichia coli* but also *Klebsiella pneumoniae, Serratia marcescens, Enterobacter* spp., *Salmonella* spp. *Pseudomonas aeruginosa, Acinetobacter* spp., and gram-positive cocci, especially *Enterococcus* spp., but also *Staphylococcus* spp., *Streptococcus* spp. Anaerobes, especially *Clostridium* spp. but also *Bacteroides* spp.
	Curved or spiral-shaped bacteria, especially *Campylobacter* spp., possibly *Helicobacter* spp. *Listeria monocytogenes* *Actinomyces* spp. *Nocardia* spp. *Bartonella* spp. (peliosis hepatis) (dogs) *Brucella* spp. *Mycobacterium* spp. (e.g., *M. avium, M. bovis*) *Leptospira* spp. *Neorickettsia helminthoeca* (dogs)
Protozoa	*Neospora caninum* *Toxoplasma gondii* *Cytauxzoon felis* (cats) *Leishmania infantum* (primarily dogs)
Fungi	*Histoplasma* spp. *Cryptococcus neoformans* *Blastomyces* spp. *Coccidioides* spp. *Candida albicans* *Aspergillus* spp. *Prototheca* spp.
Helminths	Migrating ascarids *Platynosomum illiciens* (cats) *Mesocestoides* spp. *Echinococcus* spp.

BOX 126.1 Mechanisms Contributing to Infection of the Hepatobiliary System

Reduced mechanical cleansing of the biliary tree
Impaired biliary IgA production or enteric delivery
Enhanced intestinal bacterial translocation
Impaired Kupffer cell activation and/or microbial phagocytosis
Reduced humoral immune responses
Impaired neutrophil function
Disruption of tight junctions between hepatocytes
Increased access to hepatic lymph as occurs in intrahepatic portal hypertension

some stimuli and are more easily activated. Nitric oxide released by Kupffer cells mediates a wide variety of physiologic events, including vasodilation, neutrophil chemotaxis, and adhesion of neutrophils to vascular endothelium (response to bacteria or endotoxin).[9] As potent inducers of inflammatory cytokines, Kupffer cells are implicated in pathologic events resulting in liver injury.[10] Later, during the course of an infection, other cells including hepatocytes, T lymphocytes, and immigrating phagocytes (monocytes and neutrophils) contribute cytokines to the inflammatory process. Kupffer cells have been shown to be critical in T cell priming in the liver.[3] In addition, sophisticated imaging techniques have shown T cells to populate the liver from secondary lymphoid organs, adhere to platelets, crawl along sinusoids, and interact with liver sinusoidal endothelial cells. When they encounter a pathogen, they secrete IFN-γ to eradicate the infection.[3]

Biliary Epithelial Cells (Cholangiocytes)

Cholangiocytes (biliary epithelial cells) in larger bile ducts express the polymeric IgA receptor (secretory component) that localizes secretory IgA (S-IgA) to the ductal system. Uptake from the basolateral side of the cholangiocyte is followed by transport to the luminal ductal surface, where the secretory component is cleaved from but secreted with S-IgA into bile. Cholangiocytes from larger intrahepatic bile ducts, septal bile ducts, interlobular bile ducts, and bile ductules express TLRs that bind a variety of ligands including bacterial molecules, double-stranded messenger RNA (mRNA), LPS, and flagellin. In the presence of inflammatory cytokines, cholangiocytes also can activate the (proinflammatory) NF-κB pathway. Cholangiocytes also produce the antimicrobial peptides defensin and cathelicidin, part of the innate immune system, that defend the biliary tree against gram-positive and gram-negative bacteria, mycobacteria, fungi, and viruses. Expression of cathelicidin in biliary epithelium is enhanced by exposure to endogenous and therapeutic bile salts (e.g., ursodeoxycholic acid). In biliary inflammation, cholangiocytes also recruit CD4+ T cells as well as immature dendritic cells to provide defense against antigenic and microbial challenge. Cholangiocytes also express a variety of leukocyte and vascular adhesion molecules that can facilitate tissue-specific leukocyte migration, slowing leukocyte circulation near damaged epithelium and trafficking cells to the targeted site of injury. Expression of antigen-presenting molecules on cholangiocytes also may contribute to local immune defense.

Bile

Secretory IgA is the major immunoglobulin in bile; IgG and IgM are present in much smaller quantities. Bile contains approximately twice the concentration of S-IgA as found in the upper intestinal fluid.[11] Bile and IgA each influence the enteric bacterial population (type, number of organisms, and enterocyte adherence). Normal physiologic choleresis mechanically clears the biliary pathways of microbial organisms and particulate debris. This function is thwarted in cholestatic disorders. A normal biliary-enterobacterial cycle permits rapid elimination of bacteria that have entered the biliary system where locally produced IgA prevents epithelial invasion.[12,13] Bile salts also have antibacterial action. In health, tight junctions between hepatocytes (abutting canaliculi) resist bacterial entry into canalicular bile.

Experimental models have helped clarify the physiologic significance of enteric portal bacteremia. Infusion of 10^5 to 10^7 bacteria into the splenic vein of normal adult cats significantly retards bile flow and causes bacterobilia within 30 minutes. However, in the presence of extrahepatic bile duct obstruction, only modest bacterial inocula (10^3) lead to bacterobilia within the same time frame. As bacteria enter sinusoidal blood, some are phagocytized (Kupffer cells and neutrophils) and killed while others remain viable entering bile.[14] Experimental studies confirm that any cause of cholestasis can augment development of bacterobilia, including the cholestasis resulting from endotoxemia. The presence of bacteria within choleliths also can sustain

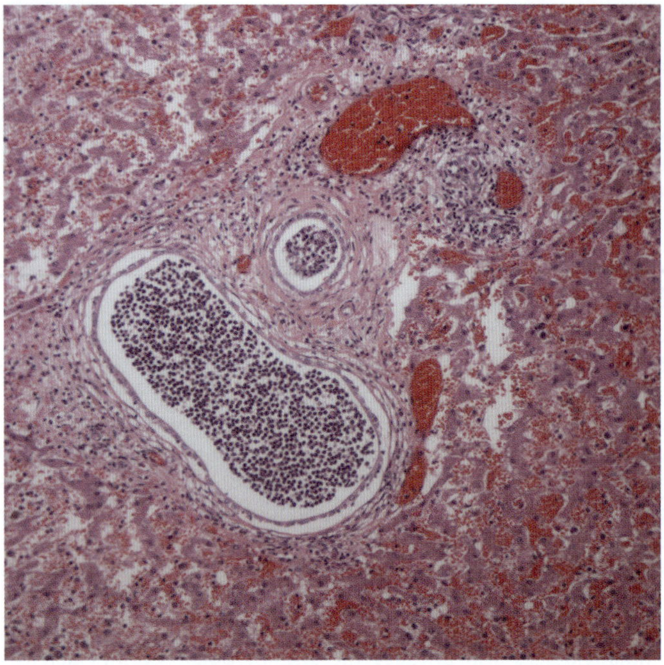

Fig. 126.1 Histopathology showing severe, acute neutrophilic cholangitis in a 20-year-old female spayed domestic shorthair. *Escherichia coli* was isolated from the liver in large numbers at necropsy. Other concurrent diseases found at necropsy were pulmonary adenocarcinoma and moderate multifocal glomerulonephritis.

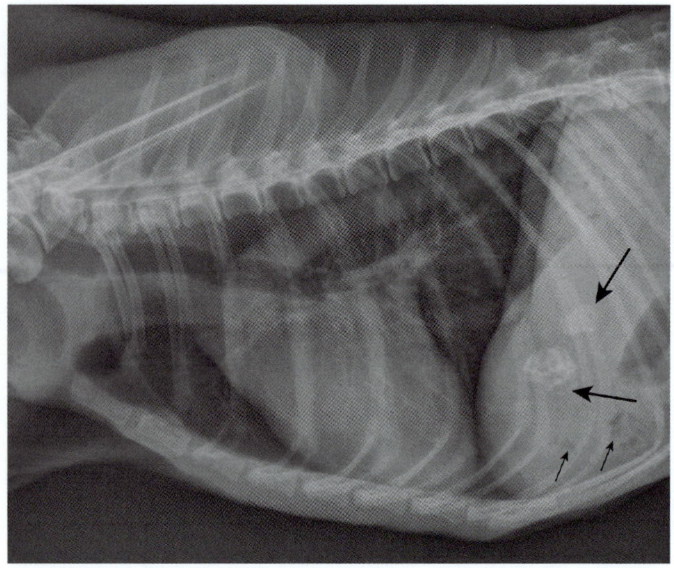

Fig. 126.2 Lateral thoracic radiograph from a 4-year-old male neutered Chihuahua with a 3-month history of vomiting, lethargy, weight loss, and progressive icterus. Within the viewable abdomen, multiple irregular mineral opacities are present in the region of the gall bladder *(large arrows)*. In this region, there are also multiple small irregular gas opacities *(small arrows)*. A diagnosis of necrotizing cholecystitis and secondary bile peritonitis was made based on ultrasound and abdominal fluid analysis. Exploratory laparotomy revealed multiple choleliths, and a cholecystectomy was performed. Histopathology revealed severe, subacute to chronic, transmural suppurative and necrotizing cholecystitis.

bacterial infections in the biliary tree.[15] Enteric organisms in bile may dehydroxylate and deconjugate bile acids, generating membranocytolytic forms that are capable of provoking cholestasis, oxidant cell injury, and cell apoptosis.

Transient or episodic portal bacteremia likely explains the unexpected isolation of bacterial organisms from liver or bile in animals with illnesses thought not to be primarily bacterial in origin, especially if specimens are collected after surgical manipulations of visceral structures. A discussion of bacterial translocation can be found in Chapter 125.

Bacterial infections can lead to suppurative cholangitis/cholangiohepatitis, cholecystitis, choledochitis, and cholelithiasis.[16-23] *Cholangitis* is inflammation of intrahepatic bile ducts, whereas *cholangiohepatitis* is inflammation of the bile ducts that has spread to the adjacent liver parenchyma. The use of the term "cholangitis" (rather than "cholangiohepatitis") has been recommended by the WSAVA Liver Diseases and Pathology Standardization Research Group, because inflammatory disruption of the limiting plate to involve hepatic parenchyma is not a consistent feature and if present, is usually an extension of a primary cholangitis. For these reasons, the term "cholangitis" will be used from this point onwards.

In cats, cholangitis has been classified histologically as *neutrophilic cholangitis, lymphocytic cholangitis*, or *chronic cholangitis associated with liver fluke infestation.*[24] Neutrophilic cholangitis may be further subclassified as acute or chronic depending on the presence of fibrosis, fibroplasia, or bile duct proliferation.[25] Neutrophilic cholangitis is thought to develop as a result of ascending bacterial infection from the GI tract, which may occur secondary to IBD and/or pancreatitis (Fig. 126.1); however, a study evaluating the utility of FISH for the detection of bacteria in feline inflammatory liver disease observed intrahepatic bacteria located predominantly within portal vessels and venous sinusoids, or the hepatic parenchyma near the capsule. This spatial distribution of bacteria within the livers of cats with inflammatory liver disease is inconsistent with an ascending bacterial infection from the GI tract, and more consistent with the translocation of enteric bacteria across the mucosal barrier into the portal circulation.[1] In contrast, bacteria that are localized within the bile ducts are more likely to have ascended secondary to pancreatic and hepatobiliary reflux in the face of intestinal inflammation, pancreatitis, and biliary disease (triaditis) as a consequence of the common entry of the pancreatic and common bile ducts into the intestine. Not all cats with cholangitis have histologic evidence of associated pancreatitis or IBD; studies have indicated that the prevalence of triaditis in cats with cholangitis is 32 to 50%.[26] Cats with acute cholangitis tend to be younger than those with chronic cholangitis.[25,27] Retrovirus infection does not appear to be a predisposing factor. The cause of lymphocytic cholangitis is unclear, although it is thought to be an immune-mediated condition.[28] Chronic cholangitis associated with liver fluke infestation is rare and is primarily reported from regions with subtropical climates such as the southeastern United States and Hawaii, but disease can occur in nonendemic areas in traveled cats. Although several different fluke species may be involved, the most prevalent appears to be *Platynosomum illiciens* (see Chapter 118).[29]

Choledochitis is inflammation of the common bile duct, whereas *cholecystitis* is inflammation of the gall bladder, and may or may not be associated with cholangitis or choledochitis. In some instances, necrotizing and/or emphysematous cholecystitis can occur, which may lead to perforation of the gall bladder wall and septic bile peritonitis. *Cholelithiasis* is stone formation within the biliary tree. In some instances, cholelithiasis or neoplasia of the biliary tree may predispose to cholangitis and necrotizing cholecystitis (Fig. 126.2).[20,21] Alternatively, it has been suggested that bacterial cholecystitis may predispose to stone formation through bacterial deconjugation of soluble bilirubin glucuronide to insoluble unconjugated bilirubin and glucuronic acid.[19]

Culture of bile is more sensitive than culture of liver parenchyma in both dogs and cats with hepatobiliary disease. In one large study, approximately 30% of biliary cultures were positive in dogs and cats, whereas hepatic cultures were positive in 14% of cats and 5% of dogs.[23] In cats, more than 80% of biliary cultures yielded a single bacterial species, whereas multiple bacterial species were isolated from approximately 50% of dogs. Bacterial species isolated from cats include anaerobes, a variety of Enterobacterales, *Enterococcus*, *Streptococcus*, or *Staphylococcus* species.[1,16,23,25] Dogs are most commonly infected with *E. coli*, *Enterococcus* spp., and/or anaerobes, primarily *Bacteroides* and *Clostridium* species.[17-21,23,30-32] *Staphylococcus* spp., other gram-negative aerobes (*Klebsiella, Enterobacter, Citrobacter,* and *Pseudomonas aeruginosa*), and *Streptococcus* spp. may also be isolated from dogs, and *Helicobacter* spp. have also been implicated as a cause of chronic hepatitis in dogs and possibly cats (see Chapter 66).[24,33] *Salmonella* in cats and *Campylobacter* in dogs may also cause cholecystitis. Although rare, emphysematous cholecystitis in dogs and cats is usually caused by *Clostridium* spp. or *E. coli*.[34]

CLINICAL FEATURES

Clinical Signs and Physical Examination Abnormalities

The most common clinical signs of hepatobiliary infection in both dogs and cats are lethargy, inappetence, vomiting, weight loss, and diarrhea, although subclinical infections can also occur.[16,17,22,25,27,30,35] Signs may be chronic, acute, and rarely peracute.[17,36] Peracute disease can occur with necrotizing cholecystitis and rupture of the gall bladder wall, and may be associated with clinical signs of septic shock. Hypersalivation may be evident in cats with neutrophilic cholangitis.[16] Physical examination may reveal fever, lethargy, dehydration, icterus, and thin body condition, with or without pain on palpation of the abdomen. Hepatomegaly may also be identified.[25] Some animals may be tachycardic or tachypneic.

DIAGNOSIS

Laboratory Abnormalities

Complete Blood Count

The CBC may show leukocytosis due to a neutrophilia, increased numbers of band neutrophils, and occasionally monocytosis.[16-18,22,25,27,36] Cats with neutrophilic cholangitis have higher segmented and band neutrophil counts compared to cats with lymphocytic cholangitis.[24] Some cats with neutrophilic cholangitis may be leukopenic with or without a left shift.[16,25] Lymphopenia and/or anemia may also be present.

Serum Biochemical Tests

Dogs with cholangitis or cholecystitis typically have increased activities of ALT, ALP, and gamma-glutamyl transferase (GGT), and hyperbilirubinemia.[30,31] At least 50% of cats with cholangitis have mild to moderate increases in the activity of ALT and/or ALP (usually < 1000 U/L). Increased activity of GGT is usually documented; however, some cats with cholangitis may have normal ALT, ALP, and GGT activity.[25] Hyperbilirubinemia is present in approximately two-thirds of cats. Along with higher neutrophil counts, cats with neutrophilic cholangitis have higher activities of ALT and higher total bilirubin concentration than cats with lymphocytic cholangitis.[24] Electrolyte abnormalities may be present secondary to GI losses in animals with vomiting or diarrhea.[16,27] Hypocholesterolemia, hyperglobulinemia, and hypoalbuminemia are uncommonly identified. Hypercholesterolemia may be present in dogs with cholestasis or bile duct obstruction, but is uncommonly present in cats.[18,20,22] Despite the differences observed in hematological and biochemical parameters in cats with neutrophilic versus lymphocytic forms of cholangitis, there is tremendous overlap in laboratory findings between the two forms of cholangitis, and caution should be heeded in relying upon the laboratory results to differentiate these forms of cholangitis.

Urinalysis

Urinalysis may be unremarkable or show evidence of bilirubinuria.[16,18,37]

Coagulation Profile

Coagulation abnormalities such as prolongations of PT and PTT may be present in dogs and cats with hepatobiliary infections, either secondary to impaired absorption of vitamin K secondary to biliary obstruction, or potentially as a result of liver dysfunction.[17,27]

Diagnostic Imaging

Plain Radiography

The most common finding on abdominal radiography of dogs and cats with cholecystitis and cholangitis is hepatomegaly, which may be variable.[22,27] Uncommonly, single or multiple radiopaque choleliths are visible, although choleliths may also be radiolucent (see Fig. 126.2).[18-20,35] Linear mineralization of the biliary tree has been described in some animals with cholelithiasis,[35] whereas other animals may reveal no abnormalities. Emphysematous cholecystitis is characterized by the presence of gas in the liver in the region of the gall bladder. Loss of abdominal detail may be present if gall bladder rupture and septic bile peritonitis has occurred.[17]

Sonographic Findings

Ultrasound examination provides important information and can influence decision-making in animals with cholangitis.[31] Findings on ultrasound in dogs and cats with cholangitis are similar and include hepatomegaly, normal or abnormal hepatic echotexture with a homogenous or heterogenous increase in echogenicity, prominent portal vasculature, ascites, a thickened and hyperechogenic gall bladder wall, and sediment within the gall bladder.[16-18,22,24,25,31,38,39] The gall bladder wall may also appear irregular and contain polypoid mass lesions. Abdominal pain in the right cranial quadrant may be evident during the procedure. Choleliths may occasionally be identified within the biliary tract as hyperechoic masses or linear structures with acoustic shadowing.[35] Distention of the biliary tract may be evident, sometimes with tortuosity of the cystic and common bile duct (Fig. 126.3).[16,17,38] Concurrent evidence of pancreatic and/or intestinal wall disease may be present in cats.[25] Ultrasound cannot be used to differentiate neutrophilic from lymphocytic cholangitis in cats. Intramural gas may be identified in animals with emphysematous cholecystitis (Fig. 126.4). Rupture of the gall bladder may also be detected using ultrasound, which is an indication for emergency surgery.[31] However, one study of 219 dogs with gall bladder mucoceles suggested that the sensitivity of abdominal ultrasound for detection of gall bladder rupture was low, only 56% (95% CI, 40–71%), whereas the specificity was 92% (95% CI, 85–96%).[40]

Microbiologic Tests

Cytologic Examination

Cytologic examination of bile collected by percutaneous ultrasound-guided cholecystocentesis (or intraoperative cholecystocentesis) may reveal increased numbers of degenerate neutrophils, small and/or large

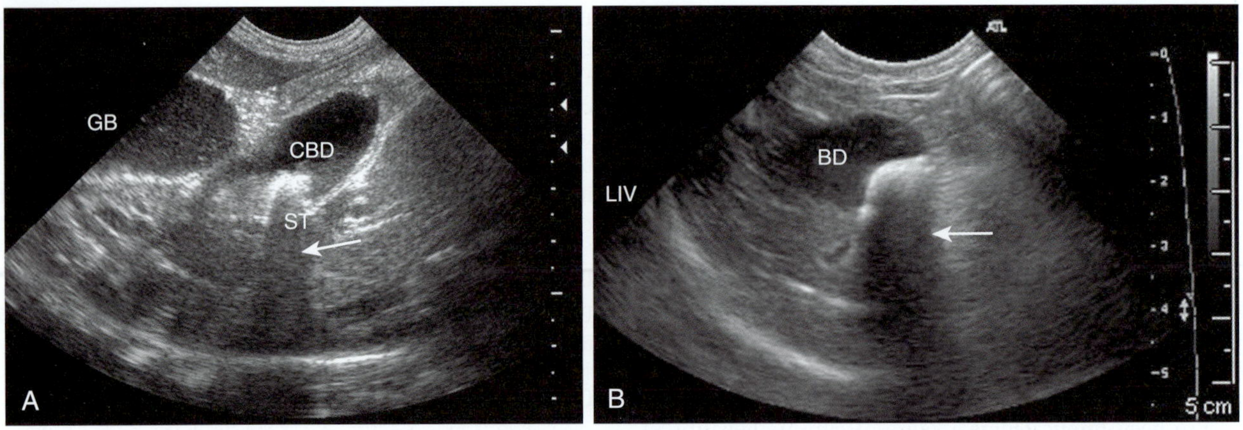

Fig. 126.3 (A) Ultrasonographic image showing a mineralized cholelith with acoustic shadowing *(arrow)* in a cat with neutrophilic cholangitis (*CBD*, distended common bile duct; *GB*, gall bladder; *ST*, stone). (B) Ultrasonographic image showing mineralized choleliths with acoustic shadowing *(arrow)* in a cat with neutrophilic cholangitis; a distended intrahepatic bile duct *(BD)* is observed to the left of the acoustic shadow. Choleliths may have led to septic inflammation or formed subsequent to infection. A cholecystectomy was performed to remove the stones, and, with antimicrobial therapy, complete recovery was achieved.

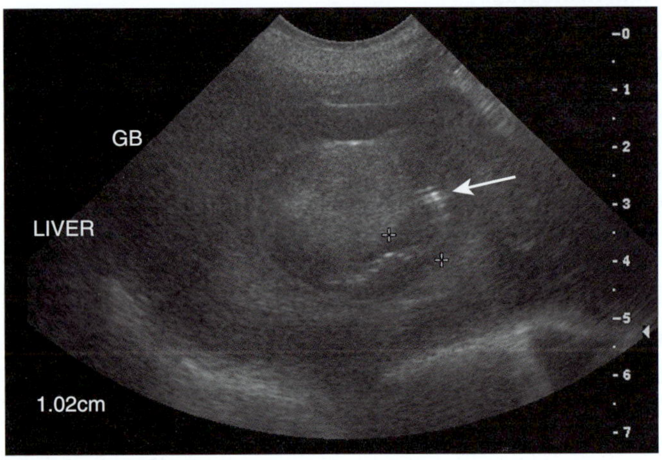

Fig. 126.4 Abdominal ultrasound image of the gall bladder of a 6-year-old female spayed American Eskimo dog with emphysematous cholecystitis. The gall bladder (*GB*) wall is markedly thickened (1 cm), is diffusely hypoechoic, and the gall bladder contains homogenous sludge. Multiple hyperechoic foci were identified tracking throughout the wall *(arrow)*. The hepatic parenchyma immediately adjacent to the gall bladder was poorly characterized because of a large amount of markedly hyperechoic inflamed mesentery within the cranial abdominal region.

mononuclear cells, and in some cases, a mixed or monomorphic bacterial population.[16,30] Identification of multilobular nuclear remnants, representing degenerate neutrophils, may be the only evidence of an inflammatory response owing to the detergent effects of bile on cell membranes. Thus, in biliary sepsis, bacterial organisms are commonly observed in biliary debris, with or without a well-defined exudative response. Examination of only the liquid partition of bile may fail to disclose bacterial organisms readily identified in the heavier biliary sediment. Thus, cholecystocentesis performed with the objective of identifying bacterobilia should include sampling of both nonparticulate and sediment portions. Standard protocol consists of introducing a 22-G needle (attached to an extension set, three-way stopcock, and 10-mL syringe) through the ventral or ventrolateral portion of the liver into the gall bladder. Cats and dogs are either heavily sedated or placed under general anesthesia for the procedure. Sampling should be done to completely empty the gall bladder to minimize postcentesis bile leakage and to optimize collection of dependent sediment. It is possible that percutaneous drainage of infected bile may also have a therapeutic benefit, although this requires further study.

Culture

Aerobic and anaerobic bacterial culture should be performed on bile collected by ultrasound-guided or intraoperative cholecystocentesis or liver biopsies. An approximately 22% isolation frequency of fastidious anaerobes among isolated bacteria from cats justifies submission of specimens for anaerobic culture.[41] Bile is more likely to yield positive results; however, bacteria are best retrieved from bile in which the gall bladder has been nearly completely emptied (3–5 mL in cats). The sensitivity of culture was also improved by combining tissue, bile, and crushed choleliths for inoculation.[41,30] Although it is generally accepted that bile is sterile in healthy dogs and cats,[2,42] transient cytologic and microbiologic evidence of bactibilia has been identified in healthy dogs.[43] Liver tissue from healthy dogs and cats can also harbor a variety of enteric bacterial species.[1,44] Thus, the results of bile culture should be interpreted in light of clinical and cytologic findings. Antibiotic resistance among bacteria isolated from the bile of dogs and cats with cholecystitis and cholangitis has been described in several studies, and so culture and susceptibility testing is suggested whenever possible.[23,31] When cholecystocentesis is undesirable because of concerns for gall bladder rupture (see Cytological Examination), blood cultures may be useful, although the utility of blood culture in dogs and cats with cholecystitis has not been studied. In human patients, bile cultures are positive in 50 to 95% of patients with acute cholecystitis, and blood cultures are positive in 30 to 40% of patients.[45]

Pathologic Findings

Neutrophilic cholangitis in cats varies considerably on histopathology in severity, chronicity, and the extent of associated hepatic parenchymal involvement.[25,37] FISH has been used to identify bacteria within the hepatobiliary system in cats; bacteria were more likely to be identified in portal vessels, venous sinusoids, and parenchyma (12 of 13 cats) than the bile duct (1 of 13 cats).[1] Concurrent hepatic lipidosis may also be present. In a small percentage of affected cats, complete or partial biliary obstruction may be identified as a result of inflammation, neoplasia, or cholelithiasis. Other findings in affected cats include acute or chronic pancreatitis (65% of cats in one study), and/or inflammatory bowel disease or intestinal lymphoma (46% of cats).[25,26] Histopathology of the gall bladder wall in both dogs and cats with cholecystitis may reveal mucosal and glandular hyperplasia, and thickening and neutrophilic or lymphoplasmacytic inflammation of the gall bladder wall.[18,22,25]

Choleliths in cats are most often composed of calcium carbonate, although they also may comprise a mixture of cholesterol, calcium bilirubinate, and calcium carbonate.[18,20] In dogs they are often composed of calcium bilirubinate, bilirubin, or a mixture of bilirubin and cholesterol. Aged female small-breed dogs (dachshunds, poodles, miniature schnauzers) were predisposed to cholelithiasis in one study.[19]

TREATMENT

Treatment of cholangitis and cholecystitis typically consists of supportive care and antibiotic administration. Dogs and cats with necrotizing or emphysematous cholecystitis require cholecystectomy. Cholecystectomy could also be considered to prevent recurrence of cholelithiasis in animals with chronic cholecystitis. Cholecystectomy, biliary stenting procedures, and/or biliary diversion surgery may be required for animals with obstructive processes such as cholelithiasis, biliary neoplasia, or obstructive cholangitis.[19,20] Because cholecystotomy or biliary diversion surgery often results in dehiscence and septic bile peritonitis if bacterial cholecystitis or choledochitis is present, cholecystectomy has been recommended for dogs with cholelithiasis as opposed to cholecystotomy.[19] When compared with other surgical biliary procedures, cholecystectomy has been associated with good clinical outcomes in dogs and cats, but any condition that requires biliary surgery carries a guarded prognosis.

Antimicrobial Drug Treatment and Supportive Care

Empirically administered antibiotics should target gram-negative enteric bacterial species, *Enterococcus* spp., and anaerobes and be concentrated in bile. Cytologic examination of bile was shown to correlate well with culture results in one study and can be used to guide initial therapy.[46] Suitable antibiotics include ampicillin-sulbactam or clavulanic acid-amoxicillin, or a fluoroquinolone with metronidazole, although resistance to clavulanic acid-amoxicillin or enrofloxacin has been documented among biliary isolates from dogs and cats.[22] Based on the results of cultures from 248 dogs and cats evaluated for hepatobiliary disease, it was concluded that broad-spectrum empirical coverage could be achieved with a combination of a fluoroquinolone, penicillin, and metronidazole (reduce dose by 50% in cats with hepatobiliary disease), or a fluoroquinolone combined with clavulanic acid-amoxicillin or clindamycin.[23] Again, because resistance can occur, culture and antimicrobial susceptibility results should then be used to adjust treatment. In human patients, specific treatment of *Enterococcus* spp. biliary infections may not be necessary when other concurrent bacterial infections are being managed, as the *Enterococcus* spp. infection tends to resolve when the other infections are treated.[45] Supportive treatments that should be considered include IV crystalloid fluids with or without colloids, glucose supplementation, antiemetics (e.g., maropitant, ondansetron), nutritional support by parenteral or enteral means (with a restricted fat diet), ursodiol, S-adenosylmethionine, and parenteral vitamin K supplementation.

PROGNOSIS

The prognosis for cats with neutrophilic cholangitis is fair to good, with mean survival times greater than 1 year.[16,27] Poor outcomes may be related to the presence of underlying disease that contributes to mortality such as neoplasia.[20,27] Among 168 cats with suppurative cholangitis-cholangiohepatitis syndrome, infection (as identified by IHC), and the presence of gram-positive bacteria by culture in conjunction with positive IHC, were associated with a significantly shorter long-term survival time of 283 days following diagnosis.[41] The presence of septic bile peritonitis was associated with mortality in one study of dogs that underwent extrahepatic biliary surgery; over 50% of dogs with septic bile peritonitis died.[21] In another study, 9 of 23 dogs with necrotizing cholecystitis died.[17]

HEPATIC ABSCESSES

Hepatic abscesses are uncommon in dogs and very rare in cats.[47,48] They may be associated with ascending bacterial infection of the biliary tree, translocation of portal bacteria, or hematogenous spread of bacteria to the liver, although the source of bacteremia in some animals is unclear. Because bacteria can be found in the liver of healthy dogs, abscessation may also develop when these bacteria proliferate secondary to compromise of normal defenses (such as hepatic necrosis).[44] Affected animals are typically middle aged to older,[47,48] and the mean age of affected dogs or cats is 10 years. The abscesses may be acute or chronic, single or multiple, and macroabscesses or microabscesses may form. Pancreatitis, diabetes mellitus, other hepatobiliary diseases, neoplasia, colonic surgery, cholelithiasis, or chronic phenobarbital or glucocorticoid administration have been involved in the histories of affected dogs.[48–50] Migrating plant awn foreign bodies may also be an underlying cause.[50] Concurrent conditions reported in cats have included IBD, pancreatitis, hepatobiliary neoplasia, chronic cholecystitis, colonic surgery, or congestive heart failure.[47] Many affected cats have concurrent bacteriuria.

The most common bacterial species isolated from hepatic abscesses in both dogs and cats is *E. coli*. In dogs, other species have included *Klebsiella pneumoniae*, *Staphylococcus*, and *Clostridium* species. In cats, *Bacteroides*, *Enterococcus*, and *Streptococcus* spp. have been isolated, often in mixed infections with *E. coli*. Blood cultures are also often positive.[47,48] Clinical signs and laboratory abnormalities are similar to those for other hepatobiliary infections, except that severe illness and signs of septic shock are often present. Evidence of bleeding diatheses may be present. Marked neutrophilia or neutropenia, bandemia, toxic neutrophils, anemia, lymphopenia, and thrombocytopenia may be present on the CBC. Hypoalbuminemia and coagulation abnormalities are common.[47,48] Abdominal radiographs may be unremarkable or they may show hepatomegaly or a hepatic mass effect, poor abdominal serosal detail, and/or pneumoperitoneum if abscess rupture has occurred (Fig. 126.5). Thoracic radiography often reveals interstitial, bronchiolar, or alveolar lung infiltrates,[47,48] which may result from associated embolic or aspiration pneumonia. Ultrasonographic examination of the abdomen reveals one or more hypoechoic, anechoic, or heteroechoic hepatic masses, with or without peritoneal effusion. In some cases, gas may be evident within the masses (see Fig. 126.5).

Antemortem diagnosis usually relies on cytologic examination of ultrasound-guided fine-needle aspirates of these masses, which reveals large numbers of degenerate neutrophils. Abscesses may also be discovered during exploratory laparotomy (e.g., in dogs and cats with bacterial peritonitis). Culture and susceptibility of aspirates of the liver abscesses, free peritoneal fluid, and/or blood should be performed. Effective treatment of solitary abscesses relies on appropriate antimicrobial drug treatment together with complete or partial liver lobectomy, or abscess drainage and omentalization. With the exception of microabscesses, antimicrobial drug therapy alone is often ineffective. Aggressive supportive care in an intensive care unit may be required. Initial antimicrobial drug treatment should be broad spectrum, after which it should be adjusted based on the results of culture and susceptibility testing. Mortality rates of 79% and 50% have been reported for cats and dogs, respectively.[47] The prognosis appears to be especially poor when multiple hepatic abscesses are present.[47,48]

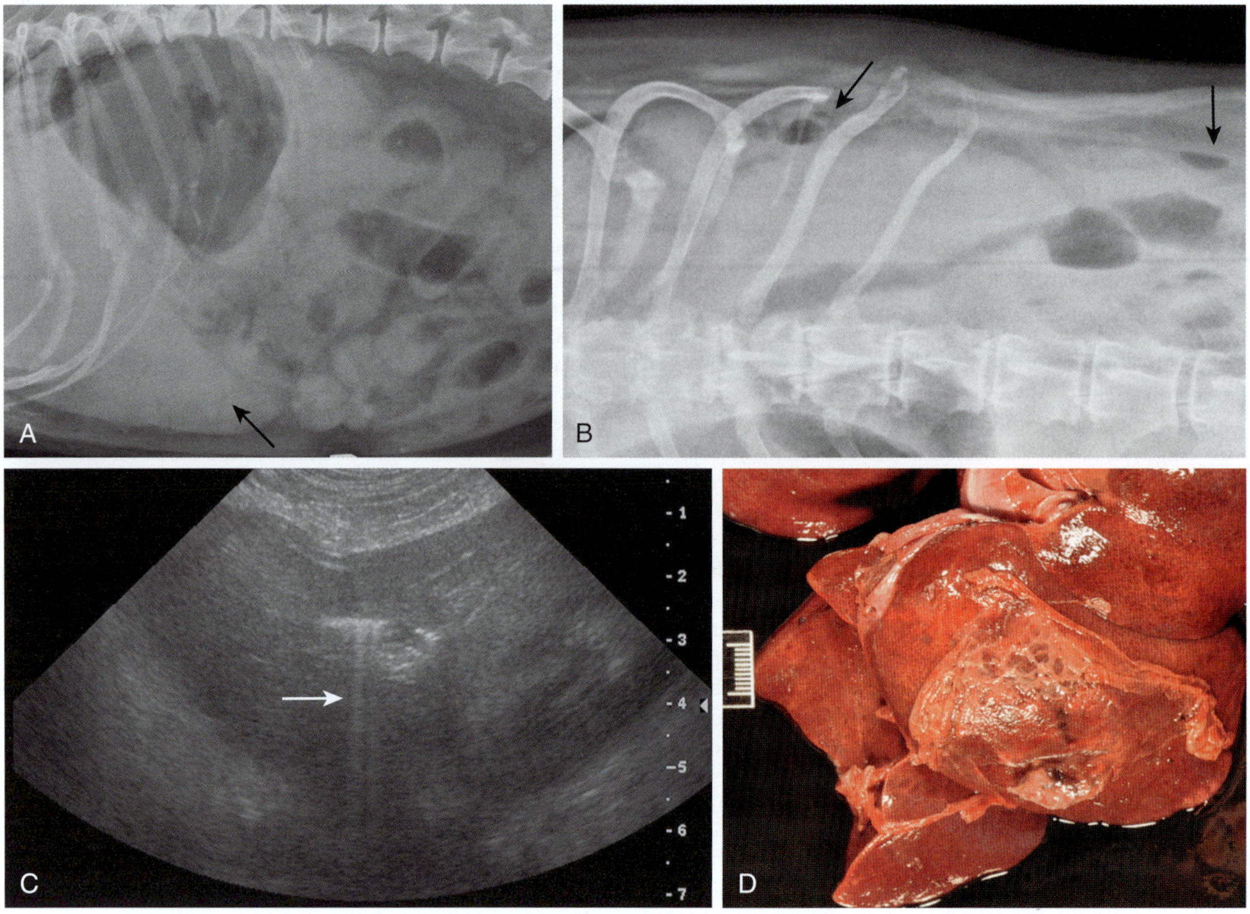

Fig. 126.5 Ruptured hepatic abscess. (A) Right lateral abdominal radiograph from a 15-year-old male neutered dachshund with acute onset of vomiting and diarrhea secondary to a ruptured hepatic abscess. There is a diffuse loss of serosal detail as well as free peritoneal gas present throughout the abdomen. The liver is enlarged. There are multiple small rounded gas opacities present over the ventral and right aspects of the liver *(arrow)*. Multiple small intestinal loops contain gas and fluid, some of which measure at the upper limits or over the upper limit of normal. (B) Free peritoneal air can be seen clearly *(arrows)* using a horizontal beam view. (C) Comet-tail artifact *(arrow)* due to the presence of gas within the liver on ultrasound examination. (D) Hepatic abscess from the same dog at necropsy.

CASE EXAMPLE

Signalment

"George," a 16-year-old male neutered domestic shorthair from northern California.

History

George was evaluated for a 2-day history of vomiting and progressive lethargy and inappetence. The owners reported that the vomiting occurred six times at the onset of illness and was associated with apparent abdominal pain, but had since resolved. The day he became ill, he was seen at an emergency clinic where a CBC showed only a mild left shift (479 band neutrophils), a chemistry panel showed mild hypokalemia (3.1 mmol/L, reference range 3.6–4.9 mmol/L), and a total serum T4 concentration was markedly increased (10.2 μg/dL, reference range, 1.1–3.3 μg/dL). Recurrent pancreatitis and hyperthyroidism were initially suspected and George was treated with subcutaneous lactated Ringer's solution (200 mL, SC, q24h), mucosal buprenorphine (0.2 mg/kg, PO, q8h to q12h), and ondansetron (0.2 mg/kg, PO, q12h). However, because George became inappetent and lethargic, he was returned for re-evaluation the following day.

Other past pertinent medical history: George had been diagnosed with pancreatitis 8 months previously. He was also diagnosed with a biliary cystadenoma via ultrasound at that time. He had been hospitalized for 9 days and treated with jejunostomy tube feeding. Since then, he had been well until this recent onset of illness.

Physical Examination

Body weight: 6.1 kg.

General: Quiet, alert, hydrated. T = 103.8°F (39.9°C), pulse = 240 beats/min, respiratory rate = 32, mucous membranes pink and moist, capillary refill time 1 s.

Eyes, ears, nose, and throat: Palpable thyroid nodule.

Integument: Full, clean haircoat.

Musculoskeletal: Body condition score 5/9. Ambulatory with normal gait.

Cardiovascular: Gallop sound with no murmurs or arrhythmias auscultated. Femoral pulses strong and synchronous.

Respiratory: Eupneic with soft breath sounds in all lung fields.

Genitourinary/GI: Soft, mildly painful abdomen. The bladder was small.

Other systems, including peripheral lymph nodes: No clinically significant findings.

Continued

CASE EXAMPLE—cont'd

Imaging Findings

Abdominal ultrasound: The margins of the kidneys were irregular and there was decreased corticomedullary distinction. In the region of the left limb of the pancreas, the mesentery was markedly hyperechoic and hyperattenuating. There was diffuse thickening of the muscularis layer of the small bowel. There was no evidence of mesenteric lymphadenomegaly. There was a small amount of free anechoic peritoneal fluid.

Thoracic radiographs: The cardiac silhouette appeared mildly enlarged. There was a mild bronchointerstitial pattern throughout the thorax. There was poor serosal detail within the viewable, cranial abdomen.

Outcome

George was treated supportively for pancreatitis with IV fluids (lactated Ringer's solution, 20 mmol/LKCl at 15 mL/h), buprenorphine (0.06 mg, IV, q6h), famotidine (0.5 mg/kg, IV, q12h), and ondansetron (0.5 mg/kg, IV, q12h). His temperature normalized, but he showed no interest in food or his surroundings. Cytologic examination of an ultrasound-guided liver aspirate on day 2 of hospitalization showed moderate vacuolated hepatocytes and mild mixed inflammation. Laboratory testing was re-evaluated, and an echocardiogram was performed on the third day of hospitalization in preparation for anesthesia and placement of an esophageal feeding tube. The echocardiogram was unremarkable and the gallop sound was suspected to result from a systolic click. New findings on the CBC were mild, nonregenerative normocytic, normochromic anemia (HCT 29.9%, RR, 30–50%), with a WBC of 11,580 cells/μL (4,500–14,000 cells/μL), 4053 neutrophils/μL (2,000–9,000 cells/μL), bandemia (3,242 cells/μL) without evidence of toxicity, and circulating metamyelocytes (232 cells/μL). Findings on the serum biochemistry panel included a bicarbonate of 24 mmol/L (15–21 mmol/L), calcium of 8.3 mg/dL (9.0–10.9 mg/dl), BUN of 20 mg/dL (18–33 mg/dL), creatinine of 0.8 mg/dL (1.1–2.2 mg/dL), glucose of 114 mg/dL (63–118 mg/dL), total protein of 5.3 g/dL (6.6–8.4 g/dL), albumin of 2.0 g/dL (2.2–4.6 g/dL), globulin of 3.3 g/dL (2.8–5.4 g/dL), ALT of 57 U/L (27–101 U/L), AST of 46 U/L (17–58 U/L), ALP of 26 U/L (14–71 U/L), GGT of < 3 U/L (0–4 U/L), cholesterol of 109 mg/dL (89–258 mg/dL), and total bilirubin of 0.4 mg/dL (0–0.2 mg/dL). Urinalysis showed a specific gravity of 1.015; pH 7.0, protein 25 mg/dL, no bilirubin, 25 erythrocytes/μL hemoprotein, 1–3 WBC/HPF, 1–6 RBC/HPF, and many lipid droplets. Serum vitamin B12 and folate concentrations were 383 ng/L (279–1254 ng/L) and 7.5 ng/mL (10.4–20.7 ng/mL), respectively.

Because of the severely left-shifted neutrophil count, bacterial cholecystitis was suspected. Findings on abdominal ultrasonography were unchanged from the previous examination. Ultrasound-guided cholecystocentesis was performed while George was under anesthesia for esophagostomy tube placement, and a small volume of the scant ascites was also collected.

Microbiologic Testing

Cytologic examination (bile): Smears had light blue backgrounds and contained a moderate amount of unidentified material. Nucleated cells were not found, but there were many short, plump coccobacilli observed. Most of the bacteria were in large clusters, but a few groups were in chains. During detailed evaluation, no inflammatory cells were recognized. Interpretation: possible severe sepsis.

Peritoneal fluid analysis: Grossly the fluid was pink and cloudy, and it had a yellow, clear supernatant. The total protein concentration was 2.8 g/dL and there were 100,000 RBC/μL. There were 5,380 nucleated cells/μL, with 70% nondegenerate neutrophils, 6% small and well-differentiated lymphocytes, 7% foamy macrophages, and 17% eosinophils. No infectious agents were identified.

Aerobic and anaerobic bacterial culture (bile): Large numbers of *Enterococcus faecium*. No anaerobes were cultured. The isolate was susceptible to clavulanic acid-amoxicillin (≤ 4 μg/mL), ampicillin (≤ 0.25 μg/mL), penicillin (0.12 μg/mL), chloramphenicol (≤ 4 μg/mL), doxycycline (≤ 2 μg/mL), and imipenem (≤ 1 μg/mL); had intermediate susceptibility to erythromycin (1 μg/mL); and was resistant to rifampin (> 2 μg/mL).

Aerobic and anaerobic bacterial culture (ascites): Very small numbers of *Enterococcus faecium*. The antibiogram was identical to the isolate from the bile.

Diagnosis

Bacterial cholecystitis and peritonitis caused by *E. faecium*; pancreatitis and secondary hepatic lipidosis. Hyperthyroidism. A concurrent chronic enteropathy was also likely present in light of the ultrasound changes (thickened muscularis layer) with concurrent hypocobalaminemia and hypofolatemia.

Treatment

Medical treatment with ampicillin-sulbactam (30 mg/kg, IV, q8h) and enrofloxacin (5 mg/kg, IV, q24h) was commenced on day 3 of hospitalization, before the results of culture and susceptibility were available. Treatment was also continued with IV fluids, buprenorphine, omeprazole, ondansetron, and nutritional support via the esophagostomy feeding tube with a slurry of a commercially available gastroenteric diet (Purina ProPlan Veterinary Diets EN Gastroenteric Feline Formula, q4h). Surgery was considered, but because George was medically stable, a decision was made to continue medical treatment with close observation and serial CBC and abdominal ultrasound examinations. Within 12 hours of antibiotic treatment, George was brighter. A repeat abdominal ultrasound showed no changes with the exception of mildly enlarged and hypoechoic mesenteric lymph nodes. The CBC showed persistent nonregenerative anemia (HCT of 26.4%), 10,181 moderately toxic neutrophils/μL, 5,553 bands/μL, 185 metamyelocytes/μL, and a normal platelet count (305,000/μL). On day 5 of hospitalization, abdominal ultrasonography showed a decrease in the amount of ascites. The enrofloxacin was discontinued when the results of culture and susceptibility became available. On day 6, the CBC showed a stable HCT, 9,366 moderately toxic neutrophils/μL, 2,810 bands/μL, and no metamyelocytes. A serum chemistry panel was unremarkable and the total bilirubin had decreased to 0.1 mg/dL. On day 8, George began eating a small amount of food on his own and the CBC showed further improvement with 6,048 neutrophils/μL with no evidence of toxicity, 336 bands/μL, and a mild monocytosis (896 cells/ μL). He was discharged from hospital the following day with instructions to continue tube feeding, ondansetron (0.3 mg/kg, PO, q24h), omeprazole (1 mg/kg, PO, q12h), and amoxicillin-clavulanic acid (15 mg/kg, PO, q12h). At a recheck 1 week later, the owner reported that George had been doing well at home, although he had vomited three times over the course of the week. Physical examination was unremarkable, apart from the thyroid nodule and evidence of mild weight loss (body weight, 5.6 kg compared with 5.9 kg at discharge). A CBC showed a HCT of 30%, 10,592 neutrophils/μL, and 132 bands/μL. A serum chemistry panel was within normal limits and the total T4 concentration was 8.2 μg/dL. Treatment with methimazole (1.25 mg q12h) was initiated for the hyperthyroidism, but because of continued vomiting, this was discontinued after three doses. George's demeanor and appetite continued to improve. A week later he was eating canned and dry food on his own with no vomiting, a CBC showed no abnormalities, and the antibiotics were discontinued. The esophagostomy feeding tube was removed 3 weeks later, and methimazole was reinstituted, after which his T4 normalized. George was still doing well at follow-up 6 months later.

Comments

In this cat, cholecystitis and bacterial peritonitis were diagnosed based on cytologic and microbiologic analysis of bile and peritoneal fluid. However, there were no ultrasonographic abnormalities within the biliary tract, and cytologic evidence of infection in the peritoneal fluid was absent. Pancreatitis or an underlying chronic enteropathy may have predisposed the cat to ascending infection of the biliary tract, or infection may have occurred secondary to bacterial translocation. The lack of an inflammatory reaction in the bile was unusual, but it may have resulted from marked neutrophil disruption in a toxic environment. Isolation of the same bacterial organism from both the bile and the peritoneal fluid and the rapid clinical response to antibiotic treatment suggested that *Enterococcus* played a role in disease in this cat, although the clinical signs and hematologic abnormalities may also have resulted from severe pancreatitis and suspected hepatic lipidosis. Surgery was postponed because the peritonitis appeared to be very mild, and there was a concern that it could exacerbate the pancreatitis. Fortunately, the cat made a complete recovery.

SUGGESTED READINGS

Callahan Clark JE, Haddad JL, Brown DC, et al. Feline cholangitis: a necropsy study of 44 cats (1986-2008). *J Feline Med Surg.* 2011;13:570–576.

Center SA, Randolph JF, Warner KL, et al. Bacterial culture and immunohistochemical detection of bacteria and endotoxin in cats with suppurative cholangitis-cholangiohepatitis syndrome. *J Am Vet Med Assoc.* 2022;260:194–211.

Li P, He K, Li J, et al. The role of Kupffer cells in hepatic diseases. *Mol Immunol.* 2017;85:222–229.

Simpson KW. Pancreatitis and triaditis in cats: causes and treatment. *J Small Anim Pract.* 2015;56:40–49.

Tamborini A, Jahns H, McAllister H, et al. Bacterial cholangitis, cholecystitis, or both in dogs. *J Vet Intern Med.* 2016;30:1046–1055.

REFERENCES

1. Twedt DC, Cullen J, McCord K, et al. Evaluation of fluorescence in situ hybridization for the detection of bacteria in feline inflammatory liver disease. *J Feline Med Surg.* 2014;16:109–117.
2. O'Neill EJ. Bacterial cholangitis in the dog. In: *Proceedings of the 21st ECVIM-CA Congress*; 2011.
3. Li L, Zeng Z. Live imaging of innate and adaptive immune responses in the liver. *Front Immunol.* 2020;11:564768.
4. Bilzer M, Roggel F, Gerbes AL. Role of Kupffer cells in host defense and liver disease. *Liver Int.* 2006;26:1175–1186.
5. Li P, He K, Li J, et al. The role of Kupffer cells in hepatic diseases. *Mol Immunol.* 2017;85:222–229.
6. Heymann F, Tacke F. Immunology in the liver: from homeostasis to disease. *Nat Rev Gastroenterol Hepatol.* 2016;13:88–110.
7. Scott-Conner CE, Grogan JB. The pathophysiology of biliary obstruction and its effect on phagocytic and immune function. *J Surg Res.* 1994;57:316–336.
8. Howe LM, Boothe DM, Boothe HW. Endotoxemia associated with experimentally induced multiple portosystemic shunts in dogs. *Am J Vet Res.* 1997;58:83–88.
9. Geier A, Fickert P, Trauner M. Mechanisms of disease: mechanisms and clinical implications of cholestasis in sepsis. *Nat Clin Pract Gastroenterol Hepatol.* 2006;3:574–585.
10. Su GL. Lipopolysaccharides in liver injury: molecular mechanisms of Kupffer cell activation. *Am J Physiol Gastrointest Liver Physiol.* 2002;283:G256–G265.
11. Chuang YH, Lan RY, Gershwin ME. The immunopathology of human biliary cell epithelium. *Semin Immunopathol.* 2009;31:323–331.
12. Scott AJ, Khan GA. Origin of bacteria in bile duct bile. *Lancet.* 1967;2:790–792.
13. Cardoso V, Pimenta A, da Fonseca JC, et al. The effect of cholestasis on hepatic clearance of bacteria. *World J Surg.* 1982;6:330–334.
14. Sung JY, Shaffer EA, Olson ME, et al. Bacterial invasion of the biliary system by way of the portal-venous system. *Hepatology.* 1991;14:313–317.
15. Hazrah P, Oahn KT, Tewari M, et al. The frequency of live bacteria in gallstones. *HPB.* 2004;6:28–32.
16. Brain PH, Barrs VR, Martin P, et al. Feline cholecystitis and acute neutrophilic cholangitis: clinical findings, bacterial isolates and response to treatment in six cases. *J Feline Med Surg.* 2006;8:91–103.
17. Church EM, Matthiesen DT. Surgical treatment of 23 dogs with necrotizing cholecystitis. *J Am Anim Hosp Assoc.* 1998;24:305–310.
18. Eich CS, Ludwig LL. The surgical treatment of cholelithiasis in cats: a study of nine cases. *J Am Anim Hosp Assoc.* 2002;38:290–296.
19. Kirpensteijn J, Fingland RB, Ulrich T, et al. Cholelithiasis in dogs: 29 cases (1980-1990). *J Am Vet Med Assoc.* 1993;202:1137–1142.
20. Mayhew PD, Holt DE, McLear RC, et al. Pathogenesis and outcome of extrahepatic biliary obstruction in cats. *J Small Anim Pract.* 2002;43:247–253.
21. Mehler SJ, Mayhew PD, Drobatz KJ, et al. Variables associated with outcome in dogs undergoing extrahepatic biliary surgery: 60 cases (1988-2002). *Vet Surg.* 2004;33:644–649.
22. O'Neill EJ, Day MJ, Hall EJ, et al. Bacterial cholangitis/cholangiohepatitis with or without concurrent cholecystitis in four dogs. *J Small Anim Pract.* 2006;47:325–335.
23. Wagner KA, Hartmann FA, Trepanier LA. Bacterial culture results from liver, gallbladder, or bile in 248 dogs and cats evaluated for hepatobiliary disease: 1998-2003. *J Vet Intern Med.* 2007;21:417–424.
24. Boland L, Beatty J. Feline cholangitis. *Vet Clin North Am Small Anim Pract.* 2017;47:703–724.
25. Callahan Clark JE, Haddad JL, Brown DC, et al. Feline cholangitis: a necropsy study of 44 cats (1986-2008). *J Feline Med Surg.* 2011;13:570–576.
26. Simpson KW. Pancreatitis and triaditis in cats: causes and treatment. *J Small Anim Pract.* 2015;56:40–49.
27. Gagne JM, Armstrong PJ, Weiss DJ, et al. Clinical features of inflammatory liver disease in cats: 41 cases (1983-1993). *J Am Vet Med Assoc.* 1999;214:513–516.
28. Warren A, Center S, McDonough S, et al. Histopathologic features, immunophenotyping, clonality, and eubacterial fluorescence in situ hybridization in cats with lymphocytic cholangitis/cholangiohepatitis. *Vet Pathol.* 2011;48:627–641.
29. Haney DR, Christiansen JS, Toll J. Severe cholestatic liver disease secondary to liver fluke (*Platynosomum concinnum*) infection in three cats. *J Am Anim Hosp Assoc.* 2006;42:234–237.
30. Harrison JL, Turek BJ, Brown DC, et al. Cholangitis and cholangiohepatitis in dogs: a descriptive study of 54 cases based on histopathologic diagnosis (2004-2014). *J Vet Intern Med.* 2018;32:172–180.
31. Tamborini A, Jahns H, McAllister H, et al. Bacterial cholangitis, cholecystitis, or both in dogs. *J Vet Intern Med.* 2016;30:1046–1055.
32. Ramery E, Papakonstantinou S, Pinilla M, et al. Bacterial cholangiohepatitis in a dog. *Can Vet J.* 2012;53:423–425.
33. Takemura LS, Marcasso RA, Lorenzetti E, et al. *Helicobacter* infection in the hepatobiliary system and hepatic lesions: a possible association in dogs. *Braz J Microbiol.* 2019;50:297–305.
34. Armstrong JA, Taylor SM, Tryon KA, et al. Emphysematous cholecystitis in a Siberian husky. *Can Vet J.* 2000;41:60–62.
35. Kanemoto H, Fukushima K, Tsujimoto H, et al. Intrahepatic cholelithiasis in dogs and cats: a case series. *Can Vet J.* 2017;58:971–973.
36. Neer TM. A review of disorders of the gallbladder and extrahepatic biliary tract in the dog and cat. *J Vet Intern Med.* 1992;6:186–192.
37. Hirsch VM, Doige CE. Suppurative cholangitis in cats. *J Am Vet Med Assoc.* 1983;182:1223–1226.
38. Hittmair KM, Vielgrader HD, Loupal G. Ultrasonographic evaluation of gallbladder wall thickness in cats. *Vet Radiol Ultrasound.* 2001;42:149–155.
39. Newell SM, Selcer BA, Girard E, et al. Correlations between ultrasonographic findings and specific hepatic diseases in cats: 72 cases (1985-1997). *J Am Vet Med Assoc.* 1998;213:94–98.
40. Jaffey JA, Graham A, VanEerde E, et al. Gallbladder mucocele: variables associated with outcome and the utility of ultrasonography to identify gallbladder rupture in 219 dogs (2007-2016). *J Vet Intern Med.* 2018;32:195–200.
41. Center SA, Randolph JF, Warner KL, et al. Bacterial culture and immunohistochemical detection of bacteria and endotoxin in cats with suppurative cholangitis-cholangiohepatitis syndrome. *J Am Vet Med Assoc.* 2022;260:194–211.
42. Savary-Bataille KC, Bunch SE, Spaulding KA, et al. Percutaneous ultrasound-guided cholecystocentesis in healthy cats. *J Vet Intern Med.* 2003;17:298–303.
43. Kook PH, Schellenberg S, Grest P, et al. Microbiologic evaluation of gallbladder bile of healthy dogs and dogs with iatrogenic hypercortisolism: a pilot study. *J Vet Intern Med.* 2010;24:224–228.
44. Niza MM, Ferreira AJ, Peleteiro MC, et al. Bacteriological study of the liver in dogs. *J Small Anim Pract.* 2004;45:401–404.
45. Sifri CD, Madoff LC. Infections of the liver and biliary system. In: Mandell GL, Bennett JE, Dolin R, eds. *Principles and Practice of Infectious Diseases.* 7th ed. Philadelphia, PA: Churchill Livingstone Elsevier; 2010:1035–1044.
46. Pashmakova MB, Piccione J, Bishop MA, et al. Agreement between microscopic examination and bacterial culture of bile samples for detection of bactibilia in dogs and cats with hepatobiliary disease. *J Am Vet Med Assoc.* 2017;250:1007–1013.
47. Sergeeff JS, Armstrong PJ, Bunch SE. Hepatic abscesses in cats: 14 cases (1985-2002). *J Vet Intern Med.* 2004;18:295–300.
48. Farrar ET, Washabau RJ, Saunders HM. Hepatic abscesses in dogs: 14 cases (1982-1994). *J Am Vet Med Assoc.* 1996;208:243–247.
49. Grooters AM, Sherding RG, Biller DS, et al. Hepatic abscesses associated with diabetes mellitus in two dogs. *J Vet Intern Med.* 1994;8:203–206.
50. Sykes JE. 2012. Unpublished observations.

127

Infections of the Genitourinary Tract

Jodi L. Westropp, Jane E. Sykes

KEY POINTS

- Causes: The most common cause of genitourinary tract infections is *Escherichia coli*, but other gram-negative bacteria, staphylococci, and streptococci may also be involved. Anaerobic bacterial infections are rare causes of genitourinary tract infections, but may be involved in pyometra.
- Geographic Distribution: Worldwide.
- Major Clinical Signs: No signs, or dysuria, hematuria, or pollakiuria may occur with lower UTI. Acute pyelonephritis, prostatitis, and pyometra may be accompanied by fever or abdominal pain. Lethargy, inappetence, vomiting, or diarrhea may occur with sepsis. Pyometra may be accompanied by abdominal distention and/or a vaginal discharge. Prostatitis may be accompanied by dyschezia, dysuria, and a purulent or hemorrhagic urethral discharge.
- Differential Diagnoses: Feline idiopathic/interstitial cystitis, bladder neoplasia, or cystolithiasis (bacterial cystitis); toxicity, leptospirosis, and fungal or protozoal pyelonephritis (pyelonephritis); pregnancy, mucometra, or hydrometra (pyometra); benign prostatic hyperplasia, paraprostatic cysts, and prostatic neoplasia (prostatitis).
- Human Health Significance: MDR uropathogens might have the potential to colonize human patients.

INTRODUCTION

Infections of the genitourinary tract include sporadic bacterial cystitis, recurrent bacterial cystitis, pyelonephritis, renal abscesses, prostatitis, epididymitis and orchitis, metritis, pyometra, and potentially bacterial vaginitis. Lower UTI can also be caused by *Candida* spp. (see Chapter 85), and some fungi, especially molds such as *Aspergillus* spp., can infect the upper urinary tract leading to fungal pyelonephritis (see Chapter 86). This chapter focuses on bacterial infections of the urogenital tract; information on infections by other types of pathogens such as protozoa and nematodes can be found in other respective chapters in this book. UTI and genital infections can occur separately or concomitantly. Terminology regarding lower UTI has been addressed in the 2019 guidelines regarding diagnosis and management of bacterial UTI in dogs and cats by the ISCAID.[1] *Sporadic bacterial cystitis* (formerly known as uncomplicated UTI), in which a bacterial infection in the bladder results in inflammation and associated lower urinary tract signs (stranguria, pollakiuria, hematuria, and dysuria), is a common reason for veterinary visits and antimicrobial administration. This often occurs in otherwise healthy nonpregnant females and to a lesser extent, castrated males and cats. While possible, comorbidities such as endocrinopathies, intervertebral disc disease, and urinary stones are rarely identified in this group. Generally, animals with sporadic bacterial cystitis have had known or suspected UTI fewer than three times in the last 12 months. Complicated bacterial cystitis has also been described in dogs and cats; however, it is often difficult to determine if the bacterial cystitis is truly uncomplicated; underlying predispositions may be present.

In human medicine, *recurrent bacterial cystitis* implies three or more bacterial cystitis events within a 12-month period, or more than two events in a 6-month period; the same definition has been adopted in veterinary medicine.[1] In this case, predisposing patient factors are often identified, such as immune suppression, kidney disease, hypercortisolism, diabetes mellitus, urolithiasis, neoplasia, micturition disorders, ectopic ureters, and other anatomic abnormalities such as urethral strictures or cystic diverticulum.[2] While clinical cystitis can occur secondary to these conditions, these co-morbidities also have been associated with subclinical bacteriuria (SBU). Recurrent bacterial cystitis may reflect refractory (or persistent) infection, relapsing infection, or reinfection (Table 127.1). Without the use of molecular techniques (e.g., pulsed-field gel electrophoresis), it may not be possible to distinguish between relapsing infection and reinfection if the same bacterial species is isolated repeatedly, because a different strain may be present. *Enterococcus* spp. and *Pseudomonas* spp. may be more commonly found in dogs with persistent or recurrent UTI than dogs with simple uncomplicated UTI.[3] Some bacteria such as *Escherichia coli* can invade and form microcolonies within the uroepithelial cells (Fig. 127.1),[4] which may contribute to persistent infection in the face of antimicrobial treatment. Bacteria may also be able to form biofilms in association with the bladder wall ("deep-seated" infections), or on

TABLE 127.1 Factors that May Predispose to (or Contribute to) Development of Bacterial Cystitis or Subclinical Bacteriuria in Dogs and Cats

Dogs	Cats
Recessed vulva with concurrent perivulvar pyoderma	Perineal urethrostomy
Diabetes mellitus	Hyperthyroidism
Hyperadrenocorticism	Diabetes mellitus
Renal failure	Chronic kidney disease
Urinary catheterization	Micturition abnormalities (urinary incontinence or urinary retention)
Ectopic ureters	Urinary catheterization
Micturition abnormalities (urinary incontinence or urinary retention)	Urolithiasis
Tube cystostomy	Urinary neoplasia (rare)
Immunosuppressive drug treatment	
Urethrostomy	
Urolithiasis	
Urinary neoplasia	

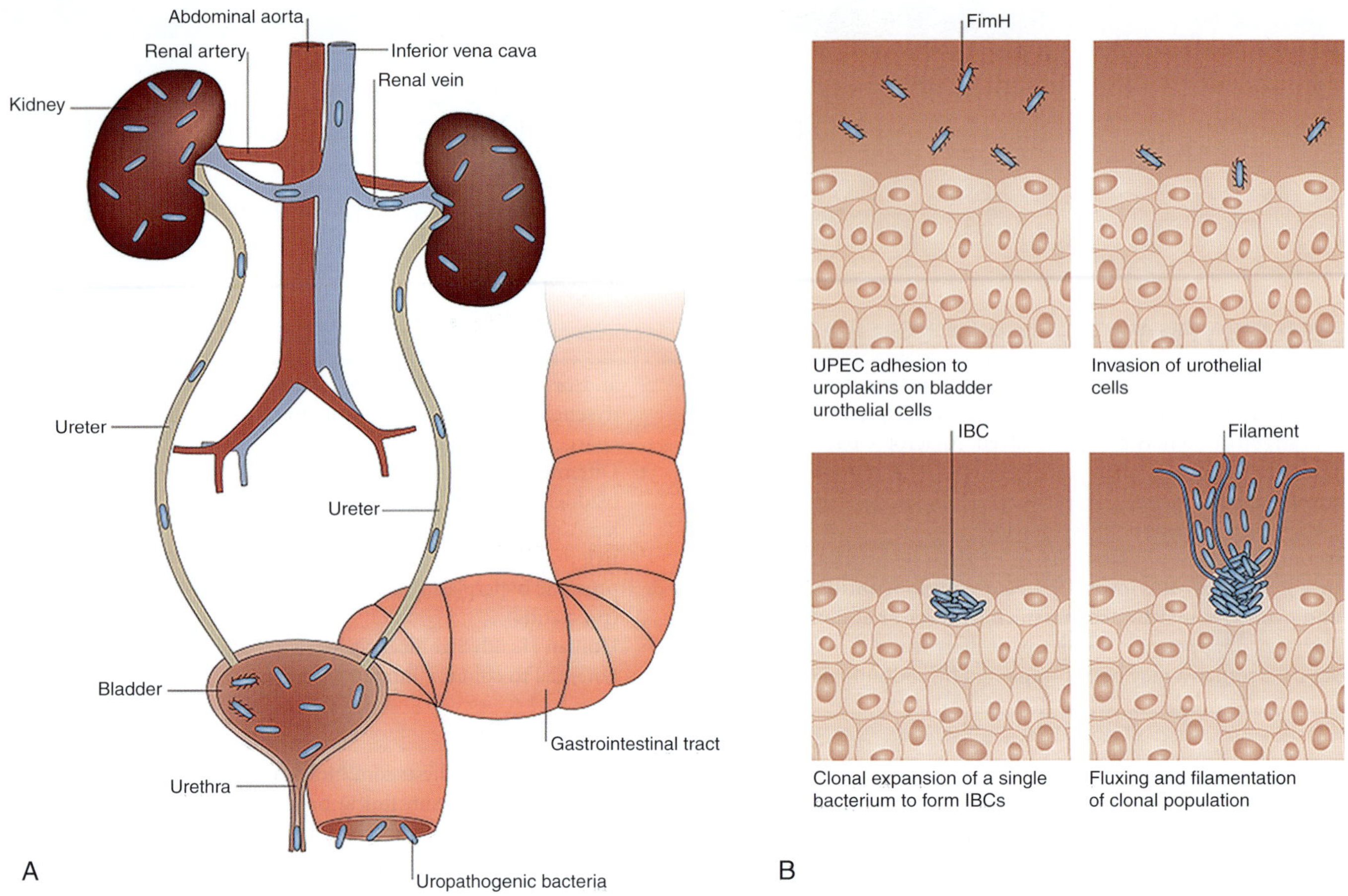

Fig. 127.1 Pathogenesis of urinary tract infection by uropathogenic *Escherichia coli* (UPEC). (A) UPEC colonizing the gastrointestinal tract, perineum, or vagina ascend into the urinary bladder to cause cystitis, which may be accompanied by lower urinary tract signs. They can also ascend into the kidneys to cause pyelonephritis. (B) In the urinary bladder, individual bacteria adhere to and invade superficial urothelial cells in a FimH-dependent manner. There they undergo clonal expansion to form biofilm-like intracellular bacterial communities (*IBCs*), where they can evade normal host mechanical and immunologic clearance mechanisms. Bacteria then form filaments that flux out of the cells into the bladder urine, where they then bind to adjacent cells and begin a new infection cycle. (From Klein RD, Hultgren SJ. Urinary tract infections: microbial pathogenesis, host-pathogen interactions and new treatment strategies. *Nat Rev Microbiol.* 2020;18:211–226.)

urinary implants such as stents and urinary catheters. *Escherichia coli* isolated from the urinary tract of dogs have been reported to frequently form biofilms; 52.6% of isolates were capable of forming biofilms in one study. Because no clinical distinguishing feature was found, biofilm formation should be considered whenever *E. coli* bacterial UTI is diagnosed. Biofilm formation was actually associated with greater susceptibility to antimicrobial drugs, suggesting that the antimicrobial tolerance may not be related to the presence of a resistance gene, but further studies are needed.[5] The use of antimicrobial-coated urinary catheters may reduce biofilm formation.[6]

Pyelonephritis can result when bacteria ascend into the renal pelvis and parenchyma from the lower urinary tract (see Fig. 127.1); less commonly, hematogenous spread to the kidney occurs. A single bacterial species (most often *E. coli*) is isolated from the urine of approximately three quarters of dogs with pyelonephritis, with two species isolated in 8% of dogs and three species from only 2% of dogs. Pyelonephritis may be acute or chronic. Strains of *E. coli* that cause pyelonephritis have greater ability to adhere to cells than strains that cause cystitis. Adhesins located on the tip of *E. coli* fimbriae adhere to glycolipid residues on tubular, collecting duct and bladder epithelial cells. In humans with pyelonephritis, both P and type I fimbriae appear to be important in colonization of the renal pelvis (Fig. 127.2).[7,8] Other *E. coli* virulence factors associated with pyelonephritis include hemolysin, cytotoxic necrotizing factor, the iron scavenger aerobactin, and a serum protease known as Sat. Fimbriae are also important in the pathogenesis of *Proteus* spp. pyelonephritis.[9] The medulla is more sensitive to colonization than the cortex, possibly owing to impaired host defenses in a high-osmolality, low-pH and low–blood flow milieu. Organisms adhere to pelvic and distal and proximal tubular epithelium, and have been observed intracellularly. Considerable renal injury results from the inflammatory response to infection. Aggregation of neutrophils within capillaries and induction of vascular spasm by bacterial toxins and/or cytokines can contribute to renal ischemia.

These infections should not be confused with SBU (also referred to as asymptomatic bacteriuria or ASB in humans). This term is used to describe the presence of bacteria in the urine, as determined by a positive bacterial culture in the absence of lower urinary tract signs (LUTS). The term "subclinical UTI" could be applied to dogs and cats if cytologic evidence of infection (e.g., pyuria or hematuria) is present,[10] but in human patients, the term SBU is used even in the presence of these abnormalities. SBU is commonly identified in dogs and cats, especially those with underlying endocrinopathies, kidney disease,

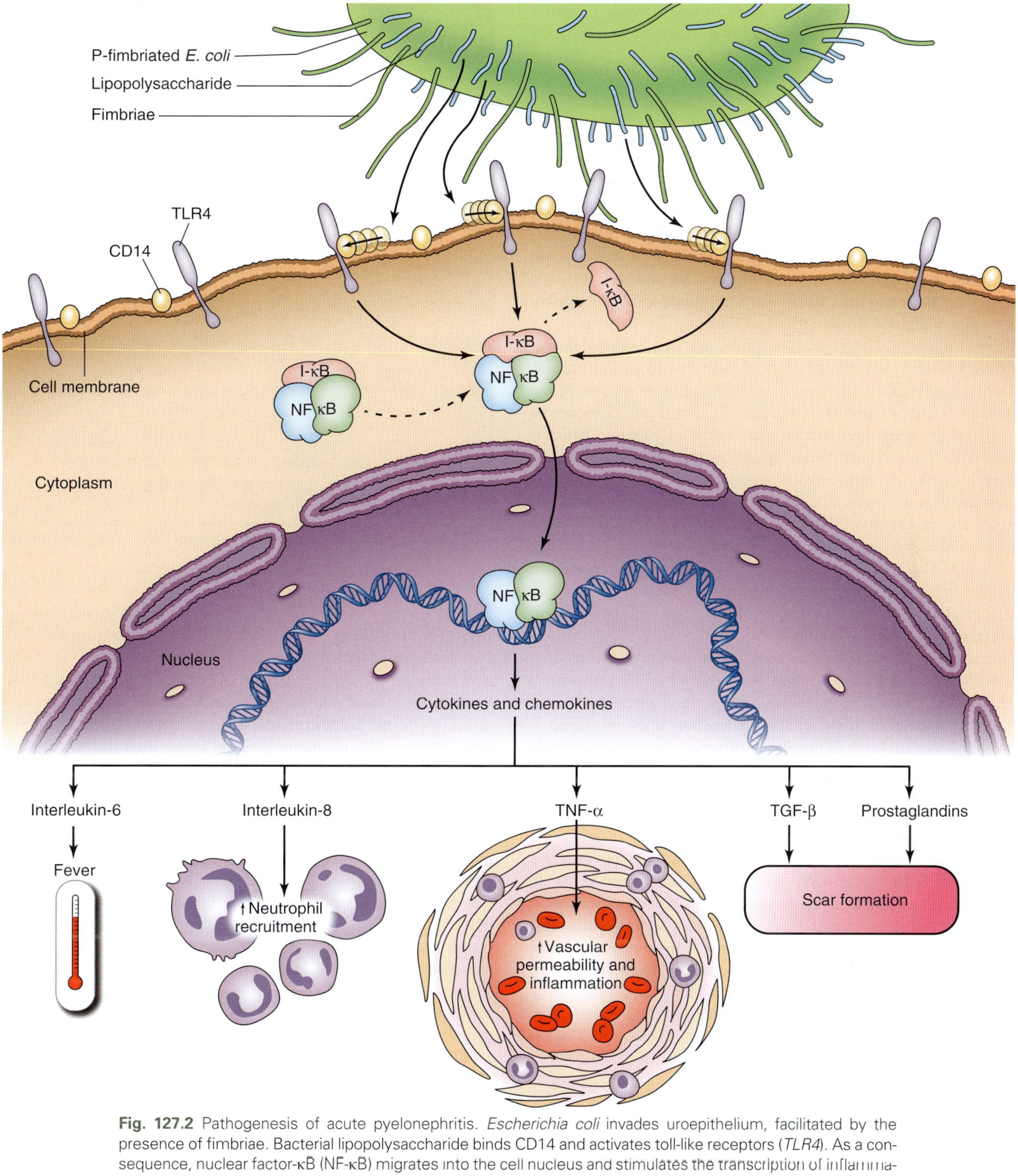

Fig. 127.2 Pathogenesis of acute pyelonephritis. *Escherichia coli* invades uroepithelium, facilitated by the presence of fimbriae. Bacterial lipopolysaccharide binds CD14 and activates toll-like receptors (*TLR4*). As a consequence, nuclear factor-κB (NF-κB) migrates into the cell nucleus and stimulates the transcription of inflammatory mediators that lead to fever, neutrophil recruitment, and increased vascular permeability. (Modified from Morello W, La Scola C, Alberici I, et al. Acute pyelonephritis in children. *Pediatr Nephrol.* 2016;31:1253 1265.)

micturition disorders, as well as dogs treated with glucocorticoids or cyclosporine.[11–15] In dogs evaluated in a primary care setting, bacteriuria was documented in 23 (12.7%) of 181 nonproteinuric specimens and 23 (8%) of the 286 proteinuric specimens. Of these 46 positive specimens, 31 were from dogs with SBU.[16] In a retrospective study that included 182 dogs with CKD, 33 (18.1%) had a positive aerobic bacterial urine culture. The highest prevalence of positive cultures was found for dogs with SBU (45%), with *E. coli* as the most frequently observed isolate.[17] In one study of dogs treated with glucocorticoids for dermatologic disorders, 18% of 127 dogs had bacteriuria in the absence of clinical signs, whereas none of 94 dogs that had not received glucocorticoids had bacteriuria.[15] SBU has a prevalence of 10%–13%

in cats; females were 21 times more likely to have a positive culture than male cats.[18] The extent to which antibiotic treatment is important in dogs or cats with SBU is not clear (see Treatment).

PATHOPHYSIOLOGY

Infections of the genitourinary tract usually follow impairment of normal host defenses and invasion by bacteria that are part of the normal flora (see Fig. 127.1). Less commonly, infection results from hematogenous spread to urogenital organs secondary to bacteremia. Specific pathogens such as *Leptospira* spp., *Borrelia* (*Borreliella* [incertae sedis]) *burgdorferi*, and *Leishmania* spp. that injure the kidneys secondary to systemic infection are described in Chapters 68, 69, and 96.

In healthy dogs and cats, bacteria are not found in upper urinary tract or prostate gland. In anestrus and diestrus, the uterus is also a sterile environment. The vagina, vestibule, prepuce, and distal urethra have a resident microflora. Normal flora should also be considered when results of aerobic bacterial cultures of urine, semen, or the preputial area are interpreted. In humans, recurrent infections can be associated with alterations in the normal vaginal microbiome, which is an important factor in host defense against pathogenic organisms. The resident microflora competes with pathogenic bacteria for nutrients and can interfere with adherence of pathogenic bacteria to vaginal epithelial receptors. Lactobacilli isolated from the vagina of dogs showed antimicrobial activity against *Proteus mirabilis, Staphylococcus aureus,* and *E. coli*.[19] The most common canine vaginal isolates reported in the dog are *E. coli* and *Staphylococcus pseudintermedius*. Vaginal lactic acid-producing bacteria were reported less often, with *Enterococcus canintestini* being the most common.[20]

Other factors that prevent bacterial colonization of the bladder include the glycosaminoglycan layer that covers bladder transitional epithelium, frequent voiding, the normal urethral microflora, antimicrobial properties of urine, an appropriate host immune response, and a functional urethral sphincter. Commensal bacteria that reside in the distal urethra, prepuce, and vagina invade opportunistically when these mechanisms are disturbed. The most common pathogen involved in all genitourinary tract infections is *E. coli*, which has a particular propensity to adhere to epithelial cells of the genitourinary tract. Others include coagulase-positive and coagulase-negative staphylococci; *Enterococcus* spp.; other aerobic gram-negative bacilli such as *Klebsiella, Proteus, Enterobacter,* and *Pseudomonas aeruginosa*; *Corynebacterium* spp.; streptococci; and mycoplasmas. Anaerobic bacteria are also found in the genital tract of female dogs, and may contribute to pyometra and metritis. In addition to impaired host defenses, a variety of bacterial virulence factors may impact the nature of the organisms that ultimately invade tissues and cause disease. The importance of virulence factors in uropathogenic *E. coli* infections is described in Chapter 53.

UPPER AND LOWER URINARY TRACT INFECTIONS

ETIOLOGY AND EPIDEMIOLOGY

Sporadic bacterial cystitis is commonly diagnosed in dogs. Although mixed bacterial infections can occur, the vast majority of these infections involve a single bacterial species.[21] The most common uropathogen isolated is *E. coli*, which accounts for approximately 50% of all isolates, followed by *Staphylococcus, Proteus, Klebsiella, Enterococcus,* and *Streptococcus* spp. Mycoplasmas have also been isolated from dogs with bacterial cystitis, although their clinical significance has been unclear because they are usually isolated from dogs that have other disorders of the lower urinary tract, such as underlying neoplasia or cystolithiasis. Spayed females and older dogs are at increased risk for infection; the mean age at diagnosis is 7 to 8 years.[3,21] As a result of breakdown in host defense mechanisms, systemic disorders such as acute or chronic kidney disease, hyperadrenocorticism, diabetes mellitus, and systemic neoplasia also predispose dogs to bacterial colonization of lower urinary tract. However, in many of these cases, SBU may be present and treatment with antimicrobials is not warranted (see later) (Table 127.2).

TABLE 127.2 Definitions Applied to Urinary Tract Infections

Term	Definition
Subclinical bacteriuria	Presence of bacteria in the urine as determined by a positive bacterial culture, in the absence of LUTS. Differentiation from subclinical UTI may be difficult
Sporadic cystitis	Bacterial infection of the lower urinary tract associated with compatible clinical signs
Complicated bacterial cystitis	UTI that occurs in the presence of an anatomic or functional abnormality or comorbidity that predisposes to persistent UTI, recurrent infection, or treatment failure
Recurrent bacterial cystitis	Three or more episodes of UTI during a 12-month period
Relapsing UTI	Isolation of the same microorganism within 6 months of apparent clearance of the infection with treatment in between positive cultures
Re-infection	Isolation of a different microorganism within 6 months of apparent resolution of a previous infection

LUTS, lower urinary tract signs; *UTI*, urinary tract infection.

In contrast, bacterial cystitis is less common in cats. Most young cats with LUTS have disorders such as feline idiopathic/interstitial cystitis (FIC), which are not associated with bacterial infection. The prevalence of sporadic cystitis in cats ranges from just 1% to 3%.[22–24] However, other studies have reported a higher prevalence of bacterial cystitis; 44/134 (33%) of cats with obstructive and nonobstructive feline lower urinary tract disease had bacteriuria from the Norwegian School of Veterinary Science.[25] As in dogs, *E. coli* is the most common pathogen. Other potential uropathogens in cats include *Streptococcus, Staphylococcus, Enterococcus, Klebsiella,* and *Pasteurella,* and *Enterobacter*.[13,21,26] Mycoplasmas are very rarely isolated from the urine of cats.[26]

While bacteriuria (clinical or subclinical) in cats is more often recognized in older cats, co-morbidities such as diabetes mellitus and CKD were reported to be associated with UTI. The prevalence of "UTI" in cats with diabetes mellitus is 11%–13%.[11,13] At referral institutions, positive aerobic bacterial urine cultures were found in 17% and 22% of cats with CKD, and 22% and 12% of cats with hyperthyroidism.[11,26] Other factors that may predispose cats to bacteriuria are breed (Persians or Abyssinians), female sex, older age, and lower body weight,[13,24,26] although some of these risk factors may also be associated with the co-morbidities mentioned above. Most recently, the prevalence of subclinical bacteriuria in cats with hyperthyroidism was reported to be low, and this did not differ from a euthyroid control group, suggesting no increased risk and no clinical benefit in routinely

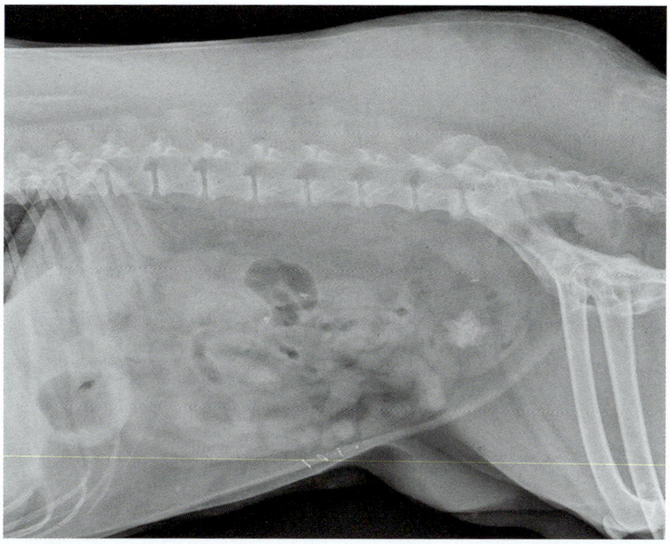

Fig. 127.3 Lateral abdominal radiograph from a 10-year-old female spayed miniature schnauzer with emphysematous cystitis and a large, irregular cystic calculus. Irregular gas densities can be seen throughout the bladder. *Escherichia coli* was cultured from a urine specimen that was obtained by cystocentesis.

performing urine cultures as a screening diagnostic in hyperthyroid cats.[27]

Uncommon forms of bacterial cystitis in dogs and cats are *encrusting cystitis* and *emphysematous cystitis.* Encrusting cystitis is caused by the gram-positive bacterium *Corynebacterium urealyticum.* Urease production by this organism leads to precipitation of large amounts of struvite and calcium phosphate within the bladder and along the bladder and urethral mucosa, and in some cases within the ureters and renal pelvis.[28–31] Most animals with *C. urealyticum* infections have severe LUTS and underlying co-morbidities such as urinary retention, urolithiasis, or ectopic ureters. Antimicrobial resistance is common and treatment should be implemented based on susceptibility testing. Use of an acidifying diet is warranted and endoscopic or surgical urothelial debridement may be required.

Emphysematous cystitis is characterized by the production of gas by bacteria within the bladder wall (Fig. 127.3). The most common cause is *E. coli*, but *Clostridium* spp. may also be involved.[32,33] The majority of dogs and cats that develop *E. coli* emphysematous cystitis have co-morbidities. In one study, diabetes mellitus was reported in 33% of 27 dogs, neurologic disease in 26%, and adrenal disease in 19%.[32] In diabetics, gas production may result from fermentation of glucose to gas products by *E. coli.* In the absence of glucose, proteins such as albumin may be fermented to gas. Emphysematous cystitis caused by *Clostridium perfringens* occurs in the absence of diabetes mellitus.[33,34]

CLINICAL FEATURES

Clinical Signs

Clinical signs of bacterial cystitis can include LUTS such as dysuria, hematuria, stranguria, and pollakiuria. Some clinical signs might be less apparent, such as subtle urinary incontinence or licking of perivulvar or prepucial area. Owners might also complain of foul-smelling urine. Cats may urinate outside the litter box (periuria or inappropriate urination). In some dogs, such as those with neurologic disorders like paraplegia, it can be difficult to ascertain if the animal is exhibiting signs of discomfort from the infection. Short-term treatment (see later) can be considered and the dog's clinical response closely monitored. Rarely, lethargy may accompany sporadic cystitis, but fever and hyporexia are not present.

Acute or acute-on-chronic pyelonephritis may result in decreased appetite, lethargy, variable fever, hematuria, and clinical signs of uremia, such as vomiting and diarrhea. Polyuria and polydipsia may also be present, or dogs with advanced disease may be anuric. Dogs and cats with chronic pyelonephritis may show no signs, or show only polyuria and polydipsia.

Physical Examination Findings

Physical examination findings in dogs or cats with bacterial cystitis may be unremarkable, or there may be mild urine staining of the perineum. Some dogs may present with urinary incontinence and evidence of urine scalding or a strong ammonia-like odor may be present. Underlying disorders that predispose to bacterial cystitis may also be apparent (such as a recessed vulva and associated vulvar fold dermatitis).

Occasionally, abdominal pain may be detected on palpation of the abdomen of dogs or cats with bacterial cystitis, but more often this is seen with acute pyelonephritis or when concurrent prostatitis is present. The bladder is often small in dogs or cats due to persistent inflammation and associated frequent voiding (pollakiuria); a thickened bladder wall may also be palpated. If a large, turgid bladder is present in dogs or cats with a UTI, urethral obstruction due to neoplasia, calculi, encrusting cystitis, or proliferative urethritis (PU) should be suspected. Fever is not present in dogs and cats with infections localized to the lower urinary tract, and is variable in dogs and cats with pyelonephritis. Dogs and cats with severe pyelonephritis may show evidence of lethargy, dehydration, and signs of severe sepsis or septic shock (e.g., tachycardia or bradycardia, tachypnea, prolonged capillary refill time).

DIAGNOSIS

Diagnosis of sporadic bacterial cystitis or pyelonephritis is based on the clinical signs present, laboratory abnormalities, imaging findings, and culture of urine. Most cases of acute pyelonephritis arise from ascension of the fecal-derived organisms. Acute pyelonephritis with *E. coli* (at least in children) is associated with type 1 and type P pili, with the latter more frequently identified. Renal scarring is noted in children due to activation of NF-κB, which perpetuates the inflammatory response, fever, and neutrophil recruitment (see Fig. 127.2).[35] The presence of fever or leukocytosis in addition to a positive bacterial urine culture should increase suspicion for concurrent bacterial pyelonephritis; prostatitis or pyometra should also be considered (see relevant sections later in this chapter). Ultrasound examination findings also can support the diagnosis and assist in the identification of predisposing disorders such as neoplasia, anatomic abnormalities, or the presence of calculi or foreign material. At a minimum, collection of urine by cystocentesis followed by complete urinalysis (with sediment examination) and quantitative aerobic bacterial urine culture are recommended to confirm the presence of bacterial UTI for dogs or cats with signs of lower urinary tract disease.[1,10] Additional diagnostics are indicated for animals that have recurrent LUTS or those with systemic signs such as fever, weight loss, or inappetence. The owners of animals that are diagnosed with a suspected sporadic bacterial cystitis should always be advised that other predisposing underlying disease may be present.

Laboratory Abnormalities

Complete Blood Count and Serum Biochemical Tests

Animals with infections localized to the lower urinary tract typically have no hematologic or serum biochemistry abnormalities. The diagnosis of pyelonephritis can be difficult. Animals with pyelonephritis may have mild anemia, leukocytosis due to a neutrophilia, increased band neutrophils, and monocytosis. A degenerative left shift, toxic neutrophils, and thrombocytopenia may also be present. The serum biochemistry panel may show azotemia. Due to the potential for renal scarring and other complications in children with acute pyelonephritis, various novel biomarkers have been evaluated to identify early kidney injury. These include CRP, IL-6, IL-8, plasma neutrophil gelatinase-associated lipocalin (NGAL),[36] kidney injury molecule-1 (uKIM -1)[37] and procalcitonin (PCT).[38] Several of these biomarkers may be useful for predicting and possibly managing acute pyelonephritis, but none are clinically available in veterinary medicine at this time. The latter (PCT) is intriguing because it is an early and reliable marker of serious bacterial infections and sepsis.[39] SDMA can be a useful marker of glomerular filtration rate (GFR) in cats and dogs and is used for screening for early detection of kidney injury. Like many of the biomarkers, it is not specific for pyelonephritis,[40] but is clinically available. Other markers such as cystatin C, NGAL, and homocysteine have also been investigated in dogs.[41]

Hypoalbuminemia and electrolyte abnormalities may be present in dogs or cats with pyelonephritis. However, pyelonephritis may be present in animals with normal CBC and serum biochemical panels. While research is underway to identify biomarkers specific for renal parenchymal infection, currently the clinician must collate all physical examination, imaging, and biochemical findings and decide if treatment for pyelonephritis is warranted.

Urinalysis

The urinalysis is usually the initial screening test for dogs with LUTS. Of 52 private practices in Denmark evaluating 151 dogs with LUTS, the veterinarian performed a urine dipstick 99% of the time and sediment examination in 80%. Only 56% of those samples were submitted for culture.[42] Findings on the urinalysis in dogs and cats with UTI can include isosthenuria, pyuria, hematuria, proteinuria, and bacteriuria. Animals with pyelonephritis may have cylindruria, and small amounts of glucose may be present in dogs with altered proximal tubular function. However, the urinalysis may also be unremarkable, even in dogs and cats with pyelonephritis. Infections with urease-producing bacteria such as staphylococci, *Proteus* spp., and *C. urealyticum* may be associated with a high urine pH and the presence of struvite crystals. The urine protein to creatinine ratio (UPCR) in dogs with pyelonephritis may be increased as a result of renal tubular or glomerular injury. However, an elevated UPCR may be noted in dogs with sporadic cystitis as well as those with SBU.[16] In patients with a high suspicion of pyelonephritis but negative urine culture, blood cultures and/or nephropyelocentesis should be considered.

Coagulation Profile

Evidence of coagulation abnormalities may be present in animals with severe pyelonephritis that develop severe sepsis or septic shock (see Chapter 123).

Diagnostic Imaging

Plain Radiography

Dogs or cats with sporadic bacterial cystitis alone generally have no radiographic abnormalities. The bladder of animals with pollakiuria may be small. Emphysematous cystitis is characterized by the presence of radiolucencies within the bladder lumen and/or in association with the bladder wall (see Fig. 127.3). Radiopaque cystic or renal ("staghorn") calculi may be visible in dogs with struvite calculi secondary to infections with *Staphylococcus* spp. or *Proteus* spp. (Fig. 127.4).

Renomegaly may be present with acute pyelonephritis, or the kidneys may be small and irregular in dogs or cats with chronic pyelonephritis.

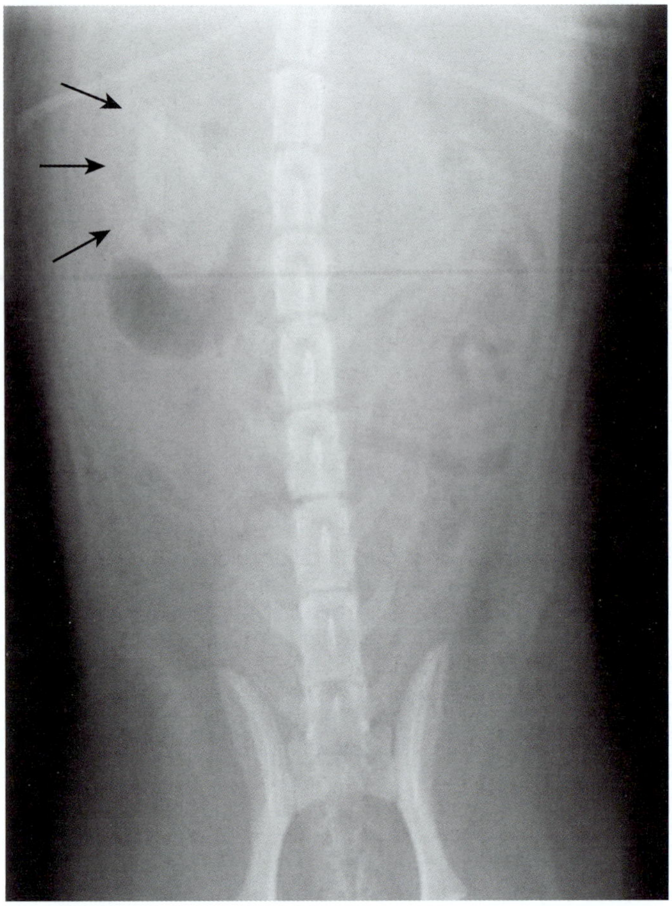

Fig. 127.4 Dorsoventral radiograph of a 6-year-old female spayed shih tzu mix with a urinary tract infection caused by *Proteus mirabilis* and *Enterococcus faecalis* and nephrolithiasis. An opacity ("staghorn" calculus) occupies the right renal pelvis *(arrows)*.

Sonographic Findings

Ultrasound examination of the urogenital tract is a noninvasive method to obtain information about the extent and severity of disease and underlying causes such as neoplasia, calculi, or foreign bodies. It does not permit visualization of the entire urethra, and urethral abnormalities (e.g., evidence of PU) may be overlooked in some animals if only ultrasound is used for imaging purposes. Ultrasound examination of the bladder may be unremarkable or show a mild to moderately thickened bladder wall in dogs or cats with bacterial cystitis. Increased echogenicity of the urine may be present. Rarely the bladder wall is severely thickened (Fig. 127.5). Animals with emphysematous cystitis may have a hyperechoic bladder wall with acoustic shadow artifacts. Shadow artifacts may also occur as a result of the presence of cystic calculi.

Dogs or cats with pyelonephritis may have a normal abdominal ultrasound examination, or blunting of the renal papilla, pyelectasia, irregularity of the renal contour, and evidence of hydronephrosis (Fig. 127.6). However, renal pelvic dilatation can occur in animals with normal renal function, diuresis, and outflow tract obstruction, and there is considerable overlap in the extent of dilatation between groups.[43] Dogs and cats with severe pyelonephritis may have hyperechoic material within the renal pelvis, or the renal pelvis may be anechoic and contain hyperechoic debris.[44] Sometimes the surrounding mesentery is hyperechoic, and perinephric anechoic fluid may be present due to localized peritonitis.

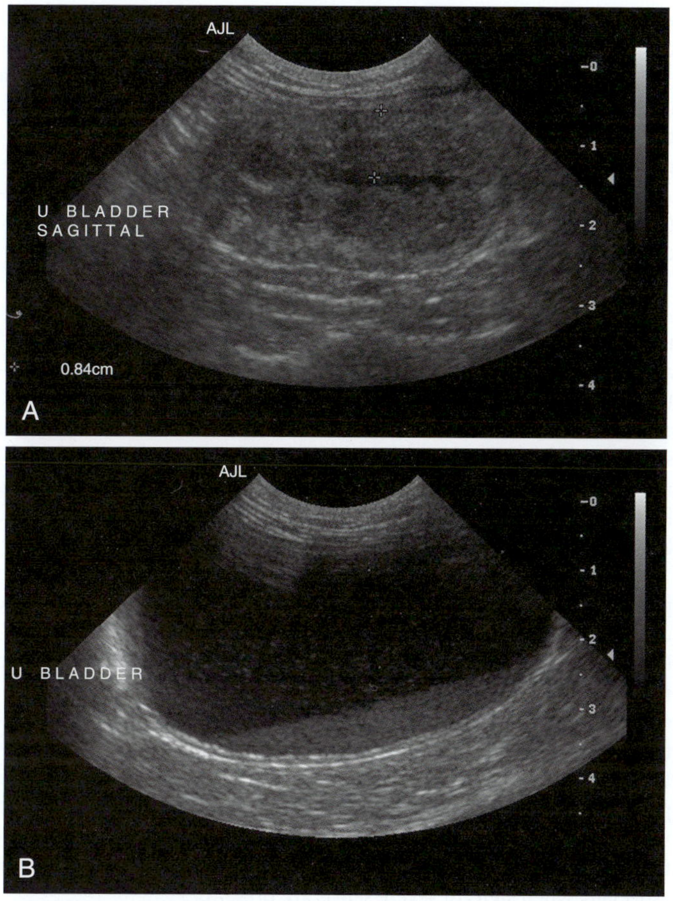

Fig. 127.5 Ultrasound images of the bladder of an 18-year old female spayed domestic shorthair cat with diabetes mellitus, generalized osteoarthritis, a myelopathy, and recurrent urinary tract infection (UTI). The cat had severe lower urinary tract signs (hematuria, pollakiuria, and stranguria) and UTI with a hemolytic *Escherichia coli* was diagnosed. (A) The bladder wall is markedly thickened. (B) Resolution of bladder wall thickening after treatment with marbofloxacin for 3 weeks, which also resolved the clinical signs.

Other nonspecific findings in pyelonephritis can include increased renal cortical echogenicity, and decreased corticomedullary definition. The diagnosis of pyelonephritis should not be made solely based on ultrasonographic findings.

Contrast Radiography and Cystoscopy

Intravenous contrast urography was utilized to identify renal pelvic enlargement and assist in the diagnosis of pyelonephritis, but has largely been replaced by abdominal ultrasonography for this purpose, which is less invasive and can be an excellent tool to identify predisposing factors such as uroliths, diverticuli, neoplasia, and polypoid cystitis. While cystoscopy can be considered for select patients with recurrent UTI, it is not often recommended for women when other imaging such as ultrasonography is normal,[45] and cystoscopy performed solely for recurrent UTI in women was reported to be low yield.[46] In 163 women with recurrent UTI, cystourethroscopy rarely (3.8%) identified a unique lesion (i.e., pertinent uroendoscopic finding) that was not previously identified by ultrasound (111 women) or contrast CT (22 women).[47] In dogs with recurrent UTI, non-specific cystourethroscopic and vaginoscopic findings such as mucosal edema, lymphoid follicles and vestibulovaginal septal remnants were noted in 45/53 (85%) dogs, but no comparisons were made in this study between endoscopic and ultrasonographic findings.[48] In addition, this study did not determine if these findings were clinically relevant or related to the LUTS for which the dog was being evaluated. Preliminary data in dogs with recurrent UTI found that cystoscopy findings were in agreement with the ultrasonographic findings in 26/30 (87%) dogs evaluated.[49] In dogs, cystoscopy can be considered if bladder or urethral biopsy is indicated for histopathology. Culture of the bladder or urethral tissue can be considered, as well as techniques such as FISH when the possibility of a deep-seated infection exists, as bladder wall infection may not be associated with positive urine cultures in some dogs.[50] Furthermore, five dogs with PU had negative urine and tissue cultures when FISH was positive. There was no association detected between the type of urethral inflammation and the results of urine and tissue culture or FISH.[51] However, if obtaining biopsy specimens for culture, it is ideal to collect these when the dog has a negative urine culture and not receiving antimicrobial therapy, which can be difficult

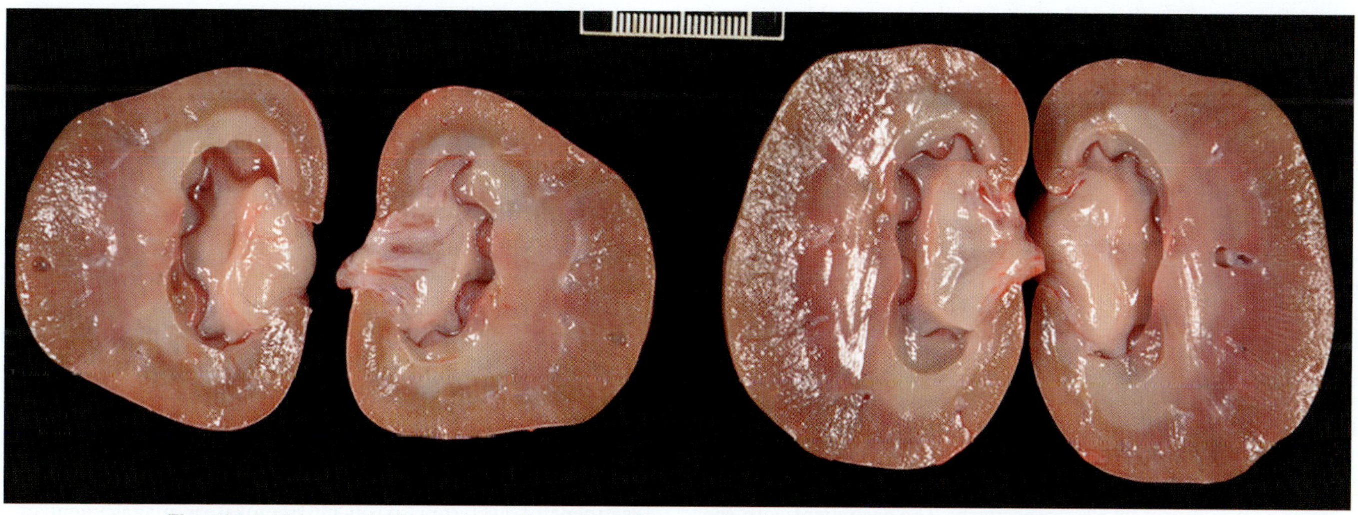

Fig. 127.6 Kidneys of a 2-year-old male neutered German shepherd with diabetes mellitus and chronic pyelonephritis secondary to *Klebsiella pneumoniae* infection. The kidneys are bilaterally asymmetrical; the right kidney is larger than the left. There are several small, cortical subcapsular cysts, and the kidneys have an irregular conformation with markedly shrunken poles. The renal parenchyma at the poles is markedly collapsed from the capsule to the pelvis and the pelvis is uniformly dilated. (Courtesy of University of California, Davis, Veterinary Anatomic Pathology Service.)

to achieve in some patients. Contrast cystourethrography can also be useful for diagnosis of anatomic abnormalities, particularly urethral lesions, when cystoscopy is not available.

Microbiologic Tests

Isolation and Identification

Quantitative aerobic bacterial culture and susceptibility testing is strongly recommended for dogs or cats with UTI before starting antimicrobial drugs, because of the possibility of antimicrobial drug resistance, which has been well recognized among *E. coli* strains isolated from dogs and cats with genitourinary tract infections.[52,53] It is especially warranted in dogs and cats with recurrent UTI that have received previous antimicrobials for UTI treatment. Isolates from dogs that had received amoxicillin, doxycycline, or enrofloxacin 30 days before culture results were obtained were significantly more likely to be resistant than those from dogs that did not receive those antimicrobials before urine cultures were obtained.[2] Guidelines for diagnosis of bacterial UTI in dogs and cats have been published.[1,10] Ideally, urine should be collected by cystocentesis; if this is not possible or contraindicated (e.g., coagulopathy or lower urinary tract neoplasia), urethral catheterization can be considered. Although any pathogens isolated from specimens collected by cystocentesis are likely significant, the presence of > 10^3 CFU/mL of bacteria is unlikely to result from skin contamination alone. If specimens are collected using catheterization, colony counts that exceed > 10^4 CFU/mL for male dogs and > 10^5 CFU/mL for female dogs are considered clinically significant.[1,10] Free-catch (midstream voiding) specimen collection is not recommended for dogs or cats because it is highly susceptible to contamination. Aerobic bacterial urine culture from a specimen collected by cystocentesis confirms the presence of bacterial infection in animals with LUTS. Culture can also help to differentiate reinfection from relapse should a UTI return.[1,10] Culture of a single organism from a mucosal swab collected from a site such as the urethra does not imply disease causation because commensal bacteria may be isolated in pure cultures from healthy dogs and cats. Specimens for culture and susceptibility testing should be refrigerated immediately and submitted to the laboratory as soon as possible. The results of culture for specimens that reach the laboratory > 24 hours after collection should be interpreted with caution because false-negative and false-positive test results can occur. For dogs and cats with recurrent UTI that undergo surgery, culture of a bladder wall biopsy or cystoliths can be considered, but a decision to treat should be based on the presence of clinical signs.

Inexpensive urine "paddles" have been marketed for in-house veterinary diagnosis of UTI, which consist of two different types of agar on either side of a plastic paddle (see also Chapter 3, Fig. 3.6). The media are inoculated with urine collected by cystocentesis and the paddles are then incubated and examined daily for growth; sensitivity and specificity of this POC test was 97.3% and 98.6%, respectively; however, the paddles do take approximately 24 hours before results are available to interpret.[54] A rapid immunoassay (RapidBac Vet, Silver Lake Research, Azusa, CA, USA) is also marketed as a POC test for detection of bacteriuria in cats and dogs with a 90% sensitivity and 96.6% specificity reported when applied to a small number of specimens. Of 200 canine urine samples, 38 (19%) were considered associated with a UTI based on the urine collection method and signifiicant bacteriuria. For these samples, the sensitivity and specificity of the rapid immunoassay was 97.8% and 98.8%, respectively. The agreement with the reference laboratory was considered substantial.[55] In another study of 22 urine specimens from dogs, sensitivity and specificity were 73% and 91%, respectively; for specimens with over 1000 CFU/mL of bacteria identified using culture, sensitivity and specificity were 80% and 91%, respectively.[56] Assay results are available in 20 minutes. These POC tests can be useful screening tools for patients with LUTS when client finances do not permit submission of specimens to a microbiology laboratory for culture. If positive results are obtained, ideally a urine specimen should then be submitted to a microbiology laboratory for culture and susceptibility testing in order to select the most appropriate antimicrobial drug. If performed in-house, bacterial culture should only be performed in clinics with appropriate laboratory facilities, proper BSL containment and waste management, and adequately trained personnel.[10]

If a urinary catheter is present, culture should be performed if clinical signs of infection are present (e.g., hematuria, suspected bacteremia).[10] The catheter should be removed and cystocentesis performed after the bladder is allowed to fill with urine. Alternatively, the catheter could be removed, replaced with a new catheter if necessary, and a urine specimen collected through the new catheter after removal of several milliliters of urine to clear the catheter. Urine culture should never be submitted from specimens collected from the urine bag because it is likely to yield growth of organisms forming biofilm on the bag or catheter; there is no indication to culture the catheter tip.

Bacteria cultured from the urine are usually those involved in pyelonephritis, when pyelonephritis is present. However, a negative urine culture does not rule out pyelonephritis. Pyonephrosis, a collection of sloughed urothelium and inflammatory cells in the dilated renal collecting system, is a complication that can be caused by partial or complete ureteral obstruction with concurrent upper tract infection. The diagnosis of pyelonephritis can be challenging clinically. Ultrasound-guided nephropyelocentesis can be considered when renal pelvic dilation is present to obtain urine for culture, but this is not usually required for effective treatment of pyelonephritis. Blood cultures should also be considered in animals with acute pyelonephritis, especially when signs of severe sepsis are present.

Laboratories that perform susceptibility testing for uropathogens should adhere to local guidelines for test performance and reporting (such as the Clinical and Laboratory Standards Institute [CLSI] in North America and the European Committee on Antimicrobial Susceptibility Testing [EUCAST] in Europe) (see Chapter 3). Breakpoints for systemic infections also apply to UTI. However, provided renal function is normal, many antimicrobials achieve much higher concentrations in urine than they do in serum. Therefore, use of some antimicrobials may eradicate the UTI despite predicted resistance. This is especially true for treatment of staphylococcal UTI with penicillins and cephalosporins. Urinary breakpoints are available for ampicillin or amoxicillin in dogs (≤8 μg/mL), amoxicillin-clavulanate in dogs and cats (<8/4 μg/mL), and nitrofurantoin. These should only be used when infection is confined to the lower urinary tract.

Pathologic Findings

Pathologic findings in dogs with bacterial cystitis and pyelonephritis depend on the chronicity of the infection, the underlying cause, and the uropathogens present. Acute infections are associated with a dense neutrophilic infiltrate on histopathology and intralesional bacteria may be identified. Chronic infections may be associated with histiocytic or lymphoplasmacytic infiltrates.

TREATMENT AND PROGNOSIS

Treatment of UTI consists of: (1) removal or management of the underlying cause of infection and (2) antimicrobial treatment. Treatment with antimicrobial drugs alone without attention to an underlying cause frequently leads to recurrent infection and selection for resistant bacteria. Because of the increasing prevalence of MDR *E. coli* and staphylococci in dogs and cats with UTI, provided the

TABLE 127.3 Suggested Initial Treatment for Stable Dogs or Cats with Genitourinary Tract Infections Pending Culture and Susceptibility Results

Disease	Drug	Dose (mg/kg)	Route	Interval (hours)
Bacterial cystitis or pyometra	Amoxicillin OR	11–15	PO	8
	Trimethoprim-sulfadiazine OR	15[a]	PO	12
	Clavulanic acid-amoxicillin	12.5–25	PO	8
Pyelonephritis, prostatitis	Enrofloxacin OR	20 (dogs)	PO	24
	Marbofloxacin OR	2.7–5.5	PO	24
	Orbifloxacin	7.5	PO	24

[a]Based on trimethoprim plus sulfadiazine concentration.
See Chapter 123 for options for severe sepsis.

patient is stable and sepsis is absent, consideration should be given to delaying antimicrobial drug treatment until the results of culture and susceptibility are available. This is especially true for dogs and cats with recurrent UTI that have a history of antimicrobial drug treatment. Empiric treatment while awaiting the results of culture and susceptibility could be considered to relieve discomfort if present in dogs that have not received previous antimicrobial treatment. The use of NSAIDs can be considered (with extreme caution in cats) to relieve clinical signs while pending susceptibility testing. When pyelonephritis or sepsis is present or suspected, treatment should commence immediately with broad-spectrum antimicrobials that have activity against MDR gram-negative bacteria (see Chapter 123).

Sporadic Bacterial Cystitis

Published guidelines provide detailed recommendations for treatment of sporadic cystitis.[1] In most situations, rational choices for initial treatment of sporadic cystitis include amoxicillin or trimethoprim-sulfonamide (Table 127.3). Amoxicillin-clavulanic acid could be considered if regional susceptibility trends suggest a high (>10%) prevalence of β-lactamase production by uropathogens isolated.[1,10] However, evidence of a need for clavulanic acid is lacking and may not be necessary due to the high urinary concentrations of amoxicillin that are achieved in most animals. Trimethoprim-sulfonamides are an excellent option, but do have a greater association with adverse events such as hepatotoxicity, and immune-mediated diseases. Resolution of clinical signs (i.e., clinical cure) is the goal of therapy, rather than elimination of bacteriuria. Once culture and susceptibility results are available, the initially chosen antimicrobial drug should either be continued (if a clinical response has occurred) for a total of 3 to 5 days or switched to an alternative drug (if clinical cure has not been achieved) with activity against the pathogen isolated and that enters urine in high concentrations. A treatment duration of 3 to 5 days has been recommended by the ISCAID Antimicrobial Working Group; however, 10 to 14 days of treatment is still routinely prescribed.[1,10] While there are numerous studies evaluating and supporting short-course therapy for UTI in humans, studies in the veterinary field are lacking. One study showed that treatment of dogs that had sporadic cystitis with high-dose enrofloxacin (20 mg/kg) for 3 days was not inferior to treatment with clavulanic acid-amoxicillin for 14 days (see Table 127.3).[57] Another study of dogs with naturally occurring UTI that evaluated short durations of treatment with trimethoprim-sulfonamide compared with longer duration of treatment with cephalosporins found that no significant difference in the microbiologic or clinical cure rates were reported between the two groups in short- or long-term (>30 days) evaluation, but long-term treatment cure rates were low in both groups.[58]

Recurrent Bacterial Cystitis

Investigation of an underlying cause is strongly recommended in animals with recurrent UTI. For animals where reinfections are confirmed (i.e., recurrent infections with differing bacterial strains or species), a thorough evaluation for micturition disorders (urinary incontinence or urine retention), perivulvar inflammation and infection, or predisposing systemic abnormalities should be performed.

Care should be taken not to overinterpret the finding of a recessed vulva. While the incidence of bacteriuria improved in 19 of 22 dogs after vulvoplasty, 59% of those dogs had perivulvar dermatitis which also improved. Moreover, 14 of 34 dogs had signs such as urinary incontinence, and perivulvar dermatitis at an older age suggesting multiple contributing factors for recurrent infections. While 16 dogs with UTI and hooded vulva improved clinically (i.e., decreased recurrence of UTI) after episioplasty, 3 of 16 had concurrent cystic calculi, and 12 of 16 dogs had concurrent perivulvar dermatitis, which also resolved.[59]

For animals with a relapsing infection (i.e., recurrent UTI with the same pathogen strain), the pathogen susceptibility should be reviewed, as well as the antimicrobial dose and duration. A thorough investigation for a nidus of infection (e.g., urinary calculi, polyp or deep-seated infection) should be considered. Referral to an internal medicine specialist should be considered for further diagnostic tests, including advanced imaging. Antimicrobial drugs should be selected on the basis of culture and susceptibility test results, and preference should be given to drugs that are excreted in the urine in active form. If excreted in the urine, drugs with intermediate susceptibility could be used to treat UTI that is resistant to other appropriate drug choices; however, a higher dose (for concentration-dependent antimicrobials) or dosing frequency (for time-dependent antimicrobials) should be considered. Nitrofurantoin should be considered for UTI that is resistant to other oral antimicrobial drugs that are excreted in the urine and only administered when the infection is isolated to the lower urinary tract. Nitrofurantoin should never be used to treat prostatitis or pyelonephritis due to poor tissue penetration. When mixed infections are present, antimicrobial drug treatment ideally should be directed at all organisms present. In mixed infections that involve *Enterococcus* spp., the *Enterococcus* spp. infection will typically resolve when other organisms present are successfully treated.[10] There is no evidence to suggest that longer antimicrobial treatment duration (10 to 14 days) is needed for animals with recurrent UTI. The primary objective for treatment is clinical cure (resolution of clinical signs); microbiologic cure is not always achievable in some patients with co-morbidities that cannot be corrected. Longer courses (14 days) can be considered for some relapsing infections, particularly for suspected deep-seated infections. Aerobic bacterial urine culture could be considered 5 to 7 days after initiating treatment, but if clinical cure is achieved, a change in treatment may not be warranted even if a positive bacterial culture is documented. If no clinical signs are present, management should be as for SBU (see later).

As mentioned earlier, urolithiasis in the urinary tract can serve as a nidus for infection and reason for relapsing infections, particularly in dogs. Stone removal is advised if appropriate (bladder, urethral stones) and consideration for a ureteral stent or subcutaneous ureteral bypass in patients presenting with ureteral obstruction. In dogs presenting with suspected struvite urolithiasis, dissolution with a calculolytic diet and concurrent antimicrobials (in dogs) should be prescribed. Traditionally, antimicrobials are recommended for the entire dissolution protocol in dogs. Shorter courses of antimicrobial therapy combined with a calculolytic diet may be efficacious; an induced canine struvite model provided limited evidence for struvite dissolution without antimicrobials[60]; however, dissolution will likely take longer utilizing this strategy. In one study, the target urinary pH appeared appropriate for struvite dissolution (pH = 5.9–6.1) at day 45 in dogs with struvite urolithiasis following only 7 days of antimicrobial administration during the first week combined with a calculolytic diet. However, radiographic evidence of struvite dissolution was not provided.[60] At this point, no definitive guidelines exist for the timing and duration of antimicrobial therapy in humans[61] or dogs with struvite uroliths. Future studies should consider this to improve antimicrobial stewardship. Recommendations for shorter course therapy have been suggested for dogs.[1] Regardless of the strategy implemented, patients should be re-evaluated on a regular basis and treatment adjusted based on clinical findings using diagnostic imaging and laboratory findings (serum chemistry, urinalysis, urine culture).

There is no evidence that direct instillation of antimicrobials, antiseptics, glycosaminoglycans, or dimethyl sulfoxide (DMSO) directly into the bladder via a urinary catheter is effective for treatment of recurrent UTI. These compounds are rapidly eliminated from the bladder during micturition and may be locally irritating, which may predispose further to infection with drug-resistant bacteria. Approaches that have been used to prevent recurrence are detailed in the Prevention section.

Subclinical Bacteriuria

In humans, there is abundant support that antimicrobial treatment is not warranted for ASB. No evidence of an association between SBU and risk of sepsis, pyelonephritis, or other complications exists. Data in veterinary medicine are limited. Of 67 nonazotemic cats that had urine cultures performed on five occasions over 3 years, the presence of SBU in cats did not adversely impact survival even though antimicrobial treatment was withheld.[18] In cats with CKD, no difference was noted in the frequency of CKD progression between cats with UTI and those with SBU or no positive urine culture. However, the impact of not treating SBU on progression of CKD or survival could not be assessed because in this group, all cats received antimicrobial treatment. When nine healthy dogs with SBU were followed for 3 months, four had persistent bacteriuria and four transient; none developed signs during this period.[62] Of 47 chronically paralyzed dogs that lacked pelvic limb pain perception, 35 had at least one positive urine culture and 13 dogs had recurrent bacteriuria.[63] Bacteriuria was not associated with survival, but the differences in antimicrobial treatment between the two groups were not clear. However, resistant bacterial isolates were cultured from 46% of dogs with recurrent positive urine cultures.

Treatment for humans with concurrent diabetes mellitus and ASB is not recommended; the authors do not advocate screening or treatment of SBU in dogs with stable diabetes mellitus or those with hypercortisolism. Identifying clinical signs of bacterial cystitis in some patients can be difficult (e.g., paralyzed dogs); if the clinician or owner is concerned for poor quality of life, a short course (3 to 5 days) of antimicrobials can be considered and the clinical signs charted during the course of therapy.

While both UTI and SBU have been described in cats and dogs that have implants such as subcutaneous ureteral bypass devices or ureteral stents,[64] whether SBU should be treated with antimicrobials requires additional study. These devices are prone to colonization with bacterial biofilms, and bacteriuria can be difficult to eradicate. Treatment should be implemented if azotemia has progressed (and no other underlying cause for the progression has been documented) and serum creatinine or SDMA re-evaluated. If no improvement is noted, further antimicrobial treatment may not be indicated.

Animals with SBU should be evaluated for potential underlying causes of SBU that need to be addressed. If no underlying conditions are evident, treatment for SBU is not warranted. The authors advise treatment for SBU only for patients that are undergoing a urologic intervention (e.g., cystotomy or laser ablation for ectopic ureter) and at least once for dogs with SBU associated with *Staphylococcus* cystitis due to its association with struvite urolithiasis. Treatment is also indicated for SBU when there is an associated new or progressive azotemia, and the response to antimicrobial therapy monitored (clinical signs, severity of azotemia). Finally, urine cultures and treatment are indicated, despite a lack of LUTS, in animals where systemic infection is suspected.

Pyelonephritis

Treatment of dogs with acute pyelonephritis should be initiated immediately, without waiting for culture and susceptibility test results. Cytologic examination of stained urine sediment may assist in initial selection of an antimicrobial drug (i.e., based on the presence of rods versus cocci). The use of a fluoroquinolone that is excreted in the urine in active form (i.e., not difloxacin) has been recommended for gram-negative bacterial pyelonephritis, provided regional susceptibility data do not show widespread resistance to fluoroquinolones.[1,10] The dosage used may need to be altered depending on the severity of renal impairment. If combination treatment is initiated and antimicrobial susceptibility test results show susceptibility to only one drug, the other drug should be discontinued. In older veterinary literature, treatment durations of 4 to 6 weeks have been recommended for pyelonephritis, but a shorter duration is likely adequate, as is recommended in human medicine. Treatment for 10–14 days is recommended by the ISCAID Working Group. Oral antimicrobial therapy is justified for animals that are otherwise systemically healthy and have a normal fluid intake without vomiting. Intravenous antimicrobials should be administered to animals that are febrile, dehydrated, hyporexic, and/or vomiting. Dogs with acute pyelonephritis may require hospitalization and supportive care with IV fluids and other medications used to treat acute kidney injury or sepsis. The patient should be re-evaluated and serum creatinine, urinalysis, and an aerobic bacterial urine culture are recommended 1 week after completion of the antimicrobial treatment. The clinical and biochemical response should be evaluated. If a microbiologic cure is not documented, the clinician should be certain the patient was evaluated properly for underlying disorders (e.g., uroliths) and decide if the isolate is associated with ongoing pyelonephritis or SBU and treated accordingly. Underlying co-morbidities should be addressed if possible.

PREVENTION AND NON-ANTIMICROBIAL THERAPIES

Prevention of lower UTI involves identification and reversal of underlying causes of disease, such as vulvar fold dermatitis or congenital abnormalities such as ectopic ureter. Urinary catheterization should only be used when necessary, and intermittent catheterization is preferred to indwelling catheterization. If indwelling catheterization is required, a closed sterile collection system should always be used, and the catheter should be removed as soon as it is no longer required, because the risk of ascending infection increases with every day the catheter is left in place. Treatment of catheterized animals with antimicrobial drugs may increase the risk of bacterial infection,[65] so catheterized animals should only be treated with antimicrobial drugs when necessary, and they should not be used in an attempt to prevent urinary catheter infection. Routine antimicrobial treatment after catheter removal is not indicated unless clinical signs of UTI develop, because colonization that follows catheterization is cleared once the catheter is removed and host defenses are restored.

Many treatments for prevention of UTI in dogs and cats with a history of recurrent disease have been considered. Currently, there is no evidence that urinary adjunct treatments such as antiseptics (e.g., methenamine), or nutritional supplements such as cranberry juice extract are effective in dogs or cats. There are numerous alternative/adjunct therapies that have been investigated for the prevention and treatment of recurrent bacterial cystitis in humans as well as animal models such as NSAIDS, estrogen compounds, intravesical glycosaminoglycans, cranberry extract, and live biotherapeutic products.[66] The efficacy of cranberry extract for treatment of recurrent UTI in women has been mixed. At the time of writing, the most recent placebo-controlled studies have shown no significant effect; however, patient selection appears critical. A reduction in UTI recurrence has been reported in other studies,[67] although it has not appeared to be as effective in patients with other co-morbidities. While cranberry has been shown to prevent adherence of *E. coli* strains in *in vitro* canine studies, no significant difference was noted in dogs with intervertebral disc disease to reduce the risk of UTI or SBU compared with placebo.[68]

Live biotherapeutic products appear promising for treatment of recurrent UTI and have the potential to reduce the need for antimicrobial therapy. Intravesicular administration of *E. coli* ASB strain 83972 in human beings with recurrent UTI reduced the symptoms of UTI and protected some patients from recurrent UTI after serial catheterizations. In a recent veterinary pilot study, intravesicular administration of ASB *E. coli* strain 212 to dogs with recurrent UTI resulted in complete or nearly complete clinical cures in four of nine dogs, and three had microbiologic cures at 2 weeks; one of these dogs had SBU after treatment (in addition to ASB *E. coli* 212) and did not require antimicrobial therapy. Long-term follow-up urine cultures were only available for two dogs. ASB *E. coli* 212 (as determined by PFGE analysis) was isolated 60 days after bacterial instillation and these two dogs remained free of LUTS for more than 6 months. Three of the four dogs had the ASB strain isolated from their urine at day 14. Further studies are underway to investigate treatment with this live biotherapeutic compared to antimicrobial administration in a larger population.[69]

PUBLIC HEALTH ASPECTS

Dogs and cats with UTI have a potential to act as a source of MDR bacteria for humans. Similarities between uropathogenic *E. coli* isolates from dogs and those from humans have been identified,[70,71] but differences also exist.[72] Owners of pets with MDR UTI should always wash their hands after handling their pets, wear gloves when medications are administered, and pets should be taken to urinate away from other people and animals.

ORCHITIS, EPIDIDYMITIS, AND PROSTATITIS

ETIOLOGY AND EPIDEMIOLOGY

Orchitis and epididymitis may occur in association with UTI in intact male dogs, but is rare. Infection with *Brucella canis* should always be suspected in dogs with epididymitis (see Chapter 71). *Escherichia coli* accounts for most cases of bacterial prostatitis in dogs, but occasionally other gram-negative and gram-positive organisms, including atypical organisms such as *Mycoplasma* spp. and *Brucella* spp., are involved. Bacterial prostatitis is extremely rare in cats.[73]

CLINICAL FEATURES

Pathophysiology and Clinical Signs

Bacterial prostatitis in dogs may be acute or chronic. It often accompanies benign prostatic hyperplasia or prostatic neoplasia, most likely as a result of ascending infection secondary to altered urinary defense mechanisms. Prostatitis should be suspected in any intact male dog that develops a UTI. Dogs with bacterial prostatitis may show infertility, fever, lethargy, decreased appetite, weight loss, LUTS, purulent or hemorrhagic urethral discharge, abdominal pain, and sometimes a stiff gait. Tenesmus, vomiting, and diarrhea may also occur in some dogs. Acute bacterial prostatitis can be accompanied by severe sepsis or septic shock (see Chapter 123). Formation of prostatic abscesses may be followed by abscess rupture and peritonitis. Dogs with chronic prostatitis may be lethargic or have no clinical signs of illness.

Physical Examination Findings

Dogs with acute bacterial prostatitis may exhibit pain on palpation of the prostate. The prostate may be normal in size and shape, or enlarged or irregularly shaped. Fluctuant regions may be palpated if abscesses are present. Palpation of genitourinary structures should always be performed cautiously when acute bacterial prostatitis is suspected so that rupture of prostatic abscesses does not occur. Hemorrhagic or purulent discharge may be seen around the urethral orifice. Dogs with severe acute prostatitis may be dehydrated, febrile, obtunded, and show other signs of severe sepsis or septic shock (e.g., tachycardia or bradycardia, tachypnea, prolonged CRT). Intact male dogs with bacterial orchitis or epididymitis may have testicular enlargement, hyperemia, and pain on palpation of the testicles. This may sometimes be present in association with prostatitis.

DIAGNOSIS

Diagnosis of prostatitis is based on clinical signs, laboratory abnormalities, imaging findings, and culture of urine or prostatic secretions. Measurement of serum canine prostate specific esterase (CPSE) has been proposed as a biomarker for prostatic disease in dogs[74]; such biomarkers may ultimately be useful to help distinguish benign prostatic hyperplasia from bacterial prostatitis.

Laboratory Abnormalities

Animals with acute prostatitis may have mild anemia, leukocytosis due to a neutrophilia, increased band neutrophils, and monocytosis. A degenerative left shift, toxic neutrophils, and thrombocytopenia may also be present. Hypoalbuminemia and electrolyte abnormalities may be present, or there may be evidence of organ dysfunction in dogs with septic shock. Hyperglobulinemia may be present in dogs with chronic prostatitis. The urinalysis may reveal abnormalities consistent with UTI.

Diagnostic Imaging

Plain and Contrast Radiography

Plain radiography is of limited value for diagnosis of bacterial prostatitis. Dogs with benign prostatic hypertrophy (BPH) or prostatic abscesses may have prostatomegaly, with ventral and cranial displacement of the bladder (defined as a prostate diameter > 70% of the distance between the pubis and the sacral promontory).[75] Prostatic mineralization can rarely accompany chronic bacterial prostatitis in intact dogs, but when present in a neutered dog, mineralization strongly supports the presence of prostatic neoplasia.[76] Extravasation of contrast material into the prostate during retrograde contrast cystourethrography supports a diagnosis of prostatitis or prostatic neoplasia.

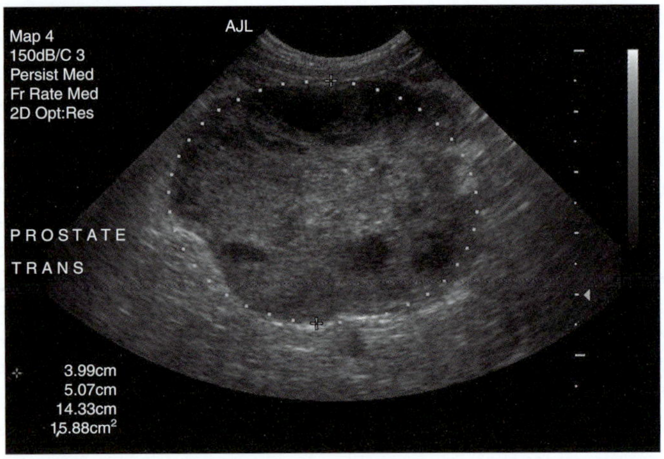

Fig. 127.7 Ultrasound image of the prostate of a 12-year-old intact male beagle dog that had acute prostatitis due to *Escherichia coli* and associated bacterial peritonitis. The dog was seen for acute onset of anorexia and vomiting and had 2,254 neutrophils/μL, 1,160 band neutrophils/μL, mild hypoalbuminemia (2.4 g/dL; reference range, 2.9–4.2 g/dL), increased serum alkaline phosphatase activity (1,338 U/L; reference range, 15–127 U/L), and increased serum total bilirubin concentration (0.5 mg/dL, reference range, 0–0.4 mg/dL). The prostate was significantly increased in size on sonographic examination and contained multiple hypoechoic nodules. There was a small quantity of ascites, which was predominantly localized in the caudal abdomen in the region of the prostate. Hemolytic *E. coli* was isolated from urine and from a prostatic aspirate. The owners elected euthanasia. Acute prostatitis and peritonitis were confirmed at necropsy.

Sonographic Findings

Sonographic abnormalities in dogs with prostatitis include prostatic irregularity, mixed echogenicity, and focal accumulations of anechoic or hypoechoic fluid, with distance enhancement (prostatic cysts or abscessation) (Fig. 127.7).[77]

Microbiologic Tests

Isolation and Identification

Many dogs with prostatitis shed bacteria into the urine; therefore, bacteria cultured from the urine are usually those involved in prostatitis (for collection methods, see Isolation and Identification section for UTI, earlier). Prostatic involvement should be suspected in any intact male dog with bacterial UTI. However, a negative urine culture does not rule out the possibility of prostatitis, and occasionally the organisms isolated from the urine may differ from those isolated from the prostate.

Collection of prostatic fluid via ejaculation, prostatic wash, or aspiration of the prostate or prostatic cysts is also recommended for diagnosis of bacterial prostatitis, particularly if the patient is refractory to treatment, neoplasia is suspected, or the urine culture is negative, and the prostate findings are suggestive for infection on ultrasonography. Aspirates of the prostate for culture and cytology (if clinically indicated) can be done in dogs with acute and chronic prostatitis; however, dogs with acute prostatitis may require sedation for patient comfort. The presence of large numbers of bacteria (>10^5 CFU/mL) together with an inflammatory response suggests infection. Cytologic examination and culture of ultrasound-guided aspirates of prostatic abscesses has been used to assist diagnosis, but there is a risk of localized peritonitis when abscessed tissues are aspirated.

Pathologic Findings

Dogs with acute prostatitis may have infiltrates of neutrophils with or without intralesional bacteria in the prostate on histopathology. Chronic infections may be associated with histiocytic or lymphoplasmacytic infiltrates. In some cases, prostatic hyperplasia or abscess formation are identified.

TREATMENT

Data are limited regarding the treatment duration for acute bacterial prostatitis, but 4 weeks of treatment with appropriate antimicrobials is recommended. For dogs with sepsis, parenteral antimicrobial administration initially may be required. If inflammation is severe, any drug appropriate for treatment of UTI may still penetrate the prostate in the acute phase.

Drug penetration is impaired in dogs with chronic prostatitis because of the blood-prostatic fluid barrier. Drugs that effectively cross the prostatic barrier of dogs include enrofloxacin, ofloxacin, marbofloxacin, trimethoprim, and chloramphenicol. Drugs such as the penicillins, cephalosporins, aminoglycosides, and tetracyclines are not able to cross an intact blood-prostate barrier and should be avoided, particularly in cases of chronic prostatitis. Ciprofloxacin should not be administered due to its variable GI absorption. Fosfomycin can be considered if an MDR gram-negative organism is isolated. Organisms may persist within the prostate of dogs with chronic prostatitis despite appropriate antimicrobial drug treatment. Because trimethoprim-sulfamethoxazole and chloramphenicol are more likely to be associated with adverse effects when administered for prolonged periods, a fluoroquinolone such as enrofloxacin is the drug of choice for initial treatment of gram-negative bacterial prostatitis. If the MIC of the organism is between 0.5 and 1.0 μg/mL, the highest dose of enrofloxacin is recommended (20 mg/kg, q24h). Clindamycin may be a reasonable choice for dogs with gram-positive bacterial prostatitis. Treatment of dogs with chronic prostatitis should continue for at least 6 weeks. Cure may not be possible without castration.

Surgical castration is recommended for dogs with prostatitis and can be considered as soon as the dog is stable to undergo anesthesia and surgery. The efficacy of drugs that cause prostatic involution, such as finasteride, is not clear, but finasteride enhanced the resolution of infection in a rat model of chronic prostatitis when administered with a fluoroquinolone.[78] Prostatic abscesses and paraprostatic or large intraprostatic cysts must also be addressed and treated using ultrasound-guided drainage or surgically if necessary. Castration and antimicrobial drug treatment alone does not effectively resolve prostatic abscesses.

Follow-up should consist of a return visit for examination 7 to 10 days after initiating treatment, and aerobic bacterial urine culture should be considered at this time if a positive urine culture was initially present. A return visit and examination should also be performed 1 week after discontinuation of treatment, at which time physical examination, urinalysis, urine culture, and prostatic fluid cytology and culture should be performed. Where available, prostatic ultrasound may also provide useful information at these follow-up times, and if possible, should be performed 1 week after discontinuation of antimicrobial drugs.

PREVENTION

Routine castration reduces the risk of prostatitis, although prostatitis can still occur in neutered animals.

VAGINITIS, METRITIS, AND PYOMETRA

ETIOLOGY AND EPIDEMIOLOGY

Bacterial vaginitis in adult bitches is usually secondary to an underlying disorder such as neoplasia, foreign bodies (e.g., grass awn), or seen

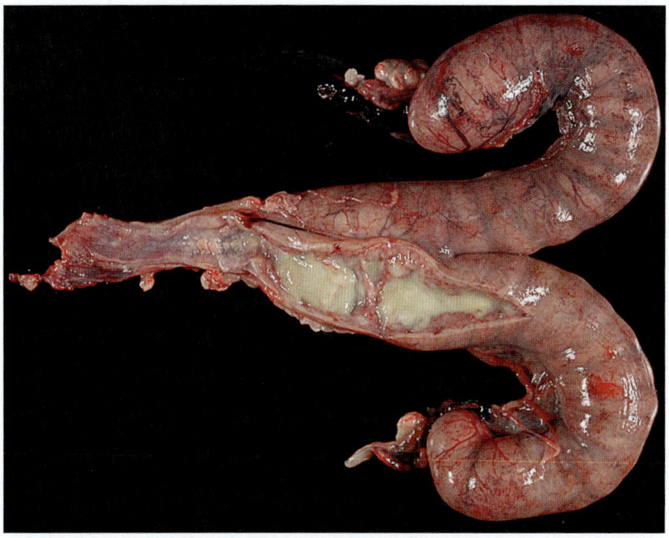

Fig. 127.8 Uterus of an 11-year-old female Pomeranian with pyometra during ovariohysterectemy. The left uterine horn was severely dilated and fluid-filled. (Courtesy of University of California, Davis, Veterinary Anatomic Pathology Service.)

concurrently with UTI or anatomic abnormalities such as strictures. Puppy vaginitis is thought to be a consequence of immaturity, rather than bacterial infection.

Metritis results from ascending infection of the uterus. It usually occurs shortly after parturition (e.g., within a week), or after obstetrical procedures, and may be associated with clinical signs of lethargy, fever, decreased appetite, and purulent vaginal discharge.

Pyometra is an accumulation of pus within the uterus (Fig. 127.8). The pathogenesis of pyometra is incompletely understood. However, in contrast to metritis, pyometra most often seems to occur as a result of increased serum progesterone concentrations, which cause cystic endometrial hyperplasia (CEH), impaired immune function, and decreased uterine contractility. The end result for at least some dogs and cats is opportunistic bacterial invasion, most often by *E. coli* strains that have virulence factors typical of uropathogenic isolates.[70,79] Bacterial biofilm may contribute to resistance to host immune defenses and antimicrobial drugs.[80] Other organisms that cause pyometra are similar to those that cause UTI, with the exception that anaerobes are more often involved, usually in mixed infections with other bacteria. CEH is not an absolute requirement for development of pyometra, and some animals with CEH never develop pyometra. Exogenous estrogen administration (used to treat mismating), as well as exogenous progesterone administration, have also been associated with pyometra.[81] Rarely, pyometra occurs in conjunction with uterine neoplasia.[82,83] Emphysematous pyometra has been reported in dogs but is uncommon; less than 10 cases have been reported in the literature.[84–87] Etiologic agents in emphysematous pyometra have included *C. perfringens*, *Citrobacter diversus*, and *P. aeruginosa*.

In dogs, pyometra usually occurs in diestrus, but it can occur in anestrus. Affected dogs are usually middle-aged to older, intact female dogs (mean age around 7 to 9 years), but pyometra has been reported in dogs as young as 8 months of age. Older dogs are likely to develop pyometra as a result of chronic and repeated exposure to progesterone with progressive cycles, whereas younger dogs may develop pyometra as a result of treatment of mismatings with estrogens. Pyometra is prevalent in regions where routine ovariohysterectomy of dogs is not widely performed; it has been estimated that 19% of all intact bitches develop pyometra before 10 years of age.[88] In a study from Scandinavia, breeds of dogs with increased risk included collies, rottweilers, Bernese mountain dogs, Cavalier King Charles spaniels, English cocker spaniels, and golden retrievers.[89,90] Bitches that have never been pregnant are at increased risk for development of pyometra compared with those that have had litters, but false pregnancy does not influence the risk for pyometra in dogs. In cats, CEH also seems to underlie pyometra. Cats with pyometra are generally > 3 years of age (mean, 5 years), but pyometra may occur in cats of any age.

CLINICAL FEATURES

Clinical Signs

Clinical signs of pyometra in dogs usually occur 2 to 10 weeks after estrus or breeding, but occasionally occur as long as 15 weeks after estrus (mean, 7 weeks). In both dogs and cats, clinical signs may be acute or chronic, and include lethargy, polyuria and polydipsia, vomiting, weight loss, decreased appetite, diarrhea, fever, and abdominal pain. Cats may have an unkempt haircoat. However, some dogs or cats show no signs of illness. Animals with *open-cervix pyometra*, the most common form of pyometra (>60% of dogs), usually have purulent vaginal discharge. The discharge may have a fetid odor, be mucopurulent, purulent, or contain blood. Dogs or cats with *closed-cervix pyometra* do not have vaginal discharge, but abdominal distention may be present. Animals with closed pyometra are more likely to have severe signs of systemic illness than those with open pyometra.[91] In one study, sepsis was more likely to occur in dogs with closed-cervix pyometra (77% of 39 dogs) than in dogs with open-cervix pyometra (51% of 71 dogs).[91] Concurrent glomerular and tubulointerstitial disease may also contribute to signs of polyuria and polydipsia.[92] In some dogs or cats, pyometra may be accompanied by severe sepsis or septic shock (see Chapter 123). Peritonitis may occur secondary to rupture of the uterus when disease is severe. Dogs with leukopenia were 18-fold more likely to have peritonitis as a complication of surgery than those that were not leukopenic.[93]

Stump pyometra is an uncommon form of pyometra. It sometimes occurs after remnants of the ovaries are inadvertently left in place after ovariohysterectomy, but this is not always identified. Stump pyometra occurs most commonly in dogs, but has been reported in the cat.[94] Clinical signs are similar to animals with pyometra. In addition, stump pyometras can contribute to recurrent lower UTI. When evaluated by ultrasound, the uterine stump was enlarged in a small group of dogs treated with estriol for urinary incontinence, without apparent adverse systemic effects.[95]

Physical Examination Findings

Purulent vaginal discharge, sometimes with a putrid odor, may be present in animals with bacterial vaginitis or open pyometra. Fever may be present in some dogs and cats with pyometra, and is more likely in closed-cervix pyometra. Abdominal pain may be present on palpation of the abdomen, which should always be performed cautiously when pyometra is suspected so that rupture of the uterus does not occur. Dogs and cats with severe pyometra may be lethargic, dehydrated, and show signs of severe sepsis or septic shock.

DIAGNOSIS

Diagnosis of vaginitis, metritis, and pyometra is based on signalment and history, clinical signs, laboratory abnormalities, imaging findings, and, in some cases, culture of the urine or uterine contents obtained during surgery.

Laboratory Abnormalities

Acute metritis or pyometra (especially closed-cervix pyometra) may be associated with anemia, leukocytosis due to a neutrophilia, increased band neutrophils, degenerate left shifts, toxic neutrophils, and monocytosis, especially if the cervix is closed.[91] Thrombocytopenia and signs of organ dysfunction (such as azotemia, increased serum ALP activity, and coagulation abnormalities) may be detected in dogs with severe sepsis or septic shock. Azotemia may also reflect the presence of concurrent pyelonephritis. Hypoalbuminemia and electrolyte abnormalities such as low serum sodium-to-potassium ratios may be present.[96,97] Dogs and cats with chronic pyometra may have few laboratory abnormalities; some animals with chronic pyometra may be hyperglobulinemic. On urinalysis, there may be abnormalities consistent with UTI. UPCRs may be increased as a result of renal tubular or glomerular injury.[92]

Diagnostic Imaging

Plain Radiography

Radiographic changes in dogs with pyometra consist of the presence of a large, coiled or tubular mass in the caudal and mid-abdomen, which displaces the small intestine cranially and dorsally. However, the uterus may not be visible in dogs with open pyometra. Differentiation of pyometra from pregnancy may require ultrasound examination. Localized or generalized loss of abdominal detail may be present in dogs with peritonitis secondary to uterine or prostatic rupture.

Sonographic Findings

Ultrasound is the imaging technique of choice for diagnosis of pyometra and differentiation of pyometra from pregnancy. However, it may not effectively distinguish pyometra from mucometra or hydrometra. Dogs with pyometra have an enlarged uterus, which is immediately dorsal to the bladder. The uterus may be thin-walled and distended with echogenic intraluminal fluid, or have a thickened wall with anechoic areas due to glandular proliferation and enlargement (CEH).[98] Assessment of uterine blood flow may help to distinguish pyometra from CEH, one study showing that dogs with pyometra had significantly higher uterine blood flow than dogs with CEH or healthy dogs.[99] In one dog with emphysematous pyometra, the uterus had a homogenously hypoechoic wall and was distended with gas, in contrast to the layered wall of the adjacent colon.[87] Stump pyometra may be recognized as a hypoechoic structure that is located dorsal and caudal to the urinary bladder (Fig. 127.9). It is important to record any concurrent estrogen exposure or administration when interpreting the uterine stump size in dogs. The maximum uterine height/aorta ratio was greater in dogs receiving estriol for urinary incontinence when compared with healthy dogs not receiving estrogen therapy. While this structure appeared ultrasonographically abnormal in these dogs, no clinical consequences were noted.[95]

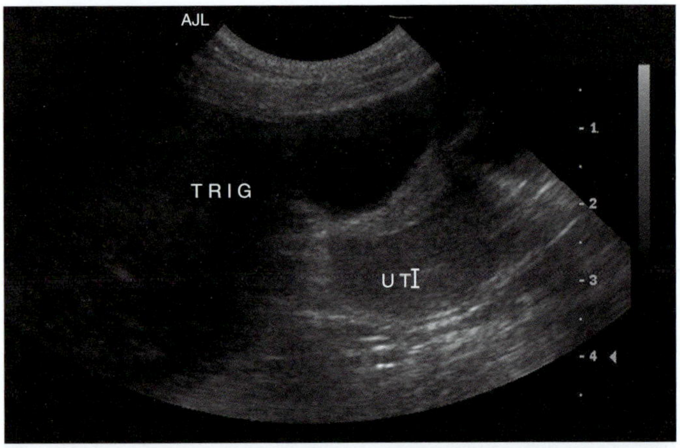

Fig. 127.9 Ultrasound image of the bladder and uterine stump in a 3-year-old female spayed mixed-breed dog that had vaginal discharge with a putrid odor due to a stump pyometra. An oval shaped structure (*UT*) that contained flocculent material is present within the pelvic inlet caudal to and dorsal to the anechoic urinary bladder. A cystic structure is seen in the region of the left ovary which represented a left ovarian remnant.

Microbiologic Tests

Isolation and Identification

Bacteria cultured from the urine are usually those involved in pyometra, although a negative urine culture does not rule out the possibility of pyometra, and occasionally the organisms isolated from the urine differ from those isolated from the uterus. Fine needle aspiration of the uterus is contraindicated because of the risk of uterine rupture. Usually, the bacteria involved are initially identified through culture of urine. Cystocentesis should always be performed with ultrasound guidance in animals suspected to have pyometra to avoid inadvertent perforation of the uterus. For animals with open pyometra, culture of a swab specimen that has been collected from the cranial aspect of the vagina could be considered, but the identity of the bacteria cultured may or may not be the same as those present within the uterus; therefore, this approach is not recommended. Tissues removed surgically can be submitted for culture and susceptibility testing, and this should be done despite the administration of broad-spectrum antimicrobial drugs before surgery, because these drugs are unlikely to penetrate pus within the uterus. If possible, both anaerobic and aerobic bacterial cultures should be performed for dogs or cats with pyometra. Blood cultures could be considered when signs of severe sepsis are present.

Pathologic Findings

As for other urogenital infections, acute pyometra is associated with a dense neutrophilic infiltrate on histopathology (Fig. 127.10) and intralesional bacteria may be identified; chronic infections may be associated with histiocytic or lymphoplasmacytic infiltrates. CEH (expansion of the endometrium with hyperplastic, dilated to cystic glands) and corpora lutea may also be identified.

TREATMENT AND PROGNOSIS

The overall prognosis for dogs with pyometra is good, with one study reporting an overall mortality rate of 10%, when euthanasias are included, to as low as 1% for surgically treated cases.[93] Sick dogs or cats with metritis or pyometra should be treated aggressively with IV fluids and broad-spectrum parenteral antimicrobial drugs that have activity against gram-negative bacteria and anaerobes, such as a combination of clindamycin and a fluoroquinolone. Ovariohysterectomy is strongly recommended for animals with pyometra, and may need to be performed on an emergency basis to resolve sepsis or septic shock. Caution is required to avoid rupture of a distended or friable uterus during surgery, because this has been associated with increased mortality (<10% to around 50%). Risk factors for peritonitis in one study were leukopenia and abnormal rectal temperature.[93] Laparoscopic approaches have been described,[100] but these should be reserved for uncomplicated cases. Reevaluation should be performed 1 week after discharge from hospital, and should include physical examination, a CBC,

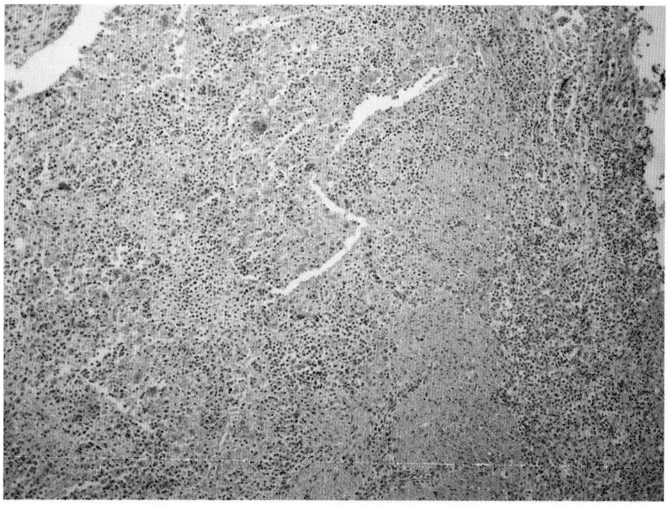

Fig. 127.10 Histopathology of the uterus from a 7-year-old female poodle with pyometra. The dog was seen for vomiting, inappetence, obtundation, nystagmus, collapse, and abdominal distention. The owner elected euthanasia. Severe, chronic, suppurative metritis with uterine perforation and septic peritonitis was found at necropsy. Aerobic and anaerobic bacterial culture of the abdominal fluid yielded mixed growth that consisted of *Escherichia coli* and a nonenteric gram-negative aerobic bacterial species, a *Bacteroides levii*-like anaerobe, *Bacteroides fragilis, Prevotella heparinolyticus, Fusobacterium nucleatum,* and *Peptostreptococcus anaerobius.* Hematoxylin and eosin stain.

biochemistry panel, and urinalysis. Usually, there is a rapid response to treatment and hematologic and biochemical abnormalities resolve within this time period. The white cell count may increase dramatically after surgery before it returns to normal. Antimicrobial drug treatment should be continued for 7 to 10 days after ovariohysterectomy.

In conjunction with antimicrobial drug treatment, medical treatment with natural or synthetic prostaglandin $F_{2\alpha}$ ($PGF_{2\alpha}$), which causes lysis of the corpora lutea, to expel uterine contents may be possible for dogs with open pyometra that are young (<6 years of age), and otherwise in good health (Table 127.4). Medical treatment for pyometra alone is not recommended for dogs that are systemically unwell, and the possibility of pregnancy must first be ruled out with ultrasound. Medical treatment is also less attractive for dogs with closed pyometra because: (1) it risks uterine rupture; (2) it is less effective than in dogs with open pyometra; and (3) dogs are often systemically unwell. However, it has been used with success in some dogs. Medical treatment is most likely to be successful in dogs that are in late diestrus (>5 weeks after the end of estrus). Improvement is generally not evident for at least 48 hours, and adverse reactions such as restlessness, hypersalivation, panting, vocalization, vomiting, diarrhea, mydriasis, and fever are common with $PGF_{2\alpha}$, so treatment should be given in the morning on an empty stomach, hospitalization and observation is recommended for at least 4 hours after the injection (or throughout the treatment period in dogs with closed pyometra), and the dose should be carefully calculated and be appropriate for the product used. Signs of shock may develop in some dogs treated with $PGF_{2\alpha}$. Walking dogs for 20 to 40 minutes after drug administration (while adverse effects

TABLE 127.4 Published Treatment Protocols for Medical Therapy of Pyometra in Dogs and Cats[101–104]

Drug	Dose[a]
Natural $PGF_{2\alpha}$ (Lutalyse)	0.1 mg/kg SC once (day 1), 0.2 mg/kg SC once (day 2), 0.25 mg/kg SC q24h (days 3 to 7)
Aglepristone	10 mg/kg SC once on days 1, 3, 6, and 9
Aglepristone and cloprostenol	Aglepristone: 10 mg/kg SC once on days 1, 2, and 8 Cloprostenol: 1 μg/kg SC for 5 days on days 3 through 7

[a]Day 1 = day of diagnosis.

occur) may lessen the adverse effects and also promotes close observation.[101] The severity of signs tends to decrease with each injection administered. Serial abdominal ultrasound examinations are recommended every 2 days during treatment for dogs with closed pyometra to evaluate for peritonitis. $PGF_{2\alpha}$ can also be used to treat postpartum metritis.

Aglepristone (RU534) is a progesterone receptor antagonist that is available in Europe for treatment of pyometra. Aglepristone appears to be a safe and effective alternative to $PGF_{2\alpha}$ in both dogs and cats.[102] Addition of low-dose cloprostenol (a synthetic $PGF_{2\alpha}$ derivative) to aglepristone in one study increased the success rate in dogs with open pyometra from 60% to 84%.[103] Aglepristone (10 mg/kg SC) has been administered at 0, 1, and 6 days after diagnosis. A modified protocol where aglepristone is administered at 0, 2, 5, and 8 days after diagnosis, together with a relatively short (6 days) duration of clavulanic acid-amoxicillin therapy was effective in all of 47 dogs, without the need for ovariohysterectomy, compared with 89% of 26 dogs using the traditional protocol.[104] No recurrence was noted in a 24-month follow-up period, and approximately 80% of dogs subsequently whelped.

All dogs treated medically should be re-evaluated 2 weeks after treatment. If signs of pyometra persist, culture of a swab specimen obtained from the cranial vaginal vault should be performed to determine if resistance to antimicrobials is present, and treatment should be repeated a second time or surgery performed. The measurement of serum progesterone to monitor effective treatment is not necessary because it does not change treatment recommendations. After successful treatment, the dog or cat should be bred at each subsequent cycle until pregnancy occurs. The chance that subsequent pregnancy will occur is over 80%, and the vast majority of dogs that respond go on to have more than one litter. Once the dog or cat is no longer required as a breeding animal, it should be neutered.

PREVENTION

Routine ovariohysterectomy reduces the risk of pyometra, although stump pyometra can still occur in neutered animals. There is no known treatment for CEH. Use of estrogens to treat mismatings is not recommended.

CASE EXAMPLE

Signalment

"Molly," a 6-year-old female spayed shih tzu mix from Sacramento, CA.

History

Molly was brought to the University of California, Davis VMTH for evaluation of recently diagnosed nephrolithiasis and hematuria. Three weeks previously, Molly's groomer noted blood on the towel she had been sitting on. The owners subsequently observed blood in Molly's urine and took her to their local veterinary clinic. There had been no stranguria, polyuria, polydipsia, or change in the frequency of urination. Blood work was performed in the clinic; the hematocrit was 56.5% and thrombocytopenia (86,000 platelets/μL) was present. A urine dipstick analysis revealed 2+ protein, a pH of 8, hematuria, and pyuria. The urine SpG was 1.014. A 3-cm opacity in the right renal pelvis that was consistent with a nephrolith was found on abdominal radiographs (see Fig. 127.4). The kidneys had a mildly irregular shape but were normal in size. Treatment with amoxicillin was initiated (23 mg/kg, PO, q12h for 10 days). After 12 days, the dog was evaluated for dental prophylaxis. A CBC showed a hematocrit of 50% and persistent thrombocytopenia (51,000 platelets/μL). An abdominal ultrasound (performed by a mobile board-certified veterinary radiologist) showed a 2.9-cm right renal pelvic calculus and a 7-mm left renal pelvic calculus. The kidneys were normal in size but had a mildly irregular shape. There was moderate thickening of the apical wall of the urinary bladder, with small (4 mm) apical polyp formation. Moderate flocculent suspended debris was present within the urine and multiple very small sand-like calculi were present. All other organs evaluated were within normal limits.

Other Medical History

There had been no history of vomiting, diarrhea, coughing, sneezing, or trauma. Molly had traveled frequently to Oregon and Nevada. There had been no change in her water consumption. She was fed a stone dissolution diet (Royal Canin Urinary SO), which had been prescribed 4 years ago when crystals were seen in her urine on urinalysis, as part of a wellness examination. She was also occasionally fed dog treats. She had been vaccinated for CDV, CAdV, CPV, and rabies; and *Bordetella bronchiseptica*, CCoV, leptospirosis, and Lyme disease. She was treated with imidacloprid and ivermectin for flea and heartworm prophylaxis, respectively, each month.

Physical Examination

Body weight: 10.8 kg.

General: Bright and alert, hydrated. T = 101.6°F (38.7°C), HR = 128 beats/minute, RR = 32 breaths/minute, mucous membranes pink and moist, CRT < 1 second.

Eyes, ears, nose, and throat: Mild epiphora bilaterally. There was mild dental calculus and gingivitis. Otherwise no clinically significant abnormalities were detected.

Integument: Abdomen clipped from previous ultrasound examination with healing clipper wounds. There was a 1-cm ecchymosis on the ventral abdomen.

Musculoskeletal: BCS 7/9. Ambulatory with normal gait.

Cardiovascular: Sinus arrhythmia. No murmurs auscultated. Femoral pulses strong and synchronous.

Genitourinary/GI: Soft, mildly painful abdomen. The bladder was moderate sized. Rectal examination was unremarkable. There was no vulvar discharge and no evidence of perivulvar dermatitis. A slightly recessed vulva was present.

Other systems, including peripheral lymph nodes: No clinically significant findings.

Laboratory Findings

CBC: HCT 49.1% (40%–55%), MCV 70.3 fL (65–75 fL), MCHC 35.0 g/dL (33–36 g/dL), nRBC 1/100 WBC, WBC 10,200 cells/μL (6,000–13,000 cells/μL), neutrophils 7,140 cells/μL (3,000–10,500 cells/μL), band neutrophils 102 cells/μL, lymphocytes 1,632 cells/μL (1,000–4,000 cells/μL), monocytes 816 cells/μL (150–1,200 cells/μL), platelets 12,000 platelets/μL (150,000–400,000 platelets/μL), MPV 21.6 fL (7–13 fL). Slight anisocytosis and many macroplatelets were reported on smear evaluation.

Serum chemistry profile: Sodium 148 mmol/L (145–154 mmol/L), potassium 4.0 mmol/L (3.6–5.3 mmol/L), chloride 111 mmol/L (108–118 mmol/L), bicarbonate 23 mmol/L (16–26 mmol/L), phosphorus 3.6 mg/dL (3.0–6.2 mg/dL), calcium 10.1 mg/dL (9.7–11.5 mg/dl), BUN 12 mg/dL (5–21 mg/dL), creatinine 0.9 mg/dL (0.3–1.2 mg/dL), glucose 92 mg/dL (64–123 mg/dL), total protein 6.1 g/dL (5.4–7.6 g/dL), albumin 3.4 g/dL (3.0–4.4 g/dL), globulin 2.7 g/dL (1.8–3.9 g/dL), ALT 42 U/L (19–67 U/L), AST 16 U/L (19–42 U/L), ALP 85 U/L (21–170 U/L), cholesterol 257 mg/dL (135–361 mg/dL), total bilirubin 0.1 mg/dL (0–0.2 mg/dL).

Urinalysis: SpG 1.013; pH 8.0, 2+ protein (SSA), 1+ bilirubin, 4+ hemoprotein, no glucose, no ketones, >100 WBC/HPF, 30–50 RBC/HPF, no crystals or casts, many rods, rafts of atypical transitional cells, many degenerated cells.

Coagulation panel: PT 9.9 seconds (7.5–10.5 seconds), PTT 8.4 seconds (9.0–12.0 seconds), fibrinogen 395 mg/dL (90–255 mg/dL).

Microbiologic Testing

Direct smear of urine: Moderate numbers of gram-negative rods and gram-positive cocci were visualized.

Aerobic bacterial urine culture and susceptibility (cystocentesis specimen): 10^5 CFU/mL *Proteus mirabilis*, *P. mirabilis* (non-swarming strain), and *Enterococcus faecalis*. Both *Proteus* spp. were resistant to ampicillin (≥256 μg/mL) but susceptible to clavulanic acid-amoxicillin (4 μg/mL), cephalexin (8 μg/mL), chloramphenicol (≤16 μg/mL), enrofloxacin (≤1 μg/mL), tetracycline (64 μg/mL), and trimethoprim-sulfamethoxazole (≤4 μg/mL). The *E. faecalis* was susceptible to ampicillin, clavulanic acid-amoxicillin (≤2 μg/mL), chloramphenicol (≤16 μg/mL), enrofloxacin (≤1 μg/mL), and tetracycline (16 μg/mL).

Diagnosis

Proteus mirabilis and *E. faecalis* cystitis and suspected pyelonephritis with nephrolithiasis, with possible secondary ITP.

Treatment

Molly was treated with enrofloxacin (7 mg/kg, PO, q24h). The following day her platelet count had increased to 31,000 platelets/μL, and by day 3 of treatment it was 64,000 platelets/μL. After 7 days of treatment, a CBC showed a neutrophil count of 5,700/μL, no band neutrophils, and the platelet count was 79,000 platelets/μL. A urine culture obtained by cystocentesis at this time showed 10^4 CFU/mL of *E. coli* and *E. faecalis*. The *E. coli* was resistant to ampicillin, cephalexin, enrofloxacin, tetracycline, and trimethoprim-sulfamethoxazole, but susceptible to clavulanic acid-amoxicillin (64 μg/mL). The susceptibility of the *E. faecalis* had not changed, with the exception that the MIC for tetracycline was 32 μg/mL. Treatment was changed to clavulanic acid-amoxicillin (23 mg/kg, PO, q12h). When re-evaluated 3 weeks later, she had no clinical signs of illness. A CBC showed only mild thrombocytopenia (146,000 platelets/μL, with an MPV of 12.6 fL). However, bacteria and large numbers of WBCs were still present in the urine sediment, the urine pH was 8.0, and *E. coli* with the same susceptibility pattern was again isolated from the urine. An extended panel showed susceptibility to amikacin (≤4 μg/mL) and imipenem-cilastatin (≤1 μg/mL), but resistance to cefazolin, cefoxitin, cefpodoxime, cephalothin, gentamicin, marbofloxacin, orbifloxacin, and ticarcillin-clavulanic acid. The dosage of clavulanic acid-amoxicillin was increased to 23 mg/kg, PO, q8h. The diet was changed to a stone dissolution diet. After an additional month, urinalysis findings were unchanged and the same *E. coli* was again isolated from the urine. The platelet count was 244,000 platelets/μL and a biochemistry panel was unremarkable. Abdominal radiographs and ultrasound showed no evidence of nephrolithiasis, but multiple small, rounded mineral opacities were present in the region of the right ureter.

Antimicrobial drug treatment was ultimately changed to amikacin (15 mg/kg, SC, q24h) 2 weeks later because an *E. coli* was isolated that was resistant to

CASE EXAMPLE—cont'd

clavulanic acid-amoxicillin. Kidney values were monitored every 2 weeks during amikacin treatment to evaluate for nephrotoxicity. The urine then became sterile and ultrasound examination showed disappearance of all urinary calculi over a 2-month period, after which antimicrobial drug treatment was discontinued and the diet was changed to a maintenance diet. Because of the recessed vulva and the dog's excess body condition, a weight loss program was discussed with the owner. Molly was diagnosed with a subclinical *Enterobacter aerogenes* UTI 2 months later, which was broadly susceptible to antimicrobial drugs and treated with enrofloxacin. The platelet count was within the reference range. Further evaluation for underlying conditions predisposing to recurrent UTI (contrast cystourethrography and cystoscopy), followed by vulvoplasty if no other abnormalities were detected, were offered to the owners but further treatment and evaluation was not pursued. The dog remained alive, untreated, and without clinical signs 4 years later, at which time hematology and biochemistry panel results were unremarkable, but MDR *E. coli* was repeatedly isolated from the urine.

Comments

This is an interesting case of bacterial cystitis and pyelonephritis associated with struvite nephrolithiasis, and probable secondary ITP. The struvite urolithiasis was likely secondary to the *P. mirabilis* infection. Months of antimicrobial treatment were necessary because of bacterial sequestration within urinary calculi. This may have explained continued isolation of bacteria from the urine in the face of antimicrobial drug treatment, although ultimately resolution of the *E. coli* infection quickly followed the change in antimicrobial drug choice. Meropenem would have been another appropriate choice based on the susceptibility of the organism isolated, but is often reserved for life-threatening infections in human patients. Fortunately, dissolution of the nephroliths occurred with antimicrobial and dietary therapy, and surgery to remove infected uroliths was not required. Continued UTI was a likely sequela in this dog in the absence of successful identification and treatment of an underlying cause. Although treatment of the UTI was necessary during nephrolith dissolution, treatment of the subclinical *E. aerogenes* infection may not have been necessary.

SUGGESTED READINGS

Weese JS, Blondeau J, Boothe D, et al. International Society for Companion Animal Infectious Diseases (ISCAID) guidelines for the diagnosis and management of bacterial urinary tract infections in dogs and cats. *Vet J.* 2019;247:8–25.

Hagman R. Canine pyometra: what is new? *Reprod Domest Anim.* 2017;52(suppl 2):288–292.

Klein RD, Hultgren SJ. Urinary tract infections: microbial pathogenesis, host-pathogen interactions and new treatment strategies. *Nat Rev Microbiol.* 2020;18:211–226.

REFERENCES

1. Weese JS, Blondeau J, Boothe D, et al. International Society for Companion Animal Infectious Diseases (ISCAID) guidelines for the diagnosis and management of bacterial urinary tract infections in dogs and cats. *Vet J.* 2019;247:8–25.
2. Wong C, Epstein SE, Westropp JL. Antimicrobial susceptibility patterns in urinary tract infections in dogs (2010-2013). *J Vet Intern Med.* 2015;29:1045–1052.
3. Seguin MA, Vaden SL, Altier C, et al. Persistent urinary tract infections and reinfections in 100 dogs (1989-1999). *J Vet Intern Med.* 2003;17:622–631.
4. Dhakal BK, Kulesus RR, Mulvey MA. Mechanisms and consequences of bladder cell invasion by uropathogenic *Escherichia coli. Eur J Clin Invest.* 2008;38(suppl 2):2–11.
5. Kern ZT, Jacob ME, Gilbertie JM, et al. Characteristics of dogs with biofilm-forming *Escherichia coli* urinary tract infections. *J Vet Intern Med.* 2018;32:1645–1651.
6. Segev G, Bankirer T, Steinberg D, et al. Evaluation of urinary catheters coated with sustained-release varnish of chlorhexidine in mitigating biofilm formation on urinary catheters in dogs. *J Vet Intern Med.* 2013;27:39–46.
7. Melican K, Sandoval RM, Kader A, et al. Uropathogenic *Escherichia coli* P and Type 1 fimbriae act in synergy in a living host to facilitate renal colonization leading to nephron obstruction. *PLoS Pathog.* 2011;7:e1001298.
8. Lane MC, Mobley HL. Role of P-fimbrial-mediated adherence in pyelonephritis and persistence of uropathogenic *Escherichia coli* (UPEC) in the mammalian kidney. *Kidney Int.* 2007;72:19–25.
9. Rocha SP, Pelayo JS, Elias WP. Fimbriae of uropathogenic *Proteus mirabilis. FEMS Immunol Med Microbiol.* 2007;51:1–7.
10. Weese JS, Blondeau JM, Boothe D, et al. Antimicrobial use guidelines for treatment of urinary tract disease in dogs and cats: Antimicrobial Guidelines Working Group of the International Society for Companion Animal Infectious Diseases. *Vet Med Int.* 2011;2011:263768.
11. Mayer-Roenne B, Goldstein RE, Erb HN. Urinary tract infections in cats with hyperthyroidism, diabetes mellitus and chronic kidney disease. *J Feline Med Surg.* 2007;9:124–132.
12. McGuire NC, Schulman R, Ridgway MD, et al. Detection of occult urinary tract infections in dogs with diabetes mellitus. *J Am Anim Hosp Assoc.* 2002;38:541–544.
13. Bailiff NL, Nelson RW, Feldman EC, et al. Frequency and risk factors for urinary tract infection in cats with diabetes mellitus. *J Vet Intern Med.* 2006;20:850–855.
14. Peterson AL, Torres SM, Rendahl A, et al. Frequency of urinary tract infection in dogs with inflammatory skin disorders treated with ciclosporin alone or in combination with glucocorticoid therapy: a retrospective study. *Vet Dermatol.* 2012;23:201–e43.
15. Torres SM, Diaz SF, Nogueira SA, et al. Frequency of urinary tract infection among dogs with pruritic disorders receiving long-term glucocorticoid treatment. *J Am Vet Med Assoc.* 2005;227:239–243.
16. Meindl AG, Lourenco BN, Coleman AE, et al. Relationships among urinary protein-to-creatinine ratio, urine specific gravity, and bacteriuria in canine urine samples. *J Vet Intern Med.* 2019;33:192–199.
17. Foster JD, Krishnan H, Cole S. Characterization of subclinical bacteriuria, bacterial cystitis, and pyelonephritis in dogs with chronic kidney disease. *J Am Vet Med Assoc.* 2018;252:1257–1262.
18. White JD, Cave NJ, Grinberg A, et al. Subclinical bacteriuria in older cats and its association with survival. *J Vet Intern Med.* 2016;30:1824–1829.
19. Delucchi L, Fraga M, Perelmuter K, et al. Vaginal lactic acid bacteria in healthy and ill bitches and evaluation of in vitro probiotic activity of selected isolates. *Can Vet J.* 2008;49:991–994.
20. Hutchins RG, Vaden SL, Jacob ME, et al. Vaginal microbiota of spayed dogs with or without recurrent urinary tract infections. *J Vet Intern Med.* 2014;28:300–304.
21. Ling GV, Norris CR, Franti CE, et al. Interrelations of organism prevalence, specimen collection method, and host age, sex, and breed among 8,354 canine urinary tract infections (1969-1995). *J Vet Intern Med.* 2001;15:341–347.
22. Buffington CA, Chew DJ, Kendall MS, et al. Clinical evaluation of cats with nonobstructive urinary tract diseases. *J Am Vet Med Assoc.* 1997;210:46–50.
23. Kruger JM, Osborne CA, Goyal SM, et al. Clinical evaluation of cats with lower urinary tract disease. *J Am Vet Med Assoc.* 1991;199:211–216.
24. Lekcharoensuk C, Osborne CA, Lulich JP. Epidemiologic study of risk factors for lower urinary tract diseases in cats. *J Am Vet Med Assoc.* 2001;218:1429–1435.

25. Eggertsdottir AV, Lund HS, Krontveit R, et al. Bacteriuria in cats with feline lower urinary tract disease: a clinical study of 134 cases in Norway. *J Feline Med Surg*. 2007;9:458–465.
26. Bailiff NL, Westropp JL, Nelson RW, et al. Evaluation of urine specific gravity and urine sediment as risk factors for urinary tract infections in cats. *Vet Clin Pathol*. 2008;37:317–322.
27. Peterson ME, Li A, Soboroff P, et al. Hyperthyroidism is not a risk factor for subclinical bacteriuria in cats: a prospective cohort study. *J Vet Intern Med*. 2020;34:1157–1165.
28. Bailiff NL, Westropp JL, Jang SS, et al. *Corynebacterium urealyticum* urinary tract infection in dogs and cats: 7 cases (1996 2003). *J Am Vet Med Assoc*. 2005;226:1676–1680.
29. Gomez A, Nombela C, Zapardiel J, et al. An encrusted cystitis caused by *Corynebacterium urealyticum* in a dog. *Aust Vet J*. 1995;72:72–73.
30. Cavana P, Zanatta R, Nebbia P, et al. *Corynebacterium urealyticum* urinary tract infection in a cat with urethral obstruction. *J Feline Med Surg*. 2008;10:269–273.
31. Maurey C, Boulouis HJ, Canonne-Guibert M, et al. Clinical description of *Corynebacterium urealyticum* urinary tract infections in 11 dogs and 10 cats. *J Small Anim Pract*. 2019;60:239–246.
32. Merkel LK, Lulich J, Polzin D, et al. Clinicopathologic and microbiologic findings associated with emphysematous cystitis in 27 dogs. *J Am Anim Hosp Assoc*. 2017;53:313–320.
33. Sherding RG, Chew DJ. Nondiabetic emphysematous cystitis in two dogs. *J Am Vet Med Assoc*. 1979;174:1105–1109.
34. Middleton DJ, Lomas GR. Emphysematous cystitis due to *Clostridium perfringens* in a non-diabetic dog. *J Small Anim Pract*. 1979;20:433–438.
35. Morello W, La Scola C, Alberici I, et al. Acute pyelonephritis in children. *Pediatr Nephrol*. 2016;31:1253–1265.
36. Sim JH, Yim HE, Choi BM, et al. Plasma neutrophil gelatinase-associated lipocalin predicts acute pyelonephritis in children with urinary tract infections. *Pediatr Res*. 2015;78:48–55.
37. Yim HE, Yim H, Bae ES, et al. Predictive value of urinary and serum biomarkers in young children with febrile urinary tract infections. *Pediatr Nephrol*. 2014;29:2181–2189.
38. van der Starre WE, Zunder SM, Vollaard AM, et al. Prognostic value of pro-adrenomedullin, procalcitonin and C-reactive protein in predicting outcome of febrile urinary tract infection. *Clin Microbiol Infect*. 2014;20:1048–1054.
39. Zhang H, Yang J, Lin L, et al. Diagnostic value of serum procalcitonin for acute pyelonephritis in infants and children with urinary tract infections: an updated meta-analysis. *World J Urol*. 2016;34:431–441.
40. Hokamp JA, Nabity MB. Renal biomarkers in domestic species. *Vet Clin Pathol*. 2016;45:28–56.
41. Palm CA, Segev G, Cowgill LD, et al. Urinary neutrophil gelatinase-associated lipocalin as a marker for identification of acute kidney injury and recovery in dogs with gentamicin-induced nephrotoxicity. *J Vet Intern Med*. 2016;30:200–205.
42. Sørensen TM, Bjørnvad CR, Cordoba G, et al. Effects of diagnostic work-up on medical decision-making for canine urinary tract infection: an observational study in Danish small animal practices. *J Vet Intern Med*. 2018;32:743–751.
43. D'Anjou MA, Bedard A, Dunn ME. Clinical significance of renal pelvic dilatation on ultrasound in dogs and cats. *Vet Radiol Ultrasound*. 2011;52:88–94.
44. Choi J, Jang J, Choi H, et al. Ultrasonographic features of pyonephrosis in dogs. *Vet Radiol Ultrasound*. 2010;51:548–553.
45. Lawrentschuk N, Ooi J, Pang A, et al. Cystoscopy in women with recurrent urinary tract infection. *Int J Urol*. 2006;13:350–353.
46. Pagano MJ, Barbalat Y, Theofanides MC, et al. Diagnostic yield of cystoscopy in the evaluation of recurrent urinary tract infection in women. *Neurourol Urodyn*. 2017;36:692–696.
47. Pagano MJ, Barbalat Y, Theofanides MC, et al. Diagnostic yield of cystoscopy in the evaluation of recurrent urinary tract infection in women. *Neurourology Urodynamics*. 2017;36:692–696.
48. Llido M, Vachon C, Dickinson M, et al. Transurethral cystoscopy in dogs with recurrent urinary tract infections: retrospective study (2011-2018). *J Vet Intern Med*. 2020;34:790–796.
49. Hsieh E, Westropp J, Palm C, et al. Diagnostic yield of cystoscopy compared to ultrasonography for evaluating lower urinary tract disorders in dogs. *J Vet Intern Med (abstr NU01)*. 2021. ACVIM Forum Research Abstract Program. p3061.
50. Gatoria IS, Saini NS, Rai TS, et al. Comparison of three techniques for the diagnosis of urinary tract infections in dogs with urolithiasis. *J Small Anim Pract*. 2006;47:727–732.
51. Borys MA, Hulsebosch SE, Mohr FC, et al. Clinical, histopathologic, cystoscopic, and fluorescence in situ hybridization analysis of proliferative urethritis in 22 dogs. *J Vet Intern Med*. 2019;33:184–191.
52. Cohn LA, Gary AT, Fales WH, et al. Trends in fluoroquinolone resistance of bacteria isolated from canine urinary tracts. *J Vet Diagn Invest*. 2003;15:338–343.
53. Ball KR, Rubin JE, Chirino-Trejo M, et al. Antimicrobial resistance and prevalence of canine uropathogens at the Western College of Veterinary Medicine Veterinary Teaching Hospital, 2002-2007. *Can Vet J*. 2008;49:985–990.
54. Ybarra WL, Sykes JE, Wang Y, et al. Performance of a veterinary urine dipstick paddle system for diagnosis and identification of urinary tract infections in dogs and cats. *J Am Vet Med Assoc*. 2014;244:814–819.
55. Jacob ME, Crowell MD, Fauls MB, et al. Diagnostic accuracy of a rapid immunoassay for point of-care detection of urinary tract infection in dogs. *Am J Vet Res*. 2016;77:162–166.
56. Sutter C, Dear J, Pires J, et al. Evaluation of a rapid immunoassay for detection of UTI in dogs. *J Vet Intern Med. (abstr NU21)*. 2021. ACVIM Forum Research Abstract Program. p3070.
57. Westropp JL, Sykes JE, Irom S, et al. Evaluation of the efficacy and safety of a high dose short duration enrofloxacin treatment regimen for uncomplicated urinary tract infections in dogs. *J Vet Intern Med*. 2012;26:506–512.
58. Clare S, Hartmann FA, Jooss M, et al. Short- and long-term cure rates of short-duration trimethoprim-sulfamethoxazole treatment in female dogs with uncomplicated bacterial cystitis. *J Vet Intern Med*. 2014;28:818–826.
59. Lightner BA, McLoughlin MA, Chew DJ, et al. Episioplasty for the treatment of perivulvar dermatitis or recurrent urinary tract infections in dogs with excessive perivulvar skin folds: 31 cases (1983-2000). *J Am Vet Med Assoc*. 2001;219:1577–1581.
60. Abdullahi SU, Osborne CA, Leininger JR, et al. Evaluation of a calculolytic diet in female dogs with induced struvite urolithiasis. *Am J Vet Res*. 1984;45:1508–1519.
61. Flannigan R, Choy WH, Chew B, et al. Renal struvite stones: pathogenesis, microbiology, and management strategies. *Nat Rev Urol*. 2014;11:333–341.
62. Wan SY, Hartmann FA, Jooss MK, et al. Prevalence and clinical outcome of subclinical bacteriuria in female dogs. *J Am Vet Med Assoc*. 2014;245:106–112.
63. Rafatpanah Baigi S, Vaden S, Olby NJ. The frequency and clinical implications of bacteriuria in chronically paralyzed dogs. *J Vet Intern Med*. 2017;31:1790–1795.
64. Kopecny L, Palm CA, Drobatz KJ, et al. Risk factors for positive urine cultures in cats with subcutaneous ureteral bypass and ureteral stents (2010-2016). *J Vet Intern Med*. 2019;33:178–183.
65. Bubenik LJ, Hosgood GL, Waldron DR, et al. Frequency of urinary tract infection in catheterized dogs and comparison of bacterial culture and susceptibility testing results for catheterized and noncatheterized dogs with urinary tract infections. *J Am Vet Med Assoc*. 2007;231:893–899.
66. Sihra N, Goodman A, Zakri R, et al. Nonantibiotic prevention and management of recurrent urinary tract infection. *Nat Rev Urol*. 2018;15:750–776.
67. Vostalova J, Vidlar A, Simanek V, et al. Are high proanthocyanidins key to cranberry efficacy in the prevention of recurrent urinary tract infection? *Phytother Res*. 2015;29:1559–1567.
68. Olby NJ, Vaden SL, Williams K, et al. Effect of cranberry extract on the frequency of bacteriuria in dogs with acute thoracolumbar disk herniation: a randomized controlled clinical trial. *J Vet Intern Med*. 2017;31:60–68.
69. Segev G, Sykes JE, Klumpp DJ, et al. Evaluation of the live biotherapeutic product, asymptomatic bacteriuria *Escherichia coli* 2-12, in healthy dogs and dogs with clinical recurrent UTI. *J Vet Intern Med*. 2018;32:267–273.
70. Chen YM, Wright PJ, Lee CS, et al. Uropathogenic virulence factors in isolates of *Escherichia coli* from clinical cases of canine pyometra and feces of healthy bitches. *Vet Microbiol*. 2003;94:57–69.

71. Kurazono H, Nakano M, Yamamoto S, et al. Distribution of the usp gene in uropathogenic *Escherichia coli* isolated from companion animals and correlation with serotypes and size-variations of the pathogenicity island. *Microbiol Immunol.* 2003;47:797–802.
72. Wilson RA, Keefe TJ, Davis MA, et al. Strains of *Escherichia coli* associated with urogenital disease in dogs and cats. *Am J Vet Res.* 1988;49:743–746.
73. Roura X, Camps-Palau MA, Lloret A, et al. Bacterial prostatitis in a cat. *J Vet Intern Med.* 2002;16:593–597.
74. Alonge S, Melandri M, Aiudi G, et al. Advances in prostatic diagnostics in dogs: the role of canine prostatic specific esterase in the early diagnosis of prostatic disorders. *Top Companion Anim Med.* 2018;33:105–108.
75. Feeney DA, Johnston GR, Klausner JS, et al. Canine prostatic disease: comparison of radiographic appearance with morphologic and microbiologic findings: 30 cases (1981-1985). *J Am Vet Med Assoc.* 1987;190:1018–1026.
76. Bradbury CA, Westropp JL, Pollard RE. Relationship between prostatomegaly, prostatic mineralization, and cytologic diagnosis. *Vet Radiol Ultrasound.* 2009;50:167–171.
77. Feeney DA, Johnston GR, Klausner JS, et al. Canine prostatic disease: comparison of ultrasonographic appearance with morphologic and microbiologic findings: 30 cases (1981-1985). *J Am Vet Med Assoc.* 1987;190:1027–1034.
78. Lee CB, Ha US, Yim SH, et al. Does finasteride have a preventive effect on chronic bacterial prostatitis? Pilot study using an animal model. *Urol Int.* 2011;86:204–209.
79. Siqueira AK, Ribeiro MG, Leite Dda S, et al. Virulence factors in *Escherichia coli* strains isolated from urinary tract infection and pyometra cases and from feces of healthy dogs. *Res Vet Sci.* 2009;86:206–210.
80. Fiamengo TE, Runcan EE, Premanandan C, et al. Evaluation of biofilm production by *Escherichia coli* isolated from clinical cases of canine pyometra. *Top Companion Anim Med.* 2020;39:100429.
81. Whitehead ML. Risk of pyometra in bitches treated for mismating with low doses of oestradiol benzoate. *Vet Rec.* 2008;162:746–749.
82. Tsioli VG, Gouletsou PG, Loukopoulos P, et al. Uterine leiomyosarcoma and pyometra in a dog. *J Small Anim Pract.* 2011;52:121–124.
83. Spoljaric B, Vince S, Folnozic I, et al. Endometrial mucinous adenocarcinoma in a bitch with pyometra: a case report. *Top Companion Anim Med.* 2019;36:16–21.
84. Hernandez JL, Besso JG, Rault DN, et al. Emphysematous pyometra in a dog. *Vet Radiol Ultrasound.* 2003;44:196–198.
85. Thilagar S, Vinita WP, Heng HG, et al. What is your diagnosis? Small intestinal and colonic obstruction; emphysematous pyometra. *J Small Anim Pract.* 2006;47:687–688.
86. Chang J, Jung J, Jeong Y, et al. What is your diagnosis? Emphysematous pyometra with a large amount of gas. *J Small Anim Pract.* 2007;48:717–719.
87. Mattei C, Fabbi M, Hansson K. Radiographic and ultrasonographic findings in a dog with emphysematous pyometra. *Acta Vet Scand.* 2018;60:67.
88. Jitpean S, Hagman R, Strom Holst B, et al. Breed variations in the incidence of pyometra and mammary tumours in Swedish dogs. *Reprod Domest Anim.* 2012;47(suppl 6):347–350.
89. Egenvall A, Hagman R, Bonnett BN, et al. Breed risk of pyometra in insured dogs in Sweden. *J Vet Intern Med.* 2001;15:530–538.
90. Niskanen M, Thrusfield MV. Associations between age, parity, hormonal therapy and breed, and pyometra in Finnish dogs. *Vet Rec.* 1998;143:493–498.
91. Jitpean S, Ambrosen A, Emanuelson U, et al. Closed cervix is associated with more severe illness in dogs with pyometra. *BMC Vet Res.* 2017;13:11.
92. Maddens B, Heiene R, Smets P, et al. Evaluation of kidney injury in dogs with pyometra based on proteinuria, renal histomorphology, and urinary biomarkers. *J Vet Intern Med.* 2011;25:1075–1083.
93. Jitpean S, Strom-Holst B, Emanuelson U, et al. Outcome of pyometra in female dogs and predictors of peritonitis and prolonged postoperative hospitalization in surgically treated cases. *BMC Vet Res.* 2014;10:6.
94. Rota A, Pregel P, Cannizzo FT, et al. Unusual case of uterine stump pyometra in a cat. *J Feline Med Surg.* 2011;13:448–450.
95. Mathews KD, Hardy B, Johnson EG, et al. Ultrasonographic evaluation of uterine stump size in ovariohysterectomized dogs receiving estriol compared to control dogs. *Top Companion Anim Med.* 2020;38:100370.
96. Roth L, Tyler RD. Evaluation of low sodium:potassium ratios in dogs. *J Vet Diagn Invest.* 1999;11:60–64.
97. Pak SI. The clinical implication of sodium-potassium ratios in dogs. *J Vet Sci.* 2000;1:61–65.
98. Bigliardi E, Parmigiani E, Cavirani S, et al. Ultrasonography and cystic hyperplasia-pyometra complex in the bitch. *Reprod Domest Anim.* 2004;39:136–140.
99. Batista PR, Gobello C, Rube A, et al. Uterine blood flow evaluation in bitches suffering from cystic endometrial hyperplasia (CEH) and CEH-pyometra complex. *Theriogenology.* 2016;85:1258–1261.
100. Wallace ML, Case JB, Singh A, et al. Single incision, laparoscopic-assisted ovariohysterectomy for mucometra and pyometra in dogs. *Vet Surg.* 2015;44(suppl 1):66–70.
101. Feldman EC, Nelson RW. Cystic endometrial hyperplasia/pyometra complex. In: *Canine and Feline Endocrinology and Reproduction.* 3rd ed. Philadelphia, PA: Elsevier Science; 2004.
102. Nak D, Nak Y, Tuna B. Follow-up examinations after medical treatment of pyometra in cats with the progesterone-antagonist aglepristone. *J Feline Med Surg.* 2009;11:499–502.
103. Fieni F. Clinical evaluation of the use of aglepristone, with or without cloprostenol, to treat cystic endometrial hyperplasia-pyometra complex in bitches. *Theriogenology.* 2006;66:1550–1556.
104. Contri A, Gloria A, Carluccio A, et al. Effectiveness of a modified administration protocol for the medical treatment of canine pyometra. *Vet Res Commun.* 2015;39:1–5.

128

Ocular Infections

Jean Stiles

KEY POINTS

- Infections of the eye can involve the ocular surface and adnexal structures, intraocular structures, or both.
- Infections of the ocular surface and adnexal structures often result from invasion by commensals when normal barriers are disrupted, and include infectious blepharitis, conjunctivitis, keratitis, dacryocystitis, and orbital infection.
- Intraocular infections may arise secondary to local injury or occur as part of a systemic process. A large number of viruses, bacteria, fungi, protozoa, and helminths can cause intraocular disease. Sometimes ocular abnormalities are the only outward clinical manifestation of systemic infectious disease.
- Examination of specimens from ocular tissues or ocular fluids can facilitate diagnosis of ocular infectious diseases, and may assist in the diagnosis of systemic infections.
- Treatment of ocular disorders typically involves topical administration of antimicrobials and anti-inflammatory drugs, as well as specific therapy that is directed at underlying causes. Systemic antimicrobial drugs or glucocorticoids are occasionally required.

INFECTIONS OF THE OCULAR SURFACE AND ADNEXA

ETIOLOGY, EPIDEMIOLOGY, AND PATHOGENESIS

Most surface bacterial infections follow other debilitating conditions that potentiate the pathogenicity of organisms that are indigenous to the ocular surface. Despite the fact that all dogs probably have indigenous bacteria in their conjunctival cul-de-sac, bacterial isolation rates of between 46% and 91% have been reported from apparently healthy dogs (Table 128.1). Variations in the type and frequency of isolates may be a result of geography, culture technique, breed, and season. Fungi are isolated from the conjunctival sac of 10 to 22% of dogs.[1,2]

Cats have a relatively lower prevalence of cultivable bacteria in their conjunctival sacs.[3] Bacteria or mycoplasmas have been isolated from 34% of conjunctival specimens and 25% of lid margin specimens. In one study of 50 cats (100 eyes), no organisms were isolated from 42% of the cats, bacteria were isolated from the conjunctival sacs of 34% of cats (47% of eyes), and fungi were isolated from 26% of the cats (14% of eyes) (Table 128.2). No anaerobes were isolated.[4]

Abnormalities that contribute to local nidi of infection, such as those of the nasolacrimal (NL) system and meibomian glands or structures adjacent to the eye (ears, lip folds), should be sought and corrected to overcome persistent or recurring infection. Control of the resident ocular flora of clinically healthy animals is maintained by rinsing of the ocular surface with tears and blinking, which directs tears into the NL system. Tears also contain IgA and other antibacterial substances such as lactoferrin and lysozyme. Competitive interactions among the indigenous flora keep the numbers of organisms lower, whereas disrupting this balance may cause an overgrowth of one species. Conditions that damage the ocular surface, such as keratoconjunctivitis sicca (KCS), ultraviolet or other radiation, immune suppression, and trauma can allow indigenous bacteria to adhere and proliferate to produce disease. To become established, bacteria must adhere, replicate, and then invade the tissue. Invasion subsequently incites inflammation. Tissue damage results from a combination of pathogen toxins and enzymes such as collagenase, elastase, and cathepsins that are liberated by the neutrophilic response.[5] Bacteria that produce proteolytic enzymes such as *Pseudomonas aeruginosa* typically cause rapidly progressive "melting" corneal ulcers.

CLINICAL FEATURES AND TREATMENT

Blepharitis

Dogs

Blepharitis (inflammation of the eyelids) can develop secondary to bacterial, fungal, or parasitic infection. Blepharitis can result from other dermatologic diseases, and sometimes may occur in conjunction with ocular diseases, such as conjunctivitis. Allergic skin disease was the most common underlying cause in 102 dogs from Germany with blepharitis (52% of dogs), followed by infectious/parasitic disease (22%), autoimmune disease (18%), and neoplasia (5%).[6] Brachycephalic breeds were at risk for blepharitis when compared to the hospital population. Infectious diseases were demodicosis, leishmaniosis, and dermatophytosis. Parasitic infection of the eyelids was always accompanied by periocular dermatitis. Secondary bacterial infection of the eyelids may occur with any of these conditions, as well as with KCS. *Staphylococcus* spp. can cause primary blepharitis and can also generate a hypersensitivity reaction. Pruritis can lead to self-trauma, which exacerbates the blepharitis. In a 2020 study, *Staphylococcus pseudintermedius* was isolated from 38 (40%) of 72 dogs and 24 cats with conjunctivitis/blepharitis, keratitis, or uveitis, and 3 (8%) of the 38 isolates were methicillin-resistant; 2 of the isolates were from dogs with conjunctivitis/blepharitis.[7]

Clinical features of blepharitis include eyelid swelling, erythema, skin ulceration, chalazia (granulomatous foci of inflammation along meibomian glands), pruritis, and ocular discharge (serous or purulent) (Fig. 128.1).

Treatment of bacterial blepharitis should include cleansing the skin with a povidone-iodine solution (1:50 dilution) and application of a broad-spectrum ophthalmic antibiotic ointment to affected skin and the eye q6-8h. If the skin is very inflamed, a product that contains an antibiotic and dexamethasone is indicated. Severe blepharitis may require systemic antibiotic therapy such as a cephalosporin

TABLE 128.1 Bacteria Isolated from the Conjunctival Sacs of Apparently Healthy Dogs[50,51]

Organism	% of Positive Specimens[a]
Staphylococcus spp.	57–70
Coagulase-positive	24–45
Coagulase-negative	46–55
Streptococcus spp.	6–43
Nonhemolytic	12–51
α-Hemolytic	4–34
β-Hemolytic	2–7
Corynebacterium spp.	30–75
Undifferentiated	11
Corynebacterium pseudodiphtheriticum	9
Corynebacterium xerosis	13
Neisseria spp.	26
Undifferentiated	4
Neisseria catarrhalis	9
Neisseria pharyngis	4
Neisseria sicca	3
Neisseria caviae	3
Neisseria lactamica	3
Neisseria flavescens	3
Pseudomonas spp.	14
Moraxella spp.	7
Bacillus spp.	6–18

[a]Percentages are based on the numbers of animals from which organisms were isolated.

TABLE 128.2 Bacterial and Fungal Isolates from Ocular Tissues of Apparently Healthy Cats[3,4]

Location	Organism	% of Positive Specimens[a]
Conjunctiva	*Staphylococcus spp.*	27
	Corynebacterium spp.	1.3–5
	Bacillus spp.	3–5
	Streptococcus spp.	2–2.5
	Mycoplasma	0–5
	Fungal isolates	13
Lids	*Staphylococcus spp.*	23–28
	Streptococcus spp.	0–2
	Bacillus spp.	2–5
	Corynebacterium spp.	1.6

[a]Percentages are based on the numbers of animals from which organisms were isolated.

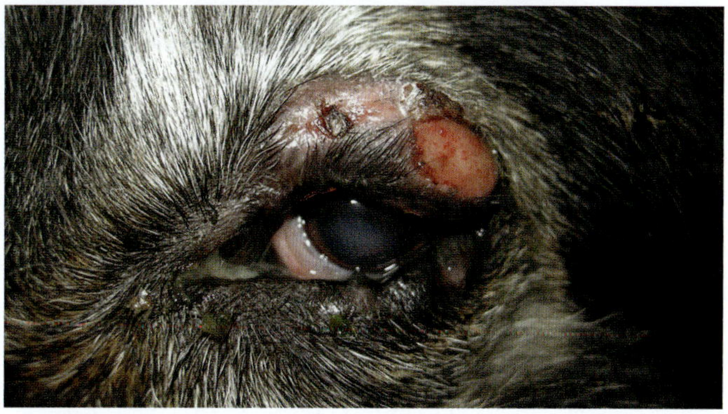

Fig. 128.1 Blepharitis in a dog. Note swelling, erythema, and ulceration of eyelids. Purulent ocular discharge is present at the medial canthus.

and possibly anti-inflammatory doses of an oral glucocorticoid. Oral prednisone at anti-inflammatory to immunosuppressive doses was not found to influence tear production in healthy dogs and those with histamine-induced conjunctivitis.[8] Any underlying condition that can be identified should be addressed. Failure of severe blepharitis to respond to antimicrobial therapy should prompt specimen collection for culture and susceptibility testing.

Canine juvenile pyoderma or cellulitis, which typically develops in puppies aged 3 to 16 weeks, often involves the conjunctiva and eyelids (Fig. 128.2). Four of the 102 dogs in the German study had juvenile cellulitis as the underlying cause of blepharitis.[6] Although the cause is unknown, the response to treatment suggests it to be immune-mediated. Pustules and pyogranulomatous inflammation develop in the eyelids, face, and ears. Conjunctivitis is usually present. Mandibular lymphadenomegaly is common. Puppies may be febrile and have generalized malaise. Swelling of joints or metaphyses may also be observed. Diagnosis is based on age, history, and clinical signs. Prednisolone (1 mg/kg PO q12h) should be administered for 2 to 3 weeks. An oral antibiotic may be used if skin infection is suspected. A topical preparation such as neomycin-polymyxin B-dexamethasone q6-8h is indicated for conjunctivitis. Lesions typically improve within a few days of beginning therapy and resolve completely within 3 weeks.

Cats

Cats appear relatively resistant to bacterial blepharitis, except when they have a traumatic injury and resulting bacterial invasion. This type of injury most commonly occurs in cat fights and can involve the head and eyelids. Abscesses near the eyelids should be drained and appropriate systemic antibiotics administered. *Leishmania infantum* can cause blepharitis in cats in endemic areas.[9]

Conjunctivitis

Dogs

Bacterial conjunctivitis can be a primary condition or secondary to another ocular condition such as KCS, entropion or trichiasis, CDV infection, parasites (e.g., *Thelazia* spp.), trauma, or foreign bodies. Primary bacterial conjunctivitis typically occurs for unknown reasons and in some cases is secondary to an insult that is no longer apparent or is merely an overgrowth of resident conjunctival microflora. Clinical signs are purulent discharge and conjunctival hyperemia with mild to moderate discomfort. Diagnosis should be based on cytologic examination of the exudate and identification of bacteria and neutrophilic inflammation. Because bacterial overgrowth occurs when tear production is low, KCS should be ruled out based on a normal Schirmer tear test result. Culture and susceptibility testing should be performed, especially if the response to therapy is poor or the problem is recurrent. A complete ocular exam, including a Schirmer tear test, fluorescein staining of the cornea, fluorescein evaluation of NL duct patency, and a search for a foreign body in the conjunctival sac and behind the third eyelid, should be performed. Therapy should include a broad-spectrum topical antibiotic such as bacitracin-neomycin-polymyxin B or tobramycin q6h until resolution.

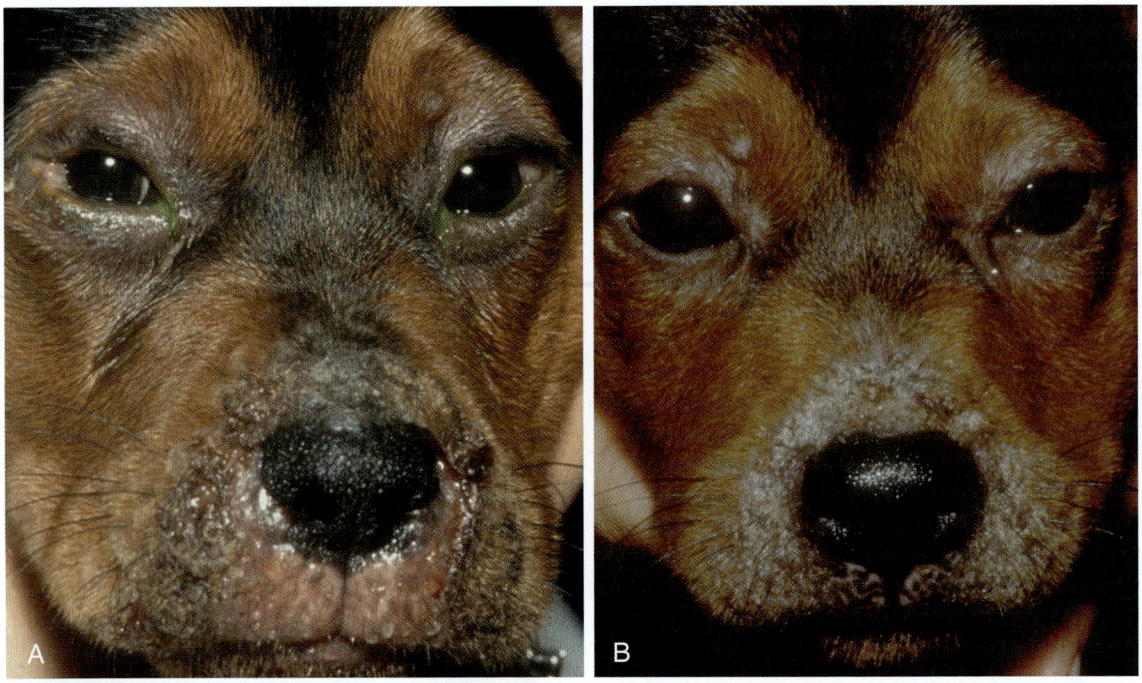

Fig. 128.2 Juvenile pyoderma in a puppy. (A) Ulcerative pyogranulomatous dermatitis of the muzzle and eyelids is evident, including conjunctivitis. (B) Appearance of lesions 2 weeks after being treated with oral prednisolone and cephalexin.

Viral conjunctivitis in dogs has been associated most often with CDV infection (see Chapter 22). The first sign of distemper is often a bilateral conjunctivitis with a serous to mucopurulent ocular discharge. Lacrimal adenitis may result in reduced tear production, which in turn results in more profound signs of conjunctivitis, corneal ulceration, and pain. The KCS typically resolves over several weeks in dogs that recover. Treatment should include regular cleaning of the eye, application of a broad-spectrum topical antibiotic to help prevent secondary bacterial infection, and, if KCS is present, topical cyclosporine or tacrolimus along with artificial tears.

CHV has been documented as a cause of severe conjunctivitis and ulcerative keratitis in a group of 3- to 4-month-old laboratory dogs following recovery from uncharacterized upper respiratory tract disease.[10] In a study of adult dogs experimentally infected with CHV using an ocular route, only self-limiting mild conjunctivitis was noted.[11] In client-owned dogs with and without idiopathic conjunctivitis, CHV or CAdV-2 were found in 23.3% of affected dogs and 0% of clinically healthy dogs.[12] Topically applied 1% prednisolone acetate solution did not reactivate latent herpes virus infection;[13] however, systemic administration of prednisolone at immunosuppressive doses resulted in reactivation of ocular illness and shedding of virus.[14] If CHV is suspected or documented as a cause of conjunctivitis, a topical antiviral agent should be used (see Table 9.5) (see also Chapter 24). Topical 1% trifluridine, topical 0.5% cidofovir, and topical 0.15% ganciclovir gel have been shown to be effective.[15–17]

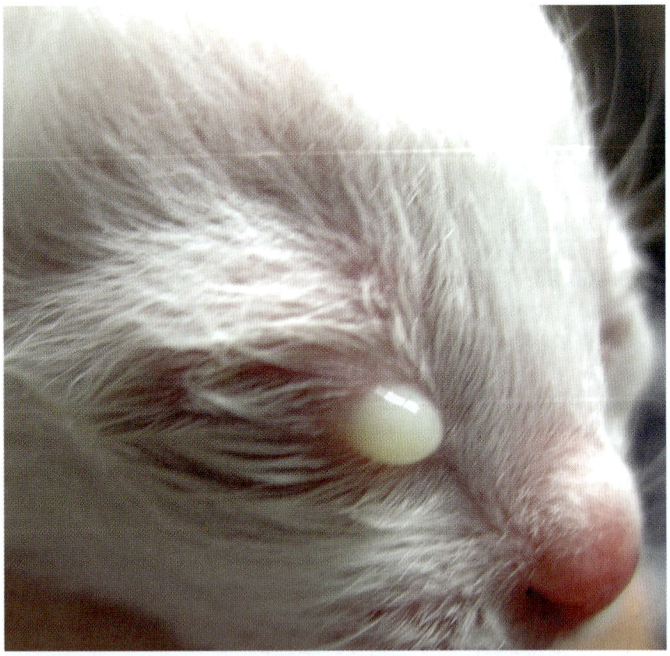

Fig. 128.3 Neonatal conjunctivitis in a 7-day-old kitten. Purulent discharge was evident as the medial-most aspect of the eyelids was opened. *Pasteurella multocida* was cultured. Virus isolation was negative.

Cats

Neonatal conjunctivitis can occur in cats secondary to bacterial or viral infection. If infection occurs before the opening of the eyelids, at approximately 10 days of age, purulent material accumulates, causing a characteristic distended appearance to the adherent eyelids. In such cases, the eyelids should be opened by inserting a small scissor blade at the medial canthus and gently sliding it along the lid margins. Copious purulent discharge usually follows (Fig. 128.3). The exudate can be submitted for cytologic examination as well as bacterial culture and PCR assays for respiratory pathogens to aid in identification of pathogens that may be present. A broad-spectrum topical antibiotic should be used several times daily. A topical antiviral agent should also be used in cases suspected to be caused by FHV-1 (see Chapters 9 and 34 and Table 9.5).

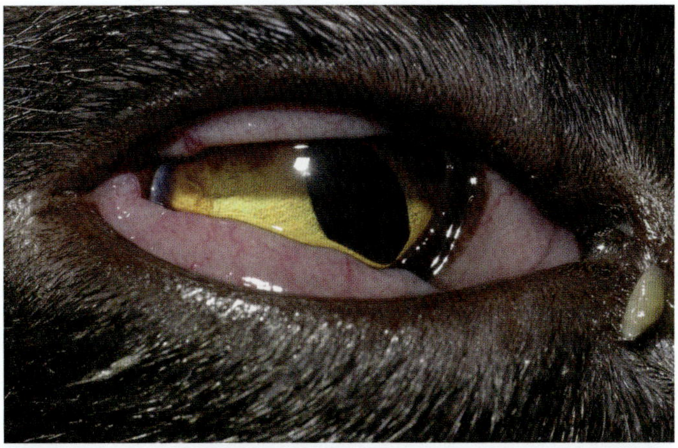

Fig. 128.4 Conjunctivitis in a cat caused by FHV-1. Note the hyperemia, chemosis, and purulent ocular discharge.

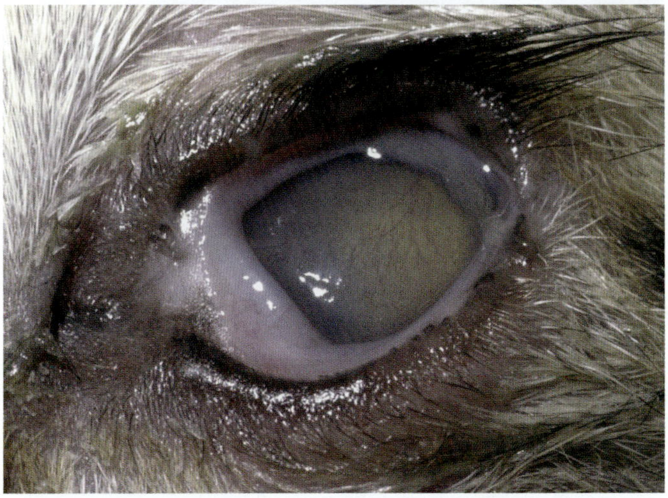

Fig. 128.5 Chronic symblepharon in a kitten secondary to FHV-1 infection. Note circumferential conjunctival adhesions and corneal vascularization.

FHV-1 is a frequent cause of ocular disease in cats. Young cats with respiratory tract disease generally have conjunctivitis with marked conjunctival hyperemia, chemosis, and serous to purulent ocular discharge (Fig. 128.4). Cats typically recover in 2 to 3 weeks. In severe cases of FHV-1 conjunctivitis, the risk of symblepharon, or adhesions of the conjunctiva to itself or the cornea, is high (Fig. 128.5). Symblepharon occurs when areas of conjunctival and corneal epithelial ulceration are present as a result of the cytopathic nature of FHV-1. Symblepharon may lead to permanent visual impairment, and an attempt to break these adhesions early should be made. After application of topical anesthesia, a cotton-tip swab or small forceps can be used to break adhesions and strip off cellular debris and fibrin. This process may need to be repeated frequently until the conjunctivitis has resolved. A topical or oral antiherpesvirus drug should be administered (see Table 9.5). In addition to general supportive care, the eyes should be cleansed frequently and a broad-spectrum topical antibiotic applied to minimize secondary bacterial infection as the conjunctival surface sloughs. Once infected, cats become latent carriers of FHV-1 and may have recurrences of ocular disease, including conjunctivitis and corneal ulcers. Many cats have transient episodes of conjunctivitis, with conjunctival hyperemia, serous or purulent ocular discharge, and blepharospasm. Mild cases that are self-limiting may not require treatment. If the conjunctivitis is painful or lasts more than a few days, antiviral therapy should be instituted.

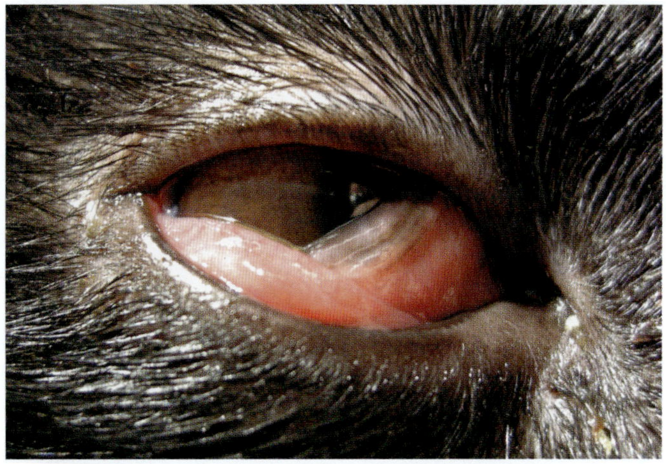

Fig. 128.6 Severe conjunctivitis in a cat associated with feline calicivirus infection.

Cats can develop chronic conjunctivitis associated with FHV-1 infection.[18] When conjunctivitis becomes chronic, the inflammation needs to be treated. Glucocorticoids should not be used because of the potential to exacerbate an underlying FHV-1 infection. A topical NSAID such as diclofenac used concurrently with a topical antiviral drug such as cidofovir appears to be both effective and safe.

IFN-α and IFN-ω have significant inhibitory effects on FHV-1 *in vitro* at relatively high doses (see Chapter 9).[19,20] High doses of topical IFNs have been used with some success in human ocular herpetic infections.[21,22] However, in a study of naturally occurring viral keratoconjunctivitis in cats, treatment with high dose (10^6 U/mL) IFNs-α and -ω q12h for 14 days failed to lessen severity or duration of clinical signs.[23] In general, studies to date have not supported a beneficial effect of IFNs for treatment of feline herpesvirus infections.[24]

The use of oral famciclovir for treating FHV-1 in cats has become more common. The drug appears to be safe at least for a short course (2 to 3 weeks), although the optimum dose remains unclear, and safety in kittens has not been determined. A retrospective study compared the clinical effects of dosing at either 40 or 90 mg/kg q8h in cats naturally infected with FHV-1.[25] While both groups showed improvement, cats in the high-dose group had greater improvement in a shorter period of time. Reduced shedding of FHV-1, but no difference in reduction in clinical signs, was noted in shelter cats treated with either 30 mg/kg or 90 mg/kg PO q12h for 7 days when compared with untreated cats.[26] Treatment of FHV-1 infections is described in detail in Chapter 34.

Feline calicivirus (FCV) is also a common cause of conjunctivitis in cats, particularly those in shelter or multicat environments. Conjunctivitis caused by FCV is indistinguishable from that caused by FHV-1 and may be severe in some cats (Fig. 128.6) (see Chapter 35). No antiviral drugs are available, so supportive care is required.

Chlamydia felis typically causes conjunctivitis in young adult cats (see Chapter 49) (Fig. 128.7). The clinical appearance of chlamydiosis is indistinguishable from conjunctivitis caused by FHV-1, and the two organisms may be present simultaneously. Chlamydial conjunctivitis can sometimes be successfully treated with topical tetracycline ointment applied to both eyes q6h until a week after resolution of clinical signs. Oral doxycycline may be preferred to clear the organism from extraocular tissues such as the intestinal tract, reproductive tract, and visceral organs. Results of one study indicated that oral doxycycline at 10 mg/kg per day for at least 28 days was necessary to ensure elimination of the organism from tissues.[27] *Hartmannella vermiformis,* an amebic

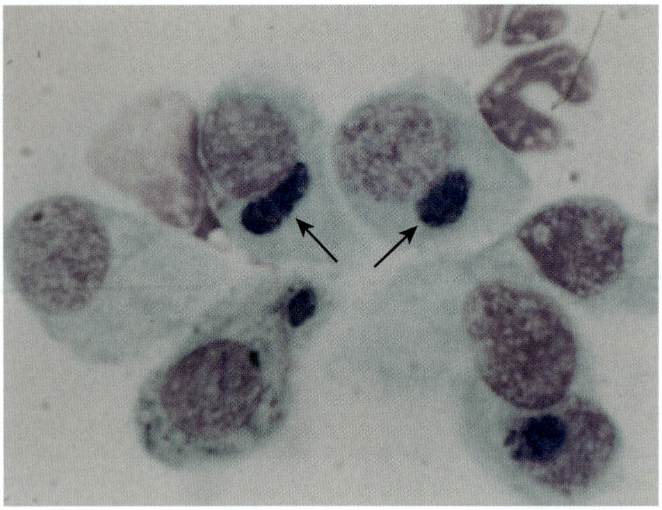

Fig. 128.7 Intracytoplasmic *Chlamydia felis* inclusions (*arrows*) in conjunctival epithelial cells of a cat with conjunctivitis (Giemsa stain, ×330).

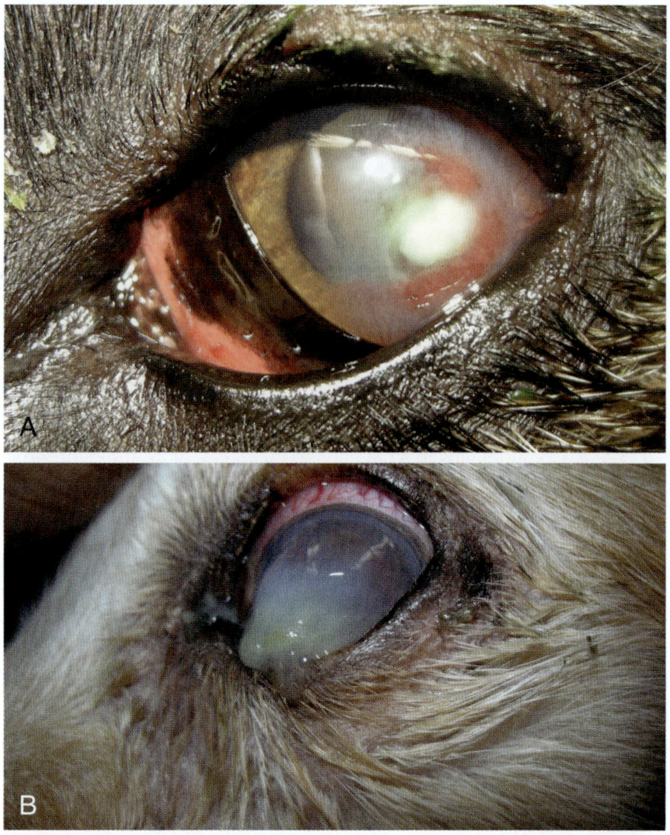

Fig. 128.8 (A) Infected corneal stromal ulcer in a dog. Note the purulent (white to yellow colored) corneal infiltrate, vascularization, and conjunctival hyperemia. (B) Keratoconus due to corneal melting secondary to an infected corneal ulcer. Note corneal edema, purulent infiltrate, and abnormal corneal contour.

endosymbiont that contains the *Chlamydia*-like agent *Neochlamydia hartmannellae,* has been isolated in greater prevalence from the ocular surfaces of cats with keratitis or conjunctivitis than from those of clinically healthy cats.[28] However, in another study, the prevalence of the organism did not differ between similar groups of cats.[29] The clinical significance of this organism is unknown (see Chapters 49 and 105).

Mycoplasma felis has been variably implicated as a cause of conjunctivitis in cats. Some studies have recovered *Mycoplasma* species as resident microflora from feline conjunctiva, whereas others have not. Similarly, experimental infections of clinically healthy, young cats have produced conjunctivitis in some studies[30] and not in others. *Mycoplasma* organisms may require a stressor such as co-infection with FHV-1 to cause disease. One study reported a slightly higher percentage of cats with conjunctivitis to have positive PCR results for *Mycoplasma* spp. DNA (9.6%) as compared to FHV-1 (6.7%) or *C. felis* (3.2%) DNA.[31] Suspected mycoplasma conjunctivitis should be treated as for chlamydiosis.

Keratitis

Dogs

Viral keratitis in dogs can be caused by CHV (see above) and CAdV-1. Bacterial keratitis in dogs develops after corneal ulceration or a traumatic wound. Resident bacterial flora inhabiting the ocular surface are those most likely to invade a corneal wound. This can lead to ulcerative keratitis or a corneal abscess. *Staphylococcus* and *Streptococcus* spp. are especially common, although infections with gram-negative bacteria may also develop. In one study of 476 dogs with ulcerative keratitis from the USA, bacteria isolated were *Staphylococcus* spp. (32%, primarily *S. pseudintermedius*), *Streptococcus* spp. (19%, primarily *Streptococcus canis*), and *Pseudomonas aeruginosa* (8%); MDR bacteria comprised 20% of the isolates and increased in prevalence from 2016 to 2020 from 5% to 34%.[32]

Bacterial keratitis usually incites a visible neutrophilic response, characterized by a yellow-to-white cellular infiltrate within the cornea. Vascular growth into the cornea also occurs but usually does not begin for several days after injury and infection. Blood vessels originate from the limbus and grow at a rate of approximately 1 mm/day toward the site of infection. Rapid corneal destruction can occur. Invading bacteria and neutrophils can release proteases and collagenases, which contribute to corneal melting (Fig. 128.8). Increased cyclo-oxygenase-2 expression has been documented in all corneal layers of affected dogs, suggesting a possible role for antiprostaglandin therapy as a treatment for inflammatory keratitis.[33] Fungal keratitis, which can have a similar clinical appearance, is less common but can be caused by penetrating injuries with plant material or prolonged topical treatment with antibiotic or glucocorticoid therapy. *Candida* spp., *Aspergillus* spp., and a variety of other molds have been implicated[34,35]; in one case report, infection with *Malassezia pachydermatis* was described.[36] Both bacterial and fungal infections can lead to corneal perforation.

Diagnosis of infectious keratitis is based on clinical findings, cytology, and culture. Fluorescein staining is used to detect epithelial loss. All corneal ulcers that are progressive or involve the stroma should be cultured. For specimen collection, a mini-tip Culturette swab with a sterile saline-moistened tip should be used to gently swab the ulcer bed. After application of topical proparacaine, a flattened spatula, the blunt end of a scalpel blade, or a cytology brush should be used to gently scrape the ulcer edge in order to obtain a specimen for cytologic examination. With bacterial keratitis, neutrophils are the predominant cell type, and bacteria can be numerous, few, or not visible. Initial antimicrobial drug selection can be based on whether cocci or rods are present. Until culture results are known, broad-spectrum antibacterial drugs should be used. A combination of chloramphenicol and a fluoroquinolone has been recommended for infected corneal ulcers.[32] To achieve broad-spectrum bactericidal activity, compounding may be required (Tables 128.3 and 128.4). Frequency of application is critical. In a rapidly progressive corneal ulcer, topical antibiotics should be applied q1-2h. To reduce the likelihood of corneal melting, serum or

TABLE 128.3 Commercially Available Ophthalmic Antibacterial Agents

Generic Name	Solution Concentration (%)	Ointment
Individual Agents		
Bacitracin	NA	500 U/g
Chloramphenicol	0.5%	1%
Azithromycin	1%	NA
Erythromycin	NA	0.5%
Gentamicin sulfate	0.3%	0.3%
Levofloxacin	0.5%	NA
	1.5%	NA
Ofloxacin	0.3%	NA
Ciprofloxacin	0.3%	0.3%
Gatifloxacin	0.3% 0.5%	NA NA
Moxifloxacin	0.5%	NA
Sulfacetamide sodium	10%	10%
Tobramycin sulfate	0.3%	0.3%
Mixtures		
Polymyxin B–bacitracin–zinc	NA	10,000 U
Polymyxin B–neomycin–bacitracin	NA	10,000 U
Polymyxin B–neomycin–gramicidin	10,000 U	NA
Polymyxin B-oxytetracycline	NA	10,000 U
Polymyxin B-trimethoprim	10,000 U/0.1%	NA

NA, not available.

plasma (autologous, homologous, or heterologous) should be applied topically q1-2h for anti-collagenolytic effect.[37,38] These blood products should be maintained in a sterile fashion and kept refrigerated. Systemic antibiotics are usually not indicated unless the cornea has a penetrating wound. Topical atropine can be used q12-24h daily if miosis is present, although it should not be used in dogs with KCS or glaucoma.

If fungal keratitis is documented or suspected, it should be treated with the application of a topical antifungal agent q2-3h. Topical 1 to 2% miconazole, 1% itraconazole, or 1% voriconazole solutions have been effective in treatment of keratomycosis in dogs (see Chapter 86).[35,36,39,40] Deep corneal ulcers in danger of perforating respond best to surgical therapy, such as placement of a conjunctival flap.

Ocular surfaces should be cleaned of discharges frequently to remove neutrophils and their proteolytic enzymes. If tear production is inadequate, topical cyclosporine or tacrolimus q12h and artificial tears several times daily should be administered to supplement and stimulate lacrimation. Closing the lids or placing a third eyelid flap should be avoided. These procedures limit drug contact with the cornea, impair discharge drainage, and increase the temperature of the environment, thus promoting bacterial growth, fungal growth, or both. They also prevent monitoring of the healing process. Systemic NSAIDs can provide analgesia and aid in the treatment of uveitis associated with deep corneal ulcers.

Cats

Bacterial keratitis in cats may develop secondary to corneal ulceration (including that initiated by FHV-1) or traumatic wounds. Appearance, diagnosis, and treatment are the same as for the dog. Fungal keratitis in cats is rare but can be treated in the same way as fungal keratitis in dogs.[41]

TABLE 128.4 Fortified and Compounded Topical Antibacterial Solution Preparations

Gentamicin (Fortified)	
Gentamicin injectable (50 mg/mL)	6 mL
Artificial tears	24 mL
TOTAL	30 mL
Final concentration = 10 mg/mL (1% solution)	
Or	
Add 2 mL of injectable gentamicin (50 mg/mL) to the 5-mL bottle of commercial ophthalmic gentamicin solution (0.3%). Final concentration: 14 mg/mL (1.4% solution). Shelf life: 30 days	
Amikacin	
Amikacin injectable (250 mg/mL)	4 mL
Artificial tears	26 mL
TOTAL	30 mL
Final concentration = 33 mg/mL (3.3% solution)	
Or	
Remove 2 mL from a 15-mL squeeze bottle of artificial tears and discard. Add 2 mL of injectable amikacin (50 mg/mL). Final concentration: 6.7 mg/mL (0.67% solution). Shelf life: 30 days	
Ampicillin	
Mix a 125-mg vial ampicillin with sterile saline or artificial tears to a concentration of 20 mg/mL	
Cefazolin	
Remove 2 mL from a 15-mL squeeze bottle of artificial tears and discard. Reconstitute a 500- or 1000-mg vial of cefazolin with sterile saline to a concentration of 250 mg/mL. Add 500 mg of the reconstituted cefazolin (2 mL) to the bottle of artificial tears. Final concentration: 33 mg/mL (3.3% solution). Shelf life: 14 days. Keep refrigerated	
Cephalothin	
Remove 6 mL from a 15-mL squeeze bottle of artificial tears and save. Add the 6 mL of tear solution to a 1000-mg vial of cephalothin. Add the entire 1000 mg of the reconstituted cephalothin (6 mL) to the bottle of artificial tears. Final concentration: 67 mg/mL (6.7% solution). Keep refrigerated	
Ticarcillin	
Reconstitute a 1-g vial of ticarcillin with 10 mL of sterile saline. Add 1.0 mL (100 mg) of this solution to a 15-mL squeeze bottle of artificial tears. Final concentration: 6.7 mg/mL (0.67% solution). Shelf life: 4 days. Keep refrigerated	
Tobramycin (Fortified)	
Add 1.0 mL of injectable tobramycin (40 mg/mL) to a 5-mL bottle of commercial ophthalmic tobramycin solution (0.3%). Final concentration: 9.2 mg/mL (0.127% solution). Shelf life: 30 days	
Vancomycin	
Remove 9 mL from a 15-mL squeeze bottle of artificial tears and discard. Reconstitute a 500-mg vial of vancomycin with 10 mL of sterile saline. Add the entire 500 mg of reconstituted vancomycin (10 mL) to the bottle of artificial tears. Final concentration: 31 mg/mL (3.1% solution). Shelf life: 4 days. Keep refrigerated	

Adapted from Whitley RD. Canine and feline primary ocular bacterial infections. *Vet Clin North Am Small Anim Pract.* 2000;30:1151-1157.

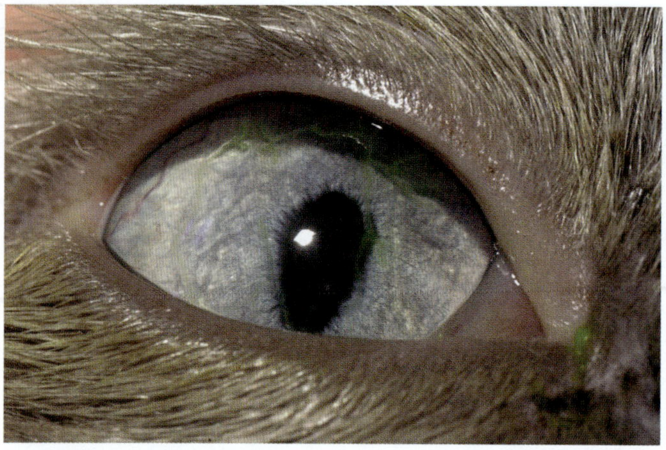

Fig. 128.9 Corneal dendritic ulceration in a cat associated with FHV-1 infection (fluorescein stain).

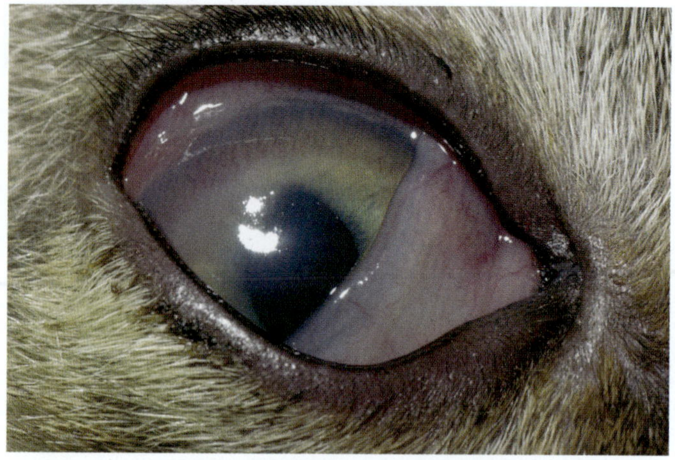

Fig. 128.10 Stromal keratitis without corneal ulceration in a kitten associated with FHV-1 infection. Note the corneal vascularization, corneal edema, and conjunctival hyperemia.

Corneal ulceration and keratitis that occur in association with FHV-1 infection are very common and begin with invasion of the corneal epithelium by the virus.[42] The most common corneal abnormality is punctate or linear (dendritic) epithelial ulcers (Fig. 128.9), which may quickly enlarge to form geographic superficial ulcers. Conjunctivitis usually accompanies corneal ulceration.[18] Mechanical debridement of any loose corneal epithelium with a cotton-tipped swab and treatment with a topical or oral antiviral agent are recommended. A topical antibiotic should also be used for bacterial prophylaxis. Grid keratotomies should not be performed in cats because this allows the virus greater access to the corneal stroma and appears to increase the risk of corneal sequestration.[43]

FHV-1 infection may also be associated with stromal keratitis in cats, which may occur with or without corneal ulceration.[44] Corneal vascularization and cellular infiltrate, often accompanied by chronic discomfort, are typical signs (Fig. 128.10). Antiviral agents alone may not improve the keratitis. Topical anti-inflammatory agents may be needed, although glucocorticoids should be avoided. Nonsteroidal topical agents such as diclofenac, and/or 0.2% cyclosporine ointment, can be used in conjunction with an antiviral agent such as cidofovir. Topical glucocorticoids predispose cats to the development of corneal ulceration and sequestration when FHV-1 is present. Topical IFN has been used in humans with herpetic keratitis and can also be considered (see Conjunctivitis in cats).

Corneal sequestration can follow chronic corneal ulcers or keratitis caused by FHV-1 in any breed of cat, but Persian and Himalayan cats are predisposed (Fig. 128.11). Corneal sequestration has occurred in cats experimentally infected with FHV-1 after topical glucocorticoid treatment, and in cats treated with grid keratotomy.[43,45] The condition is characterized by an area of corneal degeneration with a brown to black discoloration. Lesions vary from pinpoint sequestra to those that occupy more than half the cornea. Vascularization and ocular pain may be intense or absent. Like stromal keratitis, sequestra can be one of the most serious and potentially blinding sequelae of FHV-1 infection. Most ophthalmologists recommend keratectomy followed by a graft (corneal or conjunctival) as treatment for sequestra.

Dacryocystitis

Dacryocystitis, or inflammation of the NL system, is usually associated with bacterial infection (Fig. 128.12). Nasolacrimal foreign bodies such as plant material are frequently the inciting cause. Dacryocystitis is less common in cats than in dogs. Clinical manifestations of dacryocystitis include conjunctival hyperemia, especially of the ventral conjunctival sac; purulent ocular discharge; and epiphora. Blepharospasm may or

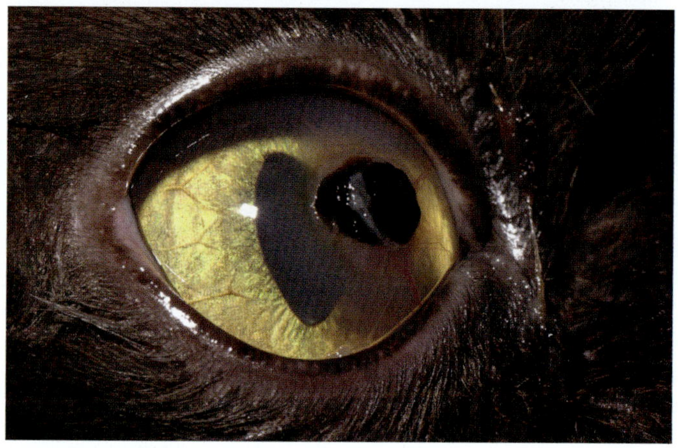

Fig. 128.11 Corneal sequestrum in a cat. Note the black plaque and corneal blood vessels.

may not be present. Palpation of the skin near the medial canthus may elicit pain and exudation of pus from the lacrimal puncta. Swelling or draining tracts in the skin near the medial canthus may also be identified.

The NL system should be flushed and purulent debris submitted for culture and susceptibility testing. Dacryocystorhinography may be necessary to identify foreign bodies or cystic structures within the NL system. If foreign bodies cannot be flushed from the system, surgical removal using dacryocystotomy may be required. Other, less invasive approaches have more recently been successful, including ultrasound-guided foreign body removal using alligator forceps inserted through the upper puncta[46] and lacrimoscopic removal.[47]

After NL flushing, a broad-spectrum topical antibiotic solution should be used q4-6h. Systemic antibiotics are usually not required if the infection is confined to the NL system. Repeated flushings may be needed to maintain patency. The NL duct can also be stented to establish and maintain patency. Stricture of the NL duct can occur with dacryocystitis, leading to chronic epiphora.

Orbital Infections

Bacterial infection of the orbit is common, especially in dogs. Fungal infections have also been reported in both dogs and cats (see Systemic Mycoses). Bacterial infection of the orbit generally has a fairly rapid onset compared with the slow progression of clinical signs seen with

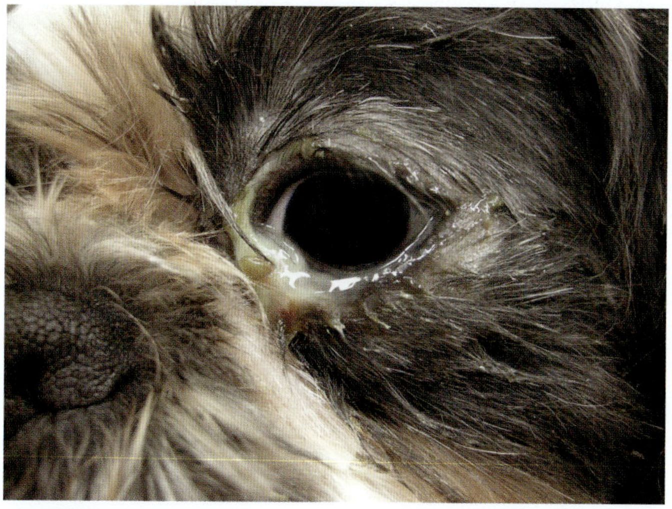

Fig. 128.12 Dacryocystitis in a dog. Purulent ocular discharge is present, particularly at the medial canthus.

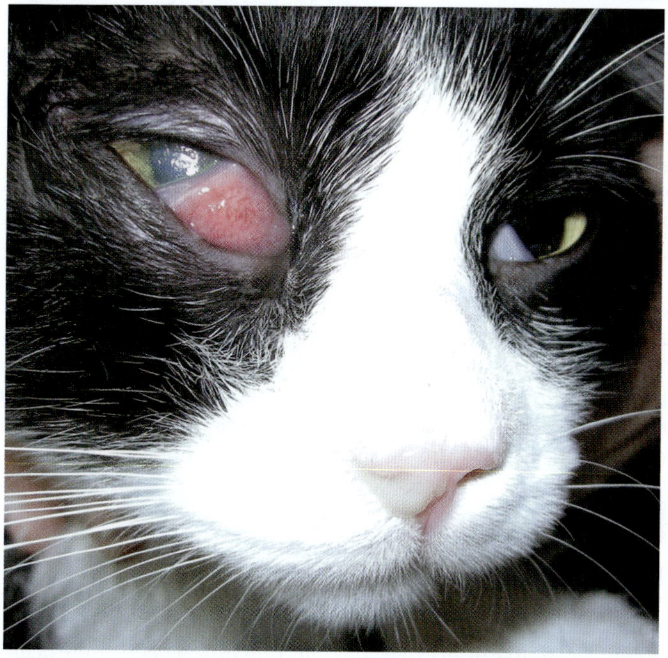

Fig. 128.13 Orbital abscess in a cat. Note the periorbital swelling, exophthalmos, and elevated third eyelid. Purulent nasal discharge is also present, an infrequent finding.

orbital neoplasia. Typical clinical signs of orbital abscess and cellulitis include periorbital swelling, exophthalmos, elevation of the nictitating membrane, conjunctival hyperemia, and pain on palpation of periorbita or when opening the mouth (Fig. 128.13). Swelling of the oral mucosa behind the last molar tooth is evident in some animals. Corneal ulceration and blindness due to exposure keratopathy and optic nerve damage, respectively, can also occur.[48]

Infectious agents may gain access to the orbit by several routes, including through the oral mucosa behind the last molar tooth, from the frontal sinus through breakdown of the medial orbital bone, by extension from tooth root abscesses, from penetrating wounds or foreign bodies of the skin or oral cavity, and through hematogenous spread from distant sites of infection.

Orbital bacterial abscesses are best diagnosed with ultrasonography. Abscesses appear as a hypoechoic area posterior to the globe (Fig. 128.14). Foreign bodies are often best visualized using ultrasonographic examination. Fungal granulomas appear hyperechoic and are not readily differentiated from neoplasia. CT or MRI may be helpful for determining the extent of infection; MRI was most often used in one retrospective study of retrobulbar cellulitis or abscesses in dogs.[48]

Drainage of orbital abscesses should be established when possible. Because only soft tissue separates the oral cavity from the ventral orbit in the dog and cat, an incision through the tissue behind the last molar can be used to access the orbit. A sterile small mosquito forceps or blunt probe should be advanced into the orbit, using gentle probing—not grasping—to attempt to enter the abscess cavity. Any purulent material should be submitted for cytologic evaluation and cultured for aerobic and anaerobic bacteria. Pending culture results, broad-spectrum systemic antibacterial therapy should be instituted. *Escherichia coli* was the most frequently isolated bacterial species in the retrospective study described earlier (9/14 isolates).[48] In other studies, anaerobes were more often isolated. Nonsteroidal agents should also be administered for analgesia and to reduce inflammation. The prognosis for bacterial orbital abscesses is generally good, whereas the prognosis for orbital fungal infections is more guarded. Occasionally, increased intraocular pressure may be so severe it can lead to irreversible blindness.[49]

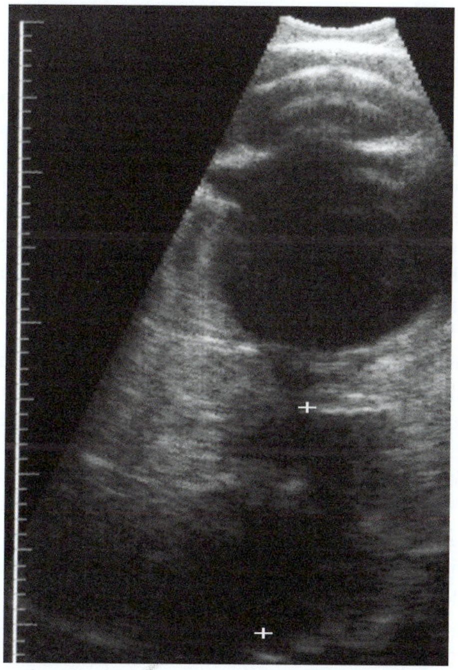

Fig. 128.14 Ultrasound image of retrobulbar abscess in a cat. Markers (+) delineate two sides of a hypoechoic structure (abscess) posterior to the globe.

DIAGNOSIS

The decision to culture the ocular surface should be made early in the examination before eye medications have been administered and manipulations performed. The use of a moist or calcium alginate swab can increase sensitivity.[50,51]

Cytologic examination of conjunctival and corneal scrapings is an important and rapid diagnostic aid. Excessive ocular discharges should be removed before scraping. Topical proparacaine should then be applied and the appropriate surface scraped with a small, flat spatula or the blunt end of a scalpel blade. Collected material should be gently spread onto glass slides and air dried. The slides can be stained with modified Giemsa or Wright stain for cytologic evaluation and Gram staining to evaluate the type of bacteria that might be present. Slides can also be made for direct IFA staining for CDV, FHV-1, and *C. felis*.

An alternate technique is to roll a small, nylon bristle brush applicator (Microbrush, Microbrush International, Grafton, WI) over the appropriate surface and then onto a slide (Fig. 128.15). Preparations made with this method have fewer cells that are dispersed better on the slide and have less crushing artifact.[52,53] This method is less traumatic and easier to perform on cats and small dogs with tight lid-globe conformations.

Small snip biopsy specimens of the conjunctiva can be readily obtained after using cotton-tipped swabs soaked in a topical anesthetic and holding it on the area to be excised for a minimum of 60 seconds. These small pieces of tissue should be spread out on a piece of paper before they are placed in fixative. Tissue should also be collected for testing using nucleic acid–based assays such as PCR; this can be submitted immediately or frozen pending the results of histopathology.

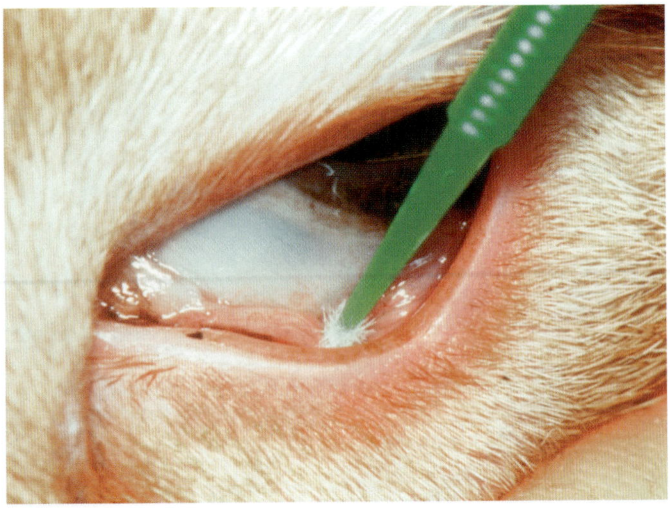

Fig. 128.15 Nylon bristle brush used to obtain a conjunctival cytology specimen.

INTRAOCULAR INFECTIONS

ETIOLOGY AND PATHOGENESIS

Intraocular bacterial infections may be exogenous or endogenous in origin. The source of an exogenous infection from a penetrating ocular injury may be obvious from the history and appearance of the eye, but injury may also be inapparent, such as a self-sealing cat claw injury through the conjunctiva and sclera. Infections that arise from exogenous sources are usually unilateral, whereas endogenous infections may be bilateral or unilateral.

Local Injury

All recent penetrating ocular injuries should be considered infected and treated aggressively with broad-spectrum antibiotics and antiinflammatory drugs, topically and systemically, until susceptibility data are obtained. Topical fluoroquinolones, especially ofloxacin, moxifloxacin, and gatifloxacin, have excellent corneal penetration and achieve therapeutic levels in the anterior segment against a wide variety of bacteria.[54] In suspected or confirmed bacterial endophthalmitis, a topical fluoroquinolone should be used every 1 to 2 hours.

Aqueous humor centesis in order to obtain specimens for cytologic examination and culture is safe when performed properly and can yield specific information to guide future therapy (see section on Diagnosis). Aqueous centesis is not as sensitive as vitreous centesis for detection of bacteria in endophthalmitis; consequently, a negative culture result from an aqueous specimen does not rule out infection.[55] The finding of nondegenerate neutrophils may indicate a sterile purulent inflammation such as that occurring with phacoclastic uveitis caused by lens capsule rupture. The prognosis for eyes with endophthalmitis is guarded. Many such eyes develop glaucoma, and enucleation is a common outcome.

Systemic Diseases

The eye is often a target organ in systemic infections. In some cases, ocular disease can be the primary owner complaint or the only sign evident in a systemic disease process. Recognition of systemic involvement is essential for prognostication and adequate therapy. Conversely, thorough ocular examination is indicated in any animals with systemic disease, because it may provide rapid diagnostic clues and prognostic information. If infectious agents access the eye, it is usually via the uveal or vascular tract. Typically, infectious agents or immune complexes become established in the uvea, producing chorioretinitis, anterior uveitis, or panuveitis.

Canine Distemper

In addition to conjunctivitis and lacrimal adenitis, CDV often produces multifocal, nongranulomatous chorioretinitis that does not usually cause blindness (see Chapter 22). As with CNS signs, whether chorioretinitis develops likely depends on the viral strain and immune competency of the host. In one study, dogs with all neurologic forms of distemper had an overall prevalence of chorioretinal lesions of 41%, but 83% of the dogs with chronic leukoencephalopathy syndromes had chorioretinal lesions.[56] Acute focal lesions in the tapetum or nontapetum have gray to white, hazy or ill-defined borders (Fig. 128.16).[40] Chorioretinal scars resulting from distemper virus infection have sharply demarcated borders, are hyperreflective in the tapetum ("gold medallion lesions"), and are depigmented in the nontapetum. Histologically, retinal changes are characterized by degeneration of the retina with perivascular cuffing in some instances. Lesions may include focal or diffuse degeneration of ganglion cells, proliferation of retinal pigment epithelium, atrophy of photoreceptors, disorganization of retinal layers, focal gliosis, and distemper inclusion bodies in glial cells. The most serious clinical ocular problem associated with CDV infection is optic neuritis, which results in acute onset of bilateral blindness and mydriasis.[57] If inflammation extends rostrally to the optic disc, ophthalmoscopic signs of peripapillary hemorrhages and edema, retinal vascular congestion, and elevation of the disc are observed (Fig. 128.17). If the neuritis remains retrobulbar, the diagnosis is made by exclusion (e.g., blind eyes with mydriasis and normal retinal function as tested by electroretinography). The optic neuritis can be isolated, prodromal, or occur in conjunction with other CNS signs. Distemper-associated blindness also may occur with inflammation of the occipital cortex or optic radiations, but pupillary light reflexes are normal under such circumstances.

Canine Adenovirus-1 Infection

CAdV-1 infection (see Chapter 23) has been estimated to produce ocular lesions in approximately 20% of dogs recovering from natural infections. The condition is bilateral in 12 to 28% of affected dogs. The most visible ocular lesion is stromal corneal edema ("blue eye") resulting from immune-complex deposition and associated inflammatory damage to the corneal endothelium (see Fig. 23.4). Fluid distention of the cornea can cause bullae to form. If the bullae rupture, corneal ulceration occurs. Occasionally, a dog has signs of uveitis (blepharospasm, miosis, hypotony, and aqueous flare) 1 to 2 days before the corneal edema is evident,

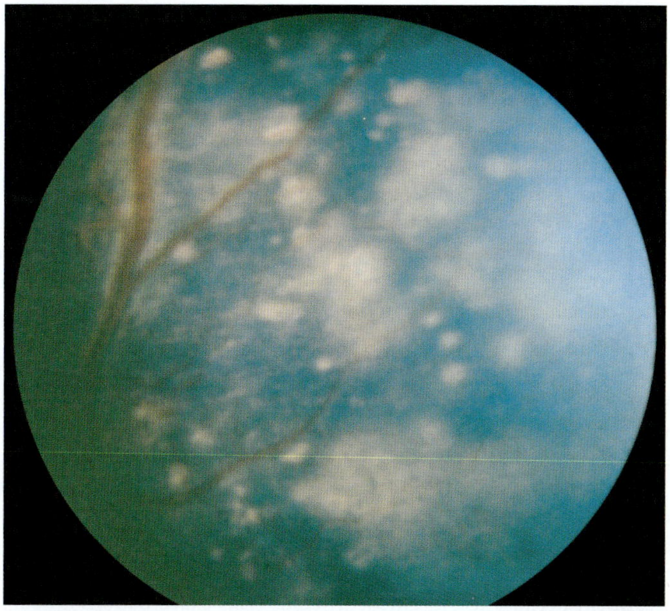

Fig. 128.16 Multifocal acute distemper lesions in the non-tapetal fundus of a dog. Active lesions are recognized by their white cellular infiltrates with hazy borders.

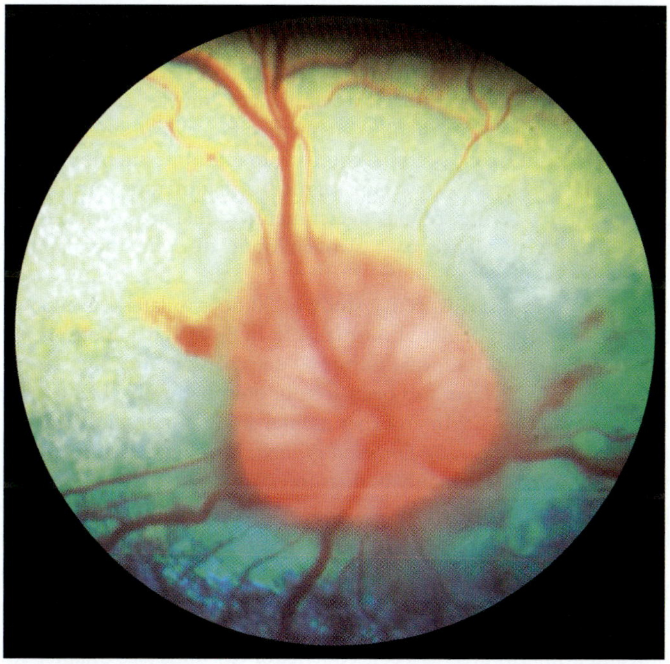

Fig. 128.17 Optic neuritis characterized by swollen and hyperemic optic disc, peripapillary hemorrhages, and loss of vision.

although most dogs do not demonstrate discomfort. Corneal edema may be focal or generalized and is usually transient. In some instances, the edema is permanent or may require several months to clear. A marked hypotony combined with altered corneal rigidity may result in a keratoconus. Other causes of corneal edema, such as congenital persistent pupillary membranes, glaucoma, corneal ulceration, and uveitis from other causes, should be ruled out.

Canine Herpesvirus Infection

Infection of adult dogs with CHV results in conjunctivitis and keratitis as described earlier in this chapter. In addition, neonatal CHV infection has been associated with a bilateral panuveitis with keratitis,

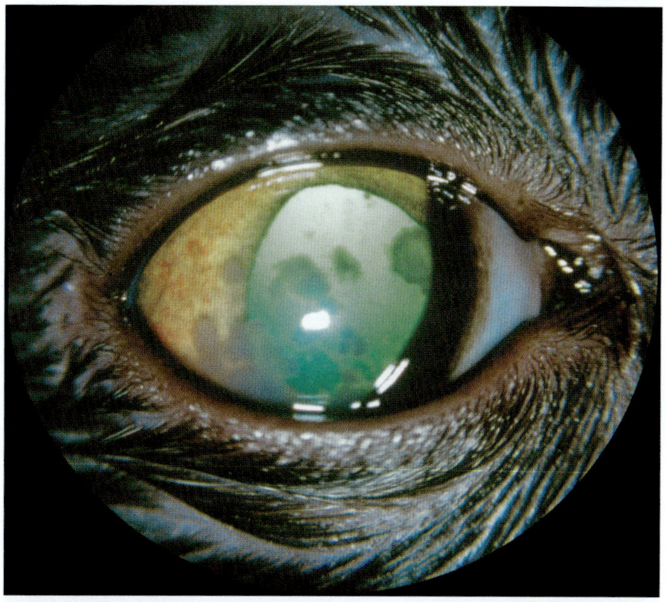

Fig. 128.18 Anterior uveitis with large keratic precipitates in a cat with feline infectious peritonitis.

synechiae, cataracts, retinal necrosis and disorganization, retinal atrophy and dysplasia, and optic neuritis and atrophy.[58]

Feline Infectious Peritonitis

The most common ocular manifestation of infection with FIP virus is bilateral granulomatous anterior uveitis, often accompanied by chorioretinitis (see Chapter 31). Frequently, large keratic precipitates and a fibrinous exudate are found in the anterior chamber (Fig. 128.18). Pyogranulomatous vasculitis, the hallmark of the disease's pathogenesis, may be evident on examination of retinal vessels (Fig. 128.19). Retinal hemorrhages and detachments may also develop. Ocular disease is more common with noneffusive FIP and may be the only sign. The use of PCR for feline coronavirus RNA on aqueous humor specimens may be helpful for diagnosis of uveitis due to FIP when positive, but sensitivity was only 36% in one study.[59] Immunocytochemistry for detection of viral antigens in aqueous humor macrophages was not recommended because of the potential for false-positive results. Topical treatment of ocular disease with glucocorticoids is supportive, and new antiviral drugs (GS441524 and remdesivir) offer promise for improved outcomes. Ocular disease may be temporarily ameliorated, but it usually recurs if the systemic disease worsens.

Feline Leukemia Virus Infection

Ocular disease in FeLV infection primarily results from FeLV-associated lymphoma (see Chapter 32). Neoplastic lymphocytes can often be found in the uveal tract as a result of hematogenous spread. Cats with ocular lymphoma may initially show signs of mild uveitis, including miosis, aqueous flare, and keratic precipitates. As the disease progresses, the iris becomes greatly thickened and distorted with the infiltration of tumor cells. Lymphoma may also initially appear as a mass within the iris in the absence of clinical signs of uveitis (Fig. 128.20). Glaucoma is a common sequela because tumor cells infiltrate the iridocorneal angle. Aqueous centesis may be helpful for diagnosis, because neoplastic lymphocytes readily exfoliate into the aqueous humor. Aggressive treatment of cats with ocular lymphoma with topical (e.g., prednisolone acetate) and systemic glucocorticoids, as well as systemic therapy with chemotherapy can result in improvement. Lymphoma may also manifest as orbital masses, with associated exophthalmos and an elevated third eyelid. Treatment for this form of

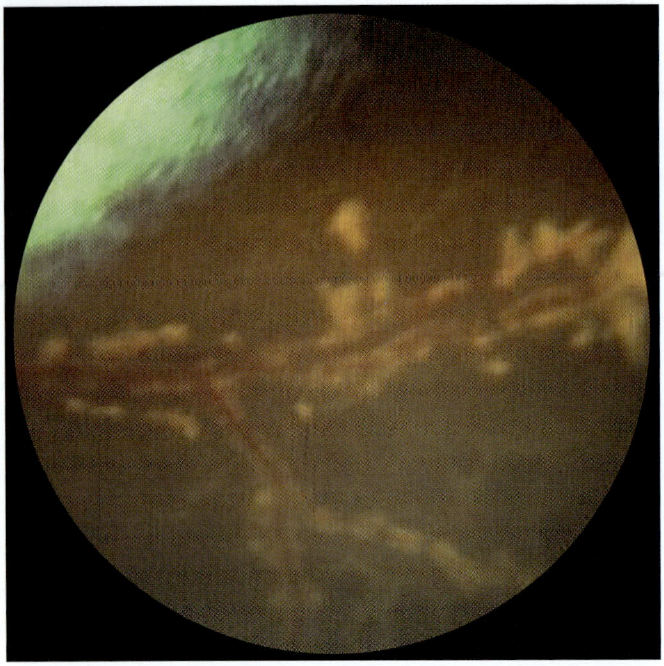

Fig. 128.19 Chorioretinitis and retinal perivascular inflammatory sheathing in a cat with feline infectious peritonitis.

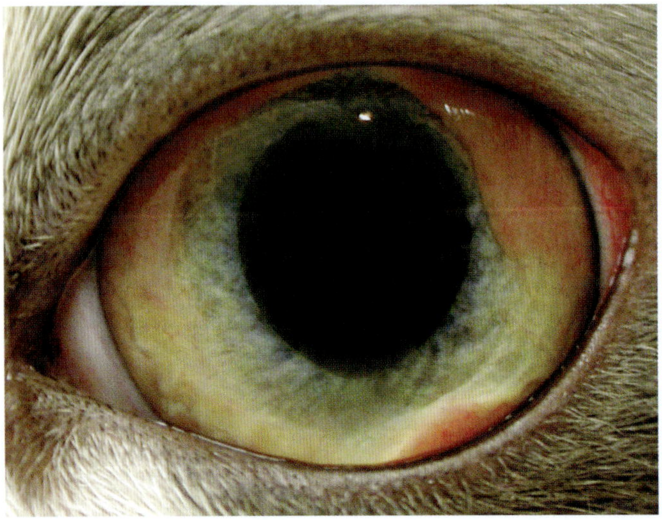

Fig. 128.20 Ocular lymphoma causing iridal masses in a cat infected with feline leukemia virus.

lymphoma should include chemotherapy and possibly orbital radiation therapy. Pupillary abnormalities, including dynamic anisocoria, have been noted in some cats with FeLV infection, as have retinal hemorrhages associated with thrombocytopenia.[60]

Feline sarcoma virus (FeSV) is a naturally occurring variant of the FeLV that has incorporated one of several oncogenes. Experimentally, the virus has caused uveal melanoma when injected into the anterior chamber of cats. Using PCR on formalin-fixed globes with uveal melanoma, one study found FeLV-FeSV DNA in 3 of 36 specimens, suggesting a possible role of the virus in tumor formation.[61] In another study of 10 globes with uveal melanoma, FeLV was not detected by PCR or immunohistochemistry.[62]

Feline Panleukopenia

Although cerebellar hypoplasia is the most common clinically apparent abnormality in cats with feline panleukopenia, kittens infected in the prenatal or neonatal period may also have retinal dysplasia and optic nerve hypoplasia or dysplasia (see Chapter 30).

Feline Immunodeficiency Virus Infection

Ocular inflammation has been associated with FIV infection in both experimentally and naturally infected cats. Anterior uveitis is most commonly reported, but conjunctivitis, pars planitis, and chorioretinitis have also been described. Ocular inflammation may result from direct viral damage, secondary immune-mediated phenomena, or opportunistic infection. In a histopathologic study of the eyes of 19 infected cats, 16 cats had lymphoplasmacytic inflammation of the iris and ciliary body.[63] Secondary opportunistic infections with FHV-1, *C. felis,* and *T. gondii* should always be considered in FIV-positive cats with ocular disease. In an experimental study of chlamydial conjunctivitis, co-infection with FIV markedly prolonged the duration of clinical signs and led to chronic conjunctivitis.[64]

If another infectious disease can be identified in an FIV-positive cat, it should be treated as specifically as possible. Uveitis that is associated with FIV infection can be a chronic problem that requires symptomatic treatment. For long-term use, a topical NSAID is preferred for treatment because use of glucocorticoids risks exacerbation of ocular FHV-1 infections. However, oral prednisolone may be required for treatment of chorioretinitis.

Ehrlichiosis

Ocular lesions occur frequently in dogs with canine monocytic ehrlichiosis (see Chapter 44). The most common lesions include unilateral or bilateral anterior uveitis characterized by conjunctival and episcleral hyperemia or hemorrhage, miosis, aqueous flare, hypopyon, keratic precipitates, hyphema, synechiae, and/or hypotony. Glaucoma can occur secondary to chronic anterior uveitis (Fig. 128.21). Signs of posterior segment inflammation can include chorioretinitis, serous retinal detachment, retinal hemorrhage, and optic neuritis. Evidence of a swollen optic disc and peripapillary hemorrhages on fundic examination suggests optic neuritis (see Fig. 128.17). In a retrospective study of 90 dogs, bilateral uveitis was the most common ocular abnormality.[65] In 30 of the 90 dogs, ocular disease was the only clinical finding; 60 dogs had systemic signs.

Anterior uveitis has also been seen in dogs naturally infected with *Ehrlichia chaffeensis*.[66] In an experimental study of dogs infected with *E. canis, E. chaffeensis*, or *Ehrlichia ewingii,* histologic examination of the eyes showed uveitis only in dogs infected with *E. canis*.[67] The lymphocytic inflammatory infiltrate was most intense in the ciliary body, becoming less intense in the choroid, iris, and retina, respectively.

Rocky Mountain Spotted Fever

Ocular lesions are frequently associated with *Rickettsia rickettsii* infection and primarily arise as a consequence of vasculitis (see Chapter 46). Lesions include conjunctival hyperemia, subconjunctival hemorrhage, hyphema, anterior uveitis, iris hemorrhage, retinal hemorrhage, retinal edema, and retinal perivascular inflammatory cell infiltrate (Fig. 128.22).[68] Lesions tend to be bilateral in affected dogs but may not be symmetrical. Fluorescein angiography in experimentally infected dogs demonstrated increased retinal vascular permeability beginning on day 6 after infection and 2 days after the onset of pyrexia.[69] Venules were affected twice as frequently as arterioles, and smaller vessels were affected more frequently than larger primary vessels. Retinal vascular lesions in this study paralleled the progression of fever, leukopenia, thrombocytopenia, and prolongation of activated partial thromboplastin time during the second week after infection.

The ocular signs of RMSF resemble those of canine ehrlichiosis. Although ocular hemorrhages are the most common ophthalmic sign of RMSF, hemorrhage can also occur with ehrlichiosis. Although

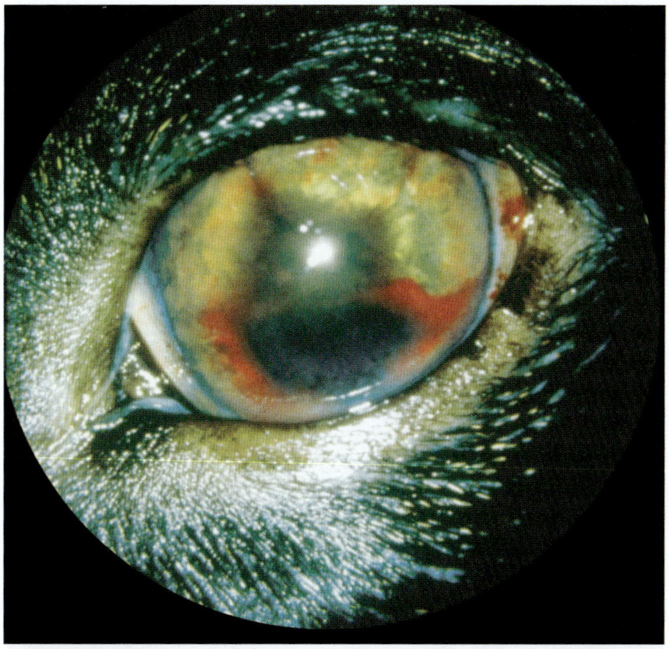

Fig. 128.21 Anterior uveitis with hyphema in a dog with *Ehrlichia canis* infection. Iris bombe and glaucoma are present.

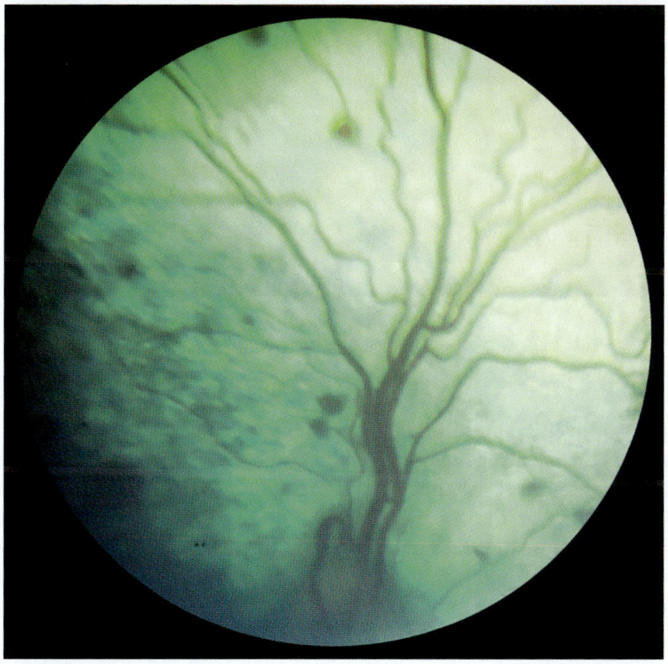

Fig. 128.22 Multifocal retinal hemorrhages in a dog with Rocky Mountain Spotted Fever.

exceptions occur, intraocular hemorrhages and inflammatory cell infiltrates tend to be less dramatic in RMSF than ehrlichiosis.[70]

Brucellosis

Brucella canis infection has been associated with unilateral or bilateral anterior uveitis or panuveitis, endophthalmitis, retinal detachment, and intraocular hemorrhage (see Chapter 71). Ocular involvement is often severe and blinding. A retrospective study of the prevalence of ocular lesions among dogs examined for brucellosis at veterinary schools in the United States and Canada found that 38 of 313 (14.2%) dogs had ocular involvement.[71] Testing for *B. canis* should be performed in dogs with unexplained uveitis or ocular hemorrhage. The prognosis for resolution of uveitis associated with brucellosis with treatment is guarded. A report of three dogs with brucellosis described resolution of unilateral endophthalmitis in each and apparent systemic clearing of the organism with a long-term multidrug treatment protocol (mean of 96 weeks) that included enrofloxacin, doxycycline, streptomycin, and rifampin.[72]

Lyme Borreliosis

In humans, ocular lesions associated with *B. burgdorferi* infection have been well described.[73,74] Uveitis is the primary manifestation, but neuro-ophthalmic disorders and surface inflammations such as episcleritis and keratitis have also been reported. Ocular manifestations are more likely to be seen in late-stage disease. A clear association between ocular disease in dogs and *B. burgdorferi* infection has not been made.

Leptospirosis

Leptospires incite vasculitis, making the eyes a potential target organ (Chapter 68). Although leptospires have been found in the eyes of infected dogs, the paucity of reports of uveitis associated with canine leptospirosis in the literature probably does not reflect the true prevalence of disease.[75] In horses and humans, the development of uveitis often occurs months after acute infection. This likely represents a delayed hypersensitivity reaction between cell-bound antibodies and persistent leptospiral antigens in the eye. Bilateral panuveitis and retinal detachments were described as the only sign of infection in a dog in association with a serovar Canicola infection.[76] Testing for leptospirosis should be included in a workup for a canine uveitis even if systemic signs are not present.

Bacteremia

Bacteremia that occurs in association with conditions such as infective endocarditis, discospondylitis, UTI, or pyometra may be associated with uveitis as a result of hematogenous spread of bacteria to the eye. If endophthalmitis secondary to bacteremia is suspected, a fluoroquinolone antibiotic should be used topically several times daily in addition to systemic antibiotic therapy. Fluoroquinolones will penetrate a normal cornea and reach therapeutic levels in the anterior segment of the eye. In addition, a topical glucocorticoid such as prednisolone acetate should be used several times daily to suppress inflammation.

Tetanus and Botulism

Ocular signs are among the most common early clinical manifestations of tetanus in the dog (Chapter 72) and were among the first signs noticed by the owner in 45% of dogs in one study.[77] Abnormalities included enophthalmos, third-eyelid protrusion, squinting, swollen eyelids, or a "strange facial expression." Miosis is the most common pupillary abnormality on physical examination. However, mydriasis may also occur (Fig. 128.23).

In botulism, autonomic nervous system dysfunction accounts for ocular abnormalities. These include mydriasis with sluggish pupillary light reflexes and a decreased palpebral reflex. Ocular surface disease such as conjunctivitis and corneal ulceration may occur if the palpebral reflex is absent, leading to lagophthalmos. Decreased tear production may also occur secondary to diminished parasympathetic nerve function to the lacrimal glands. In animals with lagophthalmos and/or tear deficiency, generous use

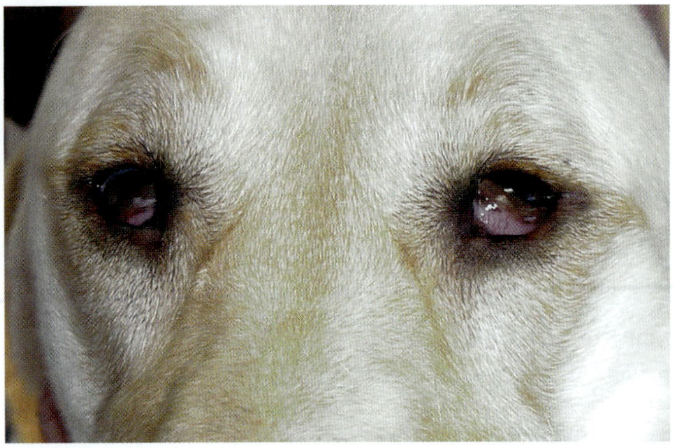

Fig. 128.23 Localized tetanus causing bilateral third-eyelid protrusion in a dog. The dog's pupils were mydriatic.

of artificial tear products should be incorporated with other treatments to avoid ocular surface drying.

Bartonellosis

Ocular complications in humans infected with *Bartonella henselae* include Parinaud's oculoglandular syndrome, neuroretinitis, and retinochoroiditis (Chapter 70).[78] In both naturally and experimentally infected cats, *B. henselae* DNA and a specific antibody have been detected in the aqueous humor, and a role of *Bartonella* in anterior uveitis has been hypothesized.[79] In a study of 366 cats with and without uveitis, the prevalence and magnitude of serum antibody titers to *B. henselae* were not higher in cats with uveitis, suggesting that serum antibody testing cannot determine whether uveitis in a cat is caused by *B. henselae*.[80] A similar lack of correlation was found between *B. henselae* isolation from blood or positive serum antibody titer results in cats with uveitis.[81] A review of our current understanding of the role of bartonellosis in feline uveitis indicates little evidence to date that this disorder is a significant cause of uveitis in cats, although further study is needed.[82] *Bartonella vinsonii* subsp. *berkhoffii* was suspected as a cause of uveitis and choroiditis in one dog,[83] but whether *Bartonella* spp. can cause ocular disease in dogs remains unknown.

Mycobacteriosis and Nocardiosis

Granulomatous to pyogranulomatous chorioretinitis, optic neuritis, and anterior uveitis may occur in disseminated mycobacterial[84-86] and nocardial infections (Sykes, unpublished observations) (Chapters 60 and 61). Granulomatous lesions have also been noted in the conjunctivae and corneas of infected cats.[87,88]

Systemic Mycoses

Systemic mycoses caused by fungi endemic to North America are frequently associated with a pyogranulomatous to granulomatous posterior uveitis. Anterior uveitis accompanies chorioretinitis in many cases. Ocular involvement occurs in up to 52% of blastomycosis cases.[89] Ocular lesions always include chorioretinitis, which may vary from a focal granuloma in the fundus to widespread subretinal infiltrates of organisms and granulomatous inflammation with retinal detachment (Fig. 128.24A).[90] Anterior uveitis is common with extensive posterior segment disease, although the organism is not usually found in these tissues or in aqueous humor aspirates. Secondary glaucoma is a frequent complication (Fig. 128.24B). Ocular involvement with histoplasmosis is relatively uncommon in dogs,[91] but is often recognized in cats and includes granulomatous chorioretinitis, retinal detachment,

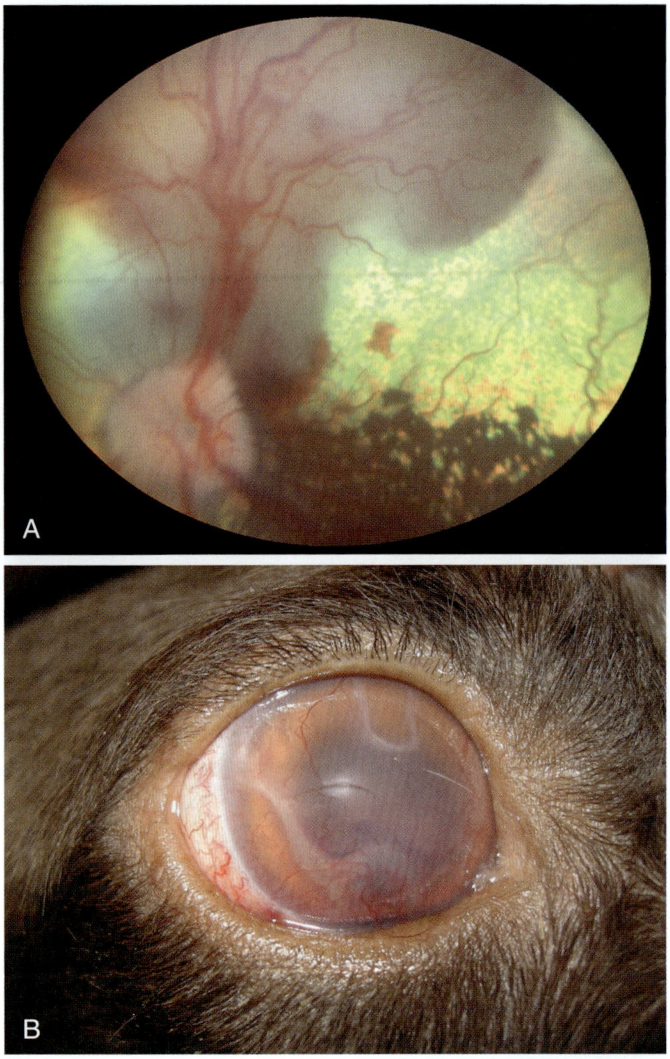

Fig. 128.24 (A) Large subretinal granuloma and retinal hemorrhages in a dog with blastomycosis. (B) Anterior uveitis and glaucoma in a dog with blastomycosis.

anterior uveitis, and secondary glaucoma.[92] Ocular adnexal structures, such as the nictating membrane and conjunctiva, may also be involved in histoplasmosis.[93] Antigen testing may be negative in animals with localized ocular disease.[94] In coccidioidomycosis, ocular lesions are similar to those of blastomycosis (granulomatous chorioretinitis, retinal detachment, anterior uveitis, and secondary glaucoma). Organisms are found predominantly in the choroid. Limited data exist regarding the prevalence of ocular lesions in dogs and cats with coccidioidomycosis; they appear to be less common than with the other endemic mycoses described here.

Chorioretinitis with granulomatous inflammation and retinal detachment is the most common manifestation in cryptococcosis; anterior uveitis is rare. Tapetal lesions are often dark gray to black in color, in contrast to the whitish appearance of most fungal granulomas (Fig. 128.25). Optic neuritis may also develop, and ocular disease is often recognized in association with cryptococcal meningitis.

Clinical signs in cats with sino-orbital aspergillosis (see Chapter 86) include exophthalmos, corneal drying with possible ulceration secondary to lagophthalmos, ocular discharge, oral cavity ulceration, pain on opening of the mouth, and nasal discharge if the infection involves the nasal cavity or sinuses.[95] Brachycephalic cats (especially Persians) appear to be predisposed. Surgical therapy alone,

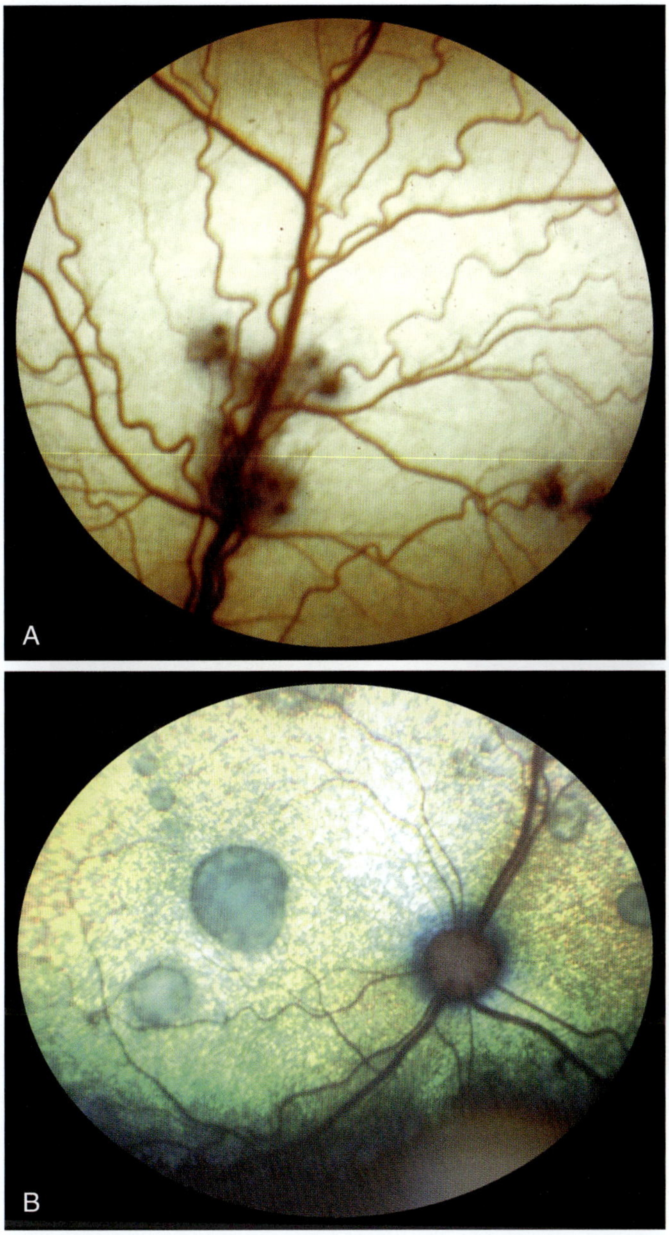

Fig. 128.25 Multifocal subretinal granulomas in a dog (A) and a cat (B) with cryptococcosis.

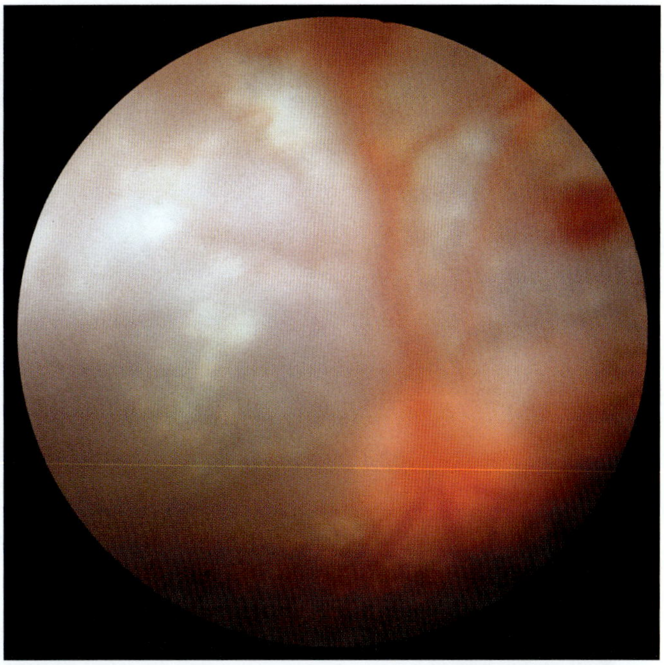

Fig. 128.26 Panophthalmitis causing retinal detachment and hemorrhage in a mixed-breed dog with disseminated aspergillosis.

including orbital exenteration, has not typically been successful. In one report, a cat was successfully treated with posaconazole after surgery and treatment with itraconazole (ITZ) and amphotericin B failed.[96] In dogs (especially German shepherd dogs), disseminated aspergillosis may also cause fungal endophthalmitis. In such cases, chorioretinitis, retinal detachment, and anterior uveitis are common (Fig. 128.26).

Chorioretinitis or endophthalmitis that appears pyogranulomatous to granulomatous should heighten the suspicion for a systemic mycosis. Associated systemic signs of fever and respiratory, skeletal, dermatologic, or CNS involvement are often present. Vitreal centesis in an eye with endophthalmitis may be helpful for diagnosis when other lesions are not present.

In many instances the ocular inflammation worsens initially with systemic antifungal therapy because of the immune reaction to the dying organisms, which can threaten vision. Short-term use of oral prednisolone at a dose of 1 to 2 mg/kg per day is recommended to dampen this reaction.[97] If anterior uveitis is present it should be treated as outlined in the section on Topical Therapy. Glaucoma is not uncommon with severe ocular involvement and should be appropriately treated.

Enucleation of blind eyes has been proposed as a means of eliminating a nidus of fungal infection that may cause relapse. Although it is justifiable to remove a blind, painful eye (such as one with intractable glaucoma), enucleation is not indicated in an animal that has been effectively treated for fungal disease and has a comfortable but blind eye.

Protothecosis

More than 50% of dogs with protothecosis have ocular involvement,[98] whereas ocular lesions have not been reported in cats (Chapter 90). Most dogs with ocular lesions also have systemic signs such as diarrhea, but in some instances systemic signs are not evident. Lesions include a granulomatous chorioretinitis, often with retinal detachment, that is similar in appearance to those associated with systemic mycoses.[99] Anterior uveitis is often present as well. Diagnosis is often possible by cytologic examination of specimens collected by vitreous centesis.

Toxoplasmosis

The most prominent ocular lesion in dogs and cats with toxoplasmosis is choroiditis with extension into the retina (Chapter 93).[100] These lesions typically appear as multifocal dark gray infiltrates in the tapetal fundus and fluffy white infiltrates in the nontapetal fundus. Anterior uveitis also occurs, and *T. gondii* bradyzoites and tachyzoites have been identified histopathologically in the irides and ciliary bodies of systemically affected cats.[101]

It is possible that *T. gondii* may incite immune-mediated uveitis in the absence of systemic disease. Several mechanisms have been proposed, including homing of activated immune cells to ocular tissues, molecular mimicry, circulating antigens or immune complexes from nonocular sites of parasite replication, and a nonspecific increase in immune response.[100,102] In kittens experimentally infected *in utero* or

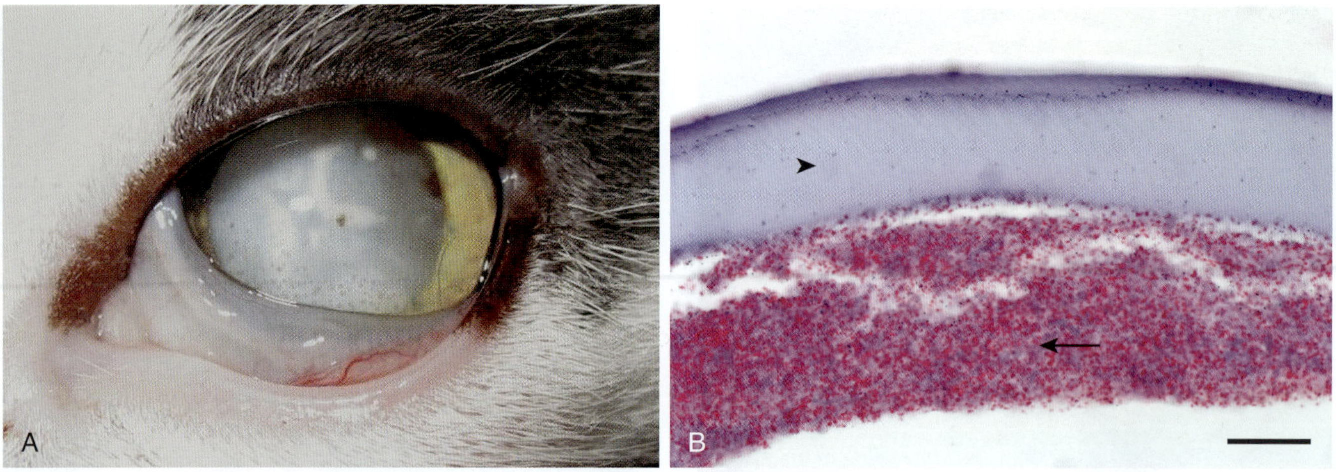

Fig. 128.27 *Encephalitozoon cuniculi* ocular disease in cats. (A) Cataract and anterior uveitis. Note keratic precipitates. (B) Histologic section of lens from an affected cat. Anterior lens capsule (*arrowhead*), and subcapsular lens cortex with many *E. cuniculi* organisms. Acid-fast trichrome stain. Bar = 30 μm. (Courtesy of Drs. Barbara Nell and Andrea Fuchs-Baumgartiner, Vienna, Austria.)

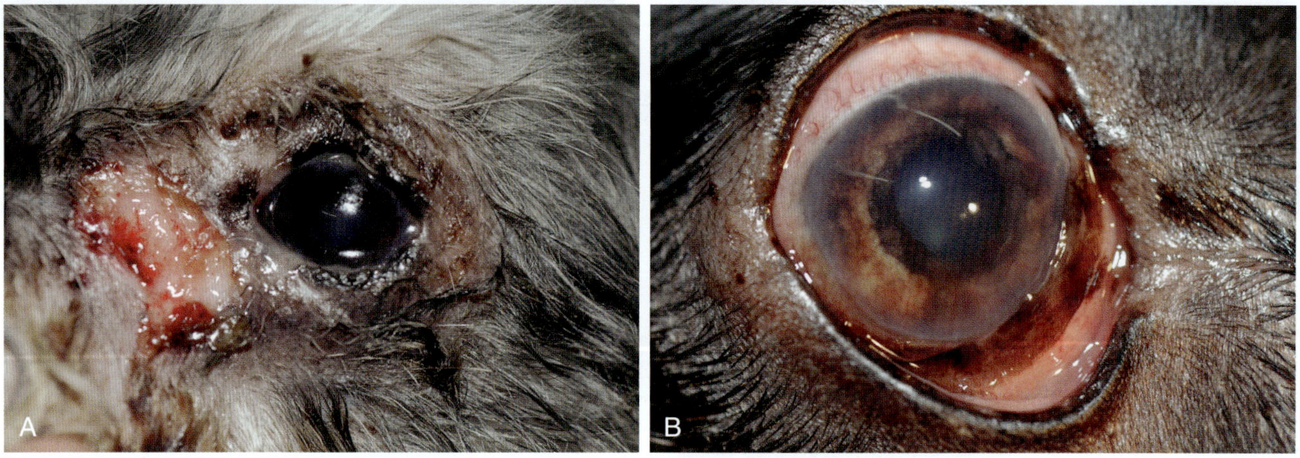

Fig. 128.28 Leishmaniosis. (A) Ulcerative blepharoconjunctivitis; (B) Granulomatous anterior uveitis. (Courtesy of Dr. Teresa Peña, Barcelona, Spain.)

in the early neonatal period, chorioretinitis and anterior uveitis developed without other evidence of clinical illness.[103]

Toxoplasma gondii–specific antibodies can be measured in aqueous humor. Antibody levels can be compared with serum levels through use of the Witmer-Goldman coefficient, or C-value. C-values greater than 3 suggest intraocular antibody production and may be more helpful than serum titers alone in diagnosing ocular toxoplasmosis. Aqueous humor can also be evaluated by PCR for the presence of *T. gondii* DNA.[104,105]

Neosporosis

Although puppies with neosporosis typically die or are euthanized because of neuromuscular signs, ocular lesions are present in some dogs (Chapter 94). Retinitis is the primary ocular lesion with extension into the choroid (retinochoroiditis). A mild anterior uveitis was also reported.[106]

Encephalitozoonosis

In many animals, including rabbits, blue fox, and mink, cataract formation with uveitis is the most common clinical problem that results from *Encephalitozoon cuniculi* infection (Chapter 92).[107-109] Vertical transmission allows the parasite to enter the lens during fetal development.[110] In one report of 11 domestic cats with cataract and uveitis, *E. cuniculi* infection was documented by serology, cytology, and PCR on aqueous humor and lens material[111] (Fig. 128.27). All cats were successfully treated with oral fenbendazole for 3 weeks in addition to undergoing phacoemulsification to remove the lens and anti-inflammatory therapy for uveitis.

Leishmaniosis

Ocular and periocular lesions associated with leishmaniosis were reported in 25% of 105 infected dogs in one study.[112] In 15% of the dogs in the study, ocular lesions were the only clinical sign. Ocular signs may include anterior uveitis, conjunctivitis, keratoconjunctivitis, periocular alopecia, diffuse blepharitis, posterior uveitis, orbital cellulitis, and optic neuritis (Fig. 128.28). In a study of 127 shelter dogs and 132 client-owned dogs in an endemic area of Italy, blepharitis predominated in shelter dogs, whereas anterior uveitis was more common in client-owned dogs.[113] In a histopathologic study of the eyes from 60 dogs from Spain with confirmed leishmaniosis, the predominant inflammatory pattern was granulomatous.[114] The organism was identified by immunohistochemical staining in 27% of globes. *Leishmania* parasites were identified in conjunctiva, cornea, iris, ciliary

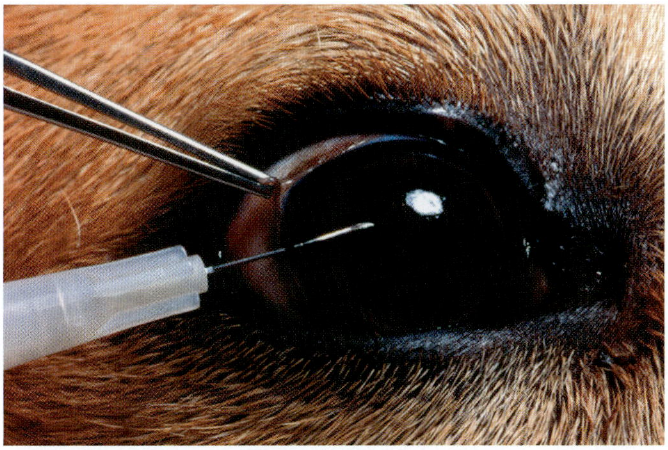

Fig. 128.29 Aqueous centesis in a dog. A 27-gauge to 30-gauge needle enters at the limbus, avoiding the iris and corneal endothelium.

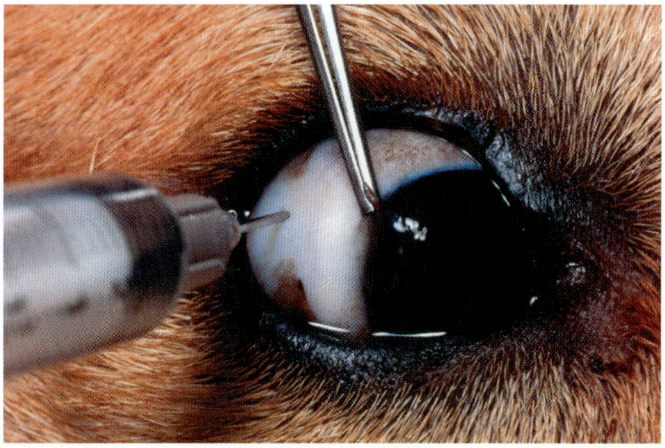

Fig. 128.30 Vitreous centesis in a dog. A 22-gauge to 25-gauge needle enters 6 mm posterior to the limbus and is directed slightly posterior and toward the center of the globe.

body, choroid, and optic nerve sheath. In dogs with blepharoconjunctivitis, scraping and cytologic examination can reveal the presence of amastigotes.

DIAGNOSIS

Aqueous Centesis

Aqueous centesis can be performed using heavy sedation or general anesthesia. A 27- to 30-gauge needle on a tuberculin syringe should be used with the "seal" broken so that movement of the plunger is smooth. Topical proparacaine should be used even with sedation. A cotton-tip swab soaked in proparacaine should be held at the site of centesis for 60 seconds before insertion of the needle. Typically the easiest location to access is the lateral limbus. Small forceps should be used to hold the conjunctiva close to the limbus to fixate the globe and apply counterpressure to the needle. The needle should enter the cornea just rostral to the limbus and parallel to the plane of the iris (Fig. 128.29). The iris, lens, and corneal endothelium should be avoided. Unless the anterior chamber is collapsed, the volume that can be removed from the dog is about 0.3 mL and from the cat is about 0.5 mL. The needle should be withdrawn slowly and a sterile cotton-tipped swab held over the site, because aqueous will leak for a brief time. An aliquot of the aspirated aqueous should be submitted in a plain tube for culture and susceptibility testing, and the remaining aliquot placed in a small EDTA tube to be centrifuged for cytologic examination. If fibrin is present or iris adhesions of less than a few days' duration are present, 25 μg of tissue plasminogen activator (tPA) may be injected to dissolve clots and break synechiae.[115]

Vitreous Centesis

Centesis of the vitreous cavity has more potential complications than aqueous centesis and is usually reserved for eyes that have lost considerable visual function. Choroidal hemorrhage and retinal tears are the two most likely complications. Topical proparacaine is not completely effective in anesthetizing the sclera; thus general anesthesia is recommended. A 22-gauge needle with a 3-mL syringe should be used. The site of entry should be 6 mm caudal to the limbus in the dorsolateral quadrant. Forceps are used to apply counter pressure, and the needle point is aimed posteriorly away from the lens and toward the center of the vitreous cavity (Fig. 128.30). The needle should be short (0.5 inch) so that it does not inadvertently pass completely across the vitreous humor and tear the opposite retina.

TABLE 128.5 Intraocular Penetration of Antibacterial Agents in the Non-inflamed Eye

	PENETRATION BY ROUTE		
Agent	**Systemic**	**Topical**	**Subconjunctival**
Penicillin	Poor	Poor	Good
Ampicillin	Poor	Poor	Good
Methicillin	Good (multiple dose)	NA	Good
Erythromycin	Poor	Good	Good
Cephalosporins	Poor	Poor	Good
Enrofloxacin	Good	NA	NR
Gentamicin	Poor	Poor	Good
Tobramycin	Poor	Poor	Good
Lincomycin	Good	NA	NA
Neomycin	NA	Poor	NA
Chloramphenicol	Fair	Good	Good
Tetracycline	Poor	Good	NA
Doxycycline	Good	NA	NA
Bacitracin	NA	Poor	Poor
Polymyxin B	NA	Poor	NA
Trimethoprim-sulfadiazine	Good	Good	Good
Sulfonamides (in general)	Good	Good	Good
Ciprofloxacin	Good	Good	NR
Ofloxacin	NA	Good	NR
Gatifloxacin	NA	Good	NR
Moxifloxacin	Good	Good	NR

NA, not available in a form for route of administration; *NR*, not recommended because of retinal toxicity.

Approximately 0.5 mL of vitreous humor can be removed for culture and cytologic examination.

TREATMENT

Ocular infection and inflammation can be treated using topical, subconjunctival, intraocular, or systemic medications. The route of administration selected depends on the location, severity of the infection, and the drug being administered. The eye has three barriers to drug penetration: the intact cornea for topical penetration and the blood-aqueous and blood-retinal barriers for systemic drug penetration. In general, drugs with a differential solubility in water and lipids and small molecular size are better able to penetrate these barriers. Inflammation or ulceration weaken these barriers to variable degrees and allow better penetration. The ability of antibiotics to penetrate the normal eye varies by drug and route (Table 128.5). The vitreous humor is a large, rather inert structure, resulting in low drug levels by any route of drug administration except direct intravitreal injection, in which the vitreous humor acts as a depot for the relatively slow release of the drug.

Topical Administration

Depending on the drug and whether the cornea is ulcerated, topical therapy may provide adequate drug concentrations only on the surface or as deep as the iris and ciliary body. Epithelial defects of 25 to 50% of the surface area increase drug penetration into the corneal stroma and aqueous humor nine-fold, but larger defects do not produce an additional increase.[116] Other variables that influence drug concentrations following topical administration are the frequency of application, drug contact time, drug concentration, and formulation. Solutions are generally easier to apply to a painful eye than ointment and, therefore, are preferred in terms of compliance. Although medications with high drug concentrations may have improved absorption, they can also increase reflex lacrimation and become diluted by osmotic influx of fluid from tissues.

When solutions are used, one drop (about 30 to 50 μL) of a preparation in the affected eye(s) is adequate. Multiple or rapidly repeated instillations of the same or different preparations simply increase the rate of loss through the NL system or mutually dilute each preparation, thereby reducing the availability of each drug. Waiting an interval of at least 5 minutes between instillation of different drugs is required to allow reflex tearing to subside and prevent dilution of the previous drop.

Treatment of routine surface infections of the conjunctiva or prophylactic antibacterial therapy of corneal ulcers should include topical broad-spectrum antibiotics such as neomycin-polymyxin B-gramicidin that are not used systemically. This rationale reduces exposure of bacteria to drugs that may be beneficial for systemic therapy (and hence reduces selection for resistant bacteria) and avoids sensitization of a patient to a topical antibiotic that might have potential in systemic therapy. Some animals develop an allergic reaction to topical neomycin, particularly when used chronically. Anaphylactic reactions in cats after administration of topical bacitracin-neomycin-polymyxin B preparations have been reported.[117] Most cases have been fatal, so this product is not recommended in cats.

Regardless of cause, treatment of uveitis requires anti-inflammatory therapy. Topical potent glucocorticoids such as 1% prednisolone acetate and 0.1% dexamethasone alcohol (the form present in neomycin-polymixin B-dexamethasone suspension) penetrate the corneal barrier well and achieve therapeutic levels in the anterior segment. Prednisolone and dexamethasone in the phosphate forms do not penetrate the cornea as well and should not be used for the treatment of uveitis. Topical NSAIDs such as diclofenac and flurbiprofen penetrate an intact cornea well and can also be used for treating uveitis. Topical NSAIDs have less potent anti-inflammatory effects and thus are better suited for treatment of mild uveitis. They can also be used in conjunction with a topical glucocorticoid for an additive effect. The frequency of use of a topical anti-inflammatory agent is dictated by the severity of the uveitis, ranging from 2 to 6 or more times daily for mild and severe uveitis, respectively.

Subconjunctival Administration

Subconjunctival administration of antibiotics or anti-inflammatory drugs is used primarily for anterior segment disease and can achieve therapeutic intraocular levels of medication. The major limitations of subconjunctival injections are drug irritation and ocular manipulation. The means by which a subconjunctivally injected drug reaches the interior of the eye are controversial, but direct diffusion through the sclera, which has no epithelial barrier as the cornea does, and leakage through the needle hole with topical absorption have been demonstrated. Except for long-acting drugs, most others must be re-administered at 12- to 24-hour intervals to maintain therapeutic levels. Typically, a single injection of a subconjunctival drug is administered, followed by topical agents, systemic agents, or both.

TABLE 128.6 Concentrations and Dosages of Locally Used Ocular Antibacterial Agents[a]

Agent	Topical	Subconjunctival	Intravitreal
Amikacin	10 mg/mL	25 mg	0.4 mg
Ampicillin	50 mg/mL	50–150 mg	5 mg
Bacitracin	10,000 U/mL	5000 U	—
Cefazolin	50 mg/mL	100 mg	2.25 mg
Ceftazidime	50 mg/mL	100 mg	2 mg
Ceftriaxone	50 mg/mL	—	—
Clindamycin	50 mg/mL	15–50 mg	1 mg
Erythromycin	50 mg/mL	100 mg	0.5 mg
Gentamicin	8–15 mg/mL	10–20 mg	0.1–0.2 mg
Kanamycin	30–50 mg/mL	30 mg	0.5 mg
Methicillin	—	20–100 mg	2 mg
Neomycin	5–8 mg/mL	125–250 mg	—
Penicillin G	100,000 U/mL	0.5–1 × 10^6 U	300 U
Polymyxin B	10,000 U/mL	100,000 U	—
Ticarcillin	6 mg/mL	100 mg	—
Tobramycin	8–15 mg/mL	10–20 mg	0.1–0.2 mg

[a]For dosage recommendations for systemic administration, see Chapter 10.

Adapted from © *Physician's Desk Reference for Ophthalmic Medicines*, ed 2009. Published by Thomson Reuters, New York. With permission.

Drugs should be injected under the bulbar conjunctiva, not the palpebral conjunctiva. The dorsal 12 o'clock position is easiest to access. Adequate topical anesthesia is required. A proparacaine-soaked cotton-tip swab should be held at the injection site for at least 60 seconds. The conjunctiva should be lifted with a small forceps to allow for proper needle placement. A 25-gauge needle should be used to slowly inject the drug. In many animals, this can be accomplished without sedation. In both dogs and cats a volume of 0.2 to 0.5 mL can be administered, creating a bleb that resolves in a few hours.

While significant posterior segment drug concentrations can be obtained when injecting near the equator of the globe, the subconjunctival route achieves inadequate concentrations for bacterial infections of the vitreous. Subconjunctival dosages vary by agent (Table 128.6).

Systemic Administration

The systemic route of therapy is indicated in cases of chorioretinitis and optic neuritis, because topical or subconjunctival application does not result in therapeutic drug concentrations in these tissues. Many drugs are unable to cross the blood-retinal or blood-aqueous barrier, although some agents have good ocular penetration (see Table 128.5). However, most drugs administered systemically do penetrate the eye when it is inflamed and the normal ocular barriers are disrupted. Of the systemically administered antifungal azole compounds, fluconazole has optimal penetration of the eye and CNS, but also is the least active azole. Itraconazole has also been effective in many animals for treating systemic mycoses such as blastomycosis with ocular involvement, and may be effective when treatment with fluconazole fails.

Some systemically administered medications may be associated with ocular adverse effects. Some cats receiving systemic enrofloxacin (oral or injectable) have developed acute retinal degeneration and permanent blindness.[118,119] This has been most notable in cats receiving greater than the recommended dose of 5 mg/kg per day. However, even lower doses may cause retinal degeneration in some cats, particularly older or debilitated animals with compromised renal function, and all systemically administered fluoroquinolones should be viewed as potentially retinotoxic in cats. However, pradofloxacin was shown to have no retinal toxicity in young healthy cats at 6 and 10 times the therapeutic dose.[120] This drug is preferred for cats when treatment with fluoroquinolones is indicated.

Treatment of moderate to severe anterior uveitis or posterior uveitis should include the use of an oral anti-inflammatory drug. Prednisone or prednisolone has the most potent effect and should be used in cases of optic neuritis, moderate to severe chorioretinitis, or retinal detachment caused by posterior uveitis. In cases of anterior uveitis without posterior segment involvement, an oral NSAID may be adequate and will also provide an analgesic effect.

Adjunctive Treatments

In addition to specific therapy, standard nursing care involves cleansing the ocular surface and lids with warm, moist wipes. Systemic analgesic drugs such as the synthetic opioid tramadol can be beneficial in treating ocular pain and can be safely used in conjunction with an oral glucocorticoid or NSAID. Topical atropine minimizes ocular pain from ciliary and iridal muscle spasm and helps prevent synechiae; however, atropine should not be used if KCS, glaucoma, or iridocorneal angle compromise are present. Injection of 25 μg of tPA into the anterior chamber is an effective and dramatic means of breaking down adhesions and dissolving fibrin clots if given within 3 to 7 days of formation. Once the clot is organized, drug efficacy is lost. If active or recent bleeding has occurred in the eye, intraocular rebleeding may occur after injection of tPA. Injections may be repeated if necessary. Injection of tPA into the vitreous humor is not as safe because of retinal toxicity.

Intraocular Administration

Intracameral or intraocular injection of antibacterial drugs is a heroic and effective means of obtaining high levels of intraocular antibiotics for the treatment of bacterial endophthalmitis. If vision is to be preserved, the decision to use the intracameral route must be made early to avoid rapidly devastating inflammation to delicate intraocular structures. Because culture and susceptibility testing results are not available for a few days, a broad-spectrum bactericidal antibiotic is usually selected. The use of intravitreal vancomycin has been common in human medicine for the treatment of bacterial endophthalmitis after injury or intraocular surgery. Prudent use of vancomycin is recommended to reduce selection for vancomycin-resistant enterococci, which represent a significant threat to human and animal health.

CASE EXAMPLE

Signalment

"Max," a 10-year-old male neutered bichon frise from northern California.

History

Max was evaluated by the University of California-Davis Veterinary Ophthalmology Service for a fleshy pink mass that had been noticed by his groomer on the outer corner of his left eye a week before the time of evaluation. The mass did not appear to be painful or pruritic, and Max had otherwise been eating well and was bright and alert. Max had been diagnosed a year previously with small B-cell lymphoma, which at that time had been detected in the right conjunctiva, peripheral lymph nodes, and GI tract. The lymphoma was treated with a combination chemotherapy protocol (cyclophosphamide, doxorubicin, vincristine, prednisone). A month later he developed a left-sided superficial corneal ulcer that was initially treated with neosporin-polymixin-bacitracin ointment, but subsequently ruptured and was treated with a conjunctival pedical flap. Topical cyclosporine and ocular lubricant were also prescribed for decreased tear production in the left eye, but because of persistently decreased tear production at a 3-month recheck, topical tacrolimus was also added. Since then, he had done well and was considered to be in complete remission. Max was up to date on vaccinations and was receiving monthly heartworm and ectoparasite prophylaxis medications.

Current Medications

Topical cyclosporine (2%, 1 drop q12h OS), tacrolimus (0.03%, 1 drop q12h OS), ocular lubricant (q6-8h OD), prednisone 1 mg/kg PO q24h.

Ophthalmic Examination

Body weight: 4.5 kg.

Eyes were open and appeared comfortable. There was moderate mucoid discharge OS. Face symmetrical, globe position and movements were normal OU. Pupil size was midrange OD. There were anterior synechia OS and the pupil could not be fully assessed due to large conjunctival flap and corneal opacity. Pupillary light reflexes (direct and consensual) were intact. The menace response was intact OU, there was a dazzle reflex, and palpebral reflexes were complete OU. Patient behaved as if sighted.

OD: Iris atrophy and nuclear sclerosis were present. All other findings were within normal limits.

OS (Fig. 128.31A): There was mild to moderate hyperemia of the third eyelid with mild diffuse thickening of the third eyelid. Mild diffuse conjunctival hyperemia and chemosis was present. There was a 7 mm × 3 mm × 3 mm smooth raised pink conjunctival mass arising from the temporal bulbar conjunctiva just posterior to the ventrotemporal limbus. The conjunctival pedicle flap was integrated into axial cornea. It appeared to be well perfused, densely pigmented, and fibrotic with extension of melanin and fibrosis forming a 2- to 3-mm rim around the incorporated flap. The anterior chamber was clear. There was a focal anterior synechia temporally. The visible iris and limited fundoscopic examination appeared normal.

STT (mm/min): OD-15, OS-5

Intraocular pressures (mmHg-rebound): OD-14, OS-10

Fluorescein stain: OU-no retention

Biopsy Procedure: Tetracaine was applied to the ocular surface OS and lidocaine 2% gel was applied to the affected conjunctiva. The conjunctiva adjacent to the mass was grasped with forceps and scissors were used to excise the conjunctival mass. Light pressure with a 4 × 4 gauze over closed lids was applied for hemostasis. Erythromycin ointment was applied OS at the conclusion of the procedure. The tissue was cut in half and submitted for histopathology and aerobic/anaerobic bacterial culture.

Histopathology Findings

The submucosa was markedly expanded by an abundant population of predominantly large foamy macrophages and plasma cells admixed with fewer neutrophils and Mott cells. Macrophages often contained phagocytosed cells, karyorrhectic debris, and occasional coccobacilli. Vascular profiles were cuffed by moderate numbers of lymphocytes and plasma cells. Gram staining revealed

CASE EXAMPLE—cont'd

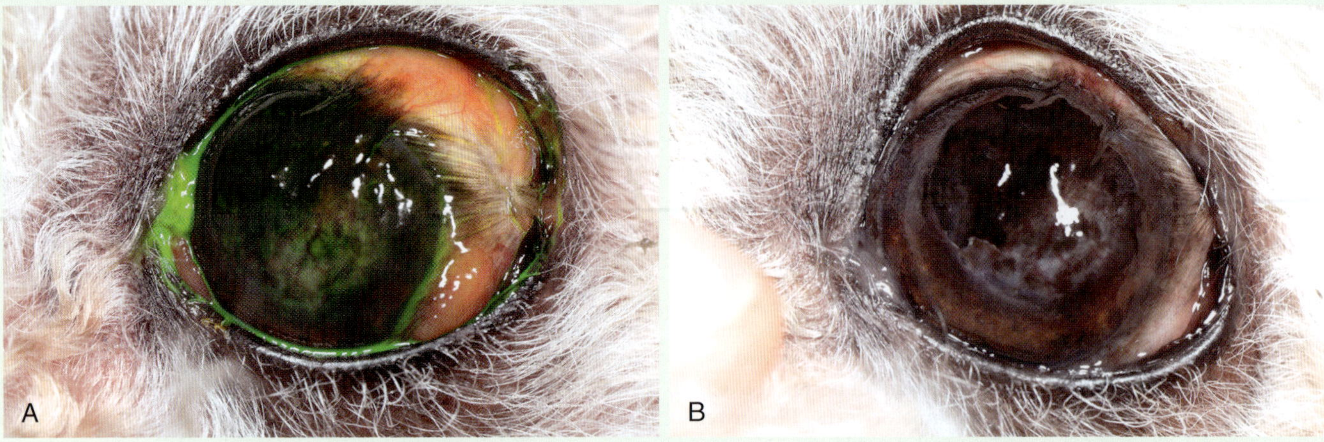

Fig. 128.31 Left eye of a 10-year-old dog with mycobacterial conjunctivitis. (A) There is a pink fleshy mass on the ventrotemporal aspect of the globe. A conjunctival pedicle graft is also present that arises from the dorsotemporal aspect of the globe. Fluorescein stain has been applied. (B) After treatment with surgical excision and topical ofloxacin, topical gentamicin, and oral doxycycline. (Courtesy of University of California-Davis Veterinary Ophthalmology Service.)

small numbers of gram-positive cocci and rare gram-negative rods scattered within histiocytes and occasionally extracellularly. Acid-fast staining revealed intrahistiocytic bundles of fibrillar to rod-shaped bacteria that were strongly acid-fast-positive. These organisms were also visible using Warthin-Starry silver stain.

Aerobic and Anaerobic Bacterial Culture

Very small numbers of mixed growth including methicillin-resistant *Staphylococcus pseudintermedius* (susceptible only to aminoglycosides, chloramphenicol, rifampin, vancomycin) and *E. coli* (susceptible to aminoglycosides, amoxicillin-clavulanic acid, ceftazidime, chloramphenicol, tetracyclines, imipenem, fluoroquinolones).

Diagnosis

Mycobacterial conjunctivitis.

Treatment

Doxycycline, 10 mg/kg PO q24h, topical gentamicin ophthalmic ointment OS q8h, and ofloxacin (0.3% ophthalmic solution, 1 drop OU q8h) in addition to continuing the other medications. At a recheck examination 1 month later, conjunctivitis had resolved and there was no evidence of mass recurrence (Fig. 128.31B). Antimicrobial treatment was discontinued. At an examination 4 months later there was still no evidence of recurrence, although the owners reported a brief period of inappetence a week before that visit. However, a month after that, Max stopped eating and began to lose weight, and the owners elected euthanasia. Necropsy was not performed.

Comments

This dog developed mycobacterial conjunctivitis, a rare infection of the ocular adnexal structures, which was likely secondary to immunosuppressive disease or medications. The lack of mycobacterial growth in culture suggests that a slow-growing or unculturable mycobacterial species was responsible, such as *Mycobacterium avium.* Bacteria cultured were likely secondary invaders and should have been inactivated with the topical antibacterial medications.

The owner was offered additional diagnostic tests to identify the *Mycobacterium* species present and determine whether there was evidence of more widespread infection, but declined. Such tests could include mycobacterial culture at a mycobacterial reference laboratory, species-specific PCR assays on paraffin-embedded biopsy tissue, and a minimum database with thoracic radiographs and abdominal ultrasound examination.

Possible reasons for the decline of this dog after treatment were recurrence of lymphoma, systemic mycobacterial disease, or another unrelated illness.

SUGGESTED READINGS

Hewitt JS, Allbaugh RA, Kenne DE, et al. Prevalence and antibiotic susceptibility of bacterial isolates from dogs with ulcerative keratitis in midwestern United States. *Front Vet Sci.* 2020;7:583965.

Weingart C, Kohn B, Siekierski M, et al. Blepharitis in dogs: a clinical evaluation in 102 dogs. *Vet Dermatol.* 2019;30:222–e269.

REFERENCES

1. Gerding PA Jr, Kakoma I. Microbiology of the canine and feline eye. *Vet Clin North Am Small Anim Pract.* 1990;20:615–625.
2. Samuelson DA, Andresen TL, Gwin RM. Conjunctival fungal flora in horses, cattle, dogs, and cats. *J Am Vet Med Assoc.* 1984;184:1240–1242.
3. Espinola MB, Lilenbaum W. Prevalence of bacteria in the conjunctival sac and on the eyelid margin of clinically normal cats. *J Small Anim Pract.* 1996;37:364–366.
4. Gerding PA, Cormany K, Weisiger R, et al. Survey and topographic distribution of bacterial and fungal microorganisms in eyes of clinically normal cats. *Feline Pract.* 1993;21:20–23.
5. Snyder R, Hyndiuk R. Mechanisms of bacterial invasion of the cornea. In: Tasman W, Jaeger E, eds. *Duane's Foundations of Clinical Ophthalmology*. Philadelphia, PA: Lippincott-Raven; 1995:1–7.
6. Weingart C, Kohn B, Siekierski M, et al. Blepharitis in dogs: a clinical evaluation in 102 dogs. *Vet Dermatol.* 2019;30:222–e269.
7. Soimala T, Lubke-Becker A, Hanke D, et al. Molecular and phenotypic characterization of methicillin-resistant *Staphylococcus pseudintermedius* from ocular surfaces of dogs and cats suffering from ophthalmological diseases. *Vet Microbiol.* 2020;244:108687.

8. Sebbag L, Yan Y, Smith JS, et al. Tear fluid pharmacokinetics following oral prednisone administration in dogs with and without conjunctivitis. *J Ocul Pharmacol Ther*. 2019;35:341–349.
9. Pimenta P, Alves-Pimenta S, Barros J, et al. Feline leishmaniosis in Portugal: 3 cases (year 2014). *Vet Parasitol Reg Stud Reports*. 2015;1–2:65–69.
10. Ledbetter EC, Kim SG, Dubovi EJ. Outbreak of ocular disease associated with naturally-acquired canine herpesvirus-1 infection in a closed domestic dog colony. *Vet Ophthalmol*. 2009;12:242–247.
11. Ledbetter EC, Dubovi EJ, Kim SG, et al. Experimental primary ocular canine herpesvirus-1 infection in adult dogs. *Am J Vet Res*. 2009;70:513–521.
12. Ledbetter EC, Hornbuckle WE, Dubovi EJ. Virologic survey of dogs with naturally acquired idiopathic conjunctivitis. *J Am Vet Med Assoc*. 2009;235:954–959.
13. Ledbetter EC, Kice NC, Matusow RB, et al. The effect of topical ocular corticosteroid administration in dogs with experimentally induced latent canine herpesvirus-1 infection. *Exp Eye Res*. 2010;90:711–717.
14. Ledbetter EC, Kim SG, Dubovi EJ, et al. Experimental reactivation of latent canine herpesvirus-1 and induction of recurrent ocular disease in adult dogs. *Vet Microbiol*. 2009;138:98–105.
15. Spertus CB, Mohammed HO, Ledbetter EC. Effects of topical ocular application of 1% trifluridine ophthalmic solution in dogs with experimentally induced recurrent ocular canine herpesvirus-1 infection. *Am J Vet Res*. 2016;77:1140–1147.
16. Ledbetter EC, Spertus CB, Pennington MR, et al. In vitro and in vivo evaluation of cidofovir as a topical ophthalmic antiviral for ocular canine herpesvirus-1 infections in dogs. *J Ocul Pharmacol Ther*. 2015;31:642–649.
17. Ledbetter EC, Nicklin AM, Spertus CB, et al. Evaluation of topical ophthalmic ganciclovir gel for the treatment of dogs with experimentally induced ocular canine herpesvirus-1 infection. *Am J Vet Res*. 2018;79:762–769.
18. Stiles J. Treatment of cats with ocular disease attributable to herpesvirus infection: 17 cases (1983-1993). *J Am Vet Med Assoc*. 1995;207:599–603.
19. Sandmeyer LS, Keller CB, Bienzle D. Effects of interferon-alpha on cytopathic changes and titers for feline herpesvirus-1 in primary cultures of feline corneal epithelial cells. *Am J Vet Res*. 2005;66:210–216.
20. Siebeck N, Hurley DJ, Garcia M, et al. Effects of human recombinant alpha-2b interferon and feline recombinant omega interferon on in vitro replication of feline herpesvirus-1. *Am J Vet Res*. 2006;67:1406–1411.
21. Sundmacher R, Mattes A, Neumann-Haefelin D, et al. The potency of interferon-alpha 2 and interferon-gamma in a combination therapy of dendritic keratitis. A controlled clinical study. *Curr Eye Res*. 1987;6:273–276.
22. Sundmacher R, Cantell K, Mattes A. Combination therapy for dendritic keratitis. High-titer alpha-interferon and trifluridine. *Arch Ophthalmol*. 1984;102:554–555.
23. Slack JM, Stiles J, Leutenegger CM, et al. Effects of topical ocular administration of high doses of human recombinant interferon alpha-2b and feline recombinant interferon omega on naturally occurring viral keratoconjunctivitis in cats. *Am J Vet Res*. 2013;74:281–289.
24. Thomasy SM, Maggs DJ. A review of antiviral drugs and other compounds with activity against feline herpesvirus type 1. *Vet Ophthalmol*. 2016;19(suppl 1):119–130.
25. Thomasy SM, Shull O, Outerbridge CA, et al. Oral administration of famciclovir for treatment of spontaneous ocular, respiratory, or dermatologic disease attributed to feline herpesvirus type 1: 59 cases (2006-2013). *J Am Vet Med Assoc*. 2016;249:526–538.
26. Cooper AE, Thomasy SM, Drazenovich TL, et al. Prophylactic and therapeutic effects of twice-daily famciclovir administration on infectious upper respiratory disease in shelter-housed cats. *J Feline Med Surg*. 2019;21:544–552.
27. Dean R, Harley R, Helps C, et al. Use of quantitative real-time PCR to monitor the response of *Chlamydophila felis* infection to doxycycline treatment. *J Clin Microbiol*. 2005;43:1858–1864.
28. von Bomhard W, Polkinghorne A, Lu ZH, et al. Detection of novel chlamydiae in cats with ocular disease. *Am J Vet Res*. 2003;64:1421–1428.
29. Richter M, Matheis F, Gonczi E, et al. *Parachlamydia acanthamoebae* in domestic cats with and without corneal disease. *Vet Ophthalmol*. 2010;13:235–237.
30. Haesebrouck F, Devriese LA, van Rijssen B, et al. Incidence and significance of isolation of *Mycoplasma felis* from conjunctival swabs of cats. *Vet Microbiol*. 1991;26:95–101.
31. Low HC, Powell CC, Veir JK, et al. Prevalence of feline herpesvirus 1, *Chlamydophila felis*, and *Mycoplasma* spp. DNA in conjunctival cells collected from cats with and without conjunctivitis. *Am J Vet Res*. 2007;68:643–648.
32. Hewitt JS, Allbaugh RA, Kenne DE, et al. Prevalence and antibiotic susceptibility of bacterial isolates from dogs with ulcerative keratitis in midwestern United States. *Front Vet Sci*. 2020;7:583965.
33. Sellers RS, Silverman L, Khan KN. Cyclooxygenase-2 expression in the cornea of dogs with keratitis. *Vet Pathol*. 2004;41:116–121.
34. Scott EM, Carter RT. Canine keratomycosis in 11 dogs: a case series (2000-2011). *J Am Anim Hosp Assoc*. 2014;50:112–118.
35. Nevile JC, Hurn SD, Turner AG. Keratomycosis in five dogs. *Vet Ophthalmol*. 2016;19:432–438.
36. Ledbetter EC, Starr JK. *Malassezia pachydermatis* keratomycosis in a dog. *Med Mycol Case Rep*. 2015;10:24–26.
37. Conway ED, Stiles J, Townsend WM, et al. Evaluation of species differences and the effects of storage duration and temperature on the anticollagenase efficacy of canine, feline, and equine serum on in vitro corneal degradation. *Am J Vet Res*. 2015;76:989–995.
38. Conway ED, Stiles J, Townsend WM, et al. Comparison of the in vitro anticollagenase efficacy of homologous serum and plasma on degradation of corneas of cats, dogs, and horses. *Am J Vet Res*. 2016;77:627–633.
39. Grundon RA, O'Reilly A, Muhlnickel C, et al. Keratomycosis in a dog treated with topical 1% voriconazole solution. *Vet Ophthalmol*. 2010;13:331–335.
40. Ben-Shlomo G, Plummer C, Barrie K, et al. *Curvularia* keratomycosis in a dog. *Vet Ophthalmol*. 2010;13:126–130.
41. Labelle AL, Hamor RE, Barger AM, et al. *Aspergillus flavus* keratomycosis in a cat treated with topical 1% voriconazole solution. *Vet Ophthalmol*. 2009;12:48–52.
42. Stiles J. Feline herpesvirus. *Vet Clin North Am Small Anim Pract*. 2000;30:1001–1014.
43. La Croix NC, van der Woerdt A, Olivero DK. Nonhealing corneal ulcers in cats: 29 cases (1991-1999). *J Am Vet Med Assoc*. 2001;218:733–735.
44. Nasisse MP, English RV, Tompkins MB, et al. Immunologic, histologic, and virologic features of herpesvirus-induced stromal keratitis in cats. *Am J Vet Res*. 1995;56:51–55.
45. Nasisse MP, Guy JS, Davidson MG, et al. Experimental ocular herpesvirus infection in the cat. Sites of virus replication, clinical features and effects of corticosteroid administration. *Invest Ophthalmol Vis Sci*. 1989;30:1758–1768.
46. Barsotti G, Mannucci T, Citi S. Ultrasonography-guided removal of plant-based foreign bodies from the lacrimal sac in four dogs. *BMC Vet Res*. 2019;15:76.
47. Strom AR, Culp WTN, Leonard BC, et al. A multidisciplinary, minimally invasive approach combining lacrimoscopy and fluoroscopically guided stenting for management of nasolacrimal apparatus obstruction in dogs. *J Am Vet Med Assoc*. 2018;252:1527–1537.
48. Fischer MC, Adrian AM, Demetriou J, et al. Retrobulbar cellulitis and abscessation: focus on short- and long-term concurrent ophthalmic diseases in 41 dogs. *J Small Anim Pract*. 2018;59:763–768.
49. Tremolada G, Milovancev M, Culp WT, et al. Surgical management of canine refractory retrobulbar abscesses: six cases. *J Small Anim Pract*. 2015;56:667–670.
50. Hacker DV, Jensen HE, Selby LA. A comparison of conjunctival culture techniques in the dog. *J Am Anim Hosp Assoc*. 1979;15:223–225.
51. Urban M, Wyman M, Rheins M, et al. Conjunctival flora of clinically normal dogs. *J Am Vet Med Assoc*. 1972;161:201–206.
52. Tsubota K, Kajiwara K, Ugajin S, et al. Conjunctival brush cytology. *Acta Cytol*. 1990;34:233–235.
53. Willis M, Bounous D, Hirsh S, et al. Conjunctival brush cytology: evaluation of a new cytological collection technique in dogs and cats with a comparison to conjunctival scraping. *Vet Comp Ophthalmol*. 1997;7:74–81.

54. Yu-Speight AW, Kern TJ, Erb HN. Ciprofloxacin and ofloxacin aqueous humor concentrations after topical administration in dogs undergoing cataract surgery. *Vet Ophthalmol.* 2005;8:181–187.
55. Forster RK, Abbott RL, Gelender H. Management of infectious endophthalmitis. *Ophthalmology.* 1980;87:313–319.
56. Thomas W, Sorjonen D, Steiss J. A retrospective evaluation of 38 cases of canine distemper encephalomyelitis. *J Am Anim Hosp Assoc.* 1993;29:129–133.
57. Fischer CA, Jones GT. Optic neuritis in dogs. *J Am Vet Med Assoc.* 1972;160:68–79.
58. Albert DM, Lahav M, Carmichael LE, et al. Canine herpes-induced retinal dysplasia and associated ocular anomalies. *Invest Ophthalmol.* 1976;15:267–278.
59. Sangl L, Felten S, Matiasek K, et al. Detection of feline coronavirus RNA, spike gene mutations, and feline coronavirus antigen in macrophages in aqueous humor of cats in the diagnosis of feline infectious peritonitis. *J Vet Diagn Invest.* 2020;32:527–534.
60. Brightman AH 2nd, Ogilvie GK, Tompkins M. Ocular disease in FeLV-positive cats: 11 cases (1981-1986). *J Am Vet Med Assoc.* 1991;198:1049–1051.
61. Stiles J, Bienzle D, Render JA, et al. Use of nested polymerase chain reaction (PCR) for detection of retroviruses from formalin-fixed, paraffin-embedded uveal melanomas in cats. *Vet Ophthalmol.* 1999;2:113–116.
62. Cullen CL, Haines DM, Jackson ML, et al. Lack of detection of feline leukemia and feline sarcoma viruses in diffuse iris melanomas of cats by immunohistochemistry and polymerase chain reaction. *J Vet Diagn Invest.* 2002;14:340–343.
63. Loesenbeck G, Drommer W, Heider HJ. Findings in the eyes of serologically FIV (feline immunodeficiency virus) positive cats. *Dtsch Tierarztl Wochenschr.* 1995;102:348–351.
64. O'Dair HA, Hopper CD, Gruffydd-Jones TJ, et al. Clinical aspects of *Chlamydia psittaci* infection in cats infected with feline immunodeficiency virus. *Vet Rec.* 1994;134:365–368.
65. Komnenou AA, Mylonakis ME, Kouti V, et al. Ocular manifestations of natural canine monocytic ehrlichiosis (*Ehrlichia canis*): a retrospective study of 90 cases. *Vet Ophthalmol.* 2007;10:137–142.
66. Breitschwerdt EB, Hegarty BC, Hancock SI. Sequential evaluation of dogs naturally infected with *Ehrlichia canis, Ehrlichia chaffeensis, Ehrlichia equi, Ehrlichia ewingii*, or *Bartonella vinsonii*. *J Clin Microbiol.* 1998;36:2645–2651.
67. Panciera RJ, Ewing SA, Confer AW. Ocular histopathology of Ehrlichial infections in the dog. *Vet Pathol.* 2001;38:43–46.
68. Davidson MG, Breitschwerdt EB, Nasisse MP, et al. Ocular manifestations of Rocky Mountain spotted fever in dogs. *J Am Vet Med Assoc.* 1989;194:777–781.
69. Davidson MG, Breitschwerdt EB, Walker DH, et al. Vascular permeability and coagulation during *Rickettsia rickettsii* infection in dogs. *Am J Vet Res.* 1990;51:165–170.
70. Greene CE, Burgdorfer W, Cavagnolo R, et al. Rocky Mountain spotted fever in dogs and its differentiation from canine ehrlichiosis. *J Am Vet Med Assoc.* 1985;186:465–472.
71. Vinayak A, Greene CE, Moore PA, et al. Clinical resolution of *Brucella canis*-induced ocular inflammation in a dog. *J Am Vet Med Assoc.* 2004;224:1804–1807.
72. Ledbetter EC, Landry MP, Stokol T, et al. *Brucella canis* endophthalmitis in 3 dogs: clinical features, diagnosis, and treatment. *Vet Ophthalmol.* 2009;12:183–191.
73. Pleyer U, Priem S, Bergmann L, et al. Detection of *Borrelia burgdorferi* DNA in urine of patients with ocular Lyme borreliosis. *Br J Ophthalmol.* 2001;85:552–555.
74. Mikkila HO, Seppala IJ, Viljanen MK, et al. The expanding clinical spectrum of ocular lyme borreliosis. *Ophthalmology.* 2000;107:581–587.
75. Dziezyc J. Canine systemic bacterial infections. *Vet Clin North Am Small Anim Pract.* 2000;30:1103–1117.
76. Townsend WM, Stiles J, Krohne SG. Leptospirosis and panuveitis in a dog. *Vet Ophthalmol.* 2006;9:169–173.
77. Burkitt JM, Sturges BK, Jandrey KE, et al. Risk factors associated with outcome in dogs with tetanus: 38 cases (1987-2005). *J Am Vet Med Assoc.* 2007;230:76–83.
78. Johnson A. Ocular complications of cat scratch disease. *Br J Ophthalmol.* 2020;104:1640–1646.
79. Lappin MR, Kordick DL, Breitschwerdt EB. *Bartonella* spp. antibodies and DNA in aqueous humour of cats. *J Feline Med Surg.* 2000;2:61–68.
80. Fontanelle JP, Powell CC, Hill AE, et al. Prevalence of serum antibodies against *Bartonella* species in the serum of cat with or without uveitis. *J Feline Med Surg.* 2008;10:41–46.
81. Sykes JE, Westropp JL, Kasten RW, et al. Association between *Bartonella* species infection and disease in pet cats as determined using serology and culture. *J Feline Med Surg.* 2010;12:631–636.
82. Stiles J. Bartonellosis in cats: a role in uveitis? *Vet Ophthalmol.* 2011;14(suppl 1):9–14.
83. Michau TM, Breitschwerdt EB, Gilger BC, et al. *Bartonella vinsonii* subspecies *berkhoffi* as a possible cause of anterior uveitis and choroiditis in a dog. *Vet Ophthalmol.* 2003;6:299–304.
84. Dietrich U, Arnold P, Guscetti F, et al. Ocular manifestation of disseminated *Mycobacterium simiae* infection in a cat. *J Small Anim Pract.* 2003;44:121–125.
85. Formston C. Retinal detachment and bovine tuberculosis in cats. *J Small Anim Pract.* 1994;35:5–8.
86. Stavinohova R, O'Halloran C, Newton JR, et al. Feline ocular mycobacteriosis: clinical presentation, histopathological features, and outcome. *Vet Pathol.* 2019;56:749–760.
87. Lamagna B, Paciello O, Ragozzino M, et al. Isolated lepromatous conjunctivo-corneal granuloma in a cat from Italy. *Vet Ophthalmol.* 2009;12:97–101.
88. Fyfe JA, McCowan C, O'Brien CR, et al. Molecular characterization of a novel fastidious mycobacterium causing lepromatous lesions of the skin, subcutis, cornea, and conjunctiva of cats living in Victoria, Australia. *J Clin Microbiol.* 2008;46:618–626.
89. Arceneaux KA, Taboada J, Hosgood G. Blastomycosis in dogs: 115 cases (1980-1995). *J Am Vet Med Assoc.* 1998;213:658–664.
90. Buyukmihci N. Ocular lesions of blastomycosis in the dog. *J Am Vet Med Assoc.* 1982;180:426–431.
91. Gwin RM, Makley TA Jr, Wyman M, et al. Multifocal ocular histoplasmosis in a dog and cat. *J Am Vet Med Assoc.* 1980;176:638–642.
92. Gionfriddo JR. Feline systemic fungal infections. *Vet Clin North Am Small Anim Pract.* 2000;30:1029–1050.
93. Ewald MM, Rankin AJ, Meekins JM, et al. Disseminated histoplasmosis with ocular adnexal involvement in seven cats. *Vet Ophthalmol.* 2020;23:905–912.
94. Smith KM, Strom AR, Gilmour MA, et al. Utility of antigen testing for the diagnosis of ocular histoplasmosis in four cats: a case series and literature review. *J Feline Med Surg.* 2017;19:1110–1118.
95. Barrs VR, Talbot JJ. Fungal rhinosinusitis and disseminated invasive aspergillosis in cats. *Vet Clin North Am Small Anim Pract.* 2020;50:331–357.
96. McLellan GJ, Aquino SM, Mason DR, et al. Use of posaconazole in the management of invasive orbital aspergillosis in a cat. *J Am Anim Hosp Assoc.* 2006;42:302–307.
97. Finn MJ, Stiles J, Krohne SG. Visual outcome in a group of dogs with ocular blastomycosis treated with systemic antifungals and systemic corticosteroids. *Vet Ophthalmol.* 2007;10:299–303.
98. Migaki G, Font RL, Sauer RM, et al. Canine protothecosis: review of the literature and report of an additional case. *J Am Vet Med Assoc.* 1982;181:794–797.
99. Shank AM, Dubielzig RD, Teixeira LB. Canine ocular protothecosis: a review of 14 cases. *Vet Ophthalmol.* 2015;18:437–442.
100. Davidson MG. Toxoplasmosis. *Vet Clin North Am Small Anim Pract.* 2000;30:1051–1062.
101. Dubey JP, Carpenter JL. Histologically confirmed clinical toxoplasmosis in cats: 100 cases (1952-1990). *J Am Vet Med Assoc.* 1993;203:1556–1566.
102. Davidson MG, English RV. Feline ocular toxoplasmosis. *Vet Ophthalmol.* 1998;1:71–80.
103. Powell CC, Lappin MR. Clinical ocular toxoplasmosis in neonatal kittens. *Vet Ophthalmol.* 2001;4:87–92.
104. Lappin MR, Burney DP, Dow SW, et al. Polymerase chain reaction for the detection of *Toxoplasma gondii* in aqueous humor of cats. *Am J Vet Res.* 1996;57:1589–1593.

105. Stiles J, Prade R, Greene C. Detection of *Toxoplasma gondii* in feline and canine biological samples by use of the polymerase chain reaction. *Am J Vet Res*. 1996;57:264–267.
106. Dubey JP, Koestner A, Piper RC. Repeated transplacental transmission of *Neospora caninum* in dogs. *J Am Vet Med Assoc*. 1990;197:857–860.
107. Stiles J, Didier E, Ritchie B, et al. *Encephalitozoon cuniculi* in the lens of a rabbit with phacoclastic uveitis: confirmation and treatment. *Prog Vet Comp Ophthalmol*. 1997;7:233–238.
108. Bjerkas I. Brain and spinal cord lesions in encephalitozoonosis in mink. *Acta Vet Scand*. 1990;31:423–432.
109. Arnesen K, Nordstoga K. Ocular encephalitozoonosis (nosematosis) in blue foxes. Polyarteritis nodosa and cataract. *Acta Ophthalmol*. 1977;55:641–651.
110. Hunt RD, King NW, Foster HL. Encephalitozoonosis: evidence for vertical transmission. *J Infect Dis*. 1972;126:212–214.
111. Benz P, Maass G, Csokai J, et al. Detection of *Encephalitozoon cuniculi* in the feline cataractous lens. *Vet Ophthalmol*. 2011;14(suppl 1):37–47.
112. Pena MT, Roura X, Davidson MG. Ocular and periocular manifestations of leishmaniasis in dogs: 105 cases (1993-1998). *Vet Ophthalmol*. 2000;3:35–41.
113. Pietro SD, Bosco VR, Crino C, et al. Prevalence, type, and prognosis of ocular lesions in shelter and client-owned dogs naturally infected by *Leishmania infantum*. *Vet World*. 2016;9:633–637.
114. Pena MT, Naranjo C, Klauss G, et al. Histopathological features of ocular leishmaniosis in the dog. *J Comp Pathol*. 2008;138:32–39.
115. Martin C, Kaswan R, Gratzek A, et al. Ocular use of tissue plasminogen activator in companion animals. *Prog Vet Comp Ophthalmol*. 1993;3:29–36.
116. Johnson DA, Johns KJ, Robinson RD, et al. The relationship of corneal epithelial defect size to drug penetration. *Arch Ophthalmol*. 1995;113:641–644.
117. Plunkett SJ. Anaphylaxis to ophthalmic medication in a cat. *J Vet Emerg Crit Care*. 2000;10:161–171.
118. Gelatt KN, van der Woerdt A, Ketring KL, et al. Enrofloxacin-associated retinal degeneration in cats. *Vet Ophthalmol*. 2001;4:99–106.
119. Wiebe V, Hamilton P. Fluoroquinolone-induced retinal degeneration in cats. *J Am Vet Med Assoc*. 2002;221:1568–1571.
120. Messias A, Gekeler F, Wegener A, et al. Retinal safety of a new fluoroquinolone, pradofloxacin, in cats: assessment with electroretinography. *Doc Ophthalmol*. 2008;116:177–191.

129

Miscellaneous Infections and Inflammatory Disorders of the Central Nervous System

Andrea Tipold, Marc Vandevelde, Renee Barber, Jane E. Sykes

KEY POINTS

Prion Diseases and Feline Spongiform Encephalopathy

- First Described: Feline spongiform encephalopathy was first recognized in 1990, but prion diseases of sheep and goats have been recognized since the 1700s and 1800s.
- Cause: Prions are small infectious agents that are resistant to inactivation by heat, formalin, glutaraldehyde, alcohol, and radiation. Infectivity is associated with a host-encoded protein, the prion protein (PrP). The mechanism of transmissible spongiform encephalopathy (TSE) involves a misfolding of the normal prion protein (PrP^c) to a new heat-resistant protein.
- Affected Hosts: Cats, humans, and a variety of other mammalian species.
- Geographic Distribution: Primarily Europe, but cases have occurred sporadically worldwide.
- Mode of transmission: The TSEs are transmissible to other animals, at least under experimental conditions. Routes of natural transmission of TSEs involve oral ingestion, skin scarification, or congenital transmission. For example, scrapie has been consistently found in the placentas of ewes. Infection has spread iatrogenically through contaminated biologic products and likely through other veterinary procedures or feeding practices.
- Major Clinical Signs: Adult cats, slowly progressive neurologic signs, behavioral changes, gait abnormalities, hypersensitivity.
- Differential Diagnoses: Degenerative diseases, neoplasia, other infectious and inflammatory diseases of the CNS.
- Human Health Significance: During the outbreak of bovine spongiform encephalopathy (BSE) in the United Kingdom, a new variant of Creutzfeldt-Jakob disease (vCJD) occurred in humans. The disease has also been reported in other countries. vCJD affected primarily young adults and was suspected of being caused by ingestion of contaminated cattle products. Not all humans are equally susceptible to the development of spongiform encephalopathy. Transmission of the agent through blood transfusions or organ donation remains a concern.

Bacterial Meningitis and Meningoencephalomyelitis

- Cause: Bacterial meningoencephalomyelitis is caused by a variety of pyogenic bacteria that enter the CSF spaces or the CNS parenchyma. Organisms are usually opportunistic microflora or enter tissues as a result of environmental contamination of penetrating objects or spread of an infection from other organs.
- Affected Hosts: Dogs and cats of all ages are affected.
- Geographic Distribution: Worldwide.
- Mode of Transmission: Bacteria can spread to the meninges from: (1) sites of infection in the nasal sinuses, retrobulbar tissues, or middle or inner ear when host immune defenses are compromised; (2) sites of traumatic focal penetration; (3) sites of infection in adjacent venous sinuses or bony structures; or (4) via hematogenous arterial dissemination.
- Major Clinical Signs: Meningitis: fever, reluctance to move, stiff gait, and muscle spasms are the most common clinical signs. Paraspinal hyperesthesia and progressive neurologic dysfunction are progressive features. Meningoencephalomyelitis: additional signs of brain and/or spinal cord lesions.
- Differential Diagnoses: Meningoencephalomyelitis caused by nonbacterial microorganisms and immune-mediated causes should be considered. Myeloid or lymphoid neoplasias may cause similar focal, multifocal, or diffuse signs of inflammation.
- Human Health Significance: None. The organisms that cause bacterial meningoencephalomyelitis are indigenous microflora or environmental contaminants. Precautions should always be taken in collecting or handling CSF potentially laden with microorganisms during diagnostic medical procedures.

Inflammatory Neurologic Diseases Previously of Suspected Infectious Origin

- First Described: Granulomatous meningoencephalitis, necrotizing encephalitis, and feline poliomyelitis were first described in the 1950s–1980s. Nonsuppurative encephalitis was reported in Ireland in 2002 and steroid-responsive meningitis-arteritis was described in 1981.
- Cause: Unknown, but uncultivable infectious agents have been suspected.
- Affected Hosts: Granulomatous meningoencephalitis, necrotizing encephalitis, greyhound nonsuppurative encephalitis and steroid-responsive meningitis-arteritis all occur exclusively in dogs. Feline poliomyelitis has been reported in domestic and wild felids.
- Geographic Distribution: Some conditions have limited distributions, whereas others can be found worldwide.
- Mode of Transmission: Mostly unknown.
- Major Clinical Signs: Depending on the localization of the lesion—spinal cord or intracranial signs, or signs may be multifocal. Cervical rigidity, and in some diseases fever can occur.
- Differential Diagnoses: The main differential diagnoses are neoplasia and a variety of infectious diseases of the CNS (viral, bacterial, fungal, protozoal, and parasitic).
- Human Health Significance: None.

PRION DISEASES AND FELINE SPONGIFORM ENCEPHALOPATHY

ETIOLOGY, EPIDEMIOLOGY AND PATHOGENESIS

Feline spongiform encephalopathy (FSE) belongs to the transmissible spongiform encephalopathies (TSEs; Table 129.1),[1] a group of neurodegenerative diseases in humans and animals characterized by a very long incubation time and degeneration of the CNS with vacuolation of the neuropil and nerve cells.[2] The infectious agent is small and resistant to inactivation by heat, formalin, glutaraldehyde, alcohol, and radiation. Infectivity is associated with a host-encoded protein, the so-called prion protein (PrP). PrP is widely distributed in the CNS, peripheral nerve, neuroendocrine and lymphatic tissues, and many other organs.[3] It is involved in neuronal development and function and in the prevention of cell death. The mechanism of TSE involves a misfolding of the normal prion protein (PrP^c) to a new heat-resistant protein known as PrP^{Sc} or PrP^{res} (*Sc* stands for scrapie, the oldest known spongiform encephalopathy [SE] in small ruminants; *res* stands for resistant to protease digestion). In its new conformation, the PrP^{Sc} is protease resistant and hence accumulates in the tissue. Misfolding of the PrP can also occur spontaneously and sporadically through genetic mutations in the PrP gene, leading to hereditary SEs, which are exceedingly rare in humans. Once formed, the modified, abnormal PrP is thought to induce additional copies of itself by interacting with normal PrP. Thus, the belief holds that this misfolded protein itself becomes an infectious agent, the prion.[3,4] The prion theory is a revolutionary concept in biology, and many questions remain. Prions are unique because they can be both inherited and infectious.

The PrP^c gene is highly conserved among different animals; however, knockout mice devoid of the protein develop normally with mild neuronal abnormalities. The presence of an abnormal PrP in the CNS is devastating. PrP^{Sc} is insoluble and aggregates as amyloid fibrils in infected brain tissue where deposits (amyloid plaques) can be observed in some SEs. Accumulation of aberrantly folded PrP^{Sc} fibrils is central in the pathogenesis of these diseases.[3] Accumulation leads to astrocytic proliferation, microglial cell activation, loss of synapses, and finally to neuronal cell death by apoptosis.[2] However, PrP^c also appears to play an important role in neurotoxicity.[5]

TABLE 129.1 Transmissible Spongiform Encephalopathies of Humans and Animals

Disease	Host[a]	First Recognized
Creutzfeldt-Jakob disease	Humans	1920
Kuru	Humans (New Guinea)	1957
Gerstmann-Straussler-Scheinker syndrome	Humans	1928
Fatal familial insomnia	Humans	1986
Variant Creutzfeldt-Jakob disease (bovine SE in humans)	Humans	1996
Sporadic familial insomnia	Humans	1999
Scrapie	Sheep	1730
	Goats	1872
Transmissible mink encephalopathy	Mink	1947
Chronic wasting disease	Mule deer	1967
	Elk	1979
Bovine SE (mad cow disease)	Cattle (Europe)	1985
SE	Eland, oryx, greater kudu (Africa)	1989
Feline SE	Domestic cats (Europe)	1990
	Exotic cats	1992
SE of captive primates	Monkeys	1996

[a]Geographic location in parentheses when restricted to a specific area. *SE*, spongiform encephalopathy.

The TSEs are transmissible to other animals, at least under experimental conditions (intracerebral inoculation), even from sheep to pigs.[6,7] Routes of natural transmission of TSEs involve oral ingestion, skin scarification, or congenital transmission. For example, scrapie has been consistently found in the placentas of ewes,[8] and in a cheetah maternal transmission was suspected.[9] Infection has spread iatrogenically through contaminated biologic products and likely through other veterinary procedures or feeding practices.[6]

During the incubation period (following mucosal exposure), which has been studied in small rodents, PrP^{Sc} accumulates on the membranes of follicular dendritic cells (FDCs) in local lymphoid tissue.[2] A crucial phase of neuronal invasion likely occurs at the interface of FDC and nerve endings in secondary lymphoid organs.[10] From the lymphoreticular tissues at the site of experimental inoculation, the prion is thought to gain access to the peripheral nervous system through local nerve endings, although the exact mechanism of transfer is unclear.[10] From there, the prion migrates to the CNS. Following exposure by ingestion, PrP^{Sc} may enter the gut-associated lymphoid tissue, then enter nerve endings in the intestinal tract, and migrate to the CNS by means of the vagus nerve. In bovine spongiform encephalopathy (BSE), there seems to be some replication in tonsils,[11] but spread appears to occur by way of the autonomic nervous system of the gut, specifically the vagus nerve to the medulla oblongata.[10,12]

Scrapie, the classic TSE of small ruminants, has been recognized for approximately 275 years. Since that time, other SEs have been recognized in humans and animals. TSEs became notorious in the late 1980s as a result of the BSE outbreak in the United Kingdom,[13] where scrapie has been endemic for centuries. BSE was spread by animal protein concentrates including scrapie-infected sheep in cattle feed. The agent present in these meats was no longer being properly inactivated because of changes in the production procedures. As a result, the scrapie agent probably became adapted to a new host and established BSE in bovines with major epidemic consequences.[14] However, BSE was not restricted to the United Kingdom. Recycling of imported live animals, processed beef, or livestock food supplements from the United Kingdom sparked new small-scale epidemics in most European countries. The United States had no reported indigenous cases because it banned the importation of beef from the United Kingdom beginning in the mid-1980s, and minimal sheep-derived products have been processed for use in feed for other animals.[15] However, cases in cattle have occurred in Canada, and two of these cattle were exported to the United States. Some infected cattle have been detected in Japan. The incidence of BSE is approaching zero in all European countries as a result of measures taken by the European Union.

FSE was first recognized during the BSE epidemic in the United Kingdom.[1] Based on strain-typing experiments, FSE is undoubtedly caused by the BSE agent.[16] Cats were probably infected by ingesting BSE-contaminated feed.[17] Cats cannot be experimentally infected by the scrapie agent directly as they can by BSE and Creutzfeldt-Jakob disease (CJD) agents, which indicates an adaptation to the new hosts.[18] The first cases of FSE were diagnosed in the early 1990s.[17,19] The outbreak was attributed to consumption of beef products contaminated by CNS tissues from infected animals.

In addition to the United Kingdom, single cases of FSE have been described in several European countries, and also worldwide.[20–23]

Captive wild species of Felidae such as lions *(Panthera leo)*, tigers *(Panthera tigris)*, cheetahs *(Acinonyx jubatus)*, and pumas *(Felis concolor)* that were fed bovine tissues have also been affected with BSE.[24,25] The number of affected cats being reported annually has sharply decreased. TSE has not been documented in the dog, most probably because of a few changes in the sequence of endogenous PrP.[26,27]

CLINICAL FEATURES

Because of the long incubation time of TSEs, the signs of FSE are observed only in adult cats (peak incidence at age 5 years). The neurologic signs develop progressively over several weeks to months and are characterized by behavioral changes such as aggressiveness and fear. Gait abnormalities include ataxia and inaccurate landing while jumping. Affected cats are hypersensitive to tactile stimulation. No focalization of the neurologic signs occurs. The disease is invariably progressive and fatal.

DIAGNOSIS

The suspicion for FSE is based on geographic location, the age of the animal, and the clinical signs. From a diagnostic standpoint, a variety of neurologic conditions have to be considered. No specific laboratory findings are present in cats with FSE. Laboratory diagnosis of TSE is based on immunohistochemical detection of the protease-resistant PrP^{Sc} in tissues obtained by biopsy or at necropsy. Tissue is subjected to proteinase K digestion to destroy PrP and selectively retain PrP^{Sc}. Several monoclonal and polyclonal antibody commercial test kits are available.[28,29] Species differences exist in reactions to these commercially available tests. In scrapie, PrP^{Sc} can be demonstrated in lymphoid tissues such as the tonsils or third eyelid.[30] Given that no replication of the BSE agent occurs in lymphatic tissues, laboratory diagnosis is possible only on brain material after slaughter. In cats, extraneural PrP^{Sc} accumulation appears to be inconsistent so that obtaining CNS tissue at necropsy has been the only absolute means of confirmation when other test results are negative.[31,32] A protein misfolding cyclic amplification technique was highly sensitive in detecting PrP^{Sc} in a cheetah.[33] Deposition was found throughout the CNS, lymphoreticular, and other tissues suggesting widespread spread of the agent throughout the body. In recent years, new assays have been developed that are based on conversion of recombinant PrP to PrP^{Sc} by PcP^{Sc} in body fluids or tissue homogenates (known as real-time quaking-induced conversion assays) (Fig. 129.1).[34] Application of these assays to CSF specimens has been useful for antemortem diagnosis of Creutzfeld-Jacob disease in humans.

Pathologic Findings

As in all other TSEs, the pathologic findings in FSE are highly characteristic. The changes consist of vacuolation in the neuropil and neurons in a bilaterally symmetric distribution, especially in the thalamus, basal ganglia, and cerebral cortex (Fig. 129.2A). Immunocytochemistry for PrP^{Sc} reveals accumulation of PrP in affected areas (Fig. 129.2B). Advanced cases have neuronal loss and gliosis. Advanced lesions are more commonly observed in human patients because affected animals are often euthanized in early stages of the neurologic disease. No inflammation is present. The neuropathologic profile varies after experimental chronic wasting disease infection.[35,36]

TREATMENT

Treatments used for TSEs must be able to cross the blood-brain barrier. A variety of compounds have been used including polyene antimicrobials,[37] analogues of Congo red, quinacrine, chlorpromazine, and inhibitors of peptide synthesis. Efforts are underway to discover more effective compounds, but to date, treatment of human SEs is largely supportive.[38] Active and passive immunization using recombinant PrP^c and antibodies to PrP^c could have some merit. TSEs are similar to Alzheimer's disease in which neurodegeneration is accompanied by massive deposition of amyloid-β-protein, and some reduction in progression occurs when immunotherapy is used. Because the incidence of TSE in humans has not risen at all as a result of the BSE epidemic that is now at its end, TSEs remain exceedingly rare diseases. Vaccine development is therefore unlikely.

PREVENTION

All TSEs are fatal diseases. Prevention of exposure is the most important control measure. Although transmitting an SE from one species to another orally is generally difficult, nonbovine species were found to be infected with BSE in the United Kingdom.[16] BSE in these other species undoubtedly resulted from oral exposure. Scrapie-infected sheep were processed into meat and bone meal supplements being fed to cattle, and tissue from sick animals was recycled through the animal food supply. However, further spread in the bovine population in Europe has been prevented by banning the feeding of animal proteins to ruminant species, and finally to all farm animals. The BSE epidemic has ended and FSE has therefore largely disappeared. Although BSE has been nearly eradicated, scrapie remains a challenge because it is a transmissible disease. Because susceptibility to scrapie is genetically controlled, PCR has been used to detect alleles of scrapie-susceptible sheep to assist selection for breeding of scrapie-resistant animals.[39]

PUBLIC HEALTH ASPECTS

In 1996, during the outbreak of BSE in the United Kingdom, a new variant of CJD (vCJD) arose in humans there.[40,41] The disease has also been reported in other countries, including the United States, often in association with a history of residence in the United Kingdom. A total of 232 cases have been reported worldwide, and although the epidemic is nearing its end, surveillance efforts continue.[40] In contrast to classical ("sporadic") CJD, vCJD affected primarily young adults and was suspected of being caused by ingestion of contaminated cattle products. Molecular typing efforts suggest that the vCJD agent is similar to the BSE agent.[42,43] Not all humans are equally susceptible to the development of SE. A higher prevalence of disease is associated with homozygosity for a polymorphism at codon 129 of the PrP gene.[3]

Transmission of the agent through blood transfusions or organ donation remains a concern. Although BSE is the only zoonotic prion disease that has been recognized to date, concerns remain about the possibility of new prion strains arising that may be capable of crossing the species barrier.[44]

BACTERIAL MENINGITIS AND MENINGOENCEPHALOMYELITIS

ETIOLOGY AND EPIDEMIOLOGY

Bacterial infections can spread into the meningeal spaces and subsequently the parenchyma of the CNS from natural orifices such as the nasal sinuses, retrobulbar tissues,[45–47] and middle or inner ear.[48,49] Bacteria that proliferate in middle or inner ear infections can enter the cranial vault and produce cranial meningitis or subdural abscess formation (empyema) and, frequently, with brain parenchymal involvement, central vestibular dysfunction.[50–53] Bacteria can also enter the

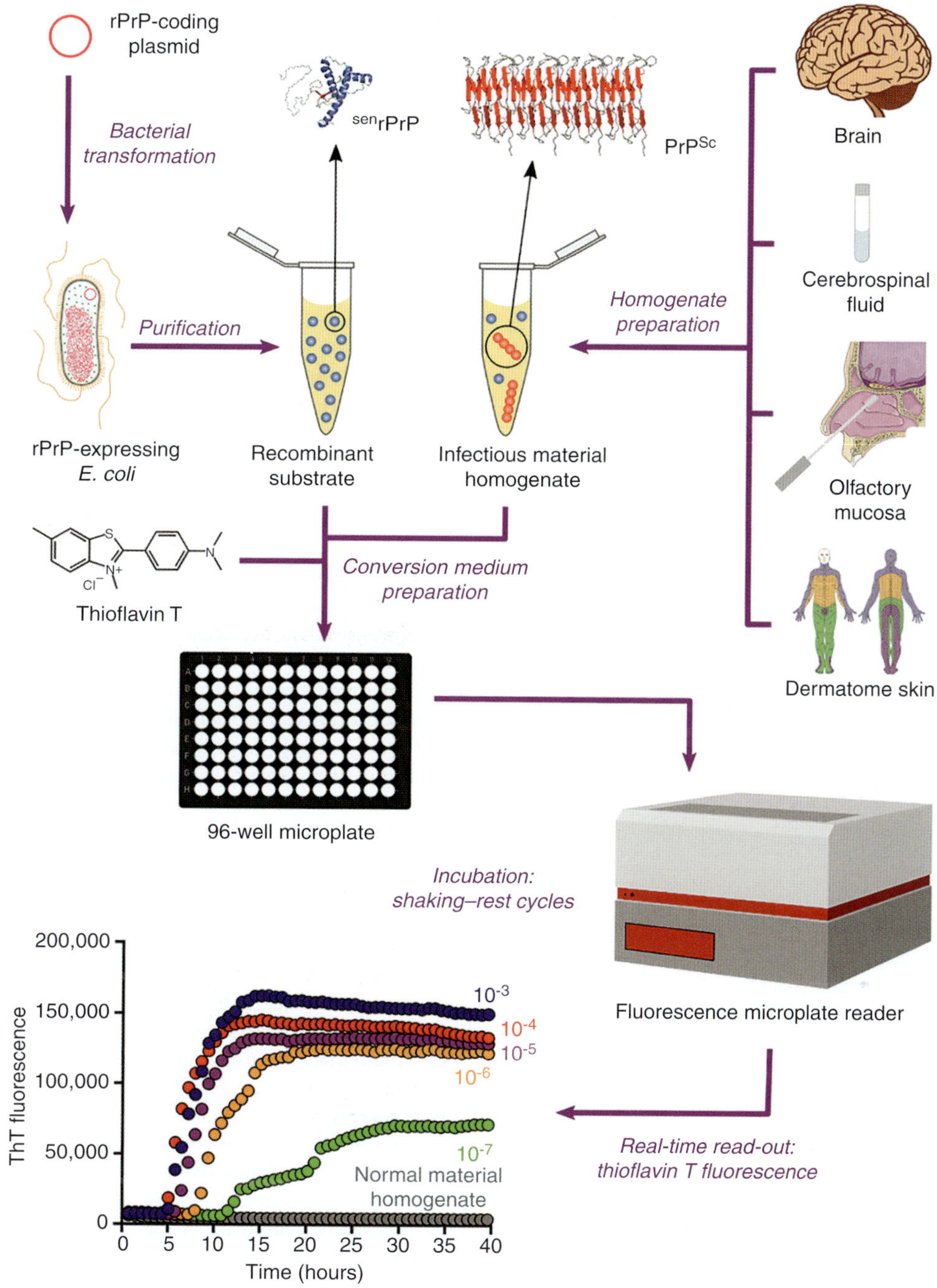

Fig. 129.1 Real-time quaking-induced conversion (RT-QuIC). Recombinant PrP (*rPrP*) is expressed in *Escherichia coli* and purified as folded protease-sensitive rPrP (^{sen}*rPrP*). Suspected infectious material (brain sections, cerebrospinal fluid, etc.), which may contain heat-resistant PrP (*PrP^{Sc}*), is mixed with ^{sen}rPrP, buffer, and thioflavin T (a fluorescent probe). The mixture is loaded into a microplate and then incubated in a fluorescence microplate reader. If PrP^{Sc} is in the sample, it triggers formation of PrP^{Sc} aggregates. The equipment records thioflavin T fluorescence emission during incubation, revealing the kinetics of aggregate formation. Sigmoidal growth in fluorescence indicates a positive transmissible spongiform encephalopathy diagnosis. If there is no PrP^{Sc} in the specimen, no fluorescence is emitted (*normal material homogenate*). (From Ascari LM, Rocha SC, Gonçalves PB, et al. Challenges and advances in antemortem diagnosis of human transmissible spongiform encephalopathies. *Front Bioeng Biotechnol.* 2020;8:1228.)

meningeal spaces through traumatic focal penetration (foreign bodies or bite wounds),[54,55] spread from sites of infection in adjacent venous sinuses or bony or cartilaginous structures, or spread via hematogenous arterial dissemination.[56,57] Vascular spread, a common pathway of entry, can result in lodgment of bacteria in the endothelial cells of capillaries or the choroid plexus, which results in bacterial invasion of the parenchyma of the CNS or colonization of the CSF, respectively. Associated vascular necrosis may be followed by hemorrhagic necrosis. In the CSF, bacteria have adequate nutrients and a paucity of phagocytes and immunoglobulin, and they can proliferate, which produces a progressive inflammatory process that can readily spread along CSF pathways.

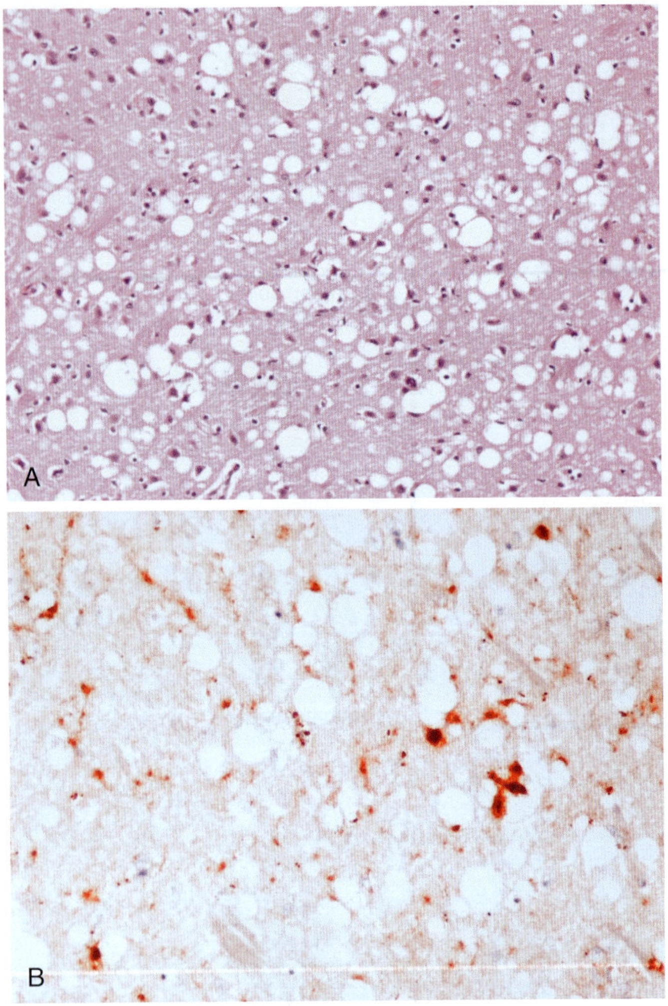

Fig. 129.2 Feline spongiform encephalopathy. (A) Area in the thalamus with many small and large vacuoles in the neuropil (hematoxylin and eosin stain, ×100). (B) Area with spongiform change. Punctate and plaque-like deposits *(red)* of the protease-resistant PrP (immunocytochemical staining with polyclonal anti-PrP; avidin biotinylated enzyme complex technique, ×250).

Bacteria that cause meningoencephalomyelitis in dogs or cats are varied and can include aerobic, microaerophilic, and anaerobic species. Staphylococci, streptococci, *Salmonella* spp., *Pasteurella* spp., *Actinomyces* spp., *Nocardia* spp., and a variety of anaerobic bacteria have been isolated.[50,58–62]

CLINICAL FEATURES

Pathogenesis and Clinical Signs

On entry into the CSF, bacteria can replicate to a moderate degree before they trigger a host protective response, because the immune response in this area is slow. The immune response of the host, rather than virulence of the pathogen, is usually responsible for most of the subsequent pathologic events. TLRs, which are present on astrocytes, neurons, microglia, and oligodendrocytes, initiate innate recognition of the microorganisms. TLR signals initiate the release of a wide variety of proinflammatory mediators including reactive intermediates, cytokines, and chemokines within the CNS tissues and CSF spaces.[63] Within the nervous tissue, inflammatory processes lead to increased expression of inflammatory cytokines such as TNF-α; thus, higher CSF concentrations of TNF-α and IL-12 have been used to distinguish bacterial from aseptic meningitis in humans.[64–66] Immunologic damage to bacteria leads to the release of breakdown products into the CSF and local CNS tissue. This further stimulates the release of cytokines and prostaglandins, which are chemotactic for leukocytes and contribute to meningeal and ependymal inflammation. Subsequent inflammation leads to vascular injury and vascular thrombosis; tissue inflammation, edema, hemorrhage, and necrosis; and increased CNS pressure within the confines of the dura mater and bony spaces. Inflammatory processes may also lead to adhesions and obstruction to CSF flow, resulting in obstructive internal or external hydrocephalus.[67]

In the rare situation of pure meningitis, hyperesthesia from nerve root irritation is an important clinical sign. The gait of animals with meningitis is often choppy and stiff. With progression or direct parenchymal destruction of the spinal cord and brain parenchyma, focal, multifocal, or diffuse neurologic deficits can occur. Manifestations of intracranial deficits include gait abnormalities, central vestibular signs, abnormal placing reactions, seizures, behavioral abnormalities, and progressive decline in mental status until coma occurs.

Physical Examination Findings

Elevated rectal temperature may be found on examination because of fever, as well as excessive muscular exertional activity. Extraneural signs may occur and depend on the site of primary infection. Animals with meningitis may walk with a short stiff or cautious stride. Often the back of affected dogs is arched and the neck is outstretched with low head carriage. Paraspinal and extremity hyperesthesia is present with limb and spinal manipulation. When inflammation is confined to the meninges, postural reactions that involve motor responses are often stilted. As the inflammation involves the CNS parenchyma, deficits in sensory and motor responses such as delayed placing reactions, paresis, and ataxia can be observed. Cranial nerve deficits are often seen on neurologic examination. Further signs of cerebral dysfunction include signs such as altered mentation (depression, aggression) or seizures. Myotatic and flexor reflexes may be difficult to elicit because of increased muscle tone from the animal's extreme tenderness and unwillingness to relax. Loss of reflex function occurs if spinal nerves or gray matter become damaged in the inflammatory process.

DIAGNOSIS

The differential diagnosis for bacterial meningoencephalomyelitis includes noninfectious CNS disease such as neoplasia, or other infectious diseases caused by viruses, rickettsiae, fungi, protozoa, algae, and helminths (Table 129.2).[68,69] FIP is probably the most common cause of meningoencephalomyelitis in cats.[70,71] When parenchymal neurologic dysfunction is apparent, then protozoal meningoencephalomyelitis and meningoencephalomyelitis of unknown origin (MUO) should be considered. Frequently, more localized hyperesthesia associated with upper or lower motor neuron deficits can be observed with epidural empyema, discospondylitis, or paraspinal osteomyelitis. Steroid-responsive meningitis-arteritis (SRMA) in dogs can mimic all the signs of bacterial meningitis.[72] Diseases associated with myositis (such as American canine hepatozoonosis and leptospirosis) can also produce clinical signs that resemble those of meningitis.

Laboratory Abnormalities

Although there are no hematologic or biochemical abnormalities that are specific for bacterial meningitis, the CBC may reveal leukocytosis, often with a left shift, especially if the process that leads to the meningitis resulted from hematogenous spread; however, an absence of neutrophilic leukocytosis is common in dogs or cats with meningitis.[60]

TABLE 129.2 Examples of Infectious Agents That Can Cause Meningitis in Dogs and Cats[a]

	Dogs	Cats
Viruses	Canine distemper virus Arboviruses Suid herpesvirus 1 (pseudorabies)	Feline infectious peritonitis virus Borna disease virus Suid herpesvirus 1 (pseudorabies)
Bacteria	*Staphylococcus* spp. *Streptococcus* spp. *Pasteurella multocida* Enterobacterales (including *Salmonella* spp.) *Actinomyces* spp. *Nocardia* spp. *Mycoplasma* spp. Anaerobes *Brucella canis* *Bartonella* spp.[b] *Borrelia* (*Borreliella* [*incertae sedis*]) *burgdorferi*[b] *Leptospira* spp.[b] *Anaplasma phagocytophilum*[b] *Rickettsia rickettsii* *Neorickettsia helminthoeca* *Ehrlichia canis*	*Streptococcus* spp. *Pasteurella multocida* *Nocardia* spp. *Mycoplasma* spp. Anaerobes
Fungi	*Blastomyces* spp.[c] *Coccidioides* spp. *Cryptococcus* spp.[c] *Aspergillus* spp.[c] *Candida* spp. *Histoplasma* spp. Phaeohyphomycoses Hyalohyphomycoses (e.g., *Paecilomyces* spp.)	*Cryptococcus* spp.[c]
Protozoa	*Toxoplasma gondii* *Neospora caninum* *Leishmania* spp. *Balamuthia mandrillaris* *Acanthamoeba* spp.	*Toxoplasma gondii*
Algae	*Prototheca* spp.	
Helminths	*Angiostrongylus vasorum* *Baylisascaris procyonis* Migrating fly larvae (e.g., *Cuterebra* spp.)	Migrating fly larvae (e.g., *Cuterebra* spp.)

[a]Many of the listed agents also cause encephalitis or encephalomyelitis in association with meningitis.
[b]Uncertain role in meningitis in dogs or cats.
[c]Via dissemination or cribriform plate destruction as a result of extension of nasal cavity disease.

Serum chemistry abnormalities are variable and nonspecific and can include increased ALT and ALP activities, hyperglycemia, and variable changes in serum electrolytes.

Definitive diagnosis of bacterial meningoencephalomyelitis requires evaluation of the CSF. Precautions should be taken not to remove too much fluid if CSF pressures could be increased. If imaging capabilities are available, they should be performed and evaluated before CSF removal since they may reveal evidence of increased intracranial pressure. However, findings on medical imaging should not be used to eliminate CNS inflammatory disease, because CSF findings have a high sensitivity for its detection.[73] Abnormalities found on CSF analysis in animals with bacterial meningitis usually consist of marked neutrophilic pleocytosis (Fig. 129.3), and CSF protein concentration is increased. CSF protein concentration (often > 100 mg/dL) and leukocyte numbers (usually > 100 cells/μL) tend to be greatest in suppurative meningitis (especially of infectious origin) as compared with other CNS diseases; however, the electrophoretic patterns of the proteins are not specific for a diagnosis.[74] Neutrophils generally predominate; however, especially in chronicity or with concurrent antimicrobial use, monocytes, lymphocytes, or eosinophils may be observed. In human bacterial meningitis, glucose levels in the CSF are reduced because of bacterial and inflammatory cell utilization, and lactic acid levels may be increased. In dogs, CSF glucose concentrations cannot be used as a distinct marker to differentiate bacterial meningitis from other inflammatory CNS diseases, especially from SRMA (which is usually accompanied by severe pleocytosis). In dogs, low CSF glucose concentrations seem to be associated with elevated CSF cell counts, rather than bacterial metabolism.[75] Finding organisms in the CSF on cytologic examination is exceedingly rare, and isolation of organisms in culture is also uncommon despite their visible presence on histopathologic examination.

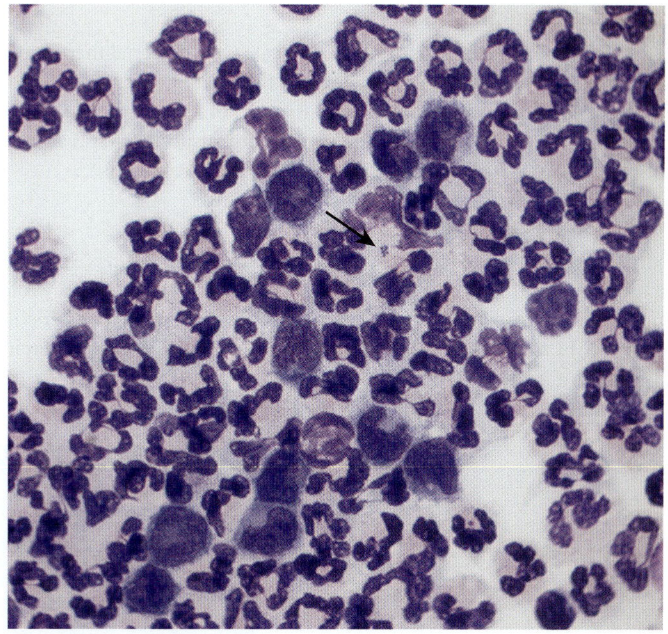

Fig. 129.3 Cytologic appearance of cerebrospinal fluid (CSF; cytospin preparation) in a 3-year-old male neutered Labrador retriever with bacterial meningitis. There is a large population of nondegenerate to moderately degenerate neutrophils. Many of the neutrophils contain intracellular cocci to pleomorphic short rod-shaped bacteria found in pairs and small aggregates *(arrow)*. Moderate numbers of foamy macrophages and reactive lymphocytes are also present. CSF analysis revealed a total protein of 402 mg/dL (reference range, <25 mg/dL), 100 red blood cells/μL, and 5,200 white cells/μL, 92% of which were neutrophils.

Diagnostic Imaging

Plain Radiography

Plain radiographic findings are unremarkable in dogs or cats with bacterial meningitis unless a bacterial osteomyelitis of paraspinal or cranial bones or discospondylitis are part of the infectious process. Bulla radiography is a valuable procedure for animals with suspected otogenic sources for their CNS infection; however, advanced imaging procedures are preferred when available.

Computed Tomography

CT of the brain or spinal cord in dogs or cats with bacterial meningitis may reveal contrast-enhancing lesions on the meningeal or ependymal surfaces. Focal areas of enhancement in areas of abscess formation or edema may also be present. In one puppy with suspected staphylococcal meningitis, CT imaging revealed external hydrocephalus.[67]

Magnetic Resonance Imaging

Purulent exudates that cover the CNS tissue may be visualized by MRI in animals with meningitis using T2-weighted (T2W) sequences while suppressing the signal from CSF (high fluid-attenuated inversion recovery [FLAIR]) (Fig. 129.4A). This method results in enhancement of signal intensity found in the meninges.[76] In more advanced cases, using postcontrast T1-weighted images, meningeal or parenchymal enhancement (signal hyperintensity) may be evident.[77] Occasionally, plaque-like densities are found that compress nervous tissue, which represent abscesses. Lentiform-shaped extra-axial collections of fluid have been described in cases of empyema.[78]

Microbiologic Tests

The main microbiologic assays used for diagnosis of bacterial meningitis in dogs and cats are aerobic bacterial culture and PCR assay of CSF. False-negative results occur because organism numbers in the CSF of dogs and cats are often low. Depending on the sensitivity of the PCR assay used and the viability of the bacteria in the specimen, culture may be positive when PCR results are negative, and vice versa.

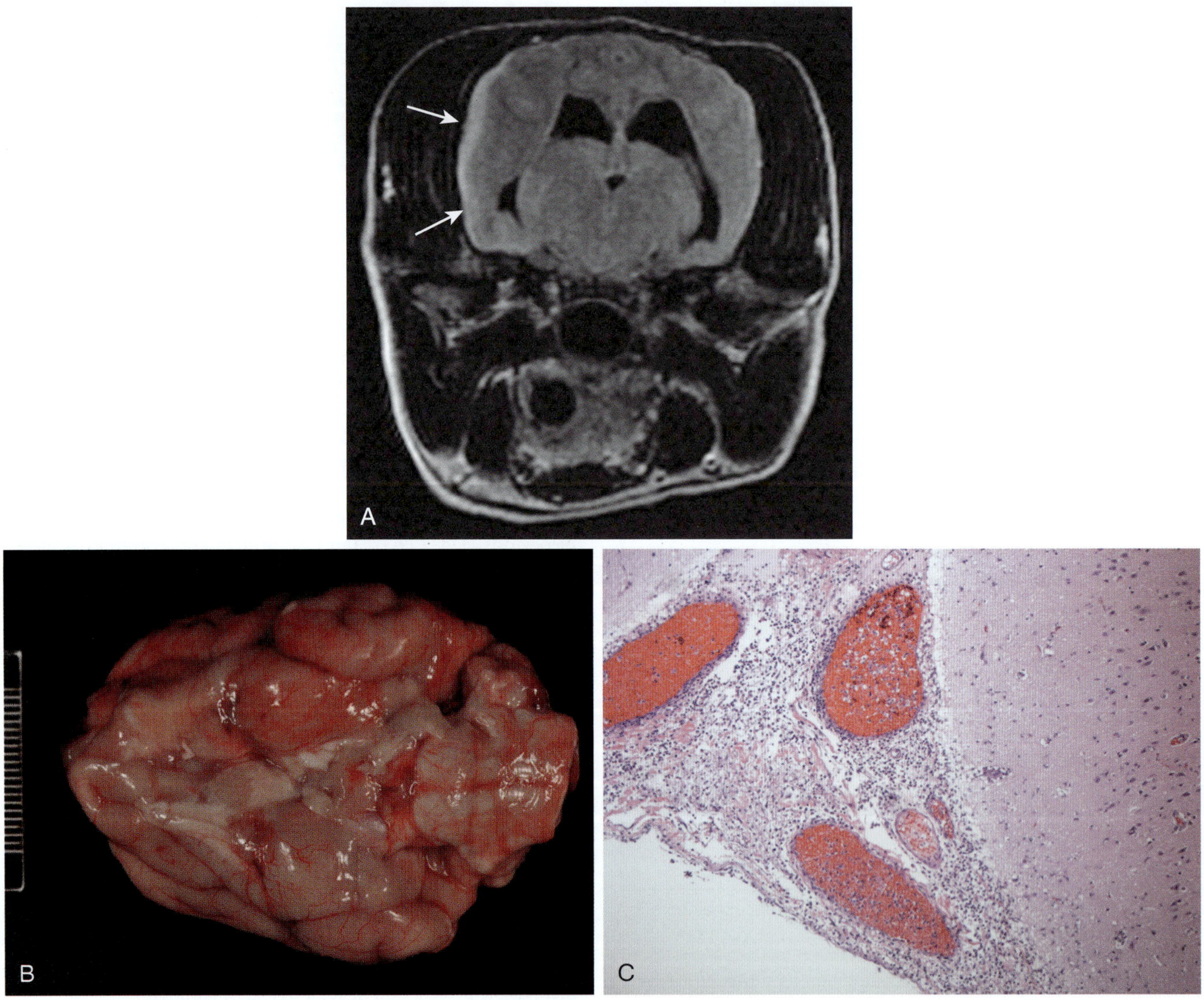

Fig. 129.4 Clinical images from a 4-year old female spayed Yorkshire terrier with bacterial meningitis. The dog had a 12-hour history of hypersalivation, generalized seizures, and vomiting. Small numbers of *Corynebacterium* spp. were isolated in culture from the meninges. (A) Magnetic resonance imaging (FLAIR image). There is marked hyperintensity of the meninges on the left side *(arrows)*. (B) Gross pathologic findings. Ventral aspect of the brain. Purulent material covered the cerebellum and left cerebral cortex and pooled on the floor of the calvarium. The right cerebral vasculature was markedly engorged *(shown)*. Cerebellar herniation was also found *(not shown)*. (C) Histopathologic appearance of meningitis. The meninges and Virchow-Robin spaces are expanded with inflammatory cells. The diagnosis was chronic, suppurative meningitis. Hematoxylin and eosin stain, 100× magnification. (Courtesy of University of California, Davis, Veterinary Anatomic Pathology Service.)

Bacterial Isolation and Identification

Bacteria may be isolated using routine aerobic and anaerobic bacterial culture media and conditions. At least 0.5 mL of CSF should be submitted for aerobic and anaerobic bacterial culture if possible. Organisms are uncommonly cultured from CSF because of their low number and the small amounts of fluid that are typically available; however, when successful, subsequent susceptibility testing assists in appropriate antimicrobial drug selection. Because of the infrequency of positive culture results despite the histopathologic presence of organisms at necropsy,[60] empiric antibacterial therapy should be employed based on a suspected site of origin of infection (see Antimicrobial Treatment, later).

Molecular Diagnosis Using Nucleic Acid–Based Testing

Sensitive and specific real-time PCR assays for detection of bacteria in the CSF have been described.[79] However, as with culture methods, their sensitivity is low. Broad-spectrum bacterial PCR assays have been used to document bacterial infection of the CSF in human medicine,[80] as well as multiplex PCR panels that are designed to simultaneously test for a number of different pathogens capable of causing meningitis or encephalitis.[81] Real-time PCR panels are widely available from commercial veterinary diagnostic laboratories for detection of CNS pathogens in CSF specimens from dogs and cats; however, the clinical sensitivity and specificity of many of the individual assays in these panels have not always been well studied. Results should always be interpreted in light of other clinical findings and diagnostic tests.

Pathologic Findings

Gross Pathologic Findings

At necropsy, sites of infection in animals with bacterial meningoencephalomyelitis may be found in organs outside the CNS, such as the skin or mucous membranes, respiratory tract, internal organs, external or middle or inner ear, or ocular tissues. Gross pathologic findings in the CNS are generally minimal in dogs or cats with early inflammatory changes. As the infection progresses in the parenchyma, the meninges may appear congested and nervous tissue parenchyma may be discolored or opaque (Fig. 129.4B). Focal accumulations of pus may occasionally be observed in the meningeal spaces or adjacent nervous tissue. In late stages, ischemic infarction of CNS tissue may occur as a result of severe vascular inflammation and necrosis. Because of vascular damage, necrosis is often hemorrhagic. Occasionally, obstructive hydrocephalus occurs if the inflammatory process occludes the mesencephalic aqueduct.

Histopathologic Findings

Microscopic findings in bacterial meningoencephalomyelitis consist of a suppurative inflammatory response that is prominent in the meningeal spaces and the penetrating sulci that contain blood vessels (Virchow-Robin spaces), with or without brain parenchymal involvement (Fig. 129.4C). With tissue Gram stains, bacteria may be observed within inflammatory cells, blood vessels, or neural tissues, in association with inflammation of the meninges and adjacent neural parenchyma.

TREATMENT

Antimicrobial Treatment

Because of the low sensitivity of culture and/or PCR assays in bacterial meningitis and the turnaround time involved, treatment must be instituted following the neurologic examination and availability of the results of CSF analysis (Table 129.3). The earlier appropriate antimicrobial therapy is administered, the better the chance that parenchymal damage will be minimized. Anti-inflammatory agents have been recommended, with some caution and on a temporary basis, to reduce intracranial pressure. Almost all drugs, either ionic or lipid-soluble, penetrate acutely inflamed meninges. However, as the inflammation subsides, only lipid-soluble drugs are effective. Where parenchymal abscesses are present, antibacterial drugs may not effectively penetrate affected tissue. In these cases, neurosurgical drainage is required in addition to systemic antibacterial therapy. One case report described the use of CT to guide drainage of a brainstem abscess in a cat on an emergency basis.[82]

Anti-Inflammatory Therapy

In addition to antimicrobial therapy, control of the immune response and resultant inflammation in CNS tissues is critical when intracranial or intraspinal pressures are elevated. Control of CNS edema is usually achieved with targeted dosages of glucocorticoids; however, therapy must be judicious since these medications are immunosuppressive and nonspecific in their effect on the host.[83]

Other Supportive Care Measures

Dogs with severe hyperesthesia may benefit from pain management and NSAIDs. Anticonvulsant medications may be needed for animals with seizures. Other supportive care measures, such as those required for hydration and nutrition, should also be considered.

PROGNOSIS

The prognosis for dogs with early acute bacterial meningoencephalomyelitis is good if minimal CNS parenchymal tissue is damaged. With severe parenchymal damage, long-term treatment might be necessary; prognosis varies depending on clinical signs and the extent of tissue destruction.

PREVENTION

Bacterial meningoencephalomyelitis is a result of exogenous or endogenous factors that allow bacterial organisms to gain access to the CNS. Although these insults cannot be completely prevented, injuries or lesions that occur close to the cranial or paraspinal spaces potentially predispose to CNS infection. Animals with wounds or infections in these areas or with systemic bacteremia should be treated appropriately, then monitored closely for CNS signs, and placed on judicious antimicrobial therapy if meningoencephalomyelitis is highly suspected or documented. Although the signs of bacterial meningoencephalomyelitis are confused with those of immune-mediated CNS disease,

TABLE 129.3 Antibacterial Drugs That Penetrate Central Nervous System Tissues and Fluids[a]

High	Intermediate	Low
Trimethoprim-sulfonamide, chloramphenicol, doxycycline, metronidazole	Third-generation penicillins, third-generation cephalosporins, fluoroquinolones	Penicillin, first-generation cephalosporins, aminoglycosides, clindamycin

[a]During acute inflammation, penetration is adequate for most drugs; however, as treatment progresses and inflammation subsides, the penetration becomes limited.

continued use of immunosuppressive drugs may lead to detrimental progression of a bacterial disease process.

PUBLIC HEALTH ASPECTS

There are minimal, if any, public health risks associated with bacterial meningitis in dogs or cats—that is, unless veterinary staff inadvertently inoculate themselves with organisms being collected for culture or PCR assays. *Haemophilus influenzae*, *Streptococcus pneumoniae*, and *Neisseria meningitidis*, which cause contagious respiratory disease and subsequent complicating hematogenous-origin meningitis in humans, do not readily infect dogs or cats.

NEUROLOGIC DISEASES OF SUSPECTED INFECTIOUS ORIGIN

The conditions described below are suspected to be caused by insidious infectious agents or immune aberrations in response to one or more stealth pathogens. The CNS is a frequent site of localization of pathogens evading host immune responses. In clinical practice, a diagnosis of MUO may be used for some of the described diseases since histologic features cannot be identified during routine clinical testing.[84–87] Unfortunately, a variety of terms have been used in the literature including "meningoencephalitis of unknown etiology" and "noninfectious inflammatory diseases of the CNS," so a common language is still missing.

GRANULOMATOUS MENINGOENCEPHALOMYELITIS AND NECROTIZING ENCEPHALITIS

Granulomatous Meningoencephalomyelitis

Granulomatous meningoencephalomyelitis (GME) has been reported in dogs in the United States,[69,88–90] Australia,[91] New Zealand,[92] Japan,[93] and several European countries (Vandevelde M, unpublished observations). It is a relatively common condition and is an angiocentric, nonsuppurative, mixed monocytic/lymphoid inflammatory process, predominately affecting the white matter of the brain and spinal cord.[89,90] Three forms of the disease have been described—disseminated, ocular, and focal; the disseminated form is the most common.

Despite its recognition as a clinical entity for over 40 years, the underlying cause and mechanism of disease production remains unclear. Genetic, autoimmune, infectious, neoplastic, and even toxic causes have been theorized. In some studies, female dogs were at greater risk for GME than male dogs; this finding is similar to other autoimmune demyelinating diseases including multiple sclerosis and experimental autoimmune encephalitis.[94] However, in another more recent study from Wisconsin, although more females than males were affected, this difference was not significant when compared to a control dog population.[95] Young to middle-aged dogs are often affected, and GME is uncommon before the age of 2 years. Smaller breeds, especially poodles, small terriers, Pekingese, and Maltese, appear to be predisposed,[88,96] although one case-control study found no breed predisposition.[95] In the latter study, more cases occurred in the spring.

GME has been proposed by some to be a DTH reaction with an autoimmune basis, supported by a predominance of major histocompatibility complex class 2 and CD3+ T cells.[97] Other investigators also noted a predominance of CD3+ T cells and a complete absence of the CD79 (B-cell marker) immunoreactivity in four cases of GME.[98] Positive immunoreactivity to IL-17 on T cells, macrophages, and microglia also has suggested an autoimmune pathogenesis, as this cytokine is often involved in the pathogenesis of other autoimmune disorders.[99] Anti-astrocytic antibodies and anti-transglutaminase 2 antibodies also have been identified in the CSF of dogs with GME.[100,101] The complete immunologic profile of GME and whether CNS autoantibodies are the cause or consequence of inflammation remain to be elucidated.

Despite the conventional view that GME is a disorder of immune dysregulation, some veterinary neuropathologists suggest that at least some cases of GME may be lymphoproliferative disorders, with features of both inflammation and neoplasia.[102] Focal GME is particularly similar to neoplasia, because lymphocytes within the perivascular cuffs often have variable degrees of pleomorphism and mitotic indices.[103] It is unclear whether the abnormal lymphocytes within brain lesions (and sometimes also CSF) are reactive inflammatory cells or representative of a true neoplastic population.

Potential viral, bacterial, and protozoal infectious triggers for GME have also been studied using PCR-based methods.[104–106] Borna disease virus was reported in dogs with meningoencephalitis in Japan and Switzerland and has been proposed as a causative agent for GME.[107,108] Borna disease virus, however, is unlikely to be a common etiology for GME given its predilection for CNS gray matter. Other investigators have demonstrated positive IHC for West Nile, CPIV, and encephalomyocarditis viruses in severe lesions of dogs with meningoencephalitides of presumed unknown origin.[109] The significance of these observations is unclear because the positive IHC may be caused by antibody cross-reactivity with endogenous proteins, as has been described with measles infections and in dogs with West Nile virus infection.[110,111] GME is most likely a nonspecific immunologic response, and multiple environmental triggers (including microbial antigens) and genetic factors are likely to play roles in the etiopathogenesis.

Necrotizing Encephalitis

Necrotizing encephalitis (NE) includes necrotizing meningoencephalitis (NME) and necrotizing leukoencephalitis (NLE). Historically referred to as "pug dog encephalitis" and "necrotizing encephalitis of Yorkshire terriers" respectively, these conditions have now been reported in various toy breeds including the pug, Maltese, Chihuahua, Yorkshire terrier, Pekingese, West Highland white terrier, Boston terrier, Japanese spitz, and miniature pinscher.[112]

Pedigree information on a large cohort of pug dogs is suggestive of a strong familial inheritance pattern for NME.[113] Disease in pugs and Maltese terriers has been strongly associated with the dog leukocyte antigen (DLA) II complex on chromosome 12 (the canine equivalent of MHCII); associations with loci on other chromosomes have also been found.[114] This association with DLAII supports an aberrant immune response as the underlying cause of disease.[115]

Although it is tempting to consider NME and NLE as distinct entities, these disorders may represent a spectrum of CNS injury with similar pathogeneses. Histopathologic differences among the NEs may result from minor genetic differences among dog breeds, modifying genes, and/or variations in antigenic exposures.

In general, attempts at virus isolation from dogs with NME have been unsuccessful. PCR screening of NME-affected brains for an extremely diverse group of DNA and RNA viruses has failed to identify viral nucleic acids.[106,113] A viral trigger for NE via molecular mimicry or the possibility that a pathogen is present in the CNS (but at undetectable levels) in the presence of a self-perpetuating immune response remain possible.

CLINICAL FEATURES

Granulomatous Meningoencephalomyelitis

In acute GME, clinical signs develop rapidly over the course of 1 to 10 days, and without treatment, it is rapidly progressive and fatal. Clinical signs also may develop more slowly over a period of 1 to 4 months. Signs are associated with the site of most extensive damage, or may be multifocal. Signs can include ataxia, dysmetria, paresis, and paralysis, and changes in mental status, with confusion, lethargy, and coma. Cranial nerve dysfunction may also be observed.

In the acute stage of the disease, more than 50% of animals have fever, and many exhibit paraspinal discomfort on palpation or signs of cervical pain.[90,116] Central vestibular signs are common, and seizures also may be observed. Clinical signs alternatively may suggest a space-occupying mass referring to a single site of involvement, most frequently the posterior fossa, with brainstem and cerebellar signs. Cerebral or spinal signs sometimes predominate. An ocular form of GME, previously called ocular reticulosis, occurs with acute unilateral or bilateral blindness and ophthalmoscopic evidence of optic neuritis.[88,117]

Necrotizing Encephalitis

The onset of neurologic signs associated with NME varies from 6 months to 7 years of age and most commonly occurs in young dogs, with a mean age of 29 months.[118] In comparison, NLE typically manifests between 4 months and 10 years of age, with a mean age of onset of 4.5 years.[119] In general, signs associated with NE typically are rapidly progressive and most commonly include seizures, depression, circling, vestibulocerebellar signs, visual deficits, and ultimately death.

DIAGNOSIS

Because histologic confirmation is required for definitive diagnosis of GME and NE, "MUO" is typically used in the list of differential diagnoses after further examinations as described here. The diagnostic approach should include consideration of potential infectious causes of inflammatory brain disease, and appropriate serologic or nucleic acid–based assays. Testing for pathogens listed in Table 129.2 should be considered based on the history, geographic location, and clinical signs. PCR assays can be used on CSF or brain biopsies in an attempt to determine an underlying infectious cause of inflammatory brain disease before starting treatment.

Laboratory Abnormalities

Laboratory abnormalities in GME and NE are nonspecific. Neutrophilia may be present in the acute phase of GME.[116] In the CSF, marked pleocytosis with cell counts of 100 to several thousand leukocytes/μL is usual. Mononuclear cells predominate, but a mixed pleocytosis can also be observed with varying numbers of neutrophils.[120] Cytologic examination of the CSF may reveal large anaplastic mononuclear cells with abundant lacy cytoplasm,[88] and up to 20% macrophages. Protein concentrations as high as 1,119 mg/dL have been reported (mean 163.2 ± 25 mg/dL).[120] CSF analysis results are abnormal in most dogs with NE, with a predominantly mononuclear pleocytosis (usually 90–600 cells/μL) and an increased protein concentration (usually 50–200 mg/dL).[121]

Diagnostic Imaging

MRI is the preferred imaging technique for dogs with suspected inflammatory brain disease. Lesions in both GME and NE are hyperintense on T2W and FLAIR images, and variably isointense to hypointense on T1W images, and have irregular margins (Fig. 129.5). Both gray and white matter may be affected.[102] Contrast enhancement on T1W images is variable. In some cases of GME, MR images may not reveal any abnormalities.[122] In the uncommon focal form of GME, mass lesions can be detected with CT and MRI.[102] Lesions associated with NME include asymmetric, multifocal prosencephalic lesions affecting the gray and white matter.[123] Loss of gray and white matter demarcation also may be discernible.[123] In NLE, multiple, asymmetric bilateral prosencephalic lesions mainly affecting the subcortical white matter have been described on MRI.[124] NLE lesions often include multiple cystic areas of necrosis. Among the most commonly affected breeds (Yorkshire terrier, French bulldog, pug dog, and Chihuahua), even breed-specific MRI characteristics of NE in dogs have been described.[125] Digital analysis of MRI images (texture analysis/radiomics) may be helpful for differentiating neoplastic and inflammatory brain lesions in dogs.[126] PET has been used on a limited basis in an attempt to distinguish NME from other inflammatory brain diseases.[127,128]

Pathologic Findings

Lesions seen on advanced imaging do not differentiate MUO from neoplasia or infectious encephalitis, so definitive antemortem diagnosis requires histopathologic examination of brain tissue. Brain biopsies can be collected using stereotactic methods that are guided by advanced imaging or an open (free-hand) technique.[129,130] Brain biopsy is associated with some risk, with one study estimating a 6% mortality and 29% with an MRI-guided free-hand technique.[129] In some cases, definitive diagnosis is made at necropsy.

In GME, lesions are found in the meninges, brain, and spinal cord, especially in the cervical segments. White matter often is more severely affected than gray matter. Although the lesions are disseminated, the cerebral hemispheres, the midbrain, and the region around the fourth ventricle are most frequently involved. The lesions, which are strictly associated with the vasculature, consist of perivascular cuffing of monocytes, lymphocytes, plasma cells, and sometimes a few neutrophils and mast cells (see Fig. 129.5). The formation of eccentrically situated nodular foci of macrophages within these cuffs is a characteristic finding in GME. The cuffs can be distinguished in three degrees of severity: small disseminated perivascular lesions, small granulomas resulting from the confluence of several perivascular cuffs, and large focal coalescing granulomas. Additionally, necrosis of the neuropil, mitosis in the perivascular cuffs, and edema may be observed. Tryptase-positive mast cells can be found in perivascular cuffs. Dogs with the acute disease have significantly more mast cells than dogs with chronic disease.[131] Special stains can be applied to help rule out potential infectious agents, and unfixed tissue should also be submitted for nucleic acid–based testing.

Histologic findings in NE are characteristic and include diffuse meningitis, choroiditis, and encephalitis, with lesions predominating in the cerebrum (Fig. 129.6). Perivascular and meningeal inflammatory infiltrates consisting of lymphocytes, plasma cells, histiocytes, and macrophages have a strong tendency to invade the adjacent parenchyma. Extensive compact subpial and subventricular lesions are present and may extend deep into the underlying brain tissue, with unusually intense microglial proliferation and destruction of tissue. In some areas, frank cerebrocortical necrosis occurs. The cerebral white matter also is severely affected, with marked perivascular cuffing and gliosis. In some areas, leukomalacia with liquefaction and cavitation of the tissue is noted.

TREATMENT

No specific therapy for GME or NE exists, although improvement frequently has been observed in GME cases after administration of glucocorticoids with or without additional immunosuppressive agents. Because glucocorticoid therapy provides only temporary improvement in many cases, a second immunosuppressive drug may also be required. Options include procarbazine, cytosine arabinoside, leflunomide, mycophenolate mofetil, cyclosporine, and lomustine.[102] In a study using prednisolone alone, or in combination with lomustine, the response to both regimens was no different.[132] Use of a combination

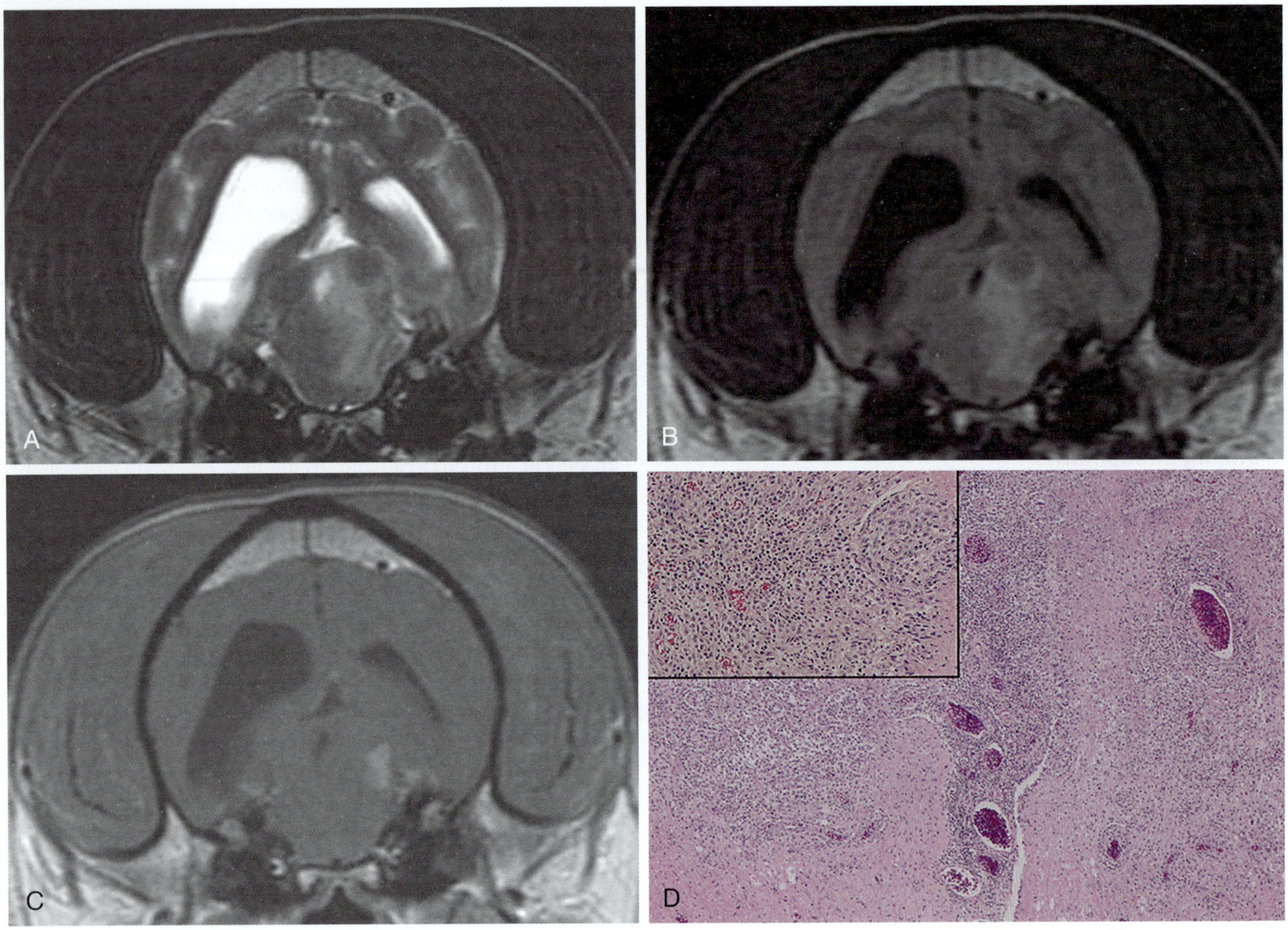

Fig. 129.5 Focal granulomatous meningoencephalomyelitis with ventriculomegaly. (A) Transverse T2-weighted (T2W) magnetic resonance image at the level of the midbrain, caudal colliculi, and cerebral cortex. Diffuse and right-sided hyperintensity involving the central gray substance, brachium of caudal colliculus, reticular formation, medial lemniscus, and mass effect of the mesencephalic aqueduct. (B) Transverse, T2W FLAIR image at the same level as in (A). Edema in the right midbrain is more conspicuous as a result of suppression of signal intensity in the mesencephalic aqueduct. (C) Transverse T1W image at the same level as in (A) after intravenous administration of a gadolinium-based contrast medium. The lesion displays variable contrast enhancement. (D) Hematoxylin and eosin staining of multifocal perivascular infiltrates consisting of macrophages, histiocytes, plasma cells, and lymphocytes. There is whorling of mixed cell infiltrates around blood vessels *(see inset)*. Original magnification x100; inset x400. (Courtesy of Gayle C. Johnson, DVM, PhD, Columbia, MO. Reprinted from Coates JR, Jeffery ND. Perspectives on meningoencephalomyelitis of unknown origin. *Vet Clin North Am Small Anim Pract.* 2014;44:1157–1185.)

of an immunosuppressive dose of prednisone and cytosine arabinoside is often used; the cytosine arabinoside is given for 2 consecutive days every 3–6 weeks on an outpatient basis. The reader is referred to the Suggested Reading list for detailed protocols.

Anticonvulsants may be needed to control seizures associated with inflammatory forebrain lesions. Glucocorticoid monotherapy does not alter the course of this NE in confirmed cases, and seizures may be refractory to anticonvulsants. However, use of anticonvulsant drugs may still prolong survival time.[118]

PROGNOSIS

The prognosis for dogs with GME is generally guarded given that many dogs develop progressive neurologic signs despite treatment, but some dogs may survive for several months.[94,122] Treatment should be attempted if possible because treated dogs have a significantly increased survival time than untreated dogs. Dogs that survive the first month appear to have an increased chance of surviving longer than a year. MRI features seem to help in establishing prognosis: loss of cerebral sulci and brain herniation were associated with a guarded prognosis.[133]

PUBLIC HEALTH ASPECTS

There is no public health significance of these conditions.

GREYHOUND NONSUPPURATIVE MENINGOENCEPHALITIS

Greyhound nonsuppurative meningoencephalitis was initially described in dogs from three different kennels in southern Ireland in 2002,[134] and cases continue to be reported from throughout the British Isles and

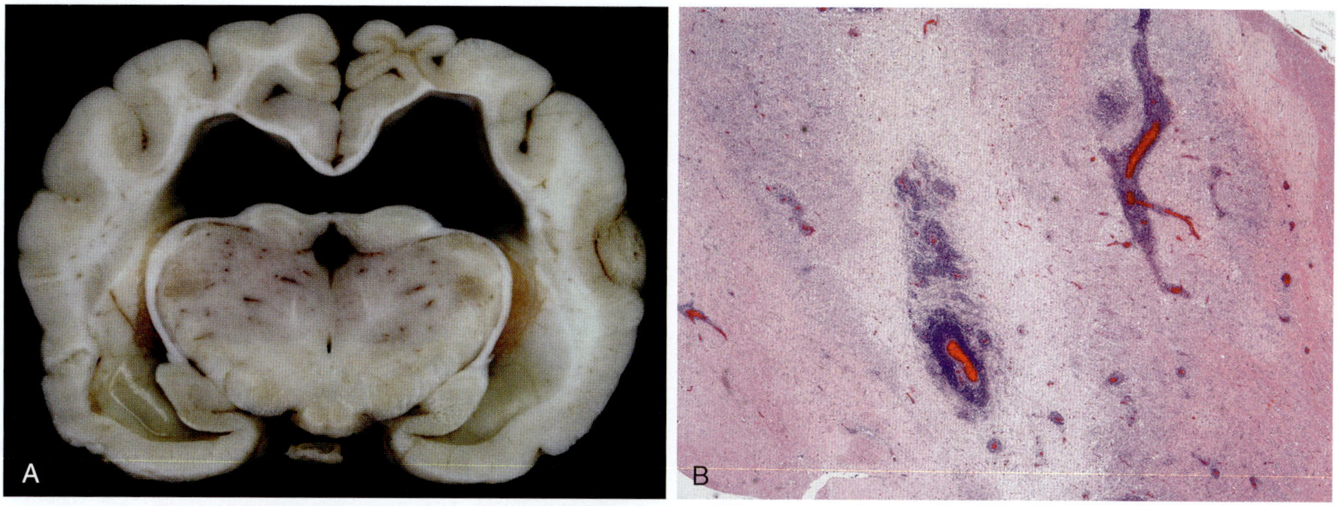

Fig. 129.6 Pathology of necrotizing encephalitis. (A) Brain of a 4-year-old intact female Yorkshire terrier. There is extensive necrosis in the dorsal subcortical white matter (with yellow discoloration) and marked atrophy with ventricular enlargement on the right side. (B) Histopathologic section of the brainstem of a 3-year-old French bulldog: there is a large area of necrosis of the nervous parenchyma with massive perivascular cuffing and intense diffuse infiltration of inflammatory cells in the necrotic tissue. Hematoxylin and eosin stain.

predominantly from Ireland.[135] The disease affects young greyhounds, usually less than 12 months of age, and frequently several littermates are affected. No evidence of underlying infectious causes has been found, but gene expression studies suggested that viral infection or autoimmunity may be involved in the pathogenesis.[136] Neurologic signs may be acute or chronic and progressive in onset and include altered mentation, head tilt, ataxia, recumbency, circling, and blindness. On MRI, lesions in four dogs predominantly affected the olfactory lobes, frontal and frontotemporal gray matter, and caudate nuclei, and were T2W hyperintense, T1W hypointense, with minimal or no contrast enhancement.[135] Histopathology reveals encephalitis with mononuclear perivascular cuffing, especially in the caudate nucleus, cortical cerebral gray matter, and periventricular gray matter of the rostral aspect of the brainstem. Results of a search for a wide range of known infectious agents has been negative.[137]

FELINE POLIOMYELITIS

Poliomyelitis in domestic cats was first reported in North Africa and Ceylon in the 1950s. Additional cases have since been described in North America and Europe.[138–140] A clinically and pathologically similar condition occurs in large Felidae (lions and tigers) held in captivity.[141,142] The disease occurs sporadically in domestic cats, but outbreaks have occurred among captive lions and tigers.[141,142] Pathologic findings indicate that poliomyelitis in cats is caused by a virus, but a search for known viruses has been unsuccessful.[142] Borna disease in cats is morphologically and clinically distinct from feline poliomyelitis, and has a different geographic distribution, so Borna virus is unlikely to be the cause.

Feline poliomyelitis has a slow onset and clinical signs progress over weeks to months. In many instances, the neurologic signs stabilize, and some animals may recover. Immature and adult cats appear to be susceptible. The predominant signs are defects in locomotion, including paresis, ataxia, and depressed placement reactions. Lower motor neuron involvement is characterized by muscle atrophy and decreased reflexes. Hyperesthesia in the thoracic and lumbar areas is apparent in some cases. Rarely, seizures, cerebellar signs, and pupillary abnormalities occur.

On histopathology, disseminated inflammatory lesions are found in the brain and spinal cord. The spinal cord and medulla oblongata are most severely affected. The lesions consist of perivascular mononuclear cuffing, gliosis, and neuronal degeneration, with the latter being most obvious in the ventral horns of the spinal cord. In chronic cases, there is minimal inflammation but substantial neuronal loss and intense astrogliosis in the cord. As a result of neuronal damage, marked diffuse Wallerian degeneration of the lateral and ventral columns also occurs, resembling a primary degenerative disorder.

Treatment is supportive. Contact between unaffected cats and those suspected to have the disease should be avoided. The prognosis is not always unfavorable because large Felidae have been known to recover.[141]

STEROID-RESPONSIVE MENINGITIS-ARTERITIS

SRMA is an immune-mediated condition of young dogs (usually < 2 years of age) that primarily involves arteries and meninges of the CNS, and one of the most common inflammatory disorders of the CNS in dogs. It has also been referred to as "beagle pain syndrome," "necrotizing vasculitis," and "sterile suppurative meningitis." In some cases, the disease occurs in combination with polyarthritis. A breed predisposition has been noted in Bernese mountain dogs, boxers, beagles, Nova Scotia duck tolling retrievers, golden retrievers, wire-haired pointing griffons, and basset hounds.[143] However, other medium- to large-breed dogs may be affected. There is no apparent sex predisposition.

A variety of studies have supported an immune-mediated pathogenesis for SRMA. Findings have included infiltration of the meninges by B cells and plasma cells, and the presence of T cells in vessel walls. Markedly increased IgA concentrations have been detected in CSF and serum, and there is an increased B cell to T cell ratio in the blood. A large portion of T cells are activated, suggesting the presence of a superantigen.[144,145] A Th2 response predominates based on an increased expression of IL-4 and reduced Th1 cytokines (IL-2 and INF-γ); other cytokines that predominate are IL-17 over a Th17-skewed immune response,[146] vascular endothelial growth factor, transforming growth factor 1, and IL-6.[147] All attempts to identify a causative infectious agent have failed. Invasion of neutrophils is facilitated through upregulation of lymphocyte antigen CD11a and matrix metalloproteinases.[148,149] Uncontrolled IgA synthesis may be the result of immune dysregulation.

Classically, clinical signs are episodic and recurrent and include cervical pain of acute onset, reluctance to move, stiff gait, resistance to neck manipulation, paraspinal hyperesthesia, and high rectal temperature. Chronically affected animals develop neurologic deficits consistent with a multifocal or spinal cord lesion; paresis, ataxia, strabismus, and anisocoria have been described. In some cases, spontaneous bleeding in the subarachnoidal space may occur; in one dog, this led to acute nonambulatory tetraparesis.[150]

Hematologic findings include a predominantly neutrophilic leukocytosis, often with a left shift.[144] The CSF may be turbid, blood tinged, or xanthochromic from hemorrhage occurring in the subarachnoidal space. Neutrophilic pleocytosis (up to several thousand cells per microliter), a high CSF protein concentration, and erythrophagocytosis are apparent in acute cases. With chronicity, mononuclear cells may predominate in the CSF. Simultaneous demonstration of high IgA levels in serum and CSF supports the diagnosis with a high sensitivity (approximately 90%), but low specificity.[151] In addition, acute-phase proteins, including CRP, have been shown to be elevated in the serum and CSF of dogs with SRMA.[152,153]

CT or MRI may reveal contrast enhancement of the meninges; evidence of extramedullary hemorrhage has also been reported.[150] In a few instances at necropsy, subarachnoid hemorrhages may be found extending over the entire length of the meninges of the spinal cord and brainstem. In chronic disease, fibrous thickening of the spinal meninges may be noted grossly. Histopathologic changes consist of necrotizing arteritis of medium- and small-sized arteries and associated leptomeningitis, predominantly in the spinal cord and to a lesser degree in the brainstem (Fig. 129.7). Chronic lesions include proliferative changes of the vascular intima with stenosis and adventitial fibrosis. Occasional vessels may be thrombosed. Extraneural arteritis is more frequently noted in affected beagles, particularly in the extramural coronary arteries and myocardium.

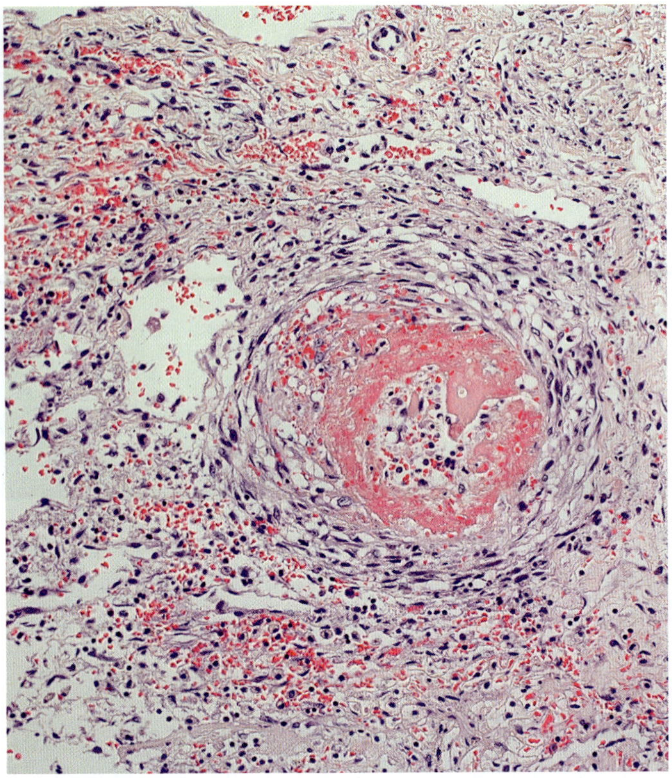

Fig. 129.7 Histopathology of cervical spinal cord meninges from a 2-year-old female intact mixed breed dog with steroid-responsive arteritis-meningitis: A large artery with acute hyaline necrosis and intense infiltration by inflammatory cells. The meninges also display diffuse infiltration by inflammatory cells and hemorrhage. Hematoxylin and eosin stain.

Spontaneous remission has been observed in some dogs. In contrast to GME and NE, the response to glucocorticoid treatment is usually dramatic. Prednisone is given as a long-term treatment starting at an immunosuppressive dose (1–2 mg/kg, PO, q12h), then tapering. Response to treatment and follow-up examinations determine the treatment protocol. The use of second immunosuppressive agents such as azathioprine[143] or cytosine arabinoside[154] may allow reduction in the prednisone dose in order to minimize glucocorticoid adverse effects. Older dogs that have experienced frequent relapses that were insufficiently treated with glucocorticoids and that have high concentrations of IgA in the CSF seem to require a longer duration of therapy and have a less favorable prognosis. Long-term treatment studies have shown relapse rates of 60% to 16%; the relapse rate with a prednisone-azathioprine protocol was 19%.[143] One study identified pathogenic involvement of the endocannabinoid system in SRMA, a potential target for new treatment strategies.[155]

CASE EXAMPLE 1

Signalment

"Maxie," a 6-year-old female Birman cat from Bern, Switzerland.

History

Maxie was evaluated by the neurology service at the University of Bern in Switzerland in June 2001. Several weeks before examination, the cat started to drink large quantities of milk, but refused water. Two weeks before examination, Maxie became progressively reluctant to have her head touched, became easily startled, and exhibited short episodes of walking in circles, ataxia, and hypersalivation. The cat had been purchased as a kitten from a local Swiss breeder, and was fed commercial cat food as well as fresh bovine and turkey meat supplemented with vitamins and minerals. The cat had traveled to other countries including England in order to participate in cat shows. She had had regular contact with other cats and a dog. The cat had had several healthy litters. Vaccinations were up to date and she was FeLV antigen negative. Treatment with glucocorticoids and vitamin B by the referring veterinarian did not improve the cat's condition.

Physical and Neurologic Examination Findings

Routine physical examination revealed no abnormalities. The cat was excited and disoriented. There was a continuous fine head and ear tremor. The cat exhibited bilateral vestibular ataxia with frequent episodes of walking in circles while hypersalivating. All postural reactions were delayed. Pupils were dilated but responsive. Menace response was strongly diminished bilaterally. There was a pronounced hyperesthesia of the head region and the cat reacted strongly to sound. Spinal reflexes were normal. A diffuse cerebral lesion with partial involvement of the brainstem was suspected. The differential diagnoses included toxic metabolic and infectious diseases.

Laboratory findings

A CBC, serum chemistry panel, and urinalysis did not reveal any abnormalities.

Occipital CSF puncture was performed under general anesthesia. Cell count and protein content were within the normal range.

(Continued)

CASE EXAMPLE 1—cont'd

Electroencephalography

EEG was performed under general anesthesia. EEG tracings revealed a generalized iso-electrical course as well as sporadic spindles of medium amplitude and episodes of slower activity.

Treatment and Outcome

The cat was hospitalized and treated with 2 mg/kg phenobarbital IV q12h. The seizures were suppressed but the cat became increasingly obtunded. The owner requested euthanasia.

Neuropathologic and Microbiologic Examination

Histopathologic examination revealed marked vacuolization of the neuropil particularly in the cerebral cortex, thalamus, and brainstem. Spongiform change was most intense in the basal nuclei. In several gray matter areas, there was intracytoplasmic neuronal vacuolation and diffuse astrogliosis. Immunocytochemical staining with anti-PrP antibodies revealed accumulations of PrP in affected areas.

Diagnosis

Feline spongiform encephalopathy.

Comments

The clinical findings in this case were similar to those in cats described in the literature. However, although rapid onset of neurologic signs is typical, rapid progression as seen in this cat is unusual. Metabolic causes were unlikely based on the normal laboratory findings, and the normal CSF was not consistent with viral, bacterial, protozoal, or fungal infection. Against the background of the BSE epidemic in Europe and the much smaller FSE epidemic in its wake at the time this case was evaluated, the history and all clinical findings raised suspicion for FSE. MRI may have been helpful for antemortem diagnosis, but this imaging technique was not yet widely used in veterinary clinics at the time of the FSE epidemic.

The most likely source of infection in this case was ingestion of contaminated feed. It is possible that the cat may have been exposed to contaminated cat feed while in the United Kingdom, but in view of the long incubation time (5 years or more) the cat could have been exposed at home to specified bovine risk materials, which were first banned from animal consumption in April 1996 in Switzerland. FSE is no longer diagnosed in Europe. However, the disease may one day reemerge, as SEs continue to occur in other animal species.

CASE EXAMPLE 2

Signalment

"Jake," a 10-month-old male Weimaraner from north Georgia, USA.

History

Jake was evaluated for a 2-week history of reluctance to move, in association with anorexia and fever. He had been treated with oral enrofloxacin and clindamycin for 2 days; however, the signs of discomfort returned 2 days after medication was discontinued. Jake also had a history of external ear inflammation and pruritic skin disease for the previous month. The dog was up to date on routine vaccinations, lived indoors and outdoors, and traveled outdoors locally with the owner.

Physical Examination

The dog was alert, but held his head down with his neck extended. He was reluctant to stand or walk, and appeared painful when his head was elevated or lifted; however, no further discomfort could be elicited by more caudal paraspinal palpation. T = 103.5°F (39.7°C), HR = 110 beats/minute, RR = 30 breaths/minute, with shallow breathing. BCS was 3/9 and body weight was 31 kg. Mild erythema of the external ear canals was present and small amount of yellow-colored exudate was noted in the ear canals bilaterally. With the exception of the neurologic examination, no other abnormalities were detected.

Neurologic Examination

The dog held its neck extended and head down and walked with a short, stiff gait. Placing reactions were present in all limbs, but initiation and follow-through were stilted. In lateral recumbency, the dog did not relax, and myotatic reflexes were difficult to elicit because of excessive muscle tone. Discomfort was elicited by paraspinal palpation and application of traction on the extremities or with deep muscle palpation. No deficits in cranial nerve responses or reflexes were observed.

Imaging Findings

Cervical spinal radiographs without anesthesia showed no detectable abnormalities.

Laboratory Findings

Hematologic and biochemical findings: The only abnormality of the CBC was a low MCV (65.5 fL; reference range 66–77 fL) and mild leukocytosis (13,200 cells/μL; reference range 5,100–13,000 cells/μL). Serum ALP activity was increased (267 IU/L; reference range 13–122 IU/L). No abnormalities were found on urinalysis.

Arthrocentesis: Synovial fluid was pink and hazy. Nucleated cell count was slightly increased (3.2×10^3 cells/μL in the stifle joint). Nondegenerate neutrophils predominated; no intracellular inclusions or LE cells observed. Impressions: Mild purulent inflammation.

CSF analysis findings (specimen collected from cisterna magna): Clear, RBC = 26 cells/μL, WBC = 462 cells/μL (reference range, <5 cells/μL), total protein 72.6 mg/dL (reference range, 15–35 mg/dL). Differential cell count: Lymphocytes 4%, macrophages 18%, neutrophils 78%, occasional RBC, no bacteria observed in this specimen. Impressions: Marked purulent inflammation.

Microbiologic Testing

Aerobic bacterial culture (CSF): Negative. Anaerobic culture was not done.

Outcome

The dog was treated with chloramphenicol (35 mg/kg, IV, q8h) for 5 days and was then discharged on oral therapy for 3 weeks. The dog made a complete recovery from the signs when monitored for over 1 year.

Diagnosis

Meningitis (antibacterial-responsive) caused by suspected unidentified bacterial organisms.

Comments

Bacterial meningitis was suspected in this dog based on the history, clinical signs, laboratory findings, and response to chloramphenicol. Systemic spread of infection from a hematogenous route was suspected based on some of the inflammatory indicators in the hematologic and biochemical profile and evidence of mild suppurative polyarthritis that was found. The original treatment with enrofloxacin and clindamycin may have been subtherapeutic since it was short-lived and may not have penetrated the CNS tissues and fluids as well as chloramphenicol. Furthermore, IV dosing with chloramphenicol for the first days of therapy allowed for very high levels of drug in the CNS (although the use of chloramphenicol is controversial because of the potential for adverse effects in humans). Although an organism was not observed or isolated, bacterial infection was suspected based on the dramatic response to antibacterial therapy alone. In bacterial meningitis of dogs and cats, organisms are not often identified by cytologic or cultural examination of CSF. Response to antibacterial therapy should be considered presumptive evidence of bacterial infection.

SUGGESTED READINGS

Coates JR, Jeffery ND. Perspectives on meningoencephalomyelitis of unknown Origin. *Vet Clin Small Anim.* 2014;44:1157–1185.

Demierre S, Botteron C, Cizinauskas S, et al. Feline spongiform encephalopathy: first clinical case in Switzerland. *Schweiz Arch Tierheilkd.* 2002;144:550–557.

Radaelli ST, Platt SR. Bacterial meningoencephalomyelitis in dogs: a retrospective study of 23 cases (1990-1999). *J Vet Intern Med.* 2002;16:159–163.

Elbert JA, Yau W, Rissi DR: Neuroinflammatory diseases of the central nervous system of dogs: a retrospective study of 207 cases (2008-2019), *Can Vet J.* 2022;63:178–186.

REFERENCES

1. Aldhous P. BSE: spongiform encephalopathy found in cat. *Nature.* 1990;345:194.
2. Aguzzi A. Prions and the immune system: a journey through gut, spleen, and nerves. *Adv Immunol.* 2003;81:123–171.
3. Collins SJ, Lawson VA, Masters CL. Transmissible spongiform encephalopathies. *Lancet.* 2004;363:51–61.
4. Levkovich SA, Rencus-Lazar S, Gazit E, et al. Microbial prions: dawn of a new era. *Trends Biochem Sci.* 2021;46:391–405.
5. Le NTT, Wu B, Harris DA. Prion neurotoxicity. *Brain Pathol.* 2019;29:263–277.
6. DeArmond SJ, Prusiner SB. Etiology and pathogenesis of prion diseases. *Am J Pathol.* 1995;146:785–811.
7. Hedman C, Bolea R, Marin B, et al. Transmission of sheep-bovine spongiform encephalopathy to pigs. *Vet Res.* 2016;47:14.
8. Race R, Jenny A, Sutton D. Scrapie infectivity and proteinase K-resistant prion protein in sheep placenta, brain, spleen, and lymph node: implications for transmission and antemortem diagnosis. *J Infect Dis.* 1998;178:949–953.
9. Bencsik A, Debeer S, Petit T, et al. Possible case of maternal transmission of feline spongiform encephalopathy in a captive cheetah. *PLoS One.* 2009;4:e6929.
10. Mabbott NA, Alibhai JD, Manson J. The role of the immune system in prion infection. *Handb Clin Neurol.* 2018;153:85–107.
11. Wells GA, Spiropoulos J, Hawkins SA, et al. Pathogenesis of experimental bovine spongiform encephalopathy: preclinical infectivity in tonsil and observations on the distribution of lingual tonsil in slaughtered cattle. *Vet Rec.* 2005;156:401–407.
12. Hoffmann C, Ziegler U, Buschmann A, et al. Prions spread via the autonomic nervous system from the gut to the central nervous system in cattle incubating bovine spongiform encephalopathy. *J Gen Virol.* 2007;88:1048–1055.
13. Smith PG, Bradley R. Bovine spongiform encephalopathy (BSE) and its epidemiology. *Br Med Bull.* 2003;66:185–198.
14. MacKnight C. Clinical implications of bovine spongiform encephalopathy. *Clin Infect Dis.* 2001;32:1726–1731.
15. Budka H, Will RG. The end of the BSE saga: do we still need surveillance for human prion diseases? *Swiss Med Wkly.* 2015;145:w14212.
16. Wyatt JM, Pearson GR, Smerdon TN, et al. Naturally occurring scrapie-like spongiform encephalopathy in five domestic cats. *Vet Rec.* 1991;129:233–236.
17. Hamir AN, Clark WW, Sutton DL, et al. Resistance of domestic cats to a US sheep scrapie agent by intracerebral route. *J Vet Diagn Invest.* 2002;14:444–445.
18. Leggett MM, Dukes J, Pirie HM. A spongiform encephalopathy in a cat. *Vet Rec.* 1990;127:586–588.
19. Bratberg B, Ueland K, Wells GA. Feline spongiform encephalopathy in a cat in Norway. *Vet Rec.* 1995;136:444.
20. Demierre S, Botteron C, Cizinauskas S, et al. Feline spongiform encephalopathy: first clinical case in Switzerland. *Schweiz Arch Tierheilkd.* 2002;144:550–557.
21. Iulini B, Cantile C, Mandara MT, et al. Neuropathology of Italian cats in feline spongiform encephalopathy surveillance. *Vet Pathol.* 2008;45:626–633.
22. Salvadori C, Lossi L, Arispici M, et al. Spongiform neurodegenerative disease in a Persian kitten. *J Feline Med Surg.* 2007;9:242–245.
23. Baron T, Belli P, Madec JY, et al. Spongiform encephalopathy in an imported cheetah in France. *Vet Rec.* 1997;141:270–271.
24. Willoughby K, Kelly DF, Lyon DG, et al. Spongiform encephalopathy in a captive puma (*Felis concolor*). *Vet Rec.* 1992;131:431–434.
25. Kirkwood JK, Cunningham AA, Flasch EJ. Spongiform encephalopathy in another captive cheetah (*Acinonyx jubatus*): evidence for variation in susceptibility or incubation periods between species? *J Zoo Wildl Med.* 1995;26:577–582.
26. Sanchez-Garcia J, Jensen K, Zhang Y, et al. A single amino acid (Asp159) from the dog prion protein suppresses the toxicity of the mouse prion protein in *Drosophila. Neurobiol Dis.* 2016;95:204–209.
27. Qing LL, Zhao H, Liu LL. Progress on low susceptibility mechanisms of transmissible spongiform encephalopathies. *Dongwuxue Yanjiu.* 2014;35:436–445.
28. Madec JY, Belli P, Calavas D, et al. Efficiency of Western blotting for the specific immunodetection of proteinase K-resistant prion protein in BSE diagnosis in France. *Vet Rec.* 2000;146:74–76.
29. Schaller O, Fatzer R, Stack M, et al. Validation of a western immunoblotting procedure for bovine PrP(Sc) detection and its use as a rapid surveillance method for the diagnosis of bovine spongiform encephalopathy (BSE). *Acta Neuropathol.* 1999;98:437–443.
30. O'Rourke KI, Baszler TV, Besser TE, et al. Preclinical diagnosis of scrapie by immunohistochemistry of third eyelid lymphoid tissue. *J Clin Microbiol.* 2000;38:3254–3259.
31. Hilbe MM, Soldati GG, Zlinszky KK, et al. Immunohistochemical study of PrP(Sc) distribution in neural and extraneural tissues of two cats with feline spongiform encephalopathy. *BMC Vet Res.* 2009;5:11.
32. Ryder SJ, Wells GA, Bradshaw JM, et al. Inconsistent detection of PrP in extraneural tissues of cats with feline spongiform encephalopathy. *Vet Rec.* 2001;148:437–441.
33. Eiden M, Hoffmann C, Balkema-Buschmann A, et al. Biochemical and immunohistochemical characterization of feline spongiform encephalopathy in a German captive cheetah. *J Gen Virol.* 2010;91:2874–2883.
34. Ascari LM, Rocha SC, Goncalves PB, et al. Challenges and advances in antemortem diagnosis of human transmissible spongiform encephalopathies. *Front Bioeng Biotechnol.* 2020;8:585896.
35. Mathiason CK, Nalls AV, Seelig DM, et al. Susceptibility of domestic cats to chronic wasting disease. *J Virol.* 2013;87:1947–1956.
36. Seelig DM, Nalls AV, Flasik M, et al. Lesion profiling and subcellular prion localization of cervid chronic wasting disease in domestic cats. *Vet Pathol.* 2015;52:107–119.
37. Koster T, Singh K, Zimmermann M, et al. Emerging therapeutic agents for transmissible spongiform encephalopathies: a review. *J Vet Pharmacol Ther.* 2003;26:315–326.
38. Giles K, Olson SH, Prusiner SB. Developing therapeutics for PrP prion diseases. *Cold Spring Harb Perspect Med.* 2017;7:a023747.
39. Yuzbasiyan-Gurkan V, Krehbiel JD, Cao Y, et al. Development and usefulness of new polymerase chain reaction-based tests for detection of different alleles at codons 136 and 171 of the ovine prion protein gene. *Am J Vet Res.* 1999;60:884–887.
40. Sanchez-Gonzalez L, Maddox RA, Lewis LC, et al. Human prion disease surveillance in Washington State, 2006-2017. *JAMA Netw Open.* 2020;3:e2020690.
41. Ironside JW, Head MW. Neuropathology and molecular biology of variant Creutzfeldt-Jakob disease. *Curr Top Microbiol Immunol.* 2004;284:133–159.
42. Collinge J, Sidle KC, Meads J, et al. Molecular analysis of prion strain variation and the aetiology of 'new variant' CJD. *Nature.* 1996;383:685–690.
43. Groschup MH, Kuczius T, Junghans F, et al. Characterization of BSE and scrapie strains/isolates. *Arch Virol Suppl.* 2000:217–226.
44. Marin-Moreno A, Huor A, Espinosa JC, et al. Radical change in zoonotic abilities of atypical BSE prion strains as evidenced by crossing of sheep species barrier in transgenic mice. *Emerg Infect Dis.* 2020;26:1130–1139.

45. Oliver JA, Llabres-Diaz FJ, Gould DJ, et al. Central nervous system infection with *Staphylococcus intermedius* secondary to retrobulbar abscessation in a dog. *Vet Ophthalmol.* 2009;12:333–337.
46. Fletcher DJ, Snyder JM, Messinger JS, et al. Ventricular pneumocephalus and septic meningoencephalitis secondary to dorsal rhinotomy and nasal polypectomy in a dog. *J Am Vet Med Assoc.* 2006;229:240–245.
47. Britton AP, Davies JL. Rhinitis and meningitis in two shelter cats caused by *Streptococcus equi* subspecies *zooepidemicus*. *J Comp Pathol.* 2010;143:70–74.
48. Fenollosa-Romero E, Taeymans O, Nelissen P, et al. Retrobulbar steatitis and meningitis/empyema secondary to right otitis media, right otitis interna and an inflammatory polyp in a cat. *Open Vet J.* 2018;8:144–148.
49. Cook LB, Bergman RL, Bahr A, et al. Inflammatory polyp in the middle ear with secondary suppurative meningoencephalitis in a cat. *Vet Radiol Ultrasound.* 2003;44:648–651.
50. Sturges BK, Dickinson PJ, Kortz GD, et al. Clinical signs, magnetic resonance imaging features, and outcome after surgical and medical treatment of otogenic intracranial infection in 11 cats and 4 dogs. *J Vet Intern Med.* 2006;20:648–656.
51. Spangler EA, Dewey CW. Meningoencephalitis secondary to bacterial otitis media/interna in a dog. *J Am Anim Hosp Assoc.* 2000;36:239–243.
52. Klopp LS, Hathcock JT, Sorjonen DC. Magnetic resonance imaging features of brain stem abscessation in two cats. *Vet Radiol Ultrasound.* 2000;41:300–307.
53. Barrs VR, Nicoll RG, Churcher RK, et al. Intracranial empyema: literature review and two novel cases in cats. *J Small Anim Pract.* 2007;48:449–454.
54. Dennis MM, Pearce LK, Norrdin RW, et al. Bacterial meningoencephalitis and ventriculitis due to migrating plant foreign bodies in three dogs. *Vet Pathol.* 2005;42:840–844.
55. Mateo I, Lorenzo V, Munoz A, et al. Brainstem abscess due to plant foreign body in a dog. *J Vet Intern Med.* 2007;21:535–538.
56. Bach JF, Mahony OM, Tidwell AS, et al. Brain abscess and bacterial endocarditis in a Kerry Blue terrier with a history of immune-mediated thrombocytopenia. *J Vet Emerg Crit Care.* 2007;17:409–415.
57. Bilderback AL, Faissler D. Medical management of a canine intracranial abscess due to a bite wound. *J Vet Emerg Crit Care.* 2009;19:507–512.
58. Dow SW, LeCouteur RA, Henik RA, et al. Central nervous system infection associated with anaerobic bacteria in two dogs and two cats. *J Vet Intern Med.* 1988;2:171–176.
59. Messer JS, Kegge SJ, Cooper ES, et al. Meningoencephalomyelitis caused by *Pasteurella multocida* in a cat. *J Vet Intern Med.* 2006;20:1033–1036.
60. Radaelli ST, Platt SR. Bacterial meningoencephalomyelitis in dogs: a retrospective study of 23 cases (1990-1999). *J Vet Intern Med.* 2002;16:159–163.
61. Andruzzi MN, Krath ML, Lawhon SD, et al. *Salmonella enterica* subspecies *houtenae* as an opportunistic pathogen in a case of meningoencephalomyelitis and bacteriuria in a dog. *BMC Vet Res.* 2020;16:437.
62. Tun AE, Benedicenti L, Galban EM. *Pasteurella maultocida* meningoencephalomyelitis in a dog secondary to severe periodontal disease. *Clin Case Rep.* 2018;6:1137–1141.
63. Hanke ML, Kielian T. Toll-like receptors in health and disease in the brain: mechanisms and therapeutic potential. *Clin Sci (Lond).* 2011;121:367–387.
64. Glimaker M, Kragsbjerg P, Forsgren M, et al. Tumor necrosis factor-alpha (TNF alpha) in cerebrospinal fluid from patients with meningitis of different etiologies: high levels of TNF alpha indicate bacterial meningitis. *J Infect Dis.* 1993;167:882–889.
65. Nelson RP Jr. Bacterial meningitis and inflammation. *Curr Opin Neurol.* 2006;19:369–373.
66. Kalchev Y, Petkova T, Raycheva R, et al. Combined testing of cerebrospinal fluid IL-12 (p40) and serum C-reactive protein as a possible discriminator of acute bacterial neuroinfections. *Cytokine.* 2021;140:155423.
67. Dewey CW. External hydrocephalus in a dog with suspected bacterial meningoencephalitis. *J Am Anim Hosp Assoc.* 2002;38:563–567.
68. Griffin JF, Levine JM, Levine GJ, et al. Meningomyelitis in dogs: a retrospective review of 28 cases (1999 to 2007). *J Small Anim Pract.* 2008;49:509–517.
69. Elbert JA, Yau W, Rissi DR: Neuroinflammatory diseases of the central nervous system of dogs: a retrospective study of 207 cases (2008-2019), *Can Vet J.* 2022;63:178–186.
70. Rand JS, Parent J, Percy D, et al. Clinical, cerebrospinal fluid, and histological data from twenty-seven cats with primary inflammatory disease of the central nervous system. *Can Vet J.* 1994;35:103–110.
71. Bradshaw JM, Pearson GR, Gruffydd-Jones TJ. A retrospective study of 286 cases of neurological disorders of the cat. *J Comp Pathol.* 2004;131:112–120.
72. Irving G, Chrisman CL. Long-term outcome of five cases of corticosteroid-responsive meningomyelitis. *J Am Anim Hosp Assoc.* 1990;26:324–328.
73. Bohn AA, Wills TB, West CL, et al. Cerebrospinal fluid analysis and magnetic resonance imaging in the diagnosis of neurologic disease in dogs: a retrospective study. *Vet Clin Pathol.* 2006;35:315–320.
74. Behr S, Trumel C, Cauzinille L, et al. High resolution protein electrophoresis of 100 paired canine cerebrospinal fluid and serum. *J Vet Intern Med.* 2006;20:657–662.
75. Weber J, Maiolini A, Tipold A. Evaluation of decreased glucose levels in the cerebrospinal fluid of dogs. *Tierarztl Prax Ausg K Kleintiere Heimtiere.* 2012;40:325–332.
76. Negrin A, Lamb CR, Cappello R, et al. Results of magnetic resonance imaging in 14 cats with meningoencephalitis. *J Feline Med Surg.* 2007;9:109–116.
77. Mellema LM, Samii VF, Vernau KM, et al. Meningeal enhancement on magnetic resonance imaging in 15 dogs and 3 cats. *Vet Radiol Ultrasound.* 2002;43:10–15.
78. Cardy TJ, Lam R, Peters LM, et al. Successful medical management of a domestic longhair cat with subdural intracranial empyema and multifocal pneumonia. *J Vet Emerg Crit Care.* 2017;27:238–242.
79. Messer JS, Wagner SO, Baumwart RD, et al. A case of canine streptococcal meningoencephalitis diagnosed using universal bacterial polymerase chain reaction assay. *J Am Anim Hosp Assoc.* 2008;44:205–209.
80. Perdigao Neto LV, Medeiros M, Ferreira SC, et al. Polymerase chain reaction targeting 16S ribosomal RNA for the diagnosis of bacterial meningitis after neurosurgery. *Clinics.* 2021;76:e2284.
81. Liesman RM, Strasburg AP, Heitman AK, et al. Evaluation of a commercial multiplex molecular panel for diagnosis of infectious meningitis and encephalitis. *J Clin Microbiol.* 2018;56:e01927–17.
82. Bersan E, Maddox T, Walmsley G, et al. CT-guided drainage of a brainstem abscess in a cat as an emergency treatment procedure. *JFMS Open Rep.* 2020;6:2055116919896111.
83. de Gans J, van de Beek D, European Dexamethasone in Adulthood Bacterial Meningitis Study Investigators. Dexamethasone in adults with bacterial meningitis. *N Engl J Med.* 2002;347:1549–1556.
84. Adamo FP, O'Brien RT. Use of cyclosporine to treat granulomatous meningoencephalitis in three dogs. *J Am Vet Med Assoc.* 2004;225:1211–1216, 1196.
85. Gonçalves R, De Decker S, Walmsley G, et al. Inflammatory disease affecting the central nervous system in dogs: a retrospective study in England (2010-2019), *Front Vet Sci.* 2022;8:819945.
86. Nessler JN, Jo WK, Osterhaus ADME, et al. Canine meningoencephalitis of unknown origin: the search for infectious agents in the cerebrospinal fluid via deep sequencing. *Front Vet Sci.* 2022;8:645517.
87. Barber RM, Li Q, Levine JM, et al. Screening for viral nucleic acids in the cerebrospinal fluid of dogs with central nervous system inflammation, *Front Vet Sci.* 2022:doi.org/10.3389/fvets.2022.850510.
88. Braund KG. Granulomatous meningoencephalomyelitis. *J Am Vet Med Assoc.* 1985;186:138–141.
89. Braund KG, Vandevelde M, Walker TL, et al. Granulomatous meningoencephalomyelitis in six dogs. *J Am Vet Med Assoc.* 1978;172:1195–1200.
90. Cordy DR. Canine granulomatous meningoencephalomyelitis. *Vet Pathol.* 1979;16:325–333.
91. Glastonbury JR, Frauenfelder AR. Granulomatous meningoencephalomyelitis in a dog. *Aust Vet J.* 1981;57:186–189.
92. Alley MR, Jones BR, Johnstone AC. Granulomatous meningoencephalitis of dogs in New Zealand. *N Z Vet J.* 1983;31:117–119.
93. Kobayashi Y, Ochiai K, Umemura T, et al. Necrotizing meningoencephalitis in pug dogs in Japan. *J Comp Pathol.* 1994;110:129–136.

94. Munana KR, Luttgen PJ. Prognostic factors for dogs with granulomatous meningoencephalomyelitis: 42 cases (1982-1996). *J Am Vet Med Assoc.* 1998;212:1902–1906.
95. Barnes Heller HL, Granick MN, Pinkerton ME, et al. Case-control study of risk factors for granulomatous meningoencephalomyelitis in dogs. *J Am Vet Med Assoc.* 2019;254:822–825.
96. Granger N, Smith PM, Jeffery ND. Clinical findings and treatment of non-infectious meningoencephalomyelitis in dogs: a systematic review of 457 published cases from 1962 to 2008. *Vet J.* 2010;184:290–297.
97. Kipar A, Baumgartner W, Vogl C, et al. Immunohistochemical characterization of inflammatory cells in brains of dogs with granulomatous meningoencephalitis. *Vet Pathol.* 1998;35:43–52.
98. Suzuki M, Uchida K, Morozumi M, et al. A comparative pathological study on granulomatous meningoencephalomyelitis and central malignant histiocytosis in dogs. *J Vet Med Sci.* 2003;65:1319–1324.
99. Park ES, Uchida K, Nakayama H. Th1-, Th2-, and Th17-related cytokine and chemokine receptor mRNA and protein expression in the brain tissues, T cells, and macrophages of dogs with necrotizing and granulomatous meningoencephalitis. *Vet Pathol.* 2013;50:1127–1134.
100. Matsuki N, Fujiwara K, Tamahara S, et al. Prevalence of autoantibody in cerebrospinal fluids from dogs with various CNS diseases. *J Vet Med Sci.* 2004;66:295–297.
101. Tanaka M, Inoue A, Yamamoto K, et al. Transglutaminase 2: a novel autoantigen in canine idiopathic central nervous system inflammatory diseases. *J Vet Med Sci.* 2012;74:733–737.
102. Coates JR, Jeffery ND. Perspectives on meningoencephalomyelitis of unknown origin. *Vet Clin North Am Small Anim Pract.* 2014;44:1157–1185.
103. Fankhauser R, Fatzer R, Luginbuhl H. Reticulosis of the central nervous system (CNS) in dogs. *Adv Vet Sci Comp Med.* 1972;16:35–71.
104. Barber RM, Porter BF, Li Q, et al. Broadly reactive polymerase chain reaction for pathogen detection in canine granulomatous meningoencephalomyelitis and necrotizing meningoencephalitis. *J Vet Intern Med.* 2012;26:962–968.
105. Barber RM, Li Q, Diniz PP, et al. Evaluation of brain tissue or cerebrospinal fluid with broadly reactive polymerase chain reaction for *Ehrlichia, Anaplasma*, spotted fever group *Rickettsia, Bartonella*, and *Borrelia* species in canine neurological diseases (109 cases). *J Vet Intern Med.* 2010;24:372–378.
106. Schatzberg SJ, Haley NJ, Barr SC, et al. Polymerase chain reaction screening for DNA viruses in paraffin-embedded brains from dogs with necrotizing meningoencephalitis, necrotizing leukoencephalitis, and granulomatous meningoencephalitis. *J Vet Intern Med.* 2005;19:553–559.
107. Weissenbock H, Nowotny N, Caplazi P, et al. Borna disease in a dog with lethal meningoencephalitis. *J Clin Microbiol.* 1998;36:2127–2130.
108. Okamoto M, Kagawa Y, Kamitani W, et al. Borna disease in a dog in Japan. *J Comp Pathol.* 2002;126:312–317.
109. Schwab S, Herden C, Seeliger F, et al. Non-suppurative meningoencephalitis of unknown origin in cats and dogs: an immunohistochemical study. *J Comp Pathol.* 2007;136:96–110.
110. Sheshberadaran H, Norrby E. Three monoclonal antibodies against measles virus F protein cross-react with cellular stress proteins. *J Virol.* 1984;52:995–999.
111. Schaudien D, Schwab S, Linke S, et al. Lack of detectable West Nile virus RNA in brains and kidneys of dogs and cats with immunohistological precipitates using virus-specific antibodies. *Vet Microbiol.* 2008;132:171–176.
112. Talarico LR, Schatzberg SJ. Idiopathic granulomatous and necrotising inflammatory disorders of the canine central nervous system: a review and future perspectives. *J Small Anim Pract.* 2010;51:138–149.
113. Greer KA, Schatzberg SJ, Porter BF, et al. Heritability and transmission analysis of necrotizing meningoencephalitis in the pug. *Res Vet Sci.* 2009;86:438–442.
114. Schrauwen I, Barber RM, Schatzberg SJ, et al. Identification of novel genetic risk loci in Maltese dogs with necrotizing meningoencephalitis and evidence of a shared genetic risk across toy dog breeds. *PLoS One.* 2014;9:e112755.
115. Tsai S, Santamaria P. MHC Class II polymorphisms, autoreactive T-cells, and autoimmunity. *Front Immunol.* 2013;4:321.
116. Sorjonen DC. Clinical and histopathological features of granulomatous meningoencephalomyelitis in dogs. *J Am Anim Hosp Assoc.* 1990;26:141–147.
117. Kitagawa M, Okada M, Watari T, et al. Ocular granulomatous meningoencephalomyelitis in a dog: magnetic resonance images and clinical findings. *J Vet Med Sci.* 2009;71:233–237.
118. Levine JM, Fosgate GT, Porter B, et al. Epidemiology of necrotizing meningoencephalitis in pug dogs. *J Vet Intern Med.* 2008;22:961–968.
119. Kuwamura M, Adachi T, Yamate J, et al. Necrotising encephalitis in the Yorkshire terrier: a case report and literature review. *J Small Anim Pract.* 2002;43:459–463.
120. Bailey CS, Higgins RJ. Characteristics of cerebrospinal fluid associated with canine granulomatous meningoencephalomyelitis: a retrospective study. *J Am Vet Med Assoc.* 1986;188:418–421.
121. Cordy DR, Holliday TA. A necrotizing meningoencephalomyelitis of pug dogs. *Vet Pathol.* 1989;26:191–194.
122. Cornelis I, Van Ham L, Gielen I, et al. Clinical presentation, diagnostic findings, prognostic factors, treatment and outcome in dogs with meningoencephalomyelitis of unknown origin: a review. *Vet J.* 2019;244:37–44.
123. Young BD, Levine JM, Fosgate GT, et al. Magnetic resonance imaging characteristics of necrotizing meningoencephalitis in pug dogs. *J Vet Intern Med.* 2009;23:527–535.
124. von Praun F, Matiasek K, Grevel V, et al. Magnetic resonance imaging and pathologic findings associated with necrotizing encephalitis in two Yorkshire terriers. *Vet Radiol Ultrasound.* 2006;47:260–264.
125. Flegel T. Breed-specific magnetic resonance imaging characteristics of necrotizing encephalitis in dogs. *Front Vet Sci.* 2017;4:203.
126. Wanamaker MW, Vernau KM, Taylor SL, et al.: Classification of neoplastic and inflammatory brain disease using MRI texture analysis in 119 dogs, *Vet Radiol Ultrasound.* 2021;62:445–454.
127. Eom KD, Lim CY, Gu SH, et al. Positron emission tomography features of canine necrotizing meningoencephalitis. *Vet Radiol Ultrasound.* 2008;49:595–599.
128. Kang BT, Kim SG, Lim CY, et al. Correlation between fluorodeoxyglucose positron emission tomography and magnetic resonance imaging findings of non-suppurative meningoencephalitis in 5 dogs. *Can Vet J.* 2010;51:986–992.
129. Flegel T, Oevermann A, Oechtering G, et al. Diagnostic yield and adverse effects of MRI-guided free-hand brain biopsies through a mini-burr hole in dogs with encephalitis. *J Vet Intern Med.* 2012;26:969–976.
130. Rossmeisl JH, Andriani RT, Cecere TE, et al. Frame-based stereotactic biopsy of canine brain masses: technique and clinical results in 26 cases. *Front Vet Sci.* 2015;2:20.
131. Demierre S, Tipold A, Griot-Wenk ME, et al. Correlation between the clinical course of granulomatous meningoencephalomyelitis in dogs and the extent of mast cell infiltration. *Vet Rec.* 2001;148:467–472.
132. Flegel T, Boettcher IC, Matiasek K, et al. Comparison of oral administration of lomustine and prednisolone or prednisolone alone as treatment for granulomatous meningoencephalomyelitis or necrotizing encephalitis in dogs. *J Am Vet Med Assoc.* 2011;238:337–345.
133. Lowrie M, Smith PM, Garosi L. Meningoencephalitis of unknown origin: investigation of prognostic factors and outcome using a standard treatment protocol. *Vet Rec.* 2013;172:527.
134. Callanan JJ, Mooney CT, Mulcahy G, et al. A novel nonsuppurative meningoencephalitis in young greyhounds in Ireland. *Vet Pathol.* 2002;39:56–65.
135. Terzo E, McConnell JF, Shiel RE, et al. Unique topographic distribution of greyhound nonsuppurative meningoencephalitis. *Vet Radiol Ultrasound.* 2012;53:636–642.
136. Greer KA, Daly P, Murphy KE, et al. Analysis of gene expression in brain tissue from greyhounds with meningoencephalitis. *Am J Vet Res.* 2010;71:547–554.
137. Shiel RE, Mooney CT, Brennan SF, et al. Clinical and clinicopathological features of non-suppurative meningoencephalitis in young greyhounds in Ireland. *Vet Rec.* 2010;167:333–337.
138. Vandevelde M, Braund KG. Polioencephalomyelitis in cats. *Vet Pathol.* 1979;16:420–427.

139. Hoff EJ, Vandevelde M. Non-suppurative encephalomyelitis in cats suggestive of a viral origin. *Vet Pathol.* 1981;18:170–180.
140. Kronevi T, Nordström M, Moreno W, et al. Feline ataxia due to nonsuppurative meningoencephalomyelitis of unknown etiology. *Nord Vet Med.* 1974;26:720–725.
141. Flir K. Encephalomyelitis in the big cats. *DTW Dtch Tierarztl Wochenschr.* 1973;80:401.
142. Melchior G. Diseases of zoo animals: meningoencephalitis in lions and tigers. In: *Proceedings of the XV International Symposium on Zoo Animal Diseases.* 1973. Berlin, Germany.
143. Giraud L, Girod M, Cauzinille L. Combination of prednisolone and azathioprine for steroid-responsive meningitis-arteritis treatment in dogs. *J Am Anim Hosp Assoc.* 2021;57:1–7.
144. Felsburg PJ, HogenEsch H, Somberg RL, et al. Immunologic abnormalities in canine juvenile polyarteritis syndrome: a naturally occurring animal model of Kawasaki disease. *Clin Immunol Immunopathol.* 1992;65:110–118.
145. Tipold A, Somberg R, Felsburg P. Is there a superantigen effect on steroid-responsive meningitis-arteritis in dogs? *Tierarztl Prax.* 1996;24:514–518.
146. Freundt-Revilla J, Maiolini A, Carlson R, et al. Th17-skewed immune response and cluster of differentiation 40 ligand expression in canine steroid-responsive meningitis-arteritis, a large animal model for neutrophilic meningitis. *J Neuroinflammation.* 2017;14:20.
147. Hilpert E, Tipold A, Meyerhoff N, et al. Steroid-responsive meningitis-arteritis in dogs in Germany: are there epidemiological or clinical factors influencing recurrence rate? *Tierarztl Prax Ausg K Kleintiere Heimtiere.* 2020;48:5–12.
148. Schwartz M, Carlson R, Tipold A. Selective CD11a upregulation on neutrophils in the acute phase of steroid-responsive meningitis-arteritis in dogs. *Vet Immunol Immunopathol.* 2008;126:248–255.
149. Schwartz M, Moore PF, Tipold A. Disproportionally strong increase of B cells in inflammatory cerebrospinal fluid of dogs with steroid-responsive meningitis-arteritis. *Vet Immunol Immunopathol.* 2008;125:274–283.
150. Wang-Leandro A, Huenerfauth EI, Heissl K, et al. MRI findings of early-stage hyperacute hemorrhage causing extramedullary compression of the cervical spinal cord in a dog with suspected steroid-responsive meningitis-arteritis. *Front Vet Sci.* 2017;4:161.
151. Maiolini A, Carlson R, Schwartz M, et al. Determination of immunoglobulin A concentrations in the serum and cerebrospinal fluid of dogs: an estimation of its diagnostic value in canine steroid-responsive meningitis-arteritis. *Vet J.* 2012;191:219–224.
152. Lowrie M, Penderis J, McLaughlin M, et al. Steroid responsive meningitis-arteritis: a prospective study of potential disease markers, prednisolone treatment, and long-term outcome in 20 dogs (2006-2008). *J Vet Intern Med.* 2009;23:862–870.
153. Bathen-Noethen A, Carlson R, Menzel D, et al. Concentrations of acute-phase proteins in dogs with steroid responsive meningitis-arteritis. *J Vet Intern Med.* 2008;22:1149–1156.
154. Gunther C, Steffen F, Alder DS, et al. Evaluating the use of cytosine arabinoside for treatment for recurrent canine steroid-responsive meningitis-arteritis. *Vet Rec.* 2020;187:e7.
155. Freundt-Revilla J, Heinrich F, Zoerner A, et al. The endocannabinoid system in canine steroid-responsive meningitis-arteritis and intraspinal spirocercosis. *PLoS One.* 2018;13:e0187197.

130

Hereditary and Acquired Immunodeficiencies

Urs Giger, Krystle L. Reagan

KEY POINTS

- Immunodeficiencies are a large heterogeneous group of hereditary (primary immunodeficiencies) and acquired (secondary immunodeficiencies) disorders of host immunity that are associated with an increased risk of infection.
- Immunodeficiencies can arise through disturbances in antigen-specific defense mechanisms mediated by lymphocytes, the nonspecific defense system (which includes phagocytes, plasma proteins, and physical barriers), or both.
- The exact pathogenesis of many canine and feline immunodeficiencies remains unknown, but the molecular defects for several hereditary immunodeficiencies have been elucidated.
- A few hereditary immunodeficiency disorders are prevalent within certain breeds of dogs and cats, whereas others have been described once and may exist only in research animal colonies. Some appear transiently in the dog population, then disappear because of screening and informed breeding.
- A definitive diagnosis of immunodeficiency often requires specific immune testing in addition to routine laboratory tests, and therapeutic interventions are limited.

INTRODUCTION

Immunodeficiencies can be divided into primary and secondary forms depending on whether they are inherited or acquired (Table 130.1).[1–3] Certain clinical features can suggest immunocompromise (Box 130.1). Specific organisms and medical conditions often implicated in immunocompromised hosts are listed in Box 130.2. A definitive diagnosis often requires specific immune testing in addition to routine laboratory tests, and therapeutic interventions are limited.

HEREDITARY OR PRIMARY IMMUNODEFICIENCIES

Many genetically determined immune defects have been described in dogs, whereas only a few are known in cats. With few exceptions, they occur rarely and are summarized in Table 130.2; some are discussed later in this chapter in more detail. They can be broadly classified according to defects of the specific or nonspecific immune system as well as combinations thereof. The innate immune system should be functional at birth and available on short notice to protect the host from invasion by all sorts of organisms. It includes physicochemical barriers, phagocytes, complement and other plasma proteins, and natural killer cells. Congenital barrier defects particularly involve the skin and mucous membrane surfaces and are associated with infections of specific organs; such infections can become systemic. A variety of hereditary skin diseases are being further defined and other immunodeficiencies are being recognized. Ehlers-Danlos syndrome, which leads to fragile, hyperextendable skin in many dogs and cats as well as the myxedematous skin and immunodeficiencies of sharpeis, predispose to pyoderma, whereas ciliary dyskinesia in dogs increases susceptibility to rhinosinusitis and pneumonia. Similarly, X-chromosomal and other ectodermal dysplasias are associated with skin problems as well as mild immunodeficiencies.

Disorders of the phagocytic system involve defects of neutrophils and monocytes as well as the complement system and can lead to pyogenic and granulomatous infections. The granulomatous reaction can occur when neutrophils malfunction and mononuclear cells are recruited. A wide variety of bacteria (e.g., staphylococci, *Escherichia coli, Klebsiella, Enterobacter*) are usually involved, most of which represent resident microflora or pathogens of relatively low virulence. Recurrent infections of the skin, respiratory tract, and oral cavity are common, and intermittent bacteremia and overwhelming sepsis are also seen. Multisystemic amyloidosis, vasculitis, and immune-complex diseases are complications that can occur as a result of chronic recurrent or persistent infections. Cyclic hematopoiesis and leukocyte adhesion deficiency (LAD) are examples of serious quantitative and qualitative phagocytic defects, respectively.

The specific immune system can be divided into humoral and CMI systems and includes lymphocytes, immunoglobulins, and cytokines. Deficiencies of B cells or humoral immunity affect the production of immunoglobulins and lead to increased susceptibility to pyogenic bacterial infections. Deficiencies of T cells or CMI are associated with viral and fungal infections, but intracellular bacterial infections may also occur. Animals with cellular immunodeficiencies may have smaller thymic and tonsillar tissues as well as intestinal and peripheral lymph nodes and decreased numbers of circulating lymphocytes.

The severity of immunodeficiency varies among defects. Infections may be systemic or restricted to a particular organ system such as the skin or respiratory tract. Some immunodeficiencies in neonates lead to overwhelming infections and death within the first few days to weeks of life, whereas others, such as morphologic leukocyte changes, are not consistently associated with any noticeable predisposition to infection. Chédiak-Higashi syndrome in smoke-colored Persian cats is characterized by abnormally large eosinophilic granules in polymorphonuclear leukocytes. It causes no immunodeficiencies, but leads to a bleeding tendency resulting from a platelet storage pool disease.[4] Similarly, Birman cats with acidophilic granulation of neutrophils and dogs and cats with various lysosomal storage diseases (e.g., mucopolysaccharidosis, gangliosidosis, mannosidosis) have granulation or

TABLE 130.1 Features of Immunodeficiency Diseases Based on the Underlying Defect

Defect	Susceptibility to Specific Infections	Diagnostic Tests to Confirm Defect
Ciliary dyskinesia	Respiratory infections	Electron microscopy of cilia
Ehlers-Danlos syndrome	Skin injury and infections	Histopathology and electron microscopy of skin
B-cell dysfunction	Pyogenic bacteria, *Giardia* spp.	Globulin, serum electrophoresis, tetanus antibody response
T-cell dysfunction	Bacterial sepsis, mycobacteria, *Candida* and *Pneumocystis* spp.	Thymic radiographs, skin testing delayed hypersensitivity, CD4 and CD8 cell quantification
Granulocyte dysfunction	Streptococci, *Pseudomonas, Nocardia, Candida,* and *Aspergillus* spp.	Neutrophil count, phagocytosis assays, molecular genetic tests[a]
Complement	Pyogenic bacteria	CH50 assay, molecular genetic tests

[a]Specific breed-specific genomic DNA mutation/variant tests are available for several hereditary defects.

BOX 130.1 Major Clinical Signs of Immunodeficiency Disorders

Recurrent infections, chronic and protracted course of infection, or both
Infection with common nonpathogenic (opportunistic) or aberrant infectious agents
Severe and often atypical infectious disease manifestations
Delayed, incomplete, or absent response to antimicrobial therapy
Adverse reactions to attenuated live virus vaccines

BOX 130.2 Infectious Agents and Medical Problems Associated with Immunocompromise

Opportunistic Pathogens

Viruses: Feline herpesvirus-1, feline infectious peritonitis virus, feline calicivirus, canine papillomavirus, canine herpesvirus
Bacteria: *Mycoplasma haemofelis, Citrobacter* spp., *Escherichia coli, Enterobacter* spp., *Klebsiella pneumoniae, Mycobacterium* spp., *Nocardia* spp., *Proteus* spp., *Pseudomonas aeruginosa, Serratia marcescens, Staphylococcus pseudintermedius*
Fungi: *Aspergillus* spp., *Candida* spp., *Cryptococcus* spp., *Histoplasma* spp., *Blastomyces* spp., *Coccidioides* spp., *Mucor* spp.
Protozoa: *Pneumocystis* spp., *Toxoplasma gondii, Neospora caninum, Cryptosporidium* spp., *Giardia* spp., *Tritrichomonas* spp., *Isospora* spp.
Mites: *Demodex canis, Ododectes* spp., *Notoedres* spp.

Medical Problems

Recurrent skin infections
Recurrent mucosal infections
Neonatal sepsis and mortality
Reactive amyloidosis
Vasculitis, arteritis, polyarthritis
Recurrent bacteremia
Granulomatous infections
Chronic hypersensitivity reactions
Autoimmune diseases
Persistent intracellular rickettsial or bacterial infections
Disproportional leukocytosis
Persistent lymphopenia

vacuolation of leukocytes without being immunocompromised; frequently they also exhibit a lymphocytosis. The Pelger-Huët anomaly, which is characterized by hyposegmentation of granulocytes, causes no immunodeficiency in animals despite the fact that the leukograms of affected dogs and cats reveal the most severe left shift with a normal leukocyte count and no toxic changes. In foxhounds, *in vitro* chemotactic response of these neutrophils was mildly diminished, whereas in basenjis no functional abnormalities have been found.[5–7]

Although an increased susceptibility to opportunistic infections develops, the type of infection varies depending on the immune system defect present. A few immunodeficiency disorders predispose animals to unusual infectious agents. Miniature dachshunds appear to be predisposed to *Pneumocystis* pneumonia (see Chapter 89), and German shepherd dogs and Hungarian vizslas may be prone to systemic aspergillosis and other systemic mold infections.[8,9] Golden and Labrador retrievers that had high serum antibody titers to *Borrelia* (*Borreliella*) *burgdorferi* were more likely to have glomerulonephritis.[10] Miniature schnauzers and basset hounds have an increased susceptibility to systemic avian mycobacteriosis, and possibly other specific infections like candidiasis.[11] Boxer dogs and German shepherds have been the predominant breeds reported with the cutaneous mycobacterial disease known as canine leproid granuloma syndrome.[12,13] Great Danes, boxers, border collies, German shepherds, Dalmatians, and Doberman pinschers (Australia)[14] and American cocker spaniels (United States)[15] have been overrepresented in retrospective studies of cryptococcosis. Boxers and French bulldogs are predisposed to granulomatous colitis secondary to adherent and invasive *E. coli*.[16] A genetic predisposition to demodicosis has been proposed in various canine breeds and families within breeds. The predisposition to develop FIP has also been suggested to have a genetic basis, more commonly in some purebred cats like Birmans. Mechanisms that predispose different breeds to specific infections remain unknown, but have been elucidated for some, such as miniature schnauzers and systemic *Mycobacterium avium* complex (MAC) infection caused by a *CARD9* variant.[11]

The mode of inheritance of primary immunodeficiencies has not yet been determined in all cases. Autosomal recessive transmission, with affected males and females born to healthy parents is usual, but a few exceptions exist. The Pelger-Huët anomaly is inherited as an autosomal dominant trait. Ectodermal dysplasia of German shepherds (but not other ectodermal dysplasias) caused by a ectodysplasin (ED) 1 gene defect, and severe combined immunodeficiency (SCID) caused by two different mutations in the common γ-chain of the IL-2 receptor in basset hounds and Cardigan Welsh corgis, are X-chromosomal recessive disorders. Thus, only males are affected, and the dams and one half of the dam's female littermates are carriers. Granulomatous colitis of boxer dogs appears to result from mutations in the gene that encodes neutrophil cytosolic factor (NCF) 2, which encodes the cytosolic subunit, $p67^{phox}$ of NAPDH oxidase.[16] Thus, the breed, sex, age of onset, type of infections, and other special characteristics can suggest a particular immunodeficiency. Furthermore, it follows that within a breed, the immunodeficiency is typically caused by the same defect and mutation, whereas different breeds can have mutations in the same or different genes.

DIAGNOSIS

Suggestive signs of infection (see Box 130.1) develop in animals with a primary immunodeficiency generally early in life. Despite receiving colostrum during the first day of life, clinically affected animals can have illness during the neonatal to juvenile period and can develop recurrent

TABLE 130.2 **Hereditary or Primary Immunodeficiencies of Dogs and Cats**

Disease (Synonym)	Inheritance	Breeds	Defect	Characterization
Barrier Defects				
Ciliary dyskinesia (immotile cilia syndrome)	AR	Many[a]	Functional and morphologic cilia abnormalities CCDC39, AKNA, NME5	Rhinosinusitis, bronchopneumonia with bronchiectasis, situs inversus, breed-specific DNA mutation test
Neutrophil Defects				
Bactericidal neutrophil defect	U	Doberman pinscher	Unknown	Upper respiratory infections, reduced bactericidal activity, ciliary dyskinesia not excluded
Cyclic hematopoiesis (cyclic neutropenia)	AR	Collie (gray), basset hound	Hematopoietic growth factor defect AP3B1	Severe neutropenia every 12–14 days, reactive amyloidosis, DNA mutation test
Chronic idiopathic neutropenia	U	Rottweiler	G-CSF deficiency	Recurrent fever, sepsis, polyarthritis, pyoderma
Leukocyte adhesion deficiency	AR	Irish setter, red and white setter, domestic medium-hair cat	CD11/18 deficiency β-chain (CD18) deficiency	Severe leukocytosis, infection with limited pus formation, lack of neutrophil adhesion, DNA mutation test
Pelger-Huët anomaly	AD	Australian shepherd, foxhound, other dog breeds, domestic shorthair cats	Unknown	No immunodeficiency, hyposegmented granulocytes
Leukocyte granulation	U	Birman cats	Unknown	No immunodeficiency, acidophilic granules
Complement component 3 deficiency (C3 deficiency)	AR	Brittany spaniel	C3 deficiency	Pyogenic infections, lack of C-mediated phagocytosis in colony of dogs with neuromuscular disease
Chédiak-Higashi syndrome	AR	Persian cats	CHS1/LYST	No immunodeficiency, large granules in phagocytes, bleeding tendency
Reactive (AA) amyloidosis	U	Abyssinian cats	Unknown	Reactive (AA) amyloidosis, renal failure
Increased susceptibility to *Pneumocystis* pneumonia	AR	Dachshund, King Charles spaniel	Unknown	*Pneumocystis*
Increased susceptibility to systemic mycobacteriosis/candidiasis	AR	Miniature schnauzers, bassets	CARD9 defect in miniature schnauzers, unknown in basset	Systemic mycobacteriosis, DNA mutation test (miniature schnauzers)
Susceptibility to fungal and rickettsial infections; pyoderma	U	German shepherd	Possible macrophage or T-cell defect	Severe ehrlichiosis, Rocky Mountain Spotted Fever, disseminated aspergillosis, deep pyoderma
Immune vasculitis, amyloidosis	U	Sharpei, Abyssinian cats, Oriental shorthair cats	Elevated IL-6	Arthritis, amyloidosis, renal failure, hepatic rupture, hypoproteinemia
Lethal acrodermatitis	AR	Bull terrier	MKLN1	Zinc deficiency, hyperkeratosis
Increased susceptibility to parvoviral infection	U	Rottweiler, Doberman pinscher	Unknown	Parvovirus infection
Vaccine-exacerbated immune disturbance	U	Akita, Weimaraner	Unknown	Variable meningitis, polyarthritis, amyloidosis
Humoral Immune Defects				
X-linked severe combined immunodeficiency (X-SCID)	XR	Basset hound, Cardigan Welsh corgi	Common γ-chain of IL-2 and other cytokines	Severe bacterial and viral infections, no IgG and IgA, deficient lymphocyte blastogenesis, DNA mutation test
SCID	AR	Jack Russell terrier	DNA-protein kinase catalytic subunit	Severe serum immunoglobulin deficiency, hypoplasia of lymphoid tissues, DNA mutation test
SCID	AR	Frisian water dog	RAG1 gene defect alters antigen recognition	Severe IgM, IgG and IgA deficiency and lymphopenia, DNA mutation test
Combined immunodeficiency	U	Sharpei	T-cell and B-cell defects, low IL-6 and IL-2	Skin, respiratory, and gastrointestinal infections
Thymic abnormalities and dwarfism	U	Weimaraner	Unknown	Reduced growth, thymosine responsive
Hypotrichosis congenita with thymic aplasia	AR	Birman	FOXN1	Nude kittens with lethal immundeficiency

In addition to the listed syndromes, bone marrow dyscrasias have been described in miniature and toy poodles and transient hypogammaglobulinemia in Samoyeds, but less is known of these disorders.

[a]For example, springer spaniel, old English sheepdog, English setter, West Highland white terrier, pointer.

AD, autosomal dominant; *AR*, autosomal recessive; *G-CSF*, granulocyte colony-stimulating factor; *IL*, interleukin; *U*, unknown; *XR*, X-linked recessive.

and overwhelming infections that lead to severe debilitation and death before 1 year of age. Some animals, but typically not all, in a litter may be affected, whereas the parents are usually clinically healthy. A genetic predisposition to infection is less commonly noted after 1 year of age (e.g., leishmaniosis in foxhounds and MAC in miniature schnauzers and basset hounds). Furthermore, animals with hereditary immunodeficiencies may have other special clinical manifestations. Hypersensitivity reactions can occur and reflect an overall dysregulation of the immune system caused by a lack of one or more components or a chronic antigen stimulation from inadequate clearance of infections. Chronic systemic infections may also impair growth. Characteristic coat color dilutions and increased tendency for surface bleeding are seen, for example, in collies with cyclic hematopoiesis, Persian cats with Chédiak-Higashi syndrome, and Weimaraners with an incompletely defined immunodeficiency. Nude Birman kittens and ectodermal dysplasia are associated with a complete lack or loss of hair and either severe or minimal predisposition to infection, respectively.

Results of a CBC, serum chemistry panel, and urinalysis can suggest a specific immunodeficiency. Results of differential leukocyte count and microscopic evaluation of a blood smear are most important. Some breeds, such as greyhounds, have low reference values for blood leukocyte counts. Neutropenia can be transient (e.g., cyclic hematopoiesis, parvovirus infection), or can be persistent (e.g., cobalamin malabsorption defects or sepsis). Lymphopenia may be observed in dogs with T-cell disorders or SCID. Although leukocytosis often accompanies infection, defects in leukocyte adhesion and egress from blood circulation at sites of infection can be associated with disproportionately high leukocytosis for the degree of infection as seen with hereditary LAD or with concurrent glucocorticoid usage. Careful review of a blood smear can reveal leukocyte abnormalities such as granulation and vacuolation resulting from lysosomal storage diseases or Chédiak-Higashi syndrome,[17] acidophilic granulation of leukocytes in Birmans,[18] phagocytized microorganisms, or toxic leukocyte changes that suggest overwhelming bacterial infections.

Serum globulin concentrations are generally increased with chronic infections. Low or normal globulin levels in infected animals can suggest major external losses or diminished production from a humoral immune defect. Indeed, specific immunoglobulin deficiencies have been recognized in dogs. Serum protein electrophoresis may identify a γ-globulin deficiency, but immunoelectrophoresis is required to detect the class and degree of immunoglobulin deficiency. Maternally derived antibodies can only be absorbed during the first day of life and influence the serum values during the first few weeks. Only IgM can be synthesized very early in life (neonatal period), whereas the development of IgA can be delayed for months. Thus, it is important to compare values with data from age-matched controls. Serum titers against specific antigens can be measured, followed by evaluation of the antibody response to vaccination against particular agents. However, despite the antibody titer, cellular immunity is not being assessed. Biopsy specimens of lymph nodes can reveal disorganization with loss of germinal centers and normal paracortical lymphocytes. Decreases in plasma cell populations can also be evident.

T-cell or combined immunodeficiencies cause defective CMI responses, which may be manifested as prolonged allograft rejection times and decreased delayed-type hypersensitivity (DTH) reactions to skin testing.[19] Reduced *in vitro* lymphocyte stimulation results can also be caused by a primary lymphocyte defect or by infection.

The identification of the nature of microbes that infect an animal is important for diagnostic as well as therapeutic reasons. Antibody titers can be used to assess response to vaccines and humoral immunity. Histopathology and cytology can assist in characterization of the architecture, morphology, maturation, and function of the immune system, including barrier systems. In ciliary dyskinesia, morphologic abnormalities of cilia may be identified by electron microscopy. Functional studies using nuclear imaging or on respiratory epithelial biopsy specimens are also indicated.

Characterization of immunodeficiencies may require special leukocyte studies. Flow cytometry can be used to differentiate between T and B cells, determine T and B cell ratios, "bacterial killing reaction," and the presence or absence of leukocyte adhesion proteins (CD11/18) or IL-2 receptors. Lymphocyte function studies include lymphocyte stimulation and plaque-forming assays that assess immunoglobulin production. Phagocyte function studies assess leukocyte adhesion, migration, chemotaxis, phagocytosis, "respiratory burst," and bactericidal activity. Functional assays must generally be performed on fresh (collected within 24 hours) blood cells and compared simultaneously with a preferably age- and breed-matched control. Infection can impair *in vitro* lymphocyte function and enhance phagocyte function. Therefore, control of infection before studying leukocyte function is preferred.

A variety of hereditary immunodeficiencies have been characterized at the molecular genetic level. This permits simple screening of affected animals or those potentially at risk. Because genetic variants (mutations) are typically breed specific, these DNA screening tests may be applied within a breed not only for detection of infected immunodeficient animals but also those potentially at risk to infection and carriers.

TREATMENT AND PREVENTION

Successful control of infection in immunodeficient animals depends on the type of infection as well as the type and severity of the immune defect. In immunocompromised patients, early and aggressive antimicrobial therapy is indicated even for mild infections with agents that are considered nonpathogenic in immunocompetent hosts. Because of the immunodeficient host's potential inability to kill infectious organisms, cidal antimicrobials are recommended for treatment if available.

Few practical treatments exist for animals with hereditary immunodeficiencies. Dogs with hereditary cobalamin malabsorption can be successfully administered parenteral cobalamin every 2–4 weeks.[20] In experimental studies, bone marrow transplantation and gene therapy corrected several canine leukocyte defects and dogs with cyclic neutropenia.[21–23] Granulocyte colony-stimulating factor (G-CSF) has been used to increase neutrophil numbers in dogs with cyclic neutropenia and G-CSF deficiency. Fresh whole blood can be transfused repeatedly to animals with overwhelming infections and neutropenia or neutrophil dysfunction, but the effect is very transient. Plasma transfusions or immunoglobulin (hyperimmune serum) injections can temporarily support animals with humoral immunodeficiencies. However, these products should not be used in animals with complete IgA deficiency, because they can experience anaphylactic reactions to the foreign IgA protein. No commercial canine or feline γ-globulin is available, and the human γ-globulin preparations do not target animal-specific infections and can cause allergic reactions on repeated use.

If an acquired immunodeficiency is present and can be corrected, the infection is often easily controlled. Administration of immunosuppressive agents should be withheld during treatment of infection, and any underlying disorder should be treated if possible. Immunocompromised animals with an infection, where the cause of immunosuppression cannot be corrected, generally have a guarded to poor prognosis. Despite aggressive antimicrobial therapy, their infections can be difficult to control, leading to overwhelming infections, protracted courses, and recurrences.

SPECIFIC HEREDITARY OR PRIMARY IMMUNODEFICIENCIES IN DOGS

Primary Ciliary Dyskinesia

Primary ciliary dyskinesia, also known as immotile cilia syndrome, is caused by various functional and ultrastructural ciliary abnormalities that include lack of outer or inner dynein arms, abnormal microtubular pattern, random ciliary orientation, and electron-dense cores in the basal body. Because of impaired mucociliary clearance, affected animals have recurrent bacterial rhinitis, sinusitis, and bronchopneumonia with bronchiectasis. Poorly motile or immotile live sperm results in male infertility. Although evidence is lacking, dysfunction of ependymal cilia can cause hydrocephalus and otitis media. The lack of coordinated cilia motility during embryogenesis is responsible for a 50% prevalence of concurrent situs inversus in some forms of primary ciliary dyskinesia. The clinical triad of rhinosinusitis, bronchiectasis, and situs inversus is known as Kartagener's syndrome.[24–26]

Primary ciliary dyskinesia is inherited by an autosomal recessive trait. It represents a heterogeneous group of defects that have been described in more than a dozen breeds.[27] Clinical signs typically begin at a young age, and recurrent respiratory infections lead to death or euthanasia before 1 year of age. However, a few dogs appear clinically healthy for months to years.[28]

A diagnosis of ciliary dyskinesia is reached through documentation of absent ciliary clearance of technetium-99m-labeled microaggregated albumin that is placed through a catheter into the nasal cavity or the tracheal bifurcation; biopsy of ciliated mucosae with ultrastructural analysis using electron microscopy; and *in vitro* motility studies.[29,30] Induction of ciliogenesis can also be determined by use of *in vitro* cell culture.[30] A likely causative mutation in the *NME5* gene encoding a sparsely characterized protein associated with ciliary function has recently been found in Alaskan malamutes with ciliary dyskinesia.[31] A deletion was found in the *AKNA* gene, encoding the AT-hook transcription factor, of rough collies with recurrent inflammatory pulmonary disease similar to ciliary dyskinesia. A mutation in the *CCDC39* gene has been found in Old English sheepdogs with axonemal disorganization and abnormal ciliary beating.[32]

Chronic recurrent respiratory infections have been observed in related Irish wolfhounds.[33,34] In wolfhound puppies, the disease begins with a serous rhinitis that later becomes catarrhal to hemorrhagic with turbinate ulceration and destruction. Pneumonia and generalized lymphadenomegaly are apparent in later stages. Although the disease is responsive to antimicrobial treatment, it can progress in intervening periods. Ciliary dyskinesia has been identified in some wolfhounds but has not been a consistent feature of the disease. Serum IgA levels were reduced in some dogs, but bronchoalveolar lavage fluid had high IgA concentrations in tested dogs, which can relate to their inflammatory response to infection.[33]

Cyclic Hematopoiesis

Cyclic hematopoiesis is characterized by a periodic production and maturation defect of hematopoietic cells in the bone marrow.[35] In human patients, the cycle is 21 days, but in dogs, severe neutropenia (<1,000 cells/μL) occurs every 12 to 14 days and lasts for 3 to 4 days (cyclic neutropenia syndrome). Serial blood counts are used to make a definitive diagnosis unless a molecular test is performed. During periods of neutropenia, dogs are very susceptible to bacterial infection. Clinical illness appears at 6 to 8 weeks of age with regular recurrence of bacterial infections. The condition culminates in sepsis or systemic amyloidosis and death from organ failure before 1 year of age. The condition may be accompanied by gingival bleeding from an associated platelet storage pool disease. Affected collies have a silver gray or light beige to tan coat color, and secondary hormonal cycling has been observed.[36]

Cyclic hematopoiesis was the first reported canine immunodeficiency observed and has only been described in hypopigmented collies, hence the term gray collie syndrome. It is inherited as an autosomal recessive trait, but no case has been reported since the 1970s outside of the research colony in this breed. Experimentally, bone marrow transplantation corrects this syndrome, including the coat color dilution. Injections of G-CSF also abolish the cycling. The defect in collie dogs is associated with a homozygous mutation of the gene encoding the dog adaptor protein complex 3 β-subunit that directs trans-Golgi export of transmembrane cargo proteins to lysosomes.[37,38] Mutations in a leukocyte elastase have been identified in humans with a similar syndrome.[35]

Leukocyte Adhesion Deficiency

LAD, originally described as canine granulocytopathy syndrome in Irish setters and cattle and more recently (2017) a cat,[51] is referred to as canine, feline or bovine LAD (or CLAD, FLAD, or BLAD).[39] It results from the absence of a family of three leukocyte integrins.[40–43] These proteins are heterodimers (CD11a-d/CD18) with a specific α-chain (CD11a-d) and a common β-chain (CD18). In LAD, the β_2-subunit is missing (CD18 deficiency), resulting in a lack of surface expression and function of all leukocyte integrins. CD11b/18 (CR3) is the most critical integrin because it is the receptor that binds leukocytes to C3bi and ICAM-1 on activated endothelium, thereby mediating tight adhesion of leukocytes (Fig. 130.1). When this is deficient, granulocytes are unable to marginate and destroy microorganisms, which is associated with an impaired inflammatory response despite marked leukocytosis (Fig. 130.2A). Furthermore, the *in vitro* lymphocyte stimulation response is reduced. A missense *ITGB2* mutation substituting a cystine with a serine has been identified in affected Irish setters and red and white setters.[40,44–48]

Dogs with LAD have a severely increased susceptibility to bacterial infections. Signs of pyogenic infections develop during the first weeks to months of life, are often recurring, and are poorly responsive to antibacterials. Omphalophlebitis and gingivitis are often the first infections and might be followed by pyoderma, pododermatitis, thrombophlebitis, pneumonia, pyometra, osteomyelitis (especially craniomandibular and metaphyseal), and fatal sepsis. Pups are often stunted or have poor body condition.[49,50] Infection sites exhibit minimal inflammation and pus formation despite a most severe persistent leukocytosis of 25,000 to 500,000/μL (Fig. 130.2B). Regional lymphadenomegaly and poor wound healing are commonly noted. Long-term therapy with bactericidal antibacterials is required.

LAD has been reported in Irish and red and white setters worldwide and is autosomal recessive. LAD due to other CD18 mutations also has been documented in Holstein cattle, humans, and one cat.[51] The diagnosis in dogs is currently made by mutation-specific DNA testing.[44,47,48,52] Carrier dogs also can be detected by genetic testing which helped to practically eliminate the disease in the affecteed breed populations.[40] In the past, demonstration of neutrophil adherence defects and deficiency of leukocyte glycoproteins CD11/CD18 by flow cytometry analysis were used (Fig. 130.2C,D). If LAD is suspected in another dog breed, leukocyte flow cytometry for CD18 is still a broad and simple screening test.

Hematopoietic stem cell transplantation of CD18+ donor cells and gene therapy can reverse the defect.[12] Mixed chimeric hematopoietic stem cell transplantation from a histocompatible littermate reversed clinical signs in an affected dog.[53]

Complement C3 Deficiency

Complement factor C3 deficiency was found in a colony of Brittany spaniels with spinal muscular atrophy.[54–56] Affected dogs have defective chemotaxis and bacterial phagocytosis from a complete deficiency of C3 (0.1%) and less than 1% plasma complement activity. The immunodeficiency is generally mild and animals live until adulthood, but serious infections can occur, including pneumonia, pyoderma, sepsis, pyometra, and septic arthritis. Affected dogs can develop renal failure with amyloidosis. This is an inherited autosomal recessive disorder, and a diagnosis can be reached by documenting a lack of serum complement activity or mutation test. However, this defect has not been noted outside the research colony.

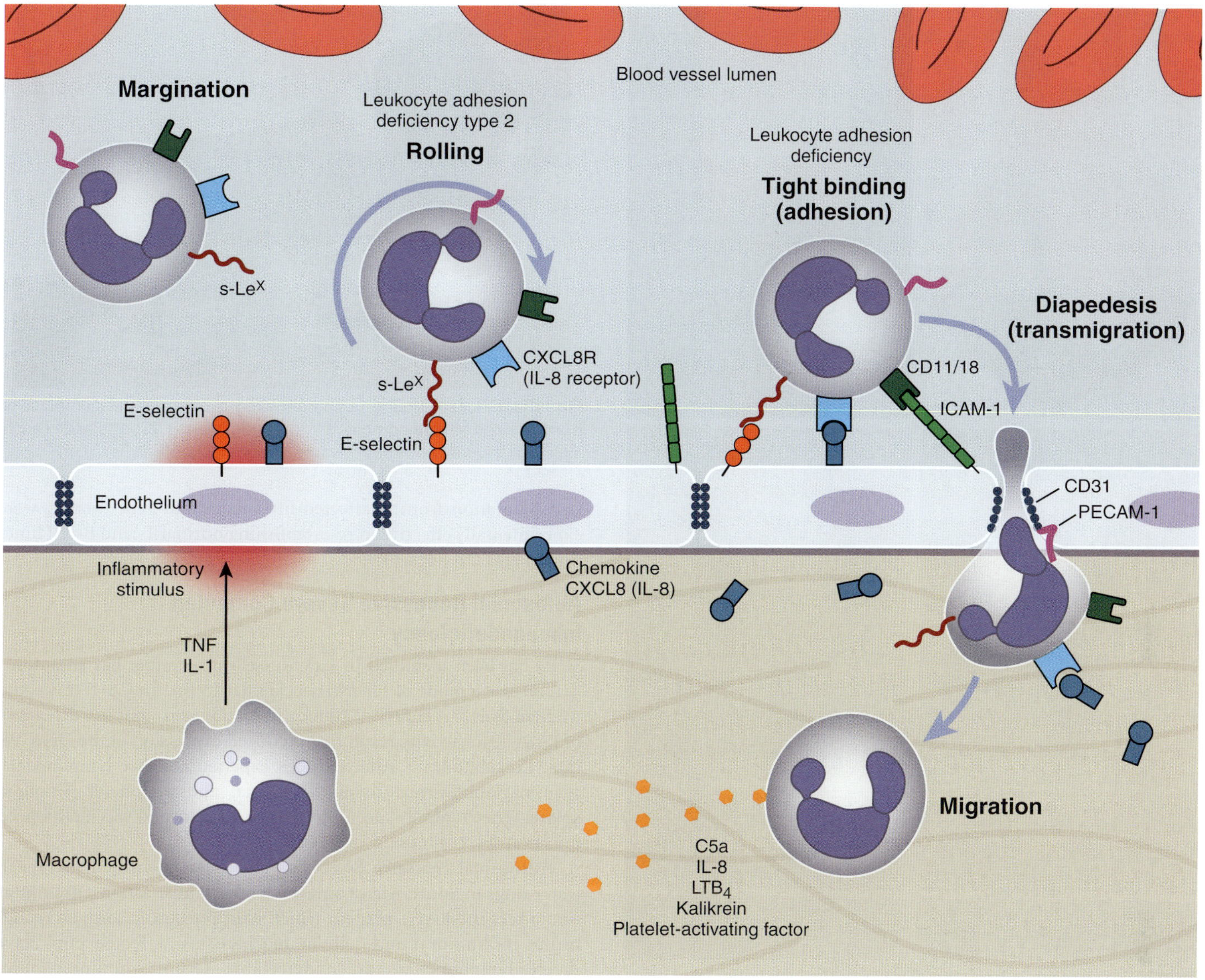

Fig. 130.1 Role of CD11/18 integrins in leukocyte migration to sites of infection.

Selective Cobalamin Malabsorption

Chronic neutropenia and megaloblastic anemia have been described in giant schnauzers, beagles, Australian shepherds, Komondors, and border collie pups.[57–59] Affected animals fail to thrive and often show lethargy, inappetence, and cachexia but are only rarely predisposed to infection accompanied by fever, lameness, or diarrhea. Blood smears show neutropenia with hypersegmented neutrophils. Affected animals have very low serum cobalamin concentrations and marked methylmalonic aciduria. A cobalamin ileal receptor defect was documented in the CUBAM complex, either due to a mutation in amnionless or cubulin.[20,59] Treatment with parenteral administration of cobalamin once or twice monthly is highly effective,[20,58] but does not resolve the very mild proteinuria.

Trapped Neutrophil Syndrome—Hereditary Neutropenia in Border Collies

Chronic neutropenia and recurrent bacterial infections have been found in certain lines of border collies in Australia and New Zealand.[60] This autosomal recessive trait (trapped neutrophil syndrome) is associated with stunted growth by 2 weeks of age and fever, anorexia, diarrhea, and lameness by 2 months of age. Metaphyseal osteomyelitis is seen radiographically, and neutropenia ($<3 \times 10^3$ cells/μL) is consistently found. Bone marrow cytologic abnormalities include granulocytic hyperplasia with a shift to the right, suggesting that the developing cells cannot enter the systemic circulation. A DNA test has been offered to screen border collies.[61,62] Puppies respond poorly to antimicrobial therapy and eventually succumb to systemic infections.

X-Linked Severe Combined Immunodeficiency

X-linked SCID (X-SCID) is characterized by a failure of humoral immunity and CMI.[63–65] It develops in various animal species when lymphocyte precursors fail to differentiate into mature lymphocytes. In dogs, defects in the γ^c chain lead to deficiency of several cytokine receptors (IL-2, IL-4, IL-7, IL-9, IL-15, and IL-21).[66] Although profound deficiencies are found in T-cell function, some B-cell activities are preserved.[67] For example, canine X-SCID B cells are capable of producing IgM but do not class-switch to the production of IgG after mitogen stimulation. The shared usage of a γ^c chain by these cytokines explains the profound immunologic abnormalities and the impaired IgG response.[68] The ability of lymphocytes to bind to IL-2 and proliferate is severely impaired, and the development of thymocytes is drastically reduced, with an increased proportion of CD4-/CD8-thymocytes.[69,70] Serum IgG and IgA concentrations are low, but IgM values are normal.[71] Because of the

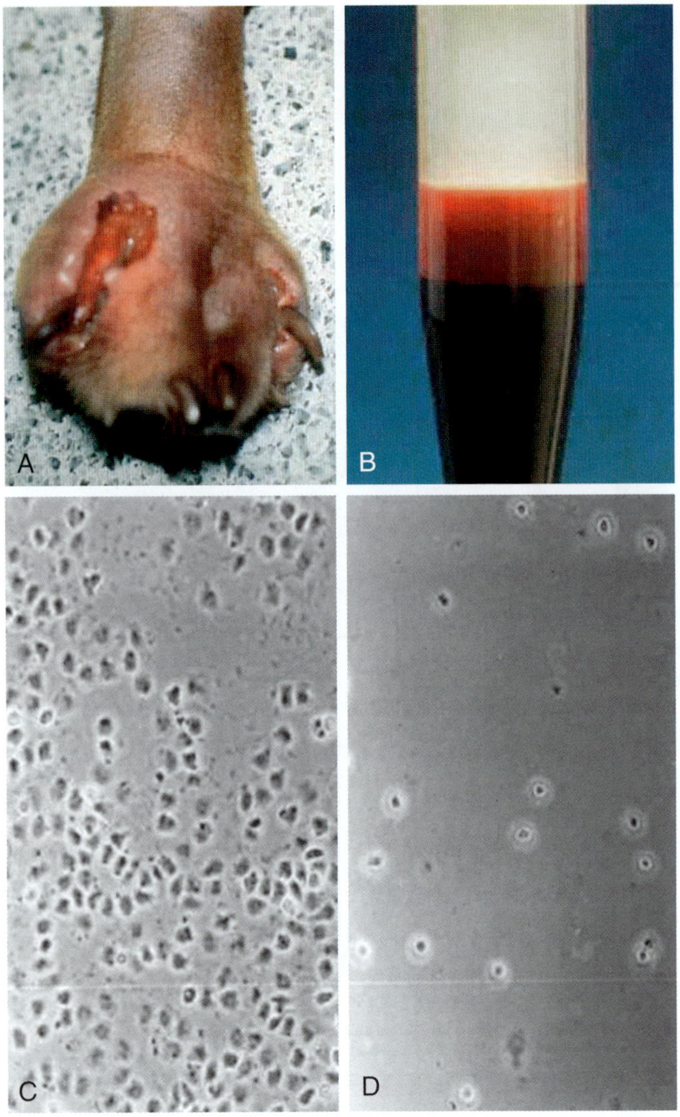

Fig. 130.2 Leukocyte adhesion deficiency in the Irish setter. (A) Lesion showing lack of pus formation. (B) Severe leukocytosis (180,000 cells/μL) as seen in visible buffy coat. Decreased neutrophil adhesion to plastic in control dog (C) and affected dog (D). (Courtesy of Teaching File, University of Pennsylvania, Philadelphia.)

X-chromosomal recessive mode of inheritance, male dogs are affected, whereas females (the dams and some littermates of those affected) are carriers. The Cardigan Welsh corgi and the basset hound have different mutations in the gene encoding the γ-chain that is common to the IL receptors in affected male basset hounds and Cardigan Welsh corgis, but both are restricted to a research colony.[63,72–74]

After the decline of maternal immunity, affected male dogs develop bacterial skin, GI, and respiratory infections (Fig. 130.3). Puppies fail to thrive and generally die within a few months. The most characteristic clinical features are a lack of lymph nodes, tonsils, Peyer's patches, and thymus. Affected basset hounds can develop vaccine-induced distemper. If they survive, affected puppies are poor doers and die by 5–6 months of age. They can survive in germ-free environments.[3] A diagnosis is reached by histopathology, immunologic testing, or molecular genetic testing (bassets and corgis); however, these mutations appear to have been eliminated from breeding populations other than those in research colonies. Bone marrow transplantation from unaffected littermates and gene therapy were experimentally effective in re-establishing normal T- and B-cell function in affected dogs.[21,67,75]

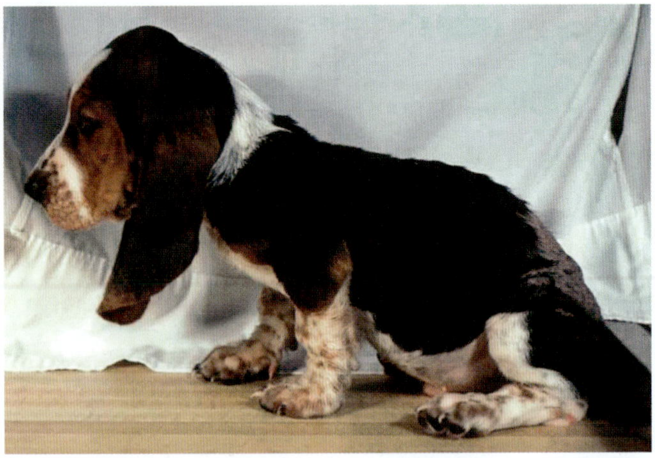

Fig. 130.3 Basset hound puppy showing pyoderma and demodicosis from X-linked severe combined immunodeficiency. (Courtesy of Teaching File, University of Pennsylvania, Philadelphia, PA.)

Autosomal Recessive Severe Combined Immunodeficiency

SCID has been identified in Jack Russell terriers that has an autosomal recessive mode of inheritance, similar to that in CB-17 mice and Arabian foals.[76] A faulty V(D)J recombination and complete deficiency of DNA-PKcs activity result from reduced expression of the DNA-PK catalytic subunit.[76,77] Affected dogs experience severe lymphopenia, agammaglobulinemia, thymic dysplasia, and peripheral lymphoid aplasia. They typically succumb to opportunistic and vaccine-induced infections by 2–4 months of age.[76]

Autosomal recessive SCID has also been identified in Frisian water dogs in South Africa and the Netherlands. A nonsense mutation alters the RAG1 protein which is important in antigen recognition by humoral and cellular mechanisms. Affected pups have severe lymphopenia and undetectable serum immunoglobulin concentrations, and die or are euthanized due to infections at 8 to 12 weeks of age.[77] Dogs develop diarrhea at 7–8 weeks of age that responds to antibacterial therapy. However, progressive neurologic signs including seizures, vestibular ataxia, and blindness ensue. Histiocytic myocarditis and hepatitis was identified in some dogs at necropsy.

Selective IgA Deficiency

Various forms of selective IgA deficiency have been described in several breeds, including beagles,[63,78] sharpeis,[79] German shepherds,[80] and others,[81] but the mode of inheritance remains unknown. The defect may be either an inherited primary defect or may arise secondary to pathologic changes within the intestinal mucosa. Serum IgA concentrations may be completely absent or markedly reduced and only very slowly developing over the first year of life. Complete deficiencies are found in sharpeis, and partial deficiencies have been found in beagles and German shepherds.[82] For diagnosis, serum IgA concentrations need to be compared with those of age-matched controls. Reduced concentrations of IgA have been found in duodenal explant cultures of some German shepherd dogs that had serum IgA values within reference limits.[83] Such assays may be more reliable than serum concentrations but are not as available for routine diagnostic purposes. Reduced secretory IgA concentrations have also been found in bronchial secretions of affected dogs.[81] IgA-deficient dogs can have positive rheumatoid factor, anti-IgA antibodies, or both, and can be predisposed to hypersensitivity and autoimmune diseases. IgA deficiency in German shepherds is not linked to their predisposition to disseminated aspergillosis, which may relate to a cell-mediated defect.[84] Although affected dogs have large polyclonal increases in serum IgG concentration, it is not directed against *Aspergillus terreus*.

Lethal Acrodermatitis in Bull Terriers

Also known as "zincers" among bull terrier breeders, the lesions of lethal acrodermatitis are similar to those of zinc deficiency in dogs, but do not respond to zinc supplementation. Affected dogs have lower plasma IgA concentrations than clinically healthy dogs.[85] The syndrome is characterized by hyperkeratosis and parakeratosis and thymus and lymph node hypoplasia, which is associated with increased susceptibility to infection, failure to thrive, and abnormal hepatic proteomic patterns.[85–87] Growth retardation, hard and cracked footpads, pyoderma around body orifices, and aggressive to unresponsive behavior are hallmark features and become apparent at a few weeks of age. Affected dogs die or are euthanized before 6 months of age. A *MKLN1* splicing defect has been recently identified and serves as screening test for this common trait in bull terriers.[88]

Susceptibility to *Mycobacterium avium* Complex Infections in Miniature Schnauzers and Basset Hounds

Increased susceptibility to *Mycobacterium avium* infection has been recognized in miniature schnauzers and basset hounds (see Chapter 61). A *CARD9* deletion has been identified in miniature schnauzers but not yet in bassets. Miniature schnauzers related to a sire born in 1986 developed progressive disseminated MAC infections at young adult age that were unresponsive to multidrug antimicrobial therapy, which led to death or euthanasia. All MAC-infected miniature schnauzers worldwide are homozygous for the mutant *CARD9* allele which results in a defective intracellular signaling pathway.[11] Occasionally, these miniature schnauzers may also develop candidiasis which is typically seen in humans with *CARD9* variants. Bassets do not seem to have a *CARD9* mutation.

Uncharacterized Breed-Associated Immunodeficiencies

Apparent breed predispositions to specific infectious diseases also have the potential to reflect underlying hereditary immunodeficiency. However, other factors also have the potential to result in breed-associated infections. For example, leishmaniosis has been identified in English and American foxhounds in the United States (see Chapter 96),[6,89] babesiosis occurs in lines of pit bulls and greyhounds (see Chapter 97), and boxers and Rhodesian ridgebacks appear to be more susceptible to neosporosis. In these cases, although a genetic susceptibility may play a role, transplacental transmission and use of these breeds for hunting or fighting practices (babesiosis) also contribute to the apparent breed predisposition.

Doberman Pinschers

Neutrophil dysfunction has been described in a family of Doberman pinschers; one young dog had chronic recurrent respiratory tract infections.[33] Oxygen radical formation and bactericidal activity of neutrophils were reduced despite normal phagocytosis of bacteria. The specific defect was not identified, and although ciliary morphology appeared normal, functional studies were not performed, so ciliary dyskinesia was not ruled out. Affected Doberman pinschers develop clinical signs of respiratory tract infections at a few weeks of age that respond to antibacterials, but prognosis is guarded.

German Shepherds

An apparent increase in susceptibility to ehrlichiosis, RMSF, pythiosis, aspergillosis, other invasive mycoses, and deep pyoderma has been described in German shepherds.[8,90,91] These predispositions likely involve different immune defects that have yet to be defined. Affected dogs with deep pyoderma have pruritus with lesions distributed primarily over the lumbosacral region.[92] *Staphylococcus pseudintermedius* is most commonly cultured from the lesions. Proposed mechanisms for this susceptibility include cell-mediated immunodeficiency associated with serum inhibitors or defective helper T cells, and hypersensitivity reactions to staphylococci.[90,91,93,94]

Miniature Dachshunds

Certain lines of miniature dachshunds are predisposed to *Pneumocystis* pneumonia by 1 year of age (see Chapter 89). Affected miniature dachshunds have hypogammaglobulinemia, with decreased serum IgA, IgG, and IgM concentrations; decreased lymphocyte transformation to phytohemagglutinin and pokeweed mitogens; and absence of B cells and presence of T cells in lymphoid tissues (stained by CD3 and CD79a cell markers).[95] The molecular defect remains unknown. This predisposition also occurs in cavalier King Charles spaniels that seem to have lower serum IgG concentrations[27]; however, additional genetic and immunologic studies in those dogs are not available.

Sharpeis

In addition to the severely abnormal skin structure, which leads to a barrier failure, two distinct syndromes have been characterized in the sharpei—one involving combined antibody and CMI defects and the other involving renal amyloidosis and swollen joints.

The combined immunodeficiency syndrome may have been confused with the selective IgA deficiency described in this breed. Juvenile to adult dogs develop recurrent infections involving respiratory, skin, and gastrointestinal asystems.[96] Chronic bronchitis, gastroduodenal or colonic ulceration, diarrhea and vomiting, adult-onset pyoderma, demodicosis, and bacterial and fungal otitis may occur. In addition, dogs are predisposed to GI neoplasia, lymphoma, and other malignancies. Single or multiple immunoglobulin class deficiencies are observed in dogs, with IgM deficiency and decreased IL-2 synthesis predominating. Dogs with GI signs or malignancy typically have had reduced serum IgM concentrations. Decreased lymphocyte stimulation test results were found in most of the dogs, suggesting a combined T- and B-cell defect.[96] In addition, peripheral blood mononuclear cells (PBMCs) had reduced expression of IL-6.

Recurrent fever of unknown origin and swelling of the tibiotarsal joints are the clinical signs of another immune-based syndrome in sharpeis, known as "sharpei fever" or "sharpei hock."[97–100] Sharpeis have been strongly selected for thick and heavily folded skin. Altered sequences within the hyaluronic acid synthase gene have been found in affected dogs.[101] Fragmentation of hyaluronan following its accumulation in the thickened skin is thought to trigger an inflammatory reaction. The lameness can be monoarticular or involve multiple joints, usually affecting the tibiotarsal joints and occasionally the carpus. Predominant mononuclear cell polyarteritis and cellulitis, with or without synovial inflammation, can develop. Clinical signs of renal failure—a result of amyloid deposition in the kidney—and nephrotic syndrome eventually develop. A majority of affected dogs have amyloid deposition in the renal medulla; 60% to 80% have glomerular amyloidosis or membranous glomerulitis.[100] Polydipsia, polyuria, weight loss, dehydration, ascites, and peripheral edema can occur. Thromboembolism can be a sudden complication in some dogs with the nephrotic syndrome. Radiographic changes are soft tissue swelling with periarticular bone erosion and bone production. Recurrent fever, joint pain, and swelling often resolve within 24 hours.[99] Postpartum metritis has developed in intact females and can be another inflammatory feature of this illness.[100] Hyperglobulinemia and increased serum IL-6 concentrations are found in affected dogs.[102] The syndrome resembles familial Mediterranean fever, a human hereditary disorder characterized by polyserositis and reactive amyloidosis. Treatment with colchicine early in the course of disease can reduce amyloid deposition in humans and has been proposed for affected dogs.

Rottweilers

In one report, a litter of rottweiler pups either died before 6 months of age from systemic inflammatory disease or subsequently developed chronic inflammatory skin disease.[103] Serum IgA and IgG concentrations were low. Secondary lymphoid tissues had reduced numbers of CD3+ T cells, although some were found within foci of B-cell follicles. Irregularities were found in plasma cell development, and plasma cells were absent from all mucosal and cutaneous sites. In inflammatory lesions, macrophages expressing major histocompatibility complex (MHC) class II molecules were present. Related unaffected dogs had reduced serum IgA concentrations; however, the spectrum of the defect in affected dogs suggests a more complex underlying defect. Rottweilers have also been considered more susceptible to parvovirus infection, oral papillomatosis, and nasal and systemic fungal infections; however, it is uncertain whether these abnormalities are interrelated.

Weimaraners

At least two distinct immunodeficiency syndromes have been observed in Weimaraners. One syndrome was reported only once, and was associated with growth hormone deficiency with dwarfism, wasting, and thymic hypoplasia.[104,105]

The second syndrome, which is similar to the common variable immunodeficiency syndromes described in humans, involves recurrent bacterial infections and inflammatory conditions in young Weimaraners, which often become systemic.[2,106–109] Some dogs outgrow their condition and do not show signs later in life. Clinical signs of those with recurrent disease start at a few months to young adult and are characterized by lethargy, anorexia, intermittent fever, lymphadenomegaly, pyogranulomatous disease, large abscesses in muscle, stomatitis, osteomyelitis, surface bleeding, and coat color dilution. Some dogs have diarrhea or vomiting. Hyperesthesia of long bones or joints (Fig. 130.4), a predisposition to local injection site reactions, and recurrent urinary infections or pyoderma have also been observed. Some dogs later develop polyarthritis or meningitis. Although dogs may respond favorably to select antibacterial therapy and/or immunosuppressive drug therapy, recurrence of systemic inflammatory disease can occur. While an immunologic deficiency is suspected, inconsistencies exist in the immunologic studies performed on these dogs. Neutrophilia, which is often marked with a left shift, has been observed. Decreased neutrophil phagocytosis of opsonized bacteria and chemiluminescence as well as slightly low serum IgG and IgM concentrations have been reported in some dogs with increased amounts of circulating immune complexes (CICs).[110] In other reports, reduced serum IgG, IgA, and IgM have been observed with no increase in CICs.[109] The lack of CICs in most reports suggests that primary decreased production rather than secondary immunoglobulin consumption is responsible for the defect. No specific diagnostic tests are available. Despite antibacterial and supportive therapy, prognosis is guarded. Some Weimaraners also appear to have an increased tendency to develop hypertrophic osteodystrophy (HOD), which has been associated with a postvaccination reaction. Whether this predisposition is only associated with this immunodeficiency syndrome is uncertain.[109] Dogs that develop HOD respond most favorably to anti-inflammatory doses of glucocorticoids, and the syndrome may be triggered by attenuated live distemper vaccination (see Chapter 20).[111]

SPECIFIC HEREDITARY OR PRIMARY IMMUNODEFICIENCIES IN CATS

Leukocyte Adhesion Deficiency

LAD (see dogs earlier for more details) was described in an adult domestic medium-haired cat with severe leukocytosis and milder signs of infection and inflammation. The disorder was associated with a β_2-integrin mutation, but not in any other cats.[51] If LAD is suspected in a cat, leukocyte flow cytometry for CD18 expression can be used for diagnosis; the gene mutation may be different and thus genetic testing is not useful.

Hypotrichosis Congenita with Thymic Aplasia

Hypotrichosis congenita with thymic aplasia is a defect that is characterized by the birth of nude athymic kittens with severe immunodeficiencies, kittens that are similar to nude research mice. This lethal syndrome has been recognized in Birmans and is autosomal recessively inherited. A deletion in *FOXN1* has been identified and can be used to screen the breed (Fig. 130.5).[112,113]

Other Defects

Abyssinians are predisposed to systemic reactive AA amyloidosis, but clinical signs are caused by renal dysfunction. A genetic basis is suspected. This syndrome is similar to amyloidosis in sharpeis and familial Mediterranean fever in humans. Splenic inflammatory diseases, often related to secondary infections from immunodeficiencies, are responsible for the amyloid deposition in reactive amyloidosis. However, in some affected cats, concurrent inflammatory disease is not detected.[114] Generalized amyloidosis has also been observed in Siamese and Oriental cats, but clinical features and amyloid protein composition differ (mostly hepatic involvement).[115,116]

A syndrome of unknown cause in ragdoll kittens is characterized by fatal infections in the neonatal to weaning period.[117] Vaccination with attenuated live feline panleukopenia vaccine may have accelerated their death. Some kittens died of panleukopenia at a younger age. By weaning, others developed numerous systemic fatal infections. Thymic, splenic, and lymphoid hypoplasia were observed in these affected kittens.

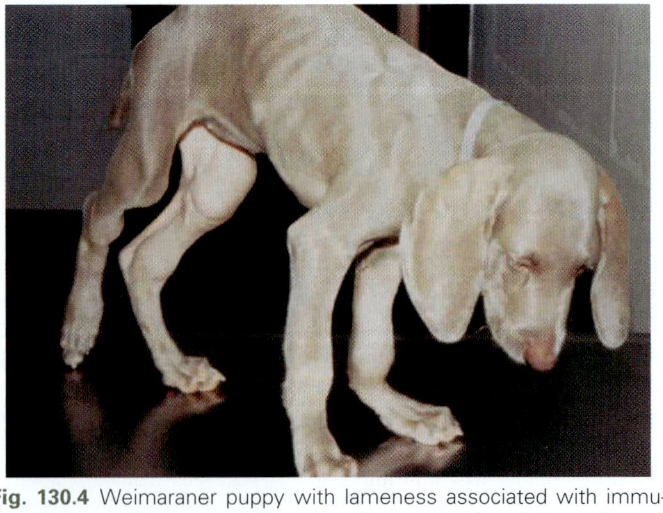

Fig. 130.4 Weimaraner puppy with lameness associated with immunodeficiency. (Courtesy of Teaching File, University of Pennsylvania, Philadelphia, PA.)

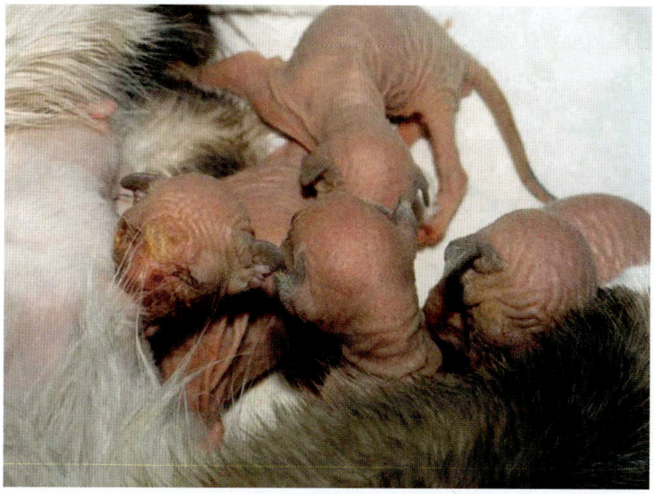

Fig. 130.5 Nude Birman kittens with congenital hypertrichosis with thymic atrophy. (Courtesy of Margret Casal, University of Pennsylvania, Philadelphia, PA.)

Neutrophil abnormalities have been observed in Birman cats with leukocyte granulation,[118] and domestic shorthaired cats with the Pelger-Huët anomaly (Fig. 130.6).[119] However, clinical immunodeficiencies with these defects have not been recognized. Historically, Persian cats with Chédiak-Higashi syndrome,[4,17] had more of a bleeding tendency and color dilution (smoked) than infections, and a large duplication was found in lysosomal trafficking regulator ((CHS1/LYST)). Loss of thymic mass has been observed in cats with GM1 gangliosidosis.[120,121]

ACQUIRED OR SECONDARY IMMUNODEFICIENCIES

Acquired or secondary immunodeficiencies encompass states of a transiently or permanently impaired immune system during or after an underlying disease condition or exposure to toxic agents. Secondary immunodeficiencies occur more commonly than primary immunodeficiencies, and, depending on the type and severity of the immunosuppression, opportunistic infections may result in localized or systemic disease.

Secondary immunodeficiencies can impact the innate or adaptive immune systems. Anatomic barrier disturbances, such as desquamation of skin or damage to the mucociliary escalator of respiratory epithelium, are types of acquired immunodeficiencies. These can also result from administration of immunosuppressive agents, exposure to toxins, nutritional deficiencies, and specific disease processes, including metabolic disorders, neoplasia, and some infectious diseases (Box 130.3). Certain infections, particularly retroviral diseases in cats, directly impair the immune system, predisposing the animals to secondary bacterial, fungal, or protozoal infections. For example, cats infected with FIV harbor more diverse fungal microflora on the hair and mucosal surfaces than non-infected cats.[122] FeLV-infected cats are also more likely to have clinical illness with hemotropic mycoplasma infections than noninfected cats.[123]

Puppies and kittens are particularly vulnerable to infections because of their incompletely developed immune systems. Transfer of maternally-derived antibody (MDA) from colostrum takes place in the first day of life and provides humoral protection during the initial weeks of life in small animals.[124,125] Failure of this transfer can lead to immunodeficiency and susceptibility to some infections. A transient hypoglobulinemia occurs after the decline of MDAs in the plasma and before immunocompetency, and this increases susceptibility to various infections.[126]

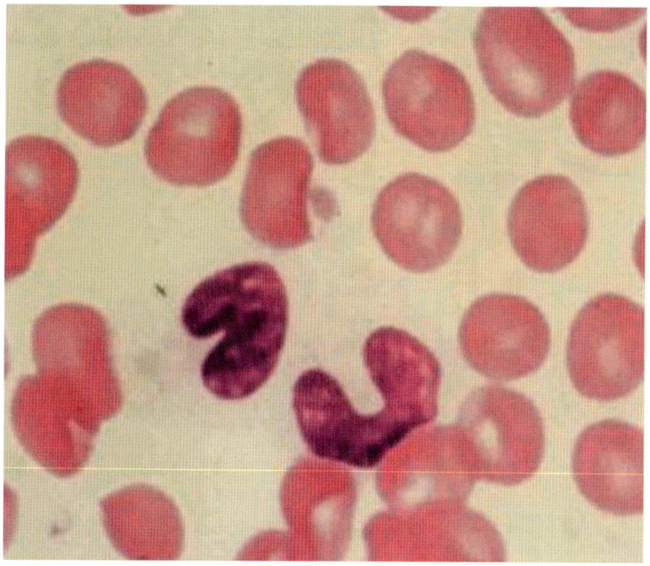

Fig. 130.6 Pelger-Huët anomaly in cat with hyposegmentation of nucleus. Despite morphologic changes, no clinical immunodeficiency was observed. (Wright stain, ×1000). (Courtesy of Teaching File, University of Pennsylvania, Philadelphia, PA.)

SPECIFIC SECONDARY OR ACQUIRED IMMUNODEFICIENCIES

Acquired or secondary immunodeficiencies can develop at any time as a result of an interference with host defense mechanisms.[127,128] Immune defects secondary to infectious diseases, metabolic disturbances, intoxications, nutritional deficiencies, and drug therapies[129,130] have been reported (Table 130.3 and see Box 130.3).

Infectious Diseases

Canine Distemper

CDV infection causes a chronic and profound inhibition and impairment of cellular and humoral immune functions characterized by lymphopenia and immunosuppression, rendering animals susceptible to opportunistic infection (see also Chapter 22). Immunosuppression is due to early virus-mediated lymphocytolysis in the spleen, lymph nodes, thymus, bone marrow, mucosa-associated lymphoid tissue (MALT), tonsils, and hepatic Kupffer cells.[128] CD4+ T cells are preferentially depleted during the acute phase, followed by CD8+ T-cell depletion.[131] In addition, CDV affects antigen presentation and lymphocyte maturation by a poorly understood mechanism.[132,133]

CDV infects cells of the immune system via viral H protein binding to CD150 (signaling lymphocyte activation molecule), a molecule expressed on B and T cells, monocytes, and mature dendritic cells.[134] The viral V protein is essential for rapid viral replication in T cells and antagonizes IFN-α, TNF-α, IL-6, IFN-γ, and IL-2 in the acute phase of infection.[134] Furthermore, viral infection leads to a diminished antigen presentation and altered dendritic cell and B-cell maturation within germinal centers. Subsequent plasma cell formation and immunoglobulin formation are reduced.[132] Thus, long-lasting immunologic abnormalities persist after viral clearance from the peripheral blood leukocytes.

Persistent suppression of CMI in neonatal puppies infected with CDV can be detected by decreased lymphocyte stimulation test results and decreased synthesis of T-cell–dependent antibodies (IgG and IgA). If thymic hypoplasia results from *in utero* infection, IgM levels may be reduced during the postnatal period. Transient depression of CMI has been reported in puppies that are infected with virulent CDV.

TABLE 130.3 Acquired Defects in Phagocyte Function

Disease	Mechanism	Site of Infection	Infecting Organisms	Predisposing Factors
Uremia	Decreased phagocytosis	Catheter sites, lungs, urinary tract, blood	Staphylococci, aerobic gram-negative organisms	Peripheral vascular disease
Diabetes mellitus	Increased adherence, variable chemotaxis, decreased phagocytosis and respiratory burst	Lungs, urinary tract, catheter sites, eyes, bone	Staphylococci, Enterbacterales, filamentous fungi	Hyperglycemia, total parenteral nutrition, skin ulcers, urinary catheterization
Hepatic cirrhosis	Increased adherence with decreased chemotaxis and phagocytosis	Urinary tract, lungs, blood, soft tissues	Staphylococci, Enterbacterales, other enteric organisms	Urinary catheterization
Systemic lupus erythematosus	Increased adherence, decreased chemotaxis, decreased phagocytosis	Lungs, blood	Gram-positive bacteria, mycobacteria, opportunistic organisms	Immunosuppressive therapy
Burns	Decreased chemotaxis and phagocytosis	Wounds, urinary tract, blood, lungs	Staphylococci, aerobic gram-negative organisms, yeasts	Extensive burns, age extremes
Traumatic injuries	Decreased chemotaxis and phagocytosis	Wounds, urinary tract, blood, lungs	Staphylococci, aerobic gram-negative organisms	Old age

Modified from Engellich G, Wright DG, Hartshorn KL. Acquired disorders of phagocyte function complicating medical and surgical illnesses. *Clin Infect Dis.* 2001;33:2040–2048.

BOX 130.3 Causes of Acquired or Secondary Immunodeficiencies

Age Related
- Impaired colostrum uptake
- Transient hypoglobulinemia associated with decline of maternal antibodies
- Weakened immune system in the very young and old

Organ Disorders
- Hyperadrenocorticism
- Hypothyroidism
- Diabetes mellitus
- Hepatic insufficiency
- Splenectomy
- Malnutrition
- Cancer, particularly hematopoietic neoplasia

Barrier Impairment
- Burns
- Invasive or indwelling catheters
- Endoscopic devices
- Splenectomy
- Aspiration of body cavities (i.e., cystocentesis)
- Pulmonary diseases
- Gastrointestinal diseases
- Skin diseases

Immunosuppressive Infections
- Feline leukemia virus infection
- Feline immunodeficiency virus infection
- Feline coronavirus infection
- Feline and canine parvovirus infection
- Canine distemper
- Canine retrovirus infection
- Demodicosis
- Ehrlichiosis
- Anaplasmosis
- Protracted bacterial infections
- Leishmaniosis
- Bartonellosis

BOX 130.3 Causes of Acquired or Secondary Immunodeficiencies—Cont'd

Physical, Chemical, or Drug-Induced
- Whole-body irradiation
- Myelosuppressive drugs
- Cytotoxic agents
- Griseofulvin
- Estrogens (dogs and ferrets)
- Immunosuppressive therapy (i.e., glucocorticoids, cyclosporine)
- Antibacterial- or antacid-induced alteration of intestinal microflora

Nutritional Disorders
- Vitamin A deficiency
- Vitamin E deficiency
- Vitamin D deficiency
- Protein-caloric restriction
- Zinc deficiency

Affected dogs can develop secondary bacterial bronchopneumonia, including *Bordetella bronchiseptica*. Other opportunistic infections reported in dogs with CDV include toxoplasmosis, salmonellosis, nocardiosis, and generalized demodicosis.[128]

Canine Parvovirus Infection and Feline Panleukopenia Virus Infection

CPV and FPV have an affinity for replicating in rapidly dividing cells, including crypt cells of the GI tract and lymphoid tissue, resulting in severe lymphopenia and immunosuppression (see Chapters 29 and 30). This combination of anatomic barrier destruction of the GI tract and leukopenia in immunologically naïve hosts leads to an increased risk of secondary bacterial infections.

In addition to virus-induced destruction of WBC precursors in the bone marrow, massive sequestration of neutrophils within the inflamed GI tract occurs resulting in both a lymphopenia and granulocytopenia. Mild depression of lymphocyte function has also been observed as a result of parvoviral infection.[135] Parvovirus-infected dogs and cats are at increased risk for bacterial translocation from the GI tract and bacteremia, leading to overwhelming sepsis.

In utero infection can lead to permanent suppression of CMI and thymic atrophy. Dogs that recover from CPV infections have had a higher prevalence of UTIs than age-matched control pups. Disseminated candidiasis has been reported in animals with parvovirus.[136] Infection with CPV has also been associated with development of postvaccinal canine distemper encephalitis.[137] There is little known about immunodeficiency that develops in cats with FPV infection, other than that associated with panleukopenia.

Canine and Feline Coronavirus Infection

Opportunistic infections are rarely reported with either enteric FCoV or FIPV infection. However, FIPV is associated with a profound, virus-induced panlymphopenia and hypergammaglobulinemia (see Chapter 31). The virus does not infect lymphocytes, so the mechanism of lymphocyte depletion is unclear, although it may be related directly to TNF-α–induced apoptosis or indirectly to the infection of antigen-presenting cells, specifically dendritic cells.[138,139]

A highly virulent strain of CCoV has been reported to cause severe systemic illness and induce a lymphopenia.[140] Depletion of the CD4+ T-cell population was observed 1 month PI in an experimental model.[141]

Feline Leukemia Virus Infection

FeLV is associated with antiproliferative (myelosuppressive) and proliferative (neoplastic) diseases of the lymphohematopoietic system, and both forms are associated with immunodeficiencies primarily due to reduced CMI competence (see Chapter 32). A reduction in CD4+/CD8+ T-cell subset ratios has been shown to develop in FeLV-infected cats.[142] FeLV-infected cats have impaired T-cell–mediated immunity as characterized by reduced *in vitro* lymphocyte stimulation, prolonged retention of cutaneous allografts, and impaired response to delayed hypersensitivity skin testing.[143–145] Lymphopenia and thymic atrophy can be observed in infected cats.[128] Secondary hyperglobulinemia and complement depletion have also been recognized.[146,147] Persistent neutropenia and decreased neutrophil microbicidal activity can also be observed as the disease progresses.[148] A panleukopenia-like syndrome can develop in cats that are co-infected with FeLV and FIV.[149]

The transmembrane viral envelope peptide p15E can mediate some of the immunosuppression.[150] This viral protein inhibits B- and T-cell function, alters monocyte morphology and distribution, and has been associated with impaired cytokine production and responsiveness.[143–145] FeLV-infected cats have increased susceptibility to concurrent infection with other organisms and severity of disease caused by those organisms, such as commensal bacteria, pathogenic fungi, hemotropic *Mycoplasma* spp., and FIP.

Feline Immunodeficiency Virus Infection

Cats naturally infected with FIV may develop fever, variable neutropenia, and chronic infections of the skin and mucosal surfaces (see Chapter 33). Experimentally inoculated cats develop generalized peripheral lymphadenopathy and transient neutropenia followed by a disease-free period that may last years. FIV infection of the bone marrow can cause blood leukopenias and myelodysplasia even in cats without clinical signs.[151] Studies of FIV infection have identified several mechanisms of innate and adaptive immune dysfunction. Defective natural killer cell proliferation and cytotoxic function occurs in chronically FIV-infected cats, and this may be due to low levels of key cytokines such as IL-2 and IL-15.[152,153] Neutropenia due to apoptosis,[154] dendritic cell dysfunction, and dysregulation of multiple cytokines have been described (e.g., decreased TNFα, IL-1, IL-2, IL-6, and IL-12 and increased IL-10 and TGF-β).[155–157] Depletion of CD4+ T cells is characteristic of the adaptive immune defect and occurs by several mechanisms including apoptosis, anergy, and thymic atrophy. Further adaptive immune dysregulation occurs due to inappropriate activation of regulatory CD4+/CD25+ T cells which in turn downregulate CD4+ and CD8+ T cells.[158–160] Alterations in the phenotype of CD8+ and other lymphocytes eventually lead to immunodeficiency.[161]

Opportunistic infections eventually occur as immunodeficiency progresses, and can include bacterial infections of the oral cavity, chronic skin infections, FCV infection, toxoplasmosis, hemotropic mycoplasma infection, and systemic fungal infections.[162–167] Affected cats tend to have increased severity of disease caused by these pathogens. Compared with noninfected cats, *Cryptococcus* spp. and *Candida albicans* are isolated more frequently from the oropharyngeal mucosa of FIV-infected cats, and *Microsporum canis* are isolated more frequently from the skin.[168]

Canine Monocytic Ehrlichiosis

Infection with *Ehrlichia canis* can be divided into acute and chronic stages (see Chapter 44). No secondary immunosuppression has been associated with acute canine ehrlichiosis.[169] Dogs with chronic ehrlichiosis can develop a marked lymphocytosis and hyperglobulinemia with antibody titers to *E. canis* occasionally exceeding 1:1,000,000. Some dogs develop pancytopenia due to bone marrow failure, and secondary bacterial infections can be attributed to neutropenia in those cases. Alternatively, some dogs can develop opportunistic infections in the absence of neutropenia; the mechanism underlying this has not been fully elucidated. These opportunistic infections, all of which rely on a robust CMI, include leishmaniosis, viral papillomatosis, generalized demodicosis, neosporosis, and opportunistic fungal infections, implying alterations in the CMI occur during chronic ehrlichiosis.[128,170,171] *In vitro* studies demonstrate downregulation of MHC class II molecules in cells infected with *E. canis*.[171] German shepherd dogs are overrepresented in cases of ehrlichiosis[172] and appear to experience a greater degree of suppression of CMI during infection than other breeds.[173] Evaluation of blood lymphocytes from dogs naturally infected with *E. canis* demonstrate higher numbers of cytotoxic T cells and lower numbers of B cells compared with healthy control dogs; however, their potential immunosuppressive effects remain unknown.[174] In fact, one study failed to demonstrate the suppression of CMI or humoral immunity in experimentally infected dogs up to 4 months PI.[169]

Canine Leishmaniosis

Dogs with leishmaniosis are prone to secondary infections and occasionally neoplasia, especially hematopoietic tumors.[175] The *Leishmania* surface protein gp63 mediates entry into macrophages and promotes survival of the parasite through inhibition of the respiratory burst and apoptosis. *Leishmania* can also decrease macrophage function and antigen presentation by inhibition of MHC class I and II molecule expression, inhibition of chemotaxis, and interference with IL-12 transcription.[176] *Leishmania* organisms promote tolerance upon infection of *in vitro* cultivated hepatic macrophages, which is reversed with leishmanicidal drug application.[177] Generalized demodicosis has been described in dogs with leishmaniosis and was associated with an absence of CD3+ cells in dermal lesions suggesting a CMI deficiency.[178]

Fungal Infections

Fungal pathogens including *Aspergillus*, *Candida*, and *Cryptococcus* spp. are capable of causing immunosuppression.[179–181] *Cryptococcus* possesses several virulent factors that suppress or orchestrate the immune response to favor fungal growth and persistence. The capsular polysaccharide inhibits phagocytosis and can interfere with leukocyte transmigration by causing these cells to shed selectin.[182] Cryptococcal urease shifts the CMI to a nonprotective Th2 immune response and promotes immature dendritic cell accumulation within the lung tissue by upregulating IL-10 production and regulatory T-cell accumulation.[183–185]

Hemophagocytic Syndrome

Pathologic proliferation of the mononuclear phagocyte system can either result from infectious diseases or contribute to immunologic dysfunction and signs of debilitation, weight loss with anorexia, splenohepatomegaly, and relapsing fever in dogs or cats.[186–188] In dogs with hemophagocytic syndrome, parvovirus infection or lymphoid or myelomonocytic leukemia and lymphoma have been described; however, the association is not understood.[189] Dogs with infection-associated hemophagocytic syndrome appeared to have better 1-month survival rates than dogs with immune-associated and idiopathic hemophagocytic syndrome.[190]

Metabolic Disturbances

Many biochemical processes that occur in noninfectious disease states interfere with normal immune mechanisms. Failure of neonates to ingest colostrum, and dysproteinemias such as multiple myeloma, are both associated with impaired humoral immune system function. Decreased complement concentration has been noted with endotoxemia and malnutrition.

Newborn puppies and kittens experience a hypothermic state during the first week of life that suppresses T-cell function. A decline in CMI in older animals may increase their susceptibility to infectious and neoplastic disorders.[191] This decline in CMI is characterized by decrease in B-cell percentages and depressed lymphocyte stimulation by various mitogens *in vitro*, with male dogs more profoundly affected than females.[192]

Protein and caloric restriction has resulted in premature thymic atrophy and decreased cell-mediated, humoral, and phagocytic responses in animals. In contrast, overfed, obese dogs have impaired T-cell function and upregulated inflammatory cytokine expression.[193,194] Ingestion of organohalogenated compounds in contaminated environments caused a reduction of serum antibody titer responses of puppies to various inoculated antigens.[195]

Vitamin E and selenium deficiencies in dogs have been associated with decreased *in vitro* lymphocyte responsiveness, decreased serologic response to vaccination, and increased susceptibility to infection with opportunistic pathogens.[196,197] The deficit can be accentuated by excessive intake of polyunsaturated fats (strong oxidants that counteract the effects of vitamin E). Vitamin E deficiency causes the animal to produce a suppressor serum factor capable of decreasing lymphocyte responsiveness to antigenic stimulation. Vitamin A deficiency can cause immunosuppression and opportunistic infections similar to those associated with vitamin E deficiency.[198] Vitamin D is important in the regulation of the innate and adaptive immune systems, and deficiency has been noted with some infections including atypical mycobacterial infection in cats.[199] Zinc deficiency during prenatal and neonatal periods can result in impaired CMI responses and thymic atrophy.

Poorly regulated or untreated diabetes mellitus in dogs is associated with weaker neutrophil adherence than in controlled diabetic and nondiabetic dogs.[200] Diabetic dogs have an increased prevalence of UTIs[201–203] and hepatic abscesses.[204] Intestinal lymphangiectasia is associated with depressed CMI because of lymphopenia.[205] Endogenous or exogenous hyperadrenocorticism is associated with a high prevalence of bacteriuria, and mechanisms have been proposed including decreased neutrophilic chemotaxis or enhanced bacterial growth in urine due to glucosuria or decreased urine osmolality.[206] Splenectomized dogs and cats are prone to clinical babesiosis, hemotropic mycoplasma infections, and bacteremia.[207]

Neutropenia

Severe neutropenia increases the risk of bacterial infection, and several infectious agents can result in neutropenia. Broadly, neutropenia can result from decreased production or increased demand with several specific causes (Box 130.4), and can range from mild to severe.[208–210]

BOX 130.4 Acquired Causes of Neutropenia

Pathologic Demand (i.e., sepsis, peritonitis, pyometra, pneumonia)

Drug-Associated
- Albendazole
- Cephalosporin
- Chemotherapy (i.e. cisplatin, carboplatin, chlorambucil, cyclophosphamide, mitoxantrone, vincristine)
- Chloramphenicol
- Diethylstilbestrol
- Methimazole
- Phenobarbital
- Phenylbutazone
- Trimethoprim/sulfamethoxazole

Bone Marrow Failure
- Aplastic marrow
- Bone marrow necrosis
- Myelophthisis
- Myelodysplasia

Infectious Agents

Dogs: Ehrlichiosis

Cats: FeLV infection, FIV infection

Dogs and cats: Parvoviral infections, histoplasmosis

Immune-Mediated
- Immune-mediated neutropenia

Primary immune-mediated neutropenia, associated with circulating antineutrophil antibodies, has also been observed in dogs and cats.[210–212] Despite the circulating neutropenia, animals have adequate or high numbers of proliferating neutrophil precursors in the bone marrow. Circulating neutrophils are typically nondegenerate and lack toxic change (which might be seen with other causes of neutropenia, such as sepsis), unless secondary bacterial infection has occurred. Rapid increases in neutrophil numbers, usually within a few days, are observed after glucocorticoids are administered. Secondary bacterial infections appear to be uncommon in animals with primary immune-mediated neutropenia when compared with neutropenias associated with other causes, such as myelosuppressive drugs.

Immunosuppressive and Myelosuppressive Therapy

Immunosuppression can be induced during treatment for immune-mediated diseases, neoplasia, or organ transplantation. Use of glucocorticoids, cyclosporine, mycophenolate, or leflunomide has been associated with an increased risk of opportunistic infections. Glucocorticoid administration increases the risk of UTI in dogs treated chronically (more than 6 months).[213,214] In one case series of 169 feline renal transplant patients being treated with cyclosporine, infection was the second most common cause of death after acute rejection of the transplant.[215] Bacterial infections were the most common, followed by viral, fungal, and then protozoal infections. Disseminated toxoplasmosis and opportunistic cutaneous fungal infections have also been reported in animals administered cyclosporine.[216–218] Recovery of T-cell function occurred within 4 days of discontinuation of cyclosporine in healthy research dogs treated for 1 week at 10 mg/kg q12h.[219]

SUGGESTED READINGS

Ghielmetti G, Giger U. *Mycobacterium avium*: an emerging pathogen for dog breeds with hereditary immunodeficiencies. *Curr Clin Microbiol Rep.* 2020;7:67–80.

Hoffman D, Amorim J, DeClue A. Immune function in critically ill dogs. *J Vet Intern Med.* 2018;32:208–216.

McAtee BB, Cummings KJ, Cook AK, et al. Opportunistic invasive cutaneous fungal infections associated with administration of cyclosporine to dogs with immune-mediated disease. *J Vet Intern Med.* 2017;31:1724–1729.

REFERENCES

1. Greene CE. Immunodeficiency and infectious disease. In: Greene CE, ed. *Infectious Diseases of the Dog and Cat.* 1 ed. Philadelphia, PA: WB Saunders; 1990:55–63.
2. Couto CG, Giger U. Congenital and acquired neutrophil function abnormalities in the dog. In: Kirk RW, ed. *Current Veterinary Therapy X.* Philadelphia, PA: WB Saunders; 1989:521–525.
3. Felsburg PJ, Somberg RL, Krakowka GS. Acute monocytic leukemia in a dog with X-linked severe combined immunodeficiency. *Clin Diagn Lab Immunol.* 1994;1:379–384.
4. Meyers KM. Chediak-Higashi syndrome. In: Feldman BF, Zinkl JG, Jain NC, eds. *Schalm's Veterinary Hematology.* 5 ed. Philadelphia, PA: Lippincott Williams & Williams; 2000:971–975.
5. Bowles CA, Alsaker RD, Wolfle TL. Studies of the Pelger-Huet anomaly in foxhounds. *Am J Pathol.* 1979;96:237–248.
6. Owens SD, Oakley DA, Marryott K, et al. Transmission of visceral leishmaniasis through blood transfusions from infected English foxhounds to anemic dogs. *J Am Vet Med Assoc.* 2001;219:1076–1083.
7. Latimer KS, Prasse KW. Neutrophilic movement of a basenji with Pelger-Huet anomaly. *Am J Vet Res.* 1982;43:525–527.
8. Krockenberger MB, Swinney G, Martin P, et al. Sequential opportunistic infections in two German Shepherd dogs. *Aust Vet J.* 2011;89:9–14.
9. Schultz RM, Johnson EG, Wisner ER, et al. Clinicopathologic and diagnostic imaging characteristics of systemic aspergillosis in 30 dogs. *J Vet Intern Med.* 2008;22:851–859.
10. Dambach DM, Smith CA, Lewis RM, et al. Morphologic, immunohistochemical, and ultrastructural characterization of a distinctive renal lesion in dogs putatively associated with *Borrelia burgdorferi* infection: 49 cases (1987-1992). *Vet Pathol.* 1997;34:85–96.
11. Ghielmetti G, Giger U. *Mycobacterium avium*: an emerging pathogen for dog breeds with hereditary immunodeficiencies. *Curr Clin Microbiol Rep.* 2020;7:67–80.
12. Malik R, Love DN, Wigney DI, et al. Mycobacterial nodular granulomas affecting the subcutis and skin of dogs (canine leproid granuloma syndrome). *Aust Vet J.* 1998;76:403–407. 398.
13. Foley JE, Borjesson D, Gross TL, et al. Clinical, microscopic, and molecular aspects of canine leproid granuloma in the United States. *Vet Pathol.* 2002;39:234–239.
14. O'Brien CR, Krockenberger MB, Wigney DI, et al. Retrospective study of feline and canine cryptococcosis in Australia from 1981 to 2001: 195 cases. *Med Mycol.* 2004;42:449–460.
15. Trivedi SR, Sykes JE, Cannon MS, et al. Clinical features and epidemiology of cryptococcosis in cats and dogs in California: 93 cases (1988-2010). *J Am Vet Med Assoc.* 2011;239:357–369.
16. Craven M, Mansfield CS, Simpson KW. Granulomatous colitis of boxer dogs. *Vet Clin North Am Small Anim Pract.* 2011;41:433–445.
17. Kramer JW, Davis WC, Prieur DJ. The Chediak-Higashi syndrome of cats. *Lab Invest.* 1977;36:554–562.
18. Hirsch VM, Cunningham TA. Hereditary anomaly of neutrophil granulation in Birman cats. *Am J Vet Res.* 1984;45:2170–2174.
19. Otto CM, Brown CA, Lindl PA, et al. Delayed hypersensitivity testing as a clinical measure of cell-mediated immunity in the cat. *Vet Immunol Immunopathol.* 1993;38:91–102.
20. Fyfe JC, Hemker SL, Frampton A, et al. Inherited selective cobalamin malabsorption in Komondor dogs associated with a CUBN splice site variant. *BMC Vet Res.* 2018;14:418.
21. Hartnett BJ, Yao D, Suter SE, et al. Transplantation of X-linked severe combined immunodeficient dogs with CD34+ bone marrow cells. *Biol Blood Marrow Transplant.* 2002;8:188–197.
22. Creevy KE, Bauer Jr TR, Tuschong LM, et al. Mixed chimeric hematopoietic stem cell transplant reverses the disease phenotype in canine leukocyte adhesion deficiency. *Vet Immunol Immunopathol.* 2003;95:113–121.
23. Dale DC, Graw RG. Transplantation of allogeneic bone marrow in canine cyclic neutropenia. *Science.* 1974;183:83–84.
24. Edwards DF, Patton CS, Kennedy JR. Primary ciliary dyskinesia in the dog. *Probl Vet Med.* 1992;4:291–319.
25. Neil JA, Canapp SO Jr, Cook CR, et al. Kartagener's syndrome in a Dachshund dog. *J Am Anim Hosp Assoc.* 2002;38:45–49.
26. Reichler IM, Hoerauf A, Guscetti F, et al. Primary ciliary dyskinesia with situs inversus totalis, hydrocephalus internus and cardiac malformations in a dog. *J Small Anim Pract.* 2001;42:345–348.
27. Watson PJ, Herrtage ME, Peacock MA, et al. Primary ciliary dyskinesia in Newfoundland dogs. *Vet Rec.* 1999;144:718–725.
28. Foodman MS, Giger U, Stebbins K, et al. Karagener's syndrome in an old miniature poodle. *J Small Anim Pract.* 1989;30:96–100.
29. Daniel GB, Edwards DF, Harvey RC, et al. Communicating hydrocephalus in dogs with congenital ciliary dysfunction. *Dev Neurosci.* 1995;17:230–235.
30. Clercx C, Peeters D, Beths T, et al. Use of ciliogenesis in the diagnosis of primary ciliary dyskinesia in a dog. *J Am Vet Med Assoc.* 2000;217:1681–1685. 1659.
31. Anderegg L, Im Hof Gut M, Hetzel U, et al. NME5 frameshift variant in Alaskan Malamutes with primary ciliary dyskinesia. *PLoS Genet.* 2019;15:e1008378.
32. Merveille AC, Davis EE, Becker-Heck A, et al. CCDC39 is required for assembly of inner dynein arms and the dynein regulatory complex and for normal ciliary motility in humans and dogs. *Nat Genet.* 2011;43:72–78.
33. Clercx C, Reichler I, Peeters D, et al. Rhinitis/bronchopneumonia syndrome in Irish wolfhounds. *J Vet Intern Med.* 2003;17:843–849.
34. Leisewitz AL, Spencer JA, Jacobson LS, et al. Suspected primary immunodeficiency syndrome in three related Irish wolfhounds. *J Small Anim Pract.* 1997;38:209–212.
35. Niemeyer GP, Lothop CD. Cyclic hematopoiesis. In: Feldman BF, Zinkl JG, Jain NC, eds. *Cyclic Hematopoiesis.* 5 ed. Philadelphia, PA: Lippincott Williams & Williams; 2000:960–964.
36. Jones JB, Lange RD. Cyclic Hematopoiesis: animal models. *Exp Hematol.* 1983;11:571–580.
37. Benson KF, Li FQ, Person RE, et al. Mutations associated with neutropenia in dogs and humans disrupt intracellular transport of neutrophil elastase. *Nat Genet.* 2003;35:90–96.
38. Katen LJ, Aprikyan AG, Dale DC, et al. Cloning and sequencing of the canine neutrophil elastase cDNA. *DNA Seq.* 2002;13:221–223.
39. Renshaw HW, Davis WC. Canine granulocytopathy syndrome: an inherited disorder of leukocyte function. *Am J Pathol.* 1979;95:731–744.
40. Debenham SL, Millington A, Kijast J, et al. Canine leucocyte adhesion deficiency in Irish red and white setters. *J Small Anim Pract.* 2002;43:74–75.
41. Giger U, Boxer LA, Simpson PJ, et al. Deficiency of leukocyte surface glycoproteins Mo1, LFA-1, and Leu M5 in a dog with recurrent bacterial infections: an animal model. *Blood.* 1987;69:1622–1630.
42. Trowald-Wigh G, Hakansson L, Johannisson A, et al. Leucocyte adhesion protein deficiency in Irish setter dogs. *Vet Immunol Immunopathol.* 1992;32:261–280.
43. Trowald-Wigh G, Johannisson A, Hakansson L. Canine neutrophil adhesion proteins and Fc-receptors in healthy dogs and dogs with adhesion protein deficiency, as studied by flow cytometry. *Vet Immunol Immunopathol.* 1993;38:297–310.
44. Foureman P, Whiteley M, Giger U. Canine leukocyte adhesion deficiency: presence of the Cys36Ser beta-2 integrin mutation in an affected US Irish Setter cross-breed dog and in US Irish Red and White Setters. *J Vet Intern Med.* 2002;16:518–523.
45. Jobling AI, Ryan J, Augusteyn RC. The frequency of the canine leukocyte adhesion deficiency (CLAD) allele within the Irish Setter population of Australia. *Aust Vet J.* 2003;81:763–765.

46. Kehrli ME, Ackermann MR, Gilbert RO. Leukocyte adhesion deficiency. In: Feldman BF, Zinkl JG, Jain NC, eds. *Schalm's Veterinary Hematology*. 5 ed. Philadelphia, PA: Lippincott Williams & Williams; 2000:995–1001.
47. Kijas JM, Juneja RK, Gafvert S, et al. Detection of the causal mutation for canine leukocyte adhesion deficiency (CLAD) using pyrosequencing. *Anim Genet.* 2000;31:326–328.
48. Kijas JM, Bauer Jr TR, Gafvert S, et al. A missense mutation in the beta-2 integrin gene (ITGB2) causes canine leukocyte adhesion deficiency. *Genomics.* 1999;61:101–107.
49. Creevy KE, Bauer Jr TR, Tuschong LM, et al. Canine leukocyte adhesion deficiency colony for investigation of novel hematopoietic therapies. *Vet Immunol Immunopathol.* 2003;94:11–22.
50. Trowald-Wigh G, Ekman S, Hansson K, et al. Clinical, radiological and pathological features of 12 Irish setters with canine leucocyte adhesion deficiency. *J Small Anim Pract.* 2000;41:211–217.
51. Bauer TR Jr, Pratt SM, Palena CM, et al. Feline leukocyte adhesion (CD18) deficiency caused by a deletion in the integrin beta2 (ITGB2) gene. *Vet Clin Pathol.* 2017;46:391–400.
52. Verfaillie T, Verdonck F, Cox E. Simple PCR-based test for the detection of canine leucocyte adhesion deficiency. *Vet Rec.* 2004;154:821–823.
53. Creevy KE, Bauer TR Jr, Tuschong LM, et al. Mixed chimeric hematopoietic stem cell transplant reverses the disease phenotype in canine leukocyte adhesion deficiency. *Vet Immunol Immunopathol.* 2003;95:113–121.
54. Blum JR, Cork LC, Morris JM, et al. The clinical manifestations of a genetically determined deficiency of the third component of complement in the dog. *Clin Immunol Immunopathol.* 1985;34:304–315.
55. Winkelstein JA, Cork LC, Griffin DE, et al. Genetically determined deficiency of the third component of complement in the dog. *Science.* 1981;212:1169–1170.
56. Winkelstein JA, Johnson JP, Swift AJ, et al. Genetically determined deficiency of the third component of complement in the dog: in vitro studies on the complement system and complement-mediated serum activities. *J Immunol.* 1982;129:2598–2602.
57. Fyfe JC, Giger U, Hall CA, et al. Inherited selective intestinal cobalamin malabsorption and cobalamin deficiency in dogs. *Pediatr Res.* 1991;29:24–31.
58. Fyfe JC. Hematology of selective intestinal cobalamin malabsorption. In: Feldman BF, Zinkl JG, Jain NC, eds. *Schalm's Veterinary Hematology*. 5 ed. Philadelphia, PA: Lippincott Williams & Williams; 2000:965–970.
59. Fyfe JC, Jezyk PF, Giger U, et al. Inherited selective malabsorption of vitamin B12 in giant Schnauzers. *J Am Anim Hosp Assoc.* 1989;25:533–539.
60. Allan FJ, Thompson KG, Jones BR, et al. Neutropenia with a probable hereditary basis in Border Collies. *N Z Vet J.* 1996;44:67–72.
61. Mason SL, Jepson R, Maltman M, et al. Presentation and management of trapped neutrophil syndrome (TNS) in UK Border collies. *J Small Anim Pract.* 2014;55:57–60.
62. Mizukami K, Yabuki A, Kawamichi T, et al. Real-time PCR genotyping assay for canine trapped neutrophil syndrome and high frequency of the mutant allele in Border collies. *Vet J.* 2013;195:260–261.
63. Felsburg PJ. Overview of the immune system and immunodeficiency diseases. *Vet Clin North Am Small Anim Pract.* 1994;24:629–653.
64. Felsburg PJ, Hartnett BJ, Henthorn PS, et al. Canine X-linked severe combined immunodeficiency. *Vet Immunol Immunopathol.* 1999;69:127–135.
65. Felsburg PJ, Somberg RL, Perryman LE. Domestic animal models of severe combined immunodeficiency: canine X-linked severe combined immunodeficiency and severe combined immunodeficiency in horses. *Immunodefic Rev.* 1992;3:277–303.
66. Felsburg PJ, Hartnett BJ, Gouthro TA, et al. Thymopoiesis and T cell development in common gamma chain-deficient dogs. *Immunol Res.* 2003;27:235–246.
67. Hartnett BJ, Henthorn PS, Moore PF, et al. Bone marrow transplantation for canine X-linked severe combined immunodeficiency. *Vet Immunol Immunopathol.* 1999;69:137–144.
68. Ozaki K, Spolski R, Feng CG, et al. A critical role for IL-21 in regulating immunoglobulin production. *Science.* 2002;298:1630–1634.
69. Somberg RL, Robinson JP, Felsburg PJ. T lymphocyte development and function in dogs with X-linked severe combined immunodeficiency. *J Immunol.* 1994;153:4006–4015.
70. Somberg RL, Tipold A, Hartnett BJ, et al. Postnatal development of T cells in dogs with X-linked severe combined immunodeficiency. *J Immunol.* 1996;156:1431–1435.
71. Jezyk PF, Felsburg PJ, Haskins ME, et al. X-linked severe combined immunodeficiency in the dog. *Clin Immunol Immunopathol.* 1989;52:173–189.
72. Henthorn PS, Felsburg PJ. X-linked severe combined immunodeficiency. In: Feldman BF, Zinkl JG, Jain NC, eds. *Schalm's Veterinary Hematology*. 5 ed. Philadelphia, PA: Lippincott Williams & Williams; 2000:984–987.
73. Pullen RP, Somberg RL, Felsburg PJ, et al. X-linked severe combined immunodeficiency in a family of Cardigan Welsh corgis. *J Am Anim Hosp Assoc.* 1997;33:494–499.
74. Somberg RL, Pullen RP, Casal ML, et al. A single nucleotide insertion in the canine interleukin-2 receptor gamma chain results in X-linked severe combined immunodeficiency disease. *Vet Immunol Immunopathol.* 1995;47:203–213.
75. Felsburg PJ, Somberg RL, Hartnett BJ, et al. Full immunologic reconstitution following nonconditioned bone marrow transplantation for canine X-linked severe combined immunodeficiency. *Blood.* 1997;90:3214–3221.
76. Meek K, Kienker L, Dallas C, et al. SCID in Jack Russell terriers: a new animal model of DNA-PKcs deficiency. *J Immunol.* 2001;167:2142–2150.
77. Bell TG, Butler KL, Sill HB, et al. Autosomal recessive severe combined immunodeficiency of Jack Russell terriers. *J Vet Diagn Invest.* 2002;14:194–204.
78. Glickman LT, Shofer FS, Payton AJ, et al. Survey of serum IgA, IgG, and IgM concentrations in a large beagle population in which IgA deficiency had been identified. *Am J Vet Res.* 1988;49:1240–1245.
79. Moroff SD, Hurvitz AI, Peterson ME, et al. IgA deficiency in shar-pei dogs. *Vet Immunol Immunopathol.* 1986;13:181–188.
80. Whitbread TJ, Batt RM, Garthwaite G. Relative deficiency of serum IgA in the German shepherd dog: a breed abnormality. *Res Vet Sci.* 1984;37:350–352.
81. Norris CR, Gershwin LJ. Evaluation of systemic and secretory IgA concentrations and immunohistochemical stains for IgA-containing B cells in mucosal tissues of an Irish setter with selective IgA deficiency. *J Am Anim Hosp Assoc.* 2003;39:247–250.
82. Day MJ, Penhale WJ. Humoral immunity in disseminated *Aspergillus terreus* infection in the dog. *Vet Microbiol.* 1988;16:283–294.
83. German AJ, Hall EJ, Day MJ. Relative deficiency in IgA production by duodenal explants from German shepherd dogs with small intestinal disease. *Vet Immunol Immunopathol.* 2000;76:25–43.
84. Day MJ, Penhale WJ. Serum immunoglobulin A concentrations in normal and diseased dogs. *Res Vet Sci.* 1988;45:360–363.
85. McEwan NA, McNeil PE, Thompson H, et al. Diagnostic features, confirmation and disease progression in 28 cases of lethal acrodermatitis of bull terriers. *J Small Anim Pract.* 2000;41:501–507.
86. Jezyk PF, Haskins ME, MacKay-Smith WE, et al. Lethal acrodermatitis in bull terriers. *J Am Vet Med Assoc.* 1986;188:833–839.
87. Grider A, Mouat MF, Mauldin EA, et al. Analysis of the liver soluble proteome from bull terriers affected with inherited lethal acrodermatitis. *Mol Genet Metab.* 2007;92:249–257.
88. Bauer A, Jagannathan V, Hogler S, et al. MKLN1 splicing defect in dogs with lethal acrodermatitis. *PLoS Genet.* 2018;14:e1007264.
89. Gaskin AA, Schantz P, Jackson J, et al. Visceral leishmaniasis in a New York foxhound kennel. *J Vet Intern Med.* 2002;16:34–44.
90. Chabanne L, Marchal T, Denerolle P, et al. Lymphocyte subset abnormalities in German shepherd dog pyoderma (GSP). *Vet Immunol Immunopathol.* 1995;49:189–198.
91. Day MJ. An immunopathological study of deep pyoderma in the dog. *Res Vet Sci.* 1994;56:18–23.
92. Rosser EJ. Jr German shepherd dog pyoderma: a prospective study of 12 dogs. *J Am Anim Hosp Assoc.* 1997;33:355–363.
93. Day MJ, Mazza G. Tissue immunoglobulin G subclasses observed in immune-mediated dermatopathy, deep pyoderma and hypersensitivity dermatitis in dogs. *Res Vet Sci.* 1995;58:82–89.

94. Wisselink MA, Bernadina WE, Willemse A, et al. Immunologic aspects of German shepherd dog pyoderma (GSP). *Vet Immunol Immunopathol.* 1988;19:67–77.
95. Lobetti R. Common variable immunodeficiency in miniature dachshunds affected with *Pneumocystis carinii* pneumonia. *J Vet Diagn Invest.* 2000;12:39–45.
96. Rivas AL, Tintle L, Argentieri D, et al. A primary immunodeficiency syndrome in Shar-Pei dogs. *Clin Immunol Immunopathol.* 1995;74:243–251.
97. Rivas AL, Tintle L, Meyers-Wallen V, et al. Inheritance of renal amyloidosis in Chinese Shar-pei dogs. *J Hered.* 1993;84:438–442.
98. Tellier LA. Immune-mediated vasculitis in a shar-pei with swollen hock syndrome. *Can Vet J.* 2001;42:137–139.
99. May C, Hammill J, Bennett D. Chinese shar pei fever syndrome: a preliminary report. *Vet Rec.* 1992;131:586–587.
100. DiBartola SP, Tarr MJ, Webb DM, et al. Familial renal amyloidosis in Chinese Shar Pei dogs. *J Am Vet Med Assoc.* 1990;197:483–487.
101. Olsson M, Meadows JR, Truve K, et al. A novel unstable duplication upstream of HAS2 predisposes to a breed-defining skin phenotype and a periodic fever syndrome in Chinese Shar-Pei dogs. *PLoS Genet.* 2011;7. e1001332.
102. Rivas AL, Tintle L, Kimball ES, et al. A canine febrile disorder associated with elevated interleukin-6. *Clin Immunol Immunopathol.* 1992;64:36–45.
103. Day MJ. Possible immunodeficiency in related rottweiler dogs. *J Small Anim Pract.* 1999;40:561–568.
104. Roth JA, Kaeberle ML, Grier RL, et al. Improvement in clinical condition and thymus morphologic features associated with growth hormone treatment of immunodeficient dwarf dogs. *Am J Vet Res.* 1984;45:1151–1155.
105. Roth JA, Lomax LG, Altszuler N, et al. Thymic abnormalities and growth hormone deficiency in dogs. *Am J Vet Res.* 1980;41:1256–1262.
106. Hansen P, Clercx C, Henroteaux M, et al. Neutrophil phagocyte dysfunction in a weimaraner with recurrent infections. *J Small Anim Pract.* 1995;36:128–131.
107. Parry AT, Penning VA, Smith KC, et al. Imaging diagnosis: necrotizing meningomyelitis and polyarthritis. *Vet Radiol Ultrasound.* 2009;50:412–415.
108. Studdert VP, Phillips WA, Studdert MJ, et al. Recurrent and persistent infections in related Weimaraner dogs. *Aust Vet J.* 1984;61:261–263.
109. Foale RD, Herrtage ME, Day MJ. Retrospective study of 25 young weimaraners with low serum immunoglobulin concentrations and inflammatory disease. *Vet Rec.* 2003;153:553–558.
110. Couto CG, Krakowka S, Johnson G, et al. In vitro immunologic features of Weimaraner dogs with neutrophil abnormalities and recurrent infections. *Vet Immunol Immunopathol.* 1989;23:103–112.
111. Abeles V, Harrus S, Angles JM, et al. Hypertrophic osteodystrophy in six weimaraner puppies associated with systemic signs. *Vet Rec.* 1999;145:130–134.
112. Abitbol M, Bosse P, Thomas A, et al. A deletion in FOXN1 is associated with a syndrome characterized by congenital hypotrichosis and short life expectancy in Birman cats. *PLoS One.* 2015;10:e0120668.
113. Casal ML, Straumann U, Sigg C, et al. Congenital hypotrichosis with thymic aplasia in nine birman kittens. *J Am Anim Hosp Assoc.* 1994;30:600–602.
114. DiBartola SP, Tarr MJ, Benson MD. Tissue distribution of amyloid deposits in Abyssinian cats with familial amyloidosis. *J Comp Pathol.* 1986;96:387–398.
115. van der Linde-Sipman JS, Niewold TA, Tooten PC, et al. Generalized AA-amyloidosis in Siamese and oriental cats. *Vet Immunol Immunopathol.* 1997;56:1–10.
116. Niewold TA, van der Linde-Sipman JS, Murphy C, et al. Familial amyloidosis in cats: Siamese and Abyssinian AA proteins differ in primary sequence and pattern of deposition. *Amyloid.* 1999;6:205–209.
117. Giger U, Pratt SM, Palena C, et al. Feline leukocyte adhesion deficiency. In: *53rd ASH Annual Meeting and Exposition.* 2011. San Diego, CA.
118. Giger U. Primäre Immundefekte beim Kleintier. *Kleintierpraxis.* 1994;39:433–438.
119. Latimer KS. Pelger-Huet anomaly. In: Feldman BF, Zinkl JG, Jain NC, eds. *Schalm's Veterinary Hematology.* 5 ed. Philadelphia, PA: Lippincott Williams & Williams; 2000:976–983.
120. Cox NR, Ewald SJ, Morrison NE, et al. Thymic alterations in feline GM1 gangliosidosis. *Vet Immunol Immunopathol.* 1998;63:335–353.
121. Buckley RM, Grahn RA, Gandolfi B, et al. Assisted reproduction mediated resurrection of a feline model for Chediak-Higashi syndrome caused by a large duplication in LYST. *Sci Rep.* 2020;10:64.
122. Sierra P, Guillot J, Jacob H, et al. Fungal flora on cutaneous and mucosal surfaces of cats infected with feline immunodeficiency virus or feline leukemia virus. *Am J Vet Res.* 2000;61:158–161.
123. George JW, Rideout BA, Griffey SM, et al. Effect of preexisting FeLV infection or FeLV and feline immunodeficiency virus coinfection on pathogenicity of the small variant of *Haemobartonella felis* in cats. *Am J Vet Res.* 2002;63:1172–1178.
124. Casal ML, Jezyk PF, Giger U. Transfer of colostral antibodies from queens to their kittens. *Am J Vet Res.* 1996;57:1653–1658.
125. Giger U, Casal M. Feline colostrum - Friend or foe: maternal antibodies in queens and kittens. *J Reprod Fertil Suppl.* 1997;51:313–316.
126. Shofer FS, Glickman LT, Payton AJ, et al. Influence of parental serum immunoglobulins on morbidity and mortality of beagles and their offspring. *Am J Vet Res.* 1990;51:239–244.
127. DeBey MC. Primary immunodeficiencies of dogs and cats. *Vet Clin North Am Small Anim Pract.* 2010;40:425–438.
128. Sykes JE. Immunodeficiencies caused by infectious diseases. *Vet Clin North Am Small Anim Pract.* 2010;40:409–423.
129. Cohn LA. Glucocorticosteroids as immunosuppressive agents. *Semin Vet Med Surg (Small Anim).* 1997;12:150–156.
130. Miller E. Immunosuppression: an overview. *Semin Vet Med Surg (Small Anim).* 1997;12:144–149.
131. Wunschmann A, Kremmer E, Baumgartner W. Phenotypical characterization of T and B cell areas in lymphoid tissues of dogs with spontaneous distemper. *Vet Immunol Immunopathol.* 2000;73:83–98.
132. Beineke A, Puff C, Seehusen F, et al. Pathogenesis and immunopathology of systemic and nervous canine distemper. *Vet Immunol Immunopathol.* 2009;127:1–18.
133. Schobesberger M, Summerfield A, Doherr MG, et al. Canine distemper virus-induced depletion of uninfected lymphocytes is associated with apoptosis. *Vet Immunol Immunopathol.* 2005;104:33–44.
134. von Messling V, Svitek N, Cattaneo R. Receptor (SLAM [CD150]) recognition and the V protein sustain swift lymphocyte-based invasion of mucosal tissue and lymphatic organs by a morbillivirus. *J Virol.* 2006;80:6084–6092.
135. Olsen CG, Stiff MI, Olsen RG. Comparison of the blastogenic response of peripheral blood lymphocytes from canine parvovirus-positive and -negative outbred dogs. *Vet Immunol Immunopathol.* 1984;6:285–290.
136. Rodriguez F, Fernandez A, Espinosa de los Monteros A, et al. Acute disseminated candidiasis in a puppy associated with parvoviral infection. *Vet Rec.* 1998;142:434–436.
137. Krakowka S, Olsen R, Axthelm M, et al. Canine parvovirus infection potentiates canine distemper encephalitis attributable to modified live-virus vaccine. *J Am Vet Med Assoc.* 1982;180:137–139.
138. de Groot-Mijnes JD, van Dun JM, van der Most RG, et al. Natural history of a recurrent feline coronavirus infection and the role of cellular immunity in survival and disease. *J Virol.* 2005;79:1036–1044.
139. Dean GA, Olivry T, Stanton C, et al. In vivo cytokine response to experimental feline infectious peritonitis virus infection. *Vet Microbiol.* 2003;97:1–12.
140. Decaro N, Campolo M, Lorusso A, et al. Experimental infection of dogs with a novel strain of canine coronavirus causing systemic disease and lymphopenia. *Vet Microbiol.* 2008;128:253–260.
141. Marinaro M, Mari V, Bellacicco AL, et al. Prolonged depletion of circulating CD4+ T lymphocytes and acute monocytosis after pantropic canine coronavirus infection in dogs. *Virus Res.* 2010;152:73–78.
142. Hoffmann-Fezer G, Mortelbauer W, Hartmann K, et al. Comparison of T-cell subpopulations in cats naturally infected with feline leukae-

mia virus or feline immunodeficiency virus. *Res Vet Sci*. 1996;61:222–226.
143. Cianciolo GJ, Copeland TD, Oroszlan S, et al. Inhibition of lymphocyte proliferation by a synthetic peptide homologous to retroviral envelope proteins. *Science*. 1985;230:453–455.
144. Mitani M, Cianciolo GJ, Snyderman R, et al. Suppressive effect on polyclonal B-cell activation of a synthetic peptide homologous to a transmembrane component of oncogenic retroviruses. *Proc Natl Acad Sci Unit States Am*. 1987;84:237–240.
145. Haraguchi S, Good RA, Day-Good NK. A potent immunosuppressive retroviral peptide: cytokine patterns and signaling pathways. *Immunol Res*. 2008;41:46–55.
146. Miro G, Domenech A, Escolar E, et al. Plasma electrophoretogram in feline immunodeficiency virus (FIV) and/or feline leukaemia virus (FeLV) infections. *J Vet Med Ser A*. 2007;54:203–209.
147. Grant CK, Pickard D, Ramaika C, et al. Complement and tumor antibody levels in cats, and changes associated with natural feline leukemia virus infection and malignant disease. *Cancer Research*. 1979;39:75–81.
148. Wardini AB, Guimaraes-Costa AB, Nascimento MT, et al. Characterization of neutrophil extracellular traps in cats naturally infected with feline leukemia virus. *J Gen Virol*. 2010;91:259–264.
149. Lutz H, Castelli I, Ehrensperger F, et al. Panleukopenia-like syndrome of FeLV caused by co-infection with FeLV and feline panleukopenia virus. *Vet Immunol Immunopathol*. 1995;46:21–33.
150. Good R, Ogasawara M, Liu W, et al. Immunosuppressive actions of retroviruses. *Lymphology*. 1990;23:56–59.
151. Fujino Y, Horiuchi H, Mizukoshi F, et al. Prevalence of hematological abnormalities and detection of infected bone marrow cells in asymptomatic cats with feline immunodeficiency virus infection. *Vet Microbiol*. 2009;136:217–225.
152. Zaccaro L, Falcone ML, Silva S, et al. Defective natural killer cell cytotoxic activity in feline immunodeficiency virus-infected cats. *AIDS Res Hum Retroviruses*. 1995;11:747–752.
153. Simões RD, Howard KE, Dean GA. In vivo assessment of natural killer cell responses during chronic feline immunodeficiency virus infection. *PLoS One*. 2012;7:e37606.
154. Sprague WS, TerWee JA, VandeWoude S. Temporal association of large granular lymphocytosis, neutropenia, proviral load, and FasL mRNA in cats with acute feline immunodeficiency virus infection. *Vet Immunol Immunopathol*. 2010;134:115–121.
155. Levy JK, Liang Y, Ritchey JW, et al. Failure of FIV-infected cats to control *Toxoplasma gondii* correlates with reduced IL2, IL6, and IL12 and elevated IL10 expression by lymph node T cells. *Vet Immunol Immunopathol*. 2004;98:101–111.
156. Taniwaki SA, Figueiredo AS, Araujo JP. Jr Virus–host interaction in feline immunodeficiency virus (FIV) infection. *Comp Immunol Microbiol Infect Dis*. 2013;36:549–557.
157. Zhang L, Reckling S, Dean GA. Phenotypic and functional analysis of CD1a+ dendritic cells from cats chronically infected with feline immunodeficiency virus. *Comp Immunol Microbiol Infect Dis*. 2015;42:53–59.
158. Tompkins MB, Tompkins WA. Lentivirus-induced immune dysregulation. *Vet Immunol Immunopathol*. 2008;123:45–55.
159. Vahlenkamp TW, Tompkins MB, Tompkins WA. Feline immunodeficiency virus infection phenotypically and functionally activates immunosuppressive CD4+ CD25+ T regulatory cells. *J Immunol*. 2004;172:4752–4761.
160. Woo JC, Dean GA, Pedersen NC, et al. Immunopathologic changes in the thymus during the acute stage of experimentally induced feline immunodeficiency virus infection in juvenile cats. *J Virol*. 1997;71:8632–8641.
161. Shimojima M, Nishimura Y, Miyazawa T, et al. Phenotypic changes in CD8+ peripheral blood lymphocytes in cats infected with feline immunodeficiency virus. *Microbes Infect*. 2003;5:1171–1176.
162. Reubel GH, Dean GA, George JW, et al. Effects of incidental infections and immune activation on disease progression in experimentally feline immunodeficiency virus-infected cats. *J Acquir Immune Defic Syndr*. 1994;7:1003–1015.
163. Davidson MG, Rottman JB, English RV, et al. Feline immunodeficiency virus predisposes cats to acute generalized toxoplasmosis. *Am J Pathol*. 1993;143:1486–1497.
164. Tenorio AP, Franti CE, Madewell BR, et al. Chronic oral infections of cats and their relationship to persistent oral carriage of feline calici-, immunodeficiency, or leukemia viruses. *Vet Immunol Immunopathol*. 1991;29:1–14.
165. Egberink H, Berrocal A, Bax H, et al. Papillomavirus associated skin lesions in a cat seropositive for feline immunodeficiency virus. *Vet Microbiol*. 1992;31:117–125.
166. Pedersen NC, Yamamoto JK, Ishida T, et al. Feline immunodeficiency virus infection. *Vet Immunol Immunopathol*. 1989;21:111–129.
167. Jacobs GJ, Medleau L, Calvert C, et al. Cryptococcal infection in cats: factors influencing treatment outcome, and results of sequential serum antigen titers in 35 cats. *J Vet Intern Med*. 1997;11:1–4.
168. Mancianti F, Giannelli C, Bendinelli M, et al. Mycological findings in feline immunodeficiency virus-infected cats. *J Med Vet Mycol*. 1992;30:257–259.
169. Hess PR, English RV, Hegarty BC, et al. Experimental *Ehrlichia canis* infection in the dog does not cause immunosuppression. *Vet Immunol Immunopathol*. 2006;109:117–125.
170. Mekuzas Y, Gradoni L, Oliva G, et al. *Ehrlichia canis* and *Leishmania infantum* co-infection: a 3-year longitudinal study in naturally exposed dogs. *Clin Microbiol Infect*. 2009;15(suppl 2):30–31.
171. Attipa C, Solano-Gallego L, Papasouliotis K, et al. Association between canine leishmaniosis and *Ehrlichia canis* co-infection: a prospective case-control study. *Parasites Vectors*. 2018;11:184.
172. Mylonakis ME, Koutinas AF, Breitschwerdt EB, et al. Chronic canine ehrlichiosis (*Ehrlichia canis*): a retrospective study of 19 natural cases. *J Am Anim Hosp Assoc*. 2004;40:174–184.
173. Nyindo M, Huxsoll D, Ristic M, et al. Cell-mediated and humoral immune responses of German shepherd dogs and beagles to experimental infection with *Ehrlichia canis*. *Am J Vet Res*. 1980;41:250–254.
174. Villaescusa A, Tesouro MA, García-Sancho M, et al. Evaluation of peripheral blood lymphocyte subsets in family-owned dogs naturally infected by *Ehrlichia canis*. *Comp Immunol Microbiol Infect Dis*. 2012;35:391–396.
175. Foglia Manzillo V, Pagano A, Guglielmino R, et al. Extranodal gammadelta-T-cell lymphoma in a dog with leishmaniasis. *Vet Clin Pathol*. 2008;37:298–301.
176. Zambrano-Villa S, Rosales-Borjas D, Carrero JC, et al. How protozoan parasites evade the immune response. *Trends Parasitol*. 2002;18:272–278.
177. Rodrigues A, Santos-Mateus D, Alexandre-Pires G, et al. *Leishmania infantum* exerts immunomodulation in canine Kupffer cells reverted by meglumine antimoniate. *Comp Immunol Microbiol Infect Dis*. 2017;55:42–52.
178. Mozos E, Perez J, Day MJ, et al. Leishmaniosis and generalized demodicosis in three dogs: a clinicopathological and immunohistochemical study. *J Comp Pathol*. 1999;120:257–268.
179. Netea MG, Sutmuller R, Hermann C, et al. Toll-like receptor 2 suppresses immunity against *Candida albicans* through induction of IL-10 and regulatory T cells. *J Immunol*. 2004;172:3712–3718.
180. Netea MG, Warris A, Van der Meer JW, et al. *Aspergillus fumigatus* evades immune recognition during germination through loss of toll-like receptor-4-mediated signal transduction. *J Infect Dis*. 2003;188:320–326.
181. Gantner BN, Simmons RM, Underhill DM. Dectin–1 mediates macrophage recognition of *Candida albicans* yeast but not filaments. *EMBO J*. 2005;24:1277–1286.
182. Yauch LE, Lam JS, Levitz SM. Direct inhibition of T-cell responses by the *Cryptococcus* capsular polysaccharide glucuronoxylomannan. *PLoS Pathog*. 2006;2:e120.
183. Osterholzer JJ, Surana R, Milam JE, et al. Cryptococcal urease promotes the accumulation of immature dendritic cells and a non-protective T2 immune response within the lung. *Am J Pathol*. 2009;174:932–943.
184. Teitz-Tennenbaum S, Viglianti SP, Roussey JA, et al. Autocrine IL-10 signaling promotes dendritic cell type-2 activation and persistence of murine cryptococcal lung infection. *J Immunol*. 2018;201:2004–2015.

185. Wiesner DL, Smith KD, Kotov DI, et al. Regulatory T cell induction and retention in the lungs drives suppression of detrimental type 2 Th cells during pulmonary cryptococcal infection. *J Immunol.* 2016;196:365–374.
186. Stockhaus C, Slappendel RJ. Haemophagocytic syndrome with disseminated intravascular coagulation in a dog. *J Small Anim Pract.* 1998;39:203–206.
187. Walton RM, Modiano JF, Thrall MA, et al. Bone marrow cytological findings in 4 dogs and a cat with hemophagocytic syndrome. *J Vet Intern Med.* 1996;10:7–14.
188. Wilkinson AR, Carr SV, Klahn SL, et al. Hemophagocytic syndrome in a cat. *JFMS Open Rep.* 2018;4:2055116918795023.
189. Suwa A, Shimoda T. Lymphoma-associated hemophagocytic syndrome in six dogs. *J Vet Med Sci.* 2018;80:1271–1276.
190. Weiss DJ. Hemophagocytic syndrome in dogs: 24 cases (1996-2005). *J Am Vet Med Assoc.* 2007;230:697–701.
191. Day MJ. Ageing, immunosenescence and inflammageing in the dog and cat. *J Comp Pathol.* 2010;142(suppl 1):S60–S69.
192. Greeley EH, Kealy RD, Ballam JM, et al. The influence of age on the canine immune system. *Vet Immunol Immunopathol.* 1996;55:1–10.
193. Van de Velde H, Janssens G, Rochus K, et al. Proliferation capacity of T-lymphocytes is affected transiently after a long-term weight gain in Beagle dogs. *Vet Immunol Immunopathol.* 2013;152:237–244.
194. Laflamme D. Companion animals symposium: obesity in dogs and cats: what is wrong with being fat? *J Anim Sci.* 2012;90:1653–1662.
195. Sonne C, Larsen HJ, Kirkegaard M, et al. Trans-generational and neonatal humoral immune responses in West Greenland sledge dogs (*Canis familiaris*) exposed to organohalogenated environmental contaminants. *Sci Total Environ.* 2010;408:5801–5807.
196. Sheffy BE, Schultz RD. Influence of vitamin E and selenium on immune response mechanisms. *Fed Proc.* 1979:2139–2143.
197. Langweiler M, Schultz R, Sheffy B. Effect of vitamin E deficiency on the proliferative response of canine lymphocytes. *Am J Vet Res.* 1981;42:1681–1685.
198. Coutsoudis A, Broughton M, Coovadia HM. Vitamin A supplementation reduces measles morbidity in young African children: a randomized, placebo-controlled, double-blind trial. *Am J Clin Nutr.* 1991;54:890–895.
199. Lalor S, Mellanby R, Friend E, et al. Domesticated cats with active mycobacteria infections have low serum vitamin D (25 (OH) D) concentrations. *Transboundary Emer Dis.* 2012;59:279–281.
200. Latimer K, Mahaffey E. Neutrophil adherence and movement in poorly and well-controlled diabetic dogs. *Am J Vet Res.* 1984;45:1498–1500.
201. Bailiff NL, Nelson RW, Feldman EC, et al. Frequency and risk factors for urinary tract infection in cats with diabetes mellitus. *J Vet Intern Med.* 2006;20:850–855.
202. Kirsch M. [Incidence of bacterial cystitis in diabetic dogs and cats at the time of diagnosis. Retrospective study for the period 1990-1996]. *Tierarztl Prax Ausg K Kleintiere Heimtiere.* 1998;26:32–36.
203. Magori E, Nakamura M, Inoue A, et al. Malate dehydrogenase activities are lower in some types of peripheral leucocytes of dogs and cats with type 1 diabetes mellitus. *Res Vet Sci.* 2005;78:39–44.
204. Grooters AM, Sherding RG, Biller DS, et al. Hepatic abscesses associated with diabetes mellitus in two dogs. *J Vet Intern Med.* 1994;8:203–206.
205. Huber X, Degen L, Muenst S, et al. Primary intestinal lymphangiectasia in an elderly female patient: a case report on a rare cause of secondary immunodeficiency. *Medicine.* 2017;96.
206. Forrester SD, Troy GC, Dalton MN, et al. Retrospective evaluation of urinary tract infection in 42 dogs with hyperadrenocorticism or diabetes mellitus or both. *J Vet Intern Med.* 1999;13:557–560.
207. Sikorski LE, Birkenheuer AJ, Holowaychuk MK, et al. Babesiosis caused by a large *Babesia* species in 7 immunocompromised dogs. *J Vet Intern Med.* 2010;24:127–131.
208. Brown CD, Parnell NK, Schulman RL, et al. Evaluation of clinicopathologic features, response to treatment, and risk factors associated with idiopathic neutropenia in dogs: 11 cases (1990-2002). *J Am Vet Med Assoc.* 2006;229:87–91.
209. Brazzell JL, Weiss DJ. A retrospective study of aplastic pancytopenia in the dog: 9 cases (1996-2003). *Vet Clin Pathol.* 2006;35:413–417.
210. Devine L, Armstrong PJ, Whittemore JC, et al. Presumed primary immune-mediated neutropenia in 35 dogs: a retrospective study. *J Small Anim Pract.* 2017;58:307–313.
211. McManus PM, Litwin C, Barber L. Immune-mediated neutropenia in 2 dogs. *J Vet Intern Med.* 1999;13:372–374.
212. Weiss DJ. Evaluation of antineutrophil IgG antibodies in persistently neutropenic dogs. *J Vet Intern Med.* 2007;21:440–444.
213. Levine JM, Levine GJ, Boozer L, et al. Adverse effects and outcome associated with dexamethasone administration in dogs with acute thoracolumbar intervertebral disk herniation: 161 cases (2000-2006). *J Am Vet Med Assoc.* 2008;232:411–417.
214. Torres SM, Diaz SF, Nogueira SA, et al. Frequency of urinary tract infection among dogs with pruritic disorders receiving long-term glucocorticoid treatment. *J Am Vet Med Assoc.* 2005;227:239–243.
215. Kadar E, Sykes JE, Kass PH, et al. Evaluation of the prevalence of infections in cats after renal transplantation: 169 cases (1987-2003). *J Am Vet Med Assoc.* 2005;227:948–953.
216. Webb JA, Keller SL, Southorn EP, et al. Cutaneous manifestations of disseminated toxoplasmosis in an immunosuppressed dog. *J Am Anim Hosp Assoc.* 2005;41:198–202.
217. Barrs VR, Martin P, Beatty JA. Antemortem diagnosis and treatment of toxoplasmosis in two cats on cyclosporin therapy. *Aust Vet J.* 2006;84:30–35.
218. McAtee BB, Cummings KJ, Cook AK, et al. Opportunistic invasive cutaneous fungal infections associated with administration of cyclosporine to dogs with immune-mediated disease. *J Vet Intern Med.* 2017;31:1724–1729.
219. Narayanan L, Mulligan C, Durso L, et al. Recovery of T-cell function in healthy dogs following cessation of cyclosporine administration. *Vet Med Sci.* 2020; 6:277-282.

131

Fever

Amy E. DeClue

KEY POINTS

- Fever may be associated with infectious, inflammatory, immune-mediated, and neoplastic disease.
- True fever is associated with a rise in the hypothalamic set point, and body temperature is increased by enhanced heat production and conservation.
- Fever of unknown origin (FUO) is defined as persistent or recurrent fever which is not responsive to treatment and for which a cause is not easily determined.
- Major endogenous pyrogens are cytokines such as IL-1β, IL-6, and TNF-α. These act to increase synthesis of prostaglandin E2 which acts on thermoregulatory neurons to raise the hypothalamic set point.
- The diagnostic approach to FUO requires consideration of a large number of differential diagnoses and a staged diagnostic investigation with thorough and repeated physical examinations.
- Therapeutic trials should be a last resort as they have the potential to mask underlying disease, contribute to adverse outcomes, and result in unnecessary expense.

Fever is a common clinical finding in patients with infectious, inflammatory, immune-mediated, or neoplastic disease. In many of these patients, fever is accompanied by other more specific or localizing clinical signs, and the cause of the fever is determined with simple diagnostic tests. In some cases, the cause of the fever is not readily apparent, but it resolves spontaneously or in response to empiric therapy, often with antibacterial drugs. In a further small subset of animals, the cause of fever is not easily determined and not therapeutically responsive, and the problem becomes persistent or recurrent. Such cases of fever of unknown origin (FUO) present a particular diagnostic challenge in both human and veterinary medicine.[1-5] This chapter outlines the pathophysiology of fever and presents an approach to the small animal patient with FUO.

ETIOLOGY OF FEVER OF UNKNOWN ORIGIN

Although fever is frequently associated with infectious diseases, the same response can be elicited by many inflammatory, immune-mediated, or neoplastic disorders, some medications and several miscellaneous disorders. Because the list of differential causes for FUO is extensive, grouping these causes into broad categories based on the underlying disease process is useful. Table 131.1 shows the causes of FUO divided into infectious and parasitic diseases, Table 131.2 summarizes inflammatory and immune-mediated causes of FUO, and neoplastic and miscellaneous causes are listed in Table 131.3. Similar tables are used in the diagnostic approach to FUO in humans. In the human medical literature, the causes of FUO are typically distributed as follows: 17% to 35% are infectious, 10% to 20% are neoplastic, 24% to 36% are inflammatory, 3% to 15% are miscellaneous, and up to 51% are undiagnosed.[5] *In general, bacterial infections are not the most common cause of fever in dogs or in cats.* In cats, fever often results from viral infection (FeLV, FIV, feline respiratory viruses, FCoV). In dogs, neoplasia and immune-mediated disease are the more common causes of fever than infectious causes. In a study of 101 dogs with fever, 22% of dogs had immune-mediated disease, 22% had primary bone marrow abnormalities (usually hemic neoplasia, but many had myelodysplasia), 16% had infectious diseases, 10% had neoplasia outside the bone marrow, 12% had miscellaneous inflammatory conditions, and 20% had pyrexia of unknown origin, where the underlying disease was never identified.[6] Variation among case series may reflect referral bias and geographic location of the study. Published case series are also exclusively or predominantly canine.[6,7] Fever needs to be distinguished from hyperthermia and dysthermia; dysthermia results from damage to the brain (hypothalamus) and is usually accompanied by other CNS signs.

PATHOGENESIS

Body temperature is determined by the set-point of the hypothalamic thermoregulatory center. Thermoregulation depends on sensory information from external and internal thermoreceptors and on physiologic and behavioral effector mechanisms that control heat production and heat loss. Body heat is lost through the skin and the respiratory tract and can be gained by transfer from the environment or generated by muscle activity or body fat catabolism. Body temperature is decreased by panting, cutaneous vasodilation, seeking shelter, and remaining inactive. In a cold environment, body temperature is maintained by shivering, postural changes, piloerection, and cutaneous vasoconstriction. In a normal animal, these mechanisms balance heat loss and heat gain and keep the body temperature as close as possible to the normal hypothalamic set-point.

In true fever, the hypothalamic set-point increases, and body temperature is increased by enhanced heat production and conservation. Heat gain and heat loss mechanisms now act to maintain body temperature at the new set-point. In nonfebrile hyperthermic conditions, the hypothalamic set-point is *not* altered, and increased body temperature is the result of increased and unregulated heat gain or heat production or impaired heat loss. Examples of nonfebrile causes of hyperthermia include heat stroke, exercise-induced hyperthermia, malignant hyperthermia, seizure activity, and hypermetabolic disorders. Hyperthermia of this type can progress to multiorgan-dysfunction syndrome caused by an interplay among circulatory disturbances, hypoxia, increased

TABLE 131.1 Infections Associated with Fever of Unknown Origin

Type of Infection	Examples
Systemic bacterial	Infective endocarditis (D), bacteremia from inapparent focus (B)
Localized bacterial	Infective endocarditis (D), pyelonephritis (B), prostatitis (D), pyometra (including stump pyometra) (B), pyothorax and bronchopneumonia (B), pancreatitis (D), visceral abscess or cholangiohepatitis (B), peritonitis (B), septic meningitis (B), septic arthritis (B), osteomyelitis (B), discospondylitis (B), tooth root abscess (B), deep pyoderma (B), other abscesses or cellulitis (B). The possibility of migrating foreign bodies should be considered
Specific bacterial	Leptospirosis (D), Lyme borreliosis (D), brucellosis (D), hemoplasmosis (B), mycobacterial infection (B), bartonellosis (B), plague (B), tularemia (B), mycoplasma and L-form infections (B), relapsing fever borreliosis (D), disease caused by certain virulent GI pathogens, such as salmonellosis (B), ehrlichiosis (B), anaplasmosis (B), neorickettsiosis (D), actinomycosis (D), nocardiosis (B)
Viral	FeLV infection (C), FIV infection (C), feline panleukopenia (C), feline infectious peritonitis (C), feline calicivirus infection (C), feline herpesvirus-1 infection, canine distemper virus infection (D), canine parvovirus infection, canine influenza virus infection (D)
Fungal/algal	Blastomycosis (B), cryptococcosis (B), coccidioidomycosis (B), histoplasmosis (B), disseminated candidiasis (D), aspergillosis (D), pythiosis (D), protothecosis (D), pneumocystosis (D)
Protozoal	Toxoplasmosis (B), neosporosis (D), hepatozoonosis (B), babesiosis (B), leishmaniosis (B), cytauxzoonosis (C), trypanosomiasis (D), sarcocystosis (D)

B, both dog and cat; *C*, predominantly cat; *D*, predominantly dog.

TABLE 131.2 Inflammatory and Immune-Mediated Diseases Associated with Fever of Unknown Origin

Type of Disease	Examples
Immune-mediated	Systemic lupus erythematosus (D, rare in C), idiopathic immune-mediated polyarthritis (B), rheumatoid arthritis (D), polymyositis (B), steroid-responsive meningitis-arteritis (D), vasculitis (B), immune-mediated hemolytic anemia (D), immune-mediated thrombocytopenia (D), sterile nodular panniculitis (D), drug reactions (B)
Inflammatory	Pancreatitis (B), hypereosinophilic syndromes (B), lymphocytic cholangitis (C), panosteitis (D), hypertrophic osteodystrophy (D)

B, both dog and cat; *C*, predominantly cat; *D*, predominantly dog.

TABLE 131.3 Neoplastic and Miscellaneous Diseases Associated with Fever of Unknown Origin

Type of Disease	Examples
Solid tumors	Several, including hepatic tumors, gastric tumors, lung tumors, bone tumors, metastatic disease, and any necrotic tumor (B)
Hematopoietic tumors	Lymphoma (B), leukemia (B), myeloma (B), malignant histiocytosis (B)

B, both dog and cat; *C*, predominantly cat; *D*, predominantly dog.

metabolic demand, cytotoxicity of high temperature, and activation of inflammatory and coagulation cascades.[8]

Fever is mediated by the action of pyrogens (Fig. 131.1). Exogenous pyrogens (infectious agents and their products such as LPS, tumors, drugs, and toxins) stimulate inflammatory cells to release endogenous pyrogens (cytokines such as interferons, IL-1β and IL-6, and TNF-α), and this leads to induction of cyclooxygenase 2 activation of the arachidonic acid cascade, with enhanced synthesis of prostaglandin E_2 (PGE_2). PGE_2 is synthesized by hypothalamic vascular endothelial cells and acts on thermoregulatory neurons to raise the hypothalamic set-point. The cytokine RANKL (receptor activator of nuclear factor kappa-B ligand), which is a member of the TNF superfamily, may also be involved in thermoregulation.[9] The thermoregulatory set-point is located in a rich vascular network called the organum vasculosum laminae terminalis in the preoptic rostral hypothalamus, which possesses little if any blood-brain barrier. Endothelial cells within this region are thought to release arachidonic metabolites themselves, and then metabolites of cyclooxygenase such as PGE_2 are thought to diffuse the short distance to the hypothalamic neurons and induce fever. PGE_2, which itself is not neurally active, can induce production of cyclic adenosine monophosphate or other neurotransmitters, which, in turn, raises the temperature set-point of the body. Additional evidence suggests that the thermoregulatory center may also be stimulated via vagal fibers that respond to release of cytokines locally released in tissues.[10] PGE_2 may also be released peripherally by hematopoietic cells in response to activation of TLR4 by bacterial LPS.[9] The increase in set-point is thought to protect the body from infection. Febrile-range temperatures have been shown to enhance the neutrophil respiratory burst; the release of neutrophils from the bone marrow; the recruitment of neutrophils to tissues; natural killer cell cytolytic activity; and the activity of macrophages and dendritic cells, with upregulation of major histocompatibility complex (MHC) Class I and MHC Class II molecules.

Cats are especially sensitive to drug-induced hyperthermia, which can result from drugs such as opioids (including buprenorphine, oxymorphone, hydromorphone) or ketamine.[11] In some cases, rectal temperatures may exceed 107°F (41.7°C). The mechanism of opioid-induced fever in cats is not fully understood.

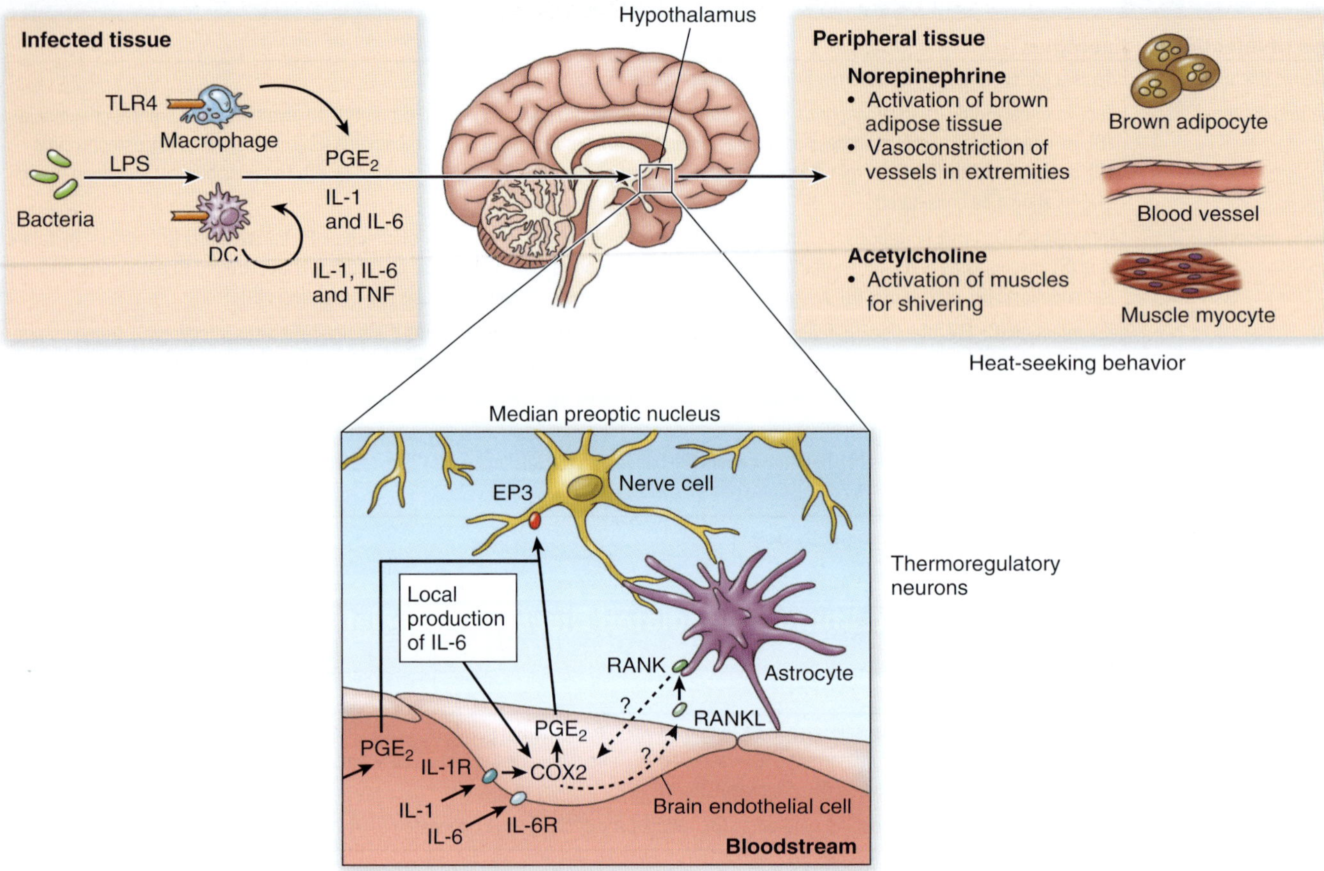

Fig. 131.1 Pathogenesis of fever. The recognition of damage-associated molecular patterns (DAMPs) or pathogen-associated molecular patterns (PAMPs), such as LPS, by TLRs and other pattern recognition receptors drives the activation of dendritic cells *(DCs)* and macrophages. These innate immune cells release prostaglandin E_2 *(PGE_2)* as well as pyogenic cytokines *(IL-1, IL-6,* and *TNF)* that act systemically to induce fever. IL-6 acts downstream of IL-1 in the median preoptic nucleus region in the hypothalamus to induce the synthesis of cyclooxygenase 2 *(COX2)*, the enzyme responsible for production of additional PGE_2. PGE_2 is the major pyogenic mediator of fever. Receptor activation of NF-κB *(RANK)* expressed by astrocytes also acts via the COX2-PGE_2 pathway to induce fever. It is not known exactly how this pathway interacts with the IL-6 pathway. Neurons that express PGE_2 receptor 3 *(EP3)* trigger the sympathetic nervous system to trigger norepinephrine release, which raises body temperature by increasing thermogenesis in brown adipose tissue and inducing vasoconstriction, which reduces heat loss. Additionally, acetylcholine contributes to fever by stimulating muscle myocytes to induce shivering. (Reprinted from Evans SS, Repasky EA, Fisher DT. Fever and the thermal regulation of immunity: the immune system feels the heat. *Nat Rev Immunol.* 2015;15:335-349.)

Another example of drug-induced hyperthermia is serotonin syndrome, which in humans is triggered by medications such as certain migraine medications, antidepressants, and ecstasy. It has also been reported in dogs with 5-hydroxytryptophan toxicosis.[12] These medications cause hyperthermia through both neuromuscular effects (muscle cramping) and a direct effect on the hypothalamus. A number of molecules can influence the hypothalamic neurons, including serotonin, norepinephrine, dopamine, acetylcholine, and prostaglandins.

Factors That Modify Fever

In some cases, fever may be masked by factors such as extremes of age, immunosuppression (e.g., immunosuppressive drugs, hyperadrenocorticism, severe malnutrition), or NSAID treatment. Renal failure can also mask a fever, because uremic toxins are considered to be endogenous cryogens; they are thought to act on the hypothalamus to reduce the set-point, although the true pathogenesis is unclear. Research into this phenomenon was stimulated by the finding that human patients that underwent dialysis often experienced an increase in rectal temperature.[13] Uremic hypothermia has been documented in dogs and cats undergoing intermittent hemodialysis, and appears to be more common in cats.[14] In this study, for dogs post dialysis, rectal temperature decreased by 0.05°F for every 1 mg/dL unit increase in serum creatinine concentration.

CLINICAL SIGNS

Rectal temperatures of 103°F to 105.5°F (39.5°C to 40.8°C) are typically identified in FUO patients and can be associated with nonspecific signs such as anorexia, lethargy, arthralgia, and dehydration.

Body temperatures above 106°F (41.1°C) can rapidly lead to CNS damage and subsequent CNS signs, disseminated intravascular coagulation and evidence of bleeding diathesis, metabolic derangements,

TABLE 131.4 Causes of Fever of Unknown Origin Grouped by Body System or Region

Body System Or Region	Appropriate Diagnostic Tests	Examples
Blood and hematopoietic	Ophthalmic examination, CBC, serum chemistry panel, urinalysis, bone marrow aspirate, bone marrow biopsy, serum protein electrophoresis, FeLV and FIV tests, vector-borne disease serology, blood culture	Leukemia, myeloma, bacteremia, drugs, ehrlichiosis, granulocytopathy, hypereosinophilic syndromes, hemotropic mycoplasmosis, babesiosis, cytauxzoonosis, metastatic neoplasia
Lymphoid	Lymph node palpation, lymph node cytology, lymph node biopsy	Lymphoma, lymphadenitis, salmon poisoning disease, plague, FIV, bartonellosis?
Cardiovascular	Auscultation, radiography, electrocardiography, echocardiography, pericardiocentesis, blood culture, biopsy, *Bartonella* serology and culture	Endocarditis, pericarditis, vasculitis
Respiratory	Radiography, transtracheal or endotracheal wash, fine-needle aspiration, biopsy, ultrasonography, bronchoscopy, bronchoalveolar lavage, CT, thoracoscopy	Bronchial foreign body, fungal or bacterial pneumonia, neoplasia
Nervous system	Fundic and neurological examination, radiography, myelography, CT, MRI, muscle biopsy, CSF analysis	Toxoplasmosis, neosporosis, fungal infection, steroid-responsive meningitis-arteritis, FIP
Musculoskeletal	Radiography, arthroscopy, blood culture, arthrocentesis, synovial membrane biopsy, bone biopsy, ANA	Immune-mediated polyarthritis, myositis, panosteitis, discospondylitis
GI	Rectal examination, fecal cytology, rectal cytology, fecal culture (*Salmonella*), radiography, barium contrast studies, ultrasonography, oral and dental radiographs, pancreatic lipase immunoreactivity, trypsin-like immunoreactivity, endoscopy, laparoscopy, exploratory surgery, biopsy	Neoplasia or abscess anywhere in GI tract, pancreatitis, fungal disease, hepatobiliary or splenic infection
Urogenital	Urinalysis, urine culture, prostatic wash and ejaculate cytology and culture, radiography, ultrasonography, IV pyelography, cystography, cystoscopy, vaginoscopy, cytology, biopsy, *Brucella* serology/blood culture	Prostatitis, stump pyometra, pyelonephritis, orchitis
Pleural or peritoneal cavity	Radiography, ultrasonography, fluid analysis, cytology, microbial culture, biopsy	Pyothorax, FIP, peritonitis, neoplasia
Skin	Physical examination, cytology, biopsy, microbial culture, ultrasound, fistulography	Abscess, fungal infection, nodular panniculitis, vasculitis, actinomycosis, nocardiosis, mycobacteriosis

ANA, antinuclear antibody.
Adapted with permission from Lunn KF. Fever of unknown origin: a systematic approach to diagnosis. *Compend Contin Educ Pract Vet.* 2001;23:976-992.

and death. Such temperatures are typically associated with hyperthermia, rather than fever. When the rectal temperature is mildly increased (< 104°F), animals that appear otherwise systemically well and active are more likely to be hyperthermic than febrile, especially if the weather is warm or the animal has a history consistent with hyperthermia (e.g., traveled in a hot car). The rectal temperature should be retaken after 20 to 30 minutes of being indoors in a cool, quiet environment to determine if the high rectal temperature is clinically relevant. In contrast to fever, hyperthermia is not responsive to treatment with antipyretics.

DIAGNOSIS

Fever (pyrexia) is defined as an increase in body temperature above 102.5°F (39.1°C) in dogs and cats, although fever is typically associated with body temperature above 103°F (39.4°C). Rarely does body temperature exceed 106°F (41.1°C). In human medicine, the following criteria are used to define FUO:

1. Prolonged fever of > 3 weeks' duration associated with vague, nonspecific signs of illness.
2. Temperature more than 1.5°F above normal on several occasions.
3. Diagnosis uncertain after 1 week of hospitalization involving repeated physical exams and routine laboratory tests.

With the availability of faster and more accurate diagnostic tests, and changing models of care (more outpatient care), this definition has changed and the requirement for a week of hospitalization is no longer considered essential.[5]

In veterinary medicine, some practitioners are quick to assign the term "FUO." Multiple definitions of FUO have been used in veterinary medicine without a clear consensus definition. FUO in both human and veterinary medicine can be most usefully defined as fever that does not resolve spontaneously in the period expected for self-limited infection and the cause of which cannot be ascertained despite considerable diagnostic effort.[1] In veterinary medicine, this diagnostic effort typically includes a complete history and physical examination, CBC, chemistry, urinalysis, aerobic bacterial urine culture, plain radiographs of the thorax and abdomen, and abdominal ultrasound examination.

Development of a Diagnostic Plan for FUO

Although some patients with FUO may have uncommon infectious, inflammatory, adverse drug reaction or neoplastic diseases, many patients are ultimately found to have an unusual or early manifestation of a common disorder. Therefore cases must be approached in a systematic fashion that allows for the detection of any potential cause of fever while avoiding unnecessary testing and minimizing invasive testing. A diagnostic plan for FUO may be based on consideration of the disease process, as outlined in Tables 131.1, 131.2, and 131.3. Similar tables are used for the approach to diagnosis of FUO in people.[5,15] A complementary approach is summarized in Table 131.4, in which the causes of FUO are grouped according to anatomic or body system location. Fever may also be classified as "high-grade" (> 104°F) or "low-grade" (≤ 104°F).

BOX 131.1 Good Practice Points in the Management of Fever of Unknown Origin

- Ensure a thorough history, meticulous examination, and baseline investigation panel (CBC, serum chemistry panel, and urinalysis) have been done
- Return to the history and physical examination at regular intervals
- Consider noninfectious causes of a fever early on in the patient's journey (this is especially important in dogs; consider viral causes of a fever in cats)
- Avoid giving empirical antimicrobial or glucocorticoid trials
- Be cautious with the interpretation of some serological tests as some perform poorly with high false-positive and false-negative rates
- Do not perform serological testing if there is no history of exposure to the pathogen you are testing for
- Ensure the client is aware that diagnostic tests may need to be repeated because findings can change over time, and that there is a possibility of no diagnosis being made

The presence of a high-grade fever can raise suspicion for viral infections, gram-negative and some gram-positive (e.g., *Streptococcus* spp.) infections, and diseases such as salmon poisoning disease, plague, and tularemia. High-grade fevers are uncommon for pathogens that replicate slowly, such as mycobacteria or fungi; or those that evade the immune system ("stealth" pathogens), such as *Bartonella* spp.

By combining a disease process and anatomic approach, the clinician can develop a comprehensive diagnostic plan for any FUO patient. In addition to including appropriate diagnostic tests, the diagnostic plan should follow a sequence that is both logical and flexible. The typical diagnostic plan will begin with tests that are safe, simple, inexpensive, easy to interpret, and high yield. Every abnormal result has to be carefully considered; the more tests that are done, the greater the number of false leads that can appear. "Good practice points" for approach to diagnosis of FUO in humans have been outlined,[5] and these can be adopted for FUO in dogs and cats (Box 131.1). A staged approach can be used to guide the selection of diagnostic tests, and examples are outlined in Box 131.2.

The results of stage 1 tests in the FUO patient will determine the tests to be performed at the next stage. If the fever has not been localized, more specialized procedures can also be introduced. Stages 2 and 3 require the repetition of earlier tests and introduce the need for advanced imaging and more invasive procedures. Ideally, the selection of the tests used in stage 3 will be based on abnormalities detected in stages 1 and 2.

An important aspect of staged testing in the FUO patient is the need to repeat the early, less invasive, and less expensive tests frequently enough to detect new changes. In animals with acute illness, fever may develop a day or two before the appearance of lesions, so withholding extensive diagnostic testing and simply repeating physical examinations should be considered in animals with a recent onset of fever to avoid wasting client financial resources and creating undue stress for the patient.

The key is not to rigidly follow a predetermined and fixed diagnostic plan but rather to review and modify the plan as new results become available. For example, if repeated CBCs demonstrate developing pancytopenia, a bone marrow aspirate and biopsy should be performed early in the diagnostic plan and not reserved for stage 3.

BOX 131.2 Staged Approach to the Diagnostic Evaluation of the Patient with Fever of Unknown Origin

Stage 1
Detailed history
Complete physical examination (repeat frequently)
Fundic examination
Neurologic examination
CBC
Serum chemistry profile
FeLV and FIV serology (cats)
Thyroxine (T4) (cats)
Complete urinalysis
Aerobic bacterial urine culture
Thoracic and abdominal radiographs

Stage 2
Repeated physical examinations
Repeat additional stage 1 tests as indicated
Referral to a specialist
Blood cultures
Arthrocentesis
Abdominal ultrasound
Bone marrow aspiration and biopsy (if unexplained cytopenia)
Lymph node aspiration
Other tissue or fluid aspirates as indicated
Fecal culture for *Salmonella* spp. (if diarrhea present)
Echocardiography (if murmur present)
Long bone and joint radiographs
Infectious disease immunoassays or PCR panels as indicated
Antinuclear antibody (only if indicated by clinical signs)

Stage 3
Repeat stage 1 and stage 2 tests as indicated
Referral to a specialist
Echocardiography (if no murmur present)
Dental radiographs
Bone marrow aspirate (with or without biopsy)
Bronchoscopy and bronchoalveolar lavage
Cerebrospinal fluid analysis
Computed tomography
Magnetic resonance imaging
Laparoscopy
Thoracoscopy
Endoscopy
Arthroscopy
Biopsies as indicated
Exploratory surgery
Scintigraphy
Trial therapy

Tests recommended in each staging column are listed in increasing order of expense or risk to animal. These tests are not indicated for initial workup and may be considered appropriate with successive workups.
Adapted with permission from Lunn KF. Fever of unknown origin: a systematic approach to diagnosis. *Compend Contin Educ Pract Vet.* 2001;23:976-992.

Client Communication

The management of the FUO patient demands flexibility, dedication, and patience from both the clinician and the client. By definition, patients with FUO will already have undergone several basic diagnostic tests, and some may have received one or more courses of antimicrobial therapy. Clients may be frustrated by the failure to reach a diagnosis or the continuation of the patient's clinical signs. Good client communication is vital to the successful resolution of the FUO case. The clinician should explain that many diagnostic tests, including repeated tests, may be necessary to reach a diagnosis, that test results

BOX 131.3 Differential Diagnosis for Antibacterial-Unresponsive Fever

Viral infections—especially young animals, e.g., CDV, FIP, FHV-1, FCV
Fungal infections
Protozoal infections
Antibiotic-resistant bacterial infections
Immune-mediated disease
Neoplasia
Pancreatitis
Central fever (dysthermia due to CNS disease)

often change over time to become more revealing, and that the process can be time-consuming and expensive. However, clients should also be reassured that a diagnosis is reached in most cases, that many causes of FUO may be treatable or even curable, and that the fever itself is rarely harmful to the patient.

History

The patient history should include details of geographic location, *any* travel history, environment and lifestyle (e.g., indoor vs. outdoor, history of wildlife exposure or ingestion, boarding, plant awn exposure, digging behavior), recent adoption from a shelter or rescue environment, other animals in the household and when they were introduced, and the possibility of exposure to ticks or other vectors. All of these factors will influence exposure to specific microorganisms. The medical history should cover diet (especially whether raw food diets are fed), vaccinations (antigens and timing), heartworm and other parasite treatment and prevention, the administration of any other medications, previous medical problems, trauma, and previous surgeries (including whether implants may be present). The response to past therapies used for the fever problem should be noted. A failure to respond to antibacterial drugs can help to narrow the differential diagnosis list (Box 131.3), and a previous response to antibacterials may suggest an underlying, inadequately treated bacterial infection or bacterial infection in association with a foreign body. Clients should be carefully questioned about the patient's urination and defecation habits and the presence of clinical signs such as lameness; neck, back, or abdominal pain; skin lesions; masses, or swellings; weakness; exercise intolerance; coughing; nasal discharge; and dyspnea. Any previous medical records should be thoroughly reviewed as the client may not be aware of or recall prescribed medications, vaccines, or procedures.

Physical Examination

All body systems should be examined in detail, and a complete physical examination should be repeated at each hospital visit for outpatients. Repeated and thorough physical examinations are one of the simplest and most rewarding things that can be done to localize the problem. Asking another clinician in the practice to perform a second physical examination may also be helpful. Inpatients should be examined twice daily. The physical examination should include careful cardiac and lung auscultation and regular and thorough examination of the oral cavity and rectum, bones and joints, lymph nodes, and skin. Thorough palpation of the entire surface of the skin, including examination of the foot pads and interdigital spaces should be performed, in an effort to identify skin lesions or painful regions of the body. Detection of a cat bite abscess or cellulitis by means of a thorough physical examination can avoid unnecessary diagnostic tests. An effort should be made to visualize as much of the oral cavity as possible. This is especially important in cats, because oral ulcerations due to viral respiratory pathogens may be located only at the base of the tongue. Musculoskeletal and neurologic examinations may reveal spinal pain or subtle neurologic deficits in dogs with discospondylitis. Repeated ocular examinations, including a fundoscopic examination, should not be overlooked because they may provide evidence of infectious, inflammatory, or neoplastic disease. Given that fever can often wax and wane in FUO, the pattern of fever in an individual patient should be determined by serial measurement of body temperature. In veterinary medicine, this measure is not of any value in elucidating the underlying cause, but it is important in monitoring the response to any subsequent therapy.

Laboratory Findings

Complete Blood Count and Serum Chemistry Panel

Fever is often accompanied by neutrophilia or a stress leukogram, and serum chemistry tests are frequently nonlocalizing in FUO patients. However, any abnormalities detected on these tests should be used to direct further testing. The CBC should always be accompanied by examination of a blood smear so as to determine blood cell morphology and look for microorganisms. Automated CBCs should be verified by manual counts. Thrombocytopenia may be a clue to an underlying vector-borne disease or immune-mediated thrombocytopenia. Neutropenia may be: (1) secondary to bacterial infection, in which case it is usually accompanied by toxic changes and bandemia, (2) an underlying cause of secondary bacterial infection and fever (e.g., because of marrow disease), or (3) an immune-mediated problem (i.e., immune-mediated neutropenia, which is uncommon to rare).[16,17] When neutropenia exists and neutrophils appear mature and nontoxic, marrow disease or immune-mediated neutropenia should be considered. For unclear reasons, dogs with immune-mediated neutropenia rarely seem to develop secondary bacterial infections.

Urinalysis and Urine Culture

Because FUO may be associated with focal urogenital infections (e.g., prostatitis, pyelonephritis), urinalysis and aerobic bacterial urine culture are mandatory in the evaluation of fever patients. Urine specimens should be obtained by cystocentesis and submitted for bacterial culture and susceptibility testing, regardless of the appearance of the urine sediment. However, because subclinical bacteriuria may be unrelated to the problem causing fever, at the same time, care should be taken not to overinterpret the finding of a positive urine culture (see Chapter 127). With the exception of *Candida*, which can cause infections localized to the urinary tract, funguria generally indicates a systemic fungal infection. However, candiduria in the presence of fever is suggestive of disseminated candidiasis.

Diagnostic Imaging

Plain Radiography

Thoracic and abdominal radiographs should be obtained during the first stage of evaluation of the FUO patient. These radiographs may provide early evidence of neoplastic disease or suggest infectious disease such as viral, bacterial, or fungal pneumonia. Attention should also be paid to each rib and the vertebral column on thoracic and abdominal radiographs for evidence of osteomyelitis or discospondylitis. In the second or third stages of diagnosis, complete spinal, long bone, joint, and dental radiographs should be considered.

Ultrasonographic Examination

A complete abdominal ultrasound examination should include examination of the liver, gall bladder, bile duct, gastrointestinal tract, spleen, pancreas, kidney, urinary bladder, prostate, uterus, abdominal lymph nodes, and adrenal glands. When lesions are present, other regions that can be investigated by ultrasonography include the thorax (particularly in the presence of effusions or masses), the retrobulbar area, and any other peripheral mass lesion or swelling. Ultrasonography can also facilitate minimally invasive acquisition of fine-needle aspirates or biopsies.

Echocardiography

Ultrasonographic examination of the pericardium, myocardium, endocardium, heart valves, and great vessels is essential in the evaluation of the patient with FUO and a heart murmur, particularly if the murmur is of recent onset, which might suggest infective endocarditis (IE) (see Chapter 122). Because IE can occur in the absence of a murmur, should other attempts to localize a cause of fever fail, echocardiography could be considered even in dogs that do not have a murmur. The results of echocardiography should be interpreted in light of the patient's signalment, clinical signs, and blood culture results. Echocardiographic evaluation is especially important in medium to large breed dogs because these breeds are overrepresented and IE is more common in dogs than in cats.[18,19]

Advanced Imaging

Advanced imaging modalities should be regarded as third-stage tests in the evaluation of the FUO patient and used when clinical signs have been localized to a particular body system. For example, CT is useful for detecting certain pulmonary lesions and for examining the nasal cavity, tympanic bullae, and pharynx. MRI is often used in evaluation of the CNS.

Nuclear medicine has provided several techniques that can be used to visualize infection or inflammation in human patients.[20] Scintigraphic imaging can demonstrate many of the steps involved in the inflammatory process and can, therefore, potentially localize some causes of FUO. For example, leukocyte infiltration of tissues can be visualized with indium-111 or technetium-99m–labeled neutrophils.[21] Other techniques in nuclear medicine include the use of radiolabeled human immunoglobulin, or gallium-67, which binds to transferrin in the blood, to nonspecifically demonstrate areas of increased fluid extravasation associated with enhanced vascular permeability in inflammation. Positron emission tomography (PET) with fluorine-18 fluorodeoxyglucose is an imaging technique used to identify areas of increased glucose metabolism such as tumors and infectious or inflammatory lesions. The combination of PET with computed tomography (PET/CT) allows for anatomic localization of the lesion which enhances diagnostic value of this technique in patients with FUO.[22,23]

Cytologic and Histopathologic Examination

Fine-needle aspirates are usually simple and safe to obtain, and touch preparations or impression smears can also be made from ulcerated lesions or discharge material. Cytologic examination of these specimens is relatively inexpensive and, depending on the skill of the clinician, can sometimes be performed in-house. For example, if blastomycosis is suspected, repeated aspirates from lymph nodes or skin nodules can be examined for *Blastomyces* organisms because they are relatively easy to identify (see Chapter 80). Ultrasound, fluoroscopy, or CT can be used to facilitate guidance. Aspirates of fluids such as pleural, pericardial, or peritoneal effusions; CSF; synovial fluid; or bile should also be submitted for bacterial and other cultures. Aspiration of peripheral lymph nodes, even if palpably normal, is recommended in the second stage of diagnostic testing if the source of the fever has not been localized.

Cisternal or lumbar puncture, bronchoalveolar lavage, transtracheal or endotracheal lavage, prostatic wash and ejaculation, and bone marrow aspiration may also be used to obtain specimens for cytologic examination and culture. Biopsy specimens may also be obtained with techniques such as thoracoscopy, laparoscopy, endoscopy, or arthroscopy, or they can be obtained percutaneously, sometimes with guidance from ultrasound or radiography.

Bone Marrow Cytology and Histology

Bone marrow disease is a relatively common cause of FUO. Reported examples include myelodysplasia, lymphoid leukemia, myeloma, hemophagocytic syndrome, and disseminated adenocarcinoma.[6,24,25] Bone marrow aspiration is indicated in the early stages of diagnostic testing if CBCs show unexplained, persistent cytopenias. Investigation of pancytopenia requires the evaluation of both cytology of a bone marrow aspirate and histopathology of a core biopsy. In cats, additional unstained bone marrow cytology smears should also be reserved for FeLV FA testing. Bone marrow aspiration is indicated in the third stage of the diagnostic plan if the FUO has not yet been localized.

Arthrocentesis

Immune-mediated polyarthritis is a common cause of FUO in dogs,[6,7,26] although only 3 of 79 dogs with polyarthritis in one study were examined because of intermittent fever.[26] The condition can be idiopathic (nondeforming and nonerosive), or it can be caused by rheumatoid arthritis or associated with other immune-mediated disorders such as systemic lupus erythematosus or steroid-responsive meningitis-arteritis (SRMA; see Chapter 129). Occasionally, nonerosive immune-mediated polyarthritis can be secondary to infection, drug therapy, or neoplasia.[27] Immune-mediated polyarthritis is rare in cats.[28]

Lameness, joint swelling, and periarticular pain can wax and wane or be inapparent in patients with immune-mediated polyarthritis. Therefore arthrocentesis should be performed in the second stage of evaluation of canine patients with FUO. Because dogs with immune-mediated polyarthritis may have fever as their only clinical sign, collection of synovial fluid by arthrocentesis should be considered. Synovial fluid specimens should be obtained from both carpi and both tarsi if possible. The fluid should be examined for color, clarity, and viscosity and submitted for cytologic examination including a differential cell count and cytologic description. The cells in synovial fluid can degrade and undergo apoptosis, quickly altering the cytologic evaluation. Ideally, joint fluid should be submitted as cytologic slide preparations; if additional fluid is available after slide preparation, that can be submitted as well. Aerobic bacterial and mycoplasma culture or mycoplasma PCR should also be performed if specimen volume is large enough. Bacterial recovery from joint fluid will be enhanced if the joint fluid is incubated in blood culture bottles immediately after collection for 24 hours before bacterial plating.

Cerebrospinal Fluid Analysis

In a retrospective study of fever in dogs, 10 of 66 patients were found to have inflammatory CNS disease.[29] This included seven dogs with SRMA (see Chapter 129). Dogs with FUO and evidence of spinal pain can also have concurrent immune-mediated polyarthritis and SRMA.[30] Therefore arthrocentesis should be considered in dogs in which this form of meningitis is suspected. If joint fluid analysis is unremarkable, CSF analysis should be performed.

Blood Culture

Blood cultures are indicated in all patients with FUO and should be especially considered where there is the presence of a cardiac murmur; spinal, long bone, or joint pain; neutropenia; or a history of immunosuppressive drug administration.

Few prospective studies have been done of blood culture techniques in veterinary patients, although this subject has been extensively reviewed in the human literature.[31] In human medicine, the likelihood of obtaining a positive culture result is directly correlated with the volume of blood drawn, regardless of whether the blood is obtained as a single blood culture set or divided into several sets over a 24-hour period. In one study, the yield from a 30-mL blood sample was found to be 62% more than that from a 10-mL sample. However, the sensitivity of blood cultures is also improved by obtaining more than one set. For example, in a study of bacteremic humans, 91.5% of bacteremic episodes were detected by the first blood culture set, and 99.3% were detected by the first two sets. Increasing the number of blood culture sets will also increase the specificity of the test because contaminants are unlikely to be present in all sets.

In dogs and cats, blood culture techniques should focus on the collection of adequately large volumes of blood, with less emphasis on the timing or periodicity of the collections. The total volume of blood that can safely be obtained will depend on patient size. If size allows, more than one blood culture set should be obtained to increase the sensitivity and specificity of the test. Detailed information on blood culture technique can be found in Chapter 3.

Serologic Testing

Tests available for the diagnosis of infectious disease include assays for specific antibodies or antigens, as well as molecular tools such as PCR-based assays. Many of these tests are performed on blood specimens; however, other body fluids can be used for detection of certain organisms. For example, urine antigen detection appears to be sensitive for the detection of some fungal diseases.[32] Consideration of the signalment, clinical signs, geographic location, and possible vector exposure of the patient should direct selection of the most appropriate tests. Vaccination history, local disease prevalence, sensitivity, specificity, etiologic predictive value, and positive and negative predictive values must be considered when interpreting the results of any diagnostic test (see Chapter 7). Ensuring that tests are only conducted when there is a reasonable likelihood of the disease in question being present will help to minimize problems associated with poor positive predictive value.

Serologic tests are also available for the diagnosis of certain immune-mediated diseases. Antinuclear antibody (ANA) can be detected in patients with systemic lupus erythematosus. However, diagnosis of this uncommon multisystem disorder requires the demonstration of multiple clinical and immunologic abnormalities and should never be based on a positive ANA assay alone.[33,34] In addition, ANA can be positive in some clinically healthy dogs and in association with other medical conditions. This disorder is more appropriately diagnosed by a combination of radiographic changes indicating an erosive polyarthritis together with joint fluid analysis and possibly synovial membrane biopsy.

In summary, extensive arrays of wide-ranging serodiagnostic tests are not recommended in the investigation of FUO, and the use of panels should be avoided if possible or each result in a panel should be interpreted with care and attention to the meaning of a positive or negative result. Ideally, serologic tests should be used to investigate a diagnosis that is suspected based on other findings.

TREATMENT

The goals of FUO therapy are to treat the underlying cause of the fever and provide supportive care to the patient. Dogs and cats with fever have the potential to develop dehydration as a result of reduced water intake and increased sensible and insensible losses. Intravenous fluid therapy can correct these conditions. While cooling measures (e.g., fans, cool water baths, colonic or gastric irritation) are indicated when body temperature is increased as a result of nonfebrile factors such as heat stroke or prolonged seizure activity, these methods should not be used for true fever unless body temperature exceeds 41.1°C (106°F) and there is concern for CNS damage, and then they should only be used to reduce body temperature sufficiently to avoid CNS damage. Fever is a *regulated* increase in body temperature; therefore any attempts to physically cool the patient will be working against the body's own thermoregulatory mechanisms. Fever is also a protective adaptive response to the effects of infection and can have beneficial effects. External cooling is the treatment of choice for hyperthermia in which core temperature exceeds the thermoregulatory set-point. Thus, when external cooling is used to treat hyperthermia, no opposition of regulatory process takes place in an attempt to increase heat gain, as is the case with fever.

Antipyretic therapies inhibit cyclooxygenase and therefore act centrally to reduce the hypothalamic set-point. However, it is extremely rare that antipyretic medications are needed for dogs or cats with FUO and like steroids, antipyretic medications have many risks such as masking disease, inducing secondary complications and preventing treatment with disease-specific appropriate therapy.

In the editor's experience, the most common cause of true FUO in dogs is immune-mediated disease. Usually, fever in cats resolves spontaneously or an underlying cause is identified.

Trial Therapy

In many cases, the investigation of the FUO patient will achieve a definitive diagnosis, and treatment of the underlying cause will lead to resolution of fever and other clinical signs. However, in some cases of true FUO, a diagnosis is not reached, and in other cases, diagnostic testing is discontinued because of client or patient factors. In these cases, therapeutic trials are undertaken in the absence of a definitive diagnosis. Antibacterial, antifungal, or glucocorticoid therapies are often used in therapeutic trials.

The goals of a therapeutic trial should be to confirm a presumptive diagnosis indirectly, control or cure the underlying disease, and resolve the patient's clinical signs, without inducing intolerable adverse effects or exacerbating an undiagnosed disease.

A therapeutic trial should be planned and monitored as rigorously as the diagnostic plan. It is important to begin with a tentative diagnosis, select safe and appropriate therapies, and implement a careful monitoring program, using predetermined criteria for success or failure of the therapeutic trial. Medication should be used at appropriate doses, and the duration of therapy should be sufficient to detect both the presence and absence of a response, particularly because fever can wax and wane independent of therapy.

Good client communication is essential in developing and monitoring a therapeutic trial, and clients should understand the risks of such an approach. Such risks include the continued progression of an undiagnosed disease if an ineffective therapy is used, development of medication adverse effects or toxicities, and the possibility of exacerbating an underlying infectious disease if immunosuppressive therapy is used. Clients should also understand that some medications, such as antifungals, can be expensive, and that initiating treatment without a diagnosis for diseases that require a long course of therapy may make attempts to make a diagnosis more difficult in the future. The risks and benefits of trial therapy should be carefully considered if the patient is likely to be referred for further diagnostic testing.[29] A therapeutic trial is unlikely to be helpful if the client abandons the plan because of expense, adverse effects, or lack of immediate response to treatment.

Many causes of FUO are inflammatory or immune mediated; therefore glucocorticoids are commonly used in patients with FUO in the absence of a specific diagnosis. Because this approach can be dangerous if infectious disease has not been ruled out first, the patient should be monitored closely for exacerbation or development of new clinical signs. The indiscriminate use of glucocorticoids can also interfere with future diagnostic testing and future more specific therapies, or worsen prognosis. This practice is a particular concern for patients with neoplasia such as lymphoma or fungal disease. Glucocorticoids can also have nonspecific antiinflammatory effects and may improve the patient's clinical signs without addressing the primary cause of the fever allowing progression of disease to go unnoticed.

Empiric antibacterial therapy is commonly used in small animal patients with fever, often with a successful outcome. Ideally, such therapy should be based on culture and susceptibility testing, although this is not always feasible. In trial therapy for FUO patients, antibacterials should be chosen based on a tentative but specific diagnosis, with consideration of spectrum of activity and an understanding of pharmacokinetics. For example, doxycycline is a reasonable choice if salmon poisoning disease, leptospirosis, or a rickettsial disease is suspected. A significant risk of indiscriminate antibacterial therapy is that it contributes to antibacterial resistance in bacterial populations. Treatment with antibiotics without attempting basic diagnostics should be avoided if possible, because serious abnormalities (especially renal failure) may be present, and if undetected and untreated, these may be life-threatening.

Trial therapy for fungal infections with antifungal drugs is rarely indicated without strong support for an underlying fungal disease. Fungal lesions respond slowly to treatment, antifungal drugs are often expensive, and prolonged treatment is typically required. Therefore the importance of investing client funds to obtain a diagnosis first cannot be overemphasized. Fortunately the advent of fungal antigen tests has facilitated diagnosis because they are relatively inexpensive and can be performed on specimens collected in a minimally invasive manner.

CASE EXAMPLE

Signalment:

"Grover," a 2-year-old male neutered Shetland sheepdog from northern California.

History:

Grover was evaluated by the University of California-Davis veterinary emergency and critical care service for fever. Six days previously, Grover vomited four to six times, and vomited up a plant awn. He was seen at a local veterinary clinic and a physical examination was unremarkable. He was treated with subcutaneous fluids and maropitant on an outpatient basis. Two days later, the owners found him shivering and reluctant to move. He was again evaluated at the local veterinary clinic and his temperature was 104.9°C (40.5°F). A CBC, serum chemistry panel, urinalysis, and thoracic radiographs were unremarkable. He was hospitalized and given IV fluids and ampicillin-sulbactam, and discharged the following day. For the following 2 days, the owners reported that he was eating normally but was quiet and still reluctant to move about the house. The owners took his temperature at home and it was 104.4°C (40.2°F).

Current Medications:

Phenobarbital 60 mg in the morning and 90 mg in the evening; levetiracetam 740 mg q 12h for previously diagnosed epilepsy. Monthly endoparasite prophylaxis (milbemycin oxime and praziquantel).

Other Medical History:

Acquired from a breeder at 9 months of age. Diagnosed with suspected idiopathic epilepsy 1 year ago. Last seizure was a week before the onset of fever.

Physical Examination

Body weight: 13.6 kg.

General: Bright, alert, responsive, hydrated. T = 102.9°C (39.4°F), HR 132 beats/min, RR 60 bpm, BCS 5/9, CRT 1–2 s, mucous membranes pink and moist.

GI and genitourinary: Tense abdomen but no apparent pain, organomegaly, or masses. No other clinically significant findings.

Laboratory Findings

CBC: HCT 40.1% (40–55%), MCV 71 fL (65–75 fL), MCHC 33.9 g/dL (33–36 g/dL), WBC 19,660 cells/μL (6000–13,000 cells/μL), neutrophils 14,015 cells/μL (3000–10,500 cells/μL), lymphocytes 2350 cells/μL (1000–4000 cells/μL), monocytes 1752 cells/μL (150–1200 cells/μL), platelets 231,000 platelets/μL (150,000–400,000 platelets/μL).

Serum chemistry profile: Sodium 143 mmol/L (143–151 mmol/L), potassium 4.3 mmol/L (3.6–4.8 mmol/L), chloride 105 mmol/L (108–118 mmol/L), bicarbonate 19 mmol/L (20–29 mmol/L), phosphorus 4.9 mg/dL (2.6–6.2 mg/dL), calcium 10.3 mg/dL (9.6–11.2 mg/dl), BUN 19 mg/dL (11–33 mg/dL), creatinine 0.9 mg/dL (0.8–1.5 mg/dL), glucose 83 mg/dL (86–188 mg/dL), total protein 6.3 g/dL (5.4–6.9 g/dL), albumin 3.4 g/dL (3.4–4.3 g/dL), globulin 2.9 g/dL (1.7–3.1 g/dL), ALT 98 U/L (21–72 U/L), AST 72 U/L (20–49 U/L), ALP 236 U/L (14–91 U/L), creatine kinase 103 U/L (55–257 U/L), GGT 4 U/L (0–5 U/L), cholesterol 426 mg/dL (139–353 mg/dL), total bilirubin < 0.2 mg/dL (0–0.2 mg/dL), magnesium 2.2 mg/dL (1.9–2.5 mg/dL).

SNAP 4Dx Plus (IDEXX Laboratories, ME, USA): negative for antibody to *Ehrlichia canis, Anaplasma platys, Anaplasma phagocytophilum*, and *Borrelia burgdorferi*. Negative for antigen to *Dirofilaria immitis*.

Imaging Findings

Abdominal ultrasound: Abdominal ultrasound examination of the liver, spleen, pancreas, GI tract, urinary tract, and adrenal glands was unremarkable. However, within the dorsal right abdominal wall, adjacent to the kidney and just deep to the last ribs, there was a gas- and fluid-containing structure. Within this structure there were one to two foreign bodies visualized that appeared to be plant awns.

Diagnosis

Suspected plant awn foreign body abscess.

Treatment

Exploratory surgery was performed using a ventral abdominal approach. This revealed significant swelling on the right side of the body wall under the last rib. The swelling was explored and purulent material as well as three plant awns were found. The area was lavaged and a drain placed to allow continuous suction. Aerobic and anaerobic cultures yielded mixed growth that included a broadly susceptible *Escherichia coli*, small numbers of a viridans streptococcus, and small numbers of *Cutibacterium acnes* (formerly *Propionibacterium acnes*). Grover was discharged on treatment with clavulanic acid-amoxicillin and carprofen. He recovered uneventfully.

Comments

This dog had fever that was associated with systemic plant awn migration. The case illustrates the value of a thorough history (as the dog had recently vomited up a plant awn) and meticulous ultrasound examination for detection of migrating foreign bodies. Plant awns often migrate to sites in the retroperitoneal region and caudal ribs, which warrants careful scanning of these regions in dogs with FUO.

SUGGESTED READINGS

Fernandez C, Beeching NJ. Pyrexia of unknown origin. *Clin Med.* 2018;18:170–174.

Evans SS, Repasky EA, Fisher DT. Fever and the thermal regulation of immunity: the immune system feels the heat. *Nat Rev Immunol.* 2015;15:335–349.

Wright WF, Auwaerter PG, Dibble EH, et al. Imaging a fever—redefining the role of 18FDG-PET/CT in FUO investigations. *Clin Infect Dis.* 2021;72:1279–1286.

REFERENCES

1. Arnow PM, Flaherty JP. Fever of unknown origin. *Lancet.* 1997;350:575–580.
2. Davies GR, Finch RG. Fever of unknown origin. *Clin Med.* 2001;1:177–179.
3. Flood J. The diagnostic approach to fever of unknown origin in cats. *Compend Contin Educ Vet.* 2009;31:26–31. quiz 31, E21-24.
4. Flood J. The diagnostic approach to fever of unknown origin in dogs. *Compend Contin Educ Vet.* 2009;31:14–20. quiz 20-11, E11-13.
5. Fernandez C, Beeching NJ. Pyrexia of unknown origin. *Clin Med.* 2018;18:170–174.
6. Dunn KJ, Dunn JK. Diagnostic investigations in 101 dogs with pyrexia of unknown origin. *J Small Anim Pract.* 1998;39:574–580.
7. Lunn KF. Fever of unknown origin: a systematic approach to diagnosis. *Compend Contin Educ Vet.* 2001;23:976–992.
8. Leon LR, Bouchama A. Heat stroke. *Compr Physiol.* 2015;5:611–647.
9. Evans SS, Repasky EA, Fisher DT. Fever and the thermal regulation of immunity: the immune system feels the heat. *Nat Rev Immunol.* 2015;15:335–349.
10. Netea MG, Kullberg BJ, Van der Meer JW. Circulating cytokines as mediators of fever. *Clin Infect Dis.* 2000;31(suppl 5):S178–S184.
11. Posner LP, Pavuk AA, Rokshar JL, et al. Effects of opioids and anesthetic drugs on body temperature in cats. *Vet Anaesth Analg.* 2010;37:35–43.
12. Gwaltney-Brant SM, Albretsen JC, Khan SA. 5-Hydroxytryptophan toxicosis in dogs: 21 cases (1989-1999). *J Am Vet Med Assoc.* 2000;216:1937–1940.
13. Kluger MJ, Turnbull AJ, Cranston WI, et al. Endogenous cryogen excreted by the kidneys. *Am J Physiol.* 1981;241:R271–R276.
14. Kabatchnick E, Langston C, Olson B, et al. Hypothermia in uremic dogs and cats. *J Vet Intern Med.* 2016;30:1648–1654.
15. Cunha BA. Fever of unknown origin: focused diagnostic approach based on clinical clues from the history, physical examination, and laboratory tests. *Infect Dis Clin North Am.* 2007;21:1137–1187 (xi).
16. Devine L, Armstrong PJ, Whittemore JC, et al. Presumed primary immune-mediated neutropenia in 35 dogs: a retrospective study. *J Small Anim Pract.* 2017;58:307–313.
17. Weiss DJ. Evaluation of antineutrophil IgG antibodies in persistently neutropenic dogs. *J Vet Intern Med.* 2007;21:440–444.
18. Sykes JE, Kittleson MD, Chomel BB, et al. Clinicopathologic findings and outcome in dogs with infective endocarditis: 71 cases (1992-2005). *J Am Vet Med Assoc.* 2006;228:1735–1747.
19. Wall M, Calvert CA, Greene CE. Infective endocarditis in dogs. *Compend Contin Educ Vet.* 2002;24:614–625.
20. Rennen HJ, Boerman OC, Oyen WJ, et al. Imaging infection/inflammation in the new millennium. *Eur J Nucl Med.* 2001;28:241–252.
21. Auletta S, Riolo D, Varani M, et al. Labelling and clinical performance of human leukocytes labelled with (99m)Tc-HMPAO Using Leukokit® with Gelofusine versus Leukokit® with HES as sedimentation agent. *Contrast Media Mol Imaging.* 2019;2019:4368342.
22. Wright WF, Auwaerter PG, Dibble EH, et al. Imaging a fever—redefining the role of 18FDG-PET/CT in FUO Investigations. *Clin Infect Dis.* 2021;72:1279–1286.
23. Grobman M, Cohn L, Knapp S, et al. ^{18}F-FDG-PET/CT as adjunctive diagnostic modalities in canine fever of unknown origin. *Vet Radiol Ultrasound.* 2018;59:107–115.
24. Weiss DJ. Hemophagocytic syndrome in dogs: 24 cases (1996-2005). *J Am Vet Med Assoc.* 2007;230:697–701.
25. Henson KL, Alleman AR, Fox LE, et al. Diagnosis of disseminated adenocarcinoma by bone marrow aspiration in a dog with leukoerythroblastosis and fever of unknown origin. *Vet Clin Pathol.* 1998;27:80–84.
26. Shaughnessy ML, Sample SJ, Abicht C, et al. Clinical features and pathological joint changes in dogs with erosive immune-mediated polyarthritis: 13 cases (2004-2012). *J Am Vet Med Assoc.* 2016;249:1156–1164.
27. Rondeau MP, Walton RM, Bissett S, et al. Suppurative, nonseptic polyarthropathy in dogs. *J Vet Intern Med.* 2005;19:654–662.
28. Tamura Y, Nagamoto T, Segawa K, et al. Successful treatment and long-term follow up of idiopathic immune-mediated polyarthritis with mycophenolate mofetil in a cat. *JFMS Open Rep.* 2020;6:2055116920963995.
29. Battersby IA, Murphy KF, Tasker S, et al. Retrospective study of fever in dogs: laboratory testing, diagnoses and influence of prior treatment. *J Small Anim Pract.* 2006;47:370–376.
30. Webb AA, Taylor SM, Muir GD. Steroid-responsive meningitis-arteritis in dogs with noninfectious, nonerosive, idiopathic, immune-mediated polyarthritis. *J Vet Intern Med.* 2002;16:269–273.
31. Mylotte JM, Tayara A. Blood cultures: clinical aspects and controversies. *Eur J Clin Microbiol Infect Dis.* 2000;19:157–163.
32. Spector D, Legendre AM, Wheat J, et al. Antigen and antibody testing for the diagnosis of blastomycosis in dogs. *J Vet Intern Med.* 2008;22:839–843.
33. Chabanne L, Rigal D, Fournel C, et al. Canine systemic lupus erythematosus. Part II. Diagnosis and treatment. *Compend Contin Educ Vet.* 1999;21:402–421.
34. Chabanne L, Monier JC, Fournel C, et al. Canine systemic lupus erythematosus. Part I. Clinical and biologic aspects. *Compend Contin Educ Vet.* 1999;21:135–141.

APPENDIX

Vaccination Schedules for Dogs and Cats

Jane E. Sykes

The schedules provided below are guidelines for immunization of dogs and cats against major viral and bacterial agents. These assume the availability of client resources and suitable products for immunization. The schedules are based on guidelines written by the WSAVA, AAHA, AAFP and ABCD,[1–11] and information available at the time of writing. These are *general guidelines*, because the vaccine types recommended and the frequency of immunization vary depending on the lifestyle of the pet being immunized, i.e., indoor versus outdoor pets, shelter animals, travel plans, kennel/boarding plans, and underlying disease conditions such as immune-mediated diseases or preexisting infections such as FIV infection. Because these factors may change over time, the vaccination plan for individual pet animals should be decided by the owner at routine annual examinations, after a discussion between the veterinarian and the client regarding the animal's lifestyle in the year ahead and the advantages and disadvantages of vaccination. This discussion should be documented in the medical record. A previous history of vaccine reactions in an individual pet will also affect recommendations for immunization. More research is required to generate optimal recommendations for vaccination of dogs and cats.

TABLE A.1 Guidelines for Vaccination of Individual Pet Dogs

	INITIAL VACCINATION			
Vaccine	**Age ≤ 16 weeks**	**Age > 16 weeks**	**Subsequent Vaccination**	**Comments**
CPV-2, CDV, CAdV-2 (A; SC); or CPV-2, recombinant CDV, CAdV-2 (A; SC)	6–8 weeks of age, then every 3–4 weeks until no sooner than 16 weeks (16–20 weeks in breeding kennels).	Two doses 3–4 weeks apart are recommended, especially for dogs at high risk of exposure, but one dose is considered protective and is sufficient in dogs seen after 6 months of age.	Consider revaccination at 6 months of age rather than 1 year of age, then every 3 years thereafter. This means an additional visit at 1 year of age for rabies and other annually required vaccines.	Core. Protection after the 12-month booster may be lifelong. The recombinant CDV vaccine may immunize in the face of maternal antibody.
CPV-2 (I; SC)				Not recommended when attenuated live vaccines are available and indicated.
Rabies (I; SC)	One dose not earlier than 12 weeks of age.	One dose.	Administer a single dose within 1 year following the initial dose, regardless of the age at the time the initial dose is administered; then every 3 years thereafter if using a 3-year-labeled vaccine or annually if using a 1-year-labeled vaccine. Local jurisdictions may dictate an alternative protocol.	Core in endemic areas or where required by local regulations.
CPiV (A; SC)	6–8 weeks of age, then every 3–4 weeks until no sooner than 14–16 weeks.	One dose.	Annual or within 6 months of boarding, and at least 1 week before boarding.	Noncore. Use as a monovalent product or in combination with other noncore vaccines for annual boosters.
CPiV, *Bordetella bronchiseptica*, CAdV-2 (A; IN)	One dose as early as 3 weeks of age; consider second dose 2–4 weeks later if initial immunization occurs at < 6 weeks of age.	One dose.	Annual or within 6 months of boarding, and second dose (or booster) at least 1 week before boarding.	Noncore. Potential to provide improved local mucosal immunity over SC products. Mucosal vaccines that contain CAdV-2 are for reduction of respiratory disease due to CAdV-2. Parenteral CAdV-2 vaccines are preferred for protection against CAdV-1.
B. bronchiseptica (I; SC)	Two doses 3–4 weeks apart as early as 6 weeks of age.	Two doses 3–4 weeks apart.	Annual or within 6 months of boarding, and at least 1 week before boarding.	Noncore.
B. bronchiseptica (cell wall antigen extract; SC)	Two doses 3–4 weeks apart starting at 8 weeks of age.	Two doses 4 weeks apart.	Annual or within 6 months of boarding, and at least 1 week before boarding.	Noncore.
B. bronchiseptica (A; IN or oral)	One dose as early as 3 weeks of age for IN vaccines, depending on product label. For oral vaccines, one dose as early as 6 or 8 weeks of age, depending on product label.	One dose.	Annual or within 6 months of boarding, and at least 1 week before boarding.	Noncore. Potential to provide improved local mucosal immunity over SC products. Never administer SC.
Borrelia burgdorferi (I or recombinant; SC)	Two doses 3–4 weeks apart starting at 9–12 weeks of age.	Two doses, 3–4 weeks apart.	Annual. Ideally revaccinate 1 month before the onset of the local *Ixodes* tick season.	Noncore.
Canine influenza H3N8 or H3N2 (I; SC)	Two doses 3–4 weeks apart starting at 6 weeks of age.	Two doses 3–4 weeks apart.	Annual.	Noncore, for dogs at risk of exposure such as co-housed dogs, or before import to certain countries. At the time of writing, canine influenza H3N8 may be extinct in the United States and the prevalence of H3N2 is low.
Leptospira (I; SC)	Two doses 3–4 weeks apart starting at 9–12 weeks of age (or earlier depending on product label).	Two doses 3–4 weeks apart.	Annual. Revaccinate 1 month before the onset of the season if disease occurs seasonally.	Author recommends as core. A 4-serovar vaccine is preferred; breakthrough infections are commonly reported with 2-serovar vaccines.
CCV (I and A; SC)				Not recommended because disease is mild and immunization of unproven benefit.

A, attenuated live; *I*, inactivated whole organism; *IN*, intranasal; *SC*, subcutaneous.

TABLE A.2 Guidelines for Vaccination of Individual Pet Cats

Vaccine	INITIAL VACCINATION ≤ 16 weeks	> 16 weeks	Subsequent Vaccination	Comments
FPV, FCV, FHV-1 (A; SC)	6–8 weeks of age, then every 3–4 weeks until no sooner than 16–20 weeks (20 weeks in breeding catteries).[4]	One or two doses 3–4 weeks apart. Two doses are recommended for cats that are at high risk of exposure.	Consider revaccination at 6 months of age rather than 1 year of age, then every 3 years thereafter. This means an additional visit at 1 year of age for FeLV and rabies vaccination.	Core. Provides cross-protection to CPV-2 strains that infect cats.[12] Administration of attenuated live vaccines to pregnant cats and kittens less than 4 weeks of age may cause cerebellar hypoplasia in the neonate. Inactivated vaccines are for pregnant cats (if absolutely necessary) and cats with advanced retrovirus infection. Administer distally in the right thoracic limb, avoiding the interscapular space.
FPV, FCV, FHV-1 (I; SC)	6–8 weeks of age, then every 3–4 weeks until no sooner than 16–20 weeks (20 weeks in breeding catteries).[4]	Two doses 3–4 weeks apart.	Consider revaccination at 6 months of age rather than 1 year of age, then every 3 years thereafter. This means an additional visit at 1 year of age for FeLV and rabies vaccination.	Core. Provides cross-protection to CPV-2.[12] Vaccine of choice for pregnant cats and cats with advanced retrovirus infection. Inactivated FPV vaccines should be avoided for routine vaccination in order to optimize protection against FPV. Administer distally in the right thoracic limb, avoiding the interscapular space. Dual-strain calicivirus vaccines may provide broader cross-protection against FCV than single-strain vaccines.
FCV, FHV-1 +/– FPV (A; IN)	6–8 weeks of age, then every 3–4 weeks until no sooner than 16–20 weeks of age.	One dose.	Yearly.	Intranasal vaccines may be associated with transient upper respiratory signs. Intranasal FPV vaccines may not provide sufficient protection against FPV in contaminated environments. Intranasal vaccines may provide rapid protection against FCV and FHV-1 which may be desirable in high-risk situations.
Rabies (I; SC or recombinant canarypox; SC)	One dose not earlier than 12 weeks of age.	One dose.	Administer a single dose within 1 year following the initial dose, regardless of the age at the time the initial dose is administered; then every 3 years thereafter if using a 3-year-labeled vaccine or annually if using a 1-year-labeled vaccine. Local jurisdictions may dictate an alternative protocol.	Core in endemic areas or where required by local regulations. Provides strong protection. AAFP/AAHA recommends administration as distal as possible in the right pelvic limb.
FeLV (I; SC)	Two doses 3–4 weeks apart starting at 8 weeks of age.	Two doses 3–4 weeks apart.	1 year, then every 2-3 years thereafter when risk is ongoing. For high-risk exposure, consider annual revaccination. Beyond 1 year of age, age-related resistance may provide additional protection.	Noncore.[a] FeLV testing before administration recommended before first administering the vaccine to kittens and if exposure was likely before booster immunization is required. Can provide strong protection.[13] Administration as distal as possible in the left pelvic limb is recommended.
FeLV (recombinant canarypox; SC)	Two doses 3–4 weeks apart starting at 8 weeks of age.	Two doses 3–4 weeks apart.	Annual when risk is ongoing.[b] Beyond 1 year of age, age-related resistance may provide additional protection.	Noncore.[a] Only for FeLV-negative cats (see above). More data are required on relative efficacy and whether it is associated with a reduced risk of injection site sarcomas. Administration as distal as possible in the left pelvic limb is recommended. Conflicting evidence exists in the literature regarding the efficacy and safety of recombinant vaccines when compared with inactivated vaccines.
FIV (I; SC) (where available)	Three doses, 3 weeks apart, starting at 8 weeks of age.	Three doses 3 weeks apart.	Annual.	Not recommended. Vaccination does not provide complete protection, can interfere with interpretation of antibody test results, and PCR is insufficiently sensitive for accurate diagnosis. Antibodies may also be passed to kittens in colostrum and interfere with testing up to 12 weeks of age.

TABLE A.2 Guidelines for Vaccination of Individual Pet Cats—cont'd

Vaccine	INITIAL VACCINATION ≤ 16 weeks	> 16 weeks	Subsequent Vaccination	Comments
FIP (A; IN)	Two doses 3–4 weeks apart starting at 16 weeks of age.	Two doses 3–4 weeks apart.	Annual.	Not recommended. Only seronegative cats have the potential to be protected. Benefit and risks currently unclear.
Chlamydia felis (I and A; SC)	Two doses 3–4 weeks apart starting at 9 weeks of age.	Two doses 3–4 weeks apart.	Annual.	Noncore. Provides incomplete protection. Could be used as part of a control program in multiple cat households where infection is confirmed using appropriate diagnostic tests as endemic. Vaccination may be associated with adverse effects and provides incomplete protection.
Bordetella bronchiseptica (A; IN)	One dose as early as 8 weeks of age.	One dose.	Annual, but young cats are most at risk.	Noncore. Provides incomplete protection. Use as part of a control program in multiple cat households where infection is confirmed using appropriate diagnostic tests as endemic. Never administer parenterally.

[a]AAFP/AAHA recommends immunization of all kittens for FeLV.[2]

[b]The ABCD, AAHA/AAFP and WSAVA suggest boosters every 2 to 3 years in view of the significant lower susceptibility of older cats, even with recombinant vaccines; annual vaccination is recommended for cats that have predominantly outdoor activities and have aggressive interactions with other cats.

A, attenuated live; *I,* inactivated whole organism; *IN,* intranasal; *SC,* subcutaneous.

GUIDELINES FOR VACCINATION OF DOGS AND CATS IN SHELTER ENVIRONMENTS

For shelter animals, attenuated live core vaccines apart from rabies should be given before or immediately on entry to the shelter. Optimally, vaccination for CPV and CDV should occur at least 3 days before entry to a shelter environment, but vaccination even hours before entry has the potential to make a difference. When outbreaks of known parvovirus disease or canine distemper are present, vaccines can be administered as early as 4–5 weeks of age, but should not be administered earlier than this because of the possibility of vaccine-induced disease and immunosuppression. In the absence of an outbreak situation, vaccination for these pathogens should be performed no earlier than 6 weeks of age. In a shelter situation, the benefits and risks of vaccination of individual pregnant animals with attenuated live vaccines must be carefully assessed. Vaccination with an inactivated vaccine is probably better than no vaccine for pregnant animals that enter a shelter, but inactivated vaccines should not be administered to other animals in the shelter environment, because the onset of immunity is slower than with attenuated live vaccines. Attenuated live vaccines should be administered if ovariohysterectomy is to be performed during pregnancy. If pregnant animals are not vaccinated, they should be strictly isolated from the rest of the shelter animal population. The use of rapid in-house serologic tests that assess for protective antibody titers may be helpful in this situation (see Chapter 20).

Revaccination should be performed no more frequently than at intervals of 2 to 3 weeks, because administration of an attenuated live vaccine within 3 to 14 days of another immunization attempt can interfere with development of immune responses. Revaccination is most important for pups and kittens younger than 16 weeks of age, and is performed to maximize the chance of immunization as soon as possible after the disappearance of maternal antibody interference. Puppies and kittens should also be physically separated from the rest of the shelter animal population and handled with strict attention to quarantine protocols.

Where affordable, vaccination for respiratory pathogens and leptospirosis is strongly recommended in shelter environments. Intranasal vaccines for respiratory pathogens are advantageous in shelter environments because of the potential for improved local immunity, the possibility of administration to very young animals, more rapid onset of protection, and improved protection in the face of maternal antibody. However, they also have been associated with vaccine-induced upper respiratory disease, which may be more severe in debilitated animals and can be difficult to distinguish from natural infection. In addition, field studies have yet not shown benefit of intranasal over parenteral vaccines for respiratory disease. Mucosal *Bordetella bronchiseptica* vaccines should never be given parenterally. This is an emergency situation that requires immediate treatment. See Chapter 20 for specific instructions on how to manage accidental parenteral administration of these vaccines. Leptospirosis vaccines are bacterins and so require 2 doses, 3-4 weeks apart, to provide protection, with annual re-vaccination. Because leptospires can be shed subclinically in the urine of dogs in shelters, vaccination should nevertheless be considered in an effort to minimize zoonotic transmission.

In endemic areas, if possible, a rabies vaccine could be administered at the time of discharge from the facility.[1] Administration of a 3-year product is preferred, but regardless of the product used, booster immunization must be performed no later than 1 year after the initial immunization. Rabies immunization must be properly documented and a veterinarian must usually be present at the time of immunization. Otherwise, the number of vaccines should be limited to those that can assist control of disease that is confirmed to exist within the shelter. This will avoid excessive immune suppression that may worsen the severity of illness due to other pathogens in the shelter for which vaccines are nonexistent.

TABLE A.3 Guidelines for Vaccination of Dogs in Shelter Environments

Vaccine	INITIAL VACCINATION Age ≤ 16 weeks	Age > 16 weeks	Recommendations for booster at exit	Comments
CPV-2, CPV, CDV or recombinant CDV (A; SC)	On entry no earlier than 4 weeks of age,[a] then every 2 weeks until no sooner than 16–20 weeks.	Two doses 2 weeks apart recommended, but one dose is considered protective.	Consider revaccination at 6 months of age rather than 1 year of age, then every 3 years thereafter. A visit at 1 year of age is necessary for vaccines requiring annual administration.	Core. Potential to provide strong protection. Do not use in pregnancy. The recombinant CDV vaccine has the potential to immunize pups in the face of maternal antibody, but protection may not be as robust as with attenuated live vaccines.
Rabies (I; SC)	One dose not earlier than 12 weeks of age	One dose.	Administer a single dose within 1 year following the initial dose, regardless of the age at the time the initial dose is administered; then every 3 years thereafter if using a 3-year-labeled vaccine or annually if using a 1-year-labeled vaccine. Local jurisdictions may dictate an alternative protocol. If local regulations or absence of veterinary oversight prevent rabies vaccination at the shelter, adopters should be encouraged to pursue rabies vaccination from another source within 4 weeks of adoption.	Use in endemic areas. Local regulations can dictate the need for rabies immunization or the ability to vaccinate in a shelter.
CPiV (A; SC)	On entry, no earlier than 4 weeks of age,[a] then every 2 weeks until no sooner than 16 weeks.	Two doses 2 weeks apart recommended, but one dose is considered protective.	Annual or within 6 months of boarding, and at least 1 week before boarding with monovalent SC or IN respiratory disease vaccines.	If the SC vaccine is used, it can be administered in shelters in combination with CDV, CPV, and CAdV-2. Administer with a vaccine for *B. bronchiseptica*.
CPiV, *Bordetella bronchiseptica*, CAdV-2 (A; IN or oral) (various combinations)	Two doses 2 weeks apart starting as early as 3 weeks (IN), or based on label recommendations (oral), although one dose may be sufficient.	Two doses 2 weeks apart, although one dose may be sufficient.	Annual or within 6 months of boarding, and at least 1 week before boarding.	Potential to provide improved local mucosal immunity over SC products. Inadvertent administration of mucosal *Bordetella* vaccines SC may cause death.
Canine influenza H3N2, H3N8 (I; SC) (subtypes available alone or in combination at time of writing)	On entry, two doses 3 weeks apart starting at 6 weeks of age.	Two doses 3 weeks apart.	Annual, if risk is ongoing.	For dogs at risk of exposure in shelters in endemic regions of the United States. At the time of writing, whether H3N8 is still circulating in the United States is controversial, and the incidence of H3N2 infection is low.

[a]Vaccination can be performed as early as 4–5 weeks in the face of an outbreak.
A, attenuated live; *I*, inactivated whole organism; *IN*, intranasal; *SC*, subcutaneous.

TABLE A.4 Guidelines for Vaccination of Cats in Shelter Environments

Vaccine	INITIAL IMMUNIZATION: Age ≤ 16 weeks	INITIAL IMMUNIZATION: Age > 16 weeks	Recommendations for booster at exit	Comments
FPV, FCV, FHV-1 (A; SC)	On entry and no earlier than 4 weeks of age, then every 2 weeks until no sooner than 16–20 weeks.[4]	Two doses 2 weeks apart recommended, but one dose is considered protective.	1 year, then every 3 years thereafter.	Potential to provide strong protection against FPV and CPV-2.[12] Use in pregnant queens may be associated with cerebellar hypoplasia in neonates. The use of inactivated FPV/FCV/FHV-1 vaccines in shelters is not recommended.
FPV, FCV, FHV-1 (A; IN) (available with or without FPV)	On entry and no earlier than 4 weeks of age, then every 2 weeks until no sooner than 16-20 weeks.	Two doses 2 weeks apart recommended, but one dose is considered protective.	1 year, then every 3 years thereafter. Annual revaccination may be indicated in contaminated environments.	Does not provide complete protection. Avoid in pregnancy. Intranasal vaccines may be associated with transient upper respiratory signs. The use of IN vaccines to protect against FPV is not recommended in shelters. Use of IN vaccines that contain FPV should be avoided in kittens < 4 weeks of age or pregnant queens. Use of IN vaccines should be accompanied by parenteral attenuated live vaccination for FPV.
Rabies (I; SC)	One dose not earlier than 12 weeks of age	One dose.	Administer a single dose within 1 year following the initial dose, regardless of the age at the time the initial dose is administered; then every 3 years thereafter if using a 3-year-labeled vaccine or annually if using a 1-year-labeled vaccine. Local jurisdictions may dictate an alternative protocol. If local regulations or absence of veterinary oversight prevent rabies vaccination at the shelter, adopters should be encouraged to pursue rabies vaccination from another source within 4 weeks of adoption.	For use in endemic areas. Local regulations may dictate the need for rabies immunization and the ability for shelters to vaccinate.

A, attenuated live; *I*, inactivated whole organism; *IN*, intranasal; *SC*, subcutaneous.

ACKNOWLEDGEMENT

The editor wishes to thank Dr. Richard B. Ford, Laurie Larson, and George Moore for their review of and contributions to portions of this Appendix.

REFERENCES

1. Day MJ, Horzinek MC, Schultz RD, et al. WSAVA guidelines for the vaccination of dogs and cats. *J Small Anim Pract*. 2016;57:E1–E45.
2. Stone AE, Brummet GO, Carozza EM, et al. 2020 AAHA/AAFP feline vaccination guidelines. *J Feline Med Surg*. 2020;22:813–830.
3. Welborn LV, DeVries JG, Ford R, et al. 2011 AAHA canine vaccination guidelines. *J Am Anim Hosp Assoc*. 2011;47:1–42.
4. Addie D, Belak S, Boucraut-Baralon C, et al. Feline infectious peritonitis. ABCD guidelines on prevention and management. *J Feline Med Surg*. 2009; 11:594–604.
5. Egberink H, Addie D, Belak S, et al. *Bordetella bronchiseptica* infection in cats. ABCD guidelines on prevention and management. *J Feline Med Surg*. 2009;11:610–614.
6. Frymus T, Addie D, Belak S, et al. Feline rabies. ABCD guidelines on prevention and management. *J Feline Med Surg*. 2009;11:585–593.
7. Gruffydd-Jones T, Addie D, Belak S, et al. *Chlamydophila felis* infection. ABCD guidelines on prevention and management. *J Feline Med Surg*. 2009;11:605–609.
8. Radford AD, Addie D, Belak S, et al. Feline calicivirus infection. ABCD guidelines on prevention and management. *J Feline Med Surg*. 2009; 11:556–564.
9. Thiry E, Addie D, Belak S, et al. Feline herpesvirus infection. ABCD guidelines on prevention and management. *J Feline Med Surg*. 2009; 11:547–555.
10. Truyen U, Addie D, Belak S, et al. Feline panleukopenia. ABCD guidelines on prevention and management. *J Feline Med Surg*. 2009;11:538–546.
11. Lutz H, Addie D, Belak S, et al. Feline leukaemia. ABCD guidelines on prevention and management. *J Feline Med Surg*. 2009;11:565–574.
12. Chalmers WS, Truyen U, Greenwood NM, et al. Efficacy of feline panleucopenia vaccine to prevent infection with an isolate of CPV2b obtained from a cat. *Vet Microbiol*. 1999;69:41–45.
13. Torres AN, O'Halloran KP, Larson LJ, et al. Feline leukemia virus immunity induced by whole inactivated virus vaccination. *Vet Immunol Immunopathol*. 2010;134:122–131.

INDEX

Page numbers that begin with *e* indicate web only material. Page numbers followed by *f* indicate figures; *t*, tables; *b*, boxes.

E

G

H

J

K

U

Abbreviations Used Throughout This Book

AAFP	American Association of Feline Practitioners
AAHA	American Animal Hospital Association
ABCD	Advisory Board on Cat Diseases
ACTH	Adrenocorticotropic Hormone
ACVIM	American College of Veterinary Internal Medicine
AE	Alveolar Echinococcosis
AGID	Agar Gel Immunodiffusion
AKI	Acute Kidney Injury
ALP	Alkaline Phosphatase
ALT	Alanine Aminotransferase
AMB	Amphotericin B
APTT	Activated Partial Thromboplastin Time
ARDS	Acute Respiratory Distress Syndrome
ASPCA	American Society for the Prevention of Cruelty to Animals
AST	Aspartate Aminotransferase
AUC	Area Under the ROC Curve
AVMA	American Veterinary Medical Association
BAL	Bronchoalveolar Lavage
BCS	Body Condition Score
BoCV	Bovine Coronavirus
BSAVA	British Small Animal Veterinary Association
BSL	Biosafety Level
BUN	Blood Urea Nitrogen
CAdV	Canine Adenovirus
CAPC	Companion Animal Parasite Council
CBC	Complete Blood Count
CCL	Chemokine Ligand
CCoV	Canine Coronavirus (Enteric or Pantropic)
CD	Cluster of Differentiation
CDC	Centers for Disease Control and Prevention
CDV	Canine Distemper Virus
CE	Cystic Echinococcosis
CFU	Colony-Forming Units
CHV	Canine Herpesvirus
CIRD	Canine Infectious Respiratory Disease
CIRDC	Canine Infectious Respiratory Disease Complex
CIV	Canine Influenza Virus
CK	Creatine Kinase
CKD	Chronic Kidney Disease
CLSI	Clinical and Laboratory Standards Institute
CMI	Cell-Mediated Immunity
CNS	Central Nervous System
CoNS	Coagulase-Negative Staphylococci
CoV	Coronavirus
COVID	Coronavirus Disease
CPE	Cytopathic Effect
CPIV	Canine Parainfluenza Virus
CPnV	Canine Pneumovirus
CPV	Canine Parvovirus[a]
CRCoV	Canine Respiratory Coronavirus
CRFK	Crandell-Rees Feline Kidney Cells
CRI	Constant Rate Infusion
CRP	C-Reactive Protein
CRT	Capillary Refill Time
CSD	Cat Scratch Disease
CSF	Cerebrospinal Fluid
CT	Computed Tomography
DIC	Disseminated Intravascular Coagulation
DLA	Dog Leukocyte Antigen
DNA	Deoxyribonucleic Acid
DOI	Duration of Immunity
dsDNA	Double-Stranded DNA
DTH	Delayed-Type Hypersensitivity
ECG	Electrocardiogram
EDTA	Ethylenediaminetetraacetic Acid
ELISA	Enzyme-Linked Immunosorbent Assay
EMG	Electromyography
EPG	Eggs Per Gram
ESBL	Extended-Spectrum Beta-Lactamase
ExPEC	Extraintestinal Pathogenic *Escherichia coli*
FA	Fluorescent Antibody
FCoV	Feline Coronavirus
FCV	Feline Calicivirus
FDA	Food and Drug Administration (United States)
FECV	Feline Enteric Coronavirus
FeLV	Feline Leukemia Virus
FeMV	Feline Morbillivirus
FFV	Feline Foamy Virus
FHV-1	Feline Herpesvirus-1
FIP	Feline Infectious Peritonitis
FIPV	Feline Infectious Peritonitis Virus
FISH	Fluorescent In Situ Hybridization
FIV	Feline Immunodeficiency Virus
FLAIR	Fluid-Attenuated Inversion Recovery
FNA	Fine-Needle Aspiration
FPV	Feline Panleukopenia Virus
FVRCP	Feline Viral Rhinotracheitis-Calicivirus-Panleukopenia
GGT	Gamma-Glutamyl Transferase
GI	Gastrointestinal
GICA	Gold Immunochromatographic Assays
GMS	Gomori's Methenamine Silver
H&E	Hematoxylin and Eosin
H2RA	Histamine-2 Receptor Antagonist
HCT	Hematocrit
HI	Hemagglutination-Inhibition
HIV	Human Immunodeficiency Virus
HLA	Human Leukocyte Antigen
HPF	High-Power Field
HR	Heart Rate
HSV	Herpes Simplex Virus
IBD	Inflammatory Bowel Disease
ID	Immunodiffusion
IFA	Immunofluorescent Antibody

[a] Refers to CPV-2 variants unless otherwise specified.

Continued

Abbreviations Used Throughout This Book—cont'd

IFN	Interferon
IHC	Immunohistochemistry
Ig	Immunoglobulin
IL	Interleukin
IM	Intramuscular
IMHA	Immune-Mediated Hemolytic Anemia
IMPA	Immune-Mediated Polyarthritis
IN	Intranasal
IRIS	International Renal Interest Society
ISCAID	International Society for Companion Animal Infectious Diseases
ISFM	International Society of Feline Medicine
ITP	Immune-Mediated Thrombocytopenia
IV	Intravenous
LAMP	Loop-Mediated Isothermal Amplification
LPG	Larvae Per Gram
LPS	Lipopolysaccharide
LRS	Lactacted Ringer's Solution
LUTS	Lower Urinary Tract Signs
MALDI-TOF MS	Matrix-Assisted Laser Desorption/Ionization-Time of Flight Mass Spectrometry
MAT	Microscopic Agglutination Test
MCHC	Mean Corpuscular Hemoglobin Concentration
MCV	Mean Corpuscular Volume
MDA	Maternally Derived Antibody
MDR	Multiple Drug Resistant
MDS	Myelodysplastic Syndrome
MHC	Major Histocompatibility Complex
MIC	Minimum Inhibitory Concentration
MIF	Microimmunofluorescence
MLST	Multilocus Sequence Typing
MLV	Modified Live Virus
MPV	Mean Platelet Volume
MRI	Magnetic Resonance Imaging
MRS	Methicillin-Resistant *Staphylococcus*
MRSA	Methicillin-Resistant *Staphylococcus aureus*
MRSP	Methicillin-Resistant *Staphylococcus pseudintermedius*
NAAT	Nucleic Acid Amplification Tests
NF-κB	Nuclear Factor κB
NGS	Next Generation Sequencing
NLM	Neural Larva Migrans
NOD	Nucleotide-Binding Oligomerization Domain
NPV	Negative Predictive Value
NSAIDs	Non-Steroidal Anti-inflammatory Drugs
OD	Oculus Dexter, Right Eye
OIE	World Organisation for Animal Health
OLM	Ocular Larva Migrans
OMP	Outer Membrane Protein
OR	Odds Ratio
OS	Oculus Sinister, Left Eye
Osp	Outer Surface Protein
OU	Oculus Uterque, Both Eyes
PABA	Para-Amino Benzoic Acid
PAMPs	Pathogen-Associated Molecular Patterns
PAS	Periodic Acid-Schiff
PBMC	Peripheral Blood Mononuclear Cell
PBP	Penicillin-Binding Protein
PCR	Polymerase Chain Reaction
PCV	Packed Cell Volume
PET	Positron Emission Tomography
PFGE	Pulsed-Field Gel Electrophoresis
PI	Post-infection
PK-PD	Pharmacokinetic-Pharmacodynamic
PLR	Pupillary Light Reflex
PO	Oral
POC	Point-of-Care
PPE	Personal Protective Equipment
PPI	Proton Pump Inhibitor
PPP	Prepatent Period
PPR	Pattern Recognition Receptor
PPV	Positive Predictive Value
PRN	As Needed
PRV	Pseudorabies Virus
PT	Prothrombin Time
qPCR	Quantitative PCR
QUAT	Quaternary Ammonium Compound
RDW	Red Cell Distribution Width
RBC	Red Blood Cells
RER	Resting Energy Requirement
RMSF	Rocky Mountain Spotted Fever
RNA	Ribonucleic Acid
ROC	Receiver Operating Characteristic
RR	Respiratory Rate
rRNA	Ribosomal RNA
RT	Reverse Transcriptase
RT-PCR	Reverse Transcriptase-Polymerase Chain Reaction
SARS-CoV-2	Severe Acute Respiratory Syndrome Coronavirus-2
SBU	Subclinical Bacteriuria
SC	Subcutaneous
SCC	Squamous Cell Carcinoma
SCT	Sedimentation and Counting Technique
SDMA	Symmetric Dimethylarginine
SIRS	Systemic Inflammatory Response Syndrome
SFG	Spotted Fever Group
SPF	Specific Pathogen-Free
SpG	Specific Gravity
SSA	Sulfosalicyclic Acid
SSI	Surgical Site Infection
STT	Schirmer Tear Test
SuHV-1	Suid Herpesvirus-1
T3SS	Type 3 Secretion System
T6SS	Type 6 Secretion System
TBRF	Tick-Borne Relapsing Fever
TDM	Therapeutic Drug Monitoring

Continued